AIIMS-MAMC-PGI's

Comprehensive Textbook of

DIAGNOSTIC RADIOLOGY

AIIMS-MAMC-PGI's

Comprehensive Textbook of DIAGNOSTIC RADIOLOGY

Third Edition

VOLUME 1

- Genitourinary Imaging
- Advances in Imaging Technology

Editors

Arun Kumar Gupta MD FAMS
Professor and Head
Department of Radiodiagnosis
All India Institute of Medical Sciences
New Delhi, India

Anju Garg MD
Director Professor and Head
Department of Radiodiagnosis
Maulana Azad Medical College
New Delhi, India

Manavjit Singh Sandhu MD FICR
CCST (UK)
Professor and Head
Department of Radiodiagnosis
Postgraduate Institute of
Medical Education and Research
Chandigarh, India

JAYPEE BROTHERS MEDICAL PUBLISHERS

The Health Sciences Publisher

New Delhi | London

JAYPEE **Jaypee Brothers Medical Publishers (P) Ltd**

Headquarter

Jaypee Brothers Medical Publishers (P) Ltd
4838/24, Ansari Road, Daryaganj
New Delhi 110 002, India
Phone: +91-11-43574357
Fax: +91-11-43574314
Email: jaypee@jaypeebrothers.com

Overseas Office

J.P. Medical Ltd
83 Victoria Street, London
SW1H 0HW (UK)
Phone: +44 20 3170 8910
Fax: +44 (0)20 3008 6180
Email: info@jpmedpub.com

Website: www.jaypeebrothers.com
Website: www.jaypeedigital.com

Inquiries for bulk sales may be solicited at: jaypee@jaypeebrothers.com

AIIMS-MAMC-PGI's Comprehensive Textbook of Diagnostic Radiology, ***Third Edition (Volumes 1 to 4)*** / *Arun Kumar Gupta, Anju Garg, Manavjit Singh Sandhu*

First Edition: 2016
Second Edition: 2019
Third Edition: 2021
Reprint: **2024**

ISBN: 978-93-90595-55-6

Printed at: Sanat Printers

ASSOCIATE EDITORS

VOLUME 1

Section 1: Genitourinary Imaging

Gaurav Shanker Pradhan DMRD DNB
Director Professor
Department of Radiodiagnosis
Maulana Azad Medical College
New Delhi, India

Alpana Manchanda MD
Director Professor
Department of Radiodiagnosis
Maulana Azad Medical College
New Delhi, India

Sapna Singh MD DNB MNAMS
Professor
Department of Radiodiagnosis
Maulana Azad Medical College
New Delhi, India

Section 2: Advances in Imaging Technology

Sanjay Sharma MD DNB MNAMS FRCR FICR
Professor
Department of Radiodiagnosis
(RP Center division)
All India Institute of Medical Sciences
New Delhi, India

Atin Kumar MD DNB MNAMS FICR
Professor
Department of Radiodiagnosis
(Trauma Centre Division)
All India Institute of Medical Sciences
New Delhi, India

Shivanand Gamanagatti MD MNAMS FICR
Professor
Department of Radiodiagnosis
(Trauma Centre Division)
All India Institute of Medical Sciences
New Delhi, India

VOLUME 2

Section 3: Paediatric Imaging

Ashu Seith Bhalla MD MAMS FICR
Professor
Department of Radiodiagnosis
All India Institute of Medical Sciences
New Delhi, India

Manisha Jana MD DNB FRCR
Additional Professor
Department of Radiodiagnosis
All India Institute of Medical Sciences
New Delhi, India

Devasenathipathy Kandasamy MD DNB FRCR
Additional Professor
Department of Radiodiagnosis
All India Institute of Medical Sciences
New Delhi, India

Priyanka Naranje MD DNB MNAMS
Associate Professor
Department of Radiodiagnosis
All India Institute of Medical Sciences
New Delhi, India

Section 4: Gastrointestinal and Hepatobiliary Imaging

Deep Narayan Srivastava MD MBA FAMS FICR
Professor
Department of Radiodiagnosis
All India Institute of Medical Sciences
New Delhi, India

Raju Sharma MD MAMS FICR
Professor
Department of Radiodiagnosis
All India Institute of Medical Sciences
New Delhi, India

VOLUME 3

Section 5: Chest and Cardiovascular Imaging

Sanjiv Sharma MD
Professor and Head
Department of Cardiovascular Radiology and Endovascular Interventions
CN Centre
All India Institute of Medical Sciences
New Delhi, India

Rashmi Dixit MD
Director Professor
Department of Radiodiagnosis
Maulana Azad Medical College
New Delhi, India

Section 6: Musculoskeletal and Breast Imaging

Mahesh Prakash MD MAMS FIACM FICR
Professor
Department of Radiodiagnosis
Postgraduate Institute of Medical Education and Research
Chandigarh, India

Anindita Sinha MD MAMS
Additional Professor
Department of Radiodiagnosis
Postgraduate Institute of Medical Education and Research
Chandigarh, India

VOLUME 4

Section 7: Neuroradiology Including Head and Neck Imaging

Paramjeet Singh MD FICR
Professor
Department of Radiodiagnosis
Postgraduate Institute of Medical Education and Research
Chandigarh, India

Shailesh B Gaikwad MD FNAMS CCST
Professor and Head
Department of Neuroimaging and Interventional Neuroradiology (CN Centre)
All India Institute of Medical Sciences
New Delhi, India

Vivek Gupta MD DM
Former Professor
Department of Radiodiagnosis
Postgraduate Institute of Medical Education and Research
Chandigarh, India

Ajay Garg MD
Professor
Department of Neuroimaging and Interventional Neuroradiology (CN Centre)
All India Institute of Medical Sciences
New Delhi, India

CONTRIBUTORS

Ajay Garg MD (Radiodiagnosis) Eur Dip in Neuroradiology (EDiNR) Eur Dip in Pediatric Neuroradiology (EDiPNR)
Professor, Department of Neuroimaging and Interventional Neuroradiology
CN Centre
All India Institute of Medical Sciences
New Delhi, India

Ajay Gulati MD MAMS
Additional Professor
Department of Radiodiagnosis
Postgraduate Institute of Medical Education and Research, Chandigarh, India

Ajay Kumar MD
Professor
Department of Radiodiagnosis
Postgraduate Institute of Medical Education and Research, Chandigarh, India

Akshay Kumar Saxena MD DNB FICR
Professor
Department of Radiodiagnosis
Postgraduate Institute of Medical Education and Research, Chandigarh, India

Alpana Manchanda MD
Director Professor
Department of Radiodiagnosis
Maulana Azad Medical College
New Delhi, India

Anil Kumar Pandey MSc PhD
Associate Professor (Medical Physics)
Department of Nuclear Medicine and PET
All India Institute of Medical Sciences
New Delhi, India

Anindita Sinha MD MAMS
Additional Professor
Department of Radiodiagnosis
Postgraduate Institute of Medical Education and Research
Chandigarh, India

Anjali Prakash DMRD DNB MNAMS
Director Professor
Department of Radiodiagnosis
Maulana Azad Medical College
New Delhi, India

Anju Garg MD
Director Professor and Head
Department of Radiodiagnosis
Maulana Azad Medical College
New Delhi, India

Ankur Goyal MD DNB MNAMS
Associate Professor
Department of Radiodiagnosis
All India Institute of Medical Sciences
New Delhi, India

Anmol Bhatia MD FPGI (Paediatric Radiology)
Assistant Professor
Department of Radiodiagnosis and Imaging
Postgraduate Institute of Medical Education and Research
Chandigarh, India

Anuj Prabhakar DNB DM (Neuroradiology)
Assistant Professor
Postgraduate Institute of Medical Education and Research
Chandigarh, India

Anupam Lal MD
Professor
Department of Radiodiagnosis
Postgraduate Institute of Medical Education and Research
Chandigarh, India

Arun Kumar Gupta MD FAMS
Professor and Head
Department of Radiodiagnosis
All India Institute of Medical Sciences
New Delhi, India

Ashu Seith Bhalla MD MAMS FICR
Professor
Department of Radiodiagnosis
All India Institute of Medical Sciences
New Delhi, India

Atin Kumar MD DNB MNAMS FICR
Professor
Department of Radiodiagnosis
(Trauma Center Division)
All India Institute of Medical Sciences
New Delhi, India

Chandan J Das MD DNB MAMS FICR FRCP
Additional Professor
Department of Radiodiagnosis
All India Institute of Medical Sciences
New Delhi, India

Chandrashekhara SH MD DNB MNAMS
Additional Professor
Department of Radiodiagnosis
Dr BRA Institute—Rotary Cancer Hospital
All India Institute of Medical Sciences
New Delhi, India

Chirag Kamal Ahuja MD DM (Neuroradiology)
Associate Professor
Department of Radiodiagnosis and Imaging
Postgraduate Institute of Medical Education and Research
Chandigarh, India

Deep Narayan Srivastava MD MBA FAMS FICR
Professor
Department of Radiodiagnosis
All India Institute of Medical Sciences
New Delhi, India

Devasenathipathy Kandasamy MD DNB FRCR
Additional Professor
Department of Radiodiagnosis
All India Institute of Medical Sciences
New Delhi, India

Ekta Dhamija MD
Associate Professor
Department of Radiodiagnosis
Dr BRA Institute—Rotary Cancer Hospital
All India Institute of Medical Sciences
New Delhi, India

Gaurav Shanker Pradhan DMRD DNB
Director Professor
Department of Radiodiagnosis
Maulana Azad Medical College
New Delhi, India

Gita Devi MD DNB
Assistant Professor
Department of Radiodiagnosis
Postgraduate Institute of Medical Education and Research
Chandigarh, India

Gurpreet Singh Gulati MD
Former Professor
Department of Cardiac Radiology
Cardio-Thoracic Sciences Centre
All India Institute of Medical Sciences
New Delhi, India

Harish Bhujade MD FVIR
Assistant Professor
Department of Radiodiagnosis
Postgraduate Institute of Medical Education and Research
Chandigarh, India

Jyoti Kumar MD DNB MNAMS FICR
Professor
Department of Radiodiagnosis
Maulana Azad Medical College
New Delhi, India

Kartik Ganga MD
Fellow
Department of Cardiovascular Radiology and Endovascular Interventions
All India Institute of Medical Sciences
New Delhi, India

Kirti Gupta MD, Neuropathology Fellowship (St Jude, USA)
Professor
Department of Histopathology
Postgraduate Institute of Medical Education and Research
Chandigarh, India

Kumble S Madhusudhan MD FRCR MAMS
Additional Professor
Department of Radiodiagnosis
All India Institute of Medical Sciences
New Delhi, India

Kushaljit Singh Sodhi MD PhD MAMS FICR
Professor
Department of Radiodiagnosis
Postgraduate Institute of Medical Education and Research
Chandigarh, India

Madhavi Tripathi MD DNB (Nuclear Medicine)
Additional Professor
Department of Nuclear Medicine and PET
All India Institute of Medical Sciences
New Delhi, India

Madhusudhan KS MD MAMS FRCR
Additional Professor
Department of Radiodiagnosis
All India Institute of Medical Sciences
New Delhi, India

Mahesh Prakash MD MAMS FIACM FICR
Professor
Department of Radiodiagnosis
Postgraduate Institute of Medical Education and Research
Chandigarh, India

Manavjit Singh Sandhu MD FICR CCST (UK)
Professor and Head
Department of Radiodiagnosis
Postgraduate Institute of Medical Education and Research
Chandigarh, India

Mandeep Garg MD FRCR
Professor
Department of Radiodiagnosis
Postgraduate Institute of Medical Education and Research
Chandigarh, India

Mandeep Kang MD MAMS FICR
Professor
Department of Radiodiagnosis
Postgraduate Institute of Medical Education and Research
Chandigarh, India

Manisha Jana MD DNB FRCR
Additional Professor
Department of Radiodiagnosis
All India Institute of Medical Sciences
New Delhi, India

Manish Modi MD DM
Professor
Department of Neurology
Postgraduate Institute of Medical Education and Research
Chandigarh, India

Manphool Singhal MD DNB MAMS FICR (India) FSCCT (USA) CMR-fellowship (London) CMR-Certification (SCMR USA and ESCVI France)
Additional Professor
Department of Radiodiagnosis
Postgraduate Institute of Medical Education and Research
Chandigarh, India

Mukesh Kumar Yadav (MD Radiodiagnosis)
Formerly Associate Professor
PGIMER, Chandigarh
Associate Professor
Department of Radiodiagnosis
All India Institute of Medical Sciences (IRCH)
New Delhi, India

Naveen Kalra MD FICR MAMS
Professor
Department of Radiodiagnosis
Postgraduate Institute of Medical Education and Research
Chandigarh, India

Nidhi Prabhakar MD DNB
Senior Research Associate
Department of Radiodiagnosis
Postgraduate Institute of Medical Education and Research
Chandigarh, India

Niraj N Pandey DM
Assistant Professor
Department of Cardiovascular Radiology and Endovascular Interventions
CN Centre
All India Institute of Medical Sciences
New Delhi, India

Niranjan Khandelwal MD Dip NBE FICR FAMS
Former Head
Department of Radiodiagnosis
Postgraduate Institute of Medical Education and Research
Chandigarh, India

Pankaj Gupta MD DNB
Assistant Professor
Department of Radiodiagnosis and Imaging
Postgraduate Institute of Medical Education and Research
Chandigarh, India

Paramjeet Singh MD FICR
Professor
Department of Radiodiagnosis
Postgraduate Institute of Medical Education and Research
Chandigarh, India

Pratik Kumar PhD (AIIMS) Dip RP (BARC)
Professor, Medical Physics Unit
BRA Institute Rotary Cancer Hospital
AIIMS, New Delhi, India

Priya Jagia MD DNB
Professor
Department of Cardiovascular Radiology and Endovascular Interventions
All India Institute of Medical Sciences
New Delhi, India

Priyanka Naranje MD DNB MNAMS
Associate Professor
Department of Radiodiagnosis
All India Institute of Medical Sciences
New Delhi, India

Punit Sharma MD
Former Senior Resident
Department of Nuclear Medicine
All India Institute of Medical Sciences
New Delhi, India

Radhika Batra MD DNB
Associate Professor
Department of Radiodiagnosis
Maulana Azad Medical College
New Delhi, India

Rajat Jain MD DNB FRCR FICR MNAMS
Assistant Professor
Department of Radiodiagnosis
Maulana Azad Medical College
New Delhi, India

Raju Sharma MD MAMS FICR
Professor
Department of Radiodiagnosis
All India Institute of Medical Sciences
New Delhi, India

Rakesh Kumar DRM DNB PhD
Professor and Head
Diagnostic Nuclear Medicine Division
Department of Nuclear Medicine and PET
All India Institute of Medical Sciences
New Delhi, India

Rakesh Kumar Vasishta MD FRCPath
Former Professor and Head
Department of Histopathology
Postgraduate Institute of Medical Education and Research
Chandigarh, India

Rashmi Dixit MD
Director Professor
Department of Radiodiagnosis
Maulana Azad Medical College
New Delhi, India

Sameer Vyas MD DM MAMS (Neuroradiology)
Additional Professor
Department of Radiodiagnosis
Postgraduate Institute of Medical Education and Research
Chandigarh, India

Sanjay Sharma MD DNB MNAMS FRCR FICR
Professor
Department of Radiodiagnosis
(Division at Rajendra Prasad Center for Ophthalmic Sciences)
All India Institute of Medical Sciences
New Delhi, India

Sanjeev Kumar MD
Associate Professor
Department of Cardiovascular Radiology and Endovascular Interventions
All India Institute of Medical Sciences
New Delhi, India

Sanjiv Sharma MD
Professor and Head
Department of Cardiovascular Radiology and Endovascular Interventions
CN Centre
All India Institute of Medical Sciences
New Delhi, India

Sapna Singh MD DNB MNAMS
Professor
Department of Radiodiagnosis
Maulana Azad Medical College
New Delhi, India

Satyam DNB MNAMS
Specialist
Department of Radiodiagnosis
Lok Nayak Hospital and Associated Maulana Azad Medical College
New Delhi, India

Shailesh B Gaikwad MD FNAMS CCST
Professor and Head
Department of Neuroimaging and Interventional Neuroradiology
CN Centre
All India Institute of Medical Sciences
New Delhi, India

Shamim Ahmed Shamim MD (Nuclear Medicine)
Associate Professor
Department of Nuclear Medicine
All India Institute of Medical Sciences
New Delhi, India

Shashi Bala Paul PhD MAMS
Senior Scientist
Department of Radiodiagnosis
All India Institute of Medical Sciences
New Delhi, India

Shivanand Gamanagatti MD MNAMS FICR
Professor
Department of Radiodiagnosis
(Trauma Center Division)
All India Institute of Medical Sciences
New Delhi, India

Smita Manchanda MD DNB MNAMS
Associate Professor
Department of Radiodiagnosis
All India Institute of Medical Sciences
New Delhi, India

Smriti Hari MD MAMS
Professor
Department of Radiodiagnosis
All India Institute of Medical Sciences
New Delhi, India

Sreedhara BC MD FVIR
Assistant Professor
Department of Radiodiagnosis
Postgraduate Institute of Medical Education and Research
Chandigarh, India

Subrat Kumar Acharya DM FNASc
FASc FNA JC Bose Fellow
Former Professor and Head
Department of Gastroenterology
All India Institute of Medical Sciences
New Delhi, India

Sudesh Prabhakar MD DM
Former Professor and Head
Department of Neurology
Postgraduate Institute of Medical Education and Research
Chandigarh, India

Sudha Suri MD
Emeritus Professor
Department of Radiodiagnosis
Postgraduate Institute of Medical Education and Research
Chandigarh, India

Surabhi Vyas MD DNB MNAMS
Additional Professor
Department of Radiodiagnosis
All India Institute of Medical Sciences
New Delhi, India

Swati Gupta MD DNB FRCR
Associate Professor
Department of Radiodiagnosis
Maulana Azad Medical College
New Delhi, India

Tulika Singh MD
Additional Professor
Department of Radiodiagnosis
Postgraduate Institute of Medical Education and Research
Chandigarh, India

Ujjwal Gorsi (MD Radiodiagnosis)
Associate Professor
Department of Radiodiagnosis
Postgraduate Institute of Medical Education and Research
Chandigarh, India

Uma Debi MD
Associate Professor
Department of Radiodiagnosis
Postgraduate Institute of Medical Education and Research
Chandigarh, India

Veenu Singla MD
Professor
Department of Radiodiagnosis
Postgraduate Institute of Medical Education and Research
Chandigarh, India

Vikas Bhatia MD DNB
DM (Neuroradiology)
Assistant Professor
Department of Radiodiagnosis
Postgraduate Institute of Medical Education and Research
Chandigarh, India

Vineeta Ojha MD DNB
DM Senior Resident
Department of Cardiovascular Radiology and Endovascular Interventions
All India Institute of Medical Sciences
New Delhi, India

Virendra Jain MD FRCR
Former Senior Resident
Department of Radiodiagnosis
Maulana Azad Medical College
New Delhi, India

Vivek Gupta MD DM
Former Professor
Department of Radiodiagnosis
Postgraduate Institute of Medical Education and Research
Chandigarh, India

PREFACE TO THE THIRD EDITION

In 1996, a unique venture was jointly initiated by the faculty of Radiodiagnosis, All India Institute of Medical Sciences (AIIMS), New Delhi; Maulana Azad Medical College (MAMC), New Delhi; and Postgraduate Institute of Medical Education and Research (PGIMER), Chandigarh, India, to organize continuing medical education (CME) programs based on a series of imaging courses. An integral part of this endeavour was publishing books covering all organ systems. The aim was to provide state-of-the-art knowledge for postgraduate students as well as the practicing radiologists along with establishing a uniform pattern of teaching in radiology across the country.

The first series of seven imaging courses was successfully completed in the year 2000. A second series of these courses was then initiated in the year 2002 and was completed in 2004. This was also highly successful. The third series of seven extremely popular and successful courses covering all the organ systems and advances in physics was started in 2008 and was completed in 2013. The fourth series started in 2016 and was completed successfuly in 2020.

Every course in each of the series has resulted in publication of a book. These books have been very popular amongst residents as well as among practicing radiologists.

Considering the popularity of these books, the editors, along with publishers, M/s Jaypee Brothers Medical Publishers (P) Ltd, New Delhi, India, had decided to combine the individual course books into three volumes— *"AIIMS-MAMC-PGI's Comprehensive Textbook of Diagnostic Radiology"*. Its first edition was released in 2016.

In keeping pace with newer developments in the field of diagnostic radiology and in order to cater to the contemporary needs of users, the second edition of *"AIIMS-MAMC-PGI's Comprehensive Textbook of Diagnostic Radiology"* was presented in 2019 after a gap of three years. It was anticipated that with such a complete coverage of all the subjects, the users will not have to refer to any other book during their routine learning of diagnostic radiology.

However by the time fourth AIIMS MAMC PGI Imaging course series was near completion in early 2021, it was felt that there is a very strong need for updating of second edition along with addition of new chapters in view of rapid advancement of knowledge in the last few years. So third edition was planned. It was also agreed that in view of increasing size of individual course books and to keep the size of individual volumes of the Textbook handy and managable the whole textbook should be divided into four volumes from its current three volumes.

We are sure that residents and radiologists will find these comprehensive four volumes easy to handle and very useful in day-to-day practice.

We are once again grateful to all the contributors from the three apex academic institutions of India, i.e. AIIMS, New Delhi; MAMC, New Delhi; and PGIMER, Chandigarh, India.

We are thankful to M/s Jaypee Brothers Medical Publishers (P) Ltd, for helping us to make our dream come true.

Arun Kumar Gupta
Anju Garg
Manavjit Singh Sandhu

PREFACE TO THE FIRST EDITION

In 1996, a unique venture was jointly initiated by the faculty of radiodiagnosis at All India Institute of Medical Sciences, Maulana Azad Medical College, New Delhi, and Postgraduate Institute of Medical Education and Research, Chandigarh, India, to organize continuing medical education programs based on a series of imaging courses. An integral part of this endeavor was publishing books covering all organ systems. The aim was to provide state of the art knowledge for postgraduate students as well as the practicing radiologists along with establishing a uniform pattern of teaching in radiology across the country.

The first series of seven imaging courses was successfully completed in the year 2000. A second series of these courses was then initiated in the year 2002 and was completed in 2004. This was also highly successful.

With the great success of the second series, we, the current editors, decided to start a third series of these courses in 2008. Seven extremely popular and successful courses covering all the organ systems and advances in physics were completed in 2013.

Every course in each of the three series have resulted in publication of a book. These books have been very popular amongst residents as well as among practicing radiologists.

Considering the popularity of these books, we, the three current editors, along with publishers M/s Jaypee Brothers Medical Publishers (P) Ltd., decided to combine the individual books published so far into a "*AIIMS-MAMC-PGI's Comprehensive Textbook of Diagnostic Radiology*" with three volumes.

We are very happy to see the end result of this great effort.

We are sure that residents and radiologists will find these comprehensive three volumes easy to handle and very useful in day-to-day practice.

We are once again grateful to all the contributors from the three apex academic institutions of India, i.e. AIIMS, MAMC, New Delhi and PGIMER, Chandigarh, India.

We are thankful to M/s Jaypee Brothers Medical Publishers (P) Ltd., for helping us to make our dream come true.

Niranjan Khandelwal
Veena Chowdhury
Arun Kumar Gupta

ACKNOWLEDGMENTS

We would like to put on record our deep appreciation and gratitude:

To Professors Manorama Berry, Sudha Suri and Veena Chowdhury (Past Editors) the three pioneers who in 1996 took a bold initiative and started a unique teaching course now popularly known as AIIMS-MAMC-PGI's imaging course. By October 2020, four series, each series comprising of seven courses, have been completed. This course series has become extremely popular and every course is followed by the publication of a book which too is highly appreciated and popular.

To Professors Sima Mukhopadhyay, Sushma Vashisht and Niranjan Khandelwal who have been the Editors of past series and who contributed to organizing the earlier courses in their capacity as Heads of Departments.

To all the Associate Editors of the different course books who put in immense effort to bring the books out on time.

To all the Authors who contributed chapters without whom we could not have collected such an outstanding content of teaching and academic material.

To our respective hospitals for giving us the privilege and unique opportunity to work, which enabled us to amass data from patients and document images of diverse diseases that provide the reader with a wide spectrum of knowledge.

Our sincere and grateful thanks to Shri Jitendar P Vij (Group Chairman), Mr Ankit Vij (Managing Director), Mr MS Mani (Group President), Dr Richa Saxena (Associate Director-Professional Publishing), Ms Nedup Denka Bhutia (Development Editor) and Other staffs of M/s Jaypee Brothers Medical Publishers (P) Ltd, New Delhi, India, for their untiring coordination efforts in the production of this book.

We are very proud indeed at the culmination of two decades of these course series, to compile and present them together in the form of these four volumes of "*AIIMS-MAMC-PGI's Comprehensive Textbook of Diagnostic Radiology*".

Arun Kumar Gupta
Anju Garg
Manavjit Singh Sandhu

CONTENTS

VOLUME 1

Section 1: Genitourinary Imaging

VOLUME 2

Section 3: Paediatric Imaging

Section 4: Gastrointestinal and Hepatobiliary Imaging

VOLUME 3

Section 5: Chest and Cardiovascular Imaging

Section 6: Musculoskeletal and Breast Imaging

VOLUME 4

Section 7: Neuroradiology Including Head and Neck Imaging

SECTION

1

Genitourinary Imaging

- Imaging Techniques and Radiological Anatomy of the Upper Urinary Tract
- Current Status of Nuclear Medicine in Urinary Tract Imaging
- Renal Calculus Disease and Obstructive Uropathy
- Renal Parenchymal Disease
- Nontubercular Infections of the Urinary Tract
- Tubercular Infection of the Urinary Tract
- Renal Cystic Diseases
- Renal Neoplasms
- Renovascular Hypertension
- Imaging of Renal Transplant
- Imaging Techniques and Radiological Anatomy of Lower Urinary Tract
- Urinary Bladder and Urethral Diseases
- Imaging Techniques and Radiological Anatomy of Female Genital Tract
- Benign Adnexal Disease
- Malignant Ovarian and Tubal Disease
- Benign Diseases of the Uterus and Vagina
- Malignant Diseases of the Uterus and Vagina
- Female Infertility
- Imaging Techniques and Radiological Anatomy of the Male Genital Tract
- Disorders of the Prostate Gland
- Scrotal Diseases
- Male Infertility and Erectile Dysfunction
- Imaging of the Adrenal Gland
- The Retroperitoneum
- Urinary Tract Trauma
- Nonvascular Interventions in the Urinary Tract
- Vascular Interventions in the Genitourinary Tract

CHAPTER

1

Imaging Techniques and Radiological Anatomy of the Upper Urinary Tract

Sapna Singh, Jyoti Kumar, Anjali Prakash

ANATOMY OF THE UPPER URINARY TRACT

The upper urinary tract consists of paired kidneys and the ureters. The kidneys develop from three structures—the pronephros, the mesonephric, and metanephric ducts in that order. The pronephros regresses by 4th to 8th week of gestation leaving no adult correlate while the mesonephric duct forms the male genital structures. The ureteric bud and the metanephric blastema arise from the metanephric duct in the 5th week of gestation. The metanephric blastema develops into Bowman's capsule, the convoluted tubules, and loop of Henle while the ureteric bud develops into ureter, the renal pelvis, calyces, and the collecting ducts. The calyces arise due to repeated divisions of the upper end of the ureteric bud and this forms the basis of the lobar structure of the kidney, each lobe consisting of a calyx and the associated collecting ducts and renal cortex. The lobar outline becomes smooth by around 5 years of age owing to multiplication of the renal cortical cells. However, in about 5% of the individuals, there is persistence of the lobar outline into adulthood.

It is during the 4th to 8th week of gestation that the kidneys migrate cranially from the pelvic region where they develop. The cranial migration is due to the lengthening of the lumbar and sacral spine during development so that the normal final position of the kidneys is upper lumbar region. They also rotate medially by around 90° so that the renal pelvis lies on the anteromedial aspect of the kidneys.[1] The lateral sacral branches of the aorta supply the pelvic kidneys but during ascent they acquire higher lateral branches of the aorta. The definitive renal arteries are seen at the first lumbar disc (L1-L2) level. If the inferior arteries do not regress, accessory renal arteries can be seen. Accessory unilateral renal arteries are seen in 30% population and bilateral are seen in 10% with a higher frequency seen with anomalies of ascent.[2]

The kidneys come to lie in the retroperitoneal space with the right kidney lower in position than the left owing to the presence of the liver on the right. The normal kidneys should be 12–14 cm in length and the difference between the two should not be more than 1 cm. In quiet respiration, the kidneys move up and down 2–3 cm and much more in deep inspiration. The renal hilum is a vertical opening on the medial aspect which contains the renal pelvis and renal vessels. The renal veins lie anterior to the renal arteries which in-turn lie anterior to the renal pelves. In addition, the hilum also contains fat, nerve fibers, and lymphatic channels which drain into the lateral aortic lymph nodal group.

Each kidney is divided into an outer renal cortex and an inner renal medulla.[3] The medulla consists of 8–16 renal pyramids **(Fig. 1)**. Each renal pyramid in-turn contains the ascending and descending limbs of the loop of Henle and the collecting ducts. The cortex contains the glomerulus and the proximal and distal convoluted tubules. The apex of the renal pyramid projects into a calyx at the renal papilla. The renal collecting system consists of 10–14 concave-shaped minor calyces. The lateral extensions of the calyces is called the forniceal angle. Two to four minor calyces join together to form the superior, middle, and inferior major calyces respectively from superior to inferior. The minor calyces drain into the major calyx by a narrow neck/infundibulum. The major calyces in-turn drain into the renal pelvis which continues as the ureter at the pelviureteric junction (PUJ).

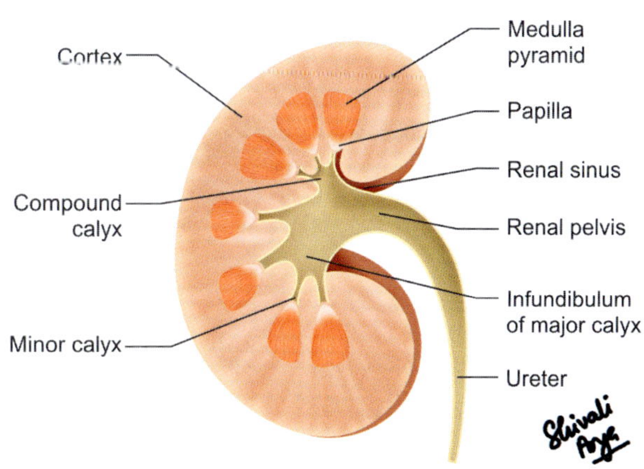

FIG. 1: Schematic diagram of the structure of the kidney.

Variants of the Calyceal Anatomy

- *Compound calyx*: Here, the multiple single calyces fail to divide and form a single large calyx known as the compound calyx. Here, several renal papillae which represent the apices of the renal pyramids drain into a single calyx. Compound calyces are usually seen at the polar region, i.e. at the upper or lower poles and are prone to reflux nephropathy.
- *Complex renal calyces and megacalycosis*: In megacalycosis, there is a greater number of calyces than normal (>15). There is dilatation of some or all renal calyces with normal renal pelvis and ureter. Renal calyces may have a blunted morphology, but this condition should not be confused with papillary necrosis in which the number of calyces is not increased and necrosis tends to be dissimilar from calyx to calyx.
- *Calyceal diverticulum*: It represents a focal extrinsic dilatation of a renal calyx. A calyceal diverticulum connects to the calyceal fornix and projects into the cortex rather than the medulla.

Retroperitoneal Spaces

The kidneys have a tough fibrous capsule closely applied to the renal cortex all around except at the hilum.

The kidneys are retroperitoneal organs and lie in a space called the *perinephric space* or the *perineal space*. The perinephric space is a space bound by layers of fascia and is an important determinant of the direction of disease spread. The fascia anterior to the kidneys is called the Gerota's fascia while the posterior fascia is called the fascia of Zuckerkandl. The space enclosed between the anterior and posterior fascia is called the *perinephric space* **(Fig. 2)**. In addition to the kidneys, the space contains the adrenal gland, the upper ureter and the perinephric fat. As the kidneys ascend from the pelvis to the abdomen, the perinephric fascia forms a cone with its apex pointing superiorly, the apex being closed.[3,4]

The transversalis fascia lines the inferior aspect of the diaphragm, the inside of the abdominopelvic cavity, anterolateral abdominal wall, the anterior aspect of the spinal column, the psoas and paraspinal muscles, and the superior aspect of the pelvic diaphragm. There is a potential space between the posterior perinephric fascia and the adjacent transversalis fascia. This space is called the *posterior pararenal space* and contains only fat **(Fig. 2)**. The posterior pararenal space is of interest to the radiologist as a guidewire may kink in this area or a drain intended for the pelvicalyceal system may be accidently positioned here. The *anterior pararenal space*, on the other hand, is the space between the anterior perinephric fascia and posterior layer of the peritoneum. In the center of the anterior pararenal space lie the pancreas and duodenum, the ascending colon lies to the right and descending colon to the left. These organs are hence in direct contact with the anterior perinephric fascia.[4]

Laterally, the anterior and posterior perirenal fascia fuse with the lateroconal fascia at the fascial trifurcation. While the posterior pararenal space is continuous laterally with the lateral extraperitoneal space (the properitoneal line) lying between the parietal peritoneum and transversalis fascia, this space is closed medially. Medially, the posterior perinephric fascia fuses with the transversalis fascia over the paraspinal muscles, that is the psoas muscle and the quadratus lumborum. The posterior perinephric space hence lies directly over the psoas muscle being separated only by the transversalis fascia. Thus, any inflammation process of the kidneys can spread rapidly into the psoas muscles and from there into the iliacus muscle, iliopsoas, and the pelvis.

Thus, superiorly the renal fascia fuses with the diaphragmatic fascia. Laterally, the renal fascia fuses with the lateroconal fascia and inferiorly with the iliac fascia blending loosely with the periureteric connective tissue. Owing to the loose blending of the fascia, the inferomedial angle adjacent to the ureter is the weakest point of the perinephric compartment through which urine or perinephric effusion escapes most easily. The posterior renal fascia fuses with the psoas and quadratus lumborum fascia medially.

The perineal spaces also communicate with each other across the midline and with the retroperitoneal vascular space. The pararenal spaces communicate caudally and with the extraperitoneal spaces including the prevesical space. Infections from one space can hence spread to the other subsequently. The *anterior interfascial or the retromesenteric space* and the *posterior interfascial or retrorenal space* are

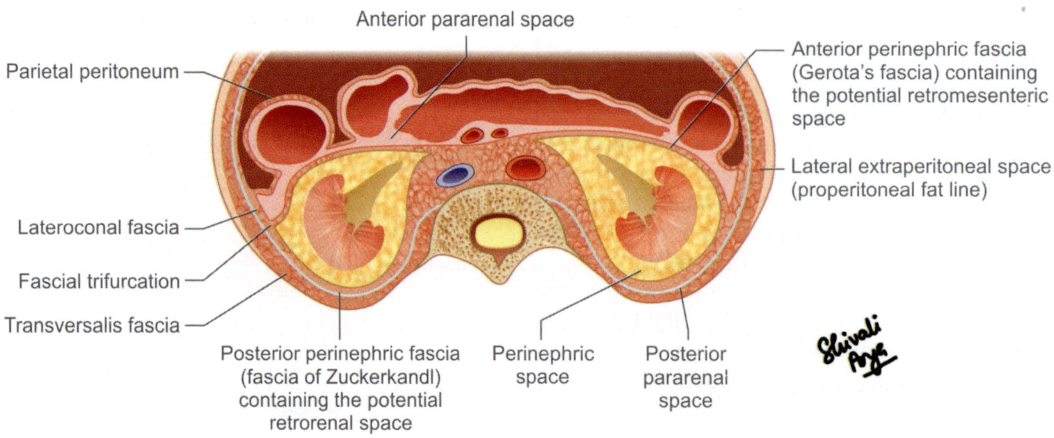

FIG. 2: Diagram showing the retroperitoneal fascial spaces.

potential spaces within the laminated anterior perinephric and posterior perinephric fasciae, respectively (*see* **Fig. 2**).[5] The perirenal space contains thin septations called the Kumin's septa. These septae may arise from the renal capsule and extend to the anterior and posterior renal fascia. Some may arise from the renal capsule and run parallel to the renal surface. The renorenal bridging septum is the most consistent which arises from the posterior renal capsule and runs parallel to the posterior surface of the kidney. These septae thicken consequent to a disease process, what is referred to as perinephric stranding. These fibrous septae act as potential conduits between the perinephric and interfascial spaces. Fluid and collections may track from any of these potential spaces to the other and also via the fascial trifurcation into the lateroconal fascia.

Relations of the Kidneys

The right kidney is related anteriorly with the inferior surface of the liver and the second part of the duodenum while the anterior relations of the left kidney are the pancreatic tail, the spleen, the stomach, the small bowel, the splenic flexure, and the left colon (**Fig. 3**).[4] Posteriorly, the diaphragm, psoas muscle, aponeurosis of the transverses abdominis muscle, and the lumbar muscles are related to the kidneys. Both the kidneys are related superiorly with the adrenal glands while inferiorly the hepatorenal pouch/Morrison's pouch separates the right kidney from the inferior surface of the liver.

Vascular Anatomy

The renal arteries arise from the aorta, slightly below the origin of the superior mesenteric artery (SMA). The right renal artery (RRA) arises from the anterolateral aspect of the aorta and then passes posterior to the inferior vena cava (IVC) as it courses toward the right renal hilum. The left renal artery (LRA) arises from the lateral or posterolateral aspect of the aorta and follows a posterolateral course to the left renal hilum. Accessory renal arteries may arise from the aorta in as many as 20% individuals, either superior or inferior to the main renal artery. The renal arteries typically divide into anterior and posterior divisions that lie anterior and posterior to the renal pelvis, respectively. These divisions give rise to the segmental arteries which branch further within the renal sinus, forming interlobar arteries that penetrate the renal parenchyma. These terminate in arcuate arteries that curve around the corticomedullary junction giving rise to cortical branches.[3,4]

Each renal vein is formed from tributaries that coalesce in the renal hilum. The left renal vein passes anterior to the aorta and posterior to SMA, to enter the left side of IVC. The right renal vein, which is shorter, extends directly to the IVC from the right renal hilum.

The lymphatic drainage is to the lateral aortic lymph nodes around the origin of the renal arteries.

Ureters

The ureter runs down the anterior aspect of the psoas muscle, the transversalis fascia separating the two. The ureters run within 1 cm of the lateral margin of the vertebral transverse processes. At the level of the sacroiliac joint, it crosses over the anterior aspect of the bifurcation of the common iliac artery as it enters the pelvis. It then runs along the lateral pelvic wall just medial to the obturator internus muscle. At the level of the ischial spine, it runs anteromedially until it enters the superolateral angle of the bladder base. In males, the vas deferens crosses over the ureter just before it enters the bladder wall. The ureters run obliquely for around 2 cm through the bladder wall.[4]

The ureters have three normal constrictions which act as points of temporary peristaltic arrest which are as follows:
1. At the ureteropelvic junction
2. Crossing the iliac vessels
3. At the pelvic inlet.

IMAGING TECHNIQUES OF THE UPPER URINARY TRACT

CONVENTIONAL RADIOGRAPHY

The conventional plain radiography of the abdomen is an imaging technique for the kidneys ureter and bladder also known as the kidney, ureter, and bladder (KUB) film.[6] The kidneys are visible on the plain radiograph due to natural contrast provided by the perirenal fat. An idea about the renal shape, margins, dimensions, and localization can be made on the plain radiograph. It can also be used to identify renal

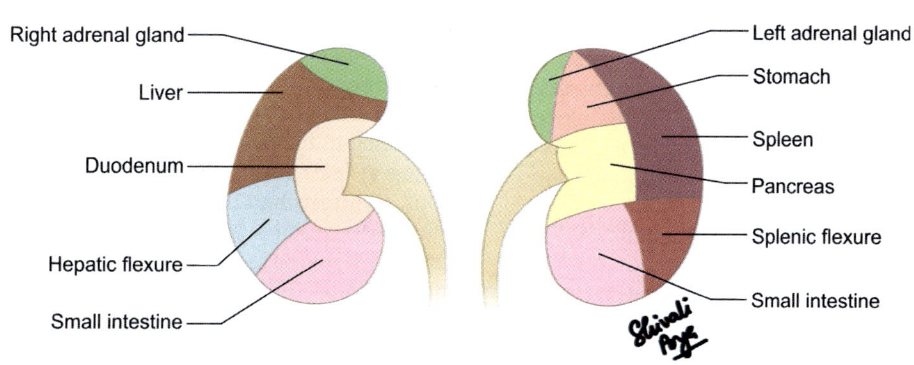

FIG. 3: Schematic diagram of the anterior relations of the right and left kidney.

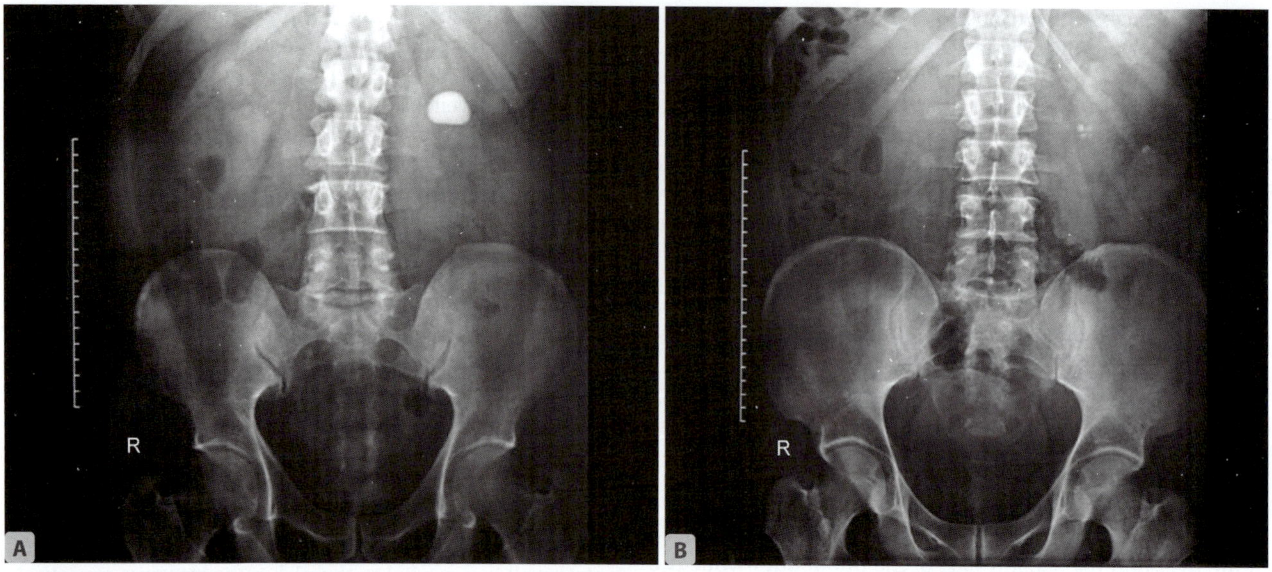

FIGS. 4A AND B: (A) Plain X-ray of kidney, ureter, and bladder (KUB) showing a large radiodensity in the left renal area suggestive of a left renal calculus; (B) Another plain film showing multiple radiopacities in the left renal area suggestive of multiple renal calculi.

TABLE 1: Calcification on the KUB.[4]

Urinary tract
Renal: Calculi, tuberculosis, renal cell carcinoma, and arterial atheroma or aneurysm *Ureter*: Calculi, tuberculosis, and schistosomiasis *Bladder*: Calculi, transitional cell carcinoma, and schistosomiasis
Outside the urinary tract
Hepatobiliary: Gallstones and hepatic granuloma *Spleen*: Granuloma *Pancreas*: Chronic pancreatitis *Adrenal*: Tuberculosis and Addison's disease *Aorta*: Atheroma and aneurysm *Venous*: Phlebolith *Musculoskeletal*: Costal cartilage calcification *Uterine*: Fibroid *Lymphatic*: Calcified lymph nodes (presumed postinfective)

(KUB: kidney, ureter and bladder)

calculi, calcifications or transparencies due to fat or gas.[7] The psoas shadow can also be seen on the plain radiograph. Radiopacities seen on the plain radiographs correspond to the renal stones or calcifications due to tuberculosis, vascular structures or traumatic lesions like hematoma **(Figs. 4A and B)**. Calcifications seen in solid or cystic neoplasms may also be seen on plain radiograph **(Table 1)**. The radiolucencies correspond to gas, e.g. emphysematous pyelonephritis or fat, i.e. large angiomyolipoma (AML) or liposarcoma.

INTRAVENOUS UROGRAPHY

Intravenous urography (IVU), also known as the excretory urogram is a time-tested technique of uroradiology providing a global view of the renal parenchyma and collecting system.[8]

Indications:

- Urolithiasis
- Ureteric fistulae/strictures
- Renal infections, e.g. tuberculosis. IVU still remains the gold standard in the imaging of renal tuberculosis. It is the only modality that can detect early changes in the renal calyces in tuberculosis, e.g. early fuzziness, irregularity of calyces, papillary necrosis, etc.
- Persistent or frank hematuria.

Normal Physiology Giving Rise to the Appearances on IVU

Intravenous urography consists of a series of plain films following intravenous injection of water soluble iodinated contrast medium.[9] The contrast reaches the renal arteries 12–20 seconds following contrast injection. The concentration of the contrast material is maximum in the vascular compartment at this stage, but it begins to fall rapidly as it enters the extracellular compartment. It also undergoes glomerular filtration and enters the renal tubules. Hence, in the first minute following contrast injection, there is a diffuse enhancement referred to as the nephrogram phase provided the kidneys are healthy with the patient having a normal cardiovascular system. The renal size and outline are best evaluated in the *nephrogram phase*, the normal renal length being at least three lumbar vertebrae and not exceeding four. Contrast then begins to appear in the calyces around 1 minute which subsequently drains into the pelvis and ureter referred to as the *pyelogram phase*. The normal ureters demonstrate continued peristalsis and it may not be possible to visualize the entire length of both (or even one) ureters in a single film. In most cases, partial visualization of the ureters is acceptable.

Technique

Traditionally, patients were deprived of fluid before an IVU examination with the belief that it would lead to a better opacification of the collecting system. However, it has long been established that dehydration is associated with an increased risk of nephrotoxicity and should be completely avoided. In fact, if the patient is dehydrated before the IVU, it needs to be corrected first. Food should be avoided 4–6 hours prior to the examination and bowel preparation (using laxatives) is preferable to avoid gases overlying the renal shadows. The patient is called fasting (4–6 hours) and with adequate bowel preparation but should be well hydrated. A plain radiograph (KUB) is must as it gives an idea of the bowel preparation and is needed to follow up a previously proven calculus. A preliminary KUB also gives an idea of exposure factors, correct positioning/centering, and any obvious pathology, most common of which is urinary tract calcification.

Blood urea and serum creatinine levels should be checked before contrast administration as the risk of contrast-induced nephropathy is increased if serum creatinine is greater than 1.5 mg/dL. Also, in patients with impaired renal function (serum creatinine greater than 3.5 mg/dL), the excretion of the contrast material and subsequent renal and ureteric visualization are limited.

If the patient is fit to undergo the examination, contrast is injected at the dose of 1 mg/kg body weight. The standard dose is usually 50 mL of 350–370 mgI/mL water soluble iodinated contrast medium. Although usually safe there is a small risk of reactions.[10] The most severe reaction that can occur following contrast administration is anaphylactoid type hypersensitivity reaction. Hence, before injection of contrast medium, a history of allergy to any previous contrast exposure should be elicited.[11] The injection should be administered through an indwelling cannula that can be kept in place for the entire duration of the investigation. This would allow any emergency treatment to be given in case of an eventuality. Also, in cases of poor contrast opacification, a further dose of contrast medium can be administered. Most contrast reactions take place within the first few minutes following contrast injection. Emergency drugs, oxygen, and resuscitation should be available in the IVU room. The radiologist should be available in the X-ray room for the entire duration of the procedure.

Sequence of films taken

Film	Purpose
5-minute film	– Opacification of the pelvicalyceal system
15-minute compression film	– Calyceal distention
15-minute release film in supine position (full length films)	– Visualization of the pelvicalyceal system and ureters
15-minute prone film (full length films)	
Post-micturition film	– Residual urine volume

Abdominal compression is applied after the 5-minute film to improve the distention of the pelvicalyceal system by inhibiting ureteric drainage. However, compression should not be applied in children, in patients of hypertension/aortic aneurysm, those with recent abdominal surgery or abdominal pain or tenderness. After 15-minute film with compression, the compression is removed and full length films are taken in the supine and prone positions, the prone position allowing a better visualization of the pelvic ureters **(Figs. 5A to C)**.

At times, a delayed film needs to be taken in cases of significant acute obstruction where there is a delay in the opacification of the pelvicalyceal system. This follow-up IVU needs to be done till a time when the contralateral kidney has completely excreted the contrast.

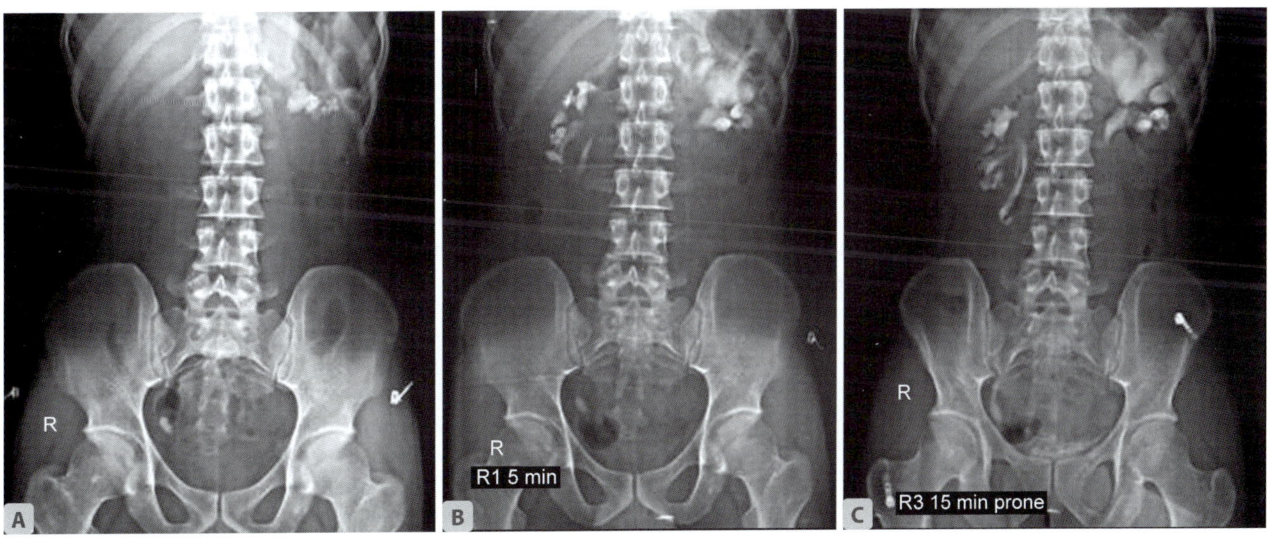

FIGS. 5A TO C: (A) Plain X-ray of kidney, ureter, and bladder (KUB) showing multiple left renal calculi and radiodensity in the line of the right ureter suggestive of left ureteric calculus; (B and C) Intravenous urography images showing renal calculi as filling defects within the opacified left pelvicalyceal system and the right ureteric calculus. Note is made of the upper ureter being dilated and tortuous with a characteristic medial angulation suggestive of retrocaval ureter.

With the advent of cross-sectional imaging, the utility of IVU is a topic of considerable debate.[12] Computed tomography (CT) scores over IVU for urolithiasis with a sensitivity of 100% versus 52–69% for IVU.[13] In one review, patient acceptability, superior diagnostic performance of CT versus IVU, equivalent radiation doses using low-dose techniques in CT were the factors for recommending CT over IVU.[14] CT is also superior to IVU for urinary tract tumor detection with sensitivities of only 21%, 52%, and 85% for masses less than 2, 2–3, and greater than 3 cm, respectively on IVU.[15] However, a blanket substitution of IVU by cross-sectional imaging is not feasible due to cost and availability factors.

DIGITAL TOMOSYNTHESIS

Digital tomosynthesis (DT) is a technique that enables visualization of stones from multiple angles rather than simply anterior to posterior. The technique involves acquisition of images at regular intervals at different angles during a single linear or arc sweep of the X-ray tube. The images can then be reconstructed providing better resolution than conventional radiography. Compared with CT, DT offers a reduced radiation exposure, higher in plane resolution, easier availability, and lower cost. In a study done to evaluate the accuracy of IVU using DT, a significant improvement was seen from 46.5% for conventional IVU to 95.5% for IVU with DT.[16] There was a dose reduction of 56% and a decrease in the length of the procedure.[16] This technique may be useful in situations such as evaluation of residual stone after percutaneous lithotripsy, that is, in situations where a detailed imaging of the renal parenchyma is not required. DT is currently an experimental technique and may play a role in KUB radiography remaining an important technique in kidney stone imaging in the future.

RETROGRADE PYELOGRAPHY

Retrograde pyelography (RGP) involves opacification of the pelvicalyceal system retrogradely by instillation of contrast medium into a ureteric catheter placed by cystoscopy. With the advent of multidetector computed tomography (MDCT) with isotropic data acquisition and multiplanar reconstruction, the role of RGP is limited.[17]

The indications include:

- As a problem-solving tool in cases of persistent diagnostic uncertainty, especially if there is hematuria and/or suspicious cytology.[18]
- To confirm or negate the presence of one or more filling defects within the collecting system.
- To demonstrate the lower end of an obstructed ureter.

Technique

Catheters are positioned within one or both ureters cystoscopically by the urologist. Under fluoroscopic screening, 5–20 mL of water-soluble iodinated contrast medium is injected via the catheter. Care should be taken so as to not inject air bubbles as these can be mistaken for filling defects. The ureters and pelvicalyceal system are hence opacified retrogradely. These should be opacified adequately but not overdistended as a forceful and excessive contrast injection can lead to reflux of contrast into the collecting ducts (pyelotubular reflux), contrast extravasation into the renal sinus (pyelosinus reflux), forniceal rupture, and even into the regional lymphatics or veins (pyelolymphatic and pyelovenous reflux).

ANTEGRADE PYELOGRAPHY

It is a simple invasive procedure used to evaluate the cause and level of ureteric obstruction where other imaging modalities have failed to do so. The technique involves positioning the patient 45° semiprone and puncturing the pelvicalyceal system with a fine (22 gauge) needle under fluoroscopy or ultrasound guidance. The puncture should be directed through the renal parenchyma into a suitable calyx and then into the pelvis.[4] Aspiration of urine can confirm the cannulation. Water-soluble contrast medium is then injected to opacify the pelvicalyceal system. A series of spot films of the ureter down to the level of obstruction can be taken.

NEPHROSTOGRAM

A nephrostomy tube is usually positioned for therapeutic purposes but contrast can be instilled through it and a nephrostogram can be performed. It is indicated to assess the continued presence of calculus or any obstructing lesion or determine the cause of obstruction if it has not been demonstrated. Nephrostogram is also done in post-operative patients of PUJ obstruction to check the patency.[4] It is used to monitor the status of fistulas. Spot films of the ureter are taken down to the level of obstruction.

GRAYSCALE ULTRASOUND

Ultrasound is a reliable technique for the evaluation of upper urinary tract. It is noninvasive, easily available, accurate, safe, and does not require exposure to ionizing radiation. It can be performed bedside for sick patients and interventions can be performed under ultrasound guidance.

Indications for sonography in upper urinary tract:[19]

- Diagnosing dilatation of the collecting system and to search for renal obstruction.
- Excellent modality for evaluation of cystic renal lesions. Their architecture including internal septations, wall thickening, calcifications, presence or absence of solid components (in order to assign a Bosniak grade) can all be evaluated on ultrasound.
- Assessment of congenital anomalies and renal infections as ultrasound is a safe method for evaluating the urinary tract particularly in pediatric patients as high resolution sonography is easily feasible and radiation can be avoided.[20,21]
- Postnatal ultrasound for the evaluation of urinary tract in documented prenatal fetal hydronephrosis.
- Characterization of renal masses.
- Detection of nephrolithiasis and resultant back pressure changes, if any.
- Painless hematuria in low- and medium-risk patients.[22]
- Guidance for therapeutic and interventional procedures.

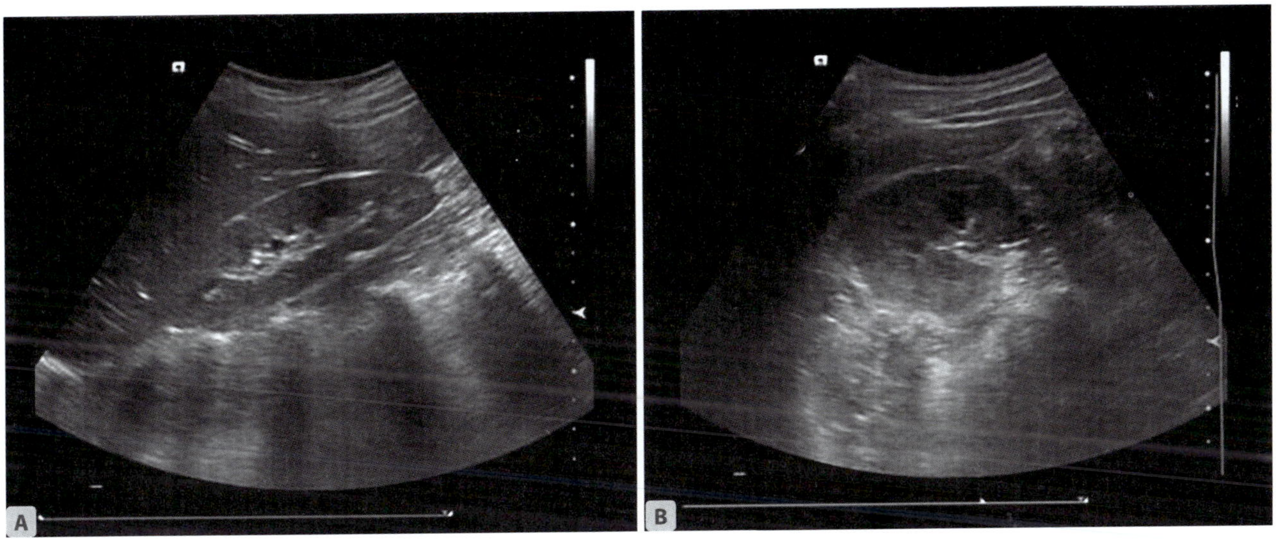

FIGS. 6A AND B: (A) Longitudinal and (B) transverse views of the kidney on ultrasound showing bright central sinus echoes, the cortex, and the hypoechoic medulla.

Technique

Positioning and Access

A 3–5 MHz curvilinear/linear transducer is used to scan the kidneys and ureter. A supine or lateral decubitus position can be adopted for kidneys. The right kidney is usually examined first where the liver is used as an acoustic window **(Figs. 6A and B)**. The transducer is placed in subcostal or intercostal position. Owing to gases from the small bowel and splenic flexure visualization of the left kidney becomes difficult at times via anterior or anterolateral approach. In such situations, a posterolateral approach can be adopted for the left kidney with the left side of the patient raised by approximately 45°.[23] The spleen provides an acoustic window on the left side. If even after raising left side of the body by 45°, visualization is not successful, a full right lateral decubitus with the pillow under the right flank and the left arm extended over the head may allow visualization of the left kidney. Prone position is usually adopted for young children for adequate visualization of the kidneys. A prone position is useful in adults in ultrasound-guided procedures.[24]

Renal Size

The longest craniocaudal length should be measured by rotating the probe around its vertical axis. The longest length should be measured as false low measurements are obtained at times due to ellipsoidal shape of the kidney. Renal length which gives an estimate of the overall renal size is quick and easy to measure. The determination of renal size with ultrasound is more accurate than with IVU because the kidney is imaged without magnification and contrast-induced osmotic diuresis. As a result renal size is approximately 15% smaller. Renal size is related to sex, age, and built of the patient. The length of the normal adult kidney is usually 10–12 cm but can range from 7 cm to 14 cm in patients with normal renal function **(Table 2)**. Length can also vary in the same individual depending on the state of hydration.

TABLE 2: Normal kidney length in adults.[25]

Adult female (cm)	Adult male (cm)
Left kidney 11 (9.9–12.1)	11.5 (10.4–12.6)
Right kidney 10.7 (9.5–12)	11.2 (10.1–12.4)

Where an absolute accurate estimate of the size of the kidneys is necessary, the renal volume can be measured. This can be achieved by measuring the area of the kidney in serial slices and calculating the volume but this method is very time consuming. A modified three-dimensional (3D) ellipsoidal formula is utilized where the length, anteroposterior diameter, and transverse diameters are multiplied by a constant which is approximately 0.5.[19] Volume measurements are done in postnephrectomy, patients to look for compensatory hypertrophy and in the assessment of renal transplants.

Emamian et al. measured the renal size in 665 healthy adult volunteers and showed that the parenchymal volume of the right kidney is smaller than the left.[26] Possible explanation for this could be: (1) The spleen is smaller than the liver and so there is more space for left kidney growth and (2) The LRA is shorter than the right and, therefore, increased blood flow on the left results in an increase in renal volume.

Cortical and Parenchymal Thickness

The cortical thickness is the distance between the renal capsule and outer margin of the renal pyramids while parenchymal thickness is the distance between renal capsule and margin of the sinus echoes **(Fig. 7)**.

Perirenal Structures

An assessment of the perirenal fat, pararenal areas, and adrenal areas should be done. At times, in case of any renal abnormality, liver, pancreas, lining of ureters, pelvis, and bladder may need to be examined.

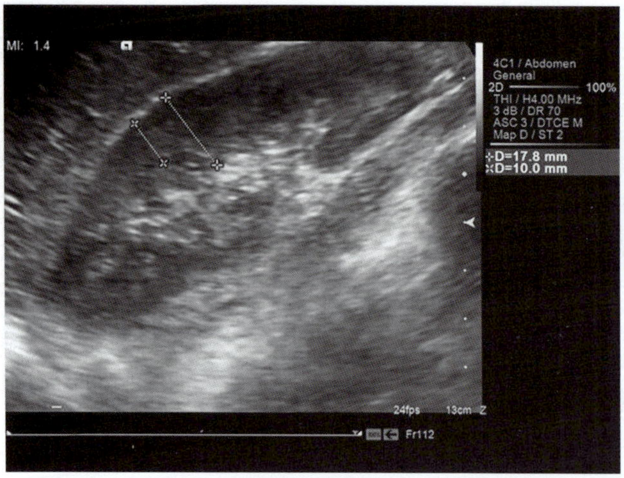

FIG. 7: Ultrasound image showing the normal cortical thickness (++) measured from the renal capsule to the outer margin of the medullary pyramids and the parenchymal thickness (xx) from the capsule to the margin of the sinus. The parenchymal thickness is more than the cortical thickness.

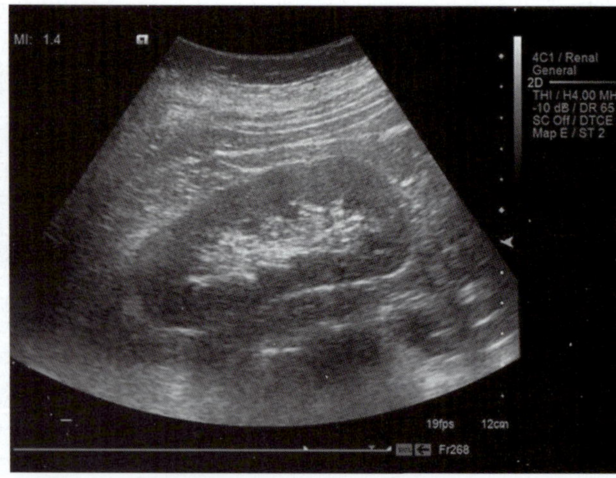

FIG. 8: Ultrasound scan of the kidney showing the corticomedullary differentiation well with the medulla seen as echopoor oval areas evenly distributed around the inner margin of the cortex. Arcuate vessels seen as echogenic foci mark the corticomedullary junction.

An important point while examining the kidneys on sonography is to take care that the whole length of the kidney is included otherwise peripheral abnormalities may be missed. When longitudinal examination is complete, turning the transducer through 90° ensures that kidney is examined in transverse plane from top to bottom. In addition to the size and shape of kidney, its cortical reflectivity as compared to the liver and spleen, the degree of corticomedullary differentiation and the appearance of medullary pyramids should be taken into account.

Normal Appearances on Ultrasound

Identification of kidneys on sonography is easy owing to the difference in reflectivity between parenchyma and surrounding fat. The outer cortical margin is well-defined due to the renal capsule, but the renal parenchyma adjacent to the renal sinus echo is less well-defined. The reflectivity of the kidneys can be compared with that of the liver and spleen on the right and left side, respectively. The renal cortex has a lower reflectivity than the adjacent liver and spleen. This difference in reflectivity may vary as it is dependent on the equipment to some extent and may be less obvious with some makes or scanners or pre- and postprocessing settings. However, if the renal cortex has a higher reflectivity, that is, it is brighter than the adjacent visceral organs, it is highly suggestive of renal parenchymal disease.[27] The medullary pyramids are seen as echo-poor oval structures evenly distributed around the inner margins of the cortical parenchyma **(Fig. 8)**. The pyramids are less reflective as compared to the cortex. The well-defined margin between the pyramids and the adjacent cortex is responsible for the corticomedullary differentiation which gets lost in the presence of generalized parenchymal inflammation and edema.

The renal sinus contains the calyces, infundibulum, a portion of the renal pelvis, fibrous tissue, fat, vessels, and lymphatics. On ultrasound, the renal sinus appears as a central hyperechoic area, largely because of its fat content.[28] When collapsed, the collecting system merges with the echoes of the renal sinus. However, in well-hydrated patients, it may be slightly distended with echo-free urine.

The *neonatal kidney* is sonographically more echogenic than that of the older infant and adults **(Figs. 9A and B)**.[29] Echogenicity is equal to or greater than the adjacent liver. It assumes the adult appearance by 2–3 months of age. Other differences are tabulated in **Table 3**.

Normal Variations

The kidneys may vary in *position* due to ptosis or an ectopic location. The most common site for the ectopic kidney is the pelvis, where it may be difficult to detect, as it can be obscured by bowel gas. *Renal duplication* is common and spans a range from complete to minimal. However, sonography may only show an elongated kidney perhaps with separation of the renal sinus into two parts. A double pelvis may be visualized when the collecting system is distended. Residual *fetal lobulations* may be seen. A *dromedary hump* can be seen sometimes which is a bulge along the lateral border of the left kidney due to molding by the adjacent spleen.

A *hypertrophied column of Bertin* is a normal variant and represents unresorbed polar parenchyma from one or both of the two subkidneys that fuse to form the normal kidney. Sonographic criteria to diagnose a hypertrophied column of Bertin include isoechogenicity and continuity with rest of the renal cortex, lack of mass effect, indentation of renal sinus laterally, generally less than 3 cm in size with a normal vascular pattern on Doppler.[32] Occasionally, it may be difficult to differentiate a small avascular tumor from a hypertrophied column of Bertin when further investigations may be required. A wedge-shaped echogenic defect or an echogenic line, the *intervesicular fissure or parenchymal junctional defect*, may sometimes be seen running obliquely from the sinus to the capsule in upper anterior or lower posterior

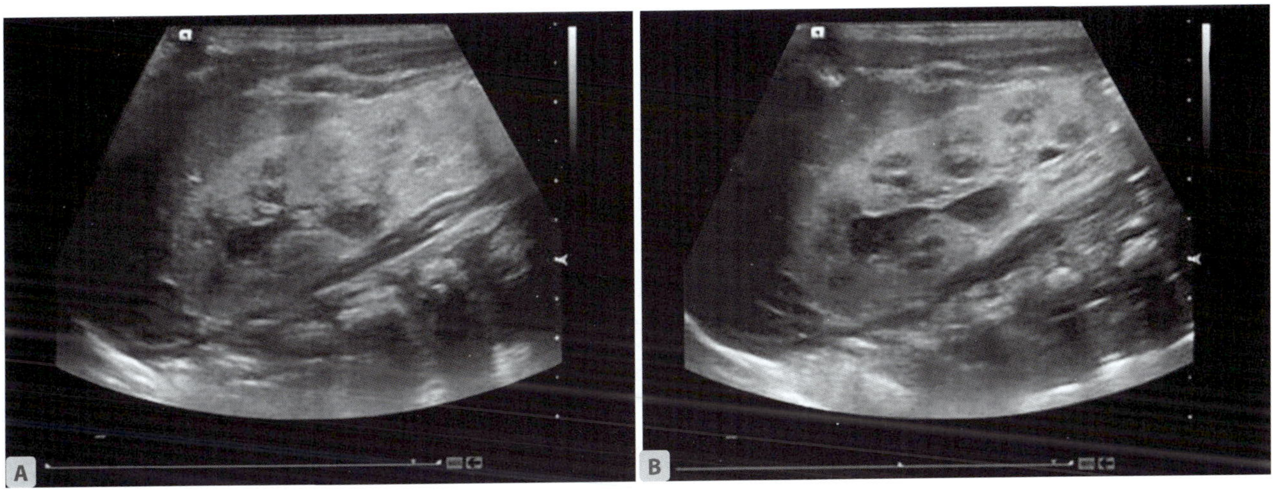

FIGS. 9A AND B: Ultrasound images showing the normal neonatal kidney. The cortex is thin and highly reflective while the medulla is large out of proportion and very poorly reflective. The renal sinus is also echopoor.

TABLE 3: Differences between neonatal and adult kidney.[30,31]

	Neonatal	Adult
Contour	Lobed	Smooth
Cortex reflectivity	++	+
Medullary reflectivity	—	—
Sinus	Echopoor	Echogenic
Collecting system	Apparent	Inapparent

part of the kidney.[33] It was thought to represent connective tissue at the junction of the development of anterior and posterior components of the kidney. However, subsequent reassessment suggests that this line represents an extension into the parenchyma of hilar/sinus fat in patients with a deep renal sinus, rather than a true plane of fusion between embryological components. It may mimic a scar or rarely a small echogenic tumor.[34]

The *renal sinus thickness* is normally equal to the parenchymal thickness. However, it may vary depending on the fat content of the sinus. An increase in fat content of the renal sinus can occur in obese individuals, in renal sinus lipomatosis, and in cases of parenchymal atrophy. It is decreased in neonates and in cachectic patients.

A mild distension of the collecting system can occur due to physiological filling. This can be seen in a fluid-loaded subject, a patient on diuretics, diabetics, recovery phase of acute tubular necrosis (ATN), single kidney, neonatal kidney, and patients with an overdistended bladder.

DOPPLER EVALUATION

Indications

- Renovascular hypertension
- Characterization of mass lesions
- Differentiation between obstructive and non-obstructive hydronephrosis
- Evaluation of transplant kidney
- Renal vein thrombosis
- Miscellaneous, e.g. trauma, arteriovenous malformation (AVM), etc.

Technique

With the patient supine, the RRA can be identified arising approximately 1 cm below the origin of the SMA. Occasionally, LRA can be identified at its origin from the posterolateral or lateral surface of aorta. Both renal veins and their junction with the IVC can usually be demonstrated in this plane. In slim patients, it is occasionally possible to follow the renal artery and vein into the hilum of the kidney.[35] The right and left posterior oblique positions can also be used to identify the vessels in the midline. Throughout the course of examination of renal vessels, color Doppler is frequently switched on to confirm the nature and direction of flow **(Fig. 10)**. The optimum pulse repetition frequency is selected to detect moderate flow velocities, although it may need to be modified to detect high velocities if a stenosis with aliasing of color signals is present.[36] With the system set to detect low or moderate flow velocities, flow can be identified in almost all patients in the vessels at the renal hilum. Angling of the probe medially from the right or left flank will allow assessment of the intrarenal vessels. Though the hilar and interlobar vessels are demonstrated in all patients, the arcuate and striate arteries may be seen only in slimmer patients. Power Doppler can show smaller vessels with slow flow, though with loss of directional information **(Fig. 11)**. Contrast-enhanced ultrasound (CEUS) can further enhance visualization of parenchymal vessels.

Normal Doppler Pattern

There is a rapid systolic upstroke, which is occasionally followed by a secondary slower rise to peak systole. Subsequently, there is a gradual diastolic decay but with persistent forward flow in diastole. Spectral indices are measured in the renal artery at proximal, middle, and at the hilum. Normal range of values is shown in **Table 4**.[36] Further, indices should also be measured in the intrarenal vessels at the superior, middle, and inferior pole of the kidney. The

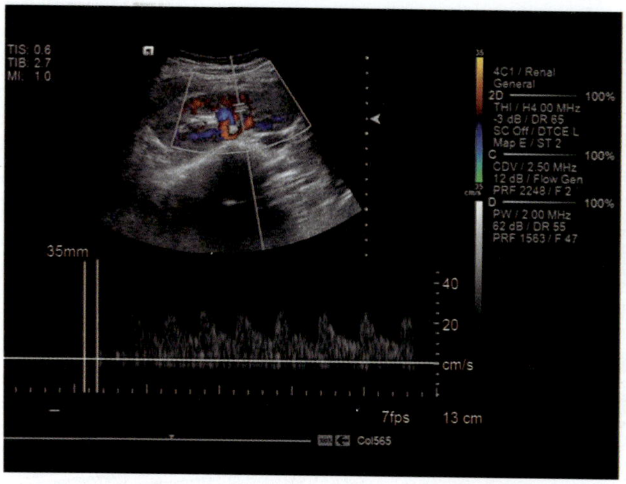

FIG. 10: Normal renal spectral pattern on color Doppler showing steep systolic peak and a good diastolic end flow.

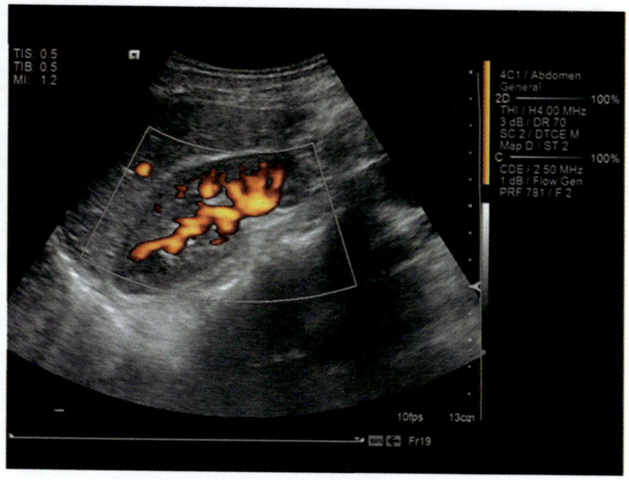

FIG. 11: Power Doppler image of the normal vasculature of the kidney.

TABLE 4: Normal renal indices.[36]

Index	Range
Pulsatility index	0.7–1.4
Resistance index	0.56–0.7
Peak systolic velocity (PSV)	60–140 cm/sec (<180)
Renal artery/aorta ratio (RAR)	< 3.5
Acceleration time	0.04–0.05 sec
Acceleration index	2.5–3.8 m/sec^2

resistive index (RI) and pulsatility index (PI) values measured in healthy subjects show a significant dependence on age and the area sampled. The values in the main artery are higher than in the more distal smaller arteries and they are lowest in the interlobular arteries.

The renal vein spectra are often different for right and left veins. The RRV is short and often mirrors the pulsatility of the IVC, while the left, particularly if it is sampled to the left of the SMA, may show only slight variability of flow velocities.

Ureters on Ultrasound

The ureter is a long (25 cm) mucosal lined tube varying in diameter from 2 mm to 8 mm. The normal ureters are usually difficult to visualize as they are thin and collapsed structures. However, dilated ureters can be imaged in their proximal and distal parts. The proximal ureters are best visualized in a coronal oblique view, using the kidney as a window. An attempt can be made to follow the ureter up to the bladder using the same approach. The distal ureters can be seen suprapubically through the full bladder.

CONTRAST-ENHANCED ULTRASOUND

Contrast-enhanced ultrasound is an emerging technology for evaluation of the genitourinary system with no known nephrotoxicity. It has a role in the characterization of indeterminate renal lesions, especially among those with chronic kidney disease (CKD). Iodinated contrast medium should be completely withheld in patients with later stages of CKD [glomerular filtration rate (GFR) <30 mL/min]. Similarly, gadolinium-based contrast agents should not be administered in severe renal insufficiency owing to the risk of nephrogenic systemic fibrosis (NSF). CEUS is safe in that it causes no nephrotoxicity. Microbubbles used in CEUS consist of a high molecular weight gas core surrounded by a lipid or albumin shell. The microbubbles are not excreted or secreted in the urinary tract but are exhaled out via the lungs and hence have no adverse effect on the kidneys. According to the 2011 European Federation for the Society of Ultrasound in Medicine and Biology Guidelines, the use of CEUS for renal indications include:[37]

- Characterization of indeterminate lesions when conventional ultrasound is equivocal
- Renal infarcts and cortical necrosis
- Abscesses
- Determination of surgical strategy for complex cystic masses
- Follow-up imaging of nonsurgical complex masses
- Tumor ablation under ultrasound guidance.

SonoVue, Optison, and Sonazoid are some of the ultrasound contrast agents available in the US for intravenous use while SonoVue is available in India. CEUS has shown promising results and its sensitivity has been reported comparable to that of contrast-enhanced CT in the characterization of renal lesions.[38] The sensitivity in detection of renal malignancy has been found to be about 90% in several studies with a moderate specificity of 79–90%.[39] An exciting new frontier in CEUS research is the use of targeted microbubbles where antibodies can be tagged to the outer shell. The antibodies get adhered to their molecular target and on imaging this is seen as persistence of enhancement. This is helpful in the detection of diseases and holds the prospect of delivering therapy specifically at these locations reducing the systemic toxic effects of the chemotherapeutic drugs.

ULTRASOUND ELASTOGRAPHY

Elastography can be used to diagnose kidney diseases and provides a more accurate estimate of the functional impairment than blood tests or kidney dimensions. Intrarenal fibrosis is a final common pathway for all chronic kidney diseases and it has been seen that the degree of fibrosis correlates with the severity of the disease. Renal biopsy can determine the degree of fibrosis and hence the severity of the renal parenchymal disease but it is invasive, is subject to sampling errors and samples a small fraction of the renal parenchyma leading to an inaccurate assessment.

Shear wave elastography (SWE) is an emerging technique which permits a noninvasive measurement of tissue stiffness. SWE uses focused acoustic energy pulses to produce shear waves which travel perpendicular to the tissue. As they progress through the tissue, they can be tracked sonographically. Stiffer the tissue, more is the shear wave velocity. Higher values of shear wave velocity thus correlate with higher degrees of renal fibrosis. Studies have shown that SWE is a low cost way to provide diagnostic information in patients with CKD and a correlation has been found between SWE, estimated renal stiffness, and renal fibrosis severity.[40] Hence, SWE-derived estimates of tissue stiffness may serve as a noninvasive biomarker of healthy and diseased renal parenchyma in the near future.

COMPUTED TOMOGRAPHY OF THE UPPER URINARY TRACT

The cross-sectional imaging modalities such as CT and magnetic resonance imaging (MRI) allow a noninvasive visualization and a better understanding of the genitourinary tract. The anatomical characteristics of the renal and perirenal regions can be visualized objectively and accurately. Perfusion characteristics of the kidney can also be studied. CT plays a vital role in evaluating patients with renal cystic diseases, renal tumors, infections, and flank pain. Lesions containing fat or calcium are best assessed on CT.

MDCT allows volumetric data acquisition and submillimeter excellent quality images can be reconstructed in any plane. MDCT with its 3D postprocessing capabilities is highly accurate in the evaluation of renal masses and a noninvasive evaluation of vascular pedicle by CT angiography. MDCT reduces the diagnosis of indeterminate masses by enabling an improved characterization of renal masses, thus allowing a better therapeutic management. The faster scanning times, improved spatial and temporal resolution, and greater volume coverage with the MDCT scanners allow detection and characterization of small renal masses, display of vasculature similar to conventional angiography, and improved visualization of the collecting system and ureters with better demonstration of both intraluminal and extraluminal pathology.[41,42] MDCT allows images to be obtained in different phases of enhancement of the renal parenchyma including the excretory phase (EP) and images simulating excretory urography can be obtained.[43] Excellent quality multiplanar reformation (MPR) images and 3D rendering of any plane is possible owing to increased temporal resolution and acquisition of thin slices with isotropic voxels.[44]

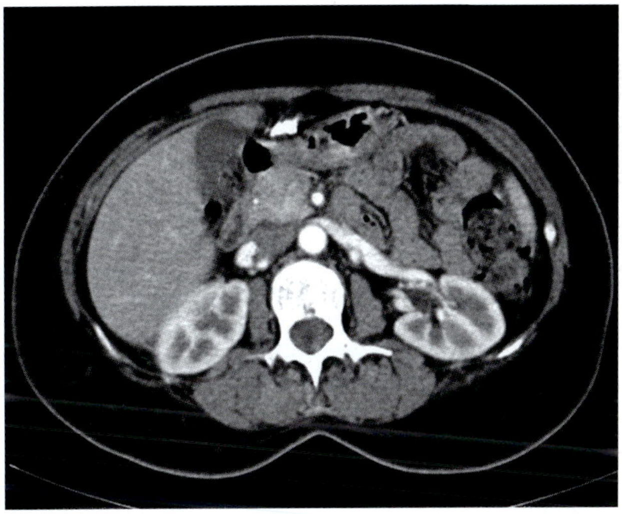

FIG. 12: Contrast-enhanced axial scans showing the kidneys as smooth and oval structures with an anteromedial break in the region of hilum where the vascular pedicle enters. The longer left renal vein is seen crossing anterior to the aorta and posterior to the superior mesenteric artery to enter the inferior vena cava at the level of the uncinate process of the pancreas.

Normal Appearance of the Upper Urinary Tract on CT

On the axial sections, the kidneys appear smooth and oval. The vascular pedicle enters the renal hilum which is seen as an anteromedial break **(Fig. 12)**. The vascular pedicle lies anterior to the renal pelvis. Differentiation between renal artery and vein may not be possible on conventional scans. The renal veins are larger than the renal artery. Of the veins, the left renal vein is larger than the right owing to the aorta and SMA pinching the left renal vein.

The ureters are best visualized after intravenous administration of iodinated contrast material. The ureters are anterior to the common iliac artery, lateral to the external iliac artery, and anteromedial to the psoas major at the level of the sacral promontory. The ureters then reach the midportion of the internal obturator muscle coursing medially and posteriorly to the external iliac arteries. They then course anteromedially to reach the trigone of the urinary bladder **(Figs. 13A to D)**.

Examination Technique and Imaging Protocols of MDCT of Kidney

A multiphasic CT is the preferred imaging technique in the evaluation of the upper urinary tract. It includes an unenhanced scan followed by scanning the kidneys in the corticomedullary, nephrographic, and EPs after rapid bolus injection of contrast (100–120 mL of 300 mgI/mL of contrast) at the rate of 3–4 mL/sec.[45] Use of dense oral contrast medium is not recommended for renal CT as the contrast in the bowel may obscure small ureteral stones making their detection difficult. The dense oral contrast medium poses a major problem in 3D-CT angiography and to avoid major overlay in the postprocessed images,[46] it is recommended that negative oral contrast medium/water should be administered.

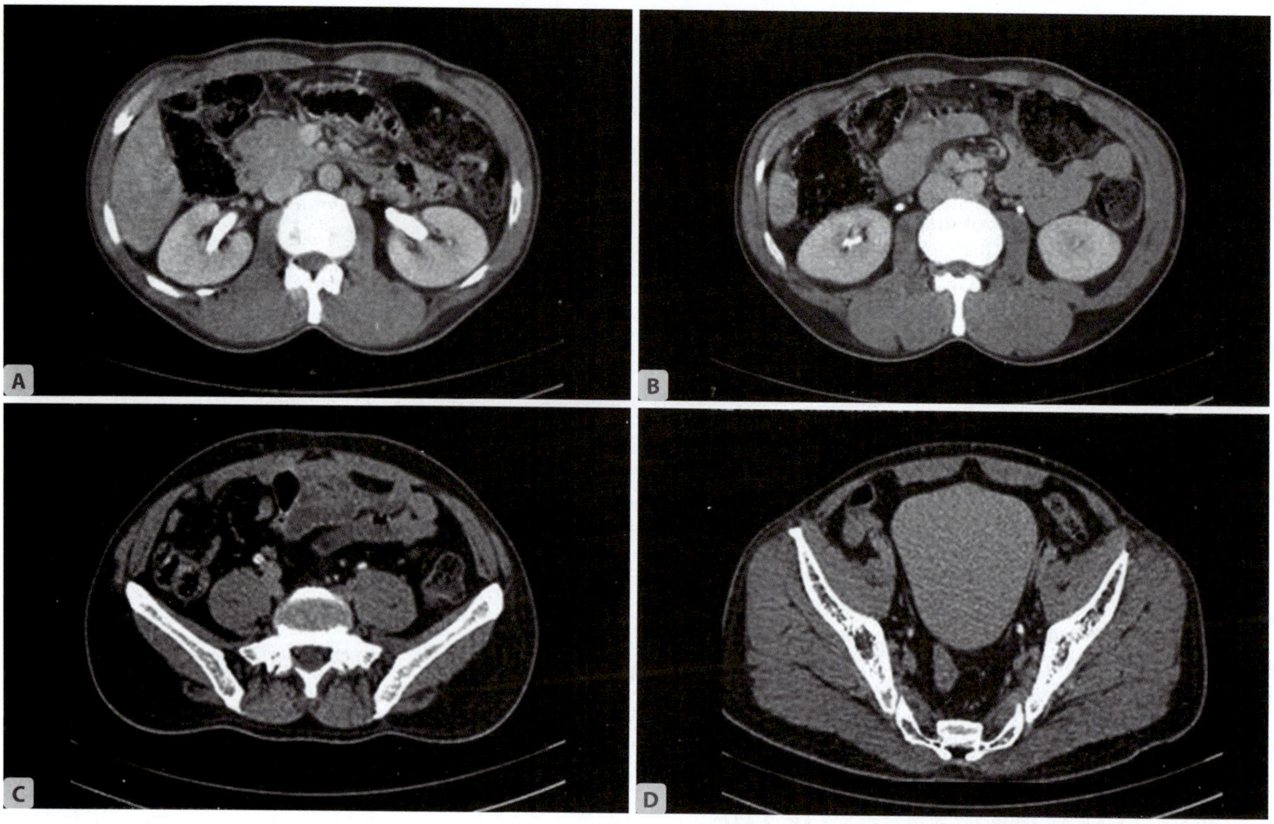

FIGS. 13A TO D: Axial CT sections showing the normal anatomy of the urinary structures from superior to inferior. (A) The renal pelvis; (B) Upper ureters; (C) Mid ureters; (D) Distal ureters.

And 500–750 mL of water can be given over a 15–20-minute period before the start of a renal CT examination.[47]

Noncontrast

This phase is useful for baseline density measurements of renal masses and diagnosis of areas of hemorrhage/renal hematoma.[48] Areas of renal parenchymal calcification, fat attenuation, and calcification in a renal mass can all be detected on the noncontrast scan. These are also helpful to differentiate a renal solid mass from hyperdense cyst. Noncontrast CT is regarded as the primary imaging modality to detect urinary tract calculi.[49] The American Association and Endourological Society Guidelines for the Surgical Management of stones specifically recommend that clinicians should obtain a noncontrast CT before performing percutaneous nephrolithotomy (PCNL) in adults and children.[50] Low-dose computed tomography (LDCT) and ultralow-dose computed tomography (ULDCT) have been proposed to reduce radiation risks for the detection of urolithiasis.[51,52]

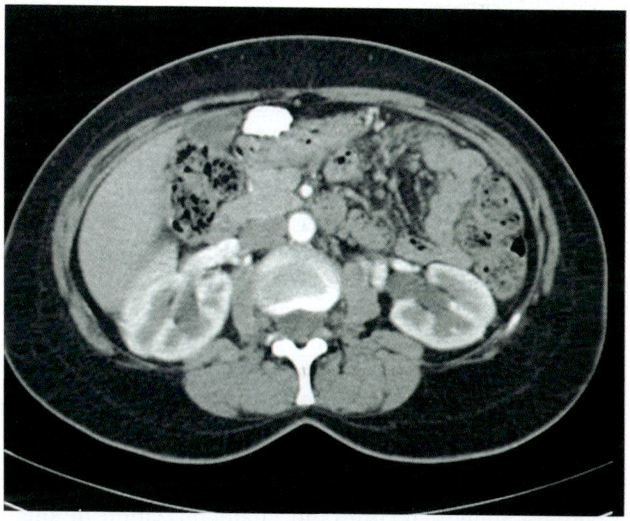

FIG. 14: Contrast-enhanced CT scan of the kidney in the corticomedullary phase showing dense cortical enhancement, the renal cortex is distinctly differentiated from the unenhanced medulla in this phase.

Normal CT Nephrogram

The first phase is the corticomedullary phase (CMP) and it is seen 25–80 seconds following contrast administration. In this phase, the lumen of the proximal tubules fills up with contrast which then enters the cortical capillaries and peritubular capillary spaces. In this phase, the renal cortex is distinctly differentiated from the unenhanced medulla (**Fig. 14**).[53] The nephrographic phase (NP) is the second phase and begins 90–120 seconds after contrast injection. The contrast passes through the renal tubules during this

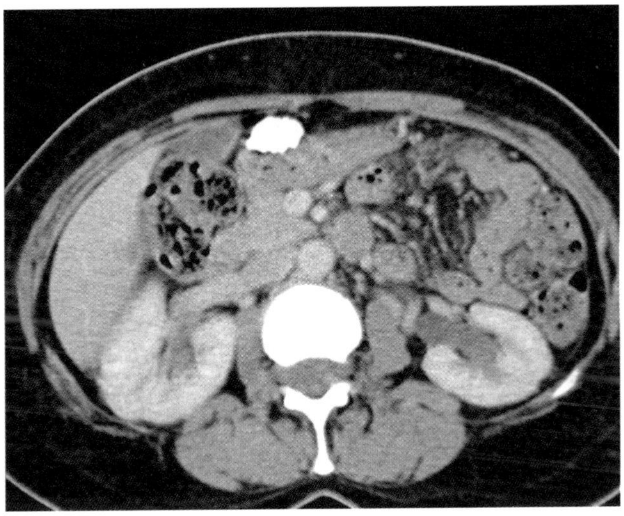

FIG. 15: Contrast-enhanced CT of the kidney in the nephrogram phase showing dense homogeneous parenchymal enhancement. The corticomedullary differentiation disappears during this phase.

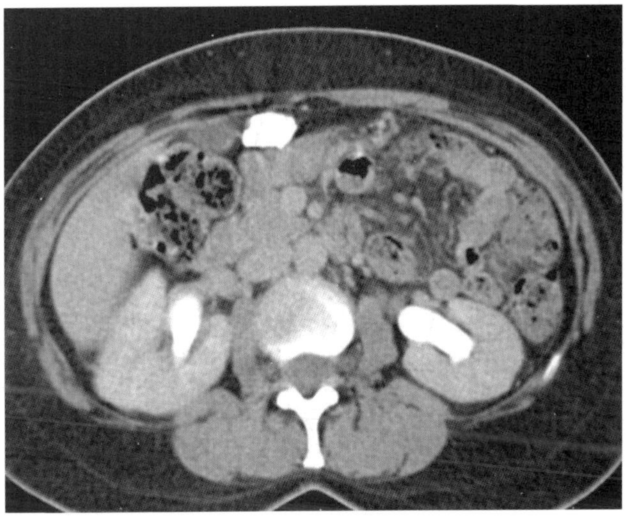

FIG. 16: Excretory phase images showing opacification of the pelvicalyceal system.

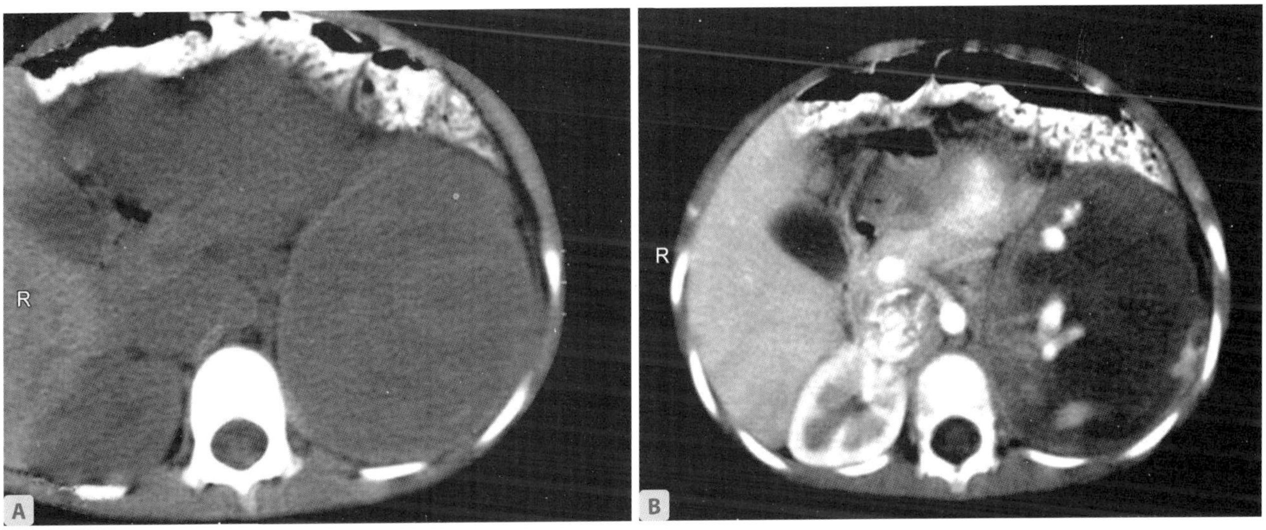

FIGS. 17A AND B: (A) Noncontrast axial CT showing a large hypodense mass replacing the left kidney. (B) The corticomedullary phase shows multiple tortuous feeder vessels depicting tumor hypervascularity. Thrombus is also seen in inferior vena cava in the case of Wilms' tumor, the corticomedullary phase being excellent for the depiction.

phase. In the nephrogram phase, there is a homogeneous enhancement of the renal parenchyma with loss of the corticomedullary differentiation **(Fig. 15)**. The excretory phase (EP) begins with the excretion of the contrast material into the collecting system and is seen best 3–5 minutes after contrast administration **(Fig. 16)**.

Corticomedullary Phase

This phase is important for the evaluation of tumor hypervascularity and differentiation of normal variants and pseudotumors from renal masses. This phase is also the best phase for the diagnosis of tumor extension in the renal vein as maximum opacification of the renal vein and arteries occur during this time **(Figs. 17A and B)**. However, scanning the kidney only in the CMP may lead to errors as hypervascular cortical renal cell carcinomas (RCCs) may enhance to the same degree as the normal cortex and thus may be obscured. Also, small hypovascular tumors of the renal medulla may not enhance sufficiently and may be missed.[54] It is therefore essential to scan the kidney in the NP following the CMP.

Nephrographic Phase

Nephrographic phase is considered as the optimum phase for not only detection but also characterization of renal masses. In this phase, there is a homogeneous enhancement of both the cortex and medulla. This phase is useful particularly for the lesions <3 cm.[55] Any enhancement >20 HU is considered suggestive of malignancy and this lesion enhancement is usually best visualized on the NP.[56] Renal infarction,

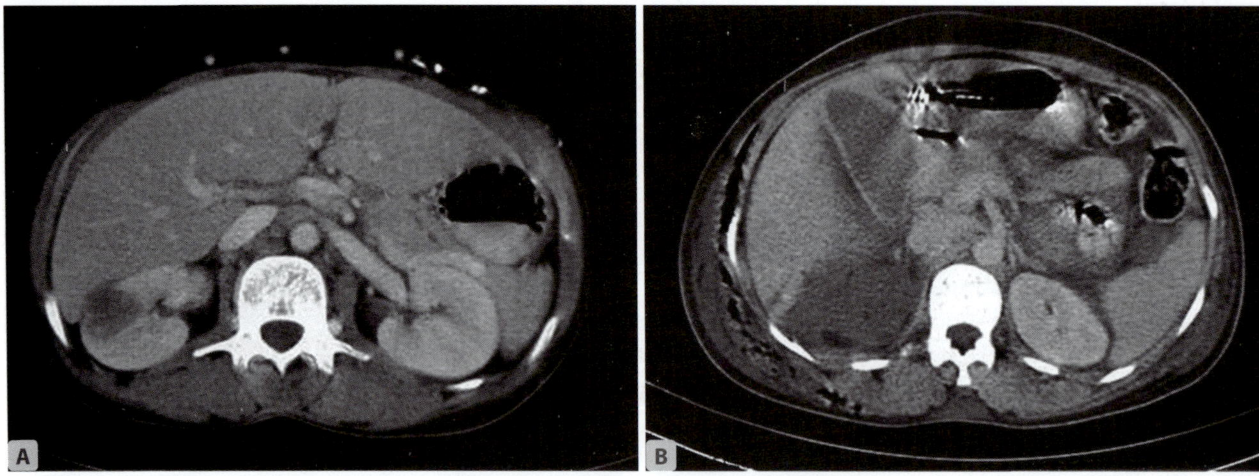

FIGS. 18A AND B: (A) Nephrogram phase showing a wedge-shaped area of hypoattenuation against the enhanced right renal parenchyma suggestive of renal infarct; (B) Image in another case showing complete lack of nephrogram suggesting devascularization of the right renal parenchyma in a case of trauma. The normal nephrogram with homogeneous enhancement of the renal parenchyma is seen on the left side.

traumatic parenchymal lesions, and acute pyelonephritis is also best visualized on the NP as the lesions stand out as hypodense areas against the enhanced renal parenchyma **(Figs. 18A and B)**.

Excretory Phase

This provides a good delineation and visualization of the pelvicalyceal system. The excretory phase (EP) images are useful for evaluation of urothelial lesions including urothelial neoplasms, calyceal deformities, papillary necrosis, and strictures and inflammatory changes of the collecting system and ureters.[57]

Pathological CT Nephrogram

Renal infarctions, blunt renal trauma, and acute pyelonephritis account for a pathological nephrogram. These conditions result in impaired renal perfusion with a focal reduction of the nephrogram. A segmental/total lack of the nephrogram is seen in cases of blunt renal trauma owing to devascularization. In acute pyelonephritis, inflammatory obstruction results in reduced tubule transit rate. The delayed perfusion of the renal tubule system is seen as a "striated nephrogram" pattern.[58] Conditions like acute ureteric obstruction, acute obstruction of the renal vein, and significant stenosis of the main renal artery result in reduced density and slowed temporal progression of the three phases of the nephrogram. Conditions like shock/severe systemic hypotension result in a bilaterally reduced density and persistence of nephrogram due to a reduced GFR and tubular stasis.

MDCT in Renal Masses

A multiphasic MDCT is necessary for optimal evaluation of renal masses.[59] Noncontrast CT is used to detect calcifications and the precontrast attenuation value allows quantification of enhancement on the postcontrast scans. The CMP best shows the extension of the tumoral tissue into the renal vein and IVC which is important for staging. A hypodense, filling defect within the renal vein which is usually dilated is suggestive of a thrombus. Heterogeneous enhancement of the thrombus with evidence of neovascularity favors a tumor thrombus over a bland thrombus. The neovascularity, arterial feeders, and the entire arterial anatomy is best seen on the CMP. Accurate demonstration of the arterial anatomy is essential to plan a nephron sparing surgery. The NP is the most useful for characterization of indeterminate masses. An enhancement value >20 HU is considered highly suggestive of a RCC as these are hypervascular and enhance on the postcontrast scans.[60] The EP is useful for demonstrating the relationship of a centrally located mass with the pelvicalyceal system. Involvement of the renal pelvis and calyces can also be best seen on the EP. Transitional cell carcinomas (TCCs) are also best detected during this phase as subtle hypodense filling defects within the renal pelvis, calyces or the ureters. A washout >15 HU seen in a mass on the EP is also highly suggestive of a RCC as these show a significant washout as well **(Figs. 19A to C)**.[61] A hyperdense renal cyst, on the contrary, will show no change in density between the corticomedullary and the excretory/delayed images.[61]

Three-dimensional CT (3DCT) along with CT angiography is useful to define the tumor and its relationship to the renal surface, the pelvicalyceal system and the adjacent organs. Viewing in multiple planes and orientations can be done to obtain all the information needed to plan a surgical resection. A display of the arterial and venous anatomy is possible prior to surgery.

MDCT in Urolithiasis and Acute Flank Pain

A noncontrast CT of the abdomen is the most sensitive and specific test for the detection of urinary tract calculi. A 98% sensitivity and 100% specificity for their detection has been reported by Fielding et al.[62] Noncontrast thin collimation scans (3–5 mm) are obtained from the upper pole of the kidneys to the pubic symphysis for the detection of urolithiasis which may be a cause of hematuria as well. Irrespective of the calcium content, almost all calculi are seen as radiopaque densities on noncontrast CT. Identification

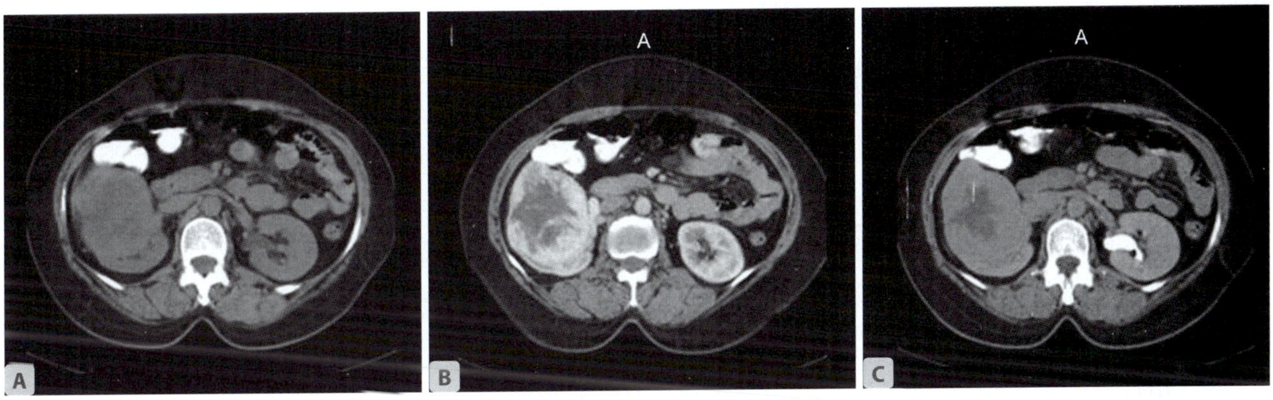

FIGS. 19A TO C: (A) Noncontrast; and (B and C) contrast-enhanced axial scans showing a large heterogeneous mass in the right kidney with enhancement >20 HU and washout >15 HU suggestive of a malignant renal mass. Areas of necrosis are also noted.

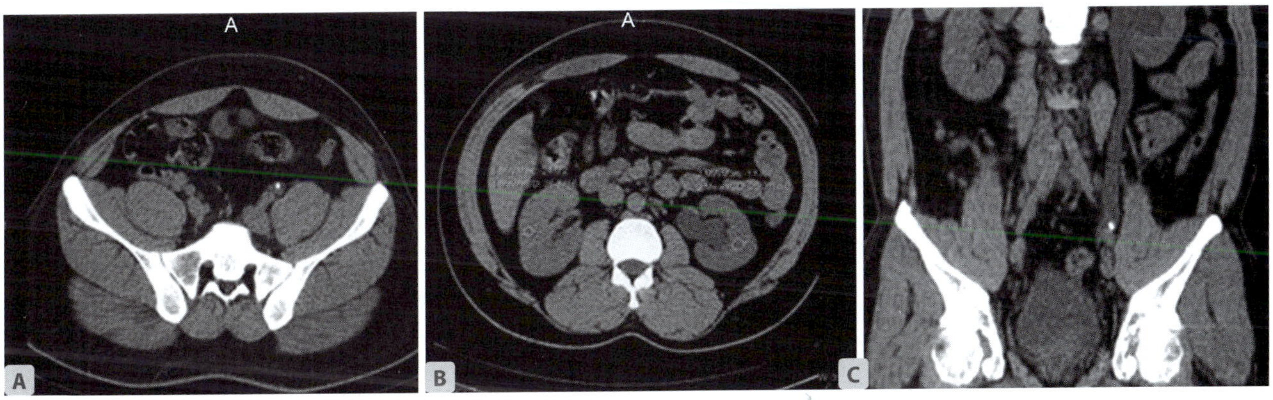

FIGS. 20A TO C: Noncontrast axial scans (A and B) of the abdomen showing a left ureteric calculus with soft tissue edema around, i.e. the rim sign (A) and the left hydronephrosis (B). The hydronephrotic left kidney has a lower attenuation than the normal right kidney. Curved multiplanar reformation displaying the left ureteric calculus, the consequent hydronephrosis, and the entire dilated left ureter proximal to it regardless of opacification (C).

of a stone within the ureter is the most specific diagnostic finding of urolithiasis. A "rim sign" may also be seen in cases of calculi owing to the ureteral wall edema that develops at the site of impaction.[63] This is seen as an area of soft tissue thickening (1–2 mm thickness) around the calculus. A decreased density of the renal parenchyma, hydronephrosis, hydroureter, and perinephric stranding are the other features seen in cases of calculi. A decreased attenuation of the renal parenchyma on the obstructed side by 5–14 HU is considered an objective finding of obstruction **(Figs. 20A to C)**.[64] CT can also differentiate calculi from phleboliths. Calculi have a dense center while phleboliths have a central lucency. A "comet tail sign" which is a linear or curvilinear soft tissue density extending from an abdominal/pelvic calcification is highly suggestive of a phlebolith.[65] MDCT is also useful for detecting the cause of pain other than stone such as appendicitis, biliary colic, diverticulitis, etc.[66]

MDCT in Blunt Renal Trauma

In patients with trauma, a noncontrast scan followed by multiphasic scanning needs to be done. The CMP is the best phase to show injuries of the renal arteries including internal injuries which are nonocclusive in nature. Renal vein thrombosis can also be seen. Contrast extravasations which occur during the CMP are due to hemorrhage as compared to contrast extravasations that occur during the EP which are due to rupture of the pelvicalyceal system **(Figs. 21A to C)**. Contained hemorrhage or pseudoaneurysm is seen as a well-defined lesion within the area of laceration. Active hemorrhage is seen as ill-defined or flame-shaped area with bright enhancement close to an artery.[67] NP is the best to demonstrate areas of renal infarction/nonperfused parenchymal injuries. EP images are the best to show contrast extravasation in urinomas indicating an injury to the collecting system.[68]

MDCT in Renal Infections

Multidetector computed tomography is a more useful modality than IVU or ultrasound in the assessment of renal infection. The nature and extent of the disease process as well as complications such as gas forming infections, abscess formation, and urinary obstruction can all be well seen on CT.[69] The most characteristic finding of acute pyelonephritis is poorly defined low attenuating areas of decreased attenuation which are wedge-shaped radiating from the medulla to the cortical surface. These wedge-shaped areas are best seen in the NP. A nephrogram pattern consisting of alternating linear bands of hyper- and hypoattenuation,

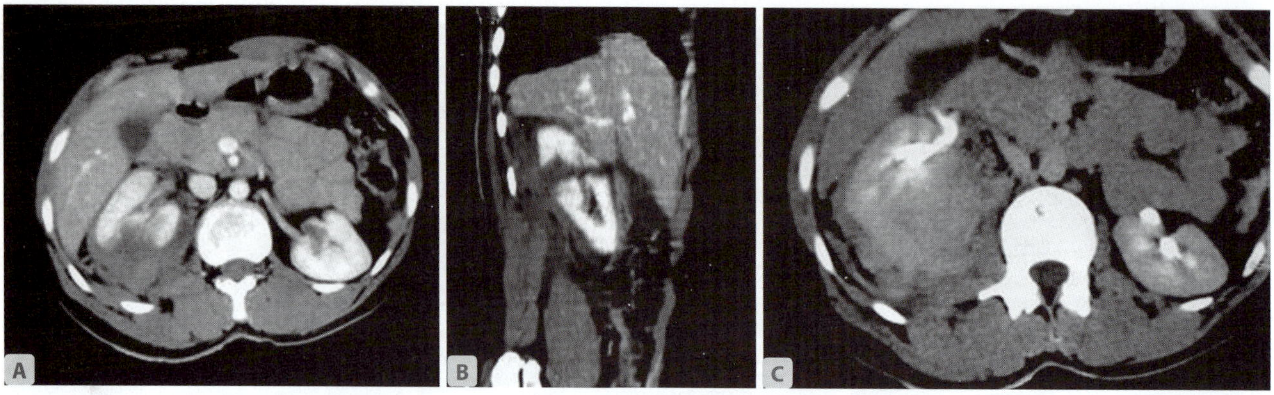

FIGS. 21A TO C: (A) Nephrogram phase image showing laceration of the right renal parenchyma with perinephric hematoma; (B) Sagittal multiplanar reformation image showing fracture of the kidney; (C) Excretory phase showing extravasation of contrast in the perinephric hematoma suggesting rupture of the pelvicalyceal system.

the so called "striated nephrogram" is another characteristic finding of acute pyelonephritis. Other findings include focal or diffuse enlargement of the kidney, diminished concentration of contrast in the tubules due to the inflammatory process, stranding of the perinephric fat, thickening of Gerota's fascia, and obliteration of renal sinus.[70] A focal thinning of the cortex may result from scarring in chronic cases.

Image Processing and Postprocessing Techniques on Computed Tomography

The various 3D visualization techniques in the evaluation of the urinary tract are MPR, maximum intensity projection (MIP), shaded surface display (SSD), and volume-rendered techniques (VRTs).

Multiplanar Reformation

Multiplanar reformation (MPR) represents a simple reordering of the image voxel. For MPR, the structures must be in the same plane, hence it cannot be generated for structures not in the same plane. Pseudostenoses are created as structures course in and out of the MPR. Curved multiplanar reformations (CPRs) are useful to overcome this problem.[71] CPR images can be obtained by drawing a line over the structure of interest, it can also be produced by a dedicated software automatically or semiautomatically. CPR is useful in the demonstration of vessels of small diameter or structures with tortuous anatomy like the ureters **(Figs. 22A to C)**.[72] The limitation, however, is the dependence on accuracy of the curve generated.

Maximum Intensity Projection

Maximum intensity projection (MIP) displays the maximum voxel intensity along a line in a given volume. Structures with high density such as the contrast opacified collecting system and vessels are well demonstrated on MIP images. Angiograms and urograms are examples where this technique is used **(Figs. 23A to C)**. However, the major limitation is obscuration of the area of interest by high density material like bone, calcium, and oral contrast medium. MIP also lacks depth orientation.[73]

Shaded Surface Display

Shaded surface display (SSD) enables an accurate 3D representation of anatomy. It relies on the gray scale to yield surface reflections of structures. Though it provides a depth orientation, its major limitation lies in the dependence on user selected threshold setting.

Volume Rendered Technique

Volume rendered technique takes the entire volume of data and displays anatomic structures with different levels of opacity/attenuation. All attenuation values within a voxel are used to obtain the final image with each voxel contributing color, brightness, and opacity to the final image. The renal parenchyma, renal vasculature, and the pelvicalyceal system have different levels of opacity and can be seen simultaneously using this technique. VRT is an excellent 3D technique that provides a roadmap to the surgeon and produces images with[72] which the clinicians are familiar with. By editing out bone and other areas that overlie the area of interest excellent 3D images can be generated in the desired orientation **(Figs. 24A and B)**.

MULTIDETECTOR CT UROGRAPHY

It is an examination of the urinary tract in the EP following intravenous contrast on MDCT. CT urography can examine the entire genitourinary tract in a single study. It is a comprehensive examination that allows evaluation of both the renal parenchyma and the urothelium. Multidetector computed tomography urography (MDCTU) can be used as a "one-stop imaging test" for the entire urinary tract.[74]

The two approaches to perform a CT urography include:

1. CT hybrid urography
2. CT—only CT urography.

CT HYBRID UROGRAPHY

This technique combines CT and IVU into a single comprehensive examination. No CT postprocessing is necessary as images are obtained in a coronal reformatted form familiar to the clinicians. CT hybrid urography may entail

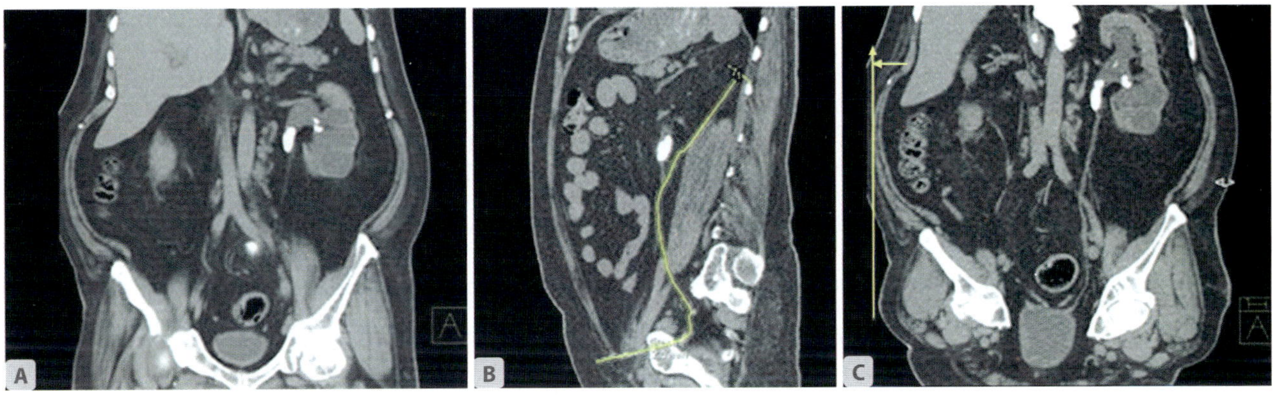

FIGS. 22A TO C: (A) Coronal multiplanar reformation (MPR) image showing a left ureteric calculus and the dilated pelvicalyceal proximal to it; (B and C) Curved multiplanar images show the left ureter in its entirety.

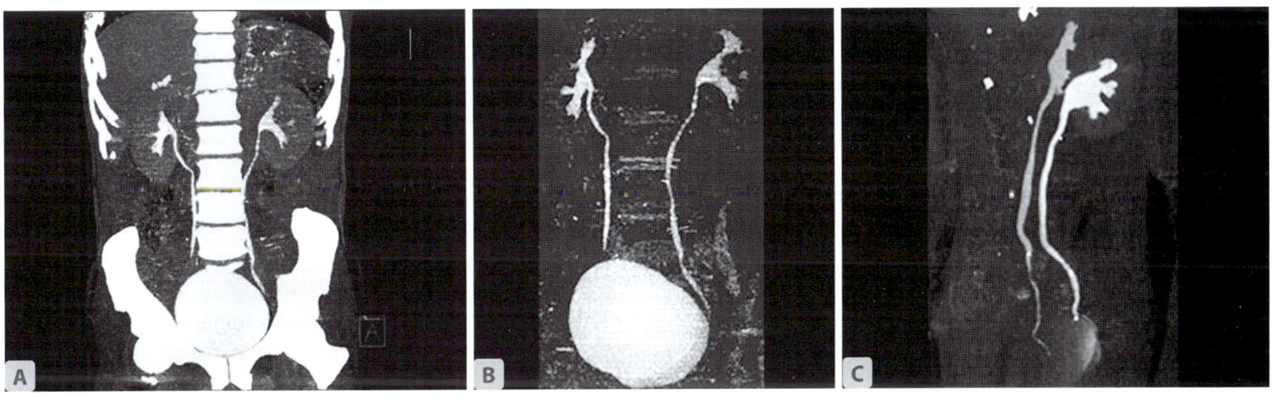

FIGS. 23A TO C: Maximum intensity projection (MIP) in the excretory phase demonstrating the normally opacified calyces, the ureters, and the bladder. This technique displays the maximum voxel value along a line of viewer and projection through a given volume and a rotational viewing of multiple projections can be done (A to C).

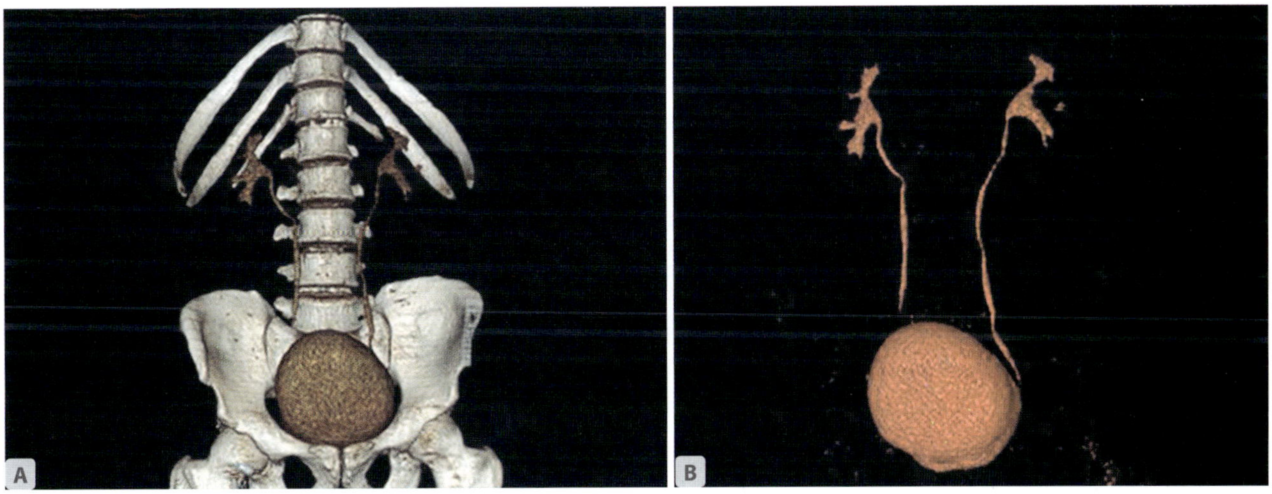

FIGS. 24A AND B: Volume-rendering technique displaying the entire urinary tract. This technique takes the entire volume of data and displays anatomic structures with different levels of opacity/attenuation.

imaging the patient in two different locations. Conventional urography images can be acquired in an IVU room followed by transferring the patient to the CT room and imaging the patient without an additional dose of contrast medium.[75] However, the disadvantages involved in moving the patient from one place to another involve longer time, additional resources, and inadequate opacification of the pelvicalyceal system during acquisition because of the time elapsed in moving the patient.[76] In some centers, this problem has been solved by installing a ceiling mounted X-ray tube above the CT table and a special tabletop that allows insertion of a screen film system beneath the patient.[77] With this technique, an abdominal radiograph, a noncontrast CT followed by a multiphasic CT followed by overhead excretory urography and postvoid films can be acquired. However, by the use of CT scanned projection radiography (CTSPR) which is also known as topogram or scannogram, the technique can be performed on any MDCT scanner.[78] CTSPR images do not require a ceiling mounted X-ray tube. In this, a combination of axial CT scans and enhanced CTSPR images are obtained. The spatial resolution of CTSPR, however, is inferior to that of conventional radiographs.

CT—Only CT Urography

This involves acquisition of unenhanced and enhanced CT scans of the abdomen and pelvis including the EP. Caoili and associated performed a four phase CT urogram comprising an unenhanced scan, NP and two EPs, one at 5 minutes and the other at 7.5 minutes.[79] However, a four phase protocol consisting of two EPs (at 5 minutes and 7.5 minutes) is usually not recommended because of radiation issues. A three phase protocol is usually followed in most institutions consisting of the unenhanced phase, a NP and an EP.[80] The NP is acquired at 90–100 sec following contrast administration (100–150 mL of 300 mg/mL iodine concentration at the rate of 2–4 mL/sec). The excretory/pyelographic phase is usually taken 12–15 minutes following contrast administration to evaluate the urothelium from the pelvicalyceal system to the bladder.

Techniques to Improve Urinary Tract Distension

- *Diuretic administration*: A diuretic like 10 mg of furosemide given 1 minute before contrast administration has been reported to increase ureteric distension. It also allows for a less dense homogeneous opacification of the collecting system.[81]
- *Oral contrast*: About 1,000 mL of water can be given orally within 15–20 minutes to cause sufficient distension of the collecting system in most cases.
- *Saline infusion*: Saline infusion technique, that is, 250 mL saline chase after administration of IV contrast helps in a better opacification of the distal ureters which are the most difficult segments to visualize.[82,83]
- *Compression*: External compression is not a part of MDCTU protocol because it causes patient discomfort and has not been shown to improve the percentage of visualized segments.[83]
- *Patient positioning*: A MDCTU performed in the prone position achieves a higher opacification of mid and distal ureters than supine position. However, being cumbersome, it is not advocated for routine use. Scanning is done in the supine position for computed tomography urography (CTU).[84]
- *Image interpretation*: MPR, MIP, and VRT images are most commonly used.[85] The reformats show the urinary tract in entirety and are useful for characterization of renal masses, presence of calculi, evaluation of ureter, and localization of the exact level of abnormality.

Split Bolus MDCT Urography with Synchronous NP and EP Enhancement

A split bolus technique has been proposed by Chow and colleagues to minimize radiation dose as well as minimize the number of images generated.[86] This is a two-phase technique in which an unenhanced series of images is followed by the "nephropyelographic phase", that is, there is a simultaneous acquisition of the nephrographic and pyelographic phases. In this technique, following the noncontrast scan, 30 cc of nonionic contrast is infused intravenously which is the first bolus. The patient is then removed from the CT table and allowed to walk around for 10 minutes. 10–15 minutes later a contrast-enhanced CT is performed following a second bolus of contrast injection. 100 cc of nonionic contrast is injected intravenously and scanning is done after a delay of 100 seconds. By allowing the contrast bolus to be split, 30 cc (1st bolus) followed by 100 cc (2nd bolus), the nephrographic and pyelographic phases can be acquired simultaneously. In this single nephropyelographic phase, both the renal parenchyma (NP) and the collecting system (pyelographic phase) can be assessed.

Triple Bolus CT Urography

In this, the bolus is split into three and then a combined corticomedullary, nephrographic, and EP is acquired.[87] The first bolus is 30 mL given at 2 mL/sec used for the opacification of the excretory system followed 7 minutes later by the second bolus of 50 mL at 1.5 mL/sec for the renal parenchyma and finally a third bolus 20 seconds later of 65 mL at 3 mL/sec for arterial information. The three phases are then acquired in a single scan, obtained some 510 seconds after start of first bolus. A triple bolus technique further reduces radiation dose as compared to the split bolus.[87,88]

Indications for CT urography are as follows:

- Hematuria
- Urothelial lesions
- Calculi
- Renal tumors
- Ureteral lesions
- Pelviureteric junction obstruction
- Congenital anomalies.

Hematuria

Computed tomography urography (CTU) has an overall sensitivity of 92.4–100% and specificity of 89–97.4% in detection of the causes of hematuria.[89,90] CTU can be justified as a first line test in hematuria patients with a high probability for TCCs.[91] For the lower risk patients, CTU is a problem-solving modality if the work-up remains negative and hematuria persists.[92]

TABLE 5: Evaluation of painless microscopic and macroscopic hematuria.[91]

ProbabilityTCC	Lowest	Low	Medium	High
Hematuria	Micro	Macro	Micro	Macro
Patient age	<40 years	<40 years	>40 years	>40 years
First line tests	CYS	CYS	CYS	CYS
	US	US	US	CTU
	↓	↓	↓	↓
Follow-up	Watch and wait If negative	IVU if US and CYS negative and symptoms persist	IVU or CTU if US and CYS negative and symptoms persist	Specialist referral

(TCC: transitional cell carcinoma; US: ultrasound; IVU: intravenous urogram; CTU: computed tomography urography; CYS: cystatin)

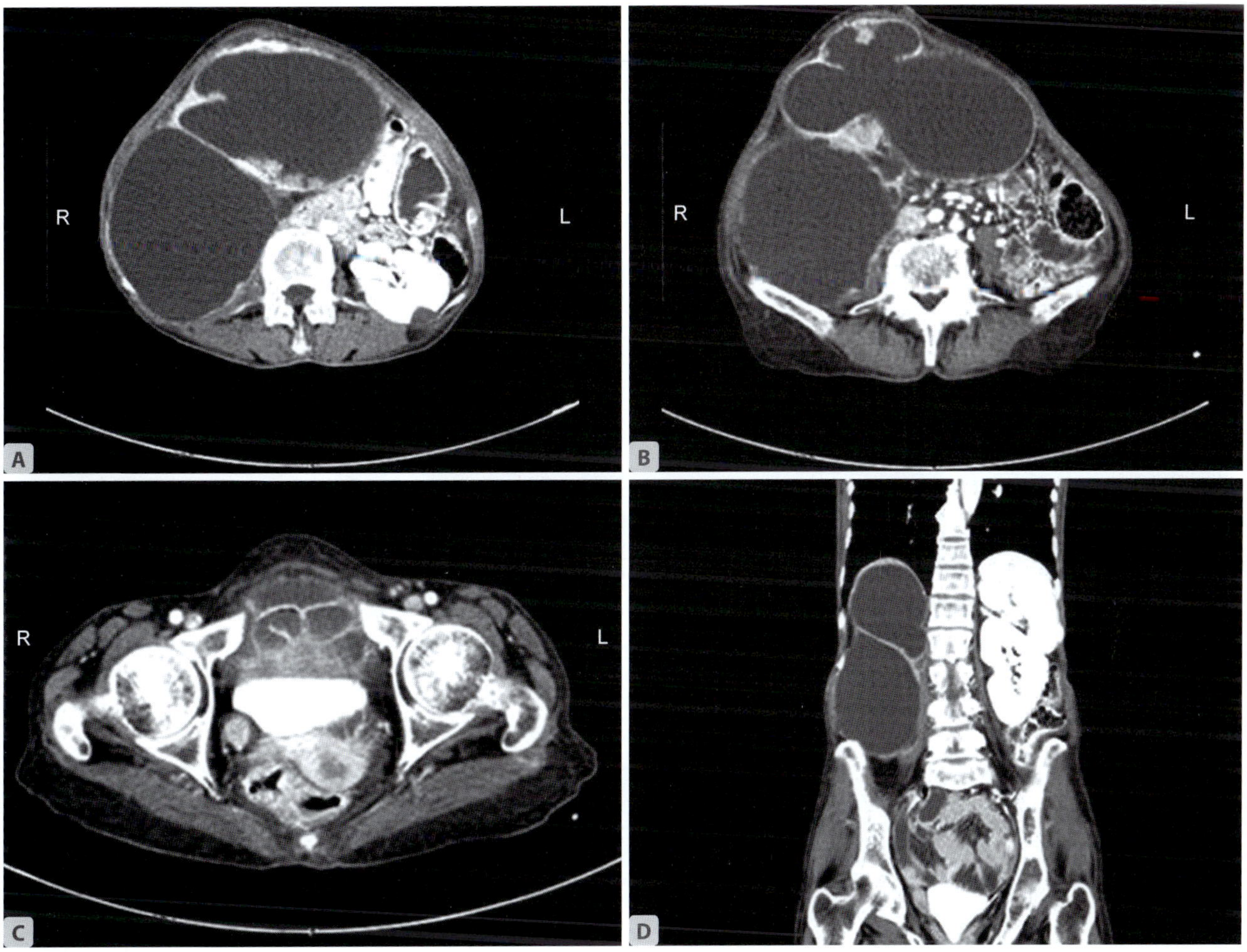

FIGS. 25A TO D: (A to C) Contrast-enhanced axial and (D) coronal images on CT scan showing a grossly hydronephrotic right kidney with small polypoidal masses within. Note is made of diffuse circumferential thickening of the right ureter at the ureterovesical junction—multifocal transitional cell carcinoma.

The algorithm for the evaluation of painless microscopic/macroscopic hematuria is given in **Table 5**.[91]

Urothelial Lesions

Computed tomography urogram is excellent in the depiction of urothelial lesions with a high sensitivity and specificity. CTU is superior not only to IVU but also to retrograde ureterography, an imaging technique considered superior to IVU in the evaluation of the pelvicalyceal system and ureters.[93] MDCTU is an accurate technique for detection and staging of TCCs of the upper urinary tract. The TCC occurs most commonly in elderly men and risk factors include chemical carcinogens, smoking, cyclophosphamide or phenacetin use. The entire urinary tract is susceptible to malignant transformation owing to the field effect of these carcinogens. As a result, TCCs are often multifocal at presentation and the entire urinary tract should be screened even if a single lesion is detected **(Figs. 25A to D)**. MDCTU is the imaging modality that provides a screening of the entire urinary tract for synchronous and metachronous lesions in TCC.[94] Synchronous lesions are discrete TCC foci identified on a single study while metachronous lesions are those detected on follow-up imaging. MDCTU is the first line imaging modality when noninvasive imaging is needed for the detection and surveillance of urothelial lesions of the upper urinary tract.[95]

Calculi

Computed tomography urogram has an advantage over intravenous urogram (IVU) in detecting extraurinary pathologies that may mimic calculi **(Figs. 26A and B)**.[96] It is more accurate than intravenous urogram in detecting presence, size, and location of the calculi, can detect calculi in unusual positions such as in a calyceal diverticulum. Like intravenous urogram, CT urogram provides physiological information about the function of kidneys. A delayed excretion of contrast which is an index of obstruction, hydronephrosis, and hydroureter can all be well seen on the CT urogram images.

Renal Tumors

A precise depiction of the tumor and its relation to the collecting system is required in cases of nephron-sparing surgery. CT urogram delineates not only the collecting system, shows distortion splaying, and amputation of the calyces in RCCs but also the renal, perirenal, and the vascular tissues **(Figs. 27A to C)**.[97]

Ureteric Lesions

Computed tomography urography has a role in the depiction of traumatic and iatrogenic ureteral injury. MDCTU scores over intravenous urogram in differentiating extrinsic from intrinsic causes of ureteric obstruction.[98] CTU can show benign ureteric strictures, short segment malignant strictures, mural thickening, retroperitoneal masses, lymphadenopathy, retroperitoneal fibrosis, and iatrogenic causes of ureteric strictures. An infiltration of the ureter due to malignant pelvic masses is also well seen on MDCTU **(Fig. 28)**.[99]

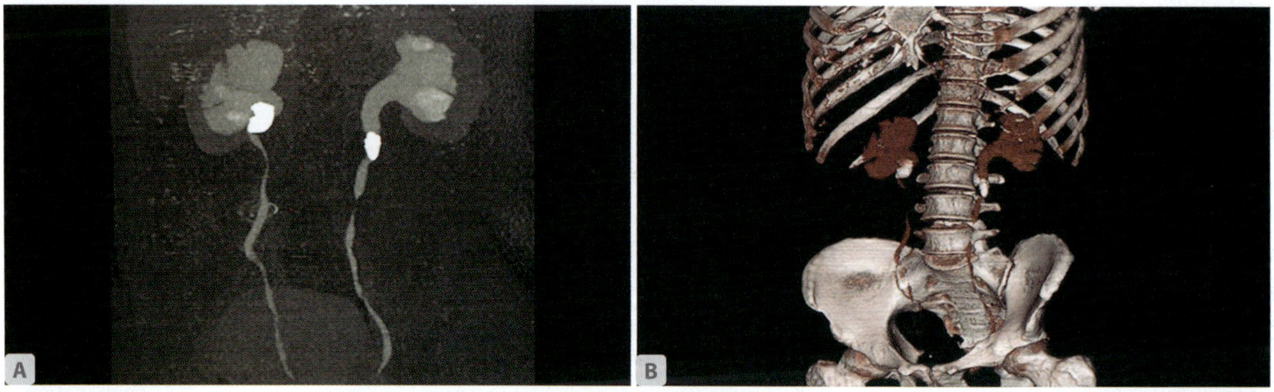

FIGS. 26A AND B: (A) CT urogram using maximum intensity projection technique depicting a calculus at the pelviureteric junction on the right side and a calculus in the proximal left ureter. There are back pressure changes on both sides; (B) Volume-rendering technique image displaying the same.

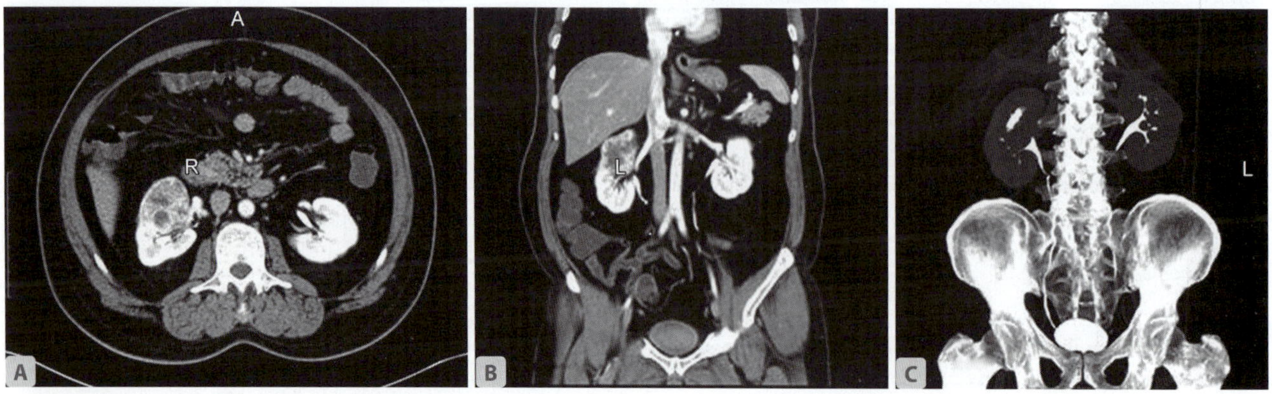

FIGS. 27A TO C: (A) Contrast-enhanced axial; and (B) coronal images showing a heterogeneous mass in the upper pole of right kidney; (C) CT urogram using maximum intensity projection technique (MIP) showing distortion and amputation of the infundibula of the calyces suggestive of a malignant mass—right renal cell carcinoma.

Pelviureteric Junction Obstruction

Visualization of crossing vessels along with narrowing of ureter in the same sets of images helps in establishing the etiology and diagnosis of PUJ obstruction.[100]

Congenital Anomalies

In a duplicated system, CT urogram shows both the functioning and nonfunctioning components in contrast to intravenous urogram which shows only the functioning moiety. It shows the entire course of both upper and lower moiety along with the ectopic opening of the upper moiety which is often hydronephrotic.[101] Crossed fused renal ectopia, horseshoe kidney, and renal ectopia are all well seen on CTU **(Figs. 29A to C)**. In cases of retrocaval ureter, CT urogram shows not only the ureteric compression but also the cause of the compression which is the IVC.

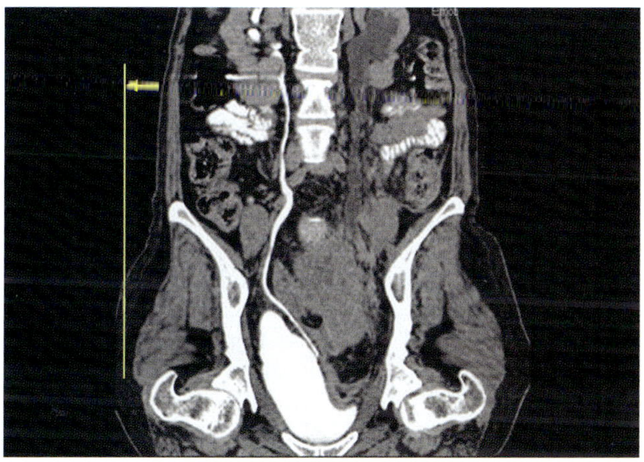

FIG. 28: Curved multiplanar reformation image depicting infiltration of left ureter via cervical mass and consequent proximal hydroureteronephrosis. Delayed opacification of the pelvicalyceal system is seen on the left as compared to the normal well-opacified pelvicalyceal system and ureter on the right side.

Radiation Dose of CT Urography

There are differing amounts of radiation exposure according to the different techniques used. While a radiation dose of 23.4 mSv is attributed to three phasic CTU, a triple bolus CTU involves lower dose of radiation about 13.2 mSv.[87] Overall a split bolus or a triple bolus technique reduces the radiation dose by 15–45% compared to a three phasic study.[102] Where dual energy computed tomography (DECT) is available, further reduction of radiation dose can be achieved by acquiring virtual nonenhanced scan from DECT and omitting unenhanced scan.[103] In several studies with CTU protocol using iterative reconstruction further reductions in radiation dosage to the tune of 6.1 mSv have been achieved.[104,105]

DUAL ENERGY CT IN THE UPPER URINARY TRACT

Acquisition of high and low energy datasets can be achieved by either a dual source dual energy scanner or a single source dual energy scanner with rapid alteration of high and low kilovoltage settings, that is, a dual energy scanner with fast kilovoltage switching, with acquisition usually at 80 kVp and 140 kVp. Two types of images are obtained on DECT which are as follows:

1. Material density images which provide material specific information.
2. Monochromatic images which provide energy selective information.

The commonly selected DECT basis material pairs are: (1) Iodine and water; (2) Iodine and calcium. Iodine has a high atomic number while water has a low atomic number. When iodine is paired with water, two sets of images are produced. One set is that of iodine density images and the other of water density. Voxels that show an attenuation similar to that of iodine attenuation are removed from the water density images and represented on the iodine density images. Virtual unenhanced images are produced which provide the same information as a noncontrast scan. The iodine density images give information about the degree of enhancement which can even be quantified by placing a region of interest (ROI)

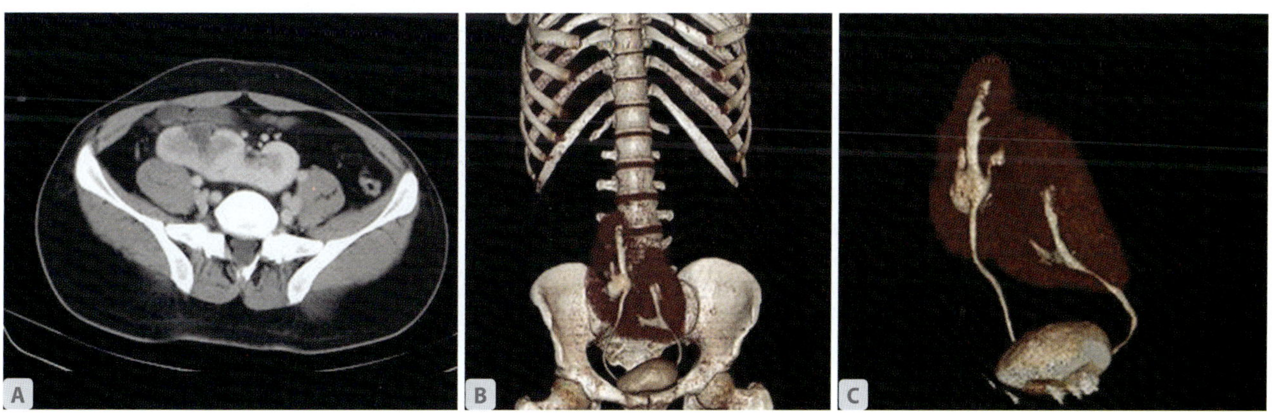

FIGS. 29A TO C: (A) Contrast-enhanced axial scans revealing a low lying ectopic kidney with fusion of renal parenchyma of both the kidneys; (B) volume-rendered image in the excretory phase depicting the fused low lying ectopic kidney; (C) Volume-rendered image with the bone edited out revealing the same—ectopic pancake kidney.

over the lesion. Color-coded overlay images can also be generated.[106] A color can be assigned to the voxels containing the selected material and the voxels can be superimposed on the monochromatic images.

Characterization of Renal Masses on Dual Energy CT

Enhancement is an important criterion for differentiating hyperattenuating renal cysts from solid masses. The attenuation measurements of the two may be quite similar on the contrast-enhanced CT images. On iodine density images, voxels containing iodine appear bright and renal masses appear brighter than proteinaceous cysts on these images. The iodine density can be measured in absolute quantitative terms (milligrams/milliliter) and the degree of enhancement in renal masses can be quantified. The water density images can be used as virtual unenhanced images and can be used to detect calcifications/hemorrhage within a renal mass.[107] Also, in cases where surgery cannot be undertaken and thermal ablation is done for renal masses a follow-up can be done by DECT since it involves a single phase of scanning and limits the radiation dose received by the patient.

Characterization of Renal Stones by Dual Energy CT

The different types of calculi cannot be differentiated when scanned at a single energy level owing to a similar attenuation. DECT helps in differentiating uric acid from nonuric acid calculi.[108] Calcium and uric acid density images can be generated depicting the respective calculi. A plot of effective atomic numbers versus monochromatic image-based attenuation values can distinguish the various types of calculi (calcium, struvite, uric acid, and cystine).[109] This differentiation is important because of the different lines of management, for example, uric acid calculi are amenable to oral medications, struvite can be managed by extracorporeal shock wave lithotripsy (ESWL) while the cysteine ones are resistant to fragmentation with lithotripsy.

Dual Energy CT in CT Urography

All CT urography protocols include an unenhanced scan to detect calculi followed by contrast-enhanced scans.[110] The generation of virtual unenhanced images on DECT urography can obviate the need for an unenhanced scan and hence reduce radiation dosages.

CT ANGIOGRAM OF RENAL ARTERIES

Indications of CT angiogram of the renal arteries include:[111]

- Evaluation of renal artery stenosis (RAS).
- Preoperative assessment of the number and course of renal arteries in renal donors.
- Assessment of renal vessels crossing the PUJ prior to repair of obstruction. It is important to know about a crossing vessel because the postsurgical outcome of endopyelotomy is worse in patients with a crossing vessel than those without it.
- Evaluation of renal artery involvement in abdominal aortic aneurysms.
- Detection of renal artery aneurysms.

Technique

The renal arteries have a small diameter and have a parallel or near parallel course to the imaging plane. Hence, nominal section thickness of 1.25 mm and overlapping reconstructions are necessary. A bolus injection of 150 mL of contrast material (300 mg Iodine/mL) with a flow rate of 4 mL/sec produces good opacification of the renal arteries. The ROI for the scan volume is determined by the initial topogram/axial scans. Conventionally, the region between the SMA and lower border of L3 is chosen. This allows the sites of origin of accessory renal arteries to be included. Delay time is determined through prior time density curves of dynamic scanning and patient is instructed to hold breath at time of acquisition. A real-time bolus tracking/care bolus technique can be adopted where acquisition is triggered with the arrival of contrast in the aorta.

Maximum intensity projection (MIP) and volume rendering (VRT) display modes are most commonly used **(Fig. 30)**.[112] Depth, surface, and relative X-ray attenuation are all conveyed with VRT. The structures adjacent to the vessels can be displayed and the 3D dataset can be modified in any orientation to optimize depiction of the renal vascular anatomy **(Figs. 31A to C)**. MIP images provide useful information about atherosclerotic burden, vascular stenosis, and vascular stents, and are used in conjunction with VRT. Perspective rendering can also be used to produce angioscopic views which are helpful in identifying a vascular orifice and stenosis.

The sensitivity of computed tomography angiogram (CTA) for determination and location of main renal artery approaches 100%.[113] Arterial branches can be identified accurately till the segmental level.[114] Limitation for detection occurs with vessels smaller than 2 mm in size. It is not only the arterial anatomy but renal venous anatomy is also well documented on CTA. The renal venous anatomy is important

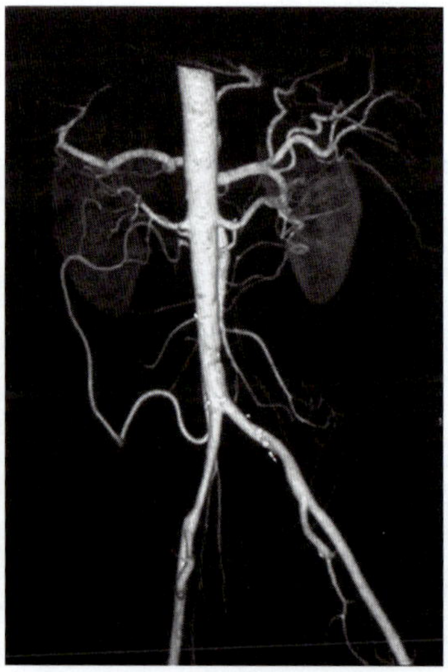

FIG. 30: CT angiogram using volume-rendering technique depicting the normal renal arteries on both sides.

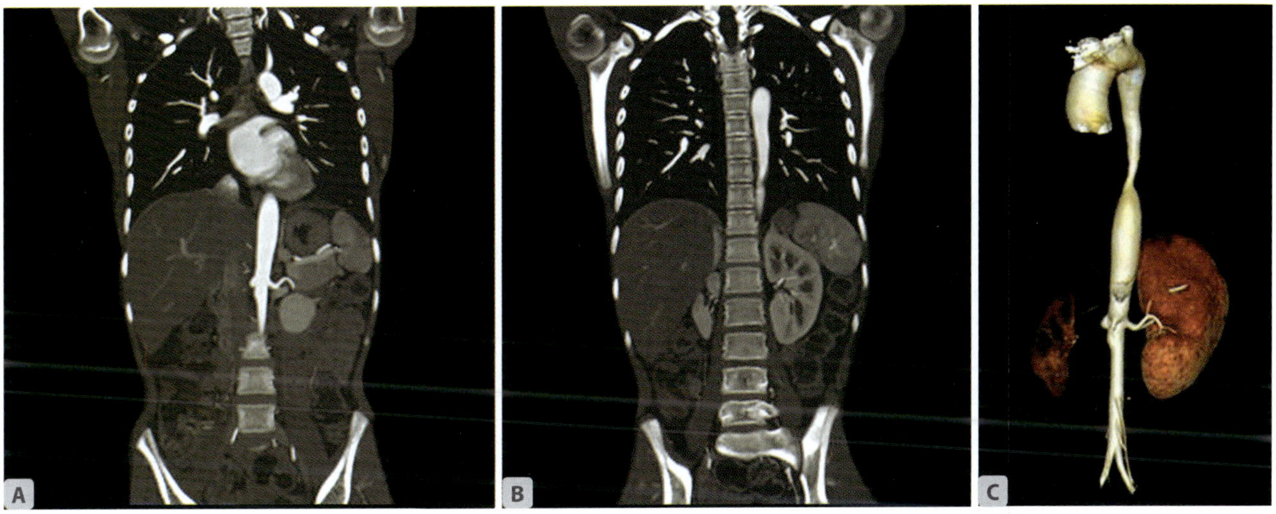

FIGS. 31A TO C: CT angiogram maximum intensity projection images (A and B) showing stenosis of the right renal artery with the left renal artery being normal in caliber. Volume-rendered image (C) showing narrowing of the abdominal aorta with stenosis of the right renal artery—involvement of the right renal artery in a case of aortoarteritis.

to document for patients undergoing laparoscopic donor nephrectomy. Tributaries into the left renal vein, especially the posterior lumbar branches, are well displayed on the CTA. If enlarged, this is of potential surgical importance.

MAGNETIC RESONANCE IMAGING OF THE UPPER URINARY TRACT

A growing need for radiation dose reduction combined with advances in MRI has led to the increasing use of MRI for assessment of the urinary tract in recent times. While contrast resolution is a major advantage of MRI over other imaging modalities, the limited temporal and spatial resolution coupled with poor sensitivity for detecting calcifications has impeded this modality to emerge as the single most important modality for evaluation of the urogenital tract.[115] However, the advent of 3 Tesla MRI has changed the scenario. And 3 Tesla MRI provides a significant improvement in signal-to-noise ratio (SNR) which can in turn be used to obtain higher spatial resolution or faster imaging, i.e. imaging times can be reduced while maintaining acceptable SNR. A two-fold increase in SNR can be achieved by 3 Tesla MRI but a major drawback is the increase in magnetic susceptibility artefacts. MRI is the preferred modality:[116,117]

- For determining the cephalic extent of an intracaval tumor in a case of RCC when the superior extent cannot be determined by CT.
- Characterization of small renal masses that are indeterminate on CT or US.
- Differentiation between hemorrhagic renal cysts and renal masses by use of subtraction imaging. In this, a nonenhanced T_1 weighted image is subtracted from a contrast-enhanced T_1 weighted sequence which cancels the native T_1 sequence and leaves behind only the enhancing portion. Thus, subtraction images are useful in identifying true enhancement in complex renal cysts.
- Evaluation of renal donors.
- Evaluation of transplanted kidneys.
- In screening patients with inherited conditions such as Von Hippel-Lindau disease which is characterized by renal cysts, angiomas, and RCC.

Technique

Patient Positioning

The patient lies supine with arms raised above the head. Phased array body coils are used. A phased array coil increases SNR, allows faster acquisitions minimizing breathing motion artefacts.[118]

Breath Holding

The motion of the kidneys during respiration leads to degradation of image quality. Hence, fast imaging techniques with rapid sequences are needed which can be acquired in a single breath hold. The preferred motion phase for breath holding is expiration as the kidney position is more constant and more reproducible in this phase. Before scanning the kidneys, it is important to ask the patient to hold his breath. The use of faster sequences such as single shot imaging, half Fourier technique helps to reduce motion artefacts. In addition, a saturation band can be placed over the subcutaneous fat of the anterior abdominal wall to reduce respiratory artefacts. Parallel imaging techniques such as sensitivity encoding and array spatial sensitivity encoding technique can also be used to reduce the acquisition time.[119] Parallel imaging not only reduces the image blurring inherent to very long echo train spin echo sequences but also lowers the specific absorption rate (SAR). A respiratory gating to limit the data acquisition to end expiration or to a particular fixed point of the respiratory cycle can be done to reduce motion artefacts. A navigator which records diaphragmatic motion can also be used to obtain motion correction.

Sequences

Usually both T_1- and T_2-weighted images are acquired in the axial, coronal, and sagittal planes. Due to shorter acquisition times, T_2 fast spin echo (FSE) imaging has almost replaced the conventional spin echo (CSE) T_2-imaging. High resolution good quality T_2-weighted images can be obtained in a short time using FSE sequences. Also, in and opposed phase breath hold T_1-weighted gradient echo sequences provide a good anatomic detail and is useful for detection of intralesional fat, e.g. in AML. Imaging of the kidneys can be done in the corticomedullary, nephrographic, and EPs following contrast administration, similar to that on MDCT. Gradient echo fast low angle shot (FLASH) sequence can be used to obtain postcontrast images. Differentiation between solid masses and complicated cystic lesions can be achieved on comparison between pre- and postcontrast images obtained in corticomedullary and NPs.[120] Delayed postcontrast images depict tumor extension in the perinephric fat and venous structures.

Gadolinium-based contrast agents (GBCAs), however, should be used with caution in patients with renal insufficiency because of risk of development of NSF.[121] Nephronic systemic fibrosis is an acquired idiopathic systemic disorder characterized by indurated plaques and papules most commonly of the extremities and trunks. Besides skin changes, NSF also results in fibrosis of other organs such as myocardium, skeletal muscles, lungs, kidneys, and testes. The condition is potentially fatal and hence gadolinium should not be administered in severe renal insufficiency (GFR < 30 mL/min).[122]

Normal Appearance of the Upper Urinary Tract on MRI

Magnetic resonance (MR) allows visualization of the corticomedullary differentiation on both T_1- and T_2-weighted images. This differentiation is best visualized on T_1 weighted MR images where the cortex has a higher signal intensity than the adjacent medulla **(Figs. 32A and B)**. The cortex has less water than the medulla and has a longer T_1-time and hence is brighter than medulla on a T_1-weighted image.[123] On T_2-weighted images, the cortex appears hypointense to the medulla **(Figs. 33A and B)**. The renal sinus fat shows a high signal on both T_1 and T_2 weighted images. The renal capsule is seen as a hypointense line while the perirenal and pararenal fat shows a bright signal on all pulse sequences.[124] The pelvicalyceal system is not seen in a nondistended state. When distended with urine, the collecting system shows a low signal on T_1- and bright on T_2-weighted images. The renal arteries, veins, aorta, and IVC are seen as flow voids. Like a contrast-enhanced CT, the corticomedullary differentiation is most accentuated *(CMP)* at 20–80 seconds following contrast. At around 90–120 seconds, there is loss of this differentiation with both cortex and medulla-enhancing intensely *(NP)*. This is followed by contrast appearing in the calyces in approximately 180 seconds *(EP)* **(Figs. 34A to C)**.[125]

MAGNETIC RESONANCE UROGRAPHY

Magnetic resonance urography (MRU) allows a complete evaluation of the urinary tract. It can be performed with a static fluid or an excretory technique.[126]

Static Fluid MR Urography

In this, no contrast is administered. This technique exploits the long T_2-relaxation time of urine. Heavily T_2-weighted sequences are used to generate high signal intensity images from static fluid in the collecting system.[127] The low signal intensity images of the background tissue are suppressed. Heavily T_2-weighted sequences such as rapid acquisition with relaxation enhancement (RARE) and half Fourier acquisition single shot turbo spin echo (HASTE) are very fast and can be acquired in a single breath-hold. The fat in the background

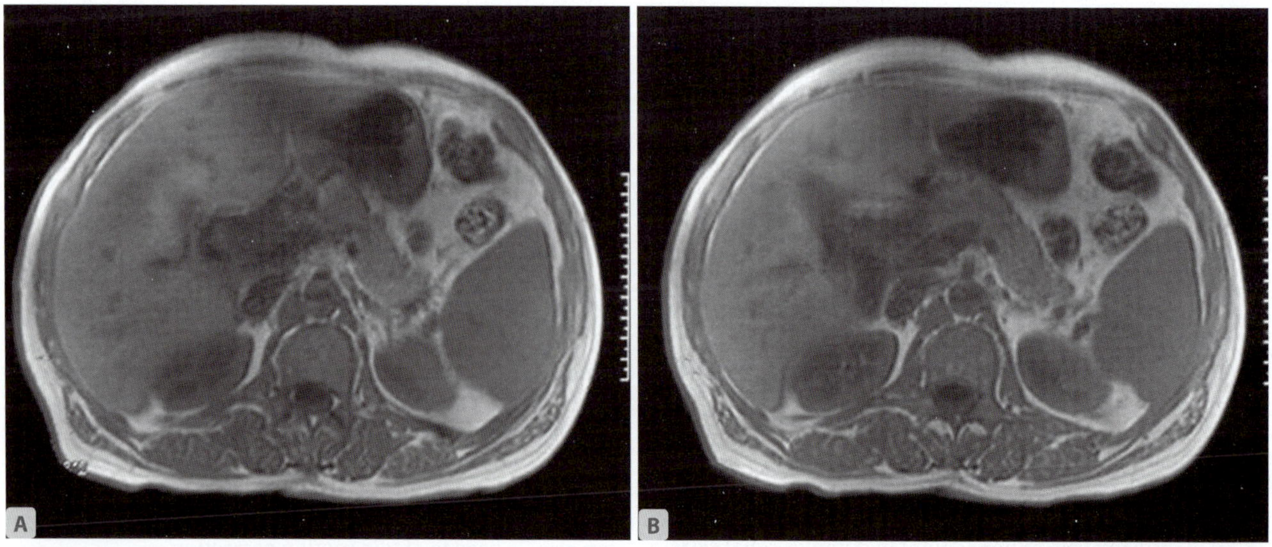

FIGS. 32A AND B: Axial T1W MR images showing the normal corticomedullary differentiation of the kidneys. The cortex appears brighter than the medulla on T1W image. The pararenal fat also has a bright signal.

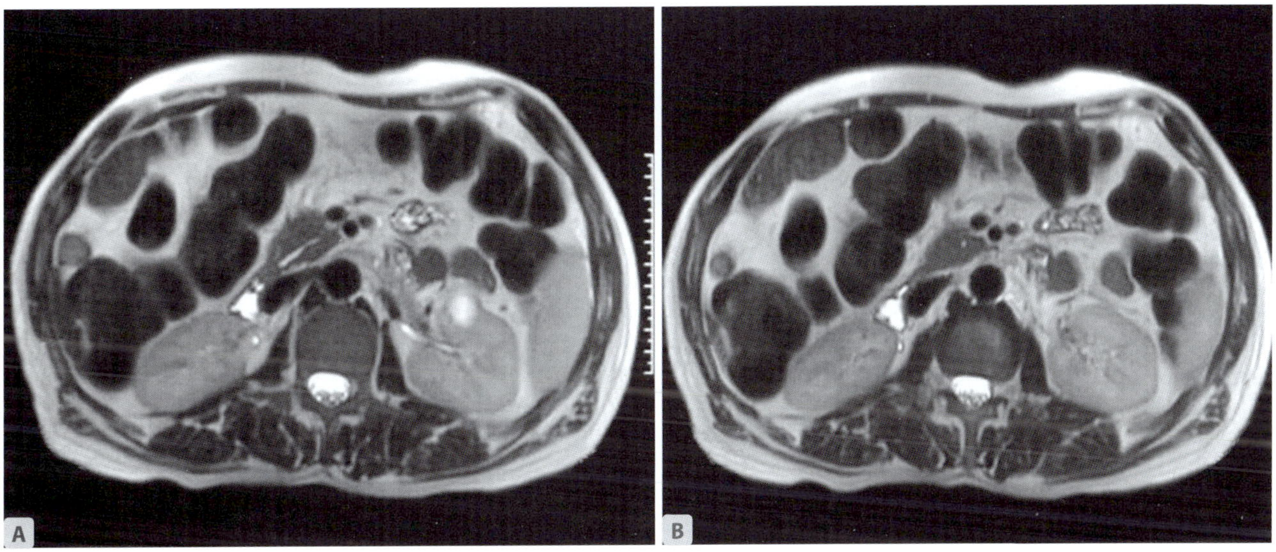

FIGS. 33A AND B: Axial T2W MR images showing the medulla to be brighter than the renal cortex. The renal sinus is also bright due to fat while the pararenal fat also shows a bright signal.

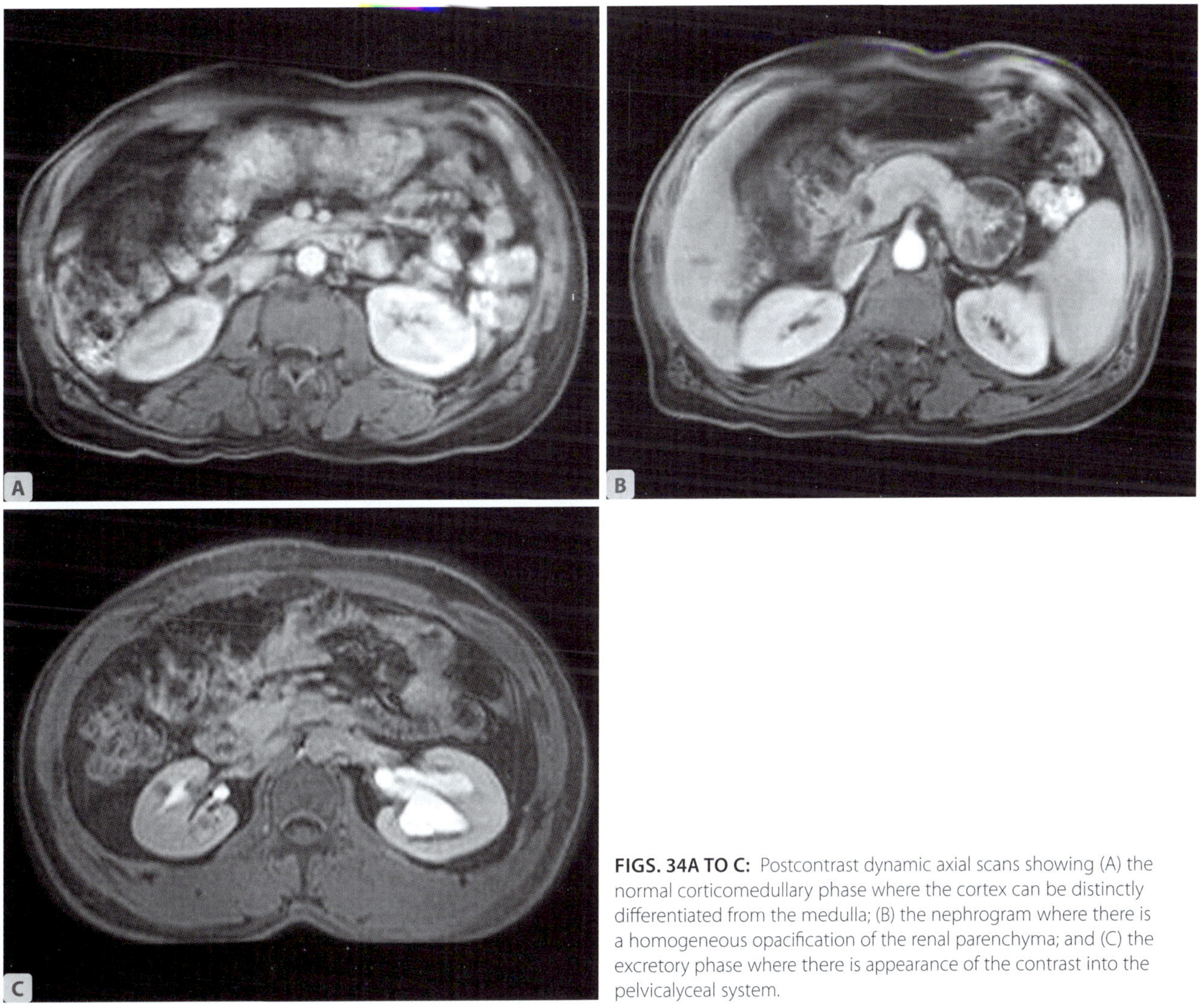

FIGS. 34A TO C: Postcontrast dynamic axial scans showing (A) the normal corticomedullary phase where the cortex can be distinctly differentiated from the medulla; (B) the nephrogram where there is a homogeneous opacification of the renal parenchyma; and (C) the excretory phase where there is appearance of the contrast into the pelvicalyceal system.

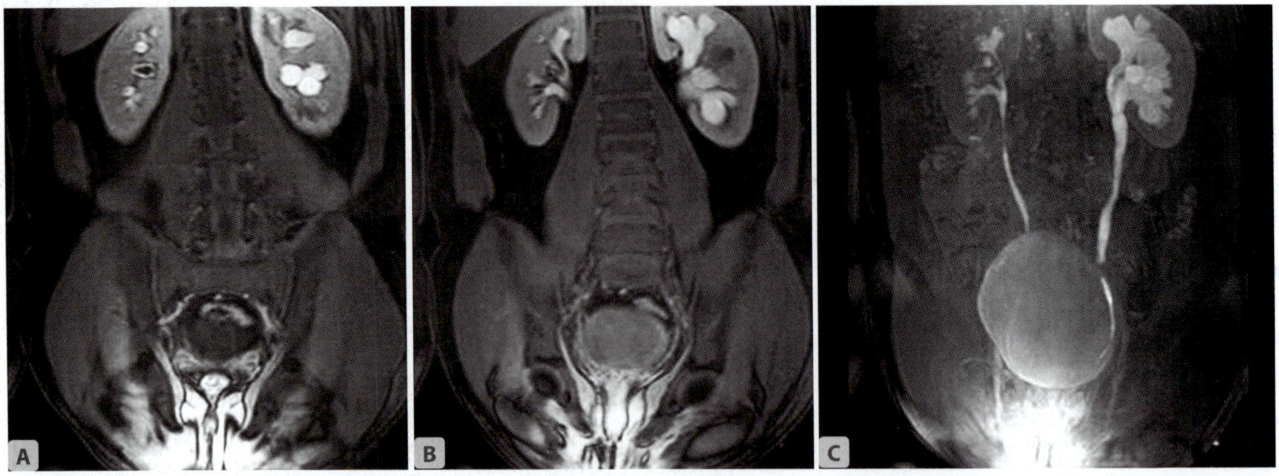

FIGS. 35A TO C: MR urogram image obtained using contrast administration showing a stricture in the left ureter with proximal hydronephrosis. A filling defect suggestive of calculus is seen in the right pelvicalyceal system—right renal calculus with left ureteric stricture.

is suppressed. 3D respiratory triggered sequences can also be used to obtain volume rendering (VR) and MIP images. For the evaluation of urinary tract peristalsis and narrowing, stenosis or stricture, multiple images obtained can be played as a cine loop. Static fluid MRU can evaluate the urinary tract course and diameter, even when the kidneys are poorly excreting or it is an obstructed system.

Excretory MR Urogram

Excretory MR urogram is performed using a T_1-weighted gadolinium-enhanced 3D gradient echo fat suppression sequence like 3D FLASH. A standard dose of gadolinium (0.1 mmol/kg) is administered intravenously. Diuretic administration (0.1 mg/kg of furosemide) enhances the urine flow and gives a better dilution and uniform distribution of the contrast agent **(Figs. 35A to C)**.[128] Oral hydration and furosemide administration improve the distension of the ureters and the collecting system. Distension of the upper urinary tracts can be improved by a full urinary bladder, provided the patient can tolerate such an approach. In order to reduce the bowel-related susceptibility effects which are a problem in the region of distal ureters and bladder dome, it is preferable to have patients fast before the examination.

Images are typically acquired in the coronal plane with a field of view that includes the kidneys, ureters, and bladder. As with intravenous urogram, oblique images or multiplanar reconstructions of the collecting system can be undertaken for a better delineation of the anatomy. Excretory MR urography is better at demonstrating a communication between the renal collecting system and a fluid collection than the static MR technique. Since this technique requires excretion of contrast into the collecting system, it is better at delineating nonobstructed ureters and does not have much role in obstructed or poorly excreting kidneys.[129] Excretory MRU is not recommended in patients with severe renal insufficiency due to the risk of NSF and also because the kidneys will not be able to excrete the contrast material.[130]

Clinical Applications of MR Urography

- Magnetic resonance urogram is useful in delineating the level of urinary tract obstruction. About 90% of ureteral stones can be detected by gadolinium-enhanced 3D gradient echo excretory MR urography combined with T_2-weighted sequences. Persistent dilatation of the ureters above a filling defect and high signal intensity perinephric edema on T_2-weighted images constitute the signs of acute calculus obstruction. Persistence of the CMP of enhancement and delayed excretion of contrast can be present when the obstruction is severe.
- Magnetic resonance urography has a role in the detection of urothelial carcinomas. Intravenous GBCAs help in delineating the extent of tumor.[131]
- Extrinsic compressions of the ureters such as in prostate or uterine carcinomas or in retroperitoneal fibrosis can be depicted on MRU.
- Magnetic resonance urography can assess the various congenital urinary tract anomalies accurately such as duplex systems, PUJ obstruction, and insertion of an ectopic ureter.[132]
- Functional data can also be obtained from excretory MRU including renal transit time, differential renal function, and estimated GFR.[133]
- Magnetic resonance urography is useful in the evaluation of potential renal transplant donors and in the assessment of urologic complications following renal transplantation as it avoids the use of potentially nephrotoxic-iodinated contrast material of CT urogram.

Limitations of MR Urograms

- Lower spatial resolution as compared to CT
- Long imaging time
- Motion sensitivity
- Lower sensitivity in detection of calcification as compared to CT.

Magnetic resonance urography is indicated in patients who cannot receive iodinated contrast material or where exposure to ionizing radiation is undesirable. Owing to these limitations of MRU, CT urography still continues to be the test of choice for evaluation of patients with hematuria though MR urography is commonly indicated in children and pregnant patients with a dilated collecting system.[134] In pregnant patients, physiological dilatations of the ureter can be distinguished from obstructive uropathy. Static fluid MRI is quick and easy to perform, does not use contrast medium and hence is well tolerated even in advanced stages of pregnancy.

MAGNETIC RESONANCE ANGIOGRAM

Magnetic resonance angiogram (MRA) can be performed without the use of contrast by techniques such as gradient time of flight (TOF), TRUFISP or the phase contrast (PC).[135] These techniques render the flowing blood bright. However, there are several limitations such as overestimation of stenosis due to turbulent jets leading to signal loss, fresh thrombus giving a bright signal, motion artefacts, nonvisualization of small vessels, and slow flow resulting in poor quality images. Hence, contrast-enhanced MRA (CEMRA) is the preferred technique as it is free of flow-related phenomenon, has high spatial resolution, and assesses the true lumen of vessels.[136] Both the arterial and venous vasculature can be well visualized on the CEMRA images. An ultrafast 3D T_1 gradient echo sequence like FLASH is used to obtain thin slices which are reconstructed as MIP to yield angiographic images **(Fig. 36)**.

Functional MRI of the Kidneys

The primary role of the kidney is to maintain homeostatic balance by filtering out metabolites and minerals from the blood and excreting them along with water in the urine. The most commonly used measure of renal function is serum creatinine. This is, however, a late marker of renal dysfunction, it is often deranged late in the course of the disease and at times when irreversible damage to the kidneys has taken place. Functional impairment occurs much before the anatomic manifestations such as atrophy in cases of renal failure and hence an early detection of functional loss allows for an early institution of therapy to halt the progression.[137] The various techniques for functional imaging include the following as described here.

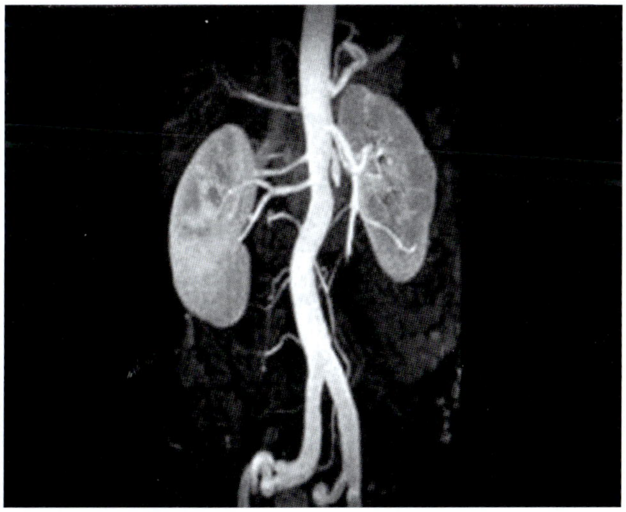

FIG. 36: MR angiogram image showing the normal renal arteries on both sides. An accessory renal artery is seen on the right side.

Contrast-enhanced MR Renography[138]

Dynamic contrast-enhanced MR of the kidneys is called MR renography. This technique measures the transit of contrast material, usually a gadolinium chelate, through the renal cortex, the renal medulla, and the collecting system. The technique involves acquiring images before, during, and after administration of the contrast material, converting the signal intensity of the renal tissues to gadolinium concentration and plotting of the time signal intensity curves.[139] As these gadolinium-contrast agents pass through capillaries and renal tubules, they cause the signal intensity of the renal tissues to increase. By analyzing the enhancement of the renal tissues as a function of time parameters such as renal blood flow, medullary blood volume GFR can be determined. Perfusion maps can then be generated.

Clinical applications of the MR renography:[140]

- *Renovascular hypertension*: Angiotensin-converting enzyme (ACE) inhibitor injection is helpful in differentiating hemodynamically significant stenosis from insignificant stenosis. Those with a significant stenosis have a decrease in GFR following administration of ACE inhibitor while no change in GFR values is noted in those with insignificant stenosis.
- *Allograft dysfunction*: The major complication in renal transplanted kidneys is ATN which is an ischemic injury to renal tubules. While acute rejection shows a reduced cortical and medullary perfusion, ATN shows a maintained perfusion. Thus, MR perfusion maps generated can help differentiate between these conditions obviating the need for an invasive renal biopsy.
- *Functional urinary obstruction*: The renal transit time which is defined as the time between tracer appearance in the kidney and in the ureter can be used to differentiate between normal and obstructed kidneys.[141]

Diffusion Weighted MRI

Diffusion weighted imaging (DWI) which measures the Brownian motion of water molecules in tissues has been historically used for stroke imaging. However, with improvements in hardware and software including parallel imaging, it is being used for abdominal applications. DWI is used for the detection and characterization of focal renal lesions as benign or malignant, in the assessment of nuclear grade and renal cancer subtype as well as in the assessment of malignant lymph nodes from urogenital tumors. It is also being used to assess treatment response in patients with renal cell cancer undergoing targeted chemotherapy. DWI is also being used in the evaluation of renal function. Single shot echoplanar imaging is the sequence most commonly used for DWI. Quantification of diffusion can be done by apparent diffusion coefficient (ADC) values. DWI has a role in:[142]

- *Renal insufficiency*: It has been seen in various studies that patient with acute and chronic renal failure showed lower ADC values in both the cortex and medulla of their kidneys as compared to normal healthy kidneys. DWI also provides split function information unlike the blood parameters which do not provide information about the function of each kidney separately though conditions like RAS and ureteric obstruction are usually unilateral. Studies have also shown that hydronephrotic kidney with impaired renal function has lower ADC values as compared to obstructed kidneys with normal function. DWI thus has a potential role in the evaluation of renal dysfunction.

- *Renal allograft*: DWI has a role in the evaluation of renal allografts. A decrease in cortical ADC value is attributed to allograft dysfunction.
- *Renal artery stenosis*: Patients with significant RAS had lower values of ADC, thus opening the possibility of it being diagnosed without the use of contrast-enhanced MR angiography.

Diffusion Tensor Imaging

The renal medulla is composed of radially oriented compactly arranged renal tubules. Fractional anisotropy (FA) can provide structural and flow information. The role of diffusion tensor imaging in renal imaging is under investigation.[143]

Blood Oxygen Level Dependent MRI

Blood oxygen level dependent (BOLD) imaging is a technique to noninvasively measure renal oxygenation. It utilizes the paramagnetic effects of deoxyhemoglobin to obtain images sensitive to local oxygen concentration. A multiple gradient recalled echo (GRE) sequence is the most widely used sequence for BOLD MRI. Deoxyhemoglobin induces a magnetic susceptibility effect that disturbs the local magnetic field and increases the spin-spin relaxation time (R_2*) of surrounding water. A high R_2* value corresponds to low tissue oxygenation.[144]

Applications of BOLD

- *Renal artery stenosis*: BOLD imaging can detect changes of renal hypoxia. It has been seen that kidneys with maintained functional reserve showed a low R_2* value (higher oxygenation) following administration of furosemide as compared to those with atrophic kidneys with total arterial occlusion.
- *Diabetic nephropathy*: A significant increase in oxygenation of renal medulla has been found in normal healthy kidney in response to water diuresis, while this response is absent in diabetic patients.
- *Renal transplant*: BOLD imaging can help differentiate cases of acute rejection from ATN.

Arterial Spin Labeling: Noncontrast Perfusion Imaging

It is a method of performing perfusion studies without the use of exogenous contrast. Arterial spin labeling (ASL) uses magnetically labeled protons in arteries and is noninvasive. The main applications are assessment of response to antiangiogenic drugs in renal tumor, differentiation between renal tumors and measurement of renal function, and perfusion in CKD.

Sodium (^{23}Na) MRI

This is a promising noninvasive method for physiologic imaging of the human kidneys. The technique allows quantification of ^{23}Na concentration of the cortex and medulla and evaluates the changes which occur under different physiologic conditions.[145]

MR Elastography

In recent years, there is a great interest in the study of tissue stiffness of the kidneys for many disease processes affecting the kidneys. It has been seen in some studies that the stiffness of the renal parenchyma is lower in a diseased kidney as compared to the normal kidneys.[146] Magnetic resonance elastography (MRE) of the kidneys is challenging and holds promise in the evaluation of chronic renal disease and renal allografts.

CONCLUSION

A clear understanding of the anatomy and physiology of the urogenital system is essential for a better understanding of the disease processes. The advanced visualization techniques do not create data over and above the cross-sections, but using the tools to display data in new ways that simulate 3D anatomy creates additional visual information about the patient. An attempt should be made by every radiologist to reach an accurate diagnosis thereby improving patient care and justifying the additional effort and expense.

REFERENCES

1. Nino-Murcia M, de Vries PA, Friedland GW. Congenital anomalies of the kidney. In: Pollack HM, McClennan BL (Eds). Clinical Urography. Philadelphia: Saunders; 2000. pp. 690-763.
2. Satyapal KS, Haffejee AA, Singh B, et al. Additional renal arteries incidence and morphometry. Surg Radiol Anat. 2001;23(1):33-8.
3. Bhatt S, Dogra VS. Kidney. In: Haaga JR, Boll DT (Eds). CT and MRI of the whole body, 6th edition. Philadelphia, PA: Elsevier; 2016. pp. 1781-861.
4. Kabala JE. The urogenital tract: Anatomy and investigations. In: Sutton D (Ed). Textbook of radiology and imaging, 7th edition. London: Churchill Livingstone; 2003. pp. 885-928.
5. Gore RM, Balfe DM, Aizenstein RI, et al. The great escape: interfascial decompression planes of the retroperitoneum. AJR Am J Roentgenol. 2000;175(2):363-70.
6. Kabala J. Attempting to increase the sensitivity of the plain film for ureteric calculi. Use of the full bladder. Br J Radiol. 1991;64(768):1151-3.
7. Levine JA, Neitlich J, Verga M, et al. Ureteral calculi in patients with flank pain: correlation of plain radiography with unenhanced helical CT. Radiology. 1997;204(1):27-31.
8. Dyer RB, Chen MY, Zagoria RJ. Intravenous urography: technique and interpretation. Radiographics. 2001;21(4):799-824.

9. Katzberg RW. Urography into the 21st century: new contrast media, renal handling, imaging characteristics and nephrotoxicity. Radiology. 1997;204(2):297-312.
10. Stacul F. Current iodinated contrast media. Eur Radiol. 2001;11(4):690-7.
11. Katayama H, Yamaguchi K, Kozuka T, et al. Adverse reactions to ionic and nonionic contrast media: a report from the Japanese Committee on the Safety of Contrast Media. Radiology. 1990;175(3):621-8.
12. Dalla Palma L. What is left of i.v. urography? Eur Radiol. 2001;11(6): 931-9.
13. Kohli A. Has the time come to write the EPITAPH for the intravenous urogram? Ind J Radiol Imaging. 2005;15(2):161-4.
14. Shine S. Urinary calculus: IVU vs CT renal stone? A critically appraised topic. Abdom Imaging. 2008;33(1):41-3.
15. Warshauer DM, McCarthy SM, Street L, et al. Detection of renal masses: sensitivities and specificities of excretory urography/ linear tomography, US, and CT. Radiology. 1988;169(2): 363-5.
16. Wells ITP, Raju VM, Rowberry BK, et al. Digital tomosynthesis: a new lease of life for the intravenous urogram. Br J Radiol. 2011;84(1001):464-8.
17. Caoili EM, Cohan RH, Inampudi P, et al. MDCT urography of upper tract urothelial neoplasms. Am J Roentgenol. 2005; 184(6): 1873-81.
18. Taylor RJ, Bennett AH, Schwentker FN, et al. Use and abuse of retrograde pyelography. Urology. 1979;14(5):536-9.
19. Paul A. The normal kidney. In: Meire HB, Cosgrove D, Dewbury KC, Tarrant P (Eds). Abdominal and General Ultrasound. Edinburgh: Churchill Livingstone; 2001. pp. 515-27.
20. Greenfield SP, Williot P, Kaplan D. Gross hematuria in children: a ten-year review. Urology. 2007;69(1):166-9.
21. Hulton SA. Evaluation of urinary tract calculi in children. Arch Dis Child. 2001;84(4):320-3.
22. Grossfeld GD, Litwin MS, Wolf JS, et al. Evaluation of asymptomatic microscopic hematuria in adults: the American Urological Association Best Practice Policy. Part I: definition, detection, prevalence and etiology. Urology. 2001:57(4):599-603.
23. Bazzocchi M, Rizzatto G. The value of the posterior oblique longitudinal scan in renal ultrasonography. Urol Radiol. 1980;1:221.
24. Thurston W, Wilson R. The Urinary Tract. In: Rumack CM, Wilson SR, Charboneau JW (Eds). Diagnostic Ultrasound, 5th edition, Maryland Heights: Elseiver Mosby; 2017. pp. 321-93.
25. Purohit K, Purohit A, Satpathy G. Measurement of normal kidney length by sonography and its relation to age, sex and body habitus. IJAR. 2017;5(4.3):4668-73.
26. Emamian SA, Nielsen MB, Pedersen JF, et al. Kidney dimensions at sonography: correlation with age, sex and habitus in 665 adult volunteers. Am J Roentgenol. 1993;160(1):83-6.
27. Marchal G, Verbeken E, Oyen R, et al. Ultrasound of the normal kidney: a sonographic, anatomic and histologic correlation. Ultrasound in Med and Biol. 1986;12:999-1009.
28. Rosenfield AT, Taylor KJ, Dembner AG, et al. Ultrasound of renal sinus: new observations. Am J Roentgenol. 1979;133(3):441-8.
29. Hricak H, Slovis TL, Callen CW, et al. Neonatal kidneys: sonographic anatomic correlation. Radiology. 1983;147(3):699-702.
30. Swischuk LE. Genitourinary Tract and Adrenal Glands. In: Imaging of the Newborn, Infant and Young Child, 5th edition. Philadelphia: Lippincott Williams & Wilkins; 2004. pp. 590-724.
31. Han BK, Babcock DS. Sonographic measurements and appearance of normal kidneys in children. Am J Roentgenol. 1985;145:611-6.
32. Lafortune M, Constantin A, Breton G, et al. Sonography of the hypertrophied column of Bertin. Am J Roentgenol. 1986;146:53-6.
33. Carter AR, Horgan JG, Jennings TA, et al. The junctional parenchymal defect: a sonographic variant of renal anatomy. Radiology. 1985;154:499-502.
34. Hoffer FA, Hanabergh AM, Teele RL. The interrenicular junction: a mimic of renal scarring on normal pediatric sonograms. Am J Roentgenol. 1985;145(5):1075-8.
35. Fine H, Keen EN. The arteries of the human kidney. J Anat. 1966;100:881-94.
36. Dubbins PA. The kidney. In: Allan PL, Dubbins PA, Pozniak M, Mc Dicken WN (Eds). Clinical Doppler Ultrasound. London: Churchill Livingstone; 2000. pp. 169-90.
37. Chang EH. An introduction to contrast-enhanced ultrasound for nephrologists. Nephron. 2018;138(3):176-85.
38. Seguel AP, Perez MM, Gonzalez TR, et al. Evaluation of upper tract urothelial carcinomas by contrast-enhanced ultrasound. Radiologia. 2018;60(6):496-503.
39. Chang EH, Chong WK, Kasoji SK, et al. Diagnostic accuracy of contrast-enhanced ultrasound for characterization of kidney lesions in patients with and without chronic disease. BMC Nephrol. 2017;18(1):266.
40. Leong SS, Wong JHD, Md Shah MN, et al. Shear wave elastography in the evaluation of renal parenchymal stiffness in patients with chronic kidney disease. Br J Radiol. 2018;91(1089):20180235.
41. Schreyer H, Uggowitzer M, Ruppert Kohlmayr A. Helical CT of the urinary organs. Eur Radiol. 2002;12:575-91.
42. Foley WD. Special focus session. Multidetector CT: Abdominal visceral imaging. Radiographics. 2002;22(3):701-19.
43. Wolin EA, Hartman DS, Olson JR. Nephrographic and pyelographic analysis of CT urography: principles, patterns and pathophysiology. Am J Roentgenol. 2013;200(6):1210-14.
44. Kocakoc E, Bhatt S, Dogra VS. Renal multidetector row CT. Radiol Clin N Am. 2005;43:1021-47.
45. Yuh BI, Cohan RH. Different phases of renal enhancement: role in detecting and characterizing renal masses during helical CT. Am J Roentgenol. 1999;173(3):747-55.
46. Wintersperger BJ, Nikolaou K, Becker CR. Multidetector row CT angiography of the aorta and visceral arteries. Semin Ultrasound CT MR. 2004;25:25-40.
47. Sheth S, Fishman EK. Multidetector row CT of the kidneys and urinary tract: techniques and applications in the diagnosis of benign diseases. Radiographics. 2004;24(2):e20.
48. Tunaci A, Yekeler E. Multidetector row CT of the kidneys. Eur J Radiol. 2004;52:56-66.
49. Villa L, Giusti G, Knoll T, et al. Imaging for urinary stones: update in 2015. Eur Urol Focus. 2016;2(2):122-9.
50. Assimos D, Krambeck A, Miller NL, et al. Surgical management of stones: American Urological Association/Endourological Society Guideline. Part I. J Urol. 2016;196(4):1153-60.
51. Lukasiewicz A, Bhargavan Chatfield M, Coombs L, et al. Radiation dose index of renal colic protocol CT studies in the United States: a report from the American College of Radiology: National Radiology Data Registry. Radiology. 2014;27(12):445-51.
52. Kluner C, Hein PA, Gralla O, et al. Does ultra-low dose CT with a radiation dose equivalent to that of KUB suffice to detect renal and ureteral calculi? J Comput Assist Tomogr. 2006;30(1): 44-50.
53. Saunders HS, Dyer RB, Shifrin RY, et al. The CT nephrogram: implications for evaluation of urinary tract disease. Radiographics. 1995;15(5):1069-85.
54. Szolar DH, Kammerhuber F, Altziebler S, et al. Multiphasic helical CT of the kidney: increased conspicuity for detection and characterization of small (<3 cm) renal masses. Radiology. 1997;202(1):211-7.
55. Urban BA. The small renal mass: What is the role of multiphasic helical scanning? Radiology. 1997;202(1):22-3.

56. Hilton S, Jones LP. Recent advances in imaging cancer of the kidney and urinary tract. Surg Oncol Clin N Am. 2014;23:863-910.
57. Cowan NC, Turney BW, Taylor NJ, et al. Multidetector computed tomography urography for diagnosing upper urinary tract urothelial tumour. BJU Int. 2007;99(6):1363-70.
58. Kawashima A, LeRoy AJ. Radiologic evaluation of patients with renal infections. Inf Dis Clin North Am. 2003;17:433-56.
59. Sheth S, Scatarige JC, Horton KM, et al. Current concepts in the diagnosis and management of renal cell carcinoma: Role of multidetector CT and three-dimensional CT. Radiographics. 2001;21:S237-54.
60. Zagoria RJ. Imaging of small renal masses: A medical success story. AJR Am J Roentgenol. 2000;175(4):945-55.
61. Macari M, Bosniak MA. Delayed CT to evaluate renal masses incidentally discovered at contrast-enhanced CT: demonstration of vascularity with de-enhancement. Radiology. 1999;213:674-80.
62. Fielding JR, Steele G, Fox LA, et al. Spiral computerized tomography in the evaluation of acute flank pain: a replacement for excretory urography. J Urol. 1997;157:2071-3.
63. Heneghan JP, Dalrymple NC, Verga M, et al. Soft tissue "rim" sign in the diagnosis of ureteral calculi with use of unenhanced helical CT. Radiology. 1997;202:709-11.
64. Georgiades CS, Moore CJ, Smith DP. Differences of renal parenchymal attenuation for acutely obstructed and unobstructed kidneys on unenhanced helical CT: a useful secondary sign. Am J Roentgenol. 2001;176:965-8.
65. Bell TV, Fenlon HM, Davison BD, et al. Unenhanced helical CT criteria to differentiate distal ureteral calculi from pelvic phleboliths. Radiology. 1998;207(2):363-7.
66. Smith RC, Verga M, McCarthy S, et al. Diagnosis of acute flank pain: value of unenhanced helical CT. Am J Roentgenol. 1996;166:97-101.
67. Willmann JK, Roos JE, Platz A, et al. Multidetector CT: Detection of active hemorrhage in patients with blunt abdominal trauma. Am J Roentgenol. 2002;179:437-44.
68. McNicholas MM, Raptopoulos VD, Schwartz RK, et al. Excretory phase CT urography for opacification of the urinary collecting system. Am J Roentgenol. 1998;170:1261-7.
69. Kundra V, Silverman PM. Impact of multislice CT on imaging of acute abdominal disease. Radiol Clin North Am. 2003;41(6):1083-93.
70. Kawashima A, Sandler CM, Goldman SM, et al. CT of renal inflammatory disease. Radiographics. 1997;17:851-66.
71. Rubin GD. 3-D imaging with MDCT. Eur J Radiol. 2003;45(Suppl 1): S37-41.
72. Lockhart ME, Smith JK. Technical considerations in renal CT. Radiol Clin North Am. 2003;41:863-75.
73. Rydberg J, Buckwalter KA, Caldemeyer KS, et al. Multisection CT: Scanning techniques and clinical applications. Radiographics. 2000;20:1787-806.
74. Dillman JR, Caoili EM, Cohan RH. Multidetector CT urography: a one stop renal and urinary tract imaging modality. Abdom Imaging. 2007;32(4):519-29.
75. Herts BR. The current status of CT Urography. Crit Rev Comput Tomogr. 2002;43(3):219-41.
76. Vrtiska TJ, King BF, LeRoy AJ, et al. CT urography: analysis of techniques and comparison with IVU (abstr). Radiology. 2000;217(P):225.
77. McCollough CH, Daly TR, King Jr BF, et al. An auxiliary CT table top for radiography at the time of CT. J Comput Assist Tomogr. 2001;25(6):876-80.
78. Kawashima A, Vrtiska TJ, LeRoy AJ. CT scanned projection radiographs (SPR) utilizing enhanced algorithms: applications in CT urography (abstr). Radiology. 2002;225(P):690.
79. Caoili EM, Cohan RH, Korobkin M, et al. Urinary tract abnormalities: Initial experience with multidetector row CT urography. Radiology. 2002;222(2):353-60.
80. Kawashima A, Vrtiska TJ, LeRoy AJ, et al. CT urography. Radiographics. 2004;24:S35-54.
81. Sanyal R, Deshmukh A, Sheorain VS, et al. CT urography: a comparison of strategies for upper urinary tract opacification. Eur Radiol. 2007;17(5):1262-6.
82. Silverman SG, Akbar SA, Mortele KJ, et al. Multidetector-row CT urography: comparison of furosemide and saline as adjuncts to contrast medium for depicting the normal urinary collecting system. Radiology. 2006;240:749-55.
83. Caoili EM, Inampudi P, Cohan RH, et al. Optimization of multidetector row CT urography: effect of compression, saline administration and prolongation of acquisition delay. Radiology. 2005;235:116-23.
84. McTavish JD, Jinzaki M, Zou KH, et al. Multidetector row CT urography: Comparison of strategies for depicting the normal urinary collecting system. Radiology. 2002;225:783-90.
85. Jinzaki M, McTavish JD, Zou KH, et al. Evaluation of small (≤3 cm) renal masses with MDCT: benefits of thin overlapping reconstructions. Am J Roentgenol. 2004;183(1):223-8.
86. Chow LC, Kwan SW, Olcott EW, et al. Split bolus MDCT urography with synchronous nephrographic and excretory phase enhancement. Am J Roentgenol. 2007;189:314-22.
87. Kekelidze M, Dwarkasing RS, Dijkshoorn ML, et al. Kidney and urinary tract imaging: triple bolus multidetector CT urography as a one stop shop: protocol design, opacification, and image quality analysis. Radiology. 2010;255(2):508-16.
88. Abedi G, Okhunov Z, Lall C, et al. Comparison of radiation dose from conventional and triple bolus computed tomography urography protocols in the diagnosis and management of patients with renal cortical neoplasms. Urology. 2014;84(4):875-80.
89. Lang EK, Thomas R, Davis R, et al. Multiphasic helical computerized tomography for the assessment of microscopic hematuria: a prospective study. J Urol. 2004;171(1):237-43.
90. Albani JM, Ciaschini MW, Streem SB, et al. The role of computerized tomographic urography in the initial evaluation of hematuria. J Urol. 2007;177(2):644-8.
91. Van Der Molen AJ, Cowan NC, Mueller-Lisse UG, et al. CT Urography Working Group of the European Society of Urogenital Radiology (ESUR). CT urography: definition, indications and techniques. A guideline for clinical practice. Eur Radiol. 2008;18(1):4-17.
92. Khadra MH, Pickard RS, Charlton M, et al. A prospective analysis of 1930 patients with hematuria to evaluate current diagnostic practice. J Urol. 2000;163(2):524-7.
93. Raman SP, Fishman EK. Upper and lower tract urothelial imaging using computed tomography urography. Urol Clin N Am. 2018;45:389-405.
94. Vikram R, Sandler CM, Ng CS. Imaging and staging of transitional cell carcinoma: part 2. Upper urinary tract. Am J Roentgenol. 2009;192(6):1488-93.
95. Chlapoutakis K, Theocharopoulos N, Yarmenitis S, et al. Performance of computed tomographic urography in diagnosis of upper urinary tract urothelial carcinoma, in patients presenting with hematuria: systematic review and meta-analysis. Eur J Radiol. 2010;73(2): 334-8.
96. Chai RY, Jhaveri K, Saini S, et al. Comprehensive evaluation of patients with haematuria on multi-slice computed tomography scanner: protocol design and preliminary observations. Australas Radiol. 2001;45:536-8.
97. Joffe SA, Servaes S, Okon S, et al. Multidetector row CT urography in the evaluation of hematuria. Radiographics. 2003;23(6):1441-55.
98. Potenta SE, D'Agostino R, Sternberg KM, et al. CT Urography for Evaluation of the Ureter. Radiographics. 2015;35:709-26.
99. Patel RC, Newman RC. Ureteroscopic management of ureteral and ureteroenteral strictures. Urol Clin North Am. 2004;31(1): 107-13.

100. Lawler LP, Jarret TW, Corl FM, et al. Adult ureteropelvic junction obstruction: insights with three dimensional multidetector row CT. Radiographics. 2005;25(1):121-34.
101. Berrocal T, López-Pereira P, Arjonilla A, et al. Anomalies of the distal ureter, bladder and urethra in children: embryologic, radiologic and pathologic features. Radiographics. 2002;22(5):1139-64.
102. Lupescu IG, Marica OL. CT urography. How when why? Rev Rom Urol. 2012;11(4):17-20.
103. Kaza RK, Platt JF, Cohan RH, et al. Dual-energy CT with single and dual source scanners: current applications in evaluating the genitourinary tract. Radiographics. 2012;32(2):353-69.
104. Juri H, Matsuki M, Itou Y, et al. Initial experience with adaptive iterative dose reduction 3D to reduce radiation dose in computed tomographic urography. J Comput Assist Tomogr. 2013;37(1):52-7.
105. Van der Molen AJ, Miclea RL, Geleijns J, et al. A survey of radiation doses in CT urography before and after implementation of iterative reconstruction. Am J Roentgenol. 2015;205(3):572-7.
106. Jepperson MA, Cernigliaro JG, Sella D, et al. Dual-energy CT for the evaluation of urinary calculi: image interpretation, pitfalls and stone mimics. Clin Radiol. 2013;68:e707-14.
107. Kaza RK, Caoili EM, Cohan RH, et al. Distinguishing enhancing from nonenhancing renal lesions with fast kilovoltage switching dual energy CT. Am J Roentgenol. 2011;197(6):1375-81.
108. Primak AN, Fletcher JG, Vrtiska TJ, et al. Noninvasive differentiation of uric acid versus non-uric acid kidney stones using dual-energy CT. Acad Radiol. 2007;14(12):1441-7.
109. Eliahou R, Hidas G, Duvdevani M, et al. Determination of renal stone composition with dual-energy computed tomography: an emerging application. Semin Ultrasound CT MR. 2010;31(4):315-20.
110. Takahashi N, Vrtiska TJ, Kawashima A, et al. Detectability of urinary stones on virtual nonenhanced images generated at pyelographic phase dual energy CT. Radiology. 2010;256(1):184-90.
111. Kim TS, Chung JW, Park JH, et al. Renal artery evaluation: comparison of spiral CT angiography to intra-arterial DSA. J Vasc Inter Radiol. 1998;9:553-9.
112. Napoli A, Fleischmann D, Chan FP, et al. Computed tomography angiography: state of the art imaging using multidetector row technology. J Comput Assist Tomogra. 2004;28:S32-45.
113. Türkvatan A, Özdemir M, Cumhur T, et al. Multidetector CT angiography of renal vasculature: normal anatomy and variants. Eur Radiol. 2009;19:236-44.
114. Yeh BM, Coakley FV, Meng MV, et al. Precaval right renal arteries: prevalence and morphologic associations at spiral CT. Radiology. 2004;230:429-33.
115. Merkle EM, Dale BM, Paulson EK. Abdominal MR imaging at 3T. Magn Reson Imaging Clin N Am. 2006;14:17-26.
116. Nikken JJ, Krestin GP. MRI of the kidney. State of the art. Eur Radiol. 2007;17:2780-93.
117. Pedrosa I, Sun MR, Spencer M, et al. MR imaging of renal masses: correlation with findings at surgery and pathologic analysis. Radiographics. 2008;28:985-1003.
118. Zhang J, Pedrosa I, Rofsky NM. MR techniques for renal imaging. Radiol Clin North Am. 2003;41:877-907.
119. Glockner JF, Hu HH, Stanley DW, et al. Parallel MR imaging: a user's guide. Radiographics. 2005;25(5):1279-97.
120. Israel GM, Bosniak MA. Pitfalls in renal mass evaluation and how to avoid them. Radiographics. 2008;28(5):1325-38.
121. Schieda N, Krishna S, Davenport MS. Update on Gadolinium Based Contrast Agent-Enhanced Imaging in the Genitourinary System. Am J Roentgenol. 2019;212(6):1223-33.
122. Perez-Rodriguez J, Lai S, Ehst BD, et al. Nephrogenic systemic fibrosis: incidence, associations and effect of risk factor assessment—report of 33 cases. Radiology. 2009;250(2):371-7.
123. Bassignani MJ. Understanding and interpreting MRI of the genitourinary tract. Urol Clin N Am. 2006;33(3):301-17.
124. Probert JL, Glew D, Gillatt DA. Magnetic resonance imaging in urology. BJU Int. 1999;83(3):201-14.
125. Prasad SR, Dalrymple NC, Surabhi VR. Cross-sectional imaging evaluation of renal masses. Radiol Clin North Am. 2008;46(1):95-111.
126. O'Connor OJ, McLaughlin P, Maher MM. MR urography. Am J Roentgenol. 2010;195(3):W201-6.
127. Leyendecker JR, Gianini JW. Magnetic resonance urography. Abdom Imaging. 2009;34(4):527-40.
128. Ergen FB, Hussain HK, Carlos RC, et al. 3D excretory MR urography: improved image quality with intravenous saline and diuretic administration. J Mag Reson Imaging. 2007;25(4):783-9.
129. Silverman SG, Leyendecker JR, Amis Jr ES. What is the current role of CT urography and MR urography in the evaluation of the urinary tract? Radiology. 2009;250(2):309-23.
130. Nolte-Ernsting CC, Staatz G, Tacke J, et al. MR urography today. Abdom Imaging. 2003;28(2):191-209.
131. Takahashi N, Kawashima A, Glockner JF, et al. Small (<2 cm) upper tract urothelial carcinoma: evaluation with gadolinium enhanced three dimensional spoiled gradient recalled echo MR urography. Radiology. 2008;247(2):451-7.
132. Dickerson EC, Dillman JR, Smith EA, et al. Pediatric MR urography: Indications, techniques and approach to review. Radiographics. 2015;35(4):1208-30.
133. Jones RA, Perez-Brayfield MR, Kirsch AJ, et al. Renal transit time with MR urography in children. Radiology. 2004;233(1):41-50.
134. Grattan Smith JD, Little SB, Jones RA. MR urography evaluation of obstructive uropathy. Pediatr Radiol. 2008;38(Suppl 1):S49-69.
135. Michaely HJ, Schoenberg SO, Rieger JR, et al. MR angiography in patients with renal disease. Magn Reson Imaging Clin N Am. 2005;13(1):131-51.
136. Leiner T, Michaely H. Advances in contrast-enhanced MR angiography of the renal arteries. Magn Reson Imaging Clin N Am. 2008;16(4):561-72.
137. Zhang JL. Functional magnetic resonance imaging of the kidneys—with and without gadolinium based contrast. Adv Chronic Kidney Dis. 2017;24(3):162-8.
138. Zhang JL, Rusinek H, Chandarana H, et al. Functional MRI of the kidneys. J Magn Reson Imaging. 2013;37(2):282-93.
139. Michaely HJ, Kramer H, Oesingmann N, et al. Intraindividual comparison of MR-renal perfusion imaging at 1.5 T and 3.0 T. Invest Radiol. 2007;42(6):406-11.
140. Chu WC, Lam WW, Chan KW, et al. Dynamic gadolinium enhanced magnetic resonance urography for assessing drainage in dilated pelvicalyceal systems with moderate renal function: preliminary results and comparison with diuresis renography. BJU Int. 2004;93(6):830-4.
141. Shokeir AA, El-Diasty T, Eassa W, et al. Diagnosis of ureteral obstruction in patients with compromised renal function: the role of noninvasive imaging modalities. J Urol. 2004;171:2303-6.
142. Mürtz P, Krautmacher C, Träber F, et al. Diffusion-weighted whole body MR imaging with background body signal suppression: a feasibility study at 3.0 Tesla. Eur Radiol. 2007;17:3031-7.
143. Notohamiprodjo M, Dietrich O, Horger W, et al. Diffusion tensor imaging (DTI) of the kidney at 3 Tesla–feasibility, protocol evaluation and comparison to 1.5 Tesla. Invest Radiol. 2010;45(5):245-54.
144. Gloviczki ML, Glockner J, Gomez SI, et al. Comparison of 1.5 and 3T BOLD MR to study oxygenation of kidney cortex and medulla in human renovascular disease. Invest Radiol. 2009;44(9):566-71.
145. Maril N, Rosen Y, Reynolds GH, et al. Sodium MRI of the human kidney at 3 Tesla. Magn Reson Med. 2006;56(6):1229-34.
146. Bensamoun SF, Robert L, Leclerc GE, et al. Stiffness imaging of the kidney and adjacent abdominal tissues measured simultaneously using magnetic resonance elastography. Clin Imaging. 2011;35(4):284-7.

CHAPTER 2

Current Status of Nuclear Medicine in Urinary Tract Imaging

Rakesh Kumar, Madhavi Tripathi

INTRODUCTION

Nuclear medicine techniques play a complimentary role in the functional evaluation of genitourinary tract. In fact, they have been effectively included in the management algorithm of conditions like congenital hydronephrosis and urinary tract infections (UTI). Radiopharmaceuticals evaluate various aspects of renal function like glomerular filtration rate (GFR) and clearance and provide a wealth of information to the nephrologist and urologist. Besides being highly sensitive, these procedures are noninvasive, simple, nontoxic, and most importantly, do not interfere with normal physiology and function. Using these techniques, it has now become possible to assess split renal function, evaluate perfusion, especially of transplant kidneys, evaluate upper urinary tract dilatation, and diagnose urinary tract obstruction, detect the presence of kidneys, which are poorly functioning and ectopic and monitor renal function in renal failure.

The nuclear medicine investigations for evaluation of nephro-urological disorders can be broadly classified into: (1) Dynamic renography, (2) renal cortical scintigraphy, (3) radionuclide cystography and voiding cystography, and (4) Clearance studies, i.e. glomerular filtration rate (GFR) estimation, effective renal plasma flow (ERPF) estimation, etc. Various interventions like Lasix diuresis and angiotensin-converting enzyme inhibitors (captopril/losartan) have further enhanced the diagnosis of obstruction and renovascular hypertension using radionuclide studies.

RENAL POSITRON EMISSION TOMOGRAPHY

Positron emission tomography (PET) radiotracers for functional renal imaging have recently been developed, in particular focusing on Fluorine-18 (^{18}F)- and Gallium-68 (^{68}Ga)-labeled agents. Several of these PET imaging probes such as ^{68}Ga ethylenediaminetetraacetic acid (^{68}Ga EDTA), ^{68}Ga-IR-Dye800-tilmanocept, and 2-deoxy-2-[^{18}F] fluorodeoxysorbitol (^{18}F-FDS) have been evaluated for assessment of GFR and the diagnostic performance of ^{68}Ga EDTA has been demonstrated in a clinical trial.[1-4] ^{68}Ga-IR-Dye800-tilmanocept shows receptor-mediated binding to glomerular mesangial cells, which in turn may allow the monitoring of progression of diabetic nephropathy. ^{18}F-FDS shows excellent kidney extraction and excretion in rats.[5] Further, due to its simple one-step radiosynthesis via the most frequently used PET radiotracer 2-deoxy-2-[^{18}F]fluoro-D-glucose, [^{18}F]FDS could be available at nearly every PET center. A new PET radiotracer for the effective assessment of plasma flow in the kidneys is Re(CO)3-N-([^{18}F]fluoroethyl) iminodiacetic acid (Re(CO)3[^{18}F]FEDA).[6] This compound demonstrates similar pharmacokinetic properties to its ^{99m}Tc-labeled analog [99mTc](CO)3(FEDA). Thus, if there is a shortage of molybdenum-99, Re(CO)3[^{18}F]FEDA would allow a direct comparison with previous ^{99m}Technetium (^{99m}Tc)-based studies. PET radiotracers for renal imaging have tremendous potential for evaluation of kidney function. Further, simultaneously acquired CT images enable precise anatomical coregistration with rapid three-dimensional imaging capability.

RADIOPHARMACEUTICALS

The various radiopharmaceuticals presently used in nephro-urology practice are classified into glomerular agents (filtered a glomerulus), and tubular agents, which are further subdivided into tubular fixation and tubular clearance agents. The prototype glomerular agent is ^{99m}Tc-diethyl triamine pentaacetic acid (DTPA), which is effectively used to measure the global GFR. Tubular clearance agents include ^{99m}Tc-L,L ethylene dicysteine (LLEC), which is the standard agent used for renography studies in India and ^{99m}Tc-mercaptoacetyltriglycine (MAG-3), which is used in the west and is not cost-effective in the Indian context. ^{99m}Tc-glucoheptonate (GHA) undergoes both glomerular filtration and tubular fixation (approximately 10–15% of the injected dose is retained in the renal parenchyma while 65% of the injected dose is eliminated in the urine within 6 hours after injection) and is an agent which can be used both for renal dynamic studies and for renal cortical scintigraphy.

The agent which is recommended for renal cortical scintigraphy is ^{99m}Tc-dimercaptosuccinic acid (DMSA) which enables detailed evaluation of the renal parenchyma.

^{99m}Technetium-L,L Ethylene Dicysteine

Currently, it is the most commonly used radiopharmaceutical for renal dynamic studies. It is a metabolite of the brain perfusion tracer ^{99m}Tc-ethylcysteinate dimer (ECD) and is cleared principally through active tubular transport. LLEC has good imaging properties and a higher renal clearance than MAG-3.[7] Labeling EC with ^{99m}Tc does not require boiling and highest labeling yield is obtained at pH of 10–12 (97%). Like ^{123}I-orthoiodohippurate (OIH) and ^{99m}Tc-MAG-3, the secretion of ^{99m}Tc-LLEC occurs in proximal tubule.[8] DD-EC has highest and faster renal clearance while LLEC has lower renal excretion and higher tissue retention.[8,9] Protein binding of DD-EC is 28% and LLEC has 50%. Production of DD-EC form, however, demands HPLC purification, a drawback for clinical use. The clearance of LLEC is about 75%. The disadvantage of EC is unknown amounts of different stereoisomers and forms produced by the different labeling kit, which have different excretion.

^{99m}Technetium-Mercaptoacetyltriglycine

Currently, ^{99m}Tc-MAG 3 is mostly used in Europe and USA. It is cleared principally through active tubular transport.[10] Plasma clearance is in the order of 300 mL/min, approximately 60% of OIH,[11,12] and after 3 hours, approximately 90% of the injected dose can be recovered in the urine. It is more extensively protein bound than ^{123}I-OIH (88% vs 65%) and therefore, its volume of distribution is lower than that of ^{123}I-OIH. Since it is eliminated by tubular secretion and has a high initial renal uptake, the kidney to background ratio provided by this tracer is high. Moreover, the rapid excretion provides good temporal resolution. ^{99m}Tc-MAG 3 is a superior agent for renal dynamic scintigraphy, but a practical limitation to its extensive use is the relatively high cost.

^{99m}Technetium-Diethyl Triamine Pentaacetic Acid

^{99m}Technetium-DTPA has been the tracer of choice for dynamic renal scintigraphy for almost three decades. However, it is has been replaced by ^{99m}Tc-LLEC and ^{99m}Tc-MAG 3 in daily clinical practice. It is excreted primarily by glomerular filtration, at a slightly lower rate than inulin, approximately 90 mL/min.[13,14] This lower rate of filtration is probably due to protein binding, the amount of which varies with the formulation. A maximum concentration in kidneys is usually achieved 3 minutes after intravenous injection. This is the best agent for in vitro GFR studies and for simultaneous renal dynamic study with estimation of GFR.

^{99m}Technetium-Dimercaptosuccinic Acid

^{99m}Technetium-DMSA is currently the agent of choice for cortical renal scintigraphy—planar and single photon emission tomography (SPECT). The renal uptake of this agent is about 50% of the injected dose at 1 hour and about 70% at 24 hours after injection.[15] One hour or more postinjection, the tracer is found principally in the proximal convoluted tubules with very minimal activity elsewhere in the kidney. In most patients, therefore, excellent images of renal cortex can be obtained approximately 4 hours after injection of ^{99m}Tc-DMSA. Here again, patients with obstructive pathology may have tracer retention within the pelvicalyceal system leading to false interpretation. In such cases, Lasix injection is recommended to allow tracer in the urine to be eliminated.

IMAGING TECHNIQUES

Renal Dynamic Scintigraphy

This refers to serial continuous imaging following intravenous injection of radio-tracer. It encompasses three principal techniques—(1) Dynamic renography, (2) diuretic renography, and (3) captopril renography.

Dynamic Renography

Patient Preparation

Patient should be well-hydrated before the study and encouraged to drink fluids ad libitum. Before the examination begins, the patients are asked to empty their bladder. In suspected cases of vesicoureteric junction obstruction, when patients cannot void completely (neurogenic bladder) or in children with vesicoureteral reflux (VUR), the study is recommended with a bladder catheter (Foley's type) in situ so that bladder drainage is maintained throughout the entire duration of the study. An intravenous line is established to avoid extravasation of tracer, which may yield erroneous interpretation.

Radiopharmaceuticals Recommended

^{99m}Tc-LLEC, or ^{99m}Tc-MAG 3, or ^{99m}Tc-DTPA (rarely): The dose administered for each tracer is given in **Table 1**.

Imaging

Patients are examined supine with the gamma-camera positioned underneath the examination table (posteriorly) viewing the kidney and bladder area. In this position, the distance from the skin to each of the kidneys is approximately the same and for calculation of the left/right renal uptake ratio, depth correction is not critical. In renal transplants, however, the camera is placed anteriorly with the patient

TABLE 1: Different radiopharmaceutical and their doses.

Radiopharmaceutical	Dose (mCi/kg)	Minimum dose (mCi)	Maximum dose (mCi)
^{99m}Tc-LLEC	0.15	1	10.0
^{99m}Tc-MAG3	0.15	1	10.0
^{99m}Tc-DTPA	0.15	1	8.0
^{99m}Tc-DMSA	0.05	0.5	3.0
^{123}I-OIH	0.010	0.1	0.5

in supine position, viewing the allograft and bladder. In children with ectopic (including fused ectopia) or horseshoe kidneys dual-head acquisition is preferred so that geometric mean can be used for calculation of the differential function of each unit. In children, appropriate immobilization should be attained during acquisition. Patient must be asked to void immediately before start of study. Once the patient is appropriately positioned, a rapid intravenous bolus of the tracer is injected and acquisition begins simultaneously. One frame per two seconds is recorded for 60 seconds (perfusion phase) followed by one frame per 15 seconds (parenchymal phase) for a total of 20–30 minutes.

Interpretation

A dynamic renal study is evaluated for the parenchymal phase, the cortical transit time, and the drainage phase. The renogram curve generated is evaluated for function and drainage pattern. A cinematic display verifies whether the patient moved during acquisition or not.

- *Parenchymal phase:* Evaluation of this phase is very critical. During the first few minutes of the dynamic study, after the initial vascular distribution of the tracer and before its appearance in the renal collecting system, the tracer is concentrated in the renal parenchyma. At this point there is progressive decrease in the blood level of the tracer with increasing concentration in the parenchyma till a peak is reached, where maximum concentration has been attained. Usual time to peak T_{max} is 2–5 minutes for normally functioning kidneys. After this, the tracer progressively decreases within the parenchyma, marking the beginning of the drainage phase. The parenchymal phase is usually visualized 60–120 seconds after the IV injection and provides the following information:
  - Relative and absolute size of the functional renal units.
  - Relative or split renal function (right vs left).
  - Overall renal morphology.
  - Position of the renal units and axis.

  The relative renal size and their placement can be estimated by simple visual observation. Renal dimensions in longitudinal and transverse planes can be measured with a measuring scale provided in the processing station. A qualitative estimate of the renal function can be obtained by visually evaluating the ratio of the renal and background activity. Normally, very little tracer activity should be present in the background, the blood pool and the liver during the parenchymal phase. If a high level of tracer activity is noted within these regions, then the renal uptake shall be low indicating a poor renal function. Split renal function can be assessed visually and also by calculating the individual renal uptake as a fraction of the total renal uptake from renal regions of interests (ROIs). Placement of ROIs should be strictly over the parenchymal region but under certain special circumstances such as hydronephrosis, this may be difficult. Background ROIs (2 pixels wide and 2 pixels away from the renal ROI) should be placed with caution since this step is usually done manually and different size and position can produce different results, a particular problem when renal function is low and/or severe hydronephrosis is present.

  Information about intrarenal distribution of radiotracer can be obtained during the parenchymal phase. Hydronephrosis is usually seen as a "photon deficient" area and depending on the severity of hydronephrosis, the cortical uptake appears as a rim of varying thickness. Reduced or absent tracer activity in a relative portion of the kidney such as a malfunctioning upper pole in a duplex kidney, trauma, tumor, or cyst can be detected.
- *Cortical transit time*: Cortical transit time is defined as the time interval between the intravenous injection of the radiotracer and its first appearance within the renal collecting system. Normally, this is about 3–6 minutes. A normal cortical transit time indicates that renal parenchymal function is not compromised, even in the presence of dilatation of the pelvicalyceal system. Conversely, therefore, the poorer the renal function, the longer is the cortical transit time. As the tracer is eliminated into the renal pelvis, there is gradual decline in the parenchymal activity. Even if the cortical transit time appears to be within the normal range, it is important to determine, if it is associated with a decrease of tracer activity from the renal cortex. Cortical retention of tracer activity indicates renal dysfunction. A number of conditions may prolong the cortical time. These include pelviureteric junction obstruction, acute and chronic pyelonephritis, nephrotoxicity, trauma, renal artery stenosis, renal vein thrombosis, acute tubular necrosis, and allograft rejection.
- *Drainage phase*: Drainage phase comprises the passage of the radiotracer from the pelvicalyceal system through the ureter into the bladder. Usually, at the end of 20 minutes of study, much of the tracer would leave the renal parenchyma. At this time, minimal or no tracer should be visible in the renal collecting system. Time activity curves (renogram) are generated from ROI over an entire kidney and reveal a peak time (T_{max}) at 2–5 minutes with subsequent decrease to 30–50% of the peak activity within 10 minutes. Time activity curves should always be interpreted along with careful evaluation of images in the parenchymal phase and drainage phase, keeping in mind the cortical transit time. It is possible to see a normal cortical transit time with complete cortical clearance of tracer by 20 minutes accompanied by a time activity curve that reveals a delayed peak and a high-residual value. Such a pattern indicates delayed drainage without parenchymal dysfunction and is almost always without any clinical significance. The possibility of a VUR of tracer during the drainage phase should also be kept in mind in order to be able to differentiate it from outflow tract obstruction.

Normal Dynamic Renal Study

There is an intense and rapid concentration of tracer in the renal parenchyma by 2–5 minutes post-injection **(Fig. 1)**. Subsequently, the tracer passes into the renal calyces and pelvis by 3–6 minutes. Ureters may be visualized during the dynamic phase in normal patients and in those with slow ureteral transit time. However, a dilated ureter with or without obstruction is always visible in the postvoid phase. The renal

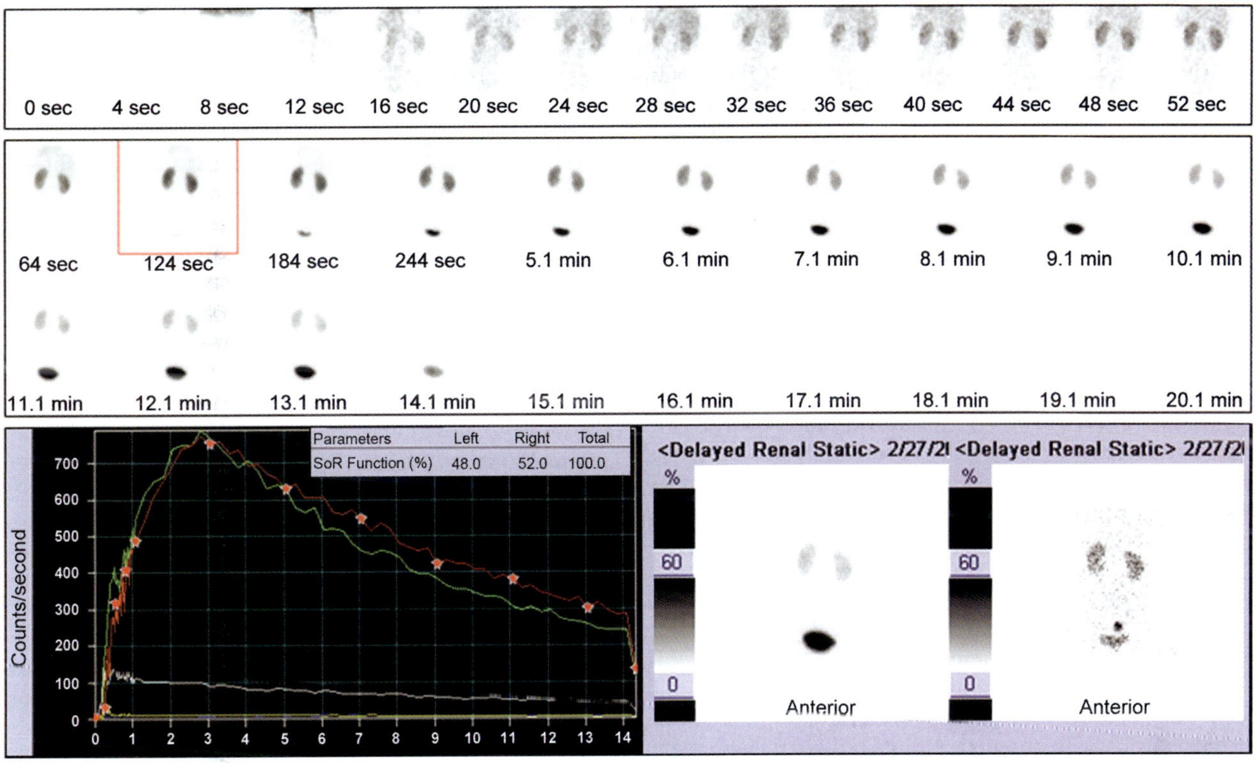

FIG. 1: Normal ^{99m}Tc-LLEC scan: Normal dynamic function images with prompt symmetric radiotracer perfusion (upper row), uptake and rapid clearance (middle row). Normal time activity curves with steep uptake slope, distinct peak, and rapid clearance (left lower row) with normal early and delayed static images (right lower row).

parenchyma is usually completely cleared of radiotracer by 20 minutes but a small residual amount may sometimes be present and is usually of no clinical significance. This residual tracer usually clears spontaneously with change in the patient's position or after the patient voids (gravity-assisted drainage). The bladder is seen 3–6 minutes after injection and there is a progressive increase in tracer concentration with time. The background activity is usually a reflection of blood clearance of tracer or rather the renal extraction of tracer from the blood pool, which rapidly decreases with time in a patient with normal renal function. The dynamic acquisition can be terminated at 15–20 minutes, when there is no retention of tracer within the pelvicalyceal system or ureters. If at the end of the initial 20 minutes, there is evidence of tracer retention, then the patient should be asked to get up and move for a few minutes (a small child should be picked up for a few minutes) to encourage postural-gravity assisted drainage (GAD). An additional postvoid image is recommended to determine the tracer clearance, which if adequate, should be considered normal, and the outflow tract not obstructed. A diuretic renogram is indicated, if an obstruction is present or suspected.

Diuretic Renography

Furosemide causes a rapid diuretic response that drains out tracer from dilated nonobstructed system. In significant outflow tract obstruction, tracer in the renal area may decrease slowly or fail to decrease or even increase in response to a diuretic challenge. The urine flow depends not only on the function and amount of renal parenchyma, but also on the ability of the parenchyma to respond to a diuretic. Drainage is directly proportional to urine flow and inversely proportional to the volume of the renal pelvis and ureters; the poorer the function, the longer is the drainage time. Compliance and volume of the pelvicalyceal system are also important; in that a large flaccid renal pelvis usually causes slow drainage of radiotracer. There are several factors that can limit the usefulness of diuretic renography. Severe hydroureteronephrosis may partly or wholly mask the effect of a diuretic on the emptying of the renal pelvis. Other factors include poor response of the renal parenchyma to the diuretic, poor delivery of the diuretic to the kidneys, bladder over distension, complex pelvic surgeries, prune-belly syndrome, dehydration, and ectopic kidney.

Imaging

Diuretic renography can be performed using the same radiopharmaceuticals mentioned earlier. It is important to ensure that tracer has filled the renal pelvis and postural drainage has not occurred before the diuretic is administered. The diuretic can be administered 15 minutes postinjection (F+15) or simultaneously with the radiotracer (F0).[16] The diuretic effect usually starts within 1–2 minutes after administration of furosemide. Patients with intermittent hydronephrosis who complain of intermittent flank pain may have reproduction of pain on administration of diuretic. It is important to note that in patients with urinary diversions, even in the absence of obstruction, flow dynamics may be slow, making the diagnosis of obstruction difficult. Overlap of kidney and an ileal or colonic diversion may give rise to confusing images. Imaging in various projections, removal or replacement of external urine collecting devices and attempts at postural drainage may sometimes be helpful.

Interpretation

Careful evaluation of the dynamic renal study preceding a diuretic administration is important during interpretation. In the absence of obstruction, rapid and complete washout of radiotracer occurs from the pelvicalyceal system **(Fig. 2)**. On the other side of the spectrum is an obstructed system with slow or no drainage of radiotracer following a diuretic challenge **(Figs. 3 and 4)**. Interpretation of equivocal diuretic renography patterns is difficult. F-15 diuresis (Lasix is administered 15 minutes prior to the tracer injection and at the start of renography) is recommended to unmask obstruction in such curves by performing study with peak diuresis.

The diuretic washout $T_{1/2}$ is estimated using an exponential interpolation between a point on the initial descent of the time activity curve and another point on the downward slope while the curve is decaying monotonically. The diuretic $T_{1/2}$ should be only one of the several factors, which are considered while assessing urinary obstruction. Although there may be many variations in the time of diuretic injection and subsequent time of acquisition following a diuretic response, the overall sensitivity of a diuretic renography for the detection of obstruction in children has been estimated at 93%.[17]

Drainage Pattern of Renogram

O' Reilly et al. (1978) classified patients on the basis of the renogram curve of ^{99m}Tc-DTPA with diuretic.[18]

Response I: Normal initial renography and remained so after diuretics.

Response II: Obstructive initial renography and remained so after diuretics.

Response IIIa: Obstructive initial renography and showed rapid clearance after diuretics.

Response IIIb: Obstructive initial renography and showed mild/partial clearance after diuretics.

Captopril Renography

Secondary hypertension is more common in children and renal disease is perhaps the most common cause in this group. In a study conducted by Londe S et al. in 1978,[19] 563 pediatric patients with secondary hypertension were evaluated. 78% had renal abnormalities and 12% had renal artery disease. Secondary hypertension may be caused less frequently by endocrinal, cardiovascular, or nervous system disorders. The renal causes of hypertension are infarction, postpyelonephritic scarring, posttraumatic lesions and renal artery stenosis. Conventional renal dynamic scintigraphy usually shows the affected kidney to be smaller with lesser uptake than the contralateral normal kidney. The more severe the affliction, the lower is the renal uptake of tracer. ^{99m}Tc-DMSA scintigraphy in patients with renovascular hypertension typically reveals renal asymmetry. The affected kidney is smaller and shows lesser tracer uptake than the normal one. In the presence of unilateral renal artery stenosis, there may be reduced renal perfusion and function on the affected side. However, sometimes the same kidney may remain adequately perfused and owing to the autoregulation mechanism, the radionuclide study may remain normal in a significant number of cases. Thus conventional radionuclide

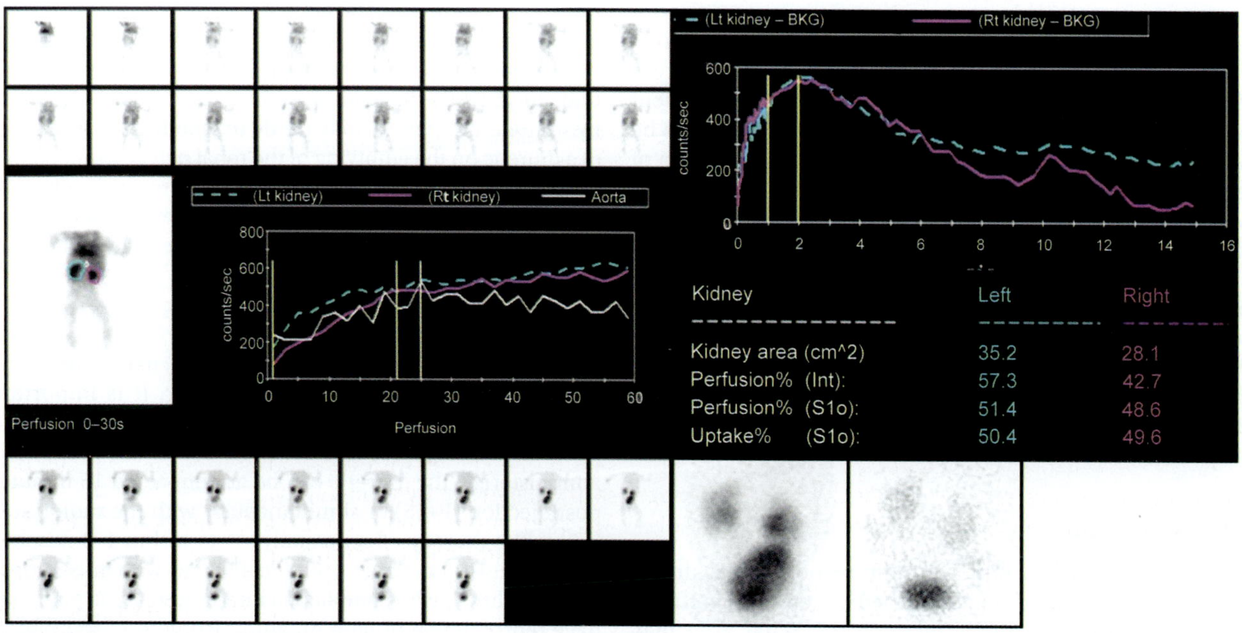

FIG. 2: ^{99m}Tc-LLEC scan in nonobstructive hydronephrosis: Dynamic and static renal images shows right-sided hydronephrosis with good clearance on delayed images; findings are consistent with nonobstructive hydronephrosis (Lt: left; Rt: right).

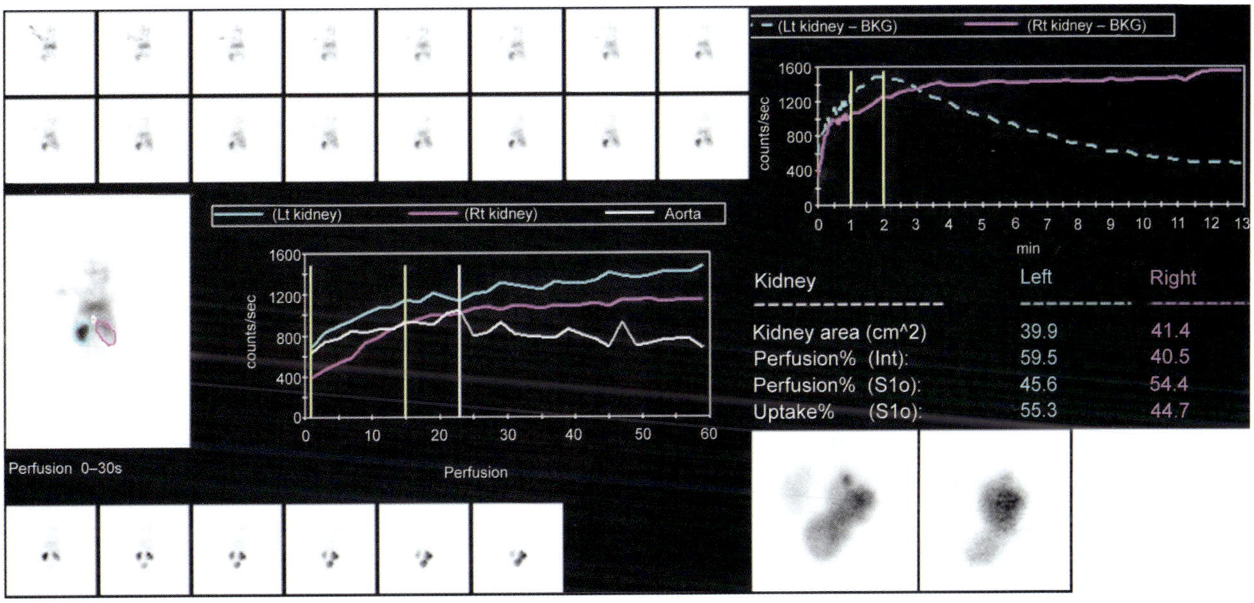

FIG. 3: ^{99m}Tc-LLEC scan in obstructive hydronephrosis: Progressive filling of dilated pelvicalyceal system (PCS) is seen on right side, whereas the left kidney clears normally. Time activity curves show washout on the left side and obstructed pattern on right side. Early and delayed static images show persistent activity in dilated PCS without any clearance on right side (Lt: left; Rt: right).

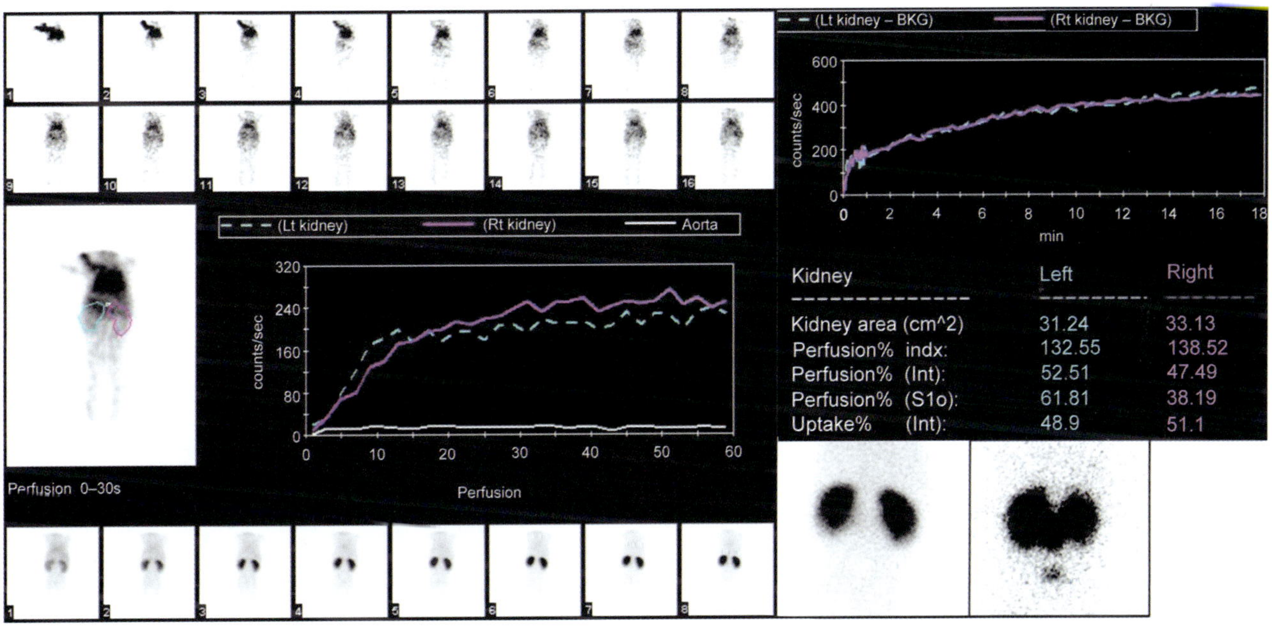

FIG. 4: ^{99m}Tc-LLEC scan in bilateral pelviureteric junction obstruction: Dynamic images shows progressive filling of dilated collecting system seen on both side. Time activity curves show obstructed pattern on both side. Early and delayed static images show persistent activity in dilated pelvicalyceal system (PCS) (Lt: left; Rt: right).

studies are not reliable screening tests for the diagnosis of renovascular hypertension and that angiotensin-converting enzyme (ACE) inhibitor renal scintigraphy is a markedly improved technique.

Angiotensin-converting enzyme inhibitors such as captopril block the formation of angiotensin II, producing dilatation of efferent arterioles and a fall in transcapillary pressure gradient. This causes a significant decrease in GFR of the kidney with renal artery stenosis that can be easily diagnosed by renography.[19-23] Initially ^{99m}Tc-DTPA was used, but presently tubular agents are used. To ensure better absorption of captopril, patients should not take solid food at least 4 hours before the study. Enalapril has a distinct advantage over captopril as this can be administered intravenously, and therefore does not depend on the variations of absorption in the gastrointestinal tract. Caution should be taken about the potentially serious hypotensive episodes following intravenous enalapril. Significant hypotension is also seen after a single dose of captopril, and therefore the patient should be well-hydrated and an intravenous access maintained throughout the study. Blood pressure should be monitored every 5–15 minutes. Diuretics may exaggerate the hypotensive effect and should not be used in conjunction with captopril renography.

A baseline study is obtained followed by a repeat examination either 1 hour after oral captopril (1 mg/kg, up to 50 mg), or 15 minutes after intravenous enalapril (0.03 mg/kg). Some authors obtain the initial study with an ACE inhibitor and repeat later without the ACE inhibitor only, if the first study is abnormal. Since the primary effect of ACE inhibitor is decreased GFR, studies using glomerular agents show decreased extraction of tracer and delayed visualization of the collecting system, whereas with tubular agents prolonged cortical tracer retention is seen. Moreover, detection of cortical retention of tracer is easier to appreciate than focal decreased extraction, tubular agents are probably more effective than glomerular agents in the detection of segmental renal artery stenosis. The typical findings of a positive captopril study (renin-dependent renovascular hypertension) are—a decrease in differential renal uptake, increase in cortical transit time, prolongation of time to peak, and retention of tracer in the renal parenchyma **(Fig. 5)**.

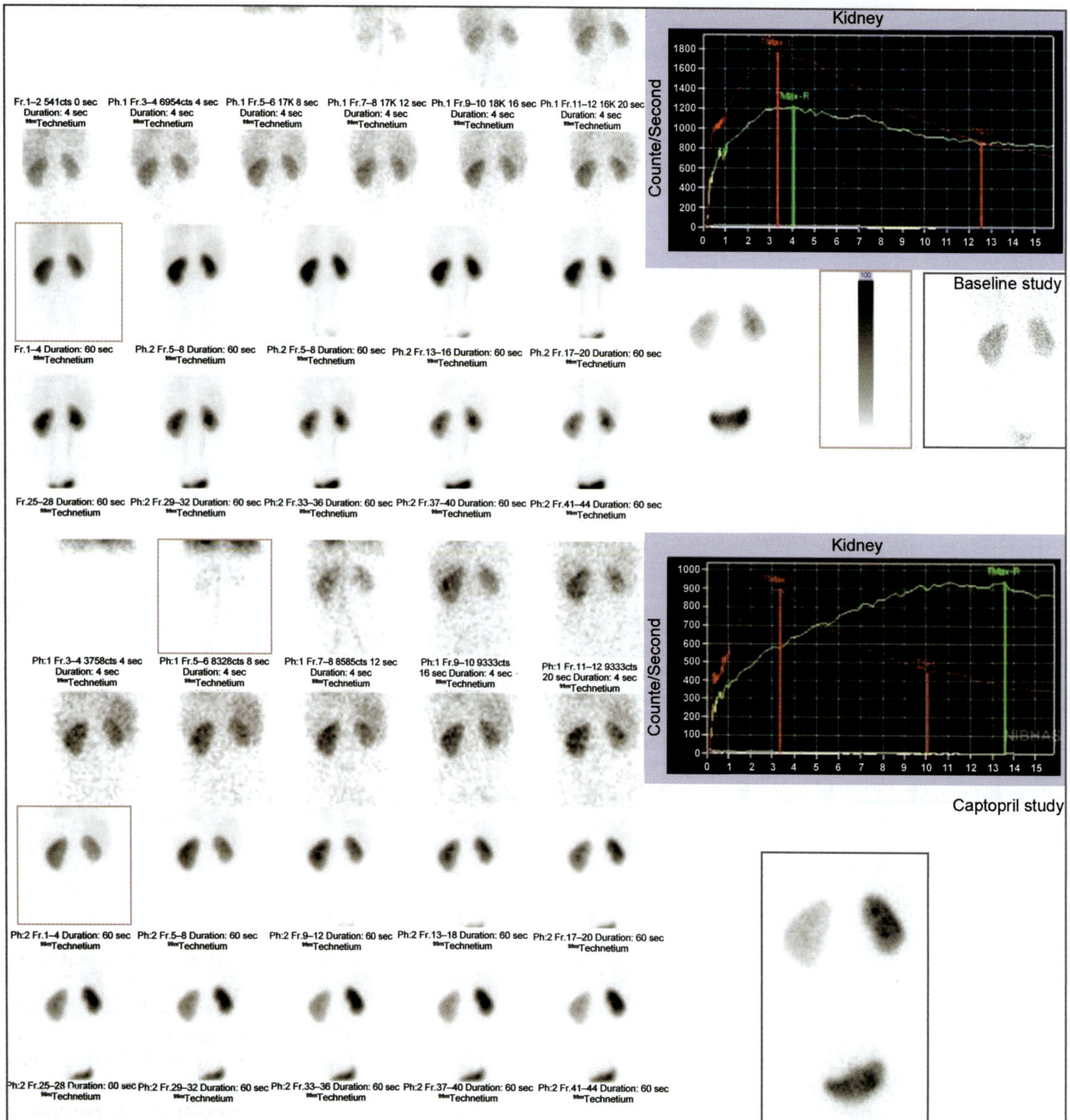

FIG. 5: Positive captopril study with ^{99m}Tc-LLEC: Baseline study (upper) shows normal functioning left kidney and slightly smaller right kidney with preserved function. Captopril study (lower) shows retention of radiotracer on right side and delayed peaking with a change in renogram pattern.

The most important parameter, however is the split renal uptake and change in renogram pattern. In patients with bilateral renal artery stenosis, the narrowing is usually asymmetrical and so is the effect of ACE inhibitor on each kidney. Cases, in which captopril does not induce scintigraphic changes, are usually associated with failure of revascularization or nephrectomy.[24-26]

RENAL CORTICAL SCINTIGRAPHY

^{99m}Technetium-DMSA is administered intravenously, dose of 0.04–0.05 mCi/kg (1.5–1.9 MBq/kg) with a minimum of 0.5 mCi (18.5 MBq) and a maximum of 3 mCi (111 MBq). Imaging is started about 3–4 hours after injection. Planar magnified images and SPECT images are acquired.

Imaging Techniques

Planar Renal Scintigraphy

Patient is examined supine with the gamma-camera positioned posteriorly and 300,000–500,000 counts are acquired in a 256 × 256 matrix using a high resolution or preferably an ultra high-resolution collimator. Left and right posterior oblique projections are acquired, which sometimes prove useful in the identification of cortical defects. Split renal uptake can be calculated by placing ROIs over posterior and anterior images and calculation of geometric mean. In cases of renal duplication, the upper and lower moieties can be outlined and differential renal function ascertained. In ectopic kidney, crossed renal ectopia and horseshoe kidneys, anterior and posterior projections are taken. Pinhole magnification or zoomed acquisition is mandatory in neonates and infants and may be useful in identification of cortical defects in older children and adults. Cortical defects following pyelonephritis, infarction, duplication and fetal lobulation can be discerned more frequently with pinhole magnification than with parallel hole high-resolution collimators since the former with an internal diameter of 2 mm provide images of higher spatial resolution than the latter.

Single Photon Positron Emission Tomography

Mapping of regional functional parenchyma is best done with ^{99m}Tc-DMSA SPECT. The surface and volume rendered SPECT images permit a superior overall view of the functional anatomy of the kidneys. Using the modern multi-headed SPECT cameras, acquiring 120 images over 360° on a 128 × 128 matrix usually requires 15–20 minutes. Proper sedation is mandatory for acquiring SPECT images.[27]

Radionuclide Cystography

This has been accepted as the technique of choice for evaluation and follow-up of children with urinary tract infection and reflux. The estimated gonadal radiation dose is one-hundredth of the voiding cystourethrography. Radionuclide cystography is more sensitive than voiding cystography in detecting vesicoureteric reflux. Other parameters like residual urine volume, bladder volume at the time of reflux and the rate of clearance of refluxed urine can also be calculated. The only disadvantage of radionuclide cystography is poor anatomical resolution of the bladder and urethra.

Clinical Applications

In urology practice, the most important clinical areas, where radionuclide studies may be of particular importance in patient management, can be considered under the following headings:

- Urinary tract obstruction
- Urinary tract infection
- Renovascular hypertension
- Congenital anomalies
- Renal failure
- Renal transplant evaluation

Urinary Tract Obstruction

Radionuclide studies may be necessary to establish or confirm the diagnosis of obstruction, to ascertain its site or level, to determine its extent or severity or to measure how well the obstructed kidney is functioning.[16,28] In addition, radionuclide studies may be needed in other situations when any change in the function or condition of the kidney, or of the site and severity of obstruction, is to be determined, if desirable clinically to assess patients prognosis and in differential diagnosis of urinary obstruction. In the differential diagnosis of urinary obstruction, diuretic renography is of immense value, especially in those patients with a nonobstructed dilated collecting system associated with indeterminate flow curve (***see* Fig. 2**). Injection of diuretic is essential, if obstruction at the pelviureteric junction is suspected, as this diagnosis can only be confirmed at high urine flow rate. However, one of the major drawbacks of diuretic renography is a large number of indeterminate results in poorly functioning kidneys. Some progress has been made in this regard by correcting furosemide response for level of renal function. Significant renal function has been reported on radionuclide studies in a large percentage of the patients with nonfunctioning kidneys seen on intravenous urography. Estimation of renal output efficacy (ROE), which is calculated by a technique independent of variations in uptake rate by the kidneys, provides an accurate diagnosis of renal outflow obstruction in patients with significantly impaired renal function.[29]

Urinary Tract Infection

Renal infection may be clinically obvious, but can be easily overlooked. Clinically, it is frequently difficult or impossible to differentiate infection of the bladder and ureters from the acute renal parenchymal infection. The lack of sensitivity of intravenous urography (IVU) and ultrasonography in the demonstration of early renal infection is well-known. ^{99m}Tc-DMSA is valuable in the identification of renal damage due to early pyelonephritis. Even in the absence of urographic or ultrasonographic abnormalities, regional parenchymal uptake of DMSA may be altered in acute pyelonephritis. ^{99m}Tc-DMSA is also useful to quantify the degree of renal damage, to follow the progress on antibiotic therapy, and to assess recovery and/or residual renal damage.

Imaging with ^{99m}Tc-DMSA facilitates, detection of cortical scarring as a sequelae of pyelonephritis **(Fig. 6)**. Unlike urography, RCS can detect cortical defects that do not deform the renal outline or the collecting system. In the detection of renal scars ^{99m}Tc-DMSA scan is more sensitive (96%) and specific (98%) as compared with IVU.[30] Besides, in patients with chronic pyelonephritis with uncontrolled hypertension, demonstration of a severe segmental scar on a DMSA scan may guide the surgeon in undertaking partial nephrectomy **(Figs. 7 and 8)**.

One of the most common and routinely employed procedures in children with urinary tract infection is the direct radionuclide cystogram (DRCG) in conjunction with RCS **(Figs. 9 to 11)**. In the diagnosis of vesicouretic reflux, this procedure is much superior and the radiation exposure to the patient is much less as compared to micturating cystourethrogram (MCU).[31]

Renovascular Hypertension

Renovascular hypertension is the most common cause of secondary and potentially curable hypertension. Regardless of the problems associated with the routine renogram, availability of gamma-camera computer system has made meaningful pre-intervention renal assessment possible in such patients. This test as a follow-up procedure for evaluating the result of percutaneous angioplasty or surgery on the function in the affected kidney of the patients with renovascular disease is an extremely important but often overlooked application.

A major approach to the nuclear medicine diagnosis of the renovascular hypertension has been the introduction of captopril, an ACE inhibitor. The concept for the use of ACE inhibitors in the differential diagnosis of the renovascular hypertension arose from the observation that patients with bilateral renal artery stenosis (RAS), or patient with solitary kidney having RAS had a tendency to develop acute renal failure when treated with these drugs. The theoretical basis for complication of ACE inhibitor therapy and the rationale for the captopril renography test are essentially the same. The renin-angiotension system is thought to be a compensatory mechanism by which the kidney maintains perfusion, when it is subjected to low perfusion pressure, as may result distal to a renal artery stenosis. ACE inhibitors act to block the step, where angiotensin I is converted to angiotensin II, and as a result prevent the subsequent increase in the efferent arteriolar tone. In the absence of this compensatory mechanism, the glomerular filtration rate (GFR) drops significantly in the affected kidney.[21-23] A normal base line study followed by unilateral decreased in split renal function are the hallmark of unilateral renovascular hypertension **(*see* Fig. 5)**. Widespread application of the captopril renography and improved surgical techniques as well as perfection of the catheter techniques for percutaneous transluminal angioplasty, has caused tremendous excitement in the field of renovascular disease, and resulted in sudden repopularization of radioisotope renography. Enalapril is presently used instead of captopril, although the procedure name remains captopril renography.

Congenital Anomalies

Renal radionuclide studies are helpful in the diagnosis and functional evaluation of a spectrum of congenital disorders. Serial evaluation of the parenchymal and drainage function may be essential in patients with polycystic kidneys, and in medullary sponge kidneys. Radionuclide investigations have a definite "functional" edge over the urography in the management of ectopic kidneys, horseshoe kidney, crossed ectopias, or malrotated kidneys.[32,33] Radionuclide studies are useful in the evaluation of regional cortical renal function in patients with duplications of the ureters and renal pelvis. Preoperative and serial postoperative functional as well as morphologic evaluation of the kidney, upper urinary tracts, and the urinary bladder can be effectively done in patients with posterior urethral valves by the dynamic renography, RCS, and DRCG studies. Functional evaluation of the kidney and the urinary bladder by radionuclide studies in patients

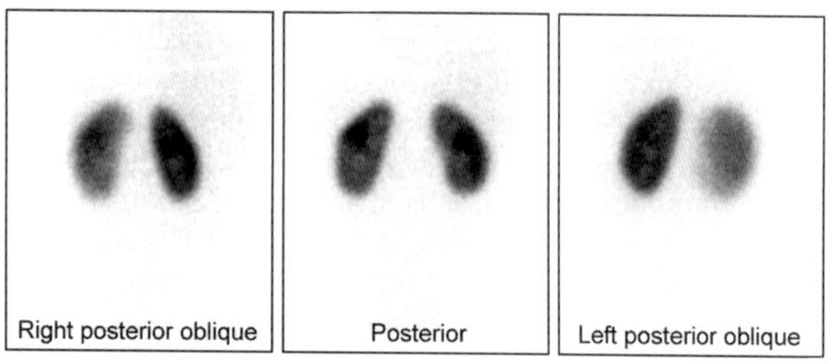

FIG. 6: Normal ^{99m}Technetium-dimer captosuccinic acid scan: Bilateral kidneys are normal in size with smooth cortical outline and normal function.

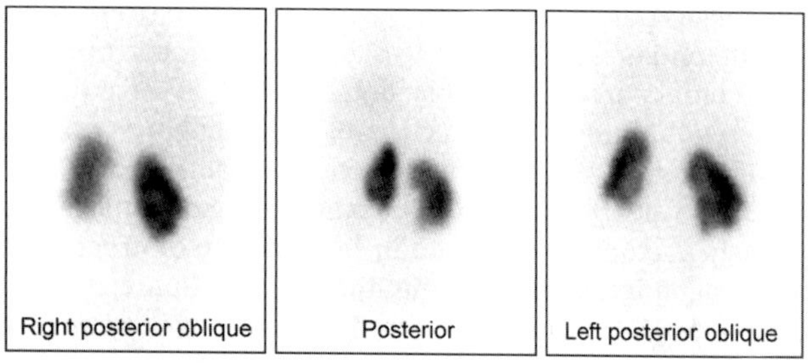

FIG. 7: ^{99m}Technetium-dimer captosuccinic acid (^{99m}Tc-DMSA) study in patient with bilateral vesicouretric reflux. All three views of ^{99m}Tc-DMSA scan show cortical break suggestive of renal scarring (multiple on left side and lower polar on right side).

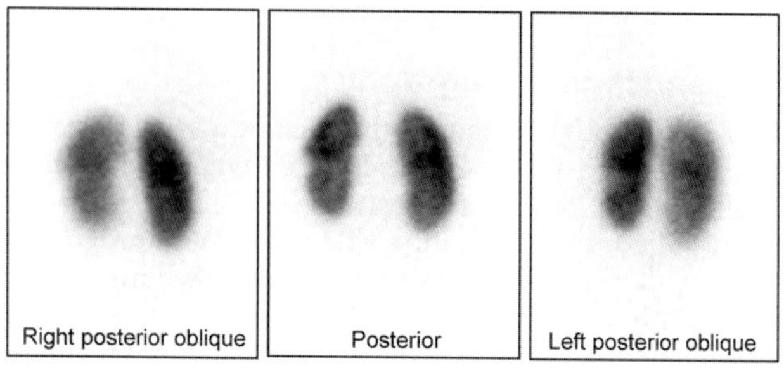

FIG. 8: ^{99m}Technetium-dimer captosuccinic acid (^{99m}Tc-DMSA) study in patient with left vesicouretric reflux. All three views of ^{99m}Tc-DMSA scan show cortical break in left kidney suggestive of left renal scarring.

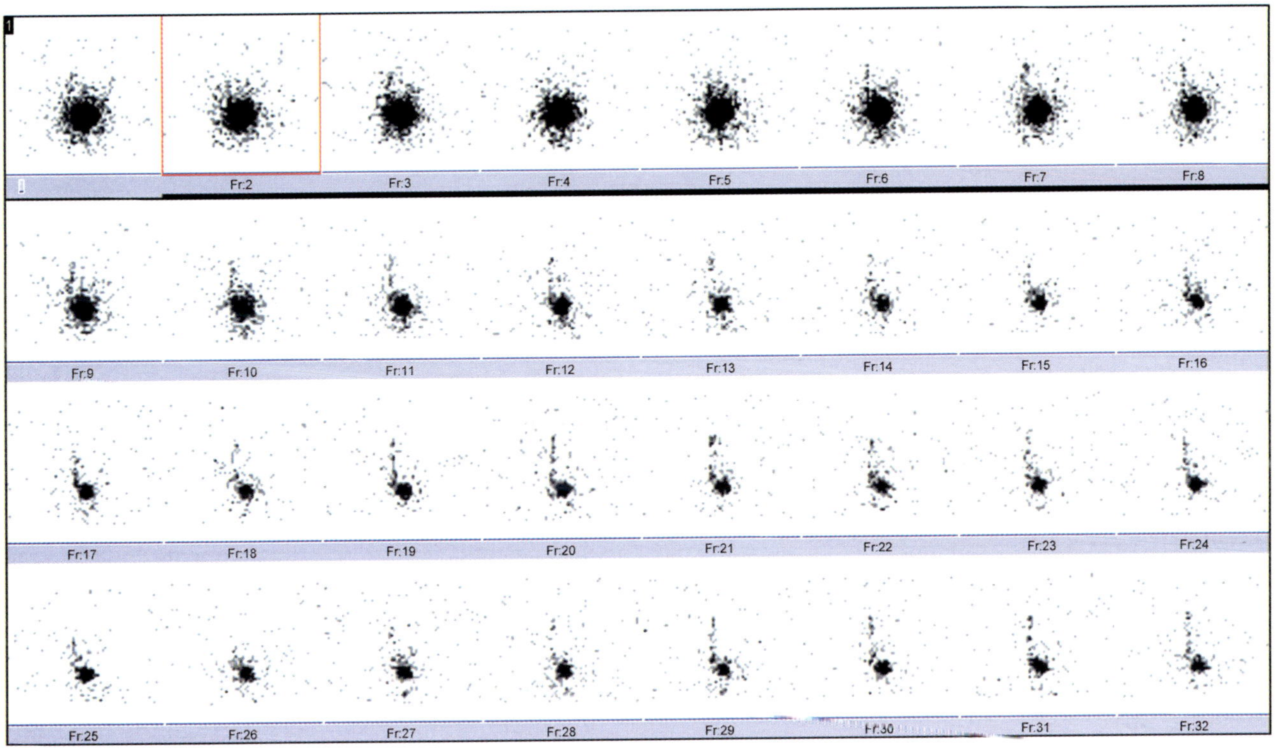

FIG. 9: Direct radionuclide cystogram study: Dynamic images show vesicoureteral reflux from bladder into left ureter (Grade-II).

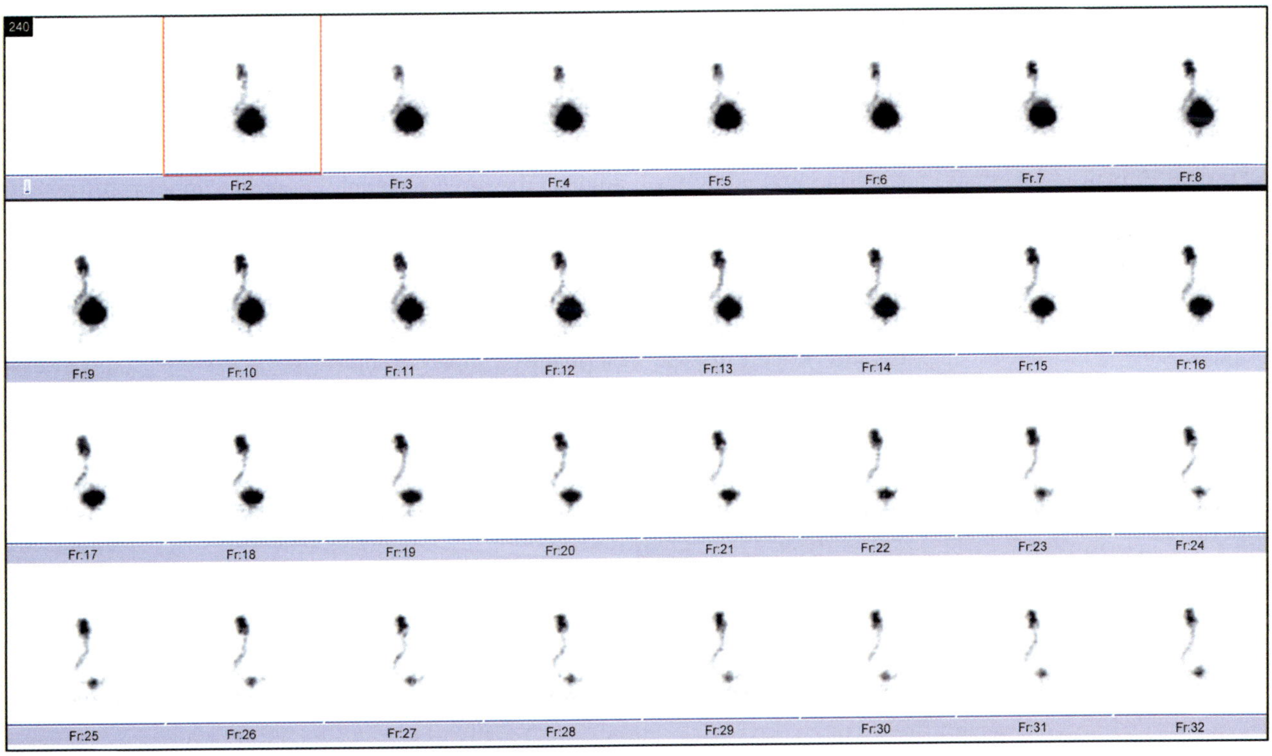

FIG. 10: Direct radionuclide cystogram study in unilateral reflux: Dynamic images show vesicoureteral reflux from bladder into left ureter (Grade-III).

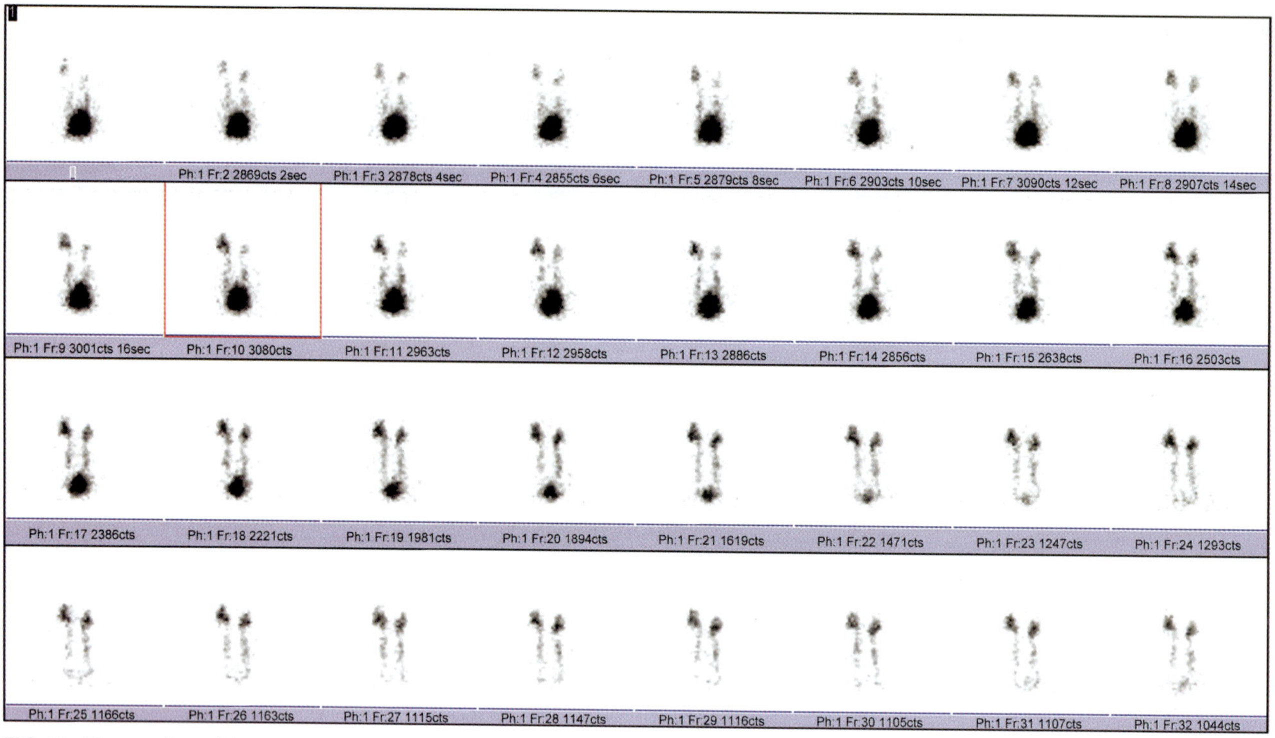

FIG. 11: Direct radionuclide cystogram study shows bilateral vesicoureteral reflux: Dynamic images showing reflux of radiotracer from bladder into both ureters (Grade-III).

with neurogenic bladder has also been very well-established. Nonfunctioning multicystic dysplastic kidneys are evaluated on DMSA scintigraphy.

Global Renal Impairment

^{99m}Tc-DMSA is used for renal imaging in chronic kidney disease (CKD) patients to establish tubulointerstitial disease as the cause for renal impairment.

Radionuclide clearance studies provide valuable information and help in monitoring glomerular or tubular function in nephropathies of various origins, the most important being the diabetic nephropathy. Kidney disease in diabetic patients has a devastating effect on survival, most evident in those with juvenile onset disease. It has been advocated that in such patients, the prospective monitoring of diminishing renal function should include precise measurement of GFR by radionuclide techniques combined with determination of fractional clearance of high molecular weight proteins. This is particular important when the effects of treatment on the early proteinuric phase of the diabetic nephropathy are being evaluated.[34,35] The considerable loss of glomerular filtration capacity at this stage is undetected by inverse creatinine measurement, which remains a valuable tool for monitoring the late stage of nephropathy, when metabolic correction is unlikely to be effective.

Renal Transplant Evaluation

Radionuclide techniques offer rapid, effective, and noninvasive means for the correct diagnosis of many of the medical and few surgical complications of the renal transplantation. Renal perfusion and function studies using ^{99m}Tc-EC or ^{99m}Tc-MAG3 offer comprehensive evaluation of the renal blood flow, function, and drainage **(Fig. 12)**. Many techniques have been described for establishing the cause of early graft dysfunction, especially for the diagnosis of acute rejection (AR) and acute tubular necrosis (ATN) **(Fig. 13)**. Some of the surgical complications like urinary obstruction, urinary extravasations, urinoma **(Fig. 14)**, nonurinary pelvic collections, e.g. hematoma or lymphocele and VUR can be diagnosed on radionuclide studies. Despite the relative merits and demerits of the radionuclide studies vis-a-vis other noninvasive diagnostic modalities, nuclear medicine has made an impact in clinical practice in at least three ways:

1. By reducing the number of invasive biopsies in transplant patients.
2. Diagnosing or confirming acute rejection very early for prompt treatment.
3. By being able to reassure the transplant surgeon regarding the viability of the allograft in uncomplicated ATN with prolonged periods of oliguria or anuria. With improved techniques and increasing availability of the renal transplantation procedures at many more centers around the country, nuclear medicine is bound to play an important role in evaluation and management of renal transplant.[36,37]

Management of a nephro-urological problem can be best done by a multidisciplinary approach. The various diagnostic modalities like X-ray, CT, US, magnetic resonance urography and nuclear medicine often support and complement each other.[38] However, radionuclide techniques have the most important "functional edge" over many other diagnostic methods. With further refinements in technology,

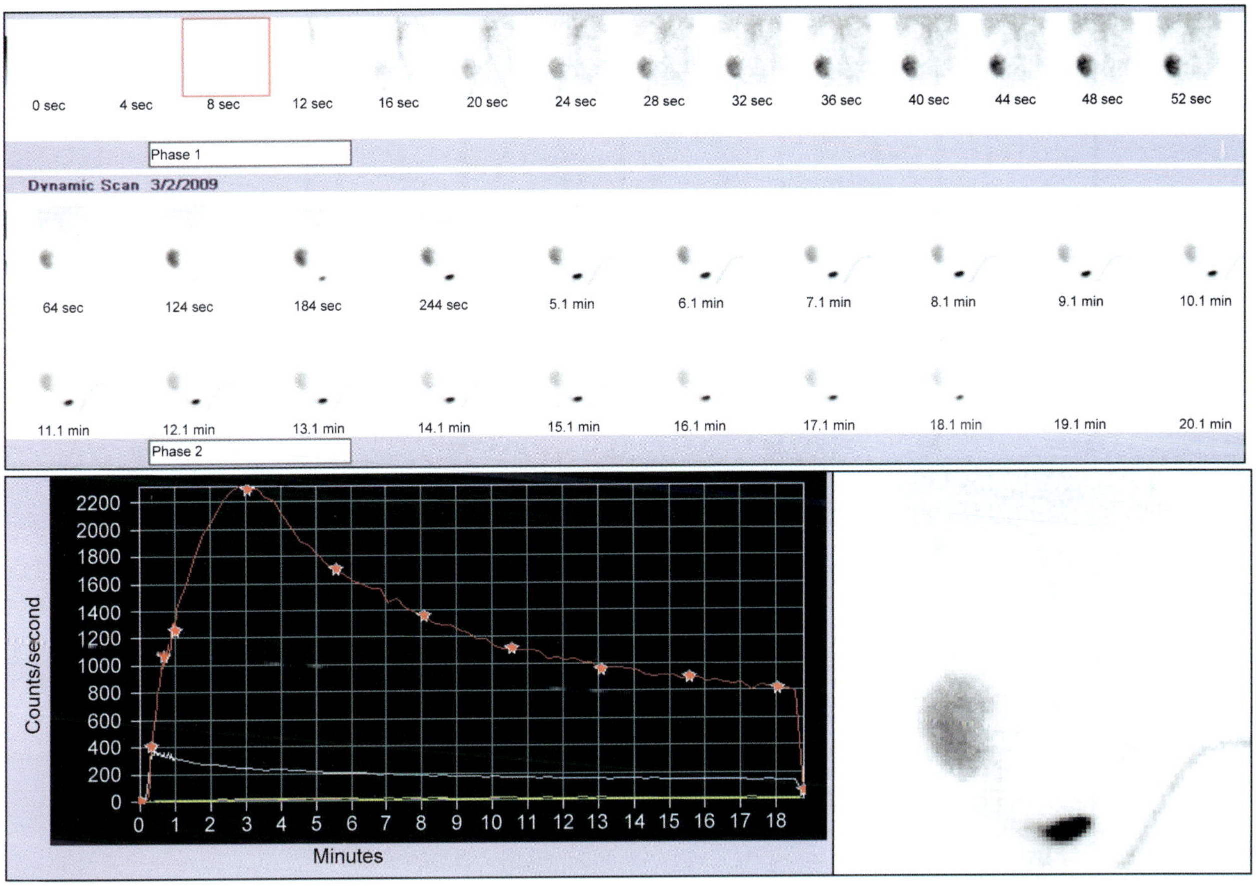

FIG. 12: ^{99m}Tc-LLEC scan in normal functioning transplanted kidney. Dynamic images show normal perfusion and uptake with prompt clearance. Time activity curves show steep uptake, distinct peak, and rapid clearance.

instrumentation, and radiopharmaceuticals, nuclear medicine is destined to improve more in the future.

Measurement of Renal Function

Glomerular Filtration Rate

Renal function can be assessed by clinical methods using blood urea nitrogen (BUN) and serum creatinine level but these are relatively crude, as significant decrease in function must occur before changes in BUN and creatinine are seen. Other factors which affect creatinine level are diet, difference in muscle mass, and certain medications.

Glomerular filtration rate is the clearance rate of substance that is excreted from the body by glomerular filtration and not secreted or reabsorbed by tubules, the ideal molecule for this is inulin. Substances which have a complete first pass extraction through kidney are used to calculate renal plasma flow (RPF). Paraamino hippurate is about 90% extracted and can be used for calculation of RPF. As it is not completely excreted, the term effective renal plasma flow (ERPF) is used.

Many radiopharmaceuticals are used to calculate GFR; these include ^{99m}Tc-DTPAand ^{51}CrEDTA. In India, ^{99m}Tc-DTPA is mainly used for GFR calculation. Though multiple blood sample techniques scan be used, presently the two blood sample techniques are most commonly used. Blood samples are taken at 1 hour and 3 hour postinjection. Normal GFR value is approximately 106 ± 27 mL/min/ 1.73 m^2 for adults. In children adult GFR levels are reached by about 2 years of age.

Effective Renal Plasma Flow (ERPF)

ERPF is another parameter of renal function and the ideal agent for this is paraaminohippuric acid (PAH). The radiolabeled form of hippuric acid, ^{131}I-OIH and ^{123}I-OIH, has been used to quantify ERPF. The urinary clearance of ^{131}I-OIH is about 85% of the PAH. ^{99m}Tc-EC or MAG-3 can be used for ERPF calculation with a single sample collected at 54 minutes and 44 minutes, respectively.

POSITRON EMISSION TOMOGRAPHY/ COMPUTED TOMOGRAPHY

State-of-art integrated positron emission tomography/ computed tomography (PET/CT) provides functional (metabolic) and structural information in the same setting. At present, 2-deoxy-2-[^{18}F]-fluorodeoxyglucose (FDG) is the workhorse agent for PET/CT imaging. ^{18}F-FDG is a radiolabeled analogue of glucose and is able to detect altered glucose metabolism in various disease conditions. There is a significant upregulation of the GLUT-1 transporters in cancer

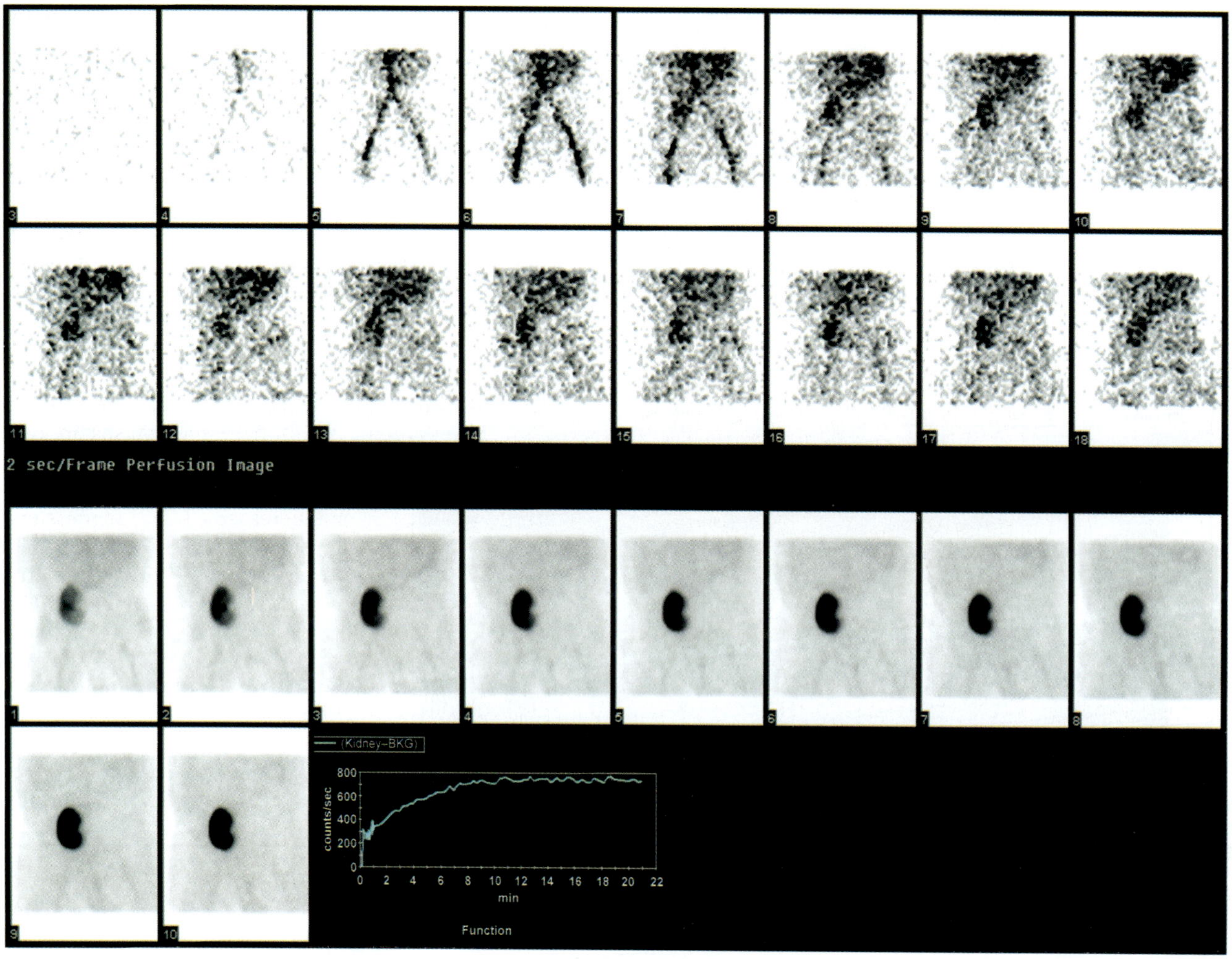

FIG. 13: ^{99m}Tc-LLEC scan in ATN. Baseline images show normal perfusion and uptake but significant retention. Time activity curve show rising trend consistent with ATN.

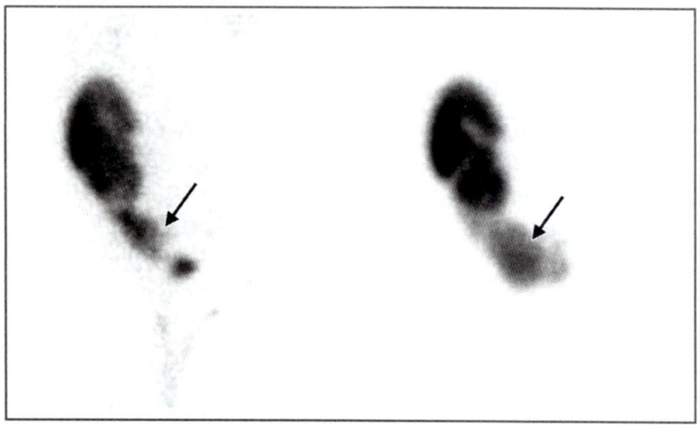

FIG. 14: Renal allograft in right iliac fossa, postvoid (left), and delayed static (right) views show an increasing collection in mid and lower ureteric regions (arrows)—suggestive of urine leak.

cells, which results in increased FDG uptake compared with the surrounding normal tissues. The role of FDG-PET in the initial staging, restaging, monitoring response to therapy, and follow-up surveillance of many cancers is well-documented.[39] There are relatively few FDG-PET reports describing its role in assessing primary urologic tumors due to the potential problem of tracer excretion through the kidneys. In recent years, however, special PET/CT techniques have evolved to make PET/CT imaging possible even in patients with primary urinary bladder cancers.[40] Moreover, the introduction of other PET radiotracers, such as ^{11}Carbon (^{11}C)-choline **(Fig. 15)**, ^{11}C-acetate, and Glu-NH-CO-NH-Lys-(Ahx) [Ga-68(HBED-CC)]) (^{68}Ga PSMA) **(Fig. 16)** has enhanced the role of this technique in patients with urologic cancers including prostate cancer.[41] ^{68}Ga PSMA 11 has emerged as a useful tracer not only as a diagnostic agent but also for therapy of metastatic castrate resistant prostate cancer with Lutetium-177 PSMA-617 therapy.[42] The main role of PET/CT in urologic malignancies is initial diagnosis and staging, restaging, evaluation of treatment response, and detection of recurrent/metastatic disease.[39]

Fluorodeoxyglucose-PET also plays a role in the evaluation of posttransplant lymphoproliferative disorders and pyrexia of unknown origin in renal transplant patients. Available studies report promising results with FDG-PET in detection, staging, and therapy evaluation of PTLD patients and PET findings can alter or guide treatment in up to 29% of cases. Concerns remain with regard to occurrence of false

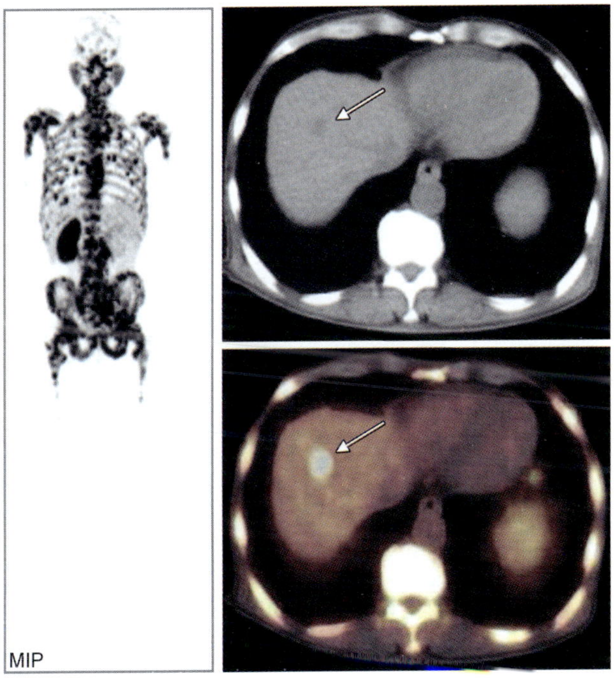

FIG. 15: ^{68}Ga PSMA positron emission tomography/computed tomography (PET/CT) in a patient with extensive skeletal metastases [maximum intensity projection (MIP)], showing in addition PSMA accumulation in a focal liver metastasis with a hypodense lesion on CT (arrow).

negatives due to physiological high background activity and early PTLD lesions as well as false positives due to inflammatory conditions.[43]

Renal Cell Carcinoma

Despite significant uptake and excretion through the kidneys, FDG has been used in the management of renal cell carcinoma (RCC). Bachor et al.[44] studied 29 patients with solid renal masses and found that PET was positive in 20 (77%) of 26 patients of RCC. PET was false positive in an angiomyolipoma, a pericytoma, and a pheochromocytoma. Ramdave et al.[45] evaluated the accuracy of FDG-PET for staging and management of 17 patients with known or suspected RCC. PET and CT had an accuracy of 94%. In addition, PET detected pulmonary metastases in two patients. Miyakita et al.[46]compared biologic characteristics of RCC with FDG and concluded that PET-positive tumors had higher tumor grade and increased GLUT-1 expression. Kumar et al.[47]showed good results with FDG PET in 28 solid renal masses of which 10 were primary (nine malignant, one benign) and 18 were metastatic renal tumors. FDG-PET accurately detected 23 of 27 (85%) malignant renal masses. Of the 10 primary renal tumors **(Fig. 17)**, FDG-PET was true positive in eight of nine (89%), true 28 negative in one and false negative in one. In addition to the characterization of primary tumors, FDG-PET was valuable in 31 primary staging and altered treatment in 30% of patients (3 of 10). Of the

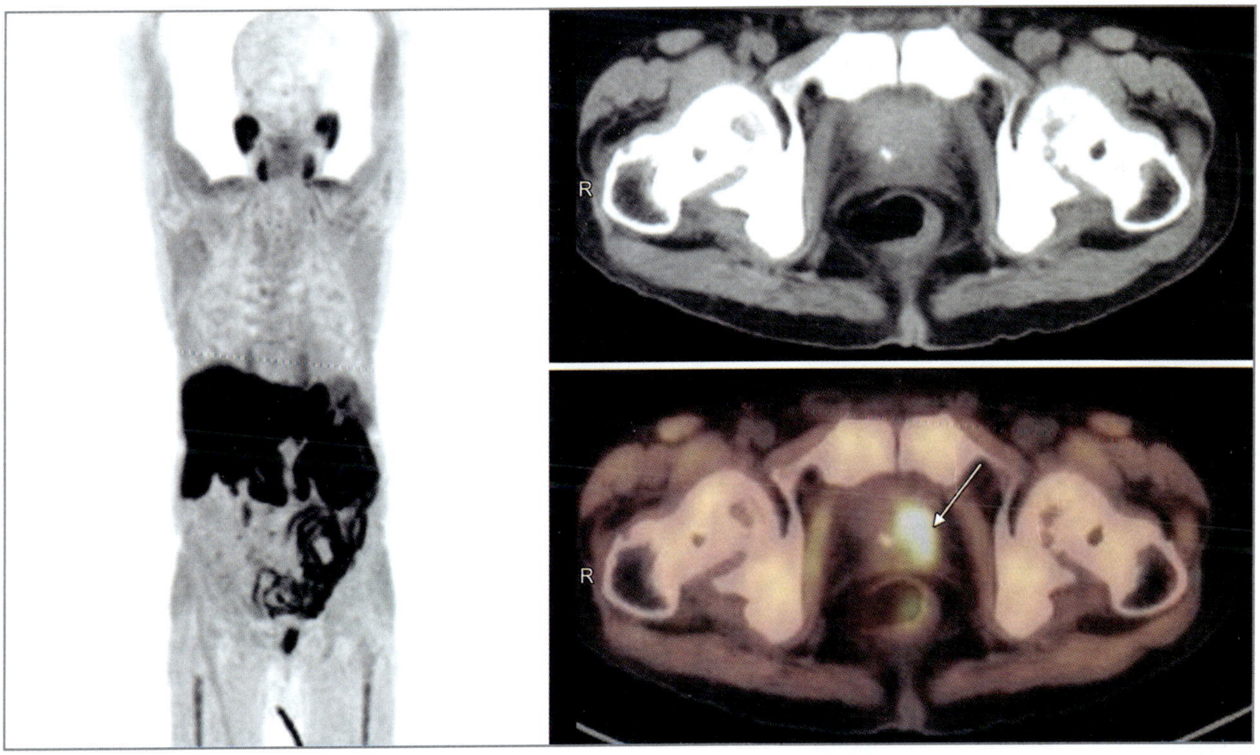

FIG. 16: ^{18}F-Fluorocholine positron emission tomography/computed tomography in a case of prostatic carcinoma with tracer accumulation in the primary in the prostate left side (arrow).

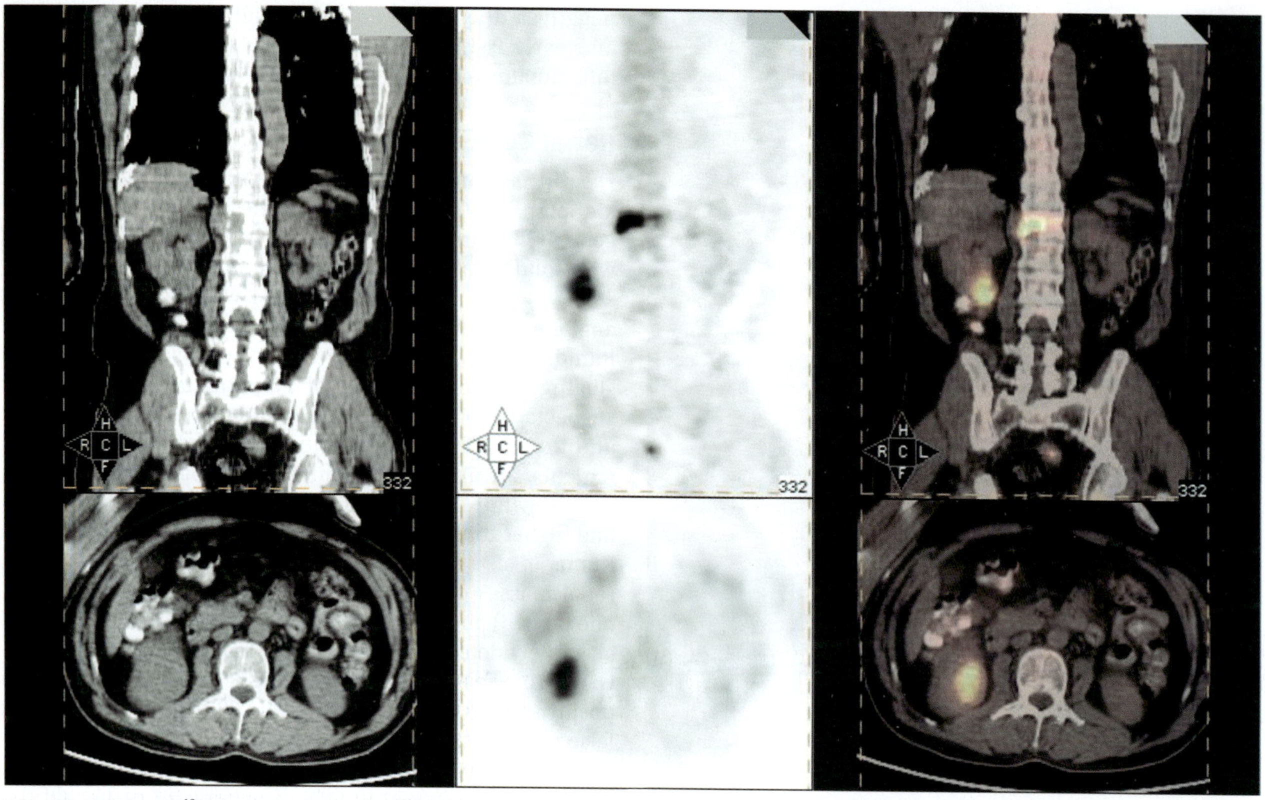

FIG. 17: 2-deoxy-2-[^{18}F]-fluorodeoxyglucose (^{18}F-FDG) positron emission tomography/computed tomography (PET-CT) study: Coronal and axial sections of CT, PET, and PET-CT showing soft tissue mass at lower pole of right kidney. Note FDG Uptake in T12.

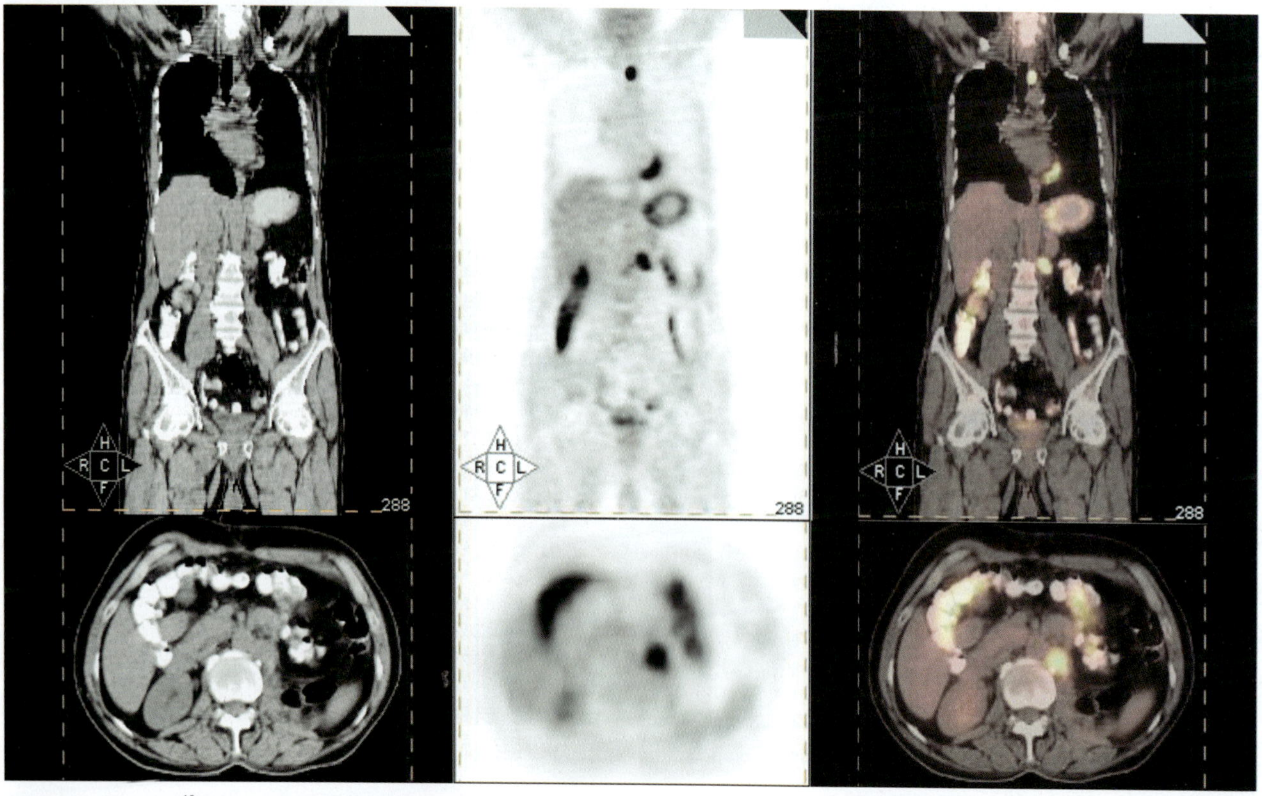

FIG. 18: 2-deoxy-2-[^{18}F]-fluorodeoxyglucose positron emission tomography/computed tomography (PET-CT) study: Coronal and axial sections of CT, PET, and PET-CT showing soft tissue mass in left renal bed suggestive of local recurrence.

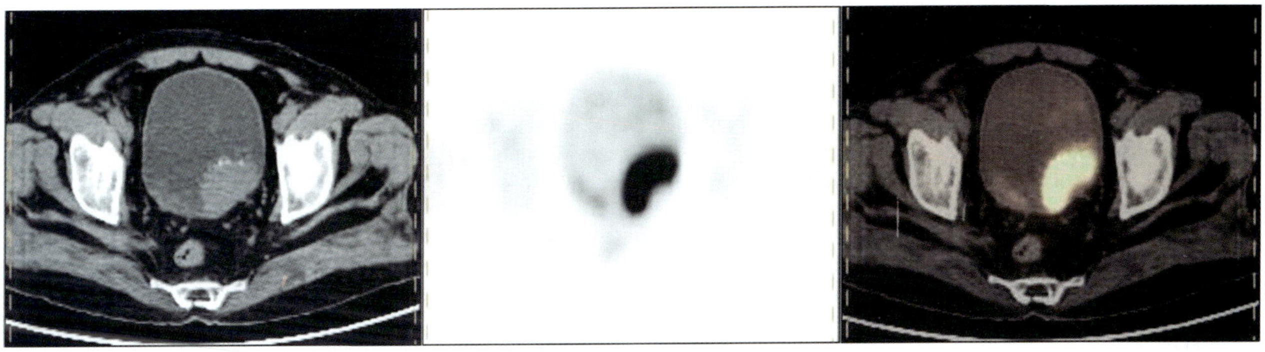

FIG. 19: 2-deoxy-2-[^{18}F]-fluorodeoxyglucose positron emission tomography/computed tomography (^{18}F-FDG PET-CT) study: Axial sections of CT, PET, and PET-CT showing soft-tissue mass in urinary bladder suggestive primary bladder cancer.

18 metastatic renal 32 masses, FDG-PET was positive in 15 (83%) masses. For detection of recurrent and distant disease, PET was found to have an accuracy of 100% in detecting local recurrence and metastases as compared CT which had accuracy of 88% **(Fig. 18)**. Majhail et al.[48]evaluated FDG-PET in the detection of distant metastases in 24 patients with RCC. FDG-PET results were compared with those abstracted with biopsy in 33 lesions. Overall sensitivity, specificity, and PPV of FDG-PET were 64%, 100% and 100%, respectively.

Urinary Bladder Cancer

Previously, FDG PET was thought to have limited use in diagnosis and management of bladder cancer. However, with modified techniques[40] (after injection of diuretic and delayed imaging) it is possible to image primary as well as recurrent urinary bladder cancer **(Fig. 19)**. Kosuda et al.[49]studied 12 patients with urinary bladder cancers with FDG PET for the evaluation of recurrent or residual disease. PET identified 100% (17 of 17) of distant metastases (lung, bones, and remote lymph nodes) and 67% (2 of 3) of local lymph nodes. Ahlstrom et al.[50] attempted to improve the accuracy of PET by using C11-methionine, which has no urinary excretion. The authors reported a sensitivity of 78% (18 of 23) and there was good correlation of tracer uptake and tumor stage.

In conclusion, PET-CT has shown very encouraging results in a limited number of studies, and has also demonstrated a good sensitivity for initial staging in patients with renal and bladder cancer. FDG-PET seems to be superior to conventional imaging modalities for detecting local disease and recurrence, and distant metastases.

REFERENCES

1. Werner RA, Chen X, Lapa C, et al. The next era of renal radionuclide imaging: novel PET radiotracers. Eur J Nucl Med Mol Imaging. 2019;46(9):1773-86.
2. Hofman MS, Hicks RJ. Gallium-68 EDTA PET/CT for renal imaging. Semin Nucl Med. 2016;46(5):448-61.
3. Wakabayashi H, Werner RA, Hayakawa N, et al. Initial preclinical evaluation of 18F-fluorodeoxysorbitol PET as a novel functional renal imaging agent. J Nucl Med. 2016;57(10): 1625-8.
4. Werner RA, Wakabayashi H, Chen X, et al. Functional renal imaging with 2-deoxy-2-(18)F-fluorosorbitol PET in rat models of renal disorders. J Nucl Med. 2018;59(5):828-32.
5. Qin Z, Hoh CK, Olson ES, et al. Molecular imaging of the glomerulus via mesangial cell uptake of radiolabeled tilmanocept. J Nucl Med. 2019;16(9):1325-32.
6. Klenc J, Taylor A, Lipowska M. Synthesis and evaluation of 99mTc(CO)3(FEDA): a new dual-purpose 99mTc/18F renal imaging agent. J Nucl Med. 2015;56(Suppl 3):654.
7. Kabasakal L. Tc-99m Ethylene dicysteine: A new renal tubular function agent. Eur J Nucl Med. 2000;27(3):351-7.
8. Gutsche HU, Scheffler M, Muller-Surr R, et al. Micropuncture study on filtration and reabsorption of technium-99m L, L-Ethylenedicysteine in rats. In: Taylor A, Nally JV, Thomsen H (Eds). Radionuclides in nephrourology. Reston, Virbinia: Society of nuclear medicine; 1997. pp. 160-64.
9. Taylor A, Hansen L, Eshima D, et al. Comparison of 99mTc-LL-EC in rats and humans. J Nucl Med. 1997;38(5): 821-26.
10. Berkhin EF, Humphreys MH. Regulation of tubular secretion of organic compounds. Kindney Int. 2001;59(1):17-30.
11. Bubek B, Brandau W, Steinbacher M. Technetium-99m labeled renal function and imaging agent: II. Clinical evaluation of Tc-99m MAG-3(99mTc mercaptoacetylglycylglycylglycine). Nucl Med Biol. 1988;15(1):109-18.
12. Jafri RA, Britton KE, Nimmon CC. Tc-99m MAG-3:A comparison with I-125 and I-131OIH, in patients with renal disorders. J Nucl Med. 1988;29:147-58.
13. Atkins HL, Cardinale KG, Eckelman WC, et al. Evaluation of Tc 99m DTPA prepared by three different methods. Radiology. 1971;98:674-77.
14. Cohen ML, Smith FGJ, Mindell RS, et al. A simple reliable method of measuring glomerular filtration rate using single low dose iothalamate I-131. Pediatrics. 1969;43(3):407-15.
15. Enlander D, Weber PM, dosRemedios LV. Renal cortical imaging in 35 patients: Superior quality with Tc99m-DMSA. J Nucl Med. 1974;15(9):743-49.
16. Tripathi M, Chandrasekhar N, Phom H, et al. Evaluation of dilated upper renal tracts by technetium-99m ethylenedicysteine F+0 diuresisi renography in infants and children. Ann Nucl Med. 2004;18(8):681-7.

17. Meller St, Eckstein HB. Renal scintigraphy: Quantitative assessment of upper urinary tract dilatation in children. J Paeditr Surg. 1981;16(2):123-26.
18. O'Reilly PH, Testa HJ, Lawson RS, et al. Diuresis renography in equivocal urinary tract obstruction. Br J Urol. 1978;50(2): 76-80.
19. Londe S. Causes of hypertension in the young. Pediatr Clin North Am. 1978;25(1):55-66.
20. Blaufox MD, Fine EJ, Heller S, et al. Prospective study of simultaneous orthoiodohippurate and diethylenetri-aminepentaacetic acid captopril renography. The Einstein/Cornell Collaborative Hypertension Group. J Nucl Med. 1998;39(3):522-28.
21. Sfakianakis GN, Sfakiankis E, Bourgoignie J. Lasix captopril renography in the diagnosis of renovascular hypertension. Contrib Nephrol. 1990;79:219-27.
22. Taylor A, Nally J, Aurell M, et al. Consensus Report on Captopril Renogram in Renovascular Hypertension. J Nucl Med. 1996;37:1876-82.
23. Wenting GJ, Tan-Tjiong HI, Derkx FH. Split renal function after captopril in unilateral renal artery stenosis. BMJ. 1984;288(6421):886-90.
24. Dondi M. Captopril renal scintigraphy with 99mTc-mercaptoacetyltriglycine (Tc99m-MAG-3) for detecting renal artery stenosis. Am J Hypertens. 1991;4(12 Pt 2):737S-40S.
25. Kumar R, Padhy AK, Machineni S, et al. Individual kidney GFR in the interpretation of non-diagnostic curves on captopril renography. Nucl Med Commun. 2000;21(7):637-43.
26. Setaro JF, Chenn CC, Hoffer PB, et al. Captopril renography in the diagnosis of renal artery stenosis and the prediction of improvement with revascularisation: The Yale vascular center experience. Am J Hypertens. 1991;4(12 Pt 2):698S-705S.
27. Tripathi M, Agarwal KK, Mukherjee A, et al. Tc-99m DMSA planar imaging versus dual-detector SPECT for the detection of renal cortical scars in patients with CKD-3. Nucl Med Commun. 2016;37(9):911-6.
28. Padhy AK, Gopinath PG, Basu AK. Role of 99mTc-DTPA renal study in children with upper urinary tract dilation. Indian J Med Res. 1985;82:238-47.
29. Chaiwatanarat T, Padhy AK, Bomanji JB, et al. Validation of renal output efficiency as an objective quantitative parameter in the evaluation of upper urinary tract obstruction. J Nucl Med. 1993;34(5):845-48.
30. Sfakianakis GN, Damoulaki-Sfakianaki E. Nuclear medicine in pediatric urology and nephrology. J Nuc1 Med. 1988;29(9): 1287-300.
31. Padhy AK, Gopinath PG, Mitra DK, et al. Direct radionuclide cystogram (DRCG) and urine flowmetry in the evaluation of patients with VUR and/or associated obstructive/neurogenic pathology of lower urinary tract in children. Indian J Paeditr. 1989;56(4):423-92.
32. Sfakianakis GN. Nuclear medicine in congenital urinary tract anomalies. In: LM Freeman (Ed). Nuclear Medicine Annua1. New York: Raven Press; 1991. pp. 129-92.
33. Kumar R, Gupta R, Malhotra A. Nephroptosis: the Tc-99m glucoheptonate scan as a diagnostic modality. Clin Nucl Med. 2000;25(6):473.
34. Bell EG, Blaufox MD. Clinical application of renal imaging. In: Gottschalk A, Potchen EJ (Eds). Diagnostic Nuclear Medicine. Baltimore: Williams and Wilkins Co.; 1976. pp. 476-91.
35. Viberti GC, Bilous RW, Mackintosh D, et al. Monitoring Glomerular function in diabetic nephropathy. A prospective study. Am J Med. 1983;74(2):256-64.
36. Padhy AK, Gopinath PG, Mehta SN, et al. Significance of transplant perfusion index in the diagnosis of acute rejection—experience in live-related renal transplant recipients. Indian J Med Res. 1989;90:113-23.
37. Hilson AJW, Maisey MN, Brown CE, et al. Dynamic renal transplant imaging with 99mTc-DTPA (Sn) supplemented by a transplant perfusion index in the management of renal transplants. J Nucl Med. 1978;19(9):994-1000.
38. Padhy AK, Gopinath PG, Mehta SN, et al. Tc-99m renal transplant scintigraphy in the diagnosis of urinoma. Clin Nucl Med. 1989;14:769-71.
39. Kumar R, Zhuang H, Alavi A. PET in the management of urologic malignancies. Radiol Clin North Am. 2004;42(6):1141-53.
40. Nayak B, Dogra PN, Naswa N, et al. Diuretic F-18 FDG PET/CT imaging for the detection and locoregional staging of urinary bladder cancer: prospective evaluation of a novel technique. Eur J Nucl Med Mol Imaging. 2013;40(3):386-93.
41. Tulsyan S, Das CJ, Tripathi M, et al. Comparison of Ga-68 PSMA PET/CT and multiparametric MRI for staging of high-rosk prostate cancer 68Ga-PSMA PET and MRI in prostate cancer. Nucl Med Commun. 2017;38(12):1094-102.
42. Yadav MP, Ballal S, Tripathi M, et al. 177Lu-DKFZ-PSMA-617 therapy in metastatic castration resistant prostate cancer: safety, efficacy and quality of life assessment. Eur J Nucl Med Mo! Imaging. 2017;44(1):81-91.
43. Montes de Jesus FM, Kwee TC, Nijland M, et al. Performance of advanced imaging modalities at diagnosis and treatment response evaluation of patients with post-transplant lymphoproliferative disorder: A systematic review and meta-analysis. Crit Rev Oncol Hematol. 2018;132:27-38.
44. Bachor R, Kotzerke J, Gottfried HW, et al. Positron emission tomography in diagnosis of renal cell carcinoma. Urologe A. 1996;35(2):146-50.
45. Ramdave S, Thomas GW, Berlangieri SU, et al. Clinical role of F-18 fluorodeoxyglucose positron emission tomography for detection and management of renal cell carcinoma. J Urol. 2001;166(3):825-30.
46. Miyakita H, Tokunaga M, Onda H, et al. Significance of 18F-fluorodeoxyglucose positron emission tomography (FDG-PET) for detection of renal cell carcinoma and immuno-histochemical glucose transporter 1 (GLUT-1) expression in the cancer. Int J Urol. 2002;9(1):15-8.
47. Kumar R, Chauhan A, Lakhani P, et al. 2-Deoxy-2-[F-18]fluoro-D-glucose-positron emission tomography in characterization of solid renal masses. Mol Imaging Biol. 2005;7(6):431-9.
48. Majhail NS, Urbain JL, Albani JM, et al. F-18 fluorodeoxyglucose positron emission tomography in the evaluation of distant metastases from renal cell carcinoma. J Clin Oncol. 2003;21(21):3995-4000.
49. Kosuda S, Kison PV, Greenough R, et al. Preliminary assessment of fluorine-18 fluorodeoxyglucose positron emission tomography in patients with bladder cancer. Eur J Nucl Med. 1997;24(6): 615-20.
50. Ahlstrom H, Malmstrom PU, Letocha H, et al. Positron emission tomography in the diagnosis and staging of urinary bladder cancer. Acta Radiol. 1996;37(2):180-5.

CHAPTER

3

Renal Calculus Disease and Obstructive Uropathy

Uma Debi, Mahesh Prakash, Mandeep Kang

UROLITHIASIS

INTRODUCTION

Urolithiasis is a common disease entity. The incidence of renal calculus in India varies between different geographical locations.[1] Maharashtra has a high incidence (7.6%). Similarly, Rajasthan reports a high incidence. Southern states, however, report a lower incidence. Recent reports suggest an increasing incidence, with more and more calculi being diagnosed at a younger age. Pregnant patients form a special subset of patients with unique diagnostic and management considerations. Calcium oxalate forms the major constituent by frequency of stones.[2] The other constituents are uric acid, magnesium ammonium phosphate (MAP or struvite), cysteine, xanthine, triamterene, and indinavir. Nephrolithiasis is also a chronic disorder. Even after treatment, the recurrence rates are very high and range from 14% to 52%.[3]

COMPOSITION

Calcium-based stones are the most common (~75%) which can include calcium oxalate (80%) and calcium phosphate (20%). Uric acid and struvite stones are the next in frequency (~10% each), followed by cysteine, indinavir, xanthine, and triamterene stones (<1% each).[4]

ETIOLOGY

Calculi have a multifactorial etiology. The cause also varies for the specific type of calculus. The proposed causative factors for calcium calculi include low urine volume, increased excretion of calcium, oxalate, uric acid, and decreased excretion of citrate. Abnormal urine pH can also lead to precipitation of calculi. For uric acid calculi, decreased urine pH is the most important cause. Surprisingly, hyperuricosuria and low urine volume are less common causes. Struvite calculi are composed of magnesium ammonium phosphate or calcium apatite. Infection with urease positive organisms leads to the development of MAP calculus. Inherited cysteine metabolism defects cause cysteine calculus.

PRESENTATION

Nonobstructive renal calculi are asymptomatic. Pain is the most common presenting symptom for any disorder involving obstruction to the urinary tract. Calculi generally get lodged at sites of narrowing in the urinary tract—the pelviureteric junction (PUJ), ureterovesical junction, and the site of crossing of iliac vessels. The pain can be very severe and incapacitating. Depending on the site of obstruction, pain is referred to the iliac fossae in the case of mid-ureteric obstruction, or may be referred to the groin in cases of obstruction at a lower level. Lower-ureteric obstruction also produces bladder symptoms like frequency, urgency and suprapubic pain.

Nausea, vomiting and rarely fever might be associated. Calculi may also produce hematuria. Calculi in the urinary tract can also predispose to infection.

DIAGNOSTIC EVALUATION

Ultrasonography

Although noncontrast computed tomography (NCCT) scan is considered to be the gold-standard imaging modality to accurately depict the calculus burden, recent studies reflect a greater role for USG in diagnosis and follow-up of stone disease. American Urological Association (AUA), American College of Radiology (ACR) and National Institute for Health and Care Excellence (NICE) guidelines advocate NCCT as the first-line imaging modality in all patients with urolithiasis, except in pediatric and pregnant patients, where USG is recommended.[5,6] However, the recent guidelines by European Association of Urology (EAU) recommend USG as the primary imaging tool in all patients, irrespective of age and gender.[7] Literature reports a wide range of sensitivities and specificities for USG as compared to NCCT. However, most recent studies report a fairly high sensitivity of approximately 60% and specificity of approximately 70–90%.[6,8]

The role of imaging in a patient presenting with symptoms of urolithiasis is to confirm the diagnosis, exclude alternate causes for flank pain/hematuria, measure the stone burden and stone size, assess the exact location of the stone, and finally to guide the subsequent management strategies.[9] In specific circumstances, an USG with kidney ureter and bladder (KUB) radiography might be sufficient to provide all the information required for subsequent management. However, in cases where more information is needed, an NCCT or CT urography is usually required. Currently, apart from calculus visualization, USG is also indicated to look for echogenic contents within the pelvicalyceal system which may suggest pyonephrosis, accurately grade hydronephrosis (HDN), suspect pyelonephritis and to detect complications of urinary tract infection (UTI) like renal/perinephric abscess. In a patient, presenting with obstruction, detection of pyonephrosis is an indication for diversion with percutaneous nephrostomy (PCN).[10]

Sonographic Technique

Ultrasonography has a high sensitivity for detecting calculi in the kidney which are more than 5 mm. Calculi appear as echogenic structures with sharp posterior acoustic shadowing **(Fig. 1A)**. Stone visualization in USG depends on a lot of factors, including patient size, positioning, probe frequency, focal zone, spatial compound imaging, bowel gases, stone size, shape, location, composition, etc. In general, the highest frequency that allows adequate penetration should be selected for imaging. The focal zone should be adjusted to lie at or just posterior to the location of calculus. Spatial compounding (obtaining an average of two or more frames obtained from different angles) should be turned off. Harmonic imaging enhances visualization of the calculus.

Color Doppler evaluation produces twinkling artifact around the calculus which can aid in diagnosis **(Fig. 1B)**. The twinkling artifact is a complex phenomenon which was first described in 1996 by Rahmouni et al.[11] The most accepted theory for the formation of this artifact involves narrow-band noise (called phase or clock jitter) in the Doppler circuitry. Highly reflective, rough surfaces are associated with this artifact. Hence, apart from calculi, these artifacts can also be produced by soft tissue/vascular calcification, ureteral stents, coils, surgical clips, gallstones, and other foreign bodies. Conversely, a very smooth calculus would not produce this artifact.[12] If the focal zone is below the calculus, twinkling artifact is more prominent. Increasing the grayscale gain, decreases whereas increasing the Doppler gain, increases visualization of the artifact. It has also been suggested that calcium oxalate or calcium phosphate calculi produced this artifact, while calcium oxalate monohydrate and calcium urate calculi did not.[13]

Ureteric stones are more difficult to detect in USG because of bowel gases. The upper ureter can usually be visualized by using the kidney as a sonographic window. Similarly, a well-distended bladder might allow evaluation of the distal ureter using a suprapubic window. A transperineal or transvaginal route may also allow evaluation of the distal ureter and vesicoureteric junction (VUJ). Complete obstruction causes ureteric dilatation which facilitates tracing using the USG probe. Alternatively, ureteric jets can be used as a diagnostic tool. Ureteric jets can be visualized both in B-mode as well as in Doppler. The frequency of ureteric jets varies from person-to-person depending on the state of hydration, but is at least one per minute. The jets are symmetric bilaterally.[14] Ureteric stone with complete obstruction produces an absence of jet on the affected side. Partial obstruction produces low level continuous jet on the affected side (as compared to intermittent bursts of high level jet on the normal side).

Ureteric calculus with complete obstruction also produces hydronephrosis which can be easily detected using USG. The resistivity index [RI = (PSV – EDV)/PSV] of intrarenal arteries has also been described as an indirect indicator of urinary tract obstruction. Acute obstruction increases the back pressure leading to elevated resistive index. An RI of more than 0.70 has been suggested as a cutoff.[15] A difference between the two kidneys of more than 0.10 is also suggestive. However, the RI being more reflective of tissue compliance, rather than tubular pressure within the nephron, is an inaccurate index for routine use.[16]

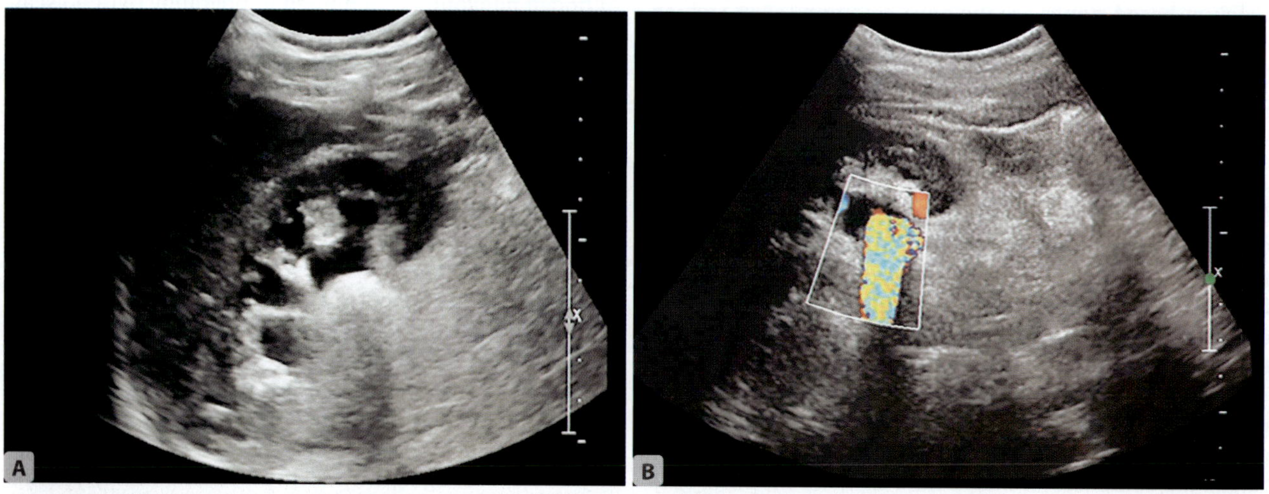

FIGS. 1A AND B: (A) Ultrasound image shows an echogenic calculus in renal pelvis with distal acoustic shadowing causing hydronephrosis. Noncontrast computed tomography (NCCT) with coronal reconstruction image shows two small hyperdense calculi in lower calyx of right kidney; (B) Color Doppler ultrasound image shows twinkling artifact.

Various disorders can mimic renal calculi in USG and reduce accuracy. These include intrarenal gas, vascular and parenchymal calcification, calcified renal cell carcinoma/transitional cell carcinoma (RCC/TCC), calcified papilla, encrusted ureteric stent, and alkaline-encrusted pyelitis.

Kidney Ureter and Bladder Radiography

Kidney ureter and bladder radiography is a low-cost, low-radiation investigation (~0.15 mSv) which is especially useful in nonemergency settings **(Fig. 2)**. It has a sensitivity of approximately 35% for stones less than 5 mm and approximately 85% for stones more than 5 mm. Uric acid, xanthine, indinavir, and triamterene stones are radiolucent and hence are not visualized in KUB radiography. Currently, KUB radiography is mainly used for follow-up of urolithiasis after treatment/medical expulsion therapy.

Computed Tomography

Noncontrast CT has the highest sensitivity among all imaging modalities for renal calculus. It can also exclude other causes of flank pain like diverticulitis, cholecystitis, pancreatitis, appendicitis, ovarian torsion, pyelonephritis, bladder outlet obstruction, etc. Hence, it is the modality of choice in urolithiasis.[9,10,17-20] All stones are visualized in CT, except indinavir stones. The Hounsfield unit (HU) value of the calculus gives a rough idea about the composition of the stone, uric acid calculi are usually 200–400 HU, while calcium oxalate calculi are 600–1200 HU **(Fig. 3)**. More importantly, a greater attenuation predicts lesser responsiveness to lithotripsy. Also, a heterogeneous appearance of the stone, with interposed areas of low and high attenuation predicts increased fragility and hence a greater susceptibility for Shockwave lithotripsy (SWL).

The various treatment modalities for urolithiasis include medical expulsion therapy, SWL, ureteroscopy (URS), percutaneous nephrolithotomy (PNL), and surgical open or laparoscopic pyelo/ureterolithotomy. Choosing one treatment modality over the other is a question of multiple considerations including the overall stone burden, size, composition, HU values and site of stone, structural and functional status of the kidneys, obstruction, hydronephrosis, presence or absence of tract infection, obesity, age of the patient, coagulopathy, pregnancy, etc. For instance, an impacted stone of 1 cm in the lower ureter can be easily dealt with using URS, whereas a similar stone in the upper polar calyx with an attenuation of 400 HU and a skin to surface distance less than 10 cm is amenable for SWL. It is hence the duty of the radiologist to give adequate information to ensure proper treatment planning. It is worth mentioning here that for measuring the size of a calculus, bone window should be used, which has a greater accuracy than soft tissue window. Recently, dual-energy CT has been used to characterize the exact composition of calculus, which has a greater potential to alter the management protocols. Uric acid stones can be easily differentiated from nonuric acid stones with 100% accuracy, thus allowing appropriate treatment strategies **(Figs. 4A to B)**.[21]

Technical and Dose Considerations

Current multidetector CT scanners allow complete scanning of the entire KUB region within 10–15 seconds, thus permitting evaluation in a single breath hold. Pitch in helical CT is the length of table fed into the scanner per gantry rotation divided by the beam collimation. If 1 cm of the table is fed per gantry rotation and the total beam collimation is 10 mm, the pitch is 1 mm. A pitch of 2 mm can be used for calculus imaging, which provides images of sufficient diagnostic quality but a reduced radiation exposure (as compared to a pitch of less than 1 mm). A calculus is a high-contrast structure. Therefore, images acquired with low-tube current can sufficiently delineate calculi. For stone imaging, the tube current can be lowered to as low as 30 mA without compromising the image quality. Current generation scanners are also equipped with automated tube modulation with automatically adjusts the tube current based on tissue attenuation. Low-dose CT is a term used for those scans with

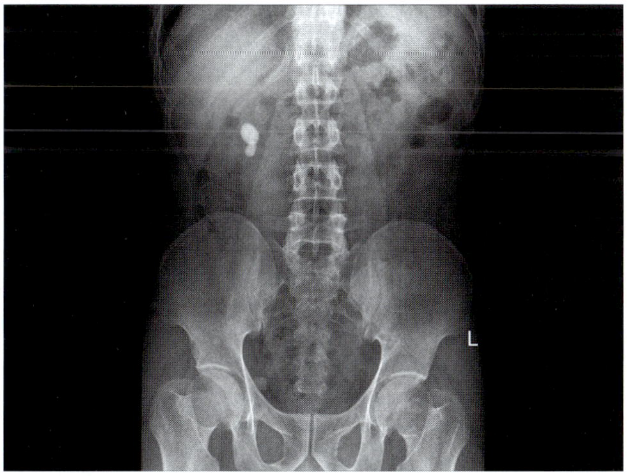

FIG. 2: Plain X-ray of abdomen shows two radiodense calculi in right kidney.

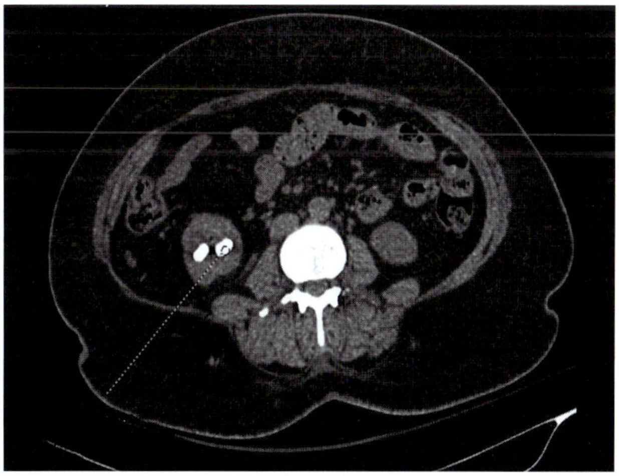

FIG. 3: Low-dose noncontrast CT scan shows two small hyperdense calculi in lower calyx of right kidney.

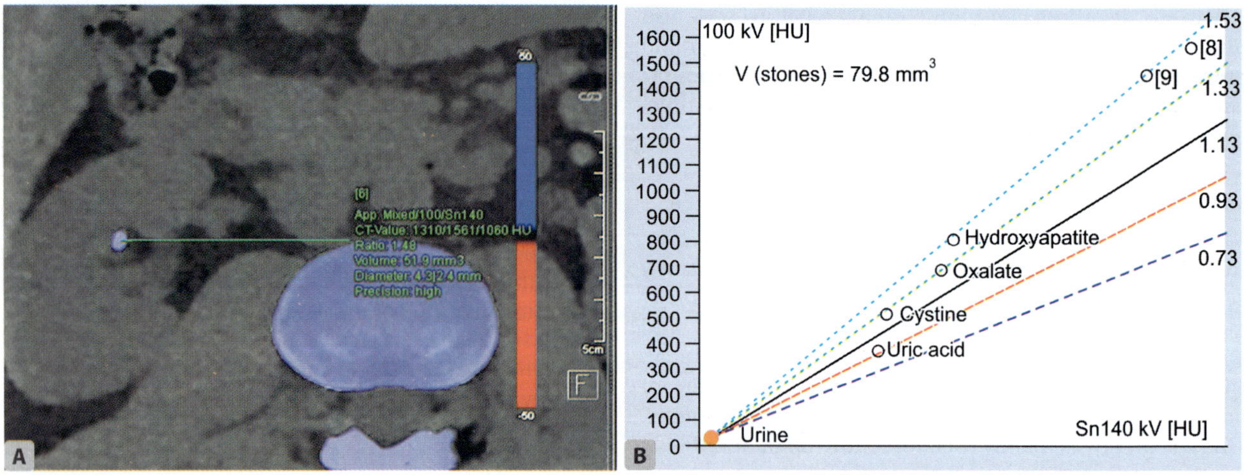

FIGS. 4A AND B: (A) Color coded axial dual-energy CT image shows a calcified calculus in the middle calyx. All calcified structure including bone of the vertebral body are color coded in blue. Color coding of the calculus is blue based on the dual-energy index. Volume of the calculus is also calculated; (B) Screenshot of the diagram used to adjust the software in the dual-energy setting. Color coding in blue above the slope indicates that it is a calcium containing calculus and in red below the slope which is consist of pure uric acid.

an effective exposure of less than 3 mSv. AUA recommends low-dose CT for all adult, nonpregnant patients with a BMI of less than 30 kg/m^2. For patients with a higher BMI a standard dose CT is recommended. An ultra-low dose CT with a radiation exposure of <1 mSv can also be used for follow- up scans (it is equivalent to ~5 KUB radiographies).

Imaging Features

The definitive sign of urolithiasis is identification of a calculus in the urinary tract. Using CT, even calculi that are less than 1 mm can be identified. The demonstration of calculus within the ureter requires tracing of the tract in contiguous sections. Soft tissue rim sign is produced due to a rim of edematous soft tissue present around an impacted ureteric calculus **(Figs. 5A to B)**. Most ureteric calculi demonstrate this sign. Phleboliths can be a problematic differential, especially in thin patients. Phleboliths are commonly seen in the pelvis. They are produced by calcification of thrombus within veins. Plain radiographs show phleboliths with a radiolucent center while this appearance is uncommon with calculi. Phleboliths demonstrate comet tail sign in CT, which is an eccentric soft tissue present around the phlebolith. The soft tissue is due to the thrombosed vein which leads up to the phleboliths.

Other indirect signs of obstruction include renal enlargement, perinephric stranding, upstream dilatation of the ureter, periureteral stranding, renal sinus fullness causing effacement of fat at the sinus **(Figs. 6A to B)**, thickening of lateroconal fascia and absence of hyperdense medullary pyramids unilaterally. Perinephric stranding is considered to be produced due to lymphatic congestion in the bridging septae. Hyperdense medullary pyramids can be seen in normal individuals as an incidental finding. Its absence on one side may indicate obstruction on that side.

Intravenous Urography

Intravenous urography (IVU) historically has been the initial technique in evaluation of possible urinary obstruction including urolithiasis. The signs indicative of acute obstructive process are: (1) prolonged dense nephrogram, (2) renal enlargement, (3) dilatation of the collecting system, (4) delayed pyelogram, (5) ureteric dilatation, and (6) pyelosinus extravasation **(Figs. 7A to D)**.

If the obstruction is mild, then the nephrogram and calyceal opacification may be normal with minimal dilatation of the ureter. With more severe obstruction, the nephrogram is delayed in onset and becomes more dense and persistent. The nephrogram may demonstrate faint radial striations due to contrast in the collecting ducts and tubules.[22] The kidney is often larger than normal. The opacification of calyces and ureter is delayed and depends upon the degree of obstruction. A completely obstructed kidney that has become anuric may not show any opacification of the collecting system, however, once the opacification of the collecting system begins, additional radiographs are required to demonstrate the site of obstruction. If no contrast appears in the collecting system by 15 minutes after injection, there is little reason to obtain next film until 2 hours later. The collecting system and ureter are mildly dilated in acute obstruction. High obstructions cause more pelvicaliectasis then low ones. Extravasation of contrast medium from the kidney is demonstrated by IVU in up to 24% of obstructed patients.[23] Forniceal rupture occurs and opacified urine dissects through the tissues of the renal sinus. Minimal extravasation of contrast causes a smudged appearance of the calyces; however, when there is extensive leakage, contrast medium tracks around the renal pelvis and along the psoas muscles causing outlining of the ureter. Rarely, pyelolymphatic and pyelosubcapsular extravasation can occur. Unrelieved obstruction with continued extravasation of urine may result to a retroperitoneal collection called urinoma.[23] These collections are best visualized on USG, CT or MRI.

There has been a significant decline in the use of IVU as the dominant imaging technique in acute obstruction. This change has been driven by fear of contrast-induced nephrotoxicity and by growth of renal sonography and

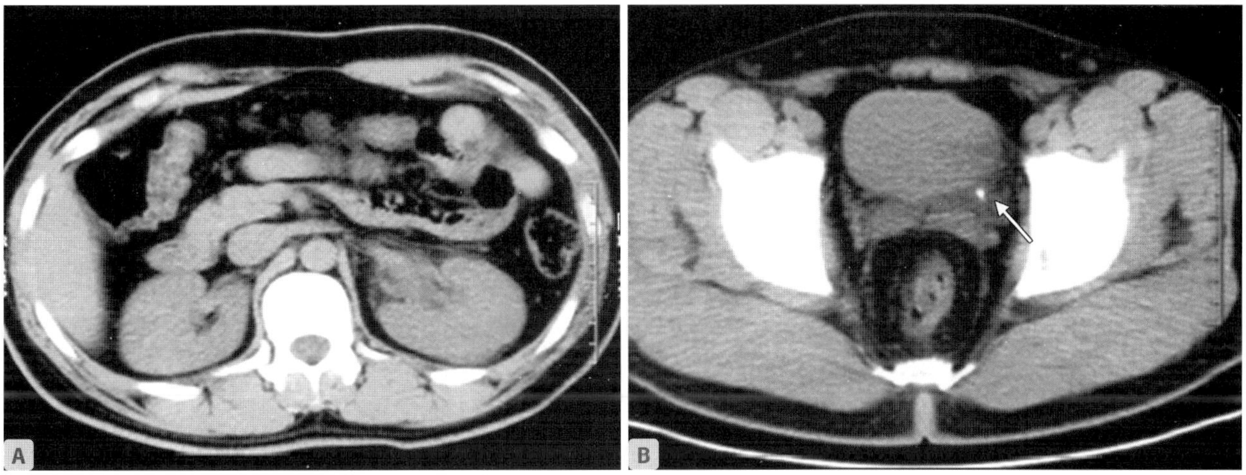

FIGS. 5A AND B: Low dose noncontrast CT scan of young male presented with acute loin pain. Axial section at the level of kidneys (A) shows minimal calyceal separation and perinephric stranding on left side and lower section at the level of bladder and (B) shows obstructed calculus in lower ureter (arrow).

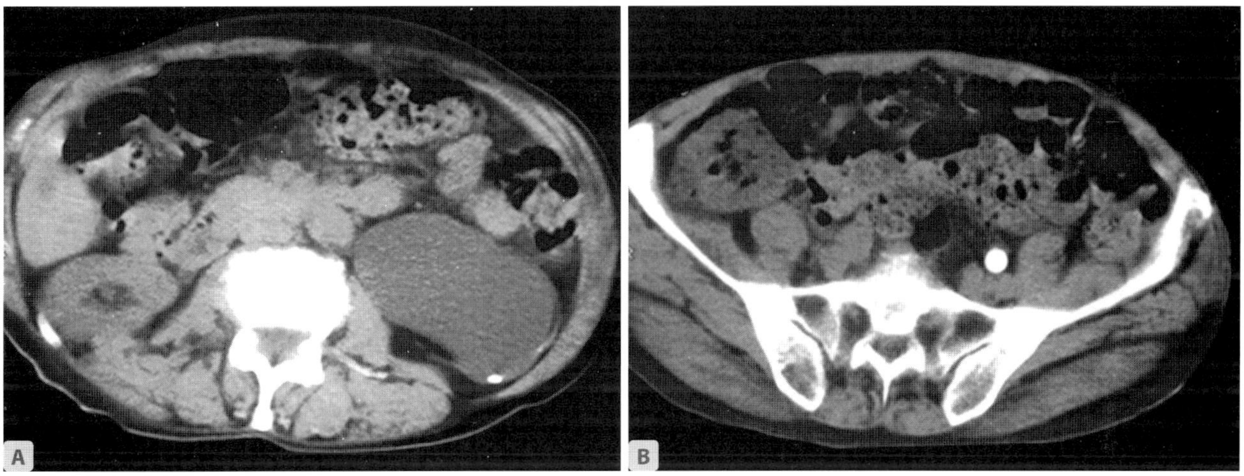

FIGS. 6A AND B: Noncontrast CT axial images (A) showing gross hydronephrosis with obstructive atrophy and left renal calculus; (B) Lower sections show obstructing calculus in lower ureter.

particularly low-dose CT. The main drawback of IVU is that it can be time consuming because of the serial delayed films which may be required to be obtained until the level of obstruction is delineated. This may require many hours and repeated films. Acute side effects of iodinated contrast and contrast-induced nephrotoxicity are also partly responsible for the decline in the use of IVU.

The urographic pattern varies in chronic obstruction. The kidney size is small in untreated complete obstruction, however, long-standing partial obstruction can result in enlargement of the collecting system and kidney. The obstructive nephrogram is usually not seen in cases of chronic obstruction as tubular concentrating ability and glomerular filtration rate (GFR) are reduced. The nephrographic density may be normal, faint or none depending upon the residual functioning parenchyma. The renal parenchyma is usually atrophied. When parenchymal thickness is reduced to 1-2 cm, but the renal function is relatively preserved then calyceal crescents are sometimes seen during nephrogram. The crescents are thin, curved collections of contrast denser than the nephrogram, located in the medulla. They represent realigned collecting tubules running perpendicular to their usual orientation.[24] They parallel the cortical margin of the ballooned calyces, located just 1-2 mm peripheral to the calyces. These crescents remain fixed regardless of patient position. The opacification of extremely thin parenchyma over the dilated calyceal sac produces a rim or shell nephrogram.

Chronic obstruction produces varying degree of pyelocalyceal dilatation. As contrast medium enters the dilated system, it glides to the dependent portion of calyces. With the patient supine, rounded puddles of contrast appear separated from the surrounding nephrogram by a boundary of non-radiopaque urine, this picture has been called the ball pyelogram **(Figs. 8A to B)**.

Chronic obstruction may lead to nonvisualized kidney on urogram. The ureter becomes dilated proximal to the

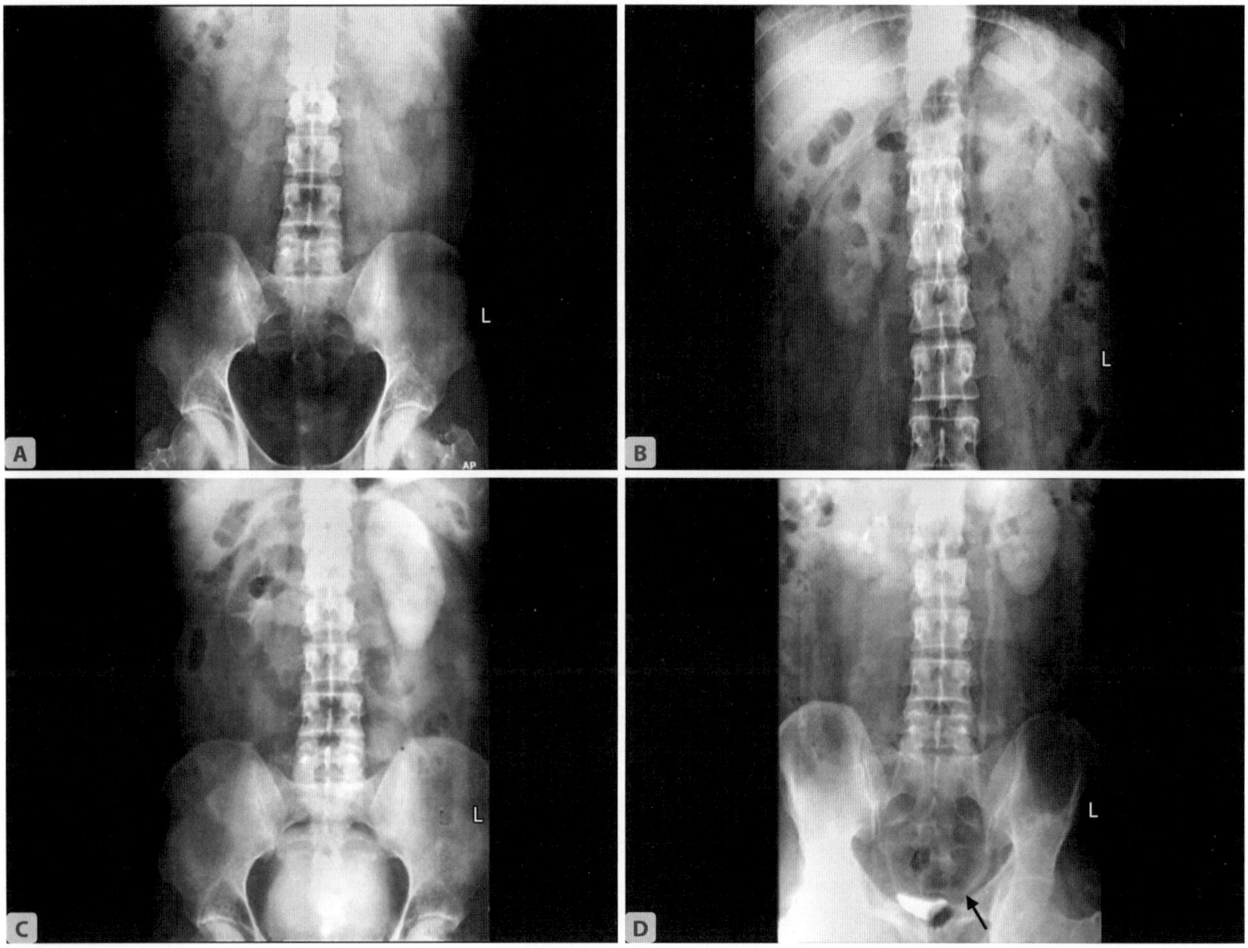

FIGS. 7A TO D: Serial intravenous urography (IVU) images of acute obstruction showing obstructing nephrogram. (A) Plain film; (B) Five-minute film; (C) 1-hour film shows increasingly dense left nephrogram; (D) Delayed film well depicted the left lower ureter calculus as the cause of obstruction (arrow).

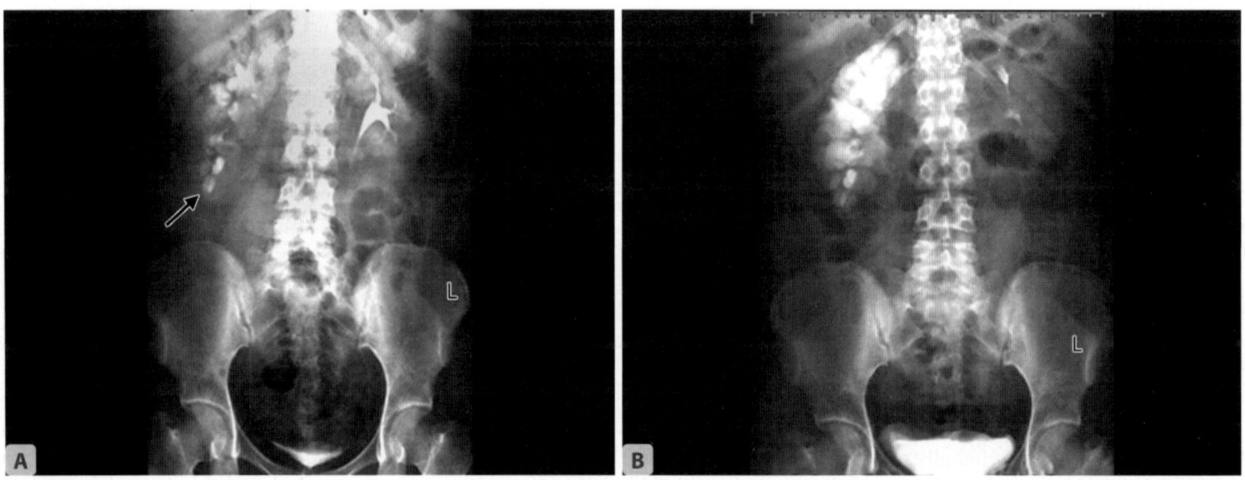

FIGS. 8A AND B: Intravenous urography study of chronic hydronephrosis due to ureteric stricture. (A) 11-minute film shows crescents (arrow); (B) 1-hour film shows ball pyelogram.

obstructing lesion, elongated and tortuous, and in extreme cases it may resemble a segment of small intestine. This is called giant hydroureter or giant megaureter.

Magnetic Resonance Imaging

At present, MRI has limited role to in the evaluation of urinary obstruction. Magnetic resonance urography (MRU) is an ideal technique in pregnancy, where there is contrast allergy, renal failure patients and if radiation dose is an issue.[25] Ureteric abnormalities are poorly defined especially if they are small.

OBSTRUCTIVE UROPATHY

INTRODUCTION

Obstructive uropathy is a general term that describes obstructive changes in any part of the urinary tract. The renal structural and functional alterations caused by obstruction are termed "obstructive nephropathy". Despite remarkable advances in diagnosis and treatment, obstruction remains a leading cause of damage to the urinary tract.[26] Urinary obstruction affects patients of all ages and is responsible for thousands of hospital admissions and surgical procedures. Obstruction predisposes to urinary tract infection and renal failure. Early diagnosis and treatment of urinary obstruction can reverse the renal damage.

PATHOPHYSIOLOGY

When the ureter is acutely obstructed, the pressure of the collecting system proximal to the obstruction rises. Over the next 6–12 hours, the renal blood flow drops due to increase of renal vascular resistance. There are two mechanisms that come into play to temporarily decompress the nephron. First is pyelosinus and pyelovenous backflow and second is enhanced absorption of fluid from the tubules. The preglomerular arteriolar resistance increases in acute obstruction. This RI measure by Doppler has been used with variable success to confirm intrarenal vascular resistance in acute obstruction **(Figs. 9A to B)**.[27] The elevated intrarenal resistance produces diminished diastolic flow eventually causing ischemia. Relief of total but short-lived obstruction leads to full restoration of the GFR. Longer period of total obstruction causes progressive nephron loss called obstructive atrophy. Relief of obstruction that has already caused renal atrophy is followed by improvement in renal function but not to normal levels. The kidney often shrinks in size with blunting of the calyces and impaired ability of urinary concentration and acidification.

These semirecovered kidneys showing the anatomical and functional sequelae are said to exhibit postobstructive atrophy. If the obstruction is partial and chronic, its effect to renal function is less predictable. Structural changes can occur in the medulla with impairment of the ability to concentrate urine. Sometimes partial obstruction can exist for years without causing any functional impairment.

CAUSES OF OBSTRUCTION AND DISEASES OF URETER

In children, obstruction is commonly due to congenital causes whereas in adults most cases are due to acquired causes. Obstruction may also be classified by location as intrarenal, postrenal, supravesical or infravesical.

Congenital Ureteric Obstruction

Primary megaureter and obstruction associated with duplication are common causes of congenital ureteric obstruction.

Ureteropelvic Junction Obstruction

Congenital obstruction of the ureteropelvic junction (UPJ) is a common anomaly of the urinary tract. The proposed etiology includes incomplete recanalization of the ureter during early gestation, aberrant vessel causing extrinsic compression, or other bands/kinks causing PUJ constriction.[28] It results due to deficiency and derangement of the ureteric smooth muscle fibers resulting in failure of normal peristalsis in the affected segment and subsequent functional obstruction.

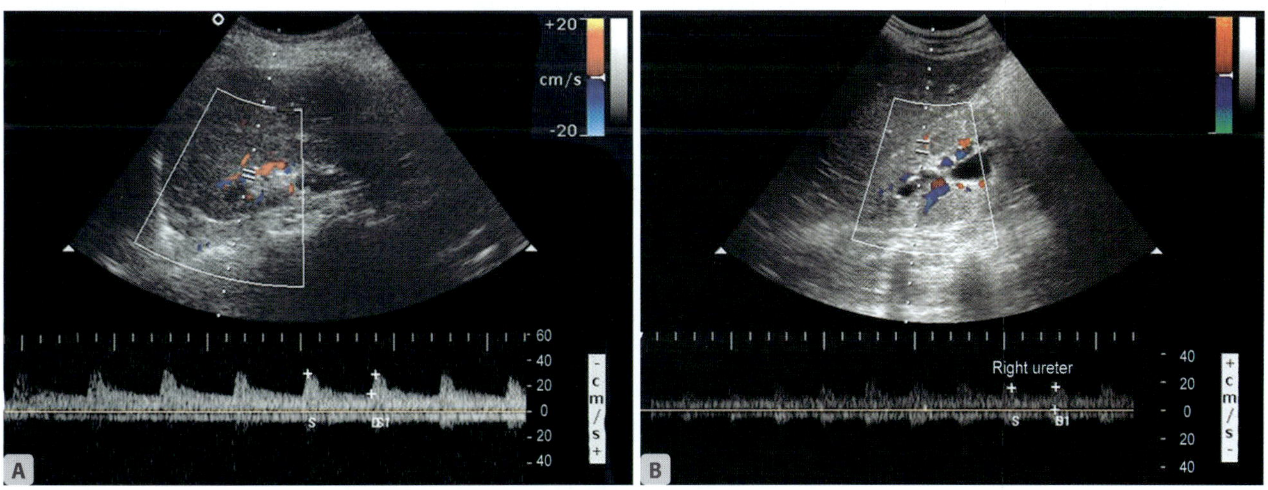

FIGS. 9A AND B: Doppler tracing of (A) normal kidney and (B) in acute obstruction. The resistive index is increased in acute obstruction.

Males and the left side are commonly affected. Dilated renal pelvis and calyces are demonstrated on urography. Delayed radiographs are usually necessary for demonstrating the point of obstruction at UPJ. With long-standing or high-grade obstruction the kidney may become nonfunctional. When there is insufficient contrast excretion or the ureter is not visualized, the diagnosis can be established by antegrade pyelography. Ultrasound usually shows hydronephrosis and dilated renal pelvis with a nondilated ureter. In patients with equivocal UPJ obstruction, diuresis renography, and Whitaker procedure may be employed to assess functional obstruction.[29]

Primary Megaureter

Primary megaureter or congenital megaureter is an uncommon entity probably caused by functional abnormality of the juxtavesical ureter, which is less distensible and fails to transmit normal peristalsis. Secondary megaureter on the other hand is secondary to causes like neurogenic bladder, vesicoureteric reflux (VUR) or posterior urethral valve (PUV).[30] The differentiation between these causes can be done using micturating cystourethrogram. Primary megaureter may be seen in both children and adults and typically remains asymptomatic in many cases. Males are affected more than females. A characteristic beak-like configuration of the distal ureteral segment is seen on urography with proximal dilatation of ureter **(Fig. 10)**. The dilatation may extend proximally to calyces. Primary megaureter may be associated with UPJ obstruction, contralateral renal agenesis, and VUR. Ultrasound readily detects PCS and ureteral dilatation. This condition is asymptomatic in majority of individuals and can be conservatively managed. Surgical intervention is indicated in cases having recurrent UTIs or falling renal function.

Ureterocele

The term ureterocele means saccular dilatation of the intramural portion of ureter as it passes through the bladder wall **(Fig. 11)**. It may be of two types—simple (orthotopic) and ectopic. The ureters of a simple ureterocele drain a nonduplex kidney and insert into the bladder at their normal position at the trigone. An ectopic ureterocele frequently occurs in a duplex kidney. In complete duplication, the ureter of the upper moiety generally inserts at a lower/ectopic location. This ureter is generally affected with ureterocele (the lower moiety, on the other hand is predisposed for VUR).[31] Morphologically, ureteroceles can be completely intravesical or extravesical—where the dilated portion extends outside the UB to involve the distal ureter. Ureterocele typically appear on urography and cystography as smooth, rounded or ovoid filling defect in the bladder. The major concern with ureterocele is obstruction, stasis, and UTI. Hence, treatment is directed toward relieving the obstruction using cystoscopy, partial nephrectomy for the nonfunctioning upper moiety and/or ureteric reimplantation for refluxing ureter of lower moiety.

Circumcaval Ureter

Circumcaval ureter results when the supracardinal vein persists and forms the major portion of the inferior vena cava (IVC). Embryonically, the subcardinal vein lies ventral to the ureter. The right ureter is carried medially by the migration of the subcardinal vein toward the developing IVC. The typical pattern on urography is a tortuous, dilated proximal right ureter, and associated hydronephrosis. The proximal ureter has a characteristic reverse-J course before it crosses behind and around the IVC and then descends medial to the ipsilateral lumbar pedicle. The confirmation of the diagnosis can be made with CT, which shows the ureter passing posterior and medial to the IVC.

Acquired Ureteric Obstruction

The causes of acquired ureteric obstruction can be intraluminal or extraluminal.

Intraluminal Causes

Abnormalities may develop within the ureteral lumen without any attachment to the uroepithelial lining. The common

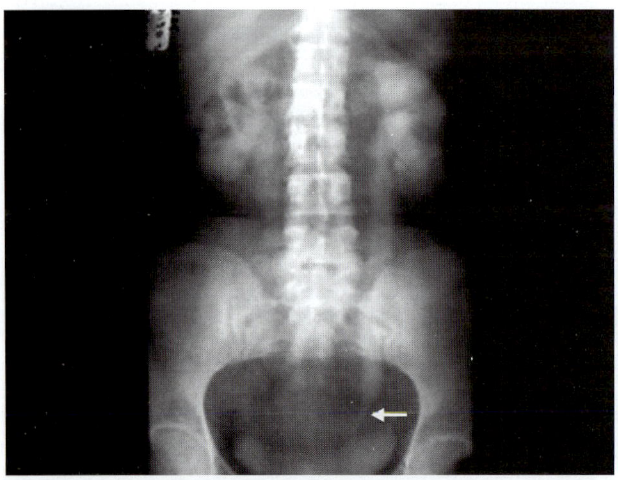

FIG. 10: Delayed intravenous urography image (1-hour film) shows bilateral hydroureteronephrosis with smooth tapering of lower ureter suggestive primary megaureter (arrow).

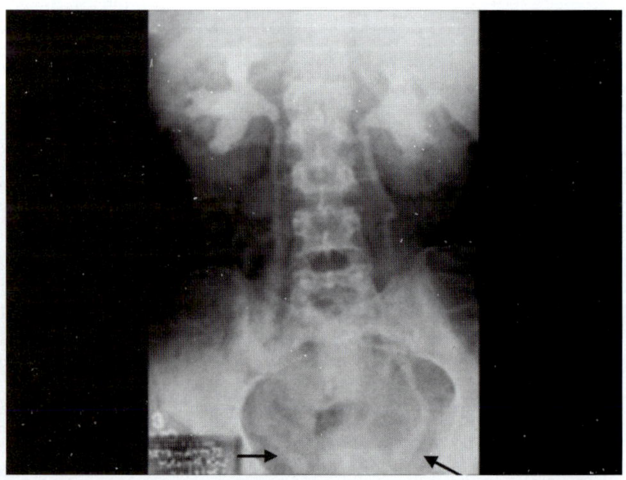

FIG. 11: Intravenous urography (IVU) (30-minute film) shows bilateral hydronephrosis with fusiform dilatation (arrows) of lower most portion of ureters suggestive of ureterocele.

causes are calculi, blood clots, tissue slough, fungus ball, and foreign material.

Ureteric Calculus

Ureteric calculus has been dealt with in the previous section on urolithiasis.

Blood Clots

Blood clots in ureter are secondary to trauma, tumors, nephritis, vasculitis and bleeding disorders. Blood clots exhibit radiographic features that are common to other non-radiopaque lesions. The location of clot varies with time or with change in position of patient. When clot persists as a mass of fibrin, calcification may develop that resembles stones or uroepithelial tumors.[32] Sonography shows a mass-like filing defect with low level echoes. The CT attenuation value of clot varies with time. When the clot is fresh, its attenuation value exceeds that of soft tissue. Within a week its attenuation decreases. Blood clot does not enhance after intravenous contrast administration.

Tissue Slough

Necrosed papilla and cholesteatoma can slough and cause obstruction of ureter with proximal dilatation. Urography shows features of nonopaque filling defect. Calcium is sometime deposited along the periphery of a sloughed papilla. Sonography and CT demonstrate hypoechoic and hyperdense mass lesion respectively.

Fungus Ball

Most fungus balls or mycetomas are caused by *Candida albicans* and *Aspergillus*. Fungal infection of the urinary tract occurs in the setting of altered host resistance like HIV, steroid intake, severe debilitating disease, and antineoplastic drug intake. The fungus balls fill the renal pelvis or ureter with a nonopaque mass. Sometime contrast material insinuates into the interstices of the mass causing lacelike radiodense pattern during IVU. The fungus ball appears as an echogenic mass on sonography while CT shows soft tissue attenuation filling defects. Neither sonography nor CT can differentiate fungus ball from other intraluminal soft tissue.

Intramural Causes

Ureteral Tumors

Primary ureteral tumors are relatively rare, accounting for approximately 1% of all urinary tract tumors. Tumors arising from epithelium are most common, however, they can arise from mesoderm. Males are affected more than females with the usual age of presentation being in the fifth to eighth decades. The most common tumor of ureter is transitional cell carcinoma. Rare tumors include squamous carcinoma, adenocarcinoma, sarcoma, and metastasis.

Transitional Cell Carcinoma

It occurs more frequently in males and has a peak incidence in the seventh decade. Certain epidemiological factors have been associated with increased risk for development of transitional cell carcinoma. These include exposure to chemicals, dye, petroleum, rubber and cable industries. Tobacco, coffee, artificial sweetener, chronic inflammation, and infection are additional risk factors. There is increased prevalence of TCC in analgesic and Balkan nephropathy. Squamous cell carcinoma occurs in older age and is generally associated with chronic infection and leukoplakia of urinary tract. Adenocarcinoma occurs in patients with severe infection and stone disease.[33]

Radiological Findings

- *Intravenous urography*: The lesion appears as a smooth or lobulated, polypoid filling defect in the ureter which maintains a constant relationship with the ureteric wall **(Fig. 12A)**. There is usually proximal obstruction dilatation of the ureter. The ureter just distal to the tumor is also often slightly dilated. The combination of distal margin of soft tissue mass invaginating into the distended

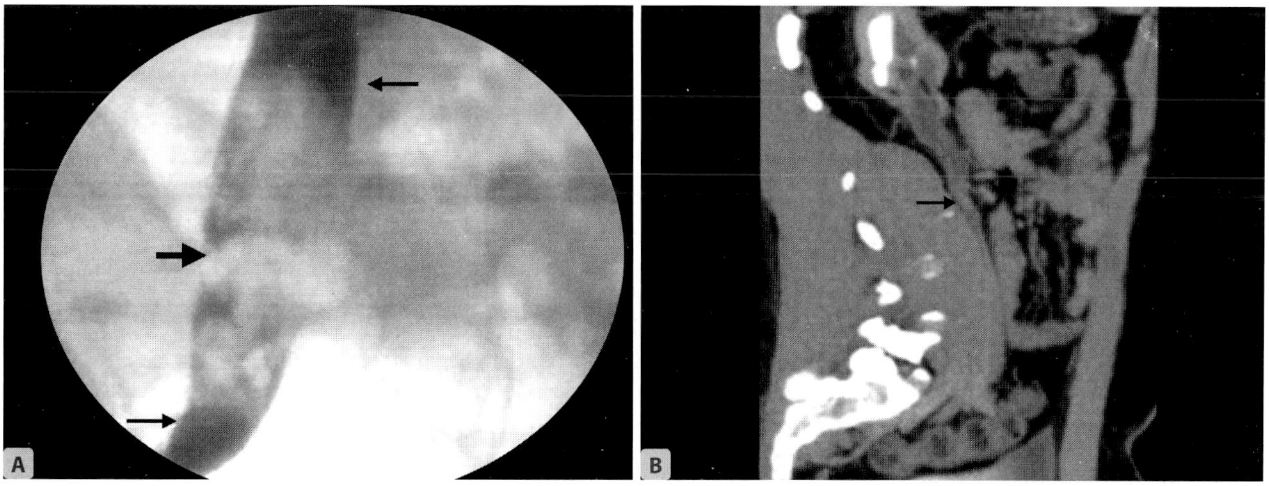

FIGS. 12A AND B: Transitional cell carcinoma (TCC) of ureter. (A) Fluoroscopic spot of nephrostogram shows irregular filling defect (thick arrow) in midureter with dilatation of ureter (thin arrows) proximal as well as distal to the lesion (Bregman's sign). Another patient with TCC: (B) Contrast-enhanced CT with sagittal reconstruction showing circumferential mural thickening (arrow) of ureter with proximal hydroureteronephrosis. These findings may mimic inflammatory lesion of ureter.

segment of opacified ureter constitutes the Chalice or Bregman's sign.[34] This sign is useful in distinguishing tumor from nonopaque stone as the ureter is not dilated distal to a stone.

- *Sonography*: Tumors of the ureter may be seen as a soft tissue mass situated at the distal end of a slightly dilated ureter.
- *Computed tomography*: CT defines the contour and mural attachment of tumor following ureteral opacification **(Fig. 12B)**. The tumor may enhance after intravenous contrast administration. The tumor may project into the ureteric lumen with circumferential or eccentric mural thickening. The lesion may infiltrate into the periureteric fat. CT is important in the staging of a documented ureteric tumor as it detects periureteral extension as well as lymph node enlargement. MR may be used in patients in whom CT cannot be done.

Benign Tumors

Benign tumors of urothelium constitute approximately 20% of ureteral neoplasms. The most common is a papilloma which presents as a solitary filling defect attached to the ureter by a stalk.

Nonepithelial Tumors

Fibroepithelial polyp is the most common nonepithelial tumor. These typically occur in patients in the 20–40 years age group. The usual location is the proximal one-third of the ureter. The lesion is usually solitary but multiple lesions can rarely be seen. The lesion can present as a mobile, smooth, cylindrical, slightly mobile, and filling defect. Sometimes the lesion can be frond like.

Secondary Tumors and Contiguous Infiltration

These are more common than primary ureteric tumors. Direct extension of the tumor from primary sites such as cervix, prostate and bladder can cause ureteric obstruction. Malignant retroperitoneal lymphadenopathy also cause obstruction to the ureter. Rarely, hematogenous malignant deposit can occur to the ureters. The common primaries responsible are melanoma, renal cell carcinoma, breast, lung, and prostate.[35]

Inflammatory Lesions of Ureter

Inflammatory conditions of the ureter include a wide variety of disorders.[36] Primary inflammation of the ureter is rare in the absence of systemic or regional disease in urinary tract, retroperitoneum, pelvis or peritoneum. Inflammation of ureteral wall may originate from inflammatory elements excreted in the urine, hematogenous embolism or contiguous spread from adjacent areas within the urinary tract and abdomen. The general responses of the ureter to inflammation are loss of ureteric peristalsis, dilatation, ulceration, irregularity, pseudopolyposis, edema, and desmoplasia leading to stricture and calcification.

Radiological Imaging

Radiology plays an important role in diagnosing and characterizing inflammatory conditions of the ureter. This information supplements that from other clinical diagnostic tools including urinalysis, urine culture, urine cytology, and cystoureteroscopy.

Malakoplakia

It is a benign chronic granulomatous disorder more commonly seen in women than men. It can be seen at any level of the urinary tract but has a predilection for the bladder and lower ureter. It is seen in association with chronic *Escherichia coli* or *Proteus mirabilis* infection and is found more frequently in diabetics and immunosuppressed patients. On urography, the lesions are rounded to flat, coalescent filling defects lending an irregular contour to the ureteral margin. Ureteric obstruction may be present. The imaging features overlap with ureteritis cystica but the lesions are usually rounder and the ureter is not dilated in the latter condition.

Ureteritis Cystica

This disease entity is usually asymptomatic but may present with hematuria or symptoms of urinary tract infection. Histologically, this condition consists of multiple, small, subepithelial, fluid-filled cysts in the ureteric wall. Ureteritis cystica does not cause ureteric obstruction. The disease has a slight predilection for the upper ureter. The typical radiographic appearance is that of multiple, small, filling defects with scalloping of the ureteral margin. The differential diagnosis include air bubbles, hemorrhage into ureteric wall, and papillary neoplasm. The condition may or may not regress with treatment of the underlying inflammatory condition.

Leukoplakia

It is a rare inflammatory condition which more commonly involves the urinary bladder than the ureter. It results from squamous metaplasia of the urothelium and is frequently associated with chronic urinary tract infection or long-standing stone disease. The imaging features include diffuse, irregular, and filling defects. There may be ridging of the mucosa with ureteric dilatation. Differentiation from malakoplakia or ureteral malignancy is difficult on imaging.

Schistosomiasis

It is a chronic indolent infestation caused by the trematode *Schistosoma haematobium*. The parasite lays its eggs in the veins of the bladder and lower ureter stimulating chronic inflammatory reaction resulting in cystitis and ureteritis and eventually scarring and calcification. Schistosomiasis commonly affects the bladder and ureteric involvement is seen in one-third of patients. The ureters are bilaterally asymmetrically involved with predominant involvement of the lower ureter. The disease usually affects a younger age group. Imaging findings are characteristic. Calcification of the ureter is seen in 75% of cases which is usually linear or tram-track in appearance. There is a characteristic deformity of the distal ureters consisting of medial and cephalic displacement which may resemble cow's horns. There is varying degree of stenosis and dilatation and the ureter may show a beaded appearance which can resemble tuberculous ureteritis.

Tuberculous Ureteritis

Tuberculosis of the urinary tract is usually due to hematogenous dissemination of *Mycobacterium tuberculosis*. Ureteral involvement is usually due to descending renal infection. The symptoms are nonspecific and include constitutional symptoms and lower urinary tract symptoms like frequency, dysuria, and suprapubic pain. The patients may present with hematuria and sterile pyuria. When the infection affects the ureteral wall, the first changes are those of ulceration and wall edema with thickening which progress to strictures and calcification. These changes may lead to proximal dilatation of the ureter and PCS. Plain films of abdomen may show evidence of ureteric calcification with or without calcification of the kidney. Characteristic urographic findings include alternating areas of dilatation and short strictures of the ureter (beaded appearance), long straight stricture (pipestem ureter) or isolated stricture. The ureter is shortened and straightened due to periureteral fibrosis **(Fig. 13)**. CT scan is useful in demonstrating ureteric wall thickening and presence of lymph nodes if any. The bladder may show poor distensibility owing to irritative spasm or fibrosis within the wall **(Figs. 14A to B)**.

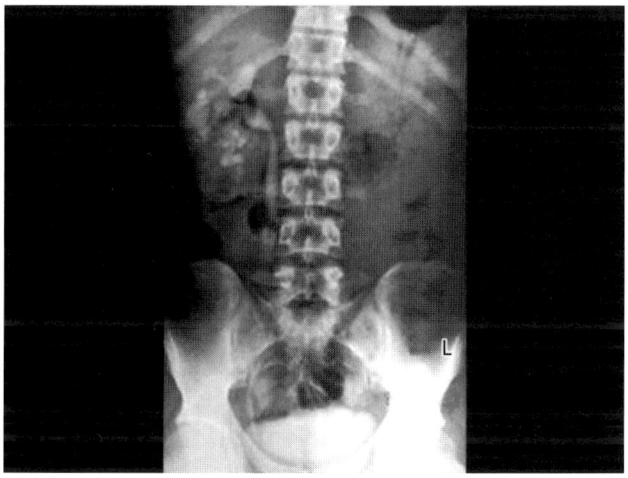

FIG. 13: Intravenous urography (15-minute film) shows hydronephrosis, forniceal stenosis, cavitary changes in right kidney with ureteric narrowing. All these features suggest tubercular involvement of urinary tract.

Radiation Ureteritis

Radiation can lead to early and late changes in the ureteric wall, ultimately leading to fibrosis and stricture. Fibrosis continues to develop long after radiotherapy has been completed. IVU may demonstrate mucosal irregularity and a short or long distal ureteric stricture. CT may demonstrate these findings as well as thickening and stranding of the wall of the ureter.

Inflammatory Bowel Disease

Genitoureteric complications may occur in up to one-fourth of patients with inflammatory bowel disease. Obstruction due to direct ureteral involvement is the second most common complication, the first being nephrolithiasis. Ureteric involvement by Crohn's disease is usually at the level of the pelvic brim and the right ureter is more commonly involved. On urography, the ureter shows a smooth area of narrowing with varying degree of obstruction. CT scan shows an inflammatory soft tissue mass with narrowing and mural thickening of the ureter.

Endometriosis

Ureteral involvement generally occurs in cases with widespread pelvic disease, however, cases of isolated ureteral involvement have been reported. Two forms of ureteral endometriosis have been described. Extrinsic involvement is four times more common than the intrinsic variety. The distal ureter is commonly involved. Ureteral involvement may result in narrowing of ureter, hydronephrosis and occasionally an intraluminal mass. The stricture is usually smooth but abruptly tapered and may show medial sharp angulation. CT may demonstrate a soft tissue mass or endometrioma causing encasement of the ureter **(Figs. 15A to D)**.

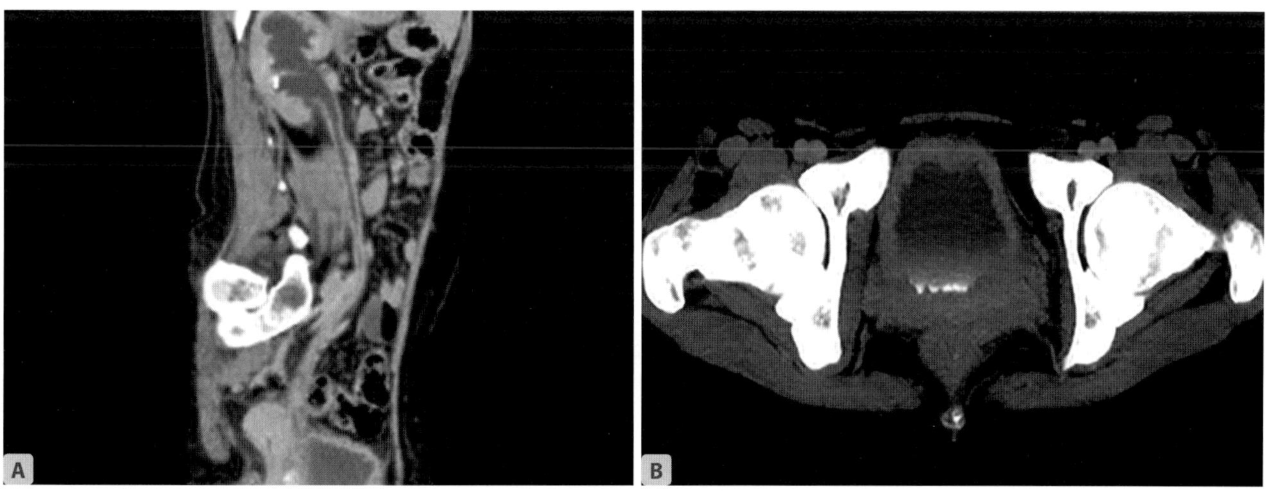

FIGS. 14A AND B: CT scan of urinary tract tuberculosis. (A) Multiplanar reconstruction (MPR) shows hydronephrosis of kidney with thickened ureteric wall; (B) Irregular thickening of urinary bladder with reduced capacity.

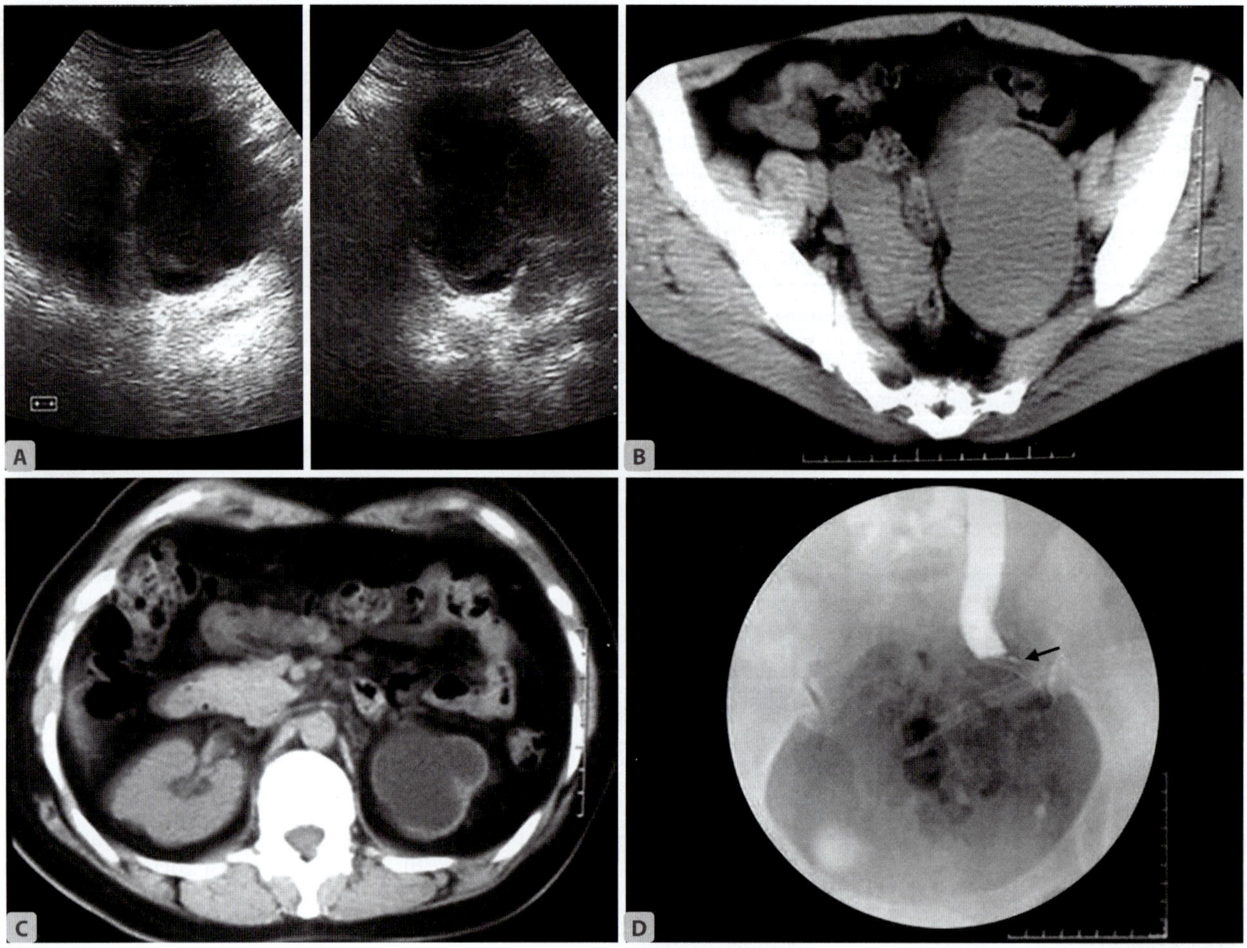

FIGS. 15A TO D: Obstructive uropathy due to endometriosis. (A) Ultrasound image shows complicated cyst within left adnexa; CT axial scan at the level of pelvis; (B) shows adnexal mass compressing and displacing lower ureter, resulting obstructive atrophy of kidney; (C) The nephrostogram of the same patients shows displacement and stricture of lower ureter (arrow); (D) of the same patients shows displacement and stricture of lower ureter (arrow).

Extrinsic Causes of Ureteral Obstruction

Retroperitoneal Fibrosis

Retroperitoneal fibrosis (RPF) is an important cause of obstructive uropathy leading to renal failure.[37] It encompasses a range of diseases characterized by the presence of fibroinflammatory tissue, which usually surrounds the abdominal aorta and iliac arteries and extends into the retroperitoneum to envelop neighboring structures including the ureters. RPF may be idiopathic (Ormond's disease) or secondary to a wide variety of stimuli which includes both benign and neoplastic causes.

The classic triad of delayed renal contrast excretion with unilateral or bilateral (60% of cases) hydronephrosis and proximal hydroureter secondary to ureteral involvement, medial deviation of the middle-third of both ureters and tapering of the ureteral lumen at the L4–L5 vertebral level, though less frequently seen than previously thought, is still useful in the identification of RPF. When there is insufficient contrast excretion on urography, retrograde or antegrade pyelography is required to demonstrate the characteristic ureteral changes. CT scan demonstrates sheet-like soft-tissue mass in retroperitoneum with encasement of ureters. CT may help in the identification of disease activity with the degree of soft-tissue enhancement correlating with the activity of the fibrotic process **(Figs. 16A to C)**. RPF has signal characteristics similar to those of other fibrotic processes, with a tendency toward diffusely low-signal intensity on T1-weighted MRI. T2 signal is a reflection of the degree of associated active inflammation (and thus edema) with high signal indicating early inflammatory phase of benign RPF or malignancy while low signal signifies chronic phase of benign RPF. Chronic, inactive fibrosis will have little edema and thus be visualized as having low signal on both T1- and T2-weighted imaging. This feature may also prove valuable in assessing a patient's response to treatment; decreasing T2-signal indicating a favorable therapeutic response.[38]

Retroperitoneal Neoplasms

Extraureteral malignancies causing obstructive uropathy are much more common than primary ureteral neoplasms.

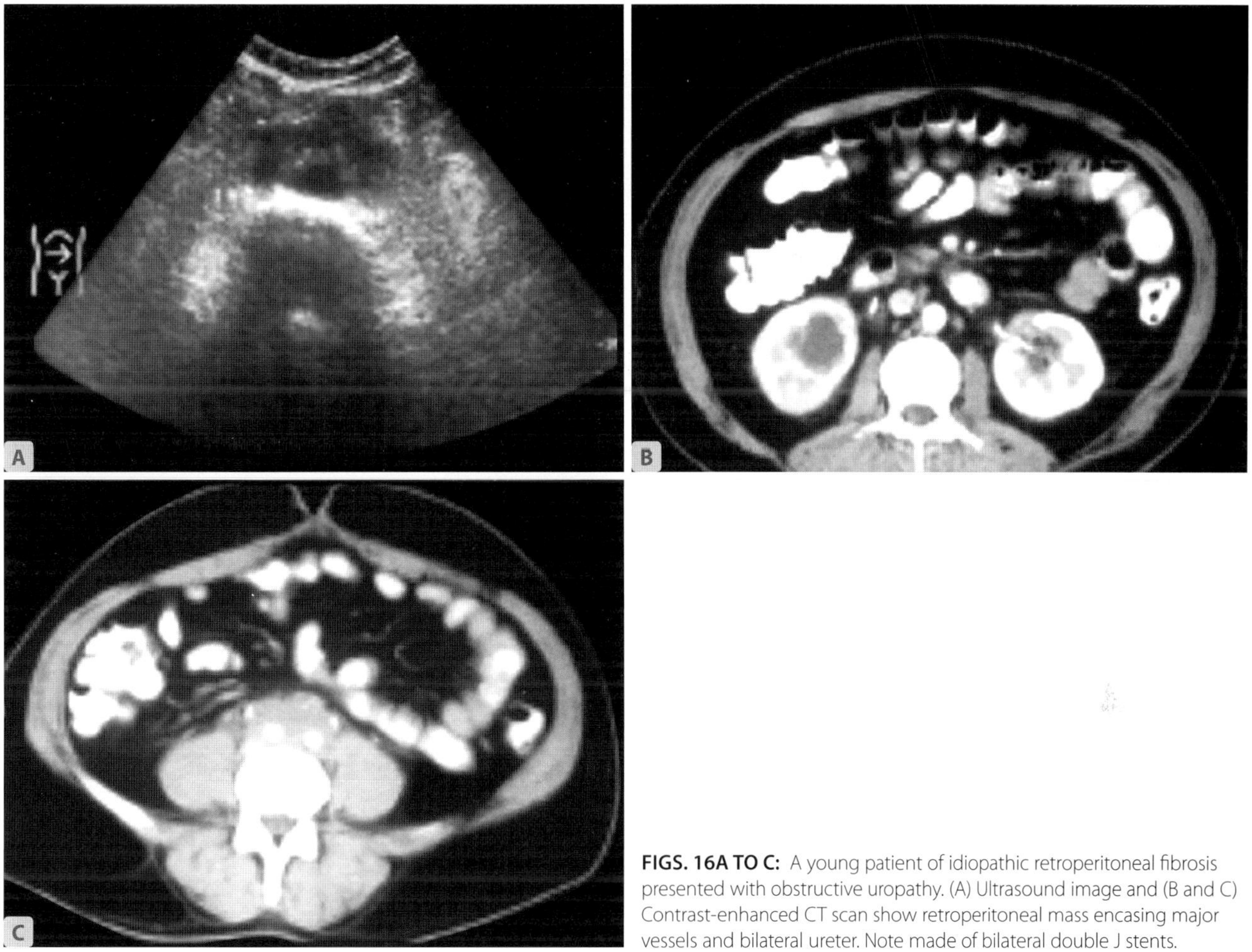

FIGS. 16A TO C: A young patient of idiopathic retroperitoneal fibrosis presented with obstructive uropathy. (A) Ultrasound image and (B and C) Contrast-enhanced CT scan show retroperitoneal mass encasing major vessels and bilateral ureter. Note made of bilateral double J stents.

The ureter is very prone to involvement as it is near many structures in the retroperitoneum that frequently harbor malignancies. In many cases, obstruction may result from direct extension of neoplasms from primary sites like the bladder, prostate, endometrium, sigmoid colon, rectum, and cervix. In other cases, there may be metastasis to the periureteral tissues especially the lymph nodes by distant tumors which causes uropathy by direct infiltration of one or both the ureters or by compression and mechanical obstruction. Bulky lymph nodes seen in lymphomas may cause similar manifestations.

Primary retroperitoneal tumors arising in the vicinity of the ureters may also lead to mechanical obstruction. CT scores over sonography in the detection and possible classification of these tumors. Malignancies may incite an intense periureteral desmoplastic reaction resembling retroperitoneal fibrosis leading to ureteral obstruction. This is especially seen in metastases from carcinomas of lung, breast, pancreas, colon, stomach, and sometimes lymphoma. Patients who have received radiation therapy in the vicinity may also experience obstructive symptoms. This was initially thought to be due to radiation-induced ureteric stricture but lately it has been realized that the ureter is relatively resistant to radiation. An obstruction in this case usually means that the tumor had involved the ureteral wall before radiation or there has been a recent relapse.

Pelvic Lipomatosis

It is an unusual disease resulting from proliferation of mature fibroadipose tissue in the pelvis. Usually seen in males, it may require surgery if it is causing obstructive uropathy by ureteral compression. Radiographic findings include relative hyperlucency of the pelvic cavity on plain radiographs. Contrast studies may show displacement and compression of rectosigmoid and urinary bladder leading to "tear drop" or "pear"-shaped bladder. The distal ends of the ureters are displaced medially in the majority of cases with presence of hydroureter or hydroureteronephrosis. Identical appearance of the bladder can also be seen with pelvic lymphadenopathy, diffuse pelvic carcinomatosis, pelvic/perivesical liposarcoma, and pelvic fibrosis (resembling retroperitoneal fibrosis).

Pregnancy-related Dilatation of Ureter

Variable degree of ureteral dilatation is often seen during pregnancy which is most marked in the third trimester with predominant involvement of the right side. In most of the cases, the dilatation progressively disappears in the postpartum period. The ureteral segments below the pelvic brim do not show dilatation indicating that partial mechanical obstruction by the gravid uterus accounts for the major changes of hydroureter seen during pregnancy.

Sonography forms the initial and mainstay imaging modality in these conditions. If the sonographic findings are equivocal, MR urography can show tapered narrowing of the lumbar portion of the ureter due to compression by the gravid uterus against the iliac artery at the sacral promontory. An obstructing calculus is usually above or below this level.

Gynecological Causes

Various gynecological disorders may cause extrinsic compression on the ureter leading to proximal dilatation of the urinary system **(Figs. 17A to B)**. Tubo-ovarian abscesses in pelvic inflammatory disease (PID) may cause extrinsic ureteric compression or surround the ureter with inflammation leading to partial obstruction with lateral displacement of the ureter below the pelvic brim. Pneumohydronephrosis may rarely develop due to fistula formation between the abscess and the ureter. Uterine and bladder prolapse are important causes of reversible and preventable renal failure. Obstruction is usually bilateral and is often associated with UTI. Sonography along with IVU helps in the easy identification of the disease. Carcinoma of urinary bladder can extend into the VUJ and distal ureter **(Figs. 18A to B)**.

Miscellaneous Diseases of Ureter

Ureteral Injury

The causes of ureteric injury can be iatrogenic and external trauma. Radical hysterectomy, gynecological surgery, and obstetric trauma are common causes of iatrogenic injury. Penetrating injury and fall from height are common causes for external trauma. Most surgically induced ureteric injuries go unsuspected at the time of injury, because they are often not a direct injury but the result of ischemia. IVU may

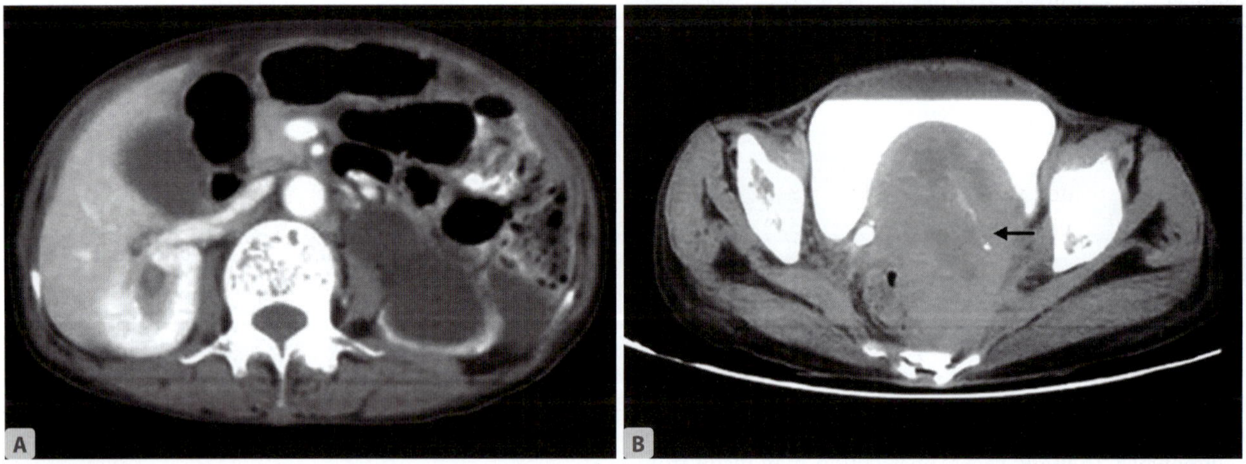

FIGS. 17A AND B: Carcinoma of cervix causing obstructive uropathy. Contrast-enhanced CT scans. (A) Axial section shows obstructive atrophy of left kidney; (B) Delayed section at the level of pelvis shows large heterogeneous cervical mass causing encasement of lower ureter (arrow).

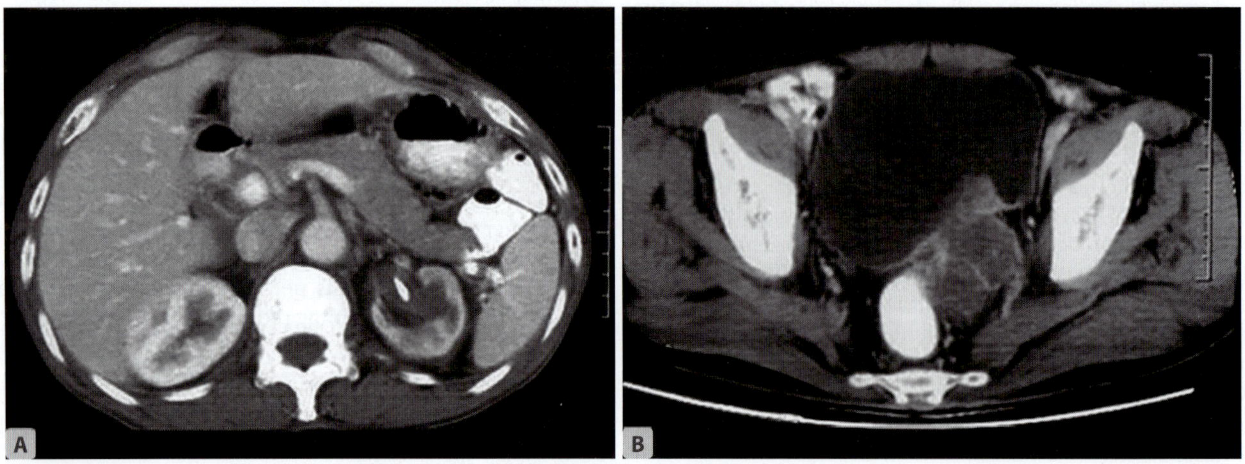

FIGS. 18A AND B: Ureteric obstruction caused by urinary bladder malignancy. Contrast-enhanced CT scans. (A) Axial section shows left hydroureteronephrosis with large calculus in renal pelvis; (B) Inferior section shows large lobulated mass arising from urinary bladder with exophytic component causing left ureteric involvement.

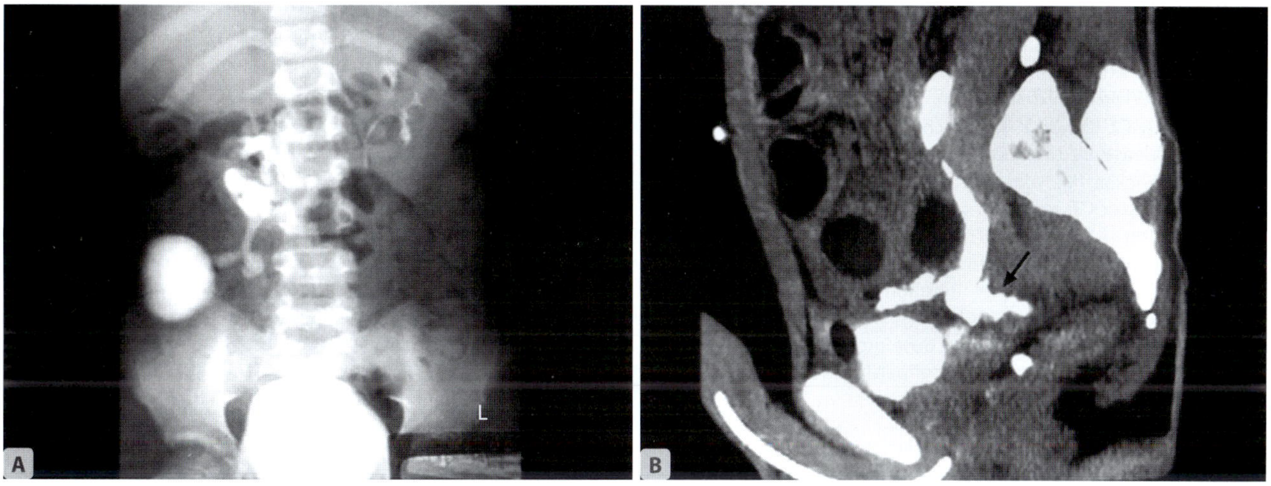

FIGS. 19A AND B: Ureteric trauma. (A) Delayed IVU film (2-hour film) shows extravasation of contrast from right upper ureter; (B) CT reformation in another patient shows contrast leak from lower ureter suggestive of ureteric trauma (arrow).

demonstrate extravasation of urine and hydronephrosis. The complications of ureteric injury include hydronephrosis/pyonephrosis secondary to stricture, calculus formation, ureteric fistula, urinomas, and renal failure **(Figs. 19A to B)**.

Ureteral Herniation

Herniation of ureter is rare. Inguinal, femoral, and sciatic hernias may include the ureter. Herniation of ureter can be recognized on urography, e.g. in sciatic herniation, the pelvic ureter extends laterally through the sacrosciatic notch, producing a hairpin-shaped redundancy.

Ureteral Fistula

The common causes of ureteral fistulae are penetrating trauma, complicated ureteral surgery and inflammatory or malignant disease. Ureteral fistula usually presents with urinary tract infection and clinical evidence of flow through the fistula. The diagnosis of fistula usually made by urography.

REFERENCES

1. Kumari A, Dokwal S, Mittal P, et al. An increase incidence in uric acid nephrolithiasis: changing patterns. J Clin Diagn Res. 2016;10(7):BC01-3.
2. Ansari MS, Gupta NP, Hemal AK, et al. Spectrum of stone composition: structural analysis of 1050 upper urinary tract calculi from northern India. Int J Urol. 2005;12(1):12-6.
3. Uribarri J, Oh MS, Carroll HJ. The first kidney stone. Ann Intern Med. 1989;111(12):1006-9.
4. Shadman A, Bastani B. Kidney calculi: pathophysiology and as a systemic disorder. Iran J Kidney Dis. 2017;11(3):180-91.
5. NICE (2019). Renal and ureteric stones: assessment and management. Guidance: Recommendations. [online] Available from https://www.nice.org.uk/guidance/ng118/chapter/Recommendations#diagnostic-imaging [Last accessed October, 2019].
6. American Urological Association (2012). Clinical Effectiveness Protocols for Imaging in The Management of Ureteral Calculous Disease: AUA Technology Assessment. [online] Available from https://www.auanet.org/guidelines/imaging-for-ureteral-calculous-disease [Last accessed October, 2019].
7. European Association of Urology. Professionals SO. EAU Guidelines: Urolithiasis [online] Available from: https://uroweb.org/guideline/urolithiasis/#3 [Last accessed October, 2019].
8. Smith-Bindman R, Aubin C, Bailitz J, et al. Ultrasonography versus computed tomography for suspected nephrolithiasis. N Engl J Med. 2014;371(12):1100-10.
9. Brisbane W, Bailey MR, Sorensen MD. An overview of kidney stone imaging techniques. Nat Rev Urol. 2016;13(11):654-62.
10. Ather MH, Jafri AH, Sulaiman MN. Diagnostic accuracy of ultrasonography compared to unenhanced CT for stone and obstruction in patients with renal failure. BMC Med Imaging. 2004;4(1):2.
11. Rahmouni A, Bargoin R, Herment A, et al. Color Doppler twinkling artifact in hyperechoic regions. Radiology. 1996; 199(1):269-71.
12. Gliga ML, Chirila CN, Podeanu DM, et al. Twinkle, twinkle little stone: an artifact improves the ultrasound performance! Med Ultrasound. 2017;19(3):272-5.
13. Alan C, Koçoğlu H, Kosar S, et al. Role of twinkling artifact in characterization of urinary calculi. Actas Urol Esp. 2011;35(7): 396-402.
14. Baker SM, Middleton WD. Color Doppler sonography of ureteral jets in normal volunteers: importance of the relative specific gravity of urine in the ureter and bladder. Am J Roentgenol. 1992;159(4):773-5.
15. Bertolotto M, Moro U, Gioulis E, et al. Changes of renal resistive index in response to hydration and diuretic administration in normal subjects and in patients with small ureteral stone. J Ultrasound Med. 1999;18(12):819-25.
16. Tublin ME, Bude RO, Platt JF. The resistive index in renal Doppler sonography: where do we stand? Am J Roentgenol. 2003;180(4):885-92.
17. Motamedinia P, Okhunov Z, Okeke Z, et al. Contemporary assessment of renal stone complexity using cross-sectional imaging. Curr Urol Rep. 2015;16(4):18.
18. Shadman A, Bastani B. Evaluation and management of kidney calculi. Iran J Kidney Dis. 2017;11(6):395-407.

19. Yamashita S, Kohjimoto Y, Iwahashi Y, et al. Noncontrast computed tomography parameters for predicting shock wave lithotripsy outcome in upper urinary tract stone cases. Biomed Res Int. 2018;2018:9253952.
20. McCarthy CJ, Baliyan V, Kordbacheh H, et al. Radiology of renal stone disease. Int J Surg Lond Engl. 2016;36(Pt D):638-46.
21. Karçaaltincaba M, Aktas A. Dual-energy CT revisited with multidetector CT: review of principles and clinical applications. Diagn Interv Radiol. 2011;17(3):181-94.
22. Bigongiari LR, Davis RM, Novak WG, et al. Visualization of the medullary rays on excretory urography in experimental ureteric obstruction. Am J Roentgenol. 1977;129(1):89-93.
23. Bernardino M, Clennan B. High dose urography: incidence and relationship to spontaneous peripelvic extravasation. Am J Roentgenol. 1976;127(3):373-6.
24. Dunbar JS, Nogrady MB. The calyceal crescent—a roentgenographic sign of obstructive hydronephrosis. Am J Roentgenol Radium Ther Nucl Med. 1970;110(3):520-8.
25. Somani BK, Dellis A, Liatsikos E, et al. Review on diagnosis and management of urolithiasis in pregnancy: an ESUT practical guide for urologists. World J Urol. 2017;35(11):1637-49.
26. Nicola R, Menias CO. Urinary obstruction, stone disease, and infection. In: Hodler J, Kubik-Huch RA, von Schulthess GK (Eds). Diseases of the Abdomen and Pelvis 2018-2021: Diagnostic Imaging—IDKD Book. Switzerland: Springer; 2018.
27. Amirthalingam U. Intrarenal Doppler indices in acute ureteric obstruction. J Clin Diagn Res. 2014;8(12):RC11-13.
28. Ramanathan S, Kumar D, Khanna M, et al. Multi-modality imaging review of congenital abnormalities of kidney and upper urinary tract. World J Radiol. 2016;8(2):132-41.
29. Johnston RB, Porter C. The Whitaker test. Urol J. 2014;11(3): 1727-30.
30. Chiodini B, Ghassemi M, Khelif K, et al. Clinical outcome of children with antenatally diagnosed hydronephrosis. Front Pediatr. 2019;7:103.
31. Merlini E, Lelli Chiesa P. Obstructive ureterocele—an ongoing challenge. World J Urol. 2004;22(2):107-14.
32. Thomas J, Steg A, Aboulker P. Calculi on blood clots. J Urol Nephrol (Paris). 1976;82(6):496-505.
33. Soria F, Shariat SF, Lerner SP, et al. Epidemiology, diagnosis, preoperative evaluation and prognostic assessment of upper-tract urothelial carcinoma (UTUC). World J Urol. 2017;35(3): 379-87.
34. Fein AB, McClennan BL. Solitary filling defects of the ureter. Semin Roentgenol. 1986;21(3):201-13.
35. Karaosmanoglu AD, Onur MR, Karcaaltincaba M, et al. Secondary tumors of the urinary system: an imaging conundrum. Korean J Radiol. 2018;19(4):742-51.
36. Moosavi B, Fasih N, Virmani V, et al. Beyond ureterolithiasis: gamut of abnormalities affecting the ureter. Clin Imaging. 2016;40(4):678-90.
37. Kawano M, Saeki T, Nakashima H. IgG4-related kidney disease and retroperitoneal fibrosis: an update. Mod Rheumatol. 2019;29(2):231-9.
38. Cronin CG, Lohan DG, Blake MA, et al. Retroperitoneal fibrosis: a review of clinical features and imaging findings. Am J Roentgenol. 2008;191(2):423-31.

CHAPTER

4

Renal Parenchymal Disease

Sreedhara BC, Anupam Lal, Anindita Sinha

Disorders of renal function are ubiquitous in contemporary practice of medicine. Kidney disease manifestations may vary from complete asymptomatic cases to life-threatening emergencies. Insight into the causes and consequences of medical renal disease has progressively increased over the last decade, and radiological imaging has played a pivotal role in this improved understanding.

DEFINITION AND CLASSIFICATION OF KIDNEY DISEASE

The term renal failure encompasses the spectrum of diseases from acute and reversible to chronic and irreversible. It is broadly divided into two categories which are described here.

Acute Kidney Injury

Acute kidney injury (AKI), also termed as acute renal failure previously is defined as a rapid deterioration in renal function, characterized by progressive azotemia (best measured by serum creatinine) which may or may not be accompanied by oliguria (urine output <400 mL/day). The cardinal feature of AKI is decline in glomerular filtration rate (GFR). According to Acute Kidney Injury Network (AKIN) criteria,[1] AKI is diagnosed if one of the following is present:

- An abrupt (within 48 hours) reduction in kidney function (defined as an absolute increase in serum creatinine of more than or equal to 0.3 mg/dL (≥26.4 μmol/L), or percentage increase in serum creatinine of more than or equal to 50% (1.5-fold from baseline).
- Reduced urine volume less than 0.5 mL/kg/h for 6 hours. There is sudden and often temporary loss of renal function, which is frequently reversible, with less than 20% cases ultimately requiring renal replacement therapy.[2] Imaging is, therefore, directed at identifying correctable causes of acute renal insult. Most common causes include acute tubular necrosis (ATN), severe dehydration, tubular blockade, infection, and obstruction.

Chronic Kidney Disease

The diagnosis of chronic kidney disease (CKD) implies a persistent abnormality in GFR with a wide range of causes. Slow progressive loss of kidney function over a span of years occurs, resulting in permanent kidney damage. CKD is defined as sustained kidney damage greater than 3 months duration resulting in a GFR of less than 60 mL/min/1.73 m^2.[2]

For purposes of diagnosis and management, renal failure can be divided into three categories which are as follows:

1. *Prerenal*: Diseases caused by any process that decreases perfusion to kidneys in which the integrity of renal parenchymal tissue is preserved.
2. *Intrarenal*: Diseases affecting renal parenchymal tissue (which can be further divided into vascular, glomerular, and tubular diseases).
3. *Postrenal*: Diseases associated with obstruction of the urinary tract or venous blood flow. It is also known as "surgical renal failure" as it is often amenable to correction.

This chapter is designed to give a contemporary insight of the intrarenal causes of acute and chronic kidney disease—"*Medical Renal Diseases*".

Various causes of acute and chronic kidney disease are enumerated in **Tables 1 and 2**.[2]

ROLE OF IMAGING IN RENAL FAILURE

Overlapping imaging findings are seen in renal failure. Comprehensive evaluation should be done in a particular case which includes clinical profile, laboratory findings, and histopathology along with imaging to arrive at a conclusive diagnosis.

The role of imaging in renal failure is to segregate the surgical and medical conditions resulting in renal insufficiency.[1] Goals for radiological studies in renal failure are as follows:

- Exclusion of correctable causes of acute renal failure (e.g. obstruction and thrombosis).
- Estimation of renal size to differentiate acute parenchymal disease from chronic parenchymal disease.

TABLE 1: Causes of acute renal failure.		
Prerenal	**Intrarenal**	**Postrenal**
• Hypovolemia • Cardiogenic shock • Anaphylaxis • Sepsis • Renal artery stenosis • Severe dehydration	• *Acute tubular necrosis:* - Hemolysis - Antibiotics - Contrast nephrotoxicity • *Glomerulopathy:* - SLE - HSP - Postinfective glomerulonephritis • Papillary necrosis • *Vascular diseases:* - PAN, scleroderma	• Renal vein thrombosis • *Obstruction due to:* - Calculi - Hemorrhage - Tumor

(SLE: systemic lupus erythematosus; HSP: Henoch-Schönlein purpura)

TABLE 2: Causes of chronic renal failure.		
Prerenal	**Intrarenal**	**Postrenal**
• Renal artery stenosis • Chronic dehydration • Congestive heart failure • Cirrhosis	• *Common causes:* - Diabetic nephropathy - Hypertensive - Glomerulosclerosis • Glomerulonephritis • Congenital ADPKD • Renal tubular acidosis • Drugs • TB • *Systemic diseases:* - FSGS - Gout - AIDS nephropathy - Scleroderma	• Posterior cortical value • Neurogenic bladder • Ureteric/bladder outlet obstruction • Retroperitoneal fibrosis • Tumor encasement

(ADPKD: autosomal dominant polycystic kidney disease; TB: tuberculosis; FSGS: focal segmental glomerulosclerosis)

Once obstruction is excluded, prerenal and postrenal causes of renal failures can be managed medically.

Radiological Approach to Renal Parenchymal Disease

Most diseases affecting the parenchyma of the kidney may produce lesions detectable only by electron or light microscopy, or by deranged renal function. However, some pathological processes manifest as renal morphological abnormalities and may be diagnosed by radiological imaging.

Morphological criteria are useful to categorize the wide spectrum of renal parenchymal diseases. Evaluation is done based on renal size, contour abnormality, and laterality of involvement **(Flowchart 1)**.

Renal size is an important diagnostic criterion. Large kidneys result from accumulation of fluid, deposition of proteins, inflammatory or neoplastic infiltrates, and hypertrophy secondary to glomerular, microvascular or cellular proliferation. Small kidneys result from loss of renal substance due to atrophy, hypoplasia, necrosis or fibrosis. Renal contour is another useful indicator. If a disease causes global reduction in renal mass, parenchymal bulk is uniformly lost and its size decreases with smooth contour. This is ascertained by preserved interpapillary line, which is a useful landmark for evaluating loss of renal parenchyma. Interpapillary line is drawn through the tips of papilla (base of the calyces) **(Fig. 1)**, the distance from this line to lateral surface of kidney is the renal parenchymal thickness which averages to 2.5–3 cm. It is greater at polar calyces ranging up to 3.5 cm. Distances less than 2 cm are suggestive of parenchymal loss while those greater than 3.5 cm indicate mass lesion or infiltration.[4]

Assessment of renal contour may show a deviation when there is focal loss or regional expansion. Laterality indicates nature of the disease. Bilateral renal lesions are usually found in systemic disorders in which total renal mass is affected.[5,6]

Radiological imaging in renal parenchymal disease is usually targeted to reach a set of differential diagnosis, with distinct morphological description. "Bilateral large smooth kidney" constitutes to the group of acute renal parenchymal disease, while "bilateral small smooth kidney" falls into description of chronic renal parenchymal disease.

FLOWCHART 1: Morphological criteria to categorize renal parenchymal disease (size, contour, and laterality).

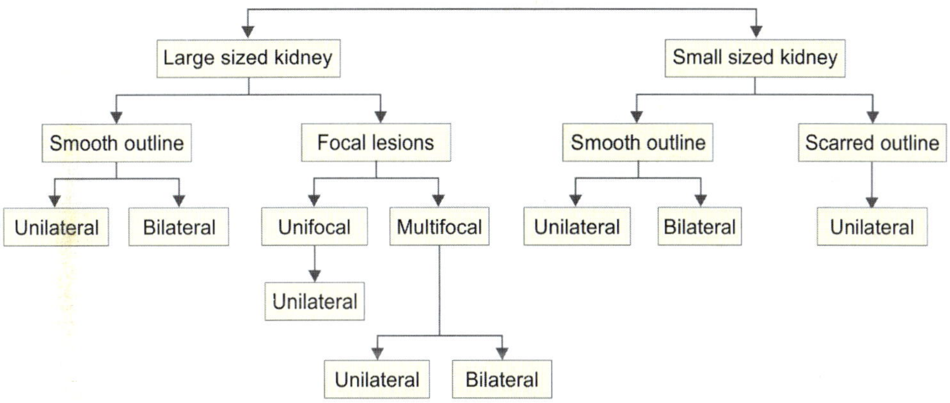

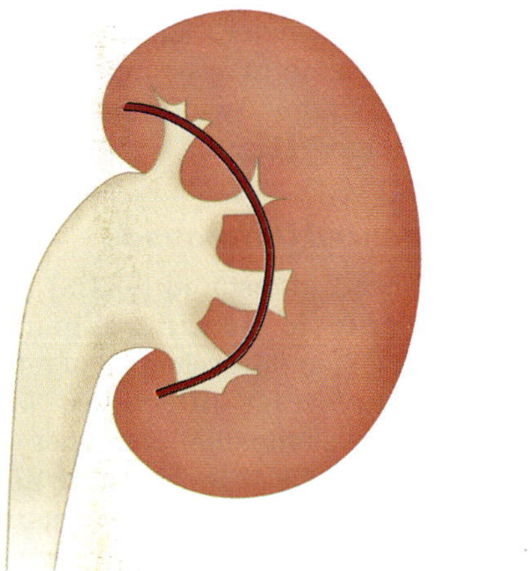

FIG. 1: Schematic diagram of normal interpapillary line. This line is drawn by joining the tips of renal papillae; smooth uninterrupted interpapillary line is seen in normal kidney.

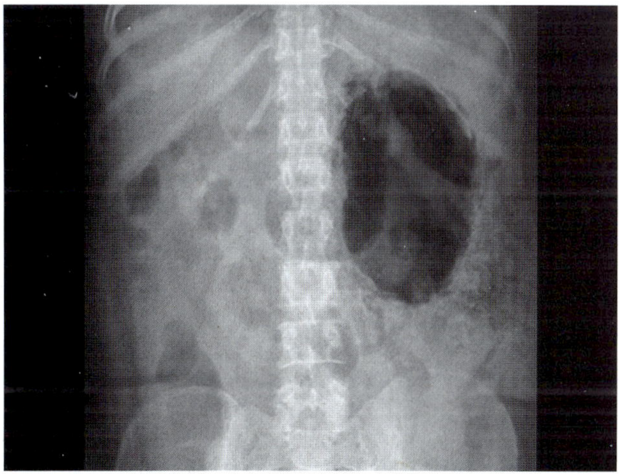

FIG. 2: Extensive gas overlying left renal parenchyma and perinephric space in a case of emphysematous pyelonephritis.

Imaging Techniques

Recent advancements in all the fields of imaging have led to better evaluation of renal diseases and their improved management. Imaging studies performed for evaluating the kidney diseases can provide anatomic, functional, and metabolic information. To reach a diagnosis for a particular case, it is important to know the benefits and the limitations along with the diagnostic yield of each modality.

Plain Radiography and Urography

The plain film also known as KUB (kidney, ureter, and bladder), has been used for years as the first step in the evaluation of the kidneys, however it gives little significant information on its own. Role of plain radiography is to detect renal parenchymal calcification and calculi. In an acute emergency setting, plain X-ray can be used to assess perinephric or retroperitoneal air foci, as seen in cases of emphysematous pyelonephritis **(Fig. 2)**. Renal size and contour may be estimated if the renal outlines can be visualized. Renal size is approximately equal to 3–4 lumbar vertebral body height. Normal kidney measures 10–14 cm in men and 9–13 cm in women on conventional radiography and 1–2 cm less on ultrasonography. Generally, right kidney is smaller than the left by about 0.5 cm. In clinical setting, discrepancy in renal size of more than 2 cm is considered significant.[3] In this era of cross-sectional imaging, urography is more of historic importance; however, interesting abnormal nephrographic patterns present in certain sets of diseases, were described by Fry and Cattell, which are as follows:[7]

- Immediate faint persistent nephrogram—chronic glomerular disease.
- Increasingly dense nephrogram—acute renal obstruction, hypotension, renal ischemia, acute glomerular disease, intratubular obstruction, and acute renal vein thrombosis **(Figs. 3A and B)**.
- Immediate dense persistent nephrogram—ATN and severe inflammatory renal disease.

Striated nephrogram is a variant of obstructive nephrogram which may also be encountered in other conditions like pyelonephritis, polyarteritis nodosa (PAN), trauma, and medullary cystic kidney disease. Prominent cortical nephrons are seen extending into the medulla as "medullary rays".

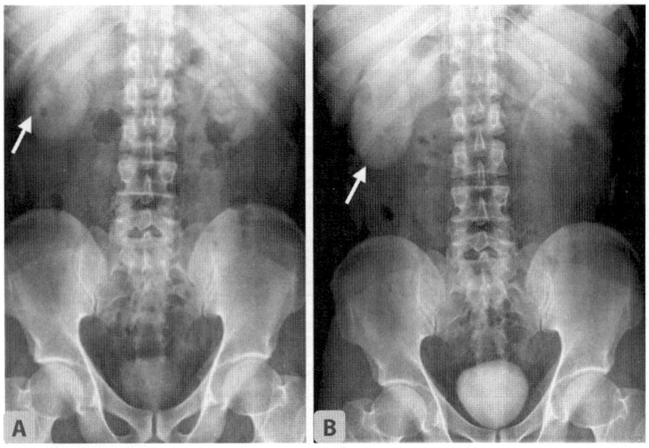

FIGS. 3A AND B: Increasing dense nephrogram. Intravenous urogram shows increased nephrographic density (arrows) on 2-hour film as compared to 5-minute nephrographic phase. Patient had right-sided urinary obstruction because of a small tumor near the right vesicoureteric junction.

Ultrasonography

Ultrasonography is initial imaging modality for azotemia as it is noninvasive and readily differentiates between obstructive (surgical) and nonobstructive (medical) causes of renal failure **(Fig. 4A)**.[6] Renal sizes, cortical thickness, echogenicity of the kidneys, and the presence or absence of hydronephrosis are easily assessed on ultrasonography. Renal size and parenchymal thickness are useful parameters to assess chronicity of renal disease **(Fig. 4B)**. Enlarged kidneys indicate an acute parenchymal lesion while contracted small kidneys suggest a chronic disease. Renal cortical echogenicity is an important indicator for the diagnosis of renal parenchymal disease. Normally the echogenicity of renal cortex is less than liver or spleen; the demonstration of increased echogenicity of the renal cortex under standard scanning techniques may be useful in suggesting the presence of renal parenchymal (medical renal) disease. Renal corticomedullary differentiation (CMD) may be preserved, obliterated or accentuated depending on the severity of renal cortical echoes **(Figs. 4C to F)**.[8,9]

Increased cortical echogenicity with preserved CMD may be seen in glomerulonephritis, nephrosclerosis, amyloidosis, acute leukemia, ATN, and Alport's syndrome while cortical echogenicity is decreased in lymphoma, acute pyelonephritis, and renal vein thrombosis. Increased medullary echotexture is found in gouty nephropathy, medullary nephrocalcinosis, and medullary sponge kidney. Interestingly, some authors recognize the altered state of hydration at the time of scanning as one of determining factors influencing the renal cortical echotexture of the patient.[9,10] An extracapsular hypoechoic rim of edema may surround the kidneys in renal failure. This finding when present is usually bilateral and is called as "kidney sweat sign".[11]

Ultrasound examination is also valuable for assessing the kidneys for follow up of renal parenchymal disease. Changes in renal size, progression as well as resolution of the disease can easily be monitored on ultrasonography.

Color Doppler

Color Doppler is a handy, easily available, and noninvasive tool for evaluation of renal blood vessels. Normal renal arterial branching pattern is well-appreciated on color flow imaging. Assessment of spectral wave pattern and flow indices of renal arteries can be done. Vascular resistance (resistive index: RI) and pulsatility (pulsatility index) along with absolute flow velocities of the main, intralobar, and arcuate arteries may be calculated. Out of these indices RI is most commonly used. It is calculated as:

$$\text{Resistive Index} = \frac{\text{Peak systolic velocity} - \text{Lowest diastolic velocity}}{\text{Peak systolic velocity}}$$

Normal RI is less than 0.7. Parenchymal diseases with tubulointerstitial or vascular involvement cause increased RI (>0.7), while glomerular diseases do not cause any significant increase in this parameter.[12] Elevated RI correlates with the severity of disease in systemic lupus erythematosus (SLE), hemolytic uremic syndrome (HUS), diabetes, and hepatorenal syndrome **(Fig. 5)**.[5]

Contrast-enhanced Ultrasound

Contrast-enhanced ultrasound (CEUS) is an alternative imaging modality to contrast-enhanced computed tomography (CECT) in the evaluation of renal parenchymal diseases, urinary tract infections, and associated complications. The elimination properties of microbubbles through lungs make CEUS an attractive nontoxic imaging modality in renal insufficiency patients. It can also be performed at the bedside in sick patients, and a useful modality in assessing claustrophobic patients and children who cannot tolerate CT or magnetic resonance imaging (MRI) without sedation.

Contrast-enhanced ultrasound showed almost equal sensitivity and specificity to CT in detecting renal parenchymal changes associated with pyelonephritis.[13] CEUS features suggestive of pyelonephritis include peripheral wedge-shaped perfusion defects and heterogeneous enhancement, similar to CECT but without the exposure to radiation. CEUS is also useful in measurement of renal perfusion in AKI, to rule out ischemic perfusion injury, and is more accurate method than Doppler. In postrenal transplant patients with acute rejection, CEUS can detect regional perfusion defects of the allograft.

Computed Tomography

Computed tomography has a specific role in evaluation of renal failure. In acute renal failure noncontrast computed tomography (NCCT) scan of kidneys may show parenchymal calcification. Renal parenchyma, however, appears homogenous in attenuation on NCCT. Various nephrographic patterns are demonstrated after the administration of contrast. Differential diagnosis of the nephrographic patterns used on urography is similarly applied to CT nephrogram. Excretory function can further be assessed on sequential dynamic imaging.[14]

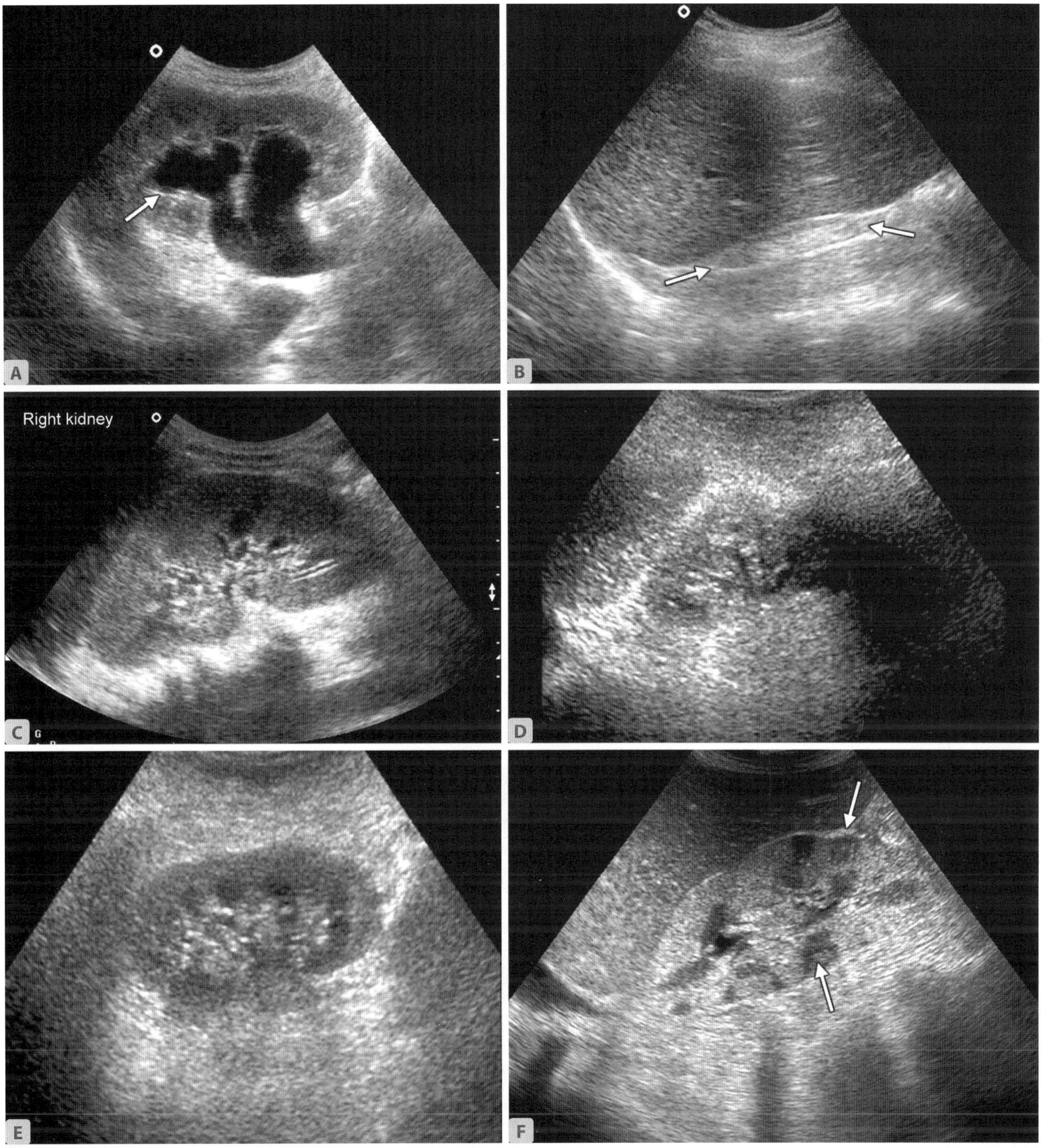

FIGS. 4A TO F: (A) Obstructive renal failure with distal ureteric calculus: Longitudinal ultrasound (US) image depicts marked dilatation of the pelvicalyceal system (arrow). Note the upper ureter is also dilated. (B) Chronic renal failure: US image shows small smooth kidney with markedly decreased renal parenchymal thickness. (C to F) Acute renal parenchymal disease US images. (C) Slightly raised cortical echogenicity and lack of renal corticomedullary differentiation. (D) Markedly increased parenchymal echoes nearing to that of renal sinus resulting in loss of corticomedullary differentiation. (E) Hyperechoic renal cortex, relatively prominent renal medulla with accentuated corticomedullary differentiation. (F) Complicated pyelonephritis with multiple renal abscesses: Severely raised cortical echoes and few hypoechoic well-defined parenchymal lesions (abscesses) (arrows) with right pleural effusion.

Magnetic Resonance Imaging

Routine MRI evaluation of the kidney includes axial and coronal T1-weighted (T1W) and T2-weighted (T2W) spin echo sequences, with or without fat suppression. CMD is distinctly seen on T1W and T2W images. In normal kidney, the cortex is slightly higher in signal intensity than the medulla on T1W images while renal medulla is hyperintense to cortex on T2W images **(Figs. 6A to D)**. In a normal well-hydrated kidney, sharp CMD is seen on T1W sequence due to high signal of cortex as compared to medulla. Wide variety of renal medical diseases cause decrease in cortical signal and subsequent loss of CMD. Loss of CMD on T1W spin echo sequences is a sensitive indicator of parenchymal diseases and correlates with elevated serum creatinine levels >3.0 mg/dL. Dynamic contrast-enhanced T1W sequences can also be done. CMD is lost on postgadolinium dynamic MRI when serum creatinine is >8.5 mg/dL.[15]

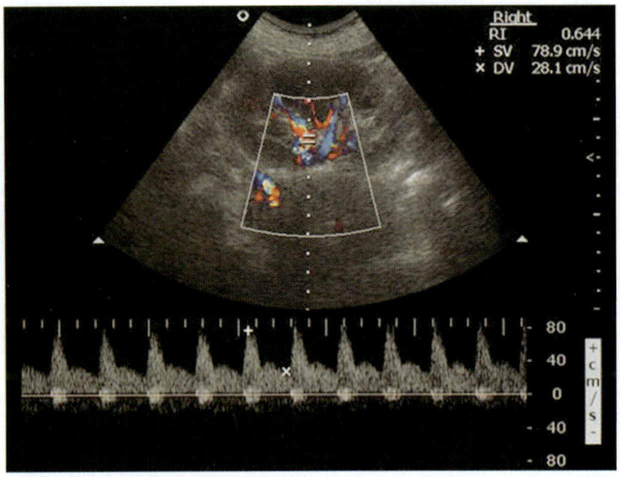

FIG. 5: Normal Doppler ultrasound. Doppler spectra obtained in the area of interlobar arteries show a sharp systolic peak and prominent antegrade flow during diastolic phase. Resistive index in this patient is 0.64, which is normal.

Diffusion-weighted imaging (DWI) is sensitive to changes in the renal interstitium during cellular infiltration or edema, renal fibrosis, and in renal perfusion. The most promising application of DWI so far is in fibrosis estimation in CKD and guidance for biopsy in acute graft dysfunction.[16] Apparent diffusion coefficient (ADC) values correlate with renal function, usually estimated by creatinine values. The cortical ADC values show good correlation with cortical fibrosis and chronic lesions (reduction in ADC values with increasing grade of CKD), however, at present no clear cut-off of ADC values can be chosen to differentiate CKD versus healthy kidney due to limitations in image resolution, protocol variability, and interindividual variability. Diffusion tensor imaging (DTI) is another noninvasive tool to assess renal function with medullary fractional anisotropy values significantly lower in patients with CKD than in healthy controls similar to ADC.[17] Arterial spin labeling (ASL) is a powerful tool for noninvasive measurement of regional renal perfusion in humans, with a typical in plane resolution of 2–3 mm. It uses magnetic labeling of water in arterial blood as an endogenous tracer to generate maps of absolute regional

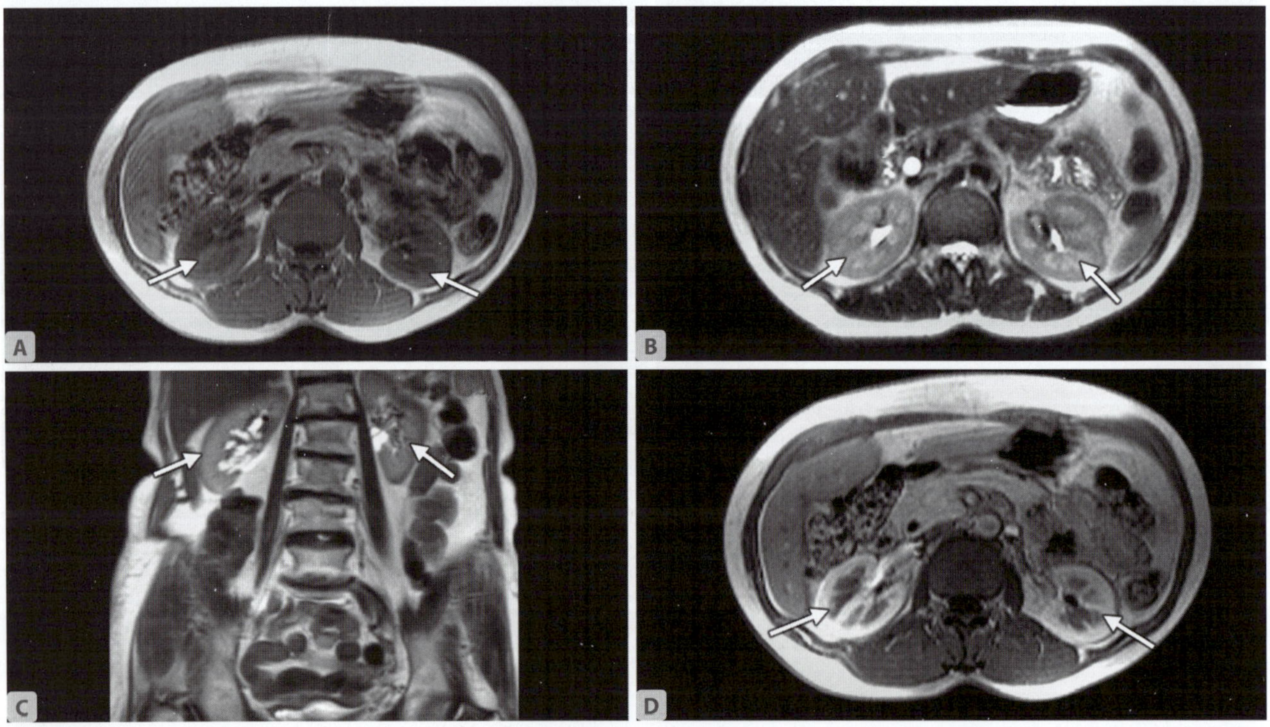

FIGS. 6A TO D: Normal spin echo magnetic resonance imaging findings. (A) T1-weighted axial image shows corticomedullary differentiation resulting from high signal intensity of normal renal cortex and lower signal intensity of renal medulla (arrows). (B and C) T2-weighted axial and coronal magnetic resonance (MR) images depict the hyperintensity of normal renal medulla as compared to renal cortex (arrows). (D) Postgadolinium dynamic MR in cortical phase reveals the striking distinction between renal cortex and medulla (arrows).

perfusion without requiring exogenous contrast. The studies performed so far have shown reproducible measurements of renal perfusion from both renal cortex and medulla, and ASL is highly suited to repeated measurements. The renal perfusion values reduce with increasing stage of CKD and correlates to estimated glomerular filtration rate (eGFR).[18]

Renal Angiography

Renal angiography has limited role in renal parenchymal disease as it is an invasive procedure and usually requires large amount of iodinated contrast medium. Characteristic appearances like aneurysmal dilatation of medium and small-sized vessels on arteriography are seen in conditions like PAN, granulomatosis with polyangiitis, and SLE. Pruned, tortuous vessels with slow flow with thinned renal cortex are demonstrated. Lucent or mottled nephrogram may be seen. Renal artery stenosis is most accurately diagnosed on angiography and can be treated by angioplasty.[19]

Radionuclide Imaging

Scintigraphy provides imaging based diagnostic information on renal structure and function. Radionuclide agents are excreted by kidneys; hence, they should be judiciously employed in patients with renal failure. ^{99m}Tc-DTPA (diethylenetriaminepentaacetic acid) is excreted solely by the glomerular filtration, therefore it should not be used frequently. Tubular secretion of ^{99m}Tc-MAG3 (mercaptoacetyltriglycine) and Hippuran I-131 occurs, hence these may be utilized in severe renal insufficiency.[20]

Contrast-induced Nephropathy

The presence of renal failure may pose some limitations on the choice of an individual imaging modality. Iodinated contrast media may cause exacerbation of renal insufficiency. Contrast-induced nephropathy (CIN) is one of the common causes of hospital-acquired acute renal failure (ARF). The exact mechanism of CIN is still unknown, but it is thought to be multifactorial.[21] CIN is defined as either 0.5 mg/dL (44 µmol/L) increase in absolute serum creatinine value within 48–72 hours or 25% increase in serum creatinine from baseline after administration of intravascular contrast material when no other cause of renal injury is readily apparent.[22] The rise in serum creatinine usually peaks at 3–5 days and return to baseline within 10–14 days. The most important risk factor is pre-existing renal insufficiency (serum creatinine >1.5–2.0 mg/dL), followed by diabetes mellitus, advancing age, congestive heart failure, dehydration, high dose of contrast media, and furosemide. Adequate hydration, dose reduction, and use of nonionic contrast media are recommended as preventive measures.

IMAGING IN RENAL PARENCHYMAL DISEASE

Acute Renal Parenchymal Disease

Radiographic appearance of "bilateral, large, smooth" kidneys is usually seen in the setting of renal failure of recent onset. When obstruction is ruled out a similar picture of enlarged smooth kidneys with normal or effaced collecting system is seen that indicates parenchymal disease of recent origin, which is possibly reversible. **Box 1** and **Table 3** enumerate the causes of renomegaly based on morphological criteria.[4]

However, in some conditions certain characteristic appearances are seen in imaging which shall be discussed in the next section of this chapter. Infections, cystic renal diseases, obstructions, renal vascular diseases, and tumors are not included here as they are covered in other chapters in this book.

Acute Tubular Necrosis

Acute tubular necrosis is the most frequent cause of AKI in the renal category. An acute clinical event with ischemic

BOX 1: Causes of bilateral large smooth kidneys.[5]

- Proliferative/necrotizing disorders
- Acute glomerulonephritis
- Polyarteritis nodosa (microscopic form)
- Systemic lupus erythematosus
- Granulomatosis with polyangiitis
- Allergic angiitis
- Diabetic glomerulosclerosis
- Lung hemorrhage and glomerulonephritis (Goodpasture's syndrome)
- Anaphylactoid purpura (Henoch-Schönlein syndrome)
- Thrombotic thrombocytopenic purpura
- Focal glomerulonephritis associated with subacute bacterial endocarditis
- Plasma cell dyscrasias
- Multiple myeloma
- Waldenstrom's macroglobulinemia
- Amyloidosis
- Abnormal glycogen deposition
- von Gierke's disease (Glycogen storage disease type-I)
- Abnormal lipid deposition
- Fabry's disease
- *Abnormal fluid accumulation:*
    - Acute tubular necrosis
    - Acute cortical necrosis
- Leukemia
- Acute interstitial nephritis
- Acute blockage of tubules
- Acute urate nephropathy
- Tamm-Horsfall protein
- Acute myeloma nephropathy
- Acromegaly
- Nephromegaly associated with cirrhosis, hyperalimentation, and diabetes mellitus
- Hemophilia
- Homozygous-S disease
- Tyrosinosis type I
- Infectious mononucleosis
- Autosomal recessive polycystic kidney disease
- Physiological response to contrast material and diuretics

TABLE 3: Large kidney with focal lesion.[5]

Unifocal unilateral	Multifocal	
	Bilateral	Unilateral
• Simple cyst • Focal hydronephrosis • *Benign neoplasm:* - Adenoma - Mesenchymal tumor - Inflammatory mass • *Malignant neoplasm:* - RCC - Sarcoma - Metastatic deposit	• Autosomal dominant polycystic kidney disease • Lymphoma • Acquired cystic kidney disease	• Multicystic kidney disease Xanthogranulomatous • Pyelonephritis • Malakoplakia

TABLE 4: Etiology of acute tubular necrosis (ATN).

Condition	Underlying mechanisms	Direct causes
Ischemic ATN	Hypovolemic state	Hemorrhage, fluid loss, burns, and fluid sequestration
	Low cardiac output	Cardiac failure and underlying conditions (arrhythmia, myocardial or pericardial diseases)
	Systemic vasodilatation	Sepsis and anaphylaxis
	Disseminated intravascular coagulation	
Nephrotoxic ATN	Exogenous agents	Aminoglycoside-related toxicity, amphotericin B related toxicity, contrast agents (CIN), cyclosporines, sulfa drugs, etc.
	Endogenous agents	Myoglobinuria (rhabdomyolysis) Hemoglobinuria (transfusion reactions) Acute crystal-induced nephropathy Multiple myeloma

(ATN: acute tubular necrosis; CIN: contrast-induced nephropathy)

cascade or nephrotoxic agents **(Table 4)** results in ATN.[23] The multicentric observational study concluded with the ischemic ATN as the presumed etiology for ~50% of patients with renal failure, ~12% related to the unresolved prerenal causes, and ~25% were related to the nephrotoxic agents.[24] Generally, ATN follows a pattern of sequential manifestations including the initiation [reduced GFR, with increased creatinine and blood urea nitrogen (BUN)], maintenance (stabilization of low GFR over 1–2 weeks with increased serum creatinine and BUN), and recovery (polyurea with return of serum creatinine and BUN to preinjury level) phases. When the hypoperfusion overwhelms the renal autoregulatory mechanisms, the tubular cell injury (especially at loop of Henle dipping into the medulla) is initiated, but not always, leading to the cellular death. Ischemia leads to the formation of apical blebs and loss of brush border membrane in proximal tubular cells followed by the loss of cell polarity and integrity of tight junctions resulting in ineffective filtration. Cellular casts block the tubular lumen and adds on to the underlying hypoperfusion complex resulting in decreased GFR. Acute tubule or cell damage resulting from the ischemic or nephrotoxic agents follows almost the similar pattern and the altered pathophysiological events.[25]

Imaging Evaluation

Blood tests and urinalysis along with renal ultrasonography findings are useful in identifying the cause for ATN. In ATN, both kidneys are enlarged (especially anteroposterior dimeter) with prominent medulla and smooth in outline. Contrast-enhanced studies are not recommended in ATN. If intravenous (IV) contrast is inadvertently given, persistent dense nephrogram is seen in neurography which may persist for more than 24 hours. As tubules are filled with cellular infiltrates, contrast leaks into the interstitium through the damaged basement membrane, hence, faint or nonopacification of pelvicalyceal system occurs.

Variable appearances of ATN on ultrasonography have been proposed by different authors, which are:[26]

- Normal cortical and medullary echogenicity—ischemic ATN.
- Increase in cortical echogenicity with maintained CMD—drug-related ATN.
- Normal cortical echogenicity with cchogenic pyramids—associated with precipitation of Tamm-Horsfall protein. Increased RI (>0.7) on Doppler imaging is present in majority of patients with ATN.[27]

Izumi et al.,[28] proved the superior role of Doppler sonography in evaluation as well as follow-up of the ATN subjects in comparison to the prerenal azotemia with the finding of raised RI (>0.75) and obvious reduction of resistive indices in ATN subjects as compared to the subjects with prerenal azotemia.

Bilateral renomegaly with patchy nephrogram is seen on CT scan. Gadolinium-enhanced MRI demonstrates compartmental renal involvement of cortex, inner and outer medulla, and give complementary information about the pathological condition of the kidney. Perfusion abnormalities were also shown in experimentally induced ATN. Blood-oxygen-level-dependent MRI (BOLD MRI) assesses intrarenal oxygen bioavailability which reflects tissue deoxyhemoglobin levels. Ischemia and hypoperfusion in ATN results in reduced tissue oxygen bioavailability which is utilized to discriminate between acute rejection and ATN that may follow renal transplantation.[29]

Acute Cortical Necrosis

Acute cortical necrosis (ACN) is a rare form of acute renal failure which is characterized by ischemic necrosis of renal cortex, including renal column of Bertin with sparing of renal medulla, and thin rim of subcapsular cortex. Both kidneys are involved either diffusely or in patchy distribution; in both instances peripheral renal cortex is spared as it is supplied by the preserved capsular vessels.[5]

More than two-thirds of cases are associated with pregnancy and its complications—abruptio placenta, septic abortion, and placenta previa. Other causes include severe trauma with shock, sepsis, transfusion reaction, severe dehydration, burns, peritonitis, and toxins (e.g. snake venom). Although large numbers of conditions are associated with ACN, the pathophysiology unfortunately remains unclear. Ischemia following vasospasm is probably the initiating event which results due to constriction of small intracortical blood vessels. This may follow exposure to toxins, circulating hormones, or neural stimuli.[30]

Diffuse involvement of both the kidneys may result in complete renal failure requiring either dialysis or transplantation for survival, whereas patchy involvement leads to renal insufficiency.

Imaging Features

Imaging findings depend on the stage of illness. In the acute stage, urographic findings are nonspecific. Kidneys are diffusely enlarged with faint opacification of collecting system. For those surviving the early phase, smooth renal shrinkage occurs over several months. Radiographically, distinctive tram-like or egg shell calcification of cortex may be seen which starts appearing as early as 24 days after the onset of disease.

On ultrasonography, enlargement of both kidneys and loss of the normal CMD with a circumferential hypoechoic zone corresponding to the necrotic cortex is seen. Ultrasound is useful for follow-up. Calcification of cortex causes dense cortical echoes with distal acoustic shadowing.

Specific appearance of ACN is described on CECT scan. The three diagnostic features are (a) enhancement of the medulla, (b) nonenhancement of the renal cortex, and (c) lack of excretion of contrast medium into the collecting system. Enhanced subcapsular cortex, the distinctive "Cortical rim sign" on CECT scan suggests the sparing of the most peripheral region of renal cortex **(Figs. 7A and B)**. "Cortical rim sign" is also seen in other conditions which result in hemodynamic derangement like renal infarction, renal vein thrombosis, and ATN.[31-33]

Magnetic resonance imaging also shows these representative findings. Kidneys are enlarged in the early phase. Low signal intensity of the inner renal cortex and the columns of Bertin on every MRI sequence is the major characteristic finding of renal cortical necrosis. Swelling of

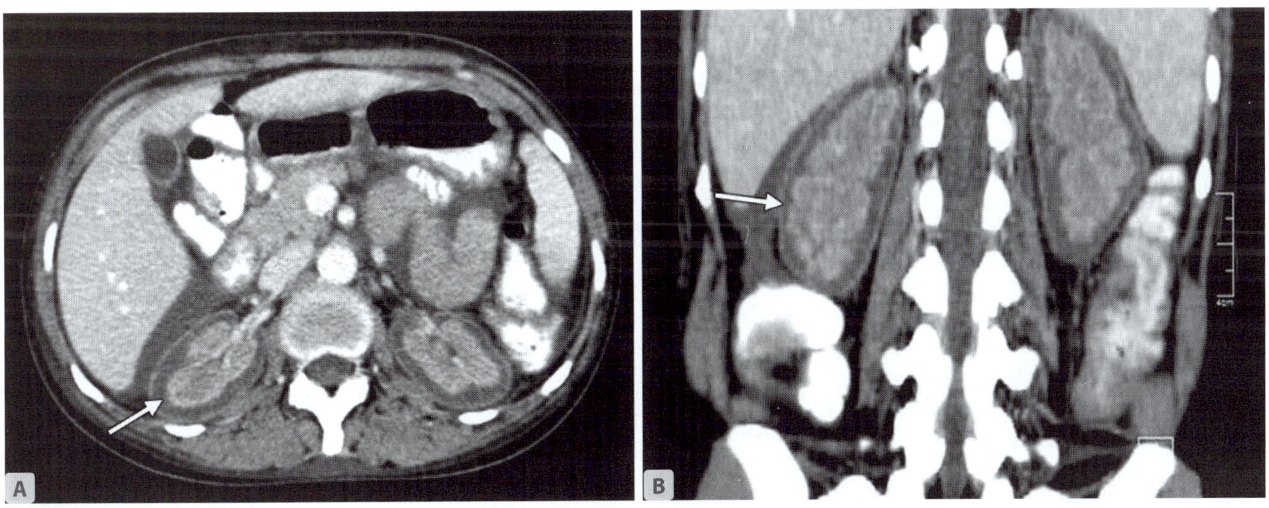

FIGS. 7A AND B: Acute cortical necrosis in a female patient with septic abortion: Axial and coronal postcontrast computed tomography scans (corticomedullary phase) demonstrate the absence of contrast enhancement in the cortex and relatively hyperdense medulla and subcapsular cortex, the characteristic "cortical rim sign".

both kidneys with increased signal intensity of the cortex on T2W images instead of T1W images is another feature of renal cortical necrosis at MRI. Later a thin rim of low signal intensity (T1WI and T2WI) may be seen along the border of kidneys due to calcification.[34]

Leukemia

Leukemia (predominantly lymphocytic leukemia) is the most common malignant cause of bilateral renal enlargement in children. Renal enlargement occurs due to infiltration of kidneys by leukemic cells. Usually, markedly large kidneys are seen, however, sometimes asymmetrical renal involvement or focal renal mass may be seen **(Figs. 8A and B)**.

Imaging Features

In leukemic infiltration of kidney, the nephrogram is faint and the collecting system is attenuated. Pelvicalyceal system is often filled with blood clots or uric acid stones which appear as filling defects.[20]

Acute Interstitial Nephritis

Acute interstitial nephritis (AIN) is an acute hypersensitivity reaction, mediated through immunologic mechanisms. It may result following an exposure to drugs, nonrenal infection (e.g. infectious mononucleosis, *legionella*, and leptospirosis), systemic autoimmune disorders (SLE, Sjögren's syndrome, and sarcoidosis), and tubulointerstitial nephritis and uveitis (TINU syndrome). However, an idiopathic variety is also described. The most common cause of AIN are drugs particularly—antibiotics (methicillin, penicillin, and amphotericin), Nonsteroidal anti-inflammatory drugs (NSAIDs), sulfonamides, phenytoin, and thiazide.[35]

Fever, skin rashes, eosinophilia, oliguria, and proteinuria are the common clinical signs and symptoms of drug-induced AIN which appear between 5 days and 5 weeks of exposure. Patient recovers with the withdrawal of the causative agent.[36]

Imaging Features

Bilateral renomegaly with diminished to normal opacification of collecting system is seen on urography. Ultrasound shows increased cortical echogenicity with renal enlargement. Enhanced uptake of Gallium citrate in the kidneys on renal scintigraphy is also reported.[35] CT shows low attenuation areas in the cortex and corticomedullary junctions **(Fig. 9)**. Kidneys may become shrunken and irregular as the disease progresses to a chronic course. Calcification of renal papillae may occur in analgesic-induced nephritis. Interstitial fibrosis leads to low signal intensity of renal cortex on T1W MRI.

Amyloidosis

Amyloidosis is a diverse group of diseases that have extracellular deposition and accumulation of an insoluble fibrillar proteinaceous substance with a beta sheath configuration, which is characteristically appreciated as

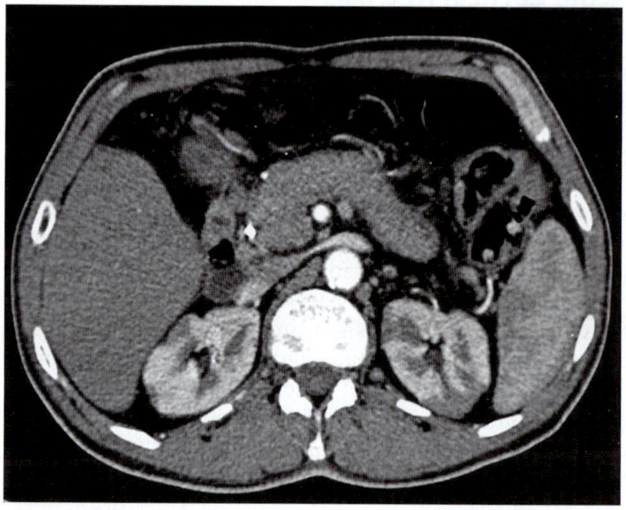

FIG. 9: Acute interstitial nephritis in a case of autoimmune pancreatitis. Multifocal hypodense areas in the cortex of bilateral kidneys.

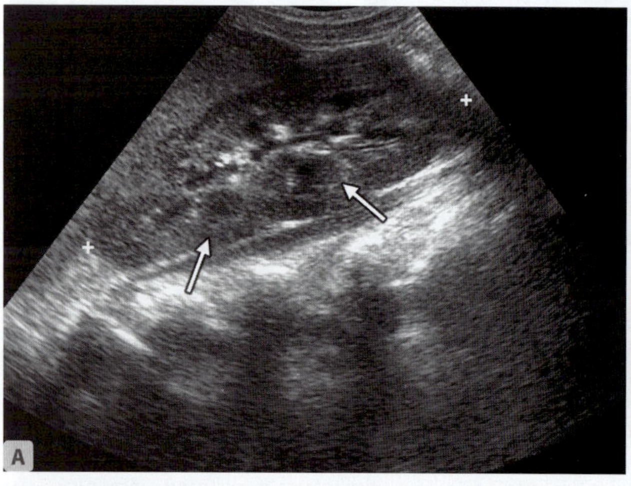

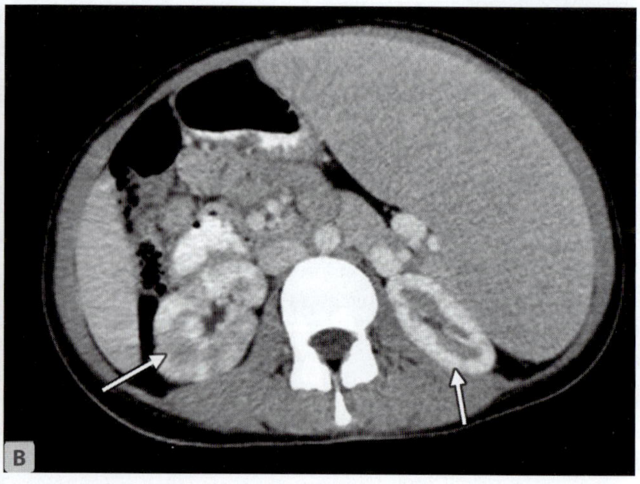

FIGS. 8A AND B: Renal manifestation of leukemia. (A) Ultrasonography of kidney shows focal, well-defined, and hypoechoic masses; (B) Contrast-enhanced CT axial image in another patient also shows bilateral, multiple, and focal hypodensities suggestive of leukemic deposits. Massive splenomegaly is also seen.

apple green birefringence on congo red staining and when viewed under polarized light.

Amyloidosis can be classified as follows:[37]

- *Primary amyloidosis*: Usually called as primary light chain (AL) amyloidosis resulting from the B-cell or plasma cell dysplasia. Usually involves renal and cardiac organs with poor prognosis. Rarely heavy chain associated amyloidosis is also seen accounting for ~4–6% with no cardiac involvement explaining the good prognosis in affected subjects.
- *Secondary amyloidosis*: Secondary amyloidosis [amyloid-associated disease (AA)] is usually associated with chronic inflammatory conditions such as rheumatoid arthritis, Crohn's disease, tuberculosis, bronchiectasis, and chronic osteomyelitis.

Secondary amyloidosis is more prevalent and more common in underdeveloped countries whereas primary amyloidosis is the most common type of amyloidosis in the Western hemisphere. Other rare familial and senile forms and dialysis-related amyloidosis have also been described.

Older men are more affected than women,[38] usually presenting with nonspecific symptoms like weight loss, fatigue, and weakness. Multiorgan involvement is present in more than 85% of cases. Kidney is affected in 80% patients with secondary amyloidosis and 35–40% patients with primary disease. Isolated involvement of the renal pelvis, ureter bladder, urethra, prostate seminal vesicle, and retroperitoneum can occur.[39]

Imaging Features

Based on the extent of involvement, amyloidosis can also be classified as systemic and localized forms of disease. In acute phase, bilateral renal enlargement is seen. Decrease in size occurs with progression of disease process, smooth outline is, however, maintained. Nephrogram is diminished with variable excretion into normal pelvicalyceal system. Cortical echogenicity is raised as seen in other parenchymal diseases. Rapid deterioration in renal function or sudden onset nephrotic syndrome indicates renal vein thrombosis, a complication of amyloidosis. Thrombosed renal vein is demonstrated on color Doppler, CT scan or MRI. Perinephric soft tissue mass with retroperitoneal and mesenteric extension is seen. CT examination depicts the extent of soft tissue involvement as well as calcification changes resulting from the amyloid proteinaceous material.

Magnetic resonance imaging shows reduced cortical signal intensity on T1W images with subsequent loss of CMD. Bilateral increased delayed uptake of Gallium 67 when other causes of abnormal gallium activity are excluded.[39]

Amyloidosis of renal pelvis-isolated involvement of renal pelvis can occur in amyloidosis. Interesting radiological appearance of calcification or ossification in the amyloid deposits may be seen. These deposits are usually located in the submucosa of the pelvicalyceal system. A lucent band of mucosa separates the IV contrast density from calcification in the pelvis on intravenous urogram (IVU). Other causes for calcification of pelvicalyceal system are tuberculosis, leukoplakia, primary carcinoma of renal pelvis, and renal calculus. Submucosal amyloid deposits appear hypointense on T1W and T2W magnetic resonance images.

Localized forms of amyloidosis are also encountered in the urinary bladder and lower ureter which may mimic chronic granulomatous (tubercular and schistosomiasis) and neoplastic conditions of these organs. It is extremely important to differentiate the systemic form of involvement from the localized variety as therapeutic approaches vary based on the involvement. Biopsy of renal tissue or extra renal tissue, bone marrow biopsy, and urinalysis will aid in establishing and guiding in management of these conditions.

Multiple Myeloma

Multiple myeloma is a plasma cell disorder which originates in the bone marrow and is characterized by involvement of the skeleton at multiple sites. The neoplastic plasma cells produce excess immunoglobulins (Igs) and Bence Jones proteins are characteristically present in the urine. Multiple pathogenic mechanisms contribute to renal injury/failure in multiple myeloma, which include abnormal protein precipitation in renal tubules, secondary to nephrotoxic monoclonal Ig and independent of paraprotein deposition. Myeloma kidney or cast nephropathy is a form of monoclonal Ig-mediated kidney disease. The mechanism of renal injury in myeloma and plasm cell dyscrasias can be broadly classified into monoclonal Ig-dependent and independent **(Table 5)**.[40]

Nausea, vomiting, anorexia, weight loss, and progressive weakness are the presenting features. Nephrocalcinosis resulting from hypercalcemia, uric acid calculi, renal infections, and amyloidosis may further complicate the illness.

Imaging Features

Imaging features are nonspecific and depends on the mechanism of renal injury. The most frequently reported renal manifestation at imaging are perinephric nodules and masses, however, can also present as focal renal masses. Positron emission tomography (PET) CT can demonstrate diffuse medullary and extramedullary (including kidneys) manifestations. Active myeloma lesions show intense FDG (fluorodeoxyglucose) activity unlike renal cell carcinomas (mild FDG activity), which helps to distinguish. Due to Ig independent mechanism of involvement in certain cases, it may present as medical renal disease on imaging, and ultrasonography shows nephromegaly with reduced cortical echotexture initially, followed by increased cortical echogenicity, progressive loss of CMD, and renal atrophy in later stages.[41] Injection of iodinated contrast media is hazardous in patients of multiple myeloma as it precipitates myeloma proteins in the renal tubules. Dehydration has to be avoided to reduce the risk of complications.

Paroxysmal Nocturnal Hemoglobinuria

Paroxysmal Nocturnal Hemoglobinuria (PNH) is a very rare, acquired hematopoietic stem cell disorder caused by an increased sensitivity to complement, resulting in intravascular hemolysis. The complement-mediated

TABLE 5: Mechanism of renal injury in myeloma and plasma cell dyscrasias.[40]

Mechanism	Details
Ig-dependent mechanisms	
Cast nephropathy (known traditionally as myeloma kidney)	Risk factors include light chain myeloma with >10 g/day monoclonal Ig excretion, volume depletion, sepsis, and medications (see below); Ig deposition is primarily in the tubules
Monoclonal Ig deposition disease	Systemic syndrome may be present; Ig deposition can be in the tubules or glomeruli but generally not both
Light chain amyloidosis (AL)	Often associated with nephrotic-range albuminuria and λ-light chains; systemic syndrome may be present, and amyloid deposition is primarily in the glomeruli
GN	Membranoproliferative, diffuse proliferative, crescentic, and cryoglobulinemic all recognized
Tubulointerstitial nephritis	May also result from non-Ig mechanisms
Thrombotic microangiopathy (TMA)	Paraprotein causes endothelial injury with resulting TMA
Hyperviscosity syndrome	More common in cases of IgA, IgG3, or IgM myeloma
Ig-independent mechanisms	
Volume depletion	Can cause prerenal azotemia and acute tubular necrosis and/or contribute to cast nephropathy
Sepsis	
Hypercalcemia	Can cause AKI directly or contribute to cast nephropathy
Tumor lysis syndrome	Uric acid or phosphate nephropathy
Direct parenchymal invasion by plasma cells	Rare cause; associated with advanced or aggressive myeloma
Pyelonephritis	Rare cause; multifactorial from immunodeficiency and deficient Ig and chemotherapy from myeloma

(Ig: immunoglobulin; GN: glomerulonephritis; AKI: acute kidney injury)

erythrocyte damage results in hemolysis with release of hemoglobin in plasma, which passes through glomeruli and reabsorbed in the proximal tubules, and stored as hemosiderin. This can result in chronic renal failure due to repeated episodes of microvascular thrombosis and tubular damage from hemosiderin deposition. Hemolysis is precipitated by infections, drugs immunization, and exercise. Patient presents with hemoglobinuria, iron deficiency anemia, and venous thrombosis.

Imaging Features

Noncontrast computed tomography may show high density of renal cortex due to hemosiderin pigments. Paramagnetic effects of hemosiderin results in markedly reduced signal in the cortex in both T1W and T2W images. Changes are more pronounced on T2W sequences with signal intensity of the renal cortex lower than that of the medulla, causing reversed CMD. Similar imaging features are seen in intravascular hemolysis like in malfunctioning prosthetic valves, sickle cell anemia, hereditary spherocytosis, and thalassemia.[42]

Chronic Renal Parenchymal Disease

In contrast to the capacity of kidney to regain back its function following acute renal insult, renal injury of more prolonged nature often leads to progressive and irreversible loss of nephrons. Such reduction in renal mass subsequently results in bilaterally small smooth kidneys. The uremic kidney shrinks globally reflecting the inherent tissue loss. Renal contour may be smooth or irregular. The echogenicity can be normal or increased. Radiological features, like those in acute renal parenchymal disease are overlapping in most of the causes of chronic renal parenchymal disease. However, some conditions show interesting radiological appearances and are discussed here. The various causes of bilateral small smooth kidneys are listed in **Flowchart 2**, the conditions leading to morphologically small, unilateral kidneys are also cited.[4] **Figures 10 to 13** show imaging in cases of chronic renal failure.

Renal Papillary Necrosis

Renal papillary necrosis is not a specific clinical entity, rather it is a manifestation of multiple renal pathological conditions resulting in prolonged sustained hypoxic injury to the medulla. Necroses of the renal papillae not only have many causes but also many radiological forms. Parenchymal diseases affecting the papillae and calyces are diagnosed on urography. In mild cases, the kidney size and function are normal, and the abnormality is limited to the papillae only. In advanced disease, there is global shrinkage of kidney with impaired renal function. Most common cause of renal papillary necrosis is analgesic abuse nephropathy. Other causes are diabetes, sickle cell nephropathy, obstruction with infection, renal vein thrombosis, dehydration, and prolonged hypotension.[5] (Pneumonic to remember causes of renal papillary necrosis—ADIPOSE: Analgesic nephropathy, diabetes, infant in shock, pyelonephritis, obstruction, sickle cell disease, and ethanol). In early papillary necrosis, ischemia occurs in the renal papillae due to compression of the medullary vessels by inflammatory changes in the interstitium. If the phase of temporary spasm passes, normal circulation is restored and the involved tissues may recover. However, if ischemia continues and perfusion is not restored, irreversible coagulation necrosis, tubular fibrosis, and lobar infarcts result.

Urographic findings during this period of early ischemic change are usually normal. On multidetector computed tomography, the ischemic changes that lead to renal papillary necrosis can be demonstrated best on nephrographic phase as small, poorly marginated areas of diminished enhancement at the tip of the medullary pyramid.

In advanced stage of necrosis, clefts originate from the fornices and extend to the medullary pyramids and papillae, ultimately causing the papillae to slough **(Fig. 14)**.

FLOWCHART 2: Causes of small kidney.

- Smooth
  - Unilateral
    - Ischemia due to focal arterial disease
    - Chronic infarction
    - Renal vein thrombosis (late)
    - Radiation nephritis
    - Congenital hypoplasia
    - Postobstructive atrophy
    - Postinflammatory atrophy
    - Reflux atrophy
    - Partial nephrectomy
  - Bilateral
    - Generalized arteriosclerosis
    - Benign and malignant nephrosclerosis
    - Atheroembolic renal disease
    - Chronic glomerulonephritis
    - Papillary necrosis
    - Hereditary nephropathies
    - Hereditary chronic nephritis (Alport's syndrome)
    - Medullary cystic disease
    - Amyloidosis (late)
    - Arterial hypotension
    - Cortical necrosis (late)
- Scarred unilateral
  - Reflux nephropathy
  - Lobar infarction

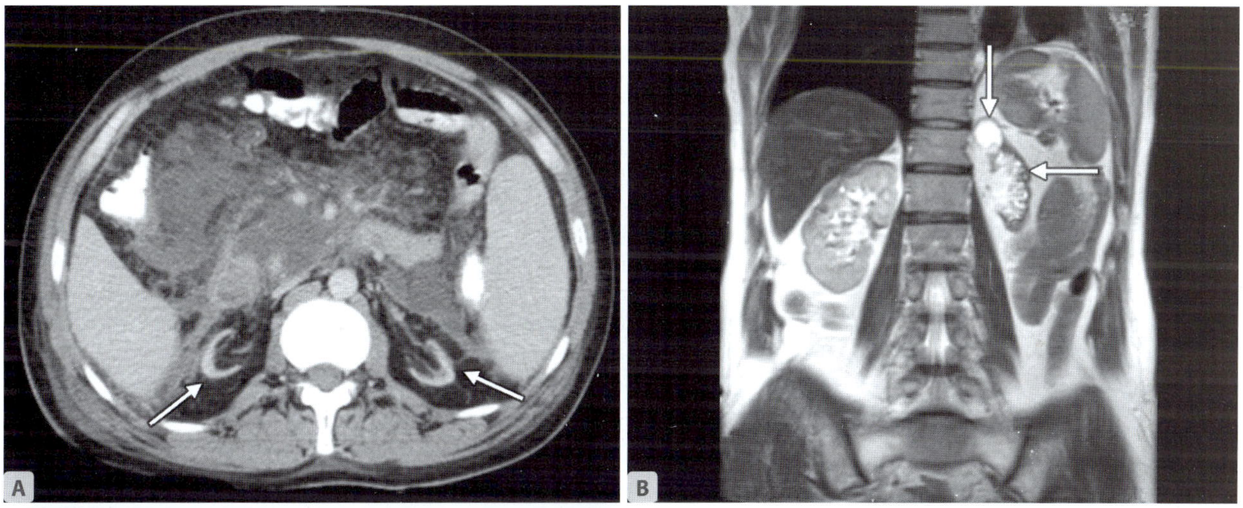

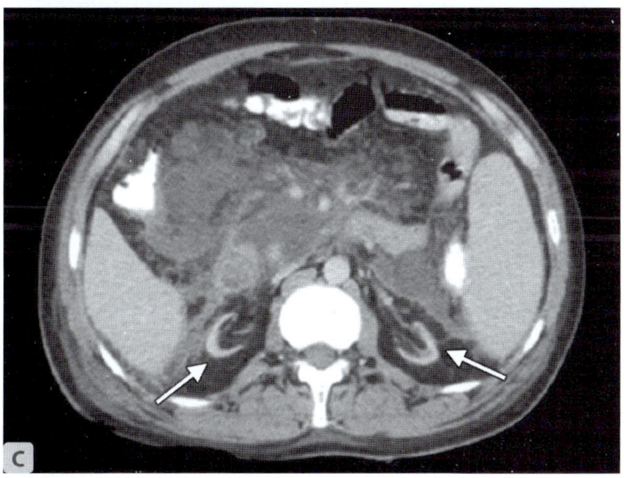

FIGS. 10A TO C: End-stage renal disease. CECT axial image shows bilateral smooth shrunken kidneys in a patient of chronic renal failure with pancreatitis. Peripancreatic inflammatory fluid collections are also present.

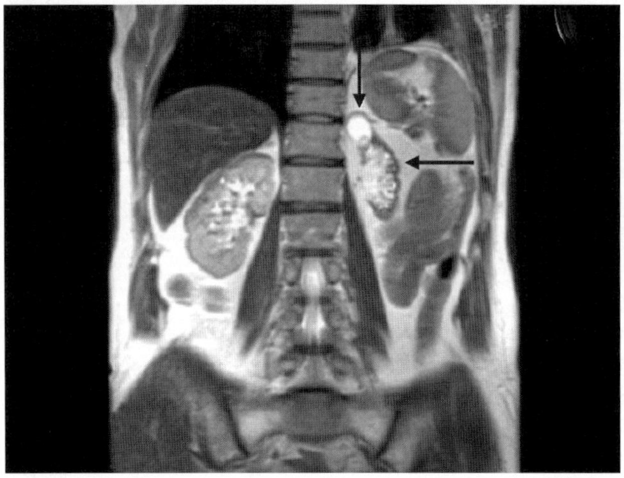

FIG. 11: Unilateral small smooth kidney. T2-weighted coronal MR image reveals small, contracted left kidney with thinned renal parenchyma and indistinct corticomedullary differentiation, subsequent to left renal artery stenosis (arrow). Note made of simple cortical renal cyst in left upper pole (short arrow).

Caliceal deformities in renal papillary necrosis occur in three forms:

1. *Medullary*: Central necrosis takes place at the tip of the pyramid. Detachment of necrotic papillae starts in the central part of the calix, opening into a round or oval cavity.
2. *Papillary*: Detachment of necrotic papillae usually begins in the region of the caliceal fornices, and the resulting defect is triangular in shape also termed as lobster claw appearance.
3. *In situ*: When papillae fail to separate (necrosis *in situ*) calyces appear normal, they later calcify to give appearance of nephrocalcinosis.

In the healing phase, the papilla may epithelialize, and its tip takes a blunted appearance. In addition, shrinkage of the kidney may occur with reduction of parenchymal thickness. This is the common sequel of renal papillary necrosis. Moreover, the loss of renal cortex is associated hypertrophy of the renal columns resulting in a typical irregular wavy renal outline.[43] In advanced disease, after the sloughing of

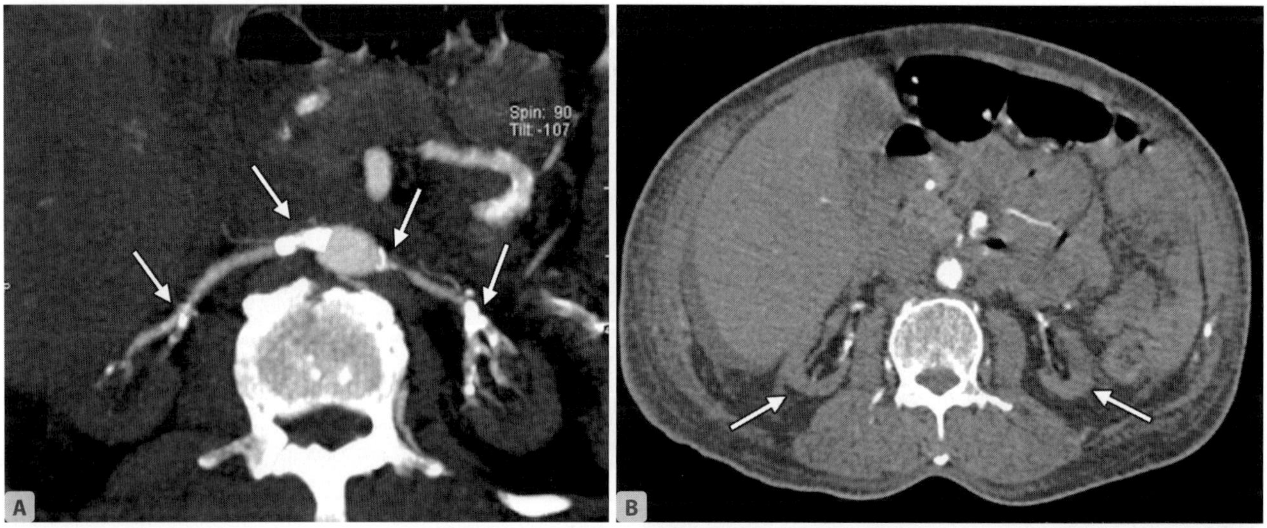

FIGS. 12A AND B: Bilateral small smooth kidneys. CT angiography. (A) shows calcified atherothrombotic plaques involving both main renal arteries and their ostia (B) smooth globally shrunken kidneys, in a patient of severe bilateral renal artery stenosis. Mild perihepatic fluid is seen.

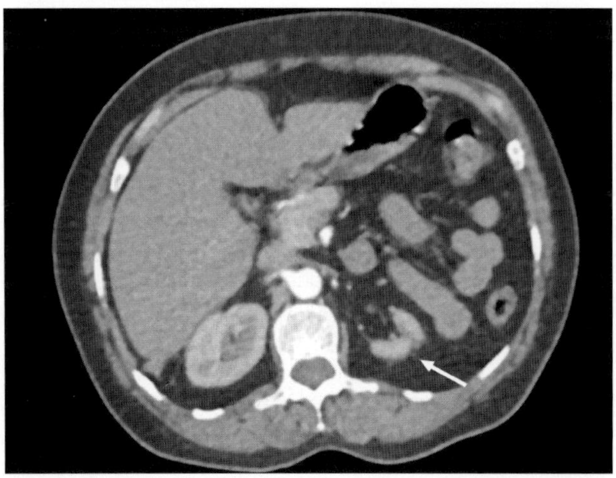

FIG. 13: Unilateral small scarred kidney. CECT axial image in cortical phase of enhancement shows small left kidney with irregular outline with parenchymal defect at interpolar region.

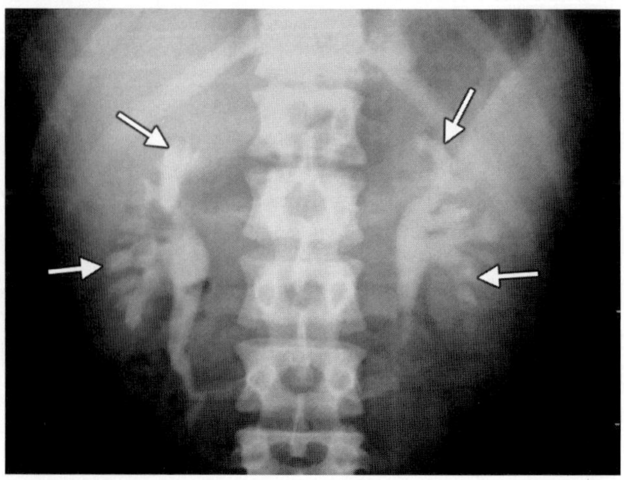

FIG. 14: Renal papillary necrosis. Intravenous urogram film showing irregular and distorted calyces of both kidneys, with contrast excavation and formation of multiple cavities. Few amputated calyces are also seen.

necrotic papillae, cavities are seen that are continuous with calyces in renal medullary areas. Their differentiation with other cystic lesions in the renal medullae should be done (like hydronephrosis, congenital megacalyces, parapelvic cysts, and caliceal diverticula).[44]

Benign and Malignant Nephrosclerosis

Nephrosclerosis affects the renal arterioles. The disease courses over many years but it rarely leads to kidney failure on its own. Malignant nephrosclerosis, however, progresses very rapidly and damages the arteries. These damaged arteries are unable to provide enough oxygen to the kidney tissues, resulting in kidney failure. The incidence of hypertensive nephrosclerosis increases with advancing age.[45]

Imaging Features

Kidneys are small and smooth in benign nephrosclerosis; occasionally shallow infarcts can be seen. Normal nephrographic opacification, and excretion into pelvicalyceal system is seen on urography.

On ultrasonography, increased central sinus echogenicity due to fat deposition may be seen. Subcapsular and perirenal hemorrhages may be detected as hypoechoic or anechoic fluid collections. High density fluid (blood) can be better detected on noncontrast CT scan. Blood degradation product may also be identified on MRI.[46]

Renal Osteodystrophy

Renal osteodystrophy is complex musculoskeletal abnormalities seen in patients with CKD. The primary radiologic bone changes reflect:

- *Deficiency in active form of vitamin D due to impaired renal function:* Rickets.
- *Impaired clearance of calcium leading to increased parathormone secretion:* Secondary hyperparathyroidism.

The spectrum consists of secondary hyperparathyroidism along with rickets, osteomalacia, osteosclerosis, and osteoporosis.

Inability of the kidney to adequately excrete phosphate, leads to hyperphosphatemia and increased osteoclastic activity. It can be categorized by resorption of bone at subperiosteal, cortical, subchondral, trabecular, endosteal, and subligamentous locations. Radiographic appearance of subperiosteal resorption has been described as a lace-like irregularity of the normal cortical margin, which may progress to areas of scalloping and spiculation. The earliest involvement is often seen along the radial aspects of the middle phalanges of the index and middle fingers, beginning in the proximal metaphyseal region. The terminal tufts may also demonstrate subperiosteal resorption **(Fig. 15)**. Additional sites of subperiosteal bone resorption include the upper medial tibia, humerus, and femur; superior and inferior ribs; and lamina dura.

Loss of trabecular sharpness occurs with trabecular resorption. This is well seen in the skull, described as a granular salt-and-pepper appearance, with loss of distinction between the inner and outer tables. Common sites of subchondral resorption are the distal clavicle and acromioclavicular joint, sacroiliac joint, sternoclavicular joint, symphysis pubis, and posterior patella **(Figs. 16A and B)**.[14] Osseous resorption may also occur at sites of ligamentous and tendinous attachments. Brown tumors are rare.

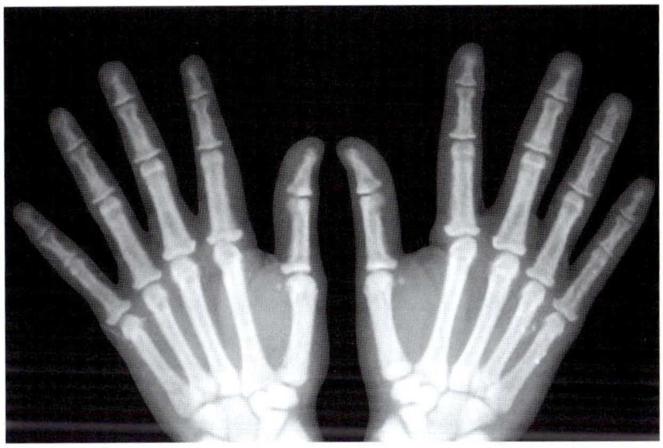

FIG. 15: Radiographs of hands in a patient of hyperparathyroidism in renal osteotrophy. Characteristic subperiosteal resorption phalanges including terminal tufts is seen. Subchondral and intracortical resorptions are also seen.

Osteosclerosis has a strong predilection for the axial skeleton, where cancellous bone predominates over cortical bone. In the vertebral bodies, band-like areas of sclerosis involving the superior and inferior end plates with intervening normal osseous density are classically seen, which resemble the stripes on rugby jerseys called as rugger jersey spine.

Changes of rickets can be seen in children with a general delay in bone age, bowing of long bones, scoliosis, diffuse concave impressions at multiple vertebral end plates, basilar invagination of the skull, "triradiate pelvis" deformity, and rachitic rosary. In children, epiphyseal displacement (slipped epiphysis) in children is also seen. Osteomalacia in adults may manifest as looser zones. Metastatic soft tissue and vascular calcification can be seen in ocular tissues, arteries, subcutaneous and periarticular soft tissues, and viscera.[47]

CONCLUSION

Imaging and management of medical renal diseases and renal failure continues to evolve with the advances in anatomical and functional imaging. Despite these achievements radiological imaging still has limitations in evaluation of renal parenchymal disease and renal failure. Radiological imaging techniques are rapidly expanding and are expected to grow even further, predominantly in advanced MRI. The future possibly holds improved methods to readily identify the causes of reversible acute renal failure and plan treatment strategies to combat chronic renal failure. The combination of better diagnostic methods and management strategies will lead to improved quality of life in patients with renal failure.

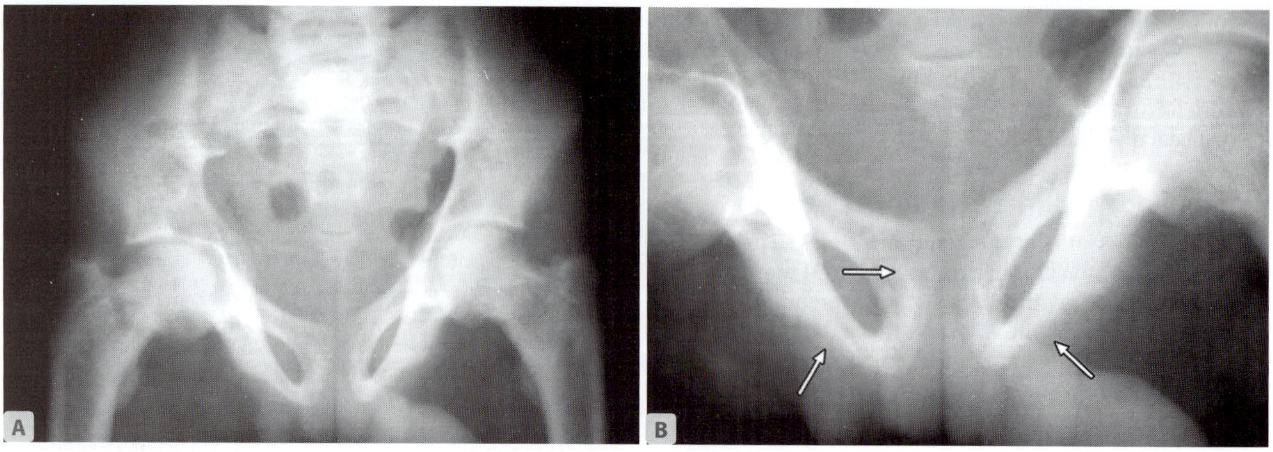

FIGS. 16A AND B: Renal osteodystrophy in a patient of tuberculosis. Anteroposterior view of pelvis shows osteopenic triradiate pelvis. Subchondral resorption of bone is seen at the pubis symphysis, ischial tuberosities, and sacroiliac joint (arrows).

REFERENCES

1. Mehta RL, Kellum JA, Shah SV, et al. Acute Kidney Injury Network: report of an initiative to improve outcomes in acute kidney injury. Crit Care. 2007;11:R31.
2. Choyke PL, Zeiessman HA. Imaging of renal failure. In: Pollack HM, McClennan BL (Eds). Clinical Urography, 2nd edition. Philadelphia, PA: WB Saunders; 2000. pp. 3029-31.
3. National Kidney Foundation: K/DOQ1 Clinical practice guidelines for chronic kidney diseases: evaluation, classification, stratification. Am J Kidney Dis. 2002;39(1):S1-266.
4. Friedenberg RM, Dunbar JS. Excretory urography. In: Pollack HM, McClennan BL (Eds). Clinical Urography, 1st edition, Philadelphia, PA: WB Saunders; 1990. pp. 2264-76, 100-245.
5. Davidson AJ, Hartman DS. A systemic approach to Radiological Diagnosis of Renal Parenchymal Disease. In: Davidson AJ, Hartman DS (Eds). Radiology of Kidney and Urinary Tract, 2nd edition. Philadelphia, PA: WB Saunders; 1990. pp. 101-243.
6. Kim SH, Kim B. Renal Parenchymal Disease. In: Pollack HM, McClennan BL (Eds), Clinical Urography, 2nd edition. Philadelphia, PA: WB Saunders; 2000. pp. 2654-84.
7. Fry IK, Cattell WR. The nephrographic pattern during excretion urography. Br Med Bull. 1972;28:227-32.
8. Ritche WW, Vick CW, Glocheski SK, et al. Evaluation of azotemic patients: diagnostic yield of initial US examination. Radiology. 1998;167:245-7.
9. Hungtington DK, Hill SC, Hill MC. Sonographic manifestations of medical renal disease. Semin Ultrasound CT MR. 1991;12:290-307.
10. Manley JA, O'Neill C. How echogenic is echogenic? Quantitative acoustics of the renal cortex. Am J Kidney Dis. 2001;37:706-11.
11. Yasa NA, Peng M, Ralls PW. Perirenal lucency ('Kidney sweat'): A new sign of renal failure. AJR. 1999;173:1075-9.
12. Platt JF, Ellis JH, Rubin JM, et al. Intrarenal arterial Doppler sonography in patients with non-obstructive renal disease: correlation of resistive index with biopsy findings. AJR. 1990;157:1223-7.
13. Mitterberger M, Pinggera GM, Colleselli D, et al. Acute pyelonephritis: comparison of diagnosis with computed tomography and contrast enhanced ultrasonography. BJU Int. 2007;101(3):341-4.
14. Saunder HS, Dyer BB, Shlfrin RY, et al. The CT nephrogram: implications of evaluation of urinary tract disease. Radiographics. 1995;15:1069-95.
15. Chung JJ, Semelka RC, Martin DR. Acute renal failure: common occurrences of preservation of corticomedullary differentiation on MR images. Magn Reson Imaging. 2001;19:789-93.
16. Caroli A, Schneider M, Friedli I, et al. Diffusion-weighted magnetic resonance imaging to assess diffuse renal pathology: a systematic review and statement paper. Nephrol Dial Transplant. 2018;33(Suppl 2):ii29-40.
17. Saini S, Kumar V, Koteshwara P, et al. Role of diffusion tensor imaging in renal parenchymal changes. Indian J Radiol Imaging. 2018;28(2):175-81.
18. Odudu A, Nery F, Harteveld AA, et al. Arterial spin labelling MRI to measure renal perfusion: a systematic review and statement paper. Nephrol Dial Transplant. 2018;33(Suppl 2):ii15-21.
19. Abrams HA, Grassi CJ. Renal angiography in hypertension. In: Baums (Ed). Abrams Angiography: Vascular and Interventional Radiology, 4th edition. Boston: Little, Brown and Company; 1997. pp. 1244-89.
20. Maisey M, Briton KE. Nuclear Imaging in Nephrology. In: Davidson AM, Cameron JS, Grunfeld JP, et al. In: Oxford Textbook of Clinical Nephrology, 2nd edition. Oxford: Oxford University Press; 1998. pp. 137-50.
21. Barrett BJ, Cariske EJ. Meta-analysis of relative nephrotoxicity of high- and low-osmolality iodinated contrast media. Radiology. 1993;188:171-8.
22. Fliser D, Laville M, Covic A, et al; Ad-hoc working group of ERBP. A European Renal Best Practice (ERBP) position statement on the Kidney Disease Improving Global Outcomes (KDIGO) clinical practice guidelines on acute kidney injury: part 1: definitions, conservative management and contrast-induced nephropathy. Nephrol Dial Transplant. 2012;27(12):4263-72.
23. Lewington A, Kanagasundaram S. Renal association clinical practice guidelines on acute kidney injury. Nephron Clin Pract. 2011;118(Suppl 1):c349-90.
24. Mehta RL, Pascual MT, Soroko S, et al. Spectrum of acute renal failure in the intensive care unit: the PICARD experience. Kidney Int. 2004;66(4):1613-21.
25. Verghese E, Ricardo SD, Weidenfeld R, et al. Renal primary cilia lengthen after acute tubular necrosis. J Am Soc Nephrol. 2009;20(10):2147-53.
26. Rosenfeld AT, Zeman RK, Cicchetti DV, et al. Experimental acute tubular necrosis: US appearance. Radiology. 1985;157:771-4.

27. Platt JH, Rubin JH, Ellis JH. Acute renal failure: Possible role of duplex Doppler US in distinction between acute pre-renal failure and acute tubular necrosis. Radiology. 1991;179:419-23.
28. Izumi M, Sugiura T, Nakamura H, et al. Differential diagnosis of prerenal azotemia from acute tubular necrosis and prediction of recovery by Doppler ultrasound. Am J Kidney Dis. 2000;35(4):713-9.
29. Han F, Xiao W, Xu Y, et al. The significance of BOLD MRI in differentiation between renal transplant rejection and acute tubular necrosis. Nephrol Dial Transplant. 2008;23: 2666-72.
30. Gormsen H, Iverson P, Raaschou I. Kidney biopsy in acute anuria: with case of acute, bilateral cortical necrosis. Am J Med. 1955;19:209-11.
31. Jordan J, Low R, Jeffrey RB Jr. CT findings in acute rena! cortical necrosis. J Comput Assist Tomogr. 1990;14:155-6.
32. Wang MT, Wu RH, Chen JC. CT findings of acute renal cortical necrosis. Chin J Radiol. 2007;32:103-6.
33. Hnn L, Pfister RC. Renal subcapsular rim sign: new etiologies and pathogenesis. AJR. 1982;138:51-4.
34. Jeong JY, Kim SH, Lee HJ, et al. Atypical low-signal intensity renal parenchyma: causes and patterns. Radiographics. 2002;22:833-46.
35. Ten RM, Torres VE, Milliner DS, et al. Acute interstitial nephritis: immunologic and clinical aspects. Mayo Clin Proc. 1988;63:921-30.
36. Davidson AJ, Hartman DS. Diagnostic set: Large smooth, bilateral. In: Davidson AJ, Hartman DS (Eds), Radiology of Kidney and Urinary Tract, 2nd edition. Philadelphia, PA: WB Saunders; 1990. pp. 157-86.
37. Sipe JD, Cohen AS. Amyloidosis. In: Fauci AS, Braunwald E, Isselbacher KJ, et al. (Eds). Harrison's Principle of Internal Medicine. New York: McGraw-Hill; 1998. pp. 1856-60.
38. Cohen AS: Amyloidosis. In: Pertersdrof RG, Adams RD, Braunwald E, et al. (Eds). Harrison's Principle of Internal Medicine. New York: McGraw-Hill; 1983. pp. 368-71.
39. Amendola RA. Amyloidosis of the urinary tract. In Pollack HM (Ed). Clinical Urography: An Atlas and Textbook of Urologic Imaging, Philadelphia, PA: WB Saunders; 1990. pp. 2493-500.
40. Heher EC, Rennke HG, Laubach JP, et al. Kidney disease and multiple myeloma. Clin J Am Soc Nephrol. 2013;8(11):2007-17.
41. Andrei SP, Antonio CW, Erick MR, et al. Imaging manifestations of hematologic diseases with renal and perinephric involvement. radiographics. 2016;36:1038-54.
42. Kim SH, Han MC, Lee JS, et al. Paroxysmal nocturnal hemoglobinuria: case report of MRI and CT findings. Acta Radiol. 1991;32:315-6.
43. Jung DC, Kim SH, Jung S, et al. Renal papillary necrosis: review and comparison of findings at multi-detector row CT and intravenous urography. Radiographics. 2006;26:1827-36.
44. Davidson A. Chronic renal failure. In: Pollack HM, McClennan BL (Eds). Clinical Urography, 1st edition. Philadelphia, PA: WB Saunders; 1990. pp. 2279-90.
45. Davidson AJ, Hartman DS. Diagnostic set: Small, Smooth, bilateral. In Davidson AJ, Hartman DS (Eds). Radiology of Kidney and Urinary Tract, 2nd edition. Philadelphia, PA: WB Saunders; 1990. pp. 135-86.
46. Ono H, Ono Y. Nephrosclerosis and hypertension. Med Clin North Am. 1997;81(6):1273-88.
47. Murphey MD, Sartoris D, Quale JL, et al. Musculoskeletal manifestations of chronic renal insufficiency. Radiographics. 1993;13:357-79.

CHAPTER

5

Nontubercular Infections of the Urinary Tract

Ujjwal Gorsi, Naveen Kalra, Ajay Kumar

INTRODUCTION

Nontubercular renal infections can be divided into acute and chronic infections. They can also be divided into uncomplicated and complicated subtypes. The infections which are not associated with permanent damage are usually referred to as uncomplicated pyelonephritis.

Common acute renal infections are acute pyelonephritis and its various complications, renal abscess, and emphysematous pyelonephritis (EPN). Chronic renal infections encountered include chronic pyelonephritis and xanthogranulomatous pyelonephritis (XGPN). In addition, various fungal and parasitic infections can also affect kidneys. Various etiologies of nontubercular renal infections are listed in **Table 1**. Spectrum of renal infections will be discussed in this chapter. Infections affecting the ureters and urinary bladder are dealt with in subsequent chapters.

The diagnosis of urinary tract infection (UTI) is based on typical clinical features and laboratory findings and usually does not warrant radiological imaging in suspected uncomplicated cases.[1-3] Indications of imaging in suspected cases of UTI include unusual severe symptoms, high-risk patients (elderly, diabetics, or immunocompromised), patient not responding to intravenous antibiotics within 72 hours and episodes of multiple repeated infections. The objectives of imaging in renal infections are: (1) to detect the conditions that must be cured immediately to preserve renal function and to avoid septic complications, e.g. pyonephrosis, EPN, and abscesses; (2) to search for primary etiological cause of UTI, i.e. calculus, obstruction, vesicoureteral reflux (VUR), and cyst infection.[1,2]

TABLE 1: Types of nontubercular renal infections.

Acute infections	Chronic infections	Others infections
Acute pyelonephritis	Chronic pyelonephritis	Fungal
Acute focal bacterial nephritis	Reflux nephropathy	Parasitic
Renal, perirenal, and pararenal abscess	Xanthogranulomatous pyelonephritis	HIV-associated nephropathy
Emphysematous pyelonephritis	Malacoplakia	
Pyonephrosis		

(HIV: human immunodeficiency virus)

With the availability of ultrasonography (USG), computed tomography (CT), magnetic resonance imaging (MRI), and advances in nuclear medicine and interventional radiology, diagnosis, and management of the renal and perirenal infections have undergone sea changes. USG and CT are most common radiological modalities used in suspected renal infections with ever- decreasing role of once indispensable plain radiograph and intravenous urography (IVU).

IMAGING MODALITIES

Ultrasonography is a sensitive modality in detecting hydronephrosis and can detect underlying stones and obstruction. USG has 98% sensitivity in detection of hydronephrosis.[4] Echogenic debris in hydronephrotic kidney suggest pyonephrosis. Renal abscess and extrarenal fluid collections are easily detected. Sonography is however less sensitive than CT in detecting the subtle changes of inflamed parenchyma, microabscesses, and small calculi. Accuracy of USG can be improved with addition of ultrasound contrast agents (UCAs). US contrast agents are of particular value in patients of renal failure in whom use of iodine-based and gadolinium-based contrast media may be hazardous.[5] USG is radiation free, relatively inexpensive, easily available, and can diagnose many of abnormalities affecting genitourinary system that require specific treatment. It is also commonly used guiding modality for various interventional procedures such as nephrostomy or cyst aspiration.

Plain X-ray may provide diagnostic information such as presence of abnormal gas collection in the renal or perirenal area in patients with EPN and renal abscess or staghorn calculus in a patient suspected to have pyonephrosis. IVU has a limited role and can exclude congenital anomalies, which are important risk factors in patients of recurrent UTIs. Certain conditions such as papillary necrosis and early tuberculosis may still be diagnosed with confidence on IVU.[6]

Contrast-enhanced computed tomography (CECT) is the gold standard for accurate diagnosis of suspected renal infections in which imaging is being contemplated. It can detect anatomic or physiologic factors associated with complicated UTI as well as delineate disease extent accurately. CT without contrast can demonstrate stones, air, hemorrhage, obstruction, and occasionally abscesses.[7] Contrast is needed to demonstrate alterations in renal perfusion, which may be subtle and become evident only after contrast administration.

Magnetic resonance imaging is being increasingly used as an effective modality for both medical and surgical diseases of kidney especially in pregnant women, children, and in diabetics. MRI may demonstrate infected regions of the renal parenchyma to enhance abnormally and to have restricted diffusion and can demonstrate obstruction and abscesses but often fails to reveal small stones. The cost and limited availability precludes its routine use, although it may provide information similar to CT.

Radionuclide studies with cortical scintigraphy agents such as ^{99m}Tc dimercaptosuccinic acid (DMSA) and glucoheptonate have been shown to be the most sensitive techniques for the diagnosis of acute pyelonephritis and detection of the renal scars in reflux nephropathy.[8]

ACUTE PYELONEPHRITIS

Acute pyelonephritis occurs when there is inflammation affecting the collecting system and the renal interstitium. Bacterial organisms such as *Escherichia coli*, *Proteus mirabilis*, and *Klebsiella pneumoniae* are the usual culprits when transmission of infection occurs by the ascending route. Hematogenous infections occur especially in drug addicts and patients with endocarditis. They are usually staphylococcal in origin. Fungal or viral infections may also be encountered. Predisposing factors for acute pyelonephritis are: obstruction, prolonged catheter drainage, reflux, congenital anomalies, pregnancy, and diabetes. 90% of UTIs occur as a single episode where as 10% are recurrent.[3] Pyelonephritis affects sexually active women commonly and a peak is also noticed in men over 60 years as a consequence of prostatic hyperplasia and resultant stasis of urine.[3]

Pathology

The affected kidney is usually increased in size due to edema. Multiple foci of inflammation, which are characteristically patchy and may lead to microabscesses, are noticed. These focal areas of inflammation usually resolve completely without any sequelae with treatment but in the presence of risk factors such as diabetes or immunocompromised status and inadequate treatment, bacterial nephritis may result which may be focal or diffuse and may lead to renal and perirenal abscesses subsequently.

Radiology

Imaging is usually not required for uncomplicated cases of acute pyelonephritis. The role of IVU in acute pyelonephritis has rapidly diminished. Positive IVU findings will be seen only in 25% of acute pyelonephritis.[1,3] IVU may show renal enlargement with decreased, delayed, and persistent nephrogram. Attenuation of the calyces or minimal dilatation of pelvicalyceal system may also be seen on IVU.

Ultrasound may show enlargement of the kidney, which can be focal or diffuse. Changes in echogenicity may mirror underlying pathological changes. Affected kidney may show hypoechoic areas due to edema or hyperechoic areas due to hemorrhage. Loss of corticomedullary differentiation and loss of renal sinus fat may also be seen **(Fig. 1)**. Unfortunately, on routine gray-scale images, interstitial nephritis is not well characterized so it is not unusual to have negative results on USG in clinically suspected pyelonephritis cases. In one prospective study, USG could reveal abnormalities in only 24% of patients whereas other studies reported abnormalities in as low as 20% of patients.[9,10]

Doppler may help in assessing areas of reduced perfusion. Extent of hypoperfusion is defined better by Power Doppler as compared to Color Doppler. Newer tools such as tissue harmonic imaging have improved sensitivities and specificities as high as 97% and 80%, respectively.[11] Areas of poor perfusion related to nephritis may be better demonstrated by US contrast agents.[5]

Multiphasic CECT is superior to both USG and IVU in demonstrating features of inflammation. The recommended phases of CT scan for evaluating renal infections are a noncontrast scan and a nephrographic phase at 50–90 seconds. Excretory phase at 2 minutes is usually acquired only if underlying obstruction is suspected.[3]

On noncontrast computed tomography (NCCT), affected areas may appear hypoattenuating as compared to normal parenchyma due to edema; less frequently, higher attenuation regions may be seen which are likely to represent hemorrhage.[12] However, it is not unusual to have nonenhanced CT images which appear completely normal. Features of acute bacterial nephritis may only be demonstrated after administration of contrast material.

Contrast-enhanced computed tomography may reveal wedge-shaped areas of decreased attenuation radiating from

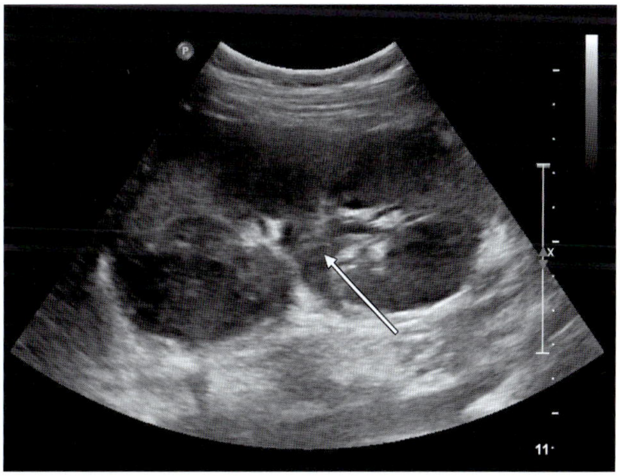

FIG. 1: *Acute pyelonephritis:* Grayscale longitudinal ultrasound scan shows diffusely enlarged kidney with heterogeneous echotexture. Both hypoechoic and hyperechoic areas are appreciated with loss of corticomedullary differentiation. Accompanying urothelial thickening (arrow) is also noticed.

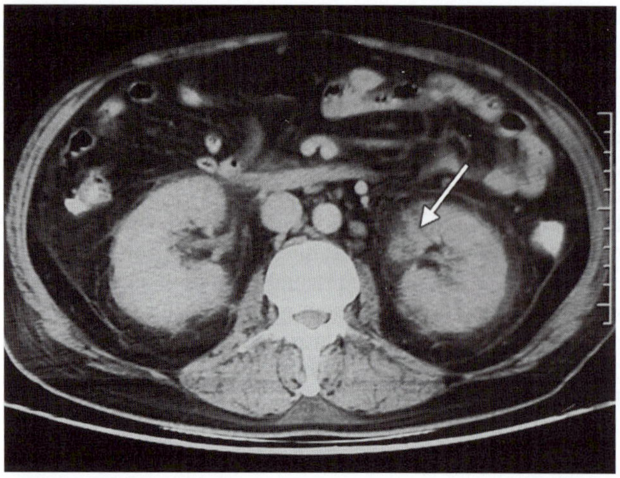

FIG. 2: Bilateral acute pyelonephritis: Contrast-enhanced computed tomography scan shows bilaterally enlarged kidneys with striated nephrogram (arrow). There is presence of perinephric stranding and thickening of Gerota's fascia and lateral conal fascia.

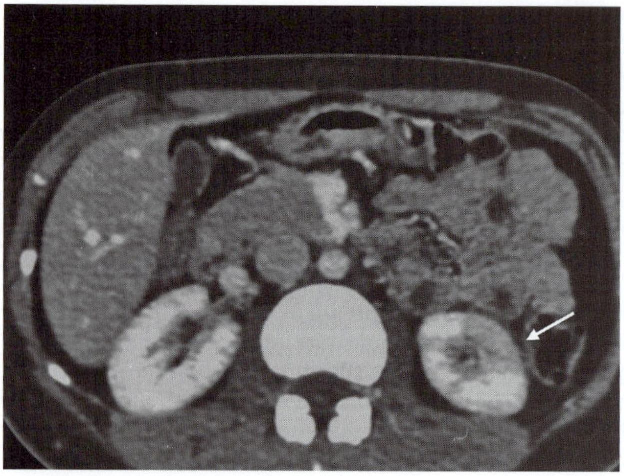

FIG. 3: Acute focal bacterial nephritis: Contrast-enhanced CT scan showing a focal wedge-shaped hypoenhancing area in left kidney reaching till renal capsule with absent cortical rim sign. Subtle perinephric stranding (arrow) is also seen.

papilla to the cortex due to hypoperfusion in an enlarged kidney **(Fig. 2)**. The transverse areas of alternate bands with increased and decreased density may also be seen and are related to underlying pathophysiology of tubular obstruction caused by inflammatory debris within the lumen, interstitial edema, and vasospasm.[13] Flow of contrast through the tubule is reduced due to these three pathophysiologic disturbances. This tubular obstruction is also the cause of persistent delayed enhancement, which usually is seen 3–6 hours after contrast injection. The wedge-shaped defects, which originally show hypoattenuation during the nephrographic phase show hyperattenuation later due to prolonged accumulation and slow transit of injected contrast through tubules which are compromised.[14]

Diffuse homogeneous involvement of the renal parenchyma in acute pyelonephritis is unusual and is seen if there is ureteric obstruction.[15] Thickening of the walls of the collecting system, which sometimes is seen in renal infections, points toward pyelitis.[15] Antibiotic therapy can alter the CT appearance of pyelonephritis. A rounded or ovoid area of decreased enhancement, which has poorly defined margins, may be seen in patients who are partially treated with antibiotics and undergo CT scan.[15]

Computed tomography is also the best modality for complete evaluation of the secondary signs of renal infections and their complications. Perinephric stranding, thickening of Gerota's fascia, renal, and perirenal abscess formation are very well demonstrated on CT.[16]

Scintigraphic techniques are superior to US and IVU for the diagnosis of acute pyelonephritis.[9] Renal cortical scintigraphy with ^{99m}Tc DMSA will reveal wedge-shaped cortical defects which are characteristic of acute pyelonephritis.

On MRI, the affected regions will have low signal on T1-weighted images (T1WI) and high signal on T2-weighted images (T2WI). Loss of corticomedullary differentiation may also be appreciated. MRI features of pyelonephritis resemble those of CECT.[16] Affected areas show diffusion restriction, and diffusion-weighted (DW) images may be more sensitive than either T2WI or contrast-enhanced T1WI for detecting regions of pyelonephritis.[15] MRI may also help in differentiating acute infection from chronic scar in problematic cases. The potential pitfalls of MRI are in patients with gas-forming infections and calculi where MRI may not be able to distinguish between the two.[3]

BOX 1: Findings in acute pyelonephritis.

- Diffuse (usually)/focal enlargement
- Striated kidney commonly seen in nephrographic phase
- Areas of increased attenuation in hemorrhagic bacterial nephritis
- Perinephric stranding
- Thickening of Gerota's fascia
- Focal involvement may mimic renal tumor

Imaging findings of acute pyelonephritis are summarized in **Box 1**.

ACUTE FOCAL BACTERIAL NEPHRITIS

Acute focal bacterial nephritis (AFBN) is a rare interstitial nephritis, which presents with focal lesions in radiological studies.[17] First described in 1978 by Rosenfield et al,[18] it was earlier known as acute lobar nephronia.

Fever and flank pain are the leading symptoms usually accompanied by leukocytosis. US reveals hypoechoic poorly defined mass, which may be echogenic if there is hemorrhage.

Computed tomography shows focal hypoattenuating area with patchy enhancement. They can be wedge-shaped occasionally and hence difficult to differentiate from acute renal infarction. The cortical rim sign when seen on CECT and contrast-enhanced magnetic resonance imaging (CEMRI) may be useful in distinguishing acute pyelonephritis from a segmental renal infarct **(Fig. 3)**. In AFBN, areas of abnormal hypoenhancement, extends from centrally located medulla to the peripheral renal capsule typically involving a complete wedge of renal parenchyma. In segmental renal infarcts by contrast, wedge-shaped areas of abnormal renal hypoenhancement spare the outermost cortex. This happens due to the fact that outer aspect of the cortex is supplied by perforating branches of the renal capsular artery, which is an early branch of the renal artery.[18,19]

Perinephric fat stranding may also be seen. AFBN can be differentiated from renal abscess by the absence of peripheral contrast enhancement and nonliquefactive center.[18]

RENAL AND PERIRENAL ABSCESSES

Renal and perirenal abscesses usually result as a complication of bacterial pyelonephritis. Other mechanisms that may lead to formation of renal and perirenal abscesses are hematogenous infection and superadded infection in a preexisting renal cyst. In addition, inflammatory conditions of colon, pancreas, and retroperitoneum may extend into perinephric space.

Plain radiograph and IVU are rarely done in suspected renal and perirenal abscesses in present era of USG and CT. Plain radiograph may show enlarged kidney, rotation and enlargement of affected kidney, presence of mottled gas in renal fossa, and loss of outline of psoas muscle. Poorly or nonfunctioning kidney with calyceal attenuation and compression due to mass affect may be seen on IVU.

Ultrasonography may reveal a well-defined focal lesion with irregular shaggy margins, good sound transmission, and no internal flow **(Fig. 4A)**. Features of accompanying pyelonephritis may also be seen. Echogenic mobile debris within the lesion may help in reaching a correct diagnosis. Cysts with superadded infection or hemorrhage or necrotic tumors may mimic renal abscess on USG.

Computed tomography is the gold standard to assess the renal abscess as well as its extrarenal extent. Changes in the renal size, contour, parenchymal attenuation, enhancement pattern, and accompanying abnormalities such as thickening of the Gerota's fascia, retroperitoneal extension, and involvement of psoas muscle are very well demonstrated on CT. During the earlier course of renal abscess, poorly marginated nonenhancing area of decreased attenuation may be seen suggestive of evolving abscess. Surrounding area may show reduced enhancement due to edema. Later in the course of the disease, as renal abscess matures, it is seen as a well-marginated area of low attenuation due to central area of necrosis with a peripheral enhancing rim **(Figs. 4B and C)**. Septations are frequent in perinephric abscess, hence they are more difficult to drain as compared to renal abscess **(Fig. 5)**.

On MRI, a renal abscess is seen as a hypointense lesion on T1WI and a hyperintense lesion on T2WI. Diffusion restriction is seen in the central necrotic area and on contrast

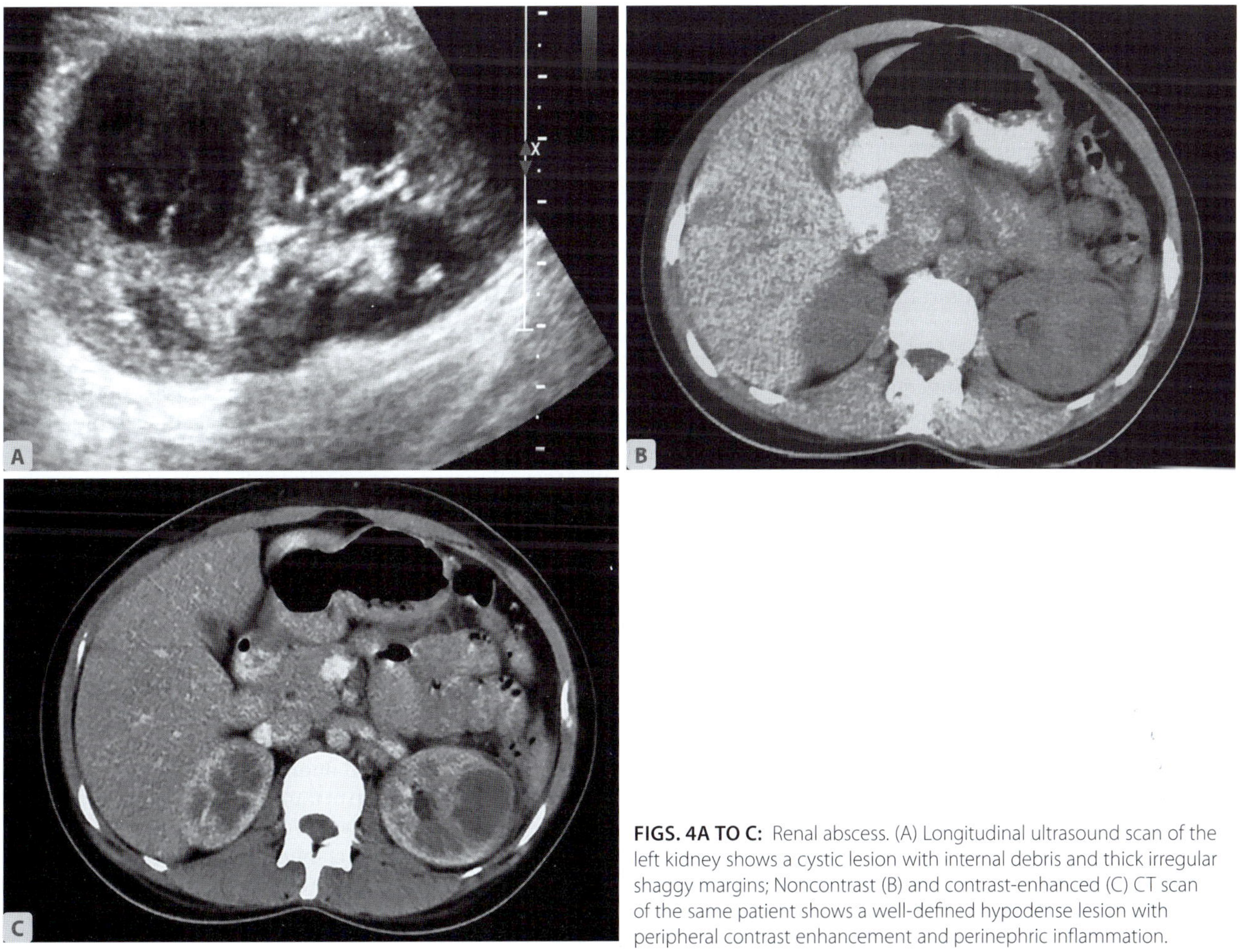

FIGS. 4A TO C: Renal abscess. (A) Longitudinal ultrasound scan of the left kidney shows a cystic lesion with internal debris and thick irregular shaggy margins; Noncontrast (B) and contrast-enhanced (C) CT scan of the same patient shows a well-defined hypodense lesion with peripheral contrast enhancement and perinephric inflammation.

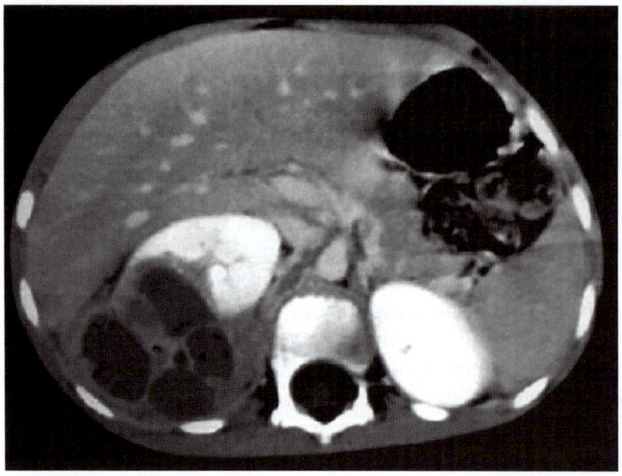

FIG. 5: Contrast-enhanced CT scan showing multiseptated hypodense lesion in the right kidney suggestive of renal abscess with extension into the perinephric space.

administration; the lesion shows peripheral rim-like enhancement **(Figs. 6A to F)**. Percutaneous drainage under USG/CT guidance has been successful in reducing mortality with a success rate of 85–95%.[20]

EMPHYSEMATOUS PYELONEPHRITIS

Emphysematous pyelonephritis is a rare but severe form of renal infection caused by gas-forming organisms. The most commonly causative organisms are *E. coli*, *K. pneumoniae* and *P. mirabilis*. Its radiological hallmark is presence of gas in the collecting system and/or renal parenchyma. Approximately 90% of patients have poorly controlled diabetes. Other predisposing factors include immunocompromised status or associated urinary tract obstruction secondary to calculus, sloughed papilla, or tumor. EPN progresses rapidly leading to fulminant sepsis. It is associated with high mortality in absence of prompt therapeutic intervention.[16,21]

Plain X-ray can reveal mottled gas in renal fossa in over 85% of cases **(Fig. 7)**. Crescentic gas collection may also be seen. The crescent-shaped air indicates the extension into perinephric space suggesting the advanced stage. IVU is rarely performed these days, but will show a poorly functioning or nonfunctioning kidney, if performed.

Ultrasound examination reveals coarse echoes with dirty shadowing in intrarenal infection **(Fig. 8A)**. The echogenic foci appear different than those seen in typical stone disease, with the distal shadowing having reverberations/ring down artefacts and low-level echoes that are nicknamed "dirty shadowing". If the gas extends into the perinephric space, kidney may not be seen at all on USG (gassed-out kidney).

Computed tomography is the imaging modality of choice to confirm the diagnosis and to see the renal as well as perirenal extent **(Fig. 8B)**. It detects the presence of air, its precise location within the kidney as well as its extension into the perirenal or pararenal compartments of the retroperitoneal space **(Fig. 9)**. The role of MRI is limited as gas appears as an area of signal loss, which cannot be differentiated from calculi, renal calcification, and flowing blood on T1 and T2WI.

Prognosis appears to correlate with two types of gaseous distribution. In Type 1 EPN, there is greater than one-third renal parenchymal destruction, which is associated with either mottled or streaky areas of gas. Intra- or extrarenal fluid collections are absent. In Type 2 EPN, renal or perirenal fluid collections are present, which are associated with loculated or bubbly gas within the collecting system. Type 1 disease has typically been found to have a more aggressive course, with a shorter duration between initial presentation and death.[22] However, recent literature reports much better results even in Type 1 disease with mortality rates for both types approximately 8%.[23] Aggressive medical treatment along with percutaneous image-guided drainage and partial or complete nephrectomy is advocated to reduce mortality due to either type of EPN.

In addition to this, the Huang-Tseng CT classification system[24] is also followed in EPN and is described in **Box 2**.

Prognosis is worse for higher classes. For localized EPN (classes 1 and 2), percutaneous drainage combined with antibiotic treatment can provide a good outcome with reduced mortality.

PYONEPHROSIS

Pyonephrosis is the term given to infection in an obstructed collecting system, which may lead to suppurative destruction of the renal parenchyma if not treated immediately. Cause of obstruction can be sloughed papilla, stone, stricture, or neoplasm. Early diagnosis is important as untreated pyonephrosis may lead to rapid and irreversible decline in renal function. In addition, patient may develop septic shock if direct, immediate intervention is not undertaken.[16]

Ultrasound is the modality of choice to detect dilated collecting system, which often shows mobile dependent echogenic debris **(Fig. 10)**. Echogenic debris (i.e. the lack of a completely anechoic collecting system) is considered the most reliable sign of pyonephrosis.[16]

On CT, high density of urine in the dilated system can suggest infection in appropriate clinical context. CT, in addition, will often reveal the underlying cause of obstruction, which USG may sometimes fail to reveal. Thickening of the urothelium can be seen both on USG or CT.

Magnetic resonance imaging will reveal findings similar to those seen at CT. Dilated pelvicaliceal system, debris within the system are usually noticed. Fluid-fluid levels are also appreciated and underlying cause may also be apparent. DW-MRI may be used as a problem-solving tool in distinguishing hydronephrosis from pyonephrosis as in pyonephrosis-restricted diffusion may be seen.[25]

Ultrasound-guided aspiration may be performed to confirm the diagnosis as well as obtain specimen for culture and sensitivity. Percutaneous nephrostomy may also be performed under USG and fluoroscopic guidance to provide immediate decompression of the collecting system and also as an adjunct prior to definitive surgery. In case of pyonephrosis due to fungal etiology, direct infusion of amphotericin B may be done through the nephrostomy tube in place of systemic amphotericin, which is more toxic.

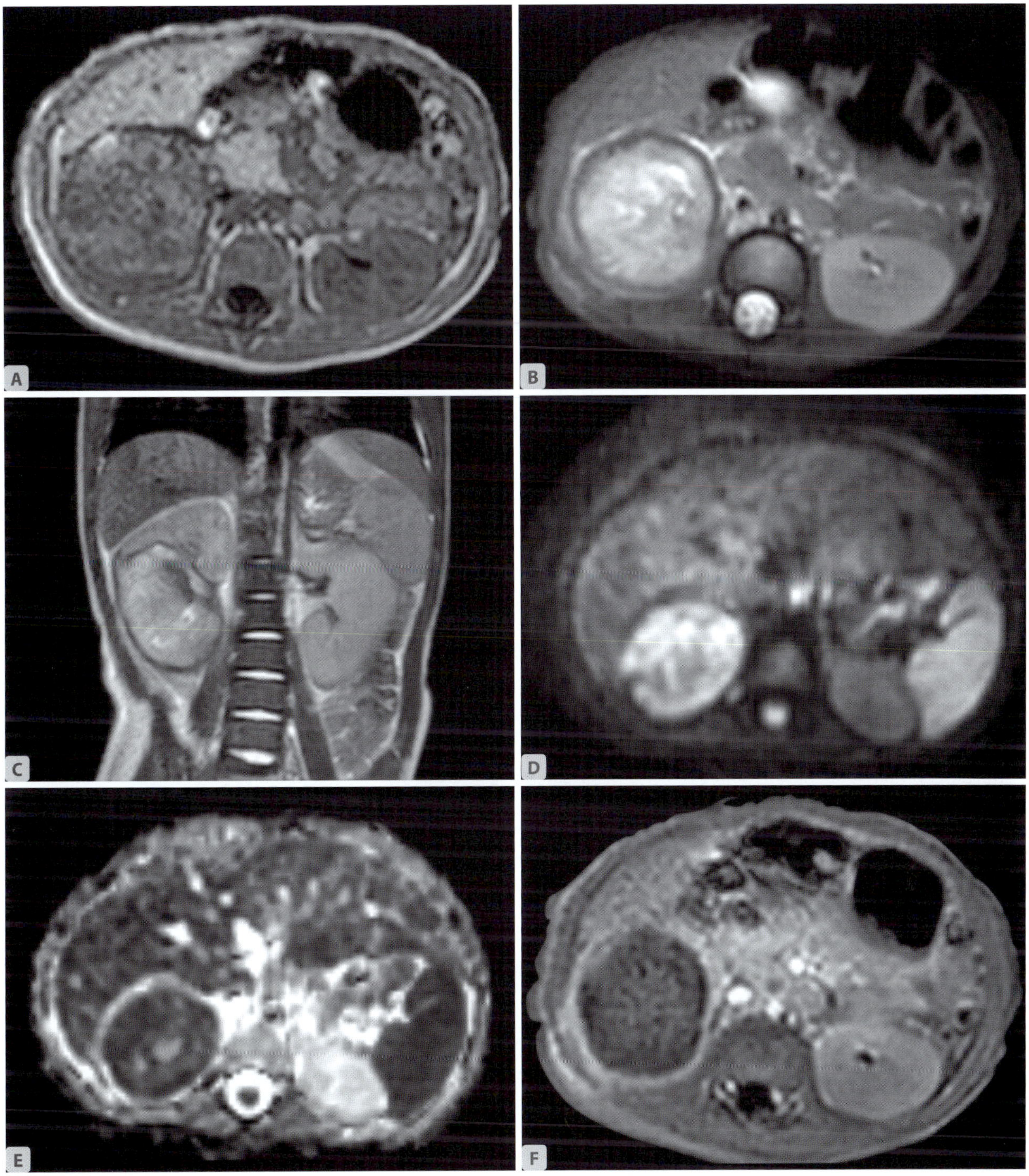

FIGS. 6A TO F: Renal abscess in a child: Axial T1-weighted image. (A) shows a large hypointense lesion in right kidney. Axial T2-weighted image (B) and coronal (C) plane shows hyperintense lesion in interpolar and lower polar region. The lesion shows diffusion restriction (D and E) Gadolinium-enhanced axial T1-weighted image (F) shows peripheral irregular rim enhancement.

CHRONIC PYELONEPHRITIS

The term chronic focal atrophic pyelonephritis refers to renal parenchymal scarring, which manifests as focal thinning of both cortex and medulla with blunting of underlying calyces.[15] This renal parenchymal scarring can be due to a number of causes, including severe focal pyelonephritis, VUR, and calyceal calculi. Once the scars have formed, the gross pathologic and radiologic appearance of the affected kidney is identical hence does not allow determination of etiology.[15] Once the radiologic manifestations of chronic pyelonephritis have been established, repeat imaging does not provide any new findings and is usually unnecessary.

The term reflux nephropathy is specifically used, if the etiology is proven to be VUR. Possible mechanism of renal scarring in reflux nephropathy is thought to be the transient

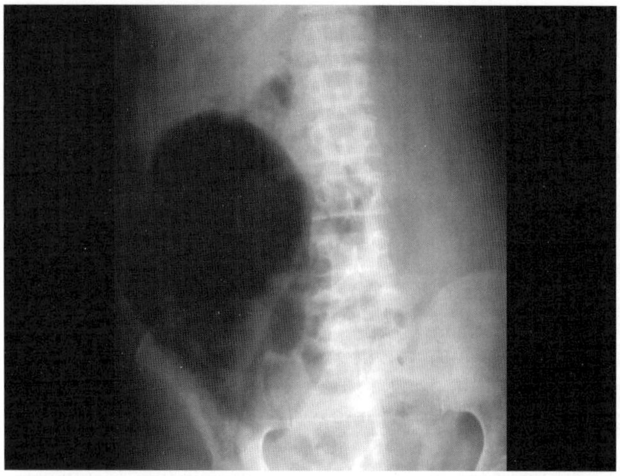

FIG. 7: Plain X-ray of abdomen showing a large loculus of air overlying the right renal fossa in a diabetic patient with extensive emphysematous pyelonephritis.

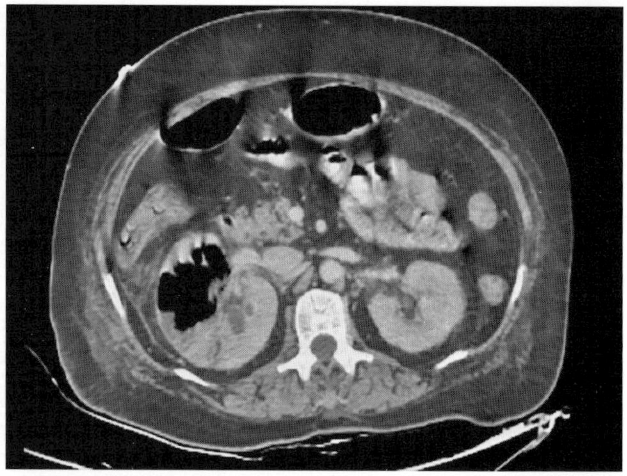

FIG. 9: Emphysematous pyelonephritis: Contrast-enhanced computed tomography scan shows large air loculus in right kidney with presence of fluid posteriorly. Thickening of perirenal fascia and associated stranding is also seen.

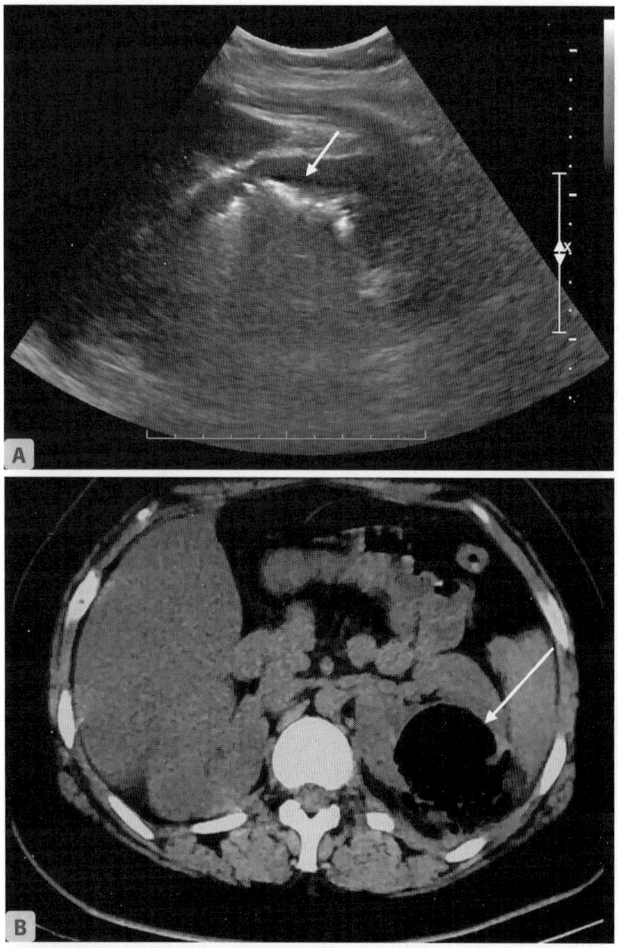

FIGS. 8A AND B: Emphysematous pyelonephritis. (A) Longitudinal ultrasound scan of the left kidney shows coarse echoes (arrow) with posterior dirty shadowing; (B) Noncontrast CT scan of the same patient shows large intraparenchymal air collection with extension into left posterior perinephric space.

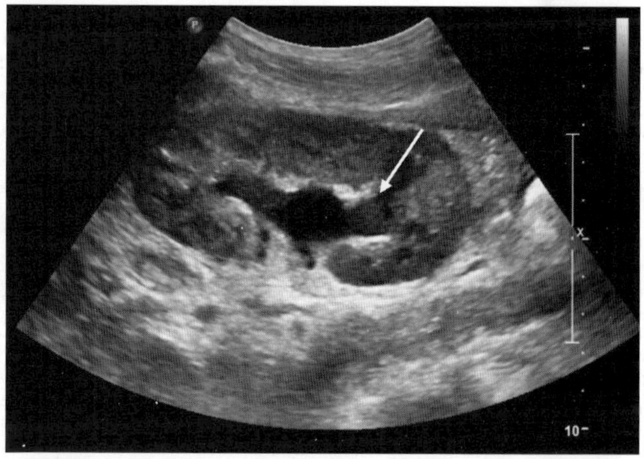

FIG. 10: Pyonephrosis: Longitudinal ultrasound scan of the kidney shows echogenic debris (arrow) in pelvicalyceal system. These debris were found to be mobile on continuous scanning. Associated features of pyelonephritis are also apparent in form of heterogeneous echotexture of kidney and poor corticomedullary differentiation.

BOX 2: Classification of emphysematous pyelonephritis.

- *Class 1*: Gas in the collecting system only
- *Class 2*: Gas in renal parenchyma only (without extrarenal extension)
- *Class 3*: Gas in renal parenchyma with extrarenal extension
  - *Class 3a*: Extension of gas or abscess to perinephric space
  - *Class 3b*: Extension of gas or abscess to pararenal space
- *Class 4*: Bilateral emphysemat ous pyelonephritis or solitary kidney with emphysematous pyelonephritis

increase in hydrostatic pressure in the collecting system due to urine reflux during contractions of urinary bladder. This often-infected urine enters into the collecting tubules of the kidney in retrograde fashion due to pyelotubular reflux. As there are local differences in the papillary openings of the collecting ducts of the renal medullae, this intrarenal reflux occurs in a patchy distribution, which is the probable cause for the focal nature of the resultant scarring.[15] Normal nephrons are replaced by dense fibrous tissue in scarred areas of renal parenchyma.

In middle-aged or elderly patients, calculi are the most common cause of chronic pyelonephritic scarring, whereas in children, reflux is the most common etiology.[15]

Intravenous urography, if done, may reveal spectrum of findings seen in chronic pyelonephritis **(Fig. 11)**. On USG, focal loss of parenchyma is usually apparent, which can be demonstrated on longitudinal or cross-sectional images. Regions of scars may show increased echogenicity due to underlying fibrosis. The central renal sinus echoes may extend to the periphery of the kidney in the area of abnormality due to underlying volume loss. The process is patchy and focal in contrast to other causes of generalized increased cortical echogenicity.[15]

The radiologic findings of chronic pyelonephritis on cross-sectional imaging whether CT, computed tomographic urography (CTU), and MRI include one or more parenchymal scars overlying a deformed calyx **(Fig. 12)**. Focal areas of compensatory hypertrophy may be apparent adjacent to the areas of cortical scarring if loss of parenchyma has been severe. These focal areas may mimic solid parenchymal tumors but can be distinguished from tumors by observing their enhancement pattern. These pseudotumors enhance to the same degree as adjacent normal parenchyma unlike true tumors.[15] Renal cortical scintigraphy is considered the best technique to detect renal scarring. Other differential diagnoses include fetal lobulation, ischemia, and hypoplastic kidney. In ischemia, the underlying calyx is usually normal. In fetal lobulation, the scars are in between the calyces and in congenital hypoplastic kidney, the number of calyces are less than five.

XANTHOGRANULOMATOUS PYELONEPHRITIS

Xanthogranulomatous pyelonephritis (XGPN) is a rare chronic granulomatous inflammation of the kidney. It is usually seen in patients who have stones and obstruction. In XGPN, there is destruction of renal parenchyma, which is replaced by para-aminosalicylic acid-positive and lipid-laden macrophages (xanthoma cells). In addition to xanthoma cells, other inflammatory cells such as leukocytes, plasma cells, and histiocytes are also present.

Three stages of XGPN have been described depending on the extent of the disease. In Stage I, only kidney is involved; in Stage II, there is extension of inflammatory process into Gerota's fascia; and in Stage III, disease extends into the perinephric spaces.

Women are more affected than men. The presenting features and signs of the disease are nonspecific and similar to any long-standing chronic inflammatory process. Patients may present with fever, malaise, weight loss, pain, or tenderness in flanks. Leukocytosis will be seen in majority of patients. Lower urinary tract symptoms such as dysuria and increased frequency are seen in only one-half of patients.[15] Active UTI is present in almost all the cases with *E. coli*, *P. mirabilis*, *K. pneumoniae*, or *Pseudomonas aeruginosa* alone or in combination being the offending agents. Triad of radiological features consists of: (1) poorly defined renal mass; (2) reduced or absent contrast excretion; and (3) staghorn calculus.[15]

Plain radiograph will reveal the calculus. IVU may show tumefactive-type focal mass or enlarged nonfunctioning kidney. USG reveals global enlargement of the kidney with a central obstructing calculus. The renal parenchyma reveals a diffuse hypoechoic pattern, which represents areas of

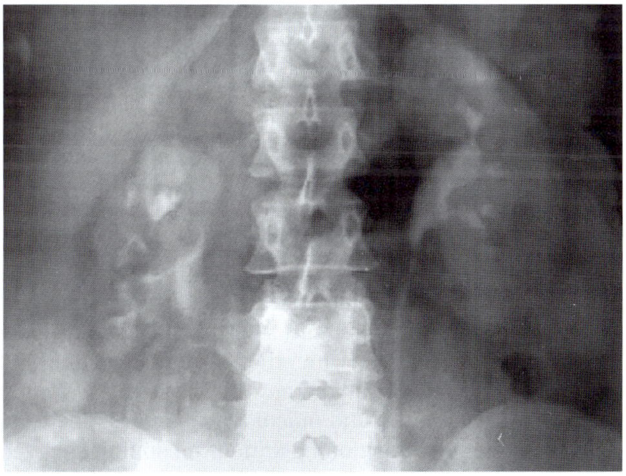

FIG. 11: Chronic pyelonephritis: Excretory urogram showing small irregular right kidney with dilated and distorted calyces and thinned out parenchyma especially opposite the polar calyces.

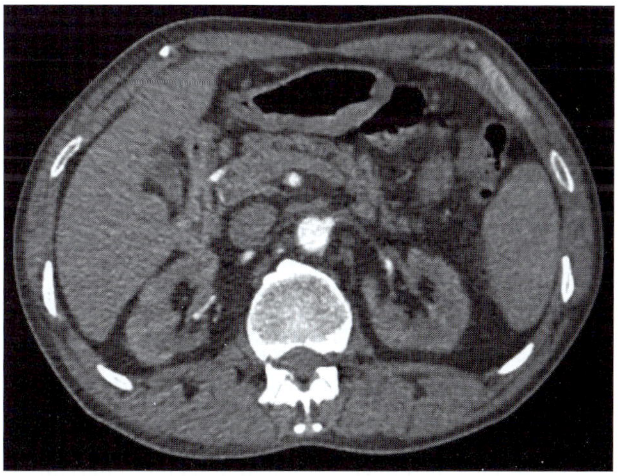

FIG. 12: Chronic pyelonephritis: Contrast-enhanced CT showing irregular outline of bilateral kidneys with multifocal areas of parenchymal scarring and distortion of underlying calyces.

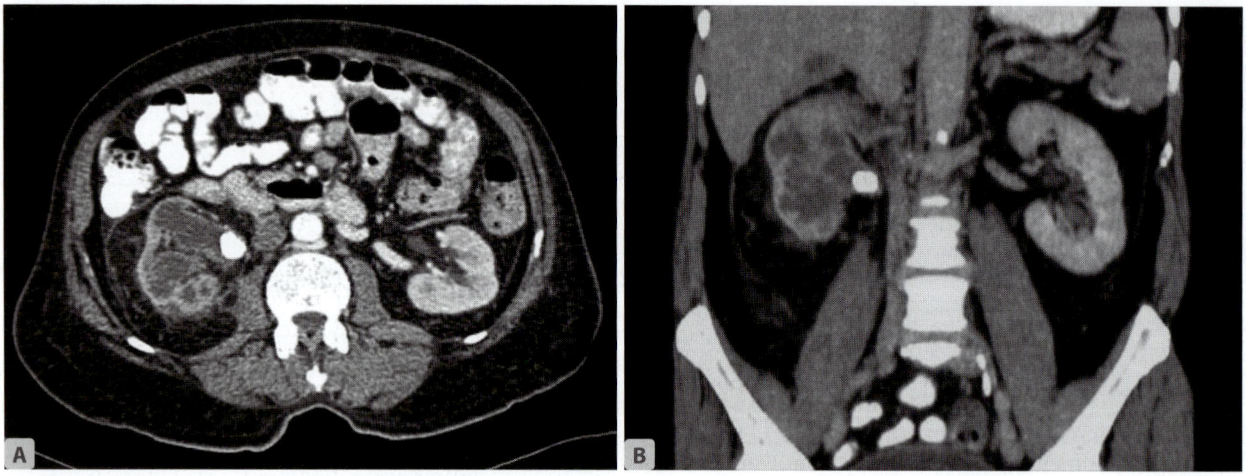

FIGS. 13A AND B: Xanthogranulomatous pyelonephritis: Contrast-enhanced CT scan in arterial phase axial plane. (A) and venous phase coronal plane; (B) shows calculus in deformed pelvis of right kidney with dilated collecting system secondary to inflammatory debris. Kidney maintains its reniform shape. Perinephric inflammation is also noted.

inflammation or abscess. The calyces may appear as multiple fluid-filled regions with echogenic debris, which may be indistinguishable from pyonephrosis.[15]

Computed tomography findings strongly point towards the correct diagnosis though are not specific. The diffusely enlarged kidney retains its reniform shape. One characteristic feature is poorly defined or normal renal pelvis, unless there is concomitant ureteropelvic junction obstruction. One or more stones are usually present **(Figs. 13A and B)**. Small areas of parenchymal calcification may also be appreciated. Atrophic parenchyma may be seen as hypoattenuating areas at the periphery of the kidneys. Hypoattenuating central areas which represent dilated calyces filled with pus and necrotic material are usually separated by renal column of Bertin. On CECT, hyperemia is seen around the calyces, at the periphery of the kidney and in the renal fascia. Extrarenal extension of inflammatory process is usually evident on CT.[15]

The common form of XGPN causes diffuse involvement of the affected kidney. In the tumefactive form of XGPN, inflammatory process is limited to a portion of the kidney. This appearance may mimic poorly enhancing renal tumor and radiological differentiation may be difficult. Both forms of XGPN usually are associated with extensive perinephric inflammation.[15]

MALACOPLAKIA

Malacoplakia is a rare granulomatous inflammatory condition seen almost exclusively in women and clinically presents as repeated attacks of UTI. Bladder and ureter are most frequently affected. Renal involvement is rare. Radiological features include enlarged poorly functioning kidney with filling defect in the ureter and bladder and may mimic pyeloureteritis cystica or transitional cell carcinoma. Strictures may also develop thus mimicking tuberculosis. Renal involvement leads to focal or multiple masses indistinguishable from renal cell carcinoma or XGPN on US, CT, or IVU. Diagnosis is confirmed on pathology, which reveals Van Hansemann cells and Michaelis–Gutmann bodies in the nodular deposits.[16]

HIV-ASSOCIATED NEPHROPATHY

Human immunodeficiency virus can affect any organ of the body and renal involvement can be seen in variety of disease processes in HIV infection. Kidneys may be involved as a collapsing glomerulopathy (HIV-associated nephropathy, HIVAN) or due to secondary infections by bacteria or opportunistic organisms such as *Pneumocystis carinii* and cytomegalovirus. HIVAN is a serious disorder, which results in rapidly progressive renal failure. It manifests histologically as focal glomerulosclerosis and as membranous, membranoproliferative, and mesangial proliferative glomerulonephritis.[25,26]

Imaging will demonstrate renal enlargement (>13 cm) with increased echogenicity on USG. Atta et al.[27] found that only renal echogenicity and not kidney size has diagnostic utility for HIVAN. On NCCT scan, hyperattenuating medulla may be seen as a result of dilated protein filled tubules. On CECT, enlarged kidneys with striated nephrogram may be evident.[28,29] Imaging findings may suggest the diagnosis of HIVAN but confirmation is on histology. *P. carinii* infection of the kidney will result in punctate areas of calcification within the renal parenchyma similar to those seen with *Mycobacterium avium* intracellulare or cytomegalovirus.[30]

FUNGAL INFECTION

Fungal infections of the kidney are rare, usually encountered in patients with deranged immunity such as diabetics, postrenal transplant patients, those with other chronic infections and those on prolonged steroid therapy. Infection by *Aspergillus*, *Candida*, *Cryptococcus*, and mucor has been described. On CT, bilateral poorly functioning or nonfunctioning enlarged kidneys with multiple hyperattenuating areas present both in the cortex and medulla should raise the possibility of the diagnosis of mucormycosis especially in diabetic patients **(Fig. 14)**.[31]

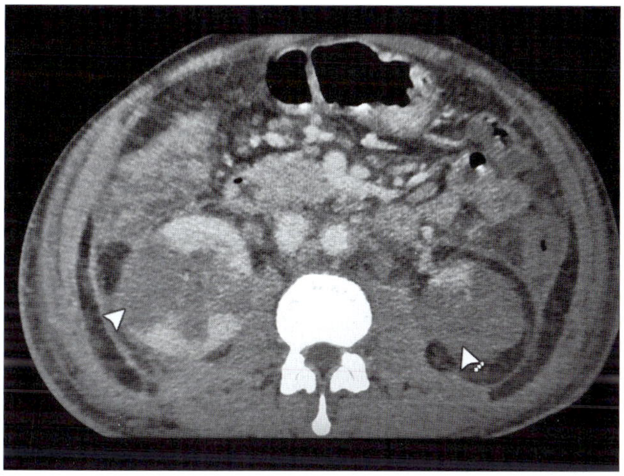

FIG. 14: Bilateral mucormycosis: Contrast-enhanced CT scan in a diabetic patient shows bilateral globular kidneys with large hypodense nonenhancing areas (arrowheads). There is extensive bilateral perinephric and mesenteric stranding and thickening of fascias. Few enlarged lymph nodes are also seen.

Both *Aspergillus* and mucor are angioinvasive fungi. These fungi cause thrombosis of the large as well as small arteries with resultant infarction and necrosis of the kidneys. The infection usually occurs by hematogenous route resulting in multiple abscesses, which may extend into perinephric space.

PARASITIC INFECTION

Schistosoma usually affects the bladder causing calcification. Renal pelvic striations may be seen. Intrarenal hydatid is rare and occurs in only approximately 2–3% of patients. Within the kidney, the worms form three-layered hydatid cyst that may grow rapidly and destroy the kidney or may progress very slowly, producing minimal clinical symptoms. USG, CT, and MRI show the lesions to be cystic and usually reveal the walls of the daughter cysts. Associated curvilinear mural calcification may be seen **(Figs. 15A to C)**. US may demonstrate internal debris. Cyst walls are of various thicknesses and may enhance slightly on CECT and CEMRI. Extensive renal destruction may result in a nonfunctioning kidney.[15]

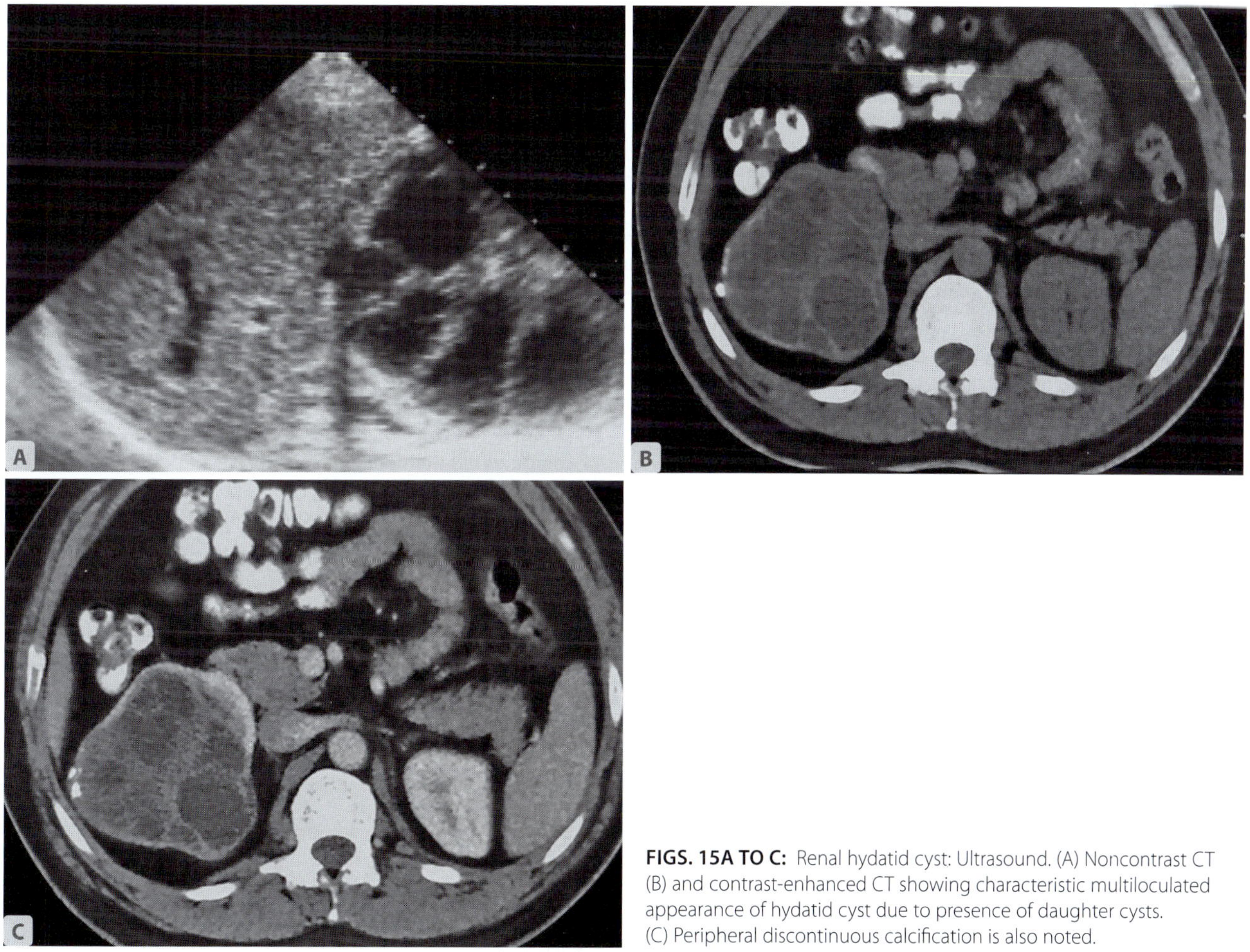

FIGS. 15A TO C: Renal hydatid cyst: Ultrasound. (A) Noncontrast CT (B) and contrast-enhanced CT showing characteristic multiloculated appearance of hydatid cyst due to presence of daughter cysts. (C) Peripheral discontinuous calcification is also noted.

REFERENCES

1. Kawashima A, Sandler CM, Goldman SM. Imaging in acute renal infection. BJU Int. 2000;86(Suppl 1):70-9.
2. Bjerklund JTE. The role of imaging in urinary tract infections. World J Urol. 2004;22(5):392-98.
3. Stunell H, Buckley O, Feeney J, et al. Imaging of acute pyelonephritis in the adult. Eur Radiol. 2007;17(7):1820-28.
4. Ellenbogen PH, Schieble FW, Talner LB, et al. Sensitivity of gray scale ultrasound in detecting urinary tract obstruction. AJR. 1978;130(4):731-3.
5. Fontanilla T, Minaya J, Cortes C, et al. Acute complicated pyelonephritis: contrast-enhanced ultrasound. Abdom Imaging. 2012;37(4):639-646.
6. Merenich WM, Popky GL. Radiology of renal infection. Med Clin N Am. 1991;75(2):425-69.
7. Kawashima A, LeRoy AJ. Radiologic evaluation of patients with renal infections. Infect Dis Clin North Am. 2003; 17(2):433-56.
8. Conway JJ. The role of scintigraphy in urinary tract infection. Semin Nucl Med. 1998;18(4):308-19.
9. June CH, Browning MD, Smith LP, et al. Ultrasonography and computed tomography in severe urinary tract infection. Arch Intern Med. 1985;145(5):841-5.
10. Vourganti S, Agarwal PK, Bodner DR, et al. Ultrasonographic evaluation of renal infections. Radiol Clin North Am. 2006; 44(6):763-75.
11. Kim B, Lim HK, Choi MH, et al. Detection of parenchymal abnormalities in acute pyelonephritis by pulse inversion harmonic imaging with or without microbubble ultrasonographic contrast agent: correlation with computed tomography. J Ultrasound Med. 2001;20(1):5-14.
12. Rigsby CM, Rosenfield AT, Glickman MG, et al. Hemorrhagic focal bacterial nephritis: findings on gray-scale sonography and CT. Am J Roentgenol. 1986;146(6):1173-7.
13. Talner LB, Davidson AJ, Lebowitz RL, et al. Acute pyelonephritis: can we agree on terminology? Radiology. 1994;192(2):297-305.
14. Dalla-Palma L, Pozzi-Mucelli R, Pozzi-Mucelli F. Delayed CT in acute renal infection. Semin Ultrasound CT MR. 1997;18(2): 122-8.
15. Dunnick NR, Newhouse JH, Cohan RH, Maturen KE, et al. Renal inflammatory disease. In: Dunnick NR, Newhouse JH, Cohan RH, Maturen KE, et al. (Eds). Genitourinary Radiology. Philadelphia: Wolters Kluwer; 2018. pp. 145-62.
16. Craig WD, Wagner BJ, Travis MD. Pyelonephritis: radiologic-pathologic review. Radiographics. 2008;28(1):255-77; quiz 327-8.
17. Sieger N, Kyriazis I, Schaudinn A, et al. Acute focal bacterial nephritis is associated with invasive diagnostic procedures: a cohort of 138 cases extracted through a systematic review. BMC Infect Dis. 2017;17(1):240.
18. Rosenfield AT, Glickman MG, Taylor KJ, et al. Acute focal bacterial nephritis (acute lobar nephronia). Radiology. 1979; 132(3):553-61.
19. Dyer RB, Chen MY, Zagoria RJ. Classic signs in uroradiology. Radiographics. 2004;24(1):247-80.
20. Van Sonnenberg E, D'Agostino HB, Sanchez RB, et al. Percutaneous abscess drainage. Radiol. 1992;184:27-9.
21. Allen HA, Walsh JW, Brewer WH, et al. Sonography of emphysematous pyelonephritis. J Ultrasound Med. 1984; 3(12):533-7.
22. Wan YL, Lee TY, Bullard MJ, et al. Acute gas-producing bacterial renal infection: correlation between imaging findings and clinical outcome. Radiology. 1996;198(2):433-8.
23. Chen MT, Huang CN, Chou YH, et al. Percutaneous drainage in the treatment of emphysematous pyelonephritis: 10-year experience. J Urol. 1997;157(5):1569-73.
24. Huang JJ, Tseng CC. Emphysematous pyelonephritis: clinicoradiological classification, management, prognosis, and pathogenesis. Arch Intern Med. 2000;160(6):797-805.
25. Cova M, Squillaci E, Stacul F, et al. Diffusion-weighted MRI in the evaluation of renal lesions: preliminary results. Br J Radiol. 2004;77(922):851-7.
26. Symeonidou C, Standish R, Sahdev A, et al. Imaging and histopathologic features of HIV-related renal disease. RadioGraphics. 2008;28(5):1329-54.
27. Atta MG, Longenecker JC, Fine DM, et al. Sonography as a predictor of human immunodeficiency virus-associated nephropathy. J Ultrasound Med. 2004;23(5):603-10.
28. Kuhlman JE, Browne D, Shermak M, et al. Retro-peritoneal and pelvic CT of patients with AIDS: primary and secondary involvement of the genitourinary tract. RadioGraphics. 1991; 11(3):473-83.
29. Miller FH, Parikh S, Gore RM, et al. Renal manifestations of AIDS. RadioGraphics. 1993;13:587-96.
30. Bray HJ, Lail VJ, Cooperberg PL. Tiny echogenic foci in the liver and kidney in patients with AIDS: not always due to disseminated *Pneumocystis carinii*. Am J Roentgenol. 1992;158(1):81-2.
31. Chugh KS, Sakuja V, Gupta KL, et al. Renal mucormycosis: computerized tomographic findings and their diagnostic significance. Am J Kidney Dis. 1993;22(3):393-7.

CHAPTER

6

Tubercular Infection of the Urinary Tract

Ashu Seith Bhalla, Priyanka Naranje, Arun Kumar Gupta

INTRODUCTION

India continues to remain a high tuberculosis (TB) burden country, with a incidence rate of 204 (140–281) per 100,000 population according to the WHO global TB report of 2018.[1] These cases comprise both pulmonary TB (PTB) and extrapulmonary TB (EPTB). TB of the urinary tract is not uncommon in India. While the lymph nodes are the most common site of EPTB, the genitourinary system is also a common site, accounting for 14–41% of cases.[2,3] Approximately 4 to 8% of patients with PTB will develop clinically significant genitourinary infection.[4] A significant number of patients (10.4%) with PTB may simultaneously, have subclinical forms of urogenital TB.[3] TB occurs in approximately 10% of patients with AIDS and involves at least one extrapulmonary site in nearly 50% of the patients, with kidneys being the most commonly involved genitourinary site.[2,5]

Urinary tract TB is an important clinical problem because of its nonspecific clinical presentation and progression to renal failure if undiagnosed and untreated. It is also a diagnostic problem because of variable imaging features which often resemble many other lesions.

PATHOGENESIS

Renal TB results from hematogenous dissemination of the tubercle bacilli from a primary infection elsewhere.[6] Past or concurrent pulmonary lesion is the most common primary lesion, followed by bone and joint TB. There is a latent period of 5 to 20 years between the pulmonary infection and initial manifestation of clinical kidney involvement. This explains the low incidence of disease in children. The organisms may involve both kidneys in the initial phase, and are lodged in the glomerular and peritubular capillary bed. The subsequent course of the infection is determined by virulence of the organisms and host-resistance factors. Most of the initial lesions heal without sequelae, and only one or a few progress to clinically or radiologically apparent abnormalities. This happens when the bacilli erode out of their initial vascular location and spill into the tubules. This results in granuloma formation along the nephron. Granuloma, caseous necrosis, and cavitation represent stages of progression of the infection. This may communicate with the pelvicalyceal system, and the infection further spreads to the ureter and urinary bladder. The pelvicalyceal and ureteral involvement appears as mucosal ulcerations, focal or generalized dilatation or cicatrization. Fibrosis and calcium depositions represent healing. The pattern of progression and healing is variable and produces asymmetric histologic, microscopic and radiological findings unique to each patient. If the hydronephrotic kidney becomes nonfunctioning, extensive dystrophic (putty like) calcification may form a cast of the kidney, referred to as autonephrectomy. Nonfunctioning kidneys in TB may be due to autonephrectomy or as a sequela of obstruction **(Flowchart 1 and Fig. 1)**. Important complications of renal TB include perinephritis, perinephric abscess, fistulae and psoas abscesses.

CLINICAL PICTURE

The disease is predominant between second and fourth decades of life being distinctly low in children, and less prevalent in fifth and sixth decades. The disease shows a male predominance. Frequency of urination, burning, dysuria or urgency are the most common presenting symptoms. Nearly 50% of the patients at sometimes during the course of the disease have hematuria.

Dull or chronic renal pain, even acute colic is not uncommon. Constitutional symptoms like fever, weight loss, and fatigue are present in about 50% of the patients. Obstructive uropathy, and chronic cystitis are not uncommon with TB.[7,8] Patients may develop fistulae particularly in lower urinary tract involvement. The physical examination is often insignificant. Diagnosis of TB should be considered in patients with recurrent urinary tract infection that is not responding to appropriate therapy for typical pathogens.

LABORATORY INVESTIGATIONS

Pyuria which is sterile when cultured on standard media is characteristic. Presence of red blood cells in urine is frequent. The diagnosis is established by demonstration of acid-fast bacilli (AFB) on microscopic examination of urine, urine

FLOWCHART 1: Pathogenesis of urinary tract tuberculosis.

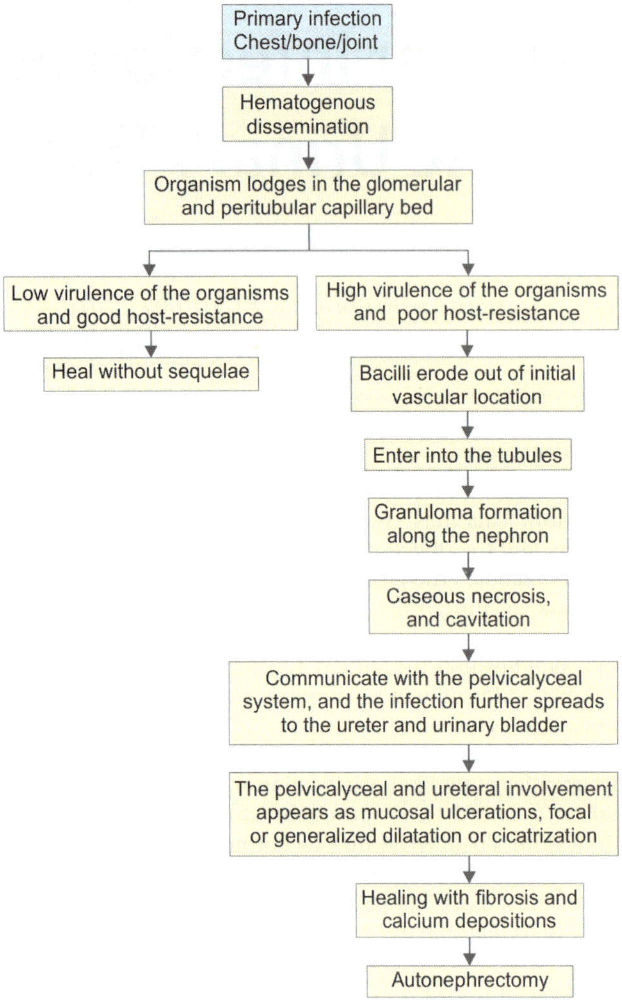

culture or growth of tubercle bacilli in inoculated guinea-pigs. However, urine culture for acid-fast bacilli is positive in nearly 33%, while soluble antigen fluorescent antibody (SAFA) test is strongly positive in only 13%, and weak or nonreactive in 87% of the patients. Also, routine AFB culture is cumbersome involving a delay of 6–8 weeks with a false negative rate of 10–20%, using LJ media. Newer techniques for recovery of mycobacteria from urine specimens include BACTEC 460 and using the automated Mycobacteria Growth Indicator Tube system (MGIT 960), with mean time of positivity of 20 days.[9] As an alternative, polymerase chain reaction (PCR) technique or US-guided fine needle aspiration cytology (FNAC) can be used. PCR is highly sensitive (up to 94%), provides a quicker diagnosis but has a relatively poor specificity.[10] FNAC is useful in those with a negative culture to define granulomatous nature of the visible lesions.

CYSTOSCOPY

Visualization of tubercle, ulcer or retracted ureteric orifice strongly suggest the diagnosis. Generalized cystitis with reduced capacity is almost diagnostic. Biopsy from ulcer, tubercle or inflammatory lesion, particularly in absence of positive urine culture may provide the only diagnostic evidence of the disease.

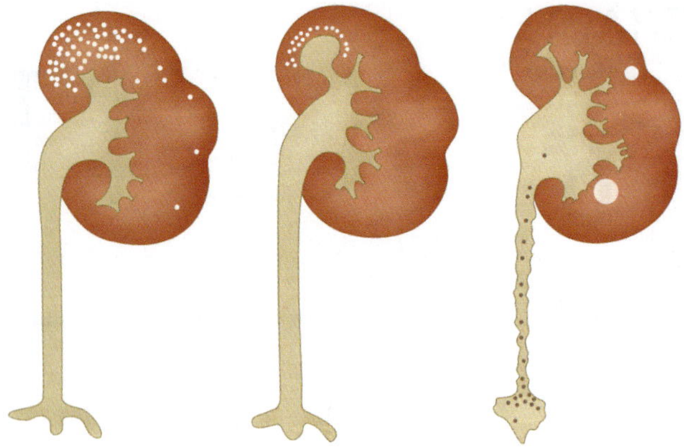

FIG. 1: Schematic diagram showing stages of progression of the disease.

IMAGING EVALUATION

A key role is often played by the radiologist in the diagnosis of the disease. The balance between local progress and healing of the disease process manifests many abnormal imaging features. Since, demonstration of the typical calyceal, ureteral and vesical abnormalities is critical to establish the diagnosis of TB, conventional radiological studies remain the procedures of choice, while ultrasonography (US) and computerized tomography (CT) have an adjunct role. Essentially, early findings are best detected on intravenous urography (IVU) while US and CT are useful for late or chronic changes. US and CT are especially valuable in the evaluation of areas of mass effect and of the nonvisualized kidney at IVU.[11] MRI had not found a place in the diagnostic protocol for evaluation till recently. However, MRI can be useful too in evaluation of the nonfunctioning kidney and focal lesions. A study by Navarro et al. found that IVU provided the diagnosis in 87.5% of cases. The average interval between onset of symptoms and diagnosis was 15 months. They in fact state that the current use of imaging studies other than urography and the finding of other microorganisms in urine culture can delay the diagnosis.[12] The most valuable radiologic feature of genitourinary TB is the multiplicity of abnormal findings. Whenever an imaging pattern of chronic renal inflammatory disease is recognized, particularly in the setting of periureteric or peripelvic fibrosis, TB must be considered.[13]

Radiographs

Plain radiograph of abdomen is an important initial examination before IVU and may provide valuable information such as calcification or evidence of skeletal involvement. Small, enlarged or normal renal size; presence of scarring or focal bulge are all nonspecific findings. Deposition of calcium in an attempt to heal and limit the pathological process often provides a diagnostic clue. Calcification is of two types: (1) Amorphous granular associated with granulomatous masses, and (2) Dense punctate calcification representing healed tuberculoma. It varies from a few minute areas to a

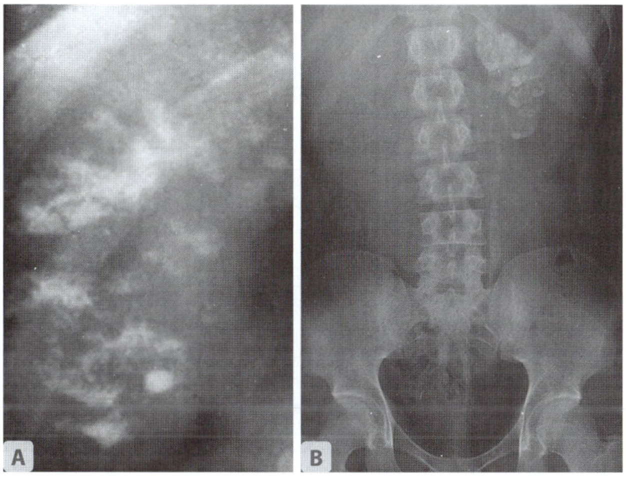

FIGS. 2A AND B: Patterns of calcification in renal tuberculosis. (A) Plain radiograph abdomen showing amorphous granular calcification involving the right kidney; (B) Extensive calcification involving the entire left kidney with ureteral calcification—autonephrectomy.

cast of entire kidney **(Figs. 2A and B)**. The lobar distribution of calcification is quite specific for renal TB. Tubercular calcification of ureter is not as common as renal calcification **(Fig. 2B)**, and calcification of bladder is relatively rare.[14] Plain films may also reveal an evidence of skeletal TB in hip, sacroiliac joint or spine with or without a paraspinal abscess and calcification of abdominal lymph nodes. A co-existing focus of extrarenal TB elsewhere, ranges from 23 to 53% in various series. Chest X-ray is abnormal in about 50% of the patients. However, active PTB is seen in only 5–10% with most patients showing sequelae of past infection.

Intravenous Urography

Even though miliary tubercles involve both kidneys, disease progression and hence radiological abnormalities are confined to a single kidney in over 70% of the patients.

Intravenous urography is a very useful modality to detect early features of urinary tract TB.[15,16] However, the diagnosis can be made with certainty on urography only if the lesion has ulcerated into the calyx. Hence, IVU may be normal in symptomatic renal TB in the initial stages when the bacilli are lodged in glomerulus and peritubular capillary bed. IVU is essential to assess the extent and severity of involvement, to monitor the response to treatment and to look for complications. The various IVU findings are summarized in **Table 1**.

Kidney

The earliest urographic abnormality is the loss of definition of a minor calyx producing an indistinct feathery outline (smudged papillae), irregularity of the surface of one or more papillae or calyces with normal renal size and contour **(Figs. 3A and B)**.[17]

Progressive involvement of renal parenchyma occurs in three forms, which occur singly or in combination. First is coalescence of granulomas leading to unifocal or multifocal mass lesions. These may enlarge overall renal length or increase thickness of renal substance and cause displacement of adjacent collecting system. Caliectasis occurs with irregularity in contour indicating erosion of the pyramids and cortical necrosis. Depending on the necrosis, a cavity with irregular walls communicates with a deformed calyx **(Figs. 4 and 5)**. Radiographic appearance of this form simulates papillary necrosis of other origins. The second form seen in advanced renal TB is parenchymal surface scarring over retracted papillae and dilated calyces. This may be focal or diffuse involving the entire kidney and occurs due to tissue loss leading to fibrosis. Associated calcification or calculi maybe seen. Radiographic identification of calcification associated with renal TB is becoming less common. Calculus disease is rapidly becoming the most frequent form of calcification associated with renal TB.[18] Due to pelvic scarring the calculi formed also tend to take on this deformed shape.

TABLE 1: Intravenous urography findings of urinary tract tuberculosis.

Region of involvement	IVU findings
Kidney	• Irregularities of surface of papillae—"Smudged" papillae • Calyceal erosion (early change)—"Moth-eaten" calyx • Irregular tract formations from calyx into papilla • Large irregular cavities communicating with deformed calyx—"papillary necrosis" • Dilated calices (hydrocalycosis) often with infundibular strictures • Renal calculi • "Hiked up pelvis" due to pelvic scarring • Marked hydronephrosis due to longstanding obstruction • "Putty kidney" extensive parenchymal and PCS calcifications • Autonephrectomy—small shrunken scarred nonfunctioning kidney ± dystrophic calcifications • Infection may extend into peri or pararenal space/psoas
Ureter	• Dilatation—due to atony and prolonged bacilluria • Long segment strictures—most commonly at distal one-third • Beaded/corkscrew ureter • "Pipe stem ureter"—rigid shortened ureter with narrow lumen • Ureteral calcifications (uncommon)
Urinary bladder	• Filling defects—due to tuberculomas in wall • "Thimble bladder"—irregular contracted bladder • Vesicoureteric reflux—fibrosis in trigone region
Urethra	• Stricture at bulbomembranous location (on MCU study)

(MCU: micturating cystourethrogram)

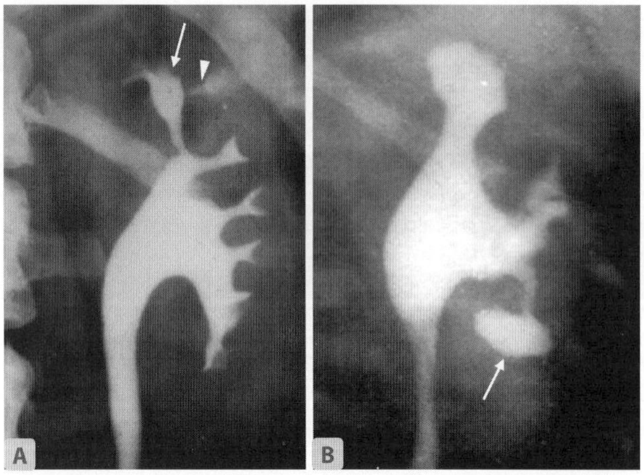

FIGS. 3A AND B: Intravenous urography findings of calyceal involvement by tuberculosis. (A) Early changes—Fuzzy, moth eaten outline of calyx (arrow) with caliectasis and irregular tracts in papilla (arrowhead); (B) Intravenous urography reveals marked dilatation of the inferior calyx with loss of sharpness and fuzziness of its outline (arrow). Rest of the calyces are also dilated.

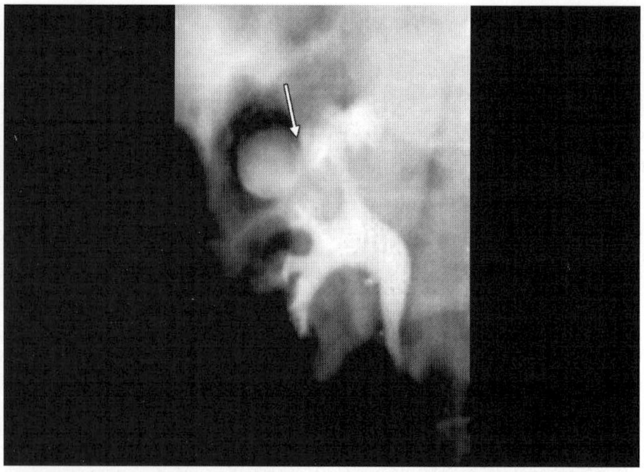

FIG. 4: Intravenous urography findings of calyceal involvement by tuberculosis. IVU shows a large cavity communicating with a dilated, irregular superior calyx (arrow).

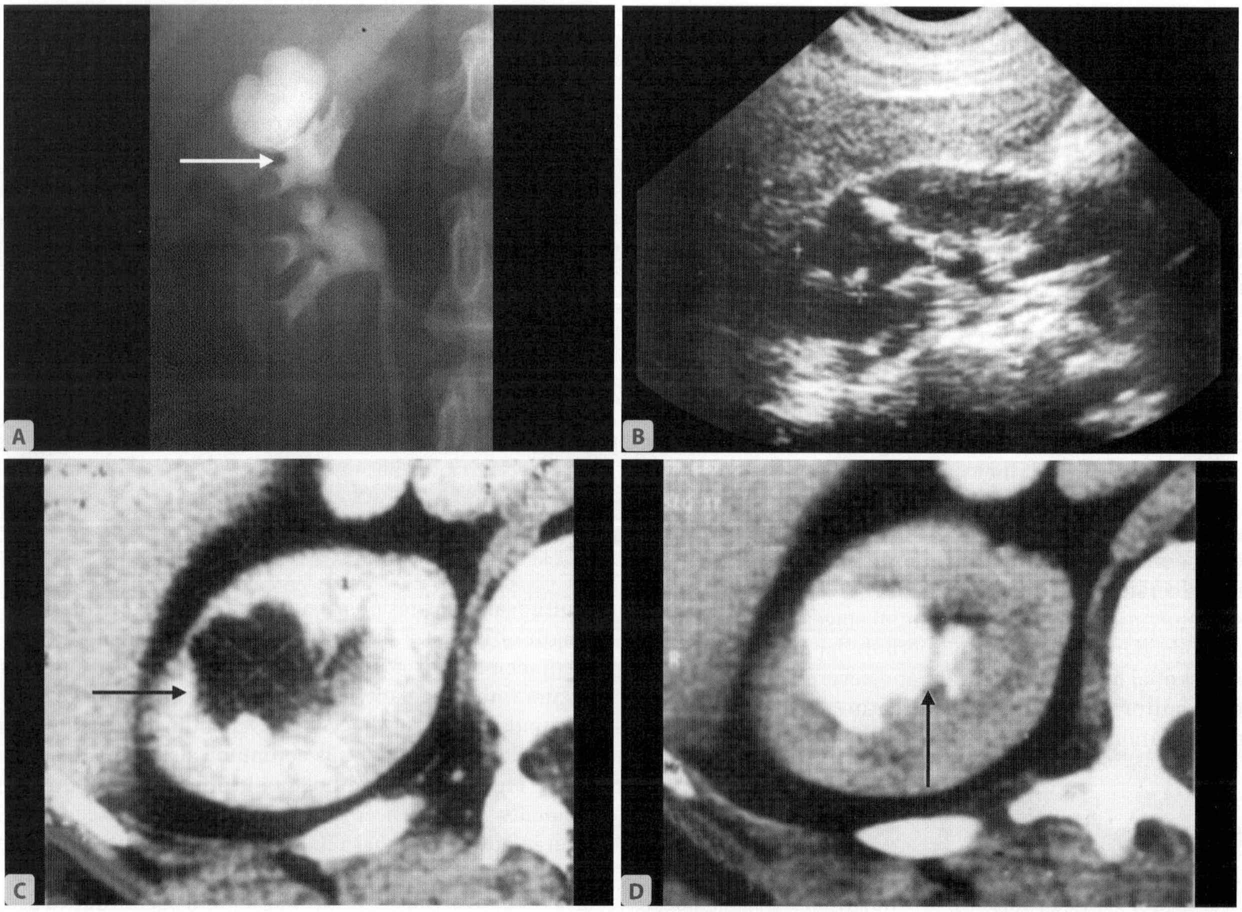

FIGS. 5A TO D: Papillary necrosis with irregular cavities. (A) IVU reveals a large cavity communicating with the superior calyx of right kidney (arrow); (B) Ultrasonography shows a hypoechoic focal lesion in the upper polar cortex with an echogenic rim; (C) CT confirms the presence of the cavity seen on IVU and US, with pooling of contrast on delayed images, (D) due to communication with the pelvicalyceal system (arrows).

Upward pointing renal pelvic calculi may be seen due to "hiked up" pelvis[18] **(Figs. 6A to C)**. Impaired excretion of contrast is seen in either of these two forms.

A third form is autonephrectomy, which represents end stage disease. It may be of two types: (1) caseo-cavernous type-enlarged sac filled with caseous material, with or without calcification[2] **(Fig. 7)**. This can simulate xanthogranulomatous pyelonephritis; (2) calcified shrunken nonfunctioning kidney.

Following the drainage of a cavity into the collecting system, there is spread of infection to other parts of the urinary tract. Subsequent stimulation of scirrhous reaction causes stenosis and obstruction of parts of the collecting system. The common sites of strictures being the neck of a calyx, pelviureteric junction and lower end of the ureter **(Figs. 8 to 10)**. Depending on the site of narrowing there is dilatation of a single calyx (hydrocalyx) or regional hydrocalycosis or generalized dilatation of the pelvicalyceal system. A completely stenosed infundibulum or calyx may lead to failure of contrast excretion by the involved parenchyma (phantom calyx). A tiny infundibular stump (amputated calyx) may be seen in such cases. The renal pelvis may be dilated or may show filling defects due to caseous debris and granulation tissue. The involvement progresses to fibrosis with scarring. If the inferior margin of the renal pelvis is involved with resultant cephalic retraction, a characteristic deformity called the "hiked up pelvis" results. In addition, deformity of the pelvicalyceal system may be caused by traction from a strictured infundibulum or parenchymal fibrosis kinking the pelvis (Kerr's kink) and involving areas not directly affected by tuberculous ulcerations. Occasionally, obstruction can be of such a high grade and so prolonged that marked hydronephrosis develops.[19]

Ureter

Ureteral involvement is almost always secondary to renal TB with spread of infection by bacilluria. In the early stages there is dilatation resulting from atony and prolonged bacilluria. With progression of the disease, irregular segments of ureter are seen due to mucosal ulcerations. Further necrosis of ureteral musculature is accompanied by fibrosis resulting in stricture formation. The ureteric segments which are more superficially involved may heal without stricture formation. This produces a beaded or corkscrew appearance of the ureter.[20] Ureteral strictures have been reported in 10–56% of patients with urinary tract TB.

The terminal segment of the ureter is most commonly involved **(Figs. 10A and B)**. However, any part may be involved with multiple strictures seen in 19% cases. In later stages, severe thickening of the wall produces a rigid shortened ureter with narrow lumen termed as "pipe stem ureter". Renal damage secondary to ureteral strictures may

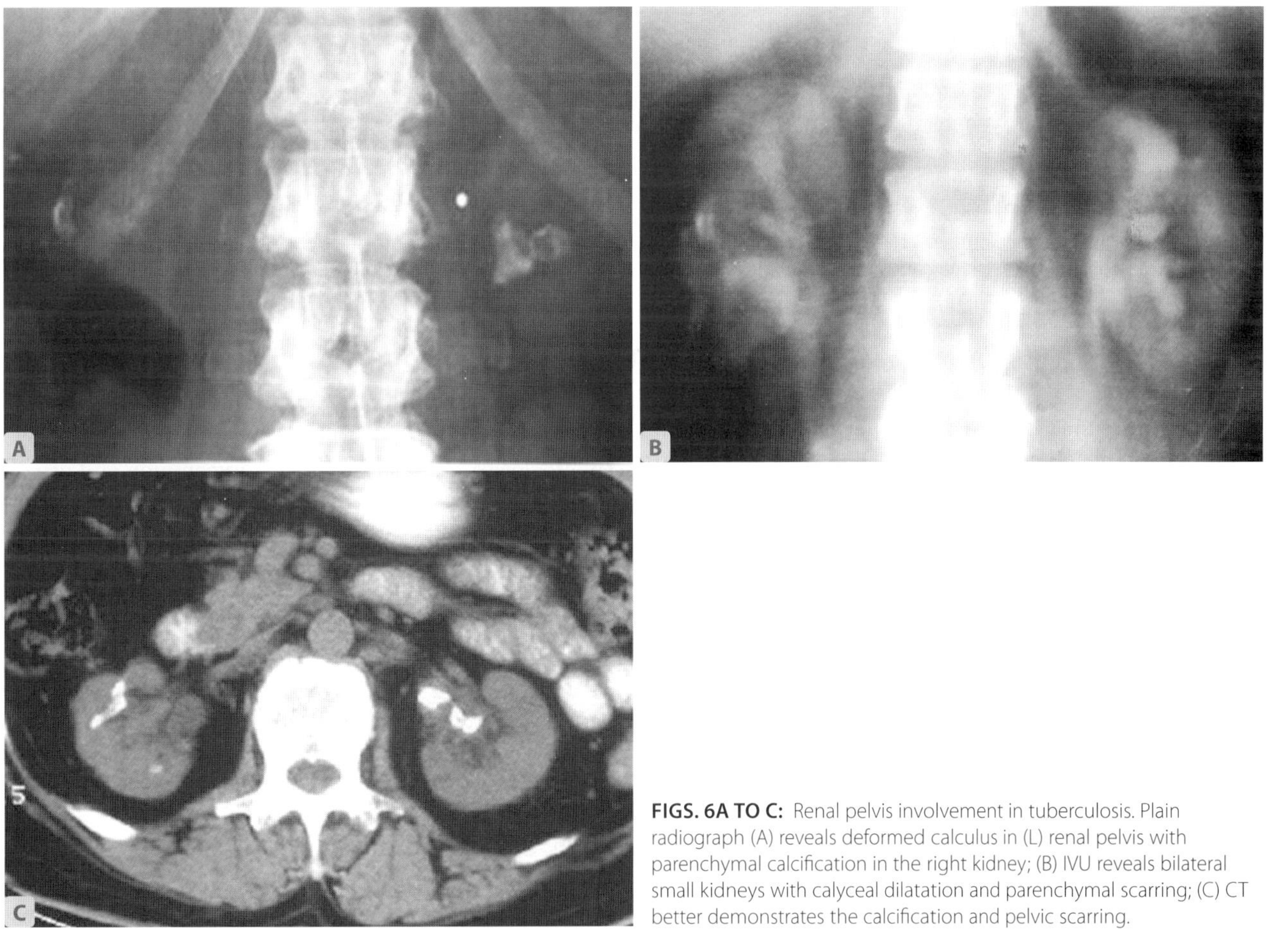

FIGS. 6A TO C: Renal pelvis involvement in tuberculosis. Plain radiograph (A) reveals deformed calculus in (L) renal pelvis with parenchymal calcification in the right kidney; (B) IVU reveals bilateral small kidneys with calyceal dilatation and parenchymal scarring; (C) CT better demonstrates the calcification and pelvic scarring.

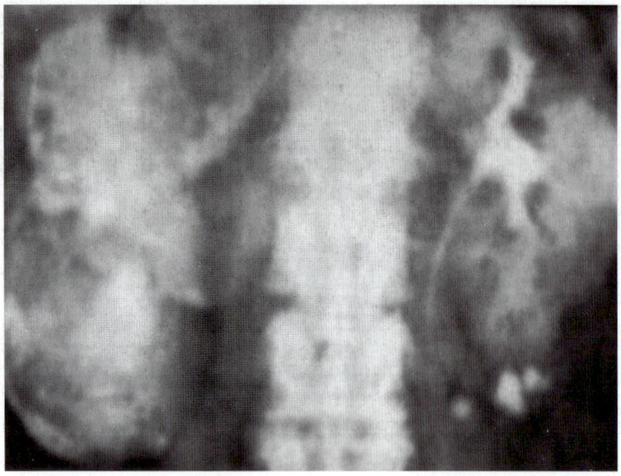

FIG. 7: Advanced disease of caseo-cavernous type. IVU slowing an enlarged, sac like poorly functioning right kidney.

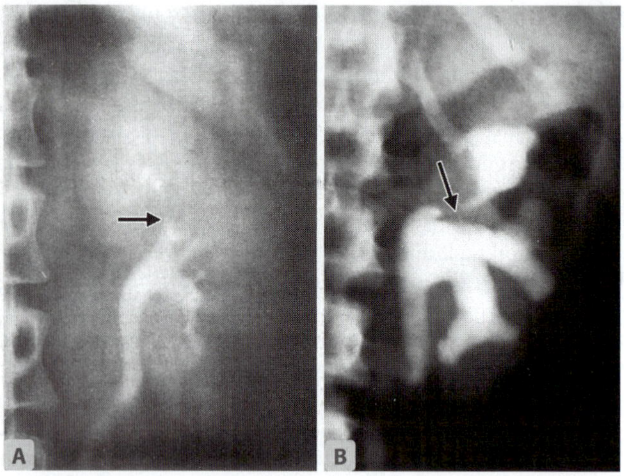

FIGS. 8A AND B: Infundibular strictures. (A) IVU shows irregularity of the superior calyx with intrarenal reflux and infundibular narrowing (arrow); (B) IVU in a different patient shows infundibular narrowing (arrow) with dilated superior calyx.

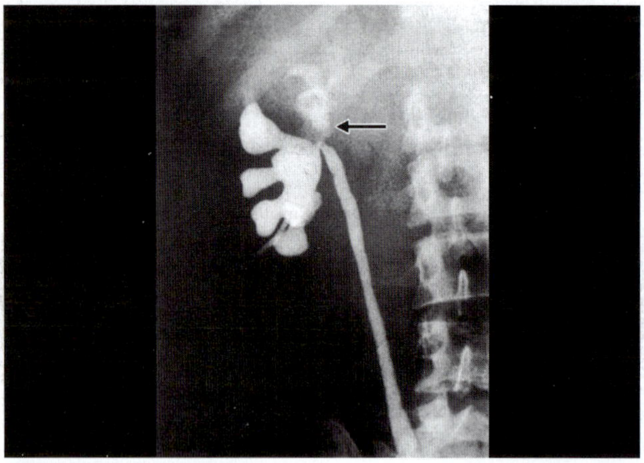

FIG. 9: Renal pelvis and Infundibular strictures. Nephrostogram showing deformed and contracted renal pelvis with proximal dilatation of the pelvicalyceal system. Superior calyx is communicating with an irregular cavity and there is infundibular stenosis (arrow). Ureter is also dilated due to lower end stricture.

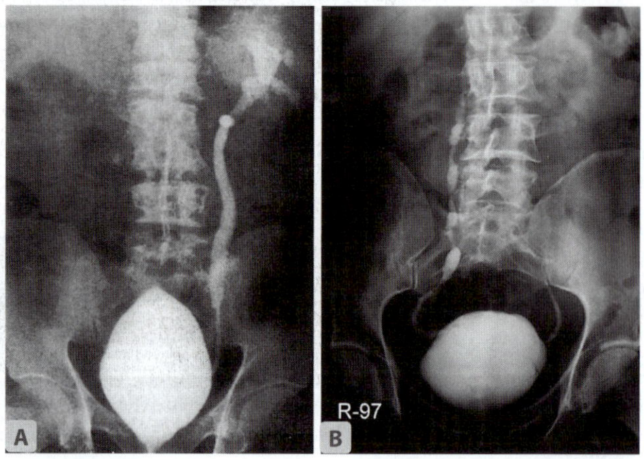

FIGS. 10A AND B: Ureteric strictures. (A) IVU showing long irregular stricture involving lower end of left ureter with hydroureter, hydronephrosis and infundibular stenosis of inferior calyx of left kidney. Also note changes of tuberculosis involving L2-L3 vertebrae; (B) Beaded appearance of right ureter.

be more severe than the effect of the original parenchymal involvement. Dilatation and stenting of the ureter may restore ureteral patency and salvage a kidney.

Urinary Bladder

Urinary bladder is involved later in the course of the disease in up to one-third of patients of urinary tract TB. Use of bacillus Calmette-Guérin therapy for bladder cancer can cause symptomatic tubercular infections of the lower genitourinary tract.[7] Tubercular cystitis leads to edema of the bladder mucosa. Large tuberculomas in vesical wall can manifest radiologically as filling defects simulating carcinoma.[21] Advanced disease leads to irregular contracture with thick walls and reduction of bladder capacity—the "thimble bladder" **(Figs. 11A to C)**. Fibrosis in the region of the trigone produces gaping of the ureterovesical junction resulting in free vesicoureteric reflux **(Fig. 12)**.

Urethral Tuberculosis

Tuberculosis of the male urethra is uncommon and usually occurs secondary to renal infection. It may also be associated with prostatic abscess, periurethral abscess or fistula formation. It may result in a nonspecific stricture almost always in the bulbomembranous urethra that is indistinguishable on imaging from strictures due to other causes.

Retrograde Pyelography

Retrograde pyelography is particularly indicated in a patient with nonfunctioning kidney to demonstrate ureteric obstruction and cavitation in the kidney.

Ultrasonography

Ultrasound is not used as the primary imaging modality for diagnosis of urinary tract TB, as it is unable to show early

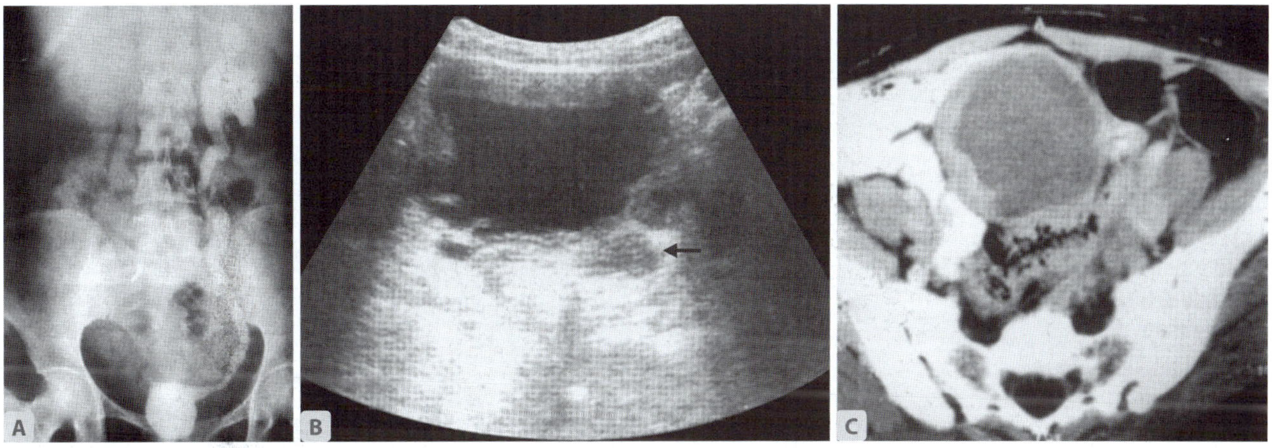

FIGS. 11A TO C: Urinary bladder TB. (A) IVU reveals a small capacity (thimble) urinary bladder, ureteral stricture with proximal hydroureter and hydronephrosis on left side. Right kidney is nonfunctioning; (B) Ultrasonography shows irregular, asymmetric wall thickening of the urinary bladder with trabeculations. A left adnexal mass is also seen posterior to the bladder (arrow) (C) CT shows a similar appearance of the urinary bladder.

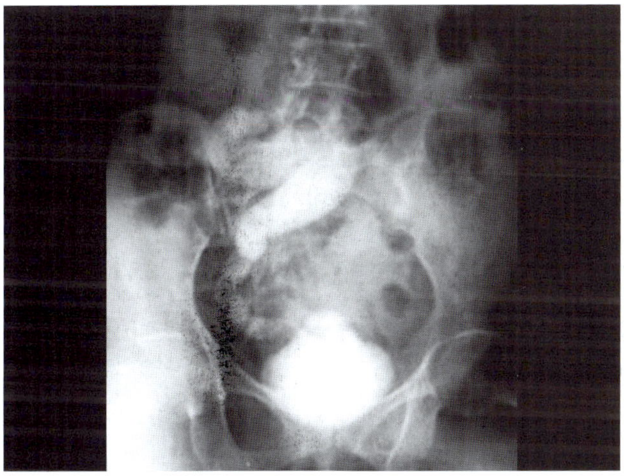

FIG. 12: Urinary bladder tuberculosis with vesicoureteric reflux (VUR). Micturating cystourethrogram (MCU) study reveals a small capacity bladder with reflux into a dilated, tortuous right ureter.

calyceal changes and does not provide information about renal functional status. However, carefully performed sonogram can show a spectrum of morphological abnormalities.[22,23] The role of sonography is also to provide guidance for the interventional procedures of percutaneous nephrostomy (PCN), antegrade dilatation of ureteral stricture and drainage of the perinephric abscess.

Kidney

A focal renal lesion of varying echogenicity is a frequently encountered sonographic abnormality. In the early stages US demonstrates papillary lesions as areas of hypoechogenicity or hypoechoic foci with echogenic walls or echogenic nonshadowing lesions (***see* Fig. 5B**).[23] A sloughed calyx is seen as an echogenic flap separated from the normal calyceal wall (**Fig. 13A**). Large liquefying conglomerate cavities or dilated calyces formed as a result of infundibular stricture appear as hypoechoic nodules or masses. The communicating tract from a cavity appears as a sonolucent track entering the dilated calyx (**Fig. 13B**). Heterogeneous echotexture of the parenchyma or normal appearing parenchyma may be seen in diffuse involvement (**Figs. 14A and B**). Such patients show poor excretory function on IVU and CT. Following pelvicalyceal system involvement, US may characteristically show uneven caliectasis without renal pelvis dilatation. It may also demonstrate hydronephrosis, parenchymal calcification, and perinephric abscess (**Figs. 15A and B**).

Xuefang Rui et al.[24] reviewed sonographic features of 258 cases of renal TB. In this series of 258 cases, 152 cases were correctly diagnosed as renal TB by B-mode ultrasonography, and these were classified under 6 types.

Type I: Nephrectasia type (23 cases); type II: Hydrops type, (21 cases); type III: Empyema type (13 cases); type IV: Inflammatory and atrophy type (15 cases); type V: Calcification type (34 cases); type VI: Mixed type (46 cases). In type I (Nephrectasia), the renal capsule was very irregular. In the renal parenchyma and renal sinus, there were one or several anechoic zones, of different sizes with irregular margins and some nebulous light spot echoes within. The type II (Hydrops type) also showed an irregular renal capsule. The renal pelvis and calyces were distended, within which there was an anechoic zone, similar to hydronephrosis. However, the inner wall was rough and uneven. In most cases, the ureter was involved and appeared thickened.

Ureter

Ultrasonography does not play a significant role in the acute phase. It is useful in assessment and follow up of back pressure changes and adjoining retroperitoneal disease.

Urinary Bladder

Ultrasonography may detect focal irregularity or thickening of the bladder wall with reduced capacity. Distension of the bladder may be necessary to gauge the bladder capacity accurately. The deformed bladder shape and focal abnormalities are also better appreciated following distension (**Fig. 11B**).

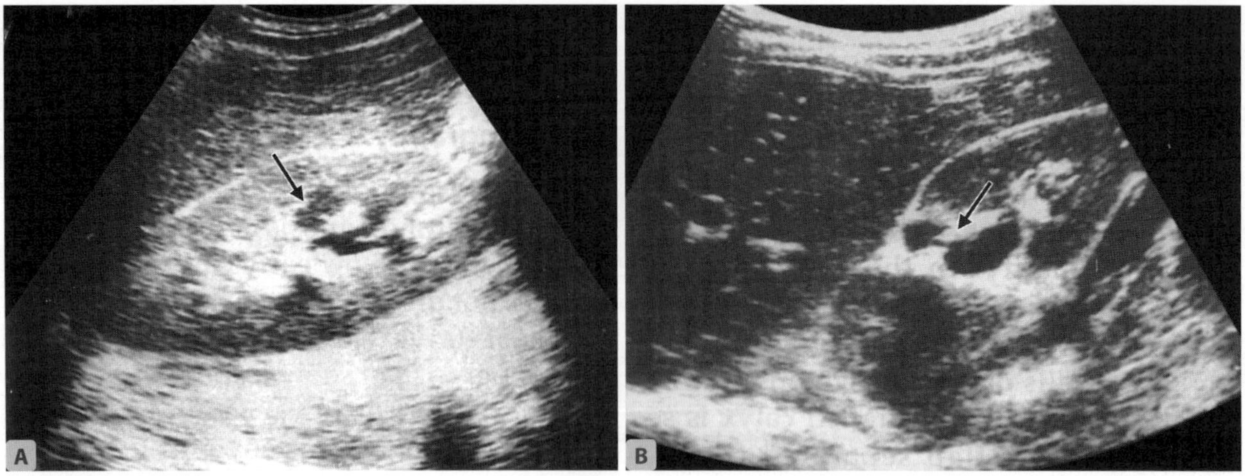

FIGS. 13A AND B: Ultrasonography findings of renal tuberculosis. (A) US showing echogenic papillary sloughing in the middle calyx of the right kidney (arrow); (B) US of another patient reveals an anechoic cavity in the renal cortex with a sonolucent track (arrow) connecting the cavity and the pelvicalyceal system.

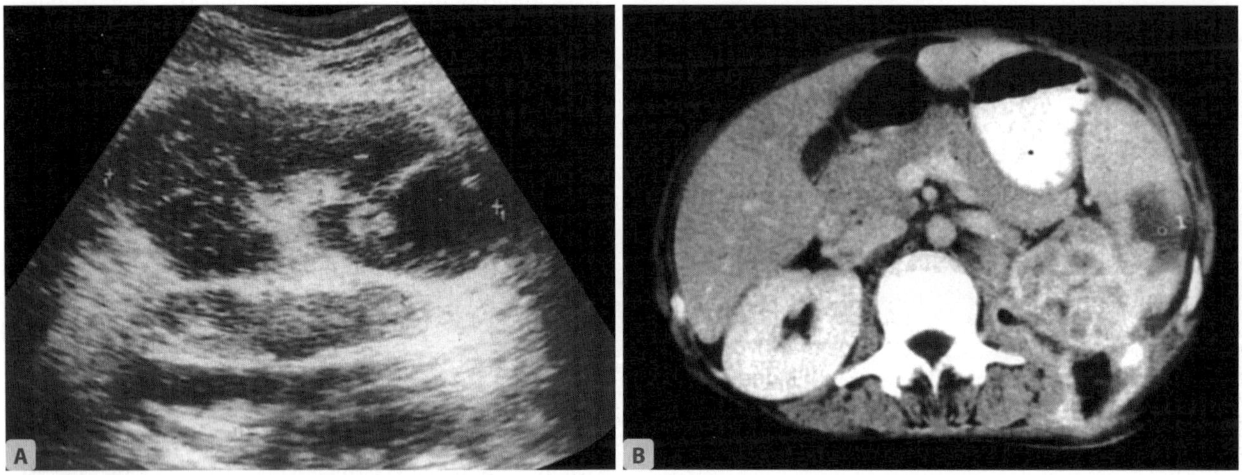

FIGS.14A AND B: Ultrasonography appearance of diffuse involvement of kidney by tuberculosis. (A) US shows an enlarged heterogeneous left kidney with an anechoic cavity in the lower pole; (B) CECT of the same patient reveals poorly functioning heterogeneous left kidney with hypodense areas within. An irregular hypoattenuating splenic abscess and inflammatory changes in the left posterior renal space, left psoas and posterior parietes are also seen.

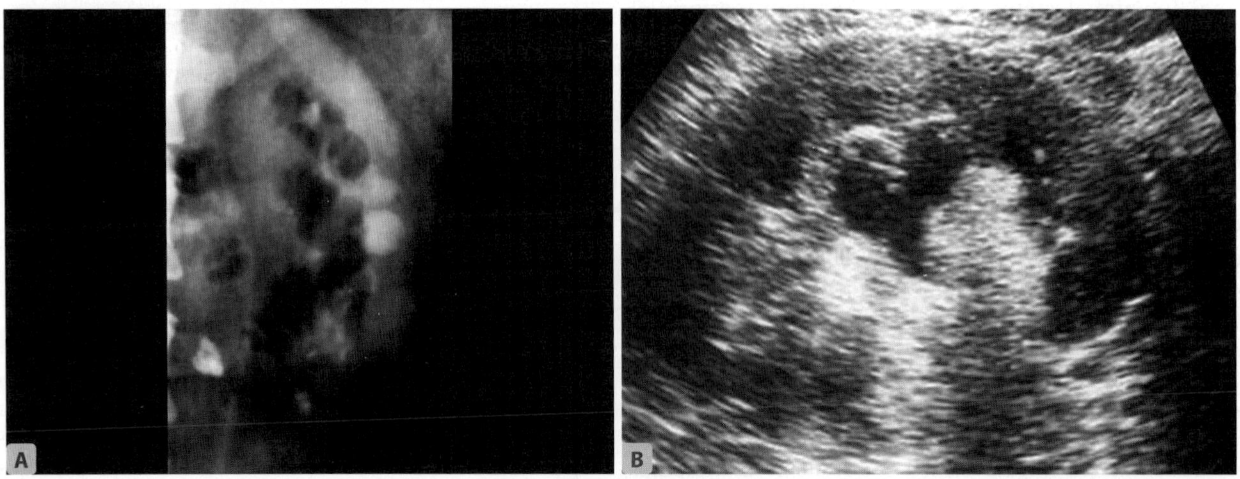

FIGS. 15A AND B: Uneven caliectasis on ultrasonography. (A) Intravenous urography; and (B) Ultrasound of left kidney of a 28 years old male reveals uneven caliectasis with calcification within.

Computed Tomography

Over the years, there has been a decrease in the number of IVUs, and a corresponding increase in the number of multidetector CT(MDCTs) being performed even in the setting of urinary tract TB. MDCT with its multiple reconstructions is useful in demonstrating the extent of involvement, length of ureteric stricture, adjoining retroperitoneal disease and associated spinal or solid organ involvement.[25] A combination of corticomedullary, nephrographic and urographic phases allows the delineation of both renal parenchymal as well as urothelial changes. However, the acquisition can be restricted to a single phase in young patients. While IVU is superior to CT in the demonstration of early calyceal changes and papillary necrosis, CT is comparable or better for most abnormalities, it also has the advantage of demonstrating involvement of other abdominal organs. Compared to US, CT is also able to provide better visualization of retroperitoneal structures, more detailed information on presence and pattern of calcification and functional status of the kidney.

Spectrum of Imaging Findings on Computed Tomography

Kidney

Computed tomography may show a spectrum of findings in renal involvement including multiple small poorly enhancing nodules, uneven caliectasis and calcification. In poorly functioning of kidneys the nephrogram effect is much better seen on CT than on IVU.

- *Solid focal lesions*: Representing granulomas, hypodense, variable size. Smaller lesions are often nonenhancing, while larger lesions show rim enhancement. **(Figs. 16A to C)** These have been reported in 12% of cases in a CT based study.[26]
- *Cystic focal lesions*: A cystic lesion adjoining a renal calyx (representing a cavity) is one of the commonest findings (reported in 68% of cases[26]). These often show multiple septations. The overlying cortex is thinned out. Granulomas which caseate and coalesce often appear as complex cystic lesions. On delayed phases, pooling of contrast is seen if the cavity is communicating with the PCS **(Fig. 5C)**. Abscesses often show peripheral enhancement and adjoining inflammation.
- *Focal areas of hypoperfusion*: These are a consequence of vasoconstriction/or small vessel narrowing resulting from active inflammation and edema. This picture resembles acute pyelonephritis.
- *Perinephric inflammation*: Abscess often spread into the perinephric space with thickening of adjoining fasciae **(Figs. 16A and B)**.
- *Urothelial involvement*:
    - Thickening of the wall of pelvis/urothelial thickening leads to narrowing **(Figs. 17 and 18)**.

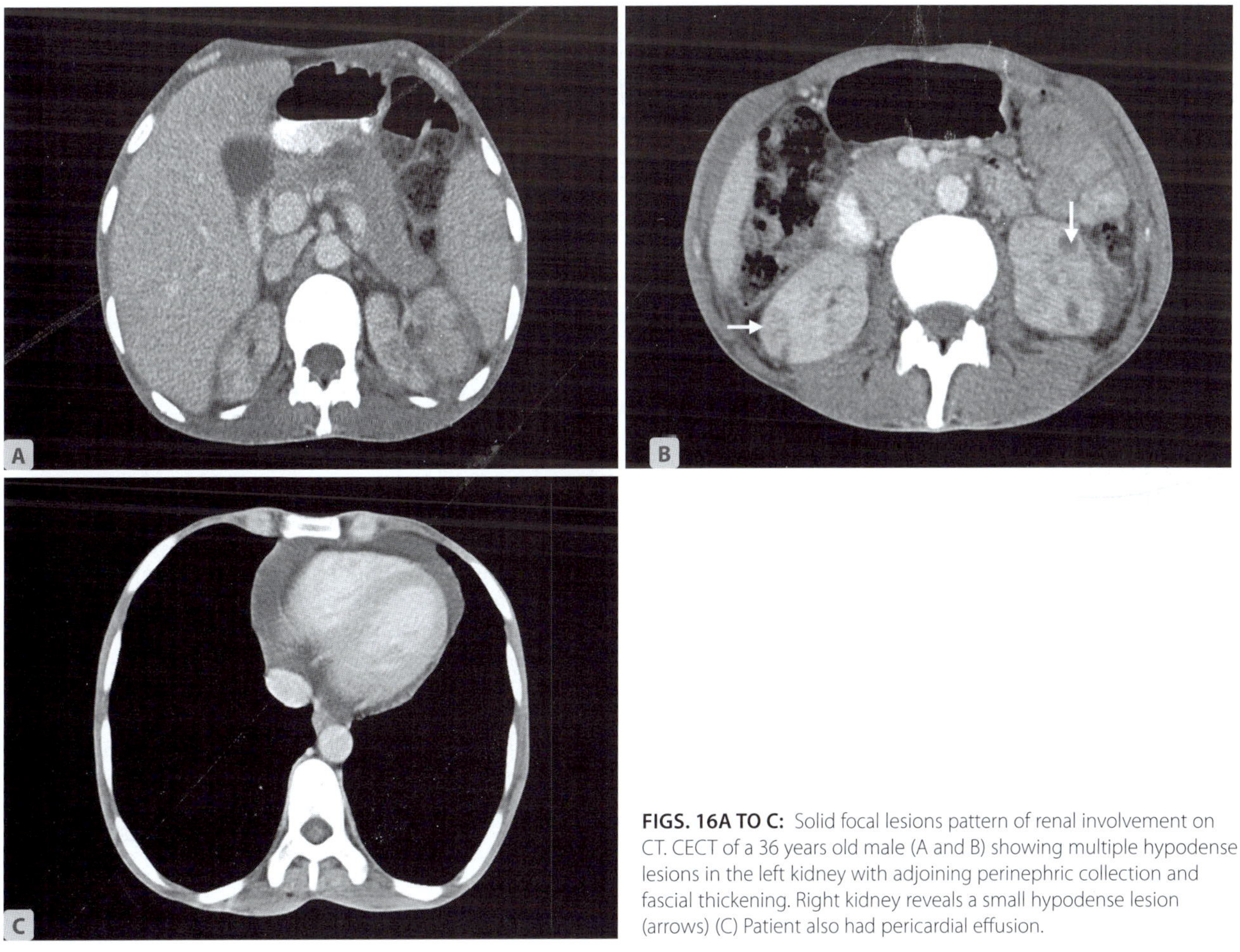

FIGS. 16A TO C: Solid focal lesions pattern of renal involvement on CT. CECT of a 36 years old male (A and B) showing multiple hypodense lesions in the left kidney with adjoining perinephric collection and fascial thickening. Right kidney reveals a small hypodense lesion (arrows) (C) Patient also had pericardial effusion.

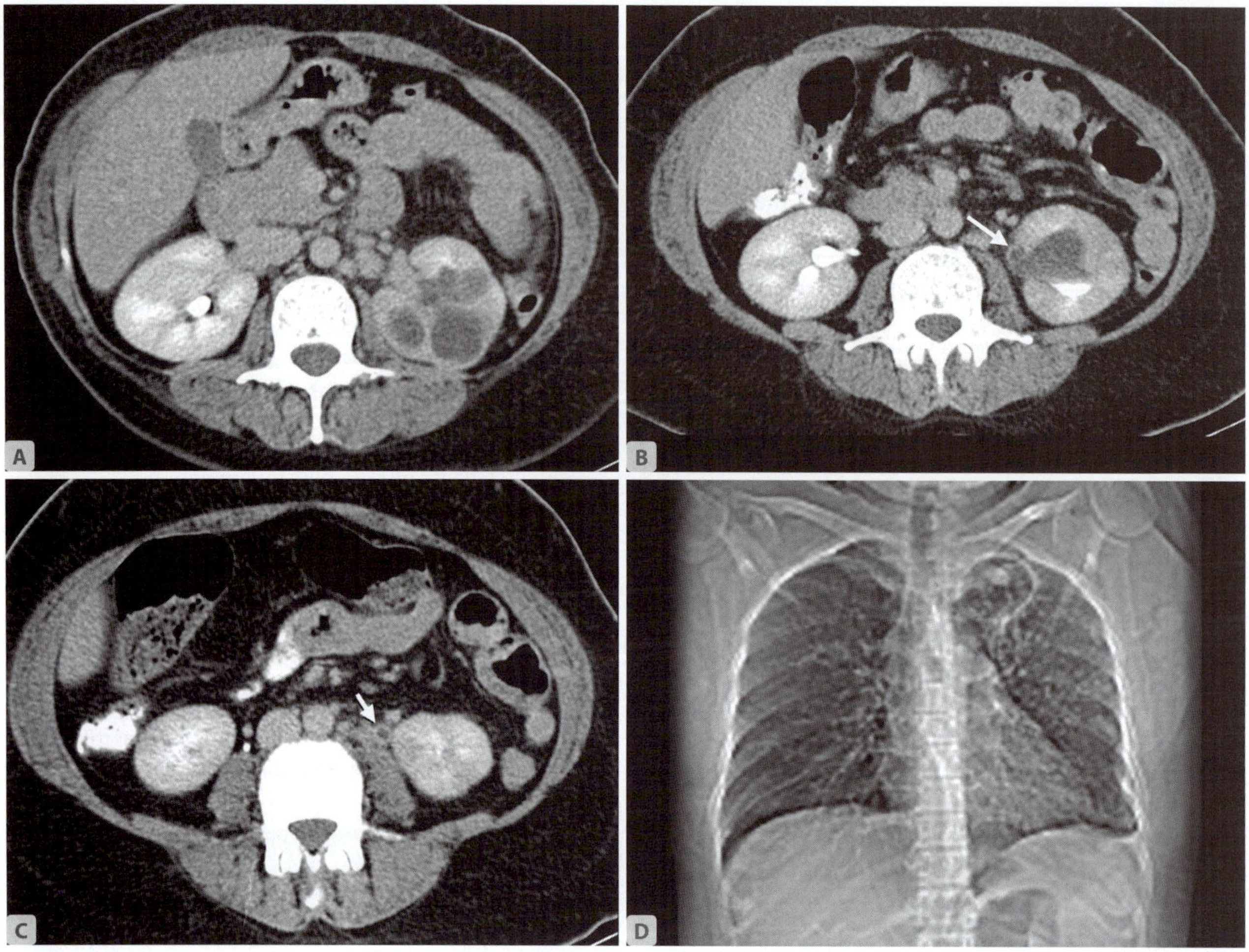

FIGS.17A TO D: Urothelial involvement. CECT of a young girl reveals a poorly functioning (L) kidney with hydronephrosis. (A) Small retroperitoneal nodes are present; (B) Renal pelvis is contracted with a thickened wall (arrow); (C) The ureteric wall is also thickened (arrow); (D) Topogram reveals a cavity in the left upper lobe of lung.

  - Calyceal irregularity and dilatation may be seen.[27]
  - Uneven caliectasis is characteristic with contracted pelvis **(Figs. 18 and 19)**.
- *Sequelae*:
  - With healing and fibrosis, parenchymal scars develop seen as focal areas of cortical thinning often overlying a dilated or distorted calyx.
  - *Calcification*: Various patterns including punctate, curvilinear, amorphous or lobar calcification are seen **(Figs. 19A to C)**.

Ureter

Thickening of the ureteric wall is highly suggestive of TB and can be readily identified on CT **(Fig. 18D)**.

Urinary Bladder

Computed tomography delineates the bladder involvement well similar to IVU/USG but offers no additional advantage except for detection of faint calcification and demonstration of adjacent genital tract disease **(Figs. 11C and 19D)**.

Magnetic Resonance Imaging

Although, there are few published studies on the use of MRI in urinary tract TB, it has in recent years evolved as a useful adjunct modality in the evaluation of these patients. MRI provides both morphological and functional information. Noncontrast scans are immensely useful in those with compromised renal functions, especially with addition of MR urography.[28] Contrast-enhanced magnetic resonance (CEMR) not only delineates the extent better, characterizes focal lesions, demonstrates urothelial thickening but can also evaluate renal function **(Figs. 20 and 21)**. Diffusion-weighted imaging (DWI) aids in characterizing the focal renal lesions, differentiates hydronephrosis from pronephrosis; and is an indicator of renal fibrosis. Time-resolved dynamic CEMR urography can be used for the evaluation of ureteral peristalsis.[29]

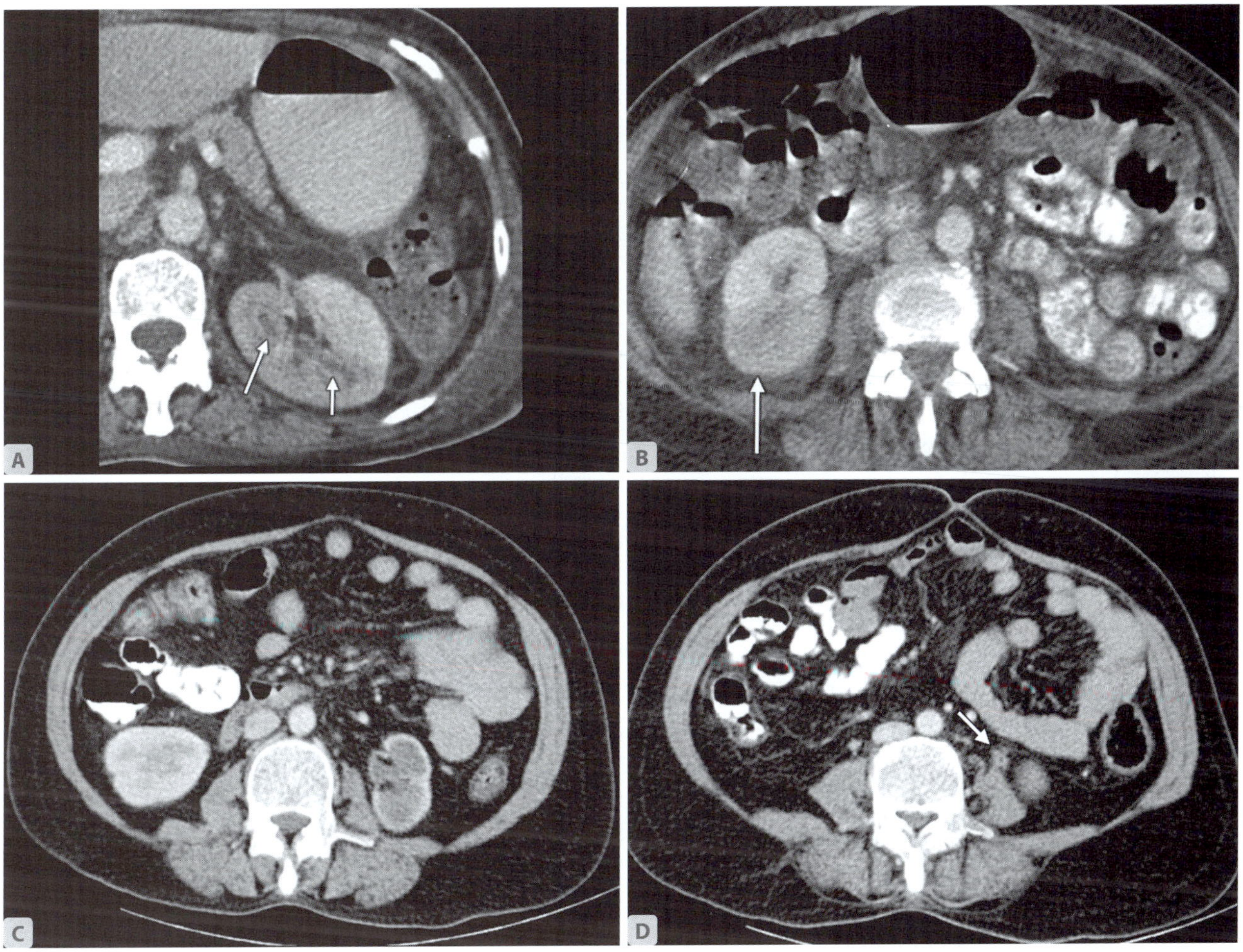

FIGS. 18A TO D: Pelvicalyceal and ureteric urothelial thickening in two different patients. (A) CECT of 61/F shows thickening of the urothelium of pelvicalyceal system (PCS) of left kidney (arrows); (B) Focal large hypodense area seen in upper pole of right kidney with perinephric stranding (focal pyelonephritis form); (C) CECT of a different patient, a 43 years old female reveals left kidney is shrunken with hydronephrosis, scarred pelvis and parenchymal thinning (C). Wall thickening of ureter (arrow) is present (D).

Key MRI findings of urinary tract TB are summarized in **Table 2**.

COMPLICATIONS

The prominent complications include perinephric inflammation/abscess formation including psoas abscesses **(Figs. 21A to E)**. Fistulae or sinus tracts may develop into adjacent tissues or viscera **(Figs. 22 and 23)**.

DIFFERENTIAL DIAGNOSIS

The differential diagnosis of urinary TB can be varied depending upon the form of involvement. Early renal TB can simulate papillary necrosis. Focal lesions resemble other infections or even neoplasms. Calcification and extensive inflammation can mimic xanthogranulomatous pyelonephritis. Similarly, urinary bladder involvement may be confused with neoplastic involvement.

GENITOURINARY TUBERCULOSIS IN HUMAN IMMUNODEFICIENCY VIRUS

The impact of human immunodeficiency virus (HIV) epidemic on the incidence and clinical presentation of genitourinary TB is largely unknown. Navarro et al.[12] evaluated clinical and epidemiological characteristics of patients diagnosed with genitourinary TB at their center over the last 10 years, found that of the 45 patients analyzed, 33% had a coexisting disease (14 were infected by HIV). In a retrospective study from USA, case records of 16 patients infected with HIV and genitourinary TB were compared with those of 8 patients without HIV infection diagnosed with genitourinary TB. Data abstracted from records included demographics, symptoms, signs, laboratory and radiologic findings, and in-hospital mortality. Of 1,282 patients with TB, 24 patients had positive urine cultures for *Mycobacterium TB*. HIV infection was present in 16 patients (75%). Patients infected with HIV were younger (mean age,

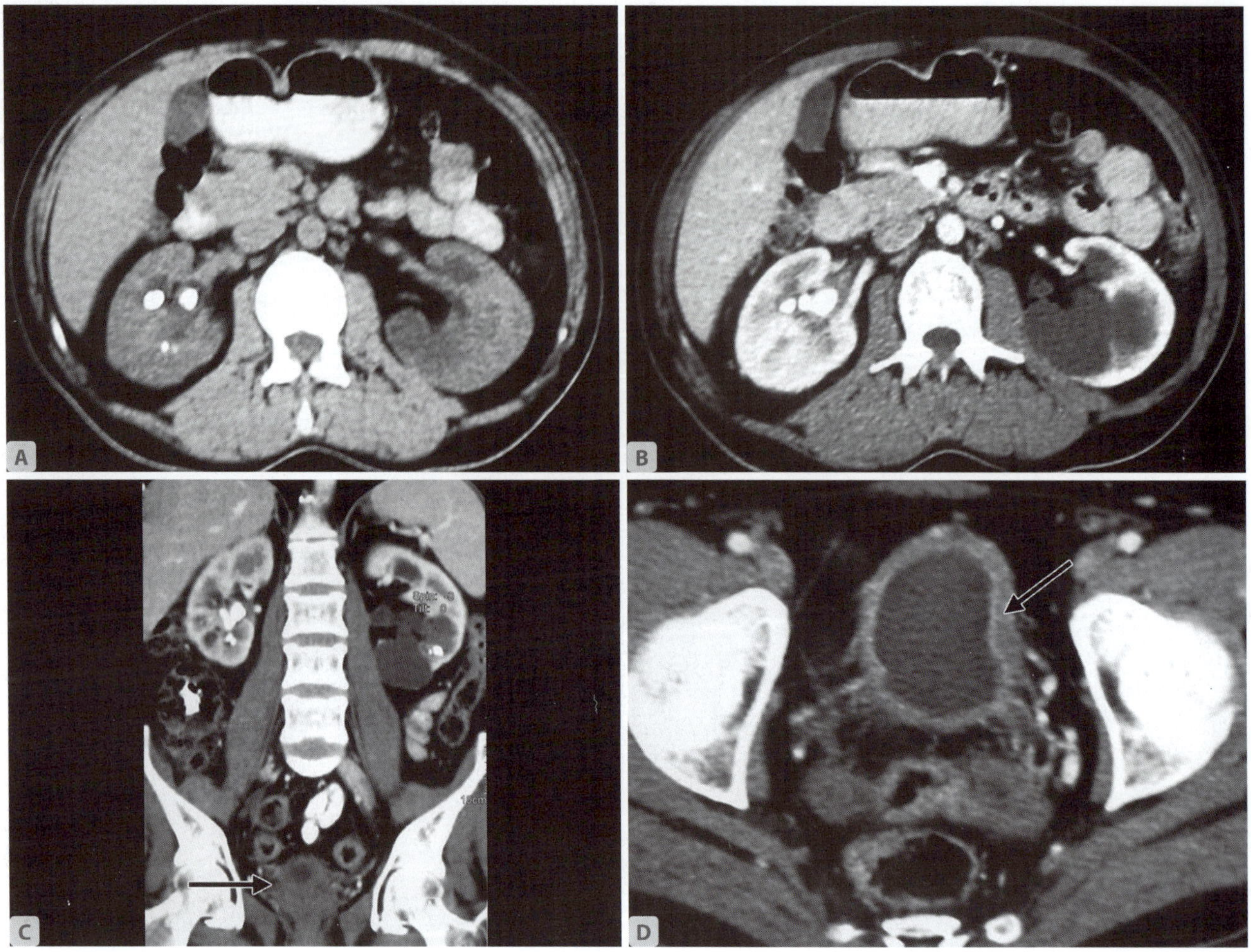

FIGS. 19A TO D: Uneven caliectasis and bladder involvement on CT. Multidetector computed tomography (MDCT) axial (A and B) and coronal; (C) Show a large cavity with irregular caliectasis and calcification involving the lower pole of left kidney. Right kidney has calculi. Scan through pelvis; (D) reveals urinary bladder wall thickening with small capacity (arrow).

39.1 ± 6.2 versus 53.9 ± 17.2, P = 0.047) but did not differ significantly in clinical presentation from patients who did not have HIV infection.[30]

TUBERCULAR INFECTION OF THE GRAFT KIDNEY

Tuberculosis is a frequent complication in solid organ transplant (SOT) recipients, due to their immunosuppressed status, especially in TB endemic regions. TB involving the transplanted kidney is however rare. TB in graft kidney may either be a consequence of preexisting infection in the donor; or a part of disseminated TB in the recipient.[31] TB in transplant kidney can result in graft rejection, and also increases mortality, 17.86% is reported in a series.[32] There are several risk factors that predispose a recipient to develop graft TB. These include: diabetes, use all cyclosporine, mycophenolate mofetil, posttransplant rejection, coexisting chronic liver disease. Renal TB in the graft is often a part of disseminated TB in the recipient, and no characteristic imaging features are described. Also, the findings are often mild and resemble other infections (nonspecific).

The main differences between TB in a graft kidney as compared to TB in an immunocompetent host are enlisted in **Box 1**.

CONCLUSION

In conclusion, diagnosis of urinary tract TB is based on a high index of clinical suspicion supported by a collective evaluation of microbiological, radiological and endoscopic features. While individual radiological features of urinary tract TB can be seen in other diseases such as papillary necrosis due to other causes, infections and neoplasms; the key to diagnosis is pattern recognition. Also, follow-up excretory urography at regular intervals is useful both for assessment of therapeutic response, and for an early detection of the complications.

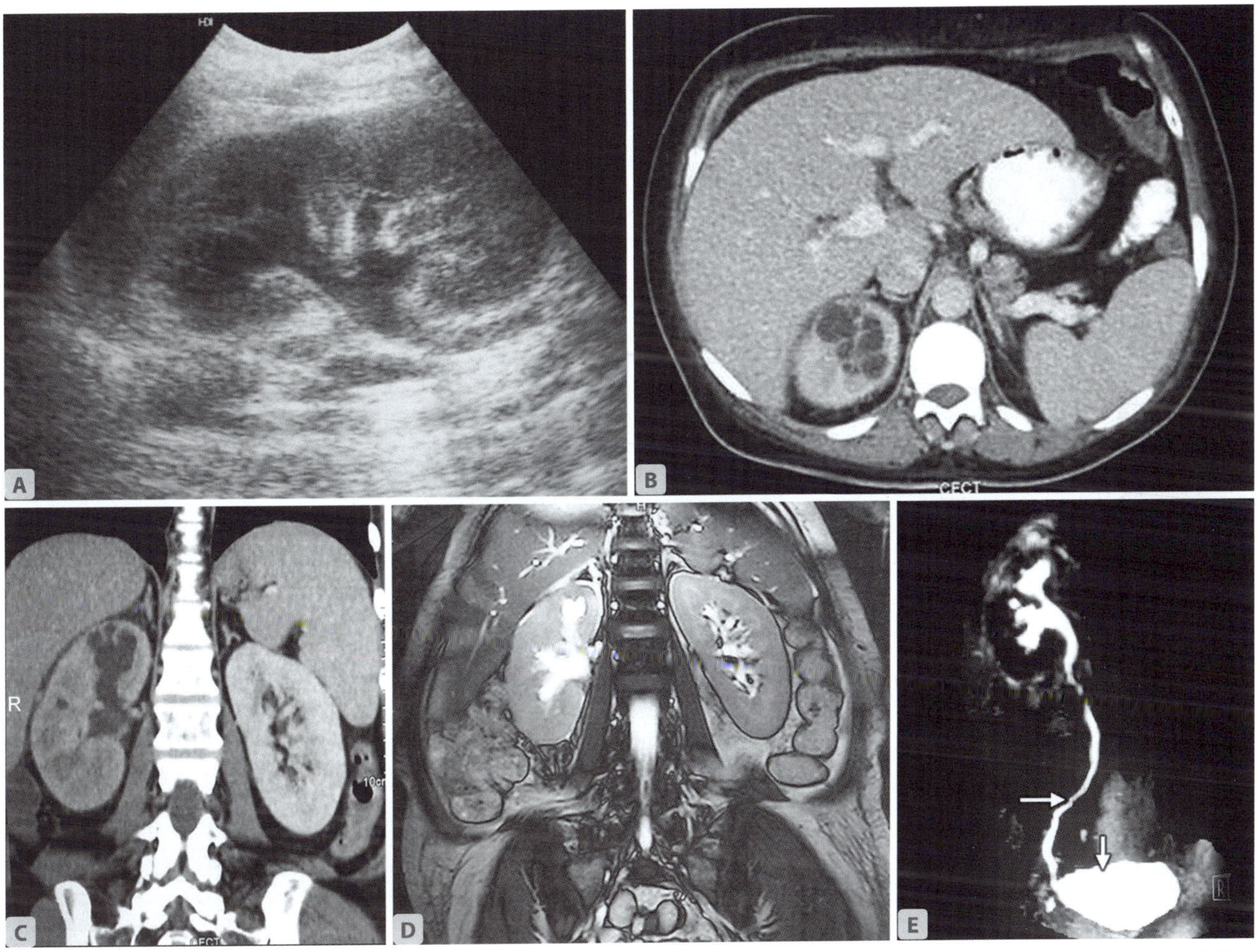

FIGS. 20A TO E: Utility of MR urography in urinary tract TB. Images of a 49 years female. US (A) reveals caliectasis of the superior calyx. Axial CECT (B) shows multiple cavities involving upper pole of the right kidney. Coronal CECT MPR (C) shows the cavities communicating with the superior calyx with parenchymal atrophy of the upper pole, and poor function of the right kidney. True-FISP coronal MRI (D) reveals increased signal intensity of the right kidney. MR urogram (E), in addition illustrates ureteric and bladder irregularity (arrows).

TABLE 2: Magnetic resonance imaging findings of urinary tract tuberculosis.

Form of involvement	MRI findings
Active inflammation	• CEMR: Focal hypoperfusion (D/D acute pyelonephritis) • Loss of interface with adjoining parenchyma • Surrounding fat tissue stranding
Chronic abscess	• Signal characteristic resembling a cyst; with thick walls and internal septae, restricted diffusion • Differential diagnosis cystic neoplasm
Granuloma (depending on size, amount of caseation and calcification)	• *Solid mass (variable size):* – Small lesions—hypointense on both T1WI and T2WI – Central hyperintensity in larger lesions • Caseation—mildly hyperintense on T2WI, fluid debris level • Calcification—hypointense
PCS involvement	• Caliectasis (MRU) • Pelvic scarring • Urothelial thickening (CEMR) • Low ADC in pyonephrosis • Ureteral strictures • Urethral strictures
TB sequelae (Interstitial fibrosis)	• Small size, irregular • Low ADC

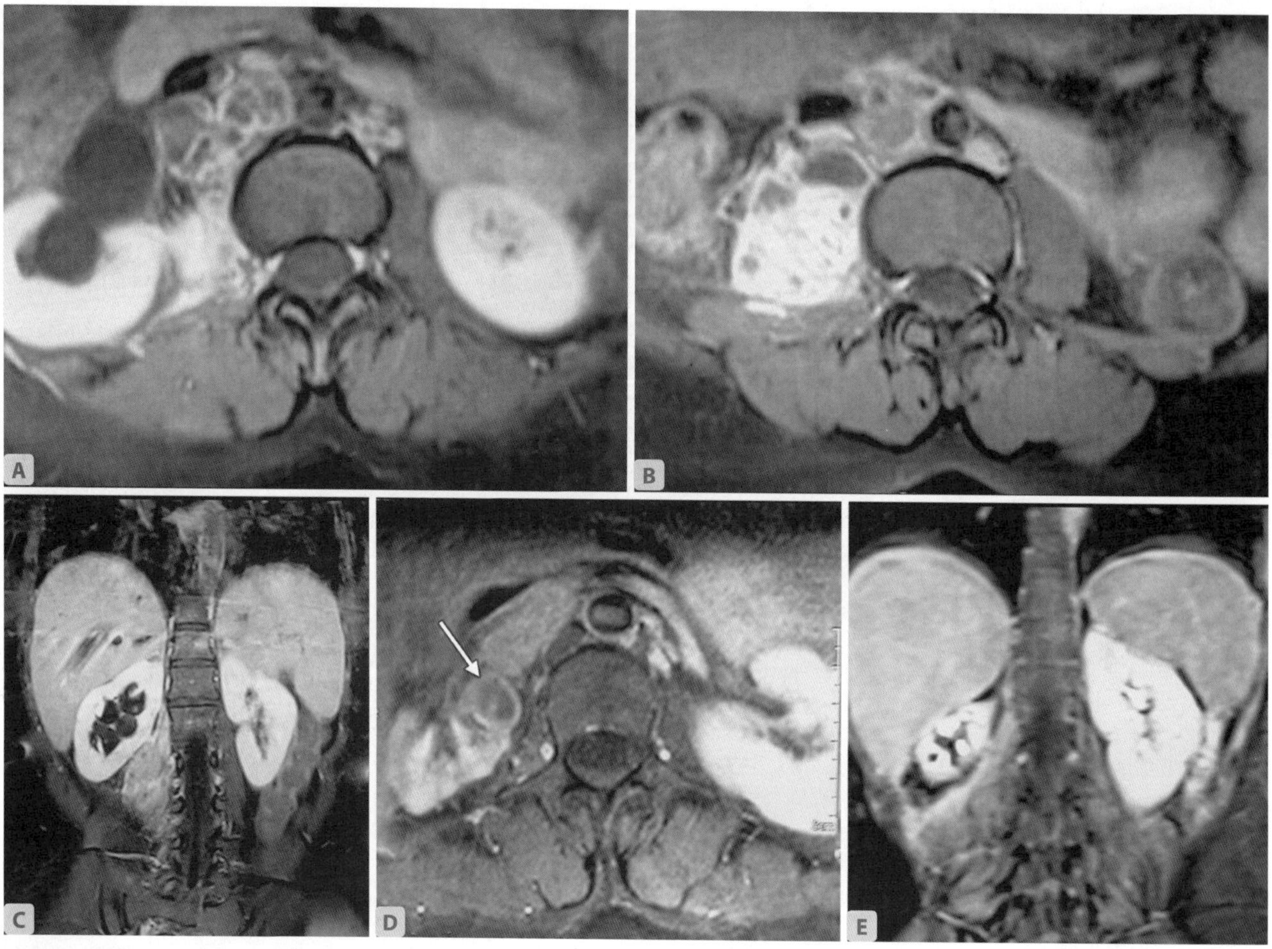

FIGS. 21A TO E: MRI characterizing focal renal lesion (chronic abscess) and retroperitoneal involvement in TB. Serial gadolinium-enhanced MR images of a 28 years old woman of multidrug resistant tuberculosis. Axial (A and B) and coronal; (C) Post-gadolinium images reveal necrotic retroperitoneal nodes with right psoas abscess encasing the ureter and causing hydronephrosis. MR scan obtained 8 months after second line antitubercular treatment (ATT); (D and E) shows reduction of the lymphadenopathy and psoas abscess. The right kidney is however shrunken and has a rim-enhancing lesion in the renal cortex suggesting an abscess (arrow).

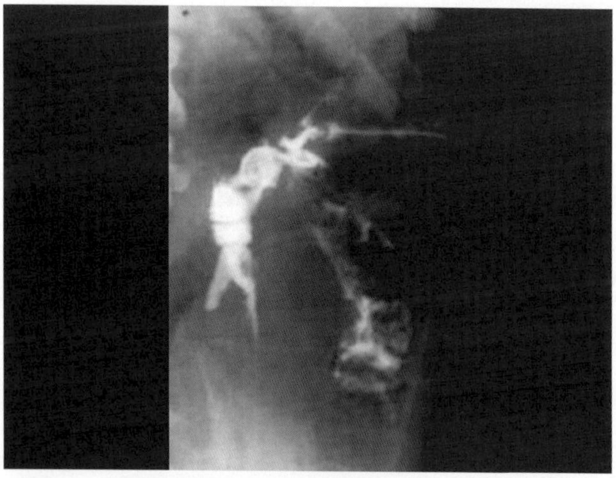

FIG. 22: Sinogram performed in a 28 years old man with a chronic discharging (L) lumbar sinus reveals opacification of the pelvicalyceal system.

BOX 1: Graft kidney tuberculosis versus tuberculosis in immunocompetent host.

- No long latency. Typical period of onset is early (often in first 6 months)
- High urine culture positivity
- Urinary tract symptoms are often absent
- Part of disseminated disease
- Imaging findings mild and nonspecific

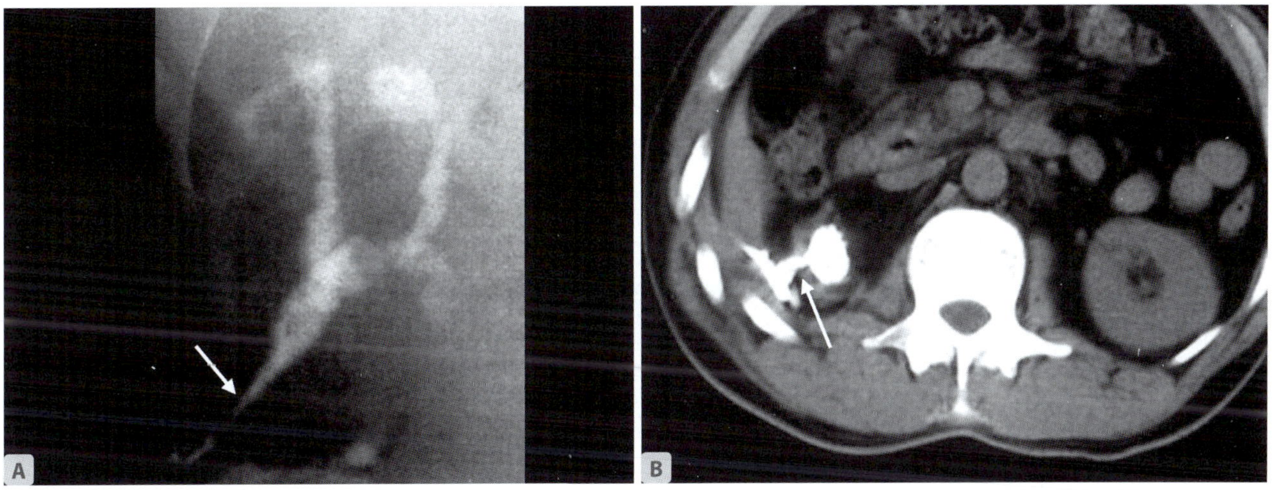

FIGS. 23A AND B: Sinogram (A) and CT sinogram; (B) of a different patient shows a shrunken right kidney, with sinus tract extending from the calyces to the skin (arrows).

REFERENCES

1. World Health Organization (2018). Global tuberculosis report 2018. World Health Organization. https://apps.who.int/irls/handle/10665/274453. License: CC BY-NC-SA 3.0 IGO.
2. Merchant S, Bharati A, Merchant N. Tuberculosis of the genitourinary system-urinary tract tuberculosis: renal tuberculosis-part I. Indian J Radiol Imaging. 2013;23(1):46-63.
3. Zachoval R, Nencka P, Vasakova M, et al. The incidence of subclinical forms of urogenital tuberculosis in patients with pulmonary tuberculosis. J Infect Public Health. 2018;11(2):243-5.
4. Leder RA, Low VH. Tuberculosis of the abdomen. Radiol Clin North Am. 1995;33(4):691-705.
5. Naidich DP, Garay SM, Leitman BS, et al. Radiographic manifestations of pulmonary disease in the acquired immunodeficiency syndrome (AIDS). Semin Roentgenol. 1987;22(1):14-30.
6. Chandan D, ankur G. Imaging in urogenital tuberculosis. 1st edition. New Delhi: Jaypee Brothers Medical Publishers; 2019.
7. Wise GJ, Shteynshlyuger A. An update on lower urinary tract tuberculosis. Curr Urol Rep. 2008;9(4):305-13.
8. Wise GJ, Marella VK. Genitourinary manifestations of tuberculosis. Urol Clin North Am. 2003;30(1):111-21.
9. Chan DS, Choy MY, Wang S, et al. An evaluation of the recovery of mycobacteria from urine specimens using the automated Mycobacteria Growth Indicator Tube system (BACTEC MGIT 960). J Med Microbiol. 2008;57(Pt 10):1220-2.
10. Hemal AK, Gupta NP, Rajeev TP, et al. Polymerase chain reaction in clinically suspected genitourinary tuberculosis: comparison with intravenous urography, bladder biopsy, and urine acid fast bacilli culture. Urology. 2000;56(4):570-4.
11. Premkumar A, Lattimer J, Newhouse JH. CT and sonography of advanced urinary tract tuberculosis. Am J Roentgenol. 1987;148(1):65-9.
12. Navarro-Vilasaro M, Font B, Sala M, et al. Genitourinary mycobacteriosis: retrospective study of 45 cases in a general hospital. Enferm Infecc Microbiol Clin. 2008;26(9):540-5.
13. Goldman SM, Fishman EK, Hartman DS, et al. Computed tomography of renal tuberculosis and its pathological correlates. J Comput Assist Tomogr. 1985;9(4):771-6.
14. Pollack HM, McClennan BL. Clinical Urography: Saunders; 2000.
15. Dalla Palma L. What is left of IV urography? Eur Radiol. 2001;11(6):931-9.
16. Kollins SA, Hartman GW, Carr DT, et al. Roentgenographic findings in urinary tract tuberculosis. A 10 year review. Am J Roentgenol Radium Ther Nucl Med. 1974;121(3):487-99.
17. Engin G, Acunas B, Acunas G, et al. Imaging of extrapulmonary tuberculosis. Radiographics. 2000;20(2):471-88.
18. Merchant S, Bharati A, Merchant N. Tuberculosis of the genitourinary system-urinary tract tuberculosis: renal tuberculosis-part II. Indian J Radiol Imaging. 2013;23(1):64-77.
19. Narayana A. Overview of renal tuberculosis. Urology. 1982;19(3):231-7.
20. Wasserman NF. Inflammatory disease of the ureter. Radiol Clin North Am. 1996;34(6):1131-56.
21. Camilien LD, Boyce JG. Diagnostic imaging of gynecological diseases: the clinician's view. Urol Radiol. 1991;13(1):3-8.
22. Das KM, Indudhara R, Vaidyanathan S. Sonographic features of genitourinary tuberculosis. Am J Roentgenol. 1992;158(2):327-9.
23. Schaffer R, Becker JA, Goodman J. Sonography of tuberculous kidney. Urology. 1983;22(2):209-11.
24. Rui X, Li XD, Cai S, et al. Ultrasonographic diagnosis and typing of renal tuberculosis. Int J Urol. 2008;15(2):135-9.
25. Gaudiano C, Tadolini M, Busato F, et al. Multidetector CT urography in urogenital tuberculosis: use of reformatted images for the assessment of the radiological findings. A pictorial essay. Abdom Radiol (NY). 2017;42(9):2314-24.
26. Lu P, Li C, Zhou X. Significance of the CT scan in renal tuberculosis. Zhonghua Jie He He Hu Xi Za Zhi. 2001;24(7):407-9.
27. Lang EK, Macchia RJ, Thomas R, et al. Improved detection of renal pathologic features on multiphasic helical CT compared with IVU in patients presenting with microscopic hematuria. Urology. 2003;61(3):528-32.
28. Leyendecker JR, Barnes CE, Zagoria RJ. MR urography: techniques and clinical applications. Radiographics. 2008;28(1):23-46.
29. Kim S, Jacob JS, Kim DC, et al. Time-resolved dynamic contrast-enhanced MR urography for the evaluation of ureteral peristalsis: initial experience. J Magn Reson Imaging. 2008;28(5):1293-8.
30. Nzerue C, Drayton J, Oster R, et al. Genitourinary tuberculosis in patients with HIV infection: clinical features in an inner-city hospital population. Am J Med Sci. 2000;320(5):299-303.
31. Nayak S, Satish R. Genitourinary tuberculosis after renal transplantation-a report of three cases with a good clinical outcome. Am J Transplant. 2007;7(7):1862-4.
32. Centers for Disease Control and Prevention (CDC). Transplantation-transmitted tuberculosis--Oklahoma and Texas, 2007. MMWR Morb Mortal Wkly Rep. 2008;57(13):333-6.

CHAPTER

7

Renal Cystic Diseases

Jyoti Kumar, Anjali Prakash, Sapna Singh

INTRODUCTION

Renal cystic lesions are a heterogeneous group of disorders characterized by multiple cysts in the kidneys. The most common cystic disease of the kidney is serous renal cyst, seen with advancing age. These may be simple or get complicated by hemorrhage, infection, or ischemia. These can then be difficult to differentiate from cystic malignancy. Bosniak classification of cysts helps categorize renal cysts to aid in management strategy based on imaging appearances. Although Bosniak classification has been currently described on contrast-enhanced computed tomography (CT) examination, contrast-enhanced ultrasound (US) and magnetic resonance (MR) are also being used to classify renal cysts.

In adults, other causes of renal cystic lesions can be focal or multifocal. Focal lesions include cystic tumors, pyelocalyceal diverticulum, and infection. Multifocal cystic disease of the kidney can also be characterized into heritable and nonheritable diseases. Since cystic lesions of kidney can have overlapping appearances, an understanding of the spectrum of this vast majority of renal cystic lesions can help reach a more specific diagnosis or suggest further relevant imaging recommendations to the clinician.

RENAL CYSTS

Serous Renal Cysts

The most common cystic disease of the kidney is serous renal cysts. These are increasingly seen with advancing age. These cysts can be multiple and variably sized.

On US examination, simple cysts are round and uniformly echo-free internally, with a well-defined posterior wall and strong acoustic shadowing. On Doppler examination, simple cysts show lack of color flow.

Computed tomographic scans show cysts to be masses of water density [0–20 Hounsfield unit (HU)] sharply defined from the adjacent renal parenchyma with no perceptible wall thickness. They are homogeneous and do not show calcification or enhancement after intravenous contrast is administered **(Fig. 1)**.

On MR imaging, simple cysts appear uniformly low-signal intensity on T1- and high-signal intensity on T2-weighted sequences with no contrast enhancement.

Atypical Cysts

Occasionally, simple cysts can get complicated by hemorrhage, infection, or ischemia. In these cysts, differentiation from cystic neoplasms, infectious diseases, and other renal cystic disorders may be difficult. In 1986, Bosniak developed a classification system to characterize cystic lesions of the kidney based on CT features. However, it does not take into account the underlying pathophysiology. Changes to this classification were made in 1990s and in 2005 and now five basic categories are recognized.

Bosniak Classification System (Table 1)

Five major categories are recognized:

1. Category I lesions are simple cysts of water density (0–20 HU), sharply defined from the adjacent renal

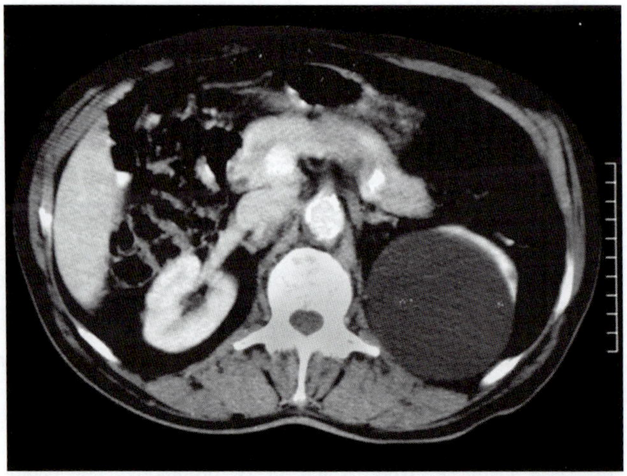

FIG. 1: Contrast-enhanced CT showing a large smoothly marginated lesion of homogeneous fluid density in left kidney with cortical "beak" sign typical of simple cyst. (CT: computed tomography).

TABLE 1: Bosniak classification.

Category of cyst	Morphology	Management
Bosniak I	• Simple cysts: No wall thickness, septae, calcification or enhancement	Benign, no follow-up
Bosniak II	• Cysts with pencil-thin wall. May have few fine internal septations (with or without perceived enhancement but no measurable enhancement); minimally thick calcification or short segment of thickened calcification • Homogeneous hyperdense cysts ≤3 cm that are well-defined and nonenhancing	Benign, no follow-up
IIF	• Cysts with mildly thickened wall/ multiple thin septations with no measurable enhancement but may have few thick or nodular calcifications • Homogeneous hyperdense nonenhancing cysts >3 cm that are completely intrarenal	Follow-up
Bosniak III	Cysts with thickened or irregular wall/septae with measurable enhancement	30–100% chances of malignancy. Surgical resection
Bosniak IV	Cyst with enhancing nodule in the wall/septum	Malignant unless proven otherwise. Surgical resection

parenchyma with no perceptible wall thickness. They are homogeneous and do not show calcification or contrast enhancement **(Fig. 1)**. Category I lesions are considered benign and do not require follow-up.

2. Category II lesions **(Fig. 2)** are minimally complicated benign cysts. These may have hairline thin septae. There may be fine calcification in the wall/septa. The septae may show perceived but no measurable enhancement. A homogeneous hyperdense cyst >20 HU or ≤3 cm in size, with some extrarenal component, is also classified as category II cysts. The extrarenal component of the cyst helps us to verify the smooth nature of the cyst wall.

   Lesions falling into category II are also considered benign and do not require follow-up.
3. *Category IIF cyst (F for follow-up):* These cysts lie in between category II and III lesions. These include cysts with multiple thin internal septations but no measurable enhancement, few nodular calcifications, or a smoothly thickened cyst wall **(Fig. 3)**. Hyperattenuating cysts which are larger than 3 cm or completely intrarenal are also included in category IIF cysts.

   The risk of malignancy in these lesions is approximately 5% and these lesions need to be followed up.

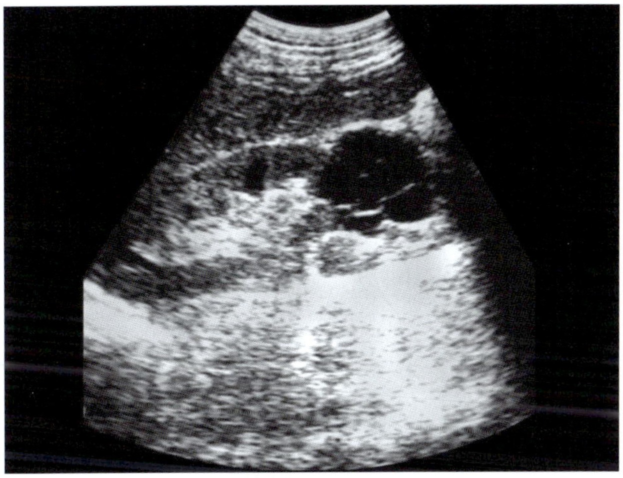

FIG. 2: Gray-scale sonogram of right kidney showing a complicated cyst with few thin internal septations (Bosniak's category II lesion) (CT: computed tomography).

   Recommendations for follow-up vary in the literature from 1 to 4 years depending upon how complex the lesion is.
4. Category III cysts have thick or irregular walls and/or septae that demonstrate measurable enhancement. There may be thick nodular calcification. As the chances of malignancy are high (30–100%), surgical resection is recommended in these lesions. Many of these lesions may prove to be benign, e.g. aggregates of simple cysts, multilocular cystic nephroma, lymphangioma, or hydatid disease.
5. Category IV cysts are cysts with a clear enhancing nodule in the wall or in the septa **(Fig. 4)**. The management is surgical resection as they are considered malignant unless proven otherwise. Several associated patient comorbidities are the only factor that warrant against surgery.

Diagnosis and management are clear in category I and IV lesions but difficult in category II and III lesions. The gold standard of surgical resection has come under the scanner owing to the increasing database that mortality rates from renal cell carcinoma (RCC) have risen over the past 20 years despite early detection and resection. Studies also suggest that more and more lesions are being treated surgically which would otherwise have no impact on patient mortality. Hence, there remains the challenge of distinguishing benign Bosniak 2F, 3, and 4 lesions from malignant Bosniak IIF, III, and IV lesions.

Although the size is not a criterion in Bosniak classification, it is believed by various researchers that small-sized lesions (<1.5 cm) in a patient with no risk factor for RCC can be considered benign.

Bosniak Classification Version 2019

In 2019, an updated Bosniak classification of cystic renal masses has been proposed to reduce inter-reader variability, more precisely predict the rate of malignancy within each Bosniak category, and minimize the number of unnecessary surgeries for otherwise benign or indolent malignant cystic

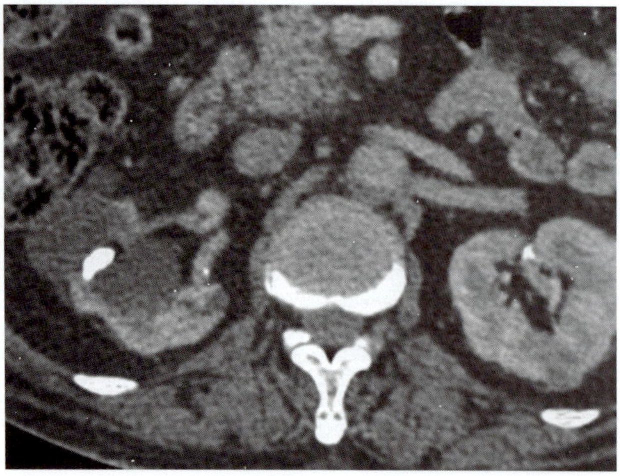

FIG. 3: Contrast-enhanced CT scan showing a cyst in the right kidney with thick nodular calcification (Bosniak's category IIF lesion). (CT: computed tomography).

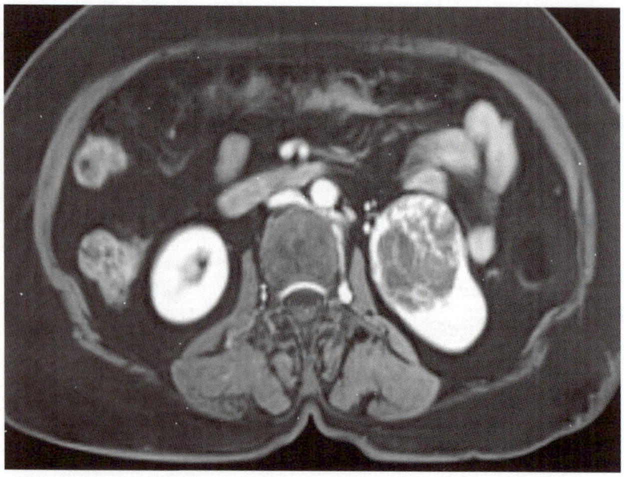

FIG. 4: Contrast-enhanced MR showing a multiloculated cystic mass arising from left kidney with nodular mural thickening and irregularity Bosniak's category IV lesion. (MR: magnetic resonance).

masses. This updated Bosniak classification incorporates MRI into the classification and gives more specific definitions for various imaging features that are ambiguous in the previous Bosniak classification. However, this new Bosniak version 2019 needs validation before it is accepted widely.

In the proposed classification, the Bosniak categories are defined as follows:

- *Bosniak version 2019, Class I*: Well-defined lesions with a thin (≤2 mm) smooth wall, which may show enhancement with homogenous internal contents (–9 to 20 HU).
- *Bosniak version 2019, Class II:* Well-defined lesions with thin (≤2 mm) smooth walls. In addition, they may have any of the following features:
    - Thin (≤2 mm) and few (1–3) septa, which may enhance; may have calcification of any type
    - Homogenous hyperattenuating mass (≥70 HU) on noncontrast CT
    - Homogenous nonenhancing mass >20 HU on renal mass protocol CT
    - Homogenous masses –9 to 20 HU at NCCT
    - Homogenous masses 21 to 30 HU at portal venous phase CT
    - Homogenous low attenuation masses too small to characterize
    - Homogenous mass markedly hyperintense on T2-weighted images (similar to cerebrospinal fluid) or markedly hyperintense on T1-weighted images (approximately 2.5 times normal renal parenchyma) on noncontrast MRI.
- *Bosniak version 2019, Class IIF*:
    - Cystic masses with minimally thickened (≥3 mm) enhancing wall or septae
    - Cystic masses with many (>4) smooth thin enhancing septa (≤2 mm).
- *Bosniak version 2019, Class III*: One or more enhancing thick (≥4 mm) septa or enhancing irregular wall/septa (≤3 mm thick protrusion with obtuse margins to the wall septa).
- *Bosniak version 2019, Class IV*: One or more enhancing nodule (≥4 mm convex thickening with obtuse margins to wall/septa or a convex protrusion of any size but with acute margin).

IMAGING MODALITIES

Conventional Radiography

Plain radiography and excretory urography (EU) are indirect imaging modalities and are relatively insensitive in detecting and characterizing renal cysts. EU may show the following imaging findings when renal cysts are present:

- Abnormality of the renal contour or adjacent fascial planes, displacement of bowel loops or splayed ribs
- Curvilinear or rim calcification in the cyst wall
- Filling defects in the opacified cortex during the nephrographic phase of urography
- Splaying and distortion of the opacified collecting system **(Fig. 5)**.

Cross-sectional imaging techniques are more appropriate for investigating a patient of renal cystic disease.

Ultrasonography

Gray-scale, real-time sonography is a noninvasive, multiplanar direct imaging modality, which requires no patient preparation, and unlike EU it shows the mass lesion itself, along with changes in the renal parenchyma and renal sinus. However, obesity and excessive bowel gas can obscure the kidneys. Gray-scale US is useful in characterizing simple cysts but is limited in evaluation of complex cysts **(Fig. 6)**. Color Doppler can aid in assessing blood flow in renal cystic lesions, however with poor sensitivity. As Bosniak classification relies on enhancement, various studies have shown promising results using contrast-enhanced US in the evaluation of renal cystic lesions based on the Bosniak classification system.

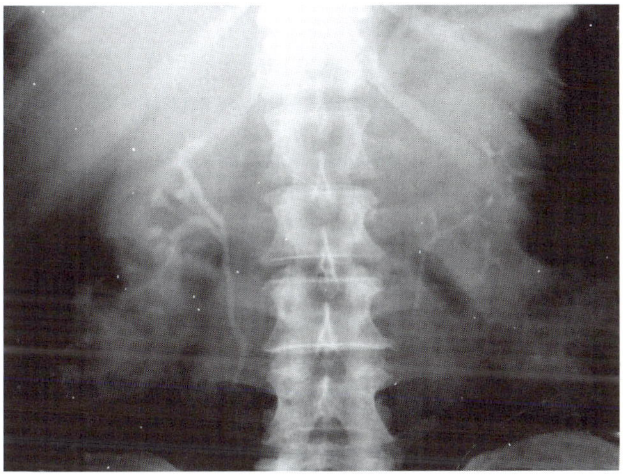

FIG. 5: Excretory urogram showing enlarged kidneys with splaying and stretching of pelvicalyceal system (spidery calyces) in a patient with polycystic kidney disease.

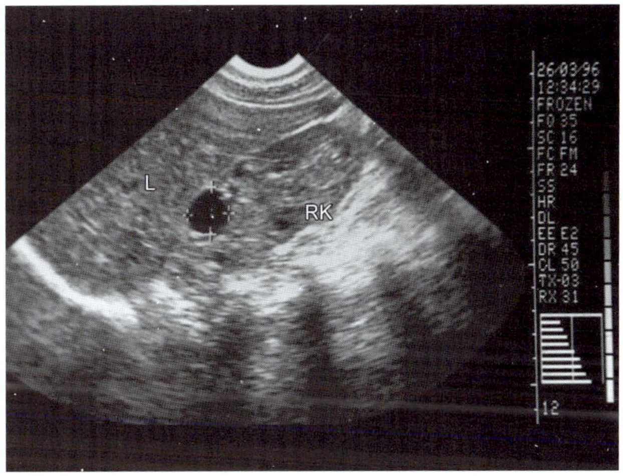

FIG. 6: US of kidney showing a well-marginated anechoic lesion with distal enhancement—simple cortical cyst. (US: ultrasonography).

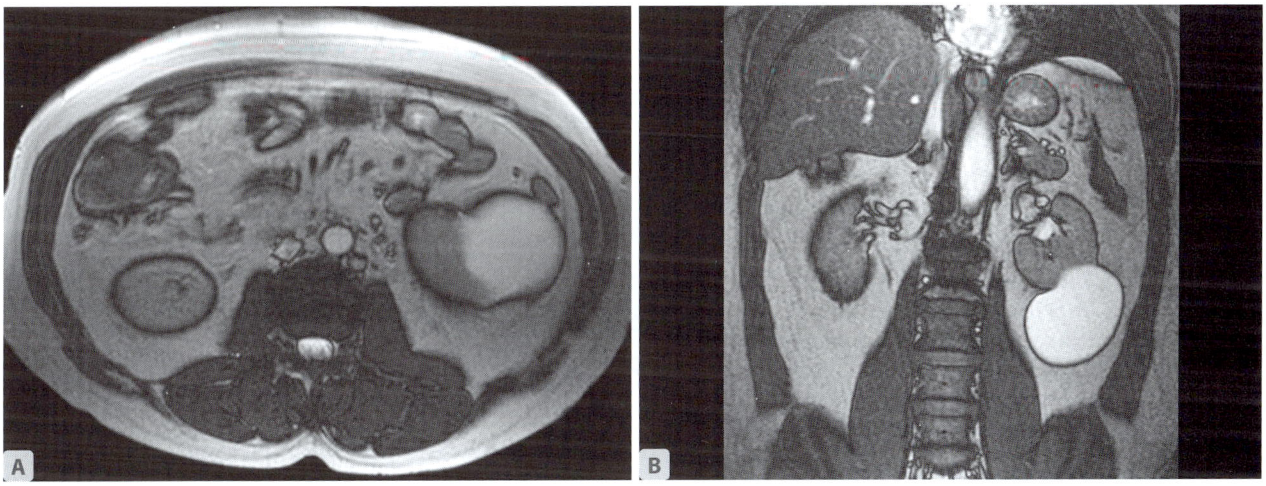

FIGS. 7A AND B: Steady state free precession sequence axial (A) and coronal (B) MR images reveal a homogenous sharply marginated lesion with imperceptible wall thickness and high signal arising exophytically from the left kidney—an exophytic simple cortical cyst. (MR: magnetic resonance).

Computed Tomography

Computed tomography is the main modality for imaging and characterizing cystic renal lesions. Multiphasic renal CT is obtained including unenhanced CT, corticomedullary phase, nephrographic phase, and excretory phase. The nephrographic phase is the most valuable for detecting mass lesions less than 3 cm which include clinically insignificant renal cysts and RCCs.

A change of less than 10 HU from pre- to postcontrast images is considered typical of a benign cyst. Very rarely, cystic tumors may enhance less than 10 HU. Majority of pathologic lesions enhance more than 15 HU. An enhancement between 10 HU and 15 HU is considered suspicious but not diagnostic of a tumor.

There are a few pitfalls on CT imaging that must be kept in mind. Pseudoenhancement that is defined as an artefactual increase in HU values of >10 on contrast-enhanced CT can result from beam hardening artifact. Also, if the lesion is smaller than twice the slice thickness used, then partial volume averaging may result in misinterpretation. Virtual monochromatic imaging on dual-energy computed tomography may completely eliminate pseudoenhancement in renal cysts larger than 1.5 cm.

Magnetic Resonance Imaging

Multiplanar imaging capability and angiographic capabilities with excellent soft-tissue contrast resolution have made MRI a useful method for evaluating the kidneys **(Figs. 7A and B)**. High-field strengths, breathhold imaging, fat suppression techniques, and use of MR-contrast agents help in differentiating tumor from cysts. The multiplanar imaging capability of MRI makes it easier to assess polar lesions and coronal images make it simple for the urologist to visualize the relative position of a small lesion if wedge resection or partial nephrectomy is to be planned.

Although the Bosniak classification has been described on CT, various researchers have proven that MR may be equivalent to CT in Bosniak classification of cystic lesions.

Calcification is however better picked up on CT than on MR. Owing to increased contrast resolution, there is increased sensitivity of MR for picking up septations and wall thickening on T2-weighted images. This can result in false upgradation of the Bosniak category of the lesion. Other pitfalls include evaluation of enhancement in hemorrhagic and calcified lesions. In these situations, subtraction imaging may be used. The subtraction imaging technique can suffer from misregistration and additional noise.

In few equivocal cases, MR can be problem solving. Postcontrast free breathing 3D fat-suppressed T1 gradient echo (T1 vibe fat sat) sequence allows better evaluation of enhancement which forms the main basis for Bosniak categorization of lesions. Diffusion-weighted imaging can also be of utility in differentiating cystic renal masses from simple cysts.

Angiography

Prior to the advent of newer imaging modalities such as US, CT, and MRI, angiography was commonly used for evaluation of renal mass lesions. However, in the present era it is mainly indicated for interventional procedures of vascular mass lesions of the kidney. Actively bleeding tumors such as angiomyolipomas (AMLs) can be treated with selective angiography by embolization of the intrarenal supply of the tumor.

Biopsy

Biopsy may not give a high yield from cystic lesions owing to paucity of cells within. It is however useful to biopsy or drain cystic lesions which are suspected to be abscesses and may be attempted in patients with suspected malignancy if they are poor surgical candidates.

ADULT RENAL CYSTIC DISEASE: CLASSIFICATION

In adults, apart from simple renal cysts, multifocal renal cystic disease comprises a diverse group of heritable and acquired disorders. Renal infections, tumors, and renal sinus cysts are other miscellaneous conditions that can present as cystic disease. Because of their diverse etiology, histology, and clinical presentation, no single universally accepted classification exists, but a practical working classification composed of major categories and the most clinically significant renal cystic diseases is shown in **Table 2**.

TABLE 2: Classification of renal cystic disease.

Multifocal	
Heritable	• Autosomal dominant polycystic kidney disease • Medullary cystic kidney disease • Von Hippel-Lindau disease • Tuberous sclerosis
Acquired	• Acquired renal cystic disease • Medullary sponge kidney disease • Glomerulocystic kidney disease • Lithium-induced nephrotoxicity • Multicystic dysplastic kidney • Localized cystic renal disease • Cyst of renal pelvis
Focal	• Mixed epithelial stromal tumor • Cystic nephroma • Cystic renal cell carcinoma • Pyelocalyceal diverticulum
Infectious causes	• Pyogenic-renal abscess • Tubercular • Parasitic-renal hydatid, echinococcosis • Fungal-renal aspergillosis

MULTIFOCAL CYSTIC RENAL DISEASE

Heritable Multifocal Cystic Renal Disease

Autosomal Dominant Polycystic Kidney Disease

Autosomal dominant polycystic kidney disease (ADPKD) is the most common of hereditary renal cystic diseases (1 in 400–1,000 live births). Mostly, it shows an autosomal dominant inheritance. Rare cases may result from a spontaneous mutation with no family history. Although multiple bilateral renal cysts are the most important manifestation, ADPKD is really a systemic hereditary disorder that is characterized by cyst formation in ductal organs, the liver being the most common site of extrarenal involvement. Other extrarenal manifestations include cysts in pancreas, spleen, and gonads. The patients may also have intracranial aneurysms, cardiac valve abnormalities, colonic diverticulae, and musculoskeletal abnormalities.

About 85% of cases are due to a dominant gene located on the short arm of chromosome 16 (the *ADPKD-1* gene) whereas 5–10% of cases are due to an abnormal gene located on the long arm of chromosome 4 (the *ADPKD-2* gene), which causes a milder form of the disorder with late onset of disease.

Patients with a positive family history of ADPKD and no imaging evidence of renal cysts can be further evaluated using gene-linkage analysis. It is proposed that the disorder results from failure of union of the branches of ureteral bud with metanephros which, deprived of the organizing influence, form cysts. There is cystic dilatation of nephrons involving all segments from the proximal convoluted tubule to the collecting duct due to epithelial hyperplasia leading to redundancy that predisposes to cyst formation. Hence, cysts may be seen in both renal cortex and medulla.

Most patients are born with normal kidneys. Only 2% patients present before 15 years of age. Most affected individuals present in the fourth or fifth decade with flank pain, palpable masses, hypertension, hematuria, urinary tract infection, proteinuria, or polycythemia. Progressive azotemia ensues as renal parenchyma is destroyed and renal failure occurs in most patients by the age of 60 years. Complications include superimposed infection, cyst hemorrhage, uric acid stones, and hypertension. Renal cell carcinoma is not a complication of ADPKD unless the patient is on prolonged dialysis.

Imaging plays an important role in diagnosis, detection of complications, and follow-up. Conventional radiograph may reveal bilateral enlarged kidneys with lobulated margins causing displacement of the surrounding structures, such as colonic flexures. Calcification may be curvilinear or amorphous and the presence of renal calculi often signifies superimposed infection. The "nephrogram" phase of the EU is characterized by numerous, smoothly marginated radiolucencies throughout the cortex and medulla, which have been likened to the appearance of "Swiss cheese." An appearance of spidery collecting system with stretched and crescentic calyces may be noted.

Ultrasound is the modality of choice for primary evaluation of most patients with suspected ADPKD. On US, cysts of varying sizes are noted in enlarged kidneys, which may result in a lobulated outline **(Figs. 8A and B)**. However, the reniform shape is maintained. Similar cysts may be seen in liver, pancreas, and spleen. Most patients develop renal cysts by their third decade. Antenatal diagnosis is sometimes also possible on demonstration of enlarged cystic kidneys, ascites, and hepatomegaly. The presence of even one cyst in a genetically predisposed child is suspicious of ADPKD.

On CT and MR, variable sized cysts which are usually ≥3 cm in diameter are seen diffusely involving bilateral enlarged kidneys. Imaging also helps to identify infection, hemorrhage, and rupture. On MRI, the renal cysts are hypointense on T1-weighted and hyperintense on T2-weighted images, with infected and proteinaceous cysts showing intermediate signal intensities **(Figs. 9 to 11)**. MRI-based renal and cyst volumetry enables assessment of disease progression. With increasing renal volume, the glomerular filtration rate may decline and the patient may present with abdominal pain, hypertension, or hematuria. Renal blood flow may also decrease suggesting progression of the disease.

Imaging is critical in evaluation of patients who have a first-degree relative with ADPKD. It is especially so in evaluation of prospective donors who plan to donate a kidney to their kin with ADPKD. Severe cases can be diagnosed easily

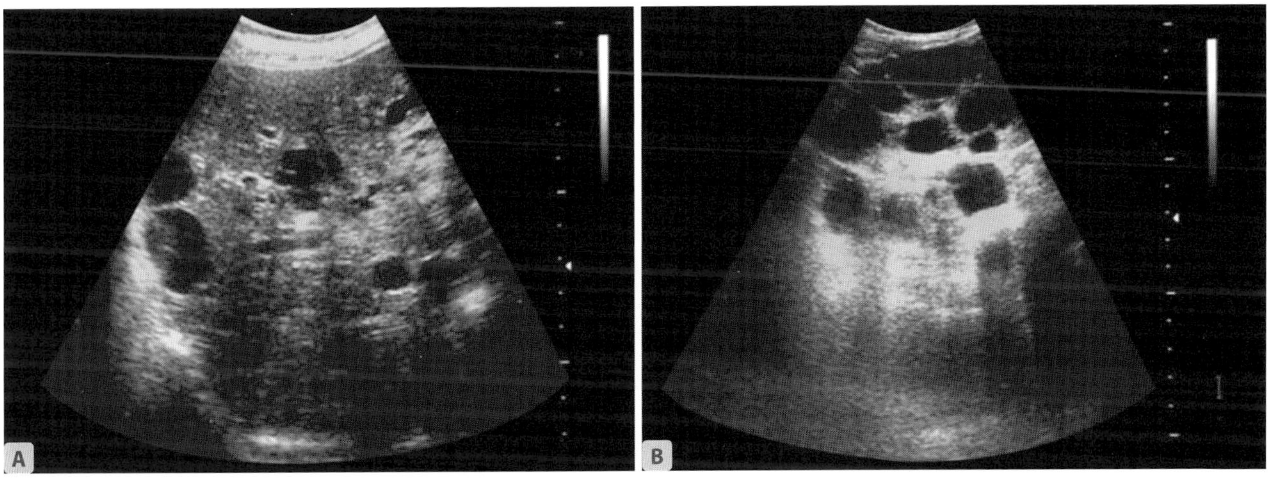

FIGS. 8A AND B: Sonography showing multiple noncommunicating cysts of varying sizes replacing the renal parenchyma and distorting the central sinus echoes—ADPKD. Cysts are also seen in the liver. (ADPKD: autosomal dominant polycystic kidney disease).

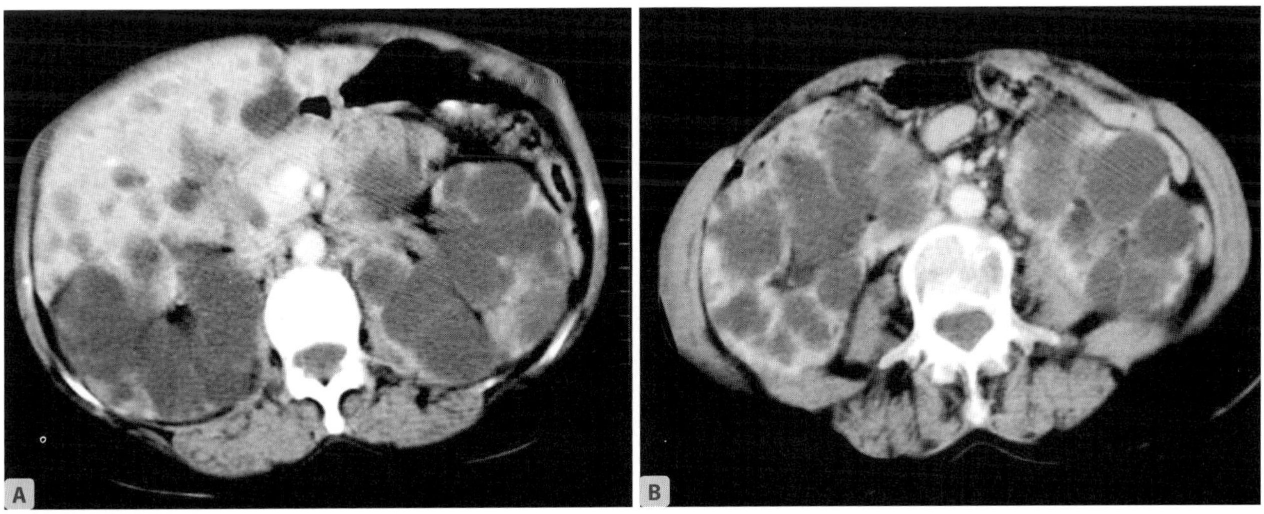

FIGS. 9A AND B: Contrast-enhanced CT scans revealing multiple noncommunicating cysts in both kidneys. Cysts are also seen in the liver—ADPKD (ADPKD: autosomal dominant polycystic kidney disease; CT: computed tomography).

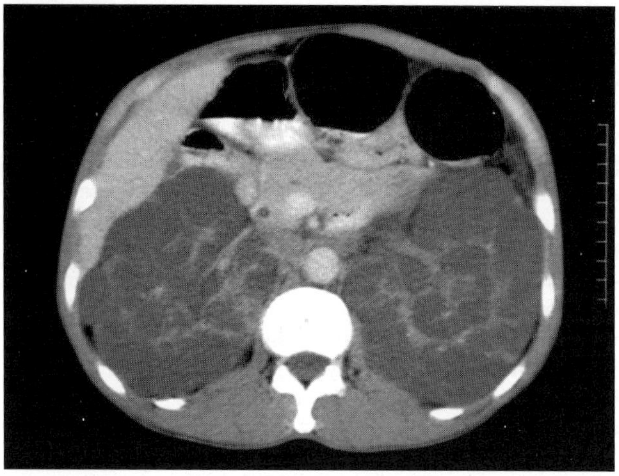

FIG. 10: Contrast-enhanced CT (CECT) scan in another case showing multiple noncommunicating cysts in both kidneys—ADPKD. (ADPKD: autosomal dominant polycystic kidney disease; CT: computed tomography).

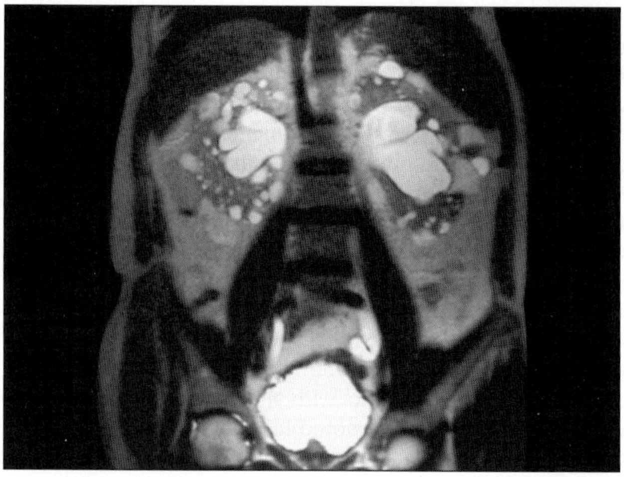

FIG. 11: T2W coronal MR image showing both kidneys to be enlarged with multiple cysts of varying sizes having fluid signal intensity studding the renal parenchyma of both kidneys consistent with polycystic kidney disease. Note is also made of bilateral hydronephrosis and back pressure changes in the bladder due to bladder outflow obstruction. (MR: magnetic resonance).

on imaging but a milder form of the disease, especially with PKD2 mutation, can be difficult to diagnose. Genetic testing helps in the diagnosis of ADPKD in only 70% cases.

The criteria for diagnosing ADPKD on US in patients with unknown genotype but at high risk of ADPKD (i.e. with a first-degree relative with the disease) are as follows:

- 15–39 years—three renal cysts
- 40–59 years—≥2 cysts in each kidney
- 60 years or more—≥4 cysts in each kidney.

The sensitivity of CT scan is greater than that of ultrasound in detecting renal cysts and thus may establish the diagnosis more definitively at an earlier age.

Nephronophthisis and Medullary Cystic Kidney Disease

Medullary cystic disease complex applies to two tubulointerstitial diseases—nephronophthisis and medullary cystic disease—which are progressive and the most common heritable cause of renal failure in children and young adults. It shows autosomal dominant inheritance. Genetic mutations result in protein derangement which further results in ciliary dysfunction and formation of medullary cysts.

Nephronophthisis has three forms—infantile, juvenile, and adolescent—based on the age of onset. The juvenile form is the most common with presentation at 4–6 years of age. Renal failure can ensue at an average age of 13 years. MCKD presents in young adults. Patients with both the forms of the disease present with polyuria, polydipsia, and salt wasting. They may also develop hyperuricemia and gout.

Imaging features are similar for both the disease entities. At US imaging, kidneys are normal to small sized with increased echogenicity and poor corticomedullary differentiation. Multiple small-sized cysts <3 cm can be seen at the corticomedullary junction and in renal medulla, but these are typically seen after the onset of end-stage renal disease. Renal cysts increase with increasing age. When present, the typical location of the cysts and characteristic clinical findings help to differentiate MCKD from other renal cystic diseases.

Patients progress to renal failure and renal transplantation is the treatment of choice. The disease does not involve the transplanted kidney.

Von Hippel-Lindau Disease

Von Hippel-Lindau (VHL) disease is a relatively rare, autosomal dominant disorder with a prevalence of 1 in 30,000–50,000. It is caused by an abnormal gene on the short arm of chromosome 3. This disorder is associated with hemangioblastomas of the central nervous system (CNS), retinal angiomatosis, pheochromocytomas, cysts and tumors of the kidney, pancreatic cysts and tumors, endolymphatic sac tumors, and papillary cystadenomas of the epididymis. Both males and females are equally affected. The diagnostic criteria include:

- >1 CNS hemangioblastoma
- 1 CNS hemangioblastoma and visceral manifestations of VHL
- Any manifestation of VHL with known family history.

Renal lesions include simple and atypical cysts, cystic RCC, and solid RCC. Clear cell RCCs are the major cause of patient morbidity and mortality, especially in Type 1 and Type 2B VHL disease.

On EU, renal cortical cysts are seen bilaterally, causing distortion of the renal architecture. Extensive disease can mimic ADPKD. USG is highly sensitive for detection of renal cysts; however, small renal tumors may not be seen. CT is more sensitive than USG for detection and characterization of renal masses and small, solid renal masses can be precisely defined **(Fig. 12)**.

MR imaging is indispensable for the diagnosis of neurological neoplasms seen in patients with VHL disease. Furthermore, small RCCs can be detected on contrast-enhanced MR. Large tumors can be evaluated and characterized on nonenhanced scans and tend to be more heterogeneous.

Although RCC in VHL disease is slower growing than in patients without VHL disease, RCC is a significant cause of mortality in VHL disease. In VHL disease, RCC may either arise de novo or within small cysts. Hence, each cyst needs to be carefully assessed in a case of VHL disease and none can be described as free of cancer cells on imaging.

In patients with VHL disease, imaging surveillance is recommended at intervals of 6–12 months. While some cysts enlarge over time, others may involute. Complex cysts and solid tumors can show progressive increase in size. The cutoff size of the solid tumor to be taken for surgery is accepted as 3 cm. When a 3 cm-sized solid nodule is seen, it needs to be resected along with other smaller solid/cystic lesions if possible. Thereafter, surveillance is maintained till a 3 cm nodule is again formed. Treatment is mostly with nephron sparing surgery.

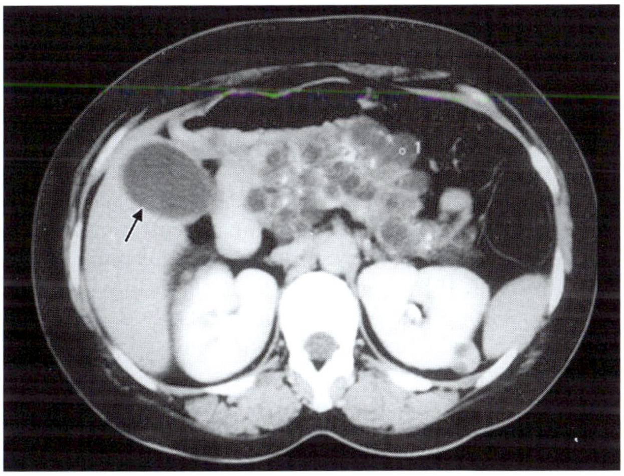

FIG. 12: Contrast-enhanced CT (CECT) sections showing a solid enhancing mass and cyst in the left kidney with multiple cysts and calcifications in the pancreas—von Hippel-Lindau disease. (CT: computed tomography).

Tuberous Sclerosis

Tuberous sclerosis (TSC) is also known as Bourneville disease. It is a genetically transmitted autosomal dominant neurocutaneous syndrome. Genetic markers have been identified at 9q34 (TSC 1) and 16p13 (TSC 2), although they account for only 50% of TSC families. Sporadic occurrence is seen in 50–60% of cases. The true incidence of TSC is difficult to measure though its birth incidence ranges from 1 per 5,800 to 1 per 10,000. It is characterized by mental retardation, seizures, and cutaneous lesions. This disorder is associated with multiple hamartomas in the brain (cortical tubers), retina, skin, heart (rhabdomyomas), kidney (AMLs), and other organs. Renal cysts and AMLs are seen in 50–60% of cases. Occurrence of both AMLs and renal cysts is virtually diagnostic of TSC. Angiomyolipomas are benign masses consisting of varying amounts of abnormal blood vessels, smooth muscle, and fat. These manifest in childhood and increase in size with age.

On abdominal radiography, lucency suggesting fat within an AML can occasionally be detected. On EU, the findings vary with the size and number of renal cysts and the presence of AMLs. Multiple nonopacifying renal masses causing distortion of the collecting system are seen.

On sonographic examination, multiple renal cysts and AMLs, showing hyperechoic reflections, may be seen owing to lesional fat. On CT, fat-containing AMLs with low attenuation values and intralesional hemorrhage may be noted along with renal cysts **(Figs. 13A and B)**. MR imaging aids in diagnosing AMLs by showing high-signal intensity on both T1- and T2-weighted images.

Although the risk of RCC in these patients is the same as that in the general population, it occurs at an earlier age. The mean age of RCC in patients with TSC is 28 years compared with 58 years in the general population. Other complications include renal failure and hemorrhage from AML rupture.

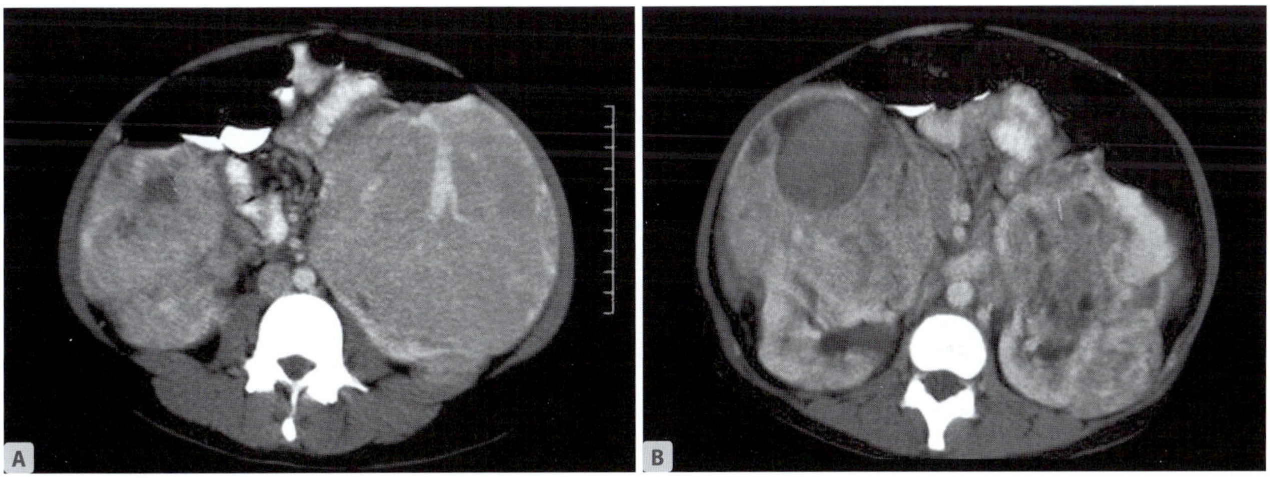

FIGS. 13A AND B: Contrast-enhanced CT scan showing heterogeneous masses involving both the kidneys. The masses show fat-attenuation values and cystic areas within. The lesions show intralesional vascularity—bilateral angiomyolipomas. (CT: computed tomography).

Lipid poor AML and RCC can be difficult to differentiate on imaging. Rapid growth and presence of calcification are features that favor RCC over AML. However, biopsy may be needed to confirm the diagnosis.

TSC2-PKD1 is a related condition which has mutations in both *TSC2* and *PKD1* genes. These patients have lesions of both TSC and ADPKD.

Acquired Multifocal Cystic Renal Disease

Acquired Cystic Kidney Disease

Acquired cystic kidney disease (ACKD) is characterized by the formation of multiple renal cysts in patients with end-stage renal disease, who have no history of hereditary cystic disease. Risk factors include male sex and increased duration of time on dialysis. These patients can have acquired cysts even before undergoing dialysis in 8–13% of patients. After 3–5 years of dialysis, the prevalence of ACKD is 40–60% while it rises to 90% after 5–10 years on dialysis. The incidence reaches nearly 100% after 10 years of dialysis. Men are affected three times more often than females. However, there is no relation with the method of dialysis, age, or race of the patient. At least three cysts in each kidney are required to make this diagnosis. US shows atrophic echogenic kidneys with small cysts of varying complexity. CT and MR show small kidneys with variably sized cysts. While US is a good modality for screening, CT and MR are useful in detecting complications. Multiple, bilateral small cysts are seen to involve both the renal cortex and the medulla **(Fig. 14)**.

ACKD is associated with an increased incidence of renal neoplasms. Risk factors for malignancy in this setting include increasing duration of dialysis, male gender, and kidney weight more than 150 g. Factors causing renal cyst and tumor formation in end-stage renal disease are unknown but the two are interrelated. It is postulated that with progressive destruction of functioning renal tissue, cystogenic substances accumulate and cause hypertrophy and hyperplasia of epithelial cells. The tubular epithelium proliferate and cystic dilatation of tubules occurs. Subsequently, there is a continuum of changes from single-layered epithelial cysts to multilayered cysts to RCCs. Tumors can be multiple and bilateral. Other complications in this setting include cyst infection, hemorrhage, rupture, and ureteral stones. Hemorrhage into cyst may result in cyst rupture leading to retroperitoneal hemorrhage. Asymptomatic patients can be followed up by US whereas complications may require nephrectomy.

In post-transplant cases, true cysts decrease in the native kidney but the risk of malignancy persists, in fact with more aggressiveness owing to ongoing immunosuppression in transplant cases.

Medullary Sponge Kidney

Medullary sponge kidney is also known as Lenarduzzi-Cacchi-Ricci disease. It was first described by Lenarduzzi in 1931. Although it is mostly sporadic, a few cases with autosomal dominant inheritance have also been described.

The most probable cause is disruption in the ureteric bud metanephros interface. It is characterized histologically by ectasia of the renal medullary and papillary collecting ducts with subcentimetric cysts in the medulla. This disease entity may be associated with congenital hemihypertrophy, Beckwith-Wiedemann syndrome, Caroli syndrome, Wilms tumor, or horseshoe kidney.

Patients usually present in the third to fifth decades of life. Although mostly asymptomatic, some patients may present with hematuria, renal colic, or urinary tract infection.

At EU **(Fig. 15)**, papillary blush is classically noted as contrast pools in the dilated medullary collecting ducts. This gives a classic "paint brush" appearance. Striated appearance of the medullary collecting ducts with calyceal distortion may also be encountered as the disease increases in severity. This entity typically involves both the kidneys. Unilateral or segmental involvement may be seen at times. US examination reveals echogenic medullary pyramids. Tiny calculi can be

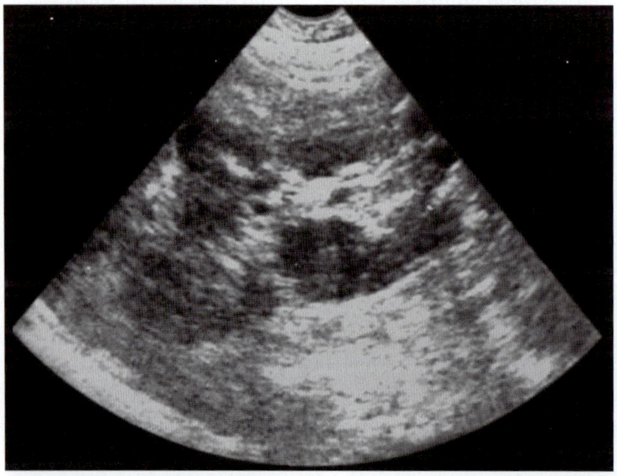

FIG. 14: US in a patient with chronic renal failure on long-term hemodialysis showing shrunken echogenic kidney with loss of corticomedullary differentiation and multiple small renal cysts—ACKD. (ACKD: acquired cystic kidney disease; US: ultrasonography).

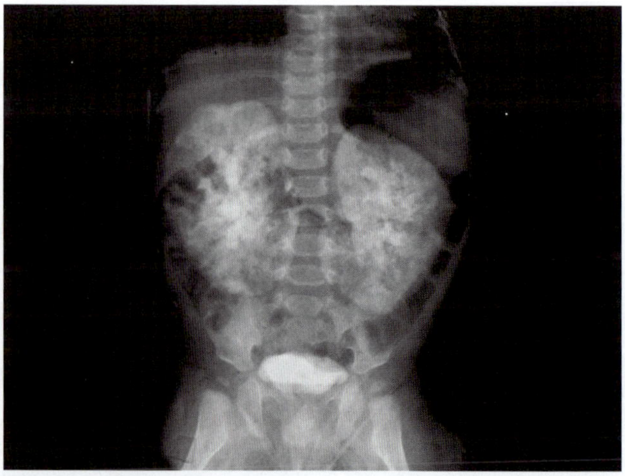

FIG. 15: Excretory urogram in a child with medullary sponge kidneys showing enlarged kidneys with and characteristic "paint brush" appearance owing to dilated medullary collecting ducts.

seen involving the medullary pyramids. On CT examination, the typical papillary blush appearance can be noted in the urographic phase with associated calculi in the dilated collecting ducts suggestive of medullary nephrocalcinosis. CT urography scores over EU in identification of dilated medullary collecting ducts, calculi, obstruction, and infection.

This is a benign disease entity. Severe complications of calculi and infection may result in renal failure in rare circumstances.

Glomerulocystic Kidney Disease

Glomerulocystic kidney disease (GCKD) is a rare cystic disease owing to cystic dilatation of Bowman's capsule. The cysts involve the subcapsular renal cortex and spare nephron tubules. Although many sporadic cases are known, autosomal dominant inheritance has also been reported. This is seen mostly in neonates and young children who may have mild renal failure.

On imaging, kidneys may be normal or small in size. Tiny cysts are seen in the subcapsular location in the cortex. These are difficult to discern on US as well as noncontrast CT. Contrast is usually not administered owing to renal failure. On US, increased cortical echogenicity may be seen owing to the extremely small size of the cysts. T2-weighted MR imaging is the most sensitive sequence in picking up these tiny cysts in the subcapsular location. This location of the cysts helps to differentiate this entity from other multifocal cystic renal diseases like ADPKD, multicystic dysplastic kidney (MCDK).

Lithium-induced Nephrotoxicity

Long-term lithium therapy can result in nephrotoxicity which can manifest in the form of acute toxicity, nephrogenic diabetes insipidus as well as chronic renal disease. While the first two are reversible, chronic interstitial nephritis is progressive and irreversible. Nephrogenic diabetes insipidus is the most common complication.

In the setting of chronic renal disease, microcyst formation results with progressive renal dysfunction in normal sized kidneys. This is seen as numerous 1–2 mm cysts scattered in cortex and medulla of normal sized kidneys. These are best seen on T2W MR images. Based on the imaging findings, the differential diagnosis is ADPKD, GCKD, and *MCKD*. Clinical history, size and distribution of the cysts help to distinguish this entity from others cystic diseases of the kidney. While clinical and laboratory data are sufficient to reach the diagnosis, renal biopsy, if performed, depicts tubular atrophy, interstitial fibrosis and distal tubular ectasia resulting in microcyst formation.

Multicystic Dysplastic Kidney

Multicystic dysplastic kidney is a developmental, nonhereditary anomaly with multiple, smooth noncommunicating cysts. It is one of the most common abdominal masses in the newborn and is typically unilateral and asymptomatic. It has an incidence of 1 in 4,300 live births. The bilateral form of MCDK is usually associated with congenital gastrointestinal and cardiac abnormalities. The bilateral form has a poor outcome due to accompanying oligohydramnios and pulmonary hypoplasia.

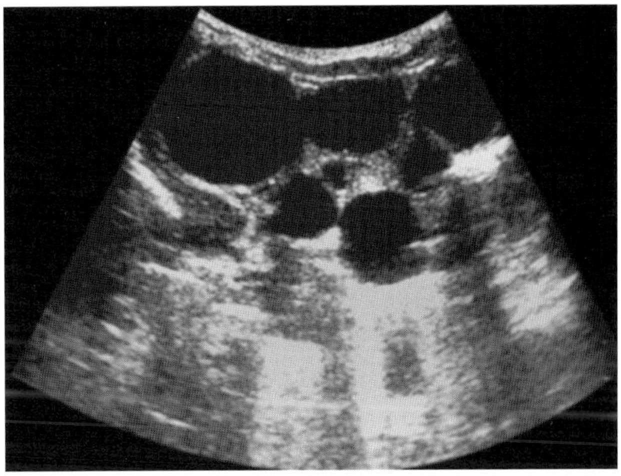

FIG. 16: US of right kidney in a 4-year-old child shows multiple cysts of varying sizes distorting the reniform contour––MCDK. (MCDK: multicystic dysplastic kidney; US: ultrasonography).

The proposed theory of this dysplastic kidney is failure of the ureteric bud to induce development of metanephric blastema. The ureteric bud may be absent or may not integrate with metanephric blastema owing to urinary tract obstruction.

In children, it is seen as a nonreniform mass which is a cluster of noncommunicating cysts replacing the renal parenchyma or sometimes only a part of the renal parenchyma **(Fig. 16)**. The contralateral kidney must be assessed to rule out associations such as vesicoureteric reflux or pelviureteric junction obstruction. It may also be picked up on antenatal USG **(Figs. 17A and B)**.

A few patients present in adulthood. The kidney regresses in size and presents as "renal agenesis" or a small central soft tissue surrounded by peripheral cysts which could be confused with cystic renal neoplasm. The findings that help to reach the correct diagnosis are nonfunctioning kidney with peripheral cysts around central soft tissue along with atrophic pelvicalyceal system, ureter, and renal vessels. With time, the affected kidney involutes and is typically not a source of clinical concern. The contralateral kidney may show compensatory hypertrophy **(Figs. 18A and B)**. There may also be a segmental form involving the upper pole of a duplex kidney and this may be associated with ureterocele of the lower moiety.

Localized Renal Cystic Disease

This is a rare disease where a cluster of tightly packed cysts replaces a portion of the kidney or rarely the entire kidney. It is also known as segmental renal cystic disease and unilateral renal cystic disease. It is a benign, nonprogressive condition. Multiple cysts are seen in one kidney with no cysts in the contralateral kidney or any other organ. Most patients are asymptomatic. Some may present with abdominal pain, hematuria, or hypertension but with intact renal function.

CT and MR show a conglomerate mass of variably sized simple renal cysts with intervening enhancing renal parenchyma involving a portion of one kidney or the entire kidney. There is no surrounding capsule **(Figs. 19A to C)**.

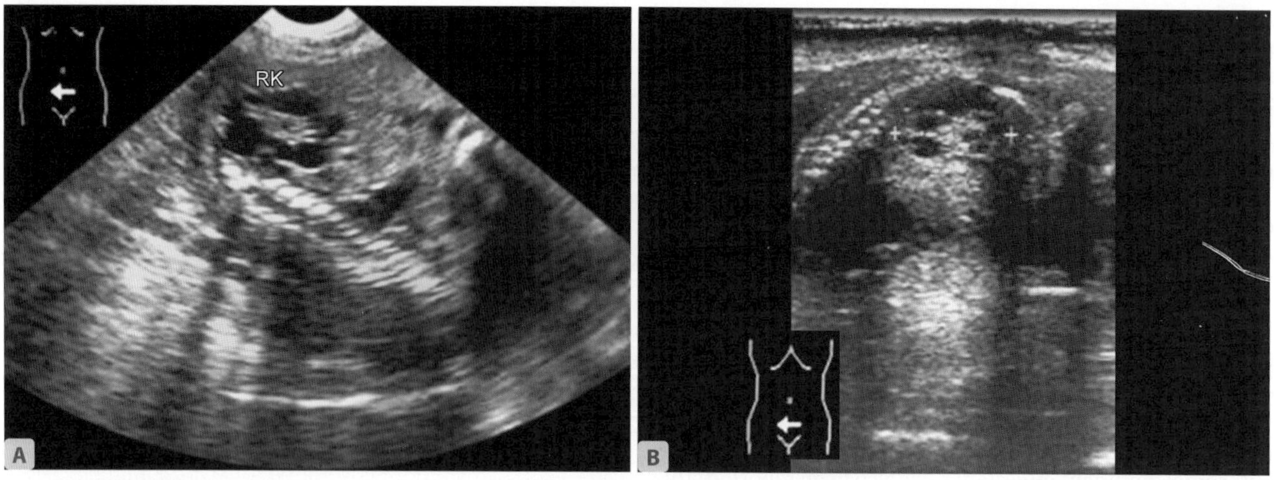

FIGS. 17A AND B: Antenatal sonogram showing multiple noncommunicating cysts in an enlarged fetal kidney—multicystic dysplasia.

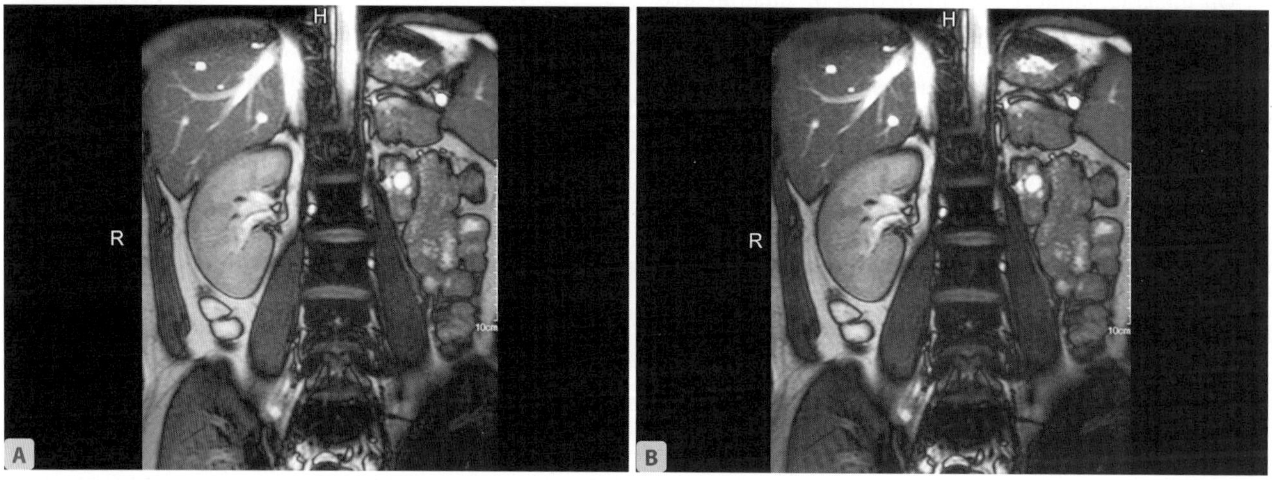

FIGS. 18A AND B: Coronal steady state MR images reveal a small dysplastic left kidney replaced by multiple noncommunicating cysts showing hyperintensity on T2W image with compensatory hypertrophy of right kidney—adult MCDK. (MCDK: multicystic dysplastic kidney).

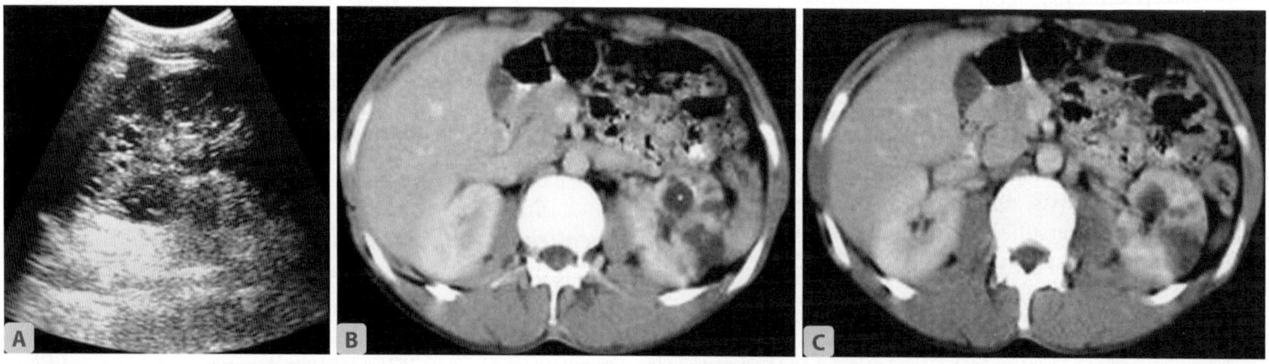

FIGS. 19A TO C: Sonogram (A) showing multiple small cysts in the upper pole of the left kidney seen as a multiloculated mass. Contrast-enhanced CT scans (B and C) revealing multiple cysts in the upper pole of the left kidney separated by enhancing bands of renal parenchyma—unilateral localized cystic disease. (CT: computed tomography).

The intervening normal parenchyma is usually normal but sometimes atrophic. Remaining renal parenchyma and contralateral kidney are generally normal but can show a few scattered cysts.

Unilateral involvement with no cysts involving other viscera distinguishes this entity from ADPKD. The presence of normal collecting system and renal vessels helps to differentiate it from multicystic dysplastic kidney. Intervening normal parenchyma and absence of capsule differentiate this nonprogressive condition from multilocular cystic RCC and cystic nephroma. As this may be difficult to discern at times, the key remains to identify at least one cyst which is surrounded by normal renal tissue.

This is a benign condition. Surveillance is however recommended if the patient is symptomatic or imaging findings are equivocal.

Cysts of Renal Pelvis

Cysts of renal pelvis can be of two types:

1. Parapelvic cyst
2. Renal sinus cyst (also called peripelvic cysts).

Parapelvic cysts are cortical cysts that extend into renal sinus **(Fig. 20)**. Mostly, these do not produce any symptoms but sometimes may result in hydronephrosis, hypertension by renal artery compression, pain, and hematuria. These are usually simple cysts on imaging.

Infection and hemorrhage are some of the unusual complications that may occur in these cysts.

Renal sinus cysts are multiple, small, and bilateral cysts in contrast to parapelvic cysts which are usually single and unilateral. These arise from renal sinus lymphatics. The differential diagnosis here is hydronephrosis which can be distinguished on the excretory phase of CT scan where there is no contrast excretion into these cysts.

FOCAL CYSTIC RENAL DISEASE

Mixed epithelial and stromal tumor (MEST) and cystic nephroma are benign cystic lesions that can have imaging

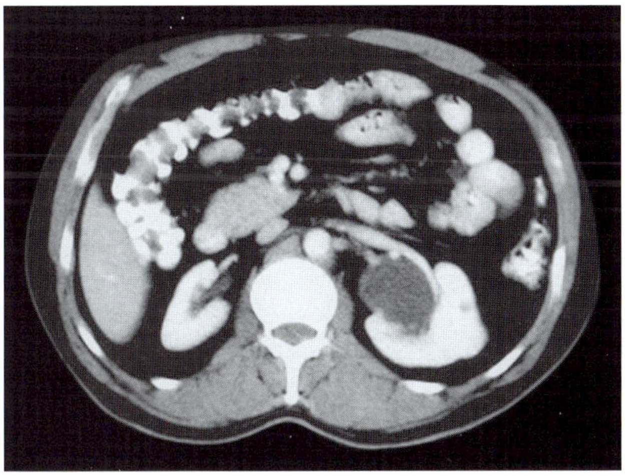

FIG. 20: Contrast-enhanced CT scan showing a solitary fluid-filled lesion in the renal sinus detected as an incidental finding in this patient—a parapelvic cyst. (CT: computed tomography).

appearance ranging from Bosniak category 2F to 4. These can appear similar to cystic RCC and hence end up being surgically treated most often.

Pelvicalyceal diverticulum is another lesion that can present as a focal cystic lesion in the renal cortex but has a distinctive feature of communication with the pelvicalyceal system.

Mixed Epithelial and Stromal Tumor

This is relatively a recently described entity that is seen most often in perimenopausal women with an average age of 50 years. Estrogen supplement/contraceptive use has been found to have an association with this tumor. Patients may present with flank mass or hematuria. However, they may also be asymptomatic in nearly one-fourth of the cases. MEST is a cystic and solid neoplasm, with both stromal elements resembling ovarian stroma and epithelial components resulting from cysts with epithelial lining.

This is seen as a multilocular cystic mass that can herniate into the renal pelvis. There may be enhancing solid component or wall calcification. The cysts may have hemorrhage within. Although the lesion is benign, it may be hard to differentiate from cystic RCC and hence is often treated surgically.

Cystic Nephroma

Cystic nephroma is also a rare benign tumor that has a bimodal age and sex distribution, the first peak occurring in boys less than 4 years of age and the second in women aged 40–60 years. In pediatric population, these present as painless abdominal masses while in the adults, they may present with pain and/or hematuria.

On imaging, these are seen as well-defined multilocular cystic masses with enhancing septae and may herniate into the pelvis like MEST. On MRI, the septae and the capsule are hypointense on both T1- and T2-weighted images owing to their fibrous nature. It is actually believed that MEST and cystic nephroma belong to the same spectrum of pathology with more cystic components in cystic nephroma than in MEST. As differentiation from RCC may be difficult on imaging, these lesions are most often treated surgically despite being benign.

Cystic Renal Cell Carcinoma

Multilocular cystic RCC is a low-grade tumor with male predominance that can look like cystic nephroma on imaging. Cystic clear cell RCC also can simulate this appearance **(*see* Figs. 8A and B)**; however, it is a more malignant lesion. This is discussed in detail elsewhere in the book.

Pyelocalyceal Diverticulum

This is a cyst within the renal cortex that has communication with the renal pelvicalyceal system. Two types have been described. Type1 is more common and seen to communicate with minor calyx while Type 2 communicates with major calyx or pelvis. These are thought to be mostly congenital in origin; however, acquired cases may result from calculi or infections.

These may be picked up on intravenous urogram studies (2.1–4.5 per 1000 IVU examinations). On US and noncontrast CT or nephrographic CT phase, these are seen as renal cysts. However, on contrast administration, these cysts show layering of contrast within them in the excretory phase. They may also be complicated by calculi or milk of calcium. These cysts then show thin layering of hyperattenuation material on noncontrast CT. Typically, these milk of calcium cysts lose connection with the collecting system and hence may not show contrast excretion within them. A large diverticulum may simulate a hydrocalyx due to obstruction. Complications of pyelocalyceal diverticulum include hemorrhage, infection, rupture, and rarely even malignancy.

INFECTIOUS CYSTS

Pyogenic Abscess

This is usually secondary to incompletely treated or untreated acute pyelonephritis. This may also result from hematogenous spread. Risk factors include pregnancy, diabetes, and other forms of immunosuppression.

Excretory urography reveals filling defects or irregular cavities that may communicate with the pelvicalyceal system. On sonography, thick-walled cystic lesions with low-level internal echoes are seen. Apart from imaging features, clinical features also help to distinguish them from renal cysts. Contrast-enhanced CT shows low attenuation masses with rim enhancement and thickening of perirenal fascia. The abscess often shows a thick halo around it. On MR, these are seen as heterogeneous mass with thick walls, hypointense on T1W and hyperintense on T2W images. Diffusion restriction is often seen. Air within the abscess results in susceptibility artifact seen on gradient echo images.

Hydatid Cyst

The kidney can also be involved by hydatid disease; the patient is usually asymptomatic until the cyst has grown large enough to cause pressure symptoms or rupture. Patients may present with flank pain/mass or dysuria. Rupture into the collecting system may result in renal colic and excretion of hydatid cysts in the urine. Hydatid cysts are typically single lesions usually located in the polar regions of either kidney.

Imaging findings are dependent on the stage of the hydatid cyst. Hydatid cysts are categorized into three types depending on the stage of the parasite:

1. *Type 1*: Unilocular cyst seen in the initial stage.
2. *Type 2*: Cyst with multiple daughter cysts seen in the intermediate stage.
3. *Type 3*: Calcified cyst suggestive of parasitic death.

Plain radiography may reveal a localized bulge on the renal contour or evidence of peripheral or curvilinear calcification which is in the pericyst. There may be complete calcification of the cyst in the third type. On EU, presence of hydatid cyst may result in distortion of the pelvicalyceal system. There may also be renal obstruction or impaired renal function.

On cross-sectional imaging, a unilocular cyst is typically seen in the first stage of the disease. In the next stage, when daughter cysts develop, they may be seen as multilocular cysts. The daughter cysts have a lower attenuation than of the mother cyst. These can have a thick enhancing wall and enhancing septae. A thick bilayered wall distinguishes type 2 cyst from multicystic renal disease. Few signs on imaging are considered characteristic of a hydatid cyst. A snowstorm sign can be seen on US when the hydatid sand disperses as the patient is rolled. The floating membrane sign results from separation of the cyst layers from pericyst. In type 3 cyst, when the parasite dies becomes quiescent, the cyst becomes calcified **(Figs. 21A to C)**.

Characteristic imaging findings along with history of stay in the endemic region is diagnostic of hydatid disease of the kidney, although the clinical findings may be nonspecific.

Tuberculosis

The genitourinary system accounts for nearly one-fifth of the extrapulmonary tubercular size. The most common route of spread of *Mycobacterium tuberculosis* to the kidney is hematogenous seeding from the lungs. A tuberculous focus is usually located in the renal cortex and may develop a communication with the tubular system and

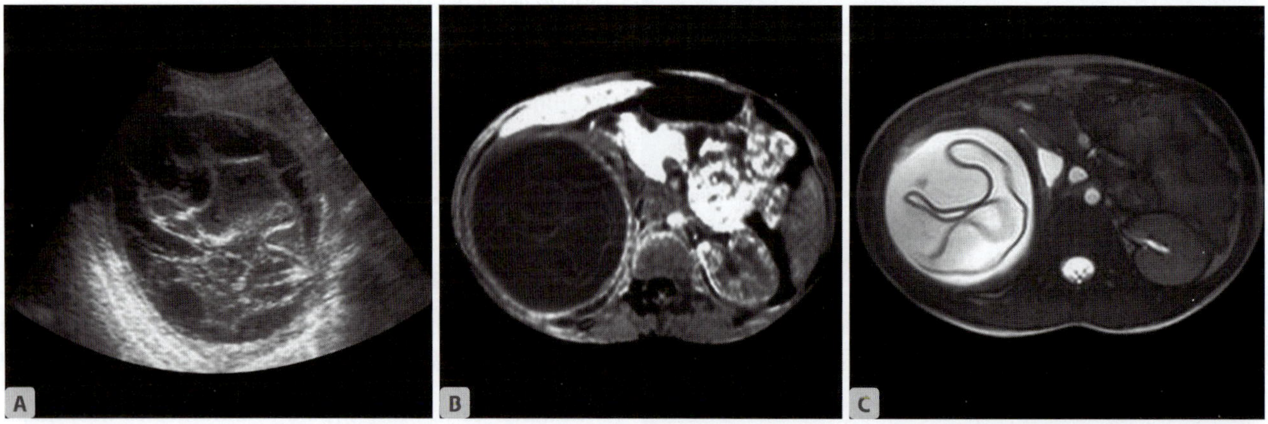

FIGS. 21A TO C: Sonogram (A) showing a cyst replacing the right kidney with multiple serpentine linear structures/membranes within s/o ruptured hydatid cyst. T1W MR axial image (B) showing the cyst replacing the right kidney. The cyst is hypointense on T1. T2W MR image (C) shows the cyst to have high signal. The membranes are seen as linear areas of low signal within—ruptured hydatid cyst of the right kidney. (MR: magnetic resonance).

the pyramids, which can rupture into the calyces. Although the route of spread to kidney is hematogenous, significant disease is usually limited to one kidney. Patients may present with flank pain, dysuria, and hematuria while constitutional symptoms are less common.

On conventional radiographs, the most common finding is that of renal calcification. Extensive calcification in a nonfunctional kidney is a characteristic finding in end-stage tuberculosis and is referred to as putty kidney. EU reveals findings dependent on the severity of infection. 10–15% patients may have normal EU. "Moth eaten" calyx is one of the early findings resulting from papillary necrosis. Papillary cavitation can then result which lead to the formation of medullary cavities that can communicate with the collecting system. These medullary cavities may be large and irregular. End-stage tubercular kidneys usually do not excrete contrast medium at urography. On US, multiple renal cavities can be seen. Focal calyceal changes are seen on CT as calyceal enlargement, pericalyceal areas of early cavitation, infundibular strictures, and loss of perirenal fat planes. Late features of calcification or hydronephrosis secondary to strictures may be seen.

Renal Aspergillosis

Renal aspergillosis is an uncommon renal infection. This is most often seen in the immunocompromised state. Infection may be acquired by the hematogenous route or ascending infection, the former being the more common route. On imaging, renal aspergillosis is difficult to differentiate from a renal abscess. It is seen as a complex cystic renal lesion with thick wall and internal septations. The kidney may show accompanying focal pyelonephritic features. Diagnosis is confirmed on either lesion aspiration or urine analysis.

CONCLUSION

Renal cystic disease in adults comprises a heterogenous group of heritable and nonheritable disorders. The Bosniak classification helps in stratification of renal cysts according to the risk of malignancy. Knowledge of imaging features of various renal cystic diseases can assist the radiologist in providing useful information to the clinician to aid patient management.

SUGGESTED READING

1. Ascenti G, Mazziotti S, Zimbaro G, et al. Complex cystic renal masses: characterization with contrast-enhanced US. Radiology. 2007;243(1):158-65.
2. Avni FE, Garel C, Cassart M, et al. Imaging and classification of congenital cystic renal diseases. Am J Roentgenol. 2012;198(5): 1004-13.
3. Chung EM, Conran RM, Schroeder JW, et al. From the radiologic pathology archives: pediatric polycystic kidney disease and other ciliopathies: radiologic-pathologic correlation. Radiographics. 2014;34(1):155-78.
4. Clevert DA, Minaifar N, Weckbach S, et al. Multislice computed tomography versus contrast-enhanced ultrasound in evaluation of complex cystic renal masses using the Bosniak classification system. Clin Hemorheol Microcirc. 2008; 39(1-4):171-8.
5. Farmer DL. Urinary tract masses. Semin Pediatr Surg. 2000;9(3):109-14.
6. Friedmann W, Vogel M, Dimer JS, et al. Prenatal differential diagnosis of cystic kidney disease and urinary tract obstruction: anatomic, pathologic, ultrasonographic and genetic findings. Eur J Obs Gyn Rep Biol. 2000;89:127-33.
7. Hindman NM. Cystic renal masses. Abdom Radiol. 2016;41:1020-34.
8. Hollenbeck BK, Taub DA, Miller DC, et al. Use of nephrectomy at select medical centers—a case of follow the crowd? J Urol. 2006;175(2):670-4.
9. Hollingsworth JM, Miller DC, Daignault S, et al. Rising incidence of small renal masses: a need to reassess treatment effect. J Natl Cancer Inst. 2006;98(18):1331-4.
10. Howlader N, Noone A, Krapcho M, et al (Eds). SEER Cancer Statistics Review, 1975–2011. Bethesda: National Cancer Institute; 2013.
11. Ignee A, Straub B, Brix D, et al. The value of contrast-enhanced ultrasound (CEUS) in the characterisation of patients with renal masses. Clin Hemorheol Microcirc. 2010;46(4):275-90.
12. Israel GM, Hindman N, Bosniak MA. Evaluation of cystic renal masses: comparison of CT and MR imaging by using the Bosniak classification system. Radiology. 2004;231(2): 365-71.
13. Katabathina VS, Kota G, Dasyam AK, et al. Adult renal cystic disease: a genetic, biological, and developmental primer. Radiographics. 2010;30:1509-23.
14. Lonergan GJ, Rice RR, Suarez ES. Autosomal recessive polycystic kidney disease: radiologic-pathologic correlation. AFIP Archives Radiographics. 2000;20:837-55.
15. Mileto A, Nelson RC, Marin D, et al. Dual-energy multidetector CT for the characterization of incidental adrenal nodules: diagnostic performance of contrast-enhanced material density analysis. Radiology. 2014;274(2):445-54.
16. Narayanasamy S, Krishna S, Shanbhogue AP, et al. Contemporary update on imaging of cystic renal masses with histopathological correlation and emphasis on patient management. Clin Radiol. 2018;74(2):83-94.
17. Park BK, Kim B, Kim SH, et al. Assessment of cystic renal masses based on Bosniak classification: comparison of CT and contrast-enhanced US. Eur J Radiol. 2007;61(2):310-4.
18. Pei Y, Obaji J, Dupuis A, et al. Unified criteria for ultrasonographic diagnosis of ADPKD. J Am Soc Nephrol. 2009;20(1):205-12.
19. Silverman SG, Israel GM, Herts BR, et al. Management of the incidental renal mass. Radiology. 2008;249(1):16-31.
20. Silverman SG, Pedrosa I, Ellis JH, et al. Bosniak classification of cystic renal masses, version 2019: an update proposal and needs assessment. Radiology. 2019;292(2):475-88.
21. Tantravahi JR, Steinman TI. Acquired cystic kidney disease. Semin Dialysis. 2000;13(5):330-4.
22. Wood III CG, Stromberg III LJ, Harmath CB, et al. CT and MR imaging for evaluation of cystic renal lesions and diseases. Radiographics. 2015;35(1):125-41.

CHAPTER

8

Renal Neoplasms

Anjali Prakash, Gaurav Shanker Pradhan, Rashmi Dixit

INTRODUCTION

Cross-sectional imaging has led not only to an increased detection of incidental renal mass, but also to a more confident diagnosis of its nature. Imaging is required to differentiate clinically significant renal masses from benign or indolent malignant conditions. Noninvasive characterization is possible in a majority of cases, which has a clinical impact by decreasing unnecessary biopsies and/or surgical interventions. A solid renal mass is aggressively pursued for a diagnosis of renal carcinoma, once infective, traumatic or vascular causes have been ruled out, solid masses are more likely than cystic masses to be malignant and management is more aggressive.

Renal tumors constitute a heterogeneous group of tumors with characteristic histology and variable clinicobiological profile.

CLASSIFICATION OF RENAL TUMORS

The World Health Organization has classified renal tumors in 2016 **(Table 1)**. This classification has divided tumors on the basis of cell/tissue of origin (renal cell, mesenchymal, metanephric, neuroendocrine tumors, etc.).[1]

Renal cell carcinoma (RCC) has been further subdivided into various subtypes based on predominant cytoplasmic features (clear cell and chromophobe RCC), architectural features (papillary RCC), anatomic location of tumors (collecting duct, renal medullary carcinoma), based on association with a specific renal disease background (acquired cystic disease-associated RCC). Certain subtypes are based on molecular alterations pathognomonic for RCC subtypes (MiT family translocation, succinate dehydrogenase-deficient renal carcinoma), and there are certain familial cancers [hereditary leiomyomatosis and RCC (HLRCC) syndrome-associated RCC].

TABLE 1: WHO classification of renal tumors (2016).

- *Renal cell tumors:*
  - Clear cell renal cell carcinoma
  - Multilocular cystic renal neoplasm of low malignant potential
  - Papillary renal cell carcinomas
  - Hereditary leiomyomatosis and renal cell carcinoma-associated renal cell carcinoma
  - Chromophobe renal cell carcinoma
  - Collecting duct carcinoma
  - Renal medullary carcinoma
  - MiT family translocation renal cell carcinomas
  - Succinate dehydrogenase-deficient renal carcinoma
  - Mucinous tubular and spindle cell carcinoma
  - Tubulocystic renal cell carcinoma
  - Acquired cystic disease-associated renal cell carcinoma
  - Renal cell carcinoma, unclassified
  - Papillary adenoma
  - Oncocytoma
- *Metanephric tumors:*
  - Metanephric adenoma
  - Metanephric adenofibroma
  - Metanephric stromal tumor
- *Nephroblastic and cystic tumors occurring mainly in children:*
  - Nephrogenic rests
  - Nephroblastoma
  - Cystic partially differentiated nephroblastoma
  - Pediatric cystic nephroma
- *Mesenchymal tumors:*
  - *Mesenchymal tumors occurring mainly in children:*
    - Clear cell sarcoma
    - Rhabdoid tumor
    - Congenital mesoblastic nephroma
    - Ossifying renal tumor of infancy
  - *Mesenchymal tumors occurring mainly in adults:*
    - Leiomyosarcoma
    - Angiosarcoma
    - Rhabdomyosarcoma
    - Osteosarcoma
    - Synovial sarcoma

Contd...

IMAGING OF RENAL MASS: MODALITIES AND TECHNIQUES

The workup of a renal mass starts with the differentiation of cystic mass from solid renal masses. Up to 90% of solid masses are malignant, with the risk increasing with size of the tumor (50% in size <1 cm to 90% in size >7 cm). The commonly

Contd...

- Ewing's sarcoma
- Angiomyolipoma
- Epithelioid angiomyolipoma
- Leiomyoma
- Hemangioma
- Lymphangioma
- Hemangioblastoma
- Juxtaglomerular cell tumor
- Renomedullary interstitial cell tumor
- Schwannoma
- Solitary fibrous tumor

- *Mixed epithelial and stromal tumor family:*
  - Cystic nephroma
  - Mixed epithelial and stromal tumor
- *Neuroendocrine tumors:*
  - Well-differentiated neuroendocrine tumor
  - Large cell neuroendocrine carcinoma
  - Small cell neuroendocrine carcinoma
  - Pheochromocytoma
- *Miscellaneous tumors:*
  - Renal hematopoietic neoplasms
  - Germ cell tumors
- *Metastatic tumors*

seen malignant solid renal masses are renal cell carcinoma, urothelial carcinoma, lymphoma, and metastasis, whereas the benign lesions seen are angiomyolipoma and oncocytoma.

Ultrasound is used as a first-line imaging test for suspected renal disease. A simple cyst can be confidently diagnosed on ultrasound as a completely anechoic structure with posterior enhancement. Septation, calcification, and solid nodular component are seen in a complicated cyst. The detection of blood flow by Doppler or lesion enhancement after intravenous contrast denotes presence of a solid component.[2]

Any solid lesion or a complicated cyst requires further evaluation by **CT or MRI**. These examinations should be performed with a protocol according meticulous attention to detail to evaluate an indeterminate mass accurately and to stage a possible renal cancer. The recommended protocols for CT and MRI for characterization of renal mass are provided in **Tables 2 and 3**.[3]

Both CT and MRI should have noncontrast imaging with contrast imaging in various phases [corticomedullary (CM), nephrographic, and delayed]. Slice thickness should be 2.5-3 mm with a reconstruction interval of not more than 3 mm.

Renal enhancement occurs in different phases at 20 seconds after administration of contrast, in the *arterial phase*, aorta, and renal arteries enhance. At 60-70 seconds starts the *CM phase*, where the differentiation of cortex and medulla is prominent, pseudotumors like dromedary hump, and hypertrophied column of Bertin can be identified. At 90-120 seconds begins the *nephrographic phase*, when enhancement of cortex fades and medulla enhances homogeneously. This is the most sensitive phase for renal mass detection. At 180 seconds appears the *excretory phase*, where contrast appears in the collecting system. Computed tomography for detection of thrombus requires thin (<5 mm) slices at level of renal vein after pressure injection of contrast. Renal vein enlargement and displacement are not accurate signs for venous invasion, as it may be enlarged due to high flow and displaced due to bulk of tumor. The flow of unenhanced blood from pelvis may be mistaken for inferior vena cava (IVC) thrombus. In these cases, delayed images may be needed for further characterization.

Precontrast imaging in MRI, should include T1 and T2 imaging, chemical shift imaging (in and opposed phase) and diffusion-weighted imaging. A fat suppression technique for detection of macroscopic fat is also required. Dynamic imaging, in at least two phases after administration of intravenous (IV) contrast completes the protocol. Subtraction imaging is required in MRI to demonstrate enhancement, especially in a T1-hyperintense lesion.

DIAGNOSTIC CRITERIA

Balls versus Beans

A useful strategy for the evaluation of renal mass is to divide them on the basis of their growth pattern into ball type or bean type masses. This concept was developed by Hartman and Ros. Most renal masses like cysts, renal cell carcinomas, angiomyolipoma, metastasis, and oncocytoma grow by expansion. These masses are shaped similarly to spheres or balls and they displace and compress the adjacent structure, rather than invade normal structure. As these masses enlarge, they expand from normal parenchymal margins, either peripherally to the kidney or into renal sinus. Other renal lesions like transitional cell carcinoma, squamous cell carcinoma, infiltrating carcinoma, lymphoma, and renal medullary carcinoma grow along the latticework of normal renal parenchyma. Infiltrating lesions do not deform the shape, with the kidney retaining the "bean" shape **(Figs. 1A and B)**. These are difficult to detect radiologically since little mass effect is associated.[4-6]

Renal Pseudotumors

It is essential to determine that the detected "mass" is actually a renal neoplasm and not a finding that mimics it. Renal pseudotumors are a diverse group, including congenital and developmental anomalies (fetal lobulations, prominent renal columns of Bertin, dromedary humps), inflammatory lesions (renal abscess, pyelonephritis), and vascular anomalies (renal artery aneurysm, arteriovenous malformation). Renal contusion and hematoma may also mimic a tumor. Many patients with chronic renal disease develop focal nodular compensatory hypertrophy which mimics a tumor. Imaging in CM phase provides the correct answer **(Figs. 2A to C)**. Enhancement, a key feature in the diagnosis of a neoplasm may be seen in infective and vascular lesions. Clinical history (e.g. pain, fever, and pyuria favor infection and not a neoplasm), multiphasic CT/MR examination, and knowledge of the pseudotumors will help to reach a correct diagnosis.[7]

Most solid renal masses measure between 20 and 70 Hounsfield units (HU) on noncontrast CT. Lesions measuring

TABLE 2: CT protocol for renal mass characterization.

Phases	Noncontrast	*Corticomedullary	Nephrographic	Excretory
Phase timing	–	40 seconds	90–120 seconds	5–7 minutes
Coverage	Kidneys	Diaphragm through kidneys	Diaphragm through kidneys	Kidneys
Field of view	Whole body	Whole body	Whole body	Whole body
Reconstructions	Axial: 3 mm	Axial: 3 mm Coronal: 2 mm Sagittal: 2 mm	Axial: 3 mm Coronal: 2 mm Sagittal: 2 mm	Axial: 3 mm Coronal: 2 mm Sagittal: 2 mm

*Contrast 100–150 mL low osmolality (LOCM) at 5 mL/second.

TABLE 3: Multiparametric magnetic resonance protocol for characterization of renal mass.

Sequences	Imaging planes
T1W dual echo gradient (in and opposed phase)	Axial
T2W HASTE	Axial, coronal, sagittal
T2W TSE with fat suppression	Axial
3D fat-saturated T1W SPGR precontrast and postcontrast DCE (corticomedullary, nephrographic, and excretory*)	Axial
Diffusion weighted (b = 50,500,800), ADC map	Axial

*Corticomedullary phase = 40 seconds, nephrographic = 90 seconds, excretory = 3 minutes after IV gadolinium at dose of 0.01 mmol/kg in patients with GFR > 60 mL/min/1.73 m^2 via pressure injector followed by a saline flush.

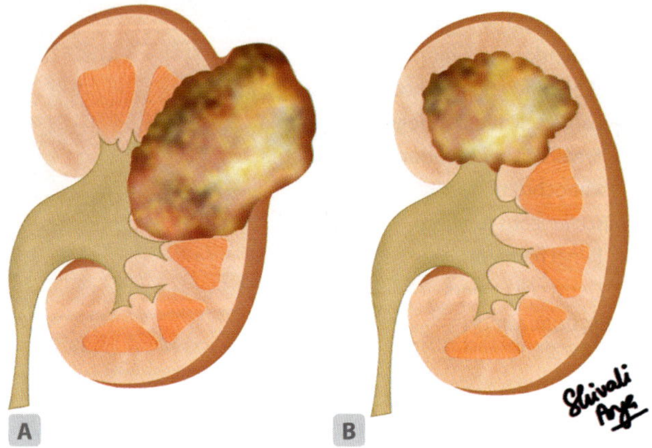

FIGS. 1A AND B: Ball versus bean concept. (A) Ball type mass grows exophytically, with a contour deformity; (B) Bean type mass uses renal parenchyma as framework for growth with maintained reniform shape. Sinus fat and collecting system elements may be destroyed.

less or more than that are cysts—simple cysts or hyperdense/hemorrhagic cysts, respectively. Indeterminate renal mass is a lesion containing areas that measure 20-70 HU on noncontrast imaging. Homogeneous lesions measuring more than 70 HU can be considered benign, whereas lesions either entirely or partially within the 20-70 HU range should be considered indeterminate and require further evaluation.

Enhancement of a renal mass is considered to be the key in determining the nature of the mass. The main criteria for diagnosing a solid renal mass is to document measurable enhancement on CT/MRI. Any nodular enhancement within a mass confirms some solid component and a high probability of a renal neoplasm. An increase of more than 20 HU on administration of IV contrast is taken as evidence of presence of solid elements while an increase of less than 10 HU is considered as no enhancement. An indeterminate enhancement is an increase of 10-20 HU and requires follow-up or imaging by MRI, which is more sensitive to contrast enhancement than CT.

Enhancement may be incorrectly identified as present on CT due to two reasons. First is *volume averaging*, which occurs when CT image averages part of mass (usually <1.5 cm in size) with the normal enhancing renal parenchyma. To prevent this, the slice thickness should not be more than half the renal mass diameter. The second reason of pseudoenhancement is *beam hardening*. This occurs in small masses or masses completely surrounded by enhancing parenchyma, leading to an increase in attenuation of less than 30 HU. This effect cannot be overcome by decreasing slice thickness.[8,9]

RENAL CELL TUMORS

Renal Cell Carcinoma

Renal cell carcinoma, also called hypernephroma, is the most common primary renal malignancy in adults. It accounts for 85% of all malignant renal tumors and about 3% of all diagnosed neoplasms. RCC is nowadays most commonly discovered incidentally (30%). These are often smaller and of lower grade and staging. RCC may however, present with symptoms like flank pain (37%), hematuria and palpable mass, weight loss, anorexia, fever, gastrointestinal or neurological symptoms, and paraneoplastic syndromes. Superficial tumors can invade and breach the renal capsule and directly involve perirenal fat, adrenal gland, and adjacent organs. Metastases often occurs in regional nodes, invasion of cisterna chyli can lead to hilar and supraclavicular nodes. RCC has a propensity for venous thrombi. Systemic dissemination can take place into liver, bone, adrenal, and opposite kidney or brain in decreasing order of frequency.

Renal cell carcinoma occurs more commonly in males, in the 5th-7th decade. Most cases are sporadic; some may

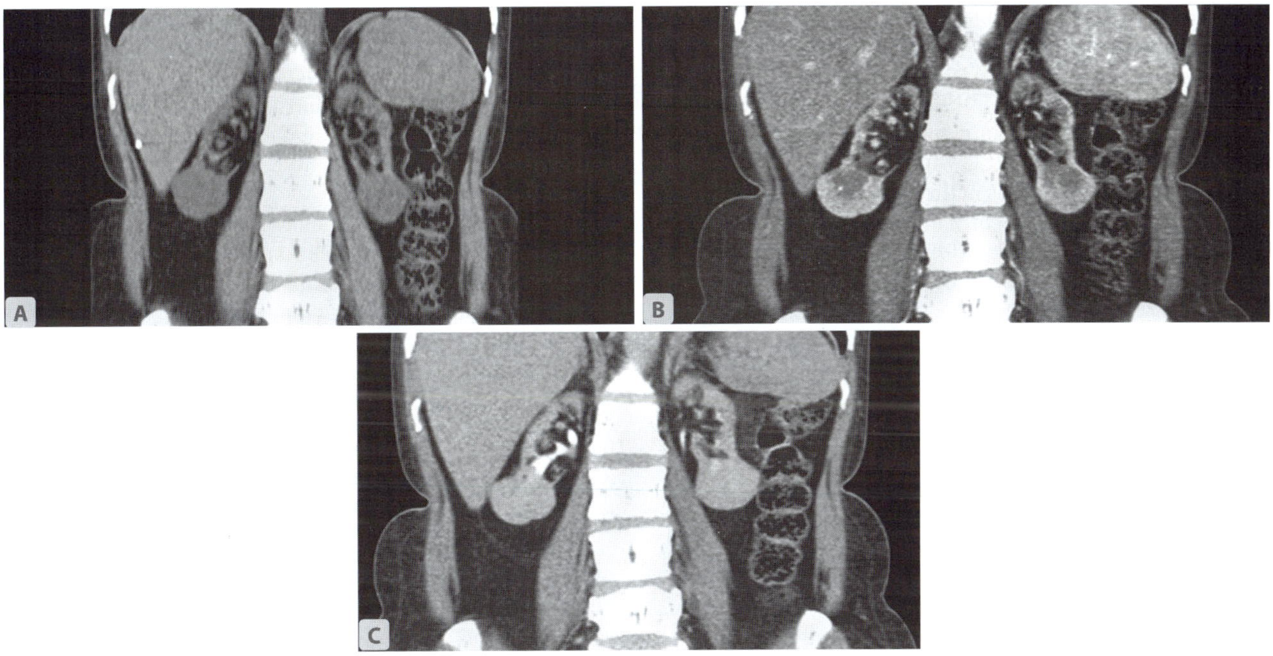

FIGS. 2A TO C: CT coronal multiphasic reconstruction (MPR). (A) Noncontrast; (B) Corticomedullary phase; (C) Nephrographic phase-focal nodular compensatory hypertrophy in a case of chronic renal disease presenting as "tumor" in lower poles of both kidneys. The true nature of these pseudotumors are appreciated on corticomedullary phase.

be associated with syndromes such as Von Hippel–Lindau disease (vHL) **(Box 1)**. Risk factors include smoking, hypertension, obesity, acquired renal cystic disease, exposure to petroleum and asbestos, and certain genetic syndromes. Usually RCC is unilateral, 2% are bilateral and 9% are multicentric in the same kidney. Bilateral and multicentric tumors arise in patients of vHL syndromic, familial RCC and in patients on long-term hemodialysis.[10]

Renal cell carcinoma is comprised of different histological subtypes with different disease progression and metastatic potential.

BOX 1: Inherited cancer susceptibility syndromes with increased risk of renal cancer.

- BAP1-mutant disease
- Birt-Hogg-Dubé syndrome
- Familial clear cell renal cancer with chromosome 3 translocation
- Hereditary leiomyomatosis and renal cell cancer
- Hereditary papillary renal cancer
- PTEN hamartoma syndrome
- SDH-associated renal cancer
- Tuberous sclerosis complex
- Von Hippel-Lindau disease

Clear Cell Renal Cell Carcinoma

Clear cell RCC is the most common subtype accounting for 75–85% of cases, which are mostly sporadic in occurrence, 5% are associated with hereditary syndromes, including vHL and tuberous sclerosis. These tumors originate from the proximal convoluted tubules. It typically appears as a variegated, expansile, cortical mass with areas of necrosis, hemorrhage, cystic change, and calcification (15%). Clear cell RCC is a hypervascular tumor and has the greatest metastatic potential with hematogenous metastasis to lung, liver, and bones. There is also a propensity of clear cell RCC for lymphatic, late, and unusual sites of metastasis.[3,11,12]

Papillary Renal Cell Carcinoma

These arise from the epithelium of the proximal convoluted tubule, and are the second most common subtype of RCC. Characterized by papillary or tubopapillary histologic architecture, they account for 10–15% of RCC. These are bilateral in I4% and multifocal in 23% cases.

Papillary RCC usually presents at 40–50 years of age and is a slow-growing tumor. Papillary RCC (pRCC) appears as homogeneous, hypovascular, soft tissue cortical mass with foci of calcification. Papillary RCCs frequently show hemorrhage.[3,11,12]

Chromophobe Renal Cell Carcinoma

It is a subtype of RCC, characterized by large, pale cells with prominent cell membranes. 5–10% of RCCs are of the chromophobe subtype, which arise from intercalated cells of the renal cortex and have the same origin as oncocytoma with overlapping histological and imaging features. They usually occur as a solitary cortical mass. Bilateral and multicentric chromophobe RCCs are found in association with oncocytomas and Birt-Hogg-Dubé syndrome. The tumor is typically large at presentation, homogeneous without necrosis or hemorrhage, and is relatively hypovascular. The chromophobe type is associated with the least malignant potential and best prognosis.[13]

Multicystic Renal Cell Carcinoma

It is a recently described, rare subtype of RCC. The term is used to describe a cystic RCC with a small volume (25% or less) of neoplastic clear cells in the cyst. Multicystic renal cell carcinoma (MCRCC) typically manifests as multiseptated cystic masses with thin septations on imaging. Distinction from other cystic masses is difficult.[14]

Other Subtypes of Renal Cell Carcinoma

Carcinoma of the Collecting Ducts (CDC) of Bellini

This is a rare subtype of RCC accounting for <1% cases. Slightly more common in males, patients are usually in the mid-50s. This tumor is characterized by its medullary location, infiltrative growth pattern and weak, heterogeneous enhancement.[15]

Renal Medullary Carcinoma

It is a rapidly growing aggressive subtype, often presenting with metastasis. Seen in young males of African descent with a sickle cell trait, this is usually seen on right side of body, presenting as an infiltrative necrotic mass with caliectasis and lymphadenopathy.[16,17]

Renal Carcinoma Associated With Xp11.2 Translocations/Tfe 3 Gene Fusions

This carcinoma affects children and young adults. Large size, cystic changes, calcification, lymph node and distant metastasis are indicative of this subtype, especially in a young female patient.[18,19]

Imaging of Renal Cell Carcinoma

Plain Radiograph

It is not used to diagnose a renal mass. Renal mass may be visible as a soft tissue shadow with displacement of retroperitoneal fat. Calcification can also be detected on plain film **(Fig. 3)**. Pattern of calcification may help in differentiating benign from malignant masses. Renal masses that contain central, irregular calcifications are usually malignant, whereas peripheral rim calcifications are seen in renal cysts.

Intravenous Urography

It is an insensitive method of detecting a renal mass, especially central placed ones. It lacks specificity for accurately characterizing a lesion. Expansile masses cause contour abnormalities calyceal splaying, stretching, and draping **(Fig. 4)**. Infiltrating renal mass produce little parenchymal mass effect, and may be seen as a filling defect in the collecting system.

Ultrasound

Ultrasound is usually the initial method of investigation in a renal mass. It can reliably differentiate solid masses from renal cysts.

Renal cell carcinoma has varied appearance on sonography. Mostly solid, RCCs can have a predominant cystic component. Usually, hypo- to isoechoic to the renal parenchyma **(Fig. 5)**, they can appear hyperechoic making differentiation from angiomyolipoma difficult. Color Doppler demonstrates neovascularity of tumor. Different patterns of flow have been demonstrated in various subtypes of RCC. High-peak systolic velocity and Doppler shift has been seen in clear cell RCC **(Fig. 6)**. Contrast-enhanced ultrasound (CEUS) is useful to demonstrate presence of vascularity in a renal mass, which is the most important feature of a possible malignant etiology. Clear cell RCC demonstrates strong uptake in arterial phase with a delayed washout. Hypovascularity of a mass compared to the renal cortex is a feature of papillary carcinoma. Presence of a vascularized capsule around a solid renal mass is another suspicious feature. CEUS helps in the workup of indeterminate lesion on CT and has proved useful in dividing these lesions as surgical or nonsurgical.[20]

Computed tomography on unenhanced CT, renal cell carcinomas may be hypodense, isodense, or hyperdense to the unenhanced renal parenchyma. They are often

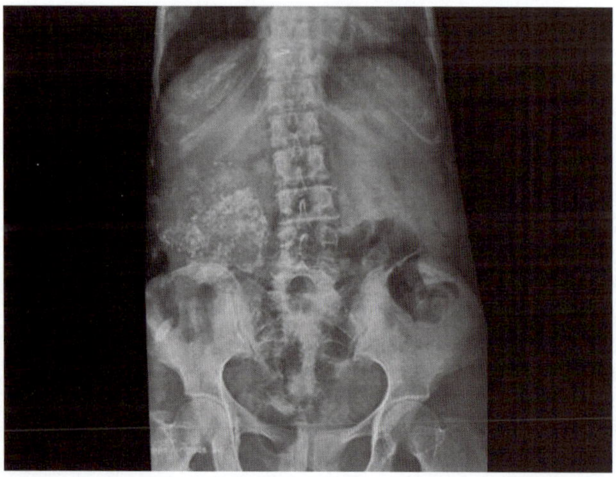

FIG. 3: X-ray abdomen showing soft-tissue mass with calcification in the right renal fossa.

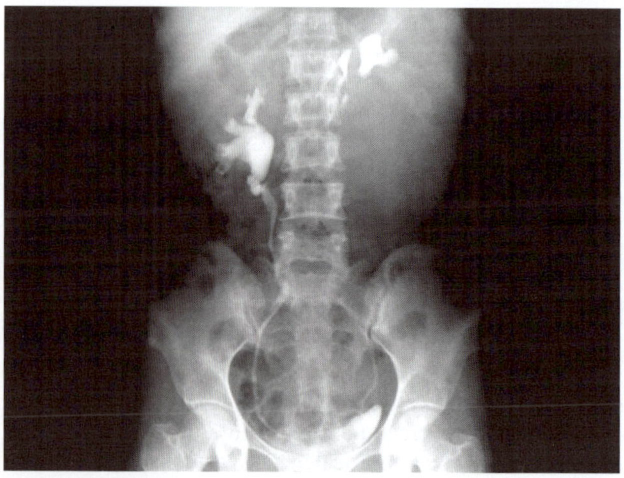

FIG. 4: Intravenous renogram—showing compression and displacement of calyces of the left kidney with focal upper pole hydrocalyx in a case of renal cell carcinoma.

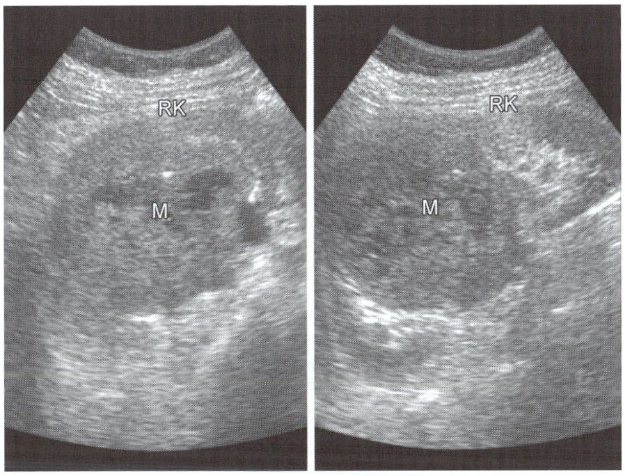

FIG. 5: US—transverse and longitudinal sonogram of the right kidney shows a large well-defined heterogeneous mass arising from the upper pole right kidney—renal cell carcinoma.

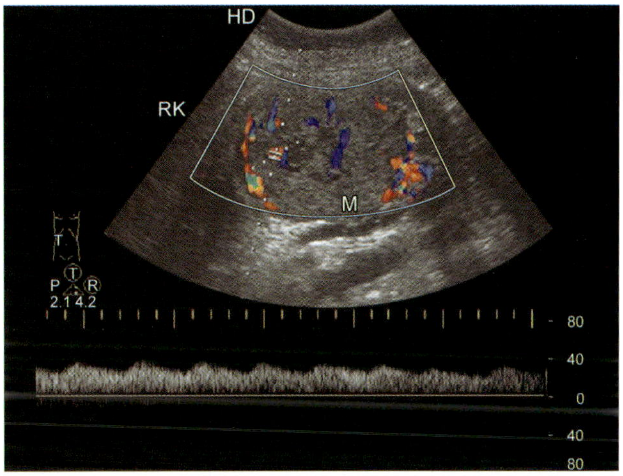

FIG. 6: CDFI shows vascularity within the mass.

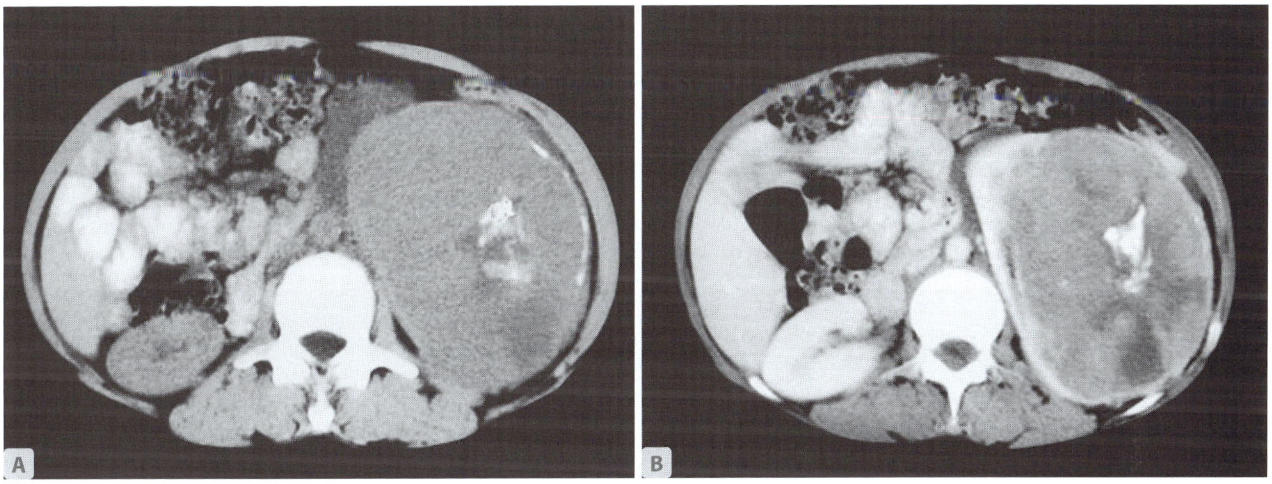

FIGS. 7A AND B: (A) Noncontrast CT; (B) Contrast-enhanced CT showing a large enhancing mass with peripheral and central coarse calcification in the left kidney.

heterogeneous in appearance with low-density necrotic areas. The renal outline is distorted in a majority (94%) of cases, irrespective of tumor size. The presence of calcification is also noted in approximately 25%, CT being the most sensitive modality for the depiction of parenchymal calcification **(Figs. 7A and B)**. Calcification in RCC may be punctate, amorphous, linear or peripheral. A zone of relative radiolucency surrounding the tumor or "Halo sign" may be noted. This represents the compressed ischemic renal parenchyma around the tumor—"pseudocapsule".

Most renal carcinomas are solid with an attenuation of at least 20 HU on precontrast scans. An increase of attenuation of more than 20 HU, post administration of IV contrast indicates a possible malignant etiology **(Figs. 8 and 9)**. Heterogeneous enhancement correlates with the presence of cellular regions within the tumor, but does not correlate with grade. Cystic and necrotic change is seen in clear cell type, whereas papillary and chromophobe are more homogeneous. Clear cell carcinomas enhance to a greater degree than other subtypes of malignant lesions, especially papillary carcinoma. A low tumor to aorta enhancement or tumor to normal renal parenchyma enhancement ratio is indicative of papillary RCC.[21,22]

The RCC shows a propensity for renal vein invasion and the thrombus may extend into the IVC, seen in almost 30% of cases. CT is specific for renal vein invasion by tumor thrombus with specificity of 98% **(Fig. 10)**. A hypodense filling defect outlined by contrast in the renal vein on a CT on CM or nephrographic phase is diagnostic for thrombus. Tumor thrombus may extend into IVC, often enlarging the caliber of the IVC. There may be bland thrombus inferior to the tumor thrombus in the IVC, as a result of occlusion of the lumen. Inadequate contrast bolus, motion and flow artefacts may cause a technically inadequate CT scan. On the right side, it may be difficult to distinguish between intraluminal tumor thrombus and extrinsic caval compression caused by a large primary tumor or enlarged lymph nodes.

Metastatic adenopathy in the retroperitoneum, associated with RCC has poor prognostic significance **(Fig. 11)**.

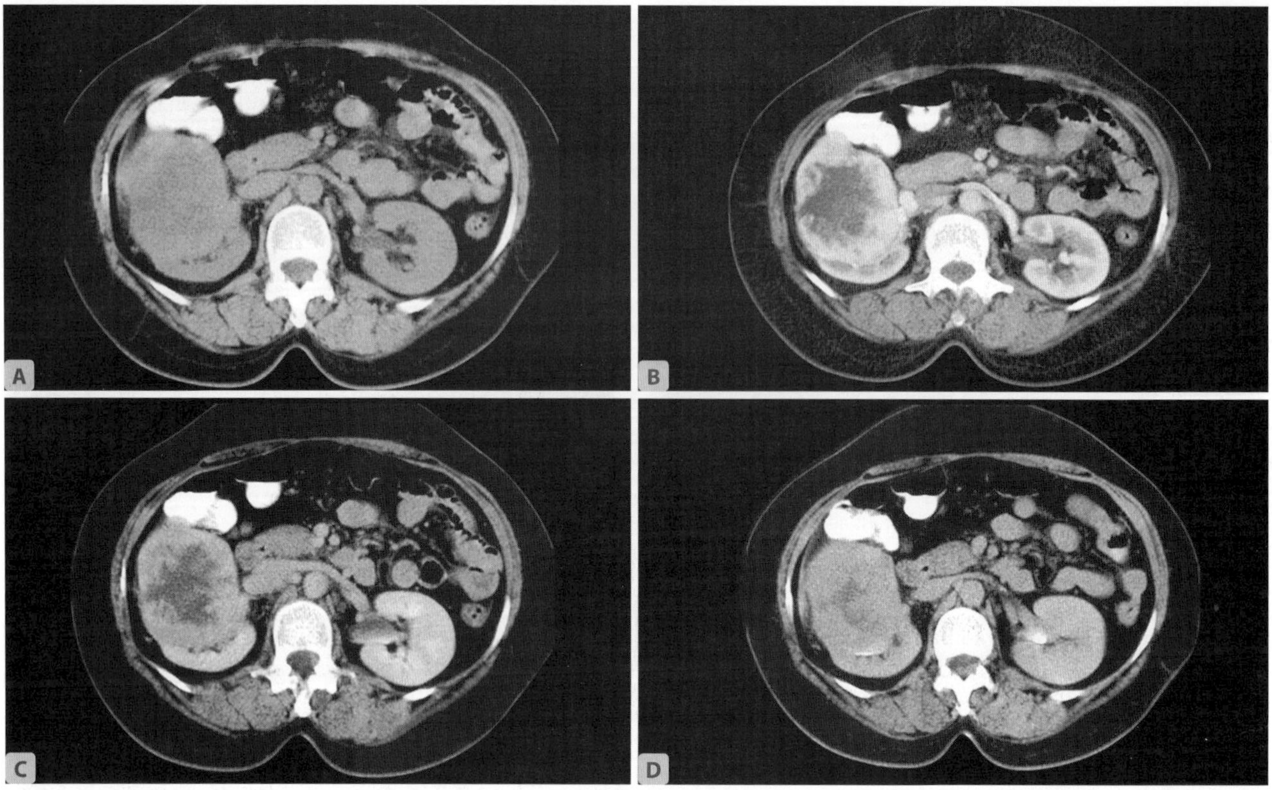

FIGS. 8A TO D: CT features of renal cell carcinomas in four phases. (A) Noncontrast; (B) Corticomedullary; (C) Nephrographic; (D) Excretory phases. Shows a right renal mass with mixed enhancement pattern containing enhancing soft tissue and low attenuation areas representing necrosis or cystic change arising from the anterior renal cortex. The mass is best demarcated on nephrographic phase and shows "de-enhancement" in the later phase.

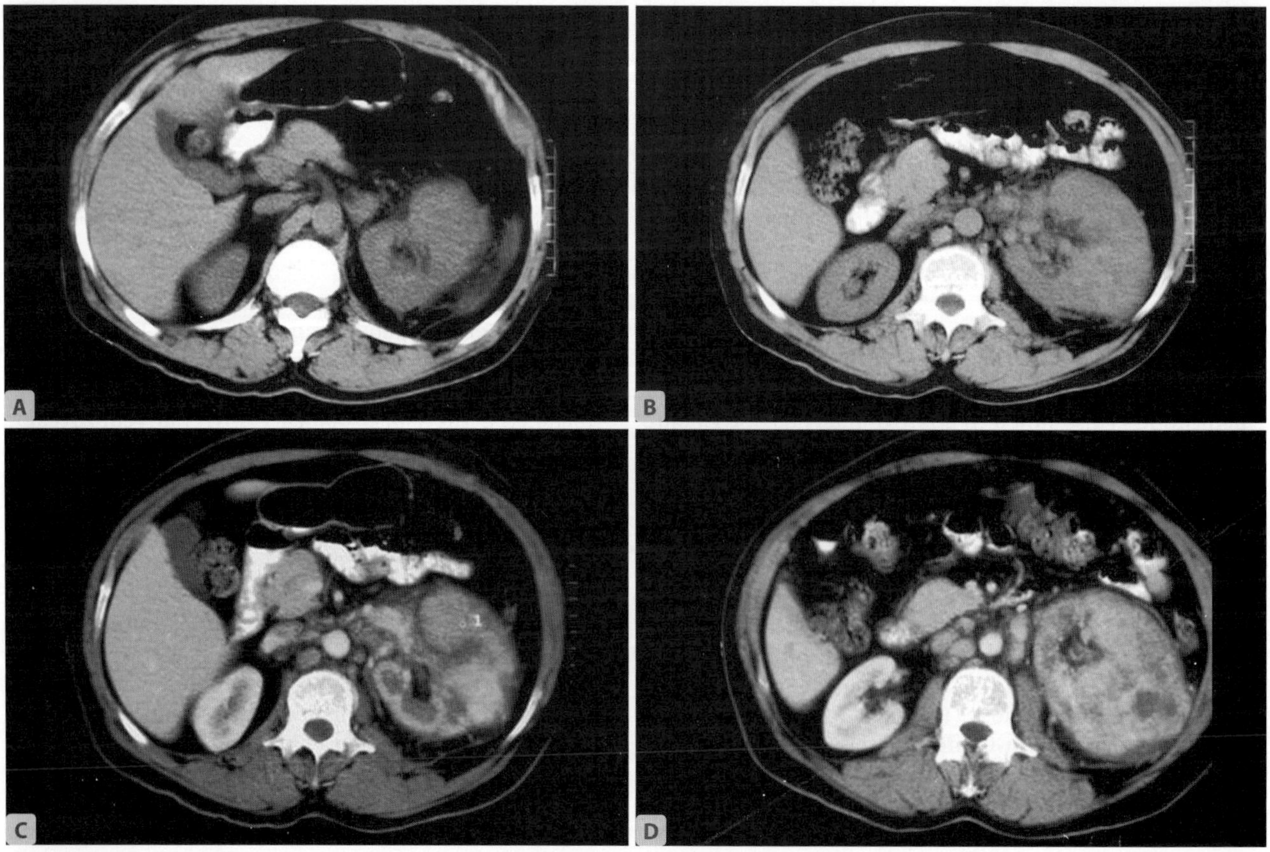

FIGS. 9A TO D: (A and B) CT precontrast; and (C and D) CT postcontrast—solid left renal mass with increase in attenuation of 20 HU—malignant etiology—renal cell carcinoma.

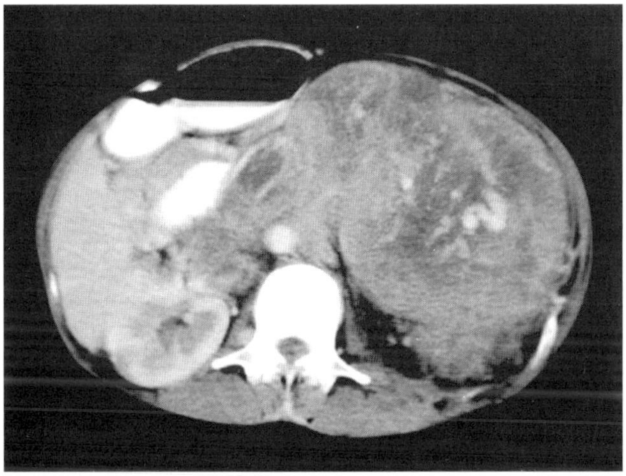

FIG. 10: Contrast-enhanced CT abdomen shows a large mass in the left kidney with neovascularity, definite extension into perinephric space, left renal vein and inferior vena cava—renal cell carcinoma.

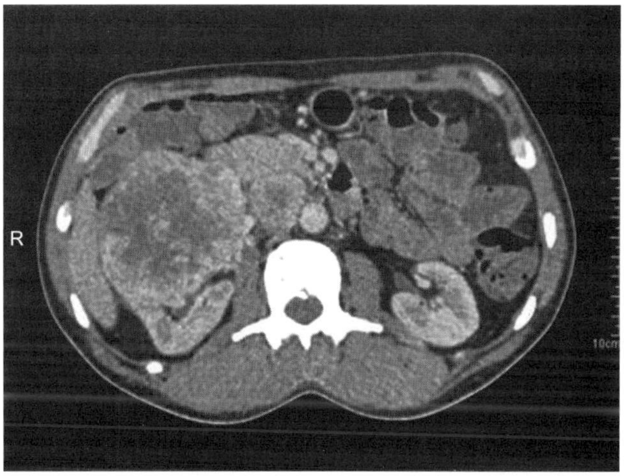

FIG. 11: Contrast-enhanced CT abdomen—right renal mass with retroperitoneal adenopathy.

The criterion of 1 cm threshold has proved to be unsuccessful in differentiating reactive nodes from metastatic adenopathy. Lymph nodes greater than 2 cm are always malignant. Nodes, less than 1 cm, may contain metastasis.

Dual-energy Computed Tomography

Dual-energy computed tomography (DECT) plays an important role in the characterization of renal masses, especially in the incidentally discovered mass. Virtual unenhanced and the water density images substitute for conventional noncontrast images, where acquisition in precontrastphasehasnotbeendone.Inpatientswhoareimaged for a multiphase renal CT, omitting noncontrast phase can lead to decrease in radiation dose. Color-coded iodine maps or iodine density maps demonstrate enhancement and can help in diagnosing nonenhancing cysts.[23]

Estimating the iodine content from a region of interest may help in the diagnosis of hyperdense cyst, complex cysts, and hypovascular renal tumor. An iodine density threshold of 0.5 mg/mL has a reported sensitivity of 100% and a specificity of 97.7% for distinguishing enhancing from nonenhancing lesions. Similarly, tumor iodine concentration of 0.9 mg/mL may serve as a threshold to differentiate between clear cell from papillary subtypes of RCC. DECT also provides virtual monochromatic data sets can help to overcome the problem of pseudoenhancement in small lesions. A recent advance of atomic number mapping can help to differentiate nonenhancing lesions from enhancing masses. DECT has a role in posttreatment imaging of renal tumors. Color-coded iodine maps can help to differentiate postoperative changes such as hyperdense foci and nodular appearance seen after ablative therapy that mimic residual changes from residual/recurrent tumor.[24,25]

Magnetic Resonance Imaging of Renal Masses

Functional imaging [diffusion-weighted imaging (DWI) and dynamic contrast-enhancement (DCE)] techniques combined with T2-weighted (T2W) and chemical-shift imaging (CSI), with or without urography, constitutes a comprehensive multiparametric (MP) MRI protocol of the kidneys.

MR imaging allows detection and characterization of renal masses. MR also helps in differentiating benign from malignant renal mass, suggests various subtypes of RCC **(Tables 4 and 5)** and possible histological grade leading to a role in management decisions. With the advent of newer treatment options and adjuvant therapies like immunotherapy with interleukin-2, interferon-α, and autolymphocytes, antiangiogenic therapy, cytotoxic chemotherapy, predicting the subtype of RCC is important in the management. Clear cell and chromophobe RCC may show response to immunotherapy, which is not useful in papillary RCC. Various studies have correlated MRI appearance of renal masses with pathology.[26-27] An MRI classification system has been proposed to predict the histological subtype and nuclear grade. This is based on certain characteristics like lesion size, peripheral vs central location, T2 signal intensity and degree of enhancement of the lesion, the presence of subvoxel fat on CSI, intratumoral necrosis, retroperitoneal vascular collaterals, and vascular thrombosis.[28]

Clear cell RCC, which demonstrates high T2 signal with heterogeneity due to associated cystic change and necrosis, are hypointense to isointense to normal renal parenchyma on T1W images. The presence of necrosis in a renal mass has been shown to correlate with tumor size and grade. Presence of intralesional microscopic fat in 60% of cases leads to a drop of signal on opposed phase imaging compared to in-phase images. A signal loss of 25% or more has predictive value. Clear cell RCC are hypervascular tumors, enhancing avidly (more than other subtypes of RCCs). A tumor pseudocapsule, representing compressed renal parenchyma, which is hypointense on both T1 and T2 may be seen. Clear cell RCCs tend to extend into the renal vein and inferior vena cava. Presence of intralesional necrosis, retroperitoneal collaterals, renal vein thrombosis interruption of pseudocapsule, large size correlate with an aggressive tumor grade[29,30] **(Figs. 12 and 13)**.

TABLE 4: MR features of various renal cell carcinoma subtypes.

Clear cell RCC	Papillary RCC	Chromophobe RCC
Hypervascular	Hypovascular	Hypovascular
Heterogeneous	Homogeneous	Homogeneous
Renal vein and IVC involvement common	Rare	Rare
Lymph nodal involvement is less	More common	Least common
Metastasis common	Less common	Least common
Hyperintense on T2WI	Hypointense on T1W1	

TABLE 5: Multiparametric MRI of renal masses.

Renal mass	MRI feature
Clear cell RCC	High SI on T2WI, microscopic fat, hypervascular
Papillary RCC	Low SI on T2WI, hypovascular, may contain hemosiderin
Chromophobe RCC	No definitive features—biopsy
Classic AML	Macroscopic fat suppresion on frequency-selective Fat Sat sequence, artefact on CSI
Lipid-poor AML	Low SI on T2WI, avid early enhancement, may contain microscopic fat
Oncocytoma	No definitive features-biopsy

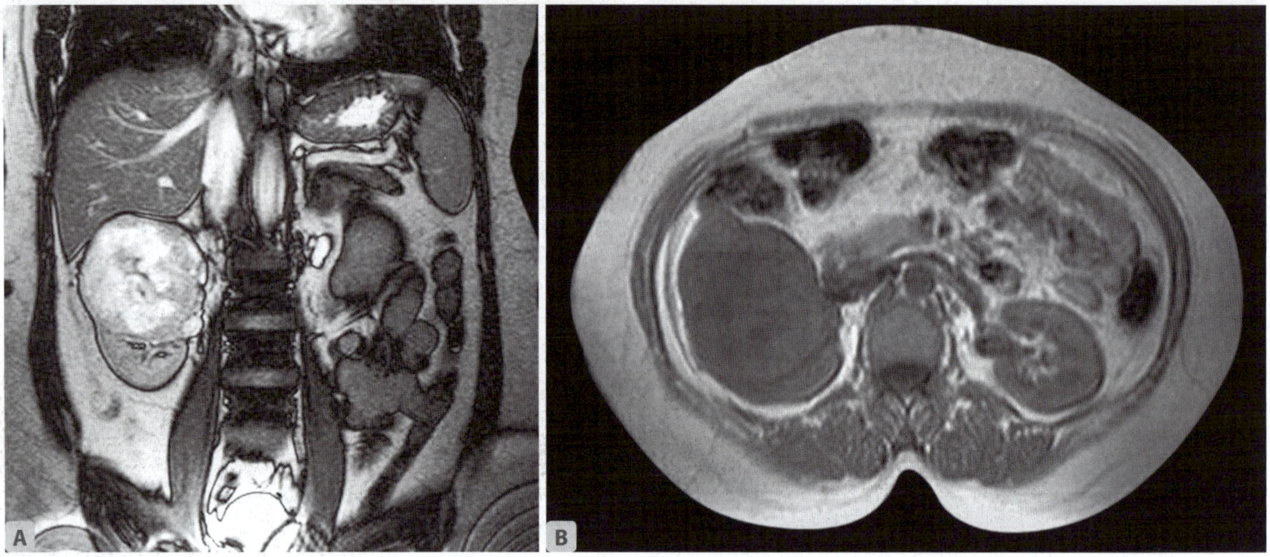

FIGS. 12A AND B: Renal cell carcinoma—(A) MRI; (B) TRUEFISP coronal T1W1 axial showing a well-circumscribed mass with necrotic change hypointense on T1 and hyperintense on T2 arising from upper pole of right kidney. Inferior vena cava appears normal. Clear cell renal cell carcinoma.

Papillary Renal Cell Carcinoma

Papillary RCC are usually well-circumscribed, peripherally located small tumors less than 3 cm. Papillary tumors are characteristically hypointense on T2W images and are hypovascular. As the tumor increases in size, internal hemorrhage may cause heterogeneous appearance **(Figs. 14A to D)**. Presence of hemosiderin due to hemorrhage leads to signal drop on in-phase images. Cystic papillary RCCs show internal papillary projections, mural nodules, and hemorrhagic fluid.

Chromophobe Renal Cell Carcinoma

No specific features are seen on MR, they may show intermediate-to-low signal on T2WI; cystic change and necrosis are uncommon. The enhancement is intermediate, more than pRCC, and less than ccRCC. In some cases, a central stellate scar and spoke wheel pattern (similar to oncocytoma) may be seen. Segmental enhancement inversion, wherby initially enhancing components of a renal mass subsequently become lower in attenuation than the initially hypoenhancing ones is another shared feature with oncocytoma.

Diffusion-weighted Imaging[31-37]

Diffusion-weighted MR imaging adds to the diagnostic ability of MRI. It is a valuable tool in evaluating pathology in patients with renal impairment in whom contrast administration is contraindicated. ADC value of renal tumor is less than normal parenchyma, a fact of utility in ruling out malignancy in pseudotumors. Solid lesions have higher cellular density, which restrict Brownian motion of water and have low ADC values whereas benign lesions lose signal with increasing b-values and have high ADC values **(Figs. 15A to E)**. In a few studies, RCCs show significantly lower ADC than benign lesions ($1.61 \pm 0.08 \times 10^{-3}mm^2/s$ vs $2.10 \pm 0.09 \times 10^{-3}mm^2/s$). Cysts have highest ADC values followed by normal renal tissue ($2.26 \pm 0.10 \times 10^{-3}mm^2/s$).

There is a difference in the reported ADC value between oncocytoma ($2.01 \pm 0.08 \times 10^{-3}mm^2/s$) and RCC, a point that can potentially help in differentiating the two. DWI helps to differentiate various subtypes of RCCs. Clear cell RCCs have significantly higher ADC values than papillary and chromophobe subtypes. ADC values are lower for high-grade clear cell RCCs compared with those of low-grade clear

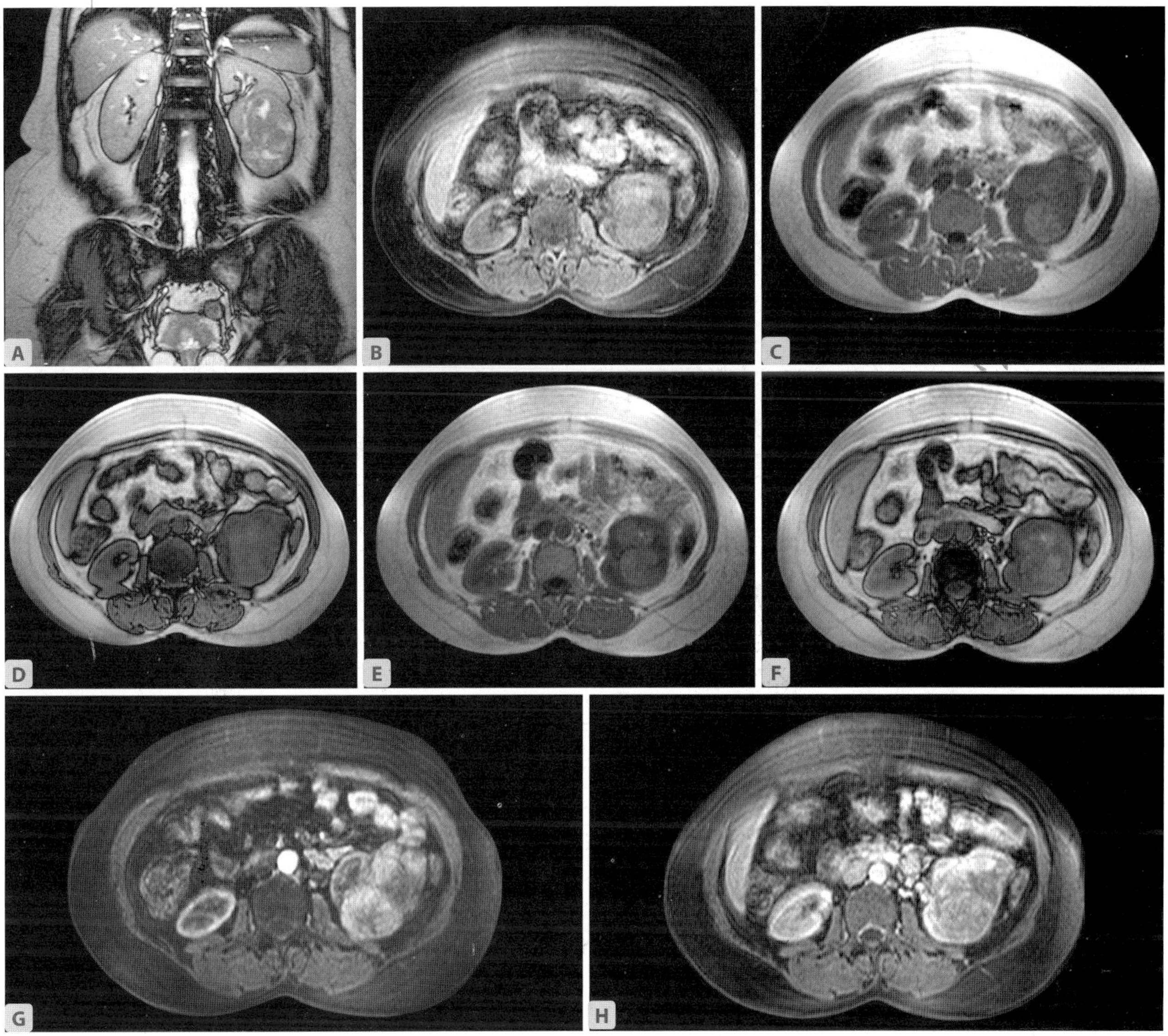

FIGS. 13A TO H: (A) MRI T2 TRUE FISP coronal; (B) TI VIBE axial; (C and E) TI in phase; and (D and F) opposed phase; (G and H) TI axial postgadolinium—a solid-enhancing mass is seen in left kidney, hypointense on T1, hyperintense on T2, with a drop in signal intensity on opposed phase images compared to in phase images. Note lack of "India ink" effect on opposed phase—clear cell renal cell carcinoma.

cell RCCs. There is a considerable overlap in ADC values between benign and malignant lesions and it cannot be used to differentiate between them. Research is going on to evaluate role of DWI as a predictor for treatment response postchemotherapy (Sorafenib in metastatic RCC).[38]

Renal Cell Carcinoma Staging

The overall accuracy of MR staging is comparable to CT. It has certain advantages over CT in the evaluation of tumor vascular extension, differentiation of perihilar vessels from nodes and the assessment of direct tumor extension into other organs. MRI is an excellent staging modality when the CT findings are equivocal.[39,40]

Currently the most commonly used staging system is the TNM system of the American Joint Committee on Cancer **(Box 2)**. The patient's overall stage is determined by the American Joint Committee on Cancer stage groupings **(Box 3)**.

The staging and histological grading affects the survival and the therapeutic approach. 5-year survival rates vary from 95% for T1 to 20% for T4.

Tumor Stage

Size of the tumor and extent of local extension determine the T stage. Tumor size is critical for staging cancer confined to the kidney **(Figs. 16A and B)**. Tumors limited to the kidney are staged T1 or T2 depending on the size. Tumors are staged T1 when they are <7 cm in size with a further subclassification into *T1a* and *T1b* at a cutoff of 4 cm. Improved survival of patients is seen with tumors measuring <4 cm compared to patients with a tumor size of 4–7 cm. Tumors confined to the kidney, measuring >7 cm are staged as *T2* **(Figs. 17A and B)**.

Stage T3, characterized by extrarenal extension of tumor, an important prognostic factor, is marked by infiltration into perinephric or renal sinus fat and venous infiltration.

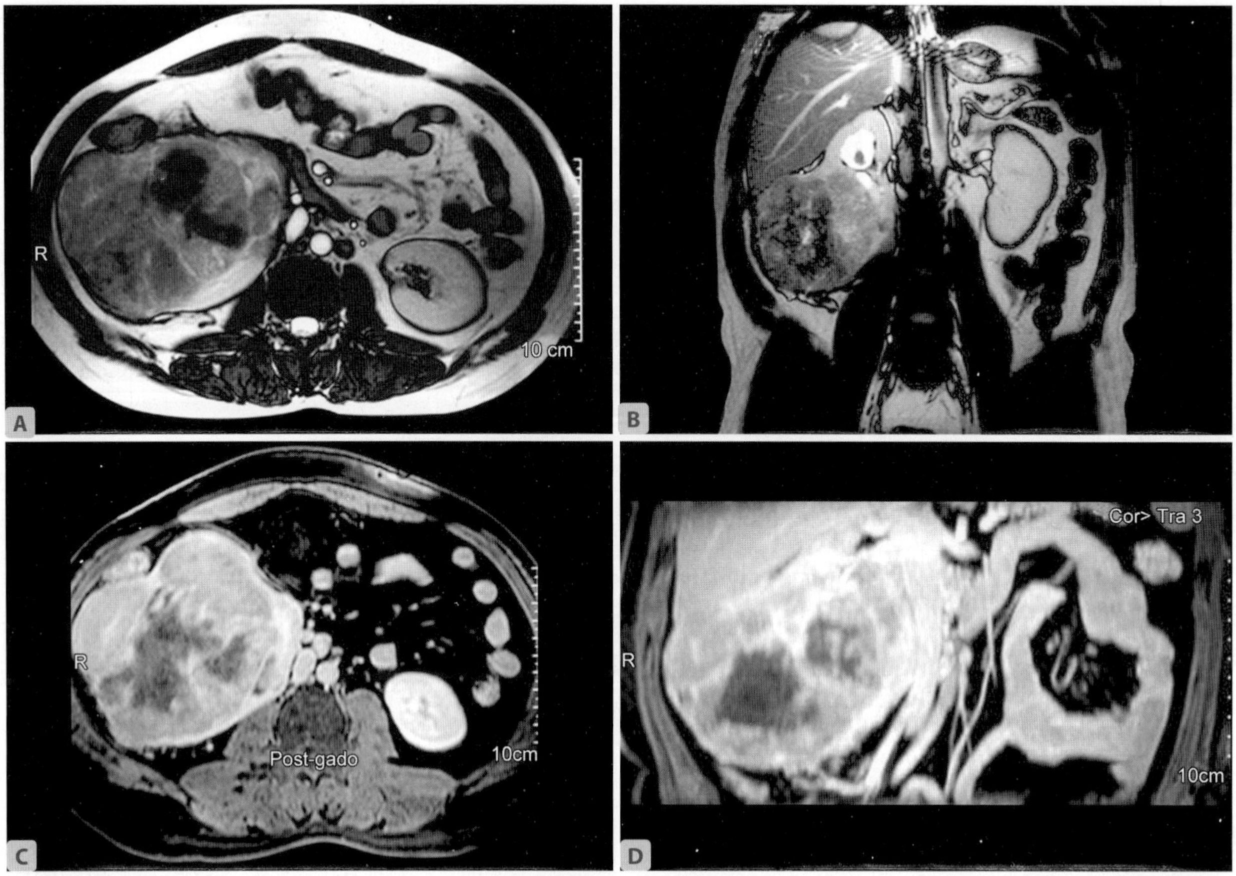

FIGS. 14A TO D: MRI TRU FISP (A) Axial; and (B) Coronal—mixed intensity right lower polar mass with areas of hemorrhage; (C) TI postgadolinium axial; and (D) Coronal maximum intensity projection (MIP) shows enhancing soft-tissue component of the mass—papillary renal cell carcinoma.

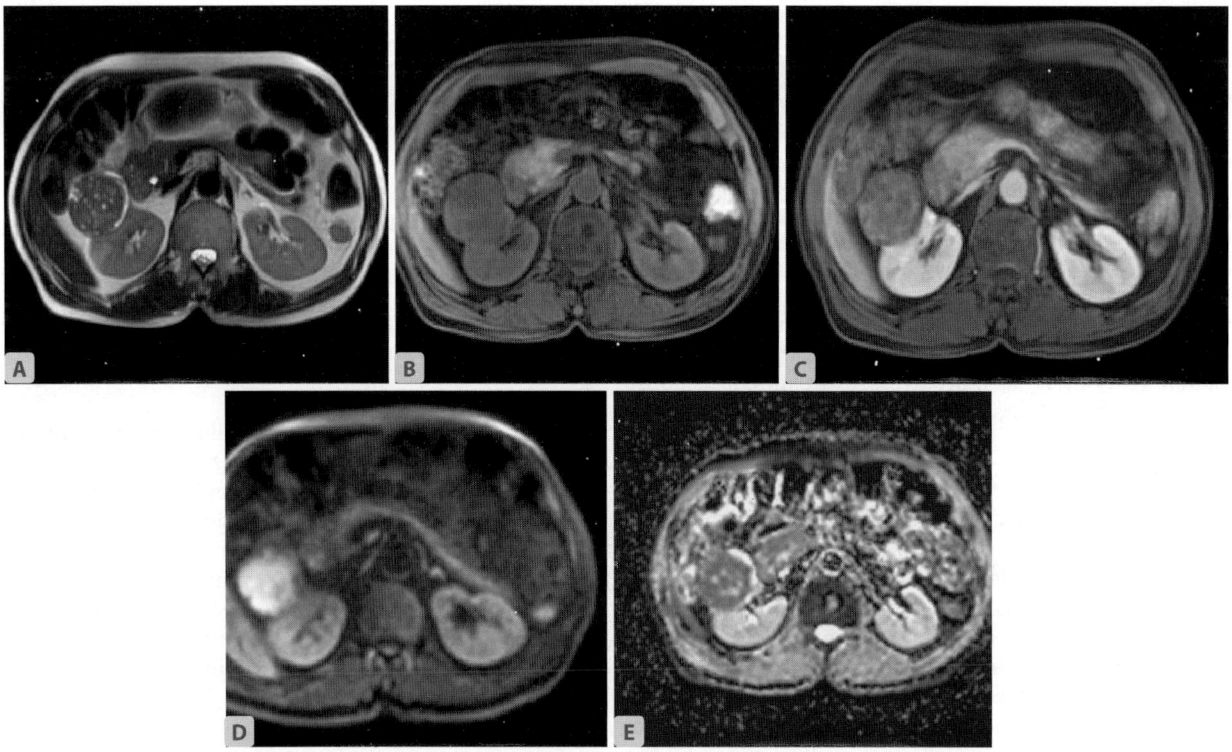

FIGS. 15A TO E: (A) T2 axial; (B) T1 axial pre; (C) Postcontrast; (D) Diffusion-weighted; and (E) Apparent diffusion coefficient (ADC) maps—well-circumscribed, peripherally located T2 hypointense, hypovascular mass with restricted diffusion—renal cell carcinoma.

Some signs like stranding of perinephric fat, fascial thickening (>3 cm), obliteration/blurring of fat, adrenal involvement, and visible collaterals are considered suggestive for extracapsular spread.

BOX 2: TNM staging for renal cell cancer.

TNM staging (7th edition)

T

- T1
  - *T1a:* Tumor confined to kidney, <4 cm
  - *T1b:* Tumor confined to kidney, >4 cm but <7 cm
- *T2:* Limited to kidney >7 cm
  - *T2a:* Tumor confined to kidney, >7 cm but not >10 cm
  - *T2b:* Tumor confined to kidney, >10 cm
- *T3:* Tumor extension into major veins or perinephric tissues, but not into ipsilateral adrenal gland or beyond Gerota's fascia
  - *T3a:* Tumor grossly extends into the renal vein or its segmental (muscle-containing) branches, or tumor invades perirenal and/or renal sinus fat but not beyond the Gerota fascia
  - *T3b:* Spread to infradiaphragmatic IVC
  - *T3c:* Spread to supradiaphragmatic IVC or invades the wall of the IVC
- *T4:* Involves ipsilateral adrenal gland or invades beyond Gerota's fascia

N

- *N0:* No nodal involvement
- *N1:* Metastatic involvement of regional lymph node(s)

M

- *M0:* No distant metastases
- *M1:* Distant metastases

BOX 3: Stage grouping for renal cancer.

- *Stage I:* T1 N0 M0
- *Stage II:* T2 N0 M0
- *Stage III:* T3 or N1 with M0
- *Stage IV:* T4 or M1

Perinephric stranding and obliteration of fat planes alone cannot be taken as a sign for extrarenal extension as it may result from edema, congestion, and mass effect. The most reliable imaging sign of RCC spread is presence of discrete perinephric mass > 1 cm in diameter **(Figs. 18 and 19)**. Presence of an intact pseudocapsule on MRI has a high accuracy in differentiating T1/T2 from T3a tumor.

Renal cancers can be staged with more than 90% accuracy; however, identification of stage T3a disease can be problematic.[21] Renal sinus fat invasion *(T3a)*, considered the most common site for extrarenal extension of RCC, is also difficult to accurately assess on CT. Presence of renal sinus fat invasion makes nephron-sparing surgery a challenge.

Tumor extension into segmental renal vein or the main renal vein is stage *T3a*. Extension of tumor thrombus into IVC must be looked for, including the cephalad extent of the thrombus **(Figs. 20A to C)**. This has management and prognostic significance with a poorer prognosis associated with supradiaphragmatic extension of IVC thrombus (T3c). Surgical planning for these patients depends on accurate preoperative staging. If tumor extends only into subdiaphragmatic cava, then a flank approach is sufficient. If it extends beyond this, then thoracoabdominal approach has to be followed.

Thrombus can be identified on the venous phase of CT. In cases, where the findings are indeterminate, MRI may be done. Noncontrast MRI has a higher sensitivity and specificity for detecting venous extension than noncontrast CT. It is more sensitive, for IVC wall invasion and to confirm tumor thrombus **(Figs. 21A and B)**. Gradient echo images may detect a low-signal defect within the high signal lumen of IVC. Bland thrombus on MRI shows a uniform signal intensity and lack of enhancement, whereas a tumor thrombus shows intermediate-to-high signal intensity, is heterogeneous and has small vessels, which enhance similar to the renal mass. Artefacts can hamper detection of venous thrombus on MRI. Contrast-enhanced MR venography is highly accurate for the detection of venous thrombus.

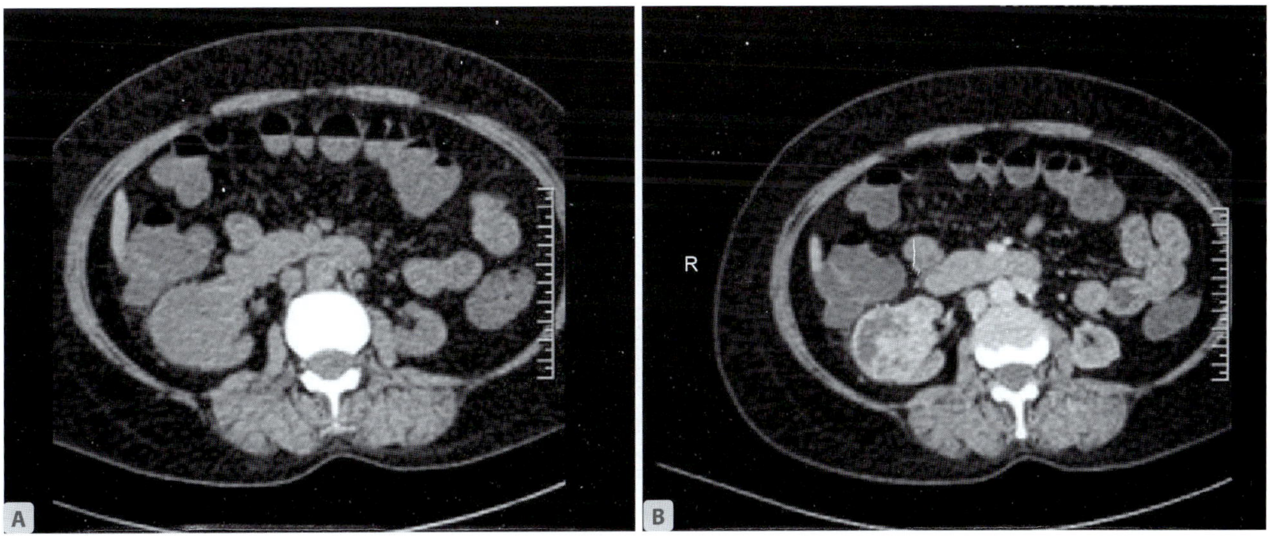

FIGS. 16A AND B: CT abdomen. (A) Precontrast; and (B) Postcontrast—an enhancing mass limited to the kidney—T1A.

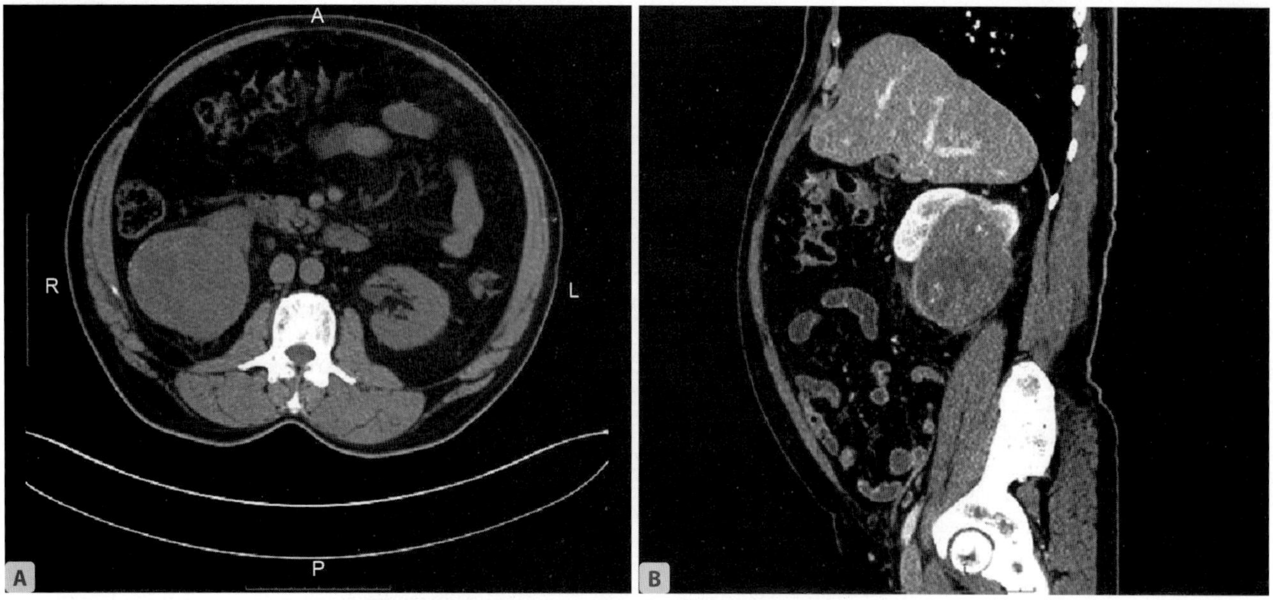

FIGS. 17A AND B: (A) Noncontrast CT axial; (B) Contrast-enhanced CT sagittal multiplanar reconstruction (MPR)—right renal solid enhancing mass measuring >7 cm, confined within Gerota's fascia. Stage T2.

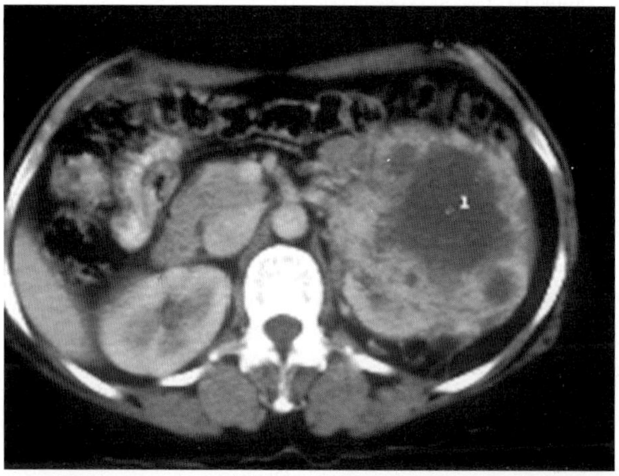

FIG. 18: CT—a large left renal mass with extension into the perinephric space.

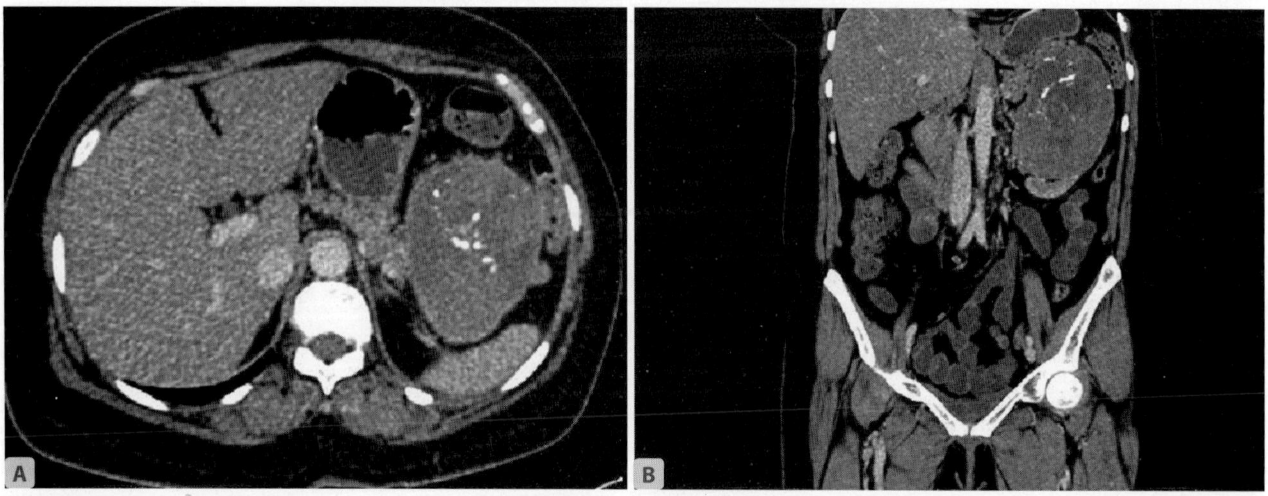

FIGS. 19A AND B: CECT abdomen: (A) Axial; (B) Coronal MPR—mass >7 cm in the left kidney with a soft tissue nodule in the perinephric region—T3.

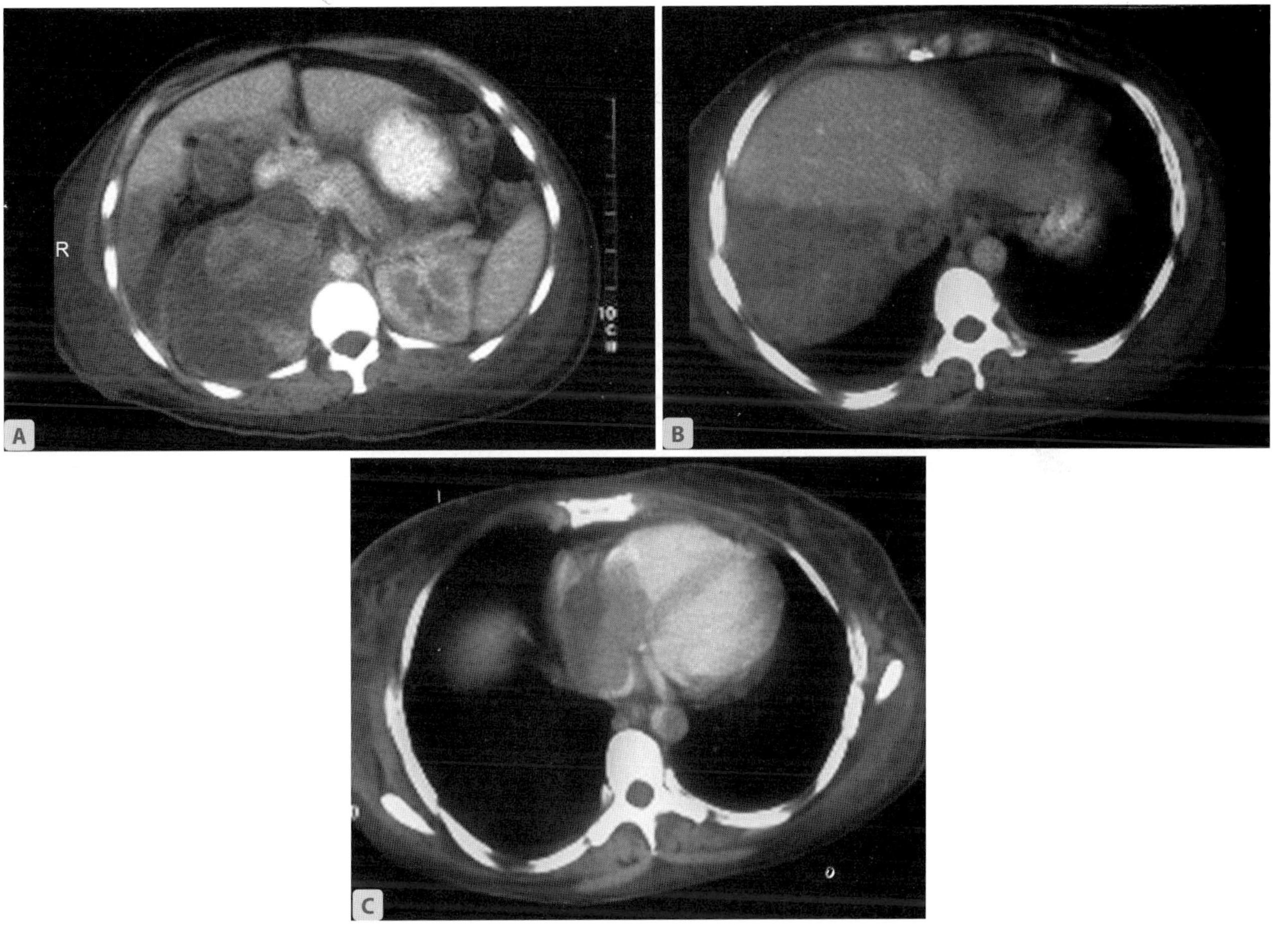

FIGS. 20A TO C: Renal cell carcinoma—CT shows (A) A complex solid cystic mass with intraluminal filling defect seen in renal vein which is enlarged; (B) A more cephlad section shows the enhancing thrombus within the inferior vena cava and a consequent to this, a perfusion deficit in liver; (C) The thrombus is seen to extend into the right atrium.

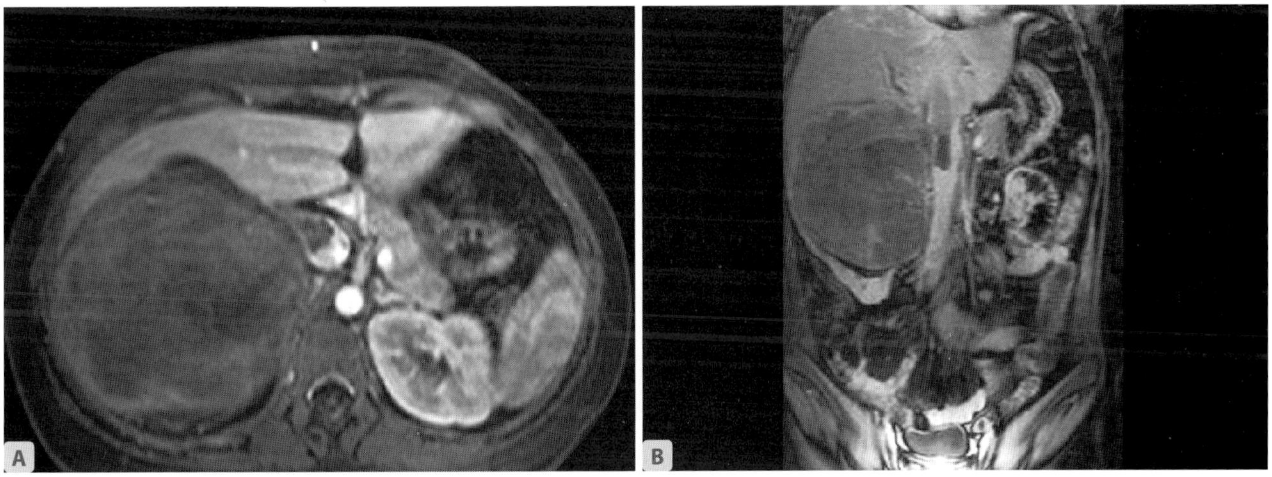

FIGS. 21A AND B: MRI abdomen postcontrast—right renal mass with venous extension into renal vein and inferior vena cava. The tumor and the thrombus are showing similar enhancement.

Contiguous invasion into adrenal, liver, diaphragm, psoas muscle, pancreas, and bowel denotes advanced *T4* stage. CT has a 100% negative predictive value in detecting contiguous spread into the adrenal gland, positive predictive value is less as it is difficult to differentiate abutment from invasion **(Figs. 22 and 23)**. It has been suggested that only when the adrenal gland is not identified, not displaced or enlarged on CT, adrenal is said to be involved.

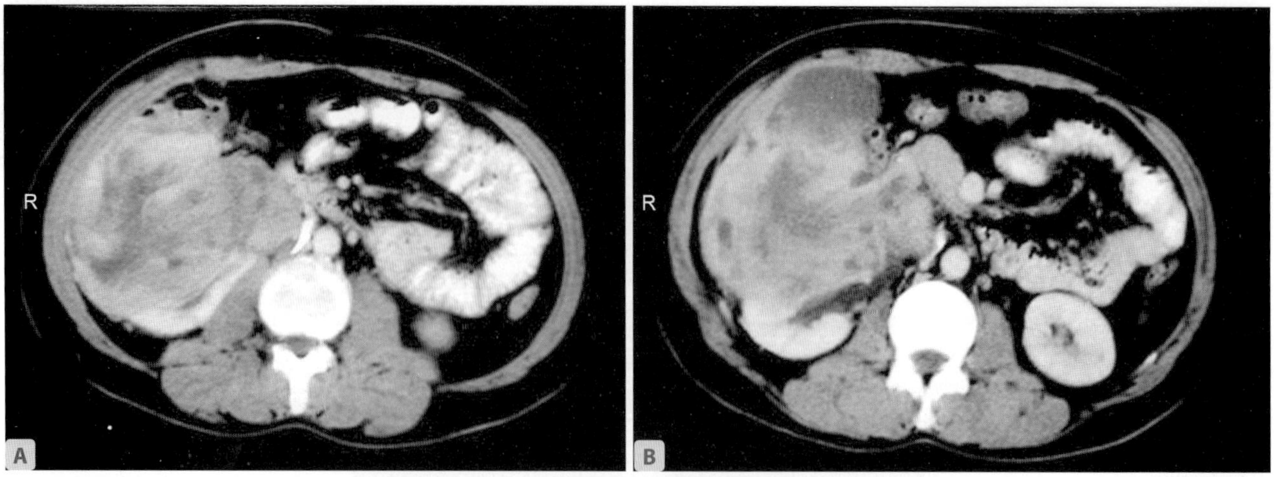

FIGS. 22A AND B: Contrast-enhanced CT abdomen. Axial—direct infiltration from right renal mass into liver, gallbladder fossa, duodeneum, and colon—stage IV.

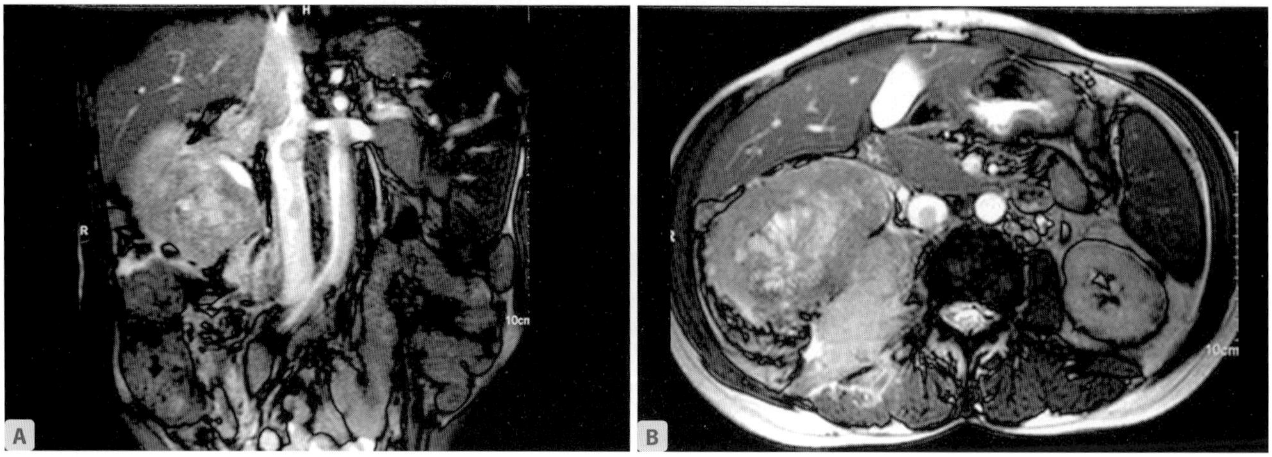

FIGS. 23A AND B: T2 TRUE FISP. (A) Coronal; (B) Axial—extension of the renal mass into right renal vein which is enlarged and into the IVC. Direct infiltration into the psoas is also noted.

Nodal Staging

Lymph node size of >1 cm and disruption of lymph node architecture are criteria for diagnosing nodal metastasis. Based on nodal size criteria alone, MRI and CT are similar in sensitivity and specificity for metastatic adenopathy. False-positive rates of 58% have been reported, however, a size criterion of 1 cm is used, owing to reactive or other benign nodal disease. These false positives are more frequent in patients with tumor involvement of the renal vein and tumor necrosis. Similar to other tumors, nodal staging for RCC by imaging is suboptimal, as up to 50% of enlarged nodes are benign and metastasis in smaller nodes is not detected.

Distant Metastases

Stage-IV renal cancer denotes distant metastases or spread to other organs, except thc adrenal. Metastatic disease involves lung, liver, bone or brain. RCC <3 cm rarely metastasize. A renal mass may appear to invade the liver or spleen, when it is actually distorting the margin without direct invasion.

Chest Radiograph

A *chest radiograph* is essential for the workup of RCC. A *chest CT* can be done if the radiograph is abnormal or the local disease is advanced. RCC is associated with hypervascular liver metastasis; particularly from clear cell RCC. Portal venous phase imaging of *abdominal CT* detects 90% of metastases. Bone metastases are usually lytic. Bone scan is performed only in patients with bone pain or raised alkaline phosphatase. *Bone scan* may be negative as the lytic metastasis produces little osteoblastic reaction. MRI may be more sensitive to CT in detection of unsuspected bony metastasis, because of bone marrow imaging capability.

Positron Emission Tomography-computed Tomography in Staging of RCC

There is no established role of PET CT in the initial staging of renal cancer. Due to high background activity of the tracer in kidney, it is difficult to detect primary renal tumor by PET scan alone. PET combined with CT has a sensitivity of 90%. 18F-fluoro-2-deoxy-2-D-glucose (FDG) uptake within a renal mass confirms that solid elements are present.

False-positive diagnosis is a problem as benign solid renal masses such as oncocytoma can be FDG avid. PET may be useful in detecting activity in metastatic lesions detected by CT and MRI bone scan.[41] The recommendations for the expert group for staging of renal malignancy is given in **Box 4**.

Treatment of Renal Cell Carcinoma

Renal cell carcinoma is managed surgically. The operative management can be radical nephrectomy or nephron-sparing surgery (partial nephrectomy). The preferred treatment of renal masses measuring 4 cm or less in maximal diameter is now *partial nephrectomy*, and *thermal ablation* in patients who are poor surgical candidates.[42] Imaging assists in planning these treatments with the least possible complications.

There is an alternative management strategy called *"active surveillance"*. This is used in biopsy proven small renal cancers (≤4 cm in size) in elderly patients who are more likely to die with, rather than of their cancer and who have a favorable histological prognosis (low-grade papillary and chromophobe) as assessed by percutaneous biopsy. Active surveillance consists of periodic imaging with no intervention till the size increases or there is rapid growth (>5 mm in 12 months).[43,44]

Renal Mass Scoring

The decision to perform partial nephrectomy was often subjective and required a standardized method to score renal mass complexity. The scoring systems, now most commonly used are nephrometry score and the Padua score.

R.E.N.A.L nephrometry score[45] **(Table 6)** was developed to categorize renal masses into low, intermediate, and high complexity, based on cross-sectional imaging findings. The score helps in decision making, patient counseling, surgical planning, and patient follow-up, as well as for academic reporting. R.E.N.A.L is an acronym for the five components of this system

1. Renal size
2. Exophyticity
3. Nearness to the collecting system or renal sinus
4. Anterior or posterior location
5. Location with respect to the renal poles. This is determined by polar lines drawn on coronal images, at the level where the medial lip of the kidney is interrupted by renal sinus fat **(Figs. 24A to C)**.

Each component, except location is graded on a scale of 1–3. All scores are summed to give a final nephrometry score.

- Score of 4–6: Low complexity
- Score of 7–9: Moderate complexity
- Score of 10–12: High complexity.

A low score of 4–6 is associated with fewer complications such as postoperative bleed or urinary fistula after partial nephrectomy. In addition to greater postsurgical complications, a higher nephrometry score of 12–14 has been shown to correlate with pathological stage and grade.

Another system to assess renal masses prior to surgery is the *PADUA classification*,[46] which is also an acronym for Preoperative Aspects and Dimensions Used for Anatomical classification. In this system, nearness to the collecting system and to renal sinus is assessed separately. The polar location of the mass is determined by drawing a renal sinus line at the first (upper pole) and the last (lower pole) axial level where pericollecting system fat is seen entirely within the kidney.

BOX 4: Recommendations for staging renal tumor.

- Contrast-enhanced multiphasic abdomen CT is the modality of choice for staging primary renal tumor. MRI is a suitable substitute when patient cannot undergo CECT abdomen
- If status of renal vein and IVC cannot be determined on CT, then contrast-enhanced multiphasic 3D MR venography can be done
- Computed tomography chest to be done in large or locally advanced tumor to look for pulmonary metastasis. Chest X-ray is sufficient for patients with small tumors
- Brain MRI and bone scan should be done in patients with suspicion of metastatic disease, based on symptoms, laboratory findings or metastasis elsewhere

Imaging Post-treatment

The imaging protocol for follow up of treated RCCs is given in **Box 5**.

Post-total/Partial Nephrectomy

In the imaging follow-up of patients after surgical excision of RCC, CT abdomen with IV contrast, CT abdomen without and

TABLE 6: R.E.N.A.L. nephrometry score.

	1 point	2 point	3 point
Radius (maximal diameter in cm)	<4	4–7	>7
Exophytic/endophytic properties	≥50%	<50%	Entirely endophytic
Nearness of the tumor to the collecting system or sinus (mm)	≥7	>4 but <7	≤4
Anterior or posterior	No points given. Mass assigned a descriptor of a, p or x		
Location relative to polar lines*	Entirely above the upper line or below the lower line	Lesion crosses polar line	>50% of mass is across polar line (a) or mass crosses the axial renal midline (b) or the mass is entirely between polar lines (c)

*Suffix "h" if mass touches the main renal artery/vein.

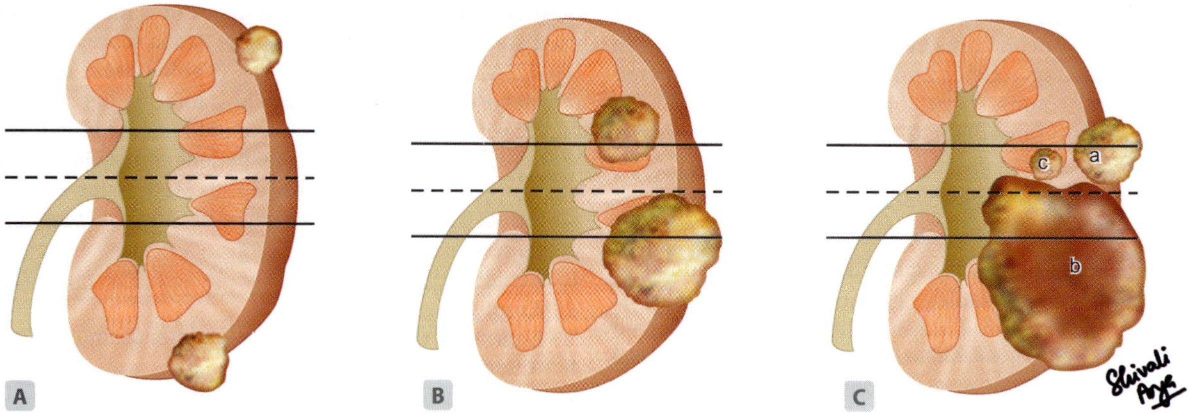

FIGS. 24A TO C: Polar lines (solid lines) and axial renal midline (dashed lines) are depicted on each coronal view of the kidney. Polar lines are determined in the coronal plane and run through the axial plane. They pass through the point where the medial renal parenchyma touches the renal sinus. Assigning location (L) score. In image (A), L = 1 because masses are above or below polar lines. In image (B), L = 2 because masses cross polar lines. In image (C), L = 3 because mass "a" crosses polar line > 50%; "b" is located between polar lines; and "c" crosses axial midline.

BOX 5: Imaging protocol for follow-up of treated RCC.

- *For low-risk/T1 tumors*:
  - Chest imaging: Every 12 to 24 months for 3–5 years
  - Abdominal imaging: Baseline between 3 months and 12 months, especially after partial nephrectomy, then yearly for 3–5 years
- *For intermediate-risk/T2 primary tumors*:
  - Chest and abdominal imaging-baseline study at 3 months, then at 6 and 12 months, followed by every 6–24 months for 5 years
- *For high-risk/T3 tumors*:
  - Chest and abdominal imaging: Baseline study at 3 months, then at 6 and 12 months, followed by every 6–12 months for 5 years

with IV contrast are recommended as equivalent alternatives for imaging. The use of MRI of abdomen and pelvis with and without IV contrast as alternative in this scenario may be appropriate, but is controversial. There is a renal parenchymal defect along with some soft tissue changes and surgical staples postpartial nephrectomy. Hemostatic packing material may look like fluid collection or residual masses gradual decrease in size will be noted, if it is normal postoperative appearance. Recurrent tumor is identified as an enhancing soft tissue nodule/mass[47] **(Fig. 25)**.

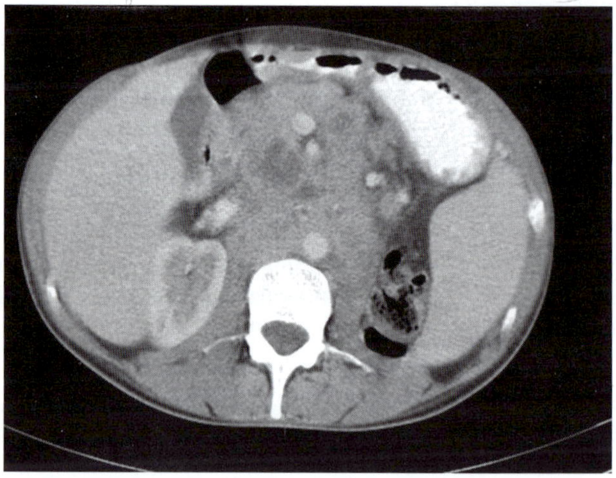

FIG. 25: CT abdomen in a postoperative case of renal cell carcinoma, presenting 1 year later with metastatic retroperitoneal lymphadenopathy.

Post-thermal Ablation

In the imaging follow-up of patients after localized RCC ablation, CT abdomen with IV contrast/CT abdomen without and with IV contrast/MRI of abdomen, and pelvis without and with IV contrast are recommended as equivalent alternatives (i.e. only one of the above procedures to be ordered).

The ablation bed may initially be significantly larger in size than the initial mass. It may take 1-2 years to decrease in size. Increased perinephric stranding with invagination of perinephric fat into the defect may be seen normally. The appearance may mimic an angiomyolipoma. A thin-enhancing rim may be seen 2-6 weeks following ablation. An enlarging ablation bed should be considered as a sign of recurrent disease.[48] Persistent areas of enhancement, especially nodular or crescentic in appearance, seen at the interface with normal renal parenchyma signifies residual/recurrent tumor. Certain procedural complications, though rare, may be seen on follow-up imaging such as hematomas, pseudoaneurysms and chyluria.

Postchemotherapy

Patients with metastasis are treated with chemotherapeutic agents like multikinase inhibitors. These produce tumor necrosis as a marker of response without decrease in size. These patients have to be evaluated for changes in enhancement along with change in size on follow-up imaging.

Active Surveillance

Active surveillance is reserved for patients with these small renal masses who are poor surgical candidates due to comorbidities or are not willing for surgery. The American Urological Association (AUA) and National Comprehensive Cancer Network (NCCN) recommend CT/MR of the abdomen CT/MR within 6 months of start of surveillance followed by imaging annually till patient is on watch.[49] In the imaging follow-up of patients who are on active surveillance of localized RCC, CT abdomen with IV contrast/CT abdomen without and with IV contrast/MRI of abdomen and pelvis without and with IV contrast/ultrasound abdomen with IV contrast are recommended as equivalent alternatives. Size has to be carefully monitored with an average growth of 0.3 cm/year. A higher growth rate is associated with unfavorable outcome.

Screening for Kidney Cancer

There are no guidelines for RCC screening in general population due to lack of a large randomized controlled trial for renal cancer screening.[50] Patients with genetic predisposition to RCC require surveillance, starting at an early age based on the syndrome. Certain syndromes like hereditary leiomyomatosis and RCC (HLRCC) require surveillance to begin at an early age, as tumors are aggressive with metastatic potential. Patients with Birt-Hogg-Dubé syndrome and von Hippel-Lindau syndrome are recommended to undergo annual or biannual surveillance, starting at 20 years of age with tumors more than 3 cm being treated. In hereditary papillary RCC, tumors develop in sixth decades onward and are slow growing, hence there is no screening protocol for these patients.

Oncocytoma

Renal oncocytoma is the most common benign, solid, nonfat-containing renal mass. It is a benign renal epithelial tumor, arising from intercalated cells of proximal tubule with many characteristics of RCCs. Oncocytomas are histologically composed of large cells (oncocytes) with mitochondria rich cytoplasm. The appearance of a typical oncocytoma cannot be reliably differentiated from RCC.[51]

Most oncocytomas are asymptomatic (80%), but few may present with hematuria, pain, or mass. The peak age of incidence is in the seventh decade with a male preponderance. The incidence of oncocytomas is higher in incidentally discovered renal masses, as compared with patients who have urinary symptoms. They may be quite large at time of presentation. Oncocytoma appears as a well demarcated, unencapsulated, fairly homogeneous renal cortical tumors.

In 10% of oncocytomas, there can be a coexistent RCC, as an incidental microscopic finding or as a hybrid tumor. Oncocytomas are multifocal in 2.5–16% and bilateral in 4–12% of cases. Multifocality can be sporadic or syndromic in Birt-Hogg-Dubé syndrome and renal oncocytosis (renal parenchyma is replaced by multiple oncocytomas, hybrid tumors, and chromophobe RCCs).[52,53]

On *ultrasound*, renal oncocytomas appear as solitary hypoechoic or isoechoic masses originating from the renal cortex with a well-defined margin. On *color Doppler imaging* blood flow signals are seen in the periphery and strip-like flow signals within the mass. Contrast-enhanced sonography, shows early enhancement, hyperenhancement, and fast washout compared to the adjacent renal cortex. Irregular nonenhanced areas may be seen within the central area corresponding to area of central fibrous scar, which may be echogenic.

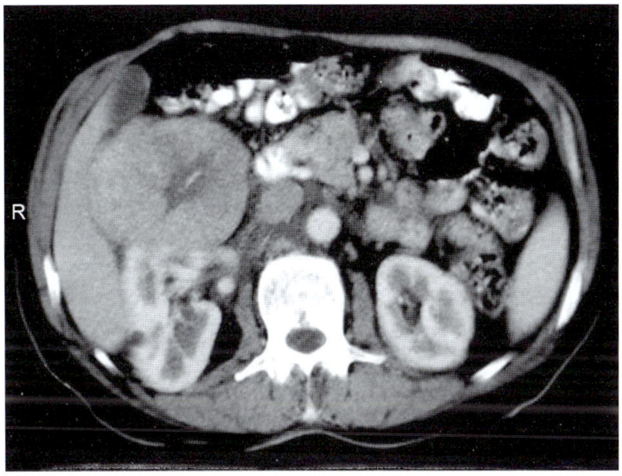

FIG. 26: CT—well-defined, homogeneously enhancing mass right renal with a central scar—oncocytoma.

On *CT*, they are solid, well-marginated tumors, slightly hypodense to renal parenchyma on unenhanced images. Some may exhibit a central low attenuation scar with a branched appearance (**Fig. 26**). However, central necrosis with RCC may mimic this. Invasion into perinephric fat occurs is 11%. There is usually no adenopathy or vascular invasion. Various patterns of enhancement have been described for oncocytomas. Segmental enhancement inversion is considered a hallmark of small (<4 cm) oncocytomas. There are two distinct zones of enhancement, which show different pattern on CM and excretory phase (EP). The zone that is hyperenhancing on CM phase becomes hypoenhancing on EP and vice versa.[54-56] Other authors found that an early heterogeneous enhancement becoming homogeneous in delayed phase is seen in small oncocytomas. The presence of a central scar, absence of calcification or necrosis and hemorrhage suggests the diagnosis, though there is no specific CT finding to differentiate oncocytoma from RCC. Surgery is usually performed for these. The MRI appearance is of a hypo- to isointense (22%) mass on T1W images with high signal on T2WI, enhancing homogeneously after IV gadolinium. It may exhibit spoke-wheel pattern of enhancement. The central scar is T1 hypointense and T2 hyperintense with delayed enhancement. A spoke-wheel pattern of feeding arteries associated with a homogeneous nephrogram is a characteristic finding on catheter angiography.

METANEPHRIC TUMORS

Renal Adenomas

Papillary adenomas are the most common renal epithelial neoplasm. According to some authors, renal adenoma is an earlier stage of evolution of renal cell carcinoma. By definition, papillary adenomas measure 5 mm or less. According to an autopsy series, approximately 40% of patients above the age of 70 harbor a renal adenoma. Papillary adenomas are also found in patients with acquired renal cystic disease and in those undergoing long-term hemodialysis. They usually occur as cortical subcapsular tumors less than 1 cm and are indistinguishable from RCCs. *Metanephric adenoma* is a benign neoplasm with a peak age in 5–6th decade. Polycythemia, a characteristic finding, is seen in 10% and disappears after surgery. Metanephric adenoma typically occurs as a well-defined, unencapsulated, solitary solid mass. Metanephric adenomas display hypovascularity and delayed, minimal enhancement.

MIXED EPITHELIAL AND STROMAL TUMORS

Cystic nephroma, mixed epithelial and stromal tumors belong to this subgroup of tumors.[57] They are seen almost exclusively in perimenopausal women, most patients receiving estrogen therapy. They usually present incidentally and are believed to be a hormonally dependent tumor. Mixed epithelial and stromal tumors (MESTs) are characterized by variegated imaging patterns including complex cysts and mixed solid cystic masses that show delayed and heterogeneous enhancement. On MR imaging, the degree of delayed enhancement and T2 hypointense signal is dependent on the amount of stromal component.

MESENCHYMAL TUMORS

Mesenchymal tumors constitute a wide spectrum of tumors with variable histology and imaging findings. Benign mesenchymal tumors include angiomyolipoma (AML), leiomyoma, lymphangioma, hemangioma, lipoma, etc. Malignant mesenchymal tumors include leiomyosarcoma, rhabdomyosarcoma, angiosarcoma, and osteosarcoma. Some mesenchymal tumors like AML, lipoma, and hemangioma may be diagnosed on imaging. Percutaneous biopsy is usually required for the diagnosis of mesenchymal tumors and to rule out RCC.

Mesenchymal renal tumors can be classified, based on the predominant tissue type **(Box 6)** or on the pattern of distribution[58] **(Box 7)**.

Angiomyolipoma

Angiomyolipoma is the most common solid benign tumor. These lesions are mesenchymal neoplasms (previously considered as hamartomas), representing excess growth of mature fat, smooth muscle and thick-walled blood vessels, the amount of each component being variable.

Angiomyolipomas are now considered to be a heterogeneous group of tumors with different imaging features, histology, and are grouped under a family of tumors characterized by the proliferation of perivascular epithelioid cells (PEComas).[59] Usually benign, a rare potentially malignant variant called epithelioid angiomyolipoma is listed separately in the WHO classification of renal tumors.

They are usually seen in women between 40 and 60 years of age. The majority being sporadic, 20% are associated with tuberous sclerosis (TS). Angiomyolipomas may rarely be associated with NF-I, Von Hippel–Lindau disease or ADPKD. TS-associated AMLs are seen in asymptomatic, young patients without sex predilection. AMLs associated with TS are often multiple, bilateral, and larger at the time of presentation. These are also likely to grow and be symptomatic. As the tumor grows, there is vessel dilatation and pseudoaneurysm formation. Tumors greater than 4 cm have an increased risk of hemorrhage (Wunderlich syndrome), potentially life-threatening and need to be prophylactically managed.

Angiomyolipoma may originate from the cortex or the medulla. The tumor is usually well defined and appears as large, heterogeneous mass with varying amount of macroscopic fat, intralesional aneurysms, and hypervascular soft tissue. As angiomyolipomas are composed of

BOX 6: Mesenchymal tumors based on tissue type.

- *Soft tissue mass:*
  - Fat-poor AML
  - Leiomyoma
  - Hemangioma
  - Schwannoma
  - Juxtaglomerular cell tumor
  - Medullary fibroma
  - Solitary fibrous renal tumor
  - Leiomyosarcoma
  - Synovial sarcoma
  - Osteosarcoma
- *Fat-containing:*
  - Classic angiomyolipoma
  - Lipoma
- *Cystic mass:*
  - Lymphangioma
- *Calcified mass:*
  - Hemangioma
  - Osteosarcoma

BOX 7: Distribution of mesenchymal tumors.

- *Capsular distribution:*
  - Leiomyoma
  - Lymphangioma
  - Solitary fibrous tumor
  - Leiomyosarcoma
  - Angiosarcoma
- *Cortical distribution:*
  - Angiomyolipoma
  - Schwannoma
  - Synovial sarcoma
- *Medullary distribution:*
  - Angiomyolipoma
  - Hemangioma
- *Renal sinus distribution:*
  - Leiomyoma
  - Hemangioma
  - Lymphangioma

thick-walled inelastic blood vessels, the risk of intratumoral and perinephric hemorrhage is higher in lesions > 4 cm diameter.

Classification of AML

There are two classifications of AML. One is based on clinical and imaging features, histological grade, and genetic features, while the second is based purely on CT and MRI features. Jinzaki et al.[60] classified AML on the basis of clinical and imaging features, histological grade, and genetic features.

Triphasic AML is a benign mesenchymal tumor consisting of three components in varying proportion—dysmorphic blood vessels, smooth muscle, and mature fat.

This is further subdivided radiologically into classic and fat-poor varieties.

Classic Angiomyolipomas

They are characterized by abundant fat and are easily diagnosed by imaging. Classical AML appears as a hyperechoic circumscribed mass (more echogenic than central fat) on ultrasound **(Figs. 27 and 28)**. 32% of renal carcinomas are also highly reflective, although there are other pointers toward RCC such as hyporeflective rim or focal small spotty areas (intratumoural cysts) of reduced central reflectivity. Another feature that helps in distinguishing an AML from a small RCC, is posterior shadowing, seen in approximately 30% of AML, but is not seen in small hyperreflective renal carcinomas.

Computed tomography is the most accurate imaging technique for detection and characterization of classic angiomyolipomas. The lesions show low attenuation, typically less than 10 HU and presence of gross fat being a typical finding[61] **(Figs. 29 to 31)**. Thin slices are necessary to demonstrate fat in small AMLs because of volume averaging. Higher specificity may be obtained with threshold measurements of –15 to –30 HU. The fat may be interposed with solid components. A subset of lesions will not meet fat attenuation criteria due to volume

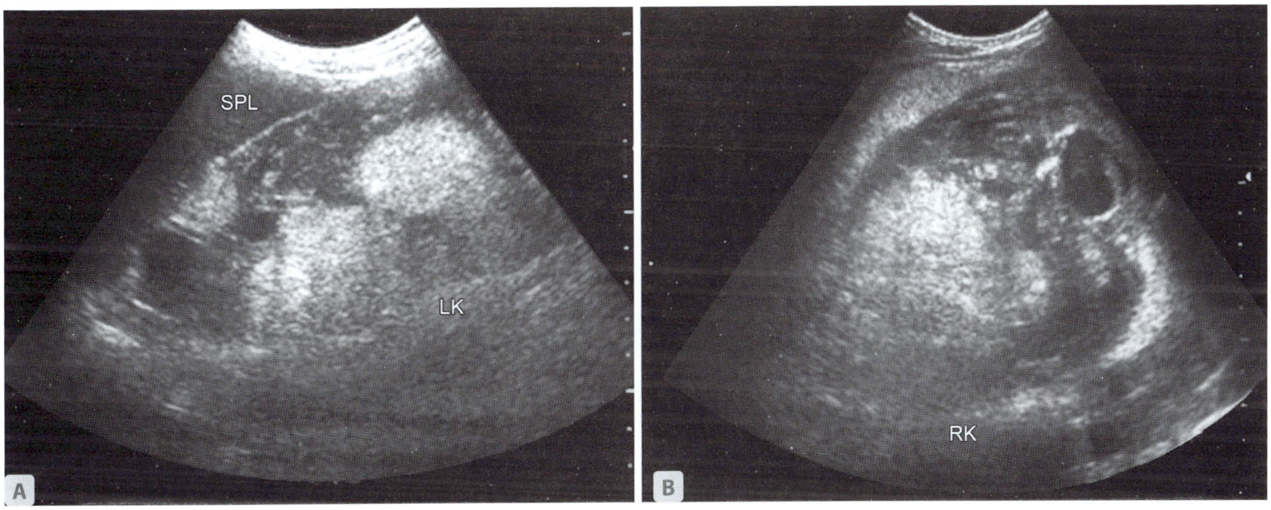

FIGS. 27A AND B: Ultrasound of the upper abdomen depicts multiple well-defined homogeneously hyperechoic lesions with no perilesional halo in both kidneys, suggestive of angiomyolipomas (AML).

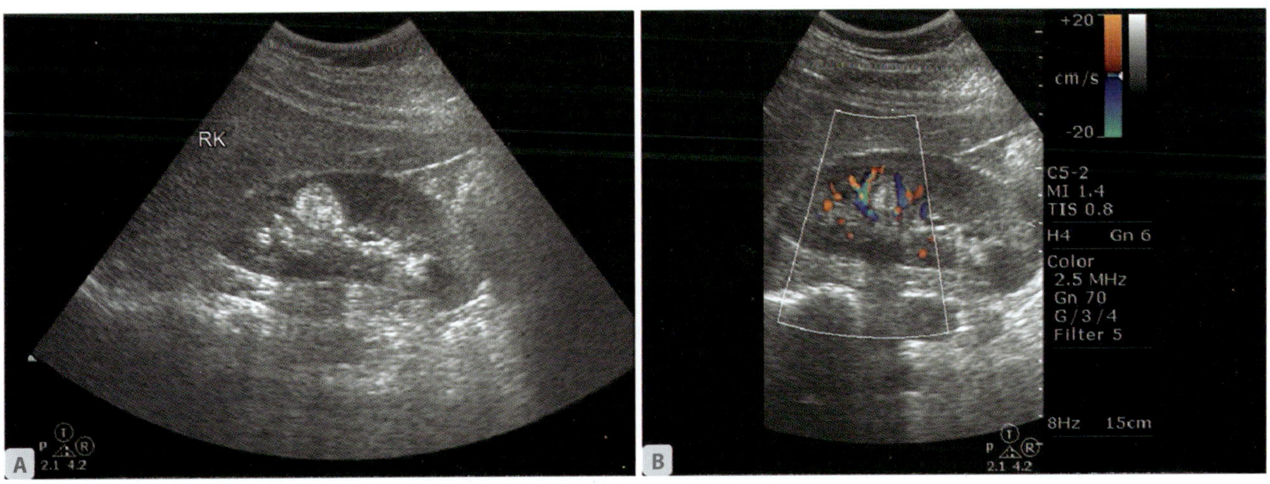

FIGS. 28A AND B: Ultrasound of the upper abdomen shows. (A) Well-defined rounded hyperechoic lesion; (B) In the right kidney with peripheral vascularity on color Doppler.

averaging or hemorrhage, others are fat-poor, and rarely, a well-differentiated RCC can mimic this appearance.

Computed tomography pixel mapping, over a region of interest within the tumor may be useful to detect small quantities of fat. With pixel mapping, three to six contiguous pixels with negative Hounsfield units averaging below -20 HU indicates intratumoral fat.[62] AMLs are usually well-marginated, but do not have a true capsule, the lesion is usually at the margin of the kidney and may expand beyond as a small hypodense wedge-shaped defect in the renal parenchyma. This wedge-shaped defect is diagnostic of angiomyolipoma. These lesions are vascular, large vessels may be identified. Intratumoral aneurysms may be present and AMLs exhibit moderate enhancement after IV contrast. Homogeneous and prolonged enhancement is a valuable predictor for differentiating AML with minimal fat from RCC.

Angiomyolipomas may have to be differentiated from a perirenal/capsular liposarcoma. Pathological differentiation between a well-differentiated liposarcoma from an angiomyolipoma may be difficult, unless radiological appearance is considered. Liposarcomas are rare, seen in older patients, are large at time of diagnosis, and are centered at perinephric space or capsule rather than intraparenchymal like AML. A renal origin of the mass seen as beak sign, presence of enlarged vessels, aneurysms, and perinephric hematoma favor a diagnosis of AML. Liposarcomas are hypovascular, without enlarged vessels and aneurysms. The renal parenchyma defect in AML as stated earlier is not seen in well-differentiated liposarcomas, which will displace, compress, and distorts the kidney, but will not invade renal parenchyma **(Figs. 32 and 33)**. Rarely RCC also contains fat, either engulfing the sinus or perinephric fat or due to metaplasia. In the latter case, presence of calcification, which is not seen in AML favors the diagnosis of RCC.[63,64]

On *MRI,* fat component of an angiomyolipoma can be detected by *Frequency-selective (FS) fat suppression technique* and *chemical shift imaging.*

Classical AMLs have a characteristic high T1 signal and fat-saturated images exhibit a drop in signal. Chemical shift

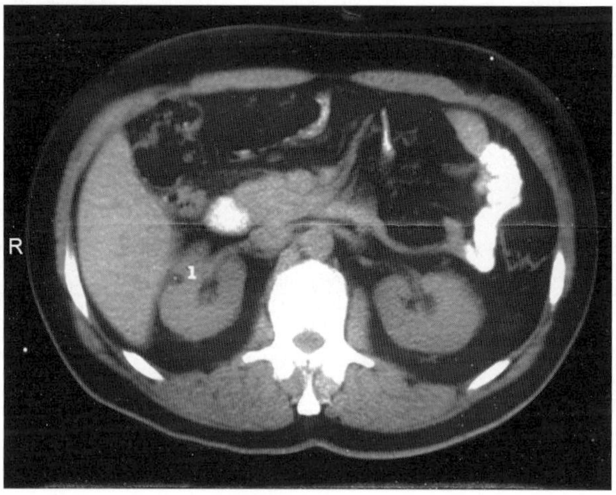

FIG. 29: CT shows a small pinhead lesion in right kidney with fat attenuation S/o angiomyolipomas (AML).

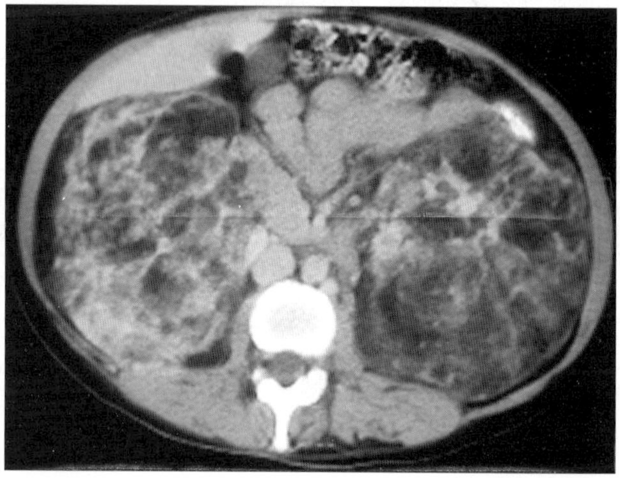

FIG. 31: CT showing bilateral large fat attenuation lesions with enhancing soft tissues —angiomyolipoma.

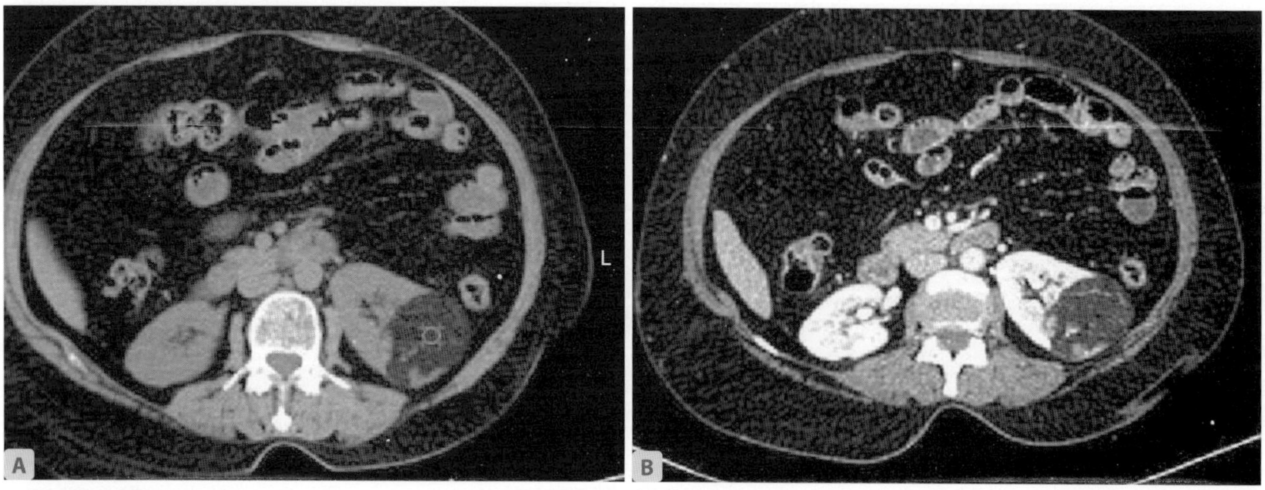

FIGS. 30A AND B: (A) Noncontrast CT; (B) Contrast-enhanced CT—mass with macroscopic fat and enhancing vessels in the left kidney—angiomyolipoma.

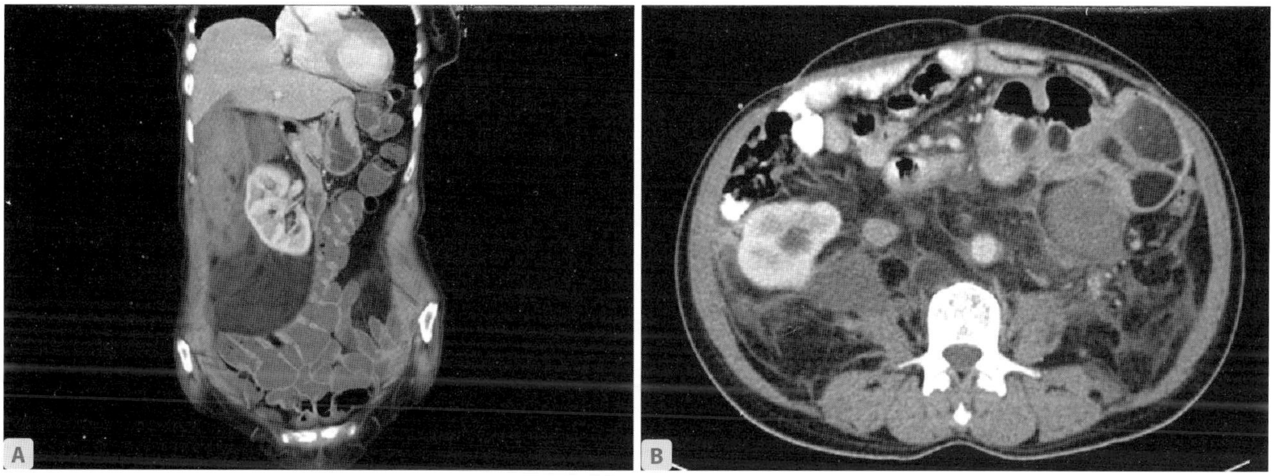

FIGS. 32A AND B: Contrast-enhanced CT abdomen. (A) Coronal MPR; (B) Axial shows a large fat-containing mass surrounding and displacing the right kidney and extending into left renal fossa—perirenal liposarcoma.

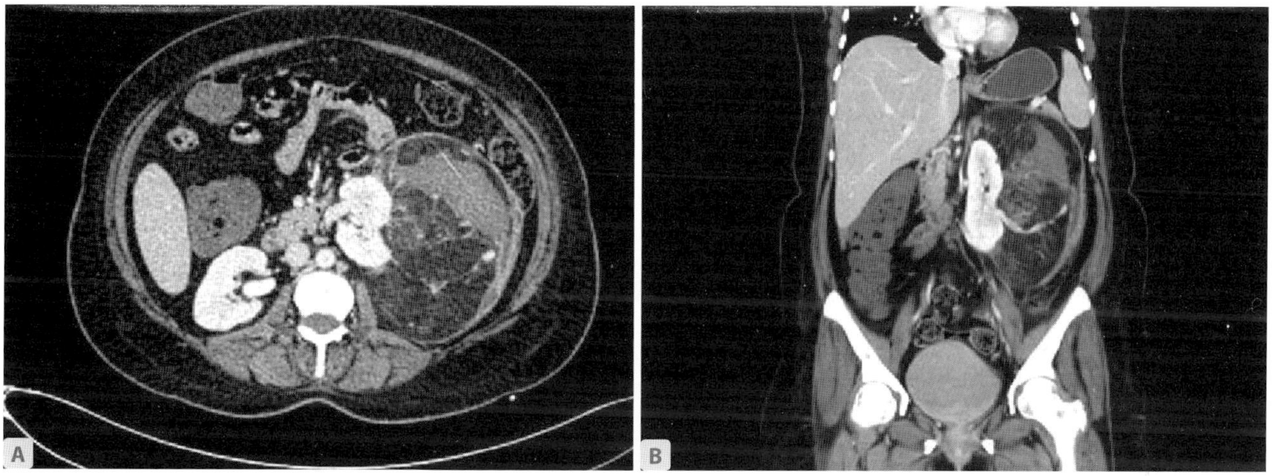

FIGS. 33A AND B: Contrast-enhanced CT abdomen. (A) Axial; (B) Coronal reformat—shows a large fat-containing mass in relation to the left kidney with a wedge-shaped defect and a vessel seen within the mass—renal angiomyolipoma.

imaging helps to detect small quantities of bulk fat. In classic AML, a characteristic *India ink artefact* is seen at the interface between the mass and the normal renal parenchyma on opposed phase T1 images, whereas the central part of the lesion does not demonstrate changes in signal intensity compared with in-phase images **(Figs. 34A to F)**. This is useful in very small lesions, where direct comparison with T1 images, with and without fat suppression may be difficult. The appearance of AML on T2-weighted images is variable and depends on bulk fat present in the lesion. An AML composed of predominantly fat would demonstrate homogeneous high signal at T2 images.

Angiography may demonstrate multiple aneurysms and onion layer appearances.

Fat-poor Angiomyolipoma (Minimal-fat AML and Lipid-poor AML)

These lesions, by definition, do not reveal fat on unenhanced CT, even on thin sections. Pathologically they are defined as containing no more than 25% fat cells per high-power field. Fat-poor AML are further divided into three subtypes based on the amount of fat cells and the distribution of the same in the mass:

1. Hyperattenuating
2. Isoattenuating
3. Epithelial cysts.

Hyperattenuating Angiomyolipoma

Usually small, they contain only 3-10% fat cells.[65] The predominant component is smooth muscle making them appear hyperdense to renal parenchyma on CT and isoechoic on ultrasound. Homogeneous enhancement is seen. On MRI, they are T1 hypointense and show no bulk fat. When a voxel contains cells with no fat or only intracytoplasmic fat, frequency-selective fat suppression will not detect fat.

Isoattenuating Angiomyolipoma

These have CT attenuation between –10 and 45 HU, with diffuse scattered fat cells and appear isodense on noncontrast CT and mildly hyperechoic on ultrasound. They are typically

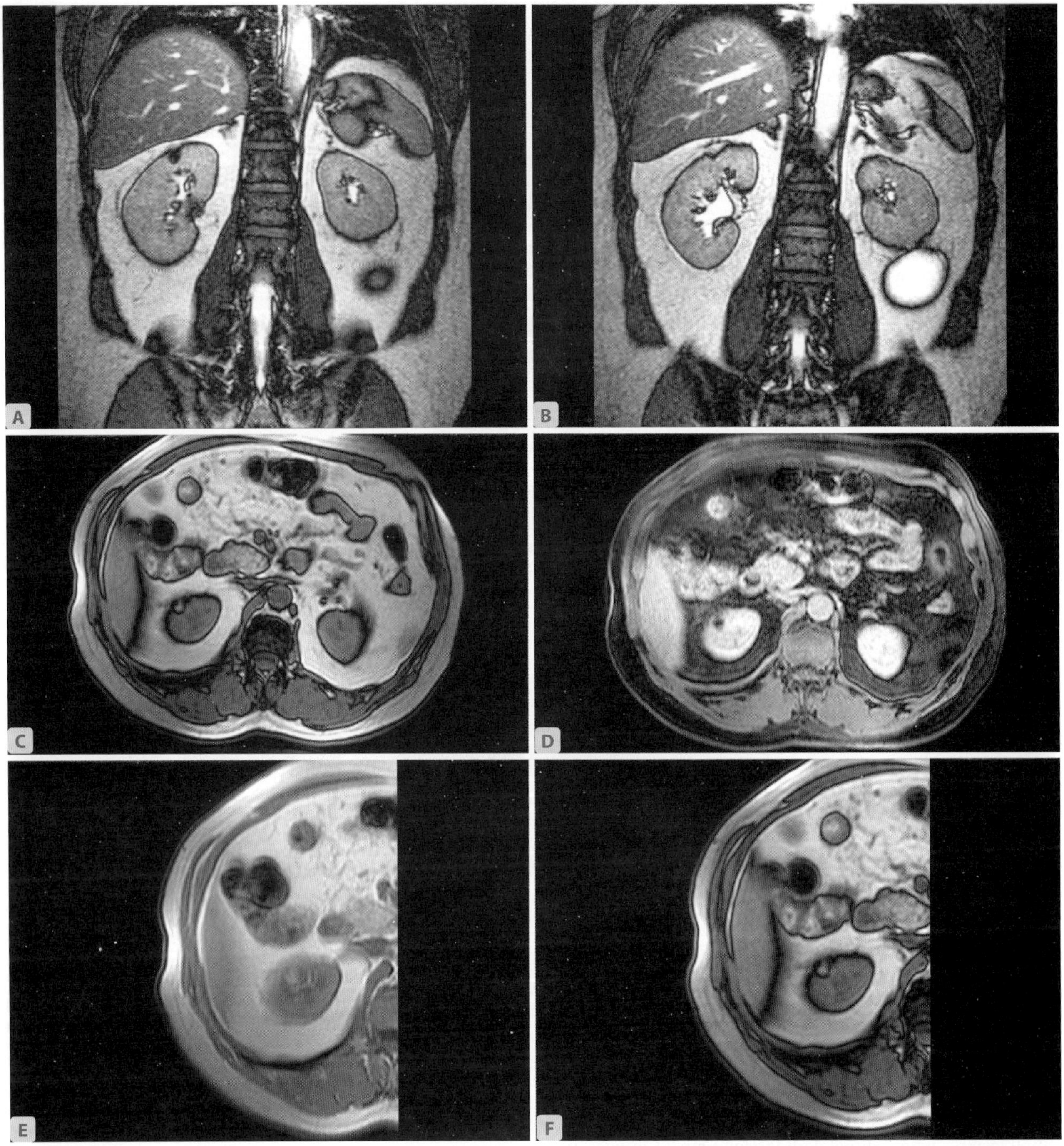

FIGS. 34A TO F: (A and B) MRI coronal TRUFISP; (C) T1 axial; (D) T1 axial fat suppressed; (E) T1 axial in phase; (F)T1 axial opposed phase. A small hyperintense lesion in right kidney with signal suppression on fat-saturated image. On opposed phase image, there is a signal drop when compared with in-phase image. An India ink artifact is also noted at lesion parenchyma interface—angiomyolipoma.

T2 hypointense and show suppression on chemical shift imaging. There is no specific feature to differentiate them from RCC.

Fat-Poor Angiomyolipoma or Renal Cell Cancer?

This continues to be a diagnostic challenge. Fat-poor AMLs are usually T2 hypointense, a feature that is not seen in clear cell RCC, but seen in papillary subtype of RCC. Chemical suppression cannot be used to differentiate small amounts of fat in AML from cells containing intracytoplasmic fat in ccRCC. AMLs have similar ADC as RCCs and this cannot be used as a point of differentiation. It has been suggested that T2 hypointensity and early enhancement with subsequent washout can be used as a marker for fat-poor AML, though in clinical practice, biopsy is indicated.[66] Certain points of differentiation are enumerated in **Table 7**.

TABLE 7: Minimal-fat AML vs RCC.

Minimal-fat AML	RCC
Lower attenuation	Higher CT number
Calcification, necrosis rare	Calcification and necrosis common
Well-defined margins	Ill-defined margins
Renal vein/IVC invasion rare	Venous involvement common
Arterial/delay enhancement ratio*>1.5	<1.5

Arterial/delay enhancement ratio* = SI (arterial-precontrast)/SI (delayed-precontrast)

Angiomyolipoma with Epithelial Cysts

This is an extremely rare subtype of AML, which contains epithelial-lined cysts.[67] These are benign lesions and are more common in women. Imaging features include a cystic component and noncystic-enhancing component. The differential diagnoses are other multilocular cystic masses such as multilocular RCC, cystic nephroma, and mixed epithelial and stromal tumor-MEST. Percutaneous biopsy may be helpful, as AML with epithelial cells and MEST stain positive for Desmin or Actin, while RCC does not.

Epithelioid Angiomyolipoma

First described in 1997, this is an extremely rare tumor, which is potentially malignant, locally aggressive, and can metastasize.[68,69] Pathologically, these are composed of numerous atypical epithelioid muscle cells and few or no fat cells. These are large masses with intratumoral hemorrhage and necrosis, with small foci of fat. Hyperattenuating on CT and T2 hypointense, they may present as enhancing solid or multilocular cystic masses.

Angiomyolipoma in Tuberous Sclerosis Complex

There is a strong association between angiomyolipoma and tuberous sclerosis. Most are the classical variety, though fat-poor AMLs are also seen. AMLs associated with TSC are usually bilateral, large with an increased rate of growth (1.25 cm/year), compared to the sporadic variety (0.19 cm/year).[70] Treatment is required in patients of angiomyolipomas with TSC. Recurrent bleeding in syndromic AML is also a notable feature. Transcatheter embolization is the preferred treatment. Patients with bilateral AMLs should be evaluated for TSC. The differences between sporadic and syndromic AML are listed in **Table 8**.

Angiomyolipoma in Lymphangioleiomyomatosis

A disease seen predominantly in young females, rarely in males and children, *angiomyolipoma in lymphangioleiomyomatosis (LAM)* is characterized by cystic changes in lung and other multisystem manifestations like renal AMLs, abdominal lymphadenopathy, chylous ascites, and cystic lymphatic masses. This disease occurs sporadically or in association with TSC. In sporadic LAM, the incidence of AML is almost 50%. The European Respiratory Society recommends screening of patients with unilateral AML, no clinical features of TSC or respiratory system to be screened for LAM.[71]

TABLE 8: Differences between sporadic and syndromic AML.

Sporadic AML	Syndromic AML
Solitary	Multiple
Unilateral	Bilateral
Female predominance (4:1)	M = F
Older	Younger
Smaller lesions	Larger lesion

In the second *classification* based purely on CT and MRI features, Song et al. have classified AML into *fat-rich, fat-poor, and fat-invisible AML* using quantitative values.[72] Fat-rich AML is a lesion with CT attenuation of ≤–10 HU. Fat-poor AML has CT attenuation >–10 HU, tumor to spleen ratio < 0.71, or a signal intensity index > 16.5%. Fat-invisible AML is defined as a lesion with CT attenuation >–10 HU, tumor to spleen ratio ≥ 0.71 and a signal intensity index of 16.5% or less **(Table 9)**.

Management of Angiomyolipoma

Conservative management is indicated for classic AMLs. Annual follow-up is recommended for asymptomatic lesions < 4 cm. For larger lesions, due to risk of hemorrhage, semiannual evaluation is suggested. Approximately 58–75% of these lesions grow with time, though a slow growth rate is seen. Growth of an isolated AML without TS is less than of those with TS and multiple lesions. For patients with larger tumors, treatment is recommended due to potential of bleeding, an intralesional aneurysm >5 mm is likely to bleed.[73] Renal artery embolization and partial nephrectomy are the treatment options available **(Box 8)**.

Leiomyosarcoma

It is an aggressive and rapidly growing tumor, which accounts for 50–60% of all renal sarcomas. Leiomyosarcoma may arise from the renal capsule, renal parenchyma, smooth muscle of the renal pelvis, or the renal vein. On CT, it appears as a large expansile heterogeneous solid mass with areas of necrosis and enhancement. It may rarely appear as a multilocular cystic mass. Leiomyosarcoma that arises from the renal capsule may envelop the entire kidney, whereas that with a parenchymal origin may replace a large part of the parenchyma and extend into perinephric fat or renal sinus. Venous extension of the tumor like RCC is also seen. On MRI, it appears T1 and T2 hypointense due to the fibrous component.

UROTHELIAL TUMOR

Transitional Cell Carcinoma

Urothelial tumors are less common in the upper urinary tract than renal cell carcinoma. However, transitional cell carcinoma (TCC) is the second most common renal neoplasm in adults. It is most common in urinary bladder, followed in frequency by ureter and the renal pelvis. They may be bilateral in 10% and multicentric in 20–44% of cases.

TABLE 9: Differentiating features of subtypes of AML.

Imaging features	Fat-rich AML	Fat-poor AML	Fat-invisible AML
Ultrasound appearance	Hyperechoic	Intermediate	Isoechoic
CT attenuation ≤ 10 HU	Present	Absent	Absent
MRI tumor to spleen ratio <0.71/ Signal intensity index >16.5%	Present	Present	Absent
Lesion management	Observation	Undetermined	Biopsy

This known multifocality warrants that the entire collecting system must be evaluated in patients with upper tract TCC because of high prevalence of an associated tumor in the lower tract.

The risk factors for TCC include nonsteroidal anti-inflammatory drug (NSAID) abuse, tobacco use or some occupational exposure. The incidence of TCC is more common is males, in the seventh decade. They commonly present with hematuria and flank pain. Hematogenous spread is less common than RCC, but lymphatic spread occurs earlier. High-grade tumors are more common in upper tract than the urinary bladder. It has been suggested that the stage rather than tumor grade is the main prognostic factor for urothelial tumor of the upper tract.

Intravenous Urography

Intravenous urography (IVU) has traditionally been used for imaging a suspected TCC before the advent of CT urography. The findings include a filling defect outlined by excreted contrast. The filling defect may be in pelvis (35%) or calyces (26%). "Stipple sign" may be seen due to trapping of contrast in the interstices of a papillary growth. There may be obstruction of kidney with nonopacification of the collecting system (phantom calyces) due to extensive areas of parenchymal infiltration. Calyces may be amputated or obliterated due to malignant infundibular stricturing. Calyces may be distended with tumor called as "oncocalcyces".

None of the signs on IVU are pathognomonic and can be simulated by a blood clot, radiolucent stone, or granuloma. Retrograde or percutaneous antegrade pyelography may be useful in such situations to delineate the site of obstruction and to obtain brush biopsy.

Ultrasonography

A large TCC is seen as an iso- to hypoechoic solid mass separating the central sinus echoes. A small TCC may not be detected on USG. Focal enlargement of renal cortex suggests infiltration of renal parenchyma. Other nonspecific findings include hydronephrosis, and pyclocalyceal wall thickening. USG can help to differentiate a radiolucent calculus from a tumor. It cannot differentiate from a blood clot unless followed up to show interval change **(Fig. 35)**.

BOX 8: Management of AML.

Indications for treatment of AML:
- Hemorrhage/pain/mass effect
- Most important predictor for hemorrhage—tumor size

Treatment of symptomatic AML:
(Irrespective of size)
- Angiogram
- Selective TCE/enucleation/partial nephrectomy

Management of asymptomatic AML:
≥4 cm—6 monthly CT/USG
<4 cm—12 monthly CT/USG.

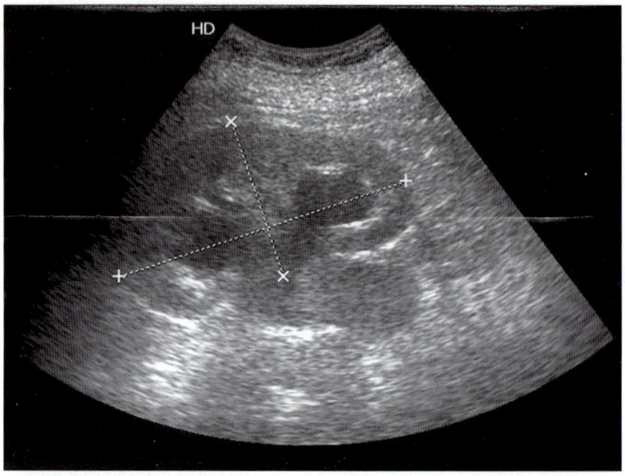

FIG. 35: Longitudinal sonogram of the left kidney shows a solid lesion in the renal pelvis and upper, a case of transitional cell carcinoma.

Computed Tomography and Magnetic Resonance Imaging

Computed tomography and MRI urography have increased the diagnostic confidence; however, mucosal detail is still best seen on IVP and RGP.[74] For CT or MRI evaluation, imaging should include excretory phase (3–5 minutes after injection) to show low attenuation mass involving the collecting system or ureter, outlined by the concentrated dense contrast.

There are three appearances on CT of a small TCC, the most common is of a small hypodense lesion in the renal collecting system, the lesion has a soft tissue attenuation (<40 HU), less than most renal calculi, slightly lower than a blood clot, but higher than urine. TCC will enhance approximately 10–50 HU, with the enhancement being less than renal parenchyma, this mild enhancement helps to differentiate it from blood clot and calculi. In the kidney, TCC is usually more central than RCC, owing to the origin in the urothelium.[75-77] TCC does not commonly involve renal vein, through rare cases of IVC involvement have been reported.[78] The central mass expands the kidney symmetrically and with centrifugal extension preserves the shape. The soft tissue component in the renal sinus obliterates and displaces intervening fat to merge with the renal parenchyma, an appearance described as "faceless" kidney **(Figs. 36A and B)**.[79]

The TCC may present as a locally aggressive infiltrative renal mass, margins being ill defined. Involvement of renal

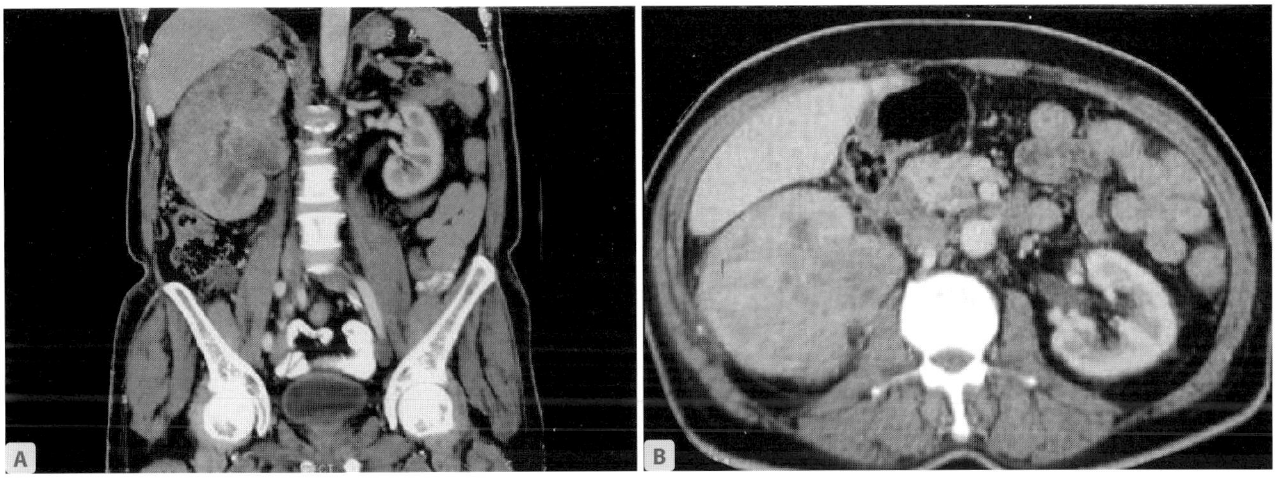

FIGS. 36A AND B: Contrast-enhanced CT abdomen—large centrally located mass in the right kidney with preserved renal shape. Renal sinus fat is obliterated giving the "faceless kidney" sign—a case of transitional cell carcinoma.

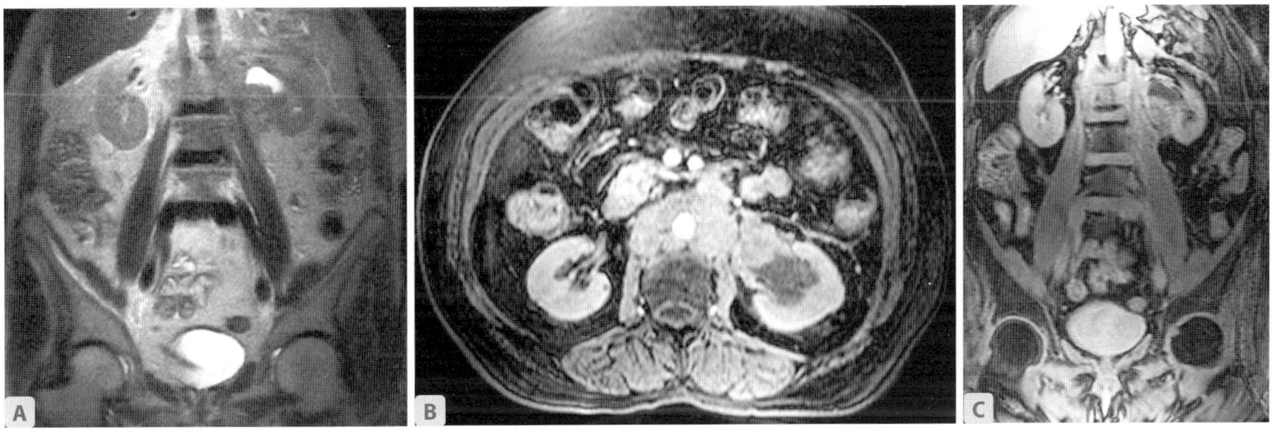

FIGS. 37A TO C: MRI T2 TRUE FISP. (A) Coronal; (B) T1 VIBE, postgadolinium axial; and (C) Coronal—enhancing mass in the renal pelvis with hydronephrosis and retroperitoneal adenopathy— transitional cell carcinoma.

parenchyma may be seen as a hypoenhancing mass involving parenchyma or heterogeneous abnormal hypoenhancement disrupting the normal parenchyma. A different appearance is thickening of collecting system urothelium or ureteral wall, the thickening may be asymmetric or eccentric. Focal infiltrative renal lesion may mimic RCC or tuberculosis. TCC tends to be more centrally located and is more likely to expand the kidney centrifugally, while preserving the shape, the coexistence of a stone is a pointer toward squamous cell carcinoma. A small area of parenchymal infiltration with papillary necrosis, is a major clue suggesting TB.

The appearance of TCC is of a small focal lesion involving renal pelvis or calyceal system. TCCs are typically isointense relative to renal medulla on T1WI, making the detection of small tumors virtually impossible. Larger infiltrative tumors may obliterate the fat in the renal sinus, this may be appreciated on T1WI. TCC is best seen on T2-weighted images due to excellent soft tissue contrast between tumor and bright signal intensity due to urine in the collecting system. Infiltrative TCCs may be seen on single shot T2WI as intermediate signal intensity mass infiltrating the renal parenchyma. A cup-shaped dilatation of the ureter just distal to a focus of TCC in the ureter may be seen called the "chalice/goblet" sign.[80] Enhancement of a focal filling defect in the collecting system is strongly suggestive of TCC **(Figs. 37A to C)**.

Staging

The TNM classification of malignant tumors (TNM) staging of TCC in upper urinary tract has different prognostic indications from bladder tumors **(Boxes 9 and 10)**. Carcinoma in situ and tumors limited to submucosa have best prognosis, tumors beyond subepithelial tissue (Stage II) and muscularis (Stage III) have worse prognosis. CT cannot accurately distinguish T1 (limited to uroepithelium and lamina propria) from T2 (extending into muscularis propria). Indications of Stage III disease

BOX 9: TNM Staging of transitional cell carcinoma of the renal pelvis.

T

- *Ta:* Noninvasive papillary tumor
- *Tis:* In situ (noninvasive flat)
- *T1:* Through lamina propria into subepithelial connective tissues
- *T2:* Into muscularis propria
- *T3:* Invasion into peripelvic fat or renal parenchyma
- *T4:* Direct invasion into adjacent structures or beyond renal capsule

N

Nodal staging is the same for TCC of any part of the urinary tract

- *N0:* No nodal involvement
- *N1:* Single node involved <2 cm
- N2
  - Single node 2–5 cm or
  - Multiple nodes all <5 cm
- *N3:* One or more nodes >5 cm

M

- *M0:* No metastases
- *M1:* Metastases identified

are parenchymal involvement or peripelvic and periureteral fat involvement.

Squamous Cell Carcinoma

Squamous cell carcinoma (SCC) of the renal pelvis is a relatively rare tumor. It is highly aggressive, with a poor clinical prognosis. Chronic infection and renal calculi are implicated in its etiology. It often involves the renal parenchyma and perinephric tissue and may present with metastasis. Intravenous urography may reveal nonfunctioning kidney, hydronephrosis, a central mass, or a pelvicalyceal filling defect seen in 83% of patients. On cross-sectional imaging, this cannot be differentiated from transitional cell carcinomas. Pointers toward the diagnosis of SCC include the fact that SCC grows fast, and rapid progression on sequential studies favors SCC. As SCC develops following metaplasia due to chronic inflammation, associated calculi are seen in 50% of cases.

LYMPHOMA

Renal lymphoma is usually *secondary* to systemic disease and associated with adenopathy or involvement of other organs such as liver and gastrointestinal tract (GIT). Contiguous involvement of retroperitoneal disease often affects the genitourinary system with the kidneys, being the most commonly involved organ. Renal involvement is more commonly seen in non-Hodgkin lymphoma than in Hodgkin lymphoma.

Renal lymphoma is often asymptomatic, with detection incidentally at imaging studies. The incidence at autopsy being as high as 41.6%. Despite the high prevalence, imaging studies demonstrate involvement in only 3–8% of patients.[81]

Malignant lymphocytes reach the renal parenchyma by means of hematogenous spread and proliferate within the interstitium, using nephrons, tubules, and blood vessels as scaffolding for further growth. If it follows this infiltrative pattern, kidneys enlarge, maintaining the reniform shape. In many cases, there is focal proliferation giving rise to single or more commonly bilateral renal expansile masses. Some tumors spread by means of contiguous extension from the retroperitoneal disease, penetrating the renal capsule. Renal involvement is usually bilateral, in form of nodules or diffuse infiltration, bulky single tumor, invasion from perirenal disease or microscopic invasion.

BOX 10: Staging groups for transitional cell CA of renal pelvis.

- *Stage 0:* Ta or Tis, N0, M0
- *Stage I:* T1, N0, M0
- *Stage II:* T2(a or b), N0, M0
- *Stage III:* T3(a or b) or T4a, N0, M0
- *Stage IV:*
  - T4b, any N, any M
  - N1-3, any T, any M

BOX 11: Renal lymphoma—patterns.

- *Multiple masses*—most common pattern (50–60%)
  - Usually 1–3 cm in size
  - Associated with enlarged retroperitoneal nodes (≥50%)
- *Single mass* (10–25%)
  - Homogeneous, hypodense without cystic change
- *Invasion from retroperitoneal nodal mass* (25–30% of cases)
  - Usually >10 cm
  - Encasement of vessels without thrombosis, +/–hydronephrosis
- *Diffuse infiltration* (up to 20% of cases)
  - No discrete mass
  - Usually bilateral
  - Seen with Burkitt lymphoma
- *Perirenal mass* (less than 10% of cases)
  - Perirenal stranding
  - Thickening of Gerota's fascia
  - Perirenal nodules.

Primary renal lymphoma (PRL) is extremely rare, due to lack of lymphatic tissue within the kidney. It should be suspected, if the disease affects only the kidney, or the patient presents with renal impairment in absence of any other cause of renal impairment; rapid improvement and decrease in renal size is noted following the initiation of chemotherapy. The tumor is aggressive and shows bilateral renal involvement in majority of cases. PRL is usually a B cell non-Hodgkin lymphoma and affects patients who are middle-aged or older. In chronic lymphatic leukemia, kidney may be involved in 90% of cases and is associated with membranous glomerulonephritis.

Imaging of Renal Lymphoma

Renal lymphoma has a variety of imaging appearances depending on the pattern of tumor spread **(Box 11)**.[81,82]

Lymphoma masses consist of large number of uniform cells. On *ultrasonography*, this results in a homogeneous,

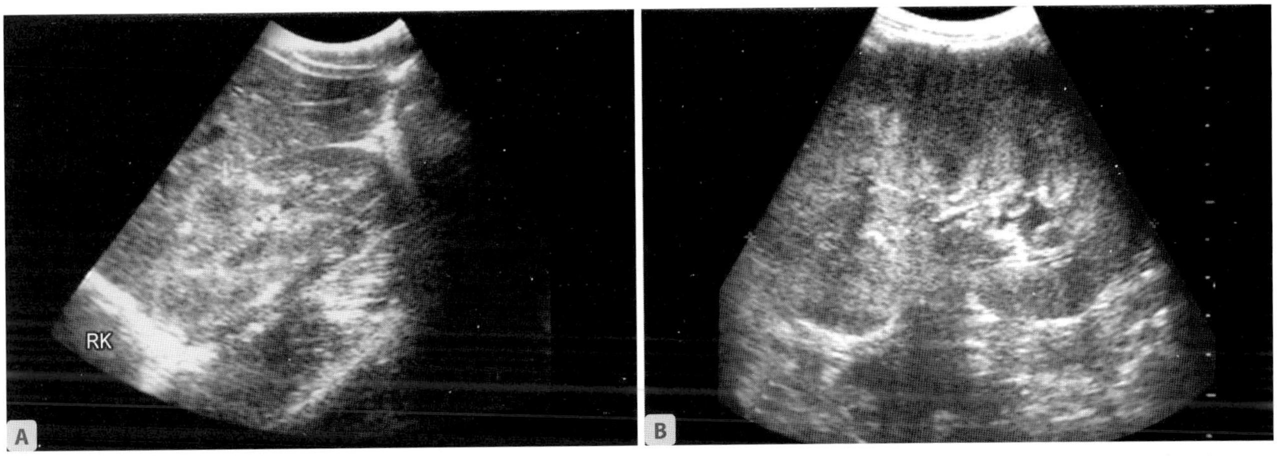

FIGS. 38A AND B: USG bilateral renal enlargement with poorly defined hypo/anechoic nodules giving a homogeneous appearance—lymphoma.

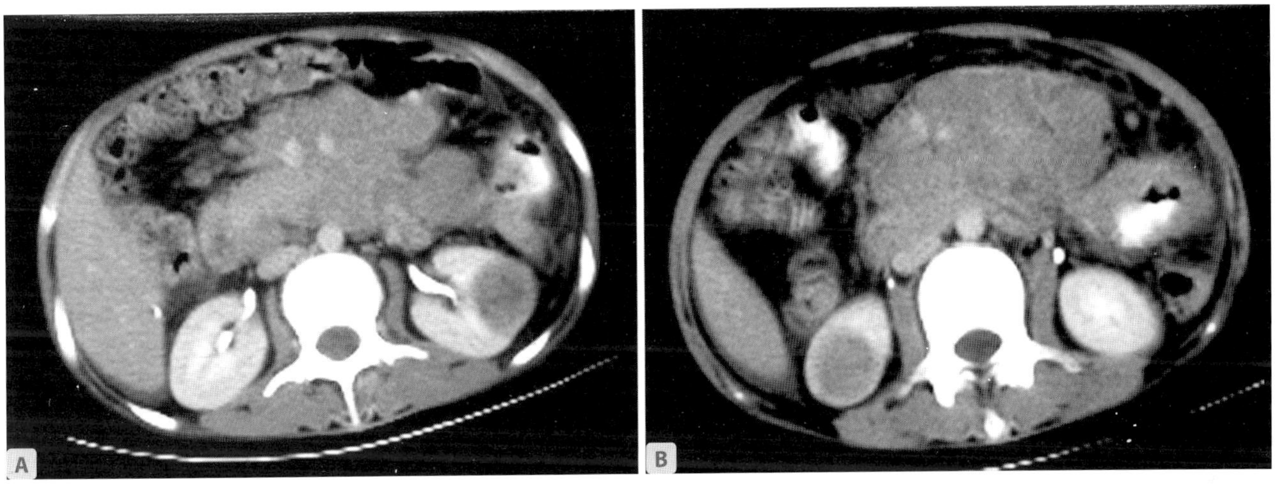

FIGS. 39A AND B: Contrast-enhanced CT showing well-defined focal hypodense masses in both kidneys with significant retroperitoneal adenopathy and bowel thickening—a case of lymphoma.

nearly anechoic appearance which may mimic renal cysts, but there is no thorough transmission and subtle low-level echoes may be seen **(Figs. 38A and B)**. The sinus fat surrounding the central pelvicalyceal echoes may completely disappear. This sonographic pattern is unique to renal lymphoma. Ultrasound may also detect hydroureteronephrosis, adenopathy and other foci in liver and spleen. Large retroperitoneal nodes may be seen encasing the vessels.[83]

Computed tomography is more sensitive than ultrasound in detection of renal lymphoma. The most common appearance, which is seen in 50–60% of cases is of multiple focal masses which have attenuation similar or only slightly less than renal parenchyma on unenhanced images (nephrographic phase-contrast CT is essential, as many lesions are small and affect the medullary part of the kidney and may be missed on CM phase). Lymphoma enhances less than normal parenchyma.[82,83] Heterogeneity and necrosis may be seen with larger lesions. Calcification is usually not seen, unless there has been therapy. Invasion into renal vein and IVC is rare.[84]

Renal lymphoma can also manifest as a solitary mass in 10–25% of patients **(Figs. 39A and B)**. It characteristically demonstrates homogeneous attenuation and low-grade enhancement, providing a point of differentiation from clear cell RCC. Biopsy may be required to differentiate from other subtypes of RCC.

Contiguous involvement to kidneys or perinephric space from large retroperitoneal nodal masses is the second most common pattern (25–30%).[85] Perinephric involvement is noted in approximately one-third of patients, most of whom also have parenchymal involvement **(Fig. 40)**.

Another appearance of renal lymphoma is a perinephric ring of soft tissue noted around the kidney without a focal parenchymal lesion; the soft tissue is of low attenuation, compresses the renal parenchyma without significant impairment of renal function. Extramedullary hematopoiesis, metastasis, and retroperitoneal sarcoma are differentials for perinephric soft tissue masses.

Diffuse renal enlargement may be seen in the infiltrative form in up to 20% of cases. It is seen as a low-attenuation mass expanding the kidney with predominant, involvement of the renal medulla, with relative sparing of cortical margins. This is more common in Burkitt lymphoma, either disseminated or limited to the kidneys **(Fig. 41)**. Heterogeneous enhancement

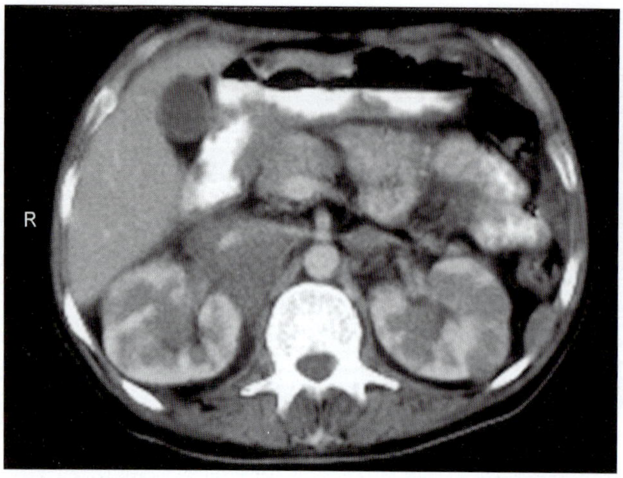

FIG. 40: Renal lymphoma—contrast-enhanced CT shows multiple nodules in both kidneys with perirenal disease on the right side.

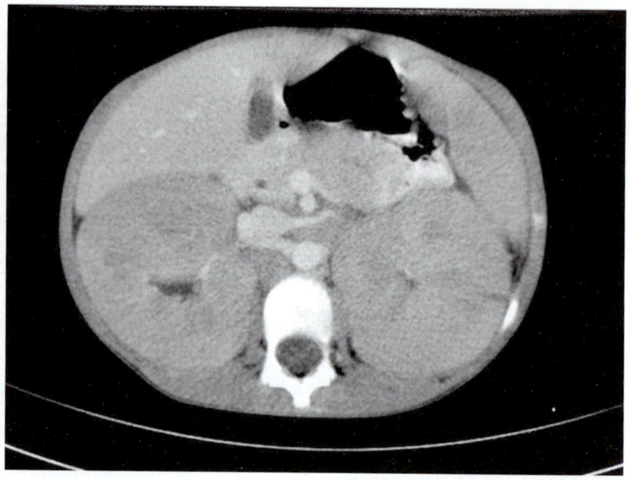

FIG. 41: CT abdomen—bilateral kidneys are enlarged with loss of corticomedullary differentiation—a case of Burkitt's lymphoma.

of the kidneys, with loss of normal differential enhancement is seen. Lymphoma can affect the renal sinus preferentially, the normal sinus fat is replaced by homogeneous soft tissue mass. The mass usually causes encasement of the renal vessels leading to poor enhancement.

The morphological appearance of lymphoma on MRI is similar to that on CT. Renal lymphoma is iso- to slightly hypointense relative to the renal cortex on T1 and iso- to mildly hyperintense on T2-weighted images. There is minimal heterogeneous enhancement on postgadolinium images, the enhancement being less than that of the normal parenchyma.

In suspected cases of lymphoma, biopsy is indicated for differentiating from other tumors. The distinction is important as lymphoma is usually treated medically.

PRIMITIVE NEUROECTODERMAL TUMOR/EXTRASKELETAL EWING'S TUMOR

This is a highly aggressive renal neoplasm, which comprises only less than 1% of all adult renal tumors, patient is usually a young adult with a median age of 27. Primitive neuroectodermal tumor (PNET) of the kidney belongs to small round cell tumors of the kidney, which include lymphoma, clear cell sarcoma, carcinoid, monophasic Wilms' tumor, synovial sarcoma, desmoplastic small round cell tumor and extraskeletal Ewing's sarcoma (EES)/PNET. It appears as solitary, large, ill-defined, irregular heterogeneous mass. Invasion of the renal cortex and renal pelvis as well as perirenal fat and adjacent organs, presence of tumor thrombus, at the time of the initial diagnosis is seen in most cases. Early metastases to liver and bone are noted. Diagnosis is based on histology and immunocytohistochemisty.[86,87]

RENAL METASTASES

The prevalence of metastatic disease to the kidney varies from 20% in autopsy series to less than 1% in clinicopathological series. The most common sites of primary tumor are lung, colon, breast, melanoma, and reproductive organs. Melanoma, when present, frequently metastasizes to the kidney. Most renal metastases are hematogenous, although a few may be due to direct invasion (adrenal, colonic, and pancreas). Usually the primary tumor is known and there is metastasis to other organs. Metastases to the kidney are usually asymptomatic, but may rarely present with hematuria.

The appearance of metastases is usually of small bilateral, multiple renal masses, an appearance not commonly seen in RCC, though solitary renal metastasis are not uncommon **(Figs. 42A and B)**. Metastases are usually at the junction of the renal cortex and medulla with ill-defined borders with poor enhancement, except those from hypervascular tumors. Direct involvement of perinephric space by metastasis, representing lymphatic spread is noted in metastasis from melanoma and lung carcinoma. Hemorrhagic renal metastases are seen in melanoma and pheochromocytomas.[88,89]

In the presence of an extrarenal malignancy that is known to metastasize to the kidney, the renal mass may represent a primary renal malignancy or metastatic disease. In patients with a history of extrarenal malignancy, 50–85% of solitary solid renal masses are metastatic. Large solitary renal metastasis that disrupt the renal cortical margins may be associated with breast, lung, or colon carcinomas. Solitary metastasis may resemble RCC, which however, has no necrosis. Hyperenhancement and renal vein involvement favors RCC. The margination of metastasis is often less well defined than RCC. Biopsy of the renal mass is indicated in the clinical dilemma of a solitary metastasis versus RCC.

RENAL MASS BIOPSY

Traditionally, percutaneous biopsy played a limited role in evaluation of all solid renal tumors. However, renal biopsy has become an accepted part of diagnostic algorithm of

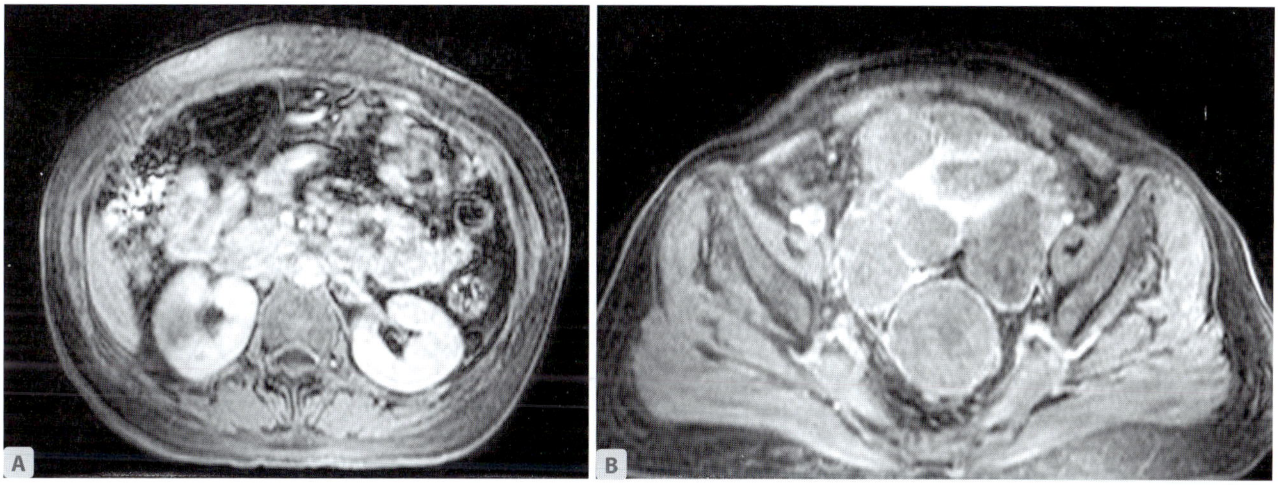

FIGS. 42A AND B: MRI T1 vibe postcontrast. (A) A focal poorly enhancing mass in the right kidney; (B) Renal metastasis from disseminated ovarian malignancy.

an indeterminate renal and in a small renal mass (<4 cm), to decide treatment options. The American Urological Association has postulated guidelines for performing renal mass biopsy. It should be offered if an alternate diagnosis is suspected such as hematological, metastatic, inflammatory or infectious etiology. Biopsy is also done for confirming RCC in certain circumstances, including prior to ablative therapies, when a solid mass is present in a solitary or transplant kidney, or when disease is either locally advanced or metastatic, when the surgical risk is high, and when the disease is locally advanced and metastatic, in the setting of a solitary/transplant kidney, and prior to ablative therapy.[90]

Renal biopsy is gaining acceptance and is increasingly used in characterizing and managing renal masses. Accepted indications include confirming an infected cyst, identifying lymphoma or a metastasis as the cause of the indeterminate renal mass, and renal mass biopsy may not be done in the older patients, who will be treated conservatively irrespective of the result, and in the young or healthy patients who may be unwilling to accept uncertainties associated with biopsy. Biopsy may underestimate aggressive features in a renal tumor.

The guidelines state that multiple core needle biopsy sampling should be done rather than fine needle aspirations. Renal mass biopsy may help predict the biological behavior of a renal tumor, its aggressive nature, and thus guide management decisions. Renal mass biopsy, done under image guidance is considered safe with a 92% diagnostic rate and a complication rate of less than 5%. No case of needle tract seeding has been reported with use of the coaxial technique.[91]

INDETERMINATE RENAL MASS

An indeterminate renal mass is one that cannot be diagnosed confidently as benign or malignant at the time it is discovered. MDCT is the most utilized imaging technique for evaluating the indeterminate renal mass, playing an important role in the characterization of both solid and cystic lesions. Presence of macroscopic fat in a renal mass marks it as benign. Enhancing solid renal masses or enhancing components in cystic masses indicate a possible malignant etiology. The small (≤1.5 cm in diameter) renal mass poses a more complex problem for CT imaging, in that volume averaging effects occur, making it difficult to assess accurately the density on noncontrast images and to evaluate for enhancement after IV-contrast administration.[92]

Magnetic resonance imaging is a rapidly evolving modality, currently valuable as a problem solving tool.[93] The addition of diffusion-weighted imaging provides additional inputs in workup of indeterminate lesions, especially in pseudotumors or in cases where IV contrast is contraindicated. The diagnostic dilemma of fat-poor AML vs RCC remains.

A diagnostic algorithm for characterization of renal masses has been suggested **(Flowchart 1)**.

Newer advances such as texture analysis may further refine the pre operative characterization of renal neoplasms.

ACKNOWLEDGMENT

Thanks to Dr Shivali Arya, MD student in the department of Radiodiagnosis, MAMC for the illustrations.

FLOWCHART 1: Diagnostic algorithm for characterization of renal mass on CT.

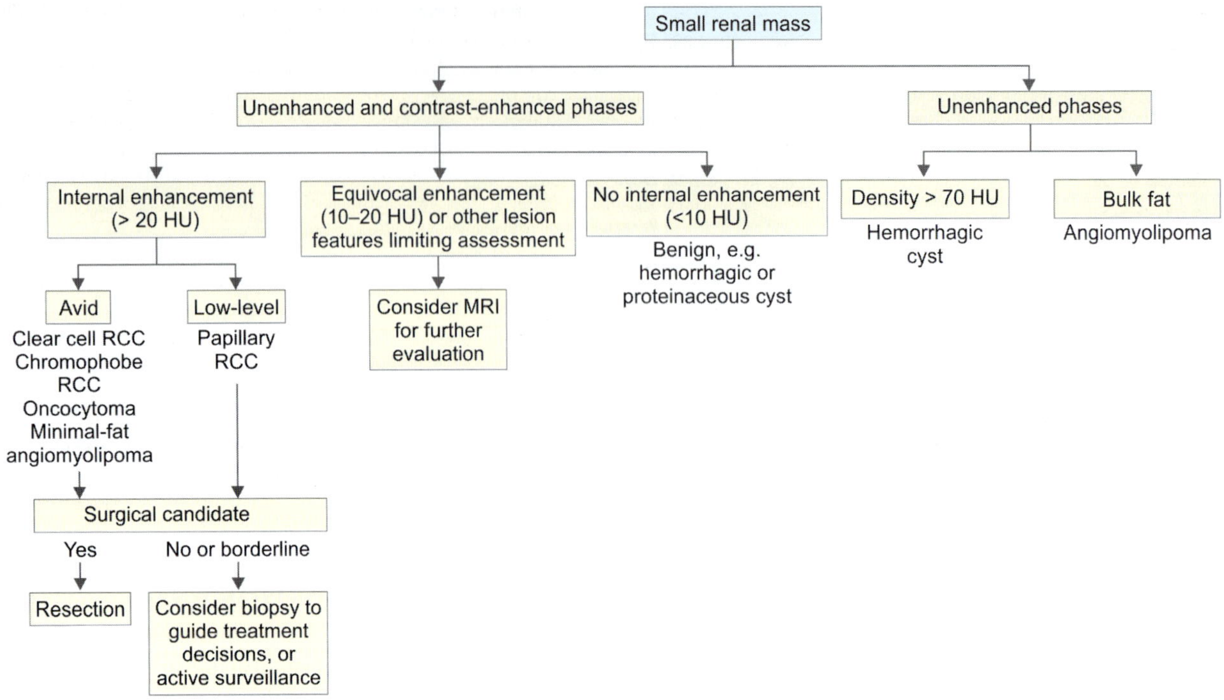

(RCC: renal cell carcinoma; HU: Hounsfield units)

REFERENCES

1. Moch H, Cubilla A, Humphrey PA, et al. The 2016 WHO Classification of Tumours of the Urinary System and Male Genital Organs—Part A: Renal, Penile, and Testicular Tumours. Eur Urol. 2016;70(1):93-105.
2. Burgan CM, Sanyal R, Lockhart ME. Ultrasound of renal masses. Radiol Clin North Am. 2019;57(3):585-600.
3. Kay FU, Pedrosa I. Imaging of solid renal masses. Radiol Clin North Am. 2017;55(2):243-58.
4. Dyer R, DiSantis DJ, McClennan BL. Simplified imaging approach for evaluation of the solid renal mass in adults. Radiology. 2008;247(2):331-43.
5. Hartman DS, Davidson AJ, Davis CJ Jr, et al. Infiltrative renal lesions: CT-sonographic-pathologic correlation. AJR Am J Roentgenol. 1988;150(5):1061-4.
6. Pickhardt PJ, Lonergan GJ, Davis CJ Jr, et al. Infiltrative renal lesions: radiologic-pathologic correlation. Radiographics. 2000;20(1):215-43.
7. Bhatt S, MacLennan G, Dogra V. Renal pseudotumors. AJR Am J Roentgenol. 2007;188:1380-7
8. Maki DD, Birhbaum BA, Chakraborty DP, et al. Renal cyst pseudoenhancement: beam hardening effects on CT numbers. Radiology. 1999;213(2):468-72.
9. Isreal GM, Bosniak MA. Pitfalls in renal mass evaluation and how to avoid them. Radiographics. 2008;28(5):1325-38.
10. Atkins MB, Choueiri TK, Richie JP, et al. (2019). Epidemiology, pathology and pathogenesis of renal cell carcinoma. [Online]. Available from: https://www.uptodate.com/contents/epidemiology-pathology-and-pathogenesis-of-renal-cell-carcinoma. [Last accessed from October, 2019]
11. Cheville JC, Lohse CM, Zincke H, et al. Comparisons of outcome and prognostic features among histological subtypes of renal cell carcinoma. Am J Surg Pathol. 2003;27(5):612-24.
12. Zhang J, Lefkowitz RA, Bach A. Imaging of kidney cancer. Radiol clin North Am. 2007;45(1):119-47.
13. Raman SP, Johnson PT, Allaf ME, et al. Chromophobe renal cell carcinoma: multiphase MDCT enhancement patterns and morphological features. AJR Am J Roentgenol. 2013;201(6):1268-76.
14. Wahal SP, Mardi K. Multilocular cystic renal cell carcinoma: a rare entity with review of literature. J Lab Physicians. 2014;6(1):50-2
15. Peyromaure M, Thiounn N, Scotte F, et al. Collecting duct carcinoma of the kidney: a clinicopathological study of 9 cases. J Urol. 2003;170(4 Pt 1):1138-40.
16. Allappan N, Marak CP, Chopra A, et al. Renal medullary cancer in a patient with sickle cell trait. Case Rep Oncol Med. 2013;2013:129813.
17. Blitman NM, Berkenblit RG, Rozenblit AM, et al. Renal medullary carcinoma: CT and MRI features. AJR Am J Roentgenol. 2005;185(1):268-72.
18. Woo S, Kim SY, Lee MS, et al. MDCT findings of renal cell carcinoma associated with Xp11.2 translocation and TFE3 gene fusion and papillary renal cell carcinoma. AJR Am J Roentgenol. 2015;204(3):542-9.
19. Sureka B, Bansal K, Arora A. Imaging hallmark of Xp 11.2 translocation renal cell carcinoma. Can Urol Assoc J. 2015;9(7-8):E572.
20. Malhi H, Grant EG, Duddalwar V. Contrast-enhanced ultrasound of the liver and kidney. Radiol Clin North Am. 2014;52(6):1177-90.
21. Cohan RH, Ellis J. Renal masses: imaging evaluation. Radiol Clin N Am. 2015;53(5):985-1003.
22. Mittal MK, Sureka B. Solid renal masses in adults. Indian J Radiol Imaging. 2016;26:429-42.
23. Kaza RK, Platt JF. Renal applications of dual energy CT. Abdom Radiol. 2016;41:1122-32.

24. Mileto A, Marin D, Ramirez-Giraldo JC, et al. Accuracy of contrast-enhanced dual-energy MDCT for the assessment of iodine uptake in renal lesions. AJR Am J Roentgenol. 2014;202(5):W466-74.
25. Mileto A, Nelson RC, Paulson EK, et al. Dual-energy MDCT for imaging the renal mass. AJR Am J Roentgenol. 2015;204(6):W640-7.
26. Vendrami CL, Villavicencio CP, DeJulio TJ, et al. Differentiation of solid renal tumors with multiparametric MR imaging. Radiographics. 2017;37(7):2026-42.
27. Pedrosa I, Chou MT, Ngo L, et al. MR classification of renal masses with pathological correlation. Eur Radiol. 2008;18(2):365-75.
28. Pedrosa I, Sun MR, Spencer M, et al. MR imaging of renal masses:correlation with findings at surgery and pathological analysis. Radiographics. 2008;28(4):985-1003.
29. Cornelis F, Tricaud E, Lasserre AS, et al. Multiparametric magnetic resonance imaging for the differentiation of low and high grade clear cell renal carcinoma. Eur Radiol. 2015;25(1):24-31.
30. Kaelo CA, Donati OF, Burger IA, et al. MR imaging of renal cortical tumours: qualitative and quantitative chemical shift imaging parameters. Eur Radiol. 2013;23(6):1738-44.
31. Choi YA, Kim CK, Park SY, et al. Subtype differentiation of renal cell carcinoma using diffusion weighted and blood oxygenation level dependent MRI. Am J Roentgenol. 2014;203(1):W78-84.
32. Rosenkrantz AB, Niver BE, Fitzgerald EF, et al. Utility of the apparent diffusion coefficent for distinguishing clear cell renal cell carcinoma of low and high nuclear grade. AJR Am J Roentgenol. 2010;195(5):W244-51.
33. Goyal A, Sharma R, Bhalla AS, et al. Diffusion weighted MRI in renal cell carcinoma: a surrogate marker for predicting nuclear grade and histological subtype. Acta Radiol. 2012:53(3):349-58.
34. Lassel EA, Rao R, Schwenke C, et al. Diffusion weighted imaging of focal renal lesions: a meta-analysis. Eur Radiol. 2014;24(1):241-9.
35. Maurer MH, Harma KH, Thoney H. Diffusion-weighted genitourinary imaging. Radiol Clin North Am. 2017;55(2):393-411.
36. Goyal A, Sharma R, Bhalla AS, et al. Diffusion-weighted MRI in inflammatory renal lesions: all that glitters is not RCC! Eur Radiol. 2013;23(1):272-9.
37. Goyal A, Sharma R, Bhalla AS, et al. Comparison of MDCT, MRI and MRI with diffusion-weighted imaging in evaluation of focal renal lesions: the defender, challenger, and winner! Indian J Radiol Imaging. 2018;28(1):27-36.
38. Jeon TY, Kim CK, Kim JH, et al. Assesment of early therapeutic response to sorafenib in renal cell carcinoma xenografts by dynamic contrast enhanced and diffusion weighted MR imaging. Br J Radiol. 2015;88(1053):20150163.
39. Johnson CD, Dunnick NR, Lohan RH, et al. Renal adenocarcinoma: CT staging of 100 tumors. AJR Am J Roentgenal. 1987;148(1):59-63.
40. Hallscheidt PJ, Bock M, Riedasch G, et al. Diagnostic accuracy of staging renal cell carcinomas using multidetector row computed tomography and magnetic resonance imaging: a prospective study with histopathological correlation. J comput Assist Tomogr. 2004;28(3):333-9.
41. Montravers F,Grahek D, Kerrou K, et al. Evaluation of FDG uptake by renal malignancies (primary tumor or metastases) using a coincidence detection gamma camera. J Nucl Med. 2000;41(1):78-84.
42. Boss A, Clasen S, Kuczyk M, et al. Image guided radiofrequency ablation of renal cell carcinoma. Eur Radiol. 2007;17(3):725-33.
43. Silverman SG, Israel GM, Herts BR, et al. Management of the incidental renal mass. Radiology. 2008;249(1):16-31.
44. Heilbrun ME, Remer EM, Casilino DD, et al. ACR Appropriateness Criteria indeterminate renal mass. J Am Coll Radiol. 2015;12(4):333-41.
45. Kutikov A, Uzzo RG. The R.E.N.A.L. nephrometry score: a comprehensive standardized system for quantitating renal tumor size, location and depth. J Urol. 2009;182(3):844-53.
46. Ficarra V, Novara G, Secco S, et al. Preoperative aspects and dimensions used for an anatomical (PADUA) classification of renal tumors in patients who are candidates for nephron-sparing surgery. Eur Urol. 2009;56(5):786-93.
47. Lall CG, Patel HP, Fujimoto S, et al. Making sense of postoperative CT imaging following laparoscopic partial nephrectomy. Clin Radiol. 2012;67(7):675-86.
48. Rutherford EE, Cast JEI, Breen DJ. Immediate and long-term CT appearances following radiofrequency ablation of renal tumours. Clin Radiol. 2008;63(32):220-30.
49. Donat SM, Diaz M, Bishoff JT, et al. Follow-up for clinically localized renal neoplasms: AUA guideline. J Urol. 2013;190(2):407-16.
50. Leon AD, Pedrosa I. Imaging and screening of kidney cancer. Radiol Clin North Am. 2017;55(6):1235-50.
51. Prasad SR, Surabhi VR, Menias CO, et al. Benign renal neoplasms in adults: cross-sectional imaging findings. AJR AM J Roentgenol. 2008;190(1):158-64.
52. Ishigami K, Jones AR, Dahmoush L, et al. Imaging spectrum of renal oncocytomas: a pictorial review with pathological correlation. Insights Imaging. 2015;6(1):53-64.
53. Dechet CB, Bostwick DG, Blute ML, et al. Renal oncocytoma: multifocality, bilateralism, metachronus tumor development and coexistent renal cell carcinoma. J Urol . 1999;162(1):40-2.
54. Woo S, Cho JY, Kim SH, et al. Segmental enhancement inversion of small renal oncocytom: differences in prevalence according to tumor size. AJR Am J Roentgenol. 2013;200(5):1054-9.
55. Kim JI, Cho JY, Moon KC, et al. Segmental enhancement inversion at biphasic multidetector CT: characteristic finding of small renal oncocytoma. Radiology. 2009;252(2):441-8.
56. McGahan JP, Lamba R, Fisher J, et al. Is segmental enhancement inversion on enhanced biphasic MDCT a reliable sign for the non invasive diagnosis of renal oncocytomas? AJR Am J Roentgenol. 2011;197(4):W674-9.
57. Wilkinson C, Palit V, Bardapure M, et al. Adult multilocular cystic nephroma: report of six cases with clinical, radio-pathologic correlation and review of literature. Urol Ann. 2013;5(1):13-7.
58. Katabathina VS,Vikram R, Nagar AM, et al. Mesenchymal Neoplasms of the kidney in adults.Imaging spectrum with radiological and pathological correlation. Radiographics. 2010;30(6):1525-40.
59. Prasad SR, Mino Kneudson M, Narra VR, et al. Neoplasms of the perivascular epithelioid cell including the abdomen and pelvis: cross sectional imaging findings. J Comput Assist Tomogr. 2007;31(5):688-96.
60. Jinzaki M, Silverman SG, Akita H, et al. Renal angiomyolipoma: a radiological classification and update on recent developments in diagnosis and management. Abdom Imaging. 2014; 39(3):588-604.
61. Bosniak MA, Meigbow AJ, Hulnick DH, et al. CT diagnosis of renal angiomyolipomas: the importance of detecting small amounts of fat. AJR Am J Roentgenol. 1988;151(3):497-501.
62. Takahashi K, Honda M, Okubo RS, et al. CT pixel mapping in the diagnosis of small angiomyolipomas of the kidneys. J Comput Assist Tomogr. 1993;17(1):98-101.
63. Israel GM, Bosniak MA, Slywotzky CM, et al. CT differentiation of large expophytic renal angiomyolipomas and perirenal liposarcomas. AJR Am J Roentgenal. 2002;179(3):769-73.

64. Ellingson JJ, Coakley FV, Joe BN,et al. Computed tomographic distinction of perirenal liposarcoma from exophytic angiomyolipoma: a feature analysis study. J Comput Assist Tomgr. 2008;32:548-52.
65. Silverman SG, Mortele KJ, Tuncali MD, et al. Hyperattenuating Renal Masses: etiologies, pathogenesis and imaging evaluation. Radiographics. 2007;27:1131-43.
66. Choi HJ, Kim JK, Ahn H, et al. Value of T2-weighted MR imaging in differentiating low-fat renal angiomyolipomas from other renal tumors. Acta Radiol. 2011;52(3):349-53.
67. Mikami S, Oya M, Mukai M. Angiomyolipoma with epithelial cysts of the kidney in a man. Pathol Int. 2008;58(10):664-7.
68. Froemming AT, Boland J, Cheville J, et al. Renal epithelioid angiomyolipoma: imaging characteristics in nine cases with radiologic-pathologic correlation and review of the literature. AJR Am J Roentgenol. 2013;200(2):W178-86.
69. Tsukada J, Jinzaki M, Yao M, et al. Epithelioid angiomyolipoma of the kidney: radiological imaging. Int J Urol. 2013;20(11): 1105-11.
70. Crino PB, Nathanson KL, Henske EP. The tuberous sclerosis complex. N Engl J Med 2006;355(13):1345-56.
71. Johnson SR, Cordier JF, Lazor R, et al. European Respiratory Society guidelines for the diagnosis and management of lymphangioleiomyomatosis. Eur Respir J. 2010;35(1):14-26.
72. Song S, Park BK, Park JJ. New radiologic classification of renal angiomyolipomas. Eur J Radiol. 2016;85:1835-42.
73. Yamakado K, Tanaka N, Nakagawa T, et al. Renal angiomyolipoma: relationships between tumor size, aneurysm formation and rupture. 2002;225(1):78-82.
74. Caoili EM, Cohan RH, Inampudi P, et al. MDCT urography of upper tract urothelial neoplasms. AJR Am J Roentgenol. 2005;184(6):1873-81.
75. Raza SA, Sohaib SA, Sahdev A, et al. Centrally infiltrating renal masses on CT:differentiating intrarenal transistional cell carcinoma from centrally located renal cell carcinoma. AJR Am J Roentgenol. 2012;198(4):846-53.
76. Gatewood OM, Goldman SM, Marshall FF, et al. Computerized tomography in the diagnosis of transitional cell carcinoma of the kidney. J Urol. 1982;127(5):876-87.
77. Parienty RA, Ducellier R, Pradel J, et al. Diagnostic valve of CT number in pelvicalcyeal filling defects. Radiology. 1982;145(3):743-7.
78. Leo ME, Petrou SP, Barrett DM. Transitional cell carcinoma of the kidney with vena caval involvement: report of 3 cases and a review of the literature. J Urol. 1992;148(2 Pt 1):398-400.
79. Hulnick DH, Bosniak MA. 'Faceless kidney' CT sign of renal duplicity. J Comput Assit Tomogr. 1986;10(5):771-2.
80. Daniels RE 3rd. The Goblet sign. Radiology. 1999;210(3):737-8.
81. Sheth S, Ali S, Fishman E. Imaging of renal lymphoma: patterns of disease with pathological correlation. Radiographics. 2006; 26(4):1151-68.
82. Ganeshan D, Iyer R, Devine C, et al. Imaging of primary and secondary renal lymphoma. Am J Roentgenol. 2013;201: W712-9
83. Ruchman RB, Yeh H-C, Mitty HA, Cohen BA, et al. Ultrasonographic and computed tomographic features of renal sinus lymphoma. J Clin Ultrasound. 1988;16(1):35-40.
84. Reznek RH, Mootoosamy I, Webb JA, et al. CT in renal and perirenal lymphoma: a further look. Clin Radiol. 1990;42(4):233-8.
85. Urban BA Fishman EK. Renal Lymphoma: CT patterns with emphasis on Helical CT. Radiographics. 2000;20(1):197-212.
86. Lee H, Cho JY, Kim SH, et al. Imaging findings of primitive neuroectodermal tumors of the kidney. J Comput Assist Tomogr. 2009;33(6):882-6.
87. Akkaya Z, Peker E, Gulpinar B, et al. CT and MRI findings in a rare case of renal primitive neuroectodermal tumor. Pol J Radiol. 2016;81:401-6.
88. Choyke PL, White EM, Zemen RK, et al. Renal metastasis: clinicopathological and radiological correlation. Radiology. 1992;159(6):1229-34.
89. Zhou C, Urbauer DL, Fellman BM, et al. Metastases to the kidney: a comprehensive analysis of 151 patients from a tertiary referral center. BJU Int. 2016;117(5):775-82.
90. Marconi L, Dabestani S, Lam TB, et al. Systematic review and meta-analysis of diagnostic accuracy of percutaneous renal tumour biopsy. Eur Urol. 2016;69(4):660-73.
91. Jason Abel E. Percutaneous biopsy facilitates modern treatment of renal masses. Abdom Radiol (NY). 2016;41(4):617-9.
92. Pahernik S, Ziegler S, Roos F, et al. Small renal tumors: correlation of clinical and pathological features with tumor size. J Urol. 2007;178(2):414-7.
93. Kang SK, Huang WC, Pandharipande PV, et al. Solid renal masses: what the numbers tell us. AJR Am J Roentgenol. 2014;202(6): 1196-206.

CHAPTER

9

Renovascular Hypertension

Sanjeev Kumar, Vineeta Ojha, Sanjiv Sharma

HYPERTENSION

Conventionally hypertension is defined as blood pressure (BP) more than or equal to 140/90 mm Hg. However, according to the latest American College of Cardiology (ACC) guidelines,[1] hypertension is defined as a blood pressures of more than or equal 130/80, measured while following proper techniques. Stage 1 hypertension is systolic BP of 130–139 mm Hg and diastolic BP of 80–89 mm Hg. Stage 2 hypertension is BP of at least 140/80 mm Hg.[1] Hypertension is a common cause of cardiovascular and neurological morbidity and mortality by the virtue of causing complications like left ventricular hypertrophy, heart failure, ischemic heart disease, chronic kidney disease (CKD), ischemic stroke, intracerebral hemorrhage. The overall prevalence of hypertension is 29.8% in India.[2] In adults, mostly (~90%) hypertension is idiopathic and is called as essential hypertension. Rest 10% have hypertension attributable to a particular cause (secondary hypertension). The incidence of hypertension in children is 1–5% and up to 10% in adolescents. Unlike adults, secondary hypertension is more prevalent (70–80%). Risk factors are age, obesity, family history, high sodium diet, alcohol, etc. In a minority of patients, a specific etiology can be identified and such patients are said to have secondary hypertension. The major etiologies implicated in this category include drugs, renovascular, renal parenchymal, obstructive sleep apnea, endocrine, and neurologic.

CAUSES OF HYPERTENSION

The major causes are:

- Primary
- Secondary
    - Renal—parenchymal, vascular
    - Other vascular—coarctation, steno-occlusive lesion of the aorta.
    - Endocrine—primary aldosteronism, Cushing's syndrome, pheochromocytoma, hypothyroidism, and primary hyperparathyroidism.
    - Drugs—oral contraceptives, nonsteroidal anti-inflammatory drugs (NSAIDs), and antidepressants.
    - CNS disease.

RENOVASCULAR HYPERTENSION

Renovascular hypertension (RVH) is a potentially correctable form of secondary hypertension. It denotes the cause and effect relationship between a renal artery stenosis (RAS) and its clinical sequelae, namely: (1) hypertension or (2) chronic ischemic nephropathy. It is also defined as hypertension that improves or resolves after correction of renal artery stenosis.[3]

Epidemiology

The prevalence of RAS in general population is unknown. It is more prevalent in people younger than 30 years and those older than 60 years of age. The prevalence of RVH among adult hypertensive patients is 1–5%.[4] Approximately 20% have bilateral disease or many a times, a single functional kidney may be affected.[5] About 70–80% of hypertension in children is secondary, out of which 5–25% is attributable to renovascular cause. The incidence of surgically correctable hypertension in children less than 5 years of age is approximately 80%, 40–45% in 6–20 years of age, and 20% in 11–18 years of age.

The prevalence of coronary artery disease, cerebrovascular disease, and peripheral vascular disease in patients with RAS is 67%, 37%, and 56%, respectively. In patients with CAD, the angiographic prevalence of RAS is 30%, of which nearly half of the cases have a stenosis greater than 50%. About 50% of patients with RAS do not have hypertension.[0,7]

Renovascular hypertension is mostly seen in younger women and older men. In young women, Takayasu's arteritis (proximal and distal renal arteries) and fibromuscular dysplasia (FMD) (distal and segmental renal artery) are common etiologies. In older men, atherosclerotic RAS affecting the ostia is common. There is no sex predilection in children.

Natural History

Atherosclerotic RAS is progressive. Risk of progression is highest with high-grade stenosis, severe hypertension, and diabetes. Less than 10% of patients with RAS progress to high-grade stenosis or occlusion within 5 years.[8] RVH in the setting of renal dysfunction is associated with the greatest mortality.

Diagnosing RVH is important because treatment of RAS may cure patient's hypertension. Renal artery stenosis is also an important cause of ischemic nephropathy and end-stage renal disease (ESRD) which can be prevented by early and appropriate intervention.[9] Also in view of the widespread use of angiotensin-converting enzyme (ACE) inhibitors, it is important to exclude the presence of RAS as these agents may precipitate renal failure in the presence of bilateral RAS or stenosis of renal artery in a solitary functioning kidney.

Pathophysiology

Renal artery stenosis causes a decrease in perfusion pressure and glomerular filtration rate (GFR) by decreasing the hydrostatic pressure in the afferent arterioles. The reduction in intrarenal arterial pressure is sensed by the juxtaglomerular apparatus of the afferent arterioles. The renin-angiotensin-aldosterone system is triggered in an attempt to maintain glomerular filtration pressure. Renin secreted by juxtaglomerular apparatus of the kidney, converts plasma angiotensinogen to angiotensin I. This is converted by ACE in the lungs to angiotensin II. Angiotensin II is a potent vasoconstrictor and increases blood pressure by direct effect on arterioles and by stimulating aldosterone secretion leading to salt and water retention. Angiotensin II also causes vasoconstriction of the efferent arterioles in an attempt to restore glomerular filtration to normal. It also leads to vascular and myocardial remodeling.

Flowchart 1 is a schematic diagram of the mechanism of RVH.

In significant unilateral RAS increased levels of angiotensin II causes not only vasoconstriction of afferent arterioles of the affected kidney but also a decrease in GFR and sodium excretion by the contralateral kidney. The normal kidney also demonstrates marked decrease in renin secretion.

FLOWCHART 1: Mechanism of renovascular hypertension.

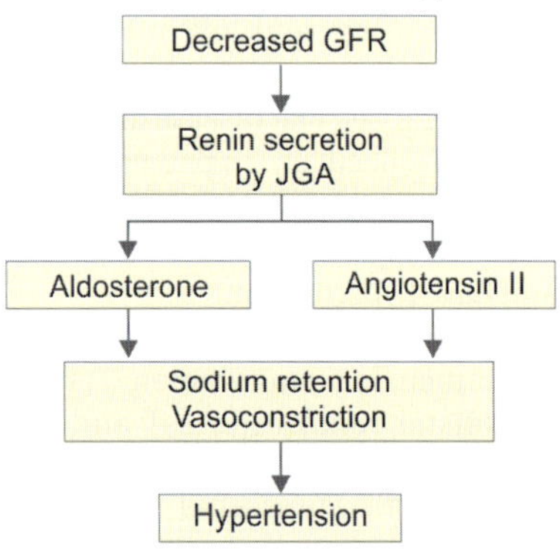

(JGA: juxtaglomerular apparatus; GFR: glomerular filtration rate)

It is called "angiotensin-dependent hypertension". Increased blood pressure ultimately results in pressure natriuresis from the contralateral kidney resulting in the classic "high renin-normal volume" pattern of unilateral RAS.[10]

In patients with bilateral stenosis or a solitary kidney with RAS the entire mass of nephrons is ischemic, resulting in increased renin, excess angiotensin II and aldosterone, which by counter regulatory mechanisms, decrease renin production. Since pressure natriuresis cannot occur from either kidney, there is volume retention. The overall picture in bilateral RAS is a mixed one with both renin and volume factors typically being involved. Because of volume overload these patients are prone to recurrent sudden "flash" pulmonary edema.[10]

Clinical Manifestations of Renovascular Disease

Flowchart 2 shows various clinical manifestations of renovascular disease. The following criteria have been proposed, in the presence of which prevalence of RVH is 20–30% **(Box 1)**.[3,11]

Laboratory tests that may indicate renovascular disease include blood urea nitrogen >20 mg/dL, serum potassium < 3.4 mEq/L, proteinuria, etc.

MAJOR CAUSES OF RENOVASCULAR HYPERTENSION

In the western literature, FMD and midaortic syndrome are the most common causes of RVH, however, in India, Takayasu (61%), FMD (26%), atherosclerosis (8%), polyarteritis nodosa (2.5%), etc. account for most of the cases, as pointed out by Chugh et al.[12]

The various causes of RVH are listed in **Box 2**.

Table 1 depicts most common causes of secondary hypertension by age.

Atherosclerotic Renal Arterial Disease

Atherosclerosis accounts for approximately two-thirds of patients of RAS in the western world. It occurs more commonly in men over the age of 50 years. Obstruction usually results from aortic plaque engulfing the renal ostium (i.e. within 4 mm of aortic lumen). Less frequently plaque develops independently in the proximal third of the renal artery. The stenosis is often circumferential but may be eccentric and is commonly associated with calcification **(Fig. 1)**. Differentiation between proximal and ostial lesions is important because of their different response to angioplasty. Because atherosclerosis is a generalized process both renal

FLOWCHART 2: Clinical manifestations of renal artery stenosis (RAS).

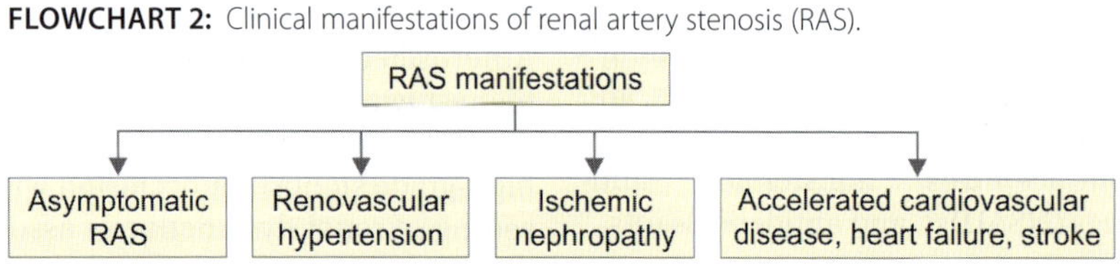

BOX 1: The various clinical criteria for suspecting RAS.

- Abdominal or flank bruit (systolic or diastolic)
- Patients presenting with accelerated/malignant hypertension
- Unilateral small kidney
- Onset of hypertension less than 20 years or more than 50 years of age
- Sudden worsening of renal function in a hypertensive patient
- Impairment of renal function after treatment with an angiotensin-converting enzyme (ACE) inhibitor
- Hypertension uncontrolled by triple-drug therapy
- Patients with hypertension and extensive arterial occlusive disease

TABLE 1: Common causes of secondary hypertension by age.

Age group	Common etiologies
Children (<12 years)	Coarctation of aorta, renovascular hypertension (including congenital renal artery stenosis), midaortic syndrome
Adolescents (12–20 years)	Renal parenchymal disease, renal artery stenosis
Young adults (20–40 years)	Vasculitis causing aortic stenosis (Takayasu's arteritis), renal artery stenosis [Takayasu's arteritis in India, fibromuscular dysplasia (FMD) worldwide], hypothyroidism, coarctation of aorta, renal parenchymal disease
Middle age (40–65 years)	Medication, vasculitis, extrinsic band, aldosteronism, obstructive sleep apnea, renal trauma, dissection, thromboembolism, thyroid dysfunction, pheochromocytoma, Cushing's syndrome
Old age (>65 years)	Atherosclerotic renal artery stenosis, chronic kidney disease (CKD), thromboembolism, dissection, radiation fibrosis, hypothyroidism

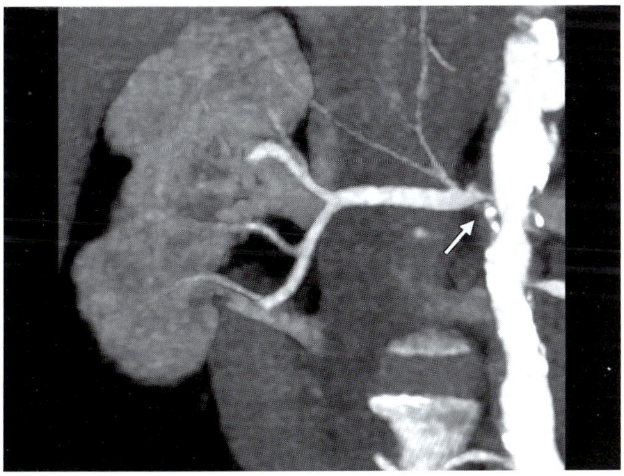

FIG. 1: Computed tomography angiography (CTA) coronal multiplanar reconstruction reveals atherosclerotic renal artery stenosis with calcific plaque at the ostium of the right renal artery (arrow).

BOX 2: Causes of renovascular hypertension.

Renal artery stenosis

- Atherosclerosis
- Nonspecific aortoarteritis/Takayasu's arteritis
- Fibromuscular dysplasia
- Vasculitis
- Dissection
- Thromboembolism
- Coarctation syndrome
- Neurofibromatosis
- Congenital RAS, supravalvular aortic stenosis
- Congenital rubella
- Syphilitic arteritis
- Tuberous sclerosis
- *Extrinsic compression*: Tumor, median arcuate ligament
- Middle aortic syndrome
- Williams syndrome

Other causes of renovascular hypertension

- Aneurysm of renal artery
- Renal artery embolus
- AVM/AVF
- Irradiation
- Renal transplant
- Trauma

(AVM/AVF: arteriovenous malformation/arteriovenous fistula; RAS: renal artery stenosis)

arteries are frequently affected. If atheromatous lesions are left untreated there is a high probability of progression to complete occlusion.[13]

Fibromuscular Dysplasia

Fibromuscular dysplasia has only been recognized for the past 30 years or so but accounts for almost a third of the patients with of RVH according to western literature. It typically occurs in young women. It comprises 10–25% of all etiologies of RAS. It may involve any layer of the artery and is classified as intimal, medial or adventitial.

- *Intimal fibroplasia*: There is concentric accumulation of collagen beneath the internal elastic membrane which causes focal smooth stenosis usually in the midportion of renal artery. It is more common in children and is progressive.
- *Medial dysplasia*: This is the most common type of dysplasia and accounts for approximately 95% cases.
    - *Medial fibroplasia*: This is the most common type of medial dysplasia in which there is replacement of smooth muscle by collagen. These alternate with small areas of dilatation due to aneurysm formation and result in the classic "string of beads" appearance. It is more common in women between 20 years and 50 years of age and is progressive. It usually responds to angioplasty **(Figs. 2A and B)**.

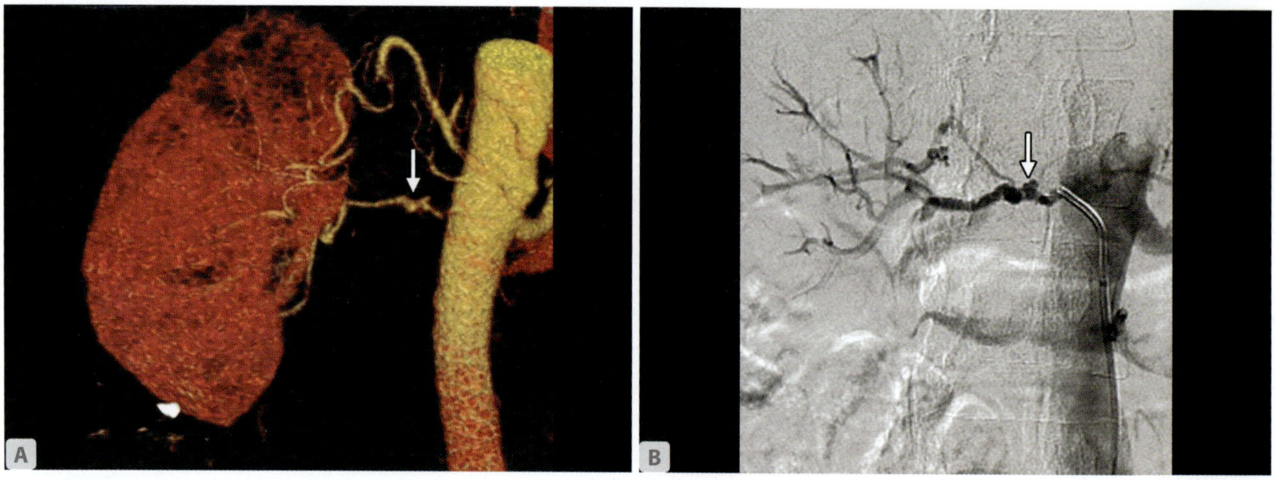

FIGS. 2A AND B: (A) Volume-rendered CTA and (B) DSA reveal multiple tandem stenoses and dilatations (string of beads appearance) in a patient with medial fibroplasia type of FMD (CTA: computed tomography angiography; DSA: digital subtraction angiography; FMD: fibromuscular dysplasia).

- *Perimedial fibroplasia*: Collagen infiltrates outer layer of media. A beaded appearance similar to medial fibroplasia is seen but the "beads" are smaller as aneurysms do not develop.
- *True medial hyperplasia:* Uncommon media is replaced by hyperplastic smooth muscle and fibrous tissue. A tubular smooth narrowing of the vessels is seen on angiography.
- *Medial dissection*: Also uncommon. A new channel is formed in the outer one-third of the media with visualization of a false channel in media on angiography.

- *Adventitial dysplasia*: Collagenous infiltrate surrounds the adventitia, producing a tubular smooth narrowing on the angiogram.

Fibromuscular dysplasia is not confined to renal arteries but is also seen in visceral and peripheral arteries. It also involves the carotid and vertebral arteries, but tends to spare the intracranial vessels. Approximately 30% progressively worsen but total occlusion is rare.

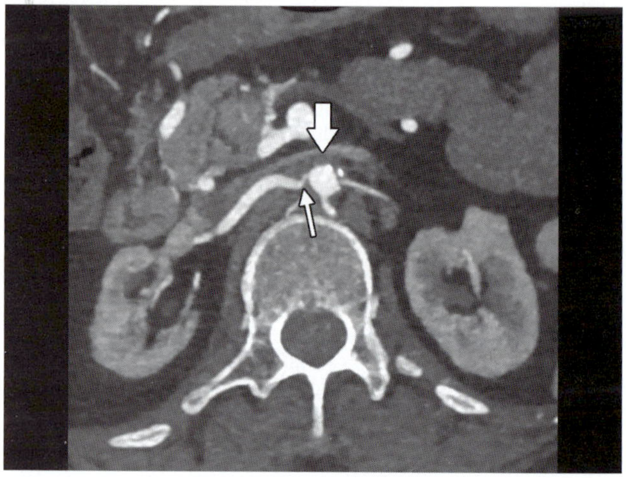

FIG. 3: Axial CTA image shows ostial stenosis of the main renal artery in a patient with Takayasu's arteritis (thin arrow). There is circumferential thickening of the aorta (thick arrow).

Nonspecific Aortoarteritis/Takayasu's Arteritis[14,15]

Nonspecific aortoarteritis, also known as Takayasu's disease is a chronic, idiopathic, granulomatous arteritis that commonly involves the aorta and its major branches and the pulmonary and coronary arteries. The disease tends to affect young females (in second and third) particularly from Southeast Asia and India. Histopathology has shown Takayasu's arteritis to be a granulomatous panarteritis characterized by infiltration of lymphocytes, macrophages and giant cells in the vessel wall. Nonspecific inflammation of the vascular wall leads to progressive adventitial fibrosis, which leads to luminal narrowing and occlusions. In the active stage, the disease is associated with clinical features like fever, carotid tenderness and increased sedimentation rate. Hypertension in Takayasu's disease may be caused by coarctation of aorta or main renal artery stenosis **(Fig. 3)**.

According to a recent classification, it can be classified into six types:[16]

1. *Type I* involves only the aortic arch branches.
2. *Type IIa* involves the ascending aorta, aortic arch, and its branches.
3. *Type IIb* affects ascending aorta, aortic arch, its branches, and descending thoracic aorta.
4. *Type III* involves the descending aorta, abdominal aorta and/or the renal arteries.
5. *Type IV* involves only the abdominal aorta and/or renal arteries.
6. *Type V* has combined features of type IIb and IV.

Type V is the most common pattern. Involvement of the coronary and pulmonary arteries is indicated as C (+) or P (+), respectively.

The morphological pattern of involvement in aortoarteritis shows racial and geographical differences.[17]

In Japan, thoracic aortic involvement is more common and neck vessels are most often involved. In most other Asian countries abdominal aorta is most often affected particularly renal and subclavian arteries. Pulmonary artery involvement is less frequently seen in Indian patients. Steno-occlusive lesions of aorta and renal arteries are the most common type of lesions found in the north Indian population, dilatative lesions are more common in Northeastern parts of India. South Indian population has mainly abdominal vessel involvement.

Other Vasculitis

Polyarteritis nodosa is a necrotizing systemic vasculitis involving medium and small sized arteries. Most cases are idiopathic. It causes approximately 2.5% of the RVH in India. Renal involvement often leads to hypertension and renal insufficiency. Imaging reveals patchy parenchymal infarcts with stenoses, microaneurysms, and post-stenotic dilatations, which can rupture and cause hematomas.

Other vasculitis that can cause RAS are systemic arterial mediolysis, scleroderma, etc.

Congenital Renal Artery Stenosis

Congenital RVH may remain asymptomatic for a long time. The RAS in neurofibromatosis usually involves the ostia and bilateral kidneys. Because of fibrotic nature, they are tough to dilate. Surgery usually shows better results than endovascular management.

Transplant Renal Artery Stenosis

It occurs in the first 6 months after renal transplant and cause graft failure or premature death in transplant recipients **(Fig. 4)**. It accounts for 1–5% cases of post-transplant hypertension. Flash pulmonary edemas can develop and is called pickering syndrome. It usually occurs at the ostium/anastomotic site as well at the external iliac artery where RA is anastomosed. It is a potentially treatable condition, usually respond to balloon dilatation. Contralateral femoral access is preferred.

Aortorenal Dissection

Dissection in renal artery, either isolated **(Fig. 5)** or that extending form concomitant aortic dissection can also cause RVH. Spontaneous RA dissection can be seen in connective tissue disorders. Therapeutic options include conservative management and revascularization. It is more frequent in middle-aged male patients.

SCREENING FOR RENOVASCULAR HYPERTENSION

Hypertension is common but RVH is not, therefore, screening should be reserved for patients at moderate-to-high risk for RVH.

Indications for Testing for Renovascular Hypertension[11,18,19]

The 2013 American College of Cardiology/American Heart Association (ACC/AHA) and 2017 European Society of Cardiology (ESC) guidelines recommend performing diagnostic studies to identify RAS in patients with any of the following (They have high likelihood of benefitting from the procedure):

1. Onset of hypertension before the age of 30 years or after age of 55 years (level of evidence, LOE-B).
2. Accelerated hypertension (sudden and persistent worsening of previously controlled hypertension) (LOE-C).
3. Resistant hypertension (failure to achieve goal BP in patients adhering to full doses of a 3-drug regimen that includes a diuretic).
4. Malignant hypertension (hypertension with coexistent end-organ damage, i.e. acute kidney injury (AKI), flash pulmonary edema, LVF, aortic dissection, new visual or neurological disturbance, and/or advanced retinopathy).

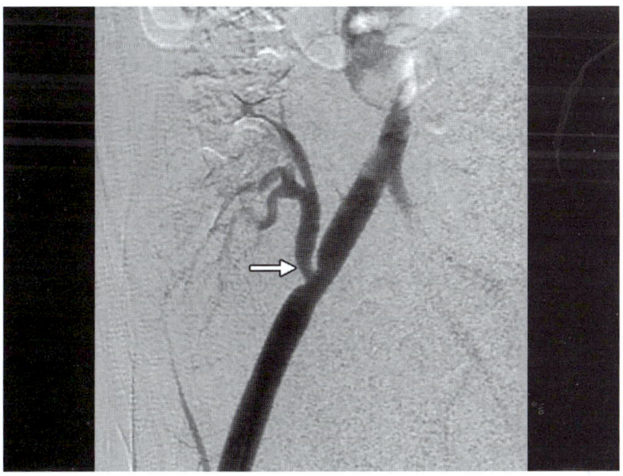

FIG. 4: Transplant renal artery stenosis: Digital subtraction angiography shows narrowing of the ostioproximal segment (arrow) of the renal artery from right external iliac artery.

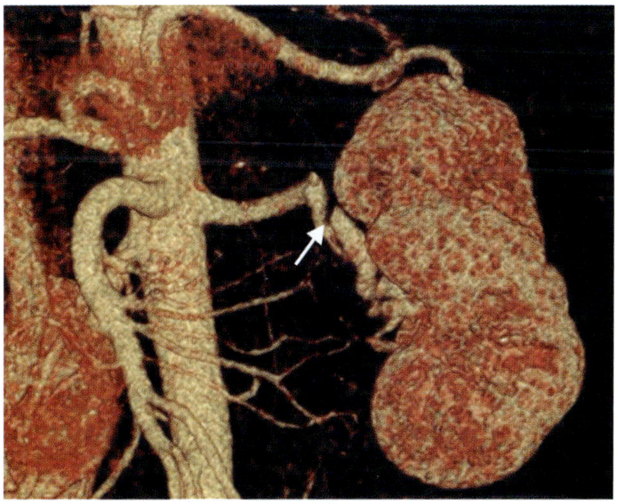

FIG. 5: Volume rendered CTA image shows isolated renal artery dissection in left main renal artery (arrow).

5. New azotemia or worsening renal function (>30% creatinine) after the administration of an ACE inhibitor or an ARB (LOE-B).
6. Unexplained atrophic kidney or size discrepancy of >1.5 cm between the kidneys (LOE-B).
7. Unexplained congestive heart failure or refractory angina (LOE-C).

The above clinical features suggest a cause of secondary hypertension rather than primary hypertension. Additionally, testing for renovascular disease is prudent if:

- Other causes of secondary hypertension such as primary kidney disease, primary aldosteronism, or pheochromocytoma, have been excluded.
- An intervention can be planned if a significant stenotic lesion is found.

Testing should not be performed if there is:

- Moderate or low likelihood of having clinically significant renovascular disease (This is because the RCTs comparing percutaneous revascularization with medical therapy primarily consisted of patients with moderate and low likelihood of clinically important renovascular disease; during 3–5 years of follow-up, they showed no evidence of benefit from adding revascularization to optimal medical therapy), or;
- In those who respond well to medical therapy.

There is no perfect screening test for the detection of RVH. The situation is further complicated by the fact that the presence of RAS may not always indicate a causal relationship. Not every RAS leads to RVH and patients with essential hypertension may also develop RAS. The degree of stenosis that causes RVH has not been established although most investigators treat stenosis measuring 50% or greater.[20] Also, there are potential risks in testing for RVH, especially in patients with impaired renal function, which include contrast-induced nephropathy and nephrogenic systemic fibrosis.

Physiologically, RAS is defined as inadequate renal blood flow leading to reduction in GFR and loss of renal parenchyma, hence it becomes prudent to establish the functional significance of RAS before proceeding to revascularization.[21]

DIAGNOSTIC MODALITIES

Clinical and Biochemical Tests

Clinical/nonradiological tests that have been used for the diagnosis of RVH include: Plasma renin activity, ACE inhibitor challenge test, aspirin challenge test and 24 hours ambulatory blood pressure monitoring.

Imaging Modalities for Assessment of Renal Artery Stenosis

In patients with clinical suspicion of RAS, noninvasive screening is required to select patients for conventional angiography and renal revascularization.[22]

An ideal renal artery imaging study should answer the following questions:[23]

- Localization and number of arteries.
- Characterization of renal stenosis, including etiology of stenosis, localization, and post-stenotic dilatation.
- Hemodynamic and functional significance of the stenosis.
- Further pathologies or variants that might have an influence on treatment planning.

The useful diagnostic tools are:

- *Noninvasive*:
  - Ultrasound/Doppler/contrast US
  - Computed tomography (CT)
  - Magnetic resonance imaging (MRI)
  - Intravascular ultrasound (IVUS)
  - Any other [nuclear imaging, optical coherence tomography (OCT)]

Invasive: Arteriography

Table 2 shows the strength of recommendations for using these tests for detection of RAS.[19]

Ultrasound and Color Doppler

A normal appearance of the kidneys on ultrasound does not exclude a significant unilateral or bilateral renal artery stenosis. Renal size and shape may be normal unless the stenosis is greater than 60% when a small decrease in size may be found.[24]

Brief Anatomy of Renal Arteries

Renal arteries arise from aorta just below the level of superior mesenteric artery, usually at L1-L2 level. There can be one or more accessory renal arteries. Stenoses in accessory renal arteries can also cause RVH. Anterior to each renal artery runs the renal vein on each side. The right renal artery has a longer course due to downward location of the right kidney. Double main renal arteries and accessory renal arteries occur in nearly 12–22% of patients.

Doppler USG is first-line imaging modality for assessment of RAS.

Advantages of Doppler ultrasound:

- Widely available
- Inexpensive
- Good sensitivity and specificity for detection of RAS.

TABLE 2: Tests for detection of RAS.

Recommendation	Class	Level
Duplex ultrasonography, computed tomography angiography (CTA) [in patients with estimated glomerular filtration rate (eGFR) >60 mL/min] and magnetic resonance angiography (MRA) (in patients with eGFR >30 mL/min) are recommended as screening tests	I	B
When the clinical index of suspicion is high and the results of the noninvasive tests are inconclusive, catheter angiography is recommended as a diagnostic test	IIB	C
Captopril renal scintigraphy, selective renal vein renin measurements and plasma renin activity are not recommended as a useful screening test	III	C

- It can be repeated to assess stenosis progression
- To exclude an obvious structural abnormality or coexistent condition.

Disadvantages of Doppler ultrasound:
- It remains operator dependent and time consuming
- It can overestimate the degree of stenosis.

Information provided by a duplex USG for assessment of severity and suitability for revascularization are:
- *Size of kidneys*: Shrunken kidneys with size <7 cm have lower chance of improvement with revascularization as kidney sizes decrease after setting in of CKD **(Figs. 6A and B)**.
- *Parenchymal cortical thickness*: Cortical thickness of at least 1 cm is necessary for considering revascularization.
- *Echogenicity*: Increased echogenicity and loss of corticomedullary differentiation are findings of CKD, and such kidneys should not be revascularized as there are minimal chances of improvement.
- Direct evaluation of the renal arteries as well as transrenal Doppler waveform analysis (as discussed below).

Two approaches are used with Doppler ultrasound. The first is the direct visualization and interrogation of the stenotic segment of the renal artery. The second is an assessment of the arterial waveform distal to the stenosis within segmental renal vessels **(Fig. 7)**.

Direct Approach

This requires evaluation of the entire main renal artery, spectral traces are then obtained from areas of stenosis identified on color Doppler. The aorta is also interrogated and peak systolic velocity (PSV) obtained at the level of renal origins. An anterior or anterolateral approach usually allows insonation of both the arteries. A coronal approach can be used when bowel gas is present. The criteria used to diagnose significant stenosis or occlusion of a renal artery is as follows:[3,25]

- An increase in PSV (thresholds commonly applied in current literature to diagnose RAS include PSV (max) in the renal artery >180 cm/ sec **(Figs. 8A and B)**.
- Renal artery/aortic ratio (RAR ratio) > 3.5 calculated as:

$$\frac{\text{PSV (max) renal arteries}}{\text{PSV aorta at the origin of renal arteries}}$$

- Turbulent flow in the post-stenotic area
- Visualization of the renal artery without detectable Doppler signal, a finding that indicates occlusion.

As main renal arteries may not be visualized in up to 42% cases, in practice, these measurements often cannot be obtained. The procedure is time consuming and operator dependent. Accessory renal arteries and branch artery stenosis cannot be diagnosed. In cases of renal artery occlusion collaterals may be sampled.

Indirect Approach

Arterial waveforms from the segmental renal arteries from the upper, mid, and lower poles are evaluated. The normal

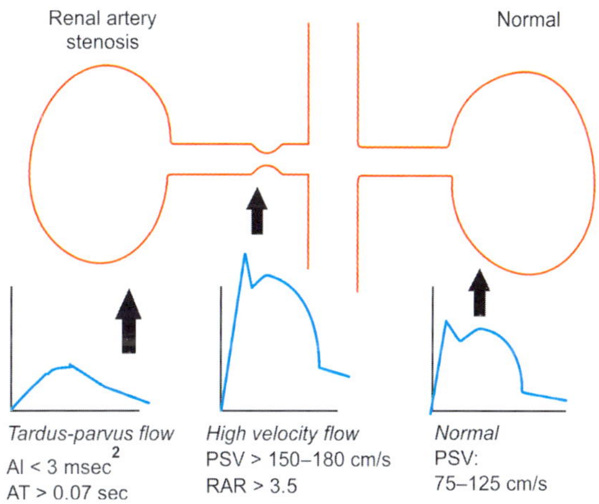

FIG. 7: Schematic diagram of the renal artery Doppler tracings showing the normal renal artery trace on the left side. On the right side high velocity at the site of stenosis and "tardus-parvus" waveform is seen distal to the stenosis (PSV: peak systolic velocity; RAR: renal-aortic ratio; AI: acceleration index; AT: acceleration time).

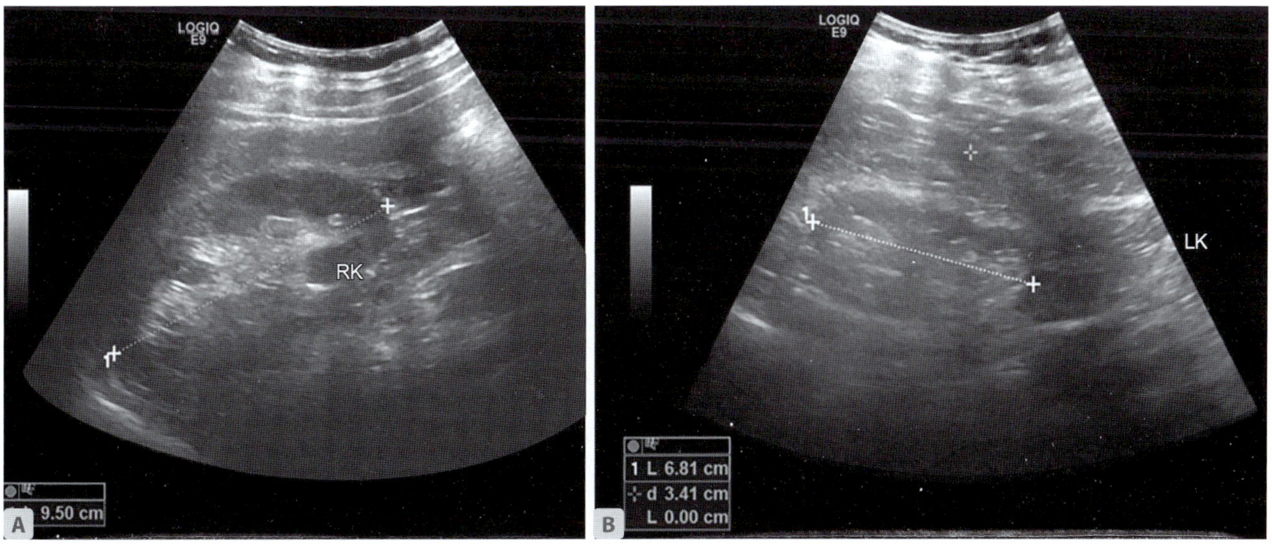

FIGS. 6A AND B: Grayscale ultrasound images show. (A) a normal-sized kidney, and (B) a shrunken kidney.

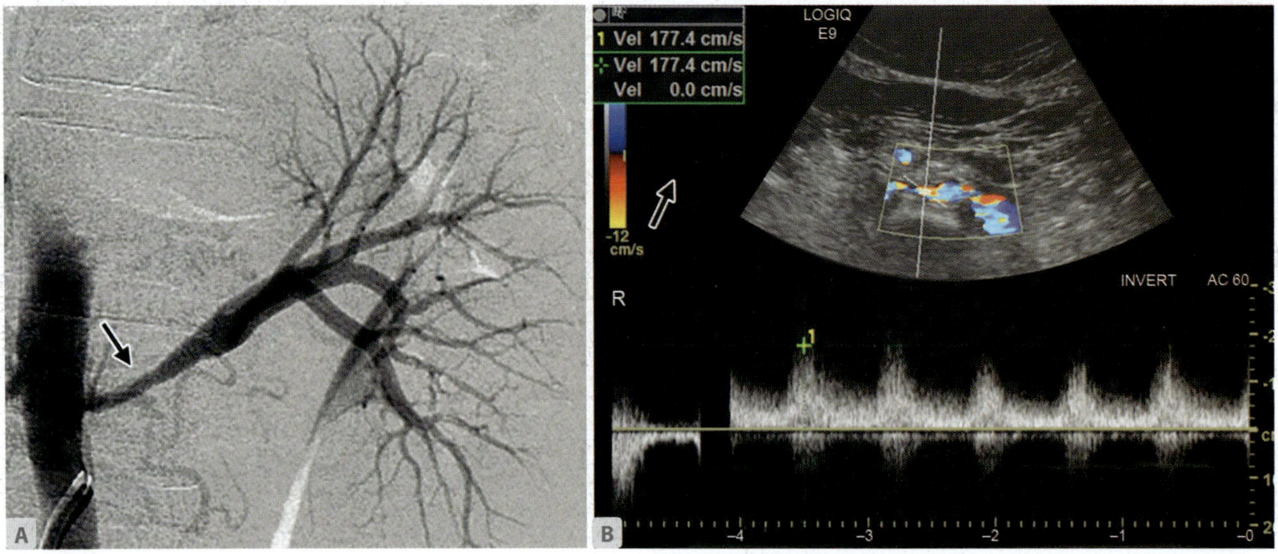

FIGS. 8A AND B: Digital subtraction angiography. (A) Frame reveals stenosis in proximal left renal artery (arrow); (B) Spectral trace with high peak systolic velocity (PSV >180 cm/s) at the site of stenosis.

waveform from these vessels shows a steep systolic upstroke with a peak in early systole referred to as early systolic peak (ESP). The early systolic acceleration seems to be the best predictor of RAS and should be measures along the initial portion of the systolic rise and should not include the late compliance peak.[26] The waveform in patients with RAS lacks both these features and is known as "tardus-parvus" waveform. Tardus refers to the slowed systolic acceleration and parvus refers to the low amplitude of the systolic peak **(Fig. 9)**.

There are two quantitative measurements that are used: (1) the acceleration time (AT) and (2) the acceleration index (AI). AT is the time from start of systole to peak systole. AI is the slope of the systolic upstroke.

Findings suggestive of significant RAS are:

- Parvus-tardus waveform
- Acceleration time greater than 0.07 sec.
- Acceleration index reduced to less than 3 m/s^2.
- Change in resistive index (RI) of greater than 5% between the right and left kidneys (RI and pulsatility index decrease).

Some authors have shown that simple pattern recognition of "tardus-parvus" waveform is more accurate than calculation of "AT" and "AI".[27] The waveform may also demonstrate a decrease in RI and pulsatility index.[28] Administration of captopril in individuals with significant RAS produces measurable changes in Doppler waveform which increases the degree of pulsus tardus and decreases the RI.[29]

These criteria only detect stenosis of greater than 70–90% reliably. A positive test is more informative than a negative test. The shape of the waveform is not simply related to the pressure drop across the stenosis but also compliance of renal arteries.[37] Coexisting parenchymal disease may also affect the waveform due to changes in peripheral resistance. The technique also cannot distinguish between high-grade stenosis and complete occlusion with collateral flow. Tardus-parvus waveform may also be produced by abdominal coarctation.[30]

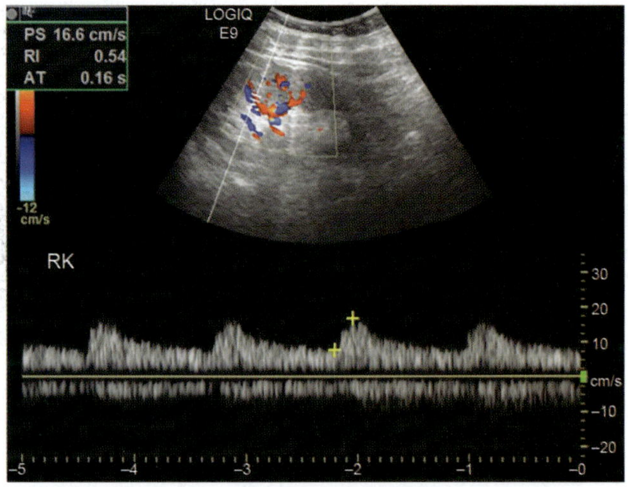

FIG. 9: Color Doppler image showing tardus-parvus waveform in intralobar artery due to main renal artery stenosis.

A meta-analysis of 88 studies including 9,974 arteries assessed the accuracy of each of these parameters and found that PSV, with a sensitivity and specificity of 85% and 92%, respectively, was more accurate than the renal aortic ratio and acceleration index.[31]

Use of Resistive Index [Ratio of (PSV–EDV) to PSV]

Normal values are 0.6–0.7. RI may also be used to predict the outcome of therapy for RAS.[32] A "RI" of more than 80 probably identifies patient with RAS in whom angioplasty or surgery will not improve renal function or blood pressure because of greater intrinsic renal damage. Other than parenchyma, RI can also be regarded as a marker of systemic vascular properties. A low (<6) RRI can reflect (in addition to RAS greater than 70%), valvular aortic stenosis, thoracic or suprarenal abdominal aortic stenosis, hypervolemia, tachycardia, and parasympathetic activation (extrarenal determinants). High RRI (>7) can reflect arteriolosclerosis, vasoconstriction, increased interstitial, and venous pressure (intrarenal determinants) or increased systemic pulse pressure, adrenergic hyperactivity, and bradycardia (extrarenal determinants).

Contrast-enhanced Ultrasound

Renal contrast-enhanced ultrasound (CEUS) is a newer method for detecting RAS noninvasively and some studies have shown it to be superior than routine duplex sonography for the same.[33] The common ultrasound contrast agents are microbubbles stabilized using sugar, albumin, lipids, or polymers. Microbubbles are smaller than 10 µm in diameter and are effective and safe agents. The most widely used agent is Levovist. It has been found to enhance the visualization of main renal vessels resulting in higher technical success rates.[34] It can be used in cases in which usual duplex Doppler is nondiagnostic or suboptimal.[35]

Computed Tomography Angiography

Computed tomography angiography (CTA) offers a noninvasive technique for obtaining angiographic images. The advent of spiral CT and more recently multidetector computed tomography (MDCT) has revolutionized CT and CTA. MDCT has made possible the acquisition of isotropic data with high spatial and temporal resolution in shorter scan times. With current generation scanners, the data can be acquired within a few seconds. We, at our institute, use a 384 slice dual source CT scanner. The protocol that we follow is as follows:

- *Arterial phase scan (including diaphragm to iliac arteries to cover potential accessory renal arteries):* The thinnest collimation is used (0.75 mm). A contrast volume of 1 mL/kg (350 mg I/mL) is injected IV at 4–6 mL/sec followed by a 20–30 mL saline chase. No oral contrast is given. Bolus tracking techniques is used to trigger the scan with ROI in the region of abdominal aorta, with trigger threshold of 100 HU.
- *Parenchymal phase scan:* Three minutes after contrast injection, only kidneys are included in scan, low-dose protocol. This scan helps in identifying the areas of hypoperfusion/infarcts and corticomedullary thicknesses.

The axial images are reconstructed in multiple planes using multiplanar reconstruction (MPR), maximum intensity projection (MIP) or real-time volume rendering techniques (VRTs) for morphological evaluation of kidneys and main renal arteries **(Figs. 10A to C)**.

The sensitivity of CTA in identifying main renal arteries has been 100%; accessory arteries are also almost always detected with any area of narrowing. The sensitivity and specificity for diagnosis of RAS has ranged between 90% and 95%.[36]

CTA is highly accurate for imaging renovascular disease due to atherosclerosis but less so for fibromuscular disease (as it involves distal arteries difficult to image).

Advantages of CTA:

- CTA can demonstrate the wall of the aorta unlike angiography which only visualizes the lumen of the vessel, important in cases of atherosclerosis and also aortoarteritis **(*see* Fig. 3)**, where the lumen may appear angiographically normal in places but may show vessel wall involvement in cross-sectional studies.
- It demonstrates the extent of plaque projecting into the vessel lumen, aiding in determining the form of intervention planned such as angioplasty versus primary stent placement.
- It has high efficacy for diagnosis of ostial stenosis.
- MDCT/CTA can also detect collaterals as well as stenoses in accessory renal arteries with great accuracy **(Figs. 11A and B)**.

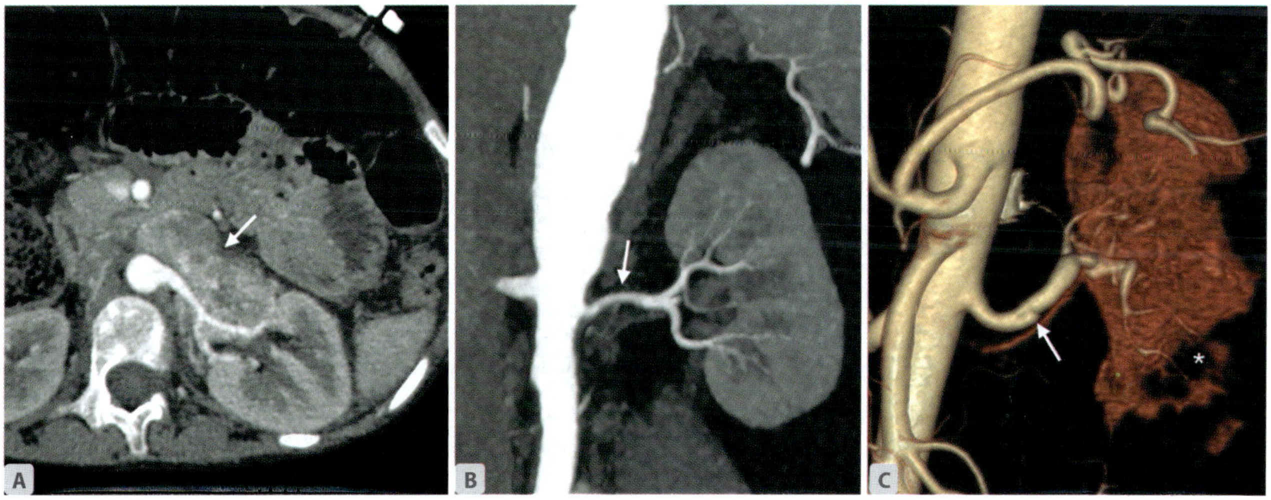

FIGS. 10A TO C: Applications of different CTA postprocessing in identifying etiologies of RVH. (A) Axial MPR shows narrowing of the main renal artery due to mass (arrow) at the perihilar region (RVH due to extrinsic compression); (B) MIP coronal image in a patient with Takayasu's arteritis shows mild stenosis (arrow) in mid left renal artery; (C) VRT image reveals left renal artery dissection (arrow) with resultant parenchymal infarcts (star) (CTA: computed tomography angiography; MIP: maximum intensity projection; MPR: multiplanar reconstruction; RVH: renovascular hypertension; VRT: volume rendering technique).

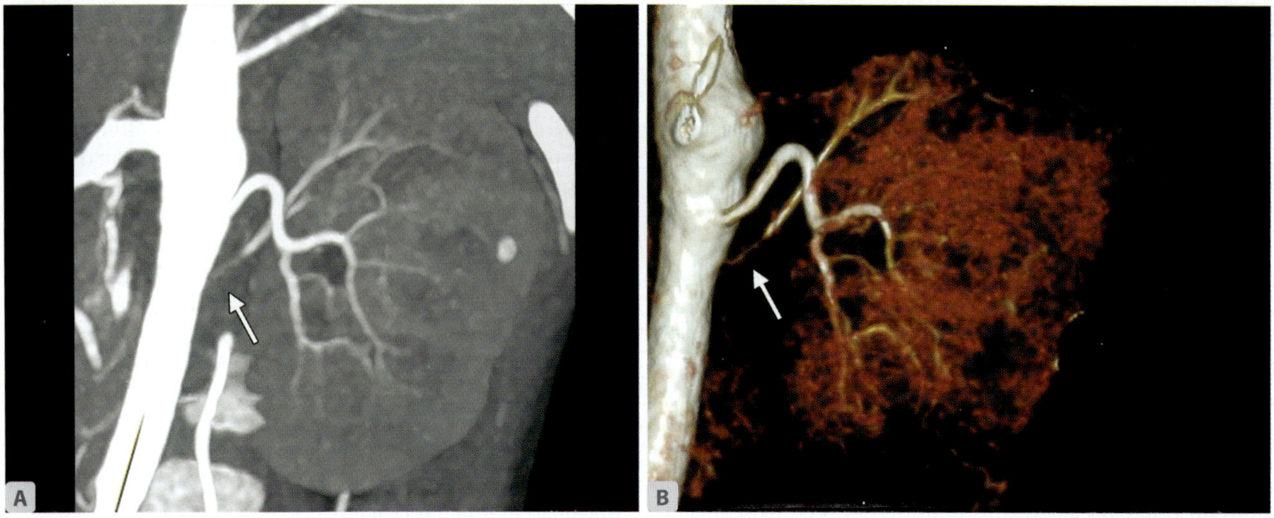

FIGS. 11A AND B: CTA MIP. (A) MPR and (B) VRT image reveal tight stenosis (arrow) of the lower accessory renal artery supplying upper pole of the left kidney.

- Unlike magnetic resonance angiography (MRA), CTA can also be used to examine the patency of vessels that have been dilated by intravascular stents.

Disadvantages of CTA:
- Relatively high cost
- Use of large amount of iodinated contrast medium precluding its use in renal insufficiency.
- Mural calcification in the aorta or renal artery may result in overestimation of stenosis.

Magnetic Resonance Angiography

After published reports of nephrogenic systemic fibrosis (NSF) following gadolinium-based contrast agent in patients with deranged renal functions, contrast-enhanced MRI as a screening test is being avoided.[37] It is of great importance that radiologists be aware of this serious disease and exercise caution when considering the use of gadolinium-based contrast media in patients with moderate (GFR <60 mL/min/1.73 m^2) to severe (GFR <15 mL/min/1.73 m^2) renal disease. In this situation various other MR techniques which can assess renal arterial morphology, perform functional measurements of arterial flow and parenchyma perfusion without the administration of gadolinium are being investigated and found useful in patients with deranged renal functions. These techniques are noncontrast studies such as time-of-flight (TOF), phase contrast (PC), steady-state free precession (SSFP), and arterial spin labeling (ASL).[37] These advancements explain why renal MRI is evolving as the first-line imaging modality for the evaluation of renovascular disease.

Most series have shown excellent correlation between conventional angiography and MRA (sensitivity > 99% and specificity >96%) for detection of RAS 50% or greater in diameter.

Contrast-enhanced MRA

Recent advances in the magnetic resonance gradient hardware with availability of 3.0 T, acquisition of isotropic data with submillimeter resolution is allowing the detection of renal artery narrowing with high sensitivities (94–97%) and specificities (85–93%). Moreover, it is now possible to demonstrate the functional consequences of RAS, such as a decline in renal perfusion and glomerular filtration.[38]

Intravenous gadolinium is used in a dose of 0.1–0.3 mmol/kg with bolus tracking. With the advent of 3.0 T, the amount of contrast can be reduced because of increase in T1 of tissue. Entire acquisition is performed during a single-breath hold. In patients unable to withhold breath for long-time parallel imaging technology provides high-resolution images with shorter acquisition times. Three-dimensional (3D) contrast MRA overcomes the limitations of noncontrast MRA. As a result, renal arteries are assessed in their entirety, including the major segmental branch vessels, as well as small accessory renal arteries **(Figs. 12A and B)**. In addition, speed, operator independence, high spatial and contrast resolution, and lack of side effects have contributed to making 3D contrast MRA a well-suited screening alterative for detection of renovascular disease. The technique has sensitivities of 93–100% and a specificity of 90–100%.

In several centers, contrast-enhanced MRA is complemented by 3D-PC acquisition. Areas of hemodynamically significant stenosis are detected by their associated turbulence seen as a signal void on 3D-PC images. The presence of a signal void at or immediately downstream from a stenosis suggests pressure drop across the stenosis. For 3D-PC MRA to be optimally sensitive to turbulent flow echo time should be approximately 8 ms and velocity encoded value (VENC) should be kept at 25–50 cm/sec.

Advantages of MRA:
- Absence of ionizing radiation.
- Production of 3D arteriogram not affected by calcific plaques.
- Phase contrast studies can provide information about blood flow velocity also (as phase is related to time).
- Multiplanar reconstructions.
- Evaluation of renal masses and renal excretion function.

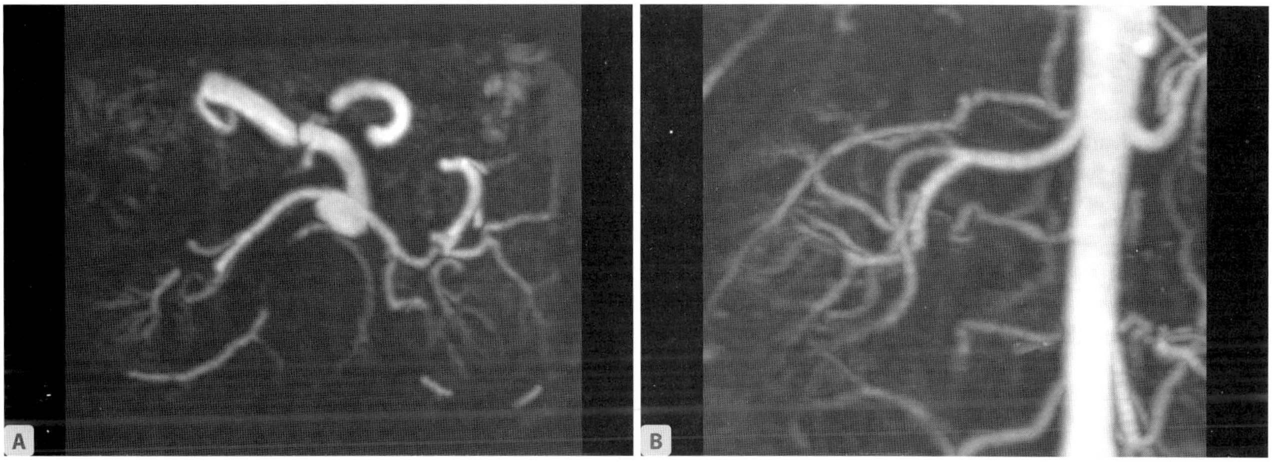

FIGS. 12A AND B: (A) 3D CE-MRA axial and (B) coronal section reveal the anatomy of main renal artery as well as segmental branches in great details (3D CE-MRA: three-dimensional contrast-enhanced magnetic resonance angiography).

Drawbacks of MRA:

- High cost
- Limited availability
- Artifacts due to bowel peristalsis.
- Evaluation of branch vessels and detection of accessory arteries are a challenge.
- Tendency toward overestimation of stenosis.
- The presence of a metallic stent also hampers evaluation.

The MRI is also being evaluated in acquiring the functional data that can provide comprehensive assessment of renal morphology and renal function prior to any intervention.[39]

Dynamic contrast-enhanced (DCE) MRI is a technique in which fast repetitious imaging of the kidney is performed using first pass of the contrast agent. In a series, significant correlations between raising serum creatinine levels and decreasing renal perfusion parameters are found indicating that renal first pass perfusion may reflect, at least to a certain degree of renal function.[40] The DCE-MRI can evaluate the kidneys after the placement of stents which otherwise cannot be assessed due to susceptibility artifacts. In such situations, demonstration of normal perfusion parameters proves the patency of stent.

Noncontrast-enhanced MRI of the Renal Arteries[37]

Various noncontrast MRA techniques have evaluated such as TOF, PC, SSFP, and ASL **(Fig. 13)**.

- *Time-of-flight MRA:* Signal in TOF MRA is produced by unsaturated blood flowing into the plane of imaging (flow related enhancement). TOF MRA is not an useful technique for the evaluation of renal arteries because of the following reasons:
  - It tends to overestimate the degree of stenosis, in particular 2D techniques do not compensate for vessel tortuosity and therefore, tend to overestimate vessels stenosis.
  - Loss of signal in slow flow when vessel is oriented in axial plane (in-plane saturation).
  - Inherently a slow technique requiring several minutes, causing breathing related degradation or extremely long scan times for signal averaging.

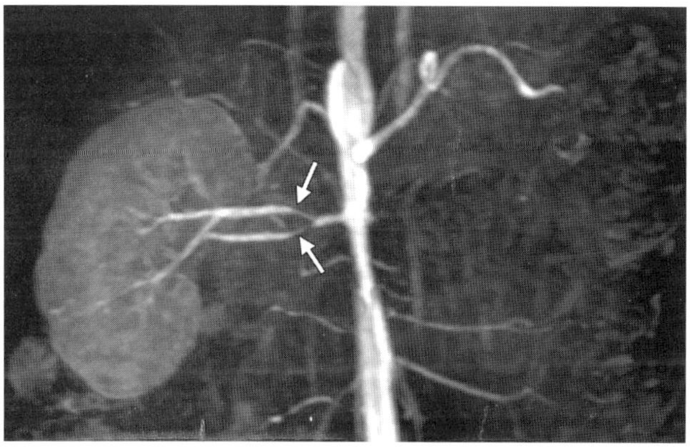

FIG. 13: Noncontrast MRA (SSFP) reveals stenosis (arrows) in both upper and lower division of the right renal artery in a patient with Takayasu's arteritis (MRA: magnetic resonance angiography; SSFP: steady-state free precession).

  - Poor visualization of the distal arterial segment where flow is slow.
- *Phase-contrast MRA*: It depicts not only the morphologic nature of a stenosis, but also provides quantitative analysis of flow dynamics in RAS. Combining PC with cardiac gating, a 2D velocity map can be obtained, which is termed as "quantitative" or "q" flow. With this flow maps similar to Doppler ultrasound can be generated and analyzed.
- *Steady-state free precession MRA*: 3D SSFP with short echo and repetition times is the most promising noncontrast bright blood technique for evaluation of renal arteries as it is intrinsically fast, high in signal-to-noise ratio (SNR), and flow compensated in all the three axis. SSFP, either breath-hold or navigator-gated can be performed as a first-line MRA technique to rule out RAS especially in patients in risk of NSF. If SSFP is negative for high-grade RAS (>50%), RAS can be excluded without using any gadolinium-based contrast agents, vice-a-versa if SSFP is positive, then further studies [contrast-enhanced MRI,

digital subtraction angiography (DSA), CTA] can be done for better delineation of stenosis.
- *Arterial spin labeling*: Arterial spin labeling uses blood as an endogenous contrast agent to obtain angiograms with an advantage to obtain tissue perfusion as well. The perfusion parameters are being investigated and initial reports suggest a good correlation with scintigraphy.

Renal Angiography

Conventional angiography (or DSA) is the gold standard for diagnosis of RAS. However, its invasiveness prevents it from becoming a screening test. All patients proceeding to percutaneous treatment of RAS initially undergo diagnostic angiography as part of the procedure.

Angiographic evaluation should include aortography and bilateral selective renal arteriography. The initial aortogram is necessary to evaluate the renal artery ostia, identifying accessory renal arteries, and avoid mistaking guidewire-induced arterial spasm for fixed disease.

Flush aortography is usually adequate to demonstrate main renal arteries and any proximal renal stenosis **(Fig. 14)**. When intrarenal or branch artery stenosis are suspected selective injections are necessary. Because the origin of right renal artery is anterolateral and left renal artery is posterolateral, an ostial lesion may be missed on an AP aortogram due to overlap by the opacified aorta, superimposition of intrarenal vessels may also mask stenosis. Depending on the site of stenosis oblique/lateral view, cranial/caudal angulation or magnification views may be required to optimally delineate stenosis.[41]

Society for Cardiovascular Angiography and Interventions (SCAI) recommends DSA as the gold standard for invasive assessment of hemodynamically significant RAS and categorizes stenosis severity as follows:
- *Mild*: <50%
- *Moderate*: 50–70%
- *Severe*: >70%—hemodynamically significant **(Fig. 15)**

Other criteria for hemodynamic significance are:
- Systolic pressure gradient >20 mm Hg across the stenosis.
- Evidence of collateral circulation into distal vessel.
- Poststenotic dilatation
- Renal fractional flow reserve (FFR) ≤0.8.

Pressure gradients are the most accurate indicator of hemodynamic significance.

Advantages of conventional angiography/DSA:
- High resolution of the technique.
- Visualizing branch renal artery stenosis.
- Pressure gradients can be measured to assess hemodynamic significance.
- Selective renal catheterization may be followed by appropriate intervention in the same sitting.
- Allows for evaluation of collaterals and intrarenal vasculature with high accuracy **(Fig. 16)**.

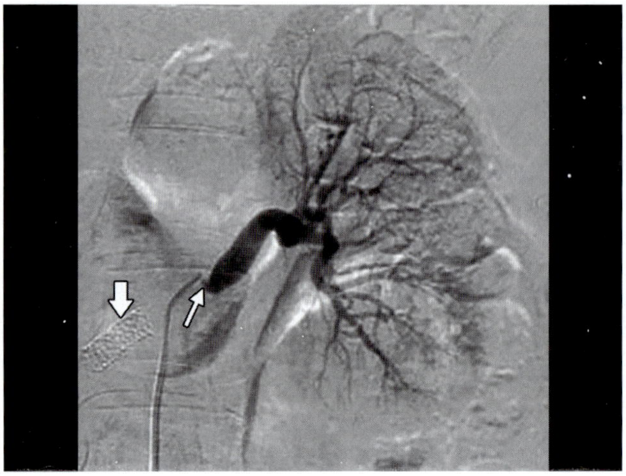

FIG. 15: Selective angiogram of left renal artery shows approximately 90% ostioproximal stenosis (thin arrow) of the left renal artery and poststenotic dilatation in a patient with atherosclerosis. Stenting (thick arrow) had previously been done for contralateral renal artery.

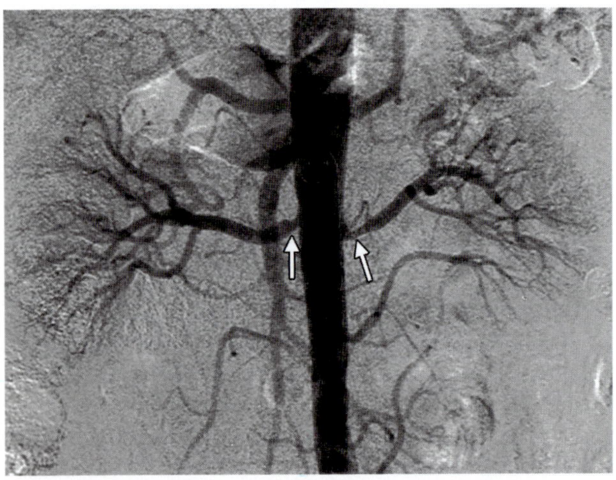

FIG. 14: Digital subtraction angiography flush aortography demonstrates bilateral proximal renal artery stenoses (RAS) in a patient with atherosclerotic RAS.

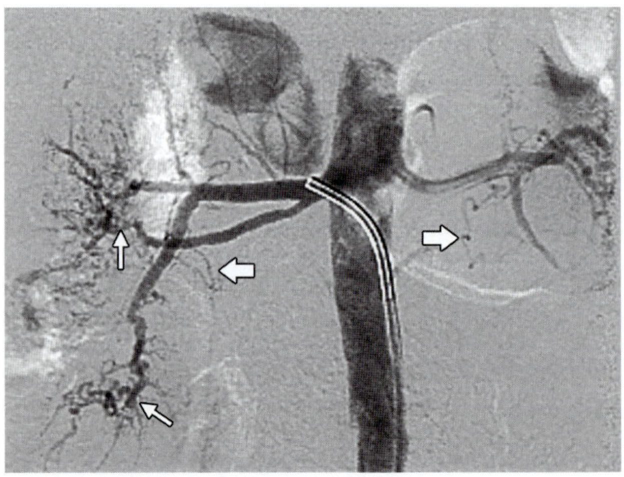

FIG. 16: Digital subtraction angiography reveals diffuse irregularities and stenoses (thin arrow) in the intrarenal vessels with multiple collaterals (thick arrows) in a patient with vasculitis.

Limitations of arteriography:
- Expensive
- Invasive
- Use of iodinated contrast
- Angiography only provides intraluminal information; no intramural information is gained about the vessel wall or plaques.
- Transient decrease in renal function may occur in up to 5% patients.
- Access site complications, RA dissection, thromboembolism.

Flowchart 3 demonstrates the diagnostic algorithm commonly followed for RVH.

Table 3 demonstrates the imaging findings in various common etiologies of RVH.

FLOWCHART 3: Diagnostic algorithm for RVH.

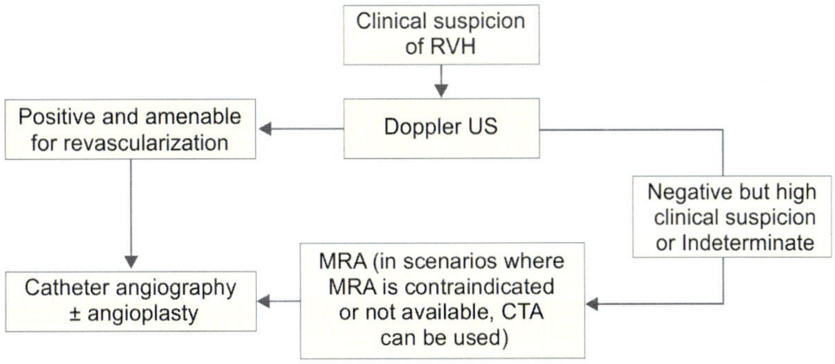

TABLE 3: Imaging findings in various common etiologies of renovascular hypertension (RVH).

Etiology	CTA	MRA	DSA
Atherosclerosis **(Figs. 1, 14, and 16)**	• Focal/segmental, eccentric stenosis • *Location*: Ostium or proximal 2 cm of RA • Bilateral disease is common • Calcifications • Infrarenal aortic involvement usually exist • Coronary, carotid involvement seen	• Limited role as calcification may cause artifacts • Same findings as CTA except that calcifications not well seen	• Irregular circumferential or eccentric narrowing of the ostium or proximal third of the renal arteries • Calcification visible • Intrarenal vessels usually not involved • Collaterals can be seen
Aortoarteritis **(Figs. 17 and 18)**	• Mural thickening of aorta, aortic arch branches and other involved vessels • Better for ostial ostioproximal involvement • Steno-occlusive or dilatative lesions depending on the type • Delayed enhancement of the vessel wall suggests active disease • Calcification sets in when there is accelerated atherosclerosis	• Useful tool • Whole body 3D MRA can reveal other vascular involvement • 3D space—can reveal wall thickening • T2 hyperintensity in wall—sensitive marker for active disease	• Involves aorta, its major branches and PAs—mainly ostioproximal segments • Intrarenal vessels may be involved • Midsegment involvement better seen
FMD **(Fig. 2)**	• Focal concentric narrowing of distal two-thirds main RA and intrarenal branches • The right kidney is affected more commonly than the left • Bilateral disease may be seen in about two-thirds of cases • Aorta is usually disease free • Calcification uncommon	• MR usually less useful as it is not an optimal modality for evaluation of distal vessels. Intrarenal stenoses can be missed • Sensitivities of only 22–28% have been noted with MRA and CTA in this setting	• Middle to distal renal arteries • Less commonly intrarenal branches • Often, poststenotic dilatation • The classic appearance of the medial fibroplasia type—String of beads. • Aneurysms can be seen
PAN **(Figs. 19A and B)**	• Vessel stenoses (renal, mesenteric, peripheral arteries) • Microaneurysms • Intra-abdominal organ infarcts, and/or bowel thickening	Not much helpful due to artifacts due to peristalsis	• Stenoses • Microaneurysms • Infarcts • In abdominal aortic branches

(CTA: computed tomography angiography; DSA: digital subtraction angiography; FMD: fibromuscular dysplasia; MRA: magnetic resonance angiography; PAN: polyarteritis nodosa RA: renal artery)

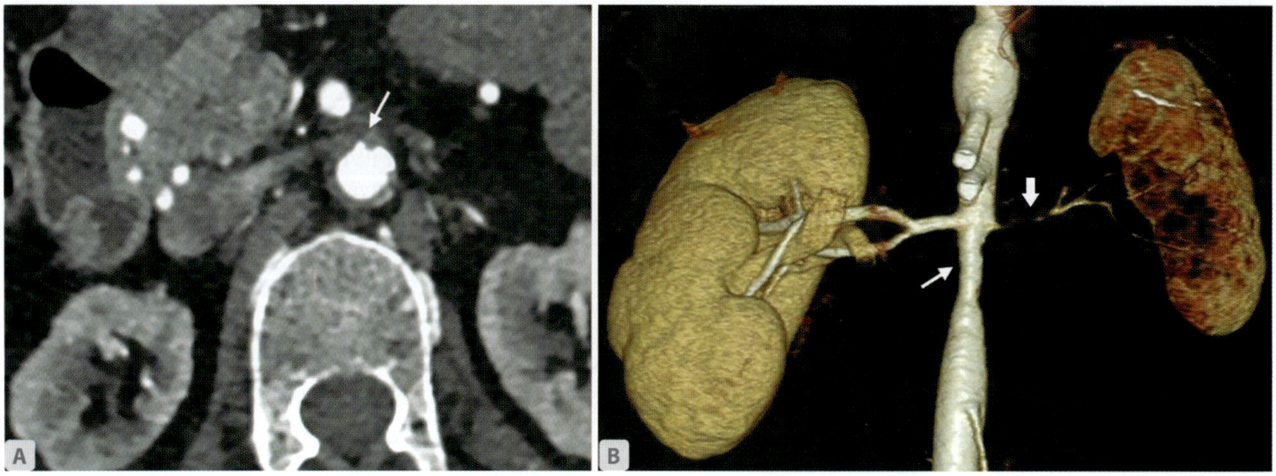

FIGS. 17A AND B: Takayasu's arteritis. (A) Axial CTA image reveals circumferential wall thickening of aorta (arrow) in a patient with Takayasu's arteritis; (B) VRT in a different patient reveals diffuse tight 99% stenosis of the left renal artery (thick arrow). Additionally, narrowing of the juxtarenal aorta (thin arrow) can also be seen in (B) (CTA: computed tomography angiography; VRT: volume-rendering technique).

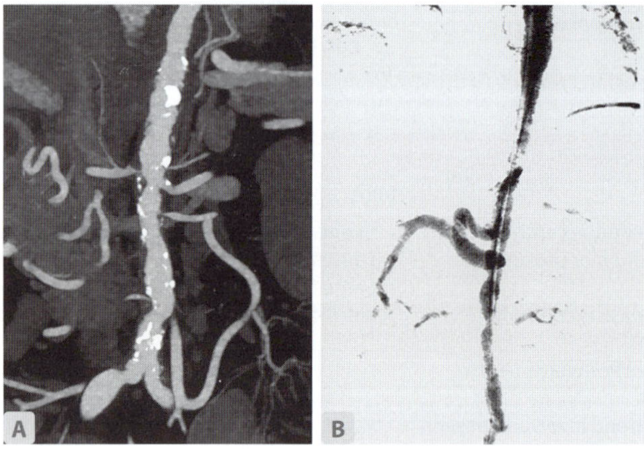

FIGS. 18A AND B: Takayasu's arteritis. (A) MIP coronal CT and (B) DSA reveal tight ostioproximal RRA stenosis approximately 50% LRA stenosis with accelerated atherosclerosis (calcifications) and diffuse involvement of abdominal aorta (DSA: digital subtraction angiography; LRA: left renal artery; MIP: maximum intensity projection).

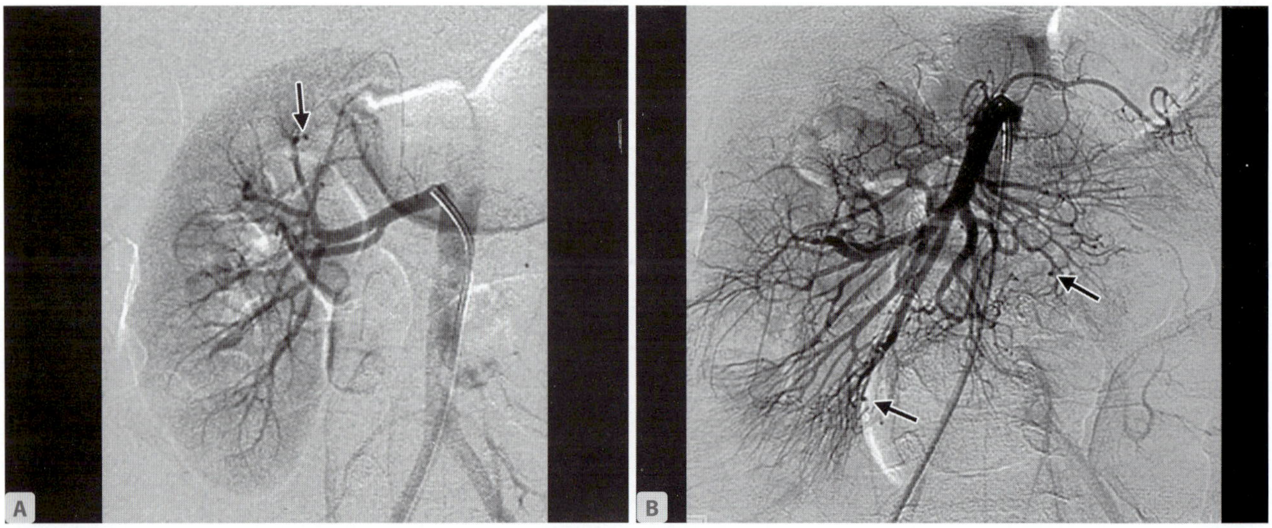

FIGS. 19A AND B: (A) Renal and (B) SMA arteriograms (DSA) reveal multiple microaneurysms in both vascular territories in a patient with PAN (DSA: digital subtraction angiography; PAN: polyarteritis nodosa; SMA: superior mesenteric artery).

Radionuclide Renal Scintigraphy

Radionuclide renal scintigraphy especially with ACE inhibitors is highly sensitive and accurate in detection of unilateral RAS but its accuracy decreases in patients suffering from bilateral RAS or azotemia and in patients with single functioning kidney.[42]

Radionuclide imaging of the kidney is the most widely performed screening test for the diagnosis of RVH I-131 orthoiodohippurate (OIH) was used in the past. Currently technetium 99m (99mTc) die-thylenetriaminepentaacetic acid (DTPA) (marker of GFR) and mercaptoacetic triglyceride (MAG 3) (secreted by proximal tubule) are commonly used for isotope renography.

The standard renogram reflects the salt and water retention on the ischemic side by demonstrating slow transit and excretion of radiotracer. The classic appearance is that of a small kidney with decreased uptake and delayed tracer transit and excretion. Captopril renal scintigraphy can be used as a screening test, to establish the hemodynamic significance of RAS, to predict the outcome of revascularization and in the follow-up after successful revascularization.

Principles of ACE Inhibitor (Captopril) Scintigraphy

In a patient with a significant RAS the efferent arterioles of the glomeruli are constricted by angiotensin II to maintain glomerular filtration pressure in the face of diminished afferent arteriolar pressure.

Administration of ACE inhibitor decreases this angiotensin related constriction of efferent arterioles which reduces glomerular filtration and hence urine flow. ACE inhibitor does not affect GFR in patients with normal renal arteries or those with essential hypertension.

Protocol

ACE inhibitor scintigraphy is performed 1 hour after the oral dose of 25 mg of captopril or 15 minutes after an intravenous dose of 0.04 mg/kg of enalapril maleate. Patients are well-hydrated, are taken off antihypertensive medication 2–5 days prior to the study according to the half-life. Resting blood pressure is monitored. After a baseline study, the scan is repeated 30 minutes after administration of ACE inhibitor. Time-activity curves are generated from renal cortex and pelvis.

Results

A positive result is said to be present if there is a decrease in uptake and delayed clearance by the affected kidney on the post-captopril study compared to the baseline study or if there is exaggeration of the baseline asymmetry between the normal and abnormal kidney in patients with unilateral RAS.

The overall sensitivity and specificity of the test exceeds 90% in most series with a few exceptions.[43] Advantages include low cost, relative reliability, and noninvasive nature. A positive captopril renography may suggest a cure or improvement in blood pressure after intervention. It may also be used in the follow-up of patients after intervention. Disadvantages and pitfalls include low sensitivity in patients with azotemia or underlying renal dysfunction and in patients with bilateral RAS. Branch artery stenosis cannot be diagnosed. It has a low spatial resolution and provides functional nonanatomic data. In patients who develop severe hypotension in response to captopril, bilateral symmetric parenchymal retention may be seen (false positive). Symmetrical retention even in the absence of hypotension is usually a false positive finding. Presence of pelvic retention may complicate interpretation of cortical retention and scintigraphy must be interpreted with caution in the presence of pelvic retention.[44]

Plasma Renin Activity (PRA)

Peripheral venous PRA is elevated in only 50–80% of patients with RVH. The predictive value of the PRA can be increased by measuring the rise in PRA 1 hour after the administration of 25–50 mg of captopril. A positive test is when postcaptopril renin level is above 12 ng/mL, increases by 10 ng/mL/h or more, and is at least 150% above the baseline value. Patients with RAS have an exaggerated increase in the PRA as perhaps due to removal of the normal suppressive effect of high angiotensin II levels.

Renal Vein Renin Measurements

It more precise estimation of "pressor kidney" renin that is ≥1.5 times the value from the contralateral kidney which is suppressed in RVH. It can be helpful in bilateral RAS in whom RV renin measurements can be used to determine which side contributes most to the hypertension or in patients considered for nephrectomy of a pressor kidney.

Newer Modalities

Intravascular ultrasound is the best modality for the correct evaluation of stenosis and plaque morphology, but it being invasive and expensive it is unlikely to become a screening modality.[35]

It allows for characterization of vessel wall layers and hence can help in identification of disease etiology.

Optical Coherence Tomography

The advantages of OCT include demonstration of the layers of arterial wall, pathological findings of the disease, and to guide percutaneous interventions. The major limitation of OCT is its lower penetration, which may cause imaging of large vessels difficult.

INDICATIONS OF REVASCULARIZATION AND TREATMENT OPTIONS

The ACC/AHA guidelines recommend percutaneous revascularization in patients with hemodynamically significant RAS and any of the following:[18]

- Recurrent congestive heart failure or sudden unexplained pulmonary edema (class I).
- Accelerated, resistant, or malignant hypertension or hypertension with unexplained unilateral small kidney and intolerance to medication (class IIa).
- Unstable angina (class IIa).
- Asymptomatic bilateral or single functioning kidney (class IIb).

- In addition, percutaneous revascularization is reasonable for patients with progressive CKD and bilateral RAS or a RAS to a single functioning kidney and can be considered for unilateral RAS with chronic renal insufficiency.

Before percutaneous transluminal renal angioplasty (PTRA) is performed the salvage ability of the procedure must be established. The commonly used criteria are:

- Residual function-single kidney GFR by radionuclide studies.
- Kidney size of 8–9 cm
- Renal biopsy showing preservation of glomeruli and tubule.
- Presence of collateral circulation to intrarenal vessels confirmed by arteriography. Revascularization is usually not beneficial in patients with severe renal failure (serum creatinine >4.0 mg/dL).

The SCAI concluded that patients with any of the following are typically not good candidates for renal artery stenting: mild or moderate blockages (less than 70%), long-standing loss of blood flow or complete blockage of the renal artery.

Atherosclerotic Renal Artery Stenosis

There are three primary modes of treatment for renovascular hypertension: (1) Medical therapy, (2) surgery, and (3) angioplasty. First-line treatment is optimal medical therapy.

Percutaneous Transluminal Renal Angioplasty and Stenting

Percutaneous transluminal renal angioplasty and stenting are justified in selected patients who have both normal renal function and normal blood pressure because of the natural history of RAS to progress and ultimately result in impaired renal function.

The ACA/AHA and ESC recommend renal stent placement for ostial atherosclerotic renal artery stenosis (ARAS) (class I). If untreated, there is high probability of progression to complete occlusion. PTRA is best suited to discrete tight concentric, short segment stenosis located away from ostium and branches of renal arteries. Eccentric, long segment and calcified lesions, occlusion in tortuous vessels, stenosis adjacent to an aneurysm and occlusion or stenosis with a thrombus increase the risk of complications and reduce the likelihood of success **(Figs. 20A and B)**.[13]

Renal Artery Stenting

Angioplasty failure is an absolute indication for stenting. The criteria for angioplasty failure include: residual stenosis of more than 30%, residual aortorenal pressure gradient of > 20 mm Hg, acute occlusive, flow limiting dissection flap and late restenosis (recurrent stenosis >50%) **(Figs. 20A and B)**.[45]

In selected patients in whom the risk of intervention or anatomic considerations make a repeat procedure in the future unlikely primary stenting is justifiable. It should be the technique of choice for ostial atherosclerotic RAS.

Outcome

Success in renal revascularization can be judged by the technical success of angioplasty and by the clinical response. Criteria for technical and clinical success are given later in this chapter. The results of PTRA depend on the type of lesion, indication for treatment, and factors such as age, coexistent essential hypertension, and nephrosclerosis.

For atherosclerotic lesions both angiographic and clinical results for nonostial stenosis are superior to those for ostial stenosis (within 2–10 mm of aortic lumen). Technical success occurs in 75–95% cases, although some authors have reported lower rates of 43% for nonostial lesions and 29% for ostial lesions. Long-term clinical benefit is seen in 76% patients with ostial lesions and 83% patients with nonostial lesions.[46]

Lesser success can be expected in patients with bilateral RAS, generalized atherosclerosis, with heavily calcified or segmental artery lesion. For renal salvage the results are less favorable and improvement is seen in 40–60% cases.

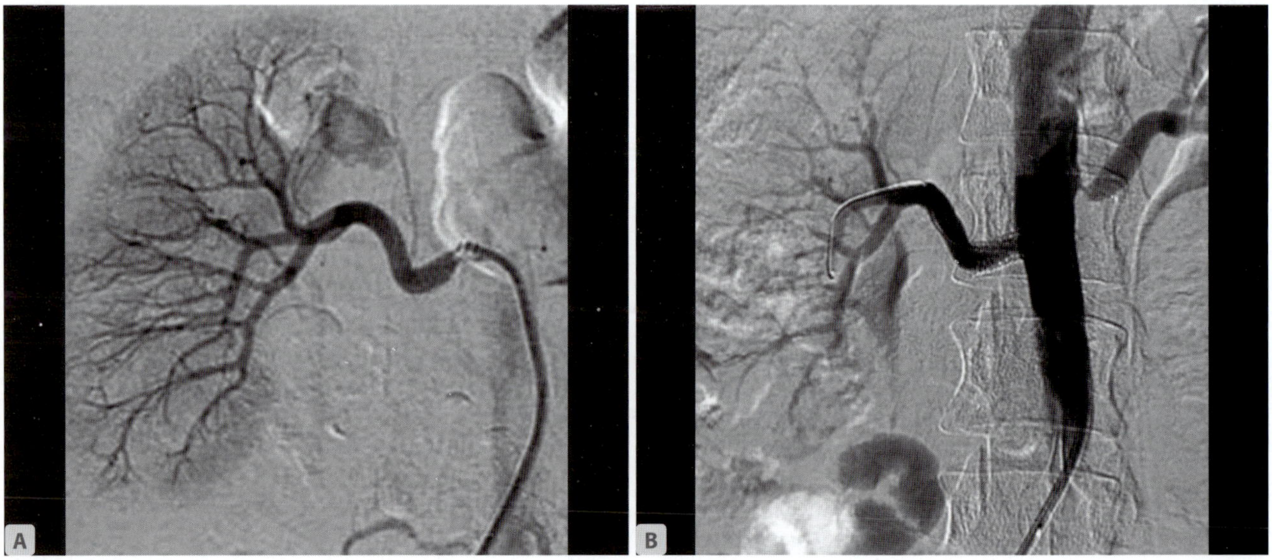

FIGS. 20A AND B: In-stent restenosis is seen on (A) DSA in a previously treated patient of atherosclerotic RAS and (B) reveals luminal opening after angioplasty within the stent (DSA: digital subtraction angiography; RAS: renal artery stenosis).

Surgical revascularization can be considered if multiple small renal arteries are present or there is a primary early branching of renal artery (class 1 ACC).

Takayasu's Arteritis/Nonspecific Aortoarteritis

The diffuse nature of the disease and complexity of pathological changes in the vessel wall make surgical revascularization difficult. Graft occlusion is also common. Hence, current guidelines recommend endovascular as the initial treatment.

Since chances of dissection or restenosis are more in active disease, endovascular treatment is not recommended unless there are absolute indications indications like:

- Refractory hypertension
- "Flash" pulmonary edema or severe left ventricular dysfunction.
- Hypertensive retinopathy, cerebropathy.

Specific technical difficulties may be encountered during PTRA for aortoarteritis because of the tough noncompliant nature of the stenosis which is difficult to cross and resists repeated prolonged balloon dilatation. Patients may also develop hypotension and backache during the procedure **(Figs. 21A to C)**.[47]

However, reports have shown high rate of technical success and frequently good clinical response. One large series including 193 patients reported technical success rate of 96%, clinical benefit of 91%, complication rate of 5.8%, restenosis rate of 17% and 5-year patency rate of 67%. Factors predicting restenosis included ostial stenosis, residual stenosis of more than 30%, residual gradient of more than 10 mm Hg after angioplasty, juxtadiaphragmatic aortic stenosis, and active disease.[48]

Following angioplasty for any cause at least 3–6 months of follow-up is required to assess durability of clinical response.

Primary stenting of renal artery stenoses is not recommended in Takayasu's arteritis as:

- Patients are young and the vessel can outgrow the stent.
- The anatomy is often complex with diffuse disease involving the aorto-ostial region and extending to the renal artery bifurcation.
- The risk of in-stent restenosis is higher.

Stenting is usually reserved as a bailout procedure for complications like obstructive dissection, arising out of angioplasty. Balloon mounted stents are preferred. If there is significant residual stenosis, cutting balloons are an option.

Surgical Therapy

Surgical revascularization is now indicated only in situations where PTRA fails or is contraindicated.

Techniques include aortorenal, lienorenal, ileorenal arterial bypass, nephrectomy, and autorenal transplantation.

Fibromuscular Dysplasia

If technically feasible, PTRA should be attempted on all patients with FMD. The ACC/AHA gives a class I recommendation for balloon angioplasty with bailout stent placement if necessary for fibromuscular dysplasia lesions. The results in FMD are uniformly good. Technical success is achieved in 90–100% patients. Hypertension is cured or improved in 98% patients. Intimal FMD may require much greater pressures than medial fibroplasia type of FMD. Restenosis is uncommon in these patients and primary patency at 15 months is 92%.

Spasm more likely during angioplasty. Liberal use of NTG is recommended. Cutting balloons can be used for intimal fibroplasia type. Stenting is only done as a bailout procedure.

Surgical revascularization is a class 1 indication for complex FMD extending into bifurcation or those with aneurysms.

Renal Artery Stenosis in Children[49]

Although RAS is uncommon in children the incidence is much higher in children with hypertension than in adults. About 4–20% of children with hypertension have RAS.

Causes

Fibromuscular dysplasia

The classical string of beads appearance is rarely seen with intimal fibroplasia being the most common type of lesion. The lesions are more often found in boys unlike adults. Branch artery stenosis is also more common.

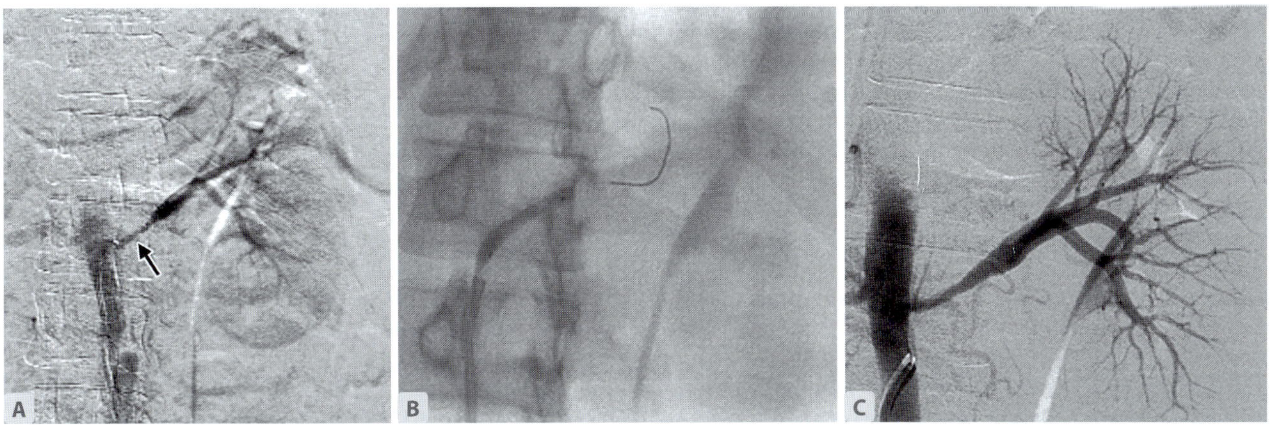

FIGS. 21A TO C: Percutaneous transluminal angioplasty for Takayasu's arteritis. (A) Initial angiogram which reveals approximately 95–99% stenosis of left renal artery (arrow); (B) Figure B shows balloon inflation at the site of stenosis; (C) Postangioplasty angiogram shows significant improvement in luminal caliber.

Neurofibromatosis

Stenosis of bilateral proximal renal arteries is the main finding in RAS associated with neurofibromatosis. This may be associated with hypoplasia of abdominal aorta.

Nonspecific aortoarteritis and middle aortic syndrome are other important causes.

Because of the higher incidence of RAS in children with hypertension patients with a strong clinical suspicion often undergo DSA.

Percutaneous transluminal renal angioplasty is being used with increasing frequency in children, however, the success rate is lower than adults for two reasons—smaller size of vessels and more frequent vasospasm make children more difficult to angiogram and dilate. Adult FMD and atherosclerosis respond well to PTRA while children have a more fibrotic process that cannot be adequately dilated.

TRIAL EVIDENCE

Numerous studies have looked into the outcomes of different therapies for renal artery stenoses.

The major studies comparing initial angioplasty without stenting with optimal medical therapy are EMMA (Essai Multicentrique Medicaments vs Angioplastie),[50] the Scottish and Newcastle Renal Artery Stenosis trial,[51] and the DRASTIC (the Dutch Renal Artery Stenosis Intervention Cooperative).[52] A meta-analysis of these trials suggested that there was a small but significant decrease in the blood pressures (mean change in systolic/diastolic pressures = 6.3/3.3 mm Hg, $p = 0.02/0.03$) in the angioplasty group when compared to those receiving only optimal medical therapy. Also, there was some decrease in serum creatinine levels as well, but it was not significant ($p = 0.06$).

Many studies have also compared the results of optimal medical therapy with angioplasty and stenting. The ASTRAL study was a randomized trial to evaluate if renal revascularization delays the decline of renal function when compared to optimal medical therapy. The study did not show any additional advantage of revascularization for rate of decline of renal function. However, this study did not include patients in whom revascularization is often required and performed, that is patients with flash pulmonary edema, critical RAS or uncontrolled hypertension. Also, it did not study the effect of revascularization in BP control.[53] Similar results were obtained from STAR trial (revascularization versus medical therapy for renal artery stenosis).[54] CORAL (Cardiovascular Outcomes in Renal Atherosclerotic Lesions) study is the most recent study which included 947 patients with RAS of at least 60% diameter, (ASTRAL and STAR studies used 40% as cutoff) and significant hypertension. These patients were randomized to receive either optimal medical therapy alone or medical therapy with renal arterial stenting. Stenting did not offer any additional benefit to prevent death from MACE, hospitalization, heart failure, progression of renal failure or need for renal replacement therapy.[55]

ENDOVASCULAR TREATMENT: TECHNICAL CONSIDERATIONS

Endovascular management of RAS includes angioplasty of the stenosed segment with or without stent placement, the procedure is known as PTRA. The procedure includes taking a vascular access, usually the common femoral route or may be brachial artery approach depending on ease of renal artery cannulation. A flush aortogram is done by a pigtail catheter which has multiple side holes, to delineate the origin of the renal arteries, any accessory renal arteries and also to rule out any other abdominal vascular involvement. Further, a double curve catheter is used to hook the ostium of each of the renal arteries and a selective angiogram is done. After establishing the diagnosis and identifying the stenosed segment, a balloon angioplasty is planned if the lesion is significantly stenosed. Significant stenosis is defined as a stenosis more than 50% for renal arteries, or that causing post-stenotic dilatation or any lesion that has a pressure gradient of 20 mm Hg across it.

For PTRA, a renal guiding catheter (usually 7Fr) is taken to provide a route for exchange of balloons and wires and also to do angiograms. Usually the balloons which are selected are compatible with 0.014'' or 0.018 guidewires and are a monorail system (common lumen for wire and balloon). Size of the balloon is decided by using distal vessel diameter as reference. The balloon is advanced via the guide catheter over the wire and put across the lesion. The position of the balloon is checked by doing a check angiogram with the guiding catheter. Balloons are inflated for 1–2 minutes at their nominal pressures. Postangioplasty, a repeat angiogram is done to look for technical success or any complications. Primary stenting is usually done in case of atherosclerotic ostial RAS.

Technical success is defined as either of:

- Increase in the luminal diameter by 50%.
- Residual stenosis of less than 30%, or
- Residual gradient of less than 20 mm Hg.

For clinical success:

- Patients are considered cured if normal BP is obtained without antihypertensive regimen.
- Improved if there is at least a 15% reduction in diastolic pressure or the diastolic pressure is less than 90 mm Hg with the patient taking less medication than before the procedure.
- Failed if there is no change in BP after the procedure.
- In patients treated for renal salvage a reduction in serum creatinine levels of >20% may be considered successful treatment.

Complications

Complication rate in PTRA varies from 3% to 6%. Complications include those related to the arteriographic procedure and those due to angioplasty and stenting. These include renal artery injury, guidewire perforation of kidney, flow limiting renal artery dissection **(Fig. 22)**, renal artery thrombosis, renal artery rupture. There may be puncture site complications such as hematoma, pseudoaneurysm or at the level of renal arteries because of selective catheterization. Stent-related complications include stent malposition, misdeployment of stent, endovascular infection, and cholesterol embolization.

CONCLUSION

The prevalence of RVH is 1–5%. Atherosclerotic renal artery disease (RAD) is the most common cause of "renovascular

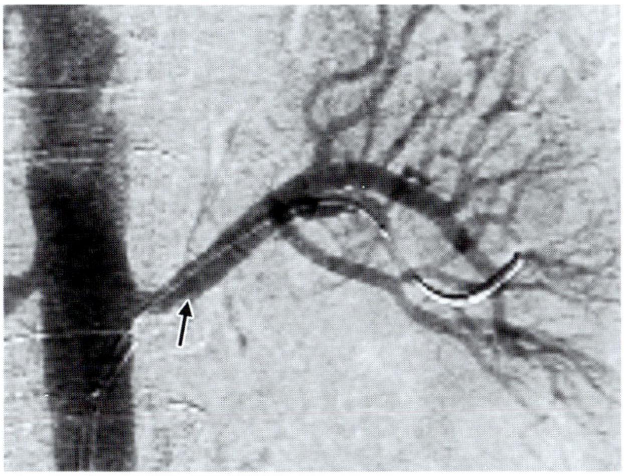

FIG. 22: Complication: Post-PTRA, small nonobstructive dissection flap is seen in LRA (arrow). (LRA: left renal artery; PTRA: percutaneous transluminal renal angioplasty).

hypertension". Renal artery stenosis should be considered in any patient with refractory or severe hypertension, or those with declining renal function or those who have atherosclerosis in other vessels. ACC/ESC suggests test only those patients who are thought to have a high likelihood of benefiting from the procedure. Initial workup includes renal function tests, ultrasound with Doppler, etc. If Doppler is positive, patients may proceed directly to noninvasive angiography. If Doppler is inconclusive or not available MRA, preferred over CTA can be used. Arteriography is gold standard for diagnosing RAS and should be done in all patients who are planned for intervention or if all other modalities are inconclusive/negative and clinical suspicion is high. Optimal medical therapy, balloon angioplasty with or without stenting or surgical revascularization can be considered in suitable patients depending on the characteristics of the lesion.

REFERENCES

1. Whelton PK, Carey RM, Aronow WS, et al. 2017 ACC/AHA/AAPA/ABC/ACPM/AGS/APhA/ASH/ASPC/NMA/PCNA Guideline for the Prevention, Detection, Evaluation, and Management of High Blood Pressure in Adults: Executive Summary: A Report of the American College of Cardiology/American Heart Association Task Force on Clinical Practice Guidelines. Hypertension. 2018;71(6):1269-324.
2. Anchala R, Kannuri NK, Pant H, et al. Hypertension in India: a systematic review and meta-analysis of prevalence, awareness, and control of hypertension. J Hypertens. 2014;32(6):1170-7.
3. Soulez G, Oliva VL, Turpin S, et al. Imaging of renovascular hypertension: respective values of renal scintigraphy, renal Doppler US, and MR angiography. Radiographics. 2000;20(5):1355-68.
4. Circulation (2005). ACC/AHA 2005 Practice Guidelines for the Management of Patients With Peripheral Arterial Disease (Lower Extremity, Renal, Mesenteric, and Abdominal Aortic). [online] Available from https://ahajournals.org/doi/10.1161/circulationaha.106.174526. [Last accessed October, 2019].
5. Mann SJ, Pickering TG. Detection of renovascular hypertension. State of the art: 1992. Ann Intern Med. 1992;117(10):845-53.
6. Olin JW, Melia M, Young JR, et al. Prevalence of atherosclerotic renal artery stenosis in patients with atherosclerosis elsewhere. Am J Med. 1990;88(1N):46N-51N.
7. American College of Physicians (1993). Annals of Internal Medicine. Atherosclerotic renovascular disease and progressive renal failure. [online] Available from https://annals.org/aim/article-abstract/706341/atherosclerotic-renovascular-disease-progressive-renal-failure. [Last accessed October, 2019].
8. Jennings CG, Houston JG, Severn A, et al. Renal artery stenosis-when to screen, what to stent? Curr Atheroscler Rep. 2014;16(6):416.
9. 1995 update of the working group reports on chronic renal failure and renovascular hypertension. National High Blood Pressure Education Program Working Group. Arch Intern Med. 1996;156(17):1938-47.
10. Brunner HR, Kirshman JD, Sealey JE, et al. Hypertension of renal origin: evidence for two different mechanisms. Science. 1971;174(4016):1344-6.
11. Textor SC, Lerman L. Renovascular hypertension and ischemic nephropathy. Am J Hypertens. 2010;23(11):1159-69.
12. Chugh KS, Jain S, Sakhuja V, et al. Renovascular hypertension due to Takayasu's arteritis among Indian patients. Q J Med. 1992;85(307-308):833-43.
13. Lao D, Parasher PS, Cho KC, Yeghiazarians Y. Atherosclerotic renal artery stenosis—diagnosis and treatment. Mayo Clin Proc. 2011;86(7):649-57.
14. Matsunaga N, Hayashi K, Sakamoto I, et al. Takayasu arteritis: protean radiologic manifestations and diagnosis. Radiogr Rev Publ Radiol Soc N Am Inc. 1997;17(3):579-94.
15. Zhu FP, Luo S, Wang ZJ, et al. Takayasu arteritis: imaging spectrum at multidetector CT angiography. Br J Radiol. 2012;85(1020):e1282-92.
16. Hata A, Noda M, Moriwaki R, et al. Angiographic findings of Takayasu arteritis: new classification. Int J Cardiol. 1996;54 Suppl:S155-63.
17. Sharma S, Rajani M, Talwar KK. Angiographic morphology in nonspecific aortoarteritis (Takayasu's arteritis): a study of 126 patients from north India. Cardiovasc Intervent Radiol. 1992;15(3):160-5.
18. Anderson JL, Halperin JL, Albert NM, et al. Management of patients with peripheral artery disease (compilation of 2005 and 2011 ACCF/AHA guideline recommendations): a report of the American College of Cardiology Foundation/American Heart Association Task Force on Practice Guidelines. Circulation. 2013;127(13):1425-43.
19. Aboyans V, Ricco JB, Bartelink MLEL, et al. 2017 ESC Guidelines on the Diagnosis and Treatment of Peripheral Arterial Diseases, in collaboration with the European Society for Vascular Surgery (ESVS). Document covering atherosclerotic disease of extracranial carotid and vertebral, mesenteric, renal, upper and lower extremity arteriesEndorsed by: the European Stroke Organization (ESO)The Task Force for the Diagnosis and Treatment of Peripheral Arterial Diseases of the European Society of Cardiology (ESC) and of the European Society for Vascular Surgery (ESVS). Eur Heart J. 2018;39(9):763-816.
20. Harden PN, MacLeod MJ, Rodger RS, et al. Effect of renal-artery stenting on progression of renovascular renal failure. Lancet Lond Engl. 1997;349(9059):1133-6.
21. Preston RA, Epstein M. Ischemic renal disease: an emerging cause of chronic renal failure and end-stage renal disease. J Hypertens. 1997;15(12 Pt 1):1365-77.

22. Watson PS, Hadjipetrou P, Cox SV, et al. Effect of renal artery stenting on renal function and size in patients with atherosclerotic renovascular disease. Circulation. 2000;102(14):1671-7.
23. Dellegrottaglie S, Sanz J, Rajagopalan S. Technology insight: Clinical role of magnetic resonance angiography in the diagnosis and management of renal artery stenosis. Nat Clin Pract Cardiovasc Med. 2006;3(6):329-38.
24. Guzman RP, Zierler RE, Isaacson JA, et al. Renal atrophy and arterial stenosis. A prospective study with duplex ultrasound. Hypertens Dallas Tex 1979. 1994;23(3):346-350. doi:10.1161/01.hyp.23.3.346.
25. Haan MW de, Kroon AA, Flobbe K, et al. Renovascular disease in patients with hypertension: detection with duplex ultrasound. J Hum Hypertens. 2002;16(7):501-507. doi:10.1038/sj.jhh.1001429.
26. Kliewer MA, Tupler RH, Carroll BA, et al. Renal artery stenosis: analysis of Doppler waveform parameters and tardus-parvus pattern. Radiology. 1993;189(3):779-87.
27. Stavros AT, Parker SH, Yakes WF, et al. Segmental stenosis of the renal artery: pattern recognition of tardus and parvus abnormalities with duplex sonography. Radiology. 1992;184(2):487-92.
28. Schwerk WB, Restrepo IK, Stellwaag M, et al. Renal artery stenosis: grading with image-directed Doppler US evaluation of renal resistive index. Radiology. 1994;190(3):785-90.
29. Oliva VL, Soulez G, Lesage D, et al. Detection of renal artery stenosis with Doppler sonography before and after administration of captopril: value of early systolic rise. Am J Roentgenol. 1998;170(1):169-75.
30. Bude RO, Rubin JM. Detection of renal artery stenosis with Doppler sonography: it is more complicated than originally thought. Radiology. 1995;196(3):612-3.
31. Williams GJ, Macaskill P, Chan SF, et al. Comparative accuracy of renal duplex sonographic parameters in the diagnosis of renal artery stenosis: paired and unpaired analysis. Am J Roentgenol. 2007;188(3):798-811.
32. Radermacher J, Chavan A, Bleck J, et al. Use of Doppler ultrasonography to predict the outcome of therapy for renal-artery stenosis. N Engl J Med. 2001;344(6):410-17.
33. Ciccone MM, Cortese F, Fiorella A, et al. The clinical role of contrast-enhanced ultrasound in the evaluation of renal artery stenosis and diagnostic superiority as compared to traditional echo-color-Doppler flow imaging. Int Angiol J Int Union Angiol. 2011;30(2):135-9.
34. Dowling RJ, House MK, King PM, et al. Contrast-enhanced Doppler ultrasound for renal artery stenosis. Australas Radiol. 1999;43(2):206-9.
35. Drelich-Zbroja A, Jargiello T, Drelich G, et al. Renal artery stenosis: value of contrast-enhanced ultrasonography. Abdom Imaging. 2004;29(4):518-24.
36. Kaatee R, Beek FJ, de Lange EE, et al. Renal artery stenosis: detection and quantification with spiral CT angiography versus optimized digital subtraction angiography. Radiology. 1997;205(1):121-7.
37. Potthast S, Maki JH. Non-contrast-enhanced MR imaging of the renal arteries. Magn Reson Imaging Clin N Am. 2008;16(4):573-84, vii.
38. Mostardi PM, Glockner JF, Young PM, et al. Contrast-enhanced MR angiography of the abdomen with highly accelerated acquisition techniques. Radiology. 2011;261(2):587-97.
39. Leiner T, Michaely H. Advances in contrast-enhanced MR angiography of the renal arteries. Magn Reson Imaging Clin N Am. 2008;16(4):561-572, vii.
40. Michoux N, Montet X, Pechère A, et al. Parametric and quantitative analysis of MR renographic curves for assessing the functional behaviour of the kidney. Eur J Radiol. 2005;54(1):124-35.
41. Verschuyl EJ, Kaatee R, Beek FJ, et al. Renal artery origins: best angiographic projection angles. Radiology. 1997;205(1):115-20.
42. Huot SJ, Hansson JH, Dey H, et al. Utility of captopril renal scans for detecting renal artery stenosis. Arch Intern Med. 2002;162(17):1981-4.
43. Jaarsveld BC van, Krijnen P, Derkx FHM, et al. The place of renal scintigraphy in the diagnosis of renal artery stenosis. Fifteen years of clinical experience. Arch Intern Med. 1997;157(11):1226-34.
44. Krijnen P, Oei HY, Claessens RA, et al. Interobserver agreement on captopril renography for assessing renal vascular disease. J Nucl Med Off Publ Soc Nucl Med. 2002;43(3):330-7.
45. Burket MW, Cooper CJ, Kennedy DJ, et al. Renal artery angioplasty and stent placement: predictors of a favorable outcome. Am Heart J. 2000;139(1 Pt 1):64-71.
46. Eldrup-Jorgensen J, Harvey HR, Sampson LN, et al. Should percutaneous transluminal renal artery angioplasty be applied to ostial renal artery atherosclerosis? J Vasc Surg. 1995;21(6):909-14; discussion 914-915.
47. Martin LG, Cork RD, Kaufman SL. Long-term results of angioplasty in 110 patients with renal artery stenosis. J Vasc Interv Radiol. 1992;3(4):619-26.
48. Sharma S, Gupta A. Visceral artery interventions in Takayasu's arteritis. Semin Interv Radiol. 2009;26(3):233-44.
49. Robinson L, Gedroyc W, Reidy J, et al. Renal artery stenosis in children. Clin Radiol. 1991;44(6):376-82.
50. Plouin PF, Chatellier G, Darné B, et al. Blood pressure outcome of angioplasty in atherosclerotic renal artery stenosis: a randomized trial. Essai Multicentrique Medicaments vs Angioplastie (EMMA) Study Group. Hypertens Dallas Tex 1979. 1998;31(3):823-9.
51. Webster J, Marshall F, Abdalla M, et al. Randomised comparison of percutaneous angioplasty vs continued medical therapy for hypertensive patients with atheromatous renal artery stenosis. Scottish and Newcastle Renal Artery Stenosis Collaborative Group. J Hum Hypertens. 1998;12(5):329-35.
52. van Jaarsveld B, Krijnen P, Bartelink A, et al. The Dutch Renal Artery Stenosis Intervention Cooperative (DRASTIC) Study: rationale, design and inclusion data. J Hypertens Suppl. 1998;16(6):S21-7.
53. ASTRAL Investigators, Wheatley K, Ives N, et al. Revascularization versus medical therapy for renal-artery stenosis. N Engl J Med. 2009;361(20):1953-62.
54. Bax L, Woittiez AJ, Kouwenberg HJ, et al. Stent placement in patients with atherosclerotic renal artery stenosis and impaired renal function: a randomized trial. Ann Intern Med. 2009;150(12):840-8, W150-1.
55. Cooper CJ, Murphy TP, Cutlip DE, et al. Stenting and medical therapy for atherosclerotic renal-artery stenosis. N Engl J Med. 2014;370(1):13-22.

CHAPTER

10

Imaging of Renal Transplant

Ajay Gulati, Manavjit Singh Sandhu, Tulika Singh

INTRODUCTION

Renal transplantation is currently the established standard treatment in patients of end-stage renal disease (ESRD), which leads to improvement of renal function, alleviation of the uremic syndrome with complete rehabilitation from the renal dysfunction. This has been made possible by advancements in the surgical techniques and availability of newer potent immune-suppressive medications and better donor-recipient matching.

Renal function impairment of the transplant kidney can be secondary to parenchymal abnormality, renal vascular causes, or due to collecting system abnormality. Depending upon the clinical findings, appropriate diagnostic studies are carried out. Renal biopsy remains the definitive way to diagnose the parenchymal abnormalities.

TECHNIQUE

The graft kidney is generally positioned extraperitoneally in patient's right lower quadrant with the pelvis lying anteriorly. In cadaveric renal transplants, an aortic patch (Carrel patch) is commonly removed with main renal artery. With live donors, the renal artery is harvested with anastomosis done commonly in end-to-side manner with recipient's external iliac artery. The donor renal vein is always anastomosed end-to-side with external iliac vein. The standard preferred method of reestablishing continuity of urinary tract is by formation of ureteroneocystostomy (commonly by using a submucosal tunnel to decrease the incidence of vesicoureteric reflux).[1,2]

Post-transplantation complications may be characterized in time frame as early or delayed. Early complications develop in the first few weeks and happen generally due to technical surgical challenges. Delayed complications manifest after few weeks and are normally due to medical causes (usually due to immunosuppression or due to drug toxicity).

Early complications include acute tubular necrosis (ATN), pyelonephritis, acute rejection, urinoma, hematoma, abscess, acute ureteral obstruction, and vascular complications. Late complications include chronic rejection, lymphocele, cyst formation, malignancies, and opportunistic infections of the transplant kidney.[3]

The greatest risk in the early post-transplant period is of early graft failure, which presents with oliguria. To diagnose this early, there is a routine policy of clinical surveillance complimented with laboratory tests and imaging.[4]

COMPLICATIONS

Various complications seen in post-transplant recipients may be broadly categorized as described here.

Vascular Complications

Renal Artery Stenosis

Well-recognized complication occurs in 0.9–8%[5] of cases, which is usually seen in the first 3 months.[5,6] It typically presents clinically as hypertension with or without deterioration of renal function. Auscultation may reveal bruit over the graft site. This is generally secondary to atherosclerotic vascular disease involving either the donor or recipient vessels and improper suture technique or iatrogenic vascular injury during graft harvesting. Color Doppler sonography is a commonly used technique, which reveals areas of focal color aliasing secondary to turbulent flow across the stenotic segments. Raised peak systolic velocity (PSV) (>200 cm/sec) is a sensitive and specific finding. Velocity gradient of >2:1 between stenotic and prestenotic segments also suggests the diagnosis. Tardus parvus waveform in distal segmental branches of the transplant kidney may be observed.[6] Computed tomography angiogram or magnetic resonance angiogram are complimentary imaging techniques which may be required in cases of technical difficulties in sonography due to vascular tortuosity or limited acoustic window.

Renal Artery Thrombosis

It is a rare complication seen in 0.4–3.5% of recipients.[5] The clinical features include oliguria and increased serum creatinine levels. Causes include vessel kinking, arterial dissection, acute rejection, and hypercoagulable states. Lack of flow with contents within the main renal artery with extension into its distal branches is seen on ultrasound (US), contrast-enhanced computed tomography, and contrast-enhanced magnetic resonance.

Renal Vein Thrombosis

It is also an uncommon complication encountered in 0.5–4% of the graft recipients.[5] Clinical presentation includes fever, pain, swelling over the transplant kidney, and or ipsilateral lower limb. It may be due to twisting or kinking at the time of surgery causing venous torsion and extrinsic compression over the vein. US shows lack of flow in main renal vein of the graft kidney.

Pseudoaneurysm

These are generally iatrogenic due to biopsy of graft kidney. These are well seen on color Doppler imaging typically showing yin yang sign and may be managed by graded compression technique. Interventional techniques such as percutaneous injection of thrombin or endovascular coils may be required in selected cases.

Arteriovenous Fistula

These also occur mainly due to iatrogenic reasons secondary to renal biopsies. They are formed when the biopsy needle accidentally hits both arterial as well as venous walls. Color Doppler along with spectral waveform analysis helps in the diagnosis. These usually follow self-limiting course and may close spontaneously. Some large fistulae may require endovascular embolization.

Nonvascular Complications

Medical Complications

Acute Tubular Necrosis

ATN occurs due to renal ischemia during transplantation and reperfusion injury. It clinically presents with anuria immediately or within first few days after an initial diuresis. The patients remain constitutionally well and urine sodium levels (Na^+) are high. It is usually self-limiting with renal parameters returning to normal in few days to weeks. It is almost exclusively seen in cadaveric transplants.[4]

Graft Rejection

Acute rejection is the most commonly encountered complication, which may be potentially serious if not managed appropriately. Currently, invasive core needle biopsy is still regarded as the gold standard for confirming the suspected acute rejection, however, carries the risk of graft injury or other vascular complications.[7]

Clinically, there are three distinct types of rejections: (1) hyperacute, (2) acute, and (3) chronic. Hyperacute rejection (due to circulating antibodies) usually occurs within hours to 1 or 2 days after the transplantation. It is characterized by the presence of fibrin thrombi in small arteries with cortical necrosis. The treatment is only the graft removal.

Acute rejection (mediated through cell-mediated immunity) is seen most frequently in first 1–3 weeks. It is characterized clinically by oliguria with flu-like symptoms, pyrexia, hypertension, graft tenderness, and swelling. The urine Na^+ is usually low (c.f. ATN in which urine Na^+ is high). If early diagnosis is made, this may be potentially reversed either by administering steroids or in some cases by antibody therapy.[4]

Chronic rejection is the most common reason for delayed graft dysfunction and usually manifests 3 months after transplant.[6] It does not respond to increased immunosuppressive therapy. Removal of the graft is required in majority of the patients.

Drug Toxicity

Calcineurin inhibitors such as cyclosporine and tacrolimus are main immunosuppressive agents given to avoid acute rejection. These drugs are potentially nephrotoxic and cause interstitial fibrosis with long-term usage.[6] Serum drug levels need to be monitored and dosage reduced if features of drug toxicity develop.

Infections

Early diagnosis is pivotal to improve patient outcome although the clinical features and early imaging features are generally variable and nonspecific. The involvement may be focal or diffuse pyelonephritis, which may progress on to abscess formation and/or pyonephrosis. US may reveal focal areas of hypo- or hyperechogenicity.[8] Abscess may have complex cystic appearance and may be treated by percutaneous drainage along with systemic antibiotics. Nuclear imaging using Gallium 67 citrate and Indium 111 tagged leukocyte may aid as a complimentary technique in diagnosing infection in equivocal cases.[9]

Neoplasms and Post-transplantation Lymphoproliferative Disorder

Immunosuppressive medications predispose the patients receiving graft kidney to increased risk of subsequently developing cancers particularly of the cervix, rectum, skin, Kaposi's sarcoma, and lymphoma (non-Hodgkin lymphoma).[8,10,11]

This risk has been estimated to be 100 times more as compared to the general population. Post-transplantation lymphoproliferative disorder (PTLD) is another uncommon malignancy, which may be seen in approximately 1% of graft recipients this is commonly secondary to Epstein-Barr virus infection, which usually involves the B cells. The frequently seen radiological manifestations are extrarenal with generalized lymphadenopathy.[7] In addition, extra nodal involvement may be seen, which can be solitary or multifocal lesions affecting the lung, liver, spleen, central nervous system (CNS), and gastrointestinal tract (GIT).[3,11,12]

Involvement of the graft kidney is not common but when present, it may present as nodular renal masses, perihilar, or perinephric soft tissue masses.

Renal cell carcinoma also shows increased prevalence in kidney graft recipients with 90% occurring in the native kidneys and 10% in the transplant kidney.[11]

Surgical Complications

Peritransplant Fluid Collections

Hematoma

They commonly occur due to inadequate surgical hemostasis, anticoagulation, coagulopathy, or after biopsy. They may be subcapsular or peritransplant in location. Significant subcapsular hematomas produce mass effect, which can alter the renal perfusion. On US, they may appear as complex hypoechoic masses with internal echoes and septation. Computed tomography (CT) and magnetic resonance (MR) are adjunct imaging techniques, which may add more confidence to the diagnosis.[8]

Urinoma

They occur from urine leaks, commonly found between kidney and the bladder. The clinical presentations may include oliguria with fullness, swelling, and tenderness over the graft. On US, they appear as well-defined hypoechoic to anechoic fluid collections making it difficult to differentiate from seroma or lymphocele.[8] Aspiration of fluid with raised creatinine levels helps to confirm the diagnosis. Percutaneous nephrostomy may be required for urinary diversion.

Abscess

They are an uncommon complication, which may present during first few weeks. The clinical features include pain, fever, tenderness over the graft kidney, and features of sepsis. On US, they appear as complex fluid collection with internal echoes and occasionally may be multiloculated. The treatment includes intravenous antibiotics, aspiration or drainage based upon the size.[8]

Lymphocele

Surgical disruption of adjacent lymphatic vessels leads to development of lymphoceles. They generally occur later (4–8 weeks after surgery).[8,13] On US, they appear as variable-sized anechoic to hypoechoic fluid collections with thin septations. Most patients are asymptomatic; symptoms may develop when they produce hydronephrosis secondary to mass effect.

Urinary Obstruction

Most commonly ureteral stenosis occurs in the distal third due to relatively less blood supply or by compression from fluid collections.[8] It manifests by increasing serum creatinine levels. US shows dilated renal pelvis and calyceal system and fluid collections, if present. CT also helps in detecting the level of and cause of obstruction. Balloon ureteroplasty or stent placement may be done for management.

IMAGING TECHNIQUES

Impaired renal allograft function during the post-transplant period warrants an immediate and thorough evaluation to distinguish between the parenchymal and surgical complications.

The various imaging techniques and their indications are as follows.

Radiography

Plain Radiography

Plain radiographs are useful in demonstrating radio-paque calculi and air within the collecting system or renal parenchyma in rare cases of emphysematous pyelonephritis.

Intravenous Urography

Intravenous urography was a useful study when ureteral obstruction or extravasation was suspected in a transplant recipient with adequate renal function. Presently, it is not indicated due to the newer advancements in various imaging technologies, which offer more comprehensive evaluation within acceptable radiation limits.

Cystography

Cystography is indicated to rule out vesicoureteral reflux in patients with persistent or recurrent urinary tract infection.

Nuclear Imaging

Radioimmunoassay is the most useful imaging technique for evaluating the renal function both qualitatively and quantitatively while screening for common complications. Obtaining a baseline scan in the immediate postoperative period is extremely important.[5] Serial radionuclide scans allow early detection of rejection and can be used to monitor the recovery from ATN. The most common technique used is dynamic renal imaging using ^{99}Tc DTPA (diethylenetriaminepentaacetic acid), which helps in assessing the renal perfusion and dimercaptosuccinic acid (DMSA) scan, which detects any morphological abnormalities.

Ultrasonography

Ultrasonography (USG) is most commonly employed imaging technique for evaluation of transplant recipients owing to its wider availability and lack of ionizing radiation. High-frequency transducers (5 MHz or higher) provide excellent details of the transplant kidney because of the superficial location. Several sonographic findings including enlargement of kidney, poor corticomedullary differentiation, reduced amplitude of sinus echoes, and enlarged pyramids may be seen in graft dysfunction, which can be due to early rejection, ATN, or infection. Real-time USG combined with duplex Doppler or color and power flow imaging techniques is the most frequently used examination to evaluate worsening renal function in the post-transplantation period[5,6,14-16] **(Figs. 1A to C)**. Vascular complications of transplantation, i.e. infarction, arteriovenous fistulae, pseudoaneurysms, arterial or venous thrombosis, and stenosis are readily identified by color and duplex Doppler sonography **(Figs. 2A and B)**.[5,6]

American College of Radiology appropriateness criteria for renal transplant dysfunction also recommend US duplex Doppler as a first-line imaging modality. Color Doppler is used to evaluate the status of graft vessels and to detect any areas of focal stenosis or thrombosis. Studies have shown that power Doppler sonography is superior to duplex Doppler sonography in screening patients with acute rejection. On spectral analysis, PSV, accelera-tion time, pulsatility index, and resistive index (RI) are assessed. The upper limit of normal PSV in renal artery is 200 cm/sec. The RI is considered to be normal if it is lesser than 0.8 **(Figs. 3A to C)**.[5,6]

Color Doppler sonography is also primary diagnostic modality for identifying various vascular complications.

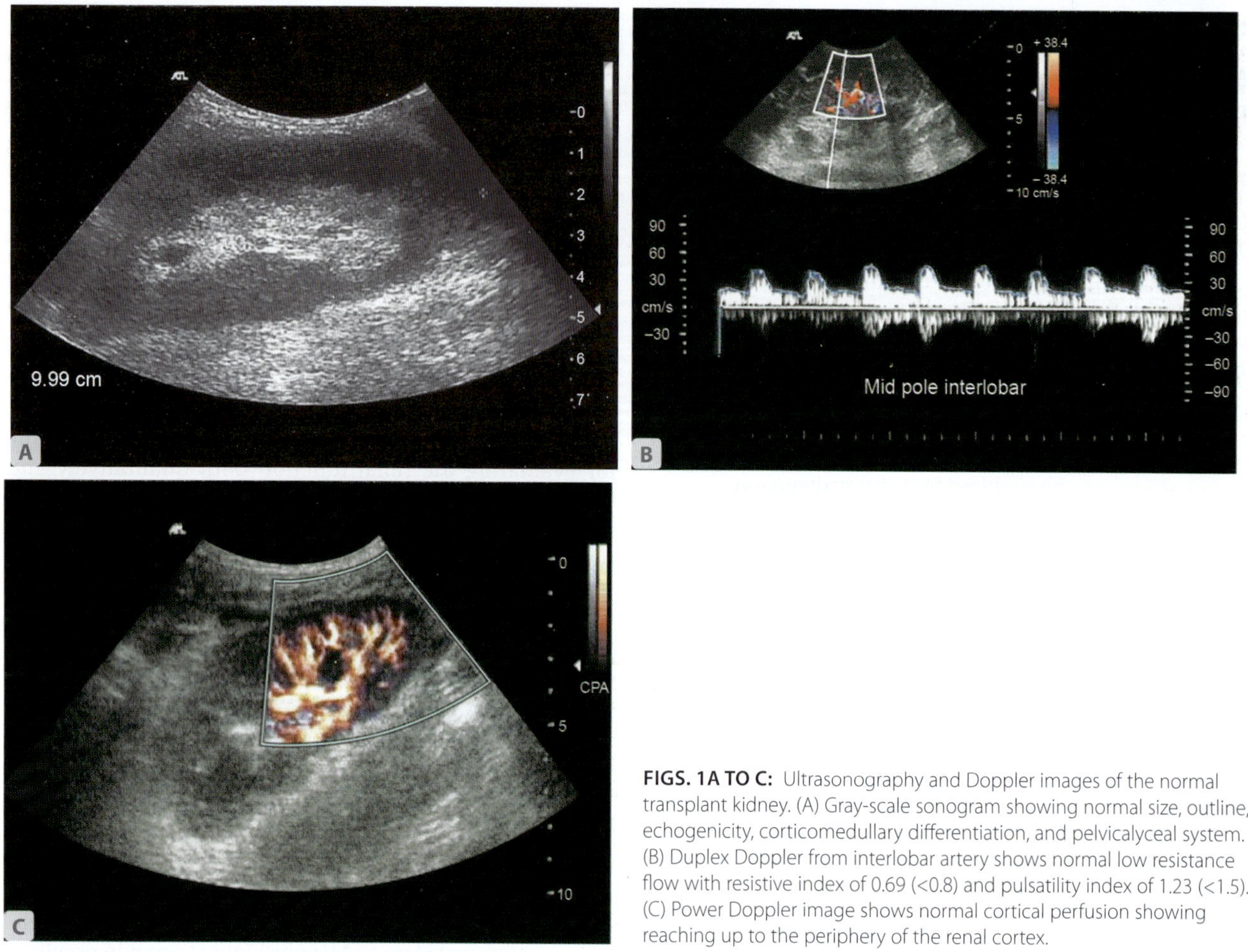

FIGS. 1A TO C: Ultrasonography and Doppler images of the normal transplant kidney. (A) Gray-scale sonogram showing normal size, outline, echogenicity, corticomedullary differentiation, and pelvicalyceal system. (B) Duplex Doppler from interlobar artery shows normal low resistance flow with resistive index of 0.69 (<0.8) and pulsatility index of 1.23 (<1.5). (C) Power Doppler image shows normal cortical perfusion showing reaching up to the periphery of the renal cortex.

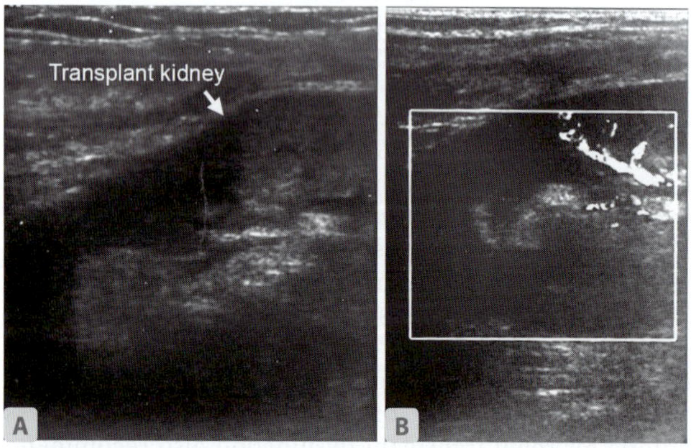

FIGS. 2A AND B: Renal infarction. (A) Ultrasound images show well-demarcated hypoechoic areas involving the renal parenchyma. (B) Power Doppler shows absence of flow in the involved renal parenchyma.

Focal stenotic segment may reveal color aliasing with velocities more than 200 cm/sec. Absent or reversed end diastolic flow is seen in severe rejection, ATN, and thrombosis in graft renal vein. Raised RI (>0.8) may also be present in acute rejection and ATN.[5,6]

Minimal dilatation of the collecting system in the immediate postoperative period is acceptable and is usually due to edema at the ureteroneocystostomy site.

Hydronephrosis may be secondary to the ureteral stricture or peritransplant fluid collections. USG is sensitive for identifying the fluid collections such as urinoma, hematoma, and abscess around the graft kidney but it is not specific for fluid type, and aspiration of the fluid collection with US guidance is helpful in the management. US guidance minimizes the risk and discomfort of the percutaneous renal transplant biopsy **(Figs. 4 and 5)**.

Recent advances in the form of contrast-enhanced ultrasound (CEUS), US elastography, and ARFI (acoustic radiation force impulse imaging) are being used to improve the diagnostic performance for early detection of graft dysfunction.

Contrast-enhanced ultrasound provides more precise information about the status of vessels and parenchymal flow; it also provides quantitative analysis of the renal perfusion thereby adding more information for identifying various causes of graft dysfunction.[17]

Another recent advancement is US elastography and ARFI for assessing early graft dysfunction. These techniques noninvasively assess the tissue's stiffness, which may help in early detection of parenchymal abnormalities, however, lack specificity for identification of precise underling disease.[7]

A novel technique for objective quantification of vascularity has been described by Gruenewald et al. This technique involves assessment of vascularity from the information obtained from Doppler cine loops, which

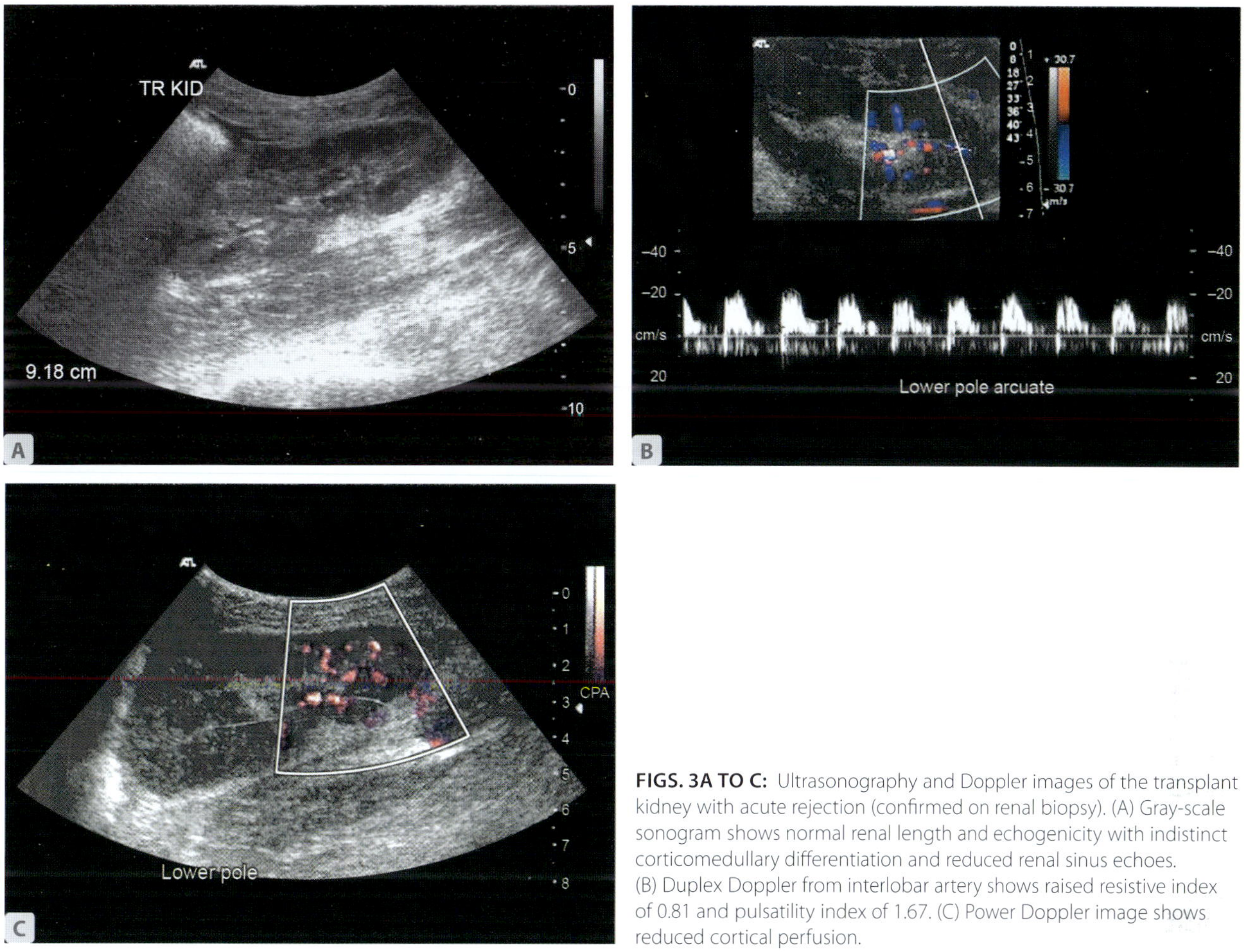

FIGS. 3A TO C: Ultrasonography and Doppler images of the transplant kidney with acute rejection (confirmed on renal biopsy). (A) Gray-scale sonogram shows normal renal length and echogenicity with indistinct corticomedullary differentiation and reduced renal sinus echoes. (B) Duplex Doppler from interlobar artery shows raised resistive index of 0.81 and pulsatility index of 1.67. (C) Power Doppler image shows reduced cortical perfusion.

are transferred to a computer for analysis. The vascularity is assessed by percentage color pixel density and mean flow velocity in mid kidney regions of interest. This technique can reliably detect allograft nephropathies.[18]

Computed Tomography

Helical CT is an accurate, noninvasive technique, which can comprehensively delineate the renal parenchyma, vasculature, pyeloureteric system, and perirenal region **(Figs. 6A to F)**. It helps to differentiate acute rejection from obstructive uropathy, urinary fistula, perinephric fluid collections, mass lesions, etc. In assessing the complex problems such as detection of malignancy such as PTLD and lymphoma or identifying sites of infection or sepsis, CT is the most useful modality **(Figs. 7 and 8)**. PTLD may present with focal lesions involving various visceral organs such as lungs, liver, spleen, CNS, and GIT **(Figs. 9 and 10)**. Dynamic CT has been used in the evaluation of physiological status of the renal transplants. It often delineates fluid collections and their anatomic relationship to adjacent structures better than USG. It can also distinguish the nature of fluid collections **(Fig. 11)**. Fresh blood in the form of hematoma has the highest attenuation value (55-66 HU), lymphoceles are between 10 HU and 20 HU, and the abscesses between 20 HU and 30 HU. In addition, drainage procedures may be performed with CT guidance when USG cannot clearly define the relationship to the collections to adjacent bowel loops. CT can reliably diagnose various infective conditions including focal or diffuse pyelonephritis or areas of abscess formation **(Figs. 12A and B)**.[8]

Computed tomography angiography with three-dimensional (3D) reformatted images allows accurate imaging of the vascular diseases such as stenosis, thrombosis, pseudoaneurysms, and arteriovenous fistulae when US studies are inconclusive. Associated parenchymal abnormalities such as infarction may be well seen with CT imaging **(Figs. 13A to C)**.

Dual Energy Computed Tomography

It is a novel technical advancement in CT technology in which acquisition is performed at two different energy levels generating two data sets, which aids in better lesion detection and characterization over traditional single-energy CT. In kidney transplant cases, it helps in differentiating hyperdense cystic lesion from an enhancing renal mass and also in characterization (differentiating uric acid stones from stones of other composition).

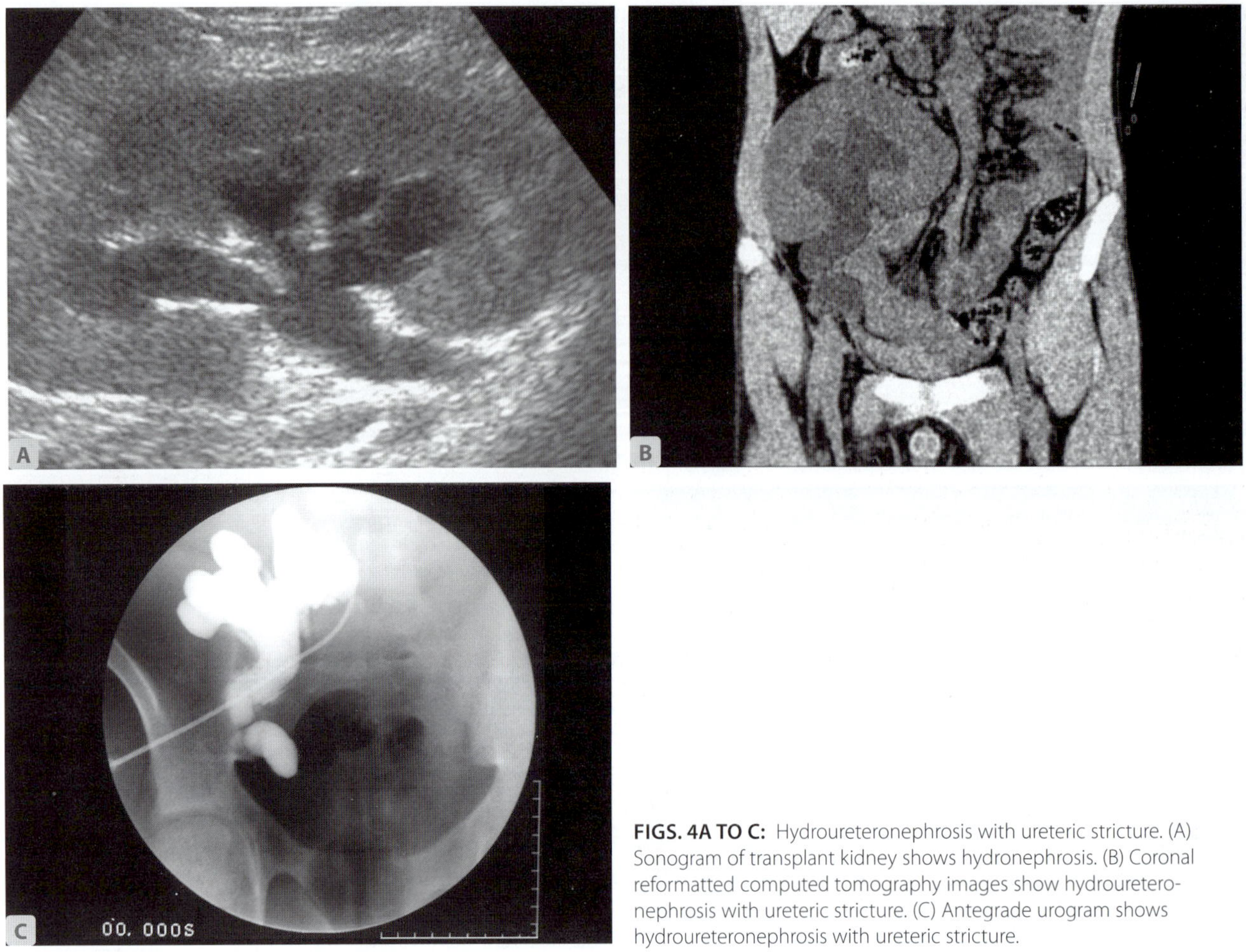

FIGS. 4A TO C: Hydroureteronephrosis with ureteric stricture. (A) Sonogram of transplant kidney shows hydronephrosis. (B) Coronal reformatted computed tomography images show hydroureteronephrosis with ureteric stricture. (C) Antegrade urogram shows hydroureteronephrosis with ureteric stricture.

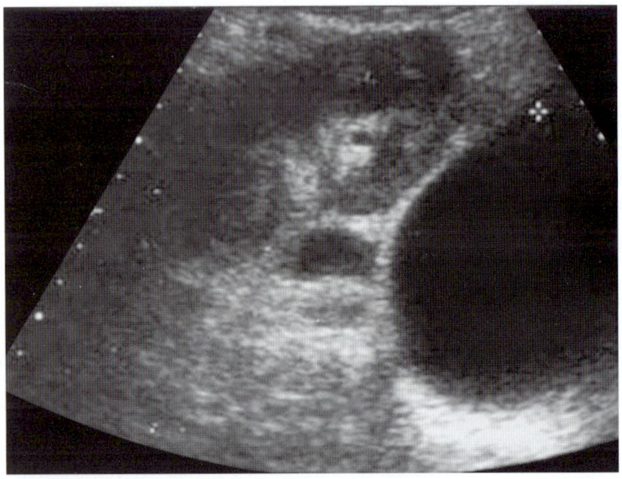

FIG. 5: Urinoma. Sagittal ultrasound image shows a large anechoic fluid collection seen posterior to the kidney. Note the dilatation of the ureter is attributable to the compression by the urinoma.

Magnetic Resonance Imaging

Magnetic resonance imaging (MRI) is employed as second-line modality for evaluation of the graft kidney as it also gives comprehensive information on the status of the renal vasculature, renal parenchyma, and peritransplant region. It can also identify or exclude various causes of renal graft dysfunction (e.g. occlusion of transplant vessels, fluid collections around the graft kidney, and ureteral obstruction).[19]

From the renal safety perspective, although the risk of renal toxicity after gadolinium injection is debatable,[20] there is added risk of nephrogenic systemic fibrosis in recipients with already compromised renal parameters.[21]

Due to high spatial resolution, nonenhanced pulse sequences may provide good details in graft recipients with compromised renal function.

A dynamic MR performed with 3D fat saturated gradient echo T1-weighted sequence provides adequate information regarding the vessels and functional status of

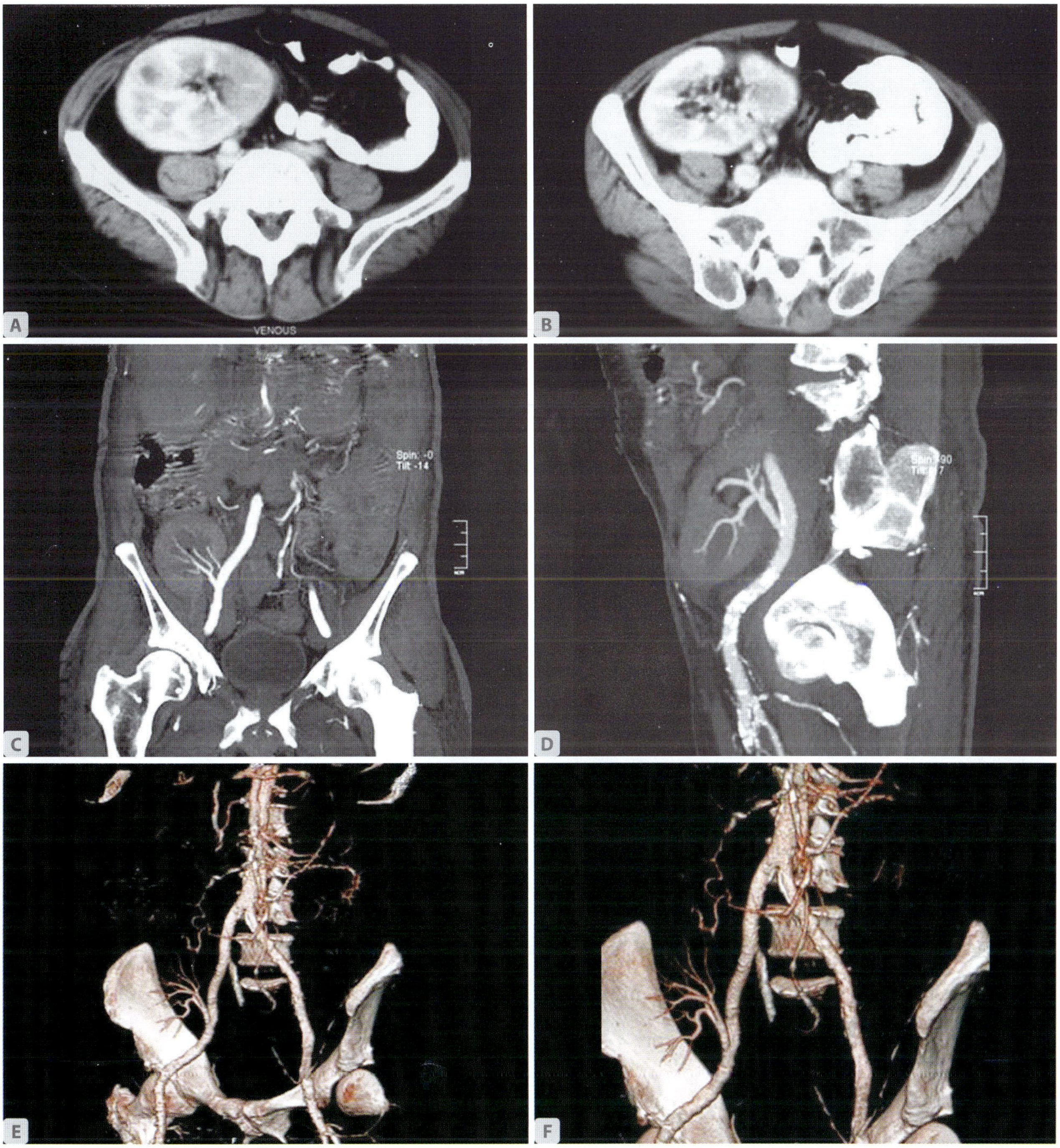

FIGS. 6A TO F: Normal transplant kidney. (A and B) Contrast-enhanced venous phase show uniformly enhanced parenchyma of the transplant kidney. Note made of a simple cyst. (C and D) Vascular myocardial infarction preformatted images depict the transplant renal artery anastomosed to the external iliac artery. (E and F) Volume-rendered images show the end-to-side anastomoses of the graft artery and the external iliac artery.

the transplant. Half-Fourier single-shot turbo spin-echo T2-weighted acquisition also provides rapid assessment of the anatomy along with the detection of hydronephrosis, perirenal collections, and malignancy, if present **(Figs. 14A and B)**.

The usefulness of MRI in renal transplant dysfunction is rapidly evolving. Decreased or absent corticomedullary differentiation on T1-weighted image is seen in majority of patients with acute rejection; however, this is nonspecific for etiology and may also be seen in allograft infection, immunosuppressant drug toxicity, and infiltrative or diffuse parenchymal diseases. On dynamic gadolinium-enhanced imaging, there is a blunted-up rise and delayed peak in the cortical signal intensity curves. The medulla also shows decreased enhancement in acute rejection.[22]

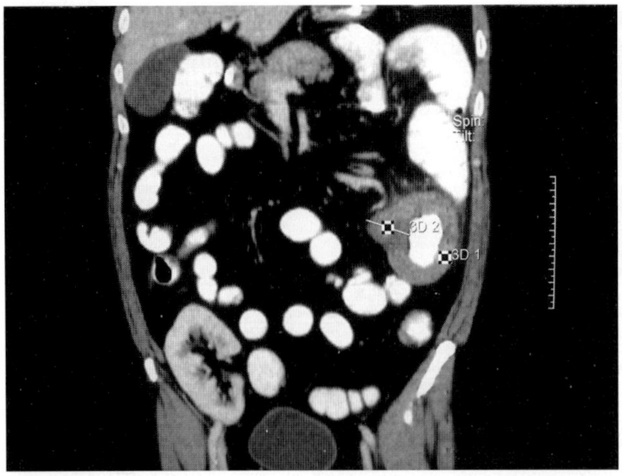

FIG. 7: Post-transplantation lymphoma. Coronal reformatted computed tomography image shows homogeneous circumferential mural thickening involving the jejunum.

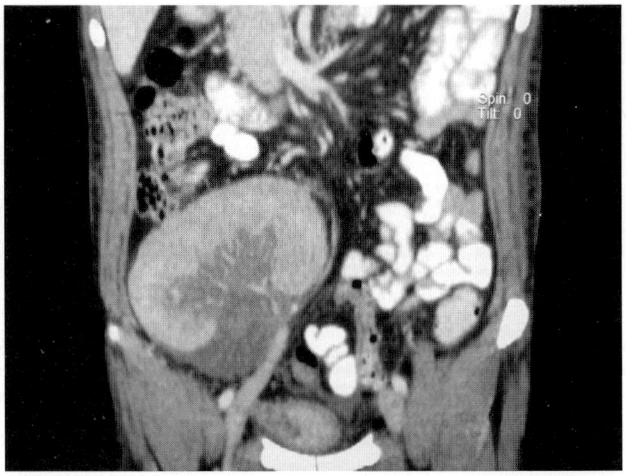

FIG. 8: Post-transplantation lymphoproliferative disorder involving renal transplant. Coronal reformatted computed tomography image shows infiltrating mass in the renal hilum surrounding the graft pedicle.

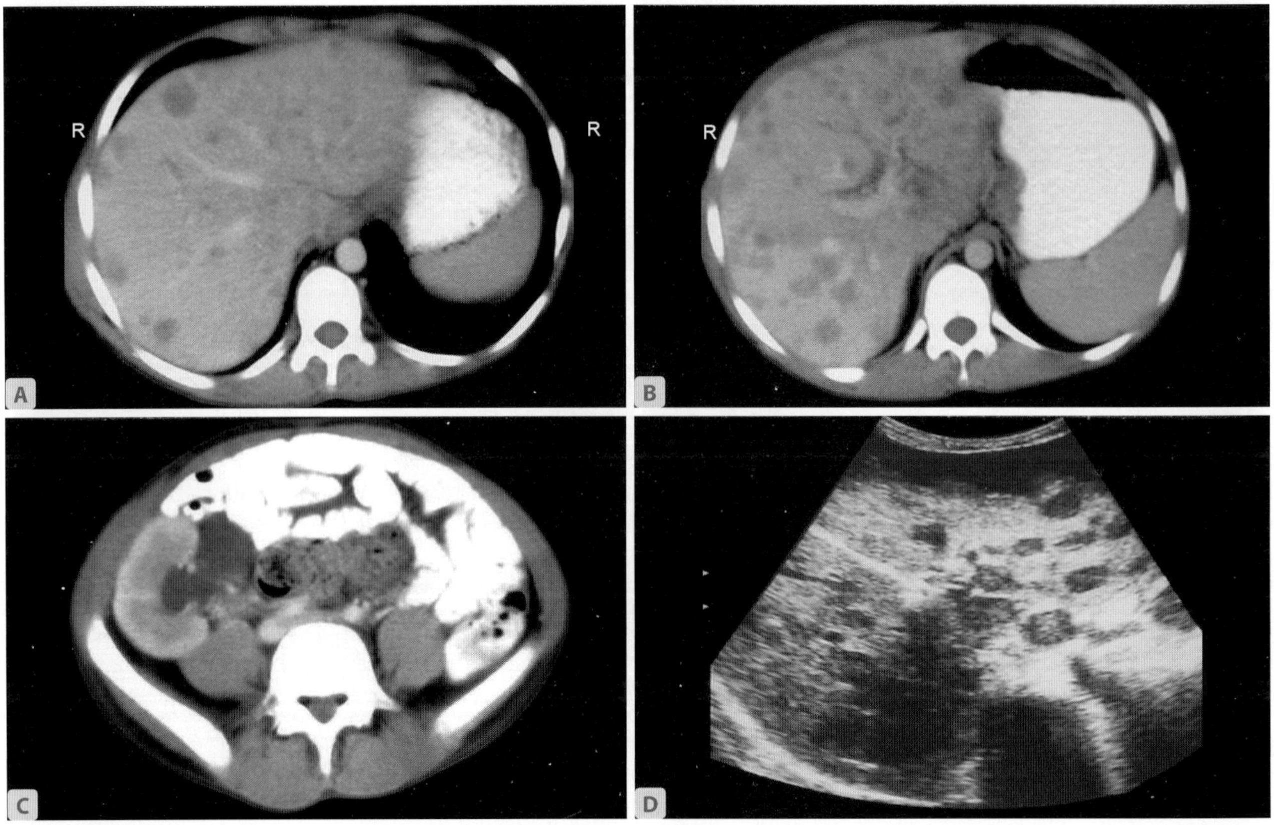

FIGS. 9A TO D: Hepatic post-transplantation lymphoproliferative disorder. (A and B) Contrast-enhanced computed tomography scan shows multiple hypodense lesions involving both the lobes. (C) Computed tomography scan at lower level shows hydronephrosis in renal transplant secondary to narrowing at ureterovesical anastomoses. (D) Ultrasound image shows multiple well-defined hypoechoic lesions in the liver parenchyma.

Preliminary published data indicate that ^{31}P-MR spectroscopy may be useful in differentiating the rejection from other causes of the renal transplant failure. The use of MR spectroscopy for evaluating the phosphorus metabolism of allografts is still under development and has been reported to be useful. The long-term assessment of post-transplant renal prognosis with ^{31}P-MR spectroscopy has been recently evaluated and a beta-adenosine triphosphate/inorganic phosphate ratio more than 1.2 will favor increased probability of 3-year renal survival, whereas a value more than 2.5 may suggest that graft kidney may survive over 5 years.[23]

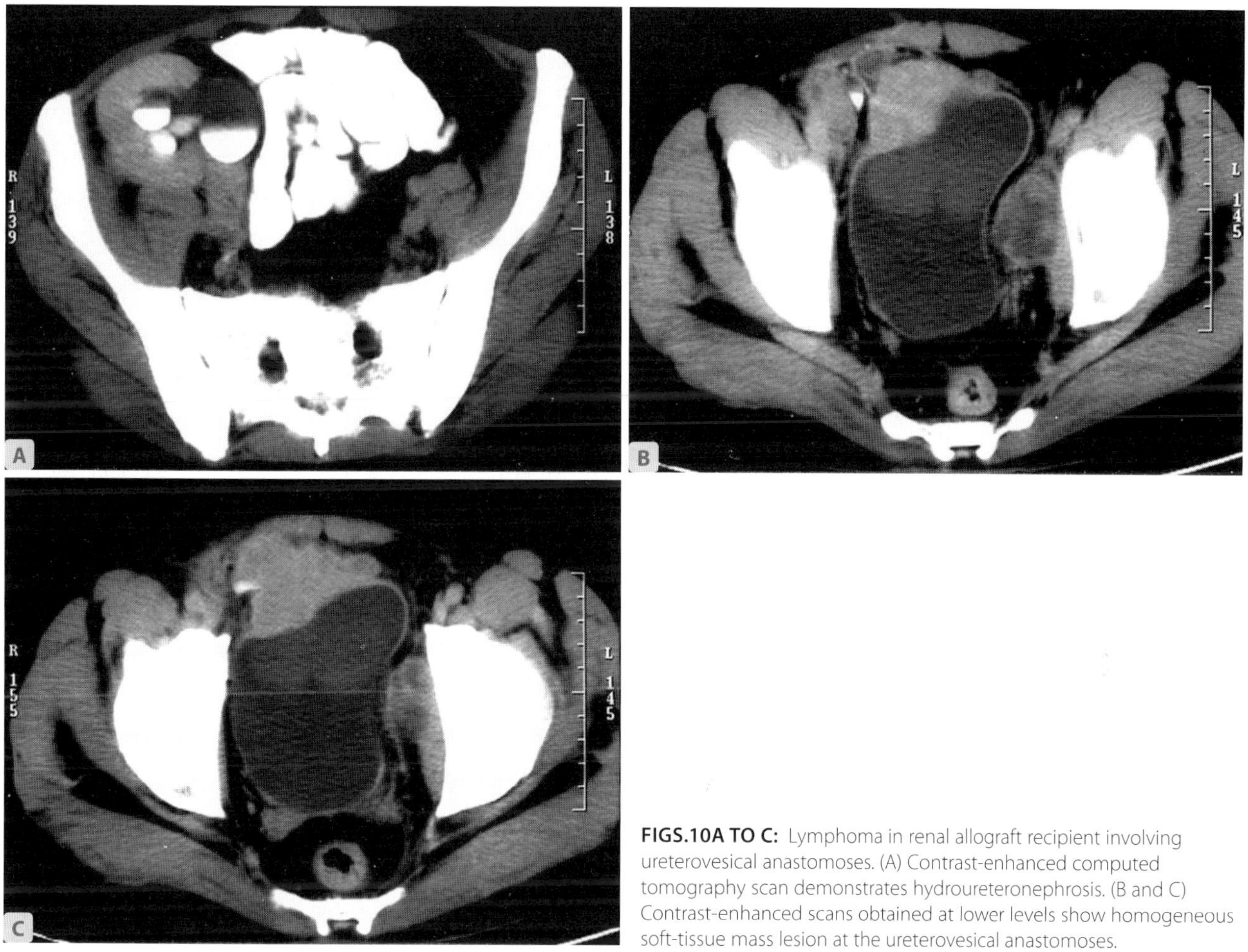

FIGS.10A TO C: Lymphoma in renal allograft recipient involving ureterovesical anastomoses. (A) Contrast-enhanced computed tomography scan demonstrates hydroureteronephrosis. (B and C) Contrast-enhanced scans obtained at lower levels show homogeneous soft-tissue mass lesion at the ureterovesical anastomoses.

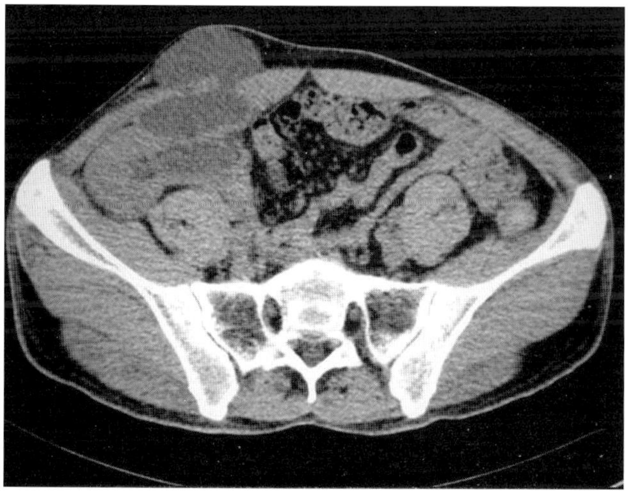

FIG. 11: Urinoma. Noncontrast computed tomography of KUB region shows hydronephrosis with perinephric urinoma extending into the anterior abdominal wall.

Recent advanced MRI techniques such as diffusion-weighted imaging (DWI) and blood oxygen level-dependent imaging has also shown promising role in detecting functional changes in kidney without intravenous contrast.[24]

By DWI, the Brownian motion can be detected, which is the random movement of the water molecule in the tissue. DWI along with quantitative apparent diffusion coefficient can detect renal allograft dysfunction wit high specificity.[25]

Blood oxygen level-dependent imaging sequence is technically obtained by altering levels of paramagnetic deoxyhemoglobin and can detect intrarenal oxygenation. This may be of benefit in differentiating between acute rejection from ATN from hypoxia caused by renal artery stenosis.[26]

Magnetic resonance is an excellent modality for screening of renal artery stenosis and other vascular complications **(Fig. 15)**. MR angiographic examination can help in avoiding unnecessary catheter angiographies in majority of cases. Noncontrast magnetic imaging angiography (NCMRA) with

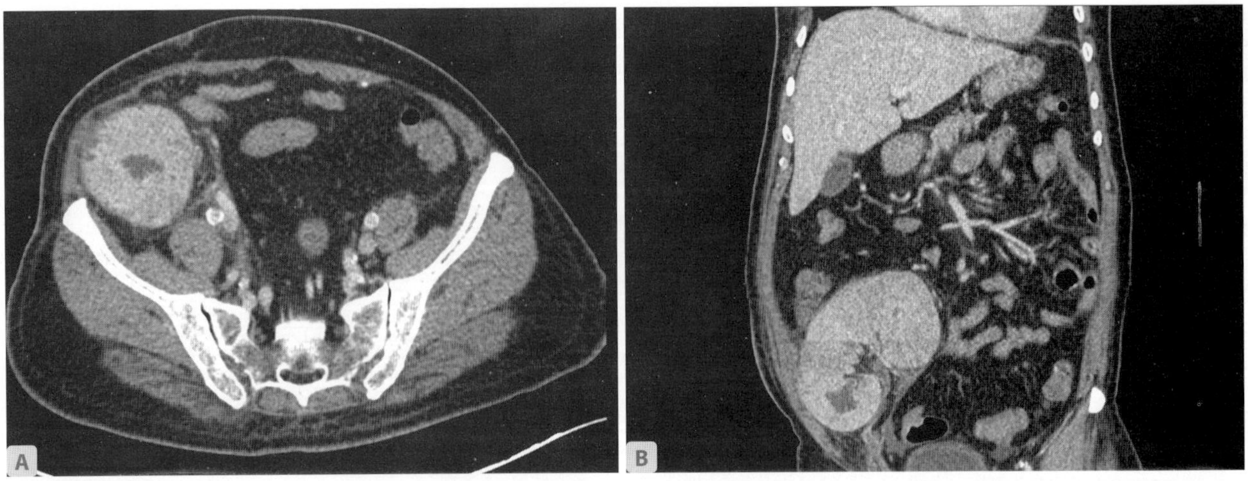

FIGS. 12A AND B: Computed tomography (axial and coronal reformatted images) showing diffuse pyelonephritis in graft kidney with focal hypodense areas of abscess formation in the lower part.

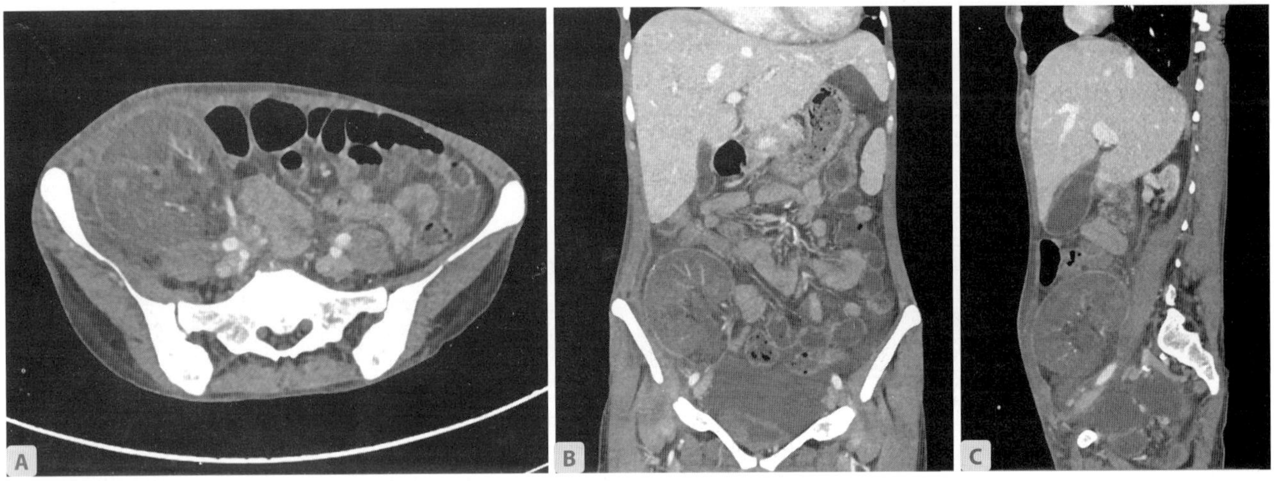

FIGS. 13A TO C: Computed tomography (axial, coronal, and sagittal reformatted images) showing globular nonenhancing graft kidney consistent with global infarction.

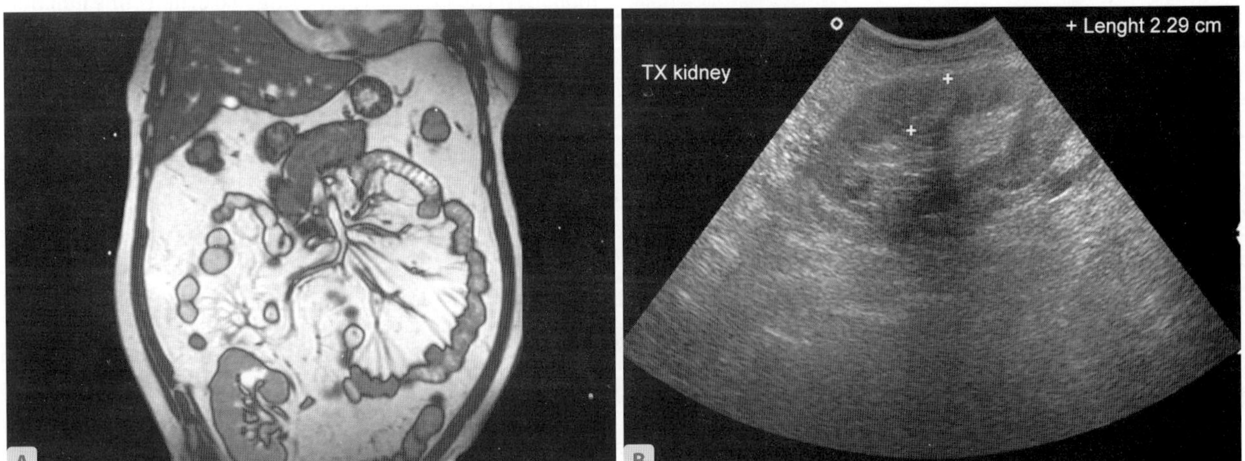

FIGS. 14A AND B: Renal cell carcinoma in renal graft. (A) Coronal MR T2WI shows focal hyperintense lesion in the transplant kidney. (B) Ultrasound image shows the lesion is iso-to-hypoechoic to the renal parenchyma.

steady-state free procession imaging can help avoiding use of MR contrast and risk of developing nephrogenic systemic fibrosis.[27]

Few studies showed that NCMRA was capable of detecting renin-angiotensin system in graft kidney with accuracy comparable to contrast-enhanced MRA.[28]

Angiography

Some important indications of renal transplant angiography are acute anuria, hypertension not responding to medication, and graft dysfunction, in which definitive diagnosis of rejection or renal artery stenosis is required order to plan subsequent appropriate management.[29,30] In acute rejection, there is a pruned-tree appearance secondary to the loss of second- and third-order branches. The arteriogram is essentially normal in ATN. In chronic rejection, arteriography demonstrates small graft size with irregularity, attenuation, and occlusion of interlobar arteries and a patchy nephrogram secondary to the areas of cortical infarction.

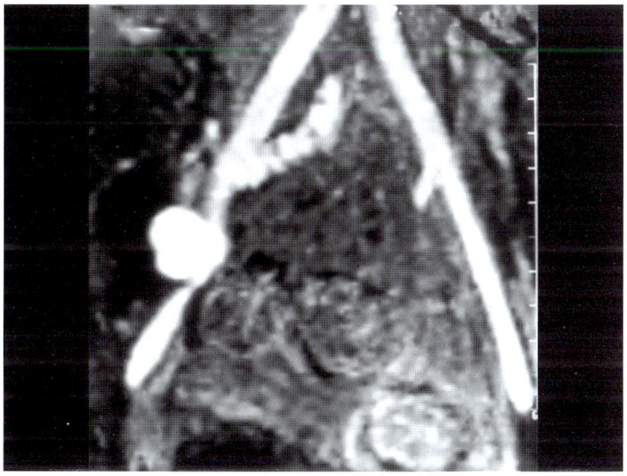

FIG. 15: Pseudoaneurysm. Maximum intensity projection reformatted magnetic resonance angiogram depicts stenosis involving the external iliac artery with a pseudoaneurysm at the anastomotic site.

Angiography is indicated in patients with hypertension not responding to the medical therapy. Angiography in such situation may demonstrate degree of renal artery stenosis. Hemodynamically significant (>50%) stenosis can be simultaneously treated with percutaneous transluminal angioplasty with covered metal stents or drug eluting stents.[31] Arteriovenous fistula (AVF) and pseudoaneurysm formation are generally iatrogenic secondary to percutaneous needle biopsy. Interventional techniques such as transcatheter embolization are the treatment of choice for both enlarging pseudoaneurysms and symptomatic AVFs. Super-selective embolization performed with metallic coils or stent grafts minimizes the loss of functioning allograft tissue and ensures long-term graft survival **(Figs. 16A to C)**. It allows selective occlusion of targeted vessels more precisely unlike particle embolization where particles may reflux into nontargeted vessels. Surgery is regarded as the treatment of last resort, with partial or total nephrectomy being two options.

Percutaneous Interventional Techniques

Percutaneous interventional radiological techniques play a pivotal role in management of the complications in the graft kidney recipients and the timely use of these techniques may obviate surgery in some cases.

Complication such as urinary obstruction or leak can occurs up to 3–10% in graft kidney patients.[32] Antegrade pyelography is the most accurate and informative examination for the demonstration of ureteral stricture as well as the site of ureteral leak (***see* Fig. 4C**). Nephrostomy drainage catheter is placed in patients with urine leak and ureteral obstruction.

Ureteral strictures can be dilated percutaneously by using angioplasty catheter, and indwelling ureteral stents left in place. Renal calculi removal through a percutaneous nephrostomy in a graft kidney recipient can also be successfully accomplished. Peri graft fluid collections such as urinoma or lymphocele are managed definitively by percutaneous drainage procedures with or without adjunct sclerosis. The commonly used sclerosing agent is dehydrated ethanol. The other agents which may be used for sclerotherapy are povidone iodine, doxycycline, bleomycin,

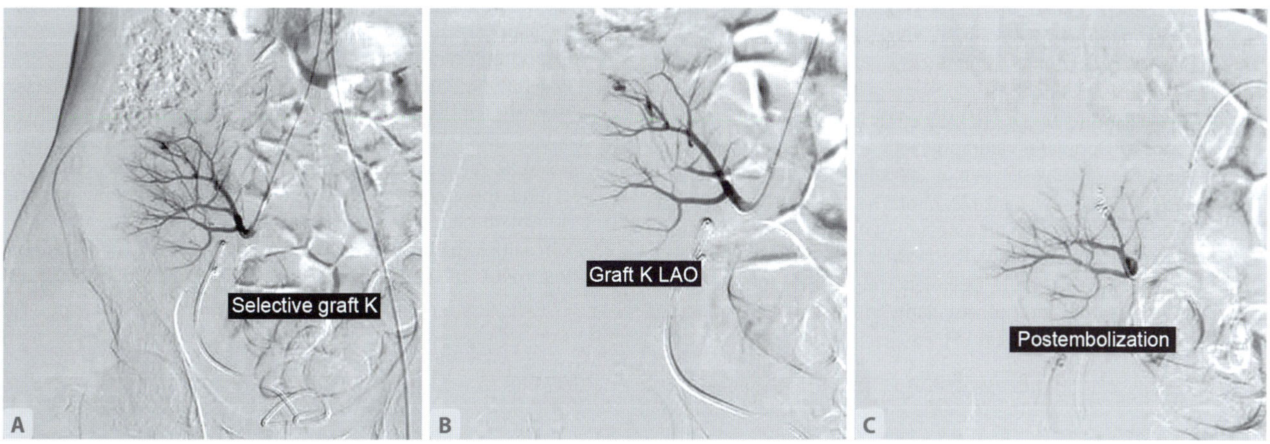

FIGS. 16A TO C: Transcatheter embolization of pseudoaneurysm. (A and B) Angiogram of transplant renal artery [anterior-posterior and left anterior oblique (LAO) projection] shows a pseudoaneurysm in upper segmental artery. (C) Angiogram obtained after coil embolization shows successful obliteration of the aneurysm with preservation of the flow in the rest of the parenchyma.

and fibrin glue.[33] Percutaneous management of postoperative hematoma is controversial and is generally avoided, however, may be helpful in subacute and chronic stages of hematoma with significant liquefied component or in case of superadded infection.

ACKNOWLEDGMENTS

Sincere thanks to Dr Hema HK, Junior Resident, Department of Radiodiagnosis, PGIMER, Chandigarh.

REFERENCES

1. Rankin S. Renal parenchymal disease, including renal failure, renovascular disease and transplantation. In: Grainger RG, Allison DJ (Eds). Diagnostic Radiology, 5th edition. London: Churchill Livingstone; 2009. pp. 851-5.
2. Oliver JH. Clinical indications, recipient evaluation, surgical considerations, and the role of CT and MR in renal transplantation. Radiol Clin N Am. 1995;33(3):435-44.
3. Sebastria C, Quiroga S, Boye R, et al. Helical CT in renal transplantation: normal findings and early and late complications. Radiographics. 2001;21(5):1103-17.
4. Kabala JE, Roobottom C. The kidneys and ureters. In: Sutton D (Ed). Textbook of Radiology and Imaging, 7th edition. London: Churchill Livingstone; 2002. pp. 982-6.
5. Moreno CC, Mittal PK, Ghonge NP, et al. Imaging complications of renal transplantation. Radiol Clin N Am. 2016;54(2):235-49.
6. Chrysafoula K, Konstantinos S, Demosthenes D. Ultrasonographic features of kidney transplants and their complications: an imaging review. ISRN Radiol. 2013;2013: 480862.
7. Thölking G, Schuette-Nuetgen K, Kentrup D, et al. Imaging-based diagnosis of acute renal allograft rejection. World J Transplant. 2016;6(1):174-82.
8. Kim N, Juarez R, Levy AD. Imaging non-vascular complications of renal transplantation. Abdom Radiol. 2018;43(10):2555.
9. Akbar SA, Jafri ZH, Amendola MA, et al. Complications of renal transplantation. Radiographics. 2005;25(5):1335-56.
10. Kumar R, Wilson DD, Santa Cruz FR. Postoperative urological complications of renal transplantation. Radiographics. 1984;3 (4):531-47.
11. Langer JE, Jones LP. Sonographic evaluation of the renal transplant. Ultrasound Clinics North Am. 2007;2:73-88.
12. Sandhu MS, Kalra N, Sidhu R. Post-transplant lymphoproliferative disorder (PTLD) localised near the allograft mimicking a collection. Indian J Radiol Imaging. 2002;12: 132-33.
13. Brown ED, Chen YM, Wolfman NT, et al. Complication of renal transplantation: evaluation with US and radionuclide imaging. Radiographics. 2000;20(3):607-22.
14. O'neill WC, Baumgarten DA. Ultrasonography in renal transplantation. Am J Kidney Dis. 2002;39:663-78.
15. Tublin ME, Dodd GD. Sonography of renal transplantation. Radiol Clin N Am. 1995;33:447-59.
16. Datta R, Sandhu M, Saxena AK, et al. Role of duplex Doppler and power Doppler sonography with acute renal parenchymal dysfunction. Australasian Radiol. 2005;49(1):15-20.
17. Álvarez RS, Hevia PV, Sanz ME, et al. The usefulness of contrast-enhanced ultrasound in the assessment of early kidney transplant function and complications. Diagnostics (Basel) 2017;7(3):pii: E53.
18. Gruenewald S, Skerrett D, Dolimier D, et al. Technique of colour Doppler quantification of vascularity in transplanted kidneys. J Clin Ultrasound. 2002;30(3):151-7.
19. Hohenwalter MD, Skowlund CJ, Erickson SJ, et al. Renal transplant evaluation with MR angiography and MR imaging. Radiographics. 2001;21(6):1505.
20. Ledneva E, Karie S, Launay-Vacher V, et al. Renal safety of gadolinium-based contrast media in patients with chronic renal insufficiency. Radiology. 2009;250(3):618-28.
21. Broome DR, Girguis MS, Baron PW, et al. Gadodiamide-associated nephrogenic systemic fibrosis: why radiologists should be concerned. Am J Roentgenol. 2007;188(2):586-92.
22. Pedrosa I, Rofsky NM, Kidneys. In; Edelman RR, Hesselink JR, Zlatkin MB, et al. (Eds). Clinical Magnetic Resonance Imaging, 3rd edition. Philadelphia: Saunders; 2007. pp. 2851-2.
23. Seto K, Ikechira H, Obata T, et al. Long-term assessment of post-transplant renal prognosis with 31 P magnetic resonance spectroscopy. Transplantation. 2001;72(4):627-30.
24. Vermathen P, Binser T, Boesch C, et al. Three-year follow-up of human transplanted kidneys by diffusion-weighted MRI and blood oxygenation level-dependent imaging. J Magn Reson Imaging. 2012;35(5):1133-8.
25. Eisenberger U, Binser T, Thoeny HC, et al. Living renal allograft transplantation: diffusion-weighted MR imaging in longitudinal follow-up of the donated and the remaining kidney. Radiology. 2014;270(3):800-8.
26. Juillard L, Lerman LO, Kruger DG, et al. Blood oxygen level dependent measurement of acute intra-renal ischemia. Kidney Int. 2004;65(3):944-50.
27. Liu X, Berg N, Sheehan J, et al. Renal transplant: nonenhanced renal MR angiography with magnetization-prepared steady-state free precession. Radiology. 2009;251(2):535-42.
28. Lanzman RS, Voiculescu A, Walther C, et al. ECG-gated nonenhanced 3D steady-state free precession MR angiography in assessment of transplant renal arteries: comparison with DSA. Radiology. 2009;252(3):914-21.
29. Orons PD, Zajko AB. Angiography and interventional aspects of renal transplantation. Radiol Clin N Am. 1995;33(3):461-71.
30. Kobayashi K, Censullo ML, Rossman LL, et al. Interventional radiologic management of renal transplant dysfunction: indications, limitations, and technical considerations. Radiographics. 2007;27(4):1109-30.
31. Beecroft JR, Rajan DK, Clark TWI, et al. Transplant renal artery stenosis: out come after percutaneous intervention. J Vasc Interv Radiol. 2004;15(12):1407-13.
32. Pollak R, Veremis SA, Maddux MS, et al. The natural history of and therapy for perirenal fluid collections following renal transplantation. J Urol. 1988; 140(4):716-20.
33. Karcaaltincaba M, Akhan O. Radiologic imaging and percutaneous treatment of pelvic lymphocele. Eur J Radiol. 2005;55(3): 340-54.

CHAPTER

11

Imaging Techniques and Radiological Anatomy of Lower Urinary Tract

Gaurav Shanker Pradhan, Satyam, Jyoti Kumar

INTRODUCTION

Radiological evaluation of the lower urinary tract was attempted in early twentieth century. John Cunningham had done urethrography for the first time in 1910 using highly dilute solution of mercuric iodide as contrast. Many contrast agents were subsequently tried to improve radiological visualization. Presently, nonionic iodinated contrast media are in widespread use because of their good radiopaque opacification and relatively less toxicity compared to other agents.

Micturating cystography is a useful technique for evaluation of bladder. Retrograde Urethrography (RGU) and Voiding Cystourethrography (VCUG) have become the gold standard for imaging of urethra. Cross-sectional imaging modalities including ultrasonography, computed tomography and magnetic resonance (MR) imaging are now frequently being used for detailed evaluation of bladder, urethral and periurethral abnormalities.

ANATOMY

Urinary Bladder

The urinary bladder is a subperitoneal musculomembranous sac which act as reservoir of urine. The size, shape, position and relation depend on the amount of fluid it contains. The empty bladder is flattened tetrahedron in shape while full bladder is round or oval in shape. The normal capacity of bladder is between 500 mL and 600 mL in adults. The empty bladder lies in the lesser pelvis and extend into the abdomen when full.

The bladder is situated posterior to symphysis pubis separated by fatty Retzius' space. Superiorly the bladder is covered by peritoneum, which continues posteriorly and is reflected on anterior surface of rectum. It is surrounded by perivesical fat and laterally bordered by obturator internus muscles and inferiorly by prostate gland. The bladder is connected to lateral pelvic wall by endopelvic fascia, which is strengthened by pubovesical and rectovesical ligaments.

It has four anatomical parts: apex, fundus, base and neck. The apex of the bladder is attached to the anterior abdominal wall by median umbilical ligament. The base of the bladder is continuous with bladder neck.

The wall of urinary bladder is smooth, regular with uniform thickness, not exceeding 6 mm in adult. The layers of the wall from inside out are serosa, smooth muscle, lamina propria, submucosa, and mucosa. The detrusor muscle has three layers: inner longitudinal, middle circular, and an outer longitudinal. Bladder is lined with a mucosal membrane consisting of the urothelium (a form of transitional epithelium), a basement membrane, and the lamina propria **(Fig. 1)**. The mucous membrane is loosely attached to the muscular layer, except in triangular area just above and behind the internal orifice of urethra, termed as trigone, where it is firmly attached. The anterior angle is formed by internal orifice and its posterolateral orifice is formed by ureters. The interureteric ridge extending between two ureteric orifices, forms the posterior aspect of trigone. The distance between two orifices is same as the distance from internal urethral orifices, 2.5 cm in contracted state and 5 cm in distended state.

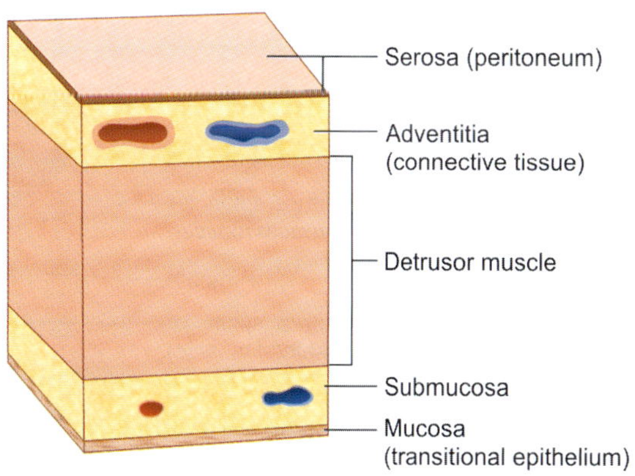

FIG. 1: Schematic diagram of constituents of wall of urinary bladder—The layers of the wall from inside out are serosa, smooth muscle, laminar propria, submucosa, and mucosa.

The arteries supplying bladder are superior, middle and inferior vesical arteries derived from anterior trunk of internal iliac artery. The inferior gluteal and obturator arteries gives a small visceral branch to the bladder and in females, additional supply is from uterine and vaginal arteries. The veins form a complicated plexus and drain into the hypogastric vein. The lymphatic drainage of bladder is primarily to external iliac lymph nodes.

Urethra

Male Urethra

The male urethra extends from the bladder to the external urethral meatus and is approximately 18 to 20 cm long. It has four parts and is divided into posterior and anterior portions **(Fig. 2)**, each of which is further divided into two parts.

The *posterior urethra* extends from the internal urethral orifice at bladder neck passing through anterior part of prostate distally to the inferior urogenital diaphragm. The posterior urethra consists of a prostatic segment and a membranous segment and is lined by transitional epithelium.

The *prostatic urethra* is surrounded by the prostate gland and measures 3 to 3.5 cm in length. It is the widest and most dilatable part of male urethra, being widest in the middle part and narrowest where it joins membranous urethra. The posterior wall of prostatic urethra has a median longitudinal ridge of smooth muscle (urethral crest) extending from bladder neck to membranous urethra. The longitudinal ridge continues into an ovoid mound known as verumontanum (15–17 mm in length and 3 mm in height). The prostatic utricle is a small saccular depression in the center of verumontanum. The ejaculatory ducts open distal and lateral to the utricle. The prostatic gland opens into prostatic urethra via prostatic sinuses.

The *membranous urethra* measures 1.5–2 cm in length and is surrounded by sphincter urethrae. It is the narrowest and least dilatable part of male urethra with the exception of external orifice. It extends from the distal end of verumontanum to the tip of cone of bulbous urethra. It runs downward and forward through the deep perineal space piercing the urogenital diaphragm about 2.5 cm below and behind the pubic symphysis. The urogenital diaphragm contains the external urethral sphincter with a Cowper gland on either side.

The *anterior urethra* extends from inferior edge of urogenital diaphragm distally to the external meatus and measures 15 cm in length. The anterior urethra consists of a bulbous segment and a penile or pendulous segment and is lined by stratified columnar epithelium.

The *bulbous urethra* is located between the inferior margin of the urogenital diaphragm and the penoscrotal junction. The bulbous urethra courses within the root of the penis and is tubular structure in the midline within the bulb of the corpus spongiosum. The proximal portion of bulbar urethra is dilated and called "sump" of bulbar urethra. It assumes a conical shape at bulbomembranous junction. The duct of Cowper glands are 2 cm long and empty into the bulbar urethral sump in midline. The periurethral Littre gland are present in anterior urethra.

The *penile urethra* extends from the penoscrotal junction to the external meatus with the distal 2 cm of dilated portion urethra known as *fossa navicularis.*

Urethral Sphincters

There are two sphincters which maintain continence of urine.

The *internal urethral sphincter* (sphincter vesicae) extends from the bladder neck through the prostatic urethra above the verumontanum and is composed of smooth muscle. It is the primary sphincter of urinary continence and involuntary in nature.

The *external sphincter* (sphincter urethrae) has both intrinsic and extrinsic components and is voluntary in nature. The *intrinsic urethral sphincter* is a concentric muscular structure that lies below the mound of the verumontanum in the distal third of the prostatic urethra and surrounds the membranous urethra. The intrinsic sphincter is composed of smooth muscle and also functions as muscle that maintains passive incontinence, along with internal sphincter. The intrinsic sphincter functions as the secondary continence sphincter. The *extrinsic sphincter* is paraurethral, composed

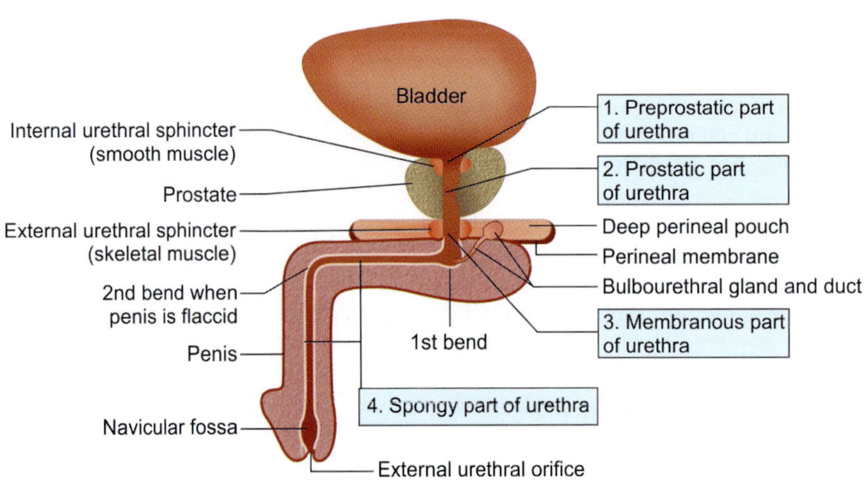

FIG. 2: Schematic diagram of male urethra.

of striated muscle with contributions from the levator ani complex and is voluntary in nature.

Female Urethra

The female urethra is a 4 cm long tubular structure, extending from the internal urethral meatus at bladder neck, 5 cm behind pubic symphysis, to external urethral meatus in the vestibule traversing through urogenital diaphragm. The external meatus opens directly in front of vaginal opening and about 2.5 cm behind glans clitoris. In the undilated stage, it is 6 mm in diameter. Numerous small submucosal paraurethral and periurethral glands opens into the urethra. The paraurethral glands of Skene secrete mucous material into either side of the distal urethra at the external meatus.

The proximal third of the urethra is lined by transitional cell epithelium and distal two-third of urethra is lined by stratified squamous epithelium. The urethropelvic and pubourethral ligaments help in maintaining urinary continence and urethral stability. The lower portion of the urethra is intimately situated next to the anterior vaginal wall and enveloped by common musculature (the urethrovaginal sphincter), which extends to the inferior pubic ramus above urogenital diaphragm.

IMAGING MODALITIES

Radiological evaluations of the urinary bladder and urethra are done by various imaging modalities such as:

- Plain radiograph
- Voiding cystourethrography
- Retrograde urethrography
- Cystography
- Retrograde pyelography
- Conduitogram
- Ultrasonography
- Computed tomography (CT)
- Magnetic resonance imaging (MRI)
- Urodynamic studies
- Radionuclide imaging.

Plain Radiographs

The plain radiograph is the primary modality for detection of radiopaque calculi in patients presenting with hematuria or foreign bodies, calcification, abnormal gas pattern and in identification of soft tissue and the bony abnormalities. **(Fig. 3)**. It is referred to as *scout film* prior to contrast studies to identify any radiopacity that may be obscured with contrast subsequently.

The plain radiograph done for evaluation of kidneys, ureters and bladder (KUB) is known by term X-ray KUB in which X-ray beam is centered in midline at level of iliac crest and exposure factors generally used are low Kvp (65–75 Kvp) and high mA (60–100 mA).

Calcification of the bladder wall may be seen in tuberculosis, hydatid disease, tumors, radiation cystitis, cyclophosphamide induced cystitis, alkaline incrustation cystitis, amyloidosis and schistosomiasis. Radiolucent foreign bodies may get encrusted with calcium.

The plain radiograph typically shows gas within the bladder lumen and wall in emphysematous cystitis. Presence of gas is seen within the ureter wall in the emphysematous pyeloureteritis or emphysematous pyelonephritis.

It is also helpful for the detection of bony abnormalities such as metastases, spinal abnormalities in cases of neurogenic bladder and diastasis of the pubic symphysis in patients with exstrophy/epispadias anomaly.

Voiding Cystourethrography

Voiding cystourethrography is the standard technique in the evaluation of the posterior urethra of male, female urethra and bladder. It allows detection of bladder neck pathology, postsurgical stenosis and urethral stricture. The main indications of VCUG include evaluation of vesicoureteric reflux (VUR), urinary leak (post-trauma, surgery) and for urodynamic study. This study is particularly useful in evaluation of posterior urethral valves and for evaluation of diverticula, false tracts and strictures in the urethra.

Technique and Normal Appearance

Voiding cystourethrography is usually performed after filling the bladder with contrast material via a transurethral or suprapubic catheter. Patient is asked to empty bladder prior to the procedure. The patient is then catheterized and Foley's bulb is inflated in bladder followed by instillation of contrast, till patient can tolerate. Once the bladder is distended, urethral catheter is withdrawn, and patient is asked to void under fluoroscopic monitoring. The spot radiographs of the bladder and urethra are then obtained after positioning the patient in right and left anterior oblique positions to avoid super imposition of the urethra on the pubic symphysis. Full KUB radiograph is taken to assess bladder anatomy and presence of any undetected VUR. This is followed by a postvoid film to evaluate residual volume of bladder (PVR).

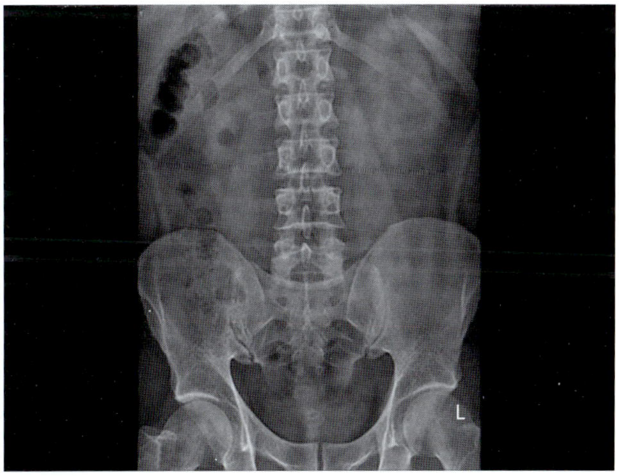

FIG. 3: X-ray Abdomen KUB- Bowel preparation is necessary. Patient micturates before examination (to see the bladder outline) and the radiograph is taken in full inspiration to include area of abdomen from adrenals to a point 2 cm below the inferior margin of pubic symphysis, with beam centering in midline at level of iliac crests.

In case clinical suspicion of vesicovaginal fistula (VVF) or rectovaginal fistula (RVF), a lateral view must also be taken.

During active voiding, the bladder neck opens widely and becomes funnel shaped in both male and female patients by means of the internal sphincter mechanism. In males, the verumontanum appears elongated and the proximal bulbar urethra has a less conical appearance. The membranous urethra remains the narrowest segment between these parts of the urethra **(Figs. 4A and B)**. During voiding, it may dilate up to 6 or 7 mm in diameter.

Voiding cystourethrography may not demonstrate certain abnormalities of the male anterior urethra because the normal anterior urethra is not fully distended. It is an invasive study and does not provide information regarding the periurethral tissues.

Retrograde Urethrography

Retrograde urethrography is considered the standard imaging technique for evaluation of *anterior urethra.* It is the primary modality indicated in the evaluation of urethral injuries, inflammatory disease, strictures and fistulas. Assessment of the location, length and severity of urethral pathologies can be done based on RGU studies.

Technique and Normal Appearance

The patient is placed in a supine 45 oblique position. The penis should be placed laterally over the proximal thigh with moderate traction. The patient should be reassured about the discomfort that is experienced during balloon inflation. A 16-F or 18-F Foley's catheter is inserted into urethra so that the balloon lies in fossa navicularis and is inflated with 2 to 3 mL of water to anchor catheter and occlude the meatus. Then, 20–30 mL of iodinated contrast material is injected in the anterior urethra under fluoroscopic guidance through the Foley's catheter till it is adequately distended **(Fig. 5)**.

After the visual confirmation of contrast material flowing into the bladder, spot radiographs are obtained. Sometimes, normal structures such as prostatic duct, Littre's gland and Cowper duct are also opacified due to intravasation of contrast.

The external urethral sphincter spasm encountered during injection can be overcome by slow and gentle pressure. Sometimes, lidocaine gel or normal saline may be used to obtain urethral distention in such cases. Sometimes, there is disruption of urethral mucosa due to increased pressure during injection, which causes opacification of corpora and draining vein due to intravasation of contrast.

Acute urinary tract infection (UTI), urethral trauma and intravasation of contrast are few *complications* of the procedure. Recent instrumentation and acute UTI are two *contraindications* of this procedure.

Cystography

Cystography (retrograde, excretory or suprapubic) is a contrast study of bladder to evaluate its position, morphology, integrity and distensibility. It allows evaluation of both intraluminal and intramural lesions and functional abnormalities. Contrast cystogram can clearly depict wall

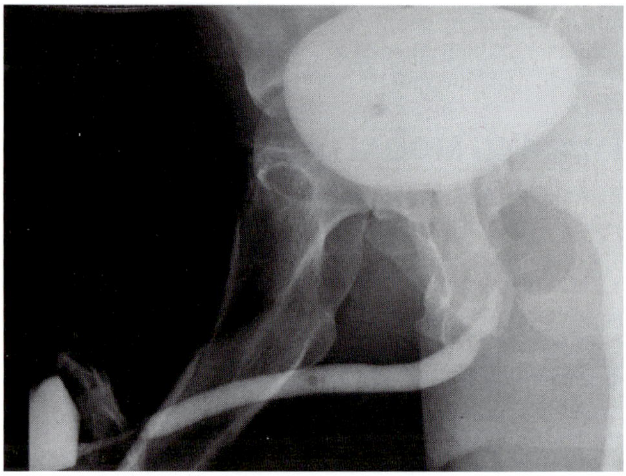

FIG. 5: For retrograde urethrography, the patient is placed in a supine 45 oblique position. 20–30 mL of iodinated contrast is injected under fluoroscopic guidance through the catheter with tip in fossa navicularis, so that the anterior urethra is filled. Spot radiographs are obtained when there is visual confirmation of contrast material flowing into the bladder.

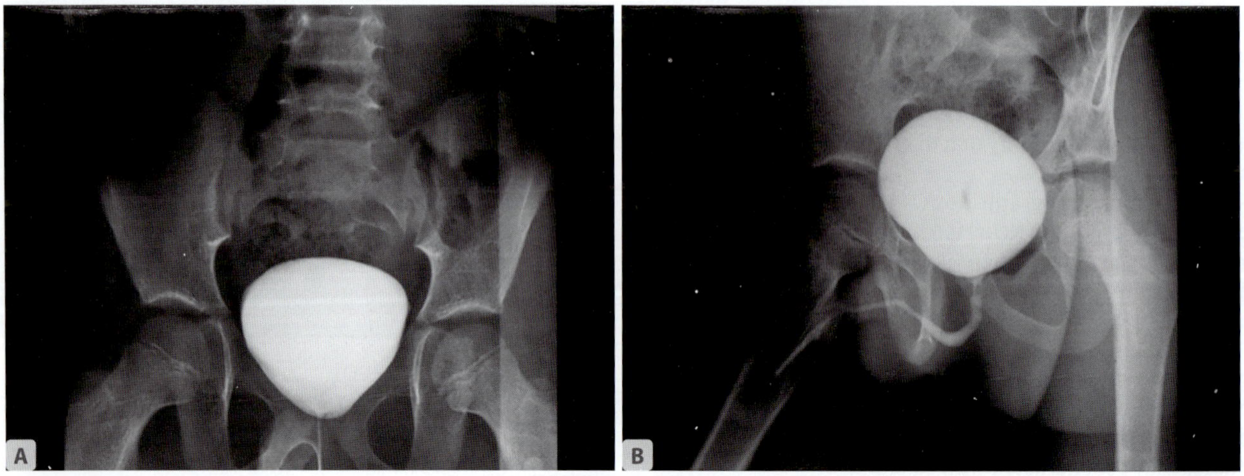

FIGS. 4A AND B: Micturating cystography involves the introduction of contrast into the urinary bladder followed by micturition urinary bladder for the evaluation of the urinary bladder and urethra.

irregularities, tumors, intraluminal calculi and hematomas. It also demonstrates the type of bladder rupture (extraperitoneal or intraperitoneal) along with pelvic fractures in traumatic injury. Extrinsic compression of the bladder produced by pelvic hematoma or lipomatosis results in "teardrop bladder" and is better evaluated on cross-sectional imaging.

Conventional retrograde cystography is considered as gold standard in suspected bladder injury and plays an important role in patients with renal failure having lesions in the bladder.

In the *excretory cystogram,* bladder is evaluated simultaneously along with upper urinary tracts in intravenous pyelography (IVP), but it is difficult to recognize reflux.

Cystography of bladder and Voiding cystourethrography are indicated for demonstration of anatomic abnormalities of the bladder neck and urethra.

About 300 to 400 mL appropriately diluted nonionic contrast is instilled in bladder using Foley's catheter. Images are then obtained under fluoroscopic guidance in various projections (AP, oblique, lateral, during rest and strain/or voiding) appropriate to the indications for the study.

Pregnancy, UTI and allergy to iodinated contrast are contraindications to the procedure.

Retrograde Pyelography

This investigation is infrequently used for evaluation of lower ureters when pathology like lower ureteric stones, mitotic process or strictures are not demonstrated by other imaging modalities. It is an invasive procedure where ureteral orifice is cannulated cystoscopically and catheter is advanced into renal pelvis and contrast is injected. The examination is performed with graded withdrawal of catheter under fluoroscopic monitoring and appropriate spot films are taken.

Conduitogram

An ileal conduit is constructed for urinary diversion after partial or complete cystectomy. One end of the ileum is brought to skin as an ileocutaneous stoma and ureters are implanted in the opposite end of the loop. Contrast material is instilled into the ileal loop through stoma. It demonstrates ureters and renal collecting system. The study is also called loopogram or an ideal conduit study. The study is useful in patient with impaired renal function and serves to exclude ureteral obstruction. It also helps to evaluate stricture or leak at the site of anastomosis of ureter and ileal conduit.

Ultrasonography

Urinary Bladder

Real-time ultrasonography (US) is the primary modality in the evaluation of bladder lesions.

Bladder US indications include:

- Evaluation of bladder wall, its base, distal ureter and urethral orifice anatomy.
- For evaluation of thickening, diverticula and trabeculations.
- Pre and post-void residual volume.
- Bladder calculi including radiolucent calculi, which may be missed on plain radiographs.
- Blood clots and sediments within the lumen.
- Intraluminal filling defects and extraluminal masses causing bladder compression.
- For guiding diagnostic and therapeutic interventions.

Technique

The urinary bladder must be examined when it is comfortably distended either by oral intake of fluid and voiding restrictions. In anuric patient, it can be retrogradely filled with normal saline through a catheter. The bladder sonography is done by transabdominal, perineal, endorectal or endovaginal approaches.

Transabdominal approach is the most common. In this approach, a 3.5–5 MHz sector scanning transducer is placed in suprapubic region and angled appropriately for longitudinal and transverse views of bladder.

Transrectal/Transvaginal transducer (frequency range from 3.5–7 MHz) is used to image bladder base, its neck and for evaluation of posterior wall masses. It is useful in defining the plane between the bladder, prostate and seminal vesicles.

Transurethral US scan provides better details of urinary bladder wall and is used to visualize and stage bladder tumor.

Normal Sonographic Appearance

The bladder is present in midline in true pelvis and appears as a sonolucent structure with smooth thin wall. Its shape is oval in the trans-axial plane and triangular in sagittal plane **(Fig. 6)**. Reverberation artefact seen during bladder scanning can be avoided by slightly changing the angle of transducer.

Bladder wall measures 3–6 mm, is comprised hyperechoic outer serosa and mucosa with hypoechoic detrusor muscle in between.

The formula used to calculate full bladder volume and postmicturition residual volume is 0.523 × length × width × height.

The ureteric orifice is seen as small focal thickening in the bladder base on either side, through which low level of echoes are seen entering bladder which are known as ureteric jets. Ureteric jets are best evaluated on Doppler and their presence rules out complete obstruction **(Fig. 7)**. In normal healthy person, ureteric jet frequency is of two or more per minute on either side. If ureteric jets are absent during steady diuresis phase for 10 more minutes of observation, it represent complete obstruction and frequency of less than two per minute may indicate partial obstruction.

Male Urethra

Urethral ultrasound plays an important role in the evaluation of urethra, periurethral tissue and for diagnosis, assessment of thickness and length of urethral strictures. It is equally efficacious as RGU in detection and characterization of anterior urethral strictures and false tracts with the added advantage of lower incidence of complications.

Voiding urethral sonography detects the bladder neck and posterior urethra pathology (anatomical and functional), postsurgical stenosis and neoplasm.

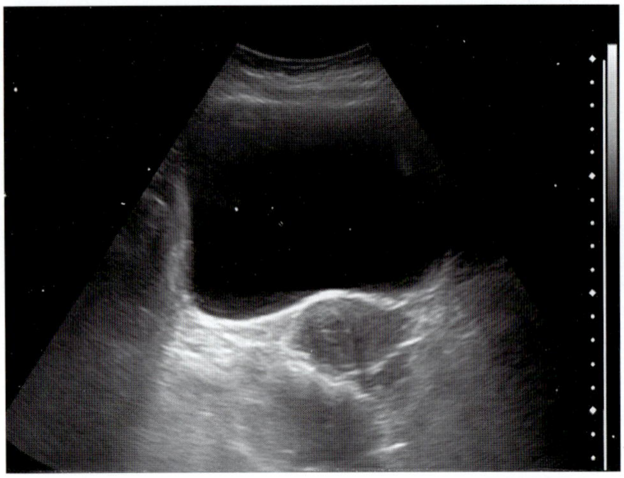

FIG. 6: Examination of the urinary bladder requires well filled bladder for its detailed evaluation for the adjoining structures and tissues.

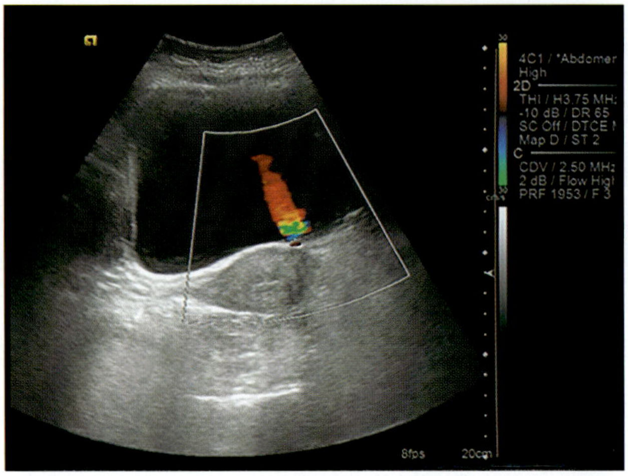

FIG. 7: For routine, transabdominal urinary bladder imaging, bladder must be full. UV junction obstruction can also be inferred by evaluation of lower ureteric jets on color Doppler.

Technique and Normal Appearance

Sonography of the urethra is usually performed using a broadband 5–10 MHz linear array for transpenile or transperineal scanning and a broadband 5–9 MHz curved array for transrectal scanning. The *posterior male urethra* can be evaluated by TRUS. Endourethral sonography is performed with a catheter (6.2-F) based transducer (12.5 MHz) on a dedicated intravascular US machine.

Penile urethra can be seen through penile shaft using the linear probe after filling the penile urethra with fluid or gel. The normal urethra is seen as an anechoic tubular structure. It is also called *ascending urethral sonography*. Subscrotal and perineal views delineate anterior urethra clearly in longitudinal and transverse scanning planes.

A modification of this technique is *descending urethral ultrasound* technique in which urethral distension is achieved during voiding, which is interrupted by gently clamping 2 cm proximal to the tip of penis. Under distension of urethra can lead to false diagnosis of stricture. This technique is useful in evaluating strictures in region of navicular fossa, pre- and postoperative patients of hypospadias repair, trauma and in planning reconstructive anterior urethroplasty.

Advances in imaging technology like extended field of view imaging have enhanced the use of this modality in clinical practice.

Female Urethra

Ultrasound allows detailed evaluation of female urethra and periurethral disease by using transabdominal, transvaginal, transperineal, and transurethral US approaches.

Technique and Normal Appearance

In transvaginal US, a 5–9 MHz curved-array transducer is used and is inserted approximately 1–2 cm into the vagina and in transperineal US, a 5–10 MHz linear-array transducer is placed on the perineum between the labia for obtaining sagittal and transverse images. For transurethral US, a catheter (6.2 F) based transducer (12.5 MHz) on an intravascular US machine is used. Axial images are obtained as catheter is withdrawn. Patients lie in the lithotomy position with partially filled bladder. The urethra is evaluated from the bladder neck to the distal urethral opening, with subsequent attention given to the periurethral area. It is used for diagnosis of urethral diverticula and strictures.

The female urethra is visualized on transabdominal scan as short anechoic channel with anteroposterior diameters just inferior to the bladder measuring 1–1.5 cm. It appears less echogenic than the surrounding connective tissue or the bladder wall.

There is an important role of dynamic US in the diagnosis and classification of pelvic floor dysfunction and pelvic organ prolapse. Dynamic US with endoluminal transducers is an emerging technique in the evaluation of pelvic floor dysfunction. It allows real-time evaluation of the displacement of pelvic floor muscles and pelvic organs during provocative maneuvers such as coughing and the Valsalva maneuver.

In women with symptoms of stress incontinence, hypermobility of the urethra or a "funnel" appearance of the proximal urethra may be noted during coughing due to laxity of connective tissues. After surgical correction of pelvic organ prolapse, endoluminal US is valuable in assessing achievement of normal genitourinary anatomy and the absence of urethral funneling and recurrent cystourethrocele.

Computed Tomography

Computed tomography urography (CTU) has emerged as a promising tool in the evaluation of urologic conditions over IVU. CT cystography is an accurate and safe means for identification of bladder injury and urine leakage following bladder or posterior urethra rupture in abdominal trauma patient.

The important indications of CTU in lower urinary tract (LUT) are:

- Evaluation of hematuria
- Identification of size and number of distal ureteric, vesicle or urethral calculi and calcification

- Staging of bladder and urethral malignancy
- Pelvic trauma and bladder rupture
- Postoperative complications
- Congenital anomalies.

Technique

Computed tomography urography is mainly done to evaluate upper tract collecting system, ureters and urinary bladder in excretory phase. The three techniques used are single bolus, split bolus and triple bolus protocols.

Single bolus technique is the most common and routinely used. In this, first noncontrast image is acquired. After full bolus of contrast injection, images are acquired in the nephrographic phase (80 to 120s), corticomedullary phase (30 to 40s) and delayed excretory phase (5 to 15 min), however, corticomedullary phase is optional for evaluation in case of bladder pathologies. The bladder tumor can be best evaluated in nephrographic or excretory phase.

In split bolus technique, the contrast is given into separate injections. After taking noncontrast scan, a part of contrast is given and corticomedullary images are obtained. The second portion of contrast is given 5 to 8 minutes after the first injection and combined nephrographic and excretory phase images are acquired. The images acquired from entire abdomen and pelvis. It is done in younger patients to reduce radiation dose.

Computed tomography cystography consists of imaging of bladder following retrograde filling of bladder with contrast up to patient tolerance (200–300 mL) followed by a CT of the pelvis. It should be followed by intravenous contrast administration and acquisition of abdomen and pelvis after that. Postdrainage scan are not required. It should be done in all patients with pelvic fracture or with gross hematuria.

Normal Computed Tomography Appearance

The urinary bladder is seen as a homogeneous midline structure of water density. The outer margin of the bladder wall is smooth and has soft tissue attenuation. It is well-delineated by the perivesical fat. The urine shows water density attenuation. The size and configuration depends on the amount of urine present **(Figs. 8A to C)**.

Noncontrast scans are useful for detection of vesicle calculi, intravesical hemorrhage, bladder wall calcification and gas in bladder wall and lumen.

In contrast enhanced CT scan, opacified urine usually occupies the dependent portion of the bladder and unopacified urine layers above it. However, this relationship may be reversed in patients with glycosuria or infectious debris in the bladder. Contrast-enhanced CT (CECT) is essential in tumor staging especially for evaluation of bladder wall and transmural extent and distinction of lymph node from vascular structures and adjacent masses compressing or displacing the bladder. CT can also reveal elevation and narrowing of the bladder (pear shaped bladder) in retroperitoneal fibrosis, pelvic lipomatosis, hematoma and lymphoceles. It also helps in the evaluation of lower ureter if thickened or inflamed as evidenced by its wall thickening and periureteral fat stranding.

Virtual Cystoscopy

Virtual cystoscopy is a diagnostic tool for evaluation of bladder pathology. It is dedicated for evaluating the mucosal surface of the bladder and therefore, can detect superficial lesion greater than 5 mm. It allows the operator to navigate the mucosal surface in various projections. The technique of virtual cystoscopy/endoscopy has been refined and clinically improved over the last few years.

It can either be done as part of the routine CTU protocol using contrast-filled bladder, or using an air-filled bladder. The contrast filled bladder protocol are more commonly used over air-filled technique as latter requires catheterization and there is possibility of leakage of air with change in position. The most commonly used multidetector computed tomography (MDCT) protocol include unenhanced scan in supine and prone and postcontrast scan as per CT urography protocol. Volumetric data set is acquired and are computer rendered to generate 3D images. Special software then allows navigation through the bladder. Virtual endoscopy techniques may provide ureteral "flythrough" allowing to have an ureteroscopic viewpoint of the urinary tract.

The main complications of air-filled technique are infection due to the use of room air and CT must be acquired in both prone and supine position and that of contrast filled technique are contrast allergy and inability to be done in renal insufficiency.

Its advantages are noninvasive nature and no risk for local infection, bladder perforation, strictures and scarring. The disadvantages include failure to detect flat lesions and to distinguish mucosal thickening due to fibrosis from neoplasm.

Magnetic Resonance Imaging

Recent technological advances in MR imaging allows more detailed evaluation of urinary bladder, urethral and periurethral abnormalities. Advances in MR imaging hardware and pulse sequences allow high-resolution, high-contrast static and dynamic imaging of the urinary bladder, urethral and periurethral region in the context of the entire pelvic floor.

Magnetic resonance images provide an excellent insight into the anatomy and pathology of the urinary bladder due to its exquisite contrast resolution and multiplanar ability. It clearly differentiates the three layers of the bladder wall and enables accurate assessment of the depth of tumor invasion and extravesical extension in patients with bladder tumors. Multiparametric MRI techniques enables better evaluation and staging of bladder cancer. It also offers functional information through pulse sequences such as diffusion weighted MRI (DW MRI) and dynamic contrast MRI (DCE MRI).

Magnetic resonance cystography is used for bladder tumor detection, complication of tumor, trauma such as leak, fistulae, or sinus tract formation and VUR. It is mainly used in a patient who have iodine allergy or contraindication to CT.

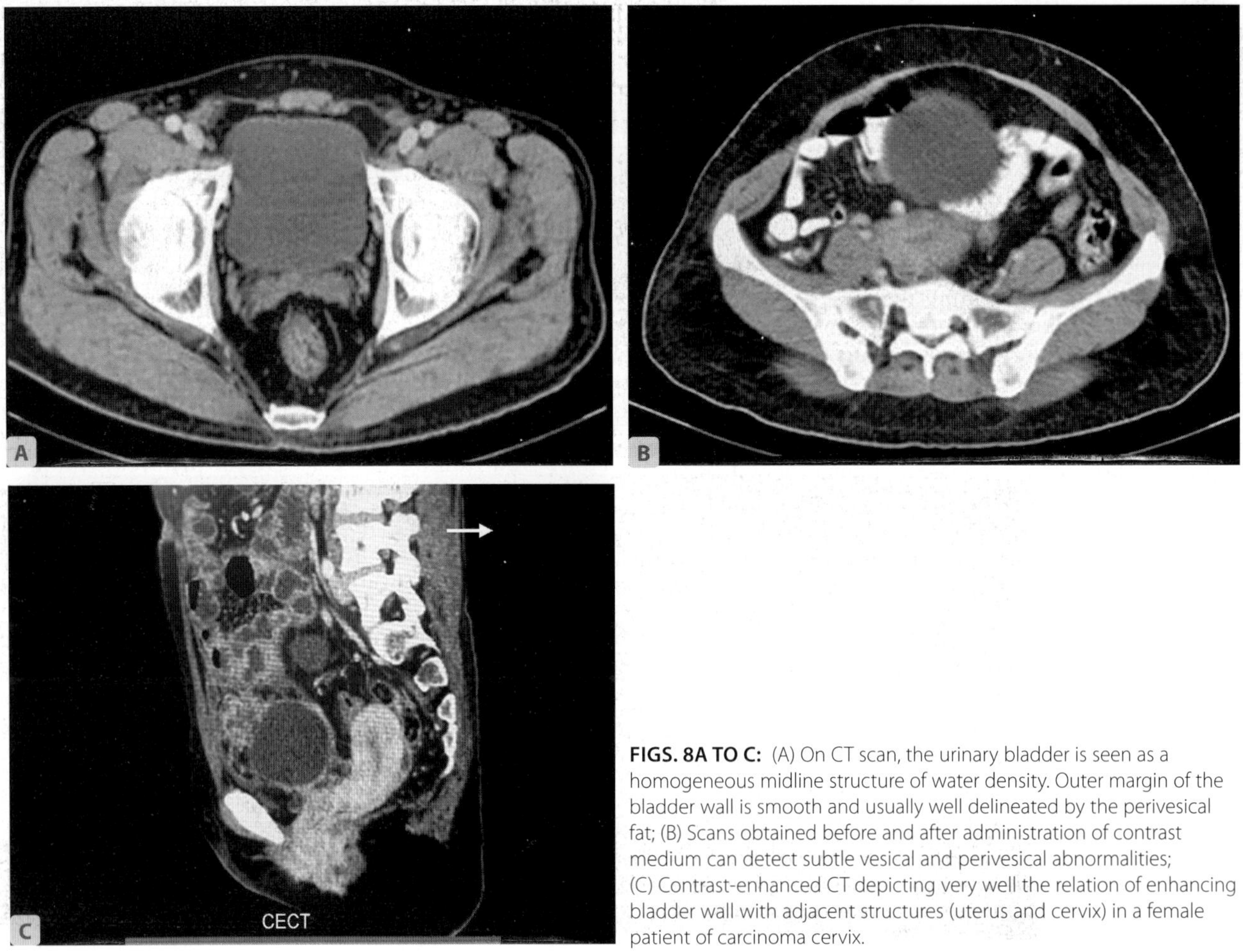

FIGS. 8A TO C: (A) On CT scan, the urinary bladder is seen as a homogeneous midline structure of water density. Outer margin of the bladder wall is smooth and usually well delineated by the perivesical fat; (B) Scans obtained before and after administration of contrast medium can detect subtle vesical and perivesical abnormalities; (C) Contrast-enhanced CT depicting very well the relation of enhancing bladder wall with adjacent structures (uterus and cervix) in a female patient of carcinoma cervix.

Technique and Recommended Sequence

The standard MRI sequences used in the bladder imaging are T1 and T2 weighted in all three axial, coronal and sagittal planes, diffusion-weighted MRI (DWI) and T1-weighted with fat saturation pre and post IV administration of gadolinium. Dedicated phased array multi coils and endorectal coils significantly improve image resolution.

Dynamic contrast-enhanced T1-weighted MRI is used for tumor staging and prognostication.

Lymphotropic nanoparticle-enhanced MRI can be used for differentiating bowel loops from lymph nodes and thus prove to be helpful in nodal staging in bladder cancer patients using MR oral intestinal contrast agents such as ferrite particles.

In MR cystogram, initially a precontrast image is taken and then imaging is done after installation of gadolinium in 1:100 concentration (5 mL in 500 mL of saline). In patients with contrast allergies gadolinium is replaced by saline solution.

Normal Magnetic Resonance Appearance

The urinary bladder is clearly demonstrated on MRI regardless of distension. Urine has low signal intensity on T1W and high on T2W. Muscle layer has low signal intensity on T2-weighted image and low to intermediate signal intensity on T1-weighted images. Both mucosa and lamina propria have higher signal intensity as compared to muscle on proton density sequences **(Figs. 9A to C)**. Lateral wall are best evaluated on axial section. Dome, base, anterior and posterior wall of the bladder are primarily evaluated on sagittal images, however, coronal images do play complimentary role. T1W Fat-Sat spin echo is helpful in evaluation of lymph node and bone.

Urethra

Magnetic resonance imaging provides detailed multiplanar evaluation of urethra and periurethral tissues. Both T1- and T2 weighted imaging are used to evaluate the male and female urethra. Dedicated phased array or endocavitary coils can be used for detailed evaluation.

Male Urethra

T2-weighted images show the course of the anterior and posterior urethras in sagittal and coronal planes. The proximal portion of the prostatic urethra and distal penile urethra is properly visualized on MR images only if an indwelling catheter is placed. Initial evaluation of the membranous urethra is done in the axial plane and images in sagittal and coronal planes are useful to assess relationship with adjoining structures, especially in cases of trauma. Contrast enhanced MR imaging can be performed in patients with mitotic or inflammatory processes involving the urethra and periurethral tissues.

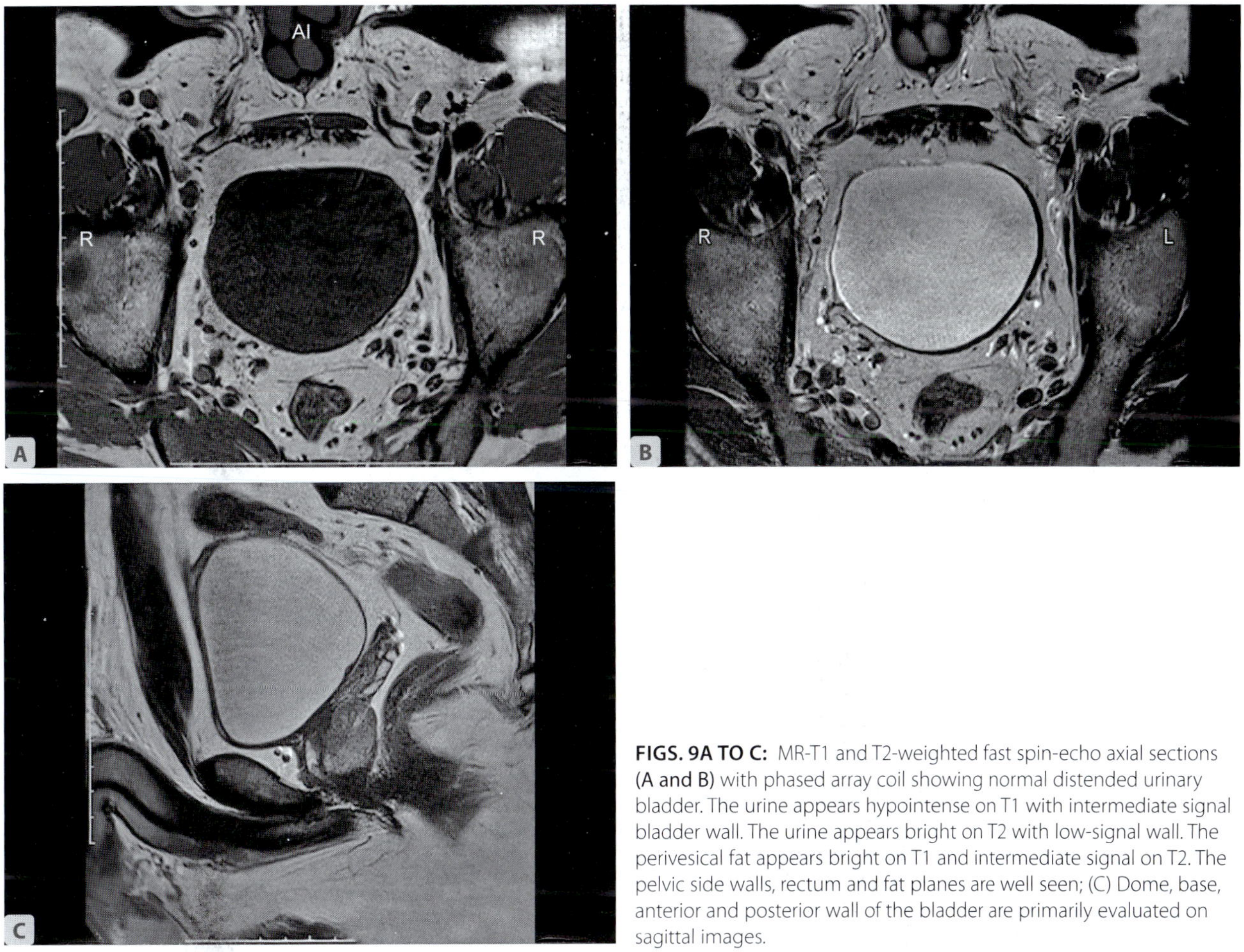

FIGS. 9A TO C: MR-T1 and T2-weighted fast spin-echo axial sections (A and B) with phased array coil showing normal distended urinary bladder. The urine appears hypointense on T1 with intermediate signal bladder wall. The urine appears bright on T2 with low-signal wall. The perivesical fat appears bright on T1 and intermediate signal on T2. The pelvic side walls, rectum and fat planes are well seen; (C) Dome, base, anterior and posterior wall of the bladder are primarily evaluated on sagittal images.

Female Urethra

Magnetic resonance imaging because of its superior temporal resolution is suitable for anatomic evaluation of various urethral and periurethral abnormalities. It is useful in local staging of urethral tumors. It can also be of help in evaluating congenital anomalies, diverticulum, inflammation, trauma, and fistula of the urethra in female patients. On MR imaging, a fistula can be seen as a direct communication channel with an adjacent organ.

Virtual Cystoscopy Magnetic Resonance

Magnetic resonance based virtual cystoscopy newer technique being increasingly used as an adjunct to conventional cystoscopy to assess bladder noninvasively. It is better than conventional cystoscopy as, it is impervious to hematuria, and anterior bladder wall lesion and urethral stricture. It has certain limitations such as time consuming, costly and require expertise. It is not possible to do biopsy with MR cystoscopy (MRC) or detect flat lesions.

Magnetic resonance cystoscopy is done by two ways: (1) 3D T1W MRI is acquired after filling the bladder with gadolinium retrogradely by catheter or intravenously, (2) 3D T2W MRI is acquired after luminal distension with urine. The 3D data sets obtained from both methods can be evaluated by multiplanar, 3D or virtual cystoscopic "fly through" reconstruction method.

Urodynamic Studies

Urodynamic studies are functional studies of urinary bladder and are considered to be the most definitive tests for determining the source of symptoms involving the lower urinary tract, including the bladder and the urethra for storing and releasing urine. These tests can help to pinpoint the anatomic or neurologic source of symptoms such as leakage, frequent urination, problem in initiating stream, dribbling, painful urination, difficulty in completely emptying the bladder and recurrent UTI.

The types of tests that are administered depend on the patient's symptoms and may include one or more of the tests like uroflowmetry, cystometry, pressure studies for stress incontinence, VCUG, video urodynamics and assessment of postvoid residual urine, etc.

Nuclear Imaging

Radionuclide cystography has been accepted as the technique of choice for evaluation and follow-up of children with UTI and reflux.

Positron emission tomography-CT (PET-CT) and PET -MR are hybrid imaging modalities that have combined both morphologic and functional imaging simultaneously for providing better information for guiding therapy.

The most commonly used PET radiotracer is 2-deoxy-2-(18F)-fluorodeoxyglucose (18F-FDG).

FDG-PET is useful in monitoring response to therapy and management urinary bladder cancer. It also helps in identification of distant metastasis. FDG PET has limited role in urologic cancer because of high urinary activity of radiotracer.

PET-CT has established its role in metastatic work up for bladder cancer. It helps in detection of primary tumor and nodal metastasis.

PET-MR due to its better soft tissue resolution and with simultaneous use of DW-MRI and DCE MRI detects local tumor, nodal and distant metastasis.

Recent advances in PET-CT/PET MR techniques and with few new radiotracer such as C11-choline and C11-acetate have increased the role of this technique in urinary bladder cancer.

CONCLUSION

The imaging techniques for evaluation of lower urinary tract have advanced seemingly in past decades. VCU and RGU remains the mainstay of conventional imaging procedures for evaluation of lower urinary tract, while ultrasound remains a promising a screening tool. Cross-sectional imaging like CT and MRI are the modality of choice for staging and follow up of urothelial malignancy. With the advent of the multiparametric MRI incorporating anatomic and functional sequences such as DWI, DCE-MRI, and lymphotropic nanoparticle-enhanced MRI, MR has become the mainstay in the diagnosis, staging, and follow-up of bladder cancer.

SUGGESTED READING

1. Arif SH, Mohammed AA. Primary hydatid cyst of the urinary bladder. BMJ Case Rep. 2018. pii: bcr-2018-226341. doi: 10.1136/bcr-2018-226341.
2. Berná-Mestre JD, Berná-Serna JD. Anterior urethral trauma: role of sonourethrography. Emerg Radiol. 2009;16(5):391-4.
3. Bernhardt TM, Rapp Bernhardt U. Virtual cystoscopy of the bladder based on CT and MRI data. Abdom Imaging. 2001;26(3):325-32.
4. Bernhardt TM, Schmidl H, Philipp C, et al. Diagnostic potential of virtual cystoscopy of the bladder. MRI vs CT preliminary report. Eur Radiol. 2003;13(2):305-12.
5. Buckley JC, Wu AK, McAninch JW. Impact of urethral ultrasonography on decision-making in anterior urethroplasty. BJU Int. 2012;109(3):438-42.
6. Chan DP, Abujudeh HH, Cushing GL Ir Novelline RAC1 cystography with multiplanar reformation for suspected bladder rupture: experience in 234 cases. AJR Am J Roentgenol. 2006;187(5):1296-302.
7. Choudhary S, Singh P, Sundar E, et al. A comparison of sonourethrography and retrograde urethrography in evaluation of anterior urethral strictures. Clin Radiol. 2004;59(8):736-42.
8. Choyke PL, Bluth EI, Bush WH Jr, et al. Radiological investigation of patients with hematuria. American College of Radiology, ACR Appropriateness Criteria, 2005.
9. Clinical Magnetic Resonance Imaging. Vol 3 2006,Elsevier Inc. Page 2889-2905.
10. Cruz J, Figueiredo F, Matos AP, et al. Infectious and inflammatory diseases of the urinary tract: role of MR imaging. Magn Reson Imaging Clin N Am. 2019;27(1):59-75.
11. David S. A Textbook of Radiology. 1993;2:1079-97.
12. Ferguson GG, Bullock TL, Anderson RE, et al. Minimally invasive methods for bulbar urethral strictures: a survey of members of the American Urological Association. Urology. 2011;78(3):701-6.
13. Gupta N, Dubey D, Mandhani A, et al. Urethral stricture assessment: a prospective study evaluating urethral ultrasonography and conventional radiological studies. BJU Int. 2006;98(1):149-53.
14. Johnin K1, Kobayashi K1, Tsuru T1, et al. Pediatric voiding cystourethrography: An essential examination for urologists but a terrible experience for children. Int J Urol. 2019;26(2):160-71.
15. Karavaş E, Gürel S, Kıyan A, et al. Effect of Prone and Supine Positioning on Computed Tomography Urography Examination. Urol Int. 2018;101(2):167-74.
16. Kawashima A, Glockner JF, King BF Jr. CT urography and MR urography. Radiol Clin North Am. 2003;41(5):945-61.
17. Kim JK, Park SY, Kim HS, et al. Comparison of virtual cystoscopy, multiplanar reformation and source CT images with contrast material filled bladder for detecting lesions. AJR Am J Roentgenol. 2005;185(3):689-96.
18. Kim JY, Harisinghani MG. MR imaging staging of pelvic lymph nodes. Magn Reson Imaging Clin N Am. 2004;12(3):581-6.
19. Kim SU, Han MC. Reversed contrast-urine levels in urinary bladder: CT findings. Urol Radiol. 1992;13(14):249.52.
20. Maher MM, Kalra MK, Rizzo S, et al. Multidetector CT urography in imaging of the urinary tract in patients with hematuria. Korean J Radiol. 2004;5(1):1-10.
21. Mallampati GK, Siegelman ES. MR imaging of the bladder. Magn Reson Imaging Clin N Am. 2004:12(3):545-55.
22. McCallum RW. The adult male urethra normal anatomy, pathology, and method of urethrography. Radiol Clin North Am. 1979;17(2):227-44.
23. Mitterberger M, Christian G, Pinggera GM, et al. Gray scale and color Doppler sonography with extended field of view technique for the diagnostic evaluation of anterior urethral strictures. J Urol. 2007;177(3):992-6.
24. Morgan DE, Nallamala LK, Kenney PJ, et al. CT cystography: Radiographic and clinical predictors of bladder rupture. AJR Am J Roentgenol. 2000;174(1):89-95.
25. Pollack HM, Banner MP Martinez LO, et al. Diagnostic considerations in urinary bladder wall calcification. AJR. 1981;136(4):791-7.
26. Price CI, Adler RS, Rubin JM. Ultrasound depiction of differences in density: Explanation of ureteral jet phenomenon and implications for new ultrasound applications. Invest Radiol. 1989;24(11):876-83.
27. Raman SP, Fishman EK. Upper and Lower Tract Urothelial Imaging Using Computed Tomography Urography. Urol Clin North Am. 2018;45(3):389-405.
28. Rickards D, Hare C. The lower urinary tract. In Meire HB, Cosgrove D, Dewbury KC, Farrant P (Eds). Abdominal and General Ultrasound. Edinburgh, Churchill Livingstone; 585-611,200
29. Silverman SG, Leyendecker JR, Amis SE Jr. What is the current role of CT urography and MR urography in the evaluation of the urinary tract? Radiology. 2009;250(2):309-23.
30. Taveras N, Demas BE, Hricak H. MR Imaging of bladder neoplasms: correlation with pathologic staging. Urol Radiol. 1990;12(1):27-33.
31. The Journal of Urology. 1932;28(4):461-76.
32. Thurston W, Wilson SR. The Urinary Tract in Rumack CM, Wilson SR, Charboneau JW (Eds) Diagnostic ultrasound. 3rd edition. Elsevier Mosby; 2005. pp. 321-93.
33. Vaccaro JP, Brody JM. CT Cystography in the Evaluation of Major Bladder Trauma. RadioGraphics. 2000;20(5):1373-81.

CHAPTER

12

Urinary Bladder and Urethral Diseases

Anupam Lal, Paramjeet Singh, Harish Bhujade

ANATOMY

Urinary Bladder

The urinary bladder is a musculomembranous sac which acts as a reservoir for the urine. Its size, shape, position, and relations vary according to the amount of fluid it contains. The empty bladder takes a form of flattened tetrahedron and when it is distended with urine, it becomes round or oval in shape. In adults, the normal bladder capacity is highly variable but is usually between 500 mL and 600 mL. The normal wall of the bladder is smooth, regular, and uniform in thickness (typically 2–3 mm in fully distended bladder) not exceeding 6 mm in adults.

The bladder lies in the anterosuperior portion of the pelvic cavity, behind the pubic ramus, with "space of Retzius" in between, which contains fat and obliterated urachus. Superiorly, the bladder is enveloped by peritoneum which continues posteriorly and is then reflected onto the anterior surface of the rectum (anterior surface of uterus in females). The bladder is surrounded by perivesical fat; and is connected to pelvic wall by the endopelvic fascia which is strengthened by the pubovesical and rectovesical ligaments. It is bordered laterally by the obturator internus muscles and inferiorly by the prostate gland. The superoanterior portion of the bladder, the apex, is attached to the anterior abdominal wall by the median umbilical ligament, a remnant of the urachus. The posteroinferior wall, referred to as the base, is continuous with the bladder neck. The urinary bladder wall consists of mucosa, lamina propria, submucosa, and smooth muscle layer.

The mucous membrane consists of multilayered transitional epithelium, which is loosely attached to the muscular coat over greater part of the viscus and appears folded/wrinkled when the bladder is contracted. Over a small triangular area, termed the "trigone," immediately behind and above the internal orifice of the urethra, the mucous membrane is firmly bounded to the muscular coat and is always smooth. The internal orifice of urethra forms the anterior angle of the trigone and its posterolateral angles are formed by the orifices of the ureters. A ridge of muscle, "the interureteric ridge," extends between the ureteral orifices and forms the posterior aspect of the trigone. In the contracted bladder the ureteric orifices are ~2.5 cm apart and at same distance from the internal urethral orifice. These measurements may be increased to about 5 cm in the distended bladder. The muscular component of the bladder wall is composed of longitudinal and circular smooth muscle bundles that form distinct layers near the bladder neck.

The arterial supply of the bladder consists of the superior, middle, and inferior vesical arteries, which are derived from the anterior trunk of the internal iliac artery. The obturator and inferior gluteal arteries also supply smaller visceral branches to the bladder; and in the female additional branches are derived from the uterine and vaginal arteries. The veins form a complex plexus on the inferior surface, and fundus near the prostate, and end in the hypogastric veins. Lymphatic drainage of the bladder is primarily to the external iliac chain of lymph nodes.

Urethra

The urethra is made up of mucous membrane, which is supported by a submucous tissue connecting it with the various other structures through which it passes.

The Male Urethra

The male urethra measures between ~17.5 cm and 20 cm in length. It is represented by a double curve in the ordinary relaxed state of penile shaft. It has anterior and posterior parts, which are further subdivided into two parts. The anterior urethra extends from the external meatus to the inferior margin of the urogenital diaphragm, courses through the corpus spongiosum. The anterior urethra is traditionally divided into the pendulous (or penile) and bulbar parts at the penoscrotal junction based on anatomical and imaging appearance. The penile segment ends in the glans penis forming a *"fossa navicularis"*, which measures ~1–1.5 cm long. The proximal part of the bulbar urethra appears dilated and termed the "sump" of bulbar urethra. The bulbar urethra has a conical shape at the bulbomembranous junction just proximal to the sump. This portion of the bulb is called as the "cone." The anterior urethra has periurethral "Littre glands," which are more in number in the bulbar urethral sump and at the dorsal side of the penile urethra. Two pea-sized glands, namely "Cowper's glands", are present within the urogenital diaphragm on either side of the membranous part of the posterior urethra. The Cowper's gland's ducts are ~2 cm long and drain into the bulbar urethral sump on each side of midline.

The posterior urethra consists of prostatic and membranous urethras. The prostatic urethra, the widest and most dilatable part of the canal, is ~3–3.5 cm long. It courses almost vertically through the prostate from its base up to apex and lies nearer to anterior surface than posterior surface. It forms spindle-shaped canal, which is wider in the middle than at either ends and narrowest where it joins the membranous part. A longitudinal ridge of smooth muscle on the posterior wall of the posterior urethra, known as "urethral crest," extends from the bladder neck to the membranous urethra. This ridge continues into "verumontanum," an ovoid mound (about ~15–17 mm in length and 3 mm in width), present in the posterior wall of the prostatic urethra.

A small saccular depression lies in the center of the verumontanum, known as "prostatic utricle." It is a vestigial remnant of the müllerian duct. The orifices of the paired ejaculatory ducts lie distally and laterally to the utricle. Prostatic glands via multiple small openings drain into the prostatic urethra which surround the verumontanum. The prostatic urethra continues into the membranous urethra, which is about ~1–1.5 cm in length, distal and it ends at lower margin of the urogenital diaphragm.

The membranous urethra, which is the shortest and least distensible, (except for external meatus), is the narrowest part of the urethra. It courses forward and downward, between the prostatic apex and the bulb of the urethra, with a slight anterior concavity. It perforates the urogenital diaphragm ~2.5 cm inferior and posterior to the pubic-symphysis.

The internal (proximal) urethral sphincter is extending between neck of bladder and the verumontanum, through the prostatic urethra. It is having different neurogenic innervation in spite of being similar to the detrusor muscle. The external (distal) sphincter has two components—intrinsic and extrinsic. The "intrinsic" urethral sphincter is a concentric muscular ring which is present in the distal one-third of the prostatic urethra that surrounds the membranous urethra and below the verumontanum. The internal sphincter and intrinsic component of external sphincter are made up of smooth muscle and maintain passive continence. The primary continence is the function of internal sphincter while secondary continence is function of intrinsic sphincter. The extrinsic component of external sphincter is a paraurethral, voluntary, striated muscle which has muscle fibers from the levator ani. Active continence is a function of sphincter surrounding membranous urethra.

The Female Urethra

The female urethra has ~4 cm length and lies from the neck of bladder at the urethrovesical junction up to the vestibule, where it forms the external urethral meatus between labia minus. It lies posterior to the pubis symphysis, confined in the anterior vaginal wall. It courses obliquely forward and downward. It is slightly curved with forward concavity. When undilated, its diameter measures ~6 mm. It penetrates the fascia of the urogenital diaphragm and its external opening is situated directly in front of the vaginal opening and 2.5 cm inferior to the clitoris. A number of small periurethral glands empty into the urethra. These glands group together on each side of the urethra ("Skene glands") distally and has two small ducts on each side of the external meatus. The proximal segment of the urethral wall consists of two layers of smooth muscle (inner longitudinal and outer circular) which are in continuation with the smooth muscle of the neck of bladder. The outer layer of the urethra is made up of striated muscle which is primarily circular in the upper two-thirds of the urethra and extends superiorly to mingle with the bladder base. The lower portion of the urethra lies closely to the vaginal wall anteriorly and is surrounded by same musculature (the urethrovaginal sphincter), above the urogenital diaphragm and extends to the inferior pubic ramus.

IMAGING MODALITIES

Various imaging modalities available for the urinary bladder and urethra include the following:

- Plain films
- Retrograde urethrography (RGU)
- Voiding cystourethrography (VCUG)
- Cystography
- Urodynamic studies
- Ultrasonography (US)
- Computed tomography (CT)
- Magnetic resonance imaging (MRI)
- Radionuclide imaging

Plain Films

The main role of plain films is in the detection of radio-paque calculi or foreign bodies, calcification, abnormal gas pattern, and in identification of soft tissue and the bony abnormalities. A plain radiograph or fluoroscopic examination is mandatory before starting the contrast studies to identify any radiopacity (calculi, calcification or foreign body) that may be obscured with contrast subsequently. Radiolucent foreign bodies can be seen if these get encrusted with calcium. Causes of bladder wall calcification include tuberculosis, tumors, radiation cystitis, cyclophosphamide-induced cystitis, alkaline incrustation cystitis, amyloidosis and schistosomiasis.[1] Bladder neoplasms may be suggested on detection of stippled calcification.

In emphysematous cystitis, the plain film typically shows gas within the lumen of bladder and streaky irregular radiolucencies within the wall of bladder. The presence of gas within the ureter may be seen in the setting of emphysematous pyeloureteritis or emphysematous pyelonephritis. Plain films may occasionally be helpful for the detection of bony metastases, spinal abnormalities in cases of neurogenic bladder and diastasis of the pubic symphysis in patients with exstrophy/epispadias anomaly.

Retrograde Urethrography

Retrograde urethrography is an initial best imaging technique for urethral and periurethral assessment in men and is useful in evaluating urethral injuries, fistulas, and strictures. The patient needs to be placed in 45° supine-oblique position. With moderate traction, the penile shaft should be pulled laterally over toward thigh. Reassurance should be given to patient regarding discomfort which may be experienced on balloon inflation. Then, under fluoroscopic guidance, ~20–30 mL of 60% iodinated-contrast material is pushed through the 16F or 18F Foley catheter (having Foley's bulb gently inflated in fossa navicularis) to fill anterior urethra with diluted contrast. Gentle, slow, gradual injection of contrast is usually required to overcome the resistance occurred due spasm of the external urethral sphincter which may prevent filling of the entire extend of urethra including posterior urethra. On fluoroscopy, when the contrast material is seen filling the bladder, the spot radiographs are obtained. During RGU, there can be the opacification of various ducts and periurethral glands (like prostatic or Cowper's ducts or periurethral Littre glands), however, this is not always associated with urethral disease.[2] Sometimes, an increased pressure due to contrast material injection may result in disruption of lining of urethral mucosa leading to intravasation of contrast medium causing opacification of the corpora and draining vein **(Fig. 1)**.

Voiding Cystourethrography

Voiding cystourethrography is radiographic study often used to evaluate the female urethra and male posterior urethra. In VCUG, urinary bladder is filled with diluted contrast through a suprapubic or transurethral catheter. After which, the transurethral catheter is removed and the patient is asked to void under fluoroscopic monitoring and spot X-rays are acquired. On active voiding, due to wide opening of neck of the bladder, funneling of urethra is seen in both male and female cases due to presence of the internal sphincteric mechanism. The verumontanum is seen elongated in male patients and the proximal bulbous urethra is less conical. The membranous urethra still appears to be the narrowest segment between these parts of the urethra, although it can regain up to ~6–7 mm diameter while voiding.[2] Voiding cystourethrography cannot be able to visualize some pathologies of the anterior urethra in male due to the fact that the distension of anterior urethra is less compared to as seen in RGU. For anterior urethra evaluation, RGU is the most appropriate and for evaluation of the posterior urethra, VCUG is the most appropriate study.

Cystography

Cystography (excretory, retrograde, and suprapubic) is a well-established modality for urinary bladder evaluation. The best cystogram is obtained by the retrograde method. Meglumine salts of diatrizoate and iothalamate are now universally used for cystography. Solution of 15% is generally adequate for cystography. In the excretory cystogram, bladder can be evaluated simultaneously along with upper urinary tracts, but it is not possible to recognize the presence of reflux.

In patients with renal failure having lesions in the bladder, retrograde cystography has a role. Cystography and micturating cystography is indicated for demonstration of the ability of the bladder to contract and control the micturition, with assessment of vesical diverticula and anatomic abnormalities of the urinary bladder neck and urethra. However, the examination is contraindicated in setting of acute infections of the bladder and urethra.

Contrast cystogram can distinctly demonstrate intraluminal calculi, hematomas, tumors **(Fig. 2)**, and wall irregularities. In traumatic injury of the bladder, cystogram depicts the type of bladder rupture (extraperitoneal or intraperitoneal), in addition to detection of pelvic fractures.

Extrinsic compression of the bladder can be produced by pelvic hematoma or lipomatosis resulting in appearance of bladder that has been referred to as "teardrop bladder". In such pathologies, ultrasound and CT play an important role in evaluating the cause of extrinsic compression.

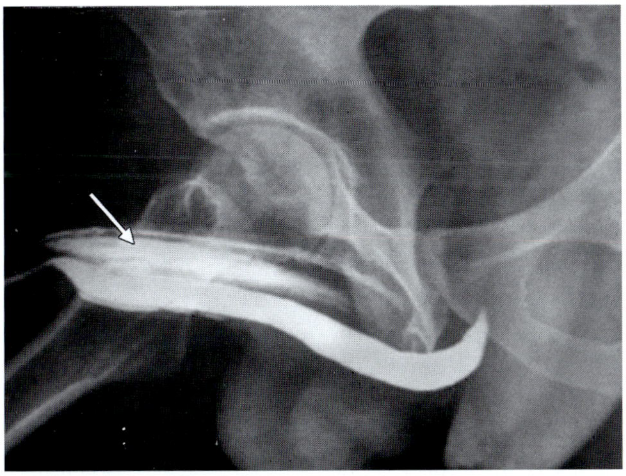

FIG. 1: Retrograde urethrography (RGU) image showing opacification of the corpora (arrow) and draining veins due to increased pressure of injection.

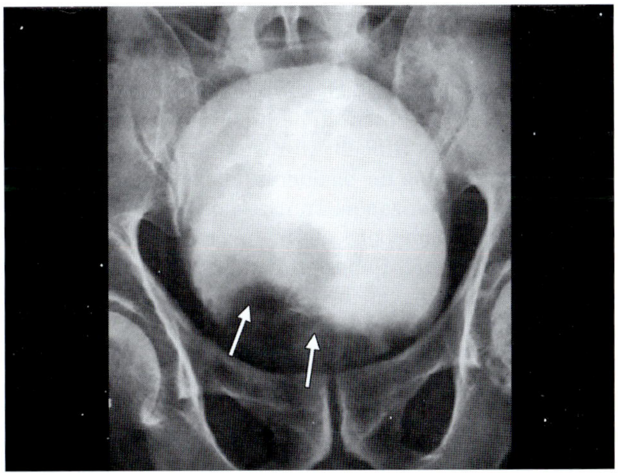

FIG. 2: Excretory cystogram showing irregular lobulated filling defect (arrows) at bladder base due to malignant growth.

Urodynamic Studies of the Lower Urinary Tract

Urodynamic studies are among the most appropriate tests to determine the source of symptoms in the lower urinary tract. A number of urodynamic tests can be useful in evaluation of the bladder and urethra and can evaluate their functioning like storing and releasing urine. These studies may be helpful to pinpoint the neurologic cause or anatomic site for source of symptoms like frequency, urgency, problems initiating a stream, dribbling, painful micturition, problems in completely emptying the bladder and recurrent urinary tract infections. Depending on the patient's symptoms, the types of tests can be done and may include one or more of the tests like uroflowmetry, cystometry, electromyelogram, pressure studies for stress incontinence, VCUG, video urodynamics, and assessment of postvoid residual urine, etc.

Ultrasonography

Real-time ultrasonography (US) is a versatile modality in the detection of bladder lesions, and is frequently employed as the first imaging tool for its assessment. US of urinary bladder can be carried out by transabdominal, endorectal or endovaginal approach. However, transabdominal approach is the simplest and the easiest. Urinary bladder should be evaluated when it is properly distended. In the majority of patients this means a volume of about ~350 mL. The bladder is seen as a smooth thin-walled anechoic structure rectangular to round in configuration on transverse scanning with no intravesical filling defects.

Ultrasonography of urinary bladder is used to evaluate the following:

- Urinary bladder wall anatomy:
    - Thickening of the wall and focal abnormalities
    - Presence of trabeculation
    - Diverticula
- Capacity of the bladder and postmicturition residual volume
- Anatomy of bladder base and urethral opening
- Distal ureteric anatomy
- Intravesical filling defects and extraluminal masses causing bladder compression.

Radiolucent calculi, which may be missed on plain radiographs, are easily picked up on US. Blood clots and sediments are usually freely mobile within the lumen. In obese patients and those with peritonitis in whom palpation of the bladder is difficult, ultrasound is very useful in determining whether the bladder is full enough to allow safe suprapubic catheterization. Transrectal US (TRUS) is useful in defining the plane between the prostate, seminal vesicle, and urinary bladder, in posterior wall masses. Ultrasound cystodynamogram can be performed in patients with symptoms of voiding disorders.

Sonography of the urethra mostly been used for diagnosis of urethral diverticula and strictures, is generally done by broad-band linear probe (5–10 MHz) for transpenile or transperineal scanning and a broad-band curved probe (5–9 MHz) for transvaginal or transrectal scanning. Endourethral USG is done with a 12.5 MHz, 6.2F, transducer based on catheter on the intravascular USG machine. However, the need for a costly intravascular USG machine is disadvantageous. A disposable urethral catheter and restricted field of view are other disadvantages for this technique.

Sonourethrography has shown good sensitivity and specificity in evaluation and diagnosis of anterior (penile and bulbous) urethral strictures. RGU and sonourethrography are equally effective in detection of penile and bulbar urethral strictures **(Fig. 3)**. Further characterization and evaluation of strictures in forms of diameter, length and periurethral pathologies, like spongiofibrosis or false tracts, is performed with more sensitivity using sonourethrography as compared to RGU, with the added benefit of radiation free modality and lower incidence of complications.[3]

Computed Tomography

The role of CT is in identification of size and number of distal ureteric, vesical or urethral calculi, pelvic trauma, and in staging of vesicle or urethral malignancy.

On CT scan, the urinary bladder appears as a homogeneous midline structure of water density. The size and configuration varies greatly which depends on the amount of urine present. The outer margin of the bladder wall is smooth and usually well-delineated by the perivesical fat. Although urine is of near water density, the bladder wall has soft tissue attenuation. In contrast-enhanced CT scan, contrast opacified urine usually gets the dependent portion of the bladder with layer of unopacified urine above it. However, this relationship may be reversed in patients with glycosuria or infectious debris in the bladder, where the unopacified urine may have higher specific gravity than the excreted opacified urine.[4] Scans obtained before and after administration of contrast medium can detect subtle vesical and perivesical abnormalities. Dense opacification of the lumen may obscure small tumors or calculi and can produce scan artifacts which degrade the image **(Figs. 4A and B)**. In the male pelvis, the seminal vesicles are seen posterior to bladder and anterior to the rectum. They are oval to tear shaped structures. A small amount of fat is usually present between posterior aspect of the bladder and the seminal vesicles. This relationship may be distorted by a distended rectum or when the patient is

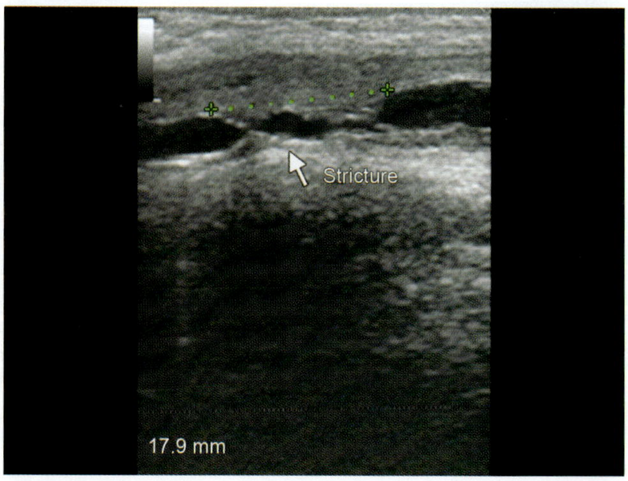

FIG. 3: Sonourethrogram showing a stricture (arrows) of penile urethra.

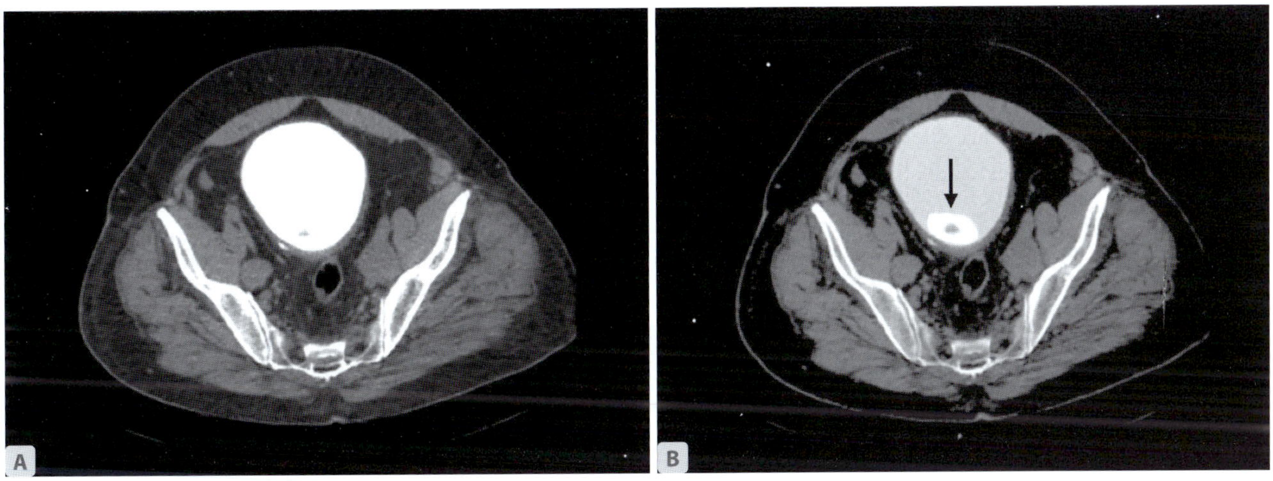

FIGS. 4A AND B: Bladder calculus: Dense opacification of bladder in CT axial image completely obscuring the calculus (A), which is visualized (arrow) in wide window setting (B).

prone. The prostate gland is located anteriorly to the rectum and just posteriorly to the symphysis pubis. Masses seen on intravenous urography compressing or displacing the bladder are readily evaluated by CT. True masses are easily distinguished from bladder impression produced by the bowel loops present in the pelvis, if the loops are adequately filled with contrast material. Alteration in the shape of the bladder can be produced by retroperitoneal fibrosis, pelvic lipomatosis, hematoma, and lymphoceles, etc. In these benign conditions, CT reveals elevation and narrowing of the bladder (pear-shaped bladder).

Contrast-enhanced CT with delayed imaging or retrograde bladder filling (CT cystography) has been shown to be highly accurate and equivalent to conventional cystography in the detection of bladder rupture.[5]

Magnetic Resonance Imaging

Magnetic resonance imaging is commonly done for cases of intersex and complex genitourinary abnormalities in patients with congenital anomalies, in which assessment of pelvic organs is very important. MRI can show diverticulum or periurethral inflammation, periurethral abscess or sinus, which are not seen on conventional radiographic modalities. In trauma cases, MRI is useful in evaluating the injuries of anterior and posterior urethra, thereby predicting the associated complications. On MRI, a fistula is seen as communicating tract with an adjacent organ. There is also important role of MRI in local staging of urethral tumors.[6]

Magnetic resonance images act as an excellent tool to delineate the anatomic structure and various pathologic conditions of the urinary bladder. Both T1-weighted and T2-weighted spin echo (SE) sequences are useful in imaging of the bladder. The muscle layer shows a T1 intermediate and T2 low signal-intensity same as of skeletal muscle **(Fig. 5)**. The mucosa and lamina propria may occasionally be differentiated from the muscle layer on proton density images, due to higher signal-intensity of the mucosa and lamina propria.

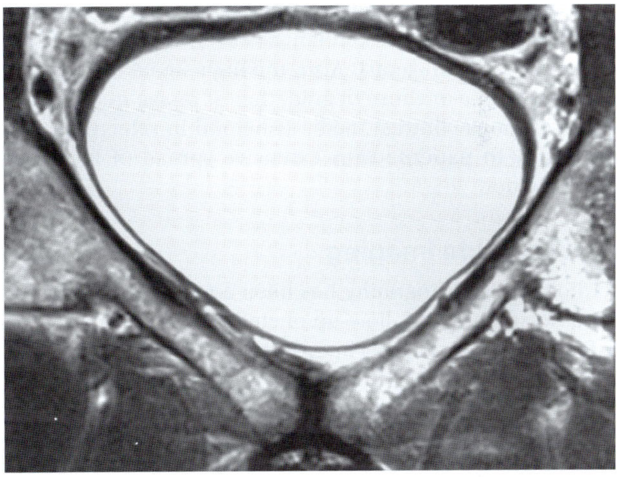

FIG. 5: MR Coronal T2 image of urinary bladder. Note low signal intensity of detrusor muscle.

Fast SE sequences provide superior quality in T2-weighted MR images with 3–5 fold less study time compared to conventional spin-echo sequences. At present, fast SE is pioneering to obtain T2W images of the pelvis. Three-dimensional (3D) techniques with offline reconstruction of high resolution images in any arbitrary plane are also very useful. The introduction of short TR (<10 msec) gradient echo sequences that use a preparation pulse, such as turbo FLASH (fast low angle shot), snapshot FLASH and MP-RAGE (magnetization prepared rapid gradient echo) and fast spin-echo (FSE) sequences significantly reduce imaging time without compromising signal to noise ratio. For T1-weighted 3D imaging, the use of an MP-RAGE sequence has been described. Also, use of phased-array multicoils and endorectal coils improves resolution. Dynamic contrast-enhanced MR provides the best information to help differentiate malignant from benign lesions.

Development of oral intestinal MR contrast agents such as ferrite particles has improved the delineation of small bowel loops and para-aortic region.

Images of the urethra may be acquired in three orthogonal planes (axial, coronal, sagittal). Alternatively, oblique images along the course of urethra can be obtained. Both T1W and T2W imaging are necessary for evaluation of the male and female urethra. In male patients, axial plane is the best for evaluation of the membranous urethra and the coronal or sagittal plane are useful for the course of the membranous and bulbous urethra (especially in traumatic cases). To obtain images of the anterior urethra, the penile shaft should be taped to the abdominal wall and positioned anteriorly in supine position under the surface coil **(Fig. 6)**. In female patients, axial images are essential.[7] A combination of imaging planes or sequences may be useful to evaluate a urethral diverticulum or local extension of urethral malignancy.

A thin slice thickness (~3–5 mm) and smaller interslice gap (~1–2 mm) are appropriate for imaging the urethra. The signal-to-noise ratio (SNR) may be improved by use of surface coils, endovaginal or endorectal coils. The endocavitary coils can give better spatial resolution; however, small field of view may be disadvantageous. Also, the high signal intensity in the near field can cause degradation of image quality. Use of intravenous contrast media is helpful in selected cases, especially in patients with extensive spread of tumor or inflammation.

Radionuclide Imaging

Radionuclide cystography has been a technique of choice for assessment and follow-up of children with urinary tract infections and reflux. The advantages being simplicity, lower radiation dose, and no catheterization needed. The sensitivity of radionuclide cystography is more than VCUG in diagnosing vesicoureteric reflux; however, this has poor anatomical resolution than the conventional VCUG. Direct and indirect radionuclide cystography can be substitute to the radiographic technique and can be incorporated into the process of diagnosis and follow-up of vesicoureteral reflux.[8]

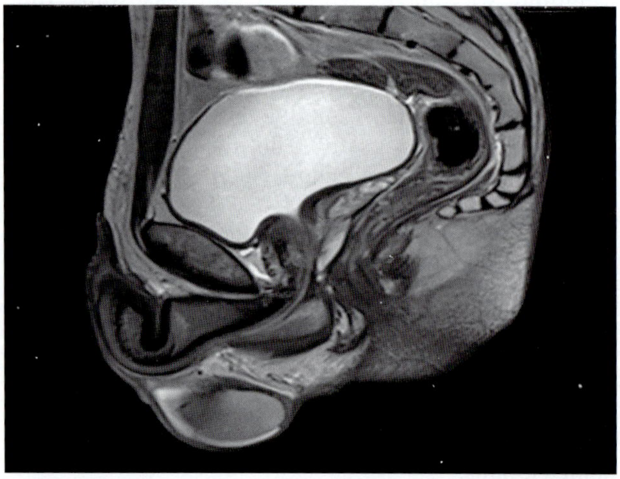

FIG. 6: MR sagittal T2 image showing the entire extent of urethra.

SPECIFIC DISEASES OF THE URINARY BLADDER

Bladder Diverticula

Bladder diverticulum refers to out-pouching of the bladder wall. These may be congenital, but are more commonly acquired as a result of bladder outlet obstruction or neurogenic bladder. Congenital bladder diverticula develop as a result of herniation or protrusion of bladder mucosa through the detrusor muscle, usually at a location slightly above and lateral to the ureteric orifice (Hutch diverticulum). These can vary from small to quite large and can cause either obstruction of, or reflux into the ipsilateral ureter. Diverticula are sites of urinary stasis and thus lead to infection, stone formation, and lower urinary tract symptoms.

On cystogram, bladder diverticula are seen as out-pouchings from the bladder which may show persistence of contrast in the postmicturition phase. On US these appear as well-defined, thin-walled fluid-containing structures communicating with the bladder lumen. The most important use of US is to detect the complications, i.e. stone or tumor in the diverticulum, which is not always possible to assess on cystography or endoscopy.

Urachal Anomalies

The urachus is developed from the superior part of the urogenital sinus and joins the allantoic duct and the dome of bladder during fetal life. It lies posterior to abdominal wall (behind transverse fascia) and anterior to parietal peritoneum, in the extraperitoneal "space of Retzius". Normally, it obliterates before birth forming a fibrous median umbilical ligament. The various congenital anomalies of urachus arise from failure to develop urachus to completely obliterate its lumen leading to the various entities given in **Table 1**.

Urachal anomalies can be delineated on US, CT, and MRI. USG is the first line and most commonly used modality with high sensitivity and diagnostic accuracy. CT and MRI are very helpful as they permit multiplanar imaging especially in the sagittal plane and are usually employed when USG fails to allow diagnosis of anomaly.

Patent urachus is often suspected in a newborn when there is leakage of urine from the umbilicus. It can be directly identified by retrograde injection of contrast into umbilical opening. It may also fill up during voiding cystourethrogram,

TABLE 1: Urachal anomalies.

Urachal anomalies	Entity
Completely patent urachus	Vesicocutaneous fistula between bladder and umbilicus
Patent caudal portion opening into the bladder	Vesicourachal diverticulum
Patent cephalic portion opening into the umbilicus	Urachal sinus
Mid-portion is patent, both cephalic and caudal ends closed	Urachal cyst

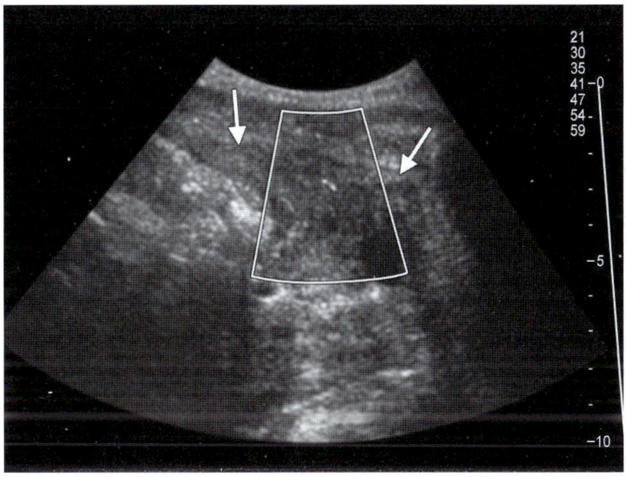

FIG. 7: Urachal diverticulum (arrows) complicated with infection: US image showing thickening of diverticular wall with increased vascularity.

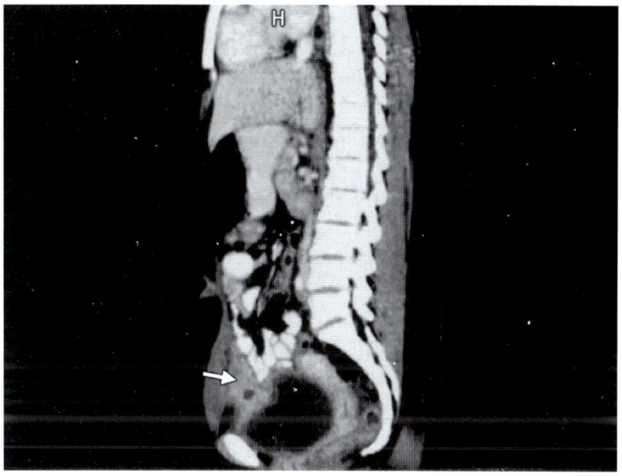

FIG. 8: Sagittal 3D reformatted CT image of the same patient as in Figure 7 showing thickening and enhancement of urachus.

best demonstrated in the lateral projection. Urachal cyst is not delineated on conventional urography studies. An urachal diverticulum is seen as urine filled anterosuperior protrusion of the dome of bladder on cystography. US reveals a tubular, anechoic structure in the lower, mid anterior abdominal wall, communicating with bladder in case of urachal fistula. Urachal cyst appears as midline homogenous fluid-filled structure in path of urachus. Urachal sinus appear as blind fusiform dilatation of urachus toward umbilical end without any communication to bladder. Urachal diverticulum is identified as a focal midline protrusion arising from dome of bladder. They can be detected incidentally or when symptomatic and suspected complications are associated with them [such as infections, stone formation, malignancy (adenocarcinoma)] **(Figs. 7 and 8)**.

Exstrophy

Exstrophy of the bladder is a spectrum of defects resulting from varying degree of failure of fusion of midline mesodermal tissue below the umbilicus with resultant defect in the formation of the anterior abdominal wall. Classical exstrophy includes epispadias, separation of pubic bones (>10 mm), and communication of bladder with the anterior skin surface **(Fig. 9)**. On excretory urography, there is a wide lateral curve of the pelvic portion of the distal ureters, which then turn upward and medially, in the shape of a hook, passing through the bladder wall in a perpendicular direction. Cystogram is performed in postoperative follow-up of these patients.

Other Anomalies

Other major anomalies include bladder agenesis and hypoplasia which are associated with other congenital anomalies, which when severe may even be incompatible with life. Duplication of bladder may be partial or complete with two separate urinary bladders, present side by side separated by a peritoneal fold (sagittal duplication). Coronal duplication of bladder is very unusual and rare. Each bladder receives the corresponding ureter and drains into a separate urethra.

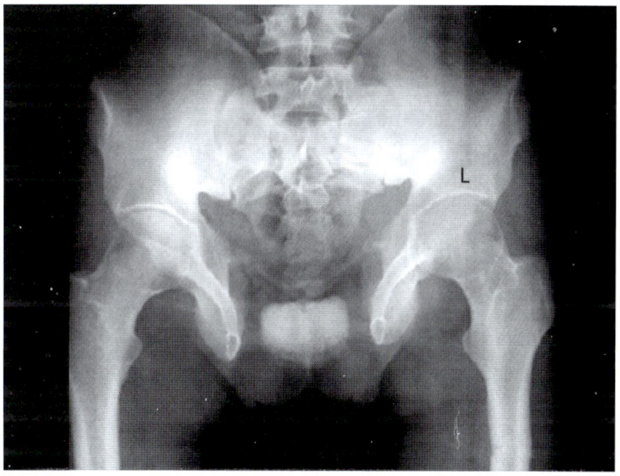

FIG. 9: Exstrophy of bladder: Radiograph showing diastasis of pubic symphysis.

This can be associated with anomalies of the gastrointestinal tract, genital system, external genitalia, and lower spine. Anatomy of duplication can be well-demonstrated on US and MRI.

Neurogenic Bladder

Neurogenic bladder dysfunction may be caused by CNS abnormalities, spinal dysraphism, cord compression or cord injury. Cystography is very helpful in diagnosis of neurogenic bladder. US is also useful to assess bladder size, shape, volume, post void residue, renal parenchymal changes, and secondary calculi.

In the condition called as detrusor-external sphincter dyssynergia (DSED), contraction of the external sphincter occurs involuntarily at the same time as detrusor contraction thus impeding urinary flow and resulting in bladder outlet obstruction. In this condition bladder is often vertically oriented, with an irregular contour with trabeculation;

frequently with multiple diverticula and is referred to as "Christmas tree" or "pine tree" bladder. On voiding cystourethrography, there may or may not be vesicoureteral reflux. In detrusor areflexia voiding cystourethrography often reveals a smooth, thin-walled bladder with increased capacity, occasionally up to several liters and extending high into the abdomen. Significant post void residue is seen in both these conditions.

Infections

Acute Cystitis

Acute cystitis due to bacterial infection is most commonly the result of transurethral infection, and is common in females due to short urethral length and proximity to anus. *Escherichia coli* is the most common pathogen. Imaging is usually advocated in complicated cystitis, recurrent infection and to diagnose upper urinary tract infection. Cystography is contraindicated in acute infection. US is the most useful modality allowing evaluation of the upper tracts as well as the bladder. On US, cystitis show thickened and less distinct bladder wall with internal echoes or debris. Cobble-stone appearance of bladder wall can be seen in severe bladder edema due to acute cystitis. Contour irregularity due to bladder mucosal edema can also be seen in radiation cystitis, cyclophosphamide cystitis, and eosinophilic cystitis, and these can be associated with hemorrhage.

Emphysematous cystitis is almost always seen in diabetic or immunocompromised patients and *E. coli* is the most common pathogen **(Fig. 10)**.

Chronic Cystitis

The hallmark of chronic cystitis is thickening, calcification, and irregularity of the bladder wall associated with trabeculation and often diminished bladder capacity. Biopsy should be done in focal mural thickening to rule out underlying malignancy. Tuberculosis of the bladder has been discussed in detail in a chapter on "Tubercular Infection of the Urinary Tract."

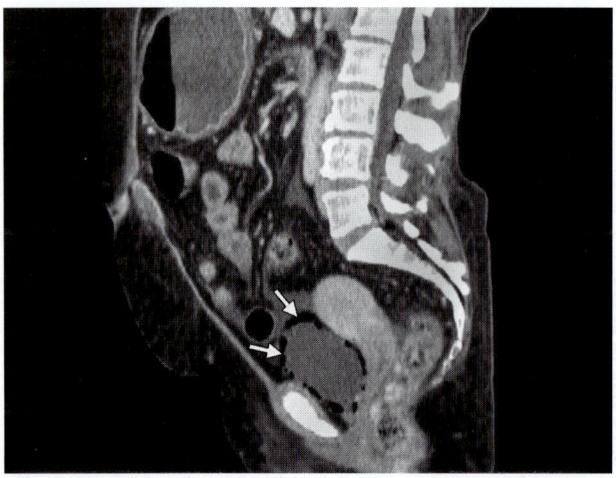

FIG. 10: Emphysematous cystitis: Sagittal reformatted CT image showing air pockets (arrows) within the bladder wall.

Cystitis Cystica and Cystitis Glandularis

Cystitis cystica and cystitis glandularis are benign inflammatory conditions commonly seen in females with recurrent or chronic cystitis, or in chronically irritated bladders such as those catheterized for long periods or with calculus disease of the bladder. Metaplasia of urothelium, with proliferation and downward extension into the connective tissue of lamina propria is seen pathologically. Cystitis glandularis is commonly associated with pelvic lipomatosis, bladder exstrophy, and bladder obstruction. On cystogram, multiple round contour defects at the bladder base can be seen in both conditions. Masses from both the conditions may vary in number and size. A hypervascular polypoidal mass has been observed on CT and MR imaging. These show low signal on T1 and T2 with central high signal on T2 with intense contrast enhancement (corresponding to vascular stalk). It is important to demonstrate intact muscular layer which differentiate these masses from malignancy.

Malakoplakia

Malakoplakia is an uncommon granulomatous response to an infection of the urinary tract, predominantly with *E. coli, especially in immunocompromised patients with female: male ratio of 4:1.* Submucosal granulomas containing macrophages with inclusion bodies known as "Michaelis-Gutmann bodies" are characteristic. It may affect any part of the urinary tract. Radiographically, these are seen as single or multiple mural filling defects due to polypoidal, vascular masses especially in the trigone and bladder base. Accompanying bladder wall thickening may also be seen, with or without perivesical extension simulating carcinoma.

Schistosomiasis

Schistosomiasis or bilharziasis is a parasitic infection caused by *Schistosoma haematobium*, producing polypoidal bladder wall thickening, which is nonspecific in appearance. In late stages, fibrosis leads to a small capacity bladder with focal or curvilinear dense wall calcification. Distal ureteric dilatation with calcification can also been seen.

Extravesical Processes

Appendicitis, diverticulitis, and pelvic abscesses may produce reactive thickening of bladder wall with mucosal irregularities. Endometriosis and inflammatory pseudotumor can also present with focal bladder lesions.

Bladder Tumors

Primary bladder tumors have mostly epithelial origin and less than 10% arises from a nonepithelial source. Almost all epithelial tumors are malignant, majority being transitional cell type with squamous cell carcinoma and adenocarcinoma being relatively uncommon. The bladder carcinoma can also be classified by growth pattern apart from histology into superficial (papillary or flat) and muscle invasive. Nonepithelial tumors may be benign (such as leiomyoma, fibroma) or malignant (such as leiomyosarcoma and rhabdomyosarcoma). The other primary tumors or masses may occur including pheochromocytoma, hemangioma, leukoplakia, and lymphoma. Metastases can be rarely seen in bladder. The staging system most often used for bladder cancer is the TNM system given in **Table 2** [The American Joint Committee on Cancer (AJCC) Staging System, 8th edition, 2017].

TABLE 2: TNM staging.

Primary tumor (T)		
Ta	Noninvasive papillary carcinoma	
Tis	Carcinoma in situ	
T1	Invades subepithelial connective tissue	
T2	Muscular invasion	T2a: Inner half
		T2b: Outer half
T3	Invades perivesical tissues	T3a: Microscopic disease
		T3b: Macroscopic disease
T4	Invades adjacent organs, pelvic–abdominal wall	T4a: Prostate, uterus or vagina
		T4b: Pelvic or abdominal wall
Regional lymph nodes (N)		
N0	No nodal metastasis	
N1	Single regional lymph node metastasis in the true pelvis (perivesical, obturator, internal and external iliac, or sacral lymph node)	
N2	Multiple regional lymph node metastasis in the true pelvis (perivesical, obturator, internal and external iliac or sacral lymph node metastasis)	
N3	Common iliac lymph node metastasis	
Distant metastasis		
M0	No distant metastasis	
M1	Distant metastasis	M1a: Distant metastasis limited to nodes beyond the common iliac lymph nodes
		M1b: Nonlymph nodal distant metastases

The clinical staging (with deep fractioned transurethral resection) is much less accurate in staging invasive (stages T2-T4) tumors. Cystogram cannot detect an early growth, extent of extravesical spread or status of the adjacent organs **(Fig. 11)**.

Although the intravesical position of many tumors can be visualized on US, an exact evaluation of depth of penetration of bladder wall cannot be done with US **(Fig. 12)**. The diagnostic accuracy of the transabdominal US for depth of infiltration ranges from 55% to 95%. Perivesical invasion cannot be frequently determined; however, extravesical spread may be recognized by the asymmetry due to infiltration.

Tumors involving the posterior bladder wall and neck, prostate and seminal vesicles may be better visualized with transrectal approach. Finally, none of the ultrasound methods optimally assesses the regional nodal status.

The important role of CT in the bladder carcinoma is to stage than detection of the primary neoplasm. However, CT is not accurate for the early stages and it is more reliable with advanced disease **(Fig. 13)**. CT cannot distinguish the different layers of urinary bladder wall; therefore, it cannot differentiate the lesions limited to the lamina propria (T1) from other lesions invading the superficial (T2) and deep (T3a) muscles. CT is useful for detecting extravesical extension which is seen by an increased density/stranding of the perivesical fat with poor definition of the outer margin of the bladder wall. Tumor involvement of the pelvic side wall is characterized by a soft tissue mass extending into the obturator internus muscle or by strands of soft tissue extending from main tumor mass to pelvic wall.

Tumor invasion of seminal vesicles should be suspected if the seminal vesicle angle gets obliterated by a soft tissue mass. However, this should be evaluated cautiously because the seminal vesicle angle may be lost if rectum is overdistended or if prone position is used for the scanning. CT is useful in detecting lymph nodal metastases; involvement being interpreted by the size of the node. Node greater than 10 mm in short axis is considered malignant. The obturator and external iliac lymph nodes are first to involve. CT has limited accuracy compared to MRI in detecting perivesical infiltration

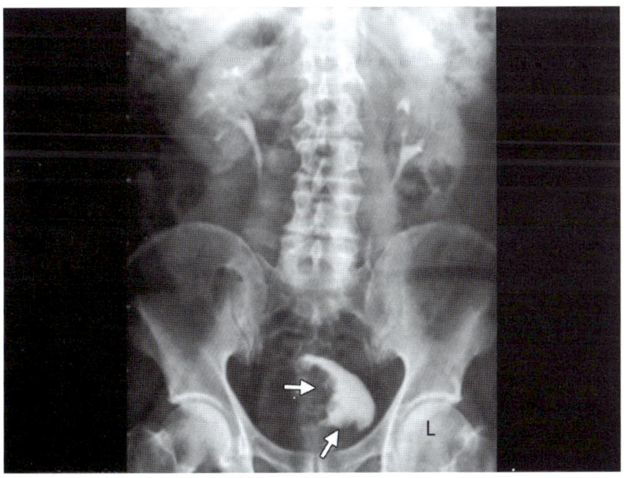

FIG. 11: Transitional cell carcinoma (TCC) of bladder: Intravenous urogram (IVU) image showing large polypoidal filling defects (arrows) within the bladder.

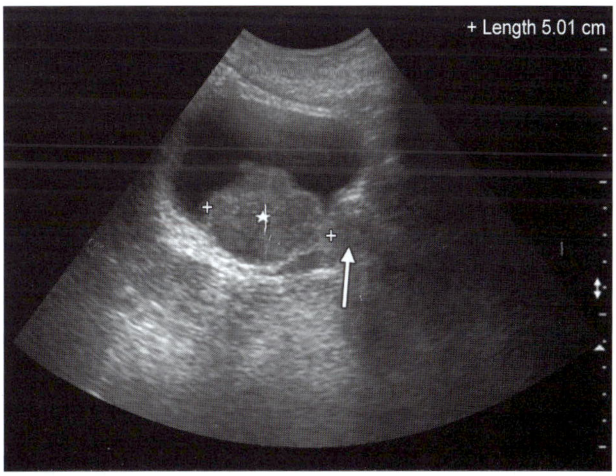

FIG. 12: Transitional cell carcinoma (TCC) of bladder: US image showing intraluminal polypoidal mass within the bladder with invasion of left ureter (arrow).

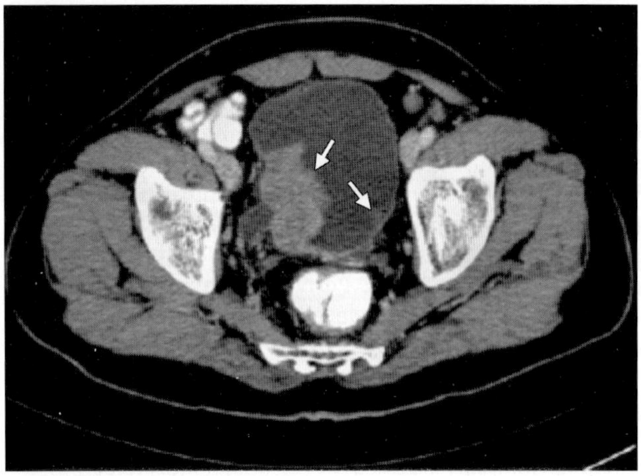

FIG. 13: Transitional cell carcinoma (TCC) of bladder: CT axial image showing a large polypoidal growth (arrow) along right lateral wall and base of bladder causing ureteric obstruction. A small tumor is also seen along left lateral wall (arrow).

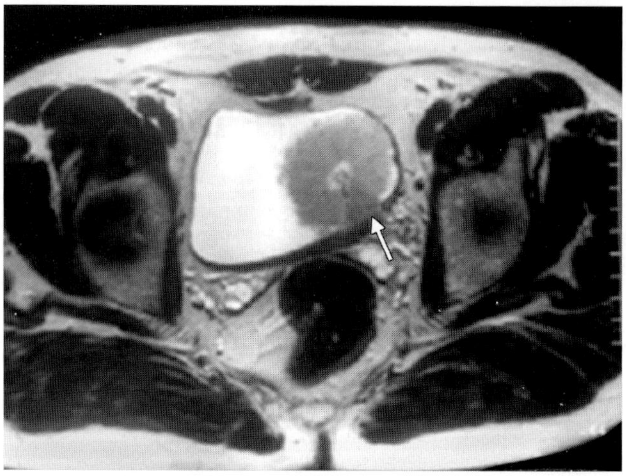

FIG. 14: Transitional cell carcinoma (TCC) of bladder: Axial T2-weighted image of a papillary transitional cell carcinoma shows an intraluminal mass which is intermediate in signal intensity. The pedicle is clearly seen (arrow). The muscle wall is not infiltrated. Perivesical enlarged vessels are noted adjacent to the tumor on left side.

and lymph nodal metastasis in invasive bladder carcinoma[9,10] (accuracy of CT varies from 40% to 90% for staging, 65–85% for detection of perivesical extension and 65–97% for lymph node detection).

On MR, T1W imaging is the best for assessing tumor spread into adjacent hyperintense fat, to detect lymph node enlargement and bone marrow evaluation.[11] There is better delineation of bladder malignancy from urine with T2W imaging. Compared to 2-dimensional T1-weighted spin echo (SE) imaging, 3-dimensional MP-RAGE imaging has improved bladder carcinoma staging by 15%.[12] When compared with conventional SE, fast SE sequences significantly have reduced acquisition time by 3-fold to 5-fold without decrease in quality of T2-weighted image.[13] Presently, fast spin-echo is pioneering for acquiring T2W images of pelvis. Contrast-enhanced study and fast dynamic imaging can improve the capability of MRI in detection and staging bladder malignancy. Most of the carcinomas show intense enhancement following intravenous contrast material administration. Tumor tissue generally enhances earlier (average ~6.5 s) than postbiopsy granulation tissue (~13.5 s).[14]

Magnetic resonance imaging is the most accurate technique in staging the invasive tumors. T2W or postcontrast T1W sequences are required to evaluate the infiltrating component of the tumor. Presence of the low intensity line on T2W images represents the uninvolved wall of bladder between tumor and perivesical fat, which is an important feature in MRI staging in differentiating stage T3a from stage T3b. Any interruption of the low signal intensity muscular layer of the urinary bladder or irregularity of the outer bladder wall and perivesical stranding suggest stage T3b **(Figs. 14 to 16)**.

The demonstration of direct tumor invasion into surrounding organs is facilitated by multiplanar imaging. A sagittal image is helpful for assessment of uterine or vaginal invasion. Assessment of invasion of the seminal vesicles is also assisted by use of sagittal image, invasion being indicated by an enlargement of vesicle, drop in signal intensity on T2W images, and loss of the angle between seminal vesicle and the posterior wall of bladder.

Infiltration of the prostate and rectum is depicted as direct tumor spread with an increase in signal intensity on T2W images. Due to multiplanar imaging capability, MR is especially useful for evaluation of tumors at dome or base of bladder.

T1W images are more suitable for assessing lymph nodes due to lower signal intensity than the adjacent fat. MRI with ultra-small super paramagnetic iron oxide agents has potential to detect metastases in normal sized node and in differentiating reactive enlargement of node from metastases.[15]

All modalities have limitation in determining extension of tumor growth in the muscular layer of the bladder wall, i.e. distinguishing between stages T2 and T3a. The imaging with endorectal surface coils or phased array multicoils in combination with IV contrast agents or T2W fast spin-echo sequences may resolve problem of distinguishing stage T2 from stage T3 tumors.

CT or MR urography (15 minute delayed image) is usually obtained with rest of the phases and sequences to increase the sensitivity or tumor detection.

Other newer imaging modalities like fluorescence cystoscopy, optical coherence tomography, and narrow-band imaging are under evaluation and may be proven useful in staging of early bladder cancer.[16] Virtual cystoscopy can help in noninvasive diagnosis, treatment planning, and surveillance. There is a promising role of diffusion weighted imaging (DWI) for evaluation of bladder tumors, differentiating benign and malignant tumor and lymph node assessment.

Because of high incidence of synchronous upper tract malignancy, kidney and ureters should also be carefully scrutinized.

Because of urinary stasis and chronic inflammation, there is ~2–10% increased incidence of carcinoma that develops

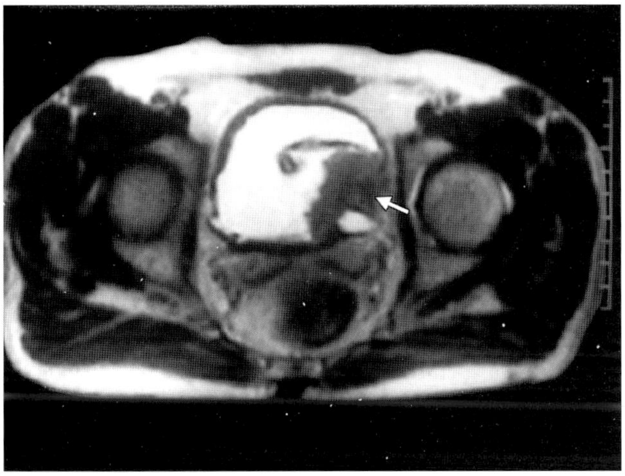

FIG. 15: Transitional cell carcinoma (TCC) of bladder: T2 axial section showing left posterolateral wall tumor (TCC) with deep muscle infiltration leading to ureteric obstruction. Early perivesical spread is seen as stranding of fat along left posterolateral aspect (arrow).

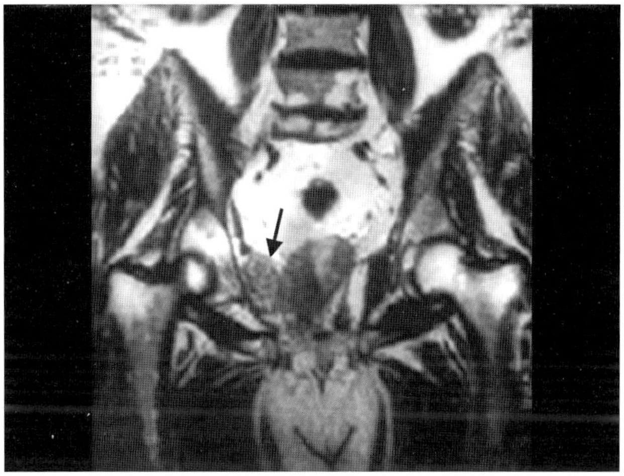

FIG. 16: Transitional cell carcinoma (TCC) of bladder: Stage T4 disease with infiltration of the right pelvic sidewall muscles (arrow) by bladder cancer. Note normal marrow signal of the pelvic bones on this T1 image.

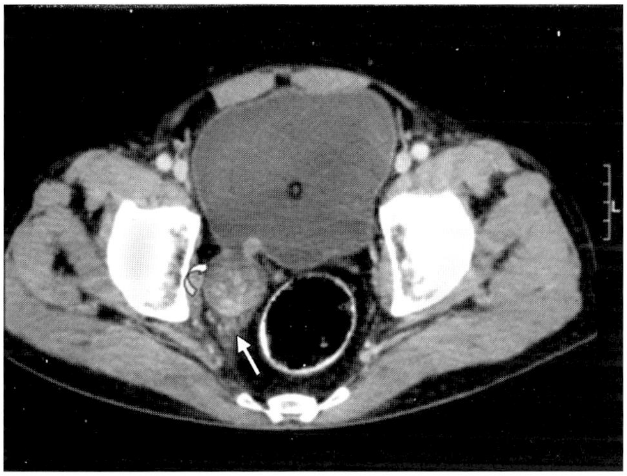

FIG. 17: Transitional cell carcinoma (TCC) of bladder diverticulum: Axial CT image shows an enhancing mass almost completely filling the bladder diverticulum (curved arrow) along right posterolateral wall. Note extravesical extension of the tumor (arrow).

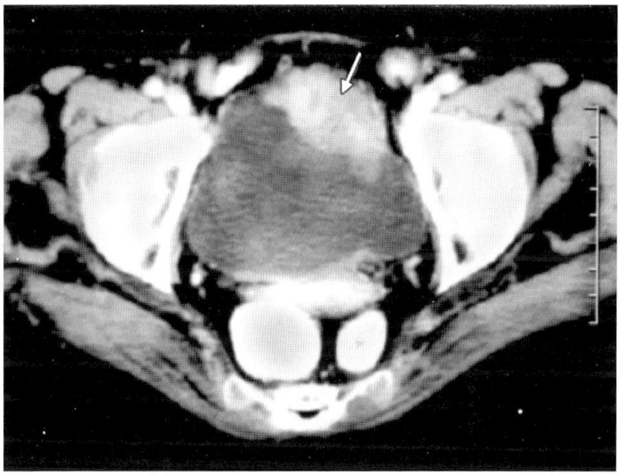

FIG. 18: Urachal carcinoma: Axial CT image showing a polypoid tumor mass (arrow) along the anterosuperior aspect of bladder.

within urinary bladder diverticulum.[17] Most of the neoplasms arising from bladder diverticulum are urothelial in origin. As the detrusor muscle is not present in diverticulum, tumors generally invade the perivesical fat **(Fig. 17)**. A narrow neck of diverticulum or unusual location can preclude adequate visualization at cystoscopy; therefore, cross-sectional imaging has an important role in detecting such occult neoplasm.

Most urachal carcinoma are mucin-producing adenocarcinomas of the juxta vesical segment of the urachus.[18] The diagnosis is commonly made by the characteristic midline location of tumor anterosuperior to the bladder, which is optimally delineated in the sagittal and coronal planes **(Fig. 18)**.

Chronic stasis and inflammation predispose to squamous cell carcinoma. Schistosomiasis (bilharziasis) is associated with an increase in incidence of vesical squamous cell carcinoma.

Benign Bladder Tumors

Epithelial (papilloma), nonepithelial (leiomyoma, fibroma, hemangioma, paraganglioma, neurofibroma), and inflammatory (nephrogenic adenoma, inflammatory myofibroblastic tumor) are common benign vesical lesions, of which leiomyoma is most common. There can be varied appearance and differentiation from malignancy can be difficult on imaging. Leiomyoma is commonly encountered in women, which is subepithelial in location, smoothly marginated and characteristically demonstrates low signal intensity on T2W image. Paraganglioma should be suspected in patient with episodic hypertension during micturition with intensely enhancing lesion in bladder.

SPECIFIC DISEASES OF URETHRA

Gonococcal and Nongonococcal Urethritis

Gonococcal urethritis is caused by Gram negative *Diplococcus, Neisseria gonorrhea. Chlamydia trachomatis* is the most commonly associated with nongonococcal urethritis, which accounts for ~30–50% of cases. Patients having gonococcal urethritis commonly manifest with purulent discharge per urethra. Nongonococcal urethritis has usually scanty urethral discharge. Acute gonococcal and nongonococcal urethritis are usually diagnosed clinically and by laboratory findings. Imaging is generally not needed in cases of noncomplicated urethritis. Urethral stricture, periurethral abscess, and periurethral fistula are complications seen with gonococcal urethritis which are more common and severe than those seen in nongonococcal urethritis.

The gonococcal urethral stricture appears as a long segment irregular narrowing of urethra **(Fig. 19)**. About ~15% of male having gonococcal urethritis develop stricture, with an interval of 2–30 years between infection and the onset of obstructive symptoms.[19] In 70% of cases, there will be hard fibrous scars at the distal part of the bulbar urethra. These scars are formed because of uneffective flushing by micturition and the preponderance of Littre glands in this area. On urethrography, there may be associated dilatation of Littre glands. When the cone shape of bulbous urethra is narrowed, elongated, asymmetric, irregular, or absent, the stricture extends into the membranous urethra in >90% of cases.[20] This imaging finding is very important to the urologist because surgical intervention may involve resection of scar tissue and, subsequently, the distal sphincter, which might lead to iatrogenic incontinence.

Periurethral abscess is developed when there is Littre gland obstruction by inspissated pus or fibrosis **(Fig. 20)**. Gram-negative rods, *Enterococci*, and anaerobes are the most common infecting organisms. Periurethral abscess can be a life-threatening infection of the urethra and periurethral tissue in male patients. These are frequently sequelae of gonococcal infection, urethral stricture disease or urethral catheterization. The urethral communication with a periurethral abscess leads to pseudodiverticulum formation. As the tunica albuginea of the penis restricts the dorsal spreading of infection, the abscess courses ventrally along the corpus spongiosum, where it is limited by the "Buck fascia". However, when there is disruption of Buck fascia, extensive subcutaneous tissue and fascia necrosis can occur. Early and quick diagnosis and treatment is necessary in such cases. Imaging technique can be needed, if diagnosis cannot be made out clinically. Urethrography may show an abscess that drains into the urethra. Ultrasonography can evaluate the presence of periurethral abscess. Cross-sectional imaging such as CT or MR is helpful for demonstrating the spread of the periurethral abscess and also complications like fasciitis and Fournier gangrene.

Urethroperineal fistulas are often seen as sequelae of a periurethral abscess. The initial abscess cavity contracts by healing fibrosis, which leads to the narrow fistulous tract from the urethra to the perineum. Consequently, micturition usually occurs through the perineal fistulas, which results in so called "watering can perineum".[21] Urethroperineal fistulas are generally the result of tuberculosis and schistosomiasis infections.

Condyloma Acuminata (Venereal Warts)

Condyloma acuminata produce soft, sessile, squamous papillomas on the glans, shaft and prepuce, are caused by viral infection. Urethral involvement occurs in 0.5–5% of male cases. Sometimes, condyloma acuminata can extend to prostatic urethra and urinary bladder. Voiding cystourethrography can help in diagnosis and is modality of choice. However, suspicion of the diagnosis is often not suspected until retrograde urethrography has been

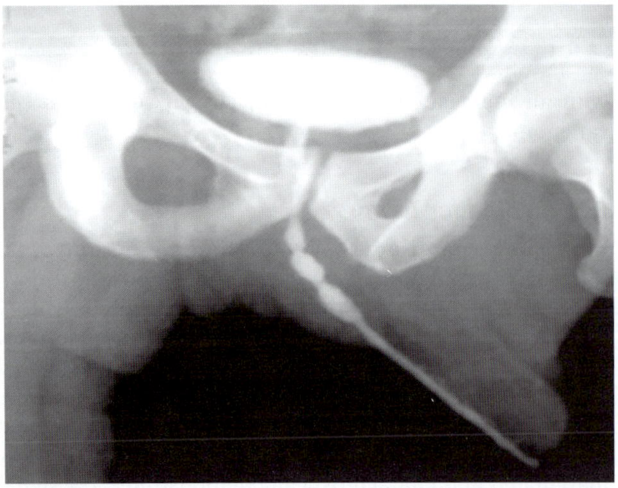

FIG. 19: Gonococcal urethral stricture: Retrograde urethrography (RGU) image showing a panurethral stricture.

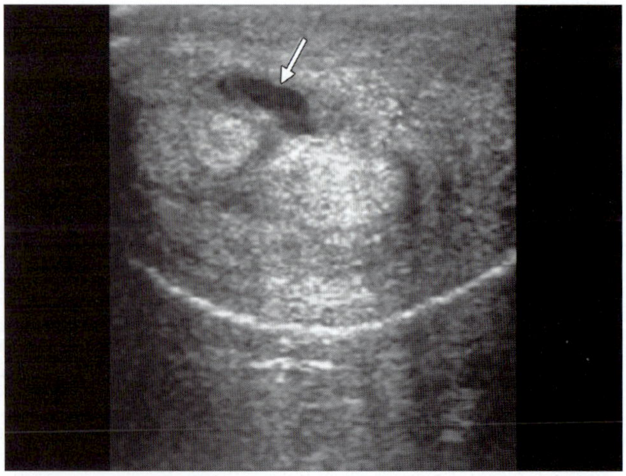

FIG. 20: Periurethral abscess: US image shows an abscess cavity (arrow) in relation to the penile urethra.

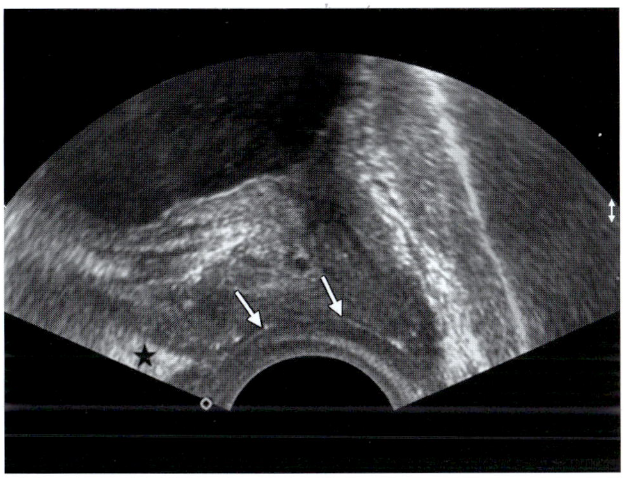

FIG. 21: Rectourethral fistula in a young male who had tuberculous prostatic abscesses and presented with pneumaturia: Transrectal US image shows the echogenic fistulous tract (arrows) between the rectum (star) and the prostatic urethra.

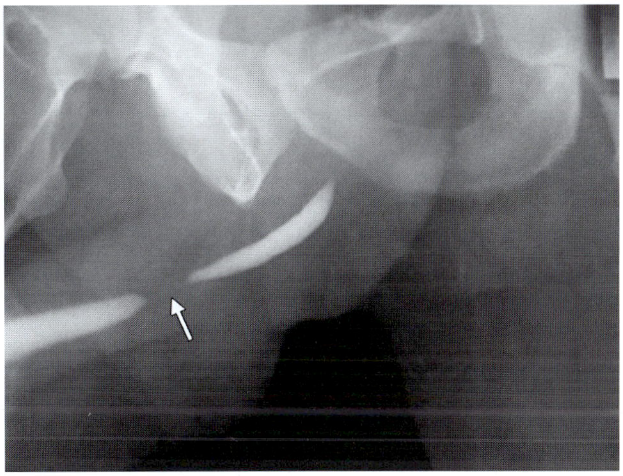

FIG. 22: Post-traumatic anterior urethral stricture: Retrograde urethrography (RGU) image showing a penile urethral stricture due to instrumentation for transurethral resection of prostate.

performed. On urethrography, anterior urethra shows typical multiple papillary filling defects.

Tuberculosis

Usually, urogenital tuberculosis is a descending infection and often present with renal tuberculosis. The prostate is involved in 70% of cases with genital tuberculosis. Abscess in prostate can rupture into surrounding structure, which may lead to prostatorectal and prostatoperineal or prostatourethral fistulas **(Fig. 21)**. In the acute phase, there is discharge perurethra with involvement of the epididymis, prostate, and other parts of the urinary system. In the chronic phase, patients have obstructive symptoms secondary to urethral strictures, therefore the diagnosis becomes difficult. Tuberculous strictures of urethra result in periurethral abscesses, which, unless treated, can lead to numerous perineal and scrotal fistulas resulting in "watering can perineum." RGU typically shows a stricture of anterior urethra associated with multiple prostatocutaneous and urethrocutaneous fistulas. In addition, fistulagraphy can be helpful for evaluating the entire urethra.

Urethral Strictures

The causes of most urethral strictures are infections, instrumentation or trauma. The anterior urethral strictures can be inflammatory (for example-infectious urethritis, balanitis xerotica obliterans), traumatic (straddle injury, iatrogenic instrumentation) or congenital. Straddle injury is the most common external cause of traumatic stricture. Iatrogenic trauma to the urethra may occur from pressure necrosis in the urethra from indwelling catheters **(Fig. 22)**. Instrumentation related strictures generally occur in the bulbomembranous part and rarely at the penoscrotal junction.

The stricture of posterior urethra is mostly an obliterative process which occurs due to disruption of urethra by trauma or surgery **(Fig. 23)**. Post-traumatic stricture of posterior urethra is generally associated with displacement of the axis

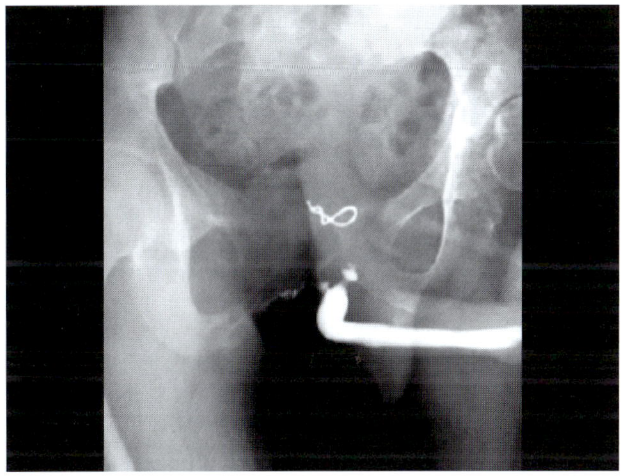

FIG. 23: Post-traumatic posterior urethral stricture: Retrograde urethrography (RGU) image showing a tight posterior urethral stricture at membranous urethra due to pelvic trauma.

of urethra from intervening fibrosis. Iatrogenic prostatic urethral stricture ("bladder neck contracture") is usually seen after transurethral resection of the prostate or open radical prostatectomy.[22]

Urethral Diverticulum

Acquired urethral diverticulum are seen more commonly in females and rarely in males. Most of the times, it involves midurethra and posterolateral wall. It is likely due to inflammation and trauma of the periurethral Skene glands and ducts, resulting in local glandular enlargement and subsequent rupture into urethra. It may be seen associated with a congenital anomaly, such as cloacal epithelium or wolffian or müllerian duct remnant. Urethral diverticulum are seen in ~1.4% of female with stress urinary incontinence.[23] Other commonly seen etiology is breach of the periurethral

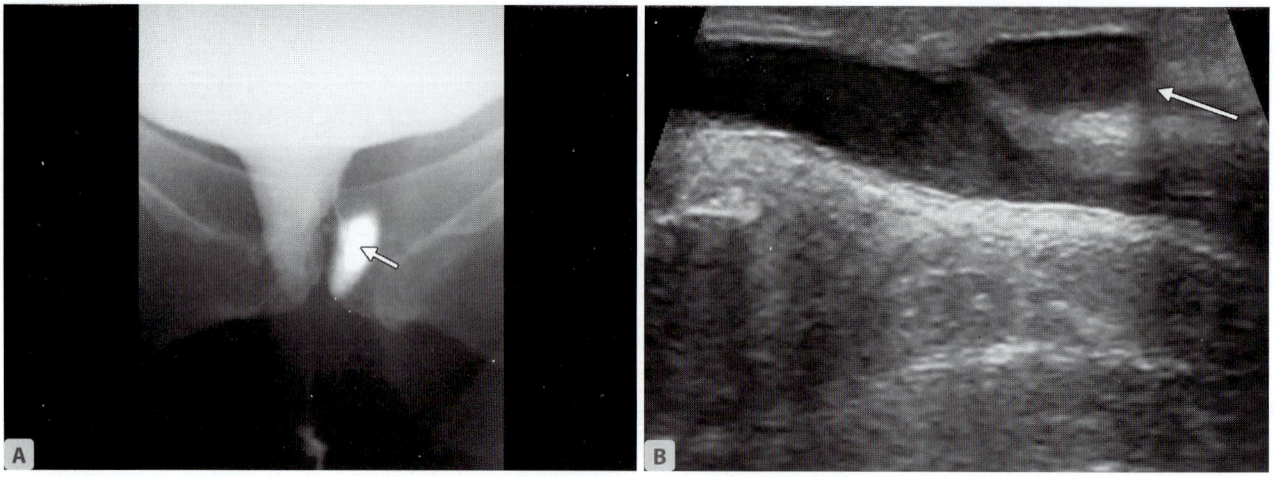

FIGS. 24A AND B: Urethral diverticulum in an elderly female. (A) Voiding cystourethrography (VCUG) image showing the urethral diverticulum (arrow). (B) Anterior urethral diverticulum in a male: Sonourethrogram showing the urethral diverticulum (arrow).

fascia during bladder neck suspension surgery for stress incontinence, which may lead to focal posterior urethral prolapse. The diagnosis is usually based on VCUG or cross-sectional imaging **(Fig. 24A)**. VCUG has an overall accuracy of ~65%.[24]

Ultrasonography can show a relatively echo-free cavitary structure adjacent to the urethra and may also show intracavitary debris or surrounding edema. MRI has more sensitivity than VCUG and double-balloon urethrography in the detecting urethral diverticulum, especially in the cases of narrow neck noncommunicating urethral diverticulum.[25] The differential diagnosis of a urethral diverticula are vaginal cyst (Gartner duct cyst, paramesonephric or müllerian duct cyst, epithelial inclusion cyst), ectopic ureterocele, endometrioma, and urethral tumors.[26]

Urethral diverticulum is often complicated by infection, stone formation, and malignant changes. Adenocarcinoma is the most commonly seen tumor in female urethral diverticulum.

Urethral diverticula in male anterior urethra, though rare, are the second most common etiology of congenital urethral obstruction in male. It typically occurs along the anterior aspect of penile urethra and on VCUG, the diverticulum of anterior urethra gets opacified with contrast media and can be seen as an oval outpouching on the ventral aspect of anterior urethra. Sonourethrogram is also useful in detecting anterior urethral diverticulum and delineating communication with urethral lumen **(Fig. 24B)**.

Megalourethra and Urethral Fistula

Megalourethra is a congenital abnormality with dilation of urethra which can be scaphoid type or fusiform type.

Urethral fistulas are commonly associated with imperforate anus and High Anorectal malformations (ARM).

Urethral Calculi

The most of urethral calculi are the small calculi coming out from the urinary bladder into the urethra during micturition (migrant calculi). Occasionally, primary (native) formation of a calculus is seen in the urethra when there is stricture or diverticulum. On a preprocedural low abdominal X-ray film, the calculus can be visualized before contrast media is injected. RGU will demonstrate a rounded filling defect in the urethra **(Figs. 25A and B)**. On sonography, the urethral calculus may be seen and appears as echogenic focus with distal shadowing within the urethral lumen **(Fig. 25 C)**.

Tumors of the Male Urethra

Benign urethral tumors are very uncommon. They can be of epithelial or mesenchymal origin with biopsy often required to establish the correct diagnosis. Malignant tumors comprise of <1% of all urologic malignancy and are generally seen after age of 50 years. At presentation, the most frequent symptom appears a palpable mass along course of the urethra or in perineum or in penile shaft with or without obstructive voiding problems. Urethral stricture or bleeding per urethra, obstructive symptoms, serosanguinous discharge, urethral fistula, periurethral abscess in an elderly man likely suggest of carcinoma of urethra.

The bulbomembranous urethra is the most common site (~60% of cases), followed by the penile urethra (~30%) and the prostatic urethra (~10%).[27] Overall, ~80% of carcinomas in male urethra are squamous cell carcinoma, ~15% are transitional cell carcinoma, and ~5% being adenocarcinoma or undifferentiated carcinoma. The histologic subtype of urethral malignancy also varies as per anatomic sites. The involvement of prostatic urethra by transitional cell carcinomas is seen in ~90% of cases and by squamous cell carcinomas in ~10%. The involvement of bulbomembranous urethra by squamous cell carcinomas is seen in ~80% of cases, by transitional cell carcinomas is seen in ~10%, and by adenocarcinomas or undifferentiated carcinomas is seen in ~10%. The penile urethral squamous cell carcinomas are seen in ~90% of cases and that of transitional cell carcinomas are seen in ~10% **(Figs. 26 and 27)**. Adenocarcinoma may originate from the Littre's or Cowper's glands. More than 50% of cases with a carcinoma of the urethra have a history of

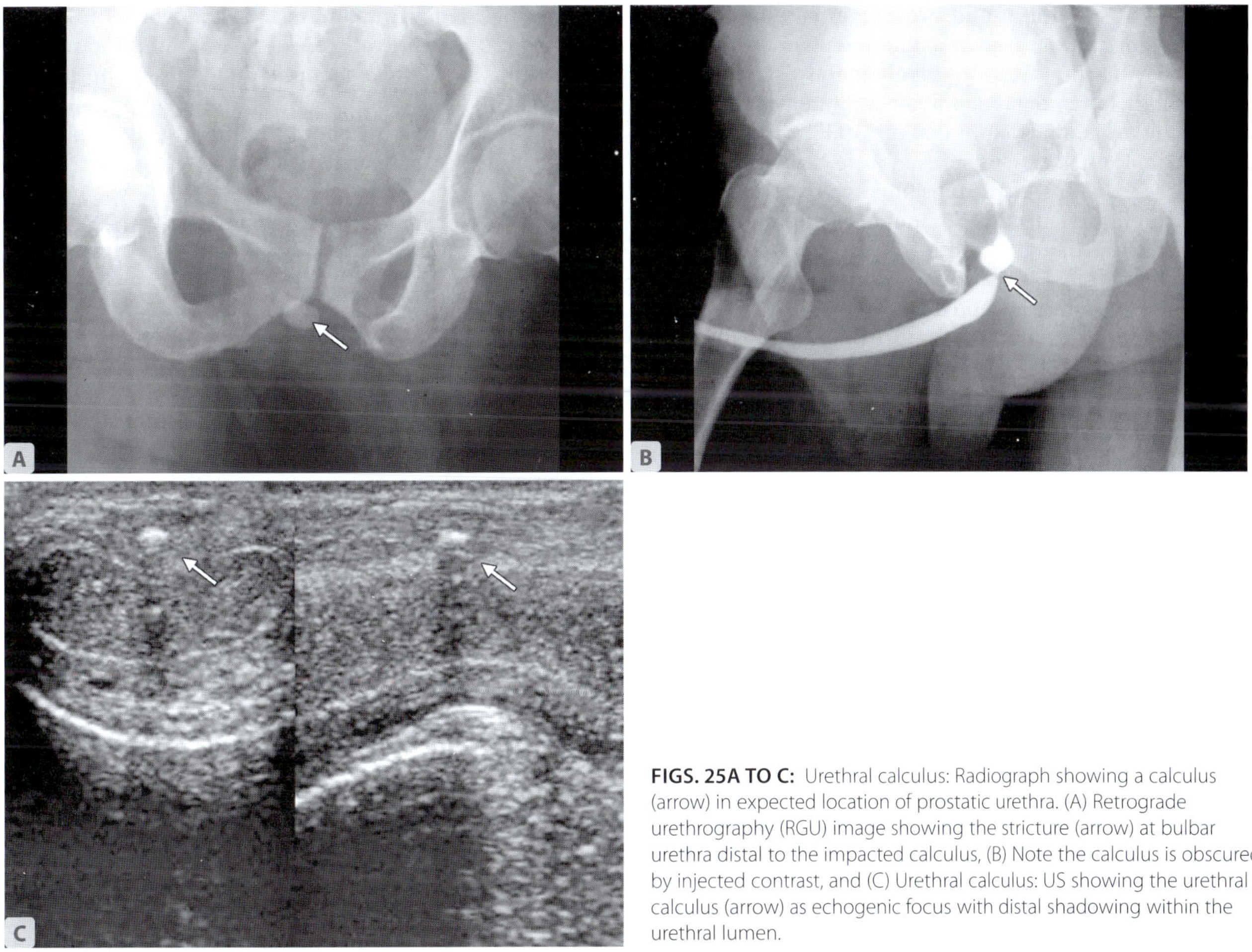

FIGS. 25A TO C: Urethral calculus: Radiograph showing a calculus (arrow) in expected location of prostatic urethra. (A) Retrograde urethrography (RGU) image showing the stricture (arrow) at bulbar urethra distal to the impacted calculus, (B) Note the calculus is obscured by injected contrast, and (C) Urethral calculus: US showing the urethral calculus (arrow) as echogenic focus with distal shadowing within the urethral lumen.

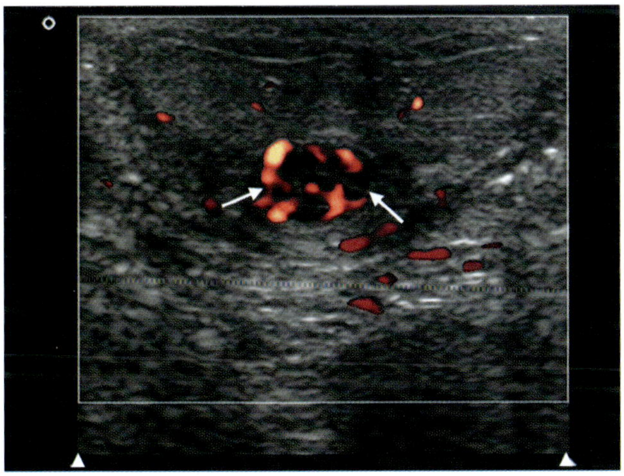

FIG. 26: Urethral transitional cell carcinoma (TCC) in an elderly male: US power Doppler image shows a hypoechoic hypervascular mass (arrows) at penile urethra.

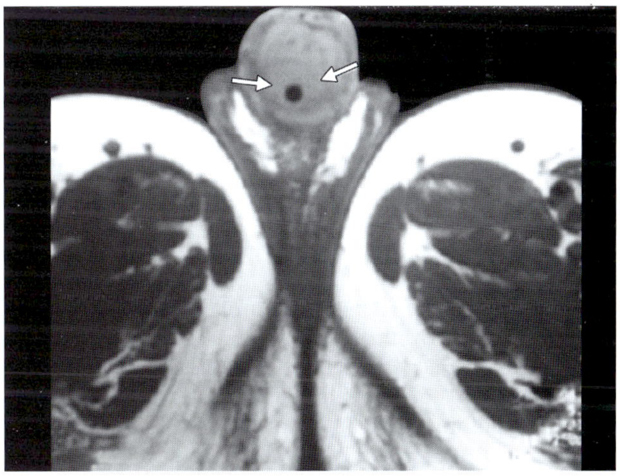

FIG. 27: Urethral squamous cell carcinoma (SCC): Contrast-enhanced magnetic resonance (CEMR) axial image showing a hypoenhancing periurethral mass (arrows) of penile urethra. Note, the urethral outline can be clearly made due to presence of urinary catheter.

urethral stricture disease and about one-fourth have a history of sexually transmitted disease.

The carcinoma of male urethra may spread by direct extension to surrounding structures or metastasize to regional lymph nodes. Stage I is confined to the subepithelial connective tissue. Stage II tumor involves the corpus spongiosum, prostate, or periurethral muscle. Stage III tumor involves the corpus cavernosum and neck of bladder or extends beyond the prostatic capsule. Stage IV tumor invades other adjacent organs. The lymphatic drainage from the anterior urethra occurs to the superficial and deep inguinal lymph nodes and sometimes, into the external iliac lymph nodes. Tumors of posterior urethra most frequently metastasize to pelvic lymph nodes. Carcinomas of bulbomembranous urethra can involve the urogenital diaphragm, prostate, perineum, and scrotal skin. Hematogenous spread is rare, seen in advanced local disease or with primary transitional cell carcinoma of the prostatic urethra. Generally, carcinoma of anterior urethra is more likely to have surgical control and has a better prognosis than carcinoma of posterior urethra, which commonly results in extensive local invasion and distant metastasis.

The diagnosis of urethral tumors is generally made by physical examination. Urethrography may be helpful in detecting urethral carcinoma, which can show an irregular focal narrowing of urethra. The MRI shows a soft tissue mass with less signal intensity compared to the normal corpora at both T1W and T2W sequences. MRI can depict invasion of the corpora cavernosa and is helpful for depicting tumor location, size, and local staging.[28]

Tumors of the Female Urethra

Urethral carcinoma in women is frequently seen than men urethra, with a women to men ratio of 4:1, however, it accounts for <0.01% of all malignancies in women. Most of these patients are >50 years of age. The various factors in association with female urethral malignancy are urinary tract infection, chronic irritation, and proliferative lesions such as adenomas, polyps, caruncles, papillomas, and leukoplakia of the urethra. Initial presentations in urethral malignancy are urethral bleeding, urinary frequency, obstructive symptoms, and at times may present as palpable mass or induration. Tumors of female urethra are divided as either "anterior" urethral or "entire" urethral tumors.[27] Anterior female urethral tumors are located exclusively in the distal one-third of the urethra and responsible for ~46% of urethral tumors. The entire urethral carcinomas are generally locally advanced and high grade in nature, most commonly with squamous cell carcinoma (60% of cases), followed by transitional cell carcinoma (20%), adenocarcinoma (10%), undifferentiated tumor and sarcoma (8%), and melanoma (2%). Local spread of primary tumors into the neck of bladder, vagina or vulva is commonly seen; hence, differentiation of the primary urethral tumors from the vulva or vagina can be troublesome.

The diagnosis of female urethral tumors are usually made clinically. Urethrography shows irregular narrowing of urethra. MRI is very accurate in assessing local urethral tumors in ~90% of patients. Tumors of urethral typically appear hypointense on T1W images and relatively hyper-intense on T2W images. Tumor extent is best evaluated on sagittal T2W sections.

Metastatic Tumors of Urethra

Metastatic tumors of the male urethra are rarely seen. Bladder transitional cell carcinomas may disseminate to anterior urethra by seeding while doing urethral instrumentation or at cystectomy; these lesions are usually identified as multiple small mucosal nodules on urethrography. Contiguous extension of carcinoma from adjacent structure (prostate, rectum, spermatic cord, and testis) can involve the corpus spongiosum, which leads to extensive urethral narrowing and irregularity. Hematogenous secondaries to the corpora cavernosa and corpus spongiosum are uncommonly seen in cases of malignant melanoma, primary prostate, bladder, colonic, testicular, and renal malignancies.

Role of Contrast-enhanced Ultrasound and Recent Advances in Lower Urinary Tract Imaging

Contrast-enhanced ultrasound involves administration of ultrasound contrast agent combined with gray scale imaging. Intravenous use is very reliable to study the dynamics of organ and lesion perfusion, demonstrating the microvascularity.[29] It is a good investigation technique for preoperative characterization of urothelial carcinoma with easy availability and being safe and noninvasive especially advantageous in patients with deranged RFT.[30] It has very good sensitivity and specificity to detect bladder malignancy (due to its hypervascular status) especially when >1 cm in size, to differentiate superficial and muscle invasive bladder malignancies.[31] By studying the contrast dynamics, high grade and low grade lesions can also be differentiated pre operatively.

Contrast-enhanced voiding urosonography is a dynamic imaging technique that enables both morphological and functional evaluation of entire urinary tract by introducing contrast into the bladder and has a major advantage of being radiation free. After emptying the bladder with Foleys or infant feeding tube, CEUS contrast (SonoVue) is instilled intravesically mixed with saline at a dose of 0.2–1% of bladder volume. Transpelvic or suprapubic placement of USG probe is used with preferable interscrotal transperineal approach in boys. It can be used to study normal variants, congenital abnormalities (megaureter, urethral diverticulum, ureteroceles), VUR, and urethral strictures.

Advances in Imaging of Lower Urinary Tract

3D ultrasound can be employed to reconstruct the tumor with visualization of bladder walls with improved rate of tumor diagnosis and staging with USG.[32]

Dual energy CT can be useful tool for CT evaluation of bladder to look calcifications, increased conspicuity of hypervascular lesions, and differentiating small posterior wall bladder carcinomas from benign prostatic hyperplasia (BPH).

Diffusion weighted imaging is a functional imaging modality and has a potential to give with qualitative and quantitative information to aid tumor detection and characterization as well as follow-up for response to chemoradiotherapy.[33]

Positron emission tomography (PET) CT/PET MRI combines both anatomical and functional imaging modalities and can improve detection accuracy of bladder cancer as well as response assessment.[32,33]

Molecular imaging with targeted agents like antibodies, peptides or small molecules thus hold a potential for real time endoscopic cancer detection.

REFERENCES

1. Pollack HM, Banner MP, Martinez LO, et al. Diagnostic considerations in urinary bladder wall calcification. AJR. 1981;136(4):791-7.
2. McCallum RW. The adult male urethra: normal anatomy, pathology, and method of urethrography. Radiol Clin North Am. 1979;17(2):227-44.
3. Choudhary S, Singh P, Sundar E, et al. A comparison of sono-urethrography and retrograde urethrography in evaluation of anterior urethral strictures. Clin Radiol. 2004;59(8): 736-42.
4. Kim SH, Han MC. Reversed contrast-urine levels in urinary bladder: CT findings. Urol Radiol. 1992;13(4):249-52.
5. Chan DP, Abujudeh HH, Cushing GL Jr, et al. CT cystography with multiplanar reformation for suspected bladder rupture: experience in 234 cases. Am J Roentgenol. 2006;187(5): 1296-302.
6. Ryu J, Kim B. MR imaging of male and female urethra. Radiographics. 2001;21(5):1169-85.
7. Tan IL, Stoker J, Zwamborn AW, et al. Female pelvic floor: endovaginal MR imaging of normal anatomy. Radiology. 1998;206(3):777-83.
8. Piepsz A, Ham HR. Pediatric applications of renal nuclear medicine. Semin Nucl Med. 2006;36(1):16-35.
9. M Jinzaki, A Tanimoto, H Shinmoto, et al. Detection of bladder tumors with dynamic contrast-enhanced MDCT. Am J Roentgenol. 2007;188(4):913-8.
10. Baltaci S, Resorlu B, Yagci C, et al. Computerized tomography for detecting perivesical infiltration and lymph node metastasis in invasive bladder carcinoma. Urol Int. 2008;81(4): 399-402.
11. Lee JK, Rholl KS. MRI of the bladder and prostate. AJR. 1986;147:732-6.
12. Barentsz JO, Jager G, Mugler JP 3rd. Staging urinary bladder cancer: value of T1-weighted three-dimensional magnetization prepared- rapid gradient echo and two dimensional spin-echo sequences. Am J Roentgenol. 1995;164(1):109-15.
13. Barentsz JO, Ruijs SH, Strijk SP. The role of MR imaging in carcinoma of the urinary bladder. Am J Roentgenol. 1993; 160(5):937-74.
14. Barentsz JO, Jager GJ, van Vierzen PB. Staging urinary bladder cancer after transurethral biopsy: value of fast dynamic contrast-enhanced MR imaging. Radiology. 1996;201(1): 185-93.
15. Deserno WM, Harisinghani MG, Taupitz M, et al. Urinary bladder cancer: preoperative nodal staging with ferumoxtran-10-enhanced MR imaging. Radiology. 2004;233(2):449-56.
16. Goh AC, Lerner SP. Application of new technology in bladder cancer diagnosis and treatment. World J Urol. 2009;27(3):301-7.
17. Dondalski M, White EM, Ghahremani GG, et al. Carcinoma arising in urinary bladder diverticula: imaging findings in six patients. Am J Roentgenol. 1993;161(4):817-20.
18. Sheldon CA, Clayman RV, Gonzalez R, et al. Malignant urachal lesions. J Urol. 1984;131(1):1-8.
19. DiSantis DJ. Inflammatory conditions of the urethra. In: Pollack AH, McClennon BL (Eds). Clinical Urography, 2nd edition. Philadelphia: Saunders; 2000. pp. 1041-57.
20. Gallentine ML, Morey AF. Imaging of the male urethra for stricture disease. Urol Clin North Am. 2002;29(2):361-72.
21. Sharfi AR, Elarabi YE. The 'watering-can' perineum: presentation and management. Br J Urol. 1997;80(6):933-6.
22. Pansadoro V, Emiliozzi P. Iatrogenic prostatic urethral strictures: classification and endoscopic treatment. Urology. 1999;53(4):784-9.
23. Fortunato P, Schettini M, Gallucci M. Diverticula of the female urethra. Br J Urol. 1997;80(4):628-32.
24. Keefe B, Warshauer DM, Tucker MS, et al. Diverticula of the female urethra: diagnosis by endovaginal and transperineal sonography. J Roentgenol. 1991;156(6):1195-7.
25. Daneshgari F, Zimmern PE, Jacomides L. Magnetic resonance imaging detection of symptomatic noncommunicating intraurethral wall diverticula in women. J Urol. 1999;161(4): 1259-61.
26. Hahn WY, Israel GM, Lee VS. MRI of female urethral and periurethral disorders. Am J Roentgenol. 2004;182(3): 677-82.
27. Donat SM, Cozzi PJ, Herr HW. Surgery of penile and urethral carcinoma. In: Walsh PC, Reitik AB, Vaughan ED Jr, Wein AJ (Eds). Campbell's Urology, 8th edition. Philadelphia: Saunders; 2002. pp. 2983-99.
28. Vapnek JM, Hricak H, Carroll PR. Recent advances in imaging studies for staging of penile and urethral carcinoma. Urol Clin North Am. 1992;19(2):257-66.
29. Nicolau C, Bunesch L, Sebastia C, et al. Diagnosis of bladder cancer: contrast-enhanced ultrasound. Abdom Imaging. 2010; 35(4):494-503.
30. Gupta VG, Kumar S, Singh SK, et al. Contrast enhanced ultrasound in urothelial carcinoma of urinary bladder: an underutilized staging and grading modality. Cent Eur J Urol. 2016;69(4):360-5.
31. Caruso G, Salvaggio G, Campisi A, et al. Bladder tumor staging: comparison of contrast-enhanced and gray-scale ultrasound. Am J Roentgenol. 2010;194(1):151-6.
32. Hafeez, Huddart. Advances in bladder cancer imaging. BMC medicine. 2013;11(1):104.
33. Srivastava A, Douglass LM, Chernyak V, et al. Advances in imaging in prostate and bladder cancer. Curr Urol Rep. 2017;18(9):69.

CHAPTER

13

Imaging Techniques and Radiological Anatomy of Female Genital Tract

Swati Gupta, Sapna Singh, Anju Garg, Satyam

INTRODUCTION

The imaging appearance of female genital tract is dynamic and changes dramatically during the lifespan of a woman.[1] Imaging plays a significant role and ultrasonography (USG) is currently the imaging modality of choice for assessing the female genital organs. Its safety has been established, and it provides excellent depiction of normal and pathologic findings in gynecologic diseases. Magnetic resonance imaging (MRI) is used to complement sonography and to answer specific pretreatment questions about malignant and benign conditions of the female pelvis. MRI allows acquisition of multiplanar images with excellent soft tissue contrast and a large field of view. Computed tomography (CT) is commonly performed in patients with acute symptoms and generally not the primary imaging modality of choice for the evaluation of suspected gynecologic disease due to low contrast of soft tissues. There has been significant advancement in nuclear imaging studies with the advent of hybrid scanners like positron emission tomography-computed tomography (PET-CT) and PET-MRI that are capable of providing both anatomical and functional information.

PLAIN FILM RADIOGRAPHY

The role of plain radiographs in the field of gynecological imaging is limited. One condition where a plain radiograph may be performed includes a radiograph to locate an intrauterine contraceptive device (IUCD) that is not visualized on ultrasound **(Figs. 1A and B)**. Pelvic calcification can be seen on an abdominal radiograph and can be due to various causes. One of the common causes is fibroids; popcorn calcification is seen in few of them. Calcification is seen in about 12% of ovarian cystadenocarcinomas.[2] Dermoid cysts may show tooth-like structure and/or a fat fluid level. Close scrutiny of pelvic bones should always be done to look for areas of erosion in suspected pelvic masses.[3]

HYSTEROSALPINGOGRAPHY

Hysterosalpingography (HSG) is an important diagnostic tool in determining anatomical contour of uterine cavity, tubal anatomy, and patency. It is indicated in cases of infertility and recurrent pregnancy loss. Rare indications include checking the completion of tubal sterilization and evaluation of tubes prior to attempted reversal of sterilization. HSG is contraindicated in patients having comorbidities such as endometriosis and pelvic inflammatory disease (PID).

Technique

Hysterosalpingography is done in the preovulatory phase of the menstrual cycle in order to ensure that the patient is not pregnant at the time when the procedure is performed, preferably between 6th day and 10th day of the cycle. Examination in the postovulatory phase of cycle is avoided also because the chances of venous intravasation and probability of false positive diagnosis of cornual occlusion are increased by thickened secretory endometrium. Routine administration of antibiotics is not recommended and decisions regarding prophylactic use of antibiotics in patients with a history of PID are left to the referring clinicians. One such specific regimen for prophylaxis is doxycycline 100 mg twice a day for 5 days, beginning 2 days prior to the procedure. It is advisable to administer a dose of nonsteroidal anti-inflammatory drug (NSAID) half an hour before the study to alleviate pain. The procedure should be explained to the patient before obtaining informed consent. Urinary bladder should be empty before the patient is positioned in lithotomy position. The perineum is prepared with povidone-iodine solution and draped with sterile towels. Cervix and vagina are exposed using speculum and cleansed with antiseptic solution. Tenaculum is used to grasp the anterior cervical lip. Leech Wilkinson cannula or a 5F HSG catheter is introduced, stabilized into the cervix and uterus retracted. A catheter is preferred as it causes less pain, is easier to perform and requires less fluoroscopic time. Nonionic water soluble contrast media in a dilution ratio of 1:1 is introduced into uterus. The first film is a scout radiograph in supine position. Spot film is taken during early filling phase after instillation of 5 mL of contrast to ensure that contrast does not obliterate the small filling defects and during early tubal filling before contrast obscures the isthmic portions. In the next step, additional 5 mL is instilled to completely

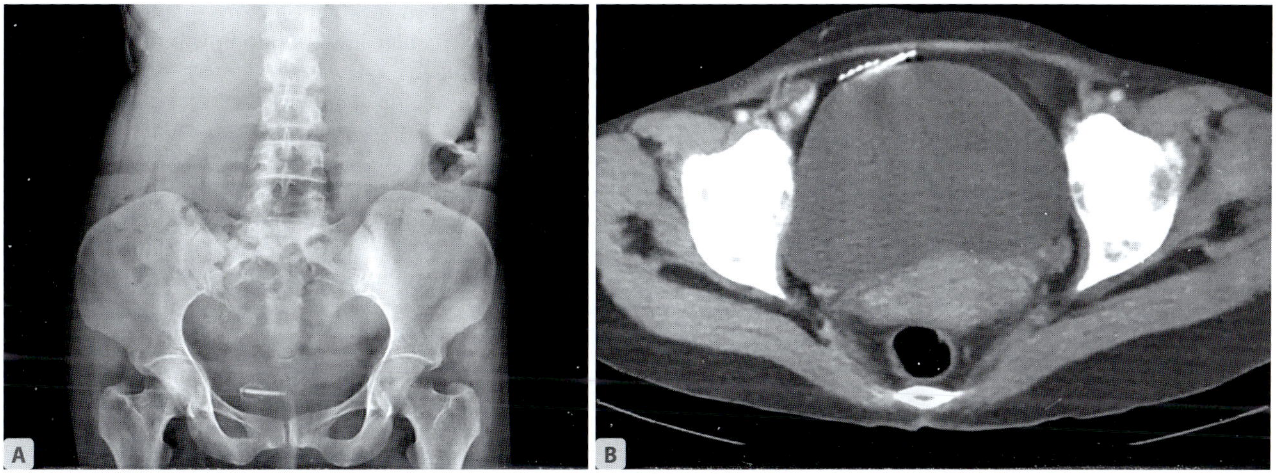

FIGS. 1A AND B: (A) Plain radiograph showing displaced intrauterine contraceptive device (IUCD); (B) Contrast-enhanced axial CT scan image of the same patient with IUCD visualized anterior to urinary bladder.

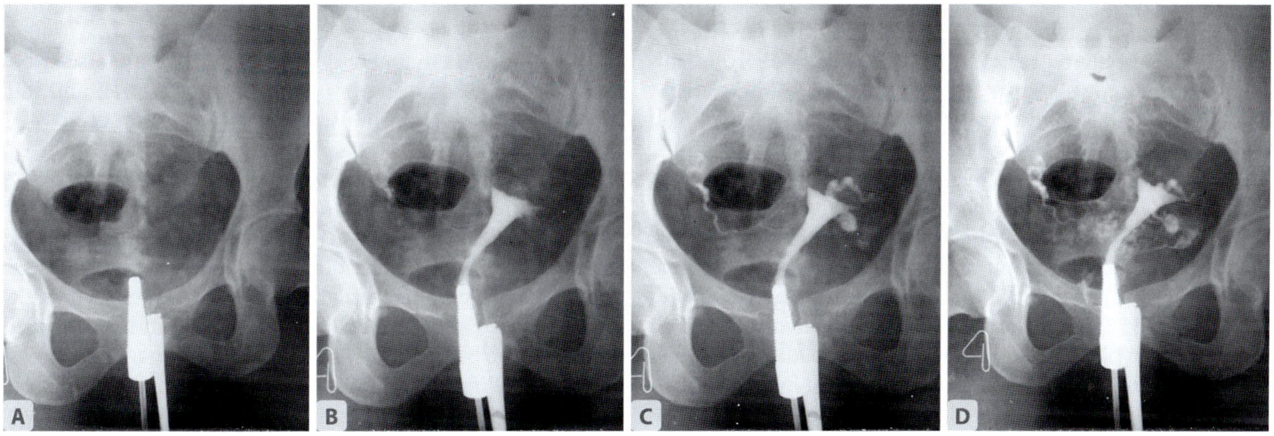

FIGS. 2A TO D: Normal hysterosalpingogram comprising scout, early uterine, early tubal and late filling phase.

fill the tube and to demonstrate free spill **(Figs. 2A to D)**. Delayed films help to study the pattern of peritoneal spillage. Additional oblique views may be taken if needed.[4]

Complications of HSG include pain, infection, vasovagal reactions, venous intravasation and allergic reaction to contrast media.

Though HSG has been used for tubal assessment since several years, meta-analysis has shown a sensitivity and specificity of 0.65 [95% confidence interval (CI): 0.50–0.78] and 0.83 (95% CI: 0.77–0.88), respectively for HSG as a test for tubal obstruction. When the HSG suggests that the tubes are patent, this can be confirmed by laparoscopy in 94% of the women. A tubal block seen on HSG will be confirmed by laparoscopy in only 38% of the women.[5] Thus, HSG is a reliable indicator of tubal patency but not of tubal block.

ULTRASOUND

Ultrasound remains the first line of investigation while evaluating the female genital tract. It gives an excellent visualization of the organs of the genital tract. With the addition of Color Doppler USG, the vascular dynamics can also be very well-evaluated. The introduction of USG contrast agents has made it possible to interrogate even the slow flow areas. Multiplanar and surface rendered images are possible with three-dimensional (3D) technology. However, it is essential to recognize that operator's skill; regardless of the equipment used, ultimately determines the final benefit of ultrasound in patient care.

Indications for Evaluation of Uterus and Adnexa

The indications for sonographic evaluation include:
- Menstrual disorders
- Postmenopausal bleeding
- Pelvic inflammatory disease
- Pelvic mass
- Infertility
- Recurrent pregnancy loss
- Lower abdominal pain
- Guided procedures.

Technique

Sonographic evaluation of the uterus and the adnexa can be done by the transabdominal and transvaginal routes. These are complementary techniques and are used extensively in evaluation of the female pelvis. The *transabdominal scan (TAS)* is performed with a 3.5–5 MHz sector transducer, with a distended bladder as an essential prerequisite. The urinary bladder is considered adequately distended when it covers the entire fundus of the uterus. Overdistension is to be avoided as it may distort the anatomy and may push the pelvic organs beyond the focal zone of the transducer. Imaging of the uterus is performed in both sagittal and axial planes. The adnexa are imaged by scanning obliquely from the contralateral side, although in many cases good visualization may be achieved by scanning directly over the adnexa.

The limitations of transabdominal scan are as follows:
- The patient may not be able to fill the bladder adequately.
- In patients with retroverted uterus, fundus may be beyond the focal zone of the transducer.
- Limited resolution.

Transvaginal scanning (TVS) affords improved resolution of the pelvic organs. Specially designed probes of 4–9 MHz frequency are used for this procedure. The urinary bladder should be empty. However, a minimal distension may be required if the uterus is severely anteflexed. The patient is positioned supine in lithotomy position with the knees flexed and hips slightly elevated. The probe is covered with a latex barrier and inserted gently into the vagina till the uterus is identified. The uterus is imaged in its longitudinal axis, first sweeping from left to right. Short-axis images are then obtained sweeping from anterior to posterior. The relative position of the uterus can be inferred by the orientation of the probe that best images the uterus, e.g. if the uterus is best imaged with a posterior inclination, the uterus is retroflexed and vice versa. For imaging the cervix, the transducer should be withdrawn to the mid-vaginal level.

The ovaries are imaged by tilting the transducer to either side of the midline in the transverse section. The internal iliac vessels can be identified as anechoic tubular structures along the pelvic side walls. The ovaries usually lie anterior and medial to these vessels; however, their position can vary.

Limitations of this technique are:
- Limited field of view
- Examination may not be possible in vaginal atrophy or when the woman is virgo intacta.

Transrectal ultrasound can be performed in patients with a contraindication to transvaginal scan. *Transperineal* scans also help in determining the origin and extent of some tumors.

DOPPLER EVALUATION

The gynecological Doppler ultrasound examination can be used to study pathological and physiological circulatory changes in the female pelvis noninvasively.

Indications

The indications for Doppler examination include:
- Characterization of uterine/ovarian masses
- Infertility and assisted reproduction.

After simultaneous evaluation of morphology and color flow, pulsed gate is placed to obtain flow information. The course of the uterine artery is suited for transvaginal assessment with ideal geometry for Doppler signal recording. It is also possible to record Doppler signals transabdominally when the uterus is anteverted. The branches of the uterine artery extending towards the ovary can be identified in the broad ligament and the superior aspect of the ovary, respectively. Because of their tortuosity, only short segments of the arteries are usually identified in any scan plane. The lowest possible filter (<50–60 Hz), with a high color gain should be used to detect slow flow. Endometrial vascularity can also be evaluated by Doppler sonography. The extent of vascular penetration into the endometrium correlates well with successful conception. Variations in the depth of vascular penetration before, during, and after the mid-cycle can be seen.

The ovarian artery is a branch of the abdominal aorta and reaches the ovary through the infundibulopelvic ligament. Signals from the ovary are identified as low Doppler shifts of a small vessel with low velocity. The waveform shape varies with state of activity of ovary.[6] Guerriero et al. demonstrated that specificity in diagnosing adnexal malignancies can be increased by association of color flow localization and the B-mode analysis of internal architectural appearance.[7]

Three-dimensional displays enable visualization of multiple overlapping vessels and their relation to other vessels, tumor, and surrounding tissues. A variation of Doppler imaging which uses the amplitude termed power Doppler imaging or color Doppler energy (CDE) is also used. The greatest advantage of CDE includes the relative angle independence and absolute lack of aliasing. It has a higher detection rate of vascularity in malignant and benign adnexal masses. The disadvantages of power imaging are high motion sensitivity and the absence of information about direction and speed of flow.

GEL SONOVAGINOGRAPHY

Regular transvaginal sonography is known to have limitations in assessing local cervical and vaginal lesions. This is due the close proximity of the vaginal and cervix walls to the transducer. In such cases, a recently described technique called gel sonovaginography is helpful. This technique involves instillation of 20 mL of ultrasound gel into the vagina followed by examination with a transvaginal transducer. The instilled gel causes a partial distension of vaginal walls and standoff resulting in increased clarity on gel sonovaginography. Disorders such as vaginal and cervical cancer, vaginal septa, deep infiltrating endometriosis, and cervical polyps can be visualized better with gel sonovaginography.[8]

THREE-DIMENSIONAL AND FOUR-DIMENSIONAL SONOGRAPHY

Three-dimensional ultrasound or volume sonography is an imaging advancement that involves acquisition of a series of two-dimensional (2D) images from a volume of the patient. They are then displayed in different planes after the acquisition **(Figs. 3A to C)**.

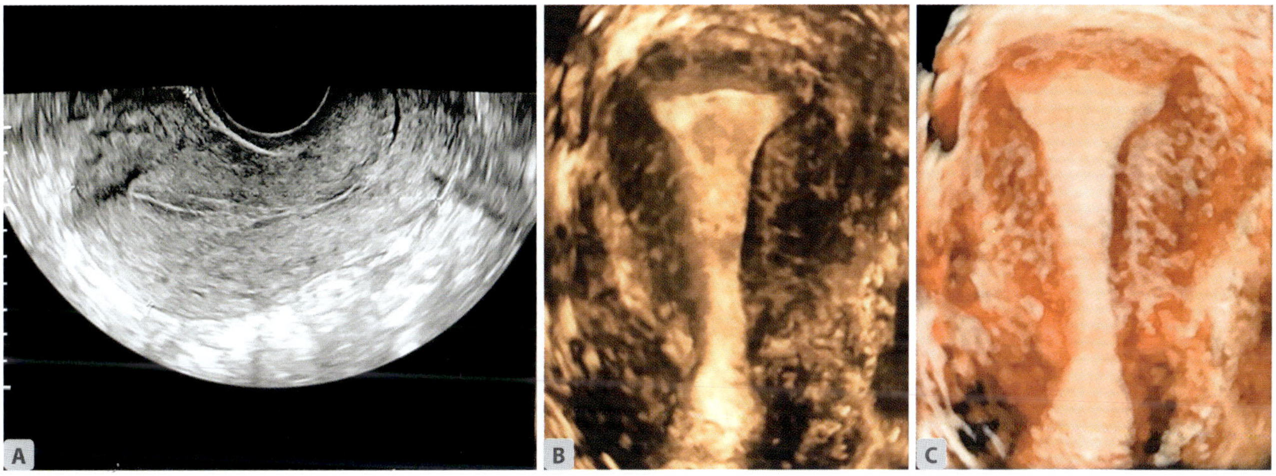

FIGS. 3A TO C: 3D ultrasound with data obtained from a volume of tissue and visualization of the third or coronal plane of the uterus with rendering techniques.

Indications

Three-dimensional ultrasound may be useful in following conditions:

- Diagnosing congenital uterine malformations **(Fig. 4)**
- Accurate volume measurement, e.g. endometrial, ovarian cysts, follicles and tumor masses
- Exact localization of pathology—intrauterine fibroid, IUCD etc
- Mapping of myomata
- Characterization of adnexal masses
- Extent of tumor infiltration into adjacent tissues/organs
- 3D power Doppler can aid in characterization of vessel morphology.

Technical Considerations

When used in conjunction with 2D ultrasound, 3D ultrasound has added clinical and diagnostic value for selected indications and circumstances in gynecologic ultrasound. 3D imaging has several obvious benefits that relate to demonstration of multiplanar views and an improved spatial orientation, of which the coronal plane is particularly useful in gynecological practice.[9] It offers a more reproducible and objective measurement of vascularity and volume of the region of interest through further postprocessing modalities. It also has the added advantages of teleconsultation, reduced scanning time, and storage of images for reevaluation. There are different types of 3D acquisitions—manual, sensor-based, and automatic. Demonstration of 3D images in real time is variously known as 4D ultrasound, real-time 3D ultrasound and live 3D ultrasound.

SALINE INFUSION SONOHYSTERO-SALPINGOGRAPHY

Saline infusion sonohysterosalpingography (SIS) involves the instillation of sterile saline into the endometrial cavity under ultrasound guidance. The saline distends the cavity, separating the walls of the endometrium. Saline infusion sonohysterosalpingography (SIS) has several advantages over HSG including simplicity, reduced cost, lack of ionizing radiation, a high level of diagnostic accuracy, and minimal invasiveness with an ability to characterize masses within the endometrial cavity. Assessment of tubes and uterine cavity is possible in presence of fluid within them. The procedure of SIS for testing tubal patency was first reported by Richman.[10]

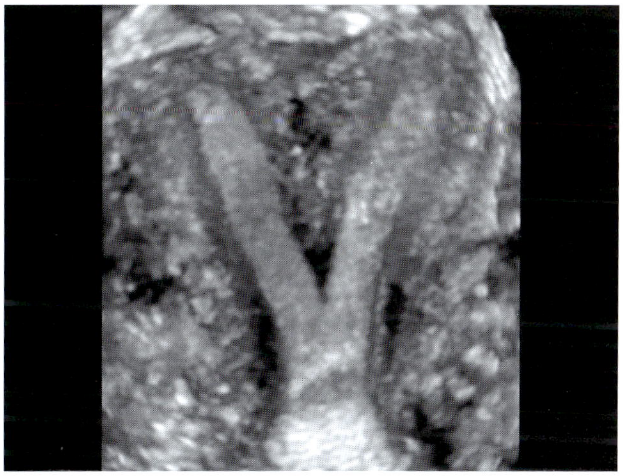

FIG. 4: 3D reconstructed coronal view showing a subseptate uterus.

Technique

Saline infusion sonohysterosalpingography is done in proliferative phase just like HSG, however, it can be done anytime in postmenopausal women. Patient's preparation is similar to that described under HSG. Initial screening using TVS probe is done to look for any pathology that may hinder successful completion of procedure.[4]

The endometrial cavity is distended with 20–40 mL normal saline introduced via a self-retaining catheter, prior to transvaginal sonography. The fluid within the cavity gives an excellent visualization of any pathology within the cavity and also differentiates between intracavitary versus extracavitary pathology **(Figs. 5A and B)**. Sonosalpingography can be done to establish the patency of the fallopian tubes by instilling

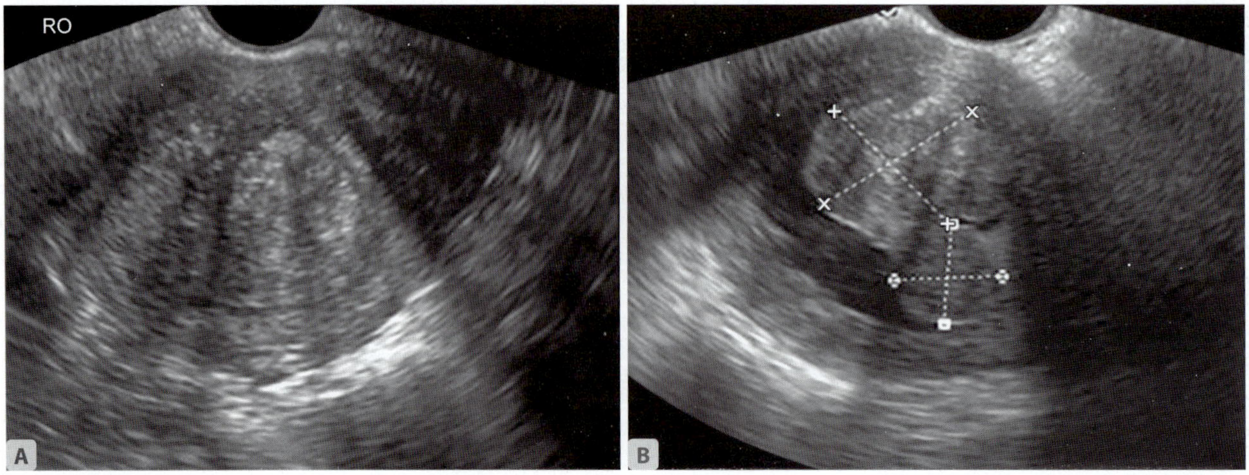

FIGS. 5A AND B: Sonohysterography. (A) Transvaginal scan shows hyperechoic masses within the uterus; it is not possible to determine their relation with the endometrium; (B) On instillation of intracavitary saline, two well-defined masses (within callipers) are seen projecting into the endometrial cavity—submucous fibroids.

fluid into the uterus and then visualizing passage of fluid through the tubes or presence of fluid in the pouch of Douglas on USG.[11] While intracavitary lesions are clearly delineated by anechoic media, very small hollow cavities, such as normal tubes are not always easily visualized using SIS.

HYSTEROSALPINGO-CONTRAST SONOGRAPHY

Deichert et al. were the first to evaluate tubal patency using injection of contrast agent and transvaginal sonography.[12] Demonstration of the lumen of tubes requires visualization of movement of fluid using highly echogenic medium. A cost-effective alternative is the use of saline mixed with air. It produces high contrast due to the presence of air bubbles; these bubbles, however, stand only for a very short period and tubal patency assessment may become difficult practically. Therefore, commercially available contrast media were launched with microbubbles that can stand longer. On ultrasound evaluation, this contrast appears echogenic. The scanning technique is the same as that for SIS. It is possible to delineate the uterine cavity along with the tubes using contrast. Total amount of contrast needed is as little as 2–3 mL/tube. The findings appreciated by conventional 2D-HyCoSy (hysterosalpingo-contrast sonography) are, however, sometimes difficult to interpret. Due to the tortuosity of the tube, the whole fallopian tube cannot be visualized in the majority of scanning planes. Furthermore, differentiation of echogenic tube from bowel becomes difficult due to the spill of the echo-positive contrast medium. This has been overcome by use of 3D and 4D imaging in conjunction with HyCoSy.[13]

A comprehensive meta-analysis was published in 2016 to assess the diagnostic value of 4D and 3D HyCoSy for detecting tubal patency and it included 23 studies. This systematic review showed a high diagnostic accuracy of 3D/4D HyCoSy for tubal patency with an overall specificity of 0.91 (95% CI: 0.89–0.93) and sensitivity of 0.92 (95% CI: 0.90–0.94). The results had a good stability among the included studies.[14]

EXTENDED FIELD-OF-VIEW IMAGING[15]

Extended field-of-view (EFOV) overcomes the drawback of limited field of view of sonography, enabling the visualization of large fields of view in a single image. This technology is now available in most of the modern equipment. The technique is relatively simple and requires only a steady sweep of the transducer over the concerned area to acquire the data. The EFOV image is then reconstructed automatically by the computer. Doppler EFOV allows a panoramic visualization of vascularity in mass lesions, helping in their characterization. Transvaginal EFOV is also possible to illustrate the relation of smaller pelvic masses with the uterus and ovaries in a single image. EFOV images are comparable to CT/MRI images as they provide a panoramic view.

ELASTOGRAPHY[16]

Elastography is an imaging method that evaluates the elasticity of tissue. All available ultrasound elastography methods employ ultrasound to measure the mechanical response resulting from an applied force. The mechanical response measured may be displacement, strain or amplitude and phase of vibration.

There are three main techniques used in sonoelastography: (1) shear wave elastography (SWE), (2)strain elastography (SE), and (3) transient elastography (TE). Both SE and SWE can be used in evaluation of uterus and cervix; however, the application in the field of gynecology has mostly been experimental and further validation requires extensive research. Stoelinga et al. and Frank et al. have investigated the use of transvaginal elastography in uterine evaluation.[17,18] Both studies concluded that transvaginal elastography could help differentiate uterine fibroids from adenomyosis. Elastography can also be used in the diagnosis of cervical malignancies. Thomas et al. have reported use of cervical elastography in 113 patients, among whom 24 had cervical malignancies. The study showed that elastography was able to differentiate malignant from normal cervical tissue.[19]

CONTRAST-ENHANCED ULTRASONOGRAPHY

Ultrasonography contrast agents can help delineate vascular structures and enhanced Doppler signals from small volumes of blood make it possible to image organ and lesion perfusion in real time.[20] These contrast agents are gas-filled microbubbles of size 2–5 µm. They are stabilized by a shell and are injected intravenously. They are capable of passing through the smallest capillaries. Microbubbles oscillate particularly at frequencies used for diagnostic imaging (1–10 MHz), reflecting a unique nonlinear echo.

The use of contrast-enhanced ultrasonography (CEUSG) in the assessment of liver lesions, renal carcinoma, and cardiac imaging is already quite established, the use of this technique is still limited in the field of gynecology. Contrast uptake and wash out can be studied subjectively or objectively by time intensity curves. These curves have a role in characterization of ovarian mass lesions. It is also possible to distinguish between endometrial hyperplasia and endometrial malignancy by analysis of intensity and time parameters recorded after contrast administration. Ultrasound contrast agents can be extremely useful in differentiating uterine fibroids from focal adenomyosis as their uptake patterns are very different.[21]

MAGNETIC RESONANCE IMAGING

Magnetic resonance imaging is now recognized as an important problem solving tool in the evaluation of female pelvis due to its multiplanar capability, lack of significant motion degradation of images, and higher soft tissue contrast resolution.

Indications

Indications for MRI include the following:

- Evaluation of congenital anomalies
- Evaluation of cervical and uterine malignancy
- Selected cases of leiomyoma, like cases that require differentiation from adnexal masses and leiomyosarcoma, treatment planning and monitoring after therapy etc.
- Assessing response to medical therapy
- Pelvic floor assessment
- Search of submucosal lesions in infertile patients
- Diagnosis of adenomyosis and endometriosis
- Problem solving modality in characterization of ovarian lesions, especially ovarian dermoid.

Patient Preparation

Imaging is performed in the supine position with a moderately full bladder after fasting for at least 4 hours to limit bowel motion. In the absence of glaucoma, 20 mg of butyl scopolamine (Buscopan) is injected intramuscularly to reduce bowel peristalsis. A variety of receiver coil (body coil allowing better coverage and endoluminal coil for better anatomical depiction) have been used for pelvic imaging but phased array coils have been found to provide the best results. Ideally, the coil position should allow imaging from mid-symphysis pubis to renal hilum. Rectal and vaginal gel contrast media can be used for specific indications.[22] Vaginal opacification has shown to be beneficial in conditions like cervical cancer, endometrial cancer, and vaginal developmental anomalies. Both rectal and vaginal opacification are recommended when imaging patients of deep pelvic endometriosis. Vaginal injection involves an average of 60 mL of sterile ultrasound gel. Rectal opacification is performed with 100–120 mL of nonsterile ultrasound gel.

Sequences

After the localizer sequence, anterior and upper saturation bands are placed to cover the subcutaneous fat for each sequence. The standard protocol for pelvic imaging comprises unenhanced T1- and T2-weighted sequences. Spoiled gradient recalled echo (GRE) and spin-echo (SE) sequences form the basis of most of the protocols. Standard sequences include the following:

- Sagittal T2-weighted sequence of the pelvis.
- One or two additional T2-weighted sequences with slice orientation based on the clinical indication and findings of the sagittal sequence (one T2 fat saturation sequence may also be acquired based on the area of interest).
- One to three T1-weighted images (the optional orientation of this native T1-weighted image depends on the slice orientation that best demonstrates the pathology and its extent).
- Fat suppressed T1 sequence whenever the lesion demonstrates hyperintensity on the T1-weighted images.
- Contrast-enhanced T1-weighted images with fat suppression—mandatory for staging of malignancies, evaluation of deep endometriosis, and characterization of adnexal masses.

Technique of MRI for Uterine and Cervical Pathologies

For uterine indications, short-axis MR images are acquired perpendicular to the hyperintense stripe of the endometrium in the uterine body. This will usually be paraxial, but in patients with extreme anteversion of the uterus, this may be closer to a true coronal plane. Long-axis MR images are acquired parallel to the stripe.

Occasionally, the uterus may be anteflexed, i.e. there may be a considerable angle between the body of the uterus and cervix. In these circumstances, the main clinical question should be answered; for example, if the procedure is being done for the assessment of a cervical carcinoma, the orientation of axial oblique T2-weighted images should be perpendicular to the hyperintense stripe of endocervical channel, permitting complete visualization of the T2 hypointense stromal ring. If this is equivocal, a fat-suppression sequence, such as short-TI inversion-recovery (STIR), may be helpful. Fat suppressed T1-weighted images should be acquired before and after gadolinium enhancement. Coronal plane imaging is occasionally helpful, particularly if disease spread to the vagina is suspected on the initial imaging sequences. Investigation of benign conditions of the uterus, such as adenomyosis and leiomyoma, will usually require a briefer protocol than imaging for preoperative staging in cases of malignancy.

Technique of MRI for Pathologies of Ovary

The axial plane is most important. Coronal imaging is often useful in clarifying the relationship of masses to vessels and the uterus. The sagittal plane is found to be of limited use.

Technique of MRI for Imaging of Vagina

T2-weighted images once again form the mainstay of the imaging technique. Layers of the vaginal can sometimes be differentiated using small field-of-view, high-resolution images. Axial, sagittal, and coronal planes are all useful in demonstrating the relationship of vagina to adjacent organs. Axial and sagittal images demonstrate the relationship to rectum and bladder while coronal images demonstrate the relationship to the levator ani muscle to its best advantage.

Nodal Survey

A common indication for pelvic MRI is staging gynecological or urological malignancy. An essential part of this investigation is surveying the retroperitoneum and pelvis for enlarged nodes. It is prudent to complete this part of the investigation first, as gut relaxation is maximum in the beginning of the procedure. Images of the pelvis are obtained using T1-weighted spoiled GRE (breath-hold) and T2-weighted sequences, in the axial plane, from the aortic bifurcation to the inguinal region just below the femoral canal. Slice thickness should be 8–10 mm using a 0–4-mm gap. This may be varied to cater to patients of varying heights. Subsequently, an evaluation of the retroperitoneum should be carried out.

Special Techniques

Various special techniques that can be added to standard protocol include the following:

- The characterization of adnexal masses may require additional in phase and out of phase sequences to allow a diagnosis of teratoma with minimal fat.
- Dynamic contrast-enhanced (DCE)-MRI involves intravenous injection of standard low-molecular weight paramagnetic intravascular contrast agents (typically gadolinium diethylenetriamine penta-acetic acid), either as a constant infusion or fast bolus injection. Serial image acquisitions are performed every few seconds over a length of few minutes, the region of interest and exact protocols depend on the tumor type being imaged. DCE-MR is useful in characterization of adnexal lesions and cases of recurrence of malignancies.[23]
- Diffusion-weighted imaging (DWI)-MRI is a robust tool for evaluation of functional status of gynecological malignancies. It has shown to have high accuracy and sensitivity for detection of nodal metastases in cervical cancer patients according to a recent meta-analysis involving 67 studies.[24] DWI-MRI is especially capable of accurate determination of the depth of myometrial invasion in patients with endometrial cancer.[25] It has also been proposed to be a potential response biomarker in cervical cancer.[26] DWI is highly sensitive for picking up peritoneal spread in gynecological malignancies and plays an important role in their management especially ovarian cancer.[27]
- Blood oxygenation level-dependent (BOLD) hypoxia imaging is an MR tool to analyze vascular functionality associated with angiogenesis. It uses deoxyhemoglobin as a natural paramagnetic contrast agent and is found to be sensitive to changes in blood flow, blood volume, and blood oxygenation. Combined physiologic and anatomic information obtained from multiparametric MRI (MPMRI) with BOLD hypoxia imaging helps in detection and grading of tumors.[28]
- Diffusion tensor imaging (DTI) has been used to quantify defects and determine direction of muscle fibers during pelvic floor assessment.[29]
- Multiphase dynamic MR defecography can be performed following intrarectal instillation of contrast to evaluate pelvic floor and defecatory dysfunction.[30]
- Magnetic resonance lymphography is performed to assess the lymph nodes. It involves intravenous injection of ultrasmall superparamagnetic particles of iron oxide (USPIO) and can detect presence of metastases in the nodes with high sensitivity and specificity.[31]
- Proton MR spectroscopy also has a role in differentiating malignant from borderline epithelial ovarian tumors (EOTs). A high Choline (CHO) peak suggests a malignant EOT and a significantly elevated N-Acetyl Aspartate (NAA) peak is highly suggestive of a borderline EOT. The NAA/Cho ratio is a reliable biomarker for differentiating malignant from borderline EOTs.[32]

COMPUTED TOMOGRAPHY

The role of CT in the evaluation of gynecologic disorders has declined due to endovaginal scanning and MRI. MRI is better than CT for staging uterine and cervical carcinoma, particularly with respect to local extent. But CT has a role in evaluation of ovarian carcinoma due to its potential to detect peritoneal deposits.[33] CT is frequently added as an imaging modality in patients with nonspecific lower abdominal symptoms such as pain.

Technique

A standard pelvic CT scan consists of continuous sections from the level of the symphysis pubis cephalad to the iliac crest. In cancer staging or abdominopelvic mass evaluation, sections are then taken from the symphysis pubis to the diaphragm. Bowel opacification achieved orally with 1,000 mL of diluted contrast medium is generally recommended. Patients are requested to drink 450 mL of water soluble contrast medium 10–12 hours before the examination to opacify the large bowel, and 450 mL 45 minutes preceding the study to opacify small bowel. In patients with suspected ovarian cancer, PID, endometriosis, 200 mL water soluble contrast enema is preferred to delineate the disease extent. Intravenous opacification is pivotal for assessing adnexal lesions, staging uterine and ovarian cancers, and assessing vascular or inflammatory diseases. A dose of 90–120 mL contrast medium with a concentration of 300–370 mg iodine/

mL administered at a rate of 2–3 mL/sec is sufficient. In multidetector computed tomography (MDCT), images are obtained in transaxial planes and reformatted in coronal and sagittal planes.

CT also plays an important role in the aspiration or drainage of fluid collections such as blood or pus.

Evaluation of the pelvic vasculature is indicated in MDCT of pelvic arteriovenous malformations after embolization and fibroids after uterine artery embolization. It is recommended to determine individual circulation time by using a bolus-tracking program for CT angiography of the pelvic arteries. The pelvis is scanned during the arterial phase after a faster injection rate (3–5 mL/sec).

PET-CT AND PET-MR

There is an increase in evidence advocating the use of PET-CT in evaluation of gynecologic malignancies. These are typically identified with increased glucose metabolism and therefore present with increased fluorodeoxyglucose (FDG) uptake, whereas benign tumors are usually negative on PET. However, common pitfalls include normal physiologic activity in bowel, endometrium, blood vessels, increased FDG uptake in normal ovaries during ovulation and focal retained activity in pelvic kidneys, ureters, bladder diverticula, and urinary diversions.

Indications

Positron emission tomography-computed tomography has been used widely in patients with advanced disease or in cases of recurrence. It is indicated in patients of ovarian and cervical carcinoma with suspected relapse. In patients of carcinoma cervix stage 2A and above, PET-CT is indicated for prognostication and treatment planning. It is also used in assessing response to therapy in patients of carcinoma cervix.[34] MRI and PET individually play important and supporting roles in assessing gynecologic malignancy. MRI is the imaging procedure of choice for assessing local extension of tumors, and PET aids in detection of distant metastases.[35]

Technical Considerations

Ideally, the bladder should be empty to avoid artifacts on PET images from high radioactivity concentration in the bladder. It is advised that the patient is scanned in a caudal to cranial direction, thereby imaging the pelvis in the beginning of the study. The CT portion of PET/CT is often important to identify focal retained activity in ureters and bladder diverticula. Pelvic imaging can be made better by intravenous injection of a diuretic agent to lessen tracer retention in the urinary system. A technique of hydration, diuretic administration, and preimaging voiding obviates the need for invasive procedures like bladder drainage in most patients.

ANATOMY

Uterus

The uterus lies between the bladder anteriorly and rectosigmoid posteriorly **(Fig. 6)**. Its size and shape vary throughout life-related to age, hormonal status, and parity **(Table 1)**. The infantile or prepubertal uterus has an inverse pear-shaped appearance with a disproportionately larger cervix occupying up to one-half to two-thirds the size of the uterus **(Fig. 7)**. In the immediate neonatal period, the uterus is slightly larger and shows an echogenic endometrium, because of residual maternal hormonal stimulation. A small amount of endometrial fluid may also be seen in 25%

TABLE 1: Normal uterine size and shape by life stage.[1]

Stage	Uterine Length (cm)	Uterine body to cervix ratio
Neonatal	3.5	2:1
Pediatric	1–3	1:1
Prepubertal	3–4.5	1–1.5:1
Pubertal	5–8	1.5–2:1
Reproductive	8–9	2:1
Postmenopausal	3.5–7.5	1.5:1

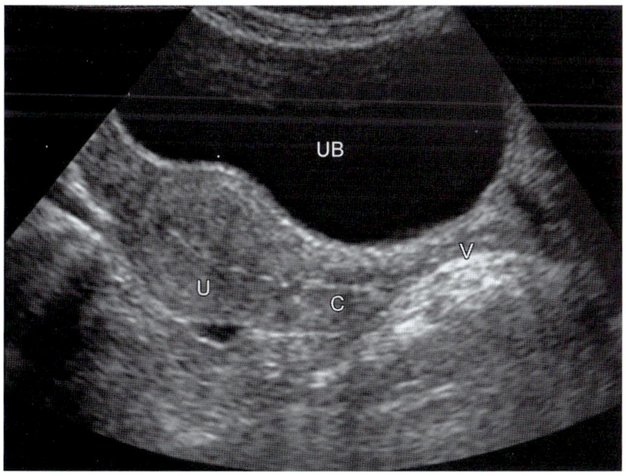

FIG. 6: Normal uterus (U), cervix (C), and vagina (V) on a transabdominal sagittal scan.

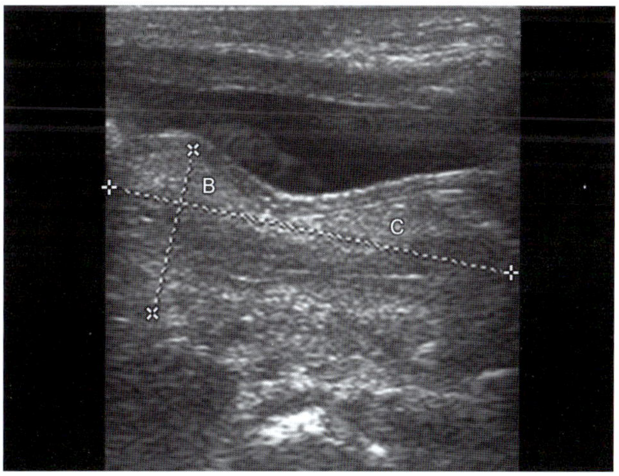

FIG. 7: Normal neonatal uterus—sagittal scans. Inverse pear shape with cervix (C) having greater width than body (B) of uterus.

of neonatal uteri.[36] There is little growth of the prepubertal uterus from infancy till about 8 years of age. The uterus gradually increases in size till puberty; when it attains a pear-shaped appearance with the body of the uterus becoming approximately double the cervix.

The normal postpubertal or adult uterus varies considerably in size. The maximal dimensions of the nulliparous uterus are approximately 8 cm in length, 4 cm in anteroposterior (AP) diameter and 5 cm in width. Parity increases the normal dimensions by more than 1 cm in each dimension.[37] After menopause, atrophy of uterus occurs, with the most rapid decrease in size occurring in the first 10 years following the cessation of menstruation. The uterus usually assumes a position that is both anteverted and anteflexed **(Fig. 8)**. The degree of bladder filling alters the lie of the uterus; with an empty bladder the uterus is angled forward from the lie of the vagina, whereas a full bladder straightens the uterus. In case of retroverted or retroflexed uterus, the fundus lies posteriorly. It is often not possible to distinguish between retroversion and retroflexion on sonography so the general term retroposition is used. On transabdominal scanning, the deeper portions of the fundus may be difficult to delineate and may even appear abnormal because of shadowing from the intervening body and cervix. Transvaginal scanning gives an excellent visualization of the retropositioned uterus as the probe can be directed posteriorly.[38]

Uterus consists of an external serosa (*perimetrium*), a middle muscle layer (*myometrium*) and the internal mucosa (*endometrium*). The perimetrium is not visible on ultrasound examination, although subserosal veins may be seen as a normal variant. *On sonography*, the myometrium has three layers: the inner myometrium (or the subendometrial halo) appears as a thin hypoechoic area surrounding the echogenic endometrium. The intermediate layer is the thickest and has a uniformly homogeneous low-to-moderate echogenicity. The thin outer layer is less echogenic and separated from the intermediate layer by the arcuate vessels, which can be visualized on ultrasound as small anechoic foci in the periphery of the uterus. Calcification may be seen in the arteries in postmenopausal women. Sometimes small highly echogenic foci may be seen in the inner layer of myometrium. These small, single or multiple, nonshadowing foci are thought to represent dystrophic calcification related to previous instrumentation like dilatation and curettage or endocervical biopsy.[39]

The endometrium is best measured on the midline sagittal scan of the uterus. The measurement is taken as the distance between the two interfaces formed by junction of subendometrial halo and the more echogenic endometrium. This is the double layer thickness **(Fig. 9)**.

The normal endometrial cavity is seen as a central echogenic line as a result of specular reflection from the interface between apposing surfaces of the endometrium. It should be straight or smoothly curved.

The cervix is better visualized by transvaginal sonography as a tubular structure of homogeneous echogenicity **(Fig. 10)**. The mucus within the endocervical canal usually appears as an echogenic interface which may become hypoechoic during the periovulatory period as the fluid content increases. Retention (nabothian) cysts of the cervix are commonly seen during routine sonography. They may vary in size from a few mm to 4 cm. They may be single or multiple and usually diagnosed incidentally, although they may be associated with chronic cervicitis.

On MRI, three distinct uterine zones can be differentiated in women of reproductive age on T2-weighted imaging. The endometrium represents the central high signal intensity portion of the uterus. The middle low signal intensity layer is the junctional zone and represents the inner myometrium.

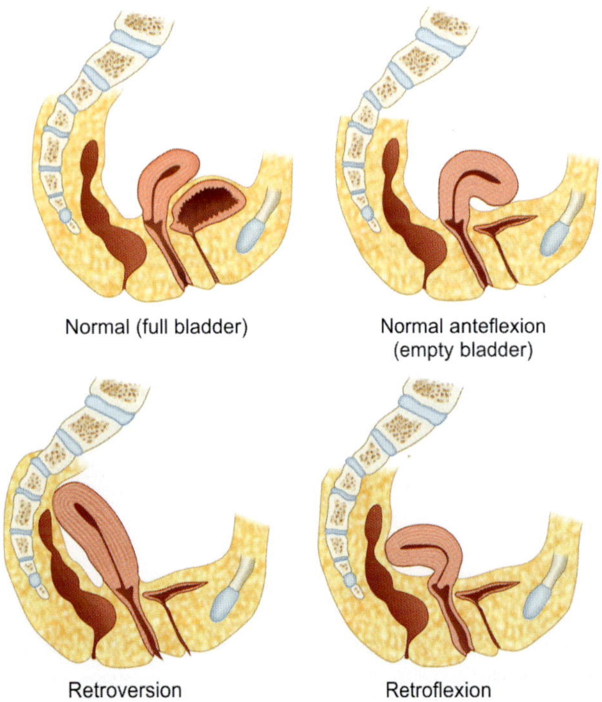

FIG. 8: Alterations in uterine position. The normal position of uterus in most women is anteverted with a mild degree of anteflexion. In retroversion, the long axis of the uterus and cervix point more posteriorly than the long axis of the vagina. In retroflexion, the body of the uterus is angled posteriorly relative to the cervix.

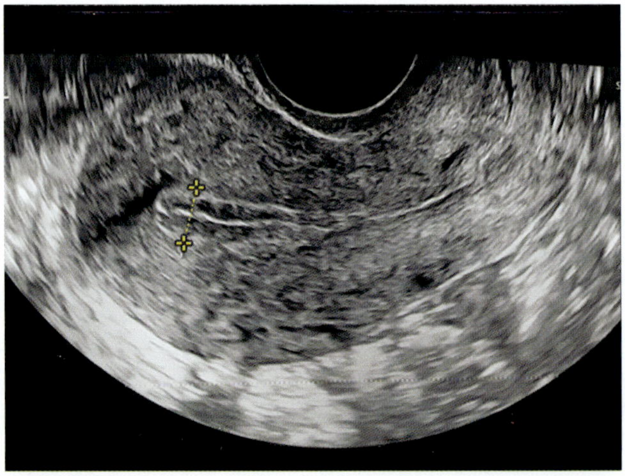

FIG. 9: Measurement of endometrial thickness on ultrasound.

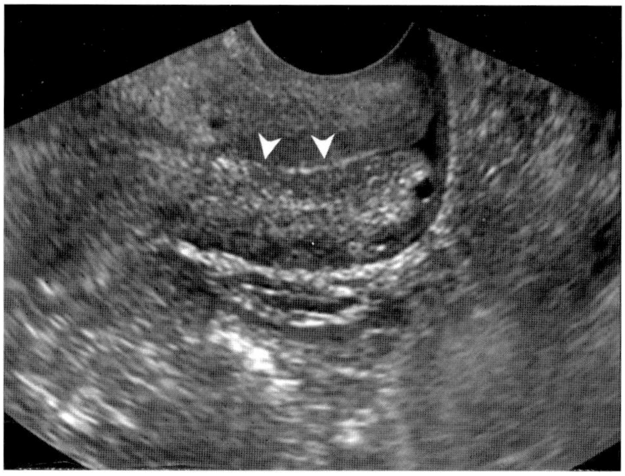

FIG. 10: The normal cervix as seen on sagittal transvaginal scan, with a central echogenic line (arrowheads) representing the cervical canal. Two small nabothian cysts are seen.

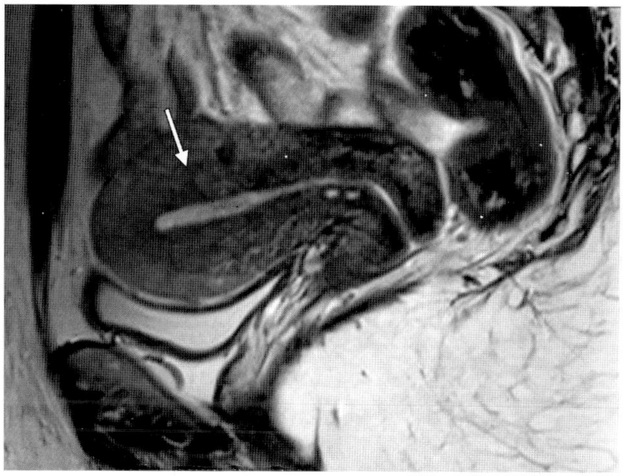

FIG. 11: T2-weighted sagittal magnetic resonance image. Outer limit of junctional zone is marked by arrow.

The thickness of normal junctional zone is less than 8 mm. The outer medium signal intensity represents the outer myometrium. Its signal intensity depends on the phase of menstrual cycle, but it usually exhibits intermediate signal intensity on T2-weighted image **(Fig. 11)**. The zonal anatomy is important to assess the depth of myometrial invasion of endometrial carcinoma. On T1-weighted images, uterus is seen as an organ with medium to low signal intensity.[40] Uterus also undergoes subtle wave-like peristalsis caused by contractions of the inner myometrium. The direction, height, and frequency of the wave vary throughout the phase of menstrual cycle, with an average of 2–3 cycles per minute. The direction is generally antegrade during menstruation and retrograde (cervicofundal) in mid-cycle. On cine mode display, wavy and subtle movement of this area can be seen, with occasional stripping movement of the endometrium. The appearance of the uterus on the DCE-MRI study is variable and depends on the time interval after intravenous contrast administration. Usually, the myometrium is homogeneous and hyperintense in the arterial and venous phase, while the endometrium enhances later and slowly, showing hypointensity when compared to myometrium. On delayed evaluation, endometrium and outer myometrium show pronounced contrast enhancement while the junctional zone is of low signal intensity, thus displaying the zonal anatomy.

The cervix shows four layers on T2-weighted MR images. The central high signal layer represents mucus, which is surrounded by high signal intensity endocervix. The hypointense stroma surrounds the endocervix and is continuous with the junctional zone of uterus. The outer intermediate signal intensity is from smooth muscle and is continuous with outer myometrium **(Fig. 12)**. Strong contrast enhancement of the endocervix and parametrium is seen on postcontrast images, whereas stroma shows initial faint enhancement with progression on delayed images.

On *CT*, the cervix and body of uterus appear as soft tissue masses, only identifiable from each other by their shape, i.e. cervix is round and uterus oval or triangular in cross section. In women of reproductive age, the endometrium exhibits hypodensity relative to the inner myometrium during most phases of contrast enhancement, a finding that might be mistaken as fluid within the uterine cavity **(Fig. 13)**.

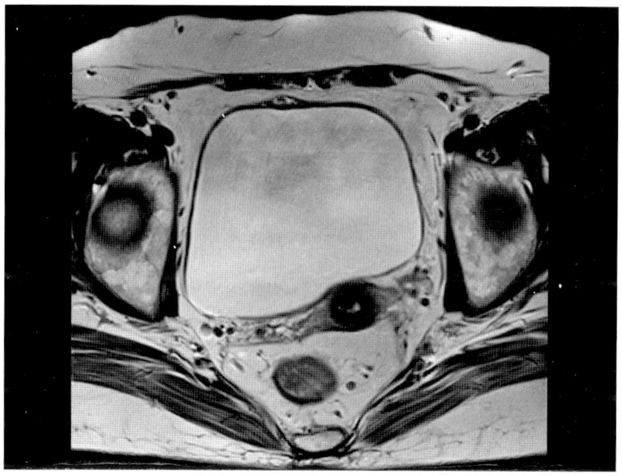

FIG. 12: Magnetic resonance appearance of cervix with T2 hypointense stroma surrounding the hyperintense endocervix.

Vagina

The vagina runs anteriorly and caudally from the cervix between the bladder and rectum. On *USG*, it is best seen on the mid-sagittal transabdominal scans as a collapsed hypoechoic tubular structure with a central hyperechoic line due to the apposed surfaces of the vaginal mucosa. A vaginal tampon can be visualized as a highly reflective structure with a strong acoustic shadow. On TVS, examining the vaginal walls is possible during slow withdrawal of the probe as they collapse around the end of probe. In patients who have had hysterectomy, the vaginal cuff should not be mistaken for a mass. The normal upper limit of the AP diameter of the vaginal cuff is 2.1 cm.[41] The vagina has three layers on T2-weighted MR images. The central high-signal intensity represents

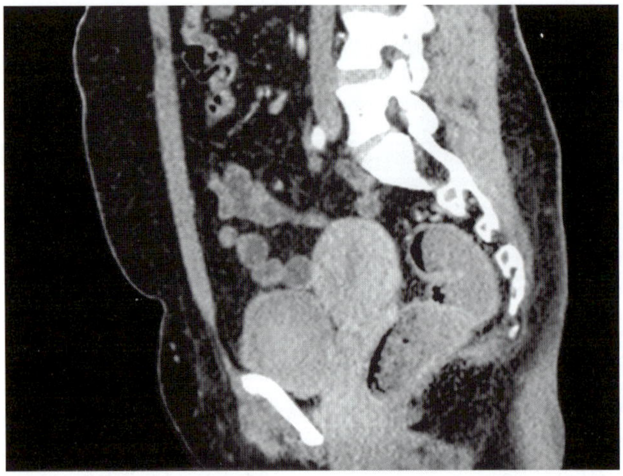

FIG. 13: Sagittal reformat of contrast-enhanced CT scan showing the normal uterus posterior to the bladder with reduced enhancement of the endometrium.

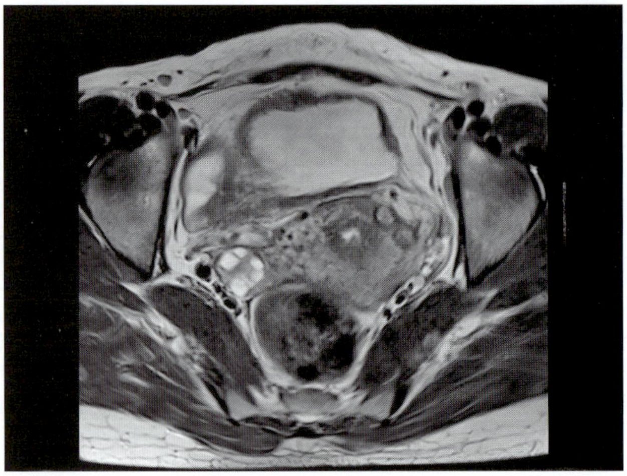

FIG. 14: Magnetic resonance appearance of ovaries. T2-weighted axial image showing multiple hyperintense follicles in ovary on the right side.

mucus; middle low-signal intensity represents submucosa and muscularis; and outer high-signal intensity representing vaginal venous plexus. On *CT axial scans*, the vagina is identified as a thin rectangular structure with an enhancing mucosa. The vulva includes the mons pubis, labia majora and minora, prepuce, frenulum, clitoris, and vestibule. A complex system of anastomoses accounts for variations in arterial, venous, and lymphatic supply.

Upper corpus and uterine fundus are drained by the common iliac and para-aortic lymph nodes. Lower and middle parts of the uterus are drained by parametrial, paracervical, and obturator nodes. In general, lymphatic drainage from the distal vagina and vulva passes along inguinal and femoral nodes. The upper two-thirds of the vagina drains to the external iliac and obturator nodes. The posterior vagina may also drain to the gluteal and anorectal lymph nodes.

Adnexae

The adnexae consist of the ovaries, the fallopian tubes, ligaments, and vessels. The *ovaries* most commonly lie lateral to the uterus (usually within a few centimeters) at about the level of the cornua. Variations are common and insignificant. A relatively constant relationship of the ovaries is their location anterior to internal iliac vessels, which serves as a useful landmark for the ovaries particularly during *TVS*.

The ovaries are typically seen as oblong structures with a relatively homogeneous echotexture. Well-defined small anechoic follicles may be seen peripherally in the cortex. The variable appearances of ovaries during different stages of life are described in **Table 2**.

Because of the variability in shape, ovarian volume is considered the best method for evaluating the ovarian size (0.523 × length × width × AP diameter). For this measurement, any cyst larger than 1 cm in diameter is excluded. The two ovaries should be approximately equal in volume; and neither should be more than twice the volume of the other. Small echogenic, nonshadowing foci may sometimes be seen in a normal ovary, which are thought to be due to specular reflection from tiny unresolved cysts below the spatial resolution of the ultrasound machine.

TABLE 2: Normal ovarian volume and appearance by life stage.[1]

Stage	Ovarian volume (cm^3)	Ovarian appearance
Neonatal	1–3.5	Follicles and cysts common
Pediatric	0.5–1.5	Fewer than six follicles; cysts uncommon
Prepubertal	1–4	Follicles and cysts common
Pubertal	2–6	Follicles and cysts common
Reproductive	4–16	Follicles and cysts common
Postmenopausal	1.3–5.8	Follicles and cysts in approximately 15–20%

On *MRI*, normal ovaries can be visualized in 85% of women of reproductive age. They are identified by following the course of the round ligament or gonadal vessels. On T1-weighted images, the ovaries are seen as low- or medium-signal intensity structures, and on T2-weighted images, they show low signal intensity in the central stroma and high signal intensity follicles and functional cysts of varying sizes **(Fig. 14)**. A low signal intensity rim around ovaries represents the fibrous capsule. On *CT images*, the ovaries are usually seen in adult premenopausal patients as soft tissue masses posterolateral to uterus; however, their position is variable **(Fig. 15)**. The normal ovary displays intense early enhancement with a secondary washout.

The nondistended fallopian tubes are difficult to see on ultrasound. Delineation of the tubes is possible if intraperitoneal fluid is present in the peritoneal cavity or if they are distended by saline/contrast agent.

The posterior cul-de-sac (pouch of Douglas) is the most posterior and inferior reflection of the peritoneal cavity located between the rectum and vagina. Small quantities of fluid (1-3 mL) in the cul-de-sac is a normal finding in asymptomatic women, and can be seen in all phases of the menstrual cycle.

The pelvic side walls are lined by psoas and iliacus muscles. Iliacus muscle arises from the iliac wings and progresses posterolateral to the psoas into the pelvis. These muscles run obliquely passing posterior to inguinal ligament and form a joint tendon to insert on greater trochanter. These muscles are visualized on ultrasound as paired hypoechoic structures separated by echogenic fascial plane. The iliac vessels lie on the psoas muscle.

Pelvic floor muscles including iliococcygeus, coccygeus, puborectalis, and pubococcygeus muscles, as well as the external and internal anal sphincter are clearly shown on MRI. Pelvic diaphragm are displayed as two layers of low signal intensity at the level of lower vagina. In addition to a precise demonstration of anatomy, dynamic MRI also helps in imaging the kinematics of pelvic organs.

The Menstrual Cycle

The appearance of the endometrium and ovaries varies during the menstrual cycle.[42] Their appearance during the various phases of the menstrual cycle has been described in **Table 3 (Figs. 16 and 17)**.

Imaging in Postmenopausal Period

In postmenopausal women, the outer myometrium displays lower signal intensity and the junctional zone is often missing or indistinctly visualized. The normal sonographic endometrial appearance varies according to absence or presence of hormonal replacement therapy (HRT). Additionally, the type of HRT (i.e. combined, sequential or continuous) is important.[43] In postmenopausal asymptomatic women not receiving HRT, several reports suggest that endometrial thickness should not exceed 4 mm, whereas others use 8 mm as the upper limit of normal value.[1] For women receiving HRT, the ultrasound appearance of the endometrium depends

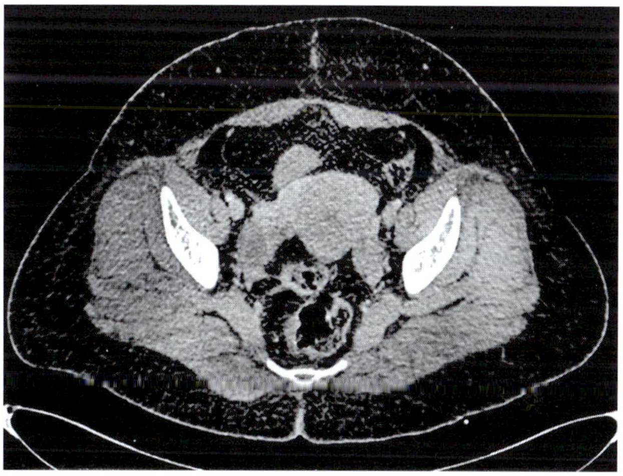

FIG. 15: Axial contrast-enhanced CT scan image showing the uterus and bilateral ovaries located posterolateral to it.

TABLE 3: Appearance of endometrium and ovaries in a normal menstrual cycle.

Day of cycle	Phase	Endometrial thickness (mm)	Ultrasound appearance of endometrium	Ultrasound appearance of ovaries	MR appearance of uterus
1–4	Menstrual phase	1–4	Small amounts of fluid may be seen endovaginally. Thin interrupted central echo	Development of a small number of follicles.	Loss of zonal appearance. Blood clot may be present in the endometrial cavity
5–14	Proliferative phase	4–8	Central hyperechoic line with surrounding thin hypoechoic band	By Day 8 or 9 of the menstrual cycle, one follicle becomes dominant, and the others become atretic. Nondominant follicles are usually less than 14 mm in diameter	Internal myometrial enhancement occurs earlier and is more intense in the proliferative than in the luteal phase of the cycle
	Periovulatory	6–10	Trilayered appearance; the hypoechoic band becomes more prominent with thin echogenic lines on either side	About Day 14, when the dominant follicle measures 18–25 mm, ovulation occurs	
15–28	Secretory phase	8–16	Thick Echogenic with through transmission.	Following ovulation, a corpus luteum develops which can commonly be seen as a hypoechoic or isoechoic structure peripherally within the ovary, but may show a very varied sonographic appearance. Sometimes, it may form a cyst and become very large. **(Fig. 18)**. A repeat scan 2–6 weeks later will usually resolve the dilemma	Signal intensity of outer myometrium increases. Increased thickness of junctional zone

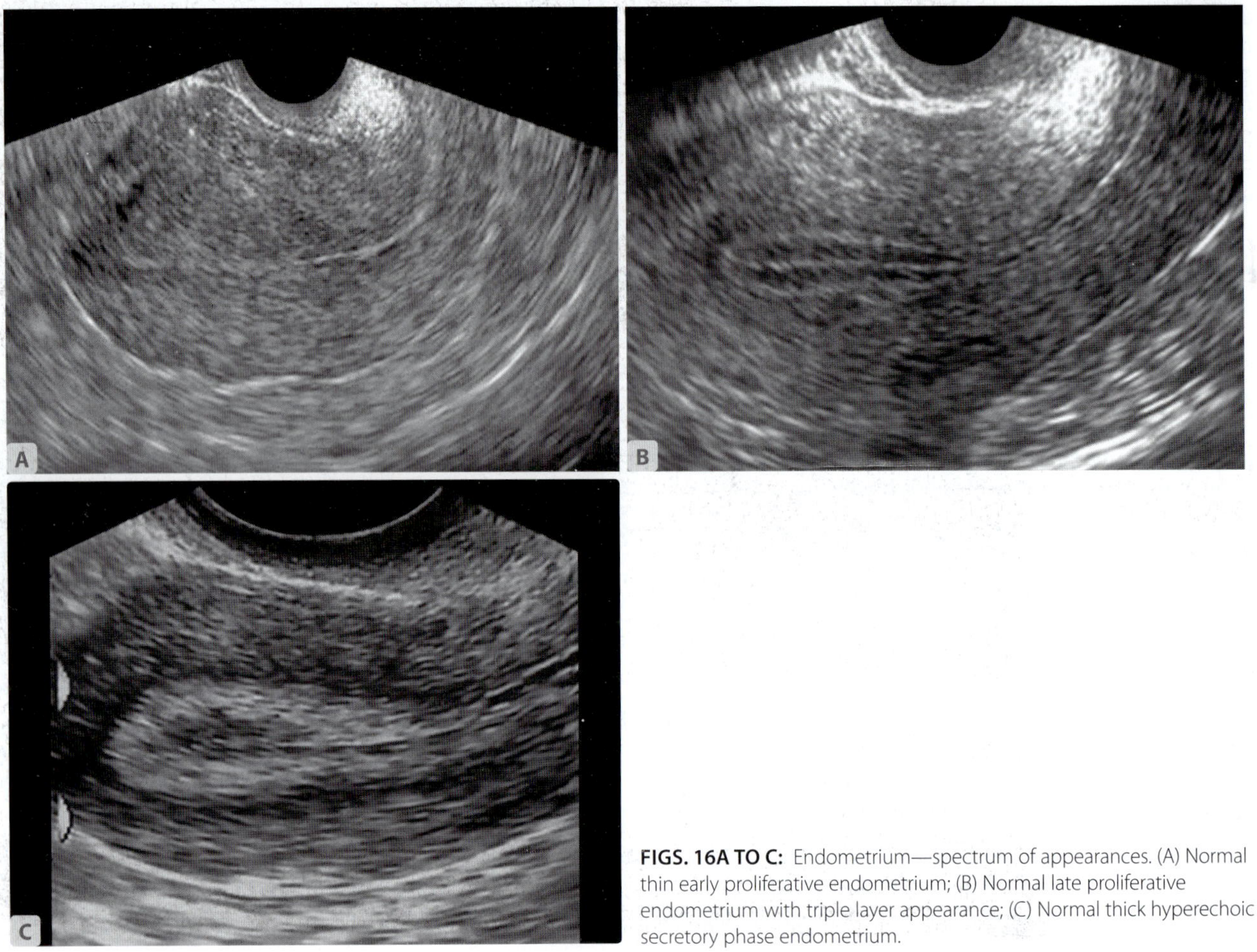

FIGS. 16A TO C: Endometrium—spectrum of appearances. (A) Normal thin early proliferative endometrium; (B) Normal late proliferative endometrium with triple layer appearance; (C) Normal thick hyperechoic secretory phase endometrium.

on whether the patient takes a combination of estrogen and progesterone (either continuously or sequentially) or continuous estrogen. Sequential HRT results in monthly cyclic endometrial thickening and withdrawal bleeding. At mid-cycle, the upper limit of maximal endometrial thickness frequently goes beyond 8 mm, and in some cases may reach up to 15 mm. In these women, it is essential to do a follow-up scan. In women taking either continuous estrogen or continuous estrogen and progesterone, the maximum endometrial thickness is 8 mm, and cyclic endometrial changes should not occur. Postmenopausal women may often have a trace of fluid (approximately 1 mm in thickness) in the endometrial cavity due to cervical stenosis.[43] The postmenopausal patients have similar internal and external myometrial enhancement which is significantly less intense than in the premenopausal patients.

The postmenopausal ovaries may be difficult to recognize sonographically as they are relatively small and do not contain follicles **(Fig. 19)**. Mean postmenopausal ovarian volume ranges between 1.2 cc and 5.8 cc with the volume decreasing in size with increasing age. An ovarian volume of more than 8 cc is definitely abnormal. Small anechoic cysts (less than 3 cm) may be seen in up to 15% of postmenopausal ovaries and are not related to age, length of time since menopause or hormone use. These cysts can disappear or change in size over time.[44] The atrophic ovaries of postmenopausal women are frequently indistinguishable from surrounding structures on CT images.

Vascular Anatomy

The blood supply to the uterus is via the *uterine artery*, a branch of the internal iliac artery. The uterine artery enters the uterus at the cervico-corporal junction and ascends along the lateral aspect of the uterine body to the cornua. At the cornua, an adnexal branch originates that supplies the ipsilateral ovary and anastomoses with the ipsilateral ovarian artery. The uterine arteries anastomose through the anterior and posterior arcuate arteries which are located in the outer one-third of the myometrium. Radial arteries arise from the arcuate vessels and extend through the myometrium up to the endometrium where they form: (1) the basal arteries which supply the basalis layer of endometrium and (2) the spiral arteries which supply the functional layer of endometrium. The spiral arteries are responsive to hormonal changes. During the reproductive years, both color and duplex Doppler patterns change concomitantly with grayscale changes.[45] The general pattern of uterine blood flow throughout the

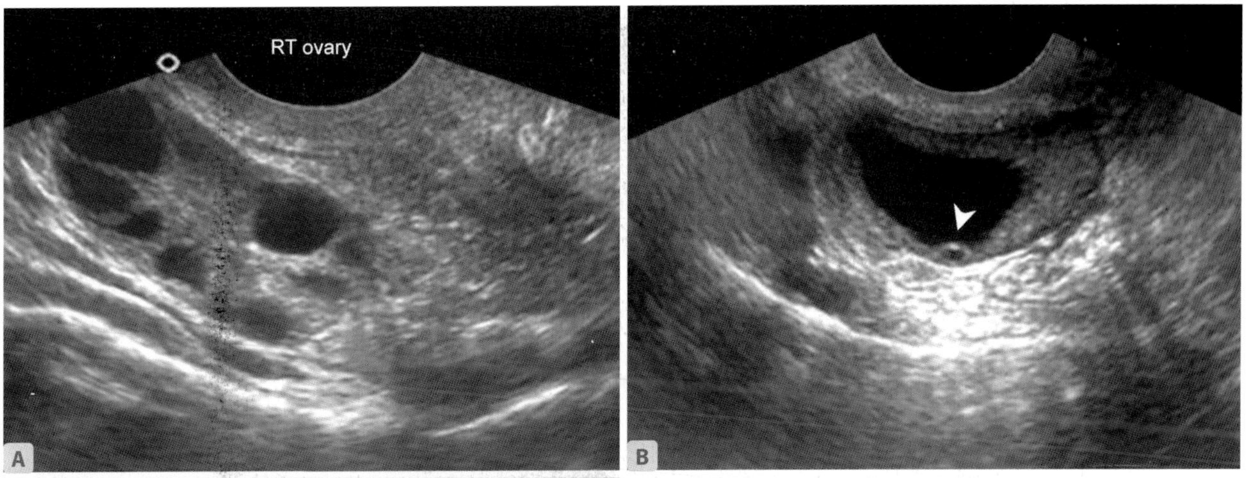

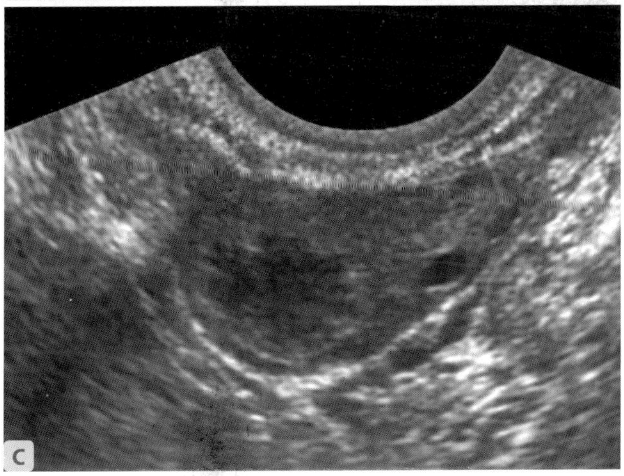

FIGS. 17A TO C: Normal ovary—transvaginal scans. (A) Ovary in proliferative phase showing multiple small follicles; (B) Dominant follicle with cumulus oophorus (arrowhead) seen just prior to ovulation; (C) Corpus luteum seen as a small hypoechoic area with crenated margins within the ovary.

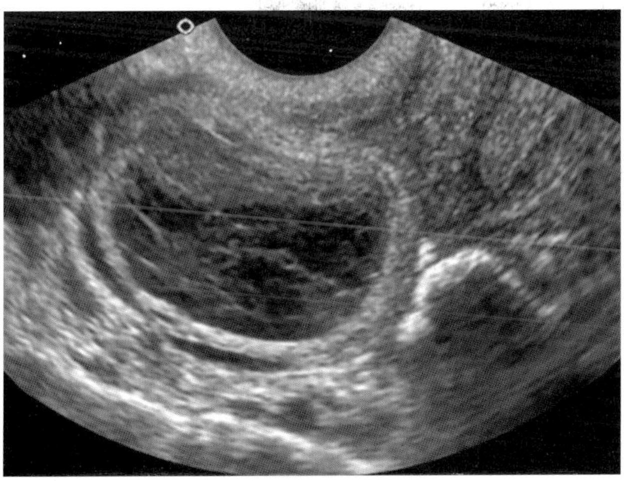

FIG. 18: Hemorrhagic corpus luteum cyst. Characteristic reticular pattern of internal echoes seen within the cyst.

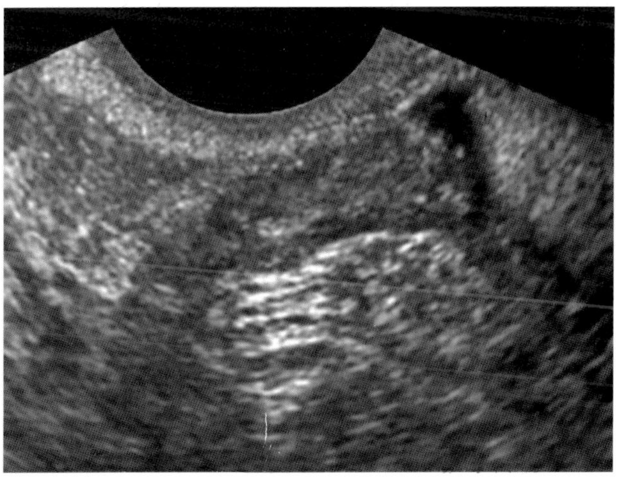

FIG. 19: Postmenopausal ovary. Small in size with no follicles, often difficult to identify.

menstrual cycle is that perfusion increases in response to rising plasma estrogen and progesterone and decreases with periovulatory fall in estrogen. The typical spectral waveform shows a high resistance pattern characterized by high flow velocity with an early diastolic notch **(Figs. 20A to C)**.

The *ovarian arteries* arise from the abdominal aorta and enter the pelvis through the infundibulopelvic ligament. They reach the ovaries through the hila via the mesovarium. After supplying the ovary, terminal branches anastomose with branches of the uterine artery. The ovarian arteries are more

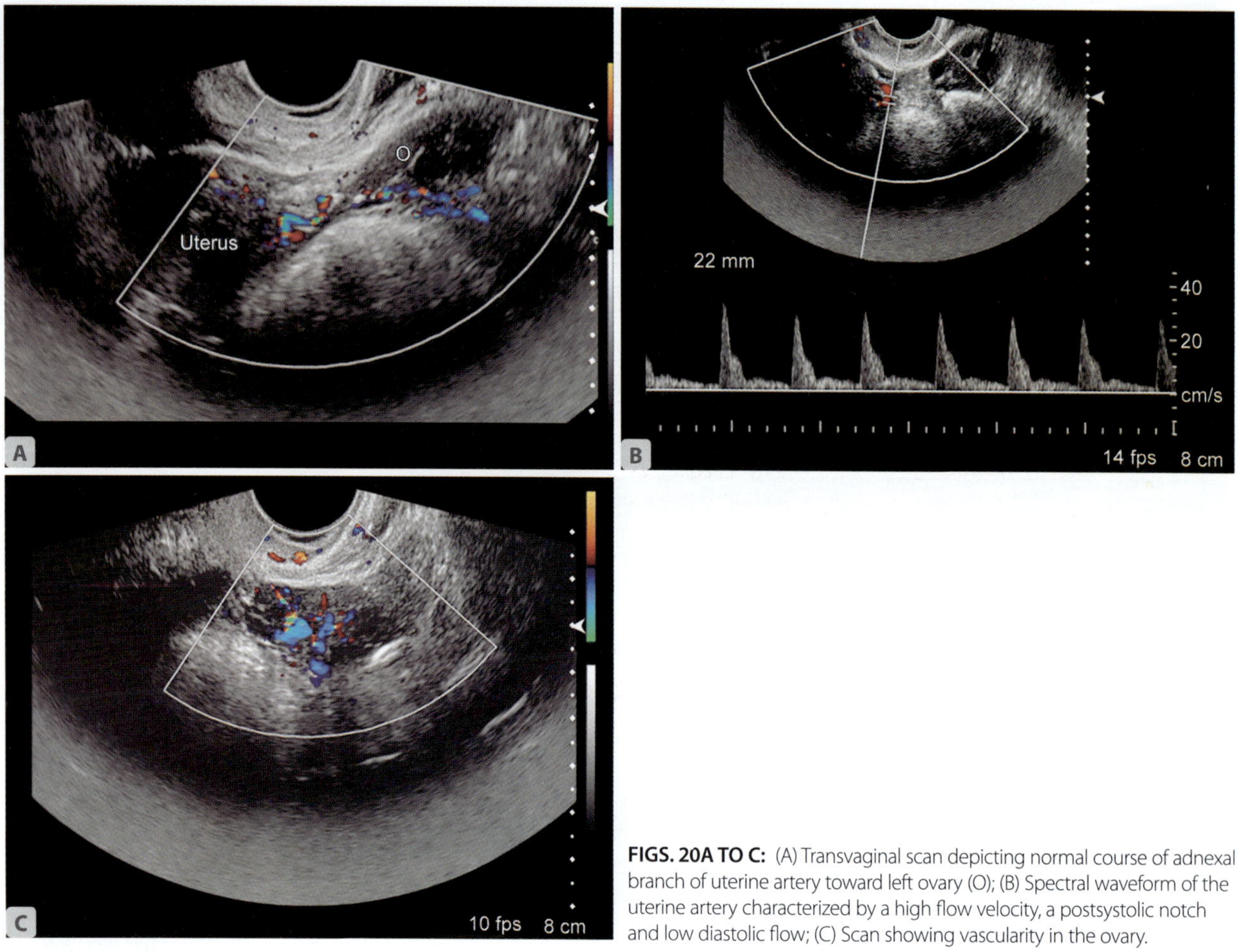

FIGS. 20A TO C: (A) Transvaginal scan depicting normal course of adnexal branch of uterine artery toward left ovary (O); (B) Spectral waveform of the uterine artery characterized by a high flow velocity, a postsystolic notch and low diastolic flow; (C) Scan showing vascularity in the ovary.

difficult to assess as they run a transverse course through the pelvis. The ovarian arterial supply also exhibits different flow characteristics during different phases of a normal menstrual cycle. In general, the index value is high during the early follicular phase which progressively decreases till the early luteal phase and then rises again in the late luteal phase **(Table 4)**.[46] Differences in flow characteristics may also be seen between the dominant and nondominant ovaries. In the ovary containing the dominant follicle, continuous diastolic flow may be seen by the early luteal phase. In contrast, both diastolic flow and cyclical changes may be absent in the nondominant ovary.

Doppler ultrasound can demonstrate neovascularity within the wall of the corpus luteum. Demonstrable color flow surrounding the developing dominant follicle becomes more apparent as the midcycle approaches and continues around the corpus luteum until the late luteal phase. In the event of pregnancy, both the low resistance flow and the color flow to the corpus luteum may remain until the 11th week of amenorrhea.[45]

The normal values are given in **Table 4**.

TABLE 4: Variation in Doppler indices in the uterine and ovarian arteries.

Phase	RI OVA	PI OVA	PI UTA
Early proliferative	0.65–0.7	1.8–2.2	1.67 ± 0.22
Late proliferative	0.55–0.6	1.0–1.3	1.89 ± 0.4
Luteal	0.6–0.65	1.3–1.8	1.23 ± 0.67
Postmenopausal	0.6–1.0	1.3–4.0	1.8–3.8

(RI: resistance index; PI: pulsatility index; OVA: ovarian artery; UTA: uterine artery)

CONCLUSION

Rapid advancements have been made in the radiologic evaluation of patients with gynecological disorders. Ultrasound forms the first line imaging modality. CT and MRI techniques have become essential tools for problem solving and in guiding presurgical treatment planning. Imaging techniques providing insights into the molecular processes in the tumor environment are gaining importance and their use is likely to expand in future.

REFERENCES

1. Langer JE, Oliver ER, Lev-Toaff AS, et al. Imaging of the female pelvis throughout the life cycle. Radiographics. 2012;32:636-9.
2. Lingley JR. The significance of psammoma body calcification in the roentgen diagnosis of papillary tumors of the ovary. Am J Roentgenol. 1942;47:563-70.
3. Sutton D. Textbook of Radiology and Imaging. 7th edition, Volume 2. Churchill Livingstone; 2003. pp. 1069-107.
4. Simpson WL Jr, Beitia LG, Mester J. Hysterosalpingography: a reemerging study. Radiographics. 2006;26(2):419-31.
5. Panchal S, Nagori C. Imaging techniques for assessment of tubal status. J Hum Reprod Sci 2014;7:2-12.
6. Kurjak A, Kupesic-Urek S, Schulman H, et al. Transvaginal color Doppler in the assessment of ovarian and uterine blood flow in infertile women. Fertil Steril. 1991;56:870-3.
7. Guerriero S, Ajossa S, Risalvato A, et al. Diagnosis of adnexal malignancies by using color Doppler energy imaging as a secondary test in persistent masses. Ultrasound Obstet Gynecol. 1998;11:277-82.
8. Sibal M. Gel sonovaginography: a new way of evaluating a variety of local vaginal and cervical disorders. J Ultrasound Med. 2016;35(12):2699-715.
9. Pretorirus DH, Borok NN, Coffler MS, et al. Three dimensional sonography in obstetrics and gynaecology, RCNA. 2001;39(3): 499-521.
10. Richman TS, Viscomi GN, deCherney A, et al. Fallopian tube patency as assessed by ultrasonogram following fluid injection. Radiology. 1984;152:507-10.
11. Lindheim SR, Sprague C, Winter TC 3rd. Hysterosalpingography and sonohysterography: lessons in technique. AJR Am J Roentgenol. 2006;186(1):24-9.
12. Deichert U, Schlief R, van de Sandt M, et al. Transvaginal hysterosalpino-contrast-sonography (Hy-Co-Sy) compared with conventional tubal diagnostics. Hum Reprod. 1989;4:418-24.
13. Zhou L, Zhang X, Chen X, et al. Value of three-dimensional hysterosalpingocontrast sonography with SonoVue in the assessment of tubal patency. Ultrasound Obstet Gynecol. 2012;40:93-9.
14. Wang Y, Qian L. Three- or four-dimensional hysterosalpingocontrast sonography for diagnosing tubal patency in infertile females: A systematic review with meta-analysis. Br J Radiol. 2016;89:20151013.
15. Henrich W, Fuchs I, Schmider A. Transvaginal and transabdominal extended field of view (EFOV) and power Doppler EFOV sonography in gynecology: advantages and applications. J Ultrasound Med. 2002;21:1137-44.
16. Ophir J, Céspedes I, Ponnekanti H, et al. Elastography: A quantitative method for imaging the elasticity of biological tissues. Ultrason Imaging. 1991;13(2):111-34.
17. Stoelinga B, Hehenkamp WJK, Nieuwenhuis LL, et al. Accuracy and reproducibility of sonoelastography for the assessment of fibroids and adenomyosis, with magnetic resonance imaging as reference standard. Ultrasound Med Biol. 2018;44:1654-63.
18. Frank ML, Schafer SD, Mollers M, et al. Importance of transvaginal elastography in the diagnosis of uterine fibroids and adenomyosis. Ultraschall Med. 2016;37:373-8.
19. Thomas A, Kümmel S, Gemeinhardt O, et al. Real-time sonoelastography of the cervix: tissue elasticity of the normal and abnormal cervix. Acad Radiol. 2007;14:193-200.
20. Burns PN. Microbubble Contrast for Ultrasound Imaging: Where, How and Why in Rumack CM, Wilson SR, Charboneau JW (Eds). Diagnostic ultrasound, 3rd edition. Maryland Heights: Elseiver Mosby; 2001. pp. 55-76.
21. Stoelinga B, Dooper AMC, Juffermans LJM, et al. Use of contrast-enhanced ultrasound in the assessment of uterine fibroids: a feasibility study. Ultrasound in Medicine and Biology. 2018;44(8):1901-9.
22. Haaga JR, Boll DT. CT and MRI of the Whole Body. 6th edition. Philadelphia, PA: Elsevier, 2017.
23. Thomassin-Naggara I, Balvay D, Rockall A, et al. Added value of assessing adnexal masses with advanced MRI techniques. Biomed Res Int. 2015;2015:785206.
24. Liu B, Gao S, Li S. A comprehensive comparison of CT, MRI, positron emission tomography or positron emission tomography/CT, and diffusion weighted imaging-MRI for detecting the lymph nodes metastases in patients with cervical cancer: a meta-analysis based on 67 studies. Gynecol Obstet Invest. 2017;82:209Y222.
25. Manoharan D, Das CJ, Aggarwal A, et al. Diffusion weighted imaging in gynecological malignancies—present and future. World J Radiol. 2016;8:288-97.
26. Makino H, Kato H, Furui T, et al. Predictive value of diffusion-weighted magnetic resonance imaging during chemoradiotherapy for uterine cervical cancer. J Obstet Gynaecol Res. 2014;40:1098-104.
27. Fujii S, Matsusue E, Kanasaki Y, et al. Detection of peritoneal dissemination in gynecological malignancy: evaluation by diffusion- weighted MR imaging. Eur Radiol. 2008;18:18-23.
28. Hallac RR, Ding Y, Yuan Q, et al. Oxygenation in cervical cancer and normal uterine cervix assessed using blood oxygenation level-dependent (BOLD) MRI at 3T. NMR Biomed. 2012;25: 1321-30.
29. Zijta FM, Lakeman MME, Froeling M, et al. Evaluation of the female pelvic floor in pelvic organ prolapse using 3.0-Tesla diffusion tensor imaging and fibre tractography. Eur Radiol. 2012;22:2806-13.
30. Colaiacomo MC, Masselli G, Polettini E, et al. Dynamic MR imaging of the pelvic floor: a pictorial review. Radiographics. 2009;29:e35.
31. Narayanan P, Iyngkaran T, Sohaib SA, et al. Pearls and pitfalls of MR lymphography in gynecologic malignancy. Radiographics. 2009;29:1057-69.
32. Ma FH, Qiang JW, Cai SQ, et al. MR spectroscopy for differentiating benign from malignant solid adnexal tumors. Am J Roentgenol. 2015;204;W724-30.
33. Iyer VR, Lee SI. MRI, CT, and PET/CT for ovarian cancer detection and adnexal lesion characterization. Am J Roentgenol. 2010;194(2):311-21.
34. Rockall AG, Cross S, Flanagan S, et al. The role of FDG-PET/CT in gynaecological cancers. Cancer Imaging. 2012;12:49-65.
35. Ohliger MA, Hope TA, Chapman JS, et al. PET/MR imaging in gynecologic oncology. Magn Reson Imaging Clin N Am. 2017;25(3):667-84.
36. Siegel MJ. Pediatric gynaecologic sonography. Radiology. 1991;170:593-600.
37. Salem S, Wilson SR. Gynaecologic ultrasound. In: Rumack CM, Wilson SR, Charboneau JW (Eds). Diagnostic Ultrasound, 3rd edition. Maryland Heights: Elsevier Mosby; 2001. pp. 527-87.
38. Coleman BG, Arger PH, Grumbach K, et al. Transvaginal and transabdominal sonography: prospective comparison. Radiology. 1988;168:639-43.
39. Burks DD, Stainken BF, Burkhard TK, et al. Uterine inner myometrial echogenic foci: relationship to prior dilatation and curettage and endocervical biopsy. J Ultrasound Med. 1991;10:487-92.
40. Aubel S, Wozney P, Edward RP. MRI of female uterine and juxta-uterine masses: clinical application in 25 patients. Magn Reson Imaging. 1991;9:485-91.

41. Schoenfield A, Levavi H, Hirsch M, et al. Transvaginal sonography in postmenopausal women. J Clin Ultrasound. 1990;18: 350-58.
42. Forrest TS, Elyaderani MK, Muilenburg MI, et al. Cyclic endometrial changes: US assessment with histologic correlation. Radiology. 1988;167:233-7.
43. Laing FC, Brown DL, DiSalvo DN, et al. Gynecologic ultrasound. RCNA. 2001;39(3):523-40.
44. Wolf SI, Gosink BB, Feldesman MR, et al. Prevalence of simple adnexal cysts in postmenopausal women. Radiology. 1991;180:65-71.
45. Applebaum M. in The menstrual cycle, menopause, ovulation induction, and in vitro fertilization. In: Copel JA, Reed KL (Eds). Doppler Ultrasound in Obstetrics and Gynecology. New York: Raven Press; 1994.pp. 71-86.
46. Dubbins PA. The female pelvis. In: Allan PL, Dubbins PA, Pozniak MA, et al. (Eds). Clinical Doppler Ultrasound. London: Churchill Livingstone; 2000. pp. 237-58.

CHAPTER

14

Benign Adnexal Disease

Anju Garg, Alpana Manchanda, Radhika Batra

INTRODUCTION

The adnexa is the region adjacent to the uterus that includes the ovary, fallopian tube, and associated structures. Pathology in this region can arise from the ovary, the fallopian tube, from adjacent organs like the uterus and less commonly from other nongynecological structures like bowel, connective tissues, etc. Benign adnexal lesions are far more common than malignant lesions and thus an accurate characterization of adnexal disease is essential for management. Imaging is an essential part of the diagnostic workup to establish the presence, identify the organ of origin, and characterize the nature of lesions in the adnexal region. This chapter deals with imaging of adnexal disease from gynecological causes.

OVARIAN DISEASE

As most of the pathological conditions of the ovary present in the form of masses, the first step after detection of a mass lesion in the adnexal region is to identify if it arises from the ovary. This can be achieved by identifying both the ovaries, seeing whether they look normal and then looking at their relation to the pathological findings. A mass arising from the ovary will deform the ovary and alter its normal shape. A positive "*beak sign*" can be identified when a mass deforms the edge of the ovary into a "beak" shape, suggesting that the mass arises from it; while an adjacent ovary with dull edges suggests that the mass compresses it but does not arise from the ovary **(Fig. 1)**. The "crescent sign" or "embedded organ sign" shows the ovarian tissue splayed around a mass which arises from the ovary. Another sign which can be used to identify a mass as of ovarian origin is to trace the ovarian vessels, especially the ovarian vein. The ovarian vein is easily identified as it lies anterior to the psoas muscle and can be followed up to the pelvic mass—the *"vascular pedicle sign"*. In a study by Lee et al., this CT finding was found to indicate that a mass was of ovarian origin, with a 91% diagnostic accuracy, 97% positive predictive value, and 69% negative predictive value.[1] The direction of displacement of other pelvic structures by the mass can also give a clue to the origin of the mass.

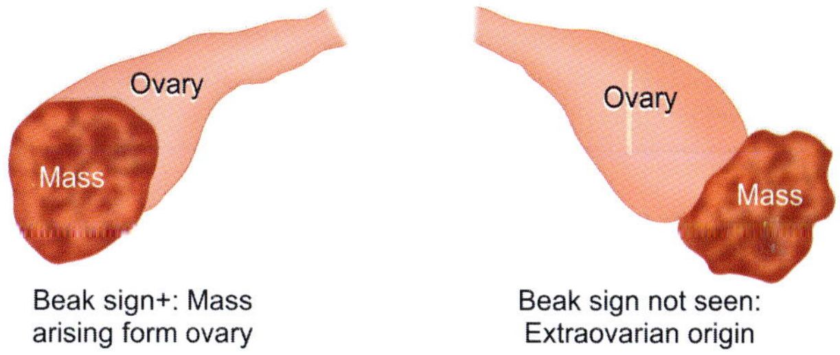

FIG. 1: Ovarian versus extraovarian origin—look at the ovary-mass interface.

The ureter is often displaced posteriorly or posterolaterally by an ovarian mass, whereas the iliac vessels are pushed laterally.

FUNCTIONAL CYSTS OF THE OVARY

Functional cysts comprise the most common benign cystic lesions of the ovary. They are formed when Graafian follicles or corpora lutea grow too large or bleed internally. They can be of three types—follicular cysts, corpus luteum cysts, and hemorrhagic cysts. Majority of these cysts are seen during the premenopausal reproductive age, however, sporadic ovulatory cycles may still occur in the postmenopausal women with occasional formation of functional cysts. Even in late menopause, 20% of women may have small simple cysts. In a study by Modesitt et al., in 3529 simple ovarian cysts of less than 10 cm, no cancers were detected in postmenopausal women. The authors estimated the risk of malignancy in simple cysts as less than 0.1%.[2]

Follicular Cyst

A follicular cyst occurs when a dominant Graafian follicle does not ovulate or fails to involute. When it becomes larger than 3 cm, it is called a follicular cyst. Most follicle cysts lose the ability to produce estrogen, however, sometimes the granulosa cells remain productive, with prolonged secretion of estrogen.

Clinical Features

Most cysts are asymptomatic and discovered incidentally. However, some patients may develop pain because of rapid enlargement of the cyst, rupture, or hemorrhage.

Imaging Features

On ultrasound (US), follicular cysts are seen as unilateral, unilocular, anechoic cysts with thin (<3 mm), smooth walls, often measuring between 3 cm and 8 cm in size. Occasionally, they may become larger.[3] A compressed rim of ovarian tissue can often be visualized around the periphery of the cyst **(Figs. 2A and B)**. They generally do not show any septations or solid components. On CT, they appear as well-defined round simple fluid collections with thin nonenhancing walls, with an attenuation generally less than 15 HU.[4] On magnetic resonance imaging (MRI), these cysts are typically homogeneously hypointense on T1-weighted image (T1WI), very high signal intensity (SI) on T2W images. Follicular cysts usually resolve spontaneously after 1–2 menstrual cycles. A follow-up US should be done on days 5–10 of a subsequent menstrual cycle to look for resolution.

Differential Diagnosis

The differential diagnosis of follicular cysts include nonfunctional cysts and cystic neoplasms like benign teratoma and simple benign epithelial neoplasms which are seen in an older age group, are larger and persistent, atypical endometrioma, and hydrosalpinx. Nonfunctional cysts include surface epithelial inclusion cysts, rete cysts, and paraovarian or paratubal cysts. Paraovarian cysts are indistinguishable from functional cysts by imaging criteria except by location. A diagnosis of paraovarian cyst can be made when the ipsilateral ovary is seen close to but separate from the cyst.

Corpus Luteum Cyst

Corpus luteum cysts form when a corpus luteum fails to regress following the release of an ovum, filling up with fluid or blood. They occur in the postovulatory phase of the menstrual cycle and grow under the influence of the luteinizing hormone. They are usually less than 2 cm in size and resolve within 1–2 menstrual cycles. Corpus luteum cysts can also occur in pregnancy, which grow under the influence of beta-human chorionic gonadotropin (β-hCG), are much larger (3–4 cm, can reach up to 15 cm), usually resolve by 12–16 weeks but may fail to involute and persist after the first trimester.

Clinical Features

These cysts are also most commonly seen in the reproductive age group. Women on birth control pills usually do not form a corpus luteum, as birth control pills prevent ovulation, and so will not have corpus luteum cysts; whereas women who are on ovulation stimulating drugs, like clomifene, have an increased incidence of corpus luteum cysts. They constitute the most common pelvic mass encountered within the first trimester of pregnancy and large cysts may present with pain.

Imaging Features

On US, they are seen as small, <3 cm sized cysts with thick, crenated margins, internal echoes, and good through transmission **(Figs. 3A to C)**. The contents are usually hyperechoic and represent some bleeding into the follicle that has ovulated. A higher fat content of the cyst wall is a likely cause for the hyperechogenic wall of the corpus luteal cyst.[3] Doppler shows peripheral vascularity—the characteristic "ring of fire" sign **(Fig. 3D)**. They need to be differentiated from a tubal ring in an ectopic pregnancy in some situations, and correct clinical interpretation is required. CT will show an irregular, low-attenuating cyst (<25 HU), with enhancing walls.[4] On MRI, these cysts are typically homogeneously hypointense on T1WI, very high SI on T2W images, and show intense wall enhancement on postcontrast scans **(Fig. 4)**. A small amount of free fluid is often seen to be associated with these cysts.

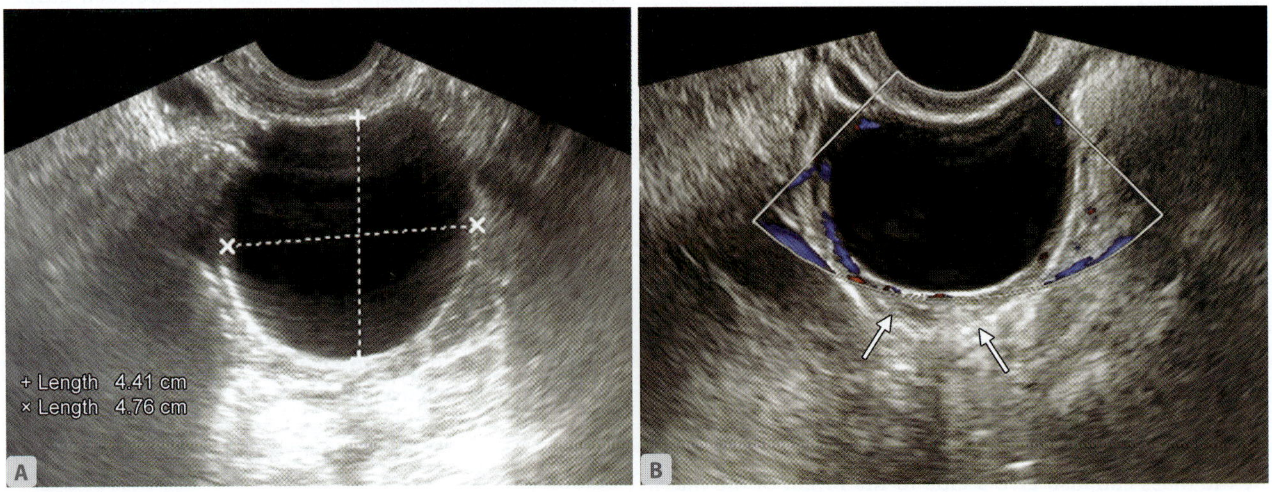

FIGS. 2A AND B: Simple follicular cyst. (A) Transvaginal scan shows a unilocular, rounded, thin-walled, anechoic cyst in the right ovary; (B) Color Doppler shows mild perifollicular color flow. Compressed ovarian rim—"crescent sign" (arrows) seen in posterior aspect of the cyst.

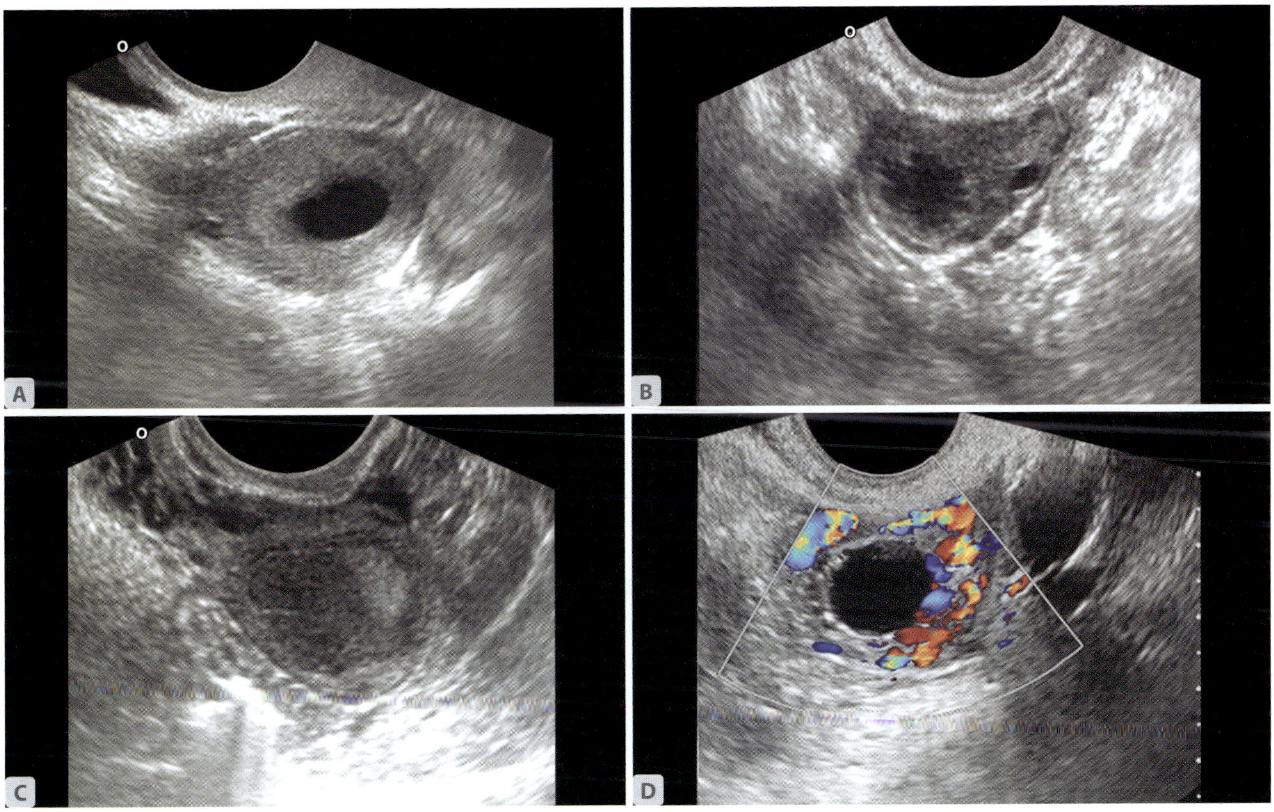

FIGS. 3A TO D: Varied appearances of corpus luteum cysts. (A) Transvaginal scan shows an anechoic corpus luteum cyst with thick echogenic walls. Ovarian tissue with follicles seen surrounding the cyst; (B) Transvaginal scan in another case shows the crenulated margins in a corpus luteum cyst with low level internal echoes; (C) Large corpus luteal cyst with differential internal echoes; (D) Peripheral vascularity seen around the corpus luteum cyst.

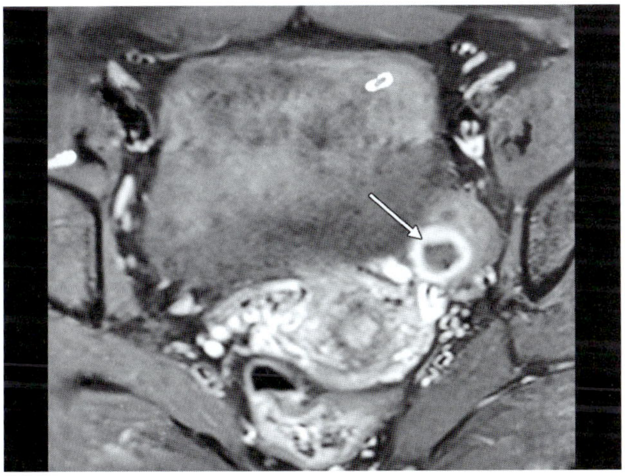

FIG. 4: Contrast-enhanced axial T1-weighted fat-suppressed MR image shows a corpus luteum cyst in the left ovary with an intensely enhancing ring (arrow).

Complications

Functional cysts may bleed leading to the formation of a hemorrhagic cyst, may rupture or cause the ovary to undergo torsion.

Hemorrhagic Ovarian Cysts

Hemorrhagic ovarian cysts (HOCs) occur due to hemorrhage into a follicle or a corpus luteum cyst. As the Graafian follicle matures, the granulosa cell layer becomes very vascular. These vessels are very fragile and rupture easily, causing bleeding into the cyst, giving rise to a hemorrhagic cyst.

Clinical Features

Patients present with sudden-onset pelvic pain, pelvic mass, or they may be asymptomatic.[5] A hemorrhagic or a ruptured ovarian cyst is the most common cause of acute pelvic pain in an afebrile, premenopausal woman presenting to the emergency room.

Imaging Features

The imaging features vary depending on the time of the radiologic evaluation, as the hemorrhagic cysts evolve through various stages of acute hemorrhage, clot formation, and clot retraction. The HOC is seen as a thin-walled cyst with an average diameter of 3.0–3.5 cm (range 2.5–8.5 cm). In the early stages, the HOC may show diffuse, low level, internal echoes (ground-glass pattern). The echogenicity decreases with time as the red cells undergo hemolysis. A whirled, spongy pattern of mixed echogenicity can be seen.

A fine reticular pattern also known variously as the "fishnet", "cobweb", "spider web" or "lacy" pattern occurs due to the fibrin strands **(Fig. 5A)**. Retracting blood clot can be seen as solid appearing, nonvascular mass within the cyst **(Fig. 5B)**. This mass may be seen to jiggle when probe pressure is applied on transvaginal scan (TVS). Sometimes a fluid-debris level may be seen within the cyst **(Fig. 5C)**. Doppler sonography helps in establishing the diagnosis as no vascularity is seen in the septae or solid nodule. On CT, HOCs are seen as unilocular cysts with a high internal attenuation of about 25–100 HU.[6] On MRI, HOCs have a characteristic appearance of blood products and the SI will vary depending on age of bleed. They are seen as intermediate or relatively high SI on T1W and intermediate to high SI on T2W images. Layering may be seen on T2W images and only mild heterogeneous signal loss will be seen as compared to T1WI, not the characteristic T2 shading of endometriomas **(Figs. 6A to E)**.

On diffusion-weighted imaging (DWI), hemorrhagic cysts may display restricted diffusion because of their blood content. HOCs can be seen to resolve spontaneously in 6–8 weeks, with follow-up US showing either complete resolution or a marked decrease in size and change in morphologic appearance **(Figs. 7A to C)**.

A hemorrhagic cyst may rupture, leading to hemoperitoneum. Patients present with acute pelvic pain. On US, the HOC can often be seen in the adnexal region along with hemoperitoneum **(Figs. 8A to E)** seen as peritoneal fluid with low-level echoes in the pouch of Douglas, Morison's pouch, or in the left upper quadrant. A close differential diagnosis is ruptured ectopic pregnancy as the clinical presentation and US imaging may be similar. A clinical history (cyst rupture occurs more often in the luteal phase, whereas ectopic pregnancy is associated with a history of delayed menstrual periods) and β-HCG levels help in differentiation.

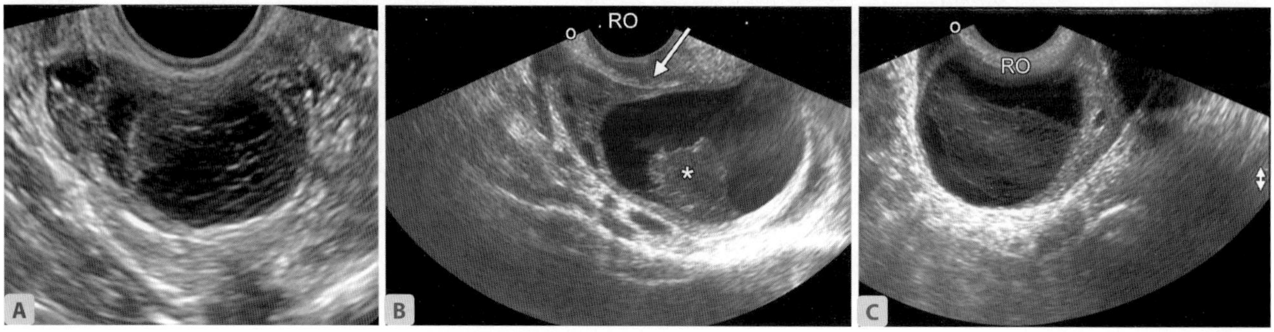

FIGS. 5A TO C: Spectrum of hemorrhagic cysts on transvaginal scan. (A) Fine reticular strands seen within the cyst—"fish net" appearance; (B) Echogenic, solid-appearing, retracted clot along dependant margin (*), did not show any vascularity on Doppler. "Beak sign" of ovarian parenchyma well seen (arrow); (C) Blood-fluid level seen in a right ovarian hemorrhagic cyst.

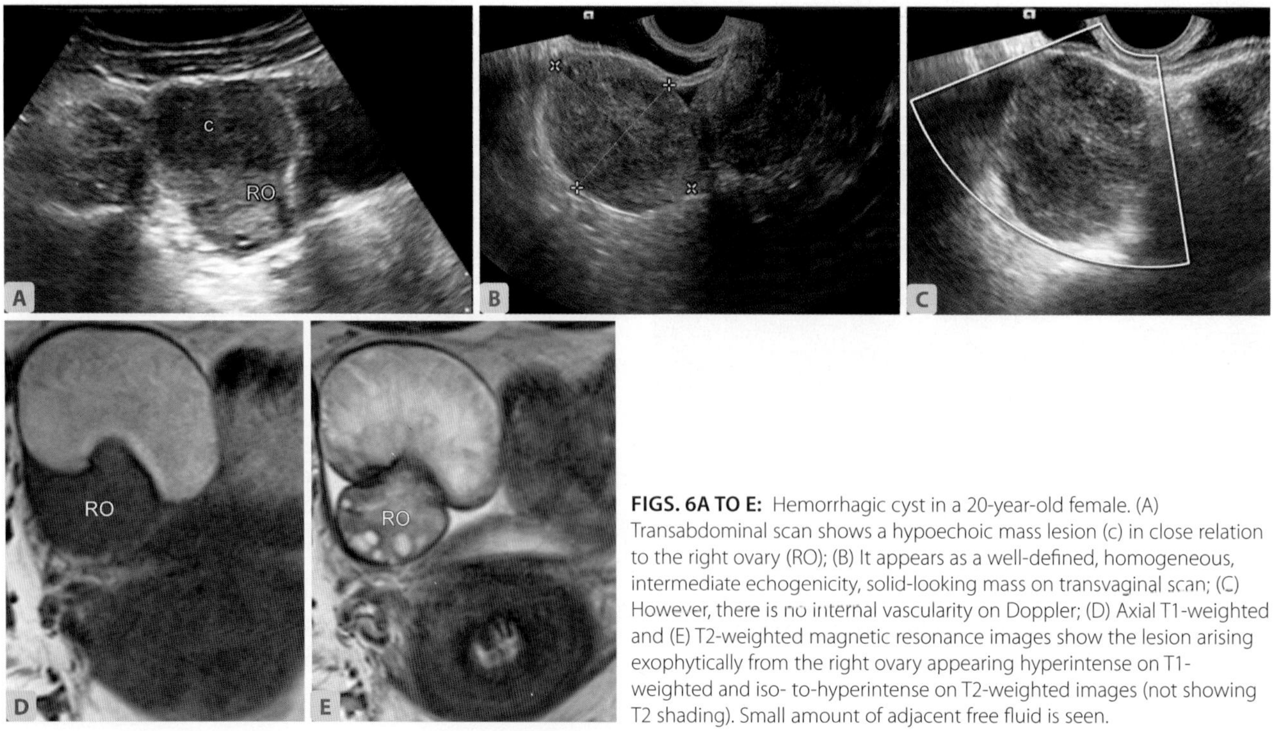

FIGS. 6A TO E: Hemorrhagic cyst in a 20-year-old female. (A) Transabdominal scan shows a hypoechoic mass lesion (c) in close relation to the right ovary (RO); (B) It appears as a well-defined, homogeneous, intermediate echogenicity, solid-looking mass on transvaginal scan; (C) However, there is no internal vascularity on Doppler; (D) Axial T1-weighted and (E) T2-weighted magnetic resonance images show the lesion arising exophytically from the right ovary appearing hyperintense on T1-weighted and iso- to-hyperintense on T2-weighted images (not showing T2 shading). Small amount of adjacent free fluid is seen.

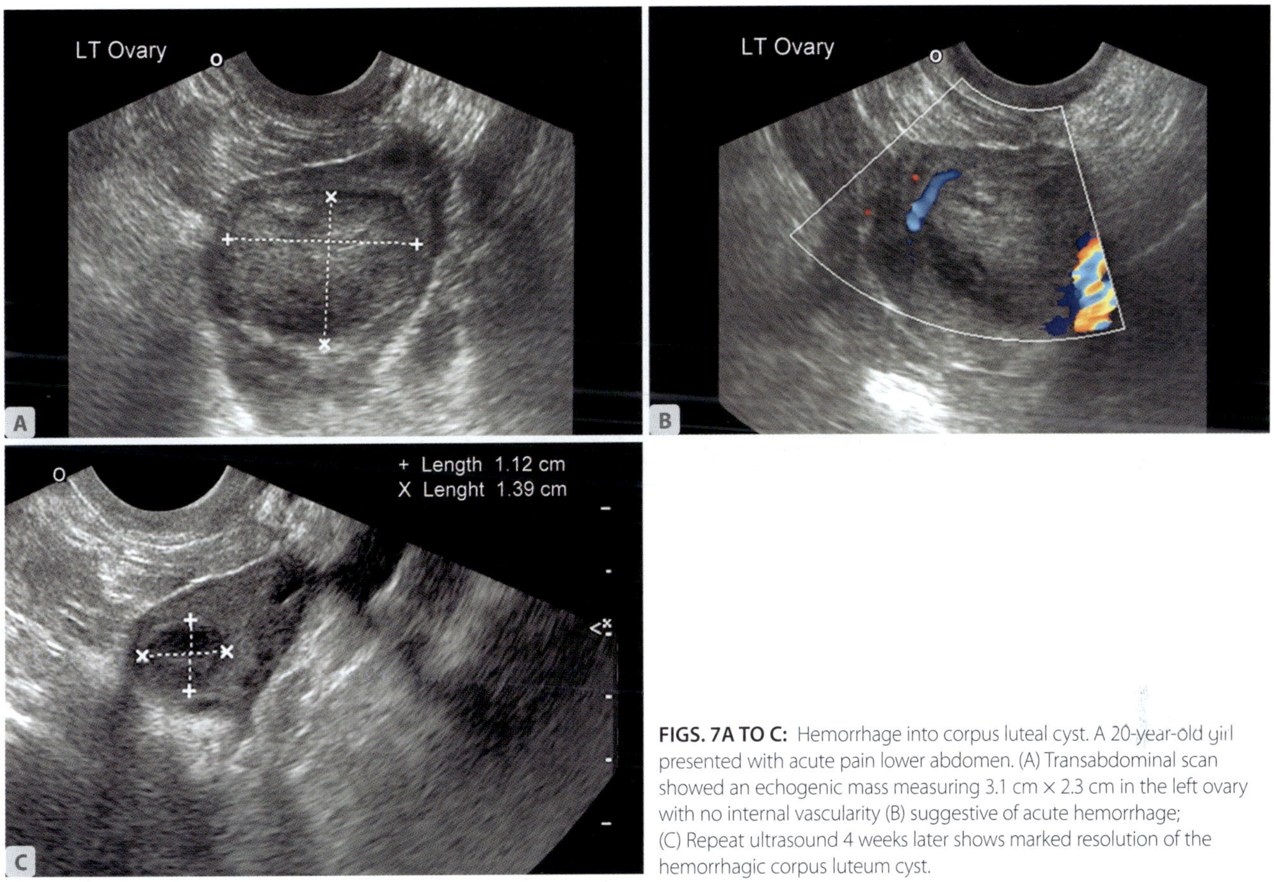

FIGS. 7A TO C: Hemorrhage into corpus luteal cyst. A 20-year-old girl presented with acute pain lower abdomen. (A) Transabdominal scan showed an echogenic mass measuring 3.1 cm × 2.3 cm in the left ovary with no internal vascularity (B) suggestive of acute hemorrhage; (C) Repeat ultrasound 4 weeks later shows marked resolution of the hemorrhagic corpus luteum cyst.

Differential Diagnosis

The most important differential diagnosis of a hemorrhagic cyst is an endometrioma, especially in the early stage. The differentiating features are discussed later in the chapter. They may also need to be differentiated from a tubo-ovarian abscess (TOA), ectopic pregnancy, and even a malignant neoplasm when a retracted solid-appearing clot resembles a malignant mural nodule. A detailed clinical history and follow-up scans which show a changing appearance, can help in clinching the diagnosis.

Follow-up Guidelines for Functional Ovarian Cysts

The most widely used guidelines for management of functional ovarian cysts imaged sonographically in asymptomatic women, are the consensus statement by the Society of Radiologists in Ultrasound 2010.[7] For simple ovarian cysts with no suspicious features on US, current follow-up guidelines are based on menopausal status, presence of any risk factors and the cyst size **(Flowchart 1)**. HOCs have a different follow-up schedule than simple cysts **(Flowchart 2)**. Patients who are symptomatic need to be managed accordingly.

Polycystic ovary syndrome (PCOS) and hyperstimulated ovarian disease have been dealt with elsewhere in this book.

ENDOMETRIOMA

Endometriomas are blood containing cysts within the ovaries formed due to endometriosis. Endometriosis is defined as presence of functional endometrial tissue (consisting of glands and stroma) outside the uterus. The common sites of involvement include ovaries (most common), uterosacral ligaments, serosal surfaces, pouch of Douglas, fallopian tubes, rectosigmoid, and urinary bladder. It is a leading cause of chronic pelvic pain and infertility in reproductive age group.

Pathophysiology

The exact etiology and pathogenesis of endometriosis is unclear and remains controversial. Three theories of pathogenesis have been proposed: (1) the *metastatic theory*, i.e. metastatic implantation of endometrial tissue from retrograde menstruation, (2) the *metaplastic theory* which is related to metaplastic differentiation of the serosal surfaces (coelomic epithelium) and remnants of Müllerian tissue, and (3) the *induction theory* which combines the first two proposed mechanisms and suggests that shed endometrium releases substances that induce undifferentiated mesenchyme to form endometrium. Circulating estradiol and estrone, which stimulate ectopic and eutopic endometrial tissue have been linked in propagation of this condition.

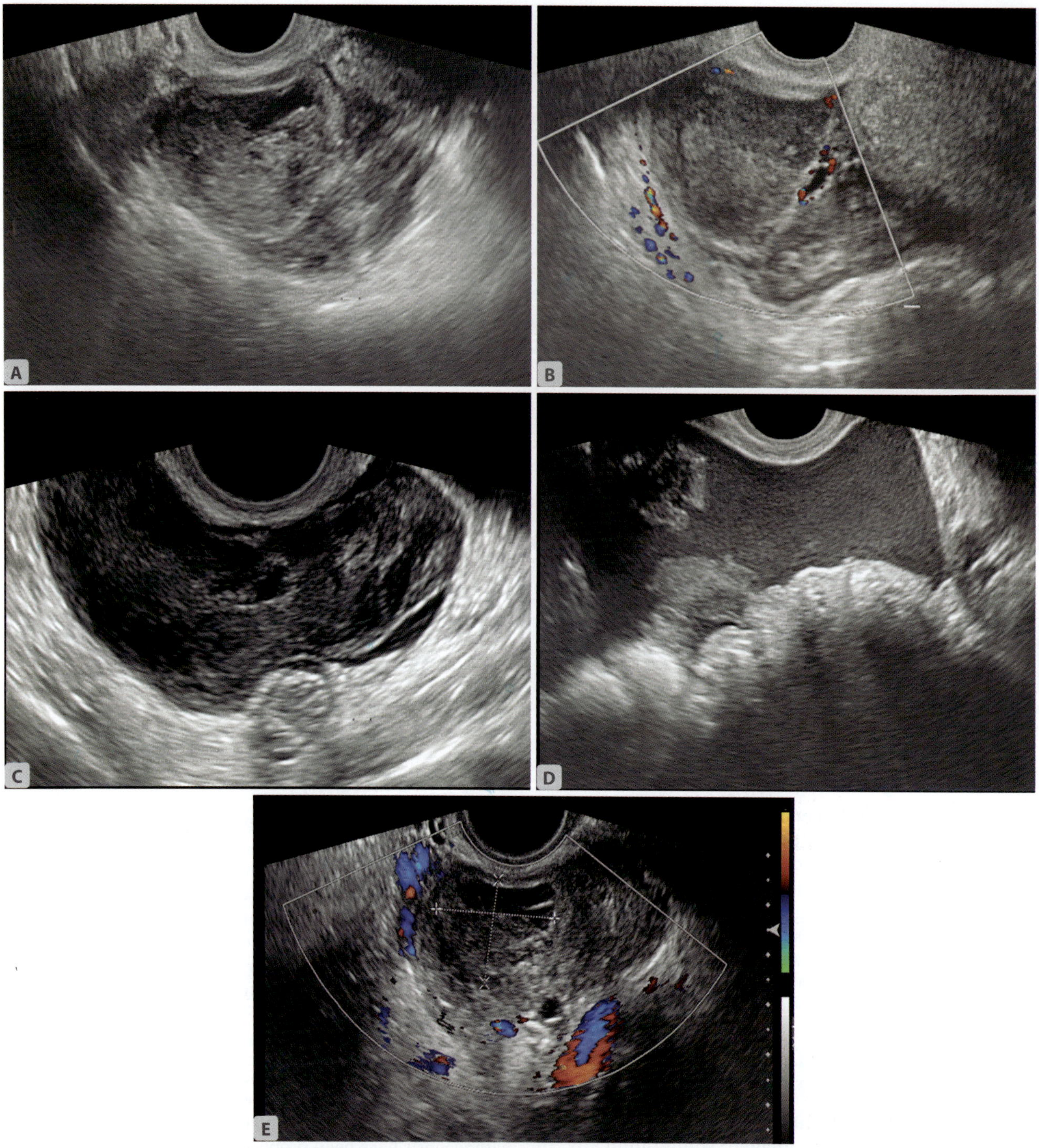

FIGS. 8A TO E: Hemorrhagic cyst in a 29-year-old female with rheumatic heart disease with mitral valve replacement and on anticoagulants. Patient presented with complaints of abdominal pain and distension since 8 days. She was premenstrual and pregnancy test was negative. Transvaginal ultrasonography (USG) reveals a well-defined heterogeneously hypoechoic lesion with hyperechoic contents within, in the right ovary. (A) showing no significant vascularity on addition of color Doppler (B). Associated pelvic hematoma (showing similar characteristics as that of hemorrhagic cyst) was also noted adjacent to the right ovary (C). Additionally, there was moderate fluid in pelvis with internal echoes within—hemoperitoneum (D). In view of above findings, a diagnosis of ruptured hemorrhagic corpus luteal cyst was suggested and patient was managed conservatively. (E) On subsequent follow-up with USG after 6 weeks, there is reduction in size of hemorrhagic cyst within the right ovary (RO) and hematoma (H) with complete resolution of hemoperitoneum. Also, note the change in morphology of hemorrhagic cyst due to evolution of the blood products within the cyst.

FLOWCHART 1: Algorithmic approach for reporting, follow-up, and management of asymptomatic ovarian cysts (Society of Radiologists in Ultrasound, 2010).[7]

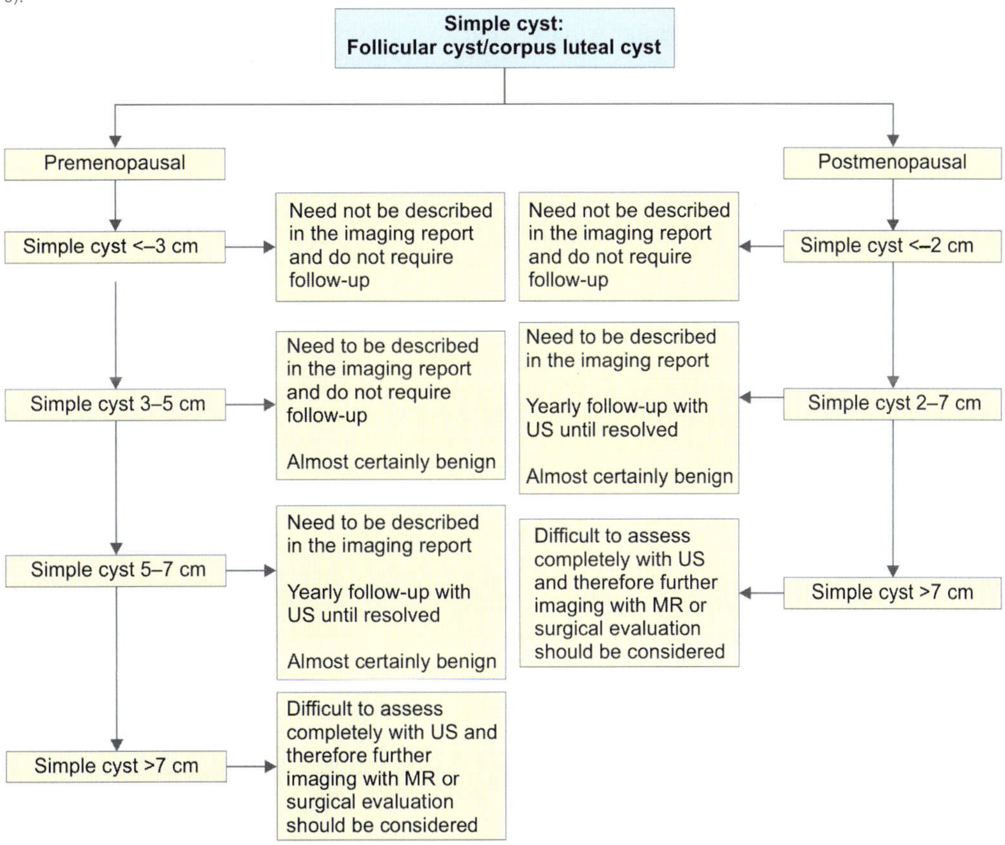

FLOWCHART 2: Algorithmic approach for reporting, follow-up, and management of asymptomatic hemorrhagic cysts (Society of Radiologists in Ultrasound, 2010).[7]

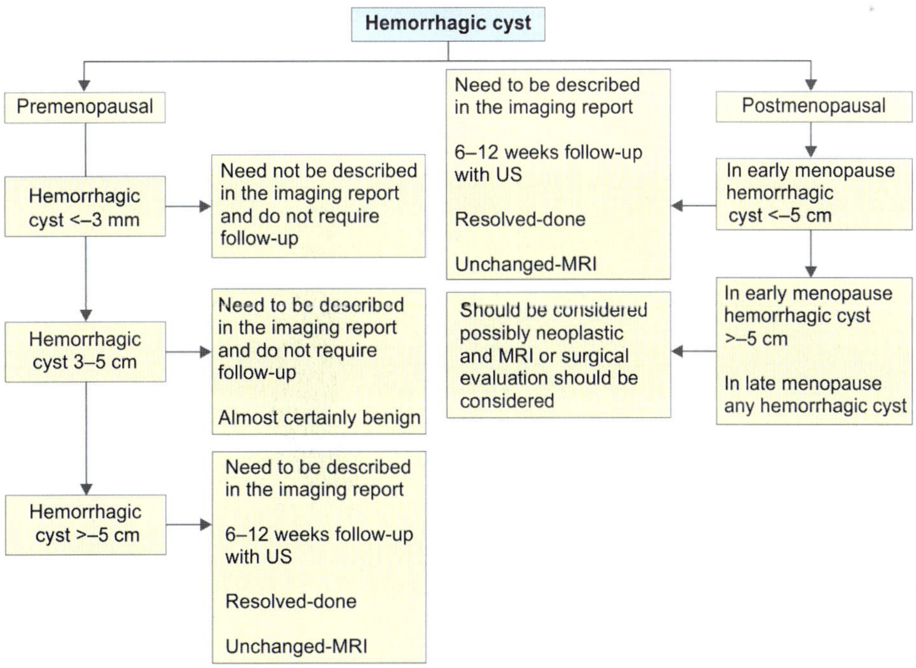

Endometriosis may present in various forms which includes endometrial nodules or plaques on the peritoneal surface, endometriotic cysts in ovaries (endometriomas), and deep infiltrative endometriosis (DIE).

Endometriomas are formed when endometrial tissue deposited in the ovaries undergoes cyclical bleeding during menstruation. With time, such repeated episodes lead to accumulation of fluid and blood products within the involved ovary with compression and peripheral displacement of rest of ovarian tissue giving rise to formation of benign chronic retention cysts or endometriomas (also known as chocolate cysts). Besides being the most common presenting form of endometriosis, they are also a marker of severity of deep infiltrating endometriosis, with the risk for multifocal and intestinal involvement in patients with endometrioma being two to three times more than those without endometrioma.[8]

Clinical Features

Patients usually present with the complaints of dysmenorrhea, dyspareunia, and chronic pelvic pain. Endometriomas are also associated with decreased ovarian function and inhibition of ovulation thus leading to infertility. In addition they can interfere with assisted reproductive technologies which are often utilized in management of infertility. In association with deep pelvic endometriosis, patients can also present with symptoms of dyschezia and dysuria. CA-125 levels (normal levels being 0–35 units/mL) are also found to be raised in patients with endometriosis but they are highly nonspecific and hence are unable to aid in diagnosis.

Imaging Features

On USG, typical endometriomas appear as well-defined, rounded, unilocular cystic lesions with regular margins which characteristically exhibit homogeneous, low level internal echoes **(Figs. 9A and B)**, and occasional fluid-fluid levels within.[9] When endometriomas are bilateral, they may be found adherent to each other above or behind the uterus, being termed as "kissing ovaries" **(Fig. 10)**. The positive predictive value of sonography in diagnosis of surgical proven typical endometriomas has been estimated to be about 97%.[10]

Endometriomas usually do not exhibit any internal vascularity on color Doppler (even if present, it is usually peripheral). As such the role of Doppler in diagnosis of endometriotic cysts has been found to be limited. A study by Alcázar et al.[11] demonstrated that the use of color or pulsed Doppler sonography did not improve the diagnostic accuracy of diagnosis of endometriomas.

Atypical forms of endometriomas, on the other hand, can have a variety of characteristics attributed to other adnexal masses thus posing a challenge for diagnosis. They may have anechoic appearance and may show irregular margins. Thin or thick septae, giving a multilocular

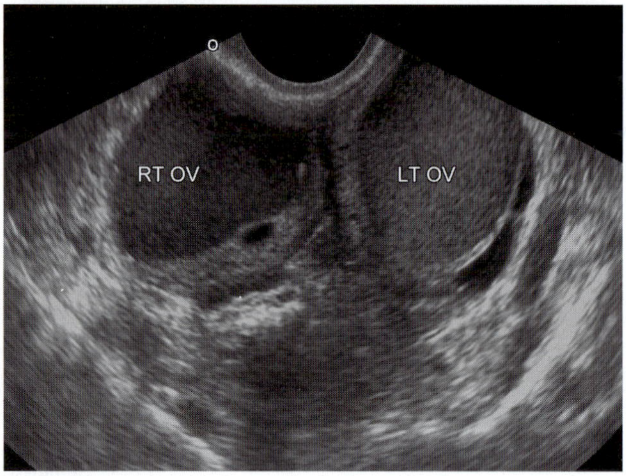

FIG. 10: Endometriomas in bilateral ovaries adherent to each other—"kissing ovaries" sign.

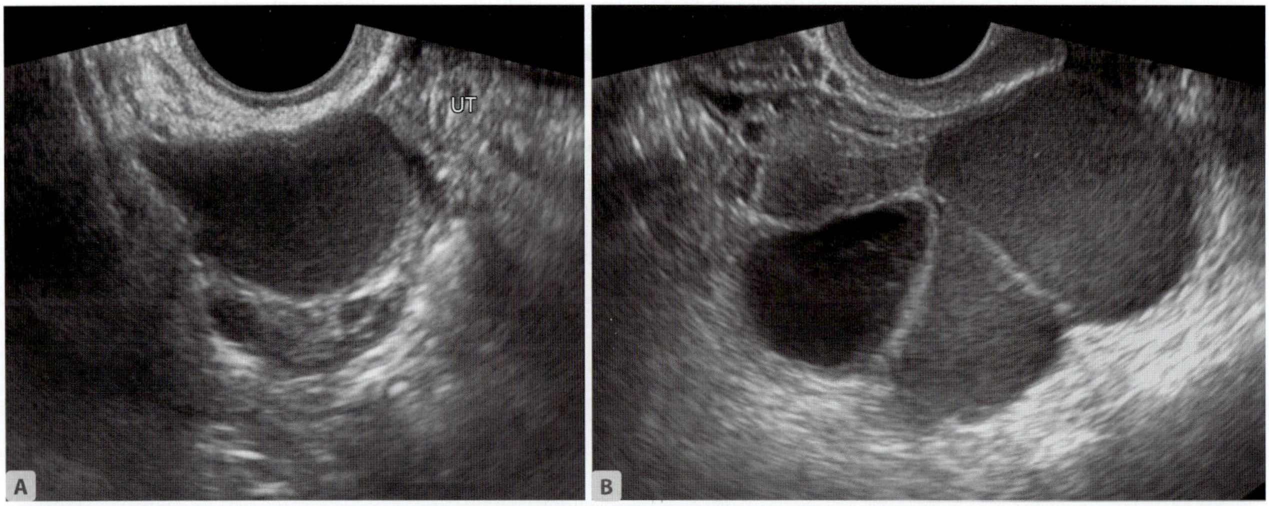

FIGS. 9A AND B: Endometriotic cysts in a 25-year-old woman with chronic pelvic pain. (A) Transvaginal scan showing the typical appearance of an endometrioma as a unilocular cyst with diffuse, low level internal echoes—"ground-glass" appearance, with a rim of normal right ovarian tissue, adherent to the uterus (UT); (B) Multiple endometriomas in the left ovary.

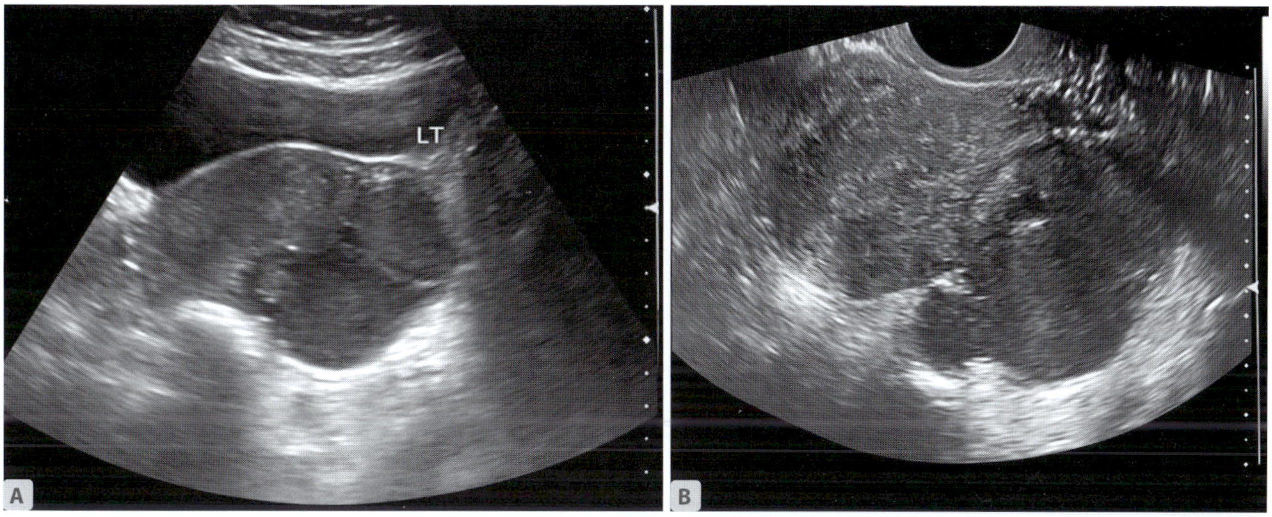

FIGS. 11A AND B: Multiloculated endometriotic cyst in a 36-year-old female. Transabdominal (A) and transvaginal (B) ultrasound images show presence of a multiloculated cystic lesion in left ovary with typical ground-glass texture.

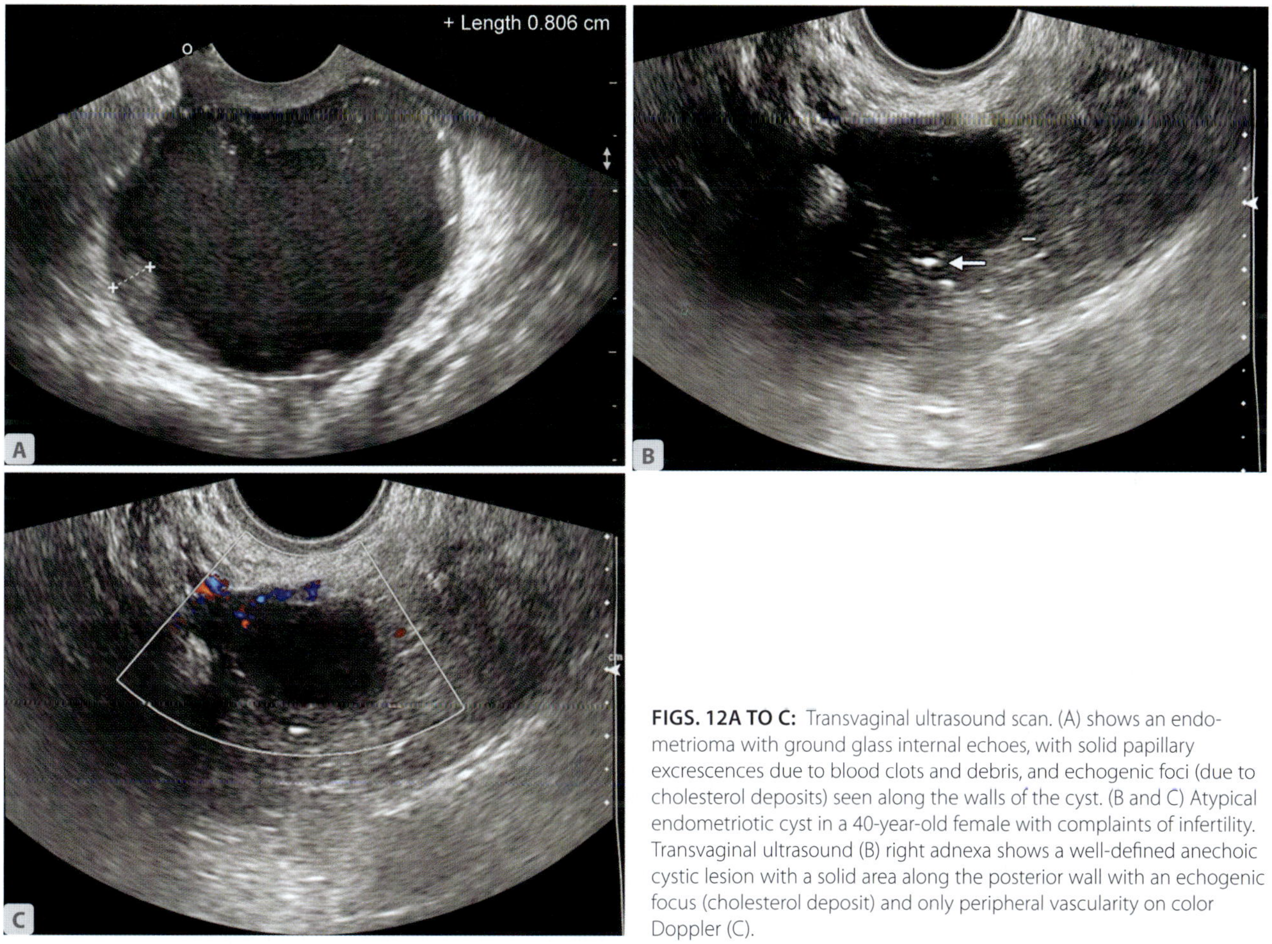

FIGS. 12A TO C: Transvaginal ultrasound scan. (A) shows an endometrioma with ground glass internal echoes, with solid papillary excrescences due to blood clots and debris, and echogenic foci (due to cholesterol deposits) seen along the walls of the cyst. (B and C) Atypical endometriotic cyst in a 40-year-old female with complaints of infertility. Transvaginal ultrasound (B) right adnexa shows a well-defined anechoic cystic lesion with a solid area along the posterior wall with an echogenic focus (cholesterol deposit) and only peripheral vascularity on color Doppler (C).

appearance **(Figs. 11A and B)** and echogenic peripheral foci (representing cholesterol deposits), may also be seen. Punctate calcifications, also seen as echogenic foci, have been described in walls of endometriomas **(Figs. 12A to C)**, they may show central calcifications which make the differentiation from teratomas difficult.

In addition, multiple solid components and papillary excrescences may be seen within thereby mimicking malignancy, however, these usually do not show vascularity on color Doppler **(Figs. 12A to C)**.

Magnetic resonance imaging is widely accepted as a highly specific imaging modality for diagnosing endometriomas due to the ability to detect aged blood. Endometriomas are characterized by blood and blood products of different ages, being particularly rich in methemoglobin. This extra- and intracellular concentration of methemoglobin results in marked T1 shortening with resultant high SI on T1W images **(Figs. 13A and B)**.[12] Additionally, this T1 shortening due to blood products persists even after addition of fat saturation and becomes much more conspicuous. Hence, use of fat-saturated T1 sequences has been recommended in imaging of endometriomas **(Fig. 13C)**. It has been found to increase the specificity and sensitivity in diagnosis especially increasing the detection rate of small endometriomas.[13]

On T2W images, endometriomas typically exhibit the characteristic "*shading sign*", being described as focal or diffuse reduction in SI due to old blood products having rich concentration of iron and proteins **(Fig. 13D)**. The wall of the endometriotic cyst is hypointense on both, T2W and T1W images, caused by hemosiderin deposition. Recently, "*T2 dark spot sign*" has been shown to be more specific than T2 shading in detecting endometriomas and differentiating them from hemorrhagic cysts.[14] These are discrete, well-defined, markedly hypointense foci seen on T2W images which can be located anywhere within the endometriotic cyst with the exception of wall of cyst **(Fig. 14)**. They are thought to occur due to long-standing accumulation of iron and protein within the lesions. Contrast-enhanced scans do not add any value to the noncontrast scans in the imaging of endometriomas **(*see* Fig. 12C)** Due to their thick proteinaceous and

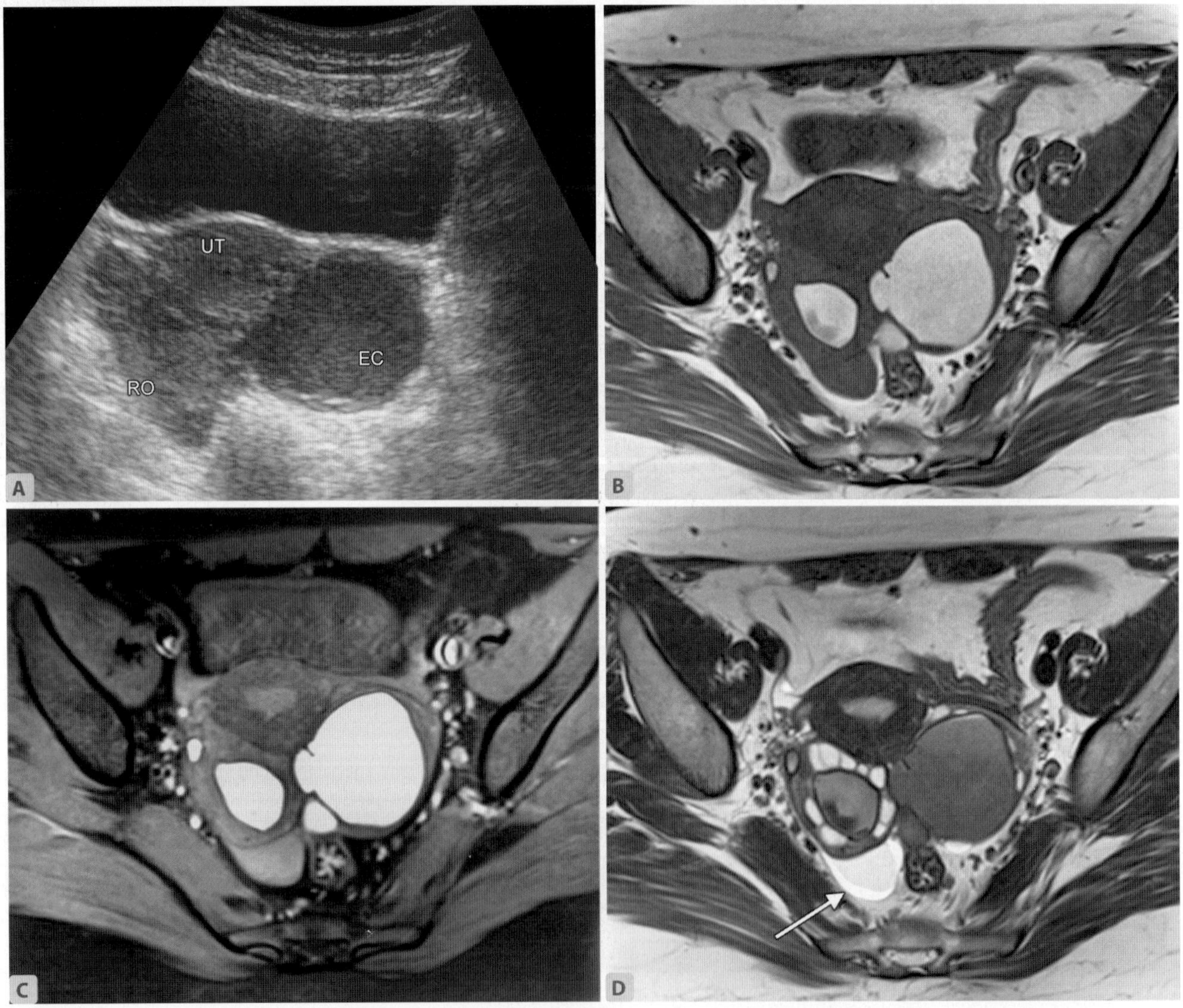

FIGS. 13A TO D: Endometriomas in a 20-year-old unmarried girl with complaints of long-standing chronic pelvic pain. (A) Transabdominal ultrasound scan shows an endometriotic cyst (EC) in the left ovary with an enlarged right ovary (RO). Both the ovaries are adherent to the uterus and to each other in the POD. Axial T1W (B) MR image shows well-defined hyperintense cystic lesions involving bilateral ovaries, which appear more hyperintense in the T1 fat-saturated image (C). They characteristically show signal drop on the axial T2W image—"shading sign" (D). In addition, both the lesions are situated in rectouterine pouch and closely abut each other in midline—"kissing ovaries". Multiple hyperintense follicles are seen in both the ovaries around the endometriomas on T2W image "embedded organ sign". The presence of loculated fluid collection is seen (arrow in D) around the right ovary appearing hyperintense on T2W image.

hemoglobin degradation products, endometriomas show a restricted diffusion pattern, exhibiting high SI on DWI at b = 1000 sec/mm^2 and low SI on apparent diffusion coefficient (ADC) maps **(Figs. 15A and B)**.[15,16]

Associations

Deep pelvic endometriosis, adenomyosis, and fibroids are found to be associated with endometriosis probably due to increased estrogen levels which are found to be increased in endometriosis.

Deep infiltrative endometriosis, which is defined as the presence of invasive endometriotic lesions that extend into the retroperitoneal space or involving the pelvic organ wall to a depth of at least 5 mm, often coexist with endometriotic cysts. These are commonly found in patients who have a long-term history of endometriosis (which may remain undiagnosed) and is responsible for symptoms like deep seated chronic pelvic pain, dysmenorrhea, dysuria, and dyschezia. Diagnosis of coexistent deep endometriotic deposits by USG/MRI is necessary for complete diagnosis and treatment. The common sites of DIE include the uterosacral ligaments, the rectosigmoid colon, the vagina, and the bladder.

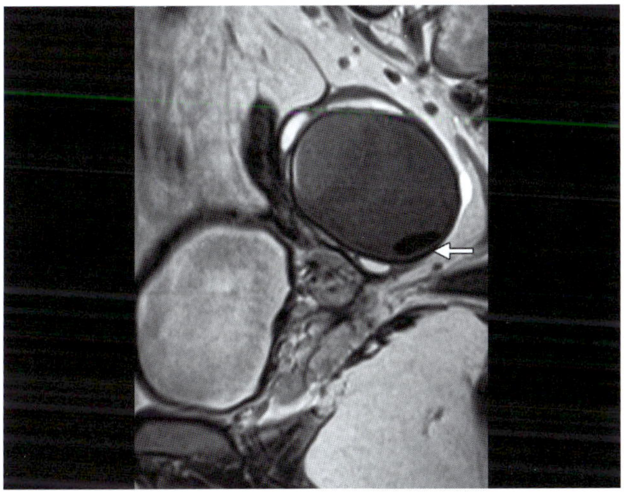

FIG. 14: Sagittal T2-weighted MR image shows the presence of a dependent hypointense focus (arrow) in left sided endometriotic cyst—*"T2 dark spot"*. This sign (although less sensitive than T2 shading sign) is highly specific for endometriotic cyst.

Recently, transvaginal sonography has been used to detect DIE of specific regions especially rectosigmoid region **(Fig. 16A)**. Sonographically, these lesions appear as solid hypoechoic masses with irregular margins involving the bowel wall which show lack of peristalsis and absent color flow. In addition, fixity of uterus and cervix with rectal wall can also be assessed with the help of sliding sign, which involves the demonstration of relative mobility of the uterus to the adjacent organs.[17]

On MRI, the diagnosis of DIE is made on a constellation of morphological and signal abnormalities. These lesions are due to fibromuscular hyperplasia surrounding ectopic endometrial glands. The regions of fibrous and smooth muscle tissue show intermediate to low SI on T1W and low SI on T2W images **(Figs. 16B and C)**. DIE may also present as soft tissue thickening involving ligaments and organ walls. Hyperintense foci on T2W images may be present representing the dilated ectopic endometrial glands. In addition, hemorrhagic foci appearing as hyperintense foci on T1W and fat-suppressed T1W images can be seen.

On CT, endometriomas have a nonspecific appearance appearing as high density cystic, or solid appearing masses with no enhancement after contrast administration. Varying degrees of adherence can be seen with the uterus, adjacent organs, and between the ovaries.

Complications

Adhesions

Endometriomas are associated with extensive adhesions leading to distortion of anatomical structures and symptoms in patients. Indirect signs of adhesions include elevation of the posterior vaginal fornix, posterior and lateral displacement of the uterus or ovaries, or both, loss of fat planes between the structures without a clear interface, hydrosalpinx or

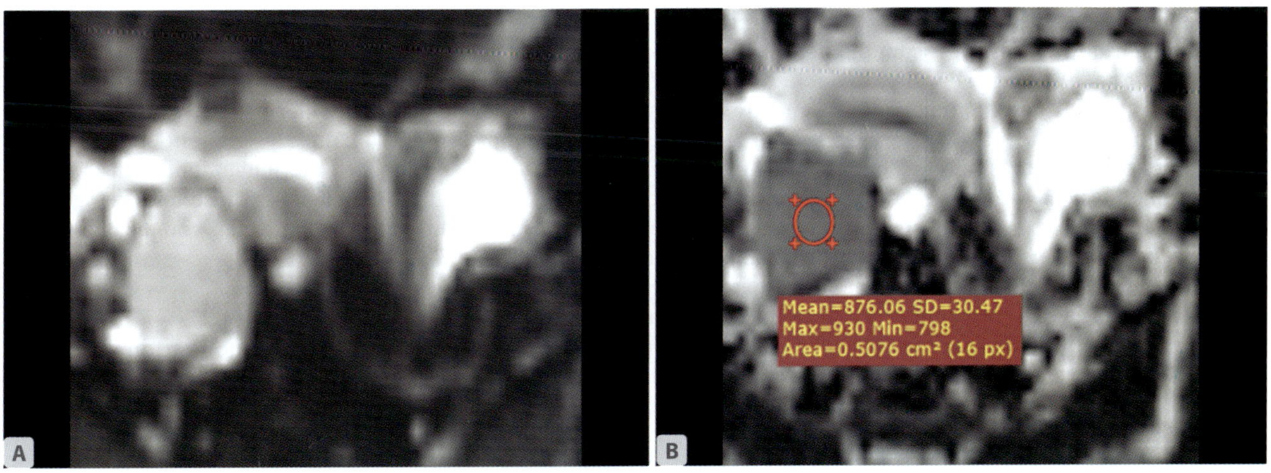

FIGS. 15A AND B: Diffusion-weighted imaging (DWI) in endometriomas. DWI (A) and corresponding apparent diffusion coefficient (ADC) map (B) demonstrating diffusion restriction (ADC value = 0.87 x 10^{-3} ± 0.03 /mm^2).

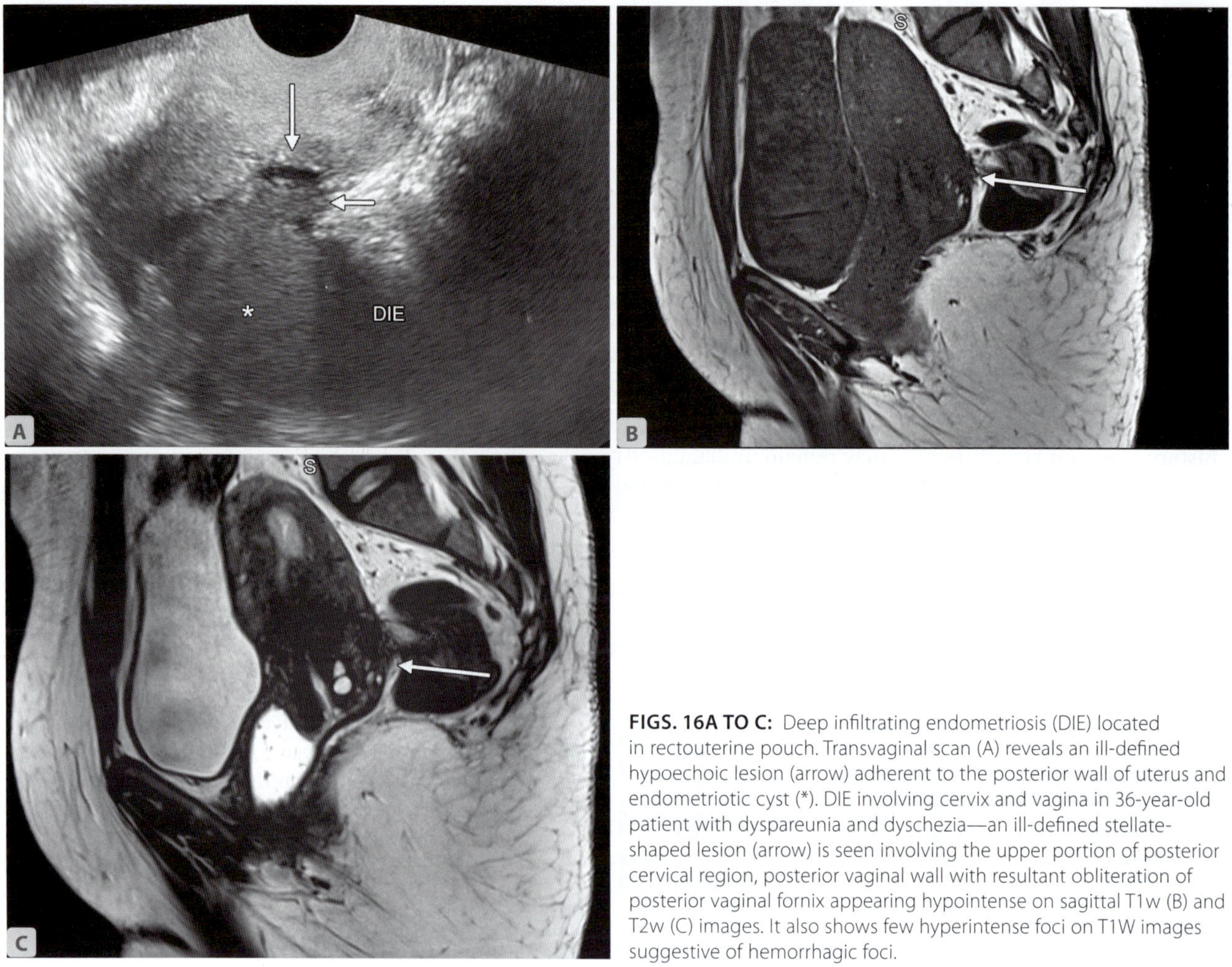

FIGS. 16A TO C: Deep infiltrating endometriosis (DIE) located in rectouterine pouch. Transvaginal scan (A) reveals an ill-defined hypoechoic lesion (arrow) adherent to the posterior wall of uterus and endometriotic cyst (*). DIE involving cervix and vagina in 36-year-old patient with dyspareunia and dyschezia—an ill-defined stellate-shaped lesion (arrow) is seen involving the upper portion of posterior cervical region, posterior vaginal wall with resultant obliteration of posterior vaginal fornix appearing hypointense on sagittal T1w (B) and T2w (C) images. It also shows few hyperintense foci on T1W images suggestive of hemorrhagic foci.

hematosalpinx, hydroureteronephrosis, angulation of bowel loops, transition points in bowel diameter, and loculated fluid collections. On MRI, adhesions may be identified as spiculated low SI strands extending between the organs on both T1W and T2W images **(Figs. 17A and B)**.

Malignant transformation of endometrioma, although rare (about 1%), is well known.[18] It may arise from within the endometriotic cyst itself or from the normal ovary. The most common histological subtypes include clear cell and endometrioid carcinoma. They are mostly seen in women older than 40 years, after several years of latency and in endometriomas larger than 9 cm. Malignant transformation is uncommon in endometriomas <6 cm.[19] Any endometrioma-exhibiting features like mural nodules or papillary components showing vascularity on Doppler should be evaluated further in view of malignancy. Other features include ascites, septal thickness >3 mm and peritoneal metastasis. Loss of T2 shading has also been described as a magnetic resonance feature of coexisting neoplasm which is attributed to dilution of hemorrhagic fluid by tumor.

Ovarian Torsion and Rupture

Due to formation of extensive adhesions, risk of torsion is rare in endometriotic cysts. Rupture of endometriotic cysts usually occurs in pregnancy due to rapid growth of endometriomas under the effects of estrogen. Endometrioma rupture is clinically indistinguishable from rupture of a hemorrhagic cyst. There may be hemoperitoneum, which becomes a surgical emergency if the patient is unstable.

Decidualization

During pregnancy, endometriomas can undergo decidual changes in the endometrial tissue lining the cysts, which can be seen as solid papillary projections with a rounded contour and increased vascularity within the ground-glass background. On MRI, the nodules may show SI and texture similar to the decidualized uterine endometrium. They can resemble malignant neoplasms. These changes generally subside in the third trimester and regress completely following pregnancy.

Differential Diagnosis

The differential diagnosis of endometriomas includes mature cystic teratomas (MCTs), hemorrhagic cysts, TOA, cystadenomas, and other ovarian neoplasms with most of the lesions being differentiated on basis of USG and MR findings.

On USG, a MCT of the ovary presents as a unilocular cystic lesion with echogenic components (representing calcification or tooth components) within. Associated posterior acoustic

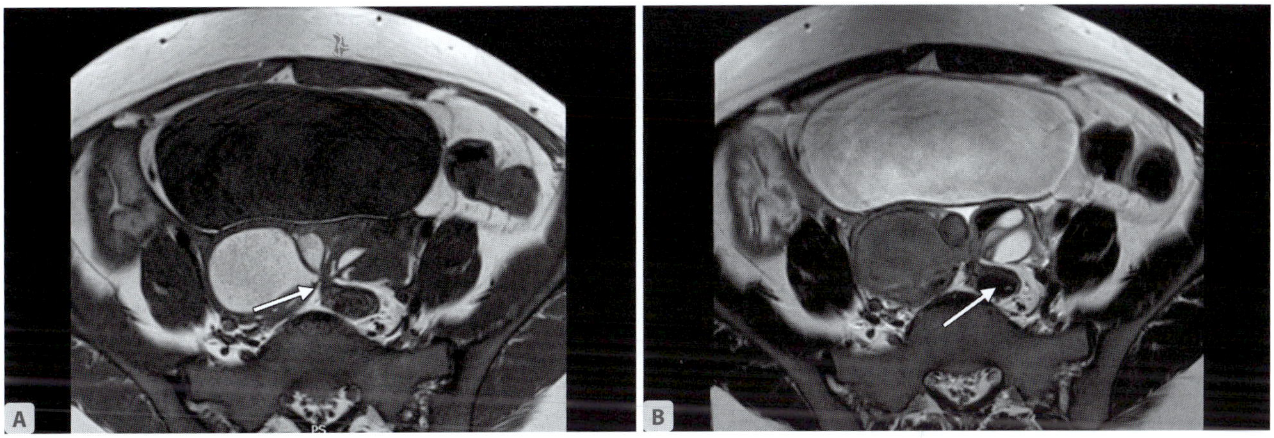

FIGS. 17A AND B: Axial T1-weighted (A) and T2-weighted (B) images reveal endometriotic cyst in right ovary with both ovaries adherent to each other in the midline—"kissing ovaries". There is tenting of the anterior wall of sigmoid colon with focal adherence to posterior aspect of ovaries (arrows).

shadowing may also be present. Like endometriomas, dermoid cysts can also depict fluid-fluid levels. However, the two may be distinguished by assessing the pattern of distribution of fluid within the cyst. In a dermoid, supernatant layer is echogenic representing fat while in endometriomas, the supernatant layer appears hypoechoic with blood and its components in the dependent hyperechoic layer.[20] MR evaluation even though reserved for doubtful cases, has a high sensitivity owing to its ability to detect presence of fat. Although both lesions may appear hyperintense on T1-weighted images, T1 fat-saturated (T1FS) MRI can easily help in distinction. Endometriotic cysts appear hyperintense on T1FS images while dermoid cysts (containing fat) appear hypointense on T1FS images, thereby aiding in differentiation between the two.

On USG, HOCs are seen as thinned-walled, cystic lesions with fine reticular network within. Echogenic foci are specific to endometriomas. On MRI, they show high signal on T1- and T2W images and show lack of T2 shading sign. However, hemorrhagic cysts of longer duration may show T2 shading like features thereby mimicking endometriomas. T2 dark spots have a higher specificity for diagnosis of endometriomas than shading sign and can help to differentiate between them. Since hemorrhagic cysts are relatively short-lived, they do not show such spots. It has been suggested that addition of DWI can help to differentiate between endometriomas and hemorrhagic cysts. However, both show restricted diffusion due to the presence of blood products, and the ADC values have not shown a consistent pattern to allow a confident differentiation.[21,22]

However, there have been variable reports on the ADC values management.

Medical treatment of endometriomas is aimed for alleviation of symptoms and reduction in size. These include the use of nonsteroidal anti-inflammatory drugs (NSAIDs) and hormonal therapy to temper estrogen levels. These include oral contraceptive pills, progesterone analogs, and gonadotropin-releasing hormone (GnRH) agonists.[21] Despite medical management, most endometriotic cysts require surgery for definitive treatment, especially in cases of infertility. However, even after complete resection, these cysts are known for recurrence.

BENIGN OVARIAN NEOPLASMS

Ovarian neoplasms can be broadly classified into epithelial tumors, germ cell tumors, sex-cord stromal tumors, and metastatic tumors **(Box 1 and Fig. 18)**.

EPITHELIAL TUMORS

Benign epithelial ovarian tumors are mainly cystic in appearance. They are seen in a younger age group as compared to their malignant counterparts. The two most common types of benign epithelial neoplasms are the serous cystadenoma and the mucinous cystadenoma.

Serous Cystadenoma

Serous cystadenomas are a commonly occurring neoplasm accounting for approximately 25% of all benign ovarian neoplasms. They are thought to arise from ovarian epithelial inclusions, which itself is derived from fallopian tube epithelium. The peak age incidence is 30–50 years with bilateral tumors seen in 12–23% cases.[22]

Pathology

Serous cystadenomas are usually unilocular (sometimes multilocular) cysts measuring 10 cm in average diameter (sometimes may be extremely large), containing thin and straw-colored fluid. Microscopically, the cyst wall is composed of a solitary layer of simple epithelium with cilia that may be columnar or flat. Psammomatous calcifications can be seen.

Clinical Features

Patients may be asymptomatic and the tumor is often discovered incidentally. In case of large tumors, patients can present with pain, abdominal fullness or distension.

Imaging Features

On US, they are often seen as unilocular cystic lesions with thin walls and anechoic internal contents **(Fig. 19)**. Some lesions may be multilocular, with thin internal septations **(Fig. 20A)**.

BOX 1: Broad classification of ovarian tumors.

Epithelial tumors—arise from surface epithelium
- *Serous epithelial tumors:*
  - Benign (serous cystadenoma/cystadenofibroma), borderline, and malignant
- *Mucinous tumors:*
  - Benign (mucinous cystadenoma/cystadenofibroma), borderline, and malignant
- *Endometroid tumors:*
  - Benign, borderline, and malignant
- *Clear cell tumors:*
  - Benign, borderline, and malignant
- *Transitional cell tumors:*
  - Brenner (benign, borderline, and malignant)
  - Transitional cell carcinoma (non-Brenner type)
- *Epithelial-stromal tumors:*
  - Adenosarcoma
  - Carcinosarcoma

Germ cell tumors—arise from the primordial germ cells
- *Teratoma:*
  - Mature teratoma (dermoid)
  - Immature teratoma
- Yolk sac tumor (endodermal sinus tumor)
- Dysgerminoma
- Embryonal cell carcinoma
- Choriocarcinoma
- *Monodermal tumors:*
  - Struma ovarii
  - Carcinoid

Sex cord–stromal tumors—arise from ovarian stroma and/or sex cord cells
- Thecoma
- Fibroma
- Fibrothecoma
- Granulosa cell tumors
- Sertoli-Leydig cell tumors
- Steroid (lipid) cell tumors

Metastatic tumors

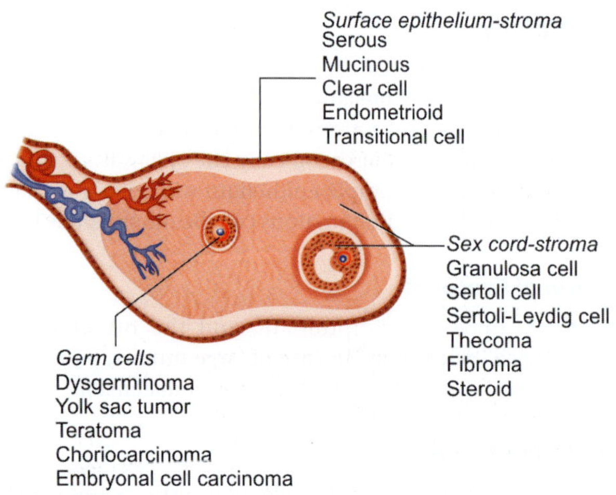

FIG. 18: Diagram to show the origin of ovarian tumors from the various cells within the ovary.

On Doppler evaluation, mild peripheral or septal vascularity may be seen **(Fig. 20B)**, which shows higher resistive and pulsatility indices on pulsed Doppler as compared to malignant neoplasms. On CT, a unilocular (typically) or multilocular cystic mass is seen with homogeneous attenuation, with thin regular walls or septae and no solid component **(Figs. 21A and B)**. On MRI, the lesions show T1W hypointense and T2W hyperintense contents on images with enhancement of the cyst wall on contrast administration. When large, these cysts can be seen to fill most of the lower pelvis and extend into the upper abdomen.

Differential Diagnosis

The common differentials are from other benign looking cystic masses in the adnexal region like functional ovarian cysts, paraovarian cysts, peritoneal inclusion cysts (PICs), and large hydrosalpinx. Presence of a solid component, even small, especially if showing internal vascularity, needs to be evaluated for malignant etiology.

Management

As these are benign lesions, they usually have a good prognosis. However, ovarian cystadenomas may evolve into cystadenocarcinomas, and thus are usually removed either by cystectomy or oophorectomy. They can also form a lead point for ovarian torsion. Cystadenomas do not recur following oophorectomy.

Mucinous Cystadenoma

Mucinous cystadenomas account for approximately 15–20% of benign ovarian neoplasms and 80% of mucinous ovarian tumors.[23] They are less common than their serous counterparts.

Pathology

They are usually multilocular cystic masses (rarely they can be unilocular), larger than their serous counterparts. Only 2–5%

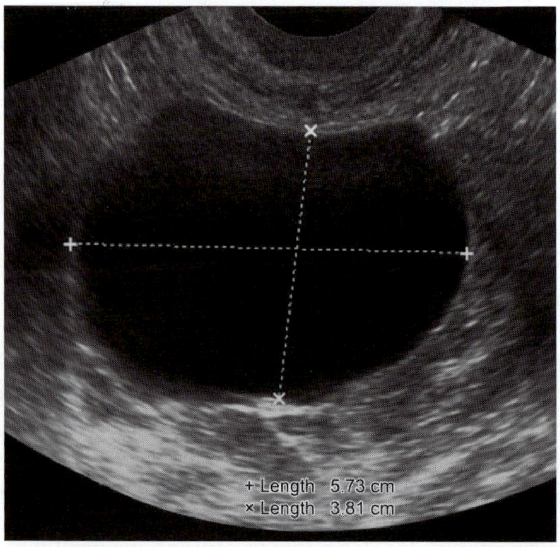

FIG. 19: Serous cystadenoma in a 70-year-old postmenopausal woman seen as a unilocular, anechoic cyst on transvaginal ultrasound.

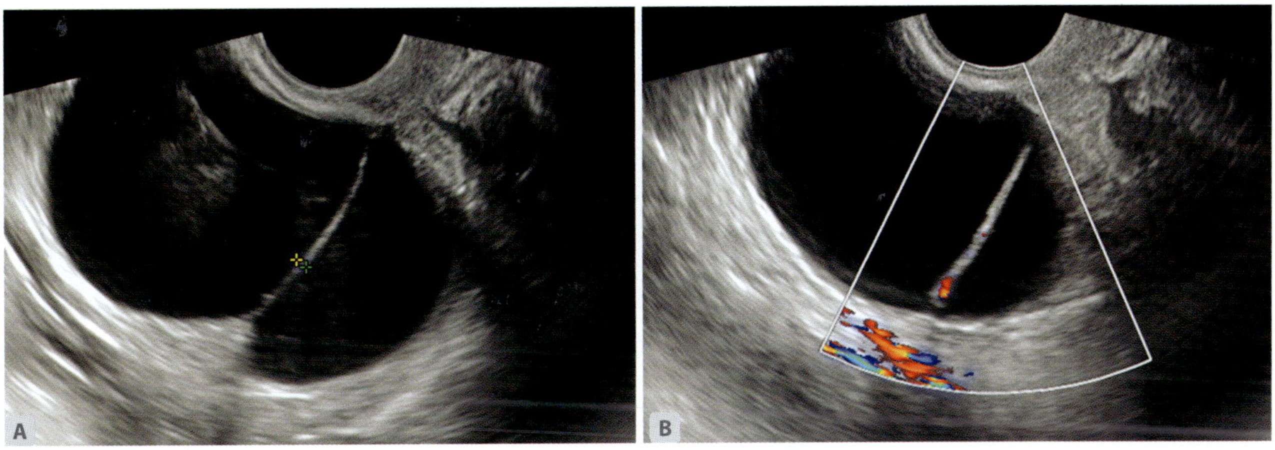

FIGS. 20A AND B: Serous cystadenoma in a 55-year-old woman. Transvaginal scan (A) shows a thin septum within a large, anechoic, cystic mass. The septum shows mild vascularity on color Doppler (B).

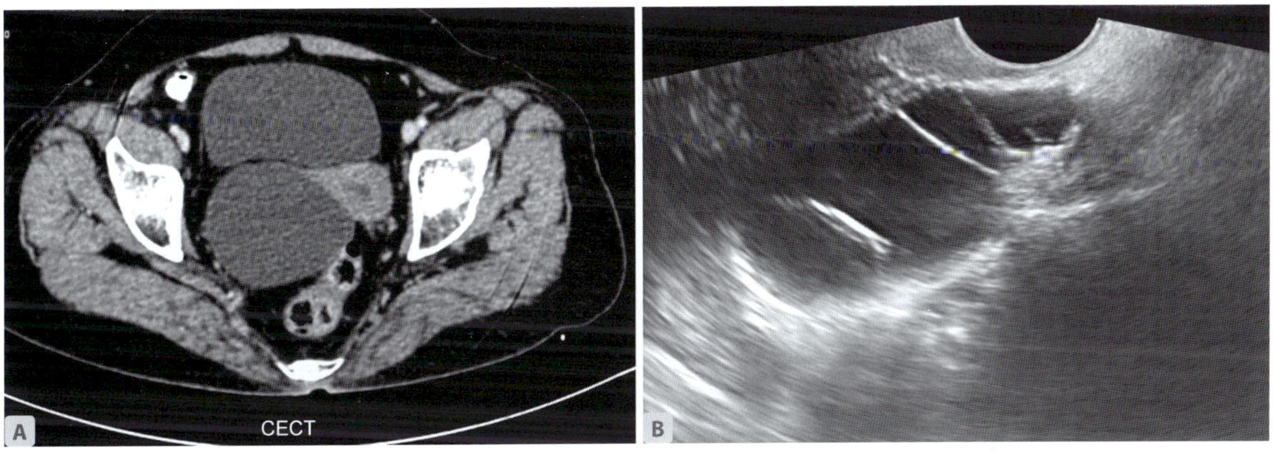

FIGS. 21A AND B: Serous cystadenoma in a 60-year-old woman. Contrast-enhanced ct scan (A) shows a unilocular, thin-walled cystic lesion in right adnexal region. On transvaginal ultrasound (B) a few, thin septae were seen within the cyst.

are bilateral. Microscopically, they are lined by columnar epithelial cells which secrete thick, gelatinous mucin which fills the locules. In 5% cases, mucinous cystadenomas may occur in association with other tumors of the ovary like Brenner tumors or dermoid cysts.

Clinical Features

Patients present with abdominal distension, pain and/or pelvic mass. In rare cases, hormonal manifestations can occur due to stromal luteinization. They commonly occur between 30 years and 50 years of age.

Imaging Features

On imaging, mucinous cystadenomas are seen as large, multilocular cystic masses with numerous thin septations which are smooth and regular **(Figs. 22A and B)**. The locules show low-level internal echogenicity on US. As the locules contain fluid of various viscosity, they often show variable density on CT and signal intensities on both T1 and T2 sequences on MRI giving a "stained glass" or "honeycomb" appearance. On T1W images, loculi with watery mucin have a lower SI than the loculi which have thicker mucin. On T2-weighted images, the loculi with watery mucin have high SI and loculi with thicker mucin appear slightly hypointense **(Figs. 23A to C)**. Lack of solid components and presence of regular smooth septa confirm the benign nature of the lesion. Small papillary projections may be present but are often difficult to visualize on imaging.[24] Mural calcification occurs more commonly than in serous tumors.[25]

Differential Diagnosis

Large cystic masses can be confused with omental or mesenteric cysts, PICs, and large serous cystadenomas. Although the "stained glass" appearance has been said to be pathognomonic for mucinous ovarian tumors, it may rarely be seen in MCT, fibrothecoma, endometrioma, Brenner tumor of the ovary, and degenerated leiomyoma of the uterus.[26]

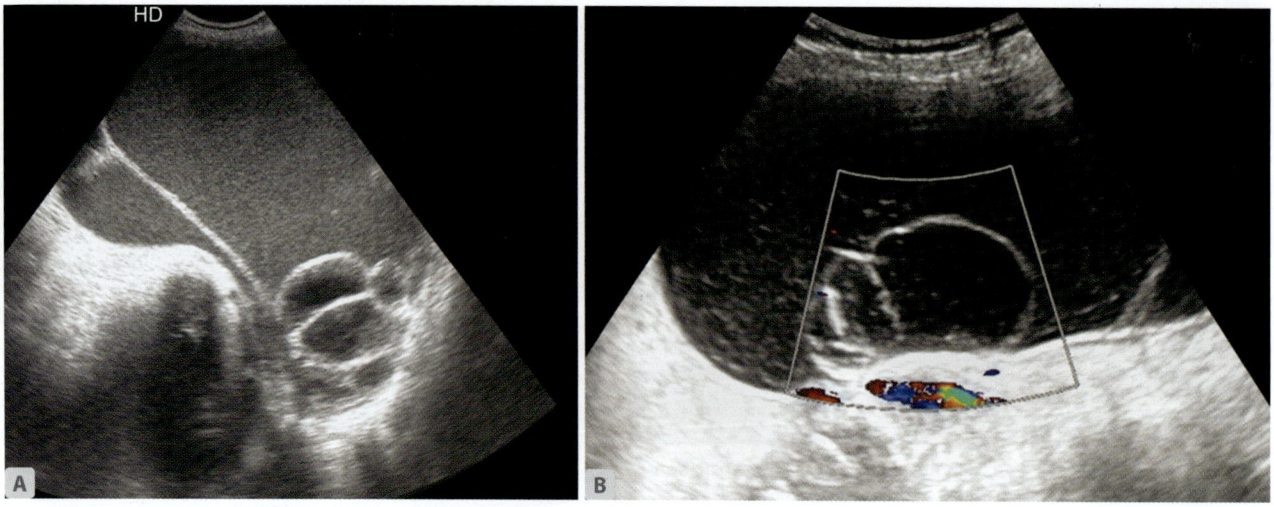

FIGS. 22A AND B: Mucinous cystadenoma in a 45-year-old woman presenting with abdominal fullness and pain. (A) Transvaginal ultrasound image shows a multiloculated cystic mass with multiple thin septae, differential internal echoes and no solid component; (B) No vascularity was seen in the septae or adjacent wall on transabdominal color Doppler scan.

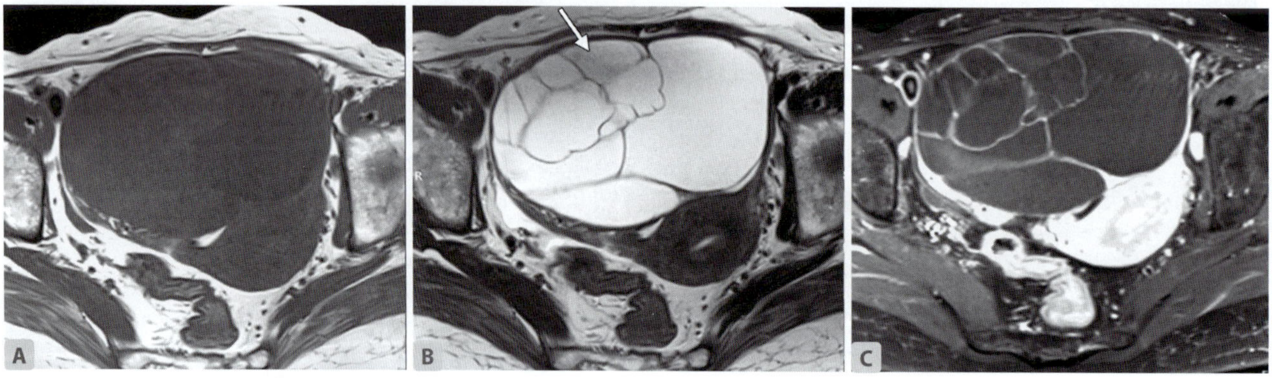

FIGS. 23A TO C: Mucinous cystadenoma. T1-weighted (A) and T2-weighted (B) axial MR images show a large multiloculated cystic mass with multiple thin, smooth septae within appearing hypointense on T1W, hyperintense on T2W images with thin, regular, hypointense septae, and cyst wall. Variable signal intensities are seen in some of the locules on T2W image (arrow). On contrast-enhanced T1W image (C) the cyst wall and septae are seen to enhance.

Management

Mucinous cystadenomas are benign masses with excellent prognosis, however, often need to be surgically removed to confirm benign histology, due to the mass effect of large tumors and potential for ovarian torsion.

Ovarian Cystadenofibroma

Cystadenofibromas of the ovary are uncommon benign neoplasms which contain both epithelial and fibrous stromal components, and account for 1.7% of all benign ovarian tumors.[27] They occur in females in the reproductive age group. Cystadenofibromas may be predominantly cystic, predominantly solid or complex cystic with variable amount of solid components and may have a serous or mucinous cystic component. Due to the presence of irregular thick septae or solid components within the lesion, they are often mistaken for malignant lesions not only on imaging, but even at surgery. A frozen section at time of surgery is necessary to make an accurate diagnosis to avoid unnecessary extensive surgery.

Imaging Features

On US, a cystadenofibroma may be seen as a solitary cyst or a multiloculated cystic mass, with solid nodules or papillary projections with some of them showing increased vascularity on Doppler evaluation. The fibrous component in the solid part may show acoustic shadowing which can give a clue to the diagnosis. On CT, a nonspecific complex cystic mass with enhancing solid component, mimics a malignant lesion.[28]

On MRI, the presence of low-SI on T2W images in the solid part of the tumor, due to its fibrous tissue component, helps in characterizing this neoplasm. A sponge-like appearance may also be seen due to multiple tiny hyperintense T2W cysts alongwith a low SI solid fibrous component. Diffuse or focal thickening of the cyst wall may be seen with low SI on T2W images. There is mild enhancement of the solid component on postcontrast images. In a study by Cho et al., 16 cases of cystadenofibromas of the ovary, presenting as complex cystic masses with solid components, were misdiagnosed as malignant ovarian neoplasms on CT scan or MRI.[27]

Differential Diagnosis

The differential diagnosis will depend on the appearance of the cystadenofibroma—whether predominantly cystic, solid or complex cystic-solid. Thus, it can vary from a serous or mucinous neoplasm to other T2W hypointense masses like fibroma, fibrothecoma, Brenner tumor, and even leiomyomas.

Brenner Tumor

Brenner tumors are surface epithelial-stromal tumors of the ovary comprising approximately 2% of all ovarian neoplasms, so-called as they were first described by Fritz Brenner in 1907.[29] They are also called "transitional cell tumors" because of their histological similarity to the urothelium. They usually occur in women between the ages of 45 years and 65 years. There may be an associated second tumor in the same ovary in about 30% of cases, which is most often a serous or a mucinous cystadenoma.

Clinical Features

Brenner tumors are unilateral masses often discovered incidentally. Symptomatic patients present with vaginal bleeding (due to excess estrogenic activity), pelvic pain or pelvic mass. Large tumors may give rise to urinary retention, ascites or even Meigs' syndrome. Histological examination shows epithelial cell nests growing in a fibrous stroma. Although 99% of Brenner tumors are benign, malignant Brenner tumors may arise from their benign counterparts, so careful histopathological examination of all Brenner tumors is essential.

Imaging Features

On US, these tumors are seen as predominantly solid masses, small in size, with few, if any, cystic areas in the benign lesions. Extensive amorphous calcification may be present. On Doppler examination, they are either avascular or show minimal vascularity. *CT* shows the calcifications better. On *MRI*, a low SI is seen on T2WI because of the solid fibrous content **(Figs. 24A and B)**. In cases where an associated cystic tumor, like mucinous or serous cystadenoma, is present along with the Brenner tumor, a lesion with both cystic (cystadenomas) and solid (Brenner) component is seen on imaging. Borderline or invasive Brenner tumors are characterized by the presence of solid-cystic or cystic appearance, with papillary structures, and mild or moderate enhancement in the solid mass.[30]

Differential Diagnosis

The important differentials include ovarian fibromas, fibrothecomas, and a pedunculated leiomyoma all of which can be seen as hypoechoic masses on US and T2 hypointense masses on MRI. Absence of a normal ipsilateral ovary helps distinguish from pedunculated leiomyomas. The presence of small follicles surrounding the mass helps identify the ovarian origin. Abundant calcification, if present, goes in favor of Brenner tumor.

GERM CELL TUMORS

Ovarian germ cell tumors arise from primordial germ cells of the ovary. The only benign germ cell tumor is the MCT.

Mature Cystic Teratoma

Mature cystic teratomas are the most common germ cell neoplasms, accounting for about 15–20% of all ovarian neoplasms.[31] These tumors arise from a single germ cell after its first meiotic division and contain mature tissue from all three germ cell layers (ectoderm, mesoderm, and endoderm) with predominance of ectodermal component. When ectodermal tissues predominate, these teratomas are called as dermoid cysts.

Pathology

Mature teratomas are usually seen as unilocular cystic masses at macroscopic examination. However, they may

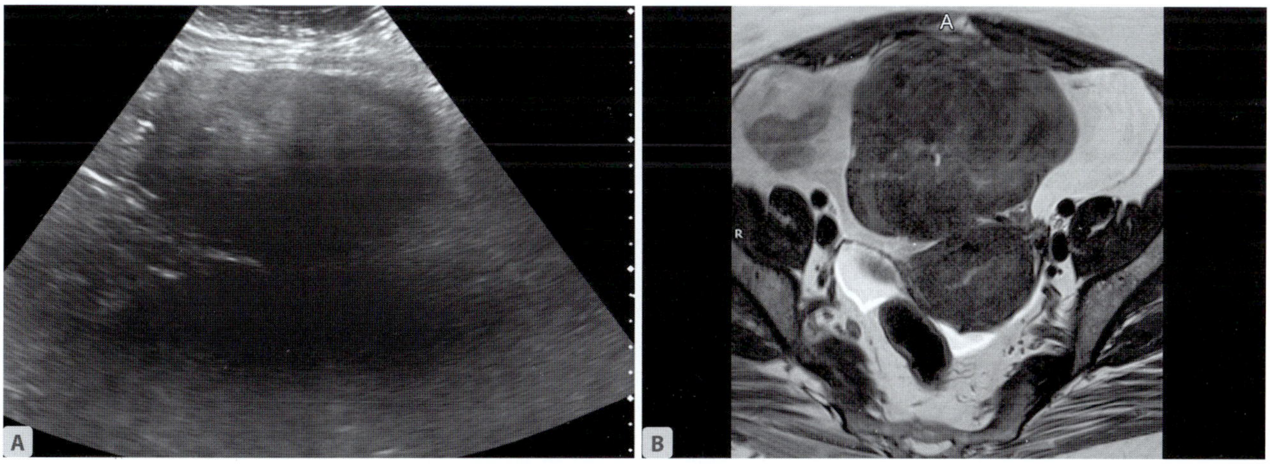

FIGS. 24A AND B: Brenner tumor in a 50-year-old patient with abdominal distension and abnormal uterine bleeding. (A) Transabdominal ultrasound image shows a hypoechoic solid mass with lobulated outer margins and some acoustic shadowing; (B) T2-weighted axial MR image shows lobulated hypointense mass anterior to the uterus with small amount of ascites.

be multilocular at times. Fat is present in more than 90% of cases,[32] either as sebum or macroscopic fat, and is the most specific finding of a mature teratoma. The cyst cavity is filled with sebaceous and keratinized material secreted by the squamous epithelial lining. Sebaceous material contains most of the lipid content whereas adipose tissue is less common. Sebum is an oily, waxy material produced by sebaceous glands in the epidermis and is primarily composed of fatty acids and triglycerides. There is usually a raised protuberance, projecting into the cyst cavity, known as the *Rokitansky protuberance or dermoid plug.* Bone and teeth tend to be located in this protuberance and most of the hair arises from it. The rare malignant transformation also occurs at this site.

Histologically, mature tissues from different cell lines are seen within the wall. Walls of the cyst are frequently lined by squamous epithelium. In an MCT, ectodermal elements are almost always present. Endodermal tissues (mucinous or ciliated epithelium) can also be seen in the majority of cases and mesodermal tissues are present in over 90% of cases.

Clinical Features

Mature cystic teratomas occur in a younger age group with mean age of 30 years, but can range between 4 months and 70 years.[33] They are the most common ovarian mass lesion found in children. The tumors are bilateral in about 10–12% of cases.[34]

They are slow growing tumors and are often discovered incidentally. Pain in the lower abdomen or other nonspecific symptoms may occur in a few cases. Complicated dermoid cysts can present with acute symptoms, the most common complication being torsion of the ovary.

Imaging Features

On *plain radiographs*, around 40% of ovarian teratomas show diagnostic characteristics with presence of teeth or fat in the pelvis.

A variety of appearances can be seen on cross-sectional imaging due to the multiple tissues within these teratomas. The classic *US* appearance is a complex cystic mass with solid mural component called *"dermoid plug" or "Rokitansky nodule"*. This is seen in almost 90% of cystic teratomas **(Figs. 25A and B)**. The dermoid plug contains hair, teeth or fat and is usually echogenic and frequently casts an acoustic shadow. Rarely, the Rokitansky nodule may appear entirely cystic.[35] The dermoid cyst may show focal or diffuse, homogeneous or heterogeneous, *hyperechogenecity* which may be associated with areas of acoustic shadowing which is due to presence of mixed sebaceous material and hair **(Fig. 26A)**.

"Tip of the iceberg" sign can be seen, on both transabdominal and transvaginal US scans, as an amorphous echogenic mass which causes posterior shadowing that obscures the posterior portion of the lesion and any structures behind it **(Fig. 26B)**.[36] This is produced by a mixture of matted hair, fatty fluid, and cellular debris which is highly echogenic because of the multiple tissue interfaces. This sign is seen. It may mimic a fecal/air-filled bowel segment and may be missed on US.

"Dot-dash" sign or *"dermoid mesh"* seen as hyperechoic lines and dots within the cyst. It occurs due to strands of hair in different orientations **(Fig. 26C)**.[37]

Fat-fluid/fluid-fluid levels can be seen when anechoic sebum layers above the hyperechoic aqueous/debris-containing layer **(Fig. 26D)**. Sometimes the supernatant

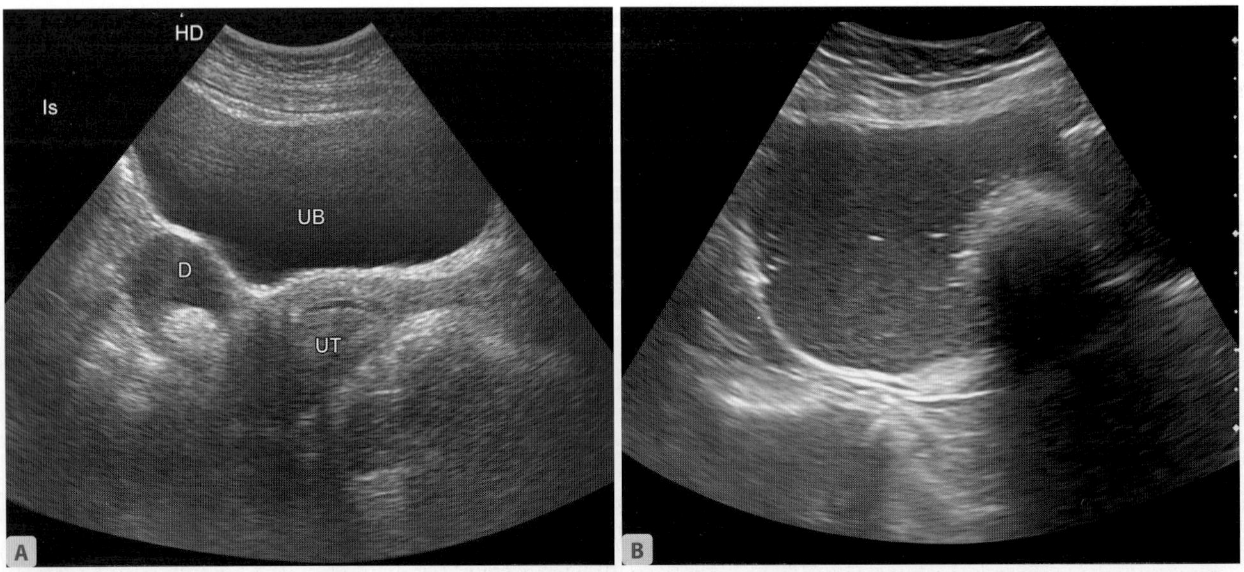

FIGS. 25A AND B: (A) Right ovarian dermoid. Transabdominal ultrasound image showing right ovarian cystic mass (D) with an echogenic nodule—Rokitansky nodule; (B) Transvaginal scan. Typical mature cystic teratoma showing a Rokitansky nodule as an echogenic nodule with marked acoustic shadowing within a cystic mass. The cyst shows low level ground-glass echoes within. Multiple hyperechoic dots and dashes seen along surface of the nodule and within the cyst represent hair. (UB: urinary bladder; UT: uterus).

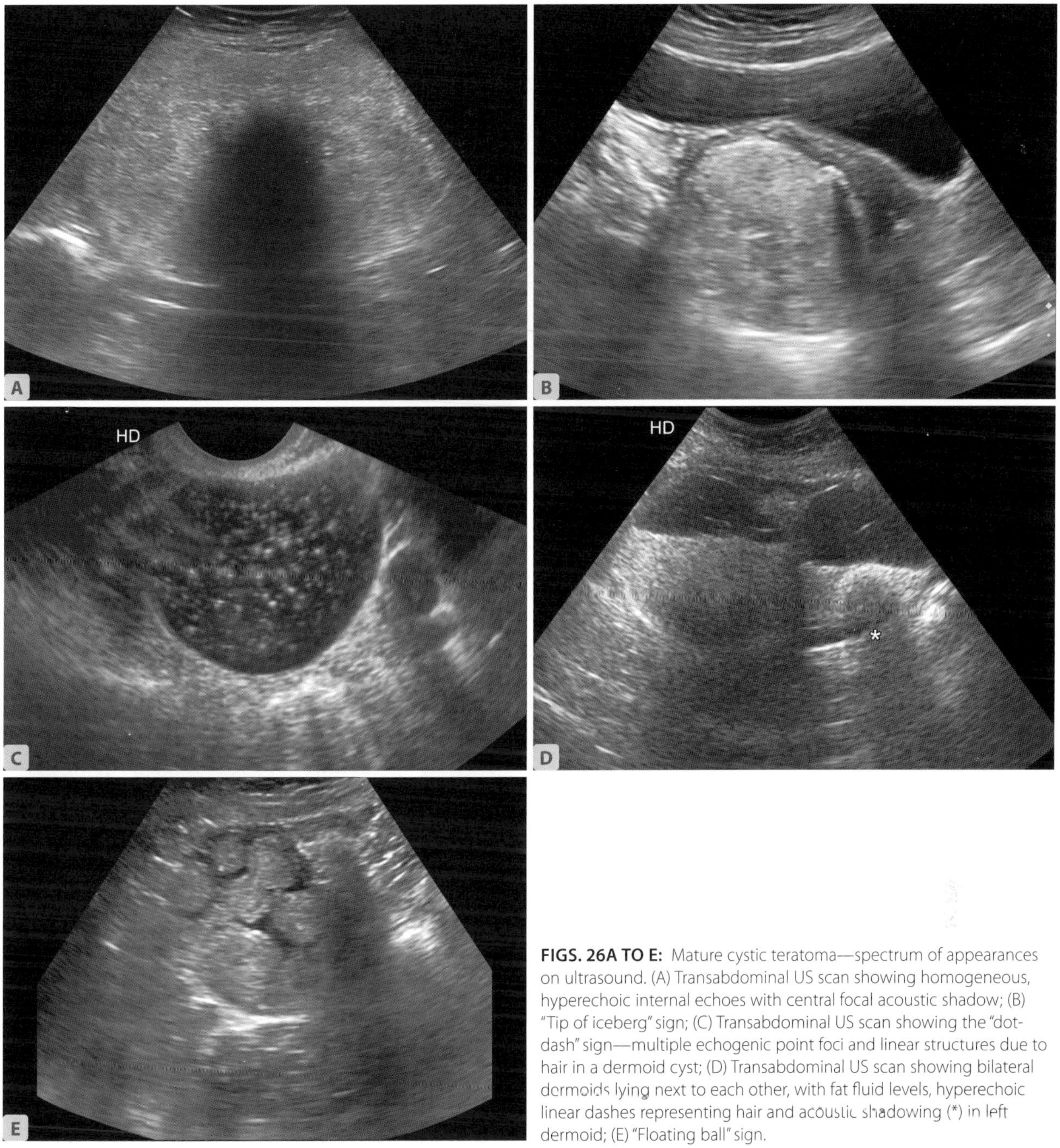

FIGS. 26A TO E: Mature cystic teratoma—spectrum of appearances on ultrasound. (A) Transabdominal US scan showing homogeneous, hyperechoic internal echoes with central focal acoustic shadow; (B) "Tip of iceberg" sign; (C) Transabdominal US scan showing the "dot-dash" sign—multiple echogenic point foci and linear structures due to hair in a dermoid cyst; (D) Transabdominal US scan showing bilateral dermoids lying next to each other, with fat fluid levels, hyperechoic linear dashes representing hair and acoustic shadowing (*) in left dermoid; (E) "Floating ball" sign.

hyperechoic sebum layers above the hypoechoic aqueous fluid.

"Floating balls" sign is seen as intracystic floating hyperechoic globules or nodules within a cystic mass **(Fig. 26E)**. This is another pathognomonic sign, but is uncommonly seen.[38]

The US appearance may vary from a very specific (when the characteristic signs can be identified), to a totally nonspecific appearance requiring further CT or MRI to confirm the nature of the mass.

Computed tomography can provide a definitive diagnosis in majority of cases due to its high sensitivity in detecting fat. The characteristic CT features include detection of fat (density <–20 HU), hair, teeth, and fat-fluid level. Rokitansky nodule is also best seen on CT, as a rounded or oval structure, generally <5 cm in diameter, protruding into the cyst. It frequently contains tooth, calcification, hair or adipose tissue **(Figs. 27A and B)**. Rarely, a Rokitansky protuberance may be seen as a mural thickening or a bridge across the cyst.[39] Curvilinear or globular calcification can be seen in the Rokitansky protuberance or in the wall of the dermoid cyst. Fat-fluid level and floating balls sign can also be well seen on CT. When a dermoid cyst does not have fat or calcification, CT may not be helpful in the differential diagnosis.[40] It may have shown

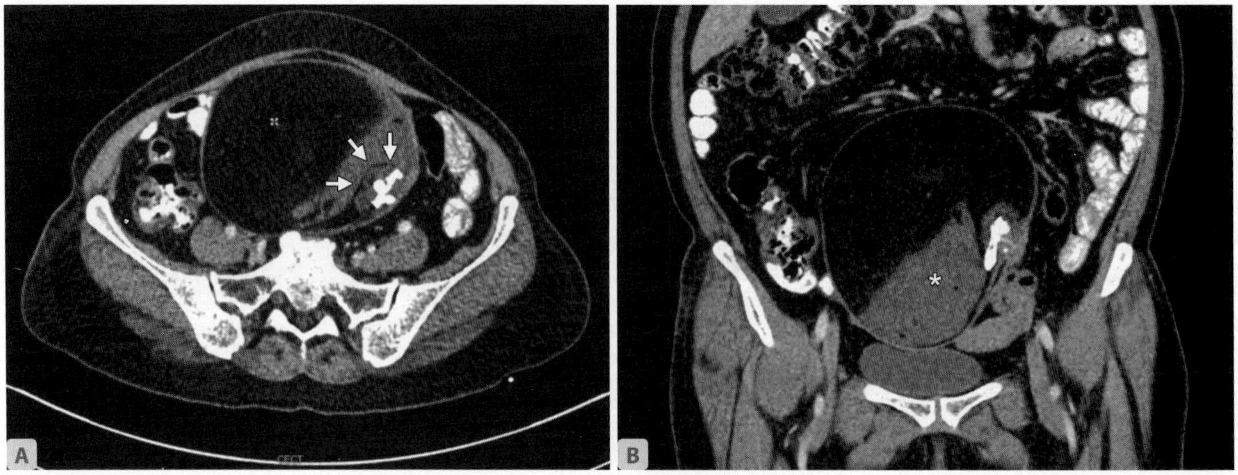

FIGS. 27A AND B: Typical mature cystic teratoma in a 45-year-old woman. (A) Axial contrast-enhanced CT shows a large, thinly encapsulated, fat containing (–113 HU) cystic mass with a rounded Rokitansky nodule (arrows) which has teeth-like structures within it. A fat fluid level is seen; (B) On the coronal CECT, the Rokitansky nodule can be seen to be arising from the soft tissue along the cyst wall. Fluid density content (*) can also be seen adjacent to the nodule within the predominantly fat-containing mature cystic teratoma.

only water density content, due to excess watery fluid or gelatinous fluid **(Fig. 28)**. Sometimes a large amount of hair maybe mixed with the fat density, resulting in a cystic density of >–20 HU. Dermoids which have undergone torsion may show a high internal density due to hemorrhage or necrosis.

Contrast administration is not really helpful in diagnosis of dermoids as most of the characteristic features are well seen on noncontrast scans. Slight enhancement may be seen in the wall, septae and the Rokitansky protuberance on delayed contrast-enhanced scans.

On *MRI*, fat within the MCT shows high intensity on T1W images with a signal drop on fat-saturated T1W images **(Figs. 29 and 30)**. This drop in signal allows a definitive diagnosis of a MCT ruling out a hemorrhagic cyst or an endometrioma which remain hyperintense on the fat saturation images. Small areas of fat maybe identified on chemical shift imaging **(Fig. 29C)**. However, MRI may fail to pick up very small fatty areas (about 1 mm) when compared with CT.[41] On T2W images the intensity can be intermediate or higher than the subcutaneous adipose tissue. Reversed chemical shift artifact (boundary artifact perpendicular to the direction of the frequency encoding gradient) may also be seen on T2W images as foci or areas of very high SI at the interface of fatty tissue and nonfatty tissue, with a low-intensity band on the opposite side **(Fig. 30D)**.[34]

The size, number, shape, and content of the Rokitansky nodule can be easily evaluated with MRI, along with its relationship to the cyst wall **(Figs. 29A to D)**.

Fat-fluid level maybe seen as layering with high SI of supernatant fatty layer on T1W images and low SI on fat suppressed TWI **(Figs. 31A and B)**. On T2WI, variable signal intensities can be seen in the supernatant and dependent layers. A ball of debris, fat, and hair may be seen floating at the interface of the fat-fluid level or layering along the dependent wall. Matted hair can layer as dependent debris

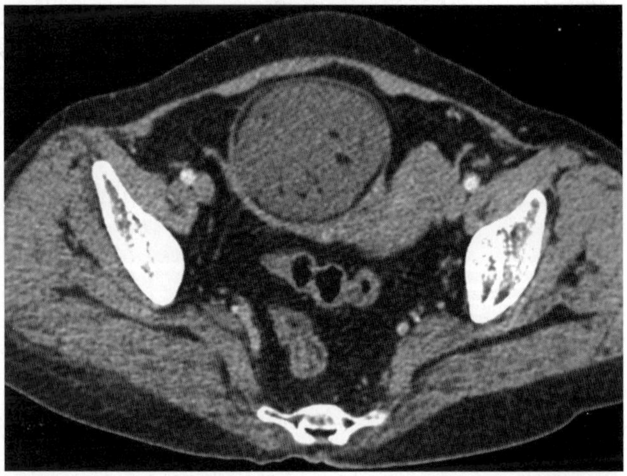

FIG. 28: Atypical mature cystic teratoma. Contrast-enhanced CT shows a well-defined, fluid density cystic lesion with a few floating fat density foci within the cystic fluid. It also shows a fatty rim along the inner margin of the wall.

and large amounts of hair lead to lower SI on T2W images.[34] Floating globules or spherules can be seen in the cyst **(Figs. 32A and B)**. These globules may also contain macroscopic or microscopic fat, which can be detected by fat-suppression techniques or in outpatient imaging.[42]

Polypoid palm tree-like protrusions maybe seen projecting into the cyst cavity **(Figs. 33A and B)**. They consist of desquamated, degenerated epithelial cells mixed with hair and the signal intensity varies according to the proportion of hair and cheese-like material.

Diffusion-weighted imaging has been used in an attempt to identify MCTs. MCTs contain a keratinoid substance, a scleroprotein, that originates from the cytoskeletal structure of the epidermis, and is a major component of skin, hair, and nails. Keratinoid is seen as low SI on T1- and high SI on T2-weighted images resembling serous fluid. However, it shows a restricted diffusion pattern on DWI, i.e. a high signal on DWI and a low ADC value **(*see* Figs. 30E and F)**. Thus, in some MCTs, particularly when fat is not obvious, DWI may serve as an accessory sequence for the correct diagnosis.[43]

Complications

The most common complication associated with MCTs is torsion. Almost 16% of ovarian teratomas will undergo torsion, and MCTs are also considered to be the most common cause of ovarian torsion. Other complications which can occur are leak or rupture (1–4%), in which the sebaceous contents enter into the peritoneal cavity and can result in a granulomatous peritonitis; malignant transformation can occur in 1–2% cases, of which squamous cell carcinoma is the most common (>80%) but other cancers such as adenocarcinomas, sarcomas, and even carcinoids may occur. The Rokitansky's nodule is the common site for malignant transformation. Malignant transformation can be suspected, if there is

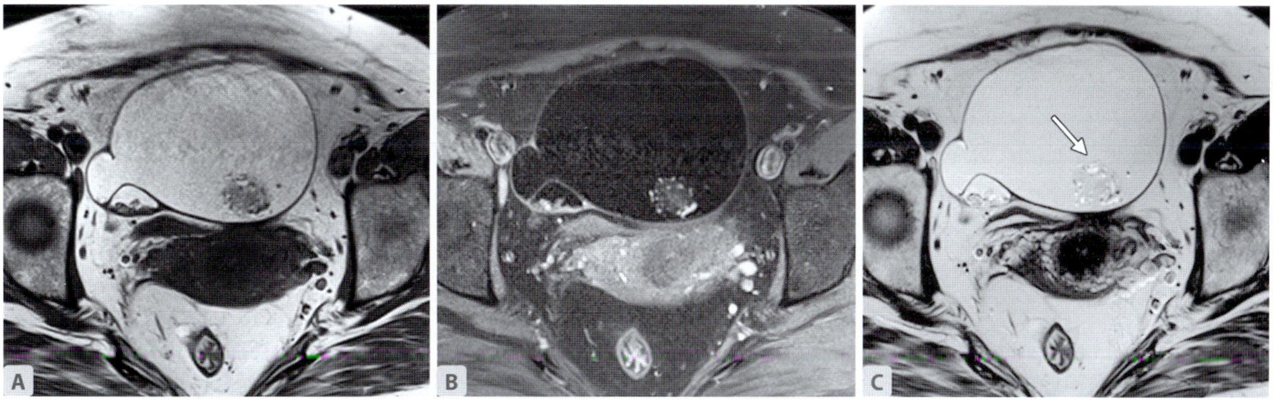

FIGS. 29A TO C: Mature cystic teratoma in a 16-year-old girl. (A) Large, thin-walled, multiloculated cystic mass, seen anterior to the uterus, homogeneously hyperintense on T1-weighted image, which is totally suppressed on the fat suppressed T1W image; (B) A Rokitansky nodule is seen on the posterior wall; (C) Axial T2-weighted image shows chemical shift artifact (arrow) at the interface of the Rokitansky nodule with the cyst fluid. It was consistent with matted hair and keratinoid material in the macroscopic specimen.

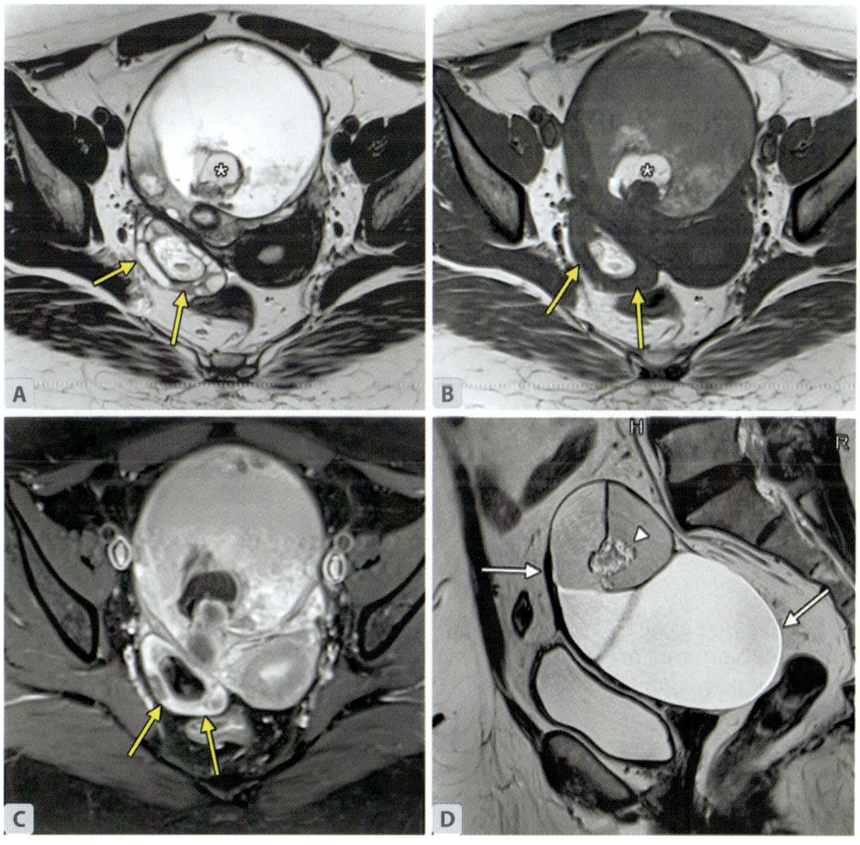

FIGS. 30A TO F: *Continued*

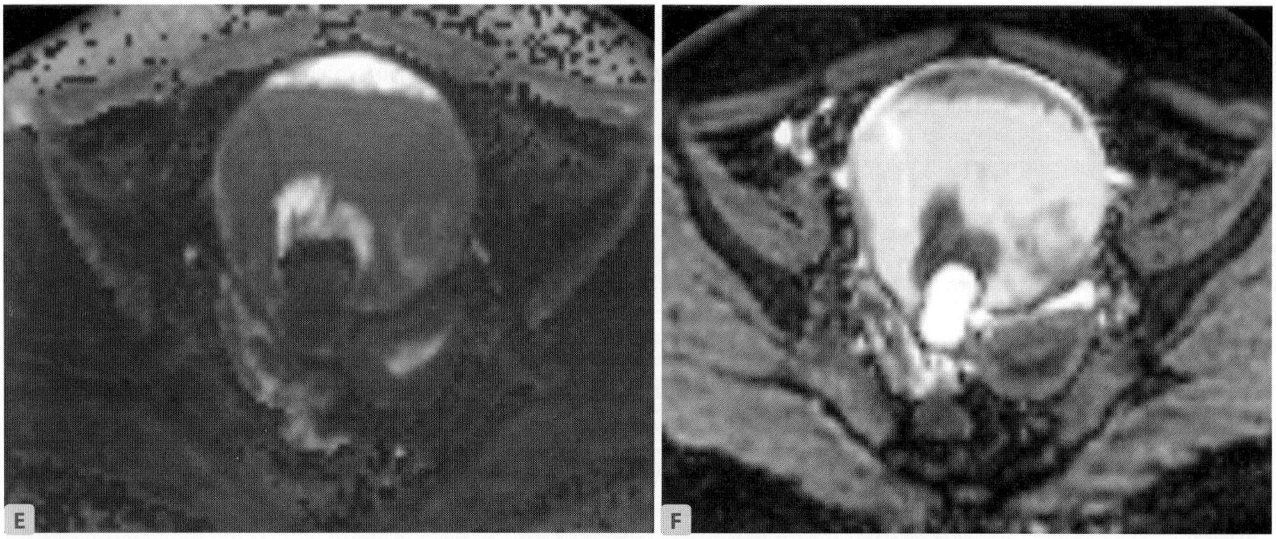

FIGS. 30A TO F: Bilateral mature cystic teratomas in a 24-year-old woman. T2-weighted (A), T1-weighted (B), and contrast-enhanced T1WFS axial MR images show a large, well-defined, hyperintense, cystic left ovarian teratoma, with a Rokitansky protuberance (*). A smaller similar mass in the right ovary (yellow arrows). Few hypointense elements seen in the protuberence on both T2- and T1-weighted images correspond to tooth/bony elements. T1-weighted image shows few scattered hyperintense foci and hyperintensity in the Rokitansky protuberance which show signal suppression on the fat-suppressed image (C). (D) On the sagittal T2W image, chemical shift artifact can be seen as a low signal intensity band (straight arrow) on the anterior border of the cyst with a high intensity band on the opposite wall (oblique arrow). The floating hair ball is also well seen in this image (arrowhead). Axial diffusion-weighted image at b = 800 sec/mm^2 (E) shows hyperintensity in few areas in the left ovarian teratoma, which appear dark on the corresponding ADC map (F) suggesting diffusion restriction in the keratin component of the teratoma.

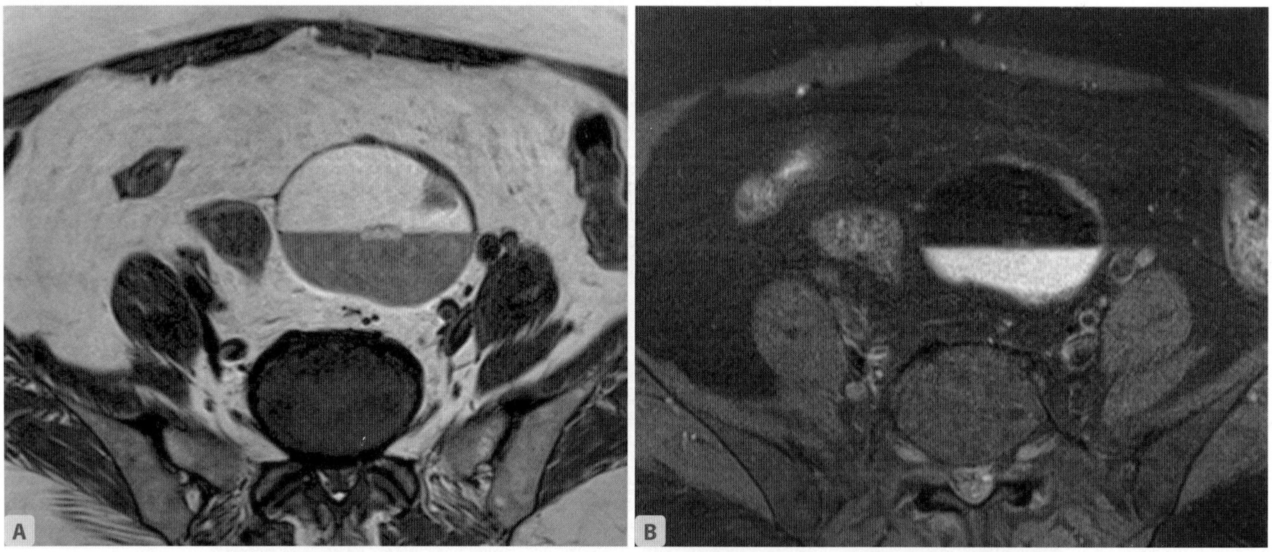

FIGS. 31A AND B: Axial T1-weighted MR image of a 60-year-old woman with mature cystic teratoma (A) shows high signal intensity of the supernatant fatty layer creating an interface with a low signal intensity aqueous layer. Fat-suppressed T1-weighted image (B) shows decreased signal intensity in the supernatant fatty layer. A free-floating ball is seen at the interface between the fat and fluid.

irregular wall thickening, enhancing solid mass within the cystic cavity, or invasion of adjacent structures.[44] Superadded infection may be seen in few cases. Autoimmune hemolytic anemia has been reported as a rare complication, occurring in <1% cases.[45] Collision tumors have been reported with MCTs, most commonly with mucinous tumors and other germ cell tumors.

Differential Diagnosis

As MCTs have a very variable appearance on imaging due to the numerous constituents, there are a large number of conditions which can mimic them. On US, endometriomas, ovarian abscesses, and mucinous cystadenomas can be confused with MCTs having homogeneous low-level internal echoes. On CT and MRI, the typical MCT with fat and

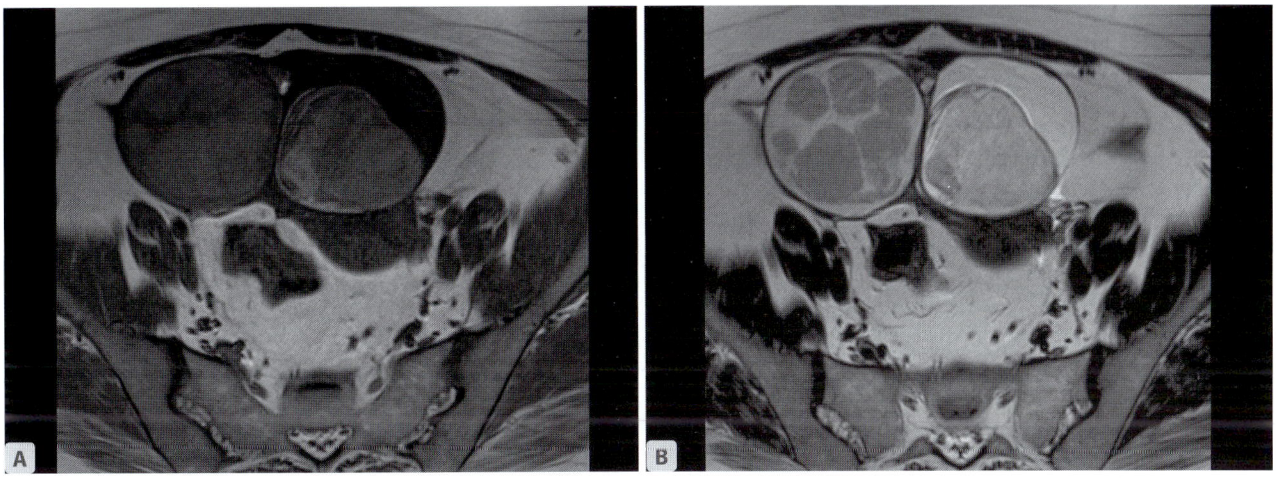

FIGS. 32A AND B: Mature cystic teratoma (MCT) in a 16-year-old girl. (A) T1-weighted and (B) T2-weighted axial magnetic resonance images. Biloculated MCT of right ovary with "floating ball sign" in the right locule and a large single heterogeneous ball within the left locule which appear hyperintense on the T1-weighted image. Normal left ovary was seen separately.

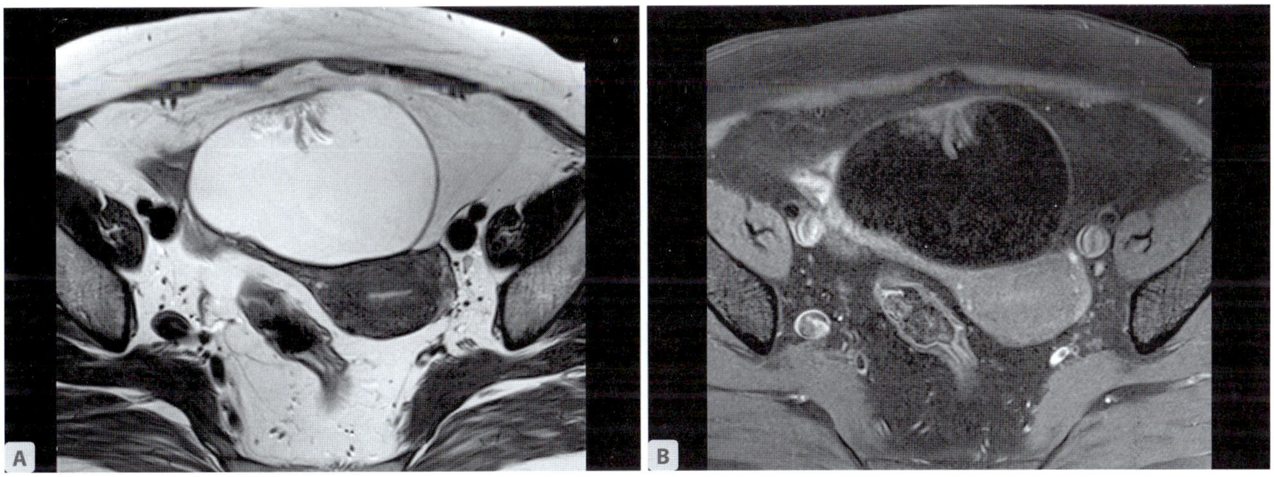

FIGS. 33A AND B: Palm tree protrusions in mature cystic teratoma (MCT). (A) Axial T2-weighted and (B) T1-weighted fat-suppressed magnetic resonance images showing the characteristic palm tree protrusions seen arising from the wall of the MCT.

calcification do not constitute a problem, however, atypical MCTs with small or no fat content may pose a diagnostic problem.

Management

Mature cystic teratomas grow slowly at an average rate of <2 mm each year, prompting a nonsurgical management of smaller tumors (<6 cm). However, due to the high rate complications, especially torsion, most clinicians advise surgical removal. MCTs requiring removal can be treated with simple cystectomy. In case a conservative approach is adopted, then a 6-monthly to annual follow-up by US is recommended, to ensure that the lesion is not changing in size or internal architecture. In case of complicated MCTs, the management will depend on nature and severity of the complication.

SEX CORD-STROMAL TUMORS

These are a subgroup of tumors derived from the *stromal* component of the ovary, i.e. from the theca cells, fibroblasts, and Leydig cells or the *gonadal primitive sex cord cells* which include granulosa cells and Sertoli cells. They form approximately 7% of all primary ovarian tumors.[46] In the recently revised WHO classification (2014) of ovarian neoplasms, these sex cord-stromal tumors were regrouped into the following clinicopathologic entities: pure stromal tumors, pure sex cord tumors, and mixed sex cord-stromal tumors.[47] As some of the cells of these types of tumors secrete ovarian steroid hormones (e.g. estrogens, androgens, and corticosteroids), sex cord-stromal tumors are often associated with various hormone-mediated syndromes and may exhibit a wide spectrum of clinical features, e.g. precocious puberty in a child, abnormal uterine bleeding, endometrial hyperplasia or carcinoma, which are signs of increased estrogen, or signs of virilization, i.e. androgen excess in association with adnexal mass.

Ovarian fibromas, thecomas, and fibrothecomas are pure stromal tumors and are thought to be variants of a single entity. They are the most common benign solid lesions of the ovaries and usually occur in middle-aged women. They are usually asymptomatic; sometimes they may be associated with ascites and pleural effusion and this condition is called Meigs' syndrome.

Fibromas contain spindle-shaped cells and secrete collagen. They do not contain thecal cells and so do not have any estrogenic activity. On US, fibromas are commonly seen as solid, hypoechoic masses. On CT, a solid homogeneous mass with delayed contrast enhancement is seen. Sometimes diffuse intratumoral calcification maybe present. MRI shows an ovarian mass which is hypointense on both T1- and T2W images **(Figs. 34A and B)**. Hyperintense areas may be seen in the T2W images due to edema and cystic degeneration. On contrast administration, a weak and delayed enhancement pattern is seen. Majority of the ovarian fibromas do not show any evidence of restricted diffusion on DWI, however, cellular fibromas may show some restriction. However, ADC measurements in the solid component may be low, possibly due to the lower mean ADCs in benign fibrous tumors associated with dense fibrous stromal proliferation. No signal increase is observed on DWI, despite their low ADCs, probably as a consequence of the T2 blackout effect. Ovarian torsion can occur with fibromas leading to infarction and necrosis. Typically fibromas are benign tumors and can be surgically excised.[2] Nevertheless, some fibromas and thecomas in this group may show restricted diffusion. For instance, functioning thecomas and cellular fibromas may show high SI on DWI and relatively low ADCs **(*see* Fig. 4)**, due to their relatively high cellularity.[35-37]

Thecomas contain lipid rich thecal cells. *Fibrothecomas*, as the name suggests, contain both thecal cells and fibrous tissue. These tumors are much rarer than fibromas and can present with hormonal features of excess estrogen. They do not have distinct US or CT features but as compared to fibromas, may be more hyperintense on T2W images and may show a greater degree of enhancement.

The differential diagnosis of these tumors is similar to that of Brenner tumors as discussed above.

Sclerosing stromal tumor is a rare benign tumor, which is more commonly seen in young adolescent girls, who present with pelvic pain and menstrual irregularity. On US, this neoplasm may mimic a malignant ovarian tumor, as it may be seen as a unilateral solid mass with multiple small hypoechoic cleft-like areas, or a multilocular mass with irregular septae may be seen with intratumoral vascularity. On MRI, it is seen as a solid heterogeneous tumor which is iso- to hyperintense on T2WI, with a spoke-wheel pattern. Dynamic contrast-enhanced (DCE) MRI shows early and avid peripheral contrast uptake, with centripetal progression on late images.[48]

Steroid cell tumors and Leydig cell tumors are other pure stromal tumors which are very rare and often manifest as virilizing tumors of the ovary.

OVARIAN TORSION

Ovarian torsion is the twisting of an ovary on its ligamentous supports resulting in a compromised blood supply. *Adnexal torsion* is a term that is inclusive of torsion of the ovary, the fallopian tube or both. Simultaneously, ovarian and tubal torsion has been shown to occur in upto 60% of cases of adnexal torsion.

Pathophysiology

Ovarian torsion proceeds in a stepwise manner. In the *early phase*, twisting of the vascular pedicle leads to the compromise of the low pressure venous system and lymphatic system first, which causes edema and enlargement of the ovary. In the *later phase*, the arterial circulation also gets compromised causing ischemia and hemorrhagic necrosis.

In more than 50% cases, an underlying mass acts as a lead point for the torsion. The mass can be a functional ovarian cyst (most common—17% of torsed ovaries), benign ovarian

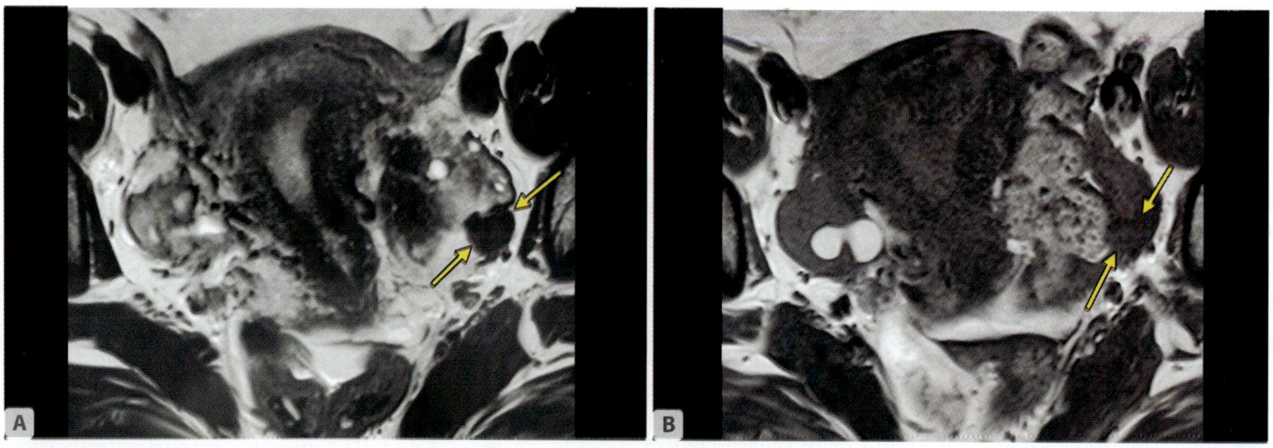

FIGS. 34A AND B: Ovarian fibroma. T2-weighted (T2W) (A) and T1-weighted (T1W) (B) axial magnetic resonance images show a small well-defined mass arising from the left ovary (yellow arrows), which is hypointense on both T2- and T1W images. Two small endometriotic cysts are also seen in the right ovary which show fluid-fluid levels on T2W image and are hyperintense on the T1W image.

neoplasms (of which most common is dermoid cyst, others can be a fibroma or cystadenoma) or a malignant ovarian neoplasm—both primary and metastatic.[49] Even extraovarian masses like a paraovarian cyst or hydrosalpinx can lead to adnexal torsion.

A normal ovary may also undergo torsion, and this is seen more frequently in the younger, adolescent age group, and has been attributed to developmental anomalies like long pelvic ligaments, mobile fallopian tube or mesosalpinx. The right ovary is more likely to torse as compared to the left, which has been attributed to the protective effect of the sigmoid colon on the left.

Clinical Features

Although torsion can occur at any age, it is seen to occur commonly in women of reproductive age, with approximately 20% cases occurring in pregnant women.[48] This could be due to the fact that both, physiological and pathologic ovarian masses, occur more commonly in this age group. Clinically, the patients present with nonspecific acute lower abdominal pain, with associated nausea, vomiting, low grade fever, and moderate leukocytosis. There may be a palpable, tender mass in the lower abdomen.

The clinical differential diagnoses include acute appendicitis, renal colic, diverticulitis, pelvic inflammatory disease (PID), rupture of corpus luteum or hemorrhagic cyst, etc.[50] Sometimes patients may present with repeated attacks of abrupt onset pain with intervening asymptomatic intervals, which occurs due to episodic torsion and detorsion.

Imaging Features

On imaging, the findings will vary depending on the phase in which the patient presents. US is often the first line imaging modality in a case of suspected ovarian torsion. In the early phase, the ovary is seen to be enlarged (>20 cc in volume, or a single maximum diameter >4 cm in premenopausal women), often lying in unusual locations—in the midline, in the pouch of Douglas or anteriorly **(Fig. 35A)**. The enlarged ovary shows hyperechoic stroma, with peripherally placed follicles (due to the follicles being pushed to the periphery by the edematous stroma). The follicles show 1–2 mm thick, hyperechoic margins—the *"follicular ring sign"* which has been described as a specific feature for torsion, and occurs due to edema and hemorrhage in the walls of the follicles. It is better visualized on transvaginal than transabdominal scans **(Fig. 35B)**.[51] When present, an associated mass, the cause of the torsion, can also be identified **(Figs. 36 and 37)**. In later stages, an infarcted or necrotic ovary may be seen as a heterogeneous mass with complete loss of architecture **(Figs. 38A and B)** real-time transvaginal probe tenderness can be elicited.

Identification of the twisted pedicle adjacent to the torsed ovary, although difficult to identify, is a specific sign for torsion. It is seen as a *"target sign"* with a central hyperechoic area with multiple concentric rings around it on cross-section, and an ellipsoid or tubular mass with heterogeneous echotexture in the longitudinal section. The *"whirlpool sign"* is seen on Doppler, when swirling vessels are seen within the twisted pedicle **(Figs. 35C and D)**.[52]

On Doppler, flow in the ovary is variable depending on the degree of vascular obstruction, intermittent torsion and presence of dual blood supply of ovary (from the ovarian and uterine artery). Abnormal Doppler flow has been reported in 35–93% of patients in many studies **(Fig. 35E)**, who have pathologically proven torsion.[50] As the flow patterns are assessed qualitatively, rather than quantitatively, it is difficult to generalize results.[53] However, it is important to remember that the presence of arterial or venous flow, does not exclude the diagnosis of ovarian torsion. Additionally, the lack of color can also be due to technical factors (especially in a transabdominal scan), and does not necessarily mean that the ovary is nonviable.

Ultrasound has a reported sensitivity of almost 100% and specificity of 97%, if there is an enlarged ovary with absent blood flow.[54]

As the clinical picture is one of nonspecific acute abdomen, a CT may often be done as first imaging investigation. MRI is not a primary imaging modality in a suspected case of torsion, but it can be helpful if sonographic findings of torsion are indeterminate. On both, CT and MRI, ovarian torsion can be seen as an enlarged ovary with or without an underlying mass and a twisted pedicle. The uterus is often deviated to the side of the torsion. The enlarged edematous ovary with peripheral follicles is best seen on contrast-enhanced CT or on fast spin-echo T2-weighted MRI **(Figs. 38A to F)**. On noncontrast CT, hemorrhagic infarction is seen as a high-density ovarian hematoma with an HU value ranging between 50 HU and 100 HU, and on T1W fat suppressed MRI, a hyperintense rim of the hematoma can be seen within an enlarged ovary **(Figs. 39A and B)**.[50] Associated free fluid and fat stranding is often seen. An underlying lead point can be identified.

Multiplanar CT reformations or MRI acquisitions can depict the twisted pedicle better as the helical configuration of the broad ligament containing the vascular pedicle and fallopian tube can be better seen on the sagittal or coronal planes **(Fig. 38G)**.

On contrast-enhanced CT and MRI, the torsed ovary may show an abnormal enhancement pattern **(Fig. 39C)**. As the ovarian ischemia progresses to infarction, there may be minimal or absent enhancement. However, as mentioned before, the presence of enhancement does not exclude torsion.

Differential Diagnosis

The differential diagnosis for ovarian torsion is long and includes ectopic pregnancy, hemorrhagic corpus luteum cyst, massive ovarian edema, hyperstimulated ovaries, oophoritis, PID, necrotic metastases, and nonepithelial primary ovarian tumors. Absence of a twisted pedicle and/or presence of a normal enhancement decreases the possibility of ovarian torsion. Sometimes torsion of a pedunculated subserosal or broad ligament fibroid may mimic ovarian torsion. Identification of both the ovaries separate from the torsed, infarcted fibroid can rule out ovarian torsion.

Management

The treatment of choice for ovarian torsion is laparoscopic untwisting of the adnexa with resection of any underlying cystic lesion. It has been found that ovaries can remain

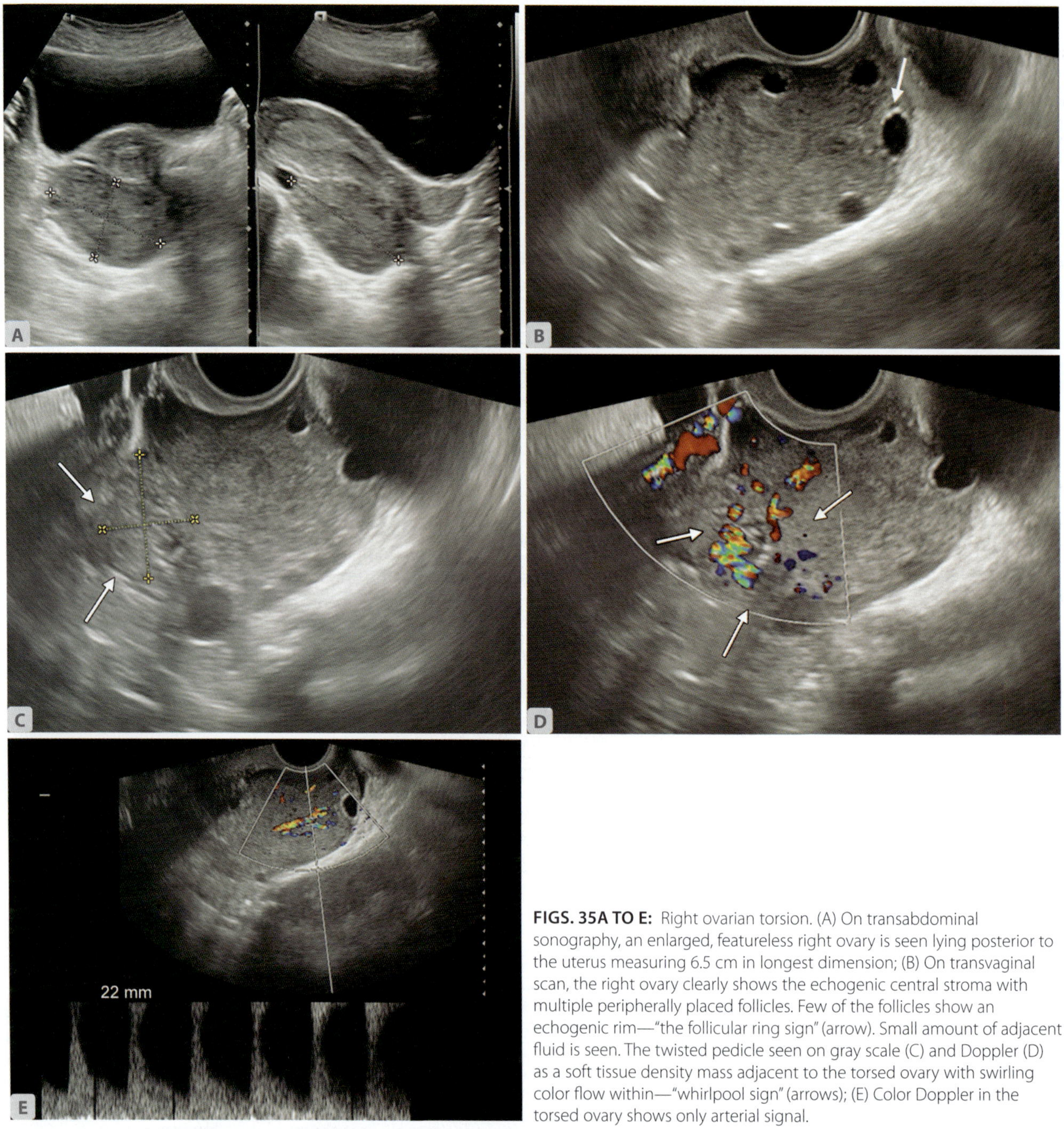

FIGS. 35A TO E: Right ovarian torsion. (A) On transabdominal sonography, an enlarged, featureless right ovary is seen lying posterior to the uterus measuring 6.5 cm in longest dimension; (B) On transvaginal scan, the right ovary clearly shows the echogenic central stroma with multiple peripherally placed follicles. Few of the follicles show an echogenic rim—"the follicular ring sign" (arrow). Small amount of adjacent fluid is seen. The twisted pedicle seen on gray scale (C) and Doppler (D) as a soft tissue density mass adjacent to the torsed ovary with swirling color flow within—"whirlpool sign" (arrows); (E) Color Doppler in the torsed ovary shows only arterial signal.

viable up to 36 hours after twisting. Multiple studies have suggested that even nonviable looking ovaries may retain ovarian function following detorsion and so oophorectomy can be avoided in majority of women. Postoperative follow-up with US has shown that over 80% of patients had a normal follicular development after detorsion.[55,56]

MASSIVE OVARIAN EDEMA

It is rare condition in which there is a marked, tumor-like enlargement of one (or rarely both) ovaries due to accumulation of edema fluid in the ovarian stroma. The right ovary is more commonly involved than the left. The etiology could be due to a partial or intermittent torsion with obstruction of venous and lymphatic supply, sparing the arterial supply, or there may be an underlying stromal proliferation complicated by torsion. It is seen in preadolescent girls, women undergoing ovulation induction or during pregnancy. Patients present with acute or intermittent lower abdominal pain of long duration. Sometimes abnormal uterine bleeding and features of masculinization may be seen due to elevated levels of androgens.

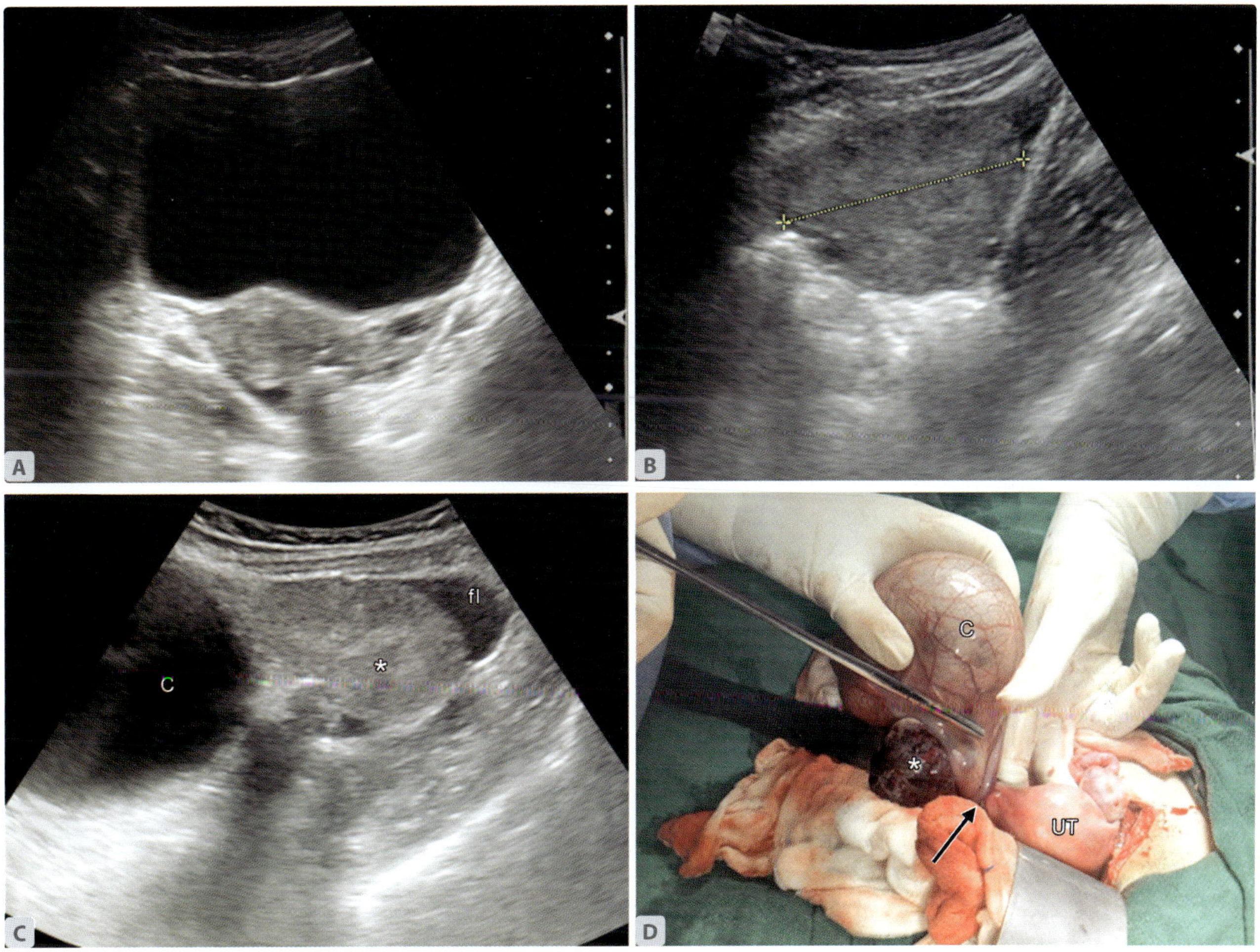

FIGS. 36A TO D: Right ovarian torsion with adjacent paraovaian cyst. A 19-year-old girl presenting with pain in right iliac fossa (RIF). Transabdominal ultrasound of pelvis (A) shows the normal uterus and left ovary. An enlarged superficially placed right ovary is seen in the RIF (B) measuring 5 cm in maximum diameter, with an echogenic groundglass stroma with few peripherally placed follicles. Longitudinal scan in the RIF shows the torsed ovary (*) with a clear, cystic mass superiorly (C); On surgery (D) the discolored, enlarged ovary is seen with its twisted pedicle (arrow) and the paraovarian cyst (C). (UT: uterus; fl: free fluid).

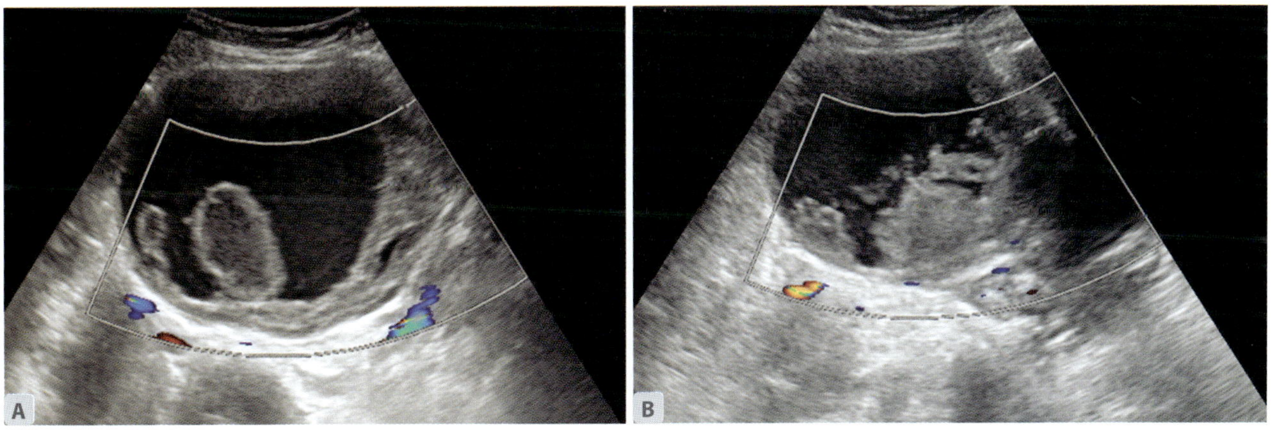

FIGS. 37A AND B: Transabdominal ultrasound scans show torsed hemorrhagic cyst of right ovary with thick walls and no color flow. Retracted clots and debris seen within the cyst.

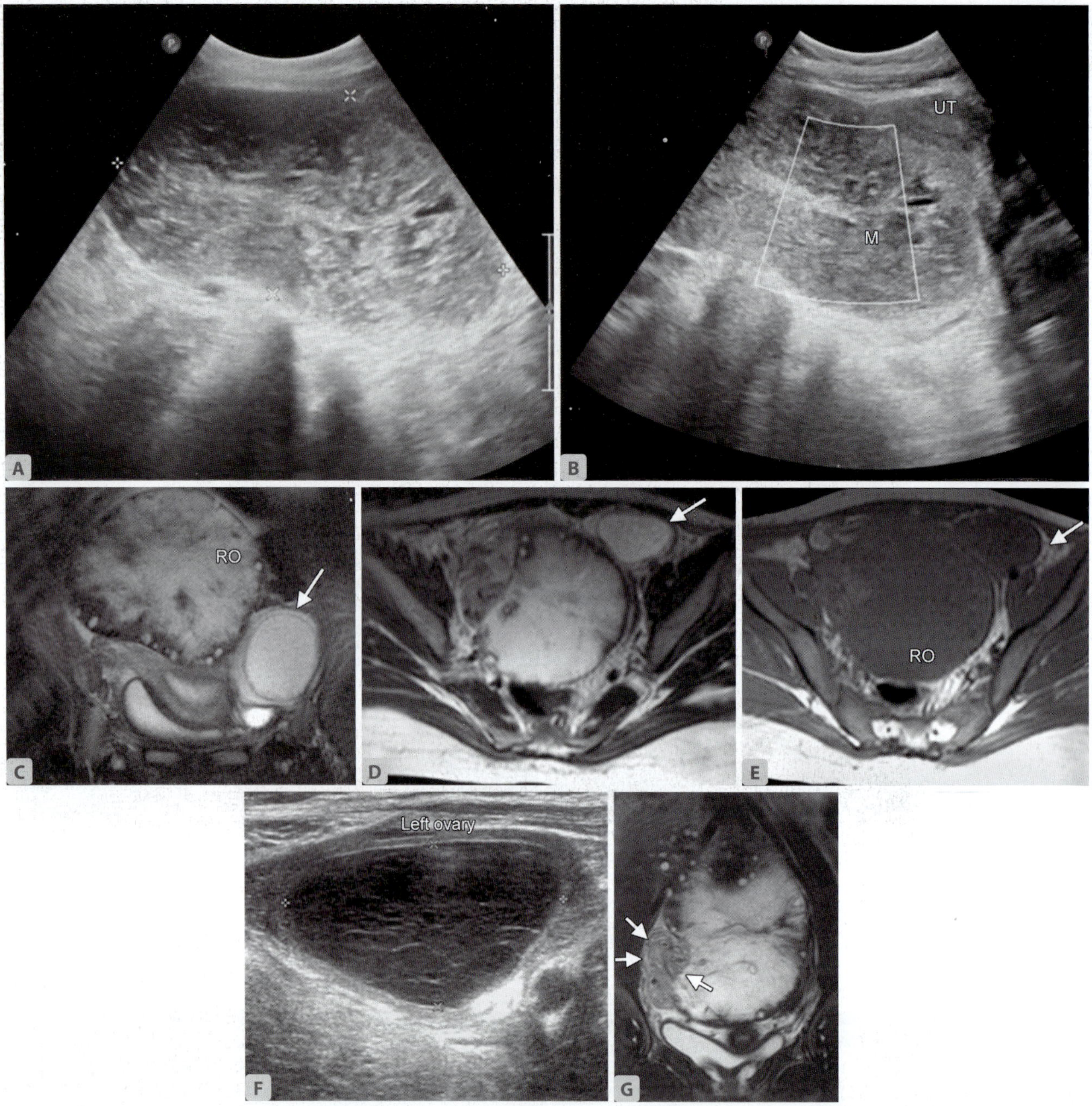

FIGS. 38A TO G: Right ovarian torsion—late stage with a left hemorrhagic cyst. Transabdominal ultrasound (A) in a 17-year-old girl with acute pain lower abdomen shows a markedly enlarged right ovary (measures 14 cm maximum dimension) with a heterogeneous internal echotexture and no flow on color Doppler (B) T2-weighted (T2W) coronal (C) and axial (D) MR images show a markedly enlarged, centrally placed right ovary with hyperintense stroma and multiple peripheral follicles (RO). The left ovary shows a hemorrhagic cyst appearing homogeneously hyperintense on the T2W images (arrows). Both appear hypointense on T1w image; (E) The characteristic internal "fish-net" appearance is better seen on a high frequency, transabdominal ultrasound (F) as the haemorrhagic cyst is superficially placed; (G) T2W coronal MR image taken more posteriorly shows the adjacent twisted pedicle (arrows) (RO: torsed right ovary; UT: uterus).

Imaging Features

On imaging, the ovary is markedly enlarged with a mean maximum diameter of 11.5 cm (range 5–40 cm) with a multicystic appearance. On US, the ovary is seen as a hypoechoic, hypovascular solid mass-like lesion. There is presence of central increased ovarian stroma, and multiple follicles arranged in the peripheral cortex with internal vascularity on color Doppler.[57] MRI shows a hypo- to isointense signal on T1W and markedly hyperintense signal on T2W images, with enhancement on postcontrast scans.[58] Long-standing ovarian edema may lead to *ovarian fibromatosis* in which case US will show a markedly hypoechoic mass, with hypointense mass on both T1 and T2W MR images.[59]

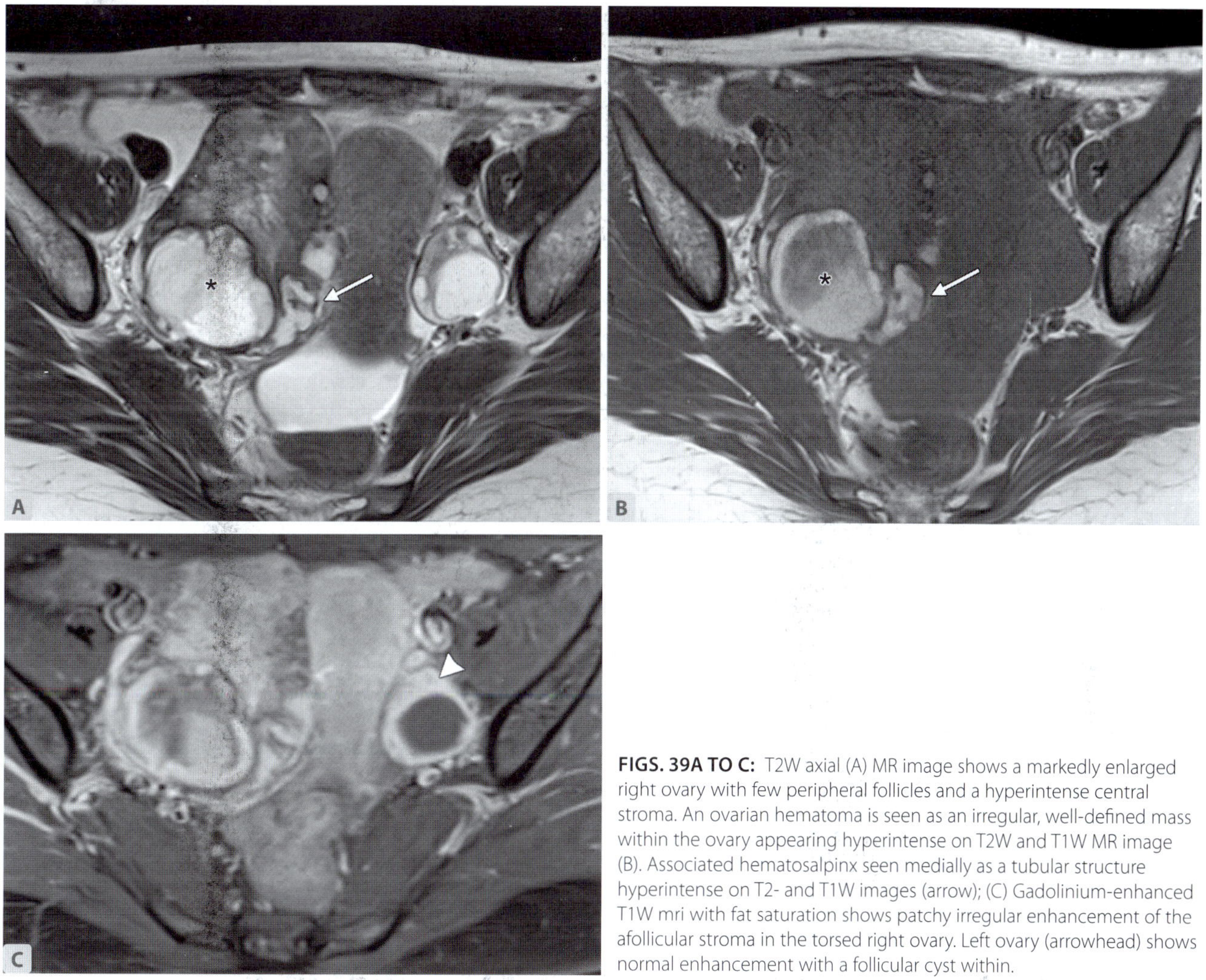

FIGS. 39A TO C: T2W axial (A) MR image shows a markedly enlarged right ovary with few peripheral follicles and a hyperintense central stroma. An ovarian hematoma is seen as an irregular, well-defined mass within the ovary appearing hyperintense on T2W and T1W MR image (B). Associated hematosalpinx seen medially as a tubular structure hyperintense on T2- and T1W images (arrow); (C) Gadolinium-enhanced T1W mri with fat saturation shows patchy irregular enhancement of the afollicular stroma in the torsed right ovary. Left ovary (arrowhead) shows normal enhancement with a follicular cyst within.

PELVIC INFLAMMATORY DISEASE

Pelvic inflammatory disease includes all upper genital tract infections including cervicitis, endometritis, salpingitis, pyosalpinx, oophoritis, TOA, and peritonitis.

Etiopathogenesis

The most frequent cause of PID is an ascending lower genital tract infection, by direct upward extension from the vagina to the cervix, uterine cavity, followed by the fallopian tubes and ovaries, and, finally, to the peritoneal cavity. Less commonly, it may occur by hematogenous spread or extension from adjacent organs. The common causative organisms are the sexually transmitted microorganisms such as *Chlamydia trachomatis, Neisseria gonorrhoeae, Mycoplasma genitalium*, and gram-negative bacteria. Mixed infections are seen in a large number of cases. Tuberculosis and actinomycosis are more often associated with chronic PID.

Acute PID of the adnexal region may manifest as isolated inflammation of one or both fallopian tubes—*salpingitis*, obstructed tube filled with pus; *pyosalpinx*, isolated inflammation of one or both ovaries; *oophoritis*, or more commonly a combined inflammation of the tube and ovary, forming a *tubo-ovarian mass*. Associated *endometritis* and *peritonitis* is often seen. Further progression of infection and inflammation results in the formation of a complex cystic and solid mass with complete destruction of the normal adnexal architecture—the *TOA*.

Clinical Features

Pelvic inflammatory disease is commonly seen in young women with a history of a prior uterine procedure, presence of intrauterine contraceptive device (IUCD) or history of multiple sexual partners.[60] Clinically, patients present with lower abdominal pain, fever, vaginal discharge, dyspareunia, leukocytosis, and other vague constitutional symptoms.

Imaging Features

In *salpingitis*, the inflamed tubes may be seen as thickened (more than 10 mm), tortuous structures with increased color flow due to hyperemia on US and marked enhancement on CT and MRI. *Pyosalpinx* is seen as a tortuous, thick-walled, tubular structure with low level internal echoes representing pus **(Fig. 40)**, with incomplete septae on longitudinal section or a "cog-wheel" appearance on cross-section due to protrusion of mucosa into the lumen. Doppler evaluation shows increased vascularity in the thickened walls and septae. On MRI, the internal contents of a pyosalpinx show an intermediate SI on T1WI and high SI on T2WI. MRI can help in the differentiation of pyosalpinx from hematosalpinx, as hematosalpinx will not show wall thickening and will show high or variable SI on T1W MR images because of the presence of blood products. On CT, the internal contents are usually higher than water density. Adjacent inflammatory fat stranding and free or loculated fluid in the peritubal region and/or the cul-de-sac are often present.

It is rare for *oophoritis* to occur in isolation, but if so, it is seen as enlarged unilateral or bilateral ovaries with hyperemia, and associated adjacent inflammatory changes.

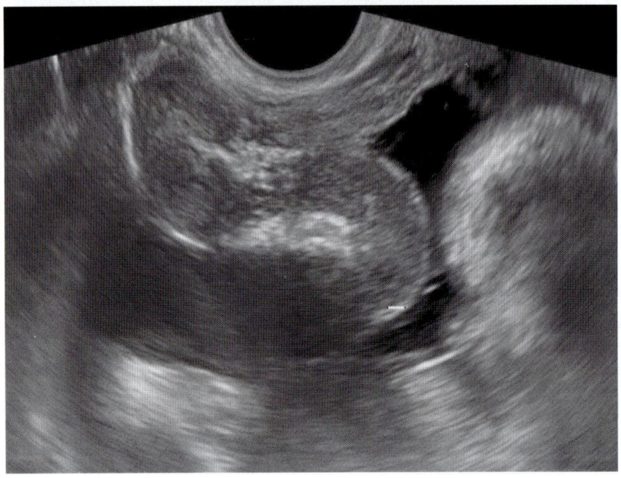

FIG. 40: Pyosalpinx. Transvaginal us shows a convoluted, tubular structure with low level internal echoes and thick walls seen in right adnexal region, with adjacent free fluid.

A *tubo-ovarian mass* is seen as a lobulated, solid or complex cystic-solid mass with increased color flow signals on Doppler interrogation. It is not possible to identify the tubes or ovaries separately **(Figs. 41A and B)**. A *TOA* has a variable appearance on sonography. Typically, it is seen as a unilocular or multilocular complex cystic-solid mass with irregular borders and thickened wall, with internal debris or fluid-debris level within the cystic component. Color Doppler shows peripheral vascularity and allows distinction of fluid from solid areas **(Figs. 42 and 43)**. Probe tenderness on US is often elicited. On CT, a complex cystic solid mass with marked enhancement of walls and septae can be seen. Presence of air within the cystic component is best seen on CT and is the most specific sign of an abscess, however, it is unusual in a TOA. On MRI, the abscess fluid has a variable signal depending on the viscosity and protein concentration. It is heterogeneous and usually low (equal to muscle) on T1WI, high on fat suppressed T1WI and T2WI. A rim of hyperintensity maybe seen along the inner margin of the wall on T1WI, which is due to a layer of granulation tissue with focal areas of hemorrhage **(Figs. 43C and D)**. On postcontrast CT and MRI, enhancement of the thickened irregular wall, septations and adjacent inflammation is a hallmark of PID **(Fig. 43E)**. Restricted diffusion with low ADC values is seen in the pus-filled abscess cavities **(Figs. 43F and G)**.

Specific Pelvic Inflammatory Disease

Tuberculosis is a very common cause of chronic pelvic inflammatory disease (PID) in our country. Infection generally spreads from an extragenital source. It can be hematogenous, via lymphatic vessels or from the peritoneal cavity. Tubercular PID often shows bilateral adnexal involvement with salpingitis, TOAs, endometritis, peritoneal spread in the form of free, and/or loculated ascites, peritoneal, mesenteric, and omental thickening. It can mimic peritoneal carcinomatosis from ovarian carcinoma **(Figs. 44 and 45)**. It is important to remember that CA-125 levels may also be

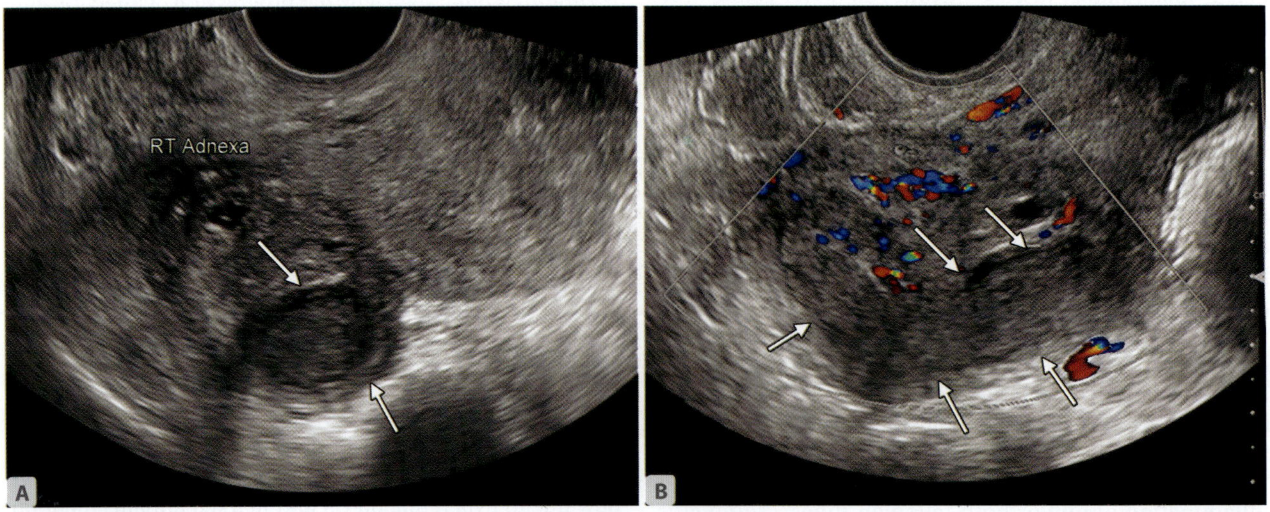

FIGS. 41A AND B: Tubo-ovarian mass. Transvaginal ultrasound transverse (A) and longitudinal Doppler (B) scans show an ill-defined hypoechoic solid mass in the right adnexal region, adherent to the uterus. A focal area of low level echoes represents the pus-filled fallopian tube (arrows). Scattered color signals are seen in the inflammatory solid mass and walls of the pyosalpinx.

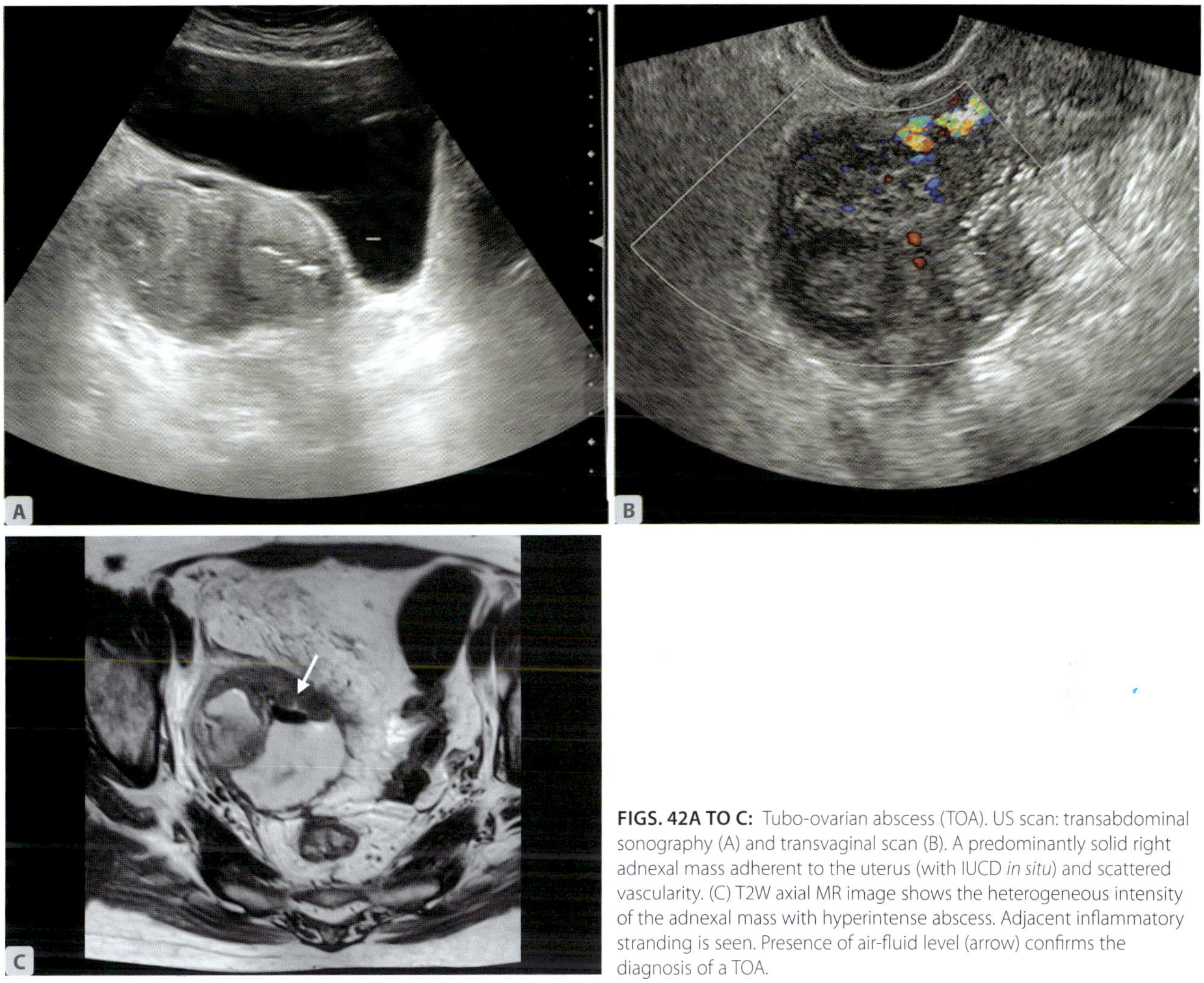

FIGS. 42A TO C: Tubo-ovarian abscess (TOA). US scan: transabdominal sonography (A) and transvaginal scan (B). A predominantly solid right adnexal mass adherent to the uterus (with IUCD *in situ*) and scattered vascularity. (C) T2W axial MR image shows the heterogeneous intensity of the adnexal mass with hyperintense abscess. Adjacent inflammatory stranding is seen. Presence of air-fluid level (arrow) confirms the diagnosis of a TOA.

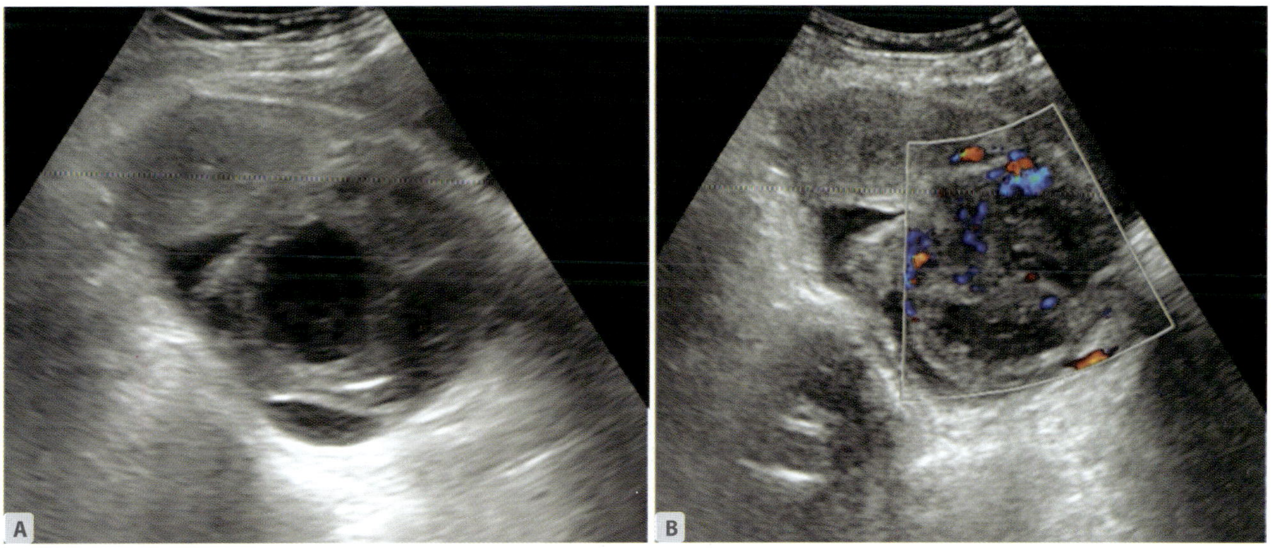

FIGS. 43A TO G: *Continued*

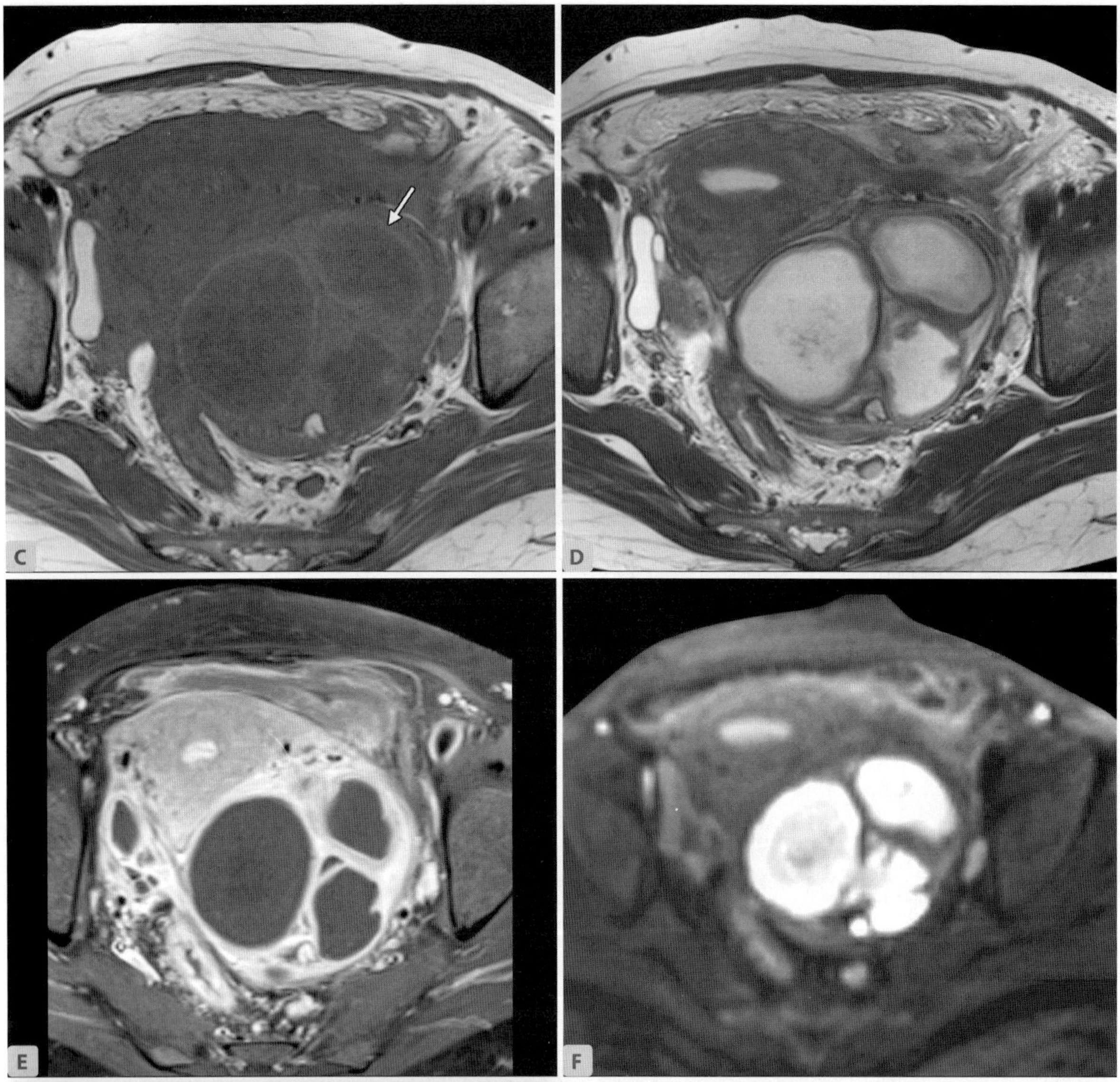

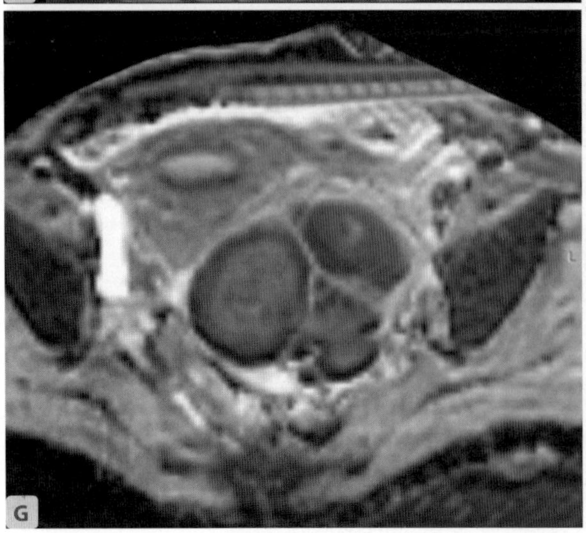

FIGS. 43A TO G: Tubo-ovarian abscess (TOA) in a 26-year-old woman with pain in lower abdomen. (A) Ultrasound shows a thick-walled multiloculated cystic left adnexal mass with thick septae. Small amount of free fluid is also seen (B) Color signals are seen in the wall and septae. T1W (C) and T2W (D) axial MR images show thick-walled tubulocystic left adnexal mass appearing iso- to hypointense on T1W and hyperintense on T2W images. A T1 hyperintense rim is seen along the inner walls of the cystic areas representing granulation tissue. (E) Intense enhancement is seen in the wall and septae and in the surrounding soft tissues. Culture of pus confirmed a tubercular TOA. (F) Axial DWI at b = 800 sec/mm^2 and corresponding apparent diffusion coefficient (ADC) map (G) shows evidence of restricted diffusion in the cystic spaces (bright on DWI, and dark on the ADC map) with a low ADC value of $<0.6 \times 10^{-3}$ mm^2/sec due to purulent material.

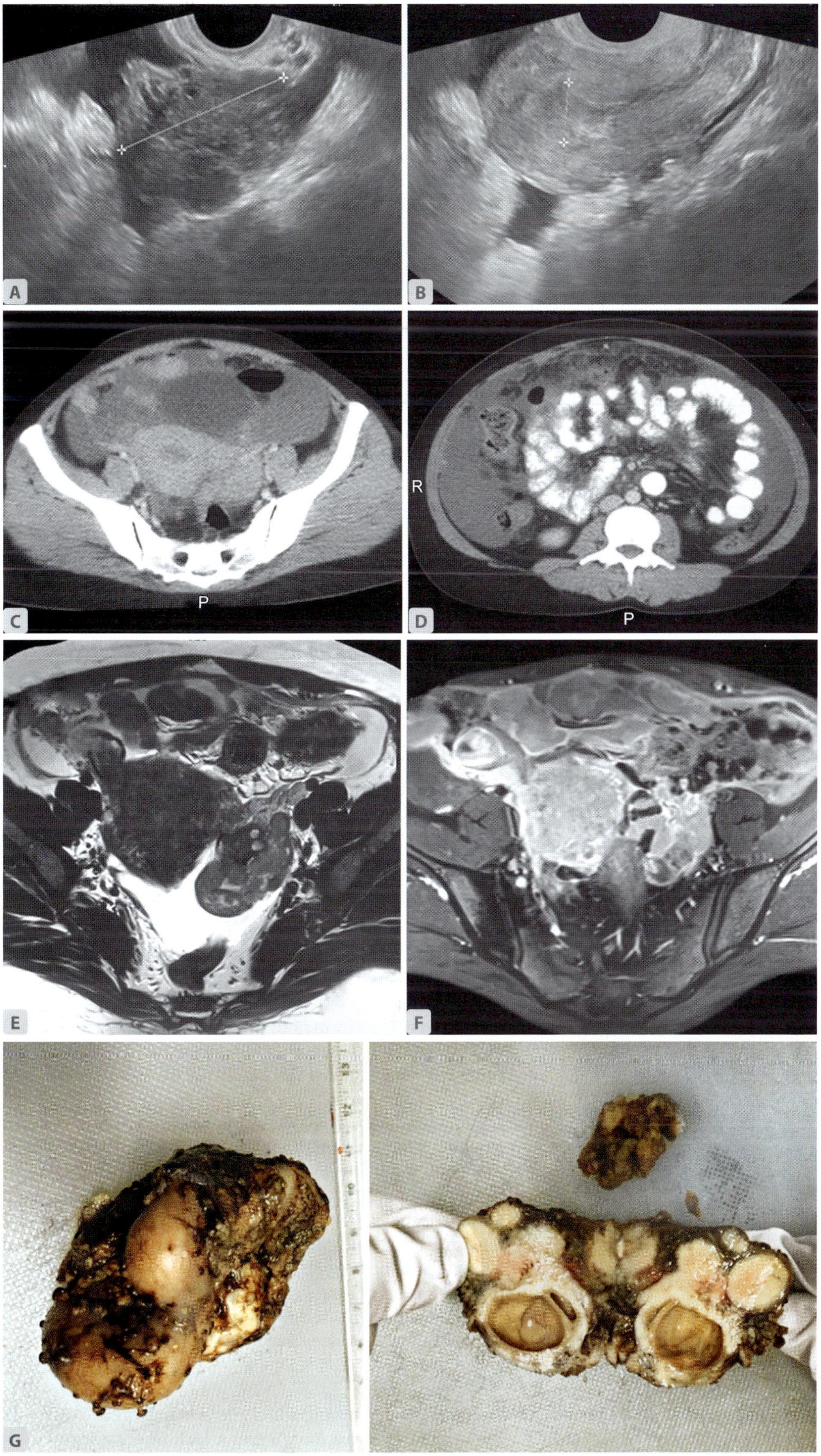

FIGS. 44A TO G: Tubercular pelvic inflammatory disease (PID). A 35-year-old woman with abdominal distension, loss of weight, and appetite. Transvaginal ultrasound (A and B) axial contrast-enhanced computed tomography (CECT) section pelvis (C) shows an irregular heterogeneous predominantly solid mass in left adnexa, with associated ascites. Ill-defined endometrial thickening is seen in the uterus—endometritis. There is peritoneal thickening and omental stranding seen in axial CECT section of abdomen (D) T2W axial MR pelvis (E) shows a predominantly hypointense left adnexal mass with ascites; Contrast-enhanced MRI (F) shows marked enhancement of the mass, uterus, and adjacent tissues; (G) On surgery, the left adnexal mass seen to be a thickened tube wrapped around left ovary with multiple small caseous nodules studding outer surface of mass and peritoneum.

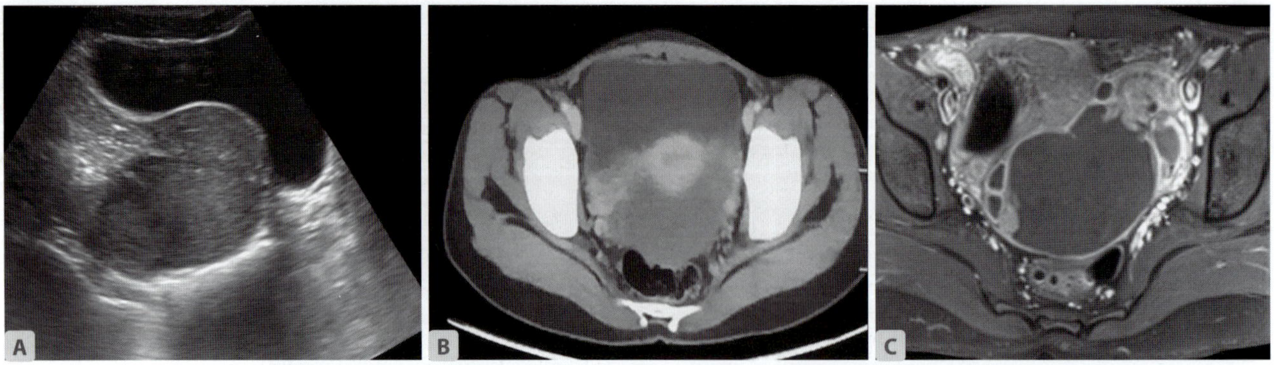

FIGS. 45A TO C: Tubercular tubo-ovarian abscess in a 16-year-old girl with low-grade fever and constitutional symptoms for 2 months. Transabdominal ultrasound; (A) CECT axial scan; (B) and CEMR scan (C) through the pelvis show a large abscess involving bilateral ovaries and tubes posterior to the uterus.

raised in tubercular PID, although not as high as in malignant carcinomatosis.

Associated lymphadenopathy, sometimes necrotic, can be seen. Generally, tubercular adnexal masses are not tender on US probe pressure. Dense adhesions with uterus and adjacent organs can occur. Calcifications maybe seen in the adnexal lesions and/or in the lymph nodes, best visualized on CT. Florid enhancement of the adnexal masses and adjacent tissues on CT and MRI, is characteristic of tubercular infection.

Actinomycosis is an uncommon pelvic infection usually seen in the presence of an intrauterine device. The findings mimic tuberculosis. The adnexal mass in actinomycosis is predominantly a solid lesion with low SI on T2-weighted images. Cystic elements are less common. There is diffuse infiltration of the uterus, adnexa, and pelvic muscles with loss of fascial planes. The presence of an IUCD further corroborates the diagnosis. Identification of sulfur granules in the aspirate is diagnos is of actinomycotic infection.[61]

Xanthogranulomatous inflammation (XGI) can also rarely involve the female genital tract. It is an uncommon form of chronic inflammation in which there is destruction of the tissues of affected organs, which are replaced by lipid-containing macrophages and lymphocytes, plasma cells, multinucleated giant cells, and neutrophils. It is more commonly seen to affect the kidney and gallbladder. The proposed causes are infection, ineffective antibiotic therapy, endometriosis, abnormality in lipid metabolism or ineffective clearance of bacteria by phagocytes. The uterus is more commonly affected. Adnexal involvement is seen as a complex adnexal mass with multiple internal cystic lesions on US and MRI. The imaging findings are nonspecific, resembling a chronic PID or even a malignant lesion. It is almost impossible to make a diagnosis of XGI on imaging, however the pathological findings show the characteristic xanthogranulomas.[62]

Complications

A common sequela of PID is damage to the fallopian tubes, due to scarring and adhesions within the lumen and in the peritubal fat, which leads to obstruction of the tubes. Tubal damage leads to ectopic pregnancies, hydrosalpinx formation and infertility. About 40–50% of cases of infertility can be attributed to previous PID.[63] There can be formation of peritoneal adhesions which can lead to small or large bowel obstruction, or ureteric obstruction. Peritoneal inclusion cysts can also occur secondary to PID.

Fitz-Hugh-Curtis syndrome is a rare complication of PID that is seen in 1–30% of cases, associated with PID caused by *N. gonorrhoeae* and *C. trachomatis.*[62] It is seen as an inflammation of the peritoneal capsule of the liver and is believed to result from peritoneal spread of pelvic infection along the right paracolic gutter. On CT, an intense enhancement and thickening of the anterior liver capsule is seen with geographic areas of variable perfusion in the subcapsular and periportal locations. Loculated perihepatic fluid may be seen and classic "violin string" adhesions may be found between the liver capsule and the anterior abdominal wall. Associated gallbladder wall thickening can occur.

Differential Diagnosis

Pelvic Endometriosis

Endometriomas can mimic ovarian abscesses, hematosalpinx can be difficult to differentiate from pyosalpinx. Associated adhesions can occur in both conditions. At MRI, the presence of T1 hyperintensity within the lesions or in the fallopian tube can help confirm the diagnosis of endometriosis and differentiate it from PID.

Hemorrhagic cysts are common mimics of PID. Clinical manifestations are frequently nonspecific and unhelpful in distinguishing between these entities. Characteristic features of hemorrhagic cysts include the presence of a unilocular adnexal cyst with a ring of peripheral contrast enhancement and an internal high-attenuation component with or without a fluid-hematocrit level.

Ovarian neoplasms can mimic the complex cystic-solid masses of PID, especially in chronic cases, where peritoneal and mesenteric involvement may also be present.

Ovarian Torsion

Distinguishing features include an enlarged ovary with a diameter of more than 5 cm, a lack of enhancement on contrast administration, and uterine deviation toward the affected side.

Other adjacent inflammatory conditions such as acute appendicitis or diverticulitis can mimic PID. An inflamed pus-filled pelvic appendix maybe impossible to differentiate from a pyosalpinx. The presence of an appendicolith, cecal origin of the tubular structure, and the presence of cecal wall thickening are helpful distinguishing features of appendicitis.

Management

In the absence of complications, PID is generally treated conservatively with a short course of oral antibiotics. However, complicated PID frequently requires hospitalization of patients with intravenous administration of antibiotics, in addition to percutaneous or surgical drainage of pelvic abscesses, if present. Specific PIDs like tubercular or actinomycotic infection have to be treated as per protocol.

EXTRAOVARIAN DISEASE

TUBAL PATHOLOGY

Tubal Dilatation/Hydrosalpinx

Tubal dilatation results from an accumulation of secretions when the tube is occluded at its distal end, fimbrial/ampullary end, or both ends, with dilatation of the proximal portion of the tube. Hydrosalpinx is used as a generic term for a dilated tube. It can contain serous fluid, blood, or pus may accumulate, depending on the cause of the dilatation. *Serous hydrosalpinx* occurs when the tube gets occluded by postinflammatory or postsurgical adhesions, or due to tubal ligation and contains serous fluid. A fallopian tube distended with blood is referred to as *hematosalpinx*, is seen commonly with endometriosis, in an ectopic tubal pregnancy, in obstructive developmental lesions in association with hematometra and rarely in association with a tubal malignancy. A tube filled with pus is referred to as *pyosalpinx* which is commonly associated with acute or chronic PID.

Clinical Features

Clinically, the patient may present with lower abdominal pain or with symptoms of the underlying cause of the tubal dilatation. In others, hydrosalpinx may be incidental finding in an asymptomatic woman.

Imaging Features

On imaging, the objective is to first recognize the tubal origin of a cystic mass in the adnexal region, and then to characterize its nature and if possible, the cause. Sonographically, dilated fallopian tubes are seen as tubular, fluid-filled structures that are folded upon themselves to form a C or S shape **(Figs. 40 and 46A)** or, at times, a multilocular mass, in the adnexal region, separate from the uterus and ovary. Incomplete septations, which result from segments of distended tube folding over/adhering to other tubal segments, are a characteristic appearance. Longitudinal folds present in a normal tube may become thickened in the presence of a hydrosalpinx, seen as small round nodules less than 3 mm in size—the characteristic *cogwheel* or *beads on a string* sign appearance when imaged in cross section **(*see* Fig. 40)**. The *waist* sign can be seen as indentations on the opposite sides of the wall and is pathognomonic of a hydrosalpinx.[64] A 3D US can depict the tubular nature of the dilated tube better than the 2D examination.

A hysterosalpingogram will show a dilated fallopian tube, filling with contrast and with absence of free spillage. It can be tubular or retort-shaped **(Fig. 46B)**.

Multiplanar imaging can be helpful in confirming the tubular nature of an adnexal mass or demonstrating incomplete septations, thus confirming it to originate from

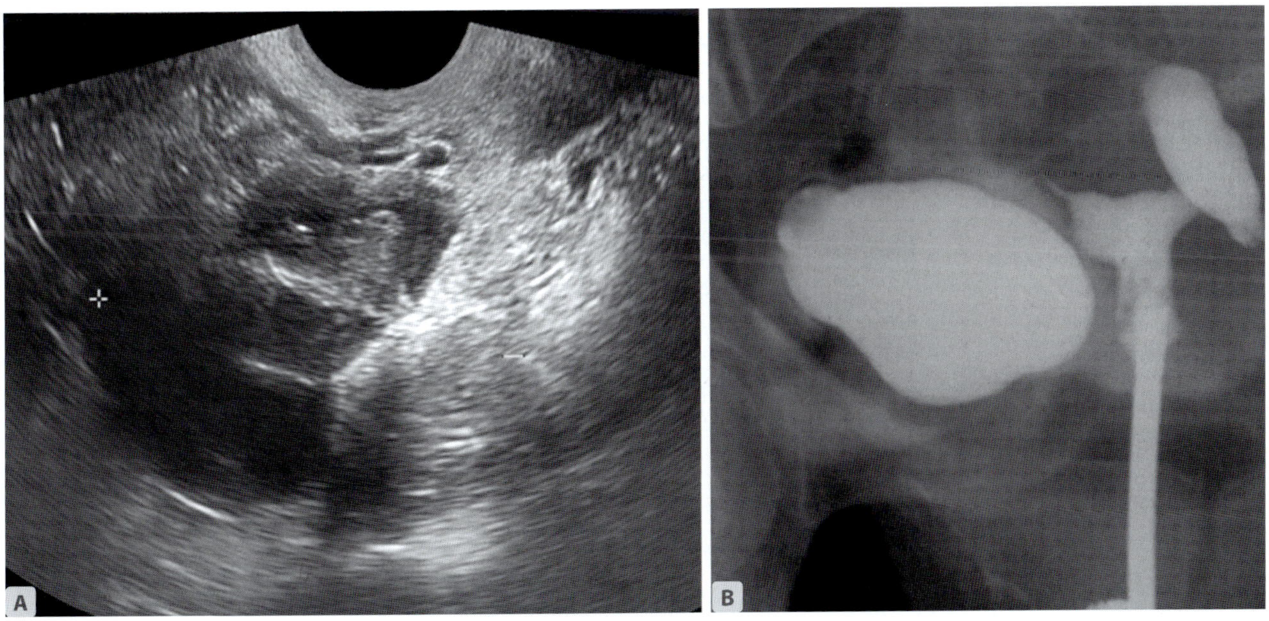

FIGS. 46A AND B: Hydrosalpinx. TVUS (A) showing fluid-filled, C-shaped tortuous dilated tube with incomplete septation; (B) HSG, in another case, showing both the fallopian tubes to be markedly dilated (right more than left), with no tubal spill.

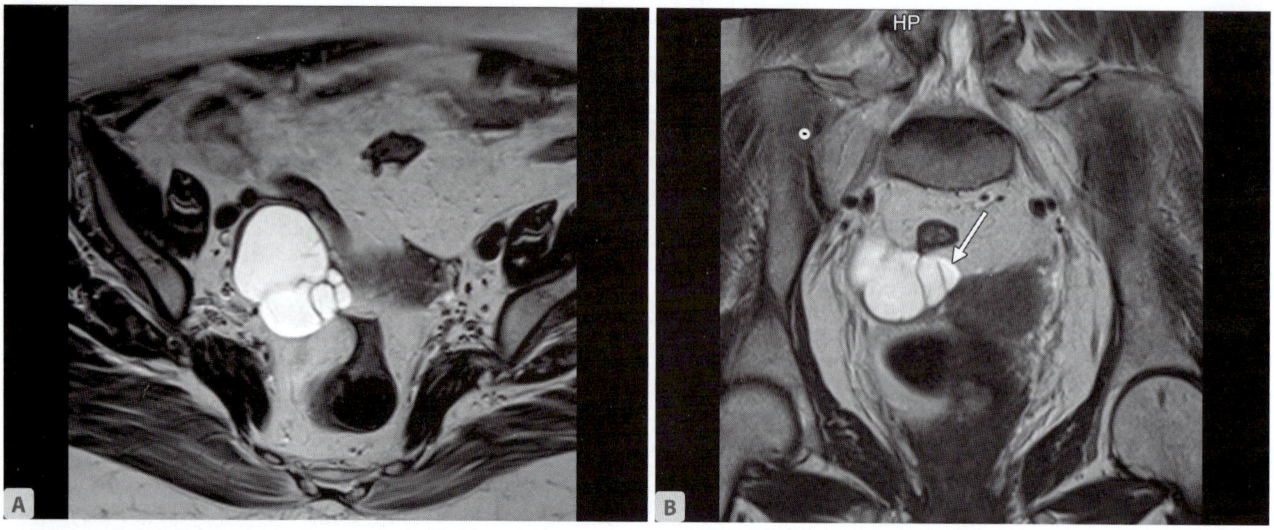

FIGS. 47A AND B: Hydrosalpinx. T2W axial (A) and coronal (B) MR images show a well-defined multiloculated cystic mass on the axial images which can be identified as a hydrosalpinx on the coronal scan, as the convoluted nature of tube with incomplete septae (arrow) can be well seen.

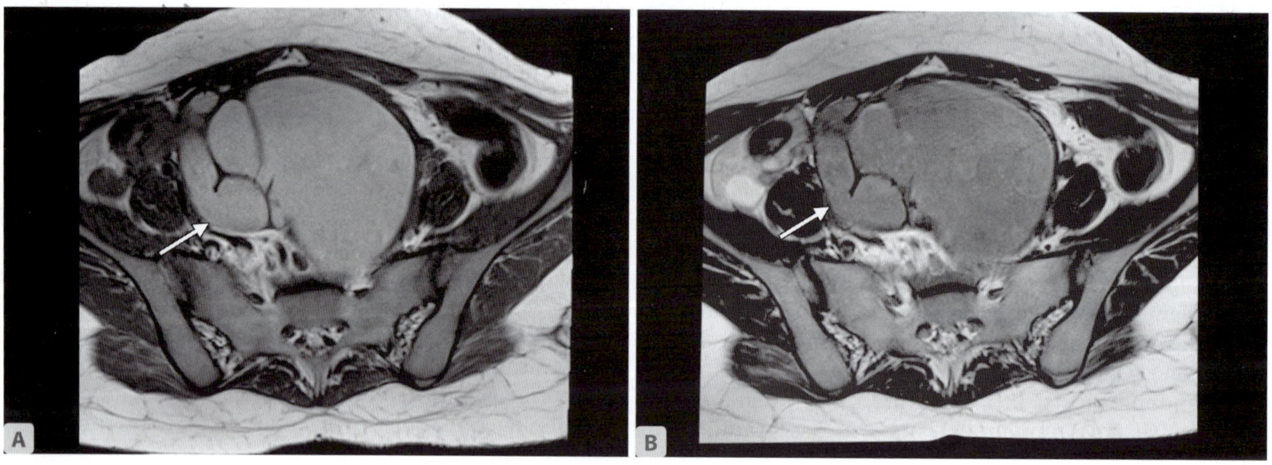

FIGS. 48A AND B: Hematosalpinx in a case of endometriosis. A dilated tortuous structure with incomplete septations appearing hyperintense on axial T1W MR image (A) and hypointense on T2W MR image (B) consistent with the dilated, blood filled left fallopian tube.

the fallopian tube **(Figs. 47A and B)**. In case of a complex cystic adnexal mass, it may not be possible to establish the tubular nature by US. MR can help to show the incomplete septations and to identify the separate normal ovary. MR can also assist in determining the etiology of the tubal dilatation. If hydrosalpinx is due to endometriosis, SI characteristics of the tubal fluid are similar to those in endometriomas, i.e. high T1 and low T2 signal intensities **(Figs. 48A and B)**. In a patient with adhesions, SI of the dilated tube follows that of simple fluid—low on T1 and high on T2W images.

Complications and Differential Diagnosis

Dilated tubes can lead to infertility due to obstruction. They can also undergo torsion. If the tubular nature of the cystic adnexal mass is not recognized, they can be confused with benign cystic neoplasms, PICs, paravarian or functional ovarian cysts. Management will depend on the cause of the tubal dilatation.

Ectopic Pregnancy

A tubal ectopic pregnancy is another very important tubal pathology that presents as an adnexal mass lesion. A detailed discussion of this topic is beyond the scope of this chapter. A few salient features are mentioned here.

The most common site for ectopic pregnancy is the fallopian tubes, occurring in up to 97% of cases of which 75–80% are located in the ampullary region.[65] The ovary, cervix, abdominal cavity, etc. are other less common sites of ectopic pregnancy. The diagnosis is usually reached by a combination of clinical presentation and correlation of last menstrual period, β-hCG levels, and findings on sonography.

The imaging findings will depend on the stage at which examined, i.e. whether there is: (1) unruptured live ectopic,

(2) early embryonic demise without rupture, or (3) ruptured ectopic with hemoperitoneum.

In an unruptured live ectopic, the most specific finding for ectopic pregnancy is seen, i.e. presence of a live extrauterine pregnancy showing a fetal pole with cardiac activity. However, it is positive in only 8–26% of ectopic pregnancies on TVS.[66] The next most specific sign is the presence of an extrauterine gestation sac containing a yolk sac, with or without an embryo. The "tubal ring" of ectopic pregnancy is another finding which has been found to be 40–68% sensitive for ectopic pregnancy.[67] The tubal ring represents an extrauterine gestation sac with trophoblastic tissue. The use of color Doppler shows a "ring of fire" pattern and a high-velocity, low-impedance flow which is compatible with placental perfusion. The most important differential diagnosis is from a corpus luteum cyst which is also very vascular and shows a similar appearance on color flow imaging. However, the most common, but less specific finding of an ectopic pregnancy is a complex adnexal mass separate from the ovary which is most often seen in a nonviable ectopic pregnancy. In the case of ruptured ectopic, a hemoperitoneum may be seen along with a complex adnexal mass.

On MRI, a heterogeneous adnexal mass separate from the ovary and/or a hematosalpinx, with or without hemoperitoneum can be seen.

Differential Diagnosis

The important considerations in the differential diagnosis are corpus luteum cyst, hydrosalpinx, endometrioma, or a ruptured hemorrhagic ovarian cyst.

Paraovarian and Paratubal Cysts

Paraovarian and paratubal cysts represent 10–20% of all adnexal masses and most commonly occur in the 3rd to 4th decade. Paraovarian cysts are remnants of the mesonephric (Wolffian) ducts and are seen close to the ovary, whereas paratubal cysts include hydatid cysts of Morgagni (fimbrial cysts), cysts arising from the paramesonephric (Müllerian) ducts and mesosalpingeal cysts, and are situated a little away from the ovary.[3]

Imaging Features

Paraovarian cysts are unilocular cysts of variable size, with an average diameter of 8 cm at diagnosis, but may reach very large sizes even occupying the whole abdomen. Sonographically, these cysts are round to oval in shape, anechoic with good sound transmission and morphologically indistinguishable from simple functional cysts. A normal ovary seen separately

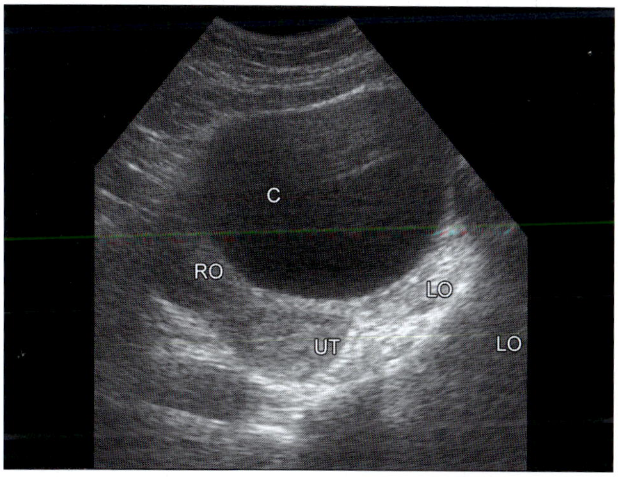

FIG. 49: Paraovarian cyst in a 22-year-old woman with right iliac fossa pain. Transabdominal US image shows a unilocular, thin-walled, cyst (C) adjacent to the right ovary (RO). Both ovaries are seen separately. (UT: uterus; LO: left ovary).

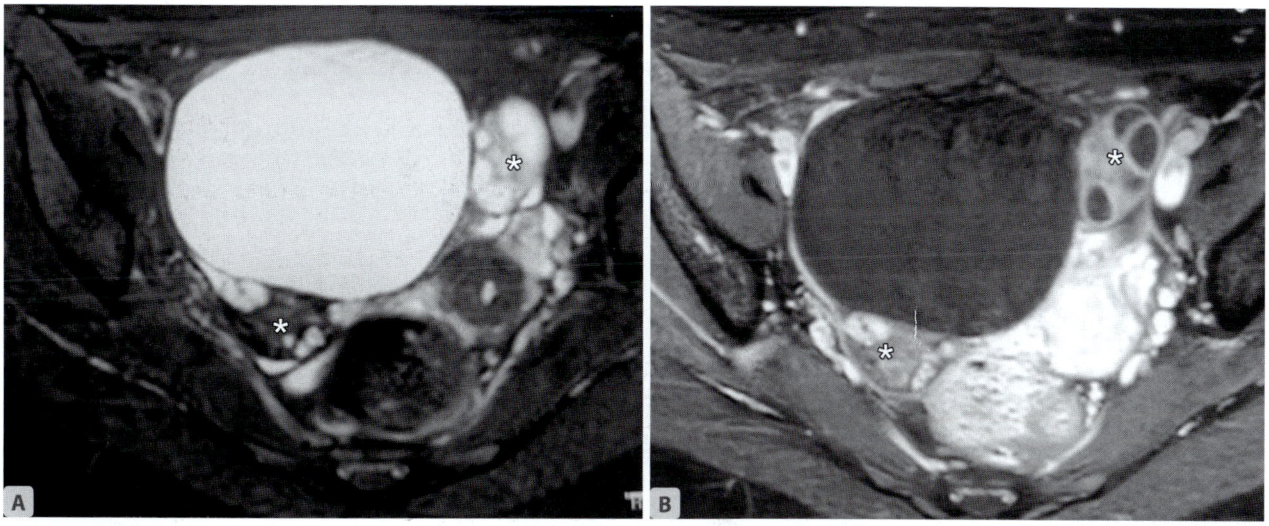

FIGS. 50A AND B: Paraovarian cyst. T2WFS (A) and T1FSCE (B) axial MR images show a large, simple cyst hyperintense on T2W and hypointense on T1W scans with no enhancing focus. Both the ovaries are seen separately (*).

from the cyst is a pointer to a paraovarian cyst **(Fig. 49)**. They may indent the ovary mimicking an intraovarian cyst, but US probe pressure may show separation from ovary. Fimbrial cysts or hydatid cysts of Morgagni can be seen as multiple, small, thin walled, anechoic cysts. Occasionally, their attachment to the fibrial end of tube may become evident in the presence of fluid in the pelvic cavity.

On CT, a round or oval cystic structure is seen close to the ovary, but separate from it. MRI shows the cyst as a well-defined homogeneous structure, with high SI on T2-wieghted images and low SI on T1-weighted images. MRI can clearly depict the independent relationship of the ovary to an adjacent paraovarian cyst **(Figs. 50A and B)**. Complicated cyst (torsion or hemorrhage) may demonstrate high SI on T1-weighted images and have thick walls.

Differential Diagnosis and Complications

Simple paraovarian cysts need to be differentiated from follicular cyst, PIC, simple benign epithelial neoplasm, benign teratoma or a hydrosalpinx. Rarely, these cysts may be complicated by torsion, infection or hemorrhage, in which case they can show thick walls and turbid internal echoes. A complicated paraovarian cyst may resemble an endometrioma, a hemorrhagic cyst or a serous cystadenoma. Malignancy is rare in cysts less than 5 cm. The presence of soft-tissue component within the cyst, which shows vascularity on US, and/or enhancement on contrast-enhanced magnetic resonance imaging (CEMRI) is indicative of a neoplasm.[67]

Management

Simple, asymptomatic paratubal or paraovarian cysts are generally managed conservatively. Surgical removal is indicated if they are symptomatic (persistent pain or pressure symptoms), undergo torsion or appear neoplastic.

Peritoneal Inclusion Cyst

Peritoneal inclusion cysts are also known as cystic mesotheliomas, peritoneal pseudocysts or inflammatory cysts of the peritoneum. They were first described by Mennemeyer and Smith in 1979.[68] They are relatively occurring lesions which are frequently misdiagnosed.

Pathophysiology

The ovary is responsible for secretion of fluid into the peritoneum, contributing to the normally occurring peritoneal fluid. This fluid, in turn, is absorbed by the normal peritoneum. When the peritoneum is damaged, its absorption properties become slower, leading to a decrease in the clearance of the ovarian fluid, which collects in the peritoneal cavity in the form of fluid containing cysts. The development of a PIC, thus depends on the presence of peritoneal adhesions and an active ovary.[69,70]

A PIC maybe a unilocular or multilocular lesion containing clear or yellow-colored serous or gelatinous fluid or sometimes even a hemorrhagic pulp-like material. Histologically, the cyst is lined by one or several layers of mesothelial cells. Although these cells may undergo squamous metaplasia, a PIC does not have any malignant potential.[71]

Clinical Features

Peritoneal inclusion cysts are most commonly seen in premenopausal women with a history of previous abdominal or pelvic surgery, trauma, PID (especially tuberculosis), inflammatory bowel disease or endometriosis.[72] Patients present with chronic or intermittent lower abdominal or pelvic pain, abdominal distension, tenderness, mass, and pressure symptoms like dyspareunia, urinary hesitancy, or constipation. Cancer antigen 125 (CA 125) is usually normal. In 10% cases, these may be detected incidentally in asymptomatic patients.

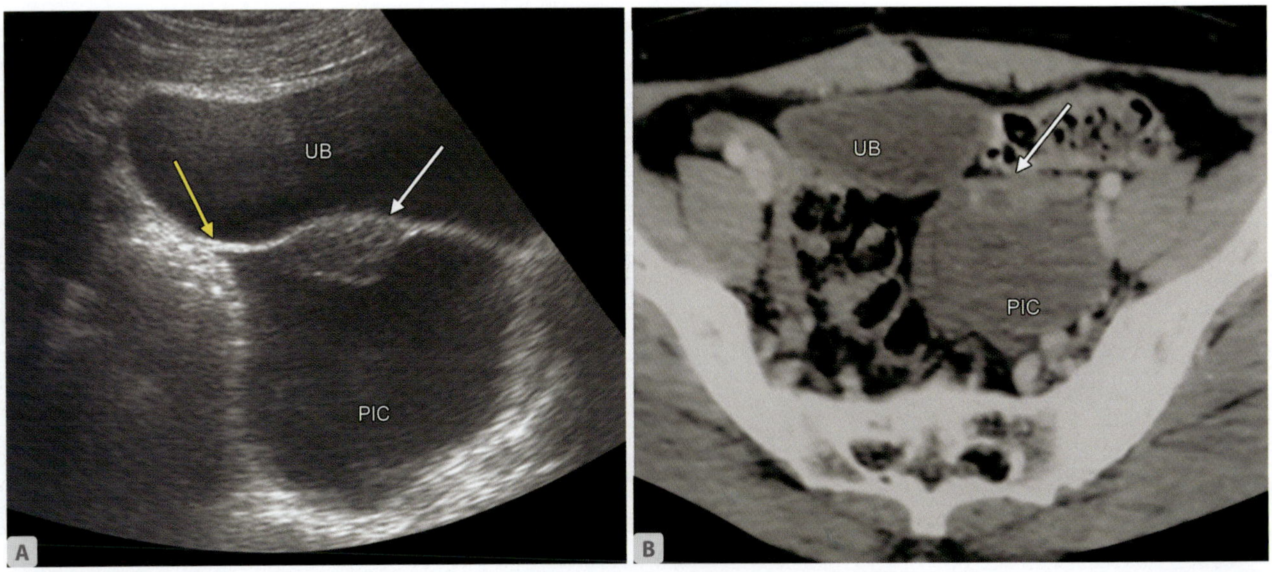

FIGS. 51A AND B: Peritoneal inclusion cyst in a 32-year-old woman with history of previous pelvic surgery. Transabdominal US (A) and axial CECT pelvis (B) show an anechoic, unilocular cystic lesion behind the bladder. The left ovary is seen to lie within the cyst along its anterior margin (white arrows). US scan shows the angular margins very well (yellow arrow). (UB: urinary bladder; PIC: peritoneal inclusion cyst).

Imaging Features

On US, they are seen as variable sized (few mm to large masses almost filling the abdominal cavity), multiseptated, cystic structures which are in close contact with the ovaries and uterus. They are frequently anechoic, but sometimes may show internal echoes due to debris or hemorrhage. The ovary may, at times, be completely surrounded by the PIC. Septations may be complete, incomplete, of varying thickness, and maybe nodular or polypoid. Unilocular and multifocal cysts may also be seen. A characteristic feature of these cysts is the irregular shape with projections around the normal structures, conforming to the peritoneal space, which is explained by the fact that these are not true cysts, but collections of fluid within peritoneal adhesions **(Figs. 51A and B)**.

Computed tomography and MR are useful in defining the exact extent of the lesion and for identifying presence of multiple cysts. Large multiseptated cysts with fluid attenuation can be seen on CT, while MR shows homogeneous fluid SI that is hypointense on T1 and hyperintense on T2W images. If the protein content of the cyst is high or hemorrhage has occurred into the cyst, intermediate to hyperintense T1 signal can be seen. The fluid can be better seen to conform to the shape of the peritoneal cavity with these imaging techniques. On contrast administration, the septations are seen to enhance **(Figs. 52A to C)**.

Differential Diagnosis

Cystic ovarian neoplasms—benign and malignant, functional cysts of the ovary, paraovarian cysts, hydro- or pyosalpinx, lymphangioma, complex loculated ascites, early stages of pseudomyxoma peritonei can all be considered in the differential diagnosis of PICs.

The diagnosis of PICs should be suspected in the right clinical setting, and depends on the presence of normal ipsilateral ovary with surrounding loculated fluid conforming to the peritoneal space. The extra-ovarian location of the lesion and identification of a normal ovary enables a definitive diagnosis. Stable imaging appearance on follow-up imaging over a period of 6 months to 1 year can also help to establish the diagnosis.[73]

Management

Peritoneal inclusion cysts tend to grow slowly, and although they are not associated with any increased mortality, they are a cause of long-term morbidity. The treatment options are varied and will depend on the clinical symptoms, imaging findings, confidence of diagnosis, and the clinician's choice: (1) Conservative approach, with use of hormonal therapy to suppress ovulation, thus reducing formation of ovarian fluid; (2) Image-guided aspiration of cyst fluid with or without sclerotherapy, if symptomatic; and (3) Surgical resection, only in selected cases as the recurrence rate ranges between 30% and 50%.[73]

UTERINE LESIONS

A few benign uterine masses can also be present in the adnexal region, the most common being a subserosal or pedunculated fibroid, a broad ligament fibroid and an obstructed or nonobstructed rudimentary horn of a unicornuate uterus. Identification of both ovaries separately, connection of fibroid with the uterus, bridging vessel sign, and the morphological characteristics of the fibroid can all help in differentiating fibroids from an ovarian mass. Multiplanar imaging capability of MRI is an important adjunct in establishing the uterine origin of the mass.

IMAGING APPROACH TO AN ADNEXAL LESION

Adnexal lesions are commonly encountered in clinical practice. It is important to determine the nature of the lesion and especially to categorize the benign or malignant potential of an adnexal lesion, to be able it to manage it properly.

Sonography is the first line of investigation for detection, establishing the origin, and for characterizing the nature of the lesion. Transvaginal US is the preferred technique, however the transabdominal route has its own advantages. Wherever possible, it is better to evaluate the lesion with both transabdominal and transvaginal routes. Over the years, various approaches have been used to categorize an adnexal mass lesion on US, including the subjective assessment or

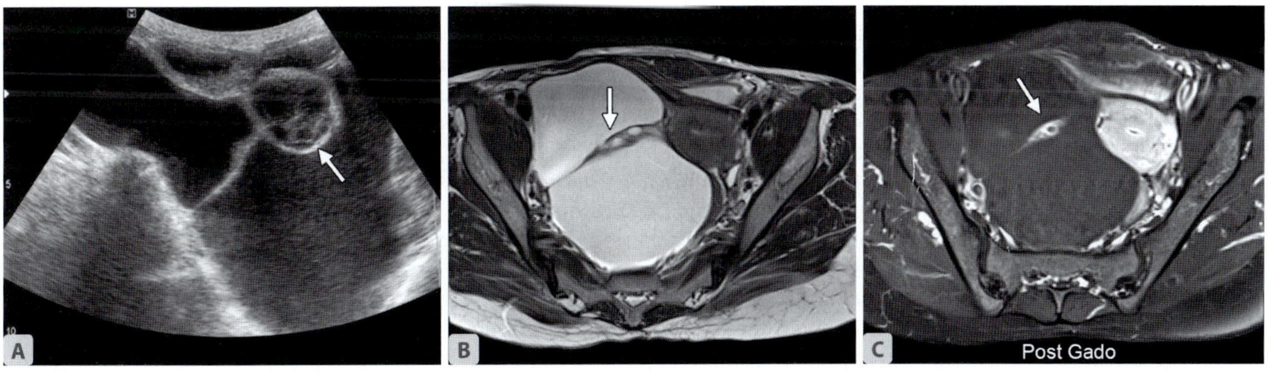

FIGS. 52A TO C: Peritoneal inclusion cyst in a 35-year-old woman with chronic pelvic pain. She had been treated 3 years back for abdominal tuberculosis. (A) Transabdominal sonogram shows a multiseptated cystic mass in the right adnexal region with thin walls, with the ovary suspended within it. The ovary shows a hemorrhagic corpus luteal cyst (arrow); (B) On T2W MRI done 6 weeks later, the large cystic mass is well seen to the right of the uterus with the ovary within (arrow). The hemorrhagic cyst in the ovary has resolved; (C) CEMR shows contrast uptake by the ovarian tissue within the cyst (arrow).

BOX 2: Morphological and color Doppler features on transvaginal sonography used by the International Ovarian Tumour Analysis group for qualitative classification of adnexal masses.[75]

Morphological characteristics
- Size of mass
- Cystic content—anechoic/low level echoes/ground-glass/hemorrhagic/mixed
- Septations—complete or incomplete
- Internal walls—smooth or irregular
- Papillary projections >3 mm
- Solid component—present or absent
- Acoustic shadow—present or absent
- Ascites present or absent

Based on above features, mass classified qualitatively into six categories
1. Unilocular cyst—no complete septum, solid component or papillary projection
2. Multilocular cyst—≥1 complete septum, no solid component or papillary projection
3. Unilocular solid cyst—unilocular cyst with solid component or ≥1 papillary projection
4. Multilocular solid cyst—multilocular cyst with solid component or >1 papillary projection
5. Solid— more than 80% solid component
6. Not classifiable—due to poor visualization

Color Doppler sonography
Score 1—no blood flow
Score 2—minimal flow
Score 3—moderate flow
Score 4—very strong flow

BOX 3: Benign and malignant features as described by the International Ovarian Tumour Analysis group.[76]

Benign features
- B1 Unilocular Cyst
- B2 Presence of solid components with largest diameter <7 mm
- B3 Presence of acoustic shadows
- B4 Smooth multilocular tumor with largest diameter <10 cm
- B5 No blood flow—color score 0

Malignant features
- M1 Irregular solid tumor
- M2 Presence of ascites
- M3 At least four papillary projections
- M4 Irregular multilocular—solid tumor with largest diameter >10 cm
- M5 Very strong blood flow—color score 4

the pattern recognition approach, simple scoring systems, probability predictors based on logistic regression analysis, etc. Of these, the pattern recognition approach has been found to be the most superior, with a sensitivity of 88–100% and specificity of 62–96% for predicting malignancy.[74] However, this approach works best in experienced hands.

A consensus opinion paper was published by the International Ovarian Tumour Analysis (IOTA) group in which objective criteria were put forward to standardize the terminology, definitions, and measurements used for describing the various morphological features of adnexal masses on gray scale and Doppler USG **(Box 2)**.[75] Using these terms and definitions, the IOTA group also described *simple rules* for categorizing the lesions into three categories—benign , malignant and indeterminate lesions on US—which has become the most used method and has shown the best validation reports. They described five benign and five malignant descriptors as elaborated in **Box 3**. In the presence of one or more benign features with no malignant feature, the mass was categorized as benign; if one or more malignant features was seen, with no benign feature, the mass was categorized as malignant; the mass was deemed indeterminate if one or more features of both benign and malignant were seen, or if no features of benign or malignant were seen.[76] Using these simple rules, about 77% of the masses could be categorized as benign or malignant with a specificity of 96% and sensitivity of 92%, while the rest were labeled as the indeterminate masses.[77]

Sonographically indeterminate masses are those masses that (1) appear complex and even after a thorough evaluation with gray scale and Doppler assessment, cannot be confidently placed into either the benign or malignant category or (2) one whose site of origin, from the ovary, uterus, or another pelvic structure cannot be established. It has been found that majority of the indeterminate masses are not malignant, but common benign adnexal conditions with a complex or unusual appearance, e.g. mature teratomas with no or little fat, hemorrhagic lesions with clot or debris mimicking a solid nodule or fibrous masses which appear solid on US and thus cause a concern for malignancy, etc.[78] Various methods have been adopted for further confirmation of the nature of the indeterminate masses including (a) a review US by an expert in the field of gynecological US, (b) MRI, (c) a diagnostic laparoscopy or (d) a "wait and watch" policy with follow-up sonography **(Flowchart 3)**. Amongst these options, MRI is the least invasive and offers the earliest solution with a high accuracy.

Magnetic resonance imaging has been found to be a useful complementary imaging modality for assessing the indeterminate lesions allowing a confident differentiation between benign and malignant etiology in majority of the cases. A number of scoring systems have been devised for systematic MR evaluation (MR ADNEX scoring system, EURAD-MR classification, etc.). The 2017 European Society of Urogenital Radiology (ESUR) recommendations for MRI incorporates the use of both conventional and functional MRI techniques.[79] As a general rule, malignant tumors show restricted diffusion on DWI, whereas benign tumors do not. However, some benign lesions can also show restricted diffusion: teratomas, endometriomas, hemorrhagic cysts, ovarian abscesses, ovarian infarction, and some benign sex cord-stromal tumors. On DCE-MRI, malignant solid components generally show a rapid rate and high level of enhancement, whereas a slow rate and low level of enhancement is seen in benign lesions.

The ESUR advocates that an initial basic series of MRI should be done in all patients, i.e. (1) A T2W sagittal sequence to look at the uterus and the position of the adnexal mass,

FLOWCHART 3: Algorithm for imaging evaluation of an adnexal mass.

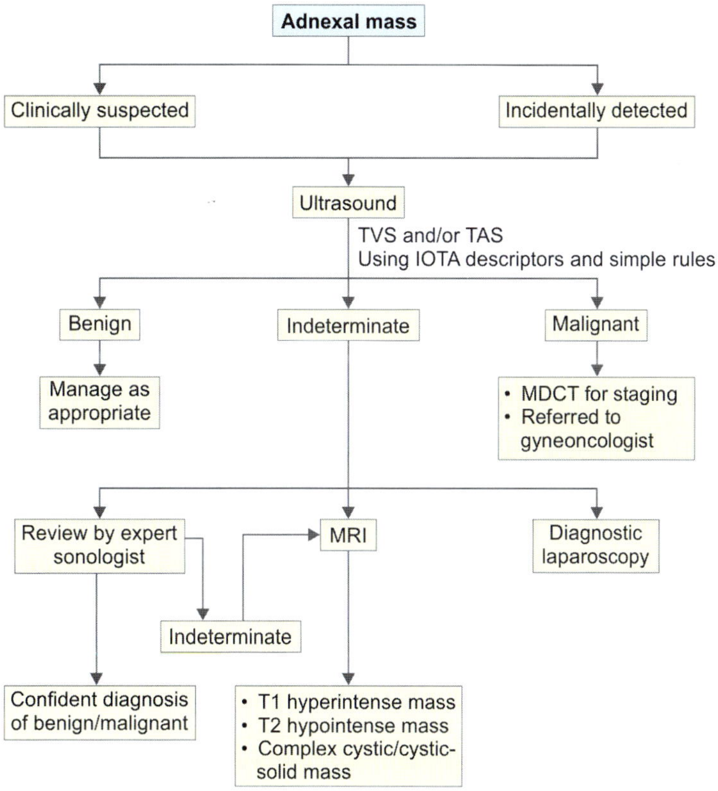

FLOWCHART 4A: MRI of sonographically indeterminate ovarian lesions—T1 "bright" mass. (ESUR recommendations, 2017).[79]

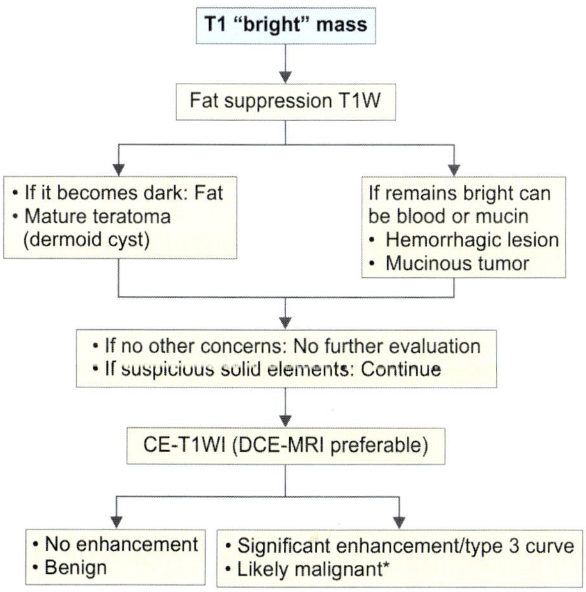

(*Mature teratoma can show enhancement at times)

FLOWCHART 4B: MRI of sonographically indeterminate ovarian lesions—T2WI "dark" or "intermediate" solid mass. (ESUR recommendations, 2017).[79]

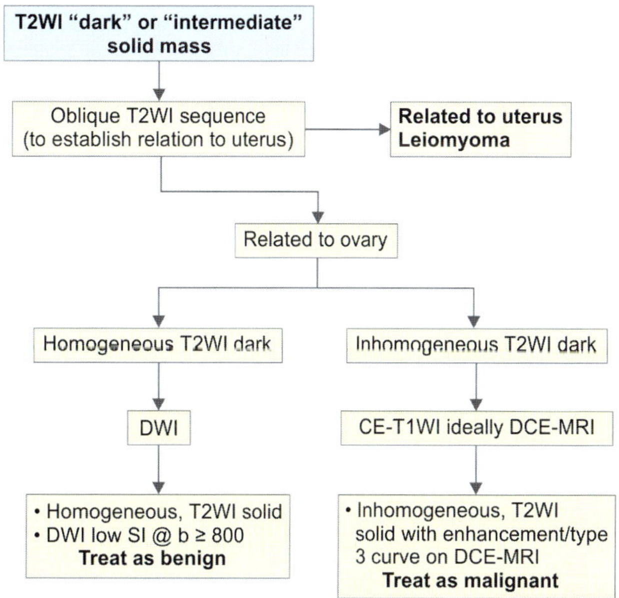

and (2) a pair of T1W and T2W sequences in an orthogonal plane for morphological evaluation of the mass. These sequences will establish the likely site and origin of the mass. At the same time, depending on the morphological characteristics on the T1- and T2W sequences, the masses can be divided into three broad categories: (1) T1W hyperintense mass, (2) the T2W low-SI mass, and (3) the complex-cystic or cystic-solid mass. Further sequences will be decided based on these categories. The subsequent algorithmic approach is given in the **Flowcharts 4A to C**, which will help in narrowing the differential diagnosis still further.

FLOWCHART 4C: MRI of sonographically indeterminate ovarian lesions—Complex cystic or cystic/solid mass. (ESUR recommendations, 2017).[79]

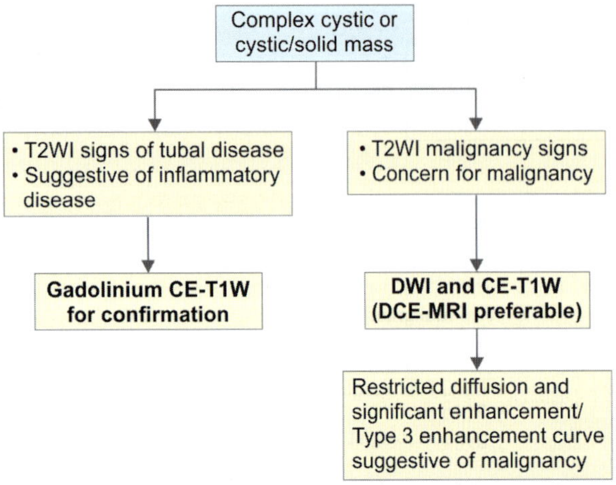

CONCLUSION

Although the large majority of adnexal lesions are benign, a significant number do turn out to be malignant. Being able to characterize the adnexal mass is important as it may lead to a more conservative management approach in benign masses, whilst ensuring an early and appropriate referral to a gynecological oncologist in the case of malignancy. Imaging plays a very significant role in establishing the origin of the lesion as well as in predicting whether it is benign or malignant. A thorough knowledge of the usual and unusual imaging appearances of the various conditions, correlation with the clinical details, laboratory parameters and use of a systematic step-by-step imaging algorithm will allow us to establish a short meaningful diagnosis or even a definitive diagnosis.

REFERENCES

1. Lee JH, Jeong YK, Park JK, et al. "Ovarian vascular pedicle" sign revealing organ of origin of a pelvic mass lesion on helical CT. Am J Roentgenol. 2003;181:131-7.
2. Modesitt SC, Pavlik EJ, Ueland FR, et al. Risk of malignancy in unilocular ovarian cystic tumors less than 10 centimeters in diameter. Obstet Gynecol. 2003;102:594-9.
3. Joshi M, Ganeshan K, Munshi HN. Ultrasound of adnexal masses. Semin Ultrasound CT MRI. 2008;29:72-97.
4. Siddall KA, Rubens DJ. Multi-detector CT of the female pelvis. RCNA. 2005;43:1097-118.
5. Jain KA. Sonographic spectrum of hemorrhagic ovarian cysts. J Ultrasound Med. 2003;21(8):879-86.
6. Potter AW, Chandrasekhar CA. US and CT evaluation of acute pelvic pain of gynecologic origin in nonpregnant premenopausal patients. Radiographics. 2008;28:1645-59.
7. Levine D, Brown DL, Andreotti RF, et al. Management of asymptomatic ovarian and other adnexal cysts imaged at US: Society of radiologists in Ultrasound Consensus. Radiology. 2010;256:943-54.
8. Chamié LP, Blasbalg R, Pereira RM, et al. Findings of pelvic endometriosis at transvaginal US, MR imaging, and laparoscopy. Radiographics. 2011;31(4):E77-100.
9. Patel MD, Feldstein VA, Chen DC, et al. Endometriomas: diagnostic performance of US. Radiology. 1999;210(3):739-45.
10. Dogan MM, Ugur M, Soysal SK, et al. Transvaginal sonographic diagnosis of ovarian endometrioma. Int J Gynaecol Obstet. 1996;52(2):145-9.
11. Alcázar JL, Laparte C, Jurado M, et al. The role of transvaginal ultrasonography combined with color velocity imaging and pulsed Doppler in the diagnosis of endometrioma. Fertil Steril. 1997;67(3):487-91.
12. Glastonbury CM. The shading sign. Radiology. 2002; 224(1): 199-201.
13. Takahashi K, Okada S, Ozaki T, et al. Diagnosis of pelvic endometriosis by magnetic resonance imaging using "fat-saturation" technique. Fertil Steril. 1994;62(5):973-7.
14. Corwin MT, Gerscovich EO, Lamba R, et al. Differentiation of ovarian endometriomas from hemorrhagic cysts at MR imaging: utility of the T2 dark spot sign. Radiology. 2013;271(1):126-32.
15. Namimoto T, Awai K, Nakaura T, et al. Role of diffusion-weighted imaging in the diagnosis of gynecological diseases. Eur Radiol. 2009;19:745-60.
16. Thomassin-Naggara I, Daraï E, Cuenod CA, et al. Contribution of diffusion-weighted MR imaging for predicting benignity of complex adnexal masses. Eur Radiol. 2009;19:1544-52.
17. Turocy JM, Benacerraf BR. Transvaginal sonography in the diagnosis of deep infiltrating endometriosis: a review. J Clin Ultrasound. 2017;45(6):313-8.
18. Bennett GL, Slywotzky CM, Cantera M, et al. Unusual manifestations and complications of endometriosis—spectrum of imaging findings: pictorial review. Am J Roentgenol. 2010;194(6):WS34-46.
19. Kobayashi H. Ovarian cancer in endometriosis: epidemiology, natural history, and clinical diagnosis. Int J Clin Oncol. 2009;14(5):378-82.
20. Asch E, Levine D. Variations in appearance of endometriomas. J Ultrasound Med. 2007;26(8):993-1002.
21. Moghissi KS. Medical treatment of endometriosis. Clin Obstet Gynecol. 1999;42(3):620-32.
22. Valentini AL, Gui B, Miccò M, et al. Benign and suspicious ovarian masses-mr imaging criteria for characterization: pictorial review. J Oncol. 2012;2012:481806.
23. Hart WR. Mucinous tumors of the ovary: a review. Int J Gynecol Pathol. 2005;24(1):4-25.
24. Imaoka I, Wada A, Kaji Y, et al. Developing an MR imaging strategy for diagnosis of ovarian masses. Radiographics, 2006;26:1431-48.
25. Okada S, Ohaki Y, Inoue K, et al. Calcifications in mucinous and serous cystic ovarian tumors. J Nippon Med Sch. 2005;72(1):29-33.
26. Tanaka YO, Nishida M, Kurosaki Y, et al. Differential diagnosis of gynaecological "stained glass" tumours on MRI. Br J Radiol. 1999;72(856):414-20.
27. Cho SM, Byun JY, Rha SE, et al. CT and MRI findings of cystadenofibromas of the ovary. Eur Radiol. 2004;14:798-804.
28. Wasnik A, Elsayes K. Ovarian cystadenofibroma: A masquerader of malignancy. IJRI. 2010;20(4):297-9.
29. Dierickx I, Valentin L, Van Holsbeke C, et al. Imaging in gynecological disease: clinical and ultrasound features of Brenner tumors of the ovary. Ultrasound Obstet Gynecol. 2012;40:706-13.
30. Zhao Y, Mao X, Yao L, et al. Computed tomography imaging features of benign ovarian Brenner tumors. Oncology letters. 2018;16(1):1141-6.
31. Rha SE, Byun JY, Jung SE, et al. Atypical CT and MRI manifestations of mature ovarian cystic teratomas. AJR. 2004;183:743-50.

32. Togashi K, Nishimura K, Itoh K, et al. Ovarian cystic teratomas: MR imaging. Radiology. 1987;162:669-73.
33. Comerci JT Jr, Licciardi F, Bergh PA, et al. Mature cystic teratoma: clinicopathologic evaluation of 517 cases and review of the literature. Obstet Gynecol. 1994;84:22-8.
34. Ismail SR. An evaluation of the incidence of right-sided ovarian cystic teratoma visualized on sonograms. JDMS. 2005;21:336-42.
35. Quinn SF, Erickson S, Black WC. Cystic ovarian teratomas: The sonographic appearance of the dermoid plug. Radiology. 1985;155:477-8.
36. Beller MJ. The "tip of the iceberg" sign. Radiology. 1998;209(2): 395-6.
37. Vyas B, Dyer RB. The "dot-dash" sign. Abdom Imaging. 2015;40:2901-2.
38. Tongsong T, Wanapirak C, Khunamornpong S, et al. Numerous intracystic floating balls as a sonographic feature of benign cystic teratoma. J Ultrasound Med. 2006;25:1587-91.
39. Guinet C, Ghossain MA, Buy J-N, et al. Mature cystic teratomas of the ovary: CT and MR findings. Eur J Radiol. 1995;20:137-43 .
40. Friedman AC, Pyatt RS, Hartman DS, et al. CT of benign cystic teratomas. AJR. 1982;138:659-65.
41. Saba L, Guerriero S, Sulcis R, et al. Mature and immature ovarian teratomas: CT, US and MR imaging characteristics. Eur J Radiol. 2009;72:454-63.
42. Sahin H, Abdullazade S, Sanci M. Mature cystic teratoma of the ovary: a cutting edge overview on imaging features. Insights Imaging. 2017;8(2):227-41.
43. Nakamaya T, Yoshimitsu K, Irie H, et al. Diffusion-weighted echo-planar MR imaging and ADC mapping in the differential diagnosis of ovarian cystic masses: usefulness of detecting keratinoid substances in mature cystic teratomas. J Magn Reson Imaging. 2005;22:271-8.
44. Outwater EK, Siegelman ES, Hunt JL. Ovarian teratomas: tumor types and imaging characteristics. Radiographics. 2001;21(2):475-90.
45. Park SB, Kim JK, Kim K, et al. Imaging findings of complications and unusual manifestations of ovarian neoplasms. Radiographics. 2008;28:969-83.
46. Haroon S, Zia A, Idrees R, et al. Clinicopathological spectrum of ovarian sex cord-stromal tumors; 20 years' retrospective study in a developing country. J Ovarian Res. 2013;6(1):87.
47. Horta M, Cunha TM. Sex cord-stromal tumors of the ovary: a comprehensive review and update for radiologists. Diagn Interv Radiol. 2015;21(4):277-86.
48. Duigenan S, Oliva E, Lee SI. Ovarian torsion: diagnostic features on CT and MRI with pathologic correlation. Am J Roentgenol. 2012;198(2):W122-31.
49. Bider D, Mashiach S, Dulitzky M, et al. Clinical, surgical and pathologic findings of adnexal torsion in pregnant and nonpregnant women. Surg Gynecol Obstet. 1991;173(5): 363-6.
50. Hibbard LT. Adnexal torsion. Am J Obstet Gynecol. 1985;152:456-61.
51. Sibal M. Follicular ring sign: a simple sonographic sign for early diagnosis of ovarian torsion. JUM. 2012;31(11):1803-9.
52. Lee EJ, Kwon HC, Joo HJ, et al. Diagnosis of ovarian torsion with color Doppler sonography: depiction of twisted vascular pedicle. J Ultrasound Med. 1998;17(2):83-9.
53. Albayram F, Hamper UM. Ovarian and adnexal torsion: spectrum of sonographic findings with pathologic correlation. J Ultrasound Med. 2001;20:1083-9.
54. Nizar K, Deutsch M, Filmer S, et al. Doppler studies of the ovarian venous blood flow in the diagnosis of adnexal torsion. J Clin Ultrasound. 2009;37(8):436-9.
55. Shalev J, Goldenberg M, Oelsner G, et al. Treatment of twisted ischemic adnexa by simple detorsion. N Engl J Med. 1989;321(8):546.
56. Huang C, Hong M-K, Ding D-C. A review of ovary torsion. Ci Ji Yi Xue Za Zhi. 2017;29(3):143-7.
57. Umesaki N, Tanaka T, Miyama M, et al. Sonographic characteristics of massive ovarian edema. Ultrasound Obstet Gynecol. 2000;16(5):479-81.
58. Coakley FV, Anwar M, Poder L, et al. Magnetic resonance imaging of massive ovarian edema in pregnancy. J Comput Assist Tomogr. 2010;34(6):865-7.
59. Takeuchi M, Matsuzaki K, Sano N, et al. Ovarian fibromatosis: magnetic resonance imaging findings with pathologic correlation. J Comput Assist Tomogr. 2008;32(5):776-7.
60. Revzin MV, Mathur M, Dave HB, et al. Pelvic inflammatory disease: multimodality imaging approach with clinical-pathologic correlation. Radiographics. 2016;36(5): 1579-96.
61. Kim SH, Kim SH, Yang DM, et al. Unusual causes of tubo-ovarian abscess: CT and MR imaging findings. Radiographics. 2004; 24:1575-89.
62. Sam JW, Jacobs JE, Birnbaum BA. Spectrum of CT findings in acute pyogenic pelvic inflammatory disease. Radiographics. 2002;22(6):1327-34.
63. Lareau SM, Beigi RH. Pelvic inflammatory disease and tubo-ovarian abscess. Infect Dis Clin North Am. 2008;22(4):693-708.
64. Patel MD, Acord DL, Young SW. Likelihood ratio of sonographic findings in discriminating hydrosalpinx from other adnexal masses. Am J Roentgenol. 2006;186(4):1033-8.
65. Eyvazzadeh AD, Levine D. Imaging of Pelvic Pain in the First Trimester of Pregnancy. Radiol Clin North Am. 2006;44:863-77.
66. Nuberg DA, Mack LA, Jeffrey RB Jr, et al. Endovaginal sonographic evaluation of ectopic pregnancy: A prospective study. Am J Roentgenol. 1987;149:1181-6.
67. Kishimoto K, Ito K, Awaya H, et al. Paraovarian cyst: MR imaging features. Abdom Imaging. 2002;27(6):685-9.
68. Mennemeyer R, Smith M. Multicystic, peritoneal mesothelioma: a report with electron microscopy of a case mimicking intra-abdominal cystic hygroma (lymphangioma). Cancer. 1979;44:692-8.
69. Sohaey R, Gardner TL, Woodward PJ, et al. Sonographic diagnosis of peritoneal inclusion cysts. J Ultrasound Med. 1995;14:913-7.
70. Kim JS, Lee HJ, Woo SK, et al. Peritoneal inclusion cysts and their relationship to the ovaries: evaluation with sonography. Radiology. 1997;204:481-4.
71. Jain KA. Imaging of peritoneal inclusion cysts. Am J Roentgenol. 2000;174:1559-63.
72. Ross MJ, Welch WR, Scully RE. Multilocular peritoneal inclusion cysts (so-called cystic mesotheliomas). Cancer. 1989;64:1336-46.
73. Vallerie AM, Lerner JP, Wright JD, et al. Peritoneal inclusion cysts: a review. Obstet Gynecol Surv. 2009;64(5):321-34.
74. Brown DL, Dudiak KM, Laing FC. Adnexal masses: US characterization and reporting. Radiology. 2010;254(2):342-54.
75. Timmerman D, Valentin L, Bourne TH, et al. Terms, definitions and measurements to describe the sonographic features of adnexal tumors: a consensus opinion from the International Ovarian Tumor Analysis (IOTA) Group. Ultrasound Obstet Gynecol. 2000;16:500-5.
76. Timmerman D, Testa AC, Bourne, T et al. Simple ultrasound-based rules for the diagnosis of ovarian cancer. Ultrasound Obstet Gynecol. 2008;31:681-90.
77. Timmerman D, Ameye L, Fischerova D, et al. Simple ultrasound rules to distinguish between benign and malignant adnexal masses before surgery: prospective validation by IOTA group. BMJ. 2010;341:c6839.
78. Ameye L, Timmerman D, Valentin L, et al. Clinically oriented three-step strategy for assessment of adnexal pathology. Ultrasound Obstet Gynecol. 2012;40:582-91.
79. Forstner R, Thomassin-Naggara I, Cunha TM, et al. ESUR recommendations for MR imaging of the sonographically indeterminate adnexal mass: an update. Eur Radiol. 2017;27(6):2248-57.

CHAPTER

15

Malignant Ovarian and Tubal Disease

Smita Manchanda, Surabhi Vyas, Manisha Jana

INTRODUCTION

Cervical cancer, endometrial cancer, and ovarian cancer constitute the spectrum of gynecologic malignancies. Ovarian malignancy is the second most common gynecologic cancer and the fourth leading cause of cancer deaths in females in the United States.[1] It accounts for 3.6% of all cases with a mortality of 4.3%.[2] It is a leading cause of mortality predominantly because of the late diagnosis. Majority of the patients present in stage III or stage IV disease as the symptoms are often nonspecific.

ETIOPATHOGENESIS

For ovarian malignancy, the etiopathogenesis appears to be multifactorial. Risk factors include a first-degree relative with ovarian cancer, nulliparity, early menarche, and late menopause. Hereditary cases are seen in the premenopausal age group usually as the breast-ovarian cancer syndrome (mutations in the *BRCA1* and *BRCA2* tumor suppressor genes).[2] Pregnancy, lactation, and the use of oral contraceptives appear to be protective factors for ovarian malignancy.

CLASSIFICATION

WHO Histological Classification

The World Health Organization (WHO) histological classification for ovarian tumors is based on the most probable tissue of origin: surface epithelial (65%), germ cell (15%), sex cord-stromal (10%), metastases (5%), and miscellaneous. Further classification is done on the basis of cell type, cellular atypia, malignant potential, and invasion. Among these, the surface epithelial tumors comprise most of the malignant tumors (around 90%). The main entities in the 2014 WHO classification[3] are given in **Table 1**.

STAGING

The 2014 revised staging system by the international Federation of Gynaecology and Obstetrics (FIGO) provides prognostic as well as personalized management guidance in the ovarian malignancies and also recognizes the heterogeneity of ovarian malignancies, which may arise from the ovaries, fallopian tubes, or peritoneum.[4,5]

Although imaging modalities like computed tomography and chest radiography, and biochemical tests like CA-125 levels in the serum, may have prognostic implications, the staging is based on the findings of surgical exploration.

The 2014 FIGO staging is summarized below:

- *Stage I*: Tumor is confined to the ovaries; limited to one ovary capsule intact (*stage IA*); tumor involves both ovaries; rest as IA (*stage IB*); tumor involves one or both ovaries (*stage IC*), with either surgical/intraoperative spill (*stage IC1*), capsule ruptured before surgery, or tumor on ovarian or fallopian tube surface (*stage IC2*) or malignant cells in the ascites or peritoneal washings (*stage IC3*).
- *Stage II*: Tumor involves one or both ovaries with pelvic or peritoneal extension; involvement of the uterus and/or fallopian tubes (*stage IIA*); involvement of other pelvic intraperitoneal tissue (*stage IIB*).
- *Stage III*: Tumor involves one or both ovaries or fallopian tubes with extension to extrapelvic peritoneum and/or retroperitoneal (RP) lymph nodes metastasis:
    - *Stage IIIA*: Positive RP lymph nodes only; if node size ≤10 mm in greatest dimension—*stage IIIA1* (i); if size >10 mm in greatest dimension *stage IIIA1* (ii). *Stage IIIA2*: There is microscopic extrapelvic peritoneal involvement with or without RP lymph node involvement.
    - *Stage IIIB*: Extrapelvic peritoneal metastasis ≤2 cm in greatest dimension, with or without RP lymph nodes metastasis.
    - *Stage IIIC*: Macroscopic extrapelvic peritoneal metastases >2 cm in greatest dimension, with or without RP lymph node metastasis, including tumor extension to liver and splenic capsules only.
- *Stage IV:* Distant metastasis, excluding peritoneal metastases; with positive pleural effusion cytology (*stage IVA*), distant metastases to parenchyma of extra-abdominal organs or inguinal lymph nodes or lymph nodes outside of the abdominal cavity (*stage IVB*).

TABLE 1: World Health Organization classification of ovarian neoplasms (2014).[3]

Histological categories	Subcategories		Individual entities
Epithelial tumors	Serous tumors	Benign	• Serous cystadenoma • Serous adenofibroma • Serous surface papilloma
		Borderline	• Serous borderline tumor/atypical proliferative serous tumor • Serous borderline tumor—micropapillary variant/noninvasive low-grade serous carcinoma
		Malignant	• Low-grade serous carcinoma • High-grade serous carcinoma
	Mucinous tumors	Benign	• Mucinous cystadenoma • Mucinous adenofibroma
		Borderline	Mucinous borderline tumor/atypical proliferative mucinous tumor
		Malignant	Mucinous carcinoma
	Endometrioid tumors	Benign	• Endometriosis cyst • Endometrioid cystadenoma • Endometrioid cystadenofibroma
		Borderline	Endometrioid borderline tumor/atypical proliferative endometrioid tumor
		Malignant	Endometrioid carcinoma
	Clear cell tumors	Benign	• Clear cell cystadenoma • Clear cell adenofibroma
		Borderline	Clear cell borderline tumor/atypical proliferative clear cell tumor
		Malignant	Clear cell carcinoma
	Brenner tumors	Benign	Brenner tumor
		Borderline	Borderline Brenner tumor/atypical proliferative Brenner tumor
		Malignant	Malignant Brenner tumor
	Seromucinous tumors	Benign	• Seromucinous cystadenoma • Seromucinous adenofibroma
		Borderline	Seromucinous borderline tumor/atypical proliferative seromucinous tumor
		Malignant	Seromucinous carcinoma
	Undifferentiated carcinoma		
Mixed epithelial and mesenchymal tumors			• Carcinosarcoma • Adenosarcoma
Sex cord—stromal tumors	Pure stromal tumors		• Fibromas • Fibrothecomas • Thecomas • Leydig cell tumors
	Pure sex cord tumors		• Adult granulosa cell tumor • Juvenile granulosa cell tumor • Sertoli cell tumors • Sex cord tumor with annular tubules
	Mixed sex cord—stromal tumors		Sertoli-Leydig cell tumors
Germ cell tumors			• Mature teratoma • Immature teratoma • Yolk sac tumor (endodermal sinus tumor) • Dysgerminoma • Nongestational choriocarcinoma • Embryonal carcinoma • Mixed germ cell tumors • Monodermal (e.g. struma ovarii, carcinoid)
Malignant not otherwise specified	Metastatic cancer from nonovarian primary		• Colonic, appendiceal • Gastric • Breast

Few salient features of the 2014 FIGO staging include:

- The ovarian and peritoneal fallopian tube origin of ovarian carcinomas are dealt collectively.
- Stage IC is subdivided into three to specify the nature and timing of capsular rupture like preoperative or intraoperative rupture or positive peritoneal washings.
- In up to 30% patients with bilateral disease, either with one-sided dominant mass or multiple small masses may be due to metastasis.
- The Stage IIC is eliminated in the 2014 FIGO staging.
- The presence of metastatic nodes rather than the number of metastatic nodes has prognostic significance.[6]
- New subdivisions of stage IV, i.e. IVA and IVB, were introduced for positive pleural cytology and distant parenchymal metastasis, respectively.

ROLE OF IMAGING MODALITIES

The role of imaging in a suspected adnexal lesion is to detect, characterize, and stage the mass. Ultrasonography (USG), computed tomography (CT), magnetic resonance imaging (MRI), and positron emission tomography CT (PET-CT) are used in various combinations to evaluate adnexal masses.

Ultrasonography

Ultrasonography, being a low-cost, noninvasive, and widely available modality, is the initial investigation of choice in the evaluation of a suspected adnexal mass. Both transabdominal and endovaginal scanning in combination with Doppler are used for adnexal mass assessment.[7,8] The morphological features **(Figs. 1A to D)** suggestive of malignancy are thick walls and septations (>2–3 mm), irregular walls/septations, and presence of solid areas/papillary projections/mural nodules. Other signs such as presence of ascites, peritoneal nodules, and metastases also indicate malignant etiology. Reported sensitivity of USG in predicting malignancy is 85–97% and specificity varies from 56% to 95%.[7,9-12]

Color Doppler

Color Doppler in the qualitative mode has greater utility to demonstrate flow within a solid component or septum. Solid component with no detectable flow likely represents a blood clot. Presence of central and strong color flow is more suggestive of malignancy. However, it is important to remember that benign lesions also show internal color flow. Spectral Doppler parameters have been used variably in the past for the prediction of malignancy in an adnexal mass with varying sensitivity and specificity. A resistive index (RI) value of 0.4 was reported by Timor-Tritsch et al. to have a sensitivity of 93.8% and specificity of 98.7% and in 2007,[13] Laban et al.[14] reported the best RI cutoff value as <0.48 with a sensitivity of 90% and specificity of 89%. *P* < 1.0 has also had low reported sensitivity and specificity (52.8% and 77.6%, respectively).[15] Since there is a significant overlap in these values in benign

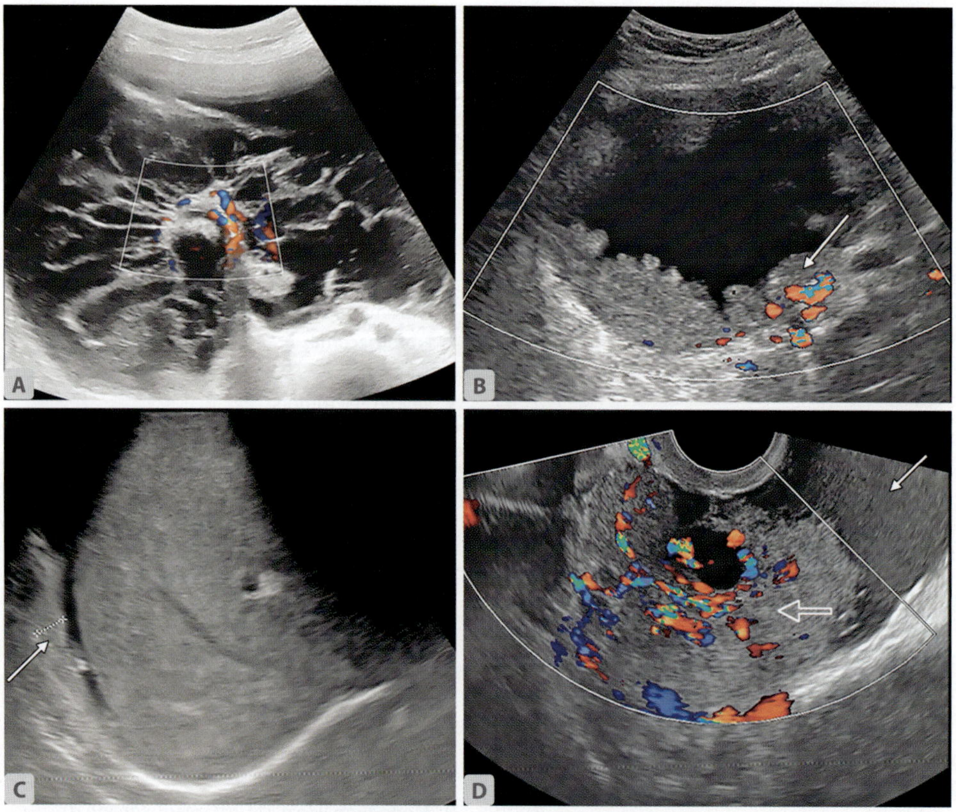

FIGS. 1A TO D: USG features of malignancy. (A) Thick septations with internal color flow. (B) Papillary projections and mural nodules (arrow). (C) Peritoneal deposits in subphrenic location (arrow). (D) Solid mass with cystic component and marked neovascularity (block arrow) with ascites (arrow).

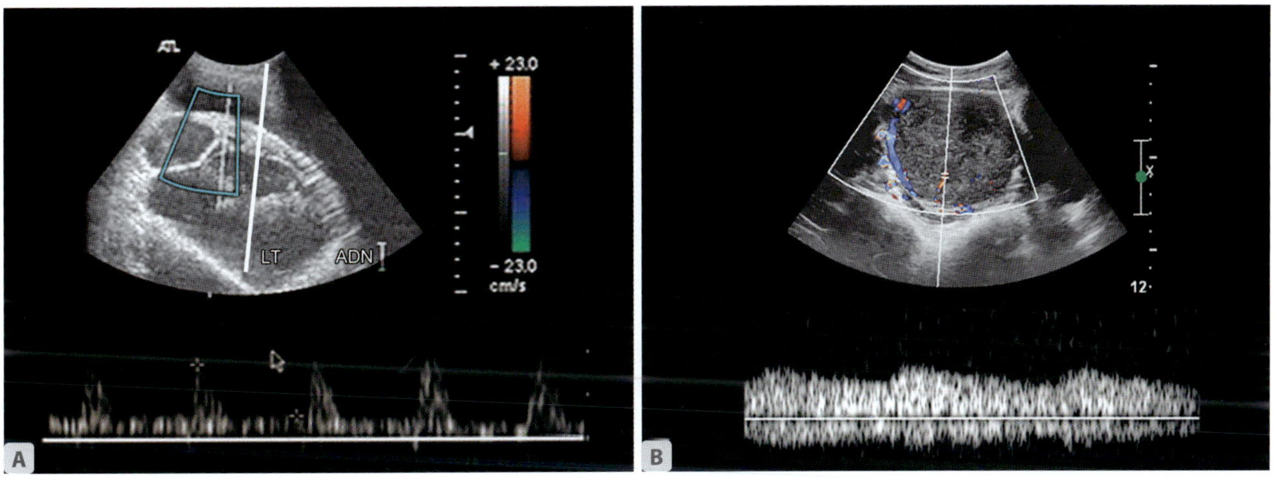

FIGS. 2A AND B: Doppler features of benign versus malignant lesion. (A) Multilocular cystic lesion with high resistance flow in septation in a case of serous cystadenoma. (B) Solid mass with low resistance internal flow in case of dysgerminoma.

and malignant masses, they are not much used in lesion characterization. In general, lower RI, lower pulsatility index (PI), and higher peak systolic velocity (PSV) suggest malignancy **(Figs. 2A and B)**.

IOTA Simple Rules

The International Ovarian Tumor Analysis (IOTA) Simple Rules (2008) consist of B-features (five features typical for benign tumors) and M-features (five features typical for malignant tumors) for preoperative classification of ovarian tumors.[16-18] These are summarized in **Table 2** and depicted in **Figures 3 and 4**. These are used to diagnose ovarian malignancy in women who have at least one persistent adnexal (ovarian, paraovarian, and tubal) tumor and are considered to require surgery.

ADNEX Model

There are various diagnostic models available for adnexal tumors [e.g. IOTA models, Risk of Malignancy Index (RMI), Risk of Ovarian Malignancy Algorithm (ROMA), Assessment of Different NEoplasias in the adneXa (ADNEX)]. However, when creating these models the patients selected for expectant management were excluded. It is therefore important to remember that these cannot be applied to adnexal tumors being conservatively treated. ADNEX is a risk model, which uses nine predictors **(Table 3)** to diagnose ovarian malignancy in females with persistent adnexal tumor (ovarian/paraovarian/tubal), which is considered to need surgical management. ADNEX estimates the probability of adnexal tumor to be benign, borderline, stage I malignancy, stage II-IV malignancy, or secondary metastatic disease (i.e. metastasis of nonadnexal tumor to the ovary). This model developed by clinicians and statisticians from the IOTA group is based on clinical and USG data from almost 6,000 women recruited at 24 centers in 10 countries (Italy, Belgium, Sweden, Czech Republic, Poland, France, UK, China, Spain, and Canada).[19]

TABLE 2: International Ovarian Tumor Analysis (IOTA) simple rules.

Benign features (B)		Malignant features (M)	
B1	Unilocular	M1	Irregular solid tumor
B2	Presence of solid components with largest diameter <7 mm	M2	Presence of ascites
B3	Presence of acoustic shadows	M3	At least four papillary structures
B4	Smooth multilocular tumor with largest diameter <100 mm	M4	Irregular multilocular—solid tumor with largest diameter >100 mm
B5	No blood flow (color score 1)	M5	Very strong blood flow (color score 4)

Benign: Only B-features apply.
Malignant: Only M-features apply.
Inconclusive: No features apply, or both B- and M-features apply.

Computed Tomography

The role of CT is primarily two-fold:

1. To stage the disease preoperatively.
2. To assess resectability and identify patients suitable for primary cytoreductive surgery vis-a-vis patients who will require neoadjuvant chemotherapy prior to surgery.

In addition, the staging CT is used to plan image-guided biopsy for histological subtyping prior to primary chemotherapy.

CT Technique

Contrast-enhanced CT (CECT) abdomen is planned with oral and intravenous contrast administration. Positive oral contrast media is used to distinguish between luminal lesions and mesenteric/serosal deposits. Some institutions prefer oral water (negative contrast medium) as the small, calcified deposits may get obscured by positive oral contrast.

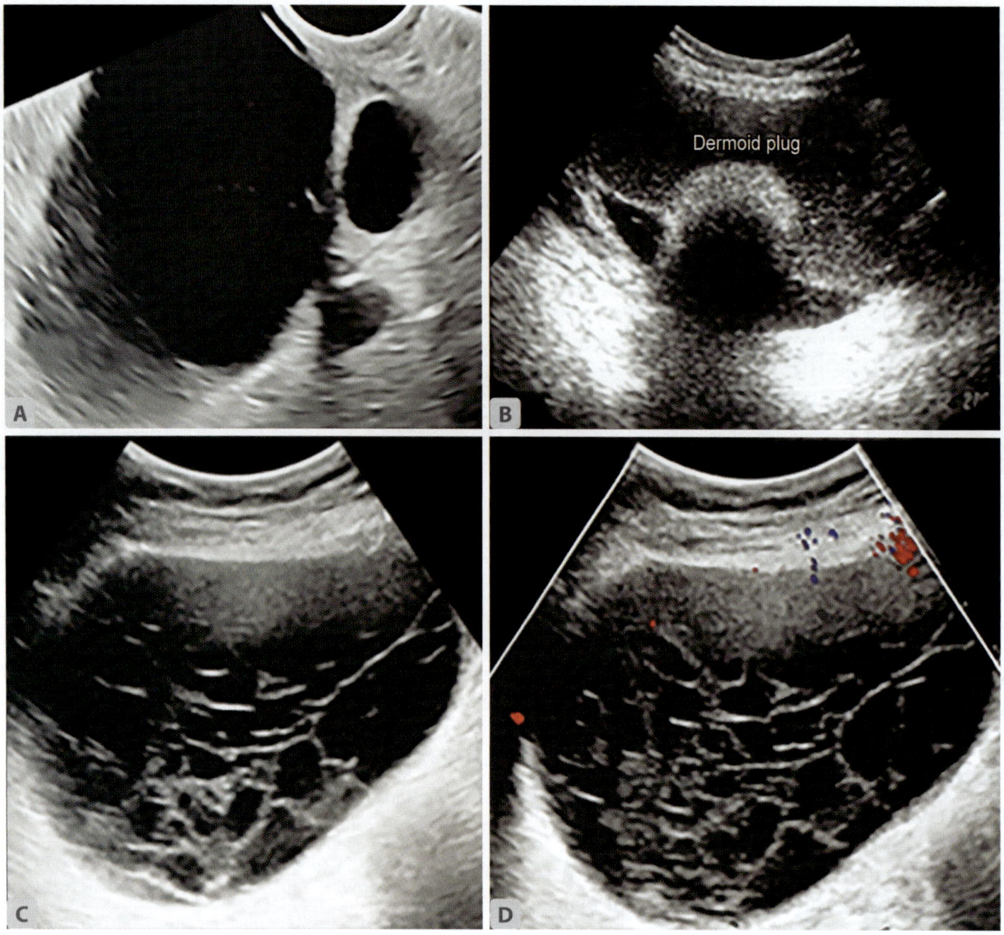

FIGS. 3A TO D: Benign features (IOTA simple rules, 2008). (A) Unilocular tumor: B1. (B) Presence of acoustic shadows: B3. (C) Smooth multilocular tumor with largest diameter <100 mm: B4. (D) No blood flow (color score 1): B5. (IOTA: International Ovarian Tumor Analysis).

Acquisition is in the venous phase 70 seconds after injection of contrast medium from the domes of diaphragm to the inguinal regions.[20] Axial thin reconstructions (1.5 mm) are then used to generate 3D coronal and sagittal multiplanar images.

CT Chest

Many centers now routinely perform CT chest to detect pleural deposits, lung metastases, paracardiac, and mediastinal lymph nodes (these findings are detected in approximately 30% of the patients at presentation). In addition, the presence of moderate or large pleural effusions or enlarged paracardiac lymph nodes is a predictor of poor post-treatment outcome.[21]

Routes of Dissemination

Direct pelvic invasion and transcoelomic peritoneal disease extension are the most common ways of dissemination.[21] **Table 4** summarizes the various routes of dissemination in ovarian malignancy.

Limitation of CT in Assessing Disease Burden

The reported accuracies for detection of disease at all stages have been in the range of 70–90% with a good CT acquisition and reading.[22]

Only limited evaluation is possible with noncontrast CT, and inability to use intravenous contrast adversely affects CT staging accuracies.

It is difficult to detect small-volume extraovarian deposits (<5 mm) on mesentery, peritoneum, and bowel serosa, especially in the absence of ascites. This emphasizes the complementary role of laparoscopy in preoperative assessment of ovarian cancer.

CECT Assessment

- *Pelvic disease*: In the pelvis, it is important to evaluate the size, location, and extent of primary disease including bladder, ureteric, and rectal invasion. Pelvic sidewall invasion is likely if the disease is less than 3 mm from the muscular sidewall and there is encasement or invasion of the iliac vessels.[21]
- *Peritoneal/omental disease*: It is important to identify peritoneal disease and document the extent of omental or peritoneal involvement. The signs of peritoneal disease are detailed in **Box 1** and depicted in **Figures 5A to D**.

Apart from the peritoneum or omentum, mesenteric disease and deposits along the *upper abdominal ligaments* **(Figs. 6A to D)** are important to document. Presence of small nodules or a misty stranded mesentery is seen in early disease whereas plaque-like thickening with retraction and distortion

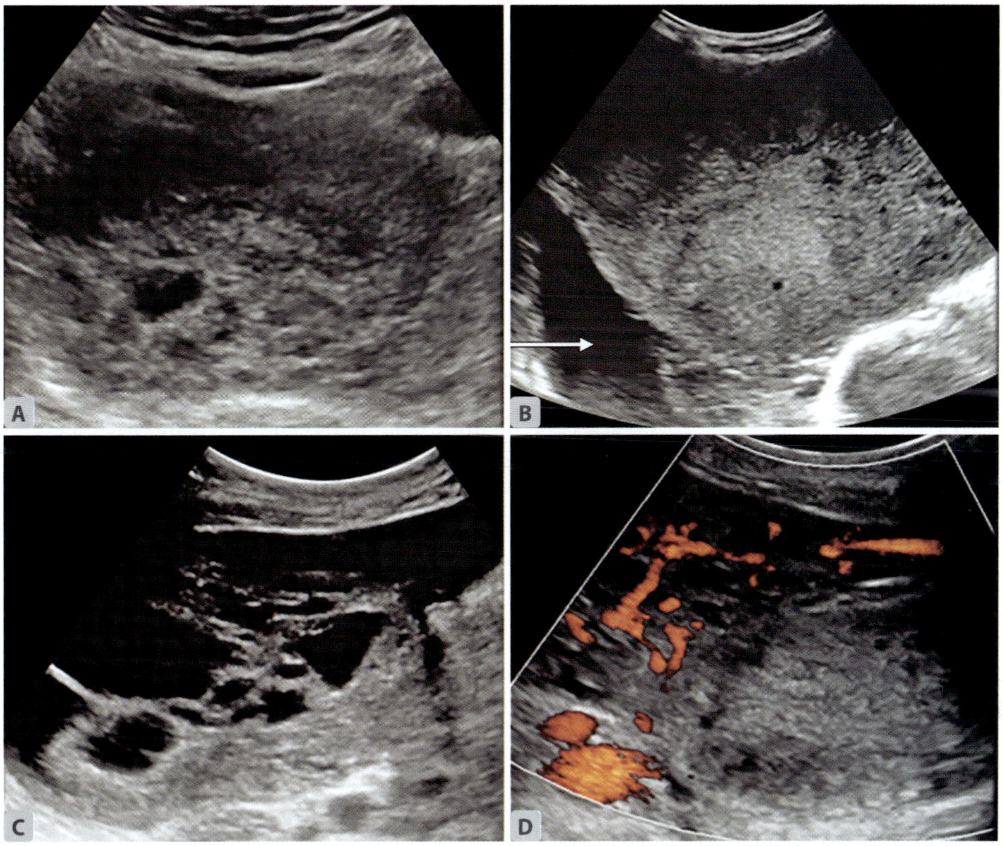

FIGS. 4A TO D: Malignant features (IOTA simple rules, 2008). (A) Irregular solid tumor: M1. (B) Presence of ascites (arrow): M2. (C) Irregular multilocular solid tumor: M4. (D) Very strong color flow: M5. (IOTA: International Ovarian Tumor Analysis).

TABLE 3: ADNEX risk model predictors.

Clinical variables	USG variables
• Age • Serum CA-125 level • Type of center (oncology referral center vs other)	• Maximal diameter of lesion • Proportion of solid tissue • >10 cyst locules • Number of papillary projections • Acoustic shadow • Ascites

TABLE 4: Routes of dissemination in ovarian malignancy.

Direct invasion in pelvis	Adnexa, uterus, pelvic side walls, bladder, and rectum
Transcoelomic spread	Peritoneal, subdiaphragmatic mesenteric and serosal surfaces
Lymphatic metastases	Pelvic, abdominal, retroperitoneal, para-aortic, paracardiac, and mediastinal lymph nodes
Hematogenous metastases (least common)	Liver, lung, bone, and brain

of the bowel loops is a feature of advanced disease. Disease in the lesser omentum, lesser sac, and perihepatic space along with the associated upper abdominal ligaments **(Table 5)** complicates surgical approach with associated increased morbidity. Nodular or plaque-like disease greater than 2 cm is considered unresectable disease.[21] Similar criteria apply for subdiaphragmatic disease extension and both the subphrenic spaces should be carefully looked for in axial and coronal planes.

- *Lymphadenopathy*: The criterion for malignant lymphadenopathy is nodal short axis diameter (SAD) of 1 cm. Pelvic, RP, and paracardiac nodal disease should be clearly documented. Diffuse RP suprarenal nodal disease and paracardiac nodes ≥1 cm may preclude surgery.
- *Visceral metastases*: Hematogenous parenchymal liver metastases are rare with invasive serosal surface implants being more common. Splenic surface implants and splenic hilar disease should also be clearly mentioned in CT report as they increase the likelihood of a splenectomy.
- *Bowel metastases*: Involvement of bowel is commonly seen in advanced disease. The mode of involvement can be:
    - Direct invasion from the pelvic carcinomas
    - Along mesenteric fascial planes
    - Intraperitoneal seeding of tumor
    - Through lymphatic channels
    - Embolic hematogenous spread

Bowel involvement is seen as nodular or plaque-like lesions along serosal surfaces and with bowel wall invasion, obstruction is a common complication.

Criteria for Nonresectability

Optimal cytoreduction is not currently defined, though at most centers less than 1 cm of residual tumor present at completion of cytoreductive surgery is considered as a better predictor of long-term survival.[23]

Table 6 summarizes the sites considered potentially nonresectable disease (may be regarded resectable at some centers with specialty surgeons) and nonresectable disease (where resection is unlikely to achieve optimal cytoreduction).[21] **Figures 7A to D** illustrate an example of nonresectable high-grade serous papillary carcinoma. Extensive surgical resections increase the risk of surgical morbidity and mortality.

Magnetic Resonance Imaging

MRI has a superior contrast resolution and can accurately characterize adnexal masses with fat/hemorrhagic/fibrotic components.

BOX 1: Signs of peritoneal disease.

- Subtle thickening of peritoneum
- Fine reticular nodular pattern along peritoneal surface
- Abnormal enhancement of peritoneum
- Large nodular deposits
- Calcified deposits in serous cystadenocarcinomas
- Omental nodularity/omental caking

Findings highly predictive of malignancy **(Figs. 8A to D)** are the demonstration of solid component, solid/cystic masses, or cystic lesions with the presence of papillary projections (vegetations) and thick septations. Secondary features of malignancy include peritoneal, mesenteric or omental involvement, pelvic side wall invasion, and lymphadenopathy.[24]

MRI features most predictive of malignancy are vegetations in a cystic lesion, tumor diameter greater than 6 cm, necrosis in a solid lesion, and the presence of ascites.[25,26] Presence of ascites anterior to the uterus or abdominal ascites is highly suggestive for malignant ascites.[24]

Imaging features for the staging of disease are similar on CT and MRI. MRI can also accurately delineate the extent of intra-abdominal and pelvic disease including involvement of peritoneum and mesentery, urinary tract, visceral and bowel metastases, lymph nodes, and ascites.

MRI Technique

For evaluation of female pelvis, patient preparation includes fasting for 4 hours, use of an antiperistaltic agent (Buscopan), and instructing the patient to void 15–30 minutes prior to imaging.[27]

The following sequences are suggested:

- Sagittal and axial non-fat-suppressed T2-weighted turbo spin-echo sequences.
- Coronal and axial non-fat-suppressed T2-weighted turbo spin-echo sequences.
- T1-weighted gradient-echo sequences with and without fat suppression in axial plane.

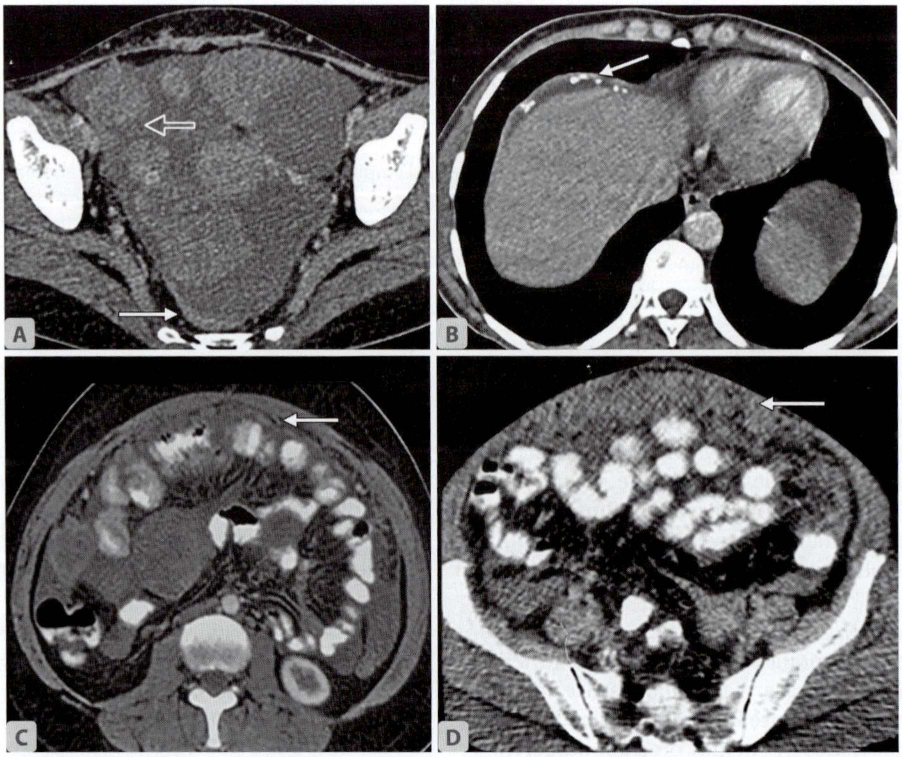

FIGS. 5A TO D: CT signs of peritoneal disease. (A) Thickening of peritoneum (arrow) and peritoneal deposits (block arrow). (B) Calcified deposits (arrow) in serous cystadenocarcinoma. (C) Omental nodularity (arrow). (D) Omental caking (arrow).

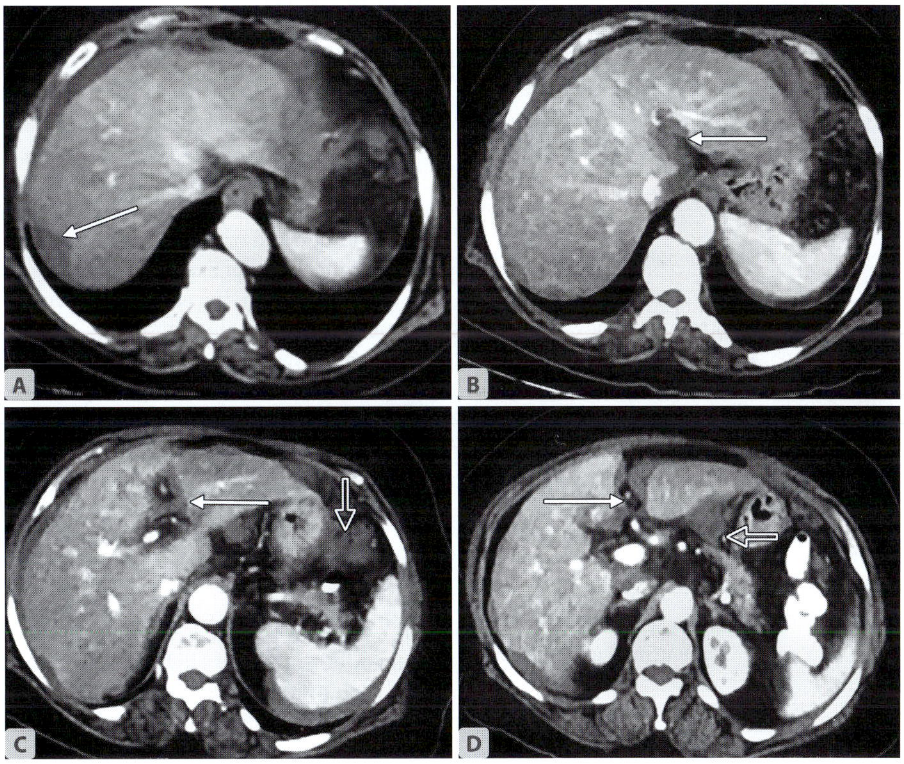

FIGS. 6A TO D: Peritoneal disease: Upper abdominal ligament involvement. (A) Large subphrenic deposit (arrow). (B) Horizontal hepatoduodenal ligament deposit (arrow). (C) Deposit along vertical gastrohepatic ligament (arrow) and lesser sac (block arrow). (D) Deposit along falciform ligament (arrow) and hepatoduodenal ligament (block arrow).

TABLE 5: Computed tomography (CT) landmarks for the upper abdominal ligaments.

Space	Abdominal ligament associated	CT identification
Lesser omentum	Horizontal hepatoduodenal ligament	• Between porta hepatis and first part of the duodenum • Contains common bile duct, portal vein, hepatic artery, lymph nodes
	Vertical gastrohepatic ligament	Identified by recognizing left gastric artery
Lesser sac	Splenorenal and splenogastric ligaments	Lies between stomach and pancreas
Perihepatic space	• Falciform ligament • Morrison's pouch • Gallbladder fossa	• Falciform ligament • Morrison's pouch: Hepatorenal space • Gallbladder fossa

- *Diffusion-weighted imaging (DWI):* Axial plane by using a single-shot echo-planar imaging sequence; b values 0 and 1000 sec/mm^2.
- *MR perfusion:* Dynamic contrast-enhanced T1-weighted gradient-echo sequence is performed with a temporal resolution of 15 seconds; through the mass at the level of "solid tissue."[28] Solid tissue[29,30] comprises vegetation/solid portion/irregular thickened septa. This sequence is performed through the mass and adjacent myometrium after injection of Gadolinium chelate (0.2 mL/kg) at a rate of 2 mL/sec, followed by 20 mL of normal saline in the optimal plane. Images are obtained successively at 2.4-second intervals starting 10 seconds before the bolus injection, for a total duration of 320 seconds.
- Delayed postcontrast axial and sagittal T1-weighted gradient-echo images are obtained.

The perfusion images are used to generate the time-intensity curve of the solid tissue.[28] These curves are defined as follows:

- *Curve type 1*: A gradual increase in the signal intensity of the solid tissue, without a well-defined "shoulder".
- *Curve type 2*: A moderate initial increase in the signal intensity of solid tissue relative to that of myometrium (enhancement of solid tissue has an initial slope less than the myometrium), followed by a plateau **(Figs. 9A and B)**.
- *Curve type 3*: An initial marked increase in the signal intensity of solid tissue steeper than that of myometrium (enhancement of solid tissue has an initial slope more than the myometrium), followed by a plateau.

MRI can be used as a problem-solving tool in sonographically indeterminate ovarian masses by providing better tissue characterization. For borderline/invasive tumors versus benign ovarian lesions the reported sensitivity of MRI is 92% and specificity is 85%.[31] Recently, the ADNEX MR scoring system **(Table 7)** was proposed which incorporates

MR perfusion and DWI sequences into an algorithm for the assessment of adnexal masses.[28] Use of the ADNEX MR scoring algorithm has increased the sensitivity to 93.5% and specificity to 96.6% for the diagnosis of ovarian cancer.[28]

TABLE 6: Criteria for nonresectability.

Potentially nonresectable disease	Nonresectable disease
• Disease in the lesser omentum, lesser sac, and perihepatic space along with the associated upper abdominal ligaments • Gastric and duodenal serosa • Rectal and sigmoid diffuse serosal, wall and luminal invasion • Vascular side wall invasion • Ureteric invasion	• Pleural infiltration • Paracardiac nodes • Subdiaphragmatic plaque-like disease greater than 2 cm • Parenchymal liver metastases • Invasive surface implants • Diffuse large volume mesenteric disease • Root of small bowel mesentery • High retroperitoneal lymph nodes • Bony and muscular side wall invasion • Diffuse presacral disease

Key Points about MRI Signal of Ovarian Lesions[2]

- T1WI with and without fat suppression are crucial for identification of fat (teratoma) or hemorrhage.
- Endometriotic cysts are usually multifocal and bilateral with high SI on T1WI and characteristic shading and layering on T2WI. However, a complex and rapidly growing mass with contrast enhancement in preexisting endometriotic cyst suggests the possibility of endometrioid or clear cell tumor.
- Varying SI is suggestive of mucinous content and presence of solid, enhancing component in such a lesion raises the possibility of malignancy.
- A very-low SI on T2WI suggests a fibrotic component (thecoma/fibroma group, Brenner tumor or cystadenofibroma).
- Bilateral complex solid/solid cystic enhancing mass is suspicious for metastases; however, serous epithelial tumors can be also be bilateral.

PET-CT

Role in Diagnosis

Fluorodeoxyglucose (FDG) PET-CT is not routinely used in the diagnosis of ovarian cancer. USG and CT remain the primary investigation modalities. While studies have

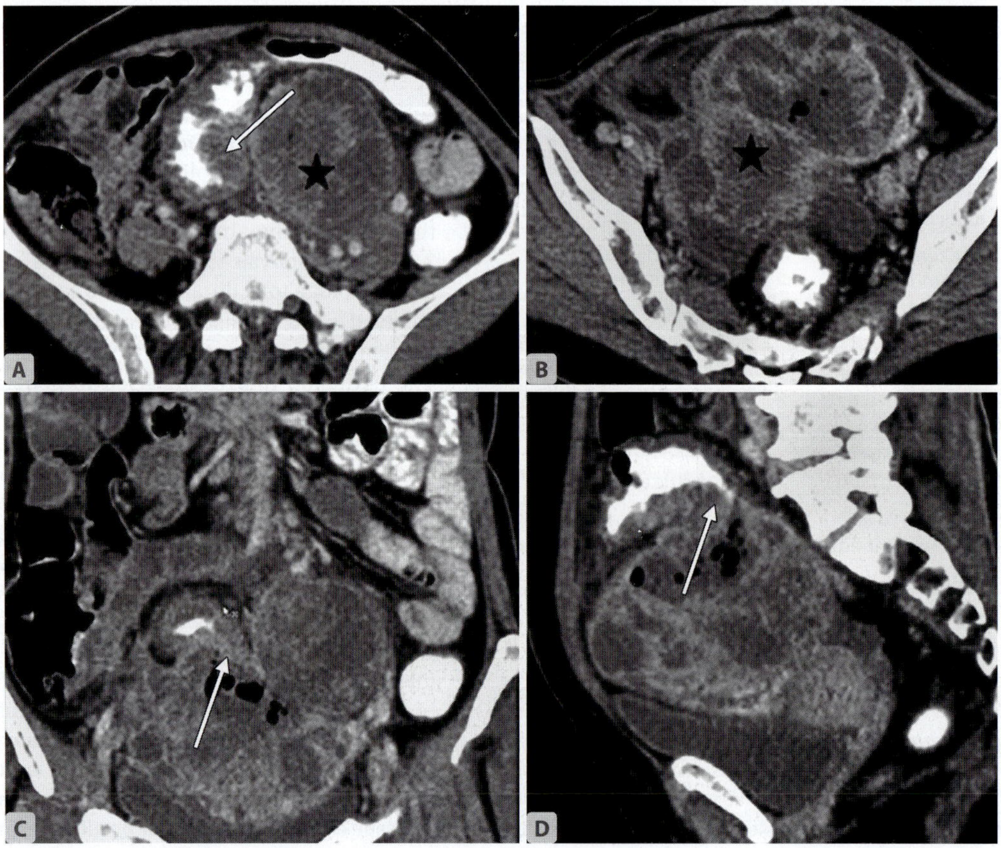

FIGS. 7A TO D: Nonresectable high-grade serous papillary carcinoma: bowel metastases. (A and B) Axial CT pelvis images reveal high-volume peritoneal disease (asterisk in A), adjacent sigmoid mural invasion (arrow in A). (C) Coronal and (D) sagittal multiplanar reconstructed images reveal infiltration of the sigmoid (arrows) by the mass, as evidenced by contiguous extension and presence of gas within the mass.

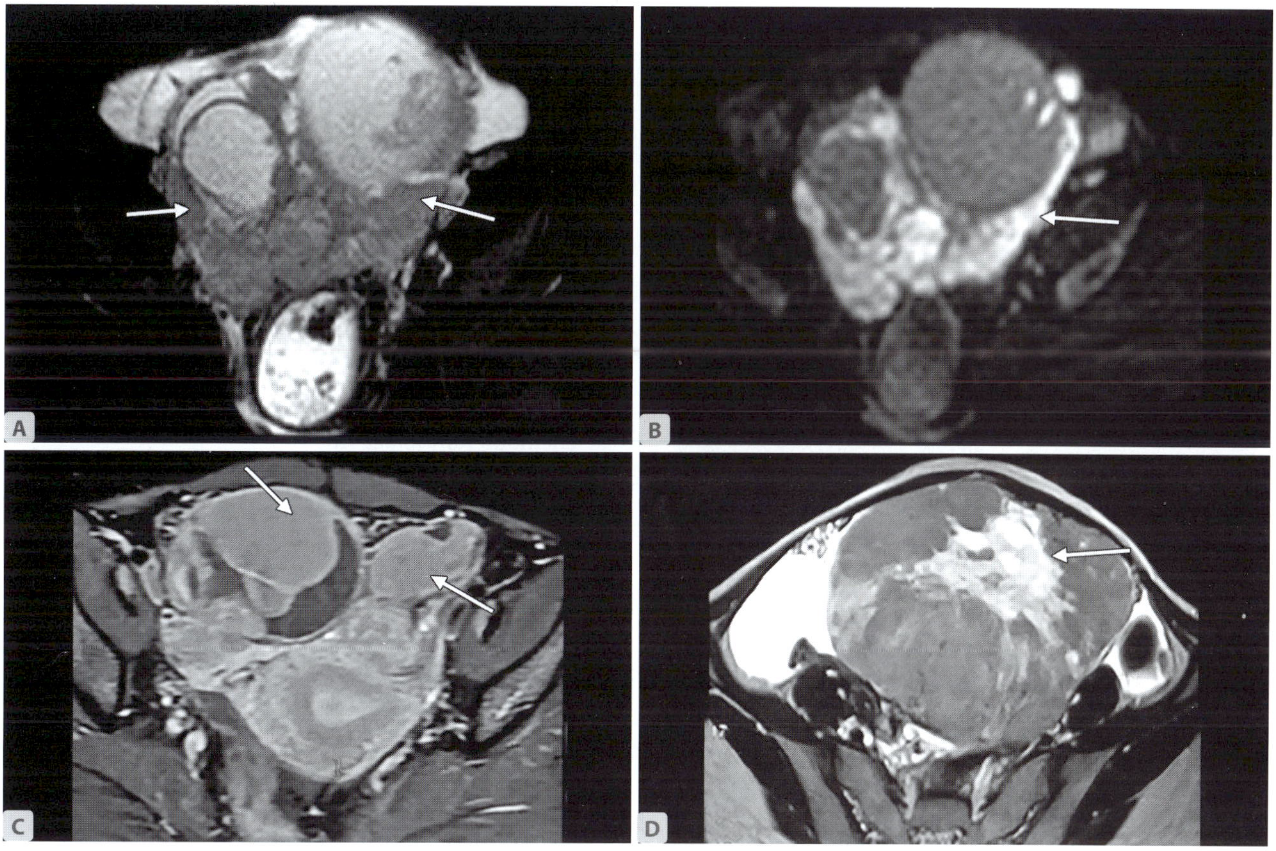

FIGS. 8A TO D: MRI features of malignant ovarian mass. (A) Bilateral complex solid cystic adnexal masses (arrows) and vegetations in a cystic lesion. (B) Diffusion restriction in the solid component (arrow). (C) Enhancing solid component (arrows) in bilateral complex solid cystic adnexal masses. (D) Large solid mass with internal necrosis (arrow) and the presence of ascites.

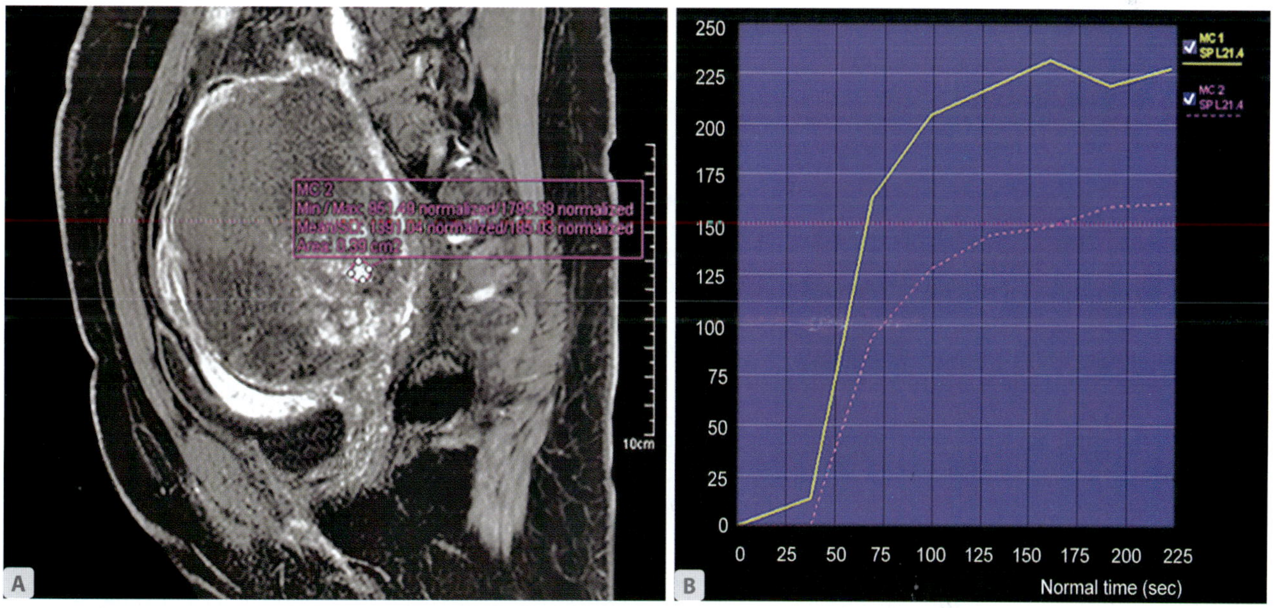

FIGS. 9A AND B: ADNEX MR score 4 (Indeterminate mass). Type 2 curve in left ovarian solid cystic complex mass. There is a moderate initial increase in the signal intensity of solid tissue (pink line) relative to that of myometrium (yellow line), followed by a plateau.

TABLE 7: ADNEX MRI scoring system.[27]

Score	Type	Definition
1	No ovarian mass	
2	Benign mass	• Unilocular cyst of any type, with no wall enhancement • Unilocular simple cyst without solid tissue; wall may enhance • Unilocular endometrioma without solid tissue; wall may enhance • Unilocular/multilocular fat-containing cystic lesion without solid tissue; wall may enhance • Cyst with solid tissue where the solid tissue is homogenously low SI on T2WI and low SI on high B-value images, with mild or moderate enhancement (type 1 or 2 curve)
3	Probably benign mass	• Unilocular hemorrhagic/ proteinaceous cyst with wall enhancement and without solid tissue • Multilocular cyst without solid tissue • Cyst with solid tissue which has intermediate SI on T2WI, is hyperintense on the high B-value DWI, and has a type 1 enhancement curve
4	Indeterminate mass	• Cyst with solid tissue which has intermediate SI on T2WI, is hyperintense on the high B-value DW image, and has a type 2 enhancement curve **(*see* Figs. 9A and B)**
5	Probably malignant mass	• Obvious peritoneal implants • Cyst with solid tissue which has intermediate T2 signal, is hyperintense on the high B-value DW image, and has a type 3 enhancement curve

reported high specificity for detection of malignancy larger than 5 mm in size, FDG PET-CT has been shown to have lower sensitivity, especially in tumors less than 5 mm.[32,33] The pitfalls in the diagnosis of ovarian carcinoma by FDG PET-CT include:

- *Normal physiological ovarian uptake:* Typically observed in the early luteal phase. In order to avoid it, scan should ideally be performed in the early few days of the menstrual cycle. The characteristic appearance of a physiological uptake is summarized in **Box 2**.
- *Small tumors <5 mm:* PET-CT has less sensitivity in small tumors.

Role in Staging

- PET-CT has high sensitivity in detecting peritoneal metastases **(Figs. 10A to D)** larger than 1 cm and lymph nodes larger than 7 mm.[34] When compared to CT alone, it increases the staging accuracy by almost 15–20%.[32]

BOX 2: Imaging appearance of physiological uptake in ovary.[34]

- Seen in premenopausal women (any ovarian uptake in postmenopausal women is abnormal)
- In early luteal phase
- Round or oval shape
- Smooth margin
- Located superior to the urinary bladder or close to the uterus
- SUV >3 is considered abnormal

(SUV: standardized uptake value)

- Another important role of PET-CT is differentiating patients who can undergo optimal debulking (FIGO stages I-IIIB) from patients who need neoadjuvant chemotherapy (stage IIIC-IV).[33]

Role in Post-treatment Follow-up

Various studies have quoted widely variable sensitivity and specificity of FDG PET-CT in recurrent ovarian cancer.[35-37] A recent study has shown that PET-CT has much higher sensitivity in detecting extrapelvic recurrence, compared to pelvic recurrence.[38] This is explained by the presence of high physiological activity in the urinary bladder and normal postoperative inflammatory changes in the pelvis. Some studies[39,40] have documented that PET-CT can change the management in a significant number of recurrent ovarian cancer; and can play an important role in determining who will benefit from optimal cytoreduction.

KEY IMAGING FEATURES OF OVARIAN MALIGNANCIES

Epithelial tumors comprise 60% of all ovarian neoplasms and 85% of ovarian malignant neoplasms.[41] They are most commonly seen in the sixth and seventh decades of life.[41] The histological subtypes include serous, mucinous, endometrioid, clear cell, and Brenner tumors and the imaging findings of these are summarized in **Table 8.**[41,42]

These can be further classified as benign (60% of cases), borderline (5%) or malignant (35%) depending on their histologic characteristics.[41-43]

Germ cell tumors are the second most common group of ovarian neoplasms, and comprise 15–20% of all ovarian tumors and <5% of malignant ovarian neoplasms.[41] These maybe associated with elevated levels of serum α-fetoprotein and human chorionic gonadotropin (βhCG). The key imaging findings of these are summarized in **Table 9.**[41-43]

Sex cord-stromal tumors are composed of cells of coelomic epithelium (sex cords) or mesenchymal cells (theca cells, granulosa cells, Leydig cells, Sertoli cells, and fibroblasts). Majority of these are benign like fibrothecoma and malignant lesions like granulosa cell tumor and Sertoli-Leydig cell tumor are also confined to the ovary at the time of diagnosis. The key imaging findings of these are summarized in **Table 10.**[2,41,42]

Collision Tumors

Collision tumor represents the simultaneous occurrence of two histologically distinct tumors with no histologic

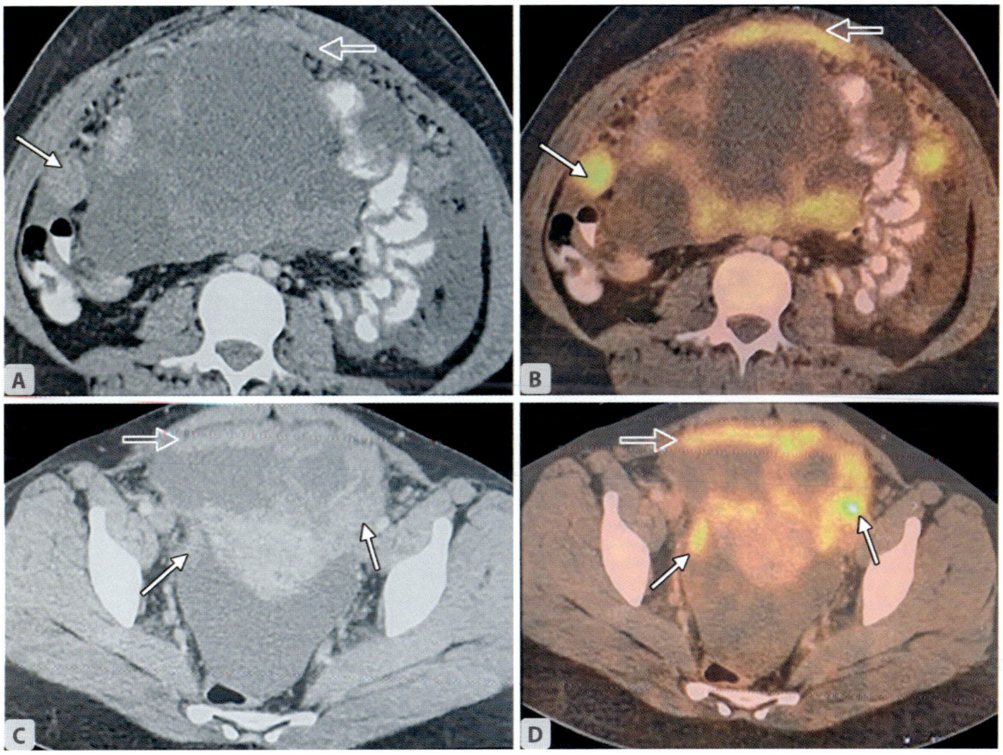

FIGS. 10A TO D: PET-CT in serous papillary cystadenocarcinoma. Axial CECT (A) and corresponding PET-CT image (B) reveal enhancing peritoneal deposits (arrow) and omental thickening (block arrow) with PET uptake. Axial CECT (C) and corresponding PET-CT image (D) show the bilateral solid adnexal masses (arrows) with diffuse peritoneal thickening (block arrow) with PET uptake. (CECT: contrast-enhanced computed tomography; PET: positron emission tomography).

TABLE 8: Key imaging features of epithelial tumors.

Histological type	Clinical	Key imaging features
Serous tumors **(Figs. 11 and 12)**	Often bilateral— 60% benign, 15% borderline, 25% malignant	• Small lesions • B-Unilocular cyst with thin regular wall, no internal septations, linear calcification (infrequent) • M-Solid component, papillary projections, peritoneal carcinomatosis
Mucinous tumors **(Figs. 13A to D)**	Often unilateral— 80% benign, 10–15% borderline, 5–10% malignant	• Large lesions • Multilocular cystic lesions with variable echoes/ density/signal intensity (stained glass appearance), psammomatous calcification • M-Solid component • Pseudomyxoma peritonei
Endometrioid tumors	Almost always malignant— Bilateral: 30–50% cases	• Complex, solid cystic mass • Associated endometrial hyperplasia/carcinoma • Most common malignancy arising from endometriosis, followed by clear cell carcinoma
Clear cell tumors	Always malignant	• Second most common malignancy arising from endometriosis • Unilocular or large cyst with solid enhancing, protrusions
Brenner tumors	• Composed of transitional cells with dense stroma • Rarely malignant • Commonly incidental lesion on imaging	• Small lesions • Usually solid mass with mild enhancement • T2 hypointense stroma • Extensive amorphous calcification may be seen

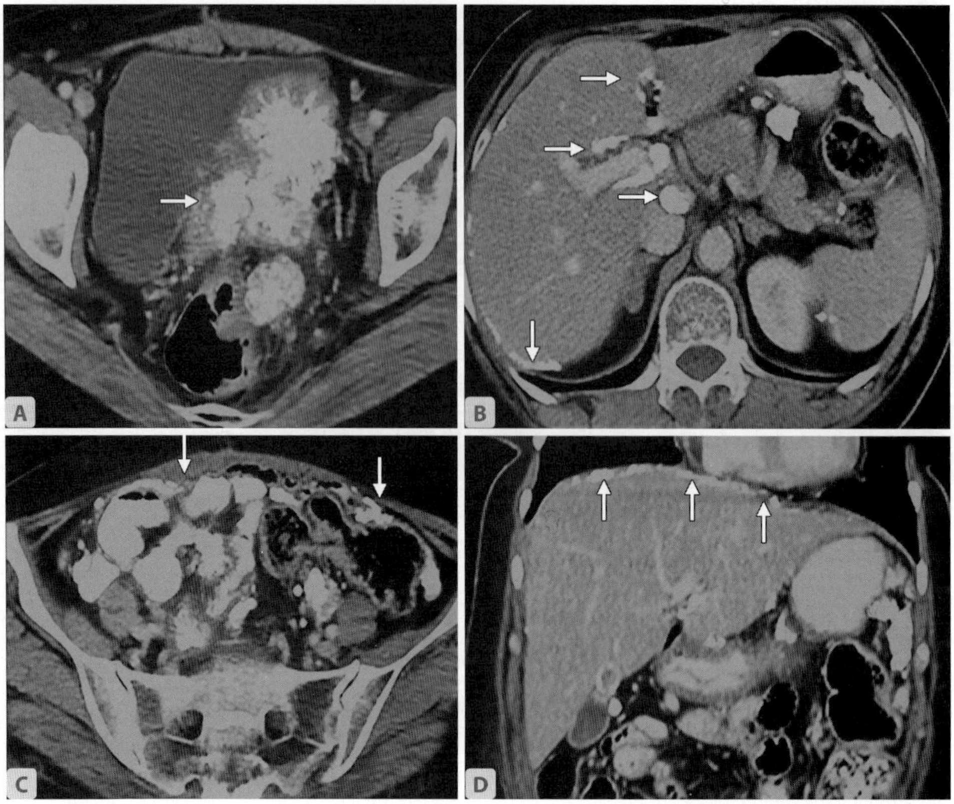

FIGS. 11A TO D: Serous cystadenocarcinoma ovary with calcified peritoneal deposits. Axial contrast-enhanced CT pelvis (A) shows left adnexal mass (arrow) with dense calcification. Calcified peritoneal deposits in upper abdomen (arrows in B) and pelvis (arrows in C). Coronal multiplanar reconstructed image (D) reveals calcified subphrenic deposits (arrows).

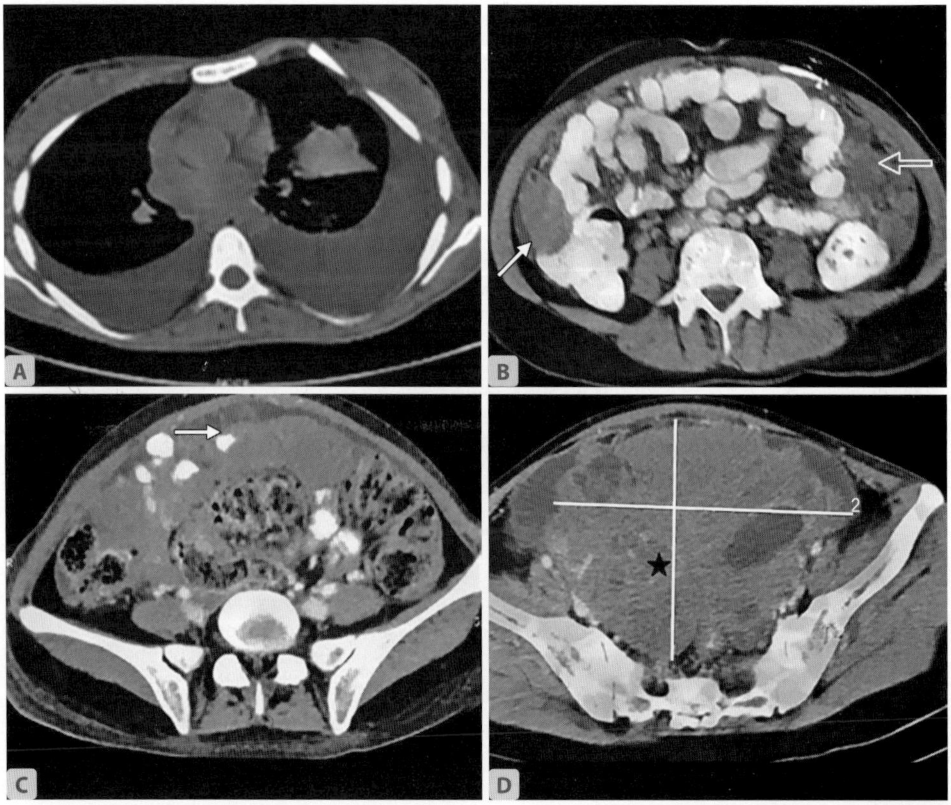

FIGS. 12A TO D: High-grade serous papillary carcinoma. (A) Axial CT chest reveals bilateral pleural effusion. (B to D) Axial contrast-enhanced CT abdomen and pelvis reveals multiple large solid peritoneal deposits (arrow in B), omental caking (block arrow in B), diffuse peritoneal thickening (arrow in C); and a large solid enhancing pelvic mass (asterisk in D).

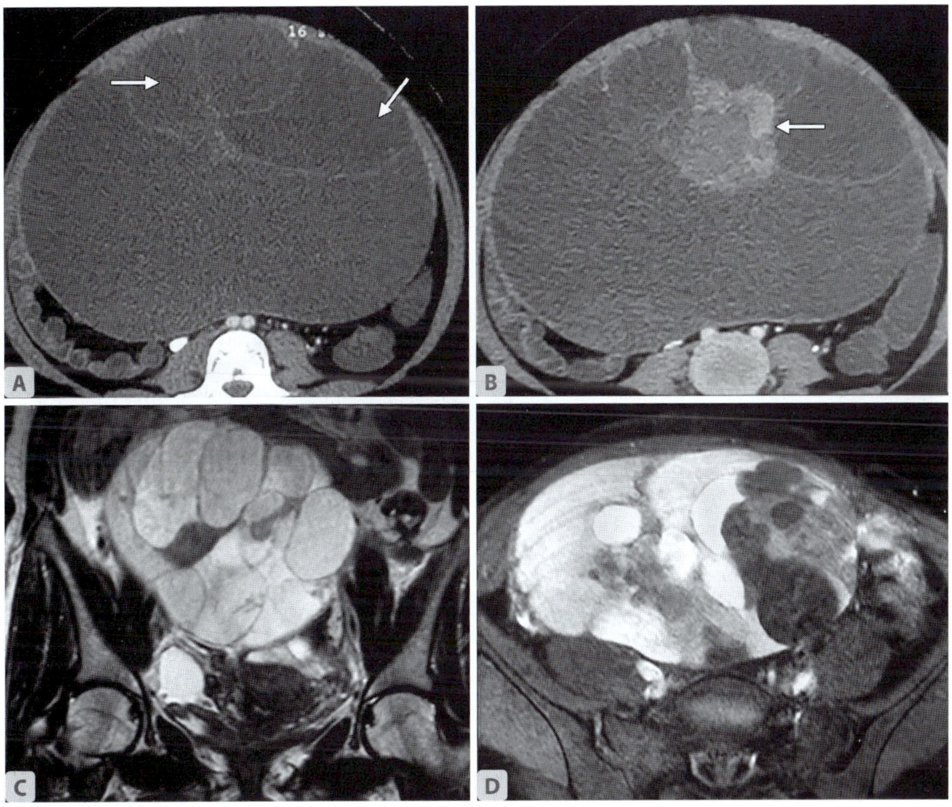

FIGS. 13A TO D: Mucinous cystadenocarcinoma ovary. (A) Axial contrast-enhanced CT shows multiloculated right adnexal cystic mass with different densities (arrows). (B) Solid-enhancing component within the lesion (arrow). (C) T2W coronal MRI shows loculi of variable signal intensities in the mass. (D) Axial T1W fat-suppressed MR image reveals multiple loculi to be hyperintense.

TABLE 9: Key imaging features of germ cell tumors.

Histological type	Clinical	Key imaging features
Mature teratoma	Most common benign ovarian tumor in <45-year-old females	• Varied spectrum (detailed in Chapter 14) • Cystic mass with fat, calcification • *Complications:* Torsion, rupture, or malignant degeneration
Immature teratoma	• First two decades of life • May have normal α-fetoprotein and βhCG levels	• Cystic solid mass with poorly defined capsule • Internal necrosis/hemorrhage • *Fat:* Small foci • *Calcification:* Small, irregular, scattered
Dysgerminoma **(Figs. 14A and B)**	• Young women • Elevated LDH • Elevated βhCG levels if syncytiotrophoblastic giant cells within the tumor	• Large, multilobulated sold mass • Fibrovascular septa characteristic
Yolk sac tumor **(Figs. 15A and B)**	• Second decade • Poor prognosis • Elevated serum α-fetoprotein • Elevated LDH may be seen	• Large solid cystic mass • "Bright dot sign" due to foci of enhancement (dilated vessels) in wall or solid component
Embryonal carcinoma	• Adolescent age group • May present as precocious puberty • Elevated βhCG and α-fetoprotein levels may be seen	• Predominantly solid mass • Nonspecific imaging features

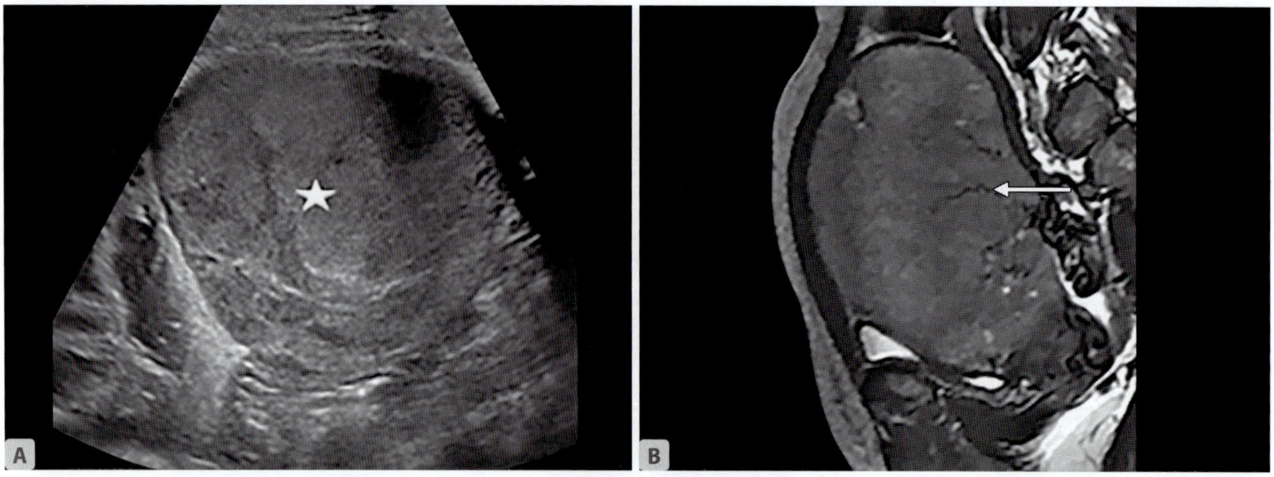

FIGS. 14A AND B: Ovarian dysgerminoma. (A) Solid echogenic mass on USG (asterisk). (B) Sagittal T2WI MRI reveals large, multilobulated solid T2 intermediate SI mass with characteristic fibrovascular septa (arrow).

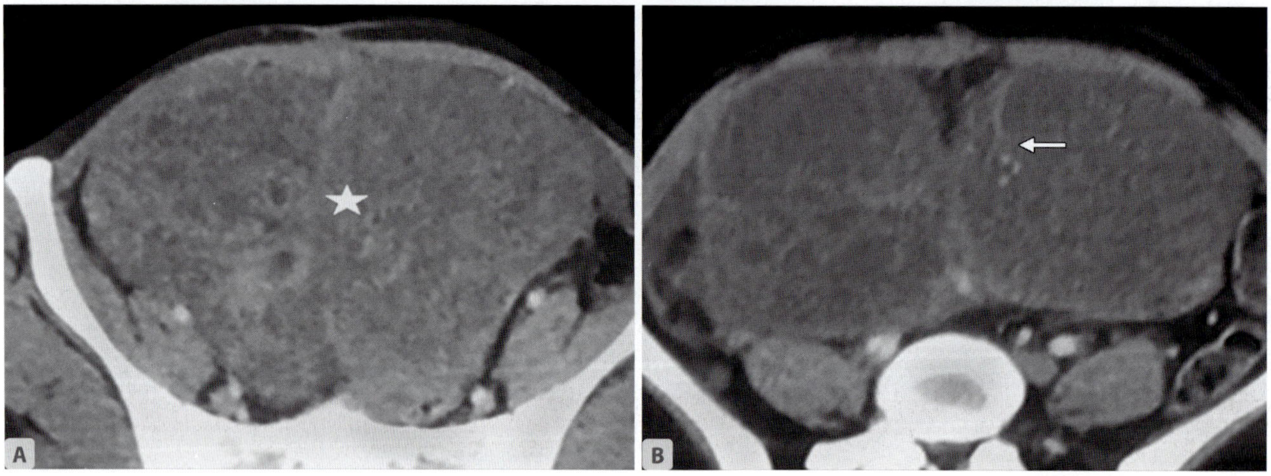

FIGS. 15A AND B: Yolk sac tumor. (A) Heterogeneously enhancing solid abdominopelvic mass (asterisk). (B) Foci of enhancing vessels: Bright dot sign (arrow).

TABLE 10: Key imaging features of sex cord–stromal tumors.

Histological type	Clinical	Key imaging features
Fibromas Fibrothecomas Thecomas	Associations: Meig syndrome	Solid masses CT: Homogenous, solid mass with delayed enhancement; dense calcifications may be seen MRI: Low SI on T1WI and markedly hypointense on T2WI
Granulosa cell tumors **(Figs. 16A and B)**	Most common estrogen producing tumor	Associated endometrial hyperplasia, polyps, or carcinoma Wide imaging spectrum: Solid masses, tumors with hemorrhage or fibrosis, multilocular cystic tumors or completely cystic tumors Compared to epithelial malignancies, these are usually confined to ovary with less peritoneal seeding and do not have intracystic papillary projections
Sertoli-Leydig cell tumors	<30 years age Most common virilizing tumor Low-grade malignancy	Well-defined, enhancing solid mass Intratumoral cysts maybe seen

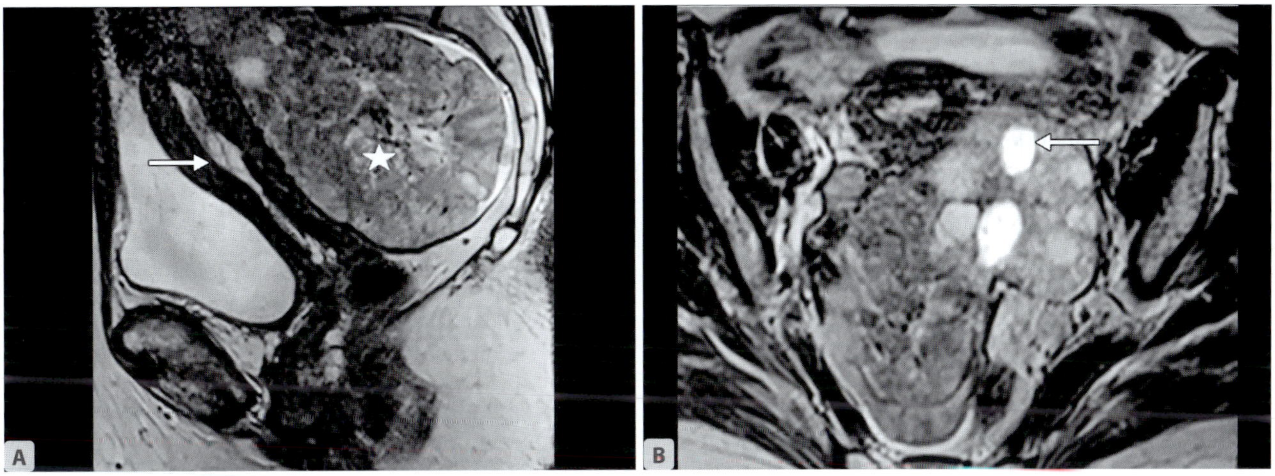

FIGS. 16A AND B: Granulosa cell tumor in 65/F. (A) Sagittal T2WI shows solid mass in pouch of Douglas (asterisk) with endometrial thickening (arrow). (B) Axial T2WI reveals lobulated, solid mass with cystic areas (arrow) in left adnexa and pouch of Douglas.

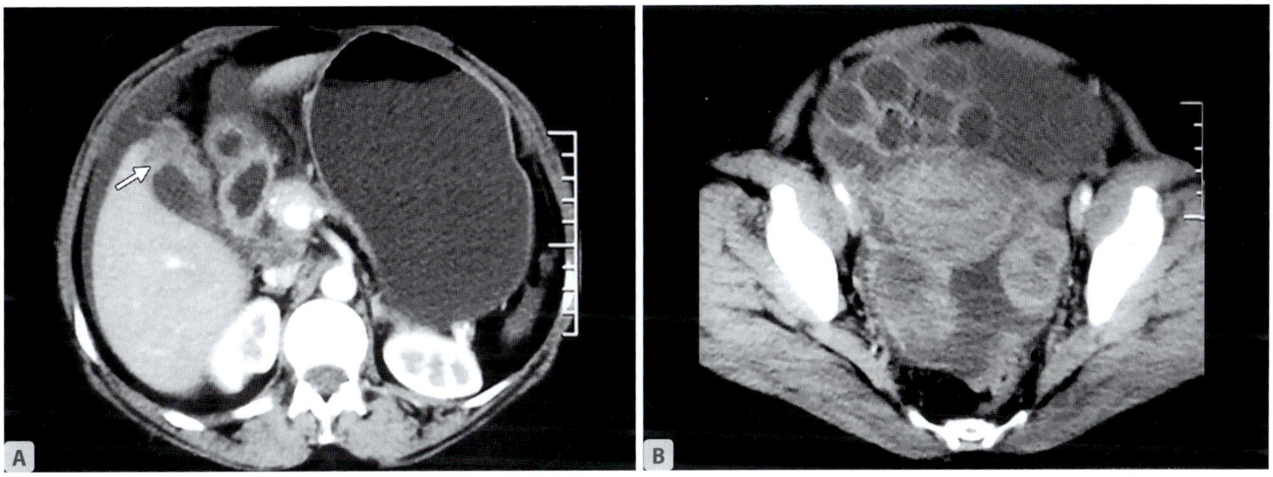

FIGS. 17A AND B: Krukenberg's tumor from carcinoma gallbladder. (A) Irregular mass-like GB wall thickening (arrow) and presence of ascites. (B) Bilateral solid ovarian masses with maintained ovarian shape.

admixture at the interface. Teratoma and cystadenoma or cystadenocarcinoma are the most common occurrence as collision tumors.[44] These should be suspected on imaging if the imaging features are not typical for any particular entity.

Metastatic Ovarian Tumors

Metastases to the ovary are most commonly from colon and stomach followed by the breast, lung, and contralateral ovary.

Imaging Findings

Nonspecific findings varying from predominantly solid masses to cystic and solid masses.

Krukenberg Tumors (Figs. 17A and B)

Metastatic tumors to the ovary containing mucin-secreting "signet ring" cells and originating in the gastrointestinal tract commonly.[45,46] On imaging, these appear as bilateral solid masses with T1 hyperintensity due to mucin and T2 hypointensity (stromal reaction).

Fallopian Tube Malignancies

These are uncommon neoplasms, seen mostly in the postmenopausal age group. Primary fallopian tube carcinomas arise from the ampulla with endoluminal growth leading to hydrosalpinx formation (because of obstruction). The classically described *Latzko's triad* of abdominopelvic mass, intermittent sudden and profuse watery serosanguineous vaginal discharge, and pelvic spasmodic pain relieved by discharge is seen in only 15% of the cases. Imaging features are indistinguishable from ovarian malignancies (typically solid cystic pelvic mass with peritoneal dissemination and lymph node metastases). Hydrosalpinx adjacent to the mass maybe seen in some cases.

Key Point

It is important to note that in the new staging FIGO classification system the ovarian, fallopian, and primary peritoneal cancers are seen as one entity. This revision takes into account the concept of a common origin of high-grade serosal tumors from tubal cells.[3]

TUMOR MARKERS IN OVARIAN NEOPLASMS

Tumor markers include various proteins and other molecules which are produced, expressed, or metabolized by tumor tissue and are characterized in blood, serum, or urine. They are utilized in early diagnosis and screening of ovarian cancers and are also useful in follow-up, treatment response evaluation, and prediction of recurrence. *The important tumor markers are discussed briefly:*

- *CA-125 (Cancer antigen 125):* Currently, it the most widely used biomarker in diagnosis and follow-up of ovarian cancer. It is a glycoprotein expressed by epithelial cells and has a sensitivity and specificity of around 85% and 66%, respectively. Normal values range from 0 U/mL to 45 U/mL.[47]
- *BRCA 1/BRCA2*: Mutation in these tumor suppressor genes is associated with 20–60% risk of ovarian cancer, in addition to the breast malignancies.
- Alpha fetoprotein (AFP)—associated with germ cell tumors (endodermal sinus tumor, embryonal carcinoma).[48]
- Beta hCG—associated with choriocarcinoma and germ cell tumor (embryonal carcinoma).
- HE4—human epididymis protein 4, associated with ovarian carcinoma, more in endometrioid and serous cancers. Increased CA-125 and HE4 levels both increase the specificity for epithelial malignancies.
- Lactate dehydrogenase—associated with germ cell tumors (dysgerminoma).
- Inhibin A/B—granulosa cell tumors.
- Carcinoembryonic antigen (CEA)—mucinous epithelial tumors.

There are multiple other biomarkers, for which initial research has suggested potential benefits in disease detection and follow-up. These are however in an experimental stage and not part of standard evaluation. These include:

Haptoglobin, osteopontin, prostatin, macrophage colony stimulating factor and OVX1, vascular endothelial growth factor (VEGF), HER 2/neu, Ras homologue member 1 (ARHI), insulin-like growth factor binding protein 3 (IGFBP-3), metastasis-related gene synuclein gamma (SNCG), p53, mesothelin, IL-6, and IL-8.[49]

RECENT ADVANCES IN IMAGING BIOLOGY

The conventional concept of considering epithelial ovarian cancer as a single disease has been replaced by the new concept of considering them as a group of different disease entities. This concept is based on new insights into tumor biology, genetic mutations, and identification of specific precursor lesions for different groups.[50-52] Whereas high-grade serous carcinoma (HGSC) is an aggressive tumor, can develop within a short span of time, and has a poor prognosis, low-grade serous carcinoma (LGSC) is much less aggressive and develops from preexisting serous cystadenoma.[50]

High-grade Serous Carcinoma

High-grade serous carcinoma is the commonest of all epithelial ovarian cancers. It presents with an advanced stage, widespread peritoneal dissemination, and a poor prognosis. *BRCA1* and *BRCA2* mutations are found in about 10% patients. The patients with the mutations have better prognosis and can have new therapeutic options.[53] Studies have shown that HGSC with *BRCA* mutation has peritoneal metastases with a "pushing" pattern whereas the tumors lacking the mutation have a more infiltrative pattern of metastases.[54] A new concept in the pathogenesis of HGSC is that it originates from serous tubal intraepithelial carcinoma (STIC). According to this new concept, HGSC, tubal carcinoma, and primary peritoneal carcinoma have the same origin from STIC.[55] Typical imaging findings in HGSC include ascites and bulky peritoneal disease. With the advances in knowledge about tumor genetics, even more detailed subtyping of HGSC has been studied. One such notable study by Vargas et al.[56] attempted to establish association CT imaging patterns and ovarian cancer subtypes based on gene signatures (*Classification of ovarian cancer; CLOVAR*). Depending on different marker gene expression, various HGSCs were divided into four groups: differentiated, immunoreactive, mesenchymal, and proliferative. The study described that the mesenchymal subtype was more often associated with diffuse peritoneal spread and poor survival. The mesenchymal subtype was also found to be more commonly associated with resistance to platinum-based chemotherapy (e.g. cisplatin).

A detailed description of these is beyond the scope of this chapter.

Low-grade Serous Carcinoma

Low-grade serous carcinoma constitutes of a small percentage of epithelial ovarian cancer and is much less aggressive in behavior compared to HGSC. It has better prognosis than HGSC and shows intermediate sensitivity to platinum-based chemotherapy.

Other Subtypes

Other subtypes of epithelial ovarian cancer include mucinous, endometrioid, and clear cell carcinoma. Mucinous cystadenoma is considered a precursor to mucinous cancer, and endometriosis a precursor to the other two variants. All of them have separate genetic mutations (similar to *BRCA1* and *BRCA2* in HGSC). An overview of the clinical, radiological, and pathological features is given in **Table 11**.

CONCLUSION

The role of imaging in ovarian malignancies is to detect, characterize, and stage the disease. It is important for the radiologist to be able to accurately characterize an adnexal mass as benign or malignant. Preoperative staging by imaging is important for definitive patient management and surgical planning.

TABLE 11: Comparison of clinico-patho-radiological features of ovarian cancer subtypes.[50,57]

	HGSC	LGSC	Mucinous	Endometrioid	Clear cell
Biological behavior	Aggressive, poor prognosis	Less aggressive, intermediate prognosis	Good prognosis	Good prognosis	Intermediate prognosis
Disease spread	Extensive peritoneal spread in the abdomen	Peritoneal spread	Localized to ovary	Spread limited to pelvis	Spread limited to pelvis
Mutation	TP53, BRCA1/2	BRAF, KRAS	KRAS	PTEN, CTNNB-1	KRAS, PTEN, PIK3CA
Precursor lesion	STIC	Serous cystadenoma	Mucinous cystadenoma	Endometriosis	Endometriosis
Radiologic appearance	Solid/cystic or solid mass	Solid-cystic mass with papillary projection and psammoma bodies	• Large solid-cystic mass with smooth outline • Different attenuations within the tumor	• Solid-cystic with smooth outline • In pre-existing endometrioma, it is seen as a solid nodule in endometrioma wall	Large thick-walled cystic mass with mural nodules

(HGSC: high-grade serous carcinoma; LGSC: low-grade serous carcinoma; STIC: serous tubal intraepithelial carcinoma)

REFERENCES

1. Iyer VR, Lee SI. MRI, CT, and PET/CT for ovarian cancer detection and adnexal lesion characterization. Am J Roentgenol. 2010;194:311-21.
2. Foti PV, Attinà G, Spadola S, et al. MR imaging of ovarian masses: classification and differential diagnosis. Insights Imaging. 2016;7:21-41.
3. Kurman RJ, Carcangiu ML, Herrington CS, et al. WHO Classification of Tumors of Female Reproductive Organs. Lyon: IARC; 2014.
4. Prat J. FIGO Committee on Gynecologic Oncology. Staging classification for cancer of the ovary, fallopian tube, and peritoneum. Int J Gynaecol Obstet. 2014;124:1-5.
5. Mutch DG, Prat J. 2014 FIGO staging for ovarian, fallopian tube and peritoneal cancer. Gynecol Oncol. 2014;133:401-4.
6. Javadi S, Ganeshan DM, Qayyum A, et al. Ovarian cancer, the revised FIGO staging system, and the role of imaging. Am J Roentgenol. 2016;206:1351-60.
7. Leibman AJ, Kruse B, McSweeney MB. Transvaginal sonography: comparison with transabdominal sonography in the diagnosis of pelvic masses. Am J Roentgenol. 1988;151:89-92.
8. Hata K, Hata T, Manabe A, et al. A critical evaluation of transvaginal Doppler studies, transvaginal sonography, magnetic resonance imaging, and CA 125 in detecting ovarian cancer. Obstet Gynecol. 1992;80:922-6.
9. Reles A, Wein U, Lichtenegger W. Transvaginal color Doppler sonography and conventional sonography in the preoperative assessment of adnexal masses. J Clin Ultrasound. 1997;25:217-25.
10. Ferrazzi E, Zanetta G, Dordoni D, et al. Transvaginal ultrasonographic characterization of ovarian masses: comparison of five scoring systems in a multicenter study. Ultrasound Obstet Gynecol. 1997;10:192-7.
11. Kurjak A, Predanic M. New scoring system for prediction of ovarian malignancy based on transvaginal color Doppler sonography. J Ultrasound Med. 1992;11:631-8.
12. Franchi M, Beretta P, Ghezzi F, et al. Diagnosis of pelvic masses with transabdominal color Doppler, CA 125, and ultrasonography. Acta Obstet Gynecol Scand. 1995;74:734-9.
13. Timor-Tritsch IE, Lerner JP, Monteagudo A, et al. Transvaginal ultrasonographic characterization of ovarian masses by means of color flow-directed Doppler measurements and a morphologic scoring system. Am J Obstet Gynecol. 1993;168:909-13.
14. Laban M, Metawee H, Elyan A, et al. Three-dimensional ultrasound and three-dimensional power Doppler in the assessment of ovarian tumors. Int J Gynecol Obstet. 2007;99:201-5.
15. Ueland FR, DePriest PD, Pavlik EJ. Preoperative differentiation of malignant from benign ovarian tumors: the efficacy of morphology indexing and Doppler flow sonography. Gynecol Oncol. 2003;91:46-50.
16. Timmerman D, Testa AC, Bourne T, et al. Simple ultrasound-based rules for the diagnosis of ovarian cancer. Ultrasound Obstet Gynecol. 2008;31:681-90.
17. Alcázar JL, Pascual MÁ, Olartecoechea B, et al. IOTA simple rules for discriminating between benign and malignant adnexal masses: prospective external validation. Ultrasound Obstet Gynecol. 2013;42:467-71.
18. Timmerman D, Van Calster B, Testa A, et al. Predicting the risk of malignancy in adnexal masses based on the simple rules from the International Ovarian Tumor Analysis group. Am J Obstet Gynecol. 2016;214(4):424-37.
19. Van Calster B, Van Hoorde K, Valentin L, et al. Evaluating the risk of ovarian cancer before surgery using the ADNEX model to differentiate between benign, borderline, early and advanced stage invasive, and secondary metastatic tumors: prospective multicentre diagnostic study. BMJ. 2014;349:g5920.
20. Forstner R, Sala E, Kinkel K, et al. ESUR guidelines: ovarian cancer staging and follow-up. Eur Radiol. 2010;20:2773-80.
21. Sahdev A. CT in ovarian cancer staging: how to review and report with emphasis on abdominal and pelvic disease for surgical planning. Cancer Imaging. 2016;16:19-27.
22. Tempany CM, Zou KH, Silverman SG, et al. Staging of advanced ovarian cancer: comparison of imaging modalities–report from the Radiological Diagnostic Oncology Group. Radiology. 2000;215(3):761-7.

23. Chang SJ, Hodeib M, Chang J, et al. Survival impact of complete cytoreduction to no gross residual disease for advanced-stage ovarian cancer: a meta-analysis. Gynecol Oncol. 2013;130: 493-8.
24. Sohaib SAA, Reznek RH. MR imaging in ovarian cancer. Cancer Imaging. 2007;7:S119-29.
25. Sohaib SA, Sahdev A, Van Trappen PO, et al. Characterization of adnexal mass lesions on MR imaging. Am J Roentgenol. 2003;180:1297-304.
26. Hricak H, Chen M, Coakley FV, et al. Complex adnexal masses: detection and characterization with MR imaging-multivariate analysis. Radiology. 2000;214:39-46.
27. Sadowski EA, Robbins JB, Rockall AG, et al. A systematic approach to adnexal masses discovered on ultrasound: the ADNEx MR scoring system. Abdom Radiol. 2018;43:679-96.
28. Thomassin-Naggara I, Aubert E, Rockall A, et al. Adnexal masses: development and preliminary validation of an MR imaging scoring system. Radiology. 2013;267:432-43.
29. Thomassin-Naggara I, Daraï E, Cuenod CA, et al. Dynamic contrast-enhanced magnetic resonance imaging: a useful tool for characterizing ovarian epithelial tumors. J Magn Reson Imaging. 2008;28(1):111-20.
30. Timmerman D, Valentin L, Bourne TH, et al. Terms, definitions, and measurements to describe the sonographic features of adnexal tumors: a consensus opinion from the International Ovarian Tumor Analysis (IOTA) Group. Ultrasound Obstet Gynecol. 2000;16(5):500-5.
31. Medeiros LR, Freitas LB, Rosa DD, et al. Accuracy of magnetic resonance imaging in ovarian tumor: a systematic quantitative review. Am J Obstet Gynecol. 2011;204:67.e61-10.
32. Castellucci P, Perrone AM, Picchio M. Diagnostic accuracy of 18F-FDG PET/CT in characterizing ovarian lesions and staging ovarian cancer: correlation with transvaginal ultrasonography, computed tomography, and histology. Nucl Med Commun. 2007;28:589-95.
33. Kitajima K, Murakami K, Yamasaki E. Diagnostic accuracy of integrated FDG-PET/contrast-enhanced CT in staging ovarian cancer: comparison with enhanced CT. Eur J Nucl Med Mol Imaging. 2008;35:1912-20.
34. Prakash P, Cronin CG, Blake MA. Role of PET/CT in ovarian cancer. Am J Roentgenol. 2010;194:W464-70.
35. Sironi S, Messa C, Mangili G, et al. Integrated FDG PET/CT in patients with persistent ovarian cancer: correlation with histological findings. Radiology. 2004;233:433-40.
36. Chung HH, Kang WJ, Kim JW, et al. Role of [18F] FDG PET/CT in the assessment of suspected recurrent ovarian cancer: correlation with clinical or histological findings. Eur J Nucl Med Mol Imaging. 2007;34:480-6.
37. Sebastian S, Lee SI, Horowitz NS, et al. PET-CT vs CT alone in ovarian cancer recurrence. Abdom Imaging. 2008;33:112-8.
38. Iagaru AH, Mittra ES, McDougall IR, et al. 18F-FDG PET/CT evaluation of patients with ovarian carcinoma. Nucl Med Commun. 2008;29:1046-51.
39. Mangili G, Picchio M, Sironi S. Integrated PET/CT as a first-line restaging modality in patients with suspected recurrence of ovarian cancer. Eur J Nucl Med Mol Imaging. 2007;34:658-66.
40. Simcock B, Neesham D, Quinn M. The impact of PET/CT in the management of recurrent ovarian cancer. Gynecol Oncol. 2006;103:271-6.
41. Jung SE, Lee JM, Rha SE, et al. CT and MR imaging of ovarian tumors with emphasis on differential diagnosis. Radiographics. 2002;22:1305-25.
42. Jeong YY, Outwater EK, Kang HK. Imaging evaluation of ovarian masses. Radiographics. 2000;20:1445-70.
43. Heo SH, Kim JW, Shin SS, et al. Review of ovarian tumors in children and adolescents: radiologic-pathologic correlation. Radiographics. 2014;34:2039-55.
44. Kim SH, Kim YJ, Park BK, et al. Collision tumors of the ovary associated with teratoma: clues to the correct preoperative diagnosis. J Comput Assist Tomogr. 1999;23:929-33.
45. Brown DL, Zou KH, Tempany CM, et al. Primary versus secondary ovarian malignancy: imaging findings of adnexal masses in the Radiology Diagnostic Oncology Group Study. Radiology. 2001;219:213-8.
46. Ha HK, Baek SY, Kim SH, et al. Krukenberg's tumor of the ovary: MR imaging features. Am J Roentgenol. 1995;164:1435-9.
47. Bast RC Jr, Badgwell D, Lu Z, et al. New tumor markers: CA125 and beyond. Int J Gynecol Cancer. 2005;15(Suppl 3):274-81.
48. Taskinen S, Fagerholm R, Lohi J, et al. Pediatric ovarian neoplastic tumors: incidence, age at presentation, tumor markers and outcome. Acta Obstet Gynecol Scand. 2015;94(4):425-9.
49. Rein BJD, Gupta S, Dada R, et al. Potential markers for detection and monitoring of ovarian cancer. J Oncol. 2011;2011:475983.
50. Forstner R, Meissnitzer M, Cunha TM. Update on imaging of ovarian cancer. Curr Radiol Rep. 2016;4:31.
51. Lawrenson K, Gyther SA. Ovarian cancer: a clinical challenge that needs some basic answers. PLoS Med. 2009;6(2e):1000025.
52. Kurman RJ, Shih IeM. Molecular pathogenesis and extraovarian origin of epithelial ovarian cancer–shifting the paradigm. Hum Pathol. 2011;42:918-31.
53. Bolton KL, Chenevix-Trench G, Goh C, et al. Association between BRCA1 and BRCA2 mutations and survival in women with invasive epithelial ovarian cancer. JAMA. 2012;307:382-90.
54. Reyes MC, Arnold AG, Kauff ND, et al. Invasion patterns of metastatic high-grade serous carcinoma of ovary or fallopian tube associated with BRCA deficiency. Mod Pathol. 2014;27(10):1405-11.
55. Nik NN, Vang R, Shih IM, et al. Origin and pathogenesis of pelvic (ovarian, tubal, and primary peritoneal) serous carcinoma. Annu Rev Pathol. 2014;9:27-45.
56. Vargas HA, Micco M, Hong SI, et al. Association between morphologic CT imaging traits and prognostically relevant signatures in women with high-grade serous ovarian cancer. A hypothesis-generating study. Radiology. 2015;274:742-51.
57. Lalwani N, Prassad SR, Vikram R, et al. Histologic, molecular, and cytogenetic features of ovarian cancers: implication for diagnosis and treatment. Radiographics. 2011;31:625-46.

CHAPTER

16

Benign Diseases of the Uterus and Vagina

Rashmi Dixit, Anju Garg, Alpana Manchanda

INTRODUCTION

A wide variety of benign lesions involve the uterus. These may be congenital or acquired. The clinical presentation is often nonspecific, hence imaging has an important role in establishing an accurate diagnosis. Ultrasound (US), especially transvaginal sonography (TVS) is the investigation of choice for initial evaluation. MRI is an excellent problem-solving tool and helps guide management decisions. The role of computed tomography (CT) is limited in the evaluation of benign disease of the female pelvis due to its poor soft tissue differentiation.

CONGENITAL ANOMALIES

The uterus arises from paired embryologic structures—the Müllerian ducts that undergo fusion and resorption, between 6 weeks and 11 weeks in utero, to give rise to the uterus, fallopian tubes, cervix, and upper two-thirds of the vagina. Disruption at any stage, i.e. ductal development, ductal fusion, or septal resorption can result in anomalies of these structures referred to as Müllerian duct anomalies (MDAs). Since the ovaries arise from the primitive yolk sac while the distal one-third of the vagina arises from the sinovaginal bud, anomalies of the external genitalia or ovary are not associated with MDAs. The reported prevalence varies widely from 1% to 5% in the general population to 13%–25% in women with recurrent pregnancy loss.[1-3]

Ultrasound, especially three-dimensional US (3D US) and MR imaging play an important role in the diagnosis and evaluation of suspected MDA. Hysterosalpingography (HSG), usually a part of the initial workup infertility, may suggest a MDA, but it cannot reliably differentiate subtypes. 3D US is recommended as the initial investigation for the diagnosis of female genital anomalies in "symptomatic" patients of the reproductive age suspected to have an anomaly of a female genital tract and for any suspicious findings on routine US.[4] It is preferable to do the US during the second half of the menstrual cycle, since the endometrium is thick and echogenic during this period, making visualization of the MDAs easier.[5] MR is generally the most preferred imaging modality especially for complex anomalies and is recommended as the first-line diagnostic procedure for symptomatic adolescents.[4] MR imaging decreases the number of invasive procedures, costs, and guides management decisions.[5] Concomitant renal anomalies like agenesis, horseshoe kidney, renal dysplasia, ectopic kidney, and duplicated collecting systems have been reported in 29% of patients. Associated skeletal anomalies may also be present.[1,3,6]

Classification

There is no universally accepted MDA classification system; each having its limitations. The system proposed by the American Society for Reproductive Medicine (ASRM)[7] has been the most widely accepted until recently.

The ASRM classification ***(Fig. 1)*** *of congenital anomalies*:

- *Class I—agenesis or hypoplasia*: Failure of development of the Müllerian ducts in the early stages (around 5 weeks' of gestation) results in varying degrees of agenesis or hypoplasia of uterus, cervix, and the proximal two-thirds of the vagina. In *agenesis*, there is no uterus or small amount of rudimentary tissue without any differentiation. This anomaly is part of the *Mayer-Rokitansky-Küster-Hauser (MRKH) syndrome*. It is the most severe type of MDA, i.e. complete agenesis of the proximal vagina, cervix, and uterus. The patients mostly manifest at puberty as primary amenorrhea with normal secondary sexual characteristics, since ovarian function is preserved. Isolated involvement of reproductive organs is classified as MRKH syndrome type 1 while if patients also have extragenital, e.g. renal, skeletal, vertebral, otologic, or cardiac anomalies, it is classified as MRKH syndrome type 2. A small but fully differentiated organ is visualized in uterine *hypoplasia*.[5,8]

  Ultrasound reveals normal-appearing ovaries and absence of a normal uterus. However, definitive diagnosis of uterine agenesis or hypoplasia is challenging since the uterine position may be variable. MR is excellent for investigating primary amenorrhea, helping to differentiate uterine hypoplasia or agenesis from other causes. On sagittal T2W images, the expected location of the cervix and uterus can be extrapolated from the position of the urethra, lower vagina, and bladder, making

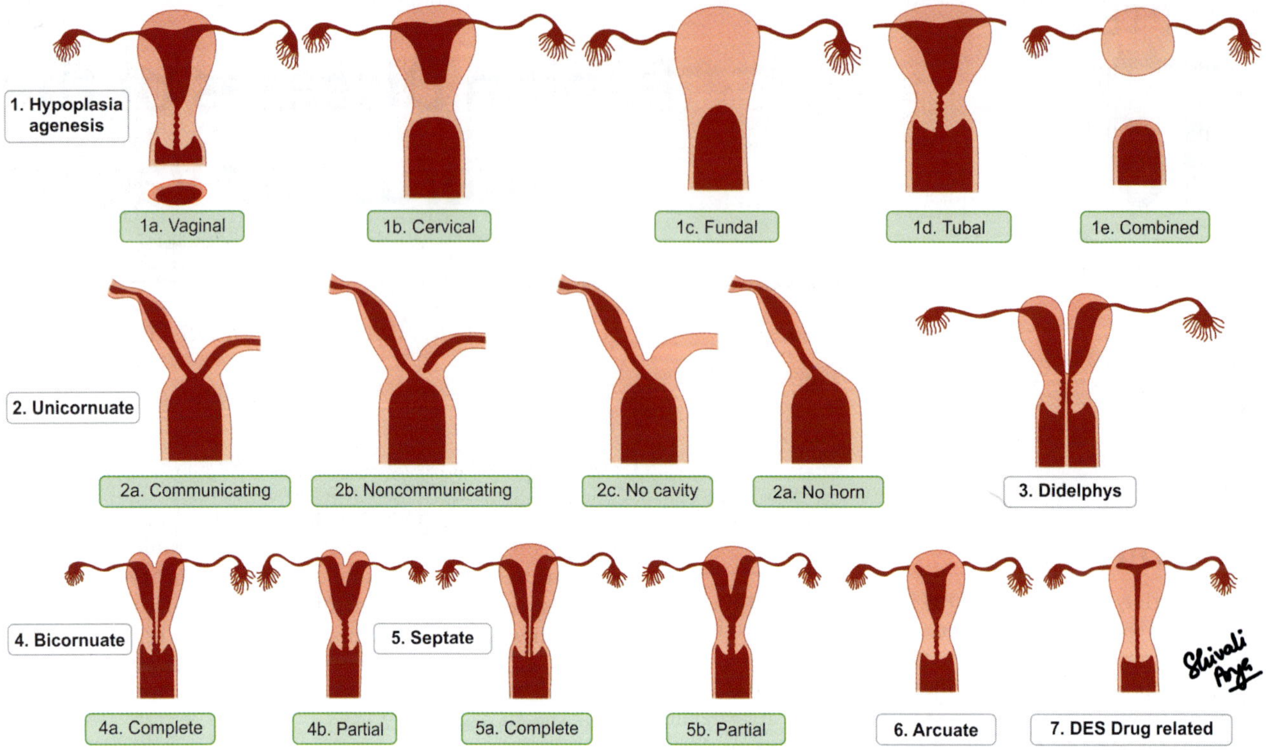

FIG. 1: The ASRM classification of female genital tract congenital anomalies (ASRM: American Society for Reproductive Medicine; DES: diethylstilbestrol).

them very useful for the diagnosis of uterine agenesis or hypoplasia. There is no identifiable uterus in complete uterine agenesis **(Figs. 2A to C)**. A hypoplastic uterus is visualized as a soft-tissue mass with signal pattern of normal myometrium, i.e. slightly hyperintense on T2-weighted images and it may be possible to identify zonal anatomy after puberty, due to the influence of female hormones. In younger females, the myometrium is T2-hypointense with poorly defined zonal anatomy.[6] In general, the endometrial cavity is small and intercornual diameter is less than 2 cm.[9] Vaginal agnesis is well seen on the axial images with no normal vaginal zonal anatomy identified between the rectum and the urethra. The length of the atretic vaginal segment may affect surgical approach in cases of isolated vaginal agenesis, and is best determined in the sagittal plane.[6]

- *Class II—unicornuate uterus*: Normal development of one Müllerian duct and near complete or complete arrest in development of the other duct results in unicornuate uterus. This can occur in four subtypes: (1) unicornuate uterus with no contralateral rudimentary horn, (2) contralateral rudimentary horn with no endometrial cavity (nonfunctioning), (3) contralateral rudimentary horn with an endometrial cavity communicating with the normal side, and (4) contralateral rudimentary horn with a noncommunicating endometrial cavity. Renal anomalies on the same side as the rudimentary horn may be seen in nearly 40% of patients with unicornuate uteri, renal agenesis accounting for most of these (67% of cases).

  The first two subtypes have minimal risk and do not require surgical management. Endometrium in a rudimentary horn is important to report. When present in a noncommunicating rudimentary horn, it can present with pelvic pain either due to an obstructed, distended horn or due to endometriosis consequent to retrograde flow of menstrual flow.[10,11] In addition, when endometrium is present in a rudimentary horn, both when it does or does not communicate with the uterine cavity, there is an increased risk of complications like ectopic pregnancy, miscarriage, preterm labor, and uterine rupture.[12]

  A fusiform, banana-shaped off midline uterine cavity is seen with a single fallopian tube on HSG. However, presence of a noncommunicating rudimentary horn cannot be excluded. A small, oblong, off-midline structure is seen on US, and the rudimentary horn may be difficult to identify. On MR, the unicornuate uterus shows normal zonal anatomy and the rudimentary horn is best delineates. When there is no endometrium in the rudimentary horn, it shows diffuse low signal intensity with no zonal anatomy, while preserved zonal anatomy is evident when endometrial tissue is present **(Fig. 3)**. A functioning rudimentary horn may become distended with blood after menarche when noncommunicating.[5,13]
- *Class III—uterus didelphys*: Complete failure of Müllerian duct fusion results in uterus didelphys producing duplication of the uterus, cervix, and proximal vagina. Vaginal duplication has been reported in 75% of patients.[14] A transverse vaginal septum on one side may be present in addition, resulting in ipsilateral obstruction.

  Two separate, elongated endometrial cavities with contrast opacification of both fallopian tubes is seen on HSG. However, if only one cervix is cannulated

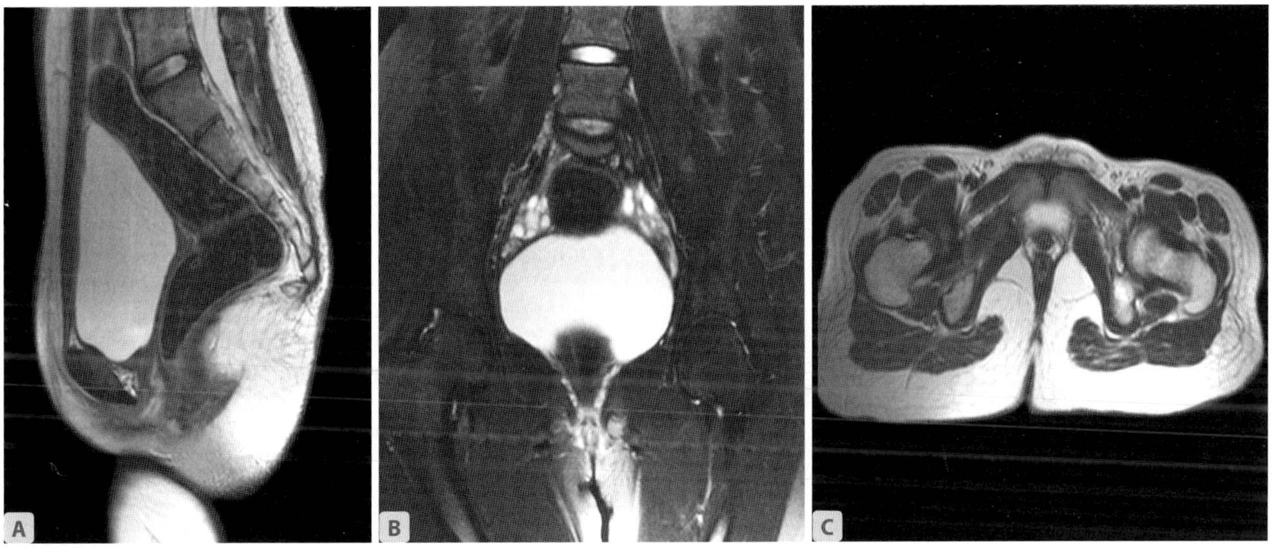

FIGS. 2A TO C: Müllerian agenesis T2W sagittal and coronal MR images. (A and B) No uterine tissue is visualized posterior to the bladder. Both ovaries are normal; (C) T2W axial image shows lower one-third of vagina between the bladder and rectum.

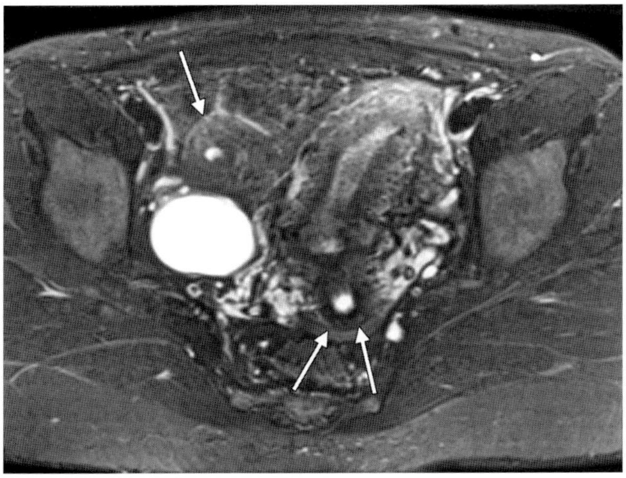

FIG. 3: Unicornuate uterus with noncommunicating functional horn. Axial T2 fat saturated MR image showing a banana-shaped uterine cavity on the left and a rudimentary horn with noncommunicating cavity on the right side (single arrow). The unicornuate uterus is seen to be continuous with the cervix posteriorly (arrows). A cyst is also seen in the right ovary. Vagina was normal—European Society of Human Reproduction and Embryology (ESHRE) class U4aC0V0.

or if one side is obstructed due to a transverse septum, nonopacification of the ipsilateral uterine horn occurs, resulting in a fallacious impression of unicornuate uterus.[15,16] On ultrasonography and MR, two widely divergent uterine horns with separate, noncommunicating endometrial cavities and two cervices are seen. Duplication of the vagina (hemivaginal septum) may not be seen on US; in such cases, differentiation between uterus didelphys and a bicornuate bicollis uterus may be difficult. Duplication of the proximal vagina is better visualized on MR, which may be aided by introduction of a viscous liquid, like US gel, into the vagina prior to imaging. If a septum obstructing one side is present, that horn will be distended with blood products producing hematometrocolpos. It is often associated with ipsilateral renal agenesis. This is referred to as **Herlyn-Werner-Wunderlich syndrome, also known as obstructed hemivagina and ipsilateral renal anomaly (OHVIRA) (Fig. 4)**.

- *Class IV—bicornuate uterus*: This is due to partial nonfusion of the Müllerian ducts accounting for nearly 10% of MDAs. The horns of the bicornuate uteri are not as fully developed and are smaller than those in the didelphys uteri.[8] The endometrial cavity is duplicated with or without cervical duplication, referred to as bicornuate bicollis and bicornuate unicollis uteri, respectively.

  Hysterosalpingography shows opacification of two symmetric fusiform uterine cavities and fallopian tubes with an intercornual angle of more than 105°. However, differentiation of the unicollis variety from a septate uterus is impossible at HSG due to overlapping features.[15,16] On MR/3D US, bicornuate uterus is characterized by the presence of a fundal cleft (>1 cm in depth) in the external contour, similar to uterus didelphys, best identified on oblique coronal images **(Figs. 5A to C)**. *This has been reported to be 100% sensitive and specific in differentiation of didelphys and bicornuate uteri, which are fusion anomalies, from septate and arcuate (reabsorption anomalies)*.[1,17] Normal zonal anatomy on MR is seen in both uterine horns. In a bicornuate bicollis uterus, the duplicated cervix gives an "owl eyes" appearance on axial section. An associated longitudinal vaginal septum may be present in one-fourth of cases, making a bicornuate bicollis uterus indistinguishable from a uterus didelphys.
- *Class V—septate uterus*: Septate uterus constitutes nearly 55% of cases, making it the most common MDA.[15,16,18-21] The septum occurs due to complete or partial failure of reabsorption of the uterovaginal septum. It arises from the midpart of the uterine fundus and is variable in length

and composition. A complete septum extends to the external cervical os and may even extend into the vagina in approximately 25% of cases.[9,22,23] It may be fibrous, myometrial, or consists of varying proportions of fibrous tissue and myometrium. Septate uterus has a strong association with repeated midtrimester miscarriage. It may at times be challenging to differentiate between a septate and bicornuate uterus. Correct diagnosis is important because the former requires surgical correction to improve reproductive outcomes. The most important difference is the appearance of the uterine fundus; a septate uterus has a normal convex external fundal contour. The external fundal contour cannot be seen on HSG hence reliable differentiation of septate from bicornuate uterus is not possible. Conventionally, an angle below 75° between the uterine horns is said to be seen in septate rather than bicornuate uterus but this is not reliable.[9,22-25]

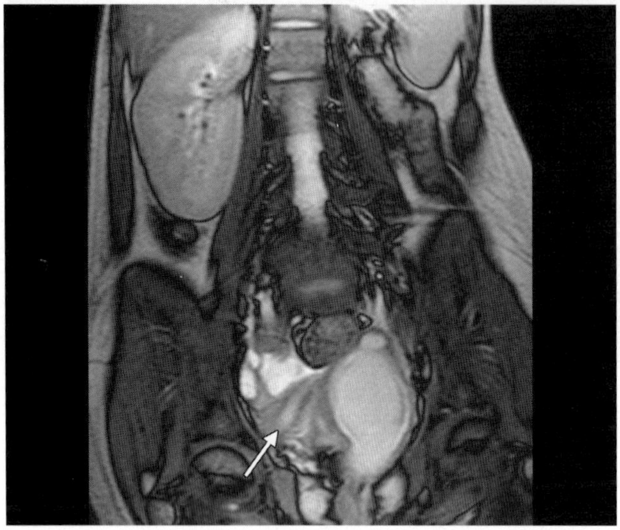

FIG. 4: OHVIRA syndrome. Coronal T2W MR image showing left hematometra and hematocolpos due to an obstructing hemivaginal septum. Note the normal right uterine cavity and cervix (arrow) and absent left kidney—ESHRE class U3bC2V2.

On US, a septum arising from fundus, dividing the endometrial cavity, is seen. The fibrous component tends to be less echogenic compared to myometrium. The external uterine contour is well-evaluated with 3D imaging, as it allows coronal views of the uterus.[22,26] The fundus either has a normal convex external contour **(Figs. 6A to D)** or a fundal cleft <1 cm deep.[27] Some authors have reported that if a line is drawn between the uterine ostia and the apex of the external fundal contour is >5 mm above this line, it suggests a septate uterus. On the other hand, if it is below or <5 mm above the interostial line, it suggests a bicornuate or didelphys uterus.[5,19]

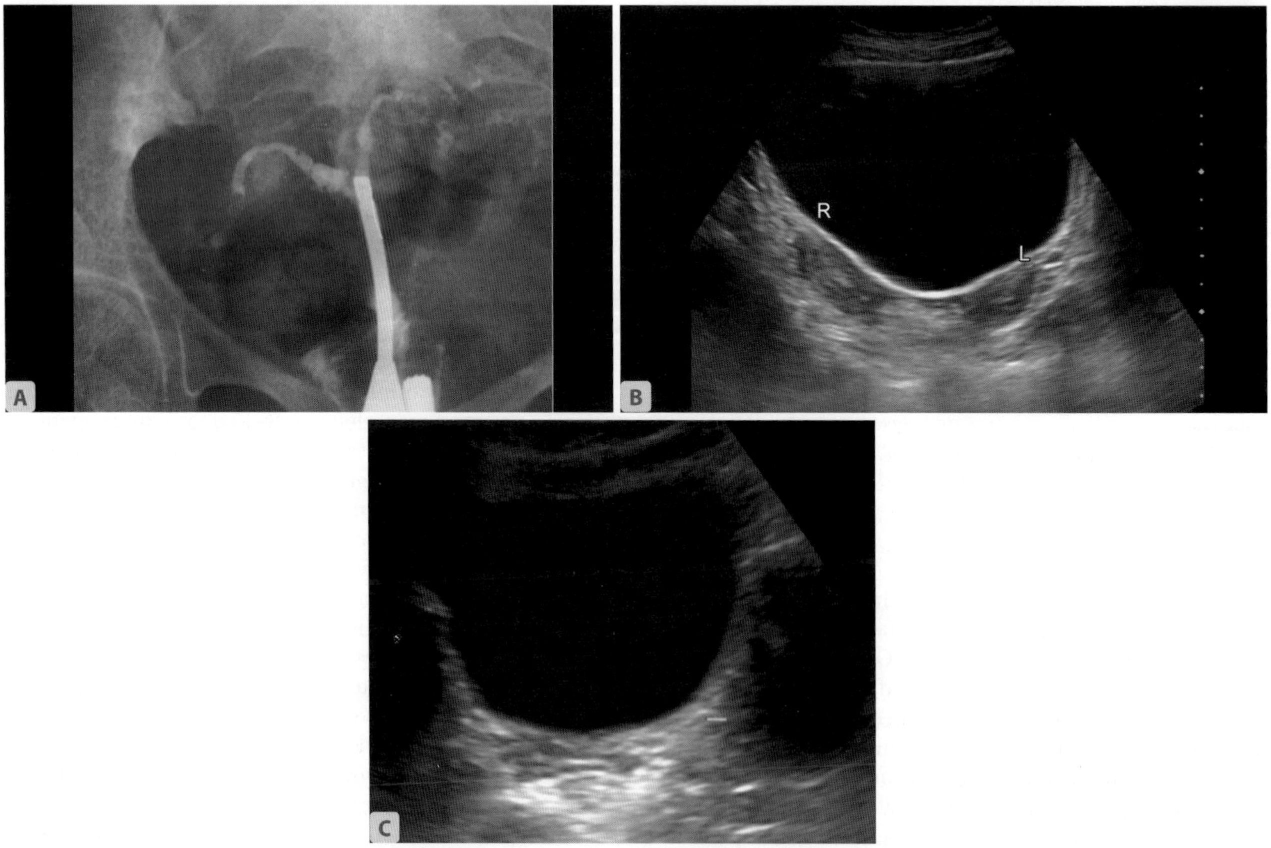

FIGS. 5A TO C: Bicornuate uterus. (A) Hysterosalpingography showing two widely divergent uterine cavities; (B) Midline transverse ultrasound image showing two widely separated uterine horns; (C) Transverse section at a lower level shows the normal vagina.

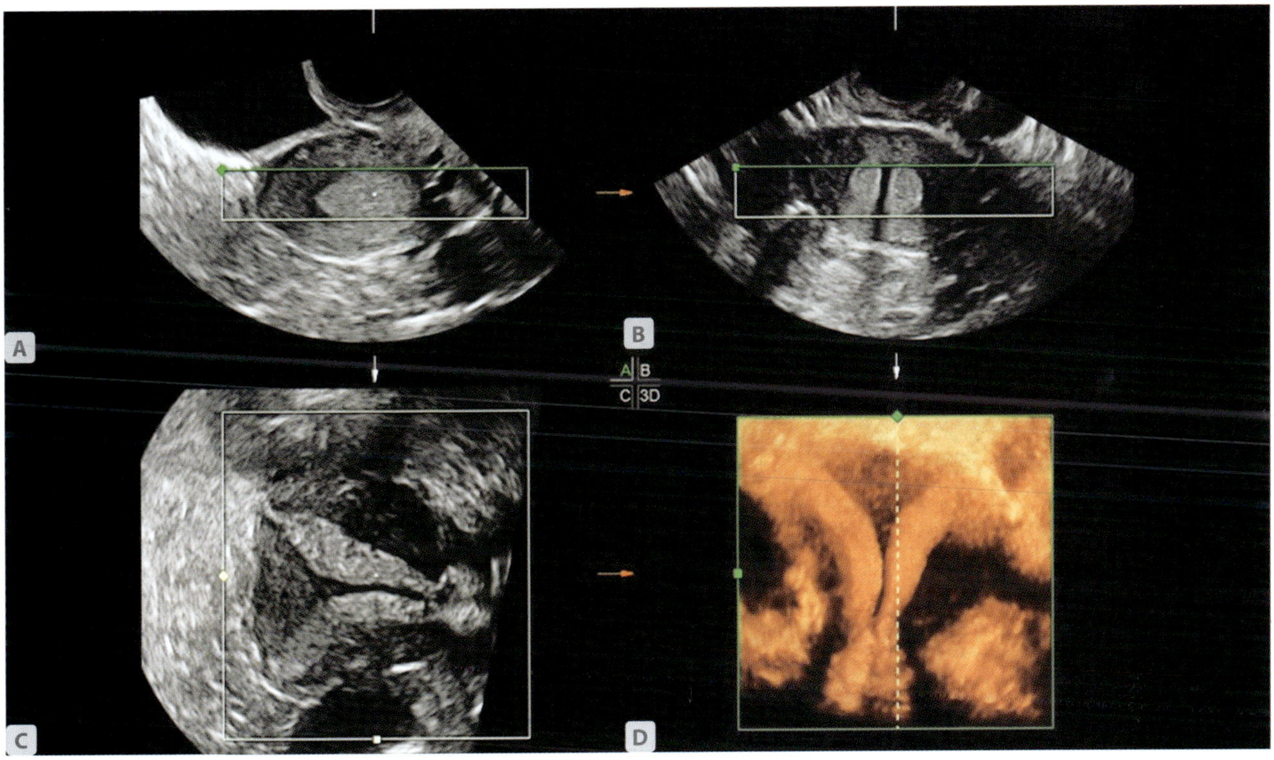

FIGS. 6A TO D: (A and B) Septate uterus on 3D USG. Normal external fundal contour is well-appreciated on the coronal images (C and D) with a hypoechoic septum arising from the fundus, dividing the endometrial cavity into two up to the level of external os—ESHRE class U2bC1V0.

On MR, the external fundal contour is well seen on oblique coronal images planned along the uterine plane. MR can also help to differentiate myometrium (which has a higher T2 signal and is usually seen closer to the fundus in a complete septum) from fibrous tissue (which has a low signal intensity). This is important as a hysteroscopic septoplasty is offered for a fibrous septum, but a transabdominal surgical approach is needed for a muscular septum **(Figs. 7A and B)**. Rarely, a complete septate uterus may also be associated with cervical duplication.[28] Careful evaluation of the outer uterine contour should be done to avoid a wrong diagnosis of a bicornuate bicollis uterus.

- *Class VI—arcuate uterus*: Arcuate uterus is characterized by only a mild indentation of the endometrium at the uterine fundus and occurs due to near complete reabsorption of the uterovaginal septum.[27] Ludwin et al. have suggested that if the distance between the interostial line and endometrial-myometrial junction at uterine fundus is >15 mm on 3D-US, it suggests a septate configuration; on the other hand, in case of arcuate uterus, this is more than 10 mm but less than 15 mm.[29] As per the modification of ASRM criteria in 2016, a septate uterus has an internal indentation of greater than 15 mm and an indentation angle less than 90° while in a normal/arcuate uterus, both the indentation depth should be less than 10 mm and angle more than 90°. Values in between these are considered to lie in the gray zone.
Hysterosalpingography reveals a single uterine cavity with a broad saddle-shaped indentation at the uterine fundus.[5,22] On US and MR imaging, the external fundal contour is normally convex with a broad-based, smooth prominence of inner myometrium, at the fundus, indenting the endometrial cavity. On MR, the signal is consistent with myometrium without low signal intensity on T2-weighted images to suggest any fibrous tissue.
- *Class VII—diethylstilbestrol (DES)-related uterus*: DES is a synthetic nonsteroidal estrogen that was used to prevent miscarriage between 1940s and 1971s. DES produces a T-shaped hypoplastic uterus or, which is now mainly of historical interest since its usage was stopped in 1975 as it was linked to vaginal clear cell carcinoma and uterine, cervical, and vaginal congenital malformations. Very rarely, the same spectrum of anomalies is noted among women without history of DES exposure **(Figs. 8A and B)**.[30,31]

It is important to classify MDAs accurately, as surgical planning differs. In case of uncertainty or presence of multiple subtypes, it is advisable to describe the anomalies and not forcibly place them in a class.[5] The major limitation of the ASRM classification is its lack of categorization of vaginal and other anomalies that bridge more than one classification.[28,32] It has also been criticized for absence of clear definitions and objective diagnostic criteria, lack of clarity on which diagnostic methods should be used introducing subjectivity in diagnosis and differential diagnosis.

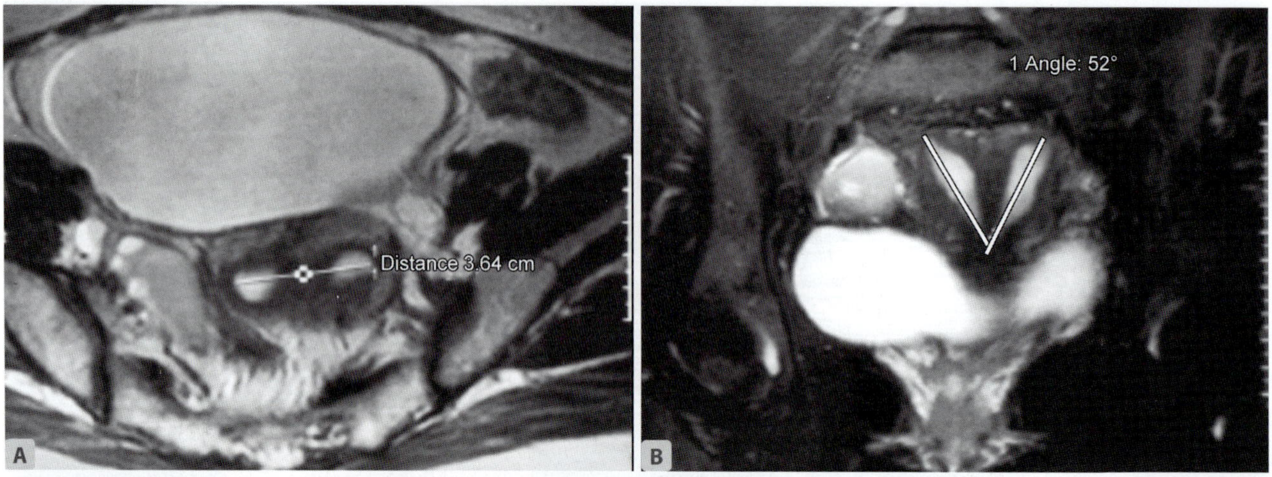

FIGS. 7A AND B: Septate uterus. (A) Axial and (B) coronal T2W MR images depict a uterus with a normal external fundal outline, well seen on the coronal image. The septum shows signal similar to the myometrium, dividing the endometrial cavity till the internal os suggesting a muscular septum.

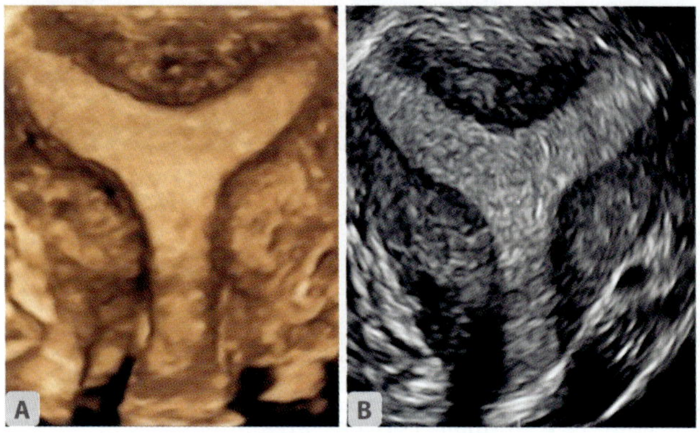

FIGS. 8A AND B: T-shaped uterus. 3D USG coronal reconstructions showing a T-shaped uterine cavity with a normal corpus-to-cervix ratio in a patient with no history of DES exposure (ESHRE: U1a).

European Society of Human Reproduction and Embryology/European Society for Gynaecological Endoscopy (ESGE) Classification System of Congenital Anomalies

The European Society of Human Reproduction and Embryology (ESHRE) and the *European Society for Gynaecological Endoscopy (ESGE)*, under a common Working Group—CONgenital UTerine Anomalies (CONUTA), have developed a new ESHRE/ESGE classification system of female genital anomalies in 2013 subsequently modified in 2015 in an attempt to overcome the limitations of the ASRM classification.[4,8] This was done mainly based on 3D US.

In the ESHRE/ESGE classification, systematic classification of anomalies into six main classes, is done primarily on anatomic basis. Deviation of uterine anatomy arising from the same embryological origin is the basis for division of the main classes. Anatomical variations of the main classes with different degrees of uterine deformity which are clinically significant are the basis of the main subclasses. The less severe variants are placed in the beginning, and the more severe ones at the end. Cervical and vaginal anomalies are classified in independent supplementary subclasses **(Fig. 9)**.

Definitions: Uterine Main Classes and Subclasses—Smaller than ESHRE/ESGE

Class U0 or Normal Uterus

A normal uterus is one with a straight or curved interostial line, with a midline internal fundal indentation not exceeding 50% of the uterine wall thickness. Uterine wall thickness is the distance between interostial line and external uterine profile on the midcoronal plane of the uterus; if a coronal plane is not feasible, the average anterior and posterior uterine wall thickness in the longitudinal plane can be used.[8] Since uterine wall thickness may vary from patient to patient, percentage measurement is used rather than absolute numbers in millimeters. The inclusion of normal uterus is useful to independently classify congenital malformations of the cervix and vagina.

Class U1 or Dysmorphic Uterus

It includes all cases with an abnormal shape of uterine cavity, except for septa and normal uterine outline. Usually, dysmorphic uteri are smaller in size. *Class I* has three subcategories:

1. *Class U1a or T-shaped uterus* has narrow uterine cavity due to thickened lateral walls with a two-thirds uterine corpus and one-third cervix ratio **(*see* Figs. 8A and B)**.
2. *Class U1b or uterus infantilis* also has a narrow uterine cavity, no lateral wall thickening, and an inversion of uterine body and cervix ratio (1/3:2/3).
3. *Class U1c or others* includes all minor deformities of the uterine cavity including those with an inner midline fundal indentation of <50% uterine wall thickness.

Class U2 or Septate Uterus

It includes all anomalies resulting from complete or partial nonabsorption of the midline septum and normal fusion.

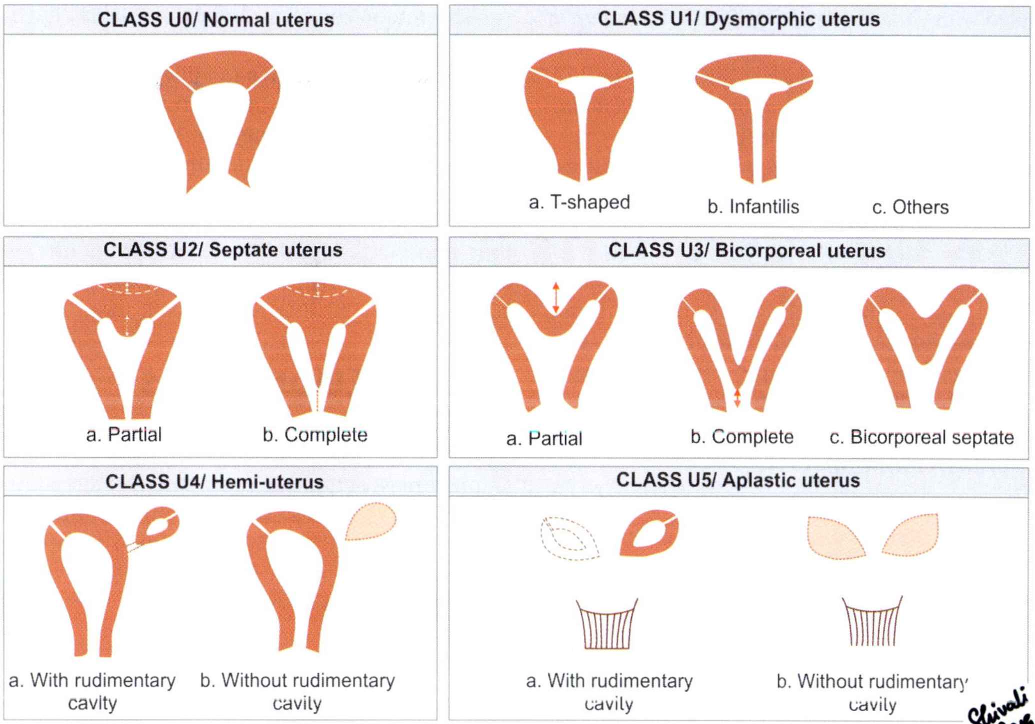

FIG. 9: Schematic representation of the ESHRE/ESGE classification of congenital uterine anomalies (ESGE: European Society for Gynaecological Endoscopy; ESHRE: European Society of Human Reproduction and Embryology).

The uterus has a normal external outline. There is an internal indentation in the midline fundal region exceeding 50% of the uterine wall thickness which is referred to as a septum. *Class U2* is divided into two subclasses:

1. *Class U2a or partial septate uterus* has a septum ending above the level of the internal cervical os dividing the uterine cavity partially.
2. *Class U2b or complete septate uterus* has a septum which completely divides the endometrial cavity up to the level of the internal cervical os. These patients (Class U2b) may or may not have cervical (e.g. bicervical septate uterus) and/or vaginal anomalies **(*see* Figs. 6 and 7)**.

Class U3 or Bicorporeal Uterus

It includes all fusion defects; it is characterized by the presence of an external indentation at the fundal midline >50% of the uterine wall thickness.

1. *Class U3a or partial bicorporeal uterus*: The external fundal indentation only partly divides the uterine corpus above the level of the cervix.
2. *Class U3b or complete bicorporeal uterus*: The external fundal indentation reaches up to the level of the cervix, completely dividing the uterine corpus. This subgroup may have coexistent cervical (e.g. double cervix or didelphys uterus of the ASRM) or vaginal anomalies (e.g. vaginal septum—obstructing or nonobstructing) **(*see* Fig. 4)**.
3. *Class U3c or bicorporeal septate uterus* has an absorption defect in addition to the fusion anomaly. In this case, the width of the midline fundal indentation exceeds the uterine wall thickness by 150%. Treatment by hysteroscopic resection of the septate component is possible to some extent.

Class U4 or Hemi-uterus

It includes all cases of unilateral uterine development; the contralateral part is absent or incompletely formed. It is a formation defect; included in a different class from aplastic uterus (also formation defect) because of the presence of a fully developed functional uterine hemi-cavity. Class U4 is divided into two subclasses depending on the presence or absence of a functional uterine cavity:

1. *Class U4a or hemi-uterus with a rudimentary (functional) cavity*: There is a functional contralateral horn which may be communicating or noncommunicating. These are clubbed together (unlike ASRM) since the presence of an endometrial cavity in the contralateral horn is the sole predictor of complications, like hematocavity or ectopic pregnancy in the rudimentary horn. Treatment is always advisable even in a communicating horn **(*see* Fig. 3)**.
2. *Class U4b or hemi-uterus with no rudimentary (functional) cavity* has either a nonfunctional contralateral uterine horn or no contralateral horn.

Class U5 or Aplastic Uterus

It includes all cases of uterine aplasia. There is absence of any fully or unilaterally developed uterine cavity. In some patients, however, there may be bilateral or unilateral rudimentary horns with cavity, or uterine remnants without cavity. The presence of a horn with cavity is used for subclassification as it is associated with clinical symptoms (cyclic pain and/or hematocavity) requiring treatment. These patients usually have concomitant defects (e.g. vaginal aplasia/MRKH syndrome).

1. *Class U5a or aplastic uterus with rudimentary (functional) cavity with* bi- or unilateral functional horn.
2. *Class U5b or aplastic uterus without rudimentary (functional) cavity* is seen as uterine remnants or full uterine aplasia.

Class U6 or Unclassified Cases

These are infrequent, subtle anomalies, or combined anomalies which cannot be allocated correctly to any other group. Duplication defects or ectopic Müllerian tissue anomalies, if present, could be put in this class.

Coexistent Cervical Anomalies

- *Subclass C0* or normal cervix.
- *Subclass C1 or septate cervix* includes cervical absorption defects. The cervix shows a normal externally rounded contour with presence of a septum.
- *Subclass C2 or double cervix* includes cases of cervical fusion anomalies. Two distinct externally rounded cervices (fully divided or partially fused) are seen. It may occur with a complete bicorporeal uterus as a Class U3b/C2 (uterus didelphys).
- *Subclass C3 or unilateral cervical aplasia* includes patients with unilateral cervix formation. The contralateral part is either incompletely formed or absent. This is obvious in Class U4 patients, and not necessary to mention in the final report (Class U4 is adequate instead of Class U4/C3). However, this gives a chance to classify other rarely seen anomalies like complete bicorporeal uterus with unilateral cervical aplasia as Class U3b/C3, a severe obstructing anomaly.
- *C4 or cervical aplasia* includes patients with complete cervical aplasia and severe cervical formation defects. There is either no cervical tissue or severely defective cervical tissue like cervical cord, obstruction, or fragmentation. This subclass may be combined with a normal or abnormal uterine corpus and helps in classification of all obstructing anomalies caused by cervical defects.

Coexistent Vaginal Anomalies

- *Subclass V0 or* normal vagina
- *Subclass V1* or longitudinal nonobstructing vaginal septum
- *Subclass V2 or* longitudinal obstructing vaginal septum
- *Subclass V3* or transverse vaginal septum and/or imperforate hymen. These vaginal anomalies classified together in this subclass as they generally present as isolated vaginal anomalies with similar clinical manifestation i.e. obstruction
- *Subclass V4 or vaginal aplasia* includes all cases of complete or partial vaginal aplasia.

Various authors have raised concerns about the clinical implications of the ESGE classifications, as specific diagnostic criteria that clearly correlate to pregnancy have not yet been validated in clinical practice by any prospective or retrospectives studies.[33]

The major concern about the ESHRE/ESGE criteria is the reclassification of the arcuate uterus into normal (U0) or septate uterus (U2), which modifies the number of diagnosed uterine septa. There is concern that it leads to overdiagnosis and perhaps overtreatment of septate uteri. Authors have reported that no significant difference was found in the past reproductive outcomes in women diagnosed with normal or partial septate uteri by these criteria. It has been suggested that clinicians should be cautious in offering surgical correction to women diagnosed to have partial septate uteri as per the new ESHRE/ESGE classification.[33]

UTERINE LEIOMYOMAS

Epidemiology

Leiomyomas, or fibroids, represent the most common benign tumors of the uterus. The incidence reported in literature varies between 25% to 50% of women of reproductive age. However, in autopsy studies, uterine leiomyomas have been found in up to 77% of women.[17,34,35]

Pathogenesis

Genetic factors, steroid hormones (i.e. estrogen and progesterone), and growth factors play a role in the development and growth of leiomyomas. They occur in women of reproductive age. They do not occur before puberty and fibroid-related symptoms reduce or resolve after menopause as a result of decreasing levels of female hormones. Early menarche and obesity are risk factors possibly due to increased estrogen exposure.[36]

Pathological Features

Leiomyomas are benign smooth muscle tumors. They usually form in the uterine corpus/fundus, less often in the cervix (<8%) and rarely in the broad ligament. Two-thirds of cases have multiple fibroids, size varying from microscopic to large tumors filling the abdomen. Leiomyomas that are no longer continuous with the uterus and develop an atypical blood supply are often referred to as parasitic leiomyomas. It is thought that a pedunculated subserosal leiomyoma becomes vascularized by the adjacent peritoneum, loses its attachment to the uterus and its vascular supply to become a parasitic leiomyoma. They are well-defined round lesions compressing the surrounding myometrium to form a pseudocapsule, which allows surgical enucleation of the tumors. Macroscopically, the cut surface has a whitish, whorled appearance, but the color (red, brown, or yellow) and texture may be different if degeneration is present. On microscopy, they are composed of intertwined smooth muscle cells, organized in fascicles, forming whorl-like patterns, embedded in a stroma of collagen fibers. The smooth muscle cells have eosinophilic cytoplasm and a centrally located cigar-shaped nucleus. Mitosis and atypia are not found in fibroids.[37-39]

As leiomyomas enlarge, they may outgrow their vascular supply. This results in different types of degeneration: hyaline, myxoid, cystic, red (hemorrhagic), or fatty degeneration and calcification, depending on the degree and rapidity of the onset of vascular insufficiency.[40,41]

Rare manifestations include diffuse leiomyomatosis of the uterus, benign metastatic leiomyomatosis, peritoneal disseminated leiomyomatosis, and intravenous leiomyomatosis, the last three being varieties that extend beyond the uterus.[42,43] These are benign leiomyomas.

Clinical Features

Most women with leiomyomas (up to 80%) are asymptomatic and require no treatment.[3] About 20–50% of women with leiomyomas present with symptoms such as menorrhagia, dysmenorrhea, urinary frequency, pelvic and back pain, dyspareunia, constipation, or obstipation depending on the size and location.[34,36]

Classification

According to their location, leiomyomas are classified as submucosal, intramural, or subserosal. This classification has clinical significance since the clinical presentation and treatment vary. *Submucosal leiomyomas* lie below the mucosal lining and protrude into the endometrial cavity. Though the least common, they are usually associated with dysmenorrhea, menorrhagia, or infertility. *Intramural leiomyomas*, the most common type, are located completely within the wall of the uterus. They are usually asymptomatic, but may occasionally produce symptoms similar to submucosal lesions. *Subserosal leiomyomas* are situated beneath the serosa, distort the outer uterine contour. They may be pedunculated, being attached to the uterus by a stalk. Subserosal leiomyomas are also mostly asymptomatic; however, pedunculated subserosal leiomyomas may undergo torsion, resulting in infarction and pain.[44,45] The FIGO classifications is often used to describe the relationship of fibroids to both the serosal and mucosal uterine surfaces and is summarized in **Figure 10**.

Imaging

Imaging of leiomyomas allows classification by location in the uterus and pretreatment planning**.** US is the first-line imaging

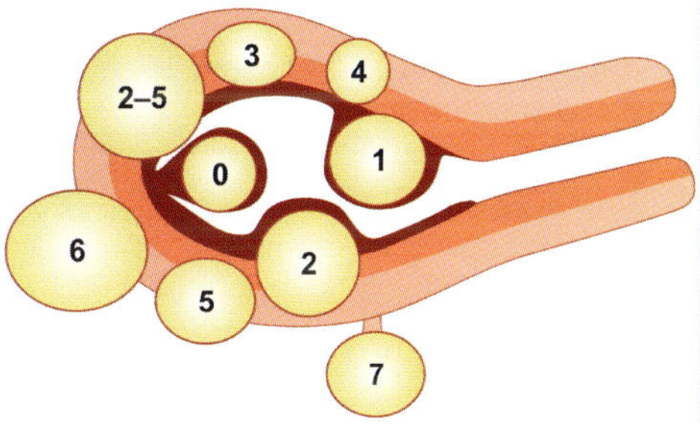

SM—Submucosal	0	Pedunculated intracavitary
	1	<50% intramural
	2	≥50% intramural
O—Other	3	Contacts endometrium; 100% intramural No distortion
	4	Intramural
	5	Subserosal ≥50% intramural
	6	Subserosal <50% intramural
	7	Subserosal pedunculated
	8	Other (specify, e.g. cervical, parasitic)
Hybrid leiomyomas	2–5	Submucosal and subserosal, each with less than half the diameter in the endometrial and pertioneal cavities, respectively

FIG. 10: The International Federation of Gynecology and Obstetrics (FIGO) classification of fibroids.

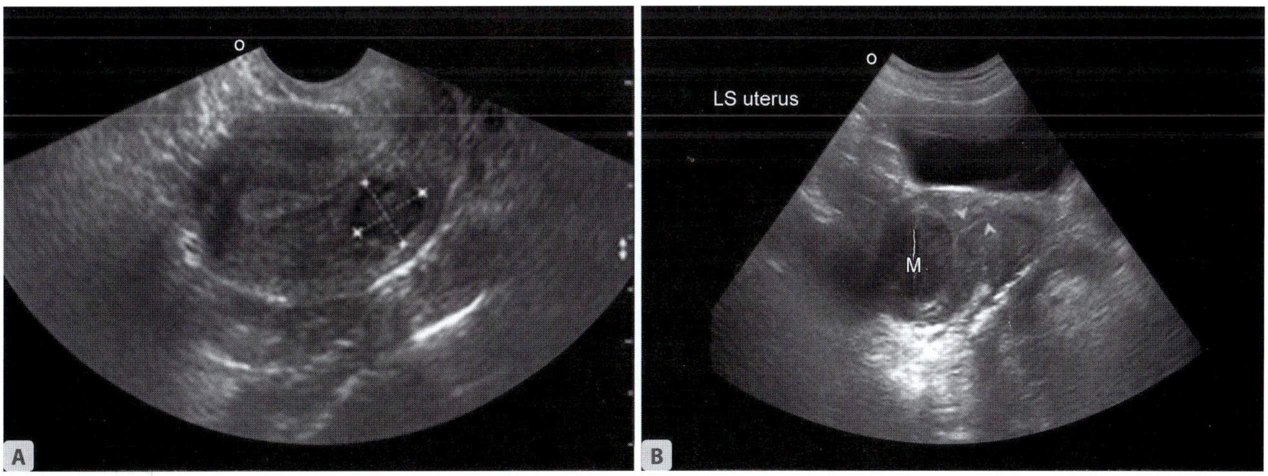

FIGS. 11A AND B: Uterine fibroids. (A) TVS shows well-defined, round, and hypoechoic mass in posterior myometrium—intramural fibroid; (B) TAS in another patient reveals homogeneous, hypoechoic well-marginated round to oval mass lesion in the uterus consistent with fibroid (TAS: transabdominal sonography; TVS: transvaginal sonography).

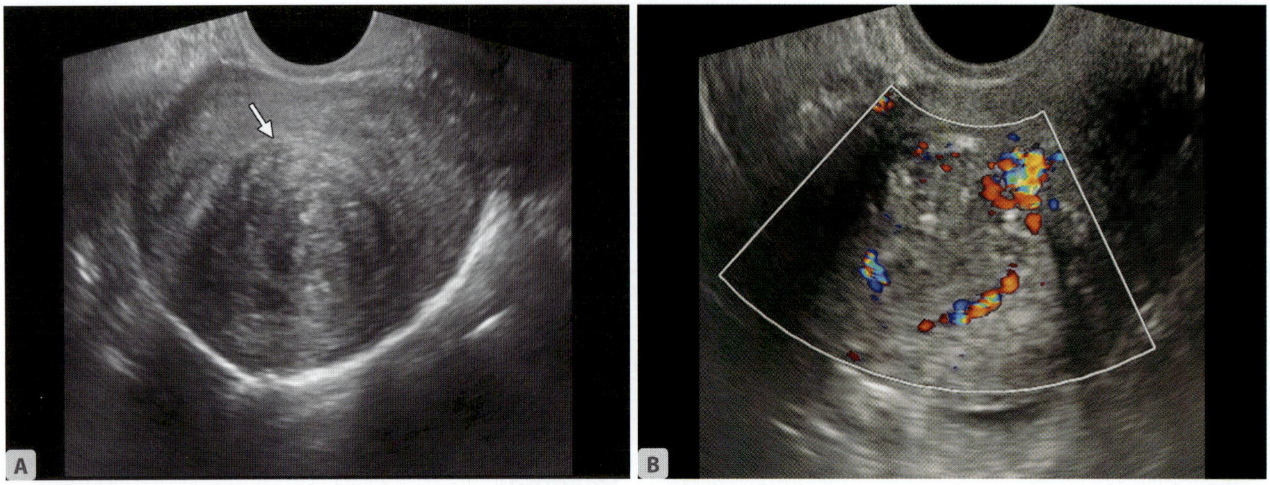

FIGS. 12A AND B: Fibroid uterus. (A) Transverse section of the uterus on transvaginal sonography shows a well-defined iso- to heteroechoic lesion displacing the endometrial echo anteriorly due to mass effect (arrow). Multiple coarse posterior acoustic shadows are well seen; (B) Color Doppler reveals peripheral vascularity.

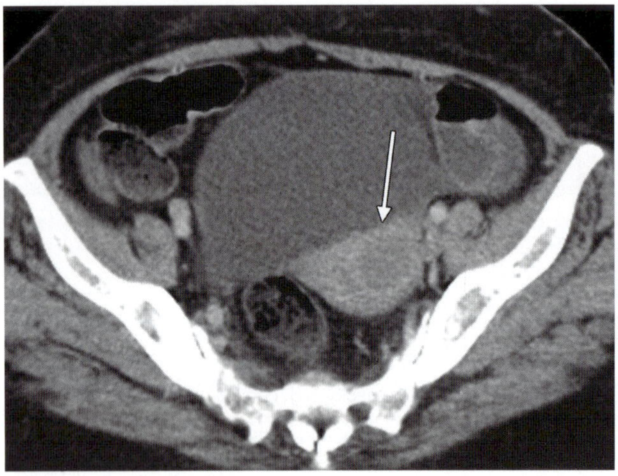

FIG. 13: Fibroid uterus. Axial contrast-enhanced CT scan shows a well-defined hypodense fibroid, enhancing less than the adjacent myometrium (arrow).

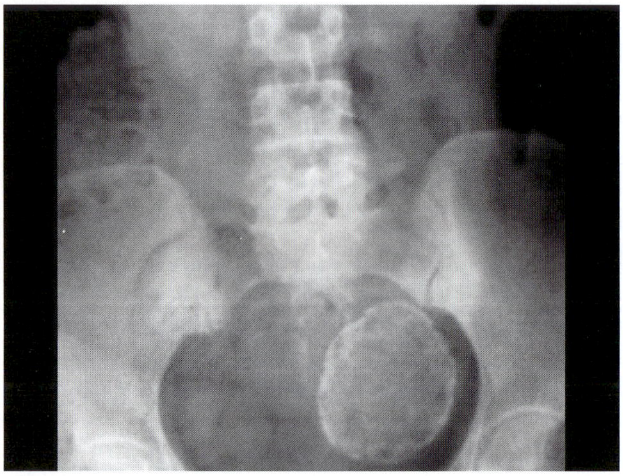

FIG. 14: Plain radiograph of pelvis shows a large fibroid with rim calcification.

and a combination of transabdominal sonography (TAS) and TVS may be required depending on size and uterine position.

Leiomyomas are round or oval well-circumscribed hypoechoic (or isoechoic) solid lesions **(Figs. 11A and B)** with associated areas of posterior shadowing at the interface of the leiomyoma with the normal myometrium or due to calcifications. Cystic areas, echo-poor foci, and heterogeneity suggest degeneration, while a hyperechoic appearance may be seen in lipoleiomyomas. Doppler US depicts tumor vascularity and typically demonstrates a marginal vascular network **(Figs. 12A and B)**.[36] Hysterosonography with the instillation of fluid/saline into the endometrial cavity can improve the accuracy of TVS in detecting and differentiating submucosal fibroids from endometrial polyps. It is also more accurate in demonstrating degree of myometrial component. 3D US is also an excellent technique to demonstrate the relationship between the fibroid and the endometrial cavity.[46-49]

CT is not a recommended imaging modality for the evaluation of leiomyomas, but they may be incidentally seen, as variably enhancing masses **(Fig. 13)**, sometimes with popcorn or rim calcifications (4%) **(Fig. 14)**.[36,46]

MRI is the most accurate and preferred tool for pretreatment planning of leiomyomas, showing the exact number, size, location, and character of leiomyomas, a process also known as (*fibroid mapping*). The excellent soft-tissue contrast enables accurate localization of lesions as submucosal, intramural, or subserosal and fibroids as small as 5 mm in diameter can be demonstrated. Nondegenerated leiomyomas are seen as well-circumscribed round or oval masses. They are isointense on T1, homogeneously low signal on T2W compared to the outer myometrium. A T2-hyperintense rim, indicating a pseudocapsule of edema, due to some degree of venous or lymphatic obstruction may be seen in some cases. On contrast-enhanced scans, fibroids usually show lesser degree of enhancement relative to the myometrium, although, occasionally they may be of the same or of higher attenuation. Routine use of gadolinium is, however, not required. Areas of calcification are poorly detected on MR but can appear as signal voids. Diffuse leiomyomatosis is characterized by the presence of many small ill-defined leiomyomas that may be confluent.[36,46-48,50]

Leiomyomas do not infiltrate surrounding structures, but show expansile growth and already have a mass effect when they are still small therefore, distorting the shape of the uterus **(Fig. 15)**. In patients with large exophytic, subserosal leiomyomas, or a markedly enlarged uterus due to multiple fibroids, it may sometimes be difficult to differentiate fibroids from extrauterine or ovarian lesions. The presence of a beak, or claw-like extension of myometrium surrounding the lesion (*claw sign*) and multiple flow voids on noncontrast images or enhancing tubular channels on contrast-enhanced T1W images, at the interface between lesion and normal uterine tissue, indicate uterine fibroids with a high degree of confidence **(Figs. 16A and B)**.[36-39] These flow voids represent the arteries arising from the uterine artery and feeding the fibroid and have been referred to as the *bridging vascular sign* (originally described on Doppler). **Table 1** summarizes the MR findings of leiomyomas.

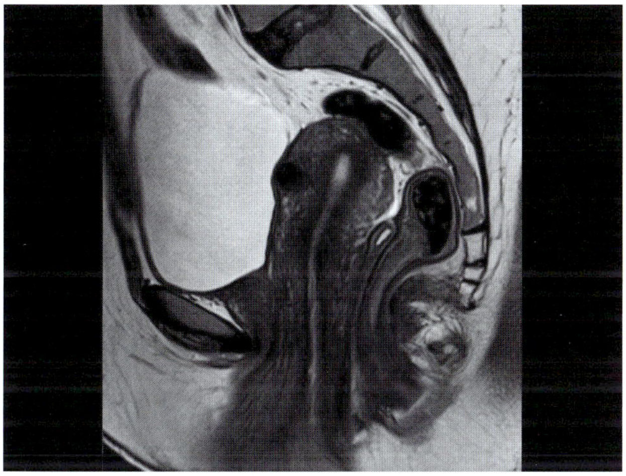

FIG. 15: T2W sagittal MR image showing a small hypointense fibroid in the anterior wall, and subserosal location. Note the subtle deformity of the uterine outline, despite the small size.

TABLE 1: MRI features of leiomyoma.

Location	Corpus, less often cervical or within uterine ligaments Subserosal, intramural, submucous
Morphology	• Spherical, sharply marginated, pseudocapsule may be present, mass effect even if small, deforming the uterine outline, and/or cavity may be singular but often numerous • Size 0.5 cm to >20 cm • Claw-like extension of myometrium surrounding the lesion
Appearance on T1	• Isointense to the myometrium • Hyperintense areas related to hemorrhage
Appearance on T2	• Variable, in general hypointense relative to myometrium • Homogeneously, high SI often seen in cellular leiomyomas • High SI rim represents dilated lymphatics in large leiomyoma
Appearance on gadolinium-enhanced T1	• hypo-, iso-, and hyperintense relative to myometrium.
Additional findings	• Flow voids in the periphery representing perifibroid plexus vessels • A vascular stalk may be seen in pedunculated leiomyomas (bridging vessel sign)

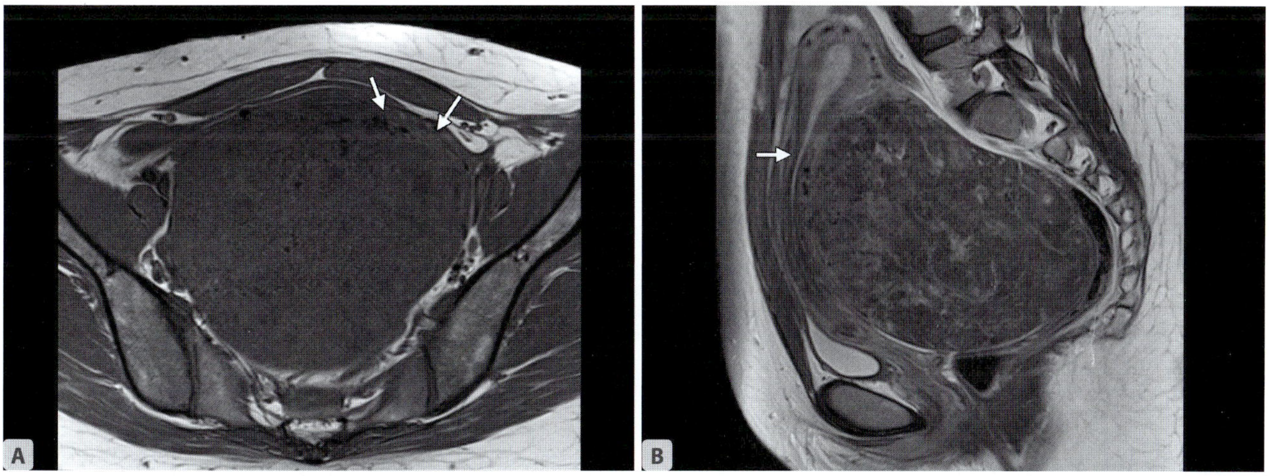

FIGS. 16A AND B: Subserosal fibroid uterus. (A) T1W axial and (B) sagittal T2W MR images depict a large posterior wall subserosal fibroid with less than 50% intramyometrial component appearing isointense on T1, hypointense on T2, stretching the myometrium and displacing the endometrial cavity anteriorly (arrow in B). Note the flow voids at the interface between the lesion and the uterus on T1W (arrows in A).

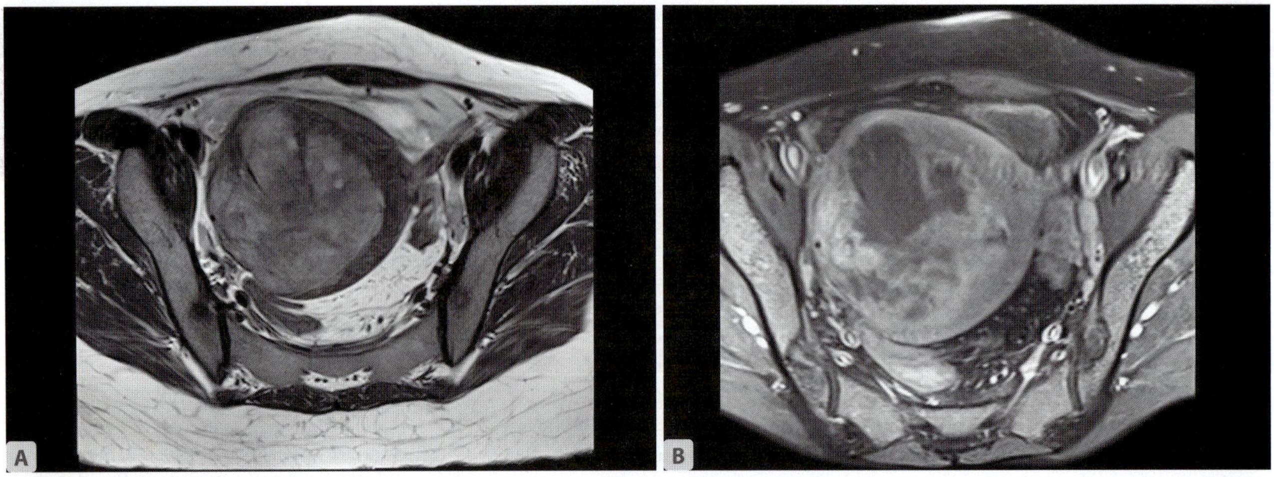

FIGS. 17A AND B: Fibroid with areas of cystic degeneration which appear hyperintense on T2 (A) and do not enhance on the postcontrast image (B).

Fibroids that have undergone degeneration show great variation in their MRI appearance.[36,44,45,49,51,52] *Hyaline degeneration* is the most common type of degeneration seen in about 60% of all leiomyomas. It is characterized by the collection of high-protein eosinophilic material, in the extracellular space, between strands of muscle cells. Hyaline degeneration produces low signal on T2W images, making it difficult to distinguish from nondegenerated fibroids, however, decreased enhancement, especially on triphasic dynamic scans has been reported with hyaline degeneration.

Other types of degeneration that can be differentiated are *cystic, myxoid, and hemorrhagic (red) degeneration. Cystic degeneration* results in internal areas of T2 hyperintensity and T1 hypointensity with no enhancement **(Figs. 17A and B)**. *Myxoid degeneration* is seen as areas of very high signal intensity on T2-weighted images, intermediate to low signal on T1-weighted images. These can be difficult to differentiate from fibroids that have undergone cystic degeneration; however, they appear as more complex cystic masses. They tend to show intense enhancement of the stroma. Minimal enhancement of the high signal areas, indicating that these are not necrotic or cystic areas, can be seen.

Hemorrhagic or carneous or red degeneration usually occurs during pregnancy or in women on oral contraceptives. It is thought to occur due to obstructed draining veins with sudden infarction and secondary intralesional hemorrhage. MRI is extremely useful to confirm the diagnosis of acute hemorrhagic degeneration of a leiomyoma, especially in conjunction with the clinical presentation of acute pain, subfebrile temperature, and leukocytosis. This is seen as a variably heterogeneous signal depending on the age of blood products. Commonly described patterns include, high signal on T1 and moderate to high signal on T2-weighted scans; there can also be a hyperintense rim on T1 and a markedly hypointense rim on T2-weighted scans. Hemorrhagic fibroids show no enhancement after contrast.

Lipoleiomyoma or fatty degeneration is rare. It is thought to be due to fatty metamorphosis of the smooth muscle cells of a leiomyoma **(Fig. 18)**. At USG, they are typically echogenic masses, unlike the usually hypoechoic appearance. If pedunculated, they can be mistaken for ovarian dermoids. On MR, they display a signal similar to subcutaneous fat on all pulse sequences due to the presence of variable amounts of fat cells. Fat suppression is useful to determine the fatty nature of these leiomyomas.

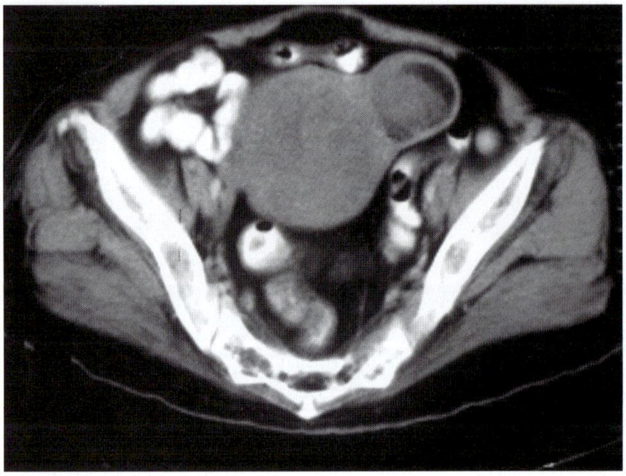

FIG. 18: CT scan of pelvis showing a lobulated uterine mass with fatty degeneration—lipoleiomyoma.

The MRI features of degenerating uterine leiomyomas are summarized in **Table 2**.

Leiomyoma Variants

Besides the ordinary leiomyomas discussed above, there are several leiomyoma variants, such as mitotically active, cellular, and atypical leiomyomas, as well as smooth muscle tumors of uncertain malignant potential (STUMP) which lie between the ordinary benign leiomyomas and the malignant leiomyosarcomas **(Box 1)**. In contrast to ordinary leiomyomas, imaging features of leiomyoma variants are neither well-studied nor understood due to their rarity.

Cellular leiomyomas, a subgroup of leiomyomas, on microscopy show compact smooth muscle cells with little

TABLE 2: MRI features of degenerated (but ordinary) leiomyomas.

Types of degeneration	T1-weighted imaging	T2-weighted imaging	IV contrast-enhanced imaging
Cystic	Hypointense relative to myometrium	Internal areas of high T2 signal intensity	With corresponding areas of nonenhancement
Hemorrhagic	Areas of high T1 signal intensity	Variable T2 signal intensity	Variable
Fatty	Moderate T1 signal intensity, which suppresses on fat-saturated sequence	Moderate	Variable
Hyaline	Isointense	Hypointense	Decreased enhancement (compared with ordinary leiomyomas)
Myxoid	iso to Hypointense	Markedly high T2 signal intensity Complex appearance	Some enhancement seen

intervening collagen. According to one study, they are more likely to be single and larger than ordinary fibroids; there is also a greater probability that the patient is symptomatic and that the indication for imaging is "enlarging lesion". Cellular leiomyomas have a homogeneously high signal intensity on T2-weighted scans, are isointense to surrounding myometrium on T1, and tend to enhance homogeneously. Studies report that cellular leiomyomas can significantly decrease in size following gonadotropin-releasing hormone (GnRH) therapy compared with degenerated leiomyomas.

Atypical leiomyomas, mitotically active leiomyomas, as well as STUMPs are very rare; hence, their imaging appearances are not well-described.[45]

Differential Diagnosis

Differential diagnostic considerations include adenomyosis, solid adnexal masses, endometrial polyp, and the rare leiomyosarcoma.

Adenomyosis may mimic intramural leiomyomas. Adenomyosis tends to be poorly marginated, with multiple cystic spaces (anechoic on US, T2 hyperfoci on MR), is mostly in contact with the junctional zone, and does not produce as much mass effect.

Submucosal leiomyomas may have to be distinguished from endometrial polyps. On color Doppler, a feeding vessel is more often seen in endometrial polyp, while fibroids tend to show circumferential vascularity. On MR, submucosal leiomyomas are differentiated from endometrial polyps by their more spherical shape, their connection to the myometrium, and lower signal intensity on T2-weighted images.

BOX 1: Uterine leiomyomas and their variants.

- *Ordinary leiomyomas—benign*:
  - Nondegenerated
  - *With degeneration*:
    - Hyaline
    - Myxoid
    - Cystic
    - Hemorrhagic (carneous)
    - Fatty (lipoleiomyoma).
- *Leiomyoma variants—in between*:
  - Cellular
  - Atypical
  - Mitotically active
  - Smooth muscle tumors of uncertain malignant potential (STUMP)
- *Leiomyosarcoma—malignant*

Solid adnexal or ovarian masses must be considered in the differential diagnosis of subserosal leiomyomas. The claw sign and/or presence of bridging vessels is useful to establish the diagnosis of leiomyoma.

Uterine contractions can appear as transient T2 hypointense lesions which may simulate leiomyomas or focal adenomyosis at MR.

Leiomyosarcomas of the uterus are rare, most are thought to arise de novo unrelated to benign leiomyomas. Due to overlapping of imaging features, differentiation of benign degenerating cellular leiomyomas and leiomyosarcomas is challenging.[52-57] The distinction, however, may be important as recently leiomyoma morcellation has been reported to have a negative impact on the survival of patients who were found to have malignant instead of benign uterine masses following the procedure (morcellation is a technique to reduce the size of the uterus or myomas by creating smaller pieces, so that they can be removed through small incisions or laparoscopically). Leiomyosarcomas occur in an older age group (6th decade) as compared with leiomyoma (4th decade/premenopausal). Traditionally, rapid enlargement of leiomyomas has been interpreted as a sign of malignancy, but the results of some large studies have not supported this. Although rapid growth is not considered, an indicator of malignancy in premenopausal women, it is suspicious in postmenopausal women. On US, the detection of hypervascularity in a large solitary uterine mass can raise the suspicion of leiomyosarcoma. According to a study, a cutoff value of 41.0 cm/s [peak systolic velocity (PSV)] on Doppler markedly increased the detection rate of uterine sarcomas.[52,53] However, there are no US findings that reliably differentiate ordinary leiomyomas from leiomyoma variants and leiomyosarcomas. Lakhman et al. recently reported four discriminative features on MR: (1) nodular borders, (2) intralesional hemorrhage, (3) T2W dark areas, and (4) central unenhanced areas. They reported that combination of more than three MR features provided a specificity of >95% **(Table 3)**.[57]

Treatment

Asymptomatic fibroids may be left alone with a wait and watch policy. Treatment of uterine fibroids is indicated when they

TABLE 3: Differentiation between leiomyoma and leiomyosarcoma.

	Leiomyoma	Leiomyosarcoma
Age	Premenopausal	Peri-/postmenopausal
Borders	Well-delineated	Often nodular*
DWI	Variable	Restricted diffusion, low ADC
Invasiveness	No	Adjacent tissues
Number	Commonly multiple	Solitary
Size	Variable	Large (>10 cm)
T2WI	Mostly low, high in degeneration, and whorled pattern	Inhomogeneous with areas of hemorrhage*, intralesional vessels; T2 dark areas*
Vascularity	Variable; often parallels myometrium	Hypervascularization, peripheral early enhancement, and central necrosis*

*Discriminative features on MR.

(ADC: apparent diffusion coefficient; DWI: diffusion-weighted imaging)

are symptomatic. Treatment depends on symptomatology, age, and patients' desire for gestation and has to be tailored on a case-to-case basis. Treatment can be medical, surgical, or interventional. *Medical therapy* is usually done to relieve abnormal menstrual bleeding, and bulk symptoms. This may include nonsteroidal anti-inflammatory drugs (NSAIDs), oral contraceptives (OCs), tranexamic acid and GnRH analogs, and the recently introduced selective progesterone receptor modulators (sPRMs) like ulipristal acetate (UPA). Levonorgestrel-releasing intrauterine device (IUD) and endometrial ablation are other techniques to reduce the severity of menstrual bleeding.

Surgical techniques include hysterectomy, hysteroscopic, or laparoscopic myomectomy.

Hysterectomy is the definitive cure, especially in patients with a symptomatic multiple fibroids not wanting to preserve fertility. *Myomectomy* is a uterus-sparing operative technique, where myomas are resected or enucleated using a laparoscopic, hysteroscopic access or via open laparotomy. Here, imaging plays an important role in accurate localization prior to myomectomy. Submucosal leiomyomas (FIGO 0, 1, and 2) with minimal intramural component can be removed by hysteroscopic resection. Hysteroscopic resection is usually considered difficult or unsuitable if the submucosal leiomyoma is larger than 5 cm in size, if there are more than three fibroids, or if the uterine cavity is very large (length of uterine probe >12 cm). A large intramural component with thin residual myometrium increases the risk of perforation during hysteroscopic resection.[58] Laparoscopic removal can be done for subserosal visible leiomyomas, but intramural tumors are not easily accessible to laparoscopic removal. Incision of the uterine cavity may be necessary for the removal of transmural fibroids which is associated with the risk of synechia. Laparotomy is primarily used in patients with one or more large fibroids.

Interventional techniques that are available include uterine artery embolization (UAE) or uterine fibroid embolization (UFE) and MRI-guided focused US. MRI can be used to both predict and assess the response of fibroids to UAE-MR prior to UAE helps in identification of tumors in which embolization is associated with a higher risk, such as subserosal pedunculated fibroids with a narrow stalk (<2 mm stalk width) or those which are likely to show poor response to embolization, e.g. those with a parasitic blood supply, cervical leiomyomas, and those with high signal on T1W images (hemorrhagic necrosis). On the other hand, high signal on T2W images and gadolinium enhancement indicating vascularity have been shown to be a predictor of good response.[36,51]

ADENOMYOSIS OF THE UTERUS

Epidemiology

According to the classical teaching, adenomyosis or endometriosis genitalis interna is mainly seen in multiparous, premenopausal women generally more than 30 years of age. Currently, however, adenomyosis is not uncommonly diagnosed between 20 years and 30 years of age, and even during adolescence with availability of hysteroscopic or laparoscopic biopsy. Hysterectomy specimens demonstrate adenomyosis in 19–63% of cases. A prevalence of 34% has been reported in nulliparous females between 18 years and 30 years, who presented for contraception advice.[59-61]

Pathogenesis

Adenomyosis is a common non-neoplastic benign uterine condition resulting from the displacement of basal endometrial glands and stroma into the underlying myometrium. While the exact reason for the displacement is unclear, estrogen-mediated and mechanical effects have been implicated. High estrogen levels in pregnancy and breakdown of the basal endometrial layer as well as inner myometrium (due to postpartum endometritis) have been postulated as possible reasons in multiparous women. Early menarche, short menstrual cycles, and high body mass index—other features associated with high estrogen levels, are also associated with an increased risk of adenomyosis. Increased incidence of adenomyosis is seen in postmenopausal women on tamoxifen, a nonsteroidal antiestrogen agent.[59-63]

Histopathology

Adenomyosis may produce focal or diffuse involvement of the uterus. It occurs more often in the posterior wall and the fundus and does not involve the uterine cervix. The cut surface has a whorled texture produced by irregular trabeculations of the thickened myometrium. Cyst-like lesions and hemorrhagic foci within the myometrium are commonly seen. On histologic examination, dispersed endometrial glandular tissue is seen in the myometrium. The pathologic diagnosis is dependent on visualization of endometrial glands and stroma in more than one low-power field, 2.5 mm from the endometrial basalis layer.[64,65]

Clinical Presentation

The clinical presentation is nonspecific and includes dysmenorrhea, menorrhagia, and pelvic pain, hence its incidence is underestimated. The uterus may be enlarged in adenomyosis but does not show distortion in its shape unlike with leiomyomas. Adenomyosis, however, often occurs along with fibroids and endometriosis.

Imaging

Ultrasound (TAS or TVS) is generally used as the initial imaging modality in suspected adenomyosis. The reported sensitivity and specificity of TAS vary between 32.5–63% and 95–97%, respectively. TVS has a higher sensitivity and specificity for diagnosing adenomyosis in the range of 53–89% and 67–98%, respectively.[60,66] Saline infusion sonohysterography (SIS) may be useful in selected cases.

Some authors have categorized the US findings into three groups, paralleling the histology of adenomyosis: (1) ectopic endometrial glands and stroma, (2) muscular hyperplasia/hypertrophy, and (3) increased vascularity.

1. *Ectopic endometrial glands* are seen as echogenic nodules or striations which radiate from the endometrium into the myometrium. Myometrial cysts, lakes, and fluid-filled striations are seen when these glands contain fluid. Myometrial cysts are generally anechoic, 1–5 mm in size, but may be variable in size or have echogenic contents representing blood. Myometrial cysts are reported to be most sensitive and specific US feature of adenomyosis. Reducing the field of view and using magnification improve the depiction of these cysts. At times, an entire striation may be fluid filled referred to as *lollipop diverticulum*. Cystic changes in the outer myometrium on gray- scale may actually be small arcuate veins and rather than myometrial cysts of adenomyosis which can be differentiated with color Doppler imaging.[64]
2. The ectopic endometrial glands are hormonally sensitive and produce a "local reaction" within the adjacent myometrium, producing *smooth muscle hyperplasia and hypertrophy*. This results in asymmetric uterine wall thickening in focal disease. A globular uterine enlargement, up to 12 cm in uterine length, is commonly associated with the diffuse variety. Thickening of the junctional zone >12 mm (seen as a hypoechoic halo surrounding the endometrium) may be seen but is less apparent than on MR. Coronal views on 3D US may allow better measurement of the junctional zone. Blurring of the normally distinct endometrial/myometrial border can be seen. There is alteration of myometrial echotexture, becoming heterogeneous and coarse, with thin vertical posterior acoustic shadows, producing a *venetian blind appearance* **(Figs. 19A and B)**. This combination of

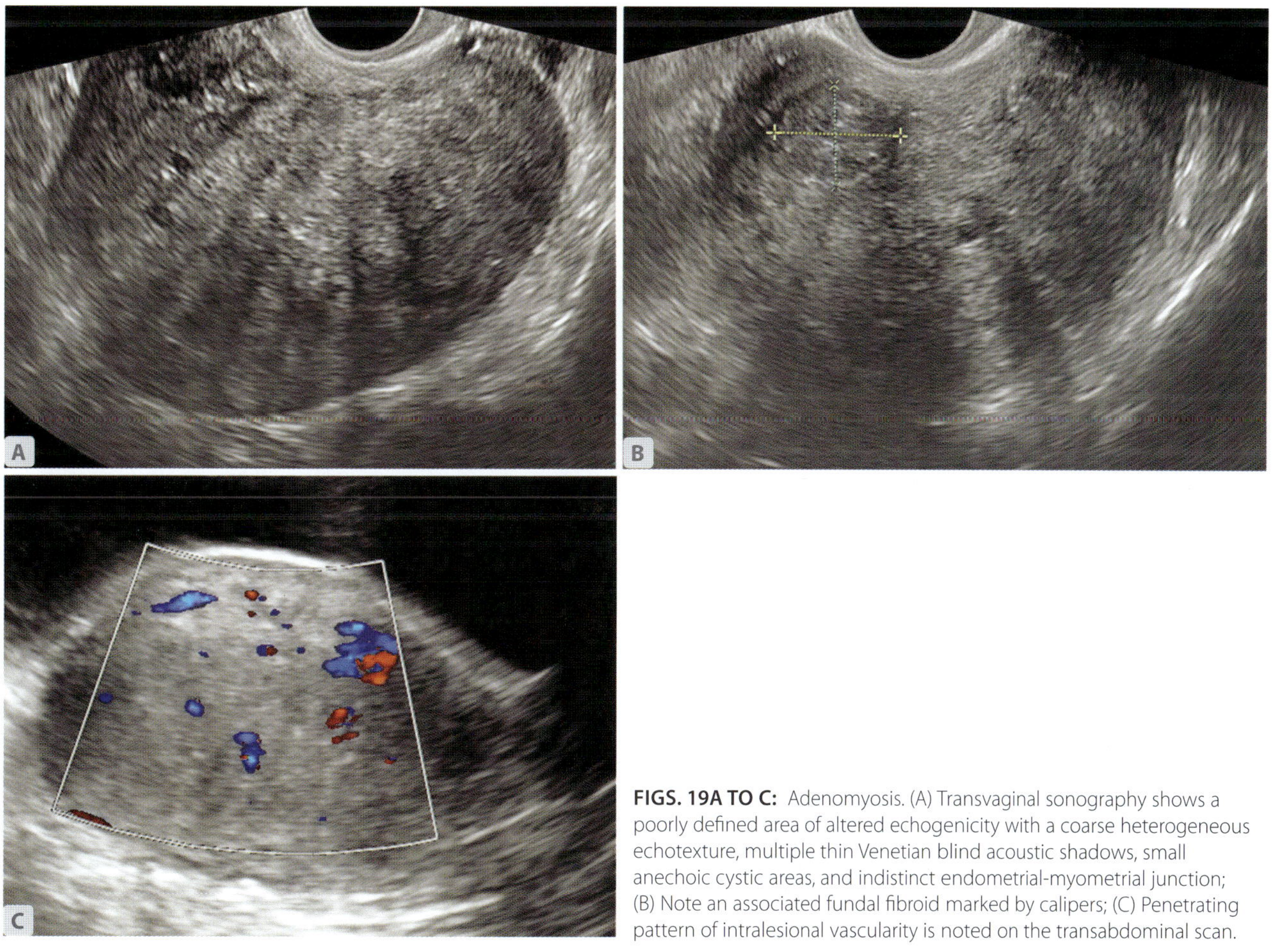

FIGS. 19A TO C: Adenomyosis. (A) Transvaginal sonography shows a poorly defined area of altered echogenicity with a coarse heterogeneous echotexture, multiple thin Venetian blind acoustic shadows, small anechoic cystic areas, and indistinct endometrial-myometrial junction; (B) Note an associated fundal fibroid marked by calipers; (C) Penetrating pattern of intralesional vascularity is noted on the transabdominal scan.

heterogeneity, thin shadows, small hyperechoic nodules, and striations gives an appearance similar to end-stage liver disease and described as *cirrhosis of the uterus* by some authors.[64]

3. *Myometrial vascularity* is generally increased due to muscular hyperplasia and hypertrophy in adenomyosis. Color Doppler demonstrates an increased number of intramural vessels, which are randomly scattered, penetrate the involved myometrium and may be tortuous. This is different from the pattern typically seen in leiomyomas, which tend to displace vessels and demonstrate peripheral vascularity rather than a penetrating pattern **(Fig. 19C)**.

MRI is an accurate technique for diagnosing adenomyosis with a high sensitivity (78–88%) and specificity (67–93%).[63-69] It may be more useful than TVS in delineating the location and extent of disease, especially in an enlarged uterus. MR is also very useful in distinguishing adenomyosis from a leiomyoma in patients with enlarged uterus and in monitoring response to hormonal therapy. Many of the features of adenomyosis, seen on US, are depicted more clearly on MR, which is superior in showing changes in zonal anatomy **(Figs. 20A and B and Table 4)**.

Adenomyosis is visualized as either diffuse or focal thickening of the junctional zone forming an ill-defined area of low signal intensity, which represents smooth muscle hyperplasia. A junctional zone thickness of >12 mm has been reported to be highly accurate for diagnosing adenomyosis. Adenomyosis can be excluded if the junctional zone thickness is 8 mm or less. Bright foci on T2-weighted images within the lesion are seen in >50% of cases, which represent islands of ectopic endometrial tissue and cystic dilatation of glands. When menstrual bleed occurs in these ectopic endometrial glands, these foci appear bright on T1-weighted images and are highly suggestive of endometriosis. In addition, striations of high signal on T2W images extending from the endometrium into the myometrium, producing pseudowidening of the endometrium, may be seen. The appearance of adenomyosis and the amount of bright foci may fluctuate with or without treatment. Contrast-enhanced imaging does not increase the accuracy in diagnosing adenomyosis although perfusion abnormalities have been reported **(Figs. 21A to C)**.[66-70]

Atypical/Unusual Patterns of Adenomyosis

Adenomyoma is a localized, circumscribed form of adenomyosis. The lesion is generally seen as a polypoid mass protruding into the endometrial cavity, or as a myometrial or subserosal mass without any connection to the junctional zone. Adenomyoma may be misdiagnosed as a leiomyoma or other tumors. An *adenomyotic cyst* is another extremely rare variation of adenomyosis which is thought to be caused by extensive hemorrhage into the ectopic endometrium. This produces a well-defined cystic myometrial lesion with different stages of blood degradation products.

Differential Diagnosis

Pseudolesions

During menstruation (especially day 1 and 2), the uterus may demonstrate marked thickening of the junctional zone (>12 mm). Thus, MR imaging should be avoided during the menstrual phase. *Myometrial contraction* is another pseudolesion. This produces focal bulging of the myometrium into the uterine cavity. The contracted area shows ill-defined or well-marginated areas of low signal intensity on T2-weighted images[71] as blood is squeezed out, reducing the water content (due to the reduced blood volume). Sequential studies demonstrate their transient nature distinguishing them from true myometrial disease although, this is not always possible on a single study.

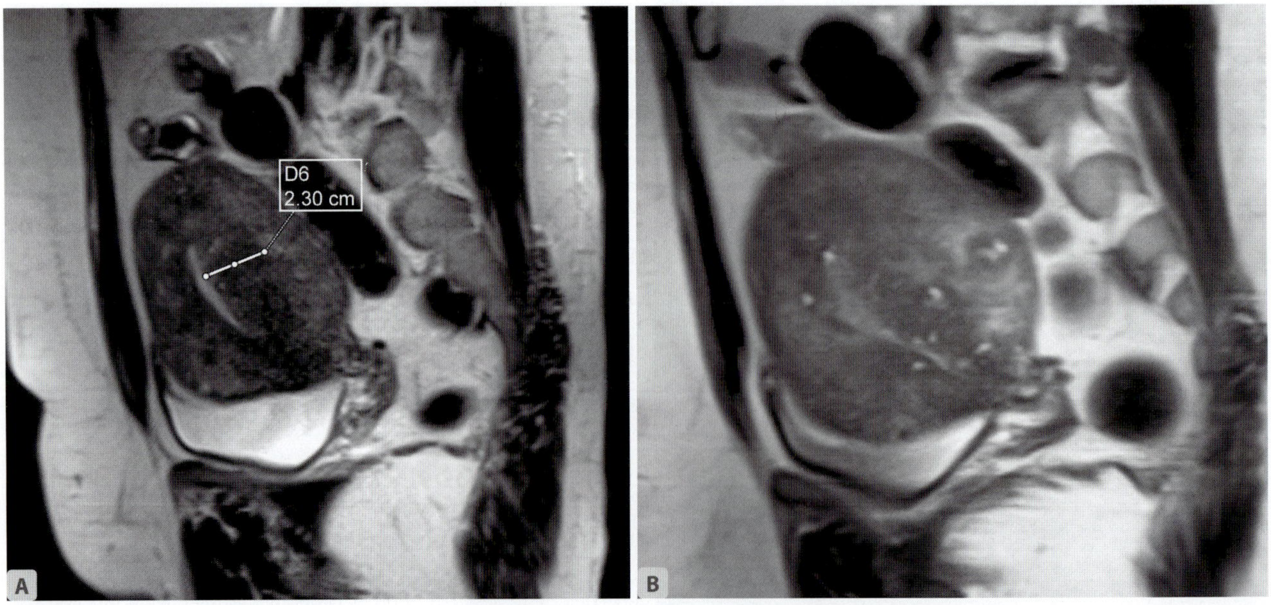

FIGS. 20A AND B: Adenomyosis. Sagittal T2W MR images of the same patient as in Figure 19 show globular enlargement of the uterus. The junctional zone is markedly widened with heterogeneous myometrium showing multiple variable-sized cystic areas.

TABLE 4: MRI criteria for adenomyosis.

Location	• Focal or diffuse widening of junctional zone >12 mm • More often found in the posterior uterine wall • Not seen in the cervix
Morphology	• Ill-defined margins blending with the surrounding myometrium • Poor definition of endomyometrial junction • *Focal:* May be globular, elliptical but usually not round or spherical • Significant mass effect missing, even if large lesion present • Mild distortion of endometrium, but marked enlargement of the uterus in diffuse adenomyosis
Appearance on T1	• Mostly isointense to the myometrium • May show hyperintense foci corresponding to small areas of hemorrhage
Appearance on T2	• Low SI uterine lesion with or without punctuate high signal intensity (SI) foci • High SI linear striations extending from the endometrium that may lead to a pseudowidening of the endometrium • Rarely large cystic spaces within a lesion (cystic adenomyosis)
Appearance on gadolinium-enhanced T1	Can appear hypo-, iso-, and hyperintense relative to myometrium
Additional findings	• No pseudocapsule • Adenomyosis is seen in combination with finding of endometriosis

Leiomyoma is the most common lesion which resembles focal adenomyosis. Focal adenomyosis produces an oval or elliptical lesion which leads to thickening of the uterine wall, but differs from leiomyoma in that there is little mass effect or distortion of the uterine cavity or outline. Unlike leiomyomas, adenomyosis shows poorly defined margins and blends with surrounding myometrium. It also lacks the pseudocapsule and dilated vessels or signal voids at the periphery that may be seen with leiomyomas. The differences have been summarized in **Table 5**.

Adenomatoid tumor, which is a relatively rare benign mesothelial tumor, resembles a leiomyoma or adenomyoma. *Metastasis* to the uterine corpus and *myometrial invasion by endometrial cancer* may also produce appearances identical to adenomyosis. *Endometrial stromal sarcoma (ESS)* which involves both endometrium and myometrium with infiltrative margins and cystic changes and *adenocarcinoma arising in adenomyosis* are other rare differential diagnostic considerations.

OTHER BENIGN MESENCHYMAL TUMORS

Fatty or mixed mesenchymal tumors such as fibromyolipoma, and lipoma of the uterus are rare benign tumors.[72] They may arise from metaplasia of connective tissue or smooth muscle cells.

On US, lipoma is seen as a rounded lesion showing increased echogenicity with a hypoechoic rim.[73] On CT, the encapsulated fat density of uterine lipoma may mimics an ovarian dermoid (benign cystic teratoma).[74] Accurate diagnosis is important because teratomas are generally managed by surgical excision, whereas lipomatous uterine tumors require no therapy unless symptomatic.

UTERINE ARTERIOVENOUS MALFORMATION

Uterine arteriovenous malformations (AVMs) may be congenital, traumatic, malignant, or idiopathic. Congenital AVMs are thought to occur due to undifferentiated vascular structures from the arrest of embryonic development. Acquired AVMs are usually secondary to trauma caused by procedures such as curettage or uterine surgery or secondary to neoplasms.[75]

On grayscale imaging, appearance of AVMs is nonspecific and includes subtle, myometrial inhomogeneity, tubular spaces within the myometrium, or prominent parametrial vessels. Doppler findings reveal a low resistance flow with high PSVs. Spectral analysis of venous flow also shows high flow velocities and systolic velocity peaks similar to arterial pattern, suggesting an arteriovenous shunting.[76]

Both computed tomography angiography (CTA) and magnetic resonance angiography (MRA) can be used to accurately assess the size, extent of AVMs and the degree of adjacent organ involved. On MRI, AVMs appear as focal uterine masses or as disruption of the junctional zones with serpiginous flow-related signal voids within the myometrium, showing intense enhancement on postgadolinium imaging with early draining veins **(Figs. 22A to D)**. Treatment of uterine AVM consists of either surgery or transcatheter embolization. The extent of involvement of adjacent pelvic viscera is important in deciding between the two treatment options.[77]

UTERINE INVERSION

Uterine inversion is most often attributed to excessive traction on the cord during delivery or a fundal location of the placenta. Nonpuerperal causes of uterine inversion include a benign or malignant uterine mass, but it is extremely rare.[78]

On longitudinal US scans, the uterine fundus is poorly seen due to the folding of the uterus on itself sometimes referred to as the *"fallen fundus"* sign. The central uterine echoes appear to have a "Y" configuration with the limbs of the "Y" formed by the inverted endometrial lining extending both anteriorly and posteriorly and the base by the noninverted endometrial lining. The miduterus gives a *"bull's eye"* appearance on transverse scans consisting of a hyperechoic ring representing the inverted endometrial lining surrounding the geographic center of the uterus. With complete inversion into the vagina, a mirror reflection of the uterus projecting into the vagina and a central pseudostripe may be seen, as the interface between the two opposing serosal surfaces may mimic an endometrial stripe. On MRI,

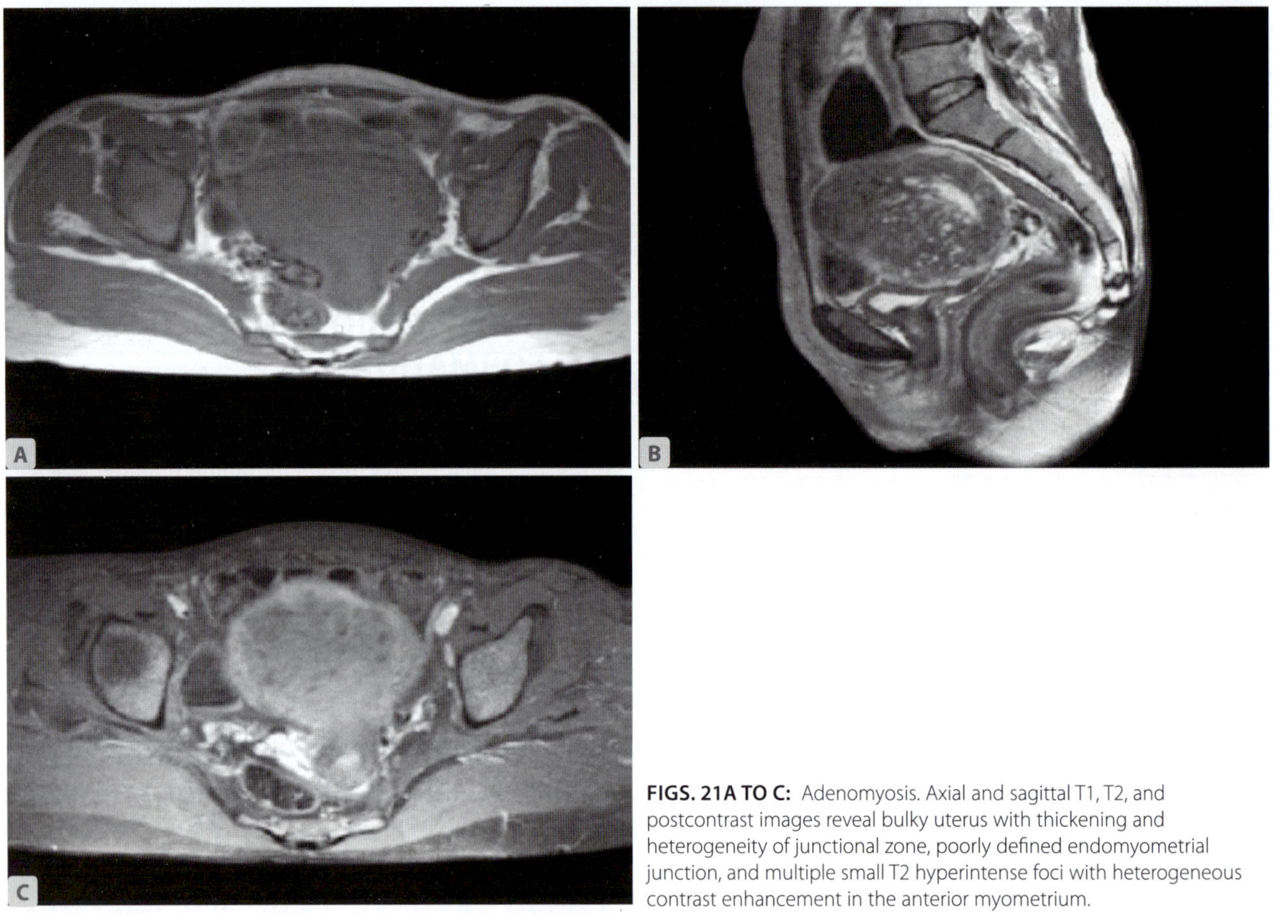

FIGS. 21A TO C: Adenomyosis. Axial and sagittal T1, T2, and postcontrast images reveal bulky uterus with thickening and heterogeneity of junctional zone, poorly defined endomyometrial junction, and multiple small T2 hyperintense foci with heterogeneous contrast enhancement in the anterior myometrium.

TABLE 5: Comparison of findings of focal adenomyosis and leiomyomas.

Categories	Adenomyosis	Leiomyomas
Borders	Indistinct	Distinct, usually round
Location	Generally contiguous with endometrium	Submucosal, intramural, or subserosal
Shadowing on US	Thin, parallel, vertical, and Venetian blind shadows	Edge shadowing; dense shadows from calcification
Mass effect	Absent	Present
Calcification	None	Common; rim and chunky
Cysts	Tiny cysts and cystic striations	Usually solid; may have macrocystic degeneration
Vascularity	Increased flow, penetrating vessels	Qualitatively variable, typically circumferential
Junctional zone	Thickened, with indistinct borders	Normal thickness

V- or U-shaped uterine cavity and an inverted uterine fundus on sagittal images, and a *bull's eye* configuration on axial images have been reported. At times, the uterine anatomy may be completely distorted.

ENDOMETRIAL PATHOLOGY

Endometrial Polyps[79-81]

Endometrial polyps usually occur in perimenopausal/postmenopausal women, and are multiple in 20% of cases. Women on tamoxifen therapy for breast cancer treatment have an increased relative risk for developing endometrial polyps. Most patients are asymptomatic; however, they may cause menorrhagia, intermenstrual bleeding, or postmenopausal bleeding.

Endometrial polyps represent localized hyperplastic overgrowth of endometrial glands and stroma, covered by endometrium. They may be sessile or pedunculated and are usually attached to the uterine fundus or cornua. They are variable in size and may be small or so large as to protrude into the endocervical canal. Histologically, they are of three types: (1) hyperplastic (resembling glands of endometrial hyperplasia), (2) atrophic (cystically dilated atrophic glands),

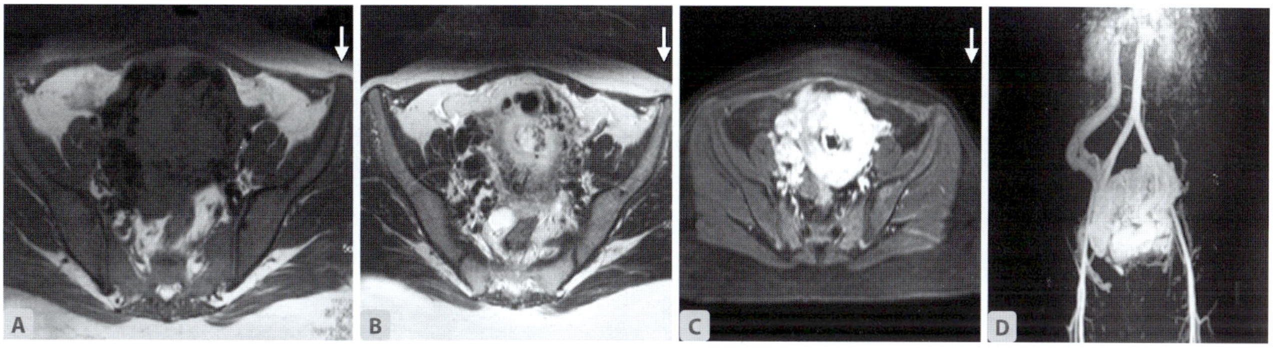

FIGS. 22A TO D: (A) T1W and (B) T2W axial MR images reveal a bulky uterus with multiple, large tortuous flow voids within the myometrium and bilateral parametrial regions; (C) Intense enhancement of the myometrium and the vascular channels is seen on postgadolinium images; (D) Magnetic resonance angiography reveals prominent arterial feeder channels arising from the internal iliac arteries. Enlarged, tortuous venous channels are seen draining into the iliac and right ovarian veins—uterine arteriovenous malformation.

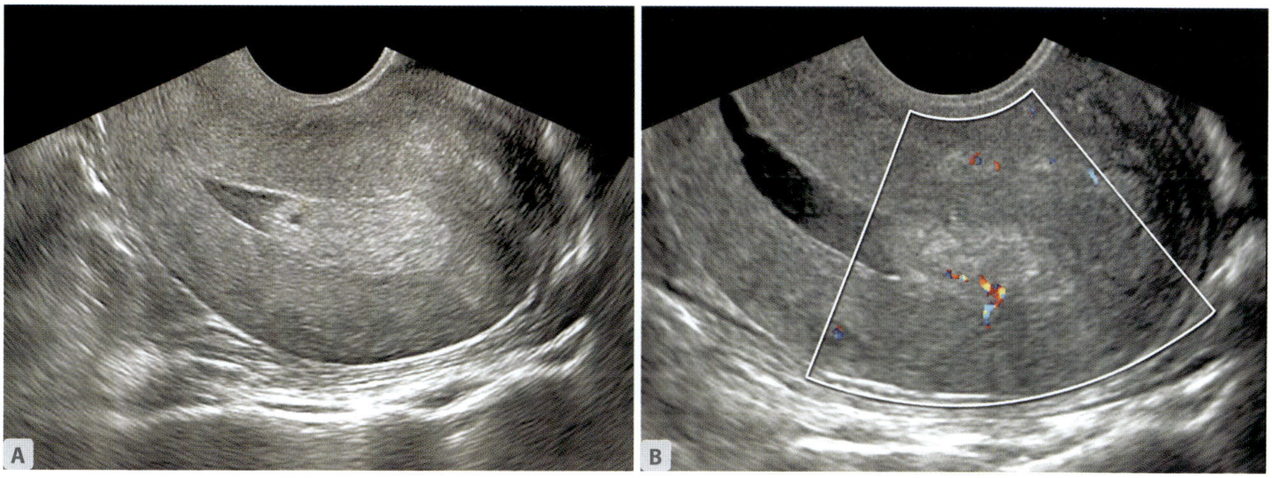

FIGS. 23A AND B: Endometrial polyp. (A) Saline infusion sonohysterography (SIS) demonstrates a well-defined echogenic mass in the endometrial cavity near the fundus; (B) A characteristic single feeding vessel is well seen on color Doppler.

and (3) functional (undergo cyclical endometrial changes). Malignancy is seen in 0.5% of endometrial polyps.

On US, endometrial polyps are visualized as nonspecific, echogenic endometrial thickening or as a focal, echogenic endometrial mass. It may be broad based and sessile or pedunculated. The point of attachment should not disrupt the endometrial lining[30] anechoic regions within the polyps may be seen and correspond histologically to dilated glands.[17] *An interrupted mucosa sign* has been described where the highly echogenic linear interface of opposing endometrial surfaces is focally interrupted by an endometrial polyp. This is best appreciated on transvaginal transverse or longitudinal images in the first half of the menstrual cycle. Color Doppler imaging demonstrates a single feeding vessel, which is reported to be fairly specific for endometrial polyps and better seen with SIS. On SIS, endometrial polyps are seen as smooth, well margined, echogenic masses protruding into the endometrial canal surrounded by fluid **(Figs. 23A and B)**.

Most commonly, endometrial polyps show a slightly hypointense signal compared to endometrium on T2-weighted MR images, but may also be isointense to endometrium, appearing as focal or diffuse thickening of the endometrium. They may show intratumoral cystic areas or have a low T2-signal intensity fibrous core or stalk, features which have been reported more often in benign lesions than malignant ones. On T1-weighted images, endometrial polyps are isointense to endometrium. On postcontrast images, moderate to strong enhancement, generally less than normal endometrium, but more than normal myometrium is seen **(Figs. 24A to D)**. On dynamic examination, early persistent enhancement or a gradually increasing enhancement has been reported. These MRI features may be useful to differentiate endometrial polyps from other endometrial lesions but overlap may be seen with hyperplasia and malignancy.

A submucosal fibroid/fibroid polyp may mimic an endometrial polyp but may be differentiated by a broader base and more irregular contour of the former on SIS. A normal layer of endometrium is seen overlying a submucosal fibroid while the polyp can be seen arising from the endometrium. A single feeding vessel as opposed to a circumferential vascular supply in fibroids is also a useful distinguishing feature. Endometrial hyperplasia may also be impossible to distinguish from a polyp, especially when the former is focal and the latter is large.

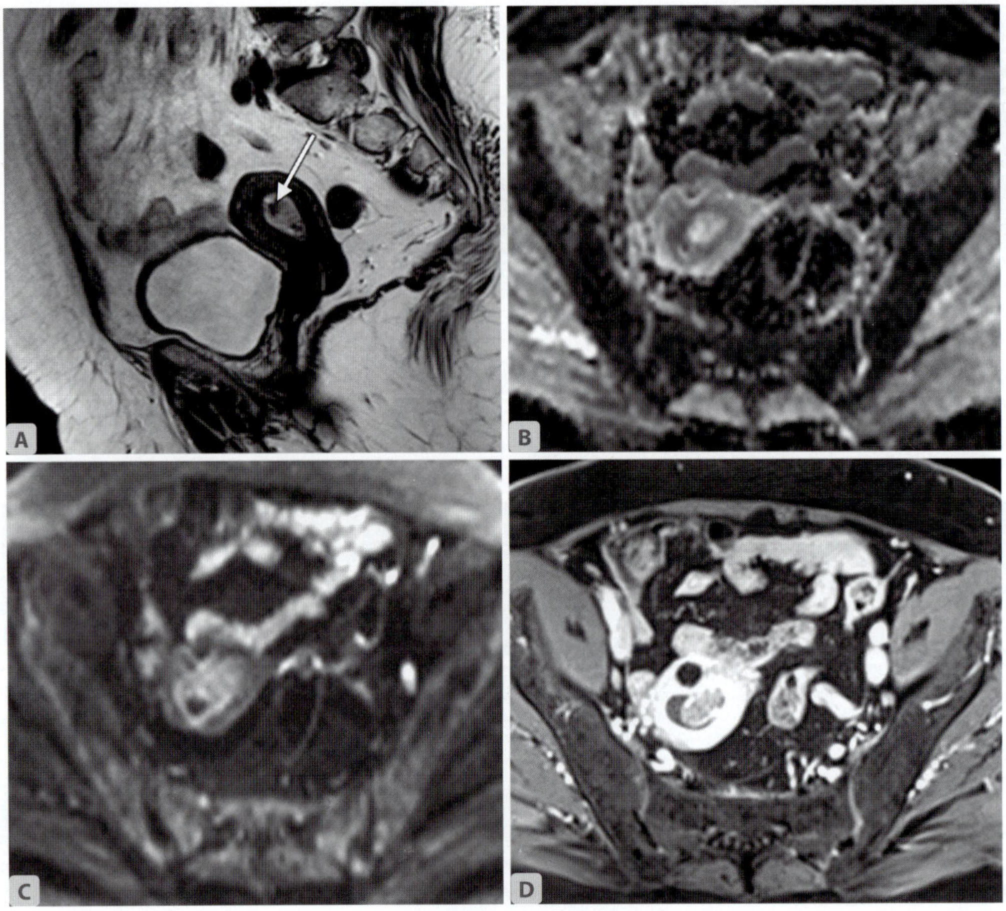

FIGS. 24A TO D: Endometrial polyp. (A) Sagittal T2W MR image reveals a focal lesion in the endometrial cavity, marginally lower in signal than expected for the normal endometrium. A few markedly hypointense areas (arrow) are also seen, representing fibrous core; (B and C) No diffusion restriction is seen on the DWI and ADC images with the lesion remaining bright on ADC; (D) Postcontrast image reveals mild enhancement of the polyp attached to the left lateral wall, well-delineated by the surrounding nonenhancing fluid. Note an incidental fibroid in the anterior myometrium (ADC: apparent diffusion coefficient; DWI: diffusion-weighted imaging).

Endometrial Hyperplasia

Excessive proliferation of the endometrial glands is termed as endometrial hyperplasia. The endometrial gland-to-stroma ratio is increased when compared with normal proliferative endometrium[82] and the glands can be cystically dilated. It may be focal or diffuse. Unopposed estrogen stimulation is the underlying cause in most cases of endometrial hyperplasia. Endometrial hyperplasia commonly presents as postmenopausal bleeding.

Two types have been described: with or without cellular atypia. Patients with cellular atypia may have foci of endometrial carcinoma in 25% of cases or develop it in future, while only approximately 2% patients without cellular atypia may develop malignancy.

On US, endometrial hyperplasia usually appears as a diffusely thickened, echogenic endometrium occasionally with small cysts representing dilated cystic glands at histology.[83] Focal, asymmetric thickening may also be seen in endometrial hyperplasia **(Fig. 25)**. The US and SIS features of endometrial hyperplasia are nonspecific and endometrial hyperplasia cannot be differentiated from endometrial carcinoma based on imaging alone.

On MRI, endometrial hyperplasia usually appears as diffuse thickening of the endometrium appearing iso- to hypointense on T2 sequences compared to normal endometrium, but the signal tends to be brighter than that in carcinoma. Small foci of increased T2 signal, attributable to cystically dilated glands, may be seen. Hyperplastic endometrium enhances less than the adjacent normal myometrium. On diffusion-weighted imaging (DWI), higher apparent diffusion coefficient (ADC) values have been reported in benign lesions as opposed to malignancy but stage 1A endometrial cancer cannot be reliably distinguished from endometrial hyperplasia based on imaging alone.

Infection

Endometritis is the most common cause of fever in the postpartum period, occurring in 2–3% of vaginal deliveries and in up to 85% of cesarean sections. The uterus and endometrium may appear normal on US, or may show a thickened, heterogeneous endometrium, intracavitary fluid, and/or intrauterine air as dirty shadowing.[84]

Tuberculosis is also an important cause of endometritis in India, usually secondary to primary infection elsewhere.

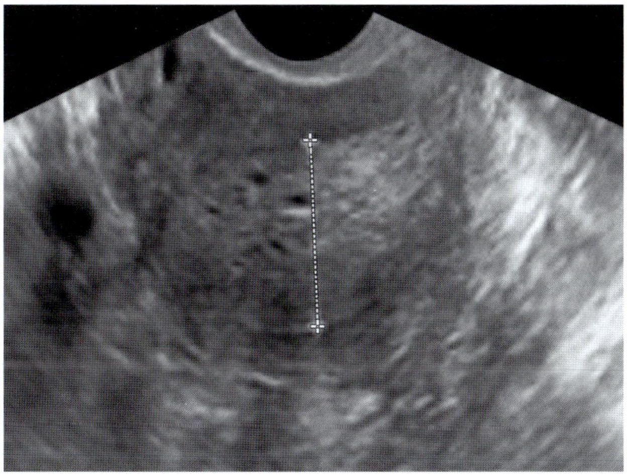

FIG. 25: Endometrial hyperplasia. Transvaginal sonography reveals diffusely thickened echogenic endometrium with small cysts within.

Tuberculosis of the genital tract may often be associated with tubo-ovarian abscesses. It has been discussed elsewhere in this text.

BENIGN VAGINAL LESIONS

Benign lesions of the vagina are very rare. Tumors occurring in other locations in the genital tract may also occur in the vagina. They usually produce no symptoms until large in size which include feeling of pressure, dyspareunia, vaginal or urethral obstruction, or vaginal bleeding. Vaginal neoplasms may be cystic or solid.

Vaginal cysts include Gartner's cysts, usually found in the anterolateral wall of upper vagina and Bartholin's cysts which occur below the pubic symphysis in the vaginal introitus posterolaterally. They are well-defined cystic lesions following fluid signal on MR unless the contents are proteinaceous.

Vaginal leiomyomas or fibromyomas are rare usually situated in the anterior vaginal wall and very few cases have been reported in the world literature.[1]

Fibroepithelial polyps of the vagina are uncommon and usually asymptomatic. They are usually small and may be multiple. During pregnancy, they may become enlarged and edematous with a bizarre in appearance. In infants and young girls, sarcoma botryoides is a differential consideration.

CONCLUSION

Benign diseases of the uterus and vagina encompass a wide variety of conditions. Uterine lesions are very common and often produce overlapping symptoms. Some of there may be extremely distressing for the patients, besides the associated morbidity. Imaging, thus, has an invaluable role in establishing an accurate diagnosis and ensuring appropriate management.

ACKNOWLEDGMENT

The authors would like to gratefully acknowledge the contribution of Dr Shivali Arya in drawing the illustrations for Figures 1 and 9.

REFERENCES

1. Chan YY, Jayaprakasan K, Zamora J, et al. The prevalence of congenital uterine anomalies in unselected and high-risk populations: a systematic review. Hum Reprod Update. 2011;17:761-71.
2. Grimbizis GF, Camus M, Tarlatzis BC, et al. Clinical implications of uterine malformations and hysteroscopic treatment results. Hum Reprod Update. 2001;7:161-74.
3. Acién P. Incidence of Müllerian defects in fertile and infertile women. Hum Reprod. 1997;12:1372-6.
4. Grimbizis GF, Gordts S, Di Spiezio Sardo A, et al. The ESHRE-ESGE consensus on the classification of female genital tract congenital anomalies. Gynecol Surg. 2013;10:199-212.
5. Behr SC, Courtier JL, Qayyam A. Imaging of Müllerian duct anomalies. Radiographics. 2012;32:E233-50.
6. Miller RJ, Breech LL. Surgical correction of vaginal anomalies. Clin Obstet Gynecol. 2008;51:223-36.
7. The American Fertility Society classifications of adnexal adhesions, distal tubal occlusion, tubal occlusion secondary to tubal ligation, tubal pregnancies, Müllerian anomalies and intrauterine adhesions. Fertil Steril. 1988;49:944-55.
8. Grimbizis GF, Gordts S, Di Spiezio Sardo A, et al. The ESHRE/ESGE consensus on the classification of female genital tract congenital malformations. Hum Reprod. 2013;28:2032-44.
9. Carrington BM, Hricak H, Nuruddin RN, et al. Müllerian duct anomalies: MR imaging evaluation. Radiology. 1990;176:715-20.
10. Uğur M, Turan C, Mungan T, et al. Endometriosis in association with Müllerian anomalies. Gynecol Obstet Invest. 1995;40:261-4.
11. Olive DL, Henderson DY. Endometriosis and Müllerian anomalies. Obstet Gynecol. 1987;69:412-5.
12. Jayasinghe Y, Rane A, Stalewski H, et al. The presentation and early diagnosis of the rudimentary uterine horn. Obstet Gynecol. 2005;105:1456-67.
13. Chandler TM, Machan LS, Cooperberg PL, et al. Mullerian duct anomalies: from diagnosis to intervention. Br J Radiol. 2009;82:1034-42.
14. Sarto GE, Simpson JL. Abnormalities of the Müllerian and Wolffian duct systems. Birth Defects Orig Artic Ser. 1978;14:37-54.
15. Ott DJ, Fayez J, Zagoria R, et al. Congenital anomalies. In: Ott DJ, Fayez JA, Zagorian RJ (Eds). Hysterosalpingography: A Text and Atlas, 2nd edition. Philadelphia: Lippincott Williams & Wilkins; 1998. pp. 59-69.
16. Zanetti E, Ferrari LR, Rossi G. Classification and radiographic features of uterine malformations: hysterosalpingographic study. Br J Radiol. 1978;51:161-70.
17. Buttram VC, Reiter RC. Uterine leiomyomata: etiology, symptomatology, and management. Fertil Steril. 1981;36:433-45.
18. Fedele L, Dorta M, Brioschi D, et al. Magnetic resonance evaluation of double uteri. Obstet Gynecol. 1989;74:844-7.
19. Homer HA, Li TC, Cooke ID. The septate uterus: a review of management and reproductive outcome. Fertil Steril. 2000;73:1-14.
20. Raga F, Bauset C, Remohi J, et al. Reproductive impact of congenital Müllerian anomalies. Hum Reprod. 1997;12:2277-81.
21. Fedele L, Bianchi S. Hysteroscopic metroplasty for septate uterus. Obstet Gynecol Clin North Am. 1995;22:473-89.

22. Pellerito JS, McCarthy SM, Doyle MB, et al. Diagnosis of uterine anomalies: relative accuracy of MR imaging, endovaginal sonography, and hysterosalpingography. Radiology. 1992;183:795-800.
23. Propst AM, Hill JA. Anatomic factors associated with recurrent pregnancy loss. Semin Reprod Med. 2000;18:341-50.
24. Zreik TG, Troiano RN, Ghoussoub RA, et al. Myometrial tissue in uterine septa. J Am Assoc Gynecol Laparosc. 1998;5:155-60.
25. Reuter KL, Daly DC, Cohen SM. Septate versus bicornuate uteri: errors in imaging diagnosis. Radiology. 1989;172:749-52.
26. Fischetti SG, Politi G, Lomeo E, et al. Magnetic resonance in the evaluation of Müllerian duct anomalies. Radiol Med. 1995;89: 105-11.
27. Brucker SY, Rall K, Campo R, et al. Treatment of congenital malformations. Semin Reprod Med. 2011;29:101-12.
28. Troiano RN, McCarthy SM. Müllerian duct anomalies: imaging and clinical issues. Radiology. 2004;233:19-34.
29. Ludwin A, Ludwin I, Kudla M. Differentiating between septate and bicornuate uterus: bi-dimensional and 3-dimensional power Doppler findings. J Minim Invasive Gynecol. 2014;21:1123-6.
30. Herbst AL, Ulfelder H, Poskanzer DC. Adenocarcinoma of the vagina: association of maternal stilbestrol therapy with tumor appearance in young women. N Engl J Med. 1971;284:878-81.
31. Rennell CL. T-shaped uterus in diethylstilbestrol (DES) exposure. Am J Roentgenol. 1979;132:979-80.
32. Olpin JD, Heilbrun M. Imaging of Müllerian duct anomalies. Clin Obstet Gynecol. 2009;52:40-56.
33. Knez J, Saridogan E, van Den Bosch T, et al. ESHRE/ESGE female genital tract anomalies classification system—the potential impact of discarding arcuate uterus on clinical practice. Hum Reprod. 2018;33:600-6.
34. Uterine leiomyomata. Number 192—May 1994. ACOG technical bulletin. Int J Gynaecol Obstet. 1994;46:73-82.
35. Cramer SF, Patel A. The frequency of uterine leiomyomas. Am J Clin Pathol. 1990;94:435-8.
36. Sue W, Scott-Barrett S. Radiological appearances of uterine fibroids. Indian J Radiol Imaging. 2009;19:222-31.
37. Kebapci M, Aslan O, Kaya T, et al. Pedunculated uterine leiomyoma associated with pseudo-Meigs' syndrome and elevated CA-125 level: CT features. Eur Radiol. 2002;12:S127-9.
38. Lurie S, Gorbacz S, Caspi B, et al. Parasitic leiomyoma: a case report. Clin Exp Obstet Gynecol. 1991;18:7-8.
39. Yeh HC, Kaplan M, Deligdisch L. Parasitic and pedunculated leiomyomas: ultrasonographic features. J Ultrasound Med. 1999;18:789-94.
40. Novak ER, Woodruff JD. Myoma and other benign tumors of the uterus. In: Novak ER, Woodruff JD (Eds). Novak's Gynecologic and Obstetric Pathology. Philadelphia: Saunders; 1979. pp. 260-79.
41. Okizuka H, Sugimura K, Takemori M, et al. MR detection of degenerating uterine leiomyomas. J Comput Assist Tomogr. 1993;17:760-6.
42. Hayasaka K, Tanaka Y, Fujii M, et al. Intravenous leiomyomatosis. J Comput Assist Tomogr. 2000;24:83-5.
43. Robboy SJ, Bentley RC, Butnor K, et al. Pathology and pathophysiology of uterine smooth-muscle tumors. Environ Health Perspect. 2000;108:779-84.
44. Gompel C, Silverberg SG. The corpus uteri. In: Gompel C, Silverberg SG (Eds). Pathology in Gynecology and Obstetrics. Philadelphia: Lippincott; 1994. pp. 163-283.
45. Arleo EK, Schwartz PE, Hui P, et al. Review of Leiomyoma Variants. Am J Roentgenol. 2015;205:912-21.
46. Gross BH, Silver TM, Jaffe MH. Sonographic features of uterine leiomyomas: analysis of 41 proven cases. J Ultrasound Med. 1983;2:401-6.
47. Dodd GD, Budzik RF. Lipomatous uterine tumors: diagnosis by ultrasound, CT, and MR. J Comput Assist Tomogr. 1990;14:629-32.
48. Vlahos N, Economopoulos K, Skarpidi E, et al. Bizarre leiomyoma of the posterior vaginal fornix. Int J Gynaecol Obstet. 2008;102: 296-7.
49. Mittl RL, Yeh IT, Kressel HY. High-signal-intensity rim surrounding uterine leiomyomas on MR images: pathologic correlation. Radiology. 1991;180:81-3.
50. Casillas J, Joseph RC, Guerra JJ. CT appearance of uterine leiomyomas. Radiographics. 1990;10:999-1007.
51. Murase E, Siegelman ES, Outwater EK, et al. Uterine leiomyomas: histopathologic features, MR imaging findings, differential diagnosis, and treatment. Radiographics. 1999;19:1179-97.
52. Exacoustos C, Romanini ME, Amadio A, et al. Can gray-scale and color Doppler sonography differentiate between uterine leiomyosarcoma and leiomyoma? J Clin Ultrasound. 2007;35: 449-57.
53. Hata K, Hata T, Maruyama R, et al. Uterine sarcoma: can it be differentiated from uterine leiomyoma with Doppler ultrasonography? A preliminary report. Ultrasound Obstet Gynecol. 1997;9:101-4.
54. Kubik-Huch RA, Weston M, Nougaret S, et al. European Society of Urogenital Radiology (ESUR) Guidelines: MR Imaging of Leiomyomas. Eur Radiol. 2018;28:3125-37.
55. Sudderuddin S, Helbren E, Telesca M, et al. MRI appearances of benign uterine disease. Clin Radiol. 2014;69:1095-104.
56. Kinkel K, Vincent B, Balleyguier C, et al. Value of MR imaging in the diagnosis of benign uterine conditions. J Radiol. 2000;81:773-9.
57. Lakhman Y, Veeraraghavan H, Chaim J, et al. Differentiation of uterine leiomyosarcoma from atypical leiomyoma: diagnostic accuracy of qualitative MR imaging features and feasibility of texture analysis. Eur Radiol. 2017;27:2903-15.
58. Wamsteker K, Emanuel MH, de Kruif JH. Transcervical hysteroscopic resection of submucous fibroids for abnormal uterine bleeding: results regarding the degree of intramural extension. Obstet Gynecol. 1993;82:736-40.
59. Parazzini F, Vercellini P, Panazza S, et al. Risk factors for adenomyosis. Hum Reprod. 1997;12:1275-9.
60. Cunningham RK, Horrow MM, Smith RJ, et al. Adenomyosis: A Sonographic Diagnosis. Radiographics. 2018;38:1576-89.
61. Struble J, Reid S, Bedaiwy MA. Adenomyosis: a clinical review of a challenging gynecologic condition. J Minim Invasive Gynecol. 2016;23:164-85.
62. Siegler AM, Camilien L. Adenomyosis. J Reprod Med. 1994;39:841-53.
63. Tamai K, Togashi K, Ito T, et al. MR Imaging findings of adenomyosis: correlation with histopathologic features and diagnostic pitfalls. Radiographics. 2005;25:21-40.
64. Sakhel K, Abuhamad A. Sonography of adenomyosis. J Ultrasound Med. 2012;31:805-8.
65. Katz VL. Benign gynecologic lesions. In: Katz VL, Lobo RA, Lentz G, Gershenson D (Eds). Comprehensive Gynecology, 5th edition. Philadelphia: Elsevier; 2007. pp. 419-71.
66. Bazot M, Cortez A, Darai E, et al. Ultrasonography compared with magnetic resonance imaging for the diagnosis of adenomyosis: correlation with histopathology. Hum Reprod. 2001;16:2427-33.
67. Reinhold C, McCarthy S, Bret PM, et al. Diffuse adenomyosis: comparison of endovaginal US and MR imaging with histopathologic correlation. Radiology. 1996;199:151-8.
68. Togashi K, Ozasa H, Konishi I, et al. Enlarged uterus: differentiation between adenomyosis and leiomyoma with MR imaging. Radiology. 1989;171:531-4.
69. Outwater EK, Siegelman ES, van Deerlin V. Adenomyosis: current concepts and imaging considerations. Am J Roentgenol. 1998;170:437-41.

70. Reinhold C, Tafazoli F, Mehio A, et al. Uterine adenomyosis: endovaginal US and MR imaging features with histopathologic correlation. Radiographics. 1999;19:S147-60.
71. Togashi K, Kawakami S, Kimura I, et al. Uterine contractions: possible diagnostic pitfall at MR imaging. J Magn Reson Imaging. 1993;3:889-93.
72. Soyer P, Harry G, Cazier A. Uterine fibromyolipoma: uncommon imaging features. Eur J Radiol. 1991;13:67-8.
73. Houser LM, Carrasco CH, Shelhan LR. Lipomatous tumour of the uterus: radiographic and ultrasonic appearance. Br J Radiol. 1979;52:992-3.
74. Lehrman BJ, Nisenbaum HL, Glasser SA. Uterine myolipoma. Magnetic resonance imaging, computed tomographic, and ultrasound appearance. J Ultrasound Med. 1990;9:665-8.
75. Dixit R, Prakash A, Chowdhury V, et al. Pelvic arteriovenous malformation. radiological quiz. GU imaging. Indian J Radiol Imaging. 2000;10:177-9.
76. Huang MW, Muradali D, Thurston WA, et al. Uterine arteriovenous malformations: gray-scale and Doppler US features with MR imaging correlation. Radiology. 1998;206:115-23.
77. Joshi M, Ganeshan K, Munshi HN. Ultrasound of adnexal masses. Semin Ultrasound CT MRI. 2008;29:72-97.
78. Rana KA, Patel PS. Complete uterine inversion: an unusual yet crucial sonographic diagnosis. J Ultrasound Med. 2009;28: 1719-22.
79. Sadro CT. Imaging the endometrium: a pictorial essay. Can Assoc Radiol J. 2016;67:254-62.
80. Kamaya A, Yu PC, Lloyd CR, et al. Sonographic evaluation for endometrial polyps: the interrupted mucosa sign. J Ultrasound Med. 2016;35:2381-7.
81. Hase S, Mitsumori A, Inai R, et al. Endometrial polyps: MR imaging features. Acta Med Okayama. 2012;66:475-85.
82. Salem S, Wilson SR. Gynaecologic ultrasound. In: Rumack CM, Wilson SR, Charbonean JW (Eds). Diagnostic Ultrasound, 3rd edition. Elsevier: Mosby; 2005. pp. 527-87.
83. Nalaboff KM, Pellerito JS, Ben-Levi E. Imaging the endometrium: disease and normal variants. Radiographics. 2001;21:1409-24.
84. DePalma R, Leveno, K, Cunningham F, et al. Identification and management of women at high risk for pelvic infection following cesarean delivery. Obstet Gynecol. 1980;55: 185S-92.

CHAPTER

17

Malignant Diseases of the Uterus and Vagina

Alpana Manchanda, Anju Garg, Gaurav Shanker Pradhan

INTRODUCTION

Gynecologic cancers consist of tumors which develop in the uterus, ovaries, cervix, vagina, vulva and rarely the fallopian tubes. The two most common uterine malignancies are endometrial cancer (arising from the glandular epithelium of the uterus) and cervical cancer. Though they both arise in the uterus, endometrial and cervical cancer differ from each other in their epidemiology, etiology and clinical features.[1,2] Uterine sarcomas are uncommon and heterogeneous tumors of the uterus arising from the mesenchymal or stromal tissue. Lymphoma, metastasis to uterus and vaginal cancers are much rarer gynecologic malignancies. Imaging has an important role in the staging, treatment planning and post-treatment evaluation of these malignancies.

ENDOMETRIAL CANCER

Epidemiology

Endometrial cancer is the most common gynecologic malignancy in developed countries. In India, its incidence is 4.3/100,000 women,[3] which is rising because of increased prevalence of obesity. A number of risk factors are associated with endometrial cancer such as nulliparity, early menarche, late menopause, exposure to unopposed estrogen therapy, obesity and polycystic ovarian disease.

The effect of long-lasting unopposed estrogen leads to endometrial hyperplasia which increases the chance of developing atypical hyperplasia, and ultimately endometrial cancer.[4] Most endometrial cancers occur sporadically, with some having a hereditary basis such as Lynch syndrome being caused by germline mutations.

Pathogenesis and Histology

The traditional histological classification of endometrial cancer based on clinical and hormonal features was proposed by Bokhman in 1983, according to which endometrial cancers are of two types: (1) Type I and (2) Type II endometrial cancers.

Type I endometrial cancer or endometrioid adenocarcinoma is the most common type, accounting for 80–85% of all endometrial cancers.[5] They are called endometrioid as they resemble the proliferative phase of endometrium. Type I tumors are estrogen-dependent, include grade 1 and 2 endometrioid adenocarcinomas, are of low malignant potential and have a good prognosis. Based on their degree of differentiation endometrioid endometrial cancer can vary from poorly-differentiated to well-differentiated cancers. In contrast, *Type II endometrial cancers or nonendometrioid adenocarcinomas* are nonestrogen-dependent, occur in older females and include clear cell carcinoma, serous papillary carcinoma, and carcinosarcoma and arise in the setting of endometrial atrophy. They are poorly differentiated, present at a higher stage, are more aggressive, have a poorer prognosis and spread-like ovarian cancer.

Table 1 outlines the differences between the two types of endometrial cancers.[5,6]

All type II and grade 3 endometrioid tumors are high-grade tumors and tend to have a poor prognosis.

The histological classification of endometrial cancer by World Health Organization (WHO) is based on tumor morphology and tumor grade. **Box 1** depicts the histological classification of endometrial cancer.[7]

Molecular Classification

The histological classification is useful in determining the appropriate surgical and adjuvant treatment. The dual classification of endometrial cancer (into type I and II) has been found to have its own limitations as all well-differentiated endometrial cancers do not have a good outcome and some poorly differentiated endometrial cancers have a good outcome. Often an overlap between histologic subtypes and grading has been seen, thereby causing a dilemma in clinical decision making. To overcome this drawback, the Cancer Genome Atlas (TCGA) in 2013 proposed a new molecular classification which by understanding the molecular alteration involved in endometrial cancer, may be useful in allowing early detection of endometrial cancer or precursor lesions and help in guiding targeted therapies.[7]

TABLE 1: Differences between type I and type II endometrial cancer.

Type I (endometrioid) endometrial cancer	Type II (nonendometrioid) endometrial cancer
• Comprises of 85% of all endometrial cancers	• Comprises of 15% of all endometrial cancers
• Premenopausal/perimenopausal age group	• Older patients (postmenopausal)
• Low-grade malignancy with endometrioid morphology (grades 1 and 2)	• High-grade malignancy with endometrioid grade 3, nonendometrioid subtypes, e.g. (Serous; Clear cell; Undifferentiated carcinoma)
• Good prognosis as diagnosed early	• Poor prognosis, account for 40% of endometrial cancer deaths
• Hormone receptor positive cancers	• Hormone receptor negative cancers
• More common in obese women, related to long-term estrogen therapy	• More common in nonobese women
• Originate from endometrial hyperplasia	• Associated with an atrophic endometrium
• Present as localized disease (low stage)	• Biologically aggressive with higher risk of metastasis
• Surgery is curative in early endometrial cancers	• Surgery with adjuvant chemoradiation
• Associated with *PTEN* or *KRAS* gene mutation	• Associated with P53 mutation
• 5-year survival is ~ 80%	• 5-year survival is ~ 40%

Sources: 1. Faria SC, Devine CE, Rao B, et al. Imaging and staging of endometrial cancer. Semin Ultrasound CT MRI. 2019;40:287-94.
2. Nougaret S, Lakhman Y, Vargas HA, et al. From staging to prognostication: achievements and challenges of MR imaging in the assessment of endometrial cancer. Magn Reson Imaging Clin N Am. 2017;25:611-33.

BOX 1: Histological classification of endometrial cancer.

- Endometrioid (~80% of all endometrial cancers)
- Serous (~10%)
- Clear cell (<6%)
- Mixed cell adenocarcinoma

Rare types:

- Mucinous adenocarcinoma
- Neuroendocrine tumor (small cell, large cell or carcinoid)
- Dedifferentiated carcinoma
- Undifferentiated carcinoma

Source: Yen TT, Wang TL, Fader AN, et al. Molecular classification and emerging targeted therapy in endometrial cancer. Int J Gynecol Pathol. 2019.

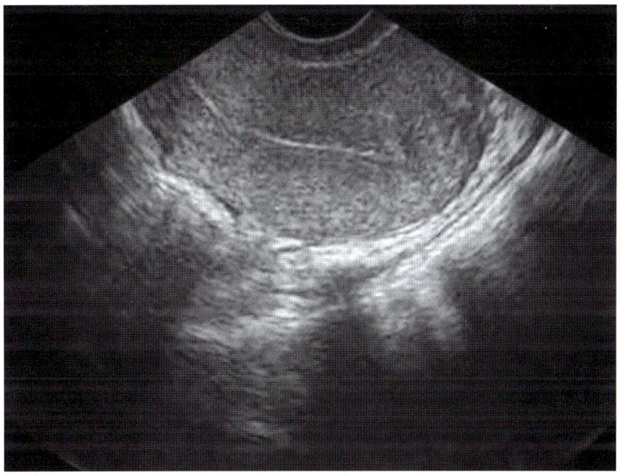

FIG. 1: Longitudinal transvaginal sonography image shows a uniformly thin (1.5 mm) well-defined endometrial echo. This appearance of the endometrium excludes malignancy in a postmenopausal woman with vaginal bleeding.

Clinical Presentation

Patients most commonly present in the 6th and 7th decades of life with history of postmenopausal bleeding. As a result, majority of endometrial cancers are diagnosed at an early stage (80% stage I) with 5-year survival > 95%.[6]

Diagnosis

The diagnosis of endometrial cancer is histopathological, by endometrial tissue sampling or aspiration. With adequate tissue sampling, detection rate of endometrial cancer is up to 99%.[4] Prognosis is affected by age of the patient, stage of disease, histological tumor grade, cell type and lymph node status. Deep myometrial and cervical invasion carry an adverse prognosis.

Imaging

Ultrasound

Transvaginal sonography (TVS) is usually the first and most common investigation performed as more than 95% women present with postmenopausal bleeding. However, only around 10% of women with postmenopausal bleeding develop endometrial cancer.[8]

Sonographic evaluation is quick, easily available and does not involve any ionizing radiation. TVS provides noninvasive, high-resolution imaging of the endometrium. The normal endometrium in postmenopausal women should be thin, homogeneous and echogenic. A cut-off value of 5 mm is considered as upper limit of normal in postmenopausal women presenting with abnormal uterine bleeding with a sensitivity and specificity of 96% and 61% respectively in diagnosing endometrial cancer **(Fig. 1)**. However, in postmenopausal women who are asymptomatic, an endometrial thickness of up to 8 mm is considered normal and biopsy should be considered only, if the endometrium is more than 11 mm thick.[8]

The margins of endometrial cancer may be well delineated on ultrasound, if it is a focal mass or thickening. The endometrial thickness should be measured in the anteroposterior dimension in the sagittal plane and a thickened endometrium must be considered as cancer until it is proven otherwise. Sonographic appearance of a uniformly thickened endometrium is the most common appearance seen **(Fig. 2)**. When the thickening is well defined, uniform and echogenic, it may be indistinguishable from endometrial hyperplasia or polyp. The diagnosis of endometrial cancer is more likely if the thickened endometrium is irregular or has poorly defined margins with a heterogeneous echotexture **(Fig. 3)**.[8] Due to overlapping features on TVS which may favor a benign or malignant etiology, an endometrial biopsy is required for a definitive diagnosis.

Ultrasound is limited in the evaluation of depth of myometrial invasion. Myometrial invasion can be suggested on TVS when there is asymmetric extension of the tumor into the myometrium, the endometrial-myometrial junction appears irregular or the subendometrial halo (inner myometrial layer) is disrupted.

On Doppler ultrasound, a normal or benign endometrium is characterized by high resistance flow, while an endometrial cancer by low resistance flow. Studies have shown that Doppler evaluation of uterine, subendometrial or intra-endometrial arteries are not reliable in the differentiation of benign and malignant endometrial processes and measurement of endometrial thickness is a better method of discrimination.

The limitations of TVS are that it is (1) operator-dependent; (2) the endometrium may not be visualized in around 10% cases; (3) it may be difficult to evaluate cervical or extrauterine extension due to its limited field of view; and (4) it may overestimate myometrial invasion in case of concomitant pathology such as adenomyosis or leiomyoma.[1]

Saline infusion sonography (SIS) or sonohysterography has been found to increase the accuracy of TVS. Endometrial cancer can appear as an intracavitary polyp or an asymmetric thickening of the endometrial lining on SIS. The depth of myometrial invasion has been found to be predicted with a greater accuracy on SIS than by TVS alone.[1]

A thin endometrium on TVS virtually excludes endometrial cancer, i.e. the negative predictive value of a thin endometrium is very high.[9]

Flowchart 1 depicts the various endometrial appearances on transvaginal sonography in postmenopausal women presenting with abnormal uterine bleeding and their workup.[10]

Such a TVS-based approach not only helps in excluding endometrial cancer, but also allows for better clinical management.

Computed Tomography

Due to its poor soft tissue differentiation, CT is not used in the local staging of endometrial cancer. On contrast- enhanced CT, endometrial cancer may be seen as a dilated endometrial cavity with a hypodense mass, which may be indistinguishable from an endometrial polyp or submucosal fibroid **(Fig. 4)**. CT has shown to have low sensitivity and specificity in evaluating myometrial invasion and cervical extension as compared to magnetic resonance imaging (MRI).[11]

Computed tomography is mainly indicated when the endometrial cancer is in a more advanced stage for assessing extrauterine spread, lymphadenopathy and extrapelvic metastasis. Lymph nodes, lungs and ovaries are the most common sites of metastasis of endometrial cancer.[5]

A recent study has shown dual energy CT to be a promising tool for assessing myometrial invasion with 50 KeV images being superior to 70 KeV images.[12]

Magnetic Resonance Imaging

Magnetic resonance imaging is the most accurate noninvasive imaging modality for preoperative assessment of endometrial cancer due to its excellent soft tissue contrast resolution. Although MR imaging is not a part of the standard

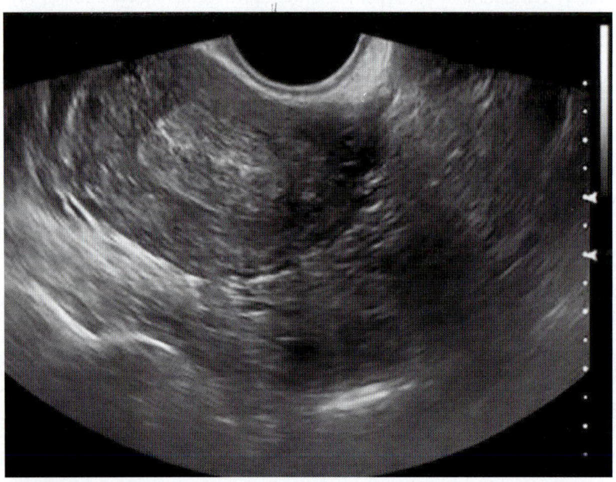

FIG. 2: Axial grayscale transvaginal sonography image reveals nonspecific diffusely thickened hyperechoic endometrium measuring 26 mm.

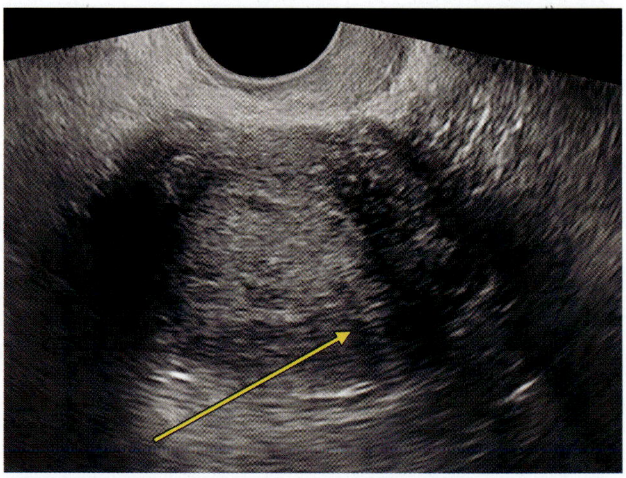

FIG. 3: Transvaginal sonography in a patient presenting with postmenopausal bleeding reveals diffuse thickening (30 mm) of the endometrium appearing heterogeneously hyperechoic with ill-defined endomyometrial junction posteriorly (arrow).

FLOWCHART 1: Endometrial assessment on TVS with history of postmenopausal bleeding.

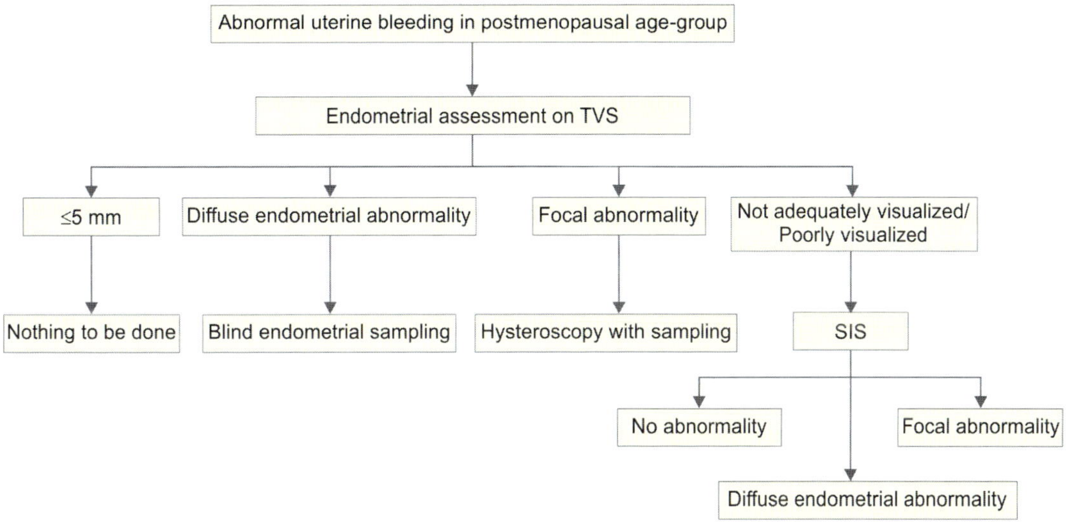

(SIS: saline infusion sonography)

Source: Rezvani M, Winter TC. Abnormal uterine bleeding: the role of ultrasound. In: Norton ME (Ed). Callen's Ultrasonography in Obstetrics and Gynecology, 6th edition. Philadelphia: Elsevier; 2017. pp. 835-45.

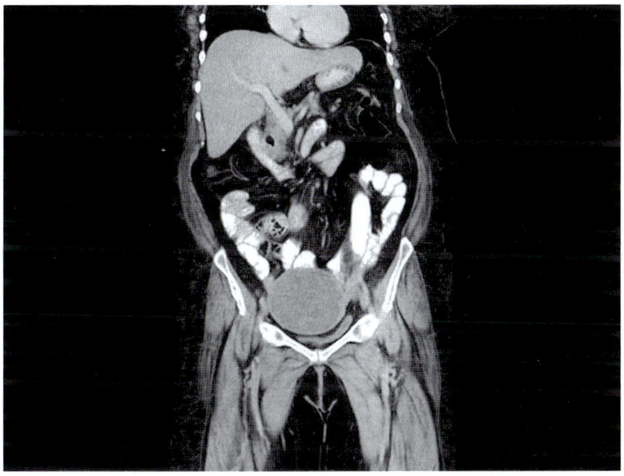

FIG. 4: Coronal contrast-enhanced CT in a 70-year-old woman with biopsy proven endometrial cancer reveals a large soft tissue mass expanding the endometrial cavity: Type II endometrial cancer.

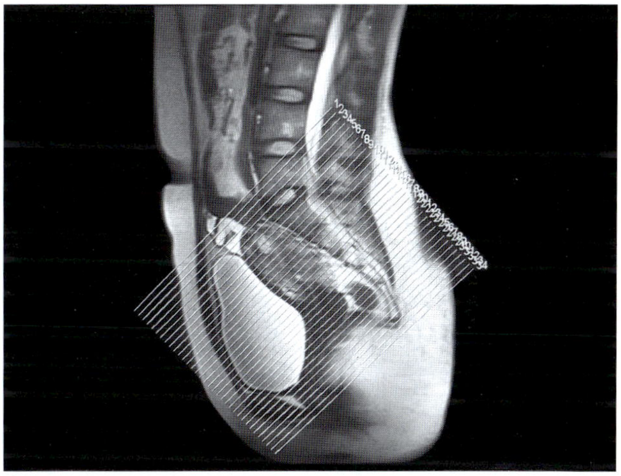

FIG. 5: Sagittal localizer image with reference lines depicting proper planning for image acquisition according to the uterine axis. The images should be acquired in a plane perpendicular to the endometrial lining.

International Federation of Gynecology and Obstetrics (FIGO) staging of endometrial cancer, MR imaging has been recommended by the National Cancer Institute of France, the European Society of Radiology guidelines and the Royal College of Radiologists.[13,14]

Technique

MRI is performed using a phased array body coil with high-resolution T2-weighted imaging being the mainstay of imaging. Nonfat suppressed images should be acquired because of the inherent contrast between the signal intensity of the uterus and surrounding fat.[15] The MRI sequences of the pelvis should be planned according to the uterine axis with the plane perpendicular to the endometrial lining to allow evaluation of depth of myometrial and cervical invasion **(Fig. 5)**. Multiparametric MR imaging is the preferred technique of MR imaging in endometrial cancer. A combination of three sequences, i.e. sagittal and axial oblique T2 weighted, diffusion-weighted imaging (DWI), and dynamic contrast-enhanced MR imaging (DCE-MRI) provides the most comprehensive evaluation by accurately delineating the extent of local disease and lymph node involvement if any. Staging of endometrial cancer by MR Imaging is found to be accurate in the range of 85–93%. By combining disease extent at MR imaging with the histologic subtype and grade obtained at endometrial biopsy, assessment of risk stratification and prognosis can be done precisely.[14]

Endometrial cancer appears hypo- to isointense mass on T1-weighted images, with intermediate signal intensity lower than the normal endometrium on T2-weighted images. On DCE-MRI, endometrial cancer enhances less than the myometrium. It shows restricted diffusion, showing high signal intensity on DWI, and low signal intensity on apparent diffusion coefficient (ADC) maps **(Figs. 6A to E)**. Both DCE-MRI and DWI increase the accuracy of T2-weighted imaging in assessment of depth of myometrial imaging. DW imaging has a role in endometrial cancer by showing the primary tumor better, depicting drop metastasis in cervix and vagina, extrauterine spread to the peritoneum and lymph nodes especially when intravenous gadolinium contrast is contraindicated and it can detect tumor when histopathology findings are inconclusive or endometrial biopsy is not possible.[16]

Diffusion-weighted imaging should always be evaluated together with the corresponding ADC maps and conventional T2-weighted images to avoid any pitfall. The ADC values of malignant lesions are found to be less than benign lesions and normal tissue. In a study by Rechichi et al., using two b values of 0 and 1,000 an ADC value of 1.05×10^3 mm^2/sec as cut-off was obtained which could differentiate endometrial cancer from normal endometrium. However a connection between ADC value and tumor grade could not be established.[17]

Bonatti et al. in 2018 documented the evidence of deep myometrial invasion and a tumor to uterus volume ratio ≥ 0.13 correlated with high-grade endometrial cancer, while ADC values were not found to be helpful in predicting the histological grade of endometrial cancer.[18]

Several features have been found to be associated with a poor prognosis in endometrial cancer, such as deep myometrial invasion (i.e. >50% depth of myometrial involvement or stage I B), cervical stromal involvement, and lymph nodal involvement.[5]

The depth of myometrial invasion is the most significant indicator for survival. The relation between depth of myometrial invasion and nodal involvement is given in **Table 2**.

Sagittal T2-weighted images depict the uterine anatomy well and are the best for optimal depiction of depth of myometrial invasion with a greater accuracy in premenopausal than postmenopausal age group.[14] This is because of poor definition of junctional zone in postmenopausal women which may also be seen in those who have any other pathology such as adenomyosis or leiomyoma. DCE-MRI should be a part of standard imaging protocol for endometrial cancer as it improves the delineation of tumor margins and enables accurate assessment of invasion as endometrial cancer enhances less than the normal myometrium.

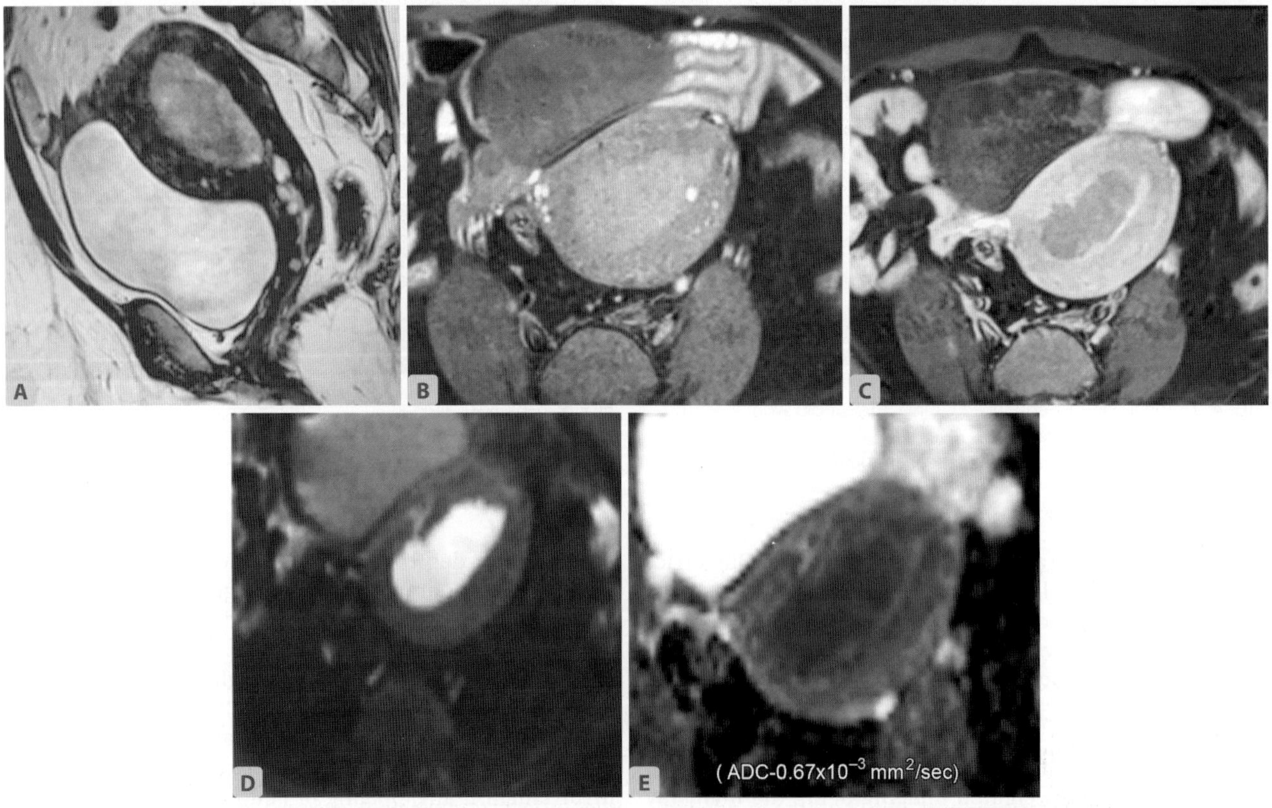

FIGS. 6A TO E: Multiparametric MR images of pelvis reveal (A) diffuse endometrial thickening of 28 mm showing intermediate hyperintense signal on T2W sagittal image (B) isointense on axial T1W image. Delayed post-contrast (3 minutes) axial T1 fat suppressed image depicts (C) endometrial lesion to be hypoenhancing to the myometrium and DWI and ADC map at the same level shows the mass to be hyperintense on DWI (D) with (E) loss of signal on corresponding ADC map with ADC value of 0.67×10^{-3} mm^2/sec. Both DWI and CEMR images depict the irregular endomyometrial junction very well: Stage IA endometrial cancer (ADC: apparent diffusion coefficient; CEMR: contrast-enhanced magnetic resonance; DWI: diffusion-weighted imaging).

TABLE 2: Relation of depth of myometrial invasion with lymph node involvement and 5-year survival in endo metrial cancer patients.[5]

Depth of myometrial invasion	Lymph node involvement	5-year survival
<50%	3–9%	95%
>50%	20–40%	68%

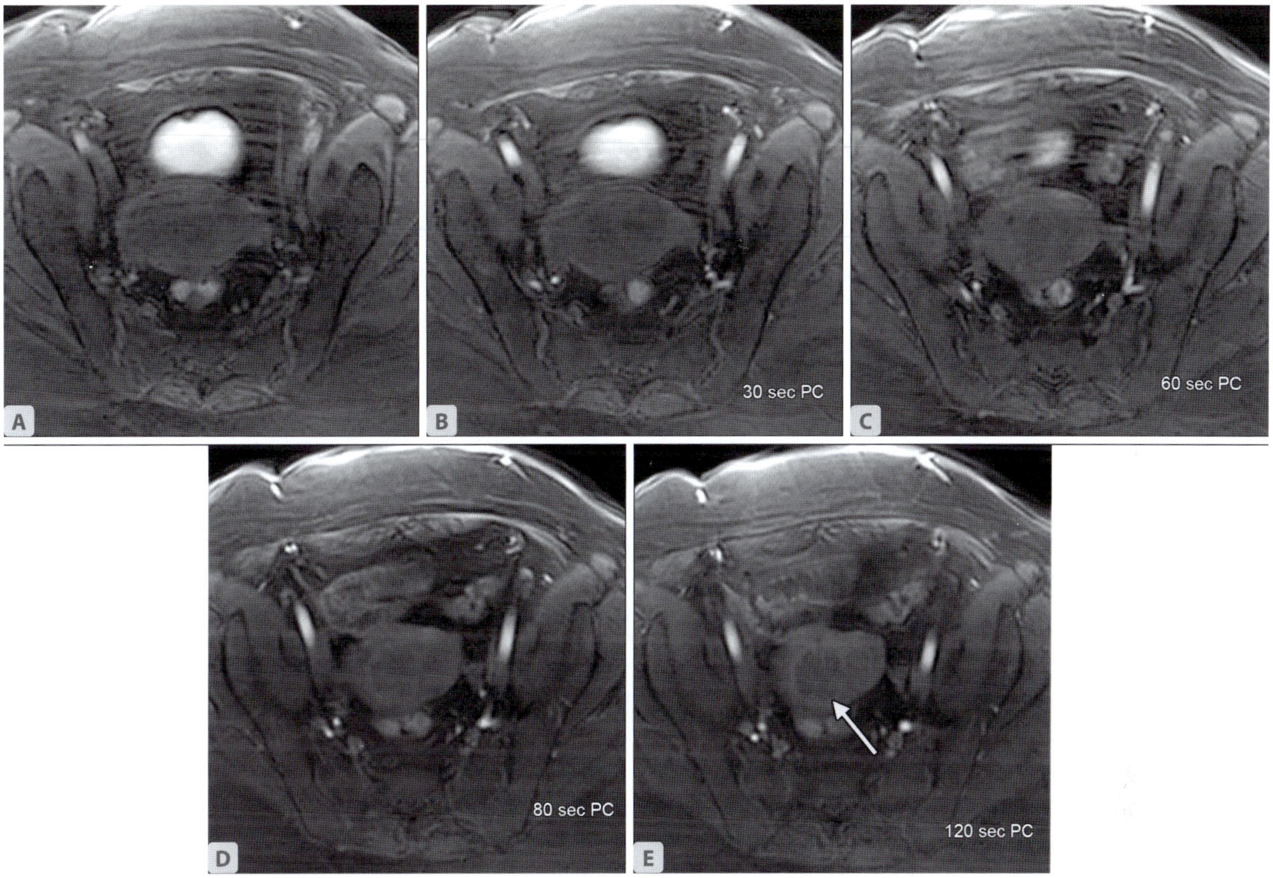

FIGS. 7A TO E: (A) Noncontrast and dynamic contrast enhanced MRI; (B to E) Axial T1-weighted fat suppressed images through the uterus reveal an endometrial mass with maximum enhancement between the mass and myometrium at 120 seconds (E) after intravenous contrast administration, appearing hypoenhancing (arrow) compared to the myometrium.

The maximum contrast between the tumor and myometrium has been described between 90 seconds and 150 seconds after intravenous contrast administration **(Figs. 7A to E)**.[19] DCE-MRI and T2-weighted imaging together have an accuracy of 98% for assessing myometrial invasion, hence are the two-key MR imaging sequences required for adequate staging of endometrial cancer.[5,13]

The presence of a smooth, uninterrupted band of early subendometrial enhancement (at 35-40 sec) on DCE-MRI helps to exclude superficial myometrial invasion. This is an important finding when fertility sparing management is being considered. Delayed DCE-MRI images (3-4 minutes after contrast administration) should be acquired to rule out cervical stromal invasion.

The presence of an intact enhancing cervical mucosa excludes cervical invasion. It is important to diagnose cervical stromal invasion as it is associated with a high risk for lymphovascular space invasion (LVSI) which thereby infers a poorer prognosis. A widened internal os with tumor protruding into the endocervical canal does not represent stromal invasion.

Staging

Staging of endometrial cancer is surgicopathological as the primary treatment is surgical. Also, clinical staging often underestimates the disease extent.[16] Staging is based on the FIGO staging system which was first established in 1958, then updated in1988. It was revised in 2009 as a result of better understanding of the clinicopathological characteristics and prognostic factors. **Table 3** gives the revised FIGO staging of endometrial cancer.[3,6]

The standard surgical procedure for staging of endometrial cancer consists of findings from exploratory laparotomy, i.e. total abdominal hysterectomy with bilateral salpingo-oophorectomy, peritoneal lavage and pelvic and para-aortic

TABLE 3: Revised FIGO staging of endometrial cancer (2009).

FIGO	Stage	Description
I	IA	Tumor confined to uterus, ≤50% myometrial invasion
	IB	≥50% myometrial invasion
II		Cervical stromal invasion
IIIA		Tumor invades serosa of uterus and/or adnexa
IIIB		Vaginal or parametrial involvement
IIIC		Metastasis to pelvic and/or para-aortic lymph nodes
	IIIC1	Pelvic node involvement
	IIIC2	Para-aortic lymph node involvement
IV	IVA	Tumor invasion of bowel and/or bladder mucosa
	IVB	Distant metastasis (including abdominal metastasis and/or inguinal lymph nodes)

Source: 1. Nougaret S, Lakhman Y, Vargas HA, et al. From staging to prognostication: achievements and challenges of MR imaging in the assessment of endometrial cancer. Magn Reson Imaging Clin N Am. 2017;25:611-33.

2. Faria SC, Sagebiel T, Balachandran A, et al. Imaging in endometrial carcinoma. Indian J Radiol Imaging. 2015;25(2):137-47.

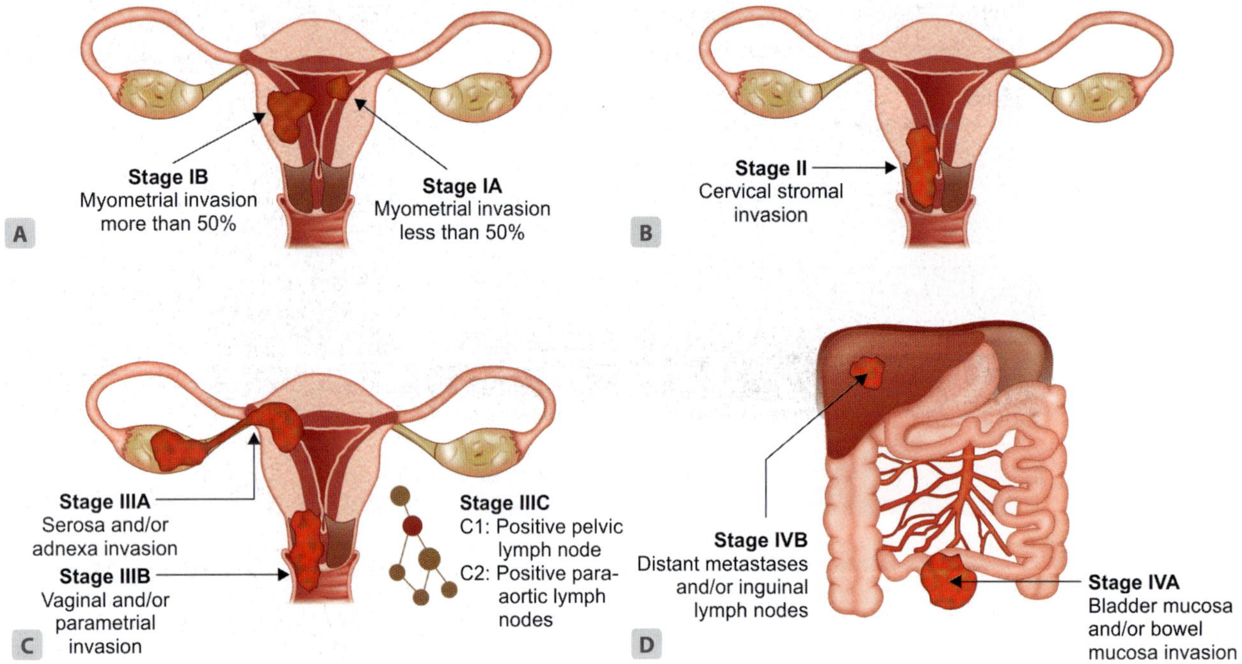

FIGS. 8A TO D: Diagrammatic representation depicting the FIGO staging of endometrial cancer.

lymphadenectomy. In patients who are at increased risk of mortality or severe morbidity, the surgical staging is not performed. Para-aortic lymphadenectomy is usually performed in patients with high-grade histologic tumor or where there is deep myometrial invasion.[3]

The five-year survival of endometrial cancer varies with the stage at which it is diagnosed. Patients in whom the tumor is confined to the uterus, the reported five-year survival rate is ≥95%.This decreases once the tumor has spread outside the uterus with five year survival rates of 69% and 17% with regional and distant metastasis, respectively.[5] **Figures 8A to D** give the diagrammatic representation of various stages of endometrial cancer.

MRI Features of Endometrial Cancer as per FIGO Staging

Stage I: Stage I endometrial cancers are confined to the uterus. Stage IA tumors appear as a focal or diffuse intermediate signal intensity lesion within the high- signal endometrial lining or involve less than 50% of the myometrium. Superficial myometrial invasion is seen as disruption or irregularity of the low signal intensity junctional zone on T2-weighted images and loss of smooth subendometrial enhancement on DCE-MR imaging. Stage IB tumors are seen as low signal intensity tumor which invade greater than 50% of the myometrial thickness but do not extend beyond the outer myometrial margin **(Figs. 9A to G)**.

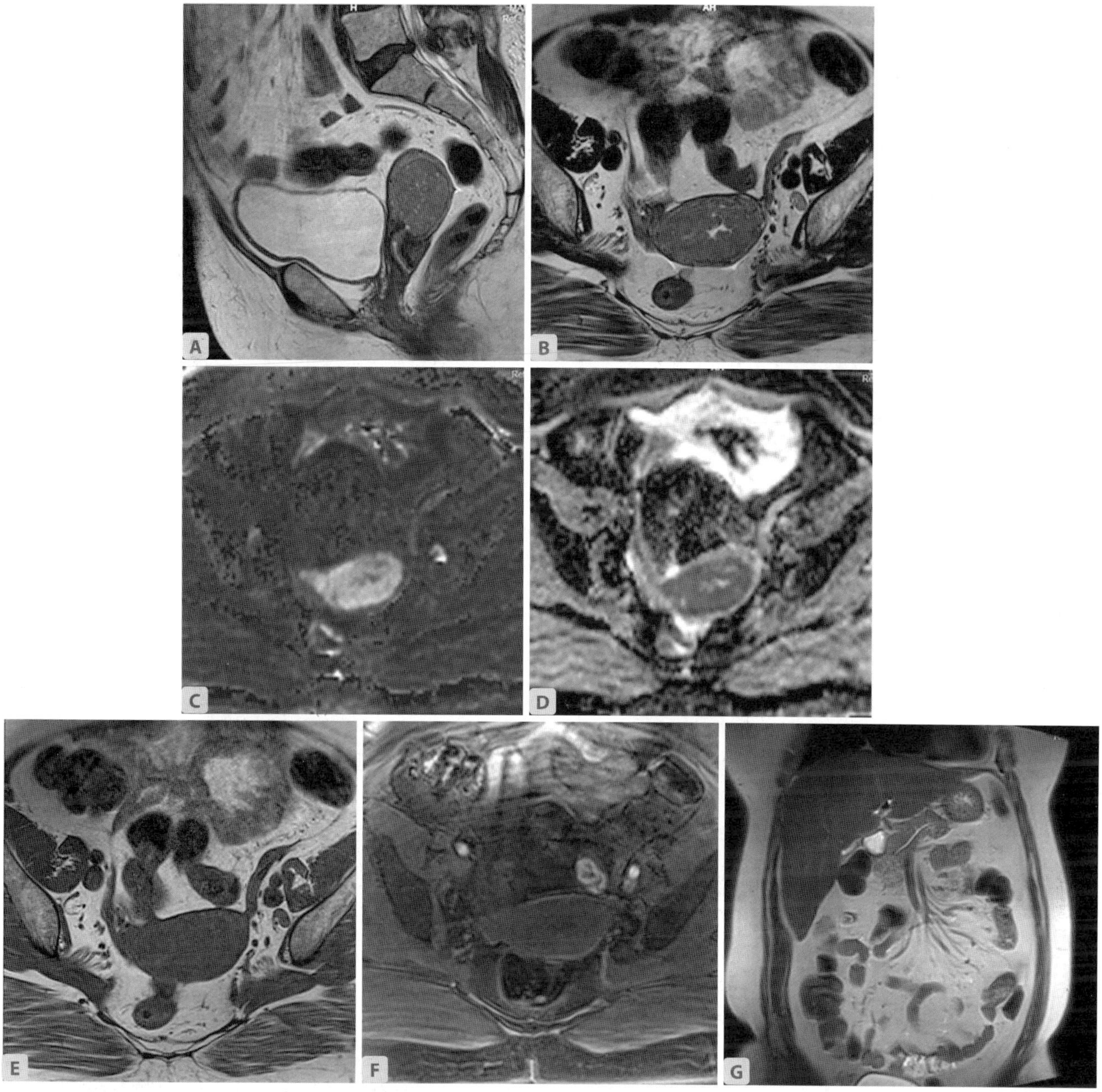

FIGS. 9A TO G: Stage IB endometrial cancer. (A and B) sagittal and axial T2-weighted images show a homogeneous mass of intermediate signal intensity expanding the endometrial cavity with thinned out myometrium. (C and D) the mass shows diffusion restriction on diffusion-weighted imaging. The mass is isointense on T1W image (E) and hypoenhancing on CE-MRI (F). (G) T2 coronal Haste sequence reveals normal liver with no evidence of any enlarged nodes or deposits (Haste: half-fourier acquisition single-shot turbo spin-echo).

It is important to differentiate stage IA from stage IB disease because stage IB is associated with high risk of LVSI which has a direct bearing with the risk of lymph node metastasis and relapse.

Accurate evaluation of depth of myometrial invasion is possible on axial oblique images on MR imaging. An objective method of assessment has been described. First a line is drawn parallel to the presumed inner edge of the myometrium. Then two perpendicular lines are drawn, one measuring the thickness of the entire myometrium and the other line measuring the maximum tumor extent within the myometrium. The ratio of the two lines described above represents the depth of myometrial invasion **(Fig. 10)**.

Stage II: Stage II endometrial cancer is characterized by the tumor invading the cervical stroma. Stromal invasion is best depicted on delayed DCE-MR images by the low signal intensity of the cervical stroma being replaced by the intermediate signal intensity tumor **(Figs. 11A to F)**.

Stage III: Stage IIIA tumors invade the serosa and/or adnexa and appear as disruption of the hypointense serosa, irregular uterine contour with or without enhancing adnexal masses.

In stage IIIB disease, the tumor extends into the upper vagina with disruption of the hypointense vaginal wall signal. Stage IIIC tumors are characterized by lymph node metastasis with involvement of pelvic nodes (IIIC1) and/or para-aortic nodes (IIIC2). This reflects the different prognosis associated with lymph node metastasis.

Risk factors for nodal metastasis consist of type 2 tumors, grade 3 tumors, lymphovascular spread invasion, and deep myometrial invasion. Lymph nodal distribution is influenced by the tumor location. The upper part of uterus drains to the common iliac and para-aortic lymph nodes while the middle and lower parts of the uterus drains to the parametrial and the paracervical and obturator nodes. Inguinal nodes are not in the regional lymphatic drainage pathway for endometrial cancer, and if present, represent stage IV disease. There is rarely direct drainage to para-aortic lymph nodes.[3]

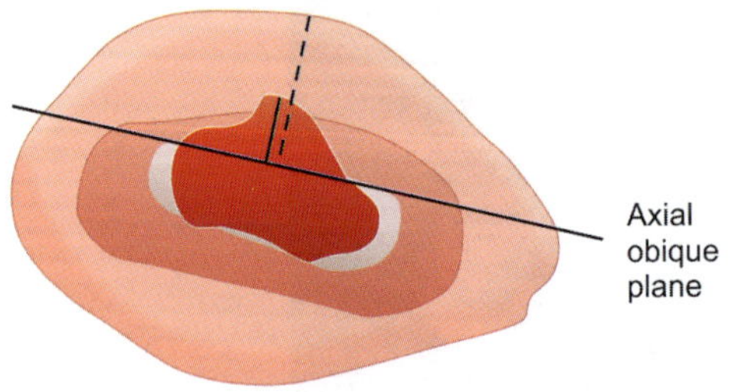

FIG. 10: Schematic diagram to show depth of myometrial invasion in axial oblique plane of uterus. A line is drawn parallel to the inner edge of the myometrium. Two perpendicular lines are drawn, one measuring the thickness of the entire myometrium and the other line measuring the maximum tumor extent within the myometrium. The ratio of the two lines described above represents the depth of myometrial invasion.

The sensitivity of CT/MRI for lymph node metastasis is low because of size cut-off. Recent studies have described an increased sensitivity of CEMRI (82–93%) compared to size (29%) using ultra small paramagnetic iron oxide (USPIO) particles which is a lymph node specific MR contrast.[6]

Magnetic resonance imaging features which are suspicious for lymph involvement are node with a short axis diameter ≥10 mm or ≥8 mm but round configuration, multiple nodes, nodes with an irregular contour, necrosis, and an abnormal signal intensity similar to the primary tumor.

Diffusion-weighted imaging can be utilized for preoperative lymph node mapping as lymph nodes can be easily detected on DWI. However as per literature, none of the studies have been able to differentiate benign from malignant lymph nodes due to an overlap in ADC values.[6]

Stage IV: In stage IVA disease, the tumor invades bladder or bowel mucosa which is seen as tumor extending directly into

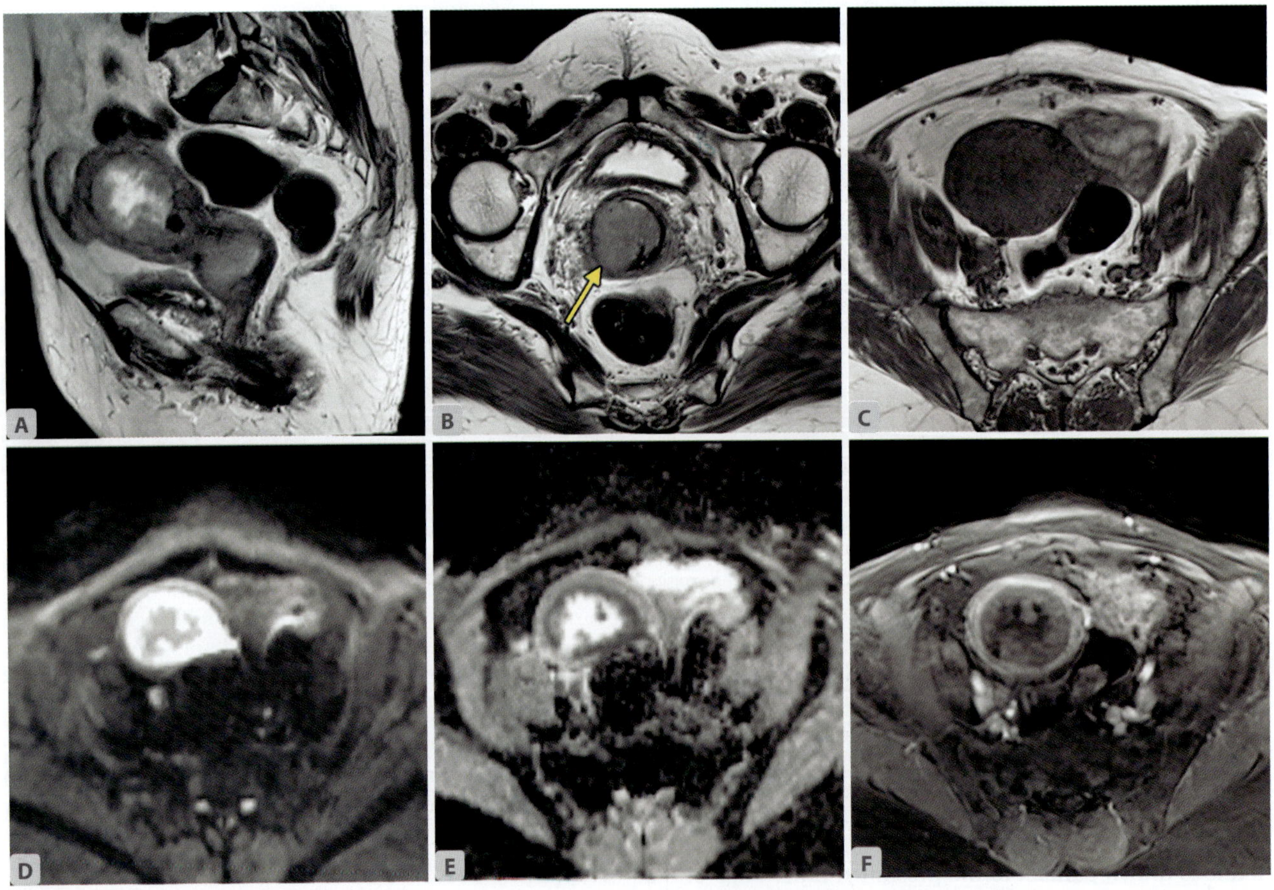

FIGS. 11A TO F: MRI pelvis in a 60-year-old woman with postmenopausal bleeding reveals a heterogeneously hyperintense mass with central necrosis expanding the endometrial cavity (A) with cervical stromal invasion (arrow in B) on T2-weighted sagittal and axial images. (C) The mass appears isointense on axial T1W image. Diffusion-weighted imaging and apparent diffusion coefficient map at the same level show diffusion restriction in the mass (D and E) and appears hypoenhancing as compared to the myometrium on contrast-enhanced-MRI (F): Stage II endometrial cancer.

the hyperintense vesical or rectal mucosa. Bullous edema (i.e. thickening of the high signal intensity mucosal layer) does not indicate mucosal invasion. Stage IVB disease is characterized by intra-abdominal metastasis and para-aortic lymph nodes above renal vessels and/or inguinal lymph nodes. Malignant ascites and peritoneal deposits are more common in type II endometrial tumors and high-grade type I tumors. Serous papillary and clear cell adenocarcinoma (both type II endometrial cancers) are characterized by omental-like and serosal deposits, a pattern of metastatic spread which is similar to that of ovarian cancer.[6]

FDG–PET

FDG–PET or PET/CT has not shown to be of value in the initial staging of patients of endometrial cancer. However, it may have a role in staging of more aggressive endometrial tumors (higher grade histology, type II endometrial cancer) such as serous papillary carcinoma, clear cell carcinoma for identifying extranodal metastatic disease in the thorax or abdomen.[20] PET-MR has been found to be comparable to PET-CT for detecting local lymph nodes and distant metastasis (i.e. N and M staging). For evaluating local tumor extent, PET-MR is superior while for evaluation of lung parenchyma PET-CT scores over PET-MR.[21]

TABLE 4: Risk stratification in endometrial cancer.

Risk category	Type of endometrial cancer
Low risk	Stage IA, endometrioid, G1 and G2, LVSI (–)
Intermediate risk	Stage IB, endometrioid G1 and G2, LVSI (–)
High intermediate risk	1. Stage IA, endometrioid G3, ± LVSI 2. Stage I A/B, endometrioid G1 and G2, LVSI (+)
High risk	1. Stage IB, endometrioid G3, ± LVSI 2. Stage II 3. Stage III, no residual disease 4. Non-endometrioid (serous, clear cell, undifferentiated carcinoma)

G: Grade of differentiation at histology

Stage: As per the revised 2009 FIGO staging of endometrial cancer

LVSI: Lymphovascular space invasion

Source: Nougaret S, Lakhman Y, Vargas HA, et al. From staging to prognostication: achievements and challenges of MR imaging in the assessment of endometrial cancer. Magn Reson Imaging Clin N Am. 2017;25:611-33.

Management of Endometrial Cancer

Stage I Endometrial Cancer

Endometrial cancer is primarily treated by surgery. The standard surgical procedure is total hysterectomy (TH) with bilateral salpingo-oophorectomy (BSO) along with cytology of peritoneal washings.

The addition of systemic lymphadenectomy to the surgical procedure in all patients is regarded as controversial as it leads to increased anesthesia and operative time with risk of development of lymphocele (7–10%) and lymphedema of the lower extremity (23%). From the various clinical trials and studies, it has been shown that only high-risk patients are likely to benefit from such an aggressive surgery. The National Comprehensive Cancer Network (NCCN) guidelines recommend sentinel lymph node mapping for the surgical staging of endometrial cancer which is confined to the uterus with no metastasis seen on imaging or no evidence of extrauterine disease at surgical exploration.[6]

Stage I endometrial cancers are stratified into four risk categories—low risk, intermediate risk, high intermediate risk, and high risk based on histology (grade and type) and depth of myometrial invasion as described in **Table 4**.[6]

As per the European Society for Medical Oncology (ESMO) Practice Guidelines, systemic/para-aortic lymphadenectomy is recommended for the intermediate- and high-risk categories. Hence, preoperative information about depth of myometrial invasion on MR imaging and histologic grade by endometrial sampling are essential to tailor the surgical approach in these patients.

Stage II Endometrial Cancer

The treatment of stage II endometrial cancer is hysterectomy, bilateral salpingo-oophorectomy, and lymphadenectomy.

Stage III and IV Endometrial Cancer

For stage III and IV cancers, extensive debulking is advocated with external radiotherapy with or without tumor directed brachytherapy.

The management of serous papillary and clear cell endometrial cancer is on the same lines as ovarian cancer with omentectomy and peritoneal biopsies in addition to TH, BSO, and lymphadenectomy.[1]

Recurrent Endometrial Cancer

Endometrial cancer is known to recur in two-thirds of patients within 2 years of surgery. The most common sites of recurrent endometrial cancer are lymph nodes, vaginal vault, peritoneum, and lungs. Patients with isolated vaginal recurrence are considered to have a better prognosis than pelvic or abdominal metastasis.[20]

Pelvic and para-aortic lymph nodes are the most common lymph nodes to be involved. Peritoneal involvement reported in 28% may be in the form of large masses, nodules or serosal implants.[20]

Patients with risk factors such as advanced age, higher grade of tumor at primary surgery, multiple sites of disease, and rapid presentation of relapse are known to have a less favorable outcome in recurrent disease. Compared to other gynecologic malignancies, endometrial cancer has the highest frequency of lung secondaries in up to 20–25%.[22]

Role of MRI in Fertility Preservation in Endometrial Cancer Patients

Around 5% of women who are diagnosed with endometrial cancer are below 40 years of age. If they wish to preserve their fertility, then MR imaging is found to be very useful by confirming that the disease is confined to the endometrium. **Box 2** shows the eligibility criteria for fertility preservation.[23]

In 2017, the European Society of Urogenital Radiology (ESUR) updated the 2009 ESUR endometrial cancer guidelines to recommend an MR imaging protocol for endometrial cancer. As per the recommendations, MR imaging should be tailored according to the tumor histology and grade, patients' desire for fertility preservation and the availability of a radiologist to monitor the MR investigation. The ESUR recommendations for MR imaging of endometrial cancer are given in the **Table 5.**[23]

UTERINE SARCOMA

Uterine sarcomas are rare, aggressive, and heterogeneous group of uterine tumors that arise from the mesenchymal or stromal elements.

They account for around 8% of uterine malignancies and have been seen to have a higher incidence than the earlier reported incidence of 2–3%, due to the longevity of the population and advancements in diagnostic techniques.[24]

Uterine sarcomas are the most malignant group of uterine tumors and differ from endometrial cancer with respect to their clinical behavior and spread. They are associated with a poorer prognosis even when detected early.

BOX 2: Eligibility criteria for fertility preservation in patients with endometrial cancer.

All criteria to be met

Histopathology:
- Histologic diagnosis with dilatation and curettage
- Grade I (well differentiated) endometrioid adenocarcinoma

Or
- Premalignant conditions such as atypical hyperplasia or endometrial intraepithelial neoplasia

MRI:

Tumor confined to the endometrium (absence of myometrial invasion, cervical stromal invasion, ovarian metastases or synchronous primary ovarian cancer, and absence of lymphadenopathy)

Clinical:

Patient compliance for close follow-up during and after conservative treatment

They comprise of malignancies which may arise from myometrial smooth muscle such as leiomyosarcoma, those arising from the endometrial stroma are endometrial stromal sarcoma (ESS) and undifferentiated endometrial sarcoma (UES) or arise from both (adenosarcoma). Carcinosarcoma (previously known as malignant mixed müllerian tumor) was earlier categorized as uterine sarcoma but is now regarded as a variant of endometrial carcinoma. This change led the FIGO to develop independent staging criteria for uterine sarcomas in 2010 which has separate staging system for leiomyosarcoma **(Table 6)** and another for endometrial stromal sarcoma and adenosarcoma **(Table 7)**. Carcinosarcomas are included in the same FIGO staging system as endometrial cancer.[25]

Clinical Presentation

The clinical presentation of uterine sarcomas is nonspecific. Patients may present with a rapidly growing pelvic mass with abdominal or pelvic pain, along with vaginal bleeding.

The various subgroups of uterine sarcoma cannot be distinguished clinically, from each other or from other uterine tumors. As uterine sarcomas arise from uterine muscle or mesenchymal tissue, they are not amenable to endometrial sampling and are difficult to diagnose preoperatively. Hence, cross-sectional imaging studies have a major role in the assessment of these tumors and in their staging.

Mixed Epithelial and Mesenchymal Tumors

Carcinosarcoma

Carcinosarcomas, also known previously as malignant mixed müllerian tumor (MMMT), constitute around 50% of all uterine sarcomas. They were originally classified as part of uterine sarcomas, but are now believed to be high grade endometrial cancers with sarcomatous/stromal differentiation due to their biological behavior being similar to high-grade endometrial cancer. Advanced age, obesity, pelvic radiation, and long-term tamoxifen use are some of the risk factors for developing uterine carcinosarcoma.[25]

Patients of carcinosarcoma are mostly postmenopausal, presenting with vaginal bleeding and bulky polypoidal mass in the endometrial cavity that prolapse through the cervical os. Elevated CA125 levels may predict myometrial invasion

TABLE 5: ESUR recommendations for MR imaging of endometrial cancer.

Type and grade of endometrial cancer (EC)/patient population	Role of MRI	MRI protocol recommendation
1. Grade 3 EC and nonendometrioid EC (carcinosarcoma, serous carcinoma, clear cell carcinoma)	To detect extrauterine disease	• DWI of whole abdomen and pelvis to be performed • DCE–MRI—not required CEMR is recommended
2. Grade 1 or 2 endometrioid EC	To evaluate myometrial invasion and cervical stromal invasion	MRI protocol depends on MR acquisition • *Unsupervised MR imaging:* DWI + CEMRI are recommended • *Supervised MR imaging:* DCE–MRI as an adjunct to DWI in challenging cases
3. Patients' of childbearing age with grade I endometrioid EC, who wish to preserve their fertility	To rule out myometrial invasion	• DCE–MRI should be added to T2WI and DWI • An intact subendometrial enhancement rules out myometrial invasion

TABLE 6: FIGO staging of uterine leiomyosarcoma.

Stage		Definition
I		Tumor confined to uterus
	IA	<5 cm
	IB	>5 cm
II		Tumor extends beyond the uterus, within the pelvis
	IIA	Adnexal involvement
	IIB	Involvement of other pelvic tissues
III		Invasion of abdominal tissues (not just protruding into the abdomen)
	IIIA	One site
	IIIB	More than one site
	IIIC	Metastasis to pelvic and/or para-aortic lymph nodes
IV	IVA	Tumor invades bladder and/or rectum
	IVB	Distant metastasis

Source: Sala E, Rockall AG, Freeman SJ, et al. The added role of MR imaging in treatment stratification of patients with gynecologic malignancies: what the radiologist needs to know. Radiology. 2013;266(3):717-40.

TABLE 7: FIGO staging of uterine endometrial stromal sarcoma and adenosarcoma.

Stage		Definition
I		*Tumor limited to uterus:*
	IA	Tumor limited to endometrium/endocervix with no myometrial invasion
	IB	<50% myometrial invasion
	IC	>50% myometrial invasion
II		*Tumor extends beyond the uterus, within the pelvis:*
	IIA	Adnexal involvement
	IIB	Involvement of other pelvic tissues
III		*Tumor invades abdominal tissues (not just protruding into the abdomen):*
	IIIA	One site
	IIIB	More than one site
	IIIC	Metastasis to pelvic and/or para-aortic lymph nodes
IV	IVA	Tumor invades bladder and/or rectum
	IVB	Distant metastasis

Source: Sala E, Rockall AG, Freeman SJ, et al. The added role of MR imaging in treatment stratification of patients with gynecologic malignancies: what the radiologist needs to know? Radiology. 2013;266(3):717-40.

or extrauterine spread and also aid in monitoring for tumor recurrence.[26]

Carcinosarcomas are aggressive tumors with nearly 60% of patients presenting with metastatic disease. As compared to other sarcomas that spread hematogenously, they show lymphatic dissemination. Lungs, peritoneum, pelvic, and para-aortic lymph nodes are the most common sites of metastases **(Fig. 12)**.[27]

On imaging, carcinosarcomas most commonly present as endometrial masses that expand the endometrial cavity and are difficult to differentiate from endometrial cancer. Certain imaging features which may help in differentiating that two are:[4]

- Carcinosarcomas are larger masses that distend endometrial cavity **(Figs. 13A to E)**. An anteroposterior tumor ratio >0.63 has been described to differentiate carcinosarcoma from endometrial cancer.[27]
- Carcinosarcomas are more heterogeneous tumors with areas of intratumoral hemorrhage and necrosis that have intermediate to high signal on T2-weighted images.
- They show significant contrast enhancement compared to endometrial cancer which are hypovascular.
- Carcinosarcomas have a poorer prognosis as they more often show deep myometrial invasion, cervical stromal invasion, and metastatic nodal disease at presentation.

Imaging feature which aids in differentiation from leiomyosarcoma is a lower incidence of hemorrhage and necrosis in carcinosarcoma.[26]

Five-year survival of carcinosarcoma is <5%. Surgery is the mainstay of treatment consisting of total hysterectomy with bilateral salpingo-oophorectomy and lymphadenectomy. Radiotherapy has shown to decrease local recurrence and chemotherapy is advocated for recurrent or metastatic disease.

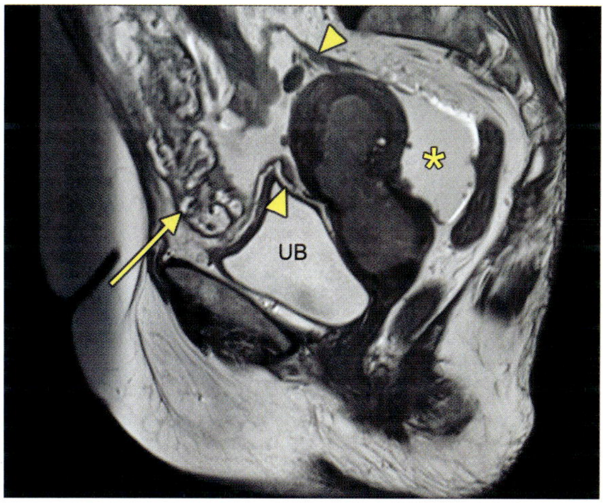

FIG. 12: T2W sagittal MRI image of pelvis shows soft tissue mass in the endometrial cavity extending into the endocervical canal. There is stranding and thickening of mesentery and omental caking (arrow). Nodular thickening also seen along peritoneal reflection (arrowheads) along with gross ascites(*): Serous papillary endometrial cancer on HPE.

Smooth Muscle Tumors

Leiomyosarcoma

Leiomyosarcoma comprises around 40% of uterine sarcoma and occur in women more than 40 years of age. Most arise de novo from uterine musculature or connective tissue of uterine blood vessels but very rarely can occur due to sarcomatous transformation of leiomyoma. They may mimic leiomyomas clinically, with a history of abnormal vaginal bleeding, pelvic mass and/or pelvic pain. Pathologically, leiomyosarcomas

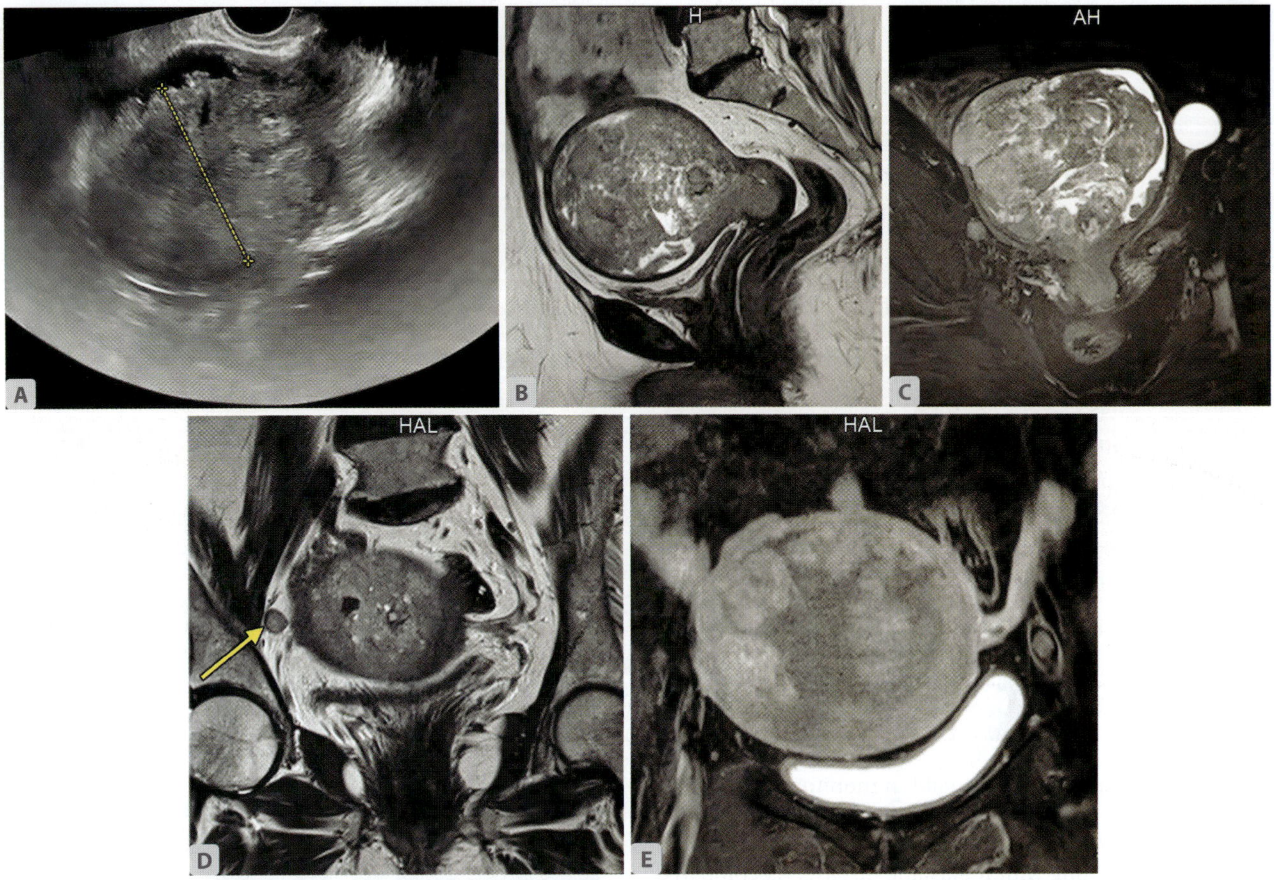

FIGS. 13A TO E: Transvaginal sonography of the uterus (A) reveals a large heterogeneous mass expanding the endometrial cavity. On T2 weighted sagittal (B) and coronal (C and D) images, the heterogeneous mass with few areas of necrosis are well visualized. A rounded lesion is seen adjacent to the uterus suggestive of nodal metastasis (arrow in D). On post-contrast MR image (E), the mass shows heterogeneous enhancement with loss of planes with the myometrium in the right lateral aspect: Carcinosarcoma on histopathology.

are large, irregular masses with hemorrhage, necrosis, extrauterine extension, and nuclear atypia.

Ultrasound may show a large heterogeneous mass with irregular margins, mixed hypo- and hyperechoic areas with distortion of endometrial cavity. Both leiomyosarcomas and degenerated/cellular leiomyoma can present as nonspecific heterogeneous solitary masses with high vascularity.[28]

On MRI, leiomyomas usually present as well-defined lesions with low-signal intensity on T1- and T2-weighted images, while sarcomas are ill-defined with irregular margins and show intermediate-to-high signal intensity on T2-weighted images. Leiomyosarcomas show presence of extensive necrosis (>50%) with hemorrhage also being common. They show heterogeneous contrast enhancement **(Figs. 14A to G)**. Features suggestive of malignancy are a large mass with rapid growth, irregular margins, and necrosis.[24]

It is important to distinguish leiomyosarcoma from leiomyoma because of difference in treatment. Leiomyomas are treated more conservatively by myomectomy, uterine artery embolization or high-intensity focused ultrasound (HIFU) while sarcomas require surgical treatment.

Diffusion-weighted imaging and ADC maps have been used for differentiating the two, with a mean ADC value of uterine sarcoma being significantly lower than that of leiomyoma (0.83×10^{-3} mm^2/sec vs 1.37×10^{-3} mm^2/sec).[28]

In patients with suspicion of uterine sarcoma on MRI, a PET-CT has been found to be effective. A SUV max >7.5 has shown to exclude leiomyoma with 100% specificity.[29] However, an overlap may occur.

Stromal Tumors

They are classified as endometrial stromal nodule (noninvasive which is benign), endometrial stromal sarcoma (low-grade), and undifferentiated endometrial stromal sarcoma (high-grade).

Endometrial Stromal Sarcoma

They account for 10–15% of all uterine myometrial tumors and affect patients in the 40–55 years age group. Their cells resemble the stromal elements of proliferative endometrium and are characterized by low cellular atypia and a low mitotic rate.[26]

Patients may be asymptomatic or present with abnormal uterine bleeding. There has been reported association of endometrial stromal sarcoma (ESS) with polycystic ovaries, estrogen use, and tamoxifen therapy.

On imaging, ESS appears as a polypoidal endometrial mass which typically shows myometrial involvement, which may be well-defined or diffuse. On MRI, they appear as low

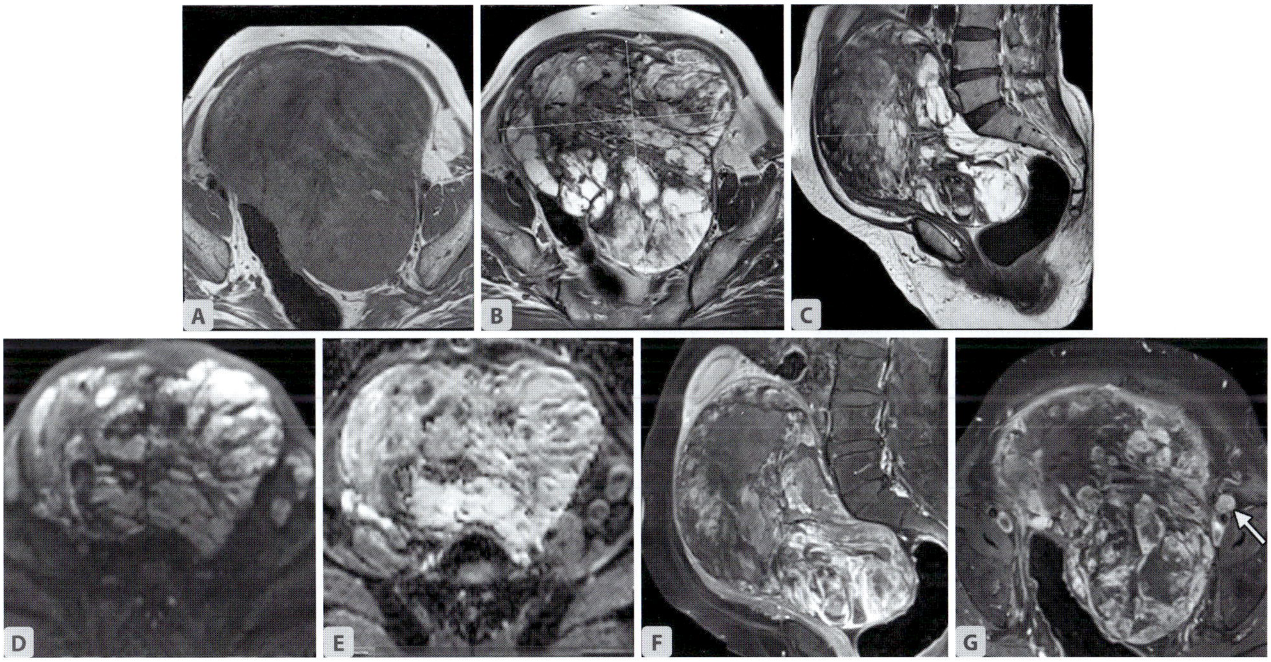

FIGS. 14A TO G: MRI of the lower abdomen and pelvis reveals (A) a large well-defined smoothly margined predominantly solid abdominopelvic mass which measures 14 × 12 × 14 cm arising from posterior myometrium. It appears hypointense on T1WI (A) and heterogeneous on T2WI (B and C) with a well-defined T2 hypointense capsule. Few foci of restricted diffusion are seen with the mass (D and E) with heterogeneous enhancement on postcontrast scans (F and G). Uterus is stretched along the anterosuperior aspect of the mass with mild fluid in endometrial cavity. The mass is compressing the cervix, vagina, and urinary bladder anteriorly and abutting the lumbar vertebrae posteriorly and rectum posteroinferiorly. An internal iliac lymph node is enlarged (arrow in G): Uterine leiomyosarcoma.

signal on T1-weighted images and have heterogeneously increased T2 signal.

These tumors have a tendency for lymphatic and vascular invasion and show mild heterogeneous contrast enhancement. When myometrial invasion is present, worm-like bands of low T2 signal intensity may be seen in the high signal tumor representing preserved normal myometrium. This "bag of worms" appearance is more common in higher grade tumors and is best seen on DWI.[30]

As compared to endometrial cancer, ESS appears larger, with greater enhancement, irregular margins, and marginal nodularity with nodular extension into myometrium. They may rarely present as a myometrial mass and mimic a leiomyoma with cystic degeneration or invasive adenomyosis.

These tumors have a favorable prognosis with metastasis and recurrence occurring late. Five-year survival is around 50–65%. Nodal metastasis is uncommon and does not affect survival. Treatment is by hysterectomy with bilateral salpingo-oophorectomy. Adjuvant hormonal therapy in patients with advanced disease and chemotherapy has also been used.

Undifferentiated Endometrial Sarcoma

They are aggressive tumors, earlier called high-grade ESS. Undifferentiated endometrial sarcomas (UES) occur in an older age group as compared to ESS and are characterized by myometrial invasion, severe nuclear polymorphism, and high mitotic activity.

On imaging, UES appear as a large polypoidal mass in an expanded endometrial cavity. They infiltrate the myometrium in a more destructive manner and are associated with areas of necrosis and hemorrhage resulting in heterogeneous signal intensity on both T1- and T2-weighted images. Due to marked lymphatic and vascular invasion, UES show extensive invasion into the myometrium with marginal irregularity and nodularity, much more frequently than seen in ESS.[30]

Adenosarcoma

Adenosarcomas are rare mixed tumors consisting of a benign epithelial component and a malignant sarcomatous stromal component. They are slow growing with a low malignant potential. Most patients present early (stage 1) with a five-year survival of approximately 80%.

At imaging, adenosarcoma are seen as predominantly endometrial based well-circumscribed, multiseptated, cystic masses with multiple well-defined cystic spaces or clefts, hemorrhage, necrosis, and heterogeneous solid component. The intervening septae give a lattice-like appearance on MRI.[30] This appearance on imaging may resemble that seen in gestational trophoblastic disease.

There is heterogeneous enhancement with septae and solid component showing enhancement similar to myometrium.

Adenosarcoma with sarcomatous overgrowth (ASSO) is said to occur when the sarcomatous component constitutes more than 25% of the tumor. On imaging, there is myometrial invasion with areas of hemorrhage and necrosis. Adenosarcomas with sarcomatous overgrowth have a poorer prognosis than adenosarcoma without sarcomatous overgrowth.[30]

CERVICAL CANCER

Cervical cancer is the second most common cancer in women in India after breast cancer and the fourth most common cancer in women in the world as per the latest data from Global Cancer Statistics 2018. Around 85% of the cases occur in developing countries such as Central and South America, parts of Africa and South Central Asia.[31] There has been a significant decrease in its incidence in developed countries due to effective screening programs which detect preinvasive disease on cervical smear.

Clinical Presentation

Cervical cancer affects women of reproductive age group, mainly in the 3rd and 4th decades. Noninvasive cancer may not produce any symptoms and may be detected by the Pap smear. Invasive cervical cancer patients typically present with a history of intermenstrual, postcoital bleeding, metrorrhagia, and/or foul swelling vaginal discharge.[32]

Etiopathogenesis

The main etiologic factor for developing cervical cancer is infection of the lower genital tract by the human papillomavirus (HPV) which is sexually transmitted. HPV 16 and 18 account for 70% of cervical cancer worldwide with HPV 16 associated with squamous cell carcinoma. HPV vaccination of adolescents has been approved to prevent persistent infection with HPV, and is recommended by major health organizations around the world with the goal of reducing the incidence of HPV related cervical cancer.[32,33] Other risk factors include low socioeconomic background, early sexual activity, multiple partners, multiparity, immunosuppression, cigarette smoking, and use of oral contraceptive pills.[1]

Histopathology

Squamous cell carcinoma (SCC) accounts for around 85% of cervical cancer and arises from the ectocervix at the squamocolumnar junction. The remaining 15% cervical cancer is of nonsquamous type which arises from the endocervix and includes adenocarcinoma, adenosquamous carcinoma, adenocystic carcinoma, small cell carcinoma, and lymphoma.

Adenoma malignum is a very rare type of cervical adenocarcinoma which has a very poor prognosis though histologically it is well differentiated.[33]

Squamous cell carcinoma of cervix spreads most commonly by direct extension to lower uterine segment and vagina. With advanced disease, the tumor invades paracervical space along the uterosacral and broad ligaments to invade adjacent organs. Lymphatic dissemination to the draining lymph nodes is the next common pattern of spread. Hematogenous spread is rare which can occur to lung, liver, and bone.

Detection and Diagnosis

Early cervical cancer is diagnosed clinically based on results of Pap smear and colposcopic-guided biopsies. Imaging alone is not adequate for the diagnosis of cervical cancer as it cannot differentiate between invasive cancer or its precursor, i.e. intraepithelial neoplasia. Hence, biopsy of suspicious lesions on colposcopy is the gold standard for diagnosis.[34]

Staging

Traditionally, the staging of cervical cancer has been clinical according to the FIGO staging system (2009) and was mainly based on tumor diameter and local extent of tumor. Unlike ovarian and endometrial cancers, it was not based on surgicopathological findings. This was because cervical cancer is more prevalent in developing countries with only clinical methods available for staging and evaluation and limited access to advanced technology. However, clinical staging was found to have several limitations. It was found to be inaccurate in evaluating important prognostic parameters such as precise evaluation of tumor size, depth of stromal invasion, and parametrial or pelvic sidewall invasion. Lymph node assessment which is an important prognostic parameter, was also not a part of FIGO (2009) staging and distant metastasis could not be assessed clinically.

Accurate tumor staging is very important not only for prognosis, but also for guiding appropriate management. Treatment of cervical cancer depends on the stage of disease, therefore, accurate staging is of prime importance.

In order to evaluate the local tumor extent and assess distant spread of disease accurately, the 2009 FIGO staging recommended the use of diagnostic imaging (CT/MRI) where available. The staging of cervical cancer has continued to be clinical but clinicians all over the world started relying more on cross sectional imaging modalities (CT/MRI) to guide treatment planning.

In 2018, the FIGO Gynecologic Oncology Committee revised the 2009 FIGO staging of cervical cancer with incorporation of imaging and pathological findings where available to assign the stage so as to maintain uniformity worldwide. The revised FIGO staging of cancer cervix is given in **Box 3**.[35]

The amendments to the staging of cancer of the cervix uteri were made by the FIGO committee for gynecologic oncology in 2018 and the general recommendations are as follows.

- It allows the use of any imaging modality (Ultrasound, CT, MRI, PET, PET-CT, PET-MRI, etc.) and pathological findings for the measurement of size of the lesion in all stages and its extent.
- Lymph nodal involvement, previously not a part of FIGO staging has been incorporated into the 2018 staging of cervical cancer. The presence of pelvic or para-aortic lymph nodes on imaging or pathological finding upstages it to stage IIIC, regardless of other findings. A notation of "*r*" or "*p*" is to be given depending on whether the staging was assigned on the basis of imaging or pathology.
- There are no recommendations for routine investigations. They are to be decided on the basis of clinical findings and standard of care.

BOX 3: FIGO staging of cancer of the cervix uteri (2018).

Stage I:

The carcinoma is limited to the cervix (extension to the uterine body should be ignored)

- *IA:* Invasive carcinoma which can be diagnosed only by microscopy, with maximum depth of invasion <5 mm[a]
  - *IA1:* Measured stromal invasion <3 mm in depth
  - *IA2:* Measured stromal invasion ≥3 mm and <5 mm in depth
- *IB:* Invasive carcinoma with measured deepest invasion ≥5 mm (greater than stage IA), lesion limited to the cervix uteri[b]
  - *IB1:* Invasive carcinoma ≥5 mm depth of stromal invasion and <2 cm in greatest dimension
  - *IB2:* Invasive carcinoma ≥2 cm and <4 cm in greatest dimension
  - *IB3:* Invasive carcinoma ≥4 cm in greatest dimension

Stage II:

The carcinoma invades beyond the uterus, but has not extended onto the lower third of the vagina or to the pelvic wall

- *IIA:* Involvement limited to the upper two-thirds of the vagina without parametrial involvement
  - *IIA1:* Invasive carcinoma <4 cm in greatest dimension
  - *IIA2:* Invasive carcinoma ≥4 cm in greatest dimension
- *IIB:* Parametrial involvement but not up to the pelvic wall

Stage III:

The carcinoma involves the lower third of the vagina and/or extends to the pelvic wall and/or causes hydronephrosis or nonfunctioning kidney and/or involves pelvic and/or para-aortic lymph nodes[c]

- *IIIA:* Carcinoma involves the lower third of the vagina, with no extension to the pelvic wall
- *IIIB:* Extension to the pelvic wall and/or hydronephrosis or nonfunctioning kidney (unless known to be due to another cause)
- *IIIC:* Involvement of pelvic and/or para-aortic lymph nodes, irrespective of tumor size and extent (with r and p notations)[c]
  - *IIIC1:* Pelvic lymph node metastasis only
  - *IIIC2:* Para-aortic lymph node metastasis

Stage IV:

The carcinoma has extended beyond the true pelvis or has involved (biopsy proven) the mucosa of the bladder or rectum

- *IVA:* Spread of the growth to adjacent organs
- *IVB:* Spread to distant organs

[a]Imaging and pathology can be used, when available, to supplement clinical findings with respect to tumor size and extent, in all stages.

[b]The involvement of vascular/lymphatic spaces does not change the staging. The lateral extent of the lesion is no longer considered.

[c]Adding notation of r (imaging) and p (pathology) to indicate the findings that are used to allocate the case to stage IIIC. For example, if imaging indicates pelvic lymph node metastasis, the stage allocation would be stage IIIC1r and, if confirmed by pathological findings, it would be Stage IIIc1p. The type of imaging modality or pathology technique used should always be documented. When in doubt, the lower staging should be assigned.

Source: Bhatla N, Berek JS, Fredes MC, et al. Revised FIGO staging for carcinoma of the cervix uteri. Int J Gynecol Obstet. 2019;143(Suppl 3): 43-991.

Imaging

Imaging is not useful for establishing diagnosis, but for staging.

Ultrasound

Ultrasound is not routinely used in assessing the primary tumor or local extent of disease. Advanced cervical cancer can be visualized on transabdominal sonography and appears as an enlarged, irregular hypoechoic mass with resultant hydrometra or hematometra if tumor obstructs the cervical canal.[36] Small masses may be visualized only on TVS **(Figs. 15A to D)**. Ultrasound can show hydronephrosis secondary to the involvement of vesicoureteric junction by the growth. However, its main limitation is that it is unable to detect the invasion of pelvic side walls and metastatic lymph nodes.

Recent studies have reported TVS and TRUS (transrectal ultrasound) as a potentially useful tool for tumor detection and parametrial invasion, comparable to MRI.[37] TRUS has shown to detect bladder invasion based on the intact mobility of bladder over cervix with accuracy greater than that of CT or MRI.[1]

Magnetic Resonance Imaging

MRI is the preferred imaging modality for staging cervical cancer as it can distinguish between early disease that can be surgically treated, from advanced disease that is treated with chemoradiotherapy. MRI accurately depicts the location (exophytic or endocervical) of tumor, the tumor size, depth of stromal invasion, parametrial and pelvic sidewall invasion, bladder or rectal involvement and lymph node metastasis, which are important prognostic parameters that determine whether treatment would be palliative or curative. The role of MR imaging in cervical cancer is well established and given in **Box 4**.

MRI Technique

The tumor extent is best assessed on T2-weighted imaging. The sagittal plane depicts the tumor extension into the body of uterus and vagina very well. The axial-oblique T2-weighted FSE (fast spin echo) sequence obtained perpendicular to the long axis of the cervix is valuable in assessing parametrial invasion.[16] DCE-MRI is not routinely recommended as part of protocol for cervical cancer. However, in the guidelines

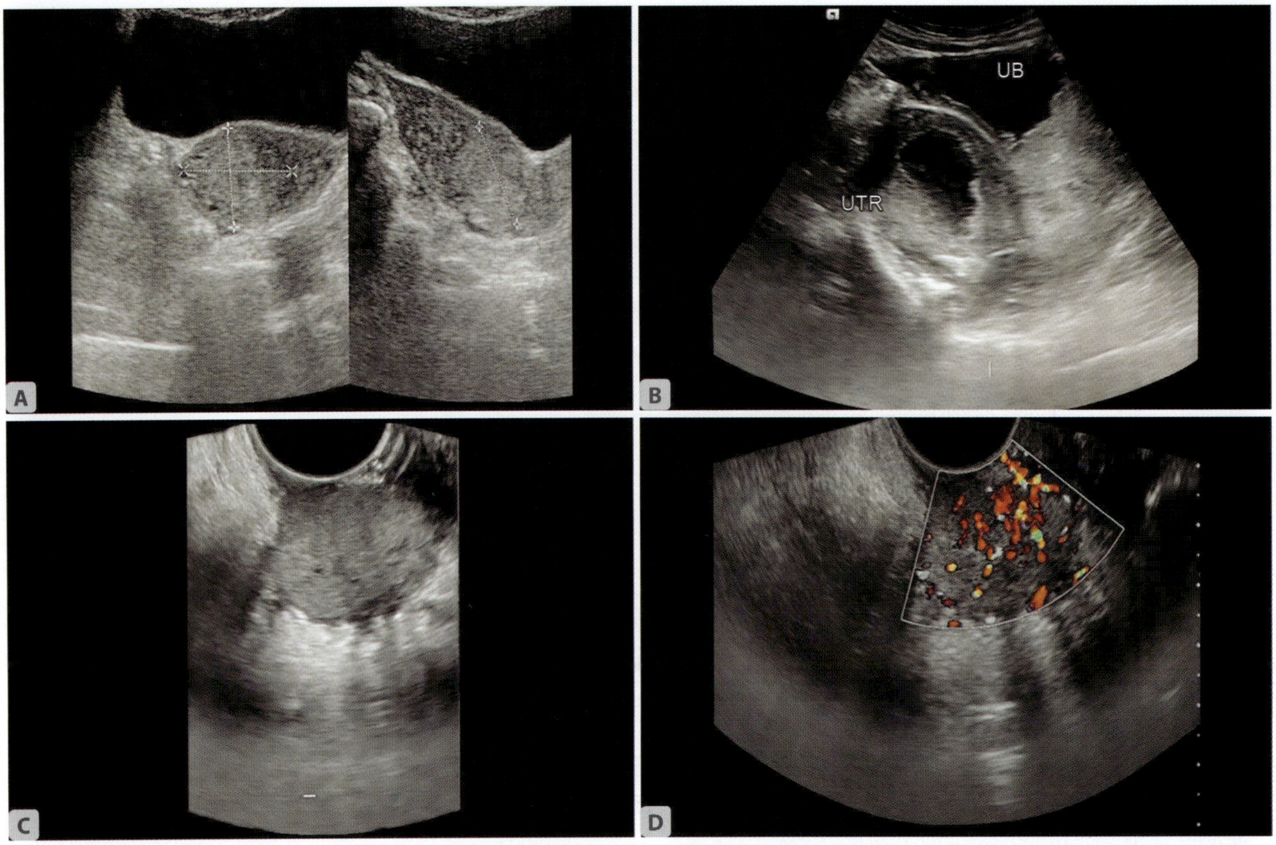

FIGS. 15A TO D: Transabdominal sonography of the pelvis reveals (A) a solid mass of 3.8 × 4.3 × 4 cm in the cervix extending into the lower uterine segment; (B) Sagittal view of the uterus depicting pyometra secondary to a cervical mass obstructing the internal os. TVS in another patient shows (C) the cervix to be replaced by a large, irregular hypoechoic mass which is (D) highly vascular on color doppler flow imaging.

given by the ESUR, contrast administration is indicated for the detection of small tumors, when findings are equivocal on T2-weighted imaging and to differentiate tumor recurrence from post-radiotherapy fibrosis. DWI is useful as it improves tumor detection and characterization and aids in visualization of small peritoneal implants. ADC values are known to precede reduction of tumor size following treatment with neoadjuvant chemotherapy.

BOX 4: Role of MR imaging in cervical cancer.

- Localization and staging the tumor
- Assess feasibility of fertility sparing surgery (trachelectomy)
- Treatment planning
- Identify complications of disease and treatment
- Monitor treatment response
- Detect recurrence

MRI Correlation with Revised FIGO (2018) Staging

Localization and Staging of Tumor

The tumor appears isointense to the normal cervix on T1-weighted images and intermediate-to-high signal intensity mass on T2-weighted images that replaces the low signal intensity cervical stroma. The tumor growth pattern may be exophytic, infiltrative or endocervical. In younger women, the tumor usually arises from the squamocolumnar junction and is exophytic, while in older women, it mostly originates from the endocervical canal and is endophytic. For an accurate size determination, the tumor should be measured in two orthogonal views in all three dimensions. Tumor size is often underestimated at clinical imaging compared with MRI, especially of endocervical lesions. The reported accuracy of MRI for determining tumor size is 93%, within 5 mm of the surgical size.[34]

Tumor size determines the type of treatment, with fertility sparing surgery (trachelectomy) possible in tumors <2 cm size, while in patients with tumors >4 cm, chemoradiation in the treatment even in the absence of parametrial spread.

- *Stage I:* Stage I cervical cancers are confined to the cervix and any extension to the body of the uterus is disregarded as it does not change the tumor stage.
    - Stage IA tumors are microinvasive with <5 mm stromal invasion which are diagnosed only by microscopy and not by any imaging modality. MRI is not indicated for their evaluation as these tumors do not show any signal alteration.
    - Stage IB tumors are defined as clinically visible tumors which are limited to the cervix. This stage has been revised and subdivided into IB1–IB3 on the basis of tumor size.

- IB1 is ≥5 mm of invasive and <2 cm in greatest dimension
- IB2 is ≥2.0 cm and <4.0 cm in greatest dimension
- IB3 is ≥4.0 cm in greatest dimension.

The above subdivisions of stage IB have been introduced based on oncologic data from fertility sparing surgery such as conization in stage IA and radical trachelectomy in stage IB.

Assessment of feasibility of fertility sparing surgery (trachelectomy): MRI helps in assessing the cervical length and distance from the internal os in patients planned for fertility sparing surgery. For undergoing trachelectomy (cervix is removed and uterine body is left intact), the tumor should be <2 cm size, length of cervix should be >2 cm and the distance from the internal os should be >1 cm. Involvement of internal os by the tumor is a contraindication to the treatment.[33]

The recurrence rates of patients with primary tumors <2.0 cm have been found to be significantly lower than those with tumors between 2.0 cm and 4.0 cm.[35]

- *Stage II:* Stage II tumors extend beyond the cervix into the upper vagina or parametrium but do not extend to the pelvic side walls or lower one-third of vagina. They are further subdivided into stage IIA and IIB according to whether parametrium is spared (IIA) or there is infiltration of tumor into the parametrium (IIB).

Stage IIA tumors show involvement of upper two-thirds of vagina which on T2-weighted images is seen as a high signal intensity lesion disrupting the low signal intensity vaginal wall **(Figs. 16A and B)**. The maximum tumor diameter has a bearing on the prognosis of patients with stage IIA tumors. Hence, they are subdivided by size into IIAI (<4 cm in greatest dimension) and IIA2 (>4 cm in greatest dimension), both having different treatment strategies.[16,36]

Stage IIB tumors are not further subdivided by size as presence of parametrial invasion itself is indicative of a poor prognosis as it precludes surgical treatment. On MRI, parametrial invasion is seen as the breech of low signal intensity stromal ring on T2-weighted imaging **(Figs. 17A to D)**. An intact stromal ring of >3 mm on MRI known as "hypointense rim sign" has a negative predictive value of >96% for parametrial invasion. Other reliable signs on MRI which suggest parametrial invasion are irregular or spiculated interface between tumor and parametrium, soft tissue extension into parametrium and uterine ligaments, encasement of parauterine vessels, and distortion of cervix with displacement to the side of parametrial invasion.[1]

Overestimation in assessment of parametrial invasion on MRI can occur due to post-biopsy stranding or hemorrhage, peripheral stromal edema in large tumors, and endometriosis or bulky intravaginal tumors. In such cases, DWI and ADC maps may help to determine the true extent of tumor.

- *Stage III:* Stage III disease occurs when there is direct extension of the tumor to the lower third of vagina (IIIA) **(Figs. 18A to E)** and /or pelvic side walls (IIIB) **(Figs. 19A to D)** which is very well-depicted on MRI. Pelvic side wall invasion is diagnosed when the tumor is within 3 mm of the obturator internus, levator ani or piriformis muscle or it encases the iliac vessels. The presence of hydroureteronephrosis due to ureteric encasement by the growth also indicates stage IIIB disease. Hence, MRI should always include a T2-weighted coronal sequence of the upper abdomen for assessment of hydronephrosis.

Stage IIIC disease which consists of lymph nodal involvement is a new subdivision which has been included in the latest revision of FIGO staging of cervical cancer. This is because nodal metastasis is one of the most important prognostic factors in cervical cancer. The five-year survival rates have found to decrease from 85–90% to 30–60% if nodal metastasis is found at surgery.[32]

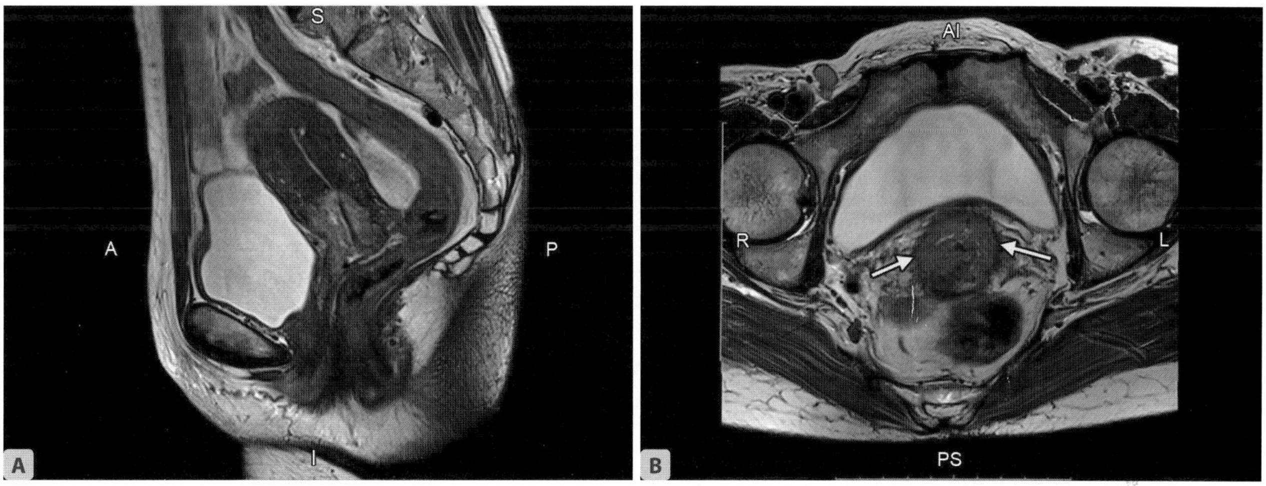

FIGS. 16A AND B: (A) Sagittal and (B) axial T2W images reveal a well-defined hyperintense mass in the cervix extending into the upper vagina and lower uterine segment. On T2W axial image, the hypointense stromal ring is intact (arrows) indicating that parametrium is spared: Stage IIA carcinoma cervix.

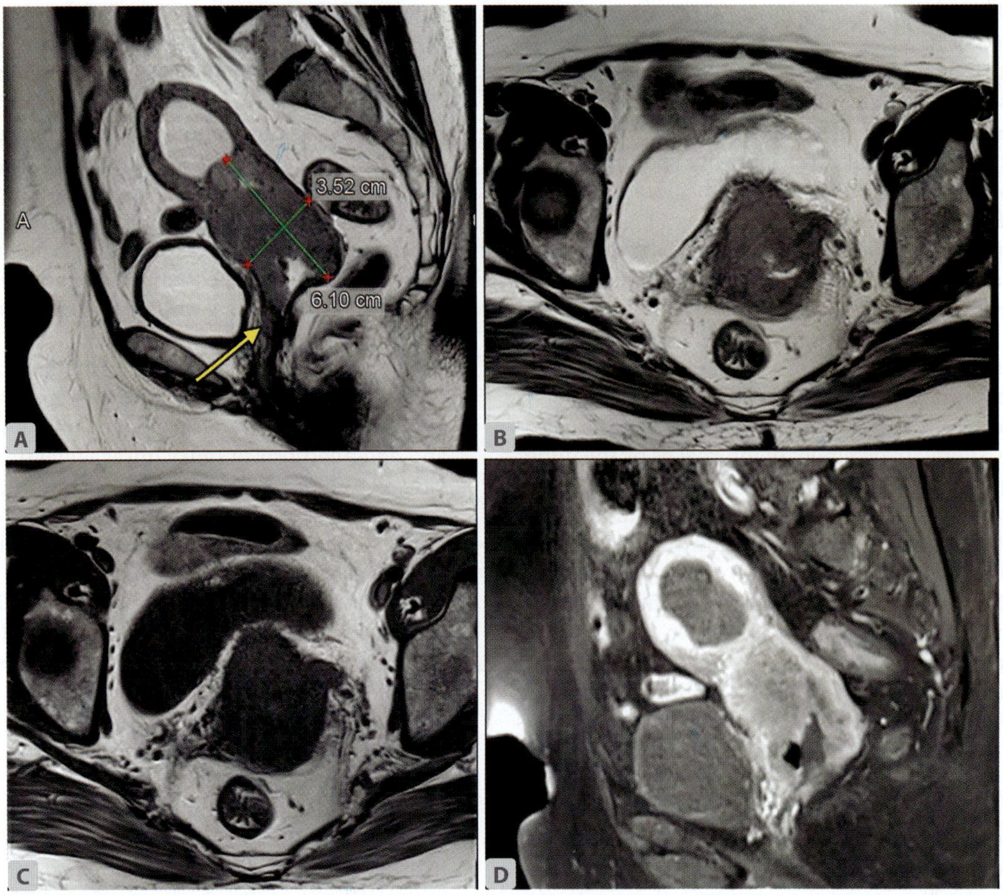

FIGS. 17A TO D: Stage IIB carcinoma cervix. (A) Sagittal and (B) axial T2W images of the pelvis reveal an infiltrating hyperintense lesion measuring 6.1 cm × 3.5 cm in the cervix extending to the upper vagina (arrow) and bilateral parametrium. The lesion appears (C) hypointense on axial T1W image and shows (D) heterogeneous enhancement and enhancing less than myometrium on postcontrast scan.

Also, presence of metastatic pelvic nodes at surgery necessitates adjuvant chemoradiation.[33]

The initial lymphatic drainage from the tumor is to the parametrial nodes. From here the lymphatic drainage proceeds to the external iliac group (laterally), internal iliac nodes (inferiorly), and along sacral nodes (posteriorly). Stage IIIC1 disease represents pelvic lymph node metastasis **(Figs. 20A to F)**. From the pelvis, there is an orderly spread to the common iliac and para-aortic nodes. Stage IIIC2 disease is indicative of para-aortic lymph node metastasis. The lymphatic spread in cervical cancer has a more orderly progression as described above, in contrast to endometrial cancer which can show a more complex lymphatic drainage with involvement of para-aortic lymph nodes without any pelvic nodal enlargement.

Metastatic lymph node involvement on MRI is mainly based on size criteria with a short-axis diameter of 10 mm or more being indicative of abnormal nodes. However, this has some limitation as larger lymph nodes may represent reactive hyperplastic nodes and small nodes may harbor microscopic foci of disease. Other imaging features of abnormal nodes suggestive of metastasis are a round shape, irregular margins, and internal heterogeneity. Malignant nodes may show signal intensity similar to the primary tumor. Central nodal necrosis on CT or MRI has been found to have 100% positive predictive value (PPV) for metastasis in cervical cancer **(Figs. 21A and B)**.[33]

- *Stage IV:* In stage IVA disease, there is tumor invasion into the urinary bladder or rectal mucosa. MRI findings which suggest bladder invasion are disruption of the normal low signal intensity of posterior wall of bladder, nodular or irregular bladder wall or mass protruding into the lumen of the bladder, best seen on T2-weighted imaging **(Figs. 22A and B)**.[38] Bladder invasion is more common than infiltration of the rectal wall due to the relative "bare area" of bladder posteriorly below the level of peritoneal reflection **(Figs. 23A to C)**.[2]

Rectal invasion is usually via the uterosacral ligaments. Direct invasion of the cervical tumor into the rectum is uncommon as the pouch of Douglas separates the posterior fornix from the rectum.[25]

The presence of a fat plane between the cervical tumor and bladder and/or rectum on MRI excludes local invasion into the urinary bladder or rectum with a NPV of 100%.[16,25] Hence, the use of invasive cystoscopic or endoscopic procedures for staging can be eliminated.

Stage IVB disease signifies distant metastasis. It is seen only in a small percentage of patients and involves spread to lungs, liver, bones, and adrenals by hematogenous route.[33] In patients of early cervical cancer, plain chest radiographs are sufficient for evaluation

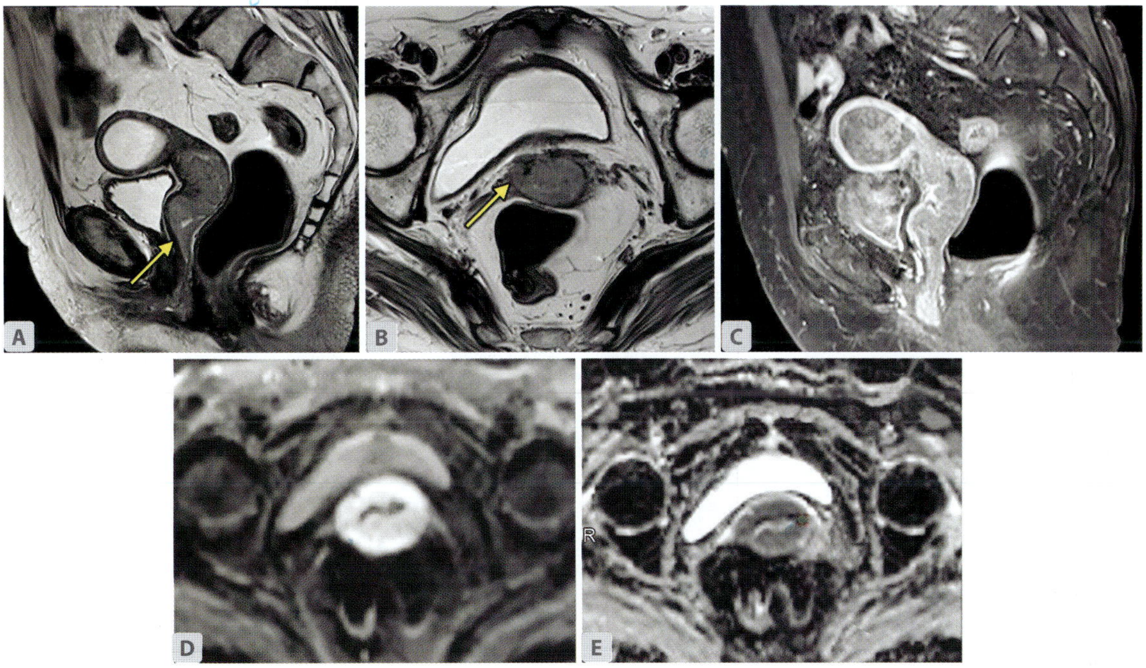

FIGS. 18A TO E: Multiparametric MR imaging in a 67-year-old presenting with foul smelling discharge and bleeding per vagina reveals (A) a well-defined hyperintense mass lesion involving the cervix and extending up to lower third of vagina (arrow in A) and parametrium (arrow in B) with associated pyometra (A). Postcontrast sagittal image (C) shows heterogeneous contrast enhancement. On diffusion-weighted image (D) and ADC map (E), the lesion shows diffusion restriction with mean ADC value 0.74×10^{-3} mm^2/sec: Stage IIIA carcinoma cervix (ADC: apparent diffusion coefficient).

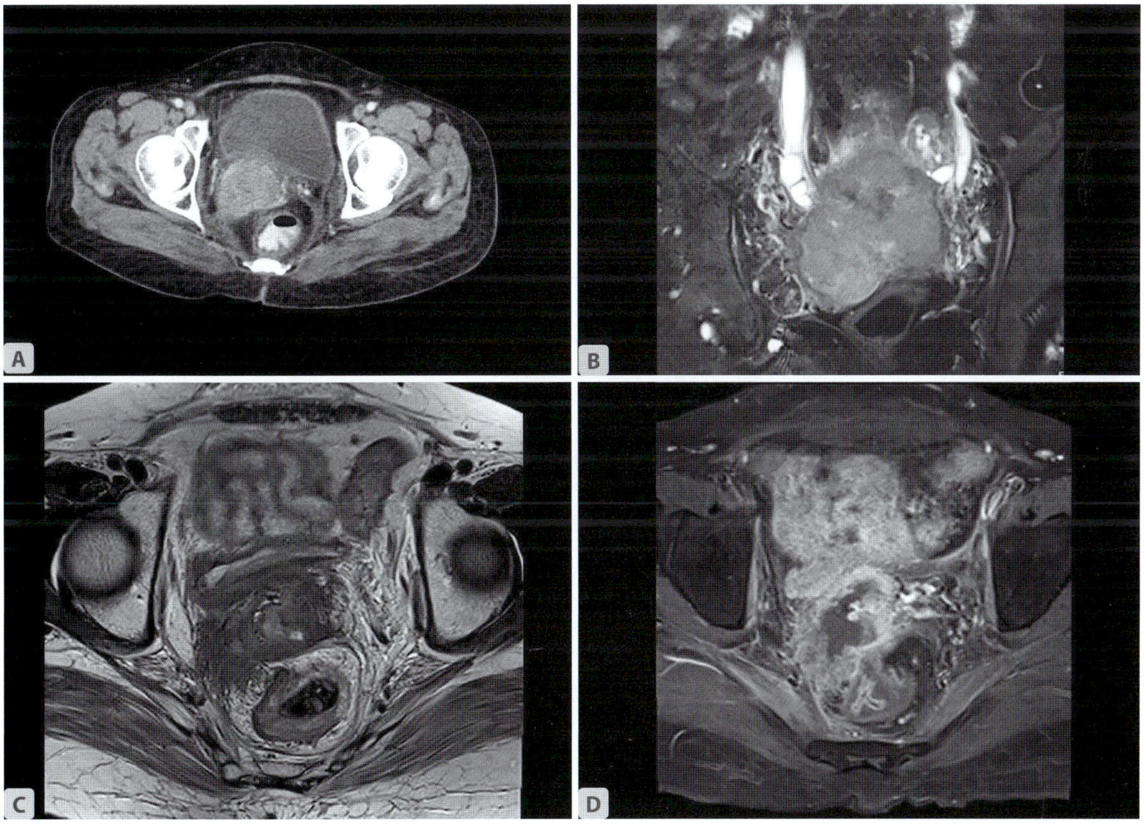

FIGS. 19A TO D: (A) Contrast-enhanced CT pelvis reveals hyperdense cervical mass extending into the right parametrium and lateral pelvic wall; (B) MRI pelvis shows bilateral hydronephrosis secondary to involvement of bilateral distal ureters; (C and D) Post-chemotherapy axial T2W image (C) depicts iso- to hypointense mass in cervix extending to right parametrium reaching till lateral pelvic wall; (D) On postcontrast axial image, the lesion shows heterogeneous enhancement with large necrotic area within.

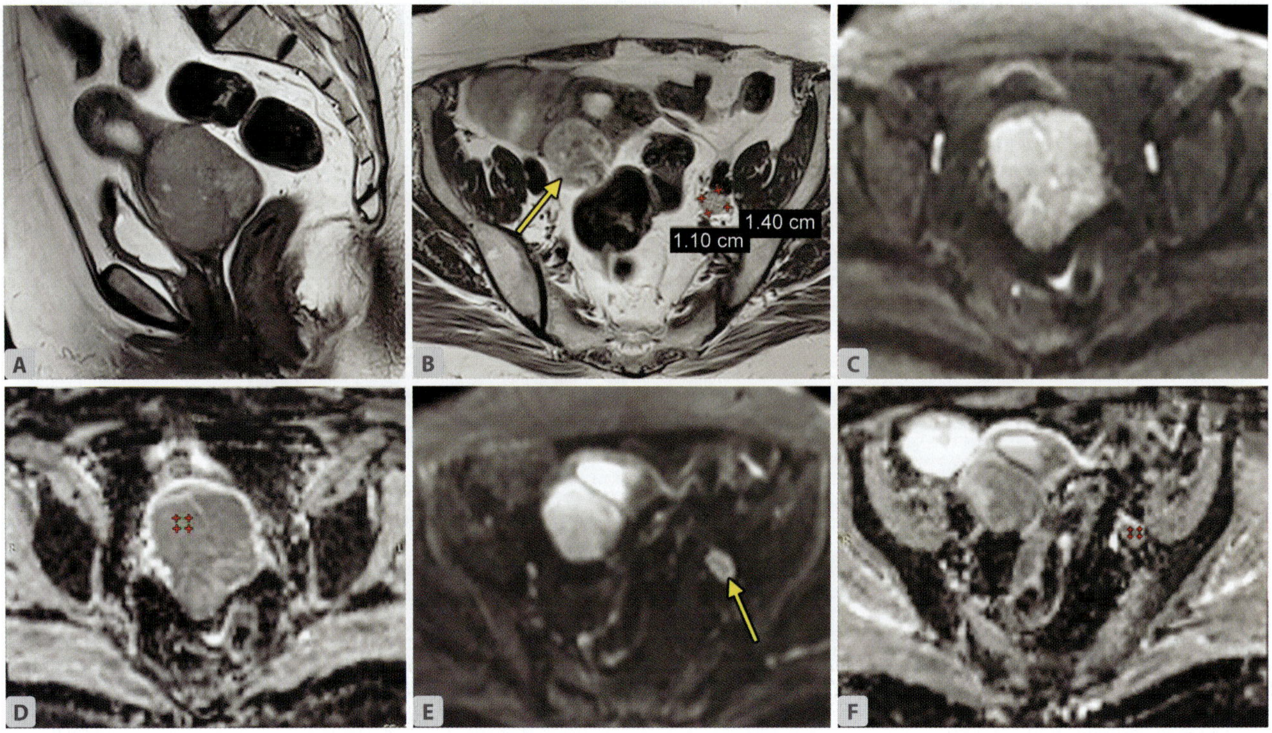

FIGS. 20A TO F: Carcinoma cervix Stage IIIC. (A) Sagittal T2W image reveals a well-defined hyperintense mass in cervix with (B) T2 axial image depicting an enlarged left external iliac lymph node measuring 1.4 cm × 1.1 cm. Note made of uterine fibroid (arrow). Cervical mass shows diffusion restriction on DWI and ADC map (C and D) with mean value 0.98 × 10^{-3} mm^2/sec; (E and F) Axial DWI and ADC map shows restricted diffusion in the left external iliac lymph node (arrow in E) with mean ADC value of 0.99 × 10^{-3} mm^2/s (ADC: apparent diffusion coefficient; DWI: diffusion-weighted imaging).

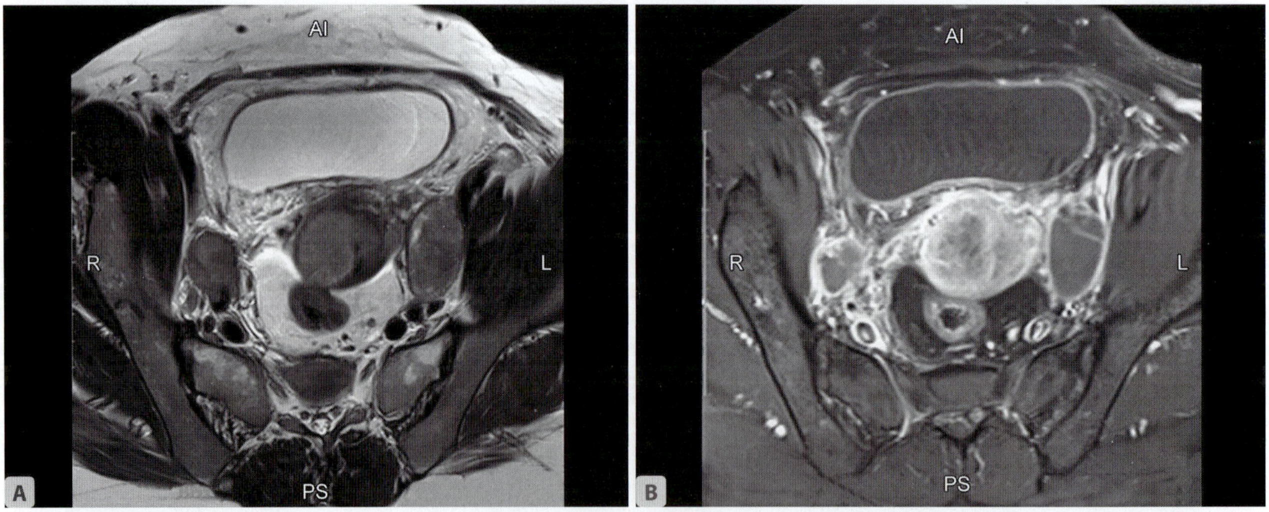

FIGS. 21A AND B: Squamous cell carcinoma cervix with bilateral internal iliac nodes. (A) Axial T2W and (B) T1FS axial images reveal an intermediate signal intensity cervical mass on T2W imaging with loss of stromal ring on right side. Bilateral low signal intensity internal iliac nodes are seen which show peripheral rim enhancement.

of any lung involvement, while chest CT should be performed in those with advanced stage of disease to rule out any lung secondaries. The metastasis of squamous cell type of cervical cancer may present as cavitating lung nodules. Bony metastasis in cervical cancer patients is rare with a reported incidence of around 1% **(Figs. 24A to E)**.[34]

Treatment

Treatment of cervical cancer depends on the stage of the disease and is stage-specific. Other factors which have an impact on treatment are age of the patient, patient's desire to have children, and overall health and accessibility to resources. Therapeutic options are available for different stages of cervical cancer as depicted in **Table 8**.[15,39]

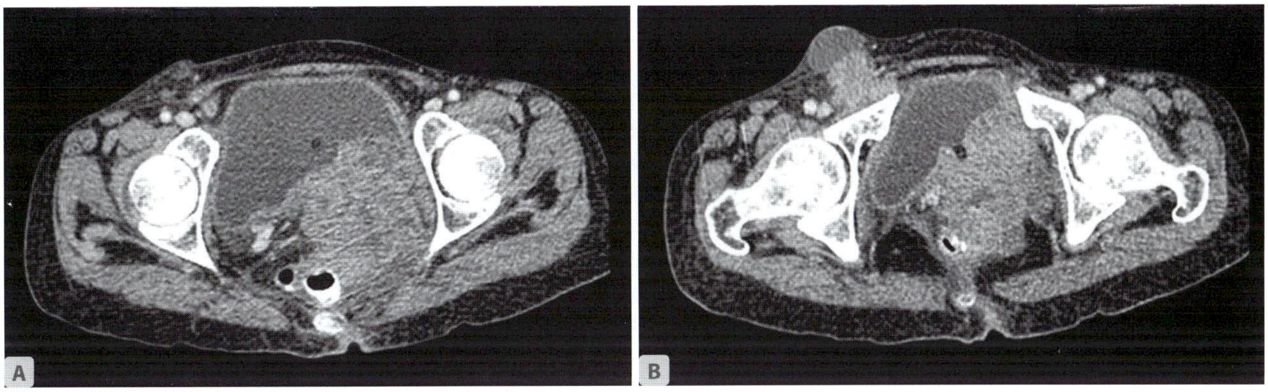

FIGS. 22A AND B: (A) CT pelvis shows a large irregular enhancing cervical mass infiltrating into urinary bladder with loss of planes with rectum and (B) There is enlargement of right inguinal node suggestive of metastasis: Stage IVB cervical cancer.

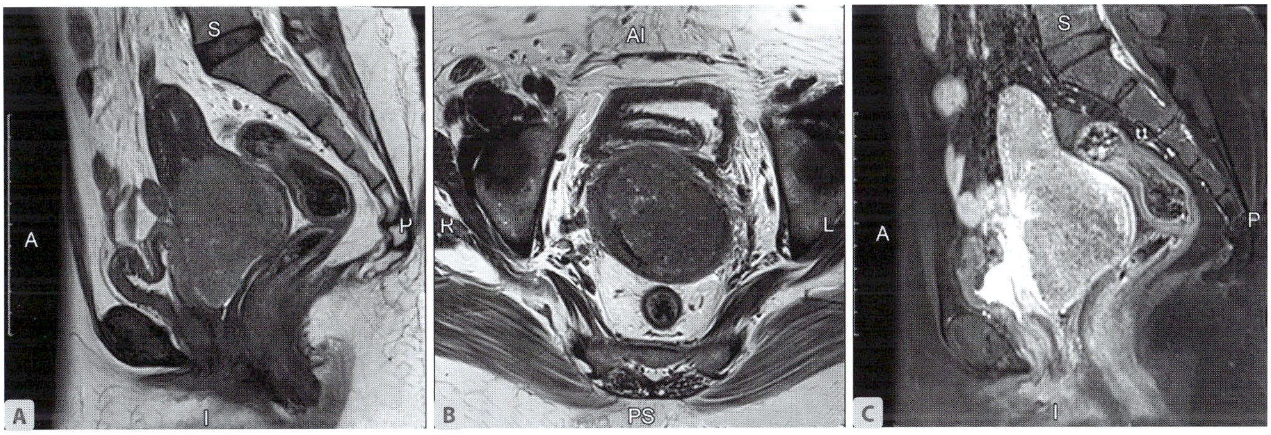

FIGS. 23A TO C: Carcinoma cervix with infiltration into urinary bladder, Stage IVA. Sagittal (A) and axial (B) T2-weighted images reveal a large well-defined hyperintense mass in the cervix extending into the vagina with parametrial involvement (B) and invasion into posterior wall of urinary bladder (A) with heterogeneous enhancement on postcontrast sagittal image (C).

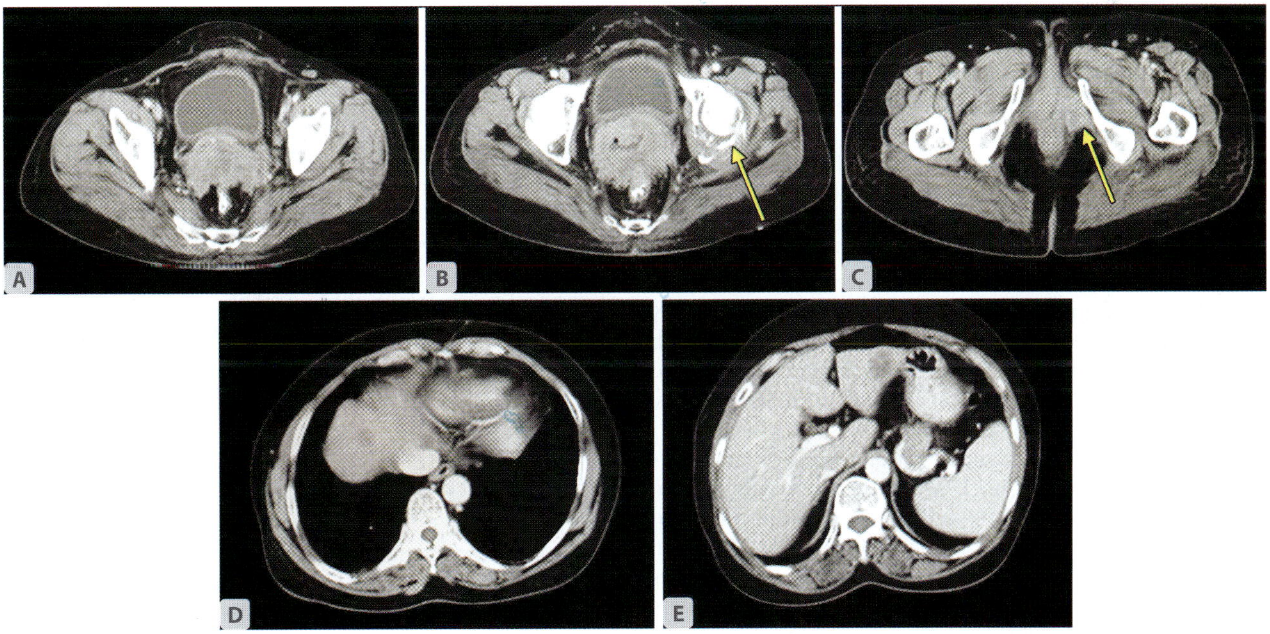

FIGS. 24A TO E: Contrast-enhanced CT of the abdomen and pelvis in a patient with advanced squamous cell carcinoma of the cervix reveals (A and B) a heterogeneous mass lesion in the cervix infiltrating into bilateral parametrium, with primary tumor showing loss of planes with rectum. A lytic lesion is noted in the left acetabulum (arrow in B). An enhancing soft tissue lesion in the perineum on the left side (arrow in C) suggestive of deposit. Sections through the upper abdomen (D and E) show hypodense lesions in the liver in segment VIII and (D) segment III (E): Carcinoma cervix with hepatic and bony metastasis.

TABLE 8: Management of cervical cancer patients.

Tumour Stage	Management
Early cancer FIGO IA1 without LVSI FIGO IA1 with LVSI	Conisation with negative margins Total extrafascial hysterectomy if family is complete Modified radical hysterectomy with pelvic lymphadenectomy. Fertility preserving procedures: • Conization with negative margins with pelvic lymphadenectomy • Radical trachelectomy with pelvic lymphadenectomy
FIGO IA2	Radical hysterectomy with pelvic lymphadenectomy, adjuvant chemoradiotherapy if required. Fertility preserving procedures: • Conization with negative margins with pelvic lymphadenectomy • Radical trachelectomy with pelvic lymphadenectomy
Invasive cancer FIGO IB1, IB2, IIA1	For tumor ≤2 cm: Radical trachelectomy with pelvic lymphadenectomy For tumor 2-4 cm: • Radical hysterectomy with pelvic lymphadenectomy, adjuvant chemoradiotherapy if required • Chemoradiation
Locally advanced cancer FIGO IB3, IIA2, IIB, III, IVA	Primary concurrent chemoradiation: CCRT (CTH + external beam RTH + brachytherapy). Chemotherapy – cisplatin or carboplatin based
FIGO IVB	Incurable – palliative treatment CTH + bevacizumab to improve survival
Recurrent cancer (Central and isolated)	Pelvic exenteration – may be curative
Non central recurrent/metastatic disease	Pelvic exenteration – not curable

(CCRT: concurrent chemoradiation therapy)

Source: Otero-Garcia MM, Mesa-Alvarez A, Nikolic O, et al. Role of MRI in staging and follow-up of endometrial and cervical cancer: pitfalls and mimickers. Insights Imaging. 2019;10:19.

Complications of Disease and Treatment

- *Tumor invasion* into pelvic side wall results in involvement of distal ureter and resultant hydronephrosis. Fistulous tract may form due to invasion of advanced tumor into urinary bladder or rectum. The most common fistulas in patients with cervical cancer are vesicovaginal or enterovaginal fistulae. MRI precisely delineates the course, extent, and complex nature of fistulae.
- *Radiation fibrosis* is a known complication of radiotherapy to the tumor and can be distinguished from recurrent disease on MR studies by typical low signal of post-radiation fibrotic tissue on T2-weighted sequences. However, this distinction can be challenging, especially within the first 6 months of radiation treatment as high signal intensity due to coexistent inflammation and edema may mimic tumor recurrence. In such instances, functional imaging like DWI, DCE-MRI, and PET/CT can aid in the diagnosis. Tumor recurrence shows restricted diffusion on DWI and early enhancement (45–90 sec) on DCE-MRI, while fibrosis either does not enhance significantly or enhances in the late phase. On DWI, both tumor recurrence and inflammatory changes may appear hypointense at a high "b" value, but only recurrent tumors will have a lower signal intensity on the ADC map.[15]

Treatment Follow-up

Evaluation of Response

In patients with locally advanced cervical cancer who are treated with chemoradiation, MRI is routinely performed during and after completion of treatment to assess tumor response. A decrease in tumor size can be seen as early as 2 months following treatment and predicts a good prognosis. DW-MRI and DCE-MRI also complement the morphological assessment based on tumor size on conventional MRI **(Figs. 25A to C)**.[25]

MR criteria for complete response consists of resolution of cervical mass, a normal low signal intensity of cervical stroma (homogeneously hypointense), and postcontrast scans showing a uniform delayed enhancement of the cervix. All follow-up MRI should be compared with pretreatment images.[33]

Recurrent Cervical Cancer

Recurrent disease is said to occur when the local tumor regrows or distant metastasis develops at least 6 months after the regression of primary tumor. Residual disease is that which is evident within 6 months of the primary treatment.[2]

Cervical cancer recurrence can be either pelvic or nodal. The prevalence varies with stage of disease, histologic type,

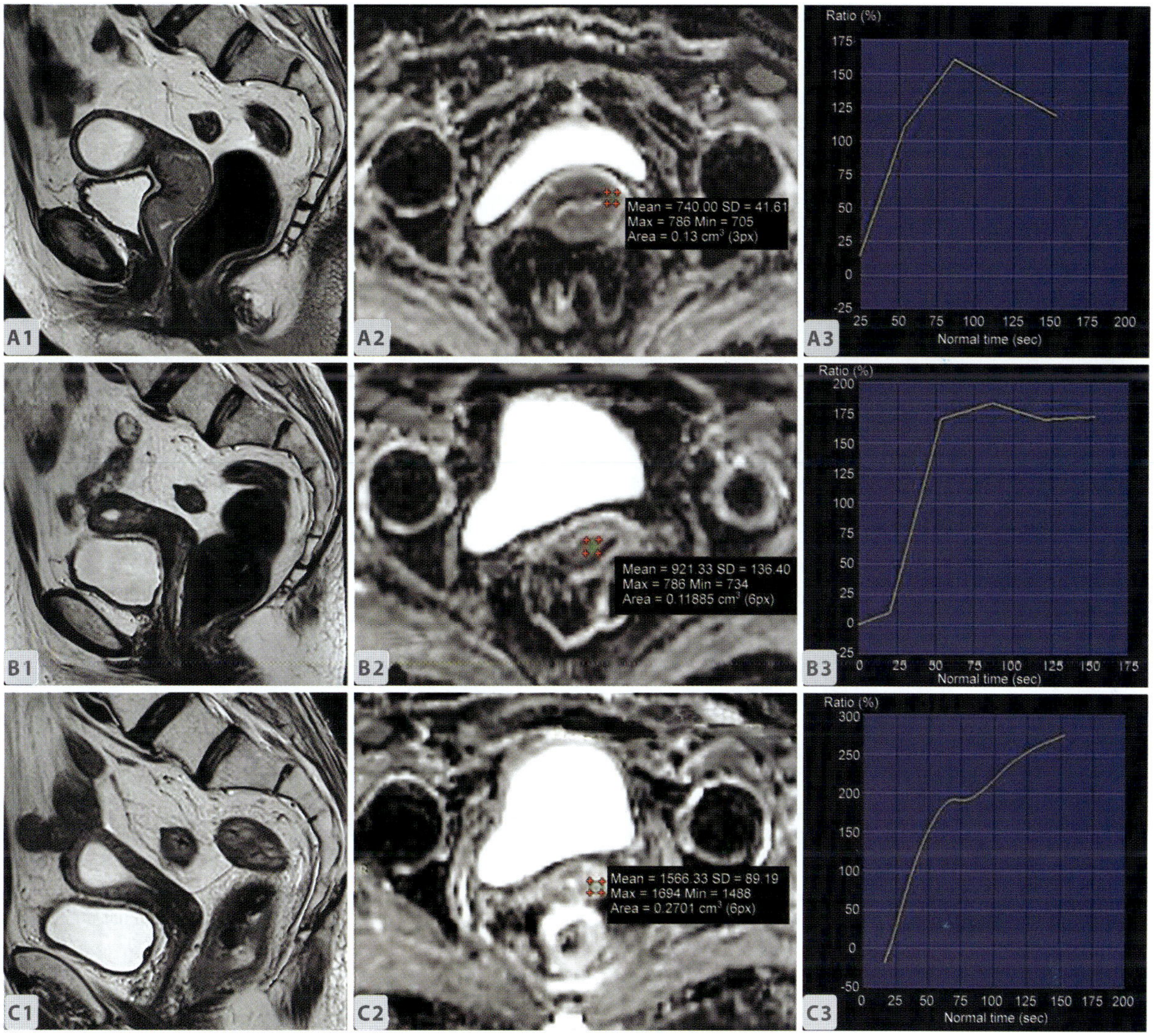

FIGS. 25A TO C: Multiparametric MRI showing post chemoradiation response: Baseline MRI (A1 to A3): T2 sagittal image (A1) of pelvis reveals well-defined hyperintense mass involving cervix extending up to lower one-third of vagina with associated pyometra. The mass shows restricted diffusion (A2) with washout pattern of enhancement (A3).
Post-chemotherapy MRI (B1 to B3): T2 sagittal image (B1) shows reduction in size of the cervical lesion. The lesion shows diffusion restriction on DWI (B2) with increase in mean ADC value to 0.92×10^{-3} mm^2/sec from baseline MRI. Time-intensity curve (TIC) (B3) shows plateau pattern of enhancement.
Post-chemoradiation therapy MRI (C1 to C3): On T2 sagittal image (C1) the cervix appears hypointense with no mass lesion seen and pyometra noted. Diffusion restriction is not seen in the cervical region on DW image (C2) with ADC value of 1.56×10^{-3} mm^2/sec. TIC (C3) depicts progressive enhancement of cervical stroma.

adequacy of therapy, and host response. Around 70% of cervical cancers are known to recur within 2 years of treatment, while 89–98% recur within 5 years of treatment. Local recurrence involves the cervix or vaginal vault after radical hysterectomy. This is well-depicted on MRI as a lobulated soft tissue mass of moderate-to-high signal intensity on T2-weighted sequences showing heterogeneous contrast enhancement, often similar to the primary mass **(Figs. 26A to F)**.

When nodal recurrence is seen in cervical cancer, the prognosis is seen to worsen when nodal involvement progresses from paracervical nodes to para-aortic nodes.

In the setting of recurrent disease, PET-CT is valuable for the evaluation of lymphadenopathy and distant metastasis.

Main factors predicting recurrence of cervical cancer are:
- Size >3 cm
- Adenocarcinoma on histology
- LVS1
- Deep stromal invasion.

Computed Tomography

On CT, cervical cancer appears as an enlarged cervix, with areas of low attenuation due to tumor necrosis. It may not be easy to distinguish tumor from normal cervix and parametrium and parametrial invasion can be overestimated on CT because of poor soft tissue resolution. Hence, CT is not indicated in assessing local

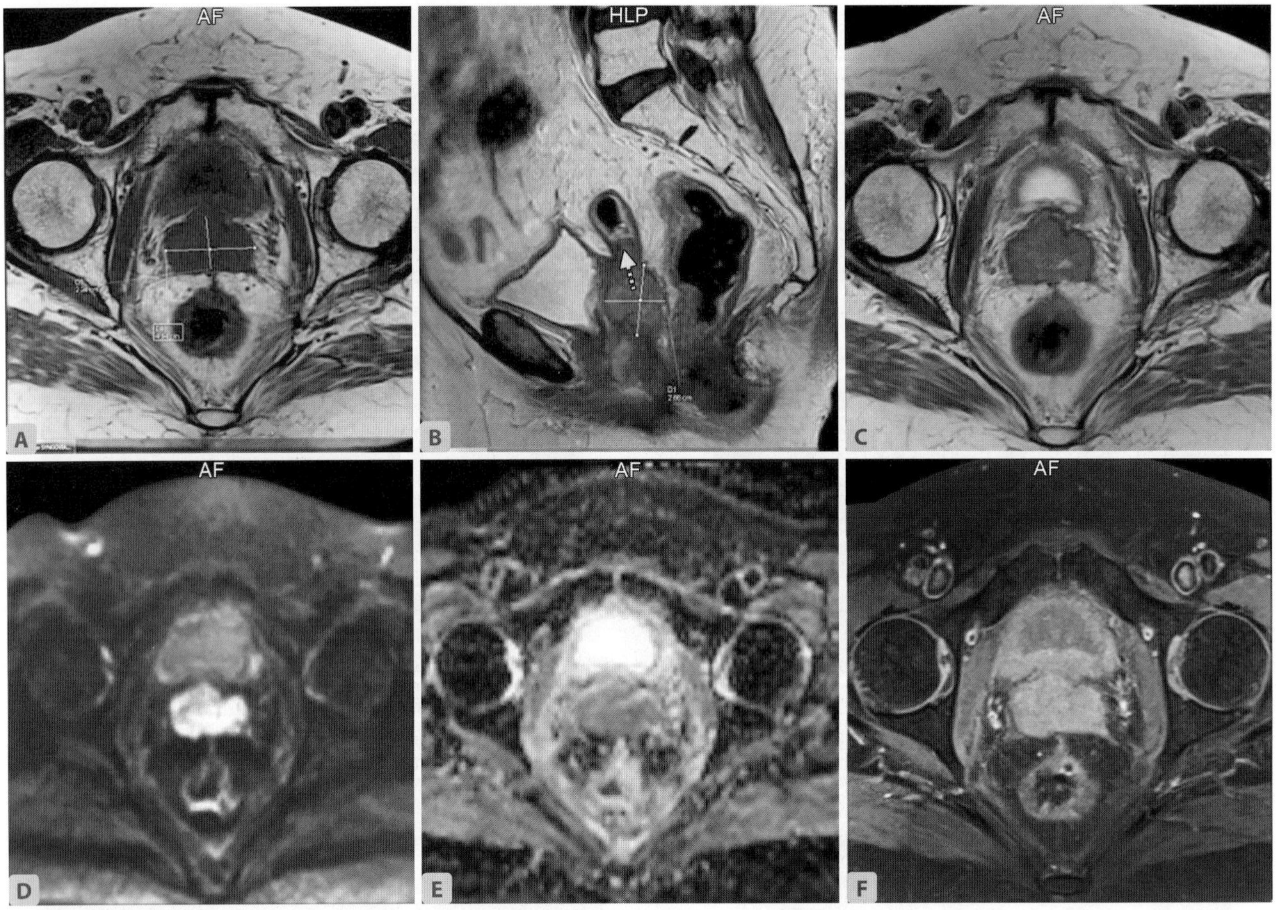

FIGS. 26A TO F: Vault recurrence in a postoperative patient of carcinoma cervix. (A to C) T1- and T2-weighted axial and sagittal images reveal a homogeneous lobulated mass isointense to muscle on T1WI and mildly hyperintense on T2WI images involving the vaginal vault abutting the urinary bladder anteriorly with loss of fat planes with sigmoid colon superiorly (arrow in B) showing restricted diffusion (D and E) homogeneous contrast enhancement (F).

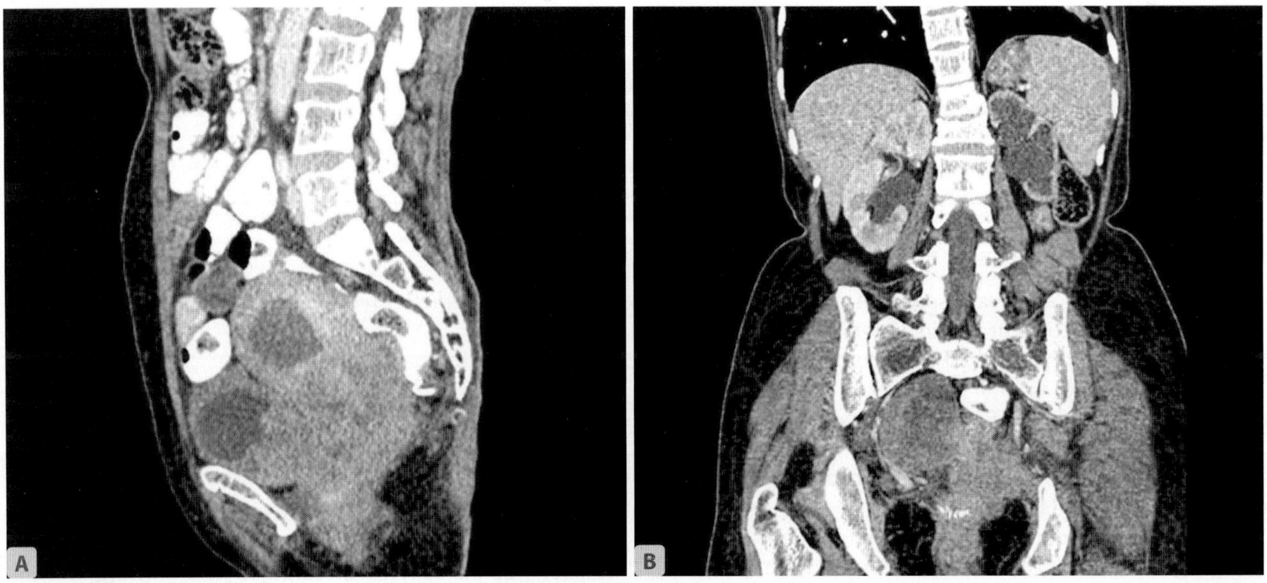

FIGS. 27A AND B: Sagittal (A) and coronal (B) CT reformations in advanced stage of cervical cancer reveal a large cervical mass infiltrating into the urinary bladder anteriorly (A) with resultant bilateral hydroureteronephrosis.

spread. CT is useful in diagnosing hydroureteronephrosis which is indicative of stage III disease or higher **(Figs. 27A and B)**. Presently, staging with CT is advocated where there is clinical evidence of advanced cervical cancer with a reported accuracy of 92% in depicting advanced disease.[26]

Hybrid Imaging (FDG–PET/CT and PET/MRI)

Fluorodeoxyglucose (FDG) PET/CT is a noninvasive tool which has a valuable role in staging, treatment planning, and assessing treatment response in cervical cancer patients. It is not indicated in early stage disease, i.e. FIGO stage IB1 or less.

PET/CT is recommended as a staging investigation in FIGO stage IIB or above disease as it helps in detecting both locoregional disease and distant metastasis in a single examination due to its wider anatomic coverage. Studies have shown FDG uptake on PET/CT to correlate with prognosis. Larger size, higher stage tumors, with parametrial invasion and nodal metastasis are seen to have higher maximum standardized uptake value (SUV). Dual phase imaging performed at 40 minutes and 3 hours after injection of tracer has enabled an increase in the sensitivity in detection of para-aortic lymph nodes from 81.6% to 100% in cervical cancer patients.

PET/MRI has evolved in recent years due to the inherent shortcoming of ionizing radiation and poor soft tissue contrast of PET/CT, especially in head and neck and gynecologic imaging. It is comparable to PET/CT in the evaluation of nodal involvement and distant metastasis and superior to PET/CT in assessment of local extent of tumor.[21]

ENDOMETRIAL VERSUS CERVICAL ORIGIN OF UTERINE CANCER WHEN BIOPSY FINDINGS ARE INCONCLUSIVE OR INDETERMINATE

Endometrial and cervical cancer can be differentiated on the basis of their clinical presentation, location, and histology of biopsy specimen. An accurate distinction between both the malignancies must be made as both of them are treated differently. About 80–90% of endometrial cancer are adenocarcinoma on histology and a similar percentage (80–90%) of cervical cancer are squamous cell cancer on histology. Around 10% of cervical cancers that arise from the endocervix are adenocarcinoma. About 10–60% of endometrial cancers can extend into the cervix and can be misdiagnosed as cervical cancer.[40] There may be difficulty in differentiating an endocervical from an endometrial origin, especially when the histopathology suggests an adenocarcinoma.

Immunohistochemical staining may be helpful in case of unclear/indeterminate findings on conventional histology. Endometrial adenocarcinoma stains positive for ER (estrogen receptor), vimentin, PR (progesterone receptor), and are negative for carcinoembryonic antigen (CEA) or p16. Endocervical adenocarcinoma stains positive for p16 and CEA.[41]

Imaging features which help in differentiating such atypical endometrial cancer from cervical cancer are based on the epicenter of the lesions and different enhancement patterns of endometrial and cervical cancers. MR imaging, with use of T2-weighted and DCE MRI, can help in differentiating primary cervical cancer from primary endometrial cancer on the basis of the epicenter of the tumor and enhancement pattern.

The bulk or epicenter of the tumor in endometrial adenocarcinoma lies in the endometrial cavity, while that of the endocervical adenocarcinoma lies in the cervix. Contrast enhancement pattern of both differ significantly. Endometrial cancers are usually hypovascular and do not enhance in the early phase. While cervical cancers are hypervascular tumors and usually show early phase contrast enhancement compared to surrounding cervical stroma **(Figs. 28A to C)**.

VAGINAL CANCER

Primary vaginal cancer is very rare and accounts for around 2% of all gynecologic malignancies. Histologically, invasive vaginal cancer is mainly of squamous cell type (<95%), followed by adenocarcinoma (<5%) and melanoma (<1%).

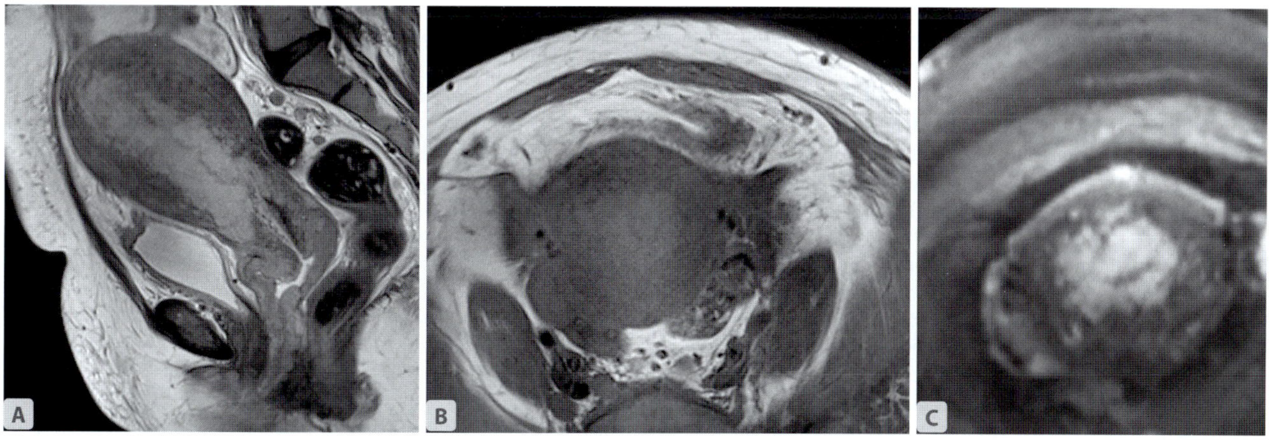

FIGS. 28A TO C: Sagittal T2W (A) and axial non-FS T1W images (B) reveal extensive intermediate signal intensity mass extending from endometrial cavity to cervix with dynamic postcontrast image revealing (C) hypervascular mass enhancing earlier than the cervical stroma: Cervical adenocarcinoma (FS: fat saturated).

TABLE 9: FIGO staging of vaginal cancer.

FIGO	Tumor spread
I	Tumor is limited to the vagina and does not involve nearby lymph nodes or distant sites
II	Tumor has infiltrated paravaginal tissue (paracolpium), but has not reached the pelvic wall
III	Tumor extends to pelvic wall
IV	Tumor extends beyond the pelvic wall or involves mucosa of bladder or rectum
IVA	Tumor invades bladder and/or rectal mucosa
IVB	Tumor spread to distant organs

It more often affects women of 70 years of age or older. The risk factors for developing squamous cell cancer of the vagina are same as that seen in cervical cancer with infection with high-risk human papilloma virus (HR-HPV) being a major risk factor.

WHO defines squamous cell cancer of the vagina as a vaginal cancer without a previous cervical or vulvar cancer in the past 10 years before the present diagnosis. Otherwise the vaginal cancer is considered to be a recurrence of the previously treated cancer.

Staging of vaginal cancer by the FIGO staging system **(Table 9)**.[42]

Staging is determined by the findings at surgery along with histopathological findings of surgical specimen. The regional lymph nodes for the cancer in the upper two-thirds of vagina are the pelvic group of nodes, i.e. obturator, internal iliac, external iliac, while cancer of lower one-third of vagina drains into the inguinofemoral lymph nodes.

The diagnostic workup of a suspicious vaginal lesion should consist of clinical, cytological, and colposcopic examination. Pelvic MRI is the imaging modality of choice for local staging of vaginal cancer of FIGO stage II and beyond. In patients with advanced vaginal cancer or if there is a suspicion of metastasis, a contrast-enhanced CT of the chest and abdomen should be carried out for complete staging.

On MRI, vaginal cancer appears as a mass which appears isointense to muscle on T1-weighted images and intermediate signal intensity on T2-weighted images, distinct from the low signal intensity of the vaginal wall, and shows enhancement on contrast administration.

Surgery is used to treat FIGO stage I tumor. Radiotherapy is the standard treatment for tumors of FIGO stage II to IV for both local and advanced squamous cell and adenocarcinoma of vagina. The five-year survival rate correlates with the tumor stage and histological subtype.

Secondary vaginal cancer accounts for more than 80% of all vaginal cancers and occur most commonly due to direct spread from carcinoma of the cervix, endometrium, ovaries, and rectum.[42]

CONCLUSION

Imaging is an essential tool in the workup of uterine malignancies. MRI, especially multiparametric MRI is the mainstay of imaging as it has an invaluable role in accurate tumor localization, evaluation of tumor extent (staging), appropriate treatment planning, and follow-up of disease. Both CT and PET/CT have important roles in advanced cancers by detecting nodal and distant metastatic disease.

It is important for the radiologists to familiarize themselves with the revised staging classification of uterine malignancies, understand the treatment options, and be aware of the diagnostic performance, advantages, and limitations of imaging modalities.

ACKNOWLEDGMENTS

We wish to thank Dr Malavika Gulati and Dr Raghavendra HK for their help; and Mohit and Dr Shivali Arya for the illustrations.

REFERENCES

1. Tirumani SH, Shanbhogue AK, Prasad SR. Current concepts in the diagnosis and management of endometrial and cervical carcinomas. Radiol Clin North Am. 2013;51:1087-110.
2. Patel S, Liyanage SH, Sahdev A, et al. Imaging of endometrial and cervical cancer. Insights Imaging. 2010;1:309-28.
3. Faria SC, Sagebiel T, Balachandran A, et al. Imaging in endometrial carcinoma. Indian J Radiol Imaging. 2015;25(2):137-47.
4. Sohaib SA, Verma H, Attygalle AD, et al. Imaging of uterine malignancies. Semin Ultrasound CT MRI. 2010;31:377-87.
5. Faria SC, Devine CE, Rao B, et al. Imaging and staging of endometrial cancer. Semin Ultrasound CT MRI. 2019;40:287-94.
6. Nougaret S, Lakhman Y, Vargas HA, et al. From staging to prognostication: achievements and challenges of MR imaging in the assessment of endometrial cancer. Magn Reson Imaging Clin N Am. 2017;25:611-33.
7. Yen TT, Wang TL, Fader AN, et al. Molecular classification and emerging targeted therapy in endometrial cancer. Int J Gynecol Pathol. 2019.
8. Salem S. Gynaecology. In: Rumack CM, Wilson SR, Charboneau JW, Levine D (Eds). Diagnostic Ultrasound, 4th edition. Philadelphia: Elsevier/Mosby; 2011. p. 4.
9. Goldstein SR. Sonography in postmenopausal bleeding. J Ultrasound Med. 2012;31:333-6.
10. Rezvani M, Winter TC. Abnormal uterine bleeding: the role of ultrasound. In: Norton ME (Ed). Callen's Ultrasonography in Obstetrics and Gynecology, 6th edition. Philadelphia: Elsevier; 2017. pp. 835-45.
11. Hardesty LA, Sumkin JH, Hakim C, et al. The ability of helical CT to preoperatively stage endometrial carcinoma. Am J Roentgenol. 2001;176:603-6.
12. Rizzo S, Femia M, Radice D, et al. Evaluation of deep myometrial invasion in endometrial cancer patients: is dual energy CT an option? La Radiologica Medica. 2018;123(1):13-9.
13. Beddy P, O'Neill AC, Yamamoto AK, et al. FIGO staging system for endometrial cancer: added benefits of MR imaging. Radiographics. 2012;32:241-54.

14. Rauch M, Kaur H, Choi H, et al. Optimization of MR imaging for pretreatment evaluation of patients with endometrial and cervical cancer. Radiographics. 2014;34(4):1082-2014.
15. Otero-Garcia MM, Mesa-Alvarez A, Nikolic O, et al. Role of MRI in staging and follow-up of endometrial and cervical cancer: pitfalls and mimickers. Insights Imaging. 2019;10:19.
16. Freeman SJ, Aly AM, Kataoka MY, et al. The revised FIGO staging system for uterine malignancies: implications for MR imaging. Radiographics. 2012;32:1805-27.
17. Rechichi G, Galimberti S, Signorelli M, et al. Endometrial cancer: correlation of apparent diffusion coefficient with tumor grade, depth of myometrial invasion, and presence of lymph node metastases. Am J Roentgenol. 2011;197(1):256-62.
18. Bonatti M, Pedrinolla B, Cybulski AJ, et al. Prediction of histological grade of endometrial cancer by means of MRI. Eur J Radiol. 2018;103:44-50.
19. Bonatti M, Stuefer J, Oberhofer N, et al. MRI for local staging of endometrial carcinoma: is endovenous contrast medium administration still needed? Eur J Radiol. 2015;84(2):208-14.
20. Kurra V, Krajewski KM, Jagannathan J, et al. Typical and atypical metastatic sites of recurrent endometrial carcinoma. Cancer Imaging. 2013;13(1):113-22.
21. Singurkar A, Poon R, Mester U. Comparison of 18F-FDG-PET/CT and 18F-FDG-PET/MR imaging in oncology: a systematic review. Ann Nucl Med. 2017;31(5):366-78.
22. Sholab SA, Houghton SL, Meroni R, et al. Recurrent endometrial cancer: patterns of recurrent disease and assessment of prognosis. Clin Radiol. 2007;62:28-34.
23. Nougaret S, Horta M, Sala E, et al. Endometrial cancer MRI staging: updated guidelines of the European Society of Urogenital Radiology. Eur Radiol. 2019;29(2):792-805.
24. Santos P, Cunha TM. Uterine sarcomas: clinical presentation and MRI features. Diagn Interv Radiol. 2015;21:4-9.
25. Sala E, Rockall AG, Freeman SJ, et al. The added role of MR imaging in treatment stratification of patients with gynecologic malignancies: what the radiologist needs to know. Radiology. 2013;266:717-40.
26. Shah SH, Jagannathan JP, Krajewski K, et al. Uterine sarcomas: then and now. Am J Roentgenol. 2012;199:213-23.
27. Sagebiel TL, Bhosale PR, Patnana M, et al. Uterine carcinosarcomas. Semin Ultrasound CT MRI. 2019;40(4): 295-301.
28. Valdes-Devesa V, Jimenez MD, Sanz-Rosa D, et al. Preoperative diagnosis of atypical pelvic leiomyoma and sarcoma: the potential role of diffusion-weighted imaging. J Obstet Gynaecol. 2019;39(1):98-104.
29. Kusunoki S, Terao Y, Ujihira T, et al. Efficacy of PET/CT to exclude leiomyoma in patients with lesions suspicious of uterine sarcoma on MRI. Taiwan J Obstet Gynecol. 2017;56:508-13.
30. Tirumani SH, Ojili V, Shanbhogue AK, et al. Current concepts in the imaging of uterine sarcoma. Abdom Imaging. 2013;38(2):397-411.
31. Bray F, Ferlay J, Soerjomataram I, et al. Global cancer statistics 2018: GLOBOCAN estimates of cancer incidence and mortality for 36 cancers in 185 countries. CA Cancer J Clin. 2018;68:394-424.
32. Bhosale P, Devine C, Gardner CS, et al. Role of magnetic resonance imaging in the evaluation of gynecologic disorders. In: Norton ME (Ed). Callen's Ultrasonography in Obstetrics and Gynecology. Philadelphia: Elsevier; 2017. pp. 1045-75.
33. Devine C, Viswanathan C, Faria S, et al. Imaging and staging of cervical cancer. Semin Ultrasound CT MRI. 2019;40(4):280-6.
34. Bourgioti C, Chatoupis K, Moulopoulos LA. Current imaging strategies for the evaluation of uterine cervical cancer. World J Radiol. 2016;8(4):342-54.
35. Bhatla N, Berek JS, Fredes MC, et al. Revised FIGO staging for carcinoma of the cervix uteri. Int J Gynecol Obstet. 2019;143(Suppl 3):43-991.
36. Sala E, Freeman S, Ascher SM, et al. Gynecological cancer. In: Adam A, Dixon A, Gillard J, Schaefer-Prokop C, Grainger R (Eds). Grainger and Allison's Diagnostic Radiology, 6th edition. London: Churchill Livingstone; 2015. pp. 957-71.
37. Moloney F, Ryan D, Twomey M, et al. Comparison of MRI and high-resolution transvaginal sonography for the local staging of cervical cancer. J Clin Ultrasound. 2016;44(2):78-84.
38. Nicolet V, Carignan L, Bordon F, et al. MR imaging of cervical carcinoma: a practical staging approach. Radiographics. 2000;20(6):1539-49.
39. Tewari KS, Agarwal A, Pathak A, et al. Meeting report, "First Indian national conference on cervical cancer management - expert recommendations and identification of barriers to implementation". Gynecol Oncol Res Pract. 2018;5:5.
40. He H, Bhosale P, Wei W, et al. MRI is highly specific in determining primary cervical versus endometrial cancer when biopsy results are inconclusive. Clin Radiol. 2013;68:1107-13.
41. Bourgioti C, Chatoupis K, Panourgias E, et al. Endometrial vs. cervical cancer: development and pilot testing of a magnetic resonance imaging (MRI) scoring system for predicting tumor origin of uterine carcinomas of indeterminate histology. Abdom Imaging. 2015;40(7):2529-40.
42. Schnürch H, Ackermann S, Alt-Radtke CD, et al. Diagnosis, therapy and follow-up of vaginal cancer and its precursors. Guideline of the DGGG and the DKG (S2k-Level, AWMF Registry No. 032/042, October 2018). Geburtshilfe Frauenheilkd. 2019;79(10):1060-78.

CHAPTER

18

Female Infertility

Radhika Batra, Rashmi Dixit, Swati Gupta

INTRODUCTION

Infertility is defined as inability to achieve pregnancy after 12 months of regular unprotected intercourse.[1] Couples are evaluated together and in around 80% of the cases the etiology is identified. A male factor is ascribed in 40% of the cases and the rest 40% cases are ascribed to the female factor. Approximately 25% couples have more than one etiology.[2]

Workup for infertility in women less than 35 years of age is indicated after 1 year of regular unprotected sexual intercourse and if the woman is more than 35 years of age, it is indicated after 6 months of unprotected intercourse.[1] The work-up may commence earlier in women with irregular menstrual cycles, endometriosis, pelvic inflammatory disease (PID), reproductive tract malformations, and prior history of multiple miscarriages. Evaluation of female infertility has greatly progressed in the last few decades with imaging playing an important role. The various causes of female infertility are listed in **Table 1**.

TABLE 1: Causes of female infertility.

Cervical factors	• Abnormal cervical mucus • Cervical stenosis • Cervicitis
Uterine factors	• Leiomyomas • Developmental anomalies • Adhesions • Infections • Tumors
Peritoneal factors	Adhesions due to infection, endometriosis or surgery
Tubal factors	• Tubal occlusion • Peritubal adhesions • Salpingitis isthmica nodosa
Ovarian factors	• Polycystic ovary syndrome • Hypothalamic amenorrhea • Luteinized unruptured follicle • Ovarian tumors or infections
Endocrine factors	• Panhypopituitarism • Hypothyroidism • Adrenal insufficiency
Others	• Idiopathic • Drugs • Radiation

RISK FACTORS FOR INFERTILITY

These include age, women's fertility rapidly drops after the age of 37 years and this is due to lower number and quality of eggs. Other factors include tobacco and alcohol use, being overweight or underweight and lack of or very strenuous exercise.

INITIAL APPROACH

It is essential to evaluate both the partners for possible causes of infertility. A thorough diagnostic evaluation should be performed to detect the underlying cause. The infertility specialist uses this information to assess the etiology and subsequently offer a treatment plan.

History

The detailed history includes the duration of infertility alongwith any results of any previous evaluation and therapy, and duration and characteristics of menstrual cycle. It is important to note any medical, surgical or gynecological history. Other aspects include previous obstetrical history, family history, and personal and lifestyle history.

Physical Examination

Patient's body mass index (BMI) should be calculated. The body habitus and secondary sexual characters are assessed. Abnormalities of thyroid gland, galactorrhea or signs of androgen excess suggest the presence of an endocrinopathy. Pelvic examination may reveal tenderness or mass in pouch of Douglas, palpable tender nodules in the cul-de-sac and uterosacral ligaments, uterine enlargement, and irregularity in leiomyoma or uterine anomaly.

Imaging Modalities

Imaging modalities used in evaluation of female infertility include the following:

- Hysterosalpingography (HSG)
- Sonography including transvaginal sonography (TVS) and sonohysterosalpingography.
- Magnetic resonance imaging (MRI).

Hysterosalpingography

Hysterosalpingography is performed during the first 6–10 days of menstrual cycle and is best performed during the second to fifth day interval just after the cessation of menstruation. This minimizes the risk of infection and avoids interference from intrauterine blood clot. It also prevents the possibility of HSG being done in a conception cycle that has not been recognized. HSG does not require any specific preparation, although pretreatment with a nonsteroidal anti-inflammatory drug (NSAID) (approximately 30 minutes before) is helpful to limit discomfort associated with the procedure. HSG is best avoided altogether for at least several weeks following any episode of acute PID to minimize risk of infectious complications. Administration of intravenous buscopan (after ruling out contraindications to buscopan such as myasthenia gravis, mechanical stenosis in gastrointestinal tract, megacolon, and prior known hypersensitivity to drug) prior to HSG is effective in relieving tubal spasm and reduces the incidence of false positive tubal occlusion due to tubal spasm.

The basic technique for performing HSG is quite standard. The study should be performed using image intensification fluoroscopy with a limited number of radiographs. The average HSG requires only 20–30 seconds of fluoroscopic time with minimal radiation exposure and has very low risk. Usually, only 3–4 basic films are required—a scout, one film during early filling, third film to document the uterine contours with the uterus fully distended and assess tubal patency, and a fourth film to detect-free intraperitoneal spill not seen earlier or any areas of contrast loculation **(Figs. 1 and 2)**. Additional films may be required when the uterus obscures the tubes or the uterine cavity appears abnormal.[3]

Contrast can be introduced using a common metal "acorn" cannula or via a balloon catheter. In general, the latter technique is preferred as it requires less fluoroscopic time and smaller volumes of contrast, produces less pain, and is easier to perform. Slow injection of contrast (typically 3–10 mL) helps to minimize the discomfort associated with HSG.[4] Water-soluble contrast media are generally used. Oil-based contrast media have also been used in the past but these are generally too viscous to reveal internal tubal architecture and disperse poorly in pelvis, so adnexal adhesions cannot be detected. They are also associated with significant risk of granulomatous reaction, venous intravasation, and embolism and are generally not used.

Complications following HSG are relatively rare but may include light spotting, infection, and pain. The light spotting usually lasts less than 24 hours after the procedure. Rarely systemic reactions to contrast media and uterine or fallopian tube perforation have been reported.[3]

Hysterosalpingography is the standard of care to look for tubal occlusion in all patients, unless laparoscopy is planned. Diagnostic laparoscopy and chromotubation are performed in women with suspicion of endometriosis or pelvic adhesions as HSG is not useful for detecting peritubal adhesions or endometriosis.

Transvaginal Sonography

Ultrasonography (USG) allows morphological characterization of the uterus and ovaries. TVS can be performed for assessing uterine contour, endometrial and myometrial abnormalities, and ovaries. While evaluating patients for infertility by TVS, especially for follicular monitoring or oocyte retrieval, normal condoms with spermicidal gels should be avoided.[5] Even ultrasound gels may have a detrimental effect on sperm and embryo and should not be used during oocyte retrieval or embryo transfers (ETs).[6]

Saline Infusion Sonohysterography

Saline infusion sonohysterography (SIS) is a technique that enables improved depiction of the endometrial lining and intrauterine cavity. Saline is instilled within the endometrial cavity under sonographic guidance and improves detection of intrauterine cavity defects. It is a sensitive technique to detect uterine synechiae, endometrial polyps and can also be used to evaluate for tubal patency. This technique allows differentiation between intrauterine, endometrial, and submucosal abnormalities without the use of contrast agents or ionizing radiation. It can be done to look for tubal patency by visualizing the passage of fluid or contrast through the tubes or presence of fluid in the cul-de-sac.[7]

Hysterosalpingo Contrast Sonography (HyCoSy)

This procedure utilizes hyperechoic contrast agents for visualization of contrast flow through the fallopian tubes.

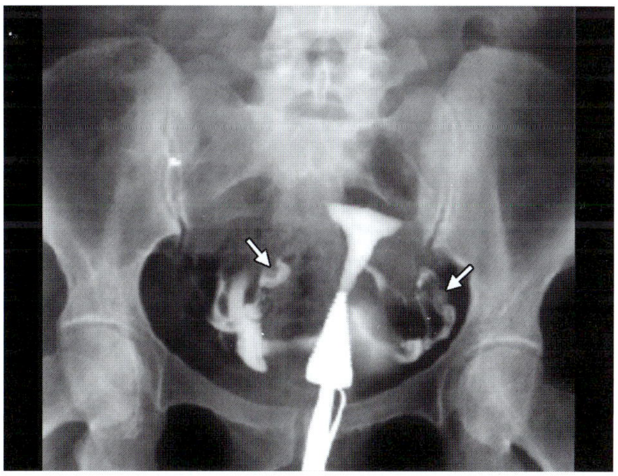

FIG. 1: Normal hysterosalpingography showing an inverted triangle-shaped smooth uterine outline. Both fallopian tubes are well outlined by contrast. Note the presence of longitudinal rugal folds in the ampullary portion (arrows). Free intraperitoneal spill is seen on both sides outlining the bowel loops.

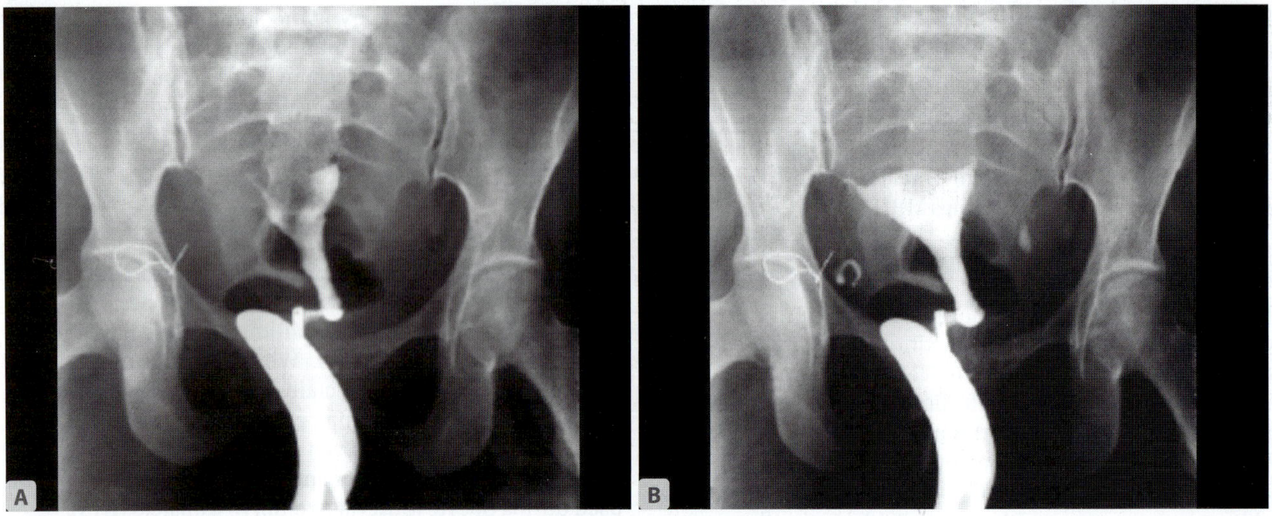

FIGS. 2A AND B: Uterine filling defect due to a fundal fibroid is much better appreciated on the early filling film (A) as compared with (B) where the uterine cavity is fully distended with contrast and the filling defect is much less apparent.

Echovist 200 has been used as a contrast agent for this technique. One of its limitations includes rapid degeneration. However, Echovist is not Food and Drug Administration approved. Another alternative used as distending media is a mixture of saline and air. "Scintillations" are rendered possible by the positive pressure flow of echogenic contrast from the uterine cavity and into the pelvis through patent fallopian tubes. Tubal patency is then distinguished by visual intratubal flow of echogenic contrast using ultrasound scanning for at least 5–10 seconds duration or flow extending from the distal end of a tube and over the adjacent ovary.[7]

Magnetic Resonance Imaging

Magnetic resonance imaging is usually performed for indeterminate cases and it provides detailed assessment of pelvic soft tissues. MRI also plays an important role in presurgical planning.

THE NORMAL MENSTRUAL CYCLE

A basic understanding of the normal menstrual cycle is important before trying to image female infertility. There are three major stages, namely the follicular/proliferative phase, the ovulation phase, and the luteal phase.

The menstrual cycle is under the control of the hypothalamic-pituitary-ovarian axis. It consists of an average 28-day cycle. Day 1 of this average 28-day cycle is the start of menstruation. In the follicular phase, the follicle-stimulating hormone (FSH) level begins to increase. This in turn stimulates the growth of the ovarian follicles. One of the follicles becomes the dominant or Graafian follicle. The developing follicles secrete estradiol, leading to endometrial proliferation. The peak of estradiol occurs 12 hours before the luteinizing hormone (LH) ovulatory surge. The estradiol peak results in an increase in the levels of LH/FSH that leads to ovulation on or around the 14th day of the cycle.

The luteal phase, also known as the secretory phase, starts after ovulation. During this phase, the ruptured Graafian follicle becomes the corpus luteum (CL). Progesterone is produced by the CL. The endometrium is primed by progesterone for the fertilized egg. The CL degenerates if conception does not occur, resulting in a decrease in estradiol/progesterone levels and shedding of the endometrial lining (menstruation).[8]

CERVICAL FACTOR

The cervical factor infertility pertains to the properties of cervical mucus and sperm transport. Imaging cannot evaluate the hospitality of the cervix to the sperm and the patient can be assessed with a postcoital test. The timing and the methodology of performing the postcoital test is a controversial topic. Most of the recommendations state doing the postcoital test as close to ovulation as possible and after at least 8 hours of intercourse.[8,9] There is limited role of imaging in this assessment. Imaging might help in monitoring of follicle development, thereby helping in optimization of the timing of the test.[1] Its utility and predictive value has seriously been questioned over the years, but it is still considered to be a useful diagnostic test by some.[10,11]

Cervical Stenosis

Cervical stenosis is clinically defined as cervical narrowing that inhibits the insertion of a 2.5 mm wide dilator.[12] Causes of cervical stenosis may be congenital or consequent to infection or trauma. Cervical stenosis leads to obstruction of menstrual flow causing amenorrhea, dysmenorrhea, and potential infertility as the sperm is unable to enter the upper genital tract. Cervical stenosis also hinders the various techniques used in the treatment of infertility including intrauterine insemination and ET.

During HSG, cervical stenosis may be seen as narrowing of the endocervical canal (normal diameter is 0.5–3 mm) or there may be complete obliteration of the cervical os with inability to insert the HSG catheter. Cervical stenosis can cause hematometra, which can be seen as a fluid-filled endometrial cavity on USG. Fluid-fluid levels may be seen within, secondary to sedimentation of red blood cells. Additional imaging with MRI may also be performed if required. Gradual dilatation of the cervix, performed with ultrasound guidance, is an effective treatment for the problem.[13] Conditions such as cervical polyps, fibroids, and neoplasms also cause narrowing of the cervical lumen.

UTERINE FACTOR

Uterine and endometrial abnormalities account for less than 10% of cases of infertility.[8,9,14] Although a relatively uncommon cause of infertility, they should be considered as they can adversely affect the outcome of pregnancies achieved by treatment of other common factors.

The abnormalities can be anatomic or physiological. The anatomic factors include uterine adhesions, leiomyomas or fibroids, and congenital uterine malformations. The physiological factors include lack of normal endometrial response to hormonal stimulation.

There are four basic methods for the assessment of the uterine cavity: HSG, standard TVS, TVS with saline contrast (sonohysterography), MRI, and hysteroscopy. The choice of the investigation needs to be assessed according to the individual patient. HSG is the traditional method and still the best initial method because it also evaluates tubal patency. However, in women with no risk for tubal disease and whose tubal status is already known (say from previous laparoscopic surgery for some other cause), TVS offers a better tolerated and simpler alternative that can also reveal suspected ovarian pathology (cyst/endometrioma) with no radiation exposure. When uterine cavity detail is critical or when congenital anomalies are suspected, sonohysterography or MRI may be used. Hysteroscopy is the most definitive method but may be safely reserved for treatment of abnormalities identified by other less invasive methods.[4]

Endometrial Adhesions or Synechiae

The adhesions or synechiae may cause infertility by two mechanisms. Firstly, they may obstruct the cervical os or fallopian tube. Secondly, the environment provided for implantation of the embryo may be suboptimal. Synechiae usually form as sequelae of infection including tuberculosis or previous history of dilatation and curettage. The association of synechiae with hypomenorrhea or amenorrhea and infertility is known as Asherman's syndrome.

The imaging modality of choice in the evaluation of synechiae is HSG. On HSG, they appear as multiple irregular filling defects in the uterine cavity.[8] They are usually linear and irregular, extending from one uterine wall to the opposite side. They allow the contrast agent to flow around them in one dimension only. Thus, these can be easily differentiated from polyps, myomas or other masses that usually allow contrast agent to flow around them in two dimensions.[15] Adhesions at the margins of the cavity may cause distortion of the uterine outline or obscure cornua **(Fig. 3)**.[4] Adhesions are tough to visualize on TVS, but when visualized, they are seen as echogenic bridges in the endometrial cavity or as irregularities of the endometrium that are surrounded by cystic spaces.[8,14] In contrast, synechiae are easier to identify on sonohysterography, appearing as linear echogenic bridges in the fluid-filled endometrial cavity.

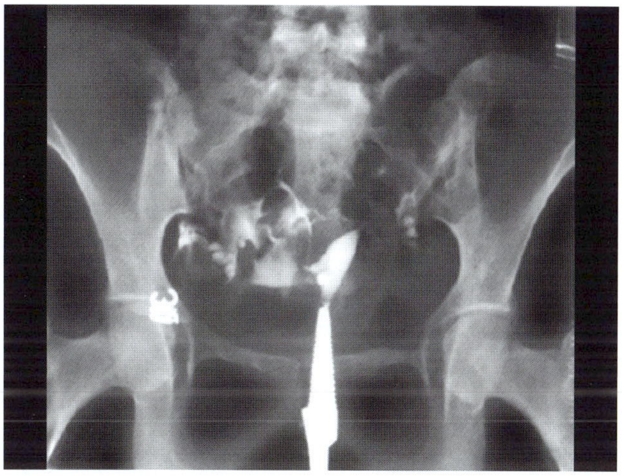

FIG. 3: Hysterosalpingography in a patient with secondary infertility following prior dilatation and curettage shows a distorted uterine cavity with irregular filling defects in the region of right cornu suggestive of intrauterine adhesions.

Leiomyoma

Leiomyoma (fibroid or myoma) is the most common neoplasm of the uterus found in up to 20–40% of women in the reproductive age group, they can be single or multiple.[16] Leiomyomas may be found in submucosal, intramural, and subserosal locations. Leiomyomas should only be considered as a primary reason of infertility after ruling out other possible causes. Pregnancy and implantation rates are significantly lower in women with submucosal myomas but not in patients with subserosal or intramural myomas that do not encroach or clearly distort the endometrial cavity, especially when modest in size (5–7 cm) **(Fig. 4)**. Suggested mechanisms by which myomas can adversely affect fertility include cornual occlusion by myomas that involve or compress the interstitial segment of the tube, dysfunctional uterine contractility interfering with ovum or sperm transport or embryo implantation and poor regional blood flow resulting in focal endometrial attenuation or ulceration.[4]

On HSG, leiomyomas are usually seen as filling defects in the endometrial cavity with enlargement of cavity when sufficiently large **(Fig. 5)**. It is essential to distinguish leiomyomas from other filling defects that include polyps, blood clots, and air bubbles. On USG, leiomyomas show a variable imaging appearance. They are usually hypoechoic, but can also be isoechoic or hyperechoic **(Fig. 6)**. Calcification causing posterior shadowing may also be seen. Limitations of USG in evaluating leiomyomas include inability to detect small lesions and difficulty in exact localization due to unfavorable uterine position, and poor uterine visualization due to patient body habitus. MRI has the highest sensitivity for picking up

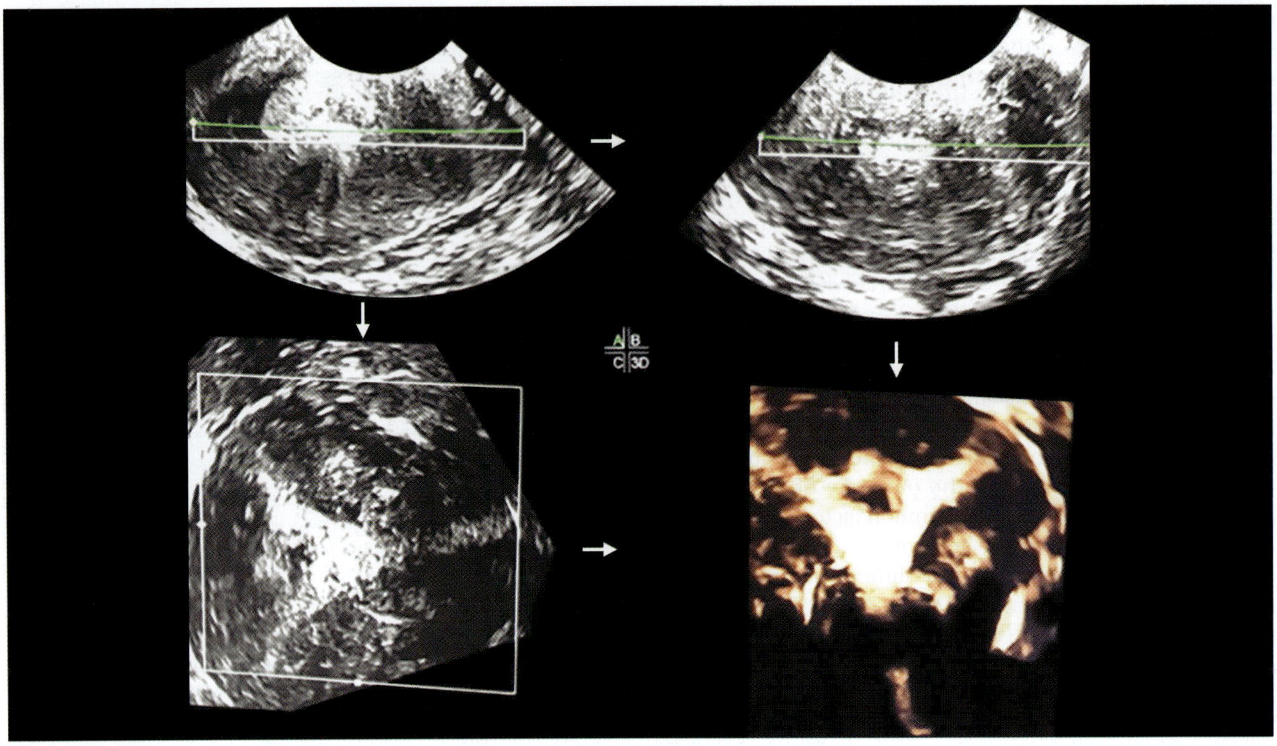

FIG. 4: Three-dimensional coronal view on ultrasound with three-dimensional reconstruction demonstrates a submucosal fibroid projecting into the mid aspect of the uterine cavity.

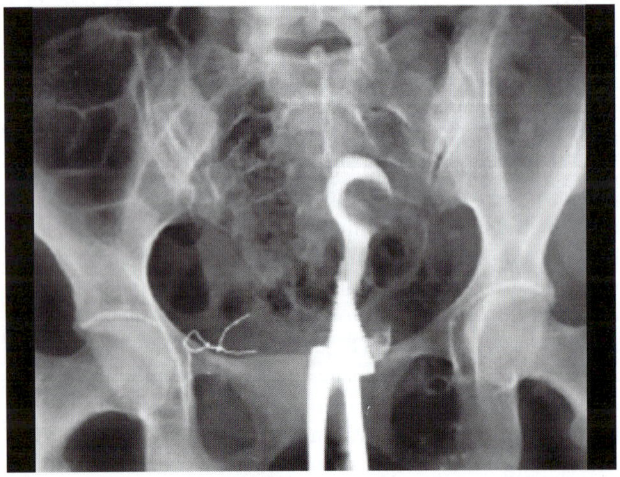

FIG. 5: A globular uterine cavity with a well-defined rounded filling defect consistent with a fibroid.

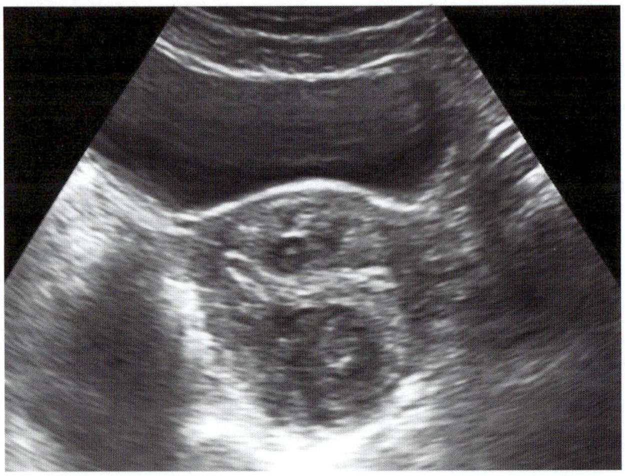

FIG. 6: Transverse ultrasound image shows few hypoechoic myomas in anterior and posterior myometrium causing mild distortion of the endometrium.

leiomyomas.[8,17] They show low to intermediate signal intensity on T1-weighted (T1W) images and low signal intensity on T2-weighted (T2W) images; however, the signal characteristics may be variable if degeneration is present **(Figs. 7A and B)**. MRI helps in distinguishing leiomyomas from adenomyosis; aids in better preoperative localization for surgical planning and better prediction of treatment outcome.

Treatment for fibroids includes myomectomy, uterine fibroid embolization, image-guided ablation, and medical management. When fertility is a concern, treatment includes myomectomy or image-guided ablation. Submucosal fibroids may be removed by a hysteroscope rather than laparotomy. When submucous myomas are single and small, the benefits of hysteroscopic myomectomy generally outweigh the few associated risks. When these are multiple and large, hysteroscopic myomectomy requires much greater technical expertise and poses greater risks including severe postoperative uterine adhesions.[8,18] Uterine fibroid embolization is not done in patients where fertility is to be preserved due to the risk of damage to the uterus and ovaries.[19]

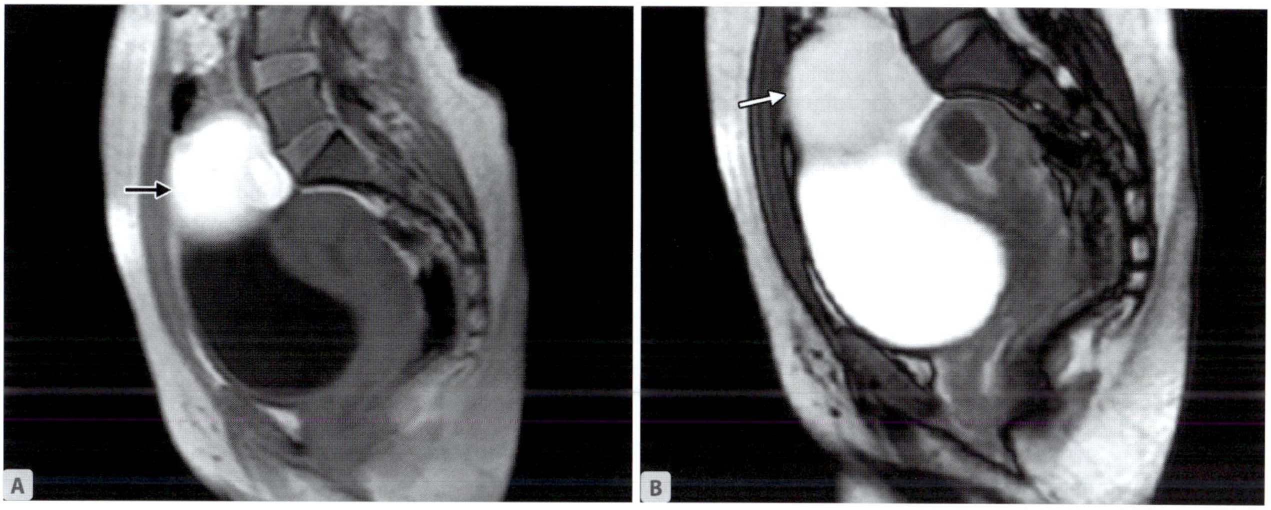

FIGS. 7A AND B: T1 (A) and T2 (B) weighted sagittal MR images reveal a small submucousal fundal fibroid appearing isointense on T1 and hypointense on T2W images causing distortion of the endometrial cavity. Note the presence of hemorrhagic cyst in one of the ovaries lying superior to the bladder and the uterus appearing hyperintense on both T1W and T2W images (arrows).

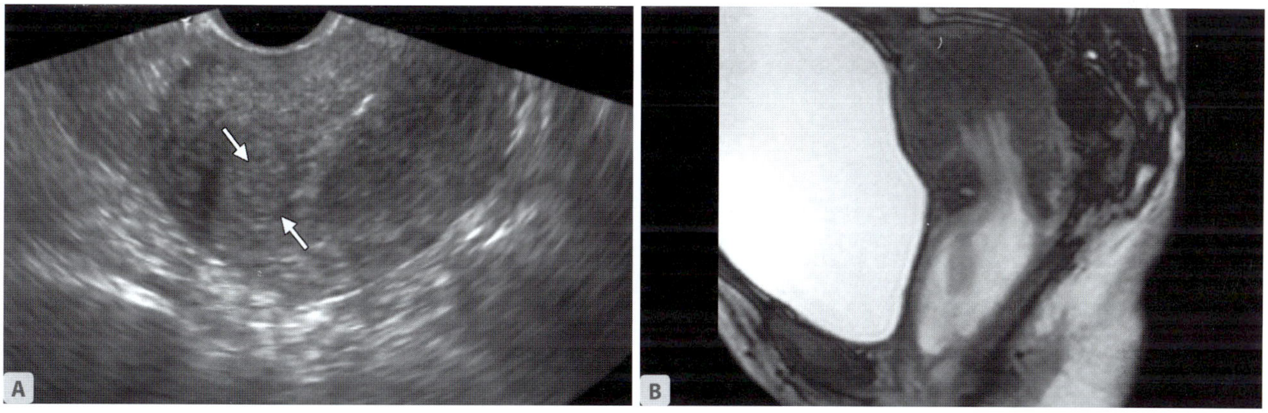

FIGS. 8A AND B: (A) TVS reveals a relatively well-defined hypoechoic mass within the upper endometrial cavity (arrows) due to an endometrial polyp which was resected hysteroscopically; (B) Sagittal T2W MR image (in another patient) reveals a large hyperintense endometrial polyp coming out through the cervix and bulging into the vagina.

Endometrial Polyps

Endometrial polyps are focal overgrowth of the endometrial glands and stroma that is surrounded by normal endometrium.[16] Endometrial polyps, even when very small, can interfere with ET and implantation. On HSG, polyps are best seen during early filling, however, differentiation from other causes, e.g. submucosal leiomyomas is limited. Endometrial lesions that are not seen on pelvic ultrasound can be picked up with SIS, the latter also helps to differentiate between endometrial polyps and submucosal leiomyomas. It also helps in an accurate assessment of the number and location of endocavitary lesions and provides guidance for their management. Endometrial polyps are seen as echogenic intracavitary masses, which may contain cystic foci. A central vascular stalk may be seen with color Doppler ultrasound. On MRI, they appear isointense to endometrium on T1W images, on T2W images, they appear hypointense with surrounding hyperintense fluid and endometrium **(Figs. 8A and B)**. Homogeneous or heterogeneous contrast enhancement may be seen on postgadolinium scans.

Müllerian Duct Abnormalities

Congenital malformations of the female genital tract are defined as deviations from the normal anatomy due to maldevelopment of the Müllerian or paramesonephric ducts with a prevalence of 4–7%.[20] Approximately 25% of females with Müllerian duct abnormalities have problems with reproduction,[21] although they have long been associated with pregnancy loss and complications, the ability to conceive is generally not affected.

As the treatment of Müllerian duct anomalies is dependent on the type of abnormality and because certain treatment options like in vitro fertilization (IVF) and super ovulation are associated with multifetal gestation which present even greater risk to women with uterine malformations, a correct diagnosis is paramount. The most accurate imaging modality for evaluation of Müllerian duct anomalies is MRI **(Fig. 9)**. Three-dimensional (3D) ultrasound is comparable in accuracy to MRI in evaluation of congenital malformations.[22,23] HSG mainly evaluates the internal morphology of the endometrial cavity and is less accurate for diagnosis.

An accurate classification system is very useful for the management and treatment of these disorders. The American Society of Reproductive Medicine (ASRM) system classified the Müllerian duct abnormalities into seven classes including class I—uterine hypoplasia or agenesis; class II—unicornuate uterus; class III—uterus didelphys; class IV—bicornuate uterus; class V—septate uterus; class VI—arcuate uterus; class VII—diethylstilbestrol (DES)-related anomalies.[21] This classification was used previously.

The European Society of Human Reproduction and Embryology (ESHRE) and the European Society for Gynecological Endoscopy (ESGE) have established a common working group called CONUTA (CONgenital UTerine Anomalies) and have formulated a new updated classification system. These criteria were proposed to eliminate the subjective diagnosis of the original ASRM classification and to allow differentiation between septate uterus and other similar conditions independent of absolute morphometric criteria.[20] This classification has been discussed in detail elsewhere in the textbook.

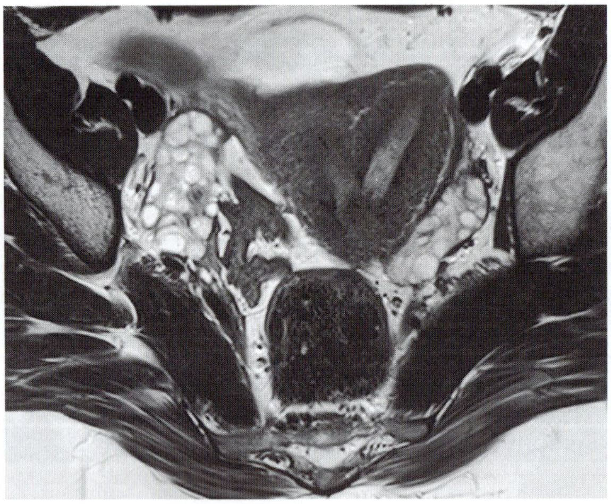

FIG. 9: Axial T2W MR image shows two uterine cavities separated by a hypointense septum—septate uterus. Bilateral polycystic ovaries are seen.

Among the Müllerian duct anomalies, the highest rate of pregnancy loss is associated with septate uterus **(Figs. 10A and B)**. According to the ESHRE/ESGE 2016, there is a high proportion of overdiagnosis of septate uterus leading to avoidable surgeries and hence risk to women and burden on healthcare systems. The ESHRE/ESGE has recommended an indentation to wall thickness (I:WT) ratio >50% for diagnosis of septate uterus. According to a study conducted by Ludwin et al, the values for defining septate uterus include indentation depth >10 mm, indentation angle <140° and I : WT ratio >110%.[24]

Adenomyosis

Adenomyosis is a benign condition in which the endometrial glands and stroma invade the myometrium. It may be diffuse in which the uterus becomes enlarged and globular in shape or focal where there is a well-circumscribed nodule known as adenomyoma. Initial imaging is performed using ultrasound, which shows the uterus to be enlarged and globular in shape with indistinct junctional zone. Increased echogenicity of the myometrium may be seen due to endometrial extension with multiple small hypoechoic myometrial cysts. Other findings include indistinct interface between the endometrium and myometrium, subendometrial echogenic nodules or linear striations, asymmetric myometrial thickening, and indistinct lesion borders **(Fig. 11)**. On HSG, adenomyosis is seen as multiple small diverticula extending into the myometrium **(Fig. 12)**. MRI reveals enlargement of uterus with thickening of the junctional zone (>12 mm), which shows poorly defined margins and low signal intensity on T2W images and small T2 bright foci secondary to dilated endometrial glands or foci of hemorrhage within the myometrium **(Figs. 13A and B)**.

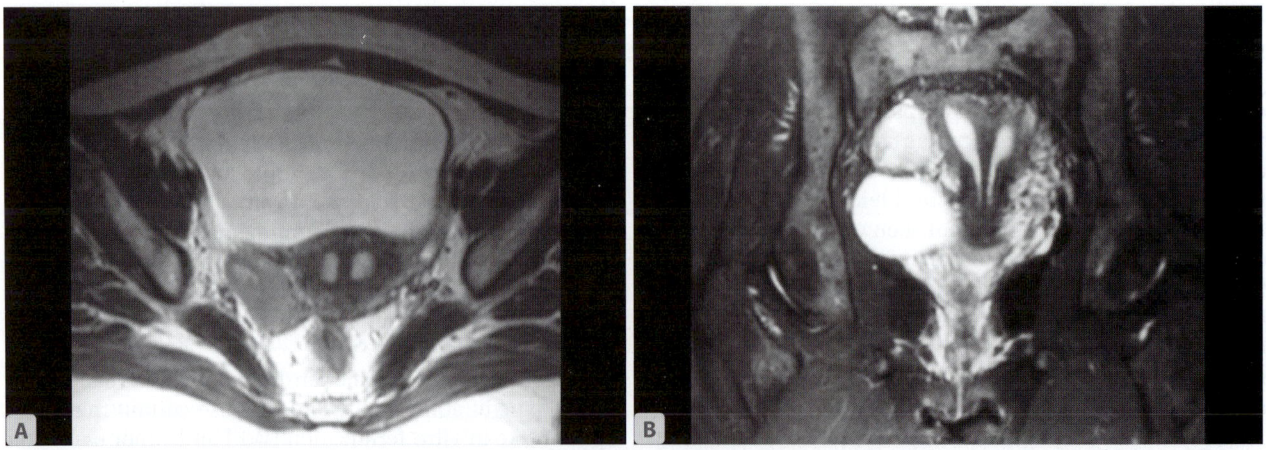

FIGS. 10A AND B: T2W axial and coronal MR images in a patient with complete uterine septum. Two uterine cavities are seen which are separated by a septum showing signal isointense to myometrium in its upper part and an inferior fibrous component which is T2 hypointense extending into the cervix, the external fundal contour is only mildly indented—septate uterus. Note the cyst in the right ovary.

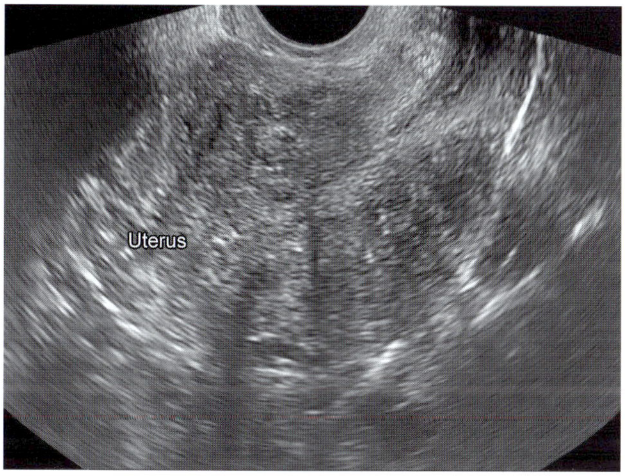

FIG. 11: Transvaginal ultrasound image shows an enlarged globular uterus with poorly defined endomyometrial interface in a case of adenomyosis.

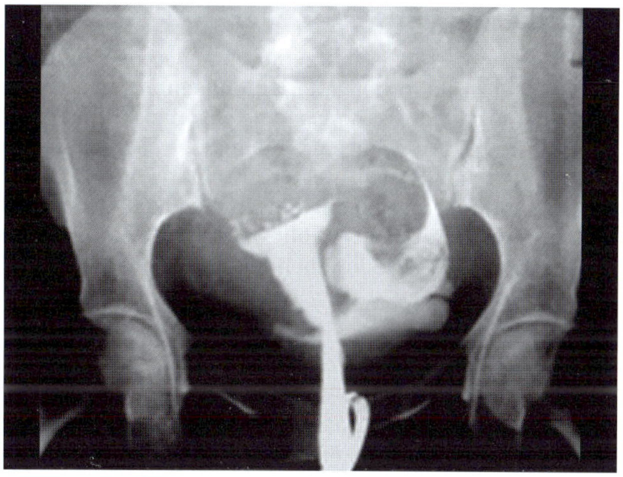

FIG. 12: HSG in a known case of adenomyosis shows multiple small irregular diverticulae in the region of fundus filling with contrast. Right-sided tube is not visualized—cornual block. Left tube is normal.

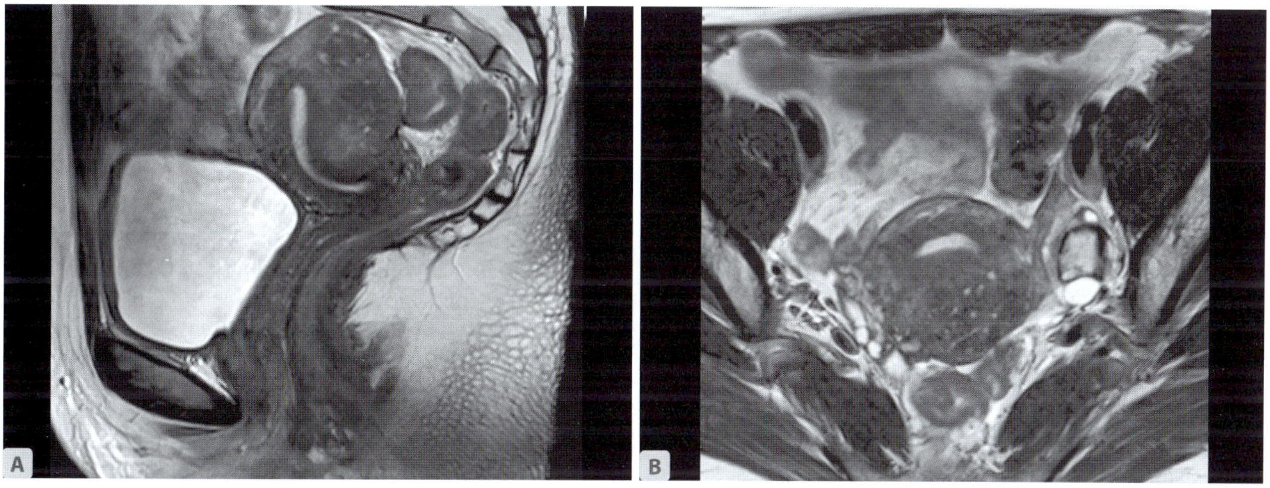

FIGS. 13A AND B: Sagittal (A) and axial (B) T2W MR images reveal ill-defined myometrial masses with indistinct margins, myometrial cysts, and widening of junctional zone—adenomyosis.

A junctional zone thickness of <8 mm rules out the diagnosis and thickness between 8 mm and 12 mm and requires additional investigations.[21] A strong association between adenomyosis and pelvic endometriosis has been found in women <36 years of age with adenomyosis being reported in approximately 90% of these patients.[25] Adenomyosis is said to be the cause of infertility in these patients. Fertility is affected by impaired uterine contractility and focal adenomyomas in submucosal location.

The only functional uterine abnormality that is of particular interest in the evaluation of infertility is chronic endometritis.

Nontubercular Chronic Endometritis

Chronic endometritis results from loss of the coexistence between microorganisms and the host immune system in the endometrium. Majority of these patients have no or mild symptoms. However, association of chronic endometritis with conditions related to infertility like implantation failure and recurrent miscarriages is of concern.[26] Chronic endometritis is diagnosed by endometrial biopsy, which shows the presence of plasma cells in endometrial stroma, but in florid cases, TVS may reveal thin echogenic endometrium that does not thicken as follicular phase advances.

Sonography has also been used to study the usual developmental response of the endometrium to try and predict implantation. During menstruation, the endometrium is seen as a thin echogenic interface, which thickens during the proliferative phase of the menstrual cycle and is relatively hypo-to isoechoic yielding a prominent trilaminar pattern. During the secretory phase, the endometrium does not thicken further but becomes more echogenic.

In a study conducted by Khan et al no pregnancy was reported with an endometrial thickness of <7 mm. They also found that average pulsatility index (PI) of the uterine artery was higher in nonconception than in conception cycles. PI value of >2.8 was associated with no conception.[27] Tekay et al reported no pregnancy when the PI was more than 3.[28]

Calcific Endometritis

Calcific endometritis is an uncommon cause of infertility. It can occur postabortion, after chronic endometritis (due to genital tuberculosis, nonspecific chronic endometritis, and pyometra). An echogenic line may be seen along the endometrial cavity with posterior shadowing. Doppler studies show increased blood flow in the myometrium and endometrium with peak systolic velocity >60 cm/sec and resistive index (RI) <0.5 in subendometrial and myometrial vessels. MRI reveals a thin hypointense line along the endometrial cavity on T2W images.[29]

TUBAL FACTOR

The fallopian tubes connect the peritoneal cavity to the external environment through the uterus, cervix, and vagina. The normal length of the fallopian tube varies from 7 cm to 16 cm, with an average length of 12 cm. Ciliated mucosal epithelial layer surrounded by three smooth muscle layers lines the tube and the tube is divided into four segments: (1) the intramural or interstitial part, which lies in the wall of the fundus, it is 1–2 cm in length; (2) the isthmic part, which is around 2–3 cm in length; (3) the ampullary portion, which is 5–8 cm in length; and (4) the infundibulum, it is the distal end of the tube which is trumpet-shaped and terminates in the fimbria.[15] Fallopian tubes help in transport of sperms from the uterine end toward the ampulla and transport of the ova in the other direction, that is from the fimbriated end to the ampulla. They also provide support to the early embryo and enable conduction of the early embryo from the ampulla to the uterus for implantation.

Fallopian tube pathology accounts for infertility in up to 40% of women and is among the most common causes of infertility. Infection or endometriosis commonly result in tubal obstruction. Salpingitis isthmica nodosa (SIN) is also a cause of tubal infertility that has commonly been described in the Western literature.[8,15]

Evaluating patency of the fallopian tube is an important part of the workup for infertility. The techniques available to evaluate the fallopian tubes include HSG, sonohysterosalpingography and laparoscopy. HSG remains the most common initial imaging technique used to evaluate the fallopian tubes. It provides exquisite depiction of the fallopian tubes and enables delineation of tubal patency, tubal occlusion, tubal irregularity, and peritubal disease. Compared with laparoscopy (which is the gold standard test for assessing tubal patency), HSG has only moderate sensitivity but relatively high specificity. The clinical implications are that when obstruction is seen on HSG, there is still a relatively high probability (approximately 60%) that the tube is in fact open, but when HSG reveals patency, there is little chance that the tube is actually blocked (approximately 5%). In these cases, contrast in a dilated tube or vaginal fornix may be mistaken for peritoneal spill.[4] Sonohysterosalpingography and 3D ultrasound and Doppler techniques have been used to evaluate the tubes. However, the techniques provide no information regarding tubal anatomy and whether one or both tubes are patent. Although 3D ultrasound and Doppler techniques have improved visualization of fluid movement through fallopian tubes, it is unlikely that they will replace traditional HSG.

On HSG, the interstitial segment of the fallopian tube may be delicate and thread-shaped or it may be funnel-shaped, taking the configuration of a small triangle or diamond. The isthmic segment is usually thread-shaped. The diameter of both these segments is around 1 mm. Proximal tubal obstruction is obstruction seen in the first 3–4 cm of the tube.[8,15] Obstruction of the proximal end of the fallopian tube is seen in 20% of cases on HSG. The cause of proximal tubal obstruction is frequently unclear, however, all reported series implicate infection and subsequent inflammation as leading causes. Histopathology of the resected proximal tubal segments reveals plugs of amorphous debris, chronic inflammation, obliterative fibrosis, and SIN. All these lesions account for majority of anatomic occlusions at the uterotubal junction. Other causes include granulomatous or "giant cell" salpingitis secondary to tuberculosis, foreign bodies, certain parasitic infestations, intraluminal endometriosis, and congenital atresia of fallopian tubes. Around 10% of tubes resected for proximal occlusion reveal intraluminal endometriosis and may exist without relation to visible lesions anywhere else in the pelvis. Müllerian anomalies of the fallopian tube are not seen frequently, but cornual occlusion is seen with variants of unicornuate uterus, where atresia of tubal segments, including the proximal isthmus, can occur.

Proximal tubal obstruction on HSG can also be seen with "tubal spasm". The cornual portion of the fallopian tube is encased by smooth muscle of the uterus. If the muscle goes into spasm during HSG, one or both tubes may not be opacified beyond the interstitial portion. A spasmolytic agent, such as glucagon or scopolamine, if administered can occasionally result in uterine muscle relaxation and consequent tube opacification. According to some authors, however, tubal spasm is the cause of proximal tubal obstruction much less often than originally proposed. They postulate that temporary nonvisualization of the tube may be due to some easily dislodged entity such as amorphous debris in the lumen of the tube.[30,31] In some cases, it may be helpful to place the patient in prone position and wait for 5 minutes before slowly reinjecting contrast. If proximal tubal obstruction persists in spite of these maneuvers, tubal catheterization with selective salpingography can be performed.

Proximal tubal obstruction can be diagnosed and treated with fluoroscopically guided selective salpingography.[15,32-34] Selective salpingography is a technique which is minimally invasive, and it involves placing the tip of the catheter in the tubal ostia and injecting contrast directly into the tube. The obstruction can usually be overcome by the injection alone. In case the obstruction is not relieved, a guidewire can be directed into the tube fluoroscopically through the catheter. Tubal recanalization may be achieved either through forceful injection of contrast or by clearing the obstruction with a guidewire. A technical success rate of 75% has been reported and in 10–22% of these patients, pregnancy is achieved without further management.[35] Traditionally, this procedure was performed for patients with bilateral proximal tubal occlusions but there is a lower threshold for considering fallopian tube recanalization in patients with unilateral occlusion. It is essential to exclude distal tubal disease especially noncommunicating hydrosalpinx. Complications include tubal perforation, infection, and tubal pregnancy. Ultrasonographic guidance has also been used for this procedure in a few cases.

Salpingitis isthmica nodosa is a tubal pathology commonly described in Western literature. An association between SIN and PID exists, however, it is unclear whether SIN is caused by pelvic inflammation or it is congenital and predisposes to inflammation. It mostly affects the isthmic portion and occasionally the interstitial and ampullary segments. On HSG, it is seen as characteristic multiple small diverticula present in the proximal two-thirds of the tube. It leads to infertility and is also associated with increased risk of ectopic pregnancy. Tuberculous salpingitis can have similar imaging appearance but may be associated with calcified lymph nodes or calcifications of the tube itself. SIN associated with tubal obstruction may be treated by tubal catheterization and recanalization under fluoroscopic guidance.[8,15]

The longest part of the fallopian tube is the ampullary segment. It measures 1–2 mm at its proximal end and widens to approximately 15 mm, where it joins the fimbriated infundibular portion. Subtle ampullary rugal folds can be seen with salpingography, and sometimes the fimbriae may be outlined by contrast material. Damage to the epithelium secondary to infection causes abnormal rugal folds and these usually coexist with a dilated and at times a distally obstructed tube. Abnormal rugal folds may be found in a patent tube, and they imply decreased chances for conception. The presence of abnormal rugal folds needs optimal tubal imaging, because the normal rugal folds are subtle. Rugal folds may be best seen before the dilated tube is fully distended with contrast, i.e. during early filling.[8]

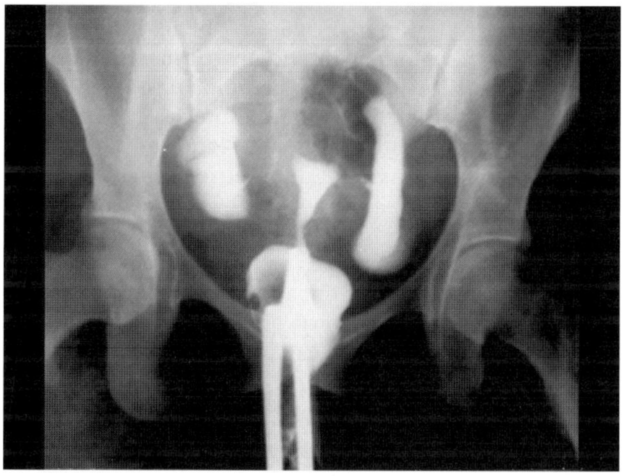

FIG. 14: HSG in a patient with bilateral fimbrial block shows markedly dilated ampullary segments (hydrosalpinx) with absence of free intraperitoneal spill.

Dilation of the ampullary portion of the tube is seen with obstruction in the fimbrial portion of the fallopian tube, which sometimes can be massive, with absence of free peritoneal spill of contrast agent in spite of adequate filling of the tubes and rolling the patient **(Fig. 14)**. It may be difficult to distinguish a dilated tube from loculated spill of contrast agent sometimes. If hydrosalpinx is seen on HSG, postprocedural antibiotic prophylaxis should be prescribed to prevent infection secondary to stasis of contrast material in the obstructed tube.

The degree of tubal dilatation does not predict results of surgery. The epithelium may be intact in a dilated tube which is soft and pliable, and thus amenable to surgery. An obstructed tube, which is mildly dilated, may not be amenable to reconstruction as the wall can be thickened and indurated. Improved chances of successful tubal reconstruction are associated with visualization of normal ampullary rugal folds. Dilatation of the ampullary part of the tube in the absence of complete occlusion suggests perifimbrial phimosis or adhesions around the fimbria that hinder egress of fluid.

Fimbrial phimosis can be mild or severe, but mostly the presence of at least a pinpoint opening in the distal tube is associated with a more favorable prognosis after surgery than complete occlusion. It also increases the risk of post-HSG peritonitis.

Although ultrasound is unable to visualize normal fallopian tubes, blockage of the fallopian tube with fluid accumulation (hydrosalpinx) is easily seen on ultrasound **(Figs. 15A and B)**. The distended tube coiled around the ovary with folds producing septa which do not completely cross the lumen. A hydrosalpinx may occasionally be visible on ultrasound, distended with fluid only at midcycle, under the estrogenic influence of a preovulatory follicle.[36]

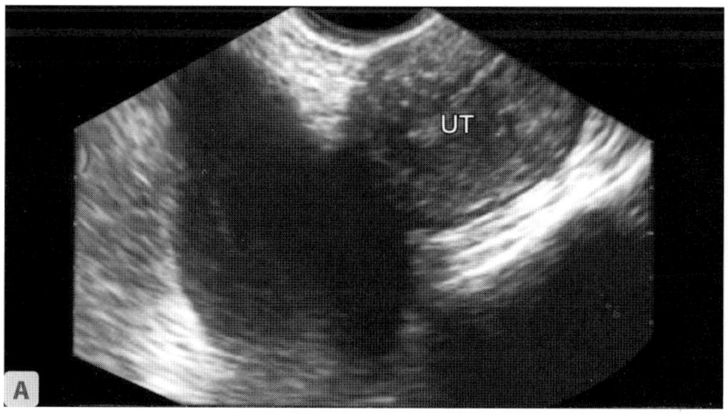

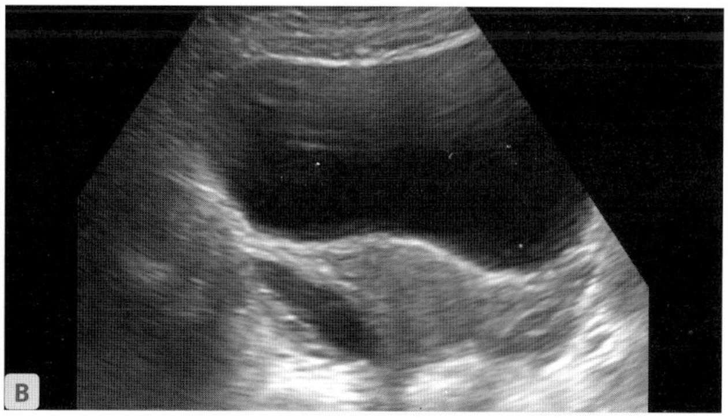

FIGS. 15A AND B: USG showing a cystic hypoechoic retort-shaped dilated tube with incomplete septations—Hydrosalpinx (A); In another case, an oblong cystic structure is seen in the right adnexa adjacent to the right ovary consistent with hydrosalpinx (B).

A woman with severely damaged fallopian tubes but a normal uterine cavity is a good candidate for IVF and ET. However, presence of hydrosalpinx in a woman being treated by IVF is associated with poor embryo uptake which may be improved after treatment of hydrosalpinx. Even a unilateral hydrosalpinx is capable of disrupting natural fertility and preventing the success of IVF.[36-38] The mechanism is as follows: Estradiol produced by the preovulatory and ovulating follicle stimulates both ampullary transudation of fluid and isthmic secretion of dense mucus which along with an estrogen mediated increase in isthmic myosalpingeal tone functionally occludes the tube's communication with the cavity of the uterus. Thus, the hydrosalpinx gathers fluid. With ovulation, increasing progesterone secretion from the luteinizing follicle relaxes the isthmus, allowing passage of accumulated hydrosalpinx fluid down the endometrial cavity just at the time that a normal tube allows passage of preembryo to the uterus. This cascade from a single tube is likely to displace any preembryos that might have reached through the contralateral patent one or through IVF and transcervical transfer. Conceptions rates following salpingostomy are less than 25% if the hydrosalpinx has a thick wall or a diameter greater than 15 mm.[5,39]

PERITONEAL FACTOR

The peritoneal factor responsible for infertility is due to pelvic adhesions resulting from previous infection, endometriosis or surgery.[8,9,15] Adhesions can cause problems in oocyte pick up and transfer due to alteration of the normal anatomy, restriction of fimbrial motility and obstruction of fallopian tubes. Imaging techniques are limited in their ability to diagnose pelvic adhesions. The gold standard for visualization of pelvic adhesions and endometriosis is laparoscopy.[8]

With HSG, the presence of peritubal adhesions and endometriosis is under diagnosed with reported sensitivities ranging from 34% to 75%. Peritubal adhesions can be suggested if loculated spill of contrast is seen in the peritoneal cavity, or it is seen to track along the outside of the tube producing "a halo effect" or double contour appearance to tubal wall.[40] Peritubal adhesions can also be diagnosed if a persistently convoluted, kinked, stretched or vertically oriented fallopian tube is seen **(Fig. 16)**. Delayed films or film obtained after rolling the patient may be useful to confirm loculated spill in doubtful cases. Normally, the contrast should flow freely to outline the bowel loops.[8,15,41] A tug and release maneuver has also been described to confirm the presence of adhesions. If traction is applied on the HSG system both a fixed laterodeviated uterus (due to adhesions) as well as a normal nonmedian uterus initially follow the traction direction, however, during the releasing phase the fixed laterodeviated uterus tends to keep the original deviated position while the nonmedian uterus keeps the pelvis midline.[40]

Ultrasound, especially TVS may also detect pelvic adhesions and loculated fluid collections in the adnexae. Adhesions may be suggested by *en masse* movement of the tethered organs when pressure is applied simultaneously by the operator's hand transabdominally and by the probe transvaginally.

Endometriosis

Endometriosis is found in 25–50% of infertile women and 30–50% of women with endometriosis are infertile.[42] Endometriosis results from ectopic foci of secretory endometrium situated outside the uterus. It can impair fertility through formation of adhesions and hormonally medicated mechanisms. Endometriosis may occur as diffuse peritoneal implants or focal endometriomas (chocolate cysts). TVS is the preferred technique to identify ovarian endometriomas which are seen as complex adnexal or cul-de-sac masses. Diffuse low level internal echoes may be seen **(Fig. 17)**. However, TVS has limited ability to identify generalized disease producing subtle changes

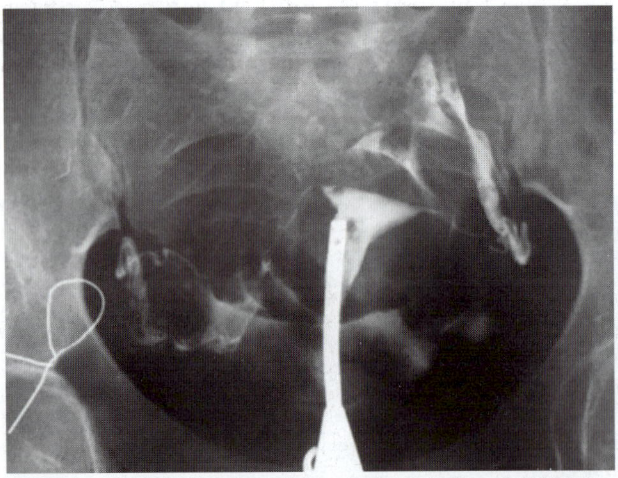

FIG. 16: HSG film reveals an irregular filling defect in the uterine body just adjacent to the cannula due to adhesions. An air bubble is seen in the right cornu. The ampullary portion of the left fallopian tube is vertically stretched with evidence of both peritubal and free spill due to peritubal adhesions.

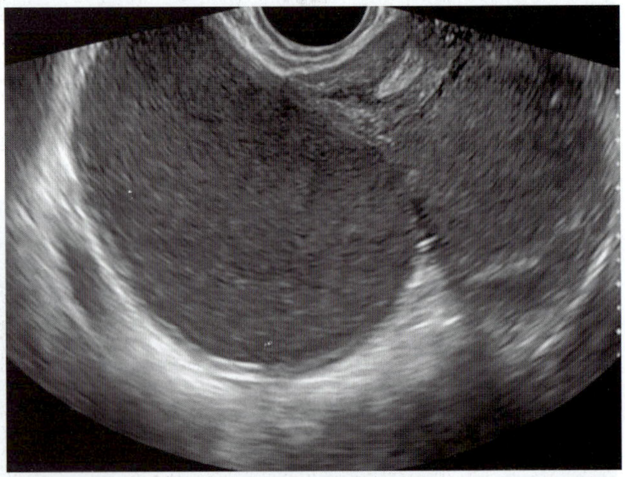

FIG. 17: Transvaginal ultrasound image shows bilateral adnexal lesions with homogeneous diffuse low level internal echoes consistent with bilateral endometriomas. The uterus is displaced anterolaterally.

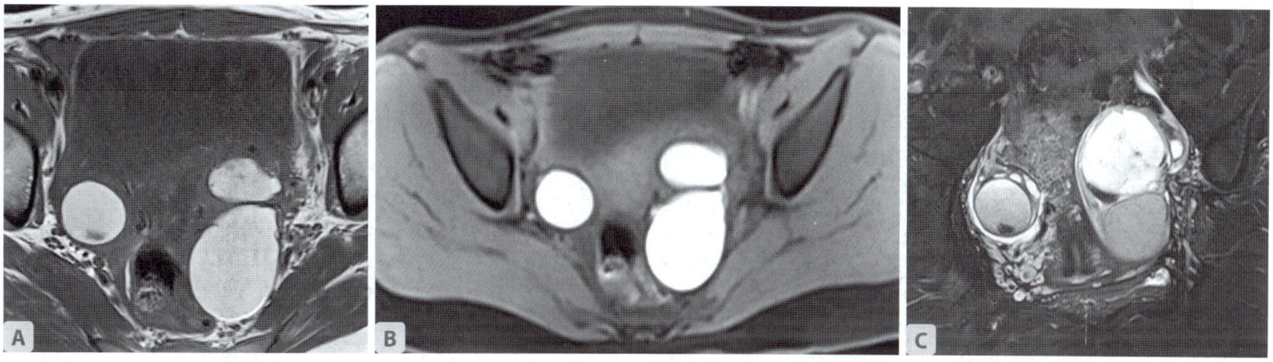

FIGS. 18A TO C: Bilateral adnexal lesions are seen appearing hyperintense on axial T1W (A) and axial T1W fat saturated (B) images. The lesions show T2 shading on T2W coronal images as well as T2 dark spots (C)—bilateral endometriomas.

such as obliteration of margins between pelvic organs and a generalized increase in echogenicity.[41,43]

On MRI, endometriomas may be seen as adnexal cysts with high signal on both T1W and T2W images or high signal on T1 and low signal on T2W images (T2 shading) with indistinct margins due to adhesions **(Figs. 18A to C)**. Evaluation of adhesions is difficult and these may be seen as low signal intensity stranding that obscures organ interfaces, posterior displacement of uterus, kissing ovaries, angulated bowel loops, an elevated posterior vaginal fornix, loculated fluid collections, and hydro/hematosalpinx **(Fig. 19)**. Hormonal therapy is occasionally used to treat endometriosis and shading on T2W images is the most important negative predictor for volume reduction with medical treatment, such therapy should be discontinued should low T2 signal be seen in a case on hormonal treatment. It is important to remember that small implants and adhesions that may cause infertility are not well visualized by any imaging technique. Laparoscopy remains the gold standard for diagnosis and staging of endometriosis and is also the mainstay for diagnosis.[10,15]

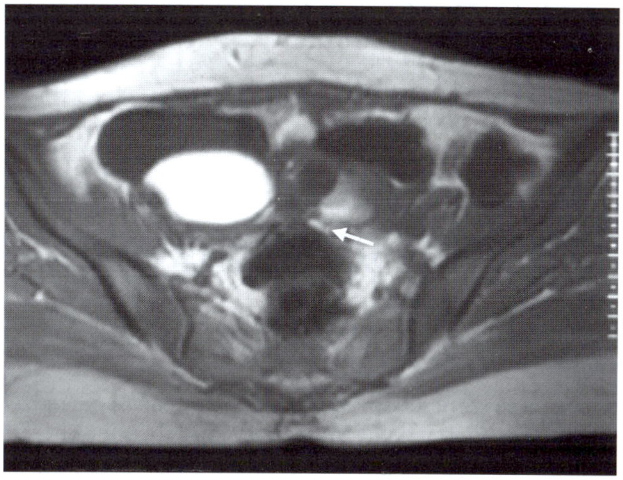

FIG. 19: T1W MR image reveals bilateral adnexal cysts with high signal due to hemorrhage and angulation of the anterior rectal surface due to adhesions (arrow).

Genital Tuberculosis

About 18% of female infertility in India is attributed to genital tuberculosis.[44] Tuberculosis commonly results in changes in the endometrium, the fallopian tubes, and pelvic peritoneum.

Scarring in uterine tuberculosis is well demonstrated by HSG. This can take few specialized forms namely: T-shaped uterus, asymmetric uterus, and pseudounicornuate uterus.[45] A significant number of patients with uterine tuberculosis show a T-shaped uterus and it is virtually diagnostic of this condition in the appropriate setting. A T-shaped uterus has usually been labelled as a DES uterus in the Western literature. The DES and the tuberculous uterus reveal irregular margins. However, tubal changes are not seen in DES uteri, but are mostly seen in T-shaped uteri due to tuberculosis. The normal uterine cavity shows a triangular configuration with straight or concave lateral walls. In tuberculous endometritis due to scarring along the long as well as the short axis of the uterus; this triangular shape is converted into a T shape.[45] DES was discontinued in the 1970s, so these cases are not seen now.

Scarring is also recognizable by the asymmetric uterine contour it produces. An asymmetric, small-sized uterine cavity is usually due to tuberculosis. Sometimes, the scarring may be more unilateral leading to obliteration of that part of the uterine cavity leading to a unicornuate uterus-like appearance—"the pseudounicornuate uterus". Comparison with previous films, laparoscopy, and awareness about this type of scarring would be essential in differentiating tuberculosis from a true unicornuate uterus. A good pointer towards endometrial tuberculosis is myometrial extravasation and/or venous intravasation. This finding in association with any other endometrial or tubal change **(Figs. 20 and 21)** is very suggestive of a tuberculous etiology of endometritis.[45]

OVARIAN FACTOR

Ovarian dysfunction accounts for up to 40% of infertility in women.[46] Adequate reproductive function requires normal ovarian follicular development, ovulation, and formation of functional CL. It is essential to evaluate these ovulatory factors while investigating infertility. TVS is an excellent imaging modality to evaluate the ovaries, which is used to detect

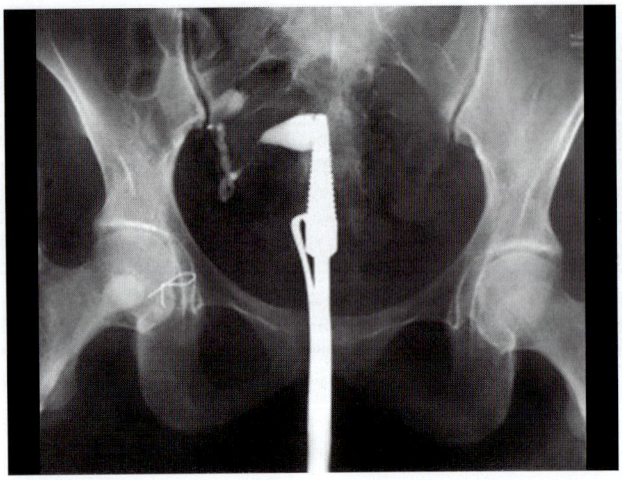

FIG. 20: A HSG showing a mildly dilated beaded right fallopian tube with evidence of loculated spill. Left tube is not visualized due to cornual block—sequelae of tuberculosis.

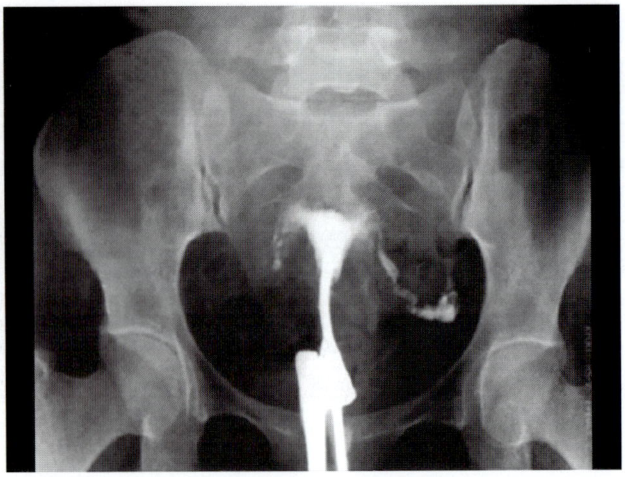

FIG. 21: HSG demonstrating a beaded left fallopian tube with no free spill. Only the proximal (isthmic and interstitial portion) of the right fallopian tube is visualized. Note the presence of myometrial extravasation suggestive of tubercular involvement.

both ovarian pathology and monitor ovulation. Functional ovarian cysts or other benign ovarian cysts and tumors like dermoid cysts or fibromata may occasionally interfere with ovarian function particularly when large. Endometriomas have already been discussed.

Gonadal Dysgenesis

Gonadal dysgenesis is a congenital condition characterized by abnormal gonadal organization and function. There is replacement of the gonadal tissue by fibrous stroma, no germ cells are present. The most common form of this condition is secondary to Turner syndrome. Diagnosis can be made on clinical, biochemical, and karyotype identification, imaging when performed demonstrates small oval to linear fibrous tissue within the broad ligament with absence of normal appearing ovaries, best seen on MRI, although detection is limited with the gonads found only in approximately 40–65% of cases.[16]

Polycystic Ovary Syndrome

Polycystic ovary syndrome (PCOS) is the most common cause of ovarian infertility. It is the most common endocrinopathy affecting women in the reproductive age group with prevalence between 8% and 13%.[47] PCOS is a complex disorder with reproductive, metabolic, and psychological features and is also known as Stein-Leventhal syndrome. Previously used criteria for PCOS on ultrasound include round, enlarged ovaries, with multiple small cysts, absence of cysts measuring more than 1.5 cm in diameter, smooth contours, and hyperechoic appearance of ovarian stroma.

The aim of imaging in PCOS is proper identification and documentation of presence of polycystic ovaries. In 2003, a joint ESHRE/ASRM meeting in Rotterdam created a definition for polycystic ovaries which was reaffirmed by the Androgen Excess and PCOS society in 2009 and then incorporated into the American College of Obstetricians and Gynecologists guidelines. Two criteria for identification of polycystic ovaries were acknowledged and these include 12 or more follicles measuring 2–9 mm in diameter in one or both ovaries and ovarian volume >10 cc.[48]

Reasons for revision of this diagnostic criteria include inadequate initial evidence, advances in ultrasound technology with greater resolution, lack of standard reporting, ill-defined cut-offs between normal ovaries and polycystic ovarian morphology, impact of approach (e.g. TVS), body habitus, and age. Natural changes in antral follicle count (AFC) occur during prepubertal and menopausal transitions and up to 70% adolescents have polycystic ovary morphology on original criteria **(Figs. 22A and B)**. Diagnosis of PCOS mandates not only polycystic ovarian morphology but presence of associated features of hyperandrogenism and/or ovulatory dysfunction. Recommendations from the international evidence-based guidelines for the assessment and management of PCOS were given in 2018. According to these, endovaginal ultrasound transducers with a frequency bandwidth that includes 8 MHz should be used and threshold for polycystic ovarian morphology should be on either ovary, a follicle number (follicle size measuring 2–9 mm) per ovary of more than or equal to 20 and/or volume more than or equal to 10 mL, ensuring no corpus lutea, cysts or dominant follicles are present **(Figs. 23 and 24)**. USG should not be used for the diagnosis of PCOS in <8 years after menarche as the incidence of multifollicular ovaries is high in this life stage. Threshold for polycystic ovary morphology should be revised regularly with advancing USG technology and age specific cut-off values for polycystic ovarian morphology should be defined.

In patients with irregular menstrual cycles and hyperandrogenism, USG is not essential for PCOS diagnosis, however, it identifies the complete PCOS phenotype. In transabdominal sonogram reporting is best focused on ovarian volume with threshold of more than or equal to 10 mL, given the difficulty of reliably assessing follicle number with this approach.

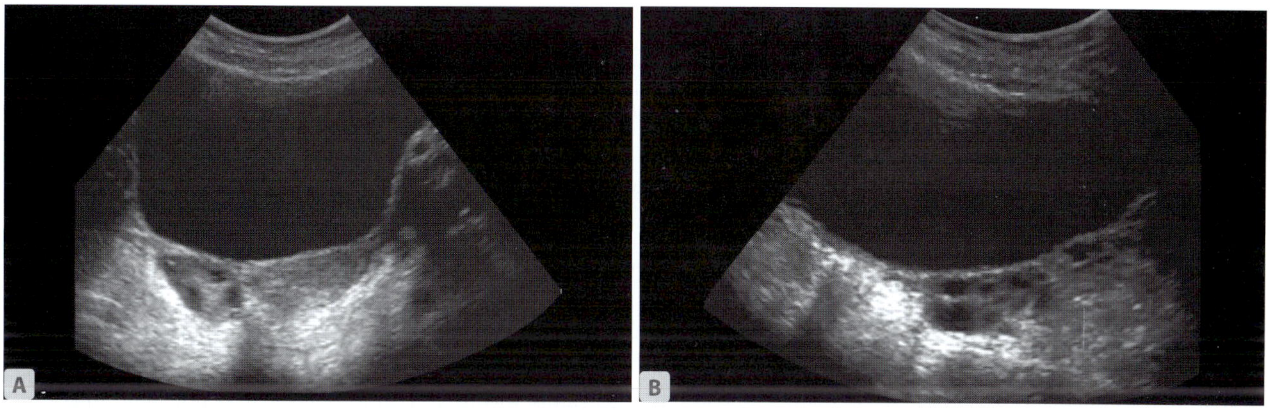

FIGS. 22A AND B: Multifollicular ovarian morphology seen in a prepubertal female.

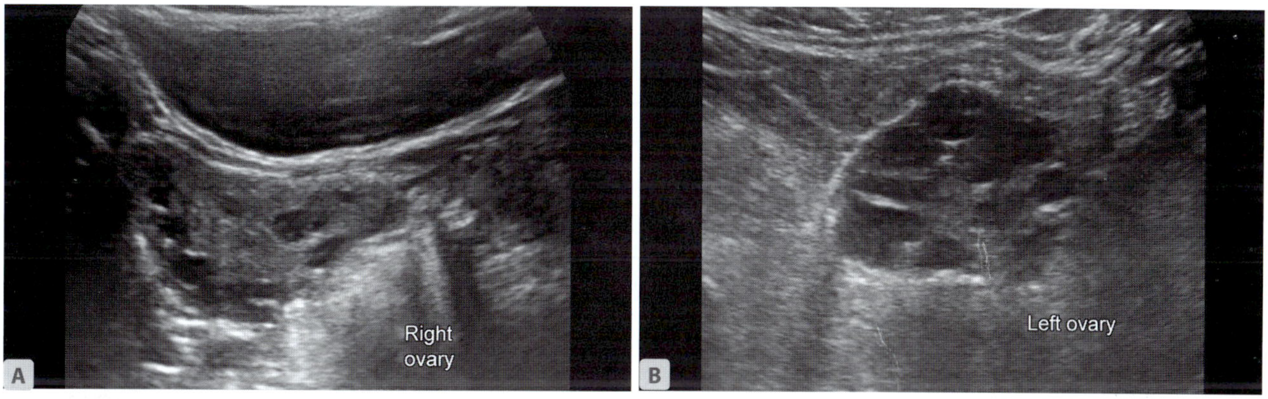

FIGS. 23A AND B: Ultrasound images reveal bilateral enlarged ovaries with multiple small follicles within. Note the peripherally arranged small follicles in the right ovary.

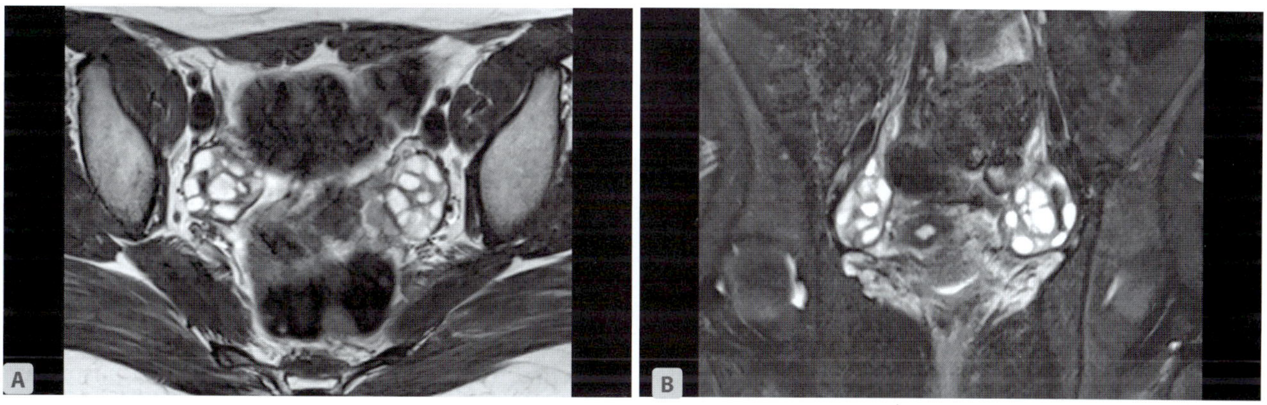

FIGS. 24A AND B: T2W (axial) and T2W fat saturated (coronal) images show bilateral enlarged ovaries showing multiple small follicles within.

The following factors are important to consider while reporting: last menstrual period, transducer bandwidth frequency, approach/route assessed, total follicle number per ovary measuring 2–9 mm, three dimensions and volume of each ovary, endometrial thickness and appearance, and other ovarian and uterine pathology. The presence of a thickened echogenic endometrium (due to estrogen excess) is also seen with PCOS.[47]

Ovulatory Function Tests

Ovulation can be monitored using basal body temperature recordings, endometrial biopsy (for documenting secretory changes in the endometrium), measurement of a serum progesterone (generally done 1 week before the expected onset of next menses), urinary LH determination using ovulation predictor kits to identify midcycle LH surge which occurs 1–2 days before ovulation and follicular monitoring using USG. The latter follows the development of the follicle till its disappearance and is the most accurate method for documentation of ovulation.

Development and Evolution of Ovarian Follicles

Ultrasonography is an excellent modality for monitoring the follicles during spontaneous and induced cycles. TVS is used for monitoring the follicles during ovarian induction using clomiphene citrate or human menopausal gonadotropin (hMG). This is done from the 7th day of the menstrual cycle and preferably on a daily basis, which can help in adjustment of the patient's medication. A follicle is considered mature when it measures 15–18 mm in mean diameter. Presence of fine echoes within the mature follicle is an indication of ovulation and is associated with serum estradiol value of 400 pg/mL or urine estrogen levels of 80–150 µg/day. Other features that help predict ovulation include sudden collapse of the preovulatory follicle, a loss of clearly defined follicular margins and increase in cul-de-sac fluid volume.

Follicular Monitoring: Spontaneous Cycles

Starting with menarche, during spontaneous cycles there is usually development of one or sometimes two dominant follicles. Sonography can show the developing follicles starting at the time measure 3–5 mm. In the spontaneous cycle, by unknown mechanisms, one or at the most two follicles develop to approximately 10 mm. At this time (about 7 days before LH surge), a dominant follicle takes over and there is a very little further growth of other follicles. Occasionally, two dominant follicles develop. During the 5 days prior to ovulation the dominant follicle grows at the rate of 2–3 mm/day. As a follicle reaches maturity, its inner dimensions range from 17 mm to 25 mm. However, within the same person the size of the mature follicle is relatively constant cycle to cycle.[5,49]

Follicular Monitoring: Induced Cycles

Ovulation induction is indicated in patients in whom infertility can be ascribed to an ovulation abnormality or anovulation. Ovulation induction or super ovulation therapy is also used in women with normal ovulation before assisted conception techniques such as IVF-ET or gamete intrafallopian transfer to increase the number of oocytes aspirated. This increases the number of fertilized conceptions that may be transferred thereby increasing the chances of pregnancy.[5,10]

Before starting treatment, a baseline scanning of the pelvis should be done. If one or more cysts, larger than approximately 2 cm in diameter are found, especially if accompanied by serum estradiol concentration of more than 100 pg/mL, it may interfere with treatment and induction may be postponed to the next cycle or cysts treated by aspiration.

The most commonly used medications for ovulation induction include clomiphene citrate, aromatase inhibitors (e.g. letrozole), and gonadotropins [FSH, LH, hMG, hCG]. Patients undergoing this treatment are usually examined every other day starting at day 10. Patients undergoing IVF-ET are examined by sonography starting earlier and usually daily in an attempt to carefully monitor their follicular development.

Clomiphene citrate is an estrogen antagonist, its action is to indirectly promote secretion of FSH and LH. In some patients ovulation occurs due to elevated serum levels of FSH and LH, without further therapy. In other patients, hCG may be required to induce ovulation. Follicular development with clomiphene citrate can be quite different from that seen in natural cycles. Each follicle seems to develop at an individual rate and at times may be accelerated or slowed down. Hence, the larger follicles on a given date may not be the same one that is the largest 2 days later and it may not even be the same one that is most mature. Furthermore, correlation of estradiol levels (E2) and follicle size is poor and maximum preovulatory diameter can range from 19 mm to 24 mm. In clomiphene stimulated cycles, the growth rate in the last few days preceding ovulation is higher.

In contrast to clomiphene citrate, treatment with hMG does not require an intact hypothalamic-pituitary axis. This contains both FSH and LH and induces follicle development. hCG is then administered to induce ovulation of mature follicles. The follicle growth can be evaluated by serial measurement of serum or urinary estradiol levels; however, multiple, small, and immature follicles may produce as much estradiol as a large mature follicle. Therefore, TVS is used to predict the optimal timing for giving an ovulation inducing dose of hCG.[8,50-52] Sonographic assessment of follicle size is critical because hCG is best administered once follicles reach 15–18 mm.[8]

Prediction of Ovulation

Follicular rupture occurs at a wide range of diameters between 2 cm and 2.7 cm. In the unstimulated ovary, follicles are approximately spherical. They may, however, be flattened in one plane by either pressure of the transducer or bladder so a mean of the maximum diameter in three planes is a better estimate of follicular size than measurements only in two planes.[5] In superovulation cycles, pressure from abutting follicles distorts the follicle so exact measurements are often difficult. Serial follicular measurement is best done by the same observer using the TVS route. In a recent study, assessment of follicular volume using 3D ultrasound was found to correlate better with oocyte retrieval than two-dimensional (2D) ultrasound alone. The authors found that a follicular size of >22 mm or a volume >5 mL was correlated with poor oocyte retrieval probably due to postmature follicle.[53]

Ovulation can also be predicted by noting collapse of a follicle that was previously seen, development of internal echoes within the follicle, crenation of follicular walls, visualization of cumulus, perifollicular halo, and visualization of fluid in the cul-de-sac (if not previously seen). However, fluid may commonly be seen in the pouch of Douglas in the periovulatory period and only a small percentage of women have a detectable increase with ovulation. Contrary to popular belief, ovulation need not alternate between two ovaries. Unfortunately, the variable appearance of ovulation makes the use these of ultrasound signs problematic in the management of infertility.[5]

Ultrasound Doppler studies reveal an increase in blood flow to the ovary carrying the dominant follicle[54-57] (and later, the CL)—an increase that precedes other indicators of follicular dominance. With maturation of the follicle, increased flow is directed to the follicle itself within the dominant ovary. Intrafollicular neovascularization occurs over the hours preceding ovulation and becomes massive after follicular collapse as blood vessels invade the luteinizing follicular (or granulosa) cells and the CL forms and impedance in intraovarian arterioles drops while velocities reach up to 40 cm/sec. These changes do not occur in nonovulatory cycles. A study was undertaken to investigate, if corpus luteal function could be improved by increasing CL blood flow in women with luteal phase defect (LPD) and high CL-RI (≥0.51).[58] They concluded that vitamin E or L-arginine treatment improved luteal function by decreasing CL blood flow impedance.

Ovarian Reserve

Ovarian reserve describes the reproductive potential as a function of the number and quality of oocytes. Diminished ovarian reserve refers to women of reproductive age group having regular menses whose response to ovarian stimulation or fecundity is reduced as compared to those women of comparable age.

Various tests utilized to assess ovarian reserve include cycle-day 3 serum FSH and estradiol measurements (high values of >10–20 IU/L have been found to be associated with poor ovarian stimulation and failure to conceive) and the clomiphene citrate challenge test (CCCT), which involves serum FSH evaluation before and after treatment with clomiphene citrate (100 mg daily, days 5–9 of cycle) on day 3 and day 10. Elevated FSH concentration after this test suggests diminished ovarian reserve.[59] Other and more frequently done tests include AFC and serum anti-Müllerian hormone (AMH) levels.

Serum AMH Level

Serum AMH is produced by the granulosa cells of the antral follicles and is a marker for ovarian reserve. Its levels remain stable throughout the menstrual cycle and therefore it can be evaluated on any day of the cycle. Low AMH levels (<1 ng/mL) have been associated with poor responses to ovarian stimulation, poor embryo quality, and poor pregnancy outcomes in IVF.[59]

Antral Follicle Count

Antral follicle count (AFC) is a good surrogate marker for evaluating ovarian reserve. AFC is used for work up of infertility and assisted reproduction techniques, prediction of risk of menopause and to raise doubt of ovulatory dysfunction secondary to hyperandrogenism anovulation.

Four different types of follicles are found in the ovary at distinct stages of development—primordial, primary, secondary, and tertiary (or antral). The first three stages are too small to be visualized on USG. The antral follicles are identified by USG when they reach 2 mm in diameter, coinciding with higher sensitivity to FSH. Antral follicles measuring between 2 mm and 10 mm are "recruitable" while antral follicles >10 mm are "dominant follicles". AFC includes follicles that have a mean diameter varying from 2 mm to 10 mm.[60]

The follicles should preferably be counted in the early follicular phase of the menstrual cycle, however, it may be performed at any time of the menstrual cycle. It is important to consider that counting follicles in the early follicular phase is simpler as this decreases the chance of presence of an ovarian cyst or CL, which may mask some of the follicles. AFC <5–7 is associated with small number of oocytes retrieved and reduced pregnancy rate, whereas AFC more than or equal to 20 is associated with risk of ovarian hyperstimulation syndrome (OHSS).[60]

Indications for counting ovarian follicles include the following:
- Woman >35 years of age attempting pregnancy for >6 months
- Risk for diminished ovarian reserve—history of cancer treatment with gonadotoxic drugs or history of irradiation
- Surgery for endometriosis.

Antral follicle count can be performed with both 2D and 3D-USG.

Real-time Two-dimensional Ultrasonography

Transvaginal sonography is performed and after centering the ovary on screen, all the follicular structures measuring between 2 mm and 10 mm in diameter are identified and counted. Only one measurement is needed for round follicles and the mean of two diameters is calculated for oval follicles. Imaging quality can be improved by using tissue harmonic imaging. Real-time 2D USG requires the presence of the patient during the entire span of examination as follicular dimensions are obtained one at a time. However, real-time imaging helps in distinguishing between a follicle and parovarian cysts/hydrosalpinx and with Doppler a vascular structure can be differentiated from a follicle. In cine loop 2D USG, a single continuous sweep of each ovary is performed and the loops are saved and images can be analyzed. This shortens the duration of examination. The loops can be replayed and assessed in case of any doubt.[60]

Three-dimensional Manual Mode

Using the 3D manual mode, AFC can be performed while visualizing three perpendicular planes simultaneously. Automatic acquisition of the ovaries occurs and the volumes are stored and studied using the three orthogonal planes simultaneously. Cross-linking of follicles in different planes provides better reliability compared with 2D methods. Volume contrast imaging (VCI) is a 3D US tool that helps to improve contrast enhancement and speckle suppression, enabling better definition between tissues and/or organs and improves the contrast between fluid and surrounding structures. Inversion mode enables visualization of 3D arrangement of follicles and all of them can be seen at the same time. However, this is time consuming and requires specifically trained observers.

Sono Automated Volume Calculations (SonoAVC)

SonoAVC is a semi-automated technique that permits counting and measuring of diameters and volumes of anechoic structures within a particular region of interest of an acquired 3D dataset. Manual postprocessing may be required to include unidentified follicles and to exclude extraovarian structures or tissue that have been inaccurately identified as follicles. This requires particular ultrasound systems and specifically trained sonologists **(Figs. 25A and B)**.[60] **Table 2** lists the interpretation of AFC.

Luteinized Unruptured Follicle

The CL formed after ovulation may have a variety of ultrasound appearances. It may be imperceptible from the surrounding ovarian stroma, it may show a small cystic component with echoes or may be large (>40 mm) and be hemorrhagic.[5]

Failure to detect follicular collapse but with infilling of the follicle suggests luteinization without ovulation. The luteinized unruptured follicle (LUF) syndrome occurs more commonly in infertile patients than in fertile patients and may be a cause of unexplained infertility. However, ultrasound diagnosis has a 15% false positive rate. Great care should be taken in diagnosing this condition because ovulation may be associated with an increase in size of follicles and these cystic corpora lutea may indicate a conception cycle.

Ovarian Hyperstimulation Syndrome

Ovarian hyperstimulation syndrome is a potentially life-threatening complication of ovulation induction or ovarian stimulation. It occurs during the luteal phase of menstrual cycle or in early pregnancy and mostly follows administration of endogenous or exogenous LH or hCG. It occurs after hCG administration to patient with a large number of immature follicles and high serum estradiol levels and is more likely to occur in those with a polycystic ovarian morphology.

Ovarian hyperstimulation syndrome results when hyperstimulation of the ovaries is associated with an aberration of the fluid balance. It is characterized by third-space fluid accumulation and electrolyte abnormalities. The severity of the syndrome is variable, but it is usually more severe if pregnancy follows ovulation. The clinical features that cause concern are: nausea, vomiting, ascites, and pleural and pericardial effusion. These worsen hemoconcentration causing hyperviscosity and hypercoagulability which predispose to thrombosis, embolism, and renal failure.

On imaging, symmetric enlargement of bilateral ovaries is seen which contain multiple cystic areas of varying sizes which represent enlarged follicles or corpus luteal cysts in the presence of ascites. The "spoke wheel" appearance has been described with peripherally located follicles surrounding a central core of ovarian stroma. The cysts are usually anechoic but may contain hemorrhage **(Figs. 26A and B)**. On MRI, the cysts are hypointense on TIW images and hyperintense on T2W images. The enlarged ovaries can be differentiated from ovarian neoplasms by absence of any abnormal enhancing soft tissue in or around the

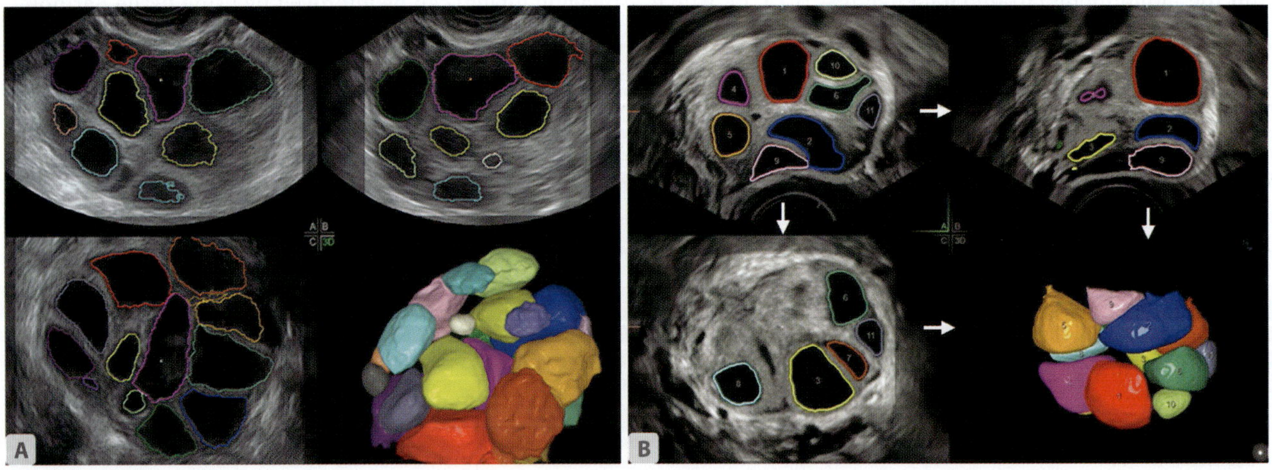

FIGS. 25A AND B: Sono AVC mode shows individual identification and automated volume calculation of the follicles, each depicted in a different color.

TABLE 2: Interpretation of AFC.

Nomenclature	Total AFC	Interpretation for ovarian stimulation
Very low functional reserve or very small number of recruitable follicles	0–4	Very high risk of poor response to ovarian stimulation and reduced chance of pregnancy
Low functional reserve or small number of recruitable follicles	5–8	High risk of poor response to ovarian stimulation
Normal functional reserve or normal number of recruitable follicles	9–19	Expected normal response to ovarian stimulation
High functional reserve or large number of recruitable follicles	>20	High risk of excessive ovarian response and OHSS

(AFC: antral follicle count; OHSS: ovarian hyperstimulation syndrome)

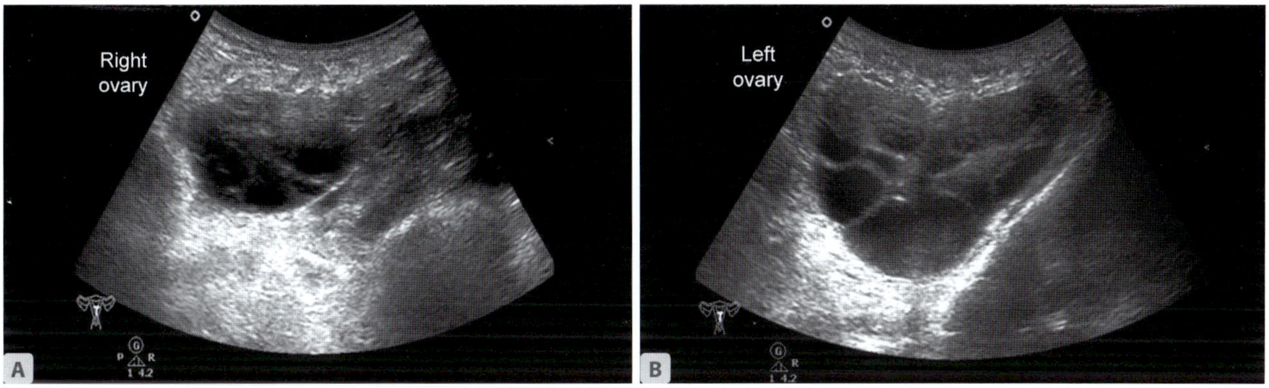

FIGS. 26A AND B: Transvaginal scans of both ovaries in a patient on ovulation induction reveals enlarged ovaries with a myriad of cysts varying in size consistent with ovarian hyperstimulation syndrome.

TABLE 3: Modified Golan classification scheme for ovarian hyperstimulation syndrome.

Category	Ovarian size (cm)	Grade	Signs and symptoms
Mild	<6	I	Abdominal distension
		II	Abdominal distension, nausea, vomiting, and diarrhea
Moderate	6–12	III	Abdominal distension, nausea, vomiting, diarrhea, ascites at USG, and weight gain
Severe	>12	IV	Ascites/hydrothorax
		V	Ascites/hydrothorax, hypovolemia, hemoconcentration, coagulation disorder, and oliguria, shock

TABLE 4: Acronyms used in assisted conception.

IVF	Recovered eggs are fertilized with prepared sperm in the laboratory and transferred back to the genital tract after usually several days' culture.
IUI	Washed and concentrated sperms are placed inside the uterus around the time of ovulation to facilitate fertilization.
GIFT	Recovered eggs are almost immediately transferred, with prepared sperm, into the fallopian tubes, so that fertilization and early development occur in the normal situation; generally, a higher pregnancy rate than after IVF, provided the tube used is normal and normal sperm function can be assumed.
ZIFT	IVF in which 1 day fertilized eggs, or zygotes, are transferred to the fallopian tube.
Uterine ET	Conventional procedure with IVF: 2-day pre-embryos are transferred through the cervix to the endometrial cavity.
FET, FrET	Transfer of IVF pre-embryos previously cryostored.
TEST	2-day IVF pre-embryos are transferred to the tube instead of the uterus.
ICSI	Laboratory refinement for IVF in cases of severely depressed sperm function, in which a single sperm is selected and microinjected into each egg.
MESA	A means of obtaining sperm for ICSI in men with obstructive azoospermia.
TESE	A means of obtaining sperm cells from testicular tubules for ICSI in some men with nonobstructive azoospermia.

IVF: *in vitro* fertilization; IUI: intrauterine insemination ; GIFT: gamete intrafallopian transfer; ZIFT: zygote intrafallopian transfer; ET: embryo transfer; FET, FrET: frozen embryo transfer; TEST: tubal embryo-stage transfer; ICSI: intracytoplasmic sperm injection; MESA: microepididymal sperm aspiration; TESE: testicular sperm extraction

cystic ovarian mass and the normal central ovarian stroma should be recognizable. Other imaging features related to complications associated with OHSS include pleural effusion, ascites, and thromboembolism. Gradual decrease in the size and number of cysts, resolution of the ascites, and pleural effusions may be seen on follow up scans.[61]

Ovarian hyperstimulation syndrome is classified according to the modified Golan classification scheme as shown in **Table 3**.

Mild and moderate OHSS is seen with clomiphene induction whereas the severe form is rarely seen in this situation.

A similar appearance of bilateral enlarged ovaries with multiple cysts resulting in a "spoke wheel" appearance can be seen with *theca lutein cysts*. They develop in response to raised levels of beta-hCG that occur with complete molar pregnancy. They may also be seen with singleton or multiple pregnancy or fetal hydrops.[62]

TREATING INFERTILITY

Increasingly assisted conception with IVF or one of its related therapeutic modalities is being used to treat infertility. These acronyms are summarized in **Table 4**.[36]

Follicle Aspiration

In the first successful IVF, oocytes were collected during laparoscopy which is an expensive procedure associated with complications such as periovarian adhesions, hemorrhage, infection, etc.

Ultrasound directed follicle aspiration (UDFA) has reduced costs considerably and can be done as an outpatient technique. Various approaches have been used in the past for follicular aspiration including direct transabdominal, transabdominal through full bladder, transvaginal, transvesical, and per-urethral approach.[5] Oocyte collection using TVS, first described by Wikland in 1985 has become the technique of choice, however, the actual method used can be tailored according to each patient depending on where the ovaries are situated. With all these aspiration techniques, a long (30 cm) 18-gauge needle is used that is scored at the tip, which results in its enhanced sonographic visualization. The procedure for follicle aspiration is performed under local anesthesia and with supplemental intravenous or intramuscular medication.

A needle guide is secured with the transvaginal transducer for aspiration through the transvaginal approach. This permits the needle to transverse in the beam path of the transducer. The cursor is seen on the scanning screen, which indicates the path of the needle. A condom containing sterile gel is placed over the transducer and a sterile needle guide is attached to it, the operator then manipulates the transducer to delineate the ovary optimally. The desired follicle is focused into the "line of sight" and the needle is introduced through the transvaginal route. After the initial aspiration, the follicle may be filled with buffered medium and flushed so that there are maximum chances of retrieving a mature oocyte. The technique has been associated with low complication rates that include vaginal hemorrhage and pelvic infection. When a transvesical or transurethral approach is used postoperative clot retention or occasionally urine extravasation may occur.

Transabdominal ultrasound-guided follicular aspiration is considered a safe option in women with ovaries that are not accessible by TVS. This approach is used in women with history of laparoscopic or pelvic laparotomy surgery, transposed ovaries, PCOS, fibroids, and Müllerian agenesis. Increased use of this approach due to increasing BMI in some populations has also been reported. No significant difference between pregnancy rates and associated complications was seen between transabdominal ultrasound and transvaginal ultrasound procedures.

Ultrasound has also been used to guide ET to the uterine cavity, to assist accurate placement of the embryos in the uterine cavity rather than cervical canal.

CONCLUSION

The causes of female infertility include abnormalities involving the uterus, cervix, tubes, peritoneum, and ovaries. Imaging plays a valuable role in evaluation of infertility and a multimodality approach is essential to establish the cause of infertility and guide further management and treatment. HSG is usually the initial investigation to be performed to assess for tubal patency, which may be followed by pelvic ultrasound, pelvic MRI or both as required. Imaging is also vital for guidance in various reproductive techniques such as oocyte collection and gamete transfer IVF programs.

REFERENCES

1. Pfeifer S, Goldberg J, Lobo R, et al. Definitions of infertility and recurrent pregnancy loss: a committee opinion. Practice Committee of American Society for Reproductive Medicine. Fertil Steril. 2013;99(1):63.
2. Jeelani R, Puscheck EE. Imaging and the Infertility Evaluation. Clin Obstet Gynecol. 2017;60(1):93-107.
3. Simpson WL, Beitia LG, Mester J. Hysterosalpingography: A reemerging study. Radiographics. 2006;26:419-31.
4. Speroff L, Fritz MA. Female Infertility. In: Speroff L, Fritz MA (Eds). Clinical gynecologic endocrinology and infertility, 7th edition. Philadelphia: Lippincott Williams and Wilkins; 2005. pp. 1013-67.
5. Steer CV, Parsons JH. Infertility. In: Dewbury K, Meire H, Cosgrove D, Farrant P (Eds). Ultrasound in Obstetrics and Gynaecology, 2nd Edition. London: Churchill Livingstone; 2001. pp. 99-122.
6. Hill LM. Transvaginal Sonography in an assisted conception program. In: Anderson JC (Ed). Gyneologic Imaging. London: Churchill Livingstone; 1999. pp. 585-99.
7. Saunders RD, Shwayder JM, Nakajima ST. Current methods of tubal patency assessment. Fertil Steril. 2011;95(7):2171-9.
8. Collins JI, Woodward PJ. Radiological evaluation of infertility. Semin Ultrasound CT MR. 1995;16(4):304-16.
9. Jaffe SB, Jewlewicz R. The basic infertility investigation. Fertil Steril. 1991;56:599-613.
10. ASRM Practice Committee. Optimal evaluation of the infertile female. Fertil Steril. 2006;86(4):264-7.
11. Glatstein IZ, Harlow BL, Hornstein MD. Practice patterns among reproductive endocrinologists: further aspects of the infertility evaluation. Fertile Steril. 1998;70:263-9.
12. Baldauf JJ, Dreyfus M, Wertz JP, et al. Consequences and treatment of cervical stenoses after laser conization or loop electrosurgical excision. J Gynecol Obstet Biol Reprod. 1997;26:64-70.
13. Christianson MS, Barker MA, Lindheim SR. Overcoming the challenging cervix: techniques to access the uterine cavity. J Low Genit Tract Dis. 2008;12:24-31.
14. Krysiewicz S. Infertility in Women: Diagnostic evaluation with hysterosalpingography and other imaging techniques. Am J Roentgenol. 1992;159:253-61.
15. Thurmond AS. Imaging of female infertility. Radiol Clin N Am. 2003;41:757-67.
16. Kaproth-Joslin K, Dogra V. Imaging of female infertility: a pictorial guide to the hysterosalpingography, ultrasonography and magnetic resonance imaging findings of the congenital and acquired causes of female infertility. Radiol Clin North Am. 2013;51(6):967-81.
17. Dudiak CM, Turner DA, Patel SK, et al. Uterine leiomyomas in the infertile patient: Preoperative localization with MR imaging versus US and hysterosalpingography. Radiol. 1988;167:627-30.
18. Woodward PJ. Wagner BJ, Farley TE. MR imaging in the evaluation of female infertility. Radiographics. 1993;13:293-310.

19. Vickramarajah S, Stewart V, Ree K, et al. Subfertility: What the Radiologist Needs to Know? Radiographics. 2017;37:1587-602.
20. Grimbizis GF, Gordts S, Sardo ADS, et al. The ESHRE/ESGE consensus on the classification of female genital tract congenital anomalies. Hum Reprod. 2013;28(8):2032-44.
21. Steinkeler JA, Woodfield CA, Lazarus E, et al. Female infertility: a Systematic approach to Radiologic Imaging and Diagnosis. Radiographics. 2009;29:1353-70.
22. Olphin JD, Heilbrum M. Imaging of Müllerian duct anomalies Clin Obstet Gynaecol. 2007;52(1):40-56.
23. Deutch TD, Abuhamad AZ. The role of 3D-USG and MR imaging in the diagnosis of MDA: a review of literature. J Ultrasound Med. 2008;27(3):413-23.
24. Ludwin A, Martins WP, Nastri CO, et al. Congenital Uterine Malformations by Experts (CUME): better criteria for distinguishing between normal/arcuate and septate uterus? Ultrasound Obstet Gynecol. 2018;51(1):101-9.
25. Kunz G, Beil D, Huppert P, et al. Adenomyosis in endometriosis: prevalence and impact on fertility. Evidence from magnetic resonance imaging. Hum Reprod. 2005;20:2309-16.
26. Park HJ, Kim YS, Yoon TK, et al. Chronic endometritis and infertility. Clin Exp Reprod Med. 2016;43(4):185-92.
27. Khan MS, Shaikh A, Ratnani R. Ultrasonography and Doppler Study to Predict Uterine Receptivity in Infertile Patients Undergoing Embryo Transfer. J Obstet Gynaecol India. 2016;66(1):377-82.
28. Tekay A, Martikainen H, Jouppilas P. The clinical value of transvaginal colour Doppler ultrasound in assisted reproductive technology procedures. Hum Reprod. 1996;11(8):1589-91.
29. Dev G, Ilyas M, Khurana A. Calcific endometritis as a cause of infertility: Ultrasonography as the main diagnostic modality. Egypt J Radiol Nucl Med. 2016;47(3):1133-6.
30. Thurmond AS, Novy MJ, Rosch J. Terburaline in diagnosis of interstitial fallopian tube obstruction. Invest Radiol. 1988;23:209-10.
31. Sulak PJ, Letterie, GS, Coddington CC, et al. Histology of proximal tubal occlusion. Fertil Steril. 1987;48:437-40.
32. Thurmond AS. Selective salpingography and fallopian tube recanalization. Am J Roentgenol. 1991;156:33-8.
33. Rösch J. Thurmond AS, Vchida BT, et al. Selective transcervical fallopian tube catherterization: Technique update. Radiol. 1988;168:1-5.
34. Thurmond AS, Rösch J. Nonsurgical fallopian tube recanalization for treatment of infertility. Radiol. 1990;174:371-4.
35. National Institute for Health and Care Excellence. (2004). Fallopian tube recanalisation by guidewire: guidance and guidelines. [online] Available from: https://www.nice.org.uk/guidance/ipg71. [Last accessed November, 2019].
36. Jansen RPS, Ramsay PA. Imaging in gynecologic infertility. In: Anderson JC (Ed). Gynecologic Imaging. London: Churchill Livingstone; 1999. pp. 567-80.
37. Strandell A, Waldenstrom U, Nilsson L, et al. Hydrosalpinx reduces *in vitro* fertilization/embryo transfer pregnancy rates. Hum Reprod. 1994;9:861-3.
38. Andersen AN, Yue Z, Meng FJ, et al. Low implantation rate after in-vitro fertilization in patients with hydrosalpinges diagnosed by ultrasonography. Hum Reprod. 1994;9:1935-8.
39. Donnez J, Casanas–Roux E. Prognostic factors of fimbrial microsurgery. Fertil Steril. 1986;46:200-4.
40. Valentini AL, Muzuil L, Marana R. Improvement of hysterosalpingographic accuracy in the diagnosis of peritubal adhesions. AJR. 2000;175:1173-6.
41. Krysiewicz S. Infertility in women: Diagnostic evaluation with hysterosalpingography and other imaging techniques. AJR. 1992;158:253-61.
42. Schenken RS. Endometriosis. In: Scott JR, Di Saia PJ, Hammona CB, Spellacy WN (Eds). Danforth's Obstetrics and Gynaecology, 8th edition. Philadelphia, PA: Lippincott Williams and Wilkins; 1999. pp. 669-75.
43. Imaka I, Wada A, Matsuo M, et al. MR imaging of disorders associated with female infertility: use in diagnosis, treatment and management. Radiographics. 2003;23:1401-21.
44. Das P, Ahuja A, Gupta SD. Incidence, etiopathogenesis and pathological aspects of genitourinary tuberculosis in India: a journey revisited. Indian J Urol. 2008;24:356-61.
45. Merchant SA. Tuberculosis of the genitourinary system. Ind J Radiol Imag. 1993;3:253-74.
46. Quaas A, Dokras A. Diagnosis and Treatment of unexplained infertility. Rev Obstet Gynecol. 2008;1(2): 69-76.
47. Teede HJ, Misso ML, Costello MF, et al. Recommendations from the international evidence-based guideline for the assessment and management of polycystic ovary syndrome. International PCOS Network. Hum Reprod. 2018;33(9):1602-18.
48. Lee TT, Rausch ME. Polycystic Ovarian Syndrome: Role of Imaging in Diagnosis. Radiographics. 2012;32:1643-57.
49. Fleischer AC, Daniell JF, Rodein J, et al. Sonographic monitoring of ovarian follicular development. J Clin Ultrasound. 1981;9:275-80.
50. Fleischer AC, Herbert CM, Hill GA, et al. Transvaginal sonography of the endometrium during induced cycles. J Ultrasound Med. 1991;10:93-5.
51. Haning RV, Zwiebel WJ. Ultrasound assistance in clinical management of infertility. Semin Ultrasound CT MR. 1983;4:226-34.
52. Hann LE, Crivello M, McArdle C, et al. In vitro fertilization: Sonographic perspective. Radiol. 1987;163:665-8.
53. Shmorgun D, Hughes E, Mohida P, et al. Prospective cohort study of three versus two dimensional ultrasound for prediction of oocyte maturity. Fertil Steril. 2010;93(4):1333-7 .
54. Campbell S, Bourne TH, Waterstone J, et al. Transvaginal colour blood flow imaging of the periovulatory follicle. Fertil Steril. 1993;60:433-8.
55. Taylor KJ, Wells PN, Conway DI, et al. Ultrasound Doppler flow studies of the ovarian and uterine arteries. Br J Obstet Gynaecol. 1985;92:240-6.
56. Deutinger J, Reinthaller A, Bernaschek G. Transvaginal pulsed Doppler measurement of blood flow velocity in the ovarian arteries during cycle stimulation and after follicle puncture. Fertil Steril. 1989;51:466-70.
57. Collins W, Jurkovic D, Bourne T, et al. Ovarian morphology, endocrine function and intrafollicular blood flow during the peri-ovulatory period. Hum Reprod. 1991;6:319-24.
58. Takasaki A, Tamura H, Taniguchi K, et al. Luteal blood flow and luteal function. J Ovarian Res. 2009;2:1.
59. Practice Committee of the American Society for Reproductive Medicine. Diagnostic evaluation of the infertile female: a committee opinion. Fertil Steril. 2015;103(6):e44-50.
60. Coelho Neto MA, Ludwin A, Borrell A, et al. Counting ovarian antral follicles by ultrasound: a practical guide. Ultrasound Obstet Gynecol. 2018;51(1):10-20.
61. Baron KT, Babagbemi KT, Arleo EK, et al. Emergent complications of assisted reproduction: expecting the unexpected. RadioGraphics. 2013;33:229-44.
62. Brown DL, Dudiak KM, Laing FC. Adnexal masses: US characterization and reporting. Radiol. 2010;254:342-54.

CHAPTER

19

Imaging Techniques and Radiological Anatomy of the Male Genital Tract

Anmol Bhatia, Paramjeet Singh, Sameer Vyas

MALE GENITAL TRACT

The male genital tract consists of the prostate, testes with epididymis, vas deferentia, seminal vesicles, and penis. The present chapter aims to discuss the various imaging techniques and the normal radiological anatomy of the organs constituting the male genital tract.

PROSTATE GLAND

Prostate gland is a pyramidal-shaped fibromuscular gland which surrounds the urethra from the bladder base up to the urogenital diaphragm. It has a thin capsule and is surrounded by fibrous sheath of pelvic fascia. Posterior to the prostate, paired seminal vesicles are present. The ejaculatory ducts penetrate the superior part along the posterior surface of the prostate gland and then open into the prostatic urethra along the lateral margin of the prostatic utricle. The prostate gland can be divided into two major zones—the peripheral and the central zones. The central gland comprises periurethral glandular tissue, and transitional and central zones.

IMAGING MODALITIES

Ultrasound

The prostate is routinely imaged using transabdominal and transrectal approaches. Transabdominally, a 3–5 MHz transducer is used with the full bladder acting as an acoustic window. The suprapubic approach allows for gross evaluation of the prostate size but does not provide images of sufficient quality to visualize the zonal anatomy **(Fig. 1)**.

Transrectal ultrasonography (TRUS) is the preferred sonological technique as it demonstrates the zonal anatomy, as well as helps in visualization of seminal vesicles and ejaculatory ducts. The most commonly used transducers (frequency ranging from 5 MHz to 8 MHz) fire from the end. The advantages of end-viewing probe designs include patient convenience, ease of use, and biopsy capability at the time of the diagnostic examination.

The patient is examined with empty bladder in the left lateral decubitus position with the knees flexed up to the abdomen. The probe is lubricated and covered by a rubber balloon or condom, and is then inserted gently into the rectum. In the sagittal plane, the gland is systematically evaluated from right to midline to left; while in the axial plane, cranial to caudal viewing is done from a plane starting cranially just superior to the prostate and extending caudally to the apex of the prostate. The central and peripheral zones form the bulk of prostate gland and appear uniformly hyperechoic with only subtle differentiation in their echogenicity. The hypoechoic periurethral area corresponds to the transitional zone **(Figs. 2A and B)**. The posterior urethra and its surrounding smooth muscle and glandular area appear relatively hypoechoic and can be quite prominent measuring up to 2 cm in diameter. Near the apex of the gland most of the tissue is the peripheral zone.

The seminal vesicles are paired, symmetric hypoechoic structures and seen cephalic to the base of prostate **(Fig. 3)**. They normally measure up to 1 cm in thickness, but sometimes may be of larger size in normal men.[1]

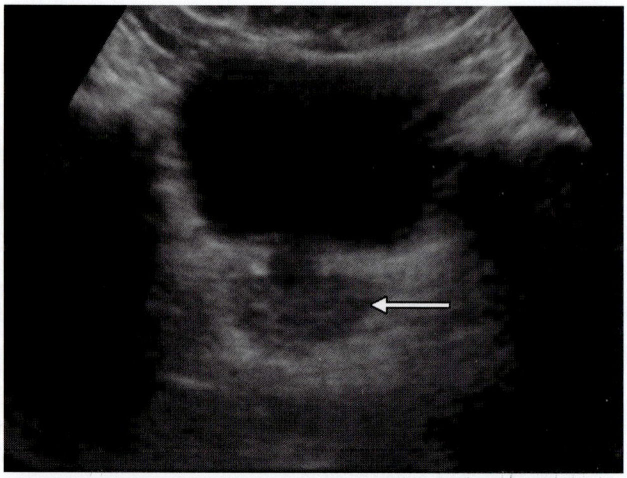

FIG. 1: Transabdominal axial scan showing a normal prostate gland (arrow) without any zonal demarcation behind the urinary bladder.

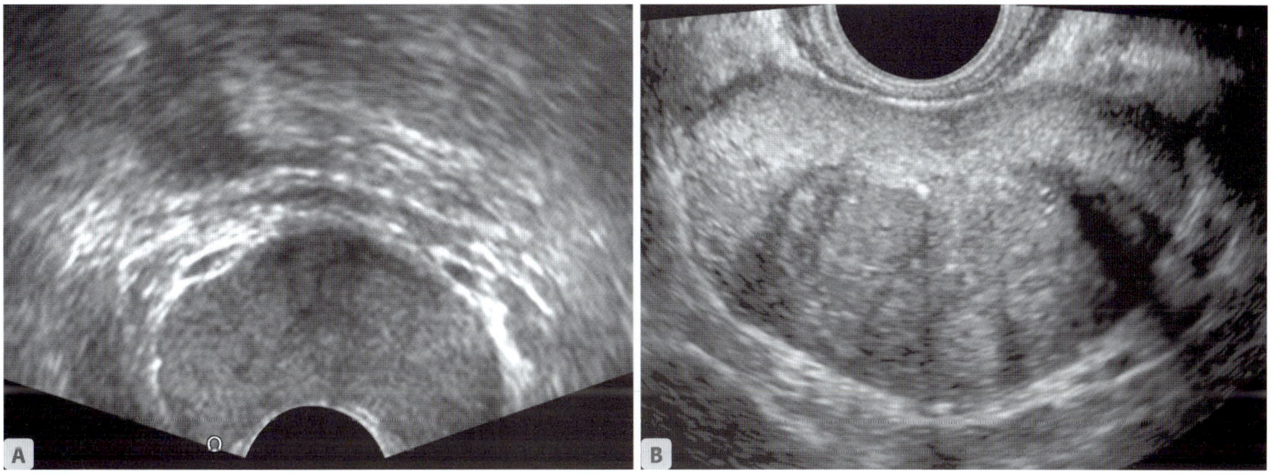

FIGS. 2A AND B: Transrectal axial images of normal prostate at midgland level in a young (A) and a middle age male (B). Demarcation of the central and peripheral zone is seen in middle age male.

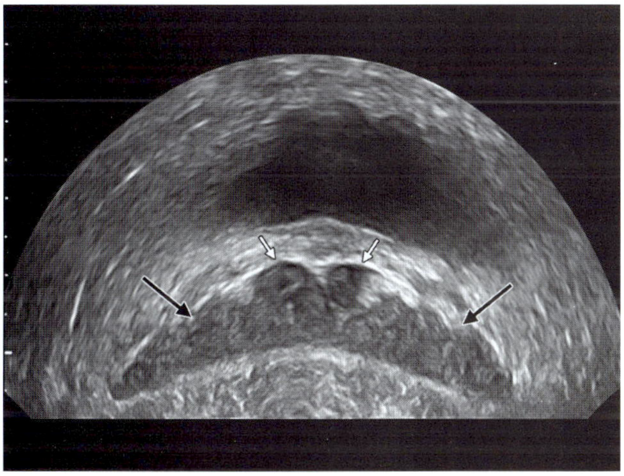

FIG. 3: Transrectal axial image showing paired seminal vesicles (black arrows) and vas (white arrows).

Prostatic volume can be calculated on transabdominal ultrasound and TRUS by using the Dodd's formula (0.523 × length × width × height).

Computed Tomography

Computed tomography is not a preferred modality to evaluate the prostate gland. A normal prostate appears as homogeneous hyperdense on CT. It is not possible to differentiate normal prostate from hyperplastic gland or detect the tumor which is limited to the prostate gland.

Magnetic Resonance Imaging

Magnetic resonance imaging (MRI) has a unique ability for delineating the zonal anatomy of the prostate gland.[2] The zonal anatomy is of clinical importance, as most carcinoma arises in the peripheral zone, while the benign hyperplasia affects the transition zone.[3] The relationship of the zones of the gland normally changes with age. The central gland predominantly consists of central zone in young population, whereas in older population with benign hyperplasia of prostate, most of the central gland is transitional zone. The prostate is described based on the division of the gland into thirds in the craniocaudal direction (base, midgland, and apex), and then into left and right side. Since surgery is potentially curable in a tumor confined to the gland, it is important to diagnose the extracapsular tumor spread, seminal vesicle, and other adjacent visceral involvement and pelvic lymphadenopathy. The primary role of MRI is not for tumor detection, but for staging diagnosed cancer. In addition, it helps in cancer localization, in treatment planning, and post-treatment follow-up.[3] MR spectroscopic examination is helpful for showing normal and altered tissue metabolism. Functional MR techniques on 3T-MRI such as diffusion-weighted images (DWI) and dynamic contrast-enhanced MRI have evolved as promising new techniques in the assessment of prostate cancer. Multimodality MRI which includes T2-weighted images (T2WI), functional imaging, and spectroscopic imaging may be able to accurately characterize and stage the carcinoma.[4]

Technique and Recommended Sequences

Magnetic resonance imaging provides one-stop examination for detailed evaluation of prostate gland, periprostatic and pelvic anatomy. The results of prostate imaging using body coil are not very satisfactory. Use of an endorectal coil along with a pelvic phased-array coil markedly improves the quality of images. A balloon-mounted endorectal coil placed in the rectum provides the best contrast and spatial resolution for prostate imaging, and the pelvic phased array coil provide good pelvic coverage and simultaneously assess pelvic side walls and lymphadenopathy.

Axial spin-echo T1-weighted images (T1WI) are taken of the entire pelvis, i.e. from the level of aortic bifurcation to the pubic symphysis for the detection of nodal disease.[5] High spatial resolution [thin sections with a small field of view (FOV)] T2W fast spin-echo (FSE) sections in the axial, coronal, and sagittal planes including prostate and seminal vesicles are useful for the detection of tumor, its localization, and staging. Axial T2WI is important in differentiating peripheral and central zones, whereas coronal and sagittal images are useful to assess the base and apex of the gland, pelvic muscles, rectum, and seminal vesicles.

Prostate imaging should not be performed for at least 4–8 weeks (preferably 6 weeks) of biopsy, as hemorrhage can lead to a false positive and negative interpretation of cancer. Routine use of gadolinium and fat suppression is not recommended. However, contrast may be used in evaluation of prostatic infections and abscesses. Enhancement of prostate cancer during the first pass of contrast during dynamic scanning has indicated its potential for the detection of cancer, especially the more aggressive ones. For dynamic contrast-enhanced MRI, the data may be evaluated in a semiquantitative (contrast arrival, time to peak, peak enhancement, and wash-in-washout gradient) or quantitative approach using pharmacokinetic modeling method. MR spectroscopy is performed by chemical shift imaging with point resolved spectroscopy voxel excitation and band selective inversion with gradient rephrasing for water and lipid suppression.[5] Diffusion imaging with value from 0 to 800 have been applied to obtain data and create apparent diffusion coefficient maps which show restriction in high cellularity of tumors.

Normal Appearance of Prostate on MRI

The appearance of prostate varies depending on the coil type and the technique used. On T1WI the zonal anatomy cannot be appreciated well and the gland is of uniform low signal intensity but postbiopsy hemorrhage is better seen in these images. T1WI also show cysts and abscesses well. The zonal anatomy is well-demonstrated on T2WI, where the peripheral zone is seen as a relatively bright area compared to the central gland[2] **(Figs. 4A and B)**. It is surrounded by a thin uninterrupted hypointense line comprising true prostatic capsule. The anterior fibromuscular stroma is dark on all pulse sequences **(Fig. 5)**. The central and transitional zones show intermediate signal due to sparse glandular elements. These cannot be differentiated from each other but in older men the transitional zone stands out due to hypertrophy. The verumontanum may be seen on T2WI, where it has high signal intensity. The anterior fibromuscular stroma is dark on all pulse sequences. The periprostatic fat is hyperintense on both T1WI and T2WI and allows easy assessment of periprostatic spread of growth. The pelvic bone marrow shows high signal. The neurovascular bundles are seen at 5 and 7 o'clock position on axial images and are outlined by periprostatic fat,

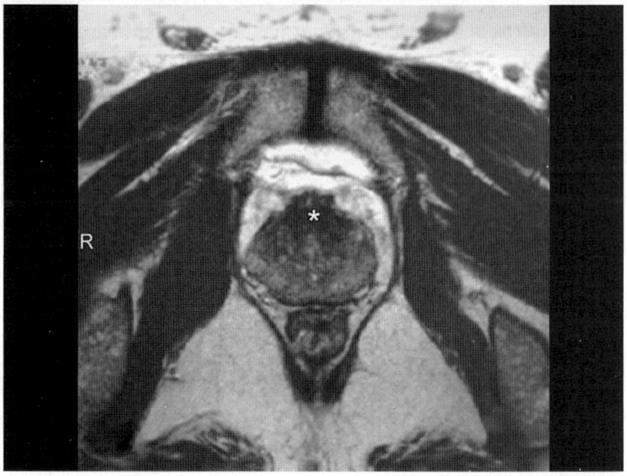

FIG. 5: T2-weighted axial section in a young adult. The gland does not show central and peripheral zone distinction or any hyperplastic central gland changes. The fibromuscular stroma anteriorly appears hypointense (*).

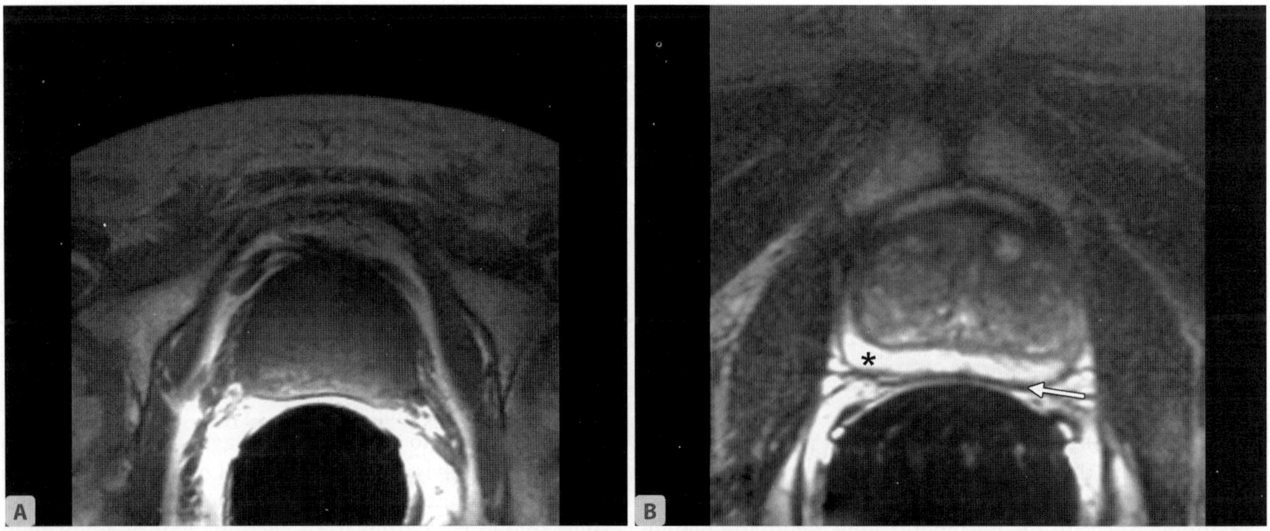

FIGS. 4A AND B: T1 (A) and T2 (B) weighted axial sections of prostate using endorectal coil. The zonal anatomy of prostate is not made out on T1 but the gland contour is well-outlined against bright periprostatic fat. The neurovascular bundle (arrow) is seen at 5 and 7 o'clock positions. T2WI (B) shows zonal anatomy, i.e. hyperintense peripheral gland (*) and heterogeneous central zone due to hyperplastic changes. The bright nodule represents glandular hyperplasia and dark areas being stromal hyperplasia. The surgical and anatomical capsules are seen as hypointense structures. The near field signal amplification is seen in proximity of the coil.

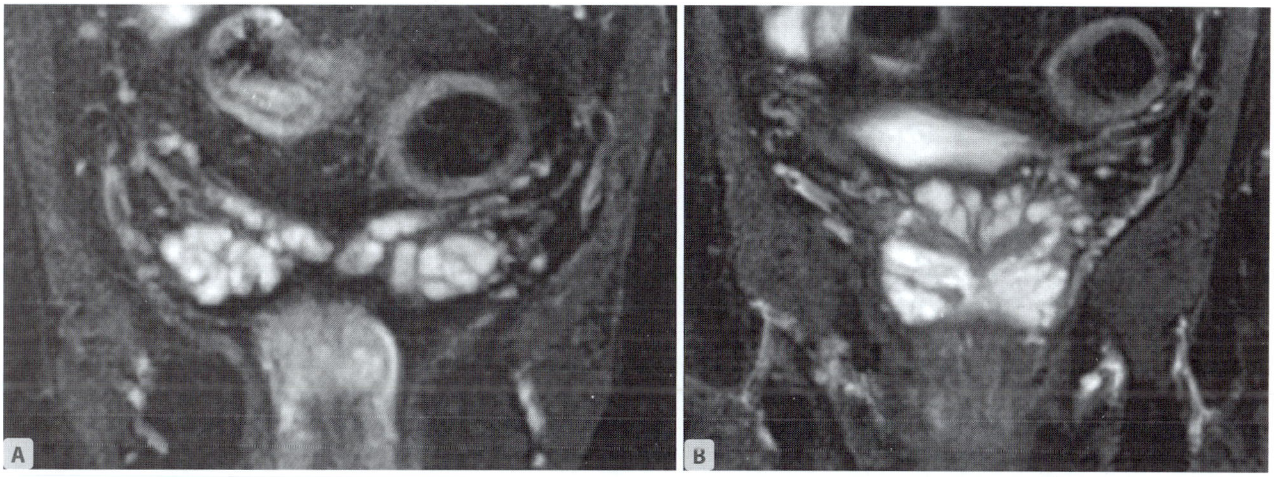

FIGS. 6A AND B: Coronal T2 images showing junction of the vas deferens and the seminal vesicle (A) both appearing normally bright due to fluid. More anteriorly (B) the ejaculatory ducts are seen approaching the verumontanum, where they open into the urethra.

pelvic fascia, and muscles.[2] The seminal vesicles and vas can be well seen on in both the axial and coronal planes **(Figs. 6A and B)**. Seminal vesicle fluid appears bright on T2WI due to water content, while the walls are hypointense. Loss of signal in these structures indicate invasion by malignancy. The prostate volume can be assessed on MR images by using the Dodd's formula.

Prostate spectroscopic examination shows relative concentrations of citrate, creatinine, choline, and polyamines inside the contiguous voxels. Normal prostate tissue shows high levels of citrate **(Fig. 7)**.[5] High field strength imaging may improve the quality of the spectra.

SCROTUM AND PENIS

The scrotum consists of skin, muscle and fascial layers, and the tunica vaginalis. The tunica vaginalis is a two-layered serous membrane which develops from the processus vaginalis during the development. The outer parietal layer forms the inner lining of the scrotum, while the inner visceral layer encloses the testis and epididymis.[6]

The penis contains paired corpora cavernosa dorsally and a midline corpus spongiosum ventrally. Tunica albuginea which is a fascial sheath surrounds both the corpus spongiosum and the corpora cavernosa. The corpora cavernosa contains venous sinusoids which are filled with blood during erection. The deep cavernosal arteries run centrally through the length of each corpus cavernosum with dorsal arteries lying superficially. The dorsal vein of the penis lies between the two dorsal arteries. The corpus spongiosum encases the penile urethra and forms the glans penis distally.[6]

IMAGING MODALITIES

Ultrasound

A high-frequency (7.5–15 MHz) linear probe is used for scanning the scrotum and penis.

Normal Appearance

The layers of the normal scrotal wall cannot be identified separately on ultrasound and are seen as a single 5–7 mm thick hyperechoic stripe. The testis is seen as an ovoid structure with homogeneous granular echotexture having medium level echoes surrounded by an echogenic capsule **(Fig. 8)**. The mediastinum testis (which is a longitudinal condensation of fibrous tissue on one side of the testis) is seen as a thin echogenic band on the same side as the epididymis with fine hypoechoic strands of septa radiating from it into the testicular parenchyma **(Fig. 9)**. The appearance of mediastinum testis depends on the amount of fibrous and fatty tissue.[7] The head of the epididymis is relatively isoechoic or slightly hyperechoic to the adjacent testis, while the main body is hypoechoic and lies along the posterolateral aspect of testis. The appendix testis is a remnant of the paramesonephric duct, and may be seen as a small ovoid structure seen along the superior pole of the testis, or in the groove between the testis and the head of the epididymis.[8]

The vas is difficult to identify and is seen as a fine hypoechoic tubular structure with a hyperechoic lumen running along the epididymis. The spermatic cord contains the vas deferens; the deferential, cremasteric and testicular arteries; pampiniform venous plexus; the lymphatics; and the nerves of the testis **(Figs. 10A and B)**. The normal spermatic cord is difficult to distinguish from the adjacent soft tissues of the inguinal canal sonologically, but its position can be identified by the pulsations of the testicular artery within it.

Examination of penis is performed in transverse and longitudinal planes. Scanning should be done from the glans to the base of the penis. A transperineal approach may be used for assessing the base of the penis.

The corpora cavernosa are seen as two circular structures adjacent to each other, of medium echogenicity with the deep arteries lying medially within them on the transverse section.[9] The corpus spongiosum is difficult to visualize optimally from the ventral aspect as it is usually compressed. It is more

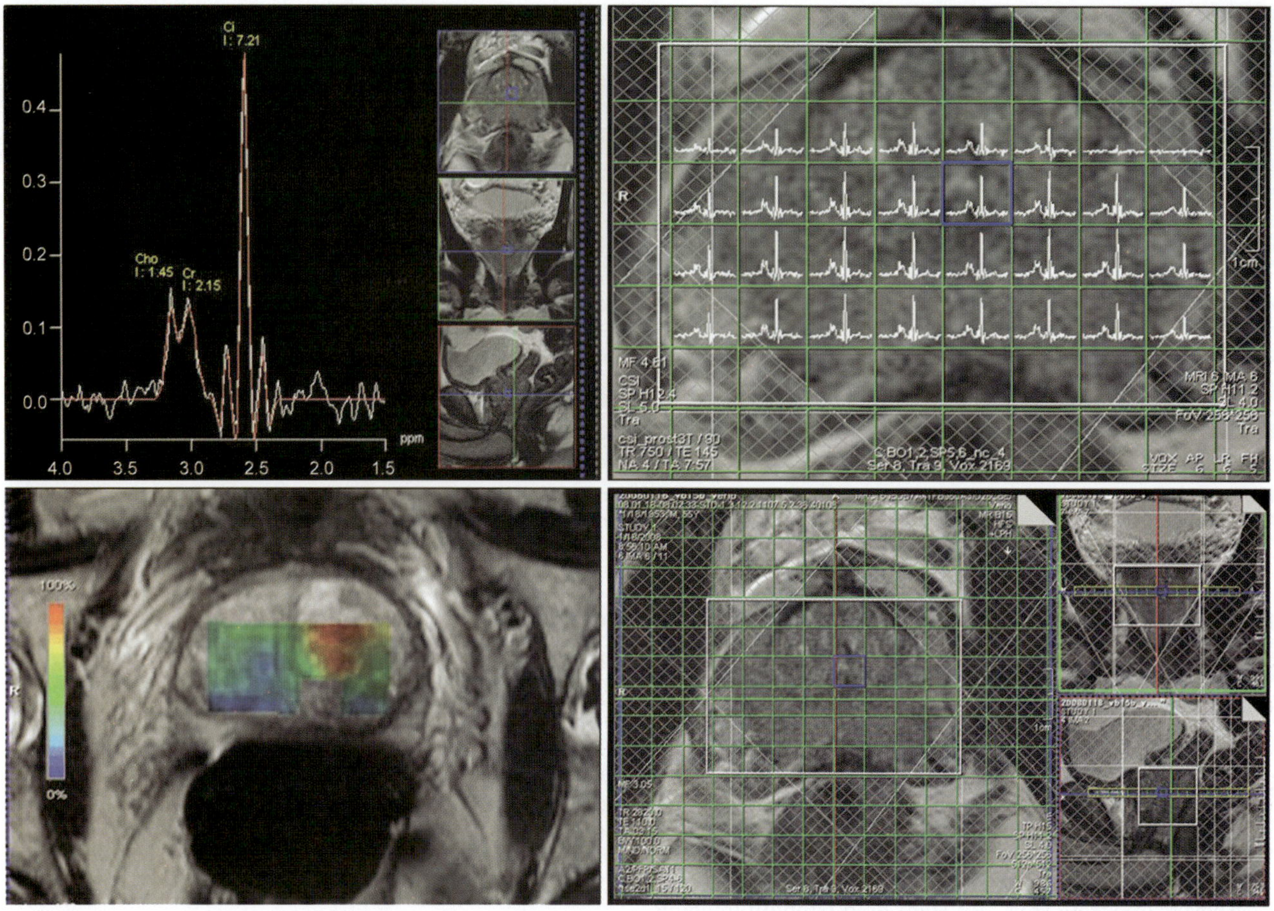

FIG. 7: Proton magnetic resonance spectroscopic imaging (3DCSI-voxel size 8 × 8 × 8, spin echo TE 145, TR 750, total acquisition time 7.57 minutes). Spectra from normal prostate tissue shows dominant citrate peak at 2.6 ppm and choline/creatinine complex at 3–3.2 ppm. Metabolite map (lower left) and spectral map (upper right) are seen over laid on the T2 axial image. Volume selection (lower right) with presaturation slabs is to suppress periprostatic fat.

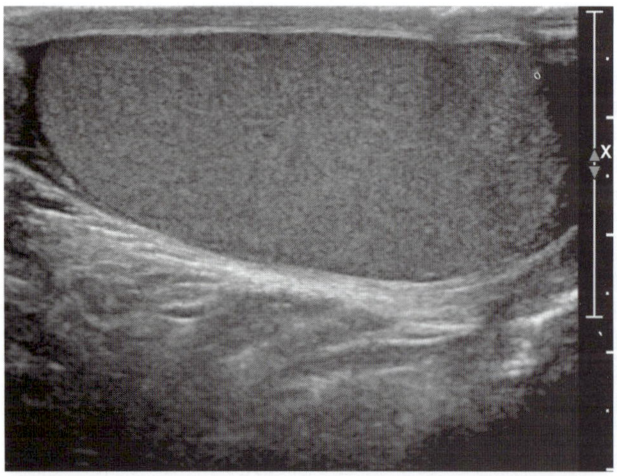

FIG. 8: Ultrasound image showing a normal testis.

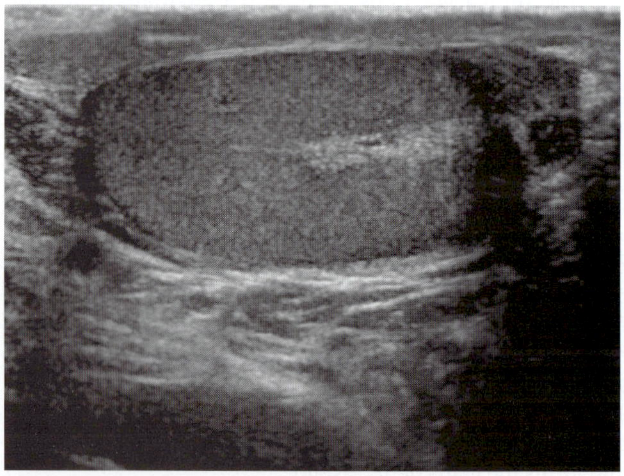

FIG. 9: Ultrasound image showing echogenic stripe of mediastinum testis.

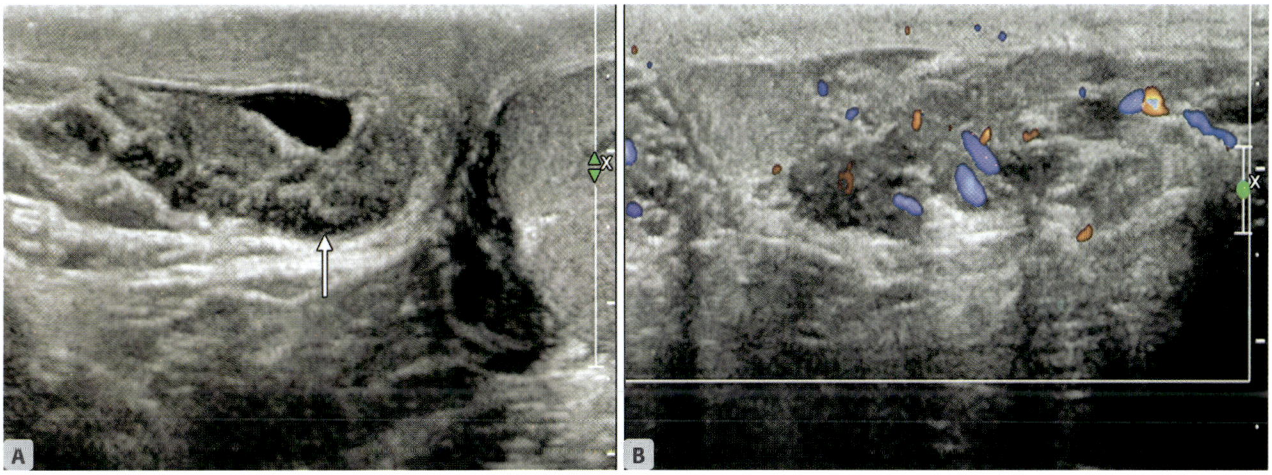

FIGS. 10A AND B: Ultrasound images showing a hypoechoic spermatic cord (arrow in A) with vascularity within on color Doppler (B).

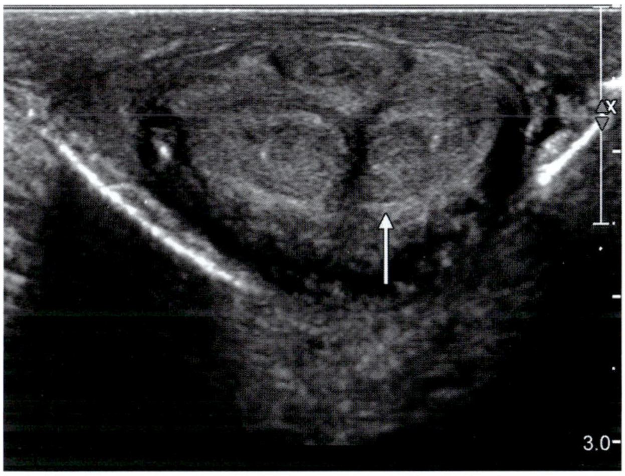

FIG. 11: Transverse ultrasound image of the penis showing corpora spongiosum and paired corpora cavernosa encased by echogenic tunica albuginea (arrow).

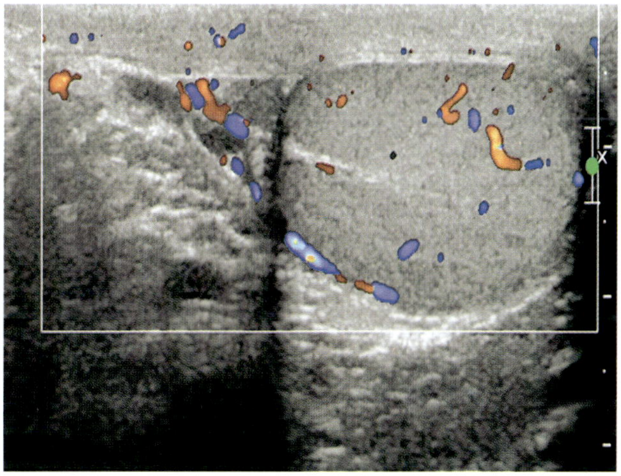

FIG. 12: Ultrasound image showing normal vascularity pattern of testis on color Doppler.

hypoechoic with the urethra seen as an anechoic central area within it. The tunica albuginea is seen as a hyperechoic capsule encasing all the three corporal structures **(Fig. 11)**.

Doppler Evaluation

On color Doppler, the normal testis shows little flow in the testicular tissue, but larger centripetal and centrifugal vessels are seen in the lobular septa and around the capsule **(Fig. 12)**. The velocity waveforms of the normal capsular and intratesticular arteries show high levels of antegrade diastolic flow, reflecting the low vascular resistance of the testis. The peak systolic flow velocities in intratesticular arteries, including capsular arteries, range from 4 cm/sec to 23.4 cm/sec (mean 10.8), end-diastolic velocities from 1.6 cm/sec to 9.2 cm/sec (mean 3.8) and resistive index (RI) from 0.46 to 0.78 (mean 0.64).[10] Supratesticular arterial waveforms vary in their appearance. Two main types of waveform exist: (1) A low resistance waveform (testicular artery and its branches) and (2) a high-resistance waveform with a sharp, narrow systolic peak and little or no diastolic flow which is believed to reflect the high vascular resistance of the extratesticular tissues (supplied by the branches of cremasteric and deferential arteries).[10]

The Doppler evaluation of the penis will be dealt in detail in the chapter on male infertility and sexual dysfunction.

Magnetic Resonance Imaging

Patients should be positioned supine, with a support placed between thighs in the upper part which will elevate the scrotum. The penis should be dorsiflexed against the anterior pelvic wall and secured using a bandage or a dressing in order to avoid its motion during the scan. A multiple phased array surface coil is used and kept covering the lower abdominopelvic wall as well as scrotum. To scan the penis and/or scrotum, a small FOV (up to 16 cm) and thin slices (4 mm) nonfat-suppressed FSE T2 should be used having a high resolution (matrix of at least 256 ×192 or higher).[9] The scan should be performed in all the three planes (sagittal, axial, and coronal). A full-FOV T2WI through the pelvis should be added in patients with known/suspected malignancy or infection. Use of dual-echo (in- and opposed-phase) spoiled Gradient Echo (GRE) T1W (11) sequence will help to identify the lesions that contain lipid, and also will improve the depiction of blood products because of the T2* effects of these substances. In cases of a suspicion of mass or a palpable abnormality, at least one FS sequence should also be included to identify macroscopic fat. Fat-suppressed FSE or short-tau inversion recovery T2WI helps in identification of fluid collections or soft-tissue edema. A three-dimensional (3D)-FS spoiled GRE T1WI should be done in the axial plane before as well as after the administration of intravenous contrast. Postcontrast 3D spoiled GRE imaging should also be done in coronal and/or sagittal planes for staging of cancer or delineating the extent of an infectious process. Axial DWI may be added in patients with suspected infection or a tumor.[9]

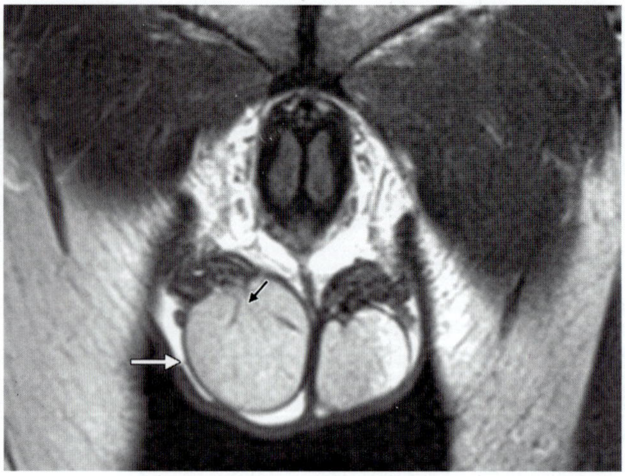

FIG. 13: T2 coronal magnetic resonance image of the scrotum showing testes as high signal intensity structures within the scrotum. Note the hypointense rim of tunica albuginea (white arrow) around the testes and the mediastinum testis (black arrow) within it.
Courtesy: Dr Anupam Lal and Dr Manphool Singhal, PGIMER, Chandigarh.

A normal adult testis is homogeneously hyperintense ovoid structure on T2WI **(Fig. 13)** and hypo- to isointense on T1WI. Tunica albuginea is seen as T1/T2 hypointense rim. The epididymis is hypointense on T2WI and isointense on T1WI compared to the testis. The testis and epididymis show enhancement following the intravenous contrast administration.[9]

The corpora spongiosum and the corpora cavernosa show bright signal on T2WI and intermediate signal on T1WI. The urethral musculature is hypointense relative to the encasing corpus spongiosum. The tunica albuginea shows hypointense signal on T1WI and T2WI. Following contrast administration, the corpora cavernosa shows a gradual enhancement with a centrifugal pattern, while early enhancement is seen in the corpora spongiosum.[9]

REFERENCES

1. Rickards D, Hare C. The lower urinary tract. In: Meire HB, Cosgrove D, Dewbury KC, Farrant P (Eds). Abdominal and General Ultrasound. Edinburgh: Churchill Livingstone; 2001. pp. 585-611.
2. Somford DM, Futterer JJ, Hambrock T, et al. Diffusion and perfusion MR imaging of the prostate. Magn Reson Imaging Clin N Am. 2008;16:685-96.
3. Akin O, Hricak H. Imaging of prostate cancer. Radiol Clin North Am. 2007;45:207-22.
4. Bonekamp D, Jacobs MA, El-Khouli R, et al. Advancements in MR imaging of the prostate: from diagnosis to interventions. Radiographics. 2011;31:677-703.
5. Rajesh A, Coakley FV. MR imaging and MR spectroscopic imaging of prostate cancer. Magn Reson Imaging Clin N Am. 2004;12:557-80.
6. Avery LL, Scheinfeld MH. Imaging of penile and scrotal emergencies. Radiographics. 2013;33:721-40.
7. Rifkin MD, Foy PM, Goldberg BS. Scrotal ultrasound: acoustic characteristics of the normal testis and epididymis defined with higher resolution superficial scanners. Med Ultrasound. 1984;8:91-7.
8. Johnson KA, Dewbury KC. Ultrasound imaging of the appendix testes and appendix epididymis. Clin Radiol. 1996;51:335-7.
9. Parker RA 3rd, Menias CO, Quazi R, et al. MR imaging of the penis and scrotum. Radiographics. 2015;35:1033-50.
10. Middleton WD, Thorne DA, Melson GL. Colour Doppler ultrasound of the normal testis. Am J Roentgenol. 1989;152: 293-7.

CHAPTER

20 Disorders of the Prostate Gland

Ujjwal Gorsi, Paramjeet Singh, Anupam Lal

INTRODUCTION

The prostate gland is a common cause of urinary symptoms in elderly men. Two most important diseases of aging men affecting the prostate gland are benign prostatic hyperplasia (BPH) and malignancy. In addition, few congenital and inflammatory pathologies also affect the gland. Imaging techniques and radiological anatomy of the prostate have been discussed in detail in Chapter 19.

BENIGN PROSTATIC HYPERPLASIA

Prostate gland enlargement is common in older men. This is the most common type of prostatic pathology. About 50–75% of men over 50 years will be affected by BPH which increases to 80% for men over 70 years of age.[1]

Pathology

In BPH, transitional zone (TZ) and periurethral region of the prostate show increased glandular epithelial cells as well as increased stromal volume. Androgens (testosterone and dihydrotestosterone) and estrogens play a major role in the proliferation of glandular epithelial elements. BPH starts in the transition zone in form of nodules which progressively enlarge in number and size, subsequently compressing the adjacent central and peripheral zones (PZs).

Clinical Features

Men usually seek medical consultation when lower urinary tract symptoms (LUTS) are caused by enlarging prostate. LUTS can be irrititative or obstructive. Urgency, frequency of urination, and nocturia are common irrititative symptoms whereas hesitancy, weak urinary stream, incomplete voiding, and straining during micturition are examples of obstructive symptoms. Although LUTS are more likely to be caused by prostate glands which are large, the gland size does not always correlate with symptoms of prostatism. Some men with severe LUTS will have only mild to moderately enlarged glands (≤50 cm)[3] whereas in others, very large glands may not be associated with significant symptoms. Left untreated, significant problems may be caused by BPH. Urinary retention, recurrent stones, recurrent infection, obstructive uropathy, and renal failure may occur in chronic long-standing nontreated BPH.

Imaging

In routine clinical practice, evaluation of men with prostatitis does not require imaging. Indications for imaging are: (1) symptoms which suggest complications of BPH, (2) if malignancy is suspected clinically or on digital rectal examination (DRE), and (3) symptomatic patients with history of previous urologic surgery.[3] Imaging usually shows enlargement and nodules of the prostate. Secondary findings of BPH are also demonstrated. In young men, whether by transrectal ultrasonography (TRUS), computed tomography (CT), or magnetic resonance imaging (MRI), the prostate gland measures about 3 cm in diameter on axial images.[2]

Primary Findings in Benign Prostatic Hyperplasia

Computed Tomography

Computed tomography can demonstrate enlarged prostate and reveal its relation with other pelvic organs. However, zonal anatomy of the prostate is not well delineated. Thus, it has limited value in patients of BPH. Changes of BPH are often detected incidentally in patients undergoing CT for unrelated indication.

Ultrasonography

Transrectal ultrasonography can show internal prostatic anatomy in detail and prostate volume can be measured accurately. However, the sonographic appearance of BPH is varied and depends on the histopathologic changes and proportion of glandular and stromal elements. Central gland can be diffused enlarged or distinct nodules may be present. The typical sonographic feature of BPH is enlargement of the inner gland, which appears relatively hypoechoic to the PZ. The border between central and peripheral gland which is indistinct in young men, becomes more distinct due to presence of BPH. Nodules can be fibroblastic, muscular, fibromuscular, hyperadenomatous, and fibroadenomatous.[4] Depending on the combination, the nodules may appear either isoechoic, hyperechoic or hypoechoic. Nodules may be

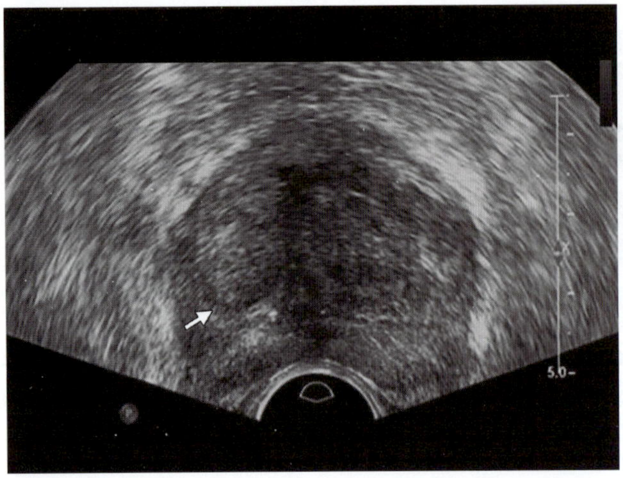

FIG. 1: *Benign prostatic hyperplasia:* Grayscale transrectal ultrasound scan shows enlarged heterogeneous central gland with variable echogenicity nodules. Hypoechoic rim (arrow) is noted around one of the nodule.

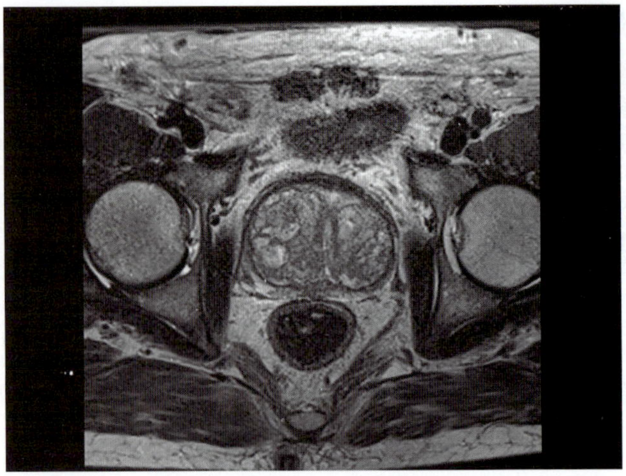

FIG. 2: Benign prostatic hyperplasia: T2-weighted axial image shows multiple nodules with varying internal signal. Well-circumscribed convex margin is noted around all nodules.

surrounded by a hypoechoic rim **(Fig. 1)** and can sometimes distort the capsule but without disrupting it. Cystic dilation of the glands of the TZ may be seen due to blockage of prostatic ducts by stromal hyperplasia.[5]

Because the growth of the gland is primarily anterior, the volume or weight cannot be estimated well by digital palpation. Prostatic ultrasound provides an accurate and reproducible method to determine the prostatic volume and the effect of the hyperplasia on the anterior urethra that correlates with the symptoms of prostatism.

Magnetic Resonance Imaging

Magnetic resonance imaging will depict enlargement of TZ clearly. The TZ will typically become heterogeneous and contain numerous nodules. The signal characteristics of BPH nodules on T2-weighted images (T2WI) are quite variable depending on the proportion of glandular and stromal elements. Glandular nodules will be hyperintense on T2WI due to accumulated secretions. They may show early enhancement and rapid washout, similar to both stromal nodules and tumors. However, because of their higher extracellular content, they typically do not show diffusion restriction.[6] Stromal nodules have lower signal on T2WI and can be very difficult to distinguish from TZ carcinoma. Like TZ carcinomas, stromal nodules may show diffusion restriction and early enhancement on dynamic postcontrast images. Due to overlapping imaging characteristics on T2WI, diffusion-weighted imaging (DWI), and postcontrast images, margins of the nodule are the key distinguishing features. BPH nodules have smooth well-defined margins with convex shapes **(Fig. 2)** whereas malignant lesions are ill-marginated and have typical erased charcoal appearance.

Secondary Findings in Benign Prostatic Hyperplasia

As the prostate enlarges, its mass effect on the bladder as well as morphologic changes of outlet obstruction may emerge.

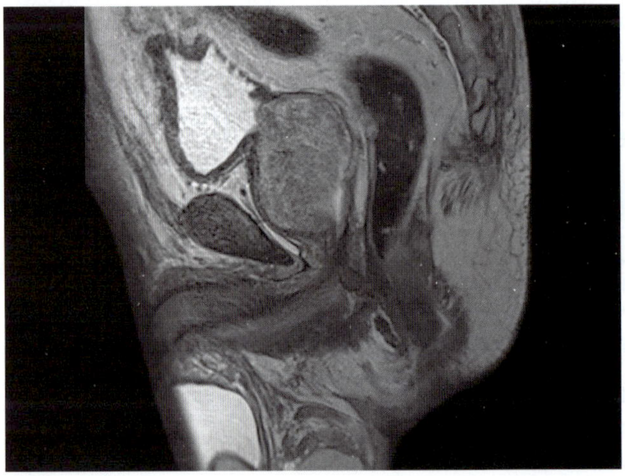

FIG. 3: Benign prostatic hyperplasia: T2-weighted sagittal image showing enlarged prostate bulging into bladder neck. Morphological changes of bladder outlet obstruction are apparent in form of bladder wall thickening and trabeculations.

Findings include indentation of the bladder base, thickening of bladder wall and formation of trabeculations **(Fig. 3)**. The bladder starts to dilate when detrusor hypertrophy cannot compensate for bladder outlet obstruction. Long-standing outlet obstruction will lead to formation of bladder calculi and diverticula.[2]

Ultrasound with combination of transabdominal and transrectal scan can demonstrate most of the secondary findings of BPH. It allows measurement of prostate size, bladder wall thickening, and postvoid residual bladder volume. Bladder wall trabeculations, diverticula, and calculi are easily demonstrated. Backpressure changes in form of bilateral hydroureteronephrosis may be seen in long-standing obstruction.

The median lobe of the prostate is particularly prone to enlargement in BPH, and may prolapse into the bladder

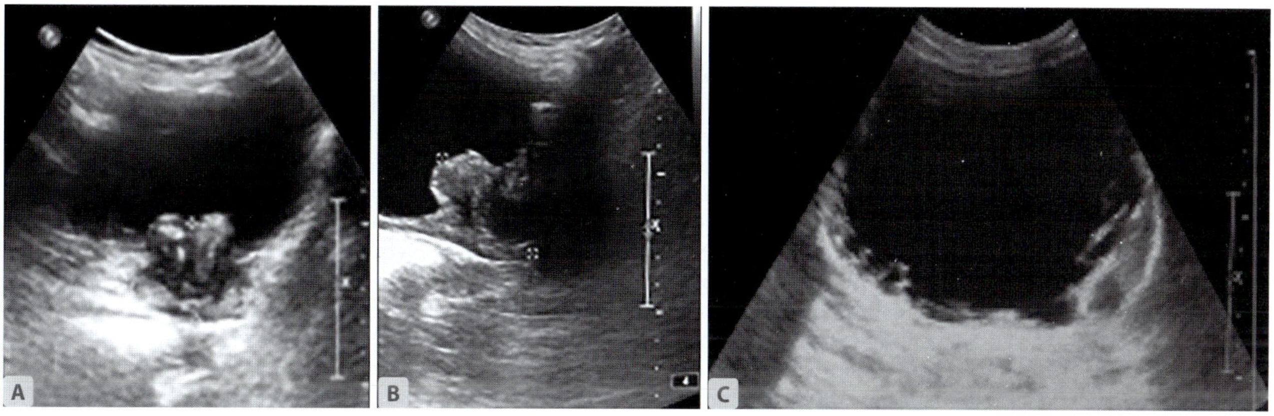

FIGS. 4A TO C: Median lobe enlargement: Transabdominal ultrasound axial (A) and sagittal (B) images show median lobe of prostate projecting into bladder base; (C) Axial image of urinary bladder shows thickening and trabeculations of bladder wall.

neck causing obstruction during voiding **(Figs. 4A to C)**. Enlargement of median lobe of the gland predicts risk of urinary retention better than overall prostate volume.

Alpha-blockers and 5α-reductase inhibitors are usually prescribed as first line of treatment in BPH. However, persistent symptoms may require surgical intervention most commonly, transurethral resection of the prostate. Open surgery is rarely performed but may be considered in situations in which the gland is very large.

PROSTATE CANCER

Introduction

Cancer of the prostate is now the second most commonly occurring malignancy affecting men and also the fifth most common cause of cancer-related deaths in men worldwide. In 2018, an estimated 1.3 million new cases were there and 359,000 deaths related to the disease. In more than 50% of the countries of the world (105 out of 185), prostate cancer (PCa) is the most common malignancy among men with highest rates of incidence seen in the Americas, Sub-Saharan Africa, Australia/New Zealand, and Northern and Western Europe.[7]

Around 10–15% of younger men who develop PCa have a positive family history. However, the etiology still remains unclear. The only established risk factors for PCa are a positive family history, ethnicity, and increasing age.[8]

Clinical Features

Many-a-time, clinical manifestations of PCa are absent when a diagnosis is made. The spectrum of clinical behavior of PCa ranges from a screen-detected asymptomatic, microscopic, well-differentiated tumor that might never become clinically significant to the rarer screen-detected or clinically symptomatic high-grade aggressive cancer that causes metastases, morbidity, and death. When symptomatic, patients usually present with nonspecific complaints such as those of LUTS, hematuria, hematospermia, pelvic pain, malaise or weight loss. In patients who have metastases at presentation, the only symptom may be bone pain as bone is the predominant site of disseminated PCa, and pain is the most common manifestation of bone metastases.

Pathology

Adenocarcinoma is the most common histologic type, encountered in approximately 95% of patients. Other prostate tumors are rare but include squamous cell carcinomas, endometrioid carcinomas arising from the prostatic utricle, carcinosarcomas, melanomas, and mesenchymal neoplasms such as rhabdomyosarcoma, leiomyosarcoma, or fibrosarcoma. Around 70% of the prostatic cancer originates in the PZ, 10–20% in the TZ, and 5–10% in the central zone. Multicentricity of the tumor is quite common. Approximately, 30–46% men above 50 years of age may harbor a cancer focus but less than 20% of those develop clinical disease which is largely related to variability in aggressiveness.

Screening

Digital rectal examination (DRE) and serum prostate-specific antigen (PSA) levels have been used in conjunction for screening men for PCa for last many decades. Neither DRE nor PSA is highly sensitive, but their combined use improves screening performance. If both DRE and PSA are positive, 60% of those patients will have PCa; if both DRE and PSA are normal, only 2% of those patients will have the disease. PSA density (obtained by dividing the PSA by the prostate size), PSA velocity (rate of increase of the PSA level), and ratio of free PSA to total PSA are found to be more useful in predicting the risk of harboring PCa as compared to single reading of serum PSA.

Studies have also found that a novel biomarker which is measured in the urine sediment attained after prostatic massage—the Prostate Cancer Antigen 3 (PCA3) may also be useful tool for screening of PCa.[9]

At present, there is no evidence of using any imaging modality in PCa screening. Broadly speaking, ultrasound, CT, MRI, scintigraphy, and positron emission tomography (PET) are insufficiently accurate and/or too expensive to be used for screening.

Diagnosis

Individuals with any abnormal findings on DRE and/or a raised (>4 ng/mL) or increasing PSA level are taken up for a standard 12-core biopsy guided by TRUS. Because accurate prognosis depends upon histologic information, tissue diagnosis is obtained prior to treatment even when disease is obviously locally advanced or metastatic clinically.

The current gold-standard investigation for the diagnosis of PCa is a 12-core TRUS-guided biopsy.[10] In a typical transrectal biopsy, passes are taken at 3 levels—the base, mid gland and apex. At each of these levels, 4 cores are to be taken—2 from the right and 2 from the left with 1 core taken medially (in parasagittal location) and the other laterally on each side. The National Comprehensive Cancer Network (NCCN) has recently suggested the concept of an "extended-pattern 12-core biopsy" which would include, apart from the standard sites, the lesion-directed palpable nodules or suspicious images as well.

The Gleason scoring system, which is based on the architectural growth patterns of adenocarcinoma of prostate was first described in 1966. Five histological patterns were described.[11] It was however observed that many adenocarcinomas of the prostate demonstrated ≥2 patterns. Because of this, the Gleason score was formulated and it was shown that this score demonstrated better correlation with the behavior of the cancer. The final Gleason score is arrived at by adding up the scores of the primary and secondary patterns. For example, if the primary pattern has a Gleason score of 3 and the secondary pattern has a Gleason score of 4, the final Gleason score will be 3 + 4 = 7. The World Health Organization has recently incorporated a new "Grade Group" system for classifying prostate cancers. According to this new system, groups have been made as follows:[12-14]

- Grade group I—Gleason scores ≤6
- Grade group II—Gleason score 3 + 4 = 7
- Grade group III—Gleason score 4 + 3 = 7
- Grade group IV—Gleason score 4 + 4 = 8
- Grade group V—Gleason score 9–10

ROLE OF VARIOUS IMAGING MODALITIES IN DIAGNOSIS OF PROSTATE CANCER

Transrectal Ultrasound

Transrectal ultrasonography alone is insufficient in diagnosing prostatic malignancy because of various reasons. Prostatic cancer can have variable appearance on gray scale mimicking benign tissue, substantial percentage of cancers are isoechoic and PCa can be multifocal.[15]

Against the background of normal PZ glandular tissue, small prostatic cancer usually appears hypoechoic because of closely packed cells in the tumor nodule. Larger tumors may appear isoechoic or hyperechoic. This appearance may be caused by a desmoplastic response of adjacent normal tissue or due to infiltration of the neoplasm into a background of BPH.[16]

The sensitivity and specificity of gray scale imaging alone is limited and has not improved the accuracy of PCa detection with an overall positive predictive value for cancer remaining <50%. TRUS is predominantly used to establish position and borders of the prostate during biopsy, rather than for lesion detection, characterization or targeting. Color Doppler, ultrasound-contrast agents, and elastography have improved diagnostic performance of TRUS for detecting and characterizing prostatic lesions.

Contrast-enhanced ultrasound (CEUS) involves the administration of an ultrasound-contrast agent (UCA) by the intravenous route which allows us to visualize the changes in vascularity (especially angiogenesis) within the prostate, some of which are characteristic for significant PCa. Shear wave elastography (SWE) is based on the measurements of the speed of shear waves through the tissue of interest. With these measurements, we can then map tissue stiffness properties (as Young's modulus). Young's modulus is significantly greater in PCa as compared to that in benign prostatic tissue as malignant tissue has more stiffness as compared to rest of gland **(Figs. 5A to C)**.

Magnetic Resonance Imaging

Indications of Magnetic Resonance Imaging

Most common situation in which MRI is requested for diagnostic work-up of suspected prostate malignancy is when repeated TRUS-guided biopsy results are negative or equivocal but occult high-risk tumor is suspected. MRI has an important role in lesion localization and risk stratification. Suspicious areas can be biopsied under direct MRI guidance or with fusion biopsy in which real-time coregistration of magnetic resonance (MR) images with TRUS guidance for biopsy is performed.

Multiparametric Magnetic Resonance Imaging

The introduction of multiparametric MRI (mp-MRI) has increased the ability of MRI in detecting and characterizing prostatic malignancies. It has also lead to improvement in lesion localization and targeted biopsy. mp-MRI combines high-resolution T2WI with ≥2 functional MRI sequences. The two sequences which we use most commonly are DWI and dynamic contrast-enhanced (DCE) perfusion imaging. Prostate imaging using a 3T magnet provides the benefit of attaining a higher signal to noise ratio, and it is not an absolute requirement to use an endorectal coil (ERC) in cancer detection protocols, but should preferably be used when working with a 1.5T magnet.

With T2WI, The PZ is seen as a T2 hyperintense area due to its high water content. Because of this, a cancerous lesion in the PZ can easily be picked up as it would appear as a low signal intensity area. This, however, is a nonspecific feature as low T2 signal may also be seen in nonmalignant conditions such as fibrosis, prostatitis, postirradiation, and also in patients with postbiopsy hemorrhage.

On DWI, a cancerous lesion can be identified by the hallmark findings of low apparent diffusion coefficient (ADC) with an associated iso-to-high signal value on DWI images (keeping b-value ≥1,400 sec/mm^2). Unlike T2WI, functional imaging (especially DWI) is very helpful in differentiating a malignant lesion from nonmalignant abnormalities (like the ones stated above) and therefore, increase the overall performance of mp-MRI in diagnosing PCa.

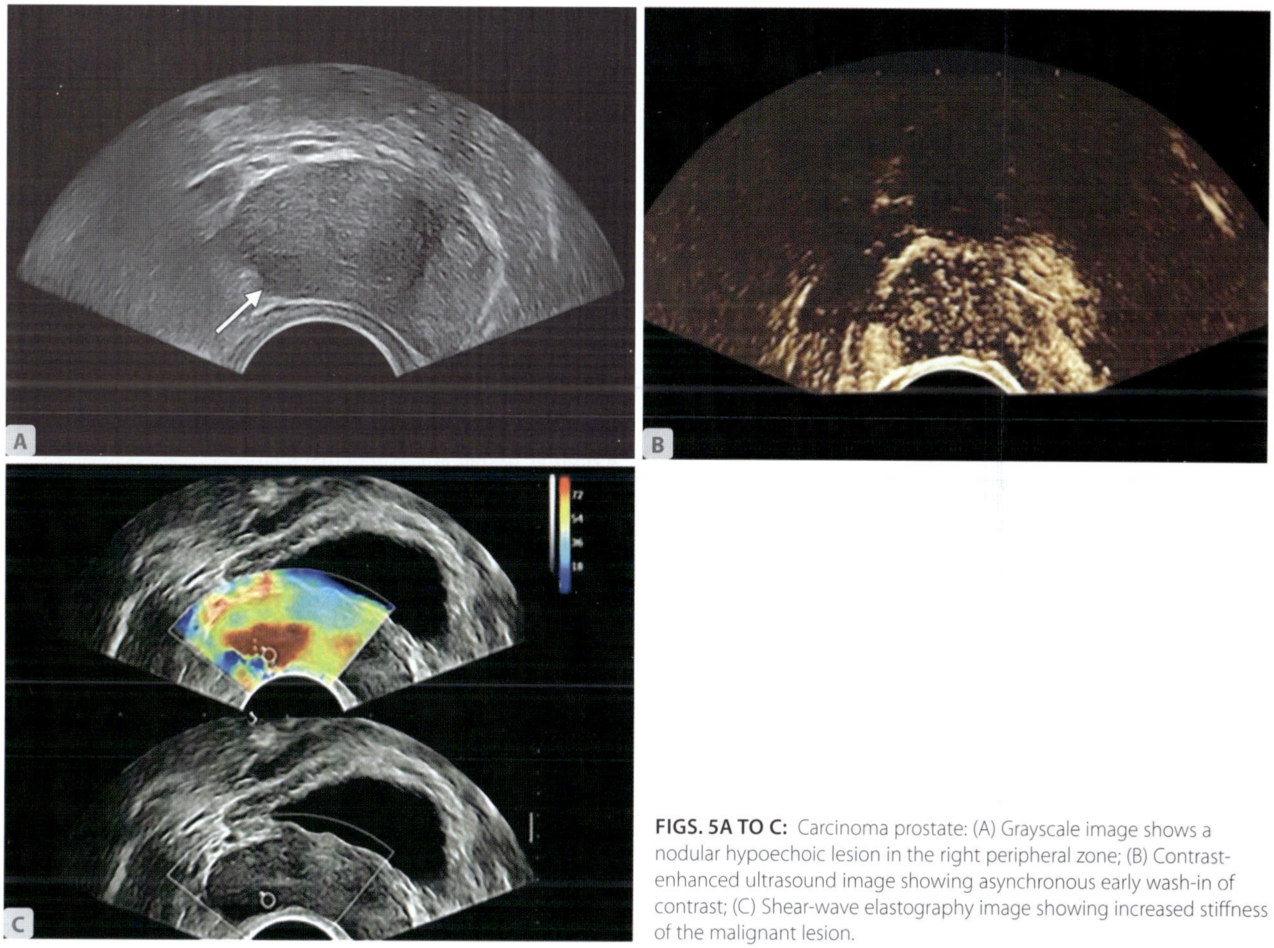

FIGS. 5A TO C: Carcinoma prostate: (A) Grayscale image shows a nodular hypoechoic lesion in the right peripheral zone; (B) Contrast-enhanced ultrasound image showing asynchronous early wash-in of contrast; (C) Shear-wave elastography image showing increased stiffness of the malignant lesion.

In DCE MRI, T1-weighted sequences are acquired before, during, and after the rapid administration of a bolus of gadolinium-based contrast agent via the intravenous (IV) route to assess tumor angiogenesis. PCa, on this sequence, may show early postcontrast enhancement (which usually has a high amplitude) followed by rapid washout. A limitation associated with this sequence is that it cannot be definitively used in isolation for diagnosing PCa because of similar enhancement patterns noted in benign conditions such as prostatitis and BPH. It however plays an important role in detecting residual/recurrent tumor following therapy.[17]

Magnetic resonance spectroscopy measures citrate, creatine, and choline to provide specific information regarding prostate metabolism. PCa is characterized by an elevated choline level and/or decreased citrate level at MR spectroscopy. Unlike the previous version, findings from MR spectroscopic imaging are not incorporated into Prostate Imaging-Reporting and Data System (PI-RADS) version 2.

Prostate Imaging-reporting and Data System

For standardizing the assessment and reporting of the mp-MRI prostate findings, the European Society of Urogenital Radiology (ESUR) published a set of guidelines, termed the Prostate Imaging-Reporting and Data System (PI-RADS).[18] In 2015, a revised version (PI-RADS version 2) was introduced which brought about a few important alterations to the original system. In the new system, T2WI and DWI-ADC combination are scored by using a 5-point scale.[19]

Newest version (Version 2.1) updated in 2019 recommends several minor adjustments which aim to simplify assessment and reduce inter-observership variability, without modifying the overall principles and scope of the original system.[20]

In PI-RADS™ v2.1, clinically significant cancer is defined on pathology/histology as the cancer with Gleason score ≥7 (including 3 + 4 with prominent but not predominant Gleason 4 component), and/or volume >0.5 cc, and/or extraprostatic extension.

PI-RADS™ v2.1 assessment uses a 5-point scale which is based on the probability that a combination of mp-MRI findings derived from T2WI, DWI, and DCE correlates with the presence of a clinically significant cancer. These assessment categories are given in **Table 1**.

Biopsy should not be considered for PI-RADS 1 or 2 lesions **(Figs. 6A and B)** but should be considered for PI-RADS 4 or 5 lesions **(Figs. 7 and 8)**. For findings with PI-RADS assessment Category 3, biopsy may or may not be considered depending on clinical scenario.

Prostate Imaging-reporting and Data System Assessment

Guidance for assignment of overall PI-RADS-v2.1 score in PZ and TZ lesions are summarized in **Tables 2 and 3**. As it is obvious in given tables, DW1 is the dominant sequence for PZ lesions whereas T2WI is the dominant sequence for TZ lesions. Detailed PI-RADS assessment for T2WI and DWI, and DCE sequences is given in **Tables 4 to 7**.

Despite various studies validating the fairly high diagnostic performance of mp-MRI in PCa, it is still not recommended as a first-line investigation in the work-up of the disease, because of its high cost, high false-positive rates, low specificity, moderate inter-reader reproducibility, and contraindications such as claustrophobia and *in situ* metallic implants.[21]

Tumor Spread and Staging

Spread of prostatic carcinoma occurs by: (1) Direct extension; (2) lymphatic spread; and (3) hematogeneous spread.

Local spread is usually to the seminal vesicles, the urethra, the urinary bladder, and rectum. Later levator muscles and pelvic wall may get involved. Lymphatic spread involves initially the obturator, the external iliac, and the internal iliac nodes. The common iliac, and para-aortic nodes may be involved in advanced disease. Hematogenous spread is to the axial skeleton or viscera. Sites of skeletal metastases are the lumbar spine, proximal femur, bony pelvis, thoracic spine, ribs, sternum, skull, and proximal humerus in order of decreasing frequency. More than 90% of prostatic metastatic lesions to bone are blastic. Spread to organs other than lymph nodes and bones is rare unless there is wide dissemination of the disease.[2]

TABLE 1: PI-RADS v2.1 assessment categories.

PI-RADS 1	Very low (clinically significant cancer is highly unlikely to be present)
PI-RADS 2	Low (clinically significant cancer is unlikely to be present)
PI-RADS 3	Intermediate (the presence of clinically significant cancer is equivocal)
PI-RADS 4	High (clinically significant cancer is likely to be present)
PI-RADS 5	Very high (clinically significant cancer is highly likely to be present)

(PI-RADS: Prostate Imaging-Reporting and Data System)

The clinical staging of PCa is based on the tumor, node, and metastasis (TNM) system given by the American Joint Committee on Cancer (AJCC). The pathological staging is performed after prostatectomy and it depends on various factors such as the status of surgical margins, extracapsular disease, tumor burden, and also on whether or not the seminal vesicles and/or pelvic lymph nodes are involved. The clinical T-staging is as follows **(Table 8)**.[22]

The 5-year survival rate among patients with localized PCa and in those with just regional spread is almost 100% while those diagnosed at a stage with distant metastasis have a relative 5-year survival of just 29.3%.

After PCa is initially diagnosed, imaging plays a definite role in staging. CT, like ultrasound, is relatively inaccurate in local staging, because it cannot detect early-stage cancers. CT may depict local invasion and lymphadenopathy.[23] Use of CT is recommended for staging in patients who have Gleason score greater than 7, PSA greater than 20 ng/mL, and cancer stage T3 or higher.[23]

Magnetic resonance imaging is by far the most accurate method for local anatomic staging of PCa. T2WI in addition to DWI and DCE are the commonly used sequences. Prostate MRI aids in the staging evaluation by verifying organ-confined status, evaluating the status of the pelvic lymph nodes, and establishing the location and local extent of the tumor in patients being considered for radiation therapy.

The ability to distinguish between organ-confined tumors (≤T2c) and those that extend beyond the prostate (≥T3a) is an important component of treatment decision-making. It is often used to define the relationship of the tumor to the neurovascular bundle and to determine the need or risk of sacrificing the nerves either unilaterally or bilaterally. The neurovascular bundle is present posterolateral to the prostate gland (at the 5 and 7 positions) on either side. It is hypointense on T1- and T2-weighted imaging and is surrounded by high-signal periprostatic fat.[23] Nerve-sparing

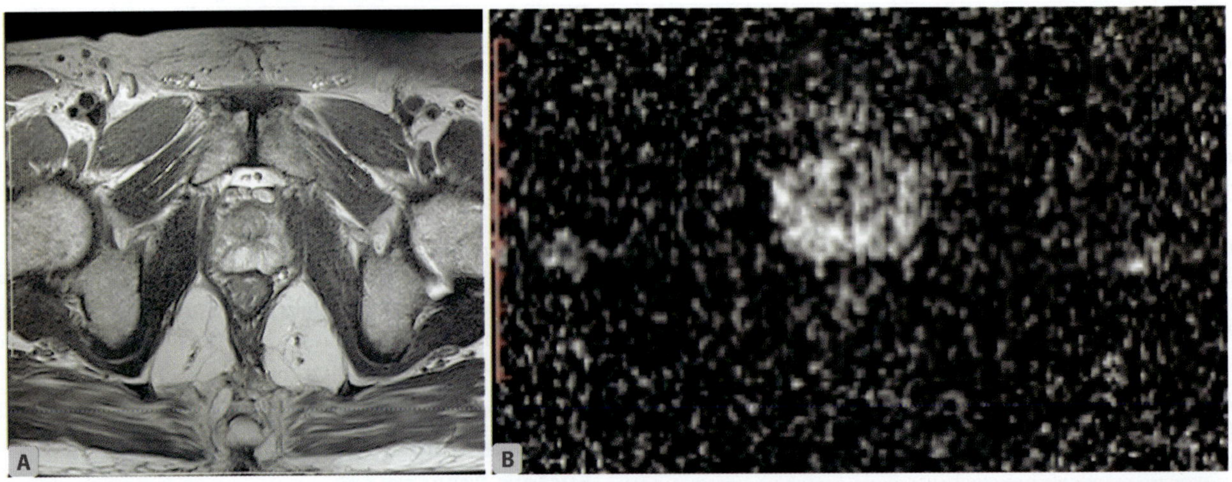

FIGS. 6A AND B: PI-RADS 2 lesion: (A) T2-weighted axial image showing multiple linear hypointensities with indistinct margin in peripheral zone; (B) On apparent diffusion coefficient map, these areas of abnormal signal appear dark.

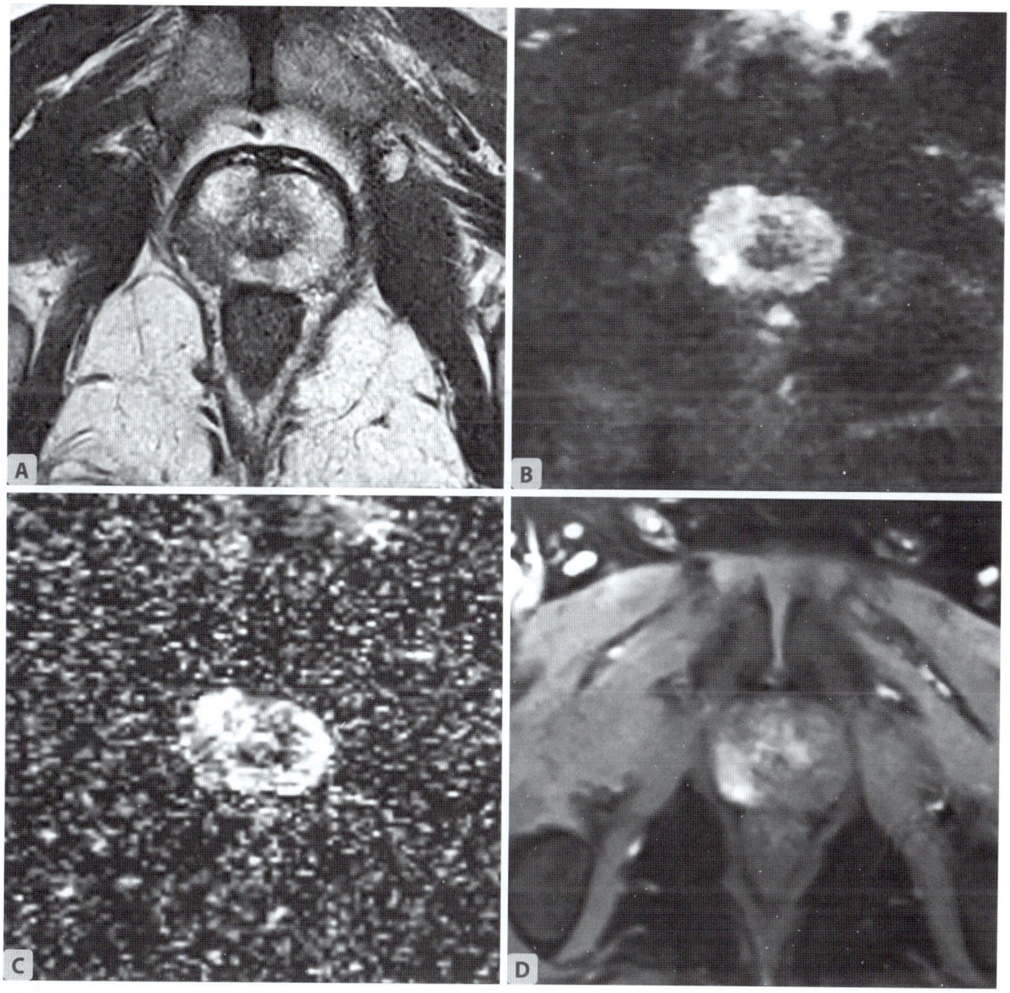

FIGS. 7A TO D: PI-RADS 5 lesion. (A) T2-weighted axial image shows a nodular hypointense lesion in the peripheral zone of the prostate on the right side; (B) On diffusion-weighted imaging, lesion shows hyperintensity and (C) on apparent diffusion coefficient map, it appears hypointense; (D) Postcontrast T1-weighted image shows early enhancement of the lesion. On biopsy, lesion turned out to be Gleason 8 adenocarcinoma.

surgery may be attempted in an effort to preserve potency if the neurovascular bundle is not involved.[24]

Few features predict extracapsular extension of PCa. These features are an irregular, spiculated, or angulated prostate margin **(Fig. 9)**, broad tumor contact with capsule, capsular retraction, tumor bulge into the periprostatic fat, asymmetry of the neurovascular bundle, and obliterated rectoprostatic angle.[23] Features of seminal vesicle involvement in a prostatic malignancy include focal hypointensity of the seminal vesicle which may be enlarged, hypointensity in ejaculatory ducts which may show increased size, obliteration of the angle between the prostate and the seminal vesicle and direct tumor extension from the prostate into seminal vesicle **(Fig. 10)**.[23] Accuracy of MRI in detecting seminal vesicle involvement in prostatic malignancy is reported as >90%. In later stages, other pelvic organs may also get infiltrated **(Fig. 11)**.

Lymph nodes are hyperintense on both T2WI and DWI and can readily be detected and measured by MRI. Nodal staging currently relies on assessment of lymph node size and shape. The relatively new technique of MR lymphangiography demonstrates potential to detect metastases in lymph nodes which are not enlarged using lymphotropic ultrasmall superparamagnetic iron oxide (USPIO) nanoparticles.[25]

Nuclear Medicine

Radionuclide bone scans have very good sensitivity but low specificity for metastatic prostate tumor. Bone scan **(Fig. 12)** and MRI spine **(Figs. 13A and B)** will reveal osteoblastic metastasis. The American College of Radiology recommends bone scintigraphy when the PSA level is greater than 10 ng/mL and the Gleason score is greater than 6.[26]

Role of 18-fluorodeoxyglucose (FDG)-PET in PCa is limited due to poor resolution and noise from the proximity to the bladder. Prostate specific membrane antigen (PSMA)-PET has shown promise in evaluation of lymph node metastasis and biochemical recurrence.

Active Surveillance and Surveillance after Treatment

Very low-risk and low-risk tumors may not need treatment at all, but may be managed by active surveillance. Active

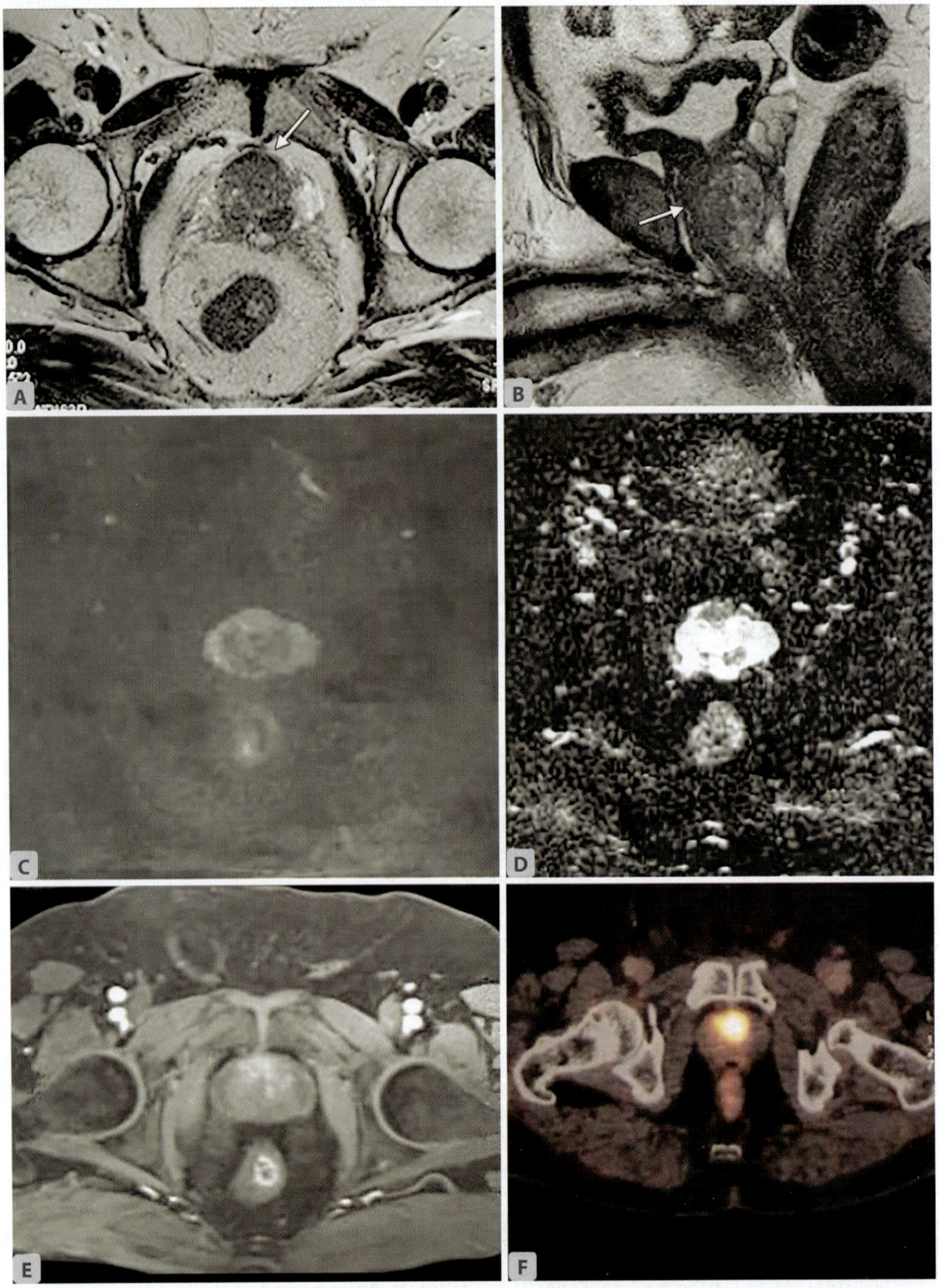

FIGS. 8A TO F: Biopsy proven transition zone Gleason 9 adenocarcinoma: T2-weighted axial (A) and sagittal (B) images demonstrating focal lenticular hypointense signal (arrows) in the anterior transitional zone of the mid-gland showing erased charcoal appearance. On diffusion-weighted imaging (C) lesion appears hyperintense and on apparent diffusion coefficient (D) it shows hypointense signal. On post-contrast T1-weighted image (E) it shows early enhancement. Prostate specific membrane antigen PET (F) done for staging shows intense uptake in the lesion. No distant metastasis, however, was seen.

surveillance may also be the preferred approach in patients with higher risk tumors but relatively short life expectancies. Active surveillance consists of periodic DRE and PSA, intermittent repeat biopsies, and MRI if suspicious findings emerge through other means of surveillance.

Localized tumors are managed with surgery (usually radical prostatectomy) or radiotherapy (brachytherapy or external beam irradiation). Tumors that are metastatic usually require antiandrogen drugs, surgery, and/or chemotherapy.[2]

After treatment for localized PCa, surveillance for recurrence is primarily performed by serial PSA determinations. If a continued rise in PSA is encountered, selection of treatment depends to a great degree upon whether the tumor has reappeared in the site of original treatment or

TABLE 2: PI-RADS score—peripheral zone.

DWI	T2W	DCE	PI-RADS
1	Any*	Any	1
2	Any	Any	2
3	Any	–	3
		+	4
4	Any	Any	4
5	Any	Any	5

* indicates 1–5.

(DWI: diffusion-weighted imaging; T2W: T2-weighted; DCE: dynamic contrast-enhanced; PI-RADS: prostate imaging-reporting and data system)

TABLE 3: PI-RADS score—transition zone.

T2W	DWI	DCE	PI-RADS
1	Any*	Any	1
2	≤3	Any	2
	≥4	Any	3
3	≤4	Any	3
	5	Any	4
4	Any	Any	4
5	Any	Any	5

*indicates 1–5.

TABLE 4: PI-RADS assessment for T2W in peripheral zone.

Score	Peripheral zone
1	Uniform hyperintense signal intensity (normal)
2	Linear or wedge-shaped hypointensity or diffused mild hypointensity, usually indistinct margin
3	Heterogeneous signal intensity or noncircumscribed, rounded, moderate hypointensity Includes others that do not qualify as 2, 4, or 5
4.	Circumscribed, homogeneous moderate hypointense focus/mass confined to prostate and <1.5 cm in greatest dimension
5	Same as 4 but ≥1.5 cm in greatest dimension or definite extraprostatic extension/invasive behavior

(T2W: T2-weighted; PI-RADS: prostate imaging-reporting and data system)

TABLE 5: PI-RADS assessment for T2W in transition zone (TZ).

Score	Transition zone
1	Normal appearing TZ (rare) or a round, completely encapsulated nodule ("typical nodule")
2	A mostly encapsulated nodule OR a homogeneous circumscribed nodule without encapsulation ("atypical nodule") OR a homogeneous mildly hypointense area between nodules
3	Heterogeneous signal intensity with obscured margins includes others that do not qualify as 2, 4, or 5
4	Lenticular or noncircumscribed, homogeneous, moderately hypointense, and <1.5 cm in greatest dimension
5	Same as 4, but ≥1.5 cm in greatest dimension or definite extraprostatic extension/invasive behavior

TABLE 6: PI-RADS assessment of DWI.

Score	Peripheral zone or transition zone
1	No abnormality (i.e. normal) on ADC and high b-value DWI
2	Linear or wedge-shaped hypointense on ADC and/or linear or wedge-shaped hyperintense on high b-value DWI
3	Focal (discrete and different from the background) hypointense on ADC and/or focal hyperintense on high b-value DWI; may be markedly hypointense on ADC or markedly hyperintense on high b-value DWI, but not both
4	Focal markedly hypointense on ADC and markedly hyperintense on high b-value DWI; <1.5 cm in greatest dimension
5	Same as 4 but ≥1.5 cm in greatest dimension or definite extraprostatic extension/invasive behavior

(PI-RADS: prostate imaging-reporting and data system; DWI: diffusion-weighted imaging; ADC: apparent diffusion coefficient)

TABLE 7: PI-RADS Assessment for DCE.

Score	Peripheral zone or transition zone
(–)	No early or contemporaneous enhancement; or diffuse multifocal enhancement NOT corresponding to a focal finding on T2WI and/or DWI or focal enhancement corresponding to a lesion demonstrating features of BPH on T2WI (including features of extruded BPH in the PZ)
(+)	Focal and earlier than or contemporaneously with enhancement of adjacent normal prostatic tissues, and corresponds to suspicious finding on T2W and/or DWI

(PI-RADS: prostate imaging-reporting and data system; DCE: dynamic contrast-enhanced; T2WI: T2-weighted image; DWI: diffusion-weighted imaging; BPH: benign prostatic hyperplasia; PZ: peripheral zone)

has produced distant metastases. CT or MRI can demonstrate local recurrence, usually evident as an enhancing soft tissue mass in the surgical bed.

Prostatic Calcifications

The PZ of the prostate gland is the seat of the corpora amylacea, where calcifications with no known etiology and without pathologic effects tend to occur. Calcification is also noted in some BPH nodules in the TZ. Prostatic calcifications have little clinical significance and are not useful in differentiating between benign and malignant diseases **(Fig. 14)**.

PROSTATITIS AND PROSTATIC ABSCESS

Acute prostatitis occurs commonly due to ascending infection from the urethra. Sometimes, it may be involved by descent of organisms from the upper urinary tract or bladder.

TABLE 8: Prostate adenocarcinoma—TNM staging classification.

TX	Primary tumor cannot be assessed
T0	No evidence of primary tumor
T1	Clinically inapparent tumor not palpable or visible by imaging
T1a	Tumor incidental histologic finding in ≤5% of tissue resected (at time of TURP)
T1b	Tumor incidental histologic finding in >5% of tissue resected (at time of TURP)
T1c	Tumor identified by needle biopsy (because of elevated PSA level)
T2	Tumor confined within prostate (*Note:* Tumors found in one or both lobes by needle biopsy but not palpable on DRE or reliably visible by imaging are classified as T1c)
T2a	Tumor involves one-half of one lobe or less
T2b	Tumor involves more than one-half of one lobe but not both lobes
T2c	Tumor involves both lobes
T3	Tumor extends through the prostatic capsule (*Note:* Invasion into the prostatic apex, or into—but not beyond—the prostatic capsule is classified as T2)
T3a	Extracapsular extension (unilateral or bilateral)
T3b	Tumor invading seminal vesicle(s)
T4	Tumor fixed or invades adjacent structures other than seminal vesicles (e.g. bladder, levator muscles, and/or pelvic wall)

(TNM: tumor, node, and metastasis; TURP: transurethral resection of the prostate; PSA: prostate specific antigen; DRE: digital rectal examination)

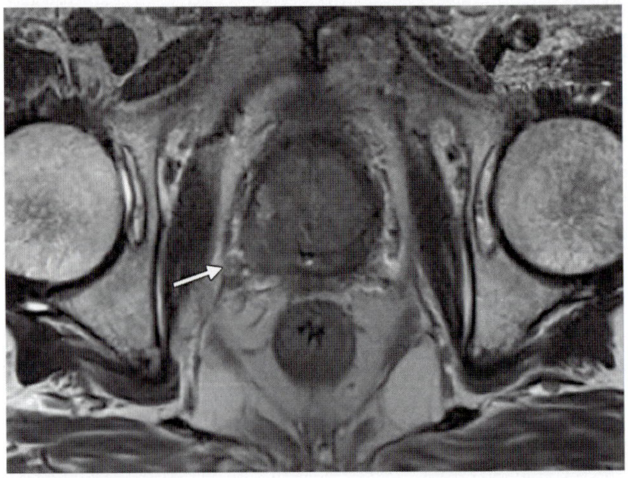

FIG. 9: Extracapsular spread: T2-weighted axial image showing focal disruption of capsule in right peripheral zone cancer with encasement of ipsilateral neurovascular bundle (arrow).

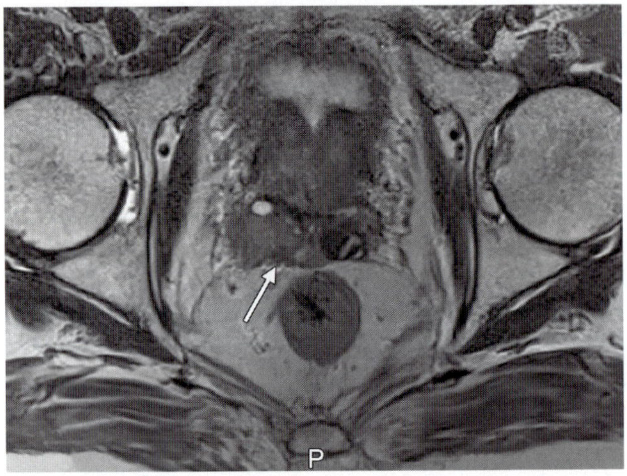

FIG. 10: Seminal vesicle involvement: T2-weighted axial image showing enlarged seminal vesicles with presence of low-signal intensity mass (arrow).

Distant focus of infection may sometimes lead to prostatitis via hematogenous or lymphogenous route. The common pathogens are those which cause urinary tract infection like *Escherichia coli*, *Klebsiella pneumoniae*, *Proteus*, *Pseudomonas*, etc.

In contrast to PCa, acute prostatitis is associated with significant symptoms. Patients may present with urinary frequency, urgency, dysuria, fever, perineal pain, and urethral discharge. DRE will reveal an extremely swollen and tender prostate.[2] In acute prostatitis, generally the glands are hypoechoic. Color Doppler shows a very vascular focus in areas of prostatitis, mimicking carcinoma.

Chronic prostatitis is caused in much the same way and by the same bacterial pathogens as acute prostatitis, however, it may be associated with certain other pathogens such as mycobacteria, chlamydia or *Mycoplasma*. A high index of suspicion for malignancy is necessary, because both PCa and prostatitis tend to occur in the PZ. Sonographic findings of chronic prostatitis include variable echogenicity focal masses, calcifications of ejaculatory duct, and irregularity and thickening of capsule. In addition, dilatation of periprostatic veins and distended seminal vesicles may be seen. Chronic granulomatous prostatitis can mimic sonographic features of prostatic carcinoma. TRUS does not reliably distinguish chronic prostatitis from cancer.

On MRI, certain morphologic features are helpful in differentiating prostatitis from malignancy. When focal, it is characteristically band-like, triangular or geographic in morphology compared with the typical nodular or mass like configuration of cancer **(Figs. 15A to D)**. When diffuse, the entire PZ may be "grayed out" or lower in signal than the very high signal expected in the PZ on T2WI. Prostatitis may be hyperintense on DWI but usually lacks the marked low-signal intensity which is seen in PCa on ADC maps. Prostatitis usually shows hyperenhancement on arterial phase DCE.[2]

On ultrasound, development of an anechoic lesion with or without internal echoes suggests the development of an abscess, which on color Doppler shows a highly vascular wall. The abscess cavity may also contain air due to gas-producing organisms. In doubtful cases, contrast-enhanced CT and MRI can show the abscess cavity with enhancement of its wall **(Figs. 16 and 17)**. TRUS guidance can be used to diagnose as well as drain these prostatic abscesses **(Figs. 18A and B)**.

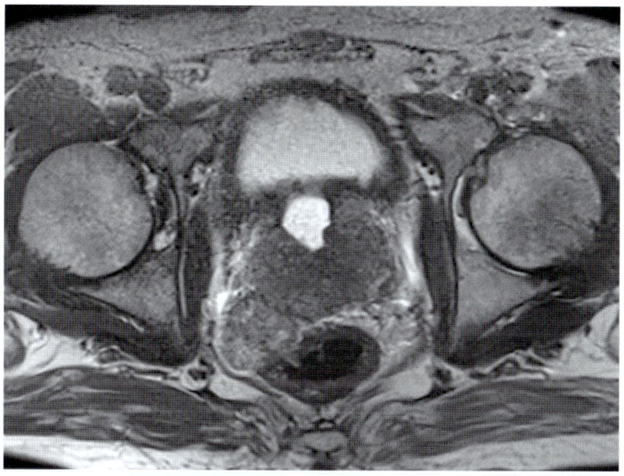

FIG. 11: Extracapsular spread: T2-weighted axial image showing lesion in right posterior peripheral zone with obvious extracapsular extension and complete encasement of right neurovascular bundle. Infiltration of anterior wall of rectum is also seen.

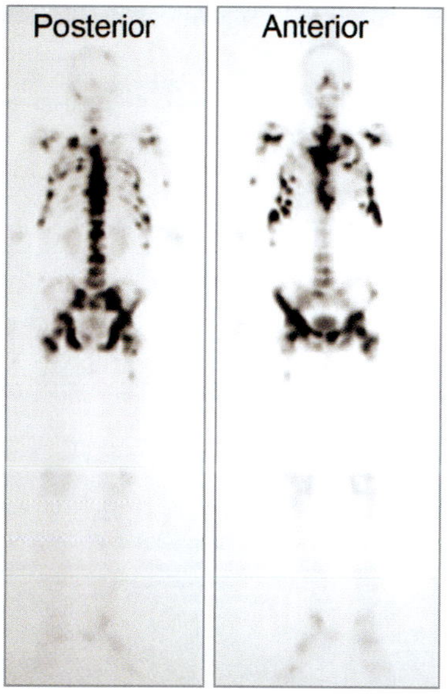

FIG. 12: Bony metastasis in carcinoma prostate: Nuclear scan anterior and posterior views showing multiple osteoblastic metastatic deposits involving axial skeleton from cancer prostate.

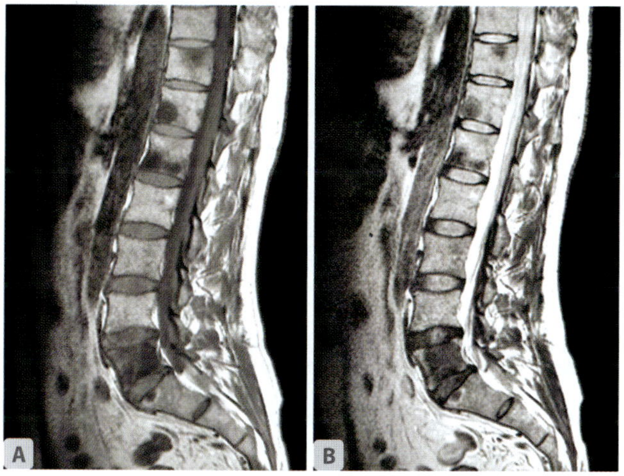

FIGS. 13A AND B: Bony metastasis from prostate cancer: T1-weighted (A) and T2-weighted (B) sagittal scans showing blastic marrow deposits appearing hypointense on T1 and T2 images involving dorsolumbar spine.

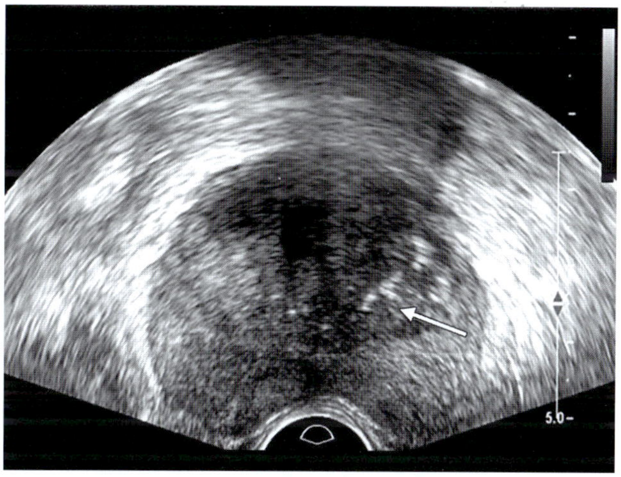

FIG. 14: Prostatic calcifications: Transrectal ultrasound scan showing areas of calcification (arrow) in transition zone.

PROSTATIC CYSTS

Midline prostatic cysts can be Müllerian duct cysts or utricle cysts. Müllerian duct cysts do not contain sperms and can cause infertility due to compression of the ejaculatory ducts. Utricle cysts contain sperms but unlike former do not extend beyond prostate **(Figs. 19 and 20)**. The paramidline cysts are Wolffian cysts, seminal vesicle cysts or ejaculatory duct cysts which contain sperms. Associated Wolffian duct anomalies, i.e. renal anomalies may be seen in these patients. Peripheral cysts are acquired retention cysts and may be associated with BPH. Cowper's gland cysts are also acquired cysts associated with urogenital diaphragm. Cystic lesions appear smooth walled, hypoechoic on USG and hyperintense on T2WI unless complicated by infection or hemorrhage.[27]

ACKNOWLEDGEMENT

Sincere thanks to Dr Prabhjyot Singh Chowhan, Department of Radiodiagnosis.

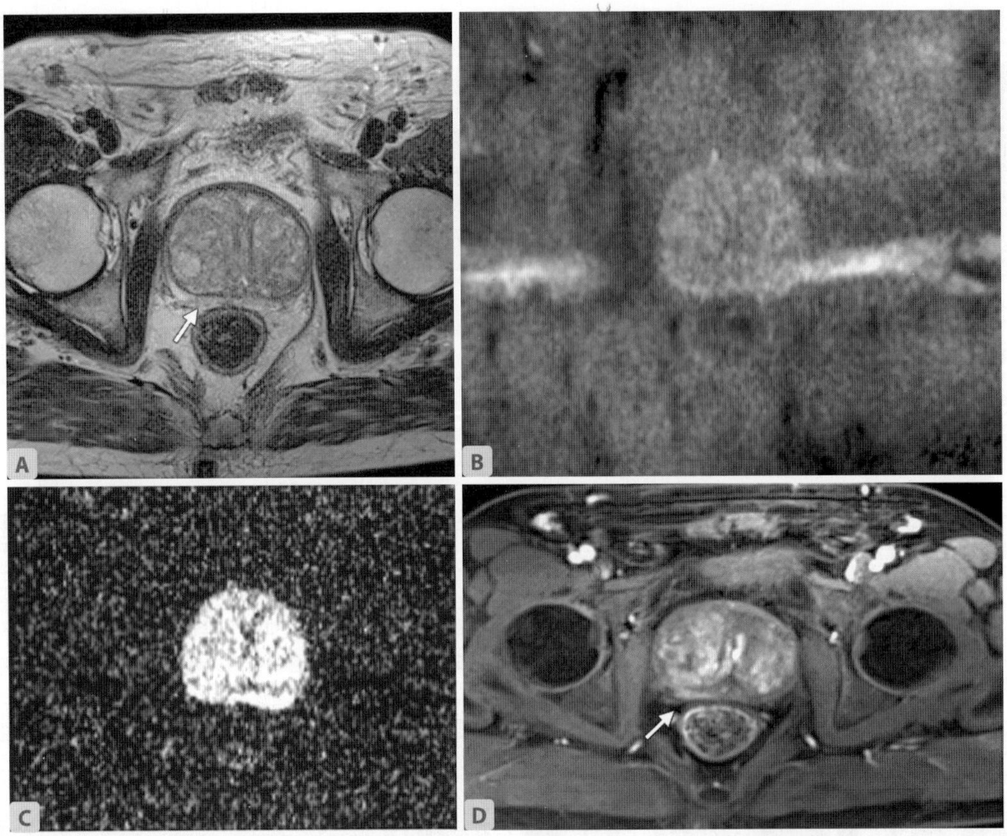

FIGS. 15A TO D: Focal prostatitis: (A) T2-weighted image shows noncircumscribed hypointense area (arrow) in right posterior peripheral zone; (B) Diffusion-weighted imaging shows mild hyperintense signal whereas on apparent diffusion coefficient; (C) corresponding area is hypointense; (D) Postcontrast T1-weighted image illustrates focal early enhancement (arrow) equal to that of the TZ. Lesion was reported as PIRADS 3 and final diagnosis of prostatitis was confirmed on biopsy.

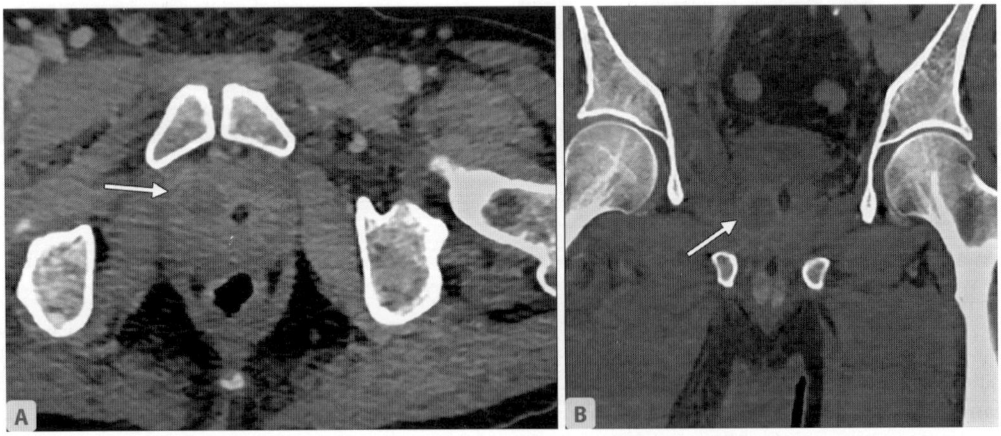

FIGS. 16A AND B: Prostatic abscess: Contrast-enhanced CT axial (A) and coronal (B) images showing hypodense collection with irregular enhancing walls (arrows).

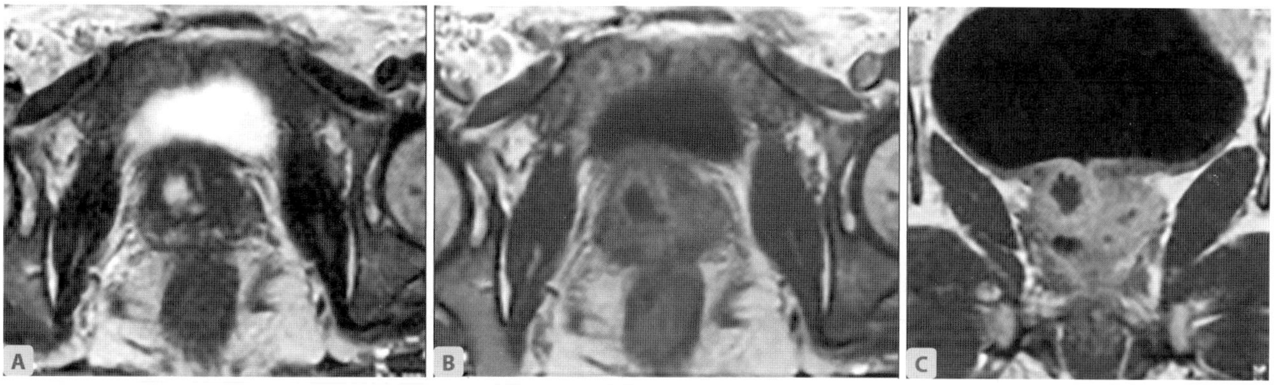

FIGS. 17A TO C: Prostatic abscess: T2 axial (A) T1 postcontrast axial (B) and coronal (C) sections show a bacterial intraprostatic abscess appearing hyperintense on T2 and showing enhancing peripheral margins in the right half of the gland.

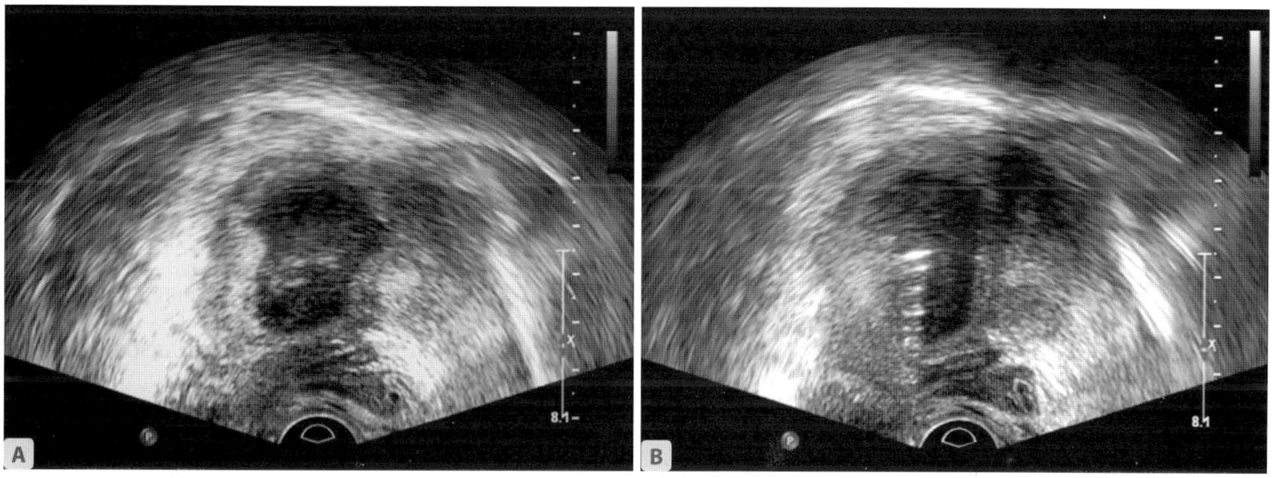

FIGS. 18A AND B: Prostatic abscess: (A) Transrectal ultrasound image showing abscess with thick irregular walls in right half of prostate; (B) Aspiration needle is seen with in the abscess.

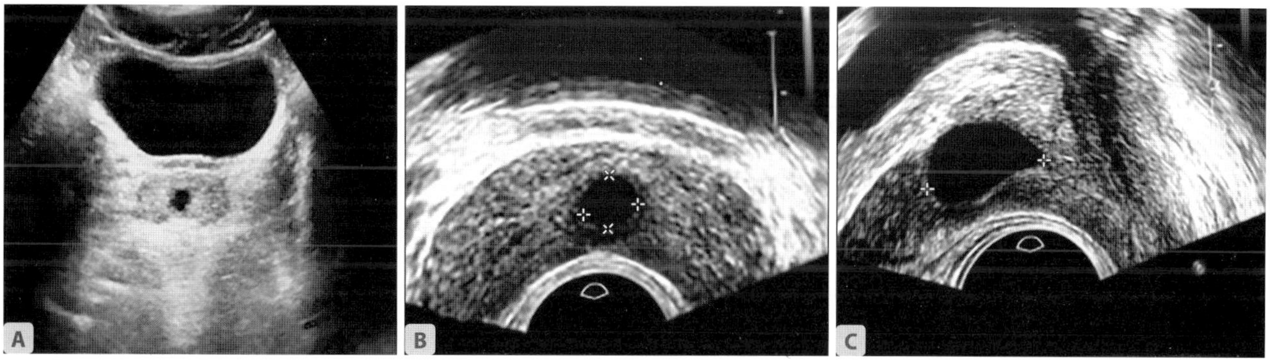

FIGS. 19A TO C: Utricle cyst: Transabdominal ultrasound (A) transrectal ultrasound axial (B) and sagittal (C) images showing small midline utricular cyst in prostate.

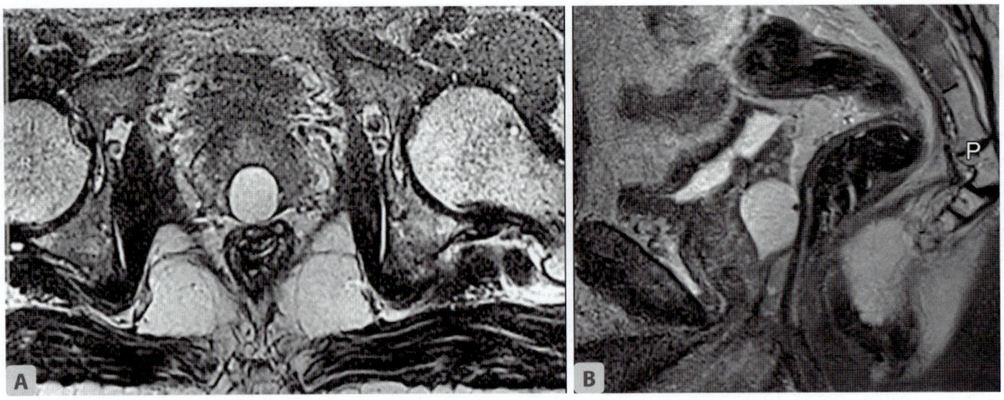

FIGS. 20A AND B: Utricle cyst: T2-weighted axial (A) and sagittal (B) images showing midline intraprostatic cyst which does not extend beyond the prostatic base.

REFERENCES

1. O'Brien WM. Benign prostatic hypertrophy. Am Fam Physician. 1991;44:162-71.
2. Dunnick NR, Newhouse JH, Cohan RH, et al. Prostate and seminal vesicles. In: Dunnick NR, Newhouse JH, Cohan RH, Maturen KE (Eds). Genitourinary Radiology. Philadelphia: Wolters Kluwer; 2018. pp. 321-38.
3. Grajo JR, Cronin C. Benign prostatic hyperplasia. In Sahani DV, Sameer AE (Eds). Abdominal Imaging. Philadelphia, Elsevier; 2017. pp. 896-904.
4. Shinohara K, Scardino PT, Carter SS, et al. Pathologic basis of the sonographic appearance of the normal and malignant prostate. Urol Clin North Am. 1989;16:675-91.
5. Kawashima A, Glockner J, King B. CT urography and MR urography. Radiol Clin North Am. 2003;41:945-61.
6. Pokharel SS, Patel NU, Garg K, et al. Multi-parametric MRI findings of transitional zone prostate cancers: correlation with 3-dimensional transperineal mapping biopsy. Abdom Imaging. 2015;40:143-50.
7. Bray F, Ferlay J, Soerjomataram I, et al. Global cancer statistics 2018: GLOBOCAN estimates of incidence and mortality worldwide for 36 cancers in 185 countries. CA Cancer J Clin. 2018;68:394-424.
8. Gann PH. Risk factors for prostate cancer. Rev Urol. 2002;4:S3-10.
9. Heidenreich A, Bellmunt J, Bolla M, et al. EAU guidelines on prostate cancer. Part 1: screening, diagnosis, and treatment of clinically localised disease. Eur Urol. 2011;59:61-71.
10. Guo G, Xu Y, Zhang X. TRUS-guided transperineal prostate 12+X core biopsy with template for the diagnosis of prostate cancer. Oncol Lett. 2017;13:4863-7.
11. Gleason DF. Histologic grading of prostate cancer: A perspective. Hum Pathol. 1992;23:237-79.
12. Kryvenko ON, Epstein JI. Changes in prostate cancer grading: Including a new patient-centric grading system. The Prostate. 2016;76:427-33.
13. Epstein JI, Egevad L, Amin MB, et al. The 2014 International Society of Urological Pathology (ISUP) Consensus Conference on Gleason Grading of Prostatic Carcinoma: Definition of Grading Patterns and Proposal for a New Grading System. Am J Surg Pathol. 2016;40:244-52.
14. Pierorazio PM, Walsh PC, Partin AW, et al. Prognostic Gleason grade grouping: data based on the modified Gleason scoring system. BJU Int. 2013;111:753-60.
15. Clements R. The role of transrectal ultrasound in diagnosing prostate cancer. Curr Urol Rep. 2002;3:194-200.
16. Yu KK, Hricak H. Imaging prostate cancer. Radiol Clin North Am. 2003;38:59-85.
17. Kitajima K, Murphy RC, Nathan MA, et al. Detection of recurrent prostate cancer after radical prostatectomy: comparison of 11C-choline PET/CT with pelvic multiparametric MR imaging with endorectal coil. J Nucl Med Off Publ Soc Nucl Med. 2014;55:223-32.
18. Barentsz JO, Richenberg J, Clements R, et al. ESUR prostate MR guidelines 2012. Eur Radiol. 2012;22:746-57.
19. Weinreb JC, Barentsz JO, Choyke PL, et al. PI-RADS prostate imaging—reporting and data system: 2015, version 2. Eur Urol. 2016;69(1):16e40.
20. Turkbey B, Rosenkrantz AB, Haider MA, et al. Prostate imaging reporting and data system version 2.1: 2019 update of prostate imaging reporting and data system version 2. Eur Urol. 2019; 76(3):340-51.
21. Mertan FV, Greer MD, Shih JH, et al. Prospective Evaluation of the Prostate Imaging Reporting and Data System Version 2 for Prostate Cancer Detection. J Urol. 2016;196:690-6.
22. Buyyounouski MK, Choyke PL, McKenney JK, et al. Prostate cancer—major changes in the American Joint Committee on Cancer eighth edition cancer staging manual. CA Cancer J Clin. 2017; 67(3):245-53.
23 Grajo JR, Lee LK, Cronin C. Benign and malignant focal prostate lesions. In: Sahani DV, Sameer AE (Eds). Abdominal Imaging. Philadelphia: Elsevier; 2017. pp. 905-22.
24. Somford DM, Hamoen EH, Fütterer JJ, et al. The predictive value of endorectal 3 Tesla multi parametric magnetic resonance imaging for extra prostatic extension in patients with low, intermediate and high risk prostate cancer. J Urol. 2013;190:1728.
25. Harisinghani MG, Barentsz J, Hahn PF, et al: Noninvasive detection of clinically occult lymph-node metastases in prostate cancer. N Engl J Med. 2003;348:2491-9.
26. Amis ES Jr, Bigongiari LR, Bluth EI, et al. Pre-treatment staging of clinically localized prostate cancer. Radiology. 2000;215 Suppl:703-8.
27. Parsons RB, Fisher AM, Bar-Chama N, Mitty HA. MR imaging in male infertility. RadioGraphics. 1997;17:627-37.

CHAPTER

21

Scrotal Diseases

Anupam Lal, Manphool Singhal, Sreedhara BC

ANATOMY

The scrotum is a cutaneous pouch which contains the testes and parts of the spermatic cords. It is formed by the fusion of two scrotal sacs separated by an inner septum that corresponds to a midline ridge or raphe on the surface, and extends anteriorly along the under surface of the penis, and posterior along the middle line of the perineum to the anus. The following structures form the wall of scrotum, from superficial to the deep layers: skin, fascia (superficial), muscle (dartos), external spermatic fascia, cremasteric fascia, and internal spermatic fascia. The testes are suspended in the scrotal sac by the spermatic cord and are anchored to scrotal wall caudally by gubernaculum testis. Gubernaculum testis is cord-like structure located caudal to the testis and guides the testicular descent. The left testis lies lower than the right, corresponding with bigger length of the left-sided spermatic cord.

Each testis is in oval form, lying obliquely in the scrotal sac; the upper pole is directed anterior and a little lateral; the lower pole is directed posterior and medial; the anterior border is convex, oriented forward and downward, and the posterior border is relatively straight oriented backward and upward, to which the spermatic cord is attached. The lateral surfaces, anterior border and extremities (both) of the testes are convex, smooth, free, and invested by the tunica vaginalis (visceral layer). There is only partial investment of tunica vaginalis along the posterior border, to which the cord is attached. Epididymis body is seen lying upon the posterior border (lateral edge). Visceral and parietal layers of tunica vaginalis surround the testis and epididymis. Between these two layers there lies vaginal cavity containing minimal amount of fluid, derived from the "saccus vaginalis" of the peritoneum. Saccus vaginalis in the fetus precedes the testis descent into the scrotum from abdomen. The testicular capsule is formed by tunica albuginea. Tunica albuginea is covered by the tunica vaginalis, except at the attachment points of the epididymis and spermatic vessels entry into the gland along its posterior border. It is attached to the tunica vasculosa, and is reflected into the interior of the gland along its posterior border, leading to formation of incomplete vertical septum, defined as mediastinum testis. From the mediastinum testis, numerous fibrous septa are seen to extend into the testis, dividing it into multiple lobules containing one to three seminiferous tubules each, supporting the Sertoli cells, spermatocytes, and "Leydig" cells within the interstitium.

All tubules drain into larger ducts called tubuli recti. These tubuli recti converge to form the rete testis, an anastomosing network of draining tubules, and enter into mediastinum testis, which carries the sperms from testis to the epididymis. The mediastinum testis consists of invagination of tunica albuginea and the rete testis. It also contains branches of testicular arteries, centripetal veins and lymphatics of the testis and hence is the anatomical hilum of the testis.

Testicular size varies with age and sexual development stage. It measures approximately 1.5 cm × 1 cm (length × width) at birth. Before 12 years of age, the average volume of testis is about 1–2 cm^3. Clinically, a male individual is considered to have reached puberty once the testis achieves a volume of 4 cm^3. The postpubertal testis of average dimensions varies from 4 cm to 5 cm in length, 2.5 cm in transverse diameter, 3 cm in the AP dimension, and 10.5–14 g in weight.

The epididymis consists of a head (globus major), body and tail (globus minor). The head lies cranial to the testis and it consists of 8–12 efferent ducts converging into a single larger duct called as vas deferens in the body and tail, which continues in the spermatic cord.

There are four testicular appendages (remnants of embryonic ducts), which have been described: (1) appendix testis, (2) appendix epididymis, (3) paradidymis and (4) vas aberrans.[1] The appendix testis and appendix epididymis can be visualized on ultrasonography (USG). The testicular appendage (hydatid of Morgagni) is a remnant of Müllerian duct, a minute oval, sessile body visualized on the upper pole of testis, and the appendix epididymis (pedunculated hydatid) is seen on the head of the epididymis. The spermatic cord is composed of arteries (the internal and external spermatics; and the artery to the ductus deferens), veins, nerves, lymphatics, and the excretory duct of the testis.

The arteries supplying the testicular coverings are: the superficial and deep external pudendal arteries, cremasteric branch from the inferior epigastric artery and superficial perineal branch of internal pudendal. The veins follow the corresponding arteries. The nerves are lumboinguinal and ilioinguinal branches from the lumbar plexus, pudendal branch of the posterior femoral cutaneous nerve and superficial perineal branches of the internal pudendal nerve.

IMAGING MODALITIES

Ultrasonography with a high-frequency (7.5–14 MHz) transducer is the imaging modality of choice to examine scrotum. Sonography combined with color Doppler and power Doppler has evolved into an all-encompassing scrotal imaging technique as both structural and perfusion abnormalities can be detected. Magnetic resonance imaging (MRI) and nuclear scan are other important complementary modalities. Computed tomography (CT) scan and MRI have important role in staging of testicular cancer and for the localization of testis in patients with cryptorchidism.

Technique of Sonography

Scrotal ultrasound (US) is performed in the supine position, with a cloth between the thighs supporting the scrotum. A high-frequency (7–14 MHz) linear array transducer is optimal for visualization of scrotal structures, and a stand-off pad is useful for superficial lesions. The testes are examined in both longitudinal and transverse axes, and dimension and echogenicity are compared with the opposite side. In acute scrotum evaluation, normal side should be scanned first in order to set the grayscale and color Doppler gain settings, which helps in comparison with the affected side. While assessing small palpable nodules, placing the finger beneath the nodule with the transducer placed directly over the nodule, or placing the finger on the nodule and the transducer opposite should be considered for optimal imaging. Scrotal skin thickness (normal 2–8 mm, depends on the cremasteric muscle contraction) should be evaluated. Additional techniques like upright positioning or Valsalva maneuver can be used for venous evaluation.

Prepubertal testes are of low to medium echogenicity, whereas pubertal and postpubertal testes are of medium homogeneous echogenicity, indicating tubular maturation and development of germ cell elements.[2] The mediastinum testis is visualized as an echogenic band (variable length and thickness) extending in a caudocranial direction **(Fig. 1)**. The small amount of fluid in the space between leaves of the tunica vaginalis is seen as thin echo-free rim adjacent to the head. This minimal amount of fluid should not be misinterpreted as hydrocele. Longitudinal view is best to evaluate epididymis, where the epididymal head (5–12 mm in length) is seen as a pyramidal structure lying above the superior pole of the testis and is usually isoechoic to the testis.[3] The body (2–4 mm in diameter) is usually indistinguishable from the surrounding peritesticular tissue, and the tail (2–5 mm) is seen as a curved structure at the inferior pole of the testis, where it becomes the ductus deferens.

The spectral waveform of the intratesticular arteries characteristically has a low-resistance pattern,[4] with a mean resistive index (RI) of 0.62 (range, 0.48–0.75);[2] however, for a testis with volume less than 4 cm^3, this may not be true,[3] as in prepubertal boys, where diastolic arterial flow may not be detectable.[5]

Contrast-enhanced US (CEUS) role in depicting minimal vascular flow, vascular morphology along with "washout" characteristics of a lesion is well established and is increasingly being used in scrotal US evaluation with focus on a particular lesion characterization. A rapid enhancement and washout of a lesion usually depicts an aggressive or malignant lesion. In case of benign vascular pattern, recommendation of monitoring with follow-up can be provided confidently.

Magnetic Resonance Imaging of Scrotum

Magnetic resonance imaging (MRI) of the scrotum is extremely valuable as a problem-solving modality. The MRI examination is performed in supine position with scrotum supported by towel. Symmetric placement of testis is important for optimal coronal scans. The scrotum is then covered by small cloth or gauze and the surface coil is placed over it in a flat position. T1-weighted (T1W) and T2-weighted (T2W) spin-echo images are obtained in coronal and axial planes. Contrast-enhancement or fat suppression sequences are also obtained when further tissue characterization is required. Optimum coverage is provided by thin (4–5 mm) slices with 1–2 mm interslice gaps and 8–20 cm field of view. The scan area must be extended to lower pole of kidneys when looking for undescended testis and up to the diaphragm when MRI is performed for staging of testicular cancer.

On MRI, the testis is seen as an oval, sharply defined structure with homogeneous intermediate signal intensity on T1W images and high-signal intensity on T2W images **(Fig. 2)**. The tunica albuginea is seen as a thin hypointense rim around the testis.

The mediastinum testis is also hypointense and it is seen as a dark stripe invaginating into the testis. The signal intensity of the epididymis is similar to testis on T1W images and much lower on T2W images. The pampiniform plexus is seen as a tortuous tubular structure extending from upper pole of testis up to the inguinal canal. Vas deferens can sometimes be seen as a low-intensity tubular structure that can be traced from epididymis to inguinal canal.

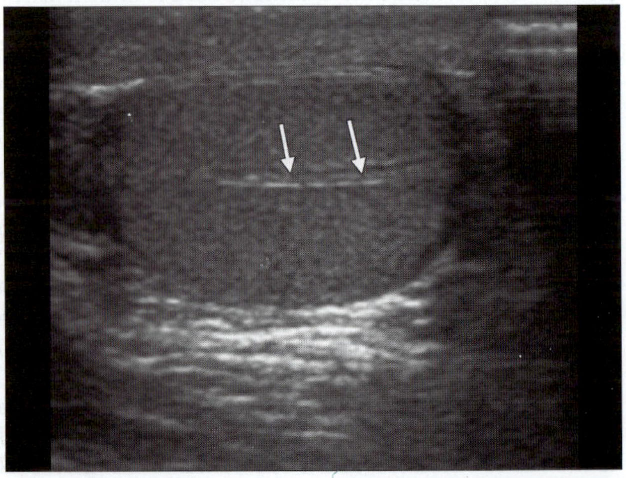

FIG. 1: US image of the test is in its long axis showing echogenic line of mediastinum testes (arrows).

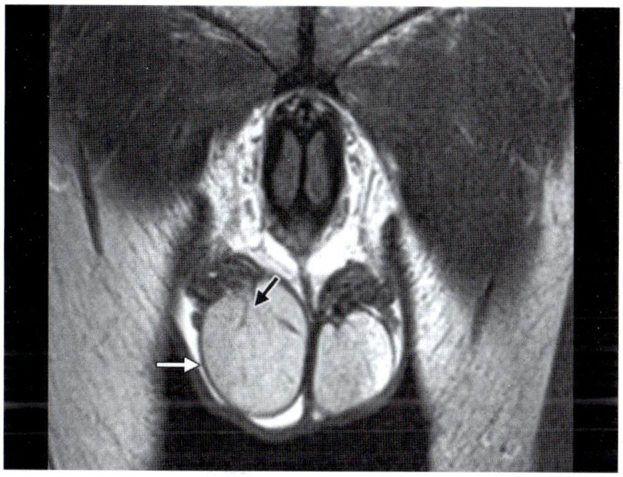

FIG. 2: T2 coronal MR image of the scrotum showing testes as high-signal intensity structures within the scrotum. Note the hypointense rim of tunica albuginea (white arrow) around the testes and the mediastinum testis (black arrow) within it.

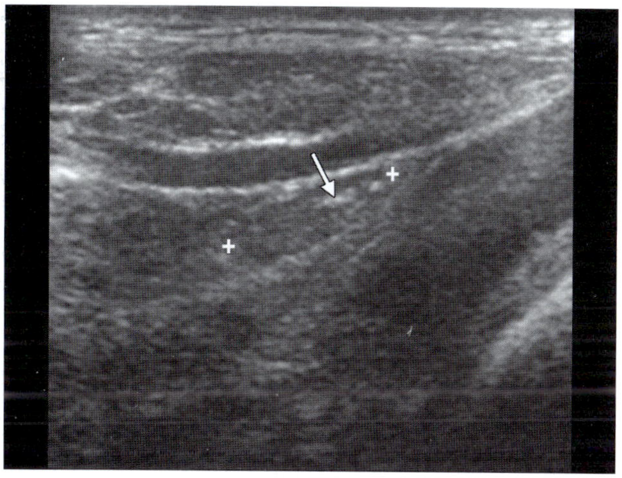

FIG. 3: US image of left undescended testis in a 24-year male: The testis is atrophic and located distal to external inguinal ring anterior to the pubic tubercle. Mediastinum testes are identified within the testis (arrow).

CONGENITAL ANOMALIES OF THE TESTIS

Cryptorchidism

Cryptorchidism is a condition where either one or both testes fails to descend to the base of the scrotum from abdomen, affects 4–5% of full-term and 9–30% of premature males at birth. In cryptorchidism, testis can be found in any position along the line of descent (abdominal, inguinal, prescrotal, or gliding); however, in about 80%, the nonpalpable undescended testis is located in inguinal canal and intra-abdominal in 20%.[6] Normal complete descent is necessary for full maturation of the testis. Complications of undescended testis include infertility, malignant degeneration, torsion and inguinal hernia. Orchiopexy performed later, even after puberty, is advocated for better surveillance of the testis. If orchiopexy is not feasible, orchidectomy is considered in patients after puberty. Recent epidemiologic studies indicate a 2.5 to 8 times greater risk of developing malignancy in cryptorchid testis.[7] Most common malignancy in the cryptorchid testis is seminoma. Orchiopexy does not reduce the risk of malignant degeneration of the once cryptorchid testis; however, it allows easier surveillance. In cases of seminoma of cryptorchid testis prompting unilateral orchiectomy, the remaining normal testis remains at a higher risk of developing cancer.

Ultrasound examination is indicated for the localization of undescended testis and also for the follow-up after orchiopexy. The undescended testis is often smaller and iso- or hypoechoic in echogenicity. Identification of mediastinum testis helps in differentiating this with other similar appearing structures like lymph nodes. The undescended testis is most commonly located distal to external inguinal ring anterior to the pubic tubercle. Even small rudimentary testis can be identified, if it is located here and hence, US is the primary imaging modality used for the localization of undescended testis **(Fig. 3)**. If testis is not located in the inguinal canal or base of the scrotum, then suprapubic, femoral and perineal regions should also be scanned. Intra-abdominal testis is difficult to locate on sonography.

Magnetic resonance imaging is an excellent modality for demonstration of penoscrotal or intracanalicular testis, but is not very satisfactory for demonstration of high intra-abdominal testis. Bladder should be emptied before the scanning. Fast T1W and T2W axial and coronal images are obtained from scrotum to the level above seminal vesicles. The examination is extended up to lower pole of the kidneys if testis is not located in the pelvis. The undescended testis can be easily identified with its characteristic signal intensity pattern. It tends to be oval in inguinal canal and round in intra-abdominal position. Sometimes the gubernaculum testis may be misdiagnosed as the undescended testis. While testis typically is hypointense on T1W and hyperintense on T2W images, the gubernaculum testis is hypointense on both T1W and T2W images. Hypertrophied inguinal lymph nodes may also have the signal characteristics similar to the testis; however, typical location of the nodes (adjacent to vessels or below the inguinal ligament) and demonstration of mediastinum in undescended testis help to differentiate testis from the lymph nodes. CT, like MRI, also allows precise identification of the undescended testis.

Miscellaneous Congenital Anomalies

Retractile or migratory testis is seen in 5- to 6-year-old boys and is due to a hyperactive reflex of cremaster muscle. The testis slides back and forth between scrotum and external inguinal ring. By puberty these usually take normal intrascrotal position and no treatment is required. The ectopic testis, i.e. location outside the descent path, is rare and is believed to be due to misdirected attachment to the scrotum. The usual sites of testicular ectopia are superficial inguinal pouch (lateral to external inguinal ring), femoral canal, suprapubic area, perineum, and contralateral scrotal pouch.[8] Unilateral absence of testis (monorchia) is usually left sided.[9] Unlike cryptorchidism, the testis in the patients with monorchia is not at increased risk of malignancy. Polyorchidism or testicular duplication is very rare.[8]

ACUTE SCROTUM

Acute scrotum is a clinical condition characterized by sudden onset of pain, swelling and redness of the scrotum that may occur alone or in any combination. It is important to differentiate surgical conditions like testicular torsion or rupture from those that can be managed conservatively (epididymo-orchitis) as early as possible. Clinical examination alone may not be helpful or it may be difficult to perform in patients with acute tender scrotum. Acute inflammation and testicular torsion are most important causes of acute scrotal pain. Other causes include torsion of appendix of testis or epididymis, trauma, tumor, incarcerated inguinal hernia and thrombophlebitis of the pampiniform plexus.

Epididymitis and Orchitis

Epididymitis is the most common cause of acute scrotum in postpubertal adults. Acute epididymitis is almost always caused by descending lower urinary tract infection. In children and older men, *Escherichia coli*, *Pseudomonas* and *Proteus* are the usual causative organisms. In young men, sexually transmitted organisms such as *Chlamydia and gonococci* are responsible. Rare causes of epididymitis and orchitis include tuberculosis, sarcoidosis,[10] brucellosis,[11] mumps and *Cryptococcus*. Chemical epididymitis can be seen due to drugs like amiodarone.[12] Direct extension of the inflammation in testis, resulting in epididymo-orchitis occurs in about 20% of patients with epididymitis.[13] Isolated orchitis is rare except when caused by viral infections such as mumps and acquired immunodeficiency syndrome (AIDS).[14] Complications of acute epididymitis include abscess, chronic pain, infarction, gangrene, atrophy, pyocele and infertility.

Patients present with insidious pain and scrotal swelling. Fever, dysuria and urethral discharge may also be present. Clinically, scrotal pain associated with epididymitis is usually relieved when the testes are elevated over the symphysis pubis (the Prehn's sign).[15] US findings of acute epididymitis include enlarged hypoechoic or hyperechoic (presumably secondary to hemorrhage) epididymis[2] **(Fig. 4)**. Indirect signs of inflammation, such as reactive hydrocele, pyocele and scrotal wall thickening can be seen. Diffuse testicular involvement is confirmed by inhomogeneous testicular echotexture and enlargement. Orchitis is characterized by heterogeneous echogenicity due to testicular edema contained within a rigid tunica albuginea.[16] It may be seen as focal or diffuse involvement, with the former manifesting as multiple hypoechoic lesions within the parenchyma **(Fig. 5)**. Lymphoma and leukemia of the testis have a similar appearance and are often bilateral (but not always), whereas infections (excluding mumps) are usually unilateral.

The sensitivity of color Doppler US (CDUS) imaging in detecting scrotal inflammation is almost 100%.[17] In acute epididymitis, there is a high-flow, low resistance pattern due to increase in the number of vessels with hyperemia.[18] In healthy volunteer, the RI in the testis is rarely less than 0.5; however, in more than 50% of epididymo-orchitis patients, the RI is less than 0.5.[19] Use of a peak systolic velocity (PSV) threshold of 15 cm/s results in a diagnostic accuracy of 93% for epididymitis and 90% for orchitis.[20] Reversal of flow during diastole is suggestive of venous infarction in acute epididymo-orchitis.[21] Follow-up sonography is necessary in patients who do not respond to therapy. However, it is not required in patients with uncomplicated epididymitis.

Contrast-enhanced US can be a problem-solving tool in acute inflammation for assessment of secondary complications like abscess formation, hemorrhage, spermatic cord thrombosis, or venous infarction. In testicular abscesses or venous infarction, CEUS demonstrates nonenhancement of a central avascular component, with enhancement of peripheral rim and septa.[22] It also shows absence of flow in the thrombosed spermatic vessels.

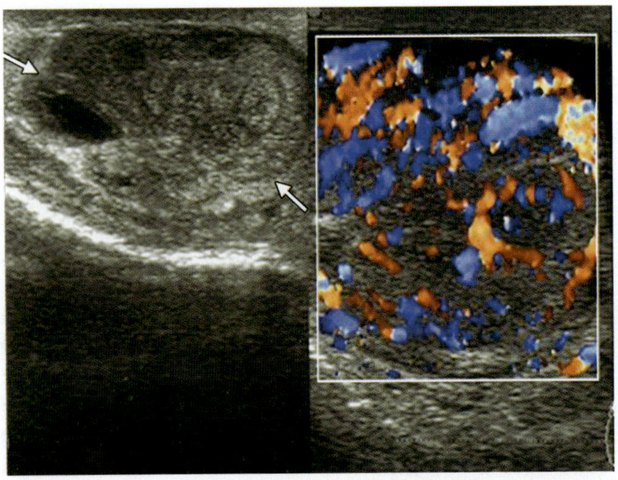

FIG. 4: US and color Doppler image of acute epididymitis showing enlarged heterogeneous epididymal head (arrows) with increased vascularity.

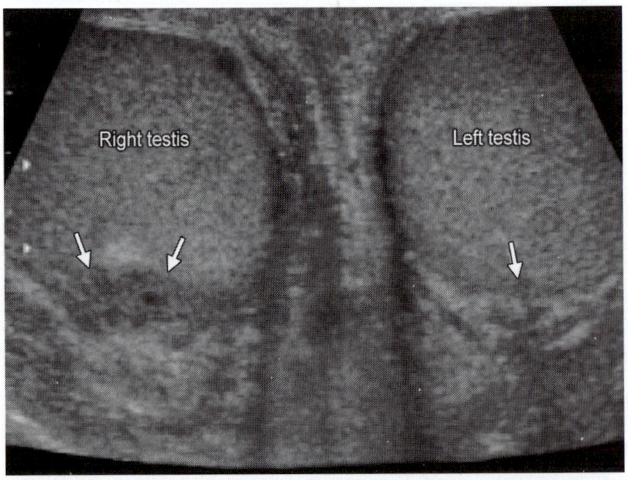

FIG. 5: Bilateral epididymo-orchitis: US image showing enlarged heterogeneous epididymis posterior to both testes and hypoechoic areas within the testes (arrows).

In acute epididymitis, enlarged epididymis with high-signal intensity on T2W images is seen on MRI. Areas of hemorrhages and hypervascularity (in the form of engorged vessels with signal void) can also be demonstrated. The inflamed epididymis shows marked enhancement on postcontrast images. Associated orchitis, if present, is seen as homogeneous or heterogeneous hypointense areas in testis on T2W images.

The sonographic findings in chronic epididymitis are nonspecific and diagnosis is usually made on the basis of clinical findings. It is characterized by persistent pain in the scrotal region and on grayscale US, an enlarged epididymis with increased echogenicity can be seen.[23] Sometimes calcifications within the epididymis can be seen. Tuberculosis, leprosy, sarcoidosis, brucellosis and syphilis can cause granulomatous epididymo-orchitis **(Fig. 6)**.

Torsion

Testicular torsion occurs due to rotation of testis along the longitudinal axis of spermatic cord. Initially, venous drainage is stopped resulting in edema and hemorrhages. Subsequently arterial flow is also impaired resulting in ischemia and hemorrhagic necrosis of the gonad. It is a surgical emergency, as delay in diagnosis and intervention leads to irreversible damage to the testis. The extent of testicular ischemia depends on the degree of torsion, which ranges from 180° to 720° or greater, and the degree of torsion and duration of ischemia determines testicular salvage rate. Nearly 100% salvage rate exists when the surgery is done in first 6 hours after the onset of symptoms; which reduces to 70% within 6–12 hours, and 20% at 12–24 hours.[24]

There are two types of testicular torsion: (1) Extravaginal; and (2) Intravaginal. Extravaginal torsion is rare and occurs almost exclusively in neonates. It occurs when testis and gubernaculum are not fixed and are free to rotate in the scrotum. The entire vaginal sac including testis rotates at the level of external inguinal ring. It often presents as a mass in the groin in newborns. Intravaginal torsion occurs within the vaginal sac. It results from anomalous suspension of testis by a long stalk of spermatic cord and most commonly occurs in boys around the puberty. There is ten-fold increased incidence of torsion in undescended testis after orchiopexy.[25]

Approximately two-thirds of the cases of torsion are seen in adolescents between 12 years and 18 years of age. Acute torsion patients present with scrotal pain of sudden onset, followed by nausea, vomiting and low-grade fever. On physical examination, swollen, edematous, tender, and inflamed hemiscrotum can be seen. US is considered the first step in evaluation, and its findings vary with the degree and duration of rotation of the cord. Grayscale images are nonspecific and often appear normal, if the torsion has just occurred. In first 4–6 hours, most commonly encountered findings are testicular swelling and decreased echogenicity **(Fig. 7)**. After 24 hours of onset, the testis shows diffusely heterogeneous echotexture due to congestion, hemorrhage, and infarction (late or missed torsion). An enlarged hypoechoic epididymal head may also be seen as the deferential artery supplying the epididymis is often involved in the torsion.[26] In the setting of complete torsion, normal echogenicity of testis on US is a strong predictor of viability. Other indicators include reactive hydrocele and scrotal wall thickening.

Torsion may be transient, incomplete or complete. Partial or transient torsion pose a diagnostic challenge, and the ability of CDUS to enable accurate diagnosis of incomplete torsion remains undetermined. The presence of color or power Doppler signal in a patient with the clinical manifestation of torsion does not exclude torsion.[27]

For accurate diagnosis the US scanner should be optimized for detection of slow flow and be adjusted for the lowest possible threshold setting and lowest repetition frequency. On color Doppler, detection of testicular torsion and ischemia in painful scrotum by using the only criteria of absence of identifiable intratesticular flow is 86% sensitive, 100% specific and 97% accurate.[17] Scintigraphy and color Doppler are comparable with regard to diagnosis of torsion in adolescent and adult populations.[17] Scintigraphy is a reasonable alternative for evaluation of acute scrotal pain

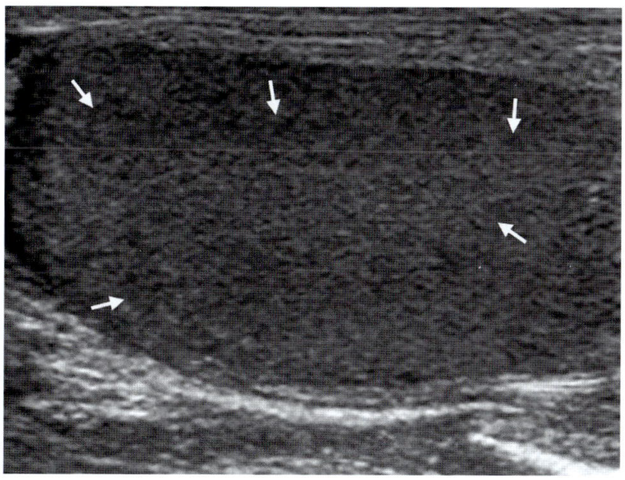

FIG. 6: Granulomatous orchitis in a case of syphilis: US image showing multiple ill-defined hypoechoic lesions (arrows) within the testis.

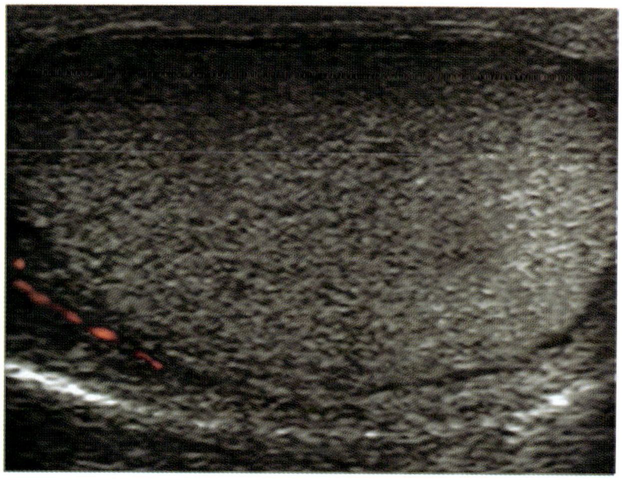

FIG. 7: Power Doppler US image showing heterogeneous appearing testis with reduced intratesticular flow in a case of torsion of testis.

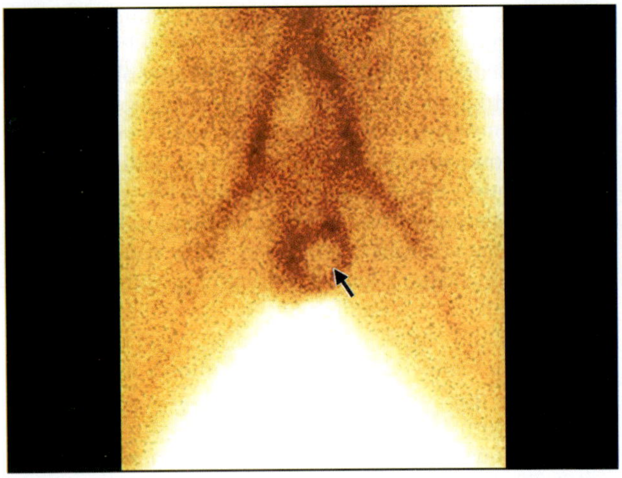

FIG. 8: Tc-99m pertechnetate scan showing photopenic area (arrow) in scrotum due to torsion of left testis.

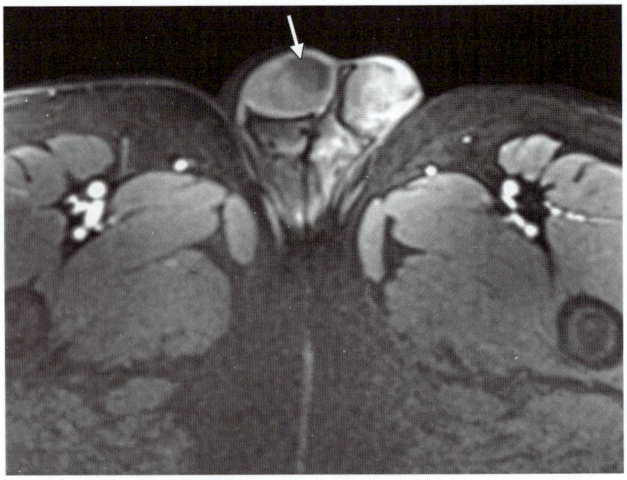

FIG. 9: Intermittent torsion: Contrast-enhanced magnetic resonance (CEMR) axial image showing hypoenhancing area within the right testis (arrow).

and should be used when diagnosis of torsion remains in question and CDUS sensitivity for low-velocity, low-volume testicular blood flow is inadequate **(Fig. 8)**.

Torsion of the testicular and epididymal appendages also present with acute scrotal pain with no other physical symptoms usually. On physical examination, a small firm nodule, palpable along the superior aspect of the testis exhibiting bluish discoloration through the overlying skin can be seen; defined as "blue dot" sign.[28] The appendix of testis is the most commonly twisted testicular appendices, seen in nearly 90% of cases and most often occur in boys of 7–14 years of age. Torsion of the appendages of the testes on US usually reveals a hyperechoic mass with a central hypoechoic area adjacent to the epididymis or testis. Skin thickening and reactive hydrocele are common in these cases. On color Doppler, increased peripheral flow may be seen around the twisted testicular appendage.[17] Management is conservative aimed at pain reduction. The pain usually subsides within 2–3 days, with atrophy of the appendix, which may calcify. The role of US examination in testicular appendage torsion is to exclude acute epididymo-orchitis and testicular torsion.

Magnetic resonance imaging in testicular torsion can show twisted cord as multiple low intensity curvilinear structures radiating in a "whirlpool" pattern. The torsion knot may be seen as an area of signal void. In patients with intermittent torsion, the testis is enlarged and hyperintense on both T1W and T2W images owing to subacute hemorrhages **(Fig. 9)**. Phosphorus magnetic resonance spectroscopy has been reported to be helpful in evaluation of acute torsion. It demonstrates decreased levels of β-ATP and phosphomonoester and increased levels of inorganic phosphorus.[13]

Scrotal Trauma

Scrotal trauma usually results from either direct injury or from straddle injuries. History is very helpful in the diagnosis; however, marked scrotal swelling, pain and open injuries limit adequate clinical examination. Patients with penetrating and open scrotal injuries undergo immediate surgery and are not candidates for US.

In cases of blunt trauma, sonography is used to confirm or exclude testicular rupture, differentiate a hematoma from hematocele and for follow-up of patients undergoing conservative management. Testicular rupture is a surgical emergency and such patients are taken up for immediate surgery whereas patients with small hematomas or hematocele are managed conservatively. Hence scrotal sonography has a decisive influence on clinical management.[29]

On sonography, intratesticular hematoma is seen as sharply defined hypoechoic space-occupying lesion (SOL). Irregularities of testicular contour and hypo- or hyperechoic heterogeneous areas suggest testicular rupture. These parenchymal areas correspond to hemorrhages and infarction. Visualization of solid and cystic intrascrotal mass and absence of testis like structure is a characteristic feature of testicular fragmentation. Sometimes a distinct fracture line may also be identified. Hematocele usually accompanies testicular rupture but its absence does not exclude the possibility of rupture.[14] Scrotal hematoma between the layers of scrotal wall is seen as nonspecific soft tissue thickening. If the urethra is injured, extravasation of urine between the layers of scrotal wall produces "onion peel" thickening of scrotal wall.

Acute hematocele or accumulation of blood in vaginal sac contains numerous small internal echoes. In chronic hematocele, thick septae and wall thickening are demonstrated.

There is good correlation of CEUS findings with extent of injury, which can clear demonstrate the fracture lines, interruption of tunica albuginea, and scrotal hematoma. It also quantifies viable parenchyma more reliably compared to conventional sonography or CDUS.[30] CEUS allows a more confident assessment of two clinically important features: (1) the presence of testicular rupture, and (2) the extent of viable testicular tissue which may influence the surgical decision.

Magnetic resonance imaging may be required in patients with scrotal injury when satisfactory sonographic examination is not possible. It is also indicated, if testicular rupture cannot be confidently excluded on the sonography. The diagnosis of testicular rupture is facilitated by unequivocal depiction of tunica albuginea on MRI.

The integrity of tunica albuginea is best assessed on T2W or contrast-enhanced T1W images. Intratesticular injuries demonstrate decreased contrast enhancement. MRI is also valuable in demonstration of hematomas.

Testicular Tumors

Testicular cancer is the most common solid malignancy affecting the young men between the age group of 18 years and 35 years, accounting for 1% of all cancers in men. Incidence of the testicular neoplasms is increasing from last decade and European men possess greater risk as compared to the other ethnicity. The germ cell tumors account for more than 90% of the testicular tumors. Risk factors for testicular cancer include cryptorchidism, testicular atrophy (e.g. mumps), testicular microlithiasis, Klinefelter's syndrome, Down syndrome, family history and maternal use of diethylstilbestrol.[31] The etiology of testicular cancer is not known till date; however; characteristic genetic alteration affecting the isochromosome of the short arm of the chromosome 12 (i(12p)) is implicated in the sporadic cases.

Localized testicular cancer presents as a painless nodule or a bump/swelling in the testicle or as a vague lower abdominal discomfort. Advanced disease or disseminated disease may present with lymphatic or hematogenous spread.

However, developments in diagnostic and therapeutic modalities during past decade have led to high cure rate, even for patients who present with metastatic disease.[16]

The main role of USG in the testicular cancer diagnosis is to distinguish between the lesions of intratesticular and extratesticular origin, as most of the extratesticular masses are benign and, intratesticular masses are more likely to be malignant.[32] Grayscale US is nearly 100% sensitive for detection of testicular tumors.[33] Many benign intratesticular processes like orchitis, abscess, hematoma, granuloma and infarction mimic malignancy and hence must considered in the differential diagnosis. Color Doppler examination demonstrates increased vascularity in the majority of malignant lesions and helps to better define testicular involvement. A suspicion of testicular cancer mandates radiological workup to ascertain the extent or spread of the disease with the help of chest and abdominopelvic cross-sectional imaging modalities. The lymph nodal metastasis into the pelvis, chest and supraclavicular nodal stations is considered as distant metastasis.

The radical inguinal orchiectomy is performed rather than a biopsy of the testis mass for histopathological evaluation as well as to achieve local tumor control. The testicular cancer stage, risk stratification and histopathological nature of tumor guide in selection of initial modality of the treatment. Definitive cure can be achieved by inguinal orchiectomy procedure alone in the patients with stage I seminoma. The adjuvant chemotherapy or radiation therapy is required in the advanced stages of the disease. With modern chemoradiation therapeutics development, it is not difficult to achieve complete cure rate even in presence of metastatic testicular cancer. Radiologists play a pivotal role in the initial detection, staging and active surveillance of the patients with testicular neoplasm.

Classification of the Testicular Tumors

Testicular cancers are broadly divided into the three categories as germ cell tumors, sex cord stromal tumors, and miscellaneous tumors **(Table 1)**. In young male, germ cell tumors account for 95% and sex cord stromal tumors for 5%, and miscellaneous tumors, including the most common entities like lymphoma or metastasis are encountered in the older age group. Among the germ cell tumors, seminoma constitutes ~50% of the prevalence and rest half is constituted by the nonseminomatous germ cell tumors which are enlisted in **Table 1** with percentage of each entity. Differentiation of seminomatous versus nonseminomatous germ cell tumor is important as treatment and prognosis is different.

Approach to Testicular Cancers

A suspected case of testicular cancer evaluation begins with complete history elicitation and systemic physical examination. The value of imaging and laboratory tests is invaluable in evaluation of testicular cancer. The USG (grayscale as well as Doppler mode), CT of chest, MRI or CT of abdomen and pelvis, MRI of brain and nuclear scans are utilized in workup of the subjects with testicular cancer based on the extent of the disease. Laboratory tests including the serum alpha-fetoprotein (AFP), serum beta-human chorionic gonadotropin (β-hCG), lactate dehydrogenase (LDH) and other chemistry profile are utilized in evaluation of patients.

TABLE 1: Classification and prevalence (germ cell tumors) of the testicular tumors.

Testicular tumor	Subtypes of testicular tumors
Germ cell tumors	• Seminoma (50%) • Mixed germ cell tumor (33%) • Embryonal carcinoma (10%) • Teratoma (4%) • Yolk sac tumor (1%) • Choriocarcinoma (0.3%)
Sex cord stromal tumors	• Leydig cell tumor • Sertoli cell tumor • Granulosa cell tumor • Thecoma
Miscellaneous	• Metastasis (8–15%) • Lymphoma • Leukemia • Sarcoma • Leiomyoma • Vascular tumor • Fibroma • Neurofibroma

Germ Cell Tumors

Germ cell tumors account for 90–95% of testicular cancer. Germ cell tumors are divided into two groups: (1) seminomatous and (2) nonseminomatous germ cell tumor (NSGCT). The later includes embryonal cell carcinoma, teratoma, choriocarcinoma, endodermal sinus tumor or mixed components of these tumors. The distinction of these tumors is primarily from the histological analysis, and immunohistochemical methods to be reserved for difficult cases. This distinction determines treatment and prognosis.

Serum tumor markers are important in diagnosis, staging and follow-up. These include LDH, AFP and hCG. LDH may increase in any type of tumor and it correlates well with the extent of the disease. The seminoma does not show elevated tumor marker AFP, if the elevated AFP in the patient with the histological analysis suggestive of seminoma warrants for consideration and treatment as for that of the nonseminomatous tumor.[34] Elevated hCG is encountered in subjects with choriocarcinoma, most of the NSGCT and a few subjects of seminomas.[31]

Seminomas

The most common tumor among the germ cell tumors is seminoma, approximately contributing to the 50% of the prevalence. Usually, it manifests in the young- and middle-aged adults in their 2nd to 3rd decade and almost never reported in the infants.[35] Best prognosis of seminomatous tumor is by virtue of its sensitivity to chemotherapeutic agents and radiation therapy.[7] The seminoma is subclassified into typical seminoma (~85%), anaplastic (~5–10%) and spermatocytic (~4–6%) histological variants. The spermatocytic variant of seminoma is seen in elderly (~60–70 years) males with excellent prognosis. On scrotal sonographic examination, seminoma of testis is visualized as a homogeneous, hypoechoic, nodule or mass, which matches the uniform appearance of gross pathological specimen **(Fig. 10)**. Infrequently, cystic changes (~10%) or calcification foci are also demonstrated in the seminoma.[36] Intralesional color uptake by the internal vascularity increases the diagnostic probability of malignant nature of the lesion of interest in appropriate clinical scenario. More advancements in the sonography modality has resulted in the advent of contrast-enhanced sonographic technique, which showed rapid uptake and washout characteristic of the seminoma lesion relative to the background parenchyma, along with the distortion of linear course of the intratesticular vascular channels.[37] Testicular mass may replace the whole of the testis in half of the cases, but still seminoma remains limited by the tunica albuginea, and rarely extends into the paratesticular substance/structures. Lymphatic and hematogenous dissemination of the seminoma is known phenomenon in testis oncology, which may be evident in the form of retroperitoneal or mediastinal lymph nodal enlargement and SOLs in the lung, liver and brain respectively, accounting for 25% of the population with seminoma.

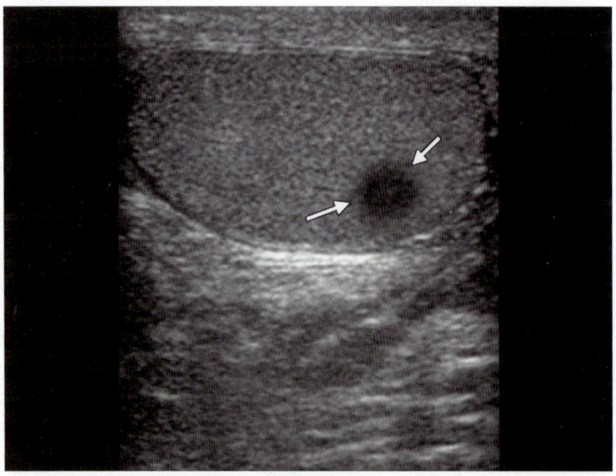

FIG. 10: US image showing a nonpalpable seminoma (arrows) of testis.

Nonseminomatous Germ Cell Tumors

The NSGCTs constitute for the rest half of the prevalence of the germ cell tumors, the mixed germ cell tumor accounts for the most common (~30–60%) single variant tumor among the other NSGCTs. The embryonal carcinoma (10%), teratoma (4%), yolk sac tumor (1%), and choriocarcinoma (0.3%) are the other components of the NSGCTs. On histology, different proportions of the mixtures of tissue components or pure composition of lesions are seen, which reflect the similar characteristics on sonography resulting heterogeneous (71%) and irregular (45%) tumor lesions in testis. These lesions also demonstrate cystic (~61%) and calcification (~35%) changes more frequently as compared to the seminoma.[36] Most of the NSGCTs population presents with advanced disease.[32]

Embryonal Carcinoma

The pure component of the embryonal cells is rarely (~2%) seen in embryonal carcinoma, rather embryonal cellular component is most frequently (~85%) expressed in the mixed germ cell tumors, accounting for the ~10% of NSGCTs. Usually, this tumor is seen in middle-aged adults in their 3rd decade and rarely seen in the prepubertal males. On sonographic evaluation, irregular, heterogeneous lesions with calcific and cystic changes are seen with testicular distortion, breach of tunica albuginea and paratesticular extension frequently.[7]

Teratoma

Teratoma constitutes for the ~3–4% of the NSGCTs, and shows the cellular components derived from all the three-germ cell layers.[32] Teratomatous tumors can be present in any group, and it is the second most common testicular tumor in prepubertal boys. The mature teratoma in children is considered as benign, where as a teratoma in adults is treated as malignant. On sonologic evaluation, teratoma may be visualized as a heterogeneous lesion **(Fig. 11)**, with echogenic contents (fat, bone and cartilage) or hypoechoic components (soft tissue or fibrotic component). As compared to other tumors in the NSGCTs, the teratoma shows frequent cystic changes.

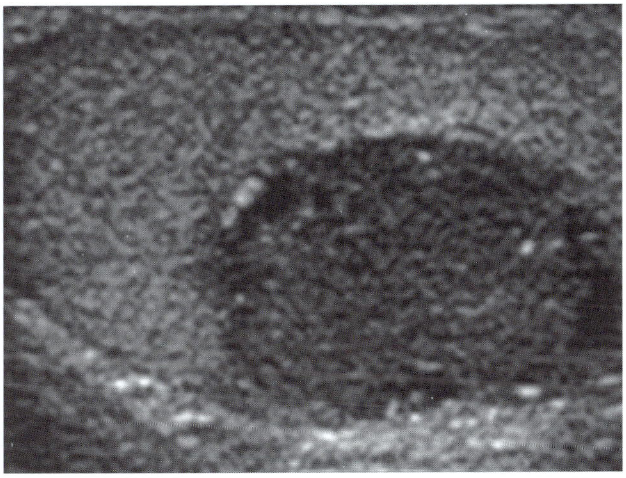

FIG. 11: US image showing teratoma of testis. Note small cystic areas and foci of calcification within the lesion.

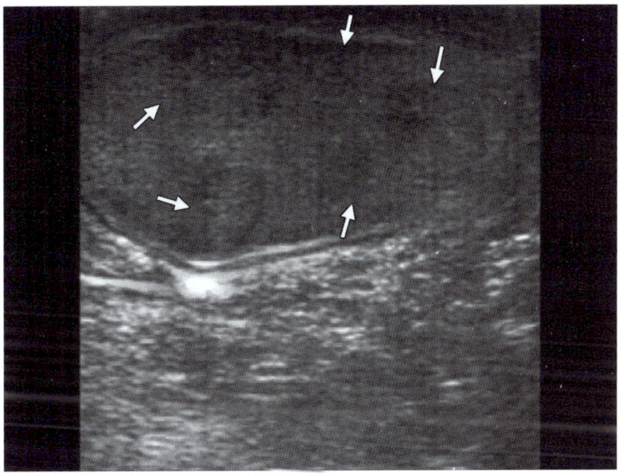

FIG. 12: US image showing multicentric rhabdomyosarcoma of testis (arrows).

Yolk Sac Tumor

Yolk sac tumors constitute ~1% of the NSGCTs, and this tumor is alternatively known an endodermal sinus tumor or infantile embryonal carcinoma. Usually, the children less than 5 year of age are most frequently involved by this tumor. Tumor marker AFP is elevated and its measurements adds in diagnosis (modest raise) as well as in prognostication of subjects with yolk sac tumor.[35] In adults, yolk sac component is encountered in the mixed germ cell tumors with associated poor prognosis. On sonographic evaluation, heterogeneous tumors with echogenic areas are seen scattered at places secondary to the hemorrhagic components.

Choriocarcinoma

The choriocarcinoma, syncytial cells containing tumor, is seen rarely, in ~0.5% subjects of NSGCTs. The choriocarcinoma is an aggressive malignant tumor, which shows microvascular invasion with early metastasis into the distant sites including the lungs and brain. Extensive tumoral hemorrhage is common in the choriocarcinoma, and exhibits poor prognosis. On US examination, mixed solid cystic mass is seen in the testis.[38] Cross-sectional imaging is warranted in the evaluation of the chest, abdominal and central nervous system metastases. The characteristic tumor marker β-hCG is used for establishing diagnosis as well as monitoring of the affected patients.

Burned-out Germ Cell Tumor

This is a biological magical phenomenon, where a rapidly growing tumor (usually the teratocarcinoma or choriocarcinoma) gets depleted of nutritional supply due to inadequate neoangiogenesis resulting the regression or vanishing of the primary tumor. The histopathological examination of such a testicular structure reveals scar or fibrotic component corresponding to the mixed echogenic or ill-defined hypoechoic lesion noted on USG.[39]

Non-germ Cell Testicular Tumors

The sex cord stromal tumors (including Leydig cell tumors, Sertoli cell tumor, granulosa cell tumors and thecoma) and miscellaneous tumors (such as lymphoma, metastasis, leukemia, and other mesenchymal tumors) are the non-germ cell tumors of testis accounting for the 5% of the testicular cancer.[40] The sex cord stromal tumors usually benign, and affect the prepubertal boys with mixed component of the tumor cells, and sometimes these tumors may biologically active with resultant secretion of endocrine substances resulting precocious puberty, scrotal enlargement and gynecomastia.

Gonadoblastoma is a rare tumor which is encountered in subjects with gonadal dysgenesis and associated intersex problems.

Sonographically, stromal tumors are seen as small, smoothly demarcated, homogeneous hypoechoic intratesticular masses[31] **(Fig. 12)**. Any lesion with rapid or aggressive growth patterns and intratumoral vascularity should suggest malignant behavior which reflects in histopathology analysis as cell atypia and high mitotic figures. Relatively newer sonological technique involving administration of US contrast agents showed persistent enhancement of the stromal tumors as opposed to the rapid enhancement and washout characteristic described in seminoma.[41]

Lymphomas constitute 5% of testicular tumors and are almost exclusively diffuse non-Hodgkin's lymphoma B-cell tumors **(Fig. 13)**. In men older than 60 years, lymphoma is the most common testicular tumor, accounting for nearly 50% of cases.[42] Sonographically, these tumors resemble seminomas but synchronous involvement of the contralateral testis and involvement of the spermatic cord and epididymis suggest lymphoma more than it does seminoma. Leukemic infiltration to the testis has been found at autopsy in 40–65% of patients with acute leukemia and in 20–35% of patients with chronic leukemia.[43] In boys with acute lymphoblastic leukemia, testicular involvement is reported in 5–10% of

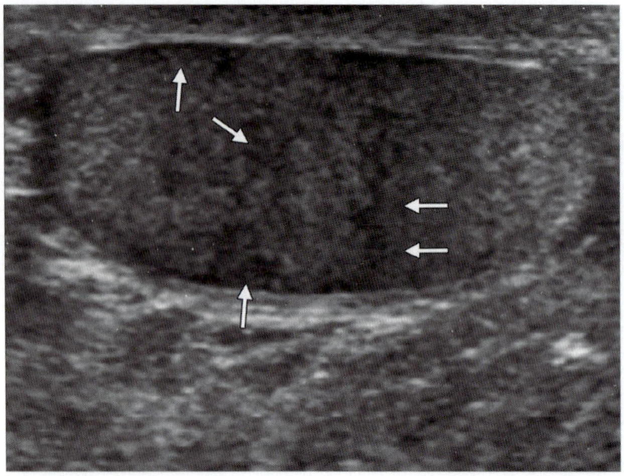

FIG. 13: US image showing sheet-like hypoechoic areas within the testis (arrows) due to lymphoma (NHL).

patients, with the majority found during clinical remission. Bilateral testicular involvement is seen in about 50% of the patients. Sonographically, lymphoma/leukemia deposits are seen as focal or diffuse hypoechoic areas. The testis is usually enlarged.

Intrascrotal metastases from tumors of other organs are rare and are usually found in older patients. Most frequent primaries are from lung, kidney, prostate and melanoma.[14] Sonographic appearances are nonspecific.

Staging of Testicular Cancer

T (Tumor) N (Node) M (Metastasis) staging by the American Joint Committee on Cancer (AJCC) is followed for testicular cancer **(Box 1)**. Extent of primary tumor (pT) is classified after radical orchiectomy, and nodal staging can be done clinically (N) or by pathological (pN) analysis.[44]

Serum Tumor Markers

Serum tumor markers(s) are also used in staging of testicular cancer. Blood tests are done before and after surgery, and for patients receiving chemotherapy, tumor markers on 1st of therapy are used for risk group determination **(Table 2)**.

BOX 1: TNM staging for testicular cancer.

TNM staging

Primary tumor

- pTx: Primary tumor cannot be assessed (if radical orchiectomy has not been performed, Tx is used)
- pT0: No evidence of primary tumor (e.g. histologic scar in testis)
- pTis: Intratubular germ cell neoplasia (carcinoma *in situ*)
- pT1: Tumor limited to the testis and epididymis without vascular/ lymphatic invasion, or tumor invasion into the tunica albuginea but not the tunica vaginalis
- pT2: Tumor limited to the testis and epididymis with vascular/ lymphatic invasion, or tumor extending through the tunica albuginea with involvement of the tunica vaginalis
- pT3: Tumor invades the spermatic cord with or without vascular/ lymphatic invasion
- pT4: Tumor invades the scrotum with or without vascular/ lymphatic invasion

Nodal staging

- NX or pNX: Regional lymph nodes cannot be assessed
- N0 or pN0: No regional lymph node metastasis
- N1 or pN1: Metastases with a lymph node mass 2 cm or less in greatest dimension; or multiple lymph nodes, none more than 2 cm in greatest dimension
- N2 or pN2: Metastases with a lymph node mass more than 2 cm but not more than 5 cm in greatest dimension; or multiple lymph nodes, any one mass greater than 2 cm but not more than 5 cm in greatest dimension
- N3 or pN3: Metastases with a lymph node mass more than 5 cm in greatest dimension

Metastasis

- MX: Distant metastasis cannot be assessed
- M0: No distant metastasis
- M1: Distant metastasis
- M1a: Nonregional nodal or pulmonary metastasis
- M1b: Distant metastasis other than to nonregional lymph nodes and lungs

(pT: primary tumor; N: clinical nodal staging; pN: pathological nodal staging)

CANCER GROUP STAGING

Considering all the above parameters [T (tumor), N (nodes), M (metastasis) and S (serum levels of tumor markers)], final staging of the tumor is done, which helps in treatment planning and prognostication of tumors **(Table 3)**.

Risk Group Classification

Another application of the TNM system is, it is used in risk stratification of advanced disease, taking into consideration of tumor markers and classifies the cancer as low, medium, and poor outlook. This helps in determining treatment plan and the likelihood of cure **(Table 4)**.

TABLE 2: Blood levels of tumor markers for staging of testicular cancer.

	LDH (U/L)	hCG (mIU/mL)	AFP (ng/mL)
Sx	Marker studies not available or not performed		
S0	Normal	Normal	Normal
S1	<1.5 × Normal	<5,000	<1,000
S2	1.5–10 × Normal	5,000–50,000	1,000–10,000
S3	>10 × Normal	>50,000	>10,000

[LDH: lactate dehydrogenase (measured in units per liter); hCG: human chorionic gonadotropin (measured in milli-international units per milliliter); AFP: alpha-fetoprotein (measured in nanograms per milliliter)]

TABLE 3: Stage grouping.

Stage	T	N	M	S
Stage 0	Tis (*in situ*)	N0	M0	S0
Stage I	T1–T4	N0	M0	Sx
Stage IA	T1	N0	M0	S0
Stage IB	T2–T4	N0	M0	S0
Stage IS	Any T	N0	M0	S1–S3
Stage II	Any T	N1–N3	M0	Sx
Stage IIA	Any T	N1	M0	S0–S1
Stage IIB	Any T	N2	M0	S0–S1
Stage IIC	Any T	N3	M0	S0–S1
Stage III	Any T	Any N	M1	Sx
Stage IIIA	Any T Any T	Any N Any N	M1a M1a	S0–S1 S1
Stage IIIB	Any T Any T	N1–N3 Any N	M0 M1a	S2 S2
Stage IIIC	Any T Any T Any T	N1–N3 Any N Any N	M0 M1a M1b	S3 S3 Any S

TABLE 4: Risk group classification.

Risk status	Nonseminoma	Seminoma
Good outlook	No nonpulmonary metastasis: • AFP <1000 ng/mL • hCG <5000 IU/mL • LDH <1.5 ULN (upper limit of normal)	• No non-pulmonary metastasis • Any tumor marker
Intermediate outlook	Nonpulmonary metastasis: • AFP: 1000–10000 ng/mL • hCG: 5000–50000 IU/mL • LDH: 1.5–10 ULN	• Nonpulmonary metastasis • Any tumor marker
Poor outlook	No nonpulmonary metastasis: • AFP >10000 • hCG >50000 • LDH >10 ULN	• None (seminoma is never classified as poor outlook)

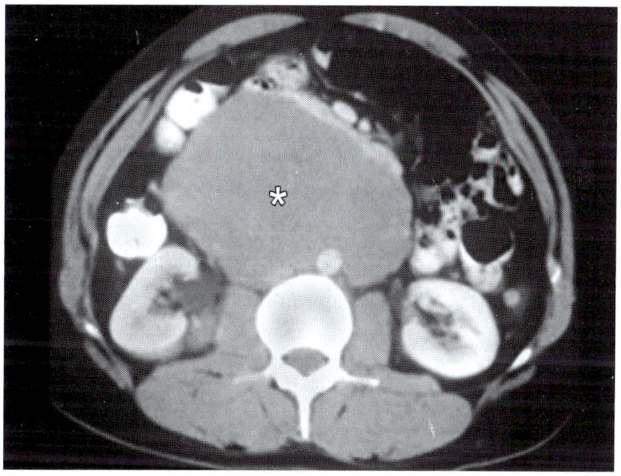

FIG. 14: Axial CECT image at the level of renal hilum showing a large metastatic homogeneous lymph nodal mass (star) in a case of seminomas testis.

Imaging in Evaluation of Testicular Cancer

Magnetic Resonance Imaging

Magnetic resonance imaging is used as a problem-solving modality. MRI of scrotum is more sensitive than sonography for detection of testicular tumors; however, the findings are variable and nonspecific. Most testicular tumors are isointense to testis on T1W images and hypointense on T2W images. On dynamic gadolinium-enhanced MRI, the tumor enhancement is often earlier and greater than the normal testicular parenchyma. Similar to their sonographic appearances, seminomas tend to be homogeneous, whereas NSGCTs are heterogeneous on MRI. Lymphoma and leukemia are characterized by testicular enlargement with diffuse, homogeneous decrease in signal intensity on T2W images. MRI is also useful in staging workup of testicular tumors when CT is inconclusive or contraindicated. It is also useful for follow-up after the treatment. In future, molecular imaging in fusion with MRI, with the help of iron oxide nanoparticles containing contrast media can aid in early and definitive, distant lymph nodal metastatic spread.

Computed Tomography

Computed tomography (CT) is the most commonly used modality in evaluation of tumor spread, staging and follow-up. CT is useful for detection of enlarged retroperitoneal or mediastinal lymph nodes as well as extranodal metastases in lungs and liver. In testicular carcinoma, lymph nodes of less than 1 cm in short-axis diameter (SAD) located in the regional nodal drainage site (e.g. renal hilum on the left or aortocaval region on right side) should be considered suspicious **(Fig. 14)**. Cut-off nodal diameter of 7 mm has been suggested as more useful for testicular cancer.[31] The enlarged lymph nodes may demonstrate necrotic center or heterogeneous contrast enhancement, particularly in NSGCTs. After completion of the treatment, some lymph nodes may not decrease in size and instead, develop more necrosis and fibrotic strands. Majority of such lymph nodal masses do not contain viable tumor; however, it cannot be ruled out on the basis of CT alone.

Positron Emission Tomography

Nuclear scans employing fludeoxyglucose-positron emission tomography (FDG-PET) in the setting of testicular malignancy is most useful in three scenarios which are described here:

1. To differentiate active disease from post-treatment changes or mature teratoma in residual component of the disease in postchemotherapy surveillance.
2. Initial staging and recurrent disease assessment in postorchiectomy period with elevation of tumor markers.
3. To predict tumor response to therapy.

The role of PET scan is invaluable in evaluation of post-treatment testicular cancer subjects for detection of residual or recurrent disease at usual or unusual sites.[45]

However, validation of the nuclear studies in routine patient care is limited due to the lack of sufficient trials and knowledge.

BENIGN INTRATESTICULAR LESIONS

Cysts

Testicular cysts are incidentally detected on sonography. These need to be differentiated from cystic tumors. Symptomatic or palpable testicular cysts or those with suspicious solid component need further evaluation and/or exploration. Others can be followed up. Two types of simple benign cysts can be identified: (1) cysts of tunica albuginea and (2) simple testicular cysts. Tunica albuginea cysts are typically small (less than 5 mm) and are usually palpated as firm nodular masses. These are located at the periphery. Simple testicular cysts are usually located near the mediastinum testis and are not palpable.

Tubular ectasia of rete testis may be mistaken for tumors. These are typically located at the mediastinum testis and consist of areas of multiple tiny cystic spaces with no flow on color Doppler flow imaging (CDFI) **(Fig. 15)**. It is usually associated with epididymal obstruction. Epidermoid and dermoid cysts of the testis are rare and these are also seen as palpable simple cysts with characteristic echogenic margins. They do not have malignant potential.

Adrenal Rests

Aberrant adrenal tissue rests may be found in testis in about 8% of patients with congenital adrenal hyperplasia. Pathogenesis may be related to the common embryonic origin of adrenals and gonads. On sonography, they are seen as multifocal and often bilateral hypoechoic lesions.

Calcifications

The consideration of testicular microlithiasis as a pre-malignant entity is a controversial topic, where multiple prospective studies failed to demonstrate the development of cancer in the surveillance of the subjects with testicular microlithiasis and at the same time ~18–75% patients with testicular malignancy are associated with the testicular microlithiasis.[45] Testicular microlithiasis is a condition where tiny calcification of the seminiferous tubules is seen, on sonographic examination these tiny calcifications fail to demonstrate posterior acoustic shadowing or rarely show in a few cases **(Fig. 16)**. Typically, testicular microlithiasis is seen as more than 5 calcific foci in single probe filed, whereas presence of less than 5 calcific foci per probe field is limited testicular microlithiasis. The self-examination or physical examination of the scrotum by the physician or regular sonological surveillance may be beneficial for those subjects with testicular microlithiasis.[46]

Scrotoliths are the loose bodies in scrotum at extra-testicular substance due to the torsion of the appendix testis and epididymis.[16] Detection of scrotoliths is easier, if fluid component is seen in the surrounding area **(Fig. 17)**. The macrocalcific changes in the testis may signify the suspicion of large cell calcifying Sertoli cell tumor, burned-out tumor or post-trauma alteration.

EXTRATESTICULAR PATHOLOGIES

Fluid Collections

Hydrocele is an abnormal accumulation of serous fluid in vaginal cavity. The congenital type is seen in infants and it is due to persistent communication between scrotal sac and the peritoneum. Acquired hydrocele is idiopathic or secondary to inflammation, torsion, trauma or tumor. Sonographically, a clear fluid is seen surrounding the testis. However, fine mobile echogenic concretions or a few thin septations can be seen

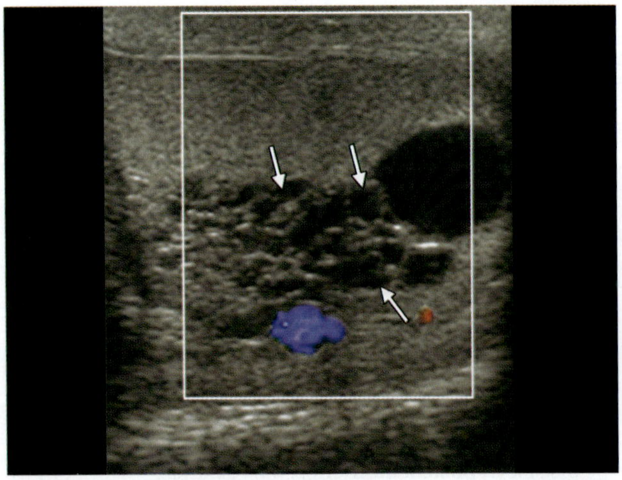

FIG. 15: US image showing tubular ectasia of rete testis (arrows). Note the absence of flow of color Doppler.

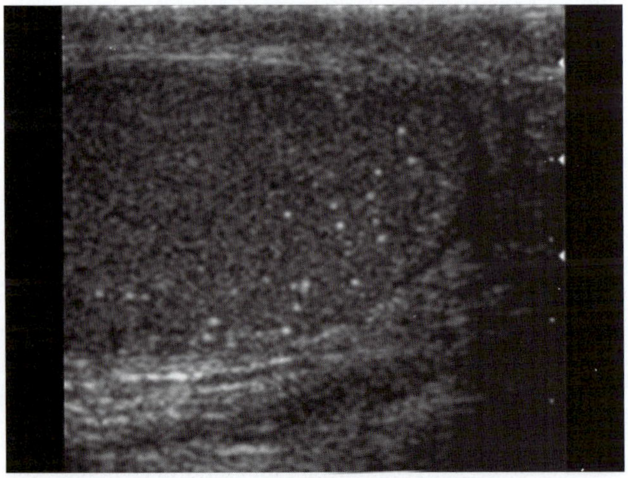

FIG. 16: US image showing multiple punctate hyperechoic non-shadowing foci of testicular microlithiasis.

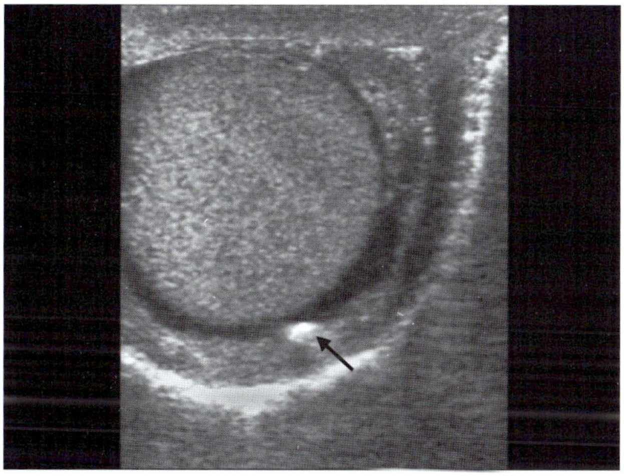

FIG. 17: US image showing a scrotal pearl (arrow).

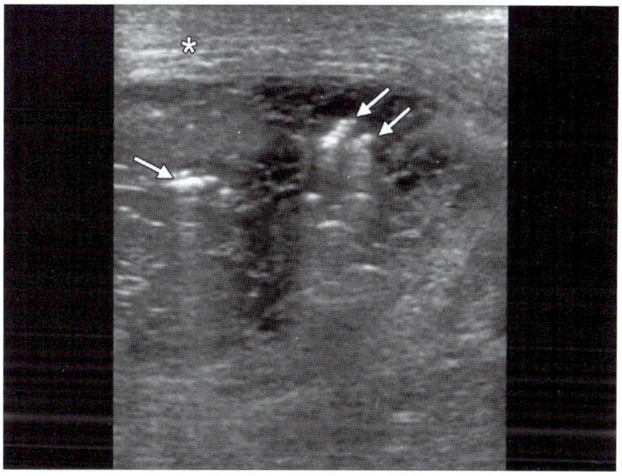

FIG. 18: Pyocele of scrotum: US image showing echogenic fluid collection within the scrotum and air foci (arrows) trapped within thin septations. Note the thickened skin of scrotum (star).

in any long-standing hydrocele and it does not necessarily suggest complicated collection. Rarely, the concretion may be fairly large when it gives a "bull's eye" appearance with central calcification surrounded by the hypoechoic layer.

Hematocele and pyocele result from hemorrhage and abscess formation respectively. Both contain multiple septations and echogenic debris. Thickening of scrotal skin and calcifications may be seen in both of these conditions[13] **(Fig. 18)**.

Inguinoscrotal hernia is usually diagnosed on the basis of clinical examination. Hernia may contain small bowel, large bowel and/or omentum.

On sonological evaluation, the inguinoscrotal hernia is appreciated as a breach in the inguinal canal fibers with abnormal protrusion of the peristaltic (bowel) or aperistaltic (omentum and other soft tissue) echogenic contents with their blood supply. The testes and appendages are localized separately from these protruded organs. Indirect inguinal hernia is more frequently associated with the bowel strangulation as compared to the direct inguinal hernia. Sonological evidence of the aperistaltic bowel loops in the hernial sac with associated dilatation and scrotum suggests bowel strangulation, which warrants immediate surgical management.[2]

Epididymal Cysts

Epididymal cysts and spermatoceles are the most common scrotal lesions and these may be encountered in up to 70% of all patients subjected to scrotal sonography.[12] Spermatoceles contain debris and sperms in addition to serous fluid and occur secondary to the obstruction of spermatic pathway. These are usually located in the head. Epididymal cysts are less common than spermatoceles and do not contain sperms. These are usually smaller in size and are located anywhere in the epididymis. Spermatoceles and epididymal cysts are identical on sonography and are seen as anechoic, well-circumscribed cysts with no or few internal echoes **(Fig. 19)**. Sperm granulomas may be found in patients with epididymal obstruction or after vasectomy.[12] On sonography, these are seen as hypoechoic epididymal lesions, sometimes with focal calcification.

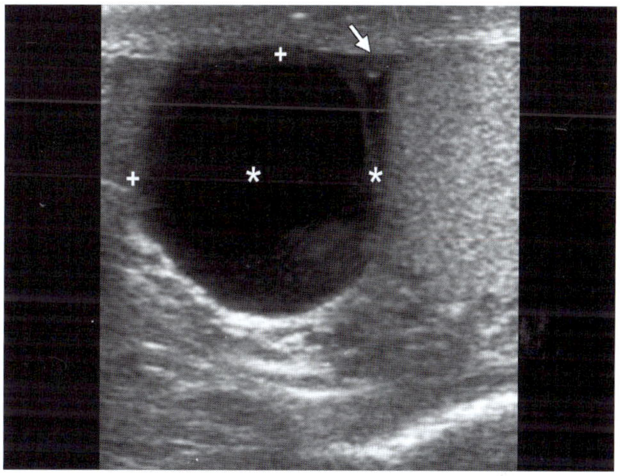

FIG. 19: US image showing an epididymal cyst. Appendix of testis (arrow) is seen between the cyst and the testis.

Postorchidectomy Scrotum

After orchidectomy, small amount of clear fluid is usually seen in the empty hemiscrotal sac, which resolves gradually. The scrotal wall appears thickened because of contraction. Hematomas are common in early postoperative period. Fresh hematomas are echogenic. These become hypoechoic or cystic as these resolve after 5–6 weeks. Tumor recurrence may be suspected if the mass develops several months after the orchidectomy.

On sonography, the recurrence is seen as a poorly defined hypoechoic lesion. Color Doppler, MRI or sonography guided biopsies are useful to differentiate recurrent tumor from hematoma.[46]

Testicular prosthesis is usually made up of silicone. On sonography, it is seen as a sharply defined, anechoic structure, frequently with excessive reverberations.[47]

Extratesticular Tumors

Extratesticular scrotal tumors are mostly benign and usually involve the epididymis. The most common is adenomatoid tumor constituting 30% of these tumors. It arises in epididymis or spermatic cord. On sonography, it is generally seen as solitary, well-defined, round to oval, small mass with variable echogenicity.[14] It may occasionally invade adjacent testicular parenchyma. Other benign paratesticular tumors include hemangioma, lipoma, neurofibroma and leiomyoma. Malignant paratesticular tumors include liposarcoma, fibrosarcoma and lymphoma in adults and rhabdomyosarcoma in children. The sonographic appearances of these tumors are nonspecific.[13]

Varicocele

Varicocele is an abnormal dilatation and tortuosity of the veins of the pampiniform plexus. It is described in detail in next chapter.

REFERENCES

1. Trainer TD. Testis and the excretory duct system. In: Sternberg S (Ed). Histology for Pathologists. New York, NY: Raven; 1992. pp. 744-6.
2. Siegel MJ. The acute scrotum. Radiol Clin North Am. 1997;35: 959-76.
3. Bree RL, Hoang DT. Scrotal ultrasound. Radiol Clin North Am. 1996;34:1183-205.
4. Middleton WD, Thorne DA, Melson GL. Color Doppler ultrasound of the normal testis. Am J Roentgenol. 1989;152:293-7.
5. Paltiel HJ, Rupich RC, Babcock DS. Maturational changes in arterial impedance of the normal testis in boys: Doppler sonographic study. Am J Roentgenol. 1994;163:1189-93.
6. Friedland GW, Chang P. The role of imaging in the management of the impalpable undescended testis. Am J Roentgenol. 1988;151:1107-11.
7. Heiken JP. Tumors of the testis and testicular adnexa. In: Pollack HM, McClennan BL (Eds). Clinical Urography. Philadelphia, PA: Saunders; 2000. pp. 1716-41.
8. Hricak H. Congenital anomalies of the testis. In: Hricak H, Hamn B, Kim B (Eds). Imaging of Scrotum. New York: Raven; 1995. pp. 37-48.
9. Levitt SB, Konyan SJ, Engel RM. The impalpable testis: a rational approach to management. J Urol. 1978;120:515-20.
10. Toyoshima M, Chida K, Masuda M. Testicular sarcoidosis. Nihon Kokyuki Gakkai Zasshi. 2000;38:63-6.
11. Bayram MM, Kervancioglu R. Scrotal gray-scale and color Doppler sonographic findings in genitourinary brucellosis. J Clin Ultrasound. 1997;25:443-7.
12. Cook JL, Dewbury K. The changes seen on high-resolution ultrasound in orchitis. Clin Radiol. 2000;55:13-8.
13. Gorman B, Carroll BA. The scrotum. In: Rummak CM, Wilson SR, Charhoneau JW (Eds). Diagnostic Ultrasound. St. Louis: Mosby; 2005. pp. 849-88.
14. Oyen RH. Scrotal ultrasound. Eur Radiol. 2002;12:19-34.
15. Noske HD, Kraus SW, Altinkilic BM, et al. Historical milestones regarding torsion of the scrotal organs. J Urol. 1998;159:13-6.
16. Dewbury KC. Scrotal ultrasonography: an update. BJU Int. 2000;86:143-52.
17. Burks DD, Markey BJ, Burkhard TK, et al. Suspected testicular torsion and ischemia: evaluation with color Doppler sonography. Radiology. 1990;175:815-21.
18. Horstman WG. Scrotal imaging. Urol Clin North Am. 1997;24:653-71.
19. Jee WH, Choe BY, Byun JY, et al. Resistive index of the intrascrotal artery in scrotal inflammatory disease. Acta Radiol. 1997;38: 1026-30.
20. Brown JM, Hammers LW, Barton JW, et al. Quantitative Doppler assessment of acute scrotal inflammation. Radiology. 1995;197:427-31.
21. Sanders LM, Haber S, Dembner A, et al. Significance of reversal of diastolic flow in the acute scrotum. J Ultrasound Med. 1994;13:137-9.
22. Lock G, Schmidt C, Helmich F, et al. Early experience with contrast-enhanced ultrasound in the diagnosis of testicular masses: a feasibility study. Urology. 2011;77(5):1049-53.
23. Rifkin MD. Inflammation of the lower genitourinary tract: the prostate, seminal vesicles, and scrotum. In: Pollack HM, McClennan BL (Eds). Clinical Urography, 2nd edition. Philadelphia, PA: Saunders; 2000. pp. 1058-87.
24. Patriquin HB, Yazbeck S, Trinh B, et al. Testicular torsion in infants and children: diagnosis with Doppler sonography. Radiology. 1993;188:781-5.
25. Williamson RC. Torsion of the testis and allied conditions. Br J Surg. 1976;63:465-76.
26. Berman JM, Beidle TR, Kunberger LE, et al. Sonographic evaluation of acute intrascrotal pathology. Am J Roentgenol. 1996;166:857-61.
27. Dogra VS, Sessions A, Mevorach A, et al. Reversal of diastolic plateau in partial testicular torsion. J Clin Ultrasound. 2001;29:105-8.
28. Skoglund RW, McRoberts JW, Ragde H. Torsion of testicular appendages: presentation of 43 new cases and a collective review. J Urol. 1970;104:598-600.
29. Kratzik C, Hainz A, Kuber W. Has ultrasound influenced the therapy concept of blunt scrotal trauma? J Urol. 1989;142: 1243-6.
30. Moschouris H, Stamatiou K, Lampropoulou E, et al. Imaging of the acute scrotum: is there a place for contrast-enhanced ultrasonography? Int Braz J Urol. 2009;35(6):692-705.
31. Hari A, Grossfeld G, Hricak A. Tumors of the scrotum. In: Bragg DG, Rubin P, Hricak H (Eds). Oncologic Imaging. Philadelphia: WB Saunders; 2002. pp. 603-28.
32. Geraghty MJ, Lee FT Jr, Bernsten SA, et al. Sonography of testicular tumors and tumor-like conditions: a radiologic-pathologic correlation. Crit Rev Diagn Imaging. 1998;39:1-63.
33. Rifkin MD, Kurtz AB, Pasto ME, et al. Diagnostic capabilities of high-resolution scrotal ultrasonography: prospective evaluation. J Ultrasound Med. 1985;4:13-9.
34. Guthrie JA, Fowler RC. Ultrasound diagnosis of testicular tumours presenting as epididymal disease. Clin Radiol. 1992;46:397-400.
35. Cotran RS, Kumar P, Collins T. The male genital tract. In: Cotran RS, Kumar V, Collins T, Robbins SL (Eds). Robbins Pathologic Basis of Disease, 6th edition. Philadelphia, PA: Saunders; 1999. pp. 1011-34.
36. Schwerk WB, Schwerk WN, Rodeck G. Testicular tumors: prospective analysis of real-time US patterns and abdominal staging. Radiology. 1987;164:369-74.

37. Huang DY, Sidhu PS. Focal testicular lesions: colour Doppler ultrasound, contrast-enhanced ultrasound and tissue elastography as adjuvants to the diagnosis. Br J Radiol. 2012;85 Spec No. 1:S41-53.
38. Comiter CV, Renshaw AA, Benson CB, et al. Burned-out primary testicular cancer: sonographic and pathological characteristics. J Urol. 1996;156:85-8.
39. Hamm B. Differential diagnosis of scrotal masses by ultrasound. Eur Radiol. 1997;7:668-79.
40. Kim I, Young RH, Scully RE. Leydig cell tumors of the testis: a clinicopathological analysis of 40 cases and review of the literature. Am J Surg Pathol. 1985;9:177-92.
41. Jaffer O, Sidhu P. Contrast-enhanced ultrasonography of the testes. Ultrasound Clinics. 2013;8(4):509-23.
42. Nonomura N, Aozasa K, Ueda T, et al. Malignant lymphoma of the testis: histological and immunohistological study of 28 cases. J Urol. 1989;141:1368-71.
43. Richie JP. Neoplasms of the testis. In: Walch PC, Retik AB, Vaughan ED, Wein AJ (Eds). Campbell's Urology, 7th edition. Philadelphia, PA: Saunders; 1998. pp. 2411-52.
44. Amin MB, Greene FL, Edge SB, et al. The Eighth Edition AJCC Cancer Staging Manual: Continuing to build a bridge from a population-based to a more "personalized" approach to cancer staging. CA Cancer J Clin. 2017;67(2):93-9.
45. Basu S, Rubello D. PET imaging in the management of tumors of testis and ovary: current thinking and future directions. Minerva Endocrinol. 2008;33:229-56.
46. Ganem JP, Workman KR, Shaban SF. Testicular microlithiasis is associated with testicular pathology. Urology. 1999;53: 209-13.
47. Eftekhari F, Smith JK. Sonography of scrotum after orchiectomy: normal and abnormal findings. Am J Roentgenol. 1993;160; 543-7.

CHAPTER

22

Male Infertility and Erectile Dysfunction

Deep Narayan Srivastava, Chandan J Das

MALE INFERTILITY

Infertility is defined as a failure to achieve pregnancy during 1 year of frequent, unprotected intercourse.[1] A multicenter study by the World Health Organization (WHO) found that in 20% of infertility cases, the male partner was the predominant cause whereas in 27% of cases abnormalities were found in both partners.[2] Hence, defects in male partner may be responsible for infertility in up to 50% of the infertile couples.[1] These defects account for a reduction in the quantity and quality of the semen. The evaluation of infertile male begins with a careful history and physical examination of the patient. This is followed by semen analysis in which ejaculate volume and its pH, sperms count, their motility, and morphology are studied. Average sperm count in normal fertile man is 70–80 million sperms per mL and it contains more than 60% motile sperms. Sperm count of less than 20 million per mL is termed as oligospermia, however, significant decrease in pregnancy rates occurs only at sperm concentration of less than 5 million per mL. Oligospermia is present in 80% and azoospermia is present in another 15–20% of the infertile men.[1,2]

Etiology

Male infertility results from many diverse conditions. Congenital anomalies include cryptorchidism, Klinefelter's syndrome, agenesis of vas deferens and/or seminal vesicles, and congenital ejaculatory duct cyst. Endocrinal abnormalities such as prolactinoma, Kallmann syndrome, Prader-Willi syndrome, and congenital adrenal hyperplasia are uncommon causes of the male infertility and these are diagnosed primarily on the basis of clinical examination and laboratory findings. Luteinizing hormone secreted by the pituitary gland regulates the *testosterone* secretion by Leydig cells of the testis. Low testosterone affects spermatogenesis, growth of the prostate, and seminal vesicle secretion.[2]

Acquired testicular abnormalities such as trauma, tumor, infection, and paratesticular abnormalities such as varicocele and epididymitis are responsible for infertility in significant number of patients. Tuberculosis and gonorrhea cause inflammation and obstruction of the ductal transport system. Other diseases such as mumps and syphilis may affect seminiferous tubules in the testicular parenchyma.[3]

IMAGING APPROACH IN MALE INFERTILITY

Male infertility is usually caused by azoospermia, which can be either due to obstructive cause [obstructive azoospermia—normal-sized testes, epididymal fullness, normal follicle-stimulating hormone (FSH)] or due to nonobstructive cause (nonobstructive azoospermia—small or soft testes, raised FSH).

Normal volume (more than 1 mL), fructose-positive ejaculate with azoospermia or oligospermia is usually caused by lesions of the testis or of paratesticular structures **(Box 1)** such as varicocele and epididymal diseases.[4] These lesions can be satisfactorily evaluated with scrotal ultrasonography, supplemented with color Doppler flow imaging. Although clinical examination is an integral part of diagnostic workup in these patients, up to 67% of scrotal pathologies detected on sonography are responsible for infertility which are not apparent clinically.[5]

Low-volume ejaculate (less than 1 mL) is caused by stenosis, obstruction, or congenital anomalies of distal sperm transport system, which include vas deferens, seminal vesicles, ejaculatory duct, and prostate. Abnormalities in these structures result in decreased semen volume and blockage of flow of sperms into the ejaculate

BOX 1: Testicular and paratesticular causes of nonobstructive azoospermia.[3]

- Cryptochidism
- Atrophy
- Torsion/Infarction
- Inflammation
- Mumps/TB
- Microlithiasis
- Hydrocele
- Varicocele
- Neoplasm
- Trauma

(TB: tuberculosis)

leading to azoospermia or oligospermia. These abnormalities include agenesis of vas deferens or seminal vesicles or both, inflammatory strictures and obstruction of seminal vesicles and vas deferens, ejaculatory duct cysts, and obstruction.[6] Transrectal ultrasonography (TRUS) is the primary imaging modality of choice for distal ductal system.[1,7] It is now widely used to diagnose congenital and other obstructive lesions that produce low-volume ejaculate and azoospermia. Magnetic resonance imaging (MRI) is indicated only if TRUS findings are inconclusive.[8]

Varicocele

Varicocele is the most common surgically correctable cause of male infertility. There is abnormal dilatation of veins of the pampiniform plexus, which is due to venous reflux in these veins. The incidence of varicocele is 15% in general population and 35–40% in men presenting with infertility.[9,10] Primary varicocele is seen in young men and is due to incompetent testicular vein. It is mostly left-sided or bilateral. Left testicular vein is maximally predisposed to develop varicocele. Various factors responsible include right-angled entry of left testicular vein into left renal vein, the intermittent compression of left renal vein between aorta and the superior mesenteric artery (nutcracker syndrome), and pressure of the left colon.[11] Secondary varicocele results from left renal vein invasion by renal cancer, compression of testicular veins by adjacent masses such as tumor, lymph nodes, or hydronephrosis.[12] Cross-communications exist between veins of the pampiniform plexus and cremasteric veins as well as external spermatic veins and veins of vas deferens. In patients, subjected to high ligation, these communications may lead to recurrence.

Although most men with varicocele are not infertile, varicocele is present in up to 40% of infertile men. Repair of varicocele improves quality of semen in majority of patients.[13] Proposed mechanisms by which varicocele causes testicular dysfunction include hormonal imbalance, hypoxia secondary to venous stasis, reflux of adrenal and renal metabolites, and elevated testicular temperature.[13] During adolescence, when the testis is growing rapidly, it may be very susceptible to harmful effects of varicocele.

The simplest and most widely used method for diagnosis of varicocele is physical examination; however, subclinical varicocele cannot be diagnosed with physical examination alone. Ultrasonography with color duplex flow imaging is the preferred imaging modality for evaluation of varicocele. The patient is examined in supine and erect position during quite breathing, deep breathing, and Valsalva maneuver before interpreting the examination as normal.[9] Vessels are scanned on each side from the scrotal neck to the lower pole of testis. As the flow in pampiniform plexus is very slow, Doppler parameters must be adjusted to detect very slow flow during color Doppler examination. On grey scale ultrasonography, visualization of three or more dilated veins with at least one of them having a diameter of 3 mm or more is suggestive of varicocele.[13] These tortuous venous channels are easily compressible as opposed to other cystic abnormalities in this region. On color Doppler study, continuous retrograde flow toward testis during Valsalva maneuver, is taken as a positive sign for varicocele **(Figs. 1A to D)**.[13,14] A brief reflux in veins of pampiniform plexus followed by cessation of flow is physiological. A further scoring system described by Chiou et al. incorporating maximal venous diameter, the sum of six venous diameters, and change of flow velocity after a Valsalva maneuver allows greater sensitivity of 93% by using a total score >4 compared to merely measuring the venous diameter **(Table 1)**.[15] Some varicoceles can be demonstrated in erect position of the patient only and hence scanning in erect position is mandatory before the study is interpreted as normal.[13] Intratesticular varicocele is rare and always associated with paratesticular varicocele. It is usually located in subcapsular location or in the mediastinum testis which measures 2 mm or more.[16]

Size of the varicocele does not correlate with degree of impairment of spermatogenesis. Thus a small varicocele detected only on radiological assessment may have a profound effect on spermatogenesis.[17] The treatment of subclinical varicocele in infertility is still controversial, however, it has been demonstrated that sperm motility improvement after varicocele surgery is comparable in patients with both clinical and subclinical varicocele.[18]

Venography is rarely performed for diagnostic purpose but may be used when embolization is used as a procedure for treating varicocele.[13] When compared with venography, color Doppler ultrasonography had a sensitivity of 93% and specificity of 80% in a group of infertile patients with normal physical examinations.[19] In addition to the diagnosis, spermatic venography has therapeutic application for embolization of varicocele. In this technique, an angiographic catheter is placed into the testicular vein via transfemoral venous route. About 5–10 mL of contrast is injected during Valsalva maneuver and radiographs of abdomen and pelvis are taken. The venography can be followed by embolization performed using coils **(Figs. 2A and B)** or sclerosants such as sodium tetradecyl sulfate foam.[13] Correct identification of all venous collaterals with their selective embolization is necessary. High technical success rate with significant improvement in semen quality can be achieved with this technique.[20] This technique is especially suitable for postsurgical recurrent varicocele.[21]

Testis

Sonographic examination of the testis is important in the evaluation of infertile male, specifically for measurement of testicular size for atrophy or for tumor identification. Normal adult testis is homogenous with low to medium echogenicity and measures 3–5 cm in length, 2–3 cm in width, and 2–3 cm in anteroposterior thickness. Testicular volume in cc can be calculated using the formula of length × width × thickness × 0.53. The normal volume of adult testis is 15–20 cc and testis is symmetrical on both sides.[21]

Cryptorchidism occurs in approximately 0.8% of all 1-year-old boys and if left untreated can represent a congenital cause of male infertility.[22] Progressive germ cell damage occurs in the cryptorchid testis secondary to the increased temperature at its extrascrotal location. Significant germ cell damage occurs by 2 years of age and untreated postpubertal undescended testis may be completely devoid of germ cells. It also has a

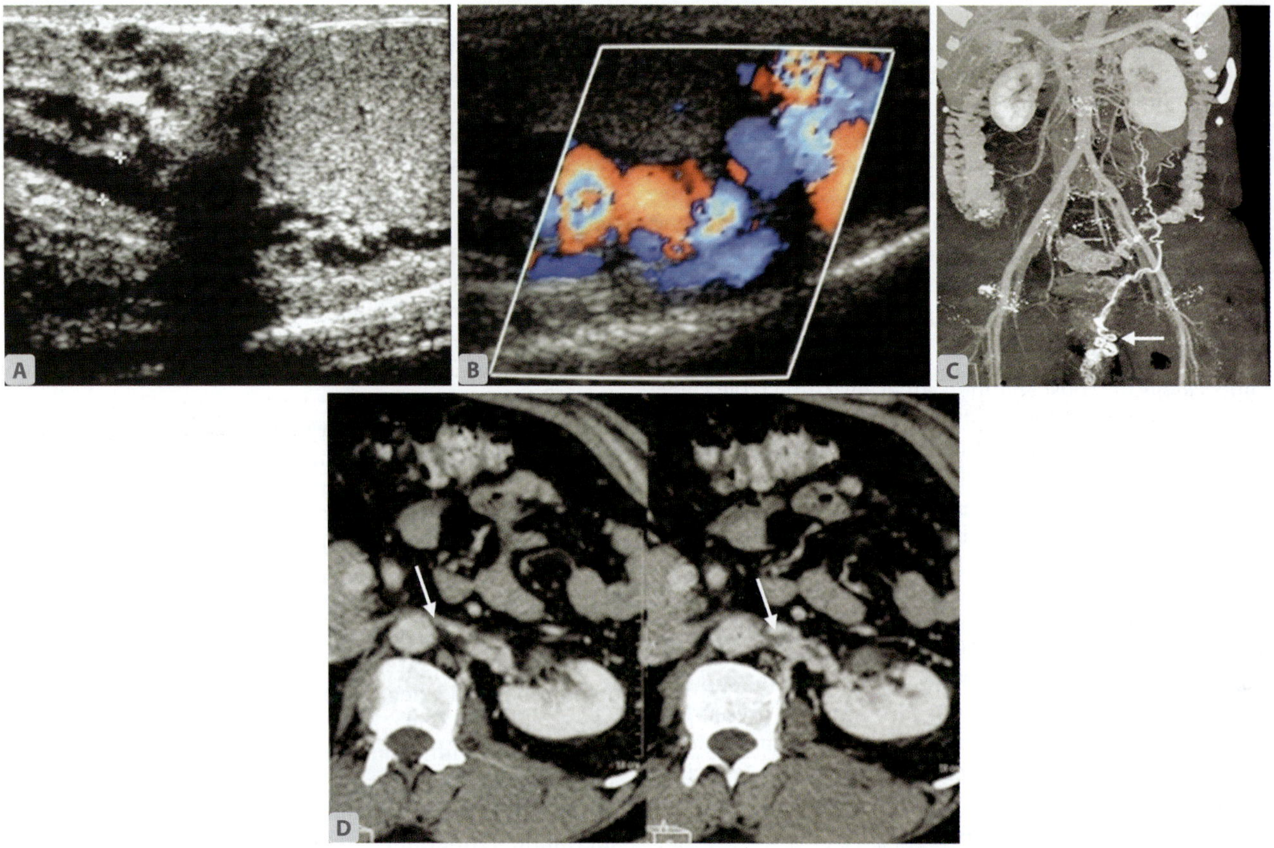

FIGS. 1A TO D: Varicocele. (A) Multiple dilated vascular channels measuring more than 3 mm on gray-scale USG at the lower pole of testes; (B) marked detectable flow is seen on this color Doppler scan which is exaggerated during Valsalva maneuver; (C) CECT coronal MIP images showing multiple dilated vessels in left scrotum (arrow) which is communicating through the left gonadal vein draining into left renal vein; (D) axial CECT showing thrombosed left renal vein (arrows) as cause of the left varicocele. (CECT: contrast-enhanced computed tomography; MIP: maximum intensity projection; USG: ultrasonography).

TABLE 1: Scoring system of Chiou et al. for color Doppler ultrasound diagnosis of varicocele.[15]

Parameter	Score
Maximum vein diameter:	
• <2.5 mm	0
• 2.5–2.9 mm	1
• 3.0–3.9 mm	2
• ≥4 mm	3
Plexus/sum of diameter of veins:	
• No plexus identified	0
• Plexus (+) with sum diameter <3 mm	1
• Plexus (+) with sum diameter 3–5.9 mm	2
• Plexus (+) with sum diameter ≥6 mm	3
Change in flow velocity of Valsalva maneuver:	
• <2 cm S^{-1} or duration <1 s	0
• 2–4.9 cm S^{-1}	1
• 5–9.9 cm S^{-1}	2
• ≥10 cm S^{-1}	3
Total score	0–9

deleterious effect on contralateral normal descended testis. Pregnancy rates in men who have undergone prepubertal treatment of unilateral cryptorchidism ranges between 65% and 80%.[22] In addition to infertility, undescended testis is highly susceptible for malignant transformation.

Most of the undescended testes are located at or close to the inguinal canal and ultrasonography is very sensitive to identify their location. Ultrasonography is less accurate in detection of undescended testis when it is located in the retroperitoneum. MRI scans of abdomen and pelvis **(Fig. 3)** from the level of inguinal rings to lower poles of the kidney are required for testicular localization in such situations. MRI is more accurate because of its high soft tissue contrast and multiplanner capabilities. The characteristic high-signal intensity of testis on T2-weighted sequences aid in easy recognition of undescended testis. MRI scores over ultrasonography (USG) in localization of atrophic undescended testis.

Testicular tumors are most common in the same age group in which fertility disorders of male are most prevalent. Testicular tumors may be identified in-patients presenting with oligospermia or azoospermia.[23] Seminomas are the most common testicular tumors and are usually homogeneously hypoechoic on sonography **(Fig. 4)**. Nonseminomatous

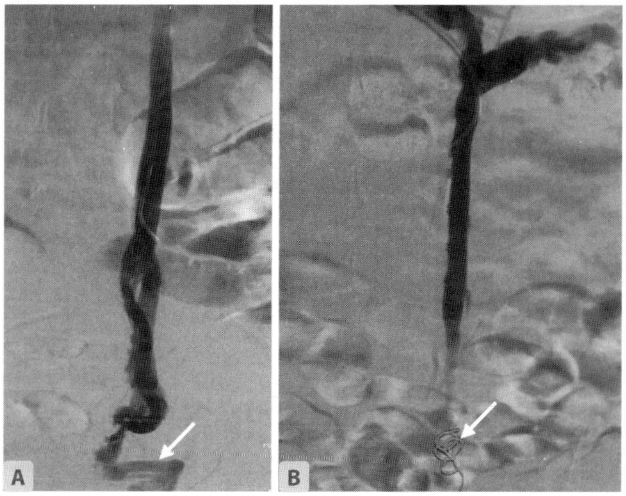

FIGS. 2A AND B: (A) Venography of left gonadal vein shows the varicocele (arrow). (B) Coil embolization (arrow) of the varicocele was performed in the same setting.

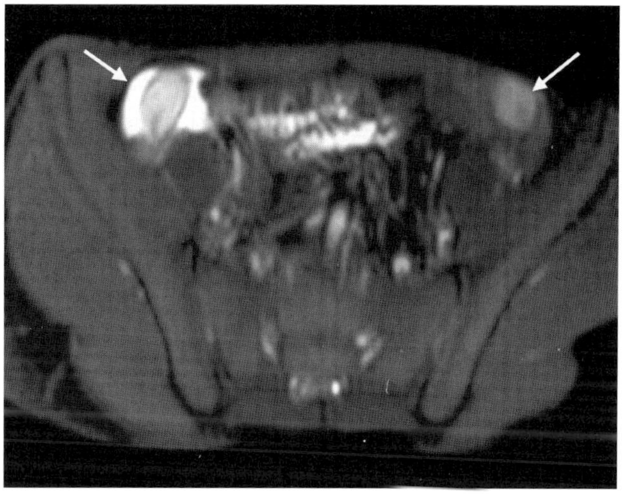

FIG. 3: T2W MRI image showing hyperintense structures (arrows) in both iliac fossa regions suggesting undescended testes. (MRI: magnetic resonance imaging).

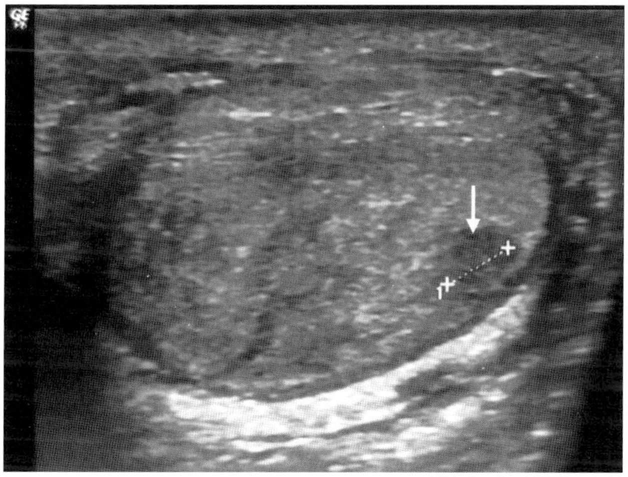

FIG. 4: USG showing a focal hypoechoic lesion in testis (arrow) and with elevated alpha-fetoprotein (AFP) level it is highly suspicious for seminoma. (USG: ultrasonography).

tumors are complex and heterogeneous in echotexture. Testicular tumors are described in details in the chapter on imaging of scrotum.

Testicular torsion occurs most frequently during adolescence and therefore has the potential impact on fertility of affected young males. Acute testicular torsion is an emergency and torsed testis must be salvaged at the earliest. There are good chances of salvage when patients are operated within 7 hours. If it is delayed for more than 24 hours, virtually all testicular function is lost. On sonography, the affected testis is hypoechoic and may be enlarged. Color Doppler shows decreased vascularity, which is best appreciated when compared with contralateral normal testis.

Testicular trauma has less impact on male fertility than the other testicular factors such as torsion or cryptorchidism.[22] Spermatogenic dysfunction may develop in testicular trauma patients, secondary to direct cell injury and the formation of antisperm antibodies from disruption of blood-testis barrier in them. Ultrasonography with color Doppler is most suitable investigation to determine the extent of testicular trauma; however, satisfactory ultrasonography examination may not be possible in acutely traumatized and painful scrotum. In such situations, MRI is more accurate to detect disruption of the testicular capsule; however, most of these patients will need surgical exploration.

Higher incidence of testicular microlithiasis is found on scrotal ultrasonography in infertile men; however, its relationship with infertility is not known.[10]

Epididymis

The epididymis is located along the posterolateral aspect of testis and runs parallel and posterior to the mediastinum testis. The head of the epididymis is pyramidal in shape and it is larger than rest of the epididymis. The head measures 5–12 mm in thickness.

Infertile man may have infection or inflammation of the epididymis. The normal epididymis has the echogenicity similar to the testis. In acute epididymitis, epididymis is enlarged and hypoechoic with increased vascularity on color Doppler **(Fig. 5)**. Adjacent increase in vascularity may be seen in testis also. Chronic inflammation results in an enlarged and heterogeneously hyperechoic epididymis, sometimes with foci of calcification.[12] Scarring in chronically inflamed epididymis may result in epididymal obstruction, which can be avoided with early and aggressive treatment of epididymitis.

Epididymal cysts and spermatoceles are usually located at the head of the epididymis and these can be easily detected on sonography. Most epididymal cysts do not cause obstruction, however, rarely, these may compress the epididymal tubules and cause epididymal obstruction, especially if large, and produce oligo- or azoospermia, very large epididymal cysts may occasionally be difficult to differentiate from hydrocele on sonography, however, compression of epididymis and adjacent testicular margin and presence of the fluid at one end of the testis instead of

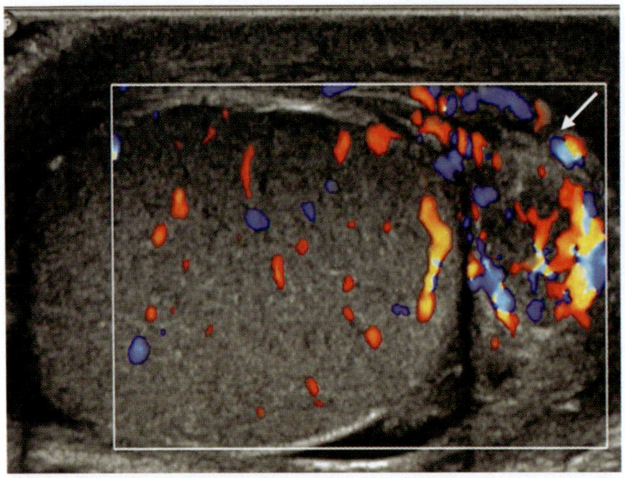

FIG. 5: USG showing enlarged epididymal head (arrow) with marked increase in vascularity in a case of acute epididymitis. Note is made of increased vascularity in adjacent testis. (USG: ultrasonography).

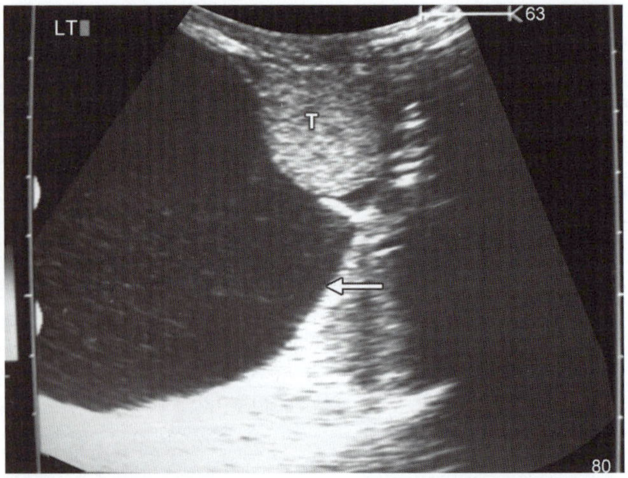

FIG. 6: Large epididymal cyst (arrow) at the upper pole of testis seen on scrotal ultrasonography pushing the testis (T) eccentrically.

surrounding the testis help to differentiate large epididymal cyst from hydrocele **(Fig. 6)**.

TRUS Evaluation of Distal Genital Ductal System

TRUS is indicated in infertile men with suspicion of obstructive pathology in distal sperm transport system. This is suggested by low-volume ejaculate with oligo- or azoospermia and palpable abnormality on digital rectal examination. The conditions that produce low-volume ejaculate with oligo- or azoospermia include agenesis of vas deferens and seminal vesicle, ejaculatory duct obstruction, and urethral strictures.[1,7] Other indications of TRUS include hematospermia, painful ejaculation, severe sperm motility defects, and azoospermia in normal-volume ejaculate without testicular atrophy.[24]

On TRUS, normal prostate is a symmetric, triangular, and ellipsoid structure with homogeneous echogenicity surrounded by a thin layer of echogenic capsule. Normal seminal vesicles are paired, well-defined, saccular, elongated hypoechoic organs, situated cranial to the prostate and posterior to urinary bladder with "bowtie" appearance on axial images. These may vary in size, shape, and degree of distention; however, usually these are symmetrical. On axial plane, ampulla of vasa deferentia are seen as round or oval tubular structures that are just cranial to prostate and medial to seminal vesicles. In sagittal plane, these can be seen behind prostate projecting medially toward seminal vesicles. Ejaculatory ducts are difficult to visualize on TRUS in normal men. These may sometimes be seen as tubular structures obliquely traversing the prostate and entering the urethra at verumontanum.[1]

Seminal Vesicles and Vas Deferens

Seminal vesicle secretions contribute about 80–90% of sperm volume. They also secrete fructose and maintain an acidic pH of semen. Congenital anomalies and obstructive lesions of seminal vesicles result in decreased semen volume, low pH, and low fructose levels.

Wolffian duct anomalies include renal agenesis, agenesis of vas deferens, agenesis or atrophy of seminal vesicles, and cysts of seminal vesicles. Seminal vesicle atrophy or agenesis may be unilateral or bilateral.[2] It occurs in all patients with agenesis of vas deferens. Bilateral absence of seminal vesicles may be seen in up to 40% of patients with low-volume azoospermia.[4] It can be diagnosed with semen analysis and clinical examination in most patients.[25] Large number of these patients also has associated renal anomalies. Another strong association is with cystic fibrosis, in which 98% of men have agenesis of seminal vesicles and vas deferens.[4] On TRUS or MRI, seminal vesicle is considered atrophic, if it measures less than 7 mm in width and dilated (as in ejaculatory duct obstruction) when it measures more than 15 mm.[2,8] Diagnosis of seminal vesicle and vas agenesis is made when these are not visualized **(Fig. 7)**.

Cysts of seminal vesicles may be congenital or acquired. Congenital cyst of seminal vesicle results from an ectopic ureter insertion into the seminal vesicle and is associated with a hypoplastic kidney on the same side. This cyst may compress ejaculatory duct and produce obstruction. Acquired cysts of seminal vesicles are secondary to infection. Chronic inflammation produces cystic dilatation with scarring and obstruction of the lumen of the seminal vesicles and causes infertility **(Fig. 8A)**. Stone formation in dilated seminal vesicles can be readily demonstrated on TRUS.[8,26] MRI also demonstrates the cystic change well due to increase in fluid content of the cyst **(Fig. 8B)**.

Ejaculatory Ducts

These are formed by confluence of seminal vesicles and terminal ampullary portion of the vas deferens and hence, ejaculatory duct obstruction results in decreased semen volume with absence of seminal fructose. TRUS may demonstrate ejaculatory duct cysts, dilatation of ejaculatory ducts, or calcification in ejaculatory ducts along with dilated seminal vesicles.[4,27] Any of these findings strongly suggest ejaculatory duct obstruction. Zinner syndrome is characterized by triad of unilateral renal agenesis, ipsilateral seminal vesicle cyst, and ejaculatory duct obstruction **(Figs. 9A to D)**.

Many of these conditions can be treated with transurethral resection of the ejaculatory duct (TURED).[27] Specificity of TRUS in the diagnosis of ejaculatory duct obstruction is unsatisfactory, hence, TRUS-guided seminal vesicle aspiration followed by vesiculography is useful before TURED.[28,29] TRUS-guided seminal vesicle aspiration is performed with a 21G needle introduced transrectally. Presence of motile sperms in seminal vesicle fluid strongly suggests ejaculatory duct obstruction because sperms are not normally seen in seminal vesicles. The aspiration is followed by injection of 5–20 mL of dilute noniodinated contrast under fluoroscopic guidance and images are obtained to study the seminal vesicles and ejaculatory ducts. Pelvic and inguinal portions of vas deferens may also be visualized with this technique.[24]

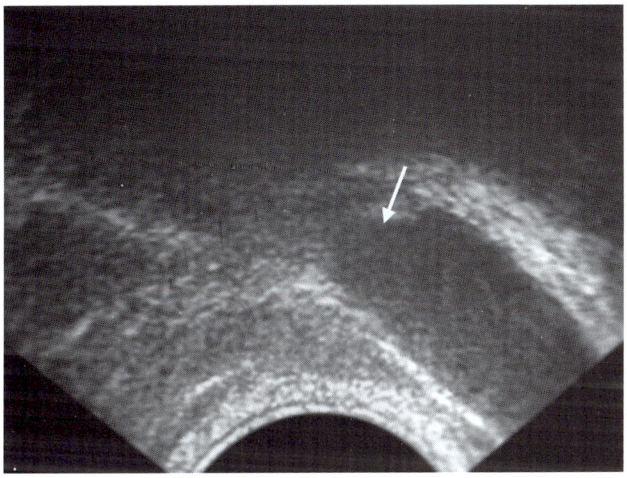

FIG. 7: Agenesis of seminal vesicle. TRUS shows absence of seminal vesicle on right side on axial scan. Normal left seminal vesicle (arrow) is seen as hypoechoic elongated structure behind the urinary bladder. (TRUS: transrectal ultrasonography).

Prostate

Müllerian duct cyst and utricle cyst are congenital prostatic cysts which may be indistinguishable from each other. When large, these may compress and produce ejaculatory duct obstruction.[2] On imaging, both are seen as midline cyst in prostate **(Figs. 10A to C)**. Müllerian duct cysts do not communicate with urethra and when large, may extend above the prostate. Utricle cysts communicate with urethra and do not extend above prostate. Acquired prostatic cysts like parasitic and prostatic retention cysts are usually located peripherally. These may produce obstruction to semen flow within the prostate and subsequent infertility. Chronic prostatitis may produce scarring, atrophy of seminal vesicles and strictures of ejaculatory duct, which may lead to infertility.[2] These can be identified on TRUS as disorganization of normal anatomy produced by scarring of prostatic tissue and occasional stone formation.[4]

Magnetic Resonance Imaging in Infertility

Scrotal MRI is the most important adjunct to ultrasonography in evaluation of testicular and paratesticular abnormalities. It is highly accurate in cryptorchidism, testicular tumors, trauma, and infection.

Magnetic resonance imaging is recommended for the evaluation of distal genital tract when TRUS findings are equivocal.[8,26] Various abnormalities of prostate and seminal vesicles such as cysts of seminal vesicles and ejaculatory duct, dilatation of vas deferens and seminal vesicles secondary to ejaculatory duct obstruction can be satisfactorily demonstrated. On MRI, absence or atrophy of seminal vesicles with very small size and loss of normal high-signal intensity is seen in up to 40% of patients.[26] Agenesis of vas may be

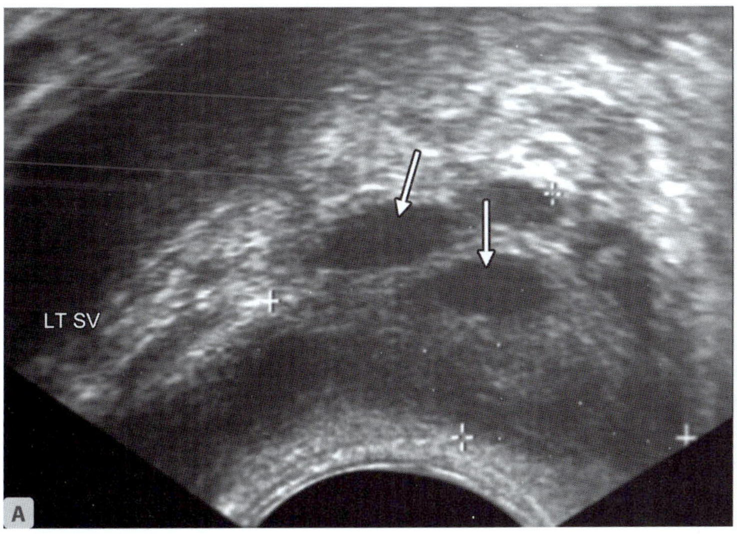

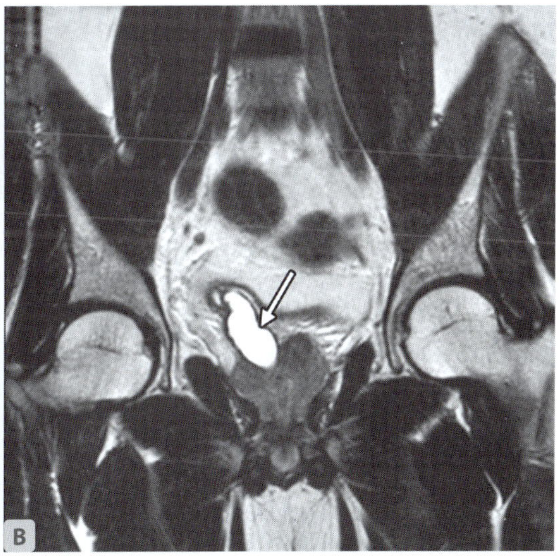

FIGS. 8A AND B: (A) Multiple postinflammatory seminal vesicle cysts (arrows) are seen on axial TRUS scan. (B) Coronal T2W image of a different patient showing a large hyperintense (arrow) right seminal vesicle cyst. (TRUS: transrectal ultrasonography).

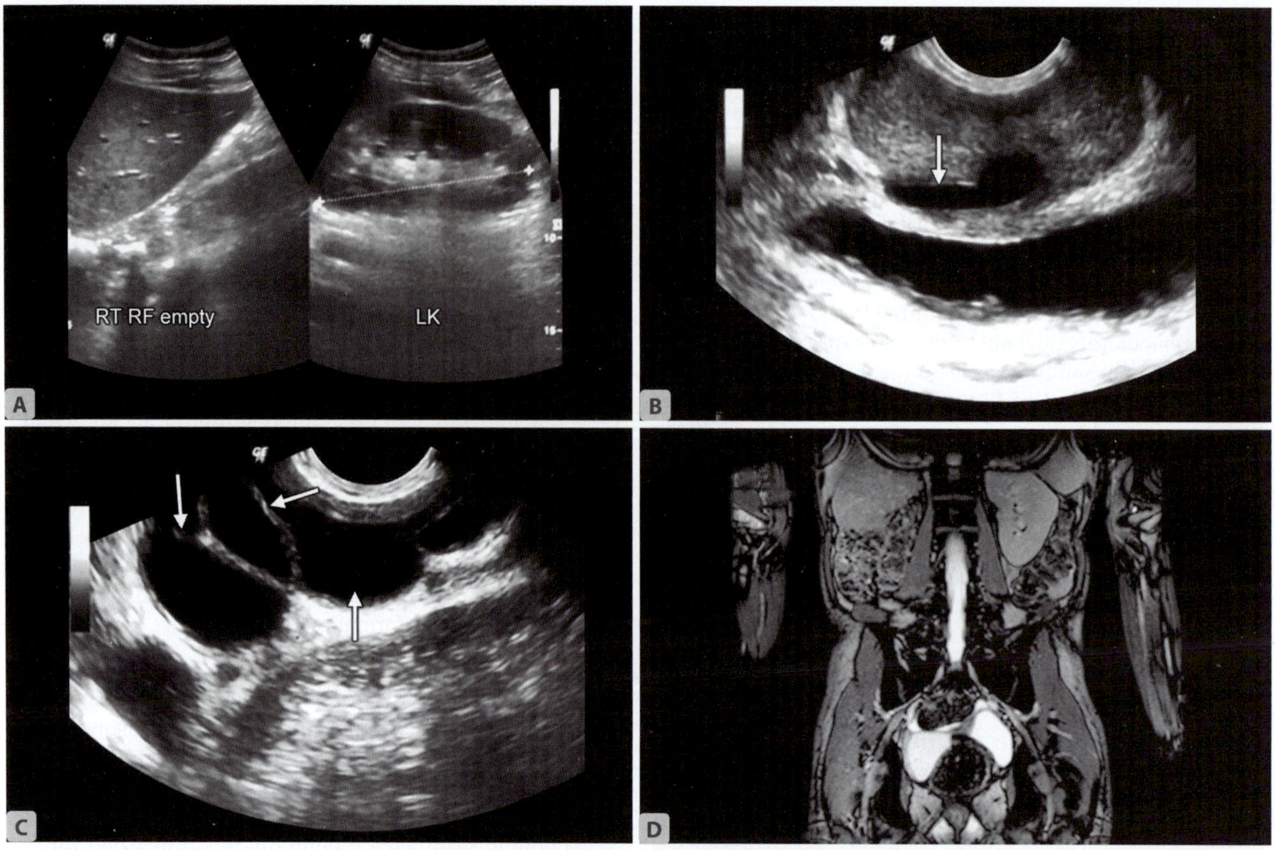

FIG. 9A TO D: Zinner syndrome. (A) USG showing empty right renal fossa. (B) USG showing obstructed ejaculatory duct leading to dilatation (arrow). (C) Multiple cysts in right seminal vesicle (arrows) is also seen. (D) Coronal TRUFISP MRI image showing absent right kidney. (MRI: magnetic resonance imaging; USG: ultrasonography).

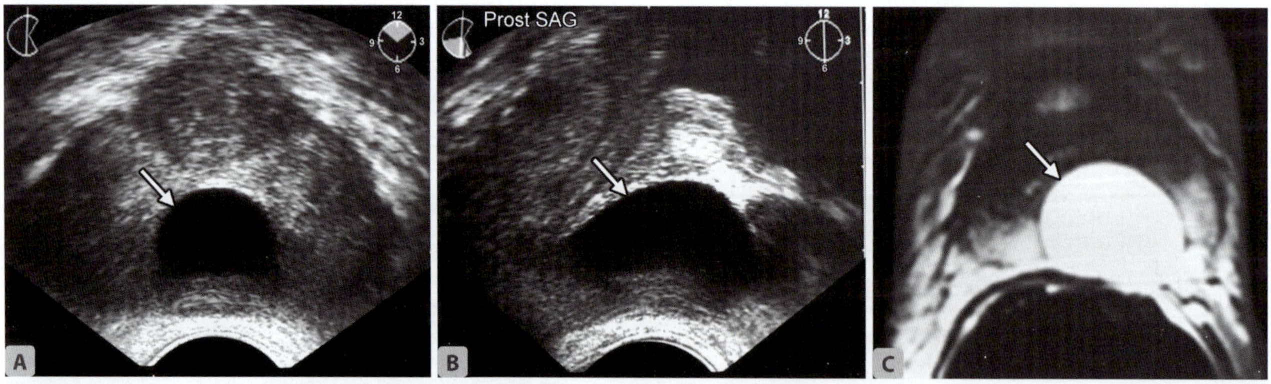

FIGS. 10A TO C: Prostatic cyst. (A and B) USG in axial and sagittal plane showing a cystic anechoic structure (arrow) in midline. (C) T2W axial image showing well-defined markedly hyperintense structure (arrow) in midline. (USG: ultrasonography).

demonstrated. MRI is particularly advantageous in suspected case of ejaculatory duct obstruction as demonstration of normal ejaculatory ducts ruling out presence of ejaculatory duct obstruction.[30]

Imaging in Assisted Fertilization

Scrotal sonography is also useful in the work-up of assisted fertilization. Testicular volume as calculated on sonography can predict the outcome of testicular biopsies for sperm retrieval. Chances of successful sperm retrieval are significantly higher in patients with testicular volume more than 12 cc.[31] Similarly, sonography-guided testicular sperm aspiration is more accurate and it has less complications when compared with the blind aspiration, as sonography allows good visualization of testicular parenchyma, easy sampling, and avoidance of prominent vessels.[32] In patients with ejaculatory duct obstruction, sperms can also be aspirated from seminal vesicles under TRUS guidance. Intraoperative use of TRUS is helpful in identification of obstructing cyst and determining the depth of resection during transurethral resection of ejaculatory duct for the treatment of ejaculatory duct obstruction.[33]

ERECTILE DYSFUNCTION

Erectile dysfunction (ED) or impotence is defined as inability to achieve and/or maintain an erection for satisfactory sexual intercourse.[34] Its prevalence increases with age and affects up to 52% men between age group of 40–69 years.[35] ED is broadly classified into two categories: Organic and psychologic. Vasculogenic impotence is the most common cause of organic impotence and may be a marker for occult cardiovascular disease.[36] Vascular ED does not rule out the presence of contributing psychological factors, but merely means that vascular factors are predominant cause of ED. Vascular ED has two different mechanisms—obstruction in penile inflow tract, termed as arterial ED and the inability to trap the incoming blood in the cavernosa, termed as veno-occlusive ED.

Anatomy and Physiology of Penile Erection

The paired internal pudendal arteries give rise to common penile arteries which divide into four branches, one each to spongiosa, cavernosa, proximal urethra, and the dorsum of the penis (deep dorsal artery). The cavernosal artery provides blood to cavernosa through multiple helicine arteries that open directly into the cavernosal sinusoids. Venules located within the subtunical space between the periphery of erectile tissue and the tunica albugenia provide venous outflow channel from corpora cavernosa via peripheral lacunae. These vein pierce tunica albuginea and drain into cavernosal and then into deep dorsal vein.

Penile erection is a neurovascular phenomenon in which neurological stimulus via parasympathetic nerves from sacral 2, 3, and 4 leads to arterial response. It is initiated by relaxation of smooth muscles of helicine arteries leading to vasodilatation. The phase of arterial response is followed by the phase of tumescence, in which relaxation of trabecular smooth muscles and increased arterial flow lead to increase in size and length of the penis. The phase of erectile response follows when subtunical venules are compressed against tunica albuginea due to dilatation of sinusoids and increase in intracavernosal pressure. If this veno-occlusive mechanism is intact, the arterial inflow leads to increase in intracavernosal pressure to the levels of mean arterial blood pressure. Perineal muscles contractions generate further increase in pressure, which leads erectile response to rigidity.

Parameters of quality of the arterial response are peak systolic velocity (PSV) and acceleration time (AT) as measured by pharmacopenile duplex ultrasonography (PPDU) and cavernosal artery occlusion pressure as measured by cavernosometry. Parameters to assess the quality of veno-occlusive mechanism are end-diastolic velocity (EDV) and resistive index (RI) on PPDU and maintenance flow and pressure loss on cavernosometry.

Evaluation of Erectile Dysfunction

Psychological factors or systemic illnesses are responsible for erectile dysfunction in majority of patients. Careful history, clinical examination, and routine laboratory tests are extremely important for the evaluation of ED as these can identify the underlying cause in up to 80% of patients.[37] Such workup may detect reversible cause of ED or unmask the systemic illness responsible for ED. With advent of effective oral pharmacotherapy, the diagnostic approach has significantly changed over past decade. A good erectile response to these drugs excludes significant arterial or vascular disease as a cause of ED. Hence, most patients are first given a therapeutic trial and only those with failure are referred for invasive diagnostic tests like PPDU, cavernosography or angiography.[34]

Pharmacopenile Duplex Ultrasonography

Pharmacopenile duplex ultrasonography is most widely used investigation to define vascular ED and to differentiate between arterial insufficiency and defective veno-occlusive mechanism.

The different vasoactive agents used for PPDU are papaverine, and combination of papaverine, phentolamine, and prostaglandin (PG) E1 (Trimix).[3,34] Papaverine may lead to false-negative erectile response in some patients and persistent painful erection (priapism) may occur in others. PGE1 has better erection rate and less incidence of priapism.[38] Genital self-stimulation, visual erotic stimulus, or application of penoscrotal tourniquet may augment the erectile response. Gadgets like virtual glasses with facility for audiovisual erotic stimulus improve the erectile response and Doppler waveform, thereby eliminating the false-positive results of PPDU examination.[39]

Technique of PPDU

The examination must be conducted in an atmosphere of privacy. The ultrasonographic evaluation begins with scanning of flaccid penile shaft in transverse plane to measure the diameter of cavernosal artery. It ranges from 0.2 mm to 1 mm.[34] Although the arterial flow in the flaccid penis is difficult to demonstrate, Doppler flowmetry of flaccid penis has the potential to detect arteriogenic ED. PSV of less than 10 cm/s in the cavernosal artery of flaccid penis is suggestive of arteriogenic ED.[40] Later, intracavernosal injection of 60 mg of papaverine is made with 30-G needle in either of the cavernosa as cross-communications exist between both sides. Care must be taken not to inject into a vessel or urethra. The erectile response is graded visually from E0 to E5 as suggested by Broderick et al.[41] **(Box 2)**. Grade E4 and E5 are sufficient for penetration.

After evaluating the erectile response, scanning is started from the base at the penoscrotal junction to distal part, both in transverse and longitudinal planes. Dorsal scanning in sagittal plane is necessary to identify cavernosal collaterals and penile deformities such as Peyronie's disease. The postinjection diameter of both cavernosal arteries is measured. Angle-corrected flow velocities are measured as proximal as possible in cavernosal arteries. Most accurate flowmetry values are obtained at the time of peak rigidity, however, this time is highly variable. Hence, flowmetry values are normally obtained at 0, 5, 10, and 20 minutes after the injection.

Postpapaverine injection, normal spectral waveform has been described to have five phases **(Figs. 11A to D)**.[42] Phase 1 is characterized by increase in both systolic and diastolic velocities. In phase 2, there is progressive decrease in EDV and appearance of a dicrotic notch. Patients with severe venous leakage do not progress beyond phase 2. In phase 3, diastolic flow approximates zero and it is reversed in phase 4. Phase 5 is characterized by eventual loss of both systolic and diastolic signals.

Various parameters studied on flowmetry are PSV, EDV, AT, and RI. Mild variations are seen in cutoff values described in different studies. PSV of more than 35 cm/s rules out arterial insufficiency and PSV of 25 cm/s is highly suggestive of the same. Lot of overlap is seen between these two values in normal and abnormal individuals.[2] Currently acceptable reference values used to interpret the examination as normal are given in **Box 3**.[34,38]

In a study of 32 men without evidence of vascular ED conducted at AIIMS, the mean PSV was 61.3 cm/s, the mean EDV was –1.2 cm (minus sign denotes flow reversal) and the mean AT was 0.06 s.[43] Mean RI was in whom diastolic flow reversal was not achieved. Another interesting observation was the linear relationship between PSV and ages of the individuals, which implies that use of single cut-off value for all ages may be debatable.

Abnormal PSV (less than 25 cm/s) and AT (more than 0.11 s) are suggestive of arterial disease. Similarly, any increase in the cavernosal artery diameter by less than 75% of the baseline diameter also indicates possibility of arterial disease. Abnormal EDV (more than 5 cm/s) and RI (<0.85) denote venous leakage. RI is considered more reliable than EDV for assessment of veno- occlusive mechanism.[43] If arterial disease is present, intracavernosal pressure remains below

BOX 2: Visual grading of penile erection during PPDU.

- E0: No response
- E1: Elongation of shaft only
- E2: Moderate tumescence, no rigidity
- E3: Full tumescence, no rigidity, easily bendable
- E4: Full erection, partial rigidity
- E5: Full rigidity for at least 20 minutes

(PPDU: pharmacopenile duplex ultrasonography)

BOX 3: Normal reference values for PPDU.

- PSV: 25 cm/s or more
- EDV: 5 cm/s or less
- AT: 0.11 s or less
- RI: 0.85 or more

(AT: acceleration time; EDV: end-diastolic velocity; PPDU: pharmacopenile duplex ultrasonography; RI: resistive index)

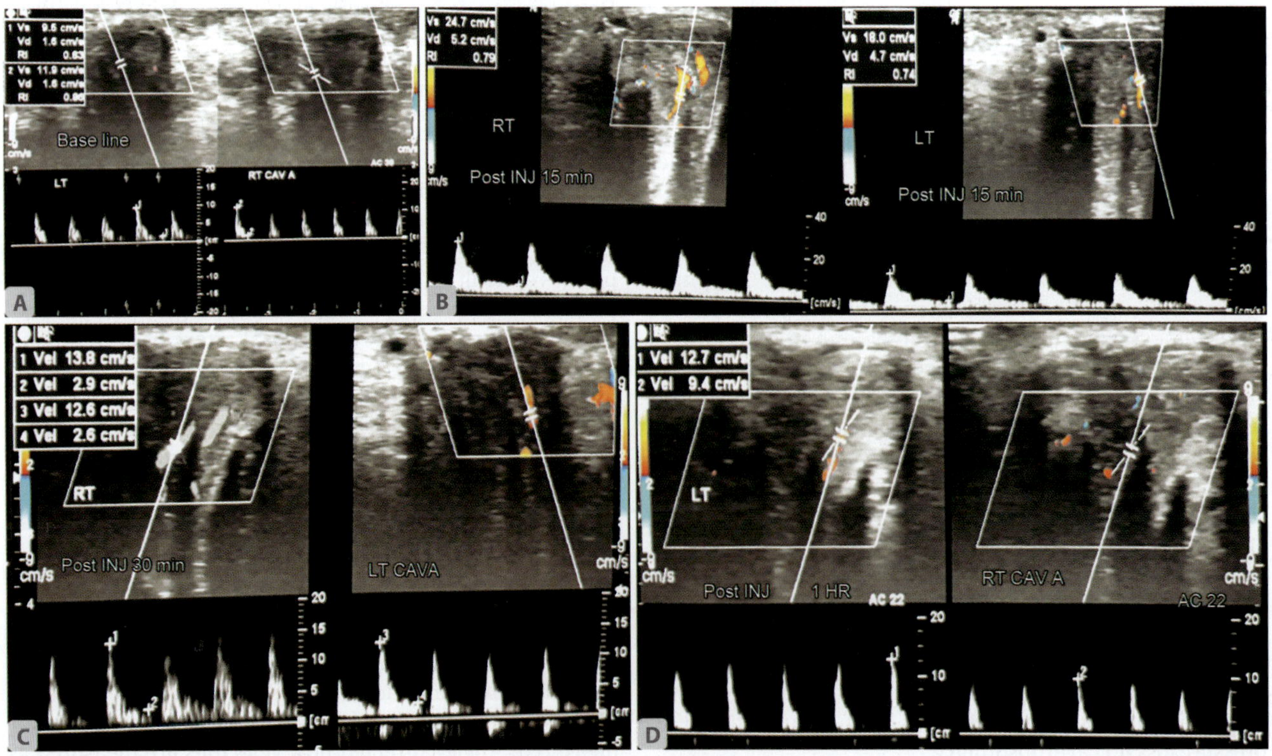

FIGS. 11A TO D: Normal spectral waveform progression of PPDU. (A) Baseline, (B) 15 minutes postinjection, (C) 30 minutes postinjection, (D) 1 hour postinjection. (PPDU: Pharmacopenile duplex ultrasonography).

systemic pressure and veno-occlusion cannot occur, even if this mechanism is intact, and diastolic flow will continue to persist. Therefore, veno-occlusive mechanism cannot be assessed with EDV and RI in presence of arterial disease.

Pharmacopenile duplex ultrasonography *with oral sildenafil:* Sildenafil citrate (Viagra) has been studied as an alternative to intracavernosal injection of vasoactive drugs for PPDU, in order to make the examination noninvasive; however, the results are inconsistent.[44,45] Oral dose of 50 or 100 mg is normally used. Unlike intracavernosal agents, sildenafil alone cannot achieve erection and it must be supplemented with audiovisual sexual stimulation. Effect of sildenafil is also slow and peak erection is usually achieved between 60 minutes and 75 minutes after its oral administration. The quality of erection and the PSV achieved with sildenafil is lower than the same parameters achieved after intracavernosal injection. This may lead to false-positive PPDU results in some patients.[45] With these limitations, oral sildenafil has failed to replace intracavernosal injections of vasoactive drugs for PPDU. A recent study has suggested that best results are obtained with combination of oral sildenafil and intracavernosal injection of trimix during PPDU.[46]

Peyronie's Disease

This is a benign condition resulting from inelastic scar of tunica albuginea, which produces curvature deformities of penis and the ED. It is traumatic in origin in majority of the patients and the ED in these patients is primarily because of penile deformities, painful erection, or associated vascular disorders.[47] On sonography, the penile plaques are seen as echogenic focal thickenings of tunica, which may displace or encase dorsal vasculature. Dense plaques may contain calcifications and cause acoustic shadowing **(Fig. 12)**, however, shadowing can be seen even without evidence of calcification on plain radiographs. Most plaques are located in the middle third of the shaft of the penis.[38]

Cavernosometry

Cavernosometry is a primary modality available for quantifying and mapping of veno-occlusive dysfunction.

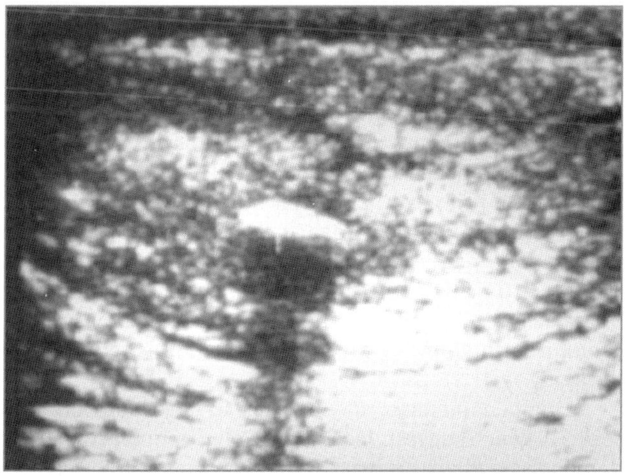

FIG. 12: Peyronie's disease: Dense echogenic plaque of tunica albuginea with distal shadowing.

However, because of its invasive nature, it is reserved for patients with suggestion of venous leakage on PPDU if surgical repair is being considered for them. In cavernosometry, venous outflow resistance is assessed by determining the intracavernosal flow rate required to sustain an erection in a state of complete sinusoidal relaxation.

In this technique, two 19-G needles are introduced, one in each cavernosa. One needle is connected to the infusion pump and the other needle to a pressure monitor. A mixture of 30 mg of papaverine and 1 mg of phentolamine is infused. The intracavernosal pressure rises gradually and then remains steady. After this, the infusion flow rate is gradually increased to demonstrate linearly proportional increase in intracavernosal pressure. Linear relationship between cavernosal pressure and infusion rate is suggestive of a state of complete sinusoidal relaxation. If a nonlinear relationship is observed, a second dose of papaverine may be given to achieve complete sinusoidal relaxation.

Maintenance flow rate is considered as the most important parameter of cavernosometry and it involves recording of minimum flow rate, which is required to maintain intracavernous pressure at 150 mm Hg. Maintenance flow rate of more than 3 mL per minute is suggestive of venous leakage. After this, the infusion is stopped and the rate of fall of cavernosal pressure is observed for 30 seconds. The rate of fall, termed as "pressure loss," of more than 1.5 mm Hg per second is considered abnormal.[38]

Gravity cavernosometry is a simple and cost-effective modification of the above technique in which the inflow needle is connected to heparinized normal saline kept at the height of 160 cm. The infusion produces increase in cavernosal pressure, which subsequently reaches at a plateau, termed as "steady state pressure." Steady state pressure of less than 97 mm Hg is considered abnormal.[48]

Cavernosography

Patient can be taken up for cavernosography after cavernosometry in the same sitting. About 40 mL of iodinated contrast is injected in infusion line while keeping intracavernosal pressure just above mean arterial pressure. Spot films of penis and pelvis are obtained under fluoroscopic guidance in AP and both oblique projections **(Figs. 13A and B)**. Normally draining veins are not opacified. In case of venous leakage, veins are visualized draining from the veins of corpus spongiosum, the deep dorsal, cavernosal, and crural veins **(Figs. 14A and B)**. More than one site is present in most patients, with deep dorsal and cavernosal veins being the most common combination.[49]

Penile Angiography

Internal pudendal angiography is indicated in younger patients with suspected isolated arterial disease, such as post-traumatic narrowing, who may benefit from surgical repair rather than in elderly patients with diffuse atheromatous involvement. Patency of common iliac, internal iliac, and internal pudendal arteries is established on initial angiographic films. Later, 60 mg of papaverine is injected in cavernosa followed by selective angiography of anterior division of internal pudendal artery. Contrast is injected

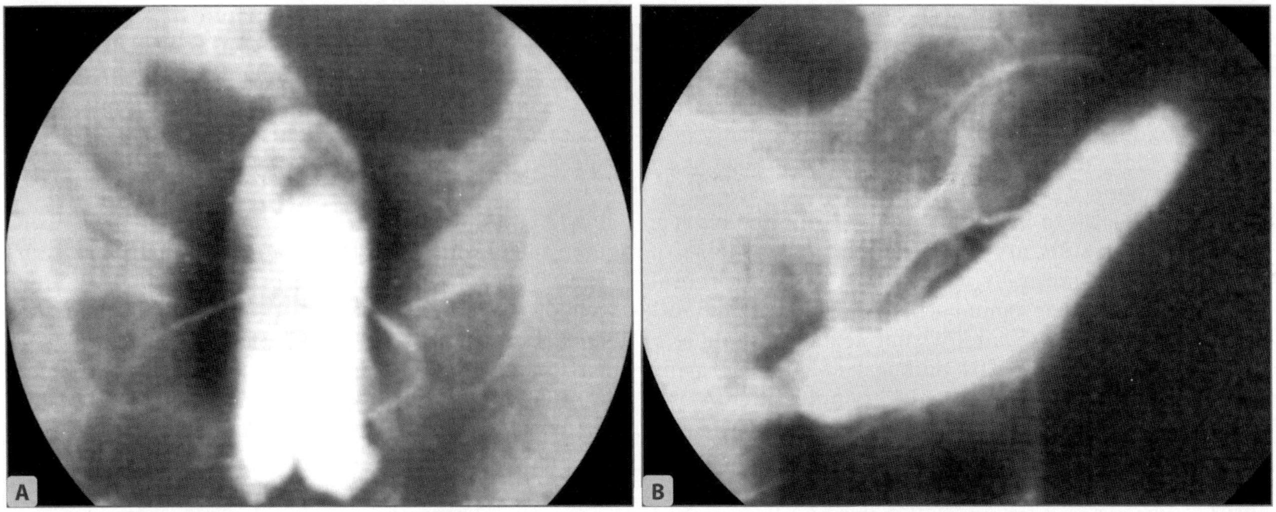

FIGS. 13A AND B: Normal cavernosogram. (A) AP and (B) oblique views show homogeneous opacification of bilateral cavernosa without visualization of any vein in vicinity. (AP: anteroposterior).

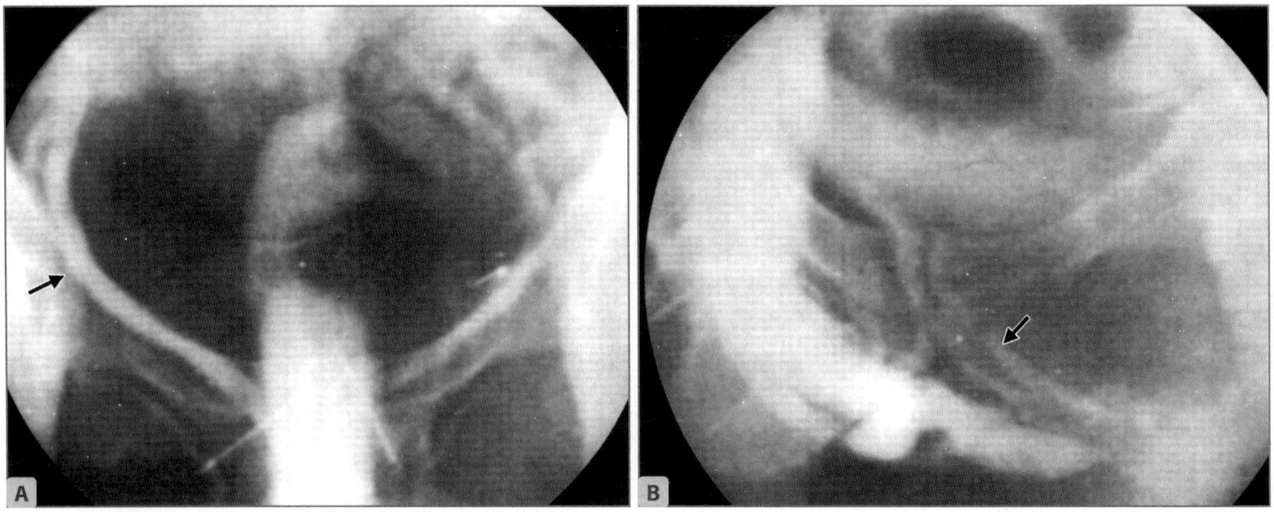

FIGS. 14A AND B: Cavernosogram: Veno-occlusive ED. (A) AP view shows venous leak into internal pudendal vein (arrow). (B) Oblique view (arrow) shows venous leak into deep dorsal vein in the cavernosogram of another patient. (ED: erectile dysfunction).

at the rate of 3–4 mL per second and images are obtained in posterior oblique projection. In majority of the patients, anatomy of the penile arterial supply and the precise location of the arterial lesion is demonstrated which allows planning of appropriate surgical approach **(Figs. 15A and B)**.

Priapism

The most common complication, during the diagnostic workup and especially during PPDU and cavernosometry, is papaverine-induced prolonged and painful erection or priapism. The incidence can be as high as 11%.[34] Chances of priapism are high if PSV of more than 66 cm/s or RI of more than 1 (diastolic flow reversal) is observed.[50] It is prudent to observe the patient for at least 2 hours after the procedure. Not all priapism cases require specific treatment as penis detumescence generally occurs within few hours. In case the duration of erection exceeds 6 hours, the corpora cavernosa are drained to decrease the pressure and 10 microgram of adrenaline is injected intracavernosally to induce cavernosal smooth muscle contraction, effective venous drainage, and restriction of arterial flow. Compression bandage is also applied for few minutes. In case of recurrence of erection, the procedure is repeated.

Broadly, priapism is divided into high-flow and low-flow priapism. High-flow priapism is usually associated with trauma. The patients have painless erection and venous outflow is usually maintained. The diagnosis of high-flow priapism is usually clinical but color Doppler US may provide useful information. No cavernosal injection is required for the study.

A hypoechoic area may be seen in cavernosa on gray scale US which suggests laceration. Color Doppler study may demonstrate the cavernosal artery tear and arterial-lacunar fistula. Selective embolization of the torn artery with blood clots, coils, or polyvinyl alcohol (PVA) is the treatment of

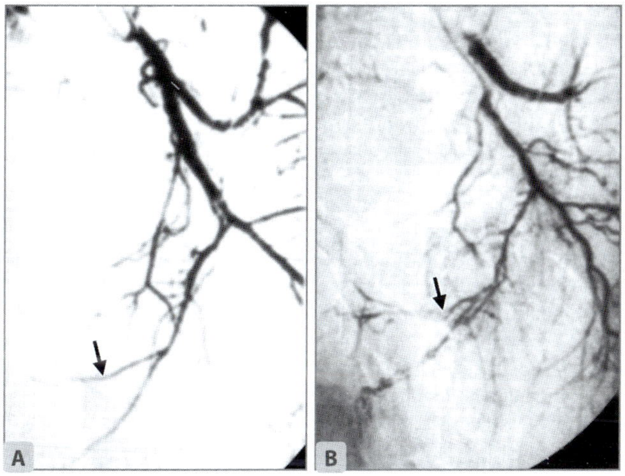

FIGS. 15A AND B: Internal pudendal angiogram. (A) Normal internal pudendal and common penile (arrow) arteries. (B) Internal pudendal angiogram of another patient shows post-traumatic narrowing of common penile artery (arrow) as a cause of arteriogenic ED. (ED: erectile dysfunction).

choice to treat these lesions.[51] Low-flow or ischemic priapism is seen as complication of intracavernosal injection of drugs or leukostasis in leukemic patients. The diagnosis is clinical and imaging is not required before surgical intervention. The condition is considered as an urologic emergency. US and color Doppler findings are same as that of normal rigid erection.

CONCLUSION

The diagnostic workup of male infertility should start at least 1 year after consummation of marriage and needs to be performed in a systematic and structured manner. Semen analysis should be complemented with a comprehensive medical history supplemented by imaging. Imaging has an important role in differentiating causes of obstructive azoospermia (investigation of choice is TRUS), which are potentially correctable causes of infertility from causes of nonobstructive azoospermia (investigation of choice is scrotal USG).

REFERENCES

1. Guttmacher AF. Factors affecting normal expectancy of conception. J Am Med Assoc. 1956;161:855-60.
2. World Health Organization. Towards more objectivity in diagnosis and management of male infertility. Int J Androl. 1987;(Suppl 7):1-53.
3. Colpi Ammar T, Sidhu PS, Wilkins CJ. Male infertility: the role of imaging in diagnosis and management. Br J Radiol. 2012;85(1):S59-68.
4. Cornund E, Amar E, Hamida K, et al. Ultrasound findings in male hypofertility and impotence. Eur Radiol. 2001;11:2126-36.
5. Pierik FH, Dohle GR, Muiswinkel JM, et al. Is routine scrotal ultrasonography advantageous in infertile men? J Urol. 1999; 162:1618-20.
6. Jarrow JP. Transrectal ultrasonography of infertile men. Fertil Steril. 1993;60:1035-9.
7. Raviv G, Mor Y, Levron J, et al. Role of transrectal ultrasonography in the evaluation of azoospermic men with low volume ejaculate. J Ultrasound Med. 2006;25:825-9.
8. Sihag P, Tandon A, Pal R, et al. Sonography in male infertility: a look beyond the obvious. J Ultrasound. 2018;21(3):265-76.
9. Dhabuwala CB, Parulkar BG. Doppler flow analysis and conventional ultrasonography for evaluation of the infertile male. In: Jafe R, Pierson RA, Abramowics JS (Eds). Imaging in Infertility and Reproductive Endocrinology. Philadelphia: JB Lippincot Co.; 1994. pp. 207-16.
10. Qublan HS, Al-Okoor K, Al-Ghoweri AS, et al. Sonographic spectrum of scrotal abnormalities in infertile men. J Clin Ultrasound. 2007;35:437-41.
11. Howards SS, Mittal PK, Little B, et al. Role of imaging in the evaluation of male infertility. Radiographics. 2017;37(3): 837-54.
12. Dambro TJ, Stewart RR, Carroll BA, et al. The scrotum. In: Rumack CM, Wilson SR, Charboneau JW (Eds). Diagnostic Ultrasound, 2nd edition. St Louis: Mosby; 1998. pp. 719-822.
13. Lorenc T, Krupniewski L, Palczewski P, et al. The value of ultrasonography in the diagnosis of varicocele. J Ultrason. 2016;16(67):359-70.
14. Kokacok E, Serhatlioglu S, Kiris S, et al. Colour Doppler sonographic evaluation of interrelations between diameter, reflux, and flow volume of testicular veins in varicocele. Eur J Radiol. 2003;47:251-6.
15. Chiou RK, Anderson JC, Wobig RK, et al. Color Doppler ultrasound criteria to diagnose varicoceles: correlation of a new scoring system with physical examination. Urology. 1997;50:953-6.
16. Dhamija E, Das CJ, Razik A. Intratesticular varicocele: a rare cause of male factor infertility. BMJ Case Rep. 2018;2018.
17. Dubin L, Amelar R. Varicocele size and results of varicocelectomy in selected infertile men with a varicocele. Fertil Steril. 1970;21: 606-9.
18. McLure R, Kho D, Dale R, et al. Subclinical varicocele—the effectiveness of varicocelectomy. J Urol. 1991;145:786-90.
19. Gonda RL Jr, Kaw JJ, Forte KA, et al. Diagnosis of subclinical varicocele in infertility. AJR. 1987;148:71-5.
20. Gandini R, Konda D, Reale CA, et al. Male varicocele: transcatheter foam sclerotherapy with sodium tetradecyl sulfate: outcome in 244 patients. Radiology. 2008;246:612-8.
21. Halden W, White RI. Outpatient embolotherapy of varicocele. Urol Clin N Am. 1987;14:137-40.
22. Thompson ST. Prevention of male infertility: an update. Urol Clin N Am. 1994;21:365-76.
23. Simon SD, Lee RD, Mulhall PP. Should all infertile males undergo urologic evaluation before assisted reproductive technologies? Fertil Steril. 2001;75:1226-7.
24. Kim Ed, Lipshultz LI. Role of ultrasound in assessment of male infertility. J Clin Ultrasound. 1996;24:437-53.
25. Kumar R, Thulkar S, Kumar V, et al. Contributions of investigations to the diagnosis of bilateral vas aplasia. ANZ J Surg. 2005;75: 807-9.
26. Kim MJ, Lee JT, Lee MS, et al. MR imaging of male infertility with an endorectal surface coil. Abdom Imaging. 1997;22: 348-53.
27. Fisch H, Lambert SM, Goluboff ET. Management of ejaculatory duct obstruction. Etiology, diagnosis and treatment. World J Urol. 2006;24:604-10.

28. Colpi GM, Negri L, Nappi RE, et al. Is transrectal ultrasonography a reliable diagnostic approach in ejaculatory duct sub obstruction? Hum Reprod. 1997;12:2186-91.
29. Purohit RS, Wu DS, Shinohara K, et al. A prospective comparison of three diagnostic methods to evaluate ejaculatory duct obstruction. J Urol. 2004;171:232-5.
30. Schnall MD, Pollack HM, Arsdalen KV, et al. The seminal tract in patients with ejaculatory dysfunction: MR imaging with an endorectal surface coil. AJR. 1992;159:337-41.
31. Toov JH, Fait G, Houser R, et al. Can Doppler ultrasonographic measurements of the testis predict spermatozoa retrieval in azoospermic patients undergoing testicular biopsy? Fertil Steril. 2001;76:1276-7.
32. Belenky A, Avrech CM, Bacher GN, et al. Ultrasound-guided testicular sperm aspiration in azoospermic patient: a new sperm retrieval method for intracytoplasmic sperm injection. J Clin Ultrasound. 2001;6:339-43.
33. Belker AM, Steinbock GS. Transrectal prostate ultrasonography as a diagnostic and therapeutic aid for ejaculatory duct obstruction. J Urol. 1990;144:356-8.
34. Mihmanli I, Kantarci F. Erectile dysfunction. Semin Ultrasound CT MRI. 2007;28:274-86.
35. Aroujo AB, Mohr BA, McKinley JB. Changes in sexual function in middle aged and older men: longitudinal data from the Massachusetts Male Aging Study. J Am Geriatr Soc. 2004;52: 1502-9.
36. Montorsi F, Briganti A, Salonia A, et al. Erectile dysfunction prevalence, time of onset, and association with risk factors in 300 consecutive patients with acute chest pain, and angiographically documented coronary artery disease. Eur Urol. 2003;44:360-4.
37. Hatzichristan D, Hatzimouratidis K, Bekas M, et al. Diagnostic steps in evaluation of patients with erectile dysfunction. J Urol. 2002;168:615-20.
38. Meuleman E, Diemont WL. Investigation of erectile dysfunction. Urol Clin N Am. 1995;22:803-19.
39. Park K, Kwon DD, Oh BR, et al. Efficacy of virtual glasses in audiovisual sexual stimulation during penile colour duplex Doppler ultrasonography. Eur Urol. 2002;41:62-5.
40. Roy C, Saussine C, Tuchman C, et al. Duplex Doppler sonography of flaccid penis: potential role in the evaluation of impotence. J Clin Ultrasound. 2000;28:290-4.
41. Broderick GA, Arger P. Duplex Doppler ultrasonography: noninvasive assessment of penile anatomy and function. Semin Roentgen. 1993;28:43-56.
42. Shwartz AM, Lawe M, Berger RE, et al. Assessment of normal and abnormal erectile function: color Doppler sonography versus conventional techniques. radiology. 1991;180:105-9.
43. Bhargava R, Srivastava DN, Thulkar S, et al. Colour duplex Doppler ultrasonography evaluation of nonvasculogenic male erectile dysfunction: an Indian perspective. Australas Radiol. 2002;44:170-3.
44. Arslan D, Esen AA, Secil M. A new method for evaluation of ED: Sildenafil plus Doppler ultrasonography. J Urol. 2001;166: 181-4.
45. Copel L, Ktz R, Blacher A, et al. Clinical and duplex US assessment of effects of sildenafil on cavernosal arteries of the penis—comparison with intracavernosal injection of vasoactive agents: initial experience. Radiology. 2005;237: 986-91.
46. Park JK, Park JS, Jeon SB, et al. Why a combined intracavernosal injection with trimix and oral sildenafil is reliable therapy in ultrasonic evaluation of erectile dysfunction. BJU Int. 2008; 102:993-7.
47. Gholami SS, Lue TF. Peyronie's disease. Urol Clin N Am. 2001;28:377-90.
48. Meulman EJ, Wijkstra H, Doesbury WH, et al. Comparison of diagnostic values of pump and gravity cavernosometry in the evaluation of cavernous veno-occlusive mechanism. J Urol. 1991;146:1266-70.
49. Shabsingh R, Fishman IJ, Toombs BD, et al. Venous leaks: anatomical and physiological observations. J Urol. 1991;146: 1260-4.
50. Metawea B, El-Nashar AR, Gad-Allah A, et al. Intracavernos papaverine phentolamine-induced priapism can be accurately predicted with colour Doppler ultrasonography. Urology. 2005;66:858-60.
51. Campliani S, Savoca G, Buttazi L, et al. High-flow priapism: treatment and long-term follow-up. Urology. 2002;59: 110-3.

CHAPTER

23

Imaging of the Adrenal Gland

Devasenathipathy Kandasamy, Raju Sharma, Arun Kumar Gupta

INTRODUCTION

Thomas Addison first described a clinical entity resulting from adrenal dysfunction in 1855, but it took nearly half a century for the scientific community to accept that adrenals are essential to life. Remarkable progress has since been made in defining the structure and function of the adrenal gland. Adrenal glands are small but their common involvement in many disease processes has made cross-sectional imaging modalities essential to detect abnormal morphological and functional alterations. With the ever-increasing volume of imaging being performed, incidental adrenal nodules are detected much more than ever. Around 4% of all abdominal computed tomography (CT) scans show adrenal nodules and this number increases to 6% in autopsy studies.[1,2] The incidence also increases with age. Imaging also plays a critical role in the characterization of adrenal mass lesions. It is important to understand the normal anatomy and functional characteristics of the adrenal gland.

ANATOMY AND PHYSIOLOGY

The adrenal gland is named for its location adjacent to the kidney. It lies within perirenal fascia, embedded in perirenal fat. Each gland measures 3–5 cm in length, 2–3 cm in width, 5.0 mm in thickness and weighs around 3.5–5.0 g. Both glands differ in shape. The right adrenal is pyramidal in shape and its relations are liver laterally, upper pole of right kidney inferiorly, right crus of diaphragm posteromedially, and inferior vena cava (IVC) anteromedially. The left adrenal gland is crescent-shaped and its relations are upper pole of left kidney posterolaterally, left crus of diaphragm posteromedially, stomach in upper two-thirds anteriorly, and pancreatic body with splenic vessels in lower one-third. Each adrenal gland receives its blood supply from three arteries, namely, superior adrenal artery, a branch of inferior phrenic artery; middle adrenal artery arising from descending aorta; and inferior adrenal artery, a branch of the renal artery. There is a single adrenal vein on either side—the right adrenal vein drains into inferior vena cava and the left one into the left renal vein.

The adrenal gland is made of an outer cortex that is derived from mesoderm and an inner medulla that is derived from neural crest. The cortex forms almost 90% of the total adrenal mass; the medulla contributes only 10%. The adrenal cortex is histologically comprised of three distinct zones—zona glomerulosa, zona fasciculata, and zona reticularis from outside to inside. The adrenal cortex secretes three groups of steroid hormones. Zona glomerulosa constitutes 10–15% of the cortex and secretes mineralocorticoids; aldosterone being the most important. Zona fasciculata constitutes 80% of the cortex and secretes glucocorticoids while zona reticularis, contributing only 5–10% of cortex, secretes androgens. Zona glomerulosa is mainly involved in aldosterone biosynthesis whereas the fasciculata-reticularis zone is the site for cortisol and androgen biosynthesis.

The adrenal medulla secretes epinephrine and norepinephrine, which form an integral part of the sympathetic autonomic nervous system and play an important role in the regulation of vital functions and many metabolic processes.

IMAGING MODALITIES

A number of imaging modalities are available for evaluation of the adrenals. Before the advent of imaging modalities like ultrasound (US), CT, and magnetic resonance imaging (MRI), the radiological techniques available for evaluation of adrenals were plain radiograph of abdomen, excretory urography, invasive techniques like perirenal air insufflation, adrenal venography, and angiography. Most of these techniques have become obsolete. Angiography may be sometimes indicated to look for extra-adrenal pheochromocytoma in situations when metaiodobenzylguanidine (MIBG) scintigraphy is not available. Adrenal venous sampling may be recommended in patients with primary hyperaldosteronism, both for distinguishing unilateral from bilateral disease and for localizing unilateral tumor. According to the recommendations of the Endocrine Society, all patients with primary hyperaldosteronism of age more than 35 years should undergo preoperative adrenal venous sampling to lateralize the lesion, irrespective of the imaging findings.[3] Both the adrenal veins are sequentially catheterized and obtained samples are tested for aldosterone and cortisol levels. The right adrenal vein drains into IVC whereas the left adrenal vein drains into the left renal vein. This technique is invasive, technically difficult to perform, and needs hospitalization. Procedural complications include adrenal infarction, adrenal vein thrombosis, adrenal hemorrhage, hypotensive crises, and adrenal insufficiency.

Ultrasound is seldom used in imaging suspected adrenal pathology. CT and MRI remain the imaging modalities of choice for the evaluation of structural changes in the diseased adrenal whereas scintigraphy provides functional assessment of the gland. ^{18}F fluorodeoxyglucose positron emission tomography (^{18}F-FDG PET) has played an important role in defining physiological and pathological conditions of the adrenal glands. Integrated information obtained from anatomic and functional imaging is essential for characterization of adrenal disease.

Percutaneous biopsy of the adrenal lesion under US/CT guidance has an accuracy of 80–90%. Minor complications include abdominal pain, hematuria, or small pneumothorax. Major ones requiring treatment occur in 3–5% of the patients and include hemorrhage and pneumothorax necessitating drainage.

Ultrasound

Despite the availability of high-resolution real-time ultrasound scanners, normal adrenal gland or small adrenal lesions remain difficult to be visualized on sonography except in infants where adrenals can be well visualized on US. Therefore, ultrasonography (USG) is seldom indicated for adrenal lesion, although large adrenal mass may be detected incidentally during abdominal US examination. USG is however, useful in evaluation of suspected adrenal hemorrhage in neonates. It may also be used as a screening modality in suspected pheochromocytoma due to the easy availability. USG guidance suffices for sampling of large adrenal lesions.

Computed Tomography

Computed tomography remains the first choice of imaging modality for evaluation of the majority of adrenal diseases. The widespread availability of CT in clinical practice makes it an ideal noninvasive technique for evaluating adrenal gland morphology owing to the speed with which examination can be performed, its superior spatial resolution, and quantification of contrast washout patterns.[4,5] The introduction of multidetector-row helical CT has allowed rapid thin-slice imaging of the adrenal glands during various phases of contrast enhancement. Small adrenal lesions can be detected and accurate density measurements of lesions can be done.

The CT technique should be tailored according to the clinical indication. In general, when CT is used to study the adrenal glands, the entire abdomen through the aortic bifurcation is scanned. This is helpful for staging or for evaluating possible ectopic adrenal lesions. Oral contrast material is helpful so that unopacified loops of bowel are not confused as adrenal lesions. A nonenhanced CT examination should be done first. This may be followed by enhanced and delayed enhanced CT examination when required in a situation, where adenoma needs to be differentiated from metastasis. Currently, adrenal protocol CT is considered more accurate and is favored over MRI for the differentiation of adenoma from metastasis, unless administration of iodinated contrast is contraindicated.[6] Thin sections along with multiplanar reconstructions need to be reviewed on a workstation.

In the search for pheochromocytoma, CT should be done from lower thorax to symphysis pubis. Pericardium is a rare site but can be easily included on CT. Large sporadic pheochromocytomas are easily detected on CT. However, syndromic pheochromocytoma may be small, multiple, and extra-adrenal. In order to optimize visualization of tumors, contrast injection is necessary. It is extremely rare for the new nonionic IV contrast agents to precipitate hypertensive crisis in patients of pheochromocytoma.

The adrenal gland has a characteristic inverted Y or V shape on CT and is seen as an anteromedial ridge with two posterior limbs, the medial limb being shorter than the lateral limb. The limbs normally have a straight or concave outline **(Figs. 1A and B)**. The adrenal measurements on CT are taken as anteroposterior diameter from the tip of the anteromedial ridge to the posterior tip of the longest limb, length by calculating the number of sequential scans in which the gland is visualized **(Fig. 2)**. The criteria for enlargement of adrenal are taken as length more than 4.0 cm, anteroposterior diameter of more than 3.0 cm, and limb thickness of more than 6.0 mm or more than adjacent diaphragmatic crus. Besides these absolute measurements, any alteration in the contour, focal bulge, calcification, pattern of enhancement, CT attenuation values on nonenhanced, enhanced and delayed-enhanced techniques, and displacement of surrounding structures should be evaluated.[7]

Another advancement in the last decade is the capability of dual-energy CT (DECT) for tissue material decomposition. One of the benefits of DECT is the generation of virtual noncontrast (VNC) CT from contrast-enhanced CT (CECT) without actually acquiring the noncontrast images. In adrenal adenoma, the VNC has been found to be equally effective as true noncontrast CT (NCCT) in diagnosis.[8-10] Besides this, it can also detect the percentage of microscopic fat within the lesion to characterize them.[11,12]

Magnetic Resonance Imaging

The intention of most MRI techniques used so far has primarily been distinction of benign from malignant disease.

The most reliable in this context is the use of in-phase and out-of-phase gradient-echo (GRE) techniques (chemical shift imaging) for adenoma versus metastasis distinction. Two different echo times (TEs) (out-of-phase TE: 2.2–2.7 ms and in-phase TE: 4.2–4.5 ms) are used in each repetition time (TR) during this sequence. The shortest echo times feasible should be used to overcome the effect of T2* decay on signal. The principle behind this sequence is the ability to highlight the presence of microscopic fat, which is typically expected in adenomas. The fat and water protons are in phase at in-phase TE when the signals add up whereas at out-of-phase

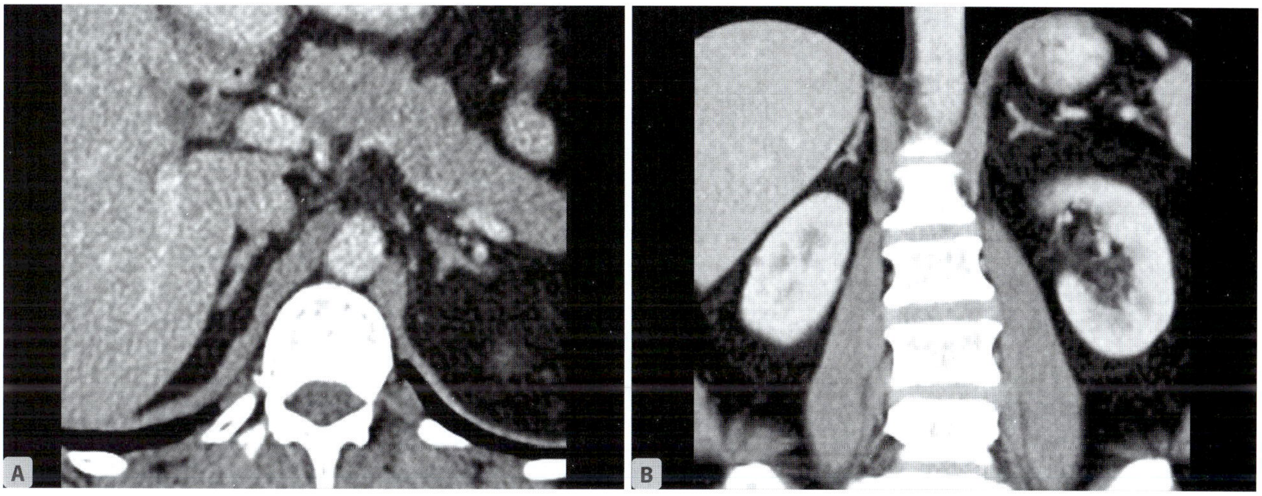

FIGS. 1A AND B: (A) Axial and (B) coronal CT images showing the normal adrenal glands.

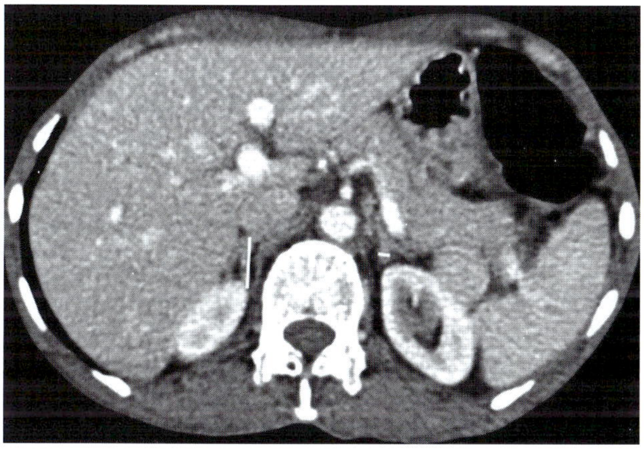

FIG. 2: Normal adrenal measurements. (1) Anteroposterior diameter and (2) limb thickness.

TE the fat and water protons are out of phase leading to cancellation of their signals. This phenomenon leads to signal drop of adenomas in out-of-phase images. It is an accurate method to diagnose adenoma, which can be helpful even when CT densitometry fails. It is because the sensitivity of MRI in detecting microscopic fat is better than CT. However, if the lipid content is very low as seen in lipopenic adenoma chemical shift imaging too will fail. CT washout technique performs better than MR chemical shift imaging in lipopenic adenomas. Another pitfall of chemical shift MRI is that it will be positive in any lesion containing microscopic fat. Metastasis from hepatocellular carcinoma and renal cell carcinoma which can have microscopic fat can show signal drop on out-of-phase imaging.[13-15] Nonetheless, both MR and CT have very high specificity (95–98%) in differentiating adenoma from metastasis.[6] The normal adrenal cortex contains abundant lipid, which however, is not enough to be demonstrated on in-phase and out-of-phase imaging.

T2-weighted images provide information on the fluid content of lesions. T2W imaging is most useful in the search for pheochromocytomas which have a high fluid content. T2W sequences also supplement benign versus malignant differentiation, although substantial overlap exists.[16] Normal adrenal gland may demonstrate corticomedullary differentiation on T2WI.

Normal adrenal glands and small adrenal masses are well demonstrated on T1-weighted fat-suppressed images **(Figs. 3A and B)**.[17] The demonstration of corticomedullary differentiation on either noncontrast T1W fat-suppressed images or immediate postgadolinium GE images is helpful in distinguishing adrenal from renal tumors.[18] The sagittal plane is more useful than coronal plane in this regard. The use of thin-section 3D-GRE sequences in one plane of acquisition allows reconstructions in other planes for defining tumor location.

Diffusion-weighted MRI provides insight into water composition and cellularity in a tumor may provide an additional tool to distinguish benign, and from malignant adrenal masses. Malignant tumors have an increased cellularity, which manifests as restricted diffusion, and a decrease in the apparent diffusion coefficient. However, even benign tumors such as adenoma and pheochromocytoma can have restricted diffusion limiting the utility of diffusion-weighted imaging (DWI) in adrenal lesion characterization.

Radionuclide Imaging

This technique is primarily used as a problem-solving modality for lesions not adequately characterized on CT and MRI. It provides functional imaging of the adrenal cortex and medulla. Radiolabeled analogs of cholesterol, e.g. 75 Se-selenomethyl-norcholesterol, NP-59 beta-iodomethyl-19-norcholesterol, can localize mass causing adrenal cortical dysfunction; the latter one is particularly useful in the workup for suspected aldosteronism. The advances in CT and MRI have largely eliminated the use of NP-59 imaging for adrenal. Iodine-131 MIBG is concentrated in sympathoadrenal tissue and is used for imaging adrenal medullary lesion, especially to evaluate for pheochromocytoma and to screen the whole body for extra-adrenal pheochromocytoma.

Positron Emission Tomography

Recently, PET has become available as a possible tool for evaluating the adrenal. ^{18}F-FDG PET imaging has been found to be a reliable noninvasive imaging technique to differentiate benign from malignant adrenal masses. It has demonstrated high sensitivity, specificity, and overall accuracy for detecting adrenal metastases in patients with malignancy. In patients with known malignancy, FDG-PET is the modality of choice to evaluate any adrenal lesion more than 4 cm.[19] At the same time, PET CT is not recommended in patients without a history of malignancy. The common causes of false-positive adrenal lesions on ^{18}F-FDG PET imaging are benign adenomas and pheochromocytoma.[20,21] All benign and malignant pheochromocytomas have been shown to accumulate ^{18}F-FDG, although uptake is found in a greater concentration in malignant as compared to benign pheochromocytoma.[20] The common causes of false-negative ^{18}F-FDG PET results are small-sized lesions, necrotic metastasis, and metastases from neuroendocrine tumors.[21] Small metastatic lesions can be missed because of the limited resolution of ^{18}F-FDG PET/PET-CT or the absence of sufficient tumor cells with increased glycolysis.

ADRENAL DISEASES

Diseases of the adrenal gland may manifest as a result of hormone excess or deficiency. The adrenal diseases may be considered under the following three groups.

- *Group I*: Adrenal hyperfunctional diseases
- *Group II*: Adrenal insufficiency
- *Group III*: Adrenal diseases with normal function.

Group I: Adrenal Hyperfunctional Diseases

Hyperfunctioning adrenal diseases occur either from the adrenal cortex (Cushing's syndrome, Conn's syndrome, and hyperandrogenism) or from the adrenal medulla (pheochromocytoma). The clinical features depend on the type of hormone produced and its manifestation on target organs.

Cushing's Syndrome

Cushing's syndrome is caused by adrenocorticotropic hormone (ACTH) overproduction in 75% of patients and by an excess of cortisol production from adrenal neoplasms in 25%. ACTH overproduction results from either pituitary adenoma or ectopic ACTH-producing nonendocrine tumors. Ectopic ACTH producing nonendocrine tumors include bronchial carcinoid tumor, neuroendocrine tumors of the pancreas, medullary carcinoma of thyroid, thymic carcinoid tumor, and pheochromocytoma **(Figs. 3A and B)**.

The diagnosis of Cushing's syndrome depends predominantly on the clinical features and biochemical findings. It presents an easily recognizable clinical picture of truncal obesity, moon facies, cutaneous striae, buffalo hump, hypertension, muscle weakness, fatigability, osteoporosis, profound emotional changes, and amenorrhea in women.

Appropriate workup of patients with Cushing's syndrome includes plasma cortisol and 24 hours' urine for cortisol estimation followed by dexamethasone suppression test. The abnormal test establishes the diagnosis of Cushing's syndrome. The purpose of imaging is to identify the source of excess ACTH from either a pituitary tumor or an ectopic source and to detect or exclude adrenal mass. The adrenal appearances in Cushing's syndrome depend on the etiology of the syndrome. CT is the primary modality used to evaluate adrenals in this setting. Visualization of adrenal pathology on CT is aided by the large amount of retroperitoneal fat that is usually present in these patients. MRI plays a secondary role.[22]

ACTH-dependent Cushing's Syndrome

This results from a pituitary cause in 85% of patients and the rest from ectopic ACTH secretion. The adrenals show changes of hyperplasia in the form of smooth thickened limbs or multiple small nodules of varying sizes involving one or both limbs.

These changes may be seen in one or both adrenals **(Figs. 4 and 5)**. MRI signal intensity in adrenal hyperplasia closely follows that of the normal adrenal gland.

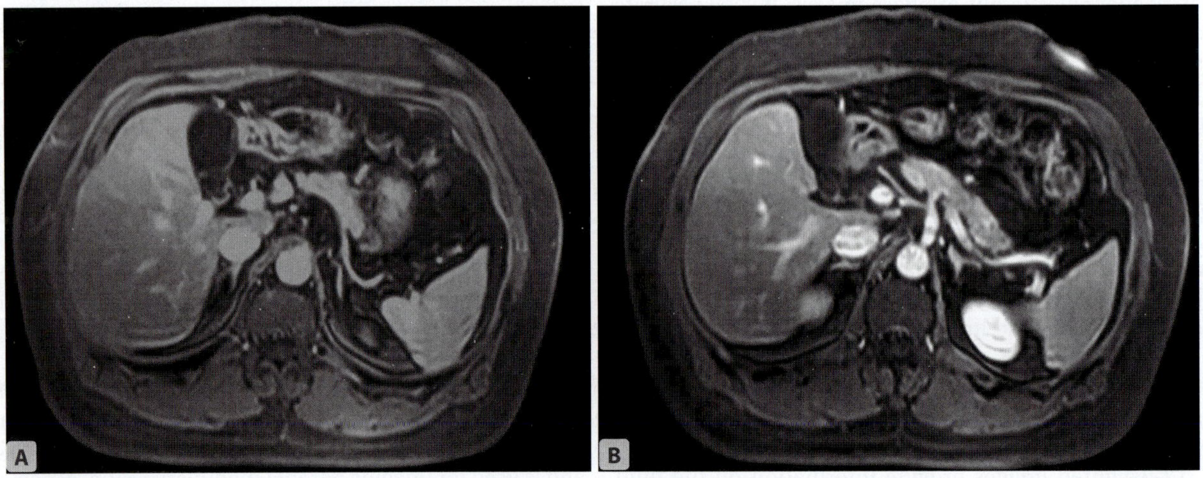

FIGS. 3A AND B: Gradient-echo T1W axial images showing the normal inverted "V" configuration of the adrenal gland.

ACTH-independent Cushing's Syndrome

Adrenocortical adenoma accounts for 10–20% of patients with Cushing's syndrome. It is seen as a solitary, well-defined homogeneous mass, usually around 2–3 cm in diameter **(Figs. 6A to C)**. However, when large, it shows focal areas of necrosis and hemorrhage. These adenomas are larger than those seen in Conn's syndrome and are usually lipid rich. The contralateral gland is normal but occasionally atrophic. Adrenal carcinoma accounts for 10–15% of patients with Cushing's syndrome. Also, only 10% of adrenal carcinomas function to a level that results in Cushing's syndrome. It is generally seen as a large mass often more than 6.0 cm, heterogeneous with areas of necrosis and calcification, with features of local invasion, regional lymphadenopathy, and distant spread **(Figs. 7 and 8)**.

Rockall et al. while reporting findings in 37 patients with primary adrenal Cushing's syndrome found that hyperfunctioning adenomas (n = 24) and functioning carcinomas (n = 10) accounted for 92% of cases.[23]

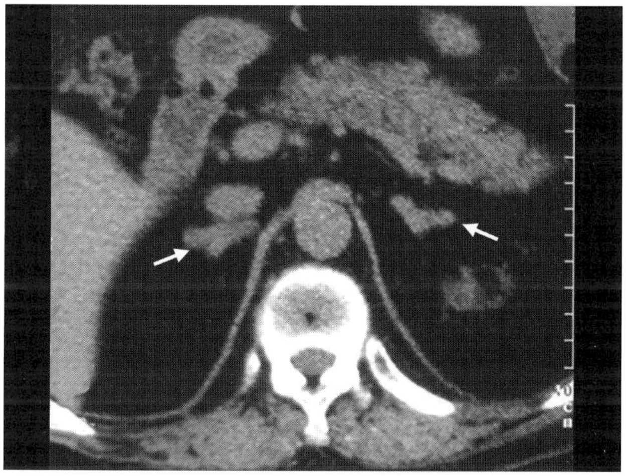

FIG. 4: Noncontrast CT of adrenal glands of a 20-year-old male patient presenting with Cushing's syndrome showing bilateral adrenal hyperplasia (arrows) with proliferation of perirenal and mesenteric fat.

Adenomas had a significantly smaller mean size (3.5 vs 14.5 cm) and lower mean unenhanced CT attenuation value [11 vs 28 Hounsfield unit (HU)] than did carcinomas. The presence of necrosis, hemorrhage, and calcification favored a diagnosis of carcinoma. Six of 10 carcinoma patients had metastases at presentation. Two adenomas were seen within a myelolipoma. Two adenomas were of uncertain malignant potential. Bilateral disease—primary pigmented nodular adrenal dysplasia (PPNAD) (n = 2) and ACTH-independent macronodular adrenal hyperplasia (AIMAH) (n = 1)—had characteristic imaging features. In PPNAD, multiple tiny (2–5 mm) nodules were visible bilaterally, with no overall glandular enlargement and normal intervening adrenal tissue. In AIMAH, both glands were grossly enlarged and contained nodules up to 3 cm in diameter.

Aldosteronism

Aldosteronism (Conn's syndrome) is associated with excess of mineralocorticoids and characterized clinically by hypertension, muscle weakness, polyuria, polydipsia, and persistent hypokalemia. It is caused by adrenal adenoma in about 80% of patients while adrenal gland hyperplasia in the rest. Adrenal carcinoma is a very rare cause of Conn's syndrome. In patients with unilateral adenoma, unilateral adrenalectomy is the treatment of choice. On the other hand, cases of bilateral adrenal gland hyperplasia are treated medically with pharmacological agents.[24] The imaging approach hence is to distinguish between these two entities. Adrenal venous sampling plays a key role in making this distinction. It is performed in all patients above 35 years to lateralize the lesion regardless of the findings on imaging.

Aldosterone-producing adenoma is small with a mean size of 1.6–1.8 cm and may have low attenuation due to high lipid content **(Fig. 9)**. A dedicated CT examination with thin sections is required for localizing the adenoma.

If CT examination is inconclusive, adrenal cortical scintigraphy with NP-59 may be done. On NP-59 scintigraphy, both adrenals are normally visualized on 5th day or later, following injection of radiopharmaceuticals. Bilateral

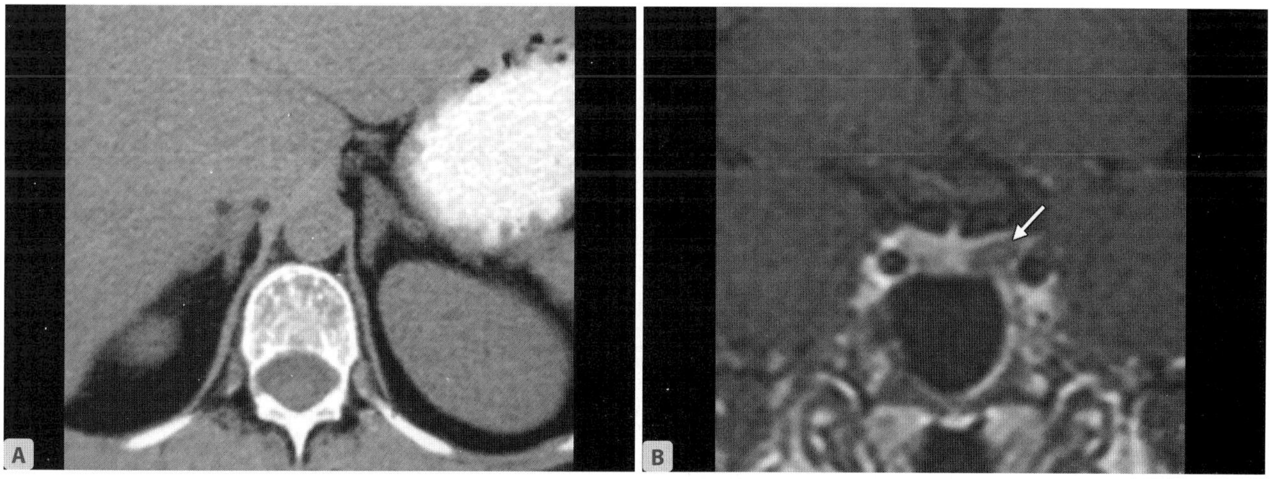

FIGS. 5A AND B: (A) Noncontrast CT of adrenal glands of a 32-year-old female patient presenting with Cushing's syndrome showing nodular, bilateral adrenal hyperplasia; (B) Postcontrast T1W coronal image of MRI sella of the same patient reveals a microadenoma on the left side of anterior pituitary (arrow).

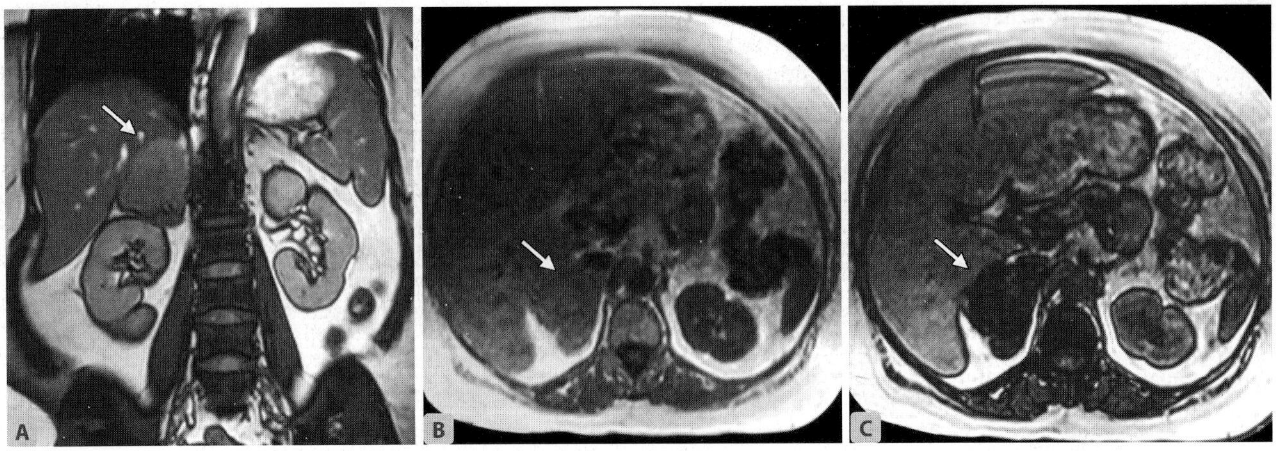

FIGS. 6A TO C: (A) MRI of a 44-year-old female with Cushingoid features. True-FISP coronal image shows an intermediate signal intensity mass in the right adrenal gland; T1 FLASH (B) in-phase and (C) opposed-phase images reveal significant signal drop in the opposed-phase images, suggesting adrenal adenoma.

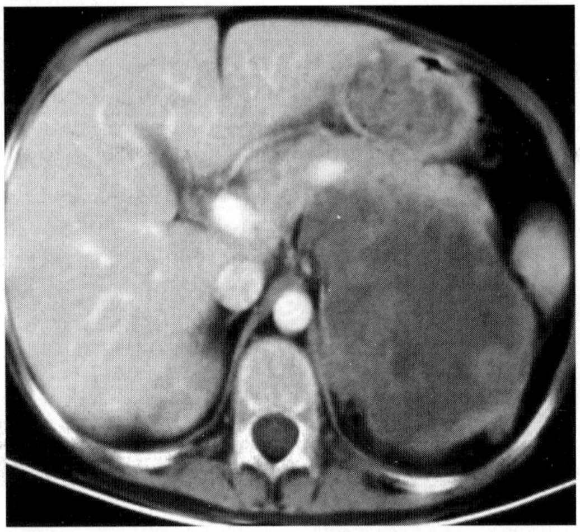

FIG. 7: Axial contrast-enhanced CT of a 12-year-old boy with Cushingoid features showing a heterogeneously enhancing mass arising from the left adrenal gland, suggesting adrenal carcinoma.

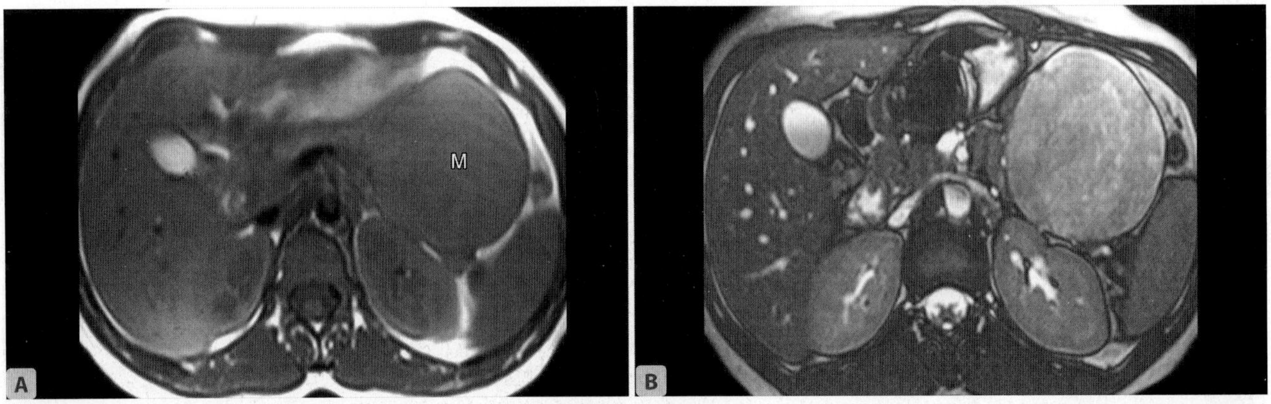

FIGS. 8A AND B: Axial (A) T1W and (B) T2W MR images of a 28-year-old female with clinical and biochemical features of Cushing's syndrome reveal a well-encapsulated mass (M), hypointense on T1W and heterogeneously hyperintense on T2W, arising from the left adrenal gland. On biopsy, it was a carcinoma.

adrenal visualization before 5th day suggests adrenal gland hyperplasia while unilateral adrenal visualization before 5th day indicates an adenoma. NP-59 scintigraphy has a long procedural time of nearly 2 weeks with an accuracy of 71% in contrast to adrenal venous sampling with an accuracy of 95–100%.

Androgenital Syndrome

Androgenital syndrome is a consequence of excessive secretion of sex hormones. It causes virilization, feminization, or precocious puberty depending upon the age and sex of the patient. The most common form is virilization, occurring in females.

The characteristic clinical features are amenorrhea, hirsutism, clitoromegaly, and deepening of voice.

The adrenal causes of androgen excess include congenital adrenal hyperplasia (CAH) in children and virilizing tumors (adenoma or carcinoma) in adults. CAH occurs due to deficiency of enzymes involved in the synthesis of steroid hormones. Each different enzyme deficiency results in a different form of CAH. The clinical manifestations are determined by the degree of deficiency of cortisol or aldosterone and by the biological properties of the biochemical intermediates that are formed and secreted in excess.

Androgen-producing tumors are rare and include adenoma or carcinoma and occur in both males and females at a later age. In general, in adults a higher proportion of malignant tumors results in adrenogenital syndrome than benign lesions.

MRI is preferred to CT to image adrenals as well as ovaries particularly in children to detect tumors because of MRI being nonionizing. CT is, however, often the initial and only modality performed in evaluation of suspected CAH, due to the easy availability and short examination times **(Figs. 10 and 11)**.[25]

The tumors are usually more than 2.0 cm in size and show imaging characteristics described above **(Figs. 12A and B)**. Occasionally, adrenal and gonadal venous sampling may be necessary to locate the source of excessive androgens.

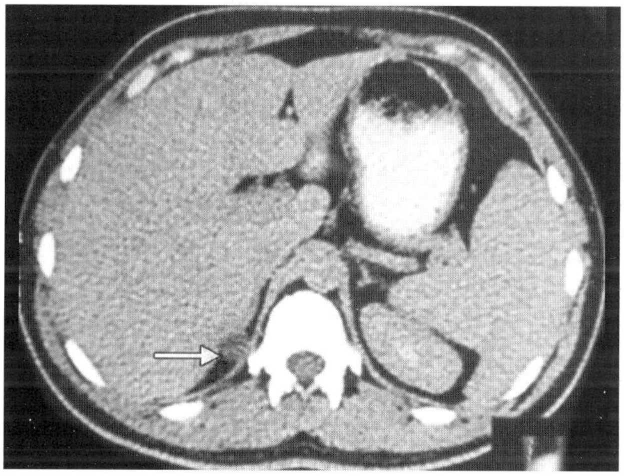

FIG. 9: Noncontrast CT of a 28-year-old male with hypertension shows a low attenuating nodule in the right adrenal (arrow) with attenuation value of 4 HU. Conn's syndrome due to adrenal adenoma.

Pheochromocytoma

Pheochromocytomas are catecholamine-producing tumors which arise from ganglion cells anywhere in the autonomic nervous system. About 90% of pheochromocytomas originate in the adrenal medulla while 10% are extra-adrenal, the common sites being paravertebral sympathetic ganglia, organ of Zuckerkandl, urinary bladder, neck, or mediastinum. About 10% of pheochromocytomas are bilateral and 10% are malignant. About 5–10% are inherited as autosomal dominant either alone or in combination with other abnormalities such as multiple endocrine neoplasia (Type II or III), neurofibromatosis, von Hippel-Lindau's retinal, and cerebellar hemangioblastomas.

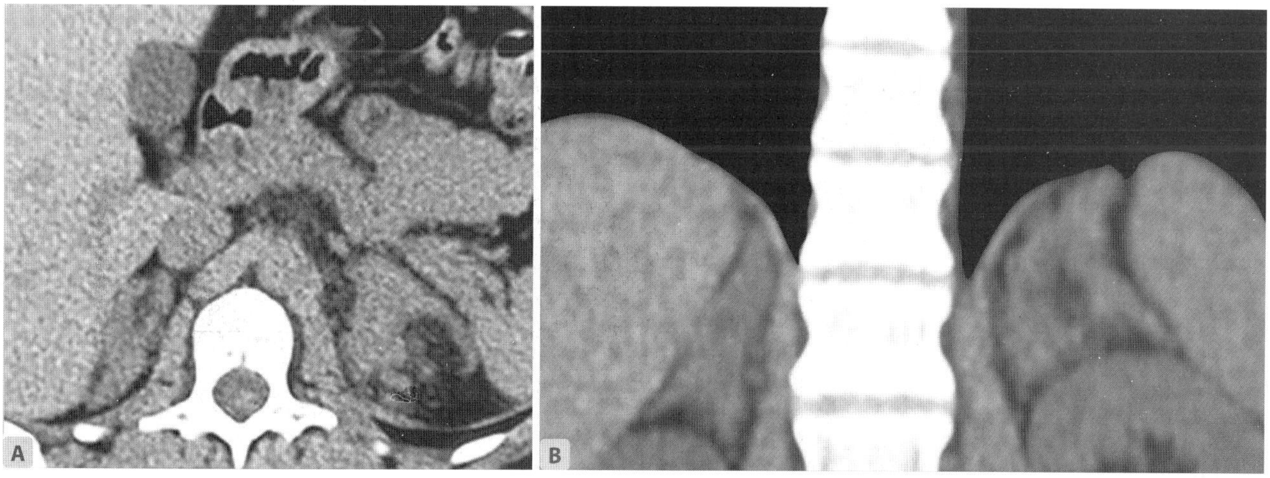

FIGS. 10A AND B: (A) Axial and (B) coronal noncontrast CT scans of a 13-year-old girl with features of virilization show bilateral nodular adrenal hyperplasia.

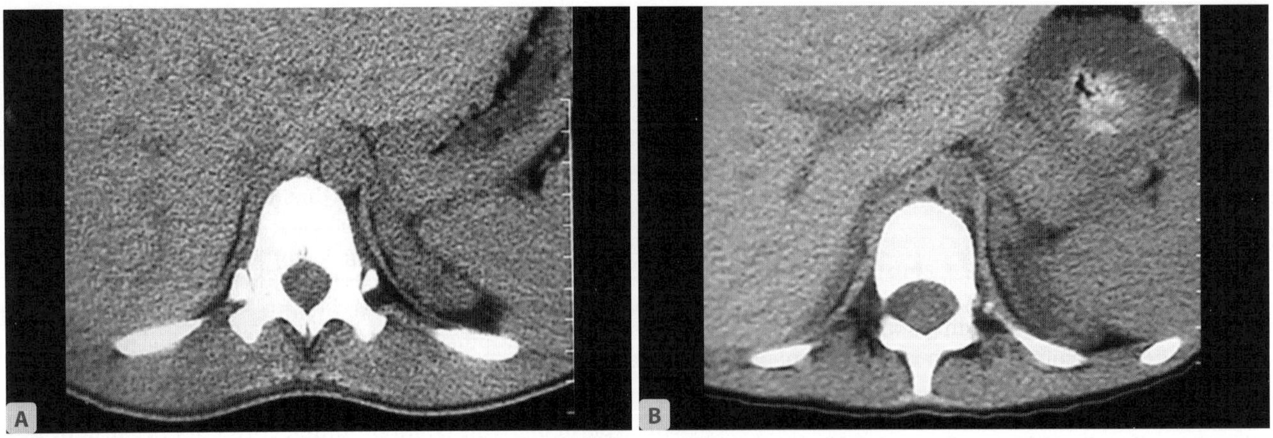

FIGS. 11A AND B: Axial noncontrast CT of an 11-year-old brother of the patient shown in Figure 10, presenting with precocious puberty (A), and 5-year-old sister with virilization (B) also show features of congenital adrenal hyperplasia.

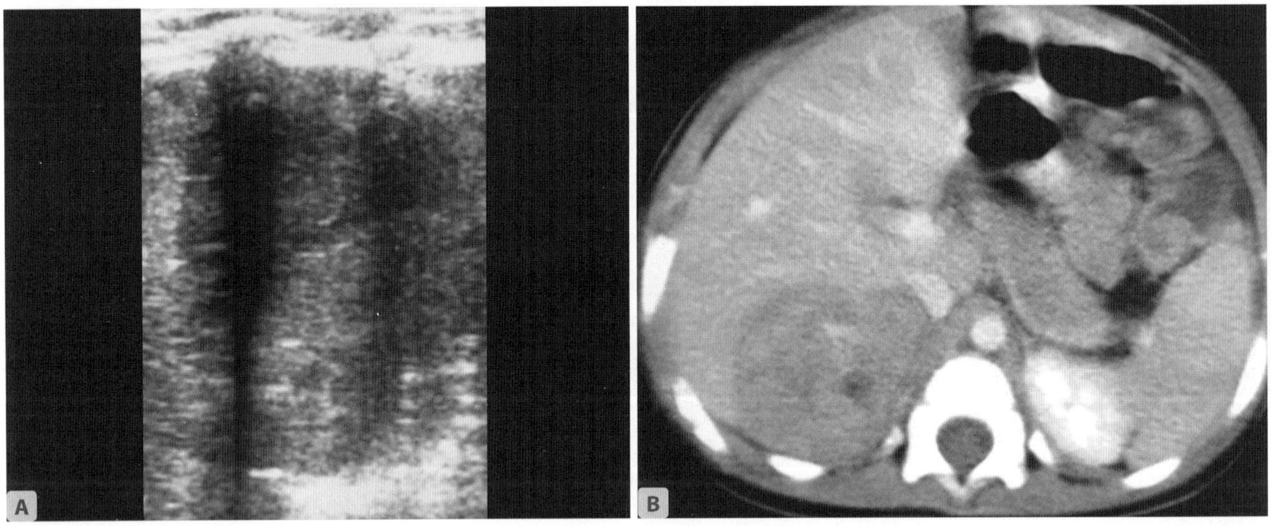

FIGS. 12A AND B: (A) Ultrasound and (B) axial contrast-enhanced CT of a 1.5-year-old girl child with features of virilization show a large heterogeneous mass arising from the right adrenal, suggesting a carcinoma.

Clinical features of hypertension, paroxysmal attacks of palpitations, headache, sweating, and biochemical tests of plasma catecholamine levels and 24-hour urine vanillylmandelic acid level can provide the diagnosis. Imaging is required to locate the tumor. CT is the technique of choice to confirm adrenal mass. It is seen as soft-tissue density mass with intense contrast enhancement on CECT **(Figs. 13A to C)**. Typically on MRI, it is isointense or hypointense on T1WI and extremely hyperintense on T2WI. Although this finding is almost universally seen with pheochromocytomas, a percentage of adrenal metastases has overlapping findings.[26] In addition, a significant number of lesions may not show this typical T2 hyperintensity. Gadolinium-DTPA (diethylenetriamine penta-acetic acid) produces marked enhancement with slower washout of contrast as compared to adenoma **(Figs. 14A to D)**.

Pheochromocytomas show insignificant signal drop on out-of-phase GRE images. It may show variable necrosis but calcification in pheochromocytoma is unusual **(Figs. 15A to D)**. The initial imaging findings in benign and malignant pheochromocytomas are nearly identical. Only the presence of metastases can clearly define a pheochromocytoma as malignant. CT and MRI can detect adrenal pheochromocytoma equally well. However, MRI is better for detecting extra-adrenal pheochromocytoma and recurrence after surgery.

On sonography, pheochromocytoma is seen as well-defined hypoechoic mass, which may show areas of necrosis or hemorrhage. The accuracy of USG in detecting pheochromocytoma is less than CT and MRI, particularly if the tumor is small and extra-adrenal.

In patients with strongly suspected pheochromocytoma, but no adrenal mass identified on CT or MRI, MIBG scintigraphy is the technique of choice to detect ectopic location and is also indicated for metastatic or locally recurrent disease. It is seen as focal area of abnormal activity. The sensitivity of MIBG scintigraphy for detecting pheochromocytoma is 80–90% with a specificity of 90–100%,

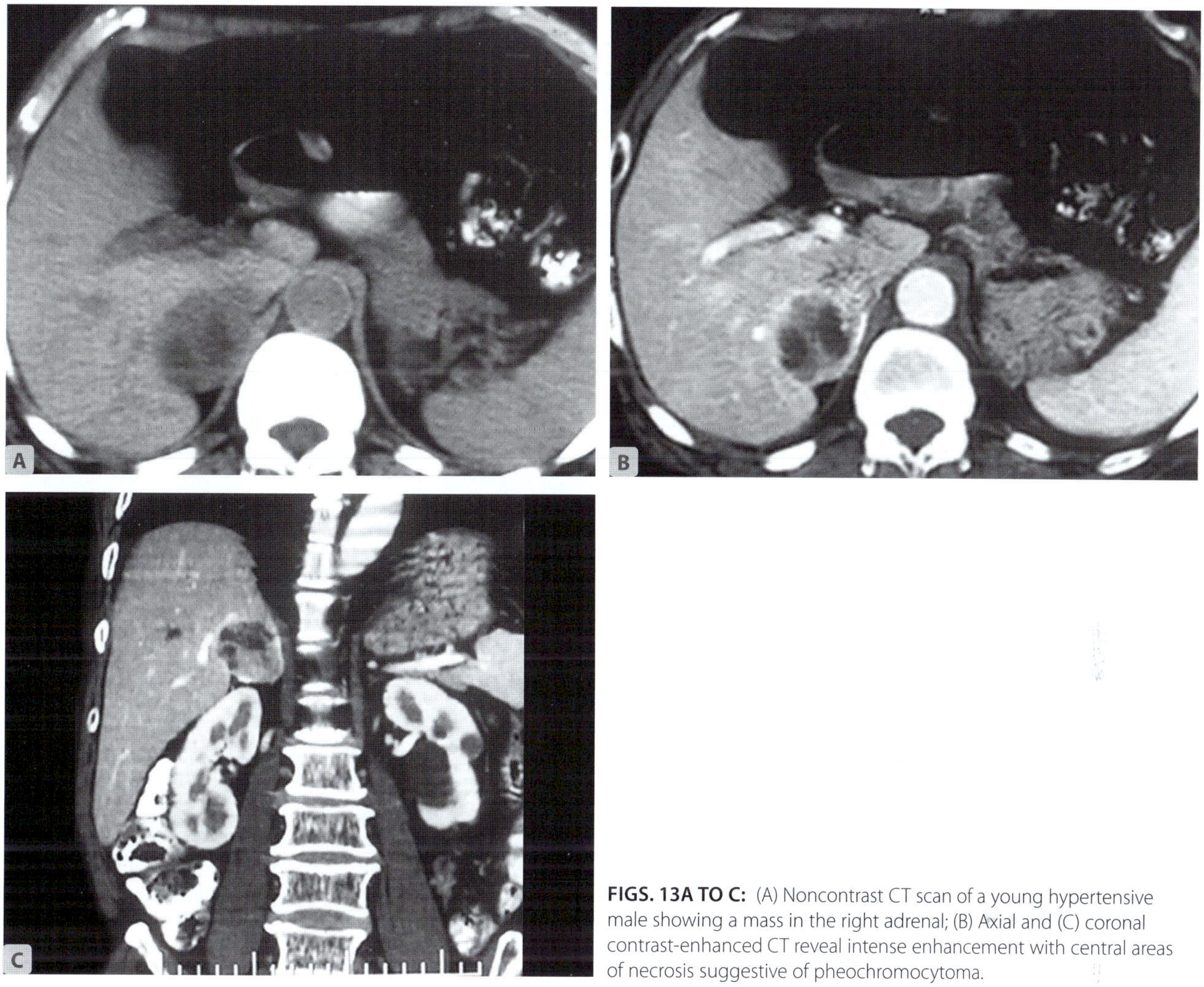

FIGS. 13A TO C: (A) Noncontrast CT scan of a young hypertensive male showing a mass in the right adrenal; (B) Axial and (C) coronal contrast-enhanced CT reveal intense enhancement with central areas of necrosis suggestive of pheochromocytoma.

but a positive MIBG scintigraphy should always be correlated with CT or MRI.

Group II: Adrenal Insufficiency

Adrenal hypofunction refers to disorders of the adrenal cortex. It is classified as primary or secondary. The primary form is due to destruction of the adrenal cortex while the secondary form results from pituitary causes. Usually 85–90% of the adrenal cortex must be destroyed before the clinical syndrome manifests. Primary adrenal insufficiency or Addison's disease presents with weakness, hypotension, weight loss with or without pigmentation.

The causes of Addison's disease include idiopathic atrophy, chronic granulomatous infections, e.g. tuberculosis, histoplasmosis, blastomycosis, and adrenal hemorrhage. Other causes include autoimmune diseases and drugs.

Of the chronic infections, tuberculosis accounts for more than 60% of patients in India. This is in contrast to the west where idiopathic adrenal insufficiency accounts for almost 90% of the patients. CT is an important imaging modality to define size and morphology.[27] In patients with idiopathic atrophy, the glands are often too small to be identified **(Fig. 16)**. The CT morphology in tuberculosis includes bilateral asymmetrical adrenal enlargement with or without calcification or necrosis, small gland with calcification involving one or both adrenals, or small gland with no calcification **(Figs. 17 to 19)**. There may be evidence of associated pulmonary tuberculosis. Follow-up studies in these patients on treatment have shown reduction in size of the adrenals and presence of calcification **(Figs. 17A and B)**.

In histoplasmosis, adrenals may show bilateral asymmetrical enlargement but often normal configuration and usually no calcification **(*see* Figs. 14A to D)**. Histoplasmosis in India is not as rare as reported in the Indian literature. Because of lack of awareness and investigative facilities, many of these patients are probably treated for tuberculosis.

Bilateral adrenal hemorrhage is usually associated with anticoagulant therapy or with stress caused by surgery, sepsis, or hypotension.

Less commonly, it is caused by trauma or hypoxia during delivery. CT may show asymmetrical adrenal enlargement with areas of high attenuation or blood-fluid level **(Fig. 20)**. Neonates, especially preterm infants, may also show bilateral adrenal hemorrhage **(Fig. 21)**. Follow-up studies after

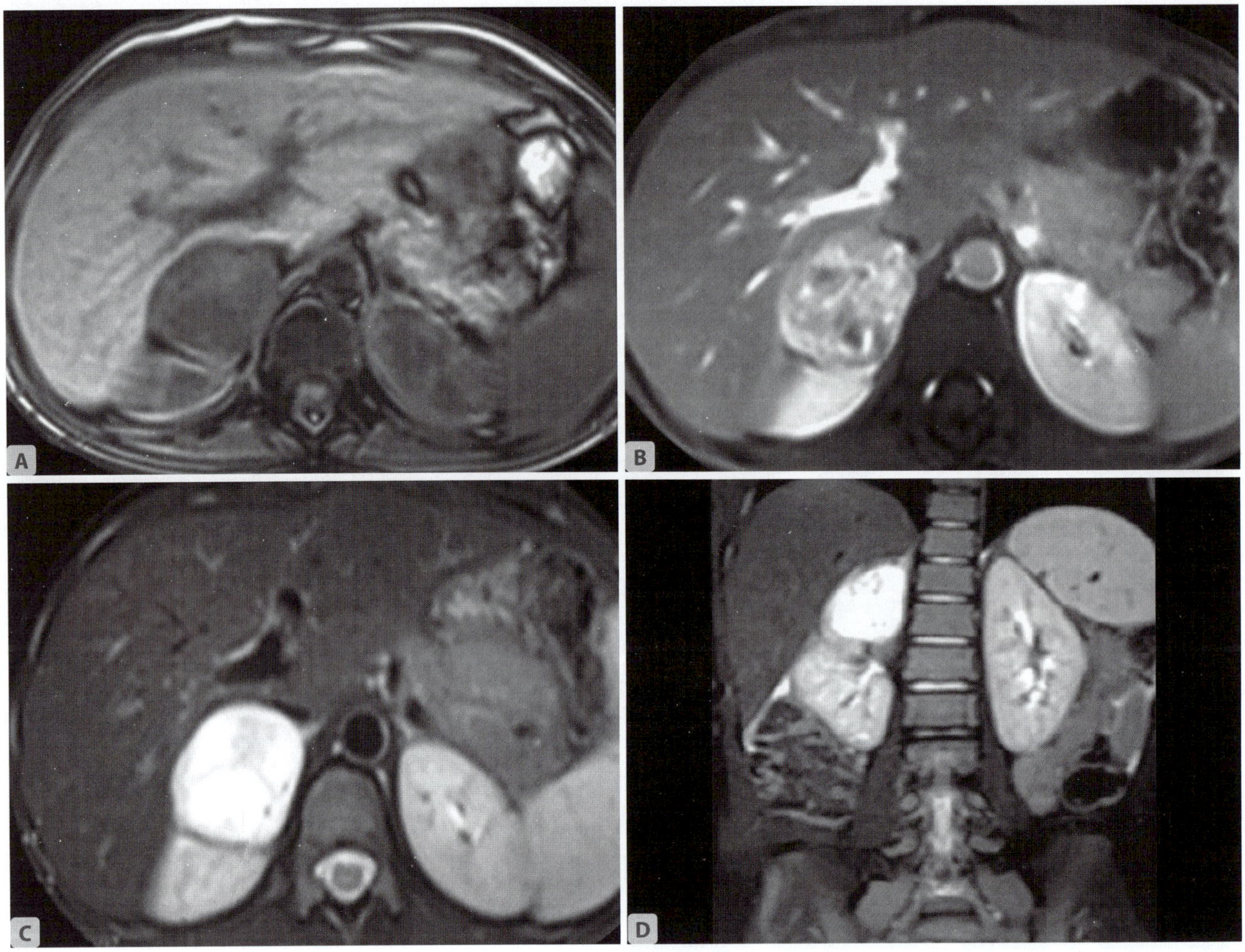

FIGS. 14A TO D: T1-weighted (A) pregadolinium and (B) postgadolinium axial images of a 15-year-old male with hypertension reveal an intensely enhancing right adrenal mass; T2-weighted (C) axial and (D) coronal images reveal the typical hyperintensity of a pheochromocytoma.

appropriate treatment show diminution in size and decrease in attenuation, thereby suggesting resorption **(Figs. 22A and B)**.

In the older child and adult, unilateral adrenal hemorrhage is usually caused by blunt abdominal trauma and often involves the right adrenal gland. Unilateral adrenal hemorrhage has also been recently reported in patients undergoing liver transplantation. The excision of a segment of the recipient's IVC necessitates ligation and division of the right adrenal vein. This may result in venous infarction and hemorrhage in the right adrenal gland. CT features are similar to those seen in bilateral hemorrhage.

Group III: Adrenal Diseases with Normal Function

A number of diseases may involve the adrenals, which do not alter the adrenal function. Most of these disease entities are detected incidentally as adrenal mass or patients may present with vague abdominal pain or discomfort. These include nonfunctional adenoma or carcinoma, metastasis, lymphoma, neuroblastoma, adrenal cyst, and myelolipoma. In some of these entities, a specific diagnosis can be made from the characteristic features on CT, e.g. adrenal cyst, myelolipoma. In some, CT may show nonspecific features but correlation with clinical features may suggest the possible etiology, e.g. neuroblastoma, metastasis.

Incidentaloma

These are adrenal nodules or masses discovered during imaging done for indications other than adrenal disease **(Figs. 23 to 26)**. They are seen in 4–7% of the imaged population, and majority of them are benign in the nononcology population.[1,28] On the other hand, almost 50% of incidentally detected adrenal lesions in patients with known malignancy represent metastatic disease.[5] Characterization of such incidental masses remains an important clinical problem when a unilateral nonfunctional adrenal mass is present; the differential diagnosis rests between adenoma and carcinoma or metastasis. In a patient with known malignancy, it is very essential to differentiate such incidental adrenal mass as adenoma or metastasis because this will greatly affect the patient's management and prognosis.

Adenoma versus Metastasis

Adenomas are thought to represent non-neoplastic overgrowth of adrenocortical cells of zona fasciculata. They

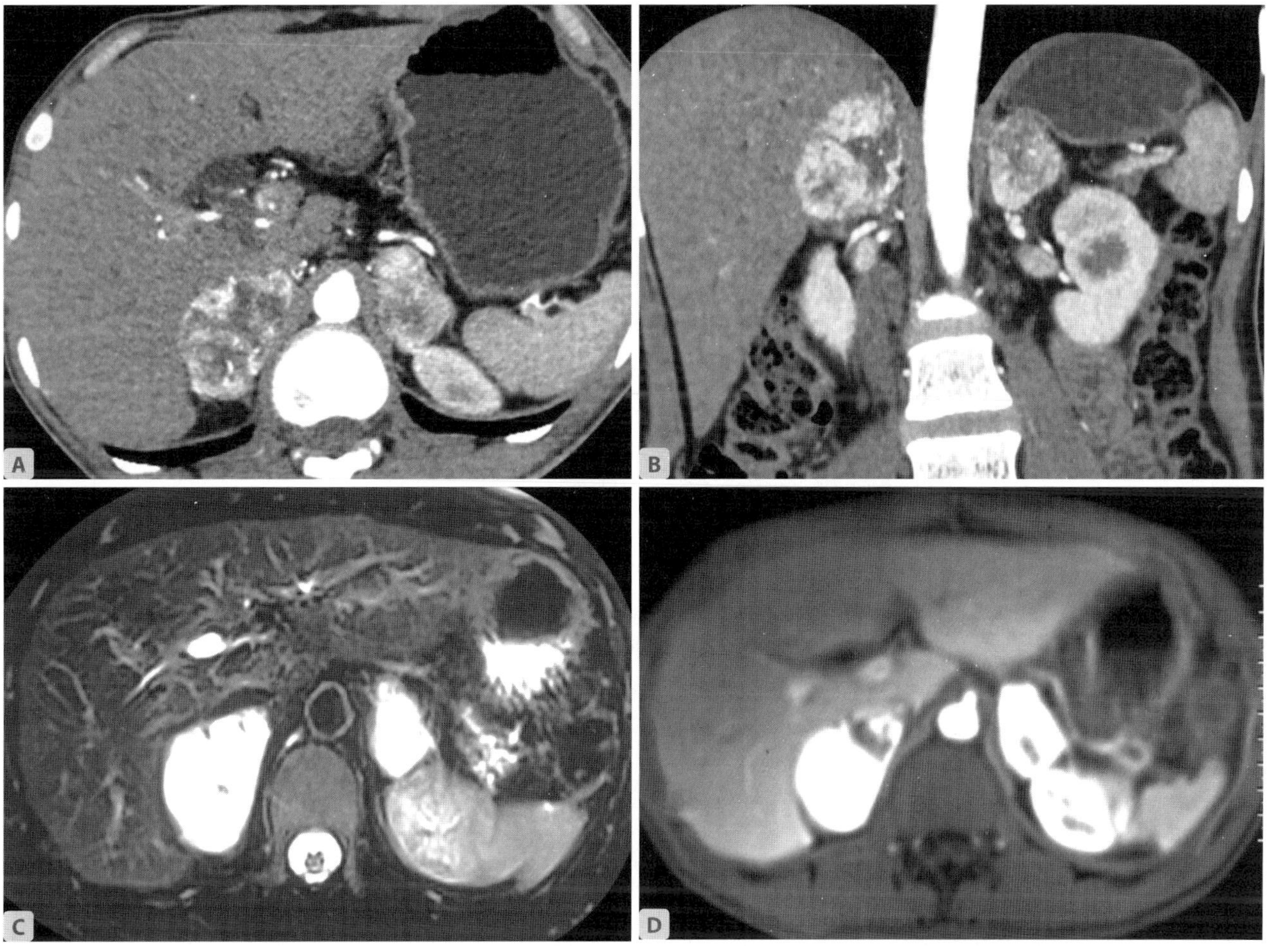

FIGS. 15A TO D: Bilateral pheochromocytoma. (A and B) Bilateral adrenal masses showing intense enhancement and variable necrosis on contrast-enhanced CT; (C and D) Bilateral hyperintense adrenal lesions on T2W image with intense postcontrast enhancement.

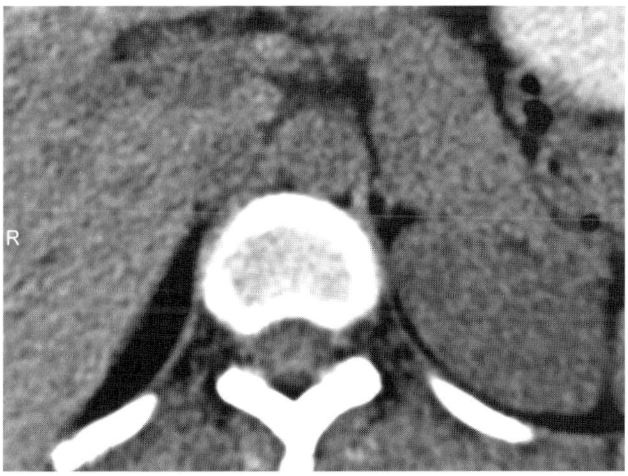

FIG. 16: Noncontrast CT scan of patient with Addison's disease showing bilateral atrophic adrenal glands.

consist of cholesterol-laden clear cells and contribute little to steroid production. The imaging features of functional and nonfunctional adenomas on CT or MRI are similar **(Figs. 23 to 26)** except that the functional tumors are usually smaller at the time of presentation than the nonfunctional ones. They account for almost 90% of all incidentalomas.[5]

Tumors of the lung, kidney, breast, digestive tract, ovary, and melanoma are the most common primary sites to metastasize to adrenals. Metastases are well-defined with heterogeneous density and a thin, irregular enhancing rim following intravenous contrast injection, commonly unilateral and usually larger than adenoma **(Figs. 27A to D)**. On MRI, they are hypointense on T1WI and hyperintense on T2WI, relative to liver intensity.

It has been reported that 27% of patients with known malignancy have microscopic adrenal metastasis. However, the detection of an adrenal mass in a patient with known malignancy does not necessarily indicate metastatic disease and it may be a nonfunctional adenoma.

CT features of adenoma include size less than 5.0 cm and well-defined margins with smooth contour **(Figs. 23 and 24)**.

Adrenal metastasis may show large mass with heterogeneous density and irregular shape **(Figs. 27A to D)**. However, these features are not specific. It has also been reported that the size alone is a poor discriminator between benign adenoma and malignant mass.

In recent years, several studies have reported two imaging criteria based on the attenuation value and differences in

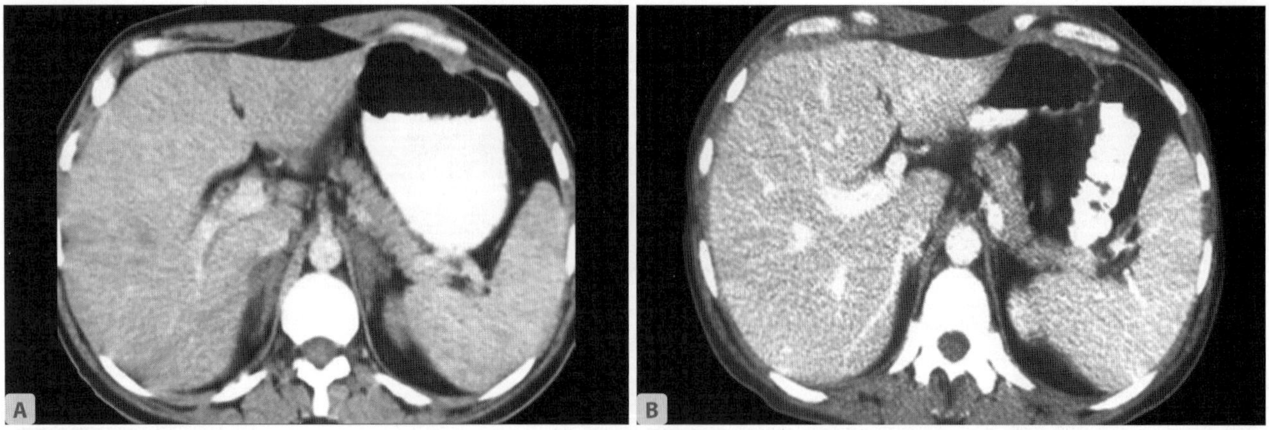

FIGS. 17A AND B: (A) Contrast-enhanced CT scan of a patient with fever and biochemical evidence of adrenal insufficiency shows bilateral asymmetric (left > right) enlargement of the adrenal glands. Few ill-defined focal areas are seen in the liver and spleen, also suggesting disseminated tuberculosis. Patient was put on anti-tubercular treatment; (B) Contrast-enhanced CT scan obtained 1 year later reveals small, atrophic adrenal glands.

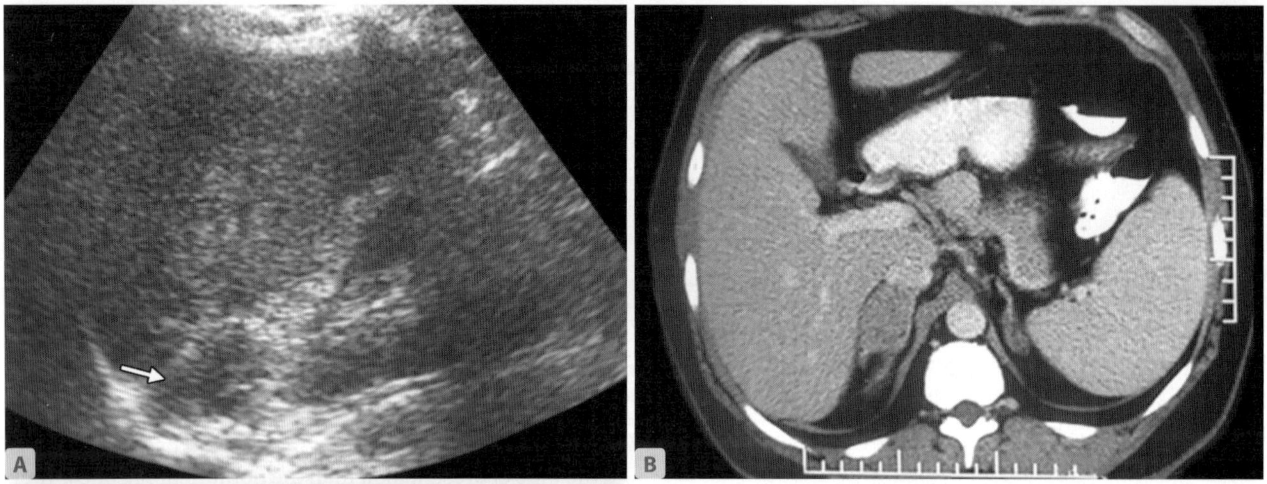

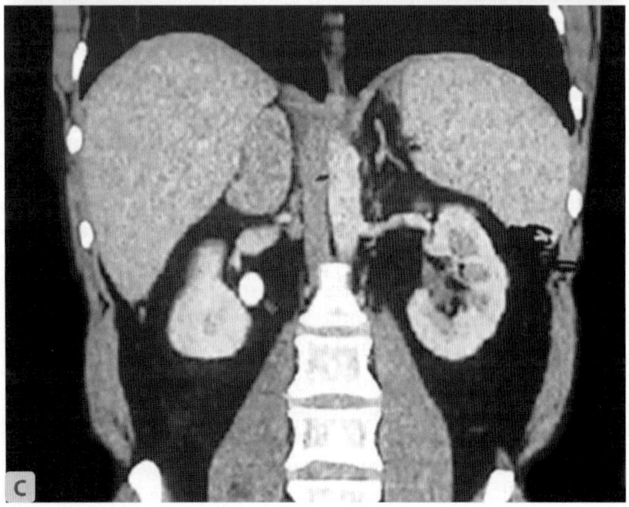

FIGS. 18A TO C: (A) Ultrasound, (B) axial contrast-enhanced CT, and (C) coronal multiplanar reconstruction images reveal an enlarged, heterogeneous right adrenal gland. Biopsy: Tuberculosis.

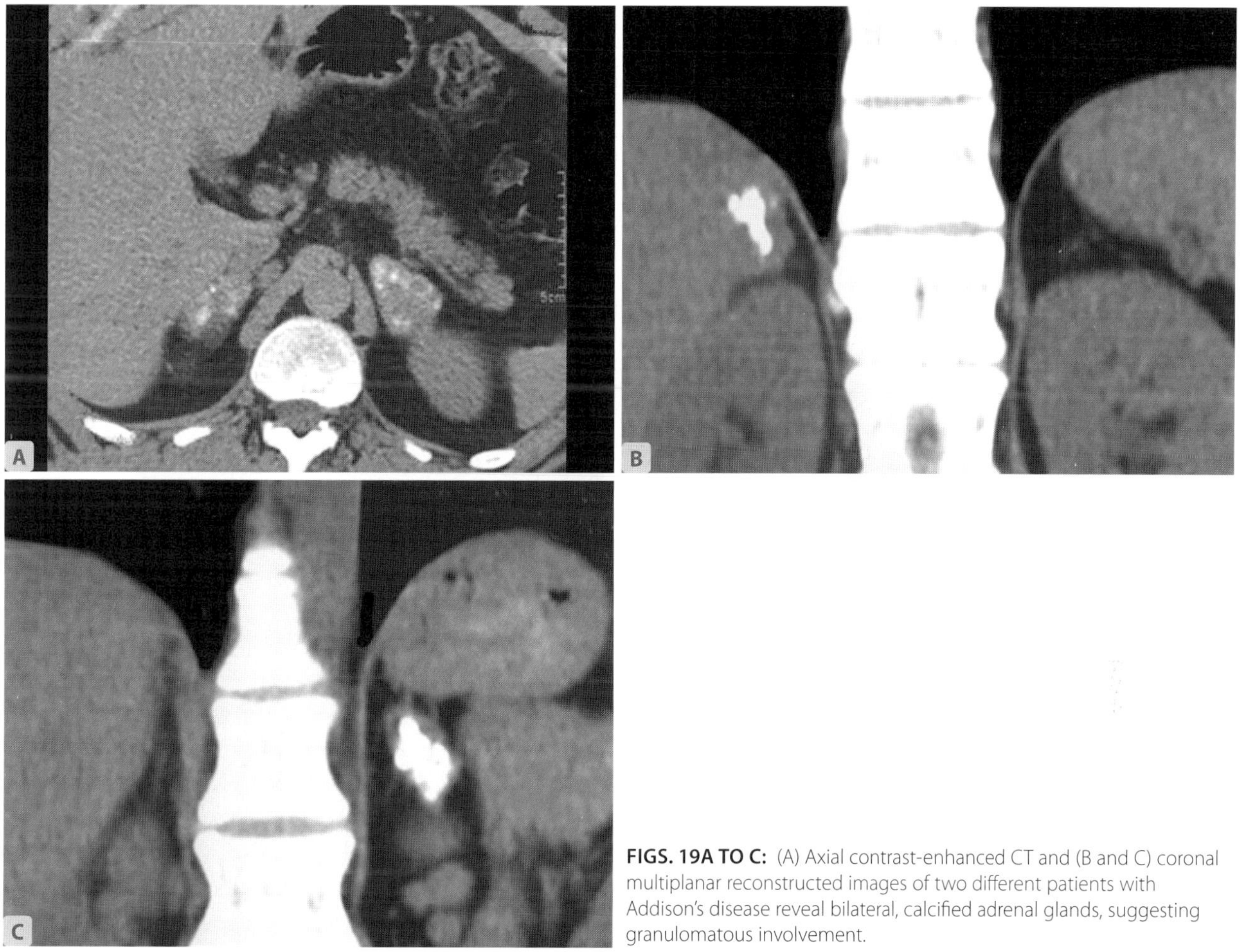

FIGS. 19A TO C: (A) Axial contrast-enhanced CT and (B and C) coronal multiplanar reconstructed images of two different patients with Addison's disease reveal bilateral, calcified adrenal glands, suggesting granulomatous involvement.

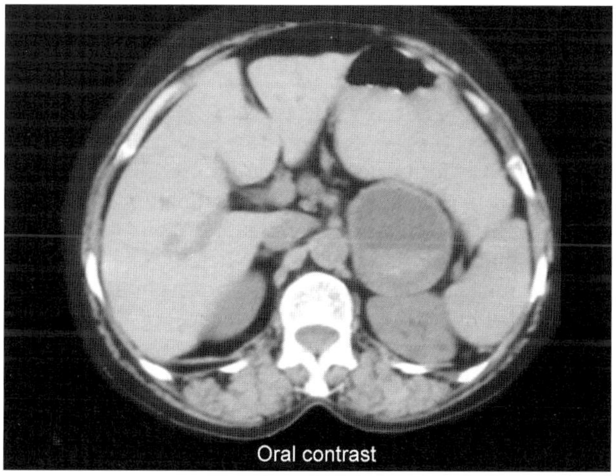

FIG. 20: Axial CT scan showing a low attenuating left adrenal mass with blood-fluid level, suggestive of adrenal hemorrhage.

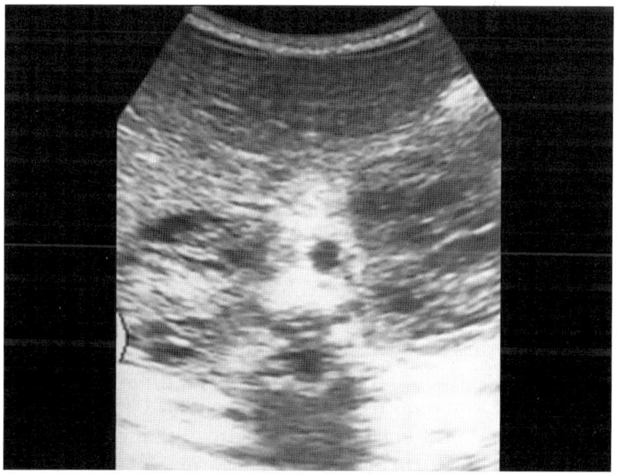

FIG. 21: Ultrasound of a preterm neonate showing bilateral enlarged adrenal glands, suggesting adrenal hemorrhage.

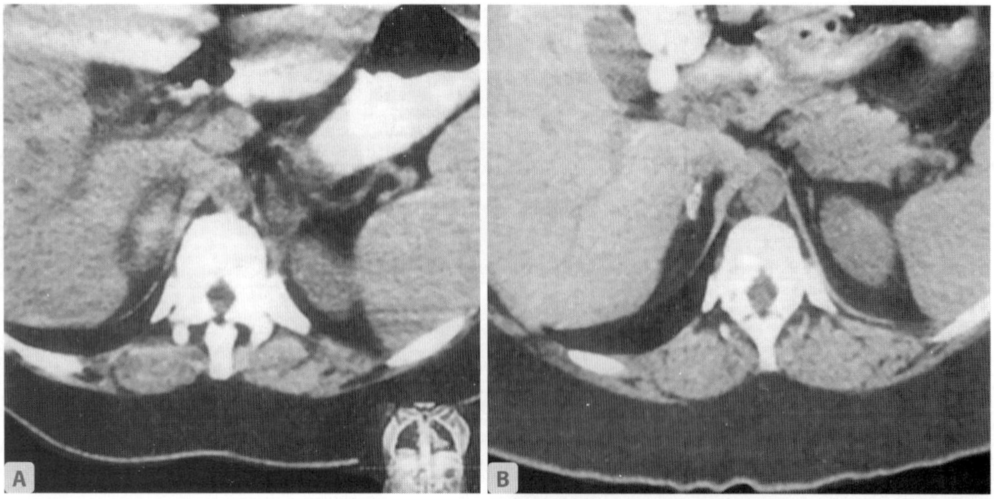

FIGS. 22A AND B: Adrenal hemorrhage. (A) CT scan shows asymmetrically enlarged adrenals with heterogeneous attenuation but no calcification; (B) Follow-up CT scan after 5 years shows small right adrenal with dense calcification and atrophic left adrenal.

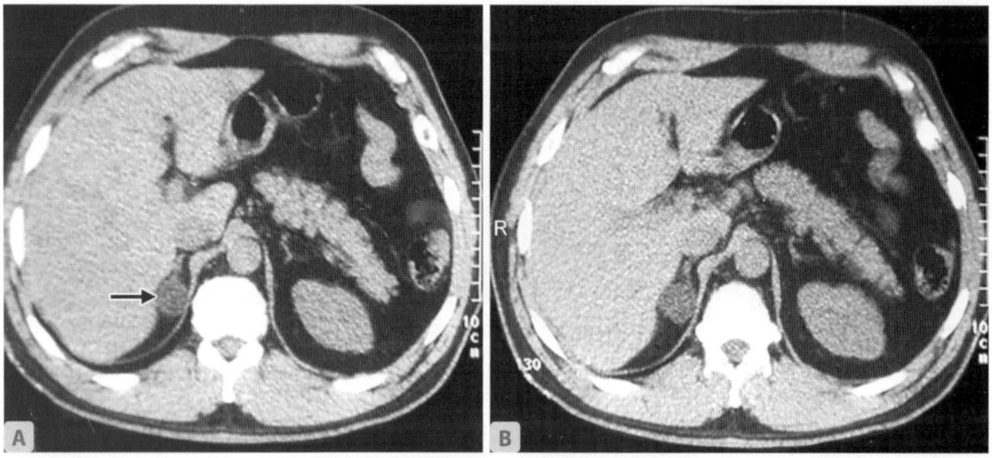

FIGS. 23A AND B: Adrenal adenoma. Noncontrast CT scan shows a low attenuating well-defined mass in the right adrenal (arrow). The attenuation value was 6 HU.

the vascular enhancement pattern to differentiate benign adenoma from adrenal metastasis.[5,28]

Adenomas have abundant intracytoplasmic fat and therefore show low attenuation on NCCT **(Figs. 23A and B)**. On the other hand, metastases have little intracytoplasmic fat and thus do not show low attenuation. A large region of interest covering the adrenal mass should be used but should not include periadrenal fat for measuring the attenuation value. It has been reported that a threshold of 10 HU has 71% sensitivity and 98% specificity for characterizing adenoma versus metastasis.[29] This specificity may be increased further if other features of size, shape, and morphology are considered. Although 70% of adenomas have abundant lipid, the remaining are lipid poor and are difficult to characterize on a noncontrast scan.

If attenuation of the adrenal mass on noncontrast CT is 10 HU or less **(Figs. 9 and 23)**, the diagnosis is lipid-rich adenoma and no further evaluation is required. If attenuation is more than 10 HU, the mass is indeterminate and requires further evaluation by portal venous phase and 15-minute delayed enhanced CT scan **(Figs. 24A to C)**.[30]

Adenomas enhance rapidly with intravenous contrast media and show rapid washout. Metastasis also enhances rapidly but the washout is delayed when compared to adenoma.[26,28] It has been speculated that this difference in enhancement washout in nonadenoma is possibly due to disturbed capillary permeability, with prolonged retention of contrast in the extracellular space.

Adrenal masses with an attenuation value less than 30–40 HU on 15-minute delayed CECT are almost always adrenal adenomas.[4,31] In addition to the delayed CT attenuation itself, it is also possible to calculate the percentage washout of initial enhancement. The patient is first scanned without contrast, then again at 70 seconds, and then 15

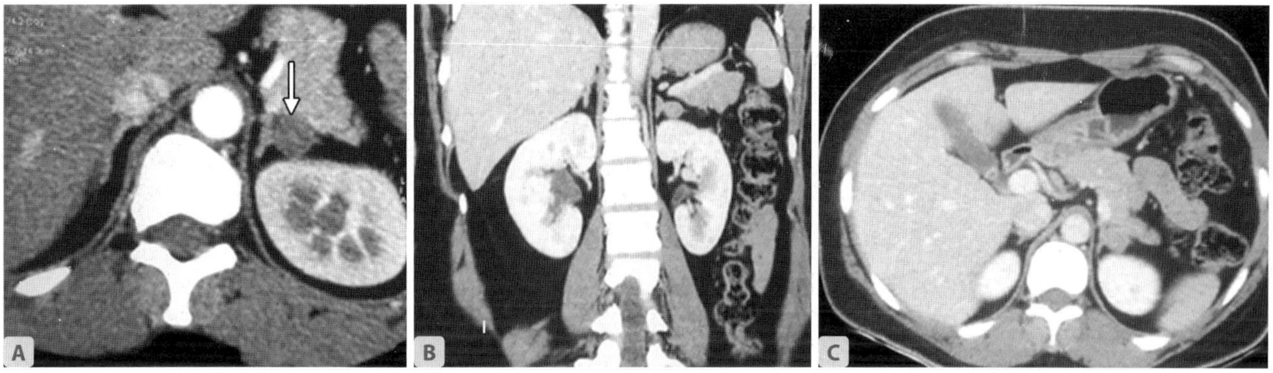

FIGS. 24A TO C: Adrenal adenoma. (A) Contrast-enhanced CT, (B) coronal multiplanar reconstruction, and (C) 15-minute delayed CT images show a mass in the left adrenal gland (arrow) which showed 65% washout on the delayed scan.

minutes after contrast administration. Contrast washout can be quantified using relative percentage washout (RPW) and absolute percentage washout (APW) as follows:

$$RPW = 100 \times (\text{Enhanced HU} - \text{Delayed HU}) / \text{Enhanced HU}$$

$$APW = 100 \times (\text{Enhanced HU} - \text{Delayed HU}) / \text{Enhanced HU} - \text{Nonenhanced HU}$$

If the APW is greater than 60% and the RPW is greater than 40%, the lesion is labeled benign.[28,30,31] This technique has a sensitivity of 88% and a specificity of 96% for the diagnosis of adenoma.[4,28] On the other hand, metastases and adrenocortical carcinoma have relative contrast retention on delayed CECT.

Dual-energy CT

The difference in CT attenuation images acquired at 140 kVp and 80 kVp is measured, and if the difference between the two kVp is more than 6 HU, it is suggestive of fat-containing lesion.[5] The cutoff values on NCCT and adrenal protocol scans are based on conventional 120 kVp scans. The values derived from VNC CT from a dual-energy scanner may not be equal to values derived from conventional scans. It has been found that the values can vary from 5 HU to 9 HU, which can be a significant confounder when the cutoff is applied.[6] However, the VNC values are usually higher than the true NCCT values which make the sensitivity lower but maintains the specificity. Hence, the traditional NCCT cutoff value of <10 HU is still valid on VNC as well irrespective of the dual-energy acquisition method (single or dual source).[8-10] It has also been found that the portal venous scan is the best phase to derive VNC for this purpose.

Magnetic Resonance Imaging

In recent years, MRI has become a problem-solving modality for the characterization of indeterminate adrenal masses. When results on CT examination are equivocal, MRI is the next imaging modality for characterizing the lesion. Due to increased fluid content in adrenal cancer and metastases, these appear bright on T2-weighted MRI images. However, there is significant overlap between T1W and T2W MRI images of adenoma and metastases. With the introduction of higher field strength magnets (3T), chemical shift imaging and dynamic gadolinium-enhanced MR imaging have shown promising results with adrenal gland lesions' characterization. Confident diagnosis of adenomas on MRI requires the addition of chemical shift imaging to the protocol.

Chemical shift MRI has been used to differentiate adenoma from metastasis. This technique is based on the different resonance frequency rates of protons in fat and water molecules in a magnetic field. The signal intensity (SI) on the in-phase image is derived from the signal of water plus fat protons while in the out-of-phase image; MR signal of water and lipid protons cancel each other out within a voxel. Therefore, a mass containing intracellular lipid and water will show loss of signal in the out-of-phase images when compared with the in-phase image **(Figs. 25A to C)**. Thus, adenoma appears darker on an out-of-phase image than on an in-phase image, while metastasis will show no significant signal loss on an out-of-phase image and the signal intensity remains unchanged.[16,17]

The sensitivity and specificity ranging from 81% to 100% and 94% to 100%, respectively, on chemical shift MR imaging for differentiating adenoma from metastasis have been reported.[17,28] The loss of signal can be assessed visually using spleen as the internal control **(Figs. 26A and B)**. The liver should not be used as the internal reference as it may also show signal loss on opposed-phase image when there is steatosis.

The chemical shift change can also be detected by quantitative methods. Two ratios have been defined in chemical shift imaging (CSI).

$$\text{SI index} = \frac{1 - [\text{SI(in)} - \text{SI(opp)}]}{\text{SI(in)}}\text{; and}$$

Adrenal-to-spleen ratio

$$= \frac{\text{SI adrenal (opp)}}{\text{SI spleen (opp)}} \Big/ \frac{\text{SI adrenal (in)}}{\text{SI spleen (in)}}$$

An SI index of >16.5% and an adrenal-to-spleen ratio of <0.71 are suggestive of adenoma or benign adrenal lesions. For a benign adrenal lesion characterization, the reported sensitivity and specificity using these two ratios were 87–100% and 92–100%, respectively, whereas the failure rate for diagnosis of lipid-poor adenomas has been 13–17%.[28]

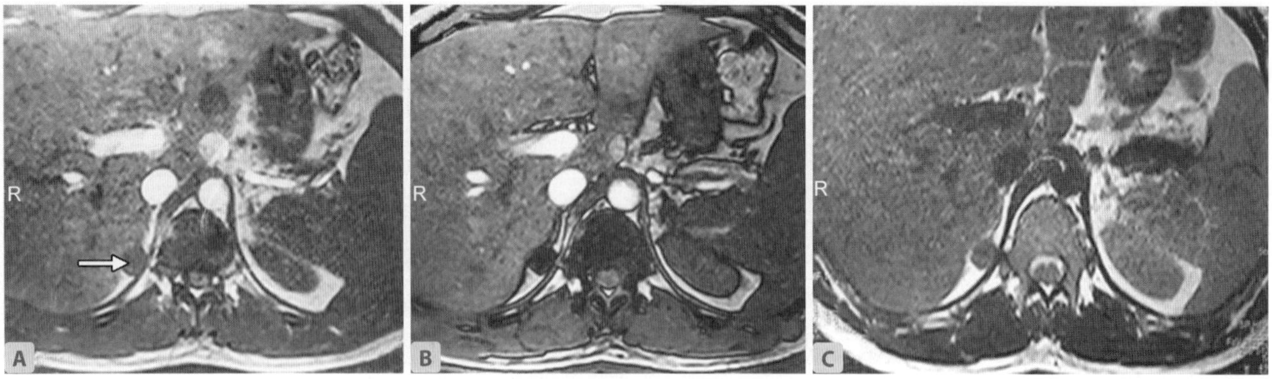

FIGS. 25A TO C: Incidentally detected adrenal adenoma. Gradient-echo T1W in-phase image (A) shows a hypointense nodule in right adrenal gland (arrow) which shows marked signal loss on the opposed-phase image (B). The lesion is hypointense on T2W scan (C) also.

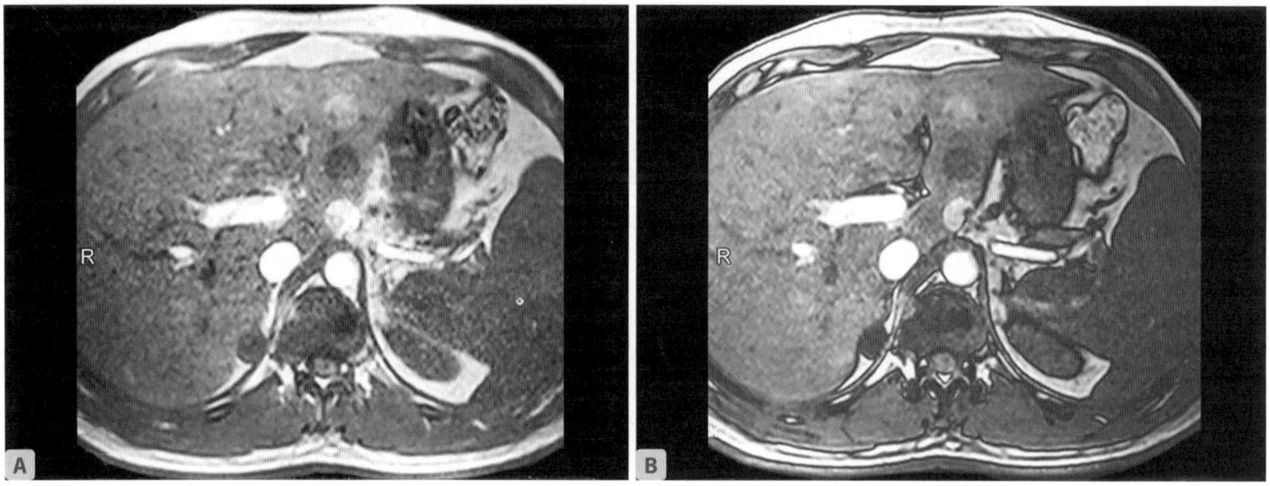

FIGS. 26A AND B: Adrenal adenoma. Gradient-echo T1W in-phase (A) and opposed-phase (B) images showing drop in the signal intensity of right adrenal lesion from 124 to 45 whereas spleen signal intensity changes from 83 to 80 only.

Positron Emission Tomography

Due to the limitations of CT and MR imaging, functional imaging modalities such as ^{18}F-FDG PET are now increasingly used for further characterization of an adrenal lesion. ^{18}F-FDG PET is an imaging modality that permits acquisition of functional information and when fused with CT imaging, it results in accurate localization and metabolic characterization of adrenal lesions. In PET-CT, ^{18}F is used as a glucose analog, which is taken up preferentially by malignant cells because of their increased glucose metabolism. Due to relative lack of glucose-6-phosphatase in the cancer cells as compared to cells of normal tissues, there is a focal intracellular accumulation of FDG, resulting in high tumor uptake values as compared to the background uptake values. The results of all these studies are encouraging and justify the use of PET for metastatic disease evaluation in cancer patients. Although PET results are encouraging, several inherent problems are associated with FDG-PET imaging, viz. small adrenal lesions are difficult to image owing to poor resolution, and uptake in other abdominal structures, such as renal pelvis, can obscure the adrenal gland.

^{18}F-FDG uptake is taken as abnormal when it is higher than background liver uptake.[21,32,33] If a lesion shows ^{18}F-FDG uptake less than that of the liver, or shows uptake that is significantly higher than the liver, the study can be interpreted with high confidence unless the patient has pheochromocytoma, which can be excluded by biochemical markers.[21]

In the evaluation of adrenal masses with ^{18}F-FDG PET/CT, combined information from the ^{18}F-FDG PET and unenhanced CT portions of a PET or CT study is more specific than ^{18}F-FDG PET information alone.[34] A standardized uptake value (SUV) cutoff of 3.1 has been used to differentiate malignant lesions and adenomas. PET data using a SUV cutoff of 3.1 to differentiate malignant adrenal masses from adenomas yielded a sensitivity, specificity, positive predictive value, and negative predictive value of 98.5%, 92%, 89.3%, and 98.9%, respectively.[34]

The current role of FDG PET is in the evaluation of adrenal lesions in a patient with known history of malignancy which is either enlarging or more than 4 cm in size.[6]

Adrenal Carcinoma

Adrenal carcinomas are rare neoplasms and are more common in women. They are usually larger than 10 cm at the time of presentation and are invasive. Unlike children

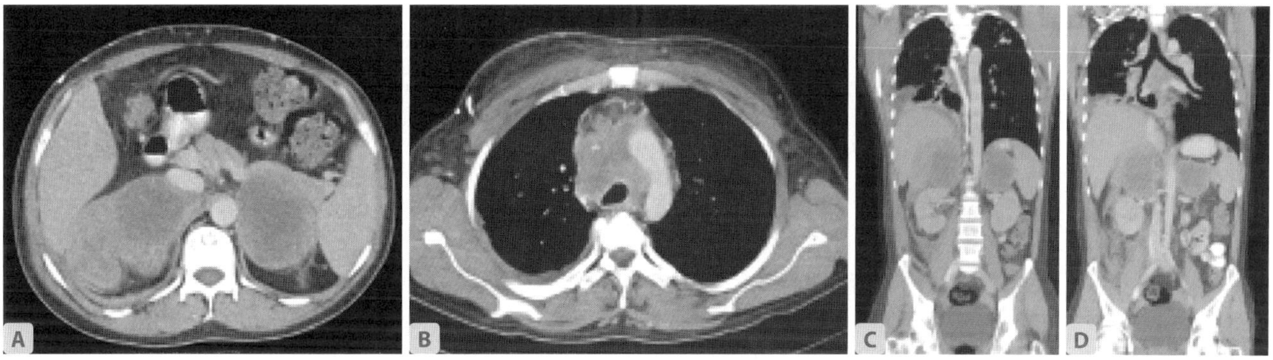

FIGS. 27A TO D: Adrenal metastases. (A and B) CECTs abdomen show bilateral solid adrenal masses; (C and D) CECT chest and coronal multiplanar reconstructed images show mediastinal adenopathy in a patient of bronchogenic carcinoma.

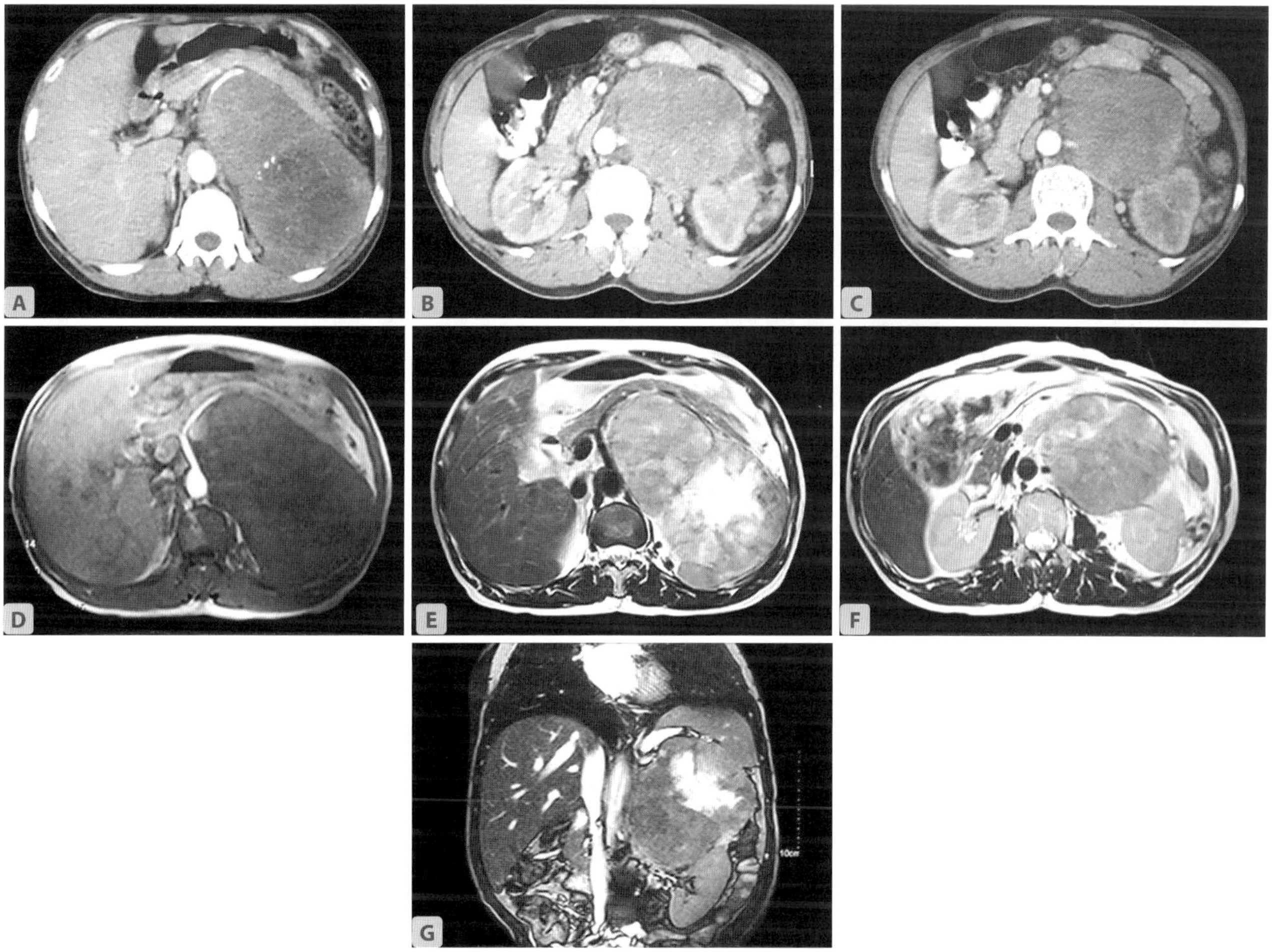

FIGS. 28A TO G: Adrenal carcinoma. Axial contrast-enhanced CT scans (A to C) show a large left adrenal mass with foci of calcification and areas of necrosis, encasing the left renal artery and displacing the left kidney laterally; (D) Axial T1W gradient-echo image shows a hypointense left-sided mass which is displacing the splenic artery anteriorly. The lesion is heterogeneously hyperintense on T2W scans (E and F); (G) True-FISP coronal image shows the left suprarenal mass displacing the left kidney inferolaterally.

where adrenal carcinomas are usually functional, only 10% of adult types are clinically functional which usually manifest as Cushing's syndrome or virilization in females. CT or MRI shows large solid masses with areas of degeneration and cystic changes, hemorrhage, and 33% contain calcification **(Figs. 28 and 29)**.[5,28] They tend to be locally invasive, especially into adrenal or renal veins and inferior vena cava. They are hypointense on T1-weighted and hyperintense on T2-weighted scans **(Figs. 28D to F)** and show variable enhancement. Differential diagnosis includes adenoma, metastases, lymphoma, exophytic liver tumors, or upper polar renal masses.

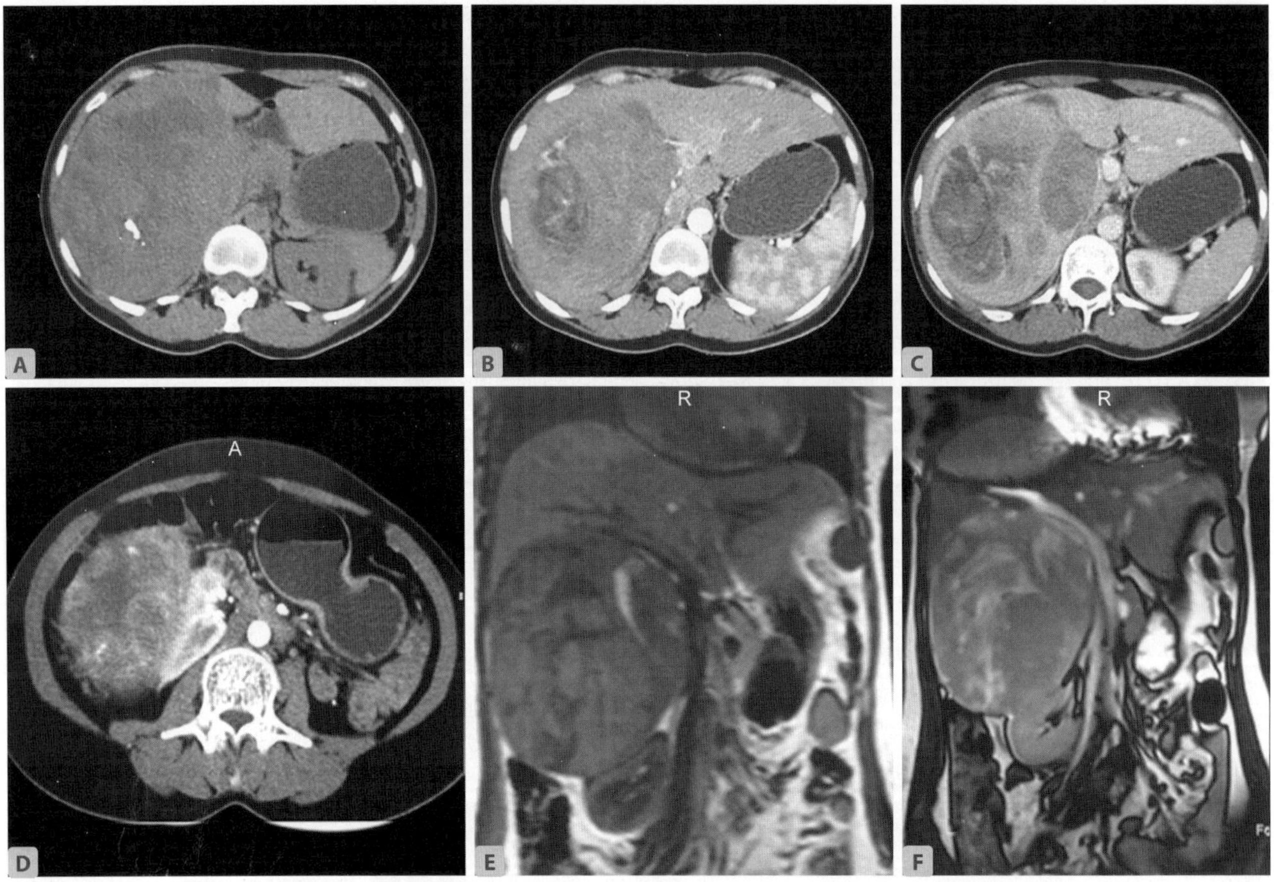

FIGS. 29A TO F: Adrenal carcinoma. Axial noncontrast CT scan (A) and contrast-enhanced CT scan (B to D) show a large right adrenal mass with foci of calcification. It mimics an exophytic liver mass. Gradient-echo T1W (E) and True FISP coronal (F) MR images of the same patient show the right adrenal mass displacing the kidney inferomedially.

Adrenal Lymphoma

Primary lymphoma of the adrenal gland is unusual, but its involvement in disseminated lymphoma is common. The latter is more often seen in non-Hodgkin's lymphoma.[35] The most common presentation is diffuse bilateral enlargement of the gland, and the shape is usually maintained **(Figs. 30A to D)**. The tumor is hypovascular and shows only mild enhancement after contrast.

Adrenal Collision Tumor

This is a very rare entity characterized by the coexistence of two contiguous but histologically different tumors. Both tumors may be malignant or one may be benign and the other malignant or both may be benign. Imaging may show two distinct morphological features within the same mass. This entity should be suspected when only a focal decrease in the signal intensity of a mass is seen on opposed-phase images or a focus of bright enhancement is seen within a mass which otherwise looks like an adenoma. Such an appearance may suggest a metastatic deposit within an adrenal adenoma.[36]

Adrenal Cyst

Adrenal cysts are rare and usually seen in females. They are derived from endothelium in 45% of patients and the rest are epithelial, parasitic, or pseudocysts from prior hemorrhage. CT shows a characteristically well-defined, round, low-attenuating lesion suggesting fluid with rim enhancement **(Fig. 31A)**. Rim calcification may be noted **(Fig. 31B)**. The attenuation values may be mixed in the presence of debris or hemorrhage. On MR, adrenal cysts are hypointense on T1W and hyperintense on T2W image. The complications of adrenal cysts include hemorrhage, infection, and rupture.[28,37]

Myelolipoma

Myelolipoma is a benign tumor of the cortex, comprised of mature fat and hematopoietic elements. Patients are usually asymptomatic and the lesion is detected incidentally. It accounts for about 7–15% of all incidentalomas. The imaging appearance may vary depending on which the histological component is dominant. USG and CT features are quite characteristic and diagnostic.

Ultrasonography shows well-defined echogenic or heterogeneous adrenal mass, which may be associated with apparent posterior displacement of the diaphragm due to propagation speed artifact resulting from slow speed of sound through the fat. CT confirms the presence of intratumoral fat **(Figs. 32A and B)**. Punctate calcification may be seen in 20% of cases. MRI can also characterize the lesion by identification of fat which appears hyperintense on both T1W and T2W

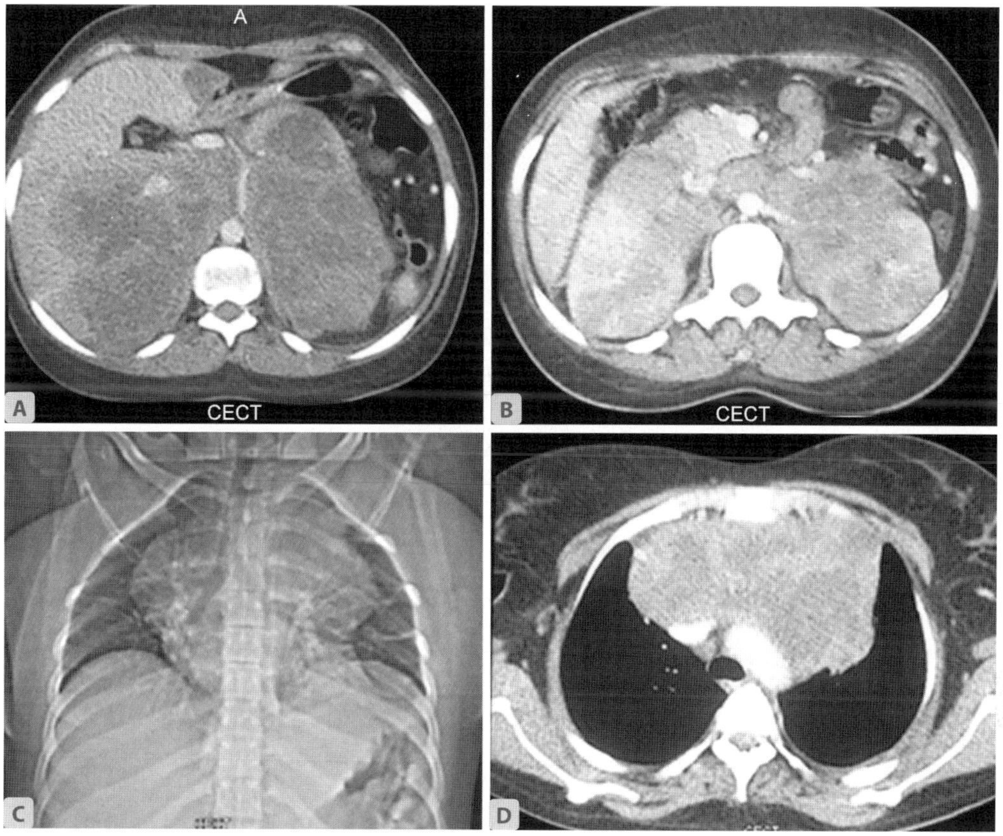

FIGS. 30A TO D: Adrenal involvement in non-Hodgkin's lymphoma. (A and B) Axial abdomen contrast-enhanced CT (CECT) scans show bilateral adrenal masses, retroperitoneal adenopathy, and focal renal lesions; (C) Chest radiograph and (D) CECT chest show bulky mediastinal adenopathy.

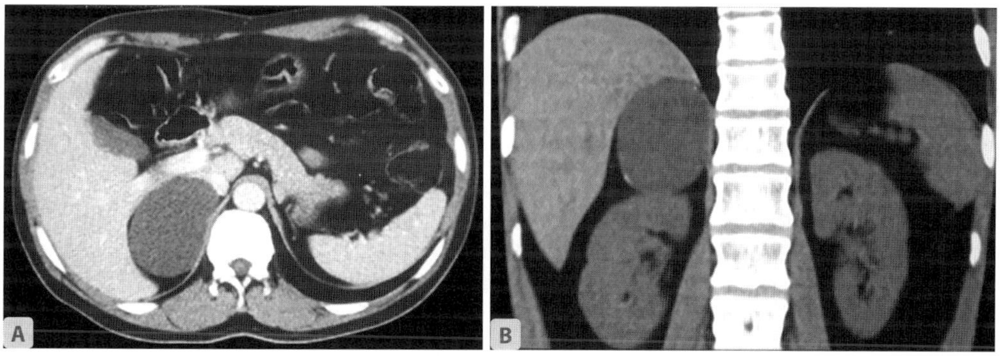

FIGS. 31A AND B: Adrenal cyst. (A) Axial CT and (B) coronal multiplanar reconstruction images show a fluid attenuating right adrenal mass with rim calcification.

images and shows loss of signal on fat suppression techniques **(Figs. 33A to D)**. Marrow elements show low signal on T1W and moderate signal on T2W images. Differential diagnosis includes adrenal adenoma and adrenal carcinoma, and large myelolipomas may mimic retroperitoneal lipoma or liposarcoma.

Neuroblastoma

Neuroblastoma is one of the most common tumors of childhood with 80% occurring below the age of 5 years. Most neuroblastomas arise from adrenal medulla but may also arise from sympathetic chain, posterior mediastinum being the second-most common site. About 75% occur in the abdomen, and two-thirds of these are in the adrenal gland. Symptoms are related to the primary tumor and metastases, which are present in more than 50% of patients at the time of diagnosis. Children can present with a palpable mass, bone pain, and opsomyoclonus. The common sites of metastases are lymph nodes, cortical bone, marrow, skin, and liver.

Ultrasonography almost always shows a mass, which must be distinguished from nephroblastoma. Neuroblastoma is seen typically as large mass with heterogeneous echogenicity with scattered hyperechoic areas due to the

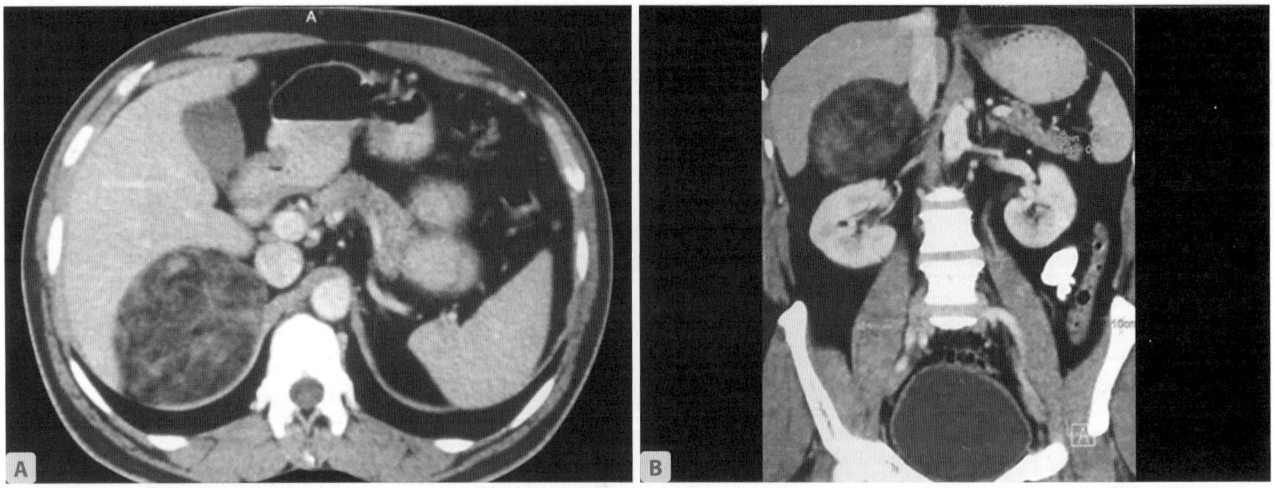

FIGS. 32A AND B: Adrenal myelolipoma. (A) Axial contrast-enhanced CT and (B) coronal multiplanar reconstruction images show a mixed attenuating right adrenal mass with fat and soft-tissue attenuation.

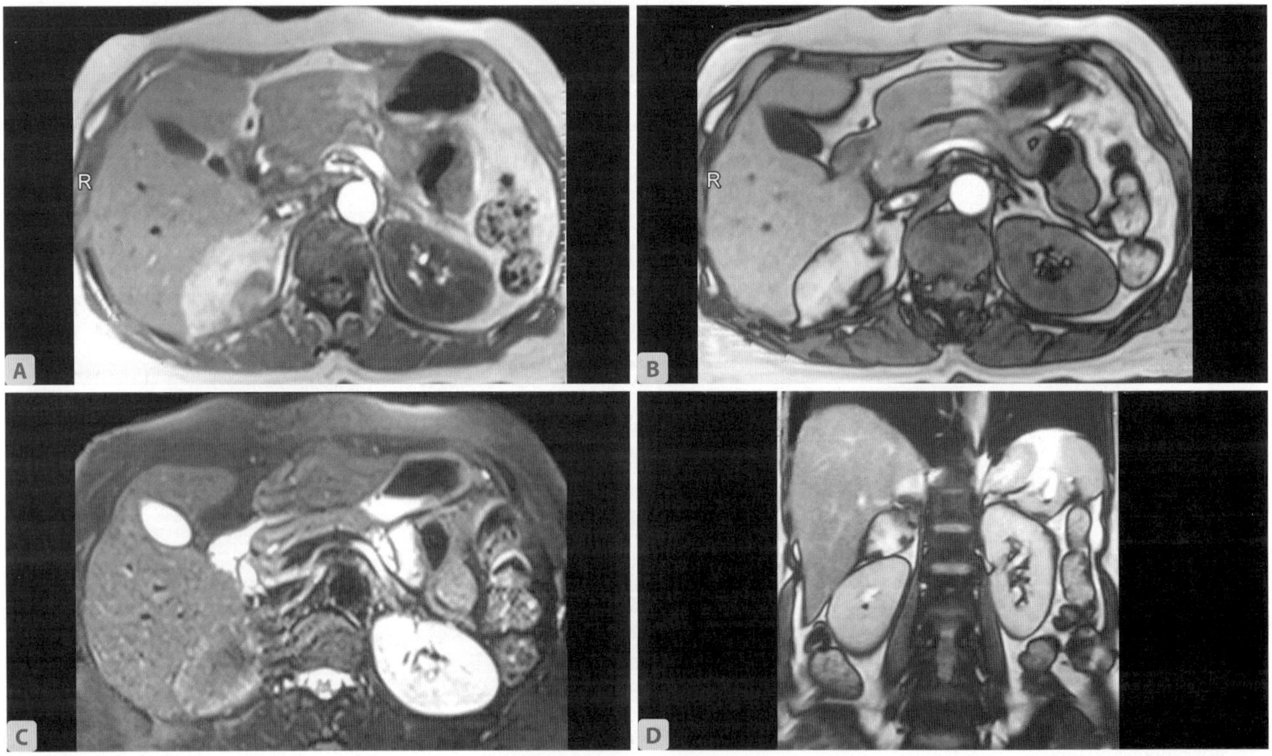

FIGS. 33A TO D: Adrenal myelolipoma. Gradient-echo T1W in-phase (A) and opposed-phase (B) images show a hyperintense right adrenal mass which shows no drop in signal intensity but is suppressed on T2W fat-suppressed image (C). Coronal true-FISP image (D) shows a hyperintense right adrenal mass.

presence of calcification. CT shows soft tissue mass with areas of low attenuation and scattered coarse or mottled calcification, seen in almost 85% of the patients. The tumor enhances with intravenous contrast. Unlike Wilm's tumor, which usually has a well-defined pseudocapsule, neuroblastoma invades adjacent structures and encases the aorta and its branches **(Fig. 34)** early in the course of the disease.

On MRI, neuroblastoma shows low signal intensity on a T1WI and increased intensity on a T2WI, relative to liver intensity. Tumor heterogeneity is seen best on T2-weighted sequence and reflects calcification and necrosis.

MRI is better than CT for defining vascular encasement, metastasis, and intraspinal extension, which occurs in 15% of patients. Therefore, MRI is the single best imaging modality for accurately staging the extent of the disease. Neuroblastoma may also take up MIBG, which may detect bony metastasis more accurately than CT or MRI. The presence of skeletal metastasis in association with an adrenal mass in a child strongly suggests the diagnosis of neuroblastoma.

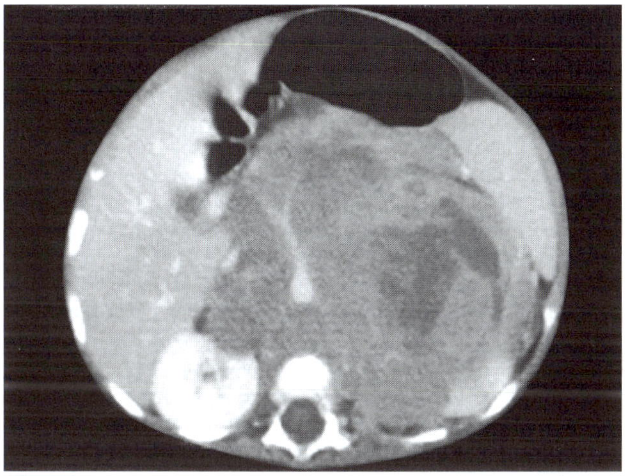

FIG. 34: Neuroblastoma. Axial contrast-enhanced CT abdomen of a 2-year-old child shows a large left adrenal mass which is extending posterior to the aorta and inferior vena cava and encasing the celiac axis.

CONCLUSION

With the widespread use of cross-sectional imaging techniques, detection of an adrenal mass has increased over the years. However, clinical and appropriate biochemical tests in adrenal lesions, especially for functional diseases, remain the most vital and initial mode of evaluation, followed by CT. The role of CT has continued to expand in both detection and characterization of an adrenal mass as benign or malignant. Based on size criteria and tumor morphology, it is not always possible to suggest benignity or malignancy. Follow-up studies are necessary in equivocal cases. Necrosis in the tumor is related directly to prognosis. More necrosis carries a worse prognosis. All attempts should be made to characterize an incidental adrenal mass as adenoma or metastasis in a patient with known malignancy. Lipid-rich adenoma can be characterized with attenuation value of 10 HU or less on NCCT. Lipid-poor adenoma can be differentiated from metastasis by studying the washout percentage on an adrenal protocol CT. Chemical shift MRI can be utilized as an alternative modality. If all these modalities still fail to characterize the lesion in a patient with known malignancy, having no other evidence of metastatic deposit, FDG PET or adrenal biopsy under CT guidance should be performed to establish a definitive diagnosis.

REFERENCES

1. Young WF. The incidentally discovered adrenal mass. N Engl J Med. 2007;356(6):601-10.
2. Schieda N, Siegelman ES. Update on CT and MRI of adrenal nodules. Am J Roentgenol. 2017;208(6):1206-17.
3. Funder JW, Carey RM, Mantero F, et al. The management of primary aldosteronism: Case detection, diagnosis, and treatment: An Endocrine Society Clinical Practice Guideline. J Clin Endocrinol Metab. 2016;101(5):1889-916.
4. Korobkin M. CT characterization of adrenal masses: The time has come. Radiology. 2000;217(3):629-32.
5. Blake MA, Holalkere N-S, Boland GW. Imaging techniques for adrenal lesion characterization. Radiol Clin North Am. 2008;46(1):65-78.
6. Glazer DI, Mayo-Smith WW. Management of incidental adrenal masses: an update. Abdom Radiol (NY); 2019. https://doi.org/10.1007/s00261-019-02149-2.
7. Azoury SC, Nagarajan N, Young A, et al. Computed tomography in the management of adrenal tumors: does size still matter? J Comput Assist Tomogr. 2017;41(4):628-32.
8. Ho LM, Marin D, Neville AM, et al. Characterization of adrenal nodules with dual-energy CT: can virtual unenhanced attenuation values replace true unenhanced attenuation values? Am J Roentgenol. 2012;198(4):840-5.
9. Glazer DI, Maturen KE, Kaza RK, et al. Adrenal incidentaloma triage with single-source (fast-kilovoltage switch) dual-energy CT. Am J Roentgenol. 2014;203(2):329-35.
10. Morgan DE, Weber AC, Lockhart ME, et al. Differentiation of high lipid content from low lipid content adrenal lesions using single-source rapid kilovolt (peak)-switching dual-energy multidetector CT. J Comput Assist Tomogr. 2013;37(6): 937-43.
11. Mileto A, Nelson RC, Marin D, et al. Dual-energy multidetector CT for the characterization of incidental adrenal nodules: diagnostic performance of contrast-enhanced material density analysis. Radiology. 2015;274(2):445-54.
12. Elsayes KM, Emad-Eldin S, Morani AC, et al. Practical approach to adrenal imaging. Radiol Clin North Am. 2017;55(2):279-301.
13. Sydow BD, Rosen MA, Siegelman ES. Intracellular lipid within metastatic hepatocellular carcinoma of the adrenal gland: A potential diagnostic pitfall of chemical shift imaging of the adrenal gland. Am J Roentgenol. 2006;187(5):W550-551.
14. Schieda N, Krishna S, McInnes MDF, et al. Utility of MRI to differentiate clear cell renal cell carcinoma adrenal metastases from adrenal adenomas. Am J Roentgenol. 2017;209(3):W152-9.
15. Adam SZ, Nikolaidis P, Horowitz JM, et al. Chemical shift MR imaging of the adrenal gland: principles, pitfalls, and applications. Radiogr Rev Publ Radiol Soc N Am Inc. 2016;36(2):414-32.
16. Reinig JW, Stutley JE, Leonhardt CM, et al. Differentiation of adrenal masses with MR imaging: comparison of techniques. Radiology. 1994;192(1):41-6.
17. Lee MJ, Mayo-Smith WW, Hahn PF, et al. State-of-the-art MR imaging of the adrenal gland. Radiographics. 1994;14(5):1015-29.
18. Bilbey JH, McLoughlin RF, Kurkjian PS, et al. MR imaging of adrenal masses: value of chemical-shift imaging for distinguishing adenomas from other tumors. Am J Roentgenol. 1995;164(3):637-42.
19. Mayo-Smith WW, Song JH, Boland GL, et al. Management of incidental adrenal masses: a white paper of the ACR Incidental Findings Committee. J Am Coll Radiol. 2017;14(8):1038-44.
20. Shulkin BL, Thompson NW, Shapiro B, et al. Pheochromocytomas: imaging with 2-[Fluorine-18]fluoro-2-deoxy-d-glucose PET. Radiology. 1999;212(1):35-41.
21. Yun M, Kim W, Alnafisi N, et al. 18F-FDG PET in characterizing adrenal lesions detected on CT or MRI. J Nucl Med Off Publ Soc Nucl Med. 2001;42(12):1795-9.
22. Lumachi F, Zucchetta P, Marzola MC, et al. Usefulness of CT scan, MRI and radiocholesterol scintigraphy for adrenal imaging in Cushing's syndrome. Nucl Med Commun. 2002;23(5):469-73.
23. Rockall AG, Babar SA, Sohaib SAA, et al. CT and MR imaging of the adrenal glands in ACTH-independent Cushing syndrome. Radiogr Rev Publ Radiol Soc N Am Inc. 2004;24(2):435-52.

24. Doppman JL, Gill JR, Miller DL, et al. Distinction between hyperaldosteronism due to bilateral hyperplasia and unilateral aldosteronoma: reliability of CT. Radiology. 1992;184(3):677-82.
25. Harinarayana CV, Renu G, Ammini AC, et al. Computed tomography in untreated congenital adrenal hyperplasia. Pediatr Radiol. 1991;21(2):103-5.
26. Mayo-Smith WW, Boland GW, Noto RB, et al. State-of-the-art adrenal imaging. Radiogr Rev Publ Radiol Soc N Am Inc. 2001;21(4):995-1012.
27. Ammini AC, Gupta R, Mukopadhyay C, et al. Computed tomography morphology of the adrenal glands of patients with Addison's disease. Australas Radiol. 1996;40(1):38-42.
28. Boland GWL, Blake MA, Hahn PF, et al. Incidental adrenal lesions: principles, techniques, and algorithms for imaging characterization. Radiology. 2008;249(3):756-75.
29. Boland GW, Lee MJ, Gazelle GS, et al. Characterization of adrenal masses using unenhanced CT: an analysis of the CT literature. Am J Roentgenol. 1998;171(1):201-4.
30. Caoili EM, Korobkin M, Francis IR, et al. Adrenal masses: characterization with combined unenhanced and delayed enhanced CT. Radiology. 2002;222(3):629-33.
31. Korobkin M, Brodeur FJ, Yutzy GG, et al. Differentiation of adrenal adenomas from nonadenomas using CT attenuation values. Am J Roentgenol. 1996;166(3):531-6.
32. Blake MA, Slattery JMA, Kalra MK, et al. Adrenal lesions: characterization with fused PET/CT image in patients with proved or suspected malignancy--initial experience. Radiology. 2006;238(3):970-7.
33. Shin YR, Kim KA. Imaging features of various adrenal neoplastic lesions on radiologic and nuclear medicine imaging. Am J Roentgenol. 2015;205(3):554-63.
34. Metser U, Miller E, Lerman H, et al. 18F-FDG PET/CT in the evaluation of adrenal masses. J Nucl Med Off Publ Soc Nucl Med. 2006;47(1):32-7.
35. Paling MR, Williamson BR. Adrenal involvement in non-Hodgkin lymphoma. Am J Roentgenol. 1983;141(2):303-5.
36. Schwartz LH, Macari M, Huvos AG, et al. Collision tumors of the adrenal gland: Demonstration and characterization at MR imaging. Radiology. 1996;201(3):757-60.
37. Tung GA, Pfister RC, Papanicolaou N, et al. Adrenal cysts: imaging and percutaneous aspiration. Radiology. 1989;173(1):107-10.

CHAPTER

24

The Retroperitoneum

Smriti Hari, Sanjay Sharma, Ekta Dhamija, Ankur Goyal

INTRODUCTION

As the name suggests, retroperitoneum (RP) is the portion of abdomen lying posterior to peritoneal cavity, located between posterior peritoneum and transversalis fascia. It extends from diaphragm superiorly to pelvis inferiorly and is divided into compartments and spaces by various fascial layers. Basic understanding of its anatomy is essential for approaching and localizing abdominal masses or collections on imaging. Computed tomography (CT) remains the workhorse of imaging of RP due to its faster acquisition and patient compliance whereas magnetic resonance imaging (MRI) serves mainly as problem solving tool. Ultrasonography (USG) on the other hand has limited role due to posterior location of the structures which get obscured by bowel gas often; however, it is the preferred modality for interventions—biopsy or fluid drainage, wherever feasible. This chapter aims to describe brief anatomy and imaging features of common retroperitoneal diseases.

ANATOMY

The RP is divided into five main compartments and three spaces by multiple fascial layers.[1,2]

- *Compartments*: There are five major compartments dividing retroperitoneal structures: (A) Lateral compartment—one on each side containing kidneys and organs; (B) Median/central or vascular compartment containing aorta, inferior vena cava (IVC), associated lymphatics, and vessels. It is located in between two perirenal spaces, anterior to the vertebra, and posterior to anterior pararenal space; and (C) Posterior compartment on both sides having psoas and iliopsoas muscles extending from T12 to lesser trochanter. It continues in pelvis bordered along transversalis fascia.
- *Spaces*: RP is divided into three spaces—the RP is divided into three spaces: An anterior pararenal space that is continuous across the midline, a perirenal space on each side, and posterior pararenal space **(Fig. 1)**.
  - The *anterior pararenal space* contains the pancreas, the second, third, and fourth segments of the duodenum, the ascending and descending colon, lymph nodes, and fat. This space is bordered anteriorly by the posterior parietal peritoneum, posteriorly by the anterior renal fascia (Gerota's fascia) and laterally by the lateroconal fascia, which is a continuation of the posterior renal fascia (Zuckerkandl fascia).[3]
  - The *perirenal space* lies between the anterior and posterior renal fascia and contains the kidney, adrenal gland, renal pelvis, proximal ureter, renal hilar vessels, lymph nodes, and fat.[4] The fascia of Gerota's blends anteriorly with the connective tissue surrounding the aorta and IVC.
  - The *posterior pararenal space* extends from the posterior renal fascia to the transversalis fascia and contains only a small amount of fat. Although it is located posterior to the kidneys, it continues anterolaterally as the properitoneal fat stripe.
- *Planes*: The renal and lateroconal fasciae are laminated, potentially expansile planes composed of apposed layers of embryonic mesentery. The *retromesenteric plane* between the leaves of the anterior pararenal fascia, the *retrorenal plane* formed by splitting of posterior pararenal fascia, and the *lateroconal plane* between the leaves of the lateroconal fascia.

  Though most collections remain confined to the retroperitoneal compartment in which they originate; CT observations and cadaveric dissections suggest that rapidly accumulating collections can dissect and decompress through these retroperitoneal fascial planes.[5]
- *Fascia*: The anterior and posterior renal fasciae fuse inferior to the cone of renal fat, effectively sealing the caudal perinephric space, and preventing the inferior extension of perirenal fluid into the pelvis.[6] The communicating retromesenteric, retrorenal, and the lateroconal fascial planes continue downward into the true pelvis anterolateral to the psoas muscle.[7] Thus, the interfascial fluid unlike perinephric fluid can spread from the abdominal RP into the pelvis.[8] Superiorly, both layers of renal fascia blend with the diaphragmatic fascia to form the cephalic limit of the RP.

The normal anterior and posterior renal fascia measure 1–3 mm in thickness and are well-visualized on CT scan,

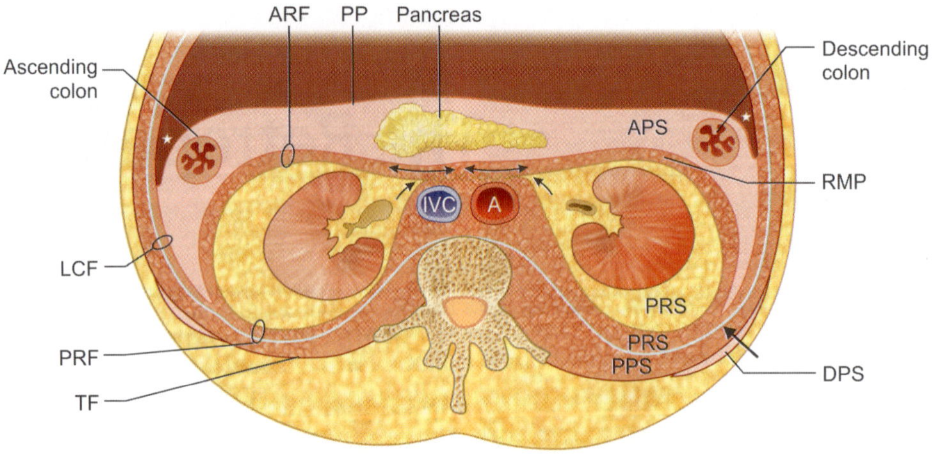

FIG. 1: Retroperitoneal and interfascial planes. Drawing at level of renal hila shows that perirenal and lateroconal fascia are laminated planes composed of apposed layers of embryonic mesentery. Note that thickness of interfascial planes is exaggerated to illustrate potentially expansile nature. Also note that perinephric spaces are closed medially (open arrows). Retromesenteric plane is continuous across midline (bidirectional arrows). Retromesenteric plane, retrorenal space, and lateroconal space communicate at fascial trifurcation (arrow). Dorsal pleural sinus may extend inferiorly to lie posterolateral to posterior pararenal space and transversalis fascia (A: aorta; APS: anterior pararenal space; ARF: anterior renal fascia; DPS: dorsal pleural sinus; IVC: inferior vena cava; LCF: lateroconal fascia; PP: parietal peritoneum; PPS: posterior pararenal space; PRF: posterior renal fascia; PRS: perinephric space; RMP: retromesenteric plane; RRS: retrorenal space; TF: transversalis fascia; *: posterior peritoneal recess).

except when abdominal fat is scanty. The posterior renal fascia is thicker and more frequently visualized than the anterior. Thickening of the retroperitoneal fascia is a sensitive but nonspecific indicator of adjacent disease, and is seen in both inflammatory **(Fig. 2)** and neoplastic disorders.

IMAGING MODALITIES

Multidetector CT is currently the preferred imaging modality for evaluating the RP. It accurately displays its anatomical limits and clearly defines individual spaces separated by various fascial layers. Isotropic multiplanar reconstructions (MPRs) of thin overlapping slices in the coronal and sagittal plane provide excellent delineation of the location and extent of retroperitoneal masses. It is a useful modality for making initial diagnosis of various pathological conditions and for follow-up. The introduction of multidetector technology has substantially improved the quality and ease of performing CT angiography. The simultaneous acquisition of multiple thin collimated slices in combination with enhanced gantry rotation speed offers thin slice coverage of extended volumes without any loss in spatial resolution. Multidetector computed tomography angiography (MDCTA) is increasingly being used for assessing diseases affecting the vasculature of the abdominal organs, for treatment planning, and post-therapy follow-up.[9] CT scanners with 16 or more detectors enable full abdominal coverage from the diaphragm to the groin with high spatial resolution. These scanners permit excellent evaluation of the whole arterial visceral vasculature (e.g. hepatic vessels, mesenteric vessels, and renal arteries) and the aortic-iliac axis in a single data acquisition **(Fig. 3)**.

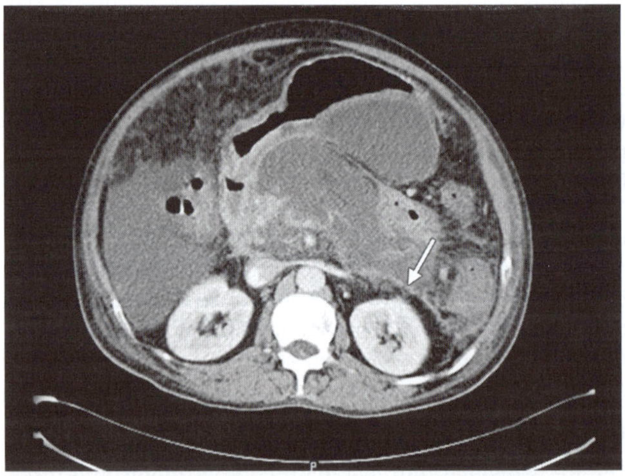

FIG. 2: Axial post contrast CT showing thickening of the left anterior renal fascia (arrow) in a patient of acute pancreatitis.

MRI may provide additional information about retroperitoneal abnormalities because of its multiplanar capability and excellent soft tissue resolution. The MRI protocol should be devised to maximize the signal intensity differences between pathologies and the background tissues. Typical sequences used are precontrast T1-weighted spoiled gradient echo (SGE), fat-suppressed T2-weighted and postgadolinium fat-suppressed T1-weighted SGE images. In the investigation of retroperitoneal hemorrhage, precontrast fat-suppressed T1-weighted SGE sequence should be obtained because it has the greatest sensitivity for subacute hemorrhage. Both T1-weighted and T2-weighted sequences are important for delineation and characterization of retroperitoneal masses, abscesses, and fibrosis. Image acquisition in two orthogonal planes permits direct evaluation of the extent of retroperitoneal disease. Applications include evaluation of patients with suspected IVC thrombosis or Budd-Chiari syndrome **(Fig. 4)**, intravascular extension of renal, adrenal, or hepatic tumors, and evaluation of anatomic anomalies of the IVC and systemic veins.[10]

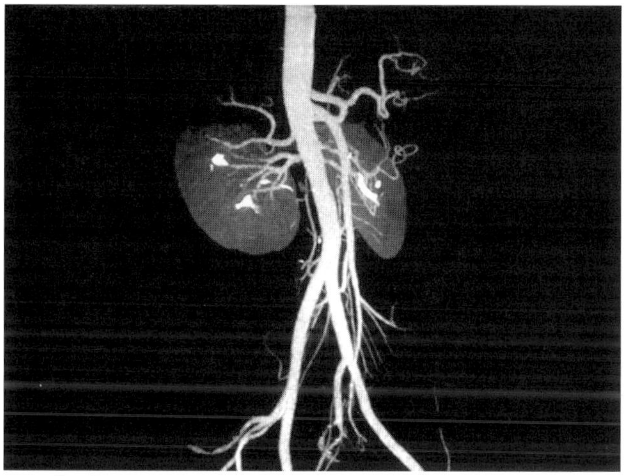

FIG. 3: Normal MDCT angiogram of the abdominal aorta. Maximum intensity projection (MIP) image shows good delineation of the entire abdominal aorta and its branches.The aorta has smooth walls and tapers gradually to the level of the aortic bifurcation.

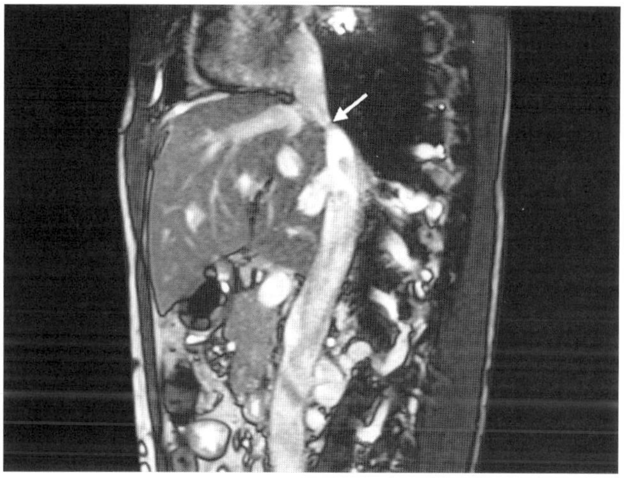

FIG. 4: Membranous obstruction of the intrahepatic IVC. Sagittal balanced steady-state (true FISP) MR image shows segmental occlusion of the IVC just below the cavoatrial junction.

Magnetic resonance angiography (MRA) has an important role to play in the imaging of aorta and IVC. Three-dimensional (3D) gadolinium-enhanced MRA can visualize the entire aorta with a single acquisition, allowing accurate determination of the extent of aneurysm, dissection, and other abnormalities. Vascular contrast is excellent and data can be viewed in any projection, which facilitates surgical planning.[11] Typically 0.1–0.2 mmol/kg body weight of gadolinium is injected intravenously as a bolus with an automatic injector at a rate of 2–4 mL/sec, followed by 20 cc of saline to clear lines and veins. For aortic imaging, the time interval between initiating contrast injection and initiating the imaging sequence can be determined using a test bolus technique. 1–2 mL of contrast is injected as a test bolus and the aorta is scanned approximately once per second. The travel time can be directly observed and then used to calculate the correct scan delay. Alternatively, automated triggering may be employed in which the aorta is continuously scanned until the contrast material bolus is directly observed or the signal intensity reaches a specified level, at which time the 3D sequence is acquired. The dataset obtained can be postprocessed either by MPRs or by 3D maximum intensity projection (MIP) **(Fig. 5)**. It is important to remember that arterial-phase MIP images demonstrate contrast material within the patent lumen and therefore may not accurately depict the true diameter of an aneurysm. The walls of vessels can usually be identified on source images or axial reformatted images. In addition, axial T1-weighted spoiled gradient-echo or spin-echo MR sequences following angiography are very useful in determining the diameter of the aneurysm and the extent of intra-arterial plaque or thrombus.

Likewise, it is important to scrutinize source images or thin-section reformatted images in patients who may have a dissection; an intimal flap can easily be missed if only MIP images are viewed.

Positron emission tomography (PET) scanning has shown very high sensitivity and specificity for detection of retroperitoneal diseases. PET with 2-(fluorine-18) fluoro-2-deoxy-D-glucose (FDG) allows detection of small malignant nodes not identified or not meeting size criteria for malignancy with CT **(Figs. 6A and B)** and tumor recurrences in surgical beds that are otherwise difficult to assess because of altered anatomy, surgical clip artifacts, and scar issue.[12] However, evaluation of retroperitoneal malignancies or adenopathy with FDG-PET can be complicated by urinary and colonic activity or anatomic variants. Urinary artifacts are avoided with intravenous (IV) hydration, administration of furosemide, and catheterization and retrograde filling of the bladder with saline solution. Colonic artifacts are avoided by cleansing the bowel with an iso-osmotic solution. FDG-PET is useful in assessing the RP for adenopathy in malignancies such as testicular cancer; lymphoma and rectal, ovarian or cervical cancer that spread along retroperitoneal lymphatics.

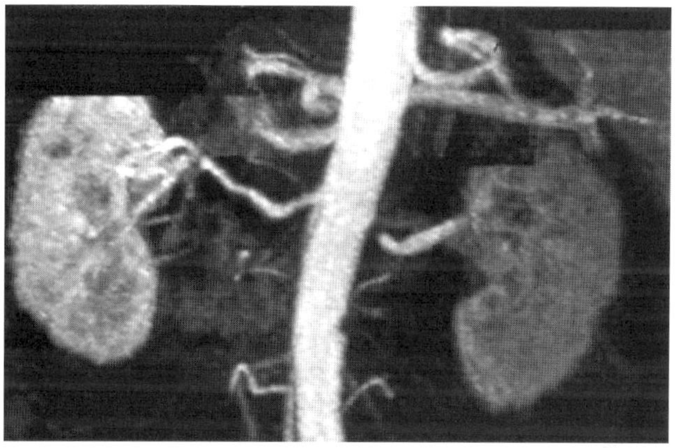

FIG. 5: Maximum intensity projection of 3D, gadolinium-enhanced MR angiogram depicting left renal artery stenosis.

Ultrasonography has role in image-guided intervention and bedside evaluation as detailed assessment of RP structures and extent of disease is limited with USG. It has advantage of portability, ease of availability, and no risk of radiation exposure.

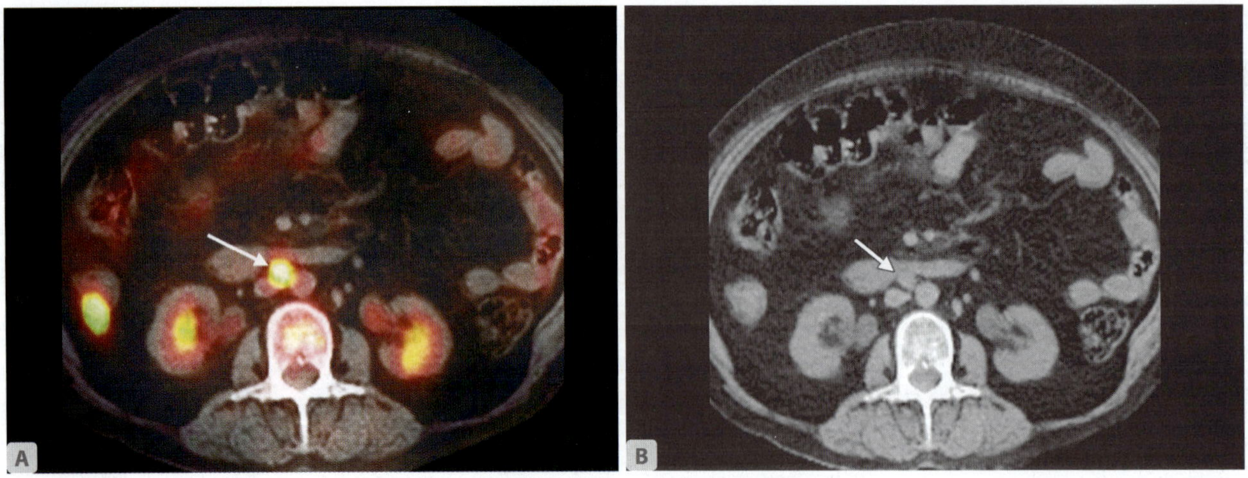

FIGS. 6A AND B: (A) FDG-PET image in a patient of carcinoma ovary shows increased uptake in a subcentimetric aortocaval lymph node (arrow); (B) Comparison CT image also shows the node (arrow), which was considered insignificant by the size criteria.

PATHOLOGIES

Retroperitoneal pathologies may broadly be classified as neoplastic or non-neoplastic conditions. Primary retroperitoneal neoplasms are rare tumors that originate in the retroperitoneal space but outside the major organs within that compartment. These can be categorized based on their origin either from mesenchymal cells, neurogenic cells, germ cell/spermatic cord or stromal, and lymphoid tissue **(Box 1)**. These can be benign or malignant. Imaging features are often overlapping and diagnosis is challenging. Imaging interpretation begins from ascertaining the location of tumor-confirming its origin from RP; followed by the organ of origin—either from a specific RP organ or primary retroperitoneal neoplasm and then recognizing specific features in terms of pattern of spread, tumor components and vascularity.[13,14]

To decide whether the tumor is located within the retroperitoneal space, it is useful to observe the displacement of normal anatomic structures. Anterior displacement of retroperitoneal organs (e.g. kidneys, adrenal glands, ureters, ascending and descending colon, pancreas, and portions of the duodenum) strongly suggests that the tumor arises in the RP **(Figs. 7A and B)**. Major vessels and some of their branches are also found in the retroperitoneal cavity, so that displacement of these vessels can be helpful as well. Before a tumor can be described as primarily retroperitoneal, the possibility that the tumor originates from a retroperitoneal organ must be excluded. Some radiologic signs that are helpful in determining tumor origin include the "beak sign", the "phantom (invisible) organ sign" and the "embedded organ sign".[15] When there is no definite sign that suggests an organ of origin, the diagnosis of primary retroperitoneal tumor becomes likely.

Beak sign—when a mass deforms the edge of an adjacent organ into a "beak" shape, it is likely that the mass arises from that organ **(Figs. 8A and B)**. On the other hand, an adjacent organ with dull edges suggests that the tumor compresses the organ but does not arise from it.

BOX 1: Common retroperitoneal pathologies.

Primary retroperitoneal neoplasms
- *Mesenchymal tumors:*
  - Liposarcoma
  - Leiomyosarcmas
  - Malignant fibrous histiocytoma
  - Desmoid
- *Neurogenic tumors:*
  - Schwannoma
  - Neurofibroma
  - Ganglioneuroma
  - Paraganglioma
  - Malignant peripheral nerve sheath tumor
- *Germ cell, sex cord or stromal tumor:*
  - Primary retroperitoneal extragonadal germ cell tumor
  - Growing teratoma syndrome
  - Primary teratoma
- *Lymphoid neoplasms:*
  - Lymphadenopathy—benign or metastatic
  - Lymphoma

Non-neoplastic conditions
- Retroperitoneal collections—infection, lymphocele, and hematoma
- Retroperitoneal fibrosis
- Erdheim-Chester disease
- Extramedullary hematopoiesis
- Lymphangioma
- Lymphangiectasis

Phantom (invisible) organ sign—when a large mass arises from a small organ, the organ sometimes becomes undetectable. This is known as the phantom organ sign. However, false-positive findings do exist, as in cases of huge retroperitoneal sarcomas that involve other small organs such as the adrenal gland.

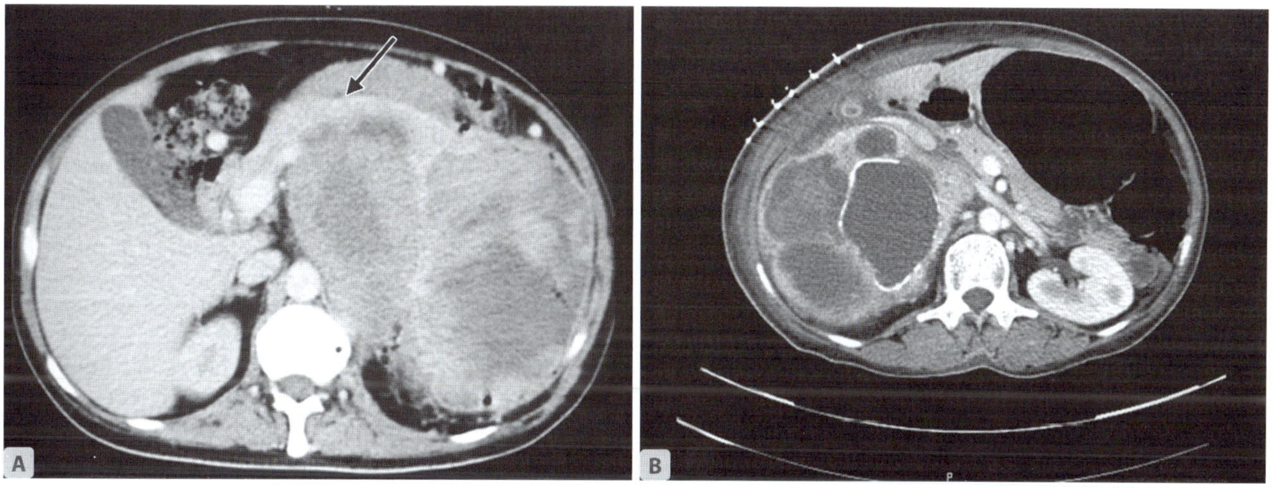

FIGS. 7A AND B: (A) Anterior displacement of pancreas. Axial CT image shows a large mass that is difficult to localize at first glance. However, anterior displacement of pancreas (arrow) confirms it to be in the retroperitoneal space; (B) Anterior displacement of the IVC. Axial CT image reveals a large, heterogeneous partially cystic right hypochondriac mass with septal calcification on the right. Its retroperitoneal location is suggested by the anterior displacement and stretching of the IVC (arrow). Histopathology revealed a diagnosis of paraganglioma.

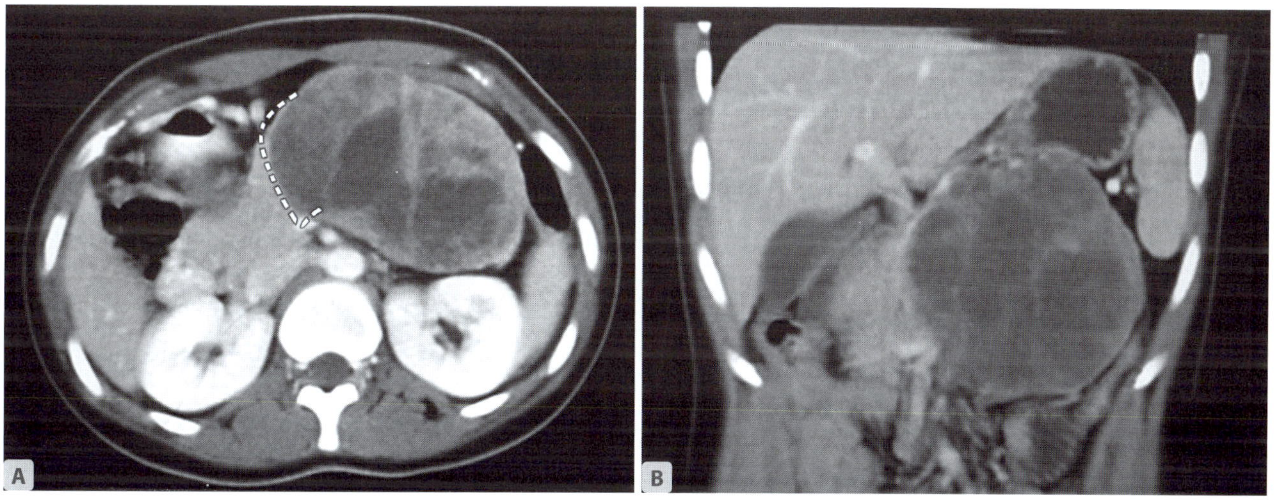

FIGS. 8A AND B: Beak sign. Axial CT image shows a large cystic tumor with the beak sign in its contact surface with the pancreas (dotted white line). This finding represents mucinous cystadenocarcinoma of the pancreas.

Embedded organ sign—when a tumor compresses an adjacent plastic organ (e.g. gastrointestinal tract and IVC) that is not the organ of origin, the organ is deformed into a crescent shape. In contrast, when part of an organ appears to be embedded in the tumor (positive embedded organ sign) at the contact surface, it is likely to be the organ of origin **(Fig. 9)**.

MESODERMAL NEOPLASMS

Soft tissue sarcomas of mesenchymal origin are rare tumor accounting for less than 1%; however, around 15% occur in RP.[16] The retroperitoneal tumors often present late and with large size due to spread along the connective tissue in RP. Role of imaging is predominantly to determine the extent, spread, and resectability of the mass along with detection of lymphadenopathy and metastases. Accurate diagnosis of the tumor is not always possible; but few imaging features may assist in narrowing the differentials, e.g. presence of fat raises suspicion of liposarcoma, cystic mass may indicate lymphangioma or lymphangiectasis, spread of mass in between vessels causing displacement but not infiltration is feature of lymphoma **(Flowchart 1)**.

Lipoma

Lipoma is a benign mesenchymal tumor that resembles normal fat. Lipomas typically demonstrate homogeneous fatty (–10 to –100 HU) attenuation on CT and homogeneous signal intensity identical to that of fat on all MRI sequences. Thin (<2 mm) fibrous septa of low signal intensity on T1- and T2-weighted images may traverse the lesion. Since, lipoma is extremely rare in RP, any fat-containing lesion in this location is considered and evaluated as liposarcoma.

Liposarcomas

CT or MRI can suggest a diagnosis of liposarcoma when fat is detected within a retroperitoneal mass. The amount of fat seen in liposarcomas varies widely and depending on the histopathology and degree of fat on imaging, RP liposarcomas can be divided into—well-differentiated liposarcoma, myxoid liposarcoma, dedifferentiated, and pleomorphic liposarcomas.[16-18]

The well-differentiated liposarcomas are predominantly of fat density with or without fine irregular strands of higher density **(Figs. 10A and B)**. These septations or soft tissue attenuation merge with fat component without any clear demarcation between the two components in contrast to dedifferentiated liposarcomas where soft tissue masses can be distinguishly and separately seen within the fatty tumor **(Fig. 11)**. Myxoid liposarcomas have cystic attenuation—seen as density less than muscle but greater than fat on CT. MRI will show high signal intensity within the soft tissue on T2-weighted image and heterogeneous enhancement postgadolinium administration due to presence of extracellular myxoid material within giving it a "pseudocystic" appearance. Pleomorphic liposarcoma has higher degree of anaplasia because of which it might not show minimal or no fat component on imaging and seen as heterogeneous retroperitoneal soft tissue mass.

The treatment and prognosis differ with each type of fat-containing retroperitoneal mass; hence, it is important to identify and observe internal imaging features. Few imaging findings like soft tissue septa more than 2 mm thick within a fatty retroperitoneal mass, septal irregularity or bulging, demarcated soft tissue mass within, and obvious enhancement help in approaching the RP mass appropriately.[19]

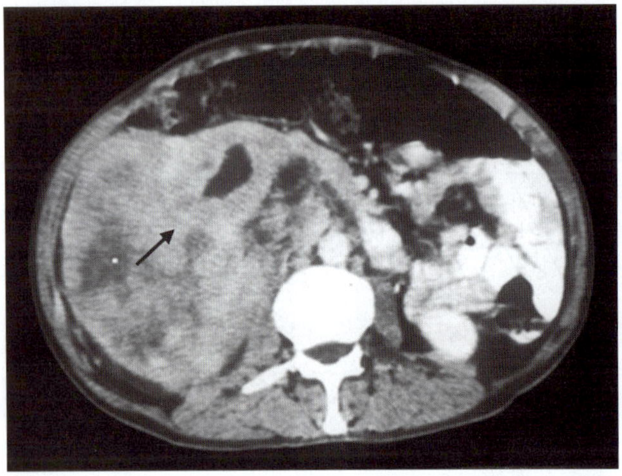

FIG. 9: Embedded organ sign. CT image shows a huge heterogeneous mass in the right side of abdomen. The lumen of the duodenum is stretched toward the mass, and the wall of the duodenum appears embedded in the mass at the contact surface (arrow). These findings represent gastrointestinal stromal tumor of the duodenum with a positive embedded organ sign.

Leiomyosarcomas

Leiomyosarcomas are the second most common retroperitoneal sarcomas with female predominance. It is the most common primary venous/IVC tumor which present as slow growing large, heterogeneous masses with foci of hemorrhage, necrosis, and cystic degeneration **(Fig. 12)**.[20] They do not contain fat or calcification. Not infrequently, retroperitoneal leiomyosarcomas extend into the adjacent veins. IVC leiomyosarcomas can have extraluminal (62%), both intraluminal as well as extraluminal (33%) and only intraluminal (5%) growth patterns from various segments of IVC.[21] Upper segment indicates extension from hepatic veins to right atrium, middle segment is from hepatic to renal veins, and lower segment involves infrarenal part of IVC.

Malignant Fibrous Histiocytomas

Malignant fibrous histiocytomas are high grade connective tissue tumors. They are multilobulated, infiltrative,

FLOWCHART 1: Brief algorithm on approach to retroperitoneal masses.

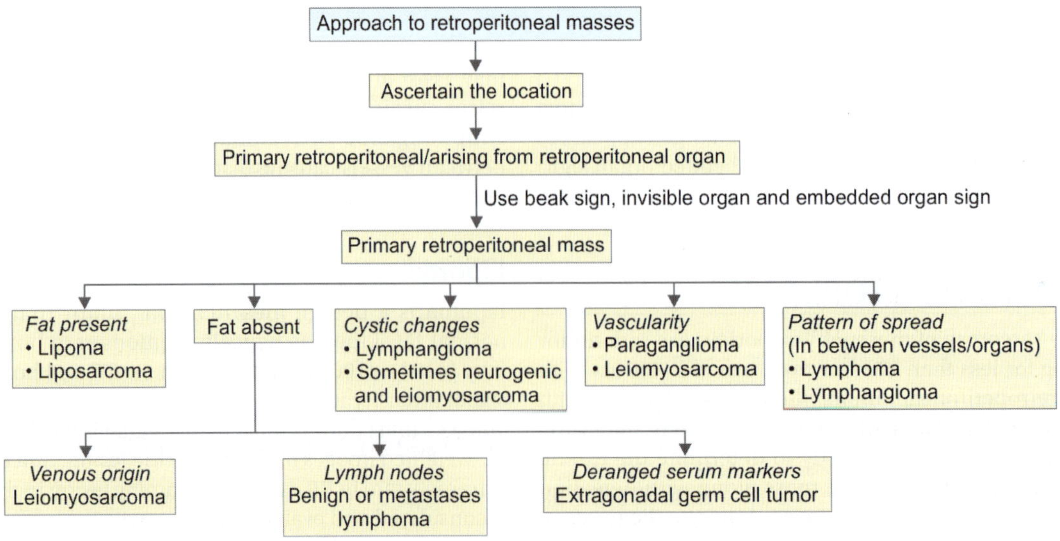

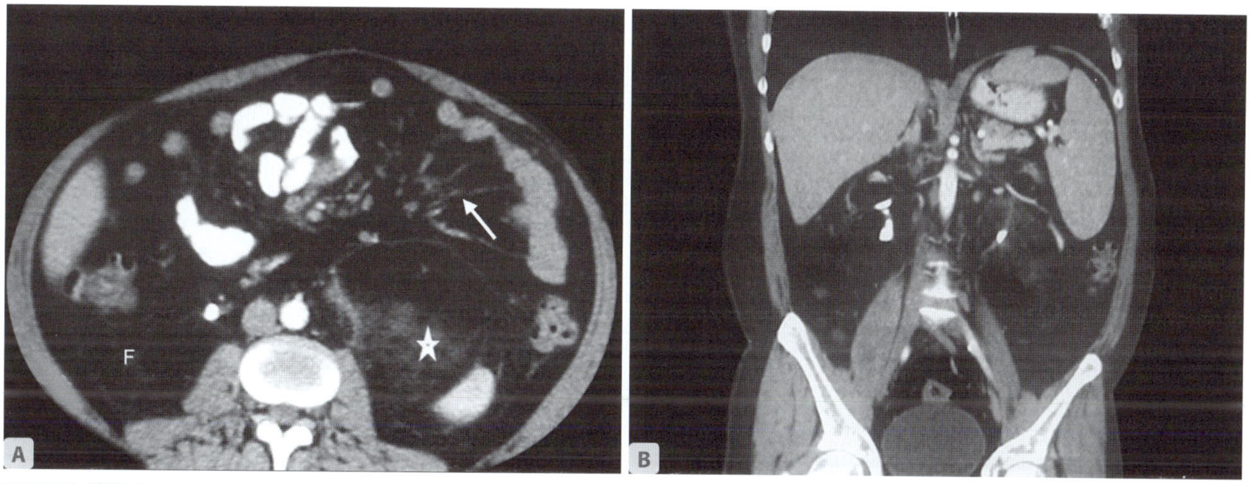

FIGS. 10A AND B: Retroperitoneal well-differentiated liposarcoma in a 60-year-old man with a history of increasing abdominal girth. Axial and coronal CT images show a diffusely infiltrative, retroperitoneal and abdominal mass composed of fat (F) with Hounsfield (HU) measurements of –80 to –120. There are multiple thick septa (arrow) and a posterior soft tissue component (star) with mildly higher attenuation.

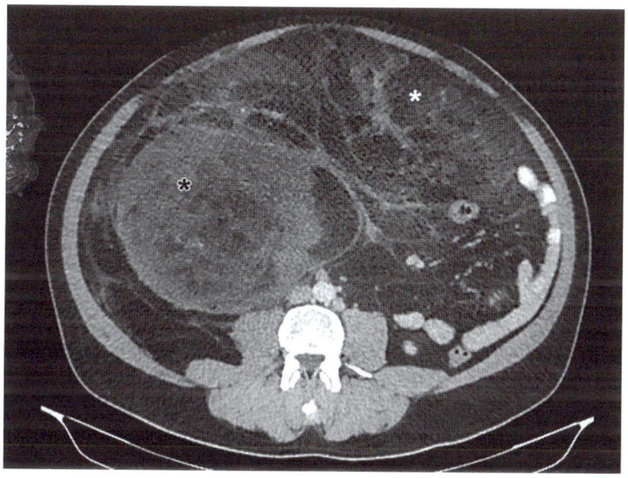

FIG. 11: Dedifferentiated liposarcoma in a 44-year-old male patient. Axial CT image shows large abdominal mass with imperceptible margins having fatty (white asterisk) as well as solid (black asterisk) component.

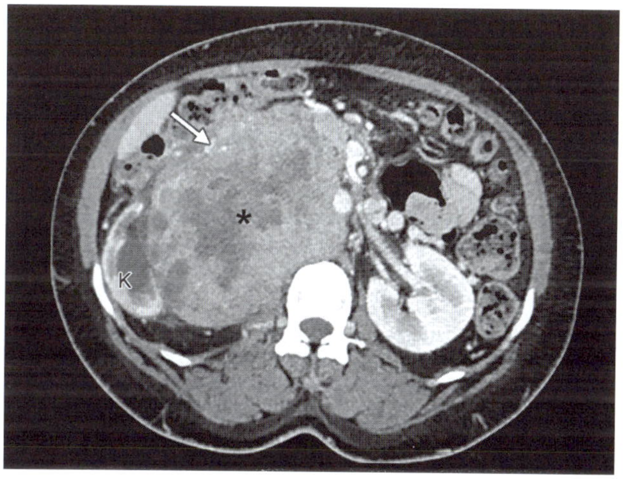

FIG. 12: Inferior vena cava (IVC) leiomyosarcoma in a 52-year-old female. Axial CT image demonstrates a large heterogeneous retroperitoneal mass (asterisk) displacing and compressing right kidney (K). The IVC is seen displaced anteriorly by the mass with luminal narrowing (arrow) indicating predominantly extraluminal component of the sarcoma.

unencapsulated but deceptively well-circumscribed masses. They may contain myxoid stroma, fibrous tissue, hemorrhage, and necrosis giving rise to a typical mosaic of mixed low, intermediate, and high signal intensity on T2-weighted MR images. Although both myxoid stroma and necrosis have similar T1 and T2 signal intensity, differentiation may be possible as myxoid stroma shows delayed enhancement in contrast to the nonenhancing necrotic areas. Up to 25% of malignant fibrous histiocytomas contain dystrophic calcification, a finding that is extremely uncommon in other retroperitoneal malignancies.[22]

Hemangiopericytomas

Hemangiopericytomas are highly vascular tumors thought to arise from blood vessel walls. They may demonstrate areas of intratumoral hemorrhage and multiple flow voids on MRI. Hemangiopericytomas enhance rapidly and intensely on dynamic contrast-enhanced CT or MRI.

Other Malignancies

Fibrosarcomas and neurofibrosarcomas are usually heterogeneous and thus identical in appearance to leiomyosarcomas, some liposarcomas, and malignant fibrous histiocytomas. Neuroblastomas and ganglioneuroblastomas often contain calcification. They are usually seen in children. Rhabdomyosarcomas are rare heterogeneous tumors also seen in pediatric patients.

NEUROGENIC NEOPLASMS

Neurogenic tumors may arise from paraganglionic cells (paragangliomas), ganglion cells (ganglioneuroma,

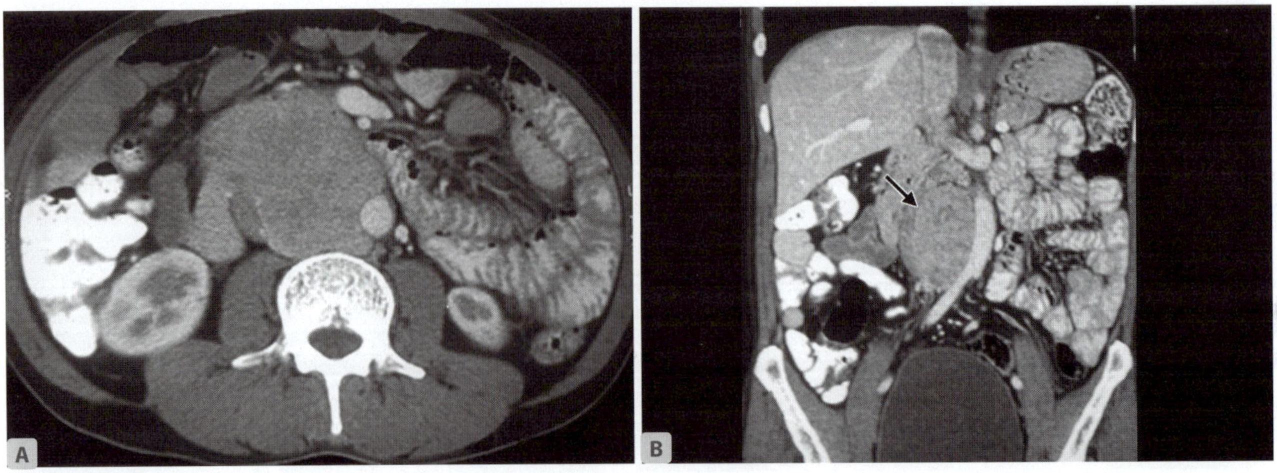

FIGS. 13A AND B: Retroperitoneal paraganglioma. (A) Axial CT image shows large homogeneous soft tissue density mass in the aortocaval region; (B) Coronal image shows the IVC draping around the right lateral margin of the mass (arrow).

ganglioneuroblastoma, and neuroblastoma), and nerve sheaths (neurofibroma and schwannoma).

Paragangliomas

Majority of paragangliomas (extra-adrenal pheochromocytoma) lie in the RP, in the immediate para-aortic region, from the level of the adrenal glands to the aortic bifurcation. Paragangliomas are well-defined soft tissue masses, usually quite large at the time of diagnosis **(Figs. 13A and B)**. Paragangliomas are homogeneous when small, but become increasingly heterogeneous as they grow due to central necrosis, hemorrhage, and even calcification.[23] On MR images, they often demonstrate extremely high signal intensity on T2-weighted images. These are generally hypervascular and most enhanced briskly after injection of IV contrast material.

Nerve Sheath Tumors

These tumors are often located adjacent to the vertebral column or deep to the psoas muscles. MRI is the imaging modality of choice for imaging of these tumors as it detects tumor extension into the neural foramina, a common feature of neurogenic tumors **(Fig. 14)**. MRI also helps in the characterization of these masses, as they tend to have high signal intensity on T2-weighted sequence due to the myxoid stroma they contain. Central low to intermediate signal intensity may be seen corresponding to fibrous tissue and is referred to as the "target sign". Sometimes, a whorled appearance consisting of linear or curvilinear structures of low signal intensity is seen on T2-weighted images. At histopathological analysis, this finding corresponds to bundles of Schwann cells and collagen fibers within the mass. Varying degrees of contrast enhancement have been reported, from slight to moderate to marked with delayed heterogeneous uptake of contrast. These enhancement features are explained by the presence of abundant myxoid material in these tumors, resulting in delayed progressive accumulation of contrast material in the extracellular space.[24]

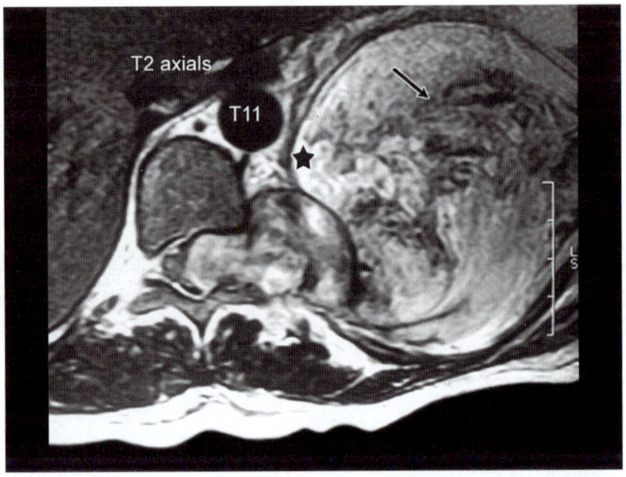

FIG. 14: Intraspinal extension of schwannoma. T2-weighted axial MR image shows a smoothly encapsulated, large heterogeneous intensity mass in the left paraspinal location. It has extended inside the extradural compartment of the spinal canal. The markedly hyperintense area (star) represents myxoid stroma. The linear, low signal intensity areas, having a somewhat whorled appearance (arrow), correspond to bundles of Schwann cells and collagen fibers within the mass.

Schwannomas usually appear as well-defined, heterogeneous soft tissue masses. Although they may contain cystic areas, they usually have large solid components. Retroperitoneal *neurofibromas* are commonly seen in patients with neurofibromatosis. On CT, neurofibromas appear as well-defined, sharply marginated, homogeneous masses that demonstrate near-water attenuation. *Ganglioneuromas* arise from sympathetic ganglia and are composed of mature Schwann cells, ganglion cells, and nerve fibers. Predominantly children and young adults (60% of cases) are affected and the prognosis is excellent, recurrence being rare after surgical resection. At CT or MRI, ganglioneuromas appear as well-circumscribed oval, crescentic, or lobulated masses. These tumors tend to partially or completely surround major blood vessels, with little or no compromise of the lumen. At unenhanced CT, the tumors appear homogeneous, with attenuation less than that of muscle. They contain calcification in about 20% of cases. The calcifications are discrete and punctate rather than amorphous and coarse as in neuroblastomas.

GERM CELL, SEX CORD OR STROMAL NEOPLASMS

Teratomas

Teratomas are congenital neoplasms containing components of all three germ layers. CT often shows calcification or even osseous elements. Fat may be seen on both CT and MRI **(Fig. 15)**. Sometimes, a dermoid plug is identifiable as a soft tissue mural nodule projecting into a cyst. The incidence of malignant degeneration is rare (<1%) and usually occurs in the dermoid plug in postmenopausal women.

Primary Extragonadal Germ Cell Tumor

Primary retroperitoneal extragonadal germ cell tumors (GCTs) arise from primordial germ cells remnants of genital ridge which fail to migrate properly. Since most of the GCTs in RP are metastases from genital primary, the patient should be evaluated for same. The retroperitoneal GCT can be seminomatous or nonseminomatous, seen as enhancing masses which are predominantly in the midline if metastasized from testicular primary neoplasm. The latter is associated with deranged serum markers and is seen as heterogeneous masses with cystic necrotic or hemorrhagic areas within. Nonseminomatous GCTs carry poor prognosis.

Growing Teratoma Syndrome

It is a rare phenomenon with documentation of 1.9–7.6% rate of occurrence in literature.[16] It refers to chemorefractory retroperitoneal teratomatous mass which shows increase in size on chemotherapy despite normalization of tumor markers. Surgical resection is the treatment of choice in such patients.

LYMPHOID NEOPLASMS

Normal lymph nodes appear as small, rounded soft tissue masses adjacent to the great vessels. Retrocrural, paraceliac, gastrohepatic, para-aortic, aortocaval, periportal, peripancreatic, and external and internal iliac groups together constitute the retroperitoneal nodes. Presently, CT is the most frequently used imaging technique for evaluation of enlarged retroperitoneal nodes. The diagnosis of lymph node abnormalities on CT is based on size and image morphology. Size of a node is best determined by measuring its short-axis diameter. The retroperitoneal lymph nodes are considered abnormal if their size is more than 10 mm, except in the retrocrural space where the upper limit is 6 mm. A variety of retro-peritoneal structures can be confused with enlarged lymph nodes like unopacified bowel loops, vascular collaterals, dilated lymphatics, and retroperitoneal fibrosis. Careful evaluation of serial CT images after oral and IV contrast is helpful in distinguishing between these structures.

Magnetic resonance sequences suited for detection of lymph nodes include precontrast T1-weighted spin-echo or SGE, fat-suppressed T2-weighted turbo spin-echo, and contrast-enhanced fat-suppressed sequences. The enlarged lymph nodes appear low in signal on precontrast SGE in a background of high-signal fat, and nodes are moderately high in signal on fat-suppressed T2-weighted and contrast-enhanced T1-weighted images. Fat- suppressed T2-weighted and diffusion weighted images are very sensitive for the detection of lymph nodes and perform better than CT, particularly in pediatric patients or other patients with paucity of retroperitoneal fat.

Benign Lymphadenopathy

Benign enlargement of lymph nodes may occur secondary to inflammatory or infectious disease; tuberculosis being the most common etiology in our country.[25]

The mesenteric, omental, and peripancreatic lymph nodes are most commonly involved. The nodes commonly demonstrate peripheral enhancement with central areas of low attenuation after IV contrast administration **(Fig. 16)**.

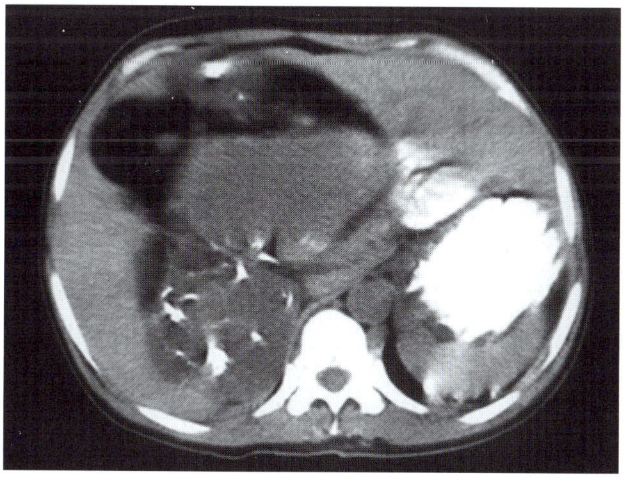

FIG. 15: Retroperitoneal teratoma. Axial CT image reveals a large heterogeneous mass containing elements that show the attenuation of fluid, fat, soft tissue and calcification.

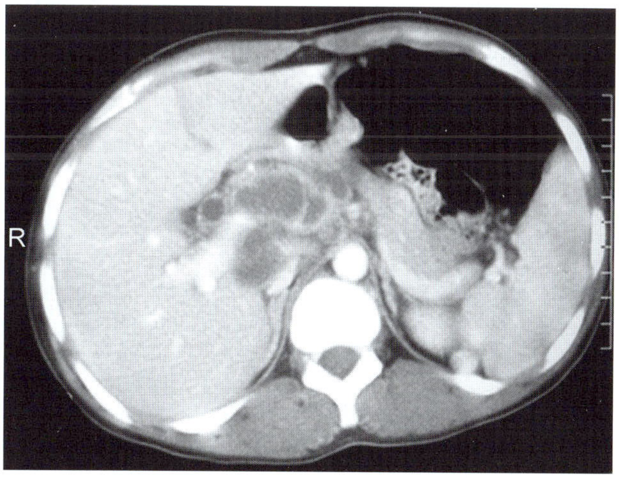

FIG. 16: Retroperitoneal tubercular lymphadenopathy. Axial CT image shows enlarged periportal and portocaval lymph nodes with characteristic central necrosis and peripheral rim enhancement.

Discrete homogeneous lymph nodes may also be seen in some cases. Calcification is frequently seen in tubercular lymph nodes. Enlarged lymph nodes with low density centers may also be seen in pyogenic infections, Whipple's disease, lymphomatous or metastatic nodes following radiotherapy and chemotherapy. Enlarged retroperitoneal nodes have also been observed in 30% of patients with sarcoidosis.[26] The periportal, paraceliac, and para-aortic groups are most often involved. On CT, the nodes affected by sarcoidosis generally show homogeneous soft-tissue attenuation and remain discrete. Nodal calcification is unusual in sarcoidosis.

Castleman disease is occasionally also associated with retroperitoneal lymph node enlargement. Mostly, the CT or MR appearance of these enlarged lymph nodes is not specific. However, identification of intense and uniform contrast enhancement in lymph nodes can suggest the diagnosis **(Fig. 17)**.[27]

Lymphangioleiomyomatosis is a rare cause of bulky retroperitoneal lymphadenopathy. This is a progressive disease involving the lung, lymphatic trunks, and lymph nodes, typically affecting young women of child-bearing age. Sometimes, it can primarily involve RP with or without subsequent development in the lungs.[28] The enlarged lymph nodes may show cystic, low-attenuation components on imaging.

Lymphoma

Abdominal lymph nodes are involved in 50% of the non-Hodgkin's lymphoma (NHL) patients as against 25% of those with Hodgkin's disease (HD) at presentation.[29] Mesenteric involvement is seen in more than half of the NHL patients (versus 5% of those with HD). The patterns of lymphadenopathy are also markedly different, slight enlargement of upper para-aortic nodes and contiguous spread being characteristic of HD. NHL on the other hand manifests with bulky lymph nodes in multiple locations.

The enlarged lymph nodes may appear as discrete masses or as confluent soft tissue mass obliterating the retroperitoneal fat **(Fig. 18)**. Lymphomas are "soft" tumors and frequently surround the adjacent vessels (floating aorta sign) and ureters without compressing their lumina. Lymphomas are homogeneous with minimal contrast enhancement and relatively low signal intensity at T2-weighted images representing densely packed cellular components. Nodes are rarely calcified (<1%) in untreated patients.[30]

Computed tomography is also used for follow-up of disease after treatment. Response to treatment is usually indicated by reduction in size and extent with or without appearance of dystrophic calcification within. In some patients, lymph nodes may become hypodense as an appropriate response to treatment with or without reduction in lymph node size.

Persistent lymph nodal masses may be seen in some patients even after treatment. These may represent residual tumor, post-treatment inflammation or fibrosis. Unfortunately, there are no reliable CT characteristics that can differentiate between malignant and benign residual masses. Several studies have suggested that MRI may be helpful in distinguishing late post-therapy fibrosis (hypointense on T2-weighted images) from viable lymph nodes (hyperintense or heterogeneous on T2-weighted images). Also, chronic fibrotic tissue shows minimal MR enhancement postcontrast while recurrence generally enhances markedly.

FDG-PET has proved to be very useful in the clinical management and follow-up of lymphomas. It is now considered the most accurate tool for the assessment of treatment response and prognosis in patients with Hodgkin's lymphoma and aggressive NHL.[31] FDG-PET can detect metabolically active disease by its increased glycolysis that is proportional to the tumor mitotic activity. It can separate high-grade from low-grade tumors and aid in prognostication. FDG-PET at the end of treatment seems to aid considerably in differentiating between residual masses with or without residual lymphoma. An early interim FDG-PET scan after 1–3 cycles of chemotherapy is a very strong predictor of outcome.[32] Like other imaging modalities, PET has its own

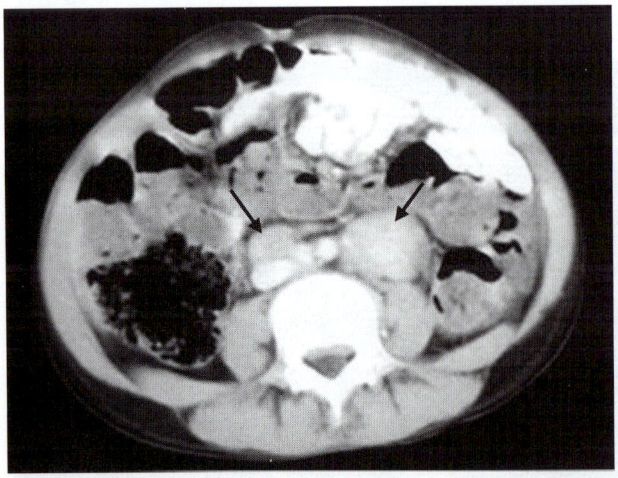

FIG. 17: Castleman disease. Contrast enhanced axial CT image shows large, well-defined, markedly enhancing para-aortic lymph nodes (arrows) compatible with the diagnosis of Castleman disease in an 8-year-old boy.

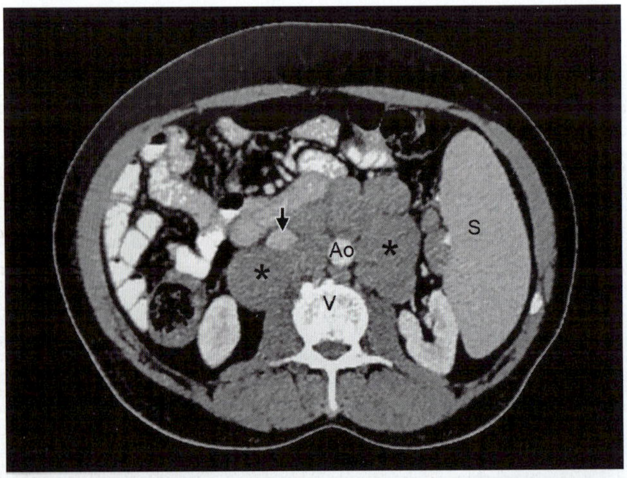

FIG. 18: Non-Hodgkin's lymphoma. Contrast-enhanced axial CT image shows large, confluent lymph nodes in pre/para-aortic, aortocaval, and retrocaval location (asterisks). Inferior vena cava (arrow) and aorta (Ao) are displaced by the mass but their patency is preserved. Note made of enlarged spleen (S) (V: vertebral body).

drawbacks including inability to detect very small lesions (<5 mm) and reduced specificity due to increased uptake in metabolically active inflammatory and infective tissues.

HIV Lymphadenopathy

Enlarged lymph node are present in most (> 60%) patients with human immunodeficiency virus (HIV) infection but in more than half of these patients, the short-axis diameter of the largest node measures only 10–15 mm.[33] Although sometimes the nodal enlargement results only from reactive hyperplasia, many other diseases may be responsible. These include disseminated mycobacterial infections **(Fig. 19)**, histoplasmosis, lymphoma, and Kaposi's sarcoma. When lymph node enlargement is massive, acquired immunodeficiency syndrome (AIDS)-related lymphoma should be suspected. Intense enhancement of lymph nodes suggests a diagnosis of Kaposi's sarcoma.

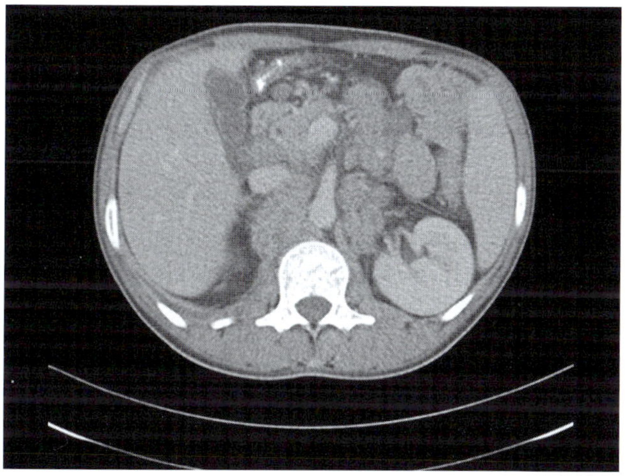

FIG. 19: Mycobacterium tuberculosis infection in a 35-year-old man with HIV infection. Axial CT image shows multiple, enlarged, low attenuation lymph nodes in the portocaval and paracelic regions.

Metastatic Lymphadenopathy

Metastatic lymph nodes show varied morphological patterns, but the diagnosis is usually straightforward due to the presence of a known primary. Neoplasms of the stomach, colon, pancreas, kidney, testis, ovary, uterus, bladder, and prostate may all metastasize to retroperitoneal lymph nodes. Calcification in the metastatic nodes suggests mucin producing primary from the ovary or gastrointestinal tract.

Testicular neoplasms tend to metastasize via lymphatics rather than via bloodstream. Lymphatics from the testes drain into ipsilateral lymph nodes, which follow the course of the gonadal veins. Typically, left-sided neoplasms spread to involve lymph nodes in the left renal hilum, as the left gonadal vein drains into the left renal vein. Right-sided neoplasms spread to paracaval lymph nodes, an area where the right gonadal vein joins the IVC. While metastatic retroperitoneal nodes from some testicular tumors appear quite homogeneous on CT, others particularly from nonseminomatous neoplasms often appear heterogeneous containing low-attenuation central areas of necrosis and rim enhancement **(Figs. 20A and B)**. Seminomas may present with bulky masses whereas nonseminomatous GCT often metastasize to normal sized nodes. On MR metastatic lymph nodes show low-intermediate signal intensity on T1-weighted images, and high signal intensity on T2-weighted images. Low signal intensity masses after treatment usually represent fibrosis.

CT and MRI use the nonspecific criterion of size and are limited in their ability to differentiate benign from malignant lymph nodes. Contrast-enhanced MR lymphography is a promising technique in differentiating benign from metastatic lymph nodes and providing information on lymph node morphology and function.

Ultrasmall super paramagnetic iron oxide (USPIO) particles with a long plasma circulation time are suitable as MR contrast agents for MR lymphography. MRI is typically performed 24–36 hours after IV infusion of USPIO particles. Normal lymph nodes decrease in signal intensity on enhanced T2-weighted and T2-weighted gradient echo images,

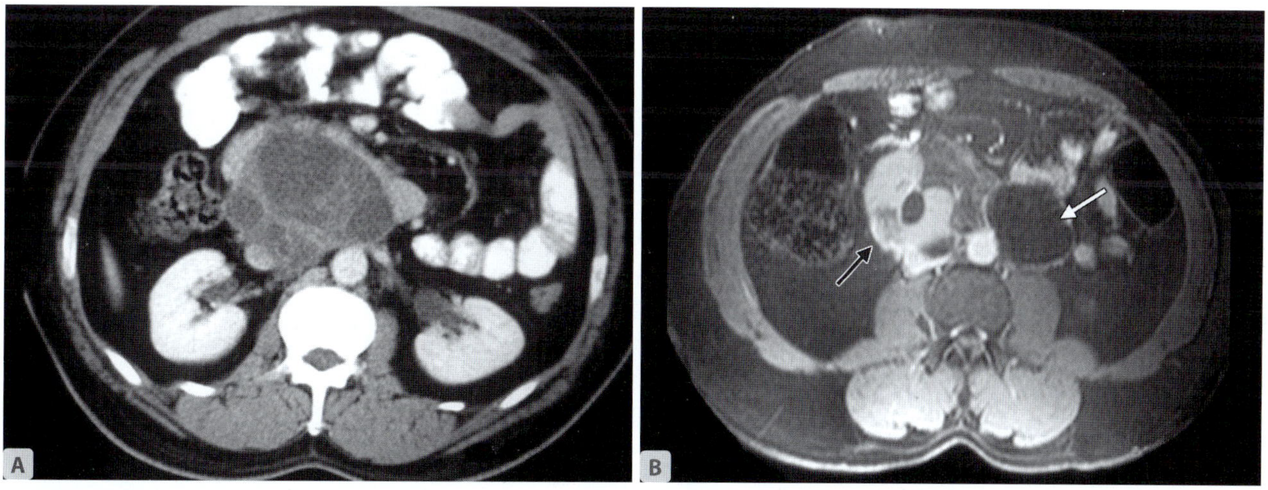

FIGS. 20A AND B: Metastatic testicular germ cell tumor. (A) Axial CT image shows massive, low attenuation retroperitoneal lymphadenopathy; (B) Postchemotherapy contrast-enhanced T1-weighted axial MR image in another patient shows enhancing viable tumor (black arrow) and the non-enhancing necrotic component (white arrow).

indicating uptake of this contrast agent. Nodes infiltrated by tumor have no appreciable USPIO uptake and thus reveal no signal change on pre- and postcontrast images.[34]

FDG-PET may be more sensitive and specific than CT for certain retroperitoneal metastases depending on the primary. Nonseminomatous GCTs with well-differentiated components are not very FDG-avid.

NON-NEOPLASTIC PATHOLOGIES

Retroperitoneal Collections

Fluid collection in the RP occurs in a variety of conditions like acute pancreatitis, urinary tract disruption with urinoma formation, hematoma, and abscess. Although the clinical presentations differ, they all share a tendency to dissect within the well-defined fascial planes in the retroperitoneal space. Most of these appear on CT as water density collections and are frequently indistinguishable from one another.

Fluid collections in the anterior pararenal space often result from acute pancreatitis **(Fig. 21)**.[35] Fluid collections arise within or adjacent to the pancreas in about 40% and resolve spontaneously without leaving any clinical sequelae in over 50% of these patients. In others, the fluid collections persist, develop a fibrous capsule, and are often associated with a variety of complications including secondary infection, perforation, and erosion into the spleen, liver or vascular system. Both infected and noninfected fluid collections and pseudocysts can be treated effectively by image-guided percutaneous catheter drainage.

Abscesses, hematomas, and urinomas can all develop in the perirenal space. Perirenal hemorrhage is usually caused by blunt trauma, rupture of an aortic aneurysm, bleeding disorders, anticoagulant therapy or spontaneous bleeding within a renal tumor **(Fig. 22)**. On CT characteristically, a hyperdense, ill-defined collection originating from the disrupted vessels and extending into the interfascial planes is seen. Loculated blood can mimic a complex cyst or neoplasm. CT attenuation of hematoma varies with time, ranging from hyperdense fresh blood, typically >50 HU to near water density within several weeks. Bleeding may be intermittent resulting in a heterogeneous appearance. MRI is more useful in determining the content of retroperitoneal fluid collections as it is more sensitive and specific for detection of blood products. An acute hematoma is isointense on T1-weighted and hyperintense on T2-weighted images. Within several days, the signal gradually becomes hyperintense on T1-weighted images and a hematoma is then hyperintense on both T1- and T2-weighted images with a developing, hypointense hemosiderin rim **(Figs. 23A and B)**.

Abnormal perirenal fluid may be in either of two locations: within the renal capsule (subcapsular) or outside the capsule in the perinephric fat. Subcapsular fluid collections usually produce distortion of the renal parenchyma whereas perinephric collections do not. Urinomas result from obstructive uropathy and less frequently from abdominal trauma and surgical or diagnostic instrumentation.

Retroperitoneal abscesses are particularly difficult to diagnose, because they may not exhibit the classic clinical features, i.e. fever, chills, and an elevated white blood cell count. When an abscess is mature, its wall is thick and generally hypervascular. On contrast-enhanced CT, there is enhancement of the wall and the fluid is usually homogeneous and does not enhance. Many abscesses contain multiple septations. There may be substantial reactive inflammation in the surrounding fat.

Abnormalities in the posterior pararenal space are much less common than abnormalities in the anterior pararenal space or the perirenal space. When present, these are most commonly the result of spread of pathologic processes in the pelvis. Causes can include hematoma, infection, and neoplasm.

Aorta

The most important abdominal aortic abnormalities are aneurysm formation and aortic dissection. MDCTA and MRA have gradually replaced conventional angiography as the procedures of choice for detailed evaluation of the aorta.

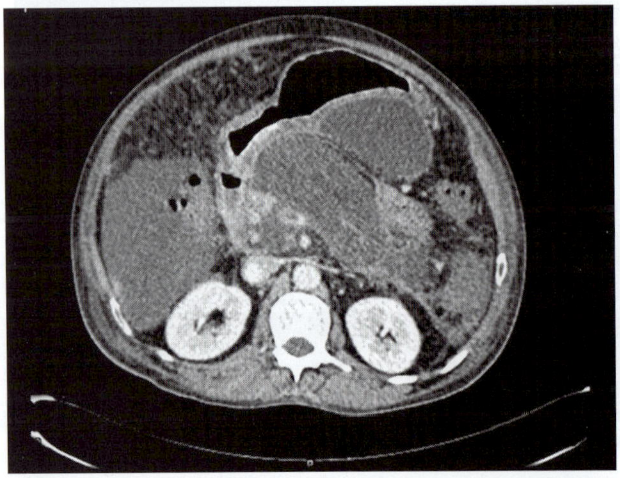

FIG. 21: Fluid collection in the anterior pararenal space. CT image in a patient with acute pancreatitis demonstrates peripancreatic fluid in the left anterior pararenal space.

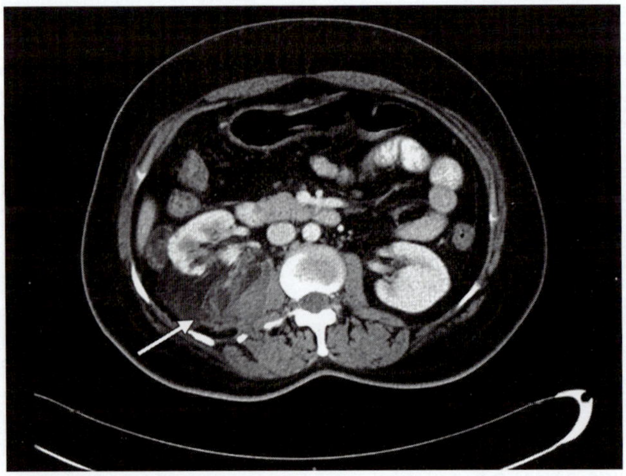

FIG. 22: Perirenal hemorrhage. Axial CT image shows right perirenal hemorrhage (arrow) that occurred spontaneously from rupture of underlying renal angiomyolipoma.

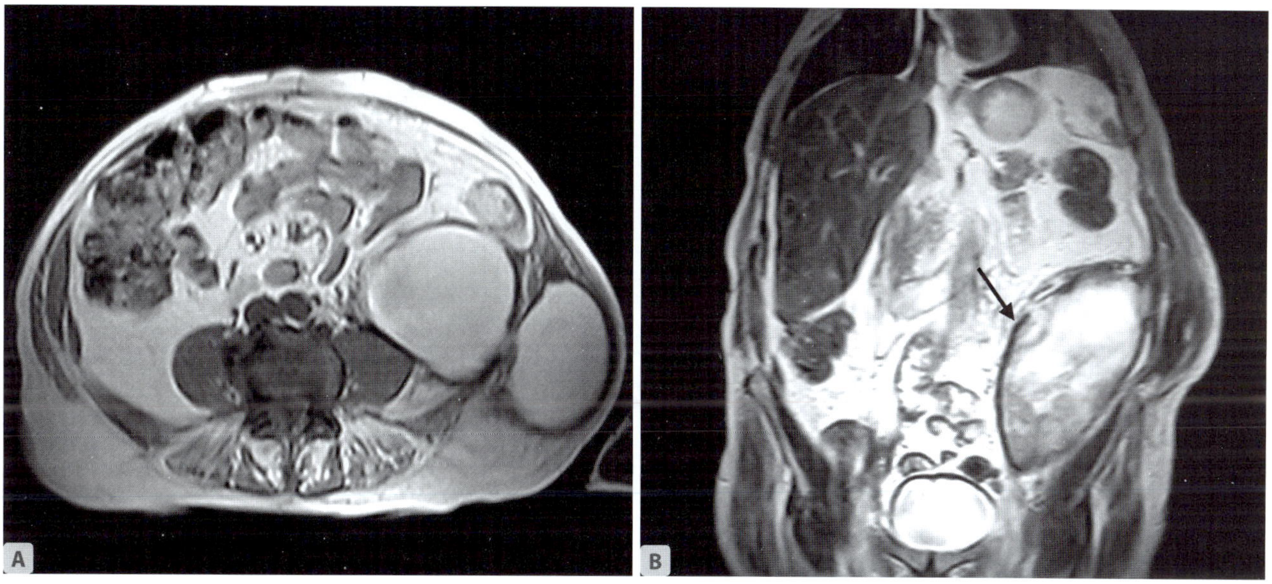

FIGS. 23A AND B: Spontaneous retroperitoneal hemorrhage in a patient on anticoagulant therapy. (A) Axial T1-weighted MR image shows a well-defined hyperintense lesion anterior to the left psoas. It is partially decompressing into the parietes; (B) Coronal T2-weighted image shows heterogeneous, predominantly high signal intensity within the mass. There is a markedly hypointense peripheral rim (arrow) due to hemosiderin deposition. These T1 and T2 signal intensities are diagnostic of a subacute hematoma.

Aortic Aneurysm

Most abdominal aortic aneurysms result from atherosclerosis. Other causes include trauma, infection, Takayasu's arteritis, cystic medial necrosis, and syphilis. The infrarenal aorta is the most common site of abdominal aortic aneurysms accounting for 95% of cases. If untreated, these aneurysms may enlarge and rupture with a mortality of 50–90%.[36]

The abdominal aortic aneurysm may show curvilinear calcification on plain abdominal radiography. On USG, CT, and MRI the aneurysm is identified as focal area of dilatation exceeding 3 cm in size. Spontaneous rupture is a frequent complication of aneurysms measuring 6 cm or more in diameter. Therefore, most aneurysms larger than 6 cm require surgery. Important diagnostic information needed for management includes location, diameter of aneurysm, its longitudinal length, its relationship to the renal, common iliac and femoral arteries, and assessment of the periaortic tissues for perianeurysmal fibrosis.[37] USG is a good modality for initial evaluation of aortic aneurysm. It may also be used for follow-up of patients who do not undergo surgical repair. However, CT and MRI are preferred techniques for evaluating the size, extent, and complications of aneurysms. At several centers, CT angiography has replaced conventional angiography because it is less invasive and can provide all the necessary information required for the management. Angiography frequently underestimates the dimensions of an aneurysm because it shows only the flowing blood in the lumen and does not show mural thrombus, which is detected on CT **(Fig. 24)**. Contrast-enhanced 3D gradient echo MRA demonstrates the full extent of the aneurysm and its relationship to aortic branches. Aneurysm rupture or leak is associated with a high morbidity and mortality, if not promptly treated. CT findings of ruptured abdominal aortic aneurysms are often straightforward.

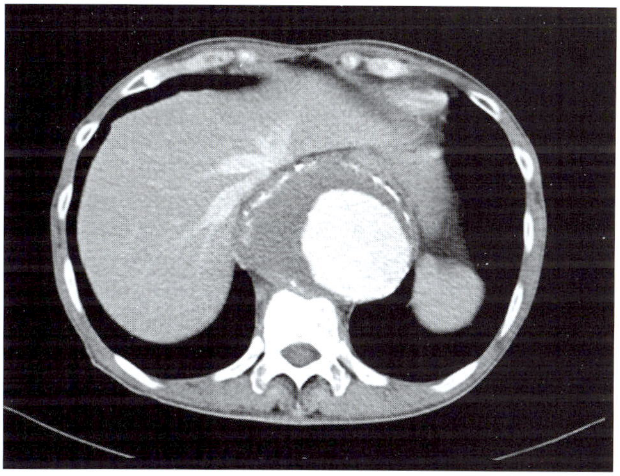

FIG. 24: Abdominal aortic aneurysm. Dynamic, contrast-enhanced axial CT image shows markedly dilated abdominal aorta with a large eccentric thrombus. A conventional angiogram on this patient would significantly underestimate the size of the aneurysm as only the patent part of the lumen containing flowing blood would be opacified.

Most ruptures are manifested as a retroperitoneal hematoma accompanied by an abdominal aortic aneurysm. Periaortic blood may extend into the perirenal space, the pararenal space, or both. Intraperitoneal extravasation may be an immediate or a delayed finding. Discontinuity of the aortic wall or a focal gap in otherwise continuous circumferential wall calcifications may point to the location of a rupture. There usually is a delay of several hours between the initial intramural hemorrhage and frank extravasation into the periaortic soft tissues. Contained or impending ruptures are more difficult to identify. A small amount of periaortic blood may be confused with the duodenum, perianeurysmal fibrosis or adenopathy. Imaging features suggestive of instability or impending rupture include increased aneurysm size, a low thrombus-to-lumen ratio, and hemorrhage into a mural thrombus. A peripheral crescent-shaped area of hyperattenuation within an abdominal aortic aneurysm represents an acute intramural hemorrhage and is another CT sign of impending rupture. Draping of the posterior aspect of an aneurysmal aorta over the vertebrae is associated with a contained rupture.[38]

The preferred surgical treatment of abdominal aortic aneurysms is an end-to-end anastomosis with aortic graft repair. Complications of abdominal aortic surgery that can be detected on CT include graft infections, aortoenteric fistulae, anastomotic aneurysms, graft leak or rupture.

Aortic Dissection

Aortic dissection usually originates in the thorax but sometimes extends into the abdomen. Mortality rate of untreated dissection is very high approaching 25% at 1 day, 50% at 1 week, and 75% at 1 month.[39] The strategy for therapy depends on the type of dissection, the site of entry, the extent of dissection, involvement of aortic branches, patency of the false lumen, and the presence of thrombus in the false lumen.

Currently, the noninvasive modalities that are most frequently used to identify aortic dissections are USG, CT, and MRI. USG including transthoracic echocardiography and transesophageal echocardiography, is widely available and can be performed quickly and easily at the bedside. Thus, USG can be used in most patients with aortic dissections, even in relatively unstable patients. However, USG has major shortcomings, namely, a limited field of view and a diagnostic accuracy that largely depends on the investigator's experience. Furthermore, USG does not provide images that can be used to plan therapy. Multidetector CT has the advantages of shorter scanning times, wide availability, and high diagnostic accuracy and has, therefore, classically been the modality of choice for the evaluation of aortic dissection. In the past, emergency MRI evaluation of aortic dissection has been impossible owing to prolonged examination times, but the advent of 3D contrast-enhanced MRA has changed this paradigm. Contrast-enhanced MRA has largely replaced unenhanced MR angiographic techniques and has dramatically shortened the total examination time required for confident diagnosis of aortic dissections; however, it is more suitable for stable patients. In principle, contrast-enhanced MRA is similar to CT angiography. Both modalities provide excellent evaluation of aortic dissections. In patients without contraindications for either modality, at most centers, the use of each modality is based on equipment availability, the personal preference of the radiologist or referring physician, and patient acceptance. Confident diagnosis and correct classification of aortic dissection is based on the detection of an intimal flap in the aorta that separates the true and false lumina **(Fig. 25)**. Such a flap manifests as a hypointense line with a linear, arc, or "S" shape in the axial plane. The true and false lumina can be differentiated on the basis of signal intensity, morphologic features, the relationship between the lumina, and the appearance of thrombosis.

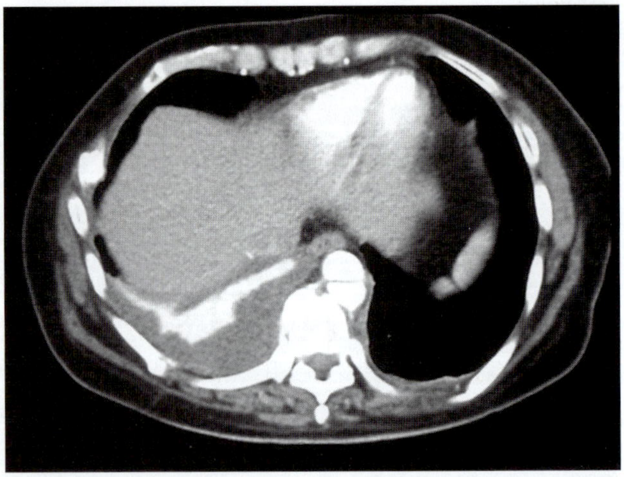

FIG. 25: Thoracoabdominal aortic dissection. Axial CT angiogram easily demonstrates the linear intimal flap between the anterior true lumen and posterior false lumen. Active extravasation into the retroperitoneum is also seen.

- *Signal intensity*: Similar to CT angiography, contrast-enhanced MRA shows the true lumen with higher signal intensity than the false lumen owing to a higher concentration of contrast material during the arterial phase.
- *Morphologic features*: The true lumen is usually smaller than the false lumen and would be thin or flat from being pressed, appearing oval in the axial plane.
- The false lumen is expanded or very large, appearing crescentic or winding around the true lumen in the axial plane.
- *Relationship between the lumina*: The lumina may be parallel to each other, the false lumen may wind around the true lumen, or the true lumen may look like a ribbon floating in the false lumen.
- *Appearance of thrombosis*: The false lumen usually contains a thrombus, especially at the retrograde end of the initial entry site, whereas the true lumen contains no thrombus in most cases.

Inferior Vena Cava

Mostly a routine CT or an MR abdominal protocol employing pre- and postcontrast SGE images provides sufficient evaluation of the IVC for patient management. At least one MR sequence should be performed in the sagittal or coronal plane, because it permits direct visualization of the longitudinal extent of IVC. However, when detailed evaluation of retroperitoneal veins is required, it is prudent to obtain CT or MR venography.

Congenital Anomalies

Congenital abnormalities of the IVC and related veins are common. Preoperative knowledge of the presence of these anomalies is helpful, particularly in patients undergoing a portosystemic shunt procedure, aortic surgery or nephrectomy, cytoreductive surgery, and reduces the risk of major venous hemorrhage associated with these anomalies.[40]

CT and MRI are well suited to determine whether rounded or tubular retroperitoneal structures are vascular in nature. Some of the developmental anomalies of IVC are: Interruption

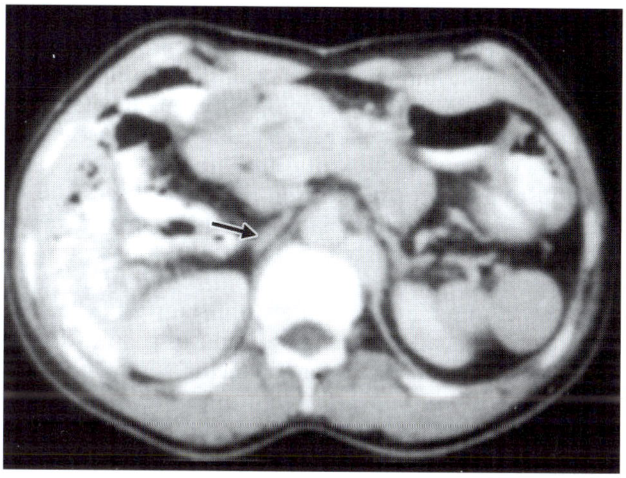

FIG. 26: Congenital polysplenia with IVC anomaly. CT scan shows multiple splenenculi and interrupted IVC with hemiazygos venous continuation. Linear density (arrow) seen lateral to the right crus is part of the right adrenal gland.

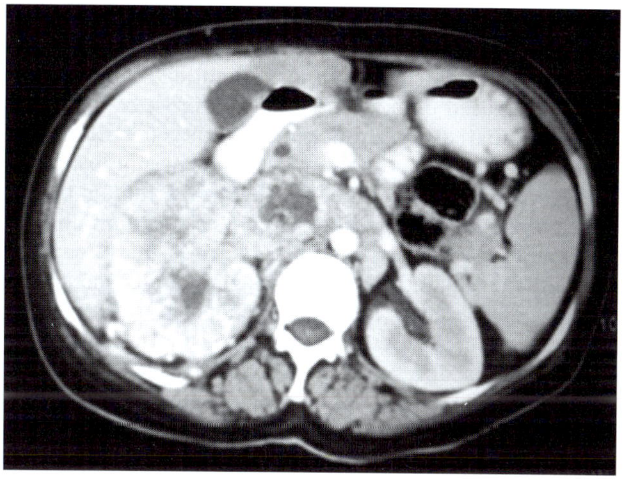

FIG. 27: IVC thrombus. Axial contrast-enhanced CT image in a 57-year-old man shows a large right renal cancer extending into the right renal vein and the IVC. The mass within the distended IVC is of the same attenuation as the primary tumor.

of IVC with azygos and hemiazygos vein continuation **(Fig. 26)**, left sided IVC, duplication of the IVC, and anomalies of the left renal vein, e.g. circumaortic or retroaortic left renal vein.[41]

Retrocaval ureter is thought to be due to persistence of right posterior cardinal vein with failure of development of the infrarenal right supracardinal vein. It occurs with a frequency of 0.2/1,000 population. In retrocaval ureter, the proximal right ureter courses medially behind the IVC, usually at L3 vertebral level and then courses anteriorly around the cava to partially encircle it. The anomaly is characterized by hydronephrosis and medial deviation (fish hook deformity) of the middle ureteral segment.

Venous Thrombosis

Inferior vena caval thrombus may result from proximal extension of thrombi from lower extremity, pelvis or renal veins. Intracaval tumor extension may occur via veins draining neoplasms such as renal cell carcinoma, hepatoma or adrenal carcinoma. CT and MRI perform well in evaluating IVC thrombosis and distinguishing tumor from bland thrombus.[42]

Tumor thrombus shows anatomic contiguity and an enhancement pattern identical to that of primary tumor **(Fig. 27)**. The bland thrombus does not enhance with contrast. Depiction of the supradiaphragmatic extent of the thrombus into the right atrium is important for surgical planning as it requires combined thoracoabdominal surgery, whereas thrombus that ends below the hepatic veins may require only an abdominal approach.[43]

In cases of chronic venous thrombosis, the affected vessel may not be identified if the thrombus is organized and contacted. In these cases careful evaluation reveals the absence of a vein in the expected location in combination with the presence of collateral vessels.

Retroperitoneal Fibrosis

Retroperitoneal fibrosis results from proliferation of fibrous tissue in the midline and para-aortic distribution. Approximately 70% cases of retroperitoneal fibrosis are idiopathic and are known as Ormond's disease. Other causes include various drugs (e.g. methysergide), previous abdominal surgery or radiation therapy, aortic hemorrhage, aortitis, aortic atherosclerosis, extravasation of urine, nonspecific gastrointestinal inflammation including appendicitis and diverticulitis, and infective pathologies including tuberculosis, histoplasmosis, syphilis, and actinomycosis. Retroperitoneal fibrosis may be a part of multifocal fibrosclerosis in which fibrous pseudotumor of the orbit, Riedel's thyroiditis, sclerosing cholangitis, and mediastinal fibrosis may also occur. Retroperitoneal malignancy especially metastases may also produce retroperitoneal fibrosis by producing a desmoplastic reaction to the tumor cells.[44]

Idiopathic retroperitoneal fibrosis most commonly occurs in patients between 40 years and 60 years of age. Males are affected twice as commonly as females. Fibrous plaque typically extends from below the level of the kidneys to the bifurcation of great vessels. The fibrous tissue may involve the IVC, aorta, ureters, and occasionally the iliac and renal veins in a symmetric or asymmetric distribution. Microscopically, collagen fibroblasts and inflammatory cells characterize idiopathic retroperitoneal fibrosis.

The clinical and laboratory findings of idiopathic retroperitoneal fibrosis are nonspecific and include fever, back pain, and raised erythrocyte sedimentation rate. Most patients have impaired renal functions. Excretory urography typically demonstrates bilateral hydronephrosis, which may be asymmetric and sometimes even unilateral. Retrograde studies demonstrate smooth tapering of the ureters that is most pronounced at the pelvic brim **(Fig. 28)**. The involvement may vary from focal to a long segment of ureter. Despite ureteral narrowing, there is no obstruction to retrograde passage of catheter in the ureter.

Ultrasonography demonstrates retroperitoneal fibrosis as a poorly demarcated periaortic mass that is typically echo-free or hypoechoic. Associated hydronephrosis may be seen. CT appearance of the fibrous plaque varies considerably—it can be midline or asymmetric, well circumscribed or poorly defined, localized or extensive **(Figs. 29A to C)**.

Contrast enhancement varies with the age of the process, while increased enhancement is seen in early stages due to vascularity of the immature fibrosis, chronic fibrosis does not enhance appreciably. MRI may permit distinction between benign or non-neoplastic retroperitoneal fibrosis and malignant retroperitoneal fibrosis. In nonmalignant retroperitoneal fibrosis low or intermediate signal intensity on T1- and T2-weighted images has been reported in contrast to higher signal intensity in most malignancies on T2-weighted images **(Fig. 30)**. However, it has been recognized that benign retroperitoneal fibrosis also can have high signal intensity on T2-weighted images when it is in the active, inflammatory stage. MRI also demonstrates effect of the fibrotic mass on the aorta and IVC.

Iliopsoas Muscle Compartment

Diseases affecting the iliopsoas muscle more commonly originate from adjacent structures and involve the muscle by direct extension. These include hemorrhage, infections, and tumors of the spine, kidneys, bowel, pancreas, and retroperitoneal lymph nodes. The iliopsoas is well evaluated by both CT and MRI. Coronal or sagittal planes provide direct evaluation of the full craniocaudal extent of the muscle.

Tuberculous spondylitis and lumbar discitis are the most common causes of an iliopsoas abscess in our country. Iliopsoas inflammatory masses display a variety of appearances, ranging from diffuse homogeneous enlargement to discrete masses containing central areas of low CT attenuation or high signal intensity on T2-weighted MR images. Postcontrast images show abscesses as expansile lesions with nonenhancing necrotic centers, intense peripheral enhancement, and enhancement of the surrounding tissues **(Figs. 31A and B)**. Calcification is detected occasionally on CT in inflammatory masses, particularly in patients with tuberculosis. MRI scores over CT in detecting intraspinal extension of the inflammatory granulation tissue and cord compression.

Neoplastic involvement of psoas muscle may occur with contiguous spread from metastatic lymph nodes from primary

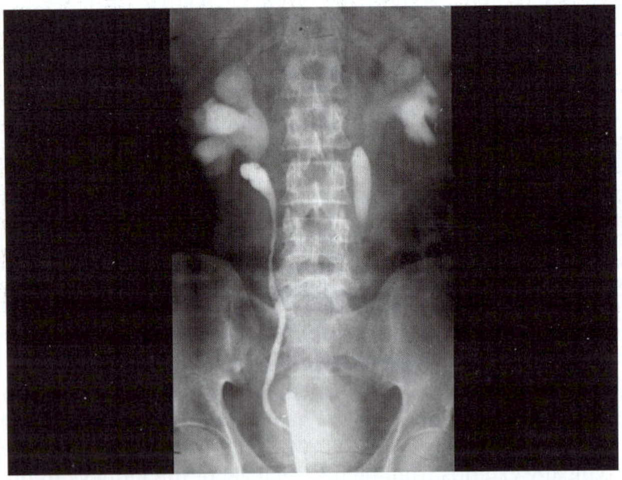

FIG. 28: Retrograde pyelography showing medial deviation of both ureters with hydroureteronephrosis in a patient with idiopathic retroperitoneal fibrosis.

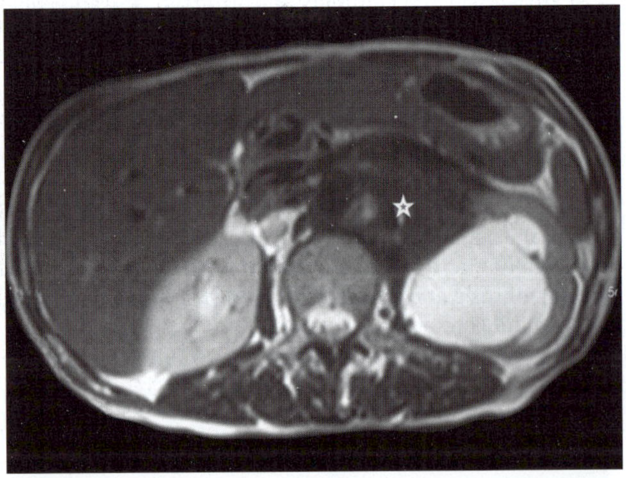

FIG. 30: Retroperitoneal fibrosis. Axial T2-weighted MR image shows a very hypointense mass (star), a finding consistent with the presence of mature fibrous tissue with little or no active inflammation.

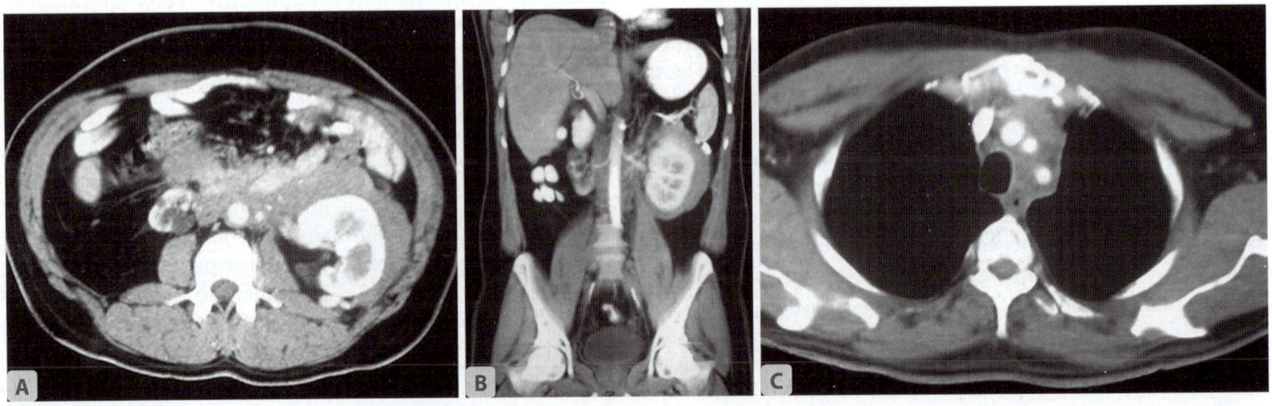

FIGS. 29A TO C: Retroperitoneal fibrosis. (A) Contrast-enhanced axial CT image shows hypodense, nonenhancing, infiltrating mass surrounding the aorta and IVC and extending into the left perirenal space. Right kidney is shrunken and hydronephrotic; (B) Coronal image shows the entire extent of the plaque like, perirenal soft tissue. Appearance is nonspecific, and differentials include malignancy such as lymphoma. Diagnosis was confirmed by biopsy; (C) CT scan though the chest shows evidence of mediastinal fibrosis, a frequent association of retroperitoneal fibrosis.

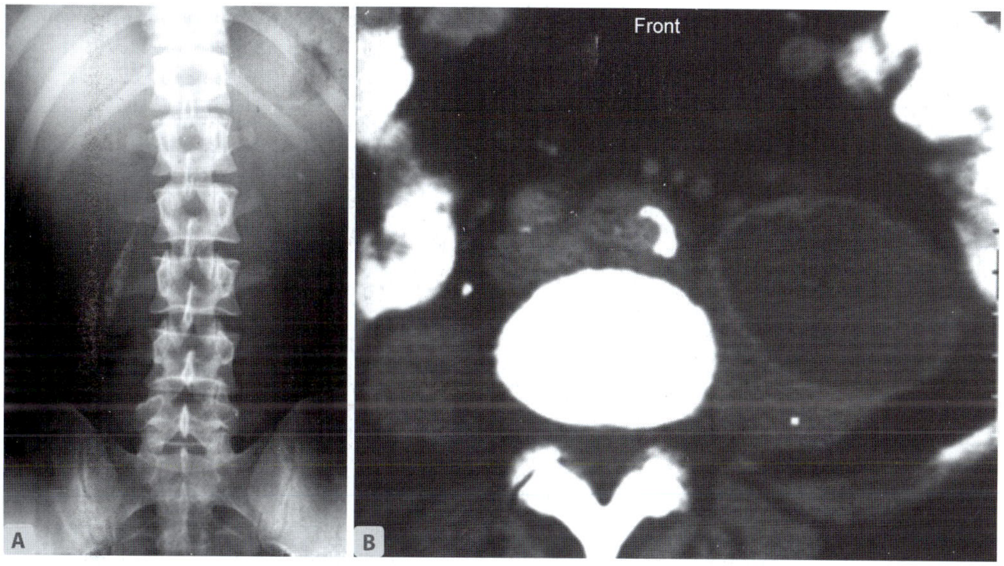

FIGS. 31A AND B: Psoas abscess. CT images show a well-defined, fluid density lesion in the left psoas muscle. It has a thin, peripheral enhancing rim and large necrotic center.

neoplasms (of kidney, testis, bladder, and cervix), lymphoma, renal cell carcinoma, and retroperitoneal sarcoma. Primary neoplasms of the psoas muscle are rare. Iliopsoas malignancies often appear similar to other pathologies on imaging. The affected muscle is usually enlarged.

As with abscesses, iliopsoas tumor may have enhancing peripheral rims and central necrosis **(Fig. 32)**. A specific diagnosis is possible only when a large solid enhancing component is seen.

To conclude, RP is complex anatomical structure composed of multiple compartments, fascias, and planes. Better understanding of its anatomy helps in approaching retroperitoneal abnormalities and thus assist in planning further management. Sarcomas is the most common primary RP neoplasm and among non-neoplastic etiologies, inflammatory collections are the most common pathology encountered.

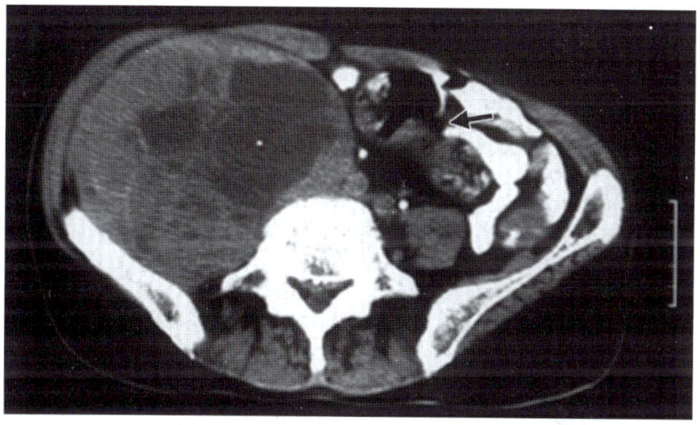

FIG. 32: Anaplastic carcinoma iliopsoas. Axial CT image shows a large heterogeneous mass involving the right iliacus muscle. The large, irregular, solid component (arrow) within the mass raises a possibility of malignancy.

REFERENCES

1. Coffin A, Boulay-Coletta I, Sebbag-Sfez D, et al. Radioanatomy of the retroperitoneal space. Diagn Interv Imaging. 2015; 96(2): 171-86.
2. Tirkes T, Sandrasegaran K, Patel AA, et al. Peritoneal and retroperitoneal anatomy and its relevance for cross-sectional imaging. Radiographics. 2012;32(2):437-51.
3. Korobkin M, Silverman PM, Quint LE, et al. CT of the extraperitoneal space: normal anatomy and fluid collections. Am J Roentgenol. 1992;159(5):933-42.
4. Raptopoulos V, Kleinman PK, Marks S, et al. Renal fascial pathway: posterior extension of pancreatic effusions within the anterior pararenal space. Radiology. 1986;158(2):367-74.
5. Molmenti EP, Balfe DM, Kanterman RY, et al. Anatomy of the retroperitoneum: observations of the distribution of pathologic fluid collections. Radiology. 1996;200(1):95-103.
6. Raptopoulos V, Lei QF, Touliopoulos P, et al. Why perirenal disease does not extend into the pelvis: the importance of closure of the cone of the renal fasciae. Am J Roentgenol. 1995;164(5):1179-84.
7. Aizenstein RI, Owens C, Sabnis S, et al. The perinephric space and renal fascia: review of normal anatomy, pathology, and pathways of disease spread. Crit Rev Diagn Imaging. 1997;38(4):325-67.
8. Gore RM, Balfe DM, Aizenstein RI, et al. The great escape: interfascial decompression planes of the retroperitoneum. Am J Roentgenol. 2000;175(2):363-70.
9. Kang PS, Spain JW. Multidetector CT angiography of the abdomen. Radiol Clin North Am. 2005;43(6):963-76, vii.
10. Kandpal H, Sharma R, Gamangatti S, et al. Imaging the inferior vena cava: a road less traveled. Radiogr Rev Publ Radiol Soc N Am Inc. 2008;28(3):669-89.
11. Glockner JF. Three-dimensional gadolinium-enhanced MR angiography: applications for abdominal imaging. Radiogr Rev Publ Radiol Soc N Am Inc. 2001;21(2):357-70.
12. Vesselle HJ, Miraldi FD. FDG PET of the retroperitoneum: normal anatomy, variants, pathologic conditions, and strategies to avoid diagnostic pitfalls. Radiogr Rev Publ Radiol Soc N Am Inc. 1998;18(4):805-23; discussion 823-824.

13. Messiou C, Moskovic E, Vanel D, et al. Primary retroperitoneal soft tissue sarcoma: Imaging appearances, pitfalls and diagnostic algorithm. Eur J Surg Oncol. 2017;43(7):1191-8.
14. Sanyal R, Remer EM. Radiology of the retroperitoneum: case-based review. Am J Roentgenol. 2009;192: S112-7.Available from: https://www.ajronline.org/doi/full/10.2214/AJR.07.7064. [Last accessed, October, 2019]
15. Nishino M, Hayakawa K, Minami M, et al. Primary retroperitoneal neoplasms: CT and MR imaging findings with anatomic and pathologic diagnostic clues. Radiographics. 2003;23(1):45-57.
16. Goenka AH, Shah SN, Remer EM. Imaging of the retroperitoneum. Radiol Clin North Am. 2012;50(2):333-55.
17. Craig WD, Fanburg-Smith JC, Henry LR, et al. Fat-containing lesions of the retroperitoneum: radiologic-pathologic correlation. Radiographics. 2009;29(1):261-90.
18. Kumar A, Suman SK, Kumar B, et al. Giant retroperitoneal liposarcoma: imaging and literature. Journal of Evolution of Medical and Dental Sciences. 2015;4(36):6315-22. Available from: https://www.jemds.com/latest-articles.php?at_id=7673. [Last accessed October, 2019]
19. Song T, Shen J, Liang BL, et al. Retroperitoneal liposarcoma: MR characteristics and pathological correlative analysis. Abdom Imaging. 2007;32(5):668-74.
20. Hartman DS, Hayes WS, Choyke PL, et al. From the archives of the AFIP. Leiomyosarcoma of the retroperitoneum and inferior vena cava: radiologic-pathologic correlation. Radiogr Rev Publ Radiol Soc N Am Inc. 1992;12(6):1203-20.
21. Monteagudo Cortecero J, Guirau Rubio MD, Payá Romá A. Leiomyosarcoma of the inferior vena cava: AIRP best cases in radiologic-pathologic correlation. Radiographics. 2015;35(2): 616-20.
22. Cohan RH, Baker ME, Cooper C, et al. Computed tomography of primary retroperitoneal malignancies. J Comput Assist Tomogr. 1988;12(5):804-10.
23. Lee KY, Oh Y-W, Noh HJ, et al. Extraadrenal paragangliomas of the body: imaging features. Am J Roentgenol. 2006; 187(2): 492-504.
24. Rha SE, Byun JY, Jung SE, et al. Neurogenic tumors in the abdomen: tumor types and imaging characteristics. Radiographics. 2003;23(1):29-43.
25. Hulnick DH, Megibow AJ, Naidich DP, et al. Abdominal tuberculosis: CT evaluation. Radiology. 1985;157(1):199-204.
26. Warshauer DM, Lee JKT. Imaging manifestations of abdominal sarcoidosis. Am J Roentgenol. 2004;182(1):15-28.
27. Gossios K, Nikolaides C, Bai M, et al. Widespread Castleman disease: CT findings. Eur Radiol. 1996;6(1):95-8.
28. Kehagias D, Pafiti A, Vaos N, et al. Retroperitoneal lymphangioleiomyomatosis: CT appearance. Eur Radiol. 1998;8(3):471-3.
29. Sheth S, Fishman EK. Non-Hodgkin lymphoma: pattern of disease at spiral CT. Crit Rev Diagn Imaging. 2001;42(6): 307-56.
30. Apter S, Avigdor A, Gayer G, et al. Calcification in lymphoma occurring before therapy: CT features and clinical correlation. Am J Roentgenol. 2002;178(4):935-8.
31. Schöder H, Moskowitz C. PET imaging for response assessment in lymphoma: potential and limitations. Radiol Clin North Am. 2008;46(2):225-41, viii.
32. Specht L. 2-[18F]fluoro-2-deoxyglucose positron-emission tomography in staging, response evaluation, and treatment planning of lymphomas. Semin Radiat Oncol. 2007;17(3):190-7.
33. Radin R. HIV infection: analysis in 259 consecutive patients with abnormal abdominal CT findings. Radiology. 1995; 197(3): 712-22.
34. Bellin MF, Lebleu L, Meric JB. Evaluation of retroperitoneal and pelvic lymph node metastases with MRI and MR lymphangiography. Abdom Imaging. 2003;28(2):155-63.
35. Ishikawa K, Idoguchi K, Tanaka H, et al. Classification of acute pancreatitis based on retroperitoneal extension: application of the concept of interfascial planes. Eur J Radiol. 2006;60(3):445-52.
36. Missiroli C, Singh AK. Nontraumatic emergencies of abdominal aorta. Semin Ultrasound CT MR. 2008;29(5): 369-77.
37. Taneja K, Sharma S, Das B, et al. Aortic aneurysm and dissection: Imaging with computerised axial tomography. Indian J Thorac Cardiovasc Surg. 1994;10(1):52-6.
38. Rakita D, Newatia A, Hines JJ, et al. Spectrum of CT findings in rupture and impending rupture of abdominal aortic aneurysms. Radiogr Rev Publ Radiol Soc N Am Inc. 2007;27(2): 497-507.
39. Anagnostopoulos CE, Prabhakar MJ, Kittle CF. Aortic dissections and dissecting aneurysms. Am J Cardiol. 1972;30(3): 263-73.
40. Aljabri B, MacDonald PS, Satin R, et al. Incidence of major venous and renal anomalies relevant to aortoiliac surgery as demonstrated by computed tomography. Ann Vasc Surg. 2001;15(6):615-8.
41. Onbaş O, Kantarci M, Koplay M, et al. Congenital anomalies of the aorta and vena cava: 16-detector-row CT imaging findings. Diagn Interv Radiol Ank Turk. 2008;14(3):163-71.
42. Cuevas C, Raske M, Bush WH, et al. Imaging primary and secondary tumor thrombus of the inferior vena cava: multi-detector computed tomography and magnetic resonance imaging. Curr Probl Diagn Radiol. 2006;35(3):90-101.
43. Lawrentschuk N, Gani J, Riordan R, et al. Multidetector computed tomography vs magnetic resonance imaging for defining the upper limit of tumour thrombus in renal cell carcinoma: a study and review. BJU Int. 2005;96(3): 291-5.
44. Cronin CG, Lohan DG, Blake MA, et al. Retroperitoneal Fibrosis: A Review of Clinical Features and Imaging Findings. Am J Roentgenol. 2008;191(2):423-31.

CHAPTER

25

Urinary Tract Trauma

Atin Kumar, Shivanand Gamanagatti

INTRODUCTION

Approximately 10% of all traumatic injuries involve the urinary tract, most often the kidney.[1] Although trauma to the urinary tract is seldom the cause of death, serious morbidity can result, if such injuries are missed. An accurate radiographic and imaging evaluation is important to determine the presence and extent of injury for the proper management of the patients. Evaluation of the urinary tract trauma should be integrated into the overall management of the trauma patient.

Blunt trauma accounts for 80–90% of all renal injuries.[1] These are primarily due to deceleration injuries in motor vehicle accidents, falls, or assault. In approximately 10–20% of the patients, penetrating injuries result due to gunshot or knife wounds. The penetrating injuries are much more likely to result in high-grade renal injuries compared with blunt trauma. Pre-existing kidney lesions, e.g. renal tumors, hydronephrosis, polycystic kidney disease, and horseshoe kidneys, make the kidney more susceptible to the injury. In 80% of the patients with penetrating trauma and 75% of blunt trauma patients, associated injuries, e.g. splenic rupture, liver laceration, and injuries to the small and large bowel, are seen.[2] In about 50% of these patients, bone fractures are present. Iatrogenic causes such as surgery, interventional procedures, and biopsies are also associated with trauma to the urinary tract.

RENAL TRAUMA

Since the late 1980s, the prevailing techniques of imaging and clinical management of renal trauma have changed dramatically. Consensus has been building toward a conservative approach and successful clinical management must be based on an accurate assessment of the extent of injury.

Imaging Work-up in a Patient with Suspected Renal Trauma

Trauma to the kidney may be suspected to be minor or significant on the basis of clinical picture, nature, and site of injury. An unstable patient may undergo no imaging work-up, if an immediate surgery is indicated on clinical grounds. In a clinically stable patient with abdominal trauma and with suspected abdominal organ injury and/or hypotension, kidneys are imaged as part of a standard abdomen and pelvic computed tomography (CT). The current globally accepted indications specifically for radiological evaluation of urinary tract in trauma patients are as follows:[2–6]

- Macroscopic hematuria (visible to human eye)
- Microscopic hematuria (>5 RBC/high power field) with hypotension (systolic BP < 90 mm Hg at any time during evaluation) or other significant abdominal injuries which necessitate imaging
- Injuries associated with renal injury such as direct contusion or hematoma of flank soft tissues, fractures of lumbar spine, lower rib, and transverse process
- Penetrating trauma with any degree of hematuria in stable patients.

Earlier, children with any degree of hematuria were also an indication for radiological evaluation, but recently there has been a trend to have an approach similar to an adult patient. Renal imaging is not required in a patient with minor trauma having microhematuria without shock.

An approach to a patient having significant trauma can be outlined as shown in **Flowchart 1**.

Role of Radiography (Plain Radiographs)

Widespread availability and use of CT and ultrasound have replaced abdominal radiography for evaluation of renal trauma. However, radiographs have a role in the setting of penetrating abdominal trauma.

Role of Ultrasound

Specific visceral injuries are poorly assessed on ultrasonography. The value of sonography lies primarily in the rapid establishment of the presence of hemoperitoneum in an unstable patient.

In the setting of abdominal trauma, it is usually done with Focused Assessment with Sonography in Trauma (FAST) protocol. It is insensitive to detect retroperitoneal blood and renal parenchymal injuries.

FLOWCHART 1: Imaging work-up in suspected renal trauma.

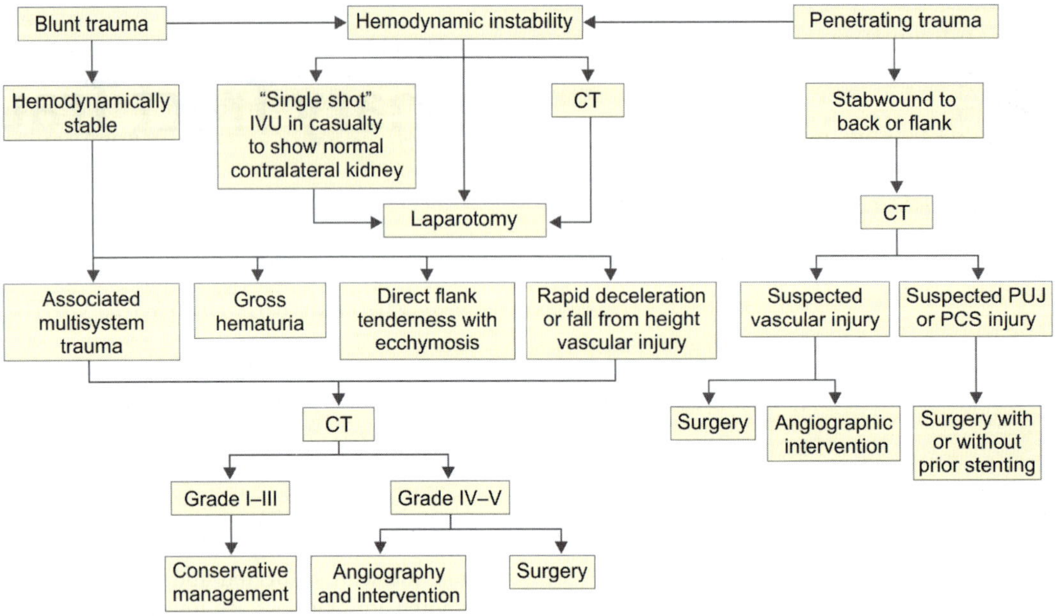

(PUJ: pelviureteric junction; PCS: postconcussion syndrome)

Role of Intravenous Urography

The role of intravenous urogram (IVU) in suspected renal trauma is limited. It has been replaced by CT which is now easily available and is more sensitive than IVU for parenchymal injuries, urinary contrast extravasation, and other abdominal injuries. However, IVU still has a role, depending on the preference of the surgeon, to establish gross function and evaluation of the uninjured contralateral kidney in hemodynamically unstable patients going for surgery and for urological evaluation of patients who are already in the operating room.[2,3] The technique followed is usually a tailored "single-shot" study with a radiograph obtained 10 minutes after administration of intravenous contrast. However, if time and condition of the patient permit, a precontrast plain radiograph, and delayed radiographs may be taken for assessment of urinary contrast extravasation and for delayed function.

Role of Computed Tomography

The contrast-enhanced CT (CECT) scan is currently the investigation of choice for radiological evaluation of patients with blunt abdominal trauma.[4,5] It has replaced IVU for evaluation of renal trauma. The current trend of conservative management of blunt renal trauma has further enhanced the role of CT because 80% of renal injuries seen on CT are self-limiting.

Computed tomography accurately assesses all the criteria essential for the management of renal trauma, viz. extent of damaged nonviable tissue, amount of perirenal hemorrhage, extravasation of urine, and evidence of renal pedicle or vascular injury.

The CT of abdomen and pelvis (along with chest) is usually done in a hemodynamically stable patient who is being evaluated for any suspected abdominal injury. Many institutions routinely do a dual-phase CECT with arterial and portal venous phase. However, some other institutions follow the practice of doing a standard portal venous phase after contrast administration with another delayed phase, if indicated, based on the findings on this phase for suspected vascular injury. At our institution which is a grade 1 trauma center, we routinely do a dual (arterial and venous) phase CT in all patients in whom the index of clinical suspicion for finding a solid organ injury is high. Essentially, these patients are those who are FAST positive with or without signs of shock. In patients with a low index of suspicion where the CT is being done for ruling out organ injuries, we routinely perform a single portal venous phase. These are most commonly FAST negative. In these patients, we acquire an immediate delayed phase after the portal venous phase if we find any suspicion of vascular injury on the portal venous phase images. In both the groups of patients who show renal lacerations extending up to the pelvicalyceal system, we acquire a 3–5 min delayed limited acquisition through the kidneys for detection of pelvicalyceal contrast extravasation.

Multiplanar reformatted images and three-dimensional images including CT urographic images can significantly aid in the evaluation.

Role of Angiography

Catheter angiography is not indicated as a diagnostic test in patients with renal trauma. However, in the last two decades, there is an increasing role of therapeutic angiographic interventions as a nonsurgical therapy in the form of transcatheter embolization of ongoing hemorrhage in renal trauma in hemodynamically stable patients. Angioembolization is indicated for vascular complications of injury including post-traumatic pseudoaneurysms and arteriovenous fistulas. In certain situations of acute traumatic main renal artery thrombosis, thrombolysis of renal artery thrombus with vascular stent placement can be done provided the time to injury is very short (less than 2 hours) or there is a solitary functioning kidney.

Role of Retrograde Pyelography

Retrograde pyelography has a role in the specific setting of suspected renal pelvic, ureteropelvic junction (UPJ), or ureteral injury, which has not been adequately excluded on CT. However, it is often not practically possible in an emergent situation and also does not characterize renal injuries.

Role of Radionuclide Renal Scintigraphy

With widespread availability of CT, radionuclide scintigraphy is rarely used in an acute trauma setting. It may have a role in demonstrating the function of an injured kidney in patients allergic to iodinated contrast and in follow-up of repair of renovascular trauma.

Role of Magnetic Resonance Imaging

Magnetic resonance imaging may have a role in patients where CT is contraindicated or not available. However, it is usually not practical in an acute trauma setting. It can demonstrate renal parenchymal injuries as well as renal function after contrast administration.

Radiological Findings

The most commonly accepted grading system of traumatic renal injuries is the Organ Injury Scale (OIS) given by the American Association for the Surgery of Trauma (AAST). The original grading scale for renal injuries was given in 1989 and has been revised in 2018.[7,8] The grading is based on the depth of injury and involvement of vessels or the collecting system.[7] The AAST 2018 OIS for renal injuries[8] classifies the renal trauma into five grades as follows.

Grade 1

Grade 1 renal injuries account for approximately 75–80% of all renal injuries. They include the following:

- *Contusion:* Focal ill-defined area of hypodensity, which shows decreased enhancement as compared to adjacent normal renal parenchyma **(Figs. 1A and B)**. These are better appreciated on the portal venous phase which corresponds to the parenchymal phase for the kidneys. On the arterial phase images (which correspond to the corticomedullary phase for the kidneys), the detection of contusion may be limited as there is suboptimal enhancement of renal pyramids. They need to be differentiated from segmental infarcts which constitute grade 4 renal injury. Contusions generally are rounded in shape with ill-defined margins and show some contrast enhancement, especially on the delayed phase. In contrast, segmental infarcts are wedge shaped with well-defined margins and do not show any contrast enhancement even on the delayed phase. A global contusion may show a striated nephrogram or spidery collecting system (due to parenchymal edema).[9,10]
- *Subcapsular hematoma:* A hyperattenuating [40–60 Hounsfield unit (HU)] fluid collection lying between the renal parenchyma and the renal capsule. It leads to mass effect over the underlying renal parenchyma resulting in flattening of its contour **(Figs. 2A and B)**. It does not enhance on contrast administration.

Grade 2

Grade 2 renal injuries include the following:

- *Perirenal hematoma:* An ill-defined hyperattenuating fluid collection in perinephric space between the renal parenchyma and Gerota's fascia **(Figs. 3A and B)**. It occurs after laceration of the renal capsule.
- *Laceration:* A superficial (<1 cm deep), irregular or linear, low-attenuation area within the renal parenchyma which may contain blood or clot. It does not enhance after contrast administration. The laceration does not extend to the collecting system.

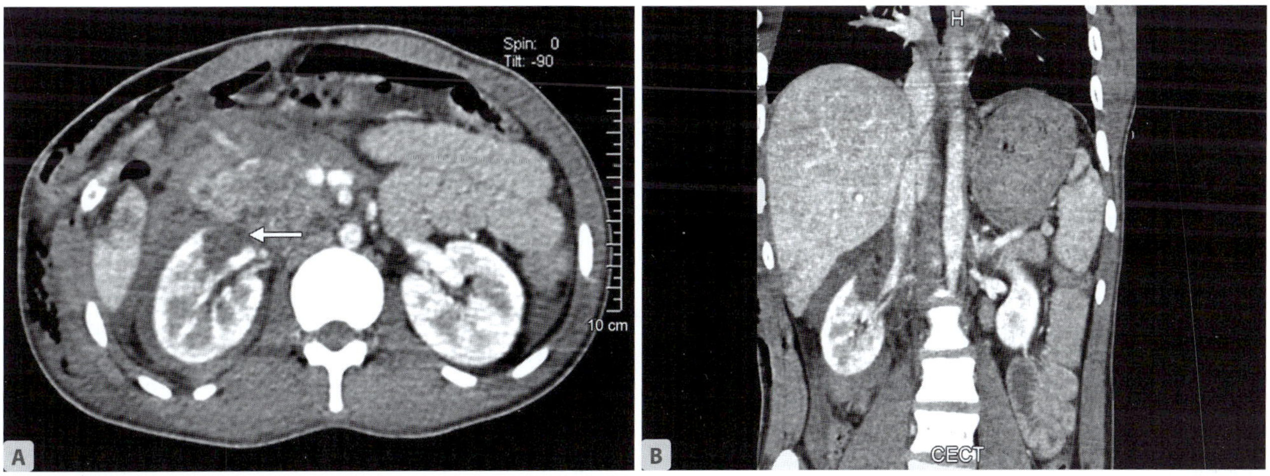

FIGS. 1A AND B: Axial (A) and multiformatted coronal (B) CECT shows a focal hypodense area (arrow) in anterior part of right kidney suggestive of contusion.

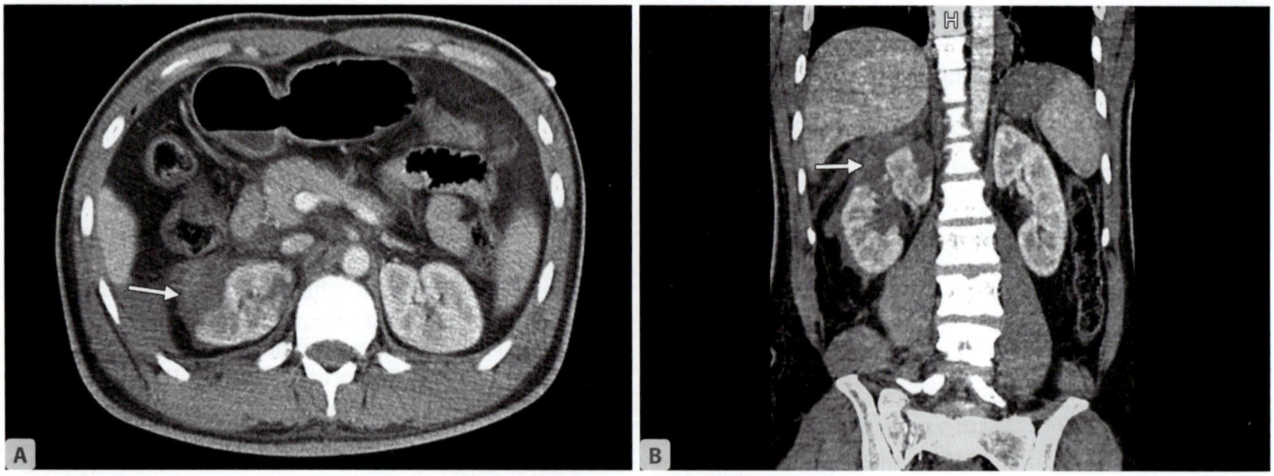

FIGS. 2A AND B: Axial (A) and multiformatted coronal (B) CECT shows a hyperdense nonenhancing subcapsular hematoma (arrows).

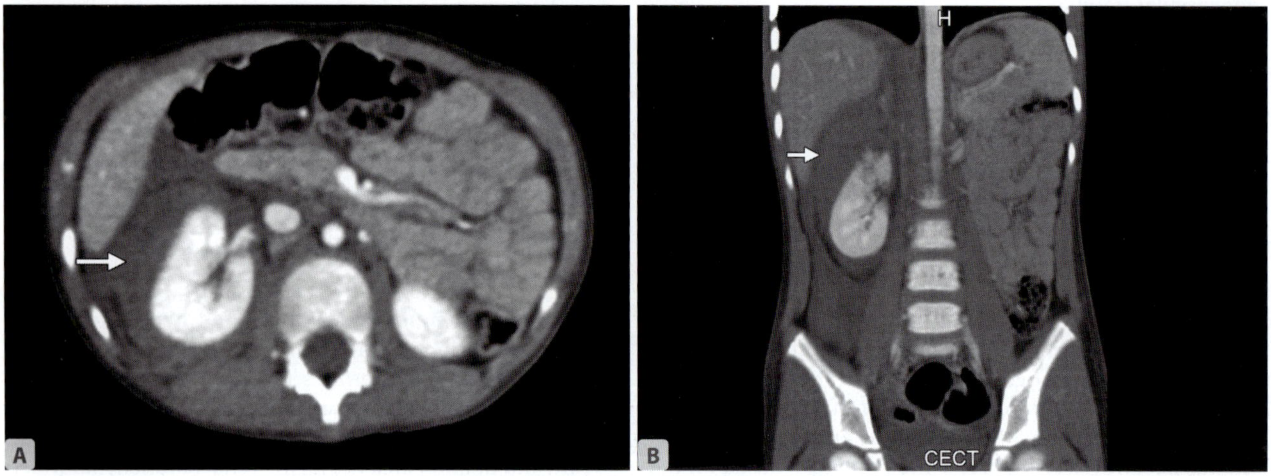

FIGS. 3A AND B: Axial (A) and multiformatted coronal (B) CECT shows perinephric hematoma (arrows) around right kidney.

Grade 3

Grade 3 renal injuries include the following:

- *Lacerations:* >1 cm in depth but do not involve the collecting system **(Fig. 4)**. The lacerations may be reaching very close to the collecting system. The integrity of the collecting system can be ascertained by evaluating the excretory phase images which do not show extravasation of urinary contrast.
- *Vascular injury:* A contained vascular injury (pseudoaneurysm or arteriovenous fistula) or active bleeding limited within Gerota's fascia. The vascular injury is classified under grade 3, if there are no other associated features to upgrade the renal injury. These injuries are included new in the revised 2018 version and were not present in an earlier version of the OIS scale.

Grade 4

Grade 4 renal injuries include the following:

- *Lacerations:* Deep lacerations extending through the kidney parenchyma into the collecting system. It leads to extravasation of urine and urinary contrast. Delayed phase CT in the excretory phase is important to demonstrate urinary contrast extravasation **(Figs. 5A to D)**. The lacerations may also involve the renal pelvis or the UPJ. If there is complete ureteropelvic avulsion, then urinary contrast extravasation is seen medial to the kidney without opacification of the ureter **(Figs. 6A and B)**. Opacification of the ureter in this setting would indicate a partial disruption of the pelviureteric junction (PUJ). Retrograde pyelography may be required for definitive diagnosis to demonstrate the distal ureter if CT or IVU fail to demonstrate distal ureteric filling.
- *Vascular injury:* Segmental renal artery or vein intimal injury/thrombus
- *Infarction:* Segmental or complete. It occurs due to dissection, thrombosis, or laceration of the segmental or main renal artery. On CT, segmental infarct is seen as a peripheral-based, well-circumscribed, wedge-shaped focal nonenhancing area through the renal parenchyma in a radial or segmental orientation **(Figs. 7A and B)**. The main renal artery thrombosis occurs due to stretching of

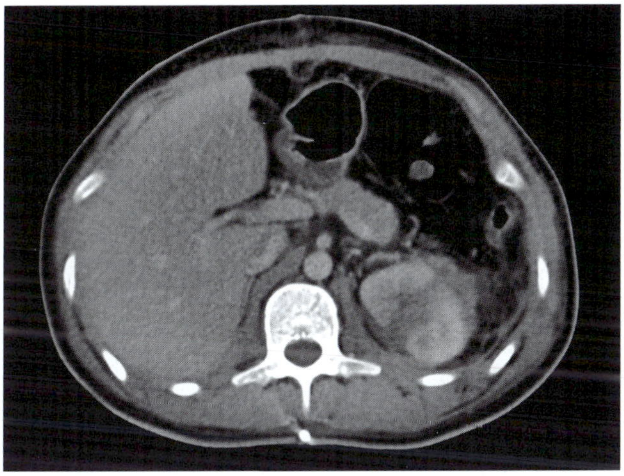

FIG. 4: Axial CECT abdomen shows a linear hypodense nonenhancing laceration involving upper pole of left kidney.

the renal artery between the artery origin anchored to aorta and mobile kidney. This leads to an intimal tear with subsequent thrombosis. CT reveals abrupt termination of the renal artery after its origin with nonenhancing renal parenchyma except for a cortical rim sign, which usually appears few days later, and retrograde opacification of renal vein from IVC **(Figs. 8A and B)**. Devascularization without active bleeding adjacent to the kidney should be classified as grade 4. The role of renal angiography with thrombolysis is not well established. It may be done in selected cases, ideally within a couple of hours after trauma.[9] The time window can be extended till 12–24 hours in a patient with only one kidney or bilateral renal artery thrombosis.

- *Active bleeding:* Uncontained hemorrhage secondary to injury of segmental or main renal vessels extending outside the confines of Gerota's fascia into the retroperitoneum or peritoneum.

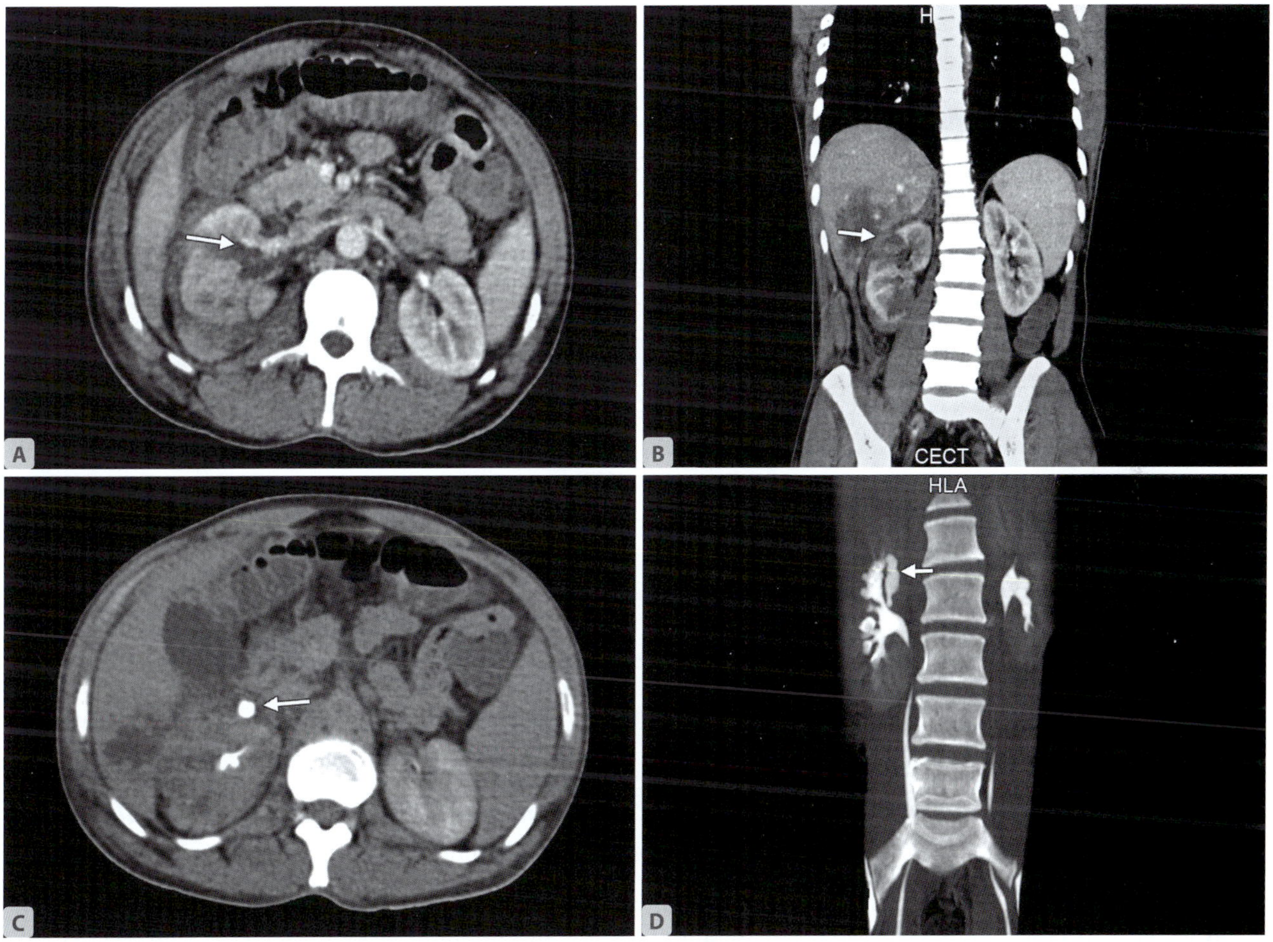

FIGS. 5A TO D: Axial (A) and multiformatted coronal (B) CECT shows a deep laceration (arrows) in upper pole of right kidney extending into pelvicalyceal system with perinephric hematoma. Delayed phase axial CT (C) shows contrast lying outside the kidney on its anterior aspect signifying urinary contrast extravasation. Reformatted coronal MIP image (D) clearly shows the extravasated contrast from upper calyceal injury.

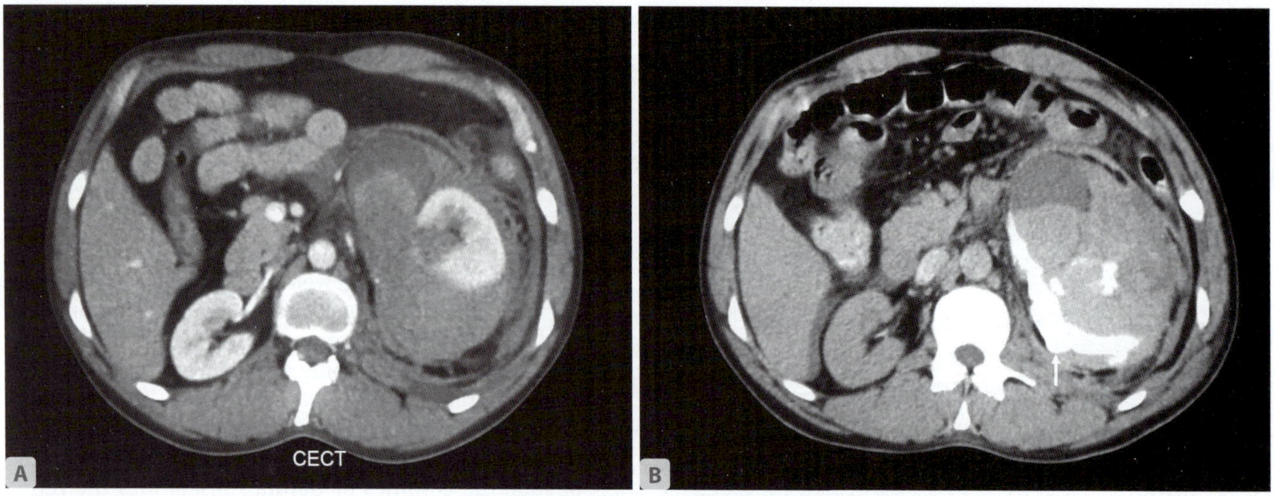

FIGS. 6A AND B: Axial CECT abdomen (A) shows extensive left perirenal hematoma/fluid collection. Delayed phase axial image (B) shows urinary contrast extravasation in medial perinephric space (arrow) signifying renal pelvic avulsion.

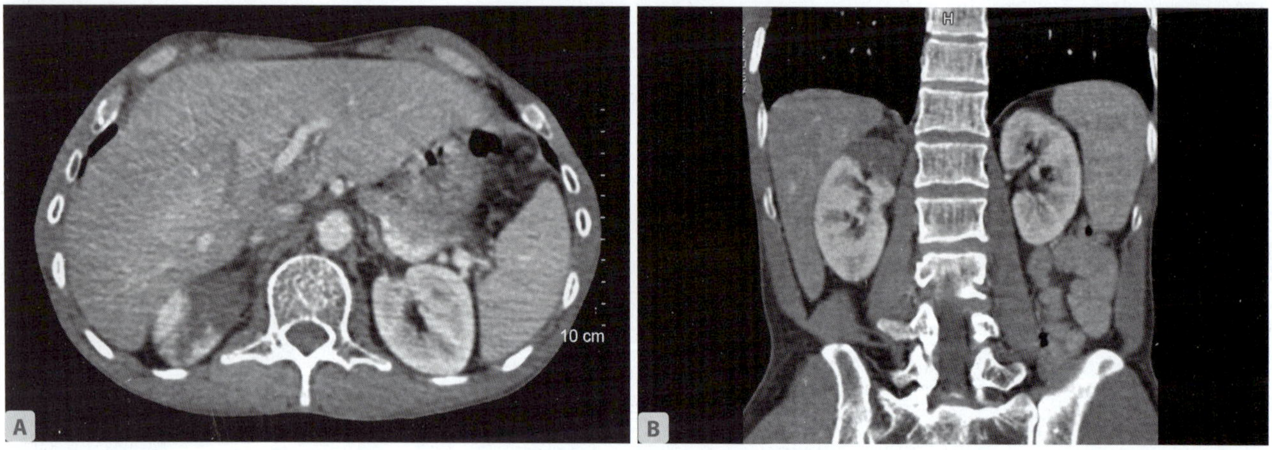

FIGS. 7A AND B: Axial (A) and multiformatted coronal (B) CECT shows a well-defined peripheral based wedge-shaped nonenhancing area in upper pole of right kidney suggestive of a segmental infarct.

Grade 5

Grade 5 renal injuries include the following:

- *Shattered kidney:* It refers to gross renal parenchymal disruption secondary to multiple renal lacerations associated with devitalized areas due to renal infarction **(Figs. 9A and B)**. There is often loss of identifiable renal parenchymal anatomy.
- Main renal artery or vein laceration or avulsion injuries at hilum.
- *Devascularized kidney with active bleeding:* It occurs secondary to the main renal arterial laceration or avulsion. This is seen on imaging as extravasation of vascular contrast into the perirenal region with a large hematoma in the medial compartment close to the hilum **(Figs. 10A to C)**. It is important to differentiate it from the main renal artery thrombosis without laceration or avulsion which also leads to devascularized kidney and is classified under grade 4 injury. Presence of active bleed/hematoma adjacent to the main renal artery signifies avulsion making it grade 5 injury. Renal vein injury is seen on CT as intraluminal thrombus with features of renal vein occlusion including increased size of kidney, diminished or delayed enhancement and delayed excretion **(Figs. 11A and B)**.

For bilateral injuries, one grade has to be advanced up to grade 3.

Renal Trauma with Pre-existing Abnormality

A kidney harboring a preexisting abnormality is at more risk for injury in blunt abdominal trauma, especially in children.[11] Hydronephrosis or extrarenal pelvis is at more risk of rupture. Cysts and tumors can also frequently hemorrhage after trauma.

An ectopic or horseshoe kidney is also more prone to trauma because it is less protected **(Figs. 12A and B)**.

Management

The classification of renal trauma into grades correlates with the need for surgery. In general, the trend is toward

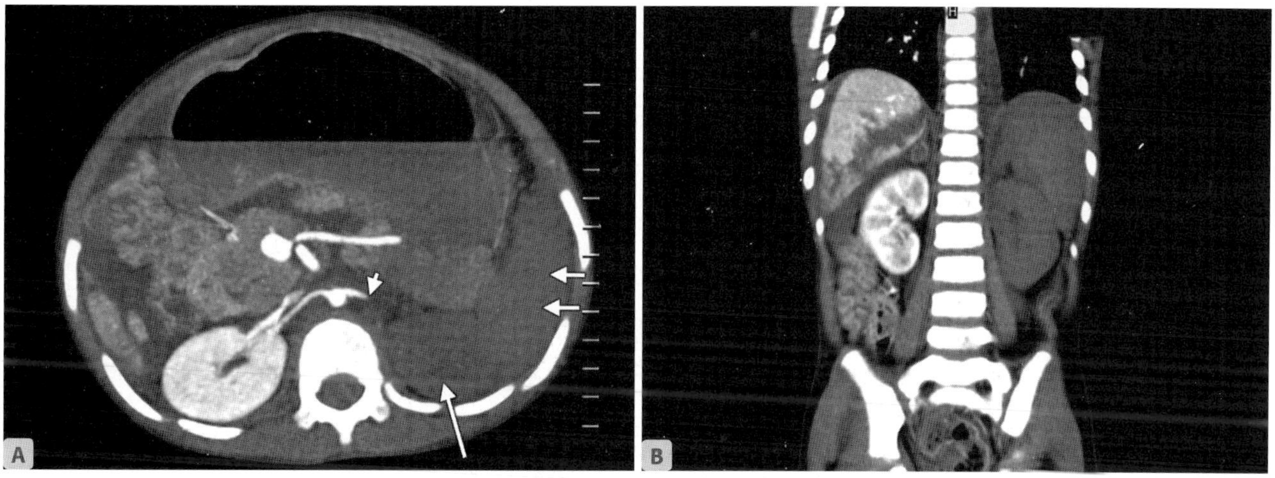

FIGS. 8A AND B: Axial MIP (A) and multiformatted coronal (B) CECT shows nonenhancing left kidney (long arrow) with abrupt termination of left renal artery (short arrow). Also note devascularized spleen [medium arrows in (A) and large liver laceration (B)].

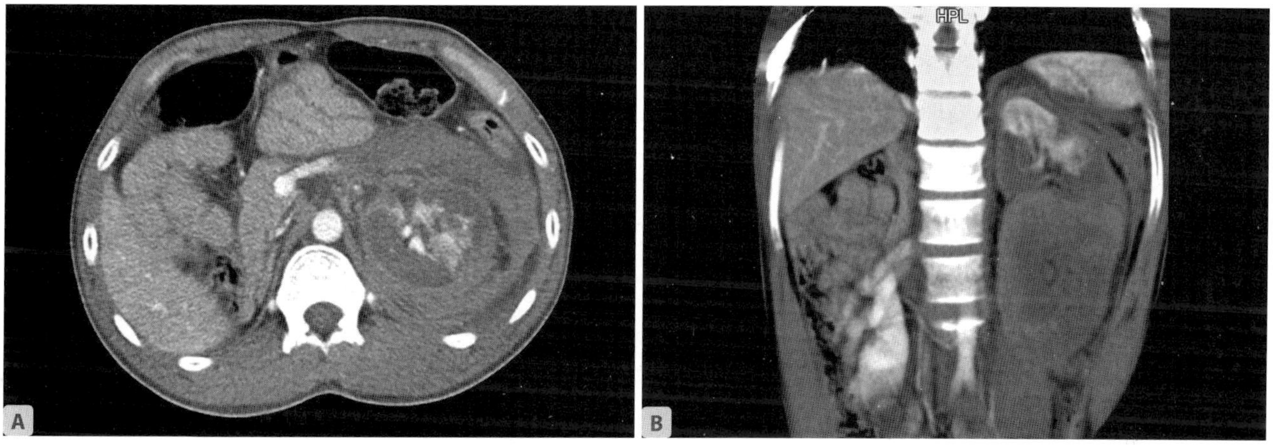

FIGS. 9A AND B: Axial (A) and multiformatted coronal (B) CECT shows completely shattered left kidney with large devitalized (nonenhancing) areas.

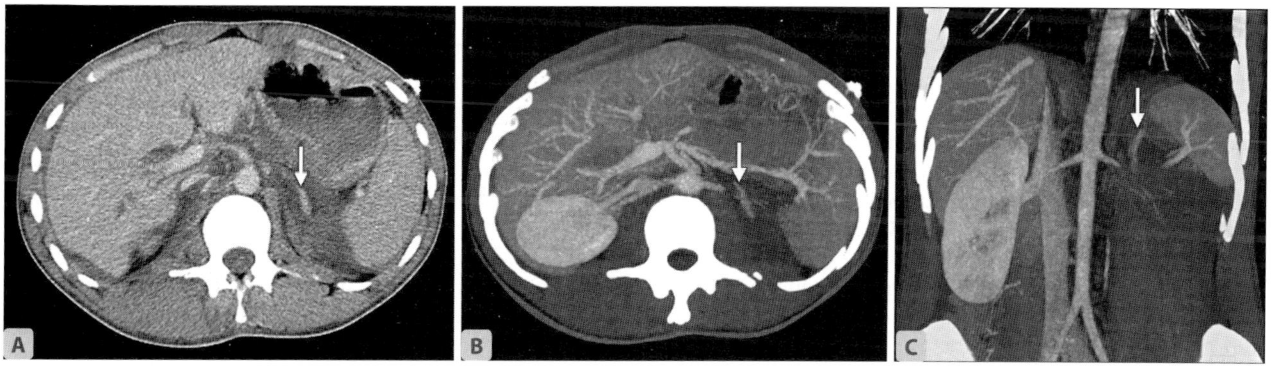

FIGS. 10A TO C: Axial CECT abdomen (A) shows a focal hyperattenuating area (arrow) in left suprarenal location within a hypodense hematoma. Axial (B) and reformatted coronal (C) MIP images clearly shows the arterial contrast extravasation (arrows) within the left perinephric hematoma. Note the abrupt termination of transected left renal artery and nonenhancing left kidney.

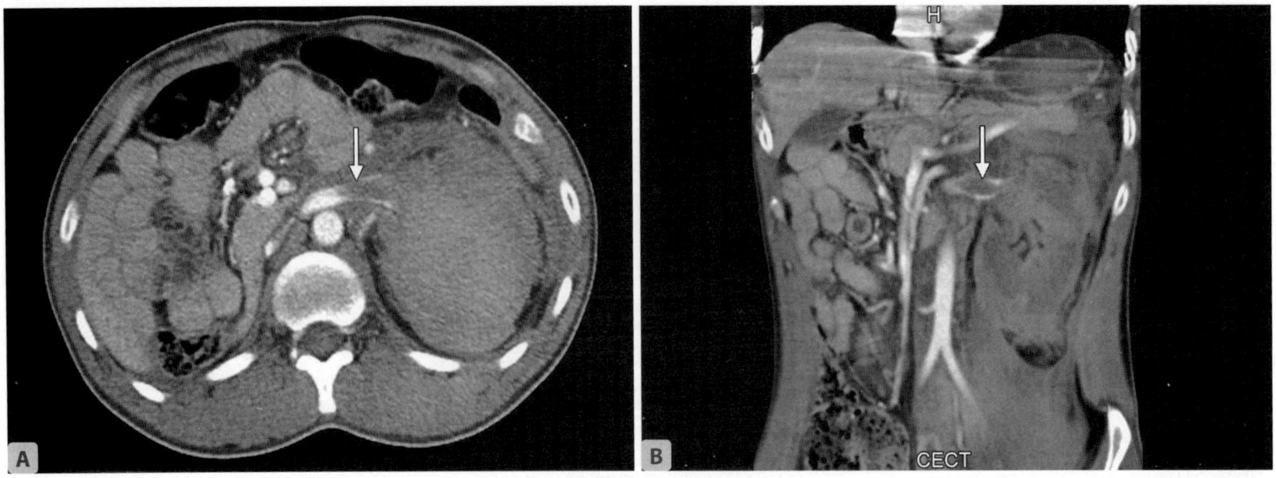

FIGS. 11A AND B: Axial (A) and multiformatted coronal (B) CECT shows an enlarged nonenhancing left kidney with large perinephric hematoma with a hypodense thrombus in the left main renal vein (arrows).

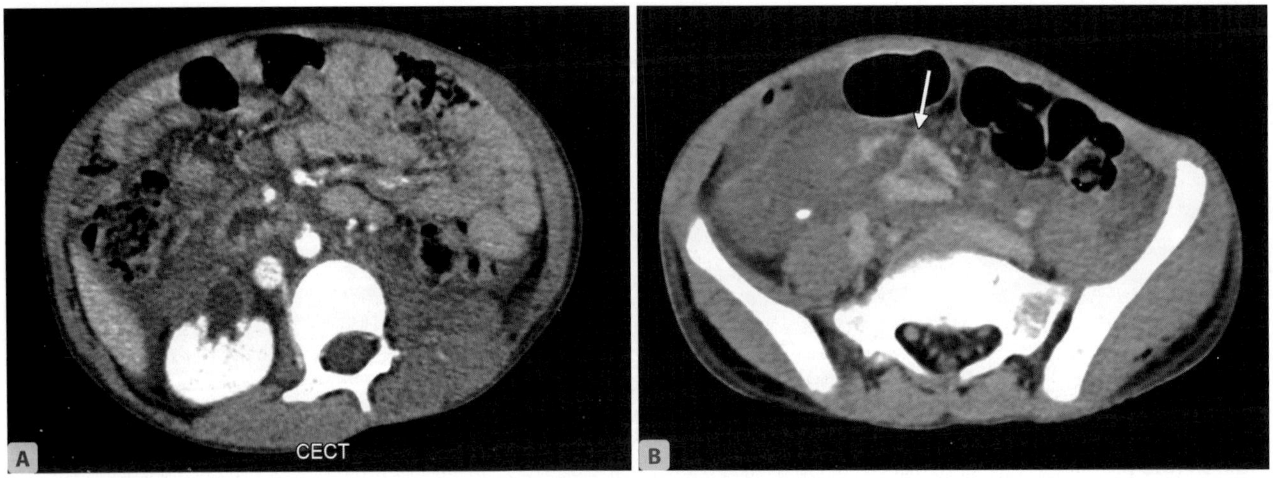

FIGS. 12A AND B: Axial CECT (A) at the level of kidneys shows left kidney is not present in left renal fossa. Axial image through the pelvis (B) shows extensive lacerations of ectopic left kidney (arrow).

nonoperative management for all but most severe injuries.[12] Grade 1–3 injuries are classified as low-grade injuries. These constitute >90% of all renal injuries and are almost always managed conservatively. The only absolute indication for active intervention in these grade patients is presence of life-threatening active hemorrhage which may be dealt with angiographic embolization **(Figs. 13A and B)** or surgical exploration.[4]

Most of grade 4 injuries can also be managed conservatively. Even large urinary extravasations resolve spontaneously on conservative management. Drainage is required in cases of increasing symptoms of pain, fever, or ileus. It is also indicated if the urinary collections are increasing in size or get infected. Ureteric stent placement is the preferred method for drainage and can be supplemented, if required, by percutaneous drainage of these collections with or without percutaneous nephrostomy.[3,13] If they fail to resolve, surgical repair may be warranted. Grade 4 injuries with significant devitalized tissue (>50%), especially with concomitant injuries or urine leak, usually require surgical debridement or repair to prevent the later development of urinoma, abscess, or infection which may warrant nephrectomy.

Active contrast extravasation limited to Gerota's fascia would often heal spontaneously due to tamponade effect. However, if there is a breach in Gerota's fascia with bleed extending beyond its confines, then angiographic embolization is often required, especially if the size of the hematoma is increasing.[6,9]

With aggressive monitoring and increasing use of angiographic embolization and percutaneous drainage, overall <10% of grade 4 injuries require surgical intervention.[13] Grade 5 injuries with complete avulsion of the ureteropelvic junction require surgical repair whereas partial tears may resolve on conservative management or stenting and proximal drainage.[2,3] Devascularization of the kidney may be managed conservatively in a stable patient but requires nephrectomy in case of active bleed or major parenchymal

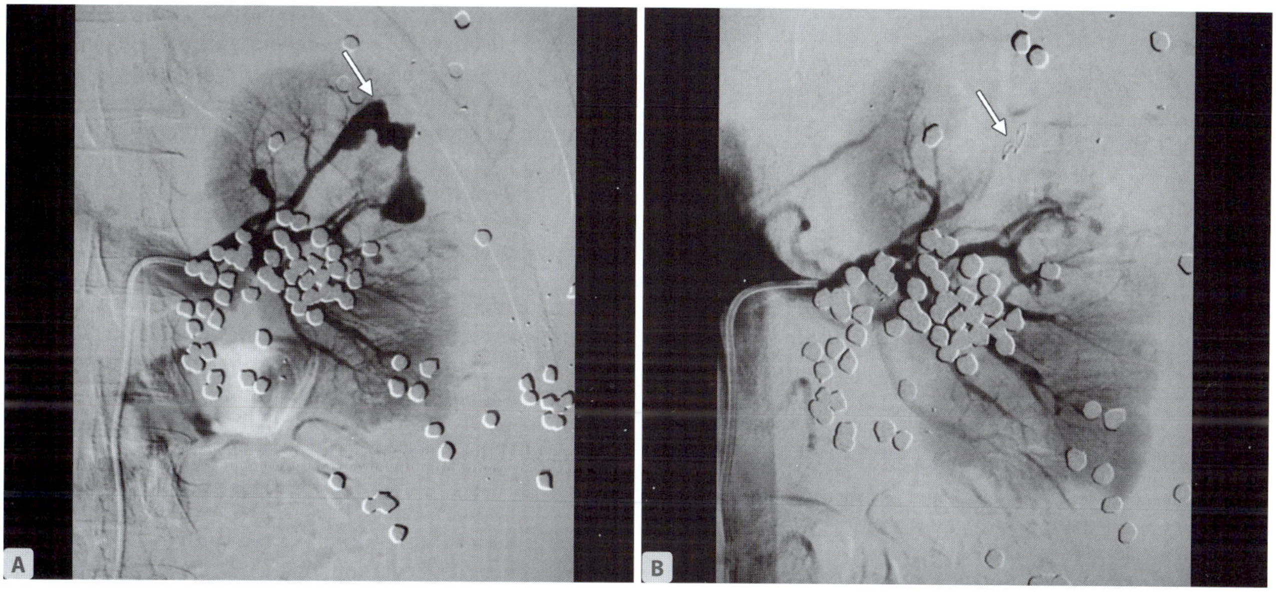

FIGS. 13A AND B: DSA image (A) of selective left renal artery injection in a patient injured with multiple pellets shows pseudoaneurysm formation with active bleed (arrow) in upper pole of left kidney. The involved upper polar segmental branch was selectively embolized with coil (arrow in B) resulting in thrombosis of pseudoaneurysm.

disruption. Surgical repair or angiographic thrombolysis of acute renal artery thrombosis can be done to try to preserve the renal function but is shown to have best results, usually within few hours of injury.[14] Renal hypertension developing weeks to months after renal trauma is a frequent finding which usually can be managed medically but may occasionally require nephrectomy.

To summarize, the only absolute indication for surgical exploration (or angiographic embolization) is life-threatening active hemorrhage.[4] Relative indications for operative management include the presence of (1) >50% of renal parenchyma devitalization, (2) arterial thrombosis, and (3) urinary extravasation which is not controlled by conservative management including proximal drainage and stenting.

Follow-up Imaging

Low-grade renal injuries do not require follow-up imaging unless there is a clinical worsening. High-grade renal injuries should be followed up with repeat imaging including the excretory phase after 48–72 hours. This has been shown to detect many urinary leaks or vascular injury, which were not detected earlier.[6]

Penetrating injuries have a lower threshold for repeat imaging and also for surgical repair.[6]

URETERAL TRAUMA

Iatrogenic surgical trauma accounts for 95% of all ureteral injuries and usually occurs in association with gynecological procedures.[15] In gynecological surgery, majority of ureteral injuries are discovered postoperatively (84%) with an average delay of 65 days after the procedure. The patients present with flank pain, fever, hematuria, and occasionally anuria. The emergence of endoscopic and laparoscopic surgery and endourological diagnostic and therapeutic interventions in the last two decades has further contributed to the increased incidence of iatrogenic ureteral trauma.[16] Iatrogenic ureteral injuries occur in 21% of patients undergoing open urological surgery and in 79% of patients undergoing endoscopic urological procedures. Recognition of the injury during surgery or the endoscopic procedure leads to immediate repair or placement of double J-stent for conservative management.

Gunshot wound, stabbing, and blunt trauma account for the remaining 5% of the ureteral injuries. Penetrating trauma to ureter is frequently associated with injuries to other organs.[17] Hematuria is usually present but may be absent. Blunt trauma in children with deceleration injury may occasionally lead to ureteral avulsion.

Imaging Work-up

Role of Intravenous Urogram

Traditionally, IVU has been used as a follow-up study to identify ureteric injury following trauma. However, with widespread availability of CT, its role has become limited. IVU still has a role in the form of one-shot study in unstable patients who require emergency surgery.[18] IVU demonstrates extravasation at the site of injury or obstruction proximal to the site of injury **(Fig. 14)**. Patients in whom ureteral injury is missed, urinary extravasation, hydronephrosis, and abscess formation can result. Demonstration of a mature fistulous tract or a large urinoma at a later stage is much more likely (90–100%). Hydronephrosis is seen at a later stage in 90% patients after ureteral injury. Ureteral avulsion may be diagnosed by contrast extravasation medial to the kidney.

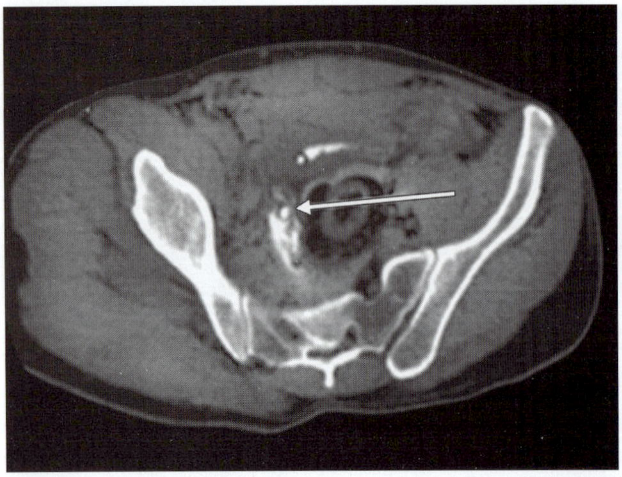

FIG. 14: Postcontrast delayed axial CT scan image at the level of pelvis shows extravasated urinary contrast material adjacent to the right ureter (arrow) suggesting ureteric injury.

Role of CT

Delayed phase CT has an important role in detection of ureter avulsion at UPJ in acute blunt trauma.[19] The diagnosis depends on the demonstration of contrast extravasation medial to the kidney and lack of distal ureter opacification. CT is also useful in accurate assessment of the size of the associated perirenal hematoma which helps the surgeon in deciding on the need for surgery.

Role of Antegrade and Retrograde Ureterograms

Ureterograms obtained *via* the antegrade or retrograde route are considered the gold standard for confirming the presence of ureteral injury. The ureterogram clearly defines the type and location of the injury as also its magnitude. Any associated fistulae and communicating urinomas are also delineated.

Classification

Ureteral injuries have been classified into the following AAST grades:[20]

- *Grade 1:* Hematoma or contusion without devascularization.
- *Grade 2:* Laceration or transection involving <50% of circumference.
- *Grade 3:* Laceration or transection involving >50% of circumference.
- *Grade 4:* Complete tear or transection with <2 cm of devascularization.
- *Grade 5:* Avulsion with >2 cm of devascularization.

Management

Injuries detected during surgery are treated immediately by either surgical repair or endourologic interventions.[20,21] Injuries recognized later are treated by percutaneous nephrostomy for urinary diversion and antegrade or retrograde stent placement. Stenting may be preceded by balloon dilatation or endoureterectomy for strictures. In ureteral avulsion, stenting is coupled with drainage of urinoma which prevents fibrosis and facilitates passage of guidewire antegradely across the dehiscence. Fistulae are also managed with nephrostomy and stenting. Disruption of the pelvic ureter can be managed by antegrade ureteroneocystostomy and stenting for 1–3 months for which a curved transjugular intrahepatic portosystemic shunt needle sheath can be used.

URINARY BLADDER TRAUMA

Urinary bladder injury is relatively rare and constitutes only 2% of all abdominal injuries that require surgical repair. It may be due to blunt, penetrating, or iatrogenic trauma. Majority of the patients of bladder trauma have associated fracture of pelvis most commonly of the anterior pubic arch.[22] A distended bladder is more prone to injury.

The patient presents with suprapubic pain or tenderness and/or hematuria. In such cases, the recommendation is to first exclude urethral injury by a retrograde urethrography (RGU) followed by insertion of Foley's catheter. If a urethral injury is found, a suprapubic cystostomy is usually done. This is followed by cystography which may be conventional technique or CT cystography. However, with increasing use of CT scan, CT cystography has become the investigation of choice which can be done at the same sitting if the patient is undergoing CT scan for abdominal injuries.[23] Delayed scanning of the bladder after intravenous contrast administration so as to allow the contrast excreted by kidneys to opacify the bladder is not a substitute for CT cystography as it has been shown to miss a significant number of bladder ruptures.[23,24] Conventional cystography may be done, if CT is not available.

Cystography

Conventional Cystography

Technique:

- 300–400 mL of dilute contrast is instilled into the bladder *via* the urethral (if urethral injury excluded) or the suprapubic route. The ideal way is by a gravity-dip infusion and not injection. It allows adequate contrast to be instilled without chances of forceful worsening of the bladder injury.
- The initial film is taken after 100 mL contrast is instilled to check gross extravasation.
- Films are then taken after the entire contrast is instilled.
- A postdrainage film excludes extravasation hidden by a distended bladder.

CT Cystography

The technique recommended is retrograde filling of the bladder with contrast (same as with conventional cystography) by gravity-dip infusion followed by a computed tomogram of the pelvis. With this technique, the diagnostic accuracy is comparable to that of conventional cystography. The CT cystography is best done as a separate phase immediately after acquisition of images of abdomen and pelvis after intravenous contrast administration. If done simultaneously with the routine phases, there may be a diagnostic pitfall in the interpretation of extravasated contrast material in the abdomen. It may be from intraperitoneal urinary bladder rupture or extravasation from vessels. Postdrainage scans are not required. According to the current recommendations, CT cystography is indicated in the following situations:

- Unexplained pelvic-free fluid with or without pelvic fractures.
- Gross or significant microscopic hematuria with nonacetabular pelvic fractures.

Classification

Blunt Trauma

The AAST classification for urinary bladder (UB) injury has five injury grades. However, it involves measuring the size of lacerations which is a potential pitfall on imaging as the size of defect varies with the distension of the bladder. Hence, the AAST classification for UB is not much used radiologically.[25] The classification based on imaging which is most widely followed was described by Sandler et al.[22]

- *Type 1:* Bladder contusion
- *Type 2:* Intraperitoneal bladder rupture
- *Type 3:* Interstitial bladder injury
- *Type 4: Extraperitoneal injury*:
  - Simple
  - Complex
- *Type 5:* Combined UB injury.

Bladder Contusion (Type 1)

This consists of a self-limiting, incomplete mural tear with localized ecchymosis. CT cystography is normal, showing a well-distended uniformly hyperattenuating thin-walled bladder with no contrast leakage. No specific therapy is required. A perivesical hematoma may be associated with major pelvic fractures even when no evidence of actual bladder tear is seen on cystography. Accumulated blood compresses upon the extraperitoneal part of the bladder narrowing it at the base. An "inverted tear drop" or "inverted pear sign" may be seen on cystogram.

Intraperitoneal Injury (Type 2)

Intraperitoneal rupture usually occurs after a blow to the lower abdomen in the presence of distended bladder. Rupture occurs at the dome due to increased intravesical pressure. This is the weakest point of the bladder and also the peritonealized portion of the bladder wall. Urine will thus enter the peritoneal cavity. On cystography, contrast material may be seen outlining the abdominal viscera, loops of bowel, mesenteric folds, paracolic gutters, or pouch of Douglas **(Figs. 15A and B)**. The contrast material may track to upper abdomen also. The locations of free intraperitoneal contrast are predictable with well-defined boundaries as compared to extraperitoneal rupture.

Interstitial Injury (Type 3)

This represents a dissecting rupture of the bladder wall without frank perforation. On CT cystography, a mural hematoma/defect may be seen. Occasionally, intramural contrast may be seen. However, there is no contrast extravasation outside the bladder. Such defects may involve both extraperitoneal and intraperitoneal portions of the bladder wall. Hence, interstitial rupture was designated as a separate category in this classification.

Extraperitoneal Injury (Type 4)

This is the most common injury to the bladder (80–90% of cases) and usually occurs in association with a fractured pelvis or in penetrating trauma. Earlier, it was thought that the tear was caused by direct penetration of the bladder by bone fragments. However, now it is postulated that this type of injury may be either a type of bursting or shearing injury resulting from the force of pelvic ring disruption.

In simple (Type 4A), extraperitoneal rupture extravasation is confined to the perivesical space.

On CT cystography, flame-shaped areas of extravasation are noted in the perivesical spaces and in the prevesical space (space of Retzius) where it can track cranially up to umbilicus. The ill-defined contrast in the prevesical space is said to have a "molar tooth" appearance.

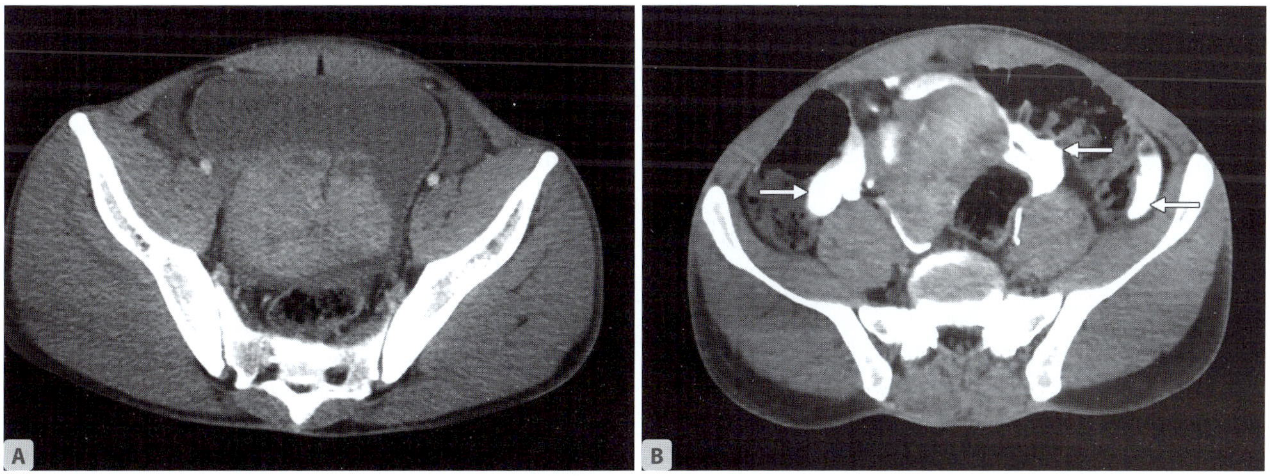

FIGS. 15A AND B: Axial CECT image (A) through urinary bladder shows a hyperdense clot within the bladder. Axial CT cystography image (B) shows extravasation of contrast outside the bladder in the peritoneal cavity outlining the bowel loops (arrows).

A complex (Type 4B) extraperitoneal rupture is diagnosed when contrast extravasation extends beyond the perivesical space into the scrotum, thigh, perineum, hip joint, and anterior abdominal wall **(Fig. 16)**. It occurs secondary to rupture of urogenital diaphragm. Contrast may also track upward into the paranephric spaces.

It is important to differentiate intraperitoneal rupture from extraperitoneal rupture of bladder because the former requires surgical repair where the latter is usually managed conservatively with Foley's catheter placement.

Combined Extra-and Intraperitoneal Bladder Injury (Type 5)

An injury may result in rupture of both intraperitoneal and extraperitoneal portions of the bladder wall. On CT cystography, both patterns of contrast extravasation may be seen.

Penetrating Bladder Trauma

Injury may result from gunshot or knife wounds and may result in extraperitoneal, intraperitoneal, or combined bladder injury. There is a high incidence of associated bowel or other visceral injury, and exploratory surgery is required in virtually every patient.

Iatrogenic Bladder Trauma

Bladder injuries may be due to urologic, gynecologic, or obstetric procedures. Bladder perforations or vesicovaginal and vesicouterine fistulae may form. Cystography and hysterosalpingography help in the diagnosis. Migration of surgical devices such as drains, catheters, contraceptives, or orthopedic prostheses can sometimes perforate the bladder.

Management

Types 1, 3, and 4 injuries are managed conservatively with placement of Foley's catheter. However, intraperitoneal rupture of bladder requires surgical repair. Hence, Types 2 and 5 injuries are managed surgically.

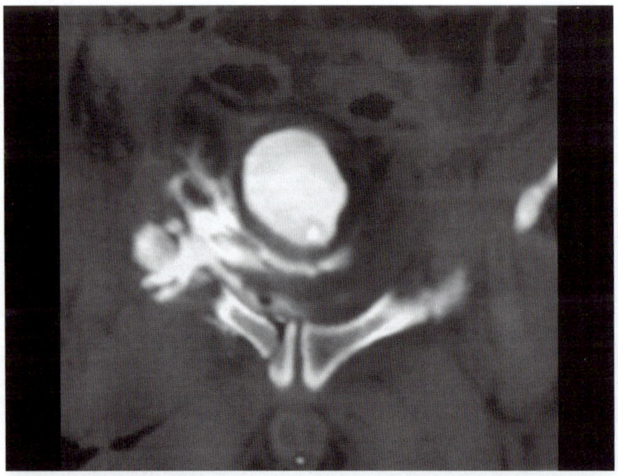

FIG. 16: Reformatted coronal MIP CT cystography image shows complex extraperitoneal rupture of urinary bladder with contrast lying in extraperitoneal spaces in perineum extending into right hip joint.

URETHRAL TRAUMA

Posterior urethral injuries result from pelvic fractures and gunshot wounds. Injury associated with pelvic fracture mostly involves the urethra near the urogenital diaphragm. Anterior urethral injuries are much less common and are more commonly due to iatrogenic cause, straddle injury, or gunshot wound. The lifelong consequences in males include incontinence, strictures, and impotence. Female urethra injury is rare.

The clinical signs suggestive of urethral injury in a male patient with pelvic trauma include gross hematuria, blood at urethral meatus, inability to void, swelling or hematoma of the perineum or penis, and a high-riding prostate on per rectal examination associated with pelvic fracture.[26] The clinical signs in a female patient include difficulty in micturition, blood at meatus, hematuria, labial edema, vaginal bleeding, or urine leak per rectum. If the above signs are present in a patient with pelvic trauma, urethrography should be done for evaluation of urethra before insertion of Foley's catheter.

Radiology

The urethra is best evaluated with RGU or voiding cystourethrography.

Technique of Urethrography

- Dynamic RGU, ideally under fluoroscopy, is used for the evaluation of urethral injury.
- Steep oblique films are obtained, at the end of injection of 25–30 mL of 50% contrast.
- If the urethra appears intact, a catheter is passed into the bladder for cystography and a voiding urethrogram is obtained.

Blunt Urethral Trauma

Urethral injuries are classified anatomically as anterior or posterior urethral injuries. Posterior urethral injury occurs in 4–14% of patients with pelvic fracture and up to 20% of these have associated bladder laceration.[27] Anterior urethral injury commonly results from straddle pelvic injury secondary to the patient falling astride a blunt object or direct blow to the perineum. However, more commonly, anterior urethral injuries may be iatrogenic due to instrumentation.

Posterior Urethral Injuries Associated with Pelvic Fracture

- Commonly, prostatomembranous urethral injury above the urogenital diaphragm results.
- A high riding urinary bladder is seen on excretory urography. This is due to disruption of puboprostatic ligaments and hematoma in retropubic and perivesical spaces.

- Contrast extravasation will be seen adjacent to the posterior urethra and sometimes into the pelvic extraperitoneal space.

Anterior Urethral Injury

Straddle injuries resulting from the patient falling astride a blunt object or direct blow to the perineum may lead to anterior, mostly bulbous, urethral injuries. More commonly, anterior urethral injuries may be iatrogenic due to instrumentation. In partial rupture, extravasation of contrast occurs on urethrogram but continuity of the urethra is preserved. In complete rupture, no contrast is seen in the proximal urethra. Venous intravasation is seen commonly. Treatment is by suprapubic urinary diversion and delayed surgery.

Classification

Based on findings of urethrography, the following types of urethral injuries have been described by Goldman, et al.[28] who have modified the initial classification given by Colapinto and McCallum.[29]

- *Type I:*
    - Stretched, but intact posterior urethra is seen **(Fig. 17)**.
    - In this type of injury, the prostate is detached from the urogenital diaphragm with an elevated bladder seen on cystography due to retropubic hematoma and rupture of puboprostatic ligaments.
    - No extravasation is seen on the urethrogram.
- *Type II:*
    - Seen in around 15% of cases.
    - Urethra is ruptured at the membranoprostatic junction above the urogenital diaphragm which is intact **(Fig. 18)**.
    - Contrast extravasation is seen into the pelvic extra-peritoneal space above the urogenital diaphragm but not in the perineum.
- *Type III:*
    - Most common type.
    - Membranobulbous urethral rupture is seen with disruption of urogenital diaphragm.
    - Contrast extravasation both above and below urogenital diaphragm, i.e. into pelvis and the perineum **(Fig. 19)**.
- *Type IV:*
    - There is bladder neck injury with extension into the posterior urethra.
    - Contrast extravasation is seen in the pelvic extra-peritoneal space with disruption of bladder neck **(Fig. 20)**.
- *Type IVa:*
    - Extraperitoneal bladder base injury simulating a bladder neck injury.
    - Radiologically indistinguishable from type IV injury
- *Type V:*
    - Caused by straddle injury.

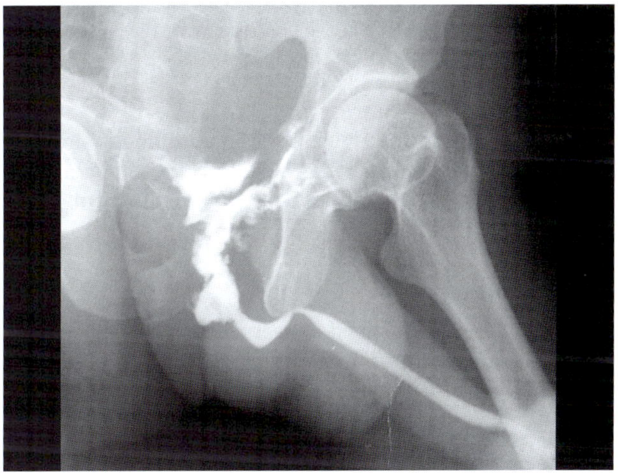

FIG. 18: RGU shows a type II urethral injury with contrast extravasation from posterior urethra above the urogenital diaphragm.

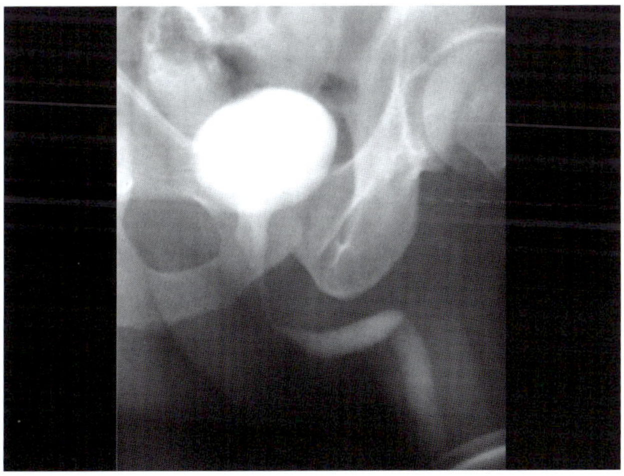

FIG. 17: MCU shows a stretched posterior urethra in a patient with multiple pelvic fractures.

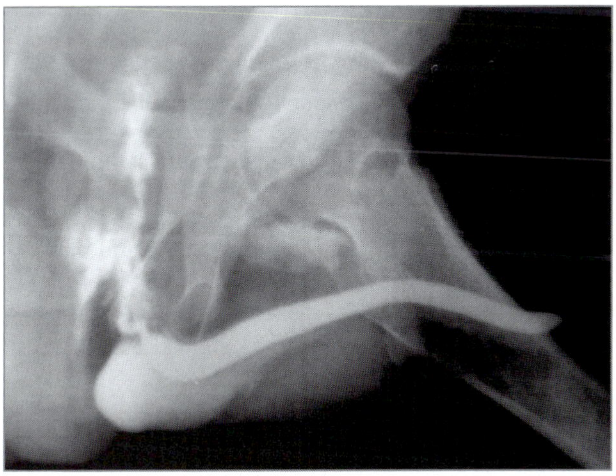

FIG. 19: RGU shows a type III urethral injury with contrast extravasation from posterior urethra both above and below the urogenital diaphragm.

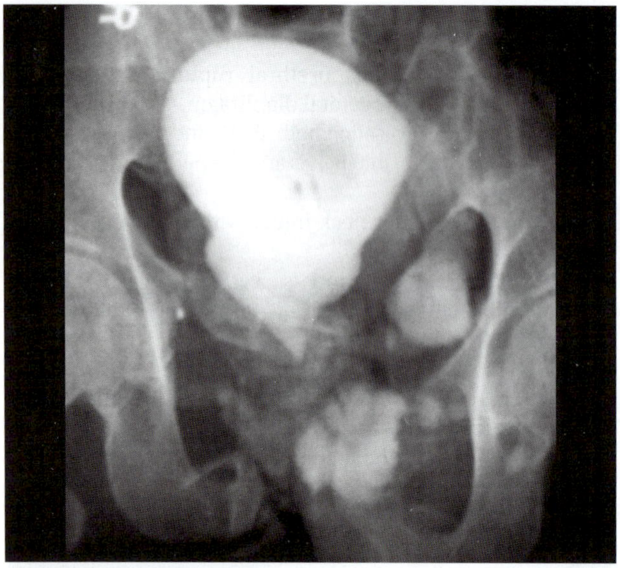

FIG. 20: MCU showing elongated injured bladder neck with contrast extravasation around the prostatic urethra.

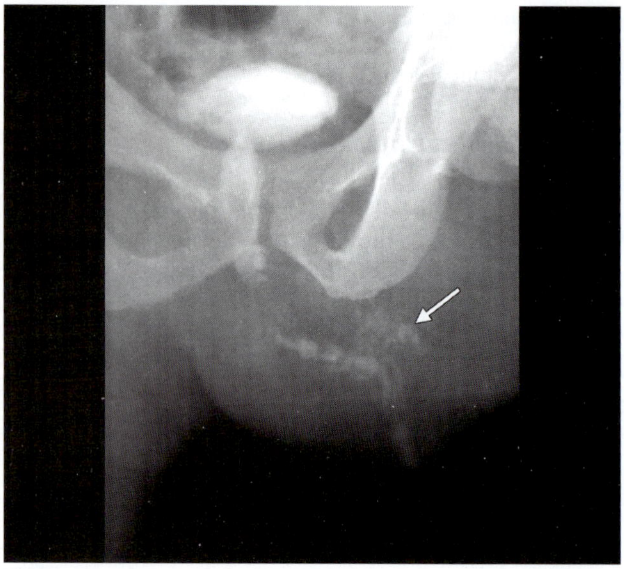

FIG. 21: RGU showing contrast extravasation in penile tissues from anterior urethral injury (arrow).

- Anterior urethra, most commonly bulbous urethra, injury is seen which may be partial or complete.
- Contrast extravasation is seen into the penile soft tissues **(Fig. 21)**.

Management

Type I injuries are managed conservatively with placement of a urethral or suprapubic catheter. In general, partial disruptions are also managed conservatively with suprapubic or urethral catheterization whereas complete disruptions of the urethra are managed either by endoscopic realignment or by delayed urethroplasty.

Bladder neck injuries involve internal sphincter and hence are treated surgically to prevent development of incontinence. However, Type IVa injury may be treated conservatively since it does not involve the bladder neck.

Evaluation before Delayed Urethroplasty

- A combined voiding cystourethrogram and a retrograde urethrogram are obtained.
- The bladder is filled with 30% dilute contrast through the suprapubic cystostomy.
- The patient is then asked to void.
- A simultaneous retrograde urethrogram is performed.
- This technique demonstrates the proximal and distal extent of the stricture. This enables the surgeon to decide between a transperineal and a transpubic approach for urethroplasty.
- Recently, reports have shown the potential of MRI to demonstrate the length of the urethral injury along with the amount of displacement of the prostatic apex. This information is helpful in preoperative planning of the surgical approach.

Penetrating Injury

Penetrating trauma to the urethra may be secondary to knife or gunshot wounds. The diagnosis is established by RGU. Early surgery is the treatment of choice.

Iatrogenic Injury

Iatrogenic urethral injury may result from pelvic surgery, urethral instrumentation, or indwelling catheters.

Female Urethra

Injury to the female urethra is rare because of its mobility. Excretory urography or cystourethrography may show extravasation of contrast at the site of rupture.

REFERENCES

1. McAninch JW. Renal injuries. In: Gillenwater JY, Grayhack JT, Howards SS, et al. (Eds). Adult and Pediatric Urology, 3rd edition. St. Louis, MO: Mosby; 1996. pp. 539-53.
2. Kawashima A, Sandler CM, Corl FM, et al. Imaging of renal trauma: a comprehensive review. Radiographics. 2001;21(3): 557-74.
3. Smith JK, Kenny PJ. Imaging of renal trauma. Radiol Clin N Am. 2003;41(5):1019-35.
4. Harris AC, Zwirewich CV, Lyburn ID, et al. CT findings in blunt renal trauma. Radiographics. 2001;21:S201-14.
5. Park SJ, Kim JK, Kim KW, et al. MDCT findings of renal trauma. Am J Roentgenol. 2006;187(2):541-7.
6. Baghdanian AH, Baghdanian AA, Armetta A, et al. Utility of MDCT findings in predicting patient management outcomes in renal trauma. Emerg Radiol. 2017;24(3):263-72.

7. Moore EE, Shackford SR, Patcher HL, et al. Organ injury scaling: spleen, liver and kidney. J Trauma. 2001;50:195-200.
8. Kozar RA, Crandall M, Shanmuganathan K, et al. Organ injury scaling 2018 update: spleen, liver, and kidney. J Trauma Acute Care Surg. 2018;85(6):1119-22.
9. Chien LC, Vakil M, Nguyen J, et al. The American Association for the Surgery of Trauma Organ Injury Scale 2018 update for computed tomography-based grading of renal trauma: a primer for the emergency radiologist. Emerg Radiol. 2019 doi: 10.1007/s10140-019-01721-z. [Epub ahead of print].
10. Dayal M, Gamanagatti S, Kumar A. Imaging in renal trauma. World J Radiol. 2013;5(8):275-84.
11. Pollack HM, Wein AJ. Imaging of renal trauma. Radiology. 1989;172:297-308.
12. Knudson MM, Maull KI. Nonoperative management of solid organ injuries: past, present and future. Surg Clin N Am. 1999;79(6):1357-71.
13. Brandes SB, McAninch JW. Reconstructive surgery for trauma of the upper urinary tract. Urol Clin N Am. 1999;26(1): 183-99.
14. Peterson NE. Genitourinary trauma. In: Feliciano DV, Moore EE, Mattox KL (Eds). Trauma, 3rd edition. Stamford, CT: Appleton & Lange; 1996. pp. 661-94.
15. Assimos DG, Patterson LC, Taylor CL. Changing incidence and etiology of iatrogenic ureteral injuries. J Urol. 1994; 152(6 Pt 2):2240-6.
16. Campbell EW, Jr, Filderman S, Jacobs SC. Ureteral injury due to blunt and penetrating trauma. Urology. 1992;40(3): 216-20.
17. Pitts JC, Peterson NE. Penetrating injuries of the ureter. J Trauma. 1981;21:978-82.
18. Lynch TH, Matnz-NL, Las, et al. European Association of urology: guidelines on urological trauma. Eur Urol. 2005;47: 1-15.
19. Kenney PJ, Panicek DM, Witanowski LS. Computed tomography of ureteral disruption. J Comput Assit Tomogr. 1987;11(3): 480-4.
20. Bent C, Iyngkaran T, Power N, et al. Urological injuries following trauma. Clin Radiol. 2008; 63(12):1361-71.
21. Lask D, Abarbanel J, Luttwak Z, et al. Changing trends in the management of iatrogenic ureteral injuries. J Urol. 1995; 154(5):1693-5.
22. Sandler CM, Hall JT, Rodriguez MB, et al. Bladder injury in blunt pelvic trauma. Radiology. 1986;158:633-8.
23. Vaccaro JP, Brody JM. CT cystography in the evaluation of major bladder trauma. Radiographics. 2000;20(5):1373-81.
24. Power N, Ryan S, Hamilton P. Computed tomographic cystography in bladder trauma: pictorial essay. Can Assoc Radiol J. 2004;55(5):304-8.
25. Joshi G, Kim EY, Hanna TN, et al. CT cystography for suspicion of traumatic urinary bladder injury: indications, technique, findings, and pitfalls in diagnosis: Radiographics Fundamentals|Online Presentation. Radiographics. 2018; 38(1):92-3.
26. Patel U. Lower urinary tract trauma. In: Patel U, Rickards D (Eds). Imaging and Urodynamics of the Lower Urinary Tract. London, Taylor & Francis; 2005. pp. 115-21.
27. Kawashima A, Sandler CM, Wasserman NF, et al. Imaging of urethral disease: a pictorial review. Radiographics. 2004;24(Suppl 1):S195-216.
28. Goldman SM, Sandler CM, Corriere JN, Jr, et al. Blunt urethral trauma: a unified anatomical mechanical classification. J Urol. 1997;157(1):85-9.
29. Colapinto V, McCallum RW. Injury to the male posterior urethra in fractured pelvis: a new classification. J Urol. 1977;118(4): 575-80.

CHAPTER

26

Nonvascular Interventions in the Urinary Tract

Mandeep Kang, Naveen Kalra, Ujjwal Gorsi, Sreedhara BC

INTRODUCTION

The past few decades have witnessed a revolution in the development of minimally invasive procedures, with interventional radiology being in the forefront of these advances. The development of percutaneous procedures under image guidance was based on the knowledge that a fine, thin needle of 21–22 gauge (G) can be safely and accurately positioned within the human body in most organ parts. Nonvascular interventions in the urinary tract are well-established procedures with the first description of a percutaneous nephrostomy (PCN) being published in literature more than 70 years ago.[1] Propelled by technological advances, minimally invasive uroradiological interventional therapies have completely changed the present day practice of urology.

PERCUTANEOUS NEPHROSTOMY

Percutaneous nephrostomy is the first step in image-guided urointerventional procedures, which secures an access into the urinary tract.[2] It involves image-guided placement of a catheter into the pelvicalyceal system.[3] Besides urinary diversion in an obstructed system, the access can be used to create large-bore tracks through which various endourological procedures can be safely performed with fewer complications than open surgical procedures.[4]

Indications

- *Supravesical urinary tract obstruction:* Obstruction of the upper urinary tract can be due to extrinsic or intrinsic causes and is the most common indication for PCN (85–90% of cases).
  Benign causes of obstruction include:
  - Calculous disease (most common)
  - Ureteral/anastomotic stricture
  - Blood clots
  - Sequestered papillae
  - Fungal balls
  - Retroperitoneal fibrosis

  Malignant causes of obstruction include neoplasms of the urinary bladder, cervix, and prostate. Percutaneous nephrostomy (PCN) should be offered to patients with tumors, which are potentially responsive to therapy or have stable disease and to improve the overall quality of life.
- Providing an alternative pathway for drainage as part of the management of urinary leaks or fistulas.
- *Access for subsequent interventions:*
  - Antegrade ureteric stenting
  - Nephrolithotomy/lithotripsy
  - Stone dissolution
  - Ureteral occlusion for treating an urinary fistula
  - Urothelial lesion: Tissue diagnosis/treatment by fulguration
  - Removal of a foreign body such as fungal ball
  - Whitaker test
  - Upper urinary tract instillation (medications or cooling pyeloperfusion for ablative procedures).

There is no absolute contraindication for PCN with the only relative contraindication being coagulopathy, which should be corrected prior to the procedure.

Anatomy for Percutaneous Renal Entry

Knowledge of anatomy of the kidneys is basic to understanding how to safely gain access to the collecting system for performing a PCN under image guidance. The main renal artery usually bifurcates into anterior and posterior divisions with further segmental branches. The anterior division supplies the anterior two-thirds of the renal parenchyma while the posterior division supplies the posterior third. A zone of relative avascularity, known as Brödel's line or zone of bloodless incision exists between these two vascular territories, which runs just posterior to the lateral convex border of the kidney **(Fig. 1)**. The best route to access the collecting system lies through this relatively avascular plane.[4] Because the kidneys are normally rotated about their horizontal axis with the pelvis facing anteromedially, the posterior calyces are directed posterolaterally with their long axis aligned with this avascular zone; these calyces should ideally be targeted at PCN. In the renal hilum, the renal artery is the most anterior structure followed by the renal vein with the renal pelvis being the most posterior structure.

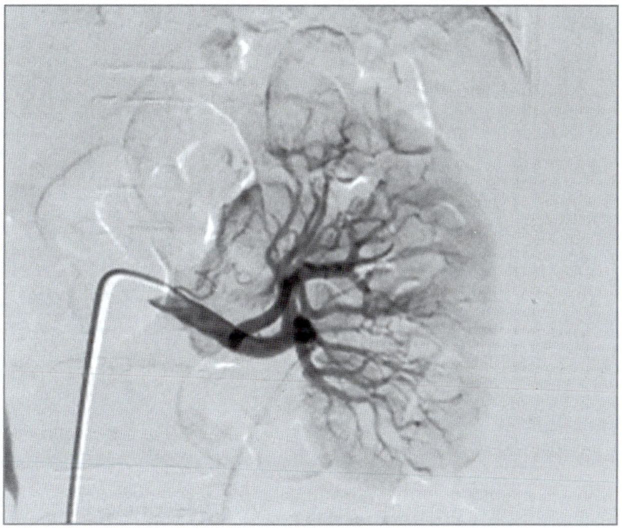

FIG. 1: Vascular anatomy of the kidney. Selective left renal arteriogram 25° left posterior oblique view shows bifurcation of the main renal artery into dorsal and ventral branches. The avascular plane of Brödel lies along the plane of division of these vascular territories.

Placement of the puncture needle centrally for accessing the collecting system should not be done, only the calyces (which anatomically are completely surrounded by renal parenchyma) should be punctured.

Central puncture can lead to two problems. First, a hilar vessel can be injured leading to severe bleeding; second, there may be urinary leakage from the catheter tract due to absence of renal tissue around the renal pelvis leading to inadequate sealing of the track.[5]

The site of access to the pelvicalyceal system depends upon the indication for nephrostomy. A lower pole posterior calyx can be safely accessed using a subcostal approach to avoid transgression of the pleura.[5] However, puncturing a posterior calyx in the upper pole or interpolar region provides the easiest access to the pelviureteric junction for subsequent ureteral interventions. In cases of complex stone disease, entry through the upper polar posterior calyx allows visualization of most parts of the collecting system.[4]

Technique

A detailed evaluation of the patient must be performed including the clinical history, laboratory parameters, and relevant radiology. The patient should also be evaluated on ultrasound (US) or fluoroscopy as body habitus can change your choice of image guidance. Coagulation parameters [prothrombin time index (PTI) >75%, international normalized ratio (INR) <1.5] and the hemogram (Hb >7 g/dL, platelet count >75,000) should be checked and abnormalities, if any, must be corrected prior to the procedure. Patients with azotemia may have profound metabolic disturbances. Any metabolic acidosis or hyperkalemia should be corrected prior to performing the intervention as these imbalances can cause systemic complications such as cardiac arrhythmias or even cardioplegia.[3] Urine analysis to screen for possible urinary infection should also be performed. Prophylactic broad-spectrum antibiotics should be started prior to the procedure in patients with known or potentially infected system (urinary conduit diversions, obstruction with or without fever, and urinary leaks). An informed consent must be obtained from the patient after explaining in detail the need for the procedure, the procedure itself, and the potential complications, which can occur.

Percutaneous nephrostomy is usually performed under fluoroscopic or US guidance. In certain cases, CT guidance may be used, for example, in emphysematous pyelonephritis when air in the collecting system obscures visualization on US. In addition, in patients with different body habitus such as kyphoscoliosis or morbid obesity, CT may be the only modality, which can provide adequate image guidance.[6] The use of MR guidance has also been described.[7]

The patient is placed prone on the fluoroscopy table with a bolster under the abdomen to fix the kidneys against the posterior abdominal wall and prevent their anterior displacement during the procedure. If the patient is unable to lie in prone position, a prone-oblique position can be used with the side to be punctured in the dependent position.

The back and flanks are cleansed and draped. The calyx to be punctured is chosen depending upon the indication. The chosen site of puncture is infiltrated with local anesthetic not only into the skin and subcutaneous tissues, but also deeper through the perirenal fat up till the renal capsule, therefore a long 9–10 cm needle maybe required.[5] This is generally adequate for pain relief during the procedure; however, conscious sedation may be required in apprehensive or noncooperative patients. Infants and young children will require general anesthesia.

The chosen calyx can be punctured with an 18-G needle under US guidance in a dilated system **(Figs. 2A and B)**. After removing the stylet, a urine sample should be aspirated for culture. A small volume of iodinated contrast is then injected to opacity the collecting system. A 0.035" stiff guidewire is then passed through the needle and negotiated into the pelvis. After a stab incision along the needle, the cannula is removed and the tract dilated using fascial dilators. For drainage of noninfected urine, catheters of 8–10 F size are usually sufficient. The catheter is placed over the guidewire and coiled in the pelvis **(Figs. 3A to D)**. A check injection of contrast should be done to confirm position of all side holes of the catheter within the collecting system.

Pigtail catheters with or without locking devices may be used. The catheter is fixed to the skin using sutures or other retention devices, connected to a urine collection bag and allowed to drain under gravity.

A variety of techniques may be used for the initial puncture. Some workers inject intravenous iodinated contrast to opacify the collecting system followed by direct puncture of the pelvis under fluoroscopic guidance with a 22-G needle. Iodinated contrast (with or without room air or carbon dioxide) is then injected under fluoroscopic control to better opacify the collecting system and find a suitable calyx. The selected calyx can then be punctured from the posterolateral aspect with an 18-G needle, with the subsequent steps being the same as described before. Another variation of this "two-stick" technique, particularly when the collecting system is only mildly dilated, is to use a 22-G needle for the second puncture as well, through

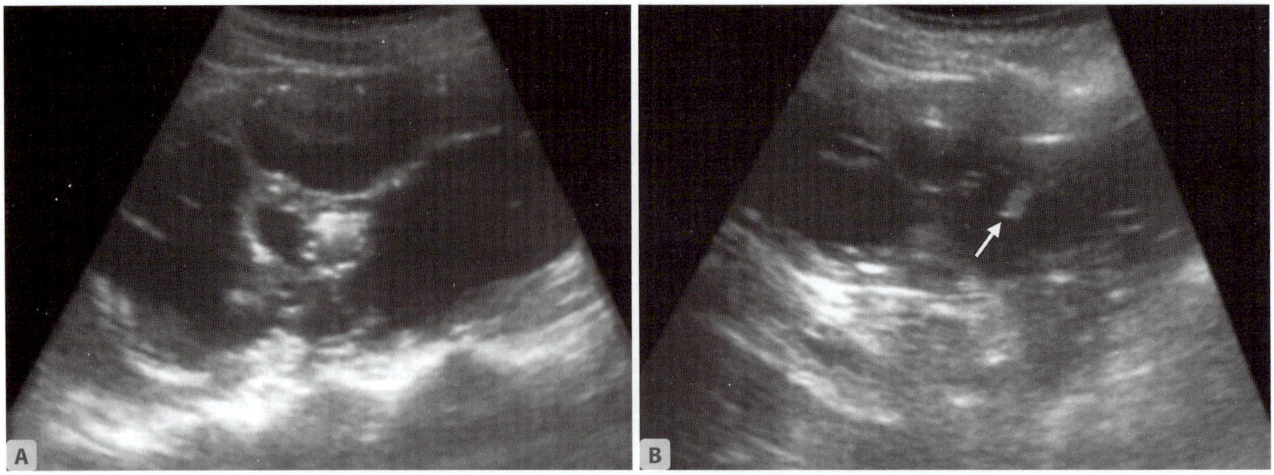

FIGS. 2A AND B: Percutaneous nephrostomy. (A) Longitudinal sonogram shows gross hydronephrosis with internal echoes suggestive of pyonephrosis. (B) The lower pole calyx has been punctured using an 18-gauge needle. Needle tip is seen *in situ* (arrow).

which a 0.014" hydrophilic guidewire can be passed, over which a 5-F percutaneous access set is placed and the guidewire exchanged for a 0.035" stiff or super-stiff Amplatz guidewire.[5,7-9] Regardless of the technique used, care has to be taken not to overdistend the collecting system so as to avoid pyelovenous reflux, particularly in infected systems.

Occasionally, external urinary diversion is necessary in nondilated collecting systems (e.g. in urinary leak or fistulas). These kidneys can be punctured using the double-stick technique with initial opacification of the collecting system with intravenous injection of iodinated contrast.[10] Alternatively, these kidneys can be accessed using sonographic guidance after intravenous injection of frusemide. Even if the calyces do not dilate adequately to be visualized on US, the renal pelvis can be seen and punctured with a skinny needle, iodinated contrast, or saline injected to distend the calyces so that a definitive calyceal puncture can be made with fluoroscopic or US guidance.[11]

Postprocedure Care

Vital signs need to be carefully monitored in the immediate postprocedure period as there is a potential for ongoing blood loss or the development of septicemic shock (due to pyelovenous reflux and bacteremia) in patients at risk. Ideally, the patient should be admitted overnight for observation after the procedure, during which time the tube should be gently flushed with saline every 4 hours. Hematuria is initially present after PCN in virtually all patients, this usually gradually settles within 24–48 hours. The PCN tube output should be recorded to assess for adequacy of drainage. Appropriate analgesics, including narcotics, if required (particularly for patients with intercostal entry), should be provided. The patients should be instructed regarding tube care, especially if long-term drainage is anticipated. The dressing around the catheter should be changed daily. The catheters need to be changed every 8–10 weeks, if long-term drainage is required.[12]

Results

Placement of a nephrostomy tube is technically successful in 84–99% of cases in dilated systems. The success rate will be lower in patients with nondilated systems, complex stone disease such as staghorn calculi, anatomical variants, and renal cysts.[3,5] Use of CT guidance may improve the technical success in patients with anatomical variants or renal cysts.[6,13]

Complications

These may be divided into systemic and local complications.

Systemic Complications

The most common systemic complication that can at times be fatal is sepsis. Every obstructed system should be considered as potentially infected. Manipulation of guidewires, catheter, and injection of contrast all lead to an increase in the pressure in the collecting system, which can lead to pyelovenous reflux. The incidence of septic complications is reported between 1% and 2.5%.[13,14] The incidence rises to 7–9% in the setting of pyonephrosis.[3] One should avoid overdistention of the system by limiting the amount of contrast injected and also keeping manipulation to a minimum in the initial procedure. Complicated or prolonged procedures should be avoided in an infected system; further manipulation should be undertaken only 48–72 hours after the initial procedure when the system is adequately decompressed.[4,5,15]

Prone positioning of the patient during the PCN procedure can lead to respiratory insufficiency, especially in infants or young children under sedation. Close patient monitoring is therefore of utmost importance.[5]

Local Complications

The most common procedure site complication is bleeding, which may occur from the renal parenchymal vessels or the intercostal vessels. Transient hematuria is observed in almost

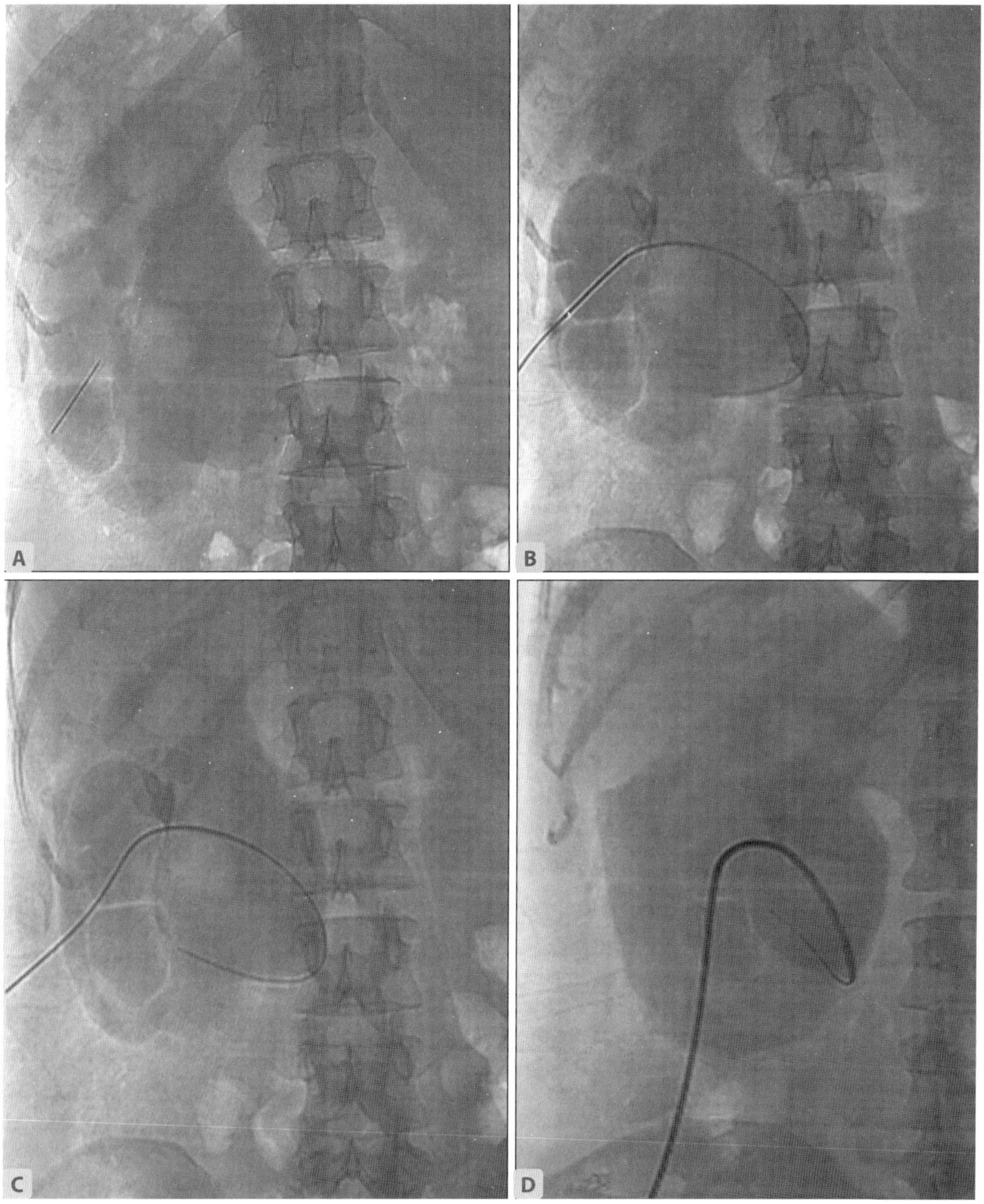

FIGS. 3A TO D: Percutaneous nephrostomy. (A) The grossly dilated calyces are opacified due to a CECT abdomen done the previous day. These have been directly punctured by an 18-gauge needle under fluoroscopic guidance. (B) A stiff guidewire has been negotiated into the pelvis. (C) The puncture needle has been withdrawn and the track is being dilated using fascial dilators. (D) An 8-F catheter is being threaded over the guidewire to coil in the pelvis. (CECT: contrast-enhanced computed tomography).

every patient. Severe bleeding that requires transfusion or further intervention is seen in 1–3% of patients.[3] Bleeding noticed at the time of PCN can often be controlled by placement of a larger-bore nephrostomy catheter to tamponade the track.[16] If bleeding persists for 2–3 days, a nephrostogram should be obtained to check for the position of the catheter. If the tip of the catheter is abutting the calyceal or pelvic wall or all the side holes are not lying within the PCN, repositioning can be done. Severe bleeding developing after catheter insertion requires further evaluation.

A track fistulogram can be obtained by exchanging the nephrostomy catheter with an introducer sheath over a stiff guidewire. The sheath is then gradually withdrawn while injecting contrast. At times, the venous or arterial source of bleed may fill with contrast. Angiographic evaluation for identification of any complication such as formation of a renal arteriovenous fistula, pseudoaneurysm, or vessel laceration should be scheduled without delay in patients with persistent or severe bleeding. Most of these vascular injuries can be managed by the endovascular route; surgical intervention is rarely necessary.[16,17] Bleeding can lead to a perinephric hematoma, which can cause a page kidney with subsequent deterioration in renal function. This should be drained percutaneously.

Adjacent organs may be inadvertently punctured. A retrorenal colon, an uncommon anatomic variant (more common on the right side), may be transgressed (0.2–0.5%) leading to a nephrocolic fistula. Treatment is conservative and consists of ensuring adequate urinary drainage by placement of an antegrade or retrograde ureteric stent, and withdrawing the nephrostomy catheter into the colon to allow the nephrocolic track to heal.[18] Pleural complications in the form of pneumothorax, pleural effusion, emphysema, or hemothorax may occur in 0.1–0.6% of cases. The incidence rises with intercostal entry or complex endourologic procedures.[5] If pleural transgression has occurred, the PCN catheter should be left in place to allow a mature track to form. The catheter can then be removed and a new access obtained into the kidney if required.[16]

Catheter blocks or dislodgements are technical complications, which may occur. The blocked catheter should be cleaned with a guidewire and changed. Replacement of a dislodged catheter is usually possible through the previous tract. Many times the whole tract can be opacified by injecting a small amount of dilute contrast via a sheath placed at the site of urine leak on the skin. A hydrophilic guidewire is then used to probe the tract which usually finds its way into the collecting system.[5,16]

Overall, considering both major and minor complications, the complication rate is around 10%. The mortality rate for PCN varies from 0.046% to 0.3%.[3-5]

Extended Applications of Percutaneous Nephrostomy

Antegrade Ureteric Stenting

The most common extended application of PCN is placement of a ureteric stent for urinary obstruction or fistula. It is often much easier to negotiate areas of narrowing, fistulae, or discontinuity in the ureter in an antegrade rather than a retrograde manner. The stenting is usually performed under local anesthesia and conscious sedation. After the initial PCN, a safety guidewire is placed through an access sheath to avoid losing renal access during the subsequent manipulation of the working guidewire. The obstructed segment is negotiated using different types of angiographic catheters and hydrophilic guidewires. Once the stricture has been negotiated, the guidewire-catheter combination can be advanced into the urinary bladder and coiled within its lumen. The hydrophilic guidewire is then exchanged for a super-stiff Amplatz wire **(Figs. 4A to D)**. Determination of the correct length of the ureteric stent required can be done by using the bent guidewire technique. Balloon dilatation of strictures, placement of ureteric stents, postprocedure drainage of the upper urinary tract, and subsequent nephrostograms can all be performed via the initial PCN tract. The percutaneous external urinary catheter is left in place for 24 hours after the procedure, after which it is capped to check for free flow of urine into the bladder. Thereafter, if there is no hydronephrosis on sonography and contrast injection shows free flow down the double J stent, the external catheter is removed under fluoroscopic control to ensure that there is no inadvertent pulling back of the proximal loop of the stent.[5,19]

Balloon dilatation of benign ureteric strictures may provide durable relief in up to 50% of cases. Following the dilatation, the ureter is buttressed with a stent. In cases where repeated entry into the ureter may be required, a percutaneous nephroureteral catheter (internal-external stent) can be placed for providing mechanical support as well as preserving percutaneous access.[12] Anastomotic strictures after cystectomy and ureteric diversion to an ileal conduit can also be managed through an antegrade percutaneous approach.[20]

Internal-external stents are also placed in cases of ureteric leaks or fistulas because of the anticipated need for multiple percutaneous ureteral interventions and prolonged urinary drainage to allow healing. One should ensure that a solid portion of the tube traverses the site of leak with side holes above and below.

In patients with fistulas of the ureters or lower urinary tract associated with advanced inoperable pelvic malignancies, external drainage with a PCN catheter and a drainage catheter placed in the associated urinoma can at times, not provide adequate urinary diversion. In such cases, ureteral occlusion can be done using stainless steel or platinum coils deployed in the ureter proximal to the leak along with a PCN to provide relief from the distressing symptoms.[21] Other materials that can be used for ureteral occlusion include gelatin sponge, *n*-butyl cyanoacrylate, detachable balloons, or radiofrequency (RF) electrocautery.[22] The major drawback is the need for a lifelong nephrostomy catheter due to the permanent occlusion.

Large-bore Track Creation

Percutaneous nephrostomy forms the first step for creation of a large-diameter track, which may be indicated for performing percutaneous stone therapy, nephroscopy, or antegrade ureteroscopy.[23] Tracks up to the size of 30F or larger can be created by using a combination of balloon dilatation systems and coaxial dilators.

SCLEROTHERAPY FOR RENAL CYSTS

Benign renal cysts (cortical or parapelvic) are found in approximately 50% of males above the age of 50 years. Renal cysts can vary greatly in size and are frequently multiple. They are usually silent, but large, infected, or hemorrhagic cysts can cause symptoms. Large cysts can also cause obstruction of the pelvicalyceal system with formation of calculi, and pressure atrophy of the adjacent renal parenchyma.[8,24]

A renal cyst that is symptomatic requires treatment. They can be managed percutaneously with a combination of sclerotherapy and drainage. Various agents can be used to induce sclerosis of the epithelial lining of the cyst. These include hypertonic dextrose or water-soluble contrast, iophandylate, absolute alcohol, tetracycline, and sodium tetradecyl sulfate. The procedure consists of puncture of the cyst under sonographic guidance and aspiration of the cyst contents. Contrast is then injected to demonstrate the internal appearance of the cyst and to rule out any communication of the cyst with the collecting system. If no communication is demonstrated and the cyst is small, sclerosant can be injected amounting to about one-third of the aspirated contents of

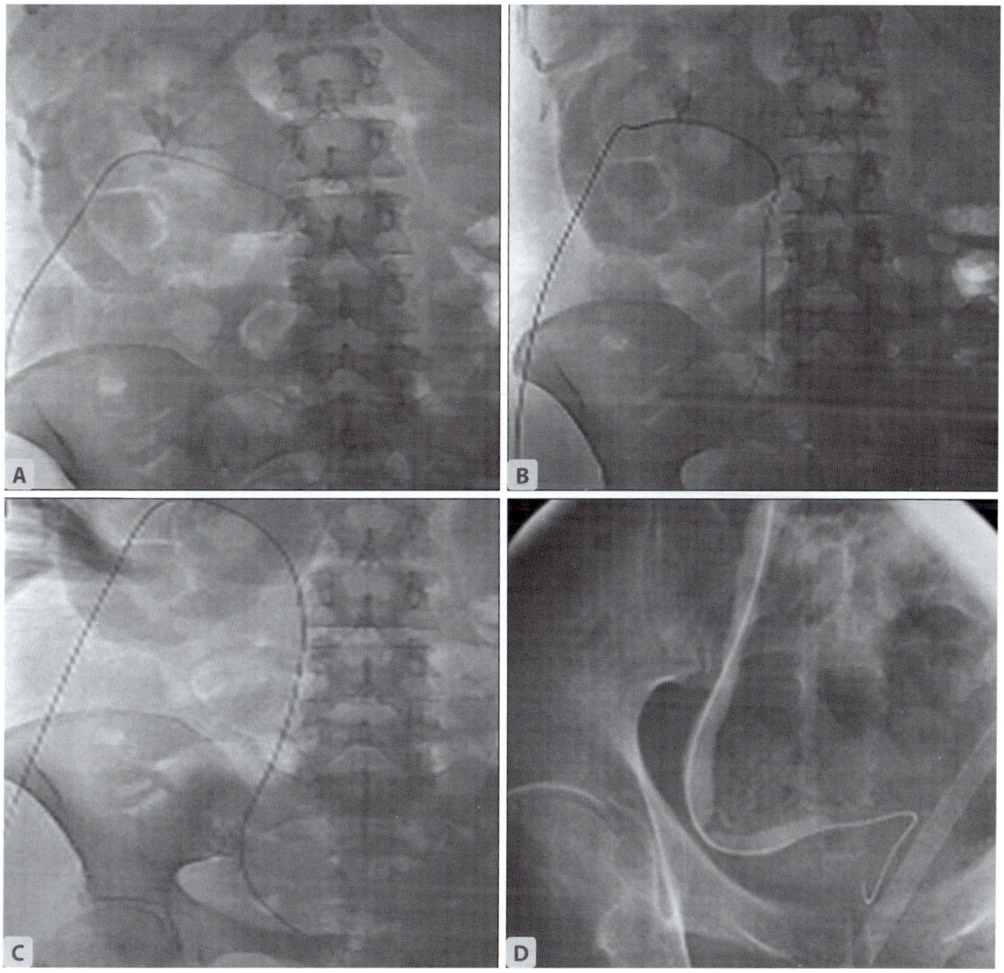

FIGS. 4A TO D: Antegrade stenting in a patient with carcinoma of the urinary bladder. (A) The PCN catheter has been exchanged for a curved angiographic catheter over a stiff guidewire. (B) A hydrophilic guidewire has been introduced through the catheter and is being negotiated down the ureter. (C) The catheter guidewire combination has been advanced into the urinary bladder. (D) The hydrophilic guidewire has been exchanged for a super-stiff Amplatz guidewire after negotiating a tight stricture at the ureterovesical junction. The ureteric stent is then placed over the stiff guidewire. (PCN: percutaneous nephrostomy).

the cyst. The sclerosant is left in place for 15–20 minutes with frequent postural changes of the patient to ensure contact with all the walls of the cyst and then reaspirated. If the cyst is larger, a 5F percutaneous drainage catheter can be placed in the cyst and left to drain for 24–48 hours before sclerotherapy. Larger cysts may require multiple sessions of sclerotherapy.

If a cyst is communicating with the renal collecting system, injection of sclerosant is not advisable as it can cause strictures in the pelvicalyceal system. An infected cyst is managed like an abscess with percutaneous catheter drainage. Good outcomes of sclerotherapy in renal cysts have been reported in literature with success rates varying between 75% and 100%.[8,24]

PERCUTANEOUS CATHETER DRAINAGE

Percutaneous catheter drainage can be done to drain renal or perirenal abscesses, collections, lymphoceles, or urinomas. The basic technique is similar to PCN consisting of needle puncture under imaging guidance, insertion and dilatation of the track followed by catheter placement **(Figs. 5A to C)**. The caliber and type of drainage catheter needs to be tailored according to the nature of fluid to be drained.

BIOPSIES

Core biopsy using automated guns is more common than fine-needle aspiration (FNA) in the genitourinary tract. Renal biopsy with a 16–18-G gun is used for identifying the cause of renal parenchymal disease. Biopsy or FNA can be performed for genitourinary tumors. Transrectal US-guided biopsy of the prostate is useful in suspected cases of prostatic carcinoma.

THE COMPLICATED RENAL TRANSPLANT

Common complications in renal transplant recipients include graft rejection, perigraft, or pelvic fluid collections (urinomas, lymphoceles, etc.), ureterovesical anastomotic

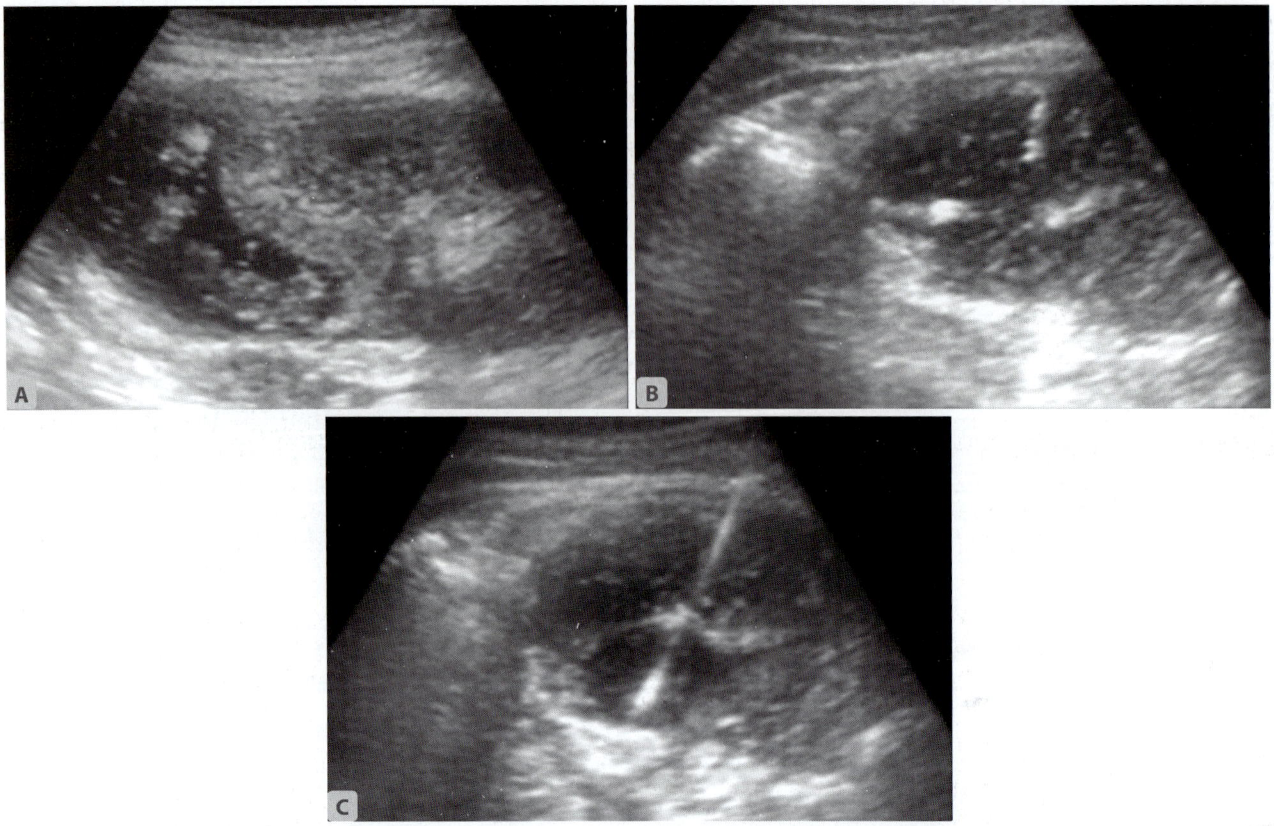

FIGS. 5A TO C: (A) An irregular collection with debris and internal echoes is seen in the upper pole of the kidney, suggestive of renal abscess. (B) The abscess has been punctured with an 18-gauge needle. (C) Guidewire is seen coiled in the abscess.

strictures and focal parenchymal lesions. The percutaneous procedures required in this group of patients are similar to those required in native kidneys. The transplant kidney is approached from the lateral aspect with the patient supine **(Figs. 6A to D)**. These patients are usually very sick and immunocompromised; therefore, meticulous attention should be paid to asepsis.

ABLATION OF RENAL TUMORS

The incidence of renal cell carcinoma (RCC) has been seen to rise over recent years. This is probably due to the increased abdominal imaging and improvements in CT and MR technology resulting in the incidental detection of small, asymptomatic renal tumors in patients undergoing imaging for other indications. Recent studies have indicated that RCC may be incidentally detected during cross-sectional imaging in up to 60% of patients.[25,26] Patients with RCC limited to renal parenchyma have an excellent prognosis for cure, if the RCC can be resected. In the past, radical nephrectomy had been the conventional treatment for RCC. However, over last three decades, nephron-sparing surgery has become a viable alternative to radical nephrectomy and shown to be equally effective curative surgery for patients with a small (<5 cm), single, and well-defined RCC with a contralateral normal kidney.[25] However, nephron-sparing surgery requires more technical skills than radical nephrectomy with higher intraoperative blood loss. Many patients may be poor surgical candidates due to presence of significant comorbidities and advanced age. In addition, some patients may have multiple, bilateral tumors or poor renal function. In these patients, minimally invasive nephron-sparing surgical techniques have been applied including laparoscopic partial nephrectomy and percutaneous ablative techniques. Percutaneous ablative techniques for the treatment of RCC include thermal ablative techniques such as radiofrequency ablation (RFA), microwave ablation (MWA), and high-intensity focused US, which are based on heating the tissue, cryoablation (based on the freezing the tissue), and non-thermal ablative technique irreversible electroporation (IRE). The first reports on the use of RFA in the treatment of renal tumors appeared in 1997 and it is widely used as an effective curative treatment option today.[27]

Indications

The American Urological Association guidelines support use of thermal ablative techniques in the treatment of T1a disease (<4 cm).[28] Indications for thermal ablation according to European Association of Urology guidelines include small renal masses in elderly comorbid patients unfit for surgery, increased risk of multiple tumors due to genetic predisposition (e.g. Von Hippel–Lindau syndrome), and in patients with tumors in both kidneys or with a single kidney and increased risk of complete loss of renal function following surgery (partial nephrectomy).[29,30]

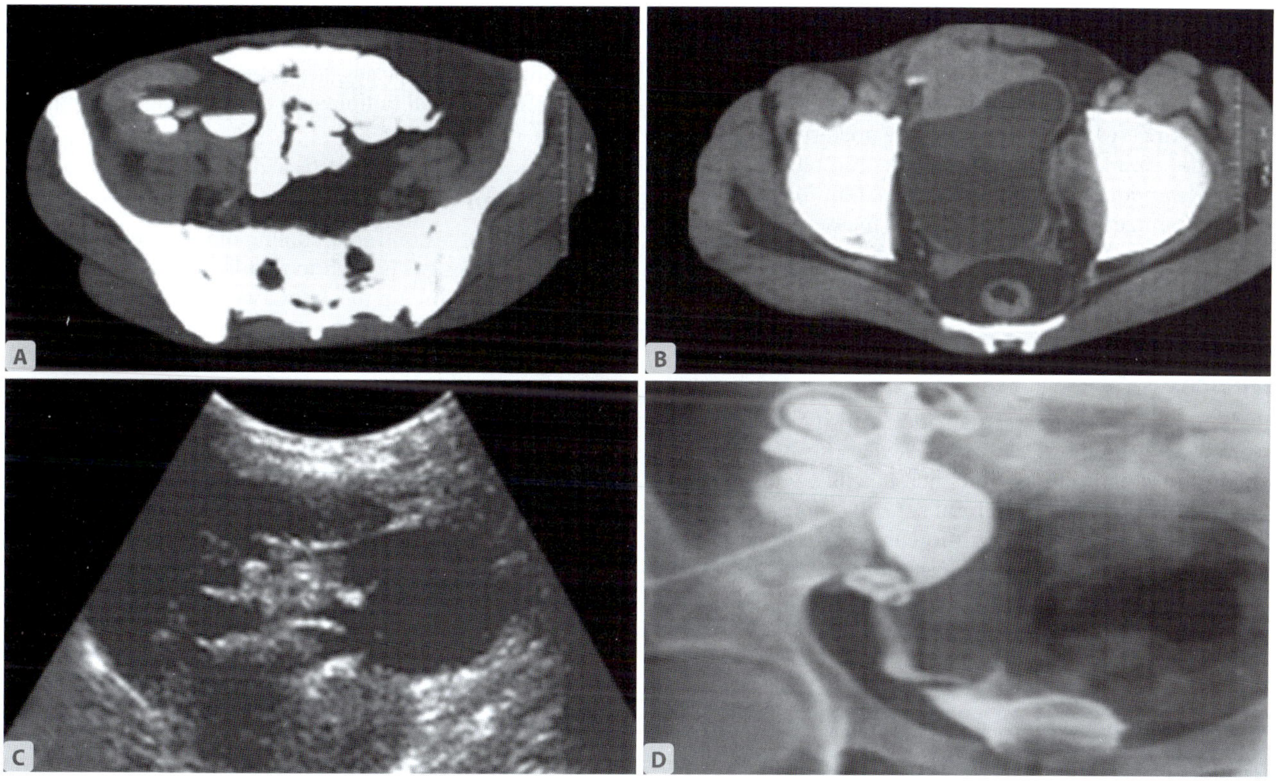

FIGS. 6A TO D: Anastomotic stricture in a transplant kidney. (A) CECT abdomen axial image showing hydroureteronephrosis in the transplant kidney. (B) There is a large, lobulated mass involving the ureterovesical anastomotic site engulfing the ureter. (C) Ultrasound image showing dilatation of the pelvis with minimal dilatation of the calyces. (D) Nephrostogram obtained after percutaneous nephrostomy demonstrates the stricture at the anastomotic site. This was successfully stented later.

The advantages of ablative therapies over surgery include decreased morbidity, better renal parenchymal volume preservation,[31] faster recovery, shorter hospital admission, and probably being the only treatment option for patients with comorbidities, unfit for surgery.[32] Meta-analysis of surgical (open or laparoscopic) and percutaneous ablative techniques reveal a lesser major complication rate for percutaneous ablative techniques.[33] The major disadvantage of ablative therapies over partial nephrectomy is higher local recurrence rate.[28] This difference may be overstatement due to a lack of significant data on long-term disease-free survival following percutaneous ablation of small RCCs. Short- and medium-term published study results[34-37] indicate that proper patient selection can yield good outcome comparable to that of partial nephrectomy, with added benefit of improved renal function preservation. The advantages and risks of each technique should be compared and contrasted with patient, and decision to ablate over surgery requires careful consideration.

Patient Selection and Preprocedure Evaluation

Large tumor size, tumors located near the hilum (renal sinus fat) or ureter were earlier not considered for ablative therapies due to the risk of complications and higher recurrence rate. However, with improved ablation devices, technical skills, and displacement of vital structures from the tumor, there has been significant increase in renal masses that are treated successfully and safely through percutaneous ablative techniques. Large tumors (up to 5 cm), central tumors, tumors in the anteromedial kidney, adjacent to bowel loops, and ureter have all been treated percutaneously, with cryoablation in particular.

Laboratory investigations to be performed prior to the procedure include serum creatinine, platelet count, and coagulation profile. Biopsy of the tumor before ablation is usually performed for tissue diagnosis, or just prior to ablation. Prophylactic antibiotics are usually administered. Contraindications are relative and include uncorrected coagulopathy and an ongoing acute illness.

All patients must undergo a contrast-enhanced CT or magnetic resonance imaging (MRI) of the abdomen before the procedure. The tumor should still be Robson's stage I or II to achieve curative results. Spread of the tumor beyond the renal fascia, into renal vein, or lymph nodes or distant metastases are contraindications for ablation. There is no absolute size criterion; however, the likelihood of complete ablation increases in smaller tumors. Tumors larger than 7 cm are unlikely to be successfully ablated and should only be considered for cytoreduction. ABLATE, a practical planning algorithm for percutaneous renal tumor ablation has been proposed, which takes into account: A—axial diameter of the tumor, B—proximity to bowel loops, L—location of the tumor within the kidney, A—adjacency or proximity to the ureter, T—touching the collecting system/

renal sinus fat, and E—exophytic or endophytic location of the tumor.[38] Another commonly used algorithm is the RENAL nephrometry score (R—radius, E—endophytic or exophytic location of tumor, N—nearness to the renal sinus or collecting system, A—anterior or posterior location of the tumor, and L—location of the tumor in relation to polar line), a standardized classification system for quantifying the anatomic characteristics of renal masses. Higher score correlates with higher tumor grade, pathological stage, and increased risk of complications.[39,40]

Technical Considerations: Different Ablation Devices

Radiofrequency ablation, cryoablation, and MWA are the most commonly used thermal ablative devices for percutaneous ablation of renal tumors, and each has its own merits and demerits, which requires careful consideration. Irreversible electroporation (IRE) and high-intensity focused ultrasound are less commonly used in clinical practice for treating renal tumors. Regardless of the procedure, the postablative goal is to achieve a predictable and complete ablation of the tumor with at least 5–10 mm tumor-free margin.[41]

Radiofrequency Ablation

In RFA, high-frequency alternating current with wavelength ranging from 350 to 500 kHz is passed through a RF electrode placed in the target tumor. Grounding pads placed around the patient's thigh complete the electrical circuit. RF energy results in the heating of cells near the RF electrode/site of energy deposition. When human tissue is heated beyond 49°C, cell death occurs within minutes due to loss of enzymatic function, destruction of cell membranes, and cytoplasm. Temperatures more than 60°C cause immediate cell death. When the temperature exceeds 100°C, the cells boil releasing gas vapors, which cause tissue charring. These in turn inhibit the dispersion of RF energy decreasing the effectiveness of the procedure. Hence, ideal RFA devices should produce prolonged heating of the target tissue between 50°C and 100°C.[27] Various modifications developed toward this purpose include: (1) Pulsed energy deployment; (2) expansion of electrode surface; (3) intraparenchymal injection of iron compounds or saline before and during RF application; and (4) internal cooling of the needle electrode with saline.

Microwave Ablation

In microwave ablation (MWA), oscillating microwave electromagnetic field causes agitation of water molecules, which increases kinetic energy and, in turn increase in temperature inducing cell death via coagulation necrosis. Unlike RFA, microwaves transmit through all types of tissues and nonmetallic materials including water vapor, dehydrated, desiccated, and charred tissues created during the ablation. Hence, microwave produces larger zone of ablation, faster ablation with relatively less heat sink effect. Microwave systems have evolved significantly over the years through generator power optimization and optimization of cooling capabilities of antenna. Performance of each MWA differs as a function of power and time, as supported by the particular system. This affects size and shape of ablation zone created by different devices, hence requires careful attention by the interventional radiologists during device and patient selection.

Cryoablation

Cryoablation relies on rapid cooling of the tissue to induce cell death. Argon gas is used to rapidly freeze cryoprobe to achieve temperature up to –140°C, with critical temperature for cell death being between –20°C and –40°C. It is followed by passive thawing and second session of freeze for over 6–10 minutes depending on the size of the lesion. Rapid cooling leads to formation of ice crystals both intra- and extracellularly, leading to cell dehydration and rupture. Thawing of this frozen tissue leads to microvascular thrombosis and occlusion, and cell hypoxia, causing indirect ischemic injury.[42]

In contrast to RFA and MWA, cryoablation allows direct visualization of the ice ball and ablation zone approximately. The shape and size of the ice ball, there by ablative area can be manipulated by using multiple cryoprobes. During real-time assessment of ablation zone, the true ablation zone of irreversible cell death is approximately 5–10 mm deep to visualized ice ball edge, with temperature at the edge of the ice ball being 0°C approximately, which is a nonlethal temperature.[43] The ice ball must extend at least 5 mm beyond the margin of tumor to avoid residual lesion. In contrast to other thermal ablative therapies, cryoablation induces the maximum postablative immunomodulatory effect by releasing proinflammatory cytokines and dendritic cells (antigen-presenting cells) activation subsequently.[44]

Choice of Ablative Therapy: Clinical Consideration

Radiofrequency ablation, MWA, and cryoablation are established thermal ablative techniques for renal tumor ablation, and success of the procedure is a function of patient selection and method used for ablation, rather than ablation technology.[45] While the merits and drawbacks within a particular patient context are considered for choice of ablative therapy, one must also consider whether cooling or heating is the most appropriate mechanism to induce cell death. Ablation with heating mechanism has lower risk of hemorrhage compared to cryoablation. Between RFA and MWA, RFA is sensitive to heat sink effect with longer ablation duration compared to MWA. Hence, MWA may be a good choice for larger tumors and exophytic tumors as fewer applicators are required for complete ablation **(Figs. 7A to D)**.[46]

Relative to the RFA and MWA, cryoablation is less painful to the patient and allows real-time visualization of the ablation zone **(Figs. 8A to D)**. Cryoablation is ideal for centrally placed tumors, as it is not associated with increased risk of bleeding from hilar vessels compared to MWA and RFA. In addition, ablation margin visualization in real time decreases the risk of ureteral damage.

All these procedures can be performed on an outpatient basis, and usually under local anesthesia with conscious

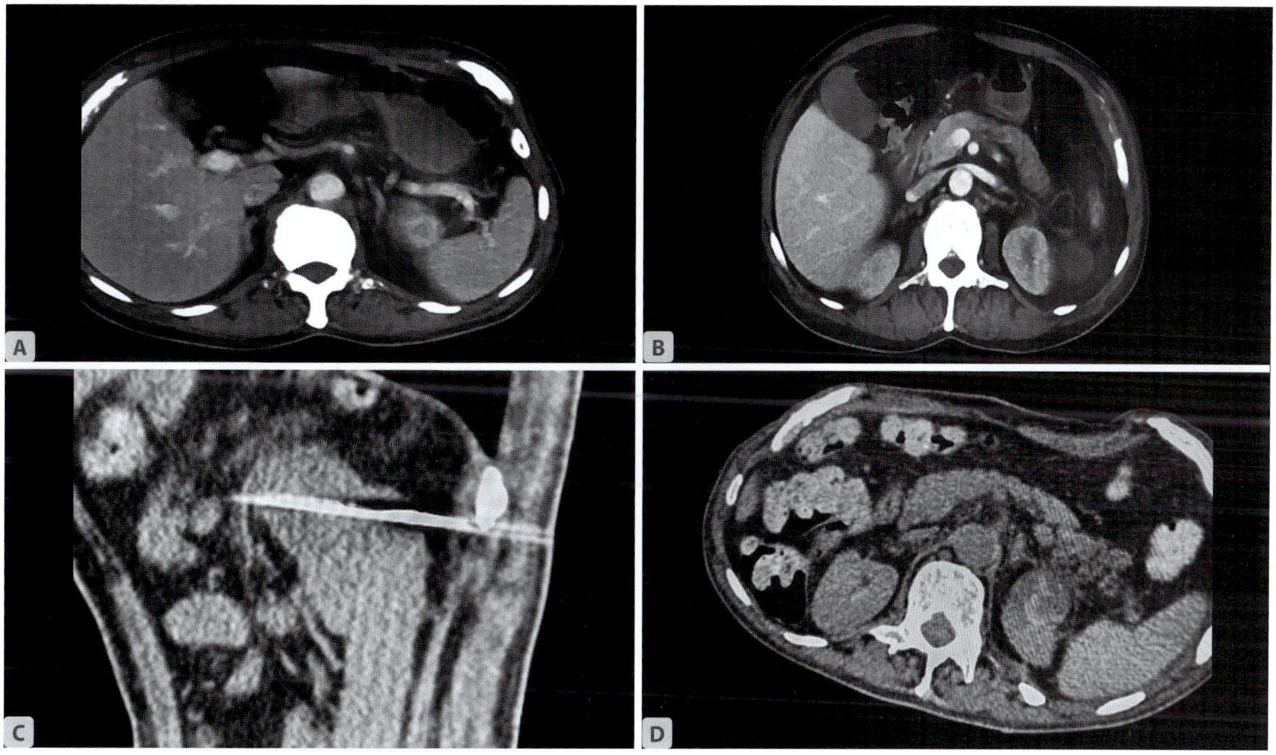

FIGS. 7A TO D: Microwave ablation (MWA) of a renal cell carcinoma. (A and B) Preprocedure axial CT image shows heterogeneously enhancing mass in upper pole of left kidney. (C) Intraprocedural CT sagittal reformatted image shows MWA probe *in situ* (D) Post-MWA ablation NCCT image shows ablated area with hemorrhage. (NCCT: noncontrast computed tomography).

sedation. General anesthesia may be required in certain cases such as deep seated, difficult to access lesions where precise respiratory control is required and large lesions where multiple probes need to be placed. The technique of placing cryoprobe or an electrode is similar to that of performing an imaging-guided biopsy of a focal lesion. The goal is to ablate the target tumor tissue as well as a 0.5–1 cm circumferential rim of adjacent normal parenchyma; therefore, an appropriate electrode size should be selected. The electrode is advanced till the deepest margin of the tumor as the ablation beyond the electrode tip is less.

Postprocedure and Follow-up

All patients should be kept under observation for 4–6 hours after the procedure. Antibiotics should be continued for at least 5 days postprocedure. Appropriate analgesics should be prescribed for ensuring adequate analgesia. Few complications have been reported after percutaneous ablation in renal lesions. Hematuria occurs rarely, is usually self-limited and commonly resolves within 1–2 days. Thermal necrosis of adjacent bowel has been reported. There should be at least 5 mm of intervening gap or fat between the target tumor and bowel to avoid injury. If bowel abuts the target, sterile water/dextrose or air can be injected for bowel loops displacement and ensure safe ablation of the tumor (hydrodissection). RFA of lesions adjacent to the adrenal gland can cause release of vasoactive catecholamines, which requires administration of alpha-blockers. Perirenal hemorrhage is common but is rarely clinically significant. Needle-track seeding and development of ureteric strictures are other rare complications.

A contrast-enhanced biphasic CT should be obtained immediately after the procedure to determine adequacy of ablation. Thereafter a contrast-enhanced CT or MRI should be obtained at 1-, 3-, 6-, and 12-month intervals to look for residual or recurrent tumor. Imaging after the first year can be done at 6–9-month intervals. CT is more often used for postablation follow-up because of its wider availability and lower cost; however, MRI may be used in patients with renal insufficiency **(Figs. 9A to C)**.

Immediately after ablation, the tumor usually appears larger because of ablation of 0.5–1 cm of adjacent normal tissue. On follow-up imaging, ablated tumors appear as focal, nonenhancing masses, which show decrease in size with time. Soft tissue stranding may be seen in the perinephric fat. At times, a curvilinear, hyperattenuating area or halo is seen surrounding the ablated lesion.[24]

Nodular enhancement in the ablated tumor or an increase in the size of lesion represent residual or recurrent tumor. On MR, the area of necrosis appears hypointense on T2-weighted images. On T1-weighted images, it usually appears hyperintense compared to the renal cortex, and occasionally it may appear iso- to hypointense. Peripheral smooth enhancement of the rim may be seen early after ablation but this gradually resolves over 3 months. Residual viable tumor tissue appears hyperintense on T2-weighted images and shows nodular enhancement postgadolinium on T1 images.[26]

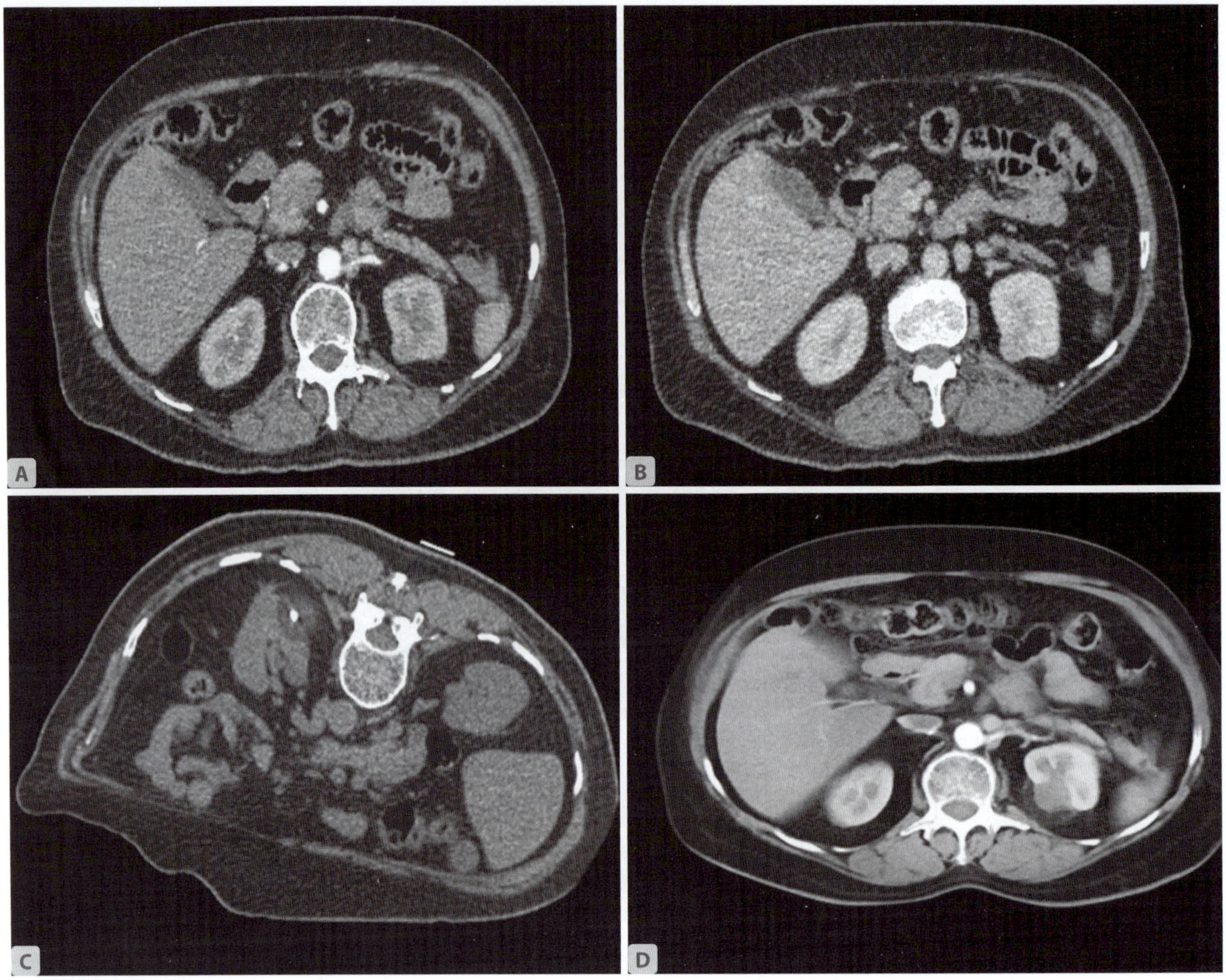

FIGS. 8A TO D: Cryoablation of a renal cell carcinoma. (A and B) Preprocedure axial CT images in arterial and venous phases show heterogeneously enhancing mass in upper pole of left kidney. (C) Intraprocedural CT image show cryoprobe *in situ* with formation of ice ball. (D) Postcryoablation arterial phase CT image shows nonenhancing ablated area.

To summarize, percutaneous ablative therapies are an effective treatment option in patients with early-stage renal cell carcinoma (RCC) who are poor surgical candidates, patients with increased risk of multiple tumors due to genetic predisposition, and in patients with bilateral tumors or with a solitary kidney. The choice of ablative technique is governed by preprocedural assessment and operative experience.

REFERENCES

1. Goodwin WE, Casey WL, Woolf W. Percutaneous trocar (needle) nephrostomy in hydronephrosis. J Am Med Asso. 1955;157(11):891-4.
2. Banner MP, Ramchandani P, Pollack HM. Interventional procedures in the upper urinary tract. Cardiovascular Intervent Radiol. 1991;14(5):267-84.
3. Pabon-Ramos WM, Dariushnia SR, Walker TG, et al. Quality improvement guidelines for percutaneous nephrostomy. J Vasc Interv Radiol. 2016;27(3):410-4.
4. Dyer RB, Regan JD, Kavanagh PV, et al. Percutaneous nephrostomy with extensions of the technique: step by step. Radiographics. 2002;22(3):503-25.
5. Hausegger KA, Portugaller HR. Percutaneous nephrostomy and antegrade ureteral stenting: technique–indications–complications. Eur Radiol. 2006;16(9):2016-30.
6. Meira MS, Barbosa PNVP, Bitencourt V, et al. Retrospective analysis of computed tomography guided percutaneous nephrostomies in cancer patients. Radiol Bras. 2019;52(3): 148-54.
7. Kariniemi J, Sequeiros RB, Ojala R, et al. MRI guided percutaneous nephrostomy: a feasibility study. Eur Radiol. 2009;19(5): 1296-301.
8. Park BK, Kim SH, Moon MH. Nonvascular interventions of the urinary tract. J Korean Med Sci. 2002;17(6):727-36.

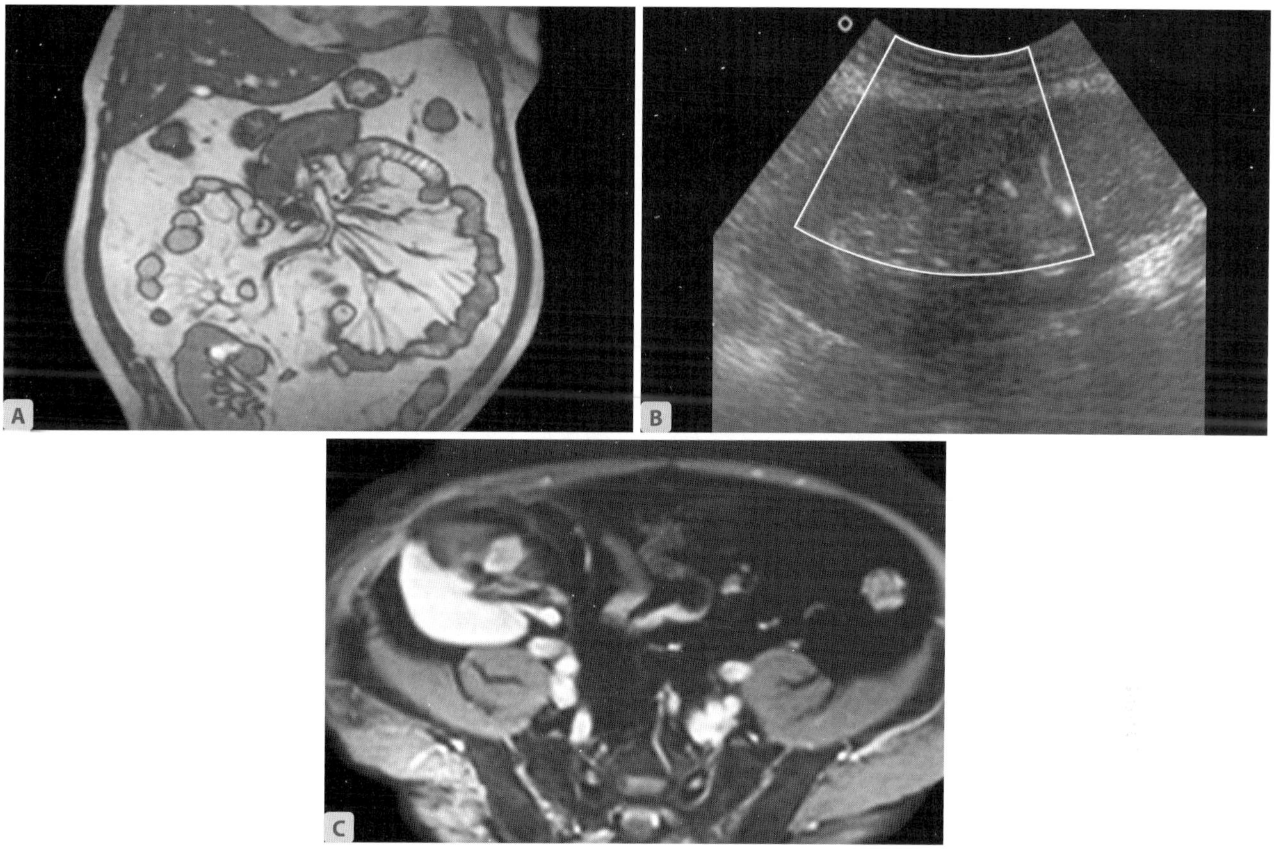

FIGS. 9A TO C: Radiofrequency ablation of a renal cell carcinoma in a transplant kidney. (A) Preprocedure MR coronal T2-weighted image shows a focal area of hyperintensity in the upper pole of the transplant kidney. (B) Follow-up Doppler image after 6 weeks shows absence of flow to the region of the ablated tumor. (C) MR axial postgadolinium T1 image 1 month after radiofrequency ablation shows absence of enhancement of the renal parenchyma in the region of ablation. Note the defect is larger than the original tumor size due to ablation of a rim of normal parenchyma around the tumor. (RFA: radiofrequency ablation).

9. Funaki B, Vatakencherry G. Comparison of single-stick and double-stick techniques for percutaneous nephrostomy. Cardiovasc Intervent Radiol. 2004;27(1):35-7.
10. Ray CR, Brown AC, Smith MT, et al. Percutaneous access of nondilated renal collecting systems. Semin Intervent Radiol. 2014;31(1):98-100.
11. Gupta S, Gulati M, Suri S. Ultrasound guided percutaneous nephrostomy in nondilated pelvicalyceal system. J Clin Ultrasound. 1998;26(3):177-9.
12. Adamo R, Saad WEA, Brown DB. Management of nephrostomy drains and ureteral stents. Tech Vasc Interv Radiol. 2009: 12(3):193-204.
13. Farrell TA, Hicks ME. A review of radiologically guided percutaneous nephrostomies in 303 patients. J Vasc Intervent Radiol. 1997;8(5):769-74.
14. Wah TM, Weston MJ, Irving HC. Percutaneous nephrostomy insertion: outcome data from a prospective multi-operator study at a UK training centre. Clin Radiol. 2004;59(3):255-61.
15. Zagoria RJ, Dyer RB. Do's and don'ts of percutaneous nephrostomy. Acad Radiol. 1999;6(6):370-77.
16. Krohmer SJ, Pillai AK, Guevara CJ, et al. Image-guided nephrostomy interventions: How to recognize, avoid, or get out. Tech Vasc Intervent Radiol. 2018;21(4):261-6.
17. Vignali C, Lonzi S, Bargellini I, et al. Vascular injuries after percutaneous renal procedures: treatment by transcatheter embolization. Eur Radiol. 2004;14(4):723-9.
18. Gerspach JM, Bellman GC, Stoller ML, et al. Conservative management of colon injury following percutaneous renal surgery. Urology. 1997;49(6):831-6.
19. Kahriman G, Ozcan N, Dogan A, et al. Percutaneous antegrade ureteral stent placement: single centre experience. Diagn Interv Radiol. 2019;25(2):127-33.
20. Tal R, Bachar GN, Baniel J, et al. External Internal nephro-ureteral-ileal stents in patients with an ileal conduit: long-term results. Urology. 2004;63(3):438-41.
21. Titton RL, Gervais DA, Hahn PF, et al. Urine leaks and urinomas: diagnosis and imaging-guided intervention. Radiographics 2003;23(5):1133-47.
22. Avritscher R, Madoff DC, Ramirez PT, et al. Fistulas of the lower urinary tract: Percutaneous approaches for the management of a difficult clinical entity. Radiographics. 2004;24(Suppl 1): S217-36.
23. Bhattacharya T, Kumaradevan J, Watkinson AF. Percutaneous nephrolithotomy: state of the art. Semin Intervent Radiol. 2000;17(4):341-9.
24. Hanna RM, Dahniya MH. Aspiration and sclerotherapy of symptomatic simple renal cysts: value of two injections of a sclerosing agent. Am J Roentgenol. 1996;167(3):781-3.
25. Kawamoto S, Permpongkosol S, Bluemke DA, et al. Sequential changes after radiofrequency ablation and cryoablation of renal neoplasms: role of CT and MR imaging. Radiographics. 2007;27(2):343-55.

26. Farrell MA, Charboneau WJ, DiMarco DS, et al. Imaging-guided radiofrequency ablation of solid renal tumours. Am J Roentgenol. 2003;180(6):1509-13.
27. Zagoria RJ. Imaging-guided radiofrequency ablation of renal masses. Radiographics. 2004;24(Suppl 1):S59-71.
28. Campbell SC, Novick AC, Belldegrun A, et al. Guideline for management of the clinical T1 renal mass. J Urol. 2009;182(4): 1271-9.
29. Ljungberg B, Bensalah K, Canfield S, et al. EAU guidelines on renal cell carcinoma: 2014 update. Eur Urol. 2015;67(5): 913-24.
30. Van Poppel H, Becker F, Cadeddu JA, et al. Treatment of localised renal cell carcinoma. Eur Urol. 2011;60(4): 662-72.
31. Woldu SL, Thoreson GR, Okhunov Z, et al. Comparison of renal parenchymal volume preservation between partial nephrectomy, cryoablation, and radiofrequency ablation. J Endourol. 2015;29(8):948-55.
32. Higgins LJ, Hong K. Renal ablation techniques: state of the art. Am J Roentgenol. 2015;205(4):735-41.
33. Hui GC, Tuncali K, Tatli S, et al. Comparison of percutaneous and surgical approaches to renal tumor ablation: metaanalysis of effectiveness and complication rates. J Vasc Interv Radiol. 2008;19(9):1311-20.
34. Katsanos K, Mailli L, Krokidis M, et al. Systematic review and meta-analysis of thermal ablation versus surgical nephrectomy for small renal tumours. Cardiovasc Intervent Radiol. 2014;37(2):427-37.
35. Chang X, Liu T, Zhang F, et al. Radiofrequency ablation versus partial nephrectomy for clinical T1a renal cell carcinoma: long-term clinical and oncologic outcomes based on a propensity score analysis. J Endourol. 2015;29(5):518-25.
36. Thompson RH, Atwell T, Schmit G, et al. Comparison of partial nephrectomy and percutaneous ablation for cT1 renal masses. Eur Urol. 2015;67(2):252-9.
37. Yu J, Liang P, Yu X, et al. US-guided percutaneous microwave ablation versus open radical nephrectomy for small renal cell carcinoma: intermediate-term results. Radiology. 2014; 270(3):880-7.
38. Schmit GD, Kurup AN, Weisbrod AJ, et al. ABLATE: a renal ablation planning algorithm. Am J Roentgenol. 2014;202(4): 894-903.
39. Kutikov A, Uzzo RG. The RENAL nephrometry score: a comprehensive standardized system for quantitating renal tumor size, location and depth. J Urol. 2009;182(2):844-53.
40. Parsons RB, Canter D, Kutikov A, et al. Renal nephrometry scoring system: the radiologist's perspective. Am J Roentgenol. 2012;199(3):W355-9.
41. Clark TWI, Millward SF, Gervais DA, et al. Reporting standards for percutaneous thermal ablation of renal cell carcinoma. J Vasc Interv Radiol. 2009;20(7 Suppl):S409-16.
42. Brian CA, Erick MR. Percutaneous cryoablation of renal tumors: patient selection, technique, and postprocedural imaging. Radiographics. 2010;30(4):887-902.
43. Georgiades C, Rodriguez R, Azene E, et al. Determination of the nonlethal margin inside the visible "ice-ball" during percutaneous cryoablation of renal tissue. Cardiovasc Intervent Radiol. 2013;36(3):783-90.
44. Jansen MC, van Hillegersberg R, Schoots IG, et al. Cryoablation induces greater inflammatory and coagulative responses than radiofrequency ablation or laser induced thermotherapy in a rat liver model. Surgery. 2010;147(5):686-95.
45. Cadeddu JA, Raman JD. Renal tumor ablation is a function of patient selection and technique—not the ablation technology. Cancer. 2008;113:2623-26.
46. Lubner MG, Brace CL, Hinshaw JL, et al. Microwave tumor ablation: mechanism of action, clinical results, and devices. J Vasc Interv Radiol. 2010;21(8 Suppl):S192-203.

CHAPTER

27

Vascular Interventions in the Genitourinary Tract

Shivanand Gamanagatti, Ankur Goyal, Deep Narayan Srivastava

INTRODUCTION

Interventional vascular radiology has grown over the past two to three decades and the radiologist has an important role to play in patient's management. With the current advances in technology allowing more accurate and controlled deployment of embolic agents, embolotherapy has now become the procedure of choice for the management of visceral and solid organ aneurysms and also percutaneous renal revascularization has become an accepted procedure of choice for renal artery stenosis (RAS).

Various vascular interventional procedures in genitourinary practice are directed toward vascular dilatation or vascular embolization. The commonly performed procedures include:

- Renal artery angioplasty
- Renal artery stenting
- Renal artery embolization
- Uterine artery embolization (UAE)
- Vaginal arteriovenous malformation (AVM) embolization
- Varicocele embolization
- Scrotal AVM embolization
- Prostatic artery embolization (PAE)
- Transjugular renal biopsy (TJRB)
- Prophylactic balloon placement in adherent placenta.

RENAL ARTERY ANGIOPLASTY

Renal artery stenosis is the most common cause of secondary hypertension, seen with a 14% prevalence among patients with chronic renal failure. Among the various causes of RAS, atherosclerosis is the most common etiology, others being fibromuscular dysplasia, Takayasu's arteritis, neurofibromatosis, etc. Medical therapy and surgical treatment including renal vascularization and nephrectomy are traditional methods of treatment for renovascular hypertension. These methods, however, have several disadvantages. The lowering of blood pressure by medical therapy further reduces renal blood flow and further deterioration of renal function even in controlled blood pressure. The surgical revascularization methods are considerably beneficial to most patients but considering the associated morbidity and operative mortality rate of 8%, surgery should be done only on carefully selected patients. Presently, percutaneous transluminal renal angioplasty (PTRA) is the first line of treatment for RAS due to its relatively lower morbidity and mortality compared to surgical methods. The Society of Cardiovascular and Interventional Radiology (SCVIR) has laid down guidelines for the renal artery angioplasty. Various pathological lesions are shown in **Table 1**.

According to the SCVIR guidelines, the above lesions can be divided into four categories as follows:[1]

- *Category I: Lesions* are those for which balloon angioplasty alone is the procedure of choice. It includes fibromuscular dysplasia of the renal artery and unilateral short (<3 cm) and nonostial atherosclerosis **(Figs. 1 and 2)**.
- *Category II: Lesions* are well suited for angioplasty and are atherosclerotic bilateral nonostial stenosis, postoperative anastomotic stenosis, and stenoses associated with worsening renal function **(Fig. 3)**.
- *Category III: Lesions* have a moderate chance of technical success or long-term benefits compared to bypass surgery and are atherosclerotic renal ostial stenosis, nonatheromatous lesions involving the proximal renal arteries.
- *Category IV: Lesions* have a low technical success rate. This includes renal artery stenoses in vessels that arise from an aneurysmal or severely diseased aortic segment or stenoses associated with renal artery aneurysm.

TABLE 1: Various pathological lesions.

Cause	Affected segment	Incidence (%)
Atherosclerosis	Ostium and proximal 1/3	90
Fibromuscular dysplasia	Mid and distal 1/3	10
Takayasu's arteritis	Ostium and proximal part	<1
NF-1	All	<1
Radiation	All	<1
Trauma	All	<1

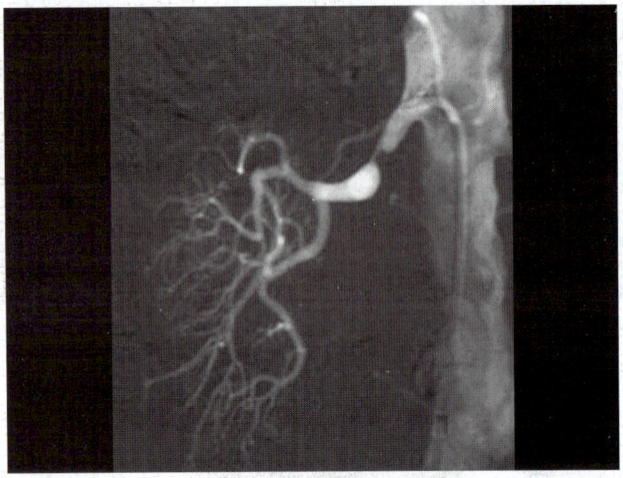

FIG. 1: Selective renal angiogram showing nonostial short segment narrowing with post-stenotic dilation of right renal artery (category I lesions).

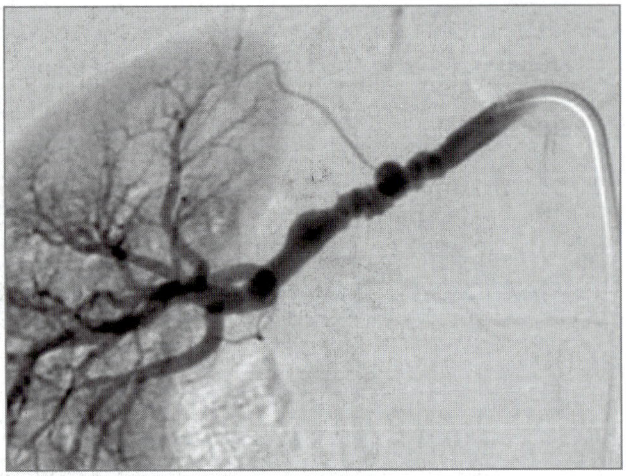

FIG. 2: Selective renal angiogram showing classic string of pearls appearance of right renal artery suggestive of fibromuscular dysplasia (category I lesions).

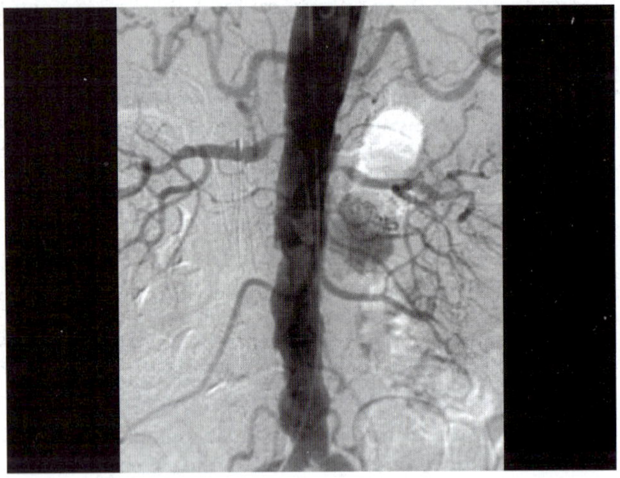

FIG. 3: Flush aortogram showing diffuse atherosclerotic abdominal aorta and ostial narrowing of bilateral renal arteries (category II lesions).

Imaging the Renal Arteries

Conventional angiography has been conventionally considered the best anatomic study for evaluating patients with RAS. Duplex ultrasonography can be very helpful and should be the first imaging study in patients suspected of having RAS. The quality of renal ultrasonography depends on the operator and on other variables such as body habitus, but even so, the sensitivity of duplex scanning has been reported to be 98%, with 98% specificity and high positive and negative predictive values.[2]

Computed tomography angiography (CTA) has now replaced conventional angiography for evaluating renal arteries. The images are comparable to those of conventional angiography, vessels can be evaluated in three dimensions, and CTA offers options for clarifying anatomy which may be better than with conventional angiography. Exposure of the patient to radiation from renal CTA is comparable to that of catheter angiography.[2]

Magnetic resonance angiography (MRA) is also used to evaluate the anatomy of the renal arteries. It has lower resolution than CTA or conventional angiography but is excellent for patients with impaired renal function, especially with the availability of noncontrast angiography sequences.[2,3]

Technique[4-6]

Endovascular treatment of RAS involves either percutaneous transluminal angioplasty or a combination of angioplasty and stent placement.

Renal Artery Angioplasty

The procedure is most commonly performed through a femoral artery approach. However, if indicated by the patient's anatomy (e.g. presence of iliac artery occlusions or a very steeply angled renal artery), the brachial approach can be used. A 6-F sheath is inserted into the femoral artery. It will be very helpful if a long (typically 35 cm) sheath is used as a guiding catheter. A preshaped catheter is then used to access the renal artery. The catheter is used in combination with a guidewire to cross the lesion. A hydrophilic guidewire such as a Terumo can be very helpful, especially in lesions that are difficult to cross, though many would also use the soft-tipped Bentson guidewire. Having crossed the lesion, heparin and an antispasmodic drug are administered. The author uses 3000 units of heparin and 300 mg of isosorbide dinitrate.

With the catheter across the stenosis, the guidewire is changed to a specialist guidewire such as the roadrunner. The guidewire itself is very stiff, providing good support for the angioplasty balloon. The atraumatic nature of the tip is very important, as it can be placed in a cortical branch without a significant danger of causing spasm. An angioplasty balloon is then introduced over the guidewire and angioplasty is performed **(Figs. 4A to E)**. After confirming the proper position of balloon, it is inflated and left for 30 seconds.

Balloons are not oversized but should instead be of the same diameter as the artery distal to the stenosis. Typical balloon diameters will vary between 5 mm and 7 mm.

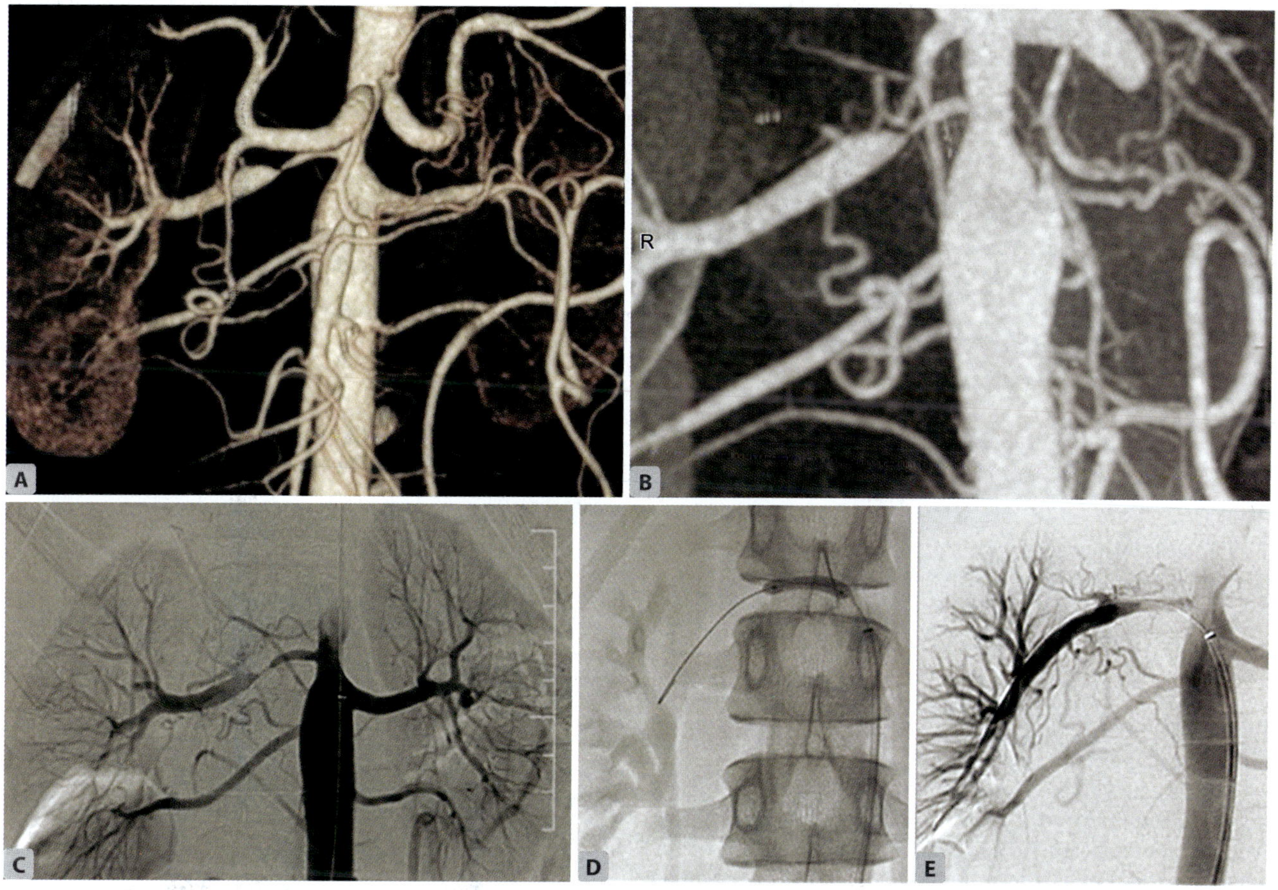

FIGS. 4A AND E: A case of renal artery stenosis treated by angioplasty: (A and B) CT images showing narrowing of juxtarenal part of abdominal aorta and right main renal artery with post-stenotic dilatation; (C) Flush aortogram confirming the CT findings of narrowing of juxtarenal part of abdominal aorta and right main renal artery; (D) Angioplasty spot image showing dilatation of narrowed segment of main renal artery using 6 mm balloon catheter; (E) Post-angioplasty angiogram showing <10% percent residual narrowing of angioplasty segment.

Loin pain with balloon inflation is common but should not be severe. In the event of the latter, vessel rupture may occur, and dilation should be stopped and a smaller balloon should be used. After dilation, the balloon is removed, the guidewire is left in place, and a check angiogram is performed through the long sheath or guiding catheter. If there has been a complication or further dilation is required, access has thus been maintained to allow additional intervention. The angioplasty is considered technically successful if after the angioplasty, the arterial lumen had less than 30% residual stenosis and the pressure gradient is less than 10 mm Hg. The clinical results can be assessed by the effect on blood pressure control and improvement of renal function.

RENAL ARTERY STENTING

The renal artery stent placement is now an established method of adjunctive treatment to renal angioplasty. Several problems related to renal angioplasty, such as flow-compromising dissection, residual stenosis greater than 30% with a trans-stenotic pressure gradient greater than 20 mm Hg or restenosis, can be successfully treated with stenting. The renal artery stenting has shown better technical results, long-term patency, and a lower rate of restenosis than that of PTRA. Stents are almost exclusively placed in the renal arteries by using an angioplasty balloon (balloon-expandable rather than self-expanding stents). In many respects, insertion of renal artery stents is performed in a similar way to renal angioplasty. However, stents are normally inserted at the ostium of the renal artery because they are used for the treatment of atheromatous disease. It is therefore essential to have a clear idea of the exact location of the ostium to facilitate accurate stent placement. Prior to stent insertion, it is of value to predilate the stenosis with a 4-mm balloon to ease the passage of the stent across the stenosis. Although many recommend the use of a guiding catheter, modern long sheaths also perform very well. Use of either allows angiograms to be performed while finally positioning the stent prior to deployment. There are no reported adverse consequences associated with leaving the stent projecting 2 mm or so into the aorta.

Positioning the stent in this manner ensures that the entire lesion is stented. Sometimes it may be necessary to perform renal arterial intervention from a brachial approach, for example, when femoral access is not possible or if the renal arteries are sharply angulated inferiorly **(Figs. 5A and B)**.

Outcome

Compared with the relatively good outcomes after angioplasty for fibromuscular dysplasia, balloon angioplasty alone

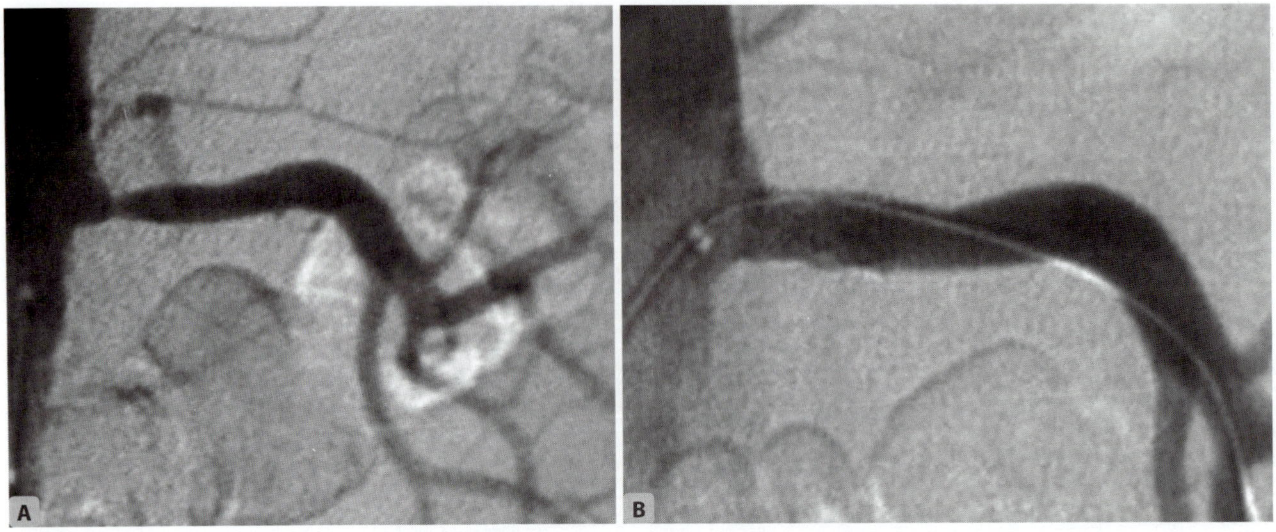

FIGS. 5A AND B: A case of renal artery ostial narrowing treated by stenting: (A) Renal angiogram showing ostial narrowing of left renal artery. (B) Post-stenting angiogram showing 0% residual stenosis.

has not been as successful in treating atherosclerotic RAS. This is most likely because of the high degree of elastic recoil in atherosclerotic arteries compared with that encountered in fibromuscular webs.

The restenosis rate after angioplasty alone varies widely but has been reported to be from 10% to 46%.[5] Angioplasty (without stent placement) has a higher technical success rate when applied to atherosclerotic lesions in the midportion of the main renal artery (72–82%) than in ostial lesions (success rate ≈ 60%).

Stents are now almost uniformly used for all ostial lesions and almost all atherosclerotic RAS. One current report quotes a technical success rate for stents of 94–100% and a restenosis rate of 11–23%, with an improvement in blood pressure control in 50–80% and stabilization of renal function in 60–70%.[5,6]

Renal function at the time of stent placement strongly predicts patency and expected survival after intervention. In patients with normal renal function, 3-year survival is 94%, 74% if serum creatinine is between 1.5 mg/dL and 2.0 mg/dL, and 52% if serum creatinine is > 2.0 mg/dL.[6] It is important to understand that though renal artery revascularization in atherosclerosis seldom cures the disease, it brings down the blood pressure and/or the requirement of antihypertensive medication modestly.

Renal Artery Intervention in Renal Transplants

Although technically angioplasty and stenting are similar in many ways to procedures in native kidneys, the management of transplant RAS involves some important differences. Cadaveric transplants are generally anastomosed to the recipient external iliac artery, because it is possible to obtain the full length of renal artery and renal vein stump. These procedures are separately described in the chapter on Imaging of Renal Transplant.

Complications

The complications can be divided into major (renal insufficiency, renal artery occlusion, renal artery damage including rupture, etc.) and minor (temporary renal insufficiency, retroperitoneal hematoma, femoral artery complications, etc).

RENAL ARTERIAL EMBOLIZATION

The various indications are embolization of renal neoplasms, renal pseudoaneurysms (secondary to either traumatic or iatrogenic injury), end-stage kidney, etc.

Technique

There are three different types of renal embolization: (1) proximal (occlusion of main or segmental renal artery), (2) distal (occlusion of lobular or arcuate arteries), and (3) capillary (occlusion of arterioles and glomeruli). Depending upon the type of embolization, the catheter is advanced into the renal artery branches. The super-selective embolization with a coaxial catheter can save part of renal parenchyma. The selection of embolizing material also depends upon the purpose of occlusion (temporary or permanent). The various materials used for embolization are particles (gelfoam, polyvinyl alcohol), liquid agents (alcohol, sclerosants), coils, and detachable balloons.

Transcatheter Embolization of Renal Neoplasms

The current role of renal embolization in carcinoma of the kidney is uncertain.

The most important aim of preoperative embolization of the renal artery is to prevent migration of tumor cells from being flooded out.

The various indications are:

- To relieve symptoms such as pain, hematuria, polycythemia, congestive heart failure
- To facilitate surgical resection by preoperative embolization to reduce the tumor vascularity
- To inhibit tumor growth and to reduce tumor mass
- To stimulate an immune response by decreasing the tumor load
- Prophylactic embolotherapy in angiomyolipomas to avoid risk of hemorrhage.

The impact of renal embolization as the palliative method of treatment on the survival time is difficult to estimate, but improvement in local symptoms such as hematuria and pain is evident.

Varieties of embolizing agents have been used such as gelatin sponge, stainless steel coil, *n*-butyl cyanoacrylate, absolute alcohol, and autologus blood clot. But the embolization material of choice is ethanol. Ethanol is widely used for permanent embolization. The optimal dose is 0.5 mL/kg of body weight with an upper limit of 1 mL/kg and at the rate of 2 mL/sec. The advantages of alcohol over other permanent embolizing material are complete tissue necroses with permanent arterial occlusion, milder postinfarction syndrome, less chances of infection, and simple to use.

The technique for delivery of absolute alcohol to renal artery includes the balloon occlusion technique and superselective technique.[7,8] The balloon occlusion technique serves several purposes like it prevents reflux of alcohol into aorta and prolongs the contact period of alcohol with endothelium.

In the superselective technique, an endhole catheter is advanced superselectively into lobar braches and the alcohol is injected to prevent reflux. This is then followed by large vessel embolization with coils. The mechanism of action of alcohol is proposed to be a combination of perivascular necrosis, sludging of erythrocytes in small arteries, and glomeruli and endothelial damage.

The rate of injection has serious impact over the success of embolization. An injection rate of 1–5 mL/sec leads to perivascular necrosis, sludging of erythrocytes in small arteries, and glomeruli indicating direct tissue toxicity. A slow rate of injection of 0.1 mL/sec causes endothelial damage and less tissue toxicity. Hence, a slow rate of injection is desirable in benign conditions such as AVM and angiomyolipomas, where permanent arterial occlusion with minimal tissue damage is desirable.[7]

All arteries smaller than major segmental arteries must be occluded. Angiographic findings of successful embolization include stagnation of flow and extravasation of contrast material into adjacent renal parenchyma **(Figs. 6A to F)**.

Care must be taken when embolizing with absolute ethanol as it causes vigorous thrombosis due to denaturing proteins. Ethanol can cause seizures and intoxication if it reaches the systemic circulation. It can also permeate the tissues and cause injury to adjacent structures such as bowel and nerves.

Transcatheter Embolization of Renal Pseudoaneurysms

Incidence

Incidence of aneurysm formation differs for the various etiologies of renal artery aneurysms. However, literature suggests that incidence ranges between 0.015% and 9.7%.[9] Poutasse have classified renal artery aneurysms into saccular, fusiform, dissecting and pseudoaneurysms.[10] The natural history of these aneurysms is not well-defined in the literature. However, the incidence of rupture rate ranges from 0% to 14%.[10] Renal artery aneurysms that are treated surgically are approached by nephrectomy, ex vivo repair and reimplantation.[9-11]

Causes

Typically, pseudoaneurysm formation in the renal artery distribution is either iatrogenic or traumatic. Other causes of aneurysm formation include fibromuscular dysplasia, polyarteritis nodosa, amphetamine abuse, angiomyolipoma (either with or without associated tuberous sclerosis) and neurofibromatosis.

Risks Posed by the Aneurysm

Rupture is a rare risk of these aneurysms. However, pregnant women are more prone to rupture which is similar to splenic artery aneurysms rupture.

Anatomic/Physiologic Considerations

The vascular supply to the kidney is considered endorgan, and hence infarction is common after embolization. Therefore, in patients with renal insufficiency or underlying diseases such as tuberous sclerosis or von Recklinghausen's disease, nephron-sparing procedures are vital. Superselective embolization is advisable in all cases of renal artery embolization unless partial or total nephrectomy is planned.

Technique

The renal arteries arise at the L2 level from the abdominal aorta. A left anterior oblique view during a flush injection of the aorta will often provide the best view of the origins. Careful examination for accessory renal arteries is necessary.

A renal double curve or Cobra catheter will easily engage the main renal ostium. A Rosen wire is an atraumatic guidewire that allows for secure exchange or upsizing to a guiding catheter or Balkin sheath. Selective injection should be performed to identify the feeding vessel or vessels. This can be done through the sheath. Many embolization techniques can be used in this setting depending on the type, number and location of the aneurysms. Commonly pseudoaneurysms are embolized superselectively by using coils **(Figs. 7A to D)**. Sometimes, aneurysms of the main renal artery maybe amenable to stent graft placement, thus allowing distal perfusion to be maintained. Alternative

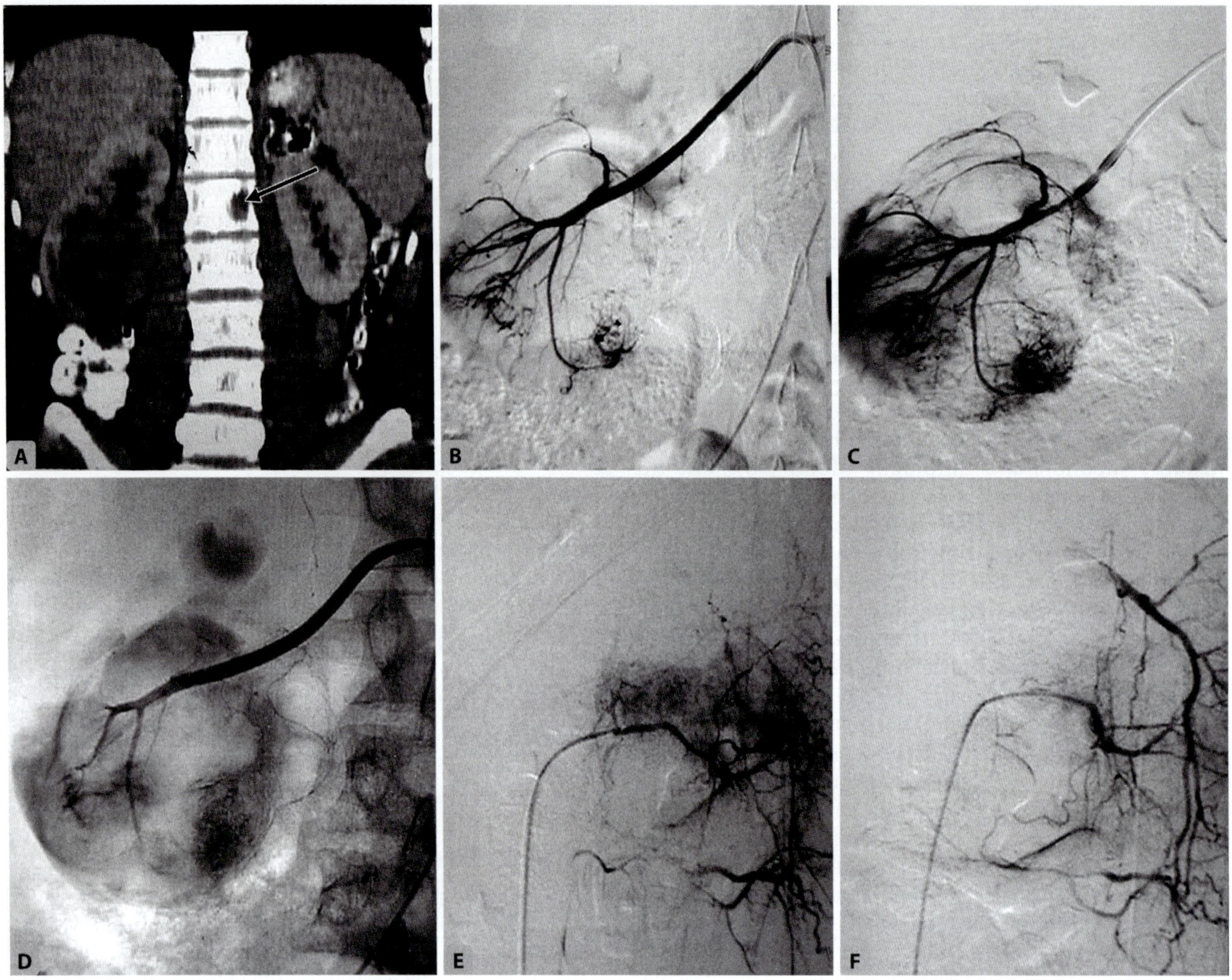

FIGS. 6A TO F: A case of renal cell carcinoma with vertebral metastasis treated by absolute alcohol. (A) Coronal MPR image showing large mass lesion in lower pole of right kidney. Note: destructive lytic lesion in L1 vertebra (arrow); (B) Selective angiogram showing tumor neovascularity in lower polar region; (C) Delayed angiogram showing tumor blush and no arteriovenous shunting; (D) Postembolization angiogram showing stasis of contrast, persistent tumor staining and obliteration of tumor vascularity; (E) Selective angiogram of paraspinal artery showing tumor blush supplying the L1 vertebral lesion; (F) Following embolization with polyvinyl alcohol (PVA) particles (500–700 μ) showing obliteration of tumor vascularity.

management options include surgical repair by resection, aneurysmorraphy and autotransplantation.

More peripherally located aneurysms can be selectively coil embolized using microcatheter technique **(Figs. 8A to F)**. Both distal and proximal control is not always possible and may not be necessary due to the vascular anatomy.

In the presence of multiple aneurysms from a lesion such as an angiomyolipoma, a combination of particle and coil embolization can be performed. If actively bleeding, the aneurysms are coiled first, followed by occlusion of the feeding vessels to the tumor with polyvinyl alcohol (PVA) or embospheres. Gelfoam can be sandwiched between coil nests to assist thrombosis.[12-15]

Results of Embolization

The technical success is quite high once the renal artery is securely accessed. If super- selective techniques are used, very little ischemia results and there is very little chance of inducing renal failure.

Complications

Although rare, dissection or perforation of the renal arteries and their branches can occur. Rupture may lead to rapid development of retroperitoneal hemorrhage. Both dissection flaps and rupture can be immediately controlled with balloon tamponade. Although dissection flaps can often be tacked down, rupture typically requires emergent surgery. Even perforation of smaller branch vessels can occur if a guidewire is passed too far into the periphery.

Embolization of End-stage Kidney

The nonfunctional kidney may manifest with pain, hypertension, albuminuria and other symptoms. In such cases

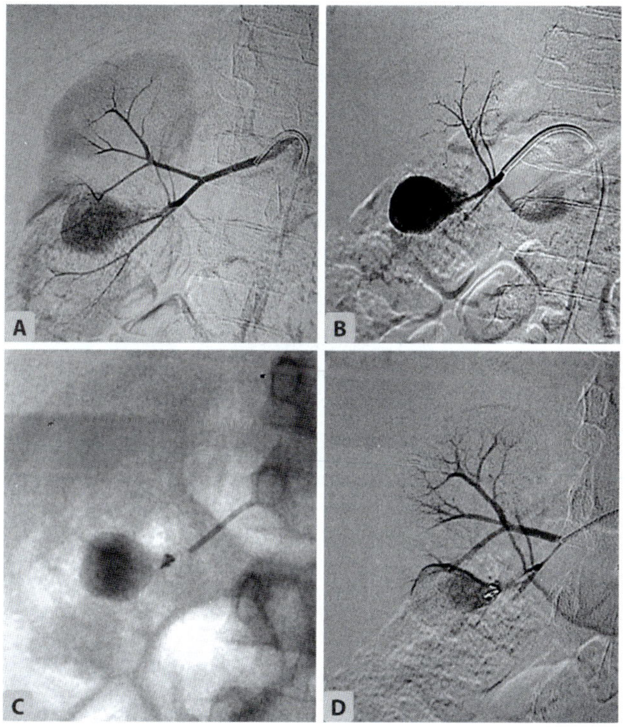

FIGS. 7A TO D: Post-percutaneous nephrolithotomy (PCNL) renal artery pseudoaneurysm treated by coil embolization. (A and B) Selective renal angiogram showing large pseudoaneurysm arising from lower polar artery; (C) Spot image showing coil at the neck of pseudoaneurysm; (D) Post-embolization angiogram showing nonfilling of pseudoaneurysm.

embolization procedure can replace surgical nephrectomy **(Figs. 9A to D)**.

Technique

Absolute alcohol is a very effective "permanent" agent for occluding capillaries. The embolization material is injected cautiously through an endhole catheter under fluoroscopic control to avoid reflux into the aorta. The embolization is considered complete when there is stasis of contrast medium in the major renal arteries without any flow of contrast material into the distal branches. There is therefore residual opacification of the parenchyma of the embolized kidney. During the embolization, patients commonly experience severe flank pain on the side of the kidney being infarcted and intravenous opiate analgesia is required for pain control. This limits the procedure to embolization of a single kidney at any one sitting. Patients must be then carefully monitored for 24 hours and kept in the hospital until their pain and any associated pyrexia has settled.[7,8]

The complications are mainly postembolization syndrome in the form of flank pain for few days, fever, nausea, vomiting, etc. There may be hypertension in the first few hours. Majority of these symptoms are self- limited and are resolve without any specific treatment. Rarely there may be major complications like renal failure, renal abscess and testicular infarction. The results of embolization are quite encouraging in most of the clinical situations.

Arteriovenous Fistulas and Malformations

Acquired arteriovenous fistulas in the kidney are usually the result of trauma, especially percutaneous biopsy. Massive renal arteriovenous (AV) fistulas can cause high-output heart failure. Congenital AVMs of the kidney are exceedingly rare. These lesions consist of numerous dilated, tortuous vessels within the subepithelium of the collecting system. When symptomatic, they usually present with gross hematuria and less commonly are associated with hypertension or an abdominal bruit. Color Doppler sonography, CT and MRI are useful in detecting some of these lesions.

At angiography, an AV fistula produces dilatation of the feeding branch and early filling of the draining vein. Numerous segmental or interlobar arteries feed the renal AVM, which is composed of dilated, tortuous channels with rapid shunting into renal vein and inferior vena cava.

Transcatheter embolization is the first-line of treatment for most of these lesions. Coils are effective for treatment of fistulas **(Figs. 10A to D)**. In AVMs, the nidus should be obliterated using a liquid agent such as cyanoacrylate (glue).[16-19]

UTERINE ARTERY EMBOLIZATION

Indications

Uterine artery embolization has become an extremely valuable therapy for patients with gynecological and obstetric diseases.

The various indications where it can be used are uterine leiomyoma, uterine AVMs, and postpartum and postoperative hemorrhage (PPH). UAE can also control bleeding following radiotherapy treatment in cases of carcinoma cervix.

Uterine Leiomyoma

Uterine artery embolization is the minimally invasive therapy in the management of uterine fibroids. The common indications for treatment are menorrhagia leading to anemia, abdominal pain, uterine enlargement with mass effect, infertility and late miscarriages. The advantages of UAE compared to operative therapies are that the patient retains the uterus, all the myomas are treated together in the same sitting and therapy is less invasive **(Figs. 11 and 12)**.

The disadvantages are vaginal expulsion of necrotic fibroid if the fibroid is submucosal, postembolization syndrome and a procedure which is not a fully curative treatment since the mean reduction of fibroid is about 40% or so.

Uterine Arteriovenous Malformations

The AVMs may either be congenital due to faulty development of arteries, veins, capillaries or are acquired as a result of intervillous space enlargement at the site of myometrial scar. The predisposing factors for acquired AVMs are previous uterine surgery, dilatation and curettage, intrauterine contraceptive devices, previous pregnancy, genital tuberculosis and trophoblastic disease.

AVMs are usually seen in women of child-bearing age with congenital ones presenting with spontaneous abortion

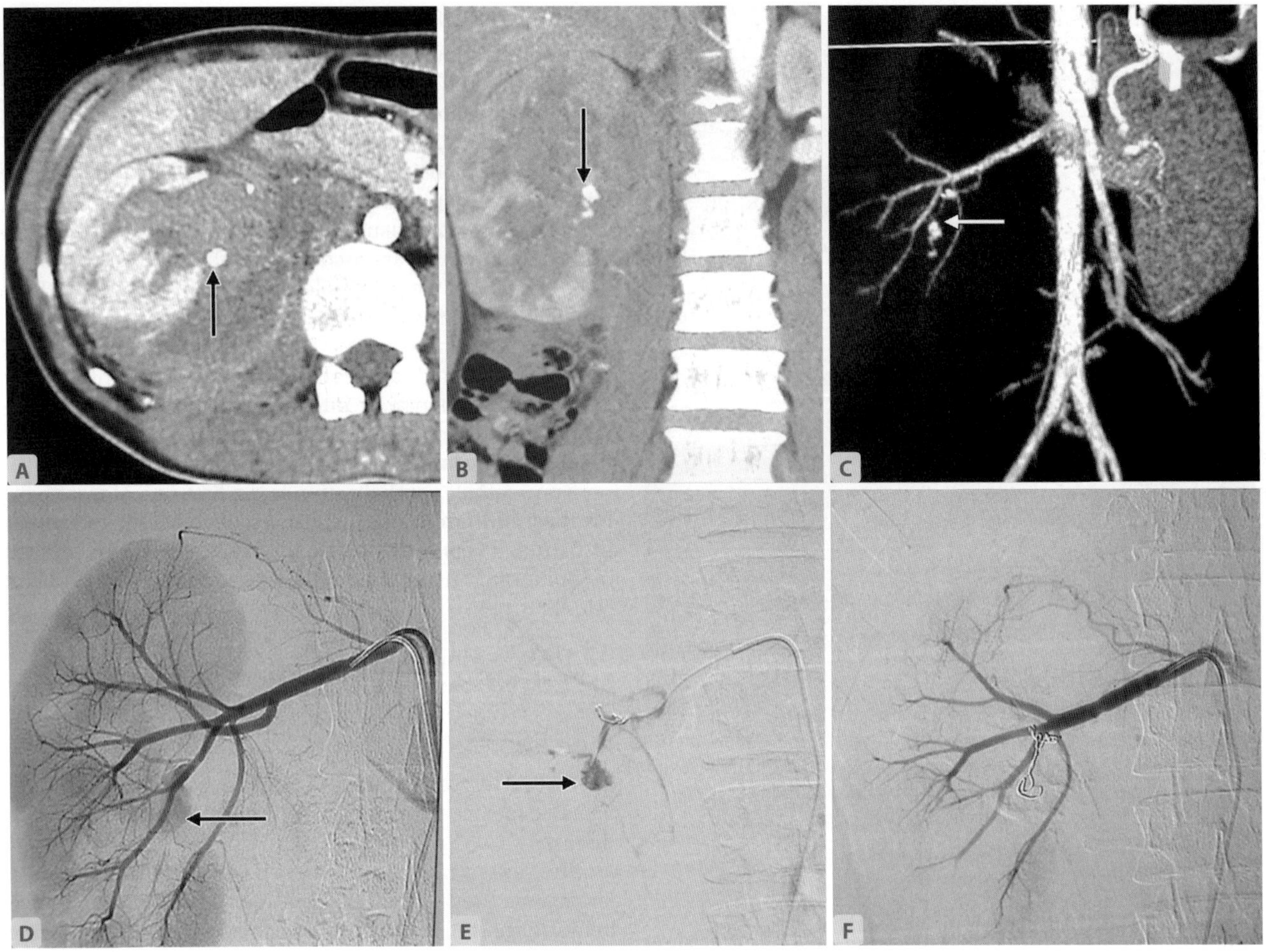

FIGS. 8A TO F: Post-PCNL renal artery pseudoaneurysm treated by microcoils using microcatheter coaxial technique. (A to C) Contrast-enhanced CT images showing small extrarenal pseudoaneurysm with surrounding large hematoma formation; (D) Selective renal angiogram showing filling of pseudoaneurysm supplied by lower polar branch of right renal artery; (E) Superselectively getting access into the branch supplying pseudoaneurysm using microcatheter; (F) Post-embolization angiogram showing nonfilling of pseudoaneurysm.

because of bleeding. The clinical presentation in acquired AVMs is profuse, intermittent repetitive bleeding.

UAE has shown good results in the treatment of these lesions with the added advantage that patient also maintains fertility **(Figs. 13A to F)**.

Postsurgical and Postpartum Hemorrhage (Figs. 14A to D)

Role of interventional radiology in the management of PPH has gained wide acceptance in the obstetric-gynecologic community as an alternative to uterine artery ligation or hemostatic hysterectomy.

The postsurgical hemorrhage due to vascular leak can be treated with gelfoam embolization of uterine or anterior division of internal iliac artery (IIA). The various causes of postpartum hemorrhage are abnormal placentation, retained products of conception, birth canal laceration, uterine atony or rupture of uterus. All such catastrophic bleeding conditions can be treated by angiographic embolization of uterine artery by using various embolizing materials.

Patient Selection

The choice between endovascular and operative treatment should be made jointly by the patient, gynecologist and intervention radiologist after the current status of all available treatment modalities has been considered and presented in a forthright fashion. Only symptomatic patients in whom other causes for disease have been excluded (including a recent Papanicolaou test) should undergo this treatment. The intervention radiologist is obligated to become the primary physician caring for the patient in preprocedure consultation, hospital recovery and all outpatient management. Adenomyosis also may respond to UAE.[20,21]

Absolute or relative contraindications include pregnancy, active or chronic pelvic infection, gynecologic malignancy (unless palliative or as an adjunct to operation), uncorrectable coagulopathy, severe contrast allergy, and prior pelvic surgery or radiation therapy. The effect of UAE on fertility has not been established, although pregnancy can occur after the procedure. Pedunculated fibroids with relatively narrow stalks are prone to detachment after UAE and may require operative removal.

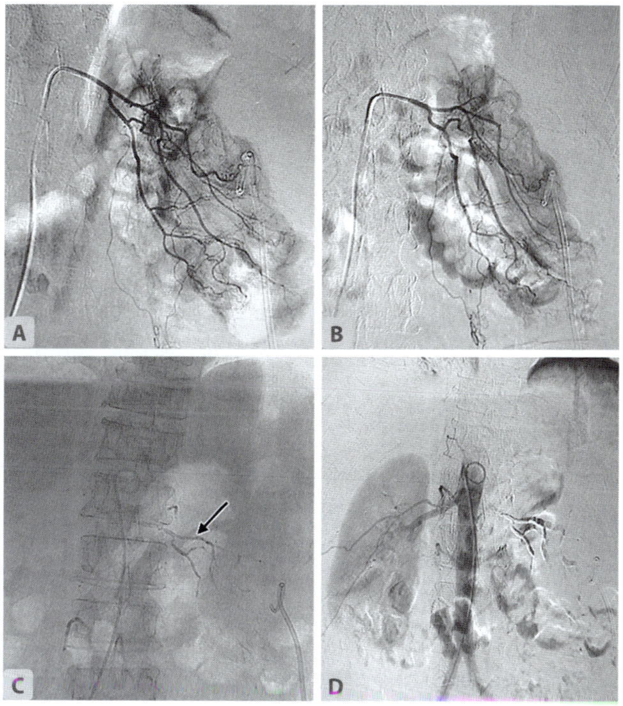

FIGS. 9A TO D: Glue embolization of nonfunctioning kidney. (A and B) Selective renal angiogram showing tortuous intrarenal branches; (C) Spot image showing glue cast in the intrarenal branches; (D) Post-embolization flush aortogram showing complete obliteration of left renal artery and no parenchymal blush seen.

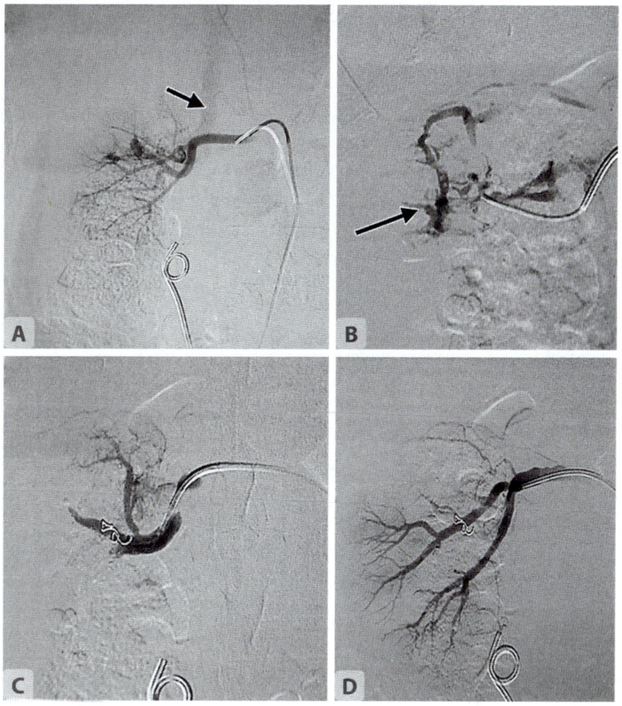

FIGS. 10A TO D: Post-PCNL arteriovenous (AV) fistula treated by coil embolization. (A) Selective right renal angiogram showing small contrast-filled structure supplied by upper polar artery with early draining vein; (B) Superselective angiogram showing getting close to the site of AV fistula (arrow); (C) Coil embolization of the AV fistula site; (D) Post-embolization angiogram showing obliteration of the AV fistula.

Technique

Uterine artery embolization for fibroids was first reported by Ravina and coworkers.[22] A pelvic arteriogram with the catheter positioned in the infrarenal abdominal aorta is obtained as a road map, especially to identify any ovarian artery supply. Selective catheterization of the anterior divisions of the IIAs is performed with a cobra or ultralong reverse-curve (e.g. Roberts) catheter.

Once the uterine artery is identified and selected, angiography shows the markedly dilated spiral arteries feeding the uterus. Tumor hypervascularity and vessel displacement is seen. In some cases, the descending portion of the uterine artery can be engaged with the 5-French diagnostic catheter. However, vasospasm may be a problem, so that coaxial placement of a microcatheter directed well into the uterine artery often is required. The preferred agents for embolization are small—caliber particulate matter, including PVA particles (500–700 μm), tris-acryl gelatin microspheres (Embospheres, 700–900 μm) and gelfoam pieces. There does not appear to be any significant difference in clinical efficacy between the two agents. Particle size <500 μm is not used because of the potential risk of crossing over to ovaries through utero-ovarian anastomoses. Proximal embolization (e.g. with coils) is inadvisable, because collateral vessels are very likely to develop and which will continue to feed the tumor. Embolization with particulate slurry (made with diluted contrast material) is continued until there is no flow in uterine artery branches ("pruned-tree" appearance). Regardless of the location of fibroids, bilateral embolization is necessary to prevent development of collateral vessels.[23-26]

Bilateral completion internal iliac arteriograms are obtained to identify any additional vessels feeding the tumors. The interventionalist should be observant of variant arterial anatomy and important collateral vessels. In most cases, the ovarian arteries contribute to fibroids through anastomoses with the main uterine artery. In about 10% of patients, the uterine artery is the major blood supply to the ovary, or the ovarian artery has significant direct communication with the fibroid. Embolization of these vessels theoretically increases the risk of ovarian infarction and infertility. Any other collateral vessels that feed the tumor must also be occluded. This is particularly true in women who have undergone prior pelvic surgery, had other tubal pathology or have fundal fibroids. Postprocedure care should be directed by the interventionalist who performed the UAE. A postembolization syndrome consisting of pain, nausea and vomiting, and low-grade fever is to be expected. Most patients require overnight hospitalization. Pain must be aggressively managed with IV, and later with oral narcotic. Antiemetics are given prophylactically or as needed. Discharge medications include anti-inflammatory drugs (e.g. ketorolac) and potent oral narcotics. Follow-up is done by the interventionalist, including routine clinic evaluation at 1–3 weeks after the procedure.[27]

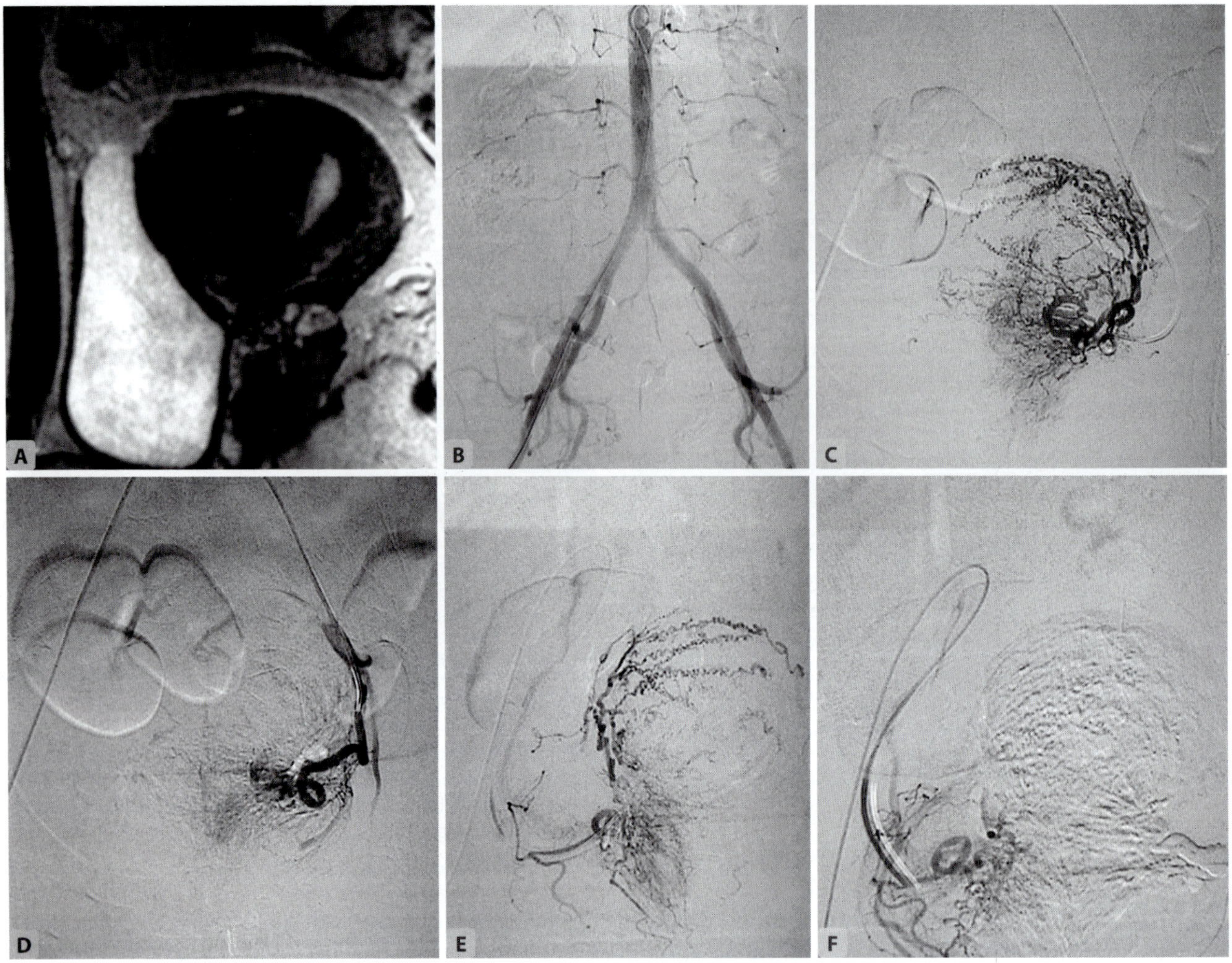

FIGS. 11A TO F: Uterine artery embolization of uterine fibroid. (A) Sagittal T2W MR image showing fibroid in fundal region; (B) Flush aortogram to look for any ovarian artery supply; (C) Selective left uterine artery angiogram showing increased vascularity supplying the fibroid; (D) Post-embolization angiogram showing reduction in vascularity following embolization with PVA particles (500–700 μ); (E and F) Right uterine angiogram followed by embolization using PVA particles and Robert's uterine catheter.

Results

Bilateral UAE is successful in about 95% of cases. Incomplete infarction of fibroids may be associated with the potential for continued growth. Clinical success with substantial improvement in symptoms is seen in about 80–90% of women. Submucosal lesions and small lesions seem to respond better than other tumors. Failure or recurrence is noted in about 6% of cases. If symptoms continue and leiomyomas persist or enlarge on imaging studies, repeat UAE (with aggressive search for collateral vessels including the ovarian arteries) is often warranted.

Complications

Intra- and postprocedure pain is a common problem after UAE. Important complications after UAE are intrauterine infection, uterine ischemia and necrosis, pulmonary embolism, and expulsion of pedunculated submucosal lesions. The overall complication rate is about 5% while major complications occur in about 1%. Most patients do not have a significant change in follicle-stimulating hormone level after the procedure though this is more likely to occur in women older than 45 years of age. Amenorrhea (which is often transient) occurs in less than 10% of cases, but it is much more likely in patients older than 45–50 years of age. Serious infections as complications are observed in 1% of treated women. Less than 2% require subsequent hysterectomy for any complications of UAE.[28-30]

The reasons for UAE failure are incomplete embolization, presence of important collaterals (e.g. ovarian arteries), large fibroids and recanalization of embolized arteries.

VAGINAL ARTERIOVENOUS MALFORMATION EMBOLIZATION

Vaginal AVMs are rare entities, and their most common presentation is vaginal hemorrhage and rarely dyspareunia. These lesions can be successfully treated by angioembolization of the supplying vessels using glue depending upon the angiographic flow dynamics. Angioembolization being safe and effective should be the first treatment of choice for symptomatic vaginal vascular malformation **(Figs. 15A to F)**.

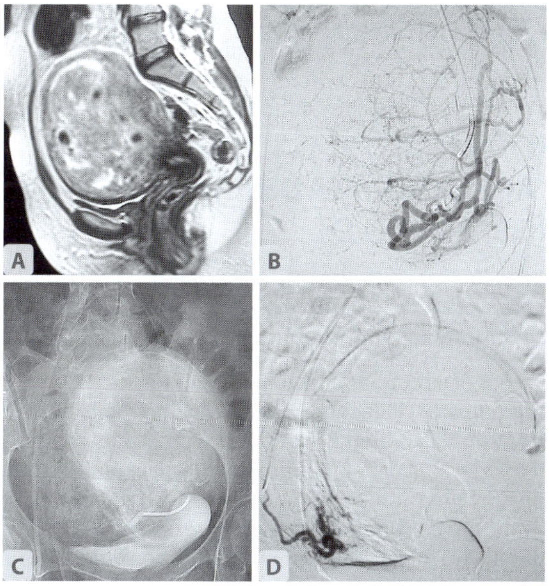

FIGS. 12A TO D: Uterine artery embolization of large uterine fibroid. (A) Sagittal T2W MR image showing large fibroid in fundal region; (B) Selective left uterine artery angiogram showing increased vascularity supplying the fibroid and splaying of branches by the large fibroid; (C) Post-embolization angiogram showing reduction in vascularity and stasis following embolization with PVA particles (500–700 μ); (D) Right uterine angiogram after the embolization showing reduction in vascularity.

SCROTAL ARTERIOVENOUS MALFORMATION AND TESTICULAR TUMOR EMBOLIZATION

Scrotal AVMs are rare entity. The scrotal AVMs and the paratesticular masses may occasionally present with uncontrollable bleeding. These lesions can be successfully treated by angioembolization of the supplying vessels using either Glue or PVA particles depending upon the situations **(Figs. 16 and 17)**. Angioembolization being safe and effective should be considered as choice of treatment for the treatment of symptomatic scrotal vascular malformation.

VARICOCELE EMBOLIZATION (FIGS. 18A TO C)

Varicocele is an important cause of male infertility. Varicocele embolization is indicated in an individual who have been infertile for at least 2 years and having oligoasthenospermia without an apparent cause of infertility. The embolization is done after placing catheter deep into the internal spermatic vein. Various embolizing materials like steel coils, PVA particles, gelfoam are used.[31-33]

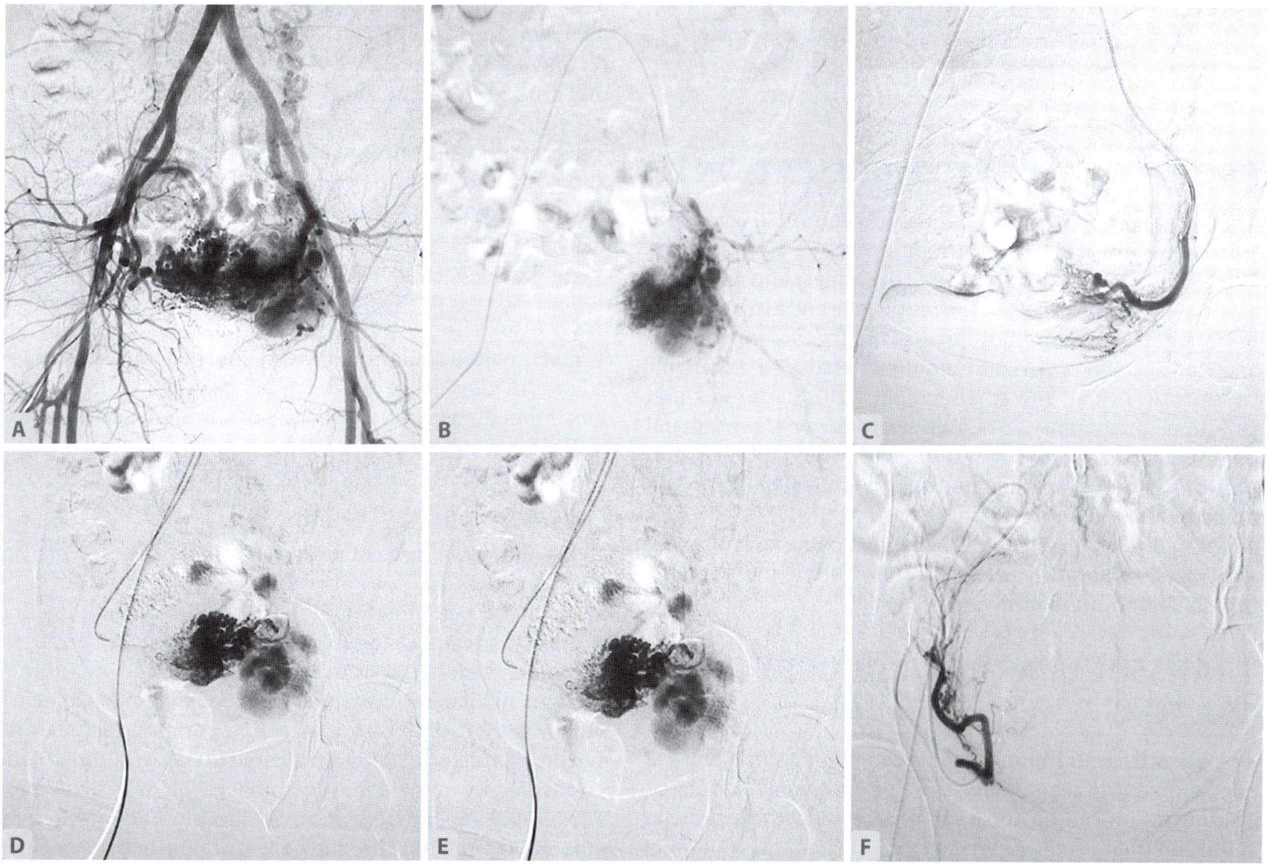

FIGS. 13A TO F: Uterine arteriovenous malformation treated by angioembolization. (A) Flush aortogram showing large vascular blush in the pelvis; (B) Selective angiogram of left uterine artery showing large vascular blush with nidus; (C) Post-embolization angiogram following embolization with PVA particles 700–1000 μ showing complete obliteration of the vascular blush on left side; (D and E) Selective angiogram of right uterine artery showing residual vascular blush with nidus which was obliterated with PVA particle embolization (F).

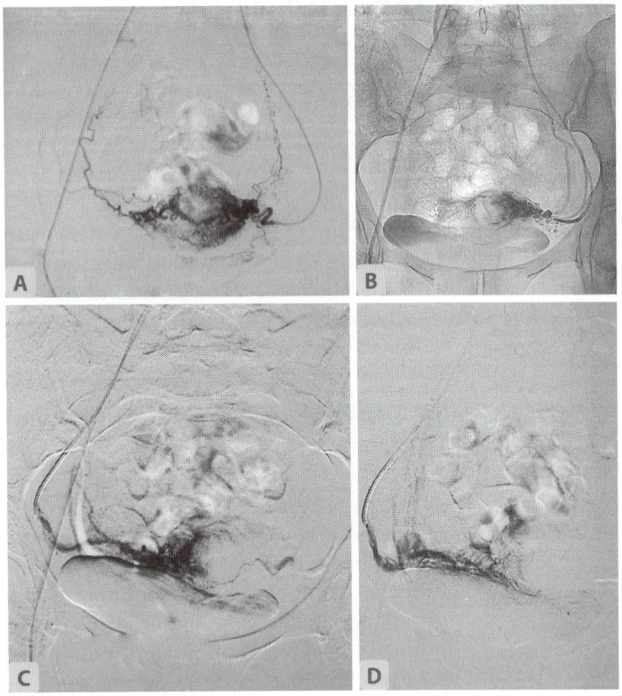

FIGS. 14A TO D: Post MTP continuous uterine bleeding treated by angioembolization. (A) Selective angiogram of left uterine artery showing vascular blush; (B) Post-embolization angiogram following embolization with PVA particles 700–1000 μ showing complete obliteration of the vascular blush and stasis of contrast; (C) Selective angiogram of right uterine artery showing vascular blush which was obliterated with PVA particle embolization (D).

PROSTATIC ARTERY EMBOLIZATION

Prostatic artery embolization is a new minimally invasive treatment modality for benign prostatic hyperplasia. Transurethral resection of prostate or surgical enucleation is associated with risk of urinary incontinence and increased risk of erectile dysfunction. The thin prostatic arteries branch from anterior division of IIAs and require expertise to selectively catheterize because of small caliber, arteriosclerosis and variations in anatomy.[34] A CT angiography or 3D rotational angiogram are often done to delineate the anatomy and oblique projections are helpful in digital subtraction angiography to identify the prostatic arteries. PVA particles of size <300 μ or gelatin microspheres are commonly used for embolization. Shrinkage of the prostate volume starts about 1 month after the embolization.

TRANSJUGULAR RENAL BIOPSY (FIGS. 19A TO C)

Transjugular renal biopsy is indicated in the presence of coagulopathy, patient unable to lie prone or small kidneys.[35] During this procedure, renal vein is accessed via transjugular route and then needle is directed into a lower pole renal vein branch, away from larger vessels into the parenchyma so that bleeding, if any, would be into the vein itself. This procedure has not got much acceptance because of technically demanding nature and high incidence of complications like arterial puncture and capsular perforation.[36]

PROPHYLACTIC BALLOON PLACEMENT IN ADHERENT PLACENTA (FIGS. 20A TO D)

Placenta accreta spectrum (PAS) is a term used to describe placenta accreta, increta and percreta. It results due to placental implantation at an area of abnormal decidualization.

Spectrum of adherent placenta:

- *Accreta vera:* Placental villi attach to myometrium
- *Increta:* Villi penetrate into the myometrium
- *Percreta:* Villi penetrate through the placental villi through the myometrium to the uterine serosa or adjacent organs.

Incidence of these entities are 79%, 14% and 7%, respectively, for accreta , increta and percreta.[6] The most important risk factor for development of PAS is placenta previa after a previous cesarean delivery.[37] It is usually asymptomatic and detected at the time of placental separation. The consequences of this is that at the time of placental separation, lack of normal cleavage plane between the uterus and placenta results in major hemorrhage and is a very common indication of peripartum hysterectomy.[38,39] After diagnosis, it is very important to develop a preoperative plan for the patient with a high likelihood of PAS. It should have a multidisciplinary team on board. The common treatment is usually cesarean hysterectomy with placenta left undisturbed *in situ* at 34–35 weeks. There are two possible management options. One is either to go for total abdominal hysterectomy with placenta *in situ*. In the other case scenario, uterus is preserved with placenta left *in situ*. Interventional radiology has an important role in both the clinical scenarios. In the first scenario of hysterectomy, balloon is placed in both IIAs and embolization is performed postcesarean delivery. As a result, there is a bloodless surgical field for hysterectomy, and it also reduces the blood loss during surgery. In the second scenario of uterine preservation, balloons are inflated in both IIA after delivery and embolization of both arteries is done immediately or the balloons can be deflated. If there is no bleeding, balloons can be removed.

Procedure (Figs. 20A to D)

On the day of delivery of patient with placenta accreta (by cesarean section), patient is first taken to interventional lab. Bilateral common femoral arteries are accessed with a 7F arterial sheath. Using minimum radiation and contrast, balloon catheters (10 mm × 4 cm) are placed in anterior divisions of bilateral IIAs (preoperative balloon placement). Patient is then shifted to maternity operation theater with sheaths and balloon catheters secured to skin by sutures. Baby is delivered by fundal incision and decision of hysterectomy is taken intraoperatively according to blood loss. Bilateral balloons are inflated after the delivery of the baby to occlude the anterior divisions of the IIAs. Hysterectomy is done with inflated balloons *in situ*. Keeping the balloons inflated,

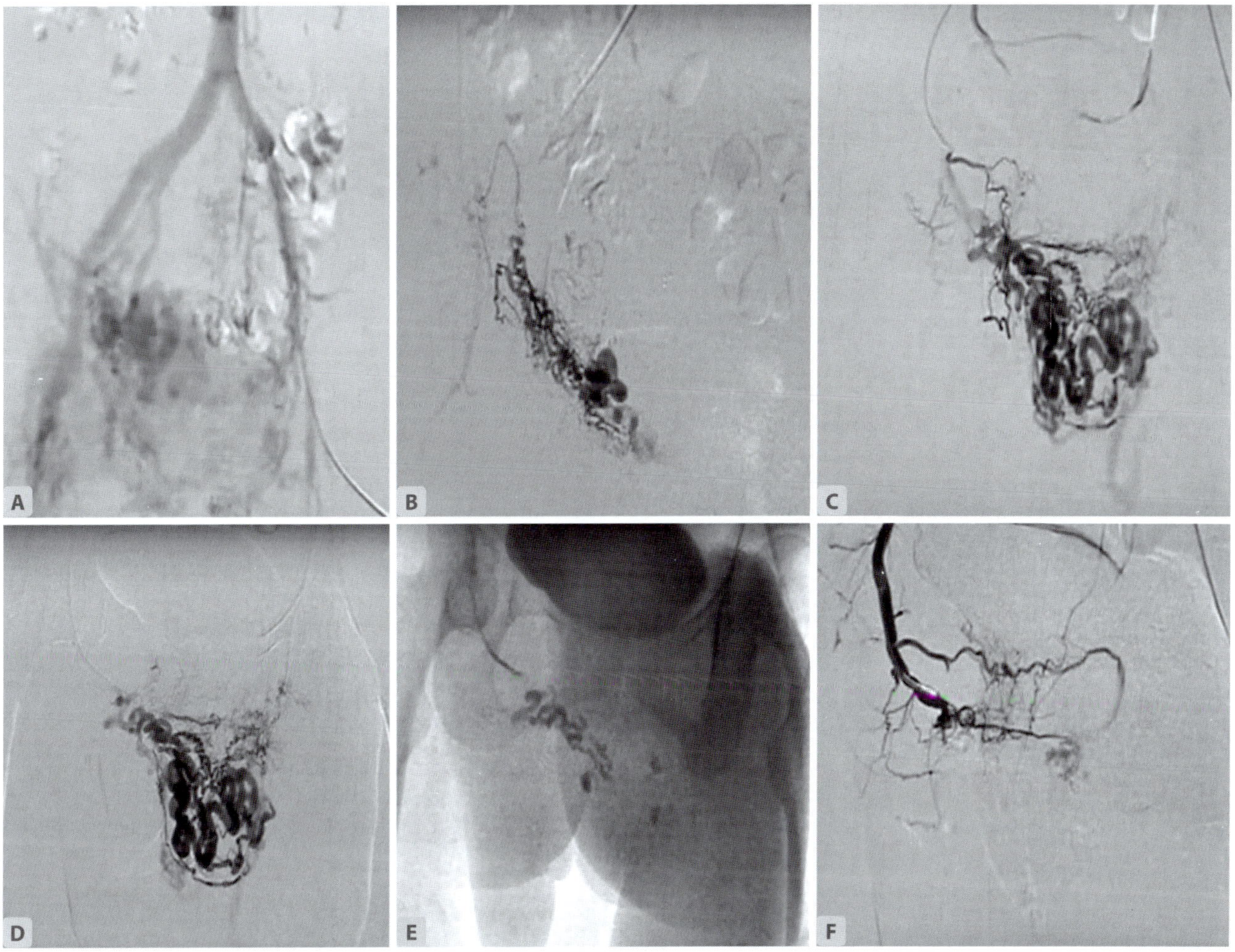

FIGS. 15A TO F: Vaginal arteriovenous malformation (AVM) treated by angioembolization. Selective angiogram of right internal pudendal artery showing multiple feeders supplying the nidus of AVM (A to D), which was obliterated using glue (E and F).

additional embolization can be done with gelfoam or coils, if the bleeding persists. Balloons are deflated after completion of hysterectomy, and the patient is shifted to the recovery room. Vascular sheaths are removed in the recovery room, if there is no persistent bleeding after a few hours. In the scenario of uterine preservation, balloons are inflated in both IIA after delivery and embolization of both arteries is done immediately or the balloons can be deflated in case there is no significant bleeding.

Many people have used infrarenal abdominal aortic balloon inflation for control of bleeding in these patients.[40,41] Apart from these, balloon placement has also been done in common iliac and uterine arteries. Other than balloon placement, postdelivery embolization of uterine arteries and IIAs can be done in case bleeding is not controlled during surgery. The primary endpoint of the procedure is estimated blood loss volume. Secondary endpoints are total number of units of packed red blood cells (PRBCs) transfused, number of patients transfused and hysterectomy rate.

CONCLUSION

In conclusion, renal artery aneurysms can be life-threatening if hemorrhage occurs. Following aneurysm rupture, surgical morbidity and mortality are fairly high. Aggressive management by the interventional radiologist, therefore is paramount since these patients are in any case too sick for major revascularization procedures, making endovascular techniques a more desirable approach. Embolization of dysfunctioning kidneys using various embolization techniques and regimens in the management of hypertension or protein wasting in end-stage renal disease has replaced surgical nephrectomy. The evolution of uterine fibroid embolization has established the role of embolotherapy as a viable alternative to hysterectomy, and undoubtedly revolutionized the management of postpartum bleeding. A variety of methods for embolization are described in the literature. The type of treatment should be tailored to each individual case as the anatomy and flow dynamics will typically dictate the therapy best suited.

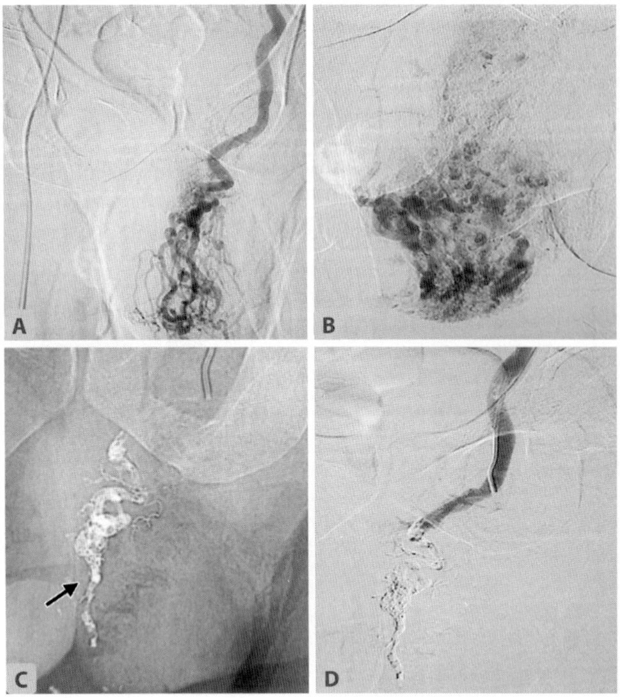

FIGS. 16A TO D: Scrotal arteriovenous malformation treated by glue embolization. (A and B) Selective left internal pudendal artery angiogram showing hypertrophied artery and large nidus; (C) Spot image showing glue cast obliterating the nidus; (D) Post-embolization angiogram showing complete obliteration of the vascular nidus.

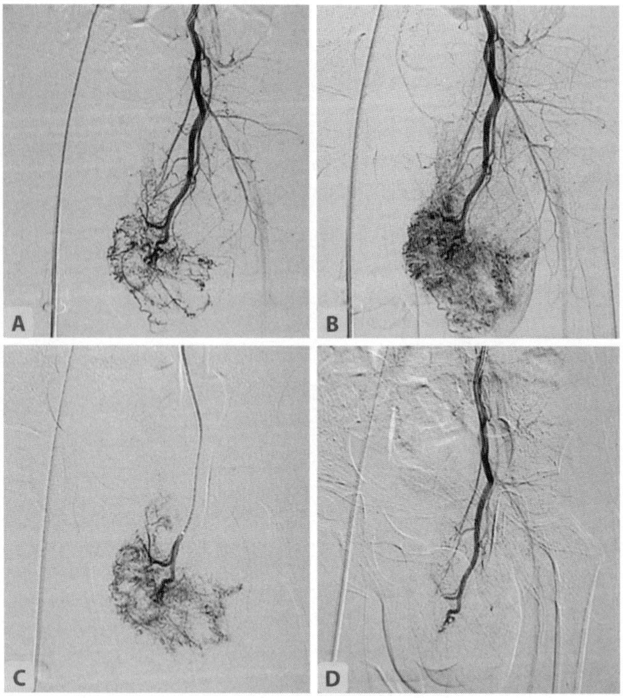

FIGS. 17A TO D: Left paratesticular mass in 5-year-old child with scrotal bleeding treated by angioembolization. (A and B) Selective left internal pudendal artery angiogram showing hypertrophied artery and large tumor blush; (C) Catheter brought close to the tumor blush; (D) Post-embolization angiogram following embolization using PVA particles 300–500 μ, showing complete obliteration of tumor blush.

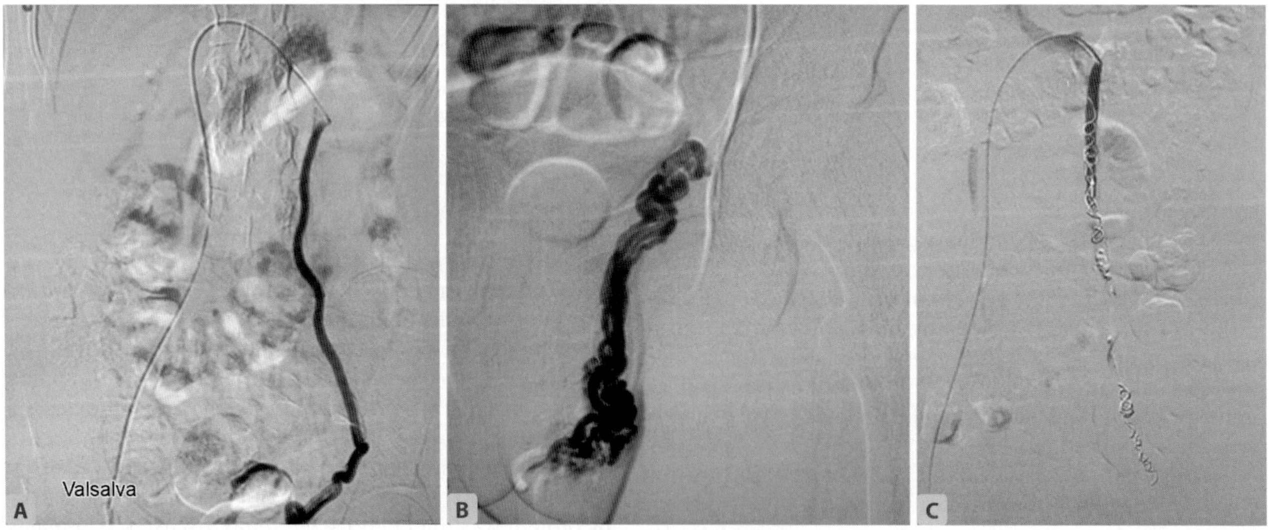

FIGS. 18A TO C: Technique of varicocele embolization: (A) Left gonadal vein was accessed through transfemoral venous route; (B) Catheter was advanced as distally as possible to the point of formation of gonadal vein from pampiniform plexus; (C) Entire left gonadal vein was embolized using combination of coils and glue till the point just proximal to draining into left renal vein.

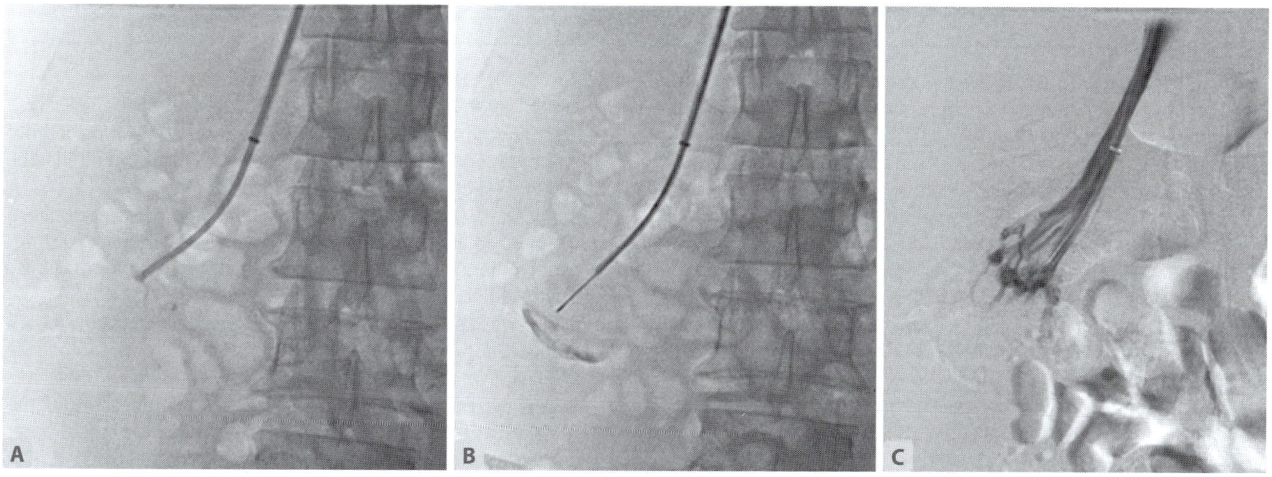

FIGS. 19A TO C: Spot images showing technique of transjugular renal biopsy (TJRB): TJLB needle placed inside lower polar branch of renal vein (A) through right transjugular route and biopsy is being taken from posterolateral cortex (B) followed by postbiopsy venogram showing free flow of contrast without any leak (C). (TJLB: transjugular liver biopsy).

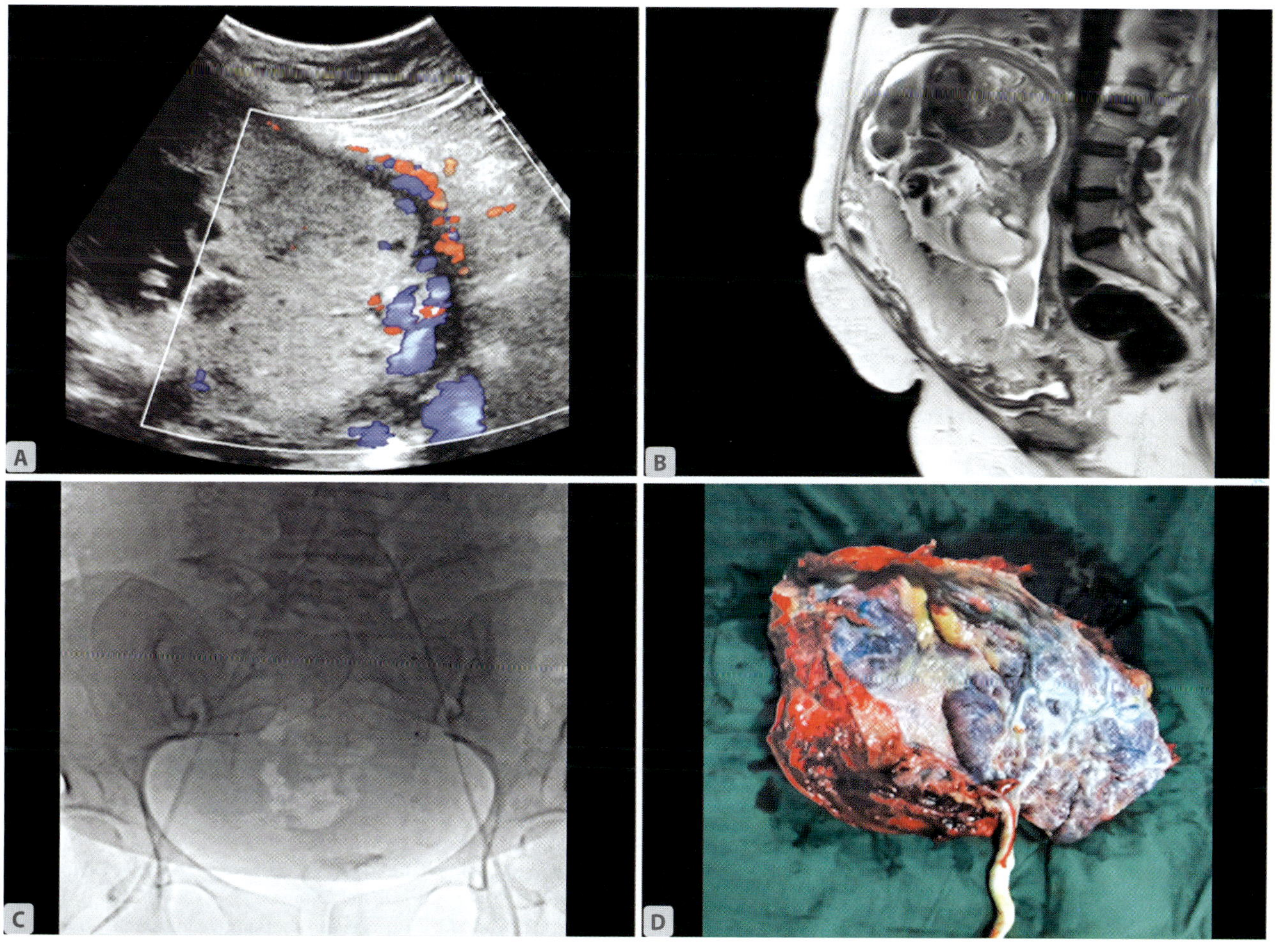

FIGS. 20A TO D: Technique of preoperative balloon placement in adherent placenta: (A) Ultrasonographic image showing low-lying heteroehoic placenta with thick interplacental bands and loss of retroplacental clear space. The planes with urinary bladder are ill defined with highly increased vascularity at bladder placenta interface; (B) T2-weighted sagittal image of same patient showing grossly heterointense placenta which is seen invading into bladder as well as scar site; (C) Patient was taken up for prophylactic balloon placement in bilateral internal iliac arteries before taking up for C-section. After delivery of baby, balloons were inflated and hysterectomy was done; (D) Image shows hysterectomy specimen showing adherent placenta attached to it. Intraoperative blood loss was 6.8 L.

REFERENCES

1. Cicuto KP, McLean GK, Oleaga JA, et al. Renal artery stenosis: Anatomical classification for percutaneous transluminal angioplasty. Am J Roentgenol. 1981;137:599-601.
2. Rountas C, Vlychou M, Vassiou K, et al. Imaging modalities for renal artery stenosis in suspected renovascular hypertension: Prospective intraindividual comparison of color Doppler US, CT angiography, GD-enhanced MR angiography, and digital substraction angiography. Ren Fail. 2007;29(3):295-302.
3. Tan KT, van Beek EJ, Brown PW, et al. Magnetic resonance angiography for the diagnosis of renal artery stenosis. A metaanalysis. Clin Radiol. 2002;57:617-24.
4. Hoffman O, Carreres T, Sapoval MR, et al. Ostial renal artery stenosis angioplasty. Immediate and mid-term angiographic and clinical results. J Vasc Interv Radiol. 1998;9:65-73.
5. Matsumoto AH, Tegtmeyer CJ, Fitzgerald EK, et al. Percutaneous transluminal angioplasty of visceral arterial stenoses: results and long-term clinical follow-up. J Vasc Interv Radiol. 1995;6:165-74.
6. Moss JG, Hamilton G. Renal and visceral artery intervention. In: Dyet JF, Nicholson AA, Ettles DF, Wilson SE (Eds), Textbook of Endovascular Procedures. Philadelphia: Churchill Livingston; 2000. pp. 151-73.
7. Park JH, Kim WS, Han MC, et al. Renal arterial embolization with absolute ethanol. J Korean Med Sci. 1987;2(1):13-8.
8. Park JH, Kim SH, Han JK, et al. Transcatheter arterial embolization of unresectable renal cell carcinoma with a mixture of ethanol and iodized oil. Cardiovasc Intervent Radiol. 1994 ;17(6):323-7.
9. Martin RS 3rd, Meacham PW, Ditesheim JA, et al. Renal artery aneurysm: selective treatment for hypertension and prevention of rupture. J Vasc Surg. 1989;9:26-34.
10. Poutasse EF. Renal artery aneurysms. Their natural history and surgery. J Urol. 1966;95:297- 306.
11. Poutasse EF. Renal artery aneurysms. J Urol. 1975;113:443-49.
12. Liguori G, Trombetta C, Bucci S, et al. Percutaneous management of renal artery aneurysm with a stent-graft. J Urol. 2002; 167:2518-19.
13. Pershad A, Heuser R. Renal artery aneurysm: successful exclusion with a stent graft. Catheter Cardiovasc Interv. 2004;61:314-16.
14. Rundback JH, Rizvi A, Rozenblit GN, et al. Percutaneous stent-graft management of renal artery aneurysms. J Vasc Interv Radiol. 2000;11:1189-93.
15. Schneidereit NP, Lee S, Morris DC, et al. Endovascular repair of a ruptured renal artery aneurysm. J Endovasc Ther. 2003;10:71-4.
16. Crotty KL, Orihuela E, Warren MM. Recent advances in the diagnosis and treatment of renal arteriovenous malformations and fistulas. J Urol. 1993;150:1355-9.
17. Takebayashi S, Aida N, Matsui K. Arteriovenous malformations of the kidneys: Diagnosis and follow-up with color Doppler sonography in six patients. Am J Roentgenol. 1991;157:991-5.
18. Allione A, Pomero F, Valpreda S, et al. Worsening of hypertension in a pregnant women with renal arteriovenous malformation: a successful superselective embolization after delivery. Clin Nephrol. 2003;60:211-3.
19. Takebayashi S, Hosaka M, Ishizuka E, et al. Arteriovenous malformations of the kidneys: Ablation with alcohol. Am J Roentgenol. 1988;150:587-90.
20. Andrews RT, Spies JB, Sacks D, et al. Patient care and uterine artery embolization for leiomyomata. J Vasc Interv Radiol. 2004;15:115-20.
21. Siskin GP, Tublin ME, Stainken BF, et al. Uterine artery embolization for the treatment of adenomyosis: clinical response and evaluation with MR imaging. Am J Roentgenol. 2001;177:297-302.
22. Ravina JH, Herbreteau D, Ciraru-Vigneron N, et al. Arterial embolisation to treat uterine myomata. Lancet. 1995;346:671-2.
23. Worthington-Kirsch RL, Andrews RT, et al. Uterine fibroid embolization: technical aspects. Tech Vasc Intent Radiol. 2002;5:17-34.
24. Banovac F, Ascher SM, Jones DA, et al. Magnetic resonance imaging outcome after uterine artery embolization for leiomyomata with use of tris-acryl gelatin microspheres. J Vasc Interv Radiol. 2002;13:681-8.
25. Pelage JP, Le Dref O, Beregi JP, et al. Limited uterine artery embolization with tris-acryl gelatin microspheres for uterine fibroids. J Vasc Interv Radiol. 2003;14:15-20.
26. Pelage JP, Le Dref O, Soyer P, et al. Arterial anatomy of the female genital tract: Variations and relevance to transcatheter embolization of the uterus. Am J Roentgenol. 1999;172: 989-94.
27. Siskin GP, Bonn J, Worthington-Kirsch RL, et al. Uterine fibroid embolization: pain management. Tech Vasc Interv Radiol. 2002;5:35-43.
28. Pelage JP, Walker WJ, Dref OL. Uterine necrosis after uterine artery embolization for leiomyoma. Obstet Gynecol. 2002;99: 676-7.
29. Spies JB, Spector A, Roth AR, et al. Complications after uterine artery embolization for leiomyomas. Obstet Gynecol. 2002;100:873-80.
30. Spies JB, Roth AR, Gonsalves SM, et al. Ovarian function after uterine artery embolization for leiomyomata: assessment with use of serum follicle stimulating hormone assay. J Vasc Interv Radiol. 2001;12:437-42.
31. Lima SS, Castro MP, Costa OF. A new method for the treatment of varicocele. Andrologia. 1978;10:103-06.
32. Trombetta C, Salisci E, Deriu M, et al. Echo-flowmetric control 6 years after percutaneous treatment of varicocele. Arch Ital Urol Androl. 1993;65:363-67.
33. Usuki N, Nakamura K, Takashima S, et al. Embolization of varicocele with ethanol. Nippon Igaku Hoshasen Gakkai Zasshi 1994;54:870-5 (Japanese).
34. Teichgräber U, Aschenbach R, Diamantis I, et al. Prostate artery embolization: indication, technique and clinical results. Rofo. 2018;190(9):847-55.
35. Rathod KR, Popat BA, Pandey A, et al. Safety and effectiveness of transjugular renal biopsy: a single center study. Indian J Nephrol. 2017;27(2):118-123.
36. Thompson BC, Kingdon E, Johnston M, et al. Transjugular kidney biopsy. Am J Kidney Dis. 2004;43(4):651-62.
37. Silver RM, Landon MB, Rouse DJ, et al. Maternal morbidity associated with multiple repeat cesarean deliveries. Obstet Gynecol. 2006;107(6):1226-32.
38. Mehrabadi A, Hutcheon JA, Liu S, et al. Contribution of placenta accreta to the incidence of postpartum hemorrhage and severe postpartum hemorrhage. Obstet Gynecol. 2015;125(4): 814-21.
39. Zelop CM, Harlow BL, Frigoletto FD, et al. Emergency peripartum hysterectomy. Am J Obstet Gynecol. 1993;168(5):1443-8.
40. Zeng C, Yang M, Ding Y, et al. Preoperative infrarenal abdominal aorta balloon catheter occlusion combined with Bakri tamponade reduced maternal morbidity of placenta increta/ percreta. Medicine (Baltimore). 2017;96(38):e8114.
41. Luo F, Xie L, Xie P, et al. Intraoperative aortic balloon occlusion in patients with placenta previa and/or placenta accreta: a retrospective study. Taiwan J Obstet Gynecol. 2017;56(2):147-52.

SECTION

2

Advances in Imaging Technology

CHAPTER

28

Ultrasound Instrumentation: Practical Applications

Ujjwal Gorsi, Anmol Bhatia, Kushaljit Singh Sodhi, Akshay Kumar Saxena

INTRODUCTION

Ultrasonography, as an imaging modality has undergone massive transformation in the last few decades. It today occupies a crucial role in practice of most of the domains of medicine. Advances in ultrasound technology include enhanced spatial, vascular and contrast resolution, besides encompassing various therapeutic options. New transducers and emerging imaging paradigms allow real time acquisition of large field of views and even three dimensional volumetric data. In sonography, transducer, is the central component, which is responsible for both, generation of ultrasound beam and detection of returning echoes.[1] It is the changes in the generation of echo signals, it's reception, analysis and display that helps to differentiate one scanner from another.[1] Safety, portability, affordability and real time application makes it one of the most widely used imaging modalities. This chapter provides a overview of practical aspects of ultrasound instrumentation which an operator must be familiar with.

PARTS OF AN ULTRASOUND MACHINE

A basic ultrasound machine consists of following parts **(Figs. 1A and B)**:

Central processing unit (CPU): The CPU can be considered the brain of ultrasound machine. It sends electric signal to the transducer and also receives electric pulses from the transducer. CPU of ultrasound machine does all calculations, data processing and also stores processed information.

Transducer probe: It is the probe that generates ultrasound beam and receives the returning echoes. Most of ultrasound machines have more than one transducers.

Transducer pulse controls: These controls are used to change the parameters of pulses emitted from transducer such as duration, amplitude and frequency.

Display monitor: Display monitor displays the images from the ultrasound data which are processed by the CPU.

Keyboard: Keyboard allows operator to add notes and takes various measurements from the images displayed.

Disk storage device: These are used to store the acquired images. These can be hard discs, compact discs, digital video discs and floppy discs.

Printer: Prints the image acquired during an ultrasound examination.

CONTROLS OF ULTRASOUND MACHINE

- *Overall gain control:* This control amplifies all received signals equally.
- *Time gain compensation:* Time gain compensation (TGC) is used to balance for attenuation of the ultrasound beam in the scanned tissue.[2] With time gain compensation, gain is applied to the echoes which is dependent on depth. Echoes originating from deeper tissue (which are attenuated to a larger degree) have much larger gain factors than those echoes which originate close to the transducer so echoes from deep structures are amplified more than signals from shallow structures.[2,3] This produces equally reflective structures which are displayed in B-mode image with the same brightness. Time gain compensation is controlled in most machines using a set of six to ten gain knobs with each knob adjusting the receiver gain at a different depth.
- *Near and far gain:* These controls equalize the differences in echo signals when they are received from various depths and displayed on the screen. Near to far gain controls (usually slide pods) should be gradually increased when compensating for sound attenuation.[2,3]
- *Compression:* This is used to vary the dynamic range of echoes signals which are displayed as shades of gray on the image. Logarithmic compression to the echo signals emerging from the receiver is applied by most of the ultrasound machines; amount of compression is under operator control.[2]

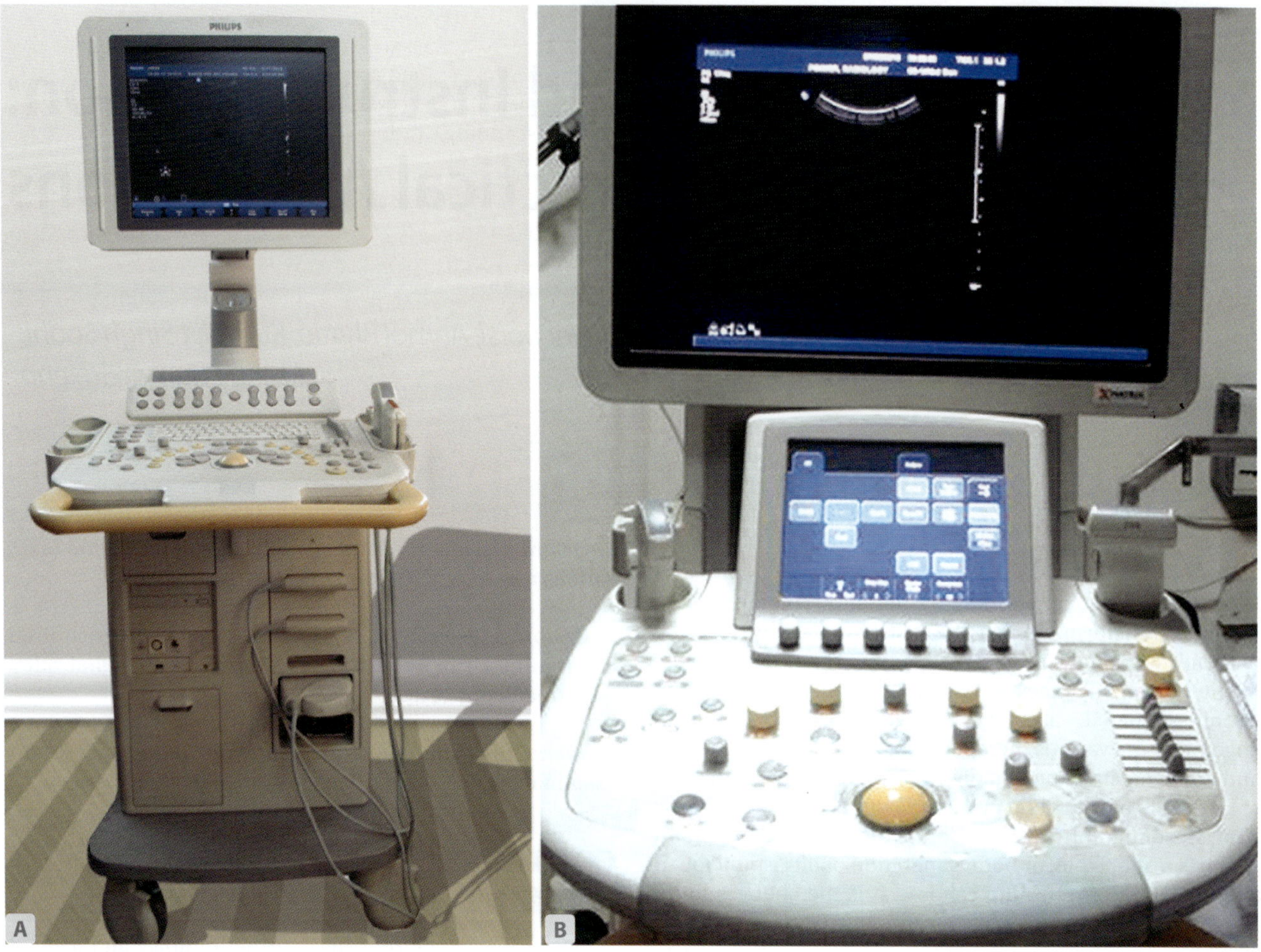

FIGS. 1A AND B: Modern ultrasound scanning unit with LCD screen.

- *Dynamic range:* Is the ratio of the largest to smallest echo signals. It decreases as signals pass through imaging system as rejection and time gain compensation remove many large and small signals.[3]
- *Depth:* Size of the image is adjusted by using this control. Which is displayed on screen. Organs, adjacent structures or regions of interest are well seen using this control.
- *Focal point:* Focal point is a control that increases the resolution at a specific point or points by choosing the level at which the ultrasound beam is focused. Focal point should be set at the posterior most aspect of the structure or organ which is being scanned[2,3]

Suboptimal image quality may result if gain control is not properly adjusted and/or focal point is not placed properly.

TRANSDUCER

The basic transducer or probe consists of the connector, the wire and the head. Most of the modern sonography machines allow sonologists to select the appropriate probe for a particular study simply by touching the probe icon on the screen.[4] Footprint is the tip of the head of the probe. This is the part of the probe which is in direct contact with the patient. Footprint acts as a transmitter and receiver of the ultrasound beam during scanning.

Footprint of the probe contains piezoelectric crystals. Synthetic plumbium zirconium titanate crystals are used as piezoelectric crystals in most of modern probes. These crystals are arranged according to the shape of the probe except for the sector probe. Image quality of ultrasound depends upon the integrity of these plumbium zirconium titanate crystals. Damage or misalignment when probe is dropped, crushed or damaged can severely affect the quality of image obtained.[4]

Most of the transducers have a marker along one side of the head of the probe which can be a linear ridge or a dot. This marker is important for orientation of the patient's anatomy while doing a scan. Orientation marker points toward either the patient's head or his right side during the scan in standard practice.[4] Type of transducer to be used for a particular study will depend upon the the fundamental principle of tissue penetration of the ultrasound beam which is expressed in megahertz.

FREQUENCY OF TRANSDUCERS

Transducer frequency can vary from 2.0 to 16.0 MHz and its selection is primarily based upon patient's body habitus and the region to be scanned.[2]

High Frequency Transducer

- Frequency range of 7.0–14.0 MHz
- Linear transducer mostly, sector transducer more suited for children
- Provides increased resolution of images, however, with reduced penetration
- Linear probes best for evaluation of superficial structure like, thyroid, scrotum, etc.

Medium Frequency Transducer

- Frequency range of 3.0–5.0 MHz
- Curvilinear or sector transducers
- Most commonly used probe for adult abdominal imaging.

Low Frequency Transducer

- Frequency of 2.0 MHz
- Transducer is sector type
- Provides increased depth of penetration but also results in loss of resolution
- More suited for ultrasound studies of obese patient.[2]

Most of ultrasonography studies can be accomplished using one of four basic types of probes: (1) Linear, (2) Curvilinear, (3) Sector/phased, and (4) Intracavity **(Fig. 2)**.

Linear Array Transducer

Linear array transducers are best for scanning superficial structures such as thyroid, scrotum, neck and extremity vessels and subcutaneous lumps. In this, image is displayed as a rectangle. In a linear array, each time only a group of elements work together to transmit or receive.[2,5] The ultrasound beam is perpendicular to the transducer surface, centered over element subset and scans a rectangular area. Size of the field of view is equal in both the far field (area of penetration farthest away from transducer) and near field (area of penetration closest to transducer).[2]

Curvilinear Array Transducer

These are commonly used for routine abdominal and pelvic imaging. In curvilinear array transducer, array of elements are arranged across a convex arc.[2,5] This fan like arrangement of elements results in a sector shaped imaging field. Compared to linear array, curved array provides a wider image at large depths (field of view is wide in far field than near field) from a narrow scanning window.

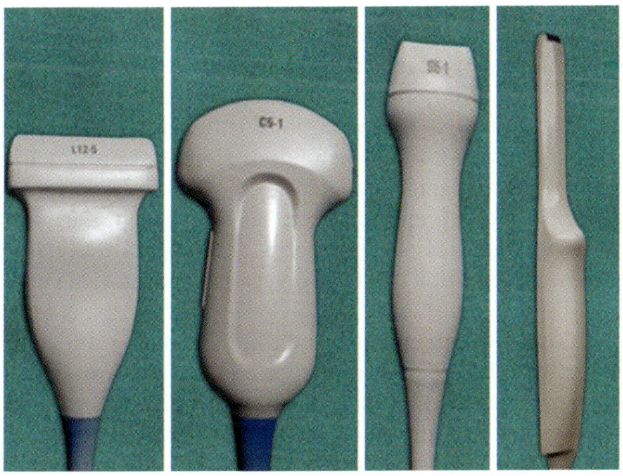

FIG. 2: Photograph showing linear, curvilinear, phased array and intracavitary transducers.

Phased Array Transducer

In contrast to linear and curved arrays, all the elements work together in phased array. All elements are used for each beam line.[5] Phase array steer the beam by applying different delay on each element, and it requires small acoustic window. Its main advantage is in providing a very broad imaged field at larger depths that too with a narrow transducer footprint. It is widely used in cardiac scanning as the transducer fits easily between the ribs.

The Intracavitary Transducer

The intracavitary transducer has much higher frequencies (8–13 MHz) as compared to other curved probes resulting in better resolution of the images. This transducer is used mainly for transvaginal scanning of female pelvis and trans rectal examination of prostate, seminal vesicle and pelvic pathologies in males.[4]

It is important to clean the head of transducer after the completion of a scan. Inability to do so cleanse may cause cracking and desiccation of the foot print resulting in damage to the crystals and subsequent degradation of images.

MODES OF SCANNING

Real-time images of the tissue anatomy and motion can be obtained by using B-mode scanning, M-mode scanning and with Doppler.

- *B-mode scanning:* B-mode scan or "brightness" mode, displays a 2D grayscale real time image of the organ being scanned on the screen.
- *M-mode scanning:* M-mode or "motion" mode acquires an image in the B-mode and displays it graphically as changes over a period of time. Scanning in this mode is useful for evaluating cardiac contractility and wall movement , pneumothorax and examining inferior vena cava for intravascular volume
- *Doppler scanning:* The Doppler effect was first described by Christian Doppler, an Austrian physicist, in 1843 and is based on the principle that, if there is relative motion between an object and an observer (receiver), the frequency of sound wave perceived by the observer (receiver) is different from that emitted/reflected by the object.[5,6]

  In radiology, Doppler effect is used to detect blood flow in peripheral vessels (e.g. lower limb) as well as those supplying different organs (renal artery, portal vein, etc.). Doppler examination gives information regarding presence or absence of blood flow, direction of blood flow, type of blood flow (arterial high resistance/venous and presence and quantification of arterial stenosis, etc.[2] In clinical practice, various Doppler techniques are utilized.[7]
  - *Continuous wave Doppler* is used for evaluation of peripheral vessels and the fetal heart. The basic

transducer for continuous wave Doppler contains an oscillator, two piezoelectric crystals and a demodulator **(Fig. 3A)**. One of these crystals acts as the transmitter while the other acts as the receiver. Both of these crystals work continuously. The two crystals are inclined at an angle to each other. The purpose of inclining the crystals is to cause overlap between the beam regions of the transmitter and receiver which in turn increases the sensitivity for detecting the returning signal (beam). The oscillator provides electrical voltage at the resonant frequency of the transducer which is converted into the transmitted ultrasound beam by the transmitter. The beam, after reflection, is received by the receiver piezoelectric crystal. The frequency of received beam is different from the transmitted frequency because of Doppler shift. The received signal is amplified and fed into the demodulator which also receives signal from the oscillator.[6] The comparison of signals from the oscillator and received beam provides Doppler shift signal. The problem with continuous wave Doppler is that all the moving objects with in the sonographic beam contribute to frequency shift. Thus, the observer cannot ascertain the depth from which the signal originates. This problem can be overcome by the use of pulsed Doppler.[8-11]

- *Pulsed wave Doppler* provides information regarding the presence, direction and depth from which the Doppler signal is coming from. In this technique, very short bursts of the sound wave are repetitively emitted by the transducer. However, a new pulse is not emitted till such time the returning signal from the previous pulse is detected by the transducer. The receiver is designed to be turned on for a short period on at a specific moment. The time at which receiver is turned on (or gated on) provides the information regarding the depth at which the signal originated. The duration for which the receiver (or the gate) is turned on determines the axial length of the beam over which the signal is received. A combination of real time imaging and pulsed Doppler is known as Duplex Doppler.
- *Colour flow Doppler:* Although pulsed Doppler and duplex scanners provide information regarding the depth from which Doppler signal originates, it is limited to a very small region of the image. As a result, the sonologist needs to sample large number of areas to evaluate the entire vessel. This limitation is overcome in the color flow Doppler imaging. Recall that in pulsed (and duplex) Doppler, the depth from which Doppler signal is recorded is determined by the time lag (after emission of sound beam) after which the gate is opened to receive the signal.[9,10] Use of multiple gates, which open after different time lags, allows detection of depths of multiple Doppler signals. A modification of this principle is utilized in color flow imaging where in electronically steered (phased array) transducers are used to detect signals at different depths of a real time image. Thus, the signal can be detected from the vessels as well as surrounding tissues. The Doppler signal is assigned color proportionate to the strength of the Doppler signal. The superimposition of such colored information on the gray scale image generates the color flow image.

- *Power Doppler* is useful for the evaluation of slow flow. Pulsed Doppler does not provide information regarding the intensity (or power) of the Doppler signal. This information can be obtained in the power Doppler mode which displays the power (or intensity) of the Doppler signal, as it changes with time in every region within the chosen area. Higher intensity Doppler signals are imparted lighter hue of color. However, there is no information available regarding the velocity. The power Doppler has superior flow sensitivity as compared to conventional color Doppler and is used to evaluate the presence and characteristics of the flow in blood vessels that are poorly imaged with conventional color Doppler **(Figs. 3B and C)**.

Tissue Harmonic Imaging

Nonlinear propagation of ultrasound waves in tissues produce harmonics. In tissue harmonic imaging (THI), information from these harmonics is used to obtain images which are of higher quality than conventional sonography.[12,15] Tissue vibration generates harmonics which are integer multiples of the transmitted frequency. In conventional grayscale sonography, image is produced by receiving the same frequency spectrum which was transmitted into the patient whereas in THI, image is produced as a result of higher harmonic frequencies which are generated as ultrasound beam propagates through the tissue. Its the second harmonic which is twice the fundamental frequency which is used for imaging. Tissue harmonic imaging gives improved signal to noise ratio, improved lateral resolution and reduced side lobe artifacts as compared to conventional imaging and thus helps in improving image quality.[12,16]

The higher harmonic may also be used but that would require extremely wide band width transducers.[14] In THI, as compared to periphery of the pulse more harmonics are generated at the center. Its the reduced width of the ultrasound beam due to which lateral resolution is improved. Ability to resolve small anatomic structures and detail by THI is attributed to increased lateral resolution. THI is especially useful in obese patients as it decreases the harmful effects of body wall. Different tissues generate harmonic waves of different intensity depending upon the the non-linearity coefficient of the tissue insonated. Highest non-linearity coefficients are generated by tissues which have higher amount of fat, which enhances the intensity of harmonic waves generated. In obese patients, whose body wall has an increased proportion of fat, lesion visibility is improved using THI.[12,16,17]

Side lobe artifacts are caused when the ultrasound beam hits an interface and is reflected back to the transducer, which produce artefactual echoes. Harmonics are produced in tissues, deep in relation to the body wall so they pass through the body wall only once, hence artifacts from body wall are reduced. As side lobe artifacts are reduced,

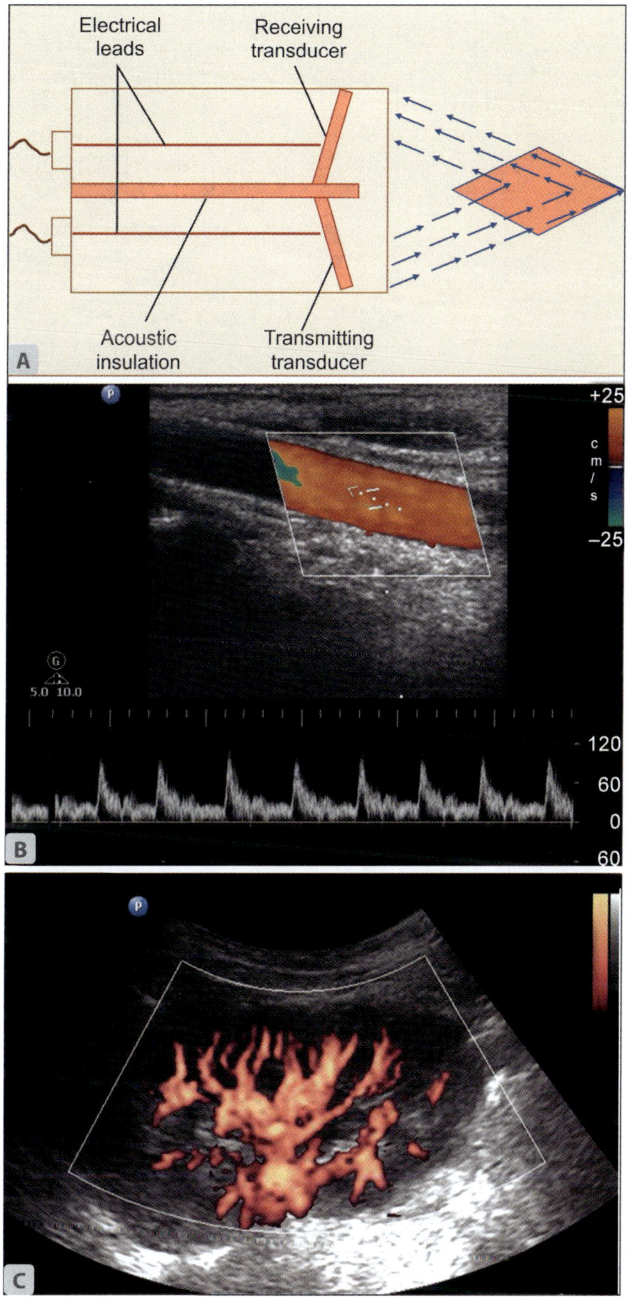

FIGS. 3A TO C: Components of a typical Doppler ultrasound transducer (A), Color Doppler and pulsed Doppler scan of common carotid artery (B), Power Doppler image showing normal Doppler signals in kidney (C).

signal-to-noise ratio is improved, resulting in an improved image in which tissues appear brighter and cavities appear darker.[18-20]

Tissue harmonic imaging provides additional information in both solid and cystic lesions **(Figs. 4 and 5)**. Harmonic imaging increases the diagnostic confidence of operator in differentiating simple from complex renal cysts. It also improves detection of gallbladder and biliary stones, improves pancreatic definition and allows distinction of cystic from solid hepatic lesions.[12,18]

1.5 harmonic imaging is another harmonic technique that has been studied.[21] This detects and visualizes echoes which are a factor of 1.5 times higher than the fundamental center frequency of the transducer. This frequency range is intermediate between the fundamental and the second harmonic frequency spectrum.[21,22] Advantage is that this frequency range is nearly free of tissue echoes and contains microbubbles echoes only. Hence, there is improvement in contrast between tissue and microbubbles of 20dB or more compared to the second harmonic technique.

Spatial Compound Imaging

Spatial compound imaging is a speckle reducing ultrasound technique, which uses electronic steering of ultrasound beams from a transducer array to obtain overlapping scans of a target object from different angles (same tissue is imaged many times by using parallel beams directed along different directions).[3,23] Resulting echoes from these multiple acquisitions are then averaged to produce a single compound image of improved quality due to reduction in image speckle. When compared to conventional B-mode imaging, in compound imaging, more time is required for acquisition of data (as here multiple ultrasound beams are used to evaluate same tissue) and frame rate is also reduced. Spatial compound imaging demonstrates reduced level of speckle, noise, refraction, reduced shadowing and enhancement artifacts and improved contrast and margin definition **(Figs. 6 and 7)**.[3,23,24]

Application of spatial compound imaging has been described in imaging of breast, peripheral vessels, and musculoskeletal system. It can also be combined with other ultrasound applications, e.g. harmonic imaging.

Extended Field of View

This technique available in most of the new scanners allows sonologists to visualize large anatomic regions in a single image. It can be performed on deep structures using a curvilinear probe as well on superficial structures using a linear array transducer, although most of its applications are in superficial structures.[3,23] Extended field of view imaging, also called panoramic imaging in some machines allows easy measurements of large lesions/structures and exact delineation of anatomical relationships in a single image **(Figs. 8A and B)**. Transducer is initially moved laterally across the area of interest being scanned and multiple images are acquired from several transducer positions.[23] Images are registered with respect to each other. This registered data is subsequently combined to form one complete large field of view image.

Elastography

Imaging of tissue stiffness or elasticity is one of the rapidly evolving ultrasound based application. The term elastography encompasses a variety of techniques that can predict a mechanical response or stiffness of tissues.[25] Introduced by Ophir et al.,[26] elastography has subsequently evolved into a real-time imaging tool. The elasticity of biological tissues depend on their constituent macromolecules (parenchyma,

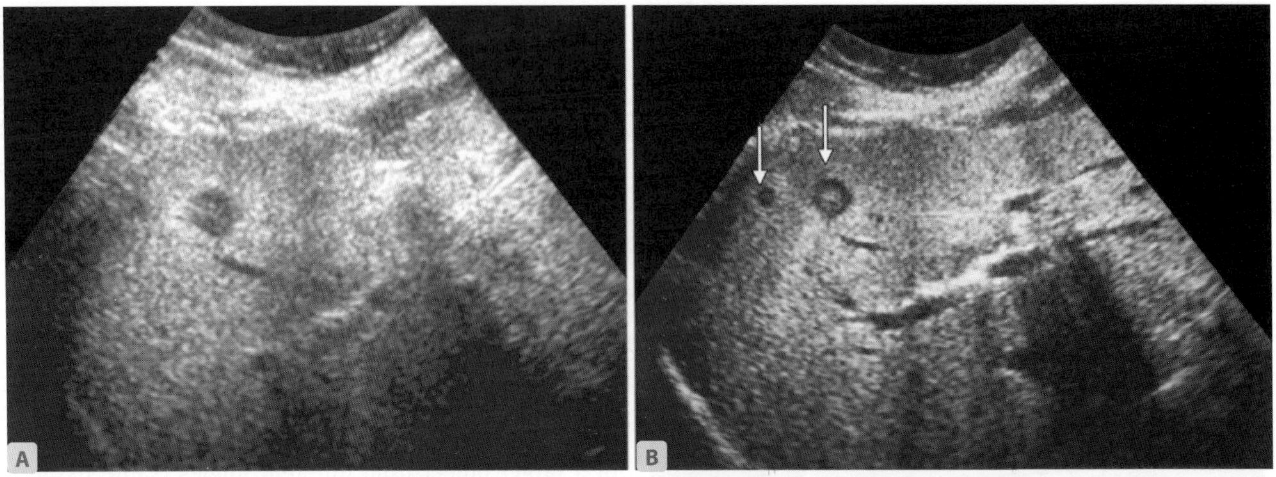

FIGS. 4A AND B: Comparison of conventional grayscale imaging (A) with tissue harmonic imaging (B) THI clearly demonstrates target lesions (indeterminate on conventional) in a metastatic liver disease. Also note that additional lesions are also detected at THI.

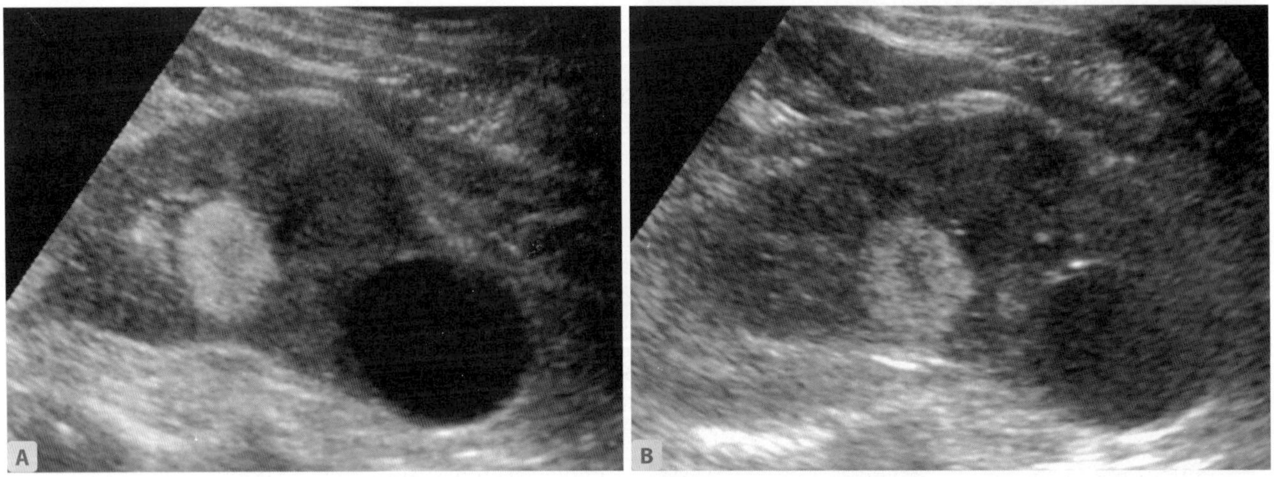

FIGS. 5A AND B: Tissue harmonic imaging (A) demonstrates much better delineation of both cystic and solid lesions in this patient of renal angiomyolipomas, when compared to conventional grayscale imaging (B).

fat, collagen, etc.) and on their structural organization.[27] Tissue elasticity is characterized by the amount of tissue's displacement or distortion in response to the application of an external load (elastic or Young's modulus). Because the echogenicity and the mechanical attributes of the tissue are generally not correlated, it is expected that imaging tissue stiffness or strain will provide new information related to tissue structure and/or pathology.[28]

Sonoelastography has been applied in the following organs:[29]

- Liver to estimate the degree of hepatic fibrosis and estimation of risk of development of HCC.
- Breast to differentiate benign and malignant breast lumps and reclassify BIRADS 4 lesions.
- Thyroid to differentiate benign and malignant nodules and to assess treatment response in malignant nodules.
- Gastrointestinal tract for characterizing bowel wall lesions, differentiating inflammatory stenosis from fibrotic stenosis and evaluation of gastric contractility.
- EUS Elastography for evaluating pancreatic head lesions, abdominal lymph nodes and anorectal lesions.
- Prostate in the differentiation of benign hypertrophy and prostate cancer.
- Musculoskeletal system in the evaluation of tendinopathies.

More details on elastography are provided subsequently in another chapter in this book.

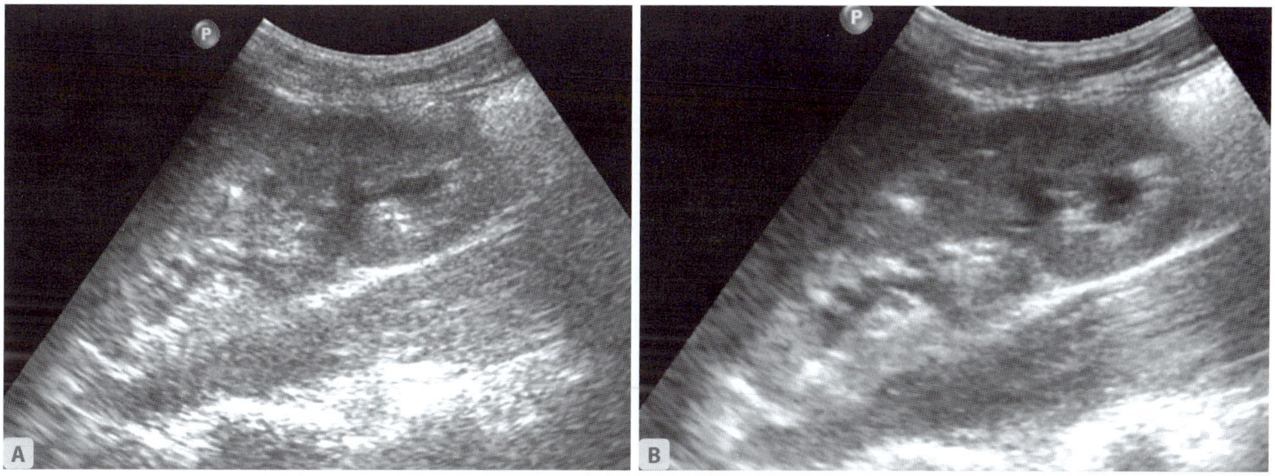

FIGS. 6A AND B: Spatial compound imaging in a patient with nephrocalcinosis. Note medullary hyperechogenicity is not well appreciated on conventional grayscale mode (A), but is clearly demonstrated on compound imaging (B).

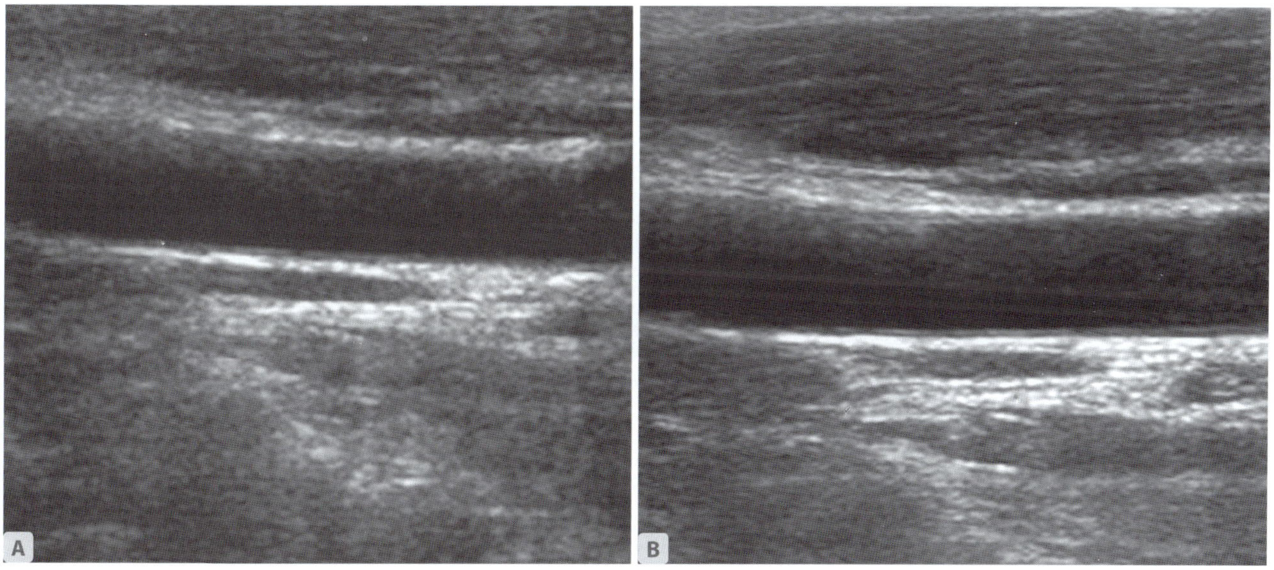

FIGS. 7A AND B: Spatial compound imaging in carotid vessels helps clear depiction of intima-media thickness for accurate measurements. (A) Refers to conventional grayscale while (B) Refers to compound imaging.

3D and 4D Ultrasound

3D ultrasonography acquires a series of sections in the region of interest from different orientations and produces a volume data set which contains the entire sonographic data of the scanned region of interest. By translation and rotation through the data set, different arbitrary planes from the volume data set can be generated. After acquisition, the volumetric data can be qualitatively and quantitatively assessed with the use of various softwares which include surface and volume rendering, multiplanar imaging, etc. Hence, similar to other cross sectional imaging like CT and MRI, the volumetric data of this 3D ultrasound can also be 'post-processed'. Because of volume imaging it is possible to display information in any orientation and any of the planes. When the 3D ultrasound is acquired and demonstrated over time, it is termed as 4D ultrasound, live 3D ultrasound or real time 3D ultrasound.[30]

Currently there are two commonly used techniques to acquire 3D volumetric data-free hand technique and automated technique. In the free hand technique the examiner requires to manually move the probe within the region of interest. In the automated technique dedicated 3D probes (also called volume probes) have to be used. In this method probe is held stationary and on activation the transducer elements within the probes automatically sweep through the 'volume box' which has been selected by the

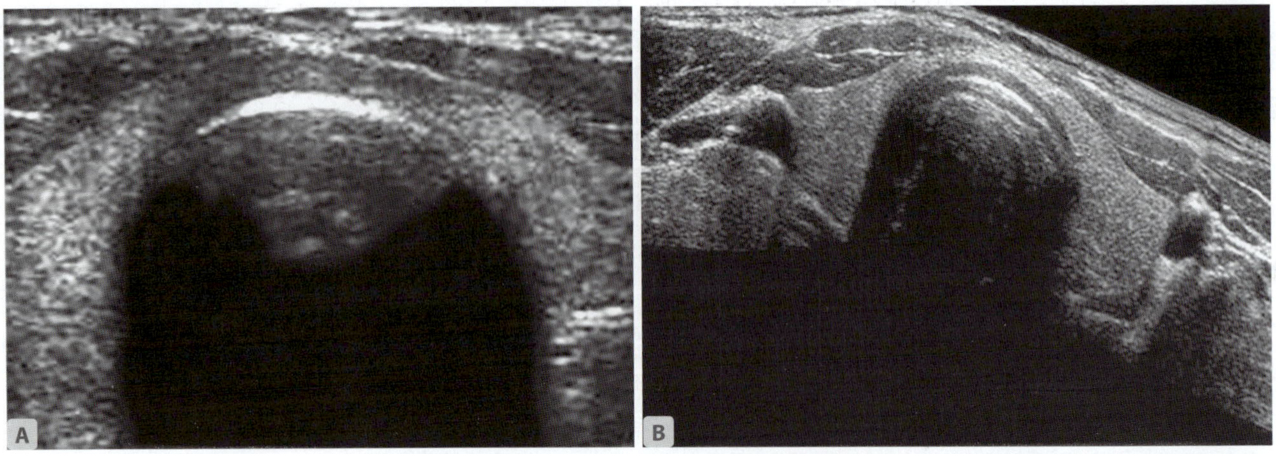

FIGS. 8A AND B: Extended field of view: Routine grayscale mode (A) is able to demonstrate only limited part of thyroid in a single image, while extended field of view mode (B) clearly demonstrates the composite image showing both lobes of thyroid, isthmus besides cervical vessels in a single image.

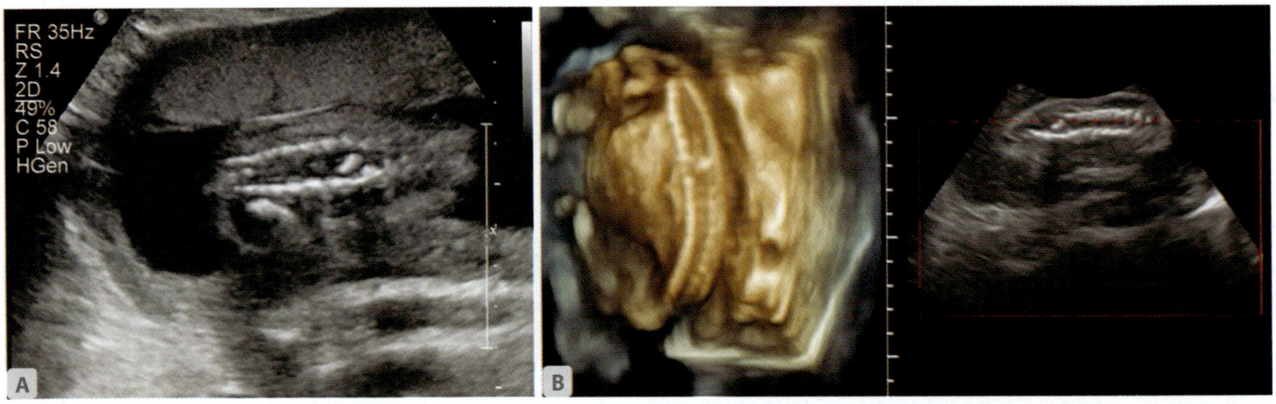

FIGS. 9A AND B: Transabdominal sonographic coronal 2D image. (A) Bony spur in a case of diastematomyelia; (B) Corresponding 3D image showing the bony spur.

operator. The resultant images are digitally stored and can be 'processed' later in various display modes for analysis.[31]

There are numerous areas in which the use of 3D and 4D can be very useful **(Figs. 9A and B)**. Few of these are as follows.[30]

Gynecology

- For assessment of congenital anomalies of uterus.[32,33]
- For evaluation of endometrial and uterine cavity.
- For preoperative localization of fibroids.
- For evaluation of possible cornual ectopic pregnancies.
- For locating intrauterine device.
- For evaluation of adnexal lesions for better differentiation of ovarian lesions from tubal or uterine lesions.
- Three dimensional guidance for interventional procedures.
- Evaluation and follow-up of patients of polycystic ovaries and tubal occlusion for infertility work-up.

Obstetrics

- For evaluation of facial anomalies like cleft palate and cleft lip.
- Evaluation of nasal bone, ears and cranial sutures.
- Detection of central nervous system anomalies like corpus callosal agenesis and Dandy-Walker cyst.
- For evaluation of ribs and intrathoracic masses.
- For evaluation of spine, e.g. vertebral abnormalities, neural, tube defect,[34,35] diastematomyelia **(Figs. 9A and B)**, etc.
- For evaluation of extremities like club feet and skeletal dysplasia, etc.
- For evaluation of heart, placenta and umbilical cord.
- For evaluation of multiple gestations for mapping of vasculature for twin transfusion syndrome.
- Telemedicine and education.
- Storing volumetric data for subsequent interpretation and review.
- For quality control by way of central monitoring, e.g. procedures done at different peripheral sites and in multicenter research studies.
- Teaching postprocessing techniques and standardized views to residents.

Studies have suggested that the mothers who are viewing the 3D images of the babies feel enhanced bonding with their fetus.[36]

With the use of 4D ultrasound various facial movements and actions such as tongue protrusion, mouth opening, etc. can be evaluated in greater details.[37-39] 4D ultrasound has also been used in the cardiac evaluation of fetus.[40-42]

Three dimensional images are very useful for demonstrating the abnormality to the referring physician as these images are better comprehended by those who are not tuned to understand grayscale format of 2D images. Similarly storage of 'volume' data allows us to reprocess the data in future for subsequent interpretation or reviews. These volume data can be sent to remote workstations for telemedicine and teaching purposes. It has also been shown in a few studies that acquisition of 3D data needs less time which can potentially increase patient through put and increase efficiency of the imaging department.[43]

Limitations

As 3D ultrasound information is dependent on reformation of acquired 2D ultrasound data, it is expected that the problems which affect the 2D ultrasound like motion and unfavorable body habitus. 3D USG evaluation may be hampered by bony or air shadowing. 3D image quality may be affected by artifacts such as reverberation artifacts, motion artifacts, and mirror artifacts.[44] Suboptimal scanning techniques also result in poor quality 3D images.[31]

Fusion Imaging

Fusion imaging or hybrid imaging means combination of two imaging techniques. This can be in the form of fusion of two anatomical techniques like ultrasound with MRI or CT; or it can be fusion of anatomical technique (ultrasound, CT or MRI) with molecular imaging technique like SPECT or PET **(Fig. 10)**.

Real-time virtual sonography (RVS) is one of the example of fusion imaging. To obtain virtual fusion images, CT/MRI data which has been previously acquired is transferred to the ultrasound machine. A point like magnetic positioning sensor unit is attached to the ultrasound probe to detect any change in position of probe during investigation. The transmitter of this sensor unit is placed onto the surface of

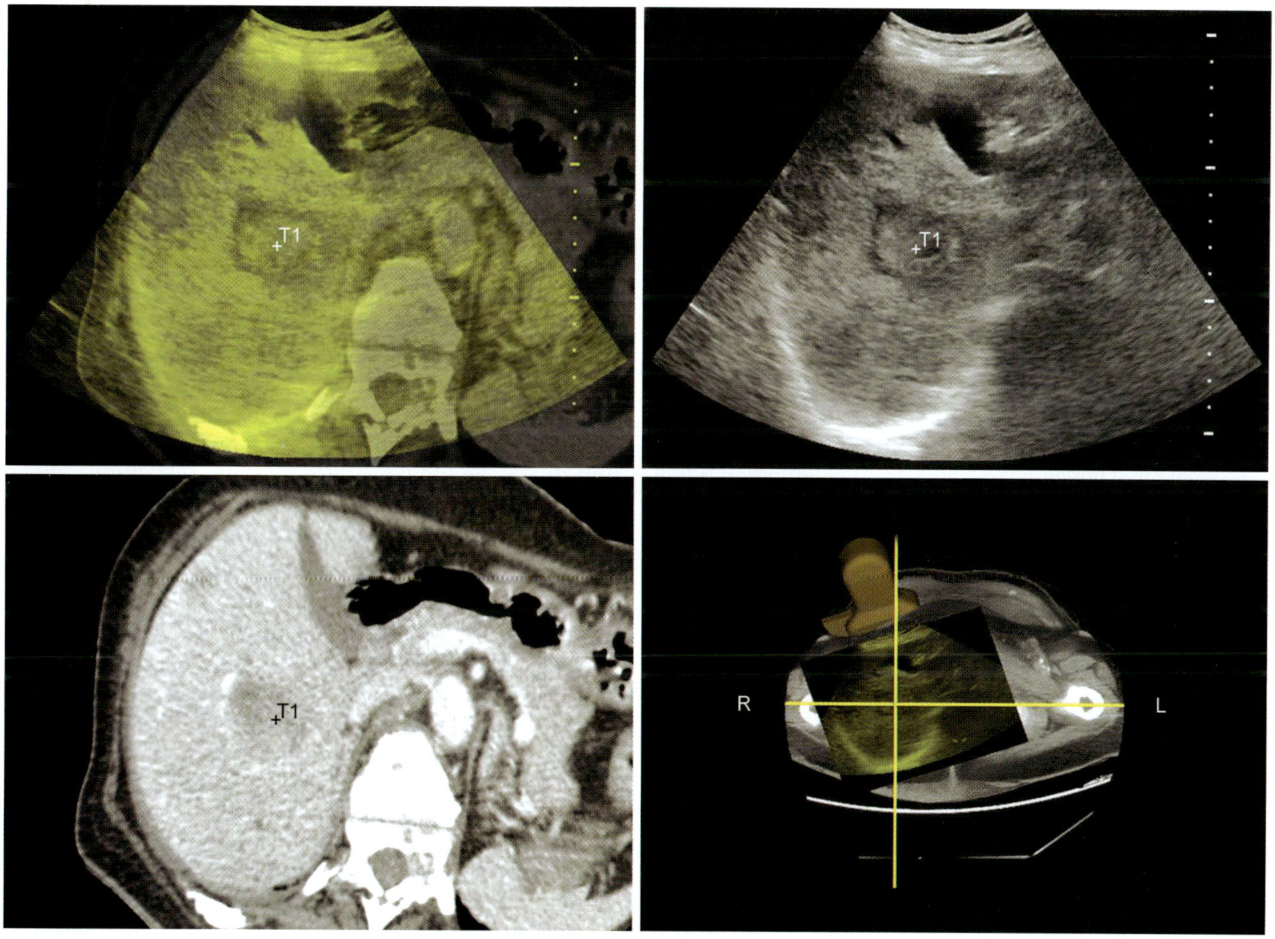

FIG. 10: Figure shows application of fusion imaging on a patient with well visualized lesion on both CT as well as on USG. Four split images seen on the screen. Image in lower left corner is a previously acquired CT images feeded in ultrasound machine. On moving the ultrasound transducer, there will be automatic reformation of these feeded images corresponding to the axis of ultrasound transducer so that the same imaging plane is matched to the ultrasound image. Right upper corner is current sonographic image. Image in left upper corner is an overlay image showing good matching of the lesions from sonographic and CT images. Right lower image shows the 3D view which is being displayed during the fusion workflow.

patient. During examination ultrasound screen is seen as split images with virtual reconstructed CT/MR image on one side and currently acquired USG image on other side of the screen. An attempt is made to match these two images with each other. This is usually done by freezing the CT or MR section with some noticeably visible anatomic landmark (e.g. portal vein bifurcation, superior most margin of kidney or the lesion itself, etc.) and identifying the same landmark by freehand USG.[45] Then these two images are matched. The real time USG image can also be superimposed on the virtual reconstructed CT image with adjustable difference in the grayness **(Fig. 10)**.

Clinical Applications of Fusion Imaging

It has been observed that there are few lesions/tumors in liver which are iso-echoic and hence not well appreciable on gray-scale ultrasound. Similarly there are subgroups of patients who have been treated with either TACE or RFA and now there is recurrence in the vicinity of the primary tumor site. These lesions are also poorly localized on grayscale USG. Hence, detection by USG or further biopsy/treatment by the local ablative therapies were difficult for such lesions. These lesions are usually clearly visible on contrast enhanced CT/MR. However, intervention is usually easier to execute with USG guidance which also avoids radiation to the operator. A combination of advantages of both the imaging techniques is achieved with RVS.[46] In one way this technique provides real time visualization of the needles in pre-procedural CT scan images. The feasibility of RVS module has been proven in many studies.[47-49] The RVS module has been shown to be compatible with B mode, color Doppler mode as well as with harmonic imaging mode.[50] However the data on accuracy and efficacy of this technique are still emerging.[51]

Limitations

Real-time virtual sonography cannot be used in those patients in whom CT/MRI are contraindicated (e.g. contrast allergy, deranged renal function tests, etc). Another limitation is that sometimes the best synchronization is not achievable hence limiting the utility.[50] It definitely prolongs the examination time and it is more expensive as it adds the cost of CT/MRI also.

Therapeutic Applications of Ultrasound

- Ultrasound-guided aspirations, drainages and biopsies form the backbone of any interventional radiology unit. With the help of ultrasound, one can easily track the needle path and perform any such interventional procedure easily. Not only it is noninvasive, radiation free, portable modality, it also offers areal time navigation facility to the interventionists.
- *High intensity focused ultrasound (HIFU):* High intensity focused ultrasound is rapidly emerging as a non invasive technique to ablate the tumors. In this, high intensity ultrasonic waves are targeted at a focal lesion with high accuracy, which results in rise of temperature in the desired target, resulting in the destruction of the tumor cells.[52] Simply put, transducers help to thermally ablate tumors without introducing needles or wires into the tumor.[53] There is absorption of high intensity energy which is converted into heat at the site of the lesion. This heat raises the temperature causing coagulative necrosis at the site.[54]
  Real-time ultrasound imaging is required for HIFU with use of multiple transducers having a range of focal lengths (90–160 mm). The most commonly used transducer has an operating frequency of 0.8 MHz and a focal length of 135 mm.[52,53] HIFU is being used for treatment of benign as well as malignant tumors. The common applications include the treatment of fibroids, osteoid osteoma, liver and prostatic cancers.

Ultrasound-based Molecular Imaging and Oncotherapy

Ultrasound molecular imaging combines the benefits of contrast enhanced ultrasound with the capability for characterizing the neoplastic process at a molecular level.[55] Ultrasound molecular imaging has enormous potential applications, which include early tumoral detection and evaluation of treatment response, as well as providing guidance for the cancer therapies.[55,56] Ultrasound contrast agents help in improving the delivery of gene therapies and chemotherapeutic agents across existing biological barriers. It involves the use of contrast microbubbles, which are emulsions (gas-liquid) of several micrometer in size and are confined to intravascular space. Much smaller newer nanoparticles are currently being investigated for future application.

Ultrasound Image Artifacts

Ultrasound artifacts result usually due to issues related to the characteristics related to ultrasound beam, the occurrence of many echo paths, and errors related to velocity errors and attenuation. The various artifacts which are commonly encountered in the clinical practice include reverberation, ring-down, shadowing, attenuation, refraction, speed displacement, side lobe, beam width, comet tail, mirror image, and increased through-transmission.[57]

Ultrasound artifacts can be grouped under:

- *Resolution-related artifacts:* Speckle occurs as a result of the use of transducer which is phase-sensitive and is seen when object being scanned is too small and is difficult to be properly resolved by the imaging system.[58] This is because of interference, i.e. small scatterers which lead to constructive as well as destructive phase interference on the receiving end. Speckle is not a desirable phenomenon as it can hide small but diagnostically important imaging findings.[59] Speckle will not change with time, so even if repeat imaging is performed across same plane and transducer orientation and position, a same speckle pattern will be seen. However, if the transducer orientation and position is changes, the speckle pattern shall also change.
- *Attenuation-related artifacts:* These include attenuation, shadowing and enhancement. It occurs when the sound cannot be transmitted through the mass lesion.

It points to internal solid consistency of the lesion. When an ultrasound beam strikes an object/ structure which attenuate the sound to a larger or smaller degree as compared to the neighboring structures, the beam strength distal to the object/structure attenuating the sound will be either less or more than that in the adjoining areas. Furthermore, the echoes which return from the tissues and structures which are far beyond the attenuating object/structure shall also get weaker. In the routine practice, this artifact is seen as a black band called as a "shadow" deep to the attenuating object/or structure **(Fig. 11A)**.

On a similar pattern, if the ultrasound beam traverses through a weakly attenuating object/structure, the beam amplitude deeper to this object/structure increases than the amplitude of the beam in the rest of the scanning field at the same depth and hence the echoes which return from the structures deep to the weakly attenuating object/structure will be of greater amplitude and will be seen as high echogenicity area or "enhancement", typically seen posterior to a cystic lesion (low attenuation lesion)[57-59] **(Fig. 11B)**.

- *Propagation related (artifacts associated with multiple echoes)* ***(Fig. 12)****:*

  This includes Reverberation, Ring down, Comet tail, Side lobe and Mirror image artifacts:[60]

  - *Reverberation:* When there are two highly reflective surfaces lying in a parallel fashion, echoes which are generated by the primary ultrasound beam might get reflected back and forth continuously before it returns back to the transducer again. This results in multiple echoes being recorded and displayed, and is seen as numerous linear reflections which lie equidistant to one another and called as reverberation artifact.[57,60] Typically, it is seen when sound beam traverses with minimal or no attenuation through a cystic (fluid) structure. These become weak as sound travels into the tissue deeper and can mimic solid component in a cystic structure (urinary bladder). This artifact can be resolved by simply changing the scanning angle.
  - *Ring down:* Its appearance is similar to the ladder-like reverberation of comet tail artifact, but it is produced by a different mechanism. The artifact is only associated with gas bubbles, and occurs when an ultrasound pulse encounters a fluid collection that is trapped between an inverted tetrahedron of 4 bubbles. The trapped fluid resonates, emitting a continuous signal back to the transducer. Whereas the transducer pulse is broad spectrum, the returning signal consists of one or more discrete (resonant) frequencies. "Beats" between these frequencies produce the variable appearance of the ring down.
  - *Comet tail:* This artifact is a type of reverberation where there are two reflective interfaces and the sequential echoes are placed in close proximity. The sequential echoes in this case may be so near that each different signal may not be perceivable. It is seen as bright, tapering echoes deep to the structure which reflects powerfully. Classic examples include metallic structures which may produce these artifacts.

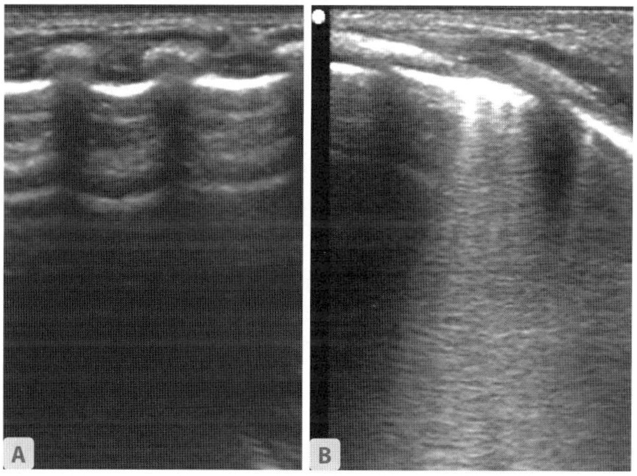

FIGS. 12A AND B: Reverberation artefacts (A) in the ultrasound image of a normal lung. Comet tail artefacts (B) in the ultrasound image of lung of a neonate with respiratory distress syndrome.

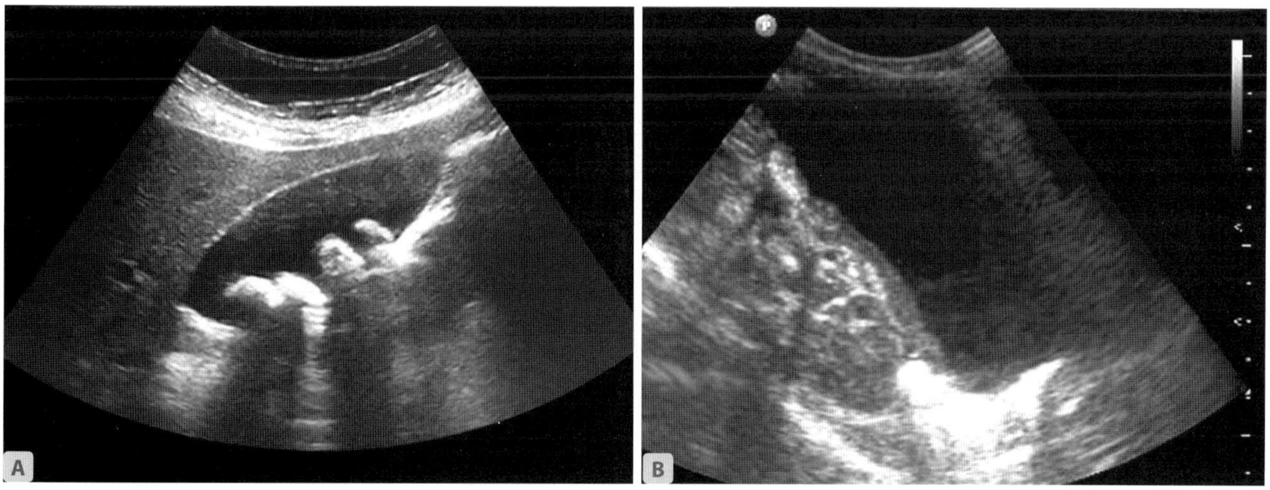

FIGS. 11A AND B: Ultrasound image artifacts: shadowing (A) due to gallbladder calculi and enhancement (B) from a large abdominal cystic lesion.

- *Side lobe:* They occur where side lobes reflect sound from strong reflector (like bowel gas adjacent to the gallbladder or urinary bladder) that is outside of the central beam, and where the echoes are displayed as if they originated from within the central beam. Ultrasound transducer crystals expand and contract to produce primary ultrasound beams in the direction of the expansion and contraction. Secondary beams also occur because the crystals also expand and contract radially. These radial beams are called side lobe beams. Side lobe beams are low-intensity beams that surround the central beam. Side lobe artifacts are echogenic, and can be linear or curvilinear in appearance.
- *Mirror image artifacts:* These are generated when the primary beam strikes upon an interface which is highly reflective. The reflected echoes then stumble upon the "back side" of that structure and then is reflected in the direction of the reflective interface again before it gets reflected towards the transducer finally for the detection.[57] This is seen as a structure which is duplicated and is seen lying equidistant from but is at a depth from the strongly reflective interface. In routine practice, this phenomenon can be seen at the level of the diaphragm, where the pleural-air interface is a strong reflector and liver can be seen on either side of the diaphragm.

- *Ultrasound beam characteristics-related artifacts:* This includes beam width artifact where a greatly reflective object which is located within the widened beam beyond transducer's margin also is able to generate detectable echoes. Ultrasound display presumes them to be generating from within narrow imaging plane and displays them in the same fashion they are detected.[57] Its clinical application can be manifested as when anechoic structure (urinary bladder) shows echoes at its periphery. This can be corrected and removed during scanning by adjusting the focal zone to the level of interest and by placing transducer at the center of the object. Side lobes are multiple beams of low amplitude ultrasound energy that project radially from the main beam axis and artifacts seen mainly with linear array transducers.[57] Similar to beam width artifact, this phenomenon is most likely to be recognized as extraneous echoes present within an expected anechoic structure such as the bladder.[61]

To conclude, knowledge of ultrasound instrumentation especially various transducers and controls is an important step for performing a successful scan. Adequate utilization of newer exciting applications enables the sonographer to play ever increasing role in patient care.

REFERENCES

1. Rizzatto G. Ultrasound transducers. Eur J Radiol. 1998; 27(Suppl 2):S188-95.
2. Cynthia Silkowski. Ultrasound Nomenclature, Image Orientation and Basic Instrumentation. In: Emergency Medicine Sonography. By Dunstan Abraham, Cynthia Silkowski, and Charles Odwin. Jones and Bartlett Publishers; 2010.pp.1-24.
3. Hangiandreou NJ. Radiographics AAPM/RSNA physics tutorial for residents. Topics in US: B-mode US: basic concepts and new technology. 2003;23(4):1019-33.
4. Enriquez JL, Wu TS. An introduction to ultrasound equipment and knobology. Crit Care Clin. 2014;30(1): 25-45.
5. Zagzebski JA. Physics and Instrumentation in Doppler and B-mode ultrasonography. In Introduction to Vascular Ultrasonography by Zwiebel & Pellerito. 5th Edn. Elsevier Saunders. Philadelphia. Chapter 2. 2005.pp.19-60.
6. Curry ST, Dowdey JE, Murry RC. Ultrasound. In Christensen's Physics of Diagnostic Radiology. 4th Edn. Lea & Febiger. 1990. pp.323-70.
7. Martinoli C, Derchi LE, Rizzatto G, Solbiati L. Power Doppler sonography: general principles, clinical applications, and future prospects. Eur Radiol. 1998;8:1224-35.
8. Kremkau F. Diagnostic ultrasound principles, Instrumentation and Exercises, 5th Edn. Orlando FL, Grune & Startton; 1993.
9. Taylor KJW, Wells PNT, Burns PN. Clinical applications of Doppler ultrasound. New York, Raven Press; 1995.
10. Evans D. Doppler ultrasound physics instrumentation and clinical applications. New York, John Wiley and Sons; 1989.
11. Rubin JM, Bude RO,Carson PL, et al. Power Doppler US: A potentially useful alternative to mean frequency-based color Doppler US. Radiology. 1994;190:853-6.
12. Sodhi KS, Sidhu R, Gulati M, Saxena A, Suri S, Chawla Y. Role of tissue harmonic imaging in focal hepatic lesions: comparison with conventional sonography. J Gastroenterol Hepatol. 2005;20(10):1488-93.
13. Shapiro RS, Wagreich J, Parsons RB, Pasik AS, Yeh HC, Lao R. Tissue harmonic imaging sonography: evaluation of image quality compared with conventional sonography. AJR. 1998;171:1203-6.
14. Yucel C, Ozdemir H, Asik E, Oner Y, Isik S. Benefits of tissue harmonic imaging in the evaluation of abdominal and pelvic lesions. Abdom. Imaging. 2003;28:103-9.
15. Ward B, Baker AC, Humphrey VF. Nonlinear propagation applied to the improvement of resolution in diagnostic medical ultrasound. J Acoust Soc Am. 1997;101:143-54.
16. Rosenthal SJ, Jones PH, Wetzel LH. Phase inversion tissue harmonic sonographic imaging: a clinical utility study. AJR 2001;176:1393-8.
17. Anvari A, Forsberg F, Samir AE. A primer on the physical principles of tissue harmonic imaging. Radiographics. 2015;35: 1955-64.
18. Hann LE, Bach AM, Cramer LD, Siegel D, Yoo HH, Gaxia R. Hepatic sonography: comparison of tissue harmonic and standard sonography techniques. AJR. 1999;173: 201-6.
19. Desser TS, Jeffrey RB. Tissue harmonic imaging techniques: physical principles and clinical applications. Semin. Ultrasound CT MR. 2001;22:1-10.
20. Lencioni R, Cioni D, Bartolozzi C. Tissue harmonic and contrast specific imaging: back to gray scale in ultrasound. Eur. Radiol. 2002;12:151-65.
21. Kollmann C. New sonographic techniques for harmonic imaging--underlying physical principles. Eur J Radiol. 2007;64(2):164-72. Epub 2007 Sep 17. Review.
22. Yamamoto K, Shiraki K, Nakanishi S, et al. The usefulness of 1.5 harmonic imaging ultrasonography with Levovlst In the diagnosis of focal hepatic tumors. Int J Oncol. 2005; 27:989-95.
23. Harvey CJ, Pilcher JM, Eckersley Rj, Blomley MJK, Cosgrove DO. Advances in Ultrasound. Clin Radiol. 2002;57:157-77.
24. Jespersen SK, Wilhjelm JE, Sillesen H. Multiangle compound imaging. Ultrason Imaging. 1998;20:81-102.

25. Sarvazyan A, Hall TJ, Urban MW, Fatemi M, Aglyamov SR, Garra BS. An overview of elastography- an emerging branch of medical imaging. Curr Med Imaging Rev. 2011; 7:255-82.
26. Ophir J, Céspedes I, Ponnekanti H, Yazdi Y, Li X. Elastography: a quantitative method for imaging the elasticity of biological tissues. Ultrason Imaging. 1991;13:111-34.
27. Sandrin L, Oudry J, Bastard C, Fournier C, Miette V, Mueller S. Non-Invasive assessment of liver fibrosis by vibration-controlled transient elastography (Fibroscan®). In: Takahashi H, editor. Liver Biopsy. Rijeka: InTech; 2011.
28. Gao L, Parker KJ, Lerner RM, Levinson SF. Imaging of the elastic properties of tissue—a review. Ultrasound Med Biol. 1996;22: 959-77.
29. Badea R, Zaro R, Opincariu I, et al. USG in the examination of the gallbladder—a holistic approach: grey scale, Doppler, CEUS, elastography, and 3D. Med Ultrason. 2014;16:345-55.
30. Benacerraf BR, Benson CB, Abuhamad AZ, et al. Three and 4-dimensional ultrasound in obstetrics and gynecology: proceedings of the American Institute of Ultrasound in Medicine Consensus Conference. J Ultrasound Med. 2005;24(12):1587-97.
31. Bega G, Lev-Toaff AS, O'Kane P, et al. Three-dimensional Ultrasonography in Gynecology Technical Aspects and Clinical Applications. J Ultrasound Med. 2003;22(11): 1249-69.
32. Raga F, Bonilla-Musoles F, Blanes J, et al. Congenital mullerian anomalies: diagnostic accuracy of three-dimensional ultrasound. Fertil Steril. 1996;65(3):523-8.
33. Wu MH, Hsu CC, Huang KE. Detection of congenital mullerian duct anomalies using three-dimensional ultrasound. J Clin Ultrasound. 1997;25(9):487-92.
34. Dyson RL, Pretorius DH, Budorick NE, et al. Three dimensional ultrasound in the evaluation of fetal anomalies. Ultrasound Obstet Gynecol. 2000;16(4):321-8.
35. Lee W, Chaiworapongsa T, Romero R, et al. A diagnostic approach for the evaluation of spina bifida by three-dimensional ultrasonography. J Ultrasound Med. 2002; 21(6):619-26.
36. Ji E, Pretorius D, Newton R, et al. Effects of ultrasound on maternal-fetal bonding: a comparison of two- and three- dimensional imaging. Ultrasound Obstet Gynecol. 2005; 25(5):473-7.
37. Kurjak A, Azumendi G, Vecek N, et al. Fetal hand movements and facial expression in normal pregnancy studied by four-dimensional sonography. J Perinat Med. 2003;31(6):496-508.
38. Kurjak A, Stanojevic M, Andonotopo W, et al. Behavioral pattern continuity from prenatal to postnatal life: a study by four-dimensional (4D) ultrasonography. J Perinat Med. 2004;32(4): 346-53.
39. Kurjak A, Stanojevic M, Azumendi G, et al. The potential of four-dimensional (4D) Ultrasonography in the assessment of fetal awareness. J Perinat Med, 2005;33(1): 46-53.
40. DeVore GR, Falkensammer P, Sklansky MS, et al. Spatio- temporal image correlation (STIC): new technology for evaluation of the fetal heart. Ultrasound Obstet Gynecol. 2003;22(4):380-7.
41. Viñals F, Poblete P, Giuliano A. Spatio-temporal image correlation (STIC): a new tool for the prenatal screening of congenital heart defects. Ultrasound Obstet Gynecol. 2003;22(4): 388-94.
42. Gonçalves LF, Lee W, Chaiworapongsa T, et al. Four-dimensional ultrasonography of the fetal heart with spatiotemporal image correlation. Am J Obstet Gynecol. 2003;189(6):1792-802.
43. Benacerraf BR, Shipp TD, Bromley B. How sonographic tomography will change the face of obstetric sonography: a pilot study. J Ultrasound Med. 2005;24(3):371-8.
44. Helge O, Thune N, Matre K. In Vitro Evaluation of Three dimensional ultrasonography in volume estimation of abdominal organs. Ultrasound Med Biol. 1994;20:157-65.
45. Sandulescu L, Saftoiu A, Dumitrescu D, Ciurea T. The role of real-time contrast-enhanced and real-time virtual sonography in the assessment of malignant liver lesions. J Gastrointestin Liver Dis. 2009;18(1):103-8.
46. Sandulescu L, Dumitrescu D, Rogoveanu I, Saftoiu A. Hybrid ultrasound imaging techniques (fusion imaging). World J Gastroenterol. 2011;17(1):49-52.
47. Minami Y, Kudo M, Chung H, et al. Percutaneous radio frequency ablation of sonographically unidentifiable liver tumors. Feasibility and usefulness of a novel guiding technique with an integrated system of computed tomography and sonographic images. Oncology. 2007; 72(Suppl 1):111-6.
48. Minami Y, Chung H, Kudo M, et al. Radiofrequency ablation of hepatocellular carcinoma: value of virtual CT sonography with magnetic navigation. AJR Am J Roentgenol. 2008;190(6):W335-W341.
49. Kitada T, Murakami T, Kuzushita N, et al. Effectiveness of real-time virtual sonography guided radiofrequency ablation treatment for patients with hepatocellular carcinomas. Hepatol Res. 2008;38(6):565-71.
50. Sandulescu L, Saftoiu A, Dumitrescu D, Ciurea T. Real-time contrast-enhanced and real-time virtual sonography in the assessment of benign liver lesions. J Gastrointestin Liver Dis. 2008;17(4):475-8.
51. Krücker J, Xu S, Venkatesan A, et al. Clinical Utility of Real-time Fusion Guidance for Biopsy and Ablation. J Vasc Interv Radiol. 2011;22(4):515-24.
52. Shehata IA. Treatment with high intensity focused ultrasound: secrets revealed. Eur J Radiol. 2012;81(3): 534-41.
53. Wu F, Wang ZB, Chen WZ, Zhu H, Bai J, Zou JZ, et al. Extracorporeal high intensity focused ultrasound ablation in the treatment of patients with large hepatocellular carcinoma. Ann Surg Oncol. 2004;11(12):1061-9.
54. Dubinsky TJ, Cuevas C, Dighe MK, Kolokythas O, Hwang JH. High-intensity focused ultrasound: current potential and oncologic applications. AJR Am J Roentgenol. 2008;190(1):191-9.
55. Kaneko OF, Willmann JK. Ultrasound for molecular imaging and therapy in cancer. Quant Imaging Med Surg. 2012;2(2):87-97.
56. Kircher MF, Willmann JK. Molecular body imaging: MR imaging, CT, and US. Part II. Applications. Radiology. 2012;264(2):349-68.
57. Feldman MK, Katyal S, Blackwood MS. US artifacts. Radiographics. 2009;29(4):1179-89.
58. Burckhardt CB. Speckle in ultrasound B-Mode scans, IEEE Trans. Sonics Ultrasonics, SU-25; 1978.pp.1-6.
59. Chen Y, Broschat SL, Flynn PJ. Phase Insensitive Homomorphic Image Processing for Speckle Reduction Ultrasonic Imaging. 1996;18:122-39.
60. Bushberg JT, Seibert JA, Leidholdt EM, Boone JM. The essential physics of medical imaging. 2nd Edn. Philadelphia, Pa: Lippincott Williams & Wilkins; 2002.pp. 469-553.
61. Laing FC, Kurtz AB. The importance of ultrasonic side-lobe artifacts. Radiology. 1982;145(3):763-8.

CHAPTER

29

Image Optimization in Ultrasound

Rashmi Dixit, Anju Garg, Alpana Manchanda, Anjali Prakash

Ultrasound imaging with its inherent flexibility, low cost and real time display plays a vital role in diagnostics. Image formation in ultrasound depends on the physics behind ultrasound pulse formation, transmission and interaction with tissues. Acoustic energy undergoes essentially three different types of interactions in the tissues-reflection (specular and diffuse), refraction, and attenuation.

Diagnostic applications of ultrasound are based on detection and display of acoustic energy reflected from interfaces within the body. The amplitude of the reflected energy is used to generate ultrasound images while frequency shifts in backscattered ultrasound provide information relating to moving targets such as blood. Real time, grayscale, B-mode display, in which variations in display intensity or brightness are used to show signals of differing amplitude, is the mainstay of ultrasound imaging. Real time ultrasound produces an impression of motion by generating a series of 2D images several times per second or frames per second.

The *quality of an ultrasound image*[1-3] depends on its spatial resolution, temporal resolution, contrast resolution and freedom from certain artifacts. **Spatial resolution** has three components *axial, lateral and elevational or azimuthal resolution. Axial resolution* is the resolution along the axis of the ultrasound beam. It is also called longitudinal or depth resolution and depends on spatial pulse length, which is the product of wavelength and number of pulses, being equal to half the spatial pulse length. As frequency increases the pulse length decreases permitting resolution of smaller details. Hence, axial resolution improves with increasing frequency (which reduces wavelength). Best axial resolution at a frequency of 3.5 MHz is approximately 0.5–1.0 mm. It does not change significantly with depth. *Lateral resolution* refers to the ability to differentiate two structures lying side by side. The width of the main beam determines the lateral resolution of the ultrasound image as objects can be resolved separately only if the beam is thinner than the distance between them. Hence in modern systems transducers are focused to reduce the beam width. Focal zone is the area where the beam is 3–4 wavelengths wide and the area where lateral resolution is highest, deteriorating rapidly beyond it. The best lateral resolution equals the minimum beam width. Focusing in the elevation plane is also possible with current technology. Importantly ultrasound resolution depends not only on the frequency but also the transducer design.

Temporal resolution refers to the ability to locate the position of a particular moving structure in time. This increases as the frame rate increases. **Contrast resolution** is the ability to show very subtle difference in echo strength. Contrast resolution improves when a system can recognize and store a wide range of echo amplitudes.

New technical developments and remarkable improvement in image quality have marked several new applications for diagnostic ultrasound. The rise of state of the art, expensive equipment has greatly eased the sonologist's job. Nonetheless, it does not by itself guarantee high quality ultrasound images. Variables, many of which are under direct user control must be managed to guarantee the production of quality studies. An accurate ultrasound diagnosis relies heavily on the experience and skill of the examiner and requires adjustment of the equipment settings from patient to patient and organ to organ. Hence, image optimization is an essential prerequisite for diagnostic ultrasound imaging.

GRAYSCALE IMAGING

Basic Guidelines[2-5]

The patient should be positioned in such a way that the area of interest can be easily accessed and the patient is comfortable during the examination. Changing the patient position to better elucidate pathology is also important, e.g. an extended neck for thyroid examination, left lateral decubitus position for gallbladder calculi, etc.

A good acoustic window improves scanning accuracy and image quality. Solid organs like the liver or spleen or fluid filled structures, which do not attenuate the sound beam, e.g. full bladder or fluid filled stomach provide a good acoustic window to see deeper structures. Use of adequate amount of coupling gel is essential as air has high acoustic impedance.

USER ADJUSTABLE PARAMETERS

Factory Presets

The more complicated machine settings are saved as presets. Presets provide a useful starting point, however, these are settings which are optimized for patients of average body habitus and further optimization of the image by manual adjustments is invariably required in order to increase diagnostic confidence and avoid artifacts. A single touch image optimization is also available on some systems however this only resets the parameters to the chosen preset.

Transducer Selection

Choosing the appropriate transducer both in terms of frequency as well as footprint is extremely important for a good examination. Higher frequencies provide a better resolution but are attenuated much more as attenuation is proportional to the fourth power of frequency. Thus a trade off has to be made between the need for penetration and resolution.

While performing superficial scans as for the thyroid, musculoskeletal system or testicular examination a linear transducer with a high frequency (7-10 MHz or even 15-17 MHz) is suitable but for deeper structures a lower frequency such as 2.5-3 MHz is used. Currently many multifrequency and broad band width transducers are available. For intercostal scanning or scanning the neonatal brain, transducers with a smaller footprint which fit into the small acoustic window are appropriate **(Figs. 1A and B)**. Sector transducers are thus useful to evaluate deeper structures through a small acoustic window, e.g. echocardiography. In sector scanning, however, resolution becomes poorer with increasing depth as the same echo lines are spread out over a wider area deeper in the tissue.

Overall Gain

Overall gain amplifies all the returning echoes/signals uniformly. An excessively high gain can result in a washed out image and can obscure many details.

Time Gain Compensation

Time gain compensation (TGC) is also referred to as distance gain compensation (DGC) or spatial time compensation (STC). Signals that arrive later, i.e. from greater depths, are amplified more than earlier signals to compensate for the attenuating effect of tissues. TGC controls permit the user to selectively amplify the signals from deeper structures or suppress signals from superficial tissues so that a smooth grayscale picture can be obtained **(Figs. 2A and B)**. Although most newer machines provide for some automatic TGC, manual adjustment by the user is one of the most important factors affecting image quality.

Depth Setting

This parameter selects the depth of the imaging field. If too much depth is selected the image will be small and the area of interest difficult to visualize, measurements may also be inaccurate. On the other hand, if the depth setting is too shallow the complete region or organ is not visualized and pathology at a deeper levels may be completely missed **(Figs. 3A and B)**. Practically, depth can be adjusted by starting at a higher depth, subsequently depths should be decreased so

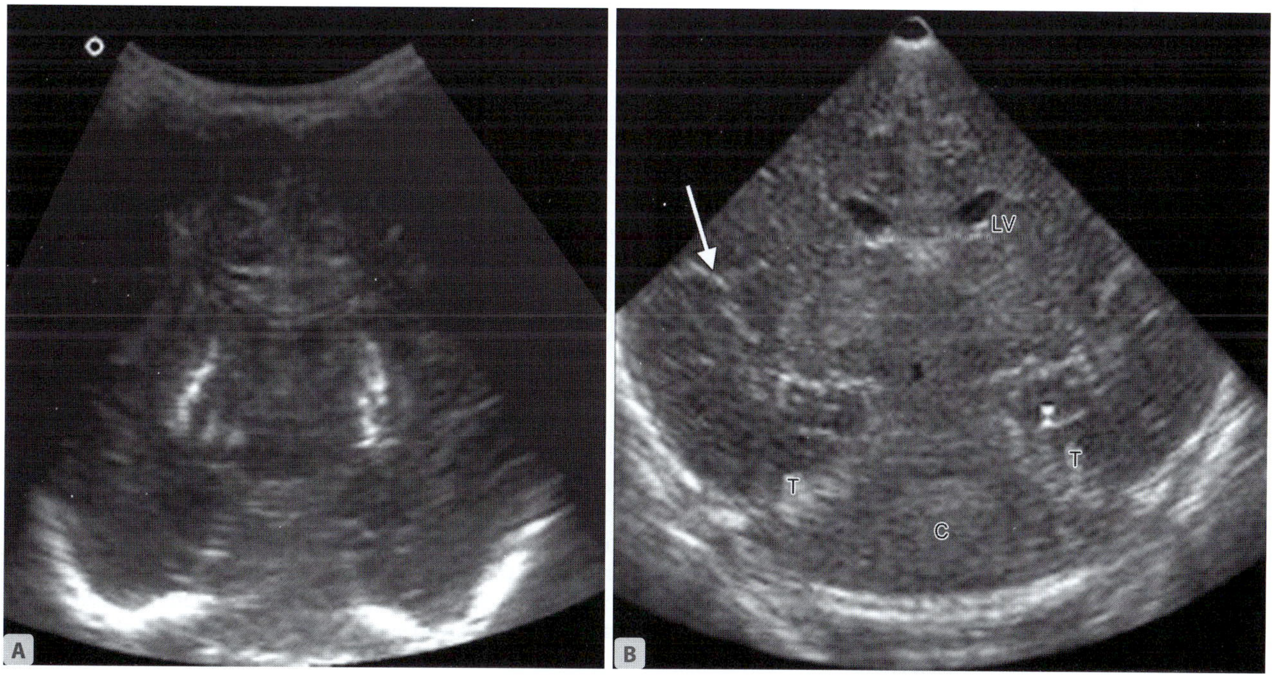

FIGS. 1A AND B: Cranial sonogram performed with a curvilinear array abdominal probe (A) shows shadowing obscuring the cerebral convexities on both sides due to mismatch between the large transducer footprint and acoustic window. The second scan (B) performed with a small foot print transducer shows good visualization of cerebral convexities. Arrow – sylvian fissure, T-tentorium, C-cerebellum.

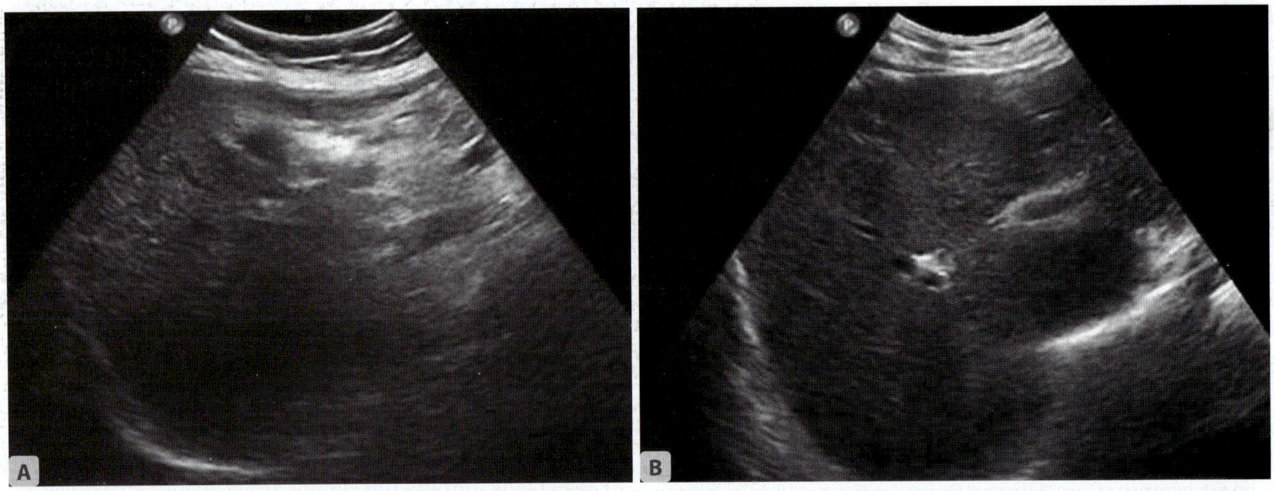

FIGS. 2A AND B: Improper TGC setting resulting in a dark band over the deep aspect of the liver (A). With the correct TGC setting the whole liver shows a uniform echopattern (B).

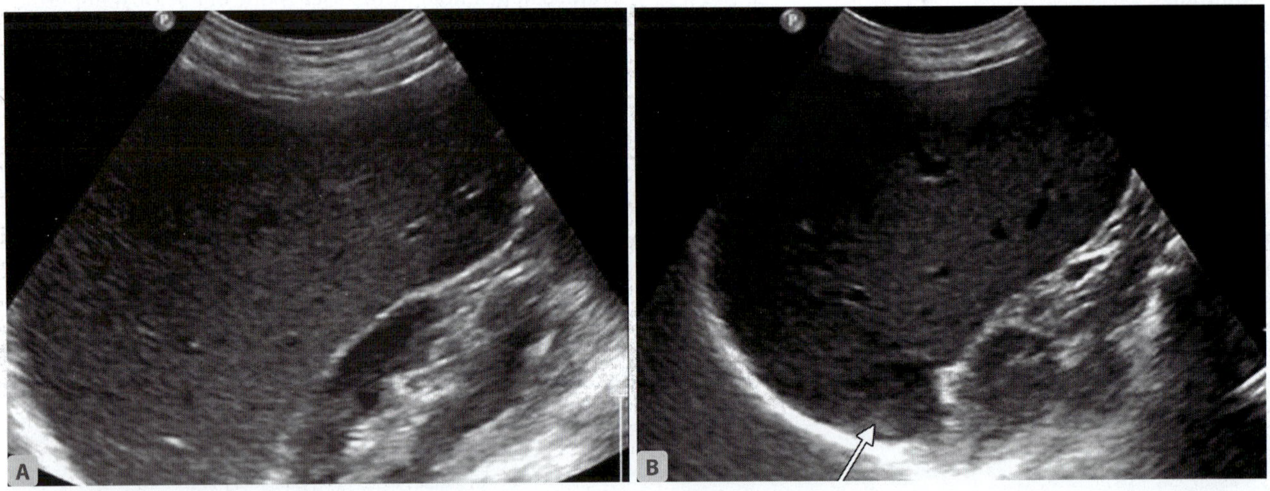

FIGS. 3A AND B: Improper depth setting in (A) results in non-visualization of posterior most portion of liver with consequently missed metastatic focus, which is easily appreciated (arrow) with proper depth setting in (B).

that the area of interest in at about three-fourths the depth of the screen. A small area should be available behind the area of interest to detect useful artifacts.

Focal Zone Setting

To improve resolution diagnostic transducers are focused electronically. As already discussed, resolution of ultrasound is best in the focal zone. The focal zone should thus be set over the area of interest. A significant difference in image resolution depending on the focal zone setting is the hallmark of a well-focused beam **(Figs. 4A and B)**. Modern scanners allow the use of multiple focal zones however this may result in decreased frame rate and hence decreased temporal resolution.

Zoom

Zoom is used to magnify the area of interest. Zoom is extremely useful for accurate measurement of small structures as the CBD.

There are two types of zoom available. *Read zoom* is used to enlarge a frozen image whereas *write zoom* is used to enlarge the display magnification, during scanning.

In *read zoom*, gray level values are read only from a small part of the computer memory and the pixels are enlarged while displaying, something like a magnifying glass. If the magnification factor is too large image matrix becomes obvious and renders the image grainy.

In *write zoom*, use is made of the fact that the echo samples are received fast enough for several samples to occur

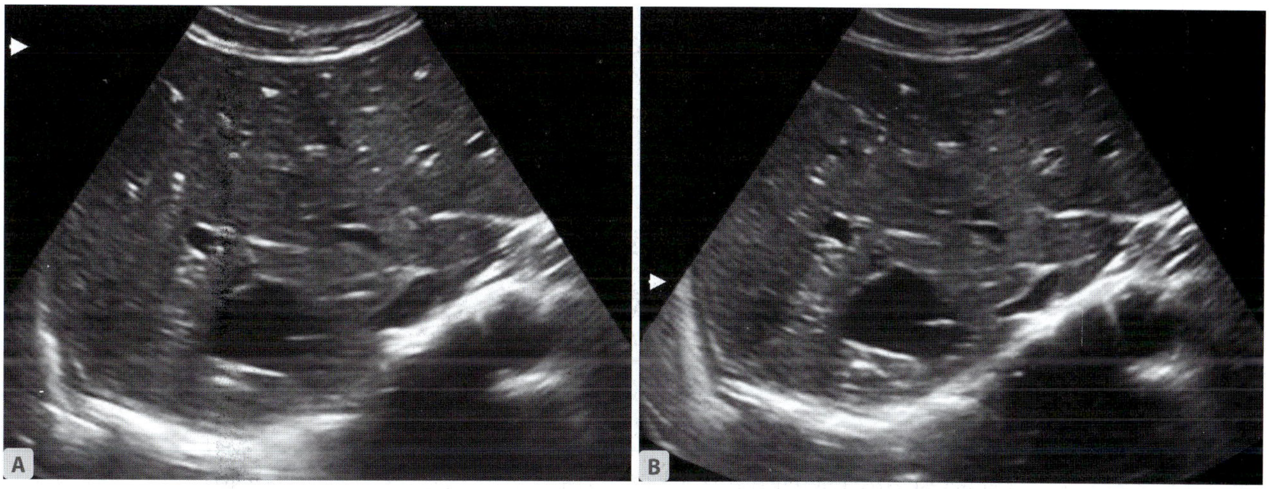

FIGS. 4A AND B: Effect of focal zone: In (A) the focal zone (denoted by the small arrowhead) is placed anteriorly resulting in a blurred appearance of the posteriorly placed hepatic cyst and diaphragm. These become more sharply defined with proper focal zone positioning over the area of interest (B).

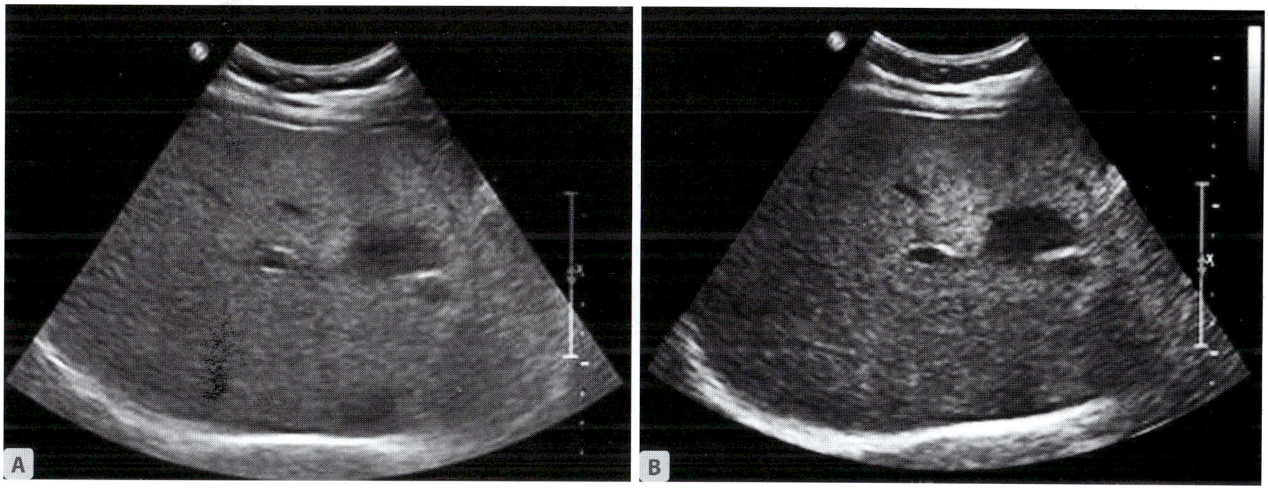

FIGS. 5A AND B: Images of the liver displayed at dynamic ranges of 70 and 36 dB are shown. The wide dynamic range (A) permits appreciation of subtle differences in echointensity between the diffusely fatty liver and a focal area of sparing. The narrow range (B) increases the conspicuity of larger echo differences with the area of focal sparing appearing darker and the diaphragm brighter than the wide dynamic range image.

in each pixel. In this situation, the image scale can be enlarged to a point where only one sample occurs in each pixel. Each pixel, whose size remains unchanged, displays less tissue. Thus, there is magnification without loss of definition. Hence one should always try to use the *write zoom*. If the scale is increased further there is a larger space between scan lines so that further interpolation and smoothening may be required to maintain an acceptable image. More real scan lines can be introduced using sophisticated signal processing so that definition is improved. One such option is referred to as high density (HD) zoom. This magnifies the region of interest while increasing line density by redistributing and reformatting all scan lines for the defined region of interest.

Dynamic Range

Dynamic range is the ratio of the highest to the lowest amplitudes that can be displayed, expressed in decibels. Dynamic range adjustment changes the contrast. The widest dynamic range that permits accurate differentiation of minor differences in echo intensity is preferred for the most applications. The narrower ranges increase the conspicuity of larger echo differences **(Figs. 5A and B)**.

ARTIFACTS IN B MODE IMAGING[3,5-7]

Artifact is a term used to describe any unwanted information generated in the process of image formation. Most artifacts interfere with image interpretation while some artifacts which contain diagnostic information are referred to as friendly artifacts.

A number of artifacts may occur during scanning. Understanding how and why a particular artifact occurs is imperative to eliminate it and avoid errors in diagnosis **(Table 1)**.

TABLE 1: Common ultrasound artifacts.

Artifact	Cause	Appearance	Correction technique/Reduction
Beam width	Poor lateral resolution due to wide beam	Lateral blurring of tiny objects, aberrant echoes from adjacent highly echogenic structures	Focal Zone (FZ) placement
Section thickness	Poor elevational resolution (beam thickness > section thickness)	Debris/internal echoes in anechoic structures, vessels	Positioning the area of interest in FZ 1.5D/2D transducer arrays allowing focusing in elevational plane
Secondary lobe Side lobes Grating lobes	Strong echoes from off axis primary beam are reflected back to transducer	Mimics debris in anechoic structures	Using tissue harmonics, decreasing gain, changing angle of insonation using multiple windows
Speckle noise	Acoustic interference causing granular appearance	Gives tissues their characteristic image texture however degrades spatial and contrast resolution	Can be reduced by SRI, SCI, THI
Reverberation	Reflections between highly reflective interfaces in parallel	Multiple bright parallel lines, mimic debris in cystic structures	Use of THI, decreasing gain, using a different window/angle of insonation
Comet tail	Reverberations from very closely placed highly reflective interfaces	Inverted echogenic triangle seen posterior to adenomyomatosis, colloid nodules, calcifications, foreign bodies	Using SCI
Ring down	Resonant vibrations in tiny air bubbles	Streak or parallel bands deep to a focus of gas Dirty shadowing	Using SCI
Mirror image	Reflections off a strong specular reflector produce a mirror image of an object	Mimics consolidated lung above diaphragm , pseudothickened bowel wall	May be reduced by decreasing gain, using a different window/angle of insonation
Speed displacement artifact	Variability of speed of sound among different tissues	Inaccurate locations and measurements of structures	Some modern US units permit manual speed of sound correction
Increased through transmission	Overcorrection of sound attenuation posterior to low attenuation structures	Increased brightness of echoes distal to a low-attenuating structure	Using SCI
Acoustic shadowing	Undercorrection of sound attenuation posterior to high attenuation structures	Decrease in echo strength distal to a highly attenuating or reflective object	Reduction with inappropriate FZ placement, and SCI

SRI: speckle reduction imaging techniques; SCI: spatial compound imaging; THI: tissue harmonic imaging.

The ultrasound machine depends on physical assumptions to determine the location and intensity of each received echo. The assumptions are:

- The echo detected arose from within the main US beam
- It has returned to the transducer after a single reflection
- The depth on an object is related only to the time taken by an ultrasound pulse to return as an echo to the transducer.
- Sound travels at a constant speed and in a straight line in human tissue
- The acoustic energy in an ultrasound field is uniformly attenuated.

While examining patients using ultrasound, these assumptions are often not maintained resulting in artifacts.

Artifacts due to Physical Characteristics of Ultrasound Beam

Beam Width Artifact

The real ultrasound beam is not of a consistently narrow, laser-like configuration which would be ideal for image resolution. A typical focused beam is of the same width as the transducer when it exits the transducer, gradually narrowing to a focus after which it spreads out rapidly in the far field, where it may be wider than the transducer width. A highly reflective object situated within the widened beam beyond the transducer edges may produce detectable echoes. The system assumes that these echoes arose from within the imaging plane and displays them accordingly **(Fig. 6)**. The more intense the reflection the further off axis its echoes will be received.

During scanning this artifact is recognized when a structure which should be anechoic has peripheral echoes. It is generally most obvious when a bony or gaseous object lies adjacent to a fluid collection **(Fig. 7)**.

This also means that a strong reflector will continue to give detectable echoes further from the central axis than a weak reflector. Hence, the resolution is better for weak reflectors than strong reflectors which tend to blur laterally and are therefore seen as cigar shaped smears or streaks so that the width is exaggerated. It also results in a tendency to fill in small anechoic regions, such as ducts producing slightly reduced measurements.

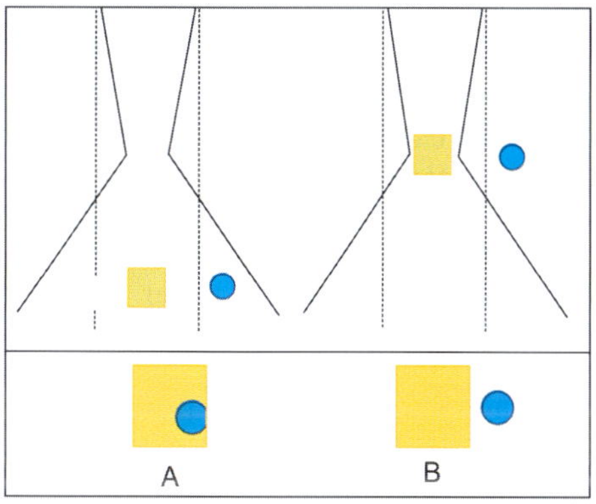

FIG. 6: Mechanism of beam width artifact. Dotted lines represent the imaging plane. Echoes from the circle are assumed to arise from within the imaging plane in A and displayed within the square. This is rectified with proper focal zone setting in B.

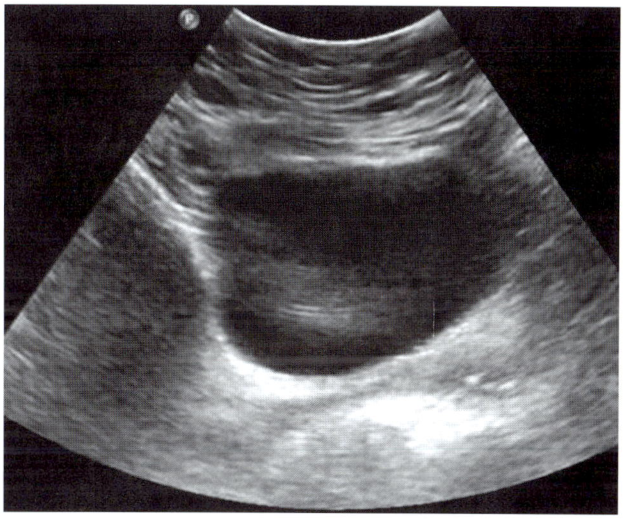

FIG. 7: Beam width artifact: strong echoes arising from a gas filled bowel loop in the pelvis smear across the bladder.

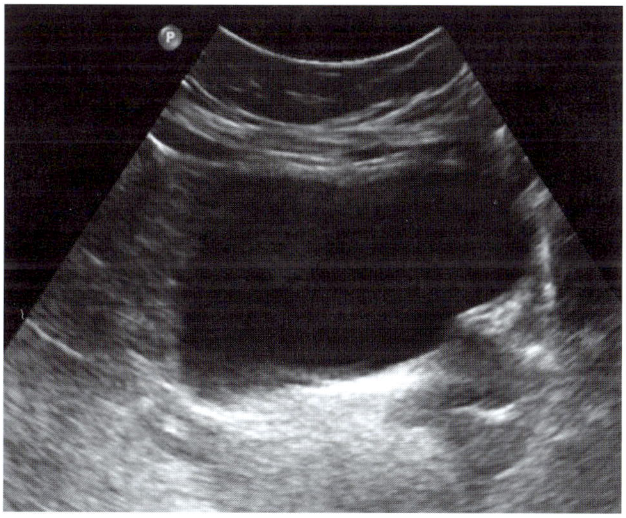

FIG. 8: Low level echoes are seen in the bladder not from debris but due to slice thickness artifact arising from gas present in the bowel in the adjacent planes.

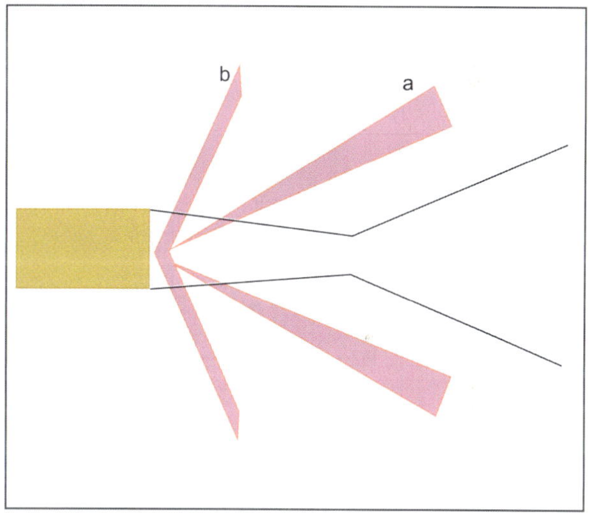

FIG. 9: Off axis beams: side lobes (a) and grating lobes (b).

This can be rectified and image quality improved by adjusting the focal zone to the area of interest and placing the transducer over the center of the object of interest.

Slice Thickness Artifact

Beam width artifacts also occur in the orthogonal plane, i.e. in the slice thickness or elevation plane. With circular transducers, either simple disc or annular array types, the beam is symmetrical in all planes but for linear and phased array transducers the beam is wider in the orthogonal plane resulting in information from adjacent planes being depicted in the image.

The beam width may be wider than a fluid collection. Some of the sound energy may hit structures outside the plane of intersection and may be projected into it. This can simulate a layer of sludge causing a simple fluid collection to appear complicated **(Fig. 8)**. Since the reflector which has caused the artifact is not visualized in the image it is more difficult to recognize it as artifactual than the same artifact occurring in the scanned plane. However, with the latest 2 D and X-matrix transducers it is possible to focus the beam in the elevation plane as well, providing a uniformly focused ultrasound beam.

Side Lobe and Grating Lobe Artifacts

These are low energy beams directed at angles away from the central line due to vibration of the edges of the transducer. The latter occur only in array transducers **(Fig. 9)**.

Highly reflective objects located in the path of these low intensity off axis beams may generate echoes detectable by the transducer. These are displayed as having originated from within the main beam usually within an anechoic structure.

They often have a convex shape and are also referred to as *Chinese hat artifacts.*

Artifacts Associated with Multiple Echoes

Reverberation Bands

A very important assumption in pulse echo ultrasound imaging is that an echo returns to the transducer after a single reflection and that the depth is related to the time taken for the echo to return. If two highly reflective surfaces lie parallel to each other, the echoes generated may be reflected back and forth before they reach the transducer. The first echo returning after a single reflection is displayed in its proper position. The later echoes returning after multiple reflections are presumed to be arising deeper to the original structure (due to the delay) and are displayed as equally spaced linear reflections in a striped pattern called *reverberation artifact* **(Figs. 10 and 11)**. The deeper echoes are weaker than the superficial ones due to loss of sound energy due to attenuation by intervening tissues and incomplete reflection so that the bands become narrower and less intense with depth.

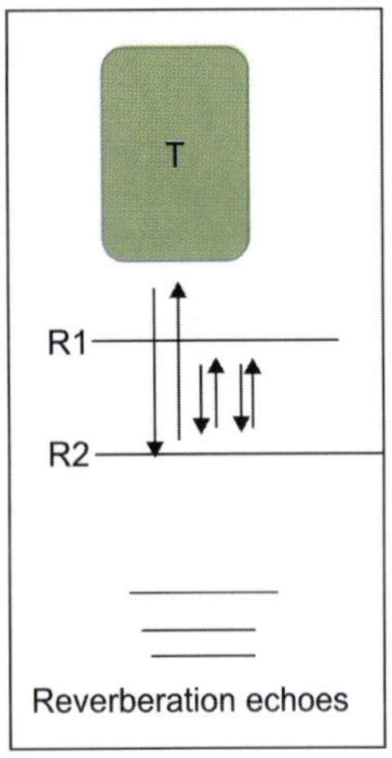

FIG. 10: Mechanism of reverberation artifact: T transducer, R1 R2 reflecting surfaces.

The distance between the reverberation bands depends on the gap between the reflectors, if the reflectors are very closely placed the sequential echoes may be so close that individual bands cannot be seen. The resulting artifact is triangular with a tapered shape resembling a comet with its bright tail hence referred to as a *comet tail artifact.* This artifact is commonly seen deep to calcifications, surgical clips, IUCD and in colloid cysts of goiter. The artifact is also diagnostic of adenomyosis of gallbladder. It is presumed that the many small fluid spaces like the Aschoff-Rokitansky sinuses in gallbladder wall in this pathology cause repeated reflections from the walls of the fluid spaces producing the comet tail artifact **(Fig. 12)**.

Another artifact, the *ring down* artifact was previously thought to be a variant of comet tail artifact because of the similar appearance of the two, however, this has a separate mechanism. The ultrasound energy is believed to cause vibrations in fluid trapped between air bubbles. These vibrations produce a continuous sound wave that is transmitted back to the receiver. This is seen as a line or series of parallel bands extending posterior to a gas collection. Ring-down artifact contributes to the occurrence of "dirty shadowing" **(Fig. 13)**. This artifact may suggest underlying pathology, such as pneumoperitoneum, portal venous gas and emphysematous (gas-forming) infections. Ring-down artifacts (B-lines) have been used in lung US for the diagnosis of interstitial conditions.

Mirror Image Artifact

This artifact is also generated by a repeat echo. It is sometimes also referred to as a multipath artifact. When the ultrasound beam encounters a highly reflective surface. The reflected echoes then reach the target on their way back and are again reflected back towards the reflective interface before being reflected to the transducer, where they are detected. This causes a delay in the return of echoes to the transducer thus the display shows a replicated structure equidistant but deep to the strongly reflective interface **(Fig. 14A)**. This artifact is commonly seen at the diaphragm with the air-pleural interface acting as a strong reflector. It is recognized

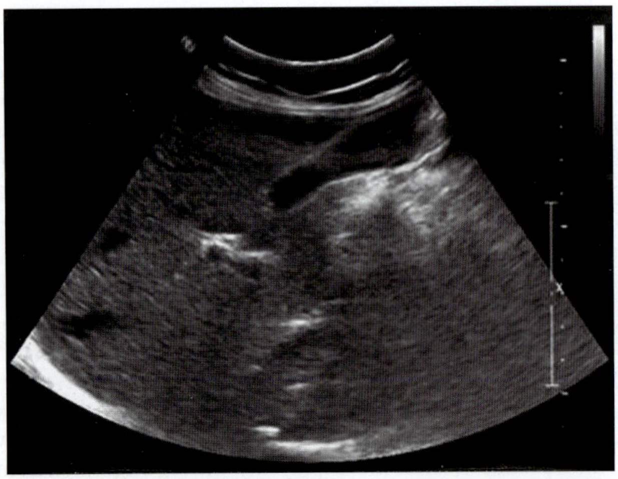

FIG. 11: Multiple equally spaced lines are seen within the gallbladder due to multiple reflections originating in the anterior abdominal wall.

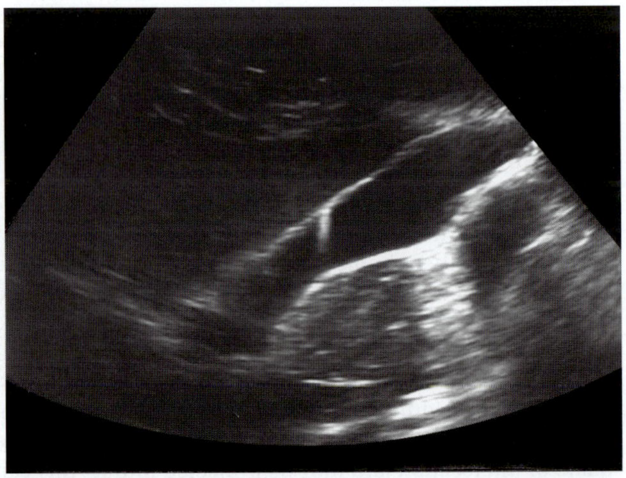

FIG. 12: Adenomyosis of the anterior wall of gallbladder producing a typical comet tail artifact.

as hepatic parenchyma seen in the expected position of the lung which should not be mistaken for consolidated lung **(Fig. 14B)**. There may also be apparent duplication of a focal hepatic lesion **(Fig. 15)**.

At this level it generally does not cause any diagnostic problem, in fact may be useful, e.g. increased through transmission behind a peripheral cyst may be seen in the mirror image which would otherwise be obscured by the hyperechoic reflection of air in the lung. However, mirror image artifact may result in pseudothickened bowel wall due to gas acting as a specular reflector. It can also produce a pelvic pseudomass at times.

Artifacts Associated with Velocity Errors

An important assumption in ultrasound imaging is that the speed of US in soft tissues is constant (1540 m/s). This is not an absolute truth in clinical sonography. Fat, for example conducts sound about 15 percent slower than most other soft tissues **(Table 2)**.

When sound travels through a tissue with a velocity significantly lower than the assumed constant of 1540 m/sec the returning echo takes longer to return to the transducer. Scanners use the amount of delay to calculate the depth of the echo (0.13 microsecond delay corresponding to ~1 cm depth on final image). The processor presumes that the delay is due to increased distance traveled by the echo and thus the object is displayed deeper on the image than it actually is. This is called *speed displacement artifact* or *propagation velocity artifact*. This geometric distortion does not affect the lateral dimension of the image as this is determined by the scanning action of the transducer rather than by the speed of sound but axial dimension may be affected. In clinical practice, this artifact is most commonly seen when an area of focal fat is encountered, e.g. areas of focal fat in the subdiaphragmatic region of the liver can result in a discontinuous appearance of

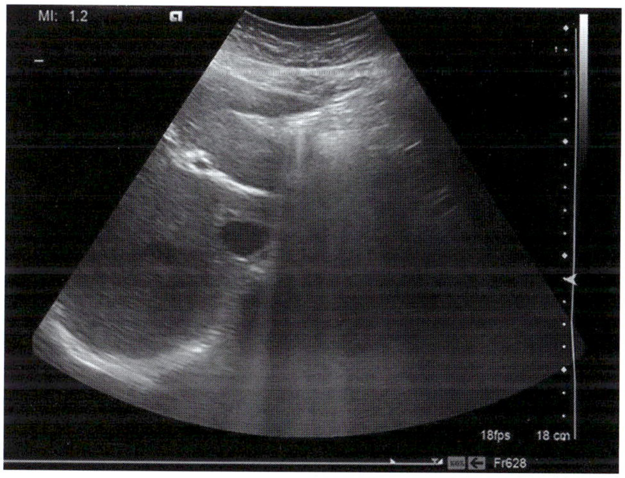

FIG. 13: Ring down artifact from the duodenum.

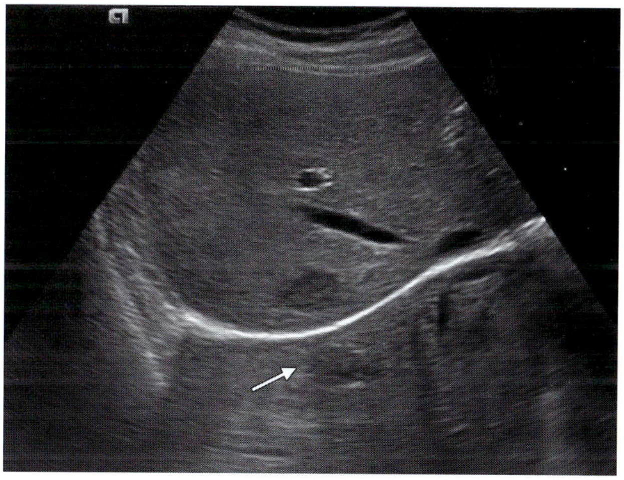

FIG. 15: Mirror image of a focal hepatic lesion seen behind the diaphragm (arrow).

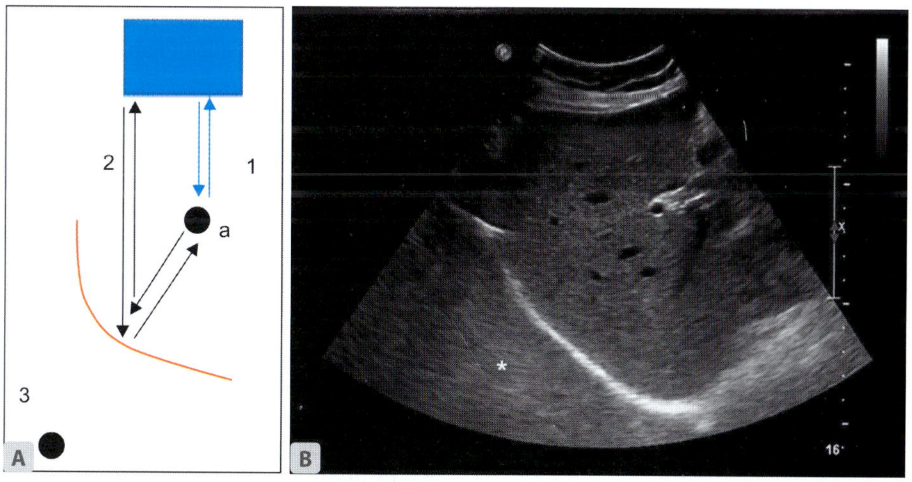

FIGS. 14A AND B: (A) Mirror image artifact due to a strong specular reflector: Without reflection (blue arrows) the beam directly encounters the target and it is appropriately imaged in the correct location. When the transmitted ultrasound beam (black arrows) reflects off the specular reflector (curved red line) and reaches the target (black circle (a), from where it is reflected back along its transmitted course and then to the transducer, because of the delay in the returning echo, the image (circle 3) appears to be deep to the reflector but at the same distance. The result is a mirror image appearance across the specular reflector; (B) Mirror reflection of the liver is seen above the diaphragm in this patient (asterix).

TABLE 2: Velocity of ultrasound in biological materials.[3]

Tissue	Velocity (m/s)
Air	330
Fat	1450
Water	1480
Brain	1565
Muscle	1580
Liver	1600
Lens of eye	1650
Soft tissue average	1540

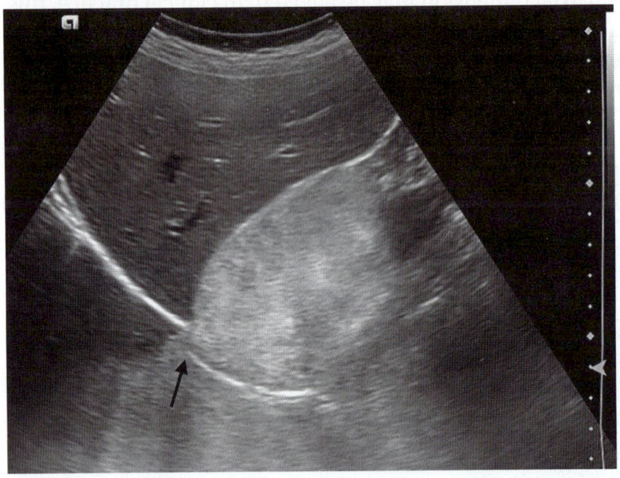

FIG. 16: Discontinuous appearance of the diaphragm (arrow) due to speed displacement artifact caused by fat in an adrenal myelolipoma.

the diaphragm because of fallacious posterior displacement of diaphragmatic segments behind the fatty change **(Fig. 16)**. Usually, imaging through tissues that differ significantly from the assumed velocity gives rise to misregistration of targets. When imaging targets through a uniform layer of fat, such as a large amount of subcutaneous fat or breast tissue, boundary distortion does not occur but the depth of all targets will be overestimated. Although minor differences in size or location are not generally important in image interpretation and may in fact provide diagnostic clues to the presence of fat within lesions, they may be important in applications such as US-guided interventions and radiation therapy, where small differences in size or location are critical.

In ophthalmic ultrasound too, where great accuracy is required distortion caused by the higher velocity in the lens can be important. The speed of sound in the lens of the eye is 1620 m/s (vs 1540 of average soft tissues) so portions of the retina imaged through the lens appear nearer than the portions imaged through the sclera producing a shelf-like anterior distortion called *Baum's bumps*.

Refractory Errors

Differences in velocity between tissues also produce refractory errors. When an obliquely incident ultrasound beam encounters an interface between two substances with different speeds of sound, it changes direction. The degree of this change and the direction depends both on the angle of incidence and the difference in velocity between the two media. If the incident beam is at 90° to the interface, no refraction will occur. The scanner working on the assumption that the US beam travels in a straight line misplaces the echoes to the side of their true location. This situation may become important clinically during transabdominal pelvic scans due to refraction occurring deep to the junction of medial margin of rectus abdominis muscle and fat in the midline. This can cause misregistration of targets and lateral stretching of pelvic structures and obstetric measurements made under these conditions may be erroneous. In more extreme cases, it may cause apparent duplication of structures, the so called ghosting. Repositioning the transducer eliminates this artifact.

TABLE 3: Attenuation coefficients for selected tissues.[6]

Material	Attenuation coefficient (dB/cm)
Water	0.0002
Soft tissue	0.3–0.8
Lipid	0.5–1.8
Osseous	13–26
Air	40

Attenuation Errors

As an ultrasound beam traverses through the tissues its energy gets attenuated due to combined effect of absorption, scattering and reflection. The greater distance the ultrasound beam travels through the tissues the more the attenuation for a beam of similar energy. To compensate for this attenuation, machines incorporate a processing technique for compensatory amplification of echoes that take longer to return i.e. arising in the deeper tissues. Attenuation also varies with different tissues depending on the attenuation coefficient which measures the loss of ultrasound intensity per unit distance travelled **(Table 3)**.

Acoustic Shadowing

Acoustic shadowing implies reduction in the strength of echoes distal to a markedly attenuating or reflective object. When the ultrasound beam traverses a tissue that attenuates sound more than the majority of the tissue in the beam, shadowing occurs. This is because the gain compensation is only set to a standard value, thus an inadequate correction will be applied to this region. Both this region and tissues deeper to it, are depicted as less echogenic than they actually are. This is visible as a dark band called an acoustic or distal shadow **(Fig. 17)**. Shadowing can also be caused by highly efficient reflectors such as gas bubbles or calcification where 99% and 80% of the incident sound beam, respectively, is reflected back. This is because very little of the sound energy passes through to insonate deeper tissues, also, any echoes from the deeper structures are unlikely to cross the reflective layer as they return, since they would be re-reflected distally.

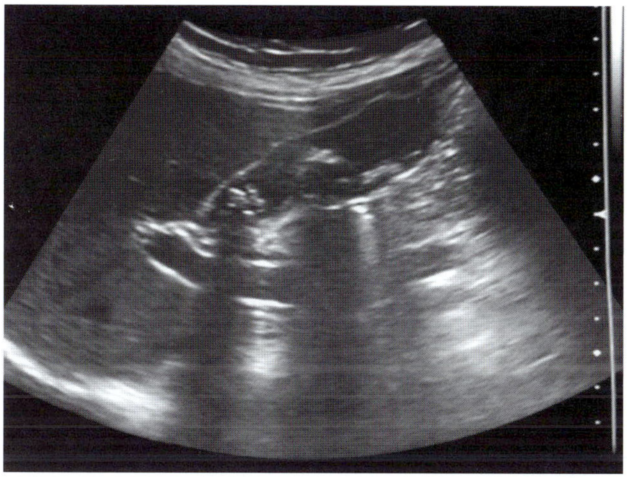

FIG. 17: Acoustic shadows: Seen as dark bands posterior to multiple gallbladder calculi.

Shadowing can be of diagnostic significance and, is usually seen with calculi, calcifications, bone, and gas, and appears as clean, partial, or dirty shadowing Clean shadowing usually occurs posterior to large calculi and bone and is seen as a dark anechoic band. Partial shadowing is visualized as a hypoechoic band and occurs posterior to highly attenuating tissues, like fat, or small stones, especially when the width of the beam is greater than the size of the calculus. Dirty shadowing is seen distal to a highly reflecting surface like gas, where multiple secondary reflections cause low-level echoes within the shadow, appearing similar to ring-down artifact. Incorrect focal zone placement, large beam widths, and spatial compound imaging decrease shadowing thus it is important to turn off spatial compounding when imaging calculi. On the other hand imaging with higher frequency probes and using tissue harmonics increase shadowing.

Edge Shadowing

Shadowing is also sometime seen deep to the edges of strongly curved surfaces, such as cyst walls, fetal skull and vessels. Fine dark lines can be seen extending deep to such edges and become even more striking in the case of a cyst due to the increased through transmission posterior to the cyst itself.

Two explanations have been offered for this: *refraction* of the ultrasound beam as it strikes a curved surface and *increased attenuation* at the edges because the ultrasound beam passing through the edge travels a larger distance through the cyst wall than that passing through the diameter of the cyst. Since, the cyst wall is presumed to be more attenuating than the surrounding tissues, the beam is attenuated more resulting in shadowing. Although acoustic shadows have diagnostic significance and are useful for diagnosis of calcification or calculi, edge shadows do not have this significance **(Figs. 18A and B)**. Edge shadowing frequently occurs in areas where shadowing may erroneously suggest calcification, e.g. vessel walls within renal sinus and Coopers ligaments in the breast. It is important to recognize them as artifactual and dismiss them.

Increased Through Transmission or Distal Bright Up

Attenuation errors also occur if a tissue attenuates less than its surrounding tissues (e.g. a full bladder or a simple cyst). In this situation the echoes from it and the tissues posterior to it are overcorrected appearing as a bright band often termed *'distal enhancement'* however since enhancing effect is also described with ultrasound contrast agents it is probably better referred to as *increased through transmission or distal bright up* **(Fig. 19)**. This artifact can be advantageously employed to diagnose cystic nature of a focal lesion, although some solid lesions such as lymphoma nodes and hepatic hemangiomas can also show posterior acoustic enhancement.

Noise

All imaging systems are prone to two types of noise *random* and *structured.* Electrical components produce random low level voltages which, when amplified, are seen as fluctuating moving grey spots on the image producing a snow storm appearance.

Speckle

Speckle is another source of noise in ultrasound images. Due to the nature of image formation in ultrasound, speckle is an inherent property of ultrasound images. Small tissue reflectors approximately the size of wavelength of sound cause scattering of sound waves which are sent out almost uniformly in all directions. Constructive and destructive interference of these acoustic fields result in speckle. Most biologic tissues appear in US images as though they are filled with tiny scattering structures. Most of the visible signal in US images results from speckle interactions. The interference pattern also gives ultrasound images a characteristic grainy appearance reducing contrast and making identification of subtle features and abnormal tissue patterns more difficult.

Clutter

Clutter results from electrical interference or beamforming artifacts, reverberations, and other acoustic phenomena. Clutter consists of fallacious echoes which can usually be seen in structures of low echogenicity, such as cysts, or amniotic fluid. Finally, another potential source of noise, especially in deep- regions, is thermal noise arising in the electronics of the transducer. All these sources of noise affect the ability to recognize tissue anomalies by interfering with the pattern recognition process in the observer's brain.

Various techniques such as temporal smoothening (i.e. frame averaging or persistence) are used to reduce noise. The real information is reinforced while noise cancels out. In addition a number of special imaging modes are available on high end scanners to deal with these problems which are discussed later.

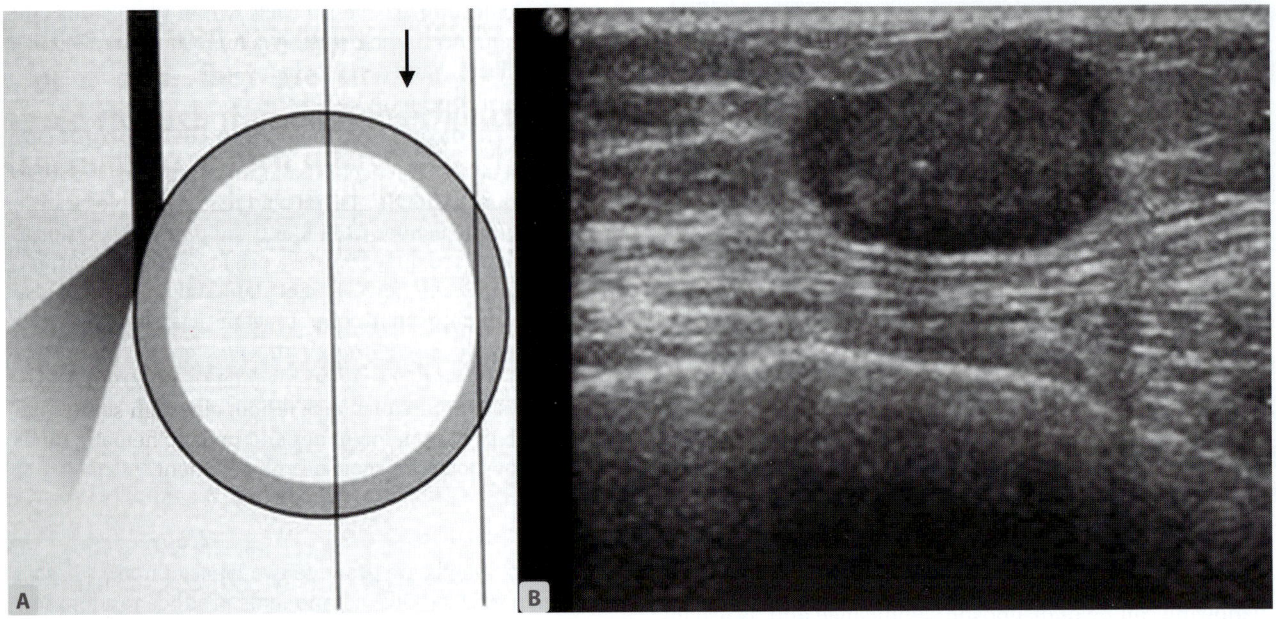

FIGS. 18A AND B: Refractive and attenuation model to explain mechanism of edge shadowing (A). Subtle edge shadowing seen along the edges of fibroadenoma breast (B).

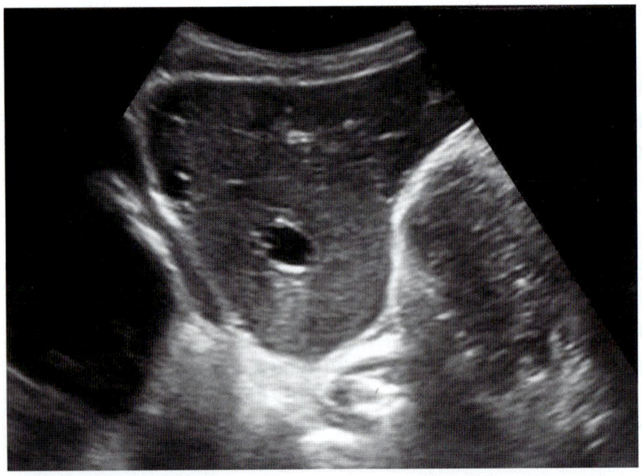

FIG. 19: A bright band is seen posterior to this hepatic cyst—increased through transmission or distal bright-up.

SPECTRAL AND COLOR DOPPLER EXAMINATION

Basic Guidelines[7]

Grayscale settings should always be optimized before color Doppler flow mapping is applied. Fine details such as small plaques or intimal thickening in vessels may be washed over by color if the grayscale image is not evaluated first.

Of the various parameters that can be controlled, the choice of correct transducer frequency is the most important, like in grayscale imaging. This is based on using different transducer frequencies till the best compromise between penetration and signal strength is achieved.

Knowledge of anatomic variants, is very important while scanning for vascular, especially venous disease, for example, failure to recognize duplication of common femoral vein can result in missing the diagnosis of deep venous thrombosis.

It is important to scan the entire length of vessel from its origin to termination when possible. If the ostium of a vessel is not evaluated, lesions at the ostia may be missed, e.g. atherosclerotic plaque commonly involve the origin of carotid and vertebral arteries. In such a situation, the elevated velocities may render evaluation of more distal stenotic lesions by velocity criteria alone difficult. Each vessel must also be examined in two planes, i.e. longitudinal and transverse to avoid missing partially occlusive eccentric thrombi, which may not be centered in the imaging plane in a longitudinal scan alone.

Optimizing Color Doppler and Spectral Doppler Settings[7-11]

Color Box or Color Doppler Sampling Window

The color box is a user adjustable area within the ultrasound image in which all color Doppler information is displayed. The angle of incidence of the color box can be changed by angling the color box to the 'right' or 'left' so called 'steering' or by angling the transducer. As the width and depth of color box increase frame rate decreases, image resolution and quality are affected. Thus, the box should be as small and superficial as possible while still providing the necessary information. This will maximize the frame rate. The frame rate refers to the rate at which complete images are produced and it affects the temporal resolution. With grayscale imaging alone the frame rate may be over 50 frames per second but the time required to produce color images is much more. The frame rate in color imaging is dependent on several factors. With increasing width of the color box more scan lines are required and it takes longer to acquire data to produce the image. Increasing the depth (or height) of the box alone will not produce any major change in the frame rate, increasing the imaging depth however will require a lower pulse repetition frequency or PRF (due to more time for the echo to travel to and fro) hence decreasing the frame rate.

Doppler or Color Gain

Gain refers to amplification of sampled information for purposes of improving the depiction of acquired data. It controls the amplitude of color signal in color or power mode and the amplitude of spectral display in pulsed Doppler mode. If the gain is set too low it is possible that no flow is depicted even when flow is present, on the other hand, an excessively high gain setting produces noise which obscures true Doppler signal and produces filling in of the spectral waveform resulting in little meaningful quantitative flow data.

For spectral Doppler the gain should be adjusted so that the tracing is continuous and easy to visualize without any low level noise band above and below baseline.

For color imaging the color gain should be set as high as possible without displaying random color speckles. This is set by turning the gain up until noise (i.e. scattered isolated color pixels overwriting grayscale pixels) appears and then turning it down until the noise just clears. The color should just reach the intimal surface of the vessel. A high color gain setting may cause bleeding of color or blooming into the wall or even outside the vessel lumen. This impairs visualization of plaques and partial thrombi **(Figs. 20A and B)**.

Velocity Scale

This is one of the most important parameters under user control during a Doppler examination. It determines the range of velocities that are accurately displayed with either the color or spectral Doppler. Pulse repetition frequency or PRF is closely related to the velocity scale hence increasing the velocity scale increases the PRF and vice versa. If the velocity setting is too low for the velocities being examined, the high velocity signals will not be displayed accurately and aliasing results. Aliasing is an incorrect and paradoxical display of the colors or spectral Doppler velocity. This is related to the fact Doppler and color flow utilize pulsed beams which are transmitted and received by the transducer. The number of such pulses sent determines the pulse repetition frequency. If the Doppler shift is higher than PRF/2 or the Nyquist limit then the display wraps around the scale and appears to change direction. For spectral Doppler, the velocity peak is cut-off at the top of the scale and written from the lowest portion of the scale back toward the top. On the color Doppler image aliasing is seen as color change from red to yellow to light blue to dark blue with the reversal being projected within central areas of higher laminar velocity. With aliasing no black border is seen from the low velocity filter between the reversed colors unlike flow reversal **(Figs. 21 and 22)**. Higher velocities require a higher PRF for accurate sampling.

Aliasing is one of the most important artifacts in Doppler. It can be useful to rapidly identify the high velocity region in the vessel and place the sample volume for velocity measurement. However, if the color velocity scale is set much lower than the average velocity of blood flow, aliasing occurs throughout the vessel lumen making it difficult to identify high velocity turbulent jets due to significant stenosis. Tortuosity of a vessel can erroneously produce the appearance of aliasing.

The options available to reduce aliasing are: (a) increasing velocity scale or PRF, (b) increasing the Doppler angle with resultant decrease Doppler shift, (c) changing the baseline (d) using a lower ultrasound frequency. Aliasing is not seen in power Doppler because it has no directional or velocity component.

Gate Size or Sample Volume Box

It is the user defined area, from where the spectral Doppler information is obtained, depicted as a pair of cross hairs within the 2D image. Although on the display it appears like a 2D rectangle, sample volume has a third dimension in and out or perpendicular to the image plane which may be up to a centimeter at times. Hence, signals may be displayed from unwanted areas of vessels or even unwanted vessels. Normally, the gate should cover approximately two-thirds of the vessel lumen **(Figs. 23A and B)**. If the sample volume encompasses the entire vessel slower velocities from the vessel margins are included resulting in spectral widening.

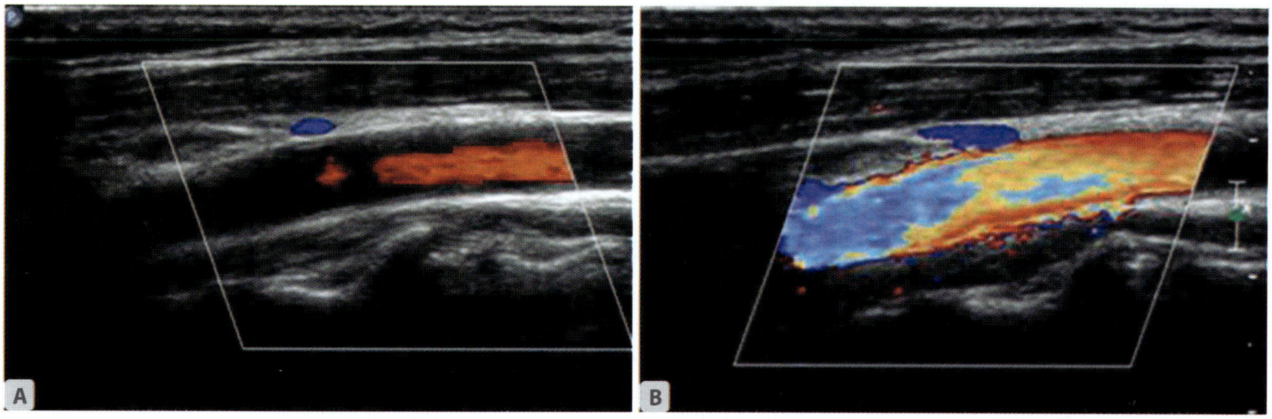

FIGS. 20A AND B: Color Doppler images of the carotid with very low color gain showing incomplete color fill in the carotid (A). Excessively high color gain resulting in bleeding of color into the wall of the carotid and some noise in the surrounding tissues (B).

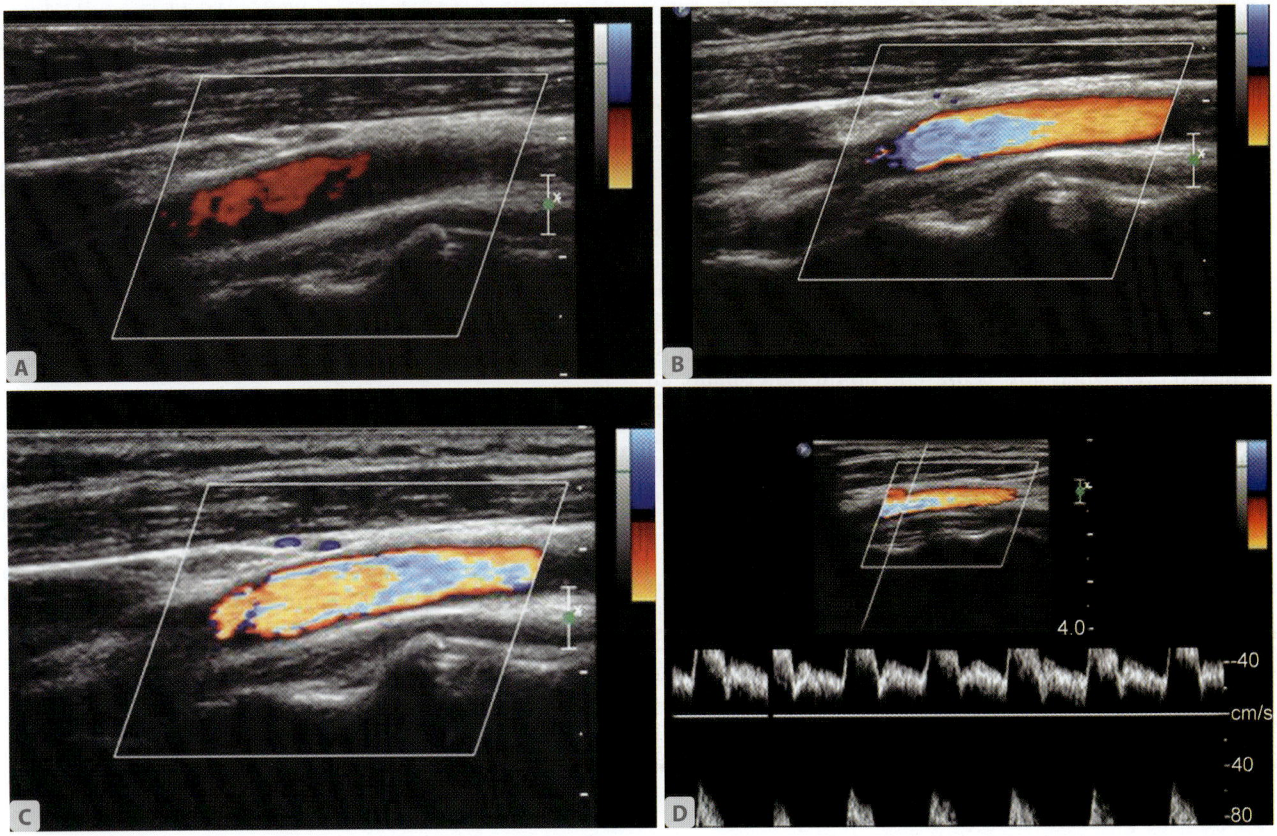

FIGS. 21A TO D: At high PRF settings of 12000 Hz only minimal flow is seen in the carotid artery (A). When the velocity scale is lowered to 4000 Hz complete wall-to-wall color fill is seen with an area of aliasing seen where the artery dips away from the transducer (B). A very low PRF results in aliasing throughout the vessel (C) Aliasing in spectral Doppler with the top of the peak being cut off and written at the bottom (D).

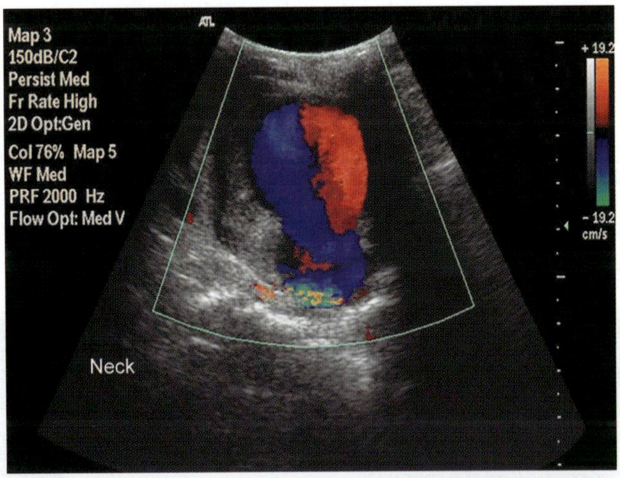

FIG. 22: Flow reversal in a pseudo aneurysm: note the dark boundary between the red and blue colors.

However, if the gate is too small no Doppler signal may be detected resulting in missed flow. In addition, if the vessel is mobile the Doppler trace may be discontinuous with loss of diastolic signal in each cycle. A wider Doppler gate is useful when looking for trickle flow or trying to obtain a Doppler signal from behind a calcified plaque.

Sample Volume or Gate Position

The optimum position of sample volume or range gate in a normal vessel is in the midposition parallel to the wall whereas in a diseased vessel there is some controversy whether the cursor should be angled parallel to the flow or parallel to the vessel wall. Whichever method is used the same technique must be used every time to allow reproducibility and standardization. If the gate is placed eccentrically too close to the vessel wall it will be degraded by signal from vessel wall motion and will also show artificial spectral broadening.

Angle Correction

In vascular applications optimal imaging of the vessel wall is obtained when the transducer is perpendicular to the vessel wall. However, this selection is not suitable for Doppler examination. In diagnostic Doppler imaging the Doppler equation is used to calculate the blood flow velocity, i.e.

$$\Delta f = (2f\,v/c)\cos\theta$$

where

Δf = change in frequency

f = original transmitted frequency

v = velocity of blood flow

c = speed of sound in tissue

θ = angle of insonation.

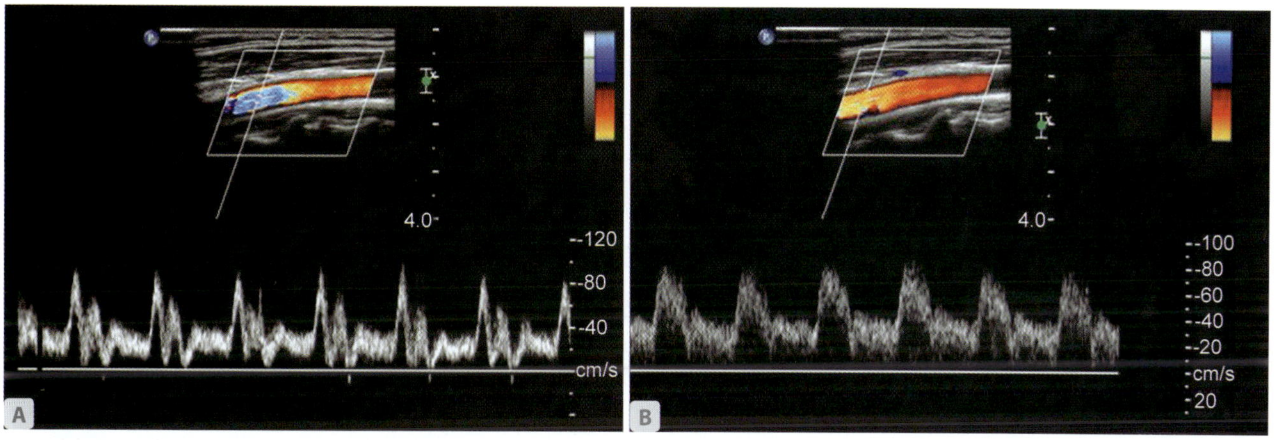

FIGS. 23A AND B: A properly positioned sample volume in the center of the vessel covering almost 2/3rd of vessel lumen results in a spectral trace with a clear window (A). An excessively large sample volume covering the entire vessel lumen results in inclusion of lower flow from the edges with consequent spectral widening (B).

Thus, the angle θ which is the angle between the direction of Doppler insonation pulses and the direction of blood flow affects the frequency shift. The maximum Doppler shift is achieved at a Doppler angle of 0° as cosine of 0° is 1. If the Doppler angle is 90° no Doppler shift will be detected because cosine of 90° is 0. Ideally a small Doppler angle, less than 60° should be used (approximately between 45° and 60°) because within this range a linear relationship exists between Doppler shifts and velocity. The cosine of Doppler angle changes rapidly for angles more than 60° hence a small change in the angle is associated with a large change in the value of Cos θ. Thus a small error in estimation of Doppler angle will result in a large change in the estimated velocity producing unreliable results.

Color Write Priority

Color write priority is a setting closely related to color gain and adjustable as a separate control on some systems. This determines whether a particular pixel is displayed in grayscale or color. While larger vessels require a low setting of color write priority, in small vessels that do not have a resolvable anechoic lumen on grayscale, color information can be suppressed by inappropriate color write priority. In such a situation color is not seen in the image even when the system has detected it. This is of particular importance in areas like the testis where the intratesticular vessels are small and Doppler is an important means of diagnosing torsion.

Baseline

The baseline is seen on both, the color bar and spectral trace. It divides the color bar into positive and negative Doppler shifts. Baseline can be adjusted to emphasize different flow velocities. Although, the overall range of depicted velocities does not change, the depicted flow that is emphasized changes. Adjustment of baseline is one method to prevent aliasing.

Wall Filters

Wall filters selectively filter out all information below a predefined frequency threshold. They are used to eliminate the low frequency-high intensity noise that may arise from vessel wall motion. These are generally preset by the manufacturer as high, medium or low which can be applied separately to spectral, color and power imaging. The aim is to eliminate low frequency noise but if it is set too high it can result in the loss of signal from slow flow. In some arteries, diastolic flow may be eliminated resulting in errors in calculation of Doppler indices, hence it should be kept as low as possible (typically in the range of 50–100 Hz). On the color bar the filter setting is indicated by a black band on both sides of the baseline separating the two colors. Increase in filter settings show up as widening of the black band. On spectral Doppler a high wall filter results in loss of spectral information just above baseline seen as a dark band separating the spectral trace from the baseline. Reducing the wall filter setting results in filling of the dark band with spectral data.

Inversion of Flow

It is possible to invert the depicted direction of flow on both color Doppler and spectral Doppler. This can result in red-blue color inversion on the color Doppler image and inversion of spectral waveform with spectral Doppler. Hence, flow direction in a vessel should never be presumed but carefully determined after comparing with the color bar. Misinterpretation of flow direction may erroneously suggest a malfunctioning shunt or result in a missed flow reversal in an artery.

Directional Ambiguity

Directional ambiguity or indeterminate flow direction implies a spectral Doppler trace in which the waveform is displayed with almost equal amplitude above and below the baseline in a mirror image pattern. Directional ambiguity usually occurs when the interrogating beam intercepts the vessel at 90° (or close to 90°). If a Doppler signal is detected it is seen as a tracing both above and below the baseline. It is worse at higher gain settings. This can be corrected by changing the angle of interrogation.

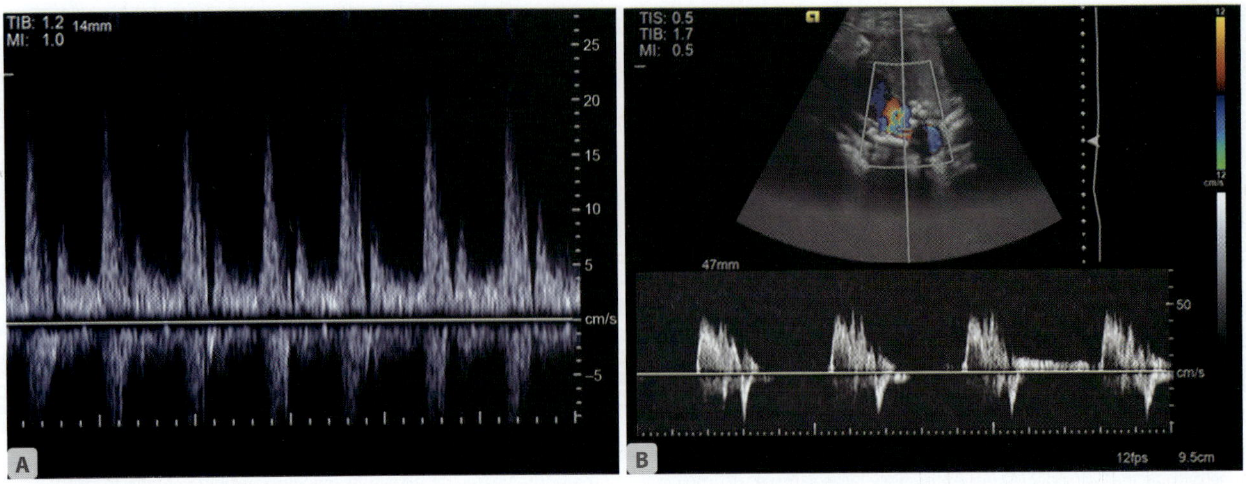

FIGS. 24A AND B: Mirror image pattern of spectral trace seen simultaneously above and below the baseline representing directional ambiguity in (A). True bidirectional flow in the neck of a pseudo aneurysm where forward flow is followed by flow reversal (B).

This should be distinguished from true bidirectional flow. In this case blood actually flows in two directions as seen in the neck of a pseudoaneurysm. The key pointer here is that flow here is first in one direction and then in the other in the same cardiac cycle and not simultaneously symmetric above and below the baseline at the same time. **(Figs. 24A and B)** Bidirectional flow can also be seen when there is high resistance organ flow such torsion, venous thrombosis etc. and is seen as diastolic reversal.

Slow Flow

If one is unable to visualize color flow in a vessel despite optimization of all Doppler parameters, the flow may be too slow for the color flow image to visualize. In such a situation use of power Doppler or spectral Doppler which are more sensitive to slow flow may help to detect flow. The power Doppler technique uses intensity or power of the Doppler signal rather than the frequency shift. Strength of a Doppler signal that exceeds a particular threshold level is displayed, hence it is less angle dependent. It is also more sensitive as more extensive dynamic range can be used than with standard color Doppler imaging because noise that would degrade the color Doppler image can be assigned a uniform background color. The spectral waveform makes use of several pulse cycles per scan line and contains qualitative and quantitative diagnostic information for interpretation. The color map, on the other hand, contains lesser pulse cycles per scan line thereby providing considerably less information than spectral Doppler. Also the color Doppler images display the mean frequency shift rather than the peak frequency shift.

DOPPLER ARTIFACTS

Appropriate settings of the above mentioned Doppler parameters eliminate or greatly reduce Doppler artifacts related to machine settings. There are certain other artifacts such as those due to anatomical factors or those unrelated to blood flow which one must be aware of to avoid misinterpreting the artifact as true flow.[7-12]

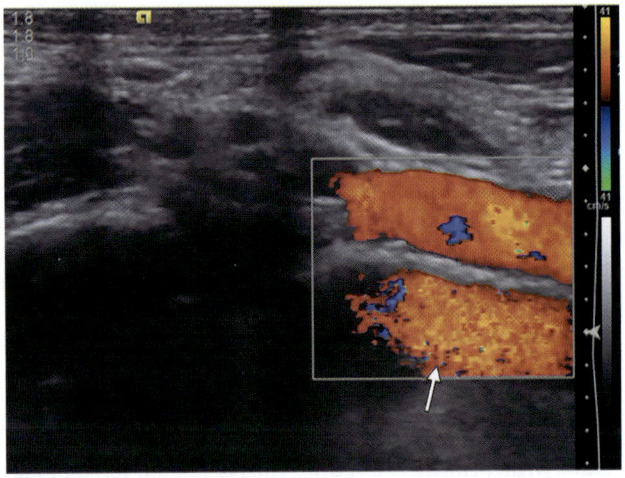

FIG. 25: Mirror image of the subclavian artery deep to the pleura (arrow).

Anatomically-related Artifacts

Mirror Image Artifact

As already discussed in the section on grayscale imaging, reflection of ultrasound by an interface between zones of high and low acoustic impedance produces an image of an object on both sides although it is located only on one side. A similar artifact can occur with color Doppler imaging most often in the supraclavicular region where mirror images of the subclavian artery or vein are caused by reflection from the pleura/lung causing apparent duplication of the vessel, with the phantom vessel being projected deeper in the image **(Fig. 25)**. Carotid and brachial arteries may also show mirror images. Changing the scanning angle will cause the mirror artifact to disappear.

Artifacts Unrelated to Blood Flow

Pseudo Flow

Pseudo flow artifact is due to motion of fluid rather than blood flow within a vessel. The signal persists as long as fluid motion continues. Pseudo flow may be caused by motion of ascites, amniotic fluid and urine from the ureteric orifice. It can mimic real blood flow on color or power Doppler. Spectral analysis reveals the presence of a Doppler signal which is atypical for a normal vessel. Some pseudo flow artifacts, such as those seen at ureteral orifice, are useful to identify the ureteric orifice and have been used to rule out complete obstruction, though not infallible (**Fig. 26**).

Twinkling Artifact

This occurs behind strongly reflecting granular interfaces such as urinary calculi or parenchymal calcification. Although primarily seen posterior to urinary calculi and parenchymal calcification it can also be seen behind any irregular highly reflective surfacelike biliary calculi, gallbladder adenomyosis and cholesterolosis Twinkling artifact is thought to be caused by a narrow band of intrinsic machine noise called phase (or clock) jitter. On a flat surface this is generally excluded by wall filters and not displayed. Rough surfaces increase the delays in measuring the signal and amplify the error which increases the spectral bandwidth of this noise above the level of wall filter.

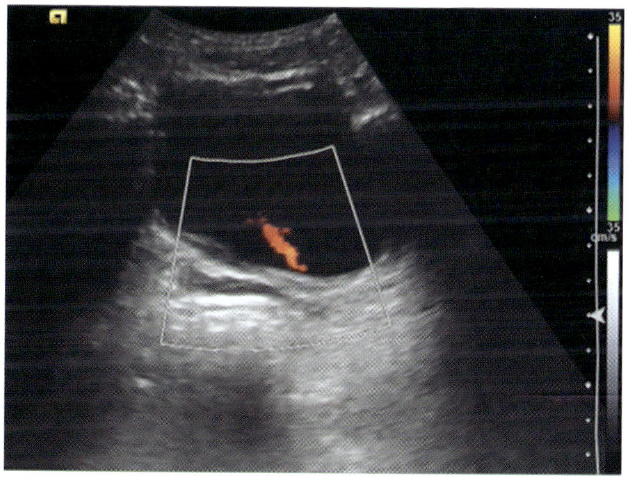

FIG. 26: Color Doppler image at the level of vesicoureteric junction shows the normal left ureteric jet. On the right side there is bladder wall thickening with non visualization of the jet.

It is seen as rapidly alternating mixture of Doppler signals, i.e. red and blue pixels which imitate turbulent flow. On spectral Doppler analysis, the tracing is absolutely flat suggestive of noise. The conspicuity of this artifact is determined by the color write priority and grayscale gain. With a decrease in color write priority twinkling artifact decreases. Twinkling artifact can be identified by the fact that color is produced behind the calcification and spectral trace depicts noise. Also, increasing the velocity scale eliminates flow signal but not twinkling (**Figs. 27A to C**).This can help to distinguish a calcified carotid plaque with twinkling from a potentially ulcerated plaque with flow in ulcer cavities.

It is also important to recognize this signal as artifactual in the gallbladder as it may mimic high velocity blood flow in a gallbladder mass erroneously suggesting the diagnosis of gallbladder carcinoma. On the other hand, the presence of twinkling artifact can be very useful for diagnosis of small stones that do not generate a strong echo. However, twinkling is not invariable. Authors suggest that calcium oxalate dihydrate and calcium phosphate calculi always produce twinkling artifact while calcium oxalate monohydrate and urate stones may lack a twinkling artifact.

Edge Artifact

This is seen with strong, smooth, specular reflectors and is visualized as steady color along the rim of calcified structures such as gall stones or cortical bone. It is more often seen with power Doppler than color Doppler. The Doppler trace is characteristically a straight line pattern equal above and below the baseline which implies noise and not true flow (**Figs. 28A and B**).

Flash Artifact

Flash artifact is a sudden burst of random color that fills the frame, obscuring the grayscale image. It can be caused by tissue motion or transducer motion. It is most often seen in hypoechoic regions like cysts or fluid collections and in the left lobe of liver (due to cardiac pulsation) (**Fig. 29**). Flash artifact occurs more commonly in power Doppler than color Doppler because of the longer time required to construct the image as more frames are averaged to form a power Doppler image than with standard color Doppler.

Flash artifact occurs due to a system setting that suppresses color pixels which would otherwise overwrite grayscale

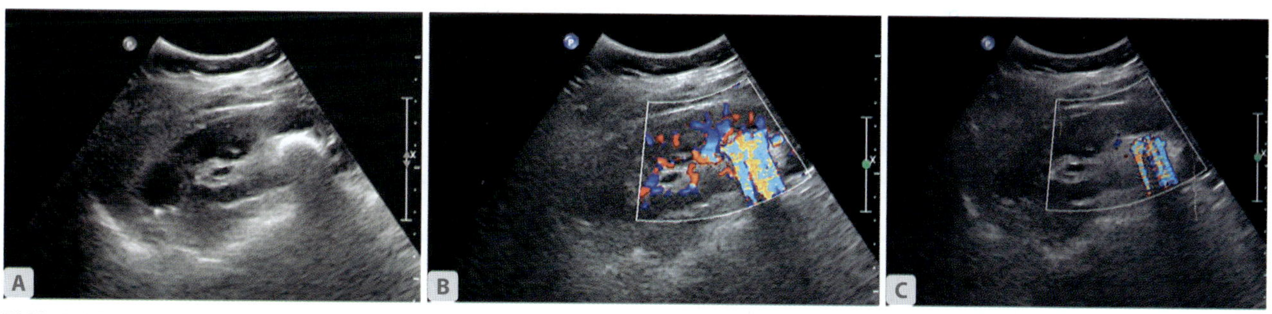

FIGS. 27A TO C: The grayscale image shows a renal calculus with distal acoustic shadowing (A). On application of color a mosaic of color is seen behind the calculus due to twinkling artifact. Note the presence of flow in the intrarenal vessels as well (B). On increasing the velocity scale the intrarenal flow disappears but the twinkling artifact persists (C).

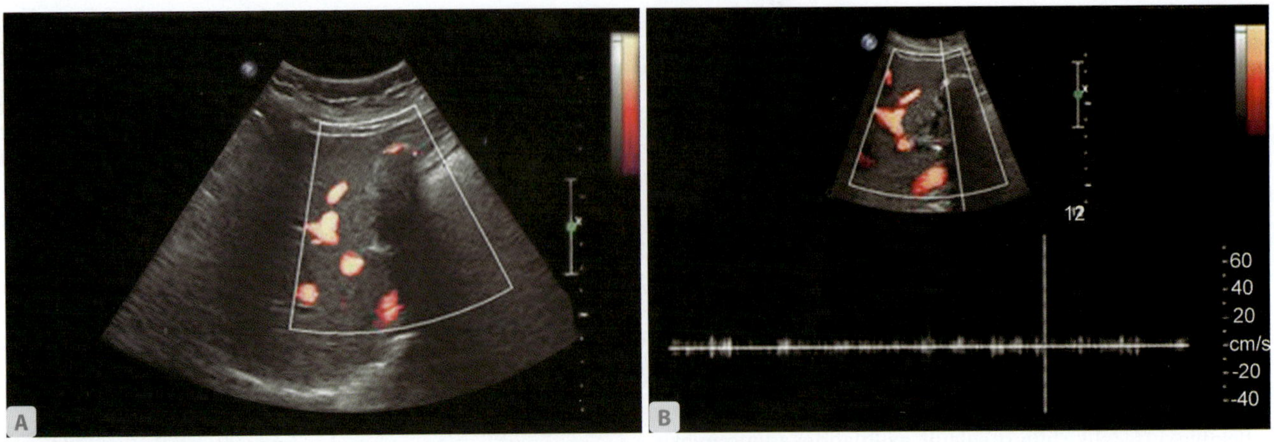

FIGS. 28A AND B: Edge artifact: Power Doppler image showing steady color along the rim of a gallbladder calculus (A). The spectral trace is characteristic of noise being a straight line pattern above and below the base line (B).

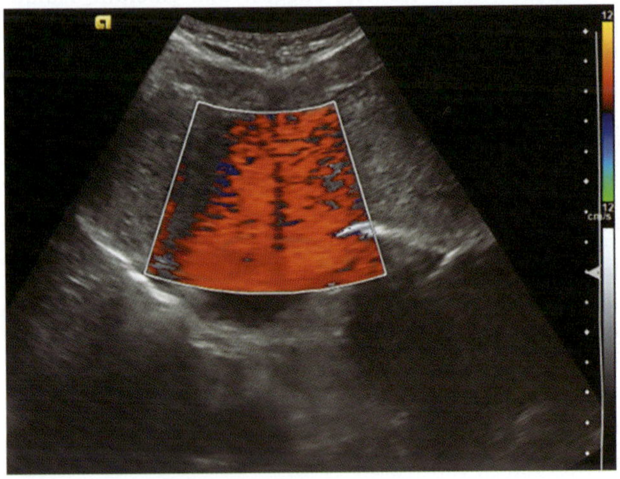

FIG. 29: Flash artifact due to cardiac motion over the left lobe liver seen as red color obscuring the frame.

echoes or the color write priority. When there is paucity of grayscale echoes, color pixels take priority so that flow is seen in nearly stationary fluid. The artifact is transient coinciding with transducer or patient movement such as respiration or cardiac pulsation and hence can be easily interpreted. In fact the flash artifact may at times be used to demonstrate fluid nature of solid appearing lesion.

Perivascular or Color Bruit Artifact

This is a tissue motion artifact in which motion is generated within an organ rather than involving an entire organ. It is seen as a color mosaic in soft tissue (not a single homogeneous color) adjacent to vessels with turbulent flow and is believed to be caused by actual vascular tissue vibration. These artifacts are more common with low PRF settings due to increased sensitivity of the system, but may also be caused by low wall filter setting.

This artifact is the imaging analogue of an auditory bruit or palpable thrill. Its prominence varies with the cardiac cycle being most obvious in systole and least in diastole. It is usually seen around anastomotic sites, stenotic arteries or arteriovenous fistulae acting as a useful pointer to their presence.

SPECIAL IMAGING MODES[1-3,10,13-17]

Modern imaging systems incorporate a number of special imaging modes involving advances in beamforming, ultrasound signal acquisition, and postprocessing to deal with inherent artifacts in ultrasound and improve image quality.

Tissue Harmonic Imaging

Difference in propagation velocity of ultrasound between tissues such as fat and other soft tissues, near the transducer results in phase aberrations that distort the ultrasound field producing noise and clutter. In addition, the focusing of the ultrasound beam depends on phase coherence of the sound waves at the focal zone and at the transducer surface during receive focusing. If the intervening tissue has heterogeneous velocities defocusing occurs as the waves no longer coincide precisely, degrading lateral resolution. Tissue harmonic imaging provides a means to reduce the effects of phase aberrations. The term harmonic refers to frequencies that are integral multiples of true frequency of the transmitted pulse which is called the fundamental frequency or first harmonic. The second harmonic has a frequency twice the fundamental.

Harmonics are generated due to the non-linear propagation of sound waves in the tissues. The wave velocity is higher for high pressure waves, i.e. compression than low pressure component, i.e. rarefaction. This causes increasing distortion of the ultrasound pulse as it travels through the tissue changing the wave pattern from a perfect sinusoidal shape to a sharper saw tooth shape. This generates waves of higher frequencies which are multiple of the fundamental frequency (2nd, 3rd, 4th, etc.) which are referred to as harmonics (**Fig. 30**). The intensity decreases as the order of the harmonics increases. In addition, the higher frequency harmonics are also attenuated more. Hence current harmonic imaging is mostly performed using the second harmonic component (Work is in progress in order to utilize higher order harmonics or the so called superharmonic imaging and frequencies lower than the transmitted frequency or subharmonic imaging for use with ultrasound contrast media) The final image is formed by the harmonic frequency bandwidth in the received signal after eliminating the transmitted frequency by frequency filtering, pulse inversion/phase cancellation or coded harmonics.

The generation of harmonics requires interaction of transmitted pulse with the propagating tissues hence harmonic generation is not important near the transducer or skin surface and becomes important only some distance away from the transducer. Harmonic images therefore show good rejection of artifacts and clutter arising from the body wall and also reduce the defocusing effect of the body wall. Artifacts are also reduced in harmonic imaging as the amplitude of the harmonic waves is relatively small reducing detection of echoes from multiple scatters. In addition, artifacts produced by the fundamental frequency and side lobes do not have sufficient energy to generate harmonic frequencies and are therefore filtered out during image formation. Penetration can be improved by using a low fundamental transmitted pulse and imaging at the higher harmonic frequency.

Other advantages include superior axial resolution due to shorter wavelength and improved lateral resolution due to better focusing with higher frequencies. Also because harmonics originate in regions of the ultrasound pulse with the greatest pressure amplitude, i.e. near the pulse center (as the amplitude at the periphery is too weak to generate harmonics) it results in a narrower beam producing images with superior lateral and elevational resolution. Harmonic images thus show less haze, noise, clutter and better cyst clearance **(Figs. 31A and B)**.

The technique is most useful in patients with thick complicated body wall structure or the so-called" difficult patients" for mid field imaging. At greater depths, harmonic signals begin to decrease substantially, relative to fundamental signal due to increased attenuation.

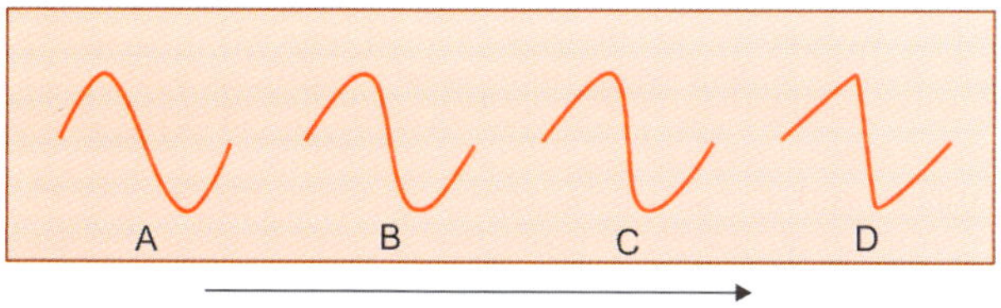

FIG. 30: Generation of harmonics: As the path length through the tissue increases the sinusoidal waveform (A). Changes to a more saw tooth pattern with higher frequency due to the compression wave traveling faster than the rarefaction wave (D).

Compound Imaging

Compound imaging is the ability to acquire multi-ple frames from different-frequencies, i.e. *frequency compound imaging* or from different angles, i.e. *spatial compound imaging*.

Frequency Compound Imaging

Frequency compounding is the combination of multiple images detected from different frequency bands into a single image. This reduces noise and speckle as the appearance of speckle varies with frequency. This is possible with the use of broad band width transducers.

Spatial Compound Imaging

In spatial compound imaging electronic steering of ultrasound beams from an array transducer is used to image the same tissue multiple times by using parallel beams oriented in different directions. Data from many such beam lines is acquired and averaged together into a single image. The appearance of speckle varies according to the beam line direction. Since speckle noise is random it cancels out during compounding while signal is reinforced making the images look less grainy.

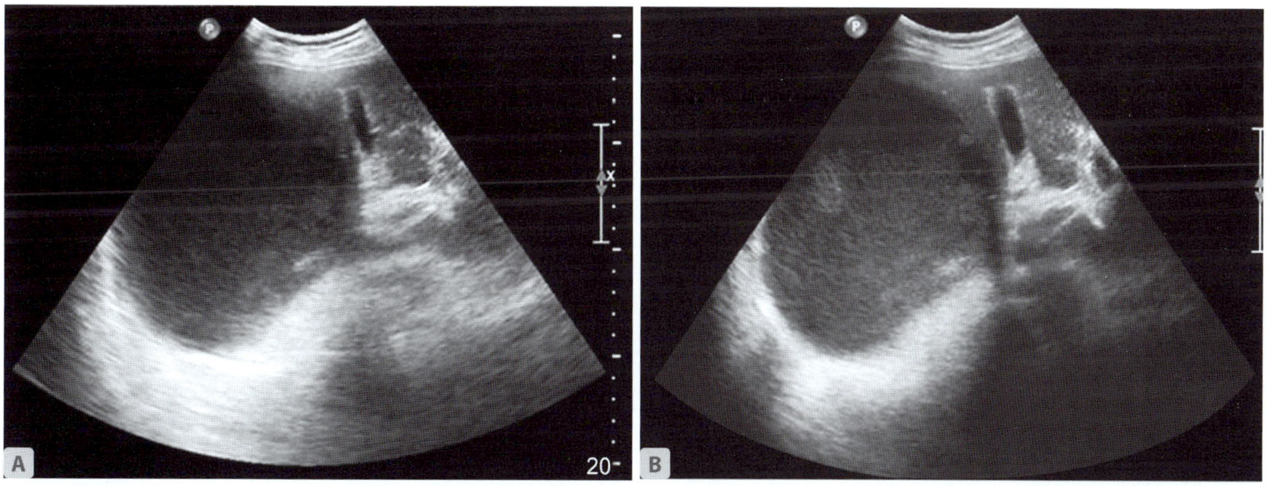

FIGS. 31A AND B: A transverse scan of the liver in a relatively obese patient with a large right lobe abscess. Although the abscess is visualized in the image without harmonics (A), the margins of the abscess, its internal echopattern and the diaphragm are much better appreciated in the harmonic imaging mode (B).

Spatial compounding is also useful to image specular reflectors. Relatively large smooth surfaces reflect sound like a mirror with angle of incidence being equal to angle of reflection. Such specular reflectors include diaphragm, wall of urinary bladder, endometrial stripe, etc. Since the ultrasound beam is not dispersed like scatters, the signals are much stronger but are highly directional. Display of specular interfaces is therefore highly dependent on angle of insonation and specular reflectors return echoes to the transducer only if the sound beam is perpendicular to the interface. As the surface is titled away from 90° the signal intensity falls rapidly (as the sound beam is reflected away from the transducer). This results in poor margin definition and less distinct boundaries for cysts and other masses in conventional imaging where each scan line used to generate the image. It is of particular importance in sonography of the *musculoskeletal system* because of the anisotropic nature of muscles and tendons. The fibrillar pattern of a tendon is best appreciated when the ultrasound beam is perpendicular to the tendon and appears relatively echo-poor at oblique angles simulating tears or tendinosis. In spatial compound imaging since the image is generated from more than one angle of insonation the chances that at at least one of these is perpendicular to the specular reflector is greater, reducing anisotropic effects improving tissue plane definition and display of curved structures.

Spatial compound images show reduction in speckle, noise, clutter and refractive shadows and improve contrast and margin definition. Acoustic enhancement and shadowing artifacts may be reduced which may be an advantage or potential drawback depending on the clinical situation **(Figs. 32A and B)**.

Another drawback is that because multiple US beams are used to image one tissue region instead of just one beam as in conventional B-mode imaging more time is required for data acquisition and processing so the compound frame rate is lower than conventional B-mode imaging depending on the processing capabilities of the imaging system.

Spatial compounding can also be achieved by using a single transmit pulse and varying the receiver crystals. This typically maintains higher frame rates as less transmit pulses are used.

Coded Pulse Excitation

Higher frequency US pulses produce images with better spatial resolution, however, increased attenuation with increasing frequency limits evaluation of deep structures with high frequencies. Coded pulse excitation is a method that can overcome this limitation and provide good penetration at higher frequencies. This technique uses longer ultrasound pulses rather than the routinely used short ultrasound pulses. These longer pulses have greater ultrasound energy, which increases the energy of echoes that return from the deeper tissues allowing use of higher frequencies. The coded pulses are produced with a very characteristic shape and the returning echoes also have a similar shape, which makes their identification from background noise easier **(Figs. 33A to C)**. The returning echoes are then processed using a pulse compression technique in which the location of the long characteristic pulse shapes are identified. These pulse shape locations may be determined with a tight spatial tolerance and correspond to the location of structures from where they are reflected. Hence, the location of reflectors is identified with good spatial resolution. This produces an image with good echo signal and good spatial resolution at greater depths.

Adaptive Image Processing

An adaptive image processing algorithm is one that is able to recognize the difference between real targets and artifacts, and to modify its processing accordingly. Multiresolution adaptive image processing algorithms to smooth speckle and enhance structural edges are now available (e.g. XRES, SRI, Ultra art, etc).

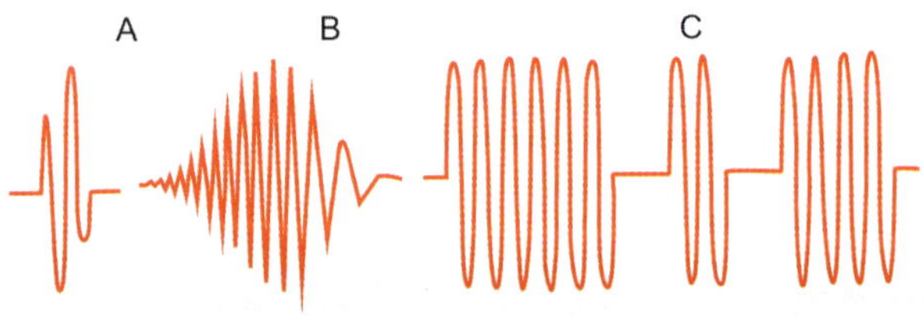

FIGS. 33A TO C: (A) Normal pulse; (B) A chirp pulse; and (C) A coded pulse.

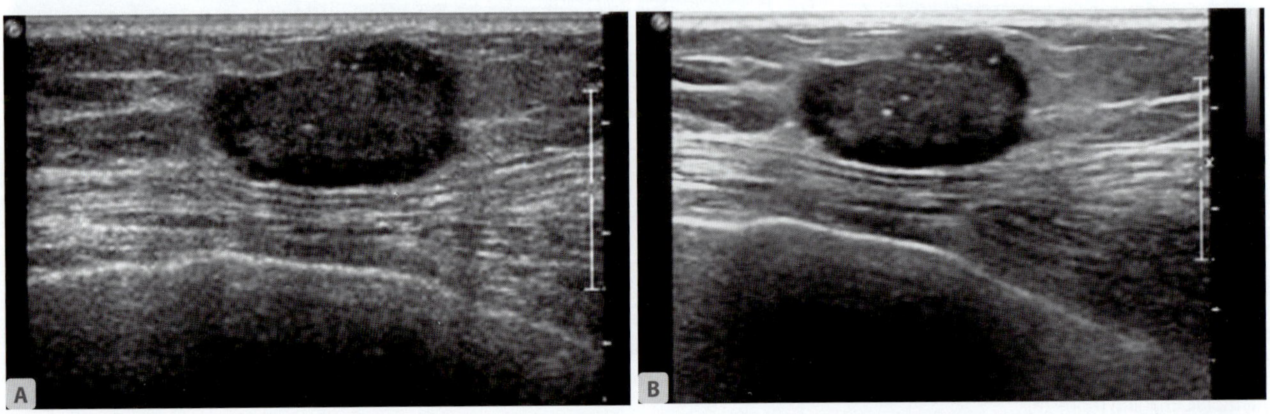

FIGS. 32A AND B: Fibroadenoma of the breast imaged without (A) and with spatial compound imaging (B). The margins of the lesion, internal architecture and calcifications are better visualized. Note the reduced edge shadows. The image appears less grainy due to reduced speckle.

It involves an analysis phase (in which artifacts and targets are identified) and an enhancement phase (in which artifacts are suppressed and targets enhanced). The analysis phase takes into account multiple characteristics of the target, such as local statistical properties, textural and structural properties. The textural and structural information in particular is vital for identifying the strength and orientation of interfaces and thus allowing directional filtering of these targets in the enhancement phase. For example, smoothing is applied along an interface to improve continuity, while edge enhancement is applied in the perpendicular direction. In regions identified by the analysis phase as being homogeneous, smoothing is applied equally in all directions.

Photopic Ultrasound Imaging

This technique can be used to optimize image contrast. Grey levels are converted to monochromatic color value, allowing very subtle structural differences to be appreciated.

Extended Field of View Imaging

Early static B-mode scanners had a large field of view (FOV) which was lost with the introduction of real time scanning. Extended FOV imaging restores the capability of visualizing large anatomic regions in a single image.

The transducer is translated across the region of interest, during which multiple images are acquired from multiple transducer positions. Image features in regions of overlap between successive images are used to determine the exact position of the multiple images relative to each other by the scanner. The images are thus registered with respect to each other accounting for both translation and in plane rotation of the transducer. The registered image data is processed in a large image buffer and combined to form the large FOV image. It is a useful image presentation format as it is easier for clinicians to understand.

B-Mode Flow Imaging

B-mode flow imaging is a new method for flow imaging available in ultrasound. This technique shows blood flow with grayscale or B-mode imaging and is not a Doppler method. For B flow imaging digitally encoded wide band pulses are transmitted and reflected from moving blood cells. The returning echoes are decoded and filtered to increase sensitivity of moving scatterers and distinguish blood from tissue. Both the surrounding stationary tissue and flowing blood are shown in shades of gray.

As this is not a Doppler technique no velocity or frequency information is provided. It is a purely visual nonquantitative method. The major advantage is that it allows precise definition of the boundary between flowing blood and vessel wall. There is no problem of blooming or over amplification of flow signals as this is a non-Doppler technique. The technique does not degrade the spatial or temporal resolution of the grayscale image unlike color Doppler and is more accurate in showing the extent of plaque and surface irregularity of the plaque as compared to color Doppler or grayscale imaging alone in superficial vessels.

The technique is, however, most useful in superficial vessels as it relies on amplification of very weak echoes from red blood cells.

CONCLUSION

With increasing technological advances, applications of ultrasound and Doppler have grown tremendously both for detection of pathology and physiology. Gaining maximum benefit from this complex technology requires a combination of skills, including knowledge of physical principles that empower ultrasound with its unique diagnostic capabilities. With this information the radiologist can gather maximum information from each examination while avoiding pitfalls and errors in diagnosis that may result from omission of information or misinterpretation of artifacts. Careful attention to technical parameters, appropriate use of special imaging features and diligence of examination technique will avoid day-to-day scanning pitfalls and result in studies with improved diagnostic accuracy.

REFERENCES

1. Hangiandreou NJ. B-mode US: basic concepts and new technology. Radiographics. 2003;23(4):1019-33. Review.
2. Merrit Christopher RB. Physics of ultrasound in Diagnostic ultrasound vol 1, 3rd edn. Rheumack Wilson SR Charboneau JW (Eds). Elsevier; 2005.pp.3-34.
3. Cosgrove D. Artefacts in B mode imaging in Abdominal and general ultrasound vol 1, 2nd edn. Meire H, Cosgrove D, Dewbury K, Farrant P (Eds). Churchill livingstone; 2001.pp.47-65.
4. Rubens DJ, Bhatt S, Nedelka S, Cullinan J. Doppler artifacts and pitfalls. Radiol Clin North Am. 2006;44(6): 805-35.
5. Farina Robrterto Saparano Amelia. Errors in ultrasonography in Errors in Radiology. Luigia Romano Antonio Pinto (Eds). Springer Verlag; 2012.pp.76-85.
6. Feldman MK, Katyal S, Blackwood MS. US artifacts. Radiographics. 2009;29(4):1179-89.
7. Acampara Ciro, Fabia Pinto, Magistris Giuseppe De Errors in color Doppler ultrasonography in Errors in Radiology. Springer Verlag; 2012.pp.86-103.
8. Tahmasebpour HR, Buckley AR, Cooperberg PL, Fix CH. Sonographic examination of the carotid arteries. Radiographics. 2005;25(6):1561-75.
9. Kruskal JB, Newman PA, Sammons LG, Kane RA. Optimizing Doppler and color flow US: application to hepatic sonography. Radiographics. 2004;24(3):657-75.
10. Zagzebski James A. Physics in Doppler and B-mode ultrasound in Introduction to vascular sonography, 6th edn. Pellirito, Polak (Eds) Elsevier; 2012.pp.20-51.
11. Campbell SC, Cullinan JA, Rubens DJ. Slow flow or no flow? Color and power Doppler US pitfalls in the abdomen and pelvis. Radiographics. 2004;24(2):497-506.

12. Rahmouni A, Bargoin R, Herment A, Bargoin N, Vasile N. Color Doppler twinkling artifact in hyperechoic regions Radiology. 1996;199(1):269-71.
13. Choudhry S, Gorman B, Charboneau JW, Tradup DJ, Beck RJ, Kofler JM, Groth DS. Comparison of tissue harmonic imaging with conventional US in abdominal disease. Radiographics. 2000;20(4):1127-35.
14. Rosenthal SJ, Jones PH, Wetzel LH. Phase inversion tissue harmonic sonographic imaging: a clinical utility study. AJR Am J Roentgenol. 2001;176(6):1393-8.
15. Desser TS, Jeffrey RB. Tissue harmonic imaging techniques: physical principles and clinical applications. Semin Ultrasound CT MR. 2001;22(1):1-10.
16. Lin DC, Nazarian LN, O'Kane PL, McShane JM, Parker L, Merritt CR. Advantages of real-time spatial compound sonography of the musculoskeletal system versus conventional sonography. AJR Am J Roentgenol. 2002;179(6):1629-31.
17. Michael Baad, Zheng Feng Lu, Ingrid Reiser, David Paushter, Clinical Significance of US Artifacts. RadioGraphics. 2017;37: 1408-23.

CHAPTER

30

Ultrasound Elastography: Principles and Application

Veenu Singla, Tulika Singh, Anindita Sinha

INTRODUCTION

Elastography images tissue stiffness noninvasively by measuring deformation of tissue on application of a small mechanical force (compression or shear wave). It is akin to "virtual palpation", which has the potential to overcome the subjectivity associated with clinical palpation. It can also provide objective and quantitative measures of tissue stiffness. It is based on the fact that pathological processes alter the elastic properties of tissue and therefore, measurement of elasticity can be used for differentiating abnormal from normal tissues.

Elastography can map the elasticity of a tissue in two ways: (i) by analysis of strain in tissues that have been put under stress, (ii) by analysis of propagation of introduced shear waves in the tissue whose propagation depends upon the tissue stiffness. The stiffer tissue resists deformation and results in faster propagation of mechanical waves.

BASIC PHYSICS

Some common terminologies like stress, strain, shear, elasticity, viscoelasticity, Hooke's law and Young's modulus are often used and a basic understanding of these is required to understand elastography. Glossary of some important definitions used in elastography is as follows.

Stress

Definition of Stress is 'force per unit area' and its unit is Pascal (Pascal = Newton/m^2) or pounds per square inch (psi).

Stress can be due to compression, which acts perpendicular to a surface and causes shortening of an object.

Shear stress acts parallel to a surface and causes deformation.

In elastography, stress can be applied exogenously by transducer compression, vibrators or acoustic radiation force. Endogenous motion of vessels, cardiac or respiratory motion can also be utilized. Although endogenous sources overcome the shortcomings of exogenous source like attenuation (e.g. due to obesity or ascites), endogenous stress is difficult to quantify.[1]

Strain

The deformation an object tends to undergo when subjected to stress is called strain.

Strain is unitless and is denoted as difference in length per unit length of the object. So, hard objects have lower strain values than softer objects. When compression is applied, lesions nearer the applied force undergo more displacement than objects lying in a deeper plane. This is similar to clinical difficulty in palpating deep seated lesions and is one of the factors which may influence efficacy of elastography.

Elasticity

The feature of materials to revert to their original form after removal of stress is called elasticity. Elastic materials strain immediately when stressed and also revert quickly back to their original position.

Viscosity

Measurement of a fluid's resistance on undergoing shear or tensile stress (compression/stretching) is called viscosity.

Viscoelasticity

This is the characteristic of materials to display both viscous and elastic properties. In viscoelastic material like soft tissue, there is a gap of time between application of force and displacement. When stress is applied, the strain escalates rapidly as free fluid in soft tissues is released. Then, the relationship of stress over strain becomes linear for small changes.

Poroelasticity

A material in which a solid material is pervaded by an interconnecting meshwork of fluid-filled pores.

Tissue may be viscoelastic, poroelastic, anisotropic (e.g. muscle fibers or nerve fibers oriented in a particular direction) or contractile or a combination of these and disease conditions may modify their character.

Elastography techniques which can estimate visco/poroelasticity give a more accurate estimate of tissue conditions than techniques where simple stress, strain or

Young's modulus is measured, as here tissue is assumed to be a homogeneous and isotropic material.

Hooke's Law

According to Hooke's law, stress is proportional to the strain, within the range of elastic limit of any object.

$\sigma = \Gamma . \varepsilon$ with stress (σ) being force/unit area, strain (ε) being expansion/unit length and elastic modulus (Γ) relating stress to strain. Since stress has kilopascals as unit and strain is dimensionless, the unit of elastic modulus is kilopascals. Softer tissues like fat undergo more deformation (strain) when stress (e.g. compression during palpation) is applied.

Harder tissues like muscle and fibrous tissue resist strain and thus have a higher elastic modulus.[2-5]

There are 3 kinds of elastic modulus according to the deformation method **(Fig. 1)**:

1. Young's modulus (*E*)—normal stress (σ_n) leads to normal strain (ε_n). Young's Modulus (E) is the ratio of stress/strain and has the same unit as stress. Young's Modulus measures the tissue's resistance to compression. In simpler terms, it is a measure of elasticity or spring like behavior, i.e. the ability of a tissue to resist deformation perpendicular to the surface.
2. Shear modulus (*G*)—shear stress (σ_s) leads to shear strain (ε_s) and shear is tangential to surface. Shear modulus is a ratio between shear stress and shear strain. It describes the capability of a tissue to withstand deformation parallel to surface.
3. Bulk modulus (*K*)—normal inward force (σ_b) causes a bulk strain or change in volume (ε_b). It measures the capability of a tissue to withstand volume change on increase in pressure. It is the inverse of compressibility.

The relationship between Young's modulus (E) and shear modulus (G) is as follows:

$E = 2 (\nu + 1) G$

$E = 3 G$ (the Poisson's ratio ν being ~ 0.5, given the high water content of soft tissue of an incompressible medium)

Poisson's Ratio (ν)*:* When exposed to stress, tissue may contract in one dimension (like width) while its length increases.

Poisson's ratio = Lateral contraction per unit breadth/longitudinal extension per unit length. Poisson's ratio of normal soft tissue is 0.5.

DIFFERENT ELASTOGRAPHY METHODS

- *Compression or static elastography:* Where static compression is imposed onto a targeted soft tissue and the resulting displacement field generated by the compressive force is directly measured by ultrasound imaging.
- *Dynamic elastography.* This further is of the following two types:
  i. Dynamic elastography with harmonic stimuli (DEHS).
  ii. Dynamic elastography with transient stimuli (DETS).

Compression Elastography

In compression elastography, an external force is applied and strain is calculated in a direction perpendicular to tissue surface. This technique is most widely used for strain elastography in different ultrasound systems and analyzes the radiofrequency pulses generated in response to external compression of a tissue.[6] Compression leads to tissue deformation and is expressed by Young's modulus of elasticity.[7] RF waveform before and after compression are windowed and the signals in the same segment are compared to calculate the displacement. Around 97% of transmitted ultrasound waves are absorbed, only 3% of energy is scattered. Scattering occurs at the tissue boundaries, especially collagenous and fat surfaces.

Tracking of displacement of this scatter in real time is the objective of strain imaging.[8] Maps of the tissues before and after the compression are acquired **(Fig. 2)**. Radiofrequency echo signals are the "map of tissue" and even very small

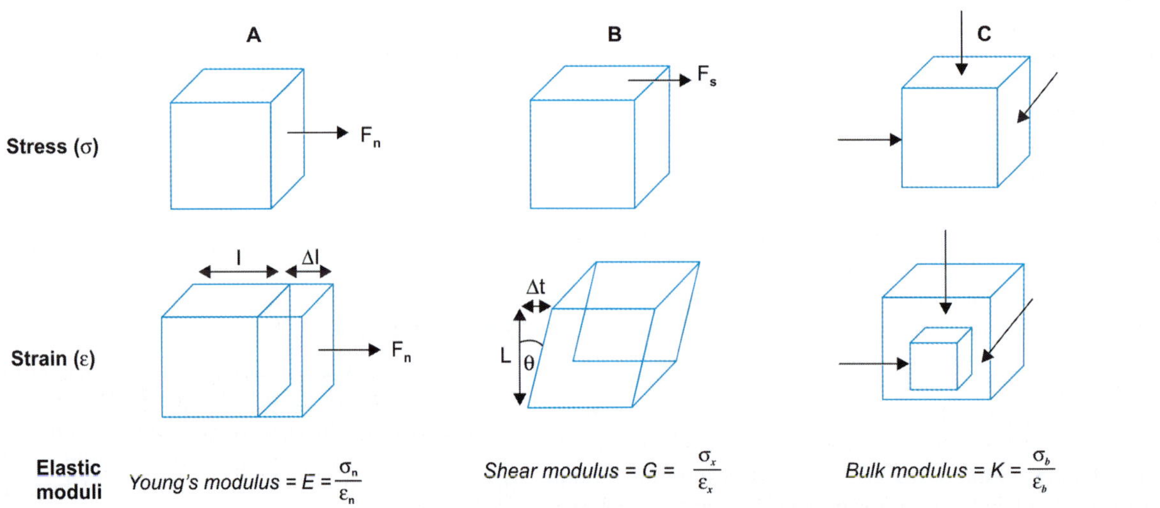

FIG. 1: Line diagrams representing ultrasound elastography physics. The static deformation of an object can be described by stress, strain and elastic moduli (stress divided by strain) as described. A, B and C represent normal (perpendicular to surface), shear (tangent to the surface) and bulk (normal inward force or pressure) forces respectively.

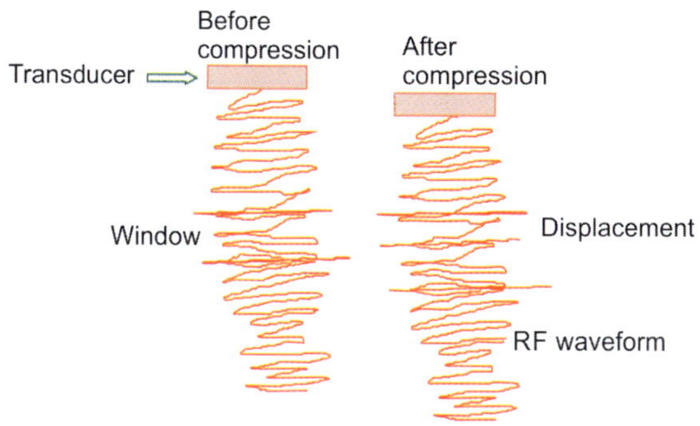

FIG. 2: The windowed segment of scattered RF waveform is cross-correlated with the waveform obtained pre- and postcompression. The amount of shift between the matching segments is equal to tissue displacement.

motion causes a change of phase of radiofrequency echoes which is tracked.[9] The change values are called strain. Relative difference in the tissue movement is calculated by software to find tissue deformation.[10]

Tissue strain is usually determined by measuring displacement at various parts of the tissue generated by application of external force, pulsation or both, and then calculating it as a spatial differential. Various methods of obtaining strain images from echo signals have been described with the three most common ones being: the spatial correlation method, phase shift tracking method and combined autocorrelation method. The spatial correlation technique is a basic method of measuring displacement which utilizes 2D matching of pattern algorithm and searches for the position that shows maximum correlation between region of interests (ROIs) selected among two images. This method, however, is not suitable for real-time processing as it requires a fairly long computation time. An alternative is the phase shift tracking method which determines longitudinal tissue motion quickly and accurately due to phase domain processing. However, the aliasing effect associated with this method prevents its application to the larger displacements that are necessary to improve the signal-to-noise ratio of the strain image.[11]

In order to overcome the drawbacks of the above-mentioned methods, the combined autocorrelation method was developed which has the advantages of producing strain images of high quality with real-time processing and being applicable to large displacements.[12] Moreover, this method is suited to free-hand compression due to wide dynamic range for strain estimation and robustness for lateral movement of tissue. Its clinical implementation typically involves freehand scanning, i.e. real time implementation for immediate feedback so that the user can control the deformation's direction.[13]

Therefore, to summarize compression elastography, hard/stiff tissues move en-piece in a wholesome way with all areas showing same amount of displacement after compression, resulting in negligible or small rate of change of displacement called as zero or no strain. Softer tissue shows bigger change of rate of displacement yielding higher strain values. The deformation/strain is mapped on elastogram with stiffer areas represented as dark and softer areas being lighter. This allows the differentiation of lesions which are otherwise isoechoic on grayscale ultrasound images.

Limitations

As tissue displacement and the rate of change in displacement vary with the quantity of compression applied, the tissue strain depends on the quantity of the compression applied and so does not represent the inherent elastic property of the given tissue. This makes it operator dependent. It is a qualitative imaging of relative stiffness, so the actual strain value cannot be compared with the next imaging.[7] However, it can be used as semi-quantitative parameter with measurement of strain ratio, which is measured as the ratio of strain between the lesion and adjoining tissue. Because it shows only differences in strain from one area to another in the same image, it is suitable for the detection and characterization of small focal lesions and not sensitive to the diffuse disease process that produces same stiffness all over in one image.

Dynamic Methods

As mentioned above, dynamic elastography can be of the following two types:

1. Dynamic elastography with harmonic stimuli (DEHS) wherein external or internal harmonic stimuli are used to generate dynamic responses in biological soft tissues. It includes sonoelastography, shear wave-induced resonance elastography (SWIRE), vibro-acoustography (VA), harmonic motion imaging (HMI) and shear wave dispersion ultrasound vibrometry (SDUV) methods.
2. Dynamic elastography with transient stimuli (DETS), wherein we use transient stimuli to deform a soft tissue and the responses of soft tissues (e.g. the shear wave velocities) are measured to extract the local elastic properties. Similar to DEHS, various external and internal stimuli may be used to generate transient shear waves within soft tissues. In recent years, DETS, in which acoustic radiation force is used to generate a transient shear wave, has attracted considerable attention.

In simpler terms, compression methods are used in strain elastography and dynamic methods are used in shear wave elastography, detailed description of which is given below. Based on elastography methods, elastography can be classified into various types **(Figs. 3A to E)**.

- Ultrasound (US) based
  - *Strain imaging:*
    - Strain elastography
    - Acoustic radiation force impulse (ARFI) strain imaging
  - *Shear wave imaging:*
    - Transient elastography (TE)
    - Point shear wave elastography (pSWE)
    - 2D shear wave elastography
- Magnetic resonance (MR) based

Our focus in this chapter will be on ultrasound based elastography.

Strain Imaging

There are two types of ultrasound strain imaging: (a) Strain Elastography and (b) ARFI strain imaging.[13]

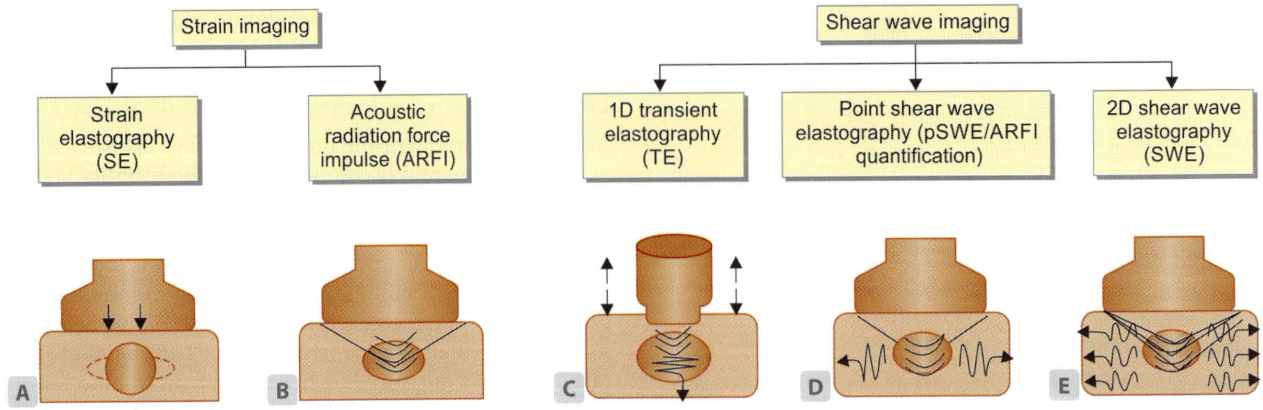

FIGS. 3A TO E: Diagram showing elastography techniques: Strain (A and B) and shear wave (C to E) elastography. Excitation method used in strain elastography (SE) is quasistatic mechanically-induced displacement by active compression. In ARFI, pSWE and 2D SWE, acoustic radiation force impulse is used for excitation. In TE, dynamic compression by thumping transducer at tissue surface is used to produce shear waves.

Strain Elastography

Principles and Technique

In strain elastography, an extrinsic force is applied to the tissue. Areas with maximum stiffness are deformed the least while areas with minimum stiffness are deformed to a greater extent. Comparison of ultrasound images is done before and after application of force. Hence, strain ratios can be calculated and no exact values are generated as the stress induced within the tissues is not quantifiable. Strain elastography can have deformation from following forces:

- *Manual compression:* May be used in superficial structures like breast and thyroid.
- *Internal physiologic motion (e.g. cardiovascular, respiratory) leading to tissue displacement:* It can be used for deeper located organs like liver.[14]

In both manual and physiological compression, applied stress is unknown. Therefore, presuming normal stress (σ_n), the measured normal strain (ε_n) is used to give qualitative Young's modulus. Semitransparent color maps called elastograms display strain elastography and these elastograms are laid on the B-mode display.[15] Usually, hard/stiff tissue having low strain is depicted as blue, and soft tissue having high strain depicted as red. But the operator should be aware that the color scale can vary between different ultrasound vendors.

Measurements

Commonly used parameters in strain elastography are *Elasticity score, Strain ratio and Distance ratio. Elasticity scores* are a qualitative method to classify color elastograms in a range from benign to malignant. A semi-quantitative measurement is *strain ratio*, which compares strain in the adjacent normal tissue with the strain in the target lesion. A strain ratio >1 denotes a stiff mass. *Distance ratio* is calculated by comparing maximum diameter of a lesion on elastography image to maximum diameter of the lesion on B-mode image.

Quantitative versus Qualitative

The results can be qualitative color coded elastograms or pseudo/semi-quantitative strain ratio measurement.

Acoustic Radiation Force Impulse Strain Imaging

It is another technique to measure strain and is used, for example, in Siemens Virtual Touch Imaging (VTI).

Principles and Technique

Acoustic radiation force impulse (ARFI) imaging involves small duration acoustic forces known as pushing pulses to create tissue displacement.

No external or physiological (pulsation or respiration) compression is needed. The cessation of force causes tissue to return to its original position. Pushing pulses can be applied by the ultrasound transducer array (frequency of 2–7 MHz) to a volume of 2 mm^3 for 1 ms per pulse resulting in a displacement of 10–20 m.

Measurements

Ultrasound pulses track these displacements by locating change in the peak along multiple tracking lines. The excitation can be performed in a sequential fashion by translating the tracking line along the tissue to assess the response. Parallel acquisition of push pulses and tracking displacements can also be done. Peak displacement, time taken to reach peak displacement and recovery time are utilized to characterize tissue response.[16]

Tissue recoil also generates shear waves, which propagate away from the focal point of excitation. The velocity of the shear waves is proportional to tissue stiffness. Shear modulus can be calculated from the shear wave velocity. Mapping shear wave velocity (cm/sec or m/sec) at multiple lateral points from the region of excitation can generate quantitative measurements of tissue stiffness.

Quantitative versus Qualitative

As in strain elastography, the displacements are depicted as an elastogram laid on the grayscale image. Quantitative analysis is required for diffuse stiffening associated with advanced liver fibrosis, differentiation of malignant and benign lesions, and monitoring response to therapy or disease progression.[17-19]

Advantages

The ARFI images are more homogeneous and have better contrast than surface displacement (compression) elastography. Deep tissues, which are not accessible by compression strain elastography can be evaluated.

Disadvantages

Physiological (respiration, pulsation) and transducer motion can degrade image quality as 1–3 ms is required per tracking line pair. Lower ultrasound frequencies and motion compensation techniques like premonitory physiological motion and subtracting this expected motion have been applied to overcome these limitations.[5,17]

Tissues >10 cm deep cannot be accurately assessed due to attenuation of the radiation force with greater depths.

Safety

Commercially available ARFI-based systems operate within accepted limits, but cavitation-based bioeffects may occur in tissues containing gas, like lungs, using MI (Mechanical Index) >0.4.[15] In addition, fetal activity has been reported to increase, so ALARA principle should be followed. The duration of pushing pulses and the frame rate are limited to keep within the standard diagnostic limits of mechanical and thermal index.[15]

Shear Wave Imaging

Principles and Technique

Shear waves travel in a direction perpendicular to the axial displacement caused by the ultrasonic pulse. Shear waves attenuate rapidly, about 10000 times faster in comparison to compression waves.[5] Due to high attenuation, shear waves enable mechanical oscillations to be induced in only a limited tissue area. Deformations by the focused ultrasound radiation are generally very small (at submicron level). Sophisticated signal processing is required to detect such motion differences. The shear wave produced is thereafter followed at lateral, spatially offset places from the radiation force excitation by a parallel tracking method **(Fig. 4)**.[5,10]

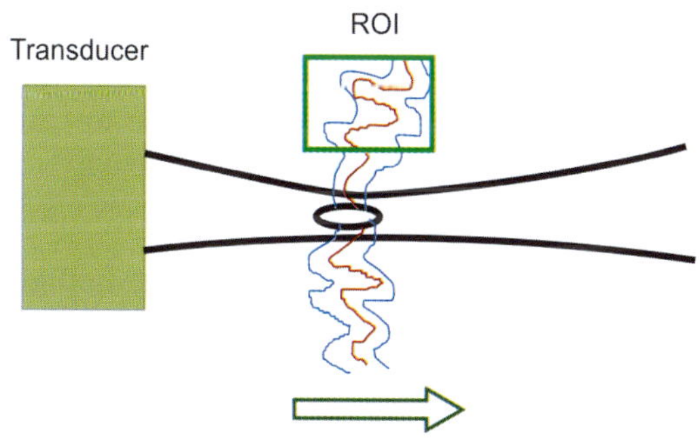

FIG. 4: Schematic diagram for shear wave sonography. Longitudinal acoustic pulse transmission causes tissue displacement. Shear waves propagate away perpendicular to transmitted pulse. Separate tracking pulses in the region of interest (ROI) track these shear waves. The stiffer the tissue, faster the shear wave velocity.

The various types of shear wave elastography are as follows:

- *Transient elastography:* In transient elastography, low frequency (50 Hz) vibrations are sent by the transducer to induce an elastic shear wave. 1D-TE system FibroScan™ (Echosens) was the first transient elastography system for assessment of the liver. It has been shown to be reliable in the assessment of liver fibrosis. However, transient elastography has its own limitations that include lack of real time imaging, difficulty in assessing obese patients and non-applicability in patients having ascites.
- *Point shear wave elastography (pSE):* In pSE, focused US pulses are used to generate a transverse wave (shear wave) at specific depths within the tissue as selected by the operator and the velocity of these shear waves are measured using tracking US pulses. Ten to twelve measurements are taken and median and average velocities are calculated automatically. The strength of this technique is that it is performed with real-time imaging with the same probe as used for B-mode ultrasound; so large vessels and dilated bile ducts can be carefully avoided. It can be done in fat patients and in patients having ascites.

  Two widely used pSWE techniques that are commercially available are: Virtual Touch Quantification or VTQ (Siemens Healthcare) and ElastPQ (Philips Healthcare).
- *Two-dimensional (2D) shear wave elastography:* Two-dimensional (2D) SWE utilizes acoustic radiation force. Rather than interrogating a solitary focal location like in ARFI strain imaging and pSWE, it interrogates many focal zones in rapid succession at a speed higher than that of speed of the shear wave. This forms a cone of shear wave and shear waves can be monitored in 2D to measure shear wave speed or Young's modulus E and also generate quantitative elastograms. The systems using 2D-SWE are:

  Virtual Touch Imaging Quantification (VTIQ/ARFI) by Siemens, Shear Wave Elastography by SuperSonic Imagine (SSI), Philips, GE Healthcare and Acoustic Structure Quantification (ASQ) by Toshiba.

Measurement

Shear wave velocity (in cms^{-1}) is used to estimate tissue stiffness and Young's modulus is calculated according to the formula: $E = 3V^2$ (E is Young's modulus in kPa, V is velocity of shear wave in cm/s).

Qualitative versus Quantitative

Shear wave elastography (SWE) gives qualitative color coded elastogram as well as quantitative maps of elasticity (in kPa) or shear wave velocity (in cm/s).

Advantages

In comparison to strain elastography, lack of tissue compression makes SWE more objective and reproducible, so, quantitative measurements are possible without the need for manual compression.

Disadvantages

Assessment of superficial structures may be difficult, as ultrasound needs certain depth to penetrate to produce shear waves.

Advances in Shear Wave Imaging

- *Spatially modulated ultrasound radiation force (SMURF):* In this technique, a linear array transducer is used to generate a radiation force beam having lateral intensity variation of a defined spatial frequency. Two pushing pulses are then transmitted and focused at the same depth laterally from the original position. This creates a shear wave of known wavelength. When this shear wave of known wavelength propagates through a tissue, we can measure its temporal frequency (by tracking the tissue motion on ultrasound, using the same transducer which was used to create the radiation force beam) and thereby derive the shear modulus of the tissue by using the equation $G = (\lambda f)^2\rho$ where f is the frequency of the propagating shear wave and ρ is the tissue density. As shear waves of a pulsed nature are used, this technique avoids interference from standing waves which are otherwise inherent in continuous wave methods. This technique therefore allows fast and accurate estimation of shear modulus with improved resolution.[20]
- *Supersonic shear wave imaging:* In supersonic shear wave imaging, the focus of the radiation force from one location is changed to multiple depths (typically five) along the beam axis. Shear waves are created at these multiple locations and these waves interfere constructively along a Mach cone to create a conical shear wave front traveling at supersonic speed. The speed of this conical shear wave is related directly to tissue stiffness and viscoelastic properties. This shear wave propagation is imaged using an ultrafast ultrasound scanner of 5000 frames/second. Single plane wave or a set of plane waves is transmitted at different angles of direction to track the shear wave. B-mode data is also acquired in real time at about 50 frames/second.
  Measurement: Shear wave propagation is measured and wave speeds are assessed to give viscoelastic moduli.[21,22]

Other Advanced Elastography Techniques

Harmonic Motion Imaging

Technique

Harmonic motion imaging (HMI) is a technique that induces dynamic tissue vibrations internally for tissue elasticity characterization. Low frequency ultrasound (10–300 Hz) produces an internal vibration that is spatially invariant. This internal vibration is then used to evaluate the tissue mechanical properties. Two separate focused ultrasound transducers are used. One transducer has a very large aperture, which is used to generate the radiation force. A small phased array transducer is placed via a hole within the larger transducer to detect motion.

HMI is different from other elastography techniques as it provides a spatially localized distribution of an oscillatory acoustic radiation force that can be applied across a wide range of frequencies. The dynamic response of the tissue at the site of interest can be related to the underlying mechanical properties, which may differentiate healthy from diseased tissue and also reliably indicate the underlying stiffness.

Applications

The same transducer, which generates the radiation force, is utilized for producing thermal lesions. This allows real time and simultaneous generation and monitoring of high intensity focused ultrasound (HIFU) therapy. Tissue stiffening signifying successful ablation can be monitored and the treatment procedure can be performed in a time-efficient manner. Real time monitoring of RF ablation of arrhythmogenic foci in the heart may help spare the surrounding healthy myocardium from ablation.[23]

Shear Wave Dispersion Ultrasound Vibrometry

Technique

This involves creating a harmonic shear wave by an extrinsic actuator or by acoustic radiation force using a time-varying radiation force. Multiple pushing pulses or excitation pulses are transmitted at a particular frequency and tissue motion stimulated at harmonic frequencies at known distances from the vibration source is detected by ultrasound tracking. The resultant phase shift is determined from the tissue motion data as a function of distance from vibration source to derive the shear wave length.

Measurement

Shear wave speed dispersion is measured from the data generated at several frequencies. Dispersion of shear wave gives a measurement of the viscoelastic properties of tissue.

Mechanical Imaging

Stress patterns of internal structures of tissue are measured by compressing the tissue by an ultrasound probe. Pressure sensors mounted on the contact surface of the probe detect the changes in stress pattern, thus providing assessment about the different elastic properties (viscosity and porosity).

Measurement

Surface stress data is recorded, allowing 2D and 3D reconstruction of tissues on the basis of elasticity. Nonlinear elasticity imaging which is most sensitive to cancerous changes can be evaluated by mechanical imaging.[24]

Applications

Detection of cancer and differentiating benign from malignant lesions.

ELASTOGRAPHY APPLICATIONS

Breast

As breast cancer is harder than the adjoining breast parenchyma because of desmoplastic reaction, characterization of breast masses to differentiate benign lesions from malignant, was an initial application of ultrasound elastography.[25] The evaluation of hardness has the same principle as that of conventional clinical palpation of any breast lump. Cancer generally appears darker than benign lesions and the adjoining normal breast tissue on elastography.[26] When used as an adjunct to grayscale USG, elastography can help the radiologist to give an appropriate category of Breast Imaging Reporting and Data System (BIRADS) classification. Lately, elasticity of breast masses is included as an adjunct feature in the 5th edition of BIRADS US lexicon.

The two commonly used elastography techniques in breast are strain elastography and shear wave elastography.

Strain Elastography

Different parameters are used to differentiate benign from malignant breast masses, with the commonly used parameter being elasticity score (Tsukuba score).[27] It is a proposed scoring system for the lesions as seen on 'color maps', which is based upon elastographic properties of the tissue.

Elastography Score (Fig. 5)

Score 1: Manifestation of chromatic tristratification (Blue/green/red).

Score 2: Manifestation of green with few, if any blue spots with non-constant locations.

Score 3: Predominantly green but with few blue spots.

Score 4: Almost completely blue, with some green points, mostly in periphery.

Score 5: Completely blue, also with a peripheral blue halo around the nodule.

When cut-off was taken between 3–4 for elastography score, there was 86.5% sensitivity, 89.8% specificity and 88.3% accuracy for diagnosis of malignant breast lesions in the initial study by Itoh et al.[27] A meta-analysis of 22 strain elastography studies which mainly used the 5-point elasticity score for the diagnosis of malignant breast lesions, revealed overall mean sensitivity of 83% and specificity 84%.[28] Elastography score, however, gives information regarding estimated strain at a particular tissue location, but is not quantitative[29] **(Figs. 6 to 9)**. Therefore, other semi-quantitative methods have been developed, one is the distance-ratio, in which the lesion is measured on elastogram and divided by measurement of the lesion on grayscale USG. Malignant lesions usually appear larger on elastography due to stromal response to breast cancer. Therefore, a distance ratio cut off >1.0 is taken as malignant and <1.0 as benign.[30] Another method of semi-quantitative assessment is 'strain ratio' between the nodule and adjoining normal breast parenchyma.[31]

As strain elastography has limitations of inter- and intraobserver variability and dependability on operator's expertise, quantitative methods of SWE are being increasingly used.

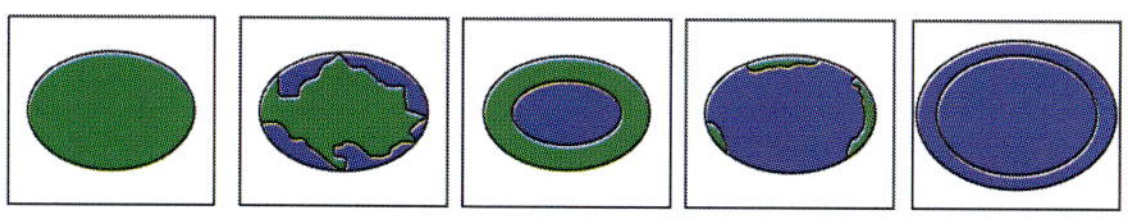

FIG. 5: Colored diagrams representing the appearance of elasticity score of breast nodule in Tsukuba scoring of 1(a), 2(b), 3(c), 4(d) and 5(e).

Shear Wave Elastography

In SWE, rather than applying mechanical external compression, the system remotely induces mechanical vibration by using acoustic radiation force created by a focused ultrasound beam. Displacement caused at the focus produces a shear wave which conveys information regarding the local viscoelastic tissue properties.[32] The interpretation and measurement of elasticity is done by Young's modulus (in kPa). It is evaluated either as a single value by a small ROI or can be taken for each point in box (FOV) displayed as a color map[33] **(Fig. 10)**. On color map, scale range from 0 to 180 kPa is used for breast masses (red-hard).[34] It is reported that mean elasticity values are noticeably greater in malignant (153.3 kPa 58.1) than in benign masses (46.1 kPa ± 42.9).[35]

With these methods, elastography can help in upgrading a mass of low suspicion, (BIRADS 3) or in down-staging a mass which is classified as BIRADS 4A (which would otherwise be sent for biopsy).[36]

Recently, elastography is also being used for assessment of neoadjuvant chemotherapy response. Breast cancers which are hard on strain elastography may less often show a complete pathological response after neoadjuvant chemotherapy than softer malignancies.[37] Few studies show correlation between histological types of breast cancer with elastography features, however, it's still an area of research and more studies are needed for validation.

Limitations

It is difficult to distinctively designate complex masses with mixed solid and cystic components. Some benign masses like hyalinized fibroadenoma, fat necrosis with fibrosis can also be stiff and some mucinous carcinomas can be soft. Posterior breast masses are difficult to assess with strain elastography.[38]

Liver

Diffuse Liver Diseases: Fibrosis, Cirrhosis, Acute Hepatitis, Nonalcoholic Fatty Liver Disease

In diffuse liver diseases, imaging modalities like B-mode ultrasound, CT and MRI have limited role in identifying liver fibrosis and early cirrhosis.

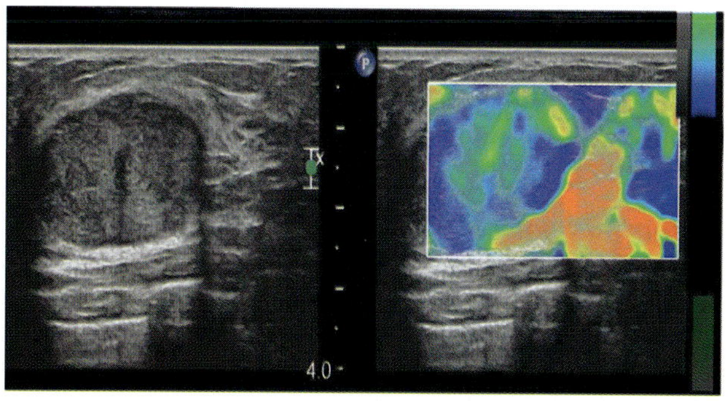

FIG. 6: Elastography image of fibroadenoma showing elastography score 2, shows it to be predominantly green, with few blue areas (spots) of no strain in the periphery. B-mode image shows well-defined ovoid hypoechoic nodule with posterior acoustic enhancement.

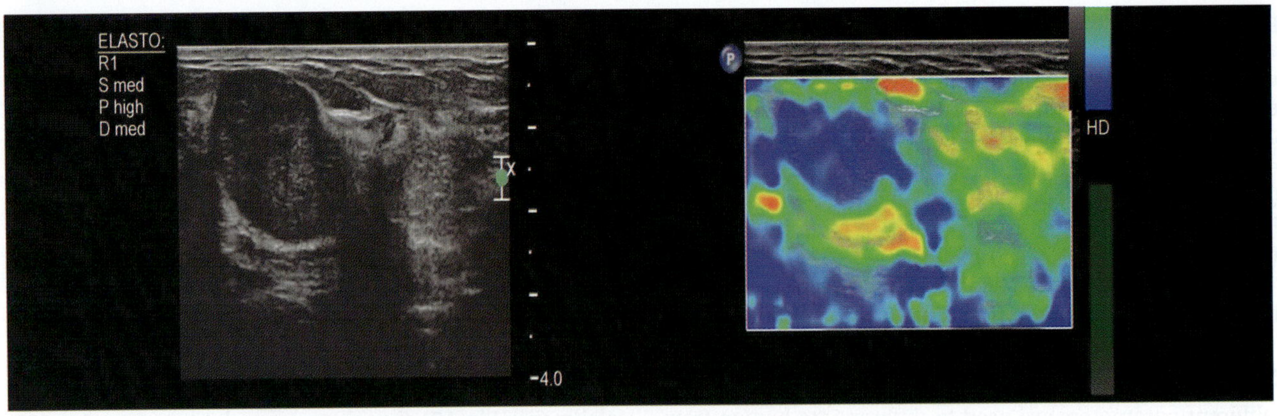

FIG. 7: Elastographic image of another fibroadenoma showing elastography score 3 with more central blue areas of no strain.

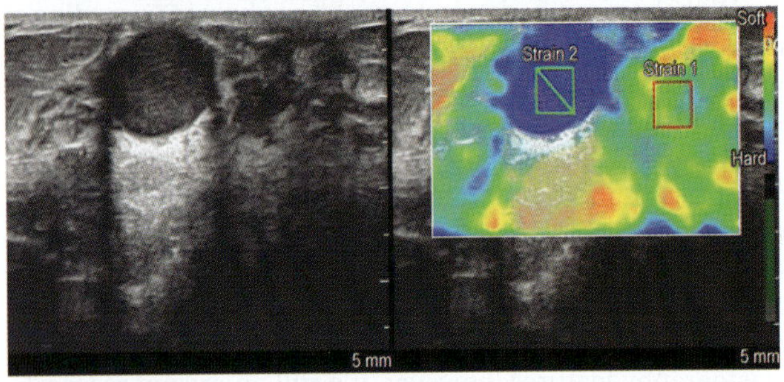

FIG. 8: Elastography image of IDC breast shows elastography score 4 with complete lesion appearing blue with no strain. It differs from elastography score 5 as there is no peripheral blue halo around the mass. There was strain ratio of 4.4 between the lesion and the adjoining normal breast.

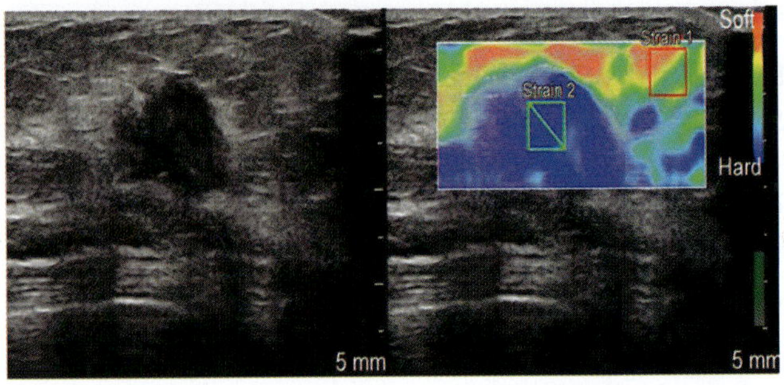

FIG. 9: Elastography image of IDC breast shows elastography score 5 with blue area of no strain in the lesion as well as in the peripheral halo.

On ultrasound, hyperechoic nodular liver may be present in both liver fibrosis as well as fatty liver. A normal CT or MRI cannot rule out cirrhosis. Liver biopsy has been the gold standard method for the diagnosis of hepatic inflammation and fibrosis. However, it is not only an invasive procedure with accompanying risks and complications, but also can have sampling errors as only a small volume of the liver is sampled.

Elastography (by ultrasound or magnetic resonance) is a noninvasive modality for assessment of fibrosis and degree of fibrosis. It is painless, reproducible and repeatable and easy to perform, allowing monitoring of disease. Although MRI elastography is sensitive for evaluation of fibrosis, it has limited availability, is time consuming and costly and therefore is not suitable for screening patients for presence or degree of fibrosis.

Factors Influencing Liver Stiffness

- Chronic liver parenchymal pathology may cause changes in liver stiffness by inducing fibrotic changes.
  On liver biopsy, fibrosis can be divided into four stages:[39]
  - *Stage 0 (normal):* No fibrosis around portal triads
  - *Stage 1 (portal fibrosis):* Fibrosis surrounds the portal triads, but is limited to these areas
  - *Stage 2 (periportal fibrosis):* Fibers begin to extend into the periportal space, but do not connect with other portal triads
  - *Stage 3 (septal fibrosis):* Fibrous connective tissue links neighboring portal triads and begins to extend to the central veins. Shape of lobule is distorted
  - *Stage 4 (cirrhosis):* Most portal triads are connected by fibrous tissue. Some portal triads and central veins are also connected.
- Necro-inflammatory activity in the setting of acute hepatitis which causes hepatocyte swelling, edema and inflammatory infiltration also may increase liver stiffness. Patients with acute hepatitis (viral, autoimmune and drug-induced) may have a discrepancy between the liver stiffness measurement (LSM) and the fibrosis grade by biopsy.
  Liver stiffness may be in the cirrhotic range (above 12.5 kPa) whereas fibrosis staging by biopsy is not more than stage 2. Similar increase in stiffness measurement is found in cases of chronic viral hepatitis who have acute increase in severity of the disease associated with rise in alanine amino transferase.[40]
- Congestive cardiac failure and extrahepatic cholestasis or congestive heart failure. Light meals also alter elastography values.[41-43]

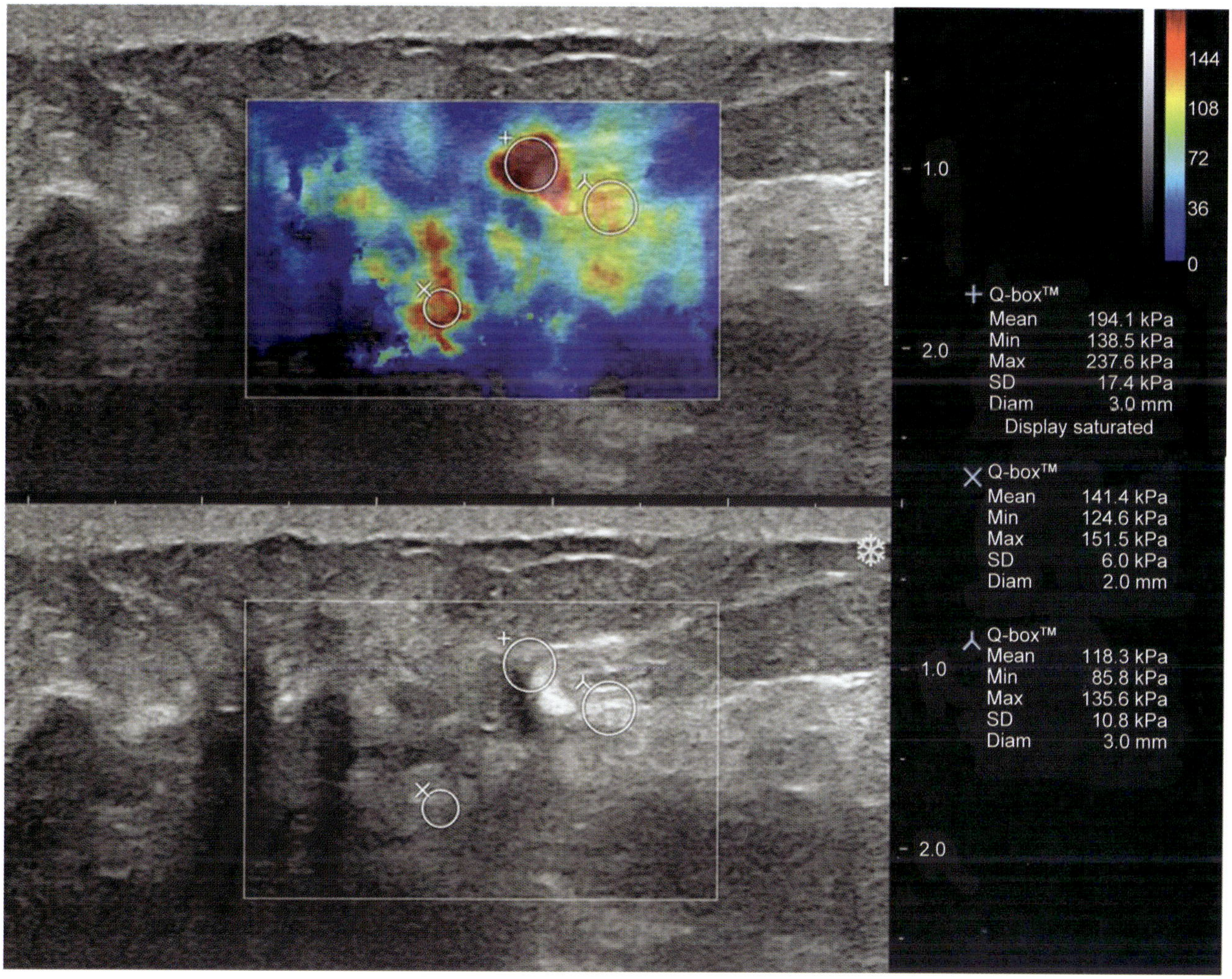

FIG. 10: Shear wave elastography image of malignant breast lesion showing red color in hard tissue with values above 130 kPa.

Ultrasound Elastography

Techniques for Liver Stiffness Measurement

Transient elastography-Fibroscan™ apparatus (Echosens, Paris, France) is a non-imaging modality which has been widely used for liver stiffness measurement **(Figs. 11A and B)**.

It uses a single cycle of low amplitude low frequency (50 Hz) vibration to induce shear wave. The shear wave velocity is faster in dense fibrotic tissue.

Transient elastography probe has a 5 MHz ultrasound probe set on a piston that acts as a vibrator. The end of the probe is kept in the space between the ribs after the patient is positioned supine with arms abducted. Under control time motion (TM) and A-mode, the sonologist chooses a part of liver in the right lobe having thickness of at least 6 cm, and which is free of large vessels as well as the gallbladder. Stiffness is measured on a cylinder of liver tissue having diameter of 1 cm and length of 2–4 cm. After ten successful acquisitions, median value in kilopascals (kPa) is taken as the liver stiffness. Measurements of 10 successful acquisitions with a success rate of at least 60%, and with Inter Quartile Range (IQR- median of the middle 50% of the values) <30% of the median value are generally considered valid.

Values vary from 2.5 to 75 kPa, with normal values about 5.5 kPa. Wide range of hepatic stiffness values are observed in patients with cirrhosis (13–75 kPa).[44] Transient elastography has excellent accuracy in diagnosing cirrhosis and significant degrees of fibrosis.

Comparison Between pSWE (ARFI), Real Time Elastography and Transient Elastography for Liver Stiffness Measurement (Table 1)

pSWE also has equal reliability in diagnosing liver fibrosis. pSWE is more sensitive for lesser degrees of fibrosis. Acute exacerbations of chronic liver disease have less influence on the liver stiffness by pSWE.[45,46]

Values for the liver stiffness measured with transient elastography cannot be directly compared with pSWE or real time (shear wave) elastography since in the former a low frequency low amplitude pulse is given. This will lead to lower values when compared with real time elastography.

The liver stiffness values with transient elastography have a wide range (2.5–75 kPa), whereas pSWE values are in a very limited range (0.5–4.4 m/s). This might make it difficult to differentiate normal form abnormal values with pSWE in

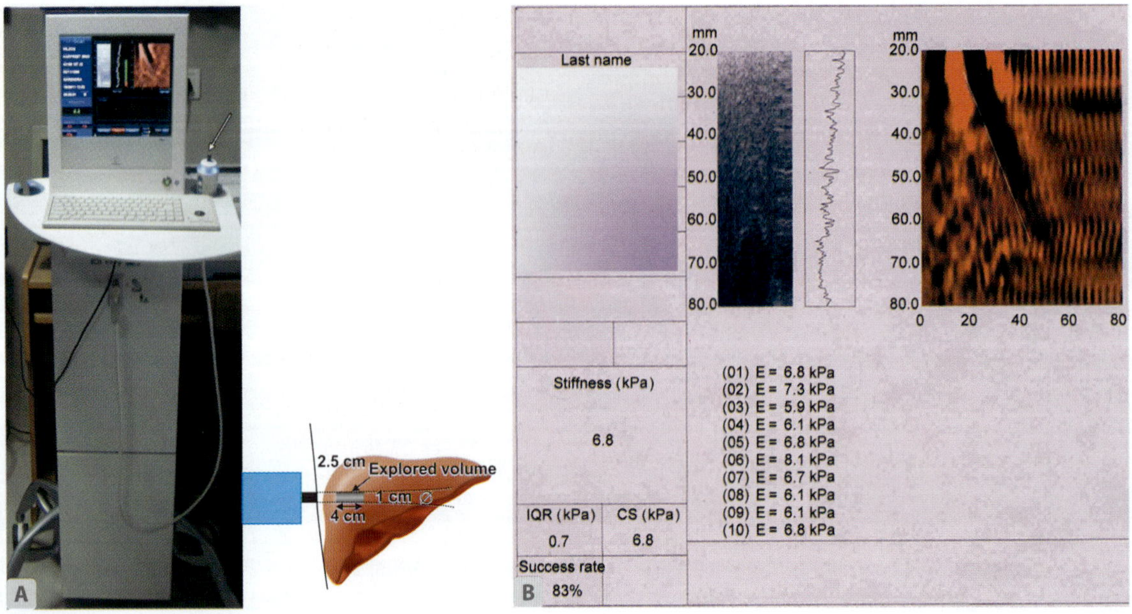

FIGS. 11A AND B: Image of the Fibroscan device (Echosens, Paris) for transient elastography. (A) The probe has a piston (arrow), which is placed in the right intercostal space. A single low frequency vibration is generated and shear wave elasticity in a cylinder of 1 cm × 4 cm of hepatic tissue is measured (inset). Measurements of 10 successful acquisitions in a normal liver (B) with a success rate of at least 60%, and with InterQuartile Range (IQR- median of the middle 50% of the values) <30% of the median are taken.

Courtesy: Dr Ajay Duseja, Professor, Department of Hepatology, PGIMER, Chandigarh.

TABLE 1: Comparison of different elastography techniques for liver diseases.

	Fibroscan (Transient elastography)	pSWE/ARFI	Shear wave elastography
Imaging	Not possible	Yes	Yes
Assessment of focal lesions	Possible for large (>5 cm) and superficial lesions. Requires prior localization with B-mode imaging. No real time image guidance	Yes	Yes Different areas within focal lesion can also be measured
Maximum depth of tissue for assessment	2.5–6.5 cm from skin	10 cm from skin	8 cm from skin
Maximum region of interest	1 cm × 5 cm	0.6 × 0.5 cm – 0.6 × 10 mm	Variable
Technique	Static –no images generated	Static images	Real time 2D evaluation
Obesity	Difficult (better with XL probe)	Less difficult	Less difficult
Ascites	Difficult to impossible	Difficult assessment	Difficult assessment
Quantification	Yes	Possible	Yes
Range of values	Large	Small	Large

a clinical setting, although values in healthy donors range between 0.85 and 1.25 m/sec.[44,47]

Post-treatment Assessment

Elastography is also used for measuring liver stiffness changes in responders and relapsers undergoing antiviral treatment with interferon and ribavirin. Liver stiffness measurements show significant decrease in patients of viral hepatitis undergoing treatment with interferon and ribavirin. Relapse after treatment also leads to increase in stiffness.[48]

Liver stiffness measurements can also predict development of hepatocellular carcinoma (HCC) in chronic hepatitis B patients.[49]

Assessment of Portal Hypertension/Varices

Hepatic venous pressure gradient (HVPG) is the reference standard for measuring portal venous pressure (values >6 mm Hg). However, it is an invasive procedure. Patients having cirrhosis and gastroesophageal varices have an HVPG of at least 10–12 mm Hg. Variceal bleed, ascites or encephalopathy may develop when HVPG increases over a threshold value of 10–12 mm Hg.

Splenic elasticity has a directly proportional relationship with HVPG and can predict the occurrence of esophageal varices in chronic liver disease.

Values of splenic stiffness above 8.7 kPa correlates with HPVG above 6 mm Hg and values above 17.6– 23 kPa correlate with severe portal hypertension (HVPG >12 mm Hg). Splenic stiffness measurements show better and linear correlation with the degree of portal hypertension than liver stiffness measurements. Combination of the liver stiffness with spleen diameter and platelet count however better correlates with degree of portal hypertension.[50]

Assessment of TIPSS

Splenic stiffness also decreases significantly with a functional TIPSS, whereas liver stiffness measurements do not show significant changes.[51]

Assessment of Liver Transplant

Regular liver stiffness measurements (LSM) after transplant can differentiate slow from rapid fibroses (fibrosis stage F2-F4 at 1st year). Liver transplant recipients with hepatitis C virus infection undergo rapid fibrosis within the first year. Serial measurements of elastography within the first year shows much higher LSM than non-HCV infected recipients; (9.9, 9.5, 12.1 kPa vs 6.9, 7.5, 6.6 kPa).[52]

Assessment of Nonalcoholic Fatty Liver Disease

Nonalcoholic fatty liver disease (NAFLD) comprises a range of disorders with hepatic steatosis without alcohol consumption, viral, or drug-related etiologies. Histologically, it can be a simple accumulation of triglyceride droplets in hepatocytes or may progress to cellular injury and inflammation with resultant fibrosis and even cirrhosis and HCC.

Fibrosis and cirrhosis due to NAFLD can be detected by transient elastography or other routine elastographic techniques. A newer technique of Controlled Attenuation Parameter (CAP) gives an estimate of the attenuation of ultrasound at 3.5 MHz and is given in decibels per meter (dB/m). CAP is assessed by the same radiofrequency data and in the same region of interest as that for transient elastography and is a non-imaging-based modality which shows promise in assessing the degree of steatosis noninvasively.[53]

Advantages

Elastography is a noninvasive, painless and repeatable procedure.

- It can evaluate a much larger liver volume than liver biopsy.
- It can be used for initial assessment, monitoring as well as diagnosis of complications (portal hypertension, esophageal varices).
- It can help in biopsy planning from stiffest regions to reduce sampling error.
- Tumor ablation monitoring is also possible real time with this procedure.

Limitations

Liver thickness of <4 cm under probe, ascites, excessive obesity, and non-availability of sufficiently wide intercostal space for probe placement limit the usage of elastography. Male sex, body mass index >30, metabolic syndrome and acute viral hepatitis are all known to cause increased liver stiffness.[54]

Focal Liver Lesions

pSWE/ARFI

Malignant and benign liver lesions were stiffer on comparison with the adjacent liver on ARFI in a study by Shuang-Ming T et al.[55] Significant differences were seen amongst malignant and benign hepatic lesions. The median values for hepatic malignant and benign lesions were 3.14 m/sec (avg 3.16 ± 0.80 m/sec, range 1.17–4.45 m/sec) and 1.35 m/sec (avg 1.47 ± 0.53 m/sec, range 0.74–3.26 m/sec) respectively.

A cut-off at 2.22 m/sec resulted in sensitivity, specificity, and accuracy for malignancy of 89.7%, 95.0%, and 92.2%, respectively.[55]

Compression Ultrasonography

Onur et al. evaluated focal benign and malignant liver lesions, viz., hemangiomas, focal nodular hyperplasia (FNH), adenomas, nodular regenerative hyperplasia, hepatocellular carcinomas, metastases, and cholangiocarcinomas. They compared the strain ratio of liver parenchyma to that of the focal lesion to give the strain index. Mean strain index of malignant lesions was significantly higher than that of benign lesions. For malignant liver lesions, mean strain index was 2.82 ± 1.82, which was much more than that of benign liver lesions which had a mean strain index of 1.45 ± 1.28. Stiffness of hemangiomas varies depending on the amount of fibrotic septa dividing the vascular spaces. Strain index as well as mean values of hemangiomas on ARFI (1.5–2.3 m/sec) are significantly low.[56,57]

Shear Wave

Shear wave values (in kPa), can distinguish between FNH and adenoma. FNH has a radial pattern of elasticity whereas adenomas and hemangiomas are homogeneous. Scars from radiofrequency ablation or healed abscesses have the highest stiffness values among benign lesions.

A significant difference was also found between HCCs and cholangiocarcinoma elasticity. Cholangiocarcinomas were the stiffest among malignant lesions (56.9 ± 25.6 kPa).

The HCC stiffness depends on the underlying liver, with lesions in cirrhotic livers appearing softer than lesions in normal or mildly cirrhotic livers. Metastasis stiffness also is highly variable and depends on the primary source. Carcinoid metastases are stiffer than colorectal metastases.[58]

Prostate

Endorectal ultrasound is most commonly used for assessing the prostate. On B-mode ultrasound, carcinoma prostate shows varying echogenicity with the ultrasound appearance of carcinoma prostate overlapping with that of benign prostatic hyperplasia (BPH) or prostatitis. So, the overall sensitivity is approximately of B-mode is only 50%.[59] This may lead to sampling of 6–12 cores without targeting the actual lesion.

On strain elastography, manual compression is produced by freehand.[60] Prostate cancers are stiff and have greater elastic modulus than the adjoining normal prostatic parenchyma.[61] Therefore, prostate cancers appear dark on elastograms. Sometimes, the malignant lesions which are very small or invisible on grayscale ultrasound may be conspicuous on elastogram as dark areas of lesser strain. Color coded elastograms depict strain differences in adjacent tissues by laying over the B-mode image **(Fig. 12)**. Most modern systems provide 'Quality Index' as a reference to the appropriateness of amount of compression/release which the ultrasonologist should take into consideration. Strain ratio gives the semi-quantitative parameter by placing ROIs in normal and abnormal areas.

Peripheral zone of a normal prostate has intermediate stiffness while elastography appearance of central zone varies with age and volume of the gland.[62] Benign prostatic hyperplasia appears as heterogeneous hypoechoic area on endorectal B-mode ultrasound. Area with benign hyperplasia also show higher stiffness than that of normal prostate tissue but less than that of carcinoma prostate. However, it may be difficult to differentiate between the two and sometimes it can give false-positive findings of cancer prostate.[62,63]

On shear wave elastography, in addition to interpreting color elastograms, quantitative parameters (mean, standard deviation, min, max) are obtained after placing ROI.[64] On SWE images, in young patients, normal peripheral and central zones appear homogenously blue, having stiffness value between 15–25 kPa and transitional zone has stiffness value <30 kPa. After benign prostatic hyperplasia develops, transitional zone shows heterogeneous color and stiffness values increase to 30–180 kPa. Prostatic cancer has stiffness value >35 kPa. SWE ratio can be calculated by comparing the mean stiffness of the lesion with the mean stiffness of normal prostate.

While interpreting elastograms, one should remember that neither all stiff lesions are cancers, nor all cancers are stiff. Presence of fibrosis and calcifications can also cause stiffness, therefore analysis of B-mode images is of utmost importance.

Elastography is also upcoming as a guiding tool for targeted prostate biopsies and therapy in addition to being used for staging of prostate cancer.[65]

Lymph Nodes

Grayscale ultrasound features for metastatic lymph nodes have been based on the size, shape, fatty hilum and thickening of cortex and sensitivity is more when all 4 features are present.[66,67] Elastography is also used as a potential additional imaging for lymph nodes in differentiating benign from malignant conditions. On elastography, metastatic lymph nodes show higher stiffness in comparison to adjoining soft tissue,[68] while benign inflammatory nodes show low elasticity value and may be the same as the adjacent tissue.[69] Elastography can also be used to detect the most appropriate lymph node for USG-guided biopsy.

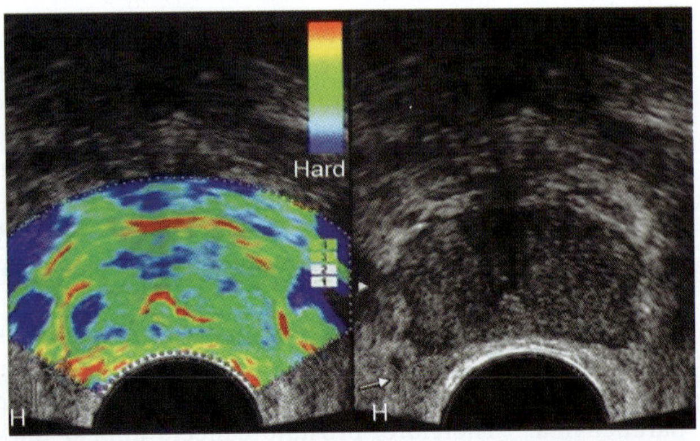

FIG. 12: Elastography image is showing hard nodule in the prostate in the right peripheral zone in blue color. Same nodule appeared hyperechoic on B-mode ultrasound image.

Lymph Node Strain Elastography

Strain elastography evaluation of lymph nodes is done by strain ratio or elasticity score in the same way as we do in breast and thyroid. For lymph nodes, we take subcutaneous fat or adjoining muscle as a reference tissue while calculating stain ratio.[69] Elasticity scores are evaluated by colored elastograms, and different scoring systems are used. 4 score pattern is widely used for axillary lymph nodes, which is as follows:

Score 1: Absent or Very Small Blue Area

Score 2: Small, scattered blue area, total blue area <45%

Score 3: Large blue area, total blue area >45%

Score 4: Blue area with or without a green rim.

Reported elasticity score of metastatic axillary lymph nodes is (3.1 ± 0.7), which is much greater than the score for reactive lymph nodes (2.2 ± 0.7; p<.001).[70] When the cut-off is taken between 2 and 3, the sensitivity and specificity is approximately 80%. Status of axillary lymph nodes is the most important prognosticating factor in patients having breast malignancy.

Similar kind of scoring has been done for cervical lymph nodes by Deng ke-teng et al in which they found that most benign lymph nodes show elasticity score 1 or 2 and most of malignant nodes show elasticity score 3 or 4 with sensitivity and specificity of 88.4% and 35.1% respectively. They also calculated the strain ratio which showed strain ratio cut-off for malignant >1.78 and for benign <1.78 with sensitivity and specificity of 98.1 % and 64.9% respectively.[71]Another study done by Alam et al to distinguish enlarged cervical lymph nodes into reactive and metastatic nodes based on elasticity score showed 100% specificity and 83% sensitivity.[72]

Shear Wave Elastography

Shear wave elastography is also now widely used for lymph node assessment especially axillary and cervical lymph nodes. Specificity of SWE for predicting malignancy in some studies has been reported to be 100%.[73] In a recent study for axillary nodes, cut-off elasticity value of 25 kPa showed 94% sensitivity and 86% specificity for categorizing nodes into benign and malignant.[74]

The main limitation in elastography evaluation is lack of standardization of reference tissue for strain ratio in strain imaging; subcutaneous fat and muscles being used in different studies. Other limitation is that some malignancies like lymphoma do not increase the stiffness of lymph nodes, which may give false negative result on elastography, thereby implying the use of elastography only as an adjunct to grayscale ultrasound.

Thyroid

Another area of potential usefulness is the evaluation of thyroid nodules because the ultrasonic and nuclear medicine features for differentiating nodules into benign and malignant are not reliable. A number of articles have shown the potential utility of nodular stiffness for characterizing them as malignant.[75,76] Similar to those in breast and other nodular lesions, the malignant thyroid nodule is stiffer than the benign thyroid nodules. Mainly semi-quantitative methods with compression elastography using strain index have been utilized. The strain index is calculated by dividing nodule strain value by the strain of adjoining normal thyroid. Good quality elastography of thyroid is challenging because of the shape of neck with sloping contour, which can cause lateral movement of thyroid and the pulsation from the adjoining carotid artery. Even with these technical difficulties as more and more results are reported, it can be used to help in deciding which nodule to be biopsied when there are many nodules present.[77] For diffuse diseases of the thyroid, quantitative or semi-quantitative elastography is used. One study with shear wave velocity analysis showed increased stiffness in case of Hashimoto's thyroiditis.[78]

Gynecology

Cervix

MR is considered to be the modality of choice for imaging in cervical cancer. However, transvaginal ultrasound (TVUS) with elastography can also be used to image cervical cancers and because of its easy availability, it can be particularly useful in follow up studies.

The strain ratios of benign cervical lesions are lower than that for malignant lesions.[79] Endophytic cervical growths, which can be missed on clinical examination as well as grayscale/Doppler USG can be picked up using elastography. Elastography can also be used for monitoring treatment response. In a study by Mabuchi et al.,[80] the Strain Ratio (SR) of treated tumors reduced significantly in patients who achieved complete response. On the other hand, in patients who had residual disease, the SR did not reduce significantly.

Transvaginal elastography of the cervix, however, lacks a proper reference tissue for comparison and strain ratio is obtained by dividing the mean strain within the lesion by the mean strain from the parametrium. In cases having infiltration of parametrial tissue by tumor, there would be errors in strain ratio measurement as parametrial tissue is taken as reference.

Moreover, normal cervix itself has heterogeneous elasticity and the portion of the cervix nearest the transducer tip is prone to compression and even the mildest movement or pressure may result in erroneous impression of softening.

Uterus

In a study by Stoelinga et al.,[81] uniform color was seen in the uterine myometrium. Fibroids were found to be stiffer than normal myometrium which in turn were stiffer than adenomyomas. Fibroids were reported to be well defined with a stiff center as compared to adenomyosis/adenomyomas which had a softer center. Fibroids with red or hyaline degeneration had lower elastic coefficients than non-degenerated fibroids.[82]

Elastography has also been used to differentiate between endometrial polyps and submucosal fibroids with the former having a lesser "Elasto Strain Ratio."[83]

Pathological endometrium is also well picked up using elastography and can be differentiated from normal endometrium. The pathological endometrium is stiffer than the normal endometrium with endometrial hyperplasia and cancer showing the highest stiffness values.[84]

Ovaries

Another interesting application of elastography was described in polycystic ovary syndrome (PCOS) by Ciraci et al.[85] They found ovaries in patients with PCOS to be stiffer than normal ovaries.

Applications in Pregnancy

The use of elastography in monitoring cervical stiffness during pregnancy has also been well described in literature.[86,87] The reported techniques have minimal inter- and intra-observer variations.[88]

Role of elastography has been studied in the prediction of success of induction of labor.[89] Significant differences have been found in the elastography indices obtained from the internal os region between the patients with successful induction as compared to patients with failed induction. Softer internal os was associated with successful induction. A soft internal os and harder external parts of the cervix are indicators of a favorable response to oxytocin during labor induction. This can also help in deciding whether prostaglandins are required. Failed induction rates were higher in patients with increased stiffness of the internal os.

Cervical elastography has also been used to predict preterm birth with good correlation.[90] In a meta-analysis by Londero et al.[91] elastography had a sensitivity of 67% and specificity of 94.4% in predicting preterm delivery. Elastography was also found to perform better than cervical length in predicting preterm delivery.

Placental elastography is also emerging as a powerful tool in predicting various maternal and fetal complications of pregnancy. Applications of placental elastography have been described in preeclampsia, gestational growth mellitus (GDM) and intrauterine growth restriction (IUGR). In patients with pre-eclampsia, placental stiffness is increased, as compared to normal patients, more so in the central regions of the cord.[92] Using a cut-off value of 7.35 KPa had a sensitivity of 90% and specificity of 92% for the diagnosis of pre-eclampsia. Thus, shear wave elastography can function as an additional diagnostic tool in such patients.

Soft Tissue Masses

Shear wave elastography has not been found to play a significant role in differentiating benign from malignant masses, although it does have an adjunct role along with ultrasound.[93,94]

However, significant differences in shear wave modulus has been found in superficial benign tumors such as epidermoid cysts, ganglion cysts and lipomatous lesions in a study by Yeoh et al.[95]

Strain ratio is lower in malignant soft tissue tumors in comparison to benign tumors and can aid in predicting malignant potential. However, some overlap exists and a single cut-off value is not possible to help in differentiation.[96]

Musculoskeletal

Compression ultrasonography has been the most commonly used technique for musculoskeletal applications. Strain of the region of interest is compared with the remaining tissue (usually fat) within the elastogram. The semi-quantitative measurement method includes the ratio of the relative strains between the area of interest and a reference area. The ARFI and shear wave elasticity imaging are being increasingly used for musculoskeletal applications **(Fig. 13)**.

Appearance of Normal Tendons

Compression Elastography

In healthy volunteers, the normal Achilles tendons were either homogeneously hard or in the majority exhibited inhomogeneity with soft areas (longitudinal bands or spots), which did not correspond to any abnormality in B-mode or Doppler ultrasound.[97]

Shear Wave

Shear wave elastography has also been used to measure mean elasticity values of muscles. There was no significant correlation between age and elasticity for the muscles. However, some differences in elasticity values were found in men and women.[98]

Tendinopathy

Symptomatic tendons showed marked softening in 57%, mild softening in 11% and no soft areas (hard structures) in 32% of cases.[99] Mild softening did not correlate with conventional ultrasound abnormalities, whereas marked softening was found mainly in cases with ultrasound evidence of disease. This could signify either a false positive finding or the increased sensitivity of elastography in early diagnosis.

Another study has found increasing stiffness in diseased tendons, probably reflecting the stage of the disease, with fibrosis being the predominant component.[100] Increased stiffness of extensor tendon has been noted in lateral epicondylitis, with elastography being more sensitive than conventional ultrasound.[101]

Zhang et al. showed a positive correlation between tendon function and elasticity, with lower elastic modulus values predictive of poor functional outcomes.[102] Ultrasound elastography also has a role in predicting post-operative failure rates in rotator cuff tendon repair. Compression ultrasonography can quantify degree of fatty infiltration and atrophy, which is a prognostic indicator of repair failure. Thus, it can help in preoperative patient selection.[103]

Normal Muscle

Relaxed muscle is inhomogeneous with intermediate or increased stiffness (green/yellow or blue color, respectively) with scattered softer and harder areas especially at the periphery near boundaries.[97]

Exercise

Elastography has also shown increase in muscle hardness (changes in strain ratio) immediately after exercise which lasted from 30 minutes to 4 days.[104,105]

Rheumatological Disorders

Soft tissue nodules: Rheumatoid nodules were significantly less elastic than tophi, indicating a possible role of this method for the investigation of soft tissue nodules.[106]

Synovitis: Benign conditions such as inflammatory synovitis due to rheumatoid arthritis were shown to be of intermediate stiffness; infectious synovitis (due to tuberculosis), fatty villous proliferations (lipoma arborescens) and pigmented villonodular synovitis were predominantly soft, while malignancies like synovial sarcoma were hard.[107]

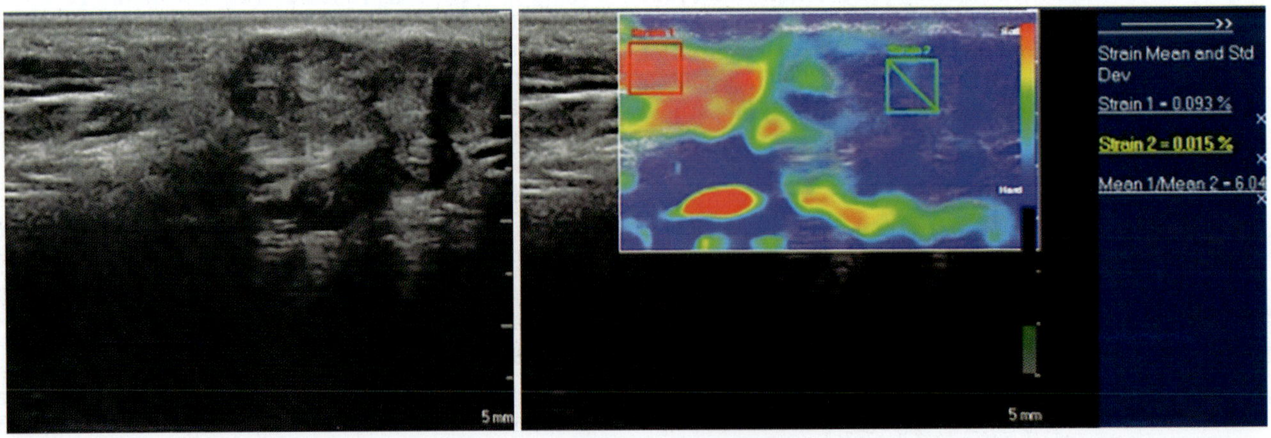

FIG. 13: A 15-year-old boy presented with painless swelling around the palmar aspect of right hand for 8 months. Ultrasound shows hypoechoic swelling on the palmar aspect of the right hand (arrow). Mean strain ratio was 4.83. Color score was 3. Histopathologically it was a benign giant cell tumor of the tendon sheath.

Skin: Elasticity of skin over the forearm in scleroderma patients has been evaluated with compression elastography showing predominantly blue areas (hard) as compared to green (intermediate) stiffness in controls.[108]

Myofascial Pain

Elastography has also been utilized in identifying active trigger points in myofascial pain, which is a major cause of non-articular pain with motor and sensory symptoms. Measurements have shown increased hardness in trigger points as compared to normal areas. This helps in objective classification instead of the subjective clinical assessment of nodular hard areas in involved muscles.[109]

Strain ratios also decreased after treatment of the trigger points, pointing to the possibility of objective assessment of treatment.[110]

Inflammatory/Dystrophic Conditions

In inflammatory myositis, increased stiffness due to fibrosis and decrease in fatty infiltration has been documented using compression strain imaging. Elastography has shown correlation with serum markers in inflammatory myopathies and could help in disease monitoring.[111]

However, although ultrasound elastography may detect abnormalities in areas of increased muscle echogenicity due to myositis, there is lack of association between ultrasound and MRI findings in patients with proven inflammatory myositis.[112]

Elastography may also be more sensitive in detecting dystrophic changes in muscle stiffness earlier than ultrasound and MRI.[113]

In spasticity due to cerebral palsy, elastography has helped to establish site of botulinum toxin injection.[114]

Hyaline Cartilage: Evaluation of elasticity of hyaline cartilage may help in evaluation prior to arthroscopy and in monitoring treatment.[115]

Standardization

Standardization is required, especially in musculoskeletal imaging. Differences in applied transducer pressure and ROI size can affect the elastic modulus even on shear wave imaging significantly. The larger the ROIs size, the higher the chance to include the muscle fascia, dense collagen fiber and/or bone. This leads to increase in the maximum value of elastic modulus, although mean values over large areas may remain the same. Increase in acquisition times may also lead to slippage of transducer from intended position.

Elastography on muscle and tendon should be performed with the lightest transducer pressure and a shorter acquisition time.[116] For the Achilles tendon, the suggested standard size for longitudinal scans is a depth of three times the tendon and about three-quarters of the screen, and for transverse scans the para-Tenon should be included.[117]

Role in Musculoskeletal Imaging

Elastography may be utilized for early diagnosis, staging and monitoring inflammatory, degenerative, myopathic or dystrophic conditions. It may also have a role in guiding interventions. However, clinical utility and validity of ultrasound elastography in musculoskeletal applications is still to be established by further studies involving larger number of patients.

OTHER APPLICATIONS

Renal Transplant Assessment

Elastography has also been utilized to diagnose allograft injury. Elastography assesses allograft stiffness, and serial increase in stiffness is an indication for biopsy even before deterioration of renal function. Stiffness shows direct correlation to the extent of interstitial fibrosis and inverse correlation to estimated glomerular filtration rate (eGFR).[118] However, detection of subclinical rejection, infection or recurrence of underlying disease poses difficulty.[119]

Cardiovascular Applications

The two main fields in cardiovascular applications are strain imaging of atheromatous plaques and of the myocardium. Vulnerable plaques are much softer than stable plaques. In a study by Kumar et al.,[120] symptomatic carotid plaques were found to have lower Young's modulus than asymptomatic patients.

Myocardial evaluation assesses focal areas of ischemia, infarction, and scarring. No extrinsic pressure or vibration is applied during elasticity evaluation. Internal physiologic myocardial and vessel wall movements during cardiac cycle are made use of. This technique was found to precisely characterize normal myocardial function throughout a whole cardiac cycle and in detecting and localizing myocardial infarction in vivo.[121]

Venous Thrombosis

Elasticity imaging is also used for evaluation of venous thrombosis.[122] As thrombi become stiff with time,[123] elasticity imaging may assess the age of thrombi. This is important because newer thrombi carry risk of embolization in comparison to old fibrotic thrombi.

Dermatological Applications

Elastography can visualize skin and soft tissue components, including the abscess cavity and surrounding induration. Some patients who do not respond to therapy might progress to more invasive infections, either by local spread to deeper tissue or by systemic spread via bacteremia. On B-mode ultrasound, contents of an abscess cavity can be distinguished from the surrounding tissue, whereas in elastography, by measuring tissue stiffness, the indurated tissue surrounding the abscess cavity can be seen. The size of the tissue indurations may predict progression to bacteremia or the time to resolution.[124]

Endoscopic Ultrasonography

Endoscopic ultrasonography (EUS) elastography is a novel advance in gastrointestinal endoscopy as it can be performed with routine EUS probes without any additional equipment needed to induce vibration or pressure. On elastography, the normal pancreas depicts an even, homogeneous green color (indicating intermediate stiffness) throughout the parenchyma. A predominantly green pattern, either homogeneous or heterogeneous, excludes malignancy with high accuracy, whereas a predominantly blue pattern points towards a malignant tumor.[125]

CONCLUSION

Elastography is a useful adjunct to B-mode ultrasound. Elastograms depict tissue stiffness in color or grayscale. Hard or low strain areas are darker gray, whereas soft tissues with high strain areas depict lighter gray. The rapidly advancing field of tissue elasticity imaging has several applications.

Current progresses in elastography include quantitative evaluation using strain ratios, acoustic radiation force impulse imaging, and shear wave velocity assessment. These are being increasingly used for characterization of focal masses and also for diagnosis of diffuse diseases, like cirrhosis. Other upcoming applications include prostate cancer detection, renal transplant evaluation, atheromatous plaque and myocardial evaluation, venous thrombus evaluation, and endoscopic elastography. Though recently magnetic resonance elastography is coming into vogue, ultrasound will always remain the preferred modality for elastography as it is less expensive and easier to use.

REFERENCES

1. Palmeri ML, Nightingale KR. What challenges must be overcome before ultrasound elasticity imaging is ready for the clinic? Imaging Med. 2011;3:433-44.
2. Duck F. Physical Properties of Tissue, A Comprehensive Reference Book. NY; Academic Press; 1990.
3. Sarvazyan A, Skovaroda AR, Emelianov SY, et al. Biophysical bases of elasticity imaging. Acoust Imaging. 1995;21: 223-40.
4. Sarvazyan, A. Handbook of Elastic Properties of Solids, Liquids and Gases. Elastic properties of soft tissue. 2001.pp. 107-27.
5. Wells PNT, Liang HD. Medical ultrasound: imaging of soft tissue strain and elasticity. JR Soc. Interface. 2011;8(64): 1521-49.
6. Garra BS. Imaging and estimation of tissue elasticity by ultrasound. Ultrasound Q. 2007;23:255-68.
7. Fehrenbach J. Influence of Poisson's ratio on elastographic direct and inverse problems. Phys Med Biol. 2007;52: 707-16.
8. Insana MF, Pellot-Barakat C, Sridhar M, Lindfors KK. Viscoelastic imaging of breast tumor microenvironment with ultrasound. J Mammary Gland Biol Neoplasia. 2004;9:393-404.
9. Sarvazyan A, Hall TJ, Urban MW, Fatemi M, Salavat R, et al. An overview of elastography: An emerging branch of medical imaging. Curr Med Imaging Rev. 2011;7: 255-82.
10. Ginat DT, Destounis SV, Barr RG, et al. US Elastography of breast and prostate lesion. Radiographics. 2009;29: 2007-16.
11. Itoh A, Ueno E, Tohno E, Kamma H, Takahashi H, Shiina T, et al. Breast disease: clinical application of US elastography for diagnosis. Radiology. 2006;239(2):341-50.
12. Shiina T, Nitta N, Ueno EI, Bamber JC. Real time tissue elasticity imaging using the combined autocorrelation method. Journal of Medical Ultrasonics. 2002;29(3): 119-28.
13. Sigrist RMS, Liau J, Kaffas AE, Chammas MC, Willmann JK. Ultrasound Elastography: Review of Techniques and Clinical Applications. Theranostics. 2017;7(5):1303-29.
14. Tang A, Cloutier G, Szeverenyi NM, Sirlin CB. Ultrasound Elastography and MR Elastography for Assessing Liver Fibrosis: Part 1, Principles and Techniques. AJR. 2015;205:22-32.
15. Shiina T. JSUM ultrasound elastography practice guidelines: basics and terminology. Med Ultrasonics. 2013;40: 309-23.
16. Shiina T, Doyley MM, Bamber JC. Strain imaging using combined RF and envelope autocorrelation processing. In: Proceedings of the IEEE Ultrasonics Symposium. Savoy, Ill: Institute of Electrical and Electronics Engineers Ultrasonics, Ferroelectrics, and Frequency Control Digital Archive. 1996;2:1331-6.
17. Zhang M, Nigwekar P, Castaneda B, Hoyt K, Joseph JV, Agnese AD, et al. Quantitative characterization of viscoelastic properties of human prostate correlated with histology. Ultrasound Med Biol. 2008;34:1033-42.
18. Nightingale K. Acoustic Radiation Force Impulse (ARFI) Imaging: a Review. Curr Med Imaging Rev. 2011;7(4): 328-39.
19. Drakonaki EE, Allen GM, Wilson DJ. Ultrasound elastography for musculoskeletal applications. Br J Radiol. 2012;85:1435-45.
20. McAleavey SA, Menon M, Orszulak J. Shear-modulus estimation by application of spatially-modulated impulsive acoustic radiation force. Ultrason Imaging. 2007;29: 87-104.
21. Bercoff J, Tanter M, Fink M. Supersonic shear imaging: a new technique for soft tissue elasticity mapping. IEEE Trans Ultrason Ferro electr Freq Control. 2004;51:396-409.
22. Bercoff J, Muller M, Tanter M, Fink M. Studying viscoelasticity in soft tissues with supersonic shear imaging. The Journal of the Acoustical Society of America. 2004;115(5):2411-2.
23. Maleke C, Konofagou EE. In vivo feasibility of real-time monitoring of focused ultrasound surgery (FUS) using harmonic motion imaging (HMI). IEEE Trans Biomed Eng. 2010;57:7-11.
24. Krouskop TA, Wheeler TM, Kallel F, Garra BS, Hall T. Elastic moduli of breast and prostate tissues under compression. Ultrason Imaging. 1998;20:260-74.
25. Cespedes I, Ophir J, Ponnekanti H, et al. Elastography: elasticity imaging using ultrasound with application to muscle and breast in vivo. Ultrasound Imaging. 1993;15: 73-88.
26. Garra BS, Cespedes EI, Ophir J, Spratt SR, Zuurbier RA, Magnant CM, Pennanen MF. Elastography of breast lesions: initial clinical results. Radiology. 1997;202:79-86.
27. Itoh A, Ueno E, Tohno E, Kamma H, Takahashi H, Shiina T, et al. Breast disease: clinical application of US elastography for diagnosis. Radiology. 2006;239(2):341-50.
28. Gong X, Xu Q, Xu Z, Xiong P, Yan W, Chen Y. Real-time elastography for the differentiation of benign and malignant breast lesions: a meta-analysis. Breast cancer research and treatment. 2011;130:11-8.
29. Burnside ES, Hall TJ, Sommer AM, et al. Differentiating Benign from Malignant Solid Breast Masses with US Strain Imaging: Radiology. 2007;245:401-10.
30. Barr RG. Real-Time Ultrasound Elasticity of the Breast: Initial Clinical Results. Ultrasound Quarterly. 2010;26(2): 61-6.
31. Zhi H, Xiao X-Y, Yang H-Y, Wen Y-L, Ou B, Luo B-M, Liang B-I. Semi quantitating stiffness of breast solid lesions in ultrasonic elastography. Academic Radiology. 2008;15: 1347-53.
32. Tanter M, Bercoff J, Athanasiou A, et al. Quantitative assessment of breast lesion viscoelasticity: initial clinical results using supersonic shear imaging. Ultrasound Med Biol. 2008;34(9):1373-86.
33. Cosgrove D, Piscaglia F, Bamber J, Bojunga J, Correas JM, Gilja OH, et al. EFSUMB Guidelines and Recommendations on the Clinical Use of Ultrasound Elastography. Part 2: Clinical Applications. Ultraschall Med. 2013;34:283-53.

34. Lee SH, Chang JM, Cho N, Koo HR, Yi A, Kim SJ, et al. Practice guideline for the performance of breast ultrasound elastography. Ultrasonography. 2014;33(1):3-10.
35. Chang JM, et al. Clinical Applications of Shear Wave Elastography (SWE) in the diagnosis of benign and malignant breast diseases. Breast Cancer Res Treat. 2011;29(1): 89-97.
36. Shiina T, Nightingale KR, Palmeri ML, Hall TJ, Bamber JC, Barr RG, et al. WFUMB guidelines and recommendations for clinical use of ultrasound elastography: Part 1: basic principles and terminology. Ultrasound in Medicine & Biology. 2015;41(5): 1126-47.
37. Hayashi M, Yamamoto Y, Ibusuki M, Fujiwara S, Yamamoto S, Tomita S, et al. Evaluation of tumor stiffness by elastography is predictive for pathologic complete response to neoadjuvant chemotherapy in patients with breast Cancer. Ann Surg Oncol. 2012;19(9):3042-9.
38. Faruk T, Islam MK, Arefin S, Zahurul Haq M. The Journey of Elastography: Background, Current Status and Future Possibilities in Breast Cancer Diagnosis. Clin Breast Cancer. 2015;15(5):313-24.
39. Emily Carey, William D Carey. Noninvasive tests for liver disease, fibrosis, and cirrhosis: Is liver biopsy obsolete? Cleaveland Clinic J Med. 2010;77:519-27.
40. Sagir A, Erhardt A, Schmitt M, Üssinger DH. Transient elastography is unreliable for detection of cirrhosis in patients with acute liver damage. Hepatology. 2008;47: 592-5.
41. Millonig G, Reimann FM, Friedrich S, Fonouni H, Mehrabi A, Buchler MW, et al. Extrahepatic cholestasis increases liver stiffness (FibroScan) irrespective of fibrosis. Hepatology. 2008;48:1718-23.
42. Millonig G, Friedrich S, Adolf S, Fonouni H, Golriz M, Mehrabi A, et al. Liver stiffness is directly influenced by central venous pressure. J Hepatol. 2010;52:206-10.
43. Berzigotti A, de Gottardi A, Delgado MG, Seijo S, Abraldes JG, Garcia-Pagan JC, et al. Liver stiffness increases after a meal in patients with cirrhosis but its change does not correlate with the changes in HVPG. Hepatology. 2010;52:1074A.
44. Castera L. Non-invasive assessment of liver fibrosis in chronic hepatitis C. Hepatol Int. 2011;5:625-34.
45. Sporea I, Bota S, Peck-Radosavljevic M, Sirli R, Tanaka H, Iijima H, et al. Acoustic Radiation Force Impulse Elastography for fibrosis evaluation in patients with chronic hepatitis C: An international multicenter study. Eur J Radiol. 2012;81(12):4112-8.
46. Rizzo L, Calvaruso V, Cacopardo B, Alessi N, Attanasio M, Petta S, et al. Comparison of transient elastography and acoustic radiation force impulse for non-invasive staging of liver fibrosis in patients with chronic hepatitis C. Am J Gastroenterol. 2011;106(12):2112-20.
47. Son CY, Kim SU, Han WK, Choi GH, Park H, Yang SC, et al. Normal liver elasticity values using acoustic radiation force impulse imaging: a prospective study in healthy living liver and kidney donors. J Gastroenterol Hepatol. 2012;27(1):130-6.
48. Martinez SM, Foucher J, Combis JM, Métivier S, Brunetto M, Capron D, et al. Longitudinal liver stiffness assessment in patients with chronic hepatitis C undergoing antiviral therapy PLoS One. 2012;7(10):e47715.
49. Wong GL, Chan HL, Wong CK, Leung C, Chan CY, Ho PP, et al. Liver stiffness-based optimization of hepatocellular carcinoma risk score in patients with chronic hepatitis B. Liver stiffness measurement using transient elastography also predicts development of hepatocellular carcinoma in chronic hepatitis B patients. J Hepatol. 2014;60(2): 339-45.
50. Castera L, Pinzani M, Bosch J. Noninvasive evaluation of portal hypertension using transient elastography. J Hep. 2012;56: 696-703.
51. Gao J, Ran HT, Ye XP, Zheng YY, Zhang DZ, Wang ZG. The stiffness of the liver and spleen on ARFI Imaging pre and post TIPS placement: a preliminary observation. Clin Imaging. 2012;36(2):135-41.
52. Carrión JA, Torres F, Crespo G, Miquel R, García-Valdecasas JC, Navasa M, Forns X. Liver stiffness identifies two different patterns of fibrosis progression in patients with hepatitis C virus recurrence after liver transplantation. Hepatology. 2010;51(1): 23-34.
53. Sasso M, Beaugrand M, de Ledinghen V, Douvin C, Marcellin P, Poupon R, et al. Controlled attenuation parameter (CAP): a novel VCTE™ guided ultrasonic attenuation measurement for the evaluation of hepatic steatosis: preliminary study and validation in a cohort of patients with chronic liver disease from various causes. Ultrasound Med Biol. 2010;36(11):1825-35.
54. Roulot D, Czernichow S, Le Clésiau H, Costes JL, Vergnaud AC, Beaugrand M. Liver stiffness values in apparently healthy subjects: influence of gender and metabolic syndrome. J Hepatol. 2008;48:606-13.
55. Shuang-Ming T, Ping Z, Ying Q, Li-Rong C, Ping Z, Rui-Zhen L. Usefulness of acoustic radiation force impulse imaging in the differential diagnosis of benign and malignant liver lesions. Acad Radiol. 2011;18(7): 810-5.
56. Onur MR, Poyraz AK, Ucak EE, Bozgeyik Z, Özercan IH, Ogur E. Semi quantitative strain elastography of liver masses. J Ultrasound Med. 2012;31(7):1061-7.
57. Gallotti A, D'Onofrio M, Romanini L, Cantisani V, PozziMucelli R. Acoustic radiation force impulse (ARFI) ultrasound imaging of solid focal liver lesions. Eur J Radiol. 2012;81:451-5.
58. Guibal A, Boularan C, Bruce M, Vallin M, Pilleul F, Walter T, et al. Evaluation of shear wave elastography for the characterisation of focal liver lesions on ultrasound. Eur Radiol. 2013;23:1138-49.
59. Kamoi K, Okihara K, Ochiai A, et al. The utility of trans rectal real-time elastography in the diagnosis of prostate cancer. Ultrasound Med Biol. 2008;34(7):1025-32.
60. Akin O, Hricak H. Imaging of prostate cancer. Radiol Clin North Am. 2007;45(1):207-22.
61. Zhang M, Nigwekar P, Castaneda B, et al. Quantitative characterization of viscoelastic properties of human prostate correlated with histology. Ultrasound Med Biol. 2008;34(7): 1033-42.
62. Ginat DT, Destounis SV, Barr RG, Castaneda B, Strang JG, Rubens DJ. US Elastography of breast and prostate lesion. Radiographics. 2009;29:2007-16.
63. Zhai L, Madden J, Foo WC, Polascik DJ, Palmeri ML, Nightingale ML. Characterizing the stiffness of Human Prostates using Acoustic Radiation Force. Ultrasound Imaging. 2010;32(4): 201-13.
64. Nightingale K, Palmeri M, Nightingale R, et al. On the feasibility of remote palpation using acoustic radiation force. JASA. 2001;110:625-34.
65. Zhai L, Polascik TJ, Foo WC, Rosenzweig S, Palmeri ML, Madden J, Nightingale ML. Acoustic radiation force impulse imaging of Human Prostate: Initial in vivo demonstration. Ultrasound Med Biol. 2012;38(1):50-61.
66. Choi YJ, Ko EY, Han BK, Shin JH, Kang SS, Hahn SY. High- resolution ultrasonographic features of axillary lymph node metastasis in patients with breast cancer. Breast. 2009;18:119-22.
67. Paterson S, Duthie F, Stanley AJ. Endoscopic ultrasound-guided elastography in the nodal staging of oesophageal cancer. World J Gastroenterol. 2012;18(9):889-95.
68. Bhatia KSS, Lee YYP, Yuen EHY, Ahuja AT. Ultrasound elastography in the head and neck. Part II. Accuracy for malignancy. Cancer imaging. 2013;13(2):260-76.
69. Dudea S, Botar Jid C, Dumitriu D, Vasilescu D, Manole S, Lenghel M. Differentiating benign from malignant superficial lymph nodes with sonoelastography. Med Ultrason. 2013;15(2):132-9.

70. Choi JJ, Kang BJ, Kim SH, Lee JH, Jeong SH, Yim HW, et al. Role of Sonographic Elastography in the Differential Diagnosis of Axillary Lymph Nodes in Breast Cancer. Journal of Ultrasound in Medicine. 2011;30(4):429-36.
71. Teng D-K, Wang H, Lin YQ, Sui GQ, Guo F, Sun LN. Value of Ultrasound Elastography in Assessment of Enlarged Cervical Lymph Nodes. Asian Pac J Cancer Prev. 2012;13(5):2081-5.
72. Alam F, Naito K, Horiguchi J, Fukuda H, Tachikake T, Ito K. Accuracy of Sonographic Elastography in the Differential Diagnosis of Enlarged Cervical Lymph Nodes: Comparison with Conventional B-Mode Sonography. AJR. 2008;191(2):604-10.
73. Cheng KL, Choi YJ, Shim WH, Lee JH, Baek J. Virtual Touch Tissue Imaging Quantification Shear Wave Elastography: Prospective Assessment of Cervical Lymph Nodes. Ultrasound Med Biol. 2016;42(2):376-82.
74. Youk JH, Son EJ, Kim JA, Gweon HM. Pre-Operative Evaluation of Axillary Lymph Node Status in Patients with Suspected Breast Cancer Using Shear Wave Elastography. Ultrasound Med Biol. 2017;42:1-6.
75. Hong Y, Liu X, Li Z, et al. Real-time ultrasound elastography in the differential diagnosis of benign and malignant thyroid nodules. J Ultrasound Med. 2009;28(7):861-67.
76. Lyshchik A, Higashi T, Asato R, Tanaka S, Ito J, Mai JJ, et al. Thyroid gland tumor diagnosis at US elastography. Radiology. 2005;237:202-11.
77. Dighe M, Kim J, Luo S, Kim Y. Utility of the ultrasound elastographic systolic thyroid stiffness index in reducing fine-needle aspirations. J Ultrasound Med. 2010;29: 565-74.
78. Bahn MM, Brennan MD, Bahn RS, Dean DS, Kugel JL, Ehman RL. Development and application of magnetic resonance elastography of the normal and pathological thyroid gland in vivo. J Magn Reson Imaging. 2009;30: 1151-4.
79. Sun L, Ning C, Liu Y, Wang Z, Wang L, Kong X, et al. Is transvaginal elastography useful in pre-operative diagnosis of cervical cancer? Eur J Radiol. 2012;81(8):e888-92.
80. Mabuchi S, Sasano T, Kuroda H, Takahashi R, Nakagawa S, Kimura T. Real-time tissue sonoelastography for early response monitoring in cervical cancer patients treated with definitive chemoradiotherapy: preliminary results. J Med Ultrason. 2015;42(3):379-85.
81. Stoelinga B, Hehenkamp WJK, Brölmann HM, Huirne JF. Real-time elastography for assessment of uterine disorders. Ultrasound Obstet Gynecol. 2013;43(2):218-26.
82. Ren Y. The value of transvaginal elastography in the diagnosis of uterine fibroids. Ultrasound Obstet Gynecol. 2017; 50(S1):391.
83. Wozniak S, Czuczwar P, Szkodziak PR, Krzyzanowski A, Wozniak A, Paszkowski T. Value of "elasto strain ratio" ultrasound elastography in the differential diagnosis of endometrial polyps and submucosal myomas: preliminary study. Ultrasound Obstet Gynecol. 2018;52(S1):261.
84. Wartecka-Zielinska K, Swiatkowska-Freund M, Preis K, Traczyk-Los A. Application of ultrasonography with elastography in women suspected of endometrial pathologies. Ultrasound Obstet Gynecol. 2016;48(S1):384.
85. Çıracı S, Tan S, Özcan AŞ, Aslan A, Keskin HL, Ateş ÖF, et al. Contribution of real-time elastography in diagnosis of polycystic ovary syndrome. Diagn Interv Radiol Ank Turk. 2015;21(2):118-22.
86. Hernandez-Andrade E, Hassan SS, Ahn H, Korzeniewski SJ, Yeo L, Chaiworapongsa T, et al. Evaluation of cervical stiffness during pregnancy using semiquantitative ultrasound elastography. Ultrasound Obstet Gynecol. 2013; 41(2):152-61.
87. Kim H, Hwang HS. Elastographic measurement of the cervix during pregnancy: Current status and future challenges. Obstet Gynecol Sci. 2017;60(1):1-7.
88. Fruscalzo A, Mazza E, Feltovich H, Schmitz R. Cervical elastography during pregnancy: a critical review of current approaches with a focus on controversies and limitations. J Med Ultrason. 2016;43(4):493-504.
89. Swiatkowska-Freund M, Preis K. Elastography of the uterine cervix: implications for success of induction of labor. Ultrasound Obstet Gynecol. 2011;38(1):52-6.
90. Schmitz R, Oturina V, Hammer K, Möllers M, Klockenbusch W, Falkenberg M, et al. Assessment of cervical elastography strain pattern and its association with preterm birth. Ultrasound Obstet Gynecol. 2017;50(S1):78.
91. Londero AP, Bertozzi S, Visentin S, Driul L, Cosmi E, Schmitz R, et al. P14.01: Diagnostic accuracy of ultrasound elastography in predicting preterm labour: a systematic review and meta-analysis. Ultrasound Obstet Gynecol. 2016;48(S1):208.
92. Kılıç F, Kayadibi Y, Yüksel MA, Adaletli İ, Ustabaşıoğlu FE, Öncül M, et al. Shear wave elastography of placenta: in vivo quantitation of placental elasticity in preeclampsia. Diagn Interv Radiol Ank Turk. 2015;21(3):202-7.
93. Tavare AN, Alfuraih AM, Hensor EMA, Astrinakis E, Gupta H, Robinson P. Shear-Wave Elastography of Benign versus Malignant Musculoskeletal Soft-Tissue Masses: Comparison with Conventional US and MRI. Radiology. 2018;Nov 27. 180950. https://doi.org/10.1148/radiol. 2018180950
94. Pass B, Jafari M, Rowbotham E, Hensor EMA, Gupta H, Robinson P. Do quantitative and qualitative shear wave elastography have a role in evaluating musculoskeletal soft tissue masses? Eur Radiol. 2017;27(2):723-31.
95. Yeoh HJ, Kim TY, Ryu JA. The feasibility of shear wave elastography for diagnosing superficial benign soft tissue masses. Ultrasonography. 2018 Jan 19 [Epub]. https://doi.org/10.14366/usg.17059
96. Hahn S, Lee YH, Lee SH, Suh JS. Value of the Strain Ratio on Ultrasonic Elastography for Differentiation of Benign and Malignant Soft Tissue Tumors. J Ultrasound Med. 2017;36:121-27.
97. EE Drakonaki, GM Allen, DJ Wilson. Elastography for musculoskeletal applications. BJR. 2012;85:1435-45.
98. Arda K, Ciledag N, Aktas E, Arıbas BK, Köse K. Quantitative Assessment of Normal Soft-Tissue Elasticity Using Shear-Wave Ultrasound Elastography. AJR. 2011;197: 532-6.
99. De Zordo T, Chem R, Smekal V, Feuchtner G, Reindl M, Fink C, et al. Real-time sonoelastography: findings in patients with symptomatic Achilles tendons and comparison to healthy volunteers. Ultraschall Med. 2010;31:394-400.
100. De Sconfienza LM, Silvestri E, Cimmino MA. Sonoelastography in the evaluation of painful Achilles tendon in amateur athletes. Clin Exp Rheumatol. 2010;28: 373-8.
101. De Zordo T, Lill SR, Fink C, Feuchtner GM, Jaschke W, Bellmann-Weiler R, et al. Real-time sonoelastography of lateral epicondylitis: comparison of findings between patients and healthy volunteers. Am J Roentgenol. 2009;193:180-5.
102. Zhang LN, Wan WB, Wang YX et al. Evaluation of elastic stiffness in healing Achilles tendon after surgical repair of a tendon rupture using in vivo ultrasound shear wave elastography. Med Sci Monit. 2016;22:1186-91
103. Beeler S, Ek ET, Gerber CA. comparative analysis of fatty infiltration and muscle atrophy in patients with chronic rotator cuff tears and suprascapular neuropathy. J Shoulder Elbow Surg. 2013;22(11):1537-1546.

104. Niitsu M, Michizaki A, Endo A, Takei H, Yanagisawa O. Muscle hardness measurement by using ultrasound elastography: a feasibility study. Acta Radiol. 2011;52(1): 99-105.
105. Yanagisawa O, Niitsu M, Kurihara T, Fukubayashi T. Evaluation of human muscle hardness after dynamic exercise with ultrasound real-time tissue elastography: a feasibility study. Clin Radiol. 2011;66(9):815-9.
106. Sconfienza LM, Silvestri E, Bartolini B, Garlaschi G, Cimmino MA. Sonoelastography may help in the differential diagnosis between rheumatoid nodules and tophi. Clin Exp Rheumatol. 2010;28:144-5.
107. Lalitha P, Reddy MCh, Reddy KJ. Musculoskeletal applications of elastography: a pictorial essay of our initial experience. Korean J Radiol. 2011;12:365-75.
108. Iagnocco AJ, Kaloudi O, Perella C, Bandinelli F, Riccieri V, Vasile M, et al. Ultrasound elastography assessment of skin involvement in systemic sclerosis: lights and shadows. Rheumatol. 2010;37(8):1688-91.
109. Ballyns JJ, Shah JP, Hammond J, Gebreab T, Gerber LH, Sikdar S. Objective Sonographic Measures for Characterizing Myofascial Trigger Points Associated with Cervical Pain Ultrasound Med. 2011;30(10):1331-40.
110. Müller CE, Aranha MF, Gavião MB. Two-dimensional ultrasound and ultrasound elastography imaging of trigger points in women with myofascial pain syndrome treated by acupuncture and electroacupuncture: a double-blinded randomized controlled pilot study. Ultrason Imaging. 2015;37(2):152-67.
111. Botar-Jid C, Damian L, Dudea SM, Vasilescu D, Rednic S, Badea R. The contribution of ultrasonography and sonoelastography in assessment of myositis. Med Ultrason. 2010;12:120-6.
112. Berko NS, Hay A, Sterba Y, Wahezi D, Levin TL. Efficacy of ultrasound elastography in detecting active myositis in children: can it replace MRI? Pediatr Radiol. 2015; 45(10):1522-8.
113. Pichiecchio A, Alessandrino F, Bortolotto C, Cerica A, Rosti C, Raciti MV, et al. Muscle ultrasound elastography and MRI in preschool children with Duchenne muscular dystrophy. Neuromuscul Disord. 2018;28(6):476-83.
114. Vasilescu D, Dudea S, Botar-Jid C, Sfrangeu S, Cosma D. Sonoelastography contribution in cerebral palsy spasticity treatment assessment, preliminary report: a systematic review of the literature apropos of seven patients. Med Ultrason. 2010;12:306-10.
115. Zheng YP, Mak AFT, Qin L, Ding CX. Ultrasound elastography of articular cartilage: a preliminary study. 20th Annual International Conference of the IEEE Engineering in Medicine and Biology Society; 1998.pp.1940-2.
116. Kot BCW, Zhang ZJ, Lee AWC, Leung VYF, Fu SN. Elastic Modulus of Muscle and Tendon with Shear Wave Ultrasound Elastography: Variations with Different Technical Settings. PLoS ONE. 2012;7(8):e44348. doi:10.1371/journal.pone.0044348.
117. Klauser AS, Faschingbauer R, Jaschke WR. Is sonoelastography of value in assessing tendons? Semin Musculoskeletal Radiol. 2010;14:323-33.
118. Nakao T, Ushigome H, Nakamura T, Harada S, Koshino K, Suzuki T, et al. Evaluation of renal allograft fibrosis by transient elastography (Fibro Scan). Transplant Proc. 2015;47(3):640-3.
119. Arndt R, Schmidt S, Loddenkemper C, Grünbaum M, Zidek W, van der Giet M, et al. Noninvasive evaluation of renal allograft fibrosis by transient elastography-a pilot study. Transpl Int. 2010;23(9):871-7.
120. Ramnarine KV, Garrard JW, Kanber B, Nduwayo S, Hartshorne TC, Robinson TG. Shear wave elastography imaging of carotid plaques: feasible, reproducible and of clinical potential. Cardiovasc Ultrasound. 2014;12(1): 49.
121. Luo J, Fujikura K, Homma S, Konofagou EE. Myocardial Elastography at Both High Temporal and Spatial Resolution for the Detection of Infarcts. Ultrasound Med Biol. 2007;33(8): 1206-23.
122. Rubin JM, Xie H, Kim K, Weitzel WF, Emelianov SY, Aglyamov SR, et al. Sonographic elasticity imaging of acute and chronic deep venous thrombosis in humans. J Ultrasound Med. 2006;25(9): 1179-86.
123. Geier B, Barbera L, Muth-Werthmann D, Siebers S, Ermert H, Philippou S, et al. Ultrasound elastography for the age determination of venous thrombi. Evaluation in an animal model of venous thrombosis. Thromb Haemost. 2005;93(2):368-74.
124. Gaspari R, Blehar D, Briones J, Dayno M. Sonoelastographic characteristics of abscess induration associated with therapy failure. J Ultrasound Med. 2012;31(9):1405-11.
125. Lee TH, Cha SW, Cho YD. EUS Elastography: Advances in Diagnostic EUS of the Pancreas. Korean J Radiol. 2012;13(Suppl 1):S12-S16.

CHAPTER

31

Computed Tomography Hardware including Dual Energy Computed Tomography: An Update

Smita Manchanda, Ashu Seith Bhalla, Priyanka Naranje

CT HARDWARE

Computed tomography (CT) scanner was invented in 1972 by a British engineer, Hounsfield.[1] Since the first clinical use of CT, this technology has made notable advances in the subsequent decades.

BASIC WORKFLOW OF CT SCANNER

The basic concept of a CT scanner is the reconstruction of structure of the imaged object from multiple projections of the absorption parameters collected by a thin X-ray beam. A CT scanner comprises of the following primary systems: gantry, patient positioning table and supports, detector assembly, X-ray tube, photodiodes, operating console **(Fig. 1)**. Earlier versions of CT employed a pencil-like X-ray beam (with single detector), and the tube-detector movement was both linear and rotary, termed as the "rotate-translate" motion (First generation). In an attempt to shorten the scan time, a fan shaped beam with multiple detectors was adopted (Second generation). The approach then shifted to "rotate-rotate" where multiple detectors are aligned as an arc, and both detector arc and X-ray tube rotate around the patient (Third generation). The quantum leap took place with the next level; wherein the detectors formed a complete ring around the patient, and only the tube rotated within the detector ring, described as "rotate-fixed" motion (Fourth generation).[2] This change was facilitated by the introduction of the "slip-ring" technology.

The first scanner had an approximate rotation time of 300 seconds. Now we have rotation times as short as 0.33 seconds in the dual energy scanners. Several vendors today offer 256-slice spiral CT scanners, and even 320 slice scanner has been available since 2008.

The recent advances in the major components will be discussed subsequently in this chapter.

DETERMINANTS OF AN OPTIMAL IMAGE

Determinants of an optimal image in CT, as in any image acquisition system are:

- Spatial resolution
- Contrast resolution
- Temporal resolution.

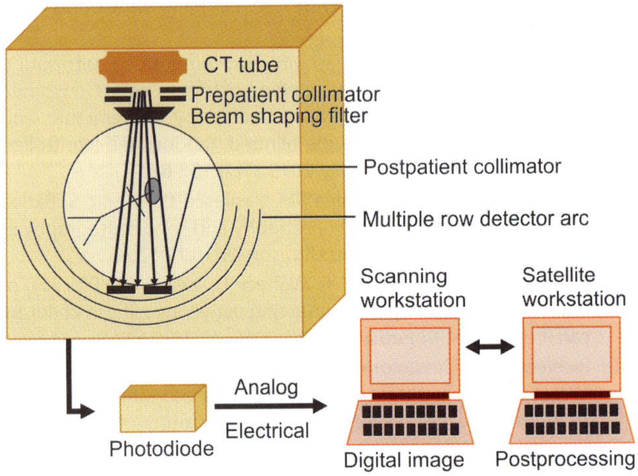

FIG. 1: Schematic diagram showing the basic components and workflow of a CT scanner.

Spatial Resolution

Spatial resolution (SR) of a CT scanner is its ability to resolve small objects within an image, and is expressed in line pairs/centimeter (lp/cm). SR is especially critical for high-resolution structures, as in temporal bone or lung. A measure of SR is Modulation Transfer Function or MTF.[3] In a CT scanner, different factors govern the spatial resolution in different planes **(Box 1)**.

Pixel Size

The scanning plane is the axial plane, i.e. the X-Y plane **(Fig. 2A and B)**, with the spatial resolution being called "in-plane" resolution. This resolution is mainly influenced by the pixel size with a smaller pixel size resulting in higher SR.

FOV—Field of View

A reduction in the FOV improves the SR, if rest of the parameters remain same.

Detector Width and Slice Thickness

The number of rows in MDCT scanner and the detector size determines the "out-of-plane" (z-axis) resolution, with a smaller detector width resulting in higher SR. There is a trade-off with increasing thickness resulting in decreasing resolution.[3,4]

Focal Spot

A smaller focal spot results in higher SR. The "flying focal spot" is a method that has been used to improve the Z-plane resolution.[3,5] In this technique, the X-ray focal spot alternates between two positions, thus acquiring 2 overlapping slices; and the z-axis resolution can then be brought down further (e.g., 0.4 mm).

Reconstruction Parameters

Kernel or filter or algorithm is a frequently used technique by clinical users to optimize image quality. A higher convolutional filter aids in sharpening the image by removing the "blurring". Blurring in the image is a consequence of the back-projection reconstruction process. There is a trade-of however of increasing noise with increasing kernel.

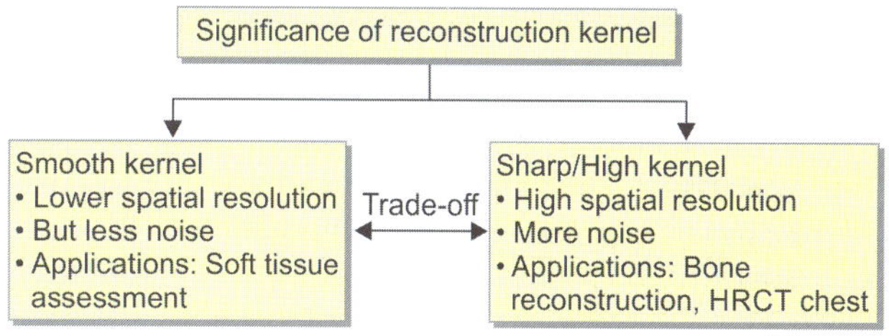

Cone beam CT uses a high-resolution two-dimensional detector and allows isotropic data acquisition and reconstruction leading to higher spatial resolution. These systems however offer poor contrast resolution as shall be discussed subsequently in the chapter.

BOX 1: Factors influencing spatial resolution.

In-plane (X-Y plane):

- Pixel size
- Ratio of scan FOV and image reconstruction matrix

Out-of-plane (z-axis):

- Width of detector row
- Minimum thickness of CT image (e.g.: if detector row width is 0.6 mm, then minimum slice thickness is 0.6 mm)
- Focal spot
- Reconstructive slice thickness (z-axis resolution)
- Reconstruction kernel

Contrast Resolution

Contrast resolution (CR) refers to the capability of a scanner to detect and differentiate subtle differences in attenuation coefficient in adjoining areas on an image; and is influenced by several factors **(Box 2)**.

"*Noise* is the consequence of statistical variation during the computation of a pixel value, and hence depicted by standard deviation." CR is inversely proportional to image noise, as noise reflects the variation in computing the pixel value. Higher image noise results in lower CR and a resultant "grainy image". The use of a soft tissue, smooth or standard algorithm during the reconstruction process enhances soft tissue and contrast resolution. Various noise reduction techniques are employed to enhance the CR.

Noise Reduction Techniques

If both CR and SR need to be improved and noise reduced, the radiation dose would increase as this can be achieved by increasing tube current and voltage.[3] Various noise reduction techniques may be applied on the projection data, or on the image. These may be in-built, being provided by the CT scan vendor, or may be available as third-party add-on products.

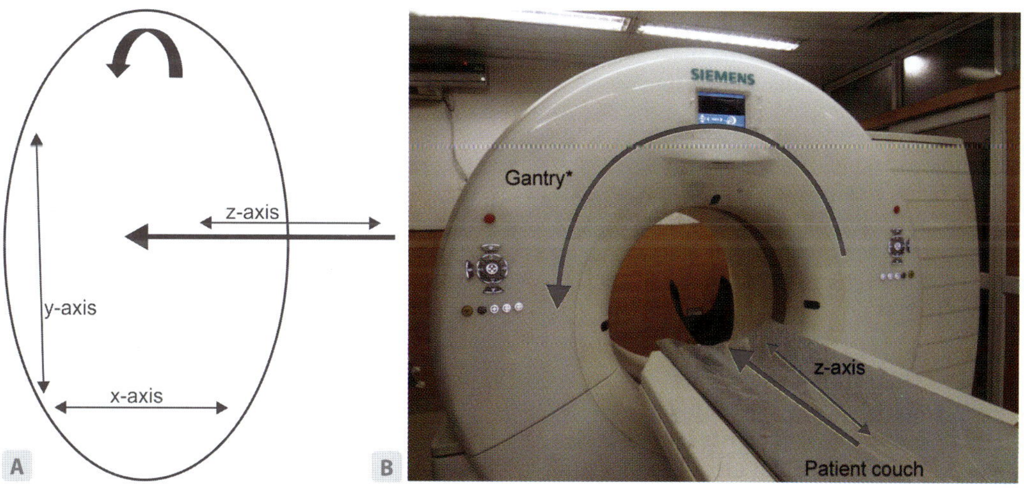

FIGS. 2A AND B: (A) Diagram showing the orientation of x, y and z-axis. (B) Photograph of a CT scanner. The gantry* houses the CT tube and the detector rows.

BOX 2: Factors influencing contrast resolution (CR).

Pixel size: CR is more with higher pixel size

FOV: CR is more with higher field of view (FOV)

Tube current (mAs): CR is better at higher mAs

Slice thickness: CR improves with increasing thickness

Reconstruction algorithm: CR is higher for smooth reconstruction algorithms

CR: contrast resolution

These include *filters*, which are often non-linear, and may be available as combinations with the different kernels. Special filters called "bow-tie filters" are used to absorb low energy photons, hence reducing the number of scattered photons in the polychromatic X-ray beam, improving the image CR. The trade-off is decreased detection of low contrast structures.

Temporal Resolution

Temporal resolution (TR) essentially reflects the ability of a scanner to capture objects that rapidly change over a period of time, and is dependent on a number of factors **(Box 3)**.

Gantry Rotation Time

Refers to the time taken for a complete 360° rotation of the detector tube assembly around the patient. Shorter rotation time results in higher temporal resolution. In single source CT, TR is approximately half the gantry rotation time; whereas in dual-source CT scanners, it becomes approximately one-fourth of a complete gantry rotation.[3]

For example, GE has introduced a wide-area detector CT (GE Revolution) with a 280-msec rotation time, which in 1 gantry rotation can scan up to 16 cm. Similarly Siemens dual-source CT (Force, Siemens) has a 250-msec rotation with a temporal resolution of 66 msec for cardiac CT.

Pitch:

$$\text{In MDCT, Pitch} = \frac{\text{Table increment in a single gantry rotation (mm)}}{\text{Total thickness of the slices acquired simultaneously (mm)}}$$

Lower pitch improves the spatial and temporal resolution but the radiation dose is also said to be inversely proportional to the pitch. This relationship is not as straightforward in modern scanners, as the automatic exposure factor (AEC) compensates for the resultant increase in dose.

ECG-gated Cardiac CT

The techniques unique to ECG-gated cardiac CT are:

- *Half scan reconstruction*: Also called short scan reconstruction. Improves temporal resolution.
- Use of very low pitch (0.2–0.3) in retrospective ECG gated techniques. This helps maintain anatomic continuity between the heart cycle.
- *ECG tube-current pulsing*: In this technique, the tube current is significantly reduced (4–20% of full current) during phases of minimal clinical interest. This strategy results in significant dose reduction.[5,6]

BOX 3: Factors influencing temporal resolution (TR).

- Gantry rotation time (TR is inversely proportional to rotation time)
- Pitch
- Mode of acquisition
- Number of X-ray sources
- Type of image reconstruction

Number of X-ray Sources

Scanners using two X-ray tubes can achieve an acquisition time (Dual Source Scanners), which is one-fourth of the gantry rotation time; unlike single source scanners where it is half. The intrinsic TR in current scanner is reduced to around 125–175 msec (single source cardiac CT Scanners) and 65–75 msec (dual source CT scanners).[6]

ADVANCES IN HARDWARE

Newer technology offers significant advantages, but different vendors have varied approaches to image acquisition. No single CT scanner offers the full range of the advanced features. This underscores the importance of understanding the properties and advancements of individual components of CT scanner.

Advances in X-ray Sources

There are several challenges and demands on the X-ray sources (generator and tubes) in modern multidetector computed tomography (MDCT) scanners. There is a need to have output tube voltages from 70 to 150 kV, high almost instantaneous power levels (50–120 kW), high tube currents at low kV and high cooling rates. The gantry now houses the CT tube, tube collimator, high voltage tank and the detector rows **(Fig. 3)**. There are mechanical challenges also as the tubes should be able to withstand phenomenal centrifugal forces resulting from high rotation speeds while keeping the designs compact and durable.

(A) CT Tubes

CT tubes are metallic rotating anode with high heat storage capacities. Some key changes that have taken place in CT tube technology are summarized below.[7]

- New tubes use less electrical energy for generating photons, as these have higher 'photon capture rates'.
- The past decade has seen marked increase in the gantry rotation speeds, and this increases the electric power requirements. Gantry speeds are in the range of 200–220 rpm.
- High rotation speeds of the tube generate mammoth centrifugal forces. This challenge is met with either using hydrodynamic anode bearings or the *Straton tube (Siemens)* strategy wherein the complete tube rotates omitting the reliance on bearings.
- To meet higher energy requirements, newer tubes use flat emitters enabling current output of over 1000 mA (at 80 kV). Better spatial resolution has been achieved with

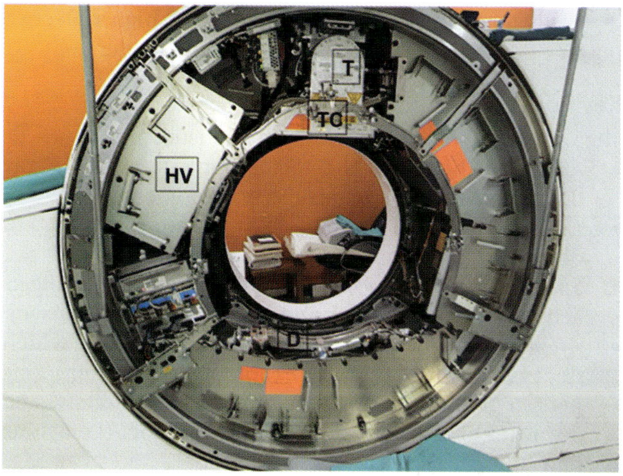

FIG. 3: Photograph of the open gantry. The gantry houses the CT tube (T) and the detector rows (D). Tube collimator is labeled as TC and the high voltage tank as HV.

decreasing the size of detector cells, as well as the focal spots. Focal track speeds are also up (up to 100 m/s).
- Due to wider coverage of detectors, the anode angle has increased.

A few specific advances are further discussed below.[7,8] Some key features of tubes of common vendors are summarized in **Table 1**.

Magnetic Dipoles for Electron Beam Positioning

Standard CT tubes position the electron beam using electrostatic methods. Recently, tubes have been developed that use magnetic dipoles instead for this purpose. Examples *Siemens Straton, Philips iMRC.*

Tube Cooling Advances

CT tubes are metallic X-ray tubes. Several innovations have been introduced in the cooling mechanism to cool down the oil to low temperatures. The *Philips iMRC* relies on heat conduction achieved by a liquid metal hydrodynamic straddle bearing which is placed within a vacuum. *Siemens Straton* is a direct cooling tube wherein the tube is placed on ball bearings directly within the oil, and the tube spins on these bearings. The principle method of heat dissipation here is again conduction.

Change in Anodes

In modern CT tubes, the anode is "grounded" and, hence the heat generated from scattered electrons does not reach back to the anode. This results in minimal off-focal radiation. The anode in most newer tubes is a metal anode (200 mm size in *Straton*, 120 mm in *iMRC*); straton anode being larger and segmented.

Graphite-backed Anodes

Another strategy that improves heat dissipation and hence heat storage capacity is the use of anodes that are graphite-backed. Herein, the principle method of heat dissipation is radiation. *GE CT* scanners, and *Toshiba Varian* have adopted this strategy. The size of the anode is 238 mm.

TABLE 1: Key features of tubes of common vendors.

SNo.	Vendor (Tube)	Features
1.	Siemens Straton X-ray tube	• Direct cooling tube, i.e. entire tube rotates, bearings thus located outside the tube (mode of heat loss-conduction) • Low inherent heat capacity • Uses flying focal spot • Magnetic dipoles for beam positioning
2.	Philips iMRC tube	• Liquid metal spiral groove or straddle bearings (mode of heat loss-conduction) • Small focal spot giving high SR • Magnetic dipoles for beam positioning
3.	GE Performix HDw tube	• Liquid bearings • Graphite backed anodes
4.	Toshiba Megacool Varian tube	• Graphite backed anodes

Measurement of Heat Storage Capacity

Conventionally, the heat storage capacity of X-ray tubes (including CT tubes) has been expressed in Million Heat Units (MHU). Modern tubes have heat storage capacities of 5-8 MHU, and heat dissipation rates of 1-5 MHU/min. In the *Straton tube*, due to its unique design features, the heat capacity is 0.8 but it achieves high heat dissipation rates (upto 5 MHU/min)

Also in 2010 the IEC 60613 standard was revised and the anode heat storage capacity and "Heat Units" were recommended to be replaced by terms like "nominal CT anode input power".[9]

(B) Generators

X-ray generators today have increased power outputs to cope up with the demands of the tubes. Parallel, substantial advancements have taken place in the *generators* also. Current generators deliver up to 120 kW/unit. These also enable rapid kVP switching. Higher frequency of inverters is also required for this rapid switching. All generator parts such as cables, capacitors handle very high currents and need concurrent improvement. In addition, modern generators are computer modulated.

Advances in Detectors

A detector essentially converts the attenuated X-rays received into electrical signal. The detectors are arranged in rows and columns and the detector array design varies with each manufacturer. The detector configuration is determined by the number of active detector rows and the z-axis width of detectors in an array.

Basic Design of Detector Array (Flowchart 1)

Detector array assembly span measures about a meter. The photodiode detector is segmented into detector elements,

FLOWCHART 1: Basic design of detectors.

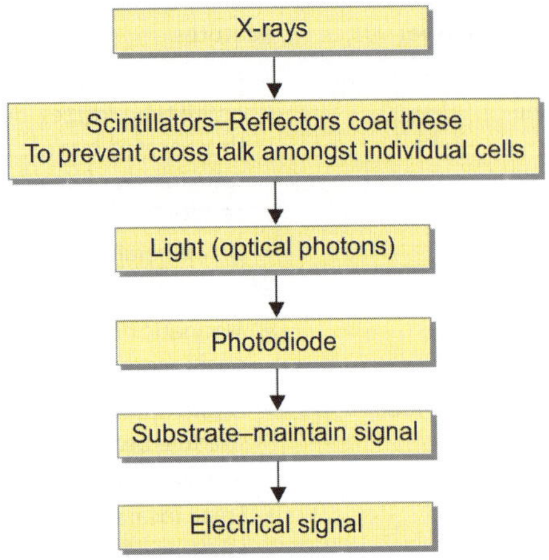

wherein scintillators and reflectors are interspersed forming a modular structure (actual photography). The reflectors are placed in between to prevent "cross-talk" between the detector elements i.e. the light that is generated by a detector element remains confined within itself.[10] To increase the number of slices, many sub-modules are created within modules, e.g., tiles concept: more tiles are added for more coverage.

Detector Design

The various common configurations of the detectors are:

- *Uniform, matrix, or mosaic*: A detector design that is subdivided into equal elements, or portions.
- *Nonuniformor Variable*: A detector design that uses variable detector size in the orthogonal direction or along the z-axis (the longitudinal axis of the patient table). In combination with a physical postpatient collimator, signals from these detectors can be combined to form various values of image thickness. The detector efficiency improves because of the smaller proportion of dead space between detector elements.
- *Hybrid*: These have a number of narrow detector elements in the center of the detector and a different number of wider detectors (usually double the width of the narrow detectors) on both sides of the span of narrow detectors **(Figs. 4A to C)**. The number of narrow and wider detectors varies among different vendors.[7]

Detector Materials

The core component of a detector is a luminescent material (scintillator material) which converts X-ray photons to visible light spectrum. A wide variety of materials have been used including single crystals/polycrystalline ceramics. Common materials employed are cadmium or gadolinium based (CdWO4), Gd2O2S: Pr, CE (GOS), garnet type gemstone. Current type of detectors in use, in most commercial CT scanners, are ceramic (solid-state) scintillation detectors coupled to photo diodes. Several new detector materials are being developed (e.g. super halides). Newer garnet-based detectors/gem stone detectors (GE Healthcare) offer higher spatial resolution and shorter after glow. The pixel size is usually around 1 mm.[10,11]

Reflector materials are fragments with high reflective power e.g. Titanium dioxide set in a polymer binder.

Key Concepts

The various important detector characteristics are:

- *Accuracy*: The ability of detector to measure small X-ray flux to detect subtle tissue density differences.
- *Dynamic range*: This refers to a variation or range of detector signals, typically more than 105.
- *Speed of response*: Speed of response of a detector affects acquisition time of a frame and is in milliseconds (msec).
- *Afterglow*: Scintillators have a luminescence, which decays over time in an exponential manner. This persistent luminescence is referred to as "afterglow" and a shorter afterglow is desirable as in garnet (gemstone detectors).
- *Resolution:* Factors affecting spatial resolution as mentioned are the focal spot size of tube and detector element size. The detector's aperture governs the in-plane (axial plane) spatial resolution of the system, i.e. the minimum slice thickness.
- *Detector Quantum Efficiency (DQE)*: This is a measure of the dose efficiency of a detector to convert the incident X-ray to electrical signal. It is taken as an indicator measure of efficiency of a detector and accounts for both signal and noise. An ideal detector is one with DQE of 1, i.e. 100% conversion of X-rays to electrical signal at all spatial frequencies.

DQE is dependent on several factors including detector material; and is represented by the equation:

$$DQE = \frac{SNR^2 \text{ out}}{SNR^2 \text{ incident}}$$

SNR^2: square of signal to noise ratio

Factors influencing DQE include radiation exposure, detector material, Modulation Transfer Function (MTF) and Noise Power Spectrum (NPS).

MTF is taken as an indicator of resolution of a detector. It is also the capability of detector to reflect the contrast of the object into the image, i.e. as different grayscale values. NPS is a measure of noise that shows variation of noise over a range of spatial frequencies, hence reflecting the "noise texture". DQE is directly proportional to MTF and inversely proportional to NPS.[12]

Advances in Reconstruction

The improvement in image reconstruction techniques has been a major advance facilitating radiation dose reduction. This is because better image quality can be achieved at the same mAs. There are two main methods for image reconstruction in CT–analytic reconstruction and iterative reconstruction (IR).[13,14]

- *Analytic reconstruction:* These are basically mathematical methods, which generate an image by using the projection data acquired by the X-ray tube at various angles while rotating around the patient. In most commercially used CT scans, the frequently employed reconstruction method is Filtered Back Projection (FBP).

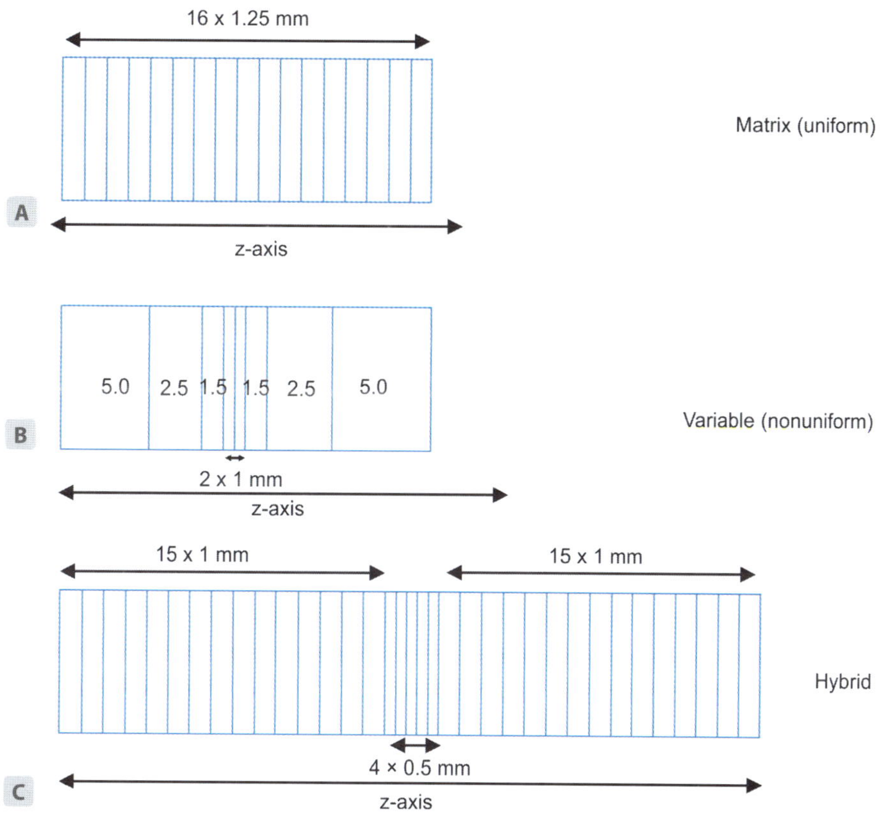

FIGS. 4A TO C: Diagram showing the basic design of matrix (A), variable (B) and the hybrid (C) detector design. The measurements indicated in the diagram are relative and not to scale.

- *Iterative reconstruction (IR):* In the IR-based techniques, multiple "iterations" or "corrections" or "optimizations" are done back and forth between the projection data and the image scan. Hence, there are repeated forward and back projections happening, which require a very high computational ability of the system. This has been commercially possible due to general advances in computer technology in recent years. 'Data fidelity' and 'Edge regularization' terms refer to method used for image optimization in IR.
- The differences between FBP and IR techniques are summarized in **Table 2**.

  There are various IR techniques commercially available.[8,14]

These include:

- *ASiR*: Adaptive statistical iterative reconstruction; GE Healthcare, Milwaukee, WI.
- *IRIS*: Iterative reconstruction in image space; Siemens, Erlangen, Germany.
- *AIDR 3D*: Adaptive iterative reconstruction 3D; Toshiba, Tochigi, Japan.
- iDose; Philips Healthcare, Best, Netherlands.
- *SAFIRE*: Sinogram-affirmed iterative reconstruction–Advanced technique employing higher number of correction loops; Siemens Healthcare.
- *MBIR*: Model based iterative reconstruction; GE Healthcare – Advanced technique that not only reduces noise but can even model the CT system geometry.

TABLE 2: Image reconstruction methods in CT.

Filtered back projections (FBP)	Iterative reconstruction (IR)
Back projects two-dimensional or three-dimensional data to form image Intervening filter is used to decrease blur	Introduction of "corrective loops" of "trial and error" type in the reconstruction Data fidelity Edge-preserving regularization
Assumes CT data to be noiseless with linear attenuation line functions throughout scan	Nonlinear processing algorithm
Does not account for scatter, beam hardening artefacts or noise	Reduces artefacts, e.g. beam hardening or metal artefacts
Can be done with lower computational ability of systems	Needs high computational ability
Simpler, less time consuming	Was initially time consuming
Higher doses for same image quality	Dose reductions (CTDI decreases from 20 to 78% with advanced reconstruction)[15] Dose reduction is least for low contrast examinations

- *FIRST*: Forward projected model based iterative reconstruction solution. Form of MBIR algorithm by Toshiba.
- A "Step-and-Shoot" sequential technique is used, which also significantly reduces doses.

SPECIAL CT SCANNERS

Cone Beam CT

Cone beam CT (CBCT) is a CT variant, which is designed to provide a compact, low radiation dose system that can be used to image *high contrast structures* as in the head and neck. CBCT uses *divergent X-rays forming a "cone" between the source and detector*, unlike the "fan-beam" geometry in conventional CT **(Figs. 5A and B)**. In CBCT multiple images are acquired during a single rotation of the gantry around the patient head producing a three-dimensional volumetric data. On the other hand, conventional CT requires both rotation as well as z-axis translation of the gantry to be able to acquire 3D data. X-ray tubes of relatively low power requirements are employed. Recent versions of the system use flat panel detectors (FPDs) of the indirect-conversion type based on a cesium iodide (CsI) scintillator.[16] These digital flat panel CBCT systems can also be mounted on a C-arm for applications in interventional radiology suites.

CBCT thus produces an entire volumetric data set in a single gantry rotation as it utilizes a two-dimensional detector system unlike the one-dimensional detector or series used in MDCT.[17,18] Depending on the variants of the system devised for various applications, several terms been used in literature to describe these new volumetric imaging techniques such as cone-beam CT, C-arm CT, cone-beam volume CT, volume CT, angiographic CT, and flat-panel CT.

Cone Beam Geometry

CBCT uses a high-resolution two-dimensional detector instead of a series of row of one-dimensional (1D) detector elements as in MDCT.[13] Images obtained by CBCT have *high isotropic spatial resolution.* This is due to the isotropic nature of acquisition and reconstruction in CBCT systems.[12] The volumetric data obtained in CBCT yield a dataset with isometric voxel size as small as 150 × 150 × 150 μm^3 at the isocenter, thus allowing high quality multiplanar reconstructions. MDCT on the other hand produces individual sections which are subsequently stacked typically yielding spatial resolution of 500 × 500 μm^2 in-plane and 500–1000-μm in the z-axis.[16]

CBCT however suffers from *poor contrast resolution* **(Fig. 6)** due to higher scatter in cone beam acquisition, lower DQE of CBCT systems and reduced temporal resolution and dynamic range of the FPDs. CBCT is thus suited for imaging of high-contrast structures. Higher scatter is a major limiting factor with the cone beam vs conventional fan-beam geometry acquisition leading to image degradation. In order to counter this effect, several anti-scatter measures are employed such as grids, software correction algorithms, beam-stop scatter map ping, and alteration of object-to-detector distance (air-gap).[17,18]

CBCT also suffers from limited anatomic coverage as it is based on acquisition of images during single gantry rotation. However this limitation has been overcome in flat panel detectors and various in-built stitching softwares. The coverage can include the entire face now, but still is much limited compared to MDCT.

Flat Panel Detector

Cone beam CT scanners use cesium iodide (CsI) scintillator detectors unlike the ceramic detectors used in MDCT. These suffer from a greater lag (afterglow) and hence scan times are much longer with CBCT relative to MDCT, thus reducing the temporal resolution of CBCT scanners. For instance, the current C-arm CBCT acquisitions take about 5 seconds. In addition, CsI detectors also have a lower quantum efficiency reducing the dynamic range of the scanner. The low dynamic range and increased also result in low contrast resolution of these systems.

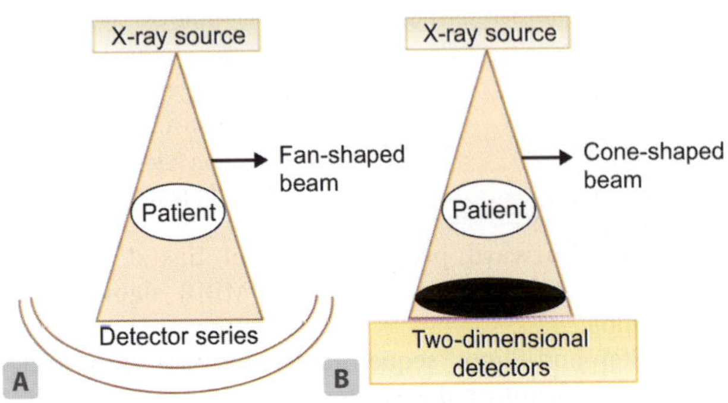

FIGS. 5A AND B: Schematic diagram showing basic design of a conventional CT (A) and a cone beam (B) CT.

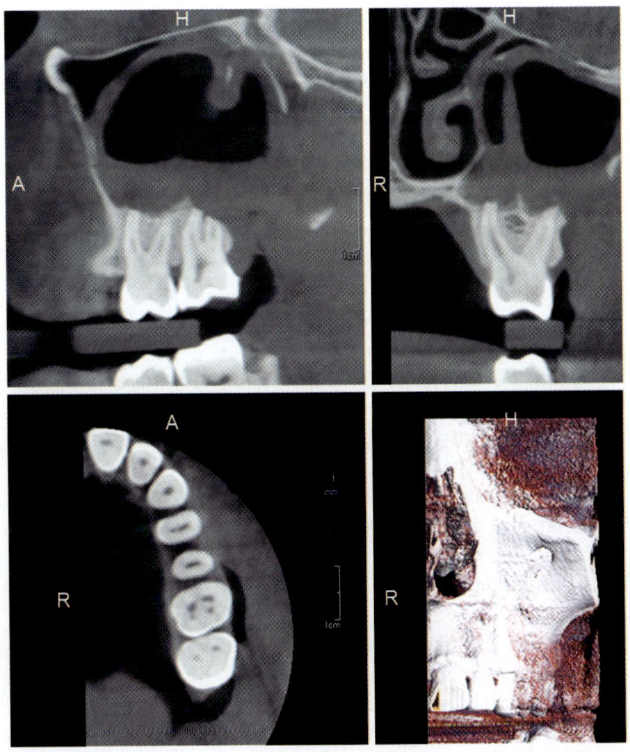

FIG. 6: Cone beam CT (CBCT) images with high spatial resolution of high contrast structures—teeth, periodontal tissues and sinuses. It has poor contrast resolution, and hence is not adequate for soft tissue evaluation.

Reconstruction

Volumetric data thus acquired in CBCT as in MDCT can subsequently be manipulated and reconstructed with software to allow multiplanar as well as panoramic reconstructions. The most commonly used reconstruction algorithm in CBCT systems is a modification of the filtered back-projection method called the Feldkamp algorithm, though the IR techniques are also available (but require more computation time). Compared to MDCT, CBCT however takes longer times for acquisition as well as reconstruction of images despite the acquisition being done in a single rotation.

Radiation Dose

The other major advantage of CBCT is reduction of radiation dose relative to MDCT. Effective dose of commercial CBCT scanner has been estimated as 0.2 mSvVs 1–2 mSv for MDCT head.[19,20] However, assessment of radiation dose during CBCT affords many challenges due to the altered beam geometry and underestimation of dose when using conventional methodology such as ion-chamber inserts. Also, conventional dosimetry metrics such as the $CTDI_w$ cannot be directly applied to CBCT imaging. It is hence suggested that the difference in absorbed dose measurements may be insignificant when FOVs and image quality parameters between CBCT and MDCT are adjusted.[21]

Applications

Cone beam CT provides a compact system wherein the scan can be performed with the patient sitting in an upright position. It has primarily found widespread applications in maxillofacial imaging including dental imaging, sinus and temporal bone imaging.

C-arm Based CBCT

The cone beam CT system is compact enough to allow it to be mounted on a C-arm. These systems allow projection radiography, fluoroscopy, digital subtraction angiography, and volumetric CT applications through a single system. This has significant utility as it eliminates the need for transporting the patient to the CT room for procedures requiring guidance of cross-sectional imaging. Currently, all commercially available C-arm mounted CBCT systems employ digital flat-panel detectors. Also, unlike MDCT as there is no z-axis translation and all acquisition occurs in a single rotation of the tube-detectors, it allows patient to remain stationary during the procedure.[21,22]

Cone beam CT has been employed for radiation therapy planning. CBCT has also been used for surgical planning particularly in orthopedic, chest, abdominal, head and neck, and neurosurgical procedures.

Portable Systems

Portable systems are now available to be used in on-the-go locations, such as bedside, emergency room and ICU setups. These mobile CT systems are optimized for scanning regions in the 25 cm field of view, primarily head and neck. These are capable of performing non-contrast CT, CT angiography and CT Perfusion. Example is CereTom by NeuroLogica Corporation (Danvers, MA); an 8-slice small bore portable CT scanner **(Figs. 7A and B)**.

Navigation Systems

Several navigation systems have recently become available to aid in CT-guided interventions. One of the methods used for this purpose is electromagnetic tracking. These systems involve interaction with previously acquired images to provide real time spatial navigation information (continuous imaging of the patient is not required). Combining electromagnetic tracking with preacquired imaging can be beneficial in guiding interventions, for instance in allowing real time targeting of lesions using previously acquired sequences in desired phase of enhancement.[23] The data from other imaging modalities can also be used with this

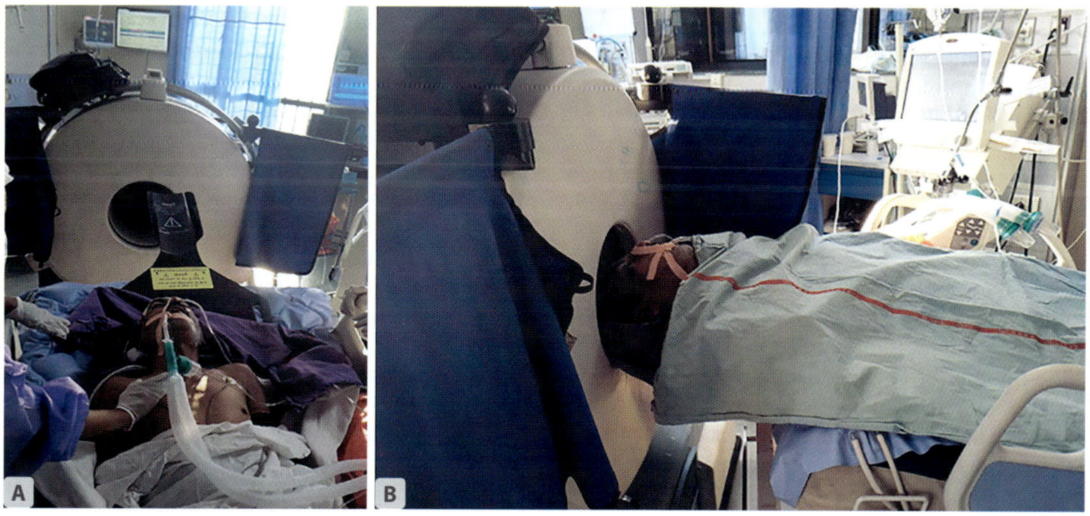

FIGS. 7A AND B: Portable CT scanner. Small bore mobile CT scanner primarily for head and neck imaging in emergency room (A) and ICU (B) setup.

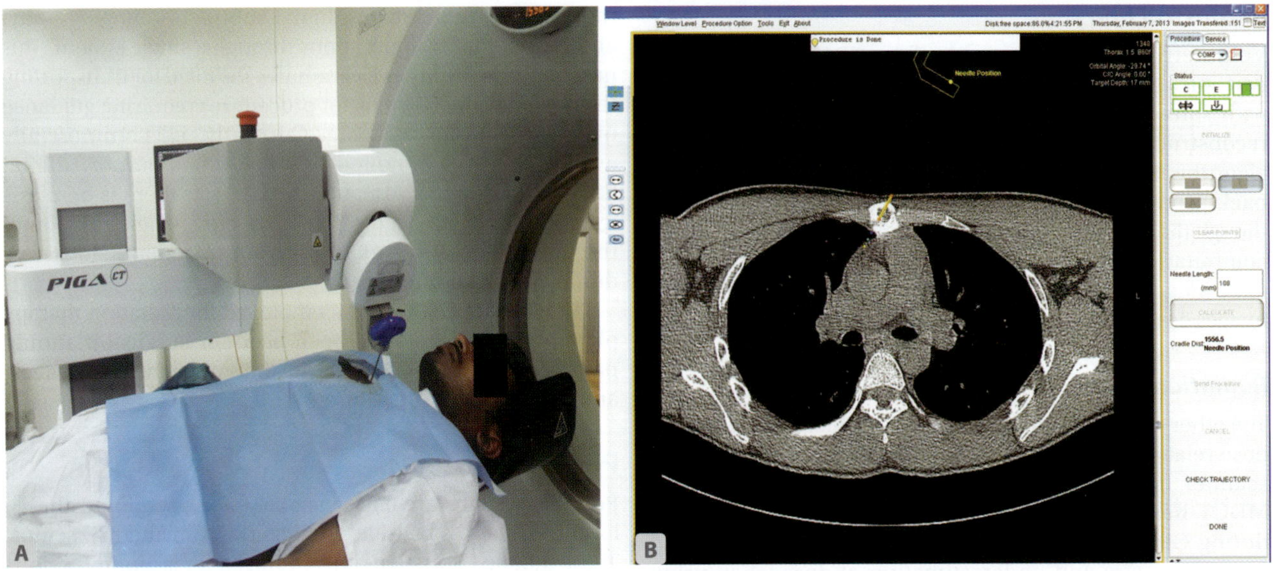

FIGS. 8A AND B: (A) Photograph showing sternal biopsy in a patient with the help of PIGA. (B) The planner image on the console projects the expected trajectory of the needle path.

technique. Similarly this technology is also being used to guide endoscopic and surgical procedures. Previously acquired CT images are loaded into proprietary software, which reconstructs 3D images as desired. These are then used to mark target locations and plan path of intervention. Real time visualization of position of the endoscope is also then available in relation to these images. Navigation devices may also be based on optical tracking systems.

Automated guiding systems for CT-guided biopsies are also available now. These typically involve the use of a robotic, electromechanical arm **(Figs. 8A and B)**. A computer interface receives the CT images and calculates coordinates on DICOM images and then guides needle placement through the arm.[24]

DUAL ENERGY CT

Dual energy CT utilizes the principle that different materials show different attenuation at varying energy levels, and this difference in attenuation can be used for tissue characterization. Since its inception, dual energy CT scanning has undergone several technical modifications. This section describes the development, principle and applications of dual energy CT.

PRINCIPLE

In clinical imaging, compton scatter and photoelectric effect are the two predominant interactions of matter with X-ray photons. The photoelectric effect occurs when an incident photon, having sufficient energy to overcome the K-shell binding energy of the electron in an atom, interacts with the atom to release the K-shell electron. The energy generated is released in the form of a photoelectron. The likelihood of photoelectric effect depends on the atomic number of the substance as well as the energy of the incident beam.[25]

TABLE 3: Atomic number and K-edges of different substances and radiographic contrast agents.

Substance	Atomic number	K-edge (keV)
Hydrogen	1	0.01
Carbon	6	0.28
Nitrogen	7	0.40
Calcium	20	4
Iodine	53	33.2
Barium	56	37.45

K-edge refers to an increased photoelectric effect and a spike in attenuation at an incident energy level just greater than the K-shell binding energy. The K-edge values of different materials are given in **Table 3.**[26]

The principle of dual energy CT imaging is based on the differential absorption of energy at variable kVp settings. For example, let us consider a substance (A) with K-edge at 60 kVp and another (B) at 130 kVp. If we image multiple combinations of A and/or B at 80 and 140 kVp, there will be differential attenuation at both these energy settings depending on the relative percentage of these substances. The object containing large amount of substance A will show higher attenuation at 80 kVp and lower attenuation at 140 kVp; whereas object containing larger amount of substance B will show higher attenuation at 140 kVp. In clinical applications, the constituents of soft tissues have a different K-edge (variable from 0.01 to 0.53), away from that of iodine (33.2) or calcium (4); hence iodine or calcium can be distinguished from soft tissues at dual energy imaging **(Fig. 9).**

In diagnostic imaging, once the datasets at 80 kVp and 140 kVp are generated, the attenuation of the enhanced structures containing iodine (vessels, highly perfused organs) are more on a 80 kVp image than on a 140 kVp image.

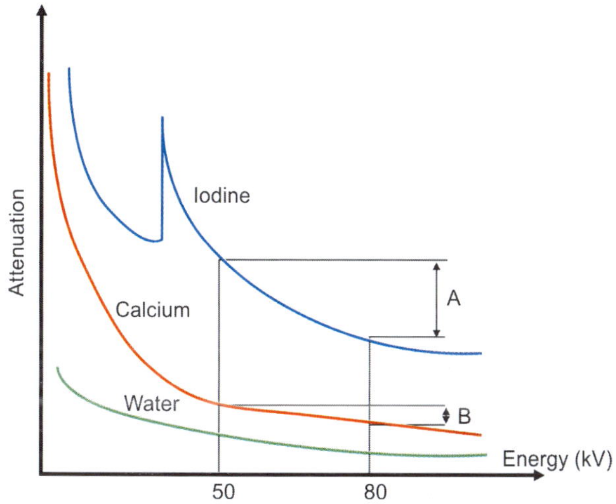

FIG. 9: Principle of dual energy CT. Change in CT attenuation of substances at different energy levels of incident beam. Iodine (k-edge 33.2 keV), shows a peak attenuation at lower energies and a rapid decrease in attenuation at higher energies. When attenuation at 50 and 80 kVp are compared; iodine shows a greater decrease (A)in attenuation at higher energy than calcium (B). Water shows very minimal change in attenuation with changes in kV. This forms the basis of material characterization in dual energy CT.

This difference in attenuation varies between different organs; for example- highly vascular organs and vessels have higher difference than muscles **(Figs. 10A to H)**. Postprocessing softwares use this information to generate a virtual non contrast image, or to calculate the material composition within a specific region of interest.

GENERATIONS OF DECT

First commercially available dual energy CT scanner that came into use in 20068 (Somatom Definition, Siemens, Erlangen, Germany) was dual source dual energy CT scanner (DS-DECT) having two X-ray tubes and two detector systems. This was followed by the development of a single-detector, single-source DECT (SS-DECT) system. DECT has evolved with numerous modifications in both DS-DECT and SS-DECT over the years.

Dual Source DECT

- There are three generations of DS-DECT, all having two tubes and two detectors.[27]
  - *First generation*: X-rays are generated by two X-ray tubes kept at 90 degrees angle to each other in the same gantry and operating at different kVp **(Fig. 11A)**. The average kVp of the higher energy tube is 120–140 and that of the lower energy tube is 80–100. The tube with larger kVp (tube A) has a larger detector of FOV 50 cm, and the lower energy tube (B) has a smaller FOV detector (26 cm). (Prototype: Siemens Definition DS 64 slice).
  - *Second generation*: the lower energy tube (tube A) is paired with a detector with FOV of 50 cm while the higher energy tube (tube B) is paired with a smaller detector with FOV of 33 cm. Higher energy tube has a selective proton shield made of tin filter. Two separate detector arrays lead to generation of two image datasets. Both the tube kVp can be modified independently and additional selective photon shield can be used. (Prototype: Siemens Flash 256 slice).
  - *Third generation*: Dual Source approach combined with tin filter is used along with dedicated set of kVp pairs and 10 kV steps availability. (Prototype: Siemens Somatom Force).
- *Spectral separation*: With its two independent tubes operated at two different voltages and the possibility to add a tin filter for the high-energy spectrum, it results in better spectral separation.[28]
- The dual energy data are acquired simultaneously with a 90° offset in projection space. Therefore the temporal coherence is very good, enabling even cardiac dual energy imaging.
- The temporal resolution of a DS-DECT is one-quarter of the rotation time as one X-ray tube acquires data during 90° of rotation.
- However, the drawback of DS-DECT is the limited dual energy FOV (33 cm), which makes it difficult to image patients with larger body habitus.

Single Source DECT

- SS-DECT scanners.[29] Use a single X-ray tube, which generates high and low energy X-ray spectra by rapid changing of the kVp settings (at an interval of 0.5 msec) in the same rotation **(Fig. 11B)**. Since the tube current cannot be changed so rapidly, in order to maximize the contrast to noise ratio, the exposure time ratio is changed between two acquisitions. For example, 65% exposure time is given for the 80 kVp beam and 35% for the 140 kVp beam.
- The SS-DECT requires a very fast detector and data acquisition system with fast sampling capability. The detector arrays used in SS-DECT are made of cerium activated garnet (Gemstone Spectral Imaging; GE Healthcare, Piscataway, NJ).[30]
- The advantage of SS-DECT over DS-DECT is a larger FOV of imaging (50 cm) and easier quantification of material density.[28]
- The disadvantage of SSDECT includes a poorer spectral separation (hence less accurate material characterization compared to DS-DECT with selective photon shielding).

The currently available dual energy CT scanners/ technology are summarized in **Table 4**, the two basic types being dual source or single source.[26,28,31]

KEY CONCEPTS IN DECT

Dual Energy Ratio

The material characterization on DECT largely depends on their dual energy ratio. The dual-energy ratio is a material-specific parameter. It depends on the atomic number, not on the material density or concentration. For experimental derivation of dual energy ratio of a given material X, the CT attenuations at any given kVp (for example, 140 kV) at different material concentrations are assessed and arranged

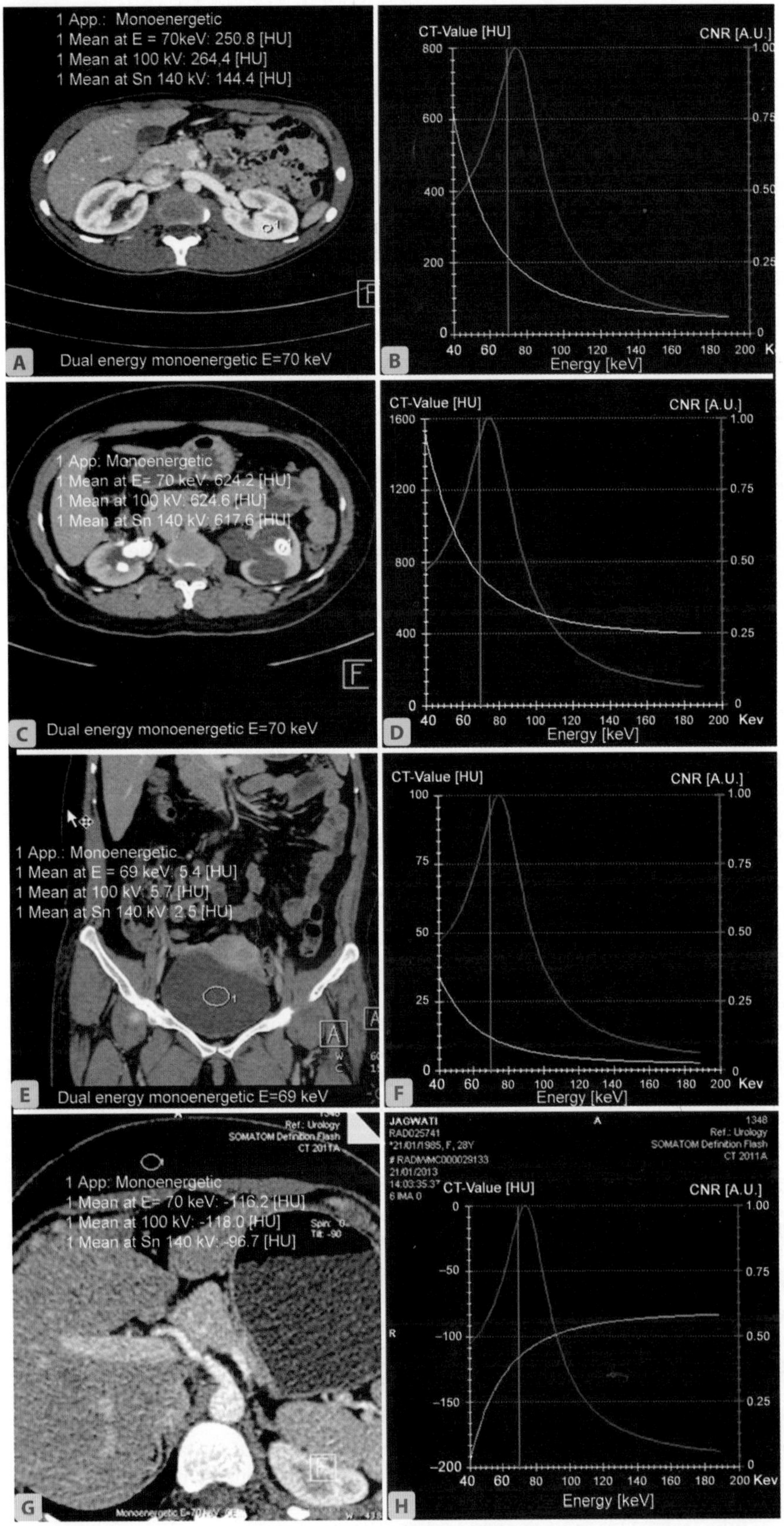

FIGS. 10A TO H: Different CT attenuation of tissues at different energy levels, based on their constituents. Highly vascular organs containing iodine on CECT shows higher attenuation at lower energy images. For example, renal parenchyma shows an attenuation of 250.8 HU at 70 kV images and 144.4 HU on 140 kV images. (A and B) Calcium shows very little variation in the attenuation values over a change of energy from 70 to 140 kV (C and D). Water also shows very little change in attenuation (E and F); 11.8 HU at 70 kV and 6.1 at 140 kV images. Fat, to the contrary, shows a minimal increase in attenuation at higher energy images (G and H); -116.2 HU at 70 kV and -96.7 HU at 140 kV.

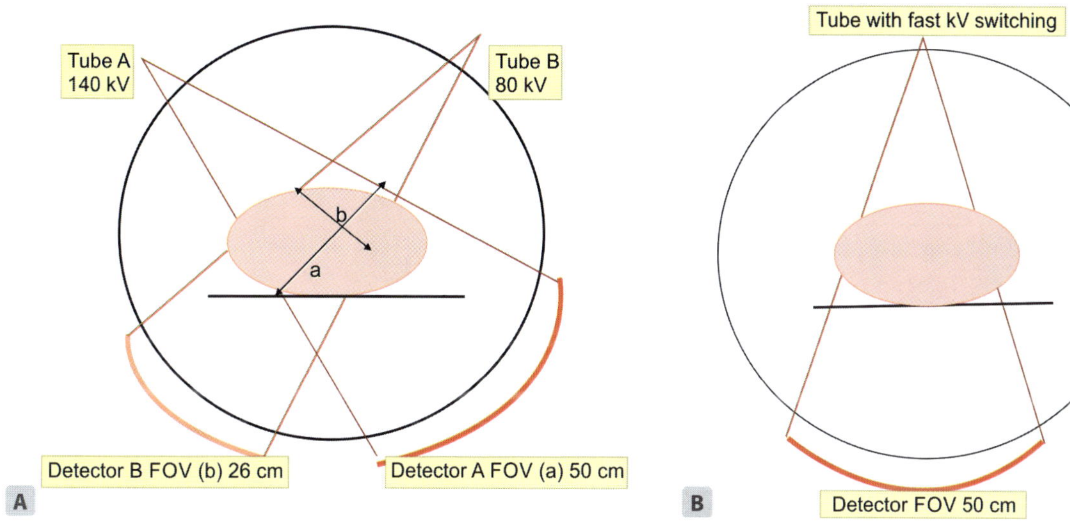

FIGS. 11A AND B: Dual energy scanners: DS-DECT scanners (A), and SS-DECT scanner (B). (A) In a first generation DS-DECT scanner, two tubes are placed in the gantry at an angle of 90° to each other. Tube A has a higher kVp (140) and had a larger detector array of FOV 50 cm. The smaller detector array (26 cm FOV) is paired against the lower energy tube (80 KV); (B) The SS-DECT scanner has a single tube and a detector array with 50 cm FOV with varied techniques (dual spiral/fast kV switching/slow kV switching/dual layer detector/twin beam).

TABLE 4: Currently available dual energy CT scanners/technology.

Type	Technology	Marketing name
Dual source dual energy	Dual source	Siemens SOMATOM Definition, SOMATOM Definition Flash, SOMATOM Force
Single source dual energy	Fast kV switching (capability for rapid alternation/fast switching between two kVp settings)	GE Gemstone Spectral Imaging (GSI or GSI Xtream)
	Slow kV switching (switch the tube voltage between two gantry rotations in a single scan)	Toshiba Aquilion ONE
	Dual spiral (two successive spiral scans at different kV and mA levels)	Siemens SOMATOM Definition Edge, SOMATOM Definition AS
	TwinBeam (split filter at the X-ray tube; two different materials positioned in z-direction of this split filter shift one part of the X-ray spectrum to lower and the other part to higher energies)	On the Siemens SOMATOM Definition Edge scanners
	Spectral CT (dual layer detector: first detector layer absorbs low energy part of the spectrum; second layer absorbs high-energy part)	Philips IQon Spectral CT

along a graph (A). Similar graph (B) is made for different material concentrations at another kVp (for example 80 kVp). The dual energy ratio of material X can be described as a ratio of the slope of the graph B to the slope of graph A.[27]

If the two incident X-ray beams have mean energies very close to each other, the difference in dual energy ratios among various component materials (for example, iodine and soft tissue) will be less and it will be difficult to differentiate them on imaging.

Spectral Separation

For efficient dual energy imaging the two incident X-ray beams should have sufficiently different energies. In reality, whenever X-ray is generated, it is emitted in the form of a continuous spectrum with photons having different energy levels (Bremsstrahlung) and a mean energy. The mean energy of an X-ray spectrum varies with the bombarding energy (kV). When two tubes with different kV are used, two spectra are generated with significant overlap between them (spectral overlap) **(Figs. 12A and B)**. As described earlier, the spectral overlap makes material characterization more difficult. Spectral overlap also reduces the dose efficiency as the 140 kVp spectrum contains significant percentage of low-energy photons also, which add to the patient dose.

Spectral separation indicates a situation when there is minimal overlap between the different energy spectra, i.e. less spectral overlap.[28] **Box 4** describes the various methods to obtain adequate spectral separation.

Temporal Resolution and Temporal Coherence

Temporal Resolution (TR)

This is the time required for collecting the data for image reconstruction, which is usually half a rotation time. It is independent of the dual energy approach, except for Dual

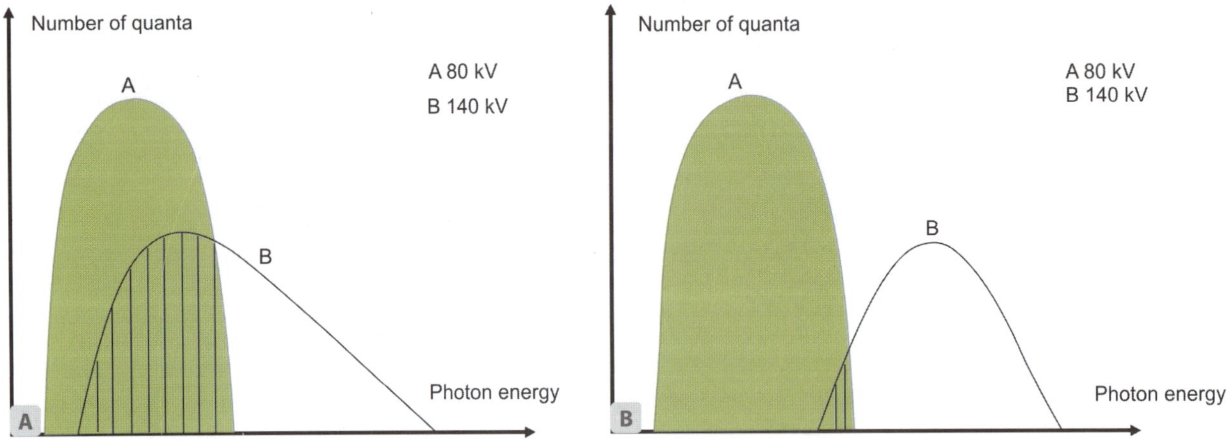

FIGS. 12A AND B: Spectral separation. When high (140 kV) and low energy X-rays (80 kV) are used, there is a significant energy overlap between them (shaded area in Figure A). Hence, generation of a true mono-energetic beam becomes difficult. After the use of a selective tin filter with the higher energy tube in second generation DS-DECT scanners (B), the lower energy X-rays from 140 kV tube are filtered; thereby reducing the overlap (shaded area in Figure B). This leads to better spectral separation, proper mono-energetic imaging and better material characterization.

BOX 4: Methods to obtain adequate spectral separation.[31,32]

- Adding separate filtration to one or more tubes in DS- DECT: Selective photon shield (Tin filter 0.5-0.8 mm added to higher energy tube) **(Fig. 12)**.
  - Improves SNR
  - Reduces dose to patient
- Adding split filtration to SS-DECT
- Sandwich (dual) detectors
- Energy discriminating, photon counting detectors

TABLE 5: Image generation with the combination of temporal resolution and temporal coherence in the context of moving objects.

Temporal resolution	Temporal coherence	Image
Low	Low	Blurred and offset
High	Low	Sharp but slightly offset
Low	High	Blurred but well registered
High	High	Sharp and well registered

Source DECT where a special algorithm allows combining 90° of data from the two systems to reconstruct images with a temporal resolution of about a quarter rotation time. The TR determines the amplitude of motion artefacts.

Temporal Coherence (TC)

This is the time delay between the acquisitions of the low and high-energy data. Ideally, this delay should be as small as possible to avoid misregistration due to motion or problems with contrast agent dynamics.

TR and TC should be differentiated from each other[28] but considered in combination for evaluation of images generated by the specific technology **(Table 5)**.

Spatial Resolution

Spatial resolution reflects the image sharpness in terms of visualization of small objects. The detector element size, focal spot size, and the number of projections per rotation mainly determine spatial resolution. However, it is important to understand that the image data should be good with respect to the spectral separation and temporal resolution also. For example, the detectability of small structures like iodine in small vessels or the characterization of small kidney stones is related to *spatial resolution and spectral separation*.

Dose Efficiency

The current DECT scanners have dose reduction features like tube current modulation or iterative reconstruction for dose neutral scanning. Spectral separation is also important, as the system with better spectral separation can achieve a certain material image quality with less dose than a system with poorer spectral separation.

PROCESSING OF DATA, IMAGE RECONSTRUCTION AND IMAGE DISPLAY IN DECT

The images generated from a DECT should have the combined morphologic data and material specific information. To obtain a material-specific image, the datasets can be processed in two ways:

1. *Image domain decomposition*: Processing after the reconstruction of low- and high energy images
   - This method is used in DS-DECT scanners and dual (sandwich) layer detector DECT scanners. In DS-DECT, images are generated by linear or non-linear sigmoidal blending of both (high and low energy) datasets.[33]

- *In linear blending*, a specific ratio of both high and low energy data are used.
- *In sigmoidal blending*, the pixels with higher attenuation are selected from the low energy datasets and the pixels with low noise are selected from high energy datasets.
- Material-specific images are obtained by calculating the difference in attenuation of varying materials between the low and high energy image datasets.
- For abdominal DS-DECT,[34] a three-material decomposition (soft tissue, fat and iodine) process is commonly used to generate virtual non-contrast images. A color-coded overlay image (usually iodine overlay in abdominal imaging) is generated by assigning a color to the voxels containing the material and overlapping them on monochromatic images.

2. *Projection-space decomposition*: Processing before the images are reconstructed from high and low energy sonograms
   - It is a more robust processing which is preferred because of greater flexibility in material decomposition, and minimizing beam-hardening artifact.
   - In this method, after data acquisition, the 100 kVp images are not routinely reconstructed.
   - The high and low energy datasets are calibrated and aligned in projection space to generate material density image and monochromatic images (providing energy-selective information).
   - Material density image reconstruction in based on the theory of *basis material decomposition*; which proposes that the attenuation coefficients of any material can be computed as a weighted sum of the attenuation coefficients of two base materials, as long as the k-edge of the material is not within the evaluated energy range.
   - The two base materials should have highly different atomic number.
   - The commonly selected dual energy base material pairs are iodine and calcium, and iodine and water. Two separate sets of material density images are generated (e.g. iodine density and water density images). The lesions containing iodine (enhanced organs, vessels) will show higher attenuation on iodine density images than on water density images.
   - *Monochromatic images* are generated during the processing of material density images by calculating the linear attenuation coefficient (μ) of an object.[35] The advantage of a monochromatic image generated from a DECT over a single energy image at the same kVp includes the reduction of beam hardening artifacts and provides accurate CT numbers.

Image Display in DECT

Images generated in DECT can have two types of display:

1. *Material density display* **(Figs. 13A and B)**. The material density display can be *iodine density display or water density display*.
   - In an *iodine density display*, the enhanced organs containing iodine appear bright whereas unenhanced areas remain dark. In abdominal imaging, iodine density display has important role in the evaluation of a hyperdense cyst on CECT.
   - The *water density display* is equivalent to *virtual unenhanced images*. Water density display can obviate the need of an additional NCCT image acquisition.
2. *Monoenergetic image display* **(Fig. 14)**. The mono-energetic or pseudomonochromatic display is an energy-specific display.

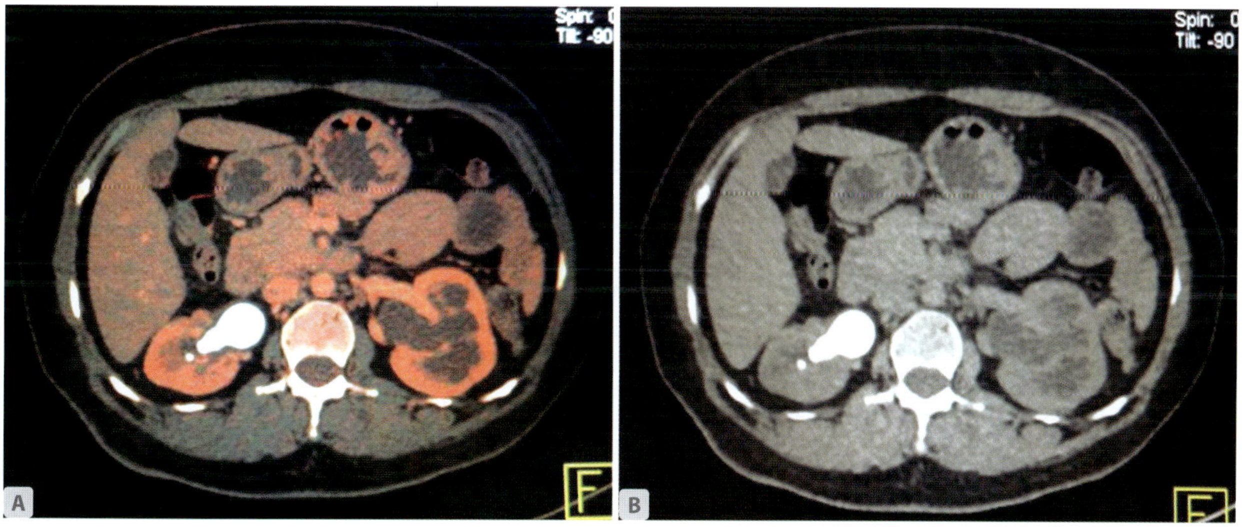

FIGS. 13A AND B: Material density display. Iodine overlay map (A), created by overlapping the iodine density images over monoenergetic image, highlight the organs containing iodine (colored red). The gradient of color varies according to the degree of enhancement of the organ. The water density display (B) is equivalent to virtual unenhanced image. Note that both calcium and iodine appear dense on a routine single energy CT, but they can be differentiated on iodine map images as calcium will not be highlighted on a iodine map image (for example, the calculus in this image).

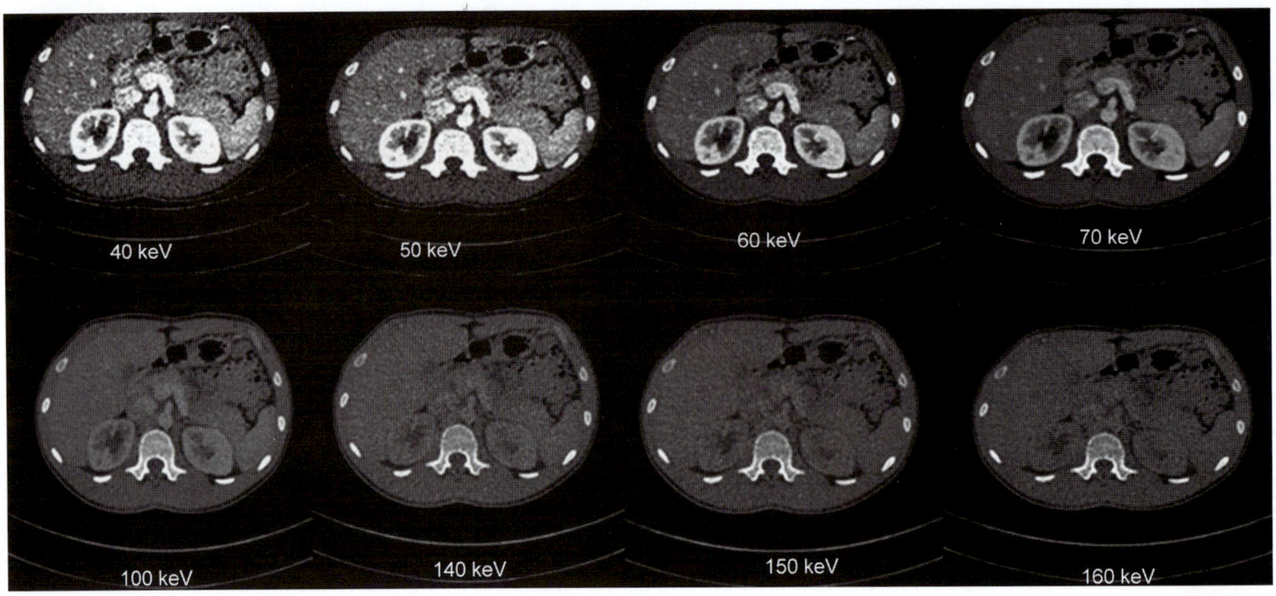

FIG. 14: Virtual monoenergetic images generated from a DS-DECT scanner. It is evident from the images that the attenuation of iodine and the image contrast are high at lower energy images, although the images appear more noisy. As the kVp increases, the contrast difference between various tissues becomes negligible and the 160 kV image becomes identical to a noncontrast image.

- Images are processed at any given kVp from the dual energy datasets, which resemble images physically acquired after scanning at that given kVp.
- Virtual monogenetic/pseudomonochromatic images at lower kVp show higher image contrast and make small enhancing lesions more conspicuous than routine display at 70 kVp.
- However, the images at lower kVp (for example 40 kV) have more noise and higher kVp images have less contrast. The optimum image contrast to noise ratio is achieved at 70 kVp.
- With monoenergetic imaging, metal artifacts can be reduced after selecting the energy level at which implants, clamps, or screws will have the smallest impact on image quality.

APPLICATIONS OF DECT

Applications in Abdomen

Renal Applications

Renal Calculi Characterization (Figs. 15A and B)

On the basis of the dominant chemical component, urinary calculi can be divided into either uric acid (UA) or nonuric acid calculi. Uric acid calculi are often associated with metabolic causes such as hyperuricemia or gout. These stones are lucent on radiograph but can be identified on CT. Nonuric acid calculi are further divided into calcium, cystine and struvite. Calcium calculi are the most common type and contains calcium oxalate monohydrate (COM), calcium oxalate dihydrate (COD), calcium phosphate and hydroxyapatite in a variable proportion. Struvite stones are composed of magnesium ammonium phosphate (triple phosphate) and are the major constituent of a stag horn calculus. Cystine calculi are rare and associated with certain metabolic conditions such as cystinuria. A calculus containing both uric acid as well as nonuric acid component is labeled as mixed calculus. Determining the composition of calculi has direct treatment implications. Uric acid stones can be treated medically whereas cystine and COM stones are resistant to extra corporeal shock wave lithotripsy (ESWL) and percutaneous nephrolithotomy (PCNL) is preferred.

Single energy NCCT is unreliable for characterizing the type of calculi since calculi of different proportions of constituents can have overlapping CT attenuation values. When imaging is done on DECT scanners, the change in attenuation between high-and low-energy scans can be used to differentiate types of calculi. UA calculi are composed of light elements whereas non-UA calculi are composed of heavy elements, hence these two groups can be differentiated on imaging. On SS-DECT, calcium and uric acid material density images are generated, uric acid calculi are depicted on uric acid material density images and calcium containing calculi on calcium density images.

DS-DECT has an added advantage of selective photon shield (tin filtration) in the 140 kVp tube for better spectral separation and more accurate composition analysis. In a DS-DECT scanner, keeping the reference dual energy ratio at 1.13, the uric acid calculi are seen to lie below the reference line and non-UA calculi above it. Several *ex vivo* studies have demonstrated the efficacy of DECT in characterizing stones, and also the advantage of additional tin filtration.[36,37]

Renal Cysts

Detecting a simple cyst with water density is not an imaging challenge. Differentiating a complex/complicated renal

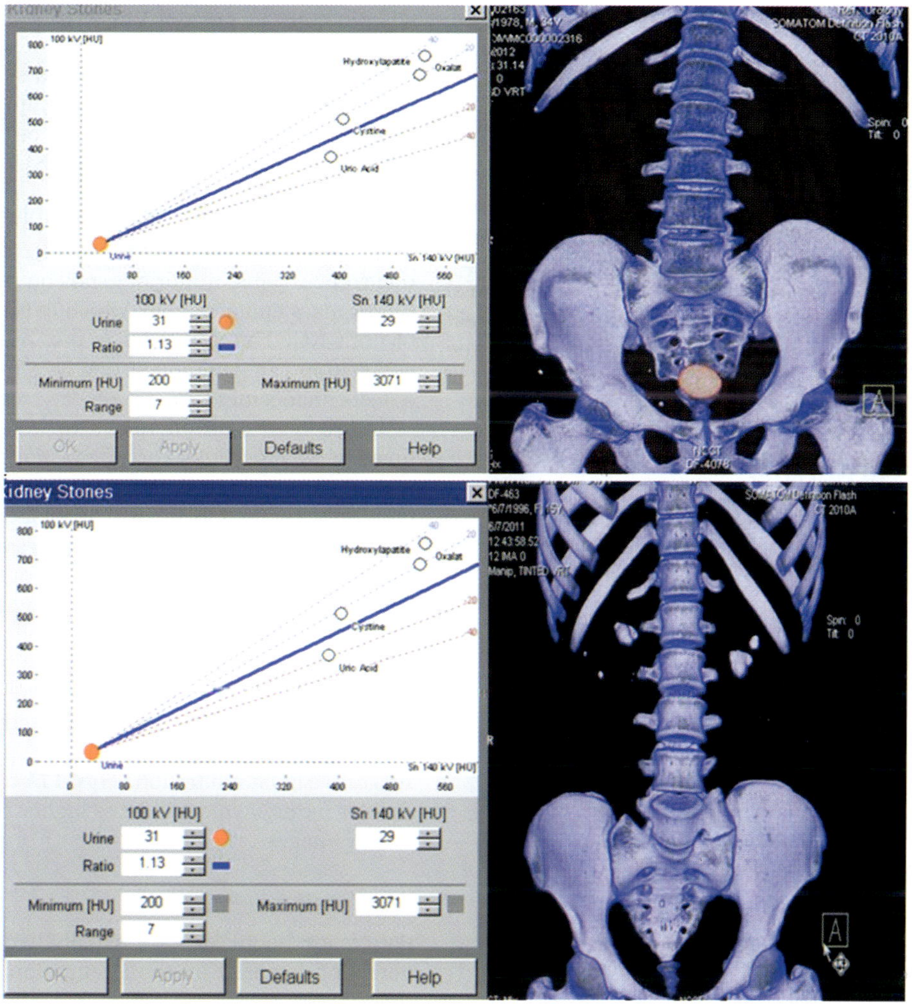

A

B

FIGS. 15A AND B: Renal calculi characterization by DECT. Images acquired at 100 and 140 kV in a DS-DECT scanner. A reference dual energy ratio of 1.13 is taken to differentiate uric acid from nonuric acid calculi. The uric acid calculus in (A) shows a dual energy ratio less than 1.13 and are colored red. The non-uric acid calculi show a dual energy ratio above the reference line and are colored blue (B).

cyst from a solid renal mass lesion is often difficult, and depends on the detection of enhancement in the lesion. Conventional single energy CT will require two acquisitions, one NCCT and another CECT. Using dual energy CT, the additional acquisition of NCCT can be avoided, as it is possible to generate virtual NCCT from the datasets. On Iodine density images, the enhancing solid mass will appear bright; whereas high-density cysts will be dark, since they do not have any iodine in them. In SS-DECT, it is not possible to calculate the HU value of the lesion, which is possible with DS-DECT.[38,39]

Hemorrhagic/complicated cysts and often pose an imaging dilemma whenever incidentally detected on a CECT. On CECT images, they appear hyperdense and require an additional NCCT scan to rule out enhancement. On iodine density display, they appear dark.

Also, in the renal cysts, it can help reduce the problem of misdiagnosis of a cyst as a solid lesion due to 'pseudo-enhancement', which refers to artifactual increase in CT numbers within a simple cyst on a single energy CECT.

Renal Mass Characterization and Follow-up after Ablation

Calcification within an enhancing renal mass can be detected on a virtual NCCT image. After thermal ablation of solid renal masses, the imaging assessment should consist of multiphase scanning with and without contrast to detect enhancement in residual tumor tissue. While imaging on DECT scanners, one contrast-enhanced acquisition can generate virtual NCCT scans and iodine overlay maps help detect the enhancement in such masses.

Both DS-DECT and SS-DECT have a few technical limitations for the evaluation of renal masses. Firstly, virtual NCCT images have more image noise than real NCCT images. Second, because of the material decomposition algorithms used, calcification in renal lesions is less conspicuous on virtual unenhanced images than on real unenhanced images. Third, smaller amounts of fat in renal masses are difficult to detect on virtual NCCT images and can be measured only on conventional thin-section unenhanced CT images.

CT Urography

On DECT imaging, virtual NCCT generated from the dual energy datasets can obviate the need for an additional NCCT acquisition during CT urography. Takahashi and colleagues[40] reported that on virtual NCCT from excretory-phase CT urography performed with a DS- DECT scanner, the rate of detection of urinary tract stones was 100% for stones larger than 7 mm but decreased significantly (29%) for stones of 1–2 mm size. Quality of the generated virtual NCCT images depends on iodine concentration within the pelvicalyceal systems, hence a highly concentrated iodinated contrast material within the PCS may lead to a 'rim artifact' at the margins and obscure small calculi. Incomplete subtraction of concentrated iodine can also be mistaken as calculi.[40]

Applications in Adrenal

Adrenal Adenoma

When an incidental adrenal nodule is detected on single-energy CECT, it becomes essential to get a delayed scan or separate NCCT scan for characterization of the nodule. On a DE-CECT acquisition, virtual NCCT images generated from the dual energy datasets help eliminate the need of another NCCT scan. The attenuation of adrenal adenoma at low and high kVp image depends on their lipid content. On several studies, there have been mixed reports related to the attenuation of adrenal adenoma on 80 and 140 kVp scans.[41]

Hepatic Mass Characterization

Characterization of Hepatic Mass Lesions

Like other organs, NCCT acquisition in liver also can be avoided by generating a virtual NCCT image from DECT acquisition of any one of the phases of multiphase CECT protocol. Secondly, hypervascular liver lesions are most conspicuous in arterial phase of examination, however detection of a hypervascular lesion on a delayed arterial phase becomes difficult. In such a scenario, on a DECT scan, the lesions can become more appreciable on a lower kVp image.[42] Nonenhancing lesions or cysts appear dark on iodine density maps **(Figs. 16A and B)**.

Follow-up After Hepatic Tumor Ablation or TACE

After tumor ablation or embolization, detection of recurrence/viable tumor depends on the demonstration of tumor mass enhancement, which in turn needs acquisition of both NCCT and a CECT scans. With DECT, single CT acquisition can generate virtual NCCT and iodine maps to detect enhancement.

A word of caution needs to be remembered while imaging hepatocellular carcinoma after chemoembolization with lipiodol. Since lipiodol contains high concentration of iodine, iodine density display images shows the lipiodol accumulation as bright spot/hyperenhancement; which should not be diagnosed as recurrent or residual tumor.[43]

Hepatic Steatosis or Iron Deposition

DECT can differentiate focal fat deposition from other hepatic mass lesion in the absence of iron deposition, which is a confounding factor. Studies[44] have described that attenuation values that are 9–13 HU lower at 80 kVp than at 140 kVp are suggestive of fat infiltration **(Figs. 17A to E)**. Iron deposition in liver parenchyma will have higher attenuation at lower energy images.

Application in Pancreas

Pancreatic neoplasms are usually hypovascular and their detection is based on the attenuation difference between the normally enhancing pancreatic parenchyma and hypoenhancing mass lesion. Pancreatic parenchymal

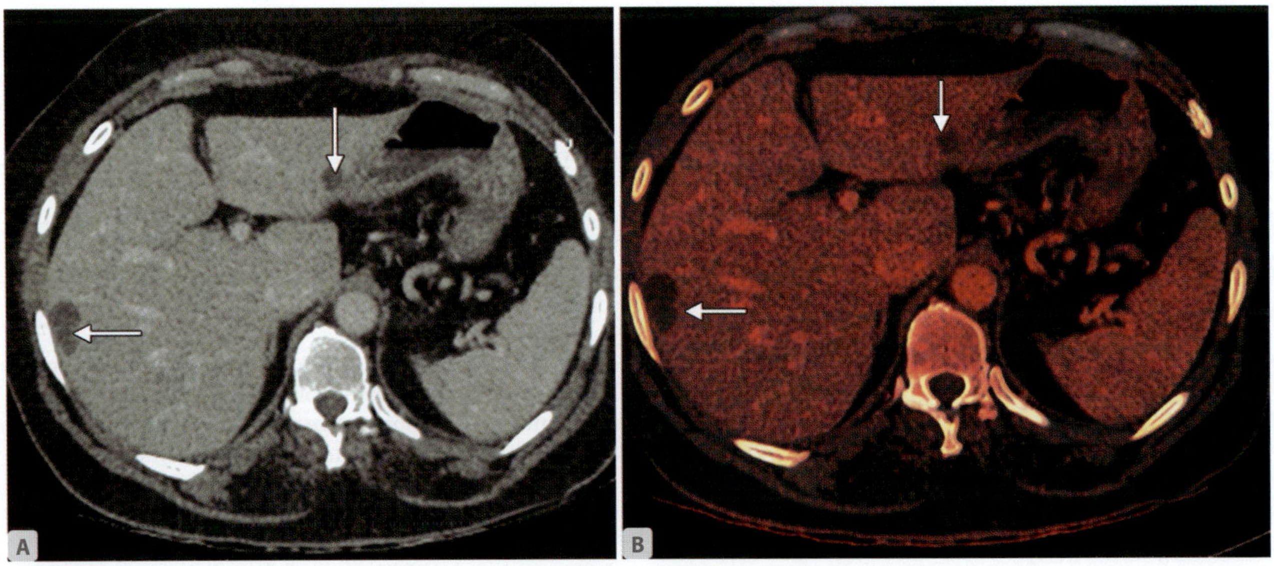

FIGS. 16A AND B: Simple hepatic cysts, imaging performed on a second generation DS-DECT scanner. Simulated monoenergetic image display at 70 kV generated from a dual energy dataset (A) shows hypodense focal lesions in segment III and V. Iodine overlay maps (B) show them to be dark (not taking up iodine).

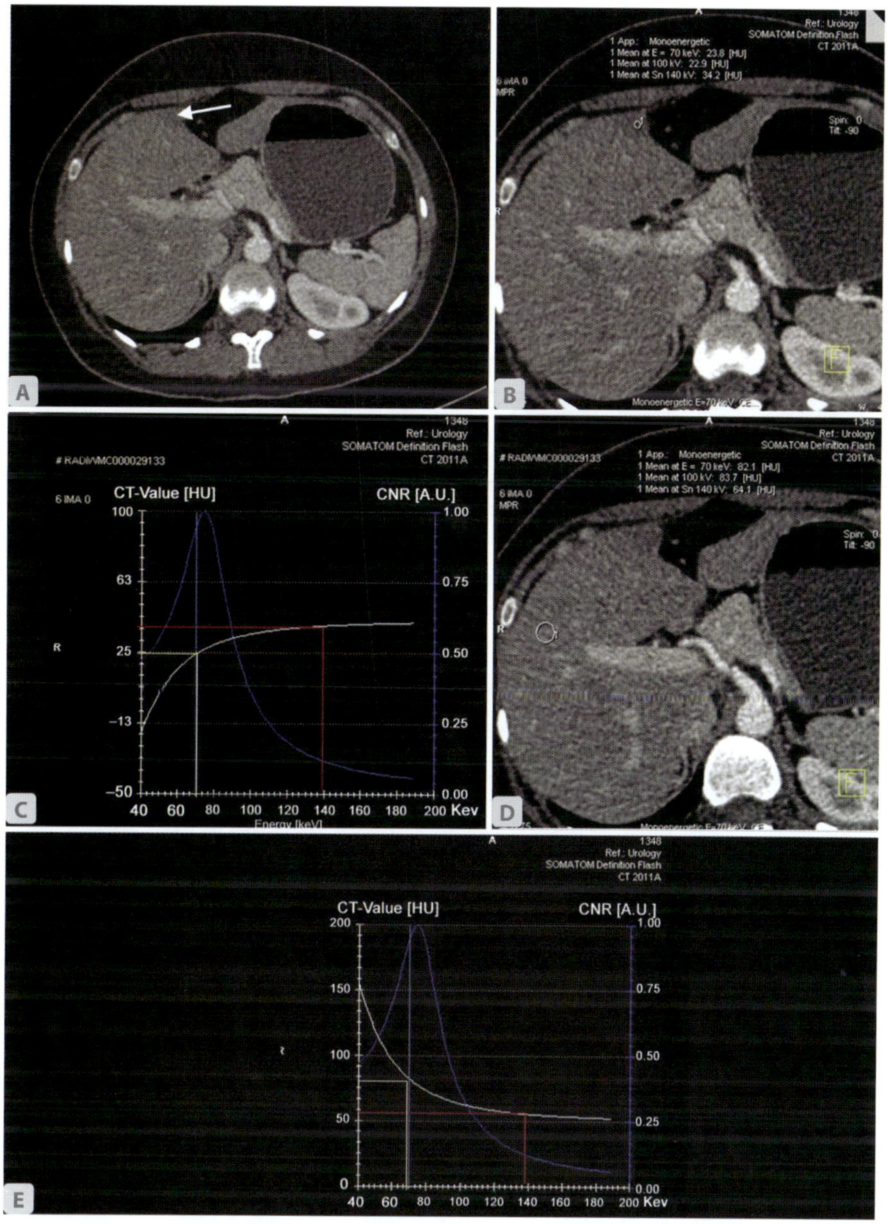

FIGS. 17A TO E: Focal hepatic steatosis. The area of focal fat deposition is seen as a hypodensity in segment 4b adjacent to the falciform ligament (arrow in A). Monoenergetic display (B) derived from a DS-DECT scanner (Somatom Definition Flash, Siemens) with tin filtration shows the increase in attenuation in higher kV images (attenuation of 23.8 at 70 kV, shown with a yellow line and 34.2 at 140 kV, shown with a red line C), which is suggestive of fatty change. In comparison, normal enhancing liver parenchyma shows a decrease in attenuation (D and E) in the higher energy images (attenuation of 82.1 at 70 kV and 64.1 at 140 kV images).

enhancement is best assessed in the pancreatic phase, 40–70 sec after injection of contrast material. However, significant percentage of pancreatic carcinomas is difficult to detect even on pancreatic phase images. With DECT, the normally enhancing pancreatic parenchyma shows higher attenuation on monochromatic lower energy display image and the iodine density display. It has been seen that the attenuation difference between the lesion and normal pancreatic parenchyma (hence the lesion detection) increases with 80 kVp image than a single energy routine 120 kVp scan.[45]

Another potential application of DECT in pancreatic imaging is the accurate identification of pancreatic necrosis; although the clinical importance is not yet established.[26]

Pulmonary Applications

Pulmonary Thromboembolism

Pulmonary thromboembolism (PTE) imaging has undergone significant change in the past few years. Pulmonary CT angiography (CTA) has been accepted as the imaging modality of choice in case of suspected high-risk population. Pulmonary CTA can detect intraluminal thrombus in segmental arteries and smaller vessels also, but smaller clots/partial occlusion in subsegmental arteries can be missed on CTA. When imaging is done on a DECT scanner, smaller clots can be detected on an iodine overlay map visible as a perfusion defect. Compared to CTA and scintigraphy, dual-energy CT has a high sensitivity and specificity for perfusion mapping for the assessment of pulmonary embolism.[46] The perfusion defects in cases of pulmonary embolism are usually peripheral and wedge-shaped **(Figs. 18A to I)**; although they can be absent in cases of very small non-occluding thrombus in smaller vessels.

For the generation of a proper iodine perfusion map of the lungs, the maximum and minimum value for material decomposition are usually kept at -600 and -960 HU. For obtaining proper parenchymal enhancement, iodinated contrast agent should be injected at a proper rate (4–4.5 mL/sec), followed by 40 mL saline chase to reduce artifacts resulting from dense contrast in SVC/brachiocephalic vein.

Perfusion defects can also be seen from non-PTE causes; for example in cases of aberrant pulmonary vascular supply,[47] or artefactual perfusion defects as in the lingual or right middle lobe (from cardiac pulsations), bilateral lower lobes near the diaphragm (from respiratory motion), in bilateral upper lobes (from streak artifacts in SVC or subclavian artery). Perfusion defects are also observed in parenchymal

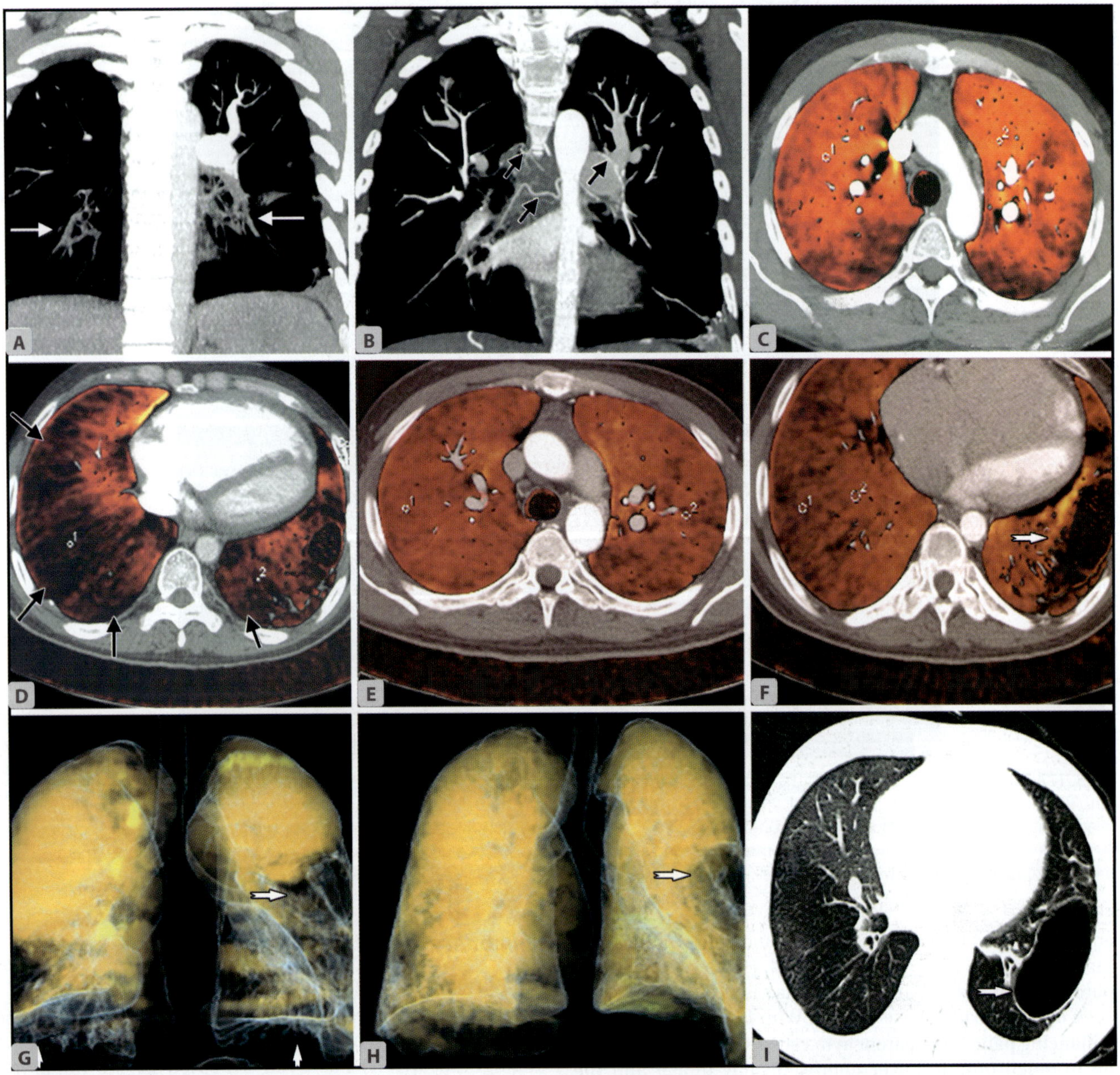

FIGS. 18A TO I: Dual energy CT perfusion in chronic pulmonary thromboembolism. Coronal reformatted CTA image acquired at pulmonary phase (A) shows nonenhancement and attenuation in caliber of the lower lobe pulmonary arteries (arrows). Aortic phase image reveals hypertrophic bronchial arteries (small arrows in B). Iodine overlay maps generated from dual energy CTA during pulmonary phase (C and D) reveal patchy areas of perfusion defect in the basal segments of both lower lobes (arrows in D). Iodine maps (E and F) generated from aortic phase images shows near complete perfusion (via bronchial collaterals) in the corresponding area. Volume rendered images generated from iodine distribution maps in pulmonary phase (G) also shows the areas of perfusion defect (block arrow); whereas aortic phase image (H) shows near complete perfusion except a small area of nonperfusion (notched arrow) secondary to a large bulla. Lung window axial image (I) confirms the presence of the bulla (notched arrow).

abnormalities such as consolidation, atelectasis or emphysema.

- *Xenon perfusion CT:* Xenon is a radioopaque gas with atomic number 54 and has photoelectric absorption characteristics similar to iodine. During xenon ventilation CT, the patient usually inhales 30% xenon through a xenon gas inhalation system (Zetron V; Anzai Medical, Tokyo, Japan). Overlay maps are generated similar to iodine perfusion CT. DE xenon ventilation CT can be used to generate a ventilation map with areas of bronchial obstruction or atresia showing reduced ventilation.[48]
- *Pulmonary nodule evaluation:* The degree of contrast enhancement on CECT is an important factor in differentiating a benign pulmonary nodule from a malignant one. DECT can generate virtual NCCT images and thereby quantify the enhancement. The differentiation of calcification from contrast enhancement is also possible.

Musculoskeletal Applications

Application in Gout

The diagnosis of gout can be made on clinical and biochemical basis, however, the definitive diagnosis of gout requires microscopic analysis of fluid aspirated from the joint with the finding of negatively birefringent monosodium urate (MSU) crystals.[49] It is challenging to aspirate an acutely inflamed joint, and it can also be negative for MSU crystals in up to 25% cases.[49,50]

On DECT, the dual energy ratio (vide supra) of uric acid varies significantly from that of calcium, hence they can be easily differentiated. DS-DECT scans can generate material specific images and keeping the reference Dual energy ratio at 1.36, the uric acid crystals lie below the line and are differently color-coded (green), whereas the calcium deposits lie above the line **(Figs. 19A to D)**. DECT not only aids in gout and also using automated volume software, the tophi volume can be quantitatively measured.[51]

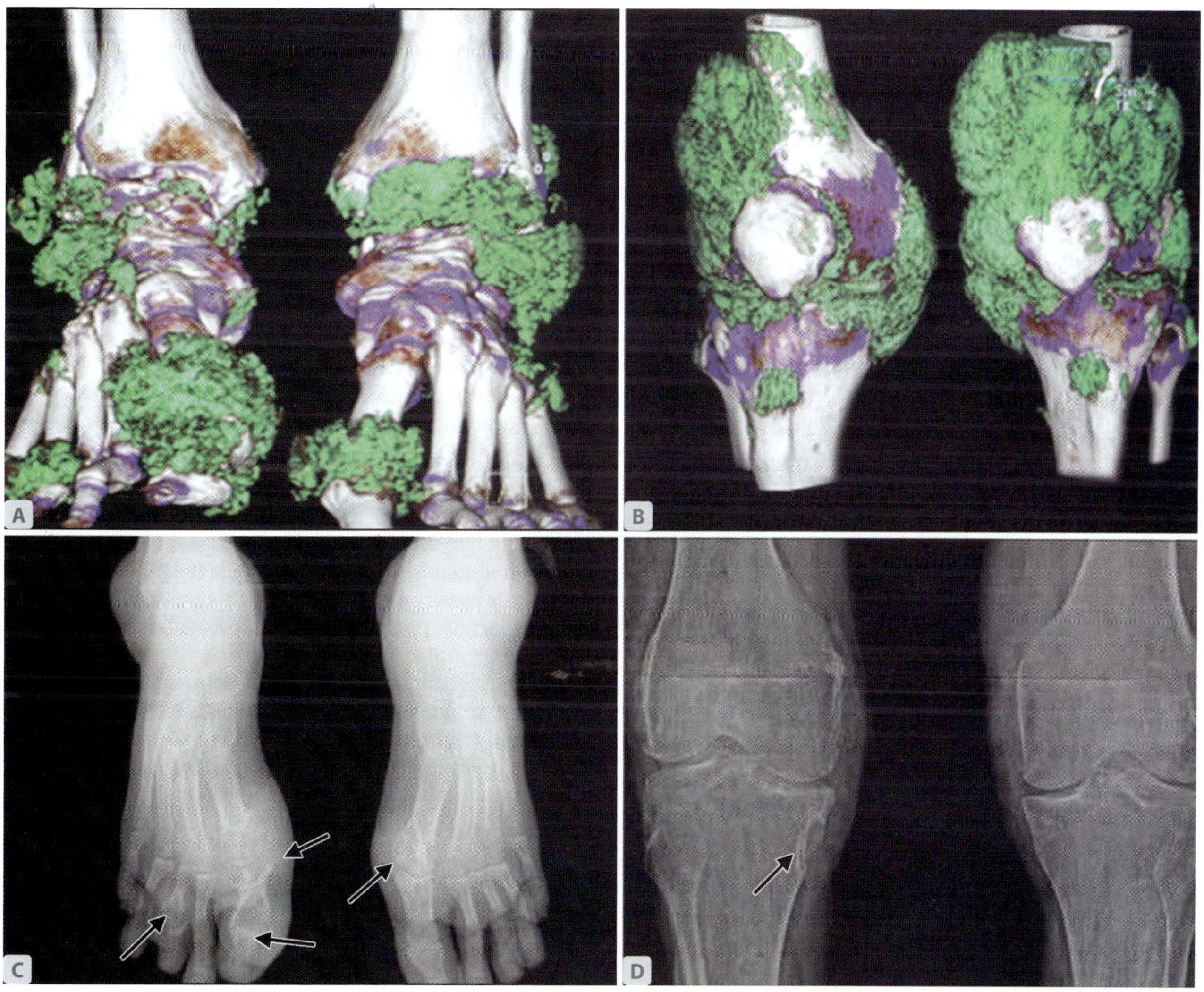

FIGS. 19A TO D: DECT in gout imaging. Scanning was performed at 80 and 140 kV in a patient with chronic gouty arthritis. Keeping a reference dual energy line at 1.36, MSU crystals are color coded green. Color coded volume rendered images of the ankle (A) and knee (B) reveal extensive MSU crystal deposition around the joints. Plain radiographs of the feet and knee reveals periarticular soft tissue swellings and corticated erosions (arrows in C and D).

Metal Artifact Reduction

Imaging of patients with metallic prosthesis remains a challenge. As the X-ray beam passes through metal prosthesis, the lower energy photons are absorbed and the character of the X-ray spectrum changes (it becomes 'harder', i.e. having higher energy photons only). This gives rise to the beam hardening artifacts around metallic prostheses which hamper the visualization of periprosthetic abnormalities.

The usual modifications to reduce metal artifact in a single energy scanner include:

- Increasing the kVp
- Increasing the mAs
- Reducing slice collimation
- Using a softer kernel for reconstruction
- Thicker slice reconstruction.

Using DECT, monoenergetic reconstruction at a higher kVp has been shown in several studies to be more effective than routine single energy CT images at 120 kVp.[52,53]

Other Musculoskeletal Applications

There are several other applications of DECT; for example, detection of bone marrow edema[55] and evaluation of ligaments and tendons. Pache et al.[54] described high sensitivity and specificity of DECT imaging in the detection of post-traumatic bone marrow edema. Using a three material decomposition (water, fat and calcium), the virtual non-calcium subtracted images can be generated to detect marrow edema.

Tendons and ligaments are made up of collagen fibrils, which have a specific dual energy ratio. In DECT, for material specific image generation a three material decomposition algorithm is used (collagen, fat and soft tissue). Several studies[55,56] have showed conflicting efficacy of DECT in the evaluation of tendons and ligaments. Thicker ligaments like anterior and posterior cruciate ligaments and patellar ligament can be adequately visualized, however visualization of thinner anatomical structures might not be appropriate.

Applications in Head and Neck

Like other parts of the body, DECT imaging in head and neck also has the advantage of generating a virtual NCCT image from the dual energy dataset, in order to quantify enhancement in a mass lesion. Iodine overlay maps can increase lesion conspicuity and improved visualization of laryngeal cartilage invasion.[57]

Vascular Applications

Dual energy CT angiography has been most widely used in aortic imaging. The advantages of DECT in aortic stent-graft imaging are multiple **(Box 5)**. In endoleak detection, single delayed DECT scanning followed by reconstruction of virtual NCCT and mono energetic low-kV images has very high sensitivity, specificity and positive predictive value (96–100%) compared with a conventional multiphase single energy CTA acquisition, thereby significantly reducing the patient dose (40–64%).[58-60]

In peripheral or neck angiography, the drawbacks of threshold based bone subtraction is that in cases of arteries lying close to bone, a part of the artery can be subtracted and may mimic stenosis or occlusion. Since the bone subtraction in DECT is based on material differentiation, it takes less time and yields more complete bone removal **(Fig. 20)**, which can reduce such artifacts.[61]

BOX 5: Advantages of DECT in aortic stent-graft imaging.

- Virtual monoenergetic high kVp images: better in metal artifact reduction
- Virtual monoenergetic low kVp images: better in detection of iodine (can pick small endoleaks)
- Iodine overlay map: detect smaller endoleaks (differentiate between blood and contrast)
- Virtual NCCT image: detect intramural hematoma
- DE subtracted angiographic images: easier to generate, more complete bone removal

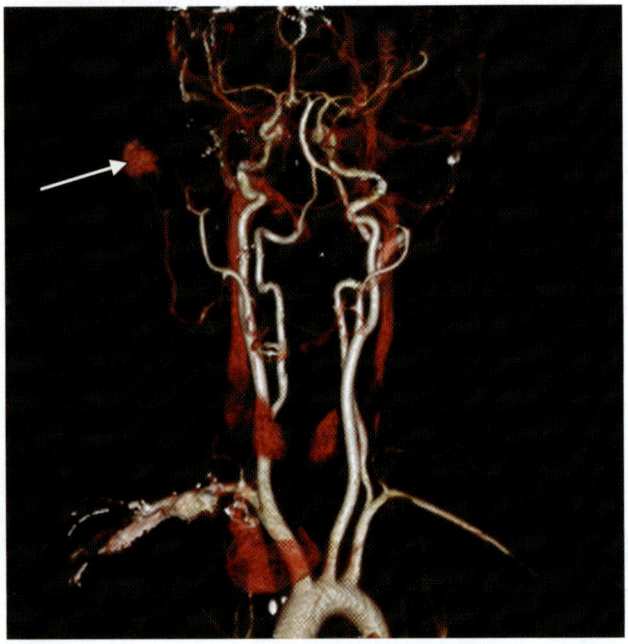

FIG. 20: Volume rendered CTA image of the head and neck in a 10-year-old male with proliferative hemangioma (arrow) on the right side of face. The bone removal in Dual energy CTA depends on material differentiation and leads to complete and quick bone subtraction compared to threshold based bone subtraction.

Also with threshold based bone subtraction, DECT CTA can remove calcified plaques also, with better visualization of vascular lumen. Compared to threshold based bone removal, DECT bone subtraction is easier, quicker and more accurate in detection of vessel stenosis.

Cardiac Applications

Coronary CT angiography in a multidetector row scanner has become an established imaging tool in the detection of significant coronary artery disease (CAD) in low to intermediate risk population.[62] However, the mere detection of an artery stenosis does not predict the hemodynamic significance of it, which can be predicted by myocardial perfusion imaging or wall motion abnormalities. Till now,

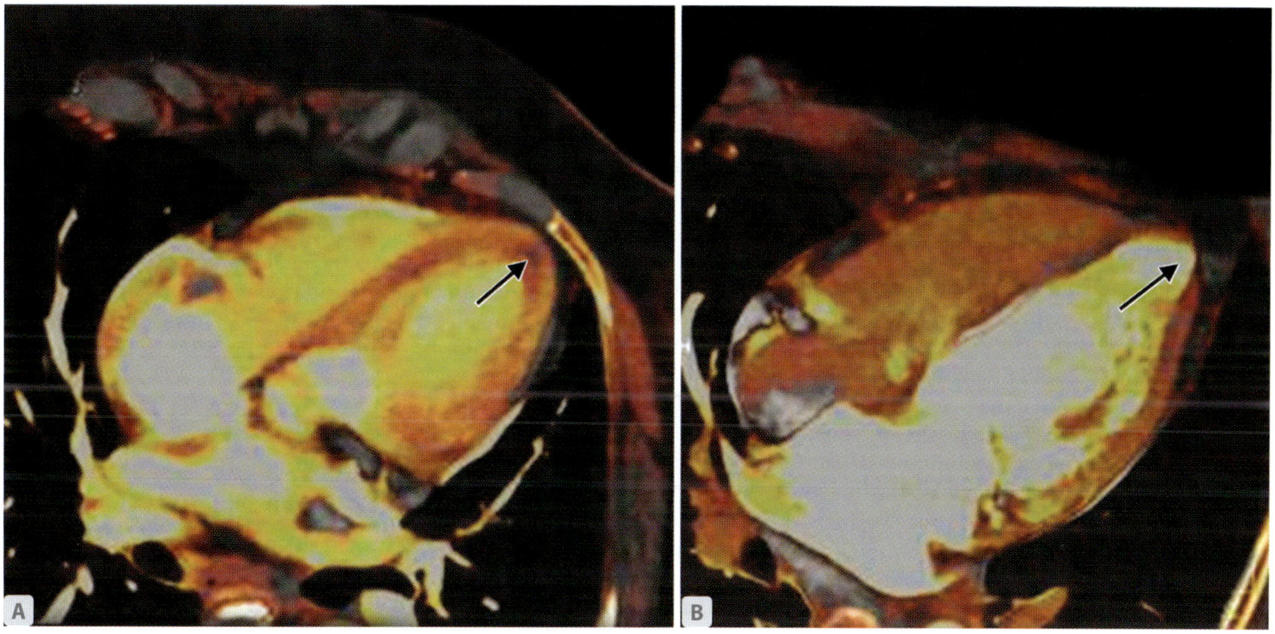

FIGS. 21A AND B: Stress myocardial perfusion imaging using DECT. A 52-year-old lady with effort intolerance. Iodine overlay maps at rest (A) shows perfusion defect (arrow) in the territory of the left anterior descending coronary artery (LAD) which is exaggerated on adenosine stress images (B); suggestive of LAD territory ischemia.

myocardial perfusion studies have been performed using nuclear medicine studies (SPECT) and MRI. However, SPECT has poor spatial resolution and is not useful for coronary artery assessment. MRI can detect myocardial perfusion and cine-MRI can detect regional wall motion abnormality; but it is time consuming and not useful for morphologic assessment of coronary artery disease.[63] With the use of DECT technology, material density (iodine) maps can be generated for the myocardium, reflecting the myocardial perfusion. Although termed 'perfusion', the map usually reflects the myocardial blood pool and is a static acquisition.

Monoenergetic low kV, high kV and iodine overlay maps are generated. Normally perfused myocardium show uniform iodine distribution **(Figs. 21A and B)**. Myocardial infarcts are visualized as perfusion defects both at rest and under stress, whereas reversible ischemia shows perfusion defect only in stress images. Nonviable myocardium will show hyperenhancement on delayed scans.[64] DECT thus can combine the benefits of superior resolution morphologic imaging in CAD coupled with detection of its hemodynamic significance in the form of ischemia/infarction, which is unique to this modality.

Material differentiation based on dual energy ratio has been tried in the characterization of plaques. Although differentiating a calcified from a noncalcified plaque is possible, but the differentiation of various types of non-calcified plaques have not been successful.[65]

Applications in Neuroimaging

As discussed for CTA elsewhere in the body, dual energy CTA of intracranial vessels also has the similar advantage of easy and quick bone removal, especially with complex bony anatomy at the base of skull. The virtual NCCT images generated from the dual energy dataset helps detect hemorrhage and can save crucial time.[66]

Studies have described dual energy CTA to be the ideal tool for evaluating an acute intracranial hemorrhage. Apart from the ease of assessment of vascular cause of hemorrhage (vide supra); iodine overlay maps can be useful in differentiating tumor bleed from a simple hematoma. Hemorrhage within a tumor will show hyperdensity on NCCT images and detection of any enhancing mass lesion in the background of hemorrhage can be an imaging challenge. Iodine overlay maps can detect the enhancing tumor tissue in the background of hematoma with greater accuracy.

Monoenergetic-imaging

This new application displays monoenergetic images in a range of 40–190 keV and helps to easily compare and quantify lesions and tissues. Also, high enhancement is observed even for low iodine concentrations at low energy levels.[67] This enables image quality enhancement and metal artifact reduction.

DOSE CONSIDERATIONS

Although DECT scanning involves imaging with two different X-ray beams, the dose is not doubled in comparison to the single energy scan. This is because the mAs are divided in the two sources; the higher energy tube operates at a lower mAs and the lower energy tube utilizes a relatively higher mAs. Till date, several experimental studies have been performed regarding dose comparisons of DECT scanning and single energy scanning. Most of the experiments are based on DS-DECT scanners. Data are sparse regarding dose issues in SS-DECT. There has been various studies comparing dose of the single and dual energy scanners, but very few of them are performed with normalization of the contrast to noise ratio (CNR) or image quality.[68]

Schenzle et al.[68] performed a study on anthropomorphic phantom equipped with TLDs, with scanning performed at 140 and 80 kVp, 14 × 1.2 collimation in a first generation DS-DECT scanner and in a second generation DS-DECT scanner at 140 and 100 kVp settings with selective photon shielding at 128 × 0.6 mm collimation. Dose comparison was done with a single energy scan at 120 kV and 64 × 0.6 mm collimation at an equivalent dose index of 5.4 mGy x cm. The respective doses were 2.61 mSv (first generation DS-DECT in dual energy mode), 2.69 mSv (second generation DS-DECT in dual energy mode), 2.70 mSv (second generation DS-DECT in single energy mode). The image noise were also similar in all these three imaging techniques. Hence, there was no significant dose difference between the imaging techniques.

In coronary CTA, the dose received by DECT imaging has been assessed by Kerl et al.[69] who compared the dose levels between DECT, first generation DS-DECT in single energy mode, and single energy single source 16 slice MDCT. The investigators reported a lower dose, higher CNR and good diagnostic image quality in DECT than single source MDCT. The increase in CNR was attributed to the low- kVp acquisition in DECT scanning by the investigators. Several other studies[70] regarding CT pulmonary angiography or CTA have shown that there is no significant increase in dose while scanning by DS-DECT scanning, compared to a single energy scanning. The added benefit of DECT scanning lies in the generation of virtual unenhanced scans, which can obviate the need of another NCCT scanning and reduce radiation dose. In renal imaging, the replacement of NCCT by virtual NCCT can result in a dose reduction of up to 35% in first generation DECT and up to 50% in second generation DECT.[71] Addition of tin filter in second generation DS-DECT reduces the dose by eliminating lower energy X-ray photons from the higher energy spectrum.

FUTURE TRENDS IN DECT IMAGING

The use of energy specific, photon-counting detector can reduce the radiation dose further, retaining the benefits of material characterization on DECT. Semiconductor materials such as cadmium telluride (CdTe) are able to convert X-rays directly into electric signal pulses. These detectors will register each photon and help to measure the energy from each individual photon.

CONCLUSION

To conclude, dual energy CT imaging adds another new dimension to conventional CT. The material-specific information gained by DECT scanning can be translated either to functional analysis of organs (for example, myocardial perfusion analysis), improvement in diagnostic confidence (noninvasive confirmation of clinical diagnosis in gout), aid in management decision-making (for example in renal calculi) or to easy image postprocessing and avoidance of unnecessary scanning.

ACKNOWLEDGMENTS

The authors sincerely acknowledge the contribution of Dr Gurpreet S Gulati for figure no. 21 and Dr Sudeep Acharya and Dr Zohra Ahmad for figure no. 15 and 19, respectively, from their MD thesis work at the Department of Radiodiagnosis, AIIMS.

REFERENCES

1. Rogalla P, Kloeters C, Hein PA, et al. CT Technology Overview: 64 –Slice and Beyond. Radiol Clin N Am. 2009;47:1-11.
2. Curry TS, Dowdey JE, Murry RC. Computed Tomography in Christensen's Physics of Diagnostic Radiology, 4th Edn. Philadelphia and London: Lea & Febiger; 1990.pp.289-322.
3. Pelc NJ. Recent and future directions in CT Imaging. Ann Biomed Eng. 2014;42(2):260-268.
4. Miraldi F, Sims MS, Wiesen EJ. Imaging Principles in Computed. Tomography in CT and MR Imaging of the Whole Body, 4th Edn. In: Haaga JR, Lanzieri CF, Gilkeson RC (Eds). United States of America: Mosby; 2003.pp.2-36.
5. Mahesh M, Cody DD. Physics of cardiac imaging with multiple-row detector CT. Radiographics. 2007;27(5):1495-509.
6. Lewis MA, Pascoal A, Keevil SF, Lewis CA. Selecting a CT scanner for cardiac imaging: the heart of the matter. Br J Radiol 2016;89:20160376.
7. Ehman EC, Yu L, Manduca A, et al. www.kau.edu.sa [cited 2019 February 26] Available from "X-Ray Tube in CT Scanner" www.kau.edu.sa/.
8. Tabari A, Gullo RL, Murugan V, Otrakji A, Digumarthy S, Kalra M. Recent Advances in Computed Tomographic Technology: Cardiopulmonary Imaging Applications. J Thorac Imaging 2017;32:89-100.
9. Behling R. Performance And Pitfalls Of Diagnostic X-Ray Sources: An Overview. Medical Physics International Journal. 2016;4: 107-114.
10. Shefer E et al. State of the Art of CT Detectors and Sources: A literature Review. Current Radiology Reports. 2013;1:76-91.
11. Yanagawa M, Tomiyama N, Honda O, et al. Multidetector CT of the lung: image quality with garnet-based detectors. Radiology. 2010;255(3):944-54.
12. Methods for Clinical Evaluation of Noise Reduction Techniques in Abdominopelvic CT. Radiographics 2014;34(4):849-62.
13. Flohr TG, Schaller S, Stierstorfer K, et al. Multi detector row CT systems and image-reconstruction techniques. Radiology. 2005;235(3):756-73.
14. Hsieh J, Nett B, Yu z, Sauer K, Thibault JB, Bouman CA. Recent Advances in CT Image Reconstruction Curr Radiol Rep. 2013;1: 39-51.
15. Ginat DT, Gupta R. Advances in Computed Tomography Imaging Technology. Annual Review of Biomedical Engineering 2014;16(1):431-53.
16. Miracle AC, Mukherji SK. Cone beam CT of the Head and Neck, Part 1: Physical Principles. AJNR. 2009;30:1088-95.
17. Orth RC, Wallace MJ, Kuo MD. For the Technology Assessment Committee of the Society of Interventional Radiology. C-arm

cone-beam CT: general principles and technical considerations for use in interventional radiology. J Vasc Interv Radiol. 2008;19:814-20.

18. Jaffray DA, Siewerdsen JH. Cone beam computed tomography with a flat-panel imager: initial performance characterization. Medical Physics. 2000;27:1311-23.
19. Bauhs JA, Vrieze TJ, Primak AN, et al. CT dosimetry: comparison of measurement techniques and devices. Radiographics. 2008;28:245-53.
20. Alspaugh J, Christodoulou E, Goodsitt M, et al. Dose and image quality of flat-panel detector volume computed tomography for sinus imaging. Med Phys. 2007;34:2634.
21. Fahrig R, Dixon R, Payne T, et al. Dose and image quality for a cone-beam C-arm CT system. Med Phys. 2006;33: 4541-50.
22. Scarfe WC, Farman AG, Sukovic P. Clinical applications of cone-beam computed tomography in dental practice. J Can Dent Assoc. 2006;72:75-80.
23. Appelbaum L, Sosna J, Nissenbaum Y, Benshtein A, Goldberg SN. Electromagnetic Navigation System for CT-Guided Biopsy of Small Lesions. AJR. 2011;196:1194-1200.
24. Chellathurai A, Kanhirat S, Chokkappan K, Swaminathan TS, Kulasekaran N. Technical note: CT-guided biopsy of lung masses using an automated guiding apparatus. Indian J Radiol Imaging. 2009;19(3):206-7.
25. Curry TS III, Dowdey JE, Murry RC. Christensen's physics of diagnostic radiology, 4th edn. Philadelphia, Pa: Lea & Febiger; 1990.pp.61-9.
26. Coursey CA, Nelson RC, Boll DT, et al. Dual-energy multi- detector CT: how does it work, what can it tell us, and when can we use it in abdominopelvic imaging? Radio Graphics. 2010;30(4): 1037-55.
27. Andrew N Primak, Juan Carlos Ramirez Giraldo, Christian D. Eusemann, Bernhard Schmidt, Birgit Kantor, Joel G. Fletcher, Cynthia H. McCollough. Dual-Source Dual-Energy CT With Additional Tin Filtration: Dose and Image Quality Evaluation in Phantoms and In Vivo. AJR. 2010;195:1164-74.
28. Faby S, Merz J, Krauss B, Kuemmel F. Spectral Imaging with Dual Energy CT; Comparison of different technologies and workflows. White paper @ siemens.com/ct.
29. Chandra N, Langan DA. Gemstone detector: dual energy imaging via fast kVp switching. In: Johnson TRC, Fink C, Schönberg SO, Reiser MF, (Eds). Dual energy CT in clinical practice. Berlin, Germany: Springer-Verlag; 2011.pp.35-41.
30. Li B, Yadava G, Hsieh J, Chandra N, Kulpins MS. Head and body CTDIw of dual-energy X-ray CT with fast-kVp switching. In: Samei E, Pelc NJ, (Eds). Proceedings of SPIE: medical imaging. Bellingham, Wash: International Society for Optical Engineering; 2010.
31. Rutt B, Fenster A. Split-filter computed tomography: a simple technique for dual energy scanning. J Comput Assist Tomogr. 1980;4:501-9.
32. Kelcz F, Joseph PM, Hilal SK. Noise considerations in dual energy CT scanning. Med Phys. 1979;6:418-25.
33. Fletcher JG, Takahashi N, Hartman R, et al. Dual-energy and dual-source CT: is there a role in the abdomen and pelvis? Radiol Clin North Am. 2009;47(1):41-57.
34. Graser A, Johnson TR, Chandarana H, Macari M. Dual energy CT: preliminary observations and potential clinical applications in the abdomen. Eur Radiol. 2009;19(1): 13-23.
35. Lehmann LA, Alvarez RE, Macovski A, et al. Generalized image combinations in dual kVp digital radiography. Med Phys. 1981;8(5):659-67.
36. Hidas G, Eliahou R, Duvdevani M, et al. Determination of renal stone composition with dual-energy CT: in vivo analysis and comparison with X-ray diffraction. Radiology. 2010;257(2):394-401.
37. Vrtiska TJ, Takahashi N, Fletcher JG, Hartman RP, Yu L, Kawashima A. Genitourinary applications of dual-energy CT. AJR. 2010;194(6):1434-42.
38. Kaza RK, Caoili EM, Cohan RH, Platt JF. Distinguishing enhancing from nonenhancing renal lesions with fast kilovoltage-switching dual-energy CT. AJR. 2011;197(6):1375-81.
39. Mendonca PRS, Bhotika R, Maddah M, et al. Multi-material decomposition of spectral CT images. In: Samei E, Pelc NJ, (Eds). Proceedings of SPIE: medical imaging 2010. Vol 7622. Bellingham, Wash: International Society for Optical Engineering; 2010.
40. Takahashi N, Vrtiska TJ, Kawashima A, et al. Detectability of urinary stones on virtual nonenhanced images generated at pyelographic-phase dual-energy CT. Radiology. 2010;256(1):184-90.
41. Gupta RT, Ho LM, Marin D, Boll DT, Barnhart HX, Nelson RC. Dual energy CT for characterization of adrenal nodules: initial experience. AJR. 2010;194(6):1479-83.
42. Marin D, Nelson RC, Samei E, et al. Hypervascular liver tumors: low tube voltage, high tube current multidetector CT during late hepatic arterial phase for detection—initial clinical experience. Radiology. 2009;251(3):771-9.
43. Silva AC, Morse BG, Hara AK, Paden RG, Hongo N, Pavlicek W. Dual energy (Spectral) CT: applications in abdominal imaging. Radiographics. 2011;31:1031-46.
44. Mendler MH, Bouillet P, Le Sidaner A, et al. Dual-energy CT in the diagnosis and quantification of fatty liver: limited clinical value in comparison to ultrasound scan and single energy CT with special reference to iron overload. J Hepatol. 1998;28(5): 785-94.
45. Spieler B, Macari M, Godoy M, et al. Dual source dual energy MDCT: comparison of 80 kVp and weighted average kVp data on pancreatic lesion conspicuity (abstr). In: Radiological Society of North America scientific assembly and annual meeting program. Oak Brook, Ill: Radiological Society of North America; 2008.p.522.
46. Thieme SF, Becker CR, Hacker M, Nikolaou K, Reiser MF, Johnson TR. Dual energy CT for the assessment of lung perfusion: correlation to scintigraphy. Eur J Radiol. 2008;68(3):369-74.
47. Boroto K, Remy-Jardin M, Flohr T, et al. Thoracic applications of dual-source CT technology. Eur J Radiol. 2008;68(3):375-84.
48. Chae EJ, Seo JB, Goo HW, et al. Xenon ventilation CT with a dual-energy technique of dual-source CT: initial experience. Radiology. 2008;248(2):615-24.
49. Monu JU, Pope TL Jr. Gout: a clinical and radiologic review. Radiol Clin North Am. 2004;42:169-84.
50. Swan A, Amer H, Dieppe P. The value of synovial fluid assays in the diagnosis of joint disease: a literature survey. Ann Rheum Dis. 2002;61:493-8.
51. Choi HK, Burns LC, Shojania K, et al. Dual energy CT in gout: a prospective validation study. Ann Rheum Dis. 2012;71(9): 1466-71.
52. Bamberg F, Dierks A, Nikolaou K, Reiser MF, Becker CR, Johnson TR. Metal artifact reduction by dual energy computed tomography using monoenergetic extrapolation. Eur Radiol. 2011;21:1424-9.
53. Zhou C, Zhao YE, Luo S, et al. Monoenergetic imaging of dual-energy CT reduces artifacts from implanted metal orthopedic devices in patients with fractures. Acad Radiol. 2011;18:1252-7.
54. Pache G, Krauss B, Strohm P, et al. Dual-energy CT virtual noncalcium technique: detecting post-traumatic bone marrow lesions—feasibility study. Radiology. 2010;256:617-24.
55. Deng K, Sun C, Liu C, Ma R. Initial experience with visualizing hand and foot tendons by dual energy computed tomography. Clin Imaging. 2009;33:384-9.
56. Sun C, Miao F, Wang XM, et al. An initial qualitative study of dual-energy CT in the knee ligaments. Surg Radiol Anat. 2008;30: 443-7.

57. Hirofumi Kuno, Hiroaki Onaya, Ryoko Iwata, Tatsushi Kobayashi, Satoshi Fujii, Ryuichi Hayashi, Katharina Otani, Hiroya Ojiri, Takeharu Yamanaka, Mitsuo Satake. Evaluation of Cartilage Invasion by Laryngeal and Hypopharyngeal Squamous Cell Carcinoma with Dual-Energy CT. Radiology. 2012;265:488-96.
58. Stolzmann P, Frauenfelder T, Pfammatter T, et al. Endoleaks after endovascular abdominal aortic aneurysm repair: detection with dual-energy dual- source CT. Radiology. 2008;249:682-91.
59. Maturen KE, Kleaveland PA, Kaza RK, et al. Aortic endograft surveillance: use of fast-switch kVp dual-energy computed tomography with virtual noncontrast imaging. J Comput Assist Tomogr. 2011;35:742-6.
60. Yamamoto S, McWilliams J, Arellano C, et al. Dual-energy CT angiography of pelvic and lower extremity arteries: dual-energy bone subtraction versus manual bone subtraction. Clin Radiol. 2009;64:1088-96.
61. Vlahos I, Chung R, Nair A, Morgan R. Dual-Energy CT: Vascular Applications AJR 2012;199:S87-97.
62. Stolzmann P, Donati OF, Scheffel H. Low-dose CT coronary angiography for the prediction of myocardial ischaemia. Eur Radiol. 2010;20:56-64.
63. Gaemperli O, Schepis T, Valenta I, et al. Functionally relevant coronary artery disease: comparison of 64-section CT angiography with myocardial perfusion SPECT. Radiology. 2008;248:414-23.
64. Arnoldi E, Lee YS, Ruzsics B, et al. CT detection of myocardial blood volume deficits: dual-energy CT compared with single-energy CT spectra. J Cardiovasc Comput Tomogr. 2011;5:421-9.
65. Henzler T, Porubsky S, Kayed H, et al. Attenuation-based characterization of coronary atherosclerotic plaque: comparison of dual source and dual energy CT with single- source CT and histopathology. Eur J Radiol. 2011;80:54-9.
66. Postma AA, Hofman PA, Stadler AA, van Oostenbrugge RJ, Tijssen MP, Wildberger JE. Dual energy CT of the brain and intracranial vessels. AJR. 2012;199(5 Suppl):S26-33.
67. Mei K et al. Dual-layer spectral computed tomography: measuring relative electron density. European Radiology Experimental. 2018;2:20.
68. Schenzle JC, Sommer WH, Neumaier K, et al. Dual energy CT of the chest: how about the dose? Invest Radiol 2010;45:347-53, Eur J Radiol. 2011;80:54-9.
69. Kerl JM et al. Dose levels at coronary CT angiography- a comparison of Dual energy Dual source and 16-slice CT. 2011;21(3):530-7.
70. De Zordo T, von Lutterotti K, Dejaco C, et al. Comparison of image quality and radiation dose of different pulmonary CTA protocols on a 128-slice CT: high-pitch dual source CT, dual energy CT and conventional spiral CT. Eur Radiol. 2012;22:279-86.
71. Graser A, Johnson TR, Hecht EM, et al. Dual-energy CT in patients suspected of having renal masses: can virtual nonenhanced images replace true nonenhanced images? Radiology. 2009;252:433-40.

CHAPTER

32

Advanced Computed Tomography Applications and Software

Mukesh Kumar Yadav, Priyanka Naranje, Ekta Dhamija

INTRODUCTION

Traditionally computed tomography (CT) has been the major work force in any imaging department. Recent times have witnessed tremendous advances in CT hardware as well as software technology. As we have seen advancement in hardware from conventional type of CT scanner to latest 512 slice CT scanner similarly there has been rapid developments in technology related to CT software.

Though it is difficult to keep pace with everyday technological advancements, this chapter focuses on brief review of recent developments in software technology related to CT. It is worthwhile to mention here that enumeration of all the advancements in CT software is beyond the scope of this chapter; we have tried to summarize advancements in commonly used clinical applications of CT. Many of these advancements are related to utilization of dual energy CT or textural analysis which have been covered elsewhere in this book. The **Table 1** enlists the technological advancements of common softwares we have included in this chapter.

TABLE.1: Advanced CT application softwares.
Lung nodule evaluation softwares
Lung parenchyma evaluation softwares
Pulmonary embolism detection softwares
CT Perfusion advanced softwares
Continuous free-breathing scans
Advanced CT angiography softwares
Advanced Cardiac application softwares
CT volumetry
Dentascan
CT cinematic rendering
Fusion imaging
Vertebral labeling
Software for oncological imaging interpretation
3D printing
Iterative reconstruction
CT colonography

LUNG NODULE EVALUATION SOFTWARES

Advanced softwares for analysis of lung nodule are useful to detect the nodule automatically and provide with the standardized measurement parameters. These applications are also convenient for follow-up. Some of the vendor specific names of such applications are Lung VCAR/Advantage ALA (GE healthcare), syngoLungCARE CT/syngoLungCAD (Syngovia, Siemens, Germany), Lung Nodule Assessment (LNA) application (Philips Healthcare, The Netherlands).

These applications can segment the nodules automatically and provide the information on volume, effective diameter, maximum area, maximum diameter, mean Hounsfield values, percentage of growth and doubling time **(Fig. 1)**. It can synchronize multiple images for nodule comparison. In addition, it can review multiple CTs and compare the nodule in any axial, coronal, sagittal, oblique planes as well as in volume-rendered images.

Clinical Applications

Accurate assessment of nodule size as well as growth on serial imaging forms the most important criterion in Lung cancer screening studies. Manual measurement of the diameter is significantly affected by nodule margin characteristics such as spiculations and lobulations. Semiautomated volume measurements provided by these softwares helps avoid such errors and hence are superior to manual measurements for objective determination of size as well as growth in the nodule.[1] Volume changes in the nodule have also shown to be more sensitive for growth assessment compared to diameter measurements.[2]

LUNG PARENCHYMA EVALUATION SOFTWARES

Lung parenchyma evaluation softwares permit the CT to quantitatively assess the lung density and structure **(Figs. 2 and 3)**. Evaluation of early parenchymal changes

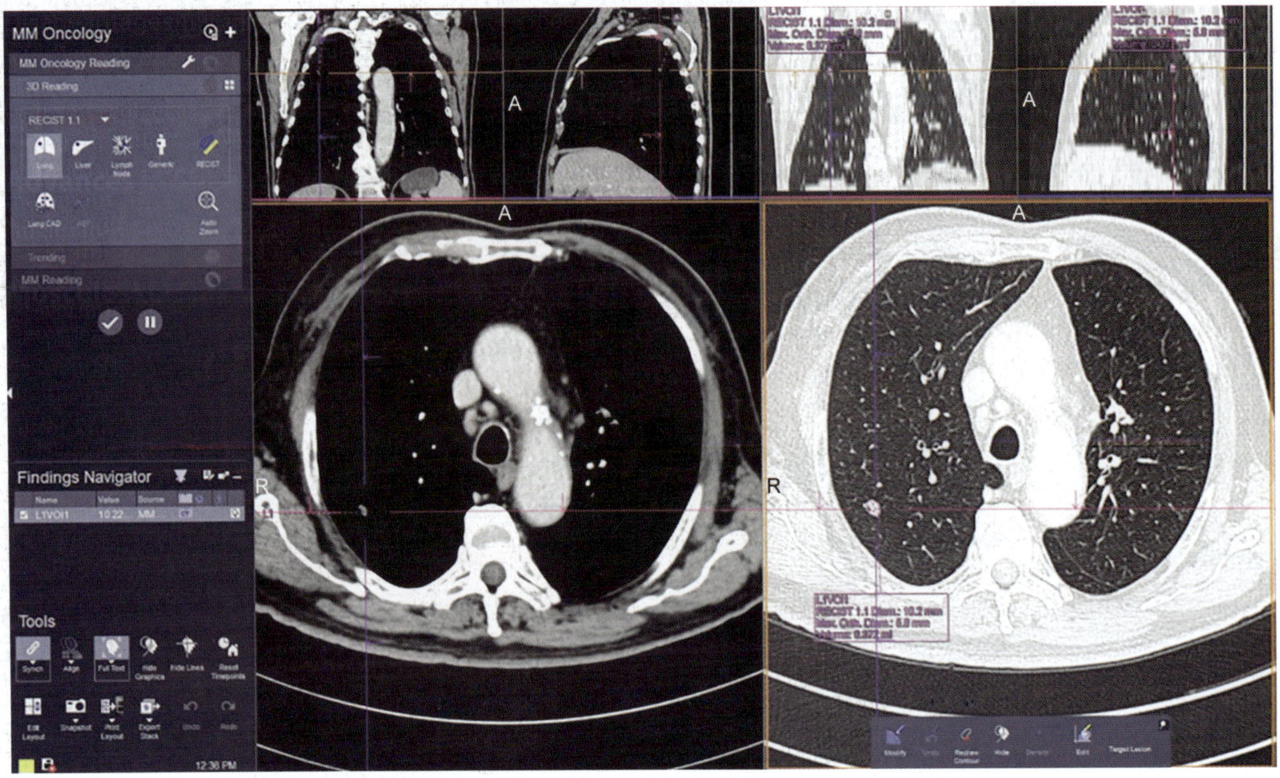

FIG. 1: Lung computer-aided detection (CAD) application. The nodule is identified by the CAD software which displays the nodule in all three planes and also various nodule characteristics such as maximum diameter and volume are displayed.

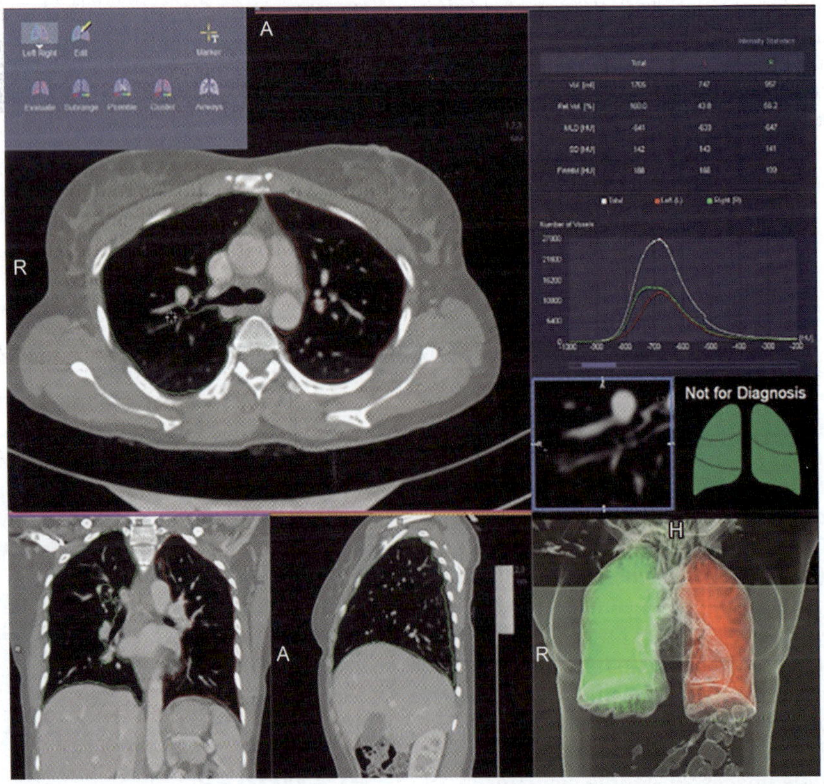

FIG. 2: Analysis of mean lung density and lung volumes using a commercially available pulmonary CT analysis software. The software automatically segments the lungs and calculates mean House field unit (HU), demonstrate relative lung volumes of left and right lung as well as total.

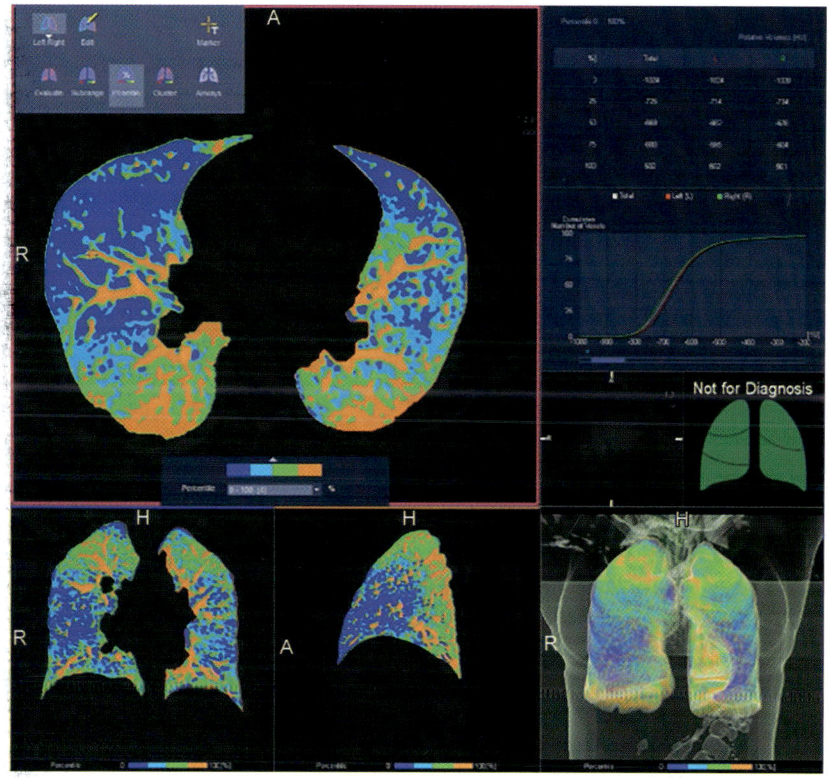

FIG. 3: Color coded maps of the distribution of HU values (in percentile) across the lung parenchyma using a commercially available pulmonary CT analysis software. Relative clustering of the number of voxels of particular HU are demonstrated in all three planes as well as graphically and tabular forms.

secondary to diffuse lung diseases such as emphysema or fibrosis help to recognize the disease as well as quantify the abnormality. These include Pulmo3D (Syngovia, Siemens, Germany), Lung density analysis (Philips Healthcare, The Netherlands) and Thoracic VCAR (GE healthcare). Some third party softwares are also available such as Osirix and Imbio. These applications help to automatically identify areas of emphysema and quantify it. Mean lung density and volume of emphysema have also been shown to correlate with pulmonary function tests (FEV1 and DLCO).[3] In addition to lung analysis, automatic airway segmentation can also be done **(Fig. 4)**. It provides automatic assessment of airway wall thickness which has a role in COPD patients. Apart from emphysema, some of the third party softwares such as CALIPER, Osirix open-source DICOM viewer software are also useful to quantify the pulmonary fibrosis.[4,5]

Clinical Applications

It has potential role in quantitative evaluation of emphysema and airway dimensions in patients with COPD. Such measurements have shown to correlate with several clinical measures of COPD such as FEV1 predicted, Body mass index, exacerbations, dyspnea score and symptoms of chronic bronchitis and hence can be useful to assess the response to therapy.[6,7]

Various semiquantitative visual scoring techniques are used to measure the burden of pulmonary fibrosis in cases of interstitial lung disease. The software based automatic quantification of such fibrosis could result in more consistent diagnosis, more sensitive disease monitoring and accurate determination of prognosis. CALIPER-derived estimates of ILD have been found to correlate significantly with pulmonary function tests.[8] CALIPER software can also estimate pulmonary vessel volume which also have been found to be a strong predictor of functional deterioration.[5]

PULMONARY EMBOLISM DETECTION SOFTWARES

Pulmonary embolism detection softwares are a computer-aided detection (CAD) tool which detects the filling defects in the pulmonary arteries automatically in CT pulmonary angiogram (CTPA) studies. These are adjunctive softwares to alert the reader towards the areas of filling defects which may have been overlooked initially. These include syngo CT PE CAD (Syngovia, Siemens, Germany) and CAD prototype software (Philips Healthcare, The Netherlands).[9]

Clinical Applications

It is useful as a second reader providing an incremental value to radiologist's interpretation of CTPA. The sensitivity of the software is comparable to radiologist, however with more false positives.[10,11]

CT PERFUSION ADVANCED SOFTWARES

CT Perfusion advanced softwares includes CT perfusion 4D multiorgans (GE healthcare), syngo Volume Perfusion CT

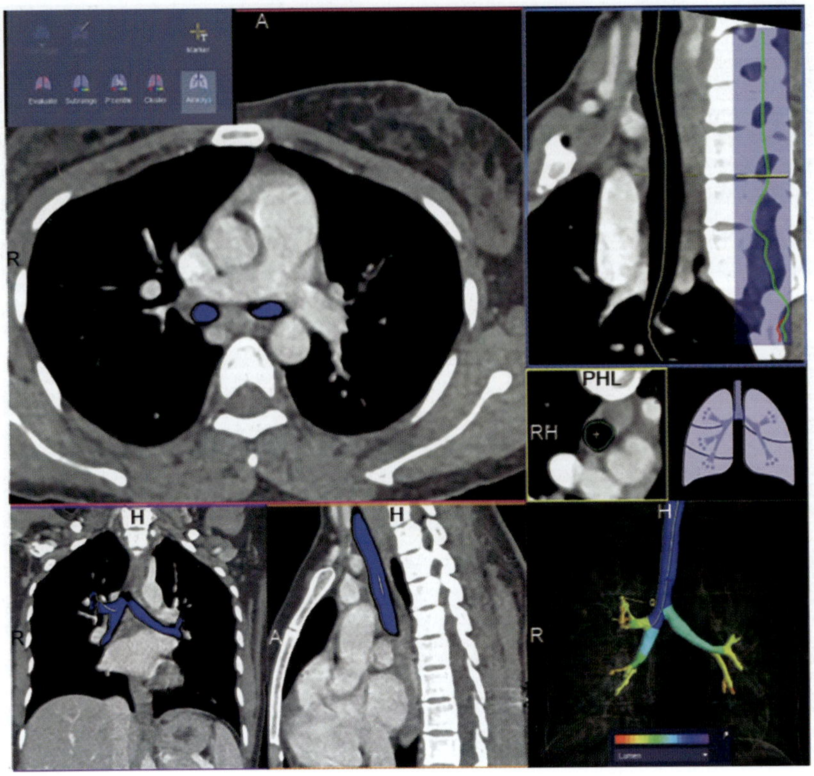

FIG. 4: Analysis of the airway tree using a pulmonary CT analysis software. Using this approach, the airway tree is reconstructed in three dimensions and the airway can be analyzed at any location. 3-dimensional reconstruction of the airway tree with the airway path of interest highlighted in colors. (Images created using the Pulmo3D software (Syngovia, Siemens, Germany).

(Syngovia, Siemens, Germany), Body Perfusion (Toshiba Medical System, Tochigi, Japan). The advancement in CT perfusion applications allows for accurate evaluation of vascular dynamics within the tumor or in cases of stroke. Various parameters of perfusion imaging such blood flow, blood volume, mean transit time and capillary permeability are also displayed in a simpler graphic formats for quick understanding. Smart Maps using the intelligent 4D noise suppression algorithm in CT perfusion 4D (GE) improves image quality of functional maps in the presence of noise.

Clinical Applications

Multiorgan analysis of perfusion parameters simultaneously have potential role in evaluating vascularity and perfusion dynamics in multiple abdominal organs such as liver, pancreas, spleen and kidneys. It can evaluate perfusion in multiple liver tumors simultaneously, thereby useful in quantitatively assessing the response to antiangiogenesis agents. Few studies have shown its utility in cirrhosis patients as well.[12]

CONTINUOUS FREE-BREATHING SCANS

Continuous free-breathing CT scans are useful to detect motion of the patient and organ distortion, such as during respiration. Prototype of such software is the Advantage 4D software (GE healthcare). These softwares efficiently analyses the respiration-induced motion of the anatomy. It displays true structural changes in the shape of the anatomical area of concern which happens during motion. It displays 4D volumes in axial, coronal, and sagittal planes for quick respiratory motion evaluation by building 4D movie loops.

Clinical Applications

Dynamic airway imaging in cases of tracheobronchomalacia,[13] tumor motion assessment for accurate targeting of radiotherapy (standard vs gated therapy planning). Feasibility of such applications in evaluation of diaphragmatic movements are also described in literature.[14]

ADVANCED CT ANGIOGRAPHY SOFTWARES

The advances in the softwares for evaluation of CT angiographies are directed towards fast routine analysis of usual CT angiography studies. CT Angiography has become the modality of choice for treatment planning in cases of aortic and peripheral vascular disease (PVD). Thoroughly analyzing the data provided by CTAs for vascular as well as non-vascular anatomy involves a considerable investment of time. Hence, these applications expedite the assessment process. These include Autobone and VesselIQxpress or dynamic shuttle (GE healthcare), syngo. CT Vascular analysis (Syngovia, Siemens, Germany) and Multimodality advanced vessel analysis (AVA) (Philips Healthcare, The Netherlands). These applications provides easy, user-friendly tools to analyze the 3D angiographic data for various parameters such as thrombus and stenosis evaluation, pre-and poststent planning procedures, and visualization of directional vessel tortuosity **(Figs. 5 and 6)**. Dynamic shuttle application allows

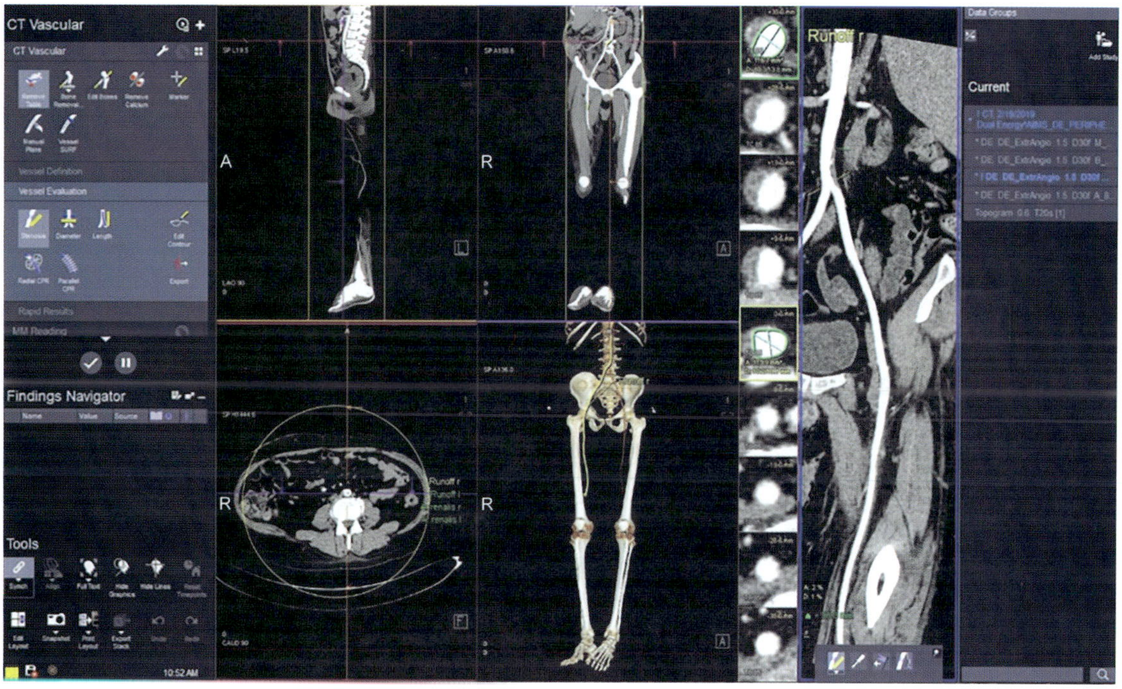

FIG. 5: Overall layout of the advanced CT vascular analysis software. Vessel evaluation for percentage of stenosis is displayed. Other parameters such as length of involvement and depiction of entire vessel along the automatic central line can also be shown on a click.

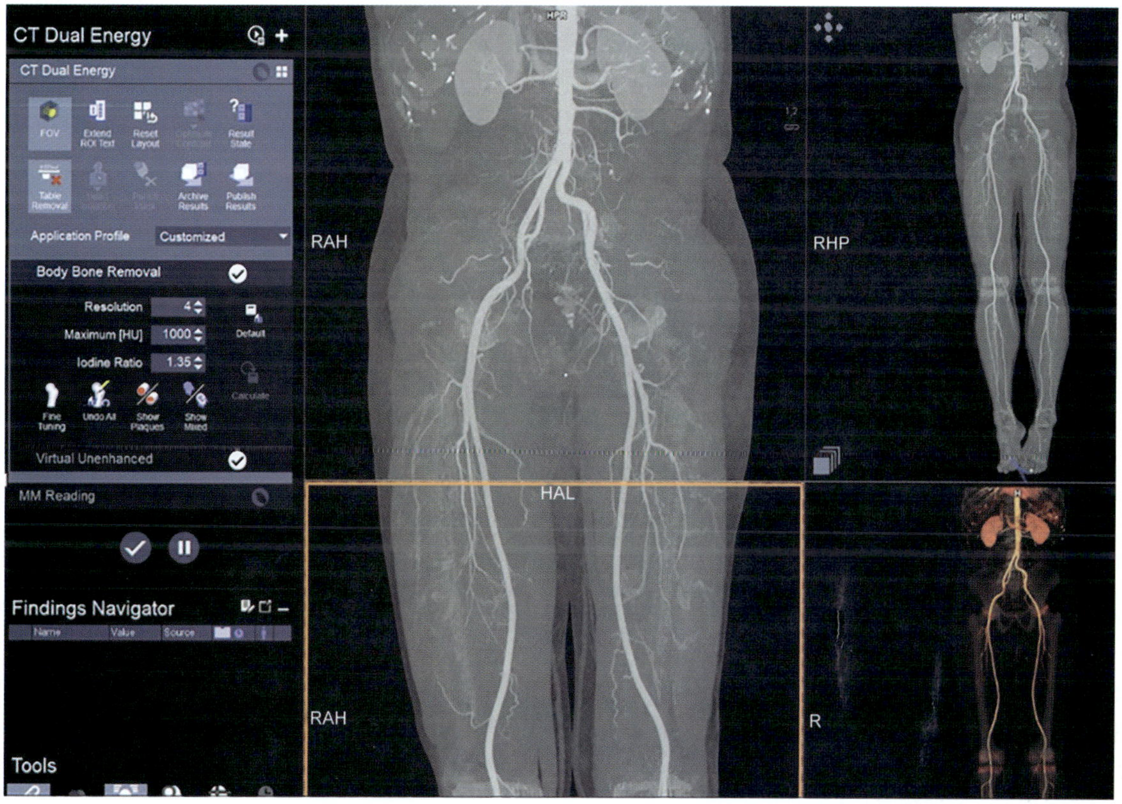

FIG. 6: Advanced bone removal software. The CT angiography shows excellent bone free visualization of the vessels.

for excellent bone free visualization of vascular anatomy and help to visualize the dynamic flow of contrast from the arteries to the veins.

Clinical Applications

The softwares have been found to be accurate in assessment of carotid artery stenosis with high rates of reproducibility as well as in saving time for interpretations.[15] Reliable sizing before endovascular aneurysm repair procedures is another advantage of using such applications.[16]

ADVANCED CARDIAC APPLICATION SOFTWARES

Advanced cardiac applications are intended to grant an optimized noninvasive application to study the cardiovascular anatomy, abnormalities as well as function to aid determine proper management. These applications constitute postprocessing software package for automatically assessing the coronary arteries including bypass graft patency, cardiac morphology, myocardial viability, relative perfusion, postintervention follow-up, and functional assessment. There are various vendor specific names of such applications such as syngo.CT cardiac function, CT TAVI planning, syngo. CT coronary analysis (Syngovia, Siemens, Germany), CardIQ Xpress 2.0 Reveal, Smart Score 4.0 for automatic coronary artery calcification scoring, TAVI planning (GE healthcare) and CT cardiac viewer (Philips Healthcare, The Netherlands). Recently, there is surge in utilizing CTA data to determine Fractional flow reserve noninvasively. FFR derived from standard coronary CT angiography (FFRCT) data sets by using several advanced computational analytic approaches enables combined anatomic and hemodynamic assessment of a coronary lesion by a single noninvasive test,[17] using a dedicated software prototype that is currently not commercially available (cFFR, version 1.4; Siemens Healthcare).[18]

Clinical Applications

These applications provides integrated anatomic and functional evaluation of the coronary vessels and myocardium in a single examination with high sensitivity and specificity[19] **(Figs. 7 and 8)**.

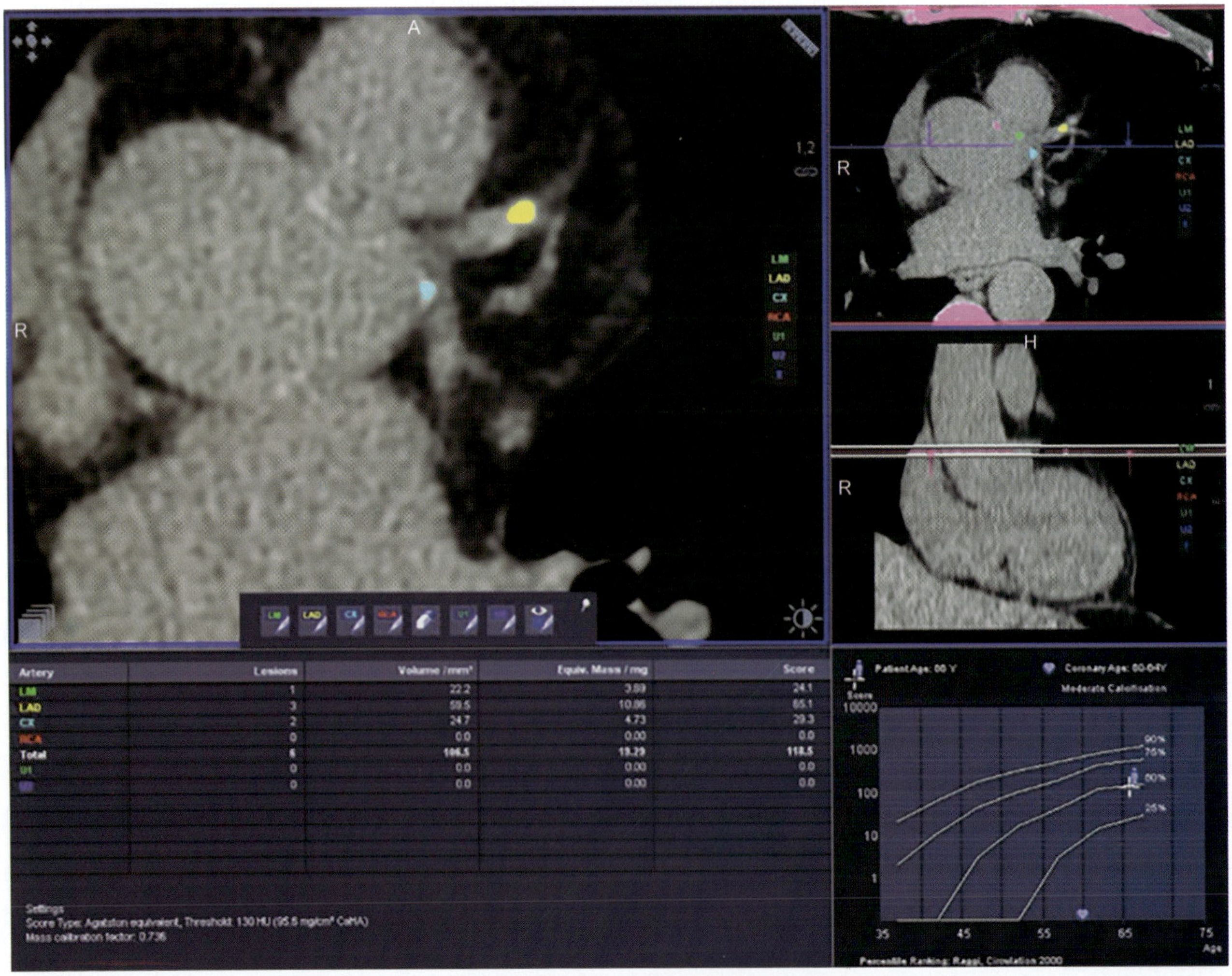

FIG. 7: Coronary calcium scoring application. The calcified coronary areas are automatically highlighted in different colors and an automatic numerical score is calculated in individual arteries as well as total score is depicted.

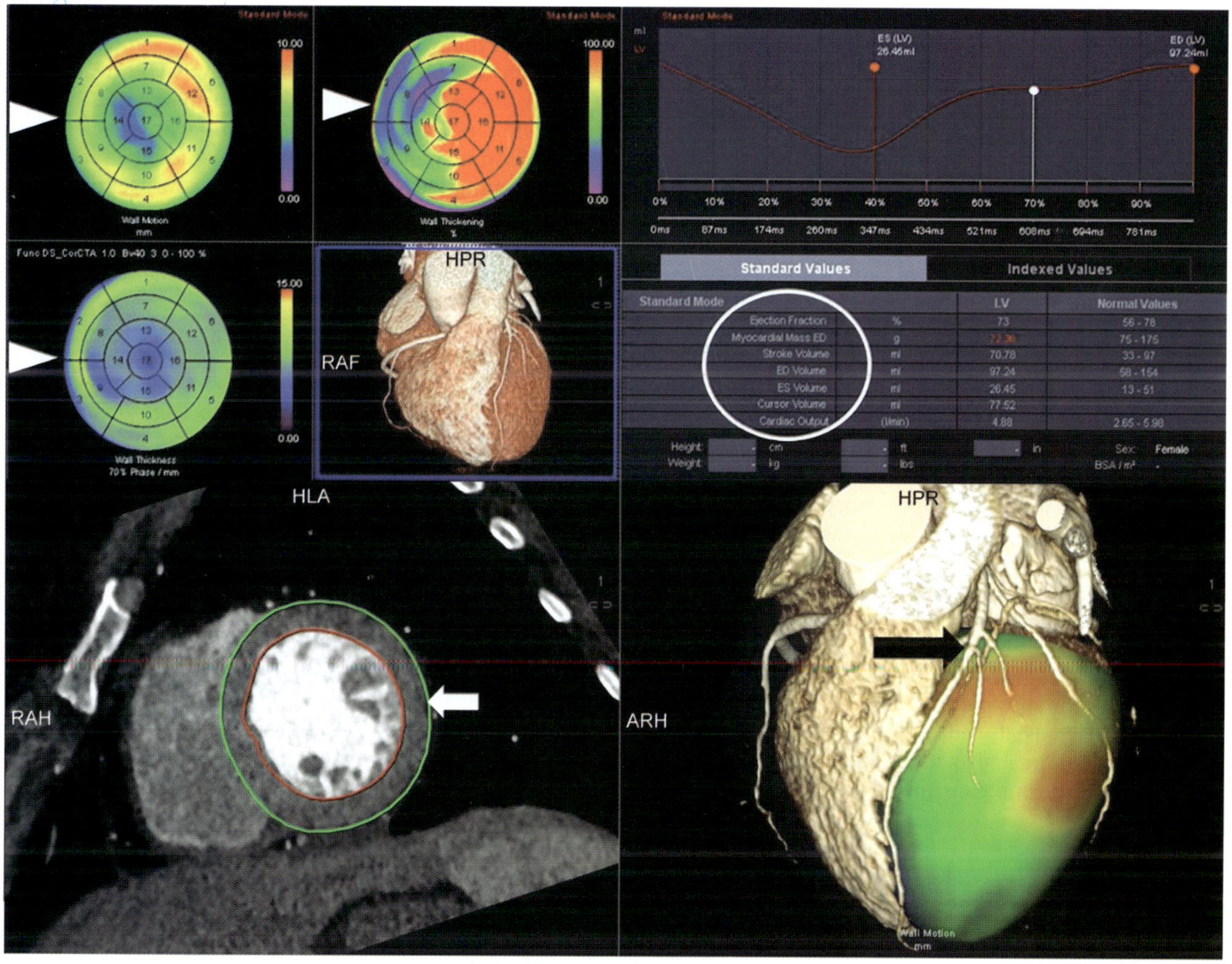

FIG. 8: CT cardiac evaluation software. Comprehensive evaluation of coronary arteries as well as myocardial perfusion can be done. Short axis view of left ventricle shows the marked area of myocardium (arrow). The application demonstrates the perfusion in the myocardium according to 17 segmental zones (arrowheads) which help to demonstrate areas of decreased perfusion and infarcts. The application also calculated various functional parameters such as ejection fraction, myocardial mass, end diastolic volume, end systolic volume as well as cardiac output (while circle). Coronary artery morphology can also be assessed simultaneously (Black arrow).

Preprocedural planning for transcatheter aortic valve implantation requires meticulous measurements which are done manually and are time consuming. The advanced softwares provides with semiautomatic measurements of multiple parameters in a significantly lower reading time.[20]

COMPUTED TOMOGRAPHY VOLUMETRY

In patients undergoing resection or transplantation, the residual volume of functioning organ has significant impact on the surgical outcome. It holds more significance in patients with underlying diseased status, for example, hepatic cirrhosis or steatosis which will have an impact on future functional status of patient. In order to obtain this volume, imaging modalities like CT and MRI have been evaluated; however most of the literature comprises of CT volumetry (CTV) as it is less costly and scan acquisition is faster. Majority of the studies are on liver volume assessment in patients planned for either resection or transplantation **(Table 2).** The future liver residual/remnant liver residual volume (FLRV) is one of the factors affecting patient outcome following surgery in addition to standard liver volume (SLV).[21-23]

TABLE 2: Indications for CT volumetry of liver.
Liver resection for liver tumor
Live donor transplantation
To increase FLRV—requirement and follow up after portal vein thrombosis
Postliver transplantation—assessment of graft regeneration

FLRV: future liver residual volume

Hence, preoperative estimation of liver volume has become part of standard work up for these patients especially in special instances where it warrants portal vein embolization in order to increase the FLRV prior to surgery.

Volumetric assessment by CT cannot be executed in clinical vacuum. It needs detailed and extensive communication with physicians with respect of type and extent of hepatectomy, variation in vascular and biliary anatomy so as to have a concrete plan and approach before surgery. It involves assessment of background liver also as patients with diseased liver will require more residual volume as compared to healthy liver. An SLV of more than 20% and FLRV of approx 26.5% is required to reduce postoperative morbidity and liver insufficiency in patients with normal liver.[23] Whereas, FLRV should be more than 50% for patients with cirrhosis and 40% in patients with high grade steatosis to improve the surgical outcome.[23] On the other hand, FLRV of 30% is the minimum threshold considered for healthy liver donors. Preoperative increase of the remnant liver volume can be achieved by performing Portal vein embolization (PVE) with or without prior transarterial chemoembolization (TACE) for liver tumor. PVE induces compensatory hypertrophy of the nonembolized lobe by reducing the vascular supply of the other lobe.

CTV is performed in axial CT sections obtained with 5–6 mm slice thickness following contrast injection in the venous phase as this phase delineates the vascular structures and tumor margins better than unenhanced scan.[24] Traditionally, manual contouring of the hepatic margins on each axial section by radiologist was done and total area was summated to obtain liver volume. The method is laborious and time consuming which led to advent of various automated methods of liver segmentation and CTV which had their own limitations.[25] Hence, semiautomated approach was proposed using interactive software tools **(Fig. 9)**. The newer automated tools OsiriX@ and iNtuition@ have shown promising and comparable results in comparison to manual as well as semiautomated modes of volume estimation significantly reducing the user time.[23,26,27]

Other imaging modalities, that is, USG and MRI have also been evaluated for volume estimation but not standardized. CTV has also been used in patients planned for nephrectomy by some authors.[28,29]

DENTASCAN

Placement of implant in patients with edentulism is one of the most important advancement in the field of dental science. Prior to the procedure, it is crucial to have detailed information about the bone in terms of its morphology, density, relationship with neurovascular structures, etc. Traditionally, this information was being acquired using panoramic radiographs. Since it is a 2D representative image, it gives limited information due to superimposition and distortion of the structures on an X-ray.[30]

In view of increase in older population and awareness about implants; role of CT has been explored.[31] Dedicated dental CT, also known as Dentascan, has now become an integral part of preprocedure evaluation of maxilla and mandible not only in the setting of implant placement but

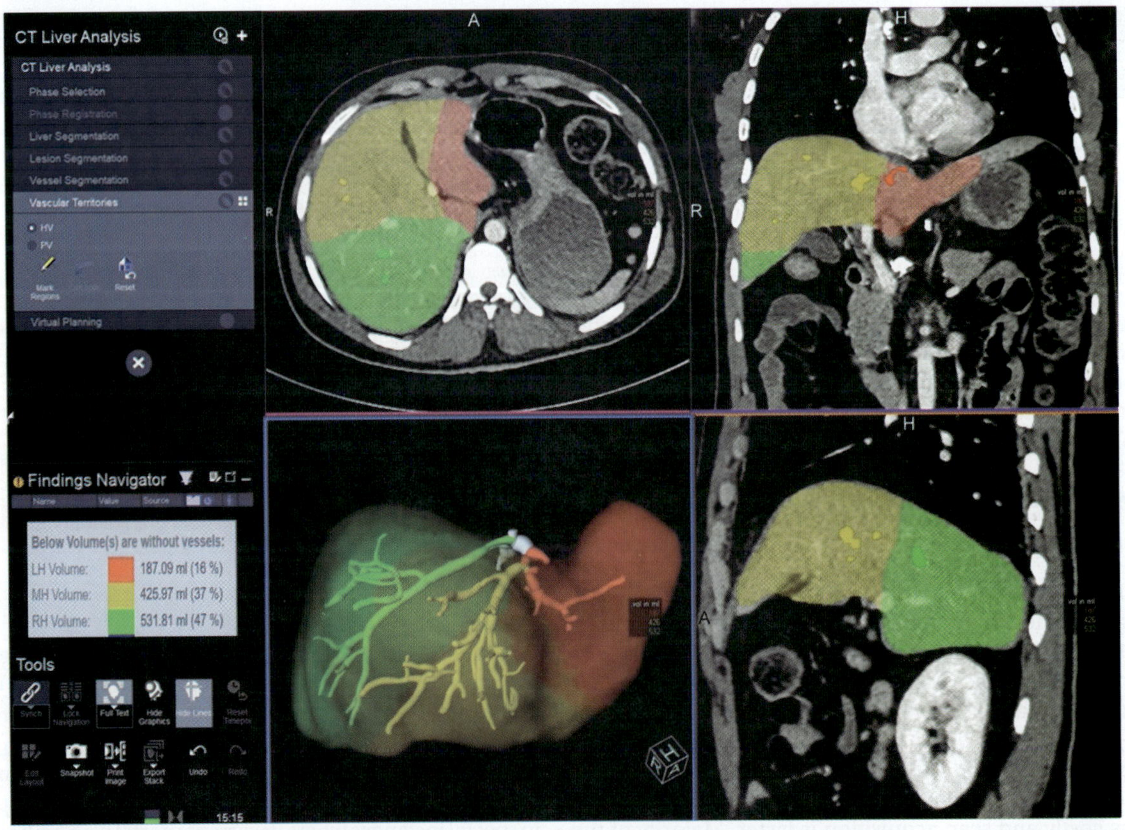

FIG. 9: CT Liver volumetry using CT liver analysis software (Siemens)—demonstrating volume of liver parenchyma drained by respective right, middle and left hepatic vein (color coded) . Note to be made of selection of hepatic veins in the left side panel of the dedicated protocol.

also in evaluation of other osseous pathologies.[32] It is a noninvasive technique providing accurate measurements of alveolar ridge along with qualitative assessment of the bones owing to its better spatial resolution.

The technique and postprocessing differs than routinely performed cross sectional imaging of chest and abdomen. Dentascan is performed in supine position with specific instructions to the patients—not to swallow, cough or move. A lateral scout image is obtained on which imaging plane is planned parallel to the alveolar ridge with image matrix 512 x 512 and an interval of 0.625 mm to 1 mm as per the configuration of gantry. Images are acquired and processed with the specific program and software on the most appropriate image selected by interpreter, demonstrating all the teeth roots and most of the contour of the arch. Freehand curved line is drawn along the curve of arch by placing atleast six cursor points. This line serves as central panoramic line along which multiple other lines are created by the software in parallel and perpendicular orientation. Coronal and sagittal reformatted images are generated; each image labeled with number correlating with corresponding tooth **(Figs. 10A to H)**.

The image interpretation includes identification of anatomical landmarks followed by qualitative and quantitative assessment of dentoalveolar ridge.[33] In maxilla, the anatomical landmarks to be identified are floor of maxillary sinuses, nasal fossa, crest of alveolar bone, nasopalatine canal and cortex of alveolar bone in maxilla. The landmarks in mandibular assessment are dental canal, mental and mandibular foraminas, lower border of mandible, buccal and lingular cortical plates of alveolar bone. The quantitative parameters are height and width of the respective alveolar bone and are measured on sagittal reformatted image. Minimum acceptable height at the implant site is 9 mm and width 5 mm with distance to adjacent cortical bone of atleast 1 mm.[34] Assessment of bone quality is also important as it indicates the strength of the bone receiving implant **(Figs. 10A to H)**. Various authors have evaluated quality of alveolar bone subjectively as well as objectively and classified in terms of morphological appearance and degree of resorption or appearance and thickness of trabecular and cortical bone or density measurement in Hounsefield unit (HU)[35] **(Table 3)**.

All this information is essential to achieve adequate osteointegration of implant and should be charted in the radiology report. In addition, the scanned images should be critically looked for any associated pathologies like infection or cysts along the teeth.[36]

Clinical Application

Dentascan is now preferred by most of the dental surgeons prior to implant placement. However, its role also extends in follow-up post implant placement to confirm position of implant and to rule out periimplantitis, other complications like perforation of maxillary sinus and mandibular canal. It is also performed in setting of impacted tooth to look for its relationship with surrounding structures and nerves/canals before intervening.[37]

COMPUTED TOMOGRAPHY CINEMATIC RENDERING

High resolution multi-detector computed tomography (MDCT) is a major revolution in the field of medical imaging as it acquires images in axial plane and enables visualization

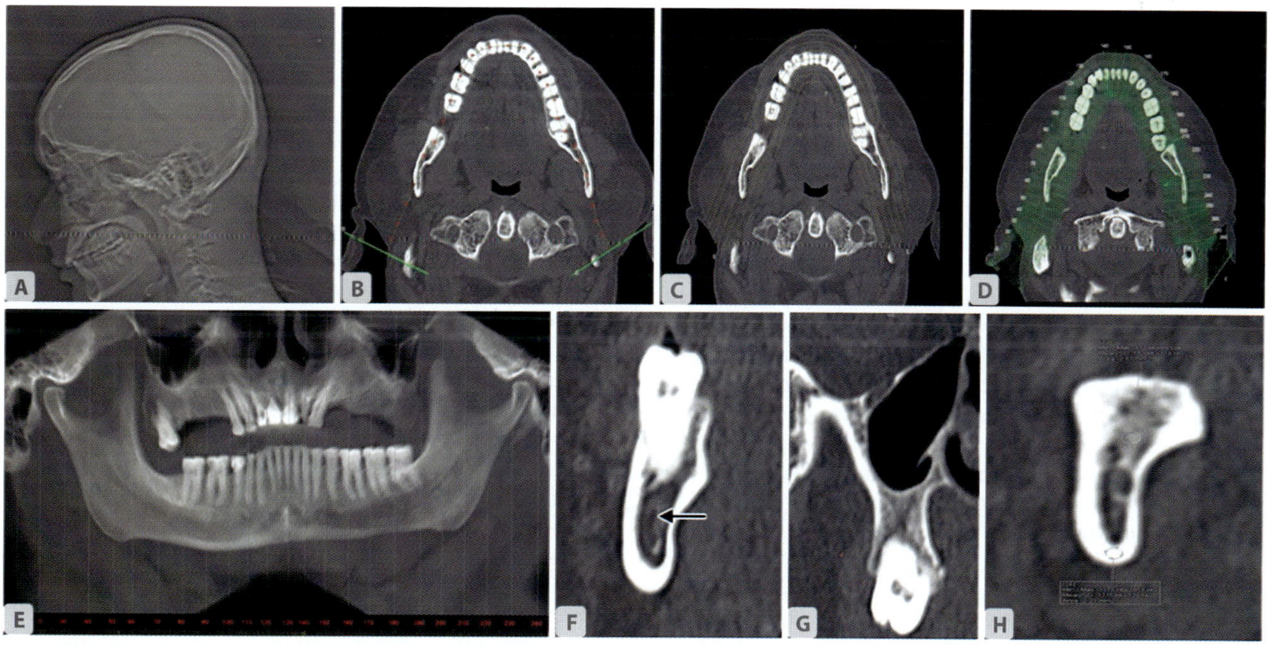

FIGS. 10A TO H: Dental scan (A to H)—after obtaining scout image in supine position (A) point cursors are placed on the selected image (B) in a contoured fashion. This image is processed by the software in parallel (C) as well as perpendicular planes (D) reformatted image with line numbers corresponding to each tooth is obtained (E). Anatomical landmarks in mandible (F, arrow showing dental canal) and maxilla (G), are identified followed by qualitative assessment in terms of Hounsefield units (H).

TABLE 3: Interpretation of Dentascan.

1. Identification of landmarks Maxilla • Floor of maxillary sinuses, nasal fossa • Crest of alveolar bone • Nasopalatine canal • Cortex of alveolar bone Mandible • Dental canal • Mandibular and mental foraminas • Lower border of mandible • Buccal and lingular cortical plates of alveolar bone
2. Quantitative assessment • Height and width of the alveolar ridge
3. Qualitative assessment[35] *In terms of osseous morphology and resorption*: Grade 1: Only dentate bone Grade 2: Alveolar crest retained with rounded shape Grade 3: Rounded crest with preserved height and width Grade 4: Normal height and width with knife-edge crest Grade 5: Flat crest with abnormal height and width Grade 6: Depressed creast with variable basal bone loss *Subjective analysis of bone* Type 1: Compact bone Type 2: Compact and trabecular bone Type 3: Thinner cortical layer with fine trabeculae Type 4: Thin cortical bone surrounded by trabecular bone of low density *Density in HU by Misch* D1: > 1250 HU D2: 850–1250 HU D3: 350–850 HU D4: 150–350 HU D5: < 150 HU *D1 represents the maximum density and D5 the minimum* *Density in HU by Norton and Gamble* Quality value 1: >850 HU Quality value 2 and 3: 500–850 HU Quality value 4: 0–500 HU

in 2D as well as 3D reconstructions which enhances the interpretation. A single volumetric parameter can be reconstructed for visualization in maximum and minimum intensity projections in 2D acquisition. More complex algorithms are used to generate 3D reconstructions. Addition of Volume rendering (VR) visualization technique in CT has been marked as another milestone in advancement as it improves visualization of complex anatomical structures. It is basically based on principle of ray casting and local lighting model wherein a single ray casting through the volume intersects a voxel; the imaging is computed with Riemann integral neglecting the complex light paths.[38]

Cinematic rendering (CR) is a new visualization technique inspired from the movie industry successful in creating realistic looking characters **(Figs. 11A and B)**. In contrast to VR, CR is based on path-tracing and global illumination models taking into account various light paths and scattering patterns, interpreted using Monte Carlo integration formula. This computes in real time the complex physics of lighting leading to natural presentation of medical data with enhanced depth and shape perception.[39,40]

Clinical Applications

Cinematic rendering (CR) is currently a research tool with its utility being evaluated in study of anatomical structures, cardiac anomalies, musculoskeletal trauma and osseous tumors. Authors have compared it with conventional VR and shown comparable results with similar shortcomings in terms of limited visualization and masking of the pathology; hence it is being used in conjunction with axial images and 2D tools at present.[41-43]

FUSION IMAGING

Imaging is an inevitable component of evaluation of any patient and the choice of imaging depends on the indication and information needed during work up. However, each modality has its own advantages and disadvantages. X-ray and Ultrasound are preferred modalities due to easy availability and short acquisition time but they provide only 2D information for which cross-sectional imaging is opted. Though CT and MRI provide detailed structural and anatomical information, these modalities are unable to illustrate the functional aspect of pathology. This limitation can be overcome by radionuclide studies like PET (positron emission tomography) which exclusively provides functional information. Hence, it is only logical that fusion of the images obtained by different sources should provide more meaningful information. Combination of PET and contrast-enhanced CT is one such example of fusion imaging which has gained wide acceptance and popularity as it yields not only anatomical but also at the same time functional information, that too in single setting **(Figs. 12A and B)**. This integration of CECT and PET have enhanced diagnostic accuracy significantly. Fusion of the imaging has become an integral part of radiotherapy planning in oncology setting where images from MRI, PET may be fused with planning CT. Its role has further extended to field of intervention radiology. Most preferred modality to conduct tissue sampling (biopsy or fine needle aspiration cytology, FNAC) is USG; however, the lesions especially when small are not well appreciated on USG. One such example is suspicious liver nodules in patients with viral or nonviral hepatitis undergoing surveillance with MRI and in patients with concerns of residual disease post treatment. In such cases where USG is indeterminate, the image of MRI can be fused with USG for further guidance and approach.[44] Contrast-enhanced ultrasound may be performed for confirmation in same setting.

Another such field which is rapidly gaining importance is transrectal ultrasound (TRUS) guided prostate biopsy with fusion of multiparametric MR images demonstrating the suspicious area. Since MR guided biopsies are technically challenging, time consuming and expensive, targeting such areas under US guidance has shown to increase the yield and accuracy of TRUS guided biopsy with reduced number of cores.[45] Vendors have this software in their recent machines

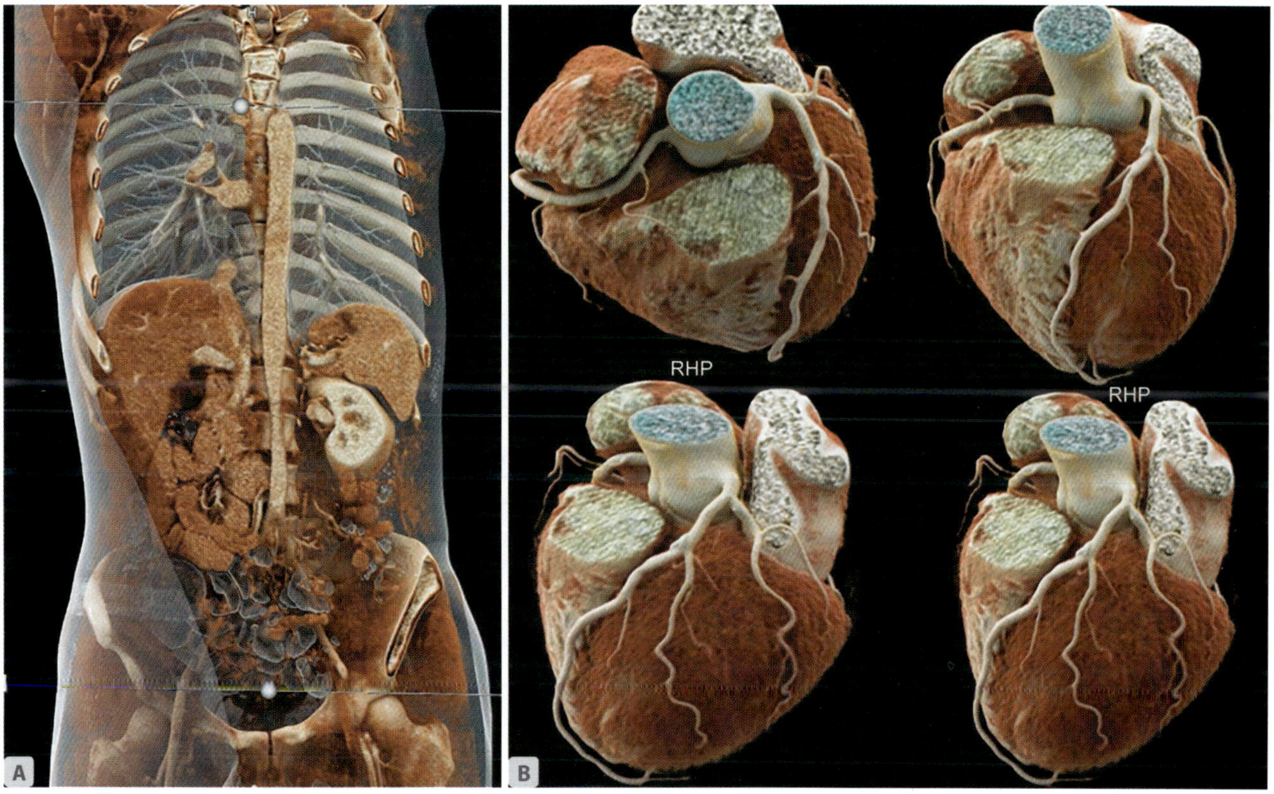

FIGS. 11A AND B: CT Cinematic rendering (CR) showing soft tissue structures, osseous profile of ribs and pelvis as well as abdominal organs in the coronal plane in a photo-realistic manner (A). Similarly, 3D-CR representation of origin and course of coronary arteries is well delineated in (B).

with enabled enhanced needle tracking ability like eSie fusion and eSieGuide (Siemens), PercuNav (Phillips) and Volume Naviagation (GE healthcare).

Clinical Application

Fusion imaging in the form of combination of PET and contrast enhanced CT or MRI to evaluate both anatomical and functional aspect of the disease. Fusion of USG and PET, PET-CT or MR images to plan radiotherapy, to guide image guided interventions by identifying and localizing normal anatomical structures and then proceeding with the desired procedure, for example biopsy or ablation.[46]

VERTEBRAL LABELING

Accurate identification and segmentation of vertebrae is essential for planning of any spinal canal surgery. Noninvasive cross sectional imaging like CT and MRI provide information about the bones and adjacent soft tissue in all three planes (axial, sagittal and coronal). The radiologist reporting routinely identifies the vertebrae by counting from C1 down. CT is the modality of choice when information about bones is being evaluated, for example, in cases of trauma and assessment of spine postfixation. In most cases, the entire spine is not included and thus counting of the vertebrae becomes difficult. Various authors have attempted to generate templates and configurations based on regression and probabilistic graphic models which assist in identification of the vertebral levels.[47,48] They classify and study morphology of vertebra-shape, length of body and transverse processes; spinal canal shape and appearance; orientation and boundary of the vertebral body; appearance of the spinous processes; edge effect, etc. Literature documents accuracy of 70–80% in identification of single vertebra which increases to more than 90% if more than six vertebrae are studied.[49,50]

Clinical Applications

Automatic detection, localization, and identification of individual vertebrae **(Fig. 13)** in computed tomography scans with limited field of view.

SOFTWARE FOR ONCOLOGICAL IMAGING INTERPRETATION

In oncological set up, there is an ever increasing demand for imaging diagnostic tests due to many factors like improved survival outcome, increasing incidence and reliance on radiology for screening, diagnosing, interventional procedures, staging, evaluation for resectability or response assessment.

Because of ever increasing availability and utilization of multiple modalities and multiple time points of imaging; the task of interpreting and then comparing this enormous data with older scans can be very labor-intensive and time consuming for radiologist. There is emergence of various softwares which help in reducing the time taken in making the comparison of all previous imaging, e.g oncoquant from GE health care or MM oncology from Siemens healthcare.

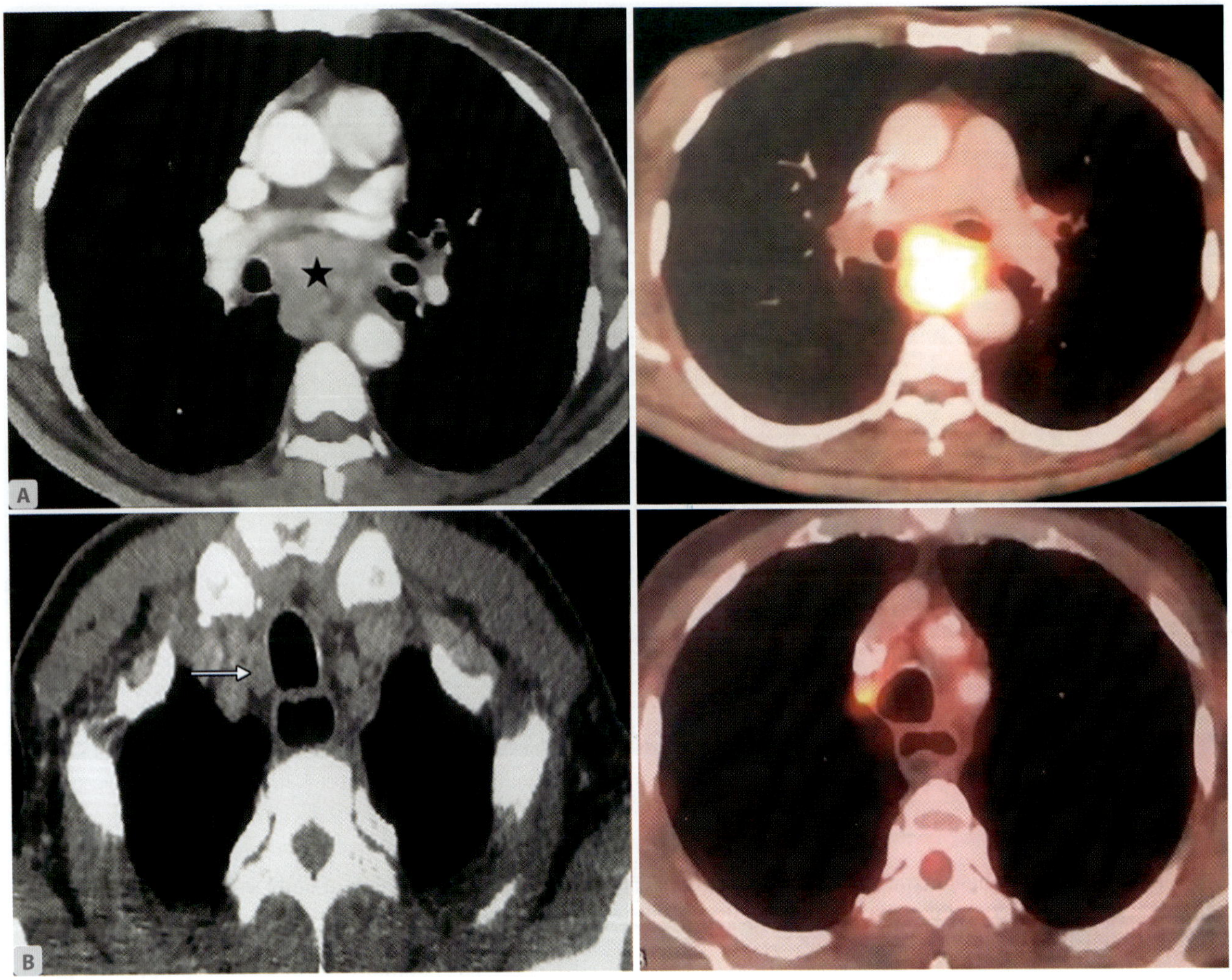

FIGS. 12A AND B: Role of fusion imaging PET-CT in a patient with carcinoma esophagus: Parallel CECT images (left side panel) with simultaneously performed PET (right-sided panel) demonstrating primary mass (asterisk) with lymph nodes in right para-tracheal (arrow in B) which are subcentimeteric in size on CT; however showing significant FDG uptake on PET modifying the N stage of tumor.

For facilitation and for quicker review these softwares help in organizing and displaying these data.

Clinical Application

By using these softwares comparison with previous imaging, even cross modality (e.g. CT Vs PET, CT vs MRI vs USG) is feasible. With the use of these, the work flow is automated and comparison with older imaging becomes easier and more efficient. These also support the standard response evaluation criteria (e.g. RECIST 1.0, RECIST 1.1 and WHO criteria) and help in comparing upto 4 (with some softwares even 8 time point data) different point time imaging. These provide result for any focal lesion comparison over time and also ability to display in interactive and intuitive comparison tables. There are features like facility to compare in a single click the comparison of up to 4 different time images showing baseline, previous imaging, nadir as well as the current examination and comparing these in tabulated form **(Fig. 14)**. Few more features to help the radiologist are the lesion contouring ability algorithm, special algorithms for long nodules, exporting DICOM, non-DICOM images, etc.

3D PRINTING

For many years the 3D reformation of the raw data acquired has been in standard use for day-to-day reporting of scans as well as communicate the findings to medical specialist and to patients for better understanding of disease process enabling them to take decisions. In last few years a new concept of actually printing the complex process into a three-dimensional structural model has emerged. This 3D printing involves image acquisition, post processing of this acquire data set and finally printing it into real 3D structure. Image acquisition is done at 1.25 mm or less isotropic voxels, then complex image post processing is done and the DICOM image data set is manipulated which involves selecting the region of interest, doing segmentation and finally converting the DICOM image to non DICOM image formats; a process which is called STL (standard tessellation language). STL

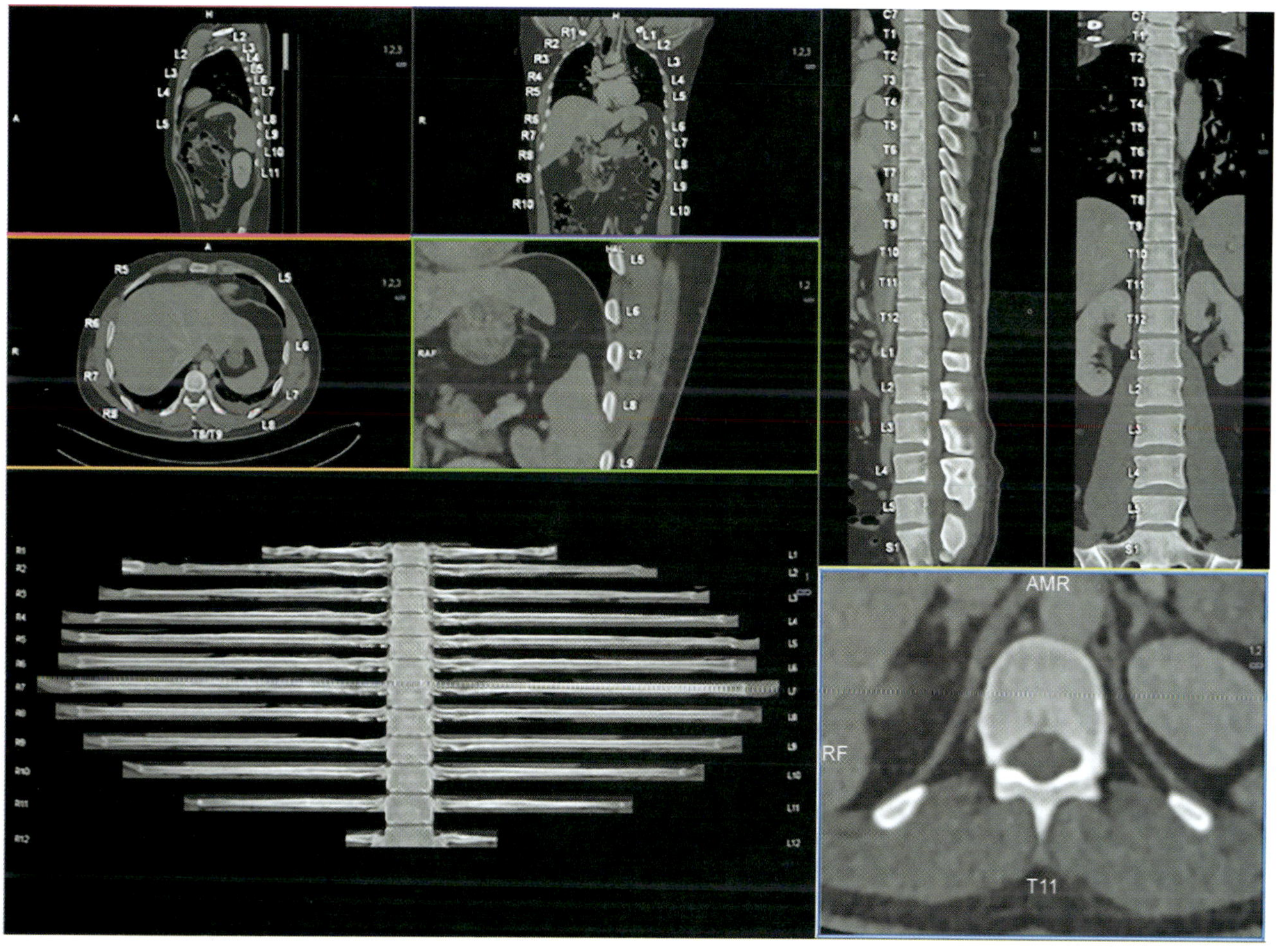

FIG. 13: Automatic vertebral as well as rib labelling demonstrated by dedicated imaging software.

format is a display method where a surface is represented by a huge collection of triangles.

This data which is represented as STL file is then printed into actual 3D structure by one of the many available printing technology **(Fig. 15)**. Which particular printing technology should be used depends upon many factors such as time needed to complete the print, cost of the material, printer, biocompatibility of materials used, sterilization capability of that material, material resistance to temperature and moisture, etc. Usually the three dimensional printing facility starts with use in surgical planning in radiology department.

Flow of work with respect to 3D printing project can be streamlined to reduce the time input by radiologist, e.g. preprocessing can be done by trained technologist which require bone subtraction, threshold setting, region growing, trimming and smoothening of the edges.

Then these initially processed images can be secondarily refined by the radiologist to ensure anatomic accuracy. The radiologist may need to edit the segmentation and sculpt/trim the actual anatomy of interest. Then tertiary processing may be done in combination with application engineers which needs engineering knowledge of the process, e.g. additional edge smoothening implantable device design, making lumen more hollow from inside, selecting materials and appropriate colour coding, etc. Thus streamlined workflow by the entire team is needed to provide excellent results of 3D printing.

Major Clinical Applications

- Craniofacial and maxillofacial region is first to develop historically and still most commonly used. It saves a lot of operating time. It has been used for full face transplantation, surgical planning and follow-up.[51-54]
- Neurosurgery
    - Highly useful for surgical planning, surgical simulation, training of residents and patient education
    - Complex spinal surgery can also be benefited by use of models produced by 3D printers.[55]
- Thorax
    - Preoperative planning and for teaching in carcinoma
    - Respiratory flow simulation of physiology
- *Cardiovascular applications*: Display of complex congenital malformations, aortic replacement, cerebral aneurysms, etc.
- *Musculoskeletal*: Formulating treatment strategy in total hip replacement, acetabular fracture, intra articular fracture, cubitus varus deformity correction, etc.

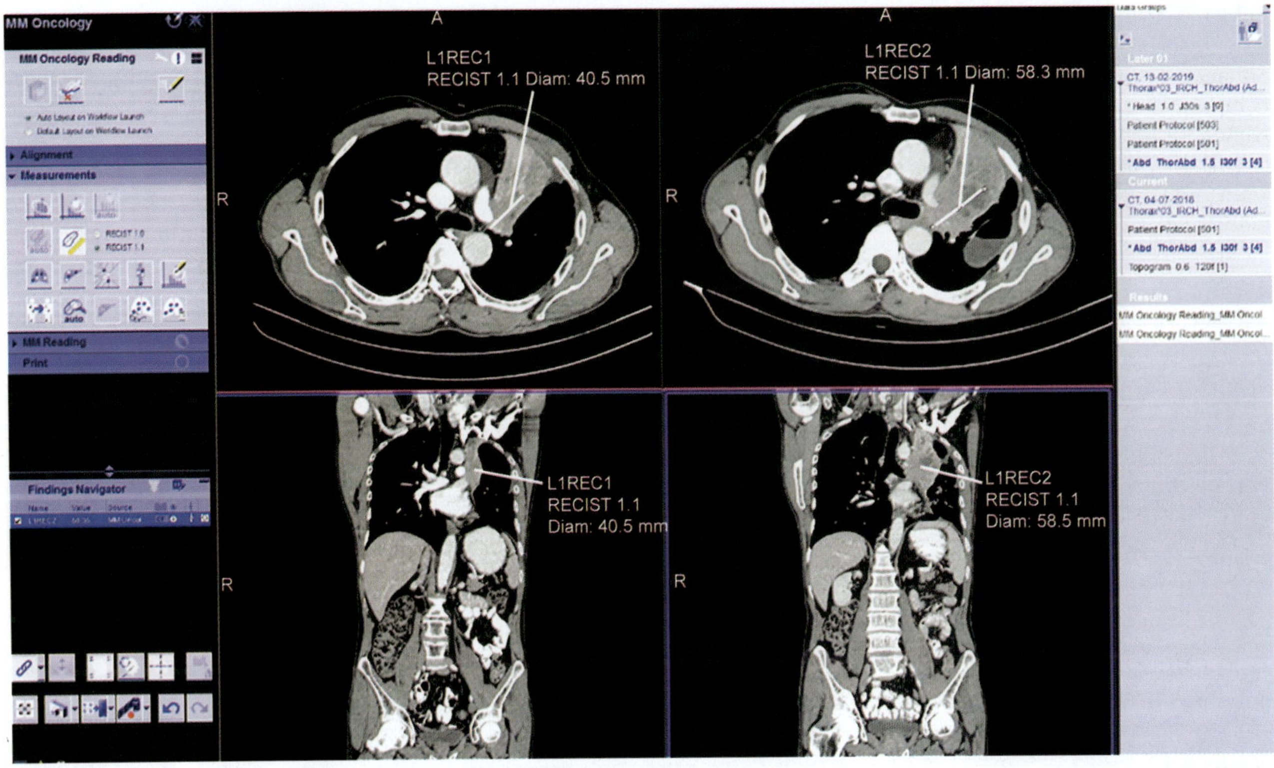

FIG. 14: Oncology reporting software—dedicated software which provides easy measurement and comparison of many time point images (images of two different timings has been compared in this image). As shown in left side panel, the software enables measurement of area of lesion, volume of lesion, diameter and comparison of successive point images and comparative interpretation according to Recist 1.1 (shown in image) for easy interpretation.

- *Education*: Very useful in teaching the complex geometrical orientation of organs facilitated by 3D visualization, physical models.

Provides optimal tool to understand anatomy and anatomical variation, 3D models can supplement or even can replace cadaveric specimen due to easier availability. Hence, a close interaction is needed between radiologist and referring physician for successful and optimal use of 3D printing technologies. Its role is expected to grow exponentially.

ITERATIVE RECONSTRUCTION

In the present era of multidetector row CT scanners the enormous amount of raw data is reconstructed for optimal display. There are two main types of reconstruction-Iterative reconstruction and analytical reconstruction (filtered back projection).

Iterative reconstruction—improves quality of images by cyclical image processing usually by reduction of noise. In 1972 Sir Godfrey Hounsfield made clinical introduction of CT scan. Since then a lot of evolution in hardware like helical CT, MDCT and dual source CT happened.

Till now faster way of reconstruction, i.e. analytical approach of filtered back projection (FBP) was used for data handling but due to significant improvement in capability of data-handling in the recent timings, there is renaissance of iterative reconstruction technique which is actually more accurate way of reconstruction.

Filtered back projection—shows significant noise particularly when patient is obese, or presence of high-density structures (metal stents, calcification or implants) or data is obtained with reduced tube output. All these drawbacks are significantly overcome by iterative methods.

Mostly iterative reconstruction algorithms are proprietary and only partial information is revealed by manufacturers.

The names of few of the vendor specific IR algorithms are as follows:

- Siemens—iterative reconstruction in space (IRIS), SAFFIRE-sinogram affirmative iterative reconstruction, Advanced model iterative reconstruction (ADMIRE) **(Figs. 16A and B)**
- G E—adaptive statistical iterative reconstruction (AS I R), Veo—more complex but quite slow in processing
- Phillips—i-Dose^4 iterative model reconstruction
- Toshiba—adaptive iterative dose reduction (AIDR), AIDR 3D.

Clinical Applications

These iterative reconstruction techniques have substantial promise for image quality improvement, artifact suppression and reduction in radiation dose.

Practical consideration: Due to incorporation of iterative reconstruction, no major changes in workflow occurs. The technologist has to simply select the appropriate IR algorithm which takes few seconds to a few minutes to generate the IR images. In some given critical scenario more aggressive noise reduction is desired for example while attempting to detect a hypovascular lesion in the liver. Sometimes decreasing artifacts and improving special resolution is more desired as compare to reduction in noise, e.g. in the CT angiography. Hence institutional preference and preference according to desired interpretation of a given examination will decide which particular advantage of IR technique is more relevant in the given examination.

Initially radiologist may feel some disliking to the IR images due to unfamiliarity of image appearances, however after initial learning curve such concerns are usually overcome. Many phantom studies have demonstrated good efficiency of IR techniques of various vendors in reducing noise and better image quality.

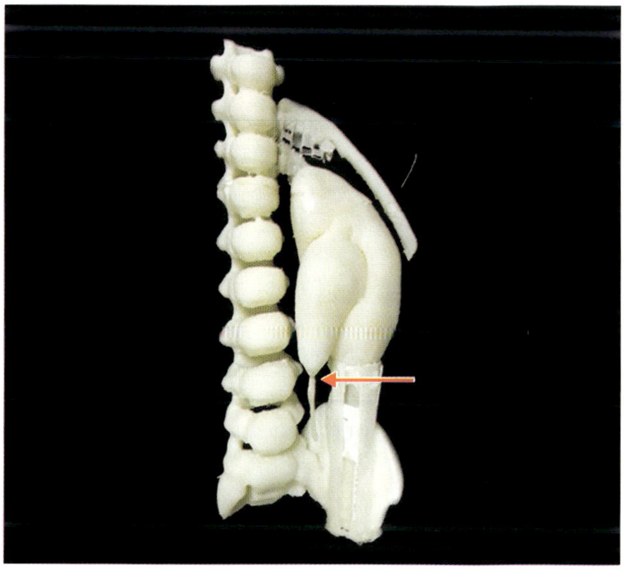

FIG. 15: 3D printing—the real 3 dimension image of kidney showing pelviureteric junction stricture (red arrow). The 3D image has been prepared with the help of a special printer which receives inputs from console. Preprocessing of the image needs inputs from radiologist in the form of segmentation, exclusion of nondesired parts as well as inputs from CT engineer for deciding the optimal material to be used for a given image to be printed. These images are useful for teaching, for explaining the disease process to patient and attendants and for better planning the surgical approach.

Few facts regarding use of IR are as follows:

Head and neck:

- *Cervical spine*: Reduced dose comparable to that of conventional radiography.[56,57] Brain CT—20-40% reduction in dose.[58-61]
- Other areas of use: Intervertebral disc and ligaments, temporal bone, better delineation of gray and white matter, reduced Streak artifacts in posterior fossa and by dental hardware .
- *Thorax-CT*: Consistently 27-80% dose reduction by various available IR products.[62]

One study showed CT constructed with the help of IR result in better visual score while compared with FBP method for assessment of interlobular septa, centrilobular region as well as small bronchi.

COMPUTED TOMOGRAPHY COLONOGRAPHY

CT colonography has been tested for many years and with many modifications it has reached a stage where it can be considered one of the best radiological diagnostic tests for the evaluation of colorectal carcinoma and polyps **(Fig. 17)**. This has many advantages over colonoscopy; for example, it is less invasive, easier to perform and it is well standardized, it also needs reduced bowel preparation. Newer ways of images reconstruction have reduced the radiation exposure, with the use of more dedicated software; the image interpretation has become easier and with the help of computer aided detection the errors of interpretation have come down in the recent times.

Few of the important points to note regarding acquisition of CT colonography are: dietary restrictions mild to moderate use of laxity versions, faecal tagging by orally taken contrast agents, use of electronic subtraction of stool

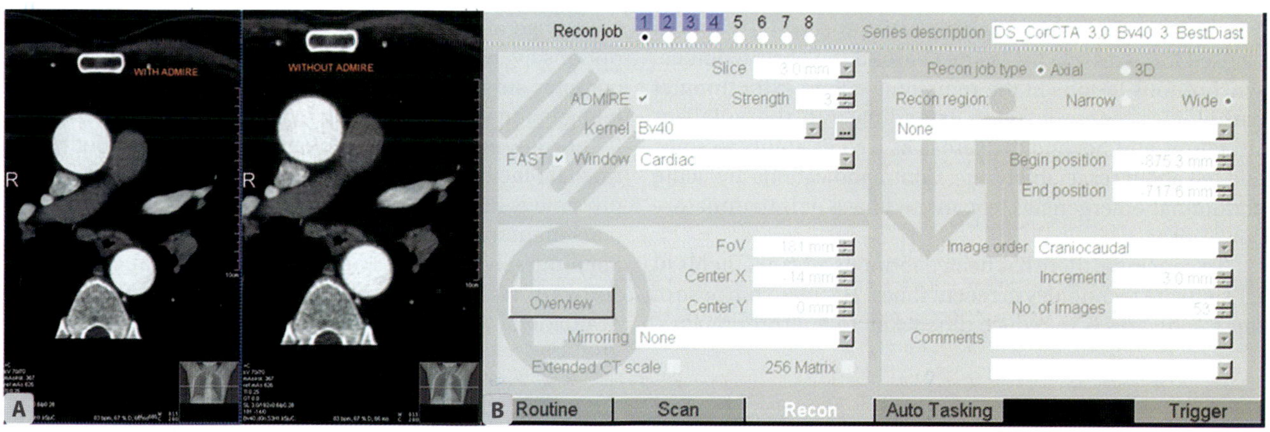

FIGS. 16A AND B: Iterative reconstruction. (A) Image acquired and processed with ADMIRE iterative reconstruction Vs image processed without iterative reconstruction. The image quality in terms of lesser blurring of margins, better anatomical details and better contrast resolution is appreciable when iterative reconstruction is employed. (B) Iterative reconstruction can be done at various strengths; in this example it is done with 3 cycles of iteration.

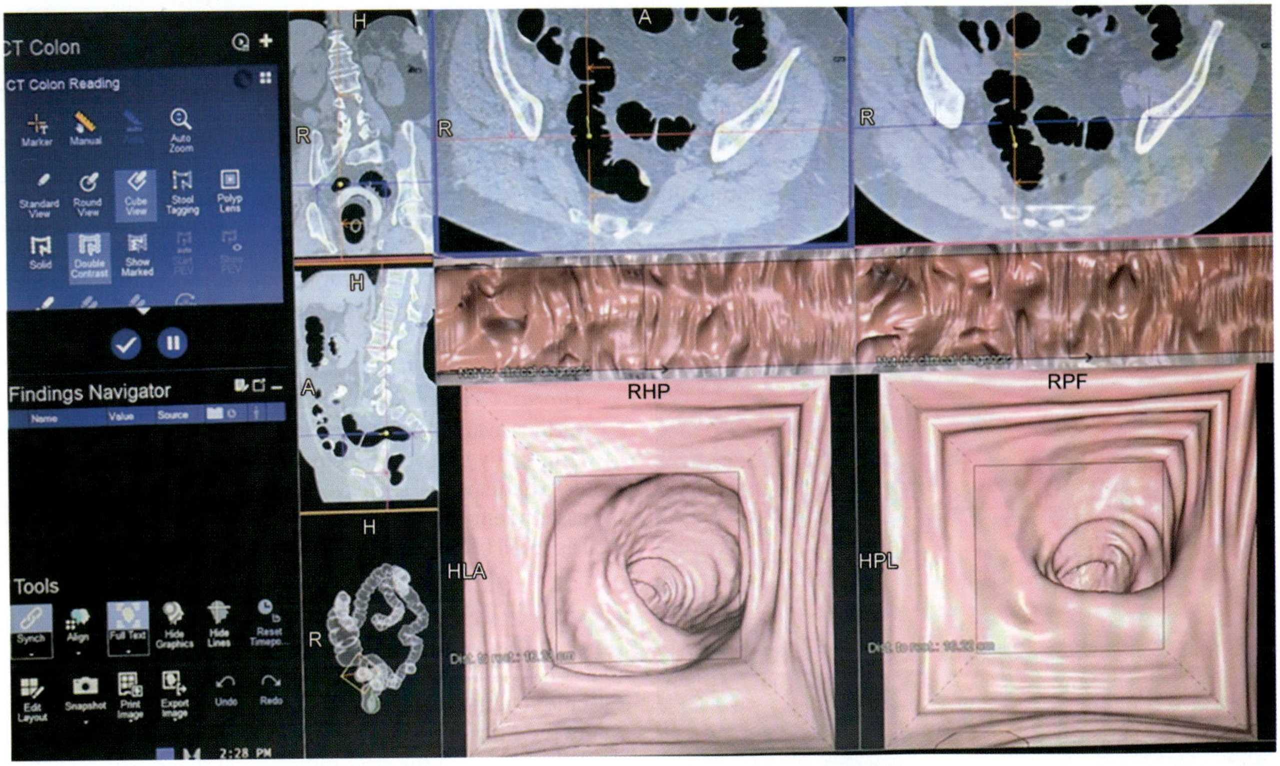

FIG. 17: Virtual CT colonoscopy: in the composite panel 'endoscopy like' images (lower panel), multiplanar reformatted images as well as translucent image of entire colon are depicted. Left side of panel shows various reading tools, e.g. marker, zoom, PAN as well as stool tagging, polyp lens and double contrast tools manipulate the images.

particles by software. Distension for CT colonoscopy is optimally achieved by use of flexible catheter and carbon dioxide by radiologist or the staff member. Multirow detector CT (MDCT) minimum 16 rows is an essential prerequisite to achieve good quality, the dose reducing reconstruction techniques should be used to reduce radiation and image analysis should be done with both two dimensional and three-dimensional images in addition to computer aided detection software. These are few of the modifications to improve the sensitivity and specificity of interpretation of CTC. Main indications of CTC is incomplete or failed colonoscopy or in case of stricture of colon by neoplastic process. CTC should be used for assessing the lesions beyond the obstruction i.e. synchronous lesions in the remaining colon; extra luminal pathologies, complications extending into the adjacent structures and beyond the serosa as well as ability to stage and tell about resectability, etc. Contra indications are acute abdominal emergencies, e.g. acute phase of inflammatory bowel disease.

To conclude, there has been enormous advancements in CT software technology in recent times. The main purpose of these softwares is to reduce time taken to interpret images, reducing the radiation doses as well as opening up possibilities of exploring newer clinical applications. Automatization of many diagnostic algorithms have really reduced the time taken for radiologist to diagnose and quantify the pathologies, increased accuracy as well as improved overall work flow in radiology department. Judicious use of various newer softwares will certainly impact patient care in near future in a positive way. Many of these applications are also useful for interventional procedures, e.g. use of fusion images for ultrasound guided procedures when originally the lesion was not visible on ultrasound. Another big advantage of newer softwares is in expanding the surgical options available to patients, e.g. 3D printing where many complex surgeries which were near impossible in past are being made feasible utilizing it. Impacts of advancement in CT not only improve the radiology work but also benefit other medical facilities like anatomical teaching, understanding physiology as well as pathology of many diseases in a more efficient manner. Hence it is very important that we should keep ourselves aware about the newer advancements in software technologies for improvement in our imaging evaluation.

REFERENCES

1. Han D, Heuvelmans MA, Vliegenthart R, Rook M, Dorrius MD, de Jonge GJ, et al. Influence of lung nodule margin on volume- and diameter-based reader variability in CT lung cancer screening. Br J Radiol. 2018;91(1090):20170405.
2. Sun Q, Huang Y, Zhao SJ, Zhang L, Tang W, Jin YJ, et al. [The volume and mass growth of persisted pulmonary nodules detected in low-dose CT screening and its influence factors]. Zhonghua Zhong Liu Za Zhi. 2018;40(4):274-9.
3. Moloney F, McWilliams S, Crush L, Laughlin PD, Kenneddy M, Henry M, et al. CT Densitometry as a Predictor of Pulmonary Function in Lung Cancer Patients. Open Respir Med J. 2012;6: 139-44.
4. Ariani A, Carotti M, Gutierrez M, Bichisecchi E, Grassi W, Giuseppetti GM, et al. Utility of an open-source DICOM viewer software (OsiriX) to assess pulmonary fibrosis in systemic sclerosis: preliminary results. Rheumatol Int. 2014;34(4):511-6.
5. Jacob J, Bartholmai BJ, Rajagopalan S, Kokosi M, Egashira R, Brun AL, et al. Serial automated quantitative CT analysis in idiopathic pulmonary fibrosis: functional correlations and comparison with changes in visual CT scores. Eur Radiol. 2018;28(3):1318-27.
6. Mair G, Maclay J, Miller JJ, McAllister D, Connell M, Murchison JT, et al. Airway dimensions in COPD: relationships with clinical variables. Respir Med. 2010; 104(11):1683-90.
7. Fernandes L, Fernandes Y, Mesquita AM. Quantitative computed tomography imaging in chronic obstructive pulmonary disease. Lung India. 2016;33(6):646-52.
8. Jacob J, Bartholmai BJ, Rajagopalan S, Kokosi M, Nair A, Karwoski R, et al. Automated Quantitative Computed Tomography Versus Visual Computed Tomography Scoring in Idiopathic Pulmonary Fibrosis: Validation Against Pulmonary Function. J Thorac Imaging. 2016;31(5):304-11.
9. Wittenberg R, Peters JF, Weber M, Lely RJ, Cobben LP, Prokop M, et al. Stand-alone performance of a computer-assisted detection prototype for detection of acute pulmonary embolism: a multi-institutional comparison. Br J Radiol. 2012;85(1014):758-64.
10. Buhmann S, Herzog P, Liang J, Wolf M, Salganicoff M, Kirchhoff C, et al. Clinical evaluation of a computer-aided diagnosis (CAD) prototype for the detection of pulmonary embolism. Acad Radiol. 2007;14(6):651-8.
11. Wittenberg R, Berger FH, Peters JF, Weber M, van Hoorn F, Beenen LF, et al. Acute pulmonary embolism: effect of a computer-assisted detection prototype on diagnosis—an observer study. Radiology. 2012;262(1):305-13.
12. Motosugi U, Ichikawa T, Sou H, Morisaka H, Sano K, Araki T. Multi-organ perfusion CT in the abdomen using a 320-detector row CT scanner: preliminary results of perfusion changes in the liver, spleen, and pancreas of cirrhotic patients. Eur J Radiol. 2012;81(10):2533-7.
13. Wielpütz MO, Eberhardt R, Puderbach M, Weinheimer O, Kauczor HU, Heussel CP. Simultaneous assessment of airway instability and respiratory dynamics with low-dose 4D-CT in chronic obstructive pulmonary disease: a technical note. Respiration. 2014;87(4):294-300.
14. Goo HW. Four-Dimensional CT of the Diaphragm in Children: Initial Experience. Korean J Radiol. 2018;19(1): 111-8.
15. Tsiflikas I, Biermann C, Thomas C, Ketelsen D, Claussen CD, Heuschmid M. Carotid artery stenosis: performance of advanced vessel analysis software in evaluating CTA. Eur J Radiol. 2012;81(9):2255-9.
16. Kaladji A, Lucas A, Kervio G, Haigron P, Cardon A. Sizing for endovascular aneurysm repair: clinical evaluation of a new automated three-dimensional software. Ann Vasc Surg. 2010;24(7):912-20.
17. Tesche C, De Cecco CN, Albrecht MH, Duguay TM, Bayer RR, Litwin SE, et al. Coronary CT Angiography-derived Fractional Flow Reserve. Radiology. 2017(10);285(1): 17-33.
18. Coenen A, Lubbers MM, Kurata A, Kono A, Dedic A, Chelu RG, et al. Fractional flow reserve computed from noninvasive CT angiography data: diagnostic performance of an on-site clinician-operated computational fluid dynamics algorithm. Radiology. 2015;274(3):674-83.
19. Seitun S, De Lorenzi C, Cademartiri F, Buscaglia A, Travaglio N, Balbi M, et al. CT Myocardial Perfusion Imaging: A New Frontier in Cardiac Imaging. Biomed Res Int. 2018;2018:7295460.
20. Horehledova B, Mihl C, Schwemmer C, Hendriks BMF, Eijsvoogel NG, Kietselaer BLJH, et al. Aortic root evaluation prior to transcatheter aortic valve implantation-Correlation of manual and semi-automatic measurements. PLoS One. 2018;13(6):e0199732.
21. D'Onofrio M, De Robertis R, Demozzi E, Crosara S, Canestrini S, Pozzi Mucelli R. Liver volumetry: Is imaging reliable? Personal experience and review of the literature. World J Radiol. 2014;6(4):62-71.
22. Gotra A, Sivakumaran L, Chartrand G, Vu KN, Vandenbroucke-Menu F, Kauffmann C, et al. Liver segmentation: indications, techniques and future directions. Insights Imaging. 2017;8(4):377-92.
23. Lim MC, Tan CH, Cai J, Zheng J, Kow AW. CT volumetry of the liver: where does it stand in clinical practice? Clin Radiol. 2014;69(9):887-95.
24. Hori M, Suzuki K, Epstein ML, Baron RL. Computed tomography liver volumetry using 3-dimensional image data in living donor liver transplantation: effects of the slice thickness on the volume calculation. Liver Transpl. 2011;17(12):1427-36.
25. Wu W, Zhou Z, Wu S, Zhang Y. Automatic Liver Segmentation on Volumetric CT Images Using Supervoxel-Based Graph Cuts. Comput Math Methods Med. 2016;2016:9093721.
26. Lodewick TM, Arnoldussen CW, Lahaye MJ, van Mierlo KM, Neumann UP, Beets-Tan RG, et al. Fast and accurate liver volumetry prior to hepatectomy. HPB (Oxford). 2016;18(9):764-72.
27. Gotra A, Chartrand G, Massicotte-Tisluck K, Morin-Roy F, Vandenbroucke-Menu F, de Guise JA, et al. Validation of a semiautomated liver segmentation method using CT for accurate volumetry. Acad Radiol. 2015;22(9):1088-98.
28. Barbas AS, Li Y, Zair M, Van JA, Famure O, Dib MJ, et al. CT volumetry is superior to nuclear renography for prediction of residual kidney function in living donors. Clin Transplant. 2016;30(9):1028-35.
29. Wahba R, Franke M, Hellmich M, Kleinert R, Cingöz T, Schmidt MC, et al. Computed Tomography Volumetry in Preoperative Living Kidney Donor Assessment for Prediction of Split Renal Function. Transplantation. 2016;100(6):1270-7.
30. Chandel S, Singh N, Agrawal A, Singh H, Nandakumar H. Feasibility of Dentascan in planning of implant surgery in posterior maxilla and mandible. J Oral Biol Craniofac Res. 2017;7(3):188-92.
31. Benington PC, Khambay BS, Ayoub AF. An overview of three-dimensional imaging in dentistry. Dent Update. 2010;37(8):494-6, 9-500, 3-4 passim.
32. Subburaj K, Ravi B, Agarwal M. Automated identification of anatomical landmarks on 3D bone models reconstructed from CT scan images. Comput Med Imaging Graph. 2009;33(5):359-68.
33. Bagchi P, Joshi N. Role of Radiographic Evaluation in Treatment Planning for Dental Implants: A Review 2012.
34. Saavedra-Abril JA, Balhen-Martin C, Zaragoza-Velasco K, Kimura-Hayama ET, Saavedra S, Stoopen ME. Dental multisection CT for the placement of oral implants: technique and applications. Radiographics. 2010;30(7):1975-91.

35. Gahleitner A, Watzek G, Imhof H. Dental CT: imaging technique, anatomy, and pathologic conditions of the jaws. Eur Radiol. 2003;13(2):366-76.
36. Kumar V, Dixit J, Lal N, Verma UP, Debnath P, Pathak AK. Dentascan an excellent tool for assessment of variations in the management of periodontal defects. Natl J Maxillofac Surg. 2017;8(2):136-42.
37. Chandak S, Shetty CM. Comparative study of dentascan and radiography for radiological evaluation of impacted teeth. J Clin Diagn Res. 2014;8(7):RC01-5.
38. Calhoun PS, Kuszyk BS, Heath DG, Carley JC, Fishman EK. Three-dimensional volume rendering of spiral CT data: theory and method. Radiographics. 1999;19(3):745-64.
39. Dappa E, Higashigaito K, Fornaro J, Leschka S, Wildermuth S, Alkadhi H. Cinematic rendering - an alternative to volume rendering for 3D computed tomography imaging. Insights Imaging. 2016;7(6):849-56.
40. Eid M, De Cecco CN, Nance JW, Caruso D, Albrecht MH, Spandorfer AJ, et al. Cinematic Rendering in CT: A Novel, Lifelike 3D Visualization Technique. AJR Am J Roentgenol. 2017;209(2):370-9.
41. Rowe SP, Fritz J, Fishman EK. CT evaluation of musculoskeletal trauma: initial experience with cinematic rendering. Emerg Radiol. 2018;25(1):93-101.
42. Rowe SP, Johnson PT, Fishman EK. Cinematic rendering of cardiac CT volumetric data: Principles and initial observations. J Cardiovasc Comput Tomogr. 2018;12(1): 56-9.
43. Yang J, Li K, Deng H, Feng J, Fei Y, Jin Y, et al. CT cinematic rendering for pelvic primary tumor photorealistic visualization. Quant Imaging Med Surg. 2018;8(8):804-18.
44. Lee MW. Fusion imaging of real-time ultrasonography with CT or MRI for hepatic intervention. Ultrasonography. 2014;33(4): 227-39.
45. Yarlagadda VK, Lai WS, Gordetsky JB, Porter KK, Nix JW, Thomas JV, et al. MRI/US fusion-guided prostate biopsy allows for equivalent cancer detection with significantly fewer needle cores in biopsy-naive men. Diagn Interv Radiol. 2018;24(3): 115-20.
46. Mallarajapatna G, Rastogi R. Fusion imaging: The current trends 2013.
47. Chen H, Shen C, Qin J, Ni D, Shi L, Cheng JCY, et al. Automatic Localization and Identification of Vertebrae in Spine CT via a Joint Learning Model with Deep Neural Networks. In: Navab N, Hornegger J, Wells WM, Frangi A, eds. Medical Image Computing and Computer-Assisted Intervention—MICCAI 2015. Cham: Springer International Publishing 2015:515-22.
48. Glocker B, Feulner J, Criminisi A, Haynor DR, Konukoglu E. Automatic Localization and Identification of Vertebrae in Arbitrary Field-of-View CT Scans. In: Ayache N, Delingette H, Golland P, Mori K, eds. Medical Image Computing and Computer-Assisted Intervention–MICCAI 2012. Berlin, Heidelberg: Springer Berlin Heidelberg 2012:590-8.
49. Ma J, Lu L. Hierarchical segmentation and identification of thoracic vertebra using learning-based edge detection and coarse-to-fine deformable model. Computer Vision and Image Understanding. 2013 2013/09/01/;117(9): 1072-83.
50. Klinder T, Ostermann J, Ehm M, Franz A, Kneser R, Lorenz C. Automated model-based vertebra detection, identification, and segmentation in CT images. Med Image Anal. 2009;13(3):471-82.
51. Pomahac B, Pribaz J, Eriksson E, Bueno EM, Diaz-Siso JR, Rybicki FJ, et al. Three Patients with Full Facial Transplantation. New England Journal of Medicine. 2011 2012/02/23;366(8):715-22.
52. Soga S, Ersoy H, Mitsouras D, Schultz K, Whitmore AG, Powers SL, et al. Surgical planning for composite tissue allotransplantation of the face using 320-detector row computed tomography. J Comput Assist Tomogr. 2010;34(5):766-9.
53. Soga S, Pomahac B, Mitsouras D, Kumamaru K, Powers SL, Prior RF, et al. Preoperative vascular mapping for facial allotransplantation: four-dimensional computed tomographic angiography versus magnetic resonance angiography. Plast Reconstr Surg. 2011;128(4):883-91.
54. Kumamaru KK, Sisk GC, Mitsouras D, Schultz K, Steigner ML, George E, et al. Vascular communications between donor and recipient tissues after successful full face transplantation. Am J Transplant. 2014;14(3):711-9.
55. Paiva W, Amorim R, Alexandre França Bezerra D, Masini M. Aplication of the stereolithography technique in complex spine surgery 2007.
56. Geyer LL, Korner M, Hempel R, Deak Z, Mueck FG, Linsenmaier U, et al. Evaluation of a dedicated MDCT protocol using iterative image reconstruction after cervical spine trauma. Clin Radiol. 2013;68(7):e391-6.
57. Maxfield MW, Schuster KM, McGillicuddy EA, Young CJ, Ghita M, Bokhari SAJ, et al. Impact of adaptive statistical iterative reconstruction on radiation dose in evaluation of trauma patients. The journal of trauma and acute care surgery. 2012;73(6):1406-11.
58. Kilic K, Erbas G, Guryildirim M, Arac M, Ilgit E, Coskun B. Lowering the dose in head CT using adaptive statistical iterative reconstruction. AJNR Am J Neuroradiol. 2011;32(9):1578-82.
59. Kilic K, Erbas G, Guryildirim M, Konus OL, Arac M, Ilgit E, et al. Quantitative and qualitative comparison of standard-dose and low-dose pediatric head computed tomography: a retrospective study assessing the effect of adaptive statistical iterative reconstruction. J Comput Assist Tomogr. 2013;37(3):377-81.
60. Korn A, Bender B, Fenchel M, Spira D, Schabel C, Thomas C, et al. Sinogram affirmed iterative reconstruction in head CT: improvement of objective and subjective image quality with concomitant radiation dose reduction. Eur J Radiol. 2013;82(9):1431-5.
61. Wu TH, Hung SC, Sun JY, Lin CJ, Lin CH, Chiu CF, et al. How far can the radiation dose be lowered in head CT with iterative reconstruction? Analysis of imaging quality and diagnostic accuracy. Eur Radiol. 2013;23(9):2612-21.
62. Laqmani A, Buhk JH, Henes FO, Klink T, Sehner S, von Schultzendorff HC, et al. Impact of a 4th generation iterative reconstruction technique on image quality in low-dose computed tomography of the chest in immunocompromised patients. Rofo. 2013;185(8):749-57.

CHAPTER

33

Magnetic Resonance Instrumentation and MRI Safety Issues: An Update

Anjali Prakash, Jyoti Kumar, Sapna Singh

Magnetic resonance image represents the relative response of specific nuclei to absorbed radiofrequency energy. The Dutch physicist CJ Gorter[1] first proposed the NMR concept in 1936, which was furthered by the work of Block and Purcell. The Nobel Prize for Physics was awarded to them in 1952. Between 1950s and 60s, it was used primarily as an analytical tool for chemists and physicists to determine the chemical structure, configuration and reactive processes.

Modern clinical use started after Paul Lauterbur's[2] suggestion in 1973, that operator controlled magnetic field gradients could be used to encode position dependent information in the NMR signal. MRI has been selected along with computed tomography (CT) as example of the benefits to society of basic research in physics. In 2003, Paul Lauterbur and Sir Peter Mansfield received the Nobel Prize in medicine for their work in the field of magnetic resonance imaging.

The main constituents of an MRI scanner are the *magnet subsystem* which produces a spatial and temporally constant magnetic field B_0, the *gradient subsystem* to produce varying magnetic field gradients for spatial encoding, *RF subsystem* to transmit and receive radiofrequency B_1 and the *computer and microprocessors* to specify and control the pulse sequence calculate, process, display, store and transfer the resultant clinical image. This includes an acquisition and control system, reconstruction system. There is viewing console for operator input of control parameters and display of imaging. In addition, magnetic and RF shielding is required. Patient table, hardware for physiological monitoring of patient (ECG and respiratory gating) and monitoring equipment is also needed[3] **(Figs. 1 and 2)**.

During imaging, patient is positioned on the MRI table placing the patient in a strong magnetic field (B_0) in a manner to place the anatomy to be imaged in the region of maximum uniformity of the field—isocenter. The magnetic field aligns along the axis of the body called the Z-axis running from head to foot. The other two short axes are X- and Y-axis. The operator selects a scan; the next step is adjustment of the amplitude and waveform of the gradient field, done by the gradient pulse generator. Gradient amplifiers increase the power required to drive the gradient coils. A RF pulse is then generated by RF transmitter which sets the required B_1 field frequency on the frequency synthesizer. Using an amplitude modulator, the carrier frequency is modulated into apodisced fine pulses. The RF amplifier increases the power of the pulse from milliwatts to kilowatts, which is used to drive the RF transmit coil. RF signal goes into the body and generates a signal which is received by a RF receive coil where it induces an alternating voltage of a few microvolts. After amplification of the signal by an RF amplifier (receiver), tuned to the resonant frequency, the amplitude or envelope of this signal is sampled, digitized and computer analyzed.

MRI system is a collection of coils **(Box 1)**.

THE MAGNET SUBSYSTEM

The magnet is the key component of the MR scanner. It determines the appearance, cost and capacity of the device. The *strength of the magnet* is measured in unit Tesla (T), research systems with a magnetic strength of 9.4[4] T4 are available for use in humans. The main magnetic field needs to be very *uniform or homogeneous for* imaging. Its strength and direction should remain unaffected by ambient temperature. The homogeneity of a magnetic field is expressed in parts per million (ppm) within a given spherical volume. The size of this volume is standardized as the *Diameter of a spherical volume (DSV)*. It defines a direction in space that is conventionally referred to as Z-direction. The Z-component of the main field at the center of the magnet is designated as B_0, Z-axis usually runs along the cylindrical axis of the main magnet and in the direction from the patients head to feet **(Fig. 3)**. Any variation of this longitudinal field Bz from its central value B_0 has a significant effect on motions of spin system. Consequently, the design of the main field coils is chosen to minimize variations in the strength of the B_0 field over the desired region of imaging.

The straightness of magnetic lines within the center needs to be perfect. Within a specified region *diameter spherical volume (DSV)* the field is uniform with a typical magnetic flux variation of 5 ppm for imaging and 1 ppm for spectroscopy. A main magnet with DSV positioned at *magnet isocenter* is called a symmetric magnet. In an asymmetric (open bore) magnet, DSV is shifted a certain distance away from the isocenter towards one end of the magnet. The magnet should have a bore size large enough to accommodate the patient.

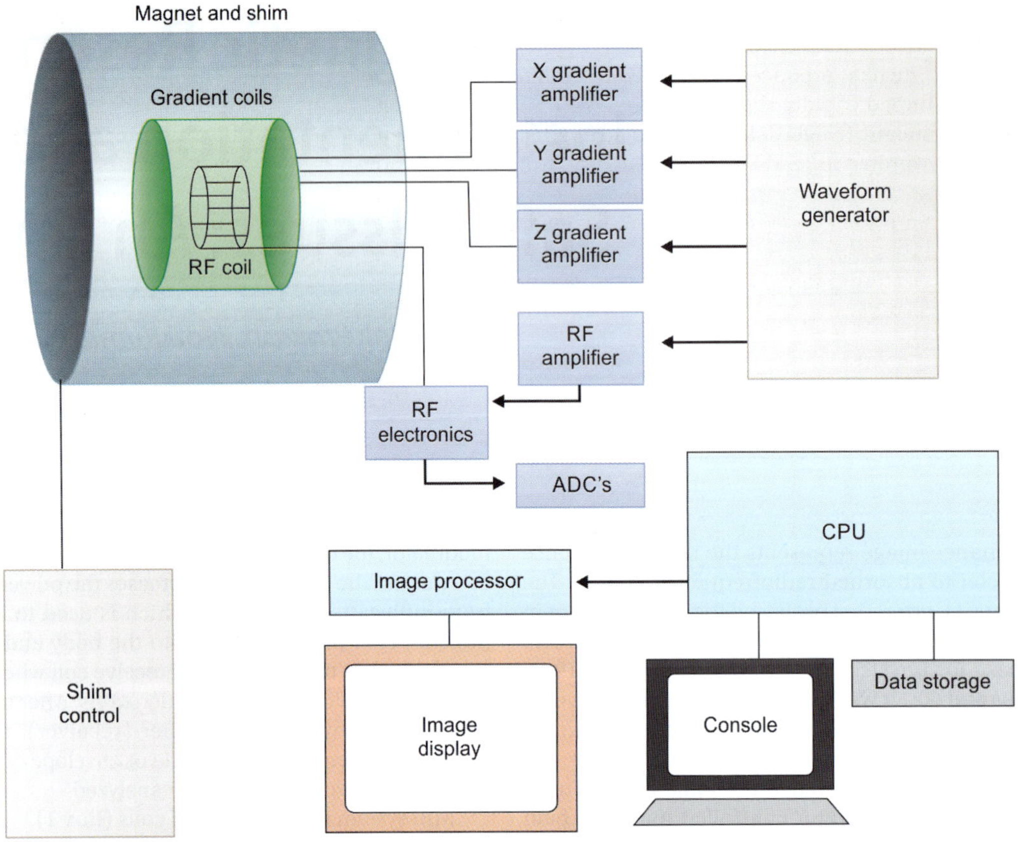

FIG. 1: Various hardware components of MRI scanner.

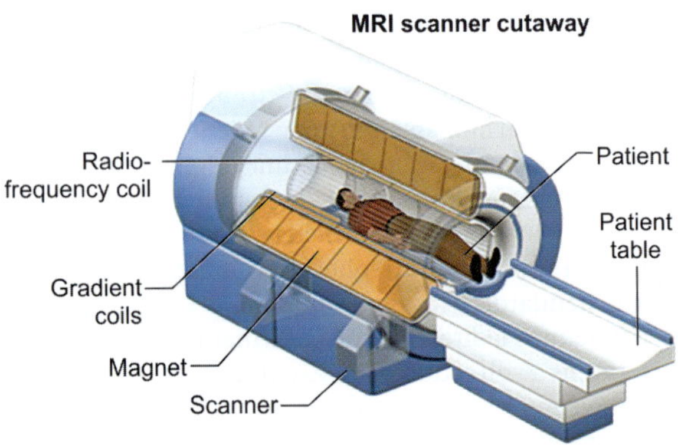

FIG. 2: Cutaway of MRI scanner indicating position of various coils.

BOX 1: Relative positions of various coils in MRI.

The relative coil positions from outside in:
- *Main field (B_0) Coils* (Principal magnet coil windings, superconducting shim and shield coils)
- *Shim coils* (to improve homogeneity)
- *Gradient coils* (for imaging, slice, frequency, and phase encoding, including their active shields)
- *Radiofrequency (RF) Body coil* (transmits B_1 field)
- *Receive coils* (primarily to detect MR signal, some coils are both transmit and receive)

The magnetic lines within the center of the bore need to be perfectly straight. The magnetic field lines form closed loops and crowd together within the magnet bore. The field lines also spread in wide area around the magnet. this is referred to as a *fringe field* **(Fig. 4)**.

There are three types of magnets used in MRI—*permanent magnet, resistive magnet and super conducting magnet:*

1. *Permanent magnet:* It consists of two opposing flat faced magnetized pole pieces made of iron and alloys of aluminum, nickel and cobalt fixed to an iron frame. Once magnetized, these maintain magnetization indefinitely without power input. Permanent magnets require no power input, and cannot be shut down. They provide low strength (0.3 T or less) vertical fields. Permanent magnets are very heavy up to 80–100 tonnes. Running costs are relatively less. Permanent magnet systems are useful in imaging of claustrophobic patients, children, obese adults and for interventional procedures. These are constructed as open access configuration unlike solenoid magnets which have a circular bore.
A newer magnetic alloy of iron neodymium and boron has been described which is of lower weight and with higher strength. Other materials used are metallic alloy alnico, ceramic barium ferrite and rare earth alloy samarium cobalt ($SmCO_3$).[5]
2. *Resistive magnet:* It is a set of DC coils with copper or aluminum conductors, passage of electric current through

the wire generates a magnetic field. It requires 50–100 KW of stable power supply to produce a homogenous magnetic field. The heat produced is removed by cooling using water pumped rapidly through the hollow coils. There are significant fringe fields and the strength of magnetic field is limited to 0.5 T. Resistive magnets are the only type of magnets which can be switched off at the end of the day. The time taken to reestablish magnetic field is 15–30 minutes. These are relatively low cost and have a small foot print of about 2 tonnes. Resistive magnets have a limited role, these days.

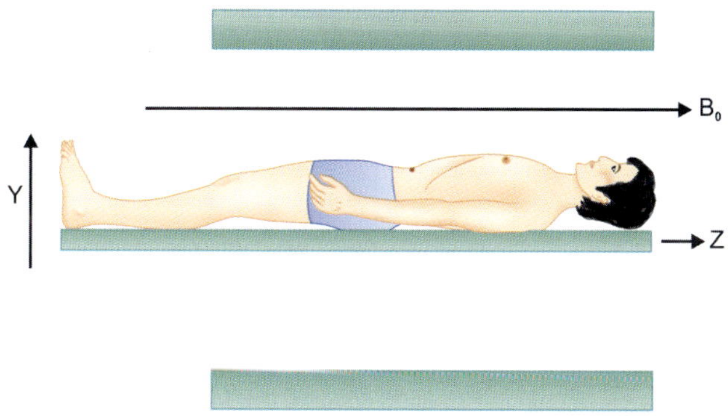

FIG. 3: Schematic depiction of the Z-axis along the main magnetic field B_0.

3. *Hybrid magnets:* Combine feature of more than one basic type. Magnet include both a permanent magnet and a set of electric coils to achieve a stronger magnetic field. In 2001, a research team at stanford university invented a new technique called prepolarized MRI/pMRI.[6] They demonstrated that two magnets can be used together, one strong, but not very uniform and the other very homogeneous, but not so strong. The magnet that is strong produces a strong magnetic field which varies in uniformity by as much as 40%. A second magnet produces a more precise magnetic field. These magnets can be ordinary copper wound magnets, lowering cost. As the magnetic field is "tuned" by the second magnet, a pMRI scan can be obtained adjacent to a metal implant.

Superconducting Magnet

Superconductivity is a property of materials, such that they lose electrical resistance at very low temperatures. Non superconductors also lose resistance at low temperatures but do not become zero resistance as superconductors do **(Fig. 5)**. Examples of such materials are some metals (Hg) and alloys—niobium/titanium, niobium/tin and vanadium/gallium.

A superconductive electromagnet is a DC solenoid about 1 m in diameter, commonly made of niobium-titanium alloy in a copper matrix **(Fig. 6)**. This becomes superconducting

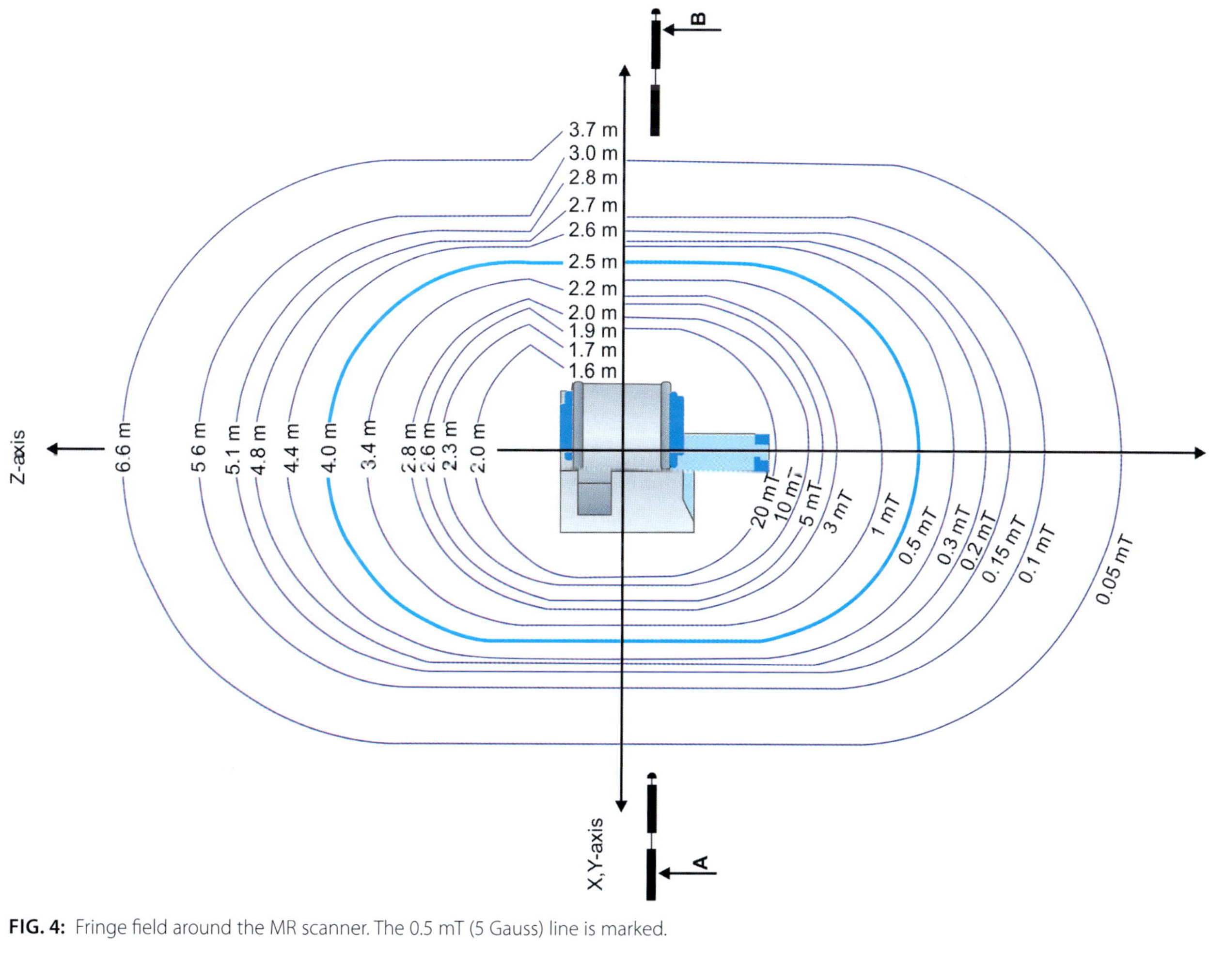

FIG. 4: Fringe field around the MR scanner. The 0.5 mT (5 Gauss) line is marked.

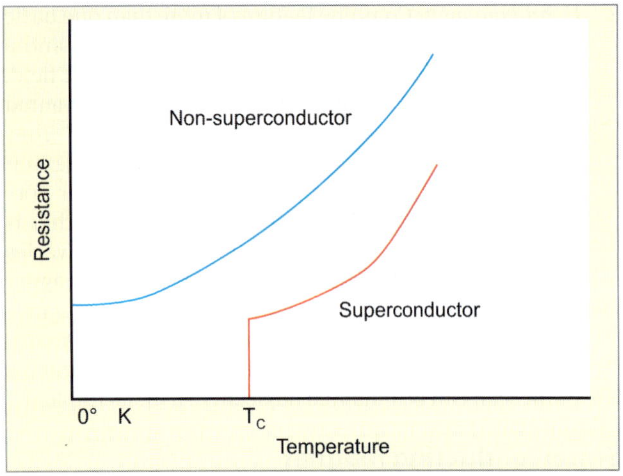

FIG. 5: Graph depicting property of superconductivity. Electrical resistence drops to zero at transition temperature (T_C) of superconductors, for other materials it decreases with lowering of temperature, but is never zero.

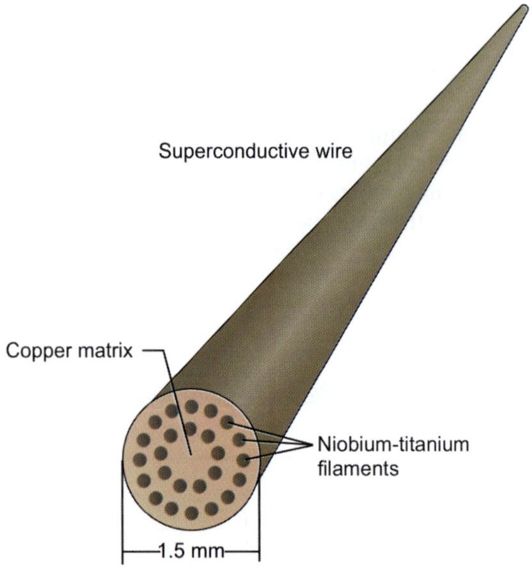

FIG. 6: Cut section of a superconductive wire made of Niobium-titanium alloy embedded in copper matrix.

at 9.2° Kelvin which is called the critical temperature. The length of the superconducting wire in the magnet is several miles long; this length of the wire has to be constructed without interruption of its superconducting properties. After the magnet is sited and ready, it is cooled to superconductive temperatures by being filled with liquid helium. The electrical terminals to charge the coil windings are located deep within the cryostat. Parallel with the main coil windings is a bypass (persistence limb) containing a component called a persistence resistor. The service engineer next attaches a power supply to circuit and begins pumping current into the system. Because the magnet coils are superconducting and have zero resistance, virtually all of the applied current flows directly through them and little or none into the persistence limb. Then the coil is short circuited and power source switched off. The time taken for the superconducting state to be reached and full field strength to be reached is, typically 2–3 days. This process is called ramping up the magnets. Once energized, the current continues in a loop as long as the temperature is maintained. The current continues to flow, while using no power like permanent magnets. They require no external power source once energized.[7-10]

Accurate temperature control is an essential requirement for maintenance of the superconductivity. The main magnet windings are immersed in liquid helium (4°K) in a structure called a *cryostat*—which contains a Dewar with ~1700 L of liquid helium. This creates a temperature gradient from the magnet core to the surrounding room to minimize thermal energy losses and stabilizes the internal core temperature. The cryostat is a multi-compartmental structure that functions like a Thermos bottle.[11] It contains not only the main magnet windings and channels for liquid helium, but also various insulating and vacuum layers to thermally shield the coils from the warm external environment **(Fig. 7)**. The cryostat also contains superconducting shim coils (to improve homogeneity) and active shielding coils

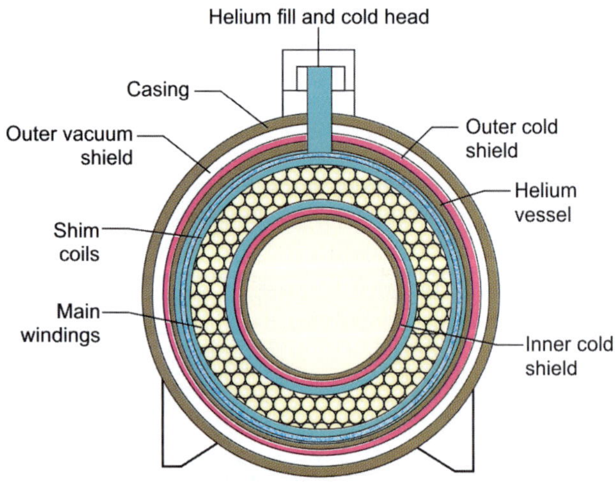

FIG. 7: Cut section of a cryostat.

(to minimize stray/fringe fields). The external casing of the cryostat as well as the helium vessel, inner and outer shells are typically made of nonmagnetic stainless steel. The walls of the vacuum chambers are constructed of either nonmagnetic stainless steel or glass-reinforced polymer. The cold shields are typically 3–10 mm thick and made from a low emissivity/high thermal conductivity material such as aluminum.

The first superconductive magnet developed in 1980's had two cryogen chambers, the inner one containing liquid helium and the outer one containing liquid nitrogen. The liquid nitrogen had to be topped up weekly and helium nearly on a monthly basis. In 1990s helium only systems were developed and by the early 2000s refrigeration system became so developed that helium filling is required once in 2–3 years.[3,7-9] *Zero boil off systems* are now standard allowing essentially unlimited normal operation without the need of helium refill.

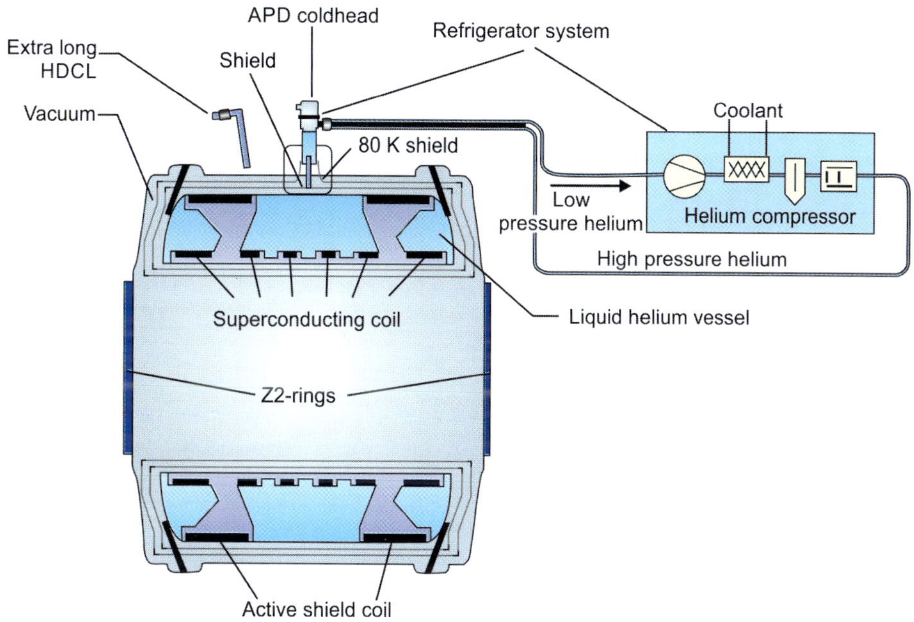

FIG. 8: The magnet assembly in a superconducting magnet is seated into an all welded stainless steel vessel filled with liquid helium.

Components of the cooling system for the MRI include a Cryocooler compressor also called as 'Cold head'/the helium pump and a heat exchanger or chiller (for gradients). Cold head is a mechanical device used for minimizing the helium boil-off by recondensing helium gas into liquid after it has cooled the magnet. This circulates liquid helium around the magnet. The cold head must be in permanent operation. Power failure will lead to stoppage of the cold head with increased helium boil off. The heat which reaches the cryo shields of the magnet is absorbed and passed via the cold head to an external heat exchanger which is part of the refrigerator system **(Fig. 8)**. A rhythmical thud that is heard in the system while it is not acquiring images is due to the operation of helium refrigeration pump. The cold head and refrigerator compressor requires service and periodic filter change as part of preventive maintenance, with some replacement of helium required at this time. In future systems may be cryogen free; this is due to the development of a new cooling system called *Gifford-McMahon (G-M) cryocoolers.*[10]

Quench

The magnet has to be kept at a temperature below the critical/ transition temperature. If a small region of wire is heated to temperature above this, it begins to dissipate heat and there is increase in temperature. This leads to a process called quench wherein the stored energy in the magnetic field is converted into heat. This raises the temperature of the liquid helium above its boiling point and magnetic field collapses, there is an explosive boil off of the cryogen. Magnets sense the onset of a quench and activate heaters that spread energy deposition throughout the coils. If this were not to happen, deposition of energy at a point could melt wire locally and destroy it.[7,8]

After a quench, magnet itself is rarely damaged and may be recooled and energized. To minimize possibility of quench due to frictional heating, magnet is 'trained' at the time of manufacture by cycling magnetic fields above the planned level of operation. Quenches are also possible if the cryostat vacuum fails or cryogenic fluid is not refilled in time. Hence, the coolant level is logged daily.

Superconducting magnets are supplied with an emergency switch system that permits a deliberate quench in case of an emergency, like a person being trapped against or inside the magnet by a ferromagnetic object. The field decreases from initial value to nearly zero in one minute (See section on MRI safety).

Magnet Geometry

MR scanners are classified on the basis of their geometry into closed- and open-bore systems. Most modern scanners are of the closed-bore cylindrical design and generate their fields by passing current through a solenoid kept at superconducting temperatures. Closed bore systems have a horizontal magnetic field, and superior magnetic field homogeneity **(Fig. 9)**. Closed bore systems can be wide bore or short bore systems. Wide bore designs have superior homogeneity for large Field of view (FOV), while short bore magnets provide relief from claustrophobia.

Open bore magnets, as the name suggests, have an air gap between two magnetic poles. These may utilize permanent magnets or electromagnets. Most *open bore* scanners utilize permanent magnets in a C-shaped or horseshoe configuration and operate at field strengths ranging from 0.2 T to 1.0 T. Most open systems have a vertical magnetic field with specially designed flat planer gradient coils. Open systems are available which can image while patient

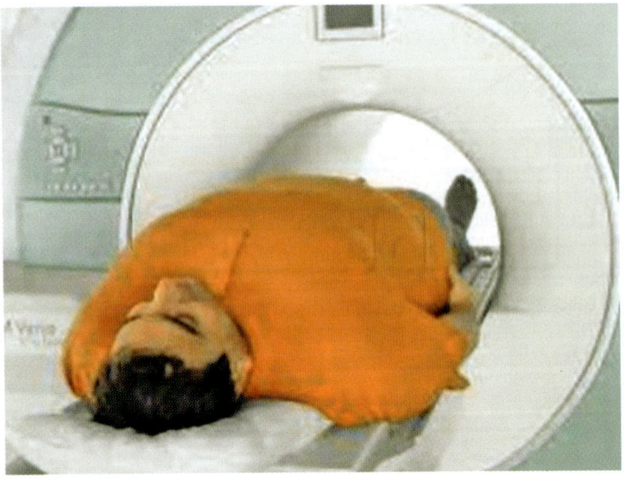

FIG. 9: Wide bore (70 cm) tunnel magnet.

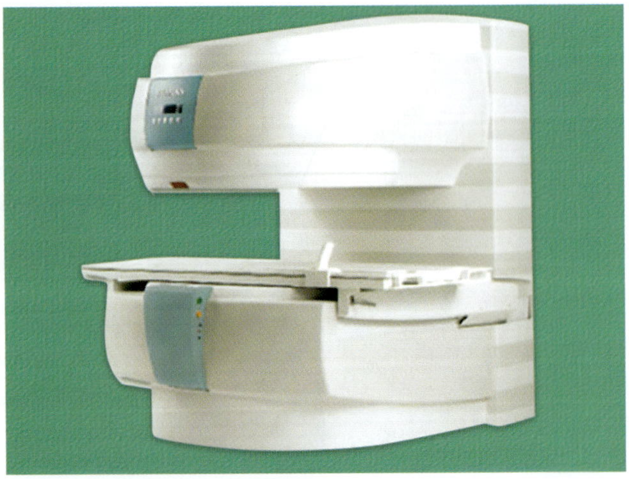

FIG. 10: Open low field MRI with a permanent magnet.

bears weight-standing or sitting instead of lying supine **(Fig. 10)**. They have smaller fringe fields and have less stringent siting requirements. The main advantage is better patient acceptability.

Another design for open magnet system comprises of a *dipolar electromagnet* configuration with coils on either side of the patient. These coils can be superconductive or resistive and range from 0.5 T to 1.2 T.[11]

Specialty magnets are specially designed for a particular type of examination usually for musculoskeletal applications. These have a superconducting/resistive magnet.[12] Dedicated RF coils (80–180 mm in diameter) are available for a range of anatomies. There is a chair/recliner so that the patient is seated comfortably **(Fig. 11)**.

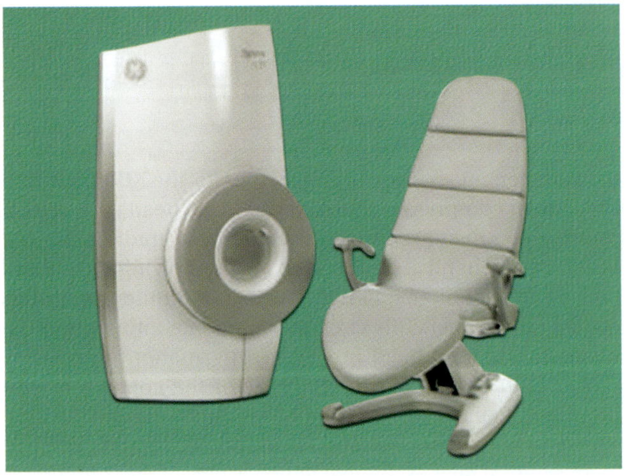

FIG. 11: Specialty magnet system used in musculoskeletal imaging.

Shim Coils

The magnetic field must be stable and not affected by temperature. Magnet homogenity has a direct impact on image quality. Problems associated with poor homogenity include shading, spatial distortion, blurring and zebra (Moire) banding artifacts. Studies with large FOV's and fas EPI sequences are more prone to these issues. MR spectroscopy requires temporal stability of the magnet. Inhomogenity also leads to incomplete fat suppression. The uniformity should be in the range of 5 ppm.

Imperfections in manufacturing of the coils lead to harmonic error field and inhomogeneity. The process of 'shimming' is required to overcome these errors. Two methods are available for shimming:

1. *Passive shimming:* It is achieved by placing small permanent magnets at strategic locations at time of installation within the scanner bore to counteract field in homogeneities.
2. *Active shimming:* A set of coils is used and current is passed through these 'shim coils'. These generate small magnetic fields gradients which are superimposed on the main magnetic field and remove the field non-uniformities. Field homogeneity is measured by examining free induction decay (FID) signal in the absence of external field gradients. The FID from a poorly shimmed sample shows a complex decay envelope with many humps. Shim currents are adjusted to provide an exponentially decaying FID which is an indicator of a homogeneous B_0 field **(Figs. 12A and B)**. Active shimming is computer optimized for each imaging volume.

The shim coils can be superconducting and located within the cryostat and maintained at low temperature. Shim coils can also be a set of resistive shim coils, when they are placed in the room temperature bore of the magnet.

GRADIENT SUBSYSTEM

Gradient coils spatially encode the position of protons by varying the magnetic field linearly across the imaging volume. The Larmor frequency will then vary as a function of position in the X, Y, Z-axis. The magnetic field gradient in the three directions are produced by three sets of orthogonally positioned coils **(Fig. 13)**. The null point at the center of the gradient coils is also the centre of the magnet and is called the isocenter. The three gradients are the slice selection, frequency encoding and the phase encoding gradients.

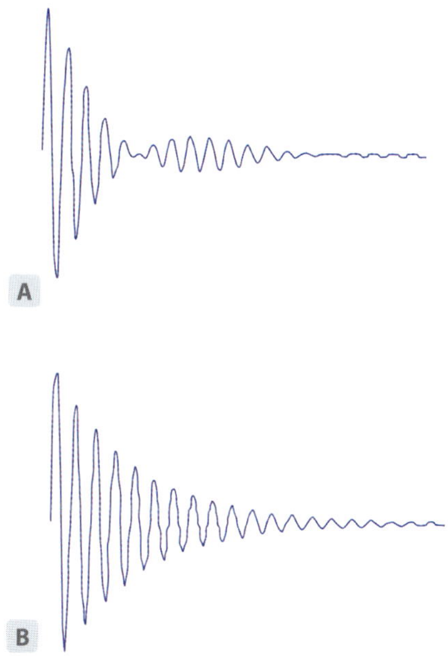

FIGS. 12A AND B: FID signal from a poorly shimmed sample. (A) Showing a complex decay envelope, while an exponentially decaying amplitude; (B) Indicates proper shim.

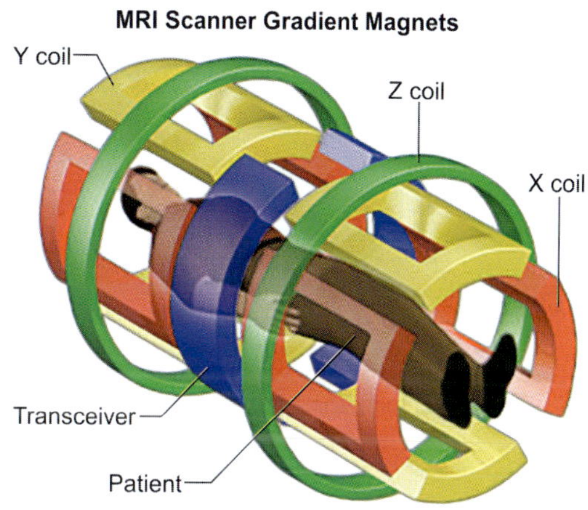

FIG. 13: Gradient coils the X, Y and Z direction.

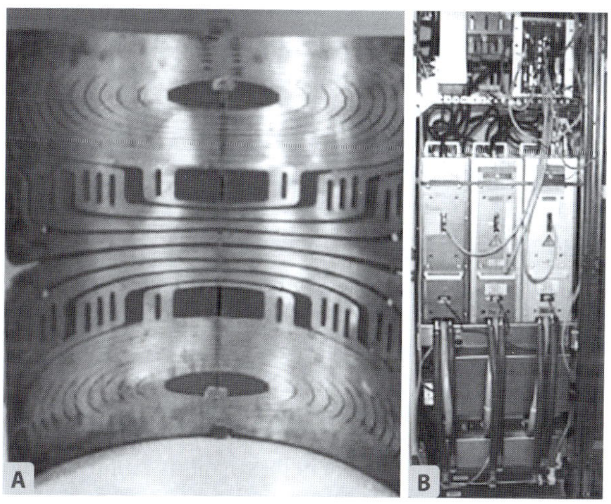

FIGS. 14A AND B: (A) Gradient coil; (B) Gradient amplifier.

The *slice selection gradient* and RF pulse define a slice, a second magnetic field gradient applied orthogonally to the slice selection gradient serves as a readout gradient or frequency encoding gradient. By repeated rotation and application of the readout gradient, spatial information in more than one direction can be obtained. A third gradient—the phase encoding gradient completes the spatial encoding of spins. The slice select or Z-axis gradient field is switched on during the application of RF pulse. The steeper the gradient, thinner the slice. In the time of a few milliseconds, when MR signal is being received, current is passed through another set of gradient coils—*frequency encoding gradient coils* XX coils. This alters the magnetic field gradient from side to side in the X direction. a steeper gradient is used for a smaller FOV. The third set of coils, the *phase encoding gradient* coils YY coils are energized, immediately after the 90° pulse, but before it is inverted by the 180° pulse. This produces a gradient from front to back of the patient. Each gradient individually produces a field in a specific direction; a gradient field in any chosen direction can be generated by activating two or all three of the gradient coils. This makes it possible to select imaging planes in any of the directions. Steeper gradients are required for finer phase matrices.

Components and Technical Parameters of Gradient Coils

Gradients coils are resistive electromagnets consisting of metallic coils driven by power amplifiers. The gradient coils are made of copper and are circular or rectangular in cross-section with a diameter of ~5 mm **(Figs. 14A and B)**. These windings are distributed in a "fingerprint" pattern consisting of multiple thin metallic strips or large copper sheets which are etched into complex patterns and applied to the cylinder. A circular *Maxwell coil* produces linear variation in field along Z-axis in other axes it is done using a *saddle-golay coil* **(Fig. 15)**. Each of the three sets of gradient coil has separate power supply, and independent computer control which alter the slope of the magnetic field. These are switched off and on frequently to allow slice selection, frequency and phase encoding. All three coils are wound on a cylinder and situated in the bore of the magnet.[13]

Gradient Amplifier

The gradient coils are connected to pulse width modulated (PWM) amplifiers that control the rise time and maximum value of the gradients. The peak power of the gradient amplifier is a key specification of this component. The increase or decrease in the field strength relative to the center is determined by the direction of the current (DC) passed through the coil. For some imaging applications like diffusion imaging, is it not unusual for peak coil driving voltages to reach 2500 V and currents to exceed 1000 A. There is a lot of heat generated, with maximum internal coil temperatures reaching 55–60°C. All modern scanners use fluidic cooling to minimize heating. This is generally accomplished by

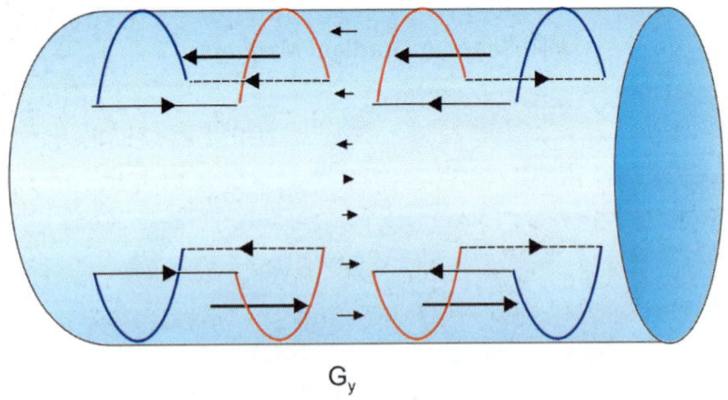

FIG. 15: Double saddle coil configuration for producing a y gradient–Golay-coil. X gradient is produced by rotating the coil along the surface of the cylinder.

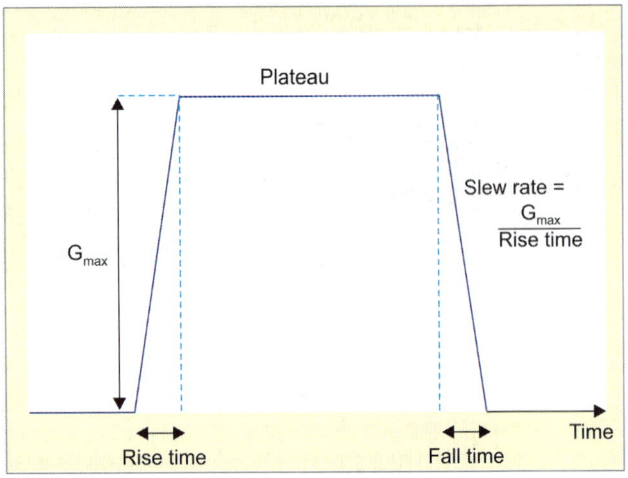

FIG. 16: Trapezoidal gradient pulse showing definitions of G_{max} (amplitude) and slew rate.

circulating de-ionized water or an ethylene glycol solution from a heat exchange pump ("chiller") located in the adjacent magnet equipment room. The water flows through tubes, jackets, or channels in close relation to the gradient coils. Some scanners use forced air cooling around the gradients. *Super G gradients* (GE) utilize hollow conductors allowing water to flow both in and around the windings.[12]

Powerful gradient amplifiers are sited in a room with restricted access adjacent to the magnet room.

Gradient Strength and Slew Rate

Gradient pulses in conventional pulse sequences have a trapezoidal shape, with a sloping rise, followed by a flat plateau and a sloping fall **(Fig. 16)**. The maximum gradient amplitude that can be generated -G_{Max} (in millitesla per meter mT/m) has a direct impact on the minimum slice thickness and FOV, and thereby on the maximum spatial resolution that is available. The current in these coils is rapidly switched on and off (on a millisecond time scale between various levels) The time required to switch between two current levels sets the limit to the minimum TR and TE values that can be achieved, and consequently the minimum acquisition time. A *slew rate* of a gradient system (in tesla per meters per second) is defined as the ratio of gradient strength divided by rise time. This is an important technical specification of the scanner capability. Slew rate depends on both the gradient coil (it takes more time to ramp up/down a large coil than a small coil) and on the performance of the gradient amplifier with significant influence on image quality. Slew rates up to 200 T/m/sec while gradient strengths up to 80 mT/m are now available.

Gradients with high amplitudes allows images to be acquired with smaller field of views and or thinner slice thickness, while maintaining short echo times or echo spacings, large peak gradient amplitudes are also required for diffusion imaging. The gradient rise time or how rapidly the gradient field changes with time from zero to the peak amplitude is usually expressed as *rise time* in microseconds with typical values of 200–1000 μs.

Gradient Linearity

Linear variation of the gradient field is required for accurate spatial encoding. The coils have a finite length hence there are nonlinear fields near the edges. The consequence of nonlinearity is misplaced signal and geometric distortion. Computer algorithms are used to compensate for gradient nonlinearities.

Duty Cycle

It represents the percentage of time the gradient is able to work at maximum amplitude during that sequence. This gradient parameter does not have a fixed value, but varies by pulse sequence. Maximum duty cycle performance of close to 100% is seen in most modern scanners.[13]

The performance of the gradient system determines the *scan speed*. Stronger gradients allow faster imaging and higher resolution. Applications such as MR angiography, cardiac MR and diffusion tensor imaging require high amplitude gradients (>20 mT/m) with a fast slew rate.

Specialized gradient coils are being developed for a variety of clinical applications. In echoplanar imaging, the requirements of gradient strengths, rise times and duty cycle have been increased as all the space is to be traversed in a single excitation. *Dual gradients* have been developed, which provides a shorter but higher performance by one gradient and the other providing the standard full region gradient.[14] Specifically, in head imaging a physically smaller gradient can be used which combines improved gradient performance with satisfactory performance.

Gradient-related Problems

Fast switching gradients can lead to induction of *eddy currents* due to the changing magnetic fields produced. These degrade imaging sequences by producing geometric distortion, blurred images and artifacts like ghosting **(Fig. 17)**. Preventing eddy currents from being formed is the way to overcome these artifacts. This is achieved by *active shielding of gradient coils,* where a second coil surrounds the primary gradient coil and carries current in the opposite direction. These cancel the eddy currents but also reduce the overall strength of the gradient fields. These shield coils cancel/minimize the distant magnetic effects of the imaging gradients, reducing

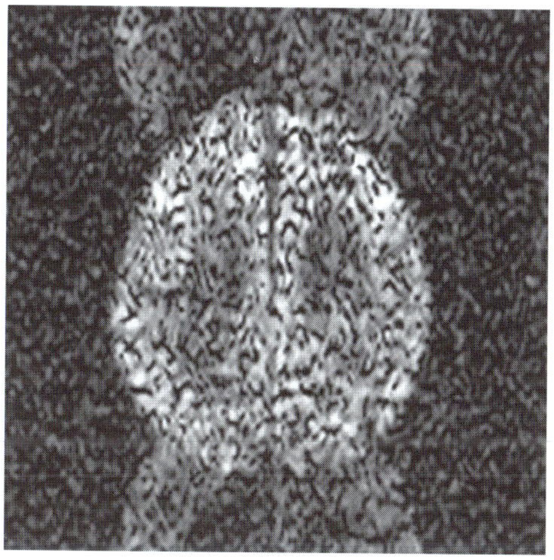

FIG. 17: "Eddy current' artifact—in homogeneities in the gradient cause distortion in the image.

eddy currents. All modern scanners have active shielding of gradients.

This characteristic noise heard and (the signature complaint) by the patient at the time of scanning arises due to the generation of Lorentz forces by the coils when current is pulsed through them in presence of static magnetic field. The noise is caused by the movement of the coils against their mountings and can be in excess of 100 db. As gradient strength is increasing, so is the noise. MR Vendors have released low noise imaging software package Silent scan (GE), QuietX (Siemens) and ComforTone (Philips) which use gentler gradient waveforms with gradual ramp up and ramp down times. These methods reduce scanner noise to within 10 d B of background but also decrease SNR, due to shorter available window for data sampling. Ultrashort TE sequences lead to nearly complete gradient silence.[11]

The switching of powerful gradients induces electrical currents in conducting tissue as per Faraday's law of Induction. The nerve depolarization threshold may be exceeded leading to *peripheral nerve stimulation*. Duration of the stimulus and the rate at which the magnetic field changes (db/dt) determine the possibility of exceeding the threshold. The shorter the stimulus the faster the magnetic field has to change to cause the stimulus (See section on MR safety).

RADIO FREQUENCY SUBSYSTEM

Radio frequency subsystem is required to perform two functions-transmitting and receiving signals at or near the Larmor frequency of the processing spins by using RF coils, which can be transmitter or receiver coils. When used as a transmitter, RF coils generate an oscillating/rotating magnetic field denoted as B_1 that is perpendicular to the static main magnetic field B_0. If the frequency of oscillation of B_1 closely matches the natural precession of nuclear spins near the Larmor frequency, energy is deposited into the spin system causing a change in its net alignment. The B_1 field is generated by the transmit coil in response to a powerful current. B_1 is typically turned on for very brief time (milliseconds) called as RF pulses. By adjusting the magnitude or duration of these B_1 pulses, the nuclear spin system can be rotated by variable flip angles. When used as receiver RF, coils are responsible for detecting the MR signal. The oscillating net magnetic flux from the excited spin system can be captured by the coil in which an induced current is generated. This current is then amplified, digitized and filtered to extract phase and frequency information.

The RF transmission system consists of RF synthesizer, amplifier and transmitter coil (usually built into the body of the scanner). The *transmitter* generates RF pulses with appropriate frequencies, bandwidths, amplitudes and phases in order to excite nuclei within the desired slices/slabs. The center frequency of the pulse is determined by the slice position and the strength of the slice select gradient at that location. The bandwidth or the range of frequencies within the pulse controls the thickness of the excited slice. The bandwidth is determined by shape and duration of the RF pulse envelope. The amplitude of the RF pulse control shows how much the magnetization has flipped by the pulse. RF pulse generation can be achieved by using an analog or digital process. In modern MR systems RF envelop is produced digitally. The transmitter must display linearity, i.e. the output of the power amplifier should be directly proportional to thc input power. This is achieved by a process called as envelope feedback. RF amplifier converts a low level RF demand signal to a high power level. RF source is combination of independent input signal and amplifiers.

RF Receiver system consists of receive coils, preamplifiers, digitisers and digital signal processors to prepare the signal for reconstruction. A *preamplifier* mounted on the coil assembly boosts the small MR signal received from the body. Amplification is used to match the voltage range of the MRI signal to the input range of the ADC, in order to engage its full dynamic range. The primary role of the receiver in an MRI scanner is to convert the analog coil signals into digital format The receive chain is responsible for detecting the tiny MR signal, amplifying and digitizing it without the addition of unwanted noise. The receiver then sends the signal to the reconstructor for image calculation and formation.

The design of a modern digital receiver is based on an analog-to-digital converter (ADC), which samples the analog MRI signal and converts it into digital format. Prior to input into the ADC, the MRI scanner signal needs to be amplified and filtered. Important characteristics of the ADC are its conversion bandwidth and resolution. The conversion bandwidth equals half the digitization rate. State-of-the-art ADCs allow conversion bandwidth of over 50 MHz at 14 bit resolution. A/D convertor is the limiting factor in the receiver chain. Each element of the receiver chain should have A/D convertor to achieve maximum SNR. In practice a multiplexer is used, with one single receive channel (A/D convertor) between two or three coil elements. The output bandwidth and center frequency can be adjusted to match those of the MRI scanner signal bandwidth. Data is collected from one or more receiver channels. This may be in analog or preferably in digital domain.

Most modern scanners use separate transmit and receive coils. Some coils like head and knee coil are both transmit and receive coils (transceive.) Transmit coils produce a uniform field B_1 at right angles to the static magnetic field. Transmit coils are usually large to encompass a large volume of tissue and to optimize their uniformity. They can also be used to receive signals using T/R switch but have poor sensitivity, hence separate receive coils are usually used. The main transmitting coil is usually the body coil which surrounds the entire patient and is built into the scanner bore, and is not generally visible. It has a uniform transmission field but is a poor receiver. There are separate receive coils usually the surface coils. A large coil (body coil) is used as a transmitter and a smaller surface coil as a receiver combining the advantage of uniform excitation of a large coil and increased SNR of a smaller coil. However, if two separate coils are used, they need to be tuned to the same frequency. Coil decoupling is necessary to prevent current in one coil to excite current in the other. Receive only and transmit only coils must be electronically isolated. When the transmitter is on, the receiver is open circuited to prevent the transmitting power from entering the receiving chain. At the time of receiving the signal, the transmitting coil is open circuited to prevent mutual coupling. When the power amplifier is not active, its output is disconnected to avoid the output noise from interfering with the sensitive signal that is being received. Most of the RF transmit and receive subsystem component such as digital to analogue converters, power amplifiers, frequency mixers are sited in the electronics/cabinet room.

RF coils are also classified as *volume* and *surface coils.* Volume coils surround the imaged object, and provide homogeneous transmission and reception over a large anatomic region. Most scanners have a built in volume coil—the body coil for whole body imaging. There are smaller volume coils like head coil **(Fig. 18)**. As the noise is nonlinearly proportional to the volume of tissue being imaged; the SNR of these is lower than the surface coils. Body coils are constructed on cylindrical coils forms—diameter of 50–60 cm and a length of 70–80 cm. These are large enough to surround the patient's chest and abdomen. Head coils are smaller 40 cm long and 28 cm in diameter.

The term *Surface coil* is used to describe a coil that fits closely over some specific anatomic region and provides better SNR. These coils include circular (e.g. for orbit and tm joint) and rectangular coils, (e.g. for lumber spine). Coils with irregular designs, e.g. for shoulder are also surface coils. These are usually receiving coils with a limited area of sensitivity from which they receive signal. Surface coils fit closely over specific anatomic region. The sensitivity of the coil is related to the radius of the coil. As the coil size is increased, noise will also increase. Surface coils are advantageous as they increase the SNR; however the sensitivity is not uniform over its field of view. These need to be positioned carefully. Surface coils can be rigid or flexible in design. Flexible coils can be closely applied to the contour of the body, are more comfortable, and however are less durable due to higher wear and tear **(Fig. 19)**.

Construction Design of an RF Coil

RF coils used in the early phase of MR imaging were all linearly polarized (LP). In this configuration, both the transmission and reception of electro-magnetic radiation took place along a single axis **(Fig. 20)**. In the transmit mode LP coils are inefficient because half of the power is wasted. In the receive mode they are incapable of extracting full phase information from the MR signal. By adding a second set of coils, perpendicular to the first and driving them with sinusoidal current phase shifted by 90°, a pure rotating B_1 field can be created. This is known as circularly polarized (CP) or *quadrature transmission* **(Fig. 21)**.

The most common type of quadrature RF-transmit coil used in MRI is the *birdcage coil* or its variant, the *transverse electromagnetic (TEM) coil.* Bird cage coil or resonator has improved B_1 homogeneity and has higher sensitivity. These are coils consisting of two circular or elliptical conducting end rings joined by conducting rings or legs **(Fig. 22)**. A common version uses 16 loops to span the cylinder. A circularly polarized birdcage resonator is called a quadrature coil. A related form of multimode resonator, referred to as TEM (transverse electromagnetic) resonator is also useful for head and neck imaging at higher field strengths. RF transmitting coils are also shielded to minimize power losses.[15-17]

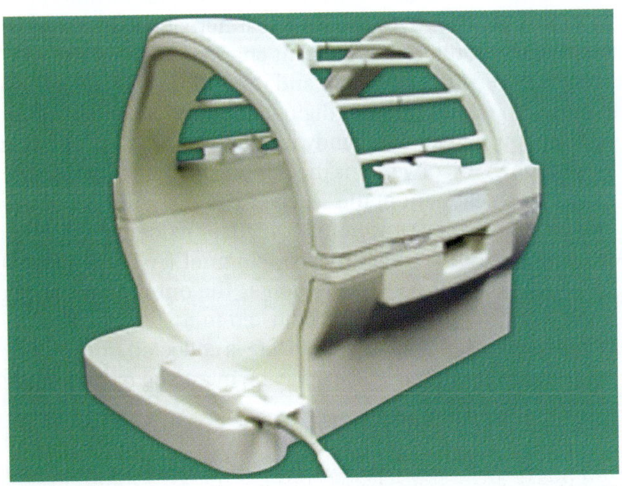

FIG. 18: Circularly polarized head coil, volume coil—both transmit and receive.

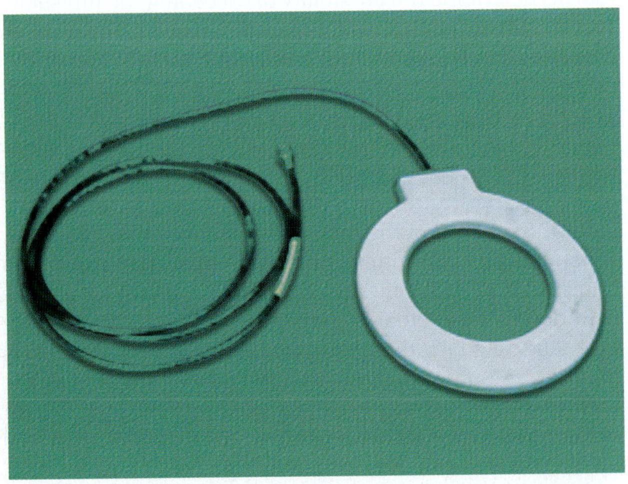

FIG. 19: Surface loop coil-receive only.

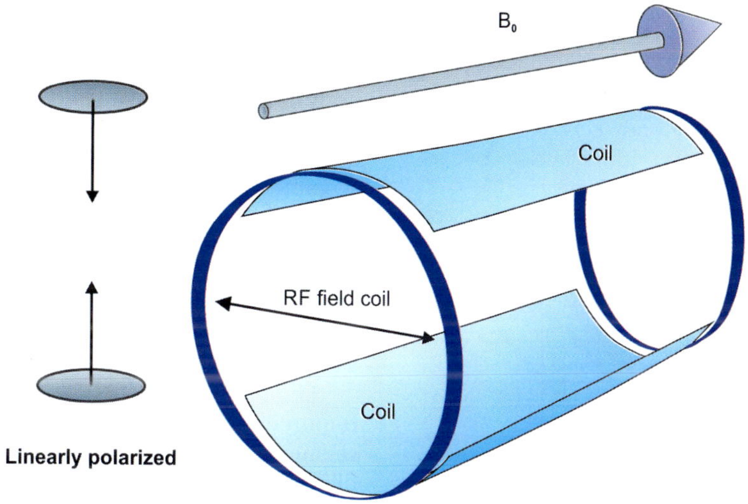

FIG. 20: Linearly polarized body coil comprising flat conductors configured in a hollow tube.

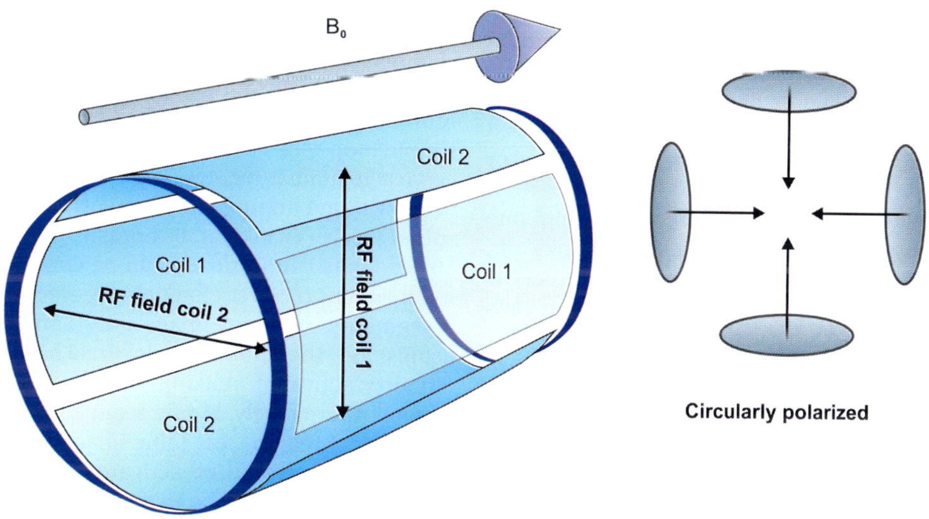

FIG. 21: Design of a circularly polarized body coil showing 2 RF fields with a phase shift.

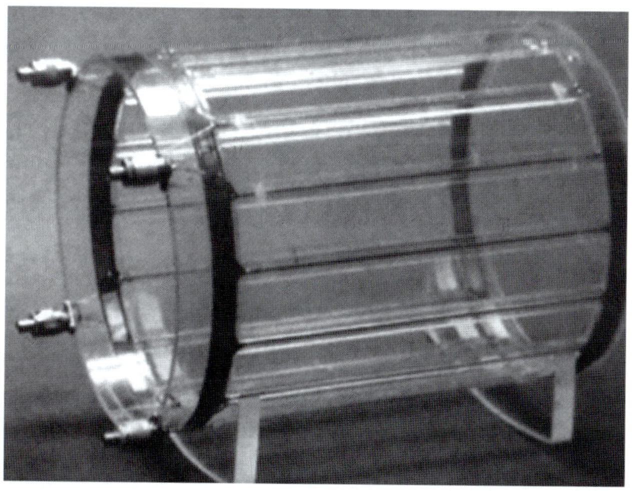

FIG. 22: Bird cage resonator.

Phased Array Coils

Surface coils detect signal based on proximity to the body and have high sensitivity but have limited FOV. Phased array coils were developed to fulfill the need for a complete spine scan. Spine imaging required a large FOV to enable complete spine scanning. Initially only single-segment coils (i.e., lumbar, thoracic, or cervical) were available, which had to be moved or changed for each spinal area imaged. Later switchable or ladder spine arrays came into use which, comprised three single-segment spine coils embedded into one long padded "CTL-coil" on which the patient would lie. Only a single spinal segment could be imaged at any one time. However, the segments could be electronically switched without moving the patient. The entire spine can be imaged without moving patient or repositioning coils with the availability of phase array coils. These coils are made of multiple small surface coils whose signals may be combined or are fed

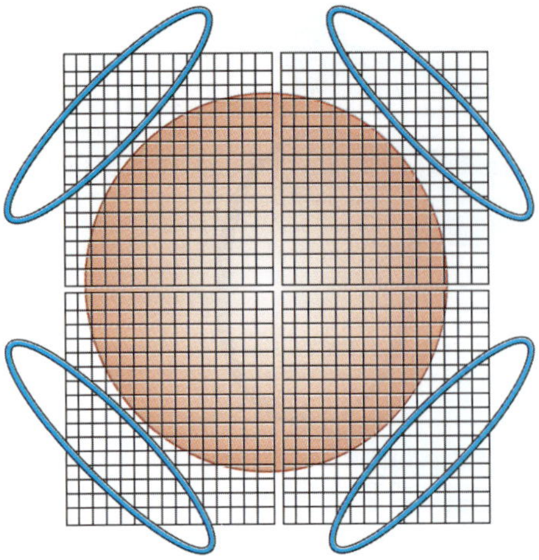

FIG. 23: Phased array coil—multiple coil elements, increasing SNR and FOV.

into independent receiver circuits. Arrays of surface coil are used to extend the effective FOV of the receiver coil while maintaining the improved SNR characteristics of a limited FOV of a single coil[18] **(Fig. 23)**.

Phased array technology is based on the principle of 'antenna', where large groups of small antennas such as used in radar installations are joined and enhance overall signal or transmission.

The coils are electromagnetically decoupled from one another by selecting the overlap between neighboring coils, so that mutual inductances disappear. This is achieved by the use of low impedance preamplifiers on the output of each individual coil or by physically overlapping the coil receiver elements. The hexagonal arrangement of coils and extent of overlap are chosen to minimize mutual inductances between coil elements. Noise is proportional to sensitivity volume of the coil, which is smaller for surface coil than for a volume coil. Phased array coils have to be positioned perpendicular to the main magnetic field. N independent phased array coils, each with their own amplifiers and receiver channels, should ideally increase signal-to-noise by a factor of $\sqrt{N}$, e.g. the signal-to-noise ratio in the 4-coil phased array should be 2X higher than that for a single coil. However, in practice such large gains are not usually achieved.

Multichannel RF Coils and Parallel Imaging

There was a need for improving the coverage, signal resolution and speed of MRI examinations.

It has been achieved by the software technique of parallel imaging, which requires multichannel RF coils.

Parallel imaging uses differential weighting of signals from multiple small surface coils to determine the spatial origin of the signal. This reduces the number of gradient encoding steps, which is a time consuming step in the imaging chain. Each small surface coil is required to have a distinct sensitivity for spatial encoding. Each coil element should have no magnetic interactions with the adjacent coil. The large overlap between coils (as seen in most phased-array configurations) is not used for parallel imaging and coil decoupling circuitry is mandatory. Thus while all parallel imaging coils are "phased arrays", not all phased array coils are suitable for parallel imaging.

Multichannel RF coil is a where each coil in the phased array has a separate receiver channel. The MRI signal used to form an image is collected by an array of separate detectors, or coil elements. Each element relays signal information along a separate channel to an image reconstruction computer. Such arrays of coil elements and receivers can improve imaging coverage and the ratio of signal-to-noise in the image.

Segments are composed of one or more basic coil elements, and are equipped with both "decoupling" and "tune and match" circuitry allowing them to be connected to a single receiver channel.

Channels are independent, complete electronic chains required for processing information received from a coil segment. Channels include amplifiers, filters, analog-to-digital conversion circuitry, demodulation/mixer devices, and image processing capability. The output of each channel is a partial view of the entire anatomy being imaged, subsequently combined with output from the other channels to produce the final MR image.

The nomenclature of coil elements, segments and channels can be understood by the example of spine array coil. For example, a total spine array coil comprises of 32 individual *elements* which are small linearly polarized simple loop receiver coils. These are distributed from the cervical to lumbar regions. These 32 elements can be paired to form 16 quadrature coil segments representing different spinal levels (4 cervical, 8 thoracic, and 4 lumbar), these 16 segments can in turn could be connected into up to 8 independent receiver channels. By electronically selecting 8 segments, one can image only half the spine in one acquisition. The 8 unused coils would have their decoupling circuitry activated, making them appear invisible to the system. Alternatively, if only a single spine region (such as the cervical region) was to be imaged, only the 4 cervical coil segments would be activated. The 12 unused lower coil segments would be detuned and 4 unused receiver channels would be turned off.[11] The clue to remember is *Coil Elements > Segments > Channels*. The number of available coil segments is generally much greater than the number of receiver channels. This is because coil elements are cheap to produce, whereas receiver channel technology is expensive, requiring a complete chain of amplifiers, digitizing circuitry, and computational engine to process the individual signals collected.

Multichannel coils are expensive and have resulted in increased complexity of the MRI system. The number of elements in the array of detectors and receivers is an important factor in characterizing an MRI scanner system upgrade to a higher number of channels is costly because a substantial expansion of the RF chain is required. Maximum number of independent receiver channels that can be used simultaneously in a single scan and a single FOV, each generating an independent partial image are now available up to 128.[19] The connection to the system of a coil with more elements than the number of channels requires complex logic switches in the coil. Phased array coil generates more data and requires more robust reconstruction techniques to keep the time less.

One major advantage of phased array coil is the applicability *of parallel imaging techniques*. This is particularly useful for high field imaging as it is another method to keep SAR low.[17] Parallel imaging technology uses complex software algorithms to reconstruct the signals from multiple channels to reduce imaging times and/or increase image resolution. Parallel imaging is useful in conditions where scan speed outweighs the need for a high SNR, e.g. cardiac imaging. Acquisition time in MRI is proportional to the number of phase encoding steps. Increasing the distance between each phase encoding lines in k space by a factor of R, reduces the acquisition time by the same factor, while keeping the spatial resolution fixed. Acquisition time is reduced by a factor (R = acceleration factor), equivalent to the number of independent coil elements (4–32). In practice, only a time reduction of 2–3 is possible as SNR is inversely proportional to $\sqrt{R}$ and at higher R, SNR becomes unacceptably low. Decreasing the phase encoding lines decreases the FOV, resulting in aliasing or wraparound. There are two techniques to remove or prevent aliasing:

1. *Simultaneous acquisition of spatial harmonics (SMASH):* The missing k space lines are restored prior to fourier transformation.[20] *GRAPPA* (generalized auto-calibrating partially parallel acquisition) is a variant of SMASH in which a small number of additional lines of k space data are acquired during the acquisition, eliminating the need for separate coil sensitivity.
2. *SENSE: Sensitivity encoding*[21]—data is first Fourier transformed, resulting in an aliased image. This is then by "unwrapped" by using the spatial information from the coil sensitivity profile.

SENSE is the most commonly used parallel imaging technique available with many vendors as ASSET (GE healthcare, Waukesha, Wisconsin), SPEEDER (Toshiba medical systems, Tokyo, Japan), SENSE (Philips medical system, Cleveland, Ohio). Siemens (Erlangen, Germany) offers both SENSE and GRAPPA as a single package under the trade name iPAT.

Digital broadband MR is a new technology that samples the MR signal directly in the coil on the patient. The fiber optic transmission of digital broadband data from the coil to the image reconstruction removes potential noise that is associated with analog RF. In conventional MR system, multiple analog coaxial cables are required (one per element/channel as digitization is performed away from the RF coil). In digital broadband system digitization is inside the RF receive coil, the number of RF channels is now determined by the coils, rather than the system. There is a single broadband fiber optic cable that is independent of number of elements/channels in an RF coil. System also is channel independent. The required data acquisition rate increases with the number of channels being sampled. The sampling frequency needs to be twice the receiver bandwidth to meet the Nyquist criteria and prevent aliasing. To account from phase errors that may occur, a sample frequency of four times the bandwidth is used. In a conventional system, an expensive upgrade is required if there is a shift from a 8 channel to a 16 channel coil. Digitization in the coil however makes number of channels required redundant.

Ongoing developments in the RF system are one of the most significant changes in MRI system development. Few of the more recent advances are listed below:

Hybrid Coil

This is a transmit/receive coil. It consists of a localized dedicated transmitter coil whose size is optimized for a target FOV and an independent set of receiver coils. As the transmitter coil is much smaller than the typical whole body transmitter coil, it requires less input power to generate the necessary B_1 with a potentially reduced SAR. Hybrid coils are thus useful for higher static magnet fields.

Multitransmit Technology

Imaging in conventional MR scanners, uses a single source to transmit a signal to the patient. Multitransmit technology uses multiple RF sources, each source individually adapted to patients anatomy. This cancels out dielectric shading seen at 3.0 T and also reduces local specific absorption rate SAR. Interleaved sequences and saline bags are not required to overcome the problem of shading. Another advantage, of using multiple RF sources is an increase in scanning speed by 40%, as claimed by the vendor.[22]

Total Imaging Matrix

Provided by one vendor, the system contains up to 102 matrix coil elements integrated seamlessly with up to 32 independent RF channels.[19] These provide high SNR associated with local coils for an FOV ranging from 5 cm to 196 cm. There is no requirement for patient/coil repositioning. This system provides a PAT factor up to 16. Tim[46] ultra high density array up to 204 coil elements with 128 RF channels increase SNR considerably **(Fig. 24)**.

Ultraflex Coils

Ultraflex coils are which adapt to anthropometric variations of the body are now available.

Biomatrix Sensors[19]

This is one of the recent technological advancement available with one vendor to increase the efficiency of scanning. Sensors are embedded in the system architecture to enable better scans. Respiratory sensors automatically detect breathing patterns as soon as the patient lies on a specially designed MR table (Biomatrix table). Respiratory scans can be performed without putting a belt or using navigator measurements. Beat sensors are also available for automatic triggering of cardiac scans without the need for ECG leads **(Figs. 25A and B)**. Kinetic sensors records head motion information and applies motion correction for high quality scans. Biomatrix tuners are additional shim elements are available on head and neck coils for improved fat saturation and homogeneity and better DWI. Online compressed sensing can fasten imaging by a factor of 10, to enable abdominal and cardiac MRI that can be done in free breathing mode.

COMPUTER SUBSYSTEM

The computer is the command center of the MRI system. It shapes and times the RF pulses, turns the gradients on and off and controls the RF receiver to collect data. After data collection, it is required for manipulation, storage and retrieval. A processor is required for computation.

Data Processing and Image Reconstruction

The two primary dedicated digital control systems are the pulse generator and the data acquisition system.

The pulse generator synchronizes the gradients and RF pulses after selection at operator console. Digital synchronization is provided for the receive channel analog to digital convertor, such that the detected signal correlate with the applied gradient and RF frequency. The *temporal positional accuracy and repeatability (TPAR)* is an important specification of the system.

Digital data processing speeds are critical in higher field magnets with larger matrix size. The complex MR signal is sampled. The data from the signal is stored in a space called k space, which is a spatial frequency domain in the computer where the signal spatial frequencies and their origin are stored. The number of lines filled in k space matches the number of encodings in the sequence.[7] Data from shallow encoding gradients, low spatial frequencies and less details, but stronger signals are stored in the central part of k space, data from the steeper gradients, high spatial frequencies, better detail but low signal intensity occupy the periphery of k space. The signal is then analyzed by a mathematical process called Fourier analysis. k space has to be completely filled with the data from the imaging sequence before the signal is analyzed and processed into the image.

The data once acquired, is filtered and is stored in a large memory array. A cached disk system is used for memory needs. Computer servers are an important component of MR hardware, rack mount servers are being used in many systems. Image reconstruction algorithms are implemented to distribute computational load and save time. The sample frequency and the number of simultaneously acquired channels determine the maximum data rates through the system. After the image is reconstructed it may be displayed for instantaneous viewing or stored in a database for review.

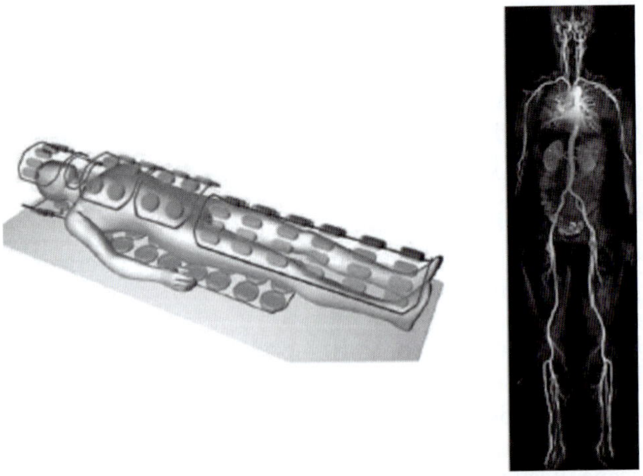

FIG. 24: Total Imaging Matrix^R—102 coil elements with 32 channels providing whole body coverage of up to 205 cm.
Courtesy: Siemens Healthineers.

INSTALLATION FOOTPRINT OF MRI

The MRI system requires careful planning before installation due to the strong magnetic field, the gradients that are used and the presence of a fringe field.

Magnet Shielding and the Fringe Field

Magnetic field shielding reduces the fringe field. Magnets can be actively or passively shielded. Active shielding is done by continuing the superconducting coil windings, carrying current in the opposite direction and positioned outside the inner main magnetic winding. This leads to partial cancellation of the field outside the main magnet. Passive shielding, is done by using an iron shroud weighing many tonnes or by the use of additional shimming coils. The fringe fields are negligible in a permanent magnet, being concentrated in the iron yoke.

Radiofrequency Shielding

Careful shielding of the MR scan room is required to prevent contamination of the weak signal arising from the patient with extraneous signal at the same frequency. These can be from broadcasting stations or operation of electronic equipment. RF interference comes from many sources, notably noise generated from nearby electrical equipment (transformers, motors, pumps) or electronic devices (computers, pulse oximeters, cardiac monitors).

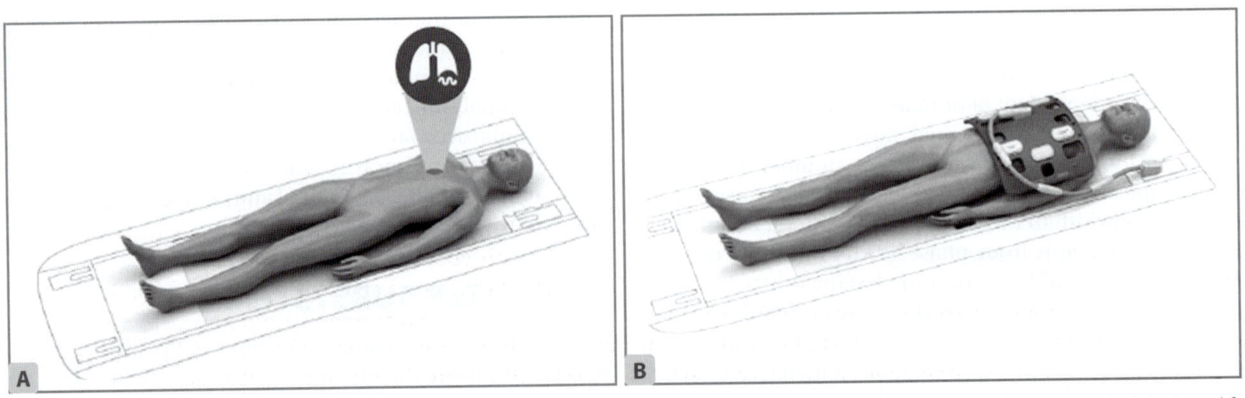

FIGS. 25A AND B: Biomatrix® sensors acquire the patients respiratory data automatically (A) and beat sensors for cardiac imaging without need for ECG leads (B).
Courtesy: Siemens Healthineers.

The RF-shield must encircle the entire room—walls, floor, and ceiling. Such a conductive box used to shield out stray electromagnetic interference is known as a *Faraday cage.* It keeps external electrical noise out and keeps the generated RF signal within the examination room. RF cage consists of a room lined by copper sheets on all six sides. All electrical connections between the magnet system and the system's electronics cabinets are connected via electrical filters through a penetration panel or filter panel in the RF shield. Special wire embedded glass is used to make windows and any doors to make an electromagnetic seal with the frame. Electronic filters are used to prevent noise from entering the scan room via wiring cables. Magnet room possesses wave guides/tubes fixed into the wall of the room, through which nonconductive tubing such as fiber optical coil passes. The examination room door should be shut while acquiring data to enable the shield to work effectively. The door must not allow any RF leakage, being sealed by a set of electrical contact strips or a continuous metallic pneumatic tube. Because of repetitive opening and closing, RF-seals around the door are frequently damaged and are a common source of RF-leakage into the room. Machine should be sited away from lifts/elevators and power cables, which may cause RF interference, distorts the image and produce linear artifacts.

Vibration Testing

Many modern MR scanners are very sensitive to environmental vibrations. Structural vibrations can result from a number of sources, including nearby motors, pumps, elevators, and vehicles passing near the building. Prior to constructing a room or installing a new MR scanner in an existing bay, it is important to perform vibration testing.

The components of a complete MR system are usually located in three adjacent rooms:

1. Magnet room
2. Equipment room
3. Control room.

Magnet room contains the MR magnet, its shell/enclosure, support footings, and patient table. It is the usually the largest of space in the installation. Most sites make it large enough to contain completely the magnetic fringe field within the room. The fringe field extends in all three directions, hence the ceiling height and floor of the magnet room have also to be also taken into consideration. Siting of the machine should be done away from steel girders and reinforced concrete, which may become manifested in the fringe field. Proximity to elevators or roads has to be taken into consideration while siting an MR unit as these may cause interference with RF field.

The walls of the magnet room are constructed in layers to enable several functions: magnetic shielding to confine the fringe field; acoustic shielding to restrict noise transmission to the control room and beyond; radio-frequency shielding to prevent electromagnetic noise from entering or leaving the room. The floor must be strong enough to e to support the weight of the magnet, table, and accessories. The weight of a typical 1.5 T cylindrical superconducting scanner is on the order of 10,000 lbs (4,500 kg) while a 3.0 T scanner may weigh up to 17,000 lbs (7,500 kg). The weight of a permanent low-field magnet may be over three times higher than a 1.5 T superconducting scanner, up to 35,000 lbs (16,000 kg). The magnet room also contains closets or storage areas for a large number of MR accessories, including phantoms, cushions, sponges, straps, wedges, cardiac leads, peripheral pulse gating devices, and respiratory bellows. Adjustable lighting is advised using current sources with less than 5% ripple. LED lighting is recommended to avoid vibration and early burnout. Florescent lighting should not be used as it causes RF interference. A window for patient monitoring is always present.

Equipment room is located immediately adjacent to the magnet room and contains devices distributed in cabinets that control and support the operation of the MRI unit, these are the gradient and radiofrequency cabinet, universal power supply, water pump/chiller and the helium pump. On the electrical side are a power cabinet (for electrical distribution), gradient cabinet (for sending currents into the gradient) and the RF cabinet (for controlling the transmission of radiofrequency pulses and the reception of the MR signal). On some scanners, the RF electronics are located immediately adjacent to the magnet under its plastic cover. Some systems may have additional cabinets to serve specialized techniques like functional MRI, and multinuclear spectroscopy. There is need for adequate cooling and uninterrupted steady electrical power to maintain temperature and humidity in the equipment room. Electronics are very sensitive to sudden loss of power, especially if one phase of the three phase power supply is lost. Powerful UPS system is a mandatory requirement.

Control room is immediately outside the magnet room, and contains the operator console, keyboard, communication devices, ECG and oxygen monitors and the computers which control the scanning.

SPECIAL TYPES OF MRI HARDWARE AND APPLICATIONS

Higher Magnet Strengths

Superconducting magnets operating at 1.5 T and 3T are now standard. Research systems of 7 T/9.4 T have been installed at a few sites; whereas individual prototypes of higher strength have been introduced. There are many advantages and challenges with the higher strength magnets. The signal to noise ratio SNR is $\propto B_1.\sqrt{NEx}.Np/BW$, where B_1 is field strength, NEx is the number of excitations, Np is the number of phase encoding lines and BW is the receiver bandwidth. The SNR at 3 Tesla should be double that at 1.5 T, however in practice is slightly less than double.[21] Improved SNR has led to powerful clinical applications of MRI like functional imaging, diffusion weighted imaging of body and multinuclear spectroscopy. Higher strength magnets have certain drawbacks which include safety considerations (See section on MR safety) and certain artifacts (See chapter on MR image optimization).

Long-Bore vs. Short-Bore 3-Tesla MR Systems. Different magnet configurations exist for commercially available 3-Tesla MR systems, including the older "long-bore" scanners and the newer "short-bore" systems. There are physical differences in the position and magnitude of the highest spatial gradient magnetic fields for different magnets and measurements of deflection angles for implants using long-bore vs. short-bore MR systems can produce substantially different results.[23]

The use of *ultrahigh field magnets* produces challenges for the RF transmitter and receiver chains and for the gradient coils. At higher field strengths, the proton operating frequency and the range of operating frequencies required for applications such as multinuclear Spectroscopy increase in proportion to the field strength. This necessitates changes in design of the amplifiers, switches and other components including RF coils. High powered RF amplifiers are required.

MR-HIFU (High Intensity Focused Ultrasound)

A noninvasive method using high intensity focused ultrasound was first used in 2008 as an alternative to surgery for treatment of uterine fibroids. MRI is used for planning and monitoring the rise in temperature during the procedure.

A focusing transducer is used to transmit ultrasound energy into a small volume at the target locations inside the body. The ultrasound energy penetrates the intact skin and soft tissue to produce a well-defined region of coagulative necrosis by producing high temperature only in the focused area. The tissue can get as hot as 150° Fahrenheit in just 20 seconds. 3-D MR provides the anatomical reference data for planning. MR imaging based temperature map acquired in real time during ablation provides monitoring support.[24] This is an outpatient procedure. Dedicated abdominopelvic coils designed for therapy applications are integrated within the table for positioning ease **(Fig. 26)**. The clinical applications of MR-HIFU are increasing to include management of bone metastasis, prostate cancer, etc.

MR Elastography

Magnetic resonance elastography (MRE) is a developing technology that assess the mechanical properties of tissue quantitatively. It is an imaging counterpart to palpation, commonly used by physicians to diagnose and characterize diseases. This is an acquisition hardware and reconstruction application that produces images with contrast related to stiffness of soft tissue. There are three steps in the technique of MRE, first, is generating shear waves in the tissue, by using an MRI compatible acoustic driver. This is followed by acquiring MR images depicting the propagation of the induced shear waves. This is followed by processing the images of the shear waves to generate quantitative color-coded anatomic maps depicting tissue stiffness in the area of interest, which are called elastograms. The hardware component is compromised of an active sound wave generator and a passive transducer that produces vibrations in the subject to be scanned. The data is reconstructed in both magnitude and phase formats, and the latter is used to produce strain wave and relative stiffness images. There are many clinical applications of this technique such as in assessment of liver fibrosis[25], breast cancer imaging, and study of skeletal muscle contractile function. Brain MRE is focus of a lot of research in neurodegenerative and demyelinating disorders.[25,26]

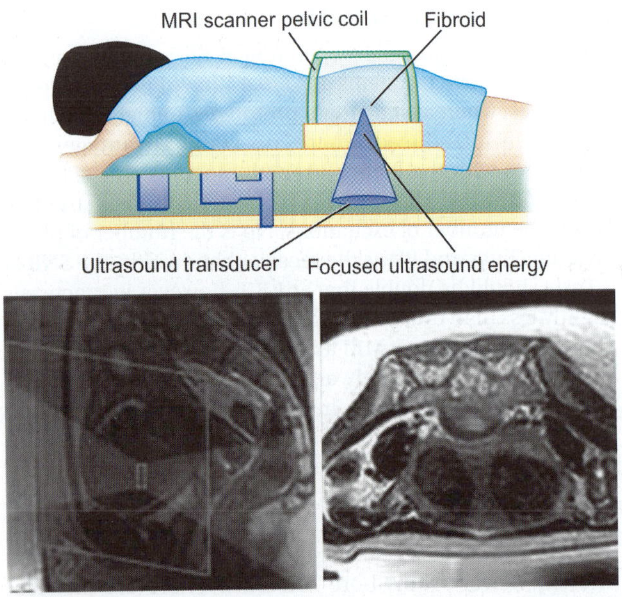

FIG. 26: MRgFUS—depicts the position of the patient, ultrasound transducer and the focused beam.

MR Surgical Suite: Interventional MRI

Interventional MRI is the use of MR techniques for guidance of both diagnostic and minimally invasive therapeutic interventions. The magnet is of the 'open' type to allow access to the patient. There is video camera and a sensor array which detects the correct location and orientation of the hand held instrument. Use of new fast gradient echo pulse sequences allows continuous MR images (0.3—7 seconds per image). These are viewed through a high resolution radiofrequency shielded monitor in the operating room. This modality is especially useful in areas of complex anatomy like skull base, retropharynx, etc.

MR-PET

Fully integrated MR-PET suite has been introduced. This has integrated cooling feature with specialized shielding to eliminate magnetic field interference in PET data processing. The detectors used in PET are MR compatible. This is dealt with in detail elsewhere in the book.

MR SAFETY

Magnetic resonance imaging is considered one of the safest imaging modality as it does not use ionising radiation. However, it has significant risks associated with it that are distinct from other imaging modalities. Each component of the MR unit-the main magnet, gradient set and the radio frequency coils has a risk associated with it.

There are no guidelines currently, in India regulating the safe use of MRI. In the United States, MR centers are subjected to regulations of US Food and drug Administration (FDA), which govern patient exposure limits (SAR, NOISE) and agency accreditations from the American college of radiology (ACR) and the joint commission. The ACR has issued safety guidelines and practices in a document which forms the basis of MR safety in the US.[27]

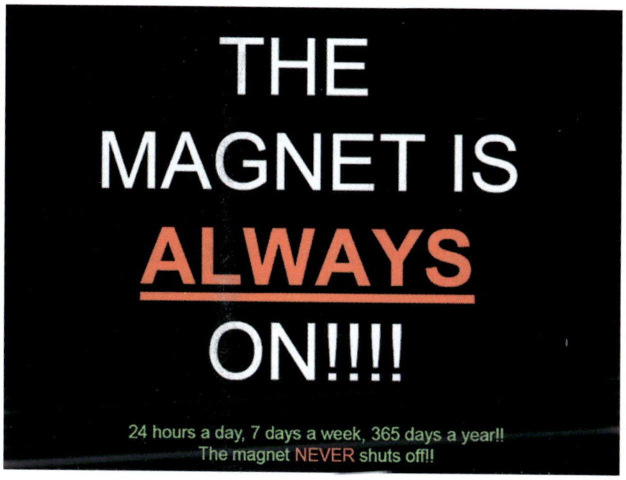

FIG. 27: The Magnet is always on. This sign must be displayed in the MR unit.

MRI Safety Risks

Risks Associated with Magnet Subsystem

The fact that a strong magnetic field is always on in a superconducting magnet has to be considered at all times **(Fig. 27)**. The main risks associated with the strong magnet are translational force and torque which can create safety issues for patients with implants and medical devices.

Translational Force and Torque

Any metallic object can interact with the static main magnetic field and the changing gradient fields and be subjected to translational and rotational force. The force increases with the mass of the ferromagnetic object and the gradient of the magnetic field strength at its location. The largest gradients are away from the isocenter of the magnet and are at the ends of the bore. This may cause the implant to move or dislodge from its position. The devices that are made of non ferromagnetic material are safe from risk of force related injury. Some devices may contain ferromagnetic material in a miniscule amount rendering them MR safe. In the case of certain implants like cardiac and vascular stents, a waiting time of few weeks prior to an MR examination is considered prudent as it may take some time for fibrous scarring to set in and for the implant/device is embedded securely.

Projectile Injury

The high magnetic field poses a risk of projectile injury due to the strong attraction of a ferromagnetic object to the static magnetic field. If a ferromagnetic object is brought into scanner room, it will be pulled into the bore. The magnetic strength is reduced outside the bore of the magnet by the process of shielding hence there may a sudden increase of the magnetic field strength as one approaches the bore. An object which does not appear to be ferromagnetic may suddenly be pulled out of one's grasp and turn into a projectile. These can cause serious injury to patients, caregivers and the staff. Fatalities have been documented. In the many incidents that have been reported, the majority involve medical support equipment. Apart from the human cost, there is huge cost of repairs as there may be extensive damage to the hardware.

Patient and Non-MR Personnel-screening

Meticulous screening of all individuals and patients entering the MR environment for magnetic objects in their bodies (e.g., shrapnel, implants, bullets), on their bodies (e.g., jewelry, hair pins) is the key to prevent such incidents as a small innocuous object can turn into a dangerous missile in the magnet room. Magnetic objects should be removed, if feasible, before the individuals enter the MR environment. All non MR personnel and patients have to undergo a safety screening process. This is done by the help of a detailed form designed to elicit any possible safety risk on or in the patient. A comprehensive screening form has been recommended by ACR.[27] The screening should be done by experienced (level 2) MR personnel. Nonambulatory patients should be brought into the MR environment using a nonmagnetic wheelchair or gurney. It has to be ensured that that no oxygen tanks, sandbags with metal shot, or other ferromagnetic objects are concealed under blankets or sheets or stowed away on the transport equipment, IV poles accompanying the patient into the MR environment should be nonferromagnetic. Patients should wear hospital gowns or scrubs without pockets and metallic fasteners for MR procedures. Patients' regular clothing can contain magnetic objects or threads (metallic) that may pose a hazard in the MR environment.

Screening by Detection

Metal Detectors

There are ferromagnetic detector systems available commercially for screening of external ferromagnetic objects. These cannot at present be used for implant screening as these have varying sensitivity and cannot detect a small potentially dangerous ferromagnetic metal fragment in an anatomically sensitive region like the orbit or near the spinal cord. The usage of conventional metal detectors which are unable to differentiate between ferrous and a non ferromagnetic material is not recommended. There are commercially available systems that can detect even small ferromagnetic objects that are external to the patient **(Fig. 28)**. The use of detectors is to be used as an adjunct to the screening process and not replace it.

Screening of patients who are unconscious or unresponsive and who cannot provide reliable history for prior exposure to surgery and trauma can be difficult. History can be obtained by family, caregivers and available medical records. It is recommended that such patients be physically examined by level 2 personnel. All areas of scars or deformities should be further examined by plain radiography.

Screening in Patients with Suspected Metallic Foreign Bodies

Plain film radiography is recommended to detect metallic foreign bodies for individuals and patients prior to admission to the MR environment. This includes screening for the presence of metallic orbital foreign bodies. The sensitivity of plain film radiography is deemed to be sufficient to identify

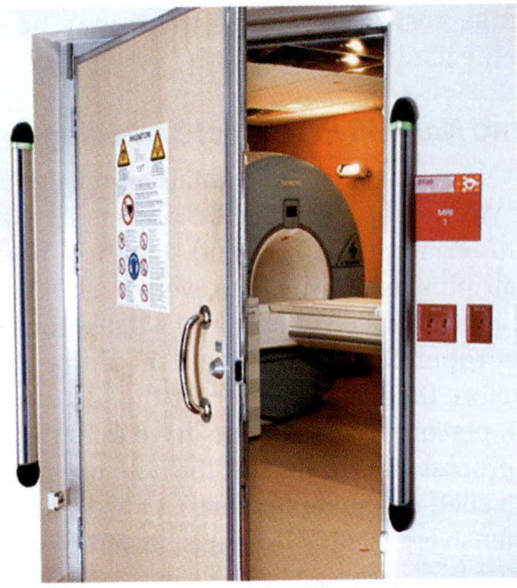

FIG. 28: Ferromagnetic sensors placed just outside the magnet room.

any metal object, large enough to present a hazard to an individual or patient in the MRI.

Risks Associated with Gradient Subsystem

Peripheral Neurostimulation

Time varying gradient fields, i.e. rate of change of the magnetic field (dB/dt) can produce electric currents perpendicular to the gradient field according to Faraday's law. This may exceed the threshold for nerve depolarization and cause peripheral neurostimulation. There is a theoretical risk of cardiac muscle depolarization. At sufficient exposure levels, peripheral nerve stimulation is perceptible as "tingling" or "tapping" sensations. At gradient magnetic field exposure levels increase, patients may become uncomfortable or experience pain. Cardiac stimulation remains a theoretical risk as it requires high level of gradient fields, not available with currently used commercial MR scanners.

Peripheral neurostimulation has the lowest threshold, though FDA does not give any recommendations about a specific value. Stimulation of motor nerves and skeletal muscle may be discomforting or even painful to the patients but does not normally occur in routine clinical scans

MR sequences that have high bandwidth readouts and rapid gradient switching such as echoplanar imaging are at particular risk for causing peripheral neurostimulation. This effect varies between patients, though particular care must be taken of patients with heart disease. Time varying gradients and the induced voltages may affect implanted devices and monitoring equipment.

Acoustic Noise

The noise in an MR imaging unit has its origin from gradient coils as they are subject to fast changing currents. Acoustic noise is associated with GRE sequences and higher magnetic field strengths. While FDA has set a limit of 140 dB for an MR system, most do not exceed 120 dB. Problems associated with acoustic noise for patients and healthcare professionals include verbal communication difficulties, anxiety, temporary hearing loss and, in extreme cases, the potential for permanent hearing impairment.[28]

Acoustic noise may affect certain patients to a greater extent than others, such as patients with psychiatric disorders who may become confused or suffer from increased anxiety. Sedated patients may experience discomfort in association with high noise levels. In addition, neonates may have adverse reactions to acoustic noise. A study was conducted to assess the impact of noise exposure of the fetus to 1.5-T MR imaging during the second and third trimesters of pregnancy and they found that it is not associated with an increased risk of substantial neonatal hearing impairment or cochlear injury.[29]

Hearing protection is recommended to prevent irreversible damage. Hearing protection used should match the frequency spectrum of the noise produced in order to be effective Earplugs reduce noise levels by 10–30 dB. Temporary hearing loss has been documented in patients who underwent routine MRI scan without the use of hearing protection devices, such as earplugs or head phones.[28]

Improvements in mounting techniques, use of damping materials and advances in materials used, placing the gradient tube in a vacuum have all been used to decrease the acoustic noise. *Quiet pulse sequences* have also been introduced to decrease noise. This is a technology that uses limited slew slew rates, less gradient resonent frequencies and 'bridging gradients.[30]

Risks Associated with RF Subsystem

Burns

Thermal injury causing burns is another risk that is associated with MRI. Although not so common, these are often unpredictable and severe. Various mechanisms can result in burn injury.[31,32] Skin contact with the RF coil and cables is often implicated, though rare due to protective insulation. Contact with bare skin can cause burn due to arcing. Cables must not touch the skin, which must be covered by a sheet and non conducting pads should be used to provide a barrier between the skin and the cables.

Another cause of burns can be due to generated currents as a result of changing magnetic fields, which may increase the local temperature. This can be sufficient to cause injury. Patients who suffer from cardiovascular disease, hypertension, diabetes, fever, old age, and obesity may not tolerate thermal challenge. In addition, certain medications like diuretics, beta-blockers, calcium blockers, amphetamines, and sedatives can alter thermoregulatory responses to a heat load. The ambient temperature, relative humidity, and airflow in the MR suite will also impact temperature change in the body that is associated with RF energy.

Patient's tissues should not come into direct contact with the inner bore of the magnet. The leads and wires should be positioned as far as possible from the inner walls of the MR Scanner, especially if body coil is being used. Vendor provided pads and insulation devices should be used for protection. It is also important that the patient does not form a conductive loop. The larger the conductive loop, the greater is the current and more is the risk of injury. Patients must be instructed not to cross their arms or legs in the scanner. Skin to skin contact should be minimized. **Box 2** summarizes safe use of RF coils.

BOX 2: How to use RF coil safely.

- Position the patient properly
- The coil should never come into contact with the patient.use the supplied coil pads with the coil at all times
- Do not allow the patient to directly touch the surface of the bore during scanning, use non conducting pads
- Do not let the coil's RF cables come in contact with the patient. position cables under a cushion whenever possible
- Do not loop or cross cables. Keep them straight, positioned down the center of the magnet, directly out of the bore
- Use only approved, undamaged RF coils
- Keep coils in good condition inspect for damage
- Position electrically conductive materials (e.g., cables, wires, etc.) to exit down the center of the MR system, not along the side of the MR system or close to the transmit RF body coil or other transmit RF coil

Extracare must be taken when dealing with circuits, wires and leads as these may resonate at the frequency of the transmitted radiofrequency power and pose a grave risk. An uncoiled wire may resonates with the electric field of the radio frequency coil -the so called *"antennae effect"*.[23] Any retained pacer wire may be subject to this and is considered a contraindication to MR imaging. All electrical connections such as surface coil leads or monitoring devices must be checked before every use to maintain the integrity of thermal and electrical insulation.

Care must be taken in patients with extensive and dark tattoos to prevent burn from RF heating due to the metallic pigment present in the tattoo. Cold compresses/ ice pack should be placed on these areas throughout the MR examination especially if the tattoos are within the volume of the body coil as a precautionary measure. There should be visual and auditory contact with the patient.

Unconscious and unresponsive patients should have any attached monitoring leads covered by ice compress to prevent burn injury.

SAR—Limits and Control

Radio frequency effects are a cause of concern due to potential bio effects. The principal effect is deposition of energy leading to heating with potential physiological effects like changing of cardiac output. Exposure metrics are available to measure how much RF energy is being deposited. One such measure is the specific absorption ratio (SAR) which is defined as the radiofrequency energy deposited per mass of tissue, expressed as watts/kg. Restricting whole body SAR in the body to an average of 1 W/kg restricts the whole body temperature rise to 0.5°.

The patient's weight is needed to calculate the temperature rise and control pulse sequences to ensure safe heating levels.[33]

FDA guidelines limit SAR whole body exposure in patients with normal thermoregulatory function to 4 W/kg in the body. The SAR increases by a factor of 4 when the magnetic field strength increases from 1.5 T to 3T. This has safety implications for the patient. The SAR is greater for large body parts than small, in pulse sequences with a 180^0 flip than that with a 90° pulse. SE pulse sequences produce more SAR than the GRE sequences. Certain tissues which have high conductivity, e.g. brain, blood, liver are subject to higher SAR than tissues with low conductivity such as fat and bone marrow.

MR systems provide an estimate of SAR by using the total radiofrequency power transmitted per unit time and the patient's weight. The scanner estimates the SAR for each sequence before scanning begins. During the scan, the scanner may compute its RF transmitter energy to calculate an average SAR.

There are certain modifications that an operator can do in order to keep SAR low are as follows:

- Using quadrature transmit coils and parallel transmission, especially on higher strength magnets
- Using a localized transmit coil for certain examinations like extremity coil
- Increasing TR
- Using fewer slices
- Decreasing echo train length, Echo train length (ETL), turbo factor in TSE sequences
- Reducing the refocusing flip angle in TSE and gradient sequences like TRUE FISP, FIESTA.

The operating modes which confine SAR and imaging gradients to certain levels for MR systems as defined by the *International Electrotechnical Commission (IEC)*[34] are, as follows:

Normal Operating Mode

Mode of operation of the MR equipment in which none of the outputs have a value that may cause physiological stress to patients.

First Level Controlled Operating Mode

Mode of operation of the MR equipment in which one or more outputs reach a value that may cause physiological stress to patients, which needs to be controlled by medical supervision.

Second Level Controlled Operating Mode

Mode of operation of the MR equipment in which one or more outputs reach a value that may produce significant risk for patients, for which explicit ethical approval is required.

RF Exposure Standards

The IEC standard[34] gives certain limits for temperature rise **(Table 1)** and SAR limits **(Table 2)** for the first and second level controlled modes. It is based upon limiting RF induced core temperature rises to 0.5° or 1°C for normal and first level controlled modes. This translates into whole body SAR limits of 2 and 4 W/kg averaged over 6 minutes.[26]

Another radiofrequency exposure metric used in magnetic resonance imaging is B_1 + RMS. This is a measure of time weighted average RF magnetic field exposure, calculated over 10 minutes intervals, measured in microtesla (μt). It is independent of the patients characteristics, but depends on flip angle, pulse type, number of echoes, slices and TR. B_1 + RMS is useful in determining compliance with implant scanning conditions.

TABLE 1: RF temperature limits.

Operating mode	Core temperature rise (degree C)	Maximum temperature core	Limits (degree C) local
Normal	0.5	39	39
First level controlled	1	40	40
Second level controlled	>1	>40	>40

TABLE 2: SAR limits averaged over 6 minutes except for short term SAR.

Operating mode	SAR W/kg	SAR W/kg	SAR W/kg	SAR W/kg	SAR W/kg	SAR W/kg
	Whole body	Partial body	Partial body	Local	Transmit	Coils
		Any	Head	Head	Trunk	Extremities
Normal	2	2–10	3.2	10	10	20
First level controlled	4	4–10	3.2	20	20	40
Second level controlled	>4	>4–10	>3.2	>20	>20	>40
Short term SAR	The SAR	Limits over any	10 s period	Should not exceed	Three times the stated	SAR average

MEDICAL DEVICE AND IMPLANT COMPATIBILITY

Standards for MR imaging device safety terminology were first issued by ASTM (American Society for Testing Materials) International in 2005.[35] These are currently documented in the ASTM International F2503 guidelines, and are required by the FDA, with devices labeled as *MR safe, MR unsafe* or *MR conditional* **(Fig. 29)**.

MR safe devices are non hazardous in all MR imaging environment and are identified with a square green label. MR unsafe devices are completely contraindicated in the MR suite and are labeled with a round red label. An MR conditional device, affixed with a triangular yellow label is safe only under certain specified operating conditions, which may include the strength of the main magnetic field, gradient strength, and maximum specific absorption rate. Heating of certain implants, which are safe at 1.5 T has been shown at 3 T and vice versa. There are differences in safety profiles of long bore and short bore 3 T MRI systems. The safety implications are primarily for magnetic field-related translational attraction. For example, the deflection angle measured for an implant on a short-bore can be substantially higher and, thus, potentially unsafe from a magnetic field interaction consideration compared to the deflection angle measured on a long-bore MR system. Safety information for measurements of magnetic field interactions for metallic objects must be considered with respect to the specific type of MR system used for the evaluation and the highest spatial gradient magnetic field that was used for the test.[36,37]

An *active implant* is one that requires electrical power either inbuilt through batteries or through an external source, e.g. pacemakers, neurostimulators. These face additional risks of malfunction, modification of operating mode, unintended stimulation or permanent damage. RF heating risks are also present with internal leads. *Any metallic or passive implant* is one that has no requirement of electrical power, e.g. titanium hip joint. This is subject to risks of static field of attraction and torque and RF heating.

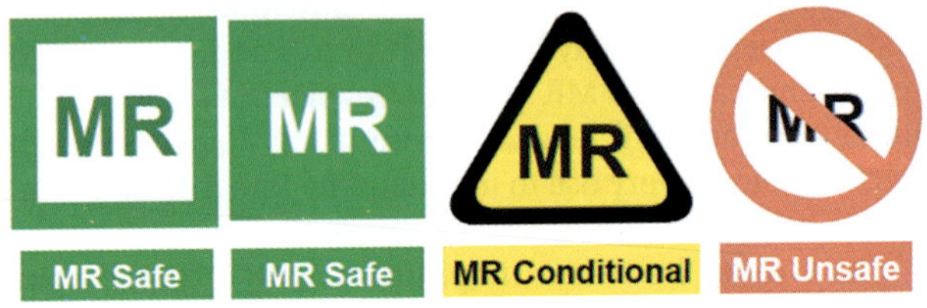

FIG. 29: Internationally recognized symbols labeling an object/device as MR safe (green square), MR conditional (yellow triangle) and MR unsafe(red circle).

All portable metallic or non metallic device on or external to the patient should be properly identified in writing and labeled as one of the three categories. All unknown devices been brought beyond zone II (see MR zoning) should be tested with a strong hand held magnet or a ferromagnetic detection device (>1000 Gauss). Any metallic and/or active electronic medical device is potentially dangerous. A comprehensive database that categories MR imaging safety ratings and recommendations for nearly all medical devices and implants is on the website *www.mrisafety.com, administered* by Frank Shellock.[23]

MRI of Patients with Cardiac Pacemakers or Implantable Cardioverter Defibrillators

MR conditional Pacemakers and implantable loop recorders are now commercially available. However, the vast majority of cardiac implantable electronic devices (CIED) are not MR conditional.

Radiologists and cardiologists must check the restrictions for each device. Unexpected program changes, transient asynchronous pacing, induction of ventricular fibrillation are a few of the complications that may occur during MRI of patients with these devices. Deaths have been documented.

There should be close coordination with the cardiologist and the manufacturer representative to determine MR safety of that device. The patients attestations regarding the device safety are not considered sufficient. Abandoned leads from a previous system have a potential for heating and should be declared MR unsafe. Each case of MRI of a patient with CIED should be reviewed on individual case by case basis. The points to be considered should include time since device insertion, region being scanned, specific device programming, residual battery power, MRI scanning parameters. Special precautions should be taken when undertaking MRI of a patient with pacemaker. The presence of a radiologist and cardiology personnel is mandatory. A fully stocked crash cart should be available. A programmer to adjust the device should be on site. Active monitoring of the patient with ECG and pulse oximetry is required. Check of the device post the scan is also needed.[38,39]

SAR has been found to be an unreliable metric to guide protocols for imaging patients with CIEDs. B_1+RMS (derived from root mean square RMS of the flip angle B+ has been reported to be a more accurate estimation of energy deposition.[40]

MRI of Patients with Intracranial Aneurysm Clips

In a patient with an intracranial aneurysm clip in place, the MR examination should not be done till it is documented in writing the model, type of clip and its compatibility with MRI. All documentation must be signed by the physician. Phone or verbal histories are not acceptable.

All intracranial aneurysm clips manufactured where labeling claims it is MR safe can be accepted for MR scanning. The fact that a patient with an aneurysm clip has undergone a prior MRI is not sufficient evidence of the implant safety and cannot be used as a sole criterion to determine the compatibility. There can be variations of field strength, magnetic field gradients and other variables.

MRI of Patients with Cochlear Implants

Cochlear implants are electronically-activated devices. MRI is contraindicated for a patient with this type of implant because of the possibility of injuring the patient and/or altering or damaging the function of the device. In general, individuals with cochlear implants should be prevented from entering the MR environment unless specific guidelines exist to ensure safety for these devices. Recently, some cochlear implants have received approval designating them as "MR Conditional".

The magnetic component of the cochlear implant should be removed prior to the MRI examination to avoid possible demagnetization and artifacts seen, if this magnet remains in place during an MRI examination. This can be replaced following the scan.

What is to be Done if a Ferromagnetic Implant or Foreign Body is Discovered during an Examination?

In case a sizable field distorting artifact is noted, the radiologist in charge should assess the situation basing it on the status of patient, location of the suspected implant relative to local anatomic structures. The further course can be continuing with scan, immobilizing the patient and removal of the patient. In this process, forces on the implant may change and slow and deliberate slow extrication of the patient from the bore should be done as less harmful forces will be there as it passes various magnetic field gradients. Patient should be removed along a straight line course parallel to the center of the magnet as far as possible from the MR magnet bore. Patient should avoid sitting up, as soon as physically out of the bore as translational or torque related forces may still be significant.

MRI in Patients with Orthopedic Implants and External Fixation Device

Most of the orthopedic implants, materials, and devices are made from nonferromagnetic materials and, therefore, are MR safe or "MR Conditional" according to the conditions specified for patients undergoing MR procedures. However, due to the length of the implant or the formation of a conductive loop, MRI-related heating may be a problem for some orthopedic implants, especially cervical fixation devices and internal or external fixation systems.

The assessment of external fixation systems for MRI is particularly challenging because of the multiple components (many of which are made from conductive materials) and configurations used for these devices. The primary concern is MRI-related heating which is dependent on particular aspects, e.g. the lengths of the component parts of the external fixation system. The MRI operating conditions (strength of the static magnetic field, frequency of the RF field, type of RF transmit coil, pulse sequence, body part imaged, position of the fixation device relative to the transmit RF coil, etc.) also impact safety. To ensure patient safety, guidelines are typically applied on a case-by-case basis and, therefore, MR professionals should always refer to product labeling.

MRI in Patients with Intrauterine Contraceptive Device

Intrauterine contraceptive devices (IUD) may be made from nonmetallic materials (e.g., plastic) or a combination of nonmetallic and metallic materials. Copper is typically the metal used in an IUD, however, stainless steel or other metals may also be utilized, copper IUDs are safe for patients in the MR environment using operating at 1.5-Tesla or less. This includes the Multiload Cu375. The Mirena intrauterine system (IUS) is made entirely from nonmetallic materials that include polyethylene, barium sulfate and silicone, therefore, the Mirena coil is safe for patients undergoing MRI at all static magnetic field strengths.

Contraindications and Cautions for MRI

MRI examinations are contradicted in patients with:

- Conventional cardiac pacemakers/implanted cardiac defibrillators
- Abandoned cardiac leads
- Cochlear implants (relative, as a few are MR conditional)
- Subcutaneous insulin pumps.

Caution to be exercised while doing MRI in the following

- Patients with implanted surgical clips or other potentially ferromagnetic objects, particularly in brain
- Patients with AIMDs-neurostimulators

- Patients with history of occupational exposure to ferromagnetic objects-military, welding
- Patients with poor thermoregulatory function-neonates, infant
- Permanent tattoos. Permanent eyeliner
- Patients with prosthetic heart valves
- Pregnancy.

MRI SAFETY PROFILE IN SPECIAL GROUPS

Pediatric Patient and MRI

MRI is the preferred cross-sectional imaging in pediatric population due to lack of ionizing radiation, however there are safety issues as in the adult population compounded by the risks of sedation and anesthesia which are often required. For the neonatal and young children special attention is required for temperature control, both hypo and hyperthermia are a risk. The accompanying parent or care giver should be screened just as any other individual entering magnet room (zone IV).

Pregnant Patient and MRI

There is no conclusive proof of any harmful effects to the fetus from MR exposure. The American college of radiology (ACR) categories MRI as a *'relatively risk free'* modality and does not recommend any special consideration in first versus any other trimester.[41] Caution is however advised and a risk benefit analysis should be undertaken.

The following may be documented in the patient's record:

- The information requested from the MR study cannot be acquired by any other means like ultrasound
- The data is needed to potentially affect the care of patient or/and fetus during pregnancy
- The referring physician believes that it is not prudent to wait till the patient is no longer pregnant.

MR contrast should not be routinely administered to pregnant patients as it does cross the placental barrier and may remain in the amniotic fluid for an indeterminate period of time. GBCAs should be considered a class C drug in pregnancy to be used if expected benefit far outweighs the potential risk and may be life saving.

Risks to Pregnant MR Personnel

Pregnant personnel are allowed to work in the MR unit during all stages of the pregnancy. They are allowed to enter the magnet room, position patients, place RF coils, inject contrast and enter the MR room in case of an emergency. It is however recommended that they do not remain near the magnet bore during data acquisition.[42]

Contrast-related Safety Issues

Gadolinium-based contrast agents have an excellent safety profile and are generally well tolerated by patients. However, there are risks associated with its use. This topic is dealt with in detail elsewhere in the book.

MR SAFETY GUIDELINES AND REGULATIONS

MR Zoning

The American College of Radiology's expert panel has conceptually divided the MR suite into zones **(Fig. 30)**. This is done to prevent ferromagnetic objects entering the MR and accidentally bypassing screening checkpoints. There are greater risks with individuals who do not work in MR Environment and may bring these dangerous items on them.

MR unit is divided into four distinct, clearly labeled zones with progressive restriction of movement and increased supervision by authorized personnel in higher zones **(Figs. 31A to C)**. This is mandatory to avoid MR related accidents. The four zones are defined as:

Zone 1: This includes areas that are freely accessible to the general public and is outside the MR unit. This is the area/ Corridor from where patients and staff enter the MR.

Zone II: This is the area of the MR reception, which is used to greet patients, obtain history and screen patients for potential MR safety risks. Patients are not free to move at will and remain under some supervision. This is an interface between the completely unsupervised zone 1 and the strictly supervised zone II and zone III.

Zone III: This is the area where entry by unscreened individual or ferromagnetic objects/equipment can lead to serious injury or death. The MR console room and the passage leading to the MR is part of this zone. Access has to strictly and physically controlled by lock or passkey supervised at all times. Only MR personnel are provided free access. Zone III, or at least the area demarcated by the 5 G line must be labeled as hazardous. Magnetic fields are three dimensional and zone III may extend through floors and ceilings. All these should be demarcated and access controlled.

Zone IV: The MR scanner room and the area of highest risk is Zone IV. This should be clearly marked as hazardous and with a sign that states that the magnet is always on. The MR technologists should be able to observe and control by visual means or with the help of monitors access and entrance to zone IV from their position.

The 5 Gauss Line

A contour of 0.5 mT (5 gauss) is used to define the outer limit or perimeter for pacemaker safety (Including MRI conditional pacemakers whose operation cannot be verified as set in MR mode). This line should usually be confined to the scan room. This line offers no protection against projectile injury. Fields above 3 mT (30 Gauss) are considered to present a projectile risk and will be within the scan room in the vicinity of the magnet. Earth's background magnetic field measures 0.05 mT (0.5 G). 5 gauss line does not protect against projectile injury.

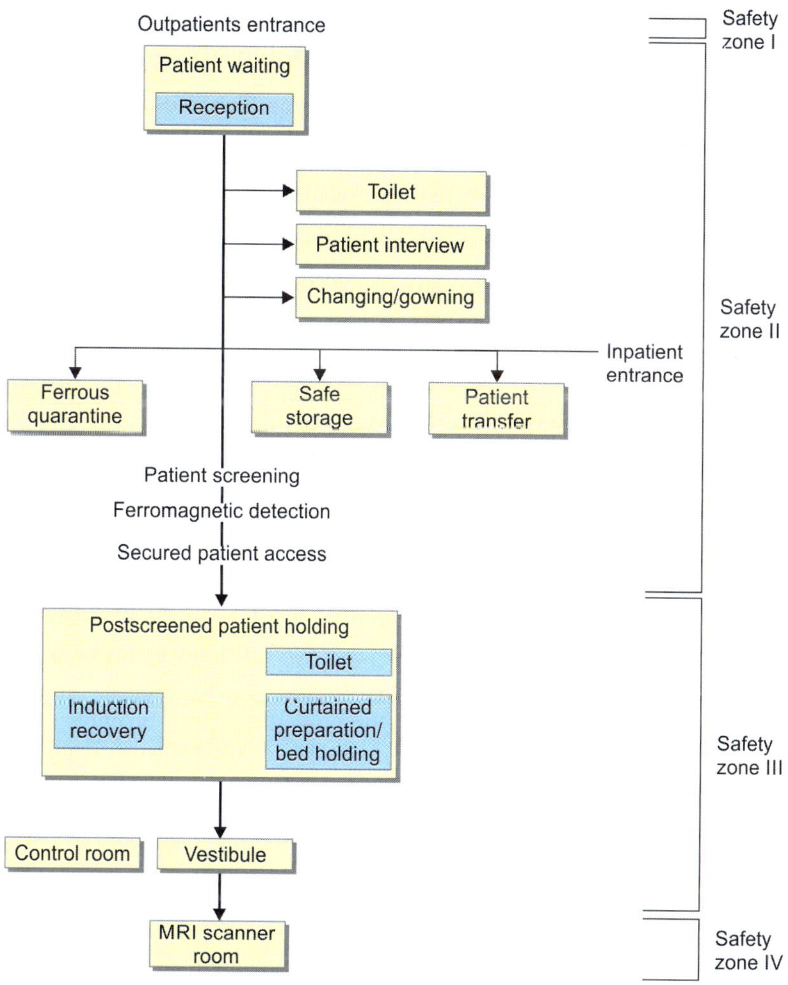

FIG. 30: Schematic diagram of MR zoning as recommended by ACR (American College of Radiology).

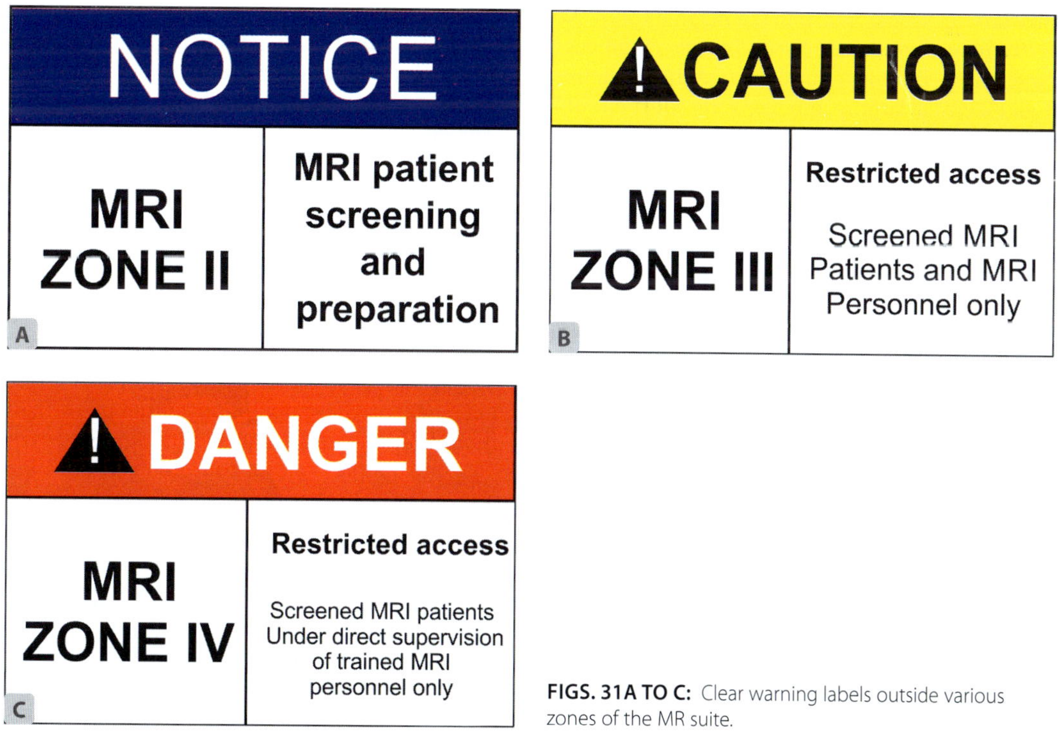

FIGS. 31A TO C: Clear warning labels outside various zones of the MR suite.

MR Personnel and Non-MR Personnel

All staff working in MR should be labeled as MR personnel and must be documented to have received MR safety education. There are two levels of MR personnel.

Level 1: Those who are educated in some safety aspects of MR to ensure their own safety as they work in MR room e.g.—nurses, technicians from anesthesia or MR housekeeping staff.

Level 2: Personnel are more extensively trained and educated in broader aspects of MR safety like thermoregulatory and neurostimulation issue. These individuals are directly responsible for all non-MR imaging personnel in zone IV. Level 2 personnel include MR technologists, radiologists who enter zone III and zone IV on a regular basis. Other staff of the radiology department must be trained to level 1 to be able to help in an emergency.

MRI EMERGENCIES

Emergencies in the MR suite include medical issues like seizure and cardiac arrest, or fire or a magnet related emergency like an uninitiated quench. The presence of a constant static magnetic field places constraints on the handling of emergencies in the MR Unit. Preplanning, safety drills and training are key in handling emergencies in MR and prevent further disasters.

In case of a medical emergency or fire in zone IV, the examination should be terminated and patient must be moved out of zone IV to a safe predetermined site for preliminary resuscitation and stabilization by trained MR personnel. Resuscitation equipment should be MR safe or MR conditional and sited in zone III or zone II. It is important that in an emergency, potential responders do not enter in a rush without screening. They may not be conversant with MR safety issues and may inadvertently bring MR unsafe equipment like laryngoscopes, etc. into the magnet room. *No code or code like procedure should be run in zone IV.* In case of fire, the emergency shutdown button should be used, this switches off all electrical supply and prevents short circuit. Fire extinguishers should be MR safe/conditional **(Fig. 32)**.

Quench occurs when the superconducting coil is heated above its critical temperature, leading to a rapid increase in electric résistance. The magnetic field collapses and there is coil heating. This leads to boil off the surrounding thousands of liters of liquid helium in an explosive manner. The Magnet room is equipped with vents/quench pipe through which the cryogen is ducted to the atmosphere. In case of failure of duct, cryogen escapes into the room, leading to safety concerns which include:

- The potential for asphyxiation as cryogenic gases replace oxygenated air.
- Frost bite due to exceedingly low temperatures.
- Fire hazards.
- Thermal expansion of the cryogens can positively pressurize the magnet room and entrap persons inside. The magnet door can be closed violently or may be swing due to pressure gradient.

Intentional quench may be required when it is life saving like a patient pinned by a projectile. Each scanner has a quench button **(Fig. 33)**. An authorized person must be identified who will be responsible for the quench. All personnel must be evacuated quickly in case of quench. At the point of cryogen discharge, a quench safety exclusion zone with a minimum clear radius of 8 feet must be established and clearly marked. This area should have no doors or windows or air vent which may allow cryogen to re-enter the building.

Are There Any Limits for Occupational Exposure?

The international commission on non ionizing radiation protection (ICNIRP) has given certain guidelines regarding occupational exposure affecting MRI **(Tables 3 and 4)**.

Studies of static field exposure have demonstrated that the peak magnetic field exposure to staff is around 40% of B_0 This translates to a time averaged exposure over an 8 hour working shift to 5 mT. Exposure to RF and time varying gradients will occur only for those working near the bore during scanning e.g. Anesthetists while monitoring a child may lean into the bore or during interventional procedures. Exposure limits that have been set are unlikely to be exceeded.[43,44]

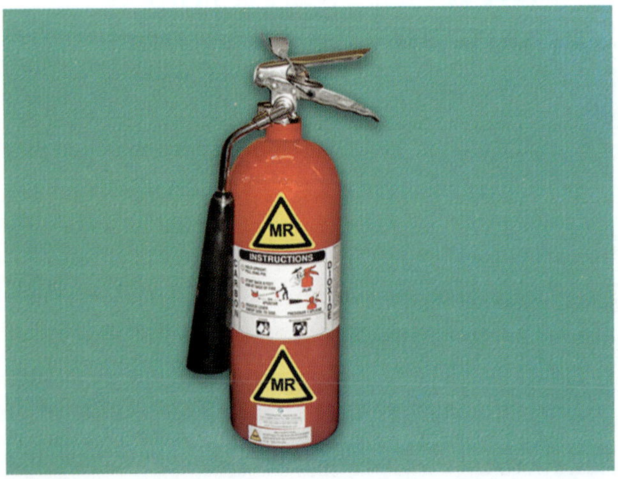

FIG. 32: MR conditional fire extinguisher.

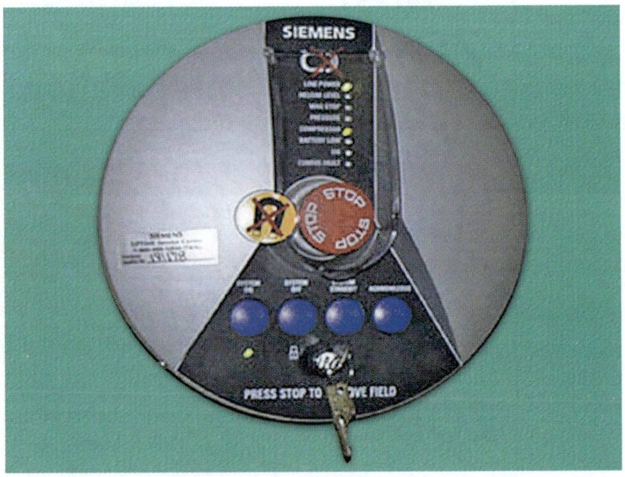

FIG. 33: The quench button—in RED.

TABLE 3: Occupational exposure limits for static magnetic fields.

	Trunk and head instantaneous ceiling (T)	Limbs (T)
IEC	8	8
ICNIRP	2	8
IEEE	0.5	0.5

IEC:[34] International Electrotechnical Commission; ICNIRP:[44] International Commission of Nonionising Radiation Protection;
IEEE:[45] The Institute of Electrical and Electronics Engineers

TABLE 4: Occupational exposure limits for RF magnetic fields.

	Frequency (MHz)	Basic restriction SAR W/kg
IEC	Any	4
ICNIRP	10–400	0.4

IEC:[34] International Electrotechnical Commission; ICNIRP:[46] International Commission of Nonionising Radiation Protection

Training and Education

The best safety net is to prevent accidents from happening. Educating oneself, MR staff, emergency responders and the patients/caregivers is the key to implement a safety program in the MR unit. There are numerous websites dedicated to this issue with a huge amount of educational material available online. Some of the important ones are listed in **Table 5**.

The safety risks relating to MRI affect not only patients and radiologists like other imaging modalities but also caregivers and other hospital staff who may come into the MR envoirnment. All radiologists, technologists have to take responsibility to prevent MR-related accidents by developing a culture of safety.

TABLE 5: Some websites dedicated to MR safety.

Resource	Link
ISMRM Safety	http://www.ismrm.org/mr-safety-links/
IMRSER MR safety videos	http://www.imrser.org/genpg.asp?pgname=videolist
MRISafety.com	http://www.mrisafety.com
ABMRS	http://www.abmrs.org/
ACR MR Safety	http://www.acr.org/Clinial-Research/Radiology -Safety/MR-Safety/

ISMRM: International Society of Magnetic Resonance in Medicine; IMRSER: Institute of Magnetic Resonance Safety, Education and Research; ABMRS: American Board of Magnetic Resonance Safety; ACR: American College of Radiology

REFERENCES

1. Gorter CJ. Negative result of an attempt to detect nuclear spins. Physica. 1936;3:995-8.
2. Lauterbur PC. Image formation by induced local interactions: examples employing nuclear magnetic resonance. Nature. 1973;242:190-1.
3. Schneck JF, Kelley DAC, Marinelli L. Instrumentation: Magnets, coils and Hardware. In Magnetic Resonance Imaging of the Brain and Spine Atlas SW, 4th edn. In: Wolters Kluwer (Ed.) Lippincott Williams & Wilkins; 2009.pp.2-24.
4. Vaughan T, DelaBarre L, Synder C, et al. 9.4 T human MRI: preliminary results. Magn Med. 2006;56:1274-82.
5. Sagawa M, Fujimura S, Togawa N, et al. New material for permanent magnets on a base of Nd and Fe. J Appl Phys. 1984;55:2083-7.
6. Scott Greig, Chronik Blaine, et al. A prepolarized MRI scanner. Proc Intl Soc Mag Med. 2001;9:610.
7. Allisy-Roberts P, Williams J. Farr's Physics For Medical Imaging, 2nd edn. Saunders Elsevier. Magnetic Resonance Imaging 189.
8. McRobbie DW, Moore EA, Graves MJ, Prince MR. MRI from picture to proton. Cambridge: Cambridge university Press; 2003.
9. Adam A, Dixon AK, Grainger RG, Allison DJ. Magnetic Resonance Imaging Basic Principles in Diagnostic Radiology; 2008.pp. 87-107.
10. CosmosTC, Parizh M. Advances in whole body magnets. IEEE. Trans applied superconductivity. 2011:21;2014-9.
11. www.mriquestions.com
12. www.gehealthcare.
13. Turner R. Gradient coil design: a review of methods. Magn Reson Imag. 1993;11:903-20.
14. Hidalgo-Tabon SS. Theory of gradient coil design methods for magnetic resonance imaging. Concepts Mag Res Part A. 2001;36A:223-42.
15. Walker KM, Tsuruda JS, Hadley JR, et al. Radiofrequency coil selection for MR imaging of the brain and skull base. Radiology. 2001;221:11-25.
16. Fujita H. New Horizons in MR Technology: RF coil designs and trends. Magn Reson Med Sci. 2007;6(1):29-42.
17. Schenck JF. Radiofrequency coils: types and characteristics. In: Bronskill MJ, Sprawls P (Eds). The Physics of MRI. Woodbury, NY: American Institute of Physics; 1993. pp.98-134.
18. Roemer PB, Edelstein WA, Hayes CE, et al. The NMR phased array. Magnetic Resonance in Medicine. 1990;16(2):192-225.
19. www.siemens.com/medical solutions.solutions
20. Sodickson DK, Manning WJ. Simultaneous acquisition of spatial harmonics (SMASH): fast imaging with radiofrequency coil arrays. Magn Reson Med. 1997;38:591-603.
21. Prussmann KP, Weiger M, Scheidegger MB, et al. SENSE: Sensitivity encoding for fast MRI. Magn Reson Med. 1999; 42: 952-62.
22. Harvey PR, et al. SAR behavior during whole-body multitransmit RF shimming at 3.0 T, Proc. ISMRM; 2009. p.4786
23. Shellock FG.MRISafety.com Web site.http://www.mrisafety.com
24. www. philips.com/healthcare/main/products/mri.
25. Mariappan YK, Glaser KJ, and Ehman RL: Magnetic resonance elastography: a review Clin Anat. 2010;23(5):497-511.
26. Venketesh S, Yin M, Ehman R. Magnetuc resonance elastography of the liver: Technique, Analysis and Clinical Applications. J Magn Reson Imaging. 2013;37(3):544-55.
27. Kanal E,Barkovich AJ,Bell C, et al. Expert Panel on MR Safety. ACR guidance document on MR safe practices: 2013 J Magn Reson Imaging. 2013;37(3):501-30.
28. Mollasadeghi A, Mehrparvar AH, Atighechi S, et al. Sensorineural hearing loss after magnetic resonance imaging. Case Rep Radiol. 2013;2013:510258.

29. Reeves MJ, et al. Neonatal cochlear function: Measurement after exposure to acoustic noise during in utero MR imaging. Radiology. 2010;257:802-9.
30. Alibek S, Vogel M, Sun W, et al. Acoustic noise reduction in MRI using silent scan: an initial experience. Diagn Interv Radiol. 2014;20(4);360-3.
31. Hardy PT 2nd, Weil KM. A review of thermal MR injuries. Radiol Technol. 2010;81(6):606-9.
32. Dempsey MF, Condon B. Thermal injuries associated with MRI. Clin Radiol. 20001;56(6):457-65.
33. Tsai LL, Grant AK, Mortele KJ, Kung JW, Smith MP. A practical guide to MR Imaging safety: what radiologists need to know. Radiographics. 2015;35:1722-37.
34. International Electrotechnical Commission (2013) Medical Electrical Equipment-part 2-33: particular requirements for the safety of Magnetic Resonance Equipment for medical diagnosis, 3rd edn. Geneva: IEC.
35. ASTM International. Standards and Publications.ASTM International web site. http://www.astm.org/standard/standards and publications.
36. US Food and Drug Administration. A primer on medical device interactions with magnetic resonance imaging systems. [FDA guidance document]. US Food and drug administration web site. http://www.fda.gov/medical devices/device regulation and guidance/guidancedocuments/ucm107721.htm.
37. Shellock FG. Reference manual for magnetic resonance safety, implements and devices: 2015 edn. Playa del ReyCalif: Biomedical research publishing group; 2015.
38. Nazarain S, Hansford R, Roguin A et al. A prospective evaluation of a protocol for magnetic resonance imaging of patients with implanted cardiac devices. Ann Intern Med. 2011;155:415-25.
39. Shulman RM, Hunt B. Cardiac implanted electronic devices and MRI safety in 2018-the state of play. European Radiology https://doi.org/10.1007/s00330-018-5396-0
40. Nazarian S, Hansford R, Rahespar AA, et al. Safety of magnetic resonance imaging in patients with cardiac devices. N Engl J Med. 2017;377:2555-64.
41. Bulas D, Egloff A. Benefits and risks of MRI in pregnancy. Semin Perinatol. 2013;37(5):301-4.
42. Kanal E, Gillen J, Evans JA, Savitz DA, Shellock FG. Survey of reproductive health among MR workers. Radiology. 1993;187:395-9.
43. McRobbie DW. Occupational exposure in MRI. Br J Radiol. 2012;85:293-312.
44. International Commission on non ionising radiation protection. Guidelines on limits to exposure from static magnetic field. Heath Physics. 2009;96:504-14.
45. The Institute of Electrical and Electronics Engineers (IEEE) (2002) IEEE Standard for safety levels with respect to human exposure to radiofrequency electromagnetic fields.0-3kHz. New York IEEE.
46. International commission on non ionising radiation protection (2010) 'Guidelines for limiting exposure to time varying electric, magnetic and electromagnetic fields (upto 100kHz)'. Health Physics 99:818-836 and Erration: Health Physics. 2011;100:112.

CHAPTER

34

Image Optimization in Magnetic Resonance Imaging

Jyoti Kumar, Anjali Prakash, Rashmi Dixit, Gaurav Shanker Pradhan

Optimizing image quality means finding a balance between the different aspects of image quality and image speed. For an image to be optimal for diagnosis, the anatomic and pathologic features within the image must be distinguishable from each other.

Ideally an image should have a high signal to noise ratio (SNR), high spatial resolution, excellent contrast, minimum artefacts and an acceptable scan time. Generally, these criteria do not go hand in hand. Knowledge about various MR parameters within the user interface that can be modified by the radiologist helps to find the most appropriate balance between image quality and scan time.

In this chapter, we shall discuss image optimization under these major headings:

1. Signal-to-noise ratio
2. Contrast to noise ratio
3. Spatial resolution
4. Scan time
5. Artefacts and their remedial measures.
6. 3T Imaging: Advantages and Limitations

SIGNAL-TO-NOISE RATIO

MR signal is the voltage received by the receiver coil from each voxel in a slice after it is stimulated by a radiofrequency pulse. This is recorded at time interval TE and at specific frequencies. Bright pixels in the image represent stronger signals, and darker pixels represent weaker signals in the image.

Noise is an unwanted occurrence in the MR image. Noise appears as a grainy random pattern superimposed on the MR image. This represents statistical fluctuations in signal intensity that are superimposed on the image and compromise image quality. Noise is not frequency specific and occurs randomly in time. The source of this noise is Brownian motion of charged particles throughout the body of the patient whereas signal comes from just the selected slice. The electronic noise of the receiver technology and the environment also contribute to the noise.

The signal-to-noise ratio (SNR) is defined as the ratio of the MR signal that can be used to create the image to the amplitude of the background noise. A high signal to noise ratio improves the quality of the image. To increase the SNR, we need to increase the signal relative to the noise. The various parameters that have an impact on the SNR are field strength, proton density, coil type and position, TR, TE, flip angle, number of signal averages, slice thickness and receiver bandwidth.

Field Strength

With higher field strength, more protons are aligned parallel to the main field (spin up nuclei) as fewer protons can now oppose this high field strength and lie antiparallel to the main field (spin down nuclei). The net magnetism of the patient (termed the net magnetization vector or NMV), reflects the balance between the parallel and antiparallel magnetic moments. In high field strengths, NMV increases and therefore the signal increases.

Proton Density

The signal strength depends on the quantity of signal generating protons in the voxel (proton density). For example, pelvis contains structures with a high proton density such as muscle and bone, giving a high signal. On the other hand, chest contains air filled lungs and vessels with low proton density, and hence imaging of chest requires measures to boost SNR.

Coil Type and Position

Imaging of small anatomical regions such as extremities (e.g. ankles, wrists), neck or the breasts require specialized surface coils to maximize both the signal-to-noise ratio and spatial resolution. Large coils such as the body coil allow coverage of larger areas but at the expense of SNR. A phased array coil combines the two advantages. This coil has multiple small coils which increase the signal to noise ratio. Also, the coverage is increased as the date from these smaller coils is combined together.

Positioning of coils is also important. To understand this, a few basic principles of MR imaging are revised here. In an external magnetic field (B0), spin up and spin down nuclei are in a state of equilibrium. Excess spins generate constant magnetization in the longitudinal plane (Z-axis). Spins are also precesssing like a wobbling top and they are out of phase with each other. NMV is zero in the transverse plane. When an RF pulse is applied, two things happen—energy absorption and phase coherence. Hydrogen nuclei absorb energy. Upon absorption of correct amount of energy, the spin up and down nuclei become equal in number. As a result the longitudinal magnetization reduces to zero. Secondly, on application of an RF pulse, the spins move into phase with each other. When parallel and antiparallel nuclei are equal in number there is no longitudinal magnetization. However protons are precessing in the transverse of XY plane. As the NMV has been moved through 90° from the direction of the main magnetic field or the Z-axis, it is called a 90° RF pulse. It is this transverse magnetization that is used to produce the signal. As the NMV rotates in the transverse plane, it induces voltage in the receiver coil which generates the MR signal. The position of the coil needs to be perpendicular to the magnetization. Hence, the coil needs to be placed either over, under, to the right or left of the area being examined. A coil positioned parallel to the transverse magnetization i.e. perpendicular to the table results in zero magnetization.

Repetition Time

Repetition time (TR) is the time between the two RF pulses. It is measured in milliseconds (msec). When the RF pulse is removed, longitudinal magnetization recovers (T1 recovery) and transverse magnetization begins to decay (T2 decay). The T1 time of a tissue is specific to the tissue. It is the time when 63% of the longitudinal magnetization gets recovered. The duration of the time is the TR. The longer the TR, the greater is the recovery of longitudinal magnetization, which can now get converted to transverse magnetization. Hence, the SNR is improved with a long TR. A short TR reduces the SNR. Although a short TR is needed to generate T1 weighting, it cannot be reduced severally as then it compromises the SNR.

Echo Time

Echo time (TE) is the duration time between an RF excitation pulse and generation of the signal. It is also measured in milliseconds (msec). The T2 decay time of a tissue is also tissue specific. It is the time it takes when 63% of transverse magnetization gets lost. Depending on the length of TE, T2 decay occurs in a particular tissue. If the TE is short, little transverse magnetization is lost. Hence there is greater residual transverse magnetization producing a higher SNR. If TE is long, SNR is reduced. Although a long TE is needed to generate T2 weighting, SNR may fall if it is increased too much.

Flip Angle

This is the angle through which NMV moves when RF pulse is applied. Greater the flip angle, greater is the NMV in the transverse plane generating greater signal. In gradient echo imaging, smaller flip angles are used which result in lower SNR. The SNR then needs to be improved using other measures.

Number of Signal Averages

Number of signal averages (NSA) refers to the number of times frequencies in the signal are sampled with the same slope of phase encoding gradient. Multiple measurements of one slice are obtained and the results are averaged in a single image. Increasing the number of excitations (NEX) increases the signal collected. When we increase the NEX, we also increase sampling of the noise. Hence the signal is not doubled on doubling the NEX but only by a square root of two. Also, when NEX is doubled the time required to obtain the scan is also doubled **(Figs. 1A and B)**.

Slice Thickness

When thicker slices are obtained, the voxel is enlarged and hence more proton spins contribute to the signal, thereby increasing the signal intensity. Noise remains the same because it is not just coming from the slice, but the patient's entire body and MR environment. Hence, SNR is directly proportional to the slice thickness. The drawback is that, increasing the slice thickness reduces the spatial resolution resulting in partial volume effects **(Figs. 2A and B)**.

Receiver Bandwidth

This is the spectrum of frequencies which are read within the FOV in the frequency encoding direction. It is measured in kiloHertz (kHz). When this is reduced, the frequencies contributing to noise adjacent to the signal are reduced, hence effectively increasing the SNR.

The drawback here is that to reduce the bandwidth, the sampling time has to be increased to satisfy the Nyquist theorem. This theorem states that the sampling rate must be at least twice the frequency of the highest frequency in the echo to accurately reflect all the frequencies in the signal. If receiver bandwidth is reduced keeping all parameters unchanged, then sampling time needs to be increased to be able to sample all frequencies accurately. Hence, TE need to be increased. Therefore, it is not suitable for T1 or proton density weighted imaging, where a low TE is used. Also, chemical shift artefact is increased when receiver bandwidth is decreased. When short TE is not required e.g. in T2 weighted sequences, receiver bandwidth can be reduced to increase the SNR. Also, when there is no fat, for example, in brain, receiver bandwidth can be reduced without increase in chemical shift artefact.

CONTRAST-TO-NOISE RATIO

MR images would have no clinical value without satisfactory image contrast which is defined as how distinguishable the signal is between two tissues in the image. A high SNR does not guarantee easy differentiation of two structures in an image. Contrast to noise ratio (CNR) is the most important image quality factor because this allows for differentiation between anatomical tissues in the image and also in differentiation between pathological and normal tissue, hence aiding in final analysis of the image. Superior soft tissue contrast is a major advantage of MR imaging versus alternative modalities such as computed radiography.

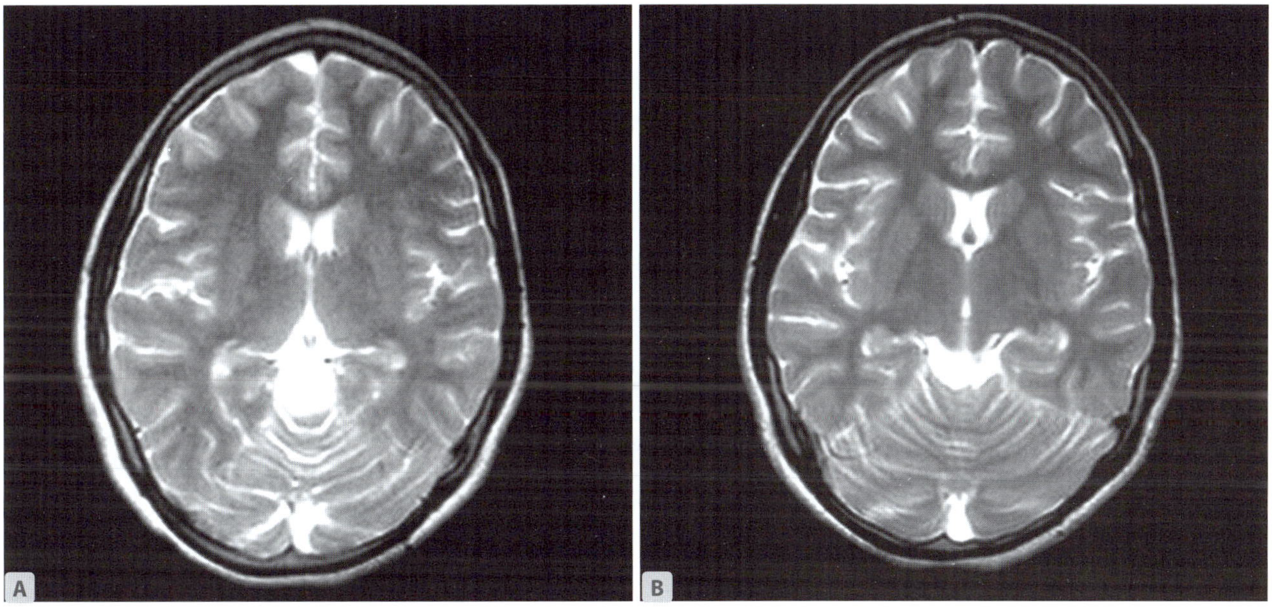

FIGS. 1A AND B: Image comparison. T2 weighted axial images of the brain acquired with one signal average (A) and four signal averages (B). The SNR of the image B was double that of A. Also, the scan time of B was four times that of A.

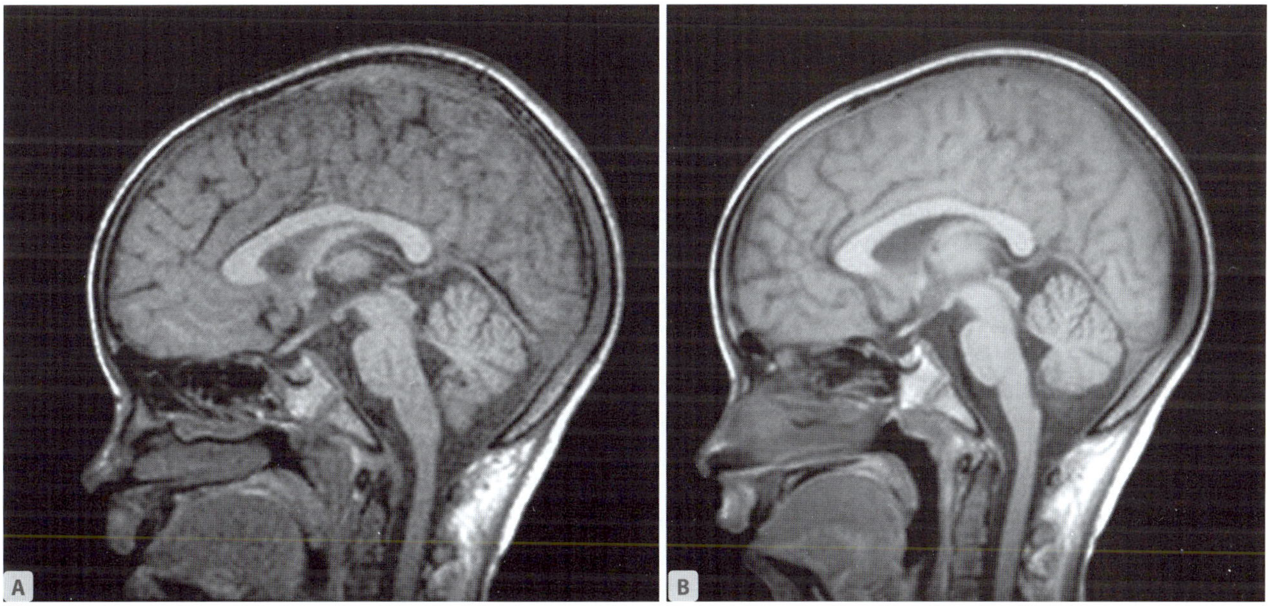

FIGS. 2A AND B: Image comparison. T1 weighted sagittal images of the brain. The image B was acquired with double the slice thickness of the image A. The SNR of the image B was double that of A. However, this occurred at the expense of spatial resolution.

Contrast in MR is a complex function of intrinsic characteristics of the structure, i.e. proton density, T1 and T2 relaxation times, magnetic susceptibility of the nuclei as well as programmable pulse sequence parameters, e.g. TR, TE, flip angle, slice thickness, etc. For example, longer TR allows more time for T1 relaxation and produces more signal from tissues with long T1 values. Longer TE, on the other hand, allows more time for T2 relaxation and produces more signal from tissues with long T2 values.

Various methods can be employed to increase CNR. Contrast administration, magnetization transfer techniques, T2 weighted sequences and fat suppression techniques can accentuate the difference between anatomy and pathology.

Administration of a Contrast Agent

A contrast agent like gadolinium shortens the T1 time of structures, especially of pathological lesions when they have a break in blood brain barrier. Enhancing tissue appears much brighter, hence boosting the CNR.

Magnetization Transfer Constant

In biological systems, protons can be described as existing in two pools. The 'free pool' consists of relatively mobile protons in free bulk water and some fat containing tissues. On standard imaging techniques, majority of the signal is provided by this free pool. The second pool or 'bound pool' of protons are restricted in proteins, cell membrane and large macromolecules. Because these have very short T2, this bound pool does not give enough signal on standard MRI.

The magnetization is a state of equilibrium between the free and bound pool for a particular tissue. When additional RF pulses are used to suppress bound protons, the magnetization of the 'bound pool' decreases and hence its equilibrium is disturbed. Magnetization is then transferred from the 'free pool' to the 'bound pool'. A new equilibrium is reached decreasing the SN ratio of a particular tissue. Hence the contrast with the surrounding tissue is accentuated. It is primarily used to suppress normal tissue.

Chemical Suppression

Signal is suppressed either from fat or water. For example, fat suppression techniques null fat and hence the lesion is better appreciated from the surrounding tissue that has fat.

Echo Train Length

In fast spin echo sequence (FSE), a train of 1800 rephasing pulses are used. The number of these pulses and resultant echoes is called the echo train length or turbo factor. Since each echo has a different TE and data from each echo are used to produce one image, the contrast of FSE is unique. On T2 FSE, fat is hyperintense as this echo train reduces spin-spin interactions in fat, hence T2 relaxation time is increased (J-coupling). Muscle appears darker because the echo train increases magnetization transfer effects that produce saturation.

Time from Inversion

The time from inversion (TI) is the crucial factor that determines the contrast in Inversion recovery sequences (IR).

These are spin echo sequences that begin with a 180° pulse which flips the NMV by 180°. At time TI after the 180° inverting pulse, a 90° pulse is applied which is then followed by 180° pulse for rephasing spins that produces echo at time TE. 90° pulse is applied after a very long TI, NMV has passed through the transverse plane already and the contrast now depends on how much saturation this 90° pulse produces. Longer is the TI, greater is the longitudinal magnetization that can be used to generate signal with 90° pulse. TIs of 300 to 700 ms result in heavy T1 weighting. Certain specific TI values result in suppression of signal from specific tissues. For example, TI of 100 to 180 ms is used in STIR sequence. 90° pulse is here applied after this TI when NMV of fat is passing exactly through transverse plane. Here, there is no longitudinal magnetization of fat and hence no transverse magnetization results on the application of 90o pulse, resulting in no signal from fat. Similarly, TIs of 1700 to 2200 ms are used to null the signal from CSF on FLAIR imaging.

SPATIAL RESOLUTION

Spatial resolution is defined as differentiation between two points lying near each other in the area being examined. The size of the voxel determines the spatial resolution. The imaging volume is divided into slices. The area of anatomy displayed in each slice is called the field of view (FOV). Depending on the matrix, the FOV is divided into a number of pixels. The FOV may be specified separately for the frequency encoding and phase encoding directions which may be the same in a square or isotropic FOV and different in an anisotropic or a rectangular FOV. Frequency and phase encoding gradients are applied to spatially locate the signal coming from each pixel in the FOV.

Voxel Volume, Field of View, Matrix

Voxel volume is a product of pixel size and slice thickness. Pixel size is in turn determined by FOV and matrix. The greater the voxel volume, more are the number of spins that contribute to MR signal, resulting in a higher SNR per voxel. However, when the voxels are larger, spatial resolution falls as it becomes more likely that two points close to one another in the patient lie in the same large voxel.

When FOV is decreased, pixel size and hence voxel volume decreases, thereby decreasing the SNR and increasing spatial resolution **(Figs. 3A and B)**. When small coils are used which boost local SNR, a small FOV may be used. However, with a large coil, when SNR is relatively less, a small FOV severely compromises the SNR further owing to small pixel size unless other measures like increasing NEX is used.

When the matrix is changed, the number of pixels in the FOV also changes. As the matrix increases, the dimension of each pixel decreases. This reduces the SNR but improves spatial resolution. In addition, as the phase matrix increases, the scan time also increases **(Figs. 4A and B)**. However, if we increase the frequency matrix only, it increases the resolution but the scan time does not increase as only the phase matrix determines scan time. A rectangular FOV where the FOV is reduced in the phase direction reduces the scan time keeping the resolution same as that of square FOV. This is especially useful when anatomy of the area examined fits into a rectangle, as in sagittal image of pelvis.

Increasing the slice thickness increases the voxel volume, hence increasing SNR at the expense of spatial resolution **(Figs. 2A and B)**.

SCAN TIME

The longer the examination time, the greater the discomfort to the patient resulting in increased chances of a bad image. Good immobilization is also essential, as a few minutes spent in making the patient comfortable can save many minutes of wasted sequences. The scan time is determined by the following factors.

Scan time = TR × number of excitations × number of phase encodings

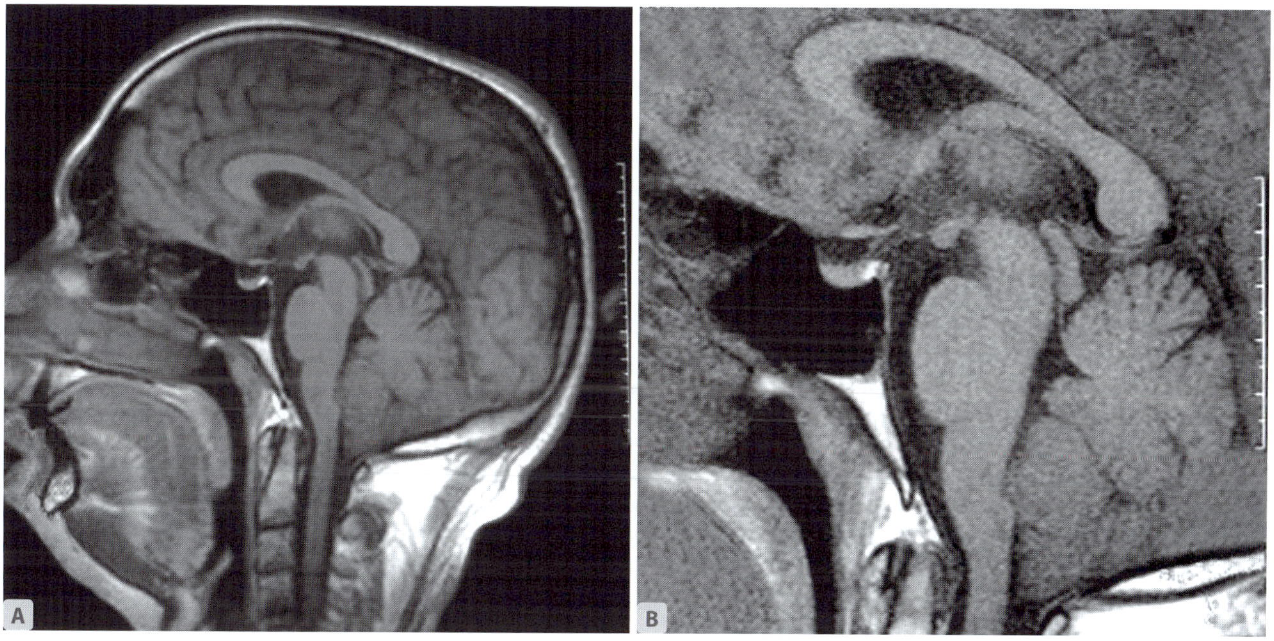

FIGS. 3A AND B: Image comparison. T1 weighted sagittal images of the brain. The image B was acquired with reduced FOV and reduced pixel size compared with image A. The spatial resolution of B was increased at the expense of reduced SNR.

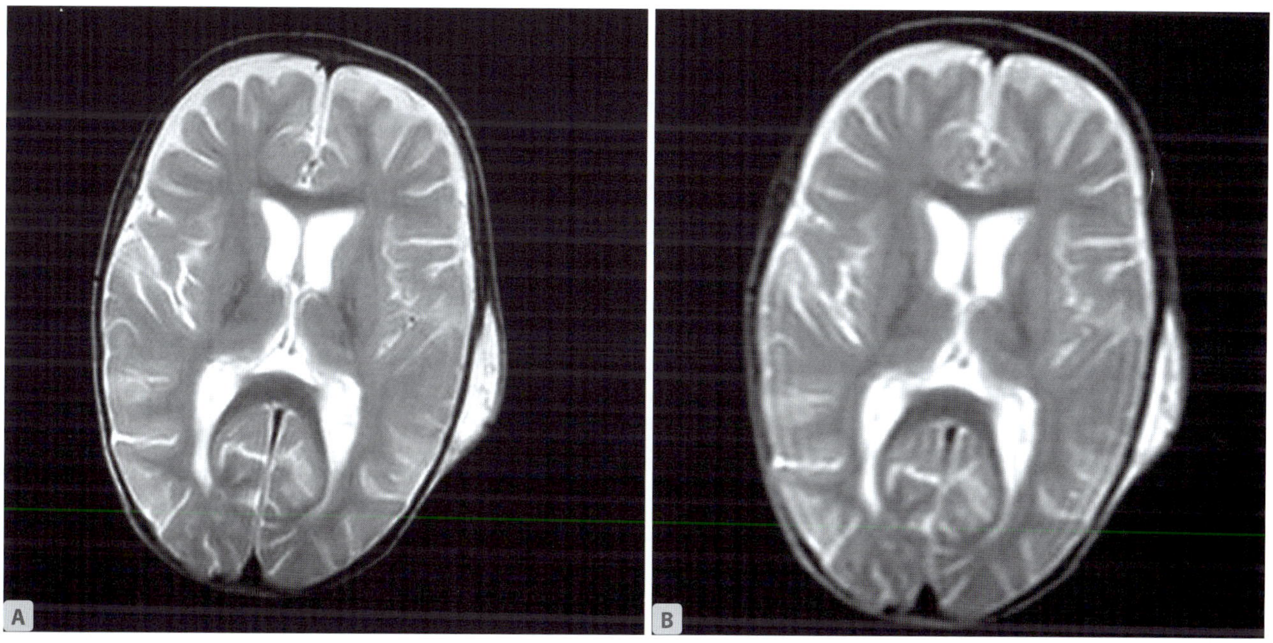

FIGS. 4A AND B: Image comparison. T2 weighted axial images of the brain. The image on the left (A) was acquired with increased matrix and hence reduced pixel size compared with right (B). The spatial resolution of A was improved. As the phase matrix was increased, the scan time was also increased.

Repetition Time

Repetition time (TR) is the time between two RF pulses. As we can understand, greater the TR, greater is the scan time. When we reduce the TR, we can reduce the scan time. However, reducing TR reduces SNR as already discussed. As when TR is short, less longitudinal magnetization recovers, the next 90° pulse flips it to beyond the transverse plane. This is called saturation and increases T1 weighting. In addition, when TR is short, the number of slices that can be excited in this reduced time also decreases.

Number of Excitations

When the Number of excitations (NEX) or signal averages is increased, more and more measurements of one slice are being obtained to average the results. This increases the scan time **(Figs. 1A and B)**. But when NEX is reduced to reduce scan time, SNR falls because now, the number of times data is stored in k-space is reduced. Since averaging of noise is also less, there is also an accompanying increase in motion artefact.

Phase Matrix

Increasing the phase matrix increases scan time **(Figs. 4A and B)**. To understand this, the basic physics behind MR gradients needs to be understood. Gradients are coils of wire which lie just inside the bore of the MR magnet. When current is passed through these coils, a secondary magnetic field is generated which slightly alters the main magnetic field. They change the precessional frequency and phase of the spins. These are employed along three orthogonal axes, XYZ, to enable us to select a slice (slice selection gradient), and to spatially locate the signal along the two dimensions of the image within a slice (frequency encoding and phase encoding gradient).

Frequency encoding gradient is switched on to locate signal along one axis of the image (usually the long axis) and produces a frequency shift. At a frequency matrix of 256, two hundred and fifty six different frequencies are mapped along the long axis of the image. Fourier transformation allows us to determine signal contribution of each frequency, enabling us to allocate this signal to the location of origin along one axis of the image. Fourier transformation is like a prism (which disperses white light into its spectra) that causes physical dispersion of the frequencies collected and assigns them to a structure in the image.

Phase encoding gradient alters the phase of the nucleus, causing a phase shift. When this gradient is switched off, the phase shift of spins remains. This phase shift is used for spatial localization of the signal along the second dimension of the image (usually the short axis). For a phase resolution of 256, we have to generate 256 signals with different phase encodings for 256 different locations. The pulse sequence has to be repeated 256 times for a phase matrix of 256. Hence, the phase matrix is an important determinant of scan time. If we reduce the phase matrix to reduce scan time, the spatial resolution of the image falls.

Number of Slice Encodings in 3D Sequences

In three dimensional fast scan sequences, scan time is also dependent on the number of slices acquired in the volume in addition to TR, NEX and number of phase encodings.

Scan time = TR × number of excitations × number of phase encodings × slice encodings

ARTEFACTS

Artefacts are features in the MR image that do not correspond to spatial distribution of tissue in the image plane. They generally degrade the image but may also be useful in certain clinical scenarios. The cause of this signal misregistration is variable; artefacts are divided into three main types based on the cause.

1. Motion artefacts
2. Artefacts related to particular measurement technique or parameters used, e.g. chemical shift, wrap around and truncation artefacts.
3. External artefacts results from either a malfunction of the MR scanner or external interference.

MOTION ARTEFACTS (PHASE MISMAPPING)

These may result from accidental patient movement, respiration, heartbeat, blood flow, eye movements or swallowing motion. These signal misregistartions occur in the direction of phase encoding gradient. The tissue is excited at one location but is mapped to a different location during readout due to its motion. This occurs in the phase encoding direction rather than the frequency encoding or readout direction because the encoding of phase by the phase encoding gradient occurs prior to signal detection, whereas frequency encoding gradient, also called the readout gradient, is applied concurrently with signal detection. For example, if the abdominal wall is at line A when the phase encoding gradient is applied, it is spatially localized to line A as per this gradient. However, during readout, although the abdominal wall has moved to line B, it is still allocated to line A resulting in ghosting artefact. Sampling along frequency encoding gradient is much faster (in order of milliseconds) while patient motion is much slower. Since time to acquire all phase encoding steps is longer and is in the order of seconds, this is another reason why motion artefacts are appreciable more along phase encoding direction.

Ghosting and Smearing

While ghosting results from periodic motion, smearing is a result of aperiodic motion.

The periodic rise and fall of thorax/abdomen during breathing produces an artefact called ghosting **(Figs. 5A and B)**. If the respiration rate is constant, then during inspiration, the abdomen is in several equidistant phase encoding steps during the inspiration phase and it is in the expiration phase in the intervening steps. This periodic motion is seen as locally offset double or multiple structures in the phase encoding direction. These ghosts are offset by the true image by an amount proportional to the respiration rate. Structures rich in signal, for example subcutaneous fat, further increase ghosting artefact. In a strictly periodic motion, the localization of the ghost can be predicted by a simple formula, describing the distance between the ghost image and the original structure.

Distance = TR × phase encoding steps × NEX × motion frequency

The higher the frequency of the motion, e.g. higher the breathing rate, the greater the distance between the original and the ghost artefact. We can increase the distance between the ghosts by increasing TR, phase matrix or NEX so that the first ghost lies outside the image; however scan time is increased by all these methods. The brightness of the ghost depends upon the magnitude of motion; larger the pulsation, more intense is the ghost.

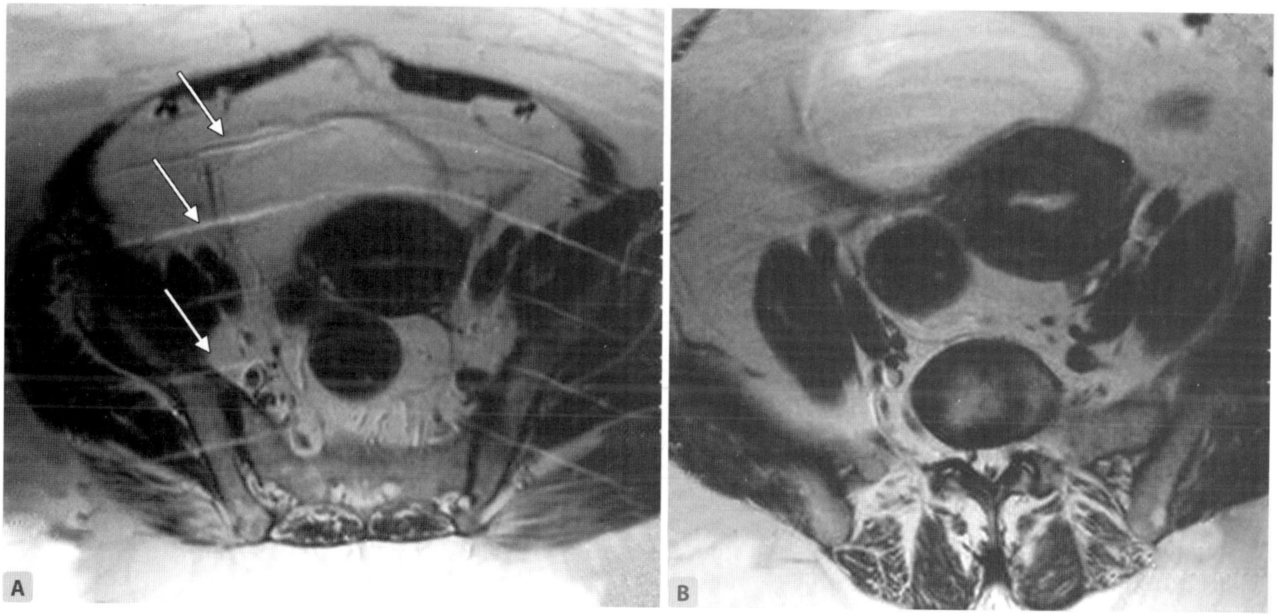

FIGS. 5A AND B: Ghosting artefact. T2 weighted image of the pelvis (A) shows marked ghosting artefact (arrows) due to periodic respiratory motion. This was reduced in (B) by increasing the number of signal averages and placing a spatial presaturation pulse in the overlying subcutaneous fat. However, both these techniques contributed to an increase in scan time.

Another type of artefact that may result from aperiodic motion like that of eyes is smearing **(Fig. 6)**. Peristalsis, which is a random movement, produces motion artefacts that result in generalized blurring of the image, which appears to be superimposed by a layer of noise.

Blood flow is a very common cause of motion artefacts in the image. Fast continuous flow in blood vessels compared to TR produces a diffuse blurring artefact throughout the FOV, as in spin echo images. In-plane flow in vessels in coronal images produces diffuse blurring. Flow in aorta and IVC affects the entire image acquired in coronal plane as these great vessels extend through the entire image. CSF flow artefacts can also degrade the image of the spine on T2 weighted images. Periodic motion due to pulsatile through plane flow (flow perpendicular to the image plane) will be discussed later.

Remedy

Various methods are employed to reduce motion artefacts, depending upon whether signal from moving tissue is desired in the image or not. While spatial presaturation pulse may be used when this signal is not desired, other remedial measures are required when signal from moving tissue is desired in the image.

Spatial Presaturation Pulse

When signal from moving tissue is not desired, spatial presaturation pulse can be used to reduce these artefacts. These are used in spine examinations to suppress cardiac and abdominal motion artefacts **(Figs. 7A to C)**. These saturation pulses are applied before the pulse sequence. Therefore, the number of slices that can be obtained per TR in multislice acquisitions is reduced. They also result in increased heat deposition.

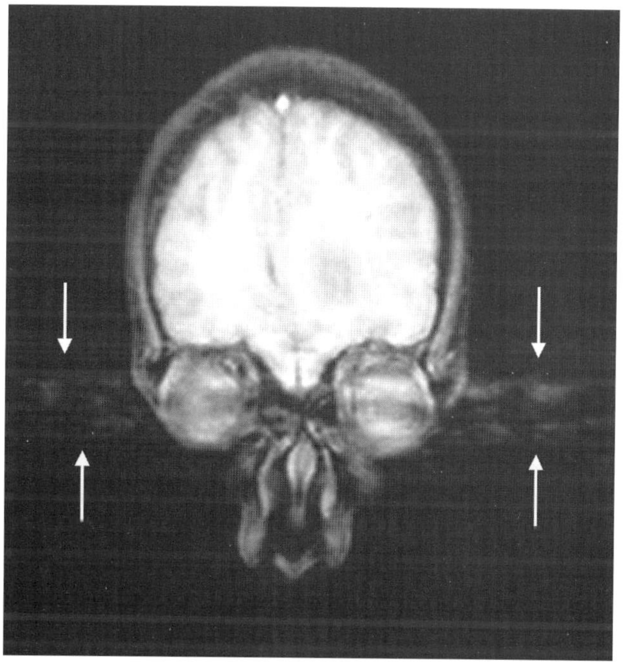

FIG. 6: Smearing artefact. T1 weighted coronal image of the brain shows smearing artefact (arrows) due to aperiodic motion of the eyes.

When signal from moving tissue is desired in the image, other methods may be used. These include use of faster sequences, modification of acquisition parameters, physiological triggering and flow compensation.

Faster Imaging

The most effective technique may be shortening of acquisition time to minimize motion artefacts. Various improvements in MR hardware, including faster and stronger gradients, multichannel coils, and higher magnetic field strengths have enabled faster acquisitions.

There are various techniques to obtain faster sequences. Fast spin echo sequences use multiple 180° refocusing pulses and allow multiple echoes to be obtained within a given TR. The number of additional echoes obtained is called the echo train length (ETL). However, excessive ETLs may blur the image and increase some flow artefacts. Sequences such as half Fourier single-shot turbo spin echo (HASTE) allow rapid acquisition by filling only half of k-space. Parallel imaging technique also reduces the scan time and hence motion artefacts. This technique uses multichannel and multicoil technology. Each coil has an individual sensitivity profile over the field of view. At least 2 coil elements are aligned in the phase encoding direction. The steps in phase encoding direction are reduced. The factor by which these steps are reduced is known as the parallel imaging factor. Only one of every X lines of k space is filled up in the phase encoding direction. The other lines are inferred from the signal amplitude and known sensitivity profile of the coils used. Several data extrapolation algorithms like GRAPPA (generalized autocalibrating partially parallel acquisition) and SENSE (sensitivity encoding) are used before and after Fourier transformation respectively. The major disadvantage is a decreased SNR. However, overall increase in SNR at 3T compensates for this loss.

Radial K Space Filling Technique

Multi-shot radial acquisition technique (e.g syngoBLADE in Siemens; PROPELLOR in GE) fills the k space radially instead of the standard rectilinear method. With this technique, multiple radial overlapping datasets are acquired. A series of low resolution images is reconstructed from each radial section which is then combined to produce a high resolution image. Because the phase encoding direction varies with each radial section, ghosting artefact from motion is not propagated in the phase encoding direction but dispersed through the radial sections. The disadvantage of this technique is its low spatial resolution. This results from sparse filling of the peripheral k space as compared to the central region.

Modification of Parameters

Parameters may be modified to alter the appearance of motion artefacts. Frequency and phase encoding direction can be swapped, which alters the position of the artefact **(Figs. 7A to C)**. These may now be relocated to image areas that do not affect image interpretation. For example, motion artefacts due to eye movement may obscure brain parenchyma if phase encoding direction is antero-posterior for an axial image. This may be overcome when phase encoding direction is made right to left and the artefact now lies outside the brain.

Increasing NEX is another method of reducing motion artefacts. Increasing the number of signal averages increases the signal from the tissue and the motion artefact signal is reduced relative to the tissue signal **(Figs. 5A and B)**.

Physiological Triggering/Gating

Physiological triggering synchronizes the data collection according to respiratory or cardiac cycle allowing normal movement of tissue. Data collection may be synchronized with ECG signal using ECG leads, pulse using pulse sensor on an extremity, respiration using pressure transducer on the patient or a navigator echo indicating diaphragmatic motion. ECG gating is used in cardiac evaluation where artefacts from cardiac motion need to be minimized. This may be prospective or retrospective gating. In the prospective method, the timing signal is first detected. The echo signal is collected at the same time following the time signal. Since the moving tissue is in the same position at this time, there is minimal misregistration of signal. This is typically used in static cardiac examinations. In prospective triggering, the data from arrhythmic beats can also be avoided. In the retrospective method, the timing signal and the echo signal are first acquired together. Data collection is done

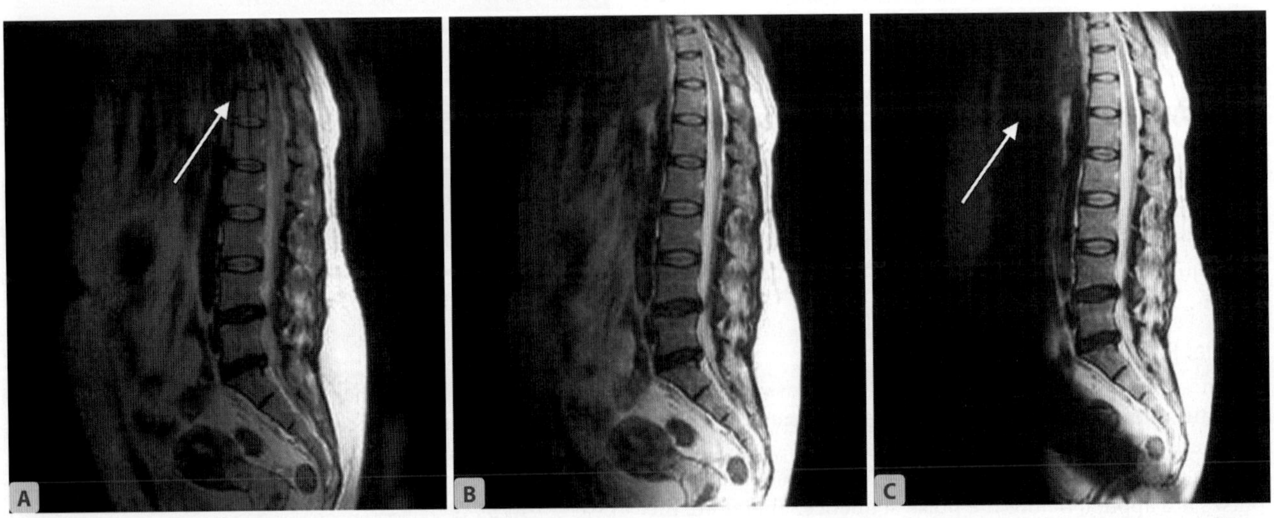

FIGS. 7A TO C: Motion artefact. T2 weighted sagittal images of the spine show marked motion artefacts degrading the image in (A) (arrow) when the phase encoding direction was anterior to posterior. On changing the phase encoding direction to head to foot in (B), the motion artefacts from the heart do not degrade the image. There is further improvement in image quality when a spatial presaturation band (arrow) is used to suppress motion artefacts from the great vessels in (C).

continuously. This is analyzed only after the completion of the scan and the data is then correlated with the cardiac cycle. This method is commonly used in cine cardiac imaging where sequential images are produced according to their time point in the cardiac cycle to allow a dynamic evaluation of cardiac function. Breath holding is another technique that allows further artefact suppression during cardiac imaging. The disadvantages of a triggered study include a longer scan time and misregistration artefacts if the trigger signal is irregular, e.g. with an irregular heart rate.

While cardiac gating is routinely done, respiratory gating is not usually employed in clinical imaging. Breath holding is the method used to avoid respiration artefacts. In pediatric population and unco-operative patients, either short sequences are used or imaging examination is divided into multiple brief sequences if the patient can hold breath for a short duration of time. However, multiple breath holds require co-operation from the patient. In respiratory gating, bellows or a belt is encircled over the abdomen and the acquisition is timed to end expiration when there is minimum motion. The disadvantages include an increased acquisition time and an additional setup time. Respiratory compensation or phase reordering [respiratory ordered phase encoding (ROPE)] is another effective way to reduce respiratory artefacts. In this technique, depending on the respiratory phase, the phase encoding steps are ordered. K space lines are reordered such that the adjacent samples in the final data have minimal differences in the respiratory phase. This works well only with regular respiratory rate. Navigator echo is a commonly used method to suppress periodic motion artefacts from breathing; it uses an additional navigator pulse. This is frequently used in imaging the abdomen where a small one dimensional spatial encoding gradient is placed perpendicular to the diaphragm **(Figs. 8A to C)**. The imaging dataset is then corrected by the navigator echo so that the data acquired at the end of expiration is what is used in reconstruction of final image, while the remaining data is discarded.

Gradient Moment Rephasing

GRE Flow compensation uses additional gradient pulses to align the phase shifts of the moving protons. It is also known as gradient motion rephasing (GMR) or motion artefact suppression technique (MAST). Using additional gradient pulses realigns the phase shifts in moving protons, bringing them back into phase but has no effect on static protons. Usually, these pulses act on protons flowing with constant velocity (first order motion compensation). As additional gradient pulses are used, there is a modest increase in TE. If short TE is desired, short duration high amplitude gradient pulses need to be used. The disadvantages of these high amplitude pulses is that the FOV then needs to be increased. For protons which are accelerating, higher order compensation needs to be done which has a further penalty on TE.

Pulsatile Flow-related Artefacts

Periodic motion due to pulsatile through plane flow (flow perpendicular to the image plane) results in ghost vessels at discrete points, frequently seen in axial abdomen gradient echo images **(Fig. 9)**. The spacing between the ghosts is dependent upon how much the heart rate and TR differ. GRE images are more prone to these ghost artefacts than spin echo sequences. In spin echo sequences, flowing blood usually appears dark. This is because after being excited to the 90° pulse in SE sequences, the moving blood protons move out of the excited slice while new non-excited protons move into the slice; hence resulting in dark signal. In contrast, bright blood phenomenon is seen on GRE sequences.

Remedy

Saturation Pulse

To reduce the pulsatile flow related artefact, a saturation band can be applied adjacent to the imaging section. The protons in this slab are saturated with the use of 90° RF pulse and then spoiled by strong gradients before image acquisition, hence resulting in no signal when spins flow into the imaging volume. These bands when placed superior and inferior to the abdominal thickness being scanned eliminate arterial and venous inflow artefacts respectively.

Advantage of Pulsation Artefacts

Pulsation artefacts from vascular lesions can help us reach the correct diagnosis, when in doubt. The vascular nature of the lesion is confirmed if we see associated pulsation artefacts.

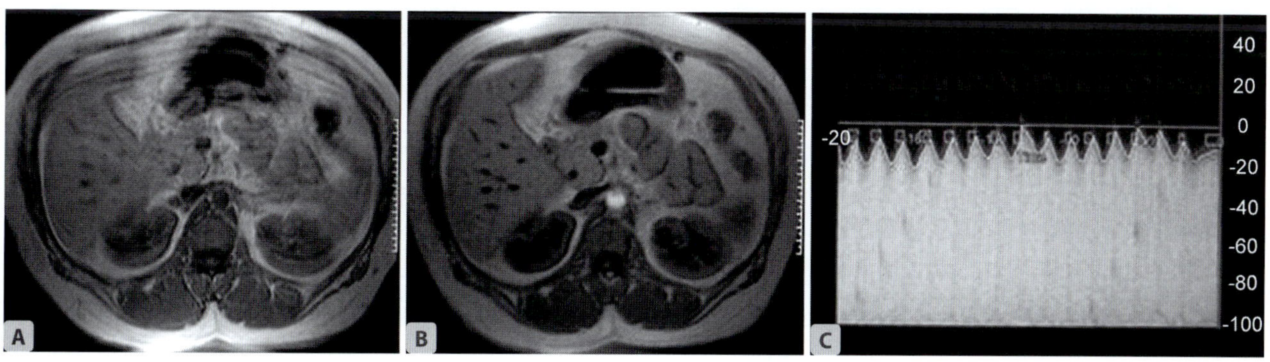

FIGS. 8A TO C: Motion artefact. Axial T1 weighted gradient echo image of the abdomen shows marked respiratory motion artefact resulting in blurring of the image (A). There is marked reduction in motion artefact (B), using a navigator echo pulse (C).

ARTEFACTS DUE TO MEASUREMENT TECHNIQUE/PARAMETERS

Aliasing

Aliasing (wraparound artefact) occurs when the imaging FOV is smaller than the anatomy being imaged. This occurs mostly in the phase encoding direction. The tissue stimulated outside the sensitive volume of the coil contains higher or lower phase and frequency information. These are misinterpreted during Fourier transformation. This tissue is misrepresented in the image on the opposite side **(Figs. 10A and B)**. To explain this, let us recapitulate that the phase of the signal originating from inside the FOV has a range from 0 to 360°. Due to the circular nature of phase, a signal from outside the FOV with a phase of 400° (=360°+40°) is not distinguishable from a phase of 40° from inside the FOV and hence is misinterpreted within the FOV during Fourier transformation. Thus, the part of the body that lies beyond the borders of the FOV is wrapped inside to the other side of the image. Hence, the normal anatomy inside the FOV gets overlapped upon.

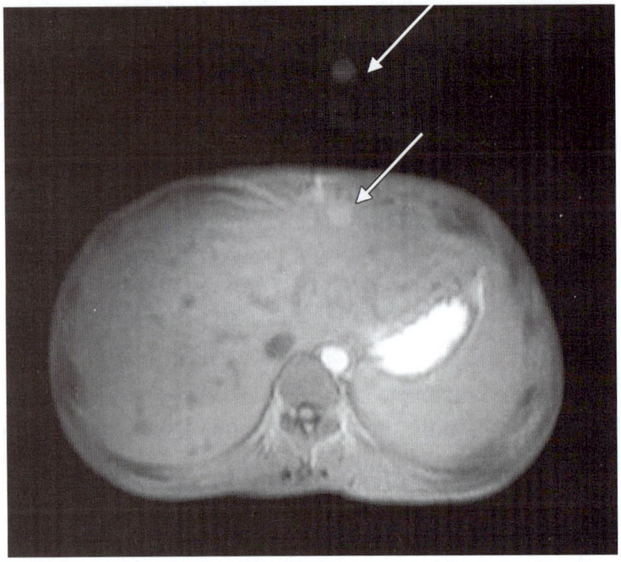

FIG. 9: Ghosting artefact from pulsatile aortic flow. Pulsatile through plane flow in the aorta is seen as ghost vessels at discrete points (arrows) on this axial gradient image.

Wraparound artefact is seldom encountered along the frequency encoding axis because the system typically oversamples along this axis. Unwanted high frequencies are filtered out by the system or a higher bandwidth is used along the frequency encoding axis. Aliasing can also occur in volume imaging along the direction of the volume acquired. The sidelobes of the RF pulse that excite the entire volume of tissue can also produce a signal form outside this slab and aliasing can occur from the first section of the slab onto the last section of the slab **(Fig. 11)**.

Remedy

Increase FOV

The phase FOV can be enlarged so that the entire anatomy is included within the FOV. Increase in FOV increases the SNR but decreases the spatial resolution.

Swapping the Phase and Frequency Encoding Direction

The phase encoding and frequency encoding directions may also be swapped if the phase encoding axis is planned along the longer axis.

Oversampling/No Phasewrap

Oversampling may be done in the phase encoding direction. This is done by increasing the sampling points; however these are not used for image creation **(Fig. 10)**. The FOV is doubled

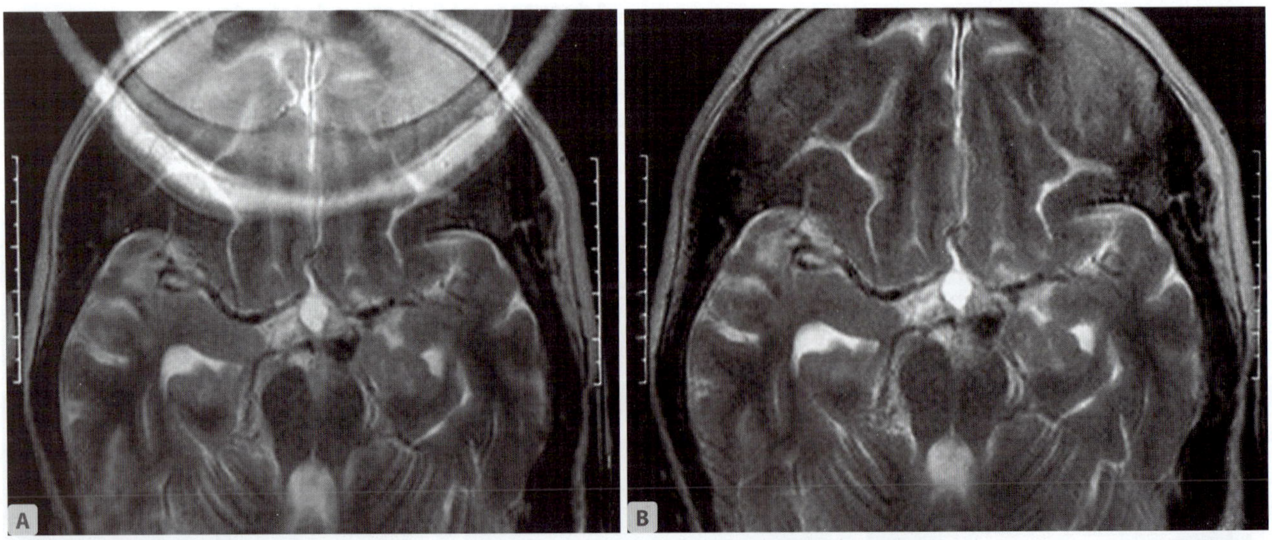

FIGS. 10A AND B: Aliasing artefact. T2 weighted axial images of the brain depict aliasing artefact when it was acquired with a reduced FOV smaller than the anatomy of the image. The tissue outside the FOV was misrepresented on the opposite side (A). This was overcome by oversampling in the phase encoding direction (B). However, there was no penalty in scan time as NEX was halved.

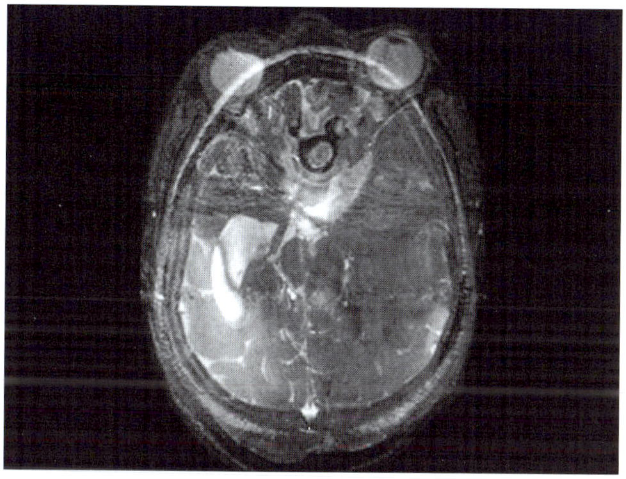

FIG. 11: Aliasing artefact in volume imaging. 3D constructive interference in steady state (CISS) GRE sequence shows overlap of information of the first and last sections of the sequence due to aliasing.

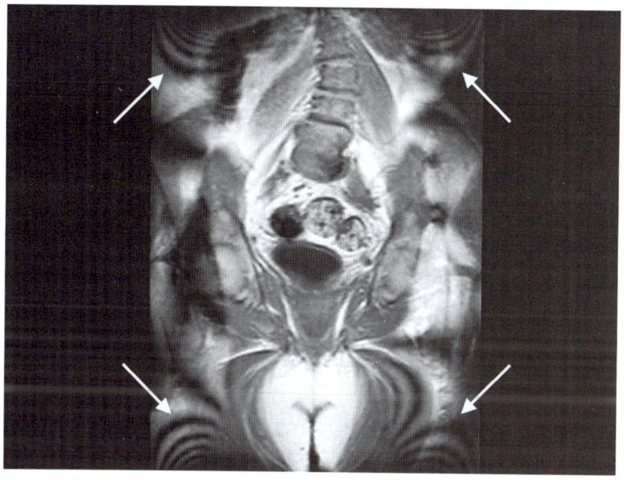

FIG. 12: Moiré artefact. T1 gradient coronal image of the abdomen in a heavy patient using a large FOV that is still smaller than the patient depicts the moiré artefact. This is seen as stripes (arrows), and occurs as a result of a combination of aliasing and field inhomogeneities between the two edges. These are especially prominent at different tissue interfaces (e.g. fat tissue interfaces).

in the phase direction along with doubling of the phase matrix to avoid any decrease in spatial resolution. Oversampling increases the scan time. Hence, the NEX is then reduced by half to overcome the time penalty while SNR and spatial resolution remain the same. This may not be possible in fast scan techniques like those in abdominal imaging, when NEX is already minimum.

Saturation Pulse/Regional Coils

Presaturation pulse or regional coils can be used to diminish the signal from outside the FOV and hence aliasing can be reduced.

In 3D sequences, aliasing can be minimized by exciting only a limited part of the volume in the Z-direction by applying a Z-gradient pulse during the RF excitation.

Moiré/Fringe Artefact

In heavy patients, a special artefact may be seen in coronal imaging when despite using a large field of view, it is still smaller than the anatomical part. This results in aliasing superimposed on phase differences between the two edges. Over large fields of view, homogeneity of the field degrades at the edges, resulting in phase differences between the protons at the edges of the FOV. Aliasing along with mismatched phases over the edges produces the moiré or fringe artefact **(Fig. 12)**. These are seen in gradient echo images.

Remedy

Use of spin echo sequences eliminates these artefacts. Another measure that may be taken to reduce these artefacts is to ensure that the arms of the patient are by the side of his/her body while positioning so that they are within the FOV while imaging chest/abdomen.

Chemical Shift Artefacts

The chemical shift phenomenon refers to the artefacts that occur due to different precessional frequencies of spins in different chemical environments. Clinically, this artefact is predominantly seen at water-fat interface. Protons in water and fat have different chemical environments as they are linked to oxygen and carbon respectively. Hence, they have slightly different precessional frequencies in the same external magnetic field (slightly lower for fat than water). Because fat and water protons have different precessional frequencies, these are allocated to different image pixels along the frequency encoding axis. Although this occurs throughout the image, this is most apparent at fat fluid interfaces, e.g. in imaging of fluid filled structures like bladder, orbits and kidneys which are surrounded by fat. This results in bright and dark bands along the frequency encoding axis towards the higher and lower parts of the frequency encoding gradient respectively.

The dark bands result from the shifting of the lipid proton signals to a lower frequency, away from the actual lipid-water interface, which causes a signal void. The bright bands result from the overlapping of water signal with "shifted" lipid signal on the high-frequency side of the interface. The bright bands, although present, may be more difficult to appreciate when the object being imaged has a curved surface.

The approximate chemical shift between lipid and water is 3.5 parts per million. At field strength of 1.5 T, precessional frequency of fat protons is approximately 220 Hz less than water protons. This difference is directly proportional to magnetic field strength. The number of pixels involved in this shift is directly proportional to the field strength and frequency matrix but inversely related to the receiver bandwidth.

$CSA = \Delta\omega . N_{freq}/BW_{rec}$

CSA = chemical sift artefact, $\Delta\omega$ = frequency difference between fat and water dependent on field strength, N_{freq} = frequency matrix, BW_{rec} = receiver bandwidth

In high field strength magnets, frequency difference between fat and water increases, resulting in greater CSA. However, higher receiver bandwidth can be used in higher field strengths owing to high inherent SNR, hence diminishing these artefacts. Use of narrow receiver bandwidths and large matrix in the frequency encoding direction can accentuate these artefacts. These artefacts were commonly seen in T2 weighted images before turbo imaging was used as the former used low bandwidths to increase the low SNR inherent in T2 weighted sequences.

Remedy

To reduce these artefacts, various measures may be taken. The phase and frequency encoding direction may be swapped. The frequency encoding direction may be used along the axis where there is narrow fluid fat interface or in a direction where this artefact does not hamper the primary area of interest. Inversion recovery sequences or spectral fat saturation technique are other means of reducing this artefact, by suppressing fat/water signal.

Receiver bandwidth is another parameter that may be altered to reduce this artefact. Receiver bandwidth is the range of frequencies which are read out in the frequency encoding direction. Higher the bandwidth, greater is the range of frequencies sampled from the same number of pixels. This reduces the chemical shift artefact. However, increasing the receiver bandwidth decreases the SNR.

Advantage/Utility

Chemical shift along the frequency axis forms the basis of MR spectroscopic imaging.

Chemical Shift in Echo-planar Imaging

These artefacts also occur with echo-planar imaging, but in the phase encoding direction. These are fast sequences where images are acquired in 50 ms to 80 ms. The receiver bandwidth is normally very large in the frequency encoding direction (greater than 100 kHz), hence chemical shift is not appreciable in this direction. However, the phase encoding occurs in a continuous fashion with a low bandwidth, resulting in pronounced chemical shift artefacts in this direction. Fat suppression is therefore necessary to minimize the artefact **(Figs. 13A and B)**.

Phase Cancellation Artefact

This is the second artefact resulting from differences between precessional frequencies of fat and water protons. It can also be referred to as *'chemical shift artefact of the second kind'*. These artefacts are observed in gradient echo images and not in spin echo sequences which use a 180° refocusing pulse, which brings back the fat and water protons in phase by the time the signal is read out at TE. As no such refocusing pulse is present in gradient-echo sequences, fat and water protons keep getting in and out of phase with respect to each other The periodicity of these protons, when they are in phase with each other, depends on the frequency shift and hence the field strength. Higher the field strength, lesser is the periodicity, i.e., the time at which fat and water protons are in phase with each other increases at low field strengths. At 3T, fat and water signals precess in phase approximately every 2.4 msec, every 4.8 msec at 1.5 T; every 7.2 ms at 1.0 T; and every 36.7 msec at 0.2 T.

This periodicity is used to obtain in-phase and opposed-phase MR images. In in-phase images, fat and water have the same phase orientation. The signal contribution of fat and water protons therefore is additive in the final image. In opposed-phase images, the transverse magnetization of fat and water cancel each other. Hence, in voxels containing equal fat and water, the signal between fat and water protons cancels each other and results in a dark ring surrounding the tissue, also known as *contour artefact* **(Figs. 14A and B)**.

Advantage/Utility

Opposed-phase images are used to detect intracellular fat and can be used in evaluation of fatty infiltration of liver, adrenal masses and in assessment of marrow infiltration.

Truncation Artefacts

Truncation or Gibbs artefacts are twin parallel lines that appear at the interface between tissues of high contrast, e.g. in T1 weighted images between high signal fat and low

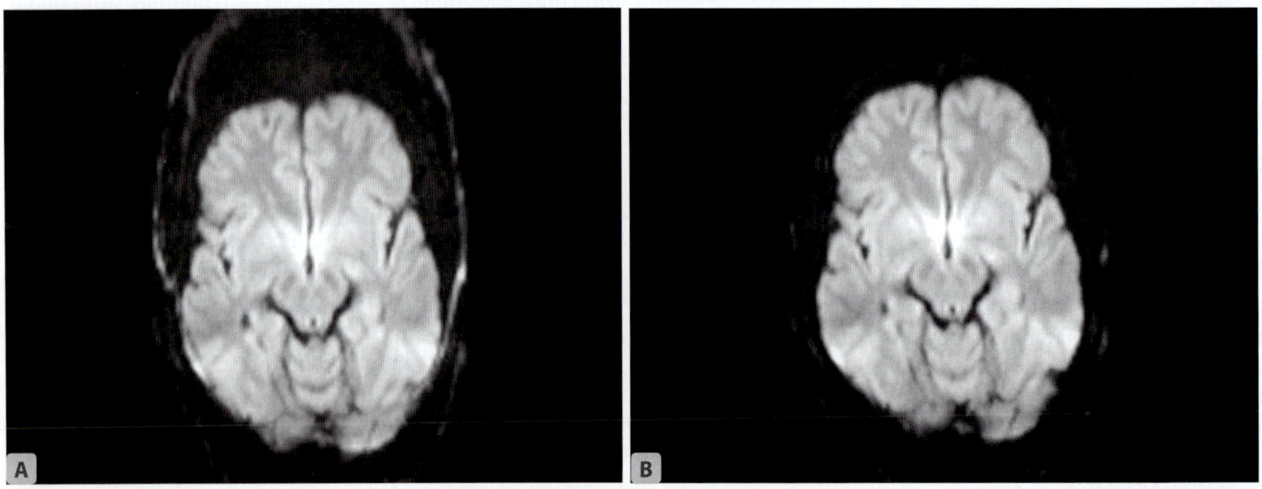

FIGS. 13A AND B: Chemical shift artefact. Echo-planar imaging depicts chemical shift artefact in phase encoding direction which is anterior to posterior (A). Fat suppression technique can be used to minimize the artefact (B).

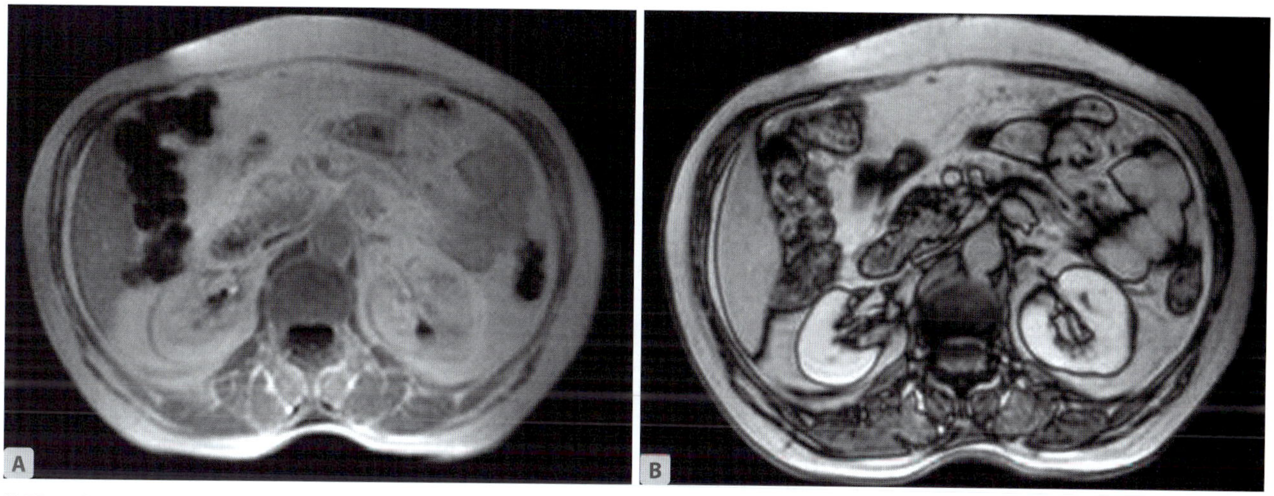

FIGS. 14A AND B: Phase cancellation artefact. In-phase (A) and opposed-phase (B) gradient echo MR images of the abdomen at TE 2.2 msec and TE 5.5 msec respectively in a 3T MR system show a dark rim surrounding the structures at fat water interfaces on the opposed phase images.

signal tissue or in T2 weighted MR images of the spine at the CSF-cord interface. These are seen as alternate high and low intensity stripes or rings in the image. These are also known as 'edge oscillations'.

These artefacts are a result of insufficient digital sampling of the echo. Since there is a limited window period available for measurement of signal, there is interruption of this measurement at certain locations and data is truncated or omitted in k- space. Approximation errors in Fourier transformation of these signals lead to truncation artefacts. As Fourier transformation is better used for estimating gradual transitions, abrupt transitions at high contrast interfaces results in these artefacts.

Since these artefacts are a result of errors in Fourier transformation, these are seen in both phase and frequency encoding direction. These are also dependent upon the matrix size. When matrix size is smaller, i.e. the pixel size gets bigger; the higher frequencies which represent these sharp interfaces are cut off resulting in the artefacts. Although seen along both phase and frequency encoding axis, they are usually seen in the phase encoding direction because usually a smaller phase matrix is used as compared to frequency matrix in order to reduce the acquisition time.

Remedy

These artefacts can be diminished by increasing the acquisition matrix. However, this results in reduced SNR and increased acquisition time. Also, various filters can be applied to reduce these artefacts. Raw data filters may be used prior to Fourier transformation (e.g. Fermi, Gaussian, Hanning filters). These filters force the signal amplitude to zero at the end of data collection period. These improve the signal to noise ratio of the image as high frequency noise is removed from the signal. However, excessive filtering may result in loss of sharpness of the image as this eliminates high frequencies responsible for edge definition, resulting in blurring. Image reconstruction of rectangular raw data matrices automatically uses a weak filter.

Magnetic Susceptibility Difference Artefacts

Magnetic susceptibility is a measure of magnetization induced in a substance by external magnetic field. The magnetic field contribution from the tissue may add to or subtract from the main magnetic field, depending upon whether the structure is paramagnetic or diamagnetic respectively. Differences in tissue susceptibility hence lead to magnetic field inhomogeneities. Most biological tissues are diamagnetic; calcium (as in cortical bone) being the most diamagnetic. Magnetic field inhomogenieties are created at the interface between regions with varying magnetic susceptibility resulting in distortion artefacts. These result from enhanced dephasing of protons located at these interfaces between tissues with very different magnetic susceptibility. These artefacts are seen as areas of signal void. The second effect is that of spatial mismapping of the signal resulting in geometric distortion of anatomy **(Figs. 15A and B)**. The paranasal sinuses, the orbits, the lungs, heart, stomach and intestinal loops are the problematic areas. These are also observed in kidneys and bladder after administration of paramagnetic contrast agent which concentrates in these organs leading to significant signal loss.

These artefacts are more pronounced with gradient echo sequences **(Fig. 15A)** and EPI imaging **(Fig. 16A)**. In gradient echo imaging, signal amplitude is a function of T2*, in which proton dephasing from magnetic field inhomogeneities is an important factor that affects image contrast. On the other hand, spin echo sequences use a refocusing 180° pulse which rephases the protons and hence minimizes these artefacts **(Fig. 15B)**. These artefacts get very pronounced in EPI imaging, when data from a single RF pulse fills the entire k space. This single shot readout using gradient refocusing over a long period is predisposed to these artefacts. Generally, high bandwidth of this sequence in frequency encoding direction protects it from these distortions in this direction. However, low bandwidth in EPI sequence in the phase encoding direction affects distortions in this direction. Therefore, the phase encoding gradient is oriented along

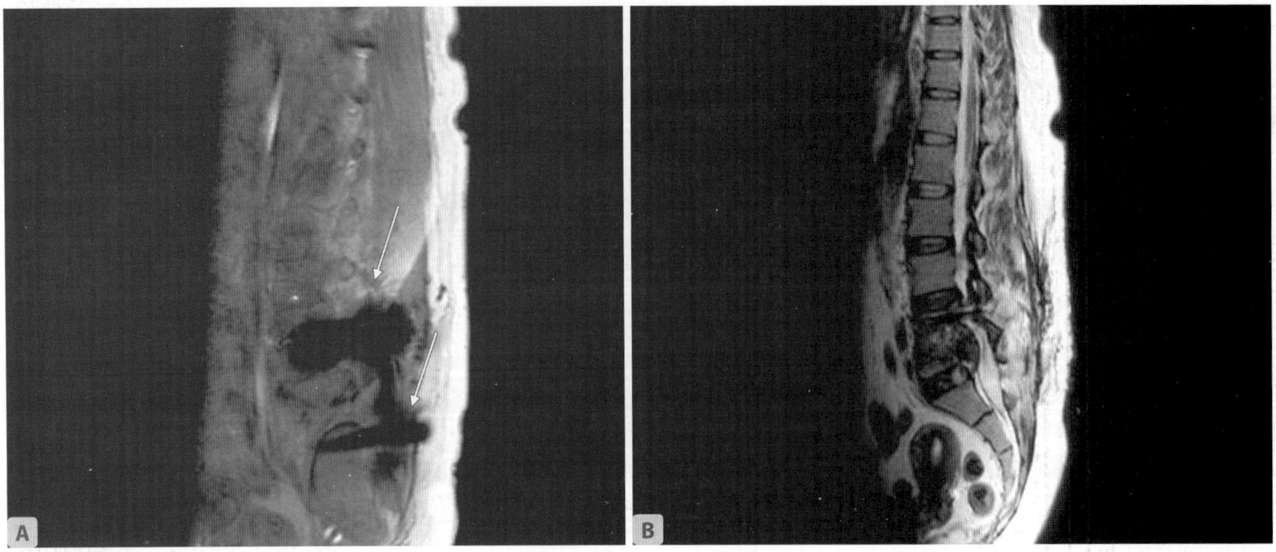

FIGS. 15A AND B: Magnetic susceptibility artefact. Gradient echo sagittal image of the spine shows magnetic susceptibility artefact due to a metal fixator, seen as areas of signal void and geometric distortion (arrows in A). Use of spin echo sequence (B) minimizes the artefact.

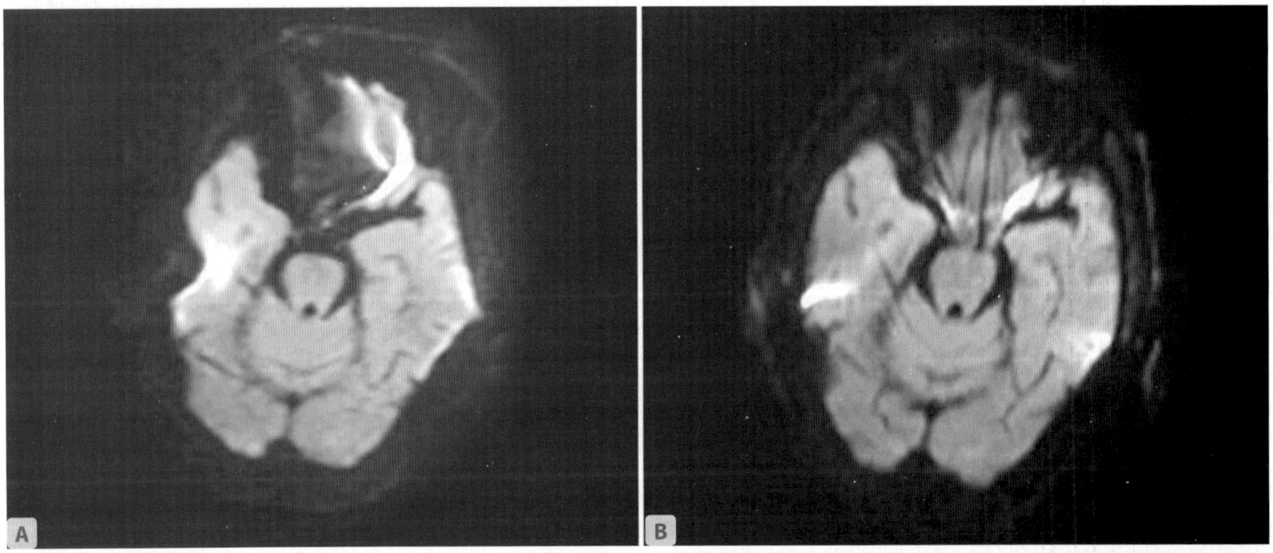

FIGS. 16A AND B: Magnetic susceptibility artefact. Echo-planar imaging shows marked distortion when the phase encoding gradient is from right to left (A). This is minimized by keeping the direction of the phase encoding gradient from anterior to posterior, and hence along the susceptibility gradient in brain (B).

the axis of the susceptibility gradient (antero- posterior direction while imaging the brain) to reduce the distortion in EPI imaging **(Fig. 16B)**. The higher the field strength of the main magnetic field, the stronger are these artefacts. Also, these artefacts are more pronounced when TE used is longer. The longer the TE, greater is the time available for dephasing of protons.

$$\text{Hence susceptibility} \propto \frac{\text{Magnetic field strength} \times \text{TE}}{\text{Receiver bandwidth}}$$

Remedy

Following remedies may be used to eliminate or reduce these artefacts. Spin echo sequences may be done which use a rephasing 180° pulse. TE may be reduced as longer the TE, greater is the time available for dephasing of protons. Both these factors together (short TE, spin echo imaging) are seen with fast spin echo sequences instead of conventional spin echo sequences. The voxel size may be reduced to reduce the local magnetic field inhomogeneities. Larger bandwidth sequences also reduce these artefacts. Although these susceptibility artefacts are more pronounced at higher field strengths, inherent improvement in SNR in 3T systems allows the use of higher bandwidth and parallel imaging to reduce these artefacts. These artefacts can be reduced in multishot EPI acquisitions, with parallel imaging and with radial k-space sampling technique.

Advantage/Utility

Presence of these artefacts proves advantageous in detection of hemorrhage, as blood products become more apparent due to magnetic susceptibility or blooming artefacts. They are also used to our advantage as they form the basis of perfusion imaging, functional imaging of the brain, quantification of liver iron content and use of reticulo-endothelial specific agents in liver imaging.

Section Cross Talk

In multisection two dimensional sequences, crosstalk artefact can result if there is no interslice gap. This is because the slice profiles obtained from RF pulses are not rectangular but slightly curved. Side lobes of RF pulses can excite part of adjacent sections. Hence these are excited twice by an RF pulse in the same TR, resulting in saturation and low signal intensity. This is seen in all sections except the first and last slices.

This is not seen in three dimensional sequences as the whole volume of tissue is excited together and gradients are used to obtain sections within this volume.

Remedy

This can be overcome by using RF pulses with sharper section profiles or by using interspace gap. If images are needed without intervening gap, then interleaving may be done i.e two separate acquisitions done in different batches involving alternate slices.

Parallel Imaging Artefact

Parallel imaging techniques such as GRAPPA and SENSE help us to reduce acquisition time by extrapolating data before and after Fourier transformation respectively. However, we must take care to avoid very high acceleration factors as the noise level increases and SNR falls with use of high acceleration factor. This noise can be seen in the center of the image **(Figs. 17A and B)**. Also, if the anatomical area is greater than the FOV used, aliasing can be seen in addition to increased noise. This aliasing artefact may also be projected in the central portion of the image. This moves outwards as the parallel imaging factor is reduced.

EXTERNAL ARTEFACTS

External artefacts are generated from sources other than the patient. These could be classified into two categories—those that are hardware related and those that are not. Improper calibration of gradients, RF transmitter and receiver system can lead to various distortions and incorrect spatial localization. The gradient system and RF transmitter system can sometimes malfunction and work in an unstable manner. This can result in amplitude and phase modulations resulting in ghosting or smearing artefacts and occur throughout the image field in the phase encoding direction. These may be indistinguishable from motion artefacts. These external artefacts could be transient owing to malfunction or these could also be due to degraded components of one or more subsystems.

Artefacts Caused by Field Distortions

Distortions artefacts may be caused by main magnetic field inhomogeneities or non linearity of the gradient field or RF field inhomogeneities.

Main Field Inhomogeneities

Despite efforts by various MR manufacturers to provide homogenous magnetic fields, some inhomogeneities still occur towards the periphery of the magnet. This is more pronounced in large bore magnets and in large field of view

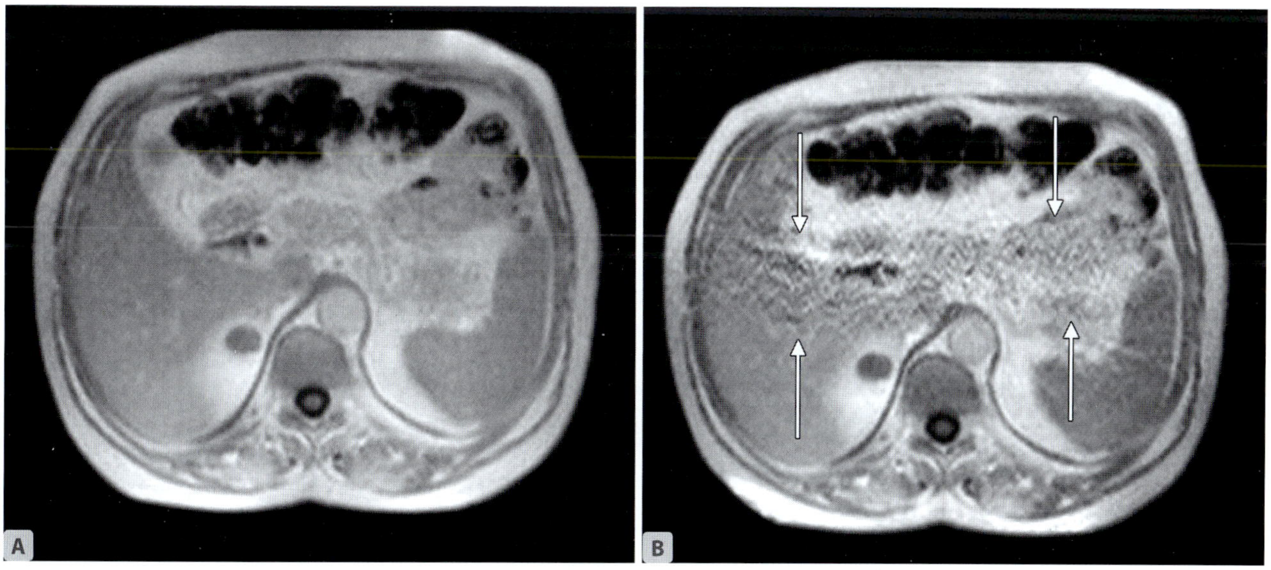

FIGS. 17A AND B: Parallel imaging artefact. Axial T1 weighted gradient image acquired without parallel imaging (A) and axial T1 gradient image acquired with a parallel imaging factor of 2 (B) shows noise and reconstruction artefacts in the middle of the FOV in the latter image (arrows in B) which limit the diagnostic quality of the image.

images at the edges. This is especially important in spectral fat suppression sequences. If the magnetic field is not homogenous, it results in poor fat saturation. To minimize the artefact, the part to be examined should be centered well within the magnet and field homogeneity correction should be done just prior to the scan, after positioning the patient within the scanner. High field homogeneity is also imperative for MR spectroscopy where protons differ by less than 1mm in their frequencies.

Distortions in the main magnetic field may also result from ferromagnetic substances like zippers, metal clips on the patient's body/clothing **(Figs. 15A and B)**. These result in magnetic susceptibility artefacts as described above, but these are more severe as metals have much higher magnetic susceptibility than body tissues. If metal cannot be removed from the patient (e.g metallic implant), the artefacts can be minimized by using fast SE sequences using a high bandwidth and decreased echo time. However, care should be taken in these cases as metallic objects can result in more energy absorption and heating as compared to normal body tissues.

Gradient Field Nonlinearity

Gradient field nonlinearity is related to a dip in the gradient owing to finite size of gradient coils. Gradient coil induces a gradient in the magnetic field that varies linearly through the centre of the magnet but falls towards the side of the magnet. This leads to distortion and loss in spatial resolution. In a large FOV image, gradient field distortion is seen as compression of the structures at the edge of the image **(Fig. 18A)**. As this is a predictable artefact, MR imaging software can correct these distortions before the final image is reconstructed. Post processing techniques can also correct the distortions but not the accompanying loss in spatial resolution **(Fig. 18B)**.

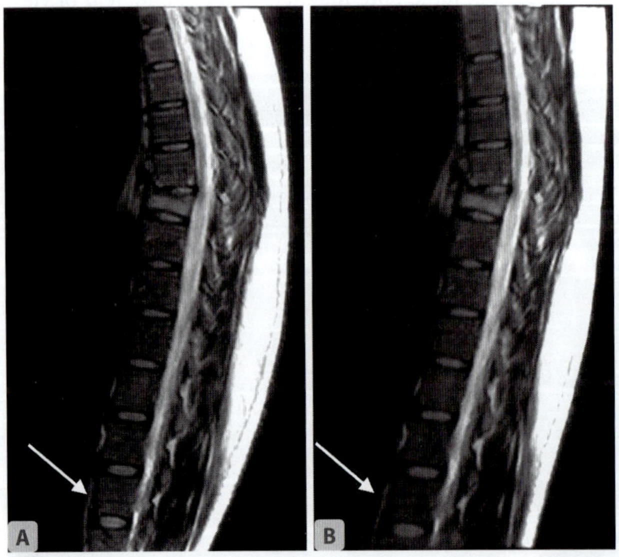

FIGS. 18A AND B: Field distortion due to gradient field nonlinearity. Sagittal T2-weighted image of the thoracic spine shows geometric distortions resulting from gradient nonlinearity, with vertebral bodies appearing progressively smaller toward the inferior edge of the FOV (arrow in A). Distortion correction software was used to correct the distortion (arrow in B).

RF Field Inhomogeneities

Inhomogeneities in RF pulse also result in artefacts. These are however signal nonuniformity rather than geometric distortions. These may be due to problems in RF construction or from dielectric (standing wave) effects. Dielectric effect is the interaction of tissues with the electric component of the electromagnetic field and is especially prominent at 3T systems because high frequency low wavelength RF pulse is required to excite protons at this high field strength because of increased Larmor frequency of protons. The wavelength of these RF pulses approximates the dimensions of the anatomic structure and standing waves may result. These waves can result in dark and bright zones on the image depending upon whether they create a destructive or constructive interference pattern. The patients' girth can be altered by using dielectric pads and hence reducing the formation of standing waves.

Remedy

RF field distortions can also lead to inhomogeneous fat suppression on STIR imaging. RF shimming can help reduce the artefact. Alternatively, spectral fat saturation may be used instead of STIR sequence to suppress fat. In STIR imaing, signal from all tissues that have a T1 equal to that of fat is saturated. Spectral fat saturation, in contrast, is a specific fat suppression technique, selectively differentiating resonant frequency of fat from water.

Spike (Herringbone) Artefact

Spikes are noise bursts of short duration that can occur randomly during data collection. These can result from loose electrical connections in an RF coil. These are more frequently encountered when gradients are applied at high duty cycle, e.g. in echo-planar imaging which can produce this spike of noise. Fourier transformation of this spike of noise results in a specific 'crisscross' or 'herringbone' pattern seen as dark stripes overlaid on the image **(Fig. 19)**. Spike noise is usually transient but can become chronic if not attended to.

Advantage/Utility

This pattern of stripes can be used to our advantage in cardiac imaging, in tagging sequence.

Zipper Artefact

Zipper artefact is an artefact that is caused by external interference resulting from external RF fields, as those caused by open doors, radios, mobile telephones, electronic controls, etc. These emit interfering electromagnetic signals that hamper MR image quality. Zipper artefact appears due to a region of increased noise as a thin line through the centre of the image that extends in the phase encoding direction in all the images of the sequence.

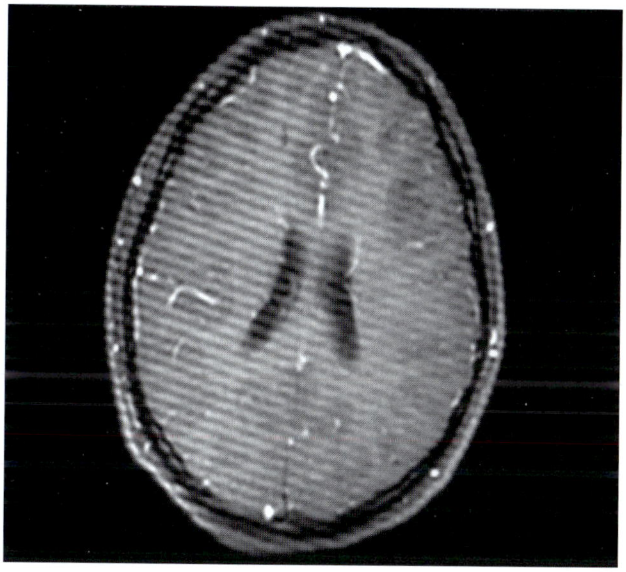

FIG. 19: Spike or herringbone artefact. Loss of data points occurring randomly due to loose electrical connections in the RF coil can lead to a "crisscross" or "herringbone" pattern of artefact.

Remedy

To prevent these artefacts, MR scanners are installed in RF-sealed rooms, also known as Faraday cage. These sealed rooms not only protect the equipment from external RF interference but also shield the environment from RF fields generated by the scanner. The door of the MR room should always be closed properly to prevent this interference. If any constructional changes take place after the installation of the MR scanner, e.g. drilling holes for cables, it may lead to interference in RF shielding. In this case, the source of interference needs to be carefully looked for. Sometimes, electrical connections from any patient monitoring device (e.g pulse oxymeters) which work on alternating current can also interfere with RF shielding. The persistence of the artefact even after the equipment is removed indicates compromise of the RF shield.

3T IMAGING: ADVANTAGES VS LIMITATIONS

Advantages

- *Signal to noise ratio*: The greater the strength of the magnetic field, greater is the number of protons aligning parallel to the field, resulting in a higher SNR. The higher SNR can be used either to increase the spatial resolution or to decrease its time of acquisition. Because of increased SNR, matrix used can now be increased, hence improving the spatial resolution.
- *CNR*: Contrast is inherently less in 3T MR system owing to altered T1, T2, T2* times. T_1 of tissues is longer on 3T as compared to 1.5T scanner. However, T_1 of gadolinium is short. Enhancing tissues stand out against the background. Hence, contrast administration markedly improves the CNR of the image on 3T imaging, hence allowing reduction in the contrast dose.
- *MRS*: MRS has improved diagnostic accuracy in 3T magnets as the SNR is better and the various metabolic peaks are more dispersed leading to its easier identification.

Limitations

- *RF field inhomogeneity*: With increasing field strength, RF field inhomogeneity increases leading to standing wave artefacts (light and dark areas, especially in obese patients) as explained earlier. In higher field strengths, highly conductive medium like ascites also dissipates the RF fields energy by acting like electromagnet. Hence, this leads to signal loss in the abdomen where ascites is present. Newer coils like transverse electromagnetic body coils and spiral configuration of coils can offset this artefact to a large extent. Specific pulse sequences especially tailored to a particular coil have also proved useful to reduce these artefacts.
- *Increased energy deposition*: Specific absorption rate (SAR) provides us with a measure of energy deposition within the tissue by RF pulses, resulting in heating. SAR depends upon the magnetic field strength, patient size, RF pulse cycle and flip angle. As per the Food and Drug administration (FDA) guidelines, total body heating cannot be greater than 10 C or 4 W/kg averaged over the whole body for 15 minutes.
  Parallel imaging reduces the time of acquisition as well as SAR in 3T systems. The drawback with parallel imaging of reduced SNR is overcome owing to enhanced inherent SNR of 3T. Also single shot sequences which employ lower bandwidth (eg. HASTE) further improve the SNR.
- *Chemical shift artefact*: Chemical shift artefact increases at higher fields strengths as described earlier. Remedial measures include increasing bandwidth, fat saturation and swapping of phases and frequency encoding direction. These concepts have been explained earlier in the chapter in detail.
- *Magnetic susceptibility artefacts*: These artefacts increase at higher strength fields. These are advantageous when looking for haemorrhage and disadvantageous when there is air or metal within the tissues. Remedial measures include shim coils and fast SE sequences instead of gradient echo sequences.

CONCLUSION

Clinical MR imaging is becoming more and more versatile and complex, making it difficult for the radiologist to grasp the physical principles underlining the changing technology. Nevertheless, knowledge of basic MR physics plays a key role in clinical imaging as its understanding can help us modify imaging protocols to obtain optimum image quality within acceptable scan time. Good quality images enable us to reach the correct clinical diagnosis with greater confidence.

SUGGESTED READING

1. Barth MM, Smith MP, Pedrosa I, Lenkinski RE, Rofsky NM. Body MR imaging at 3.0 T: understanding the opportunities and challenges. Radiographics 2007 Sep;27(5):1445-62.
2. Brown MA, Semelka RC. Artifacts. In: MRI- Basic principles and applications, 3rd edn. New Jersey: Willey Liss Inc. 2003. p.113-40.
3. Brown MA, Semelka RC. Measurement parameters and image contrast. In: MRI- Basic principles and applications, 3rd edn. New Jersey: Willey Liss Inc. 2003.p.93-102.
4. Chang KJ, Kamel IR, macura KJ, Bluemke DA. 3.0 T MR imaging of the abdomen: comparison with 1.5 T. Radiographics. 2008;28:1983-1998.
5. Chavan GB, Babyn PS, Singh M, Vidarsson L, Shroff M.MR imaging at 3T in children: Technical differences, safety issues, and initial experience. Radiographics. 2009;29:1451-1466.
6. Hood MN, Ho VB, Smirniotopoulas JG, Szumowski J. Chemical shift: the artifact and clinical tool revisited. Radiographics. 1999;19:357-71.
7. Mitchell DG, Cohen M. In: MRI principles, 2nd edn. Philadelphia, Pa: Saunders. 2004.p.416.
8. Morelli JN, Runge VM, Ai F, Attenberger U, Vu L, Schmeets SH, Nitz WR, Kirsch JE. An image based approach to understanding the physics of MR artifacts. Radiographics. 2011;31:849-66.
9. Schmitz BL, Aschoff AJ, Hoffmann MH, Grön G. Advantages and pitfalls in 3T MR brain imaging: a pictorial review. Am J Neuroradiol 2005 Oct 1;26(9):2229-37.
10. Soher BJ, dale BM, Merkle EM. Areview of MR physics: 3T versus 1.5 T. Mag Reson Imaging Clin N Am 2007;15: 277-290.
11. Stadler A, Schima W, Ba-Ssalamah A, Kettenbach J, Eisenhuber E. Artifacts in body MR imaging: their appearance and how to eliminate them. Eur Radiol. 2007;17(5):1242-55.
12. Westbrook C. Artifacts. In: MRI at a glance. 1st edn. Great Britain: Blackwell Science. 2002.p.73-78.
13. Westbrook C. Image quality. In: MRI at a glance. 1st edn. Great Britain: Blackwell Science. 2002.p.64-72.
14. Yang RK, Rith CG, Ward RJ, deJesus JO, Mitchell DG. Optimising abdominal MNR imaging: approaches to common problems. Radiographics. 2010;30:185-99.
15. Zhuo F, Gullapaali RP. MR artifacts, safety and quality control. Radiographics. 2006;26:275-97.

CHAPTER

35

Diffusion-weighted Magnetic Resonance Imaging

Devasenathipathy Kandasamy, Raju Sharma

INTRODUCTION

Magnetic resonance imaging (MRI) imaging has become an important imaging tool in the current clinical practice mainly because of its excellent contrast resolution without the risk of any ionizing radiation. This has become even more relevant with the growing concern for radiation issues in computed tomography (CT) and other imaging modalities which utilize ionizing radiation. Diffusion-weighted imaging (DWI) is a promising technique which was originally described by Le Bihan 30 years back and because of the recent developments in MR hardware this has found a place in routine clinical MR protocols. The basic principle of DWI is based on the Brownian motion of water molecules which takes place in the body and it utilizes motion sensitizing gradients to study this motion.[1,2] It provides unique information at a microstructural and functional level which can be used to characterize cellular dense lesions and this has applications in oncology. Other reasons why this technique is appealing are that it can be performed rather quickly and does not require the use of exogenous contrast agents.

Diffusion can be assessed both qualitatively and quantitatively. It is quantified by the parameter called Apparent Diffusion Coefficient (ADC) which is derived from the diffusion images. The ADC is a scalar quantity which has only magnitude without any directional information.[3] This chapter will focus on the basic principles of DWI and optimization of the technique and briefly review its clinical applications.

BASIC PRINCIPLE

Water molecules in the body undergo a random motion called "Brownian motion" which is as a result of body heat.[2]

Theoretically, these constant random motions are uniform in all directions. But the diffusion in body tissues is restricted by various organelles, membranes and tissue planes. The intracellular diffusion is more hindered than the extracellular component because of the presence of cell membrane.[4] In case of malignant tumors the cells are densely packed with large nuclei and scanty cytoplasm which results in restriction of diffusion **(Fig. 1)**. On the other hand, benign cells are loosely packed with small nucleus and abundant cytoplasm that facilitates diffusion.[5] Because of the interaction of water molecule within biological tissues which can impede the actual diffusion the measured diffusion is termed as ADC which is expressed in mm^2/s. When the diffusion is not restricted in any particular direction it is called isotropic diffusion as seen in CSF space and cystic lesions. When the diffusion occurs preferentially in a particular direction it is called anisotropic diffusion which is usually seen in white matter of brain.[6] In white matter and peripheral nerves the water diffuses preferentially along the axon.

DWI can generate images in which the contrast between the structures is based on the diffusion characteristics. There are various types of sequences with diffusion sensitizing gradients incorporated within but the basis of all of them is the technique suggested by Stejskal and Tanner in 1965 and implemented by Le Bihan in 1986.[7,8] Their technique essentially involves adding two diffusion sensitizing gradient, one on either side of 180° refocusing pulse. These gradient lobes have the same magnitude but are opposite in direction. The first gradient lobe is called dephasing gradient which will dephase the spins of water molecules and the second is called the rephasing gradient which will rephase the spins to their original state. The 180° pulse will eliminate the dephasing due to the inhomogeneity of external magnetic field. This principle has been adopted with or without slight variation even in modern day sequences.[9] The idea behind this technique is that the water molecules whose diffusion is not restricted will get dephased by the first gradient lobe and during the process the molecules will move to another location in which the water molecules will be subjected to a different magnetic environment so that the rephasing pulse will not exactly rephase them to their original state. This will cause attenuation of signal from these water molecules as they are not exactly rephased to produce a strong echo. Whereas, water molecules whose diffusion is restricted will not move and they will be subjected to the same magnetic environment and the dephasing and rephasing gradients will exactly neutralize each other and their spins will be in phase to produce a strong echo. These diffusion gradients can be applied in any of the axis (x, y, z) or in any combination and it is called diffusion sensitizing direction. This diffusion

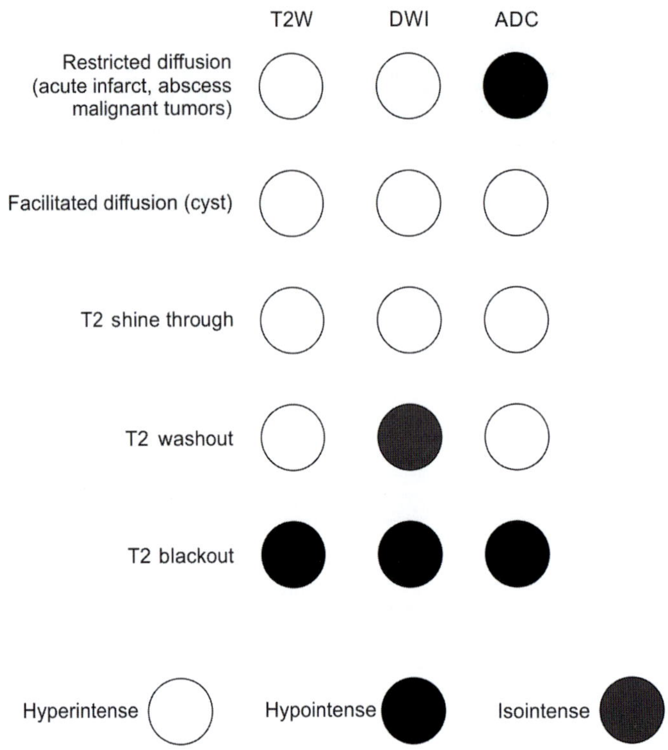

FIG. 1: Schematic representation of signal intensities on T2W, DW sequence and ADC map for disease entities and artifacts which are commonly encountered in day-to-day practice.

gradient addition can be applied in spin echo or in steady state sequences as long as they have a long TE to accommodate them and this is the reason why the diffusion sequences are T2 weighted.

B VALUE

The magnitude, duration of diffusion gradient applied and the duration between the dephasing and rephasing lobe determines the sensitivity of the sequence to water diffusion which is described by a factor called diffusion weighting factor or b factor (s/mm^2). All the above factors are directly proportional to the b value. Usually, the magnitude is kept maximal and the other two are altered to get a desired b value. At least 2 b values are needed for the calculation of ADC and multiple b values are used for more accurate quantification.[2] When multiple b values are used the TE time which is maximum for highest b value is usually kept constant for all b values for better quantification.[6] The choice of b value is very important and depends on the hardware, region of study, type of sequence and the quantitative or qualitative nature of the study. The usual thumb rule is that b value is about inverse of the expected ADC value.[9] For example if the expected ADC value of a tissue is 1.2×10^{-3} then the approximate b value is 800. The SNR of the sequence is grossly affected by the b value selection. When the b value is increased, the SNR of the sequence reduces and at very high values the SNR becomes very low so as to make the quantification unreliable. At the same time low b value will not generate an image whose contrast characteristics are truly based on diffusivity of water molecules. So optimal b value is a balance between the SNR required for quantification and the diffusion contrast of the image. High b values (>1000) are used in imaging techniques like diffusion weighted whole body imaging with background body signal suppression (DWIBS) in which background signal suppression is important. Although multiple b values increase the accuracy of quantification of diffusion it also increase the acquisition time and associated artifacts. There are several approaches developed to circumvent these issues which are discussed later in the chapter.

ADC AND EXPONENTIAL IMAGE

ADC image is a parametric map which is derived from the DW image and it is devoid of T2 shine through (vide infra). It needs images acquired at minimum of two b values to calculate ADC and in present day scanners the calculation of ADC map is automatic. The ADC value is dependent on the b value used where it is inversely proportional to the b values used even in the same patient. It is also dependent on the field strength of the scanner, gradient hardware and the type of image processing software used.[2] Since ADC map is the grayscale representation of pixel by pixel ADC values calculated from diffusion images, the artifacts associated with the diffusion sequences will also get reflected. In addition poor SNR in high b value images also adds to the deterioration of image quality. This is the reason for ADC map having poor image quality when compared to the diffusion image and in isolation it is not very useful for diagnostic purposes.

ADC values are usually inversely proportional to the degree of restriction. Area of restricted diffusion is seen as hyperintense on diffusion weighted images and hypointense on ADC and vice versa.

Another way to remove the T2 effect on the diffusion weighted image is generating an exponential image which is done by calculating the ratio of diffusion weighted image and b 0 image.[10] Contrary to ADC map, hyperintensity on the exponential image corresponds to hypointensity on ADC map and suggests diffusion restriction and vice versa.

DWI SEQUENCES AND OPTIMIZATION

Many sequences are altered to introduce the diffusion gradient pair for the development of DWI sequences. Some of the most commonly used sequences are discussed here.

Echo Planar Imaging

Although echo planar imaging (EPI) was initially proposed by Mansfield in 1978, it is the recent advancements in MR hardware and reconstruction software that made this sequence useful for clinical studies. It is an extremely fast technique which can fill the entire k space in single shot. It is robust and insensitive to motion artifacts which made it useful in DWI. After the initial excitation pulse, diffusion gradient pair, a series of fast gradient oscillations is applied for read-out and the entire k-space is filled with a long echo train **(Fig. 2)**. This can be implemented as spin echo EPI or gradient echo EPI. Typically, separate acquisition is done for 3 orthogonal axes which are averaged into one final image. One of the disadvantages of EPI is significant phase shift gets accumulated between the water and fat protons and this leads to geometric distortion along the phase encoding direction.[6] As a result the fat signals can be off-set by many pixels which will deteriorate the image quality, more so in higher field strengths. So, it is of paramount importance that all EPI sequences are done with fat suppression. There are various methods of fat suppression such as water only excitation, chemical fat suppression, short-tau inversion recovery (STIR) and spectral selection attenuated inversion recovery (SPAIR) of which the latter two are inversion recovery sequences. SPAIR is a very good method of fat suppression for small FOV in which the fat suppression is uniform along with good SNR. For larger FOV, STIR is the best method to provide uniform suppression but at the cost of reduced SNR. Another disadvantage of EPI is that in longer echo train the water protons tend to show phase shift especially in the air-soft tissue and bone-soft tissue interfaces resulting in geometric distortion in the phase encoding direction.[9] This can be reduced by using parallel imaging and high performance gradient coils which will shorten the echo train length, echo spacing and the read-out time. Another problem with single shot EPI is limited spatial resolution in the order of 128 × 128 because of the rapid signal decay and limited SNR. These problems can also be reduced by splitting the acquisition into more than one excitation. This is a challenge if it has to be implemented in body imaging where motion is an important consideration. For body diffusion several approaches are followed which are discussed here. First approach is to perform a single shot acquisition with breath-hold in which the disadvantages are the poor spatial resolution, limited number of b values, less number of averages and less anatomical coverage. Poor SNR can lead to unreliable ADC values. Second approach is acquisition across multiple excitations with respiratory/cardiac trigger. This overcomes the problems with single shot breath-hold technique. However, triggers cannot totally rule-out motion artifacts and the imaging time gets prolonged. Third approach is free breathing technique with multiple averages and can use multiple b values.[11] Regarding the choice of b values it is a balance between the accuracy of quantification and contrast resolution in the diffusion image (vide supra). One of the recent breakthroughs in EPI sequence for DWI is in the way the k space is filled during acquisition. Because of the long echo train in EPI sequence the output image suffers from artifacts due to T2* decay, susceptibility and phase shift. By segmenting the k space in to multiple columns and each column is filled by a separate shot (TR) the echo train length is considerably shortened thereby reducing the artifacts. This technique is called as read-out segmented EPI (rs-EPI).[12,13] In addition implementation of parallel imaging and compressed sensing in the sequence will have synergistic effect on better outcome. It can reduce the artifacts caused by tissue-air or tissue-bone interfaces.

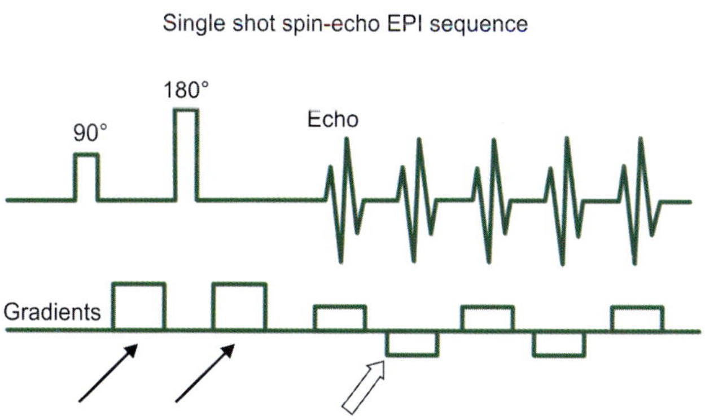

FIG. 2: Schematic representation of DW spin echo EPI sequence showing the motion probing gradients (arrows) used to detect the diffusion of water molecules and multiple gradient oscillations (outlined arrow) to generate echoes. In this single shot sequence, the entire k space is filled in single excitation.

Turbo Spin Echo Sequences or Half-fourier-acquisition Single-shot Turbo-spin-echo

This is an alternative to DW-EPI sequence and it is also relatively insensitive to motion and can perform a single shot read-out and the entire k-space is filled in single excitation. An important difference from EPI is that 180° refocusing pulse is applied during each read-out so that the phase shift accumulation because of long echo train is avoided **(Fig. 3)**. This reduces the geometric distortion and susceptibility artifacts. Apart from this it has other disadvantages of single shot EPI sequence. Parallel imaging can improve the spatial resolution and reduction of geometric distortions. This sequence can also be segmented into multishot acquisition which has similar advantages as multishot EPI.

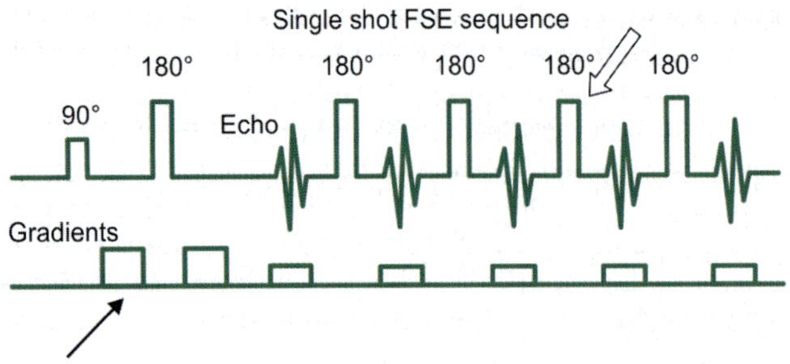

FIG. 3: Schematic representation of single shot fast spin echo sequence showing motion probing gradients (arrow) to detect the water diffusion. Multiple 180° refocusing pulses (outlined arrow) rather than gradient oscillations are used to generate echoes. In contrast to SE-EPI sequence, the use of refocusing pulses avoid the accumulation of phase shifts thereby reducing artifacts. This is also a fast sequence which is capable of acquiring the entire image in single excitation.

Steady-state Free-precession

Steady-state free-precession (SSFP) is also a fast sequence so it is relatively insensitive to motion. It is an atypical diffusion sequence in comparison to the above two with regard to the usage of diffusion sensitizing gradients. Here, both the dephasing and the rephasing gradients are not applied in the same repetition time. They are applied in different repetition times (TR) and not necessarily in the immediately following (TR). Consequently, it is almost impossible to quantitate the diffusion using this sequence. However, the contrast resolution is excellent so that it can be used for qualitative assessment of images. Recently, 3D diffusion weighted sequences have also been developed.

ARTIFACTS AND PITFALLS

There are many artifacts and pitfalls which are inherent to the technique itself, so it is very important for the radiologists and the technicians to be aware of those. In this chapter we will discuss few of the important ones which are relevant to clinical practice.

T2 Shine Through

This is one of the well-known phenomenon which can potentially lead to a wrong diagnosis when diffusion weighted images are interpreted in isolation. It is because DW sequence is based on a T2-weighted sequence and its effects are shown in the final image. It is very prominent in low b value images where the T2 effects predominate. For example, simple cysts in which diffusion is not restricted are seen as hyperintense structure on DW images. The ADC map or exponential images can help to overcome this pitfall since both of them eliminate the T2 effect in the image and represent diffusion characteristics only **(Fig. 1)**. In the above example of simple cyst the ADC map will show hyperintensity because of unrestricted diffusion. At the same time when the lesion is hyperintense on T2-weighted images and hypointense on ADC, the hyperintensity in DW images will get accentuated.[6] When multiple b value images are available then the hyperintensity which is due to T2 effect decreases with increase in b value whereas the hyperintensity due to diffusion is retained.

T2 Washout

This phenomenon is seen when the T2 hyperintensity is balanced by the increase in ADC in the DW image.[14] This is usually seen in vasogenic edema in which there is increase in ADC because of increased diffusivity and that effect is balanced by the T2 hyperintensity. Thus in the DW image the lesion appears isointense. Again this effect can be circumvented by interpreting DW images along with ADC map in which the lesion appears hyperintense **(see Fig. 1)**.

T2 Blackout

This effect is noted when the T2 hypointensity is reflected on the DW image as hypointensity **(see Fig. 1)**. It is usually seen in hematoma which is seen as T2 hypointensity because of susceptibility effect.[15,16]

Eddy Current Artifacts

Eddy current artifact is worth mentioning here because it is commonly associated with EPI sequences which is the most common sequence used for DWI. Eddy Currents are produced in the patient body and in the scanner hardware by rapidly changing magnetic gradients which are used in EPI sequence for sensing diffusion and readout. This can cause image distortion, spatial blurring and misregistration artifacts. This necessitates post processing of the data before ADC calculation to prevent quantification errors.[17] This artifact can also be reduced by using proper shielding in the hardware.

Susceptibility Artifacts

This is also commonly seen in EPI sequences at the bone-soft tissue or air-soft tissue interface like close to skull base, sinuses, mastoids, bowel and lung bases. This leads to accumulation of phase shifts which are more pronounced in the phase encoding direction. This gets even worse if the matrix size is increased because of prolonged readout time. This can be reduced by using DW-HASTE sequences in which the phase shifts are periodically corrected or by using multi-shot acquisition or by using parallel imaging so that the readout time is reduced.

Chemical Shift Artifacts

Usually in conventional spin-echo sequences the effect of difference in precession frequency of water and fat protons are seen along the frequency encoding direction. Whereas in EPI sequences the artifact is seen along the phase encoding direction and it is very prominent again because of accumulation of phase shifts during longer readouts. This can be prevented by using effective fat suppression techniques (vide supra).

Motion Artifacts

Motion artifacts are due to gross patient movement or cardiac/respiratory/bowel motion. Although the currently available single shot techniques are fast enough to avoid motion artifacts, multishot techniques suffer from motion in body imaging. This can be reduced by using cardiac/

respiratory triggered sequences, parallel imaging, propeller or high amplitude gradients.[2]

Effect of Contrast Media

The gadolinium-based contrast media used for MR imaging can have an effect on the diffusion parameters especially in kidneys where they are concentrated by causing paramagnetic effects locally. Recent evidence suggests that the ADC values of kidneys can be significantly lower in the post contrast image than the pre-contrast image. Similar effects were not found in the liver, pancreas and spleen.[18]

ADVANCED DWI TECHNIQUES

Diffusion Tensor Imaging

There are newer techniques such as diffusion tensor imaging (DTI) which have both magnitude and the directional information of diffusion also. The DTI is extensively studied in brain where it is used to show the white matter tracts. It uses the property of anisotropy of diffusion of water molecules. Because of the myelinated axons in the brain white matter, the diffusion is unhindered along the direction of the fiber which is called diffusion anisotropy. Diffusion information given by the DWI is a scalar quantity which lacks the directional component. To obtain the directional component gradient lobes are used in multiple directions and the resulting data is processed. As a result each voxel has the effective direction of diffusion which is called as Eigen vector and the value of diffusion in that direction is called as Eigen value. This information is used to reconstruct fiber tract network in the brain which is called as tractography. Although this tensor model holds good in many situations, it can be limited if there are crossing fibers with different direction of diffusion in a voxel. So there are newer approaches to overcome this limitation such as high angular resolution diffusion imaging (HARDI) which can be used to study the complex diffusion process.

Whole Body Diffusion-weighted Imaging

There is evidence that whole body diffusion weighted imaging along with anatomical images such as T1 and T2 can be very useful for the evaluation of malignant tumors.[2,19] The DWIBS is a whole body diffusion technique which is done typically using DW-EPI sequence and STIR for fat suppression. It is a free breathing technique in which the scans are usually taken from the skull base till the level of mid-thigh. Acquisition is done in multiple stations using multiple thin slices and a large number of signals are collected and averaged. Typically, b value in the range of 1000 is used which will provide good background suppression. But, more than one b value can be used if quantification is needed at the expense of time. These multiple slices are fused and usually displayed in inverted grayscale with white background similar to PET images. It can be visualized as radial projections of MIP in coronal plane. Because of the high b value, body fat muscle and most of the organs gets suppressed which highlights the abnormal areas. However, normal structures with restricted diffusion, such as spleen, lymph nodes, uterus, ovary and testis can be seen. The MIP images should always be interpreted along with the source images because improper fat suppression can lead to pseudotumor appearance. One disadvantage of this technique is long acquisition time. It has been shown to perform as well as PET/CT in the evaluation of tumors such as lymphoma and non-small cell lung cancer.[20] The DWIBS is a non-invasive technique without the use of radiation and has a huge potential in oncologic imaging.

Intravoxel Incoherent Motion

Intravoxel incoherent motion (IVIM) was initially described by Le Bihan in 1980s.[8,21] They described D* as pseudo-diffusion coefficient which is dependent on capillary perfusion. The IVIM is based on the fact that the diffusion imaging at low b values (b 0-100) will have the effect of both the tissue perfusion (pseudo-diffusion) and the true diffusion. In fact at low b values the pseudo-diffusion predominates. This effect gets reduced at high b values where the true diffusion predominates. This is one proposed reason for decrease in ADC values with increase in b value. In a normally perfused tissue at low b value the motion of water molecules because of blood perfusion in tortuous capillary network adds to the actual water diffusion. So acquiring images at increasing b values would enable us to quantify the perfusion in a tissue non-invasively. Since IVIM is very sensitive to motion and other sequence related artifacts it should be performed with single shot EPI sequence and high performance hardware. The current model available in most of the commercial scanners for the calculation of ADC is based on monoexponential function, considering that the logarithm of relative signal intensity plotted against the b value is a straight line which is not true.[22] So ADC calculated with the monoexponential fit would have a component of microcapillary perfusion in addition to true diffusion especially with low b values. The IVIM model suggests that the relationship between the signal intensity and b value is not monoexponential (Gaussian) rather biexponential (non-Gaussian). Based on the IVIM model there is evidence that shows that DWI is sensitive to tissue perfusion and this potential can be applied to obtain the tissue perfusion assessment in addition to diffusion measurement.[22-25] Although still in experimental stage, IVIM technique has been studied extensively in the last few years and has yielded promising result. It has been shown to differentiate low grade brain tumors from high grade tumors and shown to differentiate benign focal lesions from malignant lesions in liver.[26,27] In addition, it has also been used as a biomarker in assessing response to therapy in bone tumors.[28,29]

Histogram Analysis of ADC

Usually ADC value is calculated by drawing region of interest (ROI) which will typically provide mean or median ADC value of the region. Recently attempts have been made to use histogram based analysis of ADC values. In this, the ADC values across a region can be represented as histograms, i.e. frequency of voxels having the ADC values.[30] This will provide better understanding of heterogeneity of the lesion. It generally, utilizes volumetric evaluation of the lesion so that all the voxels of the lesion from different slices are evaluated rather than a selected ROI. The ADC calculation by this method is reproducible because the entire lesion is analyzed and the errors in ROI placement are reduced. Histogram analysis can provide various useful metrics, such as percentiles, kurtosis and skewness of distribution of ADC values which will provide better insights into the pattern of distribution. Comparison of these metrics based on histogram analysis between the pre- and post-treatment imaging can evaluate the response to therapy. The process of extracting quantitative data from the trace and ADC images of DWI using histogram analysis or sophisticated algorithms which can extract quantitative grayscale features is called texture analysis. These features are often based on the distribution of voxel values in the images which are not apparent to naked eye. More elaborate discussion on texture analysis will be covered elsewhere in the book.

Diffusion Kurtosis Imaging

Diffusion of water molecules in a homogeneous solution follows a Gaussian distribution whereas diffusion of water molecules in biological tissues actually follows a non-Gaussian distribution.[31] This difference in distribution is because of cellular microstructure (cell membranes and organelles) which alter the water diffusion.[16] The modern MRI scanners can generate DW images with b values more than 2000. Diffusion signals at high b values are predominated by non-Gaussian distribution which can be depicted using a sophisticated model known as diffusion kurtosis imaging (DKI). This model is getting widespread popularity and it provide unique insight into the intracellular organelles and their environment. DKI can reflect the intracellular changes such as nuclear cytoplasmic ratio and intracellular heterogeneity. They provide information which can be clinically relevant in oncological imaging. The DKI model for high b value DW images provide two quantitative parameters namely diffusion (D) and apparent diffusional kurtosis (K). Parameter D correlates with the diffusion of water molecules and it is claimed to be more accurate compared to ADC. Whereas parameter K does not have any direct biophysical correlate. It is a measure of deviation between mono-exponential model of diffusion (Gaussian) and DKI model (non-Gaussian). There are emerging applications in the field of oncoimaging. It has been used successfully to differentiate benign from malignant lesions in prostate and to differentiate low grade tumors from high grade tumors.[32-34] In addition there are emerging reports in liver, renal and breast imaging highlighting the potential benefits of DKI.[35,36] There are other few reports in the literature stating that there is no additional benefit of DKI over monoexponential model of DWI.[37]

Computed DWI

High b value diffusion weighted images have higher contrast resolution and lesser T2 shine through effect which can be helpful in lesion detection.[38] However, acquiring high b value images requires a capable scanner with high field strength and longer acquisition time. It will also lead to loss of SNR and can introduce motion artifacts. To overcome these challenges, one can compute any b value DW image with the help of the acquired low b value images and the ADC values. The principle of computed DWI is based on the mono, bi or tri-exponential model where in the assumption is that all the data points of acquired b value images fall in a straight line on the signal intensity curve. Hence, if any two b value images are available, ADC can be calculated and by simple extrapolation any high b value images can also be generated.[38] Since it is a mathematically computed image it is prone to artifacts due to misregistration (motion related) which needs proper image registration to be performed before calculation. There can be outlier values because of the artifacts in input images which needs to be taken care of. The benefits of computed DWI are that images of any arbitrary b value can be generated without actually acquiring them, provides better contrast resolution, reduces acquisition time and T2 shine through artifacts.

CLINICAL APPLICATIONS OF DWI

Although initially DWI was established and successfully used in neuroimaging, recent developments in the sequence protocols and their optimization, hardware enhancements and improvements in software have made this technique a robust tool for body imaging also.

Brain

DWI has become a gold standard in imaging of stroke to identify the infarct core mainly because of its ability to detect the infarcted area within minutes after the onset of symptoms, much earlier than other MRI sequences and CT can show changes.[39] DWI is highly sensitive (81–100%) and specific (86–100%) in detecting the ischemic area within 12 hours of symptom onset.[16] It is also superior to FLAIR and T2-weighted sequences in detecting small area of infarct and has the ability to differentiate acute infarct from old lesions and non-specific white matter changes **(Figs. 4A to C)**. Those areas which show diffusion abnormality usually progress to infarction unless early thrombolysis therapy is started. The area of diffusion abnormality also correlates well with the final clinical outcome thereby directing appropriate management for patients. The DWI and ADC parameters are used for the prediction of hemorrhagic transformation of infarct.[16] The diffusion imaging in brain is further enhanced by newer sophisticated techniques such as diffusion tensor imaging (DTI) and diffusion kurtosis imaging (DKI) (vide supra). They give additional information regarding the microstructural status of the brain tissue which will help in better understanding of the disease process.[40] It also has an important role in brain tumor imaging as well. It helps in characterization of tumors and their response assessment to treatment. Solid gliomas which show low ADC values are associated with higher grade.[41] Similarly, medulloblastoma and rhabdoid tumors have been shown to have low ADC values compared to ependymoma and astrocytoma in posterior fossa.[40] The DTI also has a proven role in the preoperative assessment of brain tumors. Response of brain tumors after chemoradiation is assessed by DWI. Changes in ADC values in the first few weeks after the therapy are found to be noninvasive biomarkers for response to therapy and it can be used for prognostication also.[42,43]

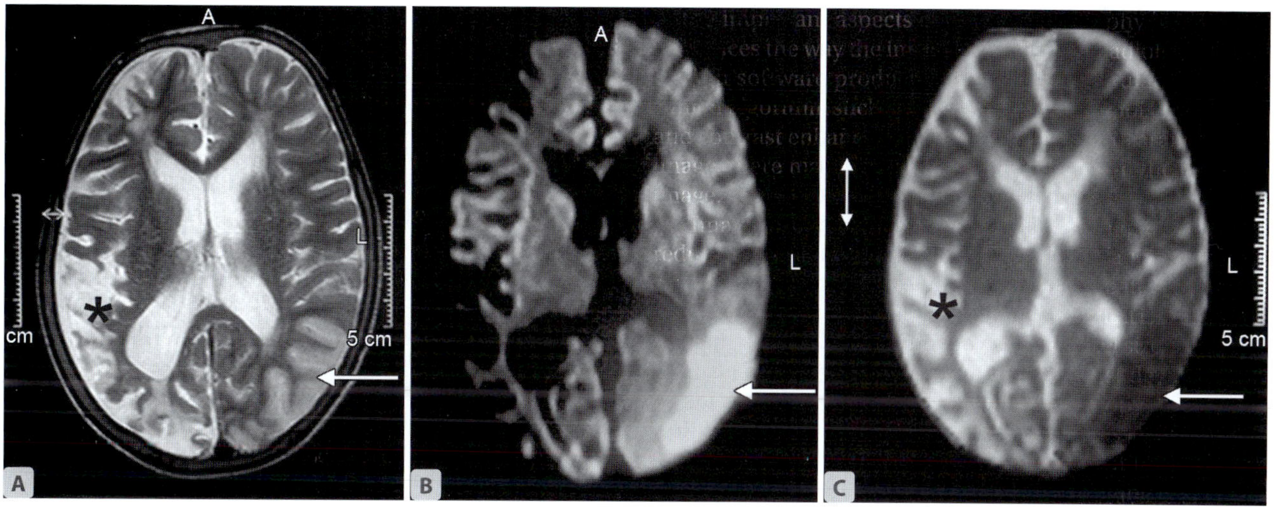

FIGS. 4A TO C: T2W axial image (A) of brain shows mild gyral hyperintensity (arrow) and swelling seen in the left parieto-occipital cortex. Multifocal areas of hyperintensities (*) seen in right cerebral hemisphere with associated volume loss suggestive of chronic infarct. DW-EPI sequence with b value of 1000 in axial plane (B) shows a brightly hyperintense area (arrow) which on ADC map (C) shows hypointensity (arrow). The above features are suggestive of acute infarct on the left side. ADC map also shows multifocal hyperintensity in right cerebral hemisphere suggestive of facilitated diffusion. As depicted in this case, DWI along with ADC can be very useful for the chronological dating of infarcts.

Head and Neck

DWI has potential to differentiate pleomorphic adenoma from other benign and malignant lesions of parotid gland.[44] Because of the presence of glandular component and fluid these tumors show significantly higher ADC value than Warthin tumors which have hypercellular stroma.[44] It can differentiate sinonasal malignant lesions from benign lesions because in the former ADC is lower. The ADC values can also be used to characterize a tumor, for instance it can differentiate squamous cell carcinoma (SCC) from lymphoma. The lymphoma usually shows low ADC values compared to SCC because of the hypercellular nature.[45,46] The limitation of its use is that some malignant lesions like chondrosarcoma can have high ADC values.[44] Prediction of tumor grading can be done by ADC values as poorly differentiated solid lesions show low ADC values compared to well differentiated lesions. By differentiating necrotic area from viable tumor it can also help to identify areas from where biopsy can be performed.[44,47] In the assessment of tumor response to therapy one of the major limitations of PET is that it is sensitive to inflammatory changes also. The DWI has the potential to overcome this difficulty because the inflammatory lesions show high ADC values whereas tumor tissue would show low ADC values. So it can be used as a surrogate marker to assess the tumor response very early during therapy. ADC values in SCC have been shown to significantly change even after the first week of treatment and the complete responders show higher increase in ADC when compared to partial responders.[48] There is a recent study which evaluated the role of DWI in the orbit and suggested that it may help to differentiate pseudotumor from lymphoma and cellulitis which is again based on the fact that lymphoma shows low ADC compared to pseudotumor and cellulitis.[49] The DWI can reliably differentiate necrosis within a tumor from abscess formation. Abscess shows very low ADC because of the presence of macromolecules and increased viscosity.

Pediatric Applications

The use of ionizing radiation in children is a concern because of long term effects, so DWI can be an alternate technique in this age group. The DWI does not involve the use of contrast media so it can be used whenever contrast enhanced imaging is not possible because of deranged renal function. Experience of DWI in pediatric imaging is limited but promising. The ADC values can be used to detect malignant tumors, characterize them and assess the treatment response. Studies have been done in variety of pediatric tumors and they found that DWI performed better or similar to conventional MR imaging.[50,51] In our experience on hepatoblastoma, it was found that MRI especially DWI performed better than multiphase CT scan in showing additional metastases in liver which influenced the management of those children.

Thorax

DWI in thorax needs faster sequences with high performance gradients and parallel imaging techniques along with phased array coils. The low proton density in lung and magnetic field inhomogeneity makes quantitative DWI even more challenging. Usually, two b values are used and STIR is used for fat suppression especially if quantification is needed. It can be done in breath-holding or free breathing with respiratory and cardiac triggers. Studies have used various methods such as qualitative, semi-quantitative and quantitative to differentiate malignant lesions from benign lesions.[4] In qualitative method the intensity of the lesion is compared with the intensity of spinal cord or chest wall muscle and the malignant lesions are usually hyperintense to spinal cord or chest wall muscles. In semi-quantitative analysis, the ratio of the signal intensity of the lesion and the signal intensity of the reference structure is used to characterize the lesion. The quantitative analysis depends on the ADC measurement of the lesion itself.

Most of the work has been done in lung carcinoma. Studies have shown that the ADC of the malignant lesions is usually lower than the benign lesions and small cell carcinoma which has closely packed cells shows lower ADC when compared to non-small cell carcinoma although overlap may occur. At the same time small metastatic nodules, inflammatory nodules and fibrotic nodules cannot be reliably differentiated.[52] In case of collapsed lung it is very difficult on routine imaging to delineate the tumor boundary. DWI has been used successfully to delineate the tumor from the collapsed lung.[53] DWI has also been used to characterize the mediastinal nodes in patients with carcinoma lung.[54,55] The ADC values of malignant nodes were significantly lower than that of benign nodes. Another potential application of DWI is in the evaluation of tumor response after therapy.

Breast

Contrast enhanced MRI of the breast is an established technique in the diagnosis of carcinoma breast with sensitivity of 89–100% and specificity of 72%.[20] Several studies have attempted to use DWI to differentiate malignant lesions from benign. There are no uniform b values or calculation methods used by the investigators which have resulted in different ADC cut-off values. Generally, the malignant lesions showed lower ADC values when compared with benign lesions **(Figs. 5A to D)**. But there is significant overlap between the two groups.[4] Lesions with fibrotic components, such as fibroadenoma and fibrocystic disease can result in low ADC values leading to diagnostic difficulty. Many optimizations were proposed including normalization of ADC of the lesion to the ADC of ipsilateral glandular parenchyma which would eliminate the ADC variations because of scanning parameters and effects of menstrual cycle.[56] This approach has been shown to improve the diagnostic accuracy. Efforts have been made to use DWI

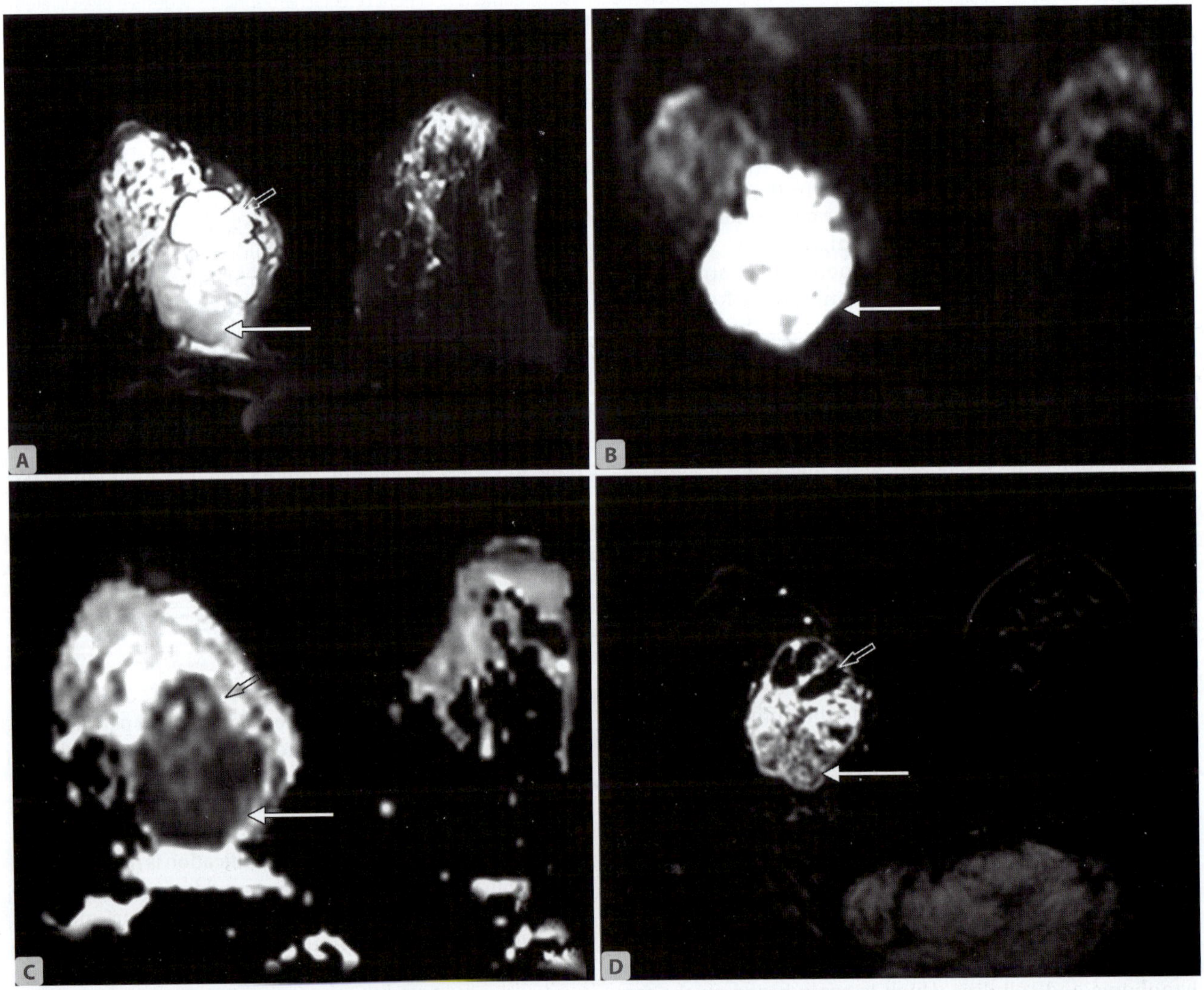

FIGS. 5A TO D: Axial T2W sequence of bilateral breasts (A) shows a hypointense mass lesion (arrow) in the right breast. It also shows areas of necrosis (outlined arrow) within. Diffusion weighted sequence with b value of 1000 (B) shows a markedly hyperintense lesion (arrow) with good background suppression of other structures making the lesion more conspicuous. ADC map (C) shows hypointensity (arrow) suggesting marked restriction of diffusion consistent with a highly cellular mass. Few areas show facilitated diffusion (outlined arrow) consistent with necrosis. These findings are also confirmed on subtracted postcontrast T1 fat suppressed image (D). Histopathology showed infiltrating ductal carcinoma.

in addition to dynamic contrast enhanced imaging and this has also been shown to improve diagnostic accuracy.[20] DWI has been used to grade the tumor, predict the histological type and to better evaluate the local extent of the tumor. Recently, many studies have been published regarding the role of DWI in the evaluation of response to treatment. Decrease in size of the lesion as response criteria is not an optimal parameter since it takes a long time to show a significant difference. Chemotherapeutic agents are toxic and they have various side effects which necessitates earlier assessment of response. Studies have shown that the increase in ADC value in comparison with the pretreatment value can be used as a non-invasive biomarker of disease response.[57,58] Using the change in ADC values, response can be evaluated as early as after the first cycle of chemotherapy and it has been found that the increase in ADC values was significantly more in responders than in non-responders.

Liver

It is challenging to apply DWI in any abdominal organ mainly because of the respiratory motion and susceptibility. The Liver is one of the most studied organs in abdomen using DWI. The Liver parenchyma shows relatively short T2 relaxation times, so the b values and the TE of the sequence should be optimized accordingly. Too high b value might cause unacceptable signal suppression which is because of long T2 time rather than diffusion characteristics itself. Usually, the recommended b values are 0, 100 and 500.[3] Presence of branching vessels within the liver parenchyma poses a difficulty in the detection of small focal lesions. In black blood DWI images, the vessels are suppressed so that the lesion detection is relatively easier especially on low b values. At the same time lesion characterization is better done on high b value images. To support this studies have shown that DWI is better than fat suppressed T2-weighted sequences.[59,60] DWI can be applied as a useful adjunct or can be used as a reasonable alternative to contrast enhanced images for the evaluation of the liver metastasis.[61,62] Hemangioma and simple cysts show significantly high ADC values that they can be reliably differentiated from hepatocellular carcinoma (HCC) and metastasis which show low ADC values **(Figs. 6 and 7)**. However, benign solid lesions like hepatic adenoma and focal nodular hyperplasia can have overlapping values which cannot be reliably differentiated from malignant lesions.[3,20] Similarly, malignant lesions which are necrotic and mucinous tumors can have high ADC values and can mimic benign lesions on DWI. Diagnosis and detection of HCC and dysplastic nodules in a cirrhotic liver is very difficult based on ADC values because the diffusion is as it is restricted in cirrhotic liver as a result of fibrosis. As in other tumors, DWI has a role in the evaluation

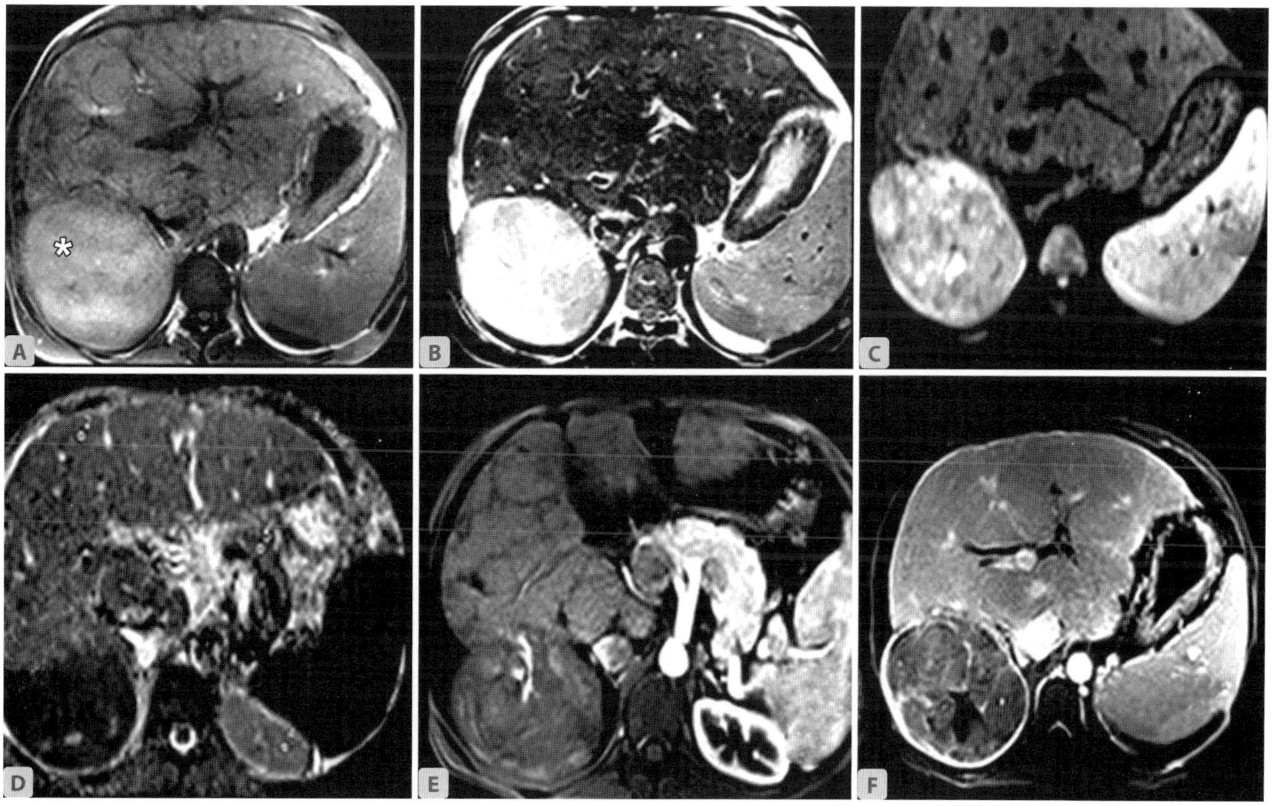

FIGS. 6A TO F: Axial T1W GRE sequence (A) shows an exophytic mildly hyperintense lesion (*) arising from the right lobe of liver. Rest of the liver is showing features of chronic liver disease. Lesion is markedly hyperintense on T2W sequence (B). DW image with b value of 500 (C) shows the hyperintense lesion which on ADC map (D) shows marked diffusion restriction suggestive of hypercellular tumor. With these findings along with arterial enhancement in post contrast T1W image (E) and capsule formation in delayed post contrast image (F), diagnosis of hepatocellular carcinoma was made.

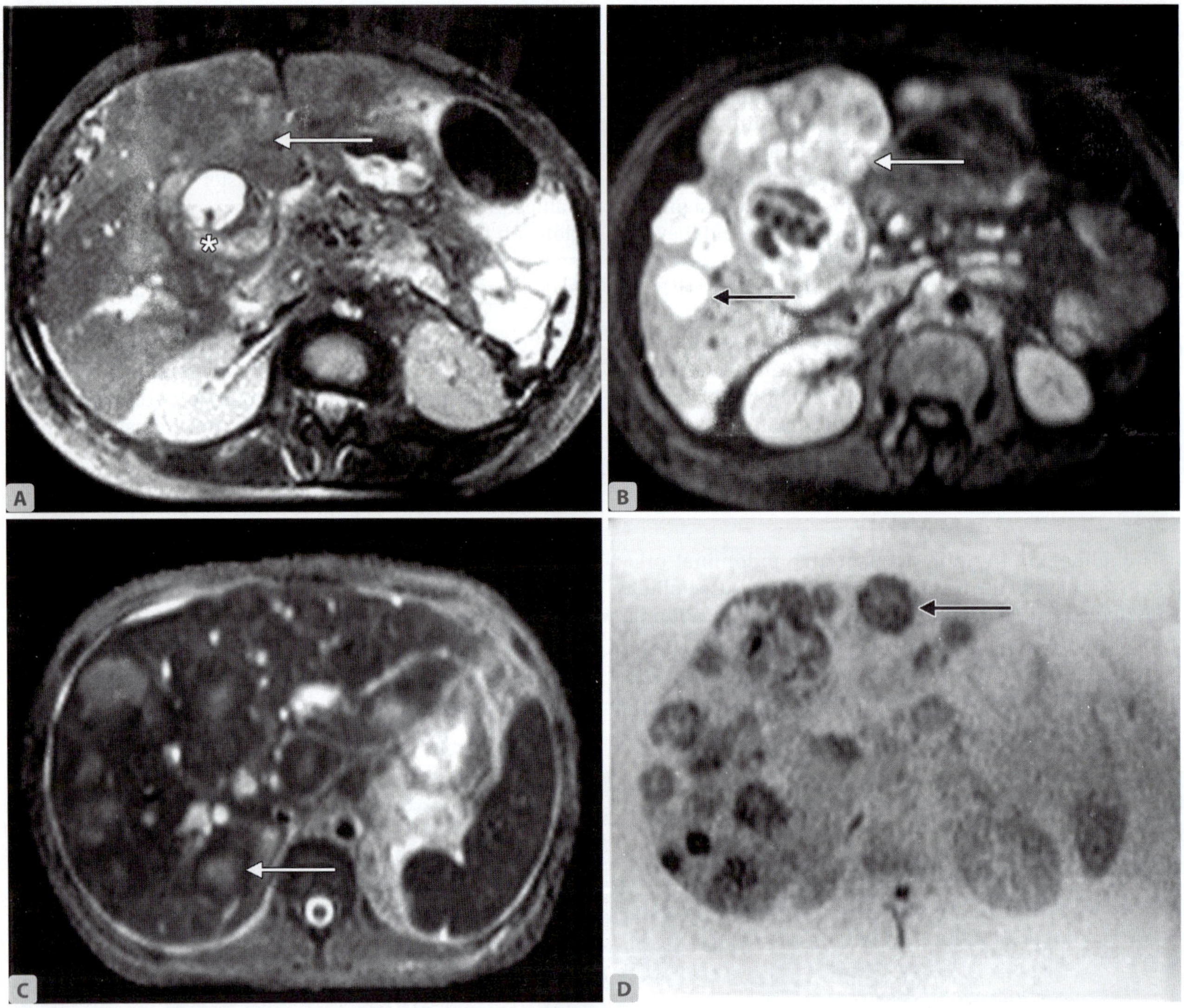

FIGS. 7A TO D: Axial T2W sequence (A) shows a mass lesion involving the gallbladder (*) with adjacent liver infiltration. Calculi were also noted in the gallbladder. Multiple subtle hyperintense lesions (arrow) in both lobes of liver seen suggestive of metastases. DW sequence with b value of 500 (B) shows these focal lesions (arrows) much better than the T2W sequence. ADC map (C) also shows multiple focal lesions (arrow) which are showing restricted diffusion in the periphery of the lesion. Most lesions on ADC map show central hyperintensity suggestive of necrosis. DW sequence with b value of 1000 displayed in inverted grayscale (D) shows multiple metastatic lesions (arrow) with very good background suppression which is comparable to positron emission tomography (PET) image.

of tumor response and it has been shown to demonstrate significantly more ADC changes in responders than in non-responders. In addition, the pretreatment high ADC values have been correlated with poorer response to therapy. It is well known that ADC values are low in cirrhotic liver and a recent study showed that ADC values correlated well with US elastography and serum markers for moderate and severe fibrosis.[63]

Gallbladder and Biliary Ducts

There is emerging evidence that DWI can be helpful in differentiating malignant gallbladder lesions from benign. Malignant lesions tend to show high signal intensity on DWI and low ADC values compared to benign lesions.[64] It can distinguish adherent or tumefactive sludge from gallbladder malignancy. A recent study has shown that DWI performed better than conventional MRCP in the detection of extrahepatic cholangiocarcinoma.[65]

Pancreas

ADC values of pancreas have been shown to vary with age of the patient and the location in pancreas. With increase in age pancreas undergoes atrophy, fatty replacement and fibrosis which is proposed to be a cause for change in ADC.[66,67] The ADC values of head and body of the pancreas is shown to be significantly more than the tail of pancreas.[67] Carcinoma of pancreas shows low ADC values compared to the rest of normal pancreas and the ADC values depend on the histological characteristics as well. However, there is overlap of ADC values of carcinoma pancreas with focal pancreatitis because of which their distinction is difficult. Cystic lesions of pancreas such as pseudocysts, simple cysts show a relatively high ADC values compared to pancreatic abscesses, hydatid cysts and cystic neoplasms.[68]

Kidneys and Adrenal

DWI has been successfully used in differentiating malignant renal lesions from benign lesions. Renal cysts show high ADC values than the normal parenchyma and other solid lesions **(Figs. 8A to E)**. Among the cysts, those with T1 hyperintensity show lower ADC than those which are T1 hypointense.[69] This has been attributed to the presence of blood or proteinaceous content which can alter diffusion and the same can be helpful in differentiating simple cysts from necrotic neoplasms. Recent studies have shown DWI can be helpful in characterization of renal malignant masses and ADC values can be used to predict the histological subtype and tumor grades of renal cell carcinoma.[70,71] The ADC values of clear cell type renal cell carcinoma were found to be significantly higher than the non clear cell type tumors.[70] Renal Abscesses and infected cysts show low ADC values than other cystic lesions.[72] According to recent studies, DWI is not useful in differentiating benign adrenal lesions from malignant lesions based on ADC values although cysts and to some extent pheochromocytoma showed higher ADC values.[73,74]

Prostate

Prostate is rich in glandular structures which facilitates free diffusion of water. Recent usage of high field strength, advancements in hardware and sequences have made DWI possible in the prostate with good SNR. Several studies have shown that prostate cancer is seen as hyperintense area on DWI and shows hypointensity on corresponding ADC maps.[75] However, there is overlap of ADC values of prostate cancer with focal chronic prostatitis and benign prostatic hyperplasia.[2] There is a significant negative correlation found between the ADC values and the Gleason score which would help in management decisions. DWI is an important component of PIRAD version 2 and it helps in the detection of clinically significant prostate cancers (Gleason score >7) which merit treatment. It is also found to be useful in loco-regional staging and lymph nodal detection.[2] It can be used as a biomarker to assess response in patients who are treated with radiation. The ADC values have been shown to increase in response to therapy.[76] DWI is so robust in prostate imaging that the importance of contrast enhanced dynamic imaging has declined in the last few years and multiparametric imaging for prostate is slowly evolving into biparametric imaging which involves a combination of T2 and DWI sequences.

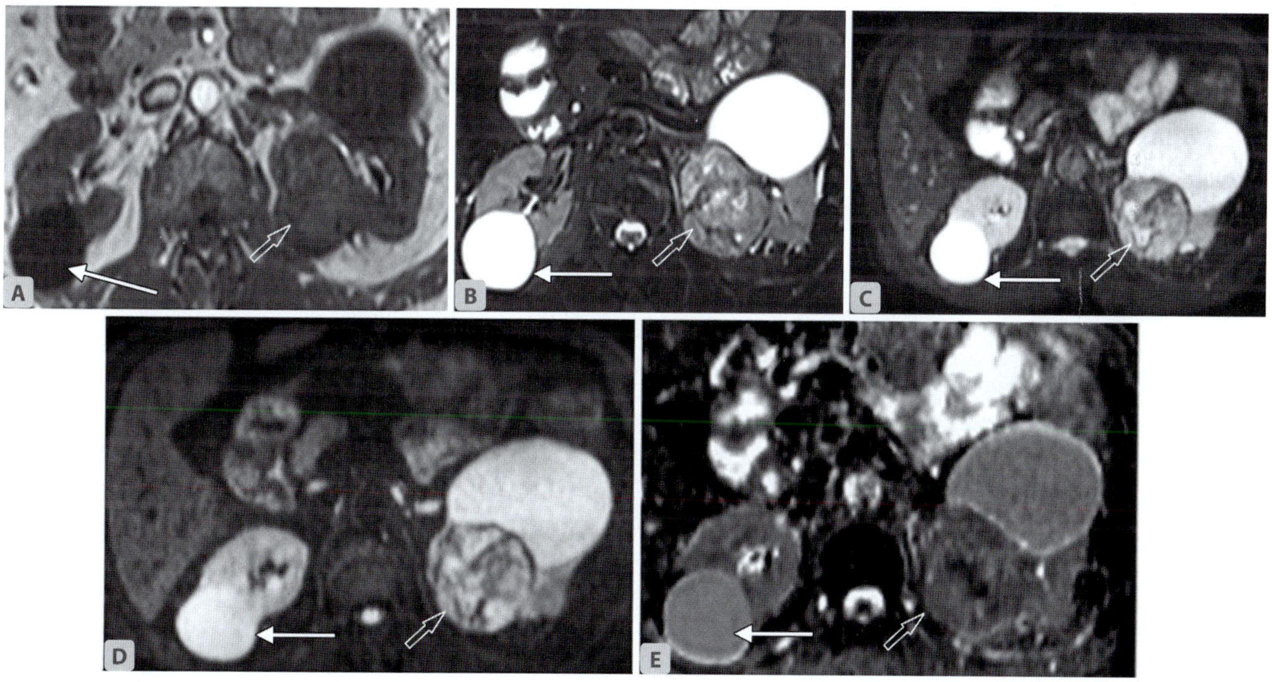

FIGS. 8A TO E: Axial T1W sequence of bilateral kidneys (A) shows hypointense exophytic lesions (arrow) in both the kidneys and an isointense lesion (outlined arrow) in the posterior cortex of left kidney. T2W fat suppressed and DW sequence with b value of 0 (B and C) shows markedly hyperintense lesions (arrow) in both kidneys suggestive of simple cysts whereas the posterior cortex lesion in left kidney (outlined arrow) is isointense to kidney parenchyma. On DW sequence with b value of 500 (D) the simple cysts are loosing signal compared to b 0 image whereas the posterior cortex lesion is retaining signal suggestive of solid nature of the lesion. ADC map (E) shows the cystic lesions as hyperintense to renal parenchyma which is consistent with simple cysts. The solid lesion in the left kidney (outlined arrow) is mildly hypointense to renal parenchyma which is consistent with a hypercellular solid tumor. Solid lesion in the left kidney was proven to be clear cell carcinoma.

Small Bowel and Rectum

MRI has many advantages over CT in terms of evaluation of activity in inflammatory bowel disease (IBD) especially Crohn's disease (CD). Currently MR enterography (MRE) has become the modality of choice along with CT enterography for the evaluation of IBD.[77] Hyperintensity on T2W images, stratified pattern of bowel wall enhancement and mesenteric changes are hallmarks of active disease in IBD. Inclusion of DWI in to MRE protocol **(Figs. 9A to D)** has several advantages such as detecting areas of disease activity and possibility of avoiding contrast administration in patients with deranged renal parameters. It is even more relevant in children and in patients who are undergoing multiple contrast MR studies because of fact that gadolinium deposition has been found in brain and marrow even in patients with normal renal function.[78,79] Another advantage of DWI in MRE is that ADC can be used to quantify inflammation which can be helpful in response evaluation. DWI is more sensitive but less specific in detecting areas of inflammation in CD.[80] DWI has shown comparable sensitivity and specificity in the detection of inflammatory disease in terminal ileum.[81] It has also been shown that ADC parameters correlate well with Magnetic resonance index of activity (MaRIA) score.[82] Apart from IBD, DWI can be used in other inflammatory pathologies such as TB, eosinophilic enteritis etc to detect inflammation.

Rectal carcinoma is another area in bowel imaging where DWI **(Figs. 10A and B)** has shown added benefits to conventional MRI. Its routine use in the restaging of rectal cancer after neoadjuvant chemo-radiotherapy has been recommended by ESGAR consensus guidelines as well.[83] Although MRI is not routinely done as a modality to detect rectal carcinoma, DWI has the capability to detect small tumors which are otherwise missed on imaging. One caveat here is that mucinous rectal cancers do not show diffusion restriction and hence they can be missed on DWI sequences.[84] There is no major role for DWI in the initial local T staging of the tumor, however its additional sensitivity in the detection of pelvic lymph nodes has been widely recognized.[85,86] At the same time the characterisation of nodal lesions is not reliably performed using DWI. DWI performs well in detecting distant metastatic lesions especially to liver. Tumor restaging using DWI has been an important area of research in the last decade and it has been well established that DWI can be used to assess response to therapy by differentiating residual tumor from radiation fibrosis.[87]

Bony Spine

MRI is the modality of choice for the evaluation of bony spine especially the vertebral marrow. The most important sequences used for the evaluation of vertebral marrow are

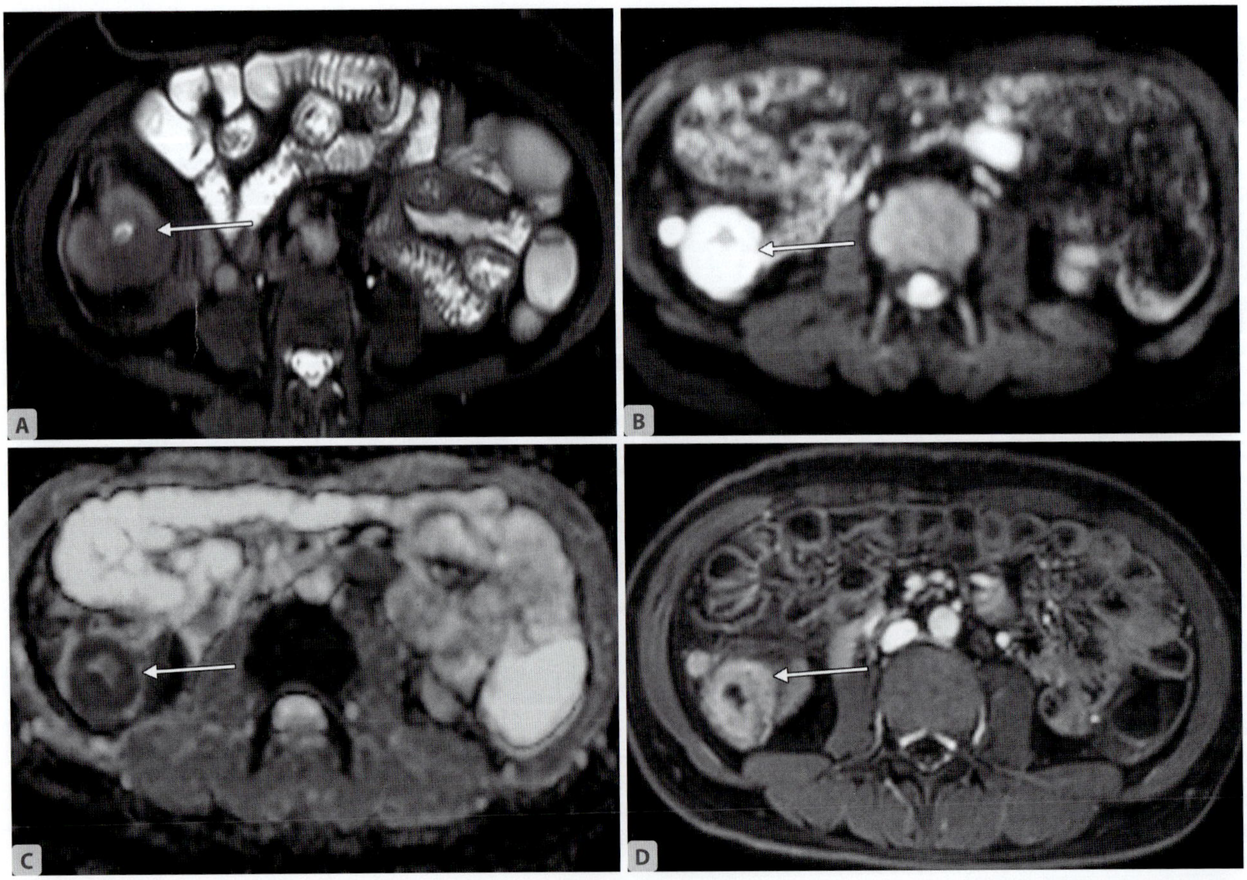

FIGS. 9A TO D: T2W fat saturated sequence (A) in a patient diagnosed with Crohn's disease showing circumferential wall thickening involving ascending colon (thick arrow) which is showing significant diffusion restriction on trace (B) as well as ADC images (C) and contrast enhancement on postcontrast image (D).

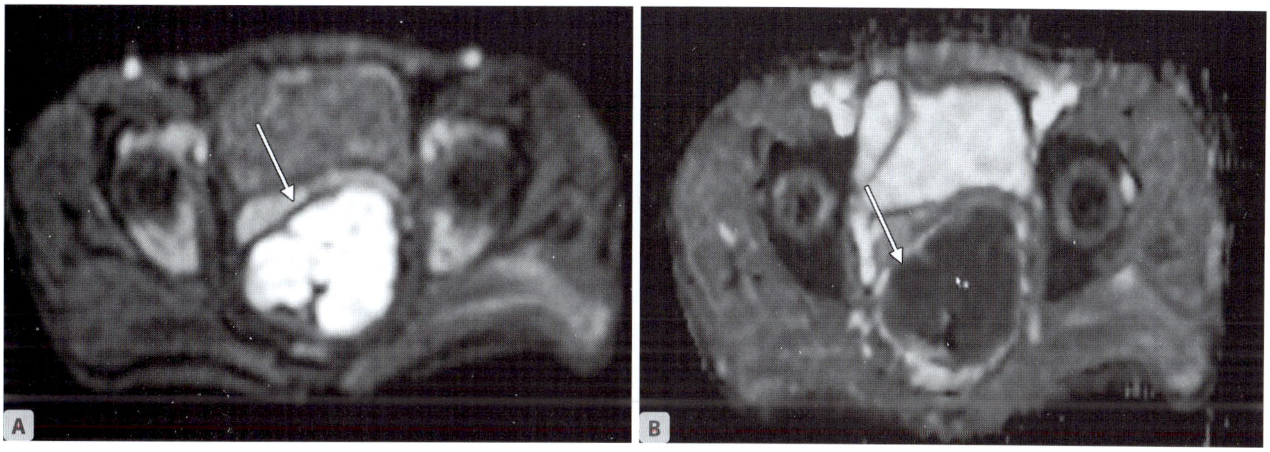

FIGS. 10A AND B: Axial high b value trace image (A) and ADC map (B) showing a rectal mass (arrow) with marked diffusion restriction. Biopsy: Adenocarcinoma.

T1W and T2 fat saturated sequence. Post contrast images have an additive role in the characterization of marrow pathology. In the last decade there has been increasing evidence that DWI can be used in bony spine evaluation. The addition of DWI to the routine sequences increased the sensitivity in the detection of focal lesions.[88] In metastatic lesions and multiple myeloma, DWI increased the lesion detectability and conspicuity compared to conventional sequences. ADC can also be used to characterize these lesions.[89] Another important area where DWI has been extensively studied is the characterization of vertebral collapse. It is challenging on imaging to differentiate osteoporotic from malignant collapse. Although there are contradicting reports regarding the utility of DWI for this purpose, there is literature supporting its role. The normal marrow shows very low ADC ($0.2 - 0.6 \times 10^{-3}$ mm/s) because of the presence of fat.[90] Both osteoporotic as well as malignant lesions show higher ADC compared to the normal marrow. However, the magnitude of rise in ADC is much higher in osteoporotic fracture compared to malignant fracture ($0.7 - 1.3 \times 10^{-3}$ mm/s for malignant and $1.2 - 2.0 \times 10^{-3}$ mm/s for osteoporotic lesions).[90] DWI has been used to assess disease activity in seronegative spondyloarthropathy where higher ADC is a marker of active disease. DWI can also be used to differentiate degenerative Modic 1 changes from infective spondylodiscitis which is otherwise difficult on conventional imaging. The claw sign on DWI trace images which is usually seen as paired hyperintensities seen between the normal and edematous marrow, when present is found to be associated with Modic change rather than spondylodiscitis.[91] DWI of bony spine is technically demanding because of the artifacts due to susceptibility. However, newer sequences such as rs-EPI can provide more reliable and artifact free images.

Female Pelvis

Conventional MRI has an important role in detection and staging of female pelvic malignancies. DWI can be used as an adjunct to it to increase its diagnostic accuracy. Normal endometrium shows varying diffusion characteristics and ADC values during different phases of menstrual cycle. Lowest ADC values are seen at the end of the cycle.[4] This variation should be taken in to account while interpreting the DW images and ADC values. Endometrial carcinoma has been shown to have significantly low ADC value compared to the normal endometrium.[4,20,92] It can show the extent of myometrial invasion which is important in the management especially if contrast media cannot be used. It can differentiate endometrial carcinoma from other benign endometrial lesions such as hyperplasia and polyp. DWI can detect the malignant nodes even though they are normal according to size criteria. Cervical carcinoma is a hypercellular tumor whose ADC values are less than the normal cervical stroma. It can clearly show the depth of invasion in cervix and can also be used for detection of involved nodes allowing to stage the disease more accurately.[93] Because of low ADC value of squamous cell carcinoma, it can be differentiated from adenocarcinoma of cervix. However, there is no clear-cut cut-off value for ADC available in the literature mainly because of variations in the technique and hardware used. There are contradicting reports regarding the potential of DWI to differentiate malignant ovarian lesions from benign lesions.[94,95] However, it improves the detection of peritoneal deposits when combined with a conventional MRI sequences than the latter alone.[96]

CONCLUSION

DWI is an evolving technique that provides a new paradigm for tissue characterization. The quality of DW images has improved significantly across vendors with the use of robust technical advancements like segmented read-out EPI. Its ability to provide both qualitative and quantitative insight in to complex diffusion mechanisms and changes at a cellular level with only a small time penalty have made this technique a valuable addition to clinical MR protocols. However, DW sequences must be interpreted in conjunction with other MR sequences to avoid the pitfalls of this technique.

REFERENCES

1. Bonekamp D, Jacobs MA, El-Khouli R, Stoianovici D, Macura KJ. Advancements in MR imaging of the prostate: from diagnosis to interventions. Radiographics. 2011;31(3):677-703.
2. Malayeri AA, El Khouli RH, Zaheer A, Jacobs MA, Corona-Villalobos CP, Kamel IR, et al. Principles and applications of diffusion-weighted imaging in cancer detection, staging, and treatment follow-up. Radiographics. 2011;31(6): 1773-91.
3. Chandarana H, Taouli B. Diffusion and perfusion imaging of the liver. Eur J Radiol. 2010;76(3):348-58.
4. Türkbey B, Aras Ö, Karabulut N, Turgut AT, Akpınar E, Alibek S, et al. Diffusion-weighted MRI for detecting and monitoring cancer: a review of current applications in body imaging. Diagn Interv Radiol. 2012;18:46-59.
5. Herneth AM, Mayerhoefer M, Schernthaner R, Ba-Ssalamah A, Czerny C, Fruehwald-Pallamar J. Diffusion weighted imaging: lymph nodes. Eur J Radiol. 2010;76(3):398-406.
6. de Figueiredo EH, Borgonovi AFNG, Doring TM. Basic concepts of MR imaging, diffusion MR imaging, and diffusion tensor imaging. Magn Reson Imaging Clin N Am. 2011;19(1):1.
7. Stejskal EO, Tanner JE. Spin diffusion measurements: Spin echoes in the presence of a time-dependent field gradient. J Chem Phys. 1965;42:288.
8. Le Bihan D, Breton E, Lallemand D, Grenier P, Cabanis E, Laval-Jeantet M. MR imaging of intravoxel incoherent motions: application to diffusion and perfusion in neurologic disorders. Radiology. 1986;161(2):401.
9. Dietrich O, Biffar A, Baur-Melnyk A, Reiser MF. Technical aspects of MR diffusion imaging of the body. Eur J Radiol. 2010;76(3): 314-22.
10. Provenzale JM, Engelter ST, Petrella JR, Smith JS, MacFall JR. Use of MR exponential diffusion-weighted images to eradicate T2" shine-through" effect. Am J Roentgenol. 1999;172(2):537-9.
11. Koh DM, Thoeny HC. Diffusion-weighted MR Imaging: Applications in the Body. Springer; 2010.p.299.
12. Xia C, Pu J, Zhang J, Peng W, Li L, Zhao F, et al. Readout-segmented echo-planar diffusion-weighted MR for the evaluation of aggressive characteristics of rectal cancer. Sci Rep. 2018;8(1):12554.
13. Xia C, Liu X, Peng W, Li L, Zhang J, Meng W, et al. Readout-segmented echo-planar imaging improves the image quality of diffusion-weighted MR imaging in rectal cancer: Comparison with single-shot echo-planar diffusion-weighted sequences. Eur J Radiol. 2016;85(10):1818-23.
14. Provenzale JM, Petrella JR, Jr LCHC, Wong JC, Engelter S, Barboriak DP. Quantitative Assessment of Diffusion Abnormalities in Posterior Reversible Encephalopathy Syndrome. Am J Neuroradiol. 2001;22(8):1455-61.
15. Hiwatashi A, Kinoshita T, Moritani T, Wang HZ, Shrier DA, Numaguchi Y, et al. Hypointensity on diffusion-weighted MRI of the brain related to T2 shortening and susceptibility effects. Am J Roentgenol. 2003;181(6):1705-9.
16. Fung SH, Roccatagliata L, Gonzalez RG, Schaefer PW. MR diffusion imaging in ischemic stroke. Neuroimaging Clin N Am. 2011;21(2):345.
17. Haselgrove JC, Moore JR. Correction for distortion of echo-planar images used to calculate the apparent diffusion coefficient. Magn Reson Med. 2005;36(6):960-4.
18. Wang CL, Chea YW, Boll DT, Samei E, Neville AM, Dale BM, et al. Effect of gadolinium chelate contrast agents on diffusion weighted MR imaging of the liver, spleen, pancreas and kidney at 3T. Eur J Radiol. 2011;80(2):e1-7.
19. Takahara T, Imai Y, Yamashita T, Yasuda S, Nasu S, Van Cauteren M. Diffusion weighted whole body imaging with background body signal suppression (DWIBS): technical improvement using free breathing, STIR and high resolution 3D display. Matrix. 2004;160(160):160.
20. Bonekamp S, Corona-Villalobos CP, Kamel IR. Oncologic applications of diffusion-weighted MRI in the body. J Magn Reson Imaging. 2012;35(2):257-79.
21. Le Bihan D, Breton E, Lallemand D. Perfusion in intravoxel incoherent motion mr imaging. Radiology. 1988;168: 497-505.
22. Koh DM, Collins DJ, Orton MR. Intravoxel incoherent motion in body diffusion-weighted MRI: reality and challenges. Am J Roentgenol. 2011;196(6):1351-61.
23. Wang Z, Su MY, Najafi A, Nalcioglu O. Effect of vasodilator hydralazine on tumor microvascular random flow and blood volume as measured by intravoxel incoherent motion (IVIM) weighted MRI in conjunction with Gd-DTPA-Albumin enhanced MRI. Magn Reson Imaging. 2001;19(8):1063-72.
24. Pickens III DR, Jolgren DL, Lorenz CH, Creasy JL, Price RR. Magnetic resonance perfusion/diffusion imaging of the excised dog kidney. Invest Radiol. 1992;27(4):287-92.
25. Lemke A, Laun FB, Simon D, Stieltjes B, Schad LR. An in vivo verification of the intravoxel incoherent motion effect in diffusion-weighted imaging of the abdomen. Magn Reson Med. 2010;64(6):1580-5.
26. Li W-F, Niu C, Shakir TM, Chen T, Zhang M, Wang Z. An evidence-based approach to assess the accuracy of intravoxel incoherent motion imaging for the grading of brain tumors. Medicine (Baltimore). 2018;97(45):e13217.
27. Wu H, Liang Y, Jiang X, Wei X, Liu Y, Liu W, et al. Meta-analysis of intravoxel incoherent motion magnetic resonance imaging in differentiating focal lesions of the liver. Medicine (Baltimore). 2018;97(34):e12071.
28. Kayal EB, Kandasamy D, Khare K, Alampally JT, Bakhshi S, Sharma R, et al. Quantitative Analysis of Intravoxel Incoherent Motion (IVIM) Diffusion MRI using Total Variation and Huber Penalty Function. Med Phys. 2017; 44(11):5849-58.
29. Fukuda T, Wengler K, de Carvalho R, Boonsri P, Schweitzer ME. MRI biomarkers in osseous tumors. J Magn Reson Imaging JMRI; 2019.
30. Downey K, Riches SF, Morgan VA, Giles SL, Attygalle AD, Ind TE, et al. Relationship Between Imaging Biomarkers of Stage I Cervical Cancer and Poor-Prognosis Histologic Features: Quantitative Histogram Analysis of Diffusion-Weighted MR Images. Am J Roentgenol. 2013;200(2):314-20.
31. Jensen JH, Helpern JA, Ramani A, Lu H, Kaczynski K. Diffusional kurtosis imaging: the quantification of non-gaussian water diffusion by means of magnetic resonance imaging. Magn Reson Med Off J Soc Magn Reson Med Soc Magn Reson Med. 2005;53(6):1432-40.
32. Suo S, Chen X, Wu L, Zhang X, Yao Q, Fan Y, et al. Non-Gaussian water diffusion kurtosis imaging of prostate cancer. Magn Reson Imaging. 2014;32(5):421-7.
33. Rosenkrantz AB. Histogram-Based Apparent Diffusion Coefficient Analysis: An Emerging Tool for Cervical Cancer Characterization? Am J Roentgenol. 2013;200(2):311-3.
34. Wang Q, Li H, Yan X, Wu C-J, Liu X-S, Shi H-B, et al. Histogram analysis of diffusion kurtosis magnetic resonance imaging in differentiation of pathologic Gleason grade of prostate cancer. Urol Oncol. 2015;33(8):337. e15-24.

35. Wu D, Li G, Zhang J, Chang S, Hu J, Dai Y. Characterization of Breast Tumors Using Diffusion Kurtosis Imaging (DKI). PLOS ONE. 2014;9(11):e113240.
36. Dai Y, Yao Q, Wu G, Wu D, Wu L, Zhu L, et al. Characterization of clear cell renal cell carcinoma with diffusion kurtosis imaging: correlation between diffusion kurtosis parameters and tumor cellularity. NMR Biomed. 2016;29(7):873-81.
37. Roethke MC, Kuder TA, Kuru TH, Fenchel M, Hadaschik BA, Laun FB, et al. Evaluation of Diffusion Kurtosis Imaging Versus Standard Diffusion Imaging for Detection and Grading of Peripheral Zone Prostate Cancer. Invest Radiol. 2015;50(8):483-9.
38. Higaki T, Nakamura Y, Tatsugami F, Kaichi Y, Akagi M, Akiyama Y, et al. Introduction to the Technical Aspects of Computed Diffusion-weighted Imaging for Radiologists. RadioGraphics. 2018;38(4):1131-44.
39. Hjort N, Christensen S, Sølling C, Ashkanian M, Wu O, Røhl L, et al. Ischemic injury detected by diffusion imaging 11 minutes after stroke. Ann Neurol. 2005;58(3):462-5.
40. Heiss WD, Raab P, Lanfermann H. Multimodality assessment of brain tumors and tumor recurrence. J Nucl Med. 2011;52(10): 1585-600.
41. Arvinda HR, Kesavadas C, Sarma PS, Thomas B, Radhakrishnan VV, Gupta AK, et al. Glioma grading: sensitivity, specificity, positive and negative predictive values of diffusion and perfusion imaging. J Neurooncol. 2009;94(1):87-96.
42. Hamstra DA, Galbán CJ, Meyer CR, Johnson TD, Sundgren PC, Tsien C, et al. Functional diffusion map as an early imaging biomarker for high-grade glioma: correlation with conventional radiologic response and overall survival. J Clin Oncol. 2008;26(20):3387-94.
43. Hamstra DA, Chenevert TL, Moffat BA, Johnson TD, Meyer CR, Mukherji SK, et al. Evaluation of the functional diffusion map as an early biomarker of time-to-progression and overall survival in high-grade glioma. Proc Natl Acad Sci USA. 2005;102(46): 16759-64.
44. Razek AAKA. Diffusion-weighted magnetic resonance imaging of head and neck. J Comput Assist Tomogr. 2010;34(6):808.
45. Maeda M, Kato H, Sakuma H, Maier SE, Takeda K. Usefulness of the apparent diffusion coefficient in line scan diffusion-weighted imaging for distinguishing between squamous cell carcinomas and malignant lymphomas of the head and neck. Am J Neuroradiol. 2005;26(5):1186-92.
46. Sumi M, Ichikawa Y, Nakamura T. Diagnostic ability of apparent diffusion coefficients for lymphomas and carcinomas in the pharynx. Eur Radiol. 2007;17(10): 2631-7.
47. Razek AAKA, Megahed AS, Denewer A, Motamed A, Tawfik A, Nada N. Role of diffusion-weighted magnetic resonance imaging in differentiation between the viable and necrotic parts of head and neck tumors. Acta Radiol. 2008;49(3):364-70.
48. Kim S, Loevner L, Quon H, Sherman E, Weinstein G, Kilger A, et al. Diffusion-weighted magnetic resonance imaging for predicting and detecting early response to chemoradiation therapy of squamous cell carcinomas of the head and neck. Clin Cancer Res. 2009;15(3):986-94.
49. Kapur R, Sepahdari AR, Mafee MF, Putterman AM, Aakalu V, Wendel LJA, et al. MR imaging of orbital inflammatory syndrome, orbital cellulitis, and orbital lymphoid lesions: the role of diffusion-weighted imaging. Am J Neuroradiol. 2009;30(1):64-70.
50. Uhl M, Altehoefer C, Kontny U, Il'yasov K, Büchert M, Langer M. MRI-diffusion imaging of neuroblastomas: first results and correlation to histology. Eur Radiol. 2002; 12(9):2335-8.
51. Humphries PD, Sebire NJ, Siegel MJ, Olsen ØE. Tumors in pediatric patients at diffusion-weighted MR imaging: apparent diffusion coefficient and tumor cellularity. Radiology. 2007;245(3):848-54.
52. Satoh S, Kitazume Y, Ohdama S, Kimula Y, Taura S, Endo Y. Can malignant and benign pulmonary nodules be differentiated with diffusion-weighted MRI? Am J Roentgenol. 2008;191(2):464-70.
53. Qi LP, Zhang XP, Tang L, Li J, Sun YS, Zhu GY. Using diffusion-weighted MR imaging for tumor detection in the collapsed lung: a preliminary study. Eur Radiol. 2009;19(2):333-41.
54. Ko\csucu P, Tekinba\cs C, Erol M, Sari A, Kavgaci H, Öztuna F, et al. Mediastinal lymph nodes: Assessment with diffusion-weighted MR imaging. J Magn Reson Imaging. 2009;30(2):292-7.
55. Nomori H, Mori T, Ikeda K, Kawanaka K, Shiraishi S, Katahira K, et al. Diffusion-weighted magnetic resonance imaging can be used in place of positron emission tomography for N staging of non-small cell lung cancer with fewer false-positive results. J Thorac Cardiovasc Surg. 2008;135(4):816-22.
56. Khouli RHEI, Jacobs MA, Mezban SD, Huang P, Kamel IR, Macura KJ, et al. Diffusion-weighted Imaging Improves the Diagnostic Accuracy of Conventional 3.0-T Breast MR Imaging1. Radiology. 2010;256(1):64-73.
57. Sharma U, Danishad KKA, Seenu V, Jagannathan NR. Longitudinal study of the assessment by MRI and diffusion-weighted imaging of tumor response in patients with locally advanced breast cancer undergoing neoadjuvant chemotherapy. NMR Biomed. 2009;22(1):104-13.
58. Park SH, Moon WK, Cho N, Song IC, Chang JM, Park IA, et al. Diffusion-weighted MR Imaging: Pretreatment Prediction of Response to Neoadjuvant Chemotherapy in Patients with Breast Cancer1. Radiology. 2010;257(1): 56-63.
59. Bruegel M, Gaa J, Waldt S, Woertler K, Holzapfel K, Kiefer B, et al. Diagnosis of hepatic metastasis: comparison of respiration-triggered diffusion-weighted echo-planar MRI and five T2-weighted turbo spin-echo sequences. Am J Roentgenol. 2008;191(5):1421-9.
60. Zech CJ, Herrmann KA, Dietrich O, Horger W, Reiser MF, Schoenberg SO. Black-blood diffusion-weighted EPI acquisition of the liver with parallel imaging: comparison with a standard T2-weighted sequence for detection of focal liver lesions. Invest Radiol. 2008;43(4):261-6.
61. Koh DM, Brown G, Riddell AM, Scurr E, Collins DJ, Allen SD, et al. Detection of colorectal hepatic metastases using MnDPDP MR imaging and diffusion-weighted imaging (DWI) alone and in combination. Eur Radiol. 2008;18(5):903-10.
62. Hardie AD, Naik M, Hecht EM, Chandarana H, Mannelli L, Babb JS, et al. Diagnosis of liver metastases: value of diffusion-weighted MRI compared with gadolinium-enhanced MRI. Eur Radiol. 2010;20(6):1431-41.
63. Lewin M, Poujol-Robert A, Boëlle P-Y, Wendum D, Lasnier E, Viallon M, et al. Diffusion-weighted magnetic resonance imaging for the assessment of fibrosis in chronic hepatitis C. Hepatology. 2007;46(3):658-65.
64. Sugita R, Yamazaki T, Furuta A, Itoh K, Fujita N, Takahashi S. High b-value diffusion-weighted MRI for detecting gallbladder carcinoma: preliminary study and results. Eur Radiol. 2009;19(7):1794-8.
65. Cui XY, Chen HW. Role of diffusion-weighted magnetic resonance imaging in the diagnosis of extrahepatic cholangiocarcinoma. World J Gastroenterol WJG. 2010; 16(25):3196.
66. Ichikawa T, Haradome H, Hachiya J, Nitatori T, Araki T. Diffusion-weighted MR imaging with single-shot echo-planar imaging in the upper abdomen: preliminary clinical experience in 61 patients. Abdom Imaging. 1999;24(5): 456-61.
67. Yoshikawa T, Kawamitsu H, Mitchell DG, Ohno Y, Ku Y, Seo Y, et al. ADC Measurement of Abdominal Organs and Lesions Using Parallel Imaging Technique. Am J Roentgenol. 2006;187(6):1521-30.

68. Inan N, Arslan A, Akansel G, Anik Y, Demirci A. Diffusion-weighted imaging in the differential diagnosis of cystic lesions of the pancreas. AJR Am J Roentgenol. 2008; 191(4):1115-21.
69. Zhang J, Tehrani YM, Wang L, Ishill NM, Schwartz LH, Hricak H. Renal Masses: Characterization with Diffusion-weighted MR Imaging—A Preliminary Experience1. Radiology. 2008;247(2):458-64.
70. Goyal A, Sharma R, Bhalla AS, Gamanagatti S, Seth A, Iyer VK, et al. Diffusion-weighted MRI in renal cell carcinoma: a surrogate marker for predicting nuclear grade and histological subtype. Acta Radiol Stockh Swed 1987. 2012; 53(3):349-58.
71. Paudyal B, Paudyal P, Tsushima Y, Oriuchi N, Amanuma M, Miyazaki M, et al. The role of the ADC value in the characterisation of renal carcinoma by diffusion-weighted MRI. Br J Radiol. 2010;83(988):336-43.
72. Goyal A, Sharma R, Bhalla AS, Gamanagatti S, Seth A. Diffusion-weighted MRI in inflammatory renal lesions: all that glitters is not RCC! Eur Radiol. 2013;23(1):272-9.
73. Miller FH, Wang Y, McCarthy RJ, Yaghmai V, Merrick L, Larson A, et al. Utility of diffusion-weighted MRI in characterization of adrenal lesions. Am J Roentgenol. 2010;194(2):W179-85.
74. Tsushima Y, Takahashi-Taketomi A, Endo K. Diagnostic utility of diffusion-weighted MR imaging and apparent diffusion coefficient value for the diagnosis of adrenal tumors. J Magn Reson Imaging. 2009;29(1):112-7.
75. Gibbs P, Pickles MD, Turnbull LW. Diffusion imaging of the prostate at 3.0 tesla. Invest Radiol. 2006;41(2):185-8.
76. Song I, Kim CK, Park BK, Park W. Assessment of response to radiotherapy for prostate cancer: value of diffusion-weighted MRI at 3 T. Am J Roentgenol. 2010;194(6): W477-82.
77. Kedia S, Sharma R, Makharia GK, Ahuja V, Desai D, Kandasamy D, et al. Imaging of the small intestine in Crohn's disease: Joint position statement of the Indian Society of Gastroenterology and Indian Radiological and Imaging Association. Indian J Gastroenterol Off J Indian Soc Gastroenterol. 2017;36(6):487-508.
78. Kandasamy D, Goyal A, Sharma R, Gupta AK. Pediatric Body Magnetic Resonance Imaging. Indian J Pediatr. 2016; 83(9): 941-51.
79. Gulani V, Calamante F, Shellock FG, Kanal E, Reeder SB. Gadolinium deposition in the brain: summary of evidence and recommendations. Lancet Neurol. 2017;16(7):564-70.
80. Kim K-J, Lee Y, Park SH, Kang B-K, Seo N, Yang S-K, et al. Diffusion-weighted MR enterography for evaluating Crohn's disease: how does it add diagnostically to conventional MR enterography? Inflamm Bowel Dis. 2015; 21(1):101-9.
81. Seo N, Park SH, Kim K-J, Kang B-K, Lee Y, Yang S-K, et al. MR Enterography for the Evaluation of Small-Bowel Inflammation in Crohn Disease by Using Diffusion-weighted Imaging without Intravenous Contrast Material: A Prospective Noninferiority Study. Radiology. 2016; 278(3):762-72.
82. Hordonneau C, Buisson A, Scanzi J, Goutorbe F, Pereira B, Borderon C, et al. Diffusion-weighted magnetic resonance imaging in ileocolonic Crohn's disease: validation of quantitative index of activity. Am J Gastroenterol. 2014; 109(1):89-98.
83. Beets-Tan RGH, Lambregts DMJ, Maas M, Bipat S, Barbaro B, Curvo-Semedo L, et al. Magnetic resonance imaging for clinical management of rectal cancer: Updated recommendations from the 2016 European Society of Gastrointestinal and Abdominal Radiology (ESGAR) consensus meeting. Eur Radiol. 2018;28(4):1465-75.
84. Nasu K, Kuroki Y, Minami M. Diffusion-weighted imaging findings of mucinous carcinoma arising in the ano-rectal region: comparison of apparent diffusion coefficient with that of tubular adenocarcinoma. Jpn J Radiol. 2012; 30(2):120-7.
85. Heijnen LA, Lambregts DMJ, Mondal D, Martens MH, Riedl RG, Beets GL, et al. Diffusion-weighted MR imaging in primary rectal cancer staging demonstrates but does not characterise lymph nodes. Eur Radiol. 2013;23(12): 3354-60.
86. Lambregts DMJ, Maas M, Riedl RG, Bakers FCH, Verwoerd JL, Kessels AGH, et al. Value of ADC measurements for nodal staging after chemoradiation in locally advanced rectal cancer—a per lesion validation study. Eur Radiol. 2011;21(2):265-73.
87. Schurink N, Lambregts D, Beets-Tan R. Diffusion-weighted imaging in rectal cancer: current applications and future perspectives. Br J Radiol [Internet]. 2018 Nov 15 [cited 2019 Feb 21]; Available from: https://www.birpublications.org/doi/abs/10.1259/bjr.20180655
88. Dietrich O, Biffar A, Reiser MF, Baur-Melnyk A. Diffusion-weighted imaging of bone marrow. Semin Musculoskelet Radiol. 2009;13(2):134-44.
89. Koutoulidis V, Fontara S, Terpos E, Zagouri F, Matsaridis D, Christoulas D, et al. Quantitative Diffusion-weighted Imaging of the Bone Marrow: An Adjunct Tool for the Diagnosis of a Diffuse MR Imaging Pattern in Patients with Multiple Myeloma. Radiology. 2016;282(2):484-93.
90. Dietrich O, Geith T, Reiser MF, Baur-Melnyk A. Diffusion imaging of the vertebral bone marrow. NMR Biomed. 2017;30(3).
91. Patel KB, Poplawski MM, Pawha PS, Naidich TP, Tanenbaum LN. Diffusion-Weighted MRI "Claw Sign" Improves Differentiation of Infectious from Degenerative Modic Type 1 Signal Changes of the Spine. Am J Neuroradiol [Internet]. 2014 Apr 17 [cited 2019 Feb 24]; Available from: http://www.ajnr.org/content/early/2014/04/17/ajnr.A3948
92. Fujii S, Matsusue E, Kigawa J, Sato S, Kanasaki Y, Nakanishi J, et al. Diagnostic accuracy of the apparent diffusion coefficient in differentiating benign from malignant uterine endometrial cavity lesions: initial results. Eur Radiol. 2008;18(2):384-9.
93. Lin G, Ho KC, Wang JJ, Ng KK, Wai YY, Chen YT, et al. Detection of lymph node metastasis in cervical and uterine cancers by diffusion-weighted magnetic resonance imaging at 3T. J Magn Reson Imaging. 2008;28(1):128-35.
94. Moteki T, Ishizaka H. Diffusion-weighted EPI of cystic ovarian lesions: Evaluation of cystic contents using apparent diffusion coefficients. J Magn Reson Imaging. 2000;12(6):1014-9.
95. Nakayama T, Yoshimitsu K, Irie H, Aibe H, Tajima T, Nishie A, et al. Diffusion-weighted echo-planar MR imaging and ADC mapping in the differential diagnosis of ovarian cystic masses: Usefulness of detecting keratinoid substances in mature cystic teratomas. J Magn Reson Imaging. 2005;22(2):271-8.
96. Low RN, Sebrechts CP, Barone RM, Muller W. Diffusion-weighted MRI of peritoneal tumors: comparison with conventional MRI and surgical and histopathologic findings—a feasibility study. Am J Roentgenol. 2009; 193(2):461-70.

CHAPTER

36

Perfusion MRI

Sameer Vyas, Pankaj Gupta, Paramjeet Singh, Niranjan Khandelwal

INTRODUCTION

Perfusion is an established physiologic and pathophysiologic measure of the volume of blood passing through the microvasculature of a mass of tissue in a given time period.[1,2] It is also referred as capillary or tissue-specific blood flow, and is a quantitative measure which can be determined with many different experimental techniques and often expressed in mL/100 gm/minute.[2] It can provide valuable information for detection, characterization and monitoring therapies in various disease processes like neoplasm, inflammations and ischemia.

The perfusion can be noninvasively measured by the use of a tracer. Depending on the characteristics of these tracers, the blood flow measures can be divided into mainly three types viz. diffusible tracers, intravascular tracers and microsphere type tracers. The diffusible tracers are those tracers which easily pass through blood vessel walls and include H_2O, or H_2O^{15} (used in positron emission tomography), and Xenon (used in computed tomography-based perfusion measures). The intravascular tracers are those tracers which remain within the vessel walls and include iodinated contrast in CT and Gadolinium and other contrast agents in magnetic resonance imaging (MRI). However these agents are partially diffusible in most tissues of the body and separating perfusion from vessel permeability effects can be a challenge. The microsphere type tracers are slightly larger than capillaries and hence they get stuck within the microvasculature indefinitely. They are widely used for invasive animal studies and are considered too risky for human studies. Clinical agents like the single photon emission computed tomography (SPECT) agent Tc-HMPAO mimic microspheres by remaining in the target tissue for a long time but they achieve this by diffusing into tissue and then undergoing a chemical transformation within the tissue that discourages diffusing back out.

As unusual nuclear species are readily detected in the body with MRI, perfusion imaging is possible with many different tracers including fluorinated compounds, deuterated water, O^{17} and hyperpolarized gas Xenon.[2] The normal concentration of these tracer agents (nuclei) in tissue is almost zero and the only signal observed in clinical MRI is due to perfusion effects as the signal from these can be well separated from the water proton signal. These techniques are interesting and potentially promising, however these agents generally produce weak signals to noise ratio, have low spatial resolution, and lack the sensitivity of the proton MRI techniques which is usually employed for clinical studies. Proton based perfusion techniques using the strong signal from water protons in tissue have been found to be useful in the clinical setting and clinical research. Perfusion imaging with the proton signal can be performed either by dynamic imaging following the bolus injection of a MR contrast agent or by labeling of the water in the inflowing arterial blood.[3-7] Methods based on contrast agents are frequently used as the effects of contrast agents in the vessels or tissue is quite strong.

Magnetic Contrast Agents in Neural Tissues

MR contrast agents (paramagnetic and superparamagnetic) are intravascular within normal brain tissue, as they are unable to cross the blood-brain barrier owing to their as large size. The signal changes resulting from alterations to the intravascular signal are relatively small because the brain blood volume is small (3–6%). However, the magnetic contrast agents within the vasculature can have effects beyond the vessels as an intravascular contrast agent and can affect tissue signal by altering the magnetic fields in the nearby tissue. In addition, spins can move between small blood vessels in the microvasculature and the tissue.

MR Imaging Techniques and Methods

The bolus tracking technique is most widely used and it is performed by injection of a bolus of magnetic contrast agent while repeatedly imaging.[8,9] It is usually performed using T2* (or T2) contrast where the signal change is due to the magnetic susceptibility of the contrast agent and is known as dynamic susceptibility contrast (DSC) MR perfusion or the T1 properties of the contrast agent, where the signal change is due to the T1 shortening effects of the contrast agent and is known as dynamic contrast enhancement (DCE) MR perfusion.[8-10] DSC imaging is mostly employed in brain whereas DCE MR perfusion is usually employed outside the brain. By selectively affecting the MRI signal from water in the inflowing arterial blood, imaging without contrast agent is possible and is known as arterial spin labeling (ASL) technique.[11-15] It produces a smaller signal change than the contrast agent methods but the lack of an injection and the use of diffusible water as the tracer make this approach an interesting alternative option.[6,10] The basic principle of these MRP techniques is repetitive serial imaging during the transit of blood, that has been labeled either with an endogenous magnetic tracer or contrast material.[11-15] The three methods of MR perfusion are compared in **Table 1**.

Dynamic Susceptibility Contrast-enhanced MR Perfusion (DSC MRP)

It is the most commonly used MR perfusion technique in day-to-day routine clinical studies of brain as it is simple to perform.

Principle

The T2* susceptibility effects of gadolinium is exploited by this technique, rather than the contrast media induced T1-shortening effects routinely used in conventional MR imaging.[16-19] The shortening of T2/T2* relaxation times is referred to as the susceptibility effect, which results into lower signal on T2- or T2*-weighted images. After the injection of a bolus of MRI contrast agent, MR signal change is measured by rapid sequential imaging.[1] The signal loss, owing to passage of the contrast agent bolus on T2* weighted images, is used for calculating the change in contrast concentration which occurs in each pixel. Contrast agent is considered as an intravascular marker and leakage of the contrast into the surrounding interstitial space is neglected or if possible eliminated. Various parameters like cerebral blood flow (CBF), cerebral blood volume (CBV), and mean transit time (MTT) are calculated from the data.

Image Acquisition

As with routine MRI, comfortable positioning of the patient is necessary with light restraining straps and adequate cushioning for reducing movement. A single or multishot echo planar imaging (EPI) based fast imaging sequence is used for data acquisition in order to achieve a temporal resolution

TABLE 1: Comparison of MR perfusion methods.

Properties	Dynamic susceptibility contrast	Dynamic contrast enhancement	Arterial spin labeling
Handling of bolus	Tracking of bolus	Passage of bolus	Tagging of bolus
Point of acquisition	First pass of contrast agent	Accumulation of contrast agent	Accumulation of tagged blood
In vitro or vivo	In vitro method	In vitro method	In vivo method
Contrast media	Intravenous gadolinium	Intravenous gadolinium	Without contrast
Tracer	Non-diffusible blood pool tracer	Flow or permeability-limited diffusible tracer	Diffusible tracer
Mechanism of relaxation	T2/T2* relaxation	T1 relaxation	Magnetic labeled blood T1 relaxation
Effect	Increased susceptibility effect	T1 shortening effect	Blood magnetization inversion
Behavior of the signal	Reduced signal	Heightened signal	Subtracted signal
Contributory signal	T2/T2* relaxation changes	T1 relaxation changes	Magnetic blood labeling
Mechanism	Magnetic field is distorted by contrast agent by virtue of its paramagnetic property, leading to more susceptibility effect and causes reduction of T2 and T2* around the vessels.	Contrast agent cause dipole-dipole interaction between the protons in the water molecules leading to T1 shortening and production of signal	Tagged blood by inversion flows into the capillary site followed by transcapillary exchange with the brain tissue and flows into the draining vein.
Types of imaging sequence	T2/T2*-w imaging	T1-w imaging	Sequence with short TE and long TR
Common sequences used	2D single-shot gradient echo EPI sequence	3D gradient echo (THRIVE/FLASH/FSPGR)	single-shot gradient echo EPI
Total duration of scan	Relatively short (<2 min)	Long (≈ 5 to 6 min)	Long with multiple averaging (≈ 4 min)
Signal-to-noise ratio	Very good	Good	Fair
Cerebral blood flow	Fair	Poor	Very good
Cerebral blood volume	Good	Very good	Poor
Transit	Very good (MTT)	Very good (k^{trans})	Fair
Coverage	Very good	Good	Good
Repeatable	Good	Fair	Very good
Pediatric application	Good	Fair	Very good
Artefacts	Fair	Very good	Good

of approximately 2 seconds. The imaging sequence used is either gradient echo, maximizing T2* weighting or a spin echo, minimizing the signal contributed by larger vessels. A series of pre-contrast images (at least five) is acquired before the bolus passage. However, for improving the estimation of the baseline signal intensity during analysis, many centers prefer to acquire for up to 1 minute in order to generate a large number of precontrast images. Most cases are acquired with a standard contrast dose (0.1 mmol/kg); however, to improve signal to noise ratio, a double dose of gadolinium (0.2 mmol/Kg) may be used. For a tight bolus of contrast material which is preferred in DSC MRP, the contrast is usually injected via an 18- or 20-gauge intravenous catheter at a high rate (3–6 mL/seconds) with a power injector. To make the bolus coherent which enters the central circulation, saline flush at the same rate of at least 25 mL (20–30 mL) should follow the bolus injection. Alternatively, manual injection technique can also be used with utmost care. The injection should be given through a wide bore cannula (at least 18 G) preferably placed into a large antecubital vein, in manual technique, to reduce the resistance of the injection system. The rate of injection should be uniform and should be immediately followed by the equal amount of normal saline administered at the same rate. Successive images of the region of interest are then acquired during the first pass of contrast material.

Data Analysis

The analysis is based on the assumption that the contrast agent acts as a blood pool marker and is confined to the vascular space throughout the examination.[19] This assumption holds true only within the brain as there is no contrast leakage owing to the presence of blood-brain barrier. A time-versus signal intensity curve is constructed based on the drop in T2* signal, secondary to the susceptibility effects of gadolinium, on a voxel-by-voxel basis. The relative concentration-time curves are obtained (delta R2 curves) **(Figs. 1A to C)** assuming that the signal drop is proportional to the concentration of gadolinium in the tissue.[20,21] By determining the area under the concentration-time curves, normalized to a contralateral uninvolved region, relative cerebral blood volume (rCBV) can be obtained. As an arterial input function (AIF) is not used for calculation of CBV, it is referred to as "relative" and thus, the exact cerebral blood volume is not quantified. Construction of rCBV map is done by repeating this process on a voxel-by-voxel basis **(Fig. 2)**. The width of the curve represents the MTT as the width at half the maximum height (full width at half maximum; FWHM). Finally, as per the central volume theorem, the blood flow is given by the formula CBF=CBV/MTT.

The observed signal change can be used to calculate local contrast concentration because the contrast concentration is linearly proportional to the T2 rate changes (ΔR2). Thus, signal intensity time course data is converted to contrast concentration time course data **(Fig. 1)**.

Problems with DSC MRI

There are several problems/errors with the DSC MRP which have to be addressed while assessment of the perfusion parameters. For accurate quantification of the perfusion parameters, many modifications of the analysis approach have been described.[20,21] Recirculation of contrast, leakage

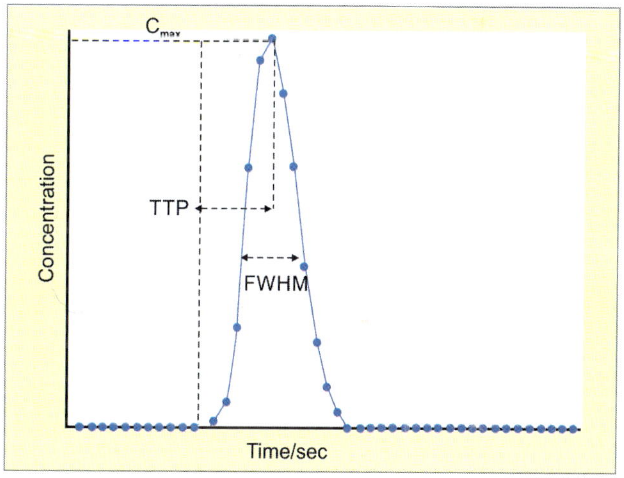

FIG. 2: Contrast (tissue concentration) versus time curve showing the different parameters. Area under curve represents cerebral blood volume, height of curve represents cerebral blood flow and area/ height of curve represents mean transit time. C^{max}, peak height and, full width half maximum (FWHM), time to peak concentration (TTP).

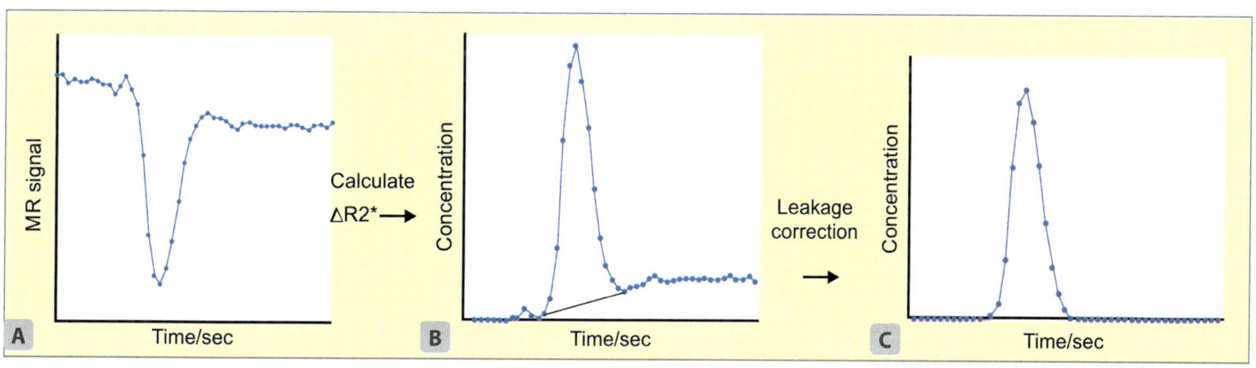

FIGS. 1A TO C: Data analysis in DSC perfusion. (A) Time-versus MR signal intensity curve where signal intensity decrease during passage of contrast agent bolus and is measured from a series of MR images. (B) Tissue concentration-versus time curve where change in the relaxation rate (ΔR2*) is calculated from signal intensity, and a baseline subtraction method is applied to measured data. (C) Corrected ΔR2* curve after leakage correction.

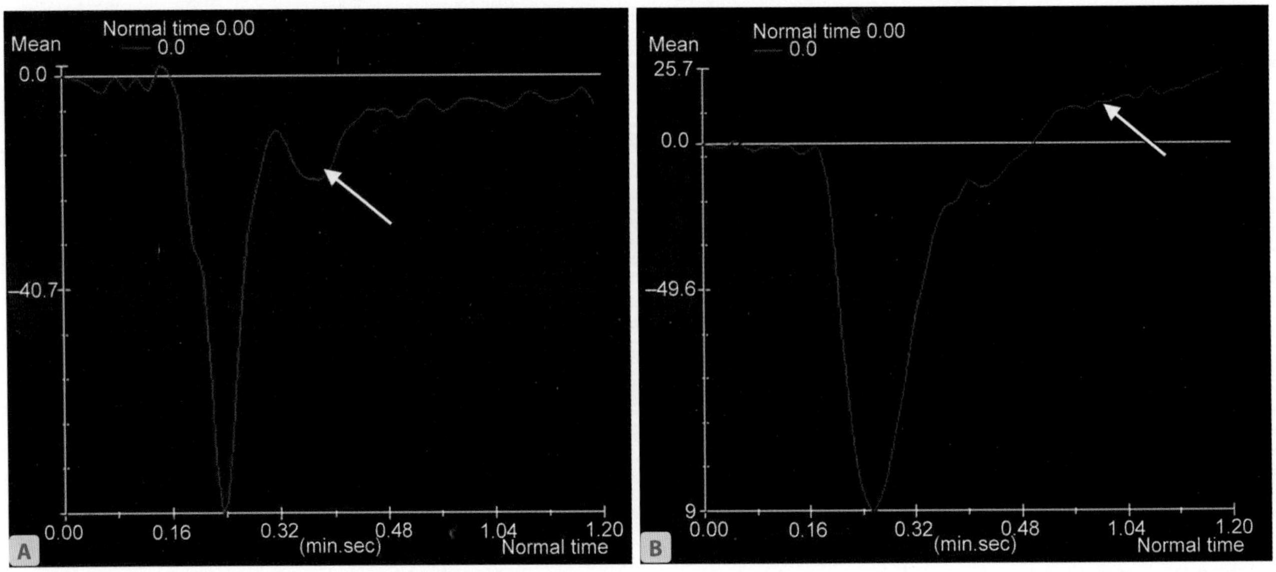

FIGS. 3A AND B: (A) Signal intensity–time curve showing marked signal intensity decrease during arrival of the contrast agent, followed by partial recovery of the signal intensity loss. A second decrease in signal intensity (arrow) is due to recirculation. (B) Signal intensity–time curve showing contrast leakage and signal above baseline due to the T1 shortening effects of gadolinium.

of contrast and dispersion of the bolus are the three major problems with this perfusion technique.

- *Contrast recirculation:* For analyzing the contrast bolus passage, it is assumed that the bolus passes through the voxel and then the contrast concentration reaches zero. However, there is re-circulation of the contrast and following the first, there is a second re-circulation peak **(Fig. 3A)**, which causes the bolus to disperse and widen. This result in the second peak to be broader and lower than the first, and then in the third re-circulation, there is even mixing of the intravascular contrast throughout the blood volume, causing a small constant baseline elevation in the contrast concentration. Errors in measurement of CBV is due to the presence of both first pass and re-circulating contrast in the vessels during the later part of the passage of the bolus. Curve fitting technique, which also smoothens the data, effectively reducing noise and eliminates contrast agent re-circulation induced contamination of the first pass bolus, can be used to minimize this error.
- *Contrast leakage and tissue enhancement:* Signal changes occur mainly by relaxivity mechanisms when the contrast agent leaks into the interstitial space. Extravasation of contrast material into the interstitial spaces can lead to signal increase above the baseline because of the T1 shortening effects of gadolinium (i.e., enhancement) in areas with severe disruption of blood-brain barrier (e.g. high-grade neoplasm) because of high permeability **(Fig. 3B)**. As a constant baseline is assumed in the algorithm for calculation of rCBV, the area above baseline is calculated by the algorithm as negative blood volume, and subtracted from the area below baseline caused by the T2* signal drop. As a result, rCBV is significantly underestimated. Separation of these relaxivity and susceptibility based effects can be done by susceptibility based imaging methods and as a result, images where the effect of contrast leakage is decreased or nullified can be produced. The use of sequences having reduced T1 sensitivity, such as low flip angle gradient echo based sequences and increased repetition time (TR), or use of a dual echo technique or use of pre-enhancement techniques preinject an additional small dose of gadolinium (0.05 mmol/Kg) for presaturating the interstitium, can effectively elevate the baseline before the dynamic acquisition; thereby effectively removing relaxivity effects. In addition, newer "blood pool" contrast agents (for example, gadobenate dimeglumine and monocrystalline iron oxide nanoparticles) may ameliorate this problem. The T1 shortening induced change in signal intensity follows a bi-exponential pattern; hence, for any particular sequence, signal intensity remains relatively constant during the plateau phase. Because of this pattern of response curve, the relaxivity based signal intensity responses to subsequent contrast doses will be reduced by pre-enhancement of tumors. However, each approach has its own benefits and characteristics, so preferred method should be individualized.
- *Bolus dispersion and the measurement of absolute CBF:* The basic assumption to calculate the absolute CBF is that the technique is able to generate accurate quantitative measurements of CBV and MTT. However, as CBV is calculated from the area under the curve and is a relative measurement which allows CBV comparison between tissues rather than producing an absolute measurement.[22,23] In addition, accurate estimation of MTT is required for the measurement of CBF. The factors which determine the width of the contrast bolus (MTT) include arterial input function (AIF), regional flow alterations and broadening of the bolus due to dispersive effects.

MRI sequence type

Gradient-echo vs. spin-echo: Either of spin echo or gradient echo sequences can be used. Theoretically, signal changes predominantly reflecting contrast passage through capillary bed and thereby tumor physiology at capillary level can be produced by spin-echo sequences. However; multiple studies have shown very minute effective benefit from the use of spin echo sequences and signal to noise ratio is significantly compromised in spin echo sequences. Selective sensitivity of spin echo sequences have been shown to small vessels, less than 20 µ in diameter. On the contrary, as signal from large tumor vessels and microvascularity are demonstrated by gradient-echo images; the GRE sequences are found to avid correlation between blood volume and pathological tumor grade.

Spatial coverage vs. time resolution: The spatial coverage and time resolution is optimized by making a tradeoff between two and depending upon the particular application and tissue of interest. As appropriate characterization of transient signal drop is necessary for accurate quantification of DSC MRP data, the tissue transit time of the bolus becomes a limiting factor for the time resolution. Typically, a repetition time (TR) of 2 seconds or lesser is required for acquisition of the fast changes occurring during the first pass. Thus, the maximum number of slices acquired within this TR becomes a limiting factor for the spatial coverage. Echo planar imaging (EPI), segmented EPI, FLASH, etc. can be used.

2D vs. 3D Sequences: Both 2D and 3D sequences can be used. 2D sequences are usually preferable; however, 3D sequences offer the advantage of increased coverage, although typically at the cost of a decreased spatial resolution or an increased TR.

Single-echo vs. dual-echo sequences: Relaxivity effects can be easily removed by using dual echo sequences; thereby allowing quantification of changes in R2* without assumption regarding the T1 behavior. However, the sampling of two echoes increases sampling time and thus, for a given TR, the maximum number of slices that can be acquired as well as the coverage is reduced. When spatial coverage is important, single-echo sequences with a pre-dose of contrast may be used as the use of a pre-enhancement approach is proven effective.

Clinical applications of DSC MR perfusion in brain:[24]

- *Brain tumors:* MRP is very useful for the diagnosis and characterization (tumor vascularity) of the brain lesions. It helps in differentiating tumor from the tumor mimic (atypical infections and tumefactive demyelination), grading of the brain tumors **(Figs. 4 and 5)**, for the surgical planning (targeting locations for biopsy or guiding resection extent) and follow-up of the patients. It is also very useful in characterizing the treatment related changes like radiation necrosis or chemo-necrosis versus recurrent or residual tumor, and pseudo-progression and pseudo-response.
- *Neurovascular disease:* MRP is helpful in assessment of ischemic penumbra in acute stroke **(Figs. 6A to E)**, assessment of vasospasm (in subarachnoid hemorrhage), and assessment of the hemodynamic significance of cervico-cranial vascular stenosis.
- Neurodegenerative disease

Dynamic Contrast-enhanced MR Perfusion (DCE MRP)

As the wash-in, plateau, and washout contrast kinetics of a given tissue can be assessed by DCE MRP, it provides an excellent insight into the tissue characteristics at the microvascular level.[25,26] It is also referred as 'permeability' MRI and is a completely different method of MR perfusion with the main objective being assessment tumor permeability.[25-32] This T1-based technique offers the main advantage that it uses tumor leakiness (enhancement) for analyzing the data rather than considering it as an artifact as in DSC MRP.

Principle

The 'relaxivity effects' of the paramagnetic contrast material i.e. the shortening of T1 relaxation time, produce higher signal on T1-weighted images and is measured by the T1-weighted technique. A two-compartmental (plasma space and extravascular-extracellular space) pharmacokinetic model is the basis of the sequence **(Figs. 7A to C)**.

Image Acquisition

The patient should be positioned as used for normal MRI. The general steps in acquisition of DCE MRP are: performing baseline T1 mapping, acquisition of DCE MRP images, converting the signal-intensity data to contrast concentration, determining the vascular input function, and performing the pharmacokinetic modeling. Pre-contrast images should be acquired for a sufficient period in the dynamic imaging sequence for accurate estimation of the extracellular space and of the contribution of renal excretion. The data is acquired by three-dimensional (3D) gradient echo sequence. A bolus injection technique as used for DSC-MRP is used. A lower dose of gadolinium is injected (typically a single dose of 0.1 mmol/Kg) at a lower rate (2–3 mL/sec) and repeated image acquisitions are then done through the lesion at longer intervals, generally every 15–30 seconds. Image acquisition is longer than DSC MRP, in order to allow the contrast leakage into the extravascular space and reach a state of equilibrium over multiple passes of the contrast bolus through the lesion.

Data Analysis

The effect of contrast enhancement can be quantified by different techniques ranging from simple measures of the rate of enhancement to complex pharmacokinetic analyses.[29-32]

Simple analysis techniques: the signal intensity curves from regions of interest can be compared directly for the quantification of enhancement. Many measurements allow this sort of analysis and are designed to minimize the patient to patient variation occurring as a result of different contrast dose, injection, scanner type and scanning techniques. T90 is one such simple measurement which refers to the time taken for the tumor tissue to acquire 90% of the maximal enhancement. Maximal intensity change per time interval ratio (MITR) is another parameter and refers to maximum rate of change of enhancement. Various curve shapes can also provide insight into the quantification and a standardized slope of the enhancement curve can be calculated. However, the enhancement curve is poorly reproducible and most of

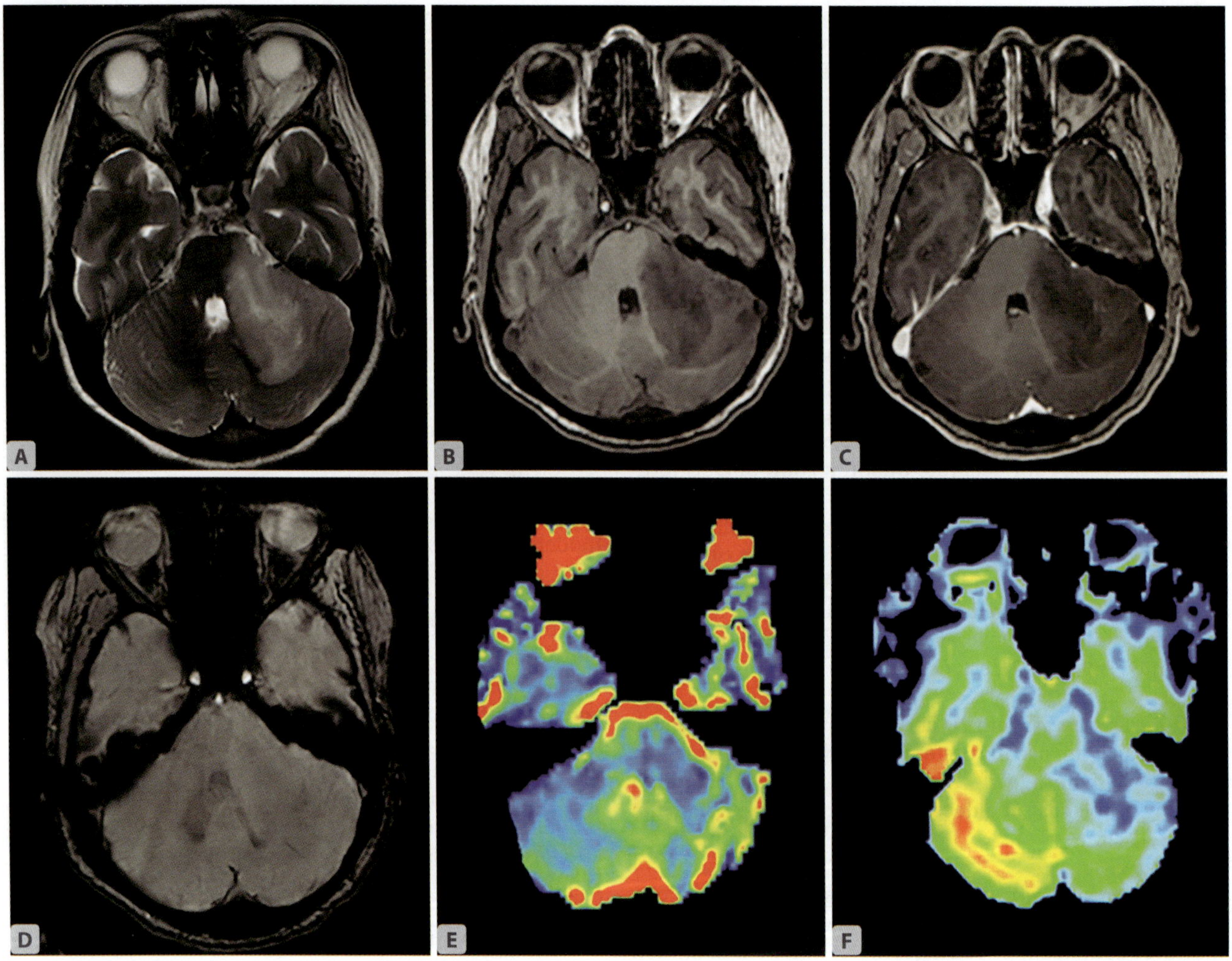

FIGS. 4A TO F: Brain MRI of a 62 years old female patient presenting with headache and vertigo, axial T2-weighted image (A), axial reformatted pre-contrast 3D T1-SPGR image (B) and axial reformatted post-contrast 3D T1-SPGR image (C) show a non-enhancing T2 hyperintense mass lesion in left cerebellar hemisphere producing mass effect in the form of effacement of 4th ventricle. Susceptibility weighted image (D) shows no intralesional susceptibility changes to suggest hemorrhage or calcification. rCBV map (E) generated from dynamic susceptibility perfusion sequence, CBF map (F) generated from arterial spin labeling perfusion sequence do not show elevated perfusion parameters within the lesion. Overall features are suggestive of low-grade glioma.

these signal intensity based methods remain sensitive to variations between acquisition system because of the non-linear relationship between signal intensity and contrast concentration.

Pharmacokinetic analysis techniques: Several metrics can be obtained with pharmacokinetic modeling of DCE MRP data: transfer constant (k^{trans}), fractional volume of the extravascular extracellular space (v_e), rate constant (k_{ep}, $k_{ep} = k^{trans}/v_e$), and fractional volume of the plasma space (v_p). These quantitative techniques are can be used for calculation of the biological characteristics like permeability and surface area of the endothelium, which are relatively independent of imaging approach (individual patient variations, scanning technique or scanner type). The most commonly employed metric in DCE MRP is k^{trans}. Depending on blood flow and permeability, it may have different interpretations. In cases with very high permeability, flow is the only limiting factor of the flux of gadolinium-based contrast agents, and thus k^{trans} mainly reflects blood flow; whereas in cases of very low permeability, k^{trans} mainly reflects permeability as the contrast agent cannot leak easily into the extravascular-extracellular space.

Problems with Quantitative Measurement of DCE MRI

The k^{trans} measurement with pharmacokinetic analysis techniques have few disadvantages which includes partial volume averaging effects, long acquisition time and flow dependency of k^{trans}.

- *Partial volume averaging effects:* The pharmacokinetic analysis technique is based on assumption that blood concentration changes are represented by sample taken from voxels in blood vessels; whereas extravascular contrast leakage is represented by voxels within the target tissue. However, this assumption is not true as the voxels within the target tissue may represent a mixture of the voxels where some will have significant intravascular

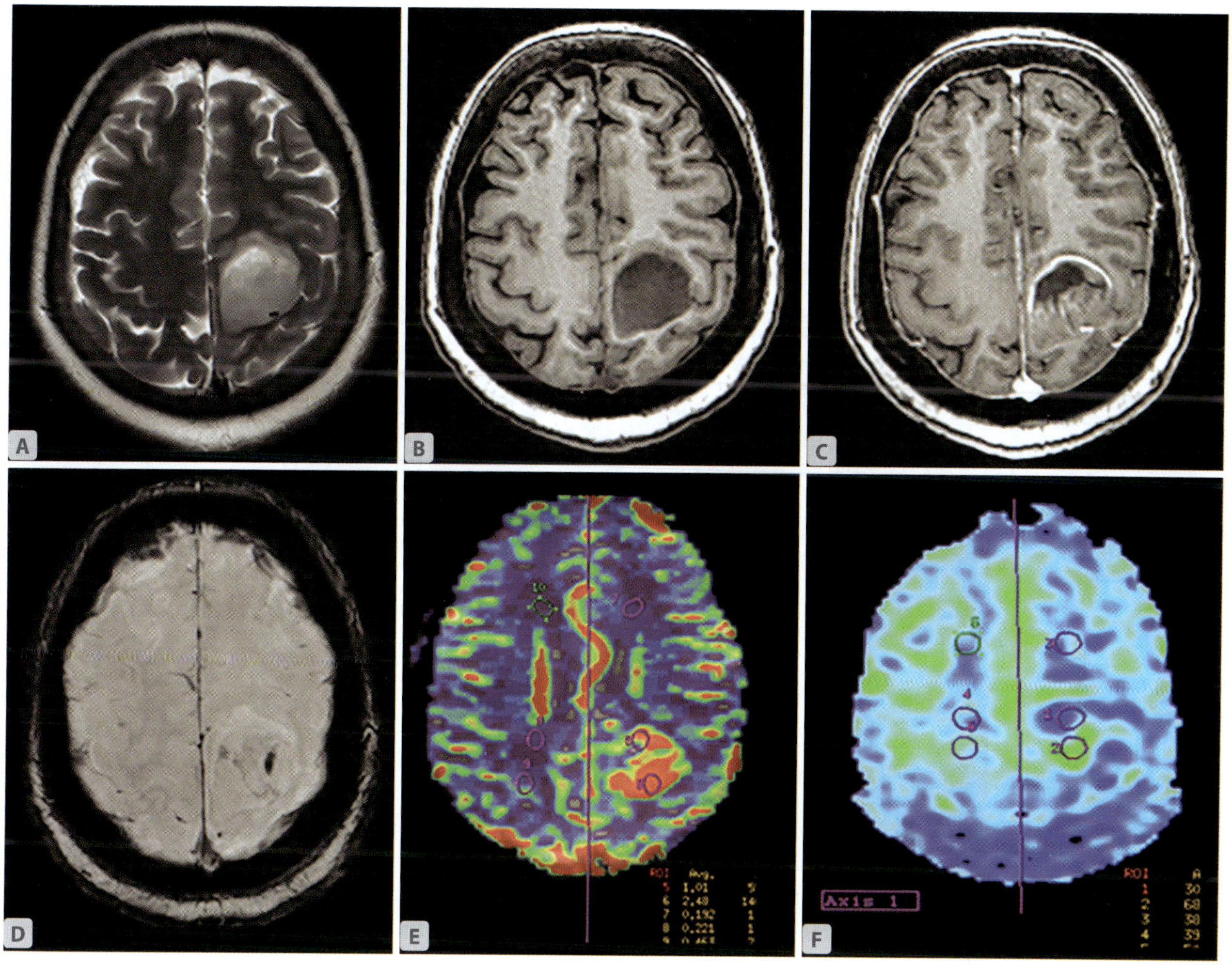

FIGS. 5A TO F: Brain MRI of a 32 years male patient presenting right hemiparesis, axial T2-weighted image (A), axial reformatted pre-contrast 3D T1-SPGR image (B) and Axial reformatted postcontrast 3D T1-SPGR image (C) show a T2 hyperintense mass lesion in left high parietal region showing peripheral enhancement. Susceptibility weighted image (D) shows few intralesional susceptibility changes suggesting hemorrhage. rCBV map generated from dynamic susceptibility perfusion sequence (E), CBF map (F) generated from arterial spin labeling perfusion sequence show elevated perfusion parameters within the lesion (as shown by the ROI drawn in the tumor and contralateral normal brain parenchyma). Overall features are suggestive of high-grade glioma.

contrast content. This leads to k^{trans} overestimation in these voxels which appear as areas of apparently high permeability in areas of normal brain. This problem can be approached by excluding any voxel which produces values above a certain threshold (1.2/min) as being vascular in origin or more complex pharmacokinetic models.

- *Long acquisition time:* Because a considerable period of time (more than 5 min) is required for the measurement, permeability imaging suffers from the drawback of longer acquisition time. There is little or no misregistration of data in brain perfusion and data co-registration can be used to remove the misregistration, if any. However, significant misregistration can occur in imaging of the body parts, affected by respiratory motion, and respiratory gating techniques significantly cripple the image acquisition strategy and the achievable temporal sampling rate. This can be approached by modifying the pharmacokinetic model and describing only the first passage of the contrast bolus. The problems with partial volume averaging described above can also be eliminated by this technique and highly reproducible parametric maps of both k^{trans} and CBV can be produced.
- *Flow dependency of k^{trans}:* k^{trans} measurement is mainly affected by flow to the voxel. In addition, the permeability and surface area of the vascular endothelium also affects the k^{trans}. For measurements of k^{trans}, it is assumed that the rate of contrast leakage will be proportional to the permeability and surface area of the vascular endothelium for any given combination of intravascular and extravascular contrast concentrations; however, it hold true only when there is sufficiently high supply of contrast to the vascular space so that the intravascular concentration is not affected by contrast leakage. There is limitation, in areas where there is contrast leakage and the blood flow is inadequate to replenish contrast at

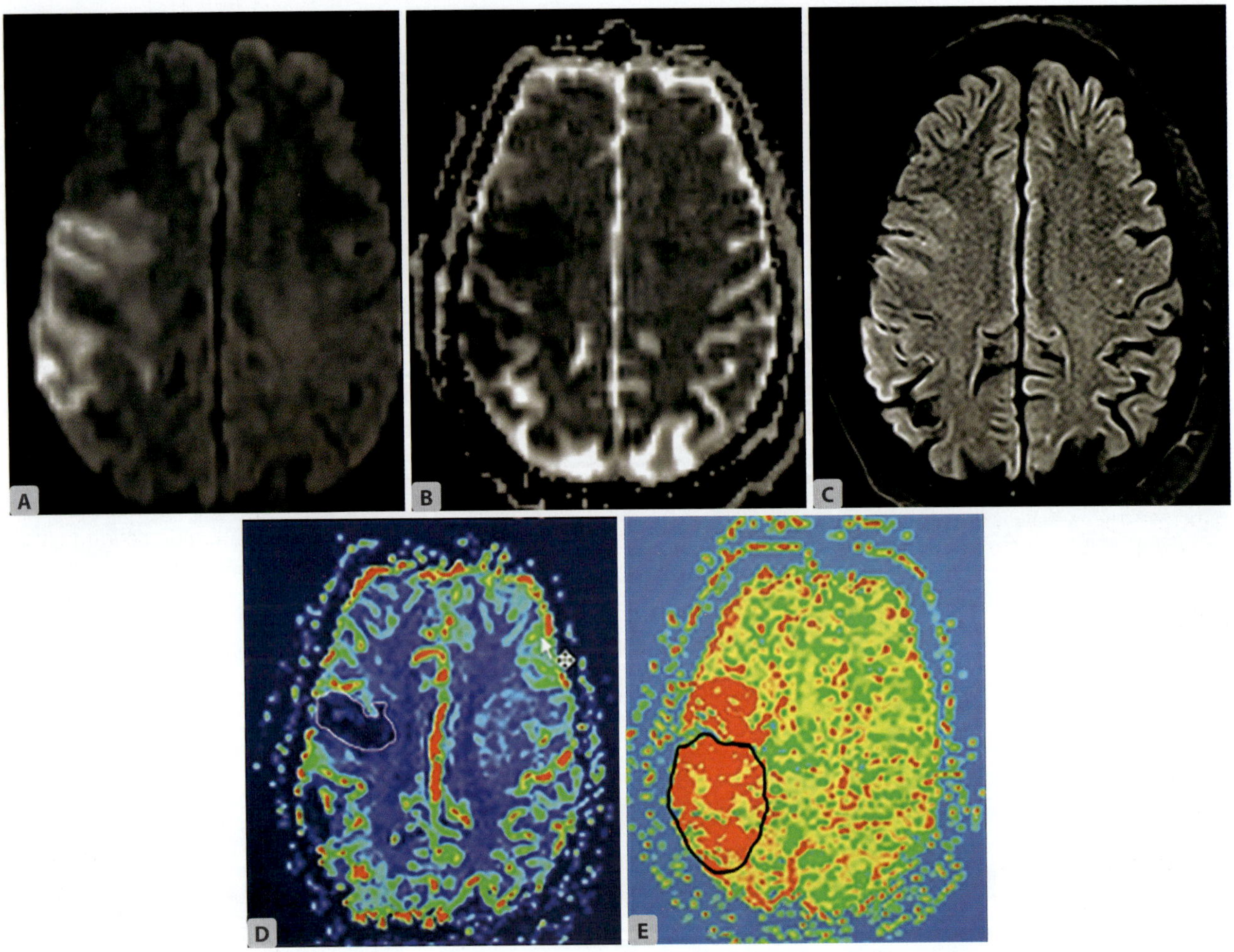

FIGS. 6A TO E: Brain MRI of a 51 years old female patient presenting left hemiparesis for 4 hours, axial DWI (A) and corresponding ADC map (B) show an area of diffusion restriction in right MCA territory. Axial FLAIR image (C) showed no signal change in the area of diffusion restriction. rCBV (D) and MTT maps (E) generated from DSC perfusion technique. Prolonged MTT is seen in the area corresponding to the area of diffusion restriction suggesting the area of ischemia. CBV map however shows area of reduced rCBV (outlined by white line in D) which is much smaller than the entire ischaemic zone suggesting infarct core. The area of CBV-MTT mismatch (outlined by black line in E) indicates the penumbra or salvageable parenchyma.

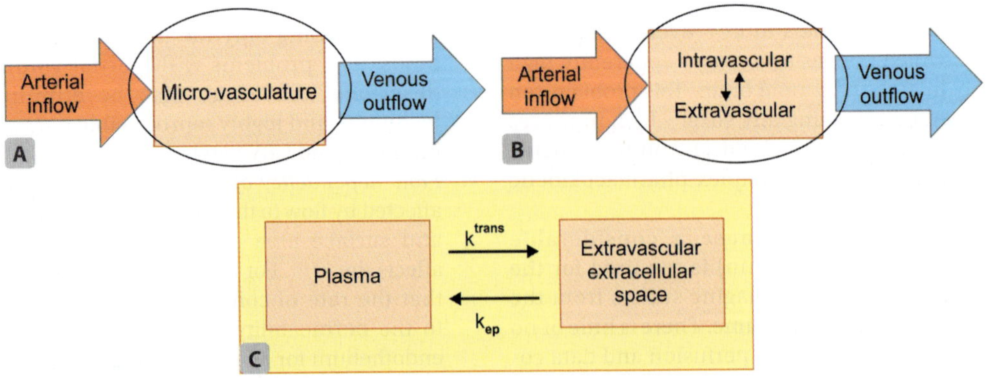

FIGS. 7A TO C: Schematic visualization of single (A) and two compartment (B) model. In dynamic contrast-enhanced MR perfusion, two-compartment model (C) demonstrates the exchange of contrast between plasma and extravascular extracellular space.

adequate rate; as a result plasma contrast concentration decreases and local blood flow is reflected by k^{trans}.

Clinical applications of DCE MR Perfusion in brain: Tough this technique is standard approach for perfusion MRI outside the brain, where it is routinely used in patients with breast, prostate, pelvic and muscles diseases for differentiation, characterizing and treatment response. It is also often used in neoplastic and inflammatory conditions of the brain. An excellent insight into neo-angiogenesis in conditions like tumor and inflammation can be obtained by quantification of contrast leakage. The technique can also be useful in monitoring the therapeutic effects of the antiangiogenic drugs.

Arterial Spin Labeling MR Imaging

Arterial spin labeling (ASL) is an alternative technique of performing perfusion MRI without using an intravenous contrast agent.[33] ASL can be thought of as a natural extension of MR angiography (MRA) and is also closely related to blood flow imaging with $H2^{15}O$ PET. Many recent studies show that ASL provides information, similar to the DSC or DCE MRP, and even have more advantages as compared to these techniques including better ASL flow maps in detecting regions of disturbed vascularity and being independent of tumor permeability, hence no corrections are required. Hitherto, limitations of ASL like long imaging times and decreased spatial resolution as compared with contrast-based techniques have excluded widespread clinical application of ASL, but with recent advancements, the ASL may cause a paradigm shift in perfusion MRI techniques.

Principle

Magnetically labeled blood is used as an endogenous contrast agent in ASL. In this technique, spatially selective excitation pulses or flow encoding gradient pulses are applied to inflowing blood to differentiate between static tissue and flowing blood. Time is allowed for the blood to move out of the vessels and into the perfused tissue, and then the signal change in tissue caused by the selective labeling of the arterial blood is measured which is closely related to the blood flow into that tissue. Calculation of CBF in ASL perfusion is done by measuring the difference of two sets of images: tag images, where the longitudinal magnetization of arterial blood is inverted or saturated, and control images where the magnetization of arterial blood is fully relaxed. The control image of the same slice is acquired where the inflowing blood is not tagged, to remove the contribution of the static tissue to the tag image. The magnetization difference ($\Delta M = M_{contr} - M_{tag}$) i.e. difference of the control and tag images provides an image that is proportional to CBF. The acquisition of tag and control images is in a temporally interleaved fashion, and a perfusion time series is formed by the difference between the control and tag images.

Image Acquisition and Labeling Techniques

Different labeling techniques of ASL, that have been described or used for in vivo studies, are very similar and differ only in subtle aspects of implementation. However they are broadly divided into spatially selective ASL and velocity-selective ASL.[34] In spatially selective ASL, a spatial separation between the imaged region and inflowing arterial blood is required to cause signal change in the image whereas in velocity-selective ASL, bipolar gradients are used to label flowing blood. Velocity-selective ASL, resemble phase contrast angiography, and can be used to label blood within the slice or slab and thus may permit labeling even closer to the capillary bed than spatially selective ASL. In most of the ASL techniques, magnetization is labeled along the main magnetic field direction (Mz). The advantage of labeling Mz is that changes in Mz return back to the equilibrium on the time scale of T1. The magnetization can also be labeled along the transverse direction (Mx or My) but since the transverse magnetization decays with T2, typically 5–10 times faster than T1 decay, the signal produced would be much smaller.

Spatially selective ASL is by far the well-developed technique and most studies have been performed using this technique. It is similar to time-of-flight angiography. Inflowing blood may be tagged intermittently or continuously and can be broadly divided into continuous ASL and pulsed ASL **(Figs. 8A to C)**. Different pulsed labeling strategies differ from each other in primarily two issues. First is what inversions are applied to other tissue, including the imaged region, and secondly what is done to insure that the differences between the two RF preparations do not cause direct effects on the image which are independent of perfusion.

Pulsed ASL

In this technique, single perturbing pulse is applied to the spins outside the slice at a single time point, and then time is given for the spins to enter the tissue **(Figs. 8B and C)**. Usually, an RF pulse is applied at a time approximately 1 s before imaging. An inversion RF pulse is usually used as it creates the largest change in the arterial magnetization and the time before imaging is referred to as TI, as in inversion recovery sequences. Two images are obtained, one with the region containing the inflowing artery inverted and one where it is not inverted. The signal change with pulsed techniques is smaller than with continuous techniques as the spins which enter the tissue later are perturbed earlier than in the continuous technique, there is additional T1 decay of the label and generally. However, this technique also have additional advantages including more traditional RF and gradient strategies, are less subject to certain types of systematic error, and can produce excellent images. Pulsed ASL methods include EPISTAR (echo planar imaging and signal targeting with alternating radiofrequency), FAIR (flow-sensitive alternating inversion recovery), STAR (Signal Targeting with Alternating Radio Frequency), TILT (Transfer Insensitive Labeling Technique) (Gobay 1999), PICORE (Proximal Inversion with a Control for Off-resonance Effect) (Wong 1997).[35]

EPISTAR (echo planar imaging and signal targeting with alternating radiofrequency) technique is the simplest pulsed inversion strategy and was first proposed by Edelman et al. In this technique a slab-selective inversion pulse is applied inferior to the imaged brain region to label arterial spins and a superior inversion slab is applied during the control image preparation. The superior inversion insures equal magnetization transfer effects from the two preparation pulses.

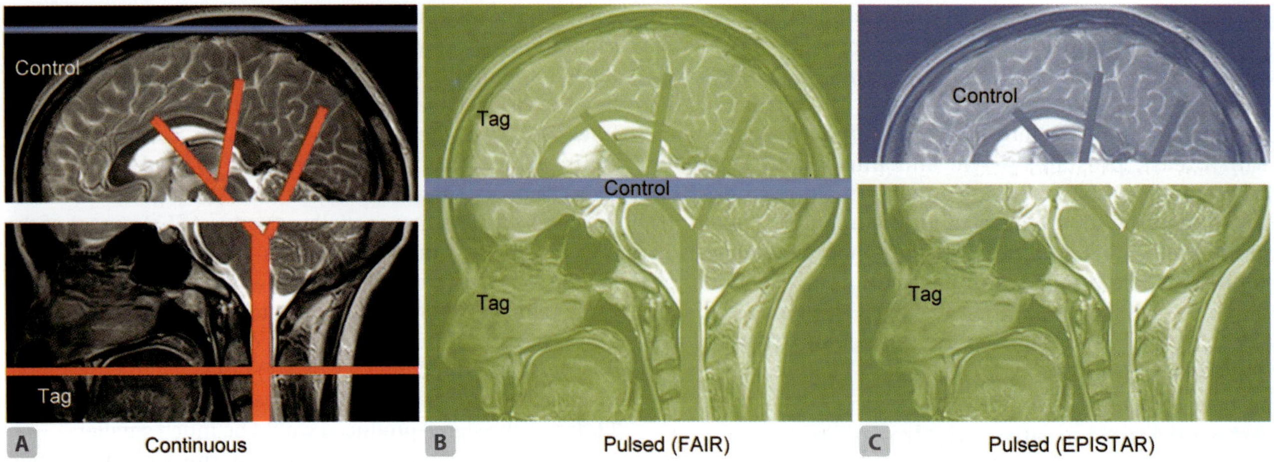

FIGS. 8A TO C: ASL techniques, schematic diagram illustrating arterial spin labeling strategies. (A) Continuous ASL (CASL) labels arterial spins as they flow through a labeling plane. (B and C) Pulsed ASL (PASL) labels arterial spins using a spatially selective labeling pulse.

Because any slight difference in the flip angle of the two pulses will have a big effect upon the measured signal, special RF pulses with low sensitivity to variations in RF amplitude and very sharp slice profiles must be employed. There are number of variations of these basic labeling techniques and most of them may provide small improvements to the results but variations in implementation and methods of assessment overshadow these small differences.

Continuous ASL

In this technique, spins are continuously inverted at a specific location before they enter the tissue.[36] Thus spins which enter the tissue first are labeled first and spins which enter later are labeled later. One can approximate continuous saturation of spins as they flow past a certain plane by applying a series of thin saturation pulses repeatedly, but trying the same strategy with inversion pulses is problematic; some spins may remain within the saturation slab for two or more inversions and get doubly inverted. Inversion pulse is considered highly desirable to use a continuous inversion technique as it provides a stronger signal change. Continuous ASL methods include Saturation, inversion (Williams 1992) with flow-driven adiabatic inversion pulse and labeling with 2nd coil. Continuous ASL usually employs a special RF labeling scheme known as flow-driven adiabatic inversion. Flow-driven adiabatic inversion is a simple technique because it requires only turning on a constant gradient and RF **(Fig. 8A)**. While the pulsed ASL experiment is essentially a decaying bolus experiment where the labeled blood transiently enters the tissue, the continuous ASL experiment can be operated as a steady-state experiment. If the labeling is left on for a long time, a balance between the inflow of newly labeled spins and the T1 decay of the labeled spins already in the tissue is reached. This makes quantification of perfusion relatively simple. As compared with pulsed ASL, the continuous ASL can achieve a signal approximately 2–3 times larger is generally more sensitive. The greatest disadvantage of the continuous labeling approach is the unusual RF requirements of the labeling. As in CASL (Flow-driven adiabatic inversion), weaker RF for an extended period of time is required, implementation may be difficult because many scanners are designed specifically for brief, widely spaced pulses of RF at high power.

Vessel Selective Labeling

This is a recent approach where arterial water is labeled selectively on the basis of the blood velocity. The main difference between this and the other ASL techniques is that the arterial water is labeled everywhere, including the volume of interest, so that the time for the blood to reach any region of interest is minimized.

Pseudo-continuous Arterial Spin Labeling (psCASL)

Pseudo-continuous arterial spin labeling (psCASL) or pulsed continuous arterial spin labeling (pCASL) is a newly proposed technique that has eased the technical restrictions of CASL and employs a train of discrete RF pulses that mimics continuous ASL.38 In pCASL, a train of rapidly repeating low tip RF pulses and alternating sign (bipolar) magnetic field gradients are used for continuous labeling. This is also ideal for MR scanners lacking continuous RF capabilities. In addition, it has been shown that pCASL can achieve better compensation of adverse MT effects than CASL.

Data analysis (Calculating Blood Flow from ASL Measurements)

The control and tag images of the ASL are acquired in an interleaved fashion and then from the running subtraction of the control and tag images, a perfusion time series is calculated. [39,40] Hence, the simple subtraction image obtained can be a good reflection of relative blood flow without any calculations. However, because differences in tissue T1 and other factors can lead to different sensitivity to blood flow across the image and quantitative measurements of blood flow can be useful for some purposes, it can be useful to convert the difference images into actual blood flow maps in physiologic units. This conversion requires some consideration of how inflow impacts tissue MR signal.

Problems with ASL

Despite its advantages, ASL imaging is limited by a large background signal and the motion artifacts. In addition, the small signal level of ASL reduces the signal-to-noise ratio of the ASL perfusion imaging. With recent advancement in MRI technology, good quality images can be obtained.

Clinical Applications of ASL Perfusion

Hitherto, ASL is mainly used in research and experimental studies; these are the potential applications of ASL in brain imaging.

- ASL perfusion may be used for early diagnosis of dementia and other neurodegenerative diseases as changes had been shown in neurocognitive decline.
- ASL perfusion can not only detect perfusion mismatch in acute stroke. It may be quiet helpful in identifying the tissue at risk in chronic cerebrovascular diseases.
- Demonstration of arteriovenous shunting in cerebral AVMs and ACFs may be possible with ASL.
- Epileptogenic foci may be identified using ASL in seizure disorder patients.
- Standard DSC perfusion may be replaced by ASL particularly in patients with gadolinium allergies or renal insufficiency or in children.
- Subtle functional changes in psychiatric disorders such as posttraumatic stress disorder or mild traumatic brain injury can be picked by ASL where standard structural MR imaging typically provides no detectable anomaly.
- Super-selective ASL to map vascular territories and cerebrovascular reserve imaging are relatively newer applications.

DYNAMIC CONTRAST-ENHANCED MAGNETIC RESONANCE IMAGING

Dynamic contrast-enhanced MR imaging (DCE-MRI) involves the acquisition of sequential MR images of the area of interest using rapid MR sequences before, during, and after intravenous injection of a gadolinium-based contrast agent.[41] This technique allows assessment of various parameters, including blood flow (BF), blood volume (BV), vascular permeability, and wash-in and washout characteristics of the tissue under study. These parameters, in turn, serve as vascular biomarkers of the tissue under evaluation. Of particular interest in this technique is the assessment of tumor tissues. This is because angiogenesis is one of the hallmark features of cancer allowing the tumor cells to grow and survive. Further, the characteristics of tumor microvasculature including the properties of the basement membrane, muscularis propria, and interendothelial junctions that contribute to the vascular permeability correlate with tumor biology.[42] Well-differentiated tumors have a normal microvasculature while poorly differentiated tumors comprise of leaky and disorganized vessels.[43]

DCE-MRI has been investigated in several clinical scenarios including for the initial diagnosis and staging of tumors.[41] In addition, it has recently been utilized as an imaging biomarker for monitoring response to various forms of treatment including chemotherapy, antiangiogenic therapy, radiotherapy and embolotherapy for various cancers.[44] Also, there is an increasing interest in non-oncologic applications of DCE-MRI.

NON-NEUROLOGY APPLICATIONS OF DCE-MRI

Head and Neck

Differentiation of Squamous Cell Carcinoma (SCC) from Lymphoma

As lymphomas have a high cell density and lower vascular permeability, they have a lower k^{trans} and V_e compared to SCCs.[43]

Detecting Metastatic Lymph Nodes

Differentiation of benign from metastatic lymph nodes allows accurate staging as well as surgical and radiotherapy planning. In a study comprising larger nodes, metastatic SCC has been shown to have a lower maximum slope, lower peak enhancement, shorter time to peak (TTP), slower washout slope, and higher k^{trans} compared to normal nodes.[45]

Evaluation of Salivary Gland Tumors

While pleomorphic adenoma shows progressive enhancement (time to peak >150 seconds), Warthin tumors show early wash-in (TTP <150 sec) and rapid wash-out (ratio >30%).[46,47] Malignant salivary gland tumors show early wash-in (TTP less than 150 sec) and slow wash-out (ratio <30%).[46,47]

Evaluation of Thyroid Gland Tumors

A delayed inflow pattern [longer time to peak and lower maximum rise slope of contrast enhancement (Type III curve)] has been shown to correlate significantly with a diagnosis of thyroid carcinoma.[48] However, in another study, rapid wash-in and wash-out (Type I curve) was shown to favor follicular malignancy over benign follicular neoplasm.[49] Other investigators have also demonstrated that plateau pattern may be seen in thyroid malignancy.[50] These different results have been attributed to some extent to the technique of DCE MRI.

Treatment Response

The application of MRI to predict treatment response in head and neck cancers has increased as there is widespread use of CRT as an alternative to surgery. This may be done at the start of therapy in order to find the most suitable agent or at the end of treatment to detect residual disease that can undergo salvage surgery. In contrast to anatomical imaging, CE-MRI based functional imaging can detect tumors that are expected to respond even before there a change in size.[51,52] This is quite relevant as CRT regimens to be changed or adapted in time.

Pre-treatment Prediction

Vascular tumors are likely to respond better to treatment as there is a better delivery of chemotherapy agents as well as a greater radiosensitivity.[52,53] The dynamic CEMRI parameter that correlated with this tumor biology most consistently is a high k^{trans}. However, a definite cut-off of k^{trans} that can predict tumor response is yet to be identified.

Early Intratreatment Assessment

Several studies suggest that CRT causes an increase in tumor perfusion. Thus, a relative rise in k^{trans} on follow up imaging predicts favorable tumor response.[54]

Post-treatment Evaluation

TIC evaluation in post-treatment response is expected to show a gradual increase in the early phase and prolonged plateau. The residual disease, on the other hand, shows rapid contrast wash-in and early wash-out. A few studies show that smaller V_e, smaller permeability surface area, and higher K_{ep} suggest residual or recurrent tumor.

Evaluation of Jaw Lesions

DCE-MRI has been utilized in the assessment of few jaw bone lesions. It has been shown that a prolonged increase in enhancement is characteristic of odontogenic myxomas.[55] However, based on the TIC pattern, the distinction could not be made between histopathological types of ameloblastomas. DCE-MRI has also been shown to be useful in distinguishing a simple bone cyst from true cysts in the jaw.[55] The role of DCE-MRI in detecting EBRT-induced changes in mandibular bone vascularity and hence radiation-induced injury has been described.[56]

Hematological Disorders

Multiple Myeloma (MM)

DCE-MRI of the spine has been demonstrated to be useful for the diagnosis of MM. The DCE-MRI parameters have also been found to be useful in follow-up after stem cell transplantation as well as evaluation of disease activity.[57] Another investigator demonstrated the ability of whole body DCE-MRI in assessing response to treatment in patients with MM. DCE-MRI was performed in 50 patients before treatment, after induction chemotherapy (n = 30) and after SCT (n = 20). Quantitative assessment of maximal percentage bone marrow enhancement (BME max) and focal lesion enhancement (FLE max) was found useful in assessing response to treatment.[58]

Leukemia

DCE-MRI measurement of vertebral bone marrow perfusion of patients with acute myeloid leukemia (AML) in remission has been demonstrated to be an indicator of outcome and survival. In a study comprising 51 patients with AML in remission, efflux rate constant (Kep) was found to significantly associated with overall survival and relapse-free survival.[59]

Musculoskeletal System

Dynamic contrast-enhanced MRI has been used for various clinical applications in musculoskeletal system including response monitoring following chemotherapy, identification of residual or recurrent tumor after treatment, differentiation of benign from malignant lesions, classification of bone lesions, detection of viable tumor prior to sampling, early detection of avascular necrosis and inflammatory spondyloarthropathy, and assessment of carpal tunnel syndrome and rheumatoid arthritis.[60-69]

Few recent applications are the assessment of disease activity in juvenile idiopathic arthritis (JIA), evaluation of bone perfusion in entities like Legg Calve Perthes disease, synovitis and arthritis, differentiation of osteoarthritis from rheumatoid arthritis, differentiation of psoriatic from rheumatoid arthritis, and monitoring of response to treatment in inflammatory arthritis.[70-75]

Chest

Due to the challenge posed by the inherent motion in the thoracic cavity, fewer studies have demonstrated the role of DCE-MRI in the evaluation of chest pathologies. In a study evaluating the additional benefit of DWI and DCE-MRI performed with 18F-FDG-PET/CT, the DCE-MRI parameters showed significant differences between benign and metastatic lymph nodes.[76] A recent study demonstrated the utility of DCE-MRI in evaluating cystic-cavitatory lung lesions. DCE-MRI obviated the need for biopsy in three patients and changed the site of biopsy in two patients when used in conjunction with CT.[77] DCE-MRI has also shown to be useful in patients with malignant pleural mesothelioma for assessing tumor microvascularity.[78,79] High pre-treatment values of K_{ep} within the tumors correlated with poor outcome. Recently DCE-MRI has also been utilized to study pulmonary perfusion.[80]

Prostate

Detection of Prostate Cancer

DCE-MRI may improve the detection of prostate cancer at biopsy **(Figs. 9A to C)**. Assessment with DCE-MRI in addition to T2-weighted MRI prior to guided repeat biopsy had a sensitivity of 83% and a 100% negative predictive value in patients with a previous negative biopsy.[81] In another study comprising patients who had elevated PSA (>4 ng/mL) and multiple inconclusive TRUS-guided biopsies, MRI-guided biopsy detected prostate cancer in 59% of the patients following a multiparametric MRI (comprising pharmacokinetic parameters and DWI).[82]

Staging of Prostate Cancer

Addition of pharmacokinetic parameters to conventional MRI is shown to be superior in the localization of prostate cancer. DCE-MRI has also been found to be superior to T2-weighted images in the demonstration of extracapsular extension of tumor.[83,84]

Detection of Recurrent Prostate Cancer

Detection of local tumor recurrence is challenging with conventional MRI, as the fibrotic changes and scar tissue after radiotherapy and prostatectomy respectively may mimic recurrence on T2-weighted MRI. DCE-MRI has a higher sensitivity for the detection of tumor recurrence after radiotherapy and prostatectomy compared with T2-weighted

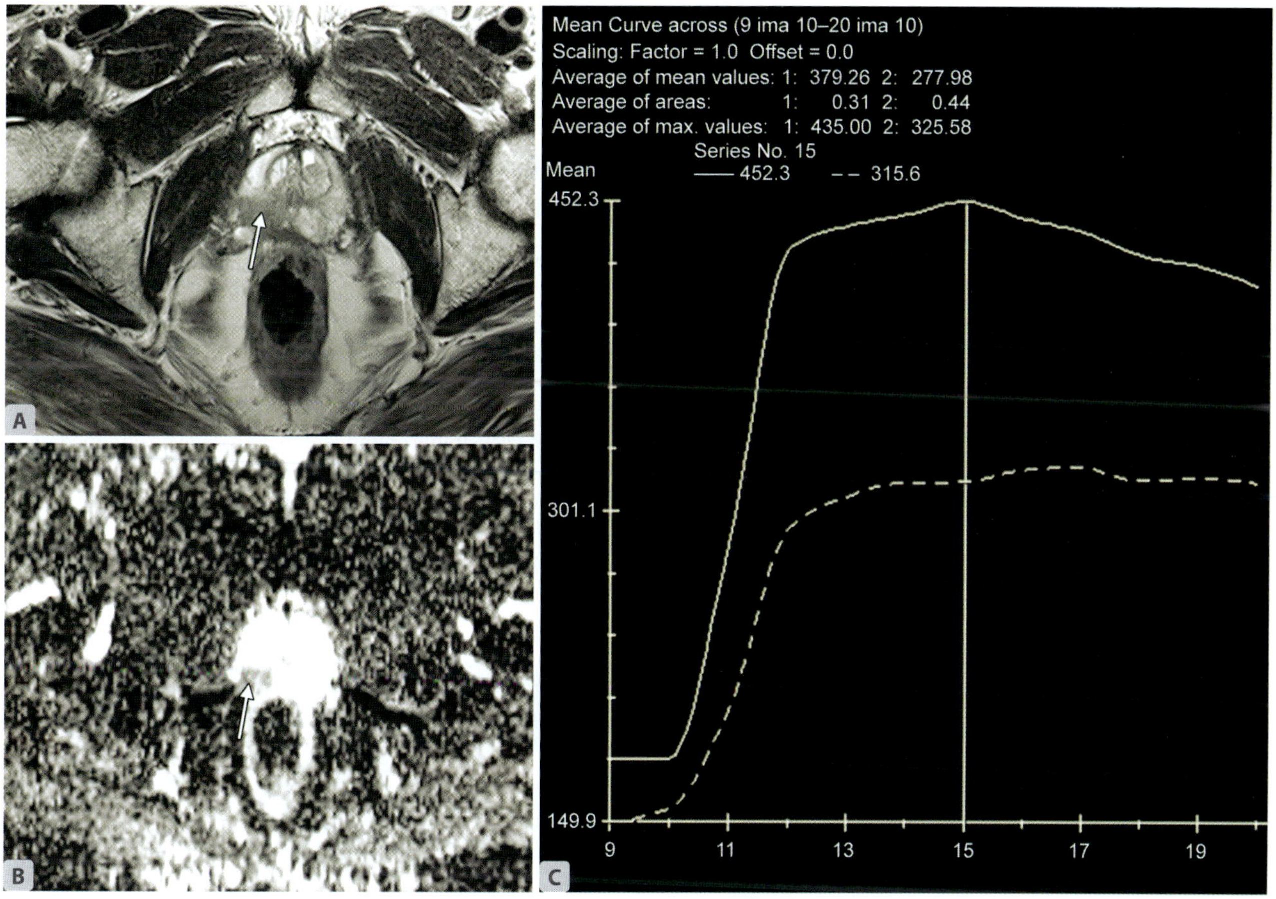

FIGS. 9A TO C: DCE-MRI of the prostate cancer. (A) Axial T2-weighted image shows a hypointense lesion in the right peripheral zone (arrow); (B) There is diffuse restriction on ADC map (arrow); (C) The time-intensity curve shows a type III curve (wash-in and wash-out).

MRI alone.[85-89] Similarly combining the pharmacokinetic parameters with the conventional MRI allows detection of recurrence after radiation with a higher positive predictive value. DCE-MRI may play a role for the detection of recurrence after high-intensity focused ultrasound (HIFU).[90]

Assessment of Biological Behavior and Prognosis

It has been shown that low-grade prostate cancers have a higher BV and higher vascular permeability compared with high-grade tumors.[91] However, studies failed to demonstrate correlation between MVD and DCE-MRI parameters.

Treatment Monitoring

Post-radiotherapy assessment of pharmacokinetic parameters on DCE-MRI has been shown to allow earlier assessment than the currently utilized methods.[92] DCE-MRI can also demonstrate a reduction in permeability following hormonal ablation therapy.[93-95]

Renal Cell Carcinoma

The primary utilization of the DCE-MRI has been as an early response biomarker following anti-angiogenic therapies or stereotactic ablative body radiotherapy.[96-98] In a study comprising 56 patients with RCC, DCE-MRI was performed following randomization to sorafenib or placebo. The initial area under curve and k^{trans} were reported as a pharmacodynamic marker of response to sorafenib.[99] However, changes in DCE-MRI parameters after four weeks were not predictive of progression-free survival (PFS). In another study comprising 17 patients with metastatic RCC, DCE-MRI demonstrated the significant reduction in k^{trans} on sorafenib therapy.[99] Moreover, it was shown that the percentage decline in k^{trans} was significantly associated with PFS.

Liver Tumors

DCE-MRI has been evaluated as a tool to differentiate hepatocellular carcinoma (HCC) from colorectal metastasis.[100] It has also been used to predict response to yttrium-90 (Y-90)-labeled octreotide (90Y-DOTATOC) treatment in patients with neuroendocrine metastases to the liver.[101] It has also been evaluated as a promising technique for response evaluation in patients with advanced unresectable HCC following chemotherapy and radiotherapy.[102-104] Similar results have been reported for anti-VEFG receptor tyrosine kinase inhibitor.[105] The decline in k^{trans} was significantly higher in patients with partial response or stable disease compared to those with disease progression. Studies have also demonstrated the role of DCE-MRI in predicting survival in patients with intrahepatic cholangiocarcinoma.[106]

Gastrointestinal Tract

DCE-MRI has been found to be beneficial in the evaluation of patients with inflammatory bowel disease and rectal cancer.[107-110] Florie et al. evaluated DCE-MRI in 48 patients with Crohn's disease.[107] The enhancement ratio was found to correlate significantly with the clinical grade and Crohn's disease activity index (CDAI). In another study, the DCE parameters were found useful in differentiating between inactive and active Crohn's disease.[108] In another study, there was a significant correlation between the DCE-MRI parameters and disease chronicity and angiogenesis. However, no correlation between these parameters and histological and clinical markers of inflammation.[109]

In a recent study, the role of DCE-MRI in the diagnosis of rectal carcinoma and tumor differentiation was assessed.[110] Forty patients and 15 controls were evaluated using DCE-MRI. The TIC showed an outflow pattern in rectal cancer. The quantitative parameters showed significantly higher values in patients compared to controls. There was a moderate correlation between k^{trans} and iAUC, and pathological differentiation.

Breast

Diagnosis of Breast Cancer and Cancer Type

DCE-MRI is an integral part of the MRI protocol for the diagnosis of breast cancer due to its high sensitivity and specificity **(Figs. 10A to F)**. DCE-MRI derived pharmacokinetic parameters, including k^{trans} and AUC as well as texture features, have been used to assess tumor characteristics.[111] In a recent study, malignant lesions had significantly higher k^{trans} and AUC values than benign tumors.[111] In a study aimed to clarify the DCE-MRI descriptors most strongly associated with a breast cancer diagnosis, mass margin on DCE, initial enhancement and delayed enhancement at DCE were found to be significantly associated with a breast cancer diagnosis.[111] A recent study found that the categorization of initial enhancement on ultra-fast DCE-MRI sequence was useful for differentiating malignant from benign breast

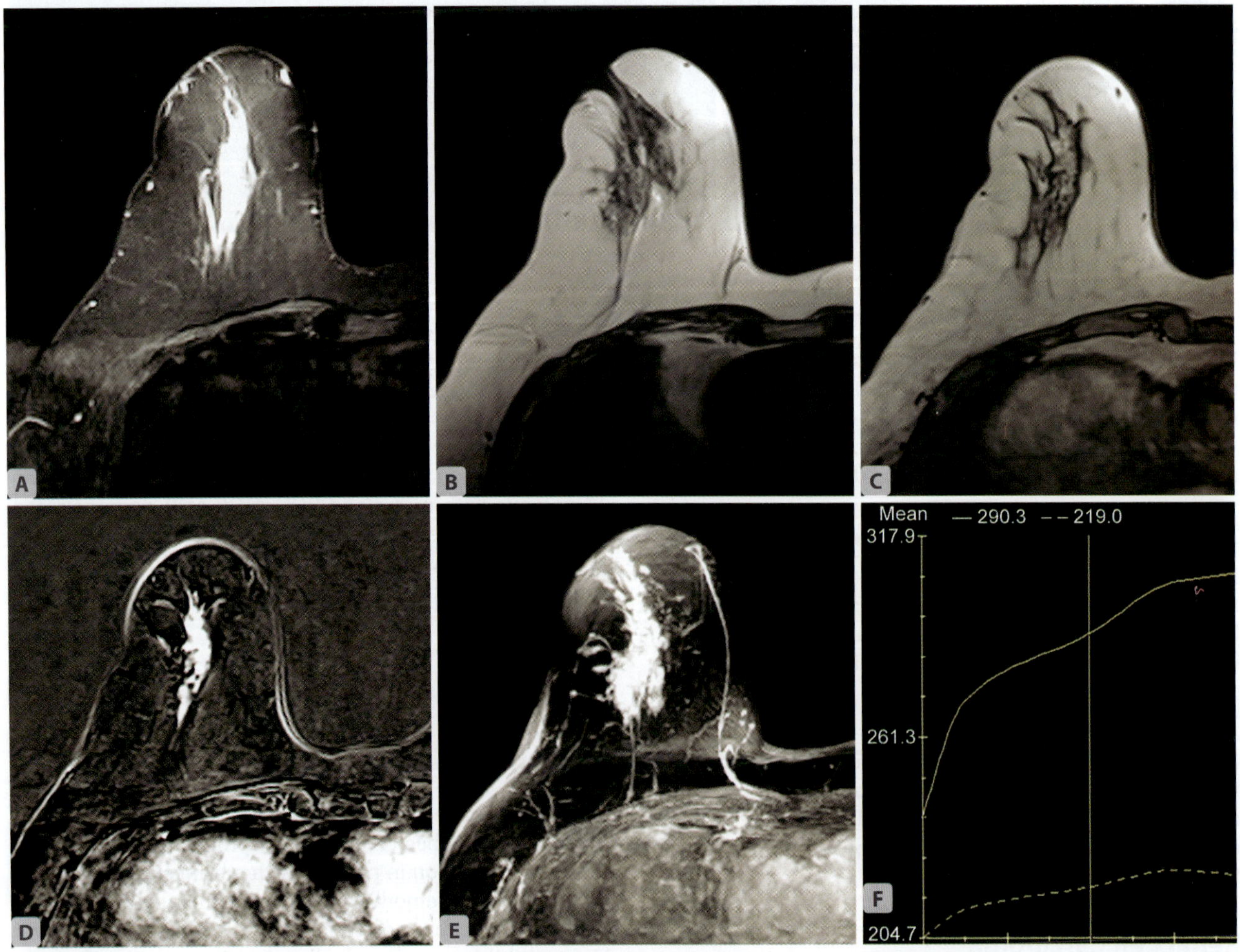

FIGS. 10A TO F: DCE-MRI of the breast cancer. (A) Axial T2-weighted fat suppressed image shows a hyperintense mass in the right breast in retro-areolar location; (B) Axial T1-weighted images shows the mass to be hypointense; (C to E) Contrast enhanced, subtracted and MIP images shows spiculated-enhancing mass; (F) The time-intensity curve shows a type I curve (persistent enhancement). Though, this type of curve is typically obtained in benign lesions, investigators have shown that qualitative assessment of the kinetic curves can misclassify certain lesions and in such cases quantitative assessment may be more useful (El Khouli, Am J Roentgen 2009).

lesions in both masses and non-mass like enhancement.[112] In the study, DCE-MRI parameters were evaluated to detect the dominant stroma-type of breast cancer.[113] V_e values were found to be significantly lower in tumors with the high tumor-stroma ratio. On the other hand, K_{ep} values were significantly lower in breast cancers that have dominant collagen type and higher in cancers with a high nuclear grade. In a recent study, delayed enhancement pattern was found to be the most reliable DCE-MRI feature in differentiating pure mucinous breast carcinoma and fibroadenoma.[114]

Response to Neoadjuvant Chemotherapy

A recent study found an associated of semi-quantitative assessment of the DCE-MRI using computer-aided detection with the response to neoadjuvant chemotherapy. Persistent type signal intensity-time curve was associated with the absence of complete pathological response to neoadjuvant chemotherapy.[115] Another study found that a decrease in blood permeability (change in k^{trans}) on DCE-MRI following bevacizumab and paclitaxel correlated with tumor regression. In yet another study, k^{trans} and K_{ep} of post-neoadjuvant chemotherapy DCE-MRI showed fair to good diagnostic performance for the prediction of response.[116]

Prognosis

DCE-MRI texture features have been found to correlate with the prognostic features of breast cancer. The expression of ER, PR and Ki-67 were found to have a significant correlation with shape, enhanced morphology type, and the edge of the cancer.[117,118] In another study, maximum enhancement, TTP, and the rate of wash-in were found to significantly correlate with various prognostic factors of breast cancer including ER status, immune profile and tumoral vascular invasion.[119]

Endometrial and Cervical Cancer

Diagnosis and Staging

In a retrospective study comprising 46 patients with cervical cancer, the authors compared the diagnostic performance of diffusion-weighted imaging (DWI) with that of DCE-MRI in the evaluation of tumor extent in stage IB cervical cancer.[120] No statistically significant difference was seen in the diagnostic performance of DCE-MRI compared to DWI. A similar study was performed to preoperative assess the myometrial invasion in patients with endometrial carcinoma.[121] The authors concluded that both DWI and DCE are good imaging techniques tools for the preoperative assessment of myometrial invasion. Another study compared the diagnostic accuracy of DWI and DCE-MRI for detecting cervical stromal invasion in endometrial cancer. DWI had a higher accuracy than DCE-MRI in the detection of cervical stromal invasion.[122] In a study comprising 22 patients with endometrial cancer, DCE-MRI was found to be more sensitive but less specific than T2-weighted MRI for the preoperative staging of early endometrial carcinoma.[123] Diagnostic accuracy of subendometrial enhancement (SEE) and peritumoral enhancement (PTE) on DCE-MRI to detect myometrial invasion was assessed in a study comprising 147 patients with endometrial carcinoma.[124] In this study, both SEE and PTE were found to be significantly correlated with myometrial invasion. **Figures 11A to D** demonstrates a case of cervical carcinoma with diffusion and DCE-MRI findings.

Assessment of Biological Behavior of Malignancy

A study compared the diagnostic accuracy of DWI and DCE-MRI for detecting cervical stromal invasion in endometrial cancer.[121] DWI had a higher accuracy than DCE-MRI in the detection of cervical stromal invasion, ADC maps had the best performance for detection of LN metastasis, and V_e maps showed the highest discriminative value for LVSI and tumor grade. In another study in patients with endometrial cancer, low blood flow and rate constant for contrast agent intravasation correlated with high-risk histological subtype and was associated with poor prognosis.[125] In another study, fast DCE-MRI was performed before and after RT in 10 patients with cervical cancer.[126] High-grade cervical cancers showed early enhancement compared with low-grade tumors. After radiotherapy, DCE-MRI parameters also differed significantly.

Response Assessment

DCE-MRI parameters have been shown to accurately assess the pathological response after preoperative combined chemo-radiotherapy in cervical carcinoma.[127] Type B TIC, maximum slope enhancement, initial AUC and k^{trans} were strongly correlated with tumor response.

Differentiation of Uterine Sarcoma from Atypical Leiomyoma

In a study evaluating the predictive value of multiparametric MRI in the differentiation of uterine sarcoma from atypical leiomyoma, besides, tumor location, ADC values, the TIC of the solid component were the factors significantly associated with accurate diagnosis.[128]

Ovarian Tumors

DCE-MRI is useful in the characterization of ovarian tumors. In a study comprising 15 benign, 28 borderline, and 66 malignant ovarian tumors, quantitative DCE-MRI parameters (k^{trans}, k_{ep}, and V_e) were evaluated.[129] The largest k^{trans} and k_{ep} values were observed in malignant tumors, followed by borderline and benign tumors. K_{ep} was found to be a better parameter for differentiating benign ovarian tumors from borderline and malignant tumors. Similar results were shown by another study comprising 102 complex ovarian tumors. In this study, the pattern of TIC allowed accurate distinction between malignant and borderline/benign tumors. Majority of the malignant tumors showed a type III TIC.[130]

Similarly, the maximal slope was significantly higher in malignant tumors compared with benign tumors. Another study evaluated the ability of the DCE-MRI features to diagnose indeterminate ovarian masses that had inconclusive MRI features of malignancy.[131] The maximum relative enhancement was found to be significantly higher in malignant masses compared with benign and borderline masses. Time to peak enhancement was shorter for malignant lesions.

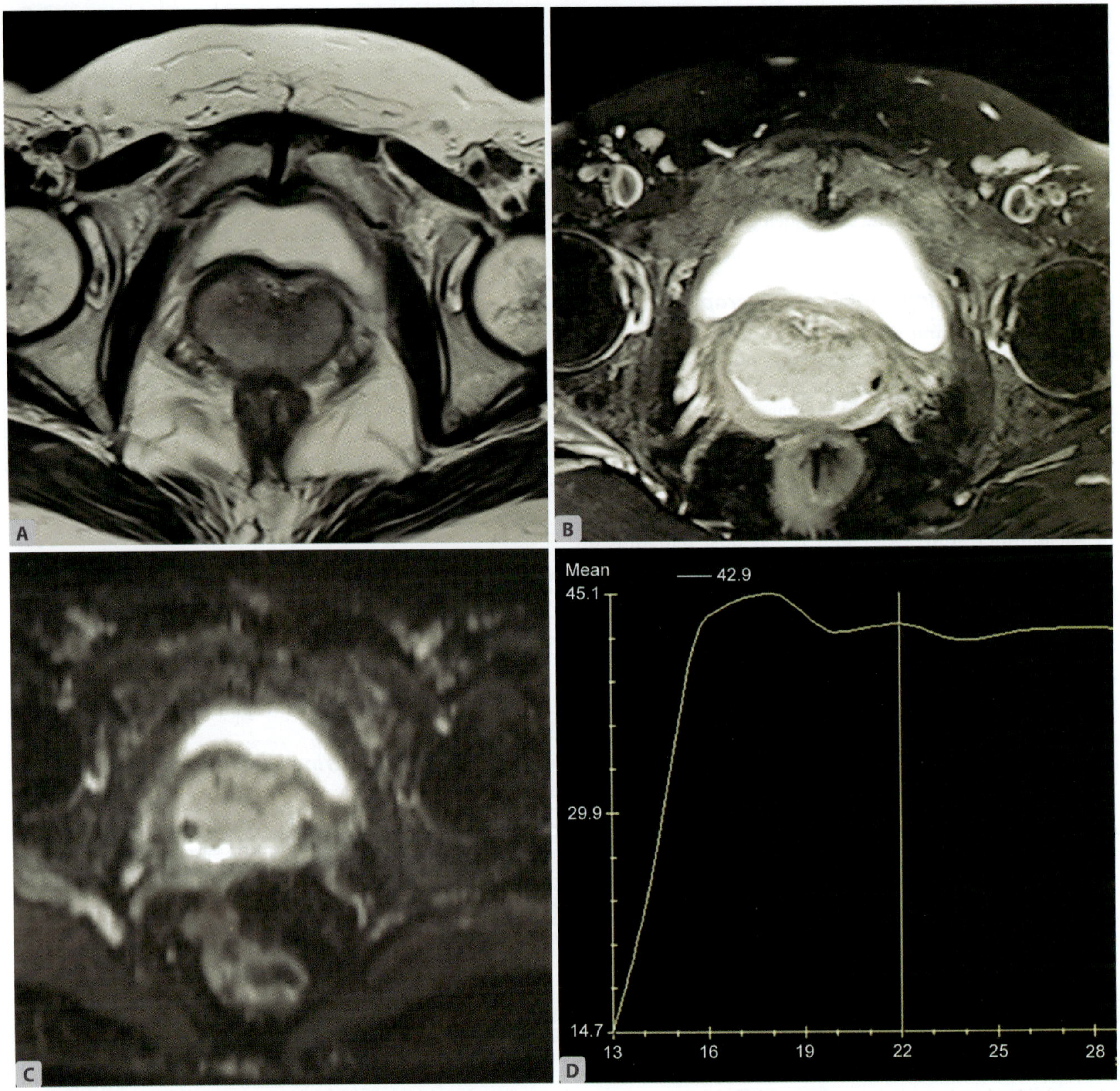

FIGS. 11A TO D: DCE-MRI of cervical cancer. (A and B) Axial T2-weighted and T2-weighted fat suppressed images shows a mass in the cervix. (C) It shows diffuse restriction. (D) The time-intensity curve shows a type II curve (plateau curve).

REFERENCES

1. Essig M, Shiroishi MS, Nguyen TB, Saake M, Provenzale JM, Enterline D, et al. Perfusion MRI: the five most frequently asked technical questions. Am J Roentgenol. 2013;200:24-34.
2. Hochberg AR, Young GS. Cerebral perfusion imaging. Semin Neurol. 2012;32:454-65.
3. Detre JA, Leigh JS, Williams DS, et al. Perfusion imaging. Magn Reson Med. 1992;23:37-45.
4. McGehee BE, Pollock JM, Maldjian JA. Brain perfusion imaging: How does it work and what should I use? J Magn Reson Imaging. 2012;36:1257-72.
5. Ostergaard. Principles of cerebral perfusion imaging by bolus tracking. J Magn Reson Imaging. 2005;22:710-7.
6. Wu, Ostergaard. Technical aspects of perfusion-weighted imaging. Neuroimaging Clin N Am. 2005;15:623-37.
7. Duyn, van Gelderen. Technological advances in MRI measurement of brain perfusion. J Magn Reson Imaging. 2005;22:751-3.
8. Rosen BR, Belliveau JW, Buchbinder BR, et al. Contrast agents and cerebral hemodynamics. Magn Reson Med. 1991;19:285-92.
9. Keston P, Murray AD, Jackson A. Cerebral perfusion imaging using contrast-enhanced MRI. Clin Radiol. 2003;58:505-13.
10. Williams DS, Detre JA, Leigh JS, et al. Magnetic resonance imaging of perfusion using spin inversion of arterial water. Proc Natl Acad Sci USA. 1992;89:212-16.

11. Sourbron S. Technical aspects of MR perfusion. Eur J Radiol. 2010;76(3):304-13.
12. Griffith B, Jain R. Perfusion Imaging in Neuro-Oncology: Basic Techniques and Clinical Applications. Magn Reson Imaging Clin N Am. 2016;24(4):765-79.
13. Jahng GH, Li KL, Ostergaard L, Calamante F. Perfusion magnetic resonance imaging: a comprehensive update on principles and techniques. Korean J Radiol. 2014;15(5): 554-77.
14. Grand S, Tahon F, Attye A, Lefournier V, Le Bas JF, Krainik A. Perfusion imaging in brain disease. Diagn Interv Imaging. 2013; 94(12):1241-57.
15. Dickerson E, Srinivasan A. Multicenter Survey of Current Practice Patterns in Perfusion MRI in Neuroradiology: Why, When, and How Is It Performed? AJR Am J Roentgenol. 2016; 207(2):406-10.
16. Petrella JR, Provenzale JM. MR perfusion imaging of the brain: techniques and applications. AJR Am J Roentgenol. 2000;175: 207-19.
17. Cha S. Perfusion MR imaging: basic principles and clinical applications. Magn Reson Imaging Clin N Am. 2003;11:403-13.
18. Covarrubias DJ, Rosen BR, Lev MH. Dynamic magnetic resonance perfusion imaging of brain tumors. Oncologist. 2004;9:528-37.
19. Chavhan GB, Babyn PS, Thomas B, Shroff MM, Haacke EM. Principles, techniques, and applications of T2*-based MR imaging and its special applications. Radiographics. 2009;29: 1433-49.
20. Levin JM, Kaufman MJ, Ross MH. Sequential dynamic susceptibility contrast MR experiments in human brain: residual contrast agent effect, steady-state, and hemodynamic perturbation. Magn Reson Med 1995;34: 655-63.
21. Barbier EL, Lamalle L, Decorps M. Methodology of brain perfusion imaging. J Magn Reson Imaging 2001;13: 496-520.
22. Calamante F, Gadian DG, Connely A. Delay and dispersion effects in dynamic susceptibility contrast MRI: simulations using singular value decomposition. Magn Reson Med. 2000;44: 466-73.
23. Lorenz C, Benner T, Lopez CJ, et al. Effect of using local arterial input functions on cerebral blood flow estimation. J Magn Reson Imaging. 2006;24:57-65.
24. Welker K, Boxerman J, Kalnin A, Kaufmann T, Shiroishi M, Wintermark M; American Society of Functional Neuroradiology MR Perfusion Standards and Practice Subcommittee of the ASFNR Clinical Practice Committee. ASFNR recommendations for clinical performance of MR dynamic susceptibility contrast perfusion imaging of the brain. AJNR Am J Neuroradiol. 2015;36(6):E41-51.
25. Tofts PS, Brix G, Buckley DL, et al. Estimating kinetic parameters from dynamic contrast-enhanced T1-weighted MRI of a diffusable tracer: standardized quantities and symbols. J Magn Reson Imaging 1999;10:223-32.
26. Dean BL, Lee C, Kirsch JE, et al. Cerebral hemodynamics and cerebral blood volume: MR assessment using gadolinium contrast agents and T1-weighted turbo-FLASH imaging. Am J Neuroradiol. 1992;13:39-48.
27. Lu H, Law M, Johnson G, Ge Y, et al. Novel approach to the measurement of absolute cerebral blood volume using vascular-space-occupancy magnetic resonance imaging. Magn Reson Med. 2005;54:1403-11.
28. Paldino MJ, Barboriak DP. Fundamentals of quantitative dynamic contrast-enhanced MR imaging. Magn Reson Imaging Clin N Am. 2009;17:277-89.
29. Tofts PS, Kermode AG. Measurement of the blood-brain barrier permeability and leakage space using dynamic MR imaging. 1. Fundamental concepts. Magn Reson Med. 1991;17:357-67.
30. Cron GO, Kelcz F, Santyr GE. Improvement in breast lesion characterization with dynamic contrast-enhanced MRI using pharmacokinetic modeling and bookend T(1) measurements. Magn Reson Med. 2004;51:1066-70.
31. Nguyen TB, Cron GO, Mercier JF, et al. Diagnostic accuracy of dynamic contrast-enhanced MR imaging using a phase-derived vascular input function in the preoperative grading of gliomas. Am J Neuroradiol. 2012;33:1539-45.
32. Jackson A. Analysis of dynamic contrast enhanced MRI. Br J Radiol. 2004;77:S154-66.
33. van Laar PJ, van der Grond J, Hendrikse J. Brain perfusion territory imaging: methods and clinical applications of selective arterial spin-labeling MR imaging. Radiology. 2008;246:354-64.
34. Wong EC, Buxton RB, Frank LR. A theoretical and experimental comparison of continuous and pulsed arterial spin labeling techniques for quantitative perfusion imaging. Magn Reson Med. 1998;40:348-55.
35. Siewert B, Bly BM, Schlaug G, et al. Comparison of the BOLD and EPISTAR technique for functional brain imaging by using signal detection theory. Magn Reson Med. 1996;36:249-55.
36. Deibler AR, Pollock JM, Kraft RA, Tan H, Burdette JH, Maldjian JA. Arterial spin-labeling in routine clinical practice, part 1: technique and artifacts. Am J Neuroradiol. 2008;29:1228-34.
37. Järnum H, Steffensen EG, Knutsson L, et al. Perfusion MRI of brain tumours: a comparative study of pseudo-continuous arterial spin labelling and dynamic susceptibility contrast imaging. Neuroradiology. 2010;52:307-17.
38. Nezamzadeh M, Matson GB, Young K, Weiner MW, Schuff N. Improved pseudo-continuous arterial spin labeling for mapping brain perfusion. J Magn Reson Imaging. 2010; 31:1419-27.
39. Werner R, Norris DG, Alfke K, et al. Continuous artery-selective spin labeling (CASSL). Magn Reson Med. 2005; 53:1006-12.
40. Warmuth C, Gunther M, Zimmer C. Quantification of blood flow in brain tumors: comparison of arterial spin labeling and dynamic susceptibility-weighted contrast-enhanced MR imaging. Radiology. 2003;228:523-32.
41. Gaddikeri S, Gaddikeri RS, Tailor T, et al. Dynamic contrast-enhanced MR imaging in head and neck cancer: techniques and clinical applications. Am J Neuroradiol. 2016;37:588-95.
42. Hayes C, Padhani AR, Leach MO. Assessing changes in tumour vascular function using dynamic contrast-enhanced magnetic resonance imaging. NMR Biomed. 2002;15:154-63.
43. Park M, Kim J, Choi YS, et al. Application of dynamic contrast-enhanced MRI parameters for differentiating squamous cell carcinoma and malignant lymphoma of the oropharynx. AJR Am J Roentgenol. 2016;206:401-7.
44. Türkbey B, Thomasson D, Pang Y, Bernardo M, Choyke PL. The role of dynamic contrast-enhanced MRI in cancer diagnosis and treatment. Diagn Interv Radiol. 2010;16: 186-92.
45. Yan S, Wang Z, Li L, et al. Characterization of cervical lymph nodes using DCE-MRI: differentiation between metastases from SCC of head and neck and benign lymph nodes. Clin Hemorheol Microcirc. 2016;64:213-22.
46. Lam PD, Kuribayashi A, Imaizumi A, et al. Differentiating benign and malignant salivary gland tumours: diagnostic criteria and the accuracy of dynamic contrast-enhanced MRI with high temporal resolution. Br J Radiol. 2015; 88(1049): 20140685.
47. Yabuuchi H, Fukuya T, Tajima T, HachitandaY, Tomita K, Koga M. Salivary gland tumors: diagnostic value of gadolinium-enhanced dynamic MR imaging with histopathologic correlation. Radiology. 2003;226:345-54.
48. Yuan Y, Yue XH, Tao XF. The diagnostic value of dynamic contrast-enhanced MRI for thyroid tumors. Eur J Radiol. 2012;81:3313-8.

49. Gupta N, Norbu C, Goswami B, et al. Role of dynamic MRI in differentiating benign from malignant follicular thyroid nodule. Auris Nasus Larynx. 2011;38:718-23.
50. Tunca F, Giles Y, Salmaslioglu A, et al. The preoperative exclusion of thyroid carcinoma in multinodular goiter: Dynamic contrast-enhanced magnetic resonance imaging versus ultrasonography-guided fine-needle aspiration biopsy. Surgery. 2007;142: 992-1002.
51. Tezelman S, Giles Y, Tunca F, et al. Diagnostic value of dynamic contrast medium-enhanced magnetic resonance imaging in preoperative detection of thyroid carcinoma. Arch Surg. 2007;142:1036-41.
52. Hoskin PJ, Saunders MI, Goodchild K, et al. Dynamic contrast enhanced magnetic resonance scanning as a predictor of response to accelerated radiotherapy for advanced head and neck cancer. Br J Radiol. 1999;72:1093-8.
53. Ng SH, Lin CY, Chan SC, et al. Clinical utility of multimodality imaging with dynamic contrast-enhanced MRI, diffusion-weighted MRI, and 18F-FDG PET/CT for the prediction of neck control in oropharyngeal or hypopharyngeal squamous cell carcinoma treated with chemoradiation. PLoS One. 2014;9(12):e115933.
54. Kim H, Hartman YE, Zhai G, et al. Dynamic contrast-enhanced MRI evaluates the early response of human head and neck tumor xenografts following anti-EMMPRIN therapy with cisplatin or irradiation. J Magn Reson Imaging 2015;42(4):936-45.
55. Yanagi Y, Asaumi J, Unetsubo T, et al. Usefulness of MRI and dynamic contrast-enhanced MRI for differential diagnosis of simple bone cysts from true cysts in the jaw. Oral Surg Oral Med Oral Pathol Oral Radiol Endod 2010;110:364-9.
56. Joint Head and Neck Radiotherapy-MRI Development Cooperative. Dynamic contrast-enhanced MRI detects acute radiotherapy-induced alterations in mandibular microvasculature: prospective assessment of imaging biomarkers of normal tissue injury. Sci Rep. 2016;6:29864.
57. Dutoit JC, Vanderkerken MA, Verstraete KL. Value of whole body MRI and dynamic contrast enhanced MRI in the diagnosis, follow-up and evaluation of disease activity and extent in multiple myeloma. Eur J Radiol. 2013;82:1444-52.
58. Lin C, Luciani A, Belhadj K, et al. Multiple myeloma treatment response assessment with whole-body dynamic contrast-enhanced MR imaging. Radiology. 2010;254:521-31.
59. Chen BB, Hsu CY, Yu CW, et al. Dynamic contrast-enhanced MR imaging measurement of vertebral bone marrow perfusion may be indicator of outcome of acute myeloid leukemia patients in remission. Radiology. 2011; 258:821-31.
60. Sujlana P, Skrok J, Fayad LM. Review of dynamic contrast-enhanced MRI: Technical aspects and applications in the musculoskeletal system. J Magn Reson Imaging. 2018;47:875-90.
61. Reddick WE, Taylor JS, Fletcher BD. Dynamic MR imaging (DEMRI) of microcirculation in bone sarcoma. J Magn Reson Imaging. 1999;10:277-85.
62. Meier R, Thuermel K, Noël PB, et al. Synovitis in patients with early inflammatory arthritis monitored with quantitative analysis of dynamic contrast-enhanced optical imaging and MR imaging. Radiology. 2014;270: 176-85.
63. Cimmino MA, Innocenti S, Livrone F, Magnaguagno F, Silvestri E, Garlaschi G. Dynamic gadolinium-enhanced magnetic resonance imaging of the wrist in patients with rheumatoid arthritis can discriminate active from inactive disease. Arthritis Rheum. 2003;48:1207-13.
64. Ktinig H, Sieper J, Wolf K. Rheumatoid arthritis: evaluation of hypervascular and fibrous pannus with dynamic MK imaging enhanced with Gd-DTPA. Radiology. 1990;176: 473-7.
65. Konig H, Sieper J, Wolf K. Dynamic MRI for the differentiation of inflammatory joint lesions. Rofo Forlschr Geh Rontgenstr Neuen Bildgeb Verfahr. 1990:153:1-5.
66. Hanna SI, Parham DM, Fairclough DL, Meyer WH, Le AH, Fletcher BD. Assessment of osteosarcoma response to preoperative chemotherapy using dynamic FLASH gadolinium-DTPA-enhanced MR mapping. Invest Radiol. 1992;27:367-73.
67. De Baere T, Vanel D, Shapeero L, Charpentier A, Terrier P. di Paola M. Osteosarcoma after chemotherapy: evaluation with contrast material-enhanced subtraction MR imaging. Radiology. 1992;185:587-92.
68. Vanel D, Tardivon A, Shapeero L. Western A, De Baere T, Guinebretiere JM. Dynamic contrast-enhanced subtraction MR imaging in follow-up of aggressive soft-tissue tumors: a prospective study of 74 patients. Radiology. 1993; 189(suppl):205.
69. Fletcher BD, Hanna SL. Fairclough DL, Gronemeyer SA. Pediatric musculoskeletal tumors: use of dynamic contrast-enhanced MR imaging to monitor response to chemotherapy. Radiology. 1992;184:243-8.
70. Schwenzer NF, Kötter I, Henes JC, et al. The role of dynamic contrast-enhanced MRI in the differential diagnosis of psoriatic and rheumatoid arthritis. Am J Roentgenol. 2010;194:715-20.
71. van der Leij C, van de Sande MG, Lavini C, Tak PP, Maas M. Rheumatoid synovial inflammation: pixel-by-pixel dynamic contrast-enhanced MR imaging time-intensity curve shape analysis—a feasibility study. Radiology. 2009;253:234-40.
72. Maijer KI, van der Leij C, de Hair MJ, et al. Dynamic Contrast-Enhanced Magnetic Resonance Imaging Using Pharmacokinetic Modeling: Initial Experience in Patients With Early Arthritis. Arthritis Rheumatol. 2016;68:587-96.
73. Vordenbäumen S, Schleich C, Lögters T, et al. Dynamic contrast-enhanced magnetic resonance imaging of metacarpophalangeal joints reflects histological signs of synovitis in rheumatoid arthritis. Arthritis Res Ther. 2014;16:452.
74. Nusman CM, Lavini C, Hemke R, et al. Dynamic contrast-enhanced magnetic resonance imaging of the wrist in children with juvenile idiopathic arthritis. Pediatr Radiol. 2017;47:205-13.
75. Malattia C, Damasio MB, Basso C, et al. Dynamic contrast-enhanced magnetic resonance imaging in the assessment of disease activity in patients with juvenile idiopathic arthritis. Rheumatology (Oxford). 2010;49:178-85.
76. Flechsig P, Zabeck H, Reubold S, et al. Impact of FDG-PET and Dynamic Contrast-Enhanced MRI in Comparison with DWI for N-Staging in Lung Cancer Patients. Iran J Radiol. 2019;16:e68638
77. Karaman A, Araz O, Durur-Subasi I, et al. Added value of DCE-MRI in the management of cystic-cavitary lung lesions. Respirology. 2016;21:739-45.
78. Coolen J, De Keyzer F, Nafteux P, et al. Malignant pleural disease: diagnosis by using diffusion-weighted and dynamic contrast-enhanced MR imaging—initial experience. Radiology. 2012;263:884-92.
79. Giesel FL, Bischoff H, von Tengg-Kobligk H, et al. Dynamic contrast-enhanced MRI of malignant pleural mesothelioma: a feasibility study of noninvasive assessment, therapeutic follow-up, and possible predictor of improved outcome. Chest. 2006;129:1570-6.
80. Ingrisch M, Maxien D, Schwab F, Reiser MF, Nikolaou K, Dietrich O. Assessment of pulmonary perfusion with breath-hold and free-breathing dynamic contrast-enhanced magnetic resonance imaging: quantification and reproducibility. Invest Radiol. 2014;49:382-9.
81. Cheikh AB, Girouin N, Colombel M, et al. Evaluation of T2-weighted and dynamic contrast-enhanced MRI in localizing prostate cancer before repeat biopsy. Eur Radiol. 2009;19:770-8.

82. Hambrock T, Futterer JJ, Huisman HJ, et al. Thirty-twochannel coil 3T magnetic resonance-guided biopsies of prostate tumor suspicious regions identified on multimodality 3T magnetic resonance imaging: technique and feasibility. Invest Radiol. 43:686-94.
83. Kim CK, Park BK, Kim B. Localization of prostate cancer using 3T MRI: comparison of T2-weighted and dynamic contrast-enhanced imaging. J Comput Assist Tomogr. 2006;30:7-11.
84. Bloch BN, Furman-Haran E, Helbich TH, et al. Prostate cancer: accurate determination of extracapsular extension with high spatial-resolution dynamic contrast-enhanced and T2-weighted MR imaging—initial results. Radiology. 2007;245:176-85.
85. Haider MA, Chung P, Sweet J, et al. Dynamic contrast-enhanced magnetic resonance imaging for localization of recurrent prostate cancer after external beam radiotherapy. Int J Radiat Oncol Biol Phys. 2008;70:425-30.
86. Akin O, Gultekin DH, Vargas HA, et al. Incremental value of diffusion weighted and dynamic contrast enhanced MRI in the detection of locally recurrent prostate cancer after radiation treatment: preliminary results. Eur Radiol. 2011;21:1970-8.
87. Donati OF, Jung SI, Vargas HA, et al. Multiparametric prostate MR imaging with T2-weighted, diffusion-weighted, and dynamic contrast enhanced sequences: are all pulse sequences necessary to detect locally recurrent prostate cancer after radiation therapy? Radiology. 2013;268: 440-50.
88. Casciani E, Polettini E, Carmenini E, et al. Endorectal and dynamic contrast-enhanced MRI for detection of local recurrence after radical prostatectomy. Am J Roentgenol. 2008;190:1187-92.
89. Sciarra A, Panebianco V, Salciccia S, et al. Role of dynamic contrast enhanced magnetic resonance (MR) imaging and proton MR spectroscopic imaging in the detection of local recurrence after radical prostatectomy for prostate cancer. Eur Urol. 2008;54:589-600.
90. Rouvière O, Girouin N, Glas L, et al. Prostate cancer transrectal HIFU ablation: detection of local recurrences using T2-weighted and dynamic contrast-enhanced MRI. Eur Radiol. 2010;20:48-55.
91. Vos EK, Litjens GJ, Kobus T, et al. Assessment of prostate cancer aggressiveness using dynamic contrast-enhanced magnetic resonance imaging at 3 T. Eur Urol. 2013;64:448-55.
92. Franiel T, Lüdemann L, Taupitz M, Bohmer D, Beyersdorff D. MRI before and after external beam intensity-modulated radiotherapy of patients with prostate cancer: the feasibility of monitoring of radiation-induced tissue changes using a dynamic contrast-enhanced inversion-prepared dual-contrast gradient echo sequence. Radiother Oncol. 2009;93:241-5.
93. Kluetz PG, Figg WD, Dahut WL. Angiogenesis inhibitors in the treatment of prostate cancer. Expert Opin Pharmacother. 2010;11:233-47.
94. Padhani AR, MacVicar AD, Gapinski CJ, et al. Effects of androgen deprivation on prostatic morphology and vascular permeability evaluated with mr imaging. Radiology. 2001;218:365-74.
95. Barrett T, Gill AB, Kataoka MY, et al. DCE and DW MRI in monitoring response to androgen deprivation therapy in patients with prostate cancer: a feasibility study. Magn Reson Med. 2012;67:778-85.
96. Reynolds HM, Parameswaran BK, Finnegan ME, et al. Diffusion weighted and dynamic contrast enhanced MRI as an imaging biomarker for stereotactic ablative body radiotherapy (SABR) of primary renal cell carcinoma. PLoS One 2018;13:e0202387.
97. Bharwani N, Miquel ME, et al. Diffusion-weighted and multiphase contrast-enhanced MRI as surrogate markers of response to neoadjuvant sunitinib in metastatic renal cell carcinoma. Br J Cancer. 2014;110:616-24.
98. Hahn OM, Yang C, Medved M, et al. Dynamic contrast-enhanced magnetic resonance imaging pharmacodynamic biomarker study of sorafenib in metastatic renal carcinoma. J Clin Oncol. 2008;26:4572-8.
99. Flaherty KT, Rosen MA, Heitjan DF, et al. Pilot study of DCE-MRI to predict progression-free survival with sorafenib therapy in renal cell carcinoma. Cancer Biol Ther. 2008;7:496-501.
100. Abdullah SS, Pialat JB, Wiart M, et al. Characterization of hepatocellular carcinoma and colorectal liver metastasis by means of perfusion MRI. J Magn Reson Imaging. 2008;28:390-5.
101. Miyazaki K, Orton MR, Davidson RL, et al. Neuroendocrine tumor liver metastases: use of dynamic contrast enhanced MR imaging to monitor and predict radiolabeled octreotide therapy response. Radiology. 2012;263:139-48.
102. Jarnagin WR, Schwartz LH, Gultekin DH, et al. Regional chemotherapy for unresectable primary liver cancer: results of a phase II clinical trial and assessment of DCE-MRI as a biomarker of survival. Ann Oncol. 2009;20: 1589-95.
103. Wang J, Chen LT, Tsang YM, Liu TW, Shih TT. Dynamic contrast-enhanced MRI analysis of perfusion changes in advanced hepatocellular carcinoma treated with an antiangiogenic agent: a preliminary study. Am J Roentgenol. 2004;183:713-9.
104. Hsu CY, Shen YC, Yu CW, et al. Dynamic contrast-enhanced magnetic resonance imaging biomarkers predict survival and response in hepatocellular carcinoma patients treated with sorafenib and metronomic tegafur/uracil. J Hepatol. 2011;55: 858-65.
105. Saito K, Ledsam J, Sugimoto K, Sourbron S, Araki Y, Tokuuye K. DCE-MRI for Early Prediction of Response in Hepatocellular Carcinoma after TACE and Sorafenib Therapy: A Pilot Study. J Belg Soc Radiol. 2018;102:40
106. Yopp AC, Schwartz LH, Kemeny N, et al. Antiangiogenic therapy for primary liver cancer: correlation of changes in dynamic contrast-enhanced magnetic resonance imaging with tissue hypoxia markers and clinical response. Ann Surg Oncol. 2011;18:2192-9.
107. Florie J, Wasser MN, Arts-Cieslik K, Akkerman EM, Siersema PD, Stoker J. Dynamic contrast-enhanced MRI of the bowel wall for assessment of disease activity in Crohn's disease. AJR Am J Roentgenol. 2006;186:1384-92.
108. Giusti S, Faggioni L, Neri E, et al. Dynamic MRI of the small bowel: usefulness of quantitative contrast-enhancement parameters and time-signal intensity curves for differentiating between active and inactive Crohn's disease. Abdom Imaging. 2010;35:646-53.
109. Taylor SA, Punwani S, Rodriguez-Justo M, et al. Mural Crohn disease: correlation of dynamic contrast-enhanced MR imaging findings with angiogenesis and inflammation at histologic examination—pilot study. Radiology. 2009; 251:369-79.
110. Shen FU, Lu J, Chen L, Wang Z, Chen Y. Diagnostic value of dynamic contrast-enhanced magnetic resonance imaging in rectal cancer and its correlation with tumor differentiation. Mol Clin Oncol. 2016;4:500-6.
111. Niu Q, Jiang X, Li Q, et al. Texture features and pharmacokinetic parameters in differentiating benign and malignant breast lesions by dynamic contrast enhanced magnetic resonance imaging. Oncol Lett. 2018;16:4607-13.
112. Goto M, Sakai K, Yokota H, et al. Diagnostic performance of initial enhancement analysis using ultra-fast dynamic contrast-enhanced MRI for breast lesions. Eur Radiol. 2019;29:1164-74.
113. Yim H, Kang DK, Jung YS, Jeon GS, Kim TH. Analysis of kinetic curve and model-based perfusion parameters on dynamic contrast enhanced MRI in breast cancer patients: Correlations with dominant stroma type. Magn Reson Imaging. 2016;34: 60-5.
114. Qu N, Luo Y, Yu T, Yu H. Differentiation between Pure Mucinous Breast Carcinomas and Fibroadenomas with Strong High-Signal Intensity on T2-Weighted Images from Dynamic Contrast-Enhanced Magnetic Resonance Imaging. Breast Care (Basel). 2018;13:32-7.

115. Kim H, Kim HH, Park JS, Shin HJ, Cha JH, Chae EY, Choi WJ. Prediction of pathological complete response of breast cancer patients undergoing neoadjuvant chemotherapy: usefulness of breast MRI computer-aided detection. Br J Radiol. 2014;87:20140142.
116. Thukral A, Thomasson DM, Chow CK, et al. Inflammatory breast cancer: dynamic contrast enhanced MR in patients receiving bevacizumab—initial experience. Radiology 2007;244:727-35.
117. Wedam SB, Low JA, Yang SX, et al. Antiangiogenic and antitumor effects of bevacizumab in patients with inflammatory and locally advanced breast cancer. J Clin Oncol. 2006;24:769-77.
118. Tao W, Hu C, Bai G, Zhu Y, Zhu Y. Correlation between the dynamic contrast-enhanced MRI features and prognostic factors in breast cancer: A retrospective case-control study. Medicine (Baltimore). 2018;97:e11530.
119. Macchini M, Ponziani M, Iamurri AP, et al. Role of DCE-MR in predicting breast cancer subtypes. Radiol Med. 2018;123:753-64.
120. Lin Y, Chen Z, Kuang F, Li H, Zhong Q, Ma M. Evaluation of international federation of gynecology and obstetrics stage IB cervical cancer: comparison of diffusion-weighted and dynamic contrast-enhanced magnetic resonance imaging at 3.0 T. J Comput Assist Tomogr. 2013;37:989-94.
121. Beddy P, Moyle P, Kataoka M, et al. Evaluation of depth of myometrial invasion and overall staging in endometrial cancer: comparison of diffusion-weighted and dynamic contrast-enhanced MR imaging. Radiology. 2012;262:530-7.
122. Lin G, Huang YT, Chao A, et al. Endometrial cancer with cervical stromal invasion: diagnostic accuracy of diffusion-weighted and dynamic contrast enhanced MR imaging at 3T. Eur Radiol. 2017;27:1867-76.
123. Zheng L, Zheng S, Yuan X, Wang X, Zhang Z, Zhang G. Comparison of dynamic contrast-enhanced magnetic resonance imaging with T2-weighted imaging for preoperative staging of early endometrial carcinoma. Onco Targets Ther. 2015;8:1743-51.
124. Fujii S, Kido A, Baba T, et al. Subendometrial enhancement and peritumoral enhancement for assessing endometrial cancer on dynamic contrast enhanced MR imaging. Eur J Radiol. 2015;84:581-9.
125. Fasmer KE, Bjørnerud A, Ytre-Hauge S, et al. Preoperative quantitative dynamic contrast-enhanced MRI and diffusion-weighted imaging predict aggressive disease in endometrial cancer. Acta Radiol. 2018;59(8):1010-7.
126. Kallehauge JF, Tanderup K, Duan C, et al. Tracer kinetic model selection for dynamic contrast-enhanced magnetic resonance imaging of locally advanced cervical cancer. Acta Oncol. 2014;53:1064-72.
127. Jalaguier-Coudray A, Villard-Mahjoub R, Delouche A, et al. Value of Dynamic Contrast-enhanced and Diffusion-weighted MR Imaging in the Detection of Pathologic Complete Response in Cervical Cancer after Neoadjuvant Therapy: A Retrospective Observational Study. Radiology. 2017;284:432-42.
128. Bi Q, Xiao Z, Lv F, Liu Y, Zou C, Shen Y. Utility of Clinical Parameters and Multiparametric MRI as Predictive Factors for Differentiating Uterine Sarcoma From Atypical Leiomyoma. Acad Radiol. 2018;25:993-1002.
129. Li HM, Qiang JW, Ma FH, Zhao SH. The value of dynamic contrast-enhanced MRI in characterizing complex ovarian tumors. J Ovarian Res. 2017;10:4.
130. Mansour SM, Saraya S, El-Faissal Y. Semi-quantitative contrast-enhanced MR analysis of indeterminate ovarian tumours: when to say malignancy? Br J Radiol. 2015; 88:20150099.

CHAPTER

37

Magnetic Resonance Angiography

Ajay Kumar, Sameer Vyas, Sreedhara BC, Naveen Kalra

HISTORY AND INTRODUCTION

The term angiography stands for the imaging depiction of vascular structures, and there are many ways to evaluate the vascular structures like Doppler, computed tomographic, catheter and magnetic resonance angiography (MRA). Over the last two decades MRA has been increasing in demand because of its physiological nature, on the contrary to CTA and catheter angiography, which involve catheterization, radiation and nephrotoxic iodinated contrast agents. However, there are many limitations of MRA such as availability, cost, time consuming and high sensitivity to motion and flow related artifacts.

The first research meeting devoted to Magnetic Resonance Angiography was hosted by Roberto Passariello in L'Aquila, Italy in 1989. Those days three-dimensional phase contrast MRA would take 19 hours from the time the patient entered the magnet until images could be seen; one hour to acquire the image and 18 hours of overnight image postprocessing. Computational capabilities of modern equipment have reduced the delay to a few seconds. Postprocessing now has taken a more central role in the communication of enormous amounts of data with less cumbersome two- or three-dimensional projections.

Many variations on the MRA theme have been presented over the ensuing 15 years. Dennis Parker developed the 3D multislab time-of-flight MRA technique which remains in routine clinical use to this day. Pulse sequence design plays a major role in the continuing advancements in the field, most notably as a consequence of more sophisticated and novel k-space filling strategies. The work of Kent Yucel and Martin Prince at the Massachusetts General Hospital in 1992 brought gadolinium-enhanced MR angiography to clinical utility. The first-pass dynamic contrast-enhanced MRA method provides robust and reproducible imaging results that have propelled the adoption of MRA into wider clinical use. This advance reliably produced images of sufficient quality to replace invasive catheter-based X-ray contrast angiography for most diagnostic purposes.

With the advent of high field clinical scanners operating at 3.0 Tesla, earlier noncontrast methods can be improved by virtue of two key benefits offered by 3.0 T MRA:

- The spatial resolution can be improved or scan time can be shortened by up to a factor of 4 because the signal to noise ratio (SNR) achieved with 3.0 T is twice that of the 1.5 T.
- The longer T1's of tissues at 3.0 T, ~20–40% higher than 1.5 T, provides better background suppression, additional inflow enhancement, and improved contrast-to-noise.

FLOW PHENOMENA AND PHASE EFFECTS IN MRA

Flow Phenomena

Flow phenomena in blood or cerebrospinal fluid (CSF) also influence the MR image contrast; in addition to inherent tissue factors like T1, T2 and proton density. Blood flow is complex and variable inside the body, so it is important to understand the various types of flow.

- Laminar flow is flow where the particles move along in concentric sheets and laminae, i.e. different but consistent velocities across the vessel. It is seen in normal vessels.
- Plug flow is flow where all fluid particles move forward in parallel lines with the same speed and has a characteristic blunt profile. It is seen in the descending thoracic aorta.
- Turbulent flow is flow at different velocities which varies, i.e. velocities across the vessel changes and is seen at vascular bifurcations.
- Vortex flow is flow after narrowing and is seen after stricture or stenosis. In it, the high velocities are seen at the center.
- Stagnant flow is flow that nearly behaves like stationary tissue and is seen in occluded vessels and large aneurysms.

The moving spins (spins that move during acquisition of data) show different contrast characteristics from the stationary spins. The moving spins cause mismapping of the signal because of the flow phenomena and result in flow motion artifacts or phase ghosting. The flow phenomena are generally categorized into time of flight, entry slice phenomenon and intra-voxel dephasing.

Outflow-related Signal Loss (Washout Effect, T2 Flow Void)

If a spin-echo (SE) pulse sequence is used to obtain the images, high velocity blood flow at a plane perpendicular to imaging plane produces weaker signal compared to adjacent stationary structures. This occurs because flowing spins get washed out from the slice during the imaging process. A sequence of slice-selective 90° and 180° radio frequency (RF) pulses are applied in spin-echo sequences. If a tissue component is affected by both the pulses, only the MR signal is produced. Flowing blood in any vessel or per se any moving material, while flowing through an excited slice at a reasonably high speed, is affected by only one of these pulses and as a result, it does not produce MR signal resulting into the so-called "flow void" **(Figs. 1A and B)**. The intensity of the vascular signal declines with decreasing slice thickness, increasing echo time (TE), and increasing flow velocity.

The vessels would appear dark when the blood flow speed is so high that all spins leave the slice between the 90° and 180° pulses ($v \geq s/(TE/2)$, as no signal is produced. This phenomenon does not affect spins flowing within the imaging plane. This effect secondary to washout phenomenon is observed only for spin echo sequences and is most marked on T2-weighted sequences as long echo times are used. On the other hand, in a gradient-echo (GRE) sequence, the echo is refocused without a 180° pulse simply by reversing the imaging gradients. The washout effect does not occur as only one RF pulse is needed to form an echo. Valuable and reliable information about blood flow can be obtained by the washout effect provided by standard SE sequences. If the flow void of a particular vessel is not visualized on T2-weighted images, it generally indicates very slow flow or even vessel occlusion. On the contrary, in presence of flow void on T2-SE sequence vessel occlusion can be excluded.

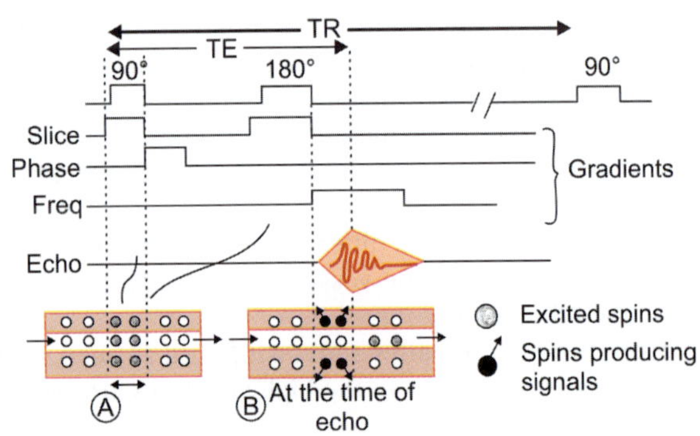

FIG. 1A: Spin echo sequence depicting the "Flow void" phenomenon (A and B) Represents the tissue sample with shaded area as stationary tissue (spins) and central nonshaded area as vessel having moving spins. (A) At the time of 90° excitation and 180° rephasing RF pulse for that particular selected slice location; (B) Same tissue with same slice location at the time of receiving signal or TE, now only stationary spins are giving signal in the selected slice however the moving spins have migrated out of selected slice with new nonexcited spins in that place giving no signals.

Inflow-related Signal Enhancement (Inflow Effect)

As already discussed, in a SE sequence, there is reduction in the signal of blood flowing rapidly out of the measured slice. Thus, an opposite effect may occur when spins flow into a slice and it is likely to generate a higher signal than the surrounding tissue- also known as "inflow enhancement". Contrast is generated on T1-weighted imaging, by applying repeated RF pulses having a time interval (repetition time, TR) which is shorter than the T1 relaxation time of the tissue (typically TR < 700 msec). Thus, it results into unequal saturation of the tissue components, depending on their individual T1 times. This is the basic principle of generation of T1-weighted image contrast. On a normal T1-weighted image, irrespective of flow effects, blood in the vessels would appear hypointense owing to its relatively long T1 time. With reduction in TR, the signal emitted by the tissue diminishes. In a GRE sequences, repetition times shorter than 50 msec can be achieved, allowing the majority of non-moving spins to become saturated; thereby, decreasing the background signal. The RF pulses do not influence the spins outside the excited slice (or volume). As a result, fully relaxed blood enters into the slice being imaged, without experiencing not more than a few excitations on its way through the slice. Consequently, significantly higher signal intensity relative to that of the saturated spins in the stationary tissue is generated by the flowing blood producing the so-called "inflow enhancement" or "flow-related enhancement". The signal intensity of flowing blood increases with decreasing slice thickness, and increasing flow velocity.

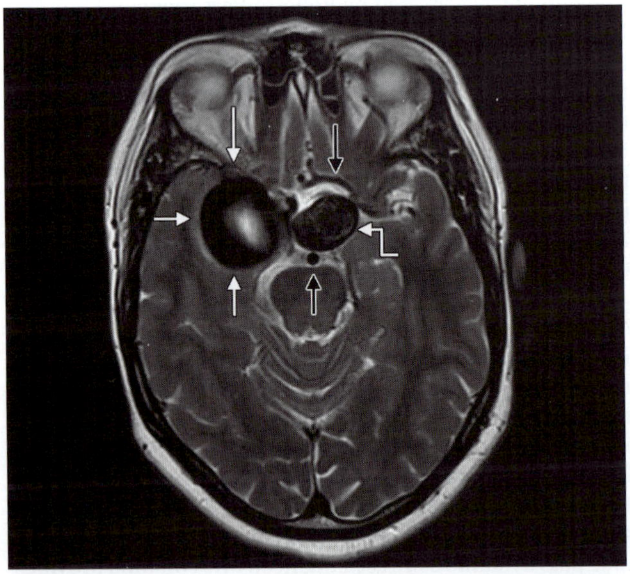

FIG. 1B: T2W axial image of the patient with bilateral ICA aneurysms shown to explain "Flow voids"–Normal arteries, i.e. left ACA and basilar arteries (black arrows) are seen hypointense due to flow void, left aneurysm (white elbow arrow) post coiling shows heterogeneous hypointense signals due to partial thrombosis. Right patent aneurysm (white arrows) reveals flow voids at periphery due to high flow however central part giving bright signals due to relative stasis of blood.

Maximal flow enhancement is achieved, if the blood flow velocity is so high that all vessel spins are replaced by unsaturated spins in the time interval TR. As a result, the vessel appears bright on a gray or black background. Although the inflow effect is seen with both SE and GRE sequences, SE sequences are not practical for the TOF method. This is because of the fact that the competing washout effect tends to overbalance the inflow effect at higher flow velocities in SE sequences, leading to decreased flow signal. Hence, production of bright blood images by virtue of flow-related enhancement using GRE sequences is the basis of time-of-flight angiography.

Phase Effects

Phase effects concern the transverse component of the magnetization. Phase effects are produced whenever spins are moving in the presence of magnetic field gradients, as are applied for spatial encoding of the MR signal. Depending on gradient strength and spin position, magnetic field gradients provoke a change in the Larmor frequency. A phase shift of the transverse magnetization can be induced by a gradient pulse of certain length and amplitude. This phase shift can be compensated by a second gradient pulse with identical strength and duration but having opposite sign. Thus, a net phase shift of zero is encountered with stationary spins. On the contrary, a non-zero phase shift is generated by the same gradients applied on a flowing spin. The first spin induced phase shift cannot be completely compensated by the second gradient pulse as the spins change their position during the bipolar gradient application. The remaining phase shift Φ is proportional to the velocity component v of the spins along the gradient direction. On standard MR imaging, this flow-induced phase shift results into a spatial mis-encoding of the signal leading to ghost artifacts, which are typically found in the phase-encoding direction. Spins in a blood vessel are moving with different velocities. Often, a parabolic flow profile is found. Larger phase shift is experienced by spins moving faster than those moving more slowly. If there is a velocity distribution inside a voxel, phase dispersion (intravoxel dephasing) occurs leading to reduced signal in the blood vessel. The strength and time interval of the gradient pulses, as well as the distribution of spin velocities are determinant for extent of spin-dephasing. A very broad spectrum of velocities within a voxel can be seen with complex flow patterns, for example in vessels with turbulent flow, leading to total signal loss in the vessel.

Using additional gradient pulses of appropriate amplitude and duration, flow-induced phase shifts can be compensated, thus eliminating any signal loss. This technique is called "gradient motion rephasing (GMR)" or just "flow compensation".[1] However, GMR is normally restricted to first-order movements, i.e. spins that move at a constant velocity. Turbulent flow and effects of acceleration cannot be completely compensated by GMR. Optimal reduction of flow-induced phase effects can be achieved by combining GMR with as short a TE as possible, in order to reduce the time available for spin dephasing. Short echo times also diminish the impact of pulsatile blood flow and turbulence **(Fig. 2)**.

Noncontrast MR Angiography (NC-MRA): Techniques

Several techniques of NC-MRA are available in current practice and they can be classified into techniques exploiting flow-related enhancement, those using the phase of MR imaging signal from moving blood, and those exploiting the physical properties of blood, independent of blood flow.[2] These techniques are shown in the **Flowchart 1** and described in detail thereafter.

FLOW-RELATED ENHANCEMENT DEPENDENT NONCONTRAST MRA TECHNIQUES

Time-of-Flight Angiography: Techniques

Inflow effect is the basis of the contrast mechanism of time-of-flight (TOF) MRA. Bright signal is produced by fully relaxed blood entering the measured volume as it behaves

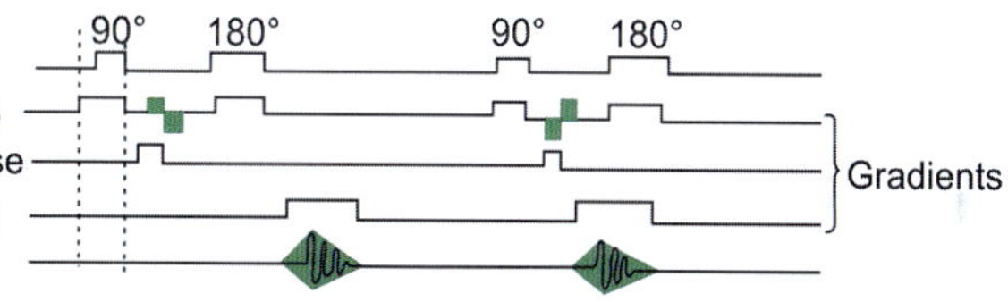

FIG. 2: Diagrammatic representation of phase-contrast MRA pulse sequence, note the velocity encoding gradient are in slice direction.

FLOWCHART 1: Noncontrast Mr angiography (Nc-Mra): Techniques.

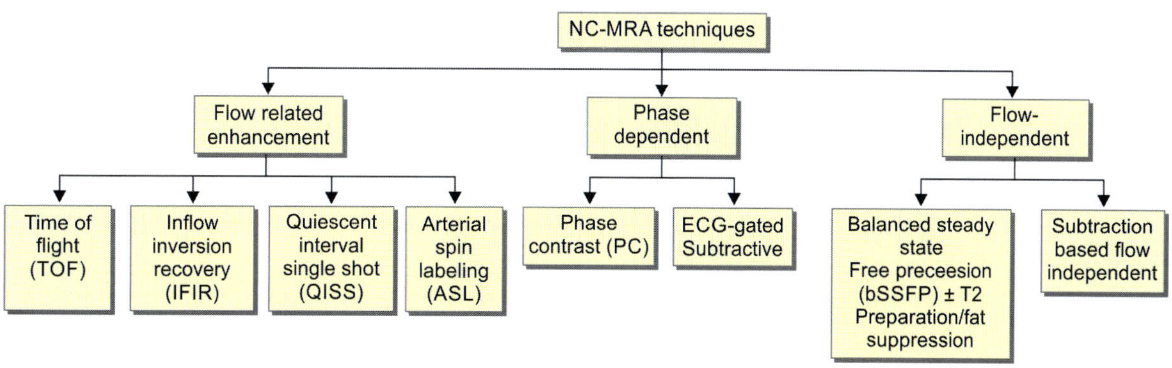

as an endogenous contrast agent. However, flow rephasing techniques (GMR) are required for the bright depiction of flowing blood, to overcome the effects of transverse magnetization induced spin dephasing. GRE sequence based TOF MRA offers several advantages:

- GRE sequences does not suffer from wash-out phenomenon which results in decreased signal of fast flowing blood as seen with SE techniques.
- A short repetition times (TR < 40 msec), necessary to efficiently saturate stationary tissue can be used in GRE techniques.
- Further reduction in spin dephasing can be done by keeping a short echo times (TE < 5 msec), In order to avoid opposed-phase effects at the vessel walls that could potentially impair the depiction of small vessels, generalized it is advisable to apply in-phase echo times
- The shorter acquisition time of GRE techniques are useful for acquiring volume (3D) datasets.

TOF techniques can be further subdivided into three groups:

1. Sequential 2D multislice method.
2. 3D single-slab method.
3. 3D multislab method.

Sequential 2D Multislice Method

Multiple thin slices are imaged sequentially in this technique for depiction of the vessels. This technique offers two advantages compared to the interleaved multislice technique:

a. The inflow effect can be boosted by the use of very short TR times.
b. The flow of partially saturated blood from one slice to another is hindered by this technique.

Even in the vessel with slow flow, sufficient inflow enhancement is guaranteed with this technique and produces good contrast vessel-background contrast in the covered area, as each slice is an entry slice.[3] However, 2D TOF MRA can be problematic in case the direction of blood flow in the vessel of interest is not perpendicular to the plane of imaging. Signal loss may occur due to the partial saturation of flow in case the vessels run partly inside the slice (in-plane) or return to the slice in a looped form **(Figs. 3A and B)**. A slice thickness of at least 2–3 mm is necessary to achieve an optimum signal-to-noise ratio, However, because of larger voxel size required, it results in increased spin dephasing and reduced spatial resolution. Because of non-rectangular profile of 2D slices, they exhibit signal variations at the edges leading to step like artifacts in maximum intensity projection (MIP) reconstructions. However, overlapping of the slices can be used to overcome this effect. The extent of inflow enhancement varies during the cardiac cycle in vessels exhibiting highly pulsatile flow. Ghost images of the vessels are produced by the periodic change of inflow enhancement. Slow flow in the diastolic phase can lead to saturation of blood spins. ECG triggered 2D TOF sequences may be used to overcome many of these problems by restricting data acquisition to the phase of maximum inflow. Thus, accentuation of blood signal and elimination of ghost artifacts can be achieved. The mapping of vessel in each slice with equal intensity can be achieved by synchronizing data acquisition with the cardiac cycle. However, this technique suffers from the drawback of longer acquisition time.

3D TOF MRA-single Slab and Multislab Methods

Simultaneous excitation the entire imaging volume, usually 30–60 mm thick, is done and then partitioned into thin slices by an additional phase encoding gradient along the slice-select direction.[4] Excellent spatial resolution coupled with high signal-to-noise ratio are the major advantages of 3D TOF MRA technique and thus it facilitates improved depiction particularly of small vessels. Isotropic voxels can be acquired easily with this technique and slice thickness of less than 1 mm

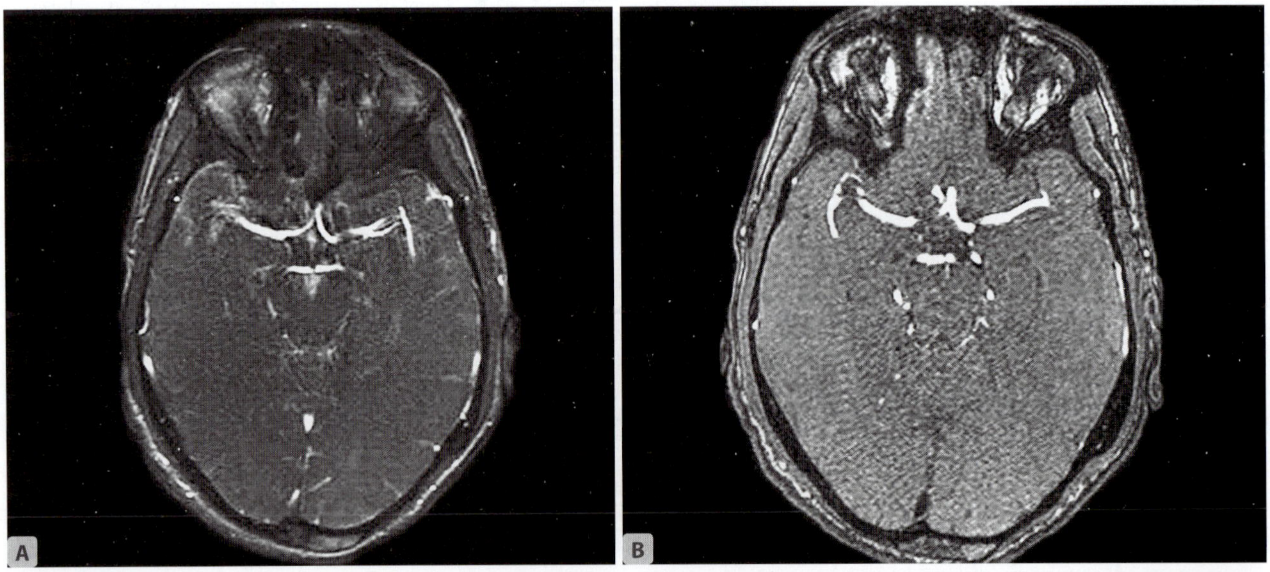

FIGS. 3A AND B: 2D TOF MRA (A) shows loss of flow-related signal in M1 segment of left MCA due to in-plane saturation however in same patient. lt MCA showing normal caliber and flow related signal on 3D TOF MRA (B).

thickness can also be achieved. However, 3D TOF suffers from the problem of progressive saturation which happens when blood flowing through the volume is subjected to repeated RF pulses. It results into continuous drop in the signal intensity in the direction of flow. The extent of saturation is determined by the length of time in which the blood stays inside the volume. In slow flow vessels, diminution of signal begins to occur after covering only a short distance. On the other hand, the signal remains visible for a greater distance in faster flowing blood. Hence, matching to the size of the vessel in the region of interest, the maximum volume thickness should be kept as small as possible. Saturation reduction can also be achieved by increasing the TR. Subdivision of the volume of interest into several thin 3D slabs that are acquired sequentially can be used for imaging Larger vessel sections **(Table 1)**.[5]

Multiple overlapping thin slab acquisition (MOTSA) is one such multislab technique, which retains the advantages of 3D TOF; however has the reduced saturation effects like 2D TOF. Generally, to avoid saturation within the slabs, the chosen slab thickness has to be small enough. However, approximately 20–30% overlap between adjacent slab are required in order to compensate for signal attenuations arising at the slab edges due to non-rectangular excitation profiles. However, in this technique time efficiency is compromised leading to a longer overall acquisition times. Frequently, owing to the high sensitivity to slow flow 2D TOF MRA is favored for imaging veins. On the contrary, for fast arterial flow and for those cases where high spatial resolution is required 3D TOF MRA is more appropriate **(Figs. 4 and 5)**.

TABLE 1: Comparison between 2D and 3D TOF.

2D TOF	3D TOF
Less susceptible to saturation effect	More susceptible to saturation effect
Visualize slow as well as fast flow	Good for high flow
Low resolution and SNR	High resolution and SNR
Better for relatively larger FOVs	Smaller FOVs
Used mainly for cerebral venographies, abdominal and peripheral angiographies	Cerebral angiography

Important Points for Optimization of TOF Angiography[6-8]

- The slices or volume should be oriented perpendicular to flow direction.
- For slow and fast flow, 2D and 3D acquisition to be done.

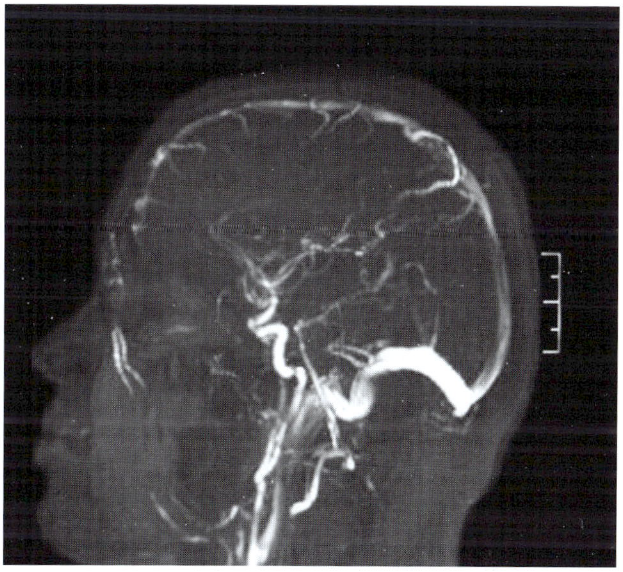

FIG. 4: 2D TOFMR venography reveals adequate visualization of cerebral venous system.

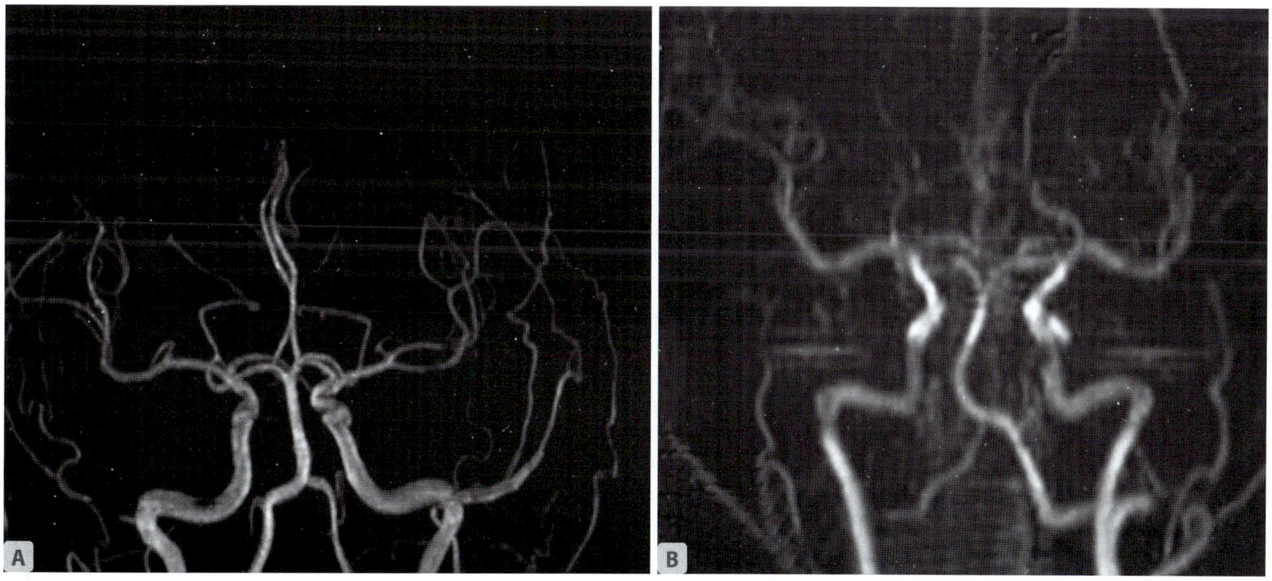

FIGS. 5A AND B: 3D TOF MRA (A) showing very good cerebral vascular anatomy with high spatial resolution and SNR in comparison to 2D TOF MRA (B) in same patient.

- 3D multislab acquisition to be done for larger vessel sections.
- For isolating, arteries and veins spatial presaturation should be applied.
- Signal loss due to spin dephasing can be minimized by use of minimum TE.
- Saturation effects in 3D TOF can be reduced by TONE pulse.
- Vessel contrast can be improved by magnetization transfer (MTC) and fat suppression.

Pitfalls with TOF MRA

- Methemoglobin in thrombosed vessels (cavernous: sinus thrombosis) may mimic blood flow (i.e. vessel patency)
- Work around—compare MIP with pre-contrast T1 images or use phase contrast MRA
- Tissue having short T1 time (blood, fat, tissue that can take up contrast) may simulate vessels
- Pulsation artifacts in CSF may mimic vessel lesions. Overestimation of stenosis and artifacts in the depiction of aneurysms can occur due to signal loss because of turbulent or very slow flow.
- Signal loss can occur due to magnetic susceptibility artifacts (coils, clips)
- Signal loss can also occur in case of in-plane flow (2D) or slow flow (3D)
- After contrast administration, overlap of arteries and veins can occur, especially in intracranial MRA.

Inflow Inversion Recovery–Magnetic Resonance Angiography (NC-MRA)

In this technique of NC-MRA, stationary background tissues are suppressed by an inversion RF pulse, while the inflow of fully magnetized arterial spins is imaged.[9,10] A slab-selective inversion pulse followed by an inflow time (TI) of several hundred milliseconds is applied in this technique. The TI is chosen to provide adequate inflow into the target vascular anatomy and a sufficient degree of background suppression. A rapid readout is then used for imaging. Chemical shift-selective fat saturation, short-tau inversion recovery, or water excitation RF pulses are different techniques used for fat suppression. TimeSLIP, NATIVE TrueFISP, Inhance Inflow IR, and B-TRANCE are few trade names for the IFIR sequence.

Vascular beds containing brisk flow are best imaged using IFIR technique as angiographic contrast depends on inflow. The imaging readout is either balanced steady-state free precession (bSSFP) or flow-compensated fast spin echo (FSE) to maintain high signal from flowing spins. The upstream edge of the inversion pulse is positioned close to the arterial bed under interrogation to minimize the inflow requirements. Respiratory motion is compensated by gating by prospective navigator or bellows.

One of the variation of IFIR technique is outflow MRA where a nonselective inversion RF pulse and then a slice-selective inversion pulse to the inflowing blood pool is applied before its entry into the target anatomy. The background signal suppression and image quality can be improved in outflow MRA in some applications compared to inflow MRA.[11] Easy execution and good image quality are main strengths of inflow inversion recovery, especially for renal angiography while poor display of vessels with slow flow is its main drawback.

Quiescent Interval Single-shot Magnetic Resonance Angiography

Another NC-MRA technique that is used for imaging lower limb arteries is Quiescent-inflow single-shot (QISS) angiography,[12] which applies:

- For suppressing the static tissue-an in-plane RF saturation pulse
- For suppressing venous signal—a tracking venous saturation RF pulse.
- A waiting period (or quiescent interval) of ~230 milliseconds needs to be applied. To ensure arterial inflow into the imaging slice-
- Fat suppression done by chemical shift-selective fat saturation and
- A single-shot Cartesian 2D bSSFP readout.

ECG gating is done in order to ensure that the systole is overlapped by the quiescent interval while data is acquired during diastole. One slice is acquired every heartbeat. Thus, a peripheral MRA from abdomen to the feet can be completed within 10 minutes using 3 mm slices.

A variant of QISS using a highly undersampled radial k-space trajectory can be used to acquire multiple slices within a single heartbeat, shortening scan times by a factor of 2–3.[13] Compared with single-slice QISS, the thickness of the in-plane saturation RF pulse is increased to span all slices that are acquired in each heartbeat. Fat saturation is applied before the bSSFP readout for each acquired slice.

Strengths of QISS MRA

- Imaging speed and ease of use, with no sequence tailoring required.
- The ability to depict slow flow.

Drawbacks

Suboptimal display of flow parallel to the imaging slice and poor display of retrograde flow is major drawback of QISS. Partial volume averaging in the slice direction can be overcome by acquiring thinner slices, at the expense of acquisition time.

Arterial Spin-labeled Magnetic Resonance Angiography

Acquisition of 2 image sets which are almost identical except for magnetization of inflowing arterial spins are required in Arterial spin labeling (ASL) MRA technique. The 2 image sets are later subtracted. The difference in arterial magnetization is imparted by a process known as labeling. Subtraction of the 2 image sets displays the labelled arterial inflow and suppresses background signal.

An inversion RF pulse is applied to achieve labeling of arterial spins during ASL MRA. This variant of ASL, commonly known as pulsed ASL, applies an inversion RF pulse to arterial spins flowing into the target vasculature, followed by a TI time to accommodate inflow, and an imaging readout. The difference between this data set and its counterpart acquired without the labeling RF pulse depicts the labeled arterial anatomy. Signal targeting with alternating RF (STAR)[14] and flow-alternating inversion recovery (FAIR),[15] are two commonly used pulsed ASL approaches.

Other ASL techniques apply a quasicontinuous or pseudocontinuous stream of RF energy to label arterial spins flowing through a thin (~1 cm thick) labeling plane.[16] The signal/noise ratio (SNR) of vessels near the labelling plane where short inversion times are realized can be improved with pseudocontinous ASL, compared with pulsed ASL.[17] The two techniques of ASL may be combined to improve SNR and vascular coverage.[18,19]

Extended, multiphase readouts can also be used in conjunction with ASL to display the temporal passage of arterial spins.[20]

Strengths

- High arterial contrast.
- The background signal can be completely eliminated.

Drawbacks

- Misregistration artifact from subtraction.
- Scan time is increased as acquisition of 2 data sets.
- Limited anatomic coverage when imaging slow flow.

PHASE DEPENDENT NONCONTRAST MRA TECHNIQUES

Phase Contrast Angiography

The other noncontrast MR angiographic technique is phase contrast MR angiography.[21-23] Velocity information can be obtained with this technique by measuring changes in the phase of protons. Currently its primary applications are in cardiovascular flow, venography, and three-dimensional (3D) vascular studies. The phase contrast study can also be used for CSF flow studies. Phase contrast angiography can provide informations that can be used in two ways: (1) for production of routine angiographic images and (2) for quantification of flow.

This technique is not routinely used in clinical practice as both TOF-MRA and contrast enhanced angiography are faster techniques. Thus, it is used in practice when the results of other angiographic studies are equivocal or physiological information about flow is required. To be precise, it is the most sensitive sequence for demonstration of slow flowing blood and it is the only MRA sequence that can provide data regarding flow, velocity and pressure.

When an MR echo is recorded, two types of information are acquired-phase and magnitude information. A corollary can be drawn with a vector where, magnitude determines the length of the vector while phase determines the direction of the vector (from 0–360°). For generating most information the phase information is not regarded and the magnitude images are displayed only; although, the phase information can be useful in some conditions. For example, phase information is frequently used to localize signal in the phase-encoding direction. Depending on their location along the gradient, protons along the phase-encoding gradient acquire different phases. Precession of a proton at the weaker end of the gradient will be slower as it experiences a 1.49-T magnetic field, compared to the precession of a proton in the middle of the gradient that experiences a 1.5-T magnetic field. The protons develop different phase shifts, owing to these differences in precession speed, which can then be used to map the location of the proton within the body. This same principle is used in phase contrast sequences, where special gradients are used to eliminate the phase differences between stagnant protons while accentuating the phase differences in moving protons. In phase contrast sequences, moving protons experiencing a changing magnetic field accumulate a phase which is different from stationary protons, experiencing a constant magnetic field. Because faster-flowing protons travel a farther distance through the gradient than slower-moving protons, their phase differences (compared with stationary protons) will be greater than those of the slower flowing protons. Thus, briefly speaking, phase differences are proportional to a proton's velocity (that can be calculated) in phase contrast imaging. Additionally, phase shift is also proportional to the magnitude of the gradient, hence, more phase shift per distance travelled is produced by larger gradients. Thus, gradient size can be adjusted to manipulate the degree of phase shift for a given velocity. As phase shifts greater than 180° result in aliasing, the ability to adjust the gradient is important.

Fortunately, manual calculation of gradient size is not required; instead a velocity encoding (VENC) value needs to be entered, using which the computer can calculate the size of the gradient. Before acquisition of any phase contrast sequence the VENC value must be defined. It is defined as the highest velocity which can be measured correctly by the sequence before aliasing takes place. In other words, the gradient is set in such a way by the computer so the VENC value (maximum projected velocity) will result in a ±180° phase shift. The closer the VENC is set to the measured velocity, the more accurate the measurement. Aliasing will occur when a too low VENC value is set. If a too high VENC value is set, accurate measurement of slow velocities will not be possible and there will be a drop in SNR. The ideal VENC value for arterial blood is usually more than 100 cm/s and can be as high as 300 or 400 cm/s, depending on the vessel being imaged and on the degree of stenosis. On the other hand, the VENC value for imaging the veins and the venous sinus should usually be set around 20 to 30 cm/s. Adjustment of the VENC value is analogous to adjustment of the maximum velocity on Doppler ultrasound. For detection of slow flowing blood, phase contrast is the most sensitive MR technique as the VENC value can be manipulated.

Bipolar gradients are used to acquire images in phase contrast sequence, which is a GRE sequence. The two lobes of the bipolar gradient, are often referred to as the dephasing and rephasing lobes. They are identical in magnitude and time; however, their directions are exactly opposite. Stationary protons experience two gradients that are exactly opposite to each other, resulting in a return to a net 0° phase and it happens irrespective of the position of the proton along the gradient. On the other hand, moving protons, will change locations in between the two lobes of the bipolar gradient, resulting into two different magnetic field strengths which influence the phase of the proton. This difference causes accumulation of a net change in phase relative to the stationary proton. In practice, magnetic field inhomogeneities, that causes unwanted phase changes in stationary protons, cannot be accounted for by a single bipolar gradient. Application of a second mirror image bipolar gradient is required to eliminate magnetic field inhomogeneities. The second gradient is identical to the first; however is in reverse order. Thus, a flow-sensitive sequence, similar to digital subtraction angiography, is generated. A stationary proton that accumulates phase during the first bipolar gradient (secondary to magnetic field inhomogeneities) will then acquire exactly the same phase during the second reversed bipolar gradient. Thus, after subtraction, the stagnant spin will have a net phase of 0°. However, the moving spin will accumulate phase of same magnitude but of opposite direction of phase during the second bipolar gradient compared with the first. When subtracted, the opposite phase shifts will result in a net doubling of the phase shift. However, the acquisition time is almost double compared to TOF-MRA as echo has to be obtained after each bipolar gradient. Moreover, only one dimensional flow (oriented parallel to the axis of the gradient) is detected. Hence, if we aim to obtain flow in all three dimensions, necessary for producing conventional angiographic image, the sequence must be repeated three times, making it prohibitively long.

As already mentioned, quantification of flow is the most common application of phase contrast. Quantification of flow can be estimated either in one dimension (through-plane flow) or two dimensions (in-plane flow). With through-plane flow, the velocity-encoding gradient is oriented along the slice selection axis (craniocaudal for an axial scan) and information is obtained about flow that is moving through the plane of the image. For in-plane flow, the gradients are along the frequency- and phase-encoding axes (e.g., transverse and anteroposterior dimensions for an axial slice). Information about flow occurring in the plane of the scan is obtained.

A characteristic angiographic appearance similar to fluoroscopic digital subtraction angiography images is generated by phase contrast images. It happens because two separate datasets are obtained and then subtracted from each other to create the flow quantification image. Intermediate gray signal is assigned to all stationary spins (0° phase shift), while based on the direction of flow the mobile protons are then assigned either hypointense or hyperintense signal, with an intensity level correlating to the velocity magnitude. Air containing body parts (which are relatively devoid of signal), like that found external to the patient, in the lungs, and in the paranasal sinuses, exhibit a static or snowstorm appearance, because of the background noise and random movement of protons. **Figures 6 and 7** demonstrate intracranial MRV and MRA acquired with phase contrast technique while **Figures 8A and B** demonstrate superiority of PCMRV over TOF MRV for depiction of intracranial venous sinuses.

Strengths

- Ability to calculate velocity and flow data is the major advantage of PC-MRA. Cardiac gated through plane images are acquired for obtaining dynamic information throughout the cardiac cycle. Both velocity and flow information in relation to time can be determined with the placement of a region of interest and the use of commercially available computer software.
  Using the Bernoulli equation these flow data can then be used determine intraluminal pressures, which can be used to evaluate the degree of a vessel stenosis (e.g., as in aortic coarctation). Finally, analysis of higher-order flow data like pulsatility and jerk can also be done using more complex gradients. Although, this application is seldom used in clinical practice.
- Good suppression of nonflowing background signal can be achieved by noise masking.

Drawbacks

- Suffers from the drawback of longer scan time (2-4 times TOF-MRA) because of need for acquisition of multiple image sets.
- Phase contrast imaging is highly sensitive to motion degradation like DSA, and usually a nondiagnostic image is produced in case of patient's movement.
- Finally, protons in the areas of turbulent flow swirl rather than having a unidirectional movement, resulting in a signal void precluding the acquisition of velocity data. Turbulent flow is encountered usually in area just distal to a site of high-grade stenosis or at the vessel bifurcation.
- Eddy currents, concomitant gradients and spatially varying background phase offsets cause phase imperfections- the other drawback of PC-MRA.[24]

Optimization

- VENC should be adapted to maximum flow velocity.
- Encoding different flow velocities (multivenc) or different flow directions.
- Flow signal can be improved by contrast agent.
- One single projection within a short scanning time can be provided by 2D acquisition technique.
- MIP postprocessing of 3D acquisition can be done.
- While dealing with pulsatile flow, ECG triggering can be applied.
- Arterial and venous separation can be done by using presaturation pulses.

Four-dimensional Phase Contrast Imaging

Blood flow in 3 spatial dimensions over the cardiac cycle can be displayed and quantified by the novel technique of 4D PC-MRA.[25] Velocity-encoding data are acquired in three directions in this technique compared to conventional phase contrast technique. Information about spatial and temporal evolution of 3D blood flow in any particular vascular bed can be assessed by this technique. However, this technique also suffers from the drawback of longer acquisition time as velocity encoding needs to be done in three directions.

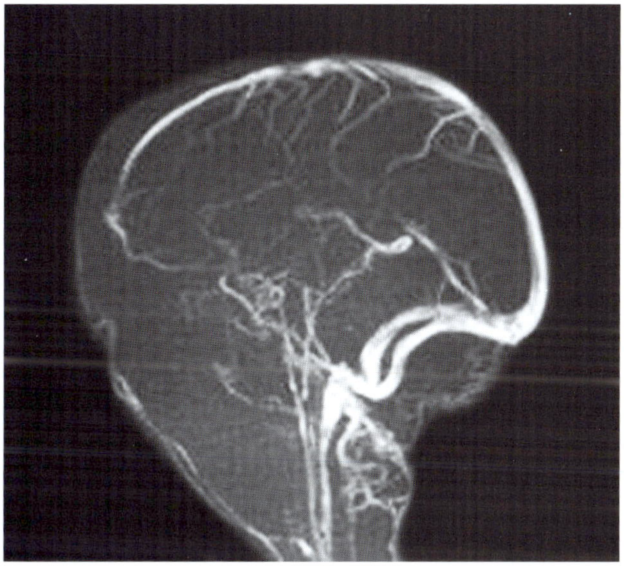

FIG. 6: Phase contrast 3D MRV showing excellent cerebral venous system.

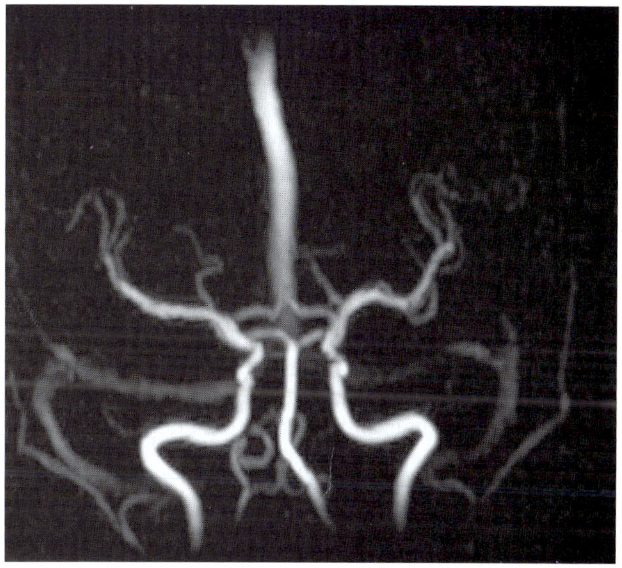

FIG. 7: Phase contrast 3D MRA giving adequate depiction of arterial anatomy.

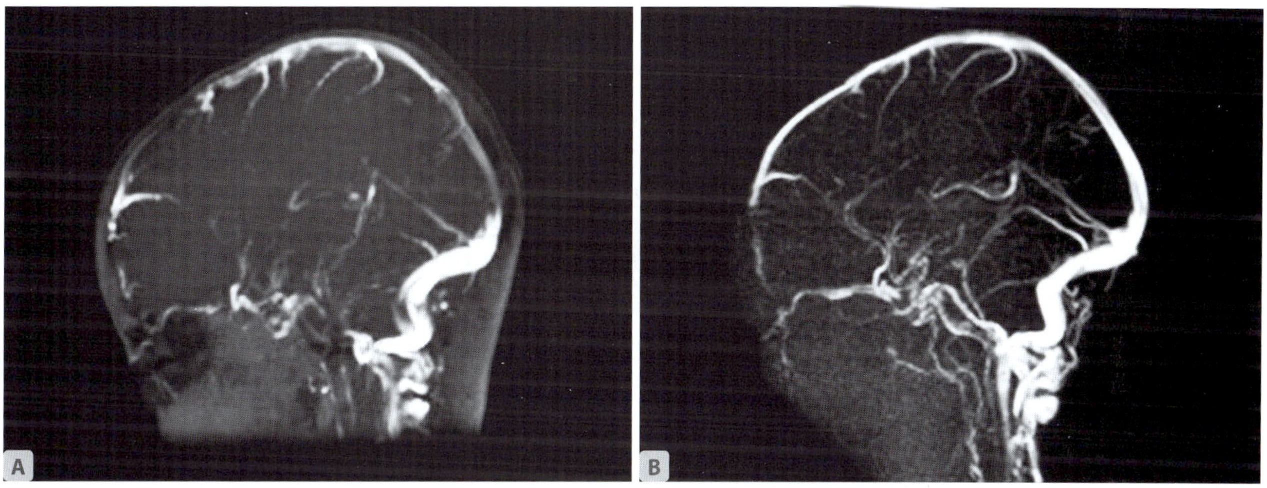

FIGS. 8A AND B: Phase contrast 3D MRV (B) showing better cerebral venous sinuses and smaller veins than 2D TOF MRV (A) in same patient.

However, novel techniques like parallel imaging and other k space undersampling techniques have made it possible to acquire 4D flow MRA at an acceptable scanning time of ~5–10 minutes for different body parts like brain, chest and abdomen.

Gated Subtractive Magnetic Resonance Angiography

The differential appearance of arteries between systole and diastole provides the angiographic contrast in this technique of NC-MRA.[26] Arteries are rendered dark at the time of systolic fast flow, because of arterial spin dephasing during the echo train. On the other hand, while imaging in slow flow during diastole arterial signal is preserved. Arterial anatomy is displayed by subtraction. The flow sensitivity of these techniques, which use FSE readouts, can be controlled by the length of the echo train, the flip angle of the refocusing RF pulses, supplementary gradient lobes for flow compensation or spoiling, and the orientation of the frequency-encoding axis.[27,28] Fresh blood imaging, Non Contrast MRA of ArTerIes and Veins (NATIVE), Sampling Perfection with Application optimized Contrast using different flip angle Evolutions (SPACE), Inhance Delta Flow, and Triggered Angiography Non-Contrast Enhanced (TRANCE) are few of the Commercially available gated subtraction techniques.

Imaging readout is used to accomplish dephasing of arterial spins in FSE-based gated subtraction MRA. However, dephasing of arterial spins during systole is achieved by applying a flow-suppressing motion-sensitized driven equilibrium (MSDE) magnetization preparation before the imaging readout, when imaging is carried out with a bSSFP readout which preserves signal from flowing arterial blood. These MSDE preparations spoil signal from arterial blood based on its velocity[29] or acceleration,[30] leaving signal from stationary or nonaccelerating tissue largely unaltered. The degree of flow spoiling depends on the timing, strength, and duration of the gradient lobes applied within the MSDE preparation, and when the preparation is applied within the cardiac cycle.

Strength

Complete suppression of nonvascular background signals.

Drawbacks

- Misregistration artefact from patient motion.
- Operator involvement to synchronize the acquisition to phases of maximal and minimal flow and tune the degree of flow spoiling (i.e. to optimize arterial dephasing and minimize venous contamination).
- Poor display of arteries with slow flow and diminished pulsatility.

FLOW INDEPENDENT NONCONTRAST MRA TECHNIQUES

Angiographic contrast is derived by using the T2 and T1 properties of the blood pool in the non flow-dependent methods of noncontrast MRA. Spin-echo and gradient-echo readouts were used in initial reports of flow-independent MRA techniques.[31,32] However, balanced steady state free precession (bSSFP) is the predominant readout for flow-independent MRA in modern practice.

Strengths

- Easy availability.
- Higher speed of acquisition.
- Efficient SNR for displaying arterial blood.

Drawbacks

High signal from fat and fluids, which may preclude routine use of standard maximum intensity projection (MIP) processing and dark band artifacts from B0 inhomogeneity. However, chemical shift-selective fat saturation can be used to achieve fat suppression. Otherwise, the phase difference between fat and water can be exploited to achieve fat suppression. Inversion-recovery and T2 magnetization preparations can be used for suppressing signal from fluids and muscle tissue respectively.

Subtraction-based bSSFP techniques may also be used for flow-independent angiography. Better extraneous nonvascular background tissue signal suppression of can be achieved with subtractive technique compared to non-subtractive technique. Signal targeting alternative RF and flow-independent relaxation enhancement (STARFIRE)[33] is one of the subtractive flow-independent MRA technique, that preferentially demonstrates blood based on its long T2 and T1. Sensitivity to subtraction artifact due to motion, and increased acquisition times caused by the need to collect 2 data sets are drawbacks of STARFIRE technique.

Contrast-enhanced MR Angiography

Contrast-enhanced MR angiography (CE-MRA) has evolved as the method of choice for vascular images. The T1shortening effect of gadolinium based contrasts are exploited by this technique contrary to the flow based TOF and PC-MRA technique relying on the inherent motion of blood flow for generating vascular signal.[34]

A gradient system with high slew rates for ultrafast acquisition is required unlike 3D TOF MRA, along with additive tools for proper scan timing with regard to the bolus arrival.[35]

The basic sequence used for CE-MRA is ultra short TR/TE 3D spoiled gradient echo sequence. The TR is made as short as possible to speed up the image acquisition and capture the first pass of contrast. The presence of Gd makes the blood immune to saturation, so the short TR tends to saturate only background tissue. In general, the highest flip angle achievable by the MRI machine is used. The TE is also made as short as possible—ideally approximately 1.0 msec, so as to limit any flow-induced dephasing effects.[36]

For achieving optimal contrast of the arteries different techniques like bolus timing, automatic bolus detection, bolus tracking and care bolus, can be are used.[37]

The peak gadolinium concentration, and hence the achievable arterial SNR is affected by the rate of injection. Generally, higher arterial SNR can be achieved with a faster injection rate, but it is associated with shorter bolus duration and earlier venous enhancement. Most CE MRA can be acquired with injection rate of 2 mL/sec with higher rates demonstrating very little advantage.[38]

Most CE MRA examinations can be optimally performed with a contrast dose of 0.15–0.2 mmol/kg (typically 20–30 mL). If good timing is achieved, optimum images can be generated using even a lower dose (0.1 mmol/kg). In general, additional advantage of prolonging the arterial phase and providing the operator with an additional buffer to compensate for errors in timing can be obtained if a larger contrast agent dose is used.[38,39]

Administration of saline flush is also an important consideration for optimum CE-MRA technique. Practically, a large saline flush (at least 30 mL) needs to be used for all CE MRA examinations. It ensures administration of the entire contrast volume beyond the tubing and bolus transit through the peripheral veins into the right heart. Thereby, sufficient gadolinium concentrations in the more distal arteries is ensured. The increase in the slope of the enhancement curve, as well as the duration of the arterial phase of the bolus (up to 50%), and delaying significant venous enhancement, the factors which are preferrable for arterial CE-MRA, can be achieved with a large saline flush.[38,40]

The goal is to record the central region of k space during the maximum enhancement of the artery. The center of k space contains the lowest (spatial) frequency wave data, so it represents the major structures of the image and thus most of the gross image form and contrast; therefore, the center of k space should be acquired during the time of highest contrast agent concentration.[41]

Also, for preventing ringing artifacts, arising in the Fourier transform, a high rate of change of the contrast agent concentration during the acquisition of central k space should be avoided.[41] So, the enhancement is maximized by timing the contrast agent injection such that the period of maximum arterial concentration corresponds to the k space acquisition.[37]

Special considerations with respect to timing must be undertaken with certain vascular problems such as aneurysms: since the flow can be much slower through an aneurysm, more time must be allowed between the injection of contrast agent and the image acquisition.[41]

A high resolution with near isotropic voxels and minimal pulsatility and misregistration artifacts should be striven for. The postprocessing with the maximum intensity projection (MIP) enables different views of the 3D data set **(Figs. 9 to 11)**.

CE-MRA Advantages[37]

- The 3D MRA can be acquired in any plane, which means that greater vessel coverage can be obtained at high resolution with fewer slices (aorta, peripheral vessels)
- The possibility to perform a time resolved examination (similarly to conventional catheter angiography)
- Most of the artifacts of time of flight angiography or phase contrast angiography can be reduced or eliminated by CE-MRA.
- Minimal invasiveness with no associated risk of neurologic complications, reduced patient discomfort and inconvenience, greater cost savings
- No use of ionizing radiation; paramagnetic agents have a beneficial safety
- The CE-MRA does not prove to be better in evaluation of carotid artery atherosclerotic stenosis[42] however it appears to give better depiction of post coiling larger residual/recurrent aneurysms[43]
- Other very important use of CE-MRA is that it differentiates between active and inactive disease in case of Takayasu arthritis by showing the intense enhancement of vessel wall.[44]

CE-MRA Disadvantages

The time window for scan acquisition is limited in the cerebral circulation, owing to the short arteriovenous transition time leading to early enhancement of venous structures. Thus, a trade-off is therefore necessary between scan time, volume coverage and spatial resolution. Another drawback is the possibility of a false neck remnant in post coiling patient with a intracranial aneurysm, which may be explained by the peripheral contrast enhancement of the organized thrombus or by the vasa vasorum within the aneurysm wall.[35,45]

Time Resolved/4D CE-MRA

Vascular malformation imaging work up always needs a dynamic depiction of the disease. However, the conventional MRA, dynamic TOF, PC and CE-MRA lacks the ability in showing the different angiographic phases as early arterial, arterial and venous. At the same time conventional angiography suffers from motion artifacts specially in unstable patients.

The time resolved CE-MRA includes combination of *k* space segmentation into central, mid, and peripheral zones with sampling the central zones of the *k* space at a more frequent rate.

Scan parameters used for rapid acquisition short TE of 0.9 ms and a short TR of 2.2 ms, fractional echo acquisition, 2.6 mm section thickness. MR contrast is injected at a rate of 2 mL/s to a total of 15 mL, followed by 30 mL of saline. Sagittal or coronal section are obtained with a FOV of about 28 × 22.4 cm, matrix of 192 × 192, NEX of 0.75, and flip angle of 20° at every 1.8 to 2.0 seconds. About 30 to 35 section are acquired **(Figs. 12A to D)**.[46]

Advantages of Time Resolved MRA

- Useful for unstable and moving patients[47]
- Better depiction of AVM feeders, nidus and venous drainages[48]
- Gives an idea about flow dynamics of AVM/AVF and aneurysms[47]

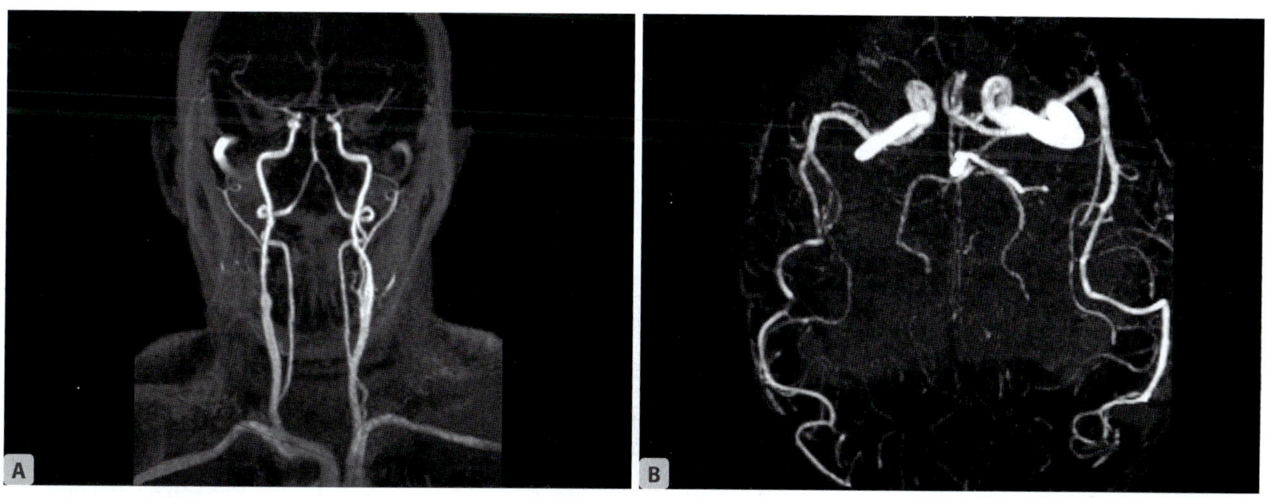

FIGS. 9A AND B: Contrast enhanced MRA showing good neck and cerebral arterial anatomy.

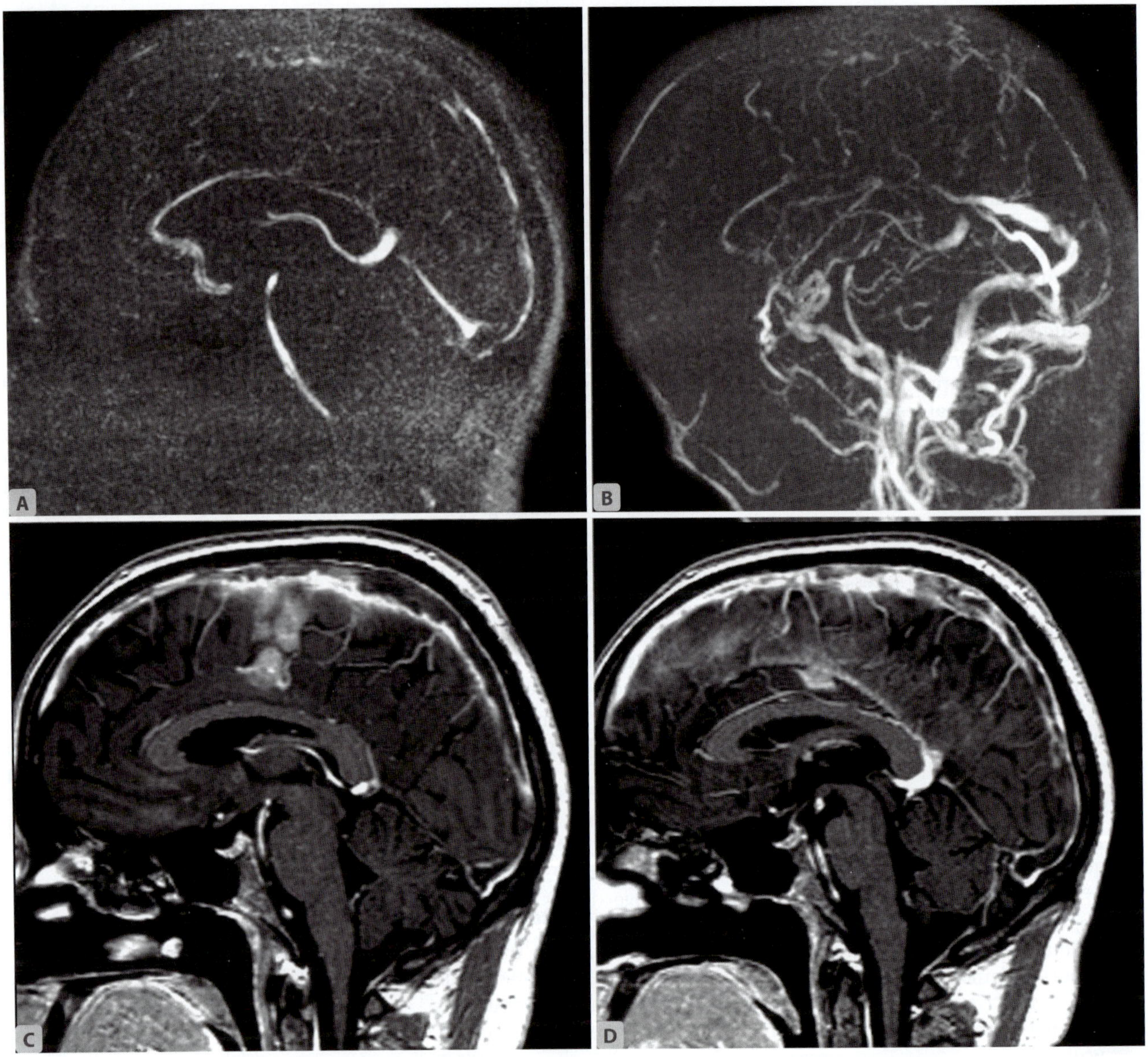

FIGS. 10A TO D: Case of superior sagittal venous sinus thrombosis showing nonvisualization of sinuses on PC 3D MRV (A and B), postcontrast T1W (C and D) confirms the filling defects in sinus.

- Good for follow-up of postembolization or gamma surgery residual AVMS.[48]

Limitations

- High dose of contrast is required
- Time taking sequences
- Nonvessel selective on the contrary to catheter angiography.

Parallel Imaging[35]

Recently developed parallel acquisition techniques (PAT) are now commonly used for vascular imaging. Multichannel coil arrays are used in PAT for shortening the measurement time by reduction of the number of phase encoding steps. Instead the sensitivity profiles of the coil elements are used to extract the spatial information.

Sensitivity encoding (SENSE), simultaneous acquisition of spatial (SMAS) harmonics, and generalized auto-calibrating partially parallel acquisitions (GRAPPA) are few of the many PAT image acquisition algorithms that have been described.

When used in intracranial 3D TOF MRA, PAT with an eight channel phased-array head coil has been used to reduce 43 percent of measurement time without comprising the image quality. However, one must be aware that use of PAT is associated with reduction of SNR, by approximately the square root of the acceleration factor. Owing to the inherently high SNR of CE-MRA, PAT is particularly suitable for CE-MRA.

In arterial CE-MRA, PAT can be exploited for accelerating the acquisition (and thus avoiding venous contamination), to increase spatial resolution and/or volume coverage, or to combine the two.[35]

Compressed sensing (CS) is another newer technique which is based on k-space undersampling[49] can also be used for acquisition of TOF-MRA at a reduced time of scan. Few studies have demonstrated the use of compressed sensing based MRA for intracranial vessels in cases of intracranial aneurysms and Moyamoya disease and shown the image quality can be comparable to that of conventional TOF MRA.[50-52] Compressed Sense (CS-SENSE) is a further development in which compressed sensing is combined with the parallel-imaging or SENSE infrastructure.[53] CS-SENSE can be used to achieve further reduction of time and can be applicable for TOF-MRA intracranial and extracranial vessels. **Figures 13A to F** show use of CS-SENSE technique for TOF MRA intracranial vessels.

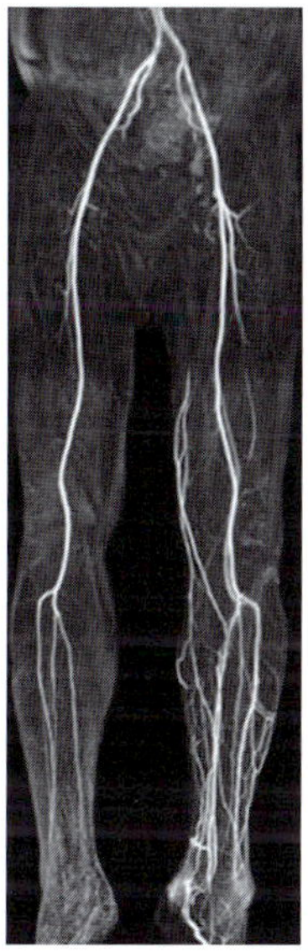

FIG. 11: CE-MRA bilateral lower limbs showing adequate visualization of lower limb arteries, early draining veins are seen on left side due to underlying vascular malformation.

APPLICATIONS OF MRA

High spatial resolution, vessel to background ratio and sufficient coverage for accurate assessment of the vessels of interest at a reasonable time of acquisition are few of the basic requirements of successful MRA in routine clinical practice. A brief review of applications of NC-MRA in different vascular bed is outlined below.

Neurovascular Imaging

Limited volumetric coverage with high spatial resolution is desired for intracranial MRA. Flow dependent techniques of MRA face the challenge of multidirectional flow in intracranial MRA as it can affect the vessel to-background contrast. TOF MRA is the predominant technique used for intracranial MRA for depicting different vascular pathologies of brain.

TOF MRA is effective in diagnosing aneurysms > 3 mm at 1.5 T.[54] Voxel volume as low as 0.08 mm^3 can be achieved with 3T systems.[55] Improved vessel contrast and diagnostic efficacy comparable to multidetector CT angiogram in aneurysm detection can also be achieved with 3T systems.[56] TOF-MRA is a useful technique for follow-up of intracranial aneurysms treated with endovascular detachable coils;[57,58] however, it performance in follow up of aneurysms less than 3 mm may not be as good.[59] Owing to susceptibility artefact associated with surgical clips, TOF-MRA is less effective in following up and accurate assessment of residual necks of aneurysms treated with titanium clips.[60] TOF-MRA may be suboptimal in evaluation of giant intracranial aneurysms because of slow and turbulent flow and CE-MRA may be more useful in evaluation of intracranial aneurysms >13 mm in size.[61] One important pitfall of TOF-MRA in the setting of intracranial hemorrhage is the potential of methaemoglobin in intracranial hemorrhage to mimic flow-related enhancement, owing to its inherent short T1 property.

Intracranial arteriovenous malformations and dural arteriovenous fistula are relatively less frequently encountered pathologies. Assessment of these disorders require high spatial as well as temporal resolution that distinguishes

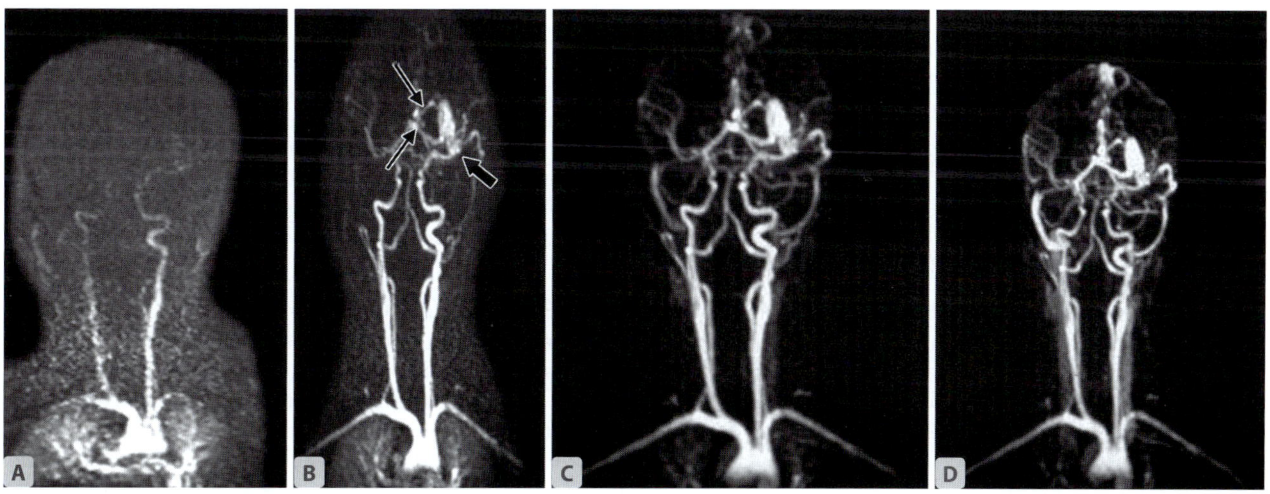

FIGS. 12A TO D: Time-resolved CE-MRA in a case of cerebral AVM demonstrating the AVM nidus, its feeders (thick arrow) and venous drainage (thin arrows) in a dynamic manner comparable to catheter angiography.

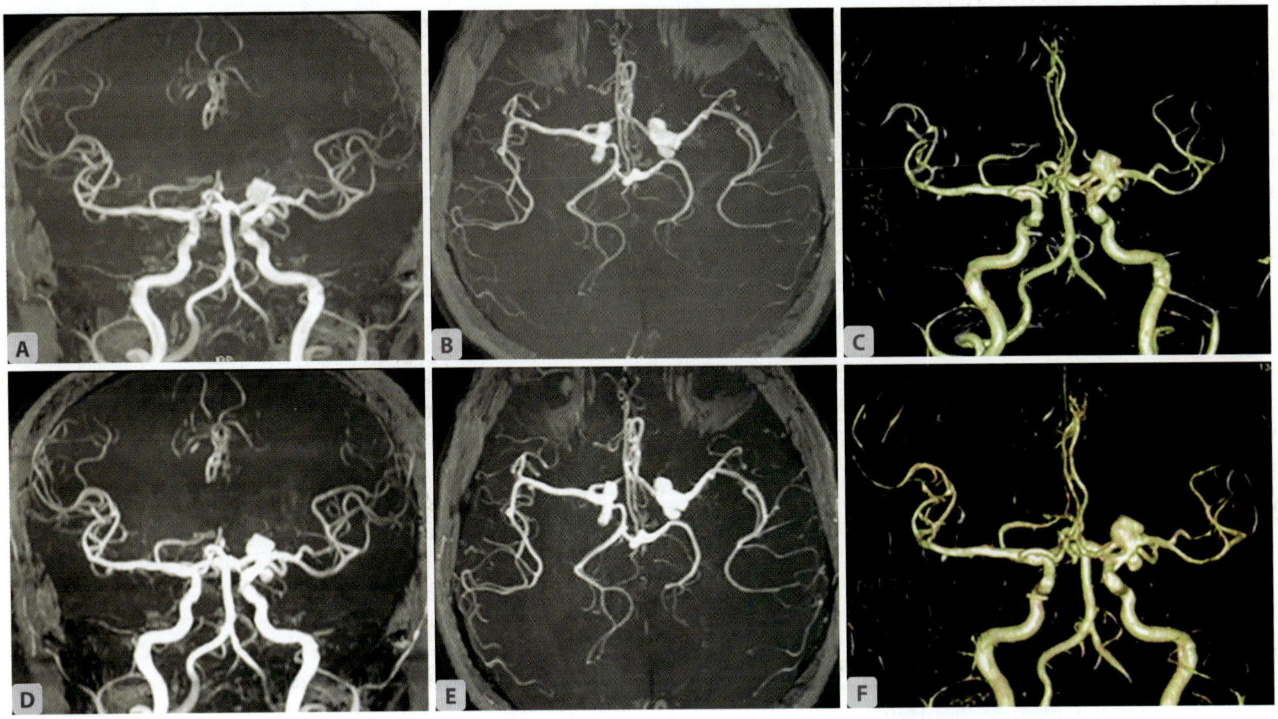

FIGS. 13A TO F: Intracranial MRA of a 62-year-old female patient presenting with headache. (A to C) MRA acquired with conventional technique (acquisition time 4 min 21 sec) and (D to F) MRA acquired with CS-SENSE with acceleration factor of 4.5 (acquisition time 2 min 34 sec). (A and B) and (D and E) coronal and axial maximum intensity projection images and (C and F) volume rendered images. The images showed a saccular aneurysm arising from left internal carotid artery bifurcation and another small aneurysm arising from communicating segment of left internal carotid artery. Both the observers considered the sets of images to have equivalent quality showing the aneurysmal morphology and bearing comparable diagnostic information.

between arterial feeders from draining veins. Although digital subtraction angiography (DSA) remains the gold standard modality for evaluating these conditions; time resolved CE MRA can provide better temporal information than non contrast MRA. TOF MRA has also been found to have lower sensitivity for evaluation of intracranial stenosis in primary CNS vasculitis.[62]

Although, requirement for spatial resolution is less exacting in extracranial MRA, problems are likely to arise from vessel tortuosity and motion related artefact from patient's swallowing. Owing to the superior speed, coverage, and low sensitivity to flow-induced artifacts CE-MRA is generally the preferred method.[63]

Magnetic resonance venography (MRV) is an important for evaluation of dural venous sinus thrombosis assessment. To minimize the in-plane flow saturation, acquisition is done in an oblique sagittal plane. 2D TOF MRV is able to depict flow as low as 2 cm/s;[64] however, a combination of TOF and contrast-enhanced MRV has been advocated for greatest sensitivity.[65] Additionally, 3D PC imaging may be used for intracranial MRV, setting a low threshold velocity encoding of approximately 15 cm/s; however, it is a slower technique.

Susceptibility weighted imaging can also be used for evaluation of intracranial veins.[66]

Abdominal Vascular Imaging

Image quality of abdominal MRA is influenced by factors like respiratory motion, bowel peristalsis and artifacts from bowel contents, which also affects subtraction in both unenhanced and contrast enhanced MRA. End expiratory breath hold techniques helps in minimizing artifacts due to cranial shift of kidneys and diaphragm seen during inspiratory breath hold. Contrast enhanced MRA is the mainstay of abdominal vascular imaging which relies on test bolus method or bolus tracking technique for timing of acquisition. Time resolved MRA allows multiphasic acquisition and useful in evaluation smaller vessels of hands and feet, and in pathologies like AVM in identifying nidus, multiple feeders and draining veins. Parallel imaging techniques deliver ultra fast imaging thereby reducing breath hold duration. In patients with impaired renal function non contrast MRA techniques like TOF and bSSFP are more commonly used.

Renovascular Hypertension

Renal artery stenosis is the most common cause of renovascular hypertension and has higher prevalence among patients with end-stage renal disease and uncontrolled hypertension. Etiological factors for RAS include atherosclerotic disease (90%) and fibromuscular

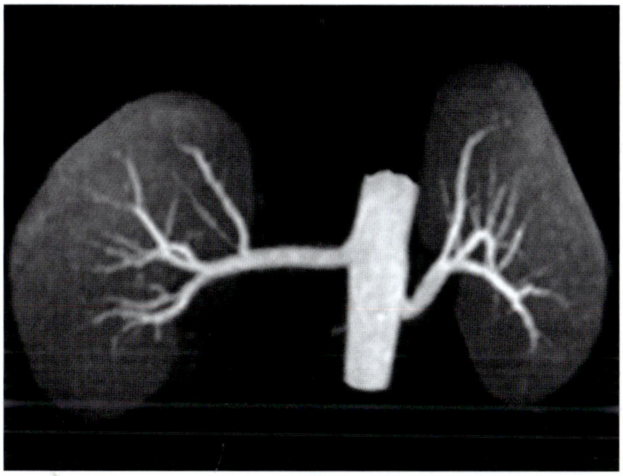

FIG. 14: Noncontrast-MRA of renal arteries showing adequate visualization of bilateral renal artery origin, course and segmental branches.

dysplasia (10%). Renal parameters being frequently impaired in these patients non contrast techniques like TOF and bSSFP are more commonly used with good specificity and sensitivity **(Fig. 14)**. Braidy et al reported 85%, 96%, 94%, and 96% sensitivity, specificity, accuracy, and NPV respectively in detecting stenosis of renal arteries using non contrast balanced SSFP sequence as compared to CE-MRA.[67] FMD, vasculitis, dissection, atheroembolic disease and post-traumatic occlusion are the other rare causes of renovascular hypertension.

Hepatic Vasculature

Recent advances in newer image reconstruction algorithms and dedicated contrast agents have enabled MR angiography to achieve higher spatial resolution and better image quality for imaging hepatic vasculature. The noncontrast technique, most effective in evaluating the hepatic arteries, is the respiratory triggered, 3-dimensional, steady-state free precession (SSFP) sequence.[68] Contrast enhanced 3D MR portography shows efficacy similar 64-slice MDCT for portal vein thrombus detection, and is able to identify portal vein anatomic variants with sensitivities and specificities of 100%.[69] CE-MRA is found to be superior to color Doppler ultrasound for the evaluation of portal hypertension as it shows evidence of thrombosis and occlusion of the main portal vein and portosystemic collaterals.[70] In cases of portal hypertension MRI can also help in assessment of liver parenchyma, focal hepatic lesions, biliary tree and vessels for shunt surgery or transplant. Phase contrast MRA can be used for quantification of increase in portal flow after transhepatic shunting or the noninvasive calculation of total hepatic blood flow rates.[71] In evaluating Budd Chiari syndrome MR venogram can be used to assess hepatic vein occlusion or stenosis, and IVC stenosis or thrombosis. Intrahepatic collaterals appear as comma-shaped enhancing vessels and bypass occlusions. The identification of level of obstruction helps to establish the cause and planning the intervention.

Peripheral Vascular Disorders

3D contrast-enhanced MRA facilitates accurate and detailed assessment of peripheral arteries without catheterization, ionizing radiation, or potentially nephrotoxic iodinated contrast agents. Unlike DSA, CE-MRA provides 3D data set that can be reformatted to produce multiplane DSA-like displays of the vessels that highlight information most relevant to prognosis and treatment planning (e.g., arterial wall inflammation, plaque composition, and mural and intramural thrombus formation).[72] MRA has advantage over CT angiography in assessment of heavily calcified arteries whereas CTA scores over MRA in assessment of in stent restenosis. Newer hybrid MRA protocols use two stage acquisition, first stage is high-spatial-resolution MRA of the calf and foot and second stage is aortoiliac and femoral bolus-chase MRA after the second injection, and are more accurate for evaluating the trifurcation and foot vessels than single-injection multistation MRA. Time resolved 3D MRA techniques eliminate the need for timing acquisitions or triggering methods, and also minimizes venous contamination. Non contrast MRA techniques are particularly useful in patients with impaired renal functions and newer techniques such as ECG-gated 3-D FSE, 3D FSE-SPACE, balanced SSFP with arterial spin labeling, and quiescent-interval single shot MRA using 2-D SSFP have good sensitivity and sensitivity in detecting stenosis, comparable to CE-MRA **(Figs. 15A and B)**.

For evaluation of vascular malformations MRI with MRA can be helpful for better characterization of lesions, assessment of high-flow versus low-flow malformations and supplying, and draining vessels. Time-resolved CE-MRA are especially useful for vessel-specific information with clear separation of the arterial and venous phases, for detection of venous shunting, and assessment of flow direction.[73]

FUTURE PERSPECTIVES

Presently MRA techniques are well established tool for vascular imaging however still there is need of decrease acquisition times, increase temporal and spatial resolution with more dynamic information. With advent of 3T MR scanner these problems has been addressed in clinical imaging. Use of high fields such as 7T are in developing and research phase and the recent studies reveals that CE-MRA at 7T demonstrates the feasibility and current constraints of ultrahigh filed contrast enhanced MRA relative to NC MRA.[74]

Also there are evidences of work under research reveals that TOF MRA at 7T have increase SNR and spatial restoration, especially for the assessment of brain AVM and high grade gliomas. Other applications like arterial

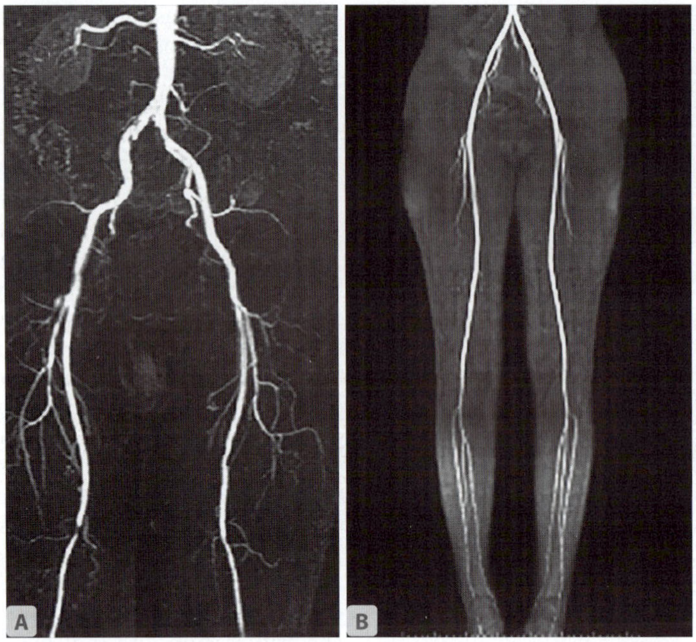

FIGS. 15A AND B: (A) Multistation CE-MRA of the abdomen, pelvis, and lower extremities reveals focal high-grade stenosis of right distal SFA and collateral formation. (B) Noncontrast-MRA of lower extremities showing adequate visualization of bilateral below knee arteries.

spin labeling are mentioned in other chapter on perfusion in this book. Newer techniques like SWI-MRA are also in developmental phase, it makes possible to image both artery as well as vein simultaneously and can be evaluated separately.[75] Veins are dark due to T2* effect with SWI processing, same time arteries are seen bright due to TOF inflow effect **(Figs. 16A to D)**. In addition, it can also provide the information about hemorrhage and calcification whether parenchymal or mural in case of atherosclerotic disease.

Lastly, there is lot more in future for MRA application due to advent of ultra-high field scanners and development of advances imaging sequences.

ACKNOWLEDGMENTS

The authors acknowledge and thank Dr Nirmalya Ray, DM resident in Neuroradiology section of department of Radiodiagnosis and imaging, PGIMER Chandigarh for writing and editing the chapter.

REFERENCES

1. Lenz G, Haacke E, Masaryk T, Laub GA. Inplane vascular imaging: pulse sequence design and strategy. Radiology. 1988;166:875-82.
2. Lim RP, Koktzoglou I. Noncontrast magnetic resonance angiography: concepts and clinical applications. Radiol Clin North Am. 2015;53:457-76.
3. Keller PJ, Drayer BP, Fram EK, Williams KD, et al. MR angiography with two-dimensional acquisition and three- dimensional display. Radiology. 1989;173:527-32.
4. Laub GA, Kaiser WA. MR angiography with gradient motion refocusing. J Comput Assist Tomogr. 1988;12:377-82.
5. Parker GL, Yuan C, Blatter DD. MR angiography by multiple thin slab 3D acquisitions. Magn Res Med. 1991;17:434-51.
6. Tkach J, Masaryk T, Ruggieri P, et al. Use of Tilted Optimized Nonsaturating Excitation. SMRM. 1992;2:3905.
7. Atkinson D, Brant-Zawadzki M, Gillan G, et al. Improved MR angiography: Magnetization transfer suppression with variable flip angles excitation and increased resolution. Radiology. 1994;190:890-4.
8. Edelman RR, Ahn SS, Chien D, et al. Improved time-of-flight MR angiography of the brain with magnetization transfer contrast. Radiology. 1992;184:395-9.
9. Wyttenbach R, Braghetti A, Wyss M, et al. Renal artery assessment with nonenhanced steady-state free precession versus contrast-enhanced MR angiography. Radiology 2007;245(1): 186-95.
10. Glockner JF, Takahashi N, Kawashima A, et al. Noncontrast renal artery MRA using an inflow inversion recovery steady state free precession technique (Inhance): comparison with 3D contrast-enhanced MRA. J Magn Reson Imaging. 2010;31:1411-8.
11. Furuta A, Isoda H, Yamashita R, et al. Non-contrastenhanced MR portography with balanced steady state free-precession sequence and time-spatial labeling inversion pulses: comparison of imaging with flow-in and flow-out methods. J Magn Reson Imaging. 2013;40:583-7.
12. Edelman RR, Sheehan JJ, Dunkle E, et al. Quiescent-interval single-shot unenhanced magnetic resonance angiography of peripheral vascular disease: technical considerations and clinical feasibility. Magn Reson Med. 2010;63:951-8.
13. Edelman RR, Giri S, Dunkle E, et al. Quiescent-inflow single-shot magnetic resonance angiography using a highly undersampled radial k-space trajectory. Magn Reson Med. 2013;70: 1662-8.

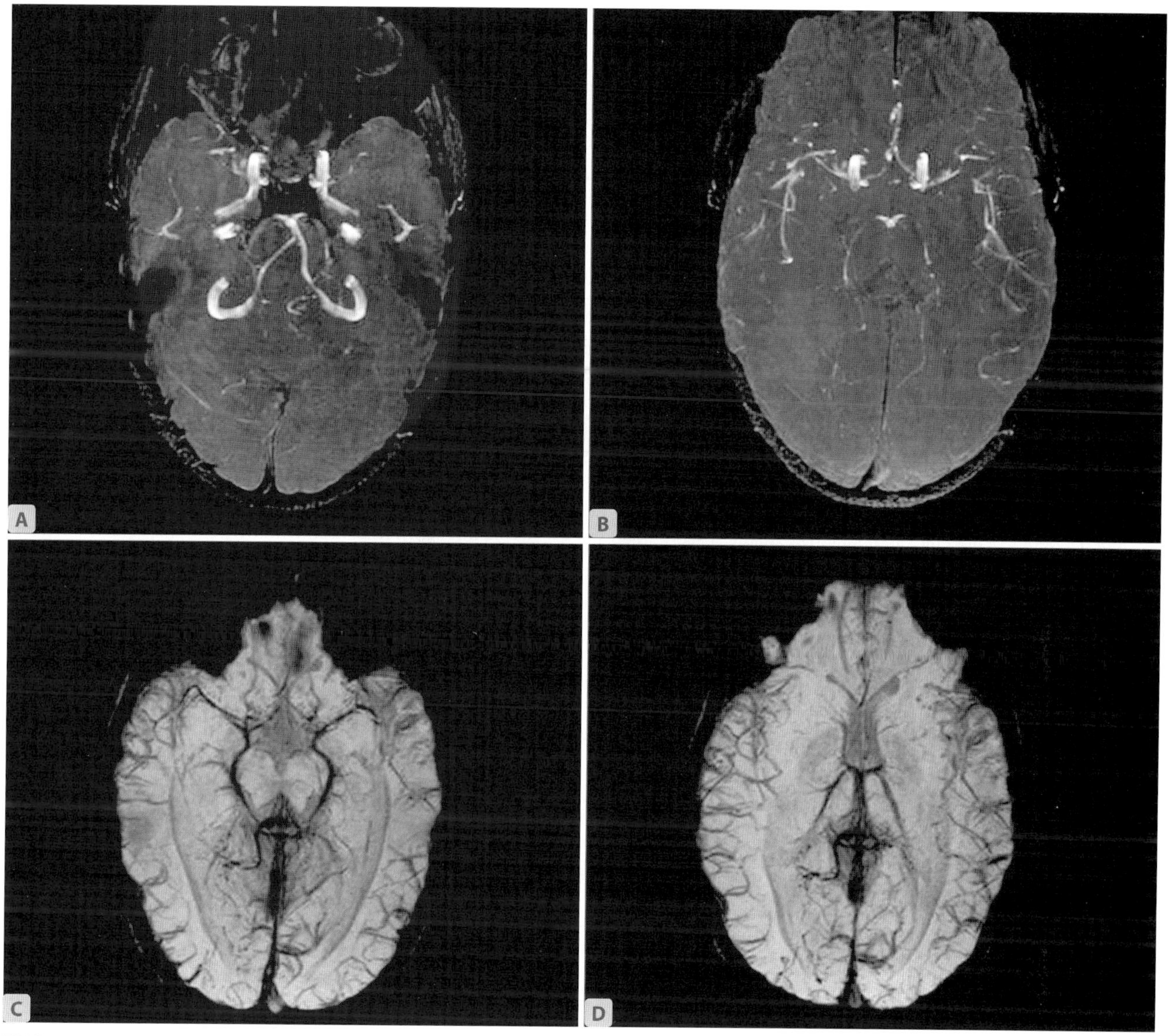

FIGS. 16A TO D: PC MRA application of SW imaging, Figures A and B are showing intracranial arterial anatomy due to TOF inflow effect and Figures C and D reveal the venous structures on SWI in same patient.

14. Edelman RR, Siewert B, Adamis M, et al. Signal targeting with alternating radiofrequency (STAR) sequences. application to MR angiography. Magn Reson Med. 1994;31: 233-8.
15. Kim SG. Quantification of relative cerebral blood flow change by flow-sensitive alternating inversion recovery (FAIR) technique: application to functional mapping. Magn Reson Med. 1995;34:293-301.
16. Dai W, Garcia D, de Bazelaire C, et al. Continuous flow-driven inversion for arterial spin labeling using pulsed radio frequency and gradient fields. Magn Reson Med. 2008;60:1488-97.
17. Koktzoglou I, Gupta N, Edelman RR. Nonenhanced extracranial carotid MR angiography using arterial spin labeling: improved performance with pseudocontinuous tagging. J Magn Reson Imaging. 2011;34(2):384-94.
18. Wu H, Block WF, Turski PA, et al. Non contrast enhanced three-dimensional (3D) intracranial MR angiography using pseudocontinuous arterial spin labeling and accelerated 3D radial acquisition. Magn Reson Med. 2013;69:708-15.
19. Koktzoglou I, Meyer JR, Ankenbrandt WJ, et al. Nonenhanced arterial spin labeled carotid MR angiography using three-dimensional radial balanced steady-state free precession imaging. J Magn Reason Imaging. 2015; 41:1150-6.
20. Bi X, Weale P, Schmitt P, et al. Non-contrast enhanced four-dimensional (4D) intracranial MR angiography: a feasibility study. Magn Reson Med. 2010;63(3):835-41.
21. Axel L, Morton D. MR flow imaging by velocity compensated/ uncompensated difference images. J Comp Assist Tomogr. 1987;11:31-4.
22. Dumoulin CL, Hart HR. Magnetic Resonance Angiography. Radiology. 1986;161:717-20.
23. Dumoulin CL, Souza SP, Walker MF, Wagle W. Three-dimensional phase contrast angiography. Magn Res Med. 1989;9:139-49.
24. Kilner PJ, Gatehouse PD, Firmin DN. Flow measurement by magnetic resonance: a unique asset worth optimising. J Cardiovasc Magn Reson. 2007;9:723-8.
25. Markl M, Frydrychowicz A, Kozerke S, et al. 4D flow MRI. J Magn Reson Imaging. 2012;36:1015-36.

26. Wedeen VJ, Meuli RA, Edelman RR, et al. Projective imaging of pulsatile flow with magnetic resonance. Science. 1985;230:946-8.
27. Miyazaki M, Takai H, Sugiura S, et al. Peripheral MR angiography: separation of arteries from veins with flow-spoiled gradient pulses in electrocardiography-triggered three-dimensional half-Fourier fast spin-echo imaging. Radiology. 2003;227:890-6.
28. Storey P, Atanasova IP, Lim RP, et al. Tailoring the flow sensitivity of fast spin-echo sequences for noncontrast peripheral MR angiography. Magn Reason Med 2010;64:1098-108.
29. Fan Z, Sheehan J, Bi X, et al. 3D noncontrast MR angiography of the distal lower extremities using flow-sensitive dephasing (FSD)-prepared balanced SSFP. Magn Reson Med. 2009;62: 1523-32.
30. Nicholas Priest A, Taviani V, John Graves M, et al. Improved artery-vein separation with acceleration dependent preparation for non-contrast-enhanced magnetic resonance angiography. Magn Reason Med. 2014;72:699-706.
31. Wright GA, Nishimura DG, Macovski A. Flow-independent magnetic resonance projection angiography. Magn Reson Med. 1991;17:126-40.
32. Brittain JH, Olcott EW, Szuba A, et al. Three-dimensional flow-independent peripheral angiography. Magn Reson Med. 1997;38:343-54.
33. Edelman RR, Koktzoglou I. Unenhanced flow independent MR venography by using signal targeting alternative radiofrequency and flow-independent relaxation enhancement. Radiology. 2009;250:236-45.
34. Schneider G, et al. Magnetic resonance angiography: Techniques, Indications and Practical Applications. Springer-Verlag Italia, 2005.
35. Papke K, Brassel F. Modern cross sectional imaging in the diagnosis of follow-up of intracranial aneurysms. Eur Radiol. 2006;16:2051-66.
36. Lohan DJ, et al. Contrast enhanced MRA vs Non enhanced MRA: Pros and Cons. Applied radiology, Journal of Practical medical imaging and Management. Supplement to May 2007.
37. Contrast Enhanced Magnetic resonance angiography; www. mr-tip.com.
38. Kopka L, Vosshenrich R, Rodenwaldt J, et al. Differences in injection rates on contrast-enhanced breath-hold three-dimensional MR angiography. AJR Am J Roentgenol. 1998; 170(2):345-8.
39. Lee VS, Rofsky NM, Krinsky GA, et al. Single dose breath-hold gadolinum-enhanced three-dimensional MR angiography of the renal arteries. Radiology. 1999;211:69-78.
40. Boos M, Scheffler K, Haselhorst R, et al. Arterial first pass gadolinium-CM dynamics as a function of several intravenous saline flush and Gd volumes. J Magn Reson Imaging. 2001;13(4):568-76.
41. Bart E Muhs, Hence JM Verhagen, Matthew G Huddle, Vinay M Pai, Elizabeth M Hecht, Alan Dardik. Theory, Technique, and Practice of Magnetic Resonance Angiography. Vascular. 2007;15(6):376-83.
42. LS Babiarz JM, Romero EK, Murphy B Brobeck. Contrast- enhanced MR angiography is not more accurate than unenhanced 2d time-of-flight mr angiography for determining >70 percent internal carotid artery stenosis. Am J Neuroradiol. 2009;30:761-8.
43. A TJ, Kaufmann J, Huston III HJ, Cloft J Mandrekar L. A Prospective Trial of 3T and 1.5T Time-of-Flight and Contrast-enhanced MR angiography in the follow-up of coiled intracranial aneurysms. Am J Neuroradiol. 2010;31:912-18.
44. Maurizio Papa, Francesco De Cobelli, Elena Baldissera. Takayasu arthritis: intravascular contrast medium for MR angiography in the evaluation of disease activity. AJR. 2012;198:W279-W284.
45. Lubicz B, et al. Is digital subtraction angiography still needle for the follow-up of intracranial aneurysms treated by embolisation with detachable coils? Neuroradiology. 2008;50:841-8.
46. RI Farb R, Agid RA, Willinsky DM Johnstone. Cranial Dural Arteriovenous Fistula: Diagnosis and Classification with Time-Resolved MR Angiography at 3T. Am J Neuroradiol. 2009;30: 1546-51.
47. Kristine A. Blackham, Matthew A. Passalacqua, Gurpreet S. Sandhu. Applications of Time-Resolved MR Angiography. AJR. 2011;196:W613-W620.
48. HK Lim, CG Choi, SM Kim. Detection of residual brain arteriovenous malformations after radio surgery: diagnostic accuracy of contrast-enhanced four-dimensional MR angiography at 3.0T. BJR. 2012;85:1064-9.
49. Lustig M, Donoho D, Pauly JM. Sparse MRI: The application of compressed sensing for rapid MR imaging. Magn Reson Med. 2007;58:1182-95.
50. Fushimi Y, Fujimoto K, Okada T, Yamamoto A, Tanaka T, Kikuchi T, et al. Compressed sensing 3-dimensional time-of-flight magnetic resonance angiography for cerebral aneurysms: optimization and evaluation. Invest Radiol. 2016;51:228-35.
51. Yamamoto T, Fujimoto K, Okada T, Fushimi Y, Stalder AF, Natsuaki Y, Schmidt M, Togashi K. Time-of-flight magnetic resonance angiography with sparse Undersampling and Iterative Reconstruction: Comparison With Conventional Parallel Imaging for Accelerated Imaging. Invest Radiol. 2016;51:372-8
52. Yamamoto T, Okada T, Fushimi Y, Yamamoto A, Fujimoto K, Okuchi S, et al. Magnetic resonance angiography with compressed sensing: An evaluation of moyamoya disease. PLoS One. 2018;13:e0189493.
53. J.E. Vranic, X N.M. Cross, X Y. Wang, X D.S. Hippe, X E. de Weerdt, and X M. Mossa-Basha. Compressed Sensing-sensitivity encoding (CS SENSE) Accelerated Brain Imaging: Reduced Scan Time without Reduced Image Quality. AJNR Am J Neuroradiol. 2019;40:92-98.
54. Huston J 3rd, Nichols DA, Luetmer PH, et al. Blinded prospective evaluation of sensitivity of MR angiograph to known intracranial aneurysms: importance of aneurysm size. AJNR Am J Neuroradiol. 1994;15:1607-14.
55. Gaa J, Weidauer S, Requardt M, et al. Comparison of intracranial 3D-ToF-MRA with and without parallel acquisition techniques at 1.5T and 3.0T: preliminary results. Acta Radiol. 2004;45:327-32.
56. Hiratsuka Y, Miki H, Kiriyama I, et al. Diagnosis of unruptured intracranial aneurysms: 3T MR angiography versus 64-channel multi-detector row CT angiography. Magn Reson Med Sci. 2008;7(4):169-78.
57. Ferre JC, Carsin-Nicol B, Morandi X, et al. Time-of flight MR angiography at 3T versus digital subtraction angiography in the imaging follow-up of 51 intracranial aneurysms treated with coils. Eur J Radiol. 2009;72:365-9.
58. Kwee TC, Kwee RM. MR angiography in the follow up of intracranial aneurysms treated with Guglielmi detachable coils: systematic review and meta-analysis. Neuroradiology. 2007;49(9):703-13.
59. Deutschmann HA, Augustin M, Simbrunner J, et al. Diagnostic accuracy of 3D time-of-flight MR angiography compared with digital subtraction angiography for follow-up of coiled intracranial aneurysms: influence of aneurysm size. AJNR Am J Neuroradiol. 2007;28:628-34.
60. Grieve JP, Stacey R, Moore E, et al. Artefact on MRA following aneurysm clipping: an in vitro study and prospective comparison with conventional angiography.Neuroradiology. 1999;41(9):680-6.
61. Cirillo M, Scomazzoni F, Cirillo L, et al. Comparison of 3D TOF-MRA and 3D CE-MRA at 3T for imaging of intracranial aneurysms. Eur J Radiol. 2013;82:e853-9.
62. Cosottini M, Canovetti S, Pesaresi I, et al. 3-T magnetic resonance angiography in primary angiitis of the central nervous system. J Comput Assist Tomogr. 2013;37:493-8.

63. Huang BY, Castillo M. Neurovascular imaging at 1.5 tesla versus 3.0 tesla. Magn Reson Imaging Clin N Am. 2009;17:29-46.
64. Pui MH. Cerebral MR venography. Clin Imaging. 2004;28:85-9.
65. Chen HM, Chen CC, Tsai FY, et al. Cerebral sinovenous thrombosis. Neuroimaging diagnosis and clinical management. Interv Neuroradiol. 2008;14:35-40.
66. Boeckh-Behrens T, Lutz J, Lummel N, et al. Susceptibility-weighted angiography (SWAN) of cerebral veins and arteries compared to TOF-MRA. Eur J Radiol. 2012;81(6):1238-45.
67. Chadi Braidy, Iskandar Daou, Abdoulay Dione Diop, et al. Unenhanced MR Angiography of Renal Arteries: 51 Patients, American Journal of Roentgenology. 2012;199:5: W629-W637.
68. Rizwan Aslam, Benjamin M. Yeh, Judy Yee, MR Imaging Evaluation of the Hepatic Vasculature. Magn Reson Imaging Clin N Am. 2010;18:515-23.
69. Heilmaier C, Sutter R, Lutz AM, et al. Mapping of hepatic vascular anatomy: dynamic contrast-enhanced parallel MR imaging compared with 64 detector row CT. Radiology. 2007;245(3):872e80.
70. Cakmak O, Elmas N, Tamsel S, et al. Role of contrast-enhanced 3D magnetic resonance portography in evaluation portal venous system compared with color Doppler ultrasonography. Abdom Imaging. 2008;33:65-71.
71. Yzet T, Bouzerar R, Baledent O, et al. Dynamic measurements of total hepatic blood flow with phase contrast MRI. Eur J Radiol. 2010;73(1):119e24
72. Hale Ersoy and Frank J Rybicki. MR Angiography of the Lower Extremities. American Journal of Roentgenology. 2008;190:1675-84. 10.2214/AJR.07.2223
73. Kramer U, Ernemann U, Mangold S, et al. Diagnostic value of high spatial and temporal resolution time-resolved MR angiography in the workup of peripheral high-flow vascular malformations at 1.5 Tesla. Int J Cardiovasc Imaging. 2012;28:823-34.
74. Umutlu L, Maderwald S, Kinner S. First- pass contrast enhanced renal MRA at 7 telsa: initial result. Eur Radiol. 2013;23:1059-66.
75. Samuel RS. Barnes, Mark Haacke. Susceptibility Weighted Imaging: Clinical angiographic applications. Magn Reson Imaging Clin N Am. 2009;17(1):47-61.

CHAPTER

38

Magnetic Resonance Imaging Pulse Sequences

Vikas Bhatia, Manphool Singhal, Mahesh Prakash

Magnetic resonance (MR) sequences are continuously evolving. From simple sequences like conventional spin echo they have increased in number as well as complexity. However, the ultimate aim of every sequence is to bring about better tissue contrast in least amount of time. Therefore, different sequences are designed to account for varied tissue characteristics. Also, with the tremendous improvement in computational powers now the sequences have become less time consuming and less prone to artifacts. It is a vast and complex topic but basic understanding of the sequences is essential to interpret the MR images they produced.

MR sequence is an array of different radiofrequency (RF) pulses, which are applied at a particular time and in a predetermined way to obtain resultant image.

A pulse sequence diagram is a schematic diagram, which depicts various pulse or gradients that are applied over a period of time.

There are minimum of four horizontal lines, which depict the excitatory RF pulse, and three representing each gradient, i.e. slice, phase and frequency gradient **(Fig. 1)**. Additional lines may be used to depict the generated echo and other pulse or gradients used.

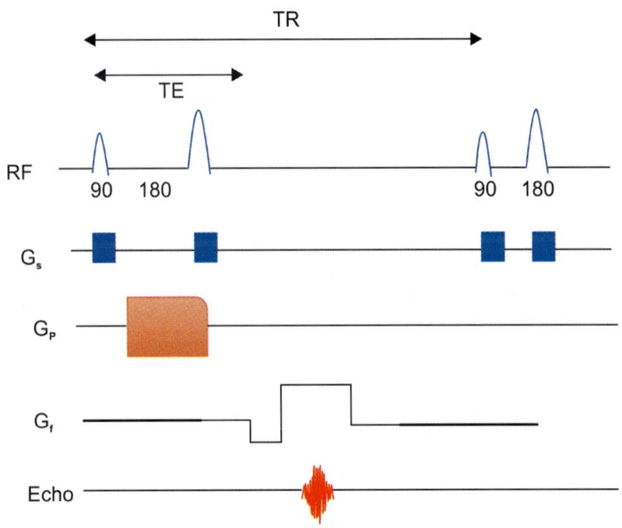

FIG. 1: A typical pulse sequence diagram for SE sequence.

BASIC TERMINOLOGIES

Image contrast is generated by variation of TR (repetition time) and TE (echo time) in any given sequence. TR is the duration of time between application of one RF excitation pulse to the start of the next RF pulse. TE is duration of time between the initial RF pulse and the peak of the echo. Both are usually in milliseconds. T1- and T2-weighting are other terms, which need to be understood. T1-weighted images would mean that though, image show all types of contrast but the T1 effect is more pronounced. T1-effect would mean that the TR and TE are both short and the difference between relaxation of longitudinal magnetization of fat and water can be detected. In T1-weighted images fat, blood products, slow flow and contrast would appear bright whereas tissues containing fluid, mineral rich content like bone and air would be dark. T2 weighting is opposite of this. Here the TR and TE and both prolonged and thus the difference in T2 decay of fat and water can be detected. At short TE this difference is not apparent. This makes high free water containing tissues bright of T2-weighted images. Another type of images are proton density images where TR is long and TE is short, thus the images are neither T1 weighted and nor T2 weighted but the image contrast produced is due to difference in proton density of the tissues with brighter signal in tissues having higher proton density.

SEQUENCE TYPES

Spin echo (SE) sequences were the first sequences to be used for MR imaging. These were closely followed by gradient echo (GRE) imaging. As more and more limitations of these classic sequences became apparent they were modified to bring about better tissue contrast in less time. This was followed by ultrafast sequences in both these groups. Finally sequences with features of both of these were created to generate hybrid sequences.

Pulse sequences can generally be categorized as shown in **Table 1**. Differences between SE and GRE are summarized in **Table 2**.

TABLE 1: Types of sequence used in MR imaging.

Spin echo pulse sequences	Gradient echo pulse sequences
Conventional SE	Coherent GRE
Fast or turbo SE	Incoherent GRE
Inversion recovery (IR)	Steady state free precession (SSFP)
	Balanced GRE/balanced dual excitation
	Fast GRE
	Echo planar imaging (EPI)

TABLE 2: Differences between a SE and GRE sequences.

Sequence	Spin echo	Gradient echo
TR	Long >2000 ms Short 300–700 ms	Long >100 ms Short <50 ms
TE	Long >70 ms Short 10–30 ms	Long >15–25 ms Short <5 ms
Flip angle	900	Small 5–20^0 Large >70^0
Scan time	More	Less
Susceptibility to magnetic field inhomogeneity	Low	Very high

TABLE 3: Parameters for obtaining different image weighting in SE sequences.

Weighting	T1W	PD	T2W
TE	Short TE (10–30 ms)	Short TE (20 ms)	Long TE (>80 ms)
TR	Short TR (300–700 ms)	Long TR (>2000 ms)	Long TR (>2000 ms)
Scan time	Scan time (4–6 min)	7–15 min	7–15 min
Echo generation	Single echo	Dual echo	Dual echo

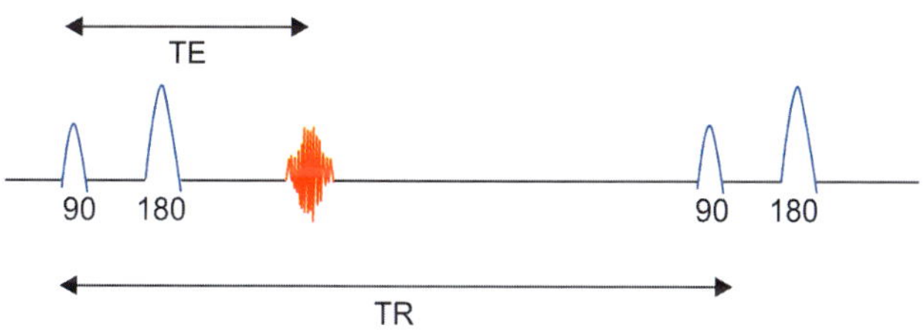

FIG. 2: Spin echo sequence.

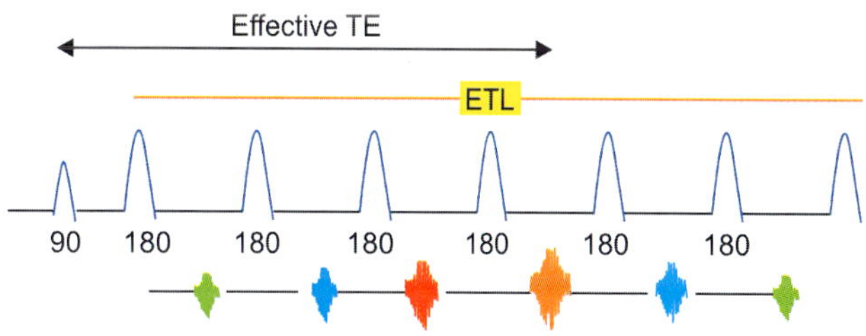

FIG. 3: Turbo or fast spin echo sequence.

The Spin Echo Pulse Sequence

Basic principle involving SE sequence is initial application of a 90° excitation pulse so as to flip the NMV into the transverse plane which induces a voltage in the receiver coil. As soon as this pulse is removed, there is generation of free induction decay (FID) signal. Immediately after this T2* effects occurs due to magnetic field inhomogeneity which result in dephasing. These cause magnetic moments of individual protons to phase out or fan out with respect to each other with some resonating faster and others resonating slower depending on the effect of inhomogeneity on the B^0. In SE sequence, a 180° radiofrequency pulse is applied to compensate for this dephasing with resultant shift in positions so that the magnetic moments which were initially trailing becomes leading and vice versa. At a particular time the spins catch up with each other and are in phase resulting in maximum signal which is known as spin echo **(Fig. 2)**. This contains predominantly information based on T1/T2 properties as T2* effects has been mitigated and appropriate time is allowed to reach T1/T2 relaxation times. The acquisition time in these sequences is longer as only one phase encoding step is applied with resultant one line of K space is filled per TR interval.

Different type of image weighting can be obtained in conventional SE sequences as shown in **Table 3**.

Fast or Turbo SE

In these sequences, a 90° pulse is closely followed by a chain of multiple 180° pulses called the *turbo factor* or the *echo train length (ETL)* **(Fig. 3)**. Here more multiple phase encoding steps are performed per TR interval with rapid filling of k space and hence resulting in reduced scan time.

Scan time is directly proportional to TR, number of excitation and phase encoding steps. In these sequences the scan time is reduced to 1/ETL due to reduction in phase encoding steps.

In these sequences echoes are generated at different TE times each having variable weighting. Operator can decide the resultant weighting and an effective TE can be selected. During each phase encoding step different slope of gradients are applied with shallow slopes resulting in maximum amplitude of resulting echo as compared to steep gradients. Thus system acquires the phase encoding steps in a way that shallow slopes corresponding to maximum signal are centered on effective TE. Different type of image weighting can be obtained in FSE sequences as shown in **Table 4**.

Single Shot FSE

In these sequences, the scan time is markedly reduced by acquiring all K space lines in one TR interval. A combination of a partial Fourier technique with FSE is used where half lines of K space are acquired in one TR and the other half are interpolated. Though the scan time is reduced, the SNR is reduced too.

TABLE 4: Parameters for obtaining different image weighting in turbo or FSE sequences.

Weighting	T1W	PD	T2W
Effective TE	Minimum	Minimum	80–140 ms
TR	Short TR	Long TR (depending on slice number)	Long TR (depending on slice number)
Turbo factor/ ETL	2–8	4–12	12–30

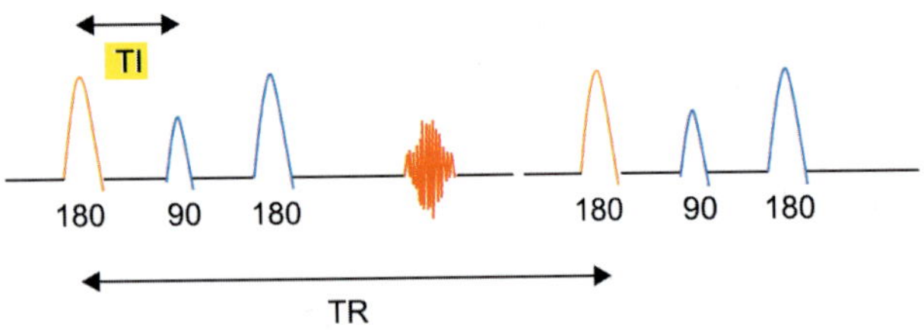

FIG. 4: Inversion recovery sequence.

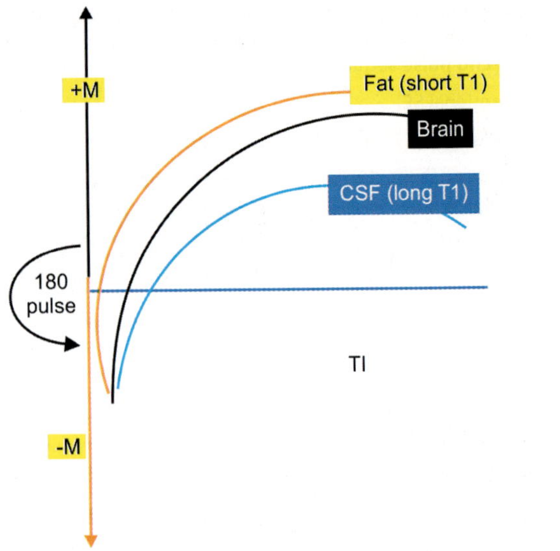

FIG. 5: Regrowth of tissue M_z for fat, brain and CSF after application of a 180° pulse.

Inversion Recovery

This is basically a SE sequence with application of another 180° inverting RF pulse is applied which inverts the net magnetizing vector (NMV) through 180°. After removal of pulse the NMV begins to recover and at a time equivalent to TI (inversion time) a 90° excitation pulse is applied followed by a 180° rephasing pulse to produce an echo at a time TE **(Fig. 4)**. TI selected is dependent on the signal which has to be suppressed, e.g. fat or CSF **(Fig. 5)**.

This sequence can be both T1 and T2 weighted.

If inversion time is sufficiently long to allow net magnetizing vector to pass through the transverse plane and then the 90° excitation pulse is applied then the contrast is predominantly T1 weighted. Here TE is to be kept short.

For T2 weighting the TE is prolonged so that T2 decay can occur and the resultant image is T2 weighted.

The TR, the interval between the two inverting 180° pulses should be kept long to allow for complete recovery of NMV to the longitudinal plane.

Different type of image weighting can be obtained in FSE sequences as shown in **Table 5**.

A. *Short T1 inversion recovery (STIR):* This sequence is predominantly used to suppress fat to delineate the structures surrounded by fatty tissues. Here inversion time is kept low and 90° excitation pulse is applied when NMV of fat is crossing the transverse plane. At this point the longitudinal component of fat is zero so it does not contribute to any signal thus is suppressed.

B. *Fluid attenuated inversion recovery (FLAIR) sequence:* This is commonly used sequence in brain to suppress the CSF signal. Here inversion time is kept long (as opposed to in STIR) and 90° excitation pulse is applied when NMV of water is crossing the transverse plane. This selectively suppresses the CSF/free fluid signal.

   Table 6 summarizes the difference between STIR and FLAIR sequences.

TABLE 5: Parameters for obtaining different image weighting in IR sequences.

Weighting	T1W	PDW	Heavy T2/ pathology weighting
TR	Long (>3000 ms)	Long (>3000 ms)	Long (>3000 ms)
TE	Short	Short	Long
TI	Medium (400–700 ms)	Long (1800 ms)	medium (400–700 ms)
Scan time	7–15 min	7–15 min	7–15 min

Double and Triple IR Prep Sequences

These are specifically used in cardiac imaging to suppress signal from blood. Double IR prep has one nonslice selective 180⁰ pulse to invert all spins in the imaged volume followed by a slice selective 180⁰ pulse to reinvert spins within a slice. The TI is selected around 800 ms to completely nulls the signal from blood in the slice resulting in black blood imaging with excellent morphological details In Triple IR another inverting pulse corresponding to TI of around 150 ms is added to suppress fat.

Gradient Echo Sequences

This is fundamentally different sequence when compared to spin echo sequence. In this type, an initial excitation pulse is applied with certain strength that it flips the NMV into transverse plane at an angle less than 90°. The angle to which it flips the NMV is called flip angle. This results in conversion of only a part of the longitudinal magnetization into transverse magnetization. After the pulse is withdrawn, the magnetic moments start to dephase due to presence of magnetic field inhomogeneities which is called as T2* decay. A gradient pulse is then applied which dephase and then rephases the

TABLE 6: Difference between STIR and FLAIR sequences.

	FLAIR	STIR
TR	Long	Long
TE	Long	Long
TI	Long (1800–2200 ms)	Short (150–180 ms)
Turbo factor	15–20	15–20
Scan time	12–20 min	5–15 min

TABLE 7: Parameters for obtaining different image weighting in GRE sequences.

Weighting	T1w	PD	T2* w
TR	Short (<50 ms)	Long (>100 ms)	Long (>100 ms)
TE	Short (1–5 ms)	Short (1–5 ms)	Long (15–25 ms)
Flip angle	Large (>70⁰)	Small (5–15⁰)	Small (5–15⁰)

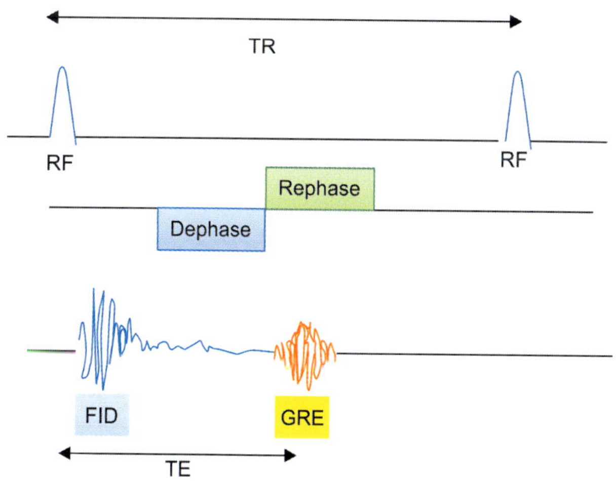

FIG. 6: Gradient echo sequence.

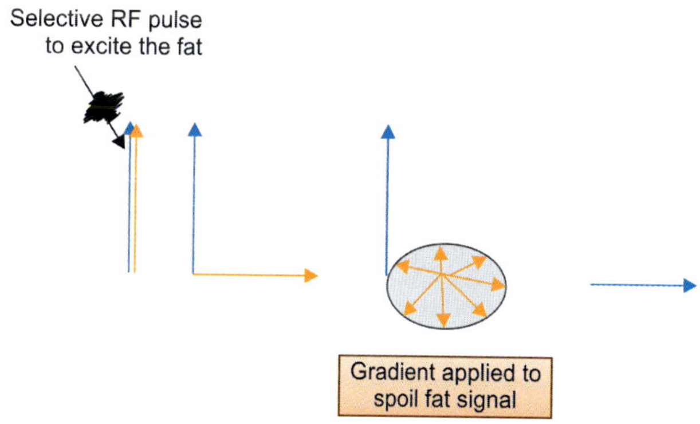

FIG. 7: CHESS sequence: Fat is selectively excited by an RF pulse to transverse plane followed by application of a gradient pulse to disperse the magnetization.

magnetic moments in the transverse component. This is followed by generation of signal called gradient echo **(Fig. 6)**. Since the rephasing by a gradient is not as effective as the RF pulse some nuclei, which are dephased (due to t2* effect) are not rephased and thus the resultant GRE image has some T2* effect.

Different type of image weighting can be obtained in GRE sequences as shown in **Table 7**.

Fat Suppression Sequences

Fat-suppression is widely used in routine MR imaging with predominant application in abdominal and musculoskeletal imaging. Principle indication for these is to enhance contrast resolution and determine their lipid content. Various commonly used fat suppression techniques are CHESS; chemical shift-selective fat suppression **(Fig. 7)**, STIR; short inversion time inversion recovery, **(Fig. 8)**, SPAIR; spectral adiabatic inversion recovery **(Fig. 9)**, water excitation **(Fig. 10)** and DIXON **(Fig. 11)**. Fat suppression enhances visualization marrow edema, can depict presence of fat in lesions, can differentiate fat from hemorrhage in certain lesions, eliminate chemical shift artifacts and leads to optimal visualization of enhancing lesions on post contrast images. A summary of various fat suppression sequences is tabulated in **Table 8**.

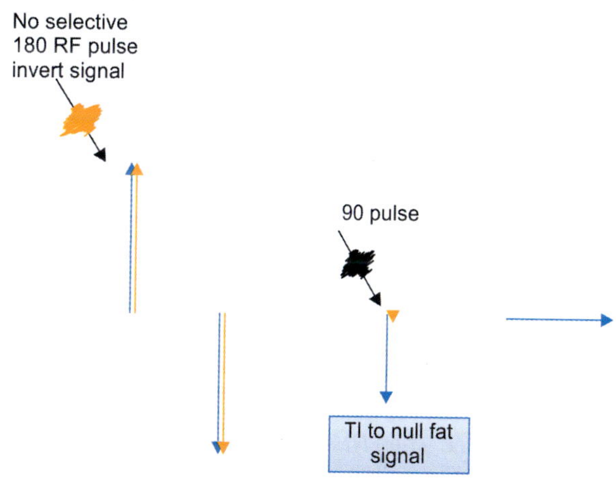

FIG. 8: STIR: Nonselective 180° pulse is applied to invert fat and water signal followed by beginning of acquisition at inversion time *(TI)* that nulls the fat signal.

STEADY STATE SEQUENCES

Concept of Steady State

After application of a RF pulse, the NMV is flipped to transverse plane and it is the sum of both longitudinal and transverse magnetization. After the pulse is switched off the transverse magnetization component begins to decrease as the magnetic

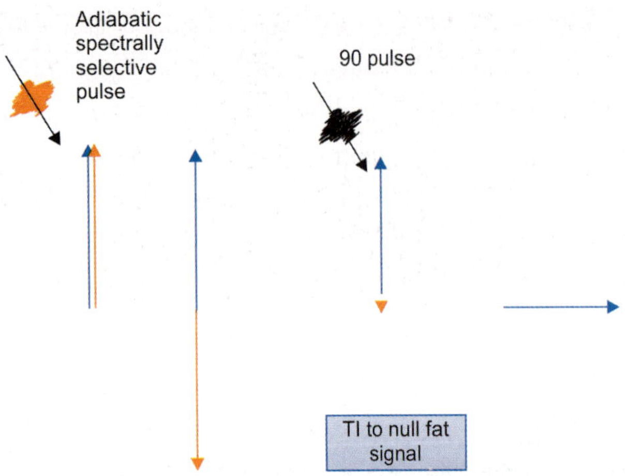

FIG. 9: SPAIR: An adiabatic spectrally selective pulse is applied to invert fat signal and acquisition is begun after the inversion time that nulls the fat signal.

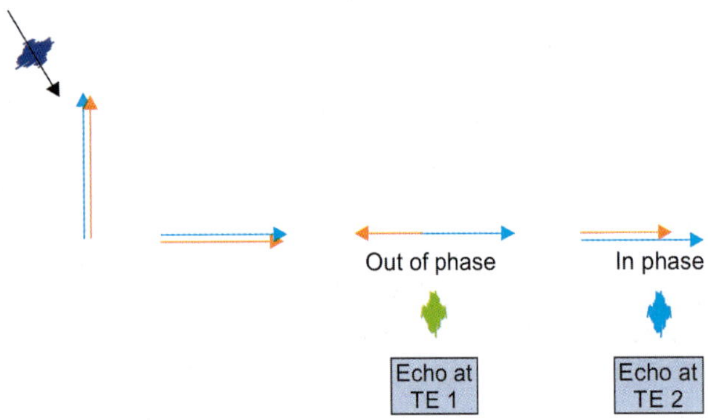

FIG. 11: Dixon technique: Both water and fat are excited with acquisition of two echoes, first when the water and fat are out of phase and second when they are in phase.

moments move out of phase. If repeat excitation pulse is applied at a TR which is shorter than T1-and T2 time of any tissue then there will be a residual transverse magnetization. This accumulates over time if repeated pulse are applied and a state is reached when NMV remains constant. This is called 'steady state'. This results in two types of signals once the steady state is achieved. First echo (s+) is due to free induction decay after the recent RF pulse of the NMV at short TE which contains both T1 and T2* weighting and the second signal (S-) is due to refocusing of the residual spin echo just before the next RF pulse is applied. This latter echo is predominantly T2 weighted. A summary of various steady state sequences is tabulated in **Table 9.**

Incoherent/Spoiled Gradient Echo Sequences

In these, the residual transverse magnetization is dephased by applying a gradient **(Fig. 12)**. Thus this does not contribute to signal. There is short TR with medium flip angle. The TE is kept very short so that T2* effect does not dominate and the resultant image is T1 weighted. (FLASH, SPGR, MPGR, T1-FFE).

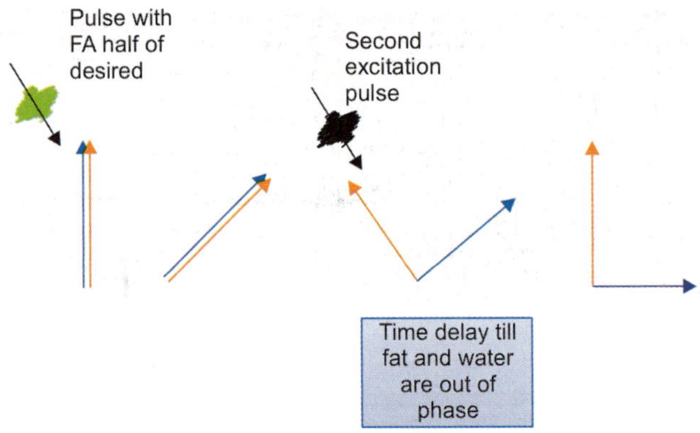

FIG. 10: Water excitation: A excitation pulse with half the desired FA is applied and after this at a time when water and fat are out of phase another excitation pulse is applied bringing the fat magnetization back to the longitudinal axis and flips the water magnetization onto the transverse plane.

Coherent Gradient Echo Sequence

In these sequences the residual transverse magnetization is utilized by applying a rephrasing gradient, which is similar to initial phase encoding gradient but is of opposite polarity. This rephases the residual magnetic moments and bring them in phase and then they contribute to signal during second excitation.

The sequences which sample the first echo (S+) are termed as postexcitation refocused steady state sequences **(Fig. 13)** and are mainly T2* weighted (FISP, GRASS, FFE, FAST).

The sequences which sample the second spin echo (S-) are pre-excitation steady state refocused sequences **(Fig. 14)** and are mainly T2 weighted (PSIF, SSFP, T2-FFE).

The sequences which sample both the first(S+) and second (S-) echoes are fully refocused steady state sequences **(Fig. 15)** and are both T1 and T2 weighted (true FISP, FIESTA, balanced FFE).

CISS/FIESTA-C

Constructive interface in steady state/fast imaging employing steady state acquisition.

These are modified fully refocused steady state sequences by different vendors. Since fully refocused steady state sequence like true-FISP is prone to 'banding artifacts', this aims to remove those. In this sequence two true-FISP sequences are acquired one with alternating phase RF pulse and second with non-alternating phase RF pulse. Combination of these two images displaces the banding artifacts. This results in high resolution 3D, T2-weighted image.

Dual Echo Steady State Sequence

This is another variation of true FISP. In true FISP being a balanced sequence S+ and S- signals are combined to form the image. In DESS images are formed with FISP (S+) and reversed FISP (S-) and are then combined. FISP component provides the T1 component and PSIF signal provides the T2 component of the image.

TABLE 8: Summarizes basic differences in various fat suppression techniques.

		Scan duration	SNR	B0/B1 sensitivity	Fat suppression with metal implants	Field strength preference
Chemical shift based	Chess	Short	High	Yes	Poor	High
	Water excitation	Short	High	B0 yes/B1 No	Poor	Medium
	DIXON	Long	High	No	Good	Medium
Inversion based	STIR	Long	Low	No	Good	Nondependent
Hybrid	SPAIR	Long	High	B0 yes/B1 No	Poor	High
	SPIR	Long	High	Yes	Poor	High

TABLE 9: Summarizes basic differences in various steady state MR sequences.

	Steady state gradient echo sequences			
		Coherent/refocused steady state		
	Spoiled/incoherent	Postexcitation refocused	Pre-excitation refocused	Fully refocused
Examples	FLASH SPGR T1FFE	FISP GRASS FFE	PSIF SSFP T2FFE	trueFISP FIESTA Balanced FFE
Steady state	LM	LM and TM	LM and TM	LM and TM
Signal for imaging	FID	FID (S+)	Spin echo (S-)	Both S+,S-
Refocusing		Phase encoding	Phase encoding	Phase, frequency and slice encoding
Image	T1W	T2*	T2	Depends on T2/T1 ratio
Motion sensitive	Yes	Yes	Yes	No

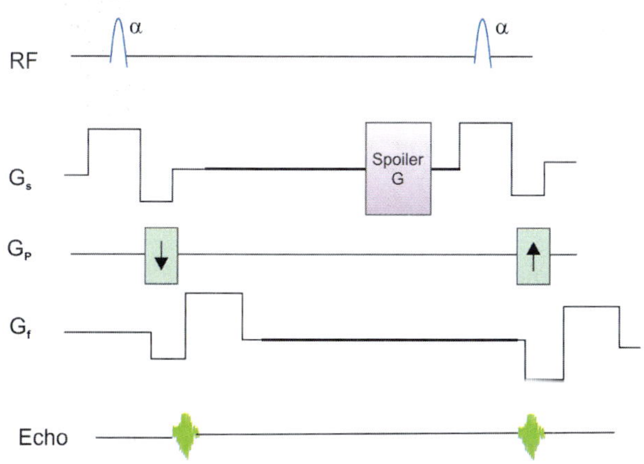

FIG. 12: Spoiled GRE sequence.

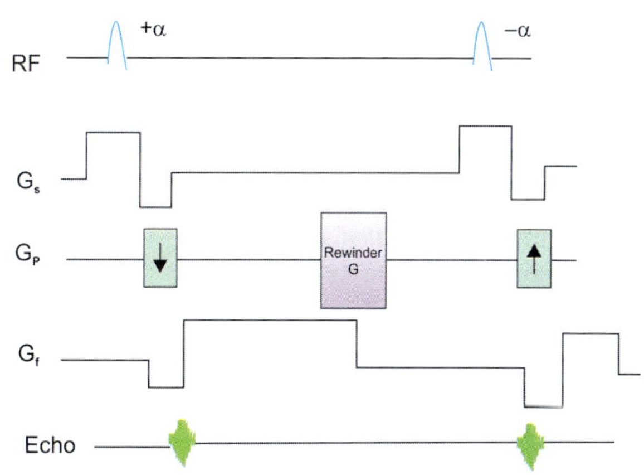

FIG. 13: Postexcitation refocused steady state sequence.

FAST GRADIENT ECHO

Very fast gradient echo sequences employ coherent or incoherent gradient echo sequences with significantly reduced TE with acquisition of required volume in a single breath hold. Here only a portion of the RF excitation pulse is applied and similarly a part of the echo is read called as partial echo resulting in reduced TE, TR and hence the scan time. Scan times are less than 1ms in these sequences and therefore acquisition can be done in a single breath hold. These sequences are also used for dynamic contrast imaging due to high temporal resolution.

Some of the fast sequences use a premagnetization pulse before the beginning of pulse sequences. Two examples are:

1. Application of a 180° pulse similar to inversion recovery and beginning of the pulse sequence after a specific delay.

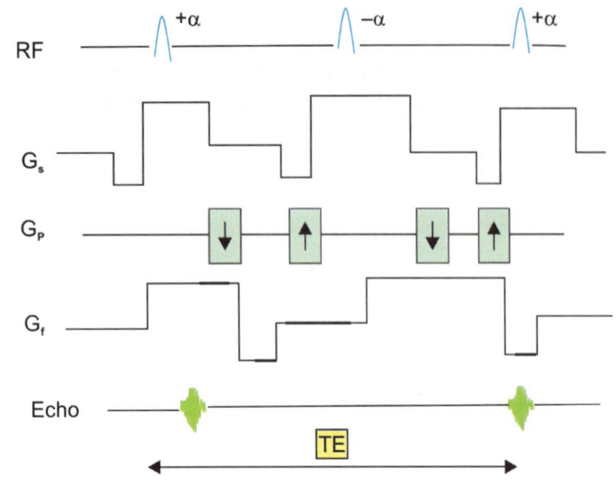

FIG. 14: Pre-excitation refocused steady state sequence.

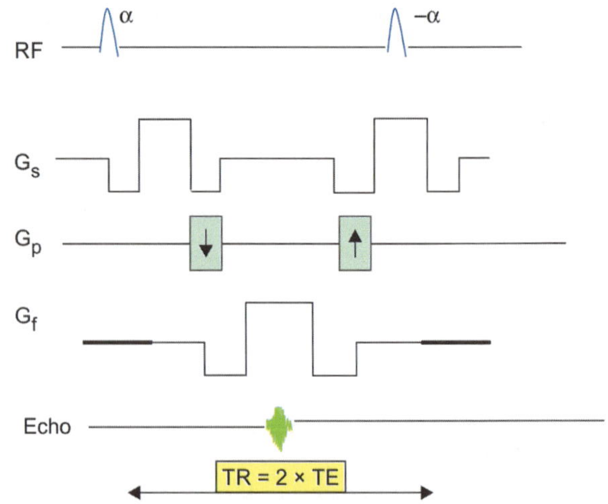

FIG. 15: Fully refocused steady state sequence.

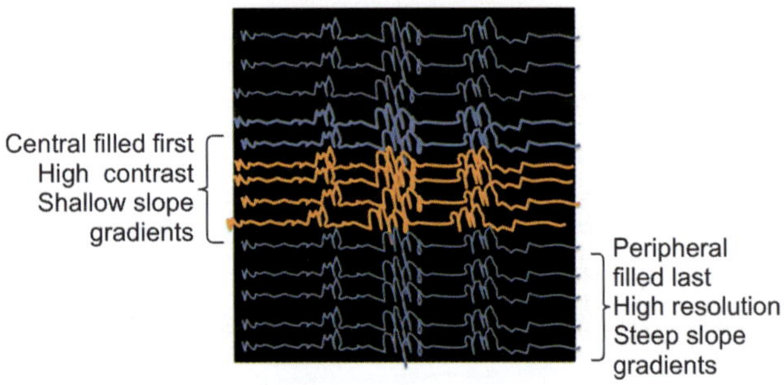

FIG. 16: Centric K space filling.

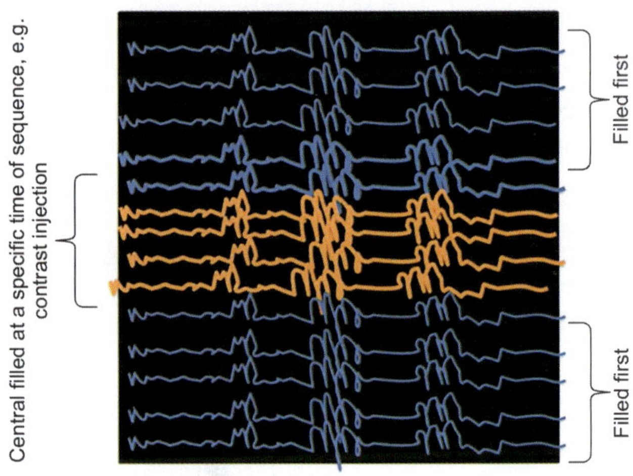

FIG. 17: Key hole K space filling.

It is used predominantly to get a T1 contrast or to null the signal from certain tissues.

2. Application of a 90°/180°/90° pulse combination to produce T2 contrast and is called as *driven equilibrium.*

K space filling in fast gradient echo sequences

Centric K space filling **(Fig. 16)**

Keyhole filling **(Fig. 17)**

Echo Planar Imaging

These are rapid MR imaging techniques which with capability of acquiring entire images in milliseconds thus reducing scan time, reducing motion artefacts and obtain dynamic and physiological information. It can be single shot or multishot. In single-shot echo planar imaging (EPI), all the spatial data is obtained after a single RF pulse. Multishot EPI produces images with high quality and SNR. Specific hardware requirements are needed for EPI with capability of rapidly switching gradients.

In EPI, gradient echoes are typically generated by oscillation of the readout gradient. Multiple echoes are generated followed by phase encoding steps to fill whole K space data within a single TR period **(Fig. 18)**. Different contrasts are generated depending on whether the beginning pulse is 90^0 (SE) or variable flip angle (GRE).

Examples of single shot are: *HASTE, SS-FSE, UFSE*

Examples of multi shot are *FSE/TSE*

K space filling in EPI:

Spiral K Space Filling (Single Shot) (Fig. 19)
Elliptical K space filling
Propeller K space filling

Multishot Methods
K space segmentation by acquisition
K space segmentation by echo

Hybrid Sequences

These combine gradient and spin echoes, such as *GRASE (gradient and spin echo)* are an effective compromise. Typically, a series of gradient rephasings are followed by an RF rephasing pulse. It has the advantage of both types of techniques: rapid acquisition of the gradient and compensation for T2* effects. These sequences increase the scan time to more than 100 ms per image but the benefits in terms of image quality are significant.

Parallel Imaging

It is a MR technique technique that utilizes the inherent spatial information within the phased-array coils that results in reduction of scan times. This is achieved byTo shorten imaging time, the number of phase-encoding steps is reduced and only half of the lines of *k*-space are acquired. Normally these will result in a reduced FOV and aliasing in the reconstructed image.

In parallel techniques, aliasing is removed by utilizing the spatial dependence of the phased-array coil elements **(Fig. 20)**. Two types of techniques are used as shown in **Table 10**.

A tabulated summary of key sequences used in MR imaging is shown in **Table 11**. A system specific imaging protocol is shown in **Table 12**.

MR Fingerprinting

Magnetic resonance fingerprinting is a new technique whose aim is to measure tissue properties through unique signals or fingerprints for different tissues. These are then matched

TABLE 10: Summarizes two basic types of techniques used in parallel imaging.

	Image based	K space based
Reconstruction	Done in the image domain with inversion procedure	Done in k-space with calculation of missing harmonic data
Examples	Philips *(SENSE)* *Siemens (mSENSE)* *GE (ASSET)*	Siemens (*GRAPPA*; GeneRalized Autocalibrating Partial Parallel Acquisition) GE (*ARC*; (Autocalibrating Reconstruction for Cartesian imaging)
Imaging time	Less	More
SNR	High	Low
Motion	SENSE, ASSET poor mSENSE good	Better
FOV	Small FOV can produce wraparound/aliasing	Better with small FOV
Susceptibility artefacts	More prone	Less prone

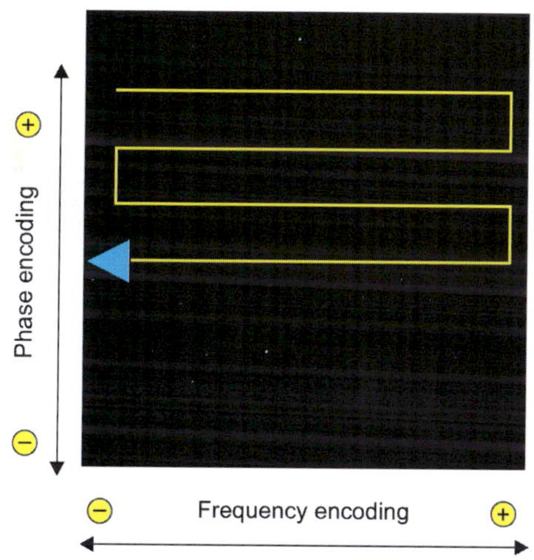

FIG. 18: Filling of K space in EPI sequence.

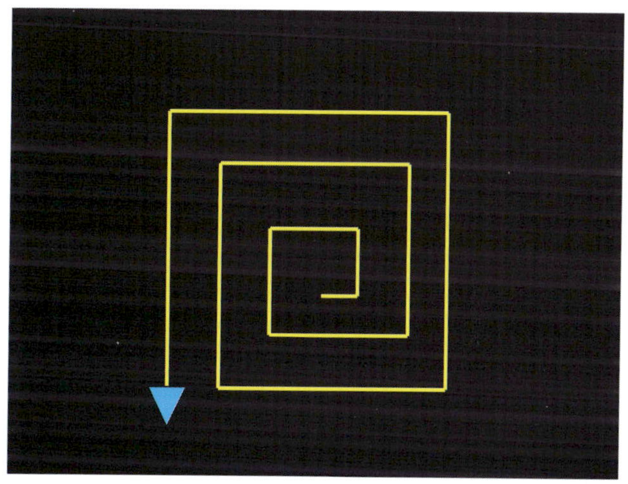

FIG. 19: Spiral K space filling.

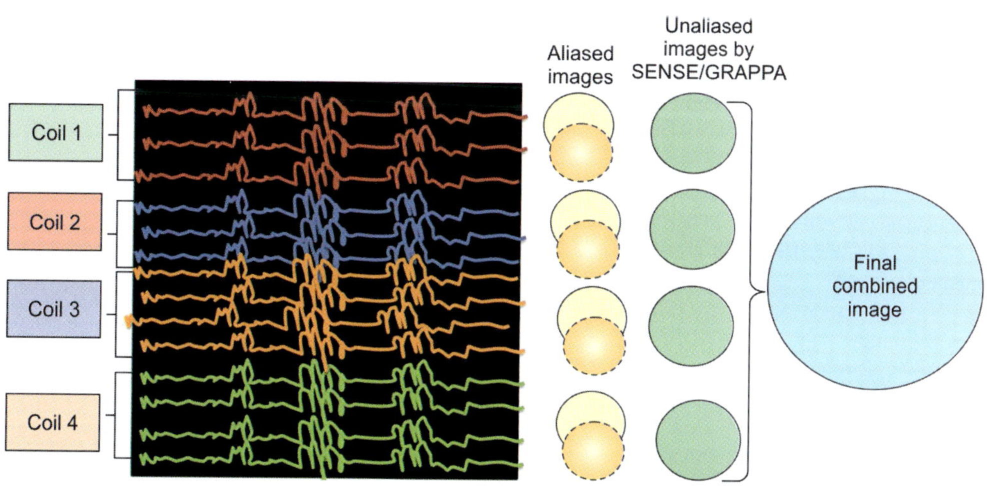

FIG. 20: Parallel imaging.

TABLE 11: Summary of various pulse sequences.

Technique	Sequences	Weighting	Features	Application
		Spin echo sequences		
Spin echo	SE	T1,T2, PD	Less susceptible to T2* effects	Mostly replaced by TSE sequences
Fast SE	RARE, TSE, FSE	T1, T2, PD	Faster Less susceptible to motion artifacts and T2* effects	High resolution neurological and orthopedic imaging. Single breath hold abdominal imaging
3D FSE	CUBE VISTA (Volume ISotropic Turbo spin echo Acquisition) SPACE (Sampling Perfection with Application optimized Contrasts using different flip angle Evolution	T1w T2w PD FLAIR	3D visualization with isotropic resolution	Brain, inner ear, joints, MRCP spinal imaging neurography
SS-FSE (single shot fast spin echo)	HASTE	T2 W	Faster	Used in MRCP, fetal imaging, urography
Inversion recovery	IR, turbo IR, TIRM (turbo IR magnitude reconstruction), IR TSE FLAIR (fluid attenuated inversion recovery) STIR (short T1 inversion recovery)	T1 W T2 W T1 and T2 W	Faster High resolution imaging Very useful in brain imaging Insensitive to susceptibility artifacts	For good contrast between white and gray matter To suppress fluid and make adjacent lesions more prominent To suppress fat signal
Incoherent/Spoiled Sequences				
2D-spoiled GRE	FLASH (fast low angle shot), T1-FFE (T1 fast field echo), SPGR (spoiled gradient echo)	T1 W	Fast imaging	MR angiography, In-out phase imaging
3D-spoiled GRE	VIBE (volumetric interpolated breath hold examination), THRIVE (T1 weighted high resolution isotropic volume examination)	T1 W	Isotropic imaging, high resolution, fast imaging	Body imaging
Ultrafast GRE	Turbo FLASH, TFE (turbo field echo)	T1W	Very fast imaging	To get rapid images like to track contrast arrival
Multiple gradient echo	MERGE ("Multiple Echo Recombined Gradient Echo") MEDIC ("Multi-Echo Data Image Combination") M-FFE ("Merged Fast Field Echo")	T2*	Excellent contrast resolution	Musculoskeletal and spine imaging
3D Ultrafast GRE	MP-RAGE (magnetization prepared rapid acquisition GE)	T1W	High resolution 3D sequence	Cerebral T1 3D imaging.
Echo planner imaging	EPI	T2*W	Ultrafast sequence	Diffusion, perfusion and functional MRI

Continued

Continued

Technique	Sequences	Weighting	Features	Application
		Coherent sequences		
Postexcitation steady state sequences	FISP (fast imaging with steady state precession), GRASS (gradient recalled acquisition in the steady state), FFE (fast field echo)	T1 and T2*	High SNR and T2* weighting, suitable for 3D imaging	Application in orthopedic imaging
Pre-excitation steady state refocused sequences	PSIF (reversed FISP), SSFP (steady state free precession)	T2W	True T2 weighting achievable, lower SNR	CSF flow studies, inner ear imaging
Fully refocused steady state sequences	True FISP, FIESTA (fast imaging employing steady state acquisition), Balanced FFE (fast field echo)	T1 And T2W	Less sensitive to motion	Cardiac, fetal imaging Abdominal imaging
Separate acquisition and combining S+ and S-	DESS (dual echo steady state) *MENSA* (Multi-Echo iN Steady-state Acquisition)	T1 and T2W		Orthopedic imaging
Combination of two fully refocused steady state sequences with and without phase alteration	CISS (constructive interference in the steady state), FIESTA-C	T2W	Less prone to banding artifacts	Inner ear 3D imaging
		Hybrid Sequences		
Gradient/spin echo hybrid	Turbo GSE (gradient spin echo), GRASE (gradient echo and spin echo)	T2/T2*	Fast imaging with low SAR	T2 weighting imaging of brain and orthopedic imaging

TABLE 12: Enumerates various pulse sequence protocols used in MR imaging of different organ systems.

System	Sequences (includes both commonly used and those in specific situations)
Cardiac imaging	Dark blood imaging: FSE or TSE Bright blood imaging: Spoiled GRE, SSFP Double or triple IR sequences Saturation recover pulse with GRE EPI for perfusion and tagging Phase contrast imaging with velocity encoding for flow assessment Postcontrast IR GRE or IR FSE EPI Parallel imaging
Breast imaging	T1 FSE T2 FSE with fat suppression Inversion recovery 3D spoiled GRE Dynamic 3D fat suppressed spoiled GRE EPI Parallel imaging DW MRS
Neuroimaging	FSE T1W FSE T2W FLAIR SWI DWI/DTI EPI/parallel imaging Ultrafast 3D GRE, e.g. MPRAGE CISS for cranial nerve evaluation MT PD Double IR 3D FSE, e.g. CUBE Inversion recovery e.g. STIR in spine SSFP for plexus imaging MRA
Abdomen/pelvis imaging	2D MRCP HASTE/RARE 3D MRCP RARE DW In and out phase GRE Inversion recovery SSFP, e.g. TruFISP 3D spoiled GRE, e.g. VIBE EPI Parallel imaging MRS Elastography
Musculoskeletal imaging	T1 FSE T2 FSE/3DFSE PD STIR/inversion recovery Multiple GRE, e.g. MERGE, MEDIC Post excitation steady state, e.g. GRASS Dual echo steady state, e.g. DESS FS T1w postcontrast Spoiled GRE T2/T2* mapping

with a dictionary to measure several unique tissue properties within a single acquisition.

Most of the MRI information is qualitative. Many times quantitative information is required, e.g. fat or iron deposition which is vital for clinical management of the patients.

While this information has proven extremely valuable for diagnosis, prognosis, and therapeutic assessment, the lack of quantification limits objective evaluation, leads to a variability in interpretation, and potentially limits the utility of the technology in some clinical scenarios.

Conventional techniques for T1 and T2 mapping are time consuming as they involve measurement of one parameter at a time. In comparison, MR fingerprinting gives simultaneous quantitative information of multiple parameters such as T1, T2, proton density and many more in a single acquisition.

Basic underlying technique in MRF is varying acquisition parameters such as FA, TR and trajectory in a pseudorandom fashion to generate a unique signal for the tissue concerned. These are then matched to a collected database known as dictionary and those that best match are then assigned to the voxel. Two vital steps for correct estimation of tissue parameters are unique signal components and accurate matching with the dictionary.

A schematic diagram showing the steps in acquisition of MR fingerprinting based maps is shown in **Figure 21**.

Clinical Applications

Predominant clinical applications have been seen in CNS and prostate imaging. MRF has shown promise to characterize and differentiate between various intra-axial brain tumors with lower mean T2 values in metastasis as compared to low grade glioma. Mean T1 values were seen higher in glioblastoma as compared low grade glioma. The mean T1, T2, and apparent diffusion coefficient in carcinoma were significantly lower than those from normal peripheral zone in prostate cancer imaging. Multiple studies are evaluating the role in abdomen, cardiac, musculoskeletal and microvasculature assessment.

MR ELASTOGRAPHY

Magnetic resonance elastography (MRE) is a new imaging technique which is analogous to physical palpation by the clinicians and provides tissue characteristic information far beyond the normal capability of conventional imaging sequences. It involves the quantification of the mechanical properties of tissues by transmitting the shear waves and then using specific resonance imaging sequence to display the maps.

Main steps that are involved in MRE technique include:

1. Production of mechanical waves in soft tissues via different types of devices positioned close to the target organ on body surface. These devices can be pneumatic, electromechanical and piezoelectric system based. These generate compression waves at skin surfaces, which are then at internal tissue generates transverse shear waves **(Fig. 22)**.
2. A specifically designed phase-contrast MR sequence is used to visualise and image this wave motion utilizing motion sensitive gradients. A wide variety of sequences such as GRE, SE, bSSFP or EPI can all be used.

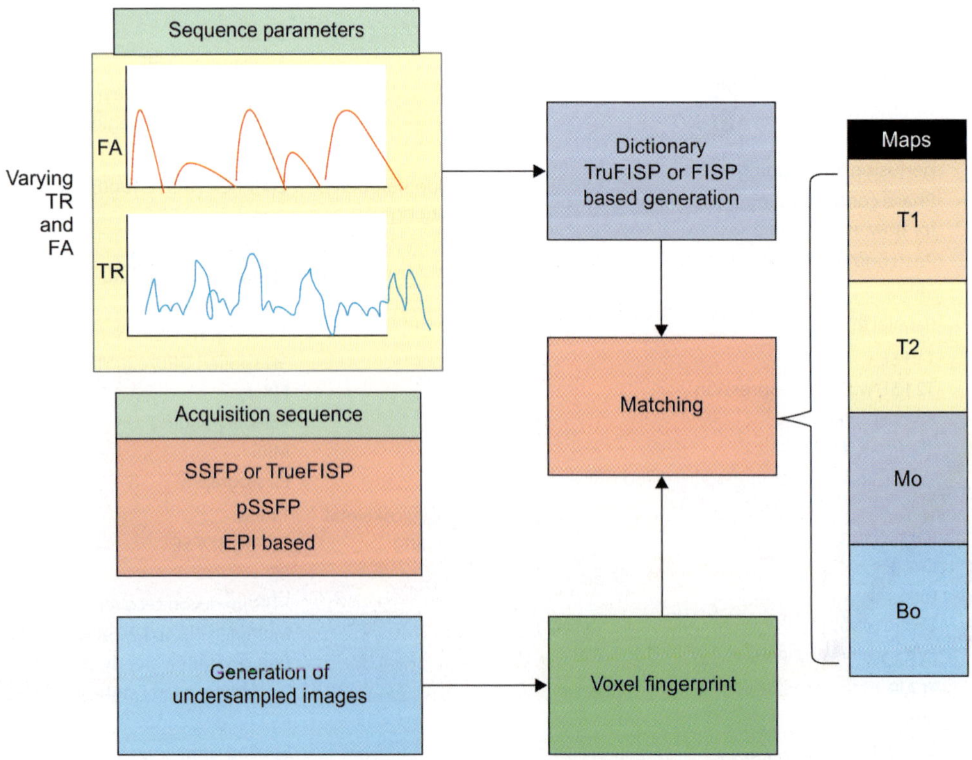

FIG. 21: Schematic diagram of MR fingerprinting acquisition.

This information is used by the MRI signal to create phase and magnitude images. A phase shift is produced based on this a wave image is generated which represents the shear wave motion in the tissues.

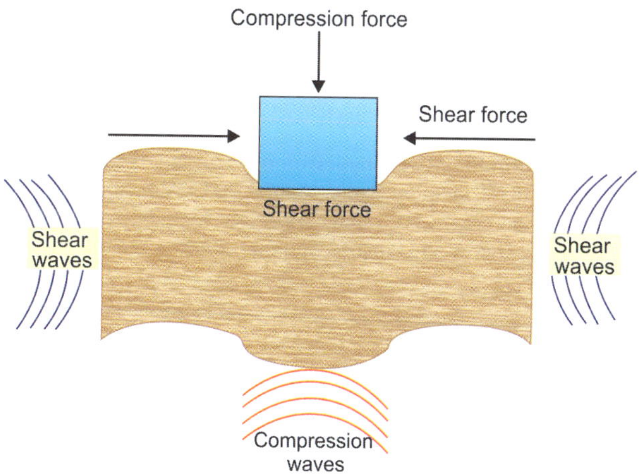

FIG. 22: Generation of compression and shear waves in MRE.

3. Inversion algorithm to convert the wave image into an elastogram via local frequency estimation and algebraic inversion of the differential equation.

Clinical applications: Principal clinical application has been seen in evaluation of patients with chronic liver disease. Multiple studies have shown excellent results in non invasive evaluation of hepatic fibrosis. Liver stiffness as shown by MRE increases with increasing severity of hepatic fibrosis **(Figs. 23A to D)**. It has been shown as an alternative to biopsy or to target areas with maximum fibrosis. Malignant lesions show higher mean stiffness as compared to benign. Multiple investigators are evaluating the role in renal, breast, brain, spleen and musculoskeletal pathologies with early promising results.

This technique has limited utility in iron overload states as it can result in generation of very small signal. This problem can be solved by utilizing SE or EPI sequences. In case of very obese and unstable patients the acquisition of MRE can be challenging. To summarize, MRE is a promising technique which is currently in evaluation to explore its full potential.

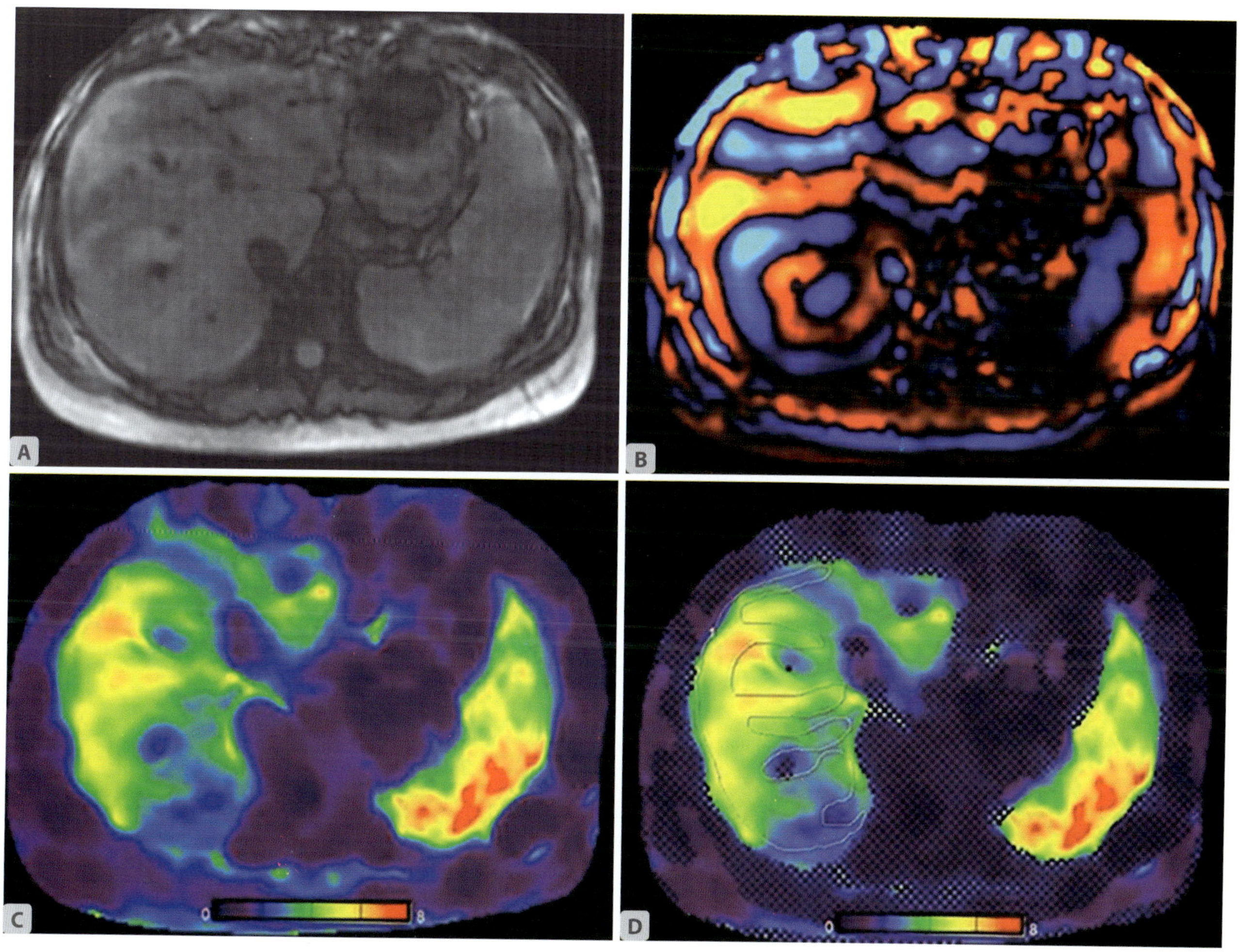

FIGS. 23A TO D: Liver stiffness measured by MRE in a 47-year-old female with auto immune hapatitis. LSM by MRE in this patient was 3.9 kPa respectively. HPE in this patient showed F2 fibrosis. (A) Magnitude image; (B) Wave image showing propagation of waves through liver parenchyma; (C) Elastogram; (D) Elastogram with superimposed confidence map and geographical ROI.

SUGGESTED READING

1. Bernstein MA, King KF, Zhou XJ. Handbook of MRI pulse sequences, Illustrated ed. Elsevier; 2004.
2. Bitar R, Leung G, Perng R, et al. MR pulse sequences: what every radiologist wants to know but is afraid to ask. Radiographics. 2006;26(2):513-37.
3. Boyle GE, Ahern M, Cooke J, Sheehy NP, Meaney JF. An interactive taxonomy of MR imaging sequences. Radiographics. 2006;26(6):e24.
4. Chavhan GB, Babyn PS, Jankharia BG, Cheng HL, Shroff MM. Steady-state MR imaging sequences: physics, classification, and clinical applications. Radiographics. 2008;28(4):1147-60.
5. Chavhan GB, Babyn PS, Thomas B, Shroff MM, Haacke EM. Principles, techniques, and applications of T2*-based MR imaging and its special applications. Radiographics. 2009;29(5):1433-49.
6. Eugene Lin. Body MRI sequences: A conceptual framework. Applied radiology. 2012;41(1).
7. Ma D, Gulani V, Seiberlich N, et al. Magnetic resonance fingerprinting. Nature. 2013;495:187-92.
8. Mariappan YK, Glaser KJ, Ehman RL Magnetic resonance elastography: a review. Clin. Anat. 2010;23:497-511.
9. MRI at a Glance. Catherine Westbrook Hoboken, 2nd Edn. NJ: Wiley-Blackwell; 2010.
10. Pooley RA. AAPM/RSNA physics tutorial for residents: fundamental physics of MR imaging. Radiographics. 2005;25(4):1087-99.
11. Vlaardingerbroek MT, Den boer JA. Magnetic Resonance Imaging: Theory and Practice. Springer; 2003.

CHAPTER

39 Digital Radiography: An Update

Alpana Manchanda, Rashmi Dixit,
Sapna Singh, Radhika Batra

Digital radiography has reshaped the field of medical imaging since it was introduced nearly four decades back. In contrast to Computed Tomography or Magnetic Resonance Imaging which were digital from the time they were first introduced, the transition of projection radiography from analog-to-digital technique was late. Nevertheless, digital radiography is now the standard technology in most institutions.

Till the past decade, the conventional film screen system was the most widely used and accepted method of recording images, wherein the film acts as an image receptor, display medium and a source of permanent record. Though these films are relatively inexpensive and provide high image quality, they have many limitations.[1]

Limitations of Film Screen Radiography

- Exposure latitude is narrow.
- Intolerant to exposure errors, resulting in frequent under and over-exposure of films.
- Image acquisition, display and storage are intrinsically nonseparable.
- Chemical processing is required
- Film quality deteriorates with time, especially if chemical processing is not optimal
- Inefficient mechanical handling
- Higher costs for film material and labor
- Incompatible with electronic transmission

Advantages of Digital Radiography[2,3]

- They have wide dynamic range.
- They are flexible, allowing image manipulation and post processing.
- Rapid image acquisition.
- Provide better image quality.
- Increased throughput possible.
- Image access at remote locations possible.
- Digital images do not deteriorate over time.
- Allow a true reproduction of image quality

The wide dynamic range and increased dose efficiency of digital detectors enable a reduction in radiation exposure to the patient. The dynamic range of digital detectors is about 400 times greater as compared to film screen radiography.[4]

EVOLUTION OF DIGITAL RADIOGRAPHY

Table 1 highlights the growth in digital radiography technology.

PHYSICS BEHIND DIGITAL RADIOGRAPHY

Digital imaging uses binary system in which information is interpreted as bits. A binary (base 2) digit can assume only

TABLE 1: Growth in digital radiography technology.[3,5]

Year	Developments in digital radiography
1980	Use of storage phosphor image plates—**first Computed radiography system developed**
1987	Amorphous selenium—based image plates
1990	First DR System introduced: Charge coupled device (CCD)
1994	Selenium drum DR system
1995	**First flat panel detector:** DR system introduced—selenium based FPD
1995	Amorphous silicon-cesium iodide (scintillator) flat-panel detector
1997	Gadolinium-based (scintillator) flat-panel detector
2001	Gadolinium-based (scintillator) portable flat-panel detector
2001	Dynamic flat-panel detectors used for digital fluoroscopy and DSA
2001	Dual side readout method for CR imaging introduced with digital mammography
2004	Dual side readout method for CR imaging with clinical radiographic system
2006	Digital tomosynthesis
2007	Portable CR system
2009	Wireless DR (flat panel detector)
2015	First twin robotic FPD X-ray system

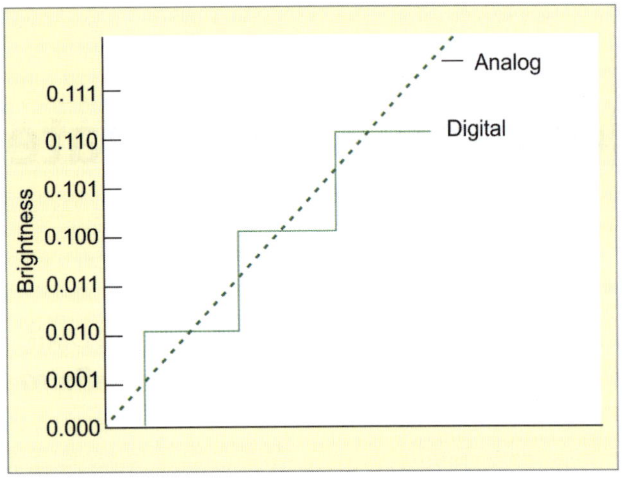

FIG. 1: Comparison of analog video voltage and digitized values.

one of two values, rather than one of ten as for decimal (base 10) system. The decimal representation of a binary number is calculated such that the digits are multiplied by power of 2 rather than power of 10.

Most digital systems handle individual pixels with eight-bit accuracy for displayed brightness. An individual pixel can therefore, have any brightness value from 0 through 255 decibel, a total of 2^8 (256) possible brightness values. Most of the information in radiology is displayed as shades of black and white.

Thus, digital information is any information that is represented in discrete units, while analog information is one that is represented in continuous rather than discrete fashion **(Fig. 1)**.[6]

PRINCIPLE OF DIGITAL RADIOGRAPHY

The digital detector is used to generate a digital image when it is exposed to X-rays. The detector absorbs the X-ray energy and transforms it into electrical energy which is then recorded, digitized and expressed as a gray scale. By use of postprocessing software the data is transformed into a useful image which can be stored on a digital medium. This is in contrast to conventional film screen radiography where the film functions both as detector and storage medium.[3]

Digital imaging involves four distinct steps, namely; image generation, image processing, image archiving and presentation of the image.

DIGITAL RADIOGRAPHY SYSTEMS

With the development and advancements in digital detector technologies in the last few decades, there has been a steady replacement of conventional film screen systems by digital radiography systems.

Digital X-ray systems can be categorized into two major types based on their difference in X-ray detection and readout process.[5] **Flowchart 1** depicts the various digital detectors.

- *Computed radiography (CR) system:* It is a cassette based X-ray system wherein a storage phosphor image plate is placed within the cassette and exposed to X-rays. The information is obtained from the exposed cassette by means of a scanner/reader technique i.e., it is an indirect conversion process, wherein image capture and image readout are done separately.
- *Digital radiography (DR) system* use detectors which convert X-rays into electrical charges by either a direct or an indirect process. In contrast to the CR system, the DR system is sometimes referred to as "cassette-less" as by this technology the latent image data is passed on directly from a flat panel detector to a monitor without any intermediary step.

On the basis of the type of X-ray conversion used, DR systems can be of two kinds:

1. *Direct conversion system:* Use amorphous selenium (aSe) as a photoconductor that converts X-ray photons into electric charge in a single step.
2. *Indirect conversion system:* It involves two steps in the conversion of X-rays into electrical charge. It has Cesium iodide (CsI) as the scintillator that converts X-rays into visible light in the first step. The second step involves the conversion of light into an electric charge by amorphous silicon photodiode array.

COMPUTED RADIOGRAPHY

Computed radiography was the first digital radiographic technology to be established in the early 1980s by Fuji. The technology consists of a photostimulable phosphor (PSP) image plate (IP) which is the detective layer that replaces the traditional film screen cassette.

The image plate is coated on one side with a thin layer of phosphor crystals which is embedded in a resin material in an unstructured way (unstructured scintillators) and enclosed in a cassette.

Europium activated barium fluoro halide ($BaFXEu^{2+}$) is the commonest phosphor material used wherein X represents bromine or iodine atoms or both. The photostimulable phosphor plates are exposed inside the cassettes. Images are obtained similar to that in the conventional film screen system. The X-ray tube and generator used in CR system is the same which is used for conventional radiography and does no necessitate any change.

CR imaging involves three steps in image formation:[5]

1. Exposure of image plate
2. Readout process
3. Erasure of residual signal.

Exposure of Image Plate

When the image plate is exposed to X-rays, the energy of incident X-ray photon is absorbed which stimulates the electrons within the phosphor layer to high energy levels of the atom. The excited electrons remain trapped in an unstable state while the energy of the absorbed X-ray photon is stored in the crystal structure of the phosphor and a latent image is created in the high energy state **(Figs. 2A and B)**.

FLOWCHART 1: Various types of digital detectors.

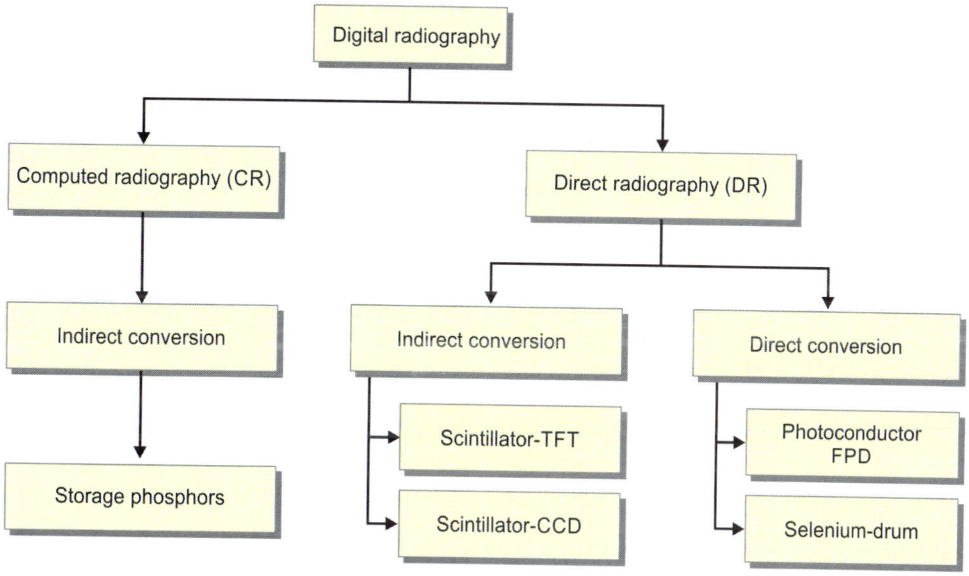

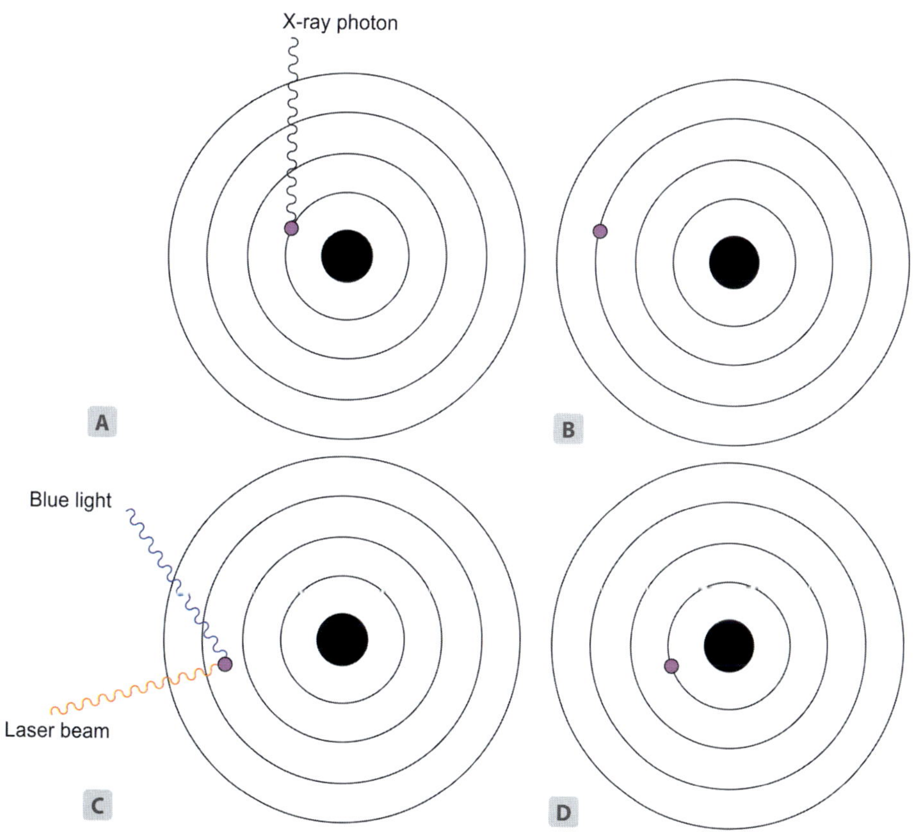

FIGS. 2A TO D: Image generation in CR system: (A) Incident X-ray photon excites an electron within phosphor layer; (B) Excitation of electron to higher unstable state. (C) Process of photostimulated luminescence by readout of latent image by laser beam. (D) Release of unstable electron to ground state.

Readout Process

This is the second step in CR imaging in which the exposed image plate is scanned by a CR reader. The latent image of high energy electrons is readout by a thinly focussed laser beam of a specific wavelength that releases the trapped electrons from their unstable state. Scanning red laser beam is used for stimulation of the phosphor (PSP plate) and the electrons emit blue light when they return to their ground state **(Figs. 2C and D)**, i.e. photostimulable luminescene. This light is then captured and digitized. The amount of blue light emitted is proportional to the intensity of the X-ray beam which exposed the plate. The light is collected by photodiodes and converted into electric charge. An analog-to-digital converter converts it to a corresponding digital image.

Figure 3 gives a schematic representation of a CR system based on storage phosphor image plates.

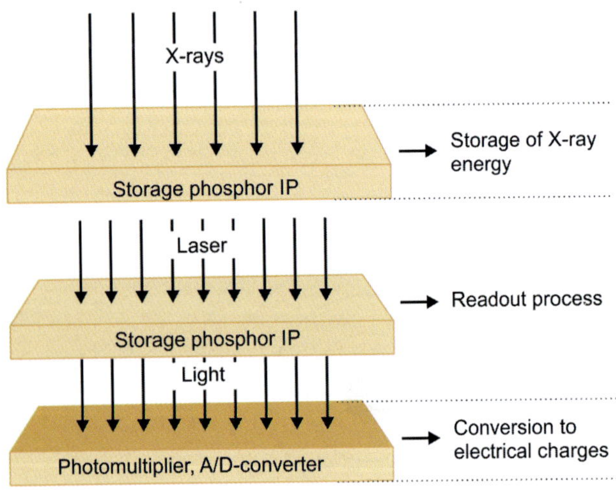

FIG. 3: Schematic representation of a CR system-based on storage phosphor image plates.

Erasure of Residual Signals

After the readout process, residual latent image electrons still remain trapped at higher energy levels which are erased in the final step of CR imaging. A high intensity white light source is used for this purpose which flushes the traps without introducing electrons from the ground energy level.

Figure 4 depicts an illustration of a CR system with a scanner.

As there is no direct electrical connection between the CR reader and the cassette, the patient information and cassette ID needs to be linked. This is done by a bar code reader or a chip embedded on the CR cassette. The PSP imaging plates are rigid, with the base in these plates being opaque or translucent. There are different types of CR cassette designs and image readers . But all cassettes from the same vendor may not be compatible with all readers. Some of the CR plate readers can process one plate while holding multiple cassettes in a queue. This is known as "drop and go" which enhances the working.[7] **Figures 5A to C** depict the various components of a CR system. A multi-slot or stacker CR reader accommodating four cassettes at one time as shown in **Figure 5B** minimizes operator waiting. The scanning speed of the image plate varies with the size of the image plate. The scanning speed of 14" × 17" cassette in approx 103 image plates/hour and for 8" × 10" cassette approx 165 IPs/hour.

CR technology thus gives a greater latitude of exposure which is useful under challenging radiographic circumstances such as the intensive case unit. It allows structures of widely differing radiographic density to be well visualized on the same image, such as the area behind the cardiac silhouette and the lung vessels or the soft tissue of the neck or cervicothoracic junction. This feature allows a reduction compared with FSR in the number of repeat images taken due to errors in selecting the correct exposure. The spatial resolution of CR is lower, i.e. 2½ line-pairs per mm than that of conventional FSR which is approximately 5 line pairs per mm. But its superior

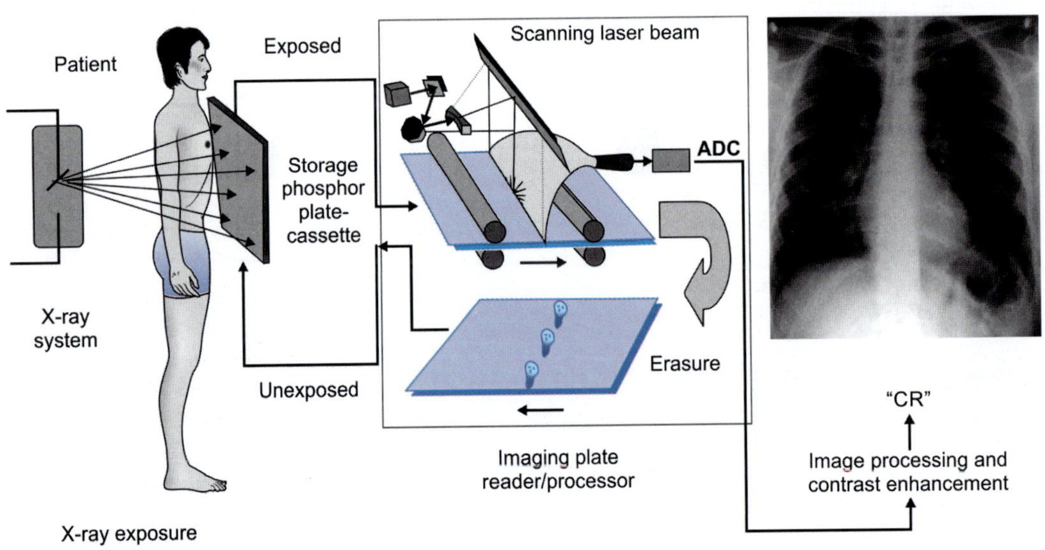

FIG. 4: Illustration of a CR imaging system with scanner.

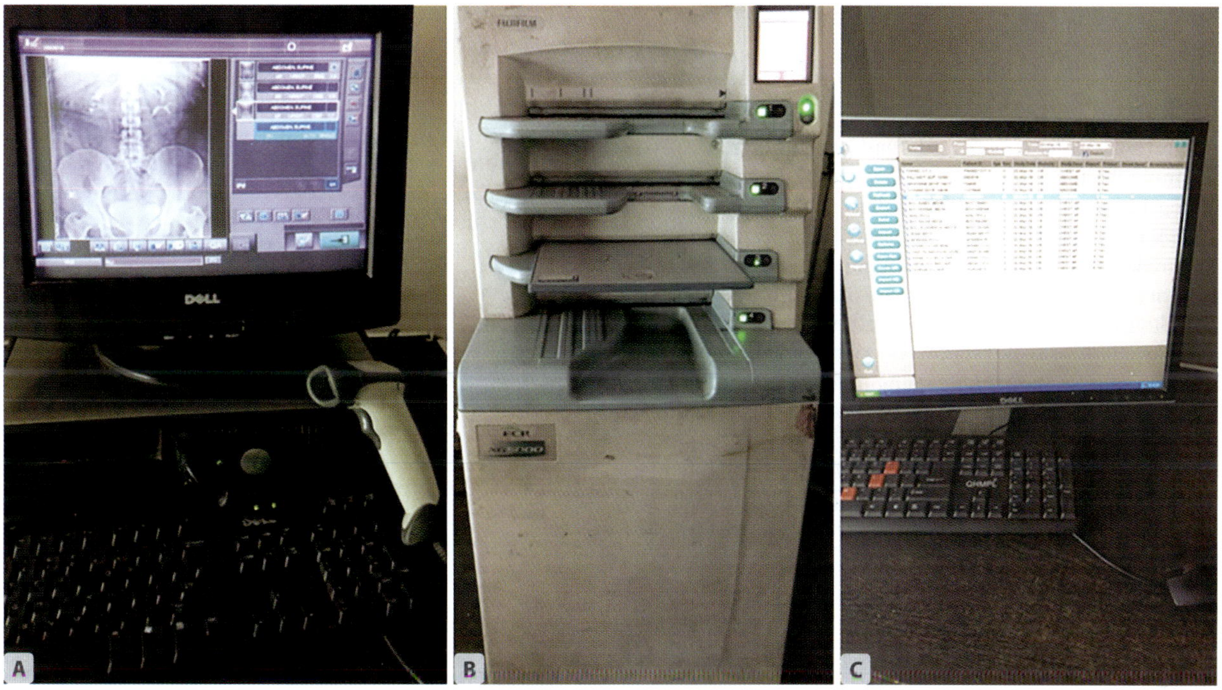

FIGS. 5A TO C: Components of a CR System. (A) Console with barcode reader; (B) 'Multi-slot' CR reader with imaging plate in one slot; (C) Workstation.

contrast resolution more than compensates for its limited spatial resolution. Phosphor plates can be reused repeatedly for a thousand or more exposures. CR equipment is cheaper than direct DR equipment, especially for mobile radiographic units.[8]

Phosphor plates have a more linear, optical density versus radiation exposure response curve than the classic sigmoid-shaped curve of the conventional film-screen combination **(Fig. 6)**.

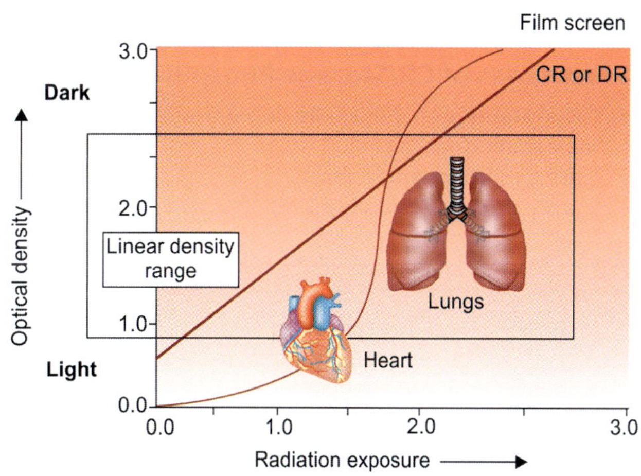

FIG. 6: Optical density vs. radiation exposure response curves.

Advances in CR

Since the introduction of computed radiography system, there has been a continuous improvement in the detector material and readout technology. Needle crystalline detectors and dual readout technology are the advancements that have led to a significant improvement in dose efficiency. The dose efficiency of newer CR system is found to approach that of direct radiography systems and found to be superior to screen film combination with a speed class of 400.[4]

Needle Crystalline CR/Channelled CR: Newer Structured Phosphor

The unstructured amorphous crystals of $BaFXEu^{2+}$ have been replaced by more efficient X-ray absorptive material consisting of $CsBr:Eu^{2+}$ which are structured in the form of needle like columns. This results in reduced lateral scattering of the emitted fluorescent light which is channelled with each needle crystal. Channelling of light permits increase in detector thickness which leads to greater X-ray absorption and dose efficiency without loss of geometric resolution. It has been seen that a thicker and high packing density of phosphor results in a dose efficiency which is of the same order of that of direct radiography systems.

Dual-sided Readout Technology

The read out efficiency of the phosphor plate has been improved by introducing the 'dual-sided read out' which consists of using new type of phosphor crystals which are transparent to the laser and phosphorescence light as well as using a transparent support material. This enables the phosphor plate to be read out from both sides resulting in an increased signal to noise ratio. As per literature, the X-ray absorption efficiency of a dual read out CR system is 50% greater than a single side read out CR system.[4]

Line Scan CR Reader

A higher read out speed and read out efficiency of the phosphor plate has been possible with the introduction of line scan mechanism of the CR reader in which a whole row of pixels is read out at the same time. This is different from the conventional point scan mechanism in which the laser reads each pixel on the imaging plate one after the other. The time taken to scan the initially developed conventional CR plates varied from 40–90 seconds depending on the plate size, resolution required and dual or single side read out.

By using a dedicated line scan CR reader it is possible to achieve a read out time of less than 10 seconds resulting in a throughput of 240 plates/hour compared to 50–80 plates/hour with conventional single cassette reader or 100–150 plates/hour with conventional reader with a provision of stacking cassettes.[4]

CR System Configuration

The initial CR systems were cassette based which are still widely used, economical; with wearing away of phosphor plates with time. The CR systems introduced later have been integrated in dedicated chest stands and bucky units and require no manual interaction with the cassettes. Options of dual readout and needle crystalline detectors are available in the cassette-based and integrated CR systems.

Advantages of CR/Storage Phosphor Systems[7]

- CR systems can be easily integrated into existing radiographic equipment.
- Have a wide dynamic range.
- Examination of bed side immobile patients is easily possible.
- CR cassettes enable flexibility for positioning for difficult views.
- Multiple cassette sizes are available.
- Any defect in the image plate can be easily replaced without specialized intervention.

Drawbacks of CR/Storage Phosphor Systems

- It is a time consuming technique.
- Takes a long time for image to be displayed by image reader, similar to that by conventional film processing.
- Spatial resolution is less as compared to film screen radiography.
- Radiation dose required is same or more than film screen radiography.
- CR cassettes need careful handling as they are delicate and can get chipped or damaged.

DIGITAL RADIOGRAPHY

The term digital radiography (DR) or direct digital radiography (dDR) is used for a digital imaging system which acquires radiographic images in a digital format almost immediately after exposure, without any additional step to extract the latent image.

Since the introduction of digital technology in the late eighties, there has been significant advancement in the detectors in terms of how the X-ray image is captured and the resultant image quality. Digital radiographic systems can be categorized into two groups depending on how the X-ray energy is converted into electric charge.

1. *Direct conversion detectors:* Are those that directly convert X-rays photons to electric charge. Amorphous selenium is the most commonly used photoconductor material used which is sensitive to X-rays.
2. *Indirect conversion detectors:* Use a two step process for conversion of X-ray energy to electrical signal.
    i. A scintillator layer in the detector converts the X-ray energy into visible light.
    ii. A light sensitive photodiode (amorphous silicon or charged coupled device-CCD) then converts the visible light into an electric charge.

An electric readout mechanism senses the electric charge pattern and an analog to digital converter produces the digital image.

Direct Conversion

Direct conversion type of detectors uses amorphous selenium as photoconductor that convert X-rays photons into electrical charge by setting electrons free. The photoconductor materials which can be used are amorphous selenium, lead iodide, thallium bromide and gadolinium compounds. Selenium is the element used typically which has a high intrinsic spatial resolution. The pixel size, matrix and spatial resolution of direct conversion detectors are not limited by the detector material itself, but only by the recording and readout devices used.[3]

Selenium-based direct conversion DR systems consist of either (a) a selenium drum or (b) a flat panel detector.

Selenium Drum-based System of Direct Conversion

In this type of direct conversion, a rotating selenium drum is exposed to X-rays which acquires a charge equivalent to the incident X-rays on the drum surface. An analog-to-digital (A/D) converter transforms the charge pattern into a digital image **(Fig. 7)**.[3]

Selenium drum detectors yield a fine image quality, superior to FSR or CR system.[9] Due to their mechanical design they are used only in dedicated chest stand systems with no mobility, and cannot be used in intensive care units. Hence, selenium drum systems are not produced anymore.

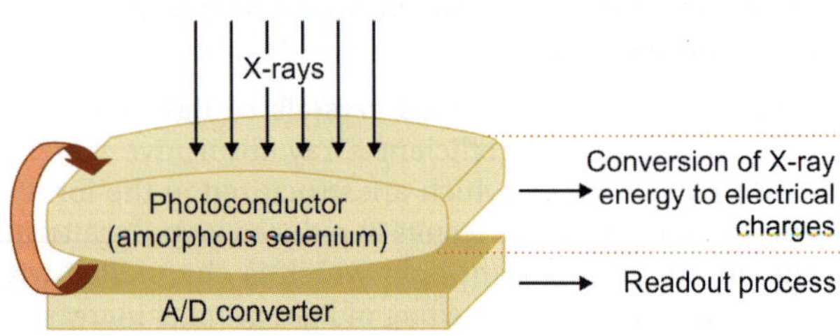

FIG. 7: Direct conversion DR system: selenium drum-based system.

But in few institutions where they are used, they are known to produce high quality chest radiography comparable to a 400 speed conventional film-screen system.[4]

Thin Film Transistor-based Flat Panel Detector Technology

1995 was a landmark year in digital radiography technology, with the development of a new class of digital detectors termed flat panel detectors (FPD). The first flat panel DR detector using amorphous selenium photoconductor was developed by Du Pont Corporation, USA.[10] As the name signifies, a radiographic flat panel detector is a slim detector panel which is digital; electronically readable and can be integrated into chest stand and bucky tables.[11] In contrast to storage phosphor based (CR) system, the readout electronics are integrated within the detector cassette i.e., direct readout mechanism.

Flat panel systems are also known as large area X-ray detectors. They blend an X-ray sensitive layer and an electronic signal based on thin film transistor (TFT) array. The TFT array is assembled on a glass substrate in multiple layers in a sandwich approach, with the charge collector arrays at the top level and read out electronics at the lowest level. Depending on the type of detector being manufactured, the top of the array is made of either X-ray sensitive or light sensitive elements or an amalgamation of both.

Direct-conversion TFT detectors are those that use an X-ray sensitive photoconductor layer and a TFT charge collector **(Fig. 8)** while detectors using a scintillator and a light sensitive TFT photodiode are called indirect conversion TFT detectors.[5]

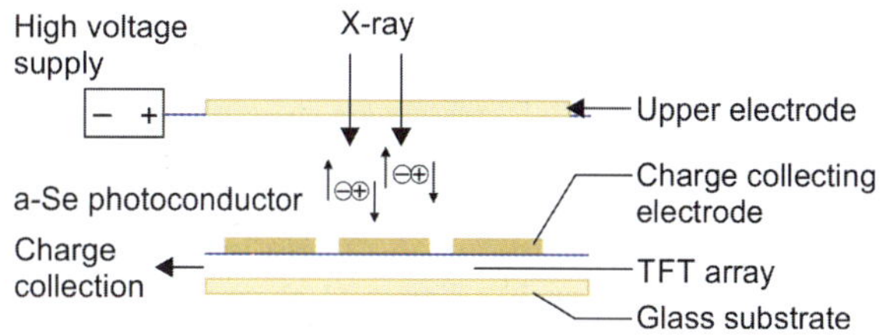

FIG. 8: Cross-section of a direct conversion TFT detector.

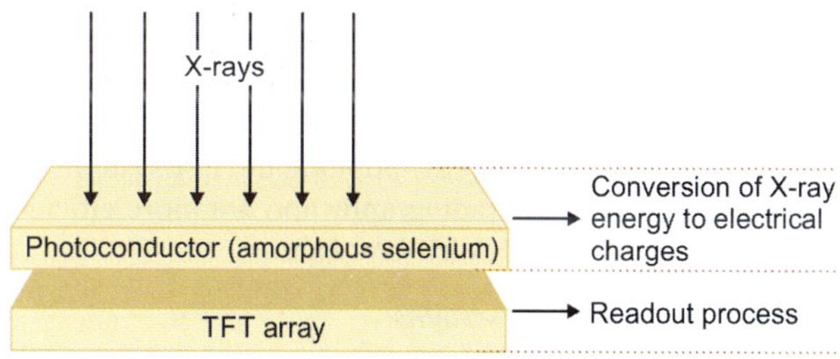

FIG. 9: Direct conversion DR system—amorphous selenium thin film transistor array.

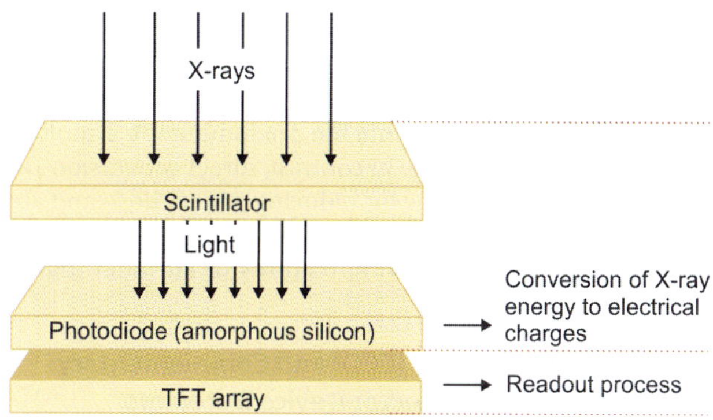

FIG. 10: Illustration of an amorphous silicon-based indirect conversion DR system.

Selenium-based FPD—Direct Conversion DR System

These direct conversion DR systems consist of a layer of selenium with a corresponding underlying array of thin film transistors. The principle of X-ray conversion to electrical charge is similar to that of the selenium drum except that the charge pattern is recorded and stored by TFT array. **Figure 9** depicts the selenium based direct conversion DR system. An advantage of Selenium FPD over selenium drum is that these detectors can be mounted on chest stands and bucky tables, hence clinically more useful. Selenium is used in amorphous form which is evaporated to make plates easily and economically.[12]

Selenium based flat panel detectors are more suited for mammography units than routine radiography because the K-edge of selenium is more suited for the diagnostic KV range required in mammography and they provide a higher dose efficiency.[13]

A limitation of these direct conversion systems is that they are not conducive to real-time imaging as there is a tendency for persistent latent images getting produced.[4]

Indirect Conversion—Thin Film Transistor Flat Panel Detector

Indirect conversion FPD consist of a scintillator layer as the top layer followed by a coating of amorphous silicon and a TFT array. When X-ray photons strike the scintillator, visible light is emitted which is proportionate to the incident X-ray energy reaching it. The emitted light is then turned into electrical charge by a line-up of silicon based photodiodes and readout by a TFT array **(Fig. 10)**. Two types of scintillators are used in indirect conversion detectors, which are (i) structured or (ii) unstructured scintillators.

Unstructured Scintillators

Unstructured scintillators scatter a large amount of light during conversion of X-ray to light, reducing its spatial resolution. Gadolinium oxysulfide (Gd_2O_2S) crystals or GOS or Gadox is an example of unstructured scintillator which has a structure similar to storage phosphors.

Portable (mobile) DR units used for bedside radiography have Gd_2O_2S as scintillator along with flexible substrate instead of glass. This makes the detector more robust and resistant to mechanical stress.[4]

Structured Scintillators

Structured scintillators have been developed to overcome the problem of lateral diffusion of light resulting in reduced sharpness and spatial resolution of the image during conversion of X-ray energy into visible light in the scintillator layer. Cesium iodide (CsI) crystals are structured scintillators that are arranged perpendicular to the detector surface. The crystals are shaped into needles, 5–10 µm wide and remarkably reduce the diffusion of light in the scintillator layer similar to fibre optics. **Figure 11** gives a diagrammatic representation of indirect conversion detectors depicting both structured and unstructured scintillators. As a result of reduced light diffusion a thicker scintillator layer can be used, thereby increasing the detective quantum efficiency (DQE) of the detector system.[3,11] The fine structure of CsI crystals in FPD make them highly vulnerable to mechanical stress. Hence, these systems cannot be used in mobile units and only used in fixed installations.[3] CsI -photodiode/TFT systems are generally used for chest radiography and are more efficient than standard CR or Gadox-TFT systems.

Applications of CsI-TFT systems:

- Wide application in chest radiography
- Skeletal radiography
- In fluoroscopy as it is amenable to real time display with high frame rate upto 30 fps.

Figures 12A and B show flat panel detector based vertical stand (A) and table top (B) DR systems.

Indirect Conversion DR detectors have a substantial capacity for improving image quality or reducing operating dose and hence, have become the predominant technology for projection radiography. In contrast, direct conversion DR detectors offers little scope for reducing patient dose and are more suited for full-field digital mammography.[4]

Schematic chart depicting features of an ideal digital detector system **(Fig. 13)**.

Charge Coupled Device (CCD) and Complementary Metal Oxide Semiconductor Device Detectors

Charge coupled devices (CCD) are light sensitive sensors which record the light emitted by the scintillators. An array of several CCD chips are needed to form a detector area similar to FPD as detector area cannot be larger than a CCD chip. Optical lenses are used to demagnify the light emitted by the scintillator to fit the CCD. A limitation of the lens type CCD is a lower signal to noise ratio and reduced image quality as only a fragment of light can be captured by them. Earlier, the CCDs were less suited for chest radiography because of their much smaller size (2–4 cm^2) compared to the chest region to be exposed. **Figure 14** depicts the lens coupled CCD based indirect conversion DR system.

However advancements in coupling mechanism by using larger CCD sensors and enhanced phosphor efficiency have made these systems more appropriate for high quality chest and large area skeletal radiography.

Slot Scan Technology

Slot scan technology uses an X-ray tube with a collimated sliding slit beam to scan the patient. This is linked simultaneously to a moving CCD detector array, with markedly reduced effect of scattered radiation on the image. It does not need demagnification and in chest imaging it is especially useful in evaluation of the mediastinum.[4]

Advances in DR

- *Wireless FPD:* A portable detector provides wireless (WiFi) transfer of data directly into the PACS network,

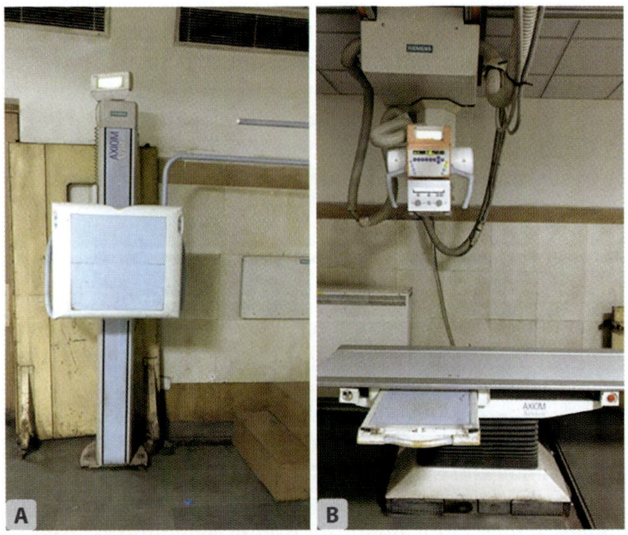

FIGS. 12A AND B: Digital radiography system with ceiling mounted X-ray tube. (A) Vertical stand; (B) Table top with integrated flat panel detector.

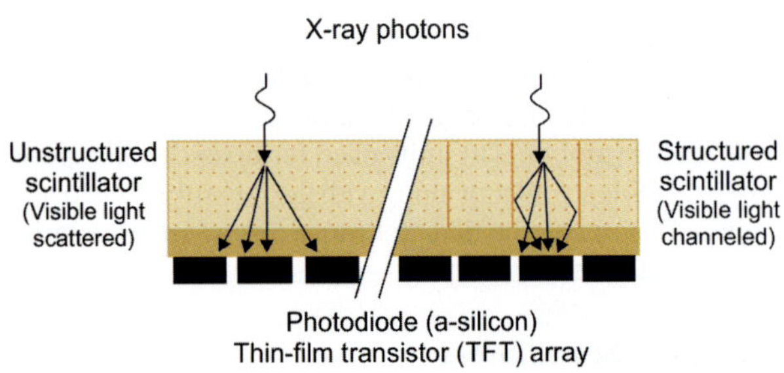

FIG. 11: Diagrammatic representation of indirect conversion detectors depicting both structured and unstructured scintillators.

Image quality		Physical design		Work flow
Superior image quality compared to the best FSR and CR systems High spatial and contrast resolution Dose efficiency	+	Solid state Robust Minimal change from existing scanning systems 14 × 17 inch (35 × 43 cm) imaging area	+	Intelligent operating console Immediate image access with high patient throughput HIS/RIS connectivity PACS connectivity DICOM compatible

FIG. 13: Depicts the features of an ideal digital detector system.

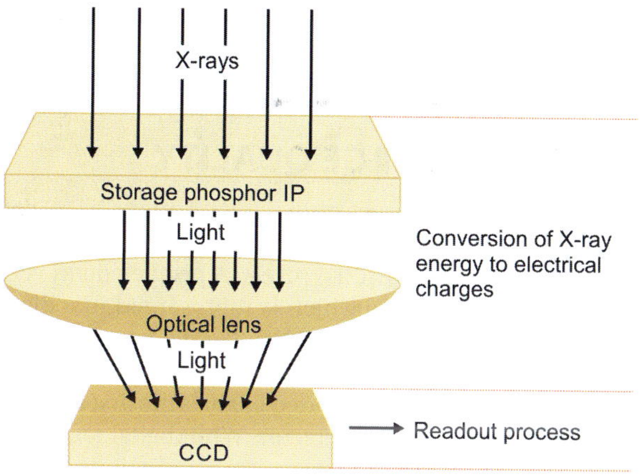

FIG. 14: Lens coupled CCD based indirect conversion DR system.

making it very useful for taking radiographs in intensive care units, wards or emergency department without use of any cable. Earlier designs of the detector used GdO_2S_2 intensifying screen and data was transferred utilizing a cable. Presently, WiFi enabled portable DR detectors have been designed to slot into a docking station that connects directly to the system and also charges the detector battery. CsI: Tl (caesium iodide doped thallium) is the primary absorber and enables reduction in patient dose in contrast to earlier designs of portable detector. A 17 × 14 inch image is ready within 3 seconds and allows radiography of difficult regions of the body like the axilla or the TM joint. Also, with wireless FPDs, radiography of a limb with limited mobility (flexed/having contractures) is possible.

- *Mobile DR:* It consists of a 17 × 14 inch flat panel detector attached by a cable to a mobile X-ray system having a monitor. The high cost and fragility of the FPDs hampers the use of mobile DR system.
- *Fluoroscopy:* Real time digital imaging clears the way for high quality radiography and fluoroscopy with up to 30 images/sec. Fluoroscopy has a role in gastroenterology, urology and vascular applications.
- *Automatic image stitching:* This feature is useful when exact measurements in long anatomical regions like the spine or lower limb are required. With use of the largest flat panel DR plates, i.e. 43 × 43 cm, only a limited portion of the body can be imaged at a time. To overcome this problem of being unable to study the whole spine or entire lower limb, multiple sequential exposures at different patient positions are acquired in a patient who is absolutely still. Automatic stitching is then performed to reconstruct a larger composite image. Earlier automatic image stitching was possible with patients in erect position. Now the automatic stitching can be performed in sick patients even when they are lying down.

IMAGE PROCESSING

After exposure and readout, the next step in digital imaging is image processing. This involves processing of the raw image data for display on the computer. Image processing is one of the important aspects of digital radiography and greatly influences the way the image appears to the radiologist. Even though software products from several manufacturers use similar algorithm such as edge enhancement, noise reduction and contrast enhancement to improve the appearance of the image, there may be considerable difference in the resulting image.[3]

Image processing helps to improve image quality by reducing noise, removing technical artifacts and optimizing contrast for viewing. One needs to know that spatial resolution cannot be effected by the processing software as it is dependent on the technical variables of the detector (pixel size).

Noise limits the ability to see low contrast detail. In real time acquisition system such as fluoroscopy, noise can be reduced by adding the signal from successive frames to give a time averaged image. This is equivalent to increasing exposure time in radiography. Frame averaging is a useful technique provided that there is no movement between frames, otherwise the image will be blurred.

Noise may also be minimised by low-pass spatial filtering. In this technique, the value of the neighboring pixels and resultant value is averaged to the gray scale value stored in each pixel. The effect is to smoothen the final image, but it blurs small details or edges.

Direct radiography systems convert X-ray image data into electronic charge which are held by the TFT array. As indirect-conversion systems depend on light, considerable scattering takes place before the energy is converted to charge which decreases signal-to-noise ratio.

The effect of edge enhancement or high pass filtering is the opposite. Rather than display a weighted average value of neighboring pixels, a high pass filter adds a proportion of the difference between the gray scale value of the pixel and that of its neighbor. The effect is to amplify the contrast at the boundary between structures, thus making the structures more visible.[14]

Image processing software is usually bundled with the detector and cannot be replaced by any other software.

Advances in Image Processing

- An optimal image density, independent of exposure can be produced by automated windowing.
- Frequency processing can increase local contrast or even selectively enhance structures of a certain size. Unsharp mask filtering is the simplest type of frequency processing, but has the drawback that stronger filter settings cause edge artifacts. Most vendors have now shifted to multifrequency processing algorithms by which there is enhancement of low density structures and subtle pathology.

Multifrequency processing makes it possible to separately enhance and suppress image structures depending on their contrast, size and background density with a resultant 'image harmonization'.

The most advanced processing algorithms are:[15]

- Computer-aided diagnosis (CAD)
- Dual energy subtraction
- Temporal subtraction
- Digital tomosynthesis

Computer-aided Diagnosis

Automated diagnostic radiographic interpretation, i.e. computer aided detection (CAD) also known as computer aided diagnosis has developed due to expanding research and a shift in focus from human perception to automated decision making. CAD systems typically depend on a combination of complex image processing, pattern recognition and artificial intelligence techniques.

Majority of applications of CAD in chest radiography involves the detection of pulmonary nodules. Its other applications in chest are in the detection of interstitial lung disease (ILD), cardiomegaly, pneumothorax, etc.[16]

The clinical role of CAD technology is highly debated and continuously evolving. It plays a complementary role in evaluating suspicious areas so that diagnostic significant findings are not overlooked.

Computer-aided diagnosis (CAD) aids the radiologist in conditions such as early detection of cancer of the lung and breast. The suspicious areas are marked by the software and alerts the radiologist so that he may not overlook diagnostic significant findings.

Dual Energy Subtraction

In dual energy subtraction radiography, two exposures are made at two different X-ray energies and bone or soft tissue are eliminated by locally weighted subtraction of the two images to create separate images of bone and soft tissue structures. Two acquisition techniques of dual energy subtraction are available. Those using single exposure technique use a stack of two detectors and the other is a dual exposure technique in which two separate exposures are made in rapid succession at low and high KVP settings. The latter is a more effective technique. It is especially useful in chest radiography where overlying ribs can be removed, aiding in better visualisation. It helps in differentiating calcified lesions from non-calcified lesions, improve detection of nodules and masses and better detection of rib lesions. A limitation of this technique is that the radiologist has to review three images, i.e. conventional, bone and soft tissues, instead of one radiograph. This can be overcome if the images are integrated in the monitor on PACS work station.

Temporal Subtraction

Temporal subtraction is a post processing method in which a follow-up radiograph is matched with a baseline image and then subtracted. The matching process is complex and can induce misregistration artifacts. The technique is good in recognising subtle interval changes and improves detection of nodules and hazy infiltrates.

Digital Tomosynthesis

Digital tomosynthesis involves multiple low dose exposures given from various angles while the X-ray tube moves in an arc and the detector remains stationary. Multiple images with different focal zones can be created by addition of these low dose images after pixel shift, which can be viewed singly or in a wire loop. Digital tomosynthesis is superior to conventional tomography as the computer processing methods can be used to minimize the contribution of the blurred out of plane structures to the images. It has been found to be helpful in evaluation of chest lesions, mammography and IVU studies.[13]

ASPECTS OF IMAGE QUALITY

The image in digital technique may appear as a conventional video or radiographic image, but it is not the case as it is formed from individual pixels. A pixel element is the smallest area of an image which is represented in a digital image. With conventional imaging, X-rays form an image directly on the receptor. Efficient detection of the spatially dependent, attenuated transmitted beam is the first and most important task of an X-ray detector. With digital technique, X-rays form an electronic image on a radiation detector and are manipulated by a computer, temporarily stored in memory and displayed as a matrix of intensities, each having a dynamic range of values.

The major factors effecting digital image quality are mentioned here.

Pixels

The pixel is the foundation block of digital imaging and is the smallest complete sample of an image. The two dimensional collection of pixels in the images is called the matrix, which is usually expressed in terms of pixels in two orthogonal directions (length x width). Maximum achievable spatial resolution is defined by pixel size and spacing. The number of pixels contained in a digital image and the distance between each pixel is known as the sampling interval. Pixel size is a measure of resolution, wherein, smaller the pixel size (or larger the matrix), greater is the resolution.

The pixel size should preferably be 150 µ or less in a FPD. The matrix size should be at least 2000 × 2000 or more, i.e. 2K × 2K matrix for chest radiography while 4K × 4K matrix is ideal for mammography.

Detector Size

The physical size of the X-ray detector has an influence on the radiographic examination performed. The detector should be adequately large to capture the desired anatomic views and sufficiently compact for all clinical applications.[7] Larger detector areas are needed for chest imaging than for imaging of the extremities. Presently, detectors integrated with table and vertical stand are manufactured wherein the X-ray tube assembly movement is automatically synchronized with the detector.

Flat panel detector size should be at least 40 × 40 cm or more so that all possible regions can be imaged. They are available in various sizes. Commonly available sizes of FPD are 43 × 43 cm(17″ × 17″), 35 × 43 cm (14″ × 17″).

Gray Scale

Gray scale refers to shades of gray available for reproducing faithfully subtle differences in densities in an accurate manner. Gray scale images are different from black and white images. Unlike the latter, which have two colors (black and white), gray scale images have a number of shades of gray in between. More the number of shades available, superior is the display. The shades of gray that compose an image range from pure black at the weakest intensity to pure white at the strongest.

For routine visual display, 2^8 or 256 intensities (shades of gray) are recorded on a nonlinear scale. However, in medical imaging more shades of gray are needed which allows 2^{16} or 65536 gray levels.

Spatial Resolution

It describes the ability to distinguish fine spatial detail and to differentiate objects in an image. In digital acquisition systems, resolution is governed by a term called spatial frequency. Resolution implies how frequently an object is sampled. As a rule of thumb:

- Increasing the sampling frequency helps to increase resolution
- Images composed with a greater number of pixels have a higher spatial resolution. However, images with higher resolution require large file sizes.[2]

Spatial resolution is effected by multiple factors:[4]

- Detector medium (needle channeled CR vs powder crystal CR)
- Detector thickness (standard vs high resolution CR)
- Size of the laser beam
- Pixel size
- Pre- and postprocessing

Increasing the radiation applied to the detector will not improve the maximum spatial resolution. In fact, scattering of X-ray and light photons with the detector influences the spatial resolution. Hence, spatial resolution for selenium-based direct conversion detectors is higher than for indirect conversion detectors. Structured scintillators are superior to unstructured scintillators.[3]

The image resolution in capturing devices is not synonymous with the image resolution of output devices such as computer monitors or printers. In general, for capturing devices, the imaging resolution is expressed as ppi (pixel per inch) and for output devices as dpi (dots per inch).[3]

Spatial resolution in digital acquisition systems is denoted as pixel size, pixels/mm, or line pairs per millimeter (lp/mm). Line pairs per millimeter are a measure of resolution wherein pairs of lines are closely approximated. The unaided human is capable of distinguishing about 10 to 14 lp/mm. More the lines placed within a millimeter, the higher the resolution.

The spatial resolution of CR and DR are comparable to each other, but less than film-screen radiography.[2] It is possible to achieve a resolution of 5 to 10 pixel/mm in general purpose CR cassettes while a resolution of 20 pixel/mm is available in most CR systems approved for mammography.[7]

Contrast Resolution and Dynamic Range

Contrast resolution refers to the amount of gray scale differentiation that exists in an image. For digital image acquisition equipment, it means the number of shades of gray that a detector can capture. Digital detectors have high contrast resolution thus enabling thousands of shades of gray to be displayed. The superior contrast resolution of digital detectors more than makes up for the reduced spatial resolution.[2]

Dynamic range is the measure of the signal response of a detector that is exposed to X-rays. In a conventional film-scan combination, the dynamic range is S-shaped with a narrow exposure range for optimal film blackening, i.e. the film has a low tolerance for exposure at higher or lower than required, resulting in failed exposures or insufficient image quality.

Dynamic range is the range of X-ray exposure over which a meaningful image can be obtained. Digital detectors have a wide and linear dynamic range **(Fig. 15)**. The dynamic range of digital radiography (CR and DR) is about 400 times wider as compared to conventional films, i.e. digital systems can obtain image information over a much wider range of entrance doses. In contrast to film screen system, the curve for digital detectors is less steep and covers a wider range. As a result an optimal signal response will occur over a wider exposure range with digital detectors than with film screen combinations. Another advantage of a wide dynamic range is that differences between specific tissue absorption (e.g. bone vs. soft tissue) can be displayed in one image without the need for additional images.[3]

Modulation Transfer Function

The performance (image quality) and efficiency (dose) of detectors and X-ray systems can be measured objectively. Measurement include frequency dependent signal transfer via the MTF(f), noise power spectrum NPS(f) and signal transfer efficiency (input to output) via the DQE metric [DQE(f)]. Different detectors have different modulation transfer characteristics.

Modulation transfer function (MTF) is the capacity of the detector to transfer the modulation of the input signal at a given spatial frequency to its output. In conventional radiography, objects having different sizes and opacity are displayed with different gray scale values in an image. MTF is responsible for converting contrast values of different sized

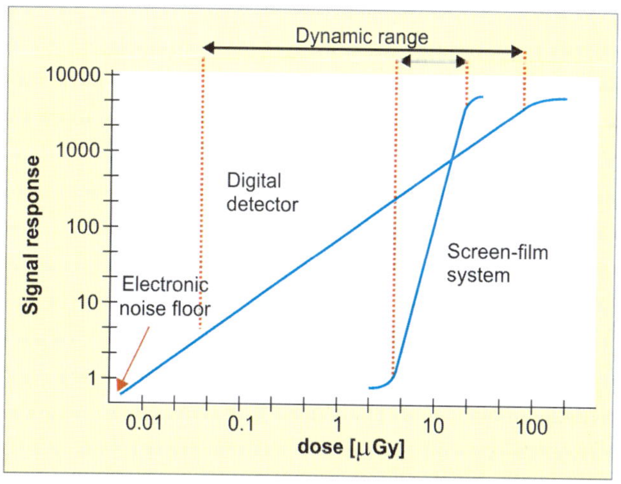

FIG. 15: Graph illustrates the dynamic range of screen-film combinations and digital detectors.

objects (object contrast) into contrast intensity levels in the image (image contrast).[14]

The ratio of the output and input modulation is known as the modulation transfer function. MTF varies with spatial frequency which generally reduces progressively from 100 percent at low spatial frequencies towards zero at higher frequencies.[14]

Higher the MTF, the smaller the details the imaging system displays with visually perceptable contrast.[4]

Detective Quantum Efficiency

The image quality/performance of digital radiographic systems is best gauged by its detective quantum efficiency (DQE). That is, it is the efficiency of a detector in converting incident X-ray energy into an image signal. It is calculated by comparing the signal to noise ratio at the detector output with that at the detector input as a function of spatial frequency. DQE depends on radiation exposure, spatial frequency, modulation transfer function, detector material and quality (voltage and current) of the radiation applied.[3]

An ideal situation is 100 percent quantum detection and conversion efficiency. Three types of materials are used and they are classified into three categories:

1. Unstructured scintillators (e.g. gadolinium oxysulphide and barium fluorobromide)
2. Structured phosphors (e.g. Cesium iodide, cesium bromide)
3. Semiconductor direct detectors (e.g. Amorphous selenium).

Digital systems with structured phosphors or semiconductors can achieve good spatial resolution. However indirect TFT technology based systems are more dose efficient.

Detectors with higher DQE will require less radiation dose than the detectors with lower DQE for similar image quality or signal-to-noise ratio, i.e., greater the value of DQE, more efficient is the detector in recording the information of the X-ray image. Both MTF and DQE are depicted in the form of a graph as a function of frequency or spatial resolution in line pairs/mm[3] (lp/mm) **(Fig. 16)**. Both are higher at low resolution and decrease with increasing spatial resolution.[7]

An ideal detector should have a DQE of 1 which means that all the radiation energy is absorbed and converted into image formation. However, in practice, the DQE of digital detectors is limited to about 0.45 at spatial frequency of 0.5 cycles/mm^3. In contrast, the maximum reported DQE for film- screen and computed radiography are typically 0.15 to 0.25 under similar conditions **(Fig. 17)**.[17]

Over the years, various methods for measuring DQE have been formulated. In 1999 the IEC62220-1 standard was established to improve the comparability of DQE measurements of digital X-ray imaging devices. The exposure level is measured at the detector surface with calibrated radiation meters after removing all protective parts including anti-scatter grid, the AEC chamber and other cover plates out of the beam. The IEC62220-1 standard enables manufacturers to specify DQE values on the basis of an internationally accepted method. This helps users to compare detectors and imaging systems and to make optimal use of the detectors.[18]

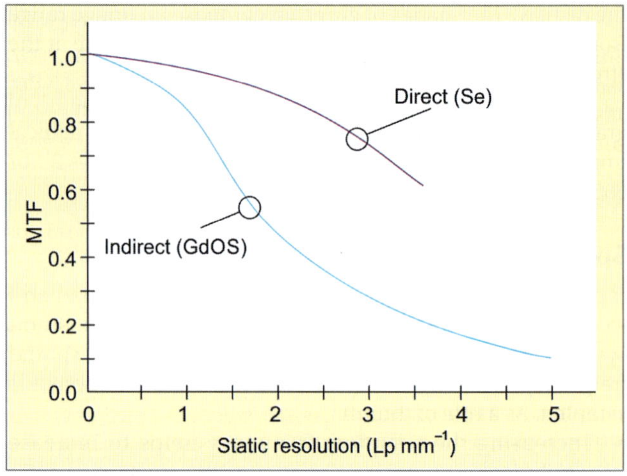

FIG. 16: Modulation transfer function (MTF) of direct and indirect digital systems.

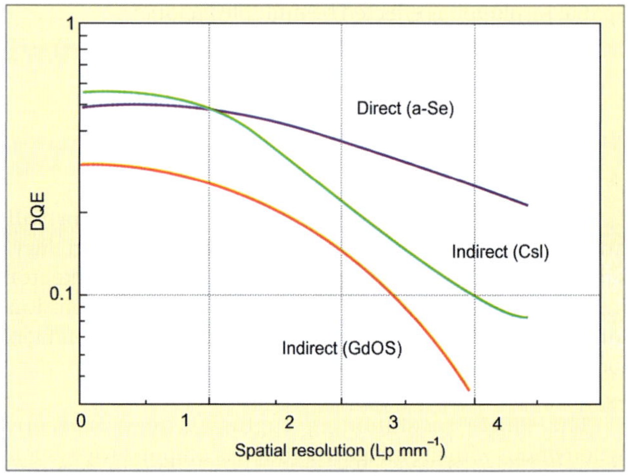

FIG. 17: Detective quantum efficiency as a function of spatial frequency for three different detector systems at 70 kVp.

RADIATION EXPOSURE

Digital detectors have the potential for substantially lowering the patient exposure. Efforts have been made to optimize both image quality and exposure in digital radiography. The most obvious way of minimizing patient exposure is to greatly reduce the number of failed exposures and requisite additional images.

In contrast to storage phosphor systems in which the possibility of exposure reduction is limited, DR systems offer a significantly higher potential for general exposure reduction because of their far superior quantum efficiency. Various studies have concluded that flat-panel detectors achieve the best results in high image quality at lower doses, followed by other DR systems such as selenium drum and CCD based systems.[3,19]

Use of CR for chest imaging leads to an increase in radiation dose, as storage phosphor plates are not suited for high KVP techniques. Moreover, storage phosphor plates are more sensitive to scatter, which makes the use of high ratio grids mandatory and thereby an increase in radiation exposure.[13] Studies show that digital system optimization is an important parameter in reducing patient dose. Hence technical requirements for digital systems should be set for achieving the same.[19]

EXPOSURE INDICATOR FOR DIGITAL RADIOGRAPHY

In contrast to FSR, where visual features such as under/overexposure help in recognizing exposure errors, digital system lack in recognizing the same. As a result, the technician needs to be familiar with and monitor the exposure indicator (EI) associated with digital imaging system. Exposure indicators have been developed by most equipment manufacturers. The purpose of the EI is to allow the technician to know the level of exposure the receptor has received and thereby determine if the correct exposure technique for the image was used. It is important to note that EIs are not measures of radiation dose to the patient but it measures the kerma (kinetic energy released in matter) in air at the detector surface i.e, it is the dose without any effect of scattering and is measured by commercial dose meters.

The exposure indicator varies among different manufactures, even having different names, symbols and units. **Table 2** shows a list of select manufacturers and details regarding their EI.[20]

ACR Practice Guideline for Digital Radiography

Radiographic examinations represent more than two-thirds of all radiologic examinations performed in both adults and children.[21] The Society for Pediatric Radiology in 2004 emphasized the need for ALARA Principle in digital imaging. The ACR developed a practice guideline of digital radiography in 2007 in "order to deliver optimal image quality at appropriate radiation doses so as to provide excellent safety and care for patients undergoing digital radiography examination".[20]

DIGITAL RADIOGRAPHIC ARTIFACTS

Radiographic artifacts in both film screen radiography as well as as digital radiography may mask or mimic abnormalities and impair image quality. Some artifacts seen on conventional films are similar to those found in CR and DR systems. However, several artifacts are unique to digital systems.

Five major categories of digital artifacts have been described according to the step during which they were created.[22]

The categories are:

1. Pre-exposure
2. Exposure
3. Post-exposure
4. Reading
5. Workstation

It is important to understand the step in which an artifact was created so as to be able to correct the error and minimise its occurrence.

Tables 3 to 7 enlist the different categories of artifacts produced in computed and digital radiography with their possible causes and preventive/remedial measures.[23]

To ensure optimum image quality in DR, when a particular part is radiographed, the correct processing menu for that region should be selected.[20]

Familiarity with the visual appearance of artifacts allows the recognition of artifacts and steps can be taken to prevent their future occurrence by proper maintenance and servicing of the digital radiography equipment.

CONCLUSION

The digital technology is here to stay and it is imperative that radiologists be familiar with the technical principles, criteria for image quality and radiation exposure issues with the various digital radiography systems that are currently available along with the technological advancements that are taking place.

TABLE 2: List of select manufacturers of digital radiography (DR) systems with details of their exposure indicator (EI).

Manufacturer	EI name	EI symbol	Units
Agfa	Log of median of histogram	1gM	Bels
Alara CR	Exposure indicator value	EIV	Mbels
Canon	Reached exposure value	REX	Unitless
Canon	EXP	EXP	Unitless
Carestream (formerly Kodak)	Exposure index	EI	Mbels
Fujifilm	S value	S	Unitless
GE	Uncompensated detector exposure	UD Exp	µGy air kerma
GE	Compensated detector exposure	CD Exp	µGy air kerma
GE	Detector exposure index	DEI	Unitless
Konica	Sensitivity number	S	Unitless
Philips	Exposure index	EI	Unitless
Siemens	Exposure index	EXI	µGy air kerma

TABLE 3: Pre-exposure related artifacts.

	Artifact	Cause	Prevention/remedial measures
CR system artifacts	• Storage scatter	Exposure to scatter and background radiation	• Proper storage of imaging plates (IP) • Erasure of IP before use
	• Cracks due to "detector drops" seen as horizontal lines or straight white band across the image **(Fig. 18)**	Dropping or damage to imaging plate	• Proper handling of Imaging plates, cleaned as per instructions[23] • Damaged plates to be replaced
	• Partial erasure	Incomplete erasure of imaging plate	• Erasure light to be cleaned and replaced as needed • Erasure with additional, exposure to UV light
	• Phantom image	Excessive time gap between erasure and exposure	Imaging plates to be erased immediately before use
DR system artifacts	• Memory	Retained charge in detector	• Proper grounding of conductive layer • Delay between radiographs
	• Dead pixels (appear as white or black spots on a radiograph)	Nonfunctional detector elements	• Map and cancel out dead pixels • Detector arrays to be replaced if required
	• Calibration mask	Variable attenuation during calibration (due to dust, contrast, etc.)	• Cleansing and recalibration of equipment • Use of table-top technique for recalibration

TABLE 4: Exposure-related artifacts.

	Artifact	Cause	Prevention/remedial measures
Artifacts exclusive to CR system	• Upside down cassette → Underexposed images	Error in cassette orientation, i.e. cassette placed upside down	• Ensuring correct orientation of cassette before use
	• Backscatter **(Fig. 19)**	• Scattering from objects behind the cassette • High exposure (kVp) settings	• Lead-backing cassettes to be used • Reduced exposure technique as possible
Artefacts created in both CR and DR systems	• Underexposed white strips on either edge of radiograph **(Fig. 20)**	Incorrect positioning or upside down orientation of focussed grid nonuniform attenuation of X-rays, i.e. greater at periphery of X-ray due to grid cut-off	Correct placement of the focussed grid before exposure
	• Double exposure **(Fig. 21)**	Multiple exposures on single imaging plate without being read or erased	Imaging plates to be erased before use Use of reliable power supply and stable data transfer
	Grainy image with reduced image quality (quantum mottle)	Use of low mA technique or increased attenuation of primary beam → decreased number of incident X-rays and a low SNR due to quantum mottle	Appropriate use of equipment specific technique charts and image filtering techniques
	• Detector saturation	Occurs when the maximal detector exposure is exceeded	Reduction of exposure levels is recommended to remain within the dynamic range of the image detector
Artifacts exclusive to DR system	• Paradoxic over exposure effect	Severe over-exposure resulting in lighter image (at edge of thick or dense regions of interest)	Reduction of exposure technique (lower mAs) may decrease the frequency of this artifact
	• Planking	Variable amplification of separate digital array sections seen alongwith paradoxic over-exposure effect.	• Routine calibration of equipment as needed • Decrease in exposure technique (lower mAs)

TABLE 5: Postexposure-related artifacts.

	Artifact	Cause	Prevention/remedial measures
CR system exclusive artifacts	Light leak	Imaging plate exposed to visible light before reading	• Images to be read as soon as possible after exposure • Avoid manual opening of cassettes after exposure
	Fading	Excessive delay in reading the imaging plate following exposure leads to an overall poor quality image which may be diffusely grainy and under exposed	• Reading imaging plate immediately after each exposure • Use of newest imaging plates having more stable forms of energy storage, less prone to fading

TABLE 6: Reading-related artifacts.

	Artifact	Cause	Prevention/remedial measures
Artifacts exclusive to CR system	• Debris	Any debris on the imaging plate blocks the emitted light from reaching the photomultiplier tube which is used to read the latent image	Imaging plates should be cleaned routinely as per the manufacturer's recommendations
	• Dirty light guide **(Fig. 22)**	Dirt on the light guide will lead to blockage of transmission of light	Light guide to be cleared routinely during maintenance and as required
	• Skipped scan-lines	• Physical jarring of the IP reader or • Fluctuations in power supply	Provisions of stable imaging plate reader mechanics and power supply
Artifacts common to both CR and DR system	• Moiré	Due to malfunction of grid oscillation or its timing mechanism	• Use of high density oscillating bucky grid • Grid should be aligned perpendicular to the detector or imaging plate readout direction

TABLE 7: Workstation-related artifacts.

	Artifact	Cause	Prevention/remedial measures
Artifacts common to both CR and DR system	Faulty transfer **(Fig. 23)**	• Loose data cables • Fluctuations in power supply • Faulty transfer error	• Use of reliable method of data transfer, stable power supply and stable connections
	Border detection	• Incorrect border detection most frequently occurs at margin of highly attenuating objects • Misalignment of cassette and field of view	• Use of semiautomatic border detection to decrease its occurrence • Align cassette with field of view • Centre area of interest
	Overall reduced image quality/ contrast/detail—diagnostic specifier artifacts	Region of interest incorrectly selected	Correct region of interest to be selected for each study
	Complete darkening of areas of higher exposure	Post processing large file size may lead to erroneous clipping of information	Modification of processing technique to include all data
	Density threshold artifact—object above the density threshold appearing entirely white	High density objects included in image analysis	Should be implemented to exclude extremely dense objects above a density threshold
	Überschwinger (metal interface artifact)—gives false impression of osteolysis/loosening of implant	• Including high density objects such as metallic implants • Use of excessive edge enhancement	Can be minimized by using moderate amounts of edge enhancement to eliminate the false lucency

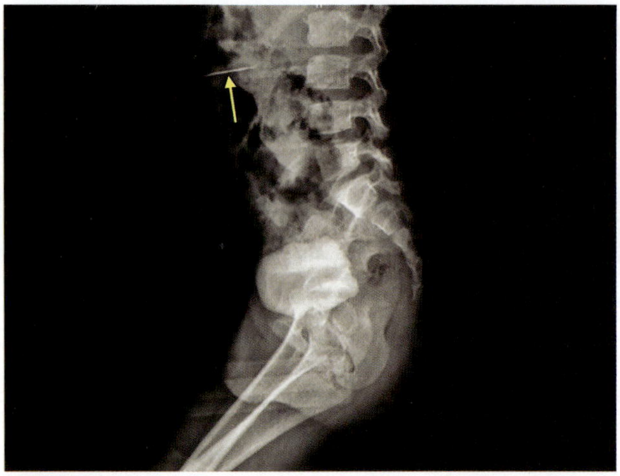

FIG. 18: Small horizontally aligned linear white line due to crack/ damage of imaging plate of CR system.

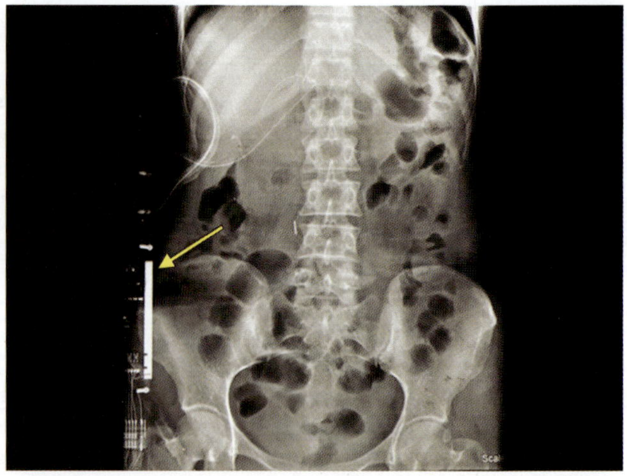

FIG. 19: X-ray KUB obtained with a CR system shows detector electronics created by backscattered X-rays along the right side of the radiograph.

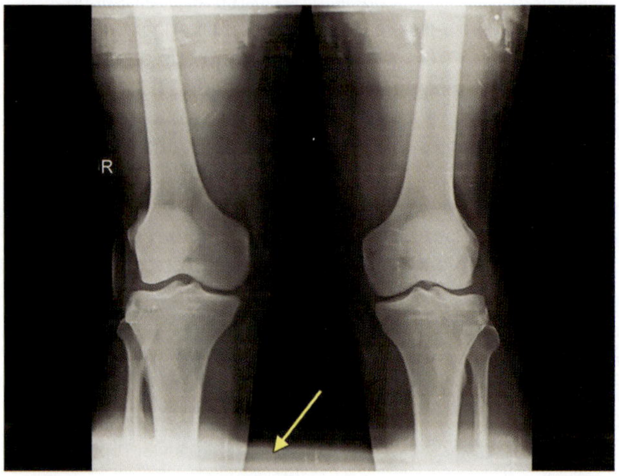

FIG. 20: Underexposed white strips on the edge of radiograph due to "grid cut-off".

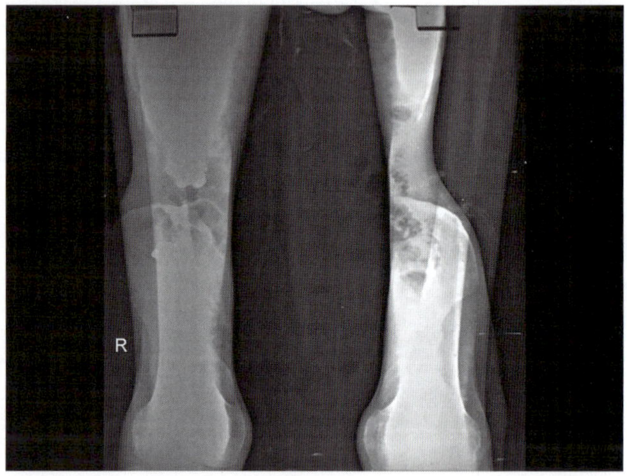

FIG. 21: 'Double exposure' artifact with CR: The radiograph shows two images of X-ray KUB and thigh summated on each other.

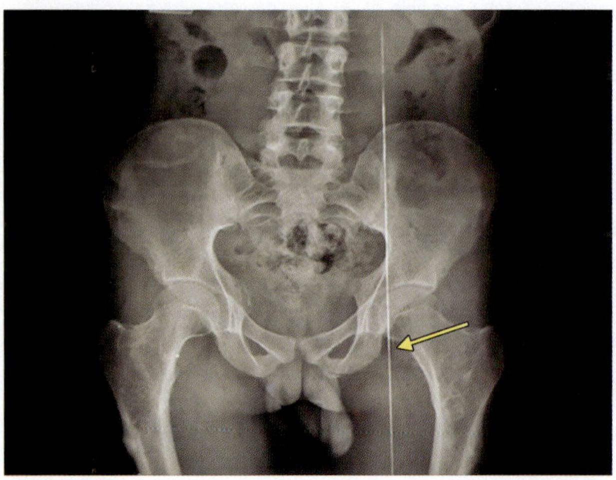

FIG. 22: "Dirty light guide" artifact—longitudinal white line towards the left of film, due to dirt on the light guide blocking transmission of light (exclusive to CR system).

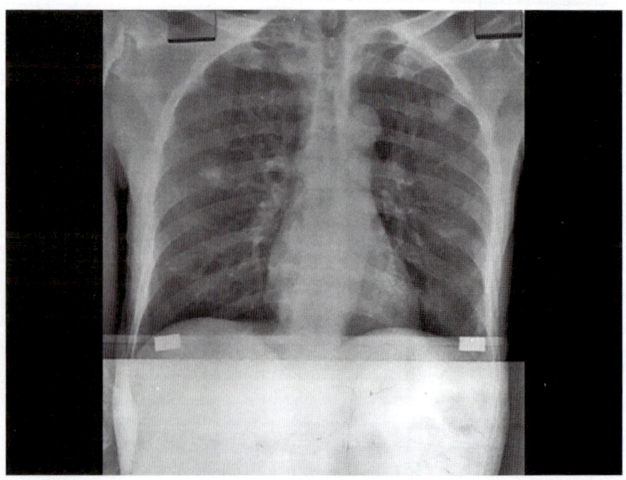

FIG. 23: 'Faulty transfer' artifact—visible as replacement of part of image by a large white band on the chest radiograph.

REFERENCES

1. Selman J. The fundamentals of X-ray and radium physics, 8th Edn. Charles C Thomas; 1994.
2. Indrajit IK, Verma BS. Digital imaging in radiology practice: An introduction to few fundamental concepts. IJRI. 2007;17(4):230-6.
3. Körner M, Weber CH, Wirth S, Pfeifer KJ, Reiser MF, Treitl M. Advances in digital radiography: physical principles and system overview. Radiographics. 2007;27(3):675-86.
4. Schaefer-Prokop CM, De Boo DW, Uffmann M, Prokop M. DR and CR: Recent advances in technology. European Journal of Radiology. 2009;72:194-201.
5. Lanca L, Silva A. Digital Radiography Detectors: A Technical Overview. Chapter 2 in Digital Imaging Systems for plain Radiography; 2013.pp.9-19.
6. Cury TS, Dowdey JE, Murry RC. Digital radiography in Christensen's Physics of Diagnostic Radiology, 4th Edn. Lea and Febiger; 1990.pp.392-431.
7. Verma BS, Indrajit IK. Advent of digital radiography: Part I. IJRI. 2008;18(2):113-6.
8. Strickland NH. Picture archiving and communication system and digital radiology. In Grainger and Allison Diagnostic Radiology. A textbook of Medical Imaging, 5th Edn, Vol I: 3-30, 2008, Edited by Adam A, Dixon AK, Chruchill Livingstone.
9. Fischbach F, Freund T, Pech M, Werk M, Bassir C, Stoever B, et al. Comparison of indirect CsI/a:Si and direct a:Se digital radiography. An assessment of contrast and detail visualization. Acta Radiol. 2003;44(6):616-21.
10. Cowen AR, Kengyelics, Davies AG. Solid-state, flat-panel, digital radiography detectors and their physical imaging characteristics. Clin Rad 2008;63:487-98.
11. Kotter E, Langer M. Digital radiography with large-area flat-panel detectors. Eur Radiol. 2002;12:2562-70.
12. Chotas HG, Dobbins JT 3rd, Ravin CE. Principles of digital radiography with large-area, electronically readable detectors: a review of the basics. Radiology. 1999;210(3):595-9.
13. Verma BS, Indrajit IK. Impact of computers in radiography: the advent of digital radiography, Part-2. IJRI. 2008;18(3): 204-9.
14. Roberts PA, Williams J. Digital radiography in Farr's Physics for Medical Imaging (2nd edn), Saunders Elsevier. 2008;79:90.
15. Schaefer-Prokop C, Netizel U, Venema HW, Uffmann M, Prokop H. Digital chest radiography: an update on modern technology, dose containment and control of image quality. Eur Radiol. 2008;(18):1818-30.
16. McAdams HP, Samei E, Dobbins III J, Tourassi GD, Ravin CE. Recent advances in Chest Radiography. 2006; 241(3):663-83.
17. Dowsett DJ, Kenny PA, Johnston RE. The digital image in The Physics of Diagnostic Imaging (2nd edn), International Thomson Publishing. 2006. pp. 313-63.
18. Illers H, Buhr E, Hoeschen C. Measurement of the detective quantum efficiency (DQE) of digital X-ray detectors according to the novel standard IEC 62220-1. Radiat Prot Dosimetry. 2005;114(1-3):39-44.
19. Neofotistou V, Tsapaki V, Kottou S, Schreiner-Karoussou A, Vano E. Does digital imaging decrease patient dose? A pilot study and review of the literature. Radiat Prot Dosimetry. 2005;117(1-3):204-10.
20. Herrmann TL, Fauber TL, Gill J, Hoffman C, et al. Best practices in Digital Radiography. White Paper (American Society of Radiologic Technologists); 2012.pp.1-26.
21. Harmon R. Realizing the full benefit of digital radiography. Imaging Economics 2001. Available from: http://www.imagingeconomics.com/issues/articles/2001_12.20asp.
22. Jiménez DA1, Armbrust LJ. Radiographic artifacts. Vet Clin North Am Small Anim 39 (2009) 689-709 Pract. 2009.
23. Walz-Flannigan AI, Brossoit KJ, Magnuson DJ, Schueler BA. Pictorial Review of Digital Radiography Artifacts. Radiographics. 2018;38(3):833-46.

CHAPTER

40

Digital Mammography

Smriti Hari, Surabhi Vyas,
Chandrashekhara SH

INTRODUCTION

Mammography is a technically challenging imaging modality as it requires excellent soft tissue contrast, high spatial resolution, and wide image latitude especially in denser breasts, with a low radiation burden. The sensitivity of mammography is reported to be ranging from 45% to 85%, with relatively poorer performance as the breast density increases.[1] However, several studies have shown an improved cancer detection with digital mammography even in younger women who have dense breasts.[2,3]

Although the requirements for optimal image acquisition for both screen film mammography (SFM) and digital mammography are same in terms of compression and positioning, there are few basic differences. Newer applications of digital mammography like digital breast tomosynthesis (DBT) and contrast enhanced mammography further increase the diagnostic accuracy of mammography.

DIGITAL MAMMOGRAPHY

In digital mammography, the image is obtained in the same manner as in SFM, using a compression plate and an X-ray tube but the screen-film cassette is replaced by a digital detector. Although images of SFM have higher spatial resolution than digital mammography, the dynamic range is narrow, leading to a lower contrast resolution.

A digital mammography system allows optimization at each step; image acquisition, image display, and archiving, which results in a significant increase in the dynamic range and contrast resolution. This compensates the effect of increasing breast density on the sensitivity of the examination.

BASIC PHYSICS OF DIGITAL MAMMOGRAPHY

Detectors

The detector is the basic unit of the digital mammography. The interaction of the X-ray beam with the detector elements forms the basis of the mammography image.[4] Detectors can be classified as direct or indirect capture. In indirect capture, X-ray photon is converted into a light photon by means of a scintillator, which then produces a digital signal. It is to be noted that with each step in digitalization, noise is introduced, which affects image quality. Examples of indirect digital detectors are charge couple devices (CCDs), photostimulable phosphors, and amorphous silicon detectors. The direct digital units on the other hand uses a photoconductive material which directly converts the X-ray photon to a digital signal, without the intervening light photon conversion step, and thus uses more of the primary beam than the indirect system. Examples of direct digital detectors are amorphous selenium detectors and crystal silicon detectors. Selenium is an optimum mammography detector material due to its high X-ray absorption efficiency, high intrinsic resolution and low noise.[5]

Another approach to digital mammography is the computed radiography (CR) approach, which uses a photostimulable phosphor plate. The plate is used to absorb X-rays just as a screen-film cassette. However, rather than emitting light immediately after exposure through fluorescence, absorption of X-ray causes electrons within the phosphor material crystal to be promoted to higher energy levels. The screen is then placed in a reader where it is scanned with the laser beam. The laser beam causes the electrons to be released and returned to their resting levels with release of higher energy (blue) light (proportional to the X-ray beam energy). The amount of blue light released is then measured by a photomultiplier tube. Problems with this system include inefficient light collection and scatter of laser light in the phosphor material resulting in loss of spatial resolution and increased noise.

Spatial Resolution

The spatial resolution of any system depends on the size of the detector (also called as "dels") and the gap between two detector elements (also called as pixel pitch). The Nyquist frequency of a detector is the smallest resolvable structure and is also equivalent to twice the size of a detector element.[6] In SFM, similar to conventional radiography, the spatial resolution is defined by the number of line pairs that can be resolved per millimeter of film.

Other factors that influence spatial resolution are focal spot size, motion and the spread of the signal in the detector. The MTF is the percentage of the signal strength entering the system relative to the signal coming out of the system, at varying frequencies and is a good measure of spatial resolution and thus indirectly of the factors affecting the spatial resolution. It is also a measure of the loss of the original signal in the system. It is known that this loss is minimal with large shapes (near perfect MTF of 1) and becomes progressively poorer for finer shapes.

Another important term is detective quantum efficiency (DQE) which is the percentage of useful signal produced to the signal lost due to noise and thus takes into consideration the signal to noise ratio (SNR).[7] Since Digital systems have a higher DQE than screen-film units, therefore these may provide a similar image quality as that of SFM systems at a lower dose or a better image quality at the same dose as SFM systems.

Analog to Digital Units

As the X-ray photons are captured by the detector, the digital signal is recorded in units known as analog to digital units (ADU). All detectors have a matrix, that is divided into rows and columns of pixels, for signal acquisition. Every time an X-ray photon reaches the pixel it is stored as an ADU. Denser the breast tissue, lower is the ADU for that pixel. For each X-ray exposure a map of ADU is created which is then converted to a gray scale map. Pixel size and matrix vary from equipment to equipment. Most available systems have pixel pitches of 50, 70 or 100 μm, however there have been no conclusive studies to show benefit of one over another.

Most digital and screen film systems come equipped with automatic exposure control (AEC) for optimum kilovolt peak (kVp), and milliamps (mA) values. In the digital system AEC ensures lower radiation exposure to an appropriate SNR.[8] This is achieved by a very low-dose fast test exposure prior to the diagnostic exposure to formulate an ADU map, which by various algorithms determines the correct exposure parameters for a given patient.

Processing Algorithms

There are various processing algorithms that are used to convert the digital signals into a readable mammographic image. These are:

- Detector correction algorithms to remove detector inhomogeneity, which is translated to the final image.
- Thickness equalization algorithms so that he thicker central tissue is as clearly seen as the thinner peripheral tissue.
- Contrast enhancement algorithms make calcifications, margin details and density differences more pronounced for easy visibility.

Dynamic Range

Dynamic range of a system refers to the range of gray scales that can be displayed and are available for viewing. It ranges from 8 to 10 bits for most systems.

Comparison between Digital Mammograms and Film/Screen Mammograms

Full-field digital mammography (FFDM) systems have spatial resolutions ranging from 5 to 10 lp/mm, whereas the screen-film mammography have a line-pair resolution of 18–20 lp/mm. In digital mammography systems, it is the size of the pixels that determines the spatial resolution. The pixel size ranges from about 50–100 microns for FFDM systems. Smaller the pixel size, more data is available for storage and display, but it increases the operational cost.[9] The lower spatial resolution of FFDM systems as compared to SFM is compensated by an increase in contrast resolution. The contrast resolution as described previously is a reflection of the dynamic range. The digital system has greater dynamic range and thus it can record and differentiate subtle variations in contrast better than SFM.

Unlike SFM, in which the image cannot be manipulated after exposure and processing, FFDM images can be optimized after image capture by image post processing and adjustment of image display. The window width and window level for all digital images viewed with soft copy display on review workstations can be adjusted, changing the contrast and brightness of the images, respectively, as well as digitally magnifying images.

Another important difference is that there is a linear relationship between the logarithm of X-ray exposure and film optical density only in the central portion of the characteristic curve for screen-film images. On the other hand, there is a linear relationship between X-ray exposure and signal over the entire dynamic range of the detector in FFDM systems, Thus, there is no loss of contrast in over or underexposed portions of the digital image and similar contrast is seen over the entire dynamic range of the detector **(Fig. 1)**. Digital mammography also eliminates the variability and noise added by film processing.

In terms of breast dose, FFDM has a mean glandular dose lower than, or comparable to, the radiation dose of SFM.

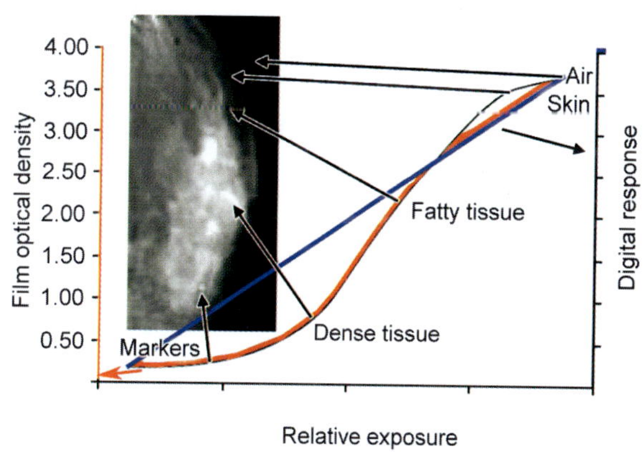

FIG. 1: Typical response curves for screen-film mammography (SFM) and digital mammography. Screen-film images demonstrate linear relationship between the film optical density and logarithm of X-ray exposure in the central portion of the characteristic curve. For FFDM systems however, there exists a linear relationship between X-ray exposure and signal over the entire dynamic range of the detector.

The average single-view mean glandular dose for FFDM is 1.86 mGy which is 22% lower than the average SFM mean glandular dose of 2.37 mGy.[10]

A number of studies have evaluated the performance of FFDM compared to SFM for screening asymptomatic women for breast cancer. Early studies showed comparable or slightly worse results for FFDM compared to SFM.[11,12] Larger studies however showed some benefits of FFDM compared to SFM. The American College of Radiology (ACR) Imaging Network Digital Mammographic Imaging Screening Trial (ACRINDMIST), which included nearly 50,000 women, showed no difference overall but found that FFDM was a better screening tool than SFM for women under age 50, for premenopausal and perimenopausal women, and for women with denser breast tissue (BIRADS density categories 3 and 4).[13]

Storage of Digital Images

The large amount of data that is available for storage and archiving with the FFDM systems presents a major challenge. The size of an image is determined by the pixel size in length and breadth, number of pixels per image and bit depth (bit depth is the number of shades of gray). A higher spatial resolution image requires a smaller pixel size and thus a greater amount of storage space. For example a screening two-view mammography examination of both breasts can take up 33–200 MB of storage space, depending on the spatial resolution of the images.

Display of Digital Images

FFDM images may be printed by dry laser printers and read on high-luminance view boxes, similar to SFM images. This approach however does not allow the viewer to utilise the benefits of digital technology. It is recommended that the images be displayed as soft copies on high-resolution (5 megapixel) special viewing monitors, to permit manipulation of resolution, contrast, and gray scale **(Fig. 2)**. Workstations need to be fast as mammography screening and diagnosis requires efficiency (i.e. ability to review old studies, magnification of areas of concern and comparison of both breasts and different views).

The workstation should be entirely compatible with PACS. Integrated multimodality workstation should be linked to the general archival system, so that different imaging modalities can be efficiently correlated to arrive at final diagnosis.

Artifacts

There can be a variety of artifacts in any radiographic imaging including digital mammography. These can be due to:

- Detector failure
- Failure in image processing
- Corruption of calibration files
- Dust particles and foreign bodies between the target and detector
- Failure of any other component like grid.

Commonly seen artifacts include ghosting, dead pixels, and flat-field inhomogeneities. Ghosting results from the leftover latent charge from the previous exposures, and is seen more with amorphous selenium direct detectors and photostimulable phosphor plates in CR imaging. This leftover charge can be cleared by putting the phosphor plate in cassette reader where clearing is achieved by the laser.

Bright white dots or white lines can be produced by dead pixels on a digital detector. Similar artifacts can also be produced if a detector array is different from its surrounding

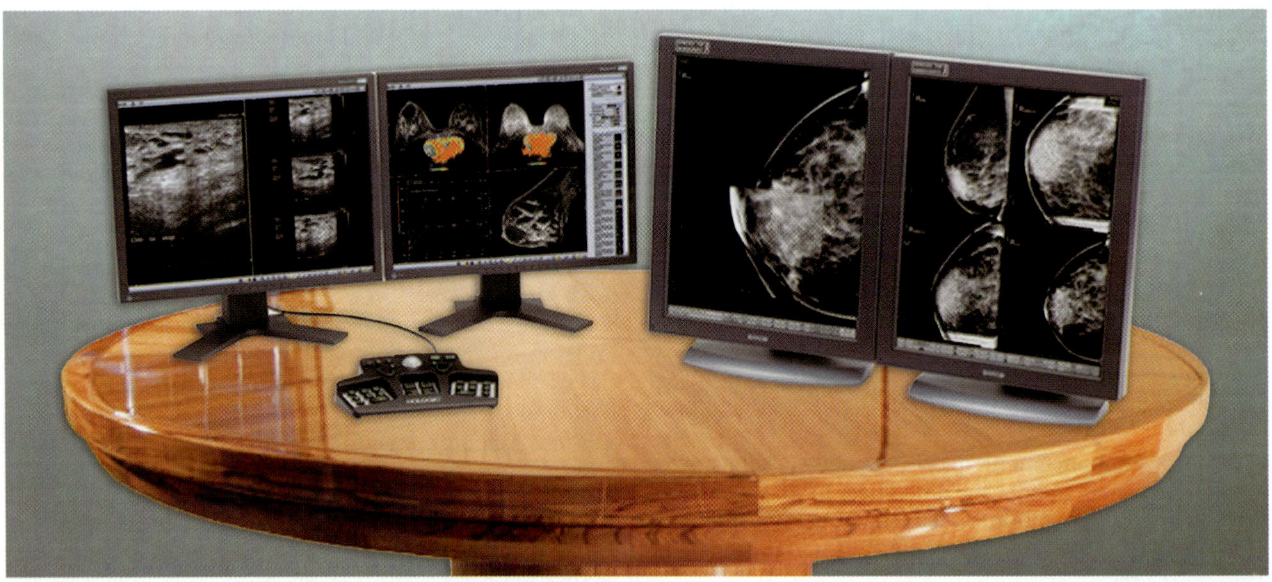

FIG. 2: Optimum soft-copy display on 5-megapixel high resolution monitors allows easy manipulations of resolution, contrast, and grayscale.

detectors in the matrix. A flat field recalibration can correct this abnormality.[14]

Failure of processing algorithms and misalignment of collimator produce straight dark lines or dark and white bands respectively on the image. Again a flat field recalibration and repositioning of collimator can correct these band like artifacts.

Mammography detectors are required to have a high spatial resolution in order to detect microcalcifications as small as 300 µm. The resultant high spatial resolution image is large enough to have more than 20 million pixels. Since mammography monitors can display around 5 million pixels, there are various modes that can be employed to sample the large data available like fit to viewport (adjacent ADUs are displayed as 1 ADU after averaging), same size (different image matrices are scaled to similar size to allow comparison with previous imaging), true size (true anatomical size scale is used to allow surgical and sterotactic planning), view actual pixels (full resolution images for margin characterization and detection of suspicious microcalcifications), and magnification (zoom or optical magnification is employed without any increase in resolution) modes. These modes can be used to create different viewing protocols to best use the expansive information available.

Magnification view where a portion of the breast parenchyma is imaged using a magnification stand or paddle can be used to increase the spatial resolution and better lesion characterization.[15]

APPLICATIONS OF DIGITAL MAMMOGRAPHY

Computer-aided Detection and Computer-aided Diagnosis

Computer-aided detection (CADe) and computer-aided diagnosis (CADx) are advanced software programs, which can assess and review mammograms for bright clustered specks representing microcalcifications and converging lines corresponding to spiculated masses. These software systems help the interpreting radiologists in identifying the subtle signs of cancer against the complex background of dense breast tissue. CAD can identify and mark all the potential abnormalities directly on the image displayed on the workstation **(Fig. 3)**. The radiologist then analyses and interprets the marked findings on CAD to decide whether the finding should be dismissed as insignificant or further worked up. It thus reduces the chances of missing cancer.[16] It acts as second reader to the experienced radiologists and may help inexperienced radiologists.[17] On the other hand, the CADe refers to those modified algorithms that simply mark areas which are to be reviewed without providing any additional information about malignancy likelihood. The CADx algorithms are little advanced programs, which provide additional information by different sizes of the mark-ups. These various marking methods are intended to help the interpretation by a radiologist and do not intend that the lesions without the CAD mark-up should be dismissed.

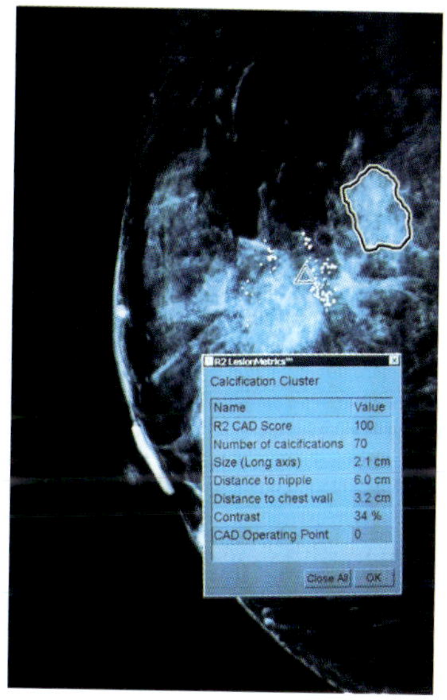

FIG. 3: CAD marks potential abnormalities directly on the image displayed on the workstation.

Dual-energy Subtraction Mammography

The principle of dual-energy subtraction mammography is that if exposures are obtained for same radiographic projection with both high and low operating tube potentials, different breast structures show different absorption of photons with some structures with greater absorption of low-energy compared with high-energy photons. Thus, image formed by the high energy photons can be electronically subtracted from the other resulting in cancelling of those structures that do not exhibit differential absorption.[18] It takes advantage of the fact that the change in attenuation is greater for calcifications than for soft tissues when the kVp is altered from high energies to low energies. Dual energy mammography system is a modified system that can produce normal mammographic images as well as images obtained at higher (45–50 kV) energy.

Contrast-enhanced Digital Mammography

Contrast-enhanced digital mammography utilizes the contrast enhancement pattern as a function of neovascularity of a malignant mass and its correlation with the anatomic features.[19] A precontrast and a postcontrast image is obtained and by subtracting the two, only the contrast image remains, making the malignant mass more evident because of its neovascularity.[19] This can be achieved in two ways: serial scanning over time and by dual energy imaging. Iodinated contrast material and modified digital mammography units are required for the technique. A noncontrast image is obtained prior to intravenous contrast injection. Then, series of images are taken after injecting the contrast. The post contrast images are subtracted from the non-contrast image making the areas of enhancement more conspicuous. Simultaneously enhancement curves can also be generated. The major limitation of this method is that only one breast can be evaluated at a time in a single projection. The dual energy technique, on the other hand, allows simultaneous evaluation of both breasts during the same contrast administration. With the dual energy technique, two exposures are made after injecting iodinated contrast, one at low and other at high kVp. Post processing creates subtraction images to highlights areas of iodine concentration or enhancement. The low energy image may be used for routine mammographic interpretation. As the scanning is done at a single time point, the kinetic assessment of enhancement curves cannot be performed.

Digital Breast Tomosynthesis

Digital breast tomosynthesis (DBT) is a technique to improve the detection and characterization of breast lesions, especially in women with dense breasts. Multiple projection images are reconstructed to allow evaluation of the breast in thin sections thus increasing the diagnostic confidence where the lesion margins are obscured by the surrounding normal fibroglandular tissue.

Technique

In conventional digital mammography, a compressed breast is exposed to ionizing radiation coming from a stationary tube and the X-rays are detected by a stationary detector. A two-dimensional image of a three dimensional breast is created, leading to overlap and obscuration. On the other hand, in DBT, the X-ray tube moves through an arc and multiple exposures are made at different angles to create several projectional images. **(Fig. 4)**. Reconstruction algorithms are applied to this projectional data and a series of tomographic images are produced. A radiologist can interpret these as a stack of images approximately 1 mm thick and read these similar to reading the CT or MRI stack of images on a workstation.

Different manufacturers have developed different methods to perform DBT with varying arc angles. The technique is not without potential constraints including total radiation dose, imaging time, patient motion, detector performance, detector motion, and ability to image the entire breast.

Radiation Dose

As the technique involves number of exposures compared to single exposure per view for digital mammography, the radiation dose is slightly increased. However all FFDM systems produce DBT images with dose below the FDA limit of 300 milirad per exposure.

Potential Benefits of Clinical Breast Imaging with Tomosynthesis

The benefits of DBT include an improved sensitivity of screening, smaller lesion detection, better image characterization, and reduced recall rates **(Figs. 5A and B)**. The primary benefit of DBT is expected to be more for masses, asymmetries, and distortion.

Clinical Tomosynthesis Evaluations

Several early studies have shown good patient acceptance, physician preference, improvement in sensitivity, improvement in characterization with DBT, with an increase in scan reading time.[20-22]

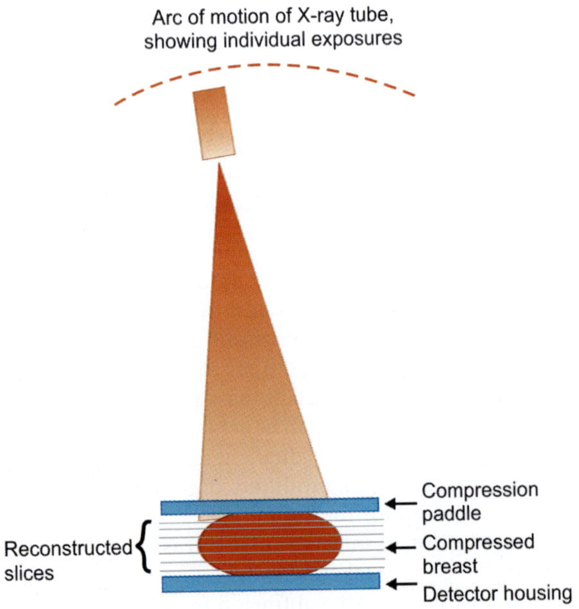

FIG. 4: Digital breast tomosynthesis: The X-ray tube moves through an arc while the breast is compressed and exposures are made after every few predetermined angles to create a series of tomographic images.

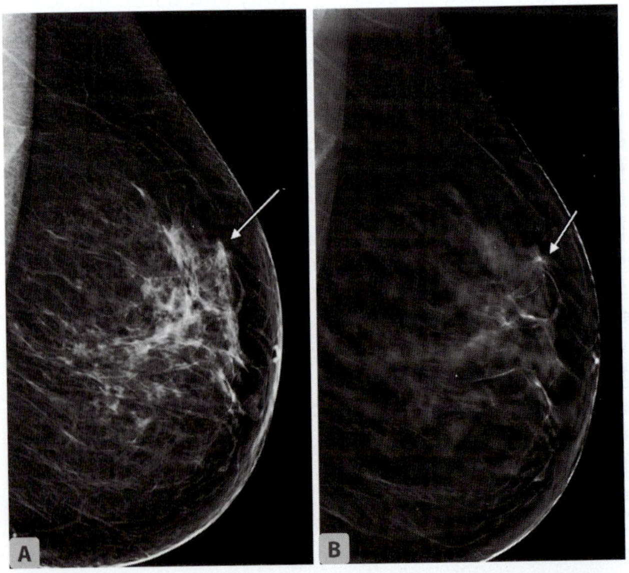

FIGS. 5A AND B: Conventional film screen mammography MLO view (A) of a patient with invasive ductal cancer. The spiculated mass is clearly visualized in the 1-mm thick tomosynthesis image (B) (arrow).

The thin DBT images may make characterization of clusters of calcification difficult, as only few from the cluster may be seen in one slice. Maximum intensity projections can be created for better evaluation of such clusters of calcifications.

Teleradiology Applications

Digital mammography has the potential to make teleradiography effective in breast imaging, as it allows rapid electronic transfer of digital data from one place to another. This is especially relevant in remote places where quality breast imaging interpretation may not be available and also in mobile units. It can also reduce recall rates for additional views and supplemental imaging. It can do away with physical transportation of the films from one center to another for a second opinion.

Stereotactic Breast Biopsy

A full-field digital mammography detector can also be used for stereotactic-breast-biopsy to allow diagnostic, interventional and follow-up evaluation with the same system.

CONCLUSION

Full-field digital mammography has significantly advanced the breast cancer diagnosis, by an improvement in the cancer detection and reduction in the X-ray dose exposure. Transition from conventional film screen mammogram to digital mammogram is quite expensive but is compensated by its numerous benefits. Radiologists face unique challenges when transitioning from SFM to digital mammography. The advanced applications of digital mammography hold great promise for early breast cancer diagnosis.

REFERENCES

1. Mandelson MT, Oestreicher N, Porter P. Breast density as a predictor of mammographic detection: comparison of interval- and screen-detected cancers. J Natl Cancer Inst. 2000;92:1081-7.
2. ED Pisano, C Gatsonis, E Hendrik. Diagnostic performance of digital versus film mammography for breast-cancer screening. N Engl J Med. 2005;353:1773-83.
3. S Vinnicombe, S Pinto Pereira, VA McCormack, et al. Full-field digital versus screen-film mammography: comparison within the UK breast screening program and systematic review of published data. Radiology. 2009;251:347-58.
4. CJ D'Orsi, MS Newell. Digital mammography: clinical implementation and clinical trials. Semin Roentgenol. 2007;42:236-42.
5. Pisano ED, Yaffe YJ. Digital Mammography. Radiology. 2005;234:353-62.
6. A Noel, F Thibault. Digital detectors for mammography: the technical challenges. Eur Radiol. 2004;14:1990-8.
7. E Samei, NT Ranger, A Mackenzie, et al. Detector of system? Extending the concept of detective quantum efficiency to characterize the performance of digital radiographic imaging systems. Radiology. 2008;249:926-37.
8. ED Pisano, MJ Yaffe. Digital mammography. Radiology. 2005;234:353-62.
9. Rowlands JA, Zhao W, Blevis IM, et al. Flat-panel digital radiology with amorphous selenium and active-matrix readout. Radiographics. 1997;17:753-60.
10. Hendrick RE, Pisano ED, Averbukh A, Moran C, Berns EA, Yaffe MJ, Herman B, Acharyya S, Gatsonis C. Comparison of acquisition parameters and breast dose in digital mammography and screen-film mammography in the American College of Radiology Imaging Network Digital Mammographic Imaging Screening Trial. AJR Am J Roentgenol. 2010;194(2):362-9.
11. Lewin JM, Hendrick RE, D'Orsi CJ, et al. Comparison of full-field digital mammography with screen-film mammography for cancer detection: results of 4,945 paired examinations. Radiology. 2001;218:873-80.
12. Skaane P, Young K, Skjennald A. Population-based mammography screening: comparison of screen-film and full-field digital mammography with soft-copy reading- Oslo I study. Radiology. 2003;229:877-84.
13. Pisano LD, Gatsonis C, Hendrick E, Yaffe M, Baum JK, Acharyya S, Conant EF, Fajardo LL, Bassett L, D'Orsi C, Jong R, Rebner M. Digital Mammographic Imaging Screening Trial (DMIST) Investigators Group. Diagnostic performance of digital versus film mammography for breast-cancer screening. N Engl J Med. 2005;353(17):1773-83.
14. RS Ayyala, MA Chorlton, RH Behrman, et al. Digital mammographic artifacts on full-field system: what are they and how do I fix them? Radio Graphics. 2008;28:1999-2008.
15. MJ Kim, EK Kim, JY Kwak. Characterization of microcalcification: can digital monitor zooming replace magnification mammography in full-field digital mammography? Eur Radiol. 2009;19:310-7.
16. Birdwell RL, Ikeda DM, O'Shaughnessy KF, et al. Mammographic characteristics of 115 missed cancers later detected with screening mammography and the potential utility of computer-aided detection. Radiology. 2001;219:192-202.
17. Karssemeijer N, Otten JD, Verbeek AL, et al. Computer-aided detection versus independent double reading of masses on mammograms. Radiology. 2003;227:192-200.
18. Lewin JM, Isaacs PK, Vance V, Larke FJ. Dual-energy contrast-enhanced digital subtraction mammography: feasibility. Radiology. 2003;229(1):261-8.
19. Jong RA, Yaffe MJ, Skarpathiotakis M, et al. Contrast-enhanced digital mammography: initial clinical experience. Radiology. 2003;228:842-50.
20. Poplack SP, Tosteson TD, Kogel CA, et al. Digital breast tomosynthesis: initial experience in 98 women with abnormal digital screening mammography. Am J Roentgenol. 2007;189:616-23.
21. Andersson I, Ikeda D, Zackrisson S, et al. Breast tomosynthesis and digital mammography: a comparison of breast cancer visibility and BIRADS classification in a population of cancers with subtle mammographic findings. Eur Radiol. 2008;18:2817-25.
22. Gur D, Abrams GS, Chough DM, et al. Digital breast tomosynthesis: observer performance study. AJR Am J Roentgenol. 2009;193:586-91.

CHAPTER

41

Fluoroscopy and Digital Subtraction Angiography

Deep Narayan Srivastava, Kumble S Madhusudhan

OVERVIEW

Fluoroscopy is an imaging technique which uses X-rays for real-time visualization of internal organs or structures of the body. A fluoroscope is used for the same which in its basic form consists of an X-ray source and a fluorescent screen between which patient is positioned. From its initial use in the early 20th century, the fluoroscope has undergone significant technological improvements with current fluoroscopic machines using larger sized flat panel detector with digital processing.[1] Digital subtraction angiography (DSA) is a fluoroscopic technique in which real-time subtraction of precontrast images is done for better visualization of contrast filled structures.[2] Fluoroscopy is used in various diagnostic and therapeutic procedures, including assessment of dynamic processes such as swallowing and cardiac function, provision of road map for positioning vascular or nonvascular catheters, evaluation of vessels using contrast in DSA and detection of gastrointestinal abnormalities in barium studies. For safe and efficient use of fluoroscopy it is essential to have adequate knowledge of these equipment and newer developments. The chapter describes principles of fluoroscopy, early fluoroscopic equipment and newer advances in fluoroscopic imaging along with safety issues.

FLUOROSCOPY

The term fluorescence means emission of light by a substance when it is exposed to electromagnetic radiation. Fluoroscope consists of this substance in the fluorescent screen which is stimulated by X-rays in a dark room. The fluorescent substance used in the initial days of fluoroscopy was barium platinocyanide which produced very dim images. Also, the substance was unstable.

This was later changed to cadmium tungstate and subsequently to zinc cadmium sulfide which though increased image brightness but still needed dark room.[1] Fluorography means serial acquisition of higher quality images for diagnosis and documentation.

In its early days, fluoroscopy was performed in a dark room (dark room fluoroscopy) as the light emitted by the fluorescent screen was dim. The radiologist would adapt his/her eyes in the room for some time to enhance visualization. The image emitted by the screen was directly viewed by the examiner **(Figs. 1A and B)**. The performance of the technique was mainly affected by the limitations of human eye at low light levels which reduced spatial and contrast resolution of the image viewed. This shortcoming was overcome by image intensifier (II) which was introduced in 1953.[3] The II amplified the brightness of the light image and improved visualization. The major problem with the initial II was small viewing angle which needed the radiologist to move his/her position frequently as and when the II moved **(Fig. 2)**. This limitation was overcome with the development of video camera for image viewing and displaying it on monitor **(Fig. 3)**. Today, the II has larger size (40 cm) compared to the older ones (15 cm). With the development of digital technique, there is improvement in the performance of the imaging chain. The latest addition is the introduction of flat panel detector which has replaced the II and video camera.

The main advantage of fluoroscopy over radiography is the use of low tube currents, in the range of 1 mA to 6 mA compared to 500–800 mA for routine conventional radiography. Typical exposure rate of fluoroscopy for an average adult is in the range of 10 to 30 mGy/min (compared

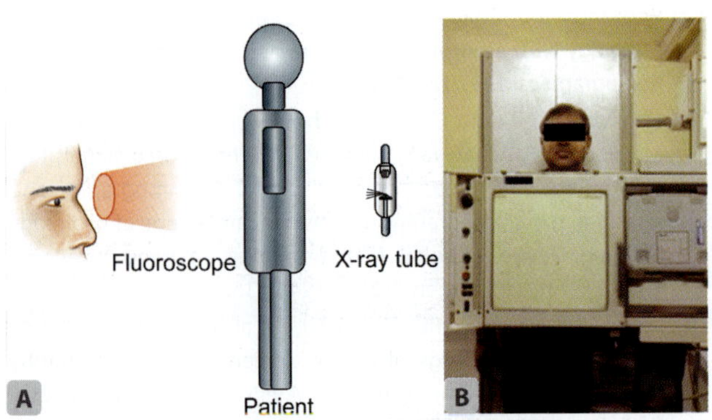

FIGS. 1A AND B: Dark room fluoroscopy. (A) Early hand held fluoroscope used in dark room for direct visualization. (B) Improvised dark room fluoroscope fixed to the table, but movable in all four directions. Here, X-ray tube is under the table.

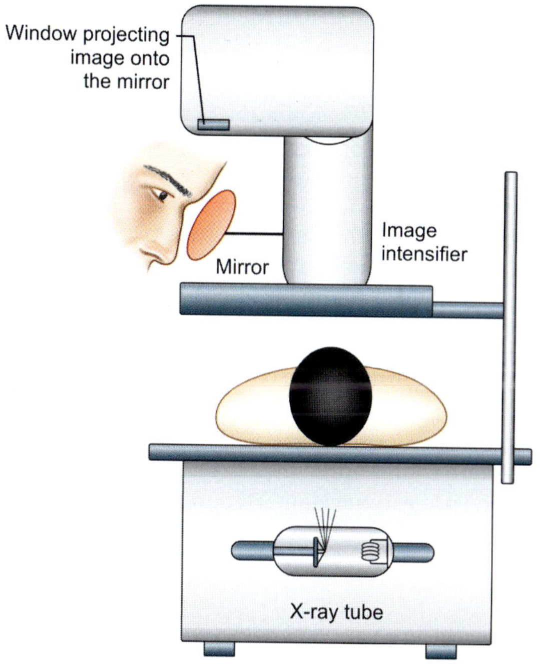

FIG. 2: First fluoroscopy machine with Image intensifier. The image formed is intensified and reflected onto the mirror for visualization by the operator.

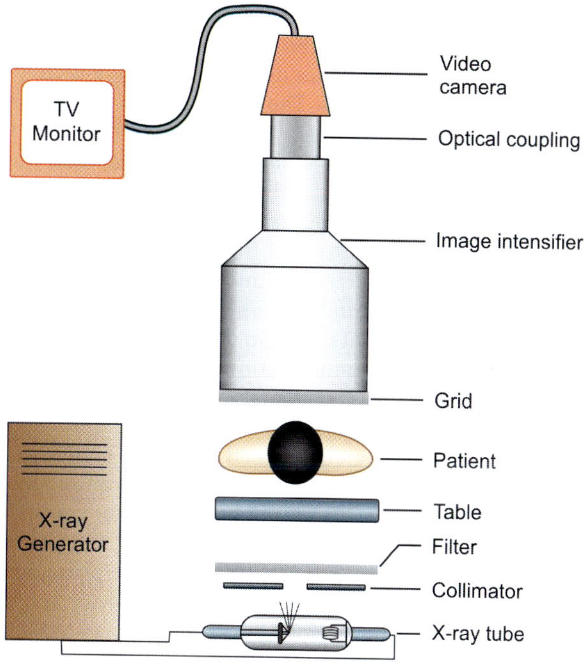

FIG. 4: Components of image intensifier fluoroscopy system.

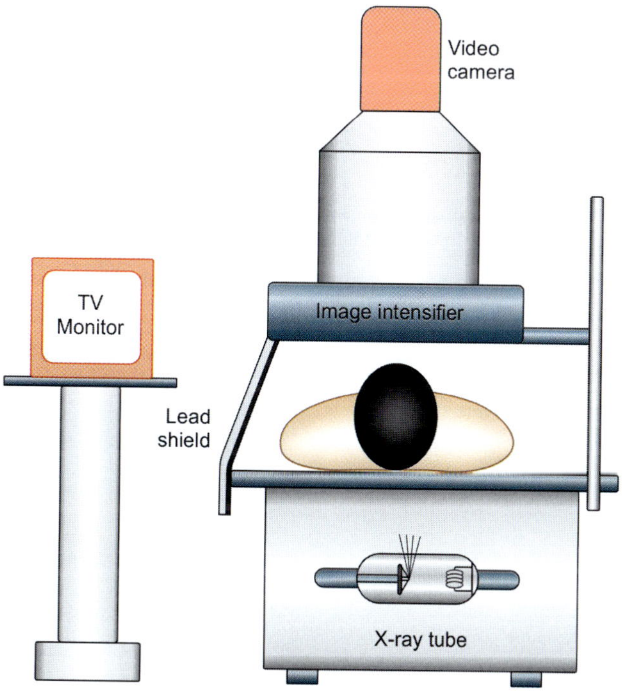

FIG. 3: Image intensifier fluoroscopy system with optical coupling system, video camera and television monitor display.

to a chest radiograph—0.3 mGy/30 msec or 600 mGy/min). But longer times may increase the risk of radiation injury. Hence, highly sensitive imaging receptors help to detect such low photon flux.

Components of Fluoroscopic System

The typical fluoroscopic imaging chain consists of a generator, X-ray tube, collimators and filters, grid, image intensifier and video camera system **(Fig. 4)**. The generator, X-ray tube, collimator and grid are similar to radiography system with few differences which are described here.

The generator used for fluoroscopy is similar to that used for radiography with an additional circuit for fluoroscopic procedure.[4] High frequency generator with faster switching is preferred due to its best exposure reproducibility (beneficial for DSA).

The X-ray tube has two focal spots: small (0.3–0.6 mm) and large (1.0–1.2 mm). Small focal spot is used for fluoroscopy as it provides sharp images. For radiographic exposure, either of them can be used. The main additional feature in the tube used for fluoroscopy is the high heat capacity (about 700 kHU) which is needed for prolonged X-ray exposure.[5] This is achieved by high speed anode rotation (above 10000 rpm), oil heat exchanger and cooling fans in the housing assembly and grid controlled exposures. Further, in the modern imaging system, the tube heat loading is constantly monitored which regulates exposure if there is tube overheating. Mobile C-arm systems incorporated with X-ray tubes having fixed anode contain single or dual focal spots (0.5 mm for fluoroscopy and 1.8 mm for radiography) and lower heat capacity (30 to 50 kHU). Modern C-arms have rotating anode for longer fluoroscopy procedures.

Collimators and filters are used to reduce unwanted radiation. One of the filters which needs special mention here is 'equalization filter'. It is used to reduce glare near the edges of the patient. They are partially radiolucent and made of lead-rubber or lead-acrylic material **(Figs. 5A and B)**. To attenuate low energy X-rays (beam hardening), copper filters are preferred over aluminum as they are more effective in filtering low energy X-rays. The grids used in fluoroscopy are of lower ratios (6:1–10:1) compared to that used for radiography (8:1 to 16:1) to limit increase in radiation dose. Some systems provide grids which can be removed when small part of the body is examined or small FOV is used and when II is positioned at a distance from the patient (for access for intervention or difficult anatomical part) which results in air gap. These modes produce less scatter and grid can be avoided to reduce patient radiation dose.

Conventional continuous fluoroscopy involves continuous production of X-rays at low mA and images are acquired at 30 frames per second (fps). Pulsed fluoroscopy (PF) is a mode of operation in which X-rays are generated in pulses (2.5–30 fps) by two methods—generator controlled and tube controlled **(Fig. 6)**. In conventional generator controlled PF the current is supplied to the X-ray tube in short pulses lasting 3–10 milliseconds. However, due to the presence of long high resistance cables between the generator and the tube the pulse has a bell shaped curve (slow rise to peak and fall to zero; **Fig. 7**). This increases the low energy X-rays which results in reduced image quality and no significant decrease in radiation dose, a limitation overcome by grid controlled PF. In grid controlled PF, a negative charge is applied between cathode and anode of X-ray tube in a pulsatile manner which regulates incidence of electrons on the anode **(Fig. 8)**. It produces uniform pulses without any low energy photons **(Fig. 7)**. The advantages of pulsed fluoroscopy are improved temporal resolution (which reduces motion blur) and reduced radiation dose. The disadvantages include increase in noise perception, flicker effect and reduced visibility of fine catheters/guidewires. The flicker effect may be reduced by interleaved image display where gap between two frames are filled by previous images from memory. The reduced radiation dose with pulsed fluoroscopy happens only when mAs remains constant. But often, vendors try to increase the mAs to compensate for increase in noise that occurs with reduced pulse rate. This may result in only modest decrease in radiation dose.

Image Intensifier

The main purpose of image intensifier is to amplify the brightness of the fluoroscopic image, thus obviating the need of dark adaptation by the radiologist. Two important functions of II are fluorescence (conversion of X-ray photons into visible light) and light signal amplification.[6] The basic elements that make an image intensifier are contained in a vacuum case and include input phosphor, photocathode, focussing lenses, anode and output phosphor **(Fig. 9)**. The vacuum case itself is covered by a protective metallic housing which is made of lead to absorb scatter radiation, mu-metal to protect electrostatic lenses from external magnetic forces and an outer aluminum shell. This aluminum shell also covers and protects the input window of the II.

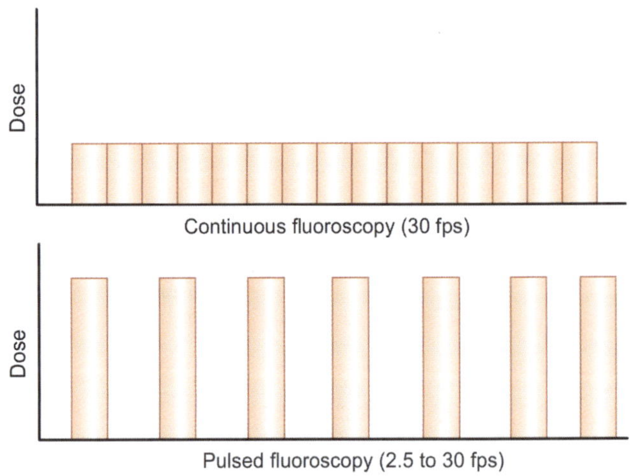

FIG. 6: Schematic diagram comparing continuous and pulsed fluoroscopy. Although there is increase in dose per pulse in the latter to maintain same image details, overall radiation dose is reduced.

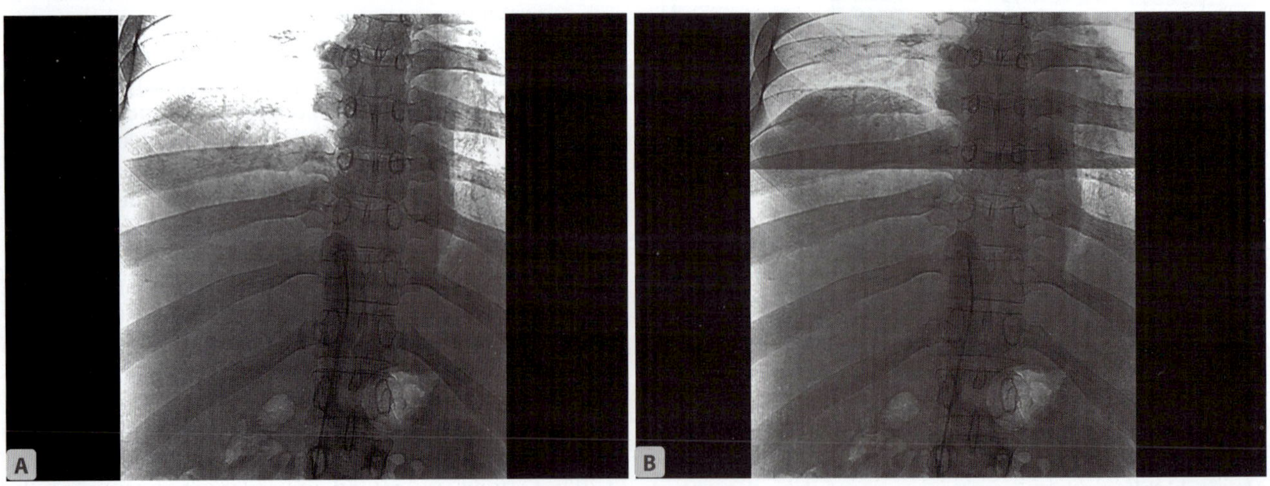

FIGS. 5A AND B: In a patient with inferior venacavogram, veiling glare is seen in the regions of lower lungs affecting the visualization of diaphragm and subdiaphragmatic regions (A). After placement of equalization filter, the glare is significantly reduced with better visualization of diaphragmatic outline (B).

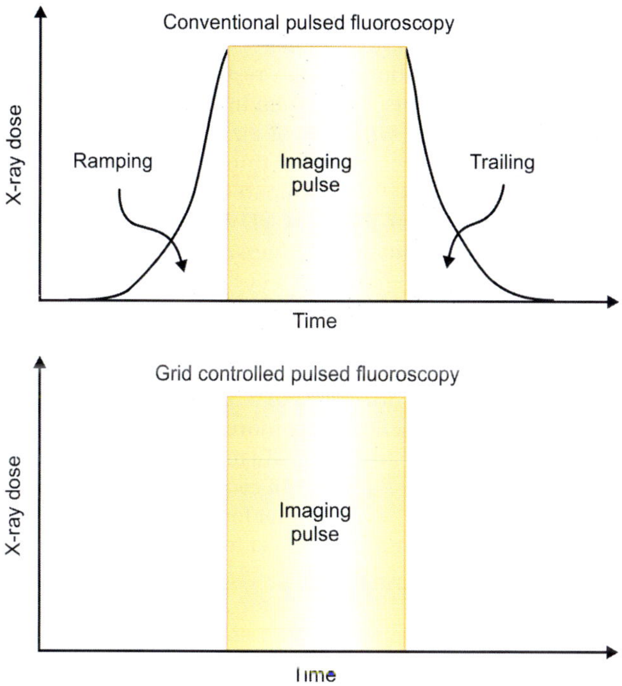

FIG. 7: The pulsing in conventional PF shows initial ramping and terminal trailing leading to generation of low energy X-rays which increases radiation dose. Grid controlled PF shows no such effect.

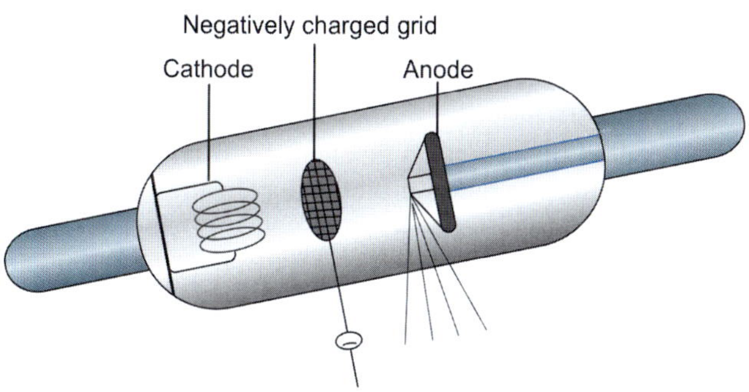

FIG. 8: Grid controlled X-ray tube shows negatively charged grid between cathode and anode which can be switched on and off to control incidence of electrons on anode.

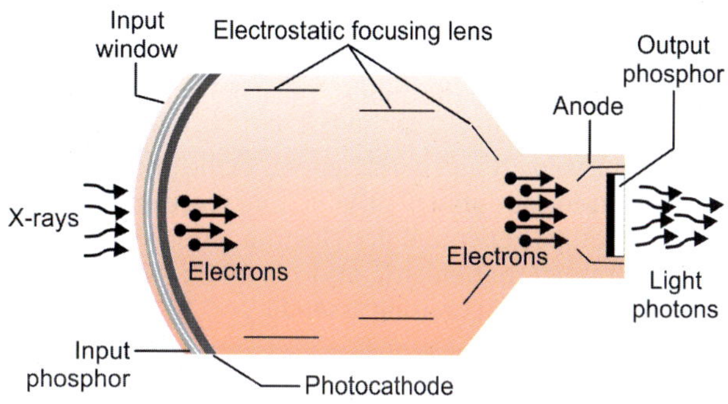

FIG. 9: Schematic diagram of image intensifier.

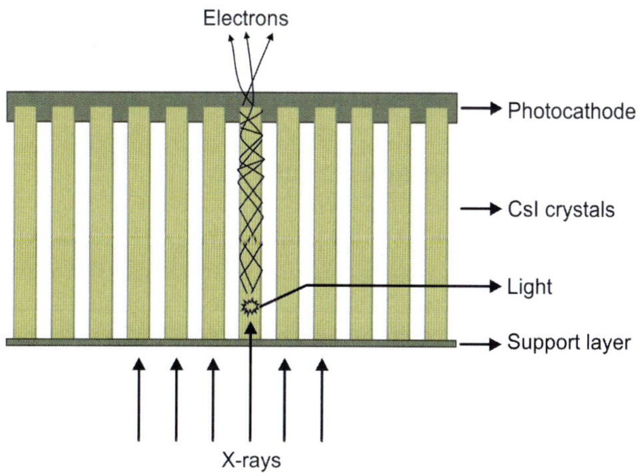

FIG. 10: Schematic diagram of input phosphor of image intensifier showing cesium iodide (CsI) crystals in needle form. This significantly reduces lateral scatter of light photons.

Input Screen

This consists of input window, supporting layer (of aluminum), input phosphor and photocathode. Input window is a part of the vacuum case of II. It is convex in shape and is made of 1 mm thick aluminum. The convex shape reduces II to patient distance and increases field of view. The support layer for input phosphor and photocathode is thin enough to allow all the X-rays to pass through.

The main function of input phosphor is to convert X-ray photons into light photons. In modern equipment, input phosphor is made of cesium iodide-sodium (CsI: Na) **(Fig. 10)**. The advantages of CsI: Na over the previously used zinc cadmium sulphide (ZnCdS) are:

a. *CsI:* Na has a mass attenuation coefficient which better matches with the radiation emitted from the patient than ZnCdS
b. It has higher atomic number resulting in higher X-ray absorption
c. It can be crystallized in needle form which reduces lateral scatter and improves spatial resolution
d. *Light emitted by CsI:* Na has a range which matches with the sensitivity spectrum of the photocathode.

The thickness of the input phosphor is a trade-off between X-ray absorption efficiency (which increases with thickness) and spatial resolution (which decreases with increased thickness due to increased lateral scatter). The thickness in the presently used II is usually between 300 μ and 500 μ with efficiency of 60–70%.

The photocathode is adjacent to the input phosphor and is made of antimony cesium ($SbCs_3$) measuring about 20 mm in thickness. Its production efficiency is about 10–15%. A single X-ray photon of 60 keV incident on the screen is converted into about 2600 light photons of which 1600 reach photocathode, which converts these into approximately 200–300 photoelectrons.

Electrostatic Lens

It consists of 3 sets of focussing electrodes which accelerate the photoelectrons to the anode. The voltage between input and output phosphor is about 25–35 keV. The electrodes increase the velocity and kinetic energy of the photoelectrons incident on output phosphor which increases the number of light photons generated per electron. The electrodes are sensitive to external electric and magnetic fields and are protected by efficient housing assembly.

Output Phosphor and Anode

The output phosphor is a fluorescent compound made of silver activated ZnCdS (ZnCdS: Ag, also called P20). It is in the form of a thin layer (4 μ–8 μ) on the inner aspect of output window of vacuum chamber. About 2000 photons are produced by the output phosphor for every 25 keV photoelectron. The anode is a thin layer of aluminum on the vacuum side of output phosphor surface.

Properties of Image Intensifier

The performance of an II is determined by various characteristics including input size, spatial resolution, brightness gain, conversion factor, contrast ratio and magnification mode.[6] Larger input size provides larger viewing field but increases the cost. Larger sized II are useful in gastrointestinal and genitourinary investigations. The spatial resolution of II is about 4–6 line pairs/mm which increases with magnification.

Brightness gain is defined as the ratio of output luminance of II to that of a fluorescent screen when both are exposed to same level of radiation. This measurement is not reproducible. Hence, actual measurement is a function of two factors: minification gain and flux gain. Minification gain is the ratio of input area to output area of II. Flux gain is defined as number of photons generated by the output phosphor for every photon generated by input phosphor. Brightness gain is the product of minification gain and flux gain. It is usually in the range of 5,000–20,000.

Conversion factor is currently used by many manufacturers for evaluating the efficiency of II. It is defined as the ratio of output luminance level (Cd/m^2) of an II to its entrance exposure rate (μGy/sec). The typical values range from 25–30 Cd-sec/μGy-m^2. The output of an II reduces over time.

Contrast ratio is the ratio of brightness of the periphery to the center of the output window when the center of the II input window is completely blocked by appropriately thick lead disc. It is the measure of veiling glare. The typical values for modern II range from 10:1 to 30:1.

Magnification is performed by collimating to the region of interest thus reducing the field of view at input screen. This however reduces minification gain. To compensate for this, there is increase in exposure at the input screen. Thus when magnification is increased, radiation dose to the patient is also increased.

Limitations of Image Intensifier System

Various drawbacks and artifacts of older II have lead to the development of better systems. However, knowledge of these is important to identify them and take adequate measures to their correction wherever possible.

The II system is bulky which results in some difficulty in positioning patients. The system includes a vacuum tube which is associated with risk of air leak. Air leak affects transmission of electrons and thus image quality. The dynamic range of II is lower compared to flat panel detector (FPD). Magnification reduces FOV and thus increases radiation dose to maintain brightness.

Defocusing is an effect which occurs when electrons do not pass through in proper plane leading to image blurring. It results from alterations in voltage of electrostatic plates which occurs in older systems or by external magnetic field. This drawback also leads to *S distortion*, where effect of the external magnetic field is more on the outer beam of electrons than the central beam. Mu metal protects the plates from external effects, although not completely.

Lag is the delay that occurs after formation of an image by II before it is ready to transmit next image. This reduces the temporal resolution of the system. Older systems had a lag of 30–40 ms, but modern systems have a lag of about 1 ms.

As the input phosphor is convex and the output phosphor is flat, the outer electrons travel a longer path compared to the central ones. This results in two artifacts: vignetting and pincushion distortion. *Vignetting* refers to increased brightness of the center of an image compared to its periphery due to higher concentration of electrons in the center than periphery. *Pincushion* distortion refers to magnification and stretching of the periphery of an image.

Veiling glare or flare occurs due to scattering of light and defocusing of electrons within the II **(Fig. 5A)**. Here, areas of low density like lungs or external air partially occupying the FOV result in high electron flux leading to saturation of the phosphor. This results in difficult visualization of adjacent structures. Glare also occurs for a short time period when image intensifier is moved from a dense area to less dense area till automatic exposure control adjusts the exposure. This can however be significantly reduced by use of pulsed fluoroscopy. Quality control should be done at regular basis to evaluate spatial and contrast resolution and radiation exposure. The resolution and brightness gain of II decrease over time and these need regular monitoring. Further details regarding quality control are described in a different chapter.

Optical Coupling and Video System

The II is optically coupled to a camera which converts light photons from II to voltage signal.[7] This signal is then transmitted to film camera or video camera for viewing. The system consists of an optical distributor and a video system.

Optical Distributor System

The main functions of optical distributor are:

- Transmission of clear focussed image from the output phosphor to all the cameras in the system
- Transmission of images of sufficient intensity/brightness to each camera, and
- Transmission of brightness information to the automatic exposure control (AEC) circuit of the X-ray generator.

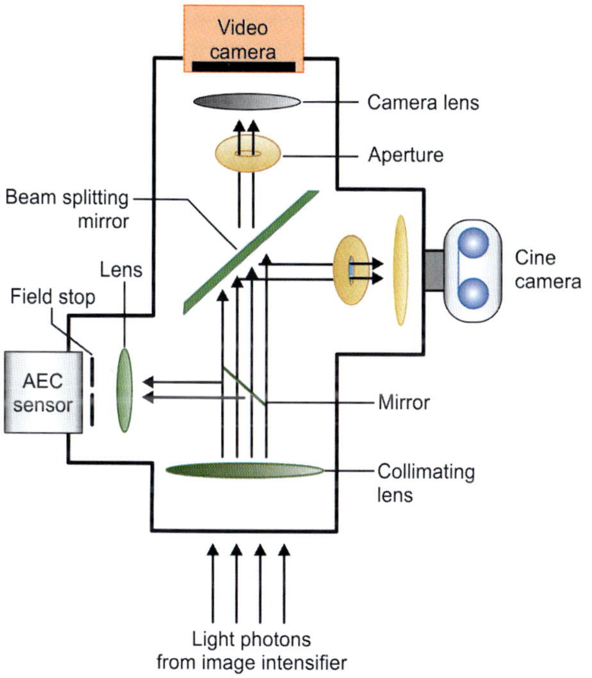

FIG. 11: Optical distributor system with its components.

The system consists of a series of mirrors, lenses and camera apertures **(Fig. 11)**.

Beam splitting mirror is partially silvered and splits the light beam exiting the output phosphor through collimating lens into two, one reaching the film camera for recording and the other to video camera for viewing. There is an additional small mirror or prism between the collimating lens and beam splitting mirror which transmits part of the light beam to AEC sensor. The AEC sensor uses a field stop between it and its lens to prevent the periphery of the light beam, which is not usually the area of interest, reaching the sensor to determine exposure.

Two types of lenses are present in the optical coupling system. The collimator lens is located at a distance from the output phosphor equal to the focal length of the lens. The light beam exiting the lens is collimated and parallel. Camera lens is present in each of the camera used in the system and is located at a distance equal to its focal length form the camera target.

The light beam reaching the camera lens is controlled by camera aperture or iris. The aperture determines the speed of the system which is a measure of total X-ray exposure needed to produce a proper image on camera. It is designated by f-number. Faster the speed, lesser is the X-ray exposure required. The apertures used can either be fixed or adjustable. Fixed apertures are usually used where detected X-ray exposure level is same across patients as in film cameras. But in video cameras, the X-ray exposure varies from low levels in fluoroscopy to high levels in angiography and thus need an adjustable aperture (motor driven iris). Sometimes, additional neutral filter may be needed to prevent overexposure at high doses.

Every region in the light beam from the collimating lens contains information from all points of output phosphor.

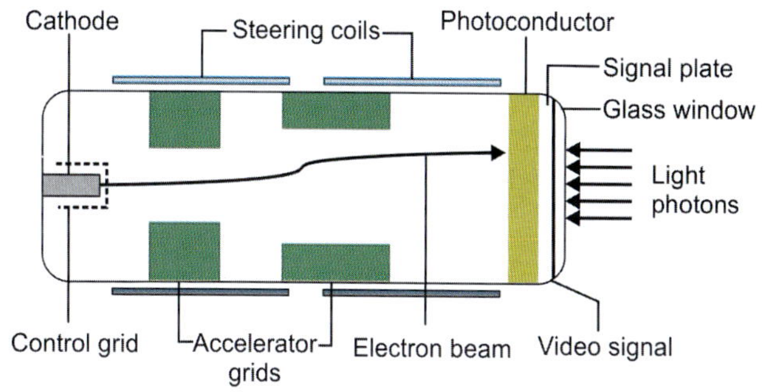

FIG. 12: Video camera pick-up tube and its components.

Hence, mirrors and apertures placed between two lenses are not visualized on the image.

Video System

This plays role in image display and recording and also provides input to the digital processor. It includes a camera head which converts light image into voltage signal and a camera control unit which process the voltage signal for display and digitization **(Fig. 12)**.

Two types of devices are used for signal generation, older vacuum tube sensor (pickup tube) and the modern CCD sensor. The pickup tube contains a photoconductor which absorbs the light photons to generate electron-hole pairs within it. The electric field placed across the target causes the holes to move towards the inner surface of the target. The hole density, which is proportional to the light image intensity, is measured by focussed electron beam and converted into voltage signal constituting the video output of the pickup tube. The photoconductor used include antimony trisulfide (SbS_3; Vidicon), lead oxide (Plumbicon) or a composite of amorphous selenium, arsenic and tellurium (Saticon). Plumbicon has very low lag time with good temporal resolution and hence used in cardiac angiography. Saticon has the advantage of linear response to light intensity. In CCD system, the target (Thallium doped Cesium Iodide) generates electron-hole pairs but the electrons accumulate in potential wells depending on the intensity of the light photons incident on it. The charge is then transferred to adjacent storage region where it is readout to generate an image. CCD is better than the pickup tube as it results in better dynamic range (12-bit depth), higher SNR and contrast resolution thus reduced patient dose. Its linear response is very useful in subtraction imaging. Further it is compact, robust, consumes less electricity, lacks maintenance and is not associated with lag phenomenon and geometric distortion. Currently, CCD cameras are available for both fluoroscopy and angiography systems.

Two operating properties of video system are lag and linearity. *Lag* refers to the time delay in the output of the video system in response to the changes in the input sensor of the video camera. CCD cameras have no lag. In pickup tubes, lag varies with high values seen in those using SbS_3 as target material. Lag is also higher in dark parts of the image than bright parts. Lag results in blurring of moving objects. One advantage of higher lag is significant reduction in image

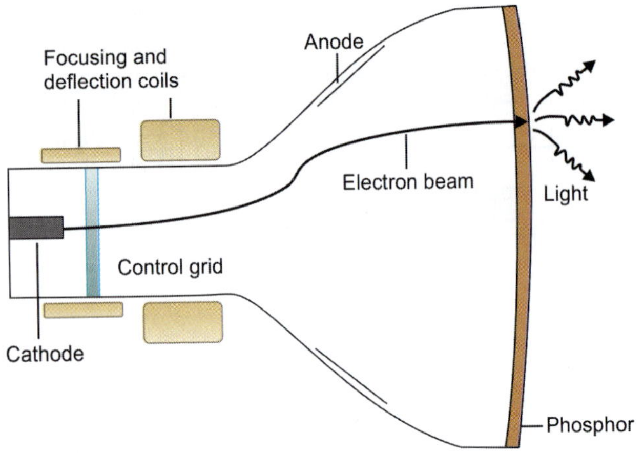

FIG. 13: Television picture tube and its operation.

noise, which is high in CCD cameras. *Linearity* indicates relationship between light input and video signal output. A nonlinear response is desirable as smaller signals are better amplified.

The video output signal from the target (pickup tube or CCD) is converted into one-dimensional voltage signal which is displayed on the monitor by raster scanning **(Fig. 13)**. Here, the voltage signal is scanned in a horizontal line from one end to the other, which is terminated by H-sync signal moving the scanning to next line. Once the whole screen is filled by horizontal lines, the V-sync signal shifts the scanning to the top of the image to restart scanning. H-sync and V-sync pulses produce dead time, equal to about 15% of the total horizontal period for the former and 7% of the total vertical period for the latter. The video scanning may be done in continuous manner (line 1, line 2, line 3 etc. in order) or interlaced manner (odd lines first followed by even lines). The standard scanning mode of a conventional video is 30 fps, 525 lines per frame and 2:1 interlaced video. Modern systems employ 60 fps and above and scan conversion for improved visualization. One has to note that this frame rate is different from the frame rate of X-ray generator.

The spatial resolution of fluoroscopic equipment is determined by the size of focal spot, the II, the digital system and the video system. The resolution of video system has two components: vertical resolution and horizontal resolution. Vertical resolution is determined by the number of horizontal lines on the screen and measured in terms of line pairs per mm. It is calculated by taking into account the size of II, magnification and number of lines of horizontal scanning. Older systems employed 525 lines per scan height but modern angiography system use 1049 lines. Horizontal resolution of video system is decided by the bandwidth of the system. A low-pass filter limits the bandwidth preventing too low or too high values thus ensuring that horizontal resolution matches vertical resolution. The bandwidth ranges from 4.5 MHz for 525 line system to 18 MHz for 1049 line system at 30 fps. Currently, many equipment use 1023-line raster line video system with liquid crystal display (LCD) monitor.

Digital Fluoroscopy

The initial fluoroscopic systems used cassettes for documentation of images. This resulted in high film usage, lag time between cassette changes and delay in viewing the spot films. Further, conventional fluoroscopic systems are associated with longer examination times, higher radiation doses, need for repetition of acquisitions due to nonavailability of postprocessing, need for multitasking (turning on fluoroscopy, cassette changes, patient positioning) by radiologist and more staff. These problems are surmounted by the development of digital fluoroscopy which is easy to use, provides better image quality by post processing, reduced examination time and radiation dose.

The main principle behind digital fluoroscopy is conversion of analog video signal into digital data using an analog-to-digital convertor (ADC).[2] Other methods of digitization are use of CCD cameras and flat panel detectors. The fundamental theory of digital imaging included binary numbers, pixels and gray levels. Binary system uses two digits i.e, 0 and 1 the values of which are determined by the number of digits (bits). A 2-bit number has 2^2 or 4 values (00, 01, 10, 11). A 3-bit number (000–111) can have 2^3 or 8 values, 4-bit number (0000–1111) 2^4 or 16 values, 8-bit number 2^8 or 256 values and so on. Each pixel in an image has a position, size and value. Pixel size is determined by field of view (FOV) and matrix size. Smaller the pixel size better is the resolution and sharper are the images. This can be done by increasing the matrix and/or reducing the FOV **(Figs. 14A to D)**. Pixel value is the gray level of the image. The range of grayscale in an image depends on the bit depth of the system. Higher the bit depth, better is the contrast resolution **(Figs. 15A to C)**.

The ADC system collects the output signal of the video camera at regular intervals and converts it into binary values (0 and 1) for storage. The range of values depends on the bit depth of the ADC (e.g. an 8-bit ADC displays 2^8 or 256 values) and are expressed as varying grayscale intensity. The resolution of ADC system is determined by the resolution of the video camera which is about 1–2 lp/mm. The digital image thus formed can be stored for subsequent printing on film. Further the images can be processed to improve visualization.

CCD cameras have substantially reduced the size of the bulky video system. As mentioned in previous section, the CCDs convert light signal from the scintillator into electrical charges which is readout and transmitted to the monitor. The CCDs have a resolution of 1.7 lp/mm. Flat panel detectors (described later) used in some of the modern fluoroscopy systems do not need a video system.[8] They directly or indirectly convert X-ray photons incident on them into electronic signals which is displayed on the monitor. The electronic signal generated varies with the intensity of incident X-ray photons. With both these systems, ADC digitizes the signal for display and storage.

Postprocessing Techniques

Last image hold (LIH) is an important feature of digital fluoroscopy. The last image/frame of cine fluoroscopy at which imaging stops, is captured and continuously displayed on the monitor even after switching-off the fluoroscopy.

This image can be transferred to reference monitor and is used for guidance without additional radiation to the patient and medical staff. This is applicable for static objects. For areas which are in motion (e.g. cardiac imaging) *fluoroscopy loop* can be captured and made available for review when needed. Here, the last 150 to 300 frames or about 10 seconds of fluoroscopy can be saved. The LIH is also used as a reference image for making adjustments in the position of the patient table or the C-arm with the outline of the image moving with movement of the equipment. This reduces the additional need of radiation.

Grayscale processing involves adjustment of brightness and contrast of the image. This is done by adjusting two values: window level and window width. Window level is the central value of the grayscale range of the image and window width is the range displayed on either sides of window level. For example, window level of 80 and window width of 50 means the central value of grayscale is 80 and 25 grayscale values can be visualized on either side of 80 (55 to 105) beyond which the image is either black or white. The level and width are adjusted depending on the region of interest with darker objects needing lower window level, brighter objects higher window level and soft tissues needing higher window width values.

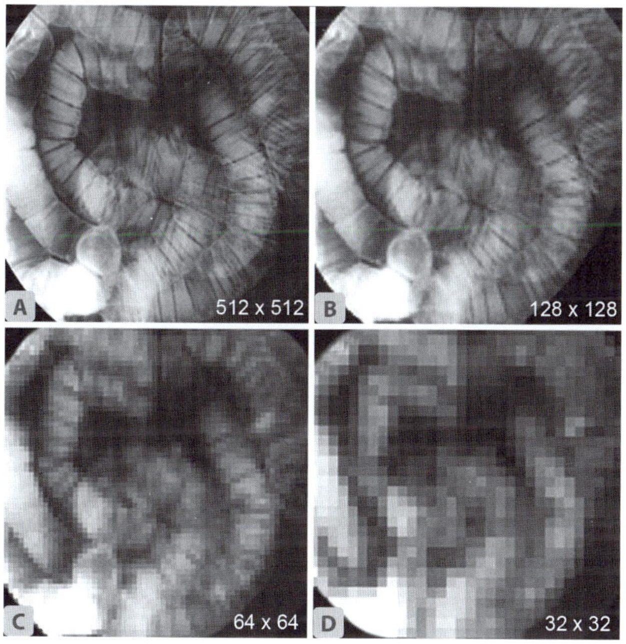

FIGS. 14A TO D: Spatial resolution of fluoroscopic image at various matrix sizes. Note the decrease in spatial resolution as matrix size is reduced.

Temporal frame averaging is a feature to reduce image noise. Here two or more images are averaged to form a single image with less noise. The drawback of this property is the image lag in dynamic fluoroscopic imaging, but may be useful for static images. *Edge enhancement* increases the sharpness of the image and may be used to make the lesion more conspicuous.

Measurement of distance of objects can be done on digital image. This usually needs calibration by measuring known dimension of a reference object (e.g. catheter) in the field of view. The machine calculates this in terms of number of pixels and uses it as reference for distance measurements on the image. Other techniques which are available include black-white reversal, image flip (horizontal/vertical), electronic shutter and annotation.

DIGITAL SUBTRACTION ANGIOGRAPHY

Digital subtraction angiography (DSA) refers to a digital imaging technique for better visualization of contrast filled vessels.[9] This technique permits use of lower amount of contrast medium. Here, the precontrast image is digitally subtracted from post-contrast image to provide background suppression. This allows better visualization of low contrast vessels, but at a cost of increase in noise. Usually the effect of noise is overcome by averaging two or more frames. Thus, this technique (subtraction) increases the noise which is countered by increased mA (compared to unsubtracted image).

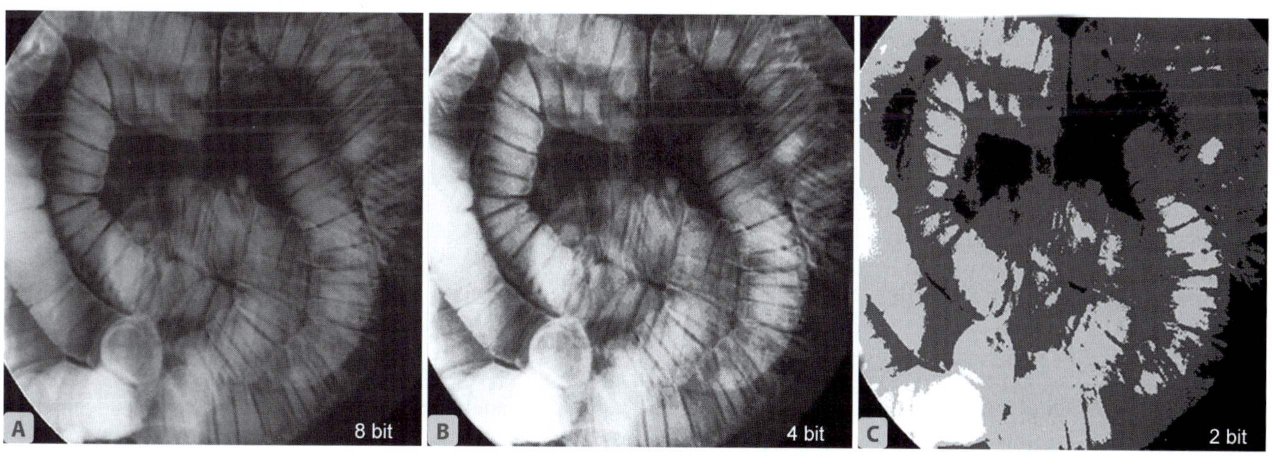

FIGS. 15A TO C: Contrast resolution of fluoroscopic image at various bit depths. Note the drastic fall in contrast resolution with reduction in bit depth (range of grayscale).

Types of Subtraction

The types of subtraction techniques include mask mode, time interval, dual energy and hybrid subtractions.

Mask-mode subtraction is the most widely used process of DSA in which temporal subtraction is done **(Figs. 16A to C)**. It involves initial acquisition of a frame of region of interest which is used to stabilize the exposure factors. Then a second image is taken and stored as mask image. This mask image is subtracted from subsequently acquired images on pixel-by-pixel basis and show only contrast filled structures. If any movement occurs after acquisition of mask image, misregistration occurs in the subtracted images. This can be overcome to some extent by pixel shifting.

Time interval difference subtraction is another mode of temporal subtraction where a consecutive previous frame is subtracted from current frame (e.g, frame 1 from frame 2, frame 2 from frame 3 and so on). This technique is very useful in cardiac imaging where there is rapid motion. The images obtained can then be stacked to provide a composite image without motion.

Dual energy subtraction is another technique in which the region of interest is exposed to higher kV (120 to 130 kV) and lower kV (70 kV) at very short interval (about 50 ms). Then, the higher kV image is subtracted from the lower kV image to produce an iodine and bone image (the soft tissue and gas shadows are eliminated). This technique has the advantage of elimination of motion artifacts. The limitations of this mode of subtraction include increased radiation dose, reduced opacity of contrast opacified structures, reduced SNR and increased complexity of the equipment.

Hybrid subtraction is a combination of dual energy and temporal subtraction.

Techniques Used in DSA

Road map is a technique in which static fluoroscopic image is subtracted from densely opacified vessel. Here, a short contrast run of the vessel is done under fluoroscopy to select the frame with maximum opacification of the vessel as the road map mask, which is stored in memory. Then subsequent live fluoroscopic image is subtracted from the road map mask for visualization of the vessel and the catheter/guide wire **(Figs. 17A and B)**. This technique is very useful in placement of catheters and guidewires in complex and small vessels. Motion after road map acquisition may affect subsequent intervention. Another similar technique is *fluoroscopy fade* in which a reference DSA image is overlaid on the real time fluoroscopic image. Dynamic 3D road mapping which is new development allows projection of 3D reconstructed vessel on live 2D fluoroscopic image. *Dynamic road map* is a new software which helps in providing real-time motion compensated images for guiding catheterization and interventions in real-time. This is helpful in regions showing motion artifacts-cardiac or respiratory. Due to motion correction, the road-map appears still allowing guidance for wires and catheters.

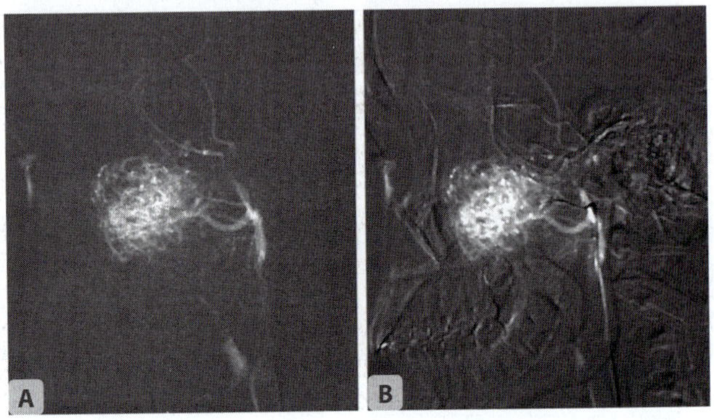

FIGS. 17A AND B: Road map in a case of preoperative embolization of nasopharyngeal angiofibroma. Subtracted fluoroscopic image with maximum contrast opacification is stored as mask image (A) and subsequent images are subtracted from mask image to visualize the guide wire/catheter within the opacified vessel (B).

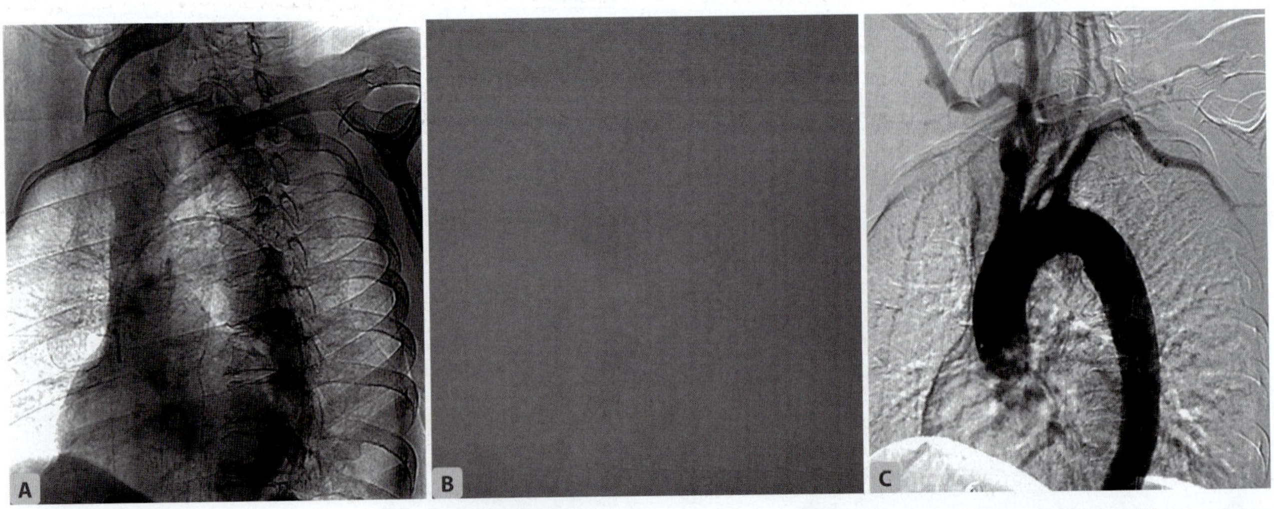

FIGS. 16A TO C: Mask mode subtraction. (A) Initial image stored as mask. (B) First subtracted image without any bones or vessels. (C) Subtracted aortogram depicting only vessels.

Peripheral DSA can be performed with single contrast injection using *stepping technique*. This is of two types. In stepping table technique, the table moves into three stations with X-ray tube and detector remaining fixed. In stepping gantry method, the tube-detector/II moves keeping the table fixed. In both methods, precontrast images are acquired at different stations and stored as mask image. Subsequently, matching postcontrast injection images are taken at same positions while chasing the bolus of contrast and subtracted from the corresponding mask image to produce clear image of peripheral arteries. The benefits of this technique are significantly reduced use of contrast and reduced examination time. The main disadvantage is increased chances of movement between precontrast and postcontrast images.

An important advancement in digital fluoroscopy is *rotational angiography* where the X-ray tube-detector system rotates through usually 90°–180° while acquiring continuous images.[10] Rotational angiography was available with II systems too. But with improvements in mechanical aspects of systems (rotation) and availability of faster detectors today they produce good quality images **(Figs. 18A and B)**. Mask images are initially acquired at 0.8° to 2° gaps followed by postcontrast rotation and acquisition at same positions. Then DSA images are produced at each angle and reconstructed to produce 3D angiograms. The same technique without subtraction is used in some systems to provide axial images (volume or cone beam CT; **Fig. 18C**). The volume data acquired is reconstructed in different planes at a predetermined thickness. This helps in accurate planning of complicated interventions, but at the cost of higher radiation dose. Also, the images have very low contrast resolution due to higher proportion of scatter radiation (due to divergent beam or cone beam).

Postprocessing in DSA

Mask pixel shift is a software modification feature used when smaller patient motion occurs after the mask image is acquired. By shifting the pixels of the mask image, reregistering of the mask with post contrast image is possible thus obviating motion artifacts **(Figs. 19A and B)**. This technique may be manual or automatic. *Remask* is a similar feature where another mask image is selected, which is temporally closer to the contrast image. This is useful when patient motion occurs prior to contrast image, but after initiation of the acquisition.

Image summation is a property in which two or more frames of a DSA acquisition are summed into a single image **(Figs. 20A to C)**. This is beneficial when rapid acquisition opacifies part of a vessel in each frame and summation adds up the frames to produce a single image showing the entire vessel. Stacking is a similar technique used in carbon dioxide angiography where the fragmented boluses of the gas are added to produce a complete picture of the opacified structure.

Land marking is a feature in which lesser intensity (10–20%, but is manually adjustable) of original image is added to the subtracted image **(Figs. 21A to C)**. This provides anatomical landmarks in subtracted images, useful in subsequent intervention.

Flat Panel Detector

Even after their availability in early 90s, the use of flat panel detectors (FPD) in fluoroscopy was delayed due to the requirement of rapid recording and read out process.

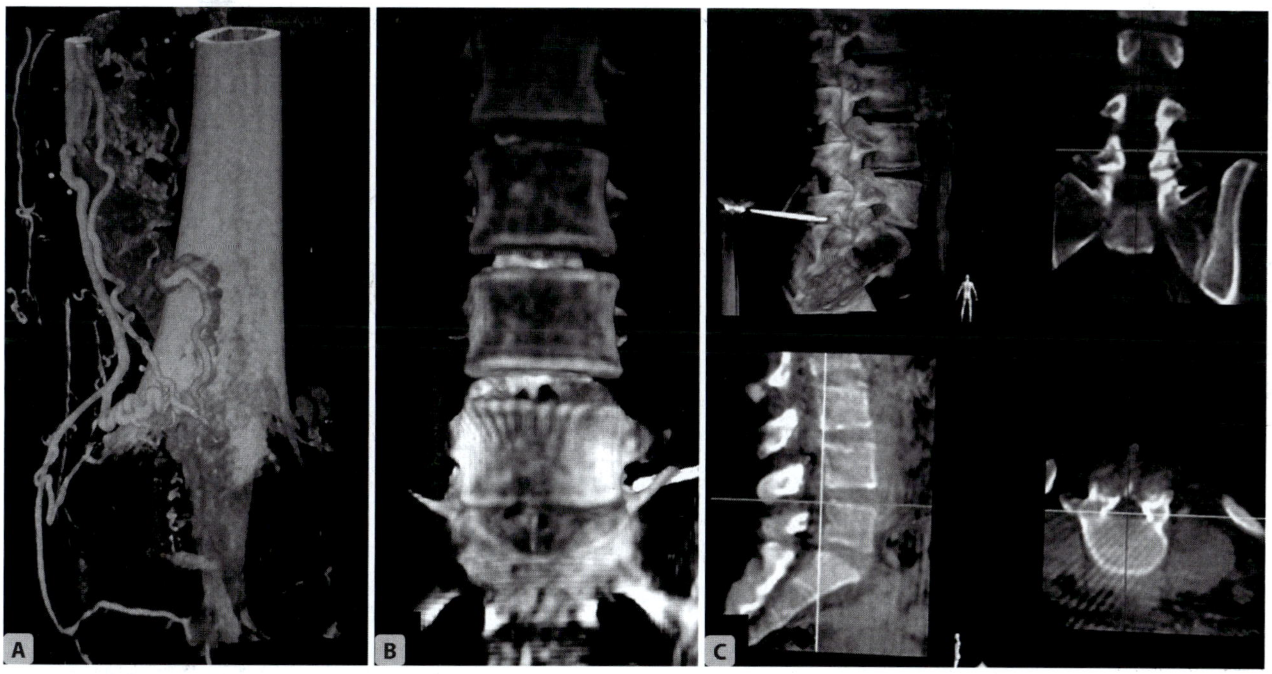

FIGS. 18A TO C: 3D rotational angiography image (A) acquired during contrast injection with rotation of the tube and detector in a case of arteriovenous fistula of lower limb. (B) lumbar spine during disc intervention. Note the images are of high contrast without soft tissue visualization. Cone beam CT (C) is similar with the ability of multiplanar reconstructions

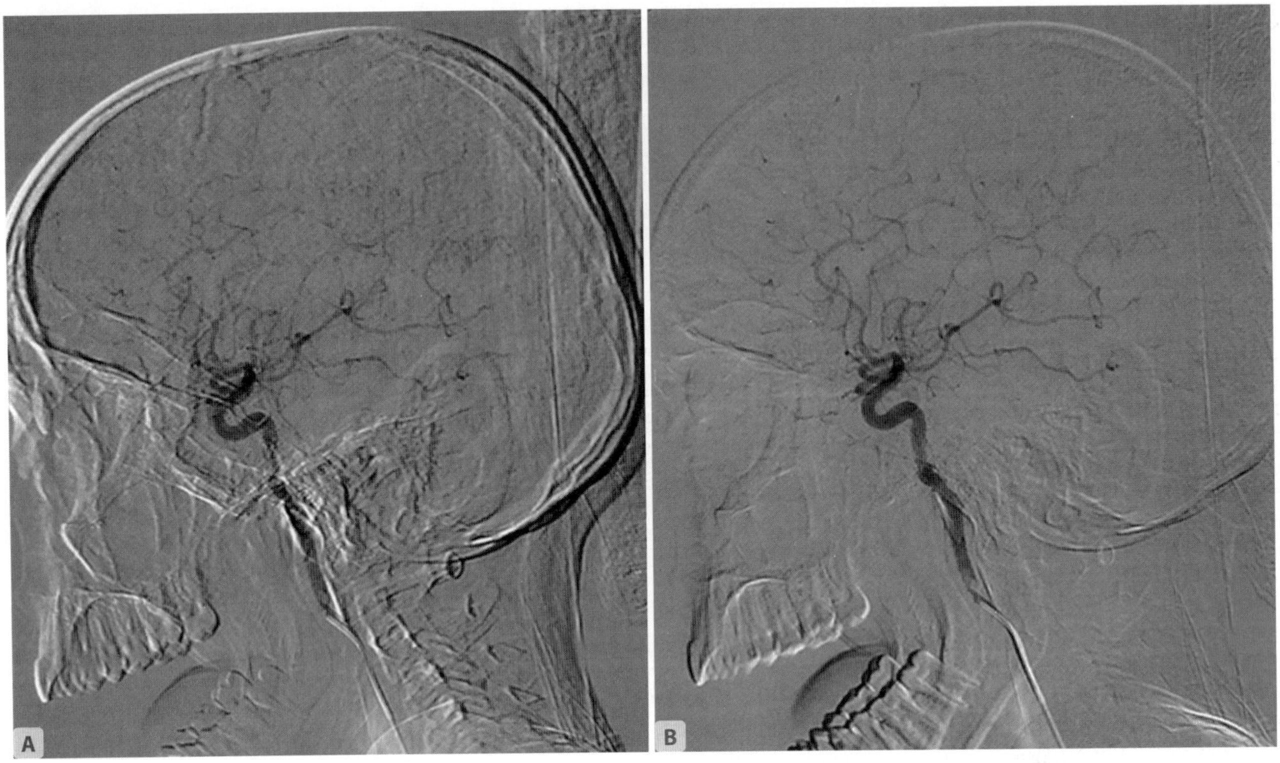

FIGS. 19A AND B: Motion after acquiring mask image results in misregistration and degradation of image quality (A). This can be partially overcome by pixel shift technique (B).

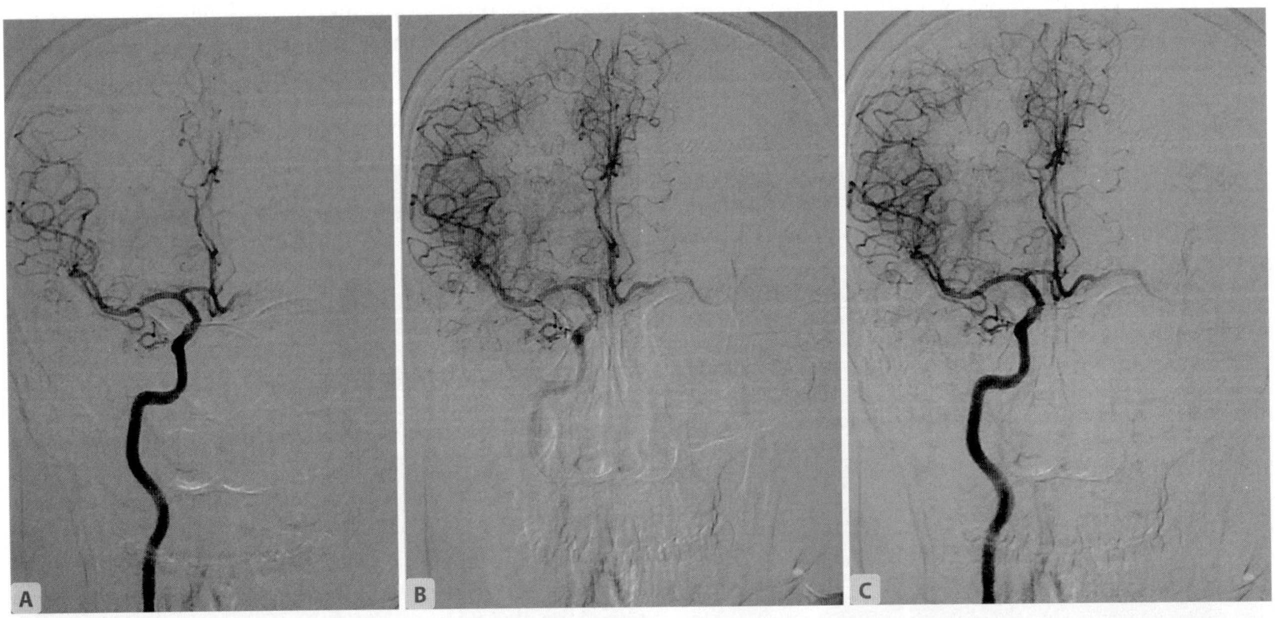

FIGS. 20A TO C: (A and B) Partial opacification of right internal carotid artery and its branches which can be overcome by summation technique (C) which adds the images to provide a composite image.

The first commercial unit was made available in 2001 intended for cardiac imaging.[11]

Flat panel detector is the modern solid-state detector array which is used as image receptor.[8] The detector consists of an array of detector elements (DELs), the size of which range from 140 µm to 200 µm. Each DEL consists of photodiodes or capacitors and thin film transistors (made of hydrogenated amorphous silicon) depending on the type of conversion. The total size of the detector varies from 25 × 25 cm to 43 × 43 cm and thus each FPD may house 1.5–5 million individual DELs. This feature is responsible for the high cost of FPD. Thus they are mainly used in interventional angiography suites and

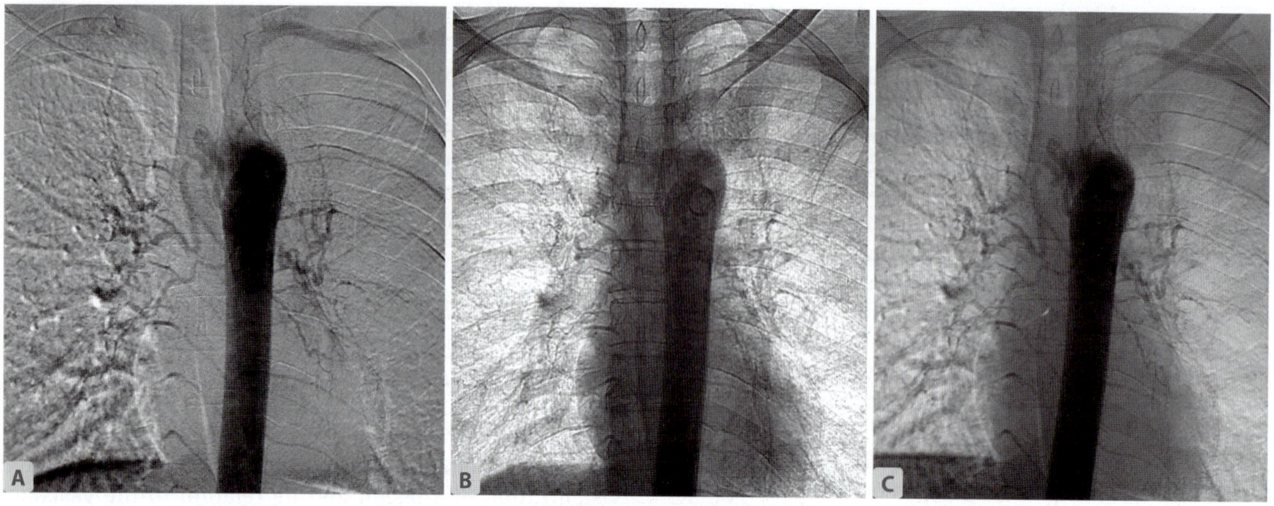

FIGS. 21A TO C: (A) Subtracted aortogram with bronchial and intercostal arteries without bony landmarks. Conventional image (B) although shows bones well, the arteries are not well seen. Land marking (C) shows both the arteries and bones.

rarely for diagnostic fluoroscopy. The X-rays passing through the patient are directly incident on the FPD and its DELs. This process generates an electronic signal either indirectly or directly **(Figs. 22A and B)**.

Indirect system FPDs consist of DELs which contain a scintillation layer made of thallium-activated cesium iodide (CsI:Tl). The CsI is arranged in the form of crystals which convert incident X-rays into light signal, intensity of which depends on the amount of incident X-ray flux. Cesium (Z = 55) and Iodine (Z = 53) have high atomic numbers and thus good X-ray absorption property. The arrangement of CsI is in the form of closely packed needle shaped crystals which reduces scatter and thus improves spatial resolution. Hence, thicker layers (550 μ–650 μ) can be used which reduced patient dose. The DQE of CsI is in the range of 60–70%. The light signal from scintillator is then transmitted to the adjacent photodiode-transistor layer (contained in thin layer of hydrogenated amorphous silicon–aSi:H) which generates electronic signal depending on the light intensity. Majority of current systems (Siemens, Philips, GE) use this type of detector in combination with grid controlled pulsed fluoroscopy.

Direct system FPDs directly convert incident X-rays into electric signal. These detectors are made of amorphous selenium (a-Se) in aSi:H matrix. Selenium has lower atomic number (Z = 34) and hence lower X-ray absorption efficiency. Thus thicker layers (up to 1000 μ) are needed to avoid increase in radiation dose. Higher thickness results in partial loss of charge as it travels to the storage material. Also, increased noise aliasing is encountered with direct conversion. Higher voltages (~10 kV) which need to be applied across the detector may damage the TFT. Shimadzu and Toshiba manufacture direct conversion fluoroscopic systems.

The process of image formation by FPDs is different from other methods. Here, each DEL is connected to a capacitor which is fully charged initially. During X-ray exposure, the capacitor discharges its stored charge, the amount of which depends on the intensity of the incident X-ray flux. Once exposure is over, the read out electronics measure the change in the charge of all the capacitors in the FPD to produce

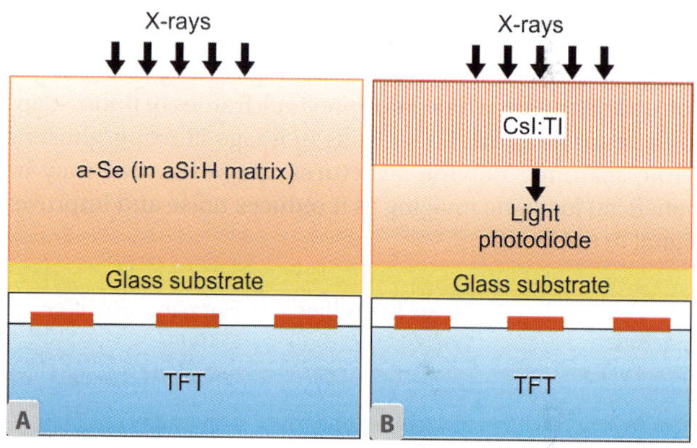

FIGS. 22A AND B: Basic structure of flat panel detector, with direct conversion (A) and indirect conversion (B).

an image. Subsequently, a light is flashed to discharge the capacitors before fully charging them again. This process is repeated many times per second.

Advantages and Limitations of FPD Systems

The FPD is small, compact and reliable. Most of the artifacts associated with image intensifier systems are not seen with FPD. As DELs are arranged in rows and columns, S-distortions and pincushion artifacts are not encountered. The digital detector system ensures excellent uniformity which obviates vignetting. The fixed positions of DELs prevent defocusing effects. The detector directly produces an electronic signal and a television camera is not needed. The digital system reduces image noise. The FPD has larger dynamic range than II (14-bit vs 4-6-bit) and hence flare or veiling glare is usually not seen. The DQE (ratio of number of detected photons to number of incident photons) of FPD is better than that of II.

The limitations of the FPD system include increased cost of the detector and difficulty in manufacturing FPD not containing defective DELs. The data from such DELs are interpolated by software which results in some artifacts.

The FPDs are temperature and mechanical shock sensitive, changes in which may damage the detector elements.

The spatial resolution of FPD is about 2.5–3.4 lp/ mm which is lower than that of II (4–6 lp/min; although the effective displayed resolution is 1–1.2 lp/mm). The resolution is limited by size of DELs (pitch) and by binning. Although reducing the size of DELs may improve spatial resolution, this happens at a cost of increase in radiation, as the effective readable surface area (which actually forms image or fill factor) is reduced. This increases image noise which is overcome by increasing radiation. Further with larger FOV, large numbers of elements are activated which substantially increases data transfer rates difficult to be handled by the system. To surmount this limitation, manufacturers carry out a process called *binning* for large FOVs where data from four DELs are grouped to form a single data (similar to single DEL). This reduces spatial resolution but also reduces noise. Further, magnification with FPD system also increases radiation dose to reduce noise, but to a lesser extent than that of II.

Another limitation of FPD system (and also II system) is 'ghosting'. This occurs because of the persistence of previous image in the scintillation crystal as a ghost and thus affects image quality. Another reason for ghosting is recursive software filtration which adds previous frames of fluoroscopy to the current frame. This results in image blurring/ghosting while scanning moving structures. However, this may be beneficial for static imaging as it reduces noise and improves signal to noise ratio.

Features	Image intensifier system	Flat panel detector system
Size	Large and bulky	Small and compact
Construction	In vacuum tube (risk of air leak)	Solid state
Cost	Cheaper	Expensive
Defocussing effect	Present	Absent
Pincushion effect	Present	Absent
S distortion	Present	Absent
Vignetting	Present	Absent
Veiling glare	Present	Absent
Resolution of II	About 5 lp/mm	2.5–3 lp/mm
Dynamic range	Lower (30:1)	Higher (14-bit or 2^{14}:1)
Television system	Needed; Low resolution (1-1.2 lp/mm)	Not needed
Image noise	High	Low

Advanced Features of FPD Systems

2D Perfusion Angiography

This is a new and evolving technique which involves assessment of temporal change in the density of a region of interest during angiography.[12] This provides quantitative information on the perfusion characteristics of the region in two dimensions without additional need of contrast or radiation. The density changes are color coded for better visualization. The quantitative values obtained are mean transit time (MTT), time to peak (TTP), peak density (PD) and area under the curve.[13] It has major role in assessing the result of an interventional procedure. Its applications are in peripheral vascular disease, neurovascular disease and oncology. Measurement of a change in the density of the tissue or tumor helps in assessing if an intervention revascularization or embolization—is successful and to what extent.

3D and 4D Digital Subtraction Angiography

The 3D-DSA is the same as rotational angiography, where the C-arm rotates around the region of interest for 200° with multiple acquisitions during contrast injection. The images are postprocessed to generate 3D volume rendered images and multiplanar reconstructions. This helps in better visualization of a lesion and its relation to the vascular structures.[14,15] Furthermore, the data can be used for 3D printing which may help the surgeon in proper planning of the treatment.[16]

An advancement over 3D DSA is the availability of 4D DSA where the acquired images are time resolved to overcome the limitation of 3D DSA, i.e. obscuration of multiple overlapping vascular structures. In 4D DSA, an algorithm allows the reconstruction of the high frame rate (up to 30/s) images obtained during 3D DSA into multiple volumes of different time points (similar to a time resolved MR angiography).[17] This helps in better visualization of the vascular structures in multiple phases. It is shown to be useful in the evaluation of arteriovenous malformations. Further, this technique can provide information on the blood flow velocity within the vessel.

Fusion Imaging

Although 3D rotational angiography technique is available in many of the current angiography systems, its utility is limited by lower soft tissue contrast. Due to this, details of smaller lesions and lesions close to bony structures may not be accurately mapped. This can be overcome by the availability of fusion imaging, wherein images of prior scans (CT scan or MRI, usually the latter) of the patient are fused with the 3D or 4D DSA images.[18-20] Further, the CT or MR images can be superimposed on the live fluoroscopy image. Similarly ultrasonography images may also be fused with the fluoroscopic images (e.g. transthoracic echocardiography with cardiac interventions). This provides a better roadmap of the lesion and assists in preforming the interventional procedure better. This has found application in neurointerventions and interventions of the aorta and peripheral arteries and in venous interventions.

Other Advanced Softwares

Embolization Guide

This helps in identification of the feeding artery of a lesion on a 3D rotational angiography. Then, with a single click, it shows the path which the catheter has to take to reach the target. This helps in embolization of an aneurysm or tumor.

Stent Live

This software greatly improves visualization of a vascular stent during deployment in areas susceptible to excessive motion, e.g. coronary stent. This allows for accurate positioning of the stent.

Further, many current systems have softwares to add different 3D angulations required to view a vessel or lesion in profile in the memory so that the same position can be obtained later when necessary at the press of a button.

Hybrid Labs

Angio-CT suite is a system where the angiography machine is integrated with a CT machine through a common patient table.[21] Here, the CT gantry slides around the patient table as and when a CT scan is necessary during angiographic procedure. This single hybrid system facilitates utilization of two modalities in a single room and avoids patient transfer. Although rotational angiography/cone beam CT provides volume information, its soft tissue contrast is lower and images are degraded by beam hardening artifacts. With hybrid lab, the CT images can be overlaid on live fluoroscopy images and thus assists in the interventional procedure.

Its applications are mainly in situations where both CT and DSA are required for optimal patient management. This is encountered in trauma patients needing imaging with angiographic intervention when both can be done on the same table without having to shift the patient. Other situations include stroke interventions and chemoembolization for liver tumors.[22]

Automatic Exposure Control

Regulation of radiation exposure to image detector is needed in fluoroscopy and image documentation.[23] Automatic exposure control (AEC) frees the operator from adjusting kVp and mA to obtain optimal penetrated and bright image. A feedback signal is provided by an ionization chamber in case of spot films or photodiode in case of cameras. The signal is then stored in a capacitor until a predefined value is reached when the exposure is terminated. This principle is followed during recording of images. For fluoroscopy, the exposure is not terminated but continuously compared with a reference value and regulated accordingly. This technique is usually referred as automatic brightness control (ABC). Another method is to use the TV video output signal as feedback to X-ray generator. The exposure rate is adjusted by varying kVp, mAs and X-ray pulse width. ABC has a response time of 1 to 1.5 sec. This can be overcome by the use of automatic gain control (AGC). In AGC, TV camera electronically increases the brightness of the image on the monitor when it is dim and noisy. This only maintains brightness and does not change radiation exposure. The lag time for AGC is in terms of milliseconds. Dynamic density optimization (DDO) is a real time pre-processing algorithm which results in uniform Grayscale distribution across the image in both fluoroscopy and DSA.

Recording Fluoroscopic Images

A number of techniques are available for recording and storing fluoroscopic images.[23] They are broadly classified into three types. They include direct film recording, indirect recording and recording of motion.

Direct Film Recording

Here, as the name suggests, the images are directly exposed on photographic films located in front of II. Two types of devices do this type of image recording.

Spot film devices use conventional screen-film cassettes for documenting images. The cassette is parked out of the way during routine fluoroscopy and during acquisition moves into the field. The images can be documented in different formats (from 1 to 6 images) on a single film, which has a resolution of about 7 lp/mm and speed of 400. The limitations include inability to use larger sized cassettes (14" × 17") and delay that occurs during acquisition for the cassette to move into the field.

Automatic film changers are mounted on II and include a supply magazine containing unexposed films (up to 30 films), pair of high speed screens, a receiving magazine which receives exposed films and a motor system for moving films (usually at a maximum rate of 4 films/second). The films have a resolution of 5 lp/mm and speed of 800 which reduces radiation dose. The disadvantages include use of only single film size, delay in documentation, motion blurring, film fogging and jamming and missed exposures.

Indirect Recording

These devices are placed behind the II and hence called indirect recording. This can be done by photofluorography and digital fluorography.

Photofluorography allows rapid filming up to an extent of 12 films per second. The photospot camera is side mounted and obtains image transmitted from beam splitting mirror. The films used are roll films which are typically 105 mm wide. Thus the images here are minified. Although, the roll films have resolution of about 200 lp/mm, this is limited by the resolution of II (4–5 lp/mm). The advantages include reduced dose, cheaper films, less storage space and less delay in exposure. The limitations include poorer resolution and smaller sized images.

Digital fluorography uses CCD cameras or FPD where the images are digitally stored. The matrix may vary from 1–9 megapixels with resolution varying from 2.4 lp/mm to 3.4 lp/mm. This limitation in resolution is surmounted by the ability of postprocessing of the images. Other benefits include option of film less system, immediate viewing of images without delay and linear response which obviates over or under exposure.

Recording Motion

Motion recording is useful in visualization and reviewing of dynamic processes of the body. Cine camera and videotapes are used for this purpose.

Cine fluorography is regularly used for recording of movement of contrast in the vessels. It uses smaller (35 mm wide) and longer (120 m) film with acquisition capacity of 90 images/second. The frame rate of exposure can be adjusted as needed. Grid controlled tubes are often used to turn X-ray exposure on and off quickly in synchrony with the camera

shutter. Since II produces a circular image, exact framing is needed to fit this image on rectangular film. The effective resolution of the system is 16 lp/mm.

Videotape recording uses super VHS (S-video) technology with its electronic bandwidth matching with that of the TV. They however produce half the resolution of cine fluorography.

Digital storage of the movements of different organ systems are now done with the increased availability of digital fluoroscopy. The images are stored in the form of cine-loop (fluoroscopic or radiographic loop) with no loss in the image quality. These can be reviewed as and when necessary.

Types of Fluoroscopic Equipment

Various configurations of fluoroscopic systems are available depending on the individual needs. Each system has its own advantages and disadvantages. The types of machines available are as follows.

Radiography-fluoroscopy Unit with Under-couch Tube

This system has an under the table X-ray tube and collimator with image intensifier or detector above the table **(Figs. 23A and B)**. The II or detector with the tube can be adjusted by the operator to the field of interest. The advantage of this machine is reduced scatter radiation and thus reduced dose to the operator and patient. The disadvantages include need for an additional X-ray tube for radiography which adds to the cost and need for the presence of operator within the examination room for positioning and fluoroscopy (which exposes the operator to radiation) as remote control switches are not available with such systems. The II/detector is fixed with a handle grip which allows effortless and smooth movement of the detector in all four directions; further it is integrated with fluoroscopic/acquisition button on it.

Radiography-fluoroscopy Unit with Over-couch Tube

Here, the tube is located above the table at a distance, which is either fixed or adjustable to some extent depending on the vendor **(Figs. 24A and B)**. The detector is under the table. The benefits include available space for patient access, option for tube angulation, remote control operation (with some units) and ability to use the same tube for radiography. The remote control operation prevents primary beam irradiating the operator. The disadvantages are increased scatter radiation, need of additional lead protection devices (additional cost) and operator away from the patient.

Fixed C-arm Fluoroscopic System

This type of system is mainly used in angiography. This consists of a C-shaped apparatus with X-ray tube assemble at one end and II or detector at other end **(Figs. 25A and B)**. The shape allows for increased mobility of tube-detector assembly. The C-arm is either ceiling mounted or floor mounted. In addition,

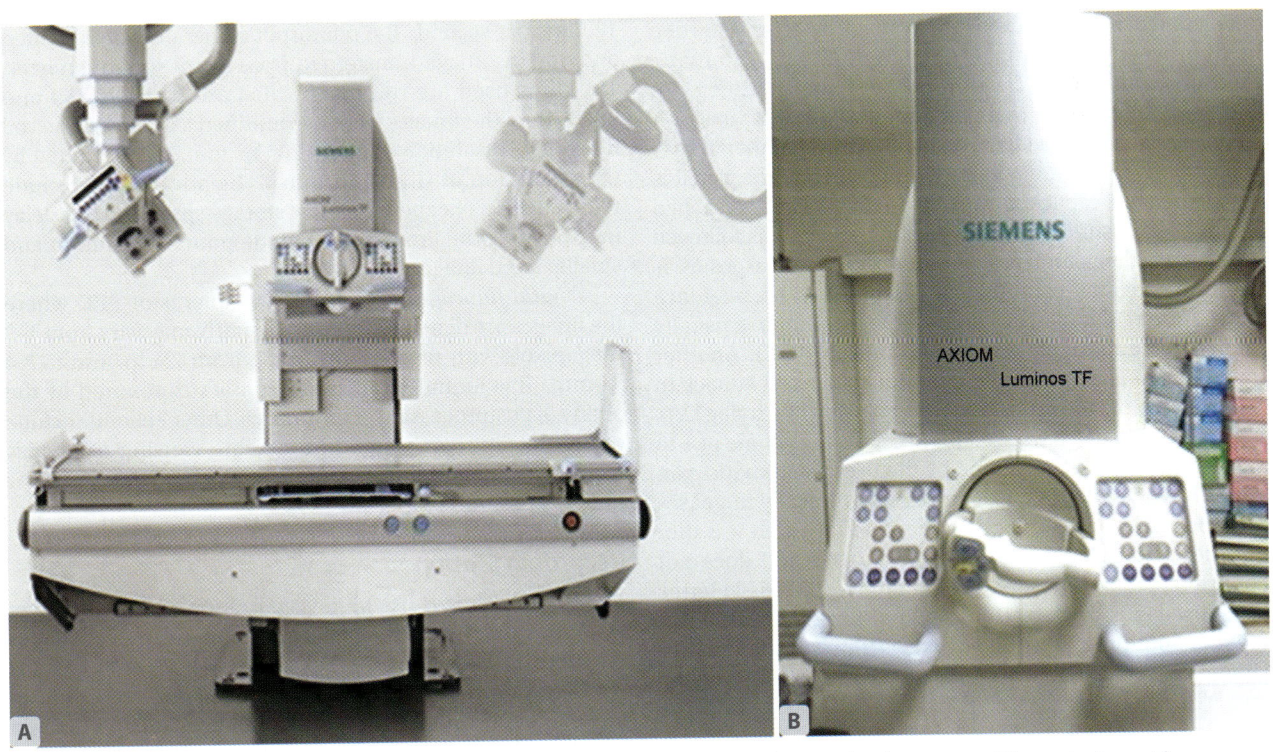

FIGS. 23A AND B: Radiography-fluoroscopy unit with under the couch X-ray tube (A). The second ceiling mounted X-ray tube is used for radiography. Close up view of the image intensifier is seen with handle grip (B).

Courtesy: Siemens Medical Systems.

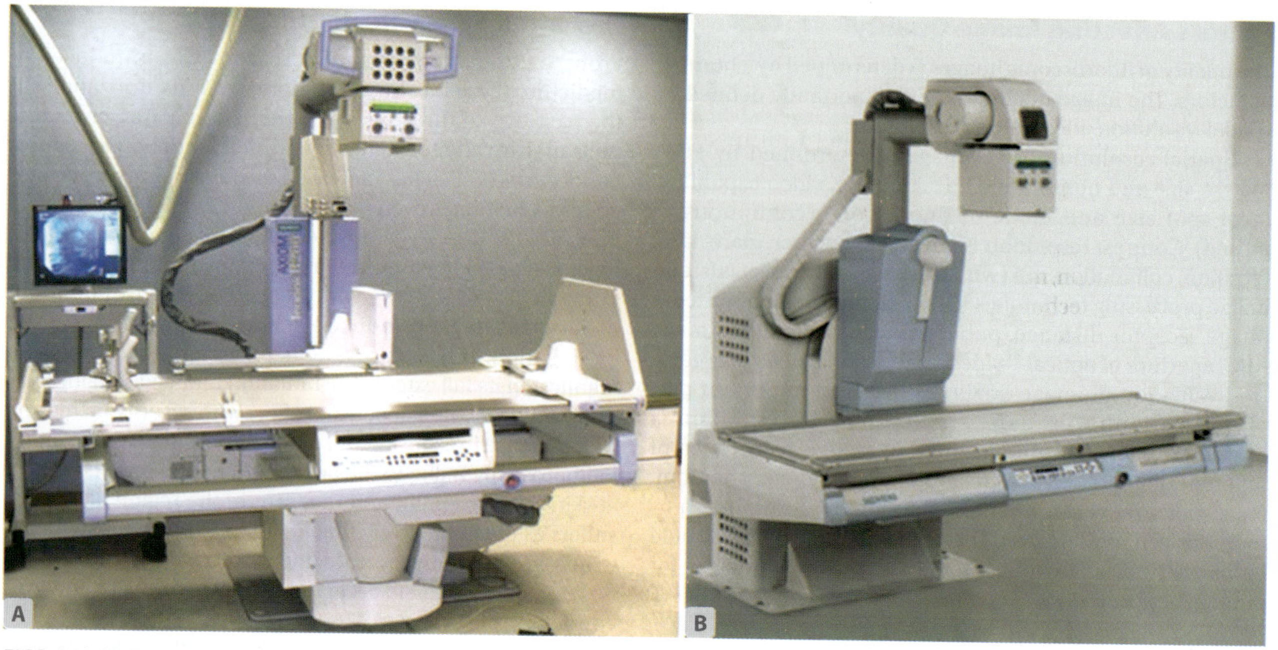

FIGS. 24A AND B: Radiography-fluoroscopy unit with over-couch X-ray tube and under the table image intensifier (A) and flat panel detector (B)
Courtesy: Siemens Medical Systems.

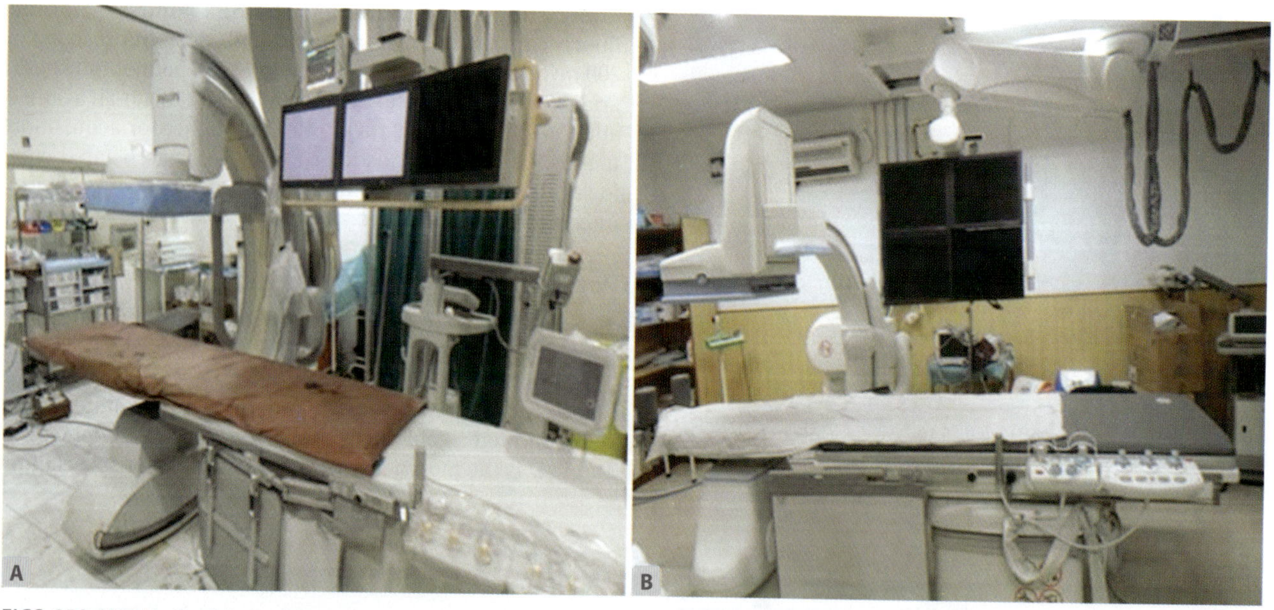

FIGS. 25A AND B: Fixed C-arm flat panel detector fluoroscopy system used for angiography with the C-arm being ceiling mounted (A; Courtesy: Philips Medical Systems) or floor mounted (B).
Courtesy: GE Medical System.

it includes a mobile floating table which is fixed to the floor at one end. Biplane C-arm system includes two C-arms, one ceiling mounted and the other floor mounted **(Fig. 26)**. This unit allows acquisition in two projections (e.g. AP and lateral) with single contrast injection.

Mobile C-arm System

This system is mainly used in operation theaters and wards to check the position of orthopedic implants, pacemakers or vascular implants **(Fig. 27A)**. This system is cheaper and mostly uses image intensifiers, usually with CCD cameras. Due to the cost involved and need of proper care, FPD C-arm systems are slowly increasing in availability. The FPD C-arms **(Fig. 27B)** are cheaper compared to a full-fledged angiography systems and can be used for most of the non-vascular diagnostic and interventional procedures. In advanced systems, even 3D rotation is possible, which is useful in image-guided surgeries.

Factors Affecting Image Quality

The quality of fluoroscopic images is determined by a number of factors. The image quality is most importantly defined by spatial resolution and contrast resolution.

Spatial resolution of an image is determined by FOV, matrix, size and number of DELs, binning, video capability, focal spot size and mode of fluoroscopy (continuous vs pulsed). Contrast resolution is affected by scatter, glare, kVp, filtration, collimation, mA (which determines noise/SNR) and image processing techniques. Other factors include source—image receptor distance, patient-image receptor distance, ABC, aperture of optical—video system and conversion gain.

Evaluation of image quality is the most important part of quality control in fluoroscopy. Contrast resolution is evaluated using an aluminum step wedge with holes of different diameter, spatial resolution by line pair phantom, focal spot size by star phantom and temporal resolution by motor driven rotating disc. These quality control tests should be carried out at regular intervals, typically annually, for optimal performance.

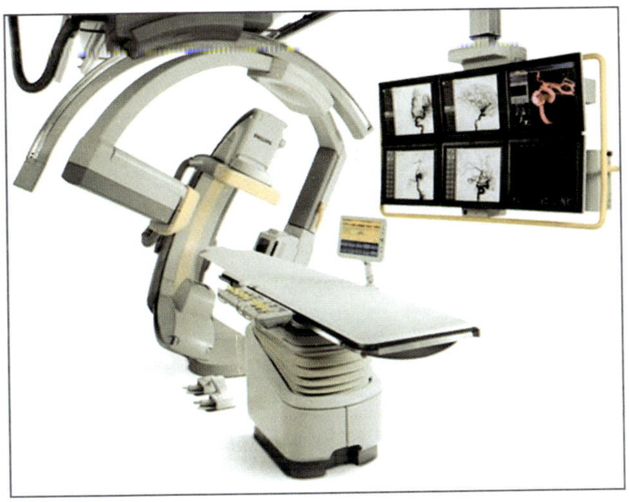

FIG. 26: Biplanar fixed C-arm system, with one arm ceiling mounted and the other floor mounted.

Courtesy: Philips Medical System.

Radiation Safety in Fluoroscopy

From the initial days when fluoroscopy was introduced in medicine, there has been an increase in its utilization. In the past two to three decades, tremendous increase in its utilization in various diagnostic and interventional procedures has occurred which has increased the total fluoroscopy times greatly, sometimes even over one hour. Availability of newer intravascular devices has further added to its growth. All these together have increased radiation exposure to patients and to medical staff working with fluoroscopy. Most important of various radiation induced effects is skin burns caused by radiation. It has an insidious onset and takes weeks to manifest in its full extent. The radiation induced skin injury is a deterministic (nonstochastic) effect with severity increasing with increase in exposure dose. The importance of skin injury in fluoroscopy is due to the fact that radiation dose is highest at skin entrance point and that skin in the region of interest suffers as the fluoroscopy time increases. The measurements which are typically used to measure radiation dose of a fluoroscopy system are receptor entrance exposure and skin entrance exposure rates.[24]

Receptor entrance exposure (REE) is defined as exposure at the entrance of image receptor required to produce a single image with grid removed. Skin entrance exposure (SEE) is the dose at entrance surface of a patient and usually measured under simulated conditions. The SEE limit for normal fluoroscopy is 100 mGy/min and high dose fluoroscopy is 200 mGy/min. The values depend on kVp, patient thickness, grid, SID etc. The typical fluoroscopic SEE rate for an average adult is about 10 to 30 mGy/min, but higher for acquisition modes. Usually, diagnostic procedures are associated with lower fluoroscopic times and exposure rates compared to interventional procedures.

Patient Dose Monitoring Methods

These methods are described in detail elsewhere. In short, they are of two types.

Direct methods use thermoluminescent dosimeters (TLD), photographic films and diodes or metal-oxide semiconductor field effect transistor (MOSFET) detectors. The TLD is the most accurate but due to smaller size cannot

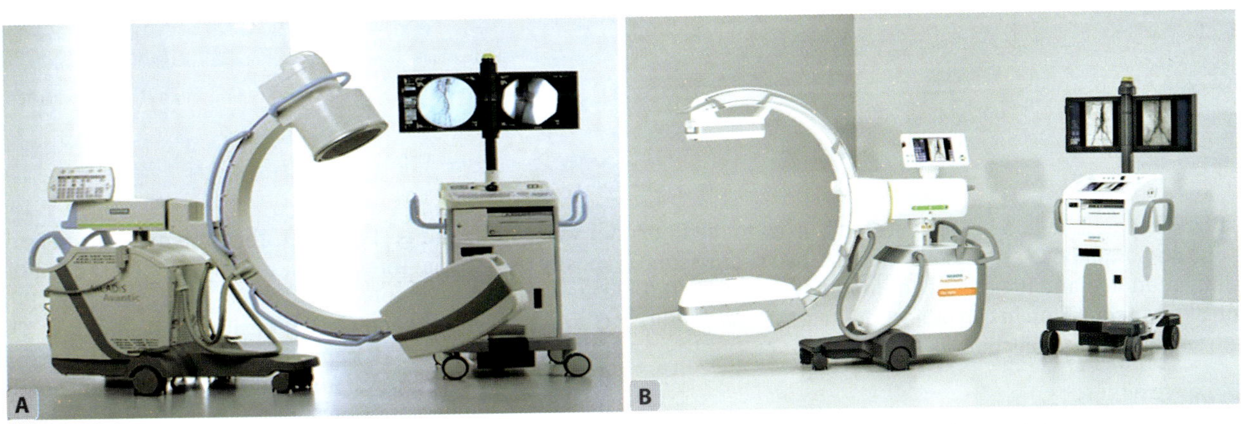

FIGS. 27A AND B: (A) Mobile C-arm fluoroscopy unit with image intensifier; (B) Mobile C-arm fluoroscopy with flat panel detector.

Courtesy: Siemens Medical Systems.

cover the entire field and may not correctly measure the peak dose field. Photographic films are inexpensive and useful in determining high dose region and the dose. But the sizes available are limited. Both these methods are associated with time delay in reading out the measured doses. The MOSFET detectors provide dynamic measurement of skin dose and are accurate.[25] They have good linear response, low detection threshold and low error percentage (10%), but are detectable in the imaging field.

Indirect method most widely used is dose area product (DAP) meter. Since it is a product of dose and area, same values can be obtained with low dose exposed to larger area and higher dose exposed to smaller area. But the skin effect of these two modes is not the same as the latter results in more skin damage. The SEE can be computed from DAP reading if dose rate and field size data is available. But this is often difficult as both, dose rate and field size change dynamically during fluoroscopy. Still, DAP meters are widely used in modern systems for dose measurement. One new system is available which dynamically measures and displays an estimate of SEE and is called PEMNET (Patient Exposure Management Network). This records patient dose from all radiation related procedures (CT, cardiac, angiography, interventions) and is available for review from any workstation in the network. Currently however there is no perfect dose monitoring system for fluoroscopy and interventional procedures.

Dose Reduction Techniques

Various dose reduction techniques include reduction of exposure time, improving collimation, reducing tube current, reducing spot exposures, using better detectors and reducing II/detector-patient distance.

Intermittent fluoroscopy is the most important due to the fact that the radiologist can control fluoroscopy time and can judiciously use it intermittently to reduce total patient and personnel dose. Last image hold (LIH) and road map have been described above. Use of reference image, especially in DSA is helpful in significantly reducing radiation dose and contrast medium. Modern systems are available with electronic collimation which can be done on LIH without additional fluoroscopy.

Pulsed fluoroscopy provides substantial reduction in patient radiation exposure. Reducing the number of pulses increases image noise and this is overcome in many models by increasing mA which increases dose. Thus instead, there is only modest reduction in dose. The radiation dose of continuous fluoroscopy and pulsed fluoroscopy at 30 fps are similar. When the pulse rate is reduced from 30 to 15, 10, and 7.5 per second, the dose is approximately reduced by 22, 38 and 49 percent respectively.[26] No significant change in image quality is seen between continuous fluoroscopy and PF at 15 fps, 7.5 fps and 3.75 fps.[27] Further, at lower frame rates and magnified fields, instead of increasing exposure, the video camera aperture can be increased to maintain brightness. Automatic dose rate and image quality (ADRIQ) control modulates kVp, mAs, pulse width and filtration as per patient characteristics to produce lowest radiation with good image quality.[28]

The use of cumulative exposure timer, typically set at 5 minutes, alerts the operator of fluoroscopy time. Further, real time display of total exposure time, kVp, mAs and total dose also helps the radiologist to regulate patient radiation exposure.

Dose spreading is a method to reduce skin dose when lengthy interventional procedures are performed. Here, the tube-detector system is rotated about the region of interest as center to spread the skin dose to different area, so that single area is not overexposed. The quality of X-ray beam can be adjusted to remove low energy X-rays (beam hardening). This can be done by increasing kVp (which reduces SEE) and use of metal filters like aluminum or copper (especially the latter as 0.1-0.3 mm of Cu reduces SEE by 30 to 50 percent).[29] Magnification, either geometric or electronic, results in increase in skin dose. Higher magnification may result in reduced spatial resolution due to focal spot blur if smaller focal spot is not used. High dose fluoroscopy mode, available in few systems, is uncommonly used for very obese patients or thick body regions and results in high skin dose.

SUMMARY

Fluoroscopy is one of the basic X-ray techniques and is widely used for various diagnostic and interventional procedures. From the initial dark room fluoroscopy considerable advancements have led to the development of image intensifiers, digital processing techniques and the present day flat panel detectors. Solid state FPD systems produce better image with less artifacts and results in less radiation dose. Radiologists, as end users, should be aware of the basic structure and function of these equipments so that judicious adjustments are made on case to case basis. A constant note has to be made of the fluoroscopic time and radiation dose to the patient during each procedure. Adequate knowledge of methods of dose reduction during fluoroscopy and DSA is important to prevent radiation effects, especially on skin. With increasing research in artificial intelligence, the future may see its potential application in the field of fluoroscopy and DSA.

REFERENCES

1. Schueler BA. The AAPM/RSNA physics tutorial for residents: General overview of fluoroscopic imaging. Radiographics. 2000;20:1115-26.
2. Pooley RA, McKinney JM, Miller DA. The AAPM/RSNA physics tutorial for residents: Digital fluoroscopy. Radiographics. 2001;21:521-34.
3. Krohmer JS. Radiography and fluoroscopy, 1920 to the present. Radiographics. 1989;9:1129-53.
4. Seibert JA. The AAPM/RSNA physics tutorial for residents: X-ray generators. Radiographics. 1997;17:1533-57.
5. Zink FE. The AAPM/RSNA physics tutorial for residents: X-ray tubes. Radiographics. 1997;17:1259-68.
6. Wang J, Blackburn TJ. The AAPM/RSNA physics tutorial for residents: X-ray image intensifiers for fluoroscopy. Radiographics. 2000;20:1471-7.
7. Van Lysel MS. The AAPM/RSNA physics tutorial for residents: Fluoroscopy: optical coupling and the video system. Radiographics. 2000;20:1769-86.
8. Nickoloff EL. The AAPM/RSNA physics tutorial for residents: Survey of modern fluoroscopy imaging: flat panel detectors versus image intensifiers and more. Radiographics. 2011;31:591-602.
9. Curry TS III, Dowdey JE, Murry RC Jr. Christensen's physics of diagnostic radiology, 4th Edn. Philadelphia, Pa: Lea & Febiger, 1990.
10. Orth RC, Wallace MJ, Kuo MD. Technology Assessment Committee of the Society of Interventional Radiology. C-arm cone-beam CT: general principles and technical considerations for use in interventional radiology. J Vasc Interv Radiol. 2008;19:814-20.
11. Cowen AR, Davies AG, Sivananthan MU. The design and imaging characteristics of dynamic, solid-state, flat-panel X-ray image detectors for digital fluoroscopy and fluorography. Clin Radiol. 2008;63:1073-85.
12. Murray T, Rodt T, Lee MJ. Two-dimensional perfusion angiography of the foot: technical considerations and initial analysis. J Endovasc Ther. 2016;23:58-64.
13. Maschke SK, Werncke T, Klöckner R, Rodt T, Renne J, Kirstein MM, Vogel A, Wacker FK, Meyer BC, Hinrichs JB. Quantification of perfusion reduction by using 2D-perfusion angiography following transarterial chemoembolization with drug-eluting beads. Abdom Radiol (NY). 2018;43(5):1245-53.
14. Wong SC, Nawawi O, Ramli N, Abd Kadir KA. Benefits of 3D rotational DSA compared with 2D DSA in the evaluation of intracranial aneurysm. Acad Radiol. 2012;19(6):701-7.
15. Tanigawa N, Komemushi A, Kojima H, Kariya S, Sawada S. Three-dimensional angiography using rotational digital subtraction angiography: usefulness in transarterial embolization of hepatic tumors. Acta Radiol. 2004;45(6):602-7.
16. Wang JL, Yuan ZG, Qian GL, Bao WQ, Jin GL. 3D pringint of intracranial aneurysm based on intracranial digital subtraction angiography and its clinical application. Medicine 2018;97:24(e11103)
17. Sandoval-Garcia C, Royalty K, Yang P, Niemann D, Ahmed A, Aagaard-Kienitz B, Başkaya MK, Schafer S, Strother C. 4D DSA a new technique for arteriovenous malformation evaluation: a feasibility study. J Neurointerv Surg. 2016;8(3):300-4.
18. Ide S, Hirai T, Morioka M, Kai Y, Yano S, Kawano T, Tochihara S, Shigematsu Y, Uetani H, Murakami Y, Watanabe K, Yamashita Y. Usefulness of 3D DSA-MR fusion imaging in the pretreatment evaluation of brain arteriovenous malformations. Acad Radiol. 2012;19(11):1345-52.
19. Tritt S, Ommer B, Gehrisch S, Klein S, Seifert V, Berkefeld J, Konczalla J. Optimization of the Surgical Approach in AVMs Using MRI and 4D DSA Fusion Technique: A technical note. Clin Neuroradiol. 2017;27(4):443-50.
20. Goudeketting SR, Heinen SG, van den Heuvel DA, van Strijen MJ, de Haan MW, Slump CH, de Vries JP. The use of 3D image fusion for percutaneous transluminal angioplasty and stenting of iliac artery obstructions: validation of the technique and systematic review of literature. J Cardiovasc Surg (Torino). 2018;59(1):26-36.
21. https://usa.healthcare.siemens.com/angio/artis-interventional-angiography-systems/miyabi/features
22. Liu FY, Li X, Yuan HJ, Guan Y, Wang MQ. Angio-Computed Tomograph-Guided Immediate Lipiodol Computed Tomograph for Diagnosis of Small Hepatocellular Carcinoma Lesions during Transarterial Chemoembolization. Chin Med J. 2018;131:2410-6.
23. Geise RA. The AAPM/RSNA physics tutorial for residents: Fluoroscopy: recording of fluoroscopic images and automatic exposure control. Radiographics. 2001;21:wwww227-36.
24. Mahesh M. The AAPM/RSNA physics tutorial for residents: Fluoroscopy: patient radiation exposure issues. Radiographics. 2001;21:1033-45.
25. Miksys N, Gordon CL, Thomas K, Connolly B. Estimating effective dose to pediatric patients undergoing interventional radiology procedures using anthropomorphic phantoms and MOSFET dosimeters. AJR Am J Roentgenol. 2010;194:1315-22.
26. Aufrichtig R, Xue P, Thomas CW, Gilmore GC, Wilson DL. Perceptual comparison of pulsed and continuous fluoroscopy. Med Phys. 1994;21:245-56.
27. Boland GWL, Murphy B, Arellano R, Niklason L, Mueller PR. Dose reduction in gastrointestinal and genitourinary fluoroscopy: use of grid-controlled pulsed fluoroscopy. AJR Am J Roentgenol. 2000;175:1453-7.
28. Lin PJ. The operation logic of automatic dose control of fluoroscopy system in conjunction with spectral shaping filters. Med Phys. 2007;34:3169-72.
29. Nicholson R, Tuffee F, Uthappa MC. Skin sparing in interventional radiology: the effect of copper filtration. Br J Radiol. 2000;73:36-42.

CHAPTER

42

Tools and Drugs in Interventional Radiology

Atin Kumar, Chandan J Das

Interventional radiology (IR) has seen a tremendous advance in the last 2 decades. It has become established as a specialized branch playing a major role in the management of various diseases. This has been helped by the availability of various tools and devices, which constitute the armamentarium of an interventional radiologist.

The common procedures performed in an interventional radiology set up could be vascular as well as nonvascular. The need of hardware starts from the giving of local anesthesia or intravenous access till the suturing or plastering of the wound of the procedure in interventional radiology. Both the procedures have some common as well as specific needs. The common requirements for both the procedures are local anesthetic agent, blades, puncture needles, wires, catheters and suturing agent.

The various tools utilized in IR practice are discussed below.

PUNCTURE NEEDLES

These are small sized needles which are used to gain access to the vessel and are therefore also called as access needles. They are also used for nonvascular indications like gaining access to bile duct, pelvicalyceal system, abscess, etc. The typical *access needle* has a sharp, beveled distal edge for puncturing the artery **(Fig. 1A)**. The guidewire is introduced through its lumen into the vessel once blood comes out from the proximal end. Some access needles have an inner stylet which protrudes slightly out of the outer lumen needle. The tip of the inner stylet is sharp to puncture the artery but the tip of the outer needle is round and blunted to prevent vessel injury. Once the vessel is punctured, the stylet is removed to allow entry of guidewire.

The size of the access needle is measured in gauges. Higher gauge number indicates smaller lumen diameter. The typical access needles are of size 18 G or 19 G.

The *seldinger needle* (Medicut 18 G) is a double lumen type of access needle commonly used in vascular puncture in which the outer lumen is soft, pliable and non-traumatic cannula with a stylet with sharp and beveled edge within its lumen **(Fig. 1B)**. Once the vessel is entered, the inner stylet is removed and the soft cannula remains within the vessel through which the guidewire can be introduced. The commonly used intravenous cannula is almost similar and can be used for the same purpose. It is important to check the compatibility of the guidewire through the lumen of the access needle before the vessel is punctured. A 19 G needle accepts a 0.035 inch guidewire.

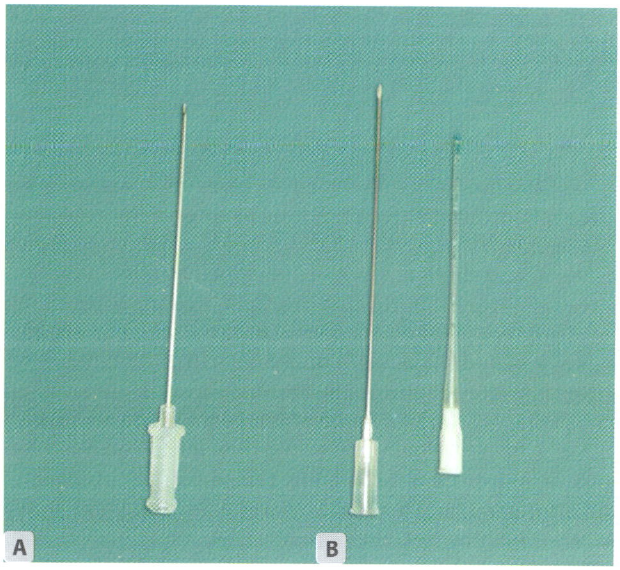

FIGS. 1A AND B: Puncture needles. Single piece needle (A) and Seldinger needle (Medicut) (B).

The vessel puncture can be single or double wall puncture.

- In the single wall technique, only the anterior wall of the artery is punctured by the advancing needle and when the tip is in the lumen (as evidenced by pulsatile backflow of blood) the guidewire is advanced within the lumen. The nonstylet access needles are preferred for this type of puncture whereas the needles with stylet are used for the double wall technique.
- In the double wall technique, the puncture needle is advanced though the vessel till it punctures the posterior wall also. Then the stylet is removed and the needle slowly withdrawn till the tip is within the lumen of the vessel. The double wall technique is comparatively easier. The single

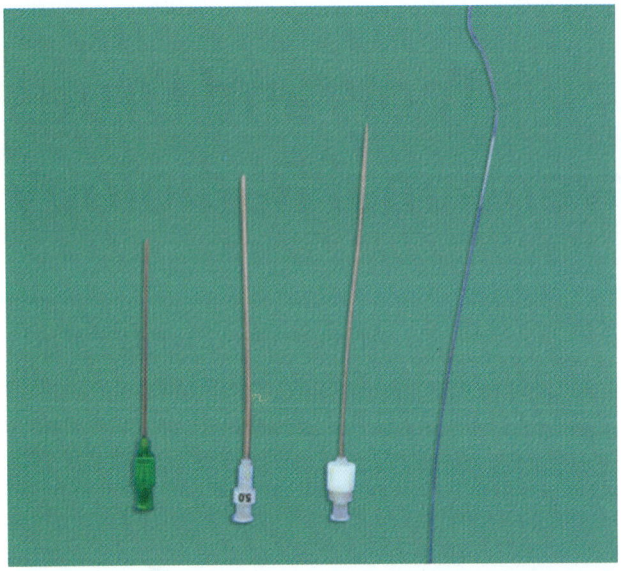

FIG. 2: Micropuncture access set. Consists of bevelled tip needle, co-axial dilators and a 0.018 guidewire.

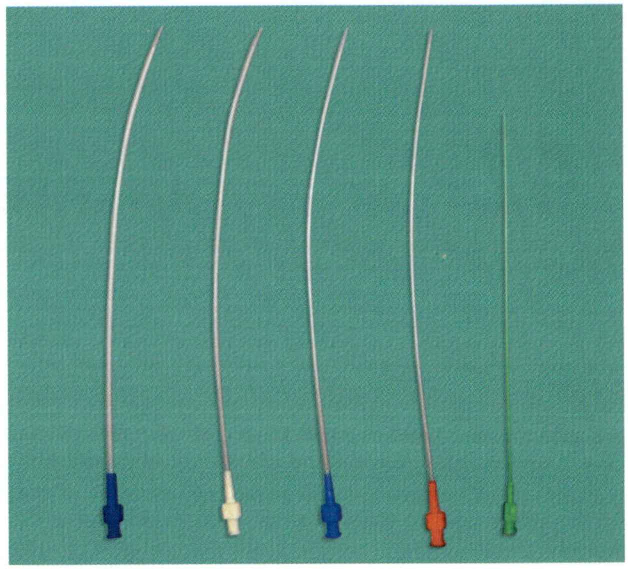

FIG. 3: Dilators of varying sizes (increasing from right to left). Each size is universally color coded.

wall technique is preferred in cases of coagulopathy or when thrombolysis is planned to prevent excessive bleeding.

Another technique of vessel puncture is by *micropuncture access set* **(Fig. 2)**. In this the needle is a sharp beveled tip needle of very small diameter (usually 21G) which is initially used to puncture the vessel. A compatible 0.018 inch guidewire is then introduced through the needle followed by removal of the needle. A co-axial dilator system with a 3 F inner dilator within a 4 F or 5 F outer dilator is then advanced over the guidewire. It is then followed by removal of the guidewire and the inner dilator to provide a large bore access within the lumen through which the normal 0.035 inch guidewire can be introduced. This technique is commonly used in situations where the access is difficult, e.g. antegrade femoral puncture, brachial artery punctures, pediatric patients, anatomically sensitive regions like jugular venous access and in conditions where thrombolysis is planned.

Seldinger technique is the systematic procedure of gaining access into the vessel. The vessel is first punctured with a needle which is followed by guidewire insertion through it. The needle is then removed over the wire and exchanged with a tapered catheter of appropriate size. This technique is also used in nonvascular procedures to gain access into biliary channels, pelvicalyceal system or into an abscess cavity.

DILATORS (FIG. 3)

Dilators are short stiff-tapered plastic catheters which are used to spread the soft tissues/fascia and the wall of the vessel so as to facilitate the subsequent passage of a catheter. Sequential use of increasing size dilators over a guidewire (preferably stiff guidewire) leads to an increase in the size of the initial percutaneous puncture. The dilators are also frequently used in nonvascular percutaneous procedures to dilate the track like in abscess drainage, percutaneous nephrostomy, percutaneous transhepatic biliary drainage, etc.

The sizes of the dilators (and access needles) are measured in Gauges. The size in inches equals 1/gauge. Hence, a 20 G needle measures 0.05 inches whereas a 25 G needle measures 0.04 inches. Smaller gauges indicate larger diameters.

SHEATHS (FIG. 4)

Introducer sheaths are small thin-walled catheters which are open at one end and are capped with a hemostatic valve or diaphragm at the other end. There is a short clear side arm which is used for flushing or injection of contrast. The distal end of the sheath is generally nontapered in contrast from normal catheters. The purpose of the sheath is to provide a continuous secured access within vessel lumen for multiple exchanges of various catheters and guidewires through a single puncture and access site. It is introduced as a co-axial system with a dilator within it to ensure smooth access. The introducer sheaths are also widely used for access in nonvascular interventions and drainage of fluid collections.

The sheaths, being slightly stiffer, are also used to improve the pushability of a diagnostic catheter through them into tortuous vessels. Long length sheaths are also available which are mainly used for interventional procedures including nonvascular procedures. The use of crossover sheaths (across the aortic bifurcation) significantly enhances the selective catheterizations of contralateral iliac/femoral vessels and use of long sheaths can enable easy and direct advancement of catheters into selective distal main vessels.

The sheath sizes are described in French (F) and represents the maximum actual size in French of the catheter which can be introduced through its lumen. Hence, a 5 F sheath size means that a 5 F catheter can be introduced through it. Note that for sheaths the size represents the inner lumen diameter

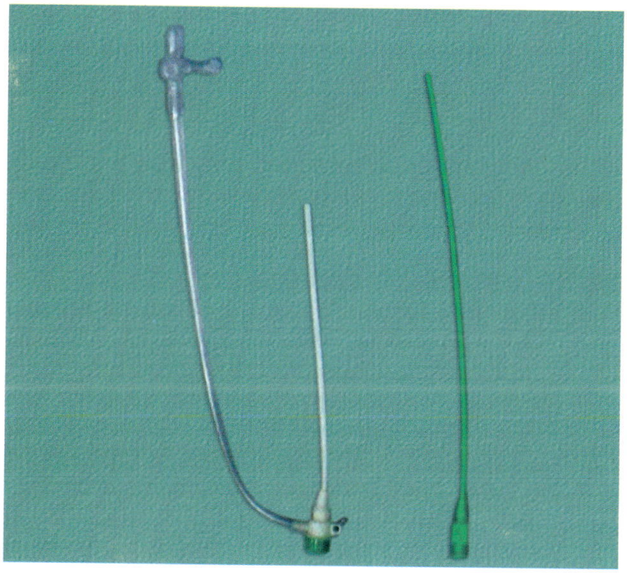

FIG. 4: Sheath. Size 6 F (green color).

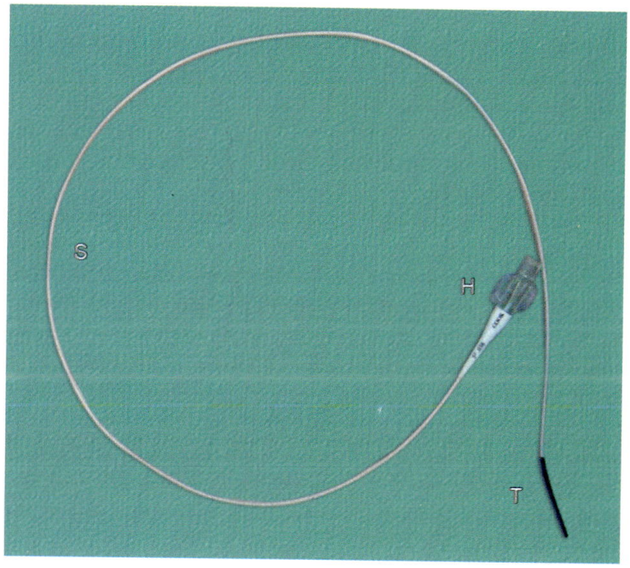

FIG. 5: Catheter parts. Hub (H), shaft (S) and tip (T).

whereas for catheters and dilators it represents the outer diameter. The sheaths are available in diameters 4–14 F with lengths ranging from 10–90 cm. There is a universal color coding system for the sizes of the sheaths. 4 F sheaths are of red color, 5 F gray, 6 F green and 7 F orange colored.

CATHETERS

The word catheter is derived from a latin word 'katheter' which means to push down. It is a hollow flexible tube that can be inserted into a body cavity, duct or vessel thereby allowing drainage or injection of fluids, distending a passageway or providing access to surgical instruments. The process of inserting a catheter is called catheterization. Catheters are the backbone of an interventional radiological procedure. They come in various shapes, sizes and material types with each serving a specific function.

Parts of Catheter (Fig. 5)

A typical catheter consists of following parts:

- Tip—the distal tapered part
- Shaft—the long tubing
- Hub—the proximal part with a plastic funnel for ease of guidewire insertions and attachment of syringes for contrasts injections.

Materials

The catheters can be made of various materials including Teflon (polytetrafluoroethylene or PTFE), polyethylene, polyurethane or nylon. The choice of the material decides the torque, stiffness, flexibility, thrombogenicity, burst pressure and the friction. Stiffness allows the pushing of the catheter while flexibility allows bending of the catheter to follow the curve of the vessel. High burst pressure measures the strength of the material and its ability to withstand the high injection rate without bursting. The ability of the catheter tip to rotate based on rotation of the catheter hub measures the torqueability. Mechanical braiding of the catheter wall by materials such as nylon or stainless steel enhances the torqueability of the catheter and facilitates selective catheterization of vessels. Decreased friction of the catheter material on the luminal surface allows higher flow rates and on the outer surface enables easier advancement of the catheter with minimal buckling and wedging. Catheters can be coated by hydrophilic polymers to allow easier trackability, e.g. slip catheter (Cook). Impregnation of the catheter wall with barium sulfate, tungsten or lead salts is often done to increase the fluoroscopic visibility as the catheters are generally faintly radiopaque.

In general, PTFE or nylon catheters are stiffer with high tensile strength and burst pressure and hence are used for purpose of flush injections requiring high flow rates and pressures. In contrast, polyethylene catheters are less stiff and more flexible and hence are used for purpose of selective catheterizations.

Sizes

The catheters can be of varying diameter and lengths.

The diameter of the catheter is conventionally measured in French size (F). 3 F = 1 mm = 0.038 inches. The catheter size in French refers to the outer diameter of the catheter. It is a factor in deciding the size of the catheter to be used based upon the size of the vessel to be catheterized. The *general use intravascular catheters* are commonly of size 4 F to 6 F. Catheters smaller than 4 F are not used for flush purpose but are required for pediatric use and for selective catheterization of tortuous or smaller vessels like intracerebral vessels. They are known as *microcatheters* and are usually of 2 F or 3 F size. Larger catheters of size 7F to 9F are used as *guiding catheters* and are mainly used to guide smaller catheters or devices within them to be used as a co-axial system. The guiding catheters are usually stiffer and firmer to allow passage of balloon catheters, PTCA wires and stent delivery system through them. Mild stiffness comes due to the wire braided design. It should be noted that for guiding catheters the size in French refers to the inner diameter of the catheter (like the introducer sheaths) in contrast to standard use catheters and hence is determinant of the size of the standard catheter which can be coaxially passed through it. For example, a 6 F guiding catheter would be able to accommodate a 6 F standard catheter.

The length of the catheter is the distance between the hub and the tip. It is conventionally measured in centimeters and usually varies between 60 and 110 cm for standard catheters. Smaller catheter lengths are required when the target vessel is close to the site of puncture (usually the femoral artery) such as contralateral iliac, renal or visceral arteries and in pediatric patients. Longer lengths measuring up to 260 cm are required for upper limb, calf, intracranial vessels selective catheterization. The microcatheters are usually of long length as they are to be used coaxially within another catheter and their tips must come out a reasonable distance out of the outer catheter.

Shapes and Holes

The shape of the catheter tip is the most essential element determining the type of use of the catheter. Depending upon the shape, the catheters are categorized as:

- *Simple straight/angled tip catheters:* These have a single curve or angle **(Fig. 6)**. The curve ranges from slightly curved (multipurpose), to more angled (hockey stick or Picard) to completely circular (pigtail). These are either used as flush catheters (pigtail) or to catheterize arteries with angled origins to the direction of catheter like aortic arch branches (picard).
- *Complex curve catheters:* These have more than one curve and are usually used for selective catheterization of branches of the descending aorta. The curve closest to the tip is known as the primary curve while the farther curves are known as secondary curves or the tertiary curves. The primary curve helps to hook a target vessel at an angle while the secondary curve hits the back wall of the main vessel (the wall opposite to the origin of target vessel) and helps to push the catheter further into the target vessel. These catheters may be of two types:
  a. The primary and secondary curves are in the same direction, e.g. Cobra, renal double curve, head hunter, etc. **(Figs. 7A to C)**. They are best used for selective catheterization of vessels which have origins angled caudally like the visceral arteries.
  b. The primary and secondary curves in opposite direction—Reverse curve catheters, e.g. Simmons (1, 2 and 3) catheters **(Fig. 7D)**. These are best used for selective catheterization of vessels which have steep obtuse angle like the left gastric artery or steep acute-angled vessels (sometimes visceral arteries, left common carotid in atherosclerotic aortic arch). These catheters are straightened over a guidewire before advancing and their curves need to be reformed within the aorta after removal of guidewire. Several techniques have been described for the formation of these curves either in the arch or at aortic bifurcation. After hooking the target vessel by the tip of the catheter over a guidewire, these catheters are advanced into the vessel till the level of apex of secondary curve by partial withdrawal of the catheter at the groin (instead of pushing as done in all standard forward curve catheters). Only after this point the catheters can be further pushed into the vessel by advancing over a stiff guidewire. Due to their shape they have increased chances of vessel wall injury while pulling out. Hence, these catheters should always be withdrawn after straightening over a guidewire under fluoroscopic monitoring.

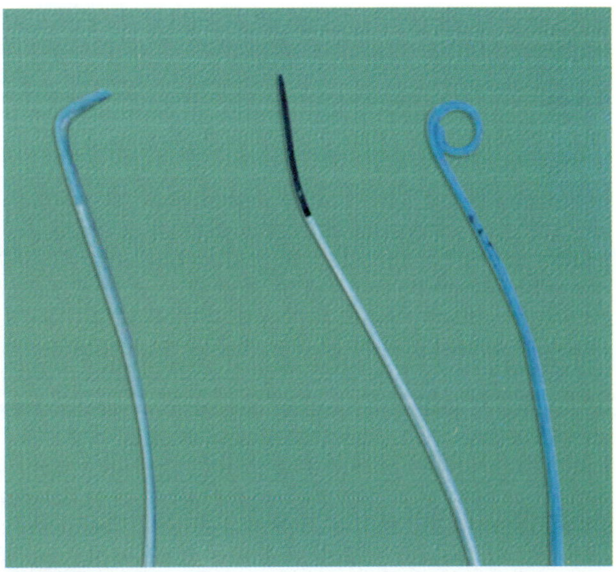

FIG. 6: Simple curve catheters. From left to right—picard, multipurpose and pigtail.

Depending upon the position and number of holes, the catheters are divided into two types:

1. *End hole catheter:* These are the standard diagnostic catheters which have a single hole at the tip of the catheter. The size of the hole is tapered to allow the maximum allowable sized guidewire to just pass through it snugly. These are used for selective catheterization. Pressure injector is not used with these catheters as it may cause plaque dislodgement and dissection.
2. *Side hole catheters:* The side holes are usually multiple with an end hole. These catheters are used as flush catheters to obtain angiograms of large vessels. The side holes vary in number with typical pigtail flush catheter having 8–12 side holes. Though the size of an individual side hole is smaller than the size of the end hole (to prevent exiting of guidewire through this hole), the combined size of the side holes is larger than the end hole allowing much larger volume of contrast dispersal through these holes than the end hole. The multiple side hole catheters are preferred for flush injections as they cause uniform dispersal of contrast in the vessel. The side hole catheters are also used for thrombolysis as they result in uniform distribution of the thrombolytic agent within the thrombus. However, these catheters are not used for embolization as the embolizing agents may either diffuse out through these holes resulting in nontarget embolization or may occlude

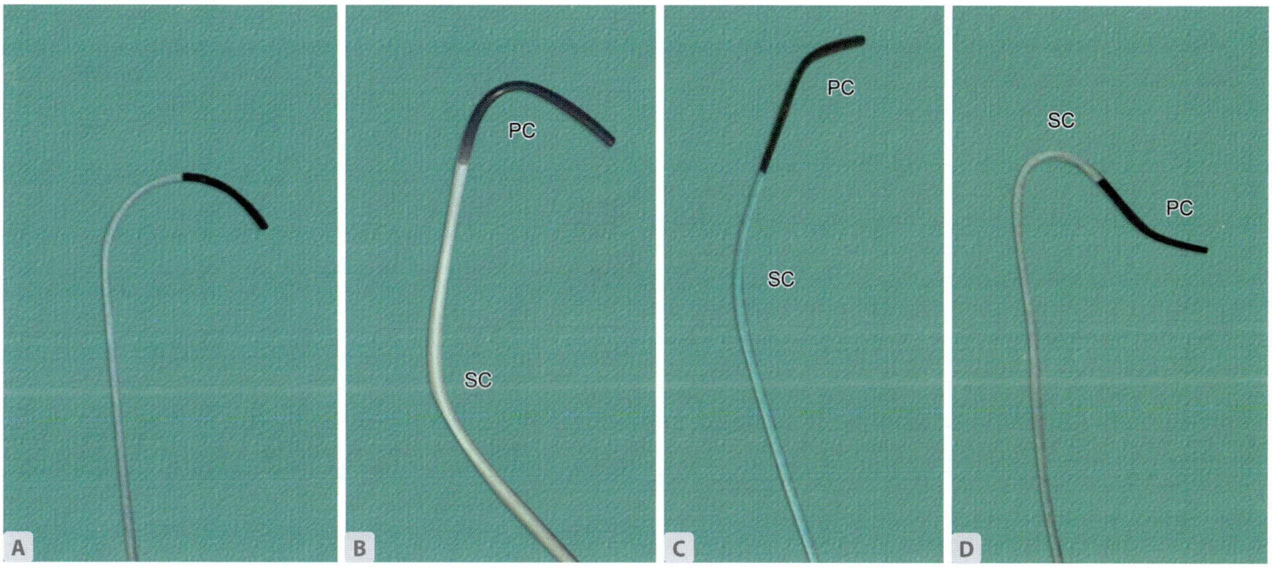

FIGS. 7A TO D: Complex curve catheters. The primary and secondary curves are in same direction in Cobra (A), renal double curve (B) and head hunter (C) catheters while in reverse curve catheters they are in opposite direction as in Simmons catheter (D). (PC: primary curve; SC: secondary curve)

the end hole at the tip due to lesser pressure delivered at the tip. The embolizing coils may also get struck within the side holes.

The commonly used catheters in clinical practice are:

- *Multipurpose* ***(Fig. 6)***: It has straight tip. It can have end hole which is used for selective catheterization of small vessels or in pediatric patients. The side holes multipurpose catheter is used for flush injections in smaller vessels which cannot accommodate the loop of pigtail catheter, e.g. iliac vessels.
- *Pigtail* ***(Fig. 6):*** It is a multiple side hole and end hole catheter with a circular shape and is used for flush injections in large lumen vessels like aorta. The pigtail shape prevents direct intimal injury and ensures much less recoil of catheter after forceful injection of contrast through a pressure injector. It is also commonly used for drainage of collections as it gets secured within the cavity.
- *Picard* ***(Fig. 6):*** It is a end hole catheter with tip angled at obtuse shape (100°). It is commonly used to selectively catheterize forward facing angled origin vessels like the arch vessels and bronchial arteries.
- *Cobra* ***(Fig. 7A):*** It is a end hole catheter with a double curve shape and is commonly used for selective catheterization of visceral vessels. It is available in three different curve shapes C1, C2 and C3 with C2 being the most commonly used.
- *Renal double curve (RDC)* ***(Fig. 7B):*** As the name suggests it has two curves and is used for catheterization of renal vessels. The secondary curve rests against the aortic wall whereas the primary curve enters the vessel.
- *Head hunter* ***(Fig. 7C):*** It has three curves. It is used for selective catheterization of the head and neck vessels.
- *Simmons* ***(Fig. 7D):*** These are reverse curved catheters which are available in three curve shapes S1, S2 and S3 with increasing length of the curved segment. They are used to catheterize vessels with very acute or obtuse angled origin.
- *Slip catheter:* These are catheters with a special hydrophilic coating to increase their pushability within the vessel. They can be of various tip shapes from straight to curved.

Balloon Catheters

These are catheters with a balloon mounted on them close to their distal end.

The balloons used in interventional radiological practice are of two types:

1. *Noncompliant, high pressure balloons:* Most often made of polyethylene terephthalate (PET) which is a relatively noncompliant polyester derivative appearing like a very thin plastic. These balloons do not get stretched beyond a maximum diameter. They are mainly used for angioplasty in lower limb, renal, visceral and internal carotid arteries. The larger sized balloons are used in aorta, veins or in valves. They may also be used for nonvascular applications like dilatation of esophagus, duodenum or colon. These balloons should not be used on calcified plaques or metal stents because of high chances of rupture.
2. *Compliant, low pressure balloons:* Made of nylon derivates like latex, silicone or polyurethane. These are softer but more scratch resistant than a PET balloon. These balloons get stretched and increase their diameter on inflation beyond a certain pressure. They are used for temporary vascular occlusion, embolectomy or mounting and molding of balloon expandable stents. The vascular occlusion by balloon may be required for the purpose of preventing reflux of embolic material proximally during embolization, or to minimize antegrade blood flow during embolization when alcohol is used as embolizing material as in embolization of renal cell carcinomas or arterio- venous malformations. The embolectomy balloon

catheters used for removing acute thrombi and clots from vessels are also compliant. The most commonly used is the Fogarty balloon catheter.

GUIDEWIRE

Medical guidewire is used to access the vascular, biliary and pelvicalyceal system for a variety of diagnostic and therapeutic medical procedures. The purpose of the guidewire is safe introduction and selective positioning of the catheter which is subsequently placed. An initial guidewire, or access wire, is first inserted through body passageways to a location where a medical procedure or treatment is to take place. In the next step, a catheter is advanced over the inserted guidewire, which enables the catheter to follow its predefined pathway to the point of treatment. Thereafter, other devices or fluids may be inserted via the catheter tubing, as needed. A guidewire is typically advanced beyond a stenosed area to allow balloon catheters and stents to treat the area.

The typical guidewires used in interventional radiology are constructed of a tightly wound fine outer wire of steel and a stiff inner "Mendrel" core wire. Addition of nitinol may be done to prevent kinking. Platinum and gold are added for better radio opacity. These wires are made in a variety of sizes and lengths but usually range from 0.010 to 0.038 inch in diameter and 50 to 300 cm in length. The outside of guidewire frequently has hydrophilic coating or Teflon coating to reduce friction and may be impregnated with heparin to reduce thrombogenicity. The hydrophilic coating works best when the wire is wet. The inner core provides the rigidity of the wire. The inner core wire is tapered towards the introduction end of the guide wire and ends at a variable distance from the tip. Varying the taper and the distance that the core extends towards the ends of guidewire allows one to vary tip flexibility and the transition zone length. Some wires have movable cores so that the flexibility of the tip can be changed at will. Most guidewires have a fine safety wire along the full length to prevent the outer wire coil from uncoiling and breaking off.

Flexible tip standard wires are generally used for routine percutaneous introduction of catheters. Tip flexibility allows the wires to buckle and avoid damaging the vessel. However, one must be aware that even a flexible guidewire may act as a sharp object when it first exits the tip of catheter. Exchange wires are long and allow enough length of the wire between the target site and external site so that a new catheter may be introduced without losing wire purchase internally.

Based on the stiffness of the guidewire, they may be classified as floppy, of normal stiffness (e.g. Terumo hydrophilic guidewire) or stiff/extra stiff (e.g. amplatz). The guidewires may also be classified as i) *steerable* - which have shaped tips with good torque control and hydrophilic coating and are used for negotiating stenosis, and ii) *non-steerable*—which are stiffer wires allowing the positioning of the catheter but not used for crossing the stenosis.

Most guidewires are fragile and can be very expensive. Care should be taken to preserve their useful life as long as possible. Guidewires should be wiped with a saline soaked gauze or lint free pad after each introduction into the body. The buildup of blood clot, fibrin, or dried contrast can render the wire useless. It may also cause it to stick inside the catheters or cause emboli. The guidewires should be stored loosely coiled in a bowl of saline. The saline can be heparinised (5000 U/L) to help prevent thrombus formation.

Selection of Guidewires

Guidewires are a tactile-based surgical tool, which means that physicians take several factors into consideration when choosing their guide wire. Some wires have tapered cores at each ends allowing both ends to be used for introduction. Some guidewires are specially made to enhance their torquibility which is the ability to translate rotational movement of the wire on the outset to the tip inside the patient. These wires can be steered into the desired location in the body.

Based on the shape of the tip, the wires are of two types—J-tip or straight tip **(Figs. 8A and B)**. The *J-tip wires* are frequently used for hooking the ostium of various arteries. *Straight tip guidewire* is used to negotiate biliary obstruction during percutaneous biliary drainage (PTBD). The hard end of the guide wire may be used to push the coil inside the catheters from the cartage where it is lodged. The *extra or superstiff guidewire* are commonly used for inserting percutaneous drainage catheters or insertion of stents into biliary system.

FNAC AND BIOPSY NEEDLE

Biopsy or fine needle aspiration cytology (FNAC) are procedures to obtain a sample of tissue from a tumor for pathological examination. FNAC is a simple and fast procedure for cytological diagnosis. The core needle biopsy is more reliable than FNAC but requires thicker needle, longer processing time and is a little more invasive than FNAC. Needle biopsy may be used to take tissue or fluid samples from muscles, bones and organs, such as the liver or lungs.

The various types of needles that are commonly used for radiologic procedures are as follows:

- *Needle size:* Fine needles (20–25 G) are ideal for cytology and can be safely introduced even through the bowel (except colon) with less chance of hemorrhage. Larger needles (14–19 G) have a better yield of tissue which can help in further subtyping. But it is more traumatic.

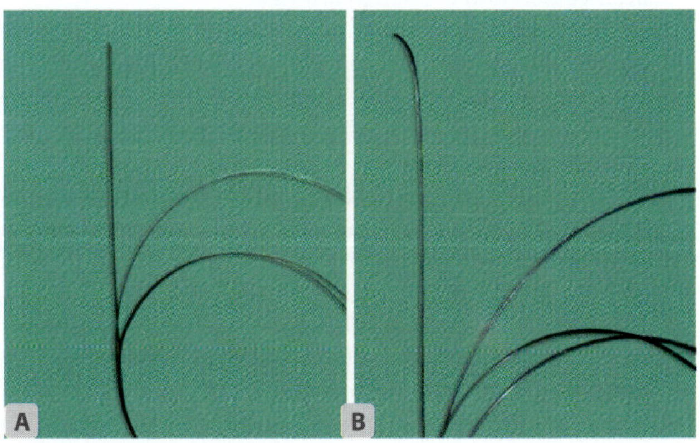

FIGS. 8A AND B: Guidewire. Straight tip (A) and J-tip (B).

- Cutting edge of the needle could be end cutting (acute bevel/ninety degree bevel) or side cutting (cannula gap/stylet gap).
- Spring loaded/automated side-cutting needles are also available.

The selection of the size of needles usually depends on the procedure, size and location of the target. Small lesions at deeper location may require 20 G needle as it stiffer than 22 G which can bend during insertion. However, 22 G needles will be optimum for FNAC of superficial lesions like thyroid or lesions located in the surface of liver. Whenever there is a need to transgress bowel (as in FNAC of pancreatic mass or mesenteric nodes) or a potential space (as in FNAC of lung mass through pleura) or in very hypervascular mass (as in kidney, thyroid), fine needles of 20–25 G need to be used for less complication. Thicker needles (14–19 G) should be used in case lymphoma as well as in equivocal fine needle aspirate in case of unknown primary. Longer needles such as Chiba (20–25 G, Cook catheter, Bloomington, IN) are used whenever samples to be taken from a deeper location.

When a single needle technique is used, multiple punctures are required to obtain multiple samples. This can be more traumatic at times. Alternatively, a coaxial needle system can be used to obtain multiple samples using a single puncture. In this system, a thinner inner needle is inserted through a larger outer needle called an introducer. True-cut-type cutting needles powered by spring-activated handles can be used to obtain a bigger core of tissue, which is of particular importance in the diagnosis of benign lesions (as in benign lung nodules-granulomas/hamartomas) and in lymphoma.

STENT

A stent is a fine tubular structure opened at both end that is usually placed into a tubular structure to keep its lumen open.

The procedure of placing a stent is called stenting. Commonly placement of stents is used in vascular, biliary and urinary system. Other reasons to use stents include keeping open a blockage in the airways. The general categories of stents are self-expanding (SE), balloon-expandable (BE), and stent-grafts (SGs).

- *SE stents* **(Fig. 9A)** are composed of nitinol or elgiloy that are compressed into a delivery catheter that is unjacketed at the point of delivery. They are flexible but are prone for foreshortening. The example of SE stents are wallstent (Boston Scientific), SMART (Cordis Endovascular) and Zilver (Cook).
- *BE stents* are manufactured premounted on a balloon and deployed by dilating with a balloon with an inflator. The BE stents possess stronger radial force but have the potential for dislodgement from the balloon. The Palmaz (Cordis Endovascular) and Express (Boston Scientific) are examples of BE stents.
- *Stent-grafts* may SE or BE which are covered with synthetic material such as Dacron or PTFE **(Fig. 9B)**. Potentially they can prevent the restenosis by their barrier effect but they are costly. Wall graft (Boston Scientific) is a self-expanding stent graft whereas iCast (Atrium Medical, Hudson) is a balloon-expandable stent graft used for aorto-iliac occlusion. These are used when the walls of the vessel need to be covered as in pseudoaneurysms and arterio-venous fistulas. The disadvantage of these stent grafts in vascular use is that if there are any branches arising from the segment of parent vessel in which graft is placed, they get blocked.

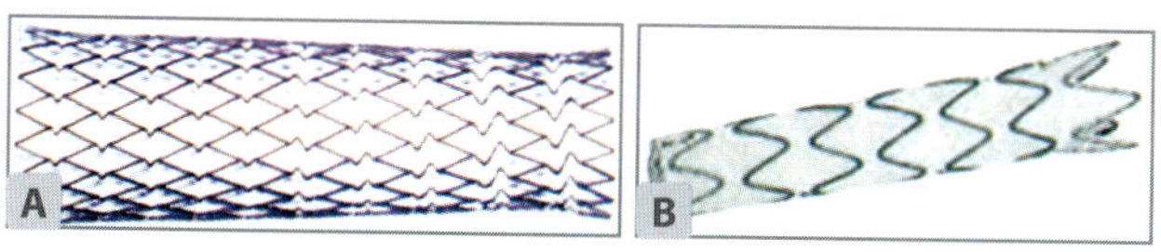

FIGS. 9A AND B: Stents. Self-expanding stent (A) and covered stent graft (B).

Commonly placement of stents is used in vascular, biliary and excretory system. Other reasons to use stents include keeping open a blockage in the airways.

Vascular Stent

The commonly performed vascular stenting is used for coronary, carotid, aorta and lower limb arteries. Vascular stenting is used after angioplasty to treat conditions that involve a narrowing or blockage of arteries or veins throughout the body, including:

- Narrowing of large arteries (aorta and its branches) due to atherosclerosis, or hardening of the arteries, a gradual process in which cholesterol and other fatty deposits, called plaques, build up on the artery walls.
- Peripheral artery disease (PAD), a narrowing of the arteries in the legs or arms. In patients with PAD, angioplasty alone or angioplasty with stenting may be used to open up a blocked artery in the pelvis, leg or arm.
- Renal vascular hypertension, high blood pressure caused by a narrowing of the kidney arteries. Angioplasty with stenting is a commonly used method to open one or both of the arteries that supply blood to the kidneys. Treating renal arterial narrowing is also performed in some patients to protect or improve the kidney function.
- Carotid artery stenosis, a narrowing of the neck arteries supplying blood to the brain.
- Coronary artery disease, a narrowing of the coronary arteries that carry blood and oxygen to the heart muscle. An intraluminal coronary artery stent is a small, self-expanding, metal mesh tube that is placed inside a coronary artery after balloon angioplasty to prevent the artery from reclosure.
- Venous narrowings involving the central veins (in the chest, abdomen or pelvis). In some cases, stenting of the narrowed vein is also needed.
- Keeping artificial communication between hepatic vein and portal vein in TIPS
- Narrowing in dialysis fistula or grafts. When there is decreased flow in the graft or fistula so that is not adequate for dialysis, angioplasty is generally the first line of treatment. Stenting or stent grafting may also be needed in some cases.

A drug-eluting stent is coated with a medicine that stops the growth of fibroblast further prevent the arteries from re-closing. It is like any other coronary artery or peripheral artery stents which is left permanently in the artery.

Biliary Stent

Biliary stents are usually placed to relieve a benign or malignant obstruction of the biliary tree. It may be plastic or metallic and the two most common methods that are used to place a biliary stent are endoscopic retrograde cholangiopancreatography (ERCP) and percutaneous transhepatic cholangiography. Biliary stenting is used to treat obstructions that occur in the bile ducts. There are a number of conditions, malignant or benign, that can cause strictures of the bile duct. Pancreatic cancer is the most common malignant cause, followed by cancers of the gallbladder, bile duct, liver, and large intestine. Noncancerous causes of bile duct stricture include injury to the bile ducts during cholecystectomy, gallstones, pancreatitis and primary sclerosing cholangitis.

An internal stent prevents the problems related to external drainage like, pericatheter leakage of bile. The disadvantage is the procedure of insertion which is invasive. Better patency rates are reported with metallic than with plastic stents in cases malignant obstruction, though no effect on survival is noted. Plastic internal stents **(Fig. 10)** are cheapest but reportedly prone to migration. Various types of plastic stents in use include the Carey-Coons stent (Percuflex; Meditech/ Boston Scientific) and silicone stents (Malecot; Cook, Inc).

Metallic stents **(Fig. 11)** are generally not used in the treatment of benign disease because studies have shown poor long-term patency rates.[1,2] The Gianturco-Rosch Z stent (Cook, Inc), a metallic stent, has been used in benign strictures, but it should not be used for primary treatment. Limited applications may include the treatment of patients who are poor surgical candidates or of those in whom surgical treatment fails. Most postoperative strictures are treated surgically, though endoscopic and (less commonly) percutaneous placement of nonmetallic stents has increasingly been used in the past few years.[3,4]

In cases of malignant obstruction, stents are placed as a palliative measure only if the tumor is unresectable. Various stents are approved for use in the biliary system, including self-expanding and balloon-mounted stents. Various self-expanding stents include the Wallstent (Boston Scientific; Natick, Mass), Luminex stent (Bard; Tempe, Ariz), and Smartstent (Cordis Endovascular; Miami, Fla).[5,6]

Ureteral Stents (Fig. 12)

Ureteral stents are used to ensure the patency of a ureter. Ureteral stents are used to relieve ureteral obstruction, promote ureteral healing following surgery, and to assist with ureteral identification during pelvic surgery. This method is sometimes used as a temporary measure to prevent damage to a blocked kidney until a procedure to remove the stone can be performed. Indwelling times of 12 months or longer are indicated to hold open ureters which have been compressed by tumors in the neighborhood of the ureter or by tumors of the ureter itself. In many cases these tumors are inoperable and the stents are used to ensure drainage of urine through

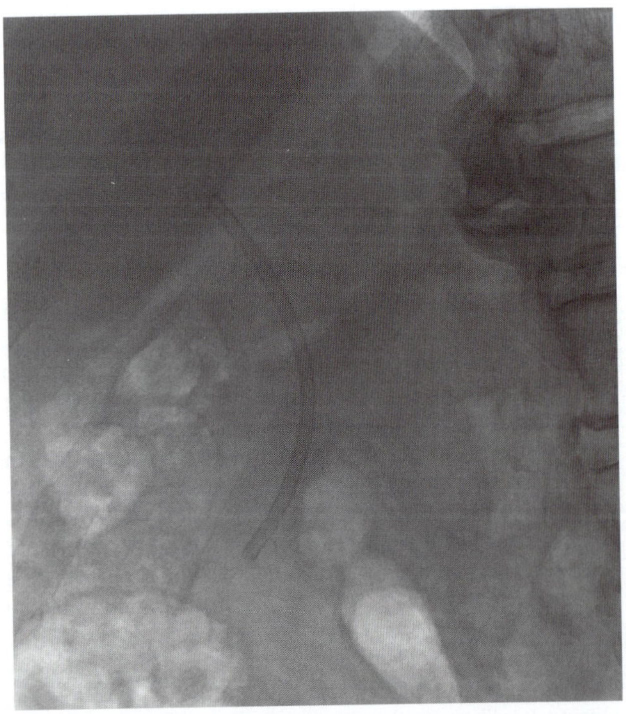

FIG. 10: Plastic stent seen within the common bile duct.

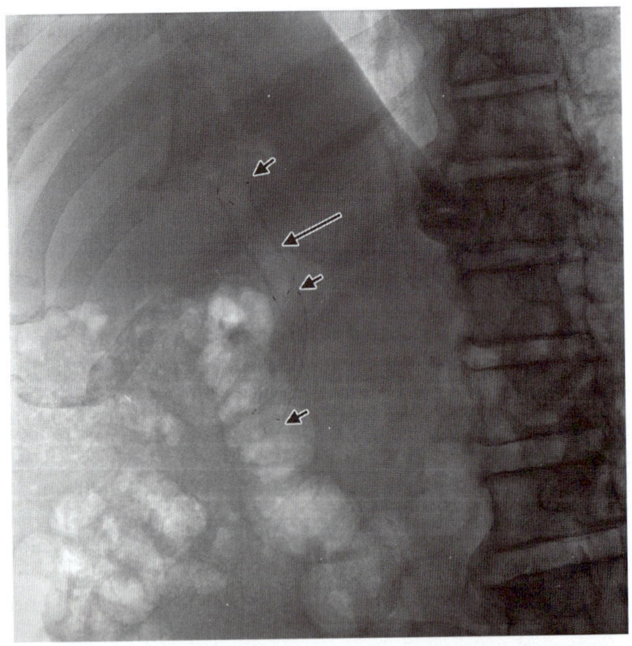

FIG. 11: Metallic stent inside the CBD—note the radiopaque markers (short arrows) in the upper, mid and lower part of the stent.

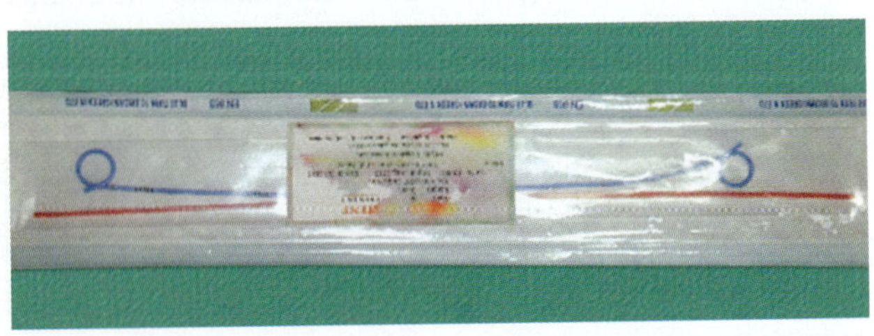

FIG. 12: Plastic double J ureteric stent with the pusher.

the ureter. If drainage is compromised for longer periods, the kidney can be damaged. The main complications with ureteral stents are dislocation, infection, and blockage by encrustation. Recently, stents with coatings (e.g., heparin) have been approved to reduce infection, encrustation and therefore the frequency of stent replacement.

EMBOLIZING AGENTS

Embolizing agents are materials used to acutely stop blood flow in a vessel by mechanical occlusion. The clinical uses are to stop hemoptysis, hematuria, hematochezia, internal bleed or a pseudoaneurysm. Embolization may also be done as an adjunct to surgery or for palliation of malignant tumors. The embolizing agents can be temporary or permanent. The embolization can be done in proximal vessel or in distal bed. Further, the embolization may or may not lead to organ/cellular death. Based on these requirements, the embolizing agents are divided into 4 main categories.

Permanent Proximal Occluders

- *Coils:* These are made of steel or platinum. They commonly have constituent thrombogenic polyester fibers. They are introduced within the vessel in straightened condition but form a spring shape when ejected out of the distal end of delivery catheter. They form a scaffolding upon which thrombus forms leading to permanent occlusion of the vessel. The coils come in various sizes depending upon the size of the wire used, the length of the coil and the diameter of the unconstrained coil. A typical example is 35-3-4. The 35 represents the diameter of the wire used to make the coil in inches which in turn determines the catheter lumen through which it will pass through. The 3 represents the length of straightened coil in cm which is chosen based on length of vessel available for deployment of coil and the 4 represents the diameter of the unconstrained coil loop in mm which is chosen based on diameter of the vessel in which the coil is to be deployed. Coils measuring 0.018 inches or less are termed microcoils and require microcatheters for their deployment. Nester coils are special fibred coils on a platinum strut which are soft and pliable. They conform to the target vessel anatomy when deployed and mainly used for filling up space in large vessels or aneurysms as they bunch up within the lumen. The coils are of two types based on method of deployment—(i) *pushable*—can be pushed out of the catheter by a guidewire or coil pushers, and (ii) *detachable*—are detached from the catheter tip in vivo by either mechanical pressure or electrolytically.
- *Amplatzer vascular plug:* Is a nitinol mesh device which is self expandable occlusive agent. It is deployed by mechanical detachment and is used to occlude vessels ranging from 4–16 mm diameter.

The other less commonly used materials in this category are detachable balloons made of latex or silicon (used for treatment of caroti-cavernous fistulas), small intestinal submucosa, suture material and bare angiographic wires.

Permanent Distal Occluders

- *Polyvinyl alcohol (PVA) particles* **(Fig. 13A)**: This is an inert plastic particle which comes in varying sizes from 100 to 1100 µm. It is available in small vials with each vial having particles of a range of sizes e.g. 300–500 µm, 500–700 µm, etc. It is in fine dry coarse powder form which needs to be suspended in saline or contrast before it is injected through the catheter. The size of the particles to be injected is chosen based on the size of the distal vessel bed to be embolized. The particles go and form clumps within the vessels to permanently occlude it. If larger size particles are chosen they may cause clumping within the catheter or proximal vessel itself to lead to their occlusion. These are most commonly used in tumor bed embolizations (often preoperatively to decrease the vascularity), bronchial artery embolizations,

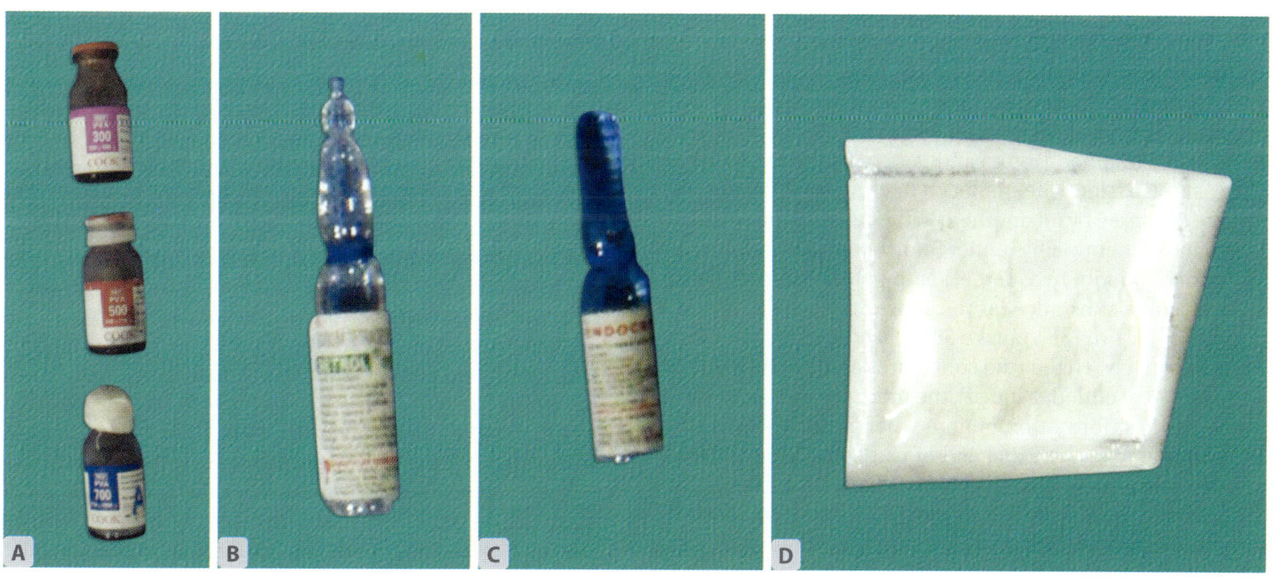

FIGS. 13A TO D: Embolizing agents. PVA particles of various sizes (A), sodium tetradecyl sulphate (B), N Butyl cyanoacrylate (C) and gelfoam (D).

uterine fibroid embolizations, etc. The end point is distal occlusion of the small arterioles without proximal vessel occlusion thereby keeping the option of future repeat embolization of the same vascular territory. PVA is also available in the form of spherical PVA which makes it more compressible and therefore facilitates the delivery. The typical examples are bead block made of hydrogel PVA or embospheres constituted from triacryl gelatin spherical hydrophilic spheres.

- *Sclerosants:* These are liquid agents which produce vascular occlusion by causing inflammation and thrombosis. Absolute alcohol and sodium tetradecyl sulfate (STS) are the two most commonly used sclerosants. Absolute alcohol, besides causing permanent vessel occlusion, also leads to cell death and tissue ablation. It is therefore reserved for use where the end organ cell death is acceptable, e.g. in renal cell carcinomas. It is a very painful procedure and thus is best performed under general anesthesia or liberal analgesia atleast. The use of protective devices like proximal balloons is often required with the use of alcohol to prevent non-target embolization. Sodium tetradecyl sulphate (STS) **(Fig. 13B)** is a relatively milder sclerosant which does not lead to cell death. A 3% concentration solution is used. It is not used intra-arterially but is mainly used for spermatic vein ablations, pelvic congestion syndrome and for venous vascular malformations. Bleomycin and polidocanol are other sclerosants which are used for same indications as above. They are comparatively of lesser efficacy but have an advantage of causing lesser inflammation and hence have lesser side effects.
- *Cyanoacrylates:* These are tissue adhesives. The most common used product is N butyl cyanoacrylate (NBCA) or glue **(Fig. 13C)**. These are in the form of clear liquids at room temperature which get instantly polymerized when they come in contact with an ionic environment. Thus, even a small amount of saline or blood leads to initiation of polymerization reaction of cyanoacrylates. For this reason, when they are to be injected via the delivery catheter, the catheter should be flushed completely with a non-ionic solution (most commonly used 20% dextrose) before and after each injection to prevent polymerization of the agent within the catheter. As soon as the agent ejects out of the distal catheter tip within the vessel, it comes in contact of blood (ionic) and gets polymerized to form a cast. Also, since the cyanoacrylates are radiolucent, they are delivered by mixing them with a radiopaque substance to make them visible under fluoroscopy. Ethiodol (brand name Lipiodol by Guerbet) is the most commonly used non-ionic substance for the same. It is usually mixed in ratio of 1:1 to 5:1 to make 50–20% concentration of glue respectively. Higher the concentration of glue (lesser the amount of ethiodol added), the more proximal and earlier is the cast formation of glue when it comes in contact with blood at the distal end of catheter within the body. A lesser concentration leads to farther delivery of the embolic agent with a slightly delayed cast formation. The embolus which ultimately forms is larger than anticipated with the amount of cyanoacrylate as the substance draws blood elements within it. It is of reasonably lower cost compared to coils.
- *Onyx:* It is a liquid embolic agent formed by combination of ethylene-vinyl alcohol copolymer, dimethyl sulfoxide and tantalum powder. It comes in the form of two vials, one containing the copolymer mixed with tantalum powder and the other containing dimethyl sulfoxide. These need to mixed and placed in a shaker for 20 minutes immediately prior to injection for the agent to become ready for use. The onyx forms a cast as soon as it gets in contact with ionic material (like glue). The cast formation starts from outer surface to inner region. The major advantage of using onyx is much better control over the injection than glue but the deterrent is the significantly higher cost compared with other agents of this category.
- *Thrombin:* It is an enzyme which participates in the coagulation pathway and converts fibrinogen to fibrin. It is mainly used for hemostasis on surgically cut surfaces in the operation theatre. Intravascularly it has been used to induce thrombosis of pseudoaneurysms. Care is required to prevent its propagation into main vessel so as to prevent its occlusion.
- *Ethiodol:* Manufactured under the brand name Lipiodol. It is an inert oil-based contrast agent which is also used as embolizing agent. The radiopaque properties of lipiodol help to make it visible during embolization procedure. Once injected into the vessel, the fat droplets get released and travel distally into smaller vessels till they cannot cross due to their size and then occlude the vessel. This level of distal embolization is at the level of small arterioles. It is commonly used mixed with glue for embolization. The radiopacity of lipiodol adds contrast to glue while the oil-based structure does not allow glue to solidify within the syringe/catheter till it comes in contact with ionic blood. Lipiodol is also used for embolization of hepatocellular carcinoma in combination with chemotherapeutic agents. It has affinity for the lesion and gets deposited in it even when injected non-selectively besides providing radio-opacity to the mixture.

Temporary Proximal Occluders

- *Gelatin sponge:* It is most commonly used in the form of gelfoam **(Fig. 13D)**. It is available as a block which is cut into small pledgets and is made as a slurry mixed with contrast agent for intravascular injection. It leads to temporary mechanical occlusion of proximal vessels for a period of one week to few months. It is used in situations where preservation of blood flow is required in the long-term, e.g. to control bleeding from liver, spleen and in immediate preoperative embolization of tumors. Being inexpensive and easy to use, it is often used as a scaffold for combined embolization with coils.
- *Autologous clot:* Used for very short-term temporary embolization as it gets lysed within few hours. May be used in coagulopathic patients to control bleeding.
- *Nondetachable occlusion balloon:* Used in specific situations like before surgery to reduce intraoperative blood loss, for precise placement of embolic material or to reduce reflux of embolizing material into parent vessel.

Temporary Distal Occluders

- *Starch microspheres:* These are produced from vegetable sources like corn and potato. They are used for very short duration (few minutes) occlusion of distal small vessels, e.g. in procedures like intra-arterial chemotherapy.
- *Gelatin-sponge powder:* It is also available in powder form. When delivered it reaches distal circulation to block it temporarily.

DRUGS IN INTERVENTIONAL RADIOLOGY

Various pharmaceuticals are used for therapeutic interventional radiology procedures. Familiarity with these drugs, and their side effects is essential for any interventional radiologists.

Vasodilators

Vasodilating drugs like nitroglycerine and verapamil relieve arterial spasm (catheter induced or following vasospasm) of distal arteries and enhance distal visualization of small arteries. *Nitroglycerine (NG)* is a short-acting vasodilator that acts instantaneously and lasts for several minutes depending on the dose. *Verapamil* is a calcium-channel blocker and exhibits peak effect within 5 minutes and actions last 10–20 minutes. 50 and 300 mg of 10 mg/ mL nitroglycerine solution is administered as an intra-arterial bolus in glass syringes or as a paste applied topically to the skin over the area of interest. Verapamil can be administered intra-arterial as a bolus of 1–10 mg, usually in a dilution of 10 mL of saline. Blood pressure of the patient should be monitored closely following drug administration. Verapamil is preferred in mesenteric angiography and treatment of cerebral arterial spasm and is contraindicated in patients with cardiac conduction abnormalities

Vasoconstrictors

Vasopressin, a potent vasoconstrictor, is useful in the setting of acute gastrointestinal bleeding. It is administered via an intra-arterial infusion with the catheter positioned selectively within the main trunk of superior mesenteric or the inferior mesenteric artery. The initial dose is usually 0.2 U/min. Repeat arteriograms are performed to assess for bleeding or vasoconstriction and the dose titrated accordingly. If the bleeding is still not controlled then alternatives, such as embolization or surgery, should be considered. Once bleeding is controlled, the infusion is continued for 12–24 hours, while tapering the dose by half every 6–12 hours if there is no further bleeding. When the continuous infusion rate reaches 0.1 U/min for 6–12 hours, the infusion is switched to normal saline; the catheter can be removed after 4–6 hours of no bleeding with normal saline infusion. With the advent of new micro catheters and new embolization agents, embolization is now considered a primary option in the treatment of both upper and lower GI bleeds. Today, vasopressin infusion is preferable in cases where embolization is technically not feasible or contraindicated, such as diffuse mucosal bleeding (e.g., inflammatory processes such as gastritis or granulomatous disease). Common adverse reactions include headache, diaphoresis, nausea/vomiting, abdominal cramps and Antidiuretic effects.

Prothrombotics

Thrombin

The most common use of intravascular thrombin is for pseudo aneurysm (PSA) repair in peripheral vessels.[11] The clinical application of thrombin (bovine and human) is to accelerate the natural clotting process. The main advantage of human recombinant over bovine thrombin is the lower dose and less risk for allergic reactions. Thrombin powder must be reconstituted with sterile normal saline immediately prior to injection. A thrombin concentration of 1000 IU/mL is standard practice. It is available in vials of 500 IU and 2500 IU **(Fig. 14)**. Usually between 0.3 and 3 mL (300–3000 IU) of thrombin is necessary for complete thrombosis. Thrombin is administered slowly into pseudo aneurysm using 19- to 25-G needle under image-guidance under ultrasound or CT guidance until the hypoechoic PSA turns to hyperechoic clot.[12] Injection should stop as soon as clot formation is visualized on duplex ultrasound. Image-guided percutaneous thrombin injection has largely replaced ultrasound-guided compression as the treatment for post catheterization PSAs.[13] True aneurysms of the splenic artery is also amenable to thrombin injection. Coils may be soaked in thrombin to facilitate vessel thrombosis.[14] Large aneurysm neck size (>10 mm) is associated with increased risk of distal embolus or thrombosis and hence needle tip should be kept away from the neck to prevent escape of clot into systemic circulation. Thrombin can also be applied topically to control surface bleeding after intra-arterial puncture, percutaneous biopsy, or dialysis access procedures. Hypersensitivity (e.g., fever, urticaria, and anaphylaxis)[15] reactions can occur with bovine thrombin. Thrombin is pregnancy should be given when benefits outweigh the risks although no contraindication in breastfeeding women.[16]

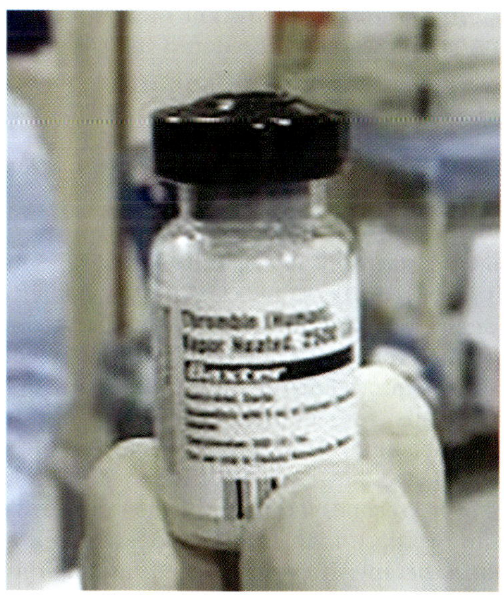

FIG. 14: Thrombin vial.

Anticoagulants

Intravascular procedures using indwelling catheters and sheaths would be impossible without inhibition of the coagulation cascade. These can be classified as:

Parenteral

- *Heparin:*
  - Unfractionated heparin (UFH)
  - Low molecular weight heparin, e.g. Enoxaparin Deltaparin, Tenzaparin
  - Heparinoids
  - Pentsaccharides- Fondoparinux
- Direct thrombin inhibitors (DTIs)—Hirudin, Bivalirudin.

Oral

- Warfarin
- Acenocumarole
- Phenindiones
- Factor Xa inhibitors—Rivaroxaban
- Thrombin inhibitors, e.g. Xemilgatron.

Heparin

Heparin in medical use are a heterogeneous population of linear polysaccharides belonging to the glycosaminoglycan family with molecular weight of 10,000–20,000. Heparin acts indirectly by activation of antithrombin (AT), leading primarily to the inactivation of clotting cascade factors Ca and thrombin(factor IIa) Thrombin is most sensitive to inhibition, and is 10 times more sensitive than factor Xa. Low dose of heparin prolong a PTT without significantly prolonging PT. High concentration of heparin prolong both aPTT and PT.

Injected IV, it acts instantaneously but after SC injection. Anticoagulant effect develops after~60 Min. Heparin does not cross blood brain barriers or placenta (the Anticoagulant of choice during pregnancy). It is metabolized in liver and excreted in urines so its half-life is longer in cirrhotics and renal failure of Patient. After IV injection of deses <100 U/kg, the average half-life is 1 hr. Monitoring of heparin dosage during intervention procedure is guided by measuring activated clotting time (ACT) taken with 2 cc of whole blood. Normal range of ACT is 91–151 and it is to be taken every 1/2 hr.

Dosage of UFM for Optimal Act values in Endovascular Procedures[7-10]

- IV bolus of 3000 U, 5000 U, and 10,000 U, or ranging from 50 U/kg to 100 U/kg. A typical dose use in intervention procedure is 80 U/kg bolus followed by 18 U/kg/hr.
- Target ACT from 150–200 seconds to 350–400 seconds.
- For low-risk procedures ACT 250–300 seconds.
- For high-risk procedures such as angioplasty and stent placement, ACT range of 300–350 seconds is recommended.
- Goal of 400 seconds for stent with filter device. Bleeding due to overdose is the most serious complication of heparin therapy. Heparin induced thrombocytopenia and osteoporosis (on long-term use) are the other adverse effects of heparin.

Heparin Antagonist

Protamine sulphate is a strongly basic low molecular weight protein obtained from the sperm of salmon fish. It is used during hemorrhage in intervention procedure (AVM, aneurysm, vessel rapture). Given IV slowly it neutralizes heparin weight for weight, i.e. 1 mg is needed of every 100 U of heparin. In absence of heparin it itself has weak anticoagulant action. Being basic in nature it can release histamine in the body and can lead to hypersensitivity reactions.

Low Molecular Weight Heparins

Low molecular weight (LMW) heparins (MW 3000–7000) have different anticoagulant profile; selectively inhibit factor Xa with little effect on factor Ia. Thrombocytopenia is less frequent. The major advantages are better subcutaneous availability with once daily s.c. administration. Dose is calculated on the body weight basis. Since aPTT is not prolonged laboratory monitoring is not needed. They are mainly used in prevention and treatment of deep venous thrombosis.

Thrombolytics

Thrombolytic agents are used for the treatment of myocardial infarction, thromboembolic strokes, deep vein thrombosis and pulmonary embolism. They may also be used to clear blocked catheters that are used in long-term medical therapy. The different agents used for thrombolysis can have varied duration of action depending upon their half life **(Table 1)**.

Classification of Thrombolytics

- *1st generation (non-fibrin specific):*
  - Streptokinase
  - Urokinase
- *2nd generation (Fibrin specific):*
  - Prourokinase
  - Recombinant tissue plasminogen activator; Alteplase (Rt.- PA)
- *3rd generation (fibrin specific):*
  - Reteplase (r-PA)
  - Tenecteplase (TNK-tPA)
  - Desmopletase.

Streptokinase is obtained from β-hemolytic Streptococci group C. It is inactive as such; combines with circulating plasminogen to form an activator complex which then cause limited proteolysis of other plasminogen molecules to plasmin. It has limited usefulness because many patients

TABLE 1: Half-life of thrombolytic agents.

Agent	Half-time (min)
Streptokinase	30–80
Urokinase	14–20
Prourokinase	20
Alteplase	3–5
Reteplase	15–18

have preformed antistreptococcal antibodies and have potential for anaphylactic reaction. It is the least expensive of all the fibrinolytics.

Dosage: Bolus 50, 000, infusion: 5000 U/hr for 12 hours.

Urokinase is an enzyme isolated from human kidney urine and mow prepared from cultured human kidney cells. It is no antigenic.

Dosage: Bolus- 30,000–60,000 U, Infusion: 4000 U/hr for 2 hours, 2000 U/hr for next 2 hours and 1000 U/hr for next 8 hours.

Alteplase is produced by recombinant DNA technology. IT is fibrin specific with little effect on circulating plasminogen. It has the drawback of lowering the levels of fibrinogen and plasminogen, leading to an increased risk of hemorrhagic complications. Presently, Rt-PA is the only agent approved by the FDA specifically for IV thrombolysis for ischemic stroke.

Dosage: It is available as 20–50 mg Lyophilized powder, to be reconstituted.

- *Intravenous:* 0.9 mg/kg, 15%-Bolus, 85%-infusion over a period of 30 minutes.
- *Bridging therapy:* 0.6 mg/kg IV (60 mg maximum over 30 minutes) followed by intra-arterially administration at the site of clot up to a total dose of 22 mg over two hours of infusion or until lysis of thrombus was obtained. 3rd generation agent offer the theoretical advantage of longer half-life and greater penetration into the thrombus matrix when compared to 2nd generation agent. Reteplase is a genetically engineered, smaller derivative of recombinant rt-PA that has increased potency and is faster acting than rt PA. Dosage: Intra-arterial: 0.5 U/hr, Intravenous: 1 U/hr, maximum dose of 24 U in 24 hours. Reversal of all thrombolytic can be done by administering fresh frozen plasma in the event of hemorrhagic complication.

Contraindications

Absolute

- Intracranial bleed
- Drug allergy

Relative

- Surgery within 10 days
- Serious GI bleed within 3 months
- Hypertension with diastolic BP≥110 mm Hg
- Active bleeding or hemorrhagic disorder
- Aortic dissection.

Adverse Effects

- Bleeding complication at catheterization site, gastro-intestinal and cerebral hemorrhages may occur.
- Re-thrombosis can occur following thrombolysis and therefore anticoagulants such as heparin are usually co-administered, and continued after thrombolytic therapy.

Antiplatelets

These drug decrease platelet aggregation and thrombus formation. They are effective in arterial circulation where anticoagulant have little effect. Antiplatelet can be classified as:

- Cyclooxygenase-1 (COX-1) Inhibitor: Aspirin
- P2Y12 inhibitors (Thienopyridines): Ticlopidine, clopidogrel, prasugrel.
- Phosphodiesterase inhibitors: Dipyridamole, cilostazol
- GPIIb/IIIa blockers: abciximab, eptifibatide, tirofiban.

Cyclooxygenase-1 Inhibitor

Aspirin induces a permanent functional defect in platelets, which can be detected clinically a prolonged bleeding time. It primarily, acts by irreversible acetylation of COX-1 responsible for the formation of prostaglandin (PG) H2, the precursor of thromboxane (TX) A2.

The nonlinear relationship between inactivation of Platelet COX-1 and inhibition of TXA-2 dependent platelet function by low-dose aspirin has important implication: (i) a substantial reduction in platelet inhibition is associated with less than maximal inactivation of COX-1; (ii) recovery of platelet function is disproportionately rapid, occurring within 3–4 days upon drug withdrawal.

Moreover, inhibition of TXA-2 dependent platelet function by aspirin leaves other platelet pathways [adenosine diphosphate (ADP)-P2Y12, thrombin-protease-activated receptor (PAR)-1] largely unaffected, thus proving a rationale for dual or triple antiplatelet therapy in high-risk settings.

Dosage: 50–325 mg oral.

REFERENCES

1. Seldinger SI. Catheter placement of needles in percutaneous arteriography: a new technique. Acta Radiol 1953;39:328-376.
2. Stavropoulos SW, Rajan D and Cope C. In Abram's angiography: vascular and interventional radiology, Baum S and Pentecost MJ (Eds), 2nd edition. Philadelphia: Lipincott Williams and Wilkins, 2006.
3. Strauss KJ, Damiano MM and Kandarpa K. In Handbook of interventional radiological procedures, Kandarpa K and Aruny JE (Eds), 3rd edition. Philadelphia: Lipincott Williams and Wilkins, 2002.
4. Bakal CW. In Image-guided interventions, Mauro MA, Murphy K, Thomson K, Venbrux AC, Morgan R and Zollikofer CL (Eds). Philadelphia: Elseviers, 2008.
5. Kaufman JA. In Image-guided interventions, Mauro MA, Murphy K, Thomson K, Venbrux AC, Morgan R and Zollikofer CL (Eds). Philadelphia: Elseviers, 2008.
6. Klein JS, Solomon G, Stewart EA. Transthoracic needle biopsy with a coaxially placed 20-gauge automated cutting needle: results in 122 patients. Radiology. 1996;198:715-20.
7. Gabelmann A, Hamid H, Brambs HJ, Rieber A. Metallic stents in benign biliary strictures: long-term effectiveness and interventional management of stent occlusion. AJR Am J Roentgenol. 2001;177(4):813-7.
8. Lopez RR Jr, Cosenza CA, Lois J, et al. Long-term results of metallic stents for benign biliary strictures. Arch Surg. 2001;136(6): 664-9.

9. Thornton K. Postprocedure clinical management for the interventional radiologist. Tech Vasc Interv Radiol. 2006; 9(3):106-12.
10. Ward E, Buckley O, Collins A, Browne RF, Torreggiani WC. The use of thrombin in the radiology department. Eur Radiol. 2009;19(3):670-8.
11. Keeling AN, McGrath FP, Lee MJ. Interventional radiology in the diagnosis, management, and follow-up of pseudoaneurysms. Cardiovasc Intervent Radiol. 2009; 32(1):2-18.
12. Sharma D, Elmore JR, Nadal LL, Sheldon DG, Franklin DP. Treatment of spontaneous lumbar artery pseudoaneurysm by computed tomography-guided thrombin injection. Vasc Endovascular Surg. 2008;42(3):284-8.
13. Lopera JE, Suri R, Cura M, Kroma G, El-Merhi F. Crural artery traumatic injuries: treatment with embolization. Cardiovasc Intervent Radiol. 2008;31(3):550-7.
14. McErlean A, Looby S, Lee MJ. Percutaneous ultrasound-guided thrombin injection as first-line treatment of pancreatic pseudoaneurysm. Cardiovasc Intervent Radiol. 2007;30(3):526-8.
15. Ward E, Doody O, Stunnell H, Torreggiani WC. Percutaneous thrombin embolization of a hepatic artery mycotic aneurysm. Acta Radiol, 2007.
16. Pelchovitz DJ, Cahill AM, Baskin KM, Kaye RD, Towbin RB. Pseudoaneurysm in children: diagnosis and interventional management. Pediatr Radiol. 2005;35(4):434-9.

CHAPTER

43

Magnetic Resonance Contrast Media

Anju Garg, Radhika Batra, Alpana Manchanda

INTRODUCTION

Contrast in magnetic resonance imaging (MRI) is largely due to the heterogeneous distribution of tissue relaxation times, and the lack of need for contrast materials was thought to be the one major advantage of MR over other imaging techniques in the early days. Excellent soft tissue contrast, without the use of any type of contrast agent, made the procedure completely noninvasive. However, it was noted that many important pathological conditions did not show enough specific changes in their relaxation times to differentiate them from surrounding healthy tissue. Exogenous MR contrast agents were therefore developed shortly after the first commercial MR system became available in the 1980's. Presently, exogenous contrast agents are frequently used in a significant proportion of MR examinations to:

- Differentiate between similar appearing structures,
- Increase the specificity in describing regions of abnormal signal,
- Highlight or specify spaces, or
- Study the vascularity and perfusion of normal or abnormal tissues.

BASIC PRINCIPLES OF MR CONTRAST AGENTS

Contrast agents for X-ray and CT show contrasting effects according to their electron-density difference, and they produce direct contrast effects on their positions. However, the contrast mechanism is more complicated for MRI, where the contrast enhancement occurs as a result of the interaction between the contrast agents and neighboring water protons, which can be affected by many intrinsic and extrinsic factors such as proton density and MRI pulse sequences.

The basic principle of MRI is based on nuclear magnetic resonance (NMR) together with the relaxation of proton spins in a magnetic field. When the nuclei of protons, i.e the body's hydrogen atoms, are subjected to a strong magnetic field, their spins align either parallel or antiparallel to the magnetic field. During this alignment, the spins process under a specified frequency, which is known as the Larmor frequency and is dependent on the strength of the magnetic field applied. These protons absorb energy and realign from a longitudinal to a transverse axis, when a 'resonance' frequency in the radio frequency (RF) range is applied. When the RF pulse disappears, the excited nuclei return to their earlier, lower-energy state by two different relaxation pathways. The first, called the longitudinal or T1 relaxation, involves the decreased net magnetization recovering to the initial state. In the second pathway, which is called the transverse or T2 relaxation, the induced magnetization in the perpendicular plane disappears by the dephasing of spins.

MR contrast agents act by altering these relaxation times and this is measured as relaxivity. The relaxivity of a contrast agent is proportional to the magnitude of its moment, its tumbling frequency in solution and its spin relaxation time. They can be classified as T1 and T2 contrast agents, based on their relaxation processes.

When placed in a magnetic field, molecules or ions with one or more unpaired electrons generate a magnetic moment, which aligns with the applied field. These ions or molecules are referred to as paramagnetic, superparamagnetic or ferromagnetic ions depending on their specific electronic configuration. Exogenous paramagnetic compounds of gadolinium, manganese and iron are the most commonly used MR contrast agents.

CLASSIFICATION OF MR CONTRAST AGENTS

Magnetic resonance contrast agents can be classified according to:

1. The magnetic property of the agent
2. The dominant effect of the agent on the signal intensity
3. The biodistribution of the agent.

Magnetic Properties

This is the most common method used to classify the contrast agents into 2 main groups, namely paramagnetic and superparamagnetic.

Paramagnetic Contrast Agents

Paramagnetic materials have their own magnetic field which leads to a reduction in the T1 and T2 relaxation times of the surrounding hydrogen nuclei, causing an increase in signal on T1-weighted images. There are many paramagnetic metal ions that could potentially be used as MR contrast agents but the transition metal gadolinium (Gd^{3+}) is the most commonly used ion. This is due to a favorable combination of seven unpaired electrons with a long electron spin relaxation time making it a very efficient relaxation enhancing agent. Manganese, having relaxation properties similar to gadolinium is also used. All paramagnetic contrast agents need to be chelated with an appropriate ligand to reduce the in vivo toxicity of free gadolinium or manganese.

Superparamagnetic Contrast Agents

Superparamagnetic agents also behave similarly to paramagnetic substances. Small or ultrasmall particles of supermagnetic iron oxide are used as contrast agents in clinical MRI. If the iron ions are magnetically ordered within the crystal, the net magnetic moment is so large that it greatly exceeds that of typical paramagnetic ions. This characteristic effect, of a large magnetic moment in the presence of an external magnetic field without any remnant magnetic moment when the field is zero, is called superparamagnetism. Depending on size and composition of their particles, these agents can also induce a strong enhancement of the T1-relaxation rate of water, but their dominant effect is on T2/T2* relaxation due to the large magnetic moment of the nanoparticles.

Image Enhancement

The contrast agent can either have a positive effect (increase in signal or T1-enhancement) or a negative effect (signal reduction or T2-enhancement) on the signal intensity. Mostly all MR agents affect both T1- and T2-relaxation times and the distinction relies on many MR specific parameters as well as contrast agent dose, e.g. gadolinium based contrast agents usually act as positive enhancers on T1-weighted images but also have a weak T2 negative enhancing effect whereas iron oxide based contrast agents are negative agents that have a predominant T2 and T2* shortening effect.

Biodistribution

The biodistribution of a contrast agent describes how the agent is distributed after intravenous administration.

Extracellular Fluid Agents

Small molecular weight (MW) paramagnetic agents are small enough to diffuse from the plasma into the interstitium and are thus distributed to the extracellular fluid. These agents are known as extracellular fluid (ECF) agents. They are not taken up by cells and are therefore eliminated by renal excretion with a half-life determined by the glomerular filtration rate, e.g. gadolinium based contrast agents.

Intravascular Fluid Agents

Intravascular agents are contrast agents with a MW large enough to prevent leakage from the vascular to the extravascular space. All iron oxide nanoparticles are intravascular agents, with a half-life in blood ranging from a few minutes to several hours. In blood, iron oxide agents with the appropriate composition can produce significant T1 shortening and several studies have reported the use of nanoparticles for MR angiography. Other types of intravascular agents are based on macromolecular gadolinium compounds. Such agents are designed either by linking Gd^{3+} ions to a macromolecular polymer during synthesis or by making the Gd^{3+} complex bind to plasma proteins after injection and thus forming macromolecules in blood.

Tissue Specific Agents

Tissue specific agents are agents which have been specifically designed to accumulate in a particular organ or tissue type. Intravascular iron oxides are taken up by the Kupffer cells present in the liver, spleen and lymphatic system. Once taken up by the liver the nanoparticles will be accumulated into larger particulate clusters in the Kupffer cells and relaxation will be completely dominated by T2/T2* effects. Iron oxides can thus be said to be both intravascular agents as well as tissue specific agents. Mangafodipir trisodium and few gadolinium chelates also act as liver specific agents as they are taken up by hepatocytes.

GADOLINIUM-BASED CONTRAST AGENTS

Copper (Cu^{2+}), Manganese (Mn^{2+}) and Gadolinium (Gd^{3+}) were identified as paramagnetic ions that could shorten the T1 of water, in the early 1980s.

Gadolinium diethyle triamine penta acetic acid salt (Gd DTPA) was found to have high tolerability in animals with preserved good relaxation properties, after extensive analysis of various paramagnetic chelates. Gadolinium DTPA was first tested in humans in 1983 and the first MR contrast medium containing the pharmaceutical product Gadopentetate dimeglumine was introduced in early 1988.[1]

Gadolinium is named after the Finnish chemist Johan Gadolin.[2] Gadolinium belongs to a series of 17 chemically inert metals known as the lanthanides and has an atomic number of 64. The presence of seven unpaired electrons makes it a paramagnetic agent. The strong paramagnetic effect interferes with the relaxivity of nearby water protons and results in a reduction of both T1 and T2 relaxation times. The decrease in the T1 relaxation time is more at low concentrations of Gadolinium and this is seen as increased signal intensity on T1-weighted spin-echo or gradient-echo images.

Free Gd^{3+} ion has high toxicity in vivo as it competes with calcium. Gadolinium has a higher binding affinity for calcium binding enzymes as compared to calcium, thus it can displace calcium and alter all biological processes catalyzed by these enzymes. Free gadolinium also interacts with calcium channels to block physiological pathways that rely on calcium influx, i.e. coagulation and neural transmission.[3] Therefore, when gadolinium is chelated to an organic ligand, it is generally considered safe for use as an MR contrast agent.

Nine GBCAs have been approved for use in the United States and/or the European Union. Most GBCAs that are available are low molecular weight polyamino-carboxylate compounds **(Table 1)**.

They can broadly be classified into two categories based on their binding to serum proteins.

1. The nonspecific extracellular gadolinium chelates or agents that do not bind to serum proteins
2. The high relaxivity agents, that bind to serum proteins.

The nonspecific extracellular GBCAs include-gadopentetate, gadoterate, gadodiamide, gadoteridol, gadobutrol and gadoversetamide. These contrast agents do not bind to any protein and their biodistribution and pharmacokinetics are similar to that of iodinated water-soluble contrast media.

After intravenous injection, they rapidly diffuse into the interstitial extravascular space. There is also reverse diffusion into the intravascular compartment and an equilibrium state between diffusion in and out is usually reached within 2 hours. They are eliminated unchanged from the intravascular compartment by passive glomerular filtration and more than 95% of the injected dose is excreted in the urine by 24 hours in patients with normal renal function. A tiny amount (less than 0.1 %) is eliminated via feces. In patients with normal renal function, the biological half-life is approximately 1.5 hours.

Three basic phases of vascular and tissue enhancement occur following administration of GBCAs: arterial, blood pool and extracellular phases. Routine post contrast images are acquired when the contrast has reached the extracellular interstitial space i.e. approximately 2 minutes after injection. As the extracellular enhancement changes little over several minutes, fast scanning techniques are not essential for imaging. Interstitial enhancement is particularly conspicuous with suppression of the lipid signal intensity and T1W, fat suppressed images give the best contrast. However, if fat is nulled via inversion recovery with a short inversion time (STIR), enhancing tissue is also nulled because of its short T1 relaxation time. Therefore, the STIR technique is not advocated after administration of T1-shortening contrast agents.

Best acquisition of the arterial phase images occurs during the first pass of contrast agents through the arterial system i.e. within 20 seconds of contrast administration. Early arterial images are best for depicting arteries, and late arterial phase images are better for depicting hypervascular tissues. Blood pool or portal venous phase occurs at 60-90 seconds after contrast administration during which contrast is typically distributed throughout the body's vessels. Maximum liver parenchymal enhancement is also achieved during this phase. Dynamic imaging for detection and characterization of lesions in the liver and other organs can be performed, similar to CT, using nonspecific extracellular GBCAs.

Interstitial contrast agent is especially prominent in neoplastic tissues and areas of inflammation. Fibrous tissue has a large interstitial space and is therefore much enhanced on extracellular phase images even though it is usually hypovascular. Many metastases also have large interstitial spaces and are hyperintense on extracellular phase images. Capillaries in brain and testicular tissue are not permeable to these contrast agents, unlike capillaries throughout the rest of the body. Hence the enhancement of the brain is minimal, owing entirely to enhancement of the blood pool. Tumors and injured brain parenchyma enhance much more because of the enhancement of their interstitial space and so the depiction of brain lesions in post contrast images is very high. In addition to diffusing across tissue capillary walls, GBCAs diffuse across glomerular walls into the renal tubules, within which they are concentrated as water is reabsorbed. This makes them highly effective for enhancing the kidneys and the urinary tract.

The high relaxivity agents include gadobenate, gadoxetate and gadofosveset. These agents bind to proteins and have a higher T1 relaxivity than the above mentioned gadolinium chelates (see **Table 1**). Immediately after the bolus injection, gadobenate and gadoxetate, act as nonspecific extracellular gadolinium chelates but later they act as liver specific agents in the delayed phase, as they are taken up by liver cells.

TABLE 1: Gadolinium-based contrast agents approved for clinical use.[6]

Generic name	Trade name/ manufacturer	T1 relaxitivity (L/mmol/s at 1.5 T)	Molecular weight	Excretion	Protein binding
Gadopentetate dimeglumine Gd-DTPA	Magnevist/Bayer Magnascan/Unijules	4.1	939.0	Renal	None
Gadoterate meglumine Gd-DOTA	Dotarem/Guerbert	3.6	558.6	Renal	None
Gadodiamide Gd-DTPA-BMA	Omniscan/GE	4.3	573.6	Renal	None
Gadoteridol Gd-HP-DO3A	ProHance/Bracco	4.1	558.7	Renal	None
Gadobutrol Gd-DO3A-butrol	Gadovist/Bayer	4.7	604.7	Renal	None
Gadoversetamide Gd-DTPA-BMEA	Optimark/Mallinckrodt	4.7	661.8	Renal	None
Gadobenate disodium Gd-BOPTA	MultiHance/Bracco	8.3	1058.2	96% Renal, 4% Hepatic	<5%
Gadoxetate disodium Gd-EOB-DTPA	Primovist, Eovist/Bayer	6.9	682.0	50% Renal, 50% Hepatic	<10%
Gadofosveset trisodium	Vasovist, Ablavar/Bayer	19	958.0	91% Renal, 9% Hepatic	>85%

Excretion occurs through both, renal and hepatobiliary pathways. Gadobenate dimeglumine has a capacity for weak and transient protein binding. Approximately 2–4% of the injected dose is taken up by liver cells and its delayed imaging time is between 90–120 minutes.

Gadoxetate disodium has the maximum biliary excretion (almost equal biliary and renal excretion) with a convenient delayed imaging time of 10–20 minutes. The liver parenchymal enhancement is more intense with gadoxetate as compared to gadobenate. These two agents act similar to other gadolinium chelates during the initial phase and are therefore useful in assessing tumor enhancement and characterization. They cause selective increase in the signal intensity of the liver (via hepatocyte uptake) in the later phases, thus helping in the detection of small tumors. This relies on degree of differentiation of tumors, as well differentiated hepatocellular carcinoma may take up the contrast and become less conspicuous. However, these agents are best used for detection of metastases. Also, due to the biliary excretion during the delayed phase, the biliary ducts can be mapped well using T1-weighted images.

Gadofosveset has 80–90% binding to serum albumin. This high protein binding has 2 effects: firstly it markedly increases the relaxivity (hence requiring lower doses and concentration) and secondly, it results in the agent being effectively confined to the vascular space. It has successfully been used as a blood pool agent for MR angiography, owing to its prolonged intravascular retention. The protein binding is reversible and gadofosevet is ultimately excreted unchanged by the kidneys through glomerular filtration.

As mentioned previously, it is essential to chelate gadolinium in order to reduce its toxicity. The chemical structure of chelators used to bind the gadolinium ion are different and may be linear or macrocyclic. The chemical structure of a typical linear and a typical macrocyclic GBCA are depicted in **Figures 1A and B**. Gadolinium chelates can also be categorized into 4 classes based on their biochemical structure-macrocyclic or linear, and ionicity-ionic or nonionic as given below:

- Linear, ionic—gadopentetate, gadobenate, gadoxetate and gadofosveset
- Linear, nonionic—gadodiamide and gadoversetamide
- Macrocyclic, ionic—gadoterate
- Macrocyclic nonionic—gadoteridol and gadobutrol

The GBCAs vary with respect to osmolality and viscosity. Their osmolality ranges between 0.63 osmol/kg to 1.97 osmol/kg **(Table 2)**. In vivo, the osmotic load of all the GBCAs is very low, compared to iodinated contrast media, as only a small amount of the contrast agent is needed to produce a diagnostic MR examination. The nonionic agents tend to have lower osmolarity and are also less viscous. Nonionic low osmolar GBCAs have lesser negative isotropic effects, which is a vital consideration for cardiac patients. Less pressure is required to inject low viscosity GBCAs and these can be administered using smaller gauge needles or catheters.

The stability of an agent describes the affinity of the gadolinium atom for its compound and is based on its thermodynamic and conditional stability. The dissociation constants **(Table 2)** can be utilized to describe the stability of the linear GBCAs. The higher the dissociation constant, greater is the stability of the agent. In contrast to the linear agents, the macrocyclic agents require a significant amount of energy to dissociate the gadolinium complexes. The kinetics of dissociation are described by the dissociation rate and the dissociation half life with these agents. In general, the ionic agents are more stable than the non-ionic agents.[4] The stability increases from nonionic linear to ionic linear to macrocyclic agents, when considering agents by class.[5,6]

Due to the toxicity of the free metal ion, many agents are bound to excess chelate **(Table 2)**. The excess chelate is considered essential because of the possibility of transmetallation with trace amounts of zinc in the blood and a consequent release of free gadolinium ion. Therefore, the least stable agents, gadodiamide and gadoversetamide, the two agents with the weakest thermodynamic stability constants, each have considerably larger amounts of excess chelate (12 mg/mL and 28.4 mg/mL respectively) as compared to the most stable agents, gadoterate and gadoteridol (0 and 0.23 mg/mL of excess chelate respectively). The presence and quantity of excess chelate can be considered as an indirect marker of the instability of the contrast agent.[6,7]

Interaction between Extracellular MRI Contrast Agents with Clinical Tests

Extracellular MRI contrast agents may cause spurious hypocalcemia as they can interfere with the assay method of calcium measurement. Knowledge of this effect on calcium measurements by some of the MRI contrast agents

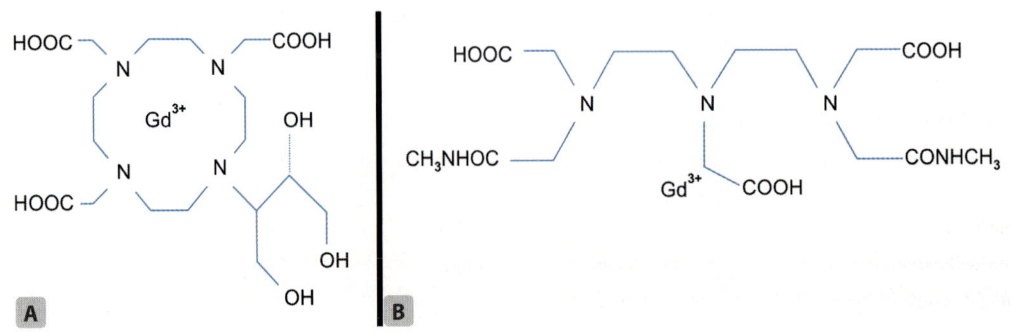

FIGS 1A AND B: Chemical structure of gadolinium-based contrast agents. (A) Typical macrocyclic agent—gadobutrol and (B) Typical linear agent—gadodiamide.

is essential in order to prevent incorrect and potentially hazardous treatment. It is prudent to be cautious when using colorimetric assays for angiotensin-converting enzyme, calcium, iron, magnesium, total iron binding capacity and zinc in serum samples of patients who have recently received GBCAs. Therefore, it is better to perform biochemical assays before the injection of contrast media, or delay them for at least 24 hours afterwards or longer in patients with renal impairment.

Dose of GBCAs

Generally the recommended dose for clinical use is 0.1 mmoL/kg body weight, but upto 0.3 mmoL/kg body weight may be used, particularly for MRA. Smaller doses can be used for the high relaxivity agents.

Adverse Effects of GBCAs

Extracellular MRI contrast agents are well tolerated and are associated with a low incidence of adverse effects. Mild adverse reactions such as nausea, vomiting and urticaria infrequently occur after GBCA administration. Other rare adverse effects include headache, taste disturbance, dizziness and paresthesia. While adverse reactions are infrequent in the general patient population, they are commoner in patients with a history of asthma or allergy, and in patients injected at a faster rate.[3]

These types of adverse effects are similar with all GBCAs, with no significant differences observed between various agents. The incidence of mild adverse effects is less than 5%. Anaphylactoid reactions have been reported, but they are very infrequent. Life-threatening reactions are very rare with an incidence around 1:100000. Fatal reactions may occur, however, are extremely rare.[8,9]

Contrast-induced Nephropathy

Extracellular MRI agents are more nephrotoxic than iodinated contrast media in equimolar doses. However, as the dose of gadolinium based contrast medium required for a diagnostic MRI examination is very small in comparison to doses of iodinated contrast media for CT and other radiographic examinations, nephrotoxicity due to these agents is uncommon even in patients with renal disease. In patients with marked reduction in renal function (particularly due to diabetes mellitus), contrast-induced nephropathy (CIN) may occur even at the standard doses of gadolinium based MR contrast agents.[10]

Gadolinium attenuates X-rays and hence its use for radiographic examinations instead of iodinated contrast media has been advocated in patients with history of serious adverse reactions to iodinated contrast media and in patients who are to undergo imminent thyroid treatment with radioactive iodine. In patients with renal impairment, GBCAs should not be used in place of iodinated contrast media as they can induce nephrotoxicity at the doses required to produce adequate radiographic enhancement.[3]

Extravasation

It can be challenging to monitor a patient for extravasation, particularly when the patient is deep in the bore of the MR unit. An extravasation may occur at a distance from the injection site. Extravasation of GBCAs into the surrounding tissues can result in edema, inflammation and necrosis. However, in majority of the cases the effect is minimal with no long term sequelae. Some patient categories like infants, young children, unconscious and debilitated patients, patients with arterial insufficiency or compromised venous/lymphatic drainage are less able to tolerate extravasation. Low osmolar, nonionic GBCAs reduce the risk of an extravasation as they tend to have lower viscosity, and because they are better tolerated, the severity is less following extravasation.[11]

Nephrogenic Systemic Fibrosis

Gadolinium enhanced MRI was considered one of the safest imaging procedures. However, the concern of associated nephrogenic systemic fibrosis (NSF) forced the radiology community to rethink this belief. The first case of NSF was described in 1997 as a skin disorder resembling scleromyxedema and was termed as nephrogenic fibrosing dermopathy.[12] Later, when systemic manifestations were identified, the nomenclature was changed to nephrogenic systemic fibrosis. NSF is characterized by scleroderma—

TABLE 2: Physicochemical properties of gadolinium-based contrast agents.[7]

Generic name/trade name	Osmolality (37°C, osmol/kg H_2O)	Viscosity (mPa at 37°C)	Thermodynamic stability constant	Conditional stability constant at pH 7.4	Metal chelates (mg/mL)	Excess chelates (mg/mL)
Gadopentetate/Magnevist	1.96	2.9	22.1	18.1	469	0.4
Gadoterate meglumine/ Dotarem	1.35	2.0	25.8	18.8	278.3	0
Gadodiamide/Omniscan	0.79	1.4	16.9	14.9	287	12
Gadoteridol/Prohance	0.63	1.3	23.8	17.1	279.3	0.23
Gadobutrol/Gadovist	1.6	4.96	21.8	14.7	605	0.5
Gadoversetamide/Optimark	1.11	2.0	16.6	15.0	330.9	28.4
Gadobenate/Multihance	1.97	5.3	22.6	18.4	334	0
Gadoxetate/Primovist/Eovist	0.688	1.19	23.5	18.7	181.4	1
Gadofosveset/Vasovist	0.825	1.8	22.1	18.9	244	0.27

like skin changes (swelling, skin induration, skin colored erythematous papules, woody skin) that mainly affect the limbs—lower limbs more than upper limbs and trunk. Fibrotic changes may also affect other organs such as muscles, heart, lungs, oesophagus, liver, kidneys and testes. The disease can be aggressive in some patients leading to severe physical deformity or even death.

The association of gadolinium with development of NSF was first described in 2006 by Grobner.[13] Since then, several studies have confirmed that gadolinium is present in the tissues of patients with NSF, thus supporting that it has a causative role in the development of this condition.[14-16] The time between the GBCA injection and onset symptoms of NSF can vary from days to months; however, in rare cases, symptoms have even appeared years after the last reported exposure.[6]

Although, the exact mechanism of NSF is not yet established, it is known to occur exclusively in patients with decreased renal function (glomerular filtration rate <30 mL/min/1.73 m^2). The most widely held hypothesis is that in patients with renal impairment there is a prolongation in the clearance time of GBCAs. This causes the gadolinium chelates to undergo transmetallation i.e the gadolinium is displaced from its chelate by other cations in the body and released in the form of free gadolinium. This free gadolinium binds with an anion such as phosphate, forming an insoluble precipitate which is deposited in various tissues leading to activation of circulating fibrocytes and subsequent fibrotic reaction in the involved tissues. The presence of gadolinium in affected tissues of NSF patients supports this theory.[15] Since the various GBCAs have varying degrees of stability in vitro and in vivo, this can help to at least partly explain why these agents differ in their apparent NSF safety profile in at-risk patients.

Currently, there is no effective treatment for NSF. Trials with corticosteroids, photopheresis, plasmapheresis, thalidomide, methotrexate, etc. have not had much success. There is also no evidence that immediate hemodialysis protects against the development of NSF. Improving renal function seems to slow or arrest progression of this condition.

Risk Factors for NSF

Patient factors: The patients at highest risk for development of NSF are those on dialysis or with acute or chronic kidney disease. It has been seen that there is a 1–7% chance of developing NSF in patients with severe chronic kidney disease (CKD4, eGFR 15–29 mL/min/1.73 m^2) and end-stage CKD (CKD5, eGFR <15 mL/min/1.73 m^2) after one or more exposures to at least some GBCAs. Only one case report of a patient with eGFR values above 30 mL/min/1.73 m^2 has been published.[17]

It has also been seen that some patients with severe CKD or acute kidney injury (AKI) develop NSF following exposure to GBCAs while others do not. In one study where 30 patients having an eGFR of under 30 mL/min/1.73 m^2 were exposed to high doses of gadodiamide (median dose of 90 mL and range of 40–200 mL), only one of the 30 patients subsequently developed NSF, an observed incidence of about 3%.[18] So it is theorized that although gadolinium is necessary for development of NSF, it is not the only trigger. A number of other possible cofactors have been postulated to play a role, including metabolic acidosis or medications that predispose patients to acidosis, increased calcium, iron, and/or phosphate levels, high-dose erythropoietin therapy, vasculopathy, immunosuppression and infection, or some other acute pro-inflammatory events.[19] As none of these have been consistently confirmed as true cofactors, routine screening for them before GBCA administration is not recommended. Hepatic disease, without the presence of AKI or severe CKD, should not considered a risk factor for NSF.[20]

Contrast medium factors: Cases of NSF have been reported for almost all GBCAs. Although it is the linear GBCAs which account for majority of NSF cases, the most commonly reported agent being gadodiamide followed by gadopentetate and gadoversetamide—NSF has also been reported for the macrocyclic formulation—gadoteridol.[21] As it is the stability of the binding of gadolinium within the chelate which is an important factor in pathogenesis of NSF (as discussed above), the macrocyclic chelates offer better protection and binding to gadolinium ion in comparison to the linear molecules. The American College of Radiology (ACR) Manual on Contrast Media states that although the differences in the number of reported cases may be explained on the basis of the different chemical properties of various GBCAs, it could be possible that other factors like amount of market share, patient population, duration of time for which the particular agent has been in use, and a possible reporting bias may, in part, also have contributed to the differences in the number of reported cases.[20]

Based on the available data, the ACR, the European Medicines Agency (EMA) and United States Food and Drug Administration (US FDA), all have classified the GBCAs into three groups **(Table 3)**, although the scheme used by each of them is not identical. There is limited data for Group III agents, although, to date, few, if any, unconfounded cases of NSF have been reported.[20] A higher incidence of NSF is also associated with high doses of GBCAs, either as a single administration or cumulatively in multiple administrations over months to years.

TABLE 3: ACR classification of GBCAs based on reported prevalence of NSF.[20]

Group I: Agents associated with the greatest number of NSF cases
• Gadodiamide (Omniscan®) • Gadopentetate dimeglumine (Magnevist) • Gadoversetamide (OptiMARK)
Group II: Agents associated with few, if any, unconfounded cases of NSF
• Gadobenate dimeglumine (MultiHance) • Gadoteridol (ProHance) • Gadoteric acid (Dotarem) • Gadobutrol (Gadovist)
Group III: Agents for which data remains limited regarding NSF risk, but for which few, if any unconfounded cases of NSF have been reported
Gadoxetate disodium (Eovist/Primovist)

In spite of differences in the incidence of NSF, there is no evidence that any of the approved GBCAs are safe in the at-risk patient population. Conversely, in patients without renal disease, all gadolinium-based contrast agents seem to be safe. As healthcare providers have been restricting their use of GBCAs in patients at risk for NSF, the incidence of NSF has dropped drastically. This reduction reflects the changes that have been implemented in MR practice since the risks of NSF have been widely publicized.[22]

Guidelines on GBCA Usage

The ACR, the US-FDA and European Commision/ European Medicines Agency (EC/EMA) have all given their recommendations on the use of GBCAs. The three groups use different words, however, there are only minor differences between their recommendations.[23] The ACR guidelines are given below:

As the risk for developing NSF varies according to the group of GBCAs being used, thus the assessment of the patients prior to contrast administration will also vary. For patients receiving *Group II agents*, in standard or lower than standard doses, the ACR committee on Drugs and Contrast Media considers that the risk of NSF is sufficiently low or possibly nonexistent such that assessment of renal function using a questionnaire or laboratory tests is optional prior to intravenous administration. Patients receiving *Group I* GBCAs should be considered at risk of developing NSF if any of the following conditions apply to the patient:

- Any form of dialysis
- Severe or end stage renal disease without dialysis
- Acute kidney injury

There is insufficient data to assess the risk of NSF after administration of *group III* agents, in spite of an alternative pathway of excretion for hepatobiliary agents. So for group I and III GBCAs renal function assessment should be done as detailed in **Table 4**.

Additionally, ACR has made recommendations for specific patient populations with compromised renal function, as given in **Table 5**.

With the recent finding of gadolinium deposition in the brain, certain additional restrictions have been imposed on the usage of GBCAs by the USFDA and EMA. These have been dealt with later in the chapter, in the section on "Gadolinium presence in brain and body".

GBCA Administration in Children

Guidelines for intravenous use of GBCAs are generally similar in the adult and pediatric population. Only few pediatric cases of NSF have been reported and no cases have been reported in children less than 6 years of age. Nevertheless, enough data is not available to demonstrate that NSF is less likely to occur in children as compared to adults. Children who are at risk for renal impairment (e.g. chronic kidney disease or acute kidney injury) or those

TABLE 5: ACR recommendations for specific groups of patients.[20]

Patient category	Recommendations
ESRD on chronic dialysis	• Consider administration of iodinated contrast media and perform CT wherever possible • If CEMRI essential—Group I agents are contraindicated, use Group II agents • Use lowest possible dose of GBCA CEMRI should be performed as closely before hemodialysis as possible
CKD 4 or 5 (eGFR <30 mL/min/1.73 m^2) not on chronic dialysis	Group I agents are contraindicated Group II agents should be used if required
CKD 3 (eGFR = 30–59 mL/min/1.73 m^2)	Development of NSF exceedingly rare in this group No special precautions required
CKD 1 or 2 (eGFR = 60–119 mL/min/1.73 m^2)	Any GBCA can be administered safely
Acute kidney injury	Group I agents should be avoided, Group II agents are preferred*

* Due to the temporal lag between eGFR and actual GFR it is not possible to determine whether a given patient has AKI based on a single eGFR determination.

TABLE 4: eGFR evaluation of renal function prior to administration of group I or group III GBCAs.[20]

Patient condition	eGFR requirement
Patient on dialysis (any type)	No eGFR required
Patient with AKI	No eGFR required
Inpatient	Obtain eGFR within 2 days of the MRI study
Outpatient/emergency with no prior eGFR at the time the MR is scheduled	If no risk factors*, no eGFR required With risk factors, obtain eGFR
Outpatient/emergency with most recent prior eGFR of 45 or above	If no risk factor and eGFR of 60 or above, no new eGFR required With risk factors and/or eGFR 45–59, if most recent prior eGFR is within 6 weeks of the MRI, no new eGFR is needed; otherwise obtain a new eGFR
Outpatient/emergency with most recent prior eGFR of 44 or below	Obtain eGFR within 2 days of the MRI study

**Risk factors*: (1) History of renal disease, including: (a) Prior dialysis, (b) Renal transplant, (c) Single kidney, (d) Kidney surgery, (e) Renal cancer; (2) Hypertension requiring medical therapy; (3) Diabetes mellitus with renal/urinary tract structural abnormalities should be identified and screened for renal function.

The eGFR values in some premature neonates and infants may be <30 mL/min/1.73 m^2 due to immature renal function, in these children cautious use of intravenous gadolinium agents is imperative. Although not based on specific evidence, some suggest avoiding use of high risk gadolinium agents in very young children (e.g. neonates <4 weeks).[20]

GBCAs During Pregnancy and Lactation

When given in clinical doses, all gadolinium based contrast agents cross the human placenta, enter the fetal circulation and are then excreted through the kidneys into the amniotic fluid. As the fetus swallows the amniotic fluid, the excreted GBCA can be absorbed and again excreted, which raises a concern of gadolinium dissociation. There are no large well-controlled teratogenic studies of the effects of these agents in pregnant women. However, small retrospective studies of women who were exposed to gadolinium chelates during their pregnancy have not reported any harmful fetal or maternal effects.[24,25]

As it is unclear how GBCAs will affect the fetus, they should be used only with extreme caution. The ACR has recommended criteria of appropriateness in using GBCAs during pregnancy. A GBCA should only be given if the referring clinician and the radiologist feel that a) the diagnosis cannot be made without its use, and would change the management, b) delaying the examination until after delivery is not possible, and c) the required information cannot be obtained by using any other imaging modality. The above should be explained to the patient, documented in the medical records of the patient and a formal consent should be taken.[20]

If it is required to perform a contrast enhanced MRI during pregnancy, then the lowest possible dose of an agent which is believed to be at low risk for development of NSF should be used. If the pregnant patient has an impaired renal function then the same precautions should be taken as in the non pregnant patient.

Only tiny amounts of GBCAs given to a *lactating mother* reach the milk.[26] In patients with normal renal function, less than 0.04% of intravenously administered GBCA is secreted into the breast milk. Less than 1% of this oral GBCA is absorbed by the baby's gastrointestinal tract (GIT), which results in exposure of less than 0.0004% of the maternal dose to the breastfeeding baby,[27] and therefore, the ACR recommends that GBCAs can be safely administered to a lactating mother. However, the EMA recommends discontinuation of breast feeding for at least 24 hours for all patients with high NSF risk GBCAs. Ultimately, an informed decision to temporarily refrain from breast feeding should be left to the mother after communication of these facts. If the mother remains concerned about any potential side effects, she may abstain from breast feeding from the time of contrast administration for a period of 12–24 hours.

Gadolinium Presence in Brain and Body

Diposition of Gadolinium in Brain

Kanda T et al. in 2014 were the first to report an association between repeated GBCA administration and increased signal intensity on noncontrast TIW images in the dentate nucleus and globus pallidus areas of the brain.[28] Since then many clinical and experimental studies have been conducted and their findings published. Autopsy studies of brain specimens have shown gadolinium deposition in the capillary endothelium and neural interstitium of dentate nucleus and globus pallidus with a significant dose-dependent relationship.[29] The increased signal intensity has been seen to occur after approximately five or more administrations of linear GBCAs with standard dose in patients with normal renal function and an intact blood brain barrier. Early studies did not show any increase in the signal intensity after repeated administrations of macrocyclic GBCAs.[30,31] However, some studies have reported that macrocyclic GBCAs can also cause gadolinium retention, although the exposure required was much higher for macrocyclic GBCAs than for linear GBCAs.[32] No clinical symptom or adverse health effects have been confirmed to be associated with the signal increase and/or the gadolinium deposition in the brain.

Deposition of Gadolinium in Other Organs

Besides brain, gadolinium has also been seen to be deposited in other organs like bone, skin, liver etc. A positive correlation was seen between the dose of administered GBCA and gadolinium concentration measured in bone.[33] Deposition of gadolinium in cortical bone occurs at much higher levels as compared to brain and there is a significant correlation between the two. Thus, it has been suggested that bone may serve as a surrogate to estimate the gadolinium in brain.

Regulatory Statements

In view of the uncertain clinical consequences of deposition of gadolinium in the brain and other organs, many official regulatory statements have been published to warn about the safe use of GBCAs. In 2017, the USFDA recommended that healthcare professionals should be careful when using a GBCA in patients with higher risk, such as those who may need repeated contrast enhanced MRI scans to monitor a chronic condition, children and pregnant patients. The FDA also recommended a new class-wide warning about gadolinium retention in the labeling of GBCAs; and a new patient medication guide that should be informed to the patient before receiving a GBCA.

The EMA has placed restrictions on using linear gadolinium agents in the Eurpopean union from November 2017. It has recommended:

- Suspension of all multipurpose intravenous linear agents (gadoversetamide, gadopentetic acid, and gadodiamide)
- Intravenous linear agents such as gadobenic acid and gadoxetic acid to be used only for liver scans when they meet an important diagnostic need
- Gadopentetic acid only to be used in intra-articular applications, as the gadolinium concentration in the formulation used for joint injections is very low.
- Macrocyclic agents (gadoteric acid, gadobutrol, and gadoteridol) can continue to be used in their current indications but at the lowest doses that enhance images sufficiently and only when unenhanced body scans are not appropriate.

Gadolinium Deposition Disease

In 2016, Semelka et al. proposed this name for a disease process observed in subjects with normal or near normal renal function who develop persistent symptoms that arise hours to 2 months after the administration of GBCAs.[34] These symptoms may include pain in the lower arms and legs, persistent headache, bone and joint pains, clouded mentation, subcutaneous soft tissue thickening and excruciating pain. In these cases, no pre-existent disease or subsequently developed disease of an alternate known process was present to account for the symptoms. The authors believe that although this is an uncommon entity, radiologists and physicians should be aware of it and not ignore severe symptoms after administration of GBCAs.[35]

MANGANESE-BASED CONTRAST AGENTS

Manganese (Mn^{2+}) like gadolinium (Gd^{3+}) is also a strongly paramagnetic substance as it has five unpaired electrons in its structure. Its compound, Mangafodipir trisodium (MnDPDP, Teslascan) is chemically similar to vitamin B_6, and so it is specifically taken up by hepatocytes. As it causes an increase in the signal intensity of normal hepatic parenchyma it gives a high lesion-to-liver contrast. Thus it improves detection and characterization of liver lesions.[36] In the later phases, MnDPDP is excreted through bile leading to excellent biliary ductal detail and helping in the diagnosis of various biliary pathologies.[37] MnDPDP was also found to collect in the pancreatic parenchyma and so has been clinically useful for the evaluation of pancreatic lesions.

Unlike the GBCAs, MnDPDP readily dissociates to yield free manganese ions after injection. The instability of the chelate raised concerns about potential toxicity. In chronic exposure, free manganese, can accumulate in the brain and cause a parkinsonism-like syndrome. It can also have a depressive action on heart function. Moreover, in patients with chronic liver failure whose ability to excrete manganese is reduced, significant neurological risk maybe associated with manganese intoxication. Hence, MnDPDP has effectively been withdrawn from the market.[7]

Mn-based nanoparticles are currently under research for use as high performance contrast agents with reduced toxicity.

IRON OXIDE-BASED CONTRAST AGENTS

Superparamagnetic iron oxide particles were suggested as potential liver specific MR contrast agents as early as 1980s. These agents contain a crystalline core of water insoluble iron oxide crystals, usually magnetite (Fe_3O_4) or maghemite (γ-Fe_2O_3) with a core diameter between 4–10 nm. These iron oxide crystals are coated by dextran or some other biodegradable polysachharide which prevents particle aggregation and makes the total size of the iron oxide particle substantially larger and also modifies their biological behavior.[38]

Each iron oxide crystal contains several thousand paramagnetic ions (Fe^{2+} and Fe^{3+}). When subjected to an external magnetic field, these particles exhibit strong magnetization which causes microscopic field inhomogeneity and activates the dephasing of protons. Thus, iron oxide nanoparticles shorten T2 and T2* relaxation times of the neighboring regions, and lead to a decrease in signal intensity in T2- and T2* weighted MR images.

Unlike low-molecular weight water soluble GBCAs, iron oxide agents do not leak into the interstitium and therefore, behave as intravascular contrast agents as long as the endothelium of the vessel wall is not altered by any pathological process. They are excreted from the blood by the reticuloendothelial system (RES) cells in liver, spleen, lymph nodes and bone marrow.[38]

The blood half-life and biological distribution of the nanoparticles is directly dependent on their size. They have been subdivided into two groups based on their mean total diameter and the distribution of particle sizes of the iron oxide agent (1) Superparamagnetic iron oxide particles (SPIOs) (2) Ultrasmall superparamagnetic iron oxide particles (USPIOs).

1. *Superparamagnetic iron oxide particles (SPIOs):* These are particles with aggregated iron oxide cores and a mean particle diameter greater than 50 nm. Two SPIOs have been approved for MR imaging:
    a. *Fexumoxide* (also known as Feridex or AMI-25) has a particle size of 50–180 nm, with a thin, incomplete dextran coating that makes individual particles form polycrystalline aggregates. These aggregates behave as large particles in solutions or within cells. They are eliminated quickly by reticuloendothelial cells and are cleared from the blood in less than an hour. Ferumoxide is administered as a slow intravenous infusion over 30-60 minutes and imaging performed 1–4 hours after the infusion. The liver appears darkest in the first 24 hours after the infusion, on T2* weighted and T2-weighted images. Complete metabolism needs 14–28 days but typically, the signal intensity of the liver returns to normal within 7–14 days. The most common complication of Feridex is acute severe low back pain, which may lead to discontinuation of the infusion in patients. This complication can be minimized with a slow infusion.[39]
    b. *Ferucarbotran* (also known as Resovist or SH U 555 A). This has a particle size of about 60 nm and the particles are coated with low molecular weight carboxydextran. Resovist is available as a ready to use formulation. It is administered as a rapid bolus and so can be used with both dynamic and delayed imaging. The most common adverse events with Resovit are vasodilation and parasthesias with an overall reported incidence of 7.1%.[7]

    As mentioned before, these iron oxide contrast agents are phagocytosed by macrophages within the body and so these agents are entrapped by the Kupffer cells in liver and spleen, leading to a reduction in the T2 relaxation time of these organs. Thus the normal liver appears dark on T2-weighted images. As most liver tumors, whether malignant or benign, are deficient in Kupffer cells, they do not take up SPIOs and appear relatively hyperintense after SPIO administration. However, tumors which are well differentiated and have not lost all their Kupffer cells, will take up SPIO agents and exhibit a reduction in signal intensity.[37,39] Some, not all, focal nodular hyperplasias show SPIO uptake. SPIO agents may also help to improve detection of HCC in cirrhotic patients. SPIO agents may also be used in combination with GBCAs to increase overall lesion detection.[39]

2. *Ultrasmall superparamagnetic iron oxide particles (USPIOs):* These are particles with non-aggregated (monodisperse) iron oxide cores with mean diameter less than 50 nm. As USPIOs are very small, they are extravasated from the blood vessels into interstitial spaces and transported to lymph nodes via the lymphatic channels. MR imaging is done 24–36 hours after contrast administration. The accumulation of the contrast within the normal nodes causes them to appear dark in T2 or T2* weighted while diseased nodes (e.g. metastatic nodes) do not show any change in signal intensity and appear uniformly or focally bright. When the hyperintense focus accounts for more than 30% of the nodal area, the node is considered metastatic. Harisinghani et al reported the successful detection of lymph-node metastases in patients with prostate cancer using USPIOs.[40] Sinerem and Combidex are two commercially available USPIO agents. USPIOs have also been tested as blood pool agents as they remain in the intravascular space for a long time.[41]

ORAL CONTRAST AGENTS

Oral contrast agents are required to: (1) delineate bowel pathology, and (2) distinguish bowel from other organs or mass lesions. An ideal oral contrast agent should have the following properties: (i) no or minimum absorption in the gastrointestinal tract, (ii) be completely excreted, (iii) should not lead to any motion or susceptibility artifacts, (iv) homogenous distribution within the GI tract, (v) good acceptance by the patient in terms of taste, amount of volume to be ingested and timing of administration, (vi) be safe and (vii) cost effective. A number of oral contrast agents have been developed to improve demarcation of the bowel in MR imaging studies. Broadly they can be classified as:

- Low-low intensity agents (proton displacement or T2 shortening) which have low signal intensity on all pulse sequences
- High-high intensity agents (T1 shortening) which have high signal intensity on all pulse sequences
- Low-high intensity agents (water based) have a low signal intensity on T1-weighted images and high signal intensity on T2-weighted images and
- High-low intensity agents (T1 and T2 shortening) which give a high signal intensity on T1-weighted images and low signal intensity on T2-weighted images

The last two categories are also known as biphasic agents.

Low-low Intensity (Dark Lumen) Agents

The signal intensity in bowel can be reduced by displacing the bowel contents with a material that contains no protons, such as air. Air can be administered by intubating the small bowel or rectum. However, due to patient discomfort and degradation of T2* weighted gradient echo images and echoplanar images by susceptibility artefacts, air is not featured as an oral contrast agent.

Perfluorocarbons are agents which do not contain protons, but they have the same susceptibility as water and thus, do not cause artefacts. Perflubron, a perfluorocarbon formulation was the first oral MR contrast agent approved for clinical use. However, as it was very expensive, it was withdrawn from the market.

SPIOs in high concentration can shorten T2 and T2* enough to eliminate signal from bowel even on so-called T1-weighted images. Their major disadvantage is the resulting distortion of the local magnetic field, which can exacerbate artefacts making fat-suppression particularly vulnerable. Ferumoxsil—a silicone-coated SPIO is commercially available as GastroMARK (Mallinckrodt) or Lumirem (Guerbert) for use as an oral contrast agent. Side effects such as nausea and vomiting, flatulence and feeling of fullness were reported in 15% of patients.[42]

Pineapple juice also shortens T2 relaxation time and hence leads to decreased T2 signal intensity on a standard magnetic resonance cholangiopancreatography (MRCP) sequence just like the commercially available negative contrast agent—Ferumoxsil due to its high manganese content (92.76 gm/dL).[43] Oral administration of 44 mL of pineapple juice, 15 minutes before acquiring MRCP sequence, gives a significant improvement in visualization of the pancreaticobiliary channels, due to suppression of the high signal intensity (SI) in the overlapping stomach and duodenum **(Figs. 2A and B)**.

Clays such as kaolin, attapulgite and helonite restrict the motion of water, thus shortening the T1 and T2 relaxation times. However, T1-weighted gradient echo images with a TE of less than 3 msec have little T2 contrast and therefore depict clay in bowel contents as high signal intensity owing to their short T1.[44]

High-high Intensity (Bright Lumen) Agents

Positive contrast agents reduce the T1 relaxation time; thus they act on T1-weighted images causing an increase in the signal intensity of bowel lumen (bright lumen). Paramagnetic materials, mainly gadolinium chelate solutions but also ferrous and manganese ions are examples of positive contrast agents. Gadolinium chelate solution was one of the first contrast agents proposed as an oral contrast for MRI. Dissolved in water at a concentration of approximately 1 mmol/L, gadolinium chelate provides sufficient reduction of the T1 relaxation time of water to generate an increase in signal intensity on T1-weighted images. Due to its low concentration, it has no T2 effect, and does not shorten the T2 relaxation time; consequently the signal intensity is high even on T2-weighted images. Gadopentetate dimeglumine solution (Magnevist Enteral) was one of the first commercially available positive oral contrasts.

Blueberry juice can be used as a positive agent due to its high content of manganese, a paramagnetic ion, which shortens the T1 relaxation time. Fat containing food materials like vegetable oils, milk and ice cream also provide a high signal on T1-weighted images as they have an intrinsically short T1.[42]

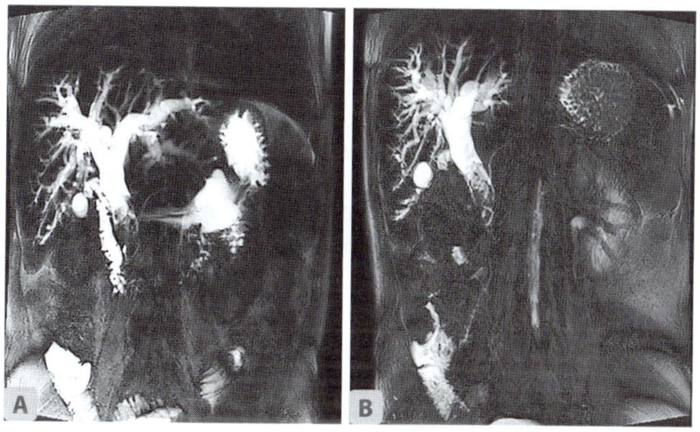

FIGS 2A AND B: T2 Half Fourier acquisition single shot-turbo spin echo (HASTE) thick slab coronal MRCP image (A) in a 60-year-old male patient shows dilatation of upper common bile duct (CBD) and intrahepatic biliary channels. Fluid filled duodenum overlaps the distal CBD. (B) T2 HASTE Thick slab coronal MRCP image in the same patient after oral ingestion of 400 mL pineapple juice shows suppression of fluid signal from duodenum and stomach. The distal CBD is now better visualized and shows a filling defect within due to calculus. Pineapple juice acts as a negative oral contrast suppressing the high signal due to fluid in upper GIT.

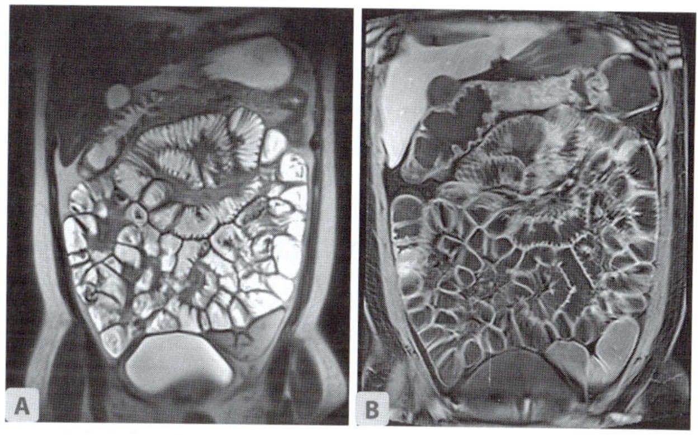

FIGS 3A AND B: Biphasic agents—low-high intensity. T2W coronal image (A) shows good distension of the small bowel, with high intraluminal signal intensity (positive effect) and hypointense bowel wall (B) On T1 fat suppressed (FS) coronal image, after administration of intravenous gadolinium, the bowel appears hypointense with enhancement of its wall by the intravenous gadolinium, allowing excellent depiction of bowel wall.

High-low Intensity Agents

These agents shorten both T1 and T2 relaxation times in such a way that the bowel contents have high signal intensity on T1-weighted images and low signal intensity on T2-weighted images. The main advantage is that the resulting signal intensity of bowel on all the pulse sequences is different from that of tumors and simple fluid collections, which tend to have low signal intensity on T1-weighted and high signal intensity on T2-weighted images. However, some T2-weighted pulse segments (e.g. fast spin echo) may depict bowel more clearly if its contents have high signal intensity, so this form of contrast is not necessarily desirable for every application.

Examples of this type of contrast agent include clay, gadolinium chelates in high concentration and compounds of manganese. Manganese is present in high concentrations in some foods such as bananas and blueberries.

Low-high Intensity Agents

The least expensive, most widely available, and best understood oral contrast agent used for MRI is water, which causes bowel to be low signal intensity on T1-weighted and high signal intensity on T2-weighted images. It provides good small bowel distension, but its main limitation is that it gets absorbed in the intestine, which leads to poor distention of the distal small bowel. For this reason, certain substances are added to the water which reduce intestinal absorbtion e.g. mannitol, sorbitrate, etc. **(Figs. 3A and B)**

Dilute suspension of barium sulphate or dilute solutions of iodinated contrast material such as those used in opacification of bowel for CT are also very useful as low-high MR oral contrast agents.

Polyethyleneglycol (PEG) is a strong hydrophilic molecule, which has the added advantage of nonabsorbability. With oral administration of 600 mL of PEG, a good distension of bowel loops can be acquired, and there are no significant side effects.[42] Low-high agents are also useful for delineating the pancreas.

However, the disadvantage of these agents is that bowel may be difficult to distinguish from simple fluid collections and tumors. High bowel signal intensity can also intensify motion artefacts.

The choice of a single agent has both, advantages and disadvantages, and so the radiologist has to choose the appropriate contrast agent according to clinical setting, availability of agent, patient tolerance and experience.

ONGOING RESEARCH AND FUTURE TRENDS

Currently most MR contrast agents are useful in improving visibility and definition of pathology, but are not suitable for extended intravascular (blood pool) or tissue/organ specific imaging and do not allow molecular imaging. There have been continuing efforts in searching for more specific contrast agents that can offer diagnosis with the accuracy approaching that otherwise only achievable with biopsy or histopathology. T1 nanoparticulate agents, target specific agents—capable of targeting organs, sites of inflammation and specific tumors , smart agents like enzyme activated agents, chemical exchange saturation transfer (CEST and PARACEST) agents, fluorinated agents, are some of the agents under research. A gadolinium free contrast agent, in view of its deposition in the body, a zwitterion coated exceedingly small superparamagnetic iron oxide nanoparticles (ZES-SPIONs) is also being developed. The majority of these agents are in pre-clinical levels of research; however, successful in vivo imaging has been reported with many pre-clinical studies.[41,45-48]

CONCLUSION

At present gadolinium chelates are the most widely used contrast agents in MR imaging and the only MR contrast agents available in India. They are easily available, have good tolerability and provide excellent lesion detection and characterization. The main concern with GBCAs was NSF, which was seen to occur only in patients with severe renal disease. Since the risks of NSF have been widely publicized leading to a change in MR practice, there has been a marked reduction in the incidence of NSF. Currently, the uncertain long term clinical consequences of gadolinium deposition in the brain, has precipitated restrictions in the use of linear GBCAs. The tissue-specific agents can be used for specific indications, depending on their availability.

REFERENCES

1. De Haen. Conception of the first magnetic resonance imaging contrast agents; a brief history. Top Mag Reson Imaging. 2001;12:221-30.
2. Wastie ML, Latief KH. Gadolimium: named after Finland's most famous chemist. Br J Radiol. 2004;77:146-7.
3. Ersoy H, Rybicki FJ. Biochemical safety profiles of gadolinium-based extracellular contrast agents and nephrogenic systemic fibrosis. J Magn Reson Imaging. 2007;26:1190-7.
4. Kei PL, Chan LP. Gadolinium chelate-associated nephrogenic systemic fibrosis. Singapore Med J. 2008;49:181-5.
5. Schmitt-Willich H. Stability of linear and macrocyclic gadolinium based contrast agents. Br J Radiol. 2007;80(955):581-2.
6. Juluru K, Vogel-Claussen J, Macura KJ. MR Imaging in Patients at risk for developing nephrogenic systemic fibrosis: protocols, practices, and imaging techniques to maximize patient safety. Radiographics. 2009;29:9-22.
7. Runge VM. Contrast Agents: Safety profile at http://cds.ismrm.org/ismrm-2008/files/Syllabus-069.pdf.
8. Muroff LR. MRI contrast: current agents issues. Appl Radiol. 2001;30(suppl):5-7.
9. Thomsen HS. Contrast media, safety issues and ESUR guidelines. Berlin Heidelberg New York, Springer, 2006.
10. Thomsen HS, Almen T, Morcos SK. The members of the contrast media safety committee of the European Society of Urogenital Radiology (ESUR): gadolinium-containing contrast media for radiographic examinations: A position paper. Eur Radiol. 2002;12:2600-5.
11. Bellin MF, Jakobsen JA, Tomassin I, et al. Contrast medium extravasation injury: guidelines for prevention and management. 2002;12:2807-12.
12. Cowper SE. Gadolinium - is it to blame? J Cutan Pathol. 2008;35:520-2.
13. Grobner T. Gadolinium—a specific trigger for the development of nephrogenic fibrosing dermopathy and nephrogenic systemic fibrosis? Nephrol Dial Transplant. 2006;21:1104-8.
14. Broome DR, Girguis MS, Baron PW, et al. Gadodiamide- associated nephrogenic systemic fibrosis: why radiologists should be concerned. AJR. 2007;188(2):586-92.
15. High WA, Ayers RA, Chandler J, et al. Gadolinium is detectable within the tissue of patients with nephrogenic systemic fibrosis. J Am Acad Dermatol. 2007;56(1):21-6.
16. Mackermann P, Skov L, Rossen K, et al. Nephrogenic systemic fibrosis: suspected causative role of gadodiamide used for contrast-enhanced MRI. J Am Soc Nephrol. 2006;17(9):2359-62.
17. Shibui K, Kataoka H, Sato N, Watanabe Y, Kohara M, Mochizuki T. A case of NSF attributable to contrast MRI repeated in a patient witrh stage 3 CKD at a renal function of eGFR > 30 mL/min/1.73 m^2. Japanese Journal of Nephrology. 2009;51:676.
18. Bridges MD, St Amant BS, McNeil RB, Cernigliaro JG, Dwyer JP, Fitzpatrick PM. High-dose gadodiamide for catheter angiography and CT in patients with varying degrees of renal insufficiency: Prevalence of subsequent nephrogenic systemic fibrosis and decline in renal function. Am J Roentgenol. 2009;192:1538-43.
19. Swaminatan S, Shah MV. New insights into nephrogenic systemic fibrosis. J Am Soc Nephrol. 2007;18:2636-43.
20. American College of Radiology. Manual on Contrast Media. Version 10.3, 2018. Available at: http://www.acr.org/~/media/ACR/Documents/PDF/QualitySafety/Resources/Contrast%20Manual/FullManual.pdf.
21. Elmholdt TR, Jorgensen B, Ramsingh M, et al. Two cases of nephrogenic systemic fibrosis after exposure to the macrocyclic compound gadobutrol. NDT Plus Advance Access. Published online On March 19, 2010. Available at: http://ndtplus.oxfordjournals.org/cgi/content/abstract/sfq028.
22. Singer RM. A review of gadolinium-based contrast agents in magnetic resonance imaging. http://www.cewebsource.com/coursePDFs/ReviewGBCAsMRI.pdf.
23. Thomsen HS. Contrast-enhanced MRI in patients with impaired renal function: Recent recommendations to minimize the risk of nephrogenic systemic fibrosis. Solutions in contrast imaging. 2010;1(2):1-8.
24. Webb JA, Thomsen HS, Morcos SK. The use of iodinated and gadolinium contrast media during pregnancy and lactation. Eur Radiol. 2005;15:1234-40.
25. Tirada N, Dreizen D, Khati NJ et al Imaging in Pregnant and Lactating Patients. Radiographics. 2015;35:1751-65
26. Hylton NM. Suspension of breast-feeding following gado-pentetate dimeglumine administration. Radiology. 2000;216:325-6.
27. Kubik-Huch RA, Gottstein-AlameNM, Frenzel T et al. Gadopentetate dimeglumine excretion into humal breast milk during lactation. Radiology. 2000:216(02):555-8.
28. Kanda T, Ishii K, Kawaguchi H, Kitajima K, Takenaka D. High signal intensity in the dentate nucleus and globus pallidus on unenhanced T1-weighted MR images: Relationship with increasing cumulative dose of a gadolinium-based contrast material. Radiology. 2014;270:834-41.
29. Kanda T, Fukusato T, Matsuda M, Toyoda K, Oba H, Kotoku J, et al. Gadolinium-based contrast agent accumulates in the brain even in subjects without severe renal dysfunction: Evaluation of autopsy brain specimens with inductively coupled plasma mass spectroscopy. Radiology. 2015;276:228-32.
30. Radbruch A, Haase R, Kieslich PJ, et al. No signal increase in the dentate nucleus on unenhanced T1W MR images after more than 20 serial injections of macrocyclic GBCAs. Radiology. 2017:282(3):699-707.
31. Kanda T, Osawa M, Oba H, Toyoda K, Kotoku J, Haruyama T, et al. High signal intensity in dentate nucleus on unenhanced T1-weighted MR images: Association with linear versus macrocyclic gadolinium chelate administration. Radiology. 2015;275:803-9
32. BANG, Bjørnerud A, Vatnehol S, Larsson C, Duetønnessen P, Hol PK, Groote IR. Signal enhancement of the dentate nucleus at unenhanced MR imaging after very high cumulative doses of the macrocyclic gadolinium-based contrast agent gadobutrol: an observational study. Radiology. 2017;285: 434–44. doi: 10.1148/radiol. 2017170391

33. Bang JG, Zhen LY, Long JZ. Gadolinium Deposition in Brain: Current Scientific Evidence and Future Perspectives Frontiers in Molecular Neuroscience. 2018;11:335. doi: 10.3389/fnmol.2018.00335.
34. Semelka RC, Ramalho J, Vakharia A, et al. Gadolinium deposition disease: Initial description of a disease that has been around for a while. Magn Reson Imaging. 2016:34(10):1383-90.
35. Semelka RC, Miguel R, Mandoh A et al. Gadolinium in Humans: A family of disorders. AJR. 2016;207(2):229-33.
36. Rofsky NM, Earls JP. Mangafodipir trisodium injection (MnDPDP): a contrast agent for abdominal MR imaging. Magn Reson Imaging Clin N Am. 1996;4:73-85.
37. Kalva SP, Blake MA, Sahani DV. MR Contrast agents. Appl Radiol. 2006;35;18-27.
38. Wang YXJ, Hussain SM, Krestin GP. Superparamagnetic iron oxide aqents; physicochemical characteristics and applications in NMR imaging. Eur Radiol. 2001;11:2319-31.
39. Gandhi SN, Brown MA, Wong JG, et al. MR contrast agents for liver imaging: What, When, How. Radiographics. 2006;26:1621-36.
40. Harsinghani MG, Barentsz J, Hahn PF, et al. Noninvasive detection of clinically occult lymph-node metastases in prostate cancer. N Engl J Med. 2003;348:2491-9.
41. Na HB, Song C, Hyeon T. Inorganic Nanopraticles for MRI Contrast Agents. Advanced Materials. 2009;21:2133-48.
42. Laghi A, Paolantonio P, Iafrate F, et al Oral contrast agents for magnetic resonance imaging of the bowel. Topics in Magnetic Reson Imaging. 2002;13:389-96.
43. Riordan RD, Khonsari M, Jeffries, et al. Pineapple juice as a negative oral contrast agent in magnetic resonance cholangiopancreatography: a preliminary evaluation. Br J Radiol. 2004;77(924):991-9.
44. Mitchell DG, Cohen MS. "Particulate and oral contrast agents" in MRI principles, 2nd edn. Elseiver. 2004.pp.295-304.
45. Laurent S, Elst LV, Muller RN. Contrast Agents for MRI: recent Advances. eMagRes. Online John Wiley & Sons, Ltd, 2009.
46. Knight JC, Edwards PG, Paisey SJ. Fluorinated contrast agents for magnetic resonance imaging; a review of recent developments. RSC Advances. 2011;1:1415-25.
47. Vithanarachchi SM, Allen MJ. Strategies for target-specific contrast agents for magnetic resonance imaging. Current Molecular Imaging. 2012;1:12-25.
48. He Wei, Oliver T. Bruns, Michael G. Kaul, Eric C. Hansen, Mariya Barch, Agata Wiśniowska, Ou Chen, Yue Chen, Nan Li, Satoshi Okada, Jose M. Cordero, Markus Heine, Christian T. Farrar, Daniel M. Montana, Gerhard Adam, Harald Ittrich, Alan Jasanoff, Peter Nielsen, Moungi G. Bawendi. Exceedingly small iron oxide nanoparticles as positive MRI contrast agents. Proceedings of the National Academy of Sciences, 2017;201620145.

CHAPTER

44

Ultrasound Contrast Agents

Shashi Bala Paul, Manisha Jana

INTRODUCTION

Ultrasound imaging technology has evolved incessantly and has come a long way since the time it was first used for medical practice.[1] Ultrasound is the most widely used imaging modality due to multiple advantages of wide availability, simple to perform, lack of radiation, real time scanning ability and above all being cost-effective. With the advent of ultrasound contrast agents (UCAs) about two decades ago, the role of diagnostic ultrasound has been revolutionized.

Contrast-enhanced ultrasound (CEUS) is a specialized form of ultrasound that uses microbubble UCAs for evaluation of the hemodynamics of the target organ and provides detailed information of its microvascularity and microperfusion on real-time scanning. Thus, CEUS has exhibited the potential of overcoming the limitations of conventional B mode ultrasound and color or power Doppler ultrasound.[2]

CEUS has twin components, the ultrasound contrast agent (UCA) and the contrast specific imaging modes on the US machine. UCAs are microbubbles of gas with a protein, lipid or polymer shell and are either reticulo endothelial or purely blood pool agents. UCAs remain confined to the intravascular space after intravenous injection as they are unable to pass through the vascular endothelium into the interstitium. Small microbubbles (1–10 um) can pass through the lung capillaries, remain in circulation for a short time and eventually get dissolved. The gas gets exhaled while the shell gets metabolized in the liver.[3-4] The UCAs, while in circulation, strongly increase the ultrasound backscatter and produce enhancement of echogenicity for the assessment of blood flow.[2] Contrast enhanced Doppler imaging is possible because the low mechanical index (MI) amplifies the Doppler signals for better characterization of tumor vascularity. Low MI of 0.07–0.2 is needed for real-time evaluation of the target organ in three vascular phases subsequent to the intravenous administration of UCAs. Detection of this flow requires the contrast specific imaging modes like the pulse inversion or amplitude modulation technology which are now available in the ultrasound machines. These sequences cancel the linear US signals from the tissue and take advantage of the nonlinear responses from the microbubbles within the ultrasound field, bringing real-time perfusion imaging of the target organs into reach.[2]

EVOLUTION OF UCAs

The first generation UCAs came into existence in the late 1960s **(Table 1)**.[2] These comprised of soluble gas and thus had a short life. Moreover, their large size prevented them from passing through the pulmonary circulation.[5] Thus; they were used primarily for right heart imaging. Evaluation of the heart and great vessels by injecting agitated liquid via a catheter was first undertaken by Gramiak et al.[6] The air bubbles within the solution greatly increased the returning echoes, but had a tendency to dissolve into the solution very quickly, resulting in short imaging window. Apart from the agitated saline, hydrogen peroxide, iodocyanine green dye, and iodinated contrast agents were also tried as ultrasound contrast media. In 1991, Echovist (Bayer Schering Pharma AG, Berlin, Germany), the first commercially available UCA, was introduced.[7] It was made of air bubbles coated with galactose and too had a very short life in the blood with minimal transpulmonary circulation limiting its clinical utility. Echovist was predominantly used for the evaluation of the cardiac shunt and the female genital tract.

Albunex (Molecular Biosystems Inc, San Diego, CA, 1994) was the first FDA approved contrast agent used clinically. It was composed of air filled albumin microspheres suspended in 5% w/v human albumin solution.[8] *In vitro*, the linear relationship of Albunex concentration with scattered power was demonstrated by De Jong.[9] It had a mean size

TABLE 1: First generation ultrasound contrast agents (UCAs).

UCAs	Gas	Stabilization
Agitated saline	Air	None
Echovist	Air	None
Levovist	Air	Palmitic acid*
Albunex	Air	sonicated albumin*

*Have transpulmonary stability

of approximately 3.5 μm. Although it was stable in albumin solution *in vitro*, it did not have significant recirculation (half-life <5 minutes) *in vivo*. It was used predominantly for the evaluation of cardiac shunts and valvular regurgitation with limited extra-cardiac applications. It is no longer manufactured.

In 1996, a relatively longer lasting UCA called Levovist came up. It contained air bubbles with a galactose/ palmitic acid surfactant coating (Schering). Main indications for use were cardiac, intracranial and abdominal. However, the Levovist bubbles easily collapsed under ultrasound emission owing to its fragile properties, therefore real time images could not be obtained for a longer period.

By now, the need to develop more stable UCAs for prolonged window period for imaging was very evident. This formed the basis for the development of the second generation UCAs.

Second generation UCAs **(Table 2)** contain insoluble gases like sulphur hexafluoride (SF6) or perfluorocarbons and have a surface shell made of different substances like phospholipids, albumin or polymers providing better stabilization. Their smaller size enables a successful transpulmonary passage to reach the various target organs. After intravenous injection, due to their low solubility in water, better stabilization and strong harmonic response, prolonged visualization of dynamic enhancement of the organ can be observed on real-time ultrasound scanning.[5]

In 1998 and 2006, Optison (GE Healthcare) and Luminity (Bristol-Myers Squibb) made of octafluoropropane coated with albumin and lipid shell respectively, were introduced. The octafluoropropane gas has low water solubility and is more stable providing longer imaging period. However, their sole indication for use has been cardiac.

In 2001, SonoVue (SonoVue, Bracco Milan, Italy) was introduced which contains sulphur hexafluoride stabilized by phospholipid shell. SonoVue is the only contrast agent available in India.

The second generation UCAs are pure blood pool agents as they are unable to destroy the vascular endothelium and thus remain exclusively intravascular resulting in prolonged enhancement of the vascular system. No extravasation into the interstitial fluid occurs. These pharmacokinetics are different from the contrast used in computed tomography (CT) and magnetic resonance imaging (MRI) which is rapidly cleared from the blood into the extra-cellular space.[2] These features make SonoVue an ideal ultrasound contrast agent for vascular phase imaging of different target organs. It is being widely used for various hepatic and non-hepatic applications.[2,10] Recently, SonoVue contrast agent has received FDA approval in the United States and is available as Lumason (Bracco Diagnostics Inc. Monroe Township, N), recommended for use in adults and pediatric population for evaluation of focal liver lesions (FLL) and vesicoureteric reflux.[11]

TABLE 2: Second generation ultrasound contrast agents (UCAs).

UCAs	Gas	Stabilizing Shell
Optison	Octafluoropropane (approved in US and Europe)	Sonicated albumin
Luminity	Octafluoropropane perflutren	Lipids
Sonovue * (Lumason in USA)	Sulphur hexafluoride (SF6)	Phospholipids
Sonazoid#	Perfluorobutane	Sonicated albumin

* The only available contrast in India

#Approved only in Japan

Sonazoid (Daiichi-Sankyo, Tokyo, Japan), is another second generation, reticulo endothelial UCA. which contains perflubutane and has a hard shell. It is available exclusively in Japan. Sonazoid has the longest window period of imaging due to the additional fourth phase called the post vascular phase or the 'Kupffer phase', starting from 10 minutes to 60 minutes. Sonazoid microbubbles are phagocytosed by the Kupffer cells in the liver and thus the contrast persists longer in the liver parenchyma than purely vascular agents aiding in better characterization.[12]

Dose of UCA has to be optimal as too high a dose could cause artefacts while too low may be sub-diagnostic in the late phase compromising the findings. Dosage varies with the type of the examination, organ to be evaluated and the age of the individual.

For intravenous use of SonoVue (4.8 mL vial), 2.4 mL (half vial) is recommended for most indications in hepatic imaging. For evaluation of Pancreas, spleen and Kidney, a low dose of 1.2 mL is used. Higher dose of 4.8 mL is needed when the high frequency transducers are used or endoscopic CEUS is to be undertaken.[13]

For intra-cavitary use, the dose of UCA ranges from 0.1–1 mL of SonoVue (a few drops diluted in 10 mL or more of 0.9% saline). If any communication between the cavities is to be documented, 1–2 mL of the dose is recommended. In situations where delineation of the anatomy of the cavity is required, a lower dose of 0.1 mL in 20 mL saline solution is important for reducing artefacts or shadowing.[2]

TECHNIQUE OF CEUS

CEUS requires an US machine equipped with low MI contrast imaging mode and the UCA. For intravenous use of UCAs, an access in the antecubital fossa using 20 gauge venflon with a three way connector is obtained. The contrast material in the vial of SonoVue is prepared in the soluble form 5 minutes prior and shaken well to be properly dissolved for use. The target organ is visualized on the B mode US and then keeping the lesion in focus, the contrast-specific imaging mode is turned on. A simultaneous display of the tissue and contrast signals can be seen on the monitor as a dual window (option in some machines) which ensures the target lesion remains in the field of view throughout the study. The freshly prepared SonoVue is administered as an intravenous bolus followed by flushing with 10 mL of 0.9% normal saline. The enhancement characteristics of the target organ is observed on real-time post-injection. The observation is recorded on the cine mode. Postprocedure, the patient is observed for about an hour for any adverse reaction if any.

SAFETY OF UCAs

UCAs are well tolerated and are safe with few non-specific side effects. Clearance of UCA is very fast and 80% to 90% of it gets eliminated through the lungs in 11 minutes. Life threatening anaphylactoid complications are very rare (0.001%).With its use in echocardiography, some fatal incidents have been reported in very ill patients.The use of UCAs mandate precautionary measures to be ready despite low incidence of side-effects. Unlike other contrast agents used for CT or MRI, the UCAs are not nephrotoxic as they have no renal excretion. Hence, CEUS can be safely performed in patients with compromised renal function.[2]

Contraindications to the use of UCAs are-cardio-pulmonary disease, use prior to extra-corporeal shock wave therapy, pregnancy, breast-feeding and severe coronary artery disease.

Advantages of CEUS Over CT/MRI

CEUS has several advantages over CT/MRI. It is a simple procedure, requires few minutes to perform and can provide immediate diagnosis obviating the need for further investigations in certain subset of patients. Being free from ionizing radiation, it can be can be safely used for repeated follow up. Unlike CT/MRI, UCAs are not nephrotoxic, thus renal function tests are not required prior to the study. Portability is another big advantage as the CEUS machine can be carried anywhere in the hospital for performing bedside procedures on immobile patients. The real time dynamic evaluation by CEUS provides highest temporal resolution for abdominal imaging in contrast to the static imaging protocols which are either predetermined or based on the aortic contrast bolus. Better assessment of arterial hyper-enhancement (early or late) is possible with CEUS whereas on CT/MRI mistiming can be a spoiler. Similarly, washout details of the onset and intensity that are crucial for the differential diagnosis, can be better elicited on real time evaluation. Claustrophobic patients who find extreme difficulty in undergoing an MRI or CT scan undergo CEUS with ease and comfort.

DIAGNOSTIC APPLICATIONS OF UCA

UCA have been in use for many years now and the recommendations and guidelines of their clinical applications have been updated periodically. The earliest CEUS application was for hepatic imaging and its guidelines and recommendations have been updated in 2013.[2] Following the FDA approval of UCA in the United states recently, the American college of Radiology (ACR) supported by other partners recommended a CEUS based diagnostic algorithm called Liver Imaging Reporting Data System (CEUS LI-RADS) for characterizing focal liver lesion in patients at risk for developing hepatocellular carcinoma (HCC). CEUS LI-RADS version 2017 is available online.[14] The recommendations for non-hepatic applications of CEUS have also been updated this year.[10]

We discuss these updated diagnostic applications of CEUS at length.

HEPATIC APPLICATIONS

CEUS of the Liver

CEUS is ideally suited for the evaluation of liver lesions. Liver has a dual blood supply comprising of the hepatic artery and the portal vein which allows evaluation of the FLL in three vascular phases in real time after the intravenous administration of UCA. The timer is started at the beginning of the saline flush to coincide with the injection of the UCA. The arterial phase (AP) lasts upto 30–45 sec, portal venous phase (PP) from 30–45 to120 sec and the late phase (LP) after 120 sec. Continuous scanning with cine recording is performed upto 60 sec to evaluate the peak of arterial enhancement, and thereafter intermittent scanning with short cine loops at about 30–60 sec intervals are taken to determine the onset of washout. In cases where the contrast continues to persists within the FLL, intermittent scanning is continued upto 6 minutes to determine the presence of late washout if any. If a second FLL needs to be evaluated in the same patient, in that case the same procedure is repeated with a fresh bolus of UCA after 10 minutes.

The enhancement pattern of the FLL is termed in relation to the adjacent liver parenchyma. It is hyper-enhancing if the enhancement is more, iso-enhancing if it is similar and hypo-enhancing if it is less enhancing than the surrounding liver parenchyma. No change in enhancement subsequent to the contrast administration is termed as no enhancement.

Detection of Focal Liver Lesions by CEUS

Traditionally, US has been the first imaging modality for the detection of FLL. However, its diagnostic accuracy is low. Based on a meta-analysis, US pooled sensitivity for detection of HCC of any stage in patients with cirrhosis is 94% and only 63% for early HCC.[15]

US is unable to detect small nodules less than a cm, isoechoic nodules in a cirrhotic liver and lesions located in the subdiaphragmatic regions. On power and color Doppler US, evaluation of vascularity of the suspicious liver nodules has limitations of detecting slow flow, evaluating deep seated vessels and invariably have associated artifacts.[16]

With CEUS, the diagnostic accuracy of a FLL has improved to 87–89% from 27–42% of conventional US.[17,18] CEUS is also superior to CT in detection of a FLL and has a comparable accuracy for the overall performance.[19,20] Improved performance is largely attributed to its capability of real time evaluation of enhancement patterns of the FLL in different vascular phases.

In contrast, for detection of HCC, CEUS using SonoVue has a relatively lower sensitivity. The short lasting AP (30–45 sec) is not enough for a thorough evaluation of the entire liver for detection of hypervascular HCC. Moreover, there is a huge variation in the appearance of HCC in the LP as most well differentiating HCCs either retain contrast or show very delayed wash out. Thus, even though the LP is relatively long, detection of HCC is quite low. Hence, CEUS is not a recommended modality for screening or staging of HCC and alternative imaging modalities of CT or MRI are mandatory.[2]

CEUS using Sonazoid performs better for HCC detection with a high sensitivity of 95% and specificity of 93%. It is primarily due to the advantage of additional post vascular or Kupffer phase. In this phase Sonazoid enters the parenchymal interstitium after being phagocytosed by the Kupfer cells, resulting in prolonged enhancement of the normal liver, allowing better detection of HCC that is seen as a hypovascular (black) defect.[21]

Characterization of FLL

FLL characterization should be undertaken with the prior knowledge of the clinical history of the patient and the availability of previous imaging if any. It is important to know whether the FLL is present in an underlying normal liver or a diseased cirrhotic liver as the probability of the types of tumors vary in the cirrhotic and non-cirrhotic livers.

CEUS can safely be considered as the first imaging modality for characterization of FLL.[22,23] It has a high sensitivity of 98% and an accuracy of 93% in differentiating benign from malignant nodules.[24]

CEUS LI-RADS

CEUS LI-RADS is the latest application recommended by ACR for characterizing the liver lesions in the 'at risk' population. It aims at standardizing the interpretation and reporting of liver observations on CEUS and providing consistent terminology for communication of findings to the clinicians.[14,25,26] CEUS LI-RADS® *v2017* is available online as a 25-page hyperlinked document. (Accessed on November 10, 2018 for details).

It is recommended for reporting findings in patients of Cirrhosis or Chronic hepatitis B viral infection, history of prior HCC, adult liver transplant candidates and post-transplant recipient. Its not recommended for use in patients less than 18 years, cirrhosis due to non-viral causes like congenital hepatic fibrosis, a vascular disorder such as hereditary hemorrhagic telangiectasia, Budd-Chiari syndrome, chronic portal vein occlusion, cardiac congestion, or diffuse nodular regenerative hyperplasia.

Prerequisite for applying CEUS LI-RADS is high expertise of the investigator, visibility of the liver nodule on B mode US (termed true nodule or observation) and the study of CEUS should be performed with either SonoVue (Lumason), Definity or Luminity.

Diagnostic algorithm of CEUS LI-RADS provides the probability of the liver nodule being an HCC based on its major features such as size, type and degree of arterial phase hyper enhancement (APHE), presence or absence of washout, timing and degree of washout if seen.[25]

APHE also called 'wash in' is termed for the enhancement of the malignant nodule compared to the adjoining hepatic parenchyma, in the AP of CEUS lasting till 30 to 45 sec, which is either partial or complete. The enhancement should neither be rim like, nor peripheral, discontinuous and globular (features of a benign nodule). Since it is mandatory for the liver nodule to be seen on prior B mode US, it is termed a true nodule. Thus, the APHE of a nodule on CEUS denotes higher significance than that seen on CT/MRI, where it could also be due to an arterio-portal shunt (APS), commonly encountered in addition to the enhancement of various benign or malignant nodules. Being a real time procedure, the exact onset and intensity of APHE is well appreciated which is vital for nodule characterization. Additionally, the morphology of the arteries within the nodule using a bubble tracking option can also be demonstrated on AP CEUS

Washout is defined as the temporal reduction in enhancement (complete or a part) of the nodule compared to the adjoining hepatic parenchyma starting from or after the AP and progressing to hypo-enhancement in the VP or LP. A nodule that does not show APHE in the AP can also depict washout in the LP. This feature is suggestive of malignancy on CEUS which may either be an HCC, Intrahepatic cholangio carcinoma (ICC) or metastases, whereas it is considered a specific feature of HCC on CT/MRI LI-ADS.[27] The degree or intensity of washout which is either mild or marked, is inferred by comparing the enhancement of the nodule with the surrounding hepatic parenchyma. Mild washout is said to occur when the nodule has mild reduction in enhancement than the adjoining liver with some retained contrast. If the nodule becomes totally devoid of contrast and looks punched out, it is termed 'marked washout'. The onset of washout is crucial for diagnosis. Washout occurring before 60 sec is called 'early onset while 'late onset' occurs after 60 sec.

Characterization of the nodules is based on the combination of the characteristics of 'wash in' or 'wash out' in the three phases along with the intensity and onset of these findings. Late phase is a vital part of the study providing the most valuable information for characterization. Benign FLL is iso to hyper-enhancing in the PP and LP, whereas the malignant is characteristically hypo-enhancing (show wash out).[2] This pattern is seen in 86% to 93% of benign and 78% to 98% of malignant liver nodules.[24, 28,29]

CEUS Patterns of Benign Focal Liver Lesions (Table 3)

Hemangioma is the most common benign liver tumor with a prevalence of 1–20%.[30] CEUS has a sensitivity of 95% and specificity of 98% in diagnosing hemangioma.[5] The commonest pattern of enhancement is the early peripheral nodular arterial enhancement with delayed centripetal fill in which is similar to that seen on CT or MRI **(Figs. 1A to C)**. It is encountered in 52–88% of the cases. Sustained enhancement during the late phase has been reported in as high as 83–100% of cases.[28,29,31-33]

The high diagnostic accuracy of hemangioma on CEUS is comparable to that of MRI., which includes even small hemangiomas. If the typical features of enhancement are seen, further confirmation of the diagnosis by any other imaging is not required.[34] Atypical features occur in very small shunts (<15 mm), very large (>4 cm) hemangiomas which have arterio-porto-venous shunts called high flow hemangiomas or shunt hemangiomas which are rapidly filling and the ones that have features of calcification, thrombosis or venoliths.[35] The chance of missing out on any rapidly enhancing hemangiomas (flash-filling) on CEUS is remote because of the advantage of continuous real time scanning.

Focal nodular hyperplasia (FNH) is the second most common benign liver tumor with a prevalence of 0.9–3%.[36]

TABLE 3: Enhancement patterns of benign focal liver lesions (FLL).

FLL	Arterial phase	Portal venous phase	Late Phase
Noncirrhotic liver			
Hemangioma Typical features	Peripheral nodular enhancement	Partial/complete centripetal fill in	Complete enhancement
Additional features (small lesion)	Complete, rapid centripetal enhancement		Nonenhancing regions
Focal nodular hyperplasia Typical features	Hyperenhancing from the centre, complete, early	Hyperenhancing	Iso-/hyperenhancing
Additional features	Spoke wheel arteries, feeding artery	Unenhanced central scar	Unenhanced central scar
Hepatocellular adenoma Typical features	Hyperenhancing, complete	Isoenhancing	Isoenhancing
Additional features	Nonenhancing regions	Hyperenhancing Nonenhancing regions	Slightly hypoenhancing Nonenhancing regions
Focal fatty infiltration/sparing	Isoenhancing	Isoenhancing	Isoenhancing
Abscess Typical features	Peripheral enhancement, no central enhancement	Hyper-/isoenhancing rim, no central enhancement	Hypoenhancing rim, no central enhancement
Additional features	Enhanced septa hyperenhanced liver segment	Hypoenhancing rim Enhanced septa Hyperenhanced liver segment	
Simple cyst	Nonenhancing	Nonenhancing	Nonenhancing
Cirrhotic liver			
Regenerative nodule (±dysplastic)			
Typical features	Isoenhancing	Isoenhancing	Isoenhancing
Additional features	Hypoenhancing		

In cirrhotic liver simple cysts, hemangiomas and abscesses may also be found and show the same enhancement pattern as in noncirrhotic livers. All other entities are rare findings in cirrhotic livers.

Source: https://www.thieme-connect.com/ejournals/pdf/10.1055/s-0032-1325499.pdf.Guidelines and good clinical practice recommendations for CEUS in liver-update 2012. Accessed on Nov 5, 2018

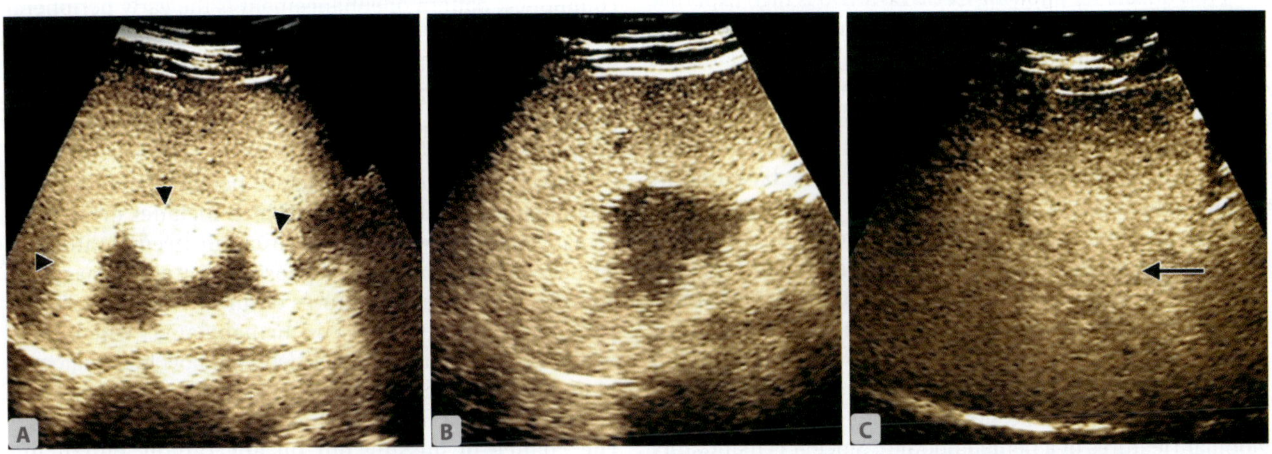

FIGS. 1A TO C: Hemangioma (CEUS LR-1) – Typical pattern. CEUS images of the FLL in segment VII showing peripheral nodular enhancement (arrowheads) in the AP at 23 sec postcontrast injection (A) with progressive centripetal enhancement (B) becoming isoenhancing (arrow) in the LP at 240 sec (C).

It results from the proliferation of abnormally arranged non-neoplastic hepatocytes as a response to an area of vascular malformation or venous thrombosis. It is commonly associated with a central fibrous scar and anamolous arteries. It is important to differentiate FNH from other entities like hepatic adenoma of carcinoma (fibro-lamellar type), because FNH is managed conservatively.

Being a hypervascular tumor, FNH shows homogeneous hyper-enhancement in the arterial phase in nearly all the cases. In the portal and late phase, it is iso-enhancing or slightly hyper-enhancing, seen in about 87% to 100% of the cases.[32,37,38]

The central scar occurs in 23% to 31% of the cases and shows two types of enhancement: (1) the stellate vascularity and (2) centrifugal filling. An anomalous artery courses in the scar in a linear and stellate fashion depicting a spoke wheel pattern, seen in 45–89% of the cases.[33,39,40]

Hepatocellular adenoma (HA) is a rare, benign liver tumor. It has a relatively non-specific pattern of enhancement on CEUS. Being hypervascular, the usual pattern is of hyper-enhancement in the AP. Small HA show homogeneous hyper-enhancement while the larger ones are heterogeneously hyper-enhancing due to the presence of intratumoral hemorrhage or necrosis. Very rarely, it may show iso- or hypo-enhancement on the portal and late phases and may thus mimic HCC posing a diagnostic dilemma. Even on histopathology, differentiation of HA from well differentiated HCC is often challenging. Similar pattern may be depicted by hypervascular metastases as well.[40]

Liver Abscess

Pyogenic abscess is most frequently encountered abscess in the liver. The CEUS findings like the conventional US, vary with the stage of the abscess. The abscess usually shows areas of hyper-enhancement. Early abscess is generally solid and shows diffuse heterogeneous enhancement in the AP persisting in the PP and LP. A transient perilesional enhancement also occurs in the AP which in very few cases may show hypo-enhancement in the PP.[41] If this rare finding is seen, this needs to be differentiated from a necrotic metastasis which appears as a punched out enhancement defects in the LP, while the abscess depicts an ill-defined area of hypo-enhancement. As the abscess matures, it develops fluid within which shows as an enhancing rim post contrast injection. The internal septations enhance on CEUS leading to a honeycomb appearance.

Liver cysts always need to be diagnosed on conventional US where they are seen as thin walled, anechoic well defined areas with posterior enhancement. They lack enhancement on any phase of CEUS. In contrast, the complex cysts often depict enhancing features, which aid in characterization and may be diagnostic. Washout differentiates a lesion from the surrounding normal liver tissue and provides information on the benign or malignant nature.

Focal fatty change (fatty infiltration or fatty sparing) may mimic masses on US. However, their location is typical-adjacent to the falciform ligament, portal veins and gall bladder. They have geographical margins with no mass effect and the vessels are seen traversing through the lesion.[42] If nodular or atypical in location, it may pose a diagnostic dilemma. After contrast enhancement, areas of focal fatty change show similar enhancement as the adjoining hepatic parenchyma in all the vascular phases.

CEUS Patterns of Malignant Focal Liver Lesions (Table 4)

CEUS has a sensitivity of 90% and specificity of 99% and an accuracy of 89% in diagnosing malignant lesions.[43] It can detect metastases, HCC in high risk patients of cirrhosis, evaluate multistep hepato-carcinogenesis, serve as a guidance procedure for biopsy or percutaneous ablative therapy and for the assessment of response to loco-regional therapy for HCC.

Metastases is the most frequent indication for performing US of the liver. The diagnosis can be simple when the patient has a known primary but very challenging if no such history is available. Conventional US has limitations in detection of metastases and its accuracy is significantly lower than CT/ MRI.[44]

Improved accuracy has been noted with the use of CEUS.[45] Metastases show variable patterns of enhancement in the AP depending upon the vascularity of the primary tumor, whereas, they are typically rapidly hypo-enhancing (within 20 sec) during the PP.[28,37] More than 85% of the metastases show very short lasting peripheral rim enhancement, diffuse or mosaic enhancement followed by rapid washout.[28,32,37] Rim enhancement with early wash out is the hallmark of metastases. Hypervascular metastasis showing complete enhancement may be mistaken for HCC in which case findings of clinical history, serum alpha-fetoprotein levels may come to rescue.

Hepatocellular Carcinoma (HCC)

HCC is the most common primary hepatic malignancy. More than 80% of HCC occur in patients with chronic liver disease of viral etiology.[46] CEUS plays a pivotal role in evaluating the multi-step hepato-carcinogenesis in patients of cirrhosis. HCC is exclusively supplied by the abnormal arteries while the regenerative nodule (RN) and the dysplastic nodule (DN) contain normal hepatic arteries and portal veins. In the process of progression of DN towards malignancy, the abnormal arterial supply increases (neo-angiogenesis) while the normal arterial and portal supply decreases.[2,47]

RN are small and seen on Conventional US as either coarse and heterogeneous liver or as multiple, tiny, hypo or hyperechoic nodules. On CEUS, most RN and DN do not show any enhancement (isoenhancing) in any phase. At times they may show transient hypo enhancement in the AP. DN may have variable and inconsistent arterial and portal supplies or significant overlaps of vascular supply leading to problems in diagnosis on all modalities (CEUS, CT, MRI). Since CEUS has the advantage of continuous real time scanning, it may pick up subtle transient patterns of enhancement in order to differentiate between HCC and DN.[47]

CEUS Patterns of HCC

About 90% of the HCCs are hypervascular and are supplied exclusively by the abnormal arteries. APHE occurs in more than 90% of them which is homogeneous and intense in small

TABLE 4: Enhancement patterns of malignant focal liver lesions (FLL).

FLL	Arterial phase	Portal venous phase	Late Phase
Noncirrhotic liver			
Metastasis			
Typical features	Rim-enhancement	Hypoenhancing	Hypo-/nonenhancing
Additional features	Complete-enhancement Hyperenhancement nonenhancing regions	Nonenhancing regions	Nonenhancing regions
HCC			
Typical features	Hyperenhancing	Isoenhancing	Hypo-/nonenhancing
Additional features	Nonenhancing regions	Nonenhancing regions	Nonenhancing regions
Cholangiocarcinoma			
Typical	Rim-like hyperenhancement, central hypoenhancement	Hypoenhancing	Nonenhancing
Additional features	Nonenhancing regions inhomogeneous/ Hyperenhancement	Nonenhancing regions	Nonenhancing regions
Cirrhotic liver			
HCC			
Typical features	Hyperenhancing, complete	Isoenhancing	Hypoenhancing (slightly or moderately)
Additional features	Nonenhancing areas (if large) Basket pattern, chaotic vessels enhancing tumor thrombus Hypo/nonenhancing	Nonenhancing regions Nonenhancing	Isoenhancing nonenhancing

Explanation: Other malignancies in cirrhosis have the same patterns as in noncirrhotic livers.

Sources: https://www.thieme-connect.com/ejournals/pdf/10.1055/s-0032-1325499.pdf.Guidelines and good clinical practice recommendations for CEUS in liver-update 2012. Accessed on Nov 5, 2018

nodules and in homogeneous in nodules larger than 5 cm due to the presence of necrosis within. Tumor capsule is an important finding present in about 5–34.6% of HCC cases and is seen as a thin, peritumoral, rim-like hyperenhancement representing blood vessels around the lesion.[37,48,49]

Detection of APHE varies with the size of the nodule and is quite low in smaller lesions. In lesions ≤1.0 cm, 1.1–2.0 cm, and 2.1–3.0 cm, APHE detection rate is 67%, 83–88%, and 92–100%, respectively.[37,49] On the late phase, 83–97% of HCCs show hypo-enhancement, classically called washout **(Figs. 2A and B)**. The washout is late (occurring after 60 sec) and of mild intensity in contrast to the washout of other malignant tumors like metastases or intrahepatic cholangiocarcinoma.

A good co-relation of the washout is seen with the histological differentiation of HCC. More the differentiation of the lesion, more slow is the wash out in the LP. Moderately differentiated HCC shows typical pattern of arterial hyper-enhancement and LP hypo-enhancement. Atypical patterns are common with well-differentiated and poorly differentiated HCC.[50] Well-differentiated HCC may or may not show wash out. If the wash out occurs, it is mild and delayed, often taking about 3 to 4 minutes **(Figs. 3A to C)**. Hence, in a patient of cirrhosis,any nodule that is isoenhancing in the PP and LP should not be considered benign as about half of the well differentiated HCCs do not show wash out.[50,51] In such cases, real time scanning should be carried out for a longer duration (>4 minutes) to increase the sensitivity of diagnosis.

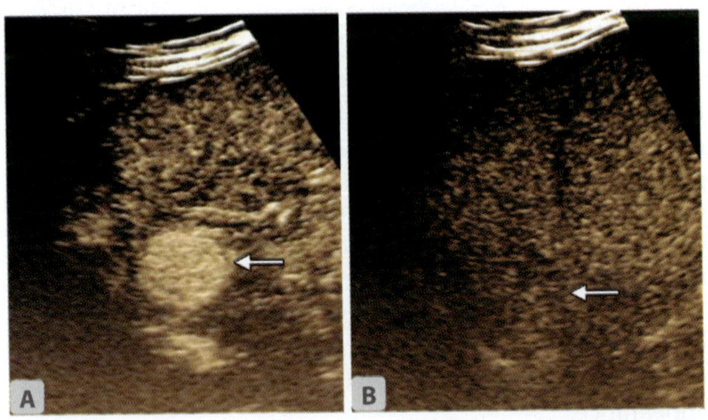

FIGS. 2A AND B: HCC—Typical pattern (CEUS LR-5): CEUS image showing a FLL in segment VII, more than one cm in size, depicting homogeneous APHE in the AP at 25 seconds (arrow, A) with mild, delayed wash out at 192 seconds (arrow, B) Findings are suggestive of HCC.

In cirrhosis patient, APHE of the nodule with late, mild wash out constitutes the typical pattern of HCC described as CEUS LI-RADS **(Figs. 2A and B)**. Nevertheless, as in many well-differentiated HCCs, APHE without washout is also highly suspicious for HCC, but not conclusive. Contrast imaging of MPCT/MRI should be recommended for atypical, inconclusive patterns of the nodule as per the CEUS LI-RADS v2017.

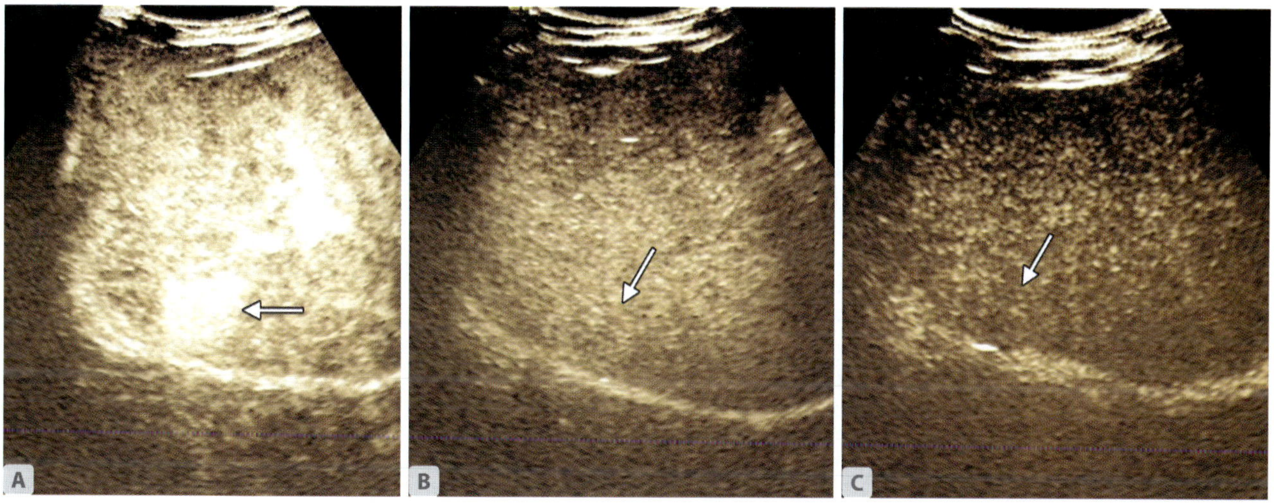

FIGS. 3A TO C: HCC—Atypical pattern (CEUS LR- 4): AP CEUS image of a known patient of cirrhosis with FLL, >1 cm, showing homogeneous APHE (arrow) at 30 sec (A) with retained contrast appearing isoenhancing (arrows) in the VP and LP at 110 and 240 sec respectively (B and C). Histopathology suggested well-differentiated HCC.

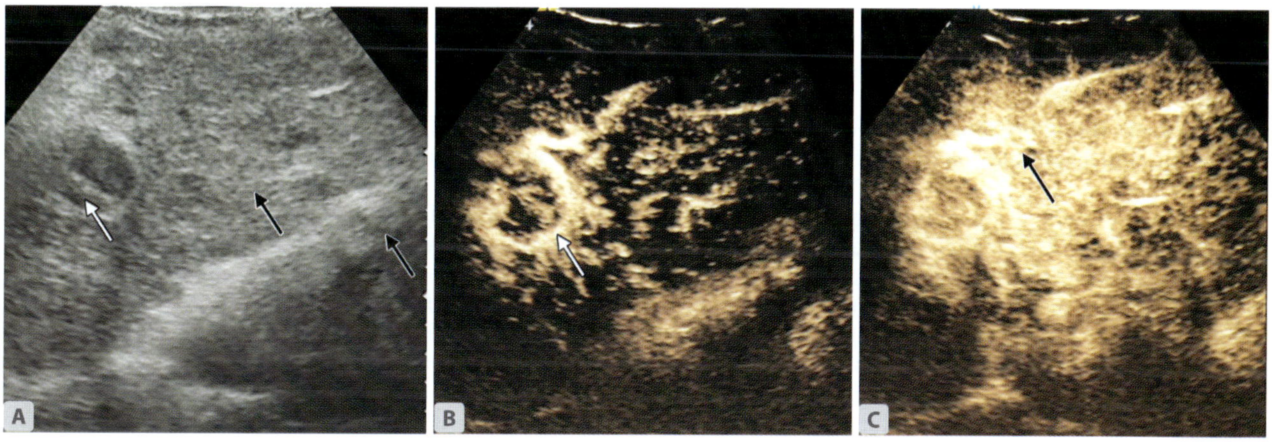

FIGS. 4A TO C: HCC with MPV thrombosis (CEUS LR-TIV): Simultaneous US display images of tissue (A) and contrast signal (B and C) in a known case of HCC, depicting a heteroechoic, ill defined, large left lobe mass (black arrows), dilated main portal vein (MPV) with a soft tissue density within (white arrow, A). On the early AP CEUS at 12 sec, there is enhancement of a part of the mass with opacification of the proximal LPV and MPV with an enhancing thrombus in the MPV (arrow, B). At 15 sec, the entire mass shows marked enhancement with encasement of the LPV (arrow, C). Findings are suggestive of HCC infiltrating the LPV, MPV thrombosis and arterio-portal shunting.

CEUS has a sensitivity of 88.8%,, specificity of 89.2%, and PPV of 91.3% in diagnosing HCC [52] and the results vary with the size of the nodules. Like CT/MRI, evaluating smaller sized nodules by CEUS is always a concern. CEUS sensitivity for 1.0–2.0, 2.1–3.0 and 3.1–5.0 cm nodules is 69%–80%, 97% and 100% respectively, and the diagnostic accuracies are 82–87%, 97% and 100% respectively.[49,53]

For evaluation of portal vein thrombosis complicating HCC, CEUS is superior to CT in detection (100% vs 68%) and characterization (98% vs 68%).[54] The malignant thrombus depicts heterogeneous enhancement or irregular linear vessels following contrast injection in the AP. In the presence of malignant portal vein thrombosis, invariably, an associated mass is seen which may have a contiguous intraluminal extension into the vein, termed as Tumor in vein (TIV) on CEUS LI-RADS **(Figs. 4A to C)**. Hence, meticulous examination of the liver is warranted. In contrast, the benign thrombus is generally avascular.

Intrahepatic Cholangiocarcinoma

ICC may occur in patients with either normal or a cirrhotic liver and is classified pathologically as an adenocarcinoma, although mixed hepatocellular-cholangiocarcinomas are also seen especially in chronic liver disease.[55]

Since the ultrasound contrast is a pure blood pool agent, ICC typically depicts early enhancement in the AP of CEUS, which is peripheral, rim like.[54,55] The onset of wash out is rapid and marked occurring in less than 60 sec. This feature helps in differentiating ICC from HCC where the later shows mild, late onset washout after 60 sec. ICC is categorized under CEUS LI-RADS-M category and final diagnosis by biopsy is recommended.

CEUS pattern of ICC on CEUS is different from the pattern of ICC seen on CT/MRI where, centripetal progressive enhancement of the tumor occurs from the AP to the LP. This is due to the difference in the kinetics of the contrast agents used in CT and MR, which are extracellular agents and thus gradually diffuse into the extracellular space causing delayed enhancement of the tumor in the LP.

CEUS for Diagnosis of HCC

Due to the high diagnostic capability of CEUS, it was accepted as a reference imaging modality for the noninvasive diagnostic algorithm of HCC by the various guidelines laid by the American Association of the Study of Liver (AASLD) in 2005, supported by other societies like APASL, JSH, EFSUMB and WFUMB. However, the updated AASLD Guidelines in 2011excluded CEUS from the recommendations due to the perceived possibility of misdiagnosing ICC by CEUS and a controversy arose.[56] Since then, multiple studies have demonstrated high specificity of 93–100% for characterization of FLL by CEUS.[57,58] Moreover, CEUS has shown similar accuracy as MPCT in diagnosing ICC with minimal likelihood of misdiagnosis.[59] Following this, CEUS is back as a part of the imaging armamentarium for diagnosis of HCC and ACR has also introduced a diagnostic algorithm of CEUS LI-RADS for patients at high risk for developing HCC.[25,26]

Categories of CEUS LI-RADS

CEUS LI-RADS diagnostic algorithm is categorized on a *five point scale* depicting different confidence levels for the diagnosis of malignancy **(Flowchart 1)**. The categories range from LI-RADS (LR)-1 (definitely benign) to LR-5 (definitely malignant) and are also linked to the recommendations for management.

Presence of certain ancillary features (AFs) facilitate diagnosis of benign and malignant nodules with increased confidence and may help in downgrading or upgrading the final index of suspicion for the nature of the nodule in doubtful cases. CEUS AF favoring malignancy in general is the presence of definite growth and that favoring HCC is the 'nodule-in-nodule' appearance or a mosaic architecture of the nodule. On the other hand, if the size of the nodule remains stable for more than two years or a reduction in size is observed, this may suggest a benign pathology. If a doubt arises about the presence of a particular finding, it is better to consider that feature as absent and characterize the nodule accordingly.

CEUS LI-RADS is indicated for more than 10 mm nodules detected on surveillance US, for assessment of LR-3, LR-4, and LR-M observations detected on CT/MRI, nodules with inconclusive histology and nodules not showing APHE due to mistiming on prior CT/MRI. Unlike CT/MRI LI-RADS, the current version of CEUS LI-RADS is not recommended for evaluating nodules that are not seen on B mode US and for the assessment of therapeutic response. Work in this regard is in progress.

- *CEUS LI-RADS-NC (Non-categorizable):* Deals with the quality of the study of CEUS and the resultant ability to interpret the findings.
  Poor quality may be an outcome of any technical failure of the equipment or the technique. Obesity, deep location or a small size nodule, affects the evaluation by CEUS. If due to any of these causes, the documentation of the enhancement pattern is not proper, it could lead to inability to assign any category to the liver nodule making it non-categorizable. In these cases, alternate imaging of multiphasic CT/MRI should be recommended.
- *CEUS LR-1 (Definitely benign):* All benign lesions like hemangiomas, focal fat deposition/sparing can also be seen in the cirrhotic liver and show similar enhancement characteristics as shown in the non-cirrhotic liver **(Figs. 1A to C)**. If the B mode as well as the CEUS findings are in agreement, these lesions can be confidently labeled as LR-1 pathologies for which 6 month surveillance is recommended.
- *CEUS LR-2 (Probably benign):* Majority of these nodules are detected incidentally while performing CEUS for some other nodule. LR-2 is a nonmass like isoenhancing nodule of any size like the regenerative nodules. These patients are advised regular 6-month surveillance.

FLOWCHART 1: Diagnostic algorithm of CEUS LI-RADS v2017.

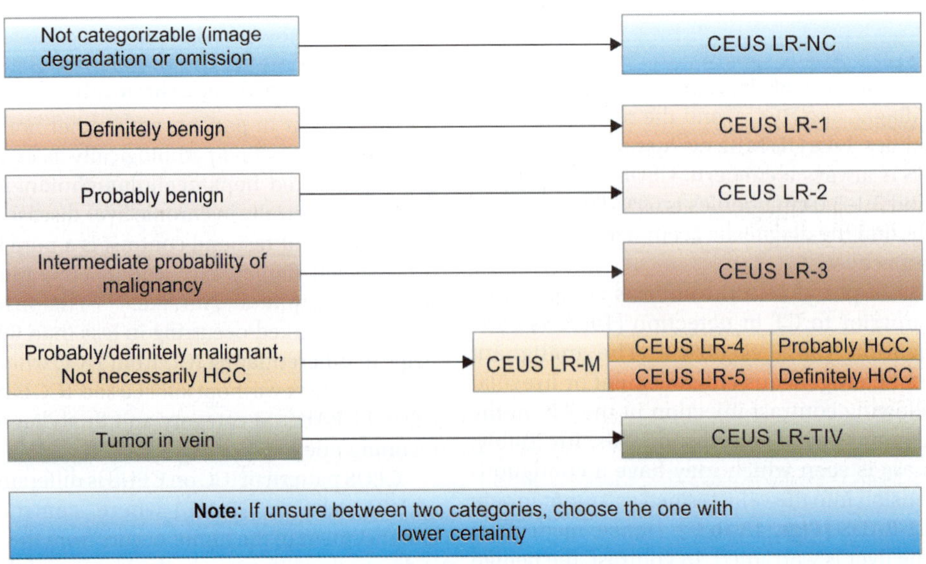

Source: http://www.acr.org/-/media/ACR/images/Clinical Resources/RADS/LI-RADS/CEUSv2017 core.png, Accessed on Nov 5, 2018.

If an LR-3 nodule shows an interval stability of more than 2 years, that particular nodule could also be downgraded to LR-2.

- *CEUS LR-M (Probably or definitely malignant, not necessarily HCC):* LR-M nodule can be of any size and would always show APHE. Any of the following features could be present: rim enhancement in the AP, early washout, occurring in less than 60 sec which is of marked intensity called punched out appearance **(Figs. 5A to C)**. LR-M nodules are always malignant but the CEUS findings lack specificity as these could be either ICC, combination tumor of hepatocholangiocarcinoma, or metastases or may even be HCC. Biopsy is mandatory for the final diagnosis.
- *CEUS LR-3 (Intermediate malignancy probability):* The nodules from categories of LR-3 onwards are in the process of hepato-carcinogenesis in the presence of chronic liver disease and have various degrees of probability of being an HCC. Accurate characterization depends on the size, APHE and washout characteristics **(Table 5)**.
There is a huge variation in the size and characteristics of APHE and washout of LR-3 nodule. It could be a nodule ≥10 mm, isoenhancing in all phases or nodule less than 10 mm size, showing APHE (not rim or peripheral discontinuous globular) but no washout. Sometimes, it may be less than 20 mm size, showing no APHE but depicting late, mild washout after 60 sec.
- *CEUS LR-4 (Probably HCC):* CEUS LR-4 nodule is highly suspicious for HCC but does not have 100% probability of being an HCC due to lack of typical characteristics for confident diagnosis of HCC. It can have a variable size and different combination of enhancement characteristics **(Table 5)**. Nodule of ≥10 mm size showing APHE (not rim or peripheral discontinuous globular) but no washout and on the contrary, size less than 10 mm but showing features of APHE (not rim or peripheral discontinuous globular) with mild, late washout after 60 sec qualifies for LR-4 **(Figs. 3A to C)**. Another category could be of a larger size nodule more than 20 mm, showing no APHE but depicting mild, late washout after 60 sec.
Significance of APHE on CEUS is paramount as it is a feature of nodules of hepatocellular origin. Unlike CEUS, APHE seen on multiphasic CT/MRI could represent a pseudo nodule due to an arterioportal shunt in a cirrhotic liver. It is thus recommended that a multi-disciplinary consensus should be obtained for undertaking either biopsy, treatment, or short interval follow-up for LR-4 nodule.
- *CEUS LR-5 (Definitely HCC):* LR-5 has 100% probability of HCC. The typical features are a nodule of ≥10 mm size, with typical combination of APHE (not rim or peripheral discontinuous globular), with mild, late washout after 60 sec **(Figs. 2A and B)**. This nodule needs treatment for HCC based on the staging of the disease and there is no requirement for tissue diagnosis.
- *LR-TIV (Tumor in vein):* CEUS can delineate the portal vein and the hepatic veins very well. A malignant tumor thrombus is seen as a soft tissue mass within the expanded lumen of the vein showing APHE with subsequent washout in the LP. LR-TIV is often associated with

TABLE 5: Diagnostic Algorithm Of CEUS LR 3 To 5 Nodules Based On The Size, Arterial Phase Hyperenhancement (APHE) And Washout.

APHE	No APHE		APHE (not rim, not peripheral discontinuous globular)	
Nodule size (mm)	<20	≥20	<10	≥10
No WO of any type	CEUS-LR-3	CEUS-LR-3	CEUS-LR-3	CEUS LR-4
Late and mild WO	CEUS-LR-3	CEUS-LR-4	CEUS-LR-4	CEUS-LR-5

If unsure about the presence of any major feature, characterize the feature as absent

Source: http://www.acr.org/-/media/ACR/images/Clinical Resources/RADS/LI-RADS/CEUSv2017 core.png, Accessed on Nov 5,2018

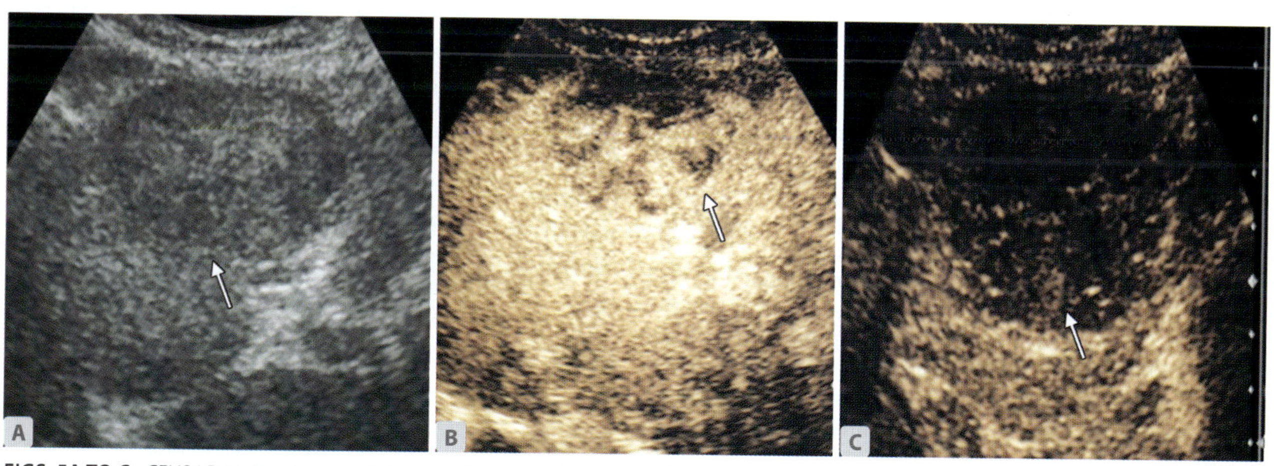

FIGS. 5A TO C: CEUS LR-M: Simultaneous US display images of tissue (A) and contrast signal (B and C), depicting a heteroechoic, well-defined segment II FLL (arrow, A), which is hetergeneously enhancing in the early AP at 12 sec (arrow) with rapid, marked early washout at 52 sec in the VP. Findings are suggestive of a malignant lesion categorized as LR-M and biopsy of the mass was advised.

malignancy like HCC, ICC, hepato-cholangiocarcinoma or other non-HCC malignancies. At times, a tumor may be seen directly infiltrating the portal vein making the diagnosis crystal clear and illustrating the underlying etiology **(Figs. 4A to C)**.

Guidance for Interventional Procedures

Ultrasound is the most commonly used modality for guiding tumour biopsy or percutaneous ablation. Conventional ultrasound fails to detect nodules that are isoechoic to liver parenchyma, with indistinct margins or infiltrative in nature. In some cases, the liver nodule may not be seen at all and management of such nodules becomes problematic.

CEUS not only depicts the nodules that are occult on US, but also facilitates accurate targeting for biopsy or ablation. It delineates the margins of the nodule well and also depicts the extent of malignant infiltration. CEUS guidance increases the diagnostic yield of biopsy by 10% and also decreases the false negative rates in large tumors with necrosis. The number of attempts needed for targeting are significantly reduced by CEUS guidance due to accurate differentiation of the viable tumor (seen as an enhancing tissue) from the necrotic tissue depicting lack of enhancement following contrast injection.[60,61]

CEUS also plays a vital role in guiding percutaneous ablative therapy for both primary and secondary liver tumors. Prior to ablation, CEUS assessment provides valuable information on the exact size, margins of the tumor and its relation with the adjoining structures, and help plan the best therapeutic strategy thereby reducing the complication rate. This baseline information of tumor characteristics serve as a guide for post treatment response assessment.

Following ablation, CEUS helps in estimating the extent of ablation. If any residual disease is detected, a repeat ablation can be performed to achieve complete response. The residual viable tumor or any local recurrence following ablation is well delineated and accurate retargeting under CEUS guidance helps in reducing the number of treatment sessions for achieving complete ablation.[62]

Assessment of Treatment Response of Malignant Tumors

Loco-regional therapy of percutaneous ablative techniques like radiofrequency ablation (RFA), ethanol (PEI) or acetic acid ablation (PAI) and microwave/laser ablation or intra-arterial therapies like transarterial chemoembolization, radio-embolization form the mainstay of therapy for nonsurgical candidates of HCC. Loco-regional therapy aims at producing coagulation necrosis of the tumor rendering it non-viable. Multiphasic CT/MRI have been the recommended imaging modalities for assessment of treatment response of HCC.[5,36] However, these cross sectional imaging modalities have their own limitations. Limited availability, high cost, hazards of ionizing radiation, mistiming of contrast bolus, prevents repetitive use of CT/MRI for follow-up imaging.

CEUS has the potential to overcome these shortcomings. Diagnostic accuracy of CEUS in differentiating between viable and non-viable tumor tissue following different types of ablative therapy is quite similar to that of CT or MRI.[63] The completely ablated tumor is hypoenhancing, well defined, shows uniform thickness margin all around with no area of hyperenhancement within or at the periphery of the hypoenhancing defect in the AP **(Figs. 6A and B)**. On the contrary, residual disease appears as an area of hyperenhancement in the AP, either at the margin or within the ablated tumor site, showing washout in PP and LP **(Figs. 7 and 8)**. CEUS can accurately assess early outcome of ablation, immediately following RFA, and the results are comparable to CT performed at 24 hours.[63,64] Being a radiation free technique, CEUS can be safely used for repeated follow up of treated patients.

Conventional TACE involves delivery of mixture of chemotherapeutic drugs with iodised oil (lipiodol) through the hepatic artery feeding the malignant liver tumor with subsequent temporary embolization causing

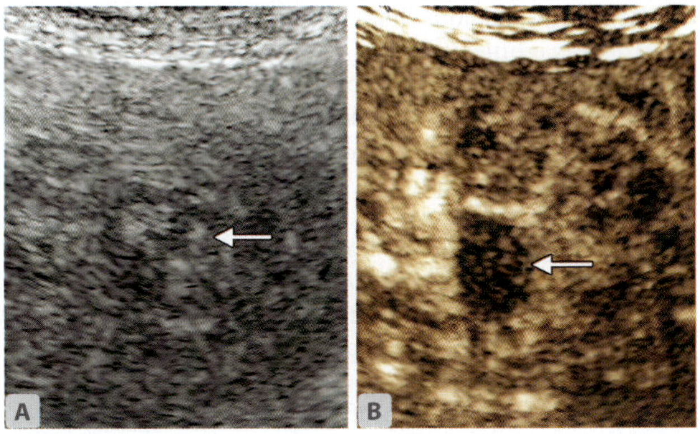

FIGS. 6A AND B: Post RFA Complete response of segment IV A HCC. Simultaneous US display images of tissue and contrast signal, showing a heteroechoic, ill-defined focal liver lesion [arrow (A)] which is seen as a well-defined hypoenhancing ablative defect with no hyperenhancing viable tissue within or at the margin on the AP image of CEUS arrow, B suggesting complete response to ablation.

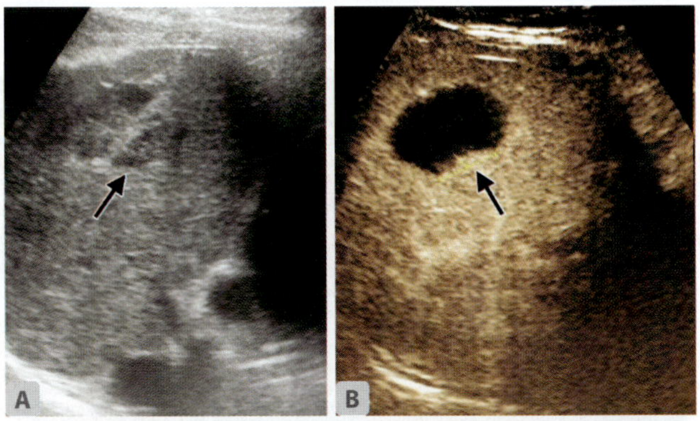

FIGS. 7A AND B: Post RFA residual disease in a patient of cirrhosis with solitary HCC. At one week post RFA, the US image showing a heterogeneous mass in the liver with no clue of the viable or non-viable tumor tissue (A). On CEUS, the mass shows a focal area of hyperenhancement along the postero-inferior margin of the RFA defect (arrow) suggesting residual disease (B). A repeat RFA was planned subsequently.

devascularization of the hypervascular HCC. Post TACE response assessment involves depiction of residual viable tumor if any. Multiphasic CT (MPCT) often has limitations in accurately detecting residual disease as immediately following TACE. Lipiodol gets deposited within the viable tumor as well as in the adjoining hepatic parenchyma. Thus, MPCT is undertaken after a minimum period of 4 weeks for proper assessment of tumor response. Moreover, both lipiodol and the viable tumor appear hyperdense on MPCT, leading to masking of the viable tumor.[65] Thus, MRI is the preferred modality for post TACE evaluation. However it is expensive and has limited availability.

CEUS is a useful alternative in this situation. CEUS assessment is not hindered by the presence of lipiodol within the tumor. Only the viable residual tumor enhances post contrast and is seen as an area of hyperenhancement in AP and washout in the PP, whereas the lipiodol gets masked leading to accurate estimation of therapeutic response **(Figs. 9 and 10)**. Thus, CEUS has a higher sensitivity than MPCT in detecting residual disease post TACE (CEUS 94% (95% CI: 81 to 99%), MPCT 50% (95% CI: 33 to 67%, P-0.0001)[66], and should be preferred over CT in such cases However, so far, the current diagnostic algorithm of CEUS-LIRADS does not include categorization of tumor response.

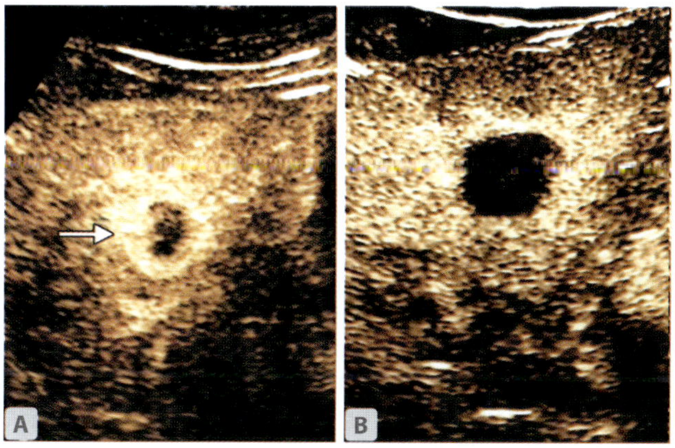

FIGS. 8A AND B: Post PAI residual disease: AP image of CEUS done at 4 weeks following PAI, depicting a hyperenhancing area all along the margin and predominantly in the supero-lateral aspect (arrow) of the segment II/III HCC suggesting residual disease (A) Repeat PAI was done and CEUS performed subsequently showing smooth margins of the ablative lesion with no enhancing tissue suggesting complete response (B).

Dynamic Contrast-enhanced Ultrasound

Quantitative assessment of the perfusion of parenchymatous organs can be done non-invasively by the use of dynamic contrast-enhanced ultrasound (DCE-US).Softwares like **VueBox**™ or SonoLiver are available for quantifying perfusion based on the contrast kinetics and generating perfusion maps. The time-to-peak (TTP), estimated perfusion (EP), peak intensity (PI) and area under the curve can be estimated.[67]

Characterizing benign and malignant liver masses can be done based on these findings. DCE-US can depict changes in perfusion within the tumor following therapy. The antiangiogenic drugs like Sorafenib, induce necrosis within the tumor without eradicating the tumor per se. DCE-US can reliably depict reduced or absent tumor vascularity following drug therapy indicating therapeutic response.[67] However, DCE-US use has still not been recommended in the CEUS guidelines so far.[68]

Hepatic Vein Transit Time Estimation

The arrival time of the UCA bolus in the hepatic artery and portal/hepatic vein can be measured and the calculation of the transit times can be done. Shortening of the transit time is encountered in cirrhosis and chronic hepatitis and this finding is quite non-specific.[69]

Liver Transplant

CEUS is a safe technique which can be performed at bedside and provides greater diagnostic confidence and additional

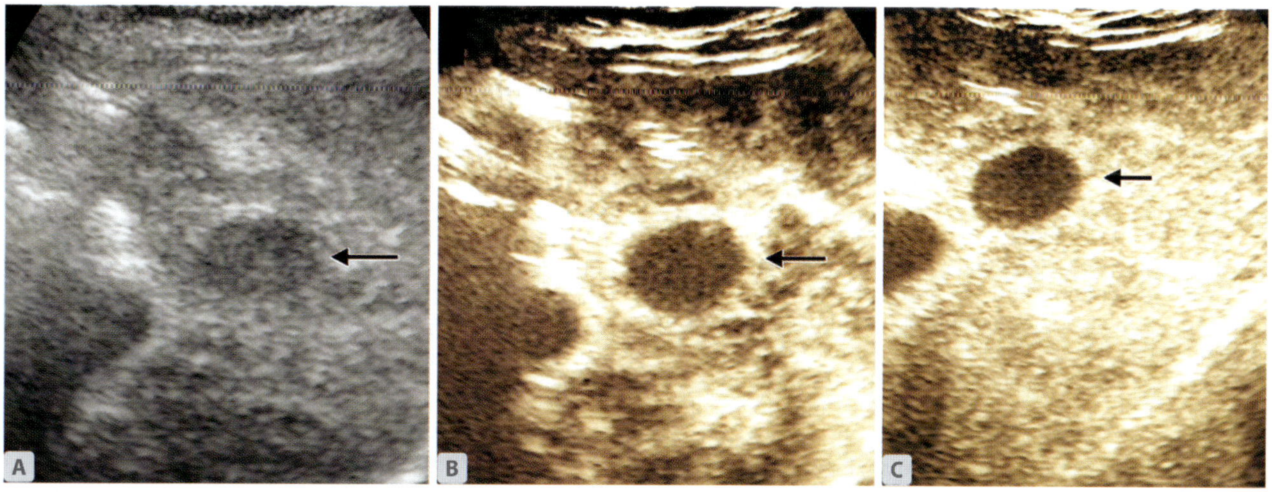

FIGS. 9A TO C: Post TACE complete response: Segment II HCC post TACE, seen as a well-defined hypoechoic lesion with slightly hyperechoic margins on US (A). On CEUS, the mass is seen as a hypoenhancing lesion with uniform hyperenhancing margins in the AP at 22 sec and DP at 62 secs suggesting complete response post TACE (B and C respectively).

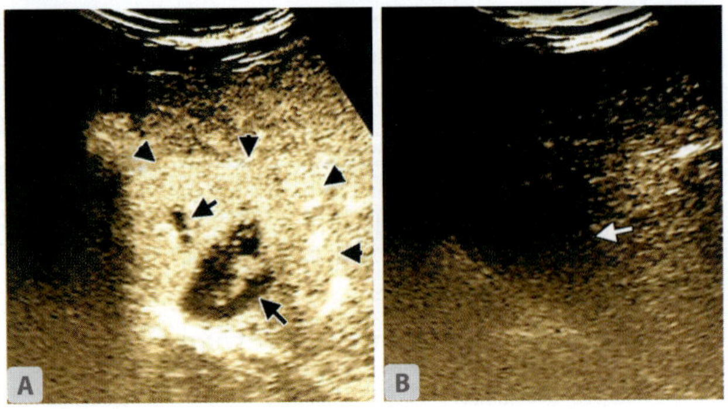

FIGS. 10A AND B: Post TACE residual disease. CEUS performed for a large segment VII HCC treated with TACE, showing, a large hyperenhancing tissue (arrowheads) with hypoenhancing necrotic areas (arrows) within, in the AP (A) and showing uniform hypoenhancement in the LP (arrow, B). Findings are suggestive of significant residual disease post TACE. A repeat session of TACE was planned.

information than conventional ultrasound. However, following liver transplant (LT), presence of surgical wound, subcutaneous emphysema, intervening bowel gas pose a huge limitation in evaluation.[70] LT is the recommended therapy for end-stage liver diseases due to multiple causes and accurate imaging evaluation is crucial for favorable outcomes. CEUS is being increasingly used for the assessment of hepatic vasculature in pre, intra and post-transplant patients

CEUS has a high diagnostic accuracy in evaluating portal venous system patency and characterizing portal vein thrombosis, hepatic vein and inferior vena cava patency in LT patients.[71,72] Intra-biliary use of UCA f or intraoperative biliary anatomy assessment has also been found to be useful.[73] 3D-CEUS can depict the biliary spatial relationship and the anatomical variations. However, further studies in larger series of patients are needed.

CEUS has paramount importance in the initial exclusion of vascular complications post LT. Compared to CT, it has a sensitivity of 89.3%, specificity of 100%, positive and negative predictive value of 100% and 91.4% respectively.[74] Hepatic artery thrombosis (HAT) is the commonest vascular complication and relatively less common entities like portal vein, hepatic vein and caval thrombosis are also encountered. Compared to conventional ultrasound, CEUS has improved diagnostic assessment of HAT and stenosis.[75,76] Hepatic vein obstruction can be better diagnosed by CEUS than the color Doppler US by identifying the middle hepatic vein tributaries.[77]

Biliary complications are severe and occur in 10% to 30% post LT. Ischemic-type biliary lesions (ITBLs) are serious, difficult to diagnose on the current available imaging techniques. Biliary tree is peculiar as it is supplied solely by the hepatic artery through a network of arterioles and capillaries termed peribiliary vascular plexus (PBP). Intravenous CEUS can depict the enhancement patterns of bile duct walls to reveal the microcirculatory changes of PBP.[78] UCAs injected into the bile ducts can produce cholangiography like images of the biliary tree (CEUSC) in LT patients, and the results are similar to conventional radiography in detection of biliary pathologies.[79]

CEUS might also be an alternative tool for evaluation of a rare complication of arterial steal syndrome following LT.[80]

Upcoming Hepatic Applications

3D-CEUS

2D-CEUS evaluates only a single slice of the lesion and is unable to display the relationship of the lesion with the surrounding issues and its perfusion. 3D-CEUS can overcome this limitation of 2D-CEUS as the volume data can be rotated to different angles to establish the best position of an image for fully analyzing a selected region. It provides detailed information of the origin, number and branches of the feeding arteries of the FLLs.[81] However, it is a static image and is unable to provide the enhancement patterns in different phases, for which 4D-CEUS is emerging as a useful option. It is a real-time 3D-CEUS with continuous data set acquisition capacity and can depict the lesion as well as the spatial relation of liver tumor blood vessels. Thus, the angiographic anatomy and the dynamic perfusion of FLLs in real-time can be illustrated by 4D-CEUS.[82] Further work is being done in this regard.

Limitations of CEUS of Liver

Despite having established itself as an important imaging tool for the evaluation of liver, CEUS has a number of limitations as well. Lesions located in the sub diaphragmatic areas are difficult to evaluate. It has limited penetration in patients of chronic liver disease and deep seated lesions may not be visualized due to steatosis and fibrosis of the liver. Small sized metastases less than 5–10 mm can often be missed being too small for detection. CEUS is not a recommended modality for staging of HCC because of the inability to examine the entire liver in the short lasting arterial phase resulting in incomplete evaluation. Moreover, one injection of UCA per nodule is required and if the nodules are present in different segments of the liver, multiple injections would be needed. This would defeat the advantage of cost-effectiveness of CEUS and thus CT/MRI would be preferred for holistic evaluation in such cases.

NON-HEPATIC APPLICATIONS

Applications in Pancreatic Imaging

The main utility of CEUS in pancreatic diseases lies in the characterization of pancreatic mass lesions and in the imaging of acute pancreatitis. After administration of UCAs, the pancreatic parenchyma shows early enhancement, immediately after aortic enhancement (10–30 sec). Maximal enhancement is reached at 60 seconds. After the AP, VP imaging should also be performed (30–100 sec).[83,84] Once the pancreatic study in completed, delayed phase imaging of the liver should also be undertaken as part of the study for ruling out metastases

Pancreatic Masses

- For pancreatic adenocarcinomas, the usual investigation modality is CECT. They are schirrhous tumors and commonly hypovascular compared to the normal pancreatic parenchyma. The detectability of small pancreatic mass lesions on CEUS is superior to US alone. Lesion size, lesion margin and relationship with adjacent vessels are better assessed with CEUS.[83,84] CEUS is essential for lesion characterization and helpful in US guided lesion biopsy.[85,86] It is also helpful in detecting changes in tumor vascularity after chemotherapy.[87,88]

- CEUS can be used to diagnose and differentiate pancreatic neuroendocrine tumors (NET) from adenocarcinoma. NETs show significant enhancement in the AP of CEUS even when it may not show significant increased vascularity on Doppler imaging.[89-91] Larger tumors may show non-enhancing necrotic internal areas.
- CEUS is very useful in making a differential diagnosis of an unilocular cystic pancreatic mass. It can differentiate a pancreatic pseudocyst from mucinous cystadenoma by demonstrating septal vascularity and nodularity.[92-96] Mucinous cystic tumors are seen as cystic lesions with contents on grey scale sonography. On CEUS, the walls and septae show enhancement, with parietal nodules. In contrast, pancreatic pseudocysts do not show any internal area of contrast enhancement. CEUS has very high sensitivity and specificity in the characterization of pseudocysts.[96]
- Intraductal papillary mucinous neoplasms (IPMN) can be of branch duct type or main duct type. CEUS can differentiate between the mucin plugs in such tumors, from a viable perfused area.[92-96]
- CEUS is useful in the differentiation of focal mass forming pancreatitis, which shows a contrast enhancement similar to pancreatic parenchyma; from an adenocarcinoma.[97]

Detection of Pancreatic Necrosis in Acute Pancreatitis

The detection of necrosis at an early stage of development is of significant clinical importance as early treatment of necrosis (either percutaneous drainage or surgical debridement) can be planned to reduce morbidity and mortality. The routine diagnostic imaging modality in acute pancreatitis is CECT. CEUS can also be used as an alternative to CECT in the follow-up of acute pancreatitis.[98,99] After administration of UCAs, the necrotic pancreatic parenchyma appears unenhanced.[98,99]

Contrast-enhanced Endoscopic Ultrasound (CE-EUS)

CE-EUS is a newer imaging modality which combines the benefit of superior resolution of EUS and assessment of enhancement characteristics (as in CEUS) in a single investigation.[100-104]

CE-EUS is useful for the differentiation of pancreatic ductal adenocarcinoma from focal pancreatitis and other focal lesions; and to differentiate cystic pancreatic tumor from pancreatic pseudocyst.[2] A few studies have described the benefit of endoscopic contrast Doppler sonography in the detection of small pancreatic adenocarcinomas and their differentiation from focal pancreatitis. Since pancreatic adenocarcinomas tend to be fibrous in nature and have a tough capsule, they show less or no venous signals, owing to increased intratumoral pressure. On the contrary, focal pancreatitis shows both arterial and venous signals. CE-EUS increases the sensitivity of EUS (from 73.2% to 91.1%) in differentiation of pancreatic adenocarcinoma from focal pancreatitis.[105]

Pancreatic Transplant

CEUS is useful in assessing the graft after pancreatic transplant. It has an advantage of assessing the microvasculature in the graft; and hence an useful addition to grey scale sonography.[106]

Applications in Renal Imaging

The main role of CEUS in renal lesions include the evaluation of a focal renal lesion, evaluation of complex cystic renal lesions,[107,108] differentiating a renal tumor from a pseudotumor,[109,110] and also in the evaluation of renal vascular lesions.[111,112] Other applications include guidance to radiofrequency ablation of renal tumors[113-117] and monitoring of renal abscesses in proven cases of urinary tract infection.[118] Kidneys are highly perfused organs and the microbubble contrast enhancement pattern of the kidneys follow a pattern similar to that seen on CECT. After administration of UCAs, the vascular pedicle of kidney enhances first, followed by the cortex and the medulla at the last. The tip of the renal medullary pyramid is the last to enhance. UCAs do not show excretion into the pelvicalyceal system.

CEUS is recommended for the following renal indications.

Characterization of Renal Masses

CECT is the usual investigation for characterization and staging of renal mass lesions. However, on a single phase CECT, it becomes difficult to differentiate complicated hyperdense cyst and a solid enhancing mass lesion. Similarly, a hypodense non-enhancing solid mass lesion may be difficult to differentiate from a cystic lesion on CECT. Since CEUS is more sensitive to detection of blood flow than CECT, it can differentiate a solid mass lesion from a cystic one with greater accuracy **(Figs. 11A and B)**. It also scores over CECT in characterization of complex cystic renal masses as it can detect the septa and solid components in Bosniak grade 2–4 cysts with better sensitivity than CECT.[107,108]

Differentiation of Renal Tumors from 'Pseudotumors'

Renal pseudotumors are proliferation of normal renal tissue which mimic tumor. US may fail to differentiate the two. After administration of UCAs, the enhancement of pseudotumors is similar to the normal renal parenchyma on all phases of enhancement.[109,110] On the contrary, the enhancement pattern of solid renal tumors differs from that of the normal renal parenchyma in at least one phase of enhancement. Although the differentiation of a benign from a malignant renal tumor cannot be done based on CEUS enhancement characteristics, it is helpful in differentiating a 'true' renal tumor from a pseudotumor.

Renal Vascular Lesions

Renal infarcts are better differentiated from ischemic areas on CEUS compared to unenhanced Doppler US or

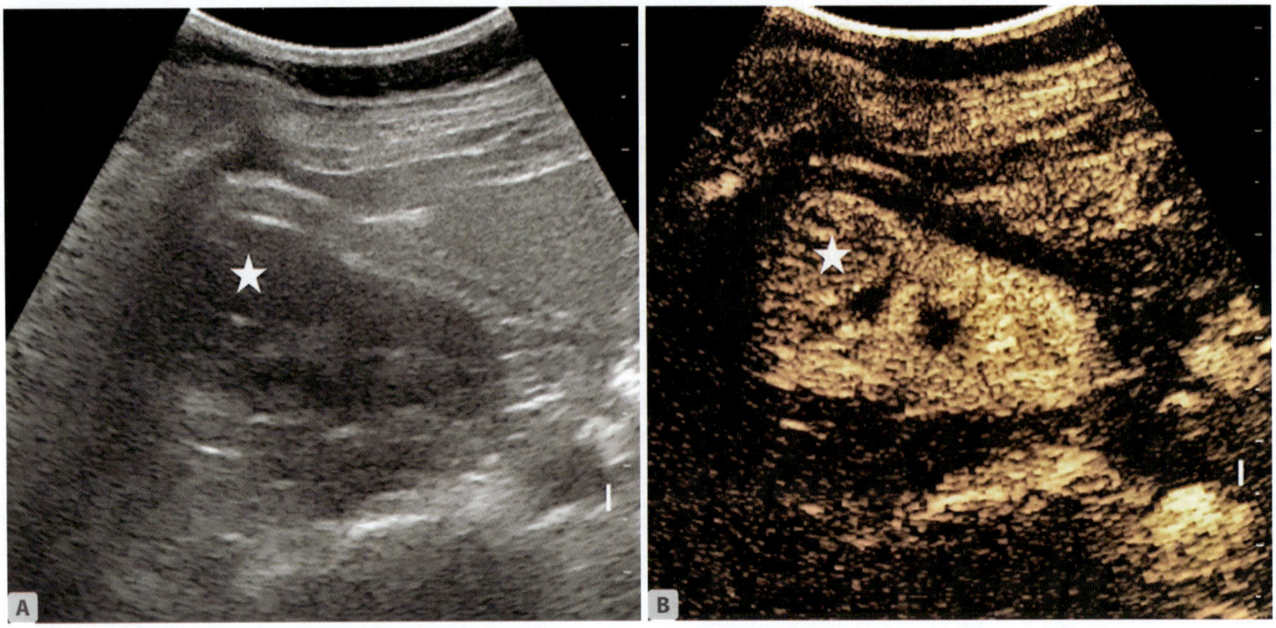

FIGS. 11A AND B: Renal cell carcinoma. Grayscale sonographic image of a focal lesion in the kidney which appears cystic (stars). CEUS image shows intralesional flow (hence a solid lesion) which is less than the normal parenchyma.

conventional US as the infarcted area shows no enhancement whereas hypoperfused area retains its blood flow, although reduced.[111,112] CEUS also differentiates renal infarct from cortical necrosis, which shows preserved hilar vascularity.

Renal Tumor Ablation under CEUS Guidance

Pre-procedure Evaluation

Traditionally, CECT or CE-MRI are used in pre and post-procedure evaluation in percutaneous renal tumor ablation. CEUS is helpful in preprocedure evaluation of renal tumors which show enhancement in early phase and wash out in LP.[113-115] If a pseudo-capsule is seen, it suggests improved ablation efficacy.[116]

Intra-procedure Monitoring

US can guide the needle path during ablation but does not provide adequate information regarding adequacy of ablation. CEUS can be used before the ablation procedure to increase tumor visibility.

Post Ablation

CEUS can be performed 10–15 minutes later (once the gas and related artifacts disappear) to look for residual viable tumor which is seen as an enhancing area whereas ablated regions appear non-enhancing.[113,114] It is also more useful than conventional US in detecting early recurrence of tumor.[117]

Monitoring in Renal Infections

In acute uncomplicated pyelonephritis, grey scale US is used to exclude the presence of calculi of urinary tract obstruction. In non-responding patients, CEUS can be used to evaluate for complications like abscesses.[118] An abscess is seen as a focal non-enhancing area inside the area of pyelonephritis, with or without septations.

Renal Transplant Evaluation

All the indications for CEUS in native kidneys also apply to a transplanted kidney. In addition, CEUS is recommended in the evaluation of graft vascularity and assessing vascular complications like arterial occlusion or venous thrombosis.[119-121]

Application in Abdominal Trauma

CECT is the gold standard imaging modality in blunt abdominal trauma. The current guidelines advocate use of CEUS in abdominal trauma in the following scenarios:[122-126]

- Hemodynamically stable isolated blunt abdominal trauma (moderate energy), especially in children as an alternative to CT
- Abdominal trauma with uncertain CT findings, for a second-look investigation
- Follow-up imaging of abdominal trauma when conservative management is followed; especially in children.

Studies have shown that CEUS can detect intra-abdominal solid organ injuries (including liver, splenic, renal lesions) with higher sensitivity and specificity than US.

The solid abdominal organs can be evaluated in a staged manner in two-part examination (once for the right hypochondrium, evaluating right kidney first, followed by adrenal, liver and pancreas) and another examination for the left hypochondrium for spleen and left kidney. Normal organs usually show homogeneous increased echogenicity in the parenchymal phase of the examination. A contusion is seen as a hypoechoic area within the enhancing parenchyma with ill-defined borders; a laceration is a more well defined, linear non-enhancing area. In hypovolemic shock, all the abdominal solid organs show reduced enhancement. Since UCAs are not excreted in the urine, they can not be used to detect the renal collecting system injury.

Applications in Gastrointestinal Tract

CEUS of the gastrointestinal tract (GIT) requires a high frequency transducer, and a higher amount of contrast (approximately 4.8 mL).[127] The arterial phase of intestinal imaging varies from 0-30 seconds, and a venous phase lasts from 30–120 seconds.[128] A high resolution US can detect all five gut layers, and hence bowel wall thickenings and mass lesions are well delineated. The main applications in bowel imaging include the following:

- Disease activity assessment in inflammatory bowel diseases, especially Crohn's disease and in children. In Crohn's disease; the bowel wall enhancement on CEUS correlates well with clinical scores like CDAI. In ulcerative colitis bowel wall enhancement correlates with histopathological markers of inflammation. Bowel wall enhancement changes during treatment, thereby making CEUS a useful tool for disease activity monitoring.[129-131]
- Differentiate between fibrous and inflammatory strictures in Crohn's disease.[132]
- CEUS can be used to detect abscesses in inflammatory bowel diseases, and to confirm and track the route of fistulae in Crohn's disease.[129-131]

Application in Peripheral Vascular System and Aorta

Major use of ultrasound contrast agents in vascular sonography lies in the evaluation of extracranial carotid arteries and the abdominal aorta. Its use in peripheral vessels is limited. For the use in aorta and carotid arteries; 1–2.4 mL of contrast agent is injected intravenously, followed by 10 mL saline injection. The recommended uses in extracranial carotid arteries and abdominal aorta include-

- Differentiating between total carotid and/or vertebral artery occlusion and residual flow in a tight stenosis. It is a superior imaging modality to Doppler US in the evaluation of re-stenosis after carotid stenting.[133]
- Diagnosis of dissection of extracranial carotid and vertebral arteries, and abdominal aorta when MRI is contraindicated.
- Carotid plaque characterization (ulceration, neovascularization, etc.) which is considered a risk factor for cerebrovascular accident.[134,135]
- In evaluating inflammatory aortoarteritis where the vessel wall enhancement can be used to monitor disease activity.[136,137]
- Follow-up of endovascular aortic repair, and detection of endoleaks.[138,139]

Miscellaneous Intravascular Applications

In spleen, UCAs can be used for focal lesion characterization, to characterize suspected accessory spleen and to confirm splenic infarction.[140-145]

While performing testicular sonography, UCAs can lead to better delineation of the infarction, a suspected segmental infarction,[146,147] better detection of fracture line in testicular trauma,[148] detecting areas of abscess formation in epididymo-orchitis[149] and differentiating a neoplastic from a nonneoplastic focal lesion.[150,151]

Endometrial and cervical tumors have also been evaluated using CEUS. Some studies have reported benefits of CEUS in the diagnosis of endometrial carcinoma, but present guidelines do not advocate the use of ultrasound contrast agents in gynecologic use.[152]

Application of CEUS in lung and pleural diseases is limited. In peripheral consolidations, CEUS can be used to differentiate embolic consolidation from an inflammatory etiology and to detect an area of abscess within a peripheral area of lung consolidation.[153-155]

CEUS can be used to detect complications in acute cholecystitis,[156,157]differentiate chronic cholecystitis from gall bladder carcinoma,[158] and differentiate polypoidal gall bladder wall lesion from a sludge (which is avascular).[158,159]

Tumor response assessment can be done in metastatic GIST.[160] CEUS is also useful in pre, intra and peri procedural evaluation of free tissue flaps.[161,162]

Intracavitary Applications

Vesicoureteric reflux: One important intracavitary application of ultrasound contrast agents is detection of vesicoureteric reflux (VUR).[163-165] Current role in VUR includes:

- Suspected VUR in girls: Contrast enhanced voiding cystourethrography should be the initial investigation.
- Follow-up of VUR in boys and girls after surgical and conservative management.
- Screening of high risk patients for VUR.

Other intracavitary uses includes Sono-hysterosalpingo-contrast sonography for tubal patency assessment,[166] CEUS guided percutaneous cholangiography,[167] T-tube cholangiogram,[168] CEUS sialography for obstructive lesions of the salivary ducts,[169] CEUS guided nephrostogram. Nonphysiologic cavities too can be evaluated by CEUS. Delineation of fistulae, abscesses and intraperitoneal collections and gastro-esophageal reflux can be done successfully by different approaches.[170-172]

Upcoming Non-hepatic Applications

Intraoperative CEUS in neurosurgery is an important use of the ultrasound contrast agents. It is helpful in neurosurgery in cases of CNS tumors,[173,174] trauma and cerebral and spinal vascular malformations.[175] CEUS guided ablation therapy is also helpful in HIFU treatment of uterine fibroid and prostatic cancer.[176,177]

In soft tissue vascular malformations, CEUS has the added advantage of superior detection of slow flow in low flow vascular malformations **(Figs. 12A to D)**. It can also detect small arteriovenous shunts within a vascular malformation which has significant treatment implications.[178]

CEUS characterization of thyroid nodules,[179,180] breast masses[181,182] and prostatic lesions[183] are areas of active research, but not recommended in current guidelines so far.

For lymph node evaluation, it has been used for evaluation of axillary sentinel lymph node sampling in cancer patients and differentiation of benign from malignant lymph nodes, is being tried but not recommended in recent guidelines yet due to certain limitations.[184]

Currently, inflammatory arthritis is also being extensively studied where CEUS has been found to improve the detection

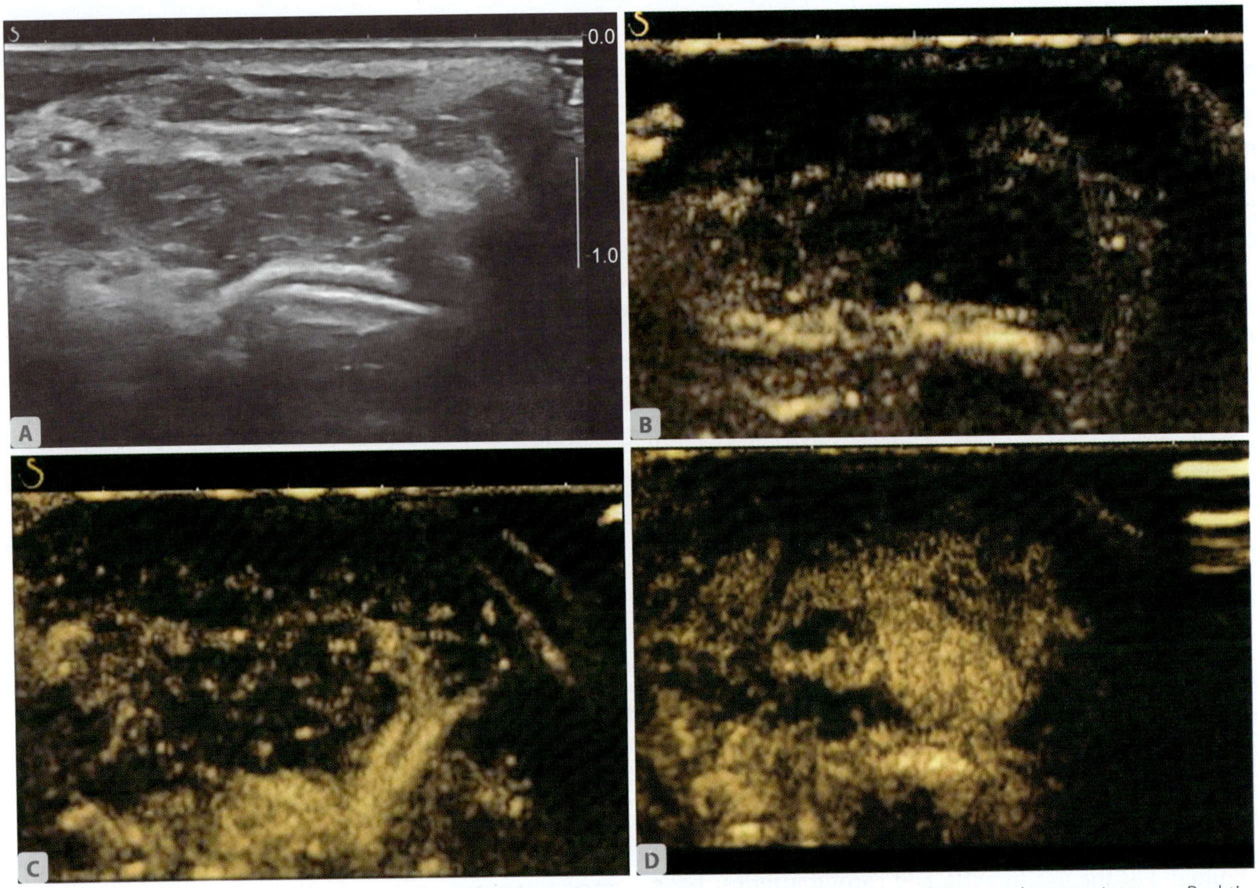

FIGS. 12A TO D: Venous malformation of upper lip. Grayscale sonography (A) shows a hypoechoic lesion without any large cystic spaces. Real-time CEUS study shows gradual contrast enhancement of the lesion, as seen in images at baseline (B), 20 seconds (C) and 80 seconds (D).

of active synovitis in rheumatoid arthritis,[185,186] differentiate active from inactive disease in juvenile idiopathic arthritis,[187,188] and can differentiate effusion from inflammatory pannus.[189]

Experience on the CEUS use for evaluating salivary glands too is limited and hence not yet included in the recommendations.[190]

FUTURE DIRECTIONS

Use of CEUS for molecular imaging is likely to develop in the near future where the targeted microbubbles may bind with ligands to tissue receptors of malignant or inflammatory tissue. Drugs and gene delivery are the futuristic therapeutic options.[191]

Applications of 3D or 4D CEUS, DCE-US are being refined to provide valuable information regarding tumor assessment in oncology patients. Future potential clinical applications of CEUS LI-RADS are likely to focus on HCC treatment response, interpretation and reporting of benign liver lesions, pediatric liver lesions and quantification imaging. Development of Radiology-Pathology consensus terminology in patients of HCC is also being considered.

To conclude, the advent of UCAs have transformed the role of US in clinical practice. CEUS combines the advantage of superior spatial resolution of US with the real time contrast kinetics assessment of target organ. New ultrasound image sequences appear to be very promising.

CEUS has become a major player in hepatic imaging. Recently introduced CEUS LI-RADS for focal liver characterization is likely to improve the integration of CEUS into the multimodality approach for evaluating patients of chronic liver disease, at risk for developing HCC. Detection and characterization of renal masses, renal transplant imaging and guided ablation of solid tumors constitute the most important non-hepatic indications.

ACKNOWLEDGMENTS

The authors sincerely acknowledge the contribution of Dr Ankur Goyal for the **Figures 11A and B**; and Dr Ankur Goyal and Dr Ankit Sangwan for **Figures 12A to D**. The latter figure was a part of the ongoing MD thesis work performed in the Department of Radiodiagnosis, AIIMS, New Delhi.

REFERENCES

1. Shampo MA, Kyle RA. Karl Theodore Dussik- pioneer in ultrasound. Mayo Clinic Proceedings. 1995;70:1136.
2. Claudon M, Dietrich CF, Choi BI, Cosgrove DO, Kudo M, Nolsøe CP et al Guidelines and Good Clinical Practice Recommendations for Contrast Enhanced Ultrasound (CEUS) in the Liver – Update 2012. A WFUMB-EFSUMB Initiative in Cooperation With Representatives of AFSUMB, AIUM, ASUM, FLAUS and ICUS. Ultraschall in Med. 2013;34:11-29.
3. Brannigan M, Burns PN, Wilson SR. Blood flow patterns in focal liver lesions at microbubble-enhanced US. Radiographics. 2004;24:921-35.
4. Cosgrove D, Blomley M. Liver tumors: evaluation with contrast-enhanced ultrasound. Abdom Imaging. 2004;29:446-54.
5. Xu HX. Contrast-enhanced ultrasound: The evolving applications. World J Radiol. 2009;1:15-24.
6. Gramiak R, Shah PM. Echocardiography of the aortic root. Invest Radiol. 1968;3:356-66.
7. Nico de Jong, Marcia Emmer, Annemieke van Wamel, and Michel Versluis Ultrasonic characterization of ultrasound contrast agents Med Biol Eng Comput. 2009;47:861-73.
8. Christiansen C, Kryvi H, Sontum PC, Skotland T. Physical and biochemical characterization of Albunex, a new ultrasound contrast agent consisting of air-filled albumin microspheres suspended in a solution of human albumin. Biotechnol Appl Biochem. 1994;19(Pt 3):307-20.
9. N. de Jong and L. Hoff, "Ultrasound scattering properties of Albunex microspheres,". Ultrasonics. 1993;31:175-81.
10. Sidhu PS, Cantisani V, Dietrich CF, Gilja OH, Saftoiu A, Bartels E, et al. The EFSUMB Guidelines and Recommendations for the Clinical Practice of Contrast-Enhanced Ultrasound (CEUS) in Non-Hepatic Applications: Update 2017 (Long Version). Ultraschall in Med. 2018;39:e2-44.
11. Seitz K, Strobel D. A Milestone: Approval of CEUS for Diagnostic Liver Imaging in Adults and Children in the USA. Ultraschall in Med. 2016;37:229-32.
12. Yanagisawa K, Moriyasu F, Miyahara T, Yuki M, Iijima H. Phagocytosis of ultrasound contrast agent microbubbles by Kupffer cells. Ultrasound Med Bio. 2007;33:318-25.
13. Dietrich CF, Averkiou M, Nielsen MB,. Barr RG, Burns PN, Calliada F, et al. How to perform Contrast-Enhanced Ultrasound (CEUS). Ultrasound Int Open. 2017;3:E2-15.
14. CEUS LI-RADS V2017 core.:http://www.acr.org/-/media/ACR/images/Clinical Resources/RADS/LI-RADS/CEUSv2017 core.png).
15. Singal A, Volk ML, Waljee A, et al. Meta-analysis: surveillance with ultrasound for early-stage hepatocellular carcinoma in patients with cirrhosis. Aliment Pharmacol Ther. 2009;30:37-47.
16. Mitchell DG. Color Doppler imaging principles, limitations, and artifacts. Radiology. 1990;177:1-10.
17. Dai Y, Chen MH, Yin SS, Yan K, Fan ZH, Wu W, et al. Focal liver lesions: can SonoVue-enhanced ultrasound be used to differentiate malignant from benign lesions? Invest Radiol. 2007;42:596-603.
18. Bartolotta TV, Taibbi A, Galia M, Runza G, Matranga D, Midiri M, et al. Characterization of hypoechoic focal hepatic lesions in patients with fatty liver: diagnostic performance and confidence of contrast-enhanced ultrasound. Eur Radiol. 2007;17:650-61.
19. Hohmann J, Albrecht T, Hoffmann CW, Wolf KJ. Ultrasonographic detection of focal liver lesions: increased sensitivity and specificity with microbubble contrast agents. Eur J Radiol. 2003;46:147-59.
20. Solbiati L, Tonolini M, Cova L, Goldberg SN. The role of contrast-enhanced ultrasound in the detection of focal liver leasions. EurRadiol. 2001;11:E15-26.
21. Hatanaka K, Kudo M, Minami Y, Maekawa K. Sonazoid-enhanced ultrasonography for diagnosis of hepatic malignancies comparison with contrast-enhanced CT. Oncology. 2008;75(Suppl 1):42-7.
22. Xu HX, Liu GJ, Lu MD, Xie XY, Xu ZF, Zheng YL, et al. Characterization of small focal liver lesions using real-time contrast-enhanced sonography diagnostic performance analysis in 200 patients. J Ultrasound Med. 2006;25:349-61.
23. Sporea I, Badea R, Martie A, Dumitru E, Ioanitescu S, Sirli R et al. Contrast enhanced ultrasound for the evaluation of Focal liver lesions in daily practice: A muticentric study. Medical Ultrasonography. 2012;14:95-100.
24. Nicolau C, Vilana R, Catalá V, Bianchi L, Gilabert R, García A, et al. Importance of evaluating all vascular phases on contrast-enhanced sonography in the differentiation of benign from malignant focal liver lesions. Am J Roentgenol. 2006;186:158-67.
25. Wilson SR, Lyshchik, A, Piscaglia F, Cosgrove D, Jang HJ, Sirlin C, et al. CEUS LI-RADS: algorithm, implementation, and key differences from CT/MRI. Abdom Radiol. 2018;43:127-42.
26. Lyshchik A, Kono Y, Dietrich CF, et al. Contrast-enhanced ultrasound of the liver : technical and lexicon recommendations from the ACR CEUS LI-RADS working group. Abdom Radiol (NY). 2018;43:861-79.
27. SchimaW and Jay Heiken J. LI-RADS v2017 for liver nodules: how we read and report. Cancer Imaging. 2018;18:1 11.
28. Von Herbay A, Vogt C, Willers R, Haussinger D. Real-time imaging with the sonographic contrast agent SonoVue differentiation between benign and malignant hepatic lesions. J Ultrasound Med. 2004;23:1557-68.
29. Wilson SR, Burns PN. An algorithm for the diagnosis of focal liver masses using microbubble contrast-enhanced pulse-inversion sonography. Am J Roentgenol. 2006;186:1401-12.
30. Mergo PJ, Ros PR. Benign lesions of the liver. RadiolClin North Am. 1998;36:319-31.
31. Ding H, Wang WP, Huang BJ, Wei RX, He NA, Qi Q, et al. Imaging of focal liver lesions low-mechanical-index real-time ultrasonography with SonoVue. J Ultrasound Med. 2005;24:285-97.
32. Leen E, Ceccotti P, Kalogeropoulou C, Angerson WJ, Moug SJ, Horgan PG. Prospective multicenter trial evaluating a novel method of characterizing focal liver lesions using contrast-enhanced sonography. AJR J Roentgenol. 2006;186:1551-9.
33. Morin SHX, Lim AKP, Cobbold JFL and Taylo-Robinson SD. Use of second generation contrast-enhanced ultrasound in the assessment of focal liver lesions.WJG. 2007;13:5963-70.
34. Burns PN, Wilson SR. Focal liver masses enhancement patterns on contrast-enhanced images--concordance of US scans with CT scans and MR images. Radiology. 2007;242:162-74.
35. Dietrich CF, Mertens JC, Braden B, Schuessler G, Ott M, Ignee A. Contrast-enhanced ultrasound of histologically proven liver hemangiomas. Hepatology. 2007;45:1139-45.
36. Nguyen BN, Flejou JF, Terris B, Belghiti J, Degott C. Focal nodular hyperplasia of the liver a comprehensive pathologic study of 305 lesions and recognition of new histologic forms. Am J Surg Pathol. 1999;23:441-54.
37. Quaia E, Calliada F, Bertolotto M, Rossi S, Garioni L, Rosa L, et al. Characterization of focal liver lesions with contrast-specific US modes and a sulfur hexafluoride-filled microbubble contrast agent diagnostic performance and confidence. Radiology. 2004;232:420-30.
38. Shortell CK, Schwartz SI. Hepatic adenoma and focal nodular hyperplasia. Surg Gynecol Obstet. 1991;173:426-31.
39. Kim TK, Jang HJ, Burns PN, Murphy-Lavallee J, Wilson SR. Focal nodular hyperplasia and hepatic adenoma differentiation with

low-mechanical-index contrast-enhanced sonography. AJR Am J Roentgenol. 2008;190:58-66.
40. Dietrich CF, Schuessler G, Trojan J, Fellbaum C, Ignee A. Differentiation of focal nodular hyperplasia and hepatocellular adenoma by contrast-enhanced ultrasound. Br J Radiol. 2005;78:704-7.
41. Catalano O, Sandomenico F, Raso MM, Siani A. Low mechanical index contrast-enhanced sonographic findings of pyogenic hepatic abscesses. Am J Roentgenol. 2004;182:447-50.
42. Kim TK, Jang HJ, Wilson SR. Benign liver masses: imaging with microbubble contrast agents. Ultrasound Q. 2006;22:31-9.
43. Von Herbay A, Westendorff J, Gregor M. Contrast-enhanced ultrasound with SonoVue differentiation between benign and malignant focal liver lesions in 317 patients. J Clin Ultrasound. 2010;38:1-9.
44. Hagspiel KD, Neidl KF, Eichenberger AC, Weder W, Marincek B. Detection of liver metastases comparison of super paramagnetic iron oxide-enhanced and unenhanced MR imaging at 1.5 T with dynamic CT, intraoperative US, and percutaneous US. Radiology. 1995;196:471-8.
45. Dietrich CF, Kratzer W, Strobe D, Danse E, Fessl R, Bunk A, et al. Assessment of metastatic liver disease in patients with primary extrahepatic tumors by contrast-enhanced sonography versus CT and MRI. World J Gastroenterol. 2006;121:699-705.
46. Pisani P, Parkin DM, Ferlay J: Estimates of the world wide mortality from eighteen major cancers in 1985: implications for prevention and projections of future burden. Int J Cancer. 1993;55:891-3.
47. Kim TK, Lee KH, Khalili K, Jang HJ. Hepatocellular nodules in liver cirrhosis: contrast-enhanced ultrasound. Abdom Imaging. 2011;36:244-63.
48. Zheng SG, Xu HX, Liu LN. Management of hepatocellular carcinoma: The role of contrast-enhanced ultrasound. World J Radiol. 2014;28:7-14.
49. Xu HX, Xie XY, Lu MD, Liu GJ, Xu ZF, Zheng YL, et al. Contrast-enhanced sonography in the diagnosis of small hepatocellular carcinoma < or =2 cm.JClin Ultrasound. 2008;36:257-66.
50. Jang HJ, Kim TK, Burns PN, Wilson SR. Enhancement patterns of hepatocellular carcinoma at contrast-enhanced US: comparison with histologic differentiation. Radiology. 2007;244:898-906.
51. Jang HJ, Yu H, Kim TK. Imaging of focal liver lesions. Semin Roentgenol. 2009;44:266-82.
52. Xu HX, Liu GJ, Lu MD, Xie XY, Xu ZF, Zheng YL, et al. Characterization of focal liver lesions using contrastenhanced sonography with a low mechanical index mode and a sulfur hexafluoride-filled microbubble contrast agent. J Clin Ultrasound. 2006;34:261-72.
53. Xu HX, Lu MD, Liu LN, Zhang YF, Guo LH, Xu JM, et al. Discrimination between neoplastic and non-neoplastic lesions in cirrhotic liver using contrast-enhanced ultrasound. Br J Radiol. 2012;85:1376-84.
54. Rossi S, Ghittoni G, Ravetta V, TorelloViera F, Rosa L, Serassi M, et al. Contrast-enhanced ultrasonography and spiral computed tomography in the detection and characterization of portal vein thrombosis complicating hepatocellular carcinoma. Eur Radiol. 2008;18:1749-56.
55. Razumilava N, Gores GJ. Classification, diagnosis, and management of cholangiocarcinoma. Clin Gastroenterol Hepatol. 2013;11:13-21.
56. Bruix J, Sherman M. Management of hepatocellular carcinoma: an update. Hepatology. 2011;53:1020-2.
57. Deng H, Shi H, Lei J, et al. A meta-analysis of contrast-enhanced ultrasound for small hepatocellular carcinoma diagnosis. J Cancer Res Ther. 2016;12:C274-6.
58. Giorgio A, Montesarchio L, Gatti P, et al. Contrast-enhanced ultrasound: a simple and effective tool in defining a rapid diagnostic work-up for small nodules detected in cirrhotic patients during surveillance. J Gastrointestin Liver Dis. 2016;25:205-11.
59. Chen LD, Xu HX, Xie XY, Lu MD, Xu ZF, Liu GJ, et al. Enhancement patterns of intrahepatic cholangiocarcinoma: comparison between contrast-enhanced ultrasound and contrast-enhanced CT. Br J Radiol. 2008;81:881-9.
60. Zheng SG, Xu HX, Liu LN. Management of hepatocellular carcinoma: The role of contrast-enhanced ultrasound.World J Radiol. 2014;28:7-14.
61. Wu W, Chen MH, Yin SS, Yan K, Fan ZH, Yang W, et al. The role of contrast enhanced sonography of focal liver lesions before percutaneous biopsy. Am J Roentgenol. 2006;187:752-61.
62. Francica G, Melonib MF, Riccardic L, Siod, ID Terraccianoe F, Caturellif E, et al. Ablation treatment of primary and secondary liver tumors under contrast enhanced ultrasound guidance in field practice of interventional ultrasound centers. A multicenter study. European Journal of Radiology. 2018;105: 96-101.
63. Lu MD, Yu XL, Li AH, Jiang TA, Chen MH, Zhao BZ, et al. Comparison of contrast enhanced ultrasound and contrast enhanced CT or MRI in monitoring percutaneous thermal ablation procedure in patients with hepatocellular carcinoma: a multi-center study in China. Ultrasound Med Biol. 2007;33:1736-49.
64. Meloni MF, Andreano A, Franza E, Passamonti M and Lazzaroni S. Contrast enhanced ultrasound: Should it play a role in immediate evaluation of liver tumors following thermal ablation. European Journal of Radiology. 2012;81:e897-902.
65. Kono Y, Lucidarme O, Choi SH, Rose SC, Hassanein TI, Alpert E, et al. Contrast-enhanced ultrasound as a predictor of treatment efficacy within 2 weeks after transarterial chemoembolization of hepatocellular carcinoma. J Vasc Interv Radiol. 2007;18: 57-65.
66. Paul SB, Dhamija E, Gamanagatti SR, Sreenivas V, Yadav DP, Jain S, et al. Evaluation of tumor response to intra-arterial chemoembolization of hepatocellular carcinoma: Comparison of contrast-enhanced ultrasound with multiphase computed tomography. Diagn Interv Imaging. 2017;98:253-60.
67. Fröhlich E, Muller R, Xin-Wu Cui, Schreiber-Dietrich D, Dietrich CF. Dynamic Contrast-Enhanced Ultrasound for Quantification of Tissue Perfusion. Ultrasound Med. 2015;34:179-96.
68. Dietrich CF, Averkiou MA, Correas JM, Lassau N, Leen E, Piscaglia F. An EFSUMB introduction into dynamic contrast-enhanced ultrasound (DCE-US) for quantification of tumour perfusion. Ultraschall Med. 2012;33:344-51.
69. Li N, Ding H, Fan P, Lin X, Xu C, Wang W, et al. Intra-hepatic transit time predicts liver fibrosis in patients with chronic hepatitis B: quantitative assessment with contrast-enhanced ultrasonography. Ultrasound Med Biol. 2010;36:1066-75.
70. Ren J, Wu T, Zheng BW, Tan YY, Zheng RQ, Chen GH. Application of contrast-enhanced ultrasound after liver transplantation: Current status and perspectives. World J Gastroenterol. 2016;22:1607-16.
71. Marshall MM, Beese RC, Muiesan P, Sarma DI, O'Grady J, Sidhu PS. Assessment of portal venous system patency in the liver transplant candidate: a prospective study comparing ultrasound, microbubble-enhanced colour Doppler ultrasound, with arteriography and surgery. Clin Radiol. 2002;57:377-83.
72. Berry JD, Sidhu PS. Microbubble contrast-enhanced ultrasound in liver transplantation. Eur Radiol. 2004;14:96-103.
73. Zheng RQ, Chen GH, Xu EJ, Mao R, Lu MQ, Liao M, et al. Evaluating biliary anatomy and variations in living liver donors by a new technique: three-dimensional contrast-enhanced ultrasonic cholangiography. Ultrasound Med Biol. 2010;36:1282-7.
74. Rübenthaler J, Paprottka KJ, Hameister E, Hoffmann K, Joiko N, Reiser M, et al. Vascular complications in liver transplantation: Beneficial role of contrast-enhanced ultrasound (CEUS) in the postoperative phase. Clin Hemorheol Microcirc. 2016;64: 475-82.

75. Fontanilla T, Noblejas A, Cortes C, Minaya J, Mendez S, Van den Brule E, et al. Contrast enhanced ultrasound of liver lesions related to arterial thrombosis in adult liver transplantation. J Clin Ultrasound. 2013;41:493-500.
76. Zheng RQ, Mao R, Ren J, Xu EJ, Liao M, Wang P, et al. Contrast-enhanced ultrasound for the evaluation of hepatic artery stenosis after liver transplantation: potential role in changing the clinical algorithm. Liver Transpl. 2010;16:729-35.
77. Park YS, Kim KW, Kim SY, Lee SJ, Lee J, Kim JH, et al. Obstruction at middle hepatic venous tributaries in modified right lobe grafts after living-donor liver Transplantation: diagnosis with contrast-enhanced US. Radiology. 2012;265:617-26.
78. Ren J, Lu MD, Zheng RQ, Lu MQ, Liao M, Mao YJ, et al. Evaluation of the microcirculatory disturbance of biliary ischemia after liver transplantation with contrast-enhanced ultrasound: preliminary experience. Liver Transpl. 2009;15:1703-8.
79. Chopra SS, Eisele R, Stelter L, Seehofer D, Grieser C, Warnick P, et al. Contrast enhanced ultrasound cholangiography via T-tube following liver transplantation. Ann Transplant 2012.
80. García-Criado A, Gilabert R, Bianchi L, Vilana R, Burrel M, Barrufet M, et al. Impact of contrast-enhanced ultrasound in the study of hepatic artery hypoperfusion shortly after liver transplantation: contribution to the diagnosis of artery steal syndrome. EurRadiol. 2015;25:196-202.
81. Lu Y, Liu B, ZhengY, Luo J, ZhangX, Huang G, et al. Application of real-time three-dimensional contrast-enhanced ultrasound using SonoVue for the evaluation of focal liver lesions: a prospective single-center study. Am J Transl Res. 2018;10(5):1469-80.
82. Wang Z, Wang W, Liu GJ, Yang Z, Chen LD, Huang Y, et al. The role of quantitation of real-time 3-dimensional contrast-enhanced ultrasound in detecting microvascular invasion: an in vivo study. Abdom Radiol. 2016;41:1973-9.
83. Faccioli N, D'Onofrio M, Malaga R et al. Resectable Pancreatic Adenocarcinoma: Depiction of Tumoral Margins at Contrast-Enhanced Ultrasonography. Pancreas. 2008;37:265-8.
84. Grossjohann HS, Rappeport ED, Jensen C et al. Usefulness of contrast enhanced transabdominal ultrasound for tumor classification and tumor staging in the pancreatic head. Scand J Gastroenterol. 2010;45:917-24.
85. Sidhu PS, Brabrand K, Cantisani V et al. EFSUMB Guidelines on Interventional Ultrasound (INVUS) Part II Diagnostic Ultrasound-Guided Interventional Procedures (Short Version). Ultraschall in Med. 2016;36:566-80.
86. Wei Y, Yu XL, Liang P et al. Guiding and Controlling Percutaneous Pancreas Biopsies with Contrast-Enhanced Ultrasound: Target Lesions Are Not Localized on B-Mode Ultrasound. Ultrasound Med Biol. 2015;41:1561-9.
87. Tawada K, Yamaguchi T, Kobayashi A et al. Changes in Tumor Vascularity Depicted by Contrast-Enhanced Ultrasonography as a Predictor of Chemotherapeutic Effect in Patients With Unresectable Pancreatic Cancer. Pancreas. 2009;38:30-5.
88. Kobayashi A, Yamaguchi T, Ishihara T et al. Evaluation of vascular signal in pancreatic ductal carcinoma using contrast enhanced ultrasonography: effect of systemic chemotherapy. Gut. 2005;54:1047.
89. D'Onofrio M, Mansueto G, Falconi M et al. Neuroendocrine pancreatic tumor. Abdom Imaging. 2004;29:246-58.
90. Malago R, D'Onofrio M, Zamboni GA et al. Contrast-Enhanced Sonographyof Nonfunctioning Pancreatic Neuroendocrine Tumors. Am J Roentgenol. 2009;192:424-30.
91. Falconi M, Bartsch DF, Eriksson B et al. ENETS consensus guidelines for the management of patients with digestive neuroendocrine neoplasms of the digestive system: well-differentiated pancreatic nonfunctioning tumors. Neuroendocrinology. 2012;95:120-34.
92. Fan Z, Yan K, Wang Y et al. Application of Contrast-Enhanced Ultrasound in Cystic Pancreatic Lesions Using a Simplified Classification Diagnostic Criterion. Biomed Res Int. 2015;2015:974621.
93. Vasile TA, Socaciu M, Stanluga R et al. Added value of intravenous contrast-enhanced ultrasound for characterization of cystic pancreatic masses: a prospective study on 37 patients. Med Ultrason. 2012;14:108-14.
94. Rickes S, Wermke W. Differentiation of cystic pancreatic neoplasms and pseudocysts by conventional and echo-enhanced ultrasound. J Gastroenterol Hepatol. 2004;19:761-6.
95. Itoh T, Hirooka Y, Itoh A et al. Usefulness of Contrast-Enhanced Transabdominal Ultrasonography in the Diagnosis of Intraductal Papillary Mucinous Tumors of the Pancreas. Am J Gastroenterol. 2005;100:144-52.
96. Pezzilli R, Serra C, Calculli L et al. Three-dimensional Contrast-enhanced Ultrasonography of Intraductal Papillary Mucinous Neoplasms of the Pancreas: A Comparison With Magnetic Resonance Imaging. Pancreas. 2013;42:1164-8.
97. D'Onofrio M, Zamboni G, Tognolini A et al. Mass-forming pancreatitis: Value of contrast-enhanced ultrasonography. World J Gastroenterol. 2006;12:4181-4.
98. Ripolles T, Martinez MJ, Lopez E et al. Contrast-enhanced ultrasound in the staging of acute pancreatitis. Eur Radiol. 2010;20:2518-23.
99. Ardelean M, Sirli R, Sporea I et al. Contrast enhanced ultrasound in the pathology of the pancreas. A monocentric experience. Med Ultrason. 2014;16:325-31.
100. Becker D, Strobel D, Bernatik T et al. Echo-enhanced color- and power- Doppler EUS for the discrimination between focal pancreatitis and pancreatic carcinoma. Gastrointest Endosc. 2001;53:784-9.
101. Bhutani MS, Hoffman BJ, van Velse A et al. Contrast-enhanced endoscopic ultrasonography with galactose microparticles: SHU508 A (Levovist). Endoscopy. 1997;29:635-9.
102. Dietrich CF, Ignee A, Frey H. Contrast-enhanced endoscopic ultrasound with low mechanical index: a new technique. Z Gastroenterol. 2005;43:1219-23.
103. Dietrich CF. Contrast-enhanced low mechanical index endoscopic ultrasound (CELMI-EUS). Endoscopy. 2009;41 (Suppl 2):E43-4.
104. Kitano M, Sakamoto H, Matsui U et al. A novel perfusion imaging technique of the pancreas: contrast-enhanced harmonic EUS (with video). Gastrointest Endosc. 2008;67:141-50.
105. D'Onofrio M, Zamboni G, Tognolini A et al. Mass-forming pancreatitis: Value of contrast-enhanced ultrasonography. World J Gastroenterol. 2006;12:4181-4.
106. Aboutaleb E, Leen E, Hakim N. Assessment of Viability of the Pancreas for Transplantation Using Contrast-enhanced Ultrasound. Transplant Proc. 2011;43:418-21.
107. Quaia E, Bertolotto M, Cioffi V et al. Comparison of contrast-enhanced sonography with unenhanced sonography and contrast-enhanced CT in the diagnosis of malignancy in complex renal masses. Am J Roentgenol. 2008;191:1239-49.
108. Clevert DA, Minaifar N, Weckbach S et al. Multislice computed tomography versus contrast-enhanced ultrasound in evaluation of complex cystic renal masses using the Bosniak classification system. Clin Hemorheol Microcirc. 2008;39:171-8.
109. Correas JM, Claudon M, Tranquart F et al. The kidney: imaging with microbubble contrast agents. Ultrasound Q. 2006;22:53-66.
110. Mazziotti S, Zimbaro F, PandolfoA et al. Usefulness of contrast-enhanced ultrasonography in the diagnosis of renal pseudotumors. Abdom Imaging. 2010;35:241-5.
111. Bertolotto M, Martegani A, Aiani L et al. Value of contrast-enhanced ultrasonographyfor detecting renal infarcts proven by contrast enhanced CT. A feasibility study. Eur Radiol. 2008;18:376-83.
112. Yusuf GT, Sellars ME, Huang DY et al. Cortical Necrosis Secondary toTrauma in a Child: Contrast-enhanced ultrasound comparable to Magnetic Resonance Imaging. Pediatr Radiol. 2014;44:484-7.

113. Meloni MF, Bertolotto M, Alberzoni C et al. Follow-Up After Percutaneous Radiofrequency Ablation of Renal Cell Carcinoma: Contrast-Enhanced Sonography Versus Contrast-Enhanced CT or MRI. Am J Roentgenol. 2008;191:1233-8.
114. Meloni MF, Smolock A, Cantisani V et al. Contrast enhanced ultrasoundin the evaluation and percutaneous treatment of hepatic and renal tumors. Eur J Radiol. 2015;84:1666-74.
115. Oh TH, Lee YH, Seo IY. Diagnostic Efficacy of Contrast-Enhanced Ultrasound for Small Renal Masses. Korean J Urol. 2014;55:587-92.
116. Ascenti G, Gaeta M, Magno C et al. Contrast-Enhanced Second-Harmonic Sonography in the Detection of Pseudocapsule in Renal Cell Carcinoma. Am J Roentgenol. 2004;182:1525-30.
117. Campbell SC, Novick AC, Belldegrun A et al. Guideline for Management of the Clinical T1 Renal Mass. J Urol. 2009;182:1271-9.
118. Fontanilla T, Minaya J, Cortes C et al. Acute complicated pyelonephritis: contrast-enhanced ultrasound. Abdominal Imaging. 2012;37:639-46.
119. Harvey CJ, Sidhu PS, Bachmann-Nielsen M. Contrast-enhanced ultrasound in renal transplants: applications and future directions. Ultraschallin Med. 2013;34:319-21.
120. Girometti R, Stocca E, Granata A et al. Impact of contrast-enhanced ultrasound in patients with renal function impairment. World J Radiol. 2017;28:10-6.
121. Granata A, Andrulli S, Fiorini F et al. Diagnosis of acute pyelonephritis by contrast-enhanced ultrasonography in kidney transplant patients. Nephrol Dial Transplant. 2011;26:715-20.
122. Catalano O, Aiani L, Barozzi L et al. CEUS in abdominal trauma: multicenter study. Abdominal Imaging. 2009;34:225-34.
123. Miele V, Piccolo CL, Galluzzo M et al. Contrast-enhanced ultrasound (CEUS) in blunt abdominal trauma. Br J Radiol. 2016;89:20150823.
124. Sessa B, Trinci M, Ianniello S et al. Blunt abdominal trauma: role of contrast-enhanced ultrasound (CEUS) in the detection and staging of abdominal traumatic lesions compared to US and CE-MDCT. Radiol Med. 2015;120:180-9.
125. Cokkinos DD, Antypa E, Stefanidis K et al. Contrast-enhanced ultrasound for imaging blunt abdominal trauma—indications, description of the technique and imaging review. Ultraschall in Med. 2012;33:60-7.
126. Durkin N, Deganello A, Sellars ME et al. Post-traumatic liver and spleen pseudoaneurysms in children: diagnosis, management and follow-up screening using contrast enhanced ultrasound (CEUS). J Pediat Surg. 2016;51:289-92.
127. Gorce JM, Arditi D, Schneider M. Influence of bubble size distribution on the echogenicity of ultrasound contrast agents: a study of Sono-Vue. Invest Radiol. 2000;35:661-71.
128. Plikat K, Klebi F, Buchner C et al. Evaluation of intestinal hyperaemia in inflammed bowel by high resolution contrast harmonic imaging (CHI). Ultraschall in Med. 2000;25:257-62.
129. Serra C, Menozzi G, Labate AMM et al. Ultrasound assessment of vascularization of the thickened terminal ileum wall in Crohn's disease patients using a low-mechanical index real-time scanning technique with a second generation ultrasound contrast agent. Eur J Radiol. 2007;62:114-21.
130. Migaleddu V, Scanu AM, Quaia E et al. Contrast-enhanced Ultrasonographic Evaluation of Inflammatory Activity in Crohn's Disease. Gastroenterology. 2009;137:43-52.
131. Girlich C, Schacherer D, Jung EM et al. Comparison between quantitative assessment of bowel wall vascularization by contrast-enhanced ultrasound and results of histopathological scoring in ulcerative colitis. Int J Colorectal Dis. 2012;27:193-8.
132. Wilson SR, Burns PN. Microbubble-enhanced US in body imaging: What role? Radiology. 2010;257:24-39.
133. Ventura CAP, da Silva ES, Cerri GG et al. Can contrast-enhanced ultrasound with second-generation contrast agents replace computed tomography angiography for distinguishing between occlusion and pseudo-occlusion of the internal carotid artery? Clinics (Sao Paulo). 2015;70:1-6.
134. ten Kate GL, Sijbrands EJ, Staub D et al. Noninvasive Imaging of the Vulnerable Atherosclerotic Plaque. Curr Probl Cardiol. 2010;35:556-91.
135. ten Kate GL, van Dijk AC, van den Oord SCH et al. Usefulness of Contrast-Enhanced Ultrasound for Detection of Carotid Plaque Ulceration in Patients With Symptomatic Carotid Atherosclerosis. Am J Cardiol. 2013;112:292-8.
136. Schinkel AFL, van den Oord SCH, van der Steen AFW et al. Utility of contrast-enhanced ultrasound for the assessment of the carotid artery wall in patients with Takayasu or giant cell arteritis. Eur Heart J Cardiovasc Imaging. 2014;15:541-6.
137. Possemato N, Macchioni P, Germano G et al. Clinical images: PET-CTand contrast-enhanced ultrasound in Takayasu GÇÖs arteritis. Rheumatology (Oxford). 2014;53:447.
138. Ten Bosch JA, Rouwet EV, Peters CTH et al. Contrast-enhanced Ultrasound versus Computed Tomographic Angiography for Surveillance of Endovascular Abdominal Aortic Aneurysm Repair. J Vasc Interv Radiol. 2010;21:638-43.
139. Gurtler VM, Sommer WH, Meimarakis G et al. A comparison between contrast-enhanced ultrasound imaging and multislice computed tomography in detecting and classifying endoleaks in the follow-up after endovascular aneurysm repair. J Vasc Surg. 2013;58:340-5.
140. Li W, Liu G, Wang W et al. Real-time contrast enhanced ultrasound imaging of focal splenic lesions. Eur J Radiol. 2014;83:646-53.
141. vonHerbay A, Barreiros AP, Ignee A et al. Contrast-enhanced ultrasonography with SonoVue. Differentiation between benign and malignant lesions of the spleen. J Ultrasound Med. 2009;28:421-34.
142. Gorg C. The forgotten organ: Contrast enhanced sonography of the spleen. Eur J Radiol. 2007;64:189-201.
143. Kim SH, Lee JM, Lee JY et al. Contrast-Enhanced Sonography of Intrapancreatic Accessory Spleen in Six Patients. Am J Roentgenol. 2007;188:422-8.
144. Menozzi G, Maccabruni V, Gabbi E et al. Contrast-enhanced Ultrasound Evaluation of Splenic Embolization in Patients with Definite Left-Sided Infective Endocarditis. Ultrasound Med Biol. 2013;39:2205–10.
145. Peddu P, Shah M, Sidhu PS. Splenic abnormalities: a comparative review of ultrasound, microbubble enhanced ultrasound and computed tomography. Clin Radiol. 2004;59:777-92.
146. Fernandez-Perez GC, Tardaguila FM, Velasco M et al. Radiologic Findings of Segmental Testicular Infarction. Am J Roentgenol. 2005;184:1587-93.
147. Bertolotto M, Derchi LE, Sidhu PS et al. Acute segmental testicular infarction at contrast-enhanced ultrasound: early features and changes during follow-up. Am J Roentgenol. 2011;196:834-41.
148. Bhatt S, Dogra VS. Role of US in testicular and scrotal trauma. Radiographics. 2008;28:1617-29.
149. Lung PF, Jaffer OS, Sellars ME et al. Contrast enhanced ultrasound (CEUS) in the evaluation of focal testicular complications secondary to epidiymitis. Am J Roentgenol. 2012;199:W345-54.
150. Isidori AM, Pozza C, Gianfrilli D et al. Differential diagnosis of nonpalpable testicular lesions: qualitative and quantitative contrast-enhanced US of benign and malignant testicular tumors. Radiology. 2014;273:606-18.
151. Huang DY, Sidhu PS. Focal testicular lesions: colour Doppler ultrasound, contrast-enhanced ultrasound and tissue elastography as adjuvants to the diagnosis. Br J Radiol. 2012;85:S41-53.
152. Sidhu PS et al. The EFSUMB Guidelines and Recommendations for the Clinical Practice of Contrast-Enhanced Ultrasound (CEUS) in Non-Hepatic Applications: Update 2017 Ultraschall in Med. 2018;39:e2-44.

153. Gorg C. Transcutaneous contrast-enhanced sonography of pleural based pulmonary lesions. Eur J Radiol. 2007;64:213-21.
154. Bertolini FA, Goerg C, Mathis G. Echo contrast ultrasound in subpleural consolidations. Echo contrast ultrasound in subpleural consolidations. 2008;18(Suppl S395): Abstract
155. Gorg C, Bert T, Gorg K. Contrast-enhanced sonography for differential diagnosis of pleurisy and focal pleural lesions of unknown cause. Chest. 2005;128:3894-9.
156. Liu LN, Xu HX, Lu MD et al. Contrast-Enhanced Ultrasound in the Diagnosis of Gallbladder Diseases: A Multi-Center Experience. PLoS ONE. 2012;7:e48371.
157. Date RS, Thrumurthy SG, Whiteside S et al. Gallbladder perforation: Case series and systematic review. Int J Surg. 2012;10:63-8.
158. Xie XH, Xu HX, Xie XY et al. Differential diagnosis between benign and malignant gallbladder diseases with real-time contrast-enhanced ultrasound. Eur Radiol. 2010;20:239-48.
159. Meacock LM, Sellars ME, Sidhu PS. Evaluation of Gall Bladder and Biliary Duct Disease Using Microbubble Contrast Enhanced Ultrasound. Br J Radiol. 2010;83:615-27.
160. Casali PG, Blay JY, On behalf of the ESMO/CONTICANET/EUROBONET Consensus Panel of Experts. Gastrointestinal stromal tumours: ESMO Clinical Practice Guidelines for diagnosis, treatment and follow-up. Ann Oncol. 2010;21:v98-102.
161. Prantl L, Fellner C, Jung ME. Evaluation of Free Flap Perfusion with Dynamic Contrast-Enhanced Magnetic Resonance Imaging. Plastic and Reconstructive Surgery. 2010;126:100e-1011e.
162. Selber JC, Garvey PB, Clemens MW et al. A Prospective Study of Transit-Time Flow Volume Measurement for Intraoperative Evaluation and Optimization of Free Flaps. Plast Reconstr Surg. 2013;131:270-81.
163. Kmetec A, Bren AF, Kandus A et al. Contrast-enhanced ultrasound voiding cystography as a screening examination for vesicoureteral reflux in the follow-up of renal transplant recipient: a new approach. Nephrol Dial Transplant. 2001;16:120-3.
164. Valentini AL, De Gaetano AM, Minordi LM et al. Contrast-enhanced Voiding US for Grading of Reflux in Adult Patients Prior to Antireflux Ureteral Implantation. Radiology. 2004;233:35-9.
165. Kenda RB, Kenig A, Novijan G et al. Cyclic voiding urosonography for detecting vesicoureteric reflux in renal transplant recipients. Nephrol Dial Transplant. 2001;16:2229-31.
166. Lanzani C, Savasi V, Leone FP et al. Two-dimensional HyCoSy with contrast tuned imaging technology and a second-generation contrast media for the assessment of tubal patency in an infertility program. Fertil Steril. 2009;92:1158-61.
167. Ignee A, Baum U, Schuessler G et al. Contrast-enhanced ultrasound-guided percutaneous cholangiography and cholangiodrainage (CEUSPTCD). Endoscopy. 2009;41:725-6.
168. Mao R, Xu EJ, Li K et al. Usefulness of contrast-enhanced ultrasound in the diagnosis of biliary leakage following T-tube removal. J Clin Ultrasound. 2009;38:38-40.
169. Zengel P, Berghaus A,Weiler C et al. Intraductally applied contrast-enhanced ultrasound (IA-CEUS) for evaluating obstructive disease and secretory dysfunction of the salivary glands. Eur Radiol. 2011;21:1339-48.
170. Henrich W, Meckies J, Friedmann W. Demonstration of a recto-vaginal fistula with the ultrasound contrast medium Echovist. Ultrasound Obstet Gynecol. 2000;15:148-9.
171. Volkmer BG, Nesslauer T, Kufer R et al. [Diagnosis of vesico-intestinal fistulas by contrast medium enhanced 3-D ultrasound]. Ultraschall in Med. 2001;22:81-6.
172. Chew SS, Yang JL, Newstead GL et al. Anal fistula: Levovist-enhanced endoanal ultrasound: a pilot study. Dis Colon Rectum. 2003;46:377-84.
173. Kanno H, Ozawa Y, Sakata K et al. Intraoperative power Doppler ultrasonographywith a contrast-enhancing agent for intracranial tumors. J Neurosurg. 2005;102:295-301.
174. Prada F, Del Bene M, Moiraghi A et al. From Grey Scale B-Mode to Elastosonography: Multimodal Ultrasound Imaging in Meningioma Surgery Pictorial Essay and Literature Review. Biomed Res Int. 2015;2015:925729.
175. Prada F, Del Bene M, Saini M et al. Intraoperative cerebral angiosonography with ultrasound contrast agents: how I do it. Acta Neurochir (Wein). 2015;157:1025-9.
176. Lei F, Jing Z, Bo W et al. Uterine myomas treated with microwave ablation: The agreement between ablation volumes obtained from contrast-enhanced sonography and enhanced MRI. Int J Hyperthermia. 2014;30:11-8.
177. Rouviere O, Glas L, Girouin N et al. Prostate Cancer Ablation with Transrectal High-Intensity Focused Ultrasound: Assessment of Tissue Destruction with Contrast-enhanced US. Radiology. 2011;259:583-91.
178. OeY, Orr L, Laifer-NarinS, HyodoE, Koczo A, Homma S et al. Contrast-enhanced sonography as a novel tool for assessment of vascular malformations. J Angiogenes Res. 2010;2:25.
179. Yu D, Han Y, Chen T. Contrast-Enhanced Ultrasound for Differentiation of Benign and Malignant Thyroid Lesions: Meta-analysis. Otolaryngol Head and Neck Surgery. 2014;151:909-15.
180. Sun B, Lang L, Zhu X et al. Accuracy of contrast-enhanced ultrasound in the identification of thyroid nodules: a meta-analysis. Int J Clin Exp Med. 2015;8:12882-9.
181. Sorelli PG, Cosgrove DO, Svensson WE et al. Can contrast-enhanced sonography distinguish benign from malignant breast masses. J Clin Ultrasound. 2010;38:177-81.
182. Jia WR, Chai WM, Tang L et al. Three-dimensional contrast enhanced ultrasound score and dynamic contrast-enhanced magnetic resonance imaging score in evaluating breast tumor angiogenesis: Correlation with biological factors. Eur J Radiol. 2014;83:1098-105.
183. Sano F, Uemura H. The Utility and Limitations of Contrast-Enhanced Ultrasound for the Diagnosis and Treatment of Prostate Cancer. Sensors (Basel). 2015;15:4947-57.
184. Sever AR, Mills P, Jones SE et al. Preoperative sentinel node identification with ultrasound using microbubbles in patients with breast cancer. Am J Roentgenol. 2010;196:251-6.
185. Hermann KG, Backhaus M, Schneider U et al. Rheumatoid arthritis of the shoulder joint: Comparison of conventional radiography, ultrasound, and dynamic contrast-enhanced magnetic resonance imaging. Arthritis Rheum. 2003;48: 3338-49.
186. Klauser A, Frauscher F, Schirmer M et al. The value of contrast-enhanced color Doppler ultrasound in the detection of vascularization offinger joints in patients with rheumatoid arthritis. Arthritis Rheum. 2002;46:647-53.
187. Doria SA, Kiss BMH, Lotito NAP et al. Juvenile rheumatoid arthritis of the knee: evaluation with contrast-enhanced color Doppler ultrasound. Pediatr Radiol. 2001;31:524-31.
188. Klauser A, Demharter J, De Marchi A et al. Contrast enhanced gray scale sonography in assessment of joint vascularity in rheumatoid arthritis: results from the IACUS study group. Eur Radiol. 2005;15:2404-10.
189. Cai XH, Yang SP, Shen HL et al. Application of contrast-enhanced ultrasonography and ultrasonography scores in rheumatoid arthritis. Int J Clin Exp Med. 2015;8:20056-64.
190. David E, Cantisani V, Vincentiis DM, Sidhu PS, Greco A, Tombolini M et al.. Contrast-enhanced ultrasound in the evaluation of parotid gland lesions: an update of the literature. Ultrasound. 2016;24:104-10.
191. Wang H, Machtaler S, Bettinger T, Lutz AM, Luong R, Bussat P, et al. Molecular imaging of inflammation in inflammatory bowel disease with a clinically translatable dual-selection-targeted US contrast agent: comparison with FDG PET/CT in a mouse model. Radiology. 2013;267:818-29.

CHAPTER

45

Iodinated Contrast Media: An Update (To Include Reactions and Management)

Gaurav Shanker Pradhan, Swati Gupta, Jyoti Kumar, Anju Garg

INTRODUCTION

Contrast medium is a substance which produces alterations in contrast in a radiographic image. This occurs due to greater photoelectric absorption of X-rays by substances with high atomic number like barium and iodine.

The development of contrast media has undergone a steady evolution over more than 50 years to achieve improvement in efficacy and safety. They are used intravenously, for most diagnostic studies, but they can also be used intra-arterially, intrathecally, orally and via direct injections in joints and indwelling catheters.

Like any other pharmaceutical agents, they are not devoid of risk. Adverse effects range from minor physiological disturbances to rare life threatening reactions. Medical personnel and radiologists involved in the use of contrast agents must be aware of risk factors for reaction to contrast media. They should use strategies to minimize adverse events and be prepared to identify and manage them promptly.[1]

DESIRABLE PROPERTIES OF AN IDEAL CONTRAST AGENT

The properties of an ideal contrast agent are:

- Water solubility
- Chemical and heat stability
- Biological inertness
- Low viscosity
- Selective excretion (i.e. through the kidney)
- Osmolality lower or equal to human serum
- Low cost
- Safety.[2-4]

HISTORY OF DEVELOPMENT OF IODINATED CONTRAST MEDIA

All research in the development of contrast media has proceeded with basic objectives of increased efficacy and reduced toxicity.

The first major breakthrough in the development of safer contrast media came when iodine was bound to organic molecules, enabling significant reduction of iodine toxicity as compared to sodium iodide (an inorganic salt). The first organic salt, uroselectan (Iopax) was developed by Moses Swick. The major disadvantage of uroselectan was lesser efficacy in terms of contrast enhancement, as each molecule was bound to only one iodine atom. Uroselectan-B (Neoiopax), which was a bisodium salt with two iodine atoms, and two particles in solution quickly replaced uroselectan. In the 1950s, sodium and meglumine salts of tri-iodinated benzoic acid (acetrizoic acid), were introduced, which were of much lower toxicity but were hyperosmolar. Acetrizoate provided adequate urograms at that time. In order to improve efficacy and safety, various modifications of this tri-iodinated contrast medium, i.e. acetrizoic acid were made.[5] Diatrizoate replaced acetrizoate in 1955-56 as sodium and meglumine salts of diatrizoic acid and proved more efficacious diagnostically and safer than earlier drugs.[6] In the 1960s, majority of the water soluble contrast media used were salts of iodinated fully substituted benzoic acid derivatives. These organic acids had 3 hydrogen atoms replaced by iodine atoms and 3 hydrogen atoms replaced by simple side chains; for every 3 iodine atoms in solution, 2 particles were produced (one anion and one cation) in the ratio of 3:2. The next major development came in the 1970s with the introduction of low osmolar contrast media (LOCM), which was achieved by converting tri-iodinated benzoic acid into a non-ionic molecule by replacing the ionizing carboxylic acid (COOH) radical with hydrophilic structures that could be covalently bound to the benzene ring, i.e. an amide (CONH2). When in solution, this molecule provided three atoms of iodine with only one active particle [ratio of 3:1]. Dr Torsten was the first to propose that nonionic molecules could reduce osmolality. Subsequently, Almen introduced metrizamide in 1977.[7-9] Low osmolar contrast media of this generation, which are now in widespread clinical use include iohexol, ioversol, iopamidol and iobitridol.[10] In the 1980s nonionic dimeric contrast media were introduced; two nonionic tri-iodinated benzoic rings were attached, giving an iodine: particle ratio of 6:1, as there are 6 iodine atoms and only one active particle in each molecule. Development of non-ionic isotonic dimers occurred in the 1980s and 1990s. A novel nonionic dimer iso-osmolar agent, Iosimenol was developed in 2002, with lower molecular weight and viscosity, is currently in trial phase and not approved for clinical use.[11]

BASIC CHEMISTRY OF ICM

Tri-iodinated benzene ring is the basic constituent of all iodinated contrast media (ICM) **(Figs. 1A to D)**. Benzene ring has 6 carbon atoms numbered 1 to 6 clockwise. Carbon 1 attachment differentiates ionic from nonionic contrast media. In ionic contrast media, acidic group with sodium or meglumine is attached at C1 whereas in non-ionic contrast media, an amide group is attached at C1.[12,13] Iodine atoms are attached at position 2, 4, 6 carbons. C3 and C5 have amide attachments to increase solubility and also to reduce protein binding. Iodine (atomic weight 127) provides excellent radiopacity.

TYPES OF ICM

Iodinated contrast media are divided based on their ionicity and osmolality.

Broadly, ICM are characterized as *ionic* or *nonionic* types. Ionic contrast media breakdown into cations (positively charged particles) and anions (negatively charged particles) in solutions such as blood.[10] On the other hand, nonionic contrast media do not break into charged particles on entering a solution.

Ionic and nonionic contrast media can be monomeric or dimeric types. Usually each benzene ring of ICM produces 3 iodine atoms. Monomer contains only one benzene ring. To deliver more iodine per molecule of contrast, 2 benzene rings may be combined to produce a dimer, which delivers 6 iodine atoms with each molecule.

In ionic monomeric agents, the iodinated benzene ring contains ionizing carboxyl groups with a cation, usually meglumine or sodium.[2] The carboxyl groups make the agents water soluble due to their ability to disassociate into ions. Since these compounds contain only one iodinated benzene ring and dissociate into ions in solution, they are described as *ionic monomeric agents*. Commonly used contrast material anions are diatrizoate and iothalamate. In a solution, ionic monomers break up into their anion and cation components, delivering 3 iodine atoms (3:2 ratio of iodine to osmolar particles). Thus, these have a relatively high osmolality (>1400 mOsm/kg at 50–76% by weight concentrations). Ionic monomer preparations are meglumine iothalamate, sodium iothalamate, meglumine and sodium diatrizoate.

Nonionic monomers are the most widely used among lower-osmolality contrast agents. In nonionic monomers, the tri-iodinated benzene ring is made water soluble by the addition of five or six hydrophilic hydroxyl groups to organic side chains placed at 1, 3 and 5 positions. These do not ionize in solution and each molecule delivers 3 iodine atoms (3:1 ratio of iodine to osmolar particles). These have relatively low osmolality (600–800 mOsm/kg) at comparable iodine concentrations. Nonionic monomer preparations currently available in India are iohexol, iopromide, ioversol, iopamidol and iomeprol.

Ionic dimers are formed by eliminating one of the carboxyl groups and joining two ionic monomers together. These would deliver 2 ionic components per 6 iodine atoms (6:2 ratio of iodine to osmolar particles). These agents have a relatively low osmolality of 600 mOsm/kg at comparable iodine concentrations. Ioxaglate (Hexabrix), an ionic dimer, that was used for peripheral arteriography, is being gradually phased out since its withdrawal in 2015 in the United States.

Nonionic dimers consist of two joined nonionic monomers. Single nonionic dimer delivers 6 iodine atoms (6:1 ratio of iodine to osmolar particles). These are iso-osmolar with plasma at approximately 60% by weight concentration.[3] However, it results in higher viscosity and greater resistance to catheter injection.[14] Nonionic dimer iodixanol (Visipaque) is currently available in India and has an osmolality of 290 mOsm/kg, which is the same as blood.

In brief, there are four classes of ICM, i.e., high osmolar ionic monomers, low osmolar nonionic monomers, low osmolar ionic dimers and iso-osmolar nonionic dimers **(Table 1)**. Hyperosmolar contrast can cause tissue damage and are responsible for the sudden drawing in of water from the cellular and interstitial spaces towards plasma, thereby producing local effects, such as heat and pain. Increased osmolality can cause systemic effects such as vasodilatation, alteration in the permeability of vessel endothelium, hyperemia and osmotic diuresis.

All ICM are distributed in the extracellular compartment and do not cross an intact blood-brain barrier, and all are excreted via glomerular filtration.[3]

The iodine concentration of an individual contrast agent determines radio-opacity of the contrast agent. Thus, more iodine ratio represents fewer particles of contrast medium, lower osmotoxic effect and better opacification.[15]

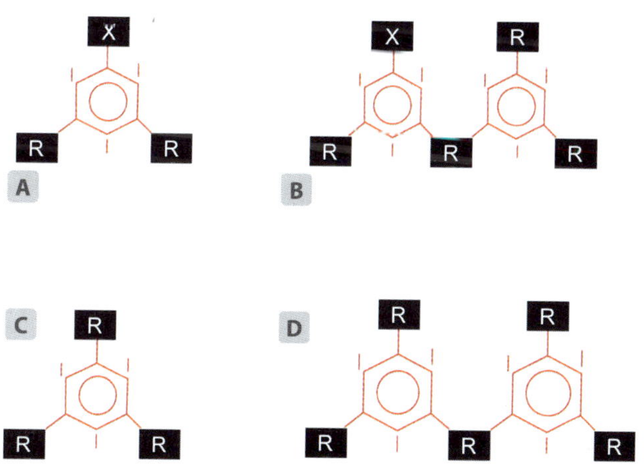

FIGS. 1A TO D: Types of iodinated contrast media. All ICM are based on tri-iodinated benzene ring. (A) Ionic monomer, (B) Ionic dimer, (C) Nonionic monomer (D) Nonionic dimer (R-Hydrophilic, nonionizing side chains; X-Ionic moiety, –COO⁻ with either sodium or meglumine cation).

ICM PHARMACOKINETICS

The salient pharmacokinetic properties of ICM are high water solubility, low lipid solubility, low plasma protein binding and molecular weight ranging from 600 to 1650. Small size of the contrast molecules and high water solubility permits free distribution of contrast across the vascular endothelium. When the contrast media molecules enter the systemic circulation, the molecules equilibrate across

TABLE 1: Most commonly available iodinated contrast media.

Name of the contrast media	Iodine/ particle ratio	Iodine concentration (mg/kg)	Osmolality (mOsm/kg)	Viscosity (cPs at 37°C)
• *Ionic monomer*				
- Diatrizoate (Hypaque 50; GE Healthcare)	3/2(1.5)	300	1,550 (high)	5.2
- Metrizoate Isopaque (Coronar 370; Nycomed A/S)		370	2,100 (high)	2.34
• *Ionic dimer*				
- Ioxaglate (Hexabrix; Guerbet lab.)	6/2(3.0)	320	580 (low)	7.5
• *Non-ionic monomer*				
- Iopamidol (Isovue-370; Bracco Diagnostics Inc.)	3/1(3.0)	370	796 (low)	3.0-9.4
- Iohexol (Omnipaque 350; GE Healthcare)		350	884 (low)	1.5–10.4
- Iomeprol (Iomeron-350,400; Bracco Intl.)		350	618 (low)	7.5
		400	726 (low)	12.6
• *Nonionic dimer*				
- Iodixanol (Visipaque 270/320; GE Healthcare)	6/1(6.0)	320	290 (iso)	6.3–11.8

capillary membranes (except an intact blood-brain barrier) and are distributed throughout the intra- and extravascular extracellular space.[16] As the contrast medium molecules pass through the capillary bed, rapid movement occurs through the capillary pores into the extracellular, interstitial space, as well as via glomerular filtration into the renal tubules. Early vascular enhancement depends on the blood flow and rate of iodine administration; whereas parenchymal enhancement depends on volume of distribution and the total iodine dose.

There is no convincing evidence of any substantial penetration of contrast media molecules through the intact cell membrane into the interior of the viable cells, except for the proximal tubular cells of the kidney.

Theoretically, the differences in the molecular weight and size between the monomeric and dimeric contrast agents could lead to slightly slower distribution rates into extracellular space for the larger dimers. This effect, however, appears to be quite small.[17,18]

All the current commercially available ICM are excreted in the kidney by glomerular filtration with no significant tubular excretion or resorption. Around 99% of the intravenous dose of contrast medium is eliminated through the kidney. Less than one percent is excreted through extrarenal routes that include hepatobiliary system, small and large intestines, sweat, tears and saliva. Vicarious excretion of contrast material occurs through extrarenal routes, in cases of renal insult or renal failure.

The half-life of iodinated contrast media is approximately 2 hours in patients with normal glomerular filtration rate whereas it can be prolonged to over 30 hours in patients with severe renal dysfunction depending on the extent of renal impairment.[9]

The biocompatibility of iodine and its physical properties allow safe and efficacious intravascular injection of large volumes at high concentration. All the other chemical elements in the molecules serve only to carry, or protect the iodine on the benzene ring. It is the iodine in the contrast and the volume distribution of the contrast material that provide contrast enhancement for imaging.[19]

Viscosity is a physical property determining the thickness or friction of the fluid as it flows. It is related to the temperature of the contrast agent, iodine concentration and the size of the molecules in a specific contrast agent. It can be significantly decreased by heating the liquid to body temperature for injection. It is largely controlled by the composition of the side chains on the molecules. Ionic monomers have reduced viscosity and high hyperosmolality; nonionic monomers have reduced viscosity and limited hyperosmolality; nonionic dimers have high viscosity and iso-osmolality. Viscosity plays a role at the level of the nervous system, as a direct correlation has been observed between viscosity of the solution and magnitude of damage to the blood-brain barrier.[20] It also determines renal clearance of an ICM.

DOSAGE OF IODINATED CONTRAST MEDIA ADMINISTRATION

High dose of ICM is considered as potential risk factor for adverse contrast reactions and nephropathy. In practice, dose is only a concern in certain situations, such as patients undergoing catheter angiography and CT on the same day. The lowest dose necessary to obtain adequate visualization should be used. Standard dose of iodinated contrast administration is 1–2 mL/kg at concentration of 300 mg/mL. The maximum limit of contrast administration is typically 200 mL of an agent with a concentration of 320 mg/mL (a total of 64 g of iodine). The maximum safe dose may also depend on individual factors, such as a patient's level of hydration. It should be noted that specific circumstances may necessitate exceeding this 200 mL guideline. This call should be taken by a radiologist after considering the risk benefit ratio.

ADVERSE REACTIONS

Adverse reactions are broadly classified into following types:

- *Acute:*
  - Allergic like
  - Physiologic
- *Delayed:*
  - Allergic like
  - Nonallergic like

Acute adverse reactions can be graded into mild, moderate, severe as follows:[1]

Grading	Description	Allergic like	Physiologic
Mild	Self-limited signs and symptoms with no obvious progression	• Sneezing/conjunctivitis/rhinorrhea • Limited urticaria/pruritis • Nasal congestion • Cutaneous edema • Limited itchy/scratchy throat	• Transient flushing/warmth/chills • Limited nausea/vomiting • Mild hypertension • Headache/dizziness/anxiety/altered taste • Vasovagal reaction that resolves spontaneously
Moderate	Reactions more pronounced and thus require medical management	• Diffuse erythema/stable vital signs • Diffuse urticaria/pruritis • Throat tightness or hoarseness without dyspnea • Facial edema without dyspnea • Wheezing/ bronchospasm, mild or no hypoxia	• Hypertensive urgency • Protracted nausea/vomiting • Vasovagal reaction responsive to treatment • Isolated chest pain
Severe	Life-threatening and can cause permanent morbidity or death if not managed appropriately	• Diffuse erythema with hypotension • Diffuse edema or facial edema with dyspnea • Anaphylactic shock (Hypotension and tachycardia) Laryngeal edema with stridor and/or hypoxia	Vasovagal reaction resistant to treatment, convulsion, hypotensive emergency, arrhythmia

Risk Factors for Adverse Reactions to ICM

Allergy

Patients who have had a reaction of unknown manifestation or a prior allergic reaction to a contrast agent are at a 5-fold increased risk of developing a reaction if exposed to the same class of contrast medium again. This history is the greatest risk factor and warrants premedication.

Patients with unrelated allergies and asthma are also at increased risk of reaction but this does not warrant premedication or restricted use.[21]

Renal Insufficiency

Contrast induced nephropathy is a nonallergic side effect of ICM administration. Its incidence is found to be increased in patients with renal insufficiency.

Cardiac Status

Patients with a severe cardiac disease like angina, severe aortic stenosis, congestive heart failure symptoms, primary pulmonary hypertension, cardiac arrhythmias and severe cardiomyopathy are at increased risk of nonallergic cardiac event. Restricting usage or premedication is however not recommended as per the latest American College of Radiology manual.

Anxiety

Contrast reactions have been found to be more common in anxious patients and mitigating anxiety by reassurance is helpful.

Other Preprocedure Considerations[1]

Age and Gender

Reaction rates are lower in infants, neonates, children and the elderly.

Beta-blockers

Some studies have suggested that beta blockers reduce threshold, increase severity and reduce response of contrast reactions to treatment. However, premedication or cessation of medicine is not recommended.

Sickle Cell Trait/Disease

Risk of sickling crisis is precipitated by ionic contrast media, but there is no evidence to suggest this with the use of modern nonionic media.

Pheochromocytoma

There is no evidence that intravenous injection of ICM increases the risk of hypertensive crisis. Effect of direct injection in renal and adrenal arteries has not been adequately assessed.

Myasthenia Gravis

The relationship between exacerbations of myasthenic symptoms and iodinated contrast medium are not clear and the condition is not a clear contraindication for administration of contrast.

Hyperthyroidism

- In a patient with Graves' disease and thyroid autonomy with multinodular goiter, iodinated contrast medium can potentiate thyrotoxicosis and hence it should be avoided.[22]
- Administration of ICM can cause interference with procedures using radioactive iodine for treatment and imaging.

Pretesting

Intradermal testing with contrast media prior to administration of full dose has not shown to be useful in minimizing reaction risk.

ACUTE ALLERGIC LIKE REACTION

Allergic reactions are uncommon (0.6%, severe-0.04%), so are associated fatalities, Caro et al.[23] documented a fatality rate of 0.9 per 100000 injections of LOCM

Mechanism[24]

Etiological manifestation of this type of reaction is poorly understood; it is however now known that 90% of these reactions are associated with release of histamine and other mediators from circulating basophils and eosinophils. Also, there is conversion of L-arginine into nitrous oxide, an activation of contact and complement systems, development of pseudoantigens and activation of XII clotting system. These reactions occur without prior sensitization. Nonionic contrast media have a lower propensity to cause these effects than the ionic contrast media.

Prevention[1]

If a patient has a previous history of reaction to contrast media, then the possibility of obtaining the necessary diagnostic information from another test without usage of iodinated contrast medium should be considered. Non-ionic, low osmolality contrast medium should be used. If there is a prior documentation of reaction from a contrast agent, then change to a different low osmolality contrast may be helpful.

12 or 13 hours oral steroid premedication is indicated in patients with a prior unknown type or allergic like contrast reaction to the same class of contrast media.

Accelerated intravenous premedication is considered in emergency department patients with a prior unknown type or allergic-like contrast reaction to the same class of contrast media, in whom oral regime is anticipated to adversely delay management decisions

Specific Recommended Premedication Regimens[1]

- Elective premedication (12 or 13 hours oral premedication)
  Prednisone—50 mg orally at 13 hours, 7 hours, and 1 hour before contrast media injection plus pheniramine—25 mg intravenously, intramuscularly, or diphenhydramine 50 mg orally 1 hour before contrast medium administration.
  Or
  32 mg methylprednisolone orally 12 hours and 2 hours before contrast medium administration. Pheniramine—25 mg intravenously, intramuscularly, or diphenhydramine 50 mg orally may be added.
  If the patient is unable to take oral medication, 200 mg of hydrocortisone intravenously may be substituted for oral prednisone
- *Emergency premedication:* Methylprednisolone sodium succinate 40 mg IV or Hydrocortisone sodium 200 mg intravenously immediately, and then every 4 hours until contrast administration plus pheniramine—25 mg intravenously, intramuscularly, or diphenhydramine 50 mg orally 1 hour prior to contrast injection.
  Or
  Dexamethasone sodium sulphate 7.5 mg immediately and then every 4 hours until contrast administration, plus pheniramine—25 mg intravenously, intramuscularly, or diphenhydramine 50 mg orally 1 hour before contrast administration. This regimen may be useful in patients with allergy to methylprednisolone.

Premedication regimens less than 4 hours in duration have not shown to be effective.

Premedication in Patients Undergoing Chronic Corticosteroid Therapy

In such patients the premedication dose may be altered by an amount equivalent to patient's chronic therapeutic dose.

Risks of Premedication

Risks of premedication include transient leucocytosis and asymptomatic hyperglycemia. Diphenhydramine may cause drowsiness. Indirect risk is related to delay in diagnosis due to long duration of premedication.

Breakthrough Contrast Reactions

Reactions occurring despite premedication are called breakthrough reactions. The chances of developing a severe breakthrough reaction are lower in patients with a mild index reaction (1%).

MANAGEMENT[1]

All patients should remain in the radiology department for at least 30 minutes after ICM administration with IV access in situ as most severe reactions occur within this period. The treatment depends on the type of reaction encountered.

- *Urticaria:*
  - No treatment needed in most cases
  - Monitor vitals and preserve IV access in moderate and severe cases
  - Give H_1-receptor blocker: Pheniramine—25 mg intravenously, intramuscularly, or diphenhydramine 50 mg orally or fexofenadine 180 mg PO.
- *Diffuse erythema:*
  - Preserve IV access, monitor vitals, 6–10 L/min oxygen by mask
  - In hypotensive patients—IV fluids 0.9% normal saline or lactated Ringer's 1000 mL rapidly
  - If unresponsive to fluids—consider epinephrine IV (preferred in hypotensive patients) or IM. The IV dose is 1 mL of 1:10,000 dilution (0.1 mg) which is administered slowly into a running IV infusion, can be repeated every few minutes as needed up to 10 mL (1 mg) total.
    IM dose is 0.3 mL of 1: 1000 dilution, can repeat every 5-15 minutes up to 1 mL. Also call emergency response team.
- *Bronchospasm:*
  - Preserve IV access, monitor vitals, 6–10 L/min O_2 by mask
  - Give beta-agonist inhalers (bronchiolar dilators, such as terbutaline, or albuterol) 2–3 puffs; repeat as

necessary up to 3 times. In moderate and severe cases, use IM or IV adrenaline in the doses as described.
  - Call for assistance (e.g., cardiopulmonary arrest response team) for severe bronchospasm.
- *Laryngeal edema:*
  - Preserve IV access, monitor vitals, 6–10 L/min O_2 by mask
  - Give alpha agonist adrenaline IV or I/M in doses as described.
  - If not responsive to therapy or if there is obvious acute laryngeal edema, seek appropriate assistance of emergency response team.
- *Hypotension with tachycardia:*
  - Elevate the legs (preferred) or Trendelenburg position.
  - Monitor: electrocardiogram, pulse oximeter, blood pressure.
  - Give O_2 6–10 L/min (via mask).
  - Rapid intravenous administration of large volumes of Ringer's lactate or normal saline.
  - If poorly responsive, administer adrenaline (1:10,000) slowly IV 1 mL. Repeat as needed up to a maximum of 1 mg
  - If still poorly responsive, seek appropriate assistance (e.g., cardiopulmonary arrest response team).

ACUTE PHYSIOLOGIC

Acute physiologic reactions are dose related and may be related to osmolality, chemotoxicity or molecular binding to certain activators.

- *Reactions unrelated to contrast media:* Pyrogenic reactions, vasovagal reactions especially in anxious or psychosomatic patients, hypoglycemia. Hypertensive attacks in patients with pheochromocytoma
- *Chemotoxic reactions:* As iodine is very firmly bound to the benzene rings, these side effects are probably due to toxicity of the contrast medium ion rather than of its iodine content. These include cardiac, neurological and renal toxicity as well as vascular manifestations.
- *Hyperosmolar reactions:* Due to very high osmolality of these compounds predominantly HOCM, adverse reactions may occur when large volumes are injected into the circulation predominantly because of erythrocyte damage, endothelial damage, blood brain barrier damage, vasodilatation, hypervolemia and cardiac decompensation.

As these reactions are predominantly related to the hyperosmolality of the contrast media and depend on the dose, concentration and volume of contrast used, they can be significantly reduced by substituting LOCM for the high osmolar contrast material. Management of few conditions is described here as recommended by the American College of Radiology.

- *Hypotension with bradycardia (Vagal reaction)*
  - Secure airway: give O_2 6–10 L/min (via mask)
  - Monitor vital signs.
  - Legs elevated 60° or more (preferred) or Trendelenburg position.
  - Secure IV access: rapid administration of Ringer's lactate or normal saline.
  - Give atropine 0.6–1 mg IV slowly, if patient does not respond quickly to steps 2–4.
  - Repeat atropine up to a total dose of 0.04 mg/kg (2–3 mg) in adult.
  - Call for assistance.
- *Hypertension, severe*
  - Give O_2 6–10 L/min (via mask).
  - Monitor electrocardiogram, pulse oximeter, blood pressure.
  - Give nitroglycerine 0.4 mg tablet, sublingual (may repeat × 3); or, topical 2% ointment, apply 1-inch strip.
  - If no response, consider labetalol 20 mg IV, then 20–80 mg IV every 10 minutes up to 300 mg.
  - Transfer to intensive care unit or emergency department.
  - For pheochromocytoma: phentolamine 5 mg IV (may use labetalol if phentolamine is not available).
- *Seizures or convulsions:*
  - Give O_2 6–10 L/min (via mask).
  - Consider lorazepam 2–4 mg IV to be administered slowly or midazolam 0.5–1 mg IV.
  - If longer effect needed, obtain consultation; consider phenytoin infusion—15–18 mg/kg at 50 mg/min.
  - Careful monitoring of vital signs required, particularly of pO_2 because of risk of respiratory depression with benzodiazepine administration.
  - Consider using cardiopulmonary arrest response team for intubation if needed.
- *Pulmonary edema:*
  - Give O_2 6–10 L/min (via mask).
  - Head end to be elevated.
  - Give diuretics: furosemide 20–40 mg IV, slow push.
  - Transfer to intensive care unit or emergency department.

POSTCONTRAST ACUTE KIDNEY INJURY

The understanding of phenomenon of deterioration in renal function after contrast injection has undergone a recent change leading to segregation of entities of postcontrast acute kidney injury (PCAKI) and contrast induced nephropathy (CIN).

PCAKI is a correlative diagnosis and describes a sudden deterioration in renal function that occurs within 48 hours following the intravascular administration of iodinated contrast medium. It may be caused by nephrotoxic event other than contrast administration. PCAKI is an umbrella term encompassing CIN and other entities that may cause reduction in renal function.

CIN is a causative diagnosis and includes a term that describes the deterioration of renal function caused by intravascular administration of contrast. It is a subgroup of PCAKI. Recent studies using appropriate control groups have demonstrated that CIN is less common than previously believed and postprocedure elevations in serum creatinine could be attributed to causes other than contrast administration.[25-28]

Pathophysiology of CIN

The mechanism of CIN involves both chemotoxic and osmotoxic events. Vasoconstriction and direct tubular toxicity are the implicated hemodynamic factors.

According to Acute Kidney Injury Network (AKIN) criteria, the diagnosis of AKI is made if one of the following occurs within 48 hours after a nephrotoxic event:

- Absolute serum creatinine increase ≥ 0.3 mg/dL (≥26.4 μmol/L).
- Urine output reduced to ≤0.5 mL/kg/hour for at least 6 hours.
- A percentage increase in serum creatinine ≥50% (≥1.5 fold above baseline)

Risk Factors

- Pre-existing renal impairment (Serum creatinine >1.3 mg/dL, GFR < 60 mL/min)—most important risk factor
- Dehydration
- Congestive heart failure
- Use of nephrotoxic drugs (NSAID, aminoglycosides)
- Hypersensitivity disease (Multiple myeloma)
- Hyperuricemia (as in active gout)
- Proteinuria (> 0.5 g/dL)
- Diuretic use
- Diabetes mellitus, age > 70 years
- Multiple iodinated contrast medium doses in short time interval (<24 hrs).

Risk Thresholds

Few studies advocate use of eGFR for risk stratification rather than serum creatinine level. However, there is no agreement on the threshold of eGFR beyond which contrast medium should never be administered. A value of eGFR<30 mL/min/1.73 cm^2 is considered a risk factor for CIN. However, in every patient risk benefit analysis is essential before deciding upon the usage of contrast media.

In anuric patients and in patients with non-functioning transplanted kidney, there is no risk of further damage on contrast administration.

In AKI, the serum creatinine level is unreliable as it may not correspond to rapidly changing renal function. Hence, in all patients of AKI, appropriate caution should be taken before contrast administration

Screening

Renal function assessment is advised in patients with the following risk factors:

- Age >60
- History of renal disease
- History of hypertension requiring medical therapy
- History of diabetes mellitus
- Metformin usage.

Prevention of contrast-induced nephropathy in high-risk patients

- *Avoidance of iodinated contrast medium:* In a high risk patient it is best to avoid use of iodinated contrast media and the possibility of obtaining the necessary diagnostic information from another test, not using iodinated contrast medium (e.g., ultrasonography, magnetic resonance imaging), must be considered. In some clinical situations where the use of intravascular iodinated contrast medium may be necessary the lowest possible dose of contrast medium to obtain the necessary diagnostic information should be used.[29-31]
- *Contrast media selection:* Increased osmotic overload on the diseased kidney is considered to be the major etiology of CIN, it can be significantly reduced by substituting LOCM for the very hypertonic HOCM.[32] Initial data showed a benefit of the iso-osmolar agent iodixanol compared to low-osmolar iohexol among patients who have diabetes and chronic kidney disease. However, it has now been demonstrated that the administration of nonionic dimer contrast agent greatly increases the urine viscosity during in vitro dialysis and delay in renal clearance of non-ionic dimeric contrast, as compared to non-ionic monomeric contrast.[33] A 2009 meta-analysis using data pooled from 25 trials found no difference in the rate of PC-AKI between iodixanol and low osmolality agents after intravenous administration.[34]
- *Hydration:* Adequate hydration is considered to be the single most effective way to prevent CIN. The ideal infusion rate and volume is unknown, but isotonic fluids are preferred (Lactated Ringer's or 0.9% normal saline). One possible protocol would be 0.9% saline at 100 mL/hr, beginning 6 to 12 hours before and continuing 4–12 hours after intravascular iodinated contrast medium administration. Oral hydration has also been utilized, but with less demonstrated effectiveness. Pediatric infusion rates are variable and should be based on patient weight.[35,36]
- *Sodium bicarbonate:* It has been found to be useful in prevention from CIN according to some studies.[37,38] The short-duration treatment consists of intravenous bolus 3 mL/kg/h of 166 mEq/L sodium bicarbonate for 1 hour immediately before the injection of the radiocontrast, with subsequent treatment with the same fluid at a rate of 1 mL/kg/h during the contrast exposure and for 6 hours after the procedure.
- *N acetyl cystine:* The role is controversial. There is evidence that it reduces serum creatinine in normal volunteers without changing cystatin-C (cystatin-C is reported to be a better marker of GFR than serum creatinine). This raises the possibility that *N*-acetylcysteine might be simply lowering serum creatinine without actually preventing renal injury. *N*-acetylcysteine should not be considered a substitute for appropriate preprocedural patient screening and adequate hydration.[39,40]
- *Diuretics:* There is no reported benefit and neither mannitol nor furosemide is recommended for CIN risk reduction.[41]
- *Other agents:* The evidence for other theoretically renal-protective medications, such as endothelin-1, theophylline and fenoldopam is even less convincing. Use of these agents to reduce the risk of CIN is not recommended.

Renal Dialysis Patients and the Use of Iodinated Contrast Medium[1]

Contrast agents are readily cleared by dialysis as they have low molecular weight and are not protein-bound. The requirement of emergent dialysis after contrast administration has been debated in renal failure patients. Though the concentration of contrast medium can be effectively reduced with dialysis, it has not shown to offer protection against contrast induced nephropathy in high risk patients.[42]

Nevertheless, the dose of contrast medium administered should be as low as possible because the patients receiving dialysis are also at an increased risk for osmotic overload due to inability to clear excess volume.

SAFE INJECTION

Method of injection depends on the type of vascular access, the type of required diagnostic information and imaging examination type. Admixture of contrast media with any medication should be avoided (only heparin can be used), open vials discarded after 24 hours of opening and regular quality check should be done during storage of contrast media.

Technique

To avoid potential complications like extravasation and air embolism, certain injection practices should be followed. Patient's cooperation should be sought and injection should be discontinued if the patient reports pain or sensation of swelling. A 20G or larger cannula is preferable for flow rates above 3 mL/sec, although 22G cannula may be able to tolerate rates up to 5 mL/sec.

For pressure injection, antecubital or large forearm vein is preferred. During pressure injection, clearance of syringe and tubing of air should be ensured. Flexible plastic cannula should be used for connection with the tubing directed downward during injection. Injection should be preceded by saline test flush. Direct or indirect communication between the patient and technologist should be possible at all times.

Pressure injection of contrast medium should not be performed in small bore, peripheral access central venous catheter unless permitted by manufacturer's specifications.

AIR EMBOLISM

Air embolism can occur on inadvertent injection of large amount of air in the venous system. The patient may present with dyspnea, cough, chest pain, pulmonary edema, tachycardia, wheezing and/or hypotension. Treatment of venous air embolism includes administration of 100% oxygen and placing the patient in left lateral decubitus position.

EXTRAVASATION

It refers to the escape of contrast material from the vessel into the surrounding tissue or body cavity. It occurs with a frequency of about 0.1–1.2%, in patients getting contrast injections. It is more common in patients having atherosclerotic peripheral vascular disease, diabetic vascular disease, Raynaud's disease, venous thrombosis, prior radiation therapy or extensive surgery, severely ill or debilitated patients, injection through indwelling peripheral intravenous lines & multiple punctures into the same vein.

Clinical Features

- *Mild:* Tissue edema, erythema, stinging, tenderness
- *Severe:* Compartment syndromes, skin ulceration and tissue necrosis.

A well-secured intravenous access reduces the incidence. Extravasation detectors present in some of the modern automatic pressure injectors prevent excess of contrast extravasation.

Treatment of Contrast Extravasation

After an initial evaluation of the patient, treatment includes elevation of the affected extremity. The usage of cold compresses for initial use has been recommended. Aspiration of contrast medium and use of hyaluronidase is no longer recommended.

Surgical consultation is sought if the patient complains of features like progressive swelling and pain, altered sensation, altered perfusion, reduced mobility in the affected part, ulceration or blistering.

DELAYED ADVERSE REACTIONS TO CONTRAST MEDIA

Delayed adverse effects can occur after 30 minutes to 1 week following contrast administration. Their mechanism is believed to be different from acute reactions and at least some of them occur due to T-cell mediated hypersensitivity. These reactions are more common in patients treated on IL2 therapy. The incidence of delayed allergic like reactions has been reported to be 0.5–14%.[43,44] Schild et al. demonstrated an increased incidence of delayed cutaneous reactions to non-ionic dimeric contrast agent.[45]

These reactions can vary in severity ranging from symptoms like rash, urticaria, pruritis to features similar to Stevens-Johnson syndrome, toxic epidermal necrolysis or vasculitis. Rarely fatalities have been reported. This spectrum can be severe in patients of systemic lupus erythematosus.

Noncutaneous delayed adverse reactions include nausea, vomiting, fever, drowsiness, headache. In severe cases hypotension may also occur. Other delayed reactions that can occur more commonly in patients with renal dysfunction include iodide mumps (salivary gland swelling) and acute polyarthropathy.

Treatment and Prophylaxis

These reactions are usually self-limiting, but may require supportive treatment in some cases. Supportive treatment includes antihistaminics and corticosteroids in cutaneous symptoms. Antiemetics, antipyretics and fluid resuscitation may be administered depending on the symptoms. Consultation with a specialist may be sought in severe cases.

The rate of recurrence of reactions has been reported to be around 25%.[46] The efficacy of corticosteroid and antihistamine prophylaxis is however not known and not advocated for patients with history of mild delayed cutaneous reactions.

CONTRAST MEDIA WARMING

Few studies have investigated the effect of warming of contrast media to human body temperature (37°) before administration on the flow kinetics and adverse effect profile. It results in reduction of resistance and reduction in injection pressure through thin catheters. One of the largest studies published in 2012 investigated the effect of warming on adverse events following injections of iopamidol 300 and iopamidol 370.[47] They reported an increase in extravasation rates and allergic like events following discontinuation of warming of Iopamidol 370. Based on the available literature, it is recommended that practice of warming may be considered in the following cases:

- For high rates of injection (>5 mL/s)
- For contrast of high viscosity
- Arterial injections through thin catheters and intravenously injected arterial studies.

Needless to say, a strict regular maintenance of temperature is required in departments practising extrinsic warming.

CONTRAS ADMINISTRATION IN PATIENTSON METFORMIN

Metformin is an oral hypoglycemic agent used for non-insulin diabetes mellitus. Lactic acidosis is the most significant side effect of metformin in susceptible patients and it has an estimated occurrence of 0–0.084 cases per 1000 patient years. It is essential to understand the pharmacokinetics of this drug. It is excreted unchanged by the kidney, probably by both tubular excretion and glomerular filtration. So, factors that decrease its excretion or increase production of lactic acid can cause acute lactic acidosis. Other conditions like cardiac failure, sepsis, alcohol abuse and liver disease also increase chances of lactic acidosis. Iodinated contrast media are not an independent risk factor for a patient taking metformin, but may cause lactic acidosis if acute kidney injury occurs. The suggested management protocol is divided into two categories:

	Management protocol
Category 1	No evidence of acute kidney injury with GFR >30 mL/min/1.73 m. No reason to discontinue metformin or reassess renal function after procedure
Category 2	Patient with acute kidney injury, severe chronic kidney disease with GFR<30 mL/min/1.73 m^2, patients undergoing arterial catheter studies. In these patients, metformin is to be discontinued prior to or at the time of procedure, up to 48 hrs after the procedure and restarted only after assessment of renal function

SPECIAL CONSIDERATIONS AND RISK FACTORS

Contrast Administration and Pregnancy

Diagnostic iodinated contrast media have been shown to enter the fetus when given in usual clinical doses after crossing the human placenta.[48,49]

Whether or not ICM pose a risk to the fetus is still debatable. Consequently, the Committee on Drugs and Contrast Media recommends the following:

- The radiologist should confer with the referring physician and document in the radiology report or the patient's medical record the following:
  - That the information needed affects the care of the fetus and patient during the pregnancy.
  - It is not possible to acquire the requested information without contrast administration (e.g. ultrasonography).
  - That the referring physician is of the opinion that it is not advisable to wait to obtain this information until after the patient is no longer pregnant.
- It is recommended that pregnant patients undergoing a diagnostic imaging examination with iodinated contrast media and ionizing radiation provide informed consent to document that they understand the benefits and risk of the procedure to be performed and the alternative diagnostic options available to them (if any), and that they wish to proceed.

Contrast Administration and Lactation

Less than 1% of contrast media are secreted in human milk and <1% of ingested contrast is absorbed by gut; thus it appears safe to continue breast-feeding after receiving such an agent.[50,51] In case the mother remains concerned about any potential ill effects to the infant, she may abstain from breast-feeding for 24 hours with active expression and discarding of breast milk from both breasts during that period. Breast milk expressed prior to contrast study may be used during this period.

RECOMMENDATIONS FOR THE DEPARTMENTS PERFORMING CONTRAST-RELATED INVESTIGATIONS

- Only authorized persons, i.e. technologists and registered nurses should inject ICM under the supervision of radiologist.
- The dose and technique of ICM injection is decided under the guidance of radiologist. The smallest dose of contrast media that will give reliable, comprehensive diagnostic results should be used.
- The radiologist must always weigh the benefit of the diagnostic procedure against the very small but ever-present risk of a severe adverse reaction to the contrast medium.

- Adequate hydration must be ensured in all patients receiving contrast media particularly if there is previous renal impairment and those patients receiving large quantities of contrast media, in order to excrete the contrast media as completely and quickly as possible.
- In high-risk patients it is best to avoid use of iodinated contrast media and the possibility of obtaining the necessary diagnostic information from another test not using iodinated contrast medium (e.g. ultrasonography, magnetic resonance imaging), must be considered.
- In the presence of risk factors, the referring clinician should be consulted and advised. The patient should also be informed, consulted and reassured. The discussion and result should be recorded in the patient's notes.
- In high-risk patients, premedication is strongly advised according to the protocols.
- Before administering the injection, the emergency trolley, alarm system and availability of experienced assistance must be confirmed.
- An individual trained in recognizing and treating severe contrast reactions, including anaphylaxis, should be available in the department.
- Patient should remain in the premises for 30 minutes after contrast administration as most of the contrast reactions occur during this period only.
- All contrast reactions, with details of their severity, nature and the agent used, should be included in the radiological report and updated in the patient's hospital notes.
- Multidose bottles of iodinated contrast media should not be used for intravascular injection if not used within 8 hours after being opened. All multidose contrast containers/vials should be properly labelled along with the time they were opened.
- All ICM stock should be monitored by designated nursing and CT staff. All radiologists/technologists/nurses should personally inspect contrast containers/vials for integrity, signs of contamination and also check expiry date.
- Ongoing quality assurance and quality improvement program for technologist, radiologist and requisite equipment.

CONCLUSION

Radiographic contrast media like any drug are useful for the patient but are not free from side effects, and minor to severe life-threatening side effects can occur with their use. Hence, radiologists and other medical personnel involved in the use of contrast agents should be aware of and use strategies to minimize adverse events and be prepared to promptly identify and manage them.

FUTURE DIRECTIONS

The current nonionic dimers are highly viscous. High viscosity has been a real problem in injection through thin catheters and as cause of nephrotoxicity. In future, a low viscous nonionic, iso-osmolar dimer may find place in the market. New contrast media including organ specific agents are also expected in near future. Alternate high atomic number elements such as gold, tantalum, platinum and bismuth are also being explored.[52]

REFERENCES

1. ACR Committee on Drugs and Contrast Media; ACR Manual on Contrast Media. 2018;Version 10.3.
2. Katzberg RW. Acute reactions to urographic contrast medium: incidence, clinical characteristics, and relationship to history of hypersensitivity states—a commentary. AJR. 2008;190(6):1431-2.
3. Cohan RH, Ellis JH. Iodinated contrast material in uroradiology-choice of agent and management of complications. Rad Clin North Am. 1997;24(3):471-91.
4. Henrik S Thomsen, Judith AW Webb. Contrast Media: Safety Issues and ESUR Guidelines, 2nd revised Edition. Springer publications; 2009.
5. Contrast media-a multifactorial approach. In: Carlo Del Favero-Intramed communications; 1997.
6. Lesser E, Farr RS, Fusjimagari T, et al. The significance of protein binding of contrast media in roentgen diagnosis. AJR. 1962;87:338-60.
7. Almen T. Contrast agent design: some aspects on the synthesis of water soluble contrast agents of low osmolality. J Theor Biol. 1969;24:216-26.
8. Almen T. Development of nonionic contrast media. Invest Radiol. 1985;20:52-9.
9. Almén T, Boijsen E, Lindell SE. Metrizamide in angiography I. Femoral angiography. Acta Radiol Diagn (Stockh). 1977;18(1):33-8.
10. Katzberg RW. Urography into the 21st century: new contrast media, renal handling, imaging characteristics, and nephrotoxicity. Radiology. 1997;204(2):297-312.
11. Meurer K, Kelsch B, Hogstrom B. The pharmacokinetic profile, tolerability and safety of the iodinated, non-ionic, dimeric contrast medium Iosimenol 340 injection in healthy human subjects. Acta Radiol 2015;56(5):581-6.
12. Costa N. Understanding contrast media. J Infus Nurs. 2004;27:302-12.
13. Bettmann MA, Morris TW. Recent advances in contrast agents. Radiol Clin North Am. 1986;24:347-57.
14. Peter Dawson. Adverse reactions to intravascular contrast agents. BMJ. 2006;333(7570):663-4.
15. Almen T. Visipaque—a step forward. A historical review. Acta Radiol Suppl. 1995;399:2-18.
16. Rapport SI, Levitan H. Neurotoxicity of X-ray contrast media: relation to lipid solubility and blood-brain barrier permeability. Am J Roentgenol. 1974;122:186-94.
17. Dobrato M, Powell CJ, Holtz E. Biochemical and morphological effects of contrast media on the kidney. Acta Radiol. 1995;36:196-203.
18. Jakobsen JA. Renal effects of iodixanol in healthy volunteers and patients with severe renal failure. Acta Radiol. 1995;36:196-203.
19. McClennan BL, Stolbery HO. Intravascular contrast media. Ionic versus nonionic: current status. Radiol Clin North Am. 1991;29(3):437-54.
20. Segal AJ. Optimizing urography. World J Urolol. 1998;16(1):3-8.
21. Katayama H, Yamaguchi K, Kozuka T, Takashima T, Seez P, Matsuura K. Adverse reactions to ionic and non-ionic contrast media. A report from the Japanese committee on the safety of contrast media. Radiology. 1990;175:621-8.

22. van der Molen AJ, Thomsen HS, Morcos SK. Contrast media safety committee, European Society of Urogenital Radiology (ESUR). Effect of iodinated contrast media on thyroid function in adults. Eur Radiol. 2004;14(5):902-7.
23. Caro JJ, Trindade E, McGregor M. The risks of death and of severe nonfatal reactions with high- vs low-osmolality contrast media: a meta-analysis. AJR. 1991;156:825-832.
24. European Society of Urogenital Radiology Guidelines on Contrast Agents. 2018; Version 10.0.
25. Davenport MS, Khalatbari S, Cohan RH, Dillman JR, Myles JD, Ellis JH. Contrast material-induced nephrotoxicity and intravenous low-osmolality iodinated contrast material: risk stratification by using estimated glomerular filtration rate. Radiology. 2013;268(3):719-28.
26. Davenport MS, Khalatbari S, Dillman JR, Cohan RH, Caoili EM, Ellis JH. Contrast material-induced nephrotoxicity and intravenous low-osmolality iodinated contrastmaterial. Radiology. 2013; 267(1):94-105.
27. McDonald JS, McDonald RJ, Carter RE, Katzberg RW, Kallmes DF, Williamson EE. Risk of intravenous contrast material- mediated acute kidney injury: a propensity score-matched study stratified by baseline-estimated glomerular filtration rate. Radiology. 2014;271(1):65-73.
28. McDonald RJ, McDonald JS, Bida JP, et al. Intravenous contrast material-induced nephropathy: causal or coincident phenomenon? Radiology. 2013;267(1):106-18.
29. Hartman GW, Hattery RR, Witten DM, Williamson B. Mortality during excretory urography: Mayo Clinic experience. Am J Roentgenol. 1982;139:919-22.
30. Shehadi WH. Death following intravascular administration of contrast media. Acta Radiol Diagn. 1985;26:457-61.
31. Thompson HS, Webb JAW. Contrast media; Safety issues and ESUR Guidelines. 2nd revised edition; 2009.pp.40-9.
32. Barrett BJ, Carlisle EJ. Meta-analysis of the relative nephrotoxicity of high- and low-osmolality iodinated contrast media. Radiology. 1993;188:171-8.
33. Jost G, Lengsfeld P, Lenhard DC, Pietsch H,Hütter J, Sieber MA. Viscosity of iodinated contrast agents during renal excretion. European Journal of Radiology. 2011;80(2):373-7.
34. Heinrich MC, Haberle L, Muller V, Bautz W, Uder M. Nephrotoxicity of iso-osmolar iodixanol compared with nonionic low-osmolar contrast media: meta-analysis of randomized controlled trials. Radiology. 2009;250(1):68-86.
35. Weisbord SD, Palevsky PM. Prevention of contrast-induced nephropathy with volume expansion. Clin J Am Soc Nephrol. 2008;3:273-80.
36. Taylor AJ, Hotchkiss D, Morse RW, McCabe J. Preparation for Angiography in Renal Dysfunction: a randomized trial of inpatient vs outpatient hydration protocols for cardiac catheterization in mild-to-moderate renal dysfunction. Chest. 1998;114:1570-4
37. Merten GJ, Burgess WP, Gray LV, et al. Prevention of contrast-induced nephropathy with sodium bicarbonate: a randomized controlled trial. JAMA. 2004;291:2328-34.
38. Navaneethan SD, Singh S, Appasamy S, Wing RE, Sehgal AR. Sodium bicarbonate therapy for prevention of contrast- induced nephropathy: a systematic review and meta-analysis. Am J Kidney Dis. 2009;53:617-27.
39. Stenstrom DA, Muldoon LL, Armijo-Medina H, et al. N-acetylcysteine use to prevent contrast medium-induced nephropathy: premature phase III trials. J Vasc Interv Radiol. 2008;19:309-18.
40. Vaitkus PT, Brar C. N-acetylcysteine in the prevention of contrast-induced nephropathy: publication bias perpetuated by meta-analyses. Am Heart J. 2007;153:275-80.
41. Solomon R, Werner C, Mann D, D'Elia J, Silva P. Effects of saline, mannitol, and furosemide to prevent acute decrease in renal function induced by radiocontrast agents. N Engl J Med. 1994;331:1416-20.
42. Deray G. Dialysis and iodinated contrast media. Kidney International. 2006;69(100):S25-9.
43. Christiansen C, PichlerWJ, Skotland T. Delayed allergy-like reactions to X-ray contrast media: mechanistic considerations. Eur Radiol. 2000;10:1965-75.
44. Loh S, Bagheri S, Katzberg RW, Fung MA, Li CS. Delayed adverse reaction to contrast-enhanced CT: a prospective single- center study comparison to control group without enhancement. Radiology. 2010;255:764-71.
45. Schild HH, Kuhl CK, Hubner-Steiner U, Bohm I, Speck U. Adverse events after unenhanced and monomeric and dimeric contrast-enhanced CT: a prospective randomized controlled trial. Radiology. 2006;240:56-64.
46. Webb JA, Stacul F, Thomsen HS, Morcos SK. Late adverse reactions to intravascular iodinated contrast media. Eur Radiol. 2003;13:181-4.
47. Davenport MS, Wang CL, Bashir MR, et al. Rate of contrast media extravasations and allergic-like reactions: effect of extrinsic warming of low-osmolality iodinated CT contrast media to 37°C. Radiology. 2012;262:475-84.
48. Dean PB. Fetal uptake of an intravascular radiologic contrast medium. Rofo. 1977;127(3):267-70.
49. Moon AJ, Katzberg RW, Sherman MP. Transplacental passage of iohexol. J Pediatr. 2000;136(4):548-9.
50. Bettman MA. Frequently asked questions: Iodinated contrast agents. Radiographics. 2004;24:S3-S10.
51. Webb JAW, Thomsen HS, Morcos, et al. The use of iodinated and gadolinium contrast media during pregnancy and lactation. Eur Radiol. 2005;15:1234-40.
52. Lusic H, Grinstaff MW. X-ray-computed tomography contrast agents. Chem Rev 2013;113(3):1641-66.

CHAPTER 46

Radiology Information System and Picture Archiving and Communication System

Devasenathipathy Kandasamy, Shivanand Gamanagatti, Arun Kumar Gupta

INTRODUCTION

Imaging informatics is a well-recognized subspecialty of radiology which enable information to be collected, managed, used and shared to support the delivery of healthcare and promote health, from person to other or one place to other.[1,2] It covers every aspect of radiologists' and technicians' day-to-day work in any digital radiology department. Modality, radiology information system (RIS) and picture archiving and communication system (PACS) form the important components for reliable running of the radiology service. The concept of PACS was envisioned in 1980's by the members of radiology community and since then it has grown in to a robust entity. In the last decade there have been numerous PACS installations worldwide. It greatly reduces the turn-around time which is the time interval between the acquisition and preparation of report. After the acquisition, the images are available instantaneously for the radiologists to report and the previous imaging studies can be pre-fetched for comparison. This increases the efficiency of the workflow in a department and decreases the manual filing and entries. Security issues are paramount regarding the patient data which is transferred across networks for various purposes. Security implementations are easier and robust in a digital environment than in analog environment because they provide application level security and tiered access to data. With digital environment, clinicians can place an order, which can be tracked. Once the reports are ready, they can access both the images and report. This makes PACS and RIS more clinician friendly and helps them to use their time efficiently. RIS and PACS are considered to the heart of a digital radiology department and it is set to become more popular and the standard of care in near future because of numerous advantages and improvements in computer technology. Current industry standards and important aspects of RIS and PACS will be discussed in this chapter.

INDUSTRY STANDARDS

Earlier, transmission of textual or image data across network used to be very difficult because of the differences in the vendor, operating system and application environment. To facilitate the free flow of information across modalities and networks in the healthcare, industry standards have been developed. By this way, images and data from various vendors can be handled in an organized manner. Currently, Health Level 7 (HL7) is the industry standard for the transmission of textual information. Digital Imaging and Communications in Medicine (DICOM) is the industry standard for the image data and communication protocols. Vendors have quickly adopted these industry standards. Because of their conformance to these standards it is possible to seamlessly transmit data across Hospital Information System (HIS), RIS and PACS and even between hospitals.

Health Level 7

HL7 standard was established in 1987 by a committee formed by the vendors and the users.[3] They established the standard of exchange of electronic information in healthcare systems. It uses the highest level, i.e. application layer in Open Systems Interconnection (OSI) model and is independent of other lower layers. The information is exchanged as messages in HL7 format. Whenever there is an event such as admission, discharge or transfer, HIS sends a message containing key details. RIS parses these messages and updates its database. RIS can also send messages carrying key information in HL7 format to PACS. Since then, there have been improvements and updates in HL7 versions 2 and 3.

Digital Imaging and Communications in Medicine

It was also necessary to standardize the format of images and communication protocols used in imaging, so as to facilitate flow of information across the hospital regardless of the involved vendors. A standard was developed together by American College of Radiology (ACR) and National Electrical Manufacturers Association (NEMA) to promote exchange of information among equipment from various vendors. This was aimed to integrate various equipment used in radiology such as radiography machines, CT scanners, MRI, printers, digitizers etc. with PACS. The first version was released in 1985 which was called as ACR-NEMA version 1.[4] Later in 1988 the second, enhanced version namely ACR-NEMA 2.0 was introduced. Subsequently in 1993, a newer version DICOM 3.0 was released with major improvements.[4]

RADIOLOGY INFORMATION SYSTEM

In the modern digital radiology department, RIS forms the backbone controlling almost all aspects of radiology workflow **(Fig. 1)**. RIS drives the workflow and transfer of information across the department. It deals with non-image text based computing functions such as scheduling of an appointment, generation of worklist, order tracking, billing and reporting.[5] The orders can come from HIS which can be scheduled by RIS. RIS is responsible for collecting the patient demographic data and send it to the respective modality in the form of worklist. The modality can use the worklist and proceed with the study acquisition. In this way manual entry of patient data in the modality is avoided as it is a common cause of error. The accuracy of the patient data is very important to automatically pre-fetch older studies from the archive and for the billing procedures. For comparison with older studies, pre-fetching of images can be done from the Long Term Storage (LTS) or a list of patients can be generated which can be taken out manually from the record room. The scheduling can be done automatically by the software based on a set of rules or manually. Once the scheduling is done the status of the exam can be tracked by any user with proper credentials till the generation of report.

After the scheduling, RIS will prepare the worklist and provide necessary data to the radiologist and technician performing the study. This worklist can be either in paper format or electronic format. Besides the patient data and the clinical information it can also provide information regarding the patients ambulatory condition, sensitivity to drugs and contrast etc. which is important for proper completion of the exam. Since the patient data is fetched electronically by the modality there is no scope for manual entry errors. Once the study is completed the images are sent to PACS after which RIS and PACS interact to validate the available image information by matching with the order placed. Then RIS generates a list of studies and sends it to appropriate specialty or the radiologist in the department. The reports are then sent to the destined department for viewing and the information is also updated at the billing department via HIS depending on the workflow. RIS archives the order, exam data and report. Thus, RIS controls the entire workflow in the radiology department.

PICTURE ARCHIVING AND COMMUNICATION SYSTEM

The PACS is an important aspect in the digital radiology department which handles the images generated by various digital modalities and is generally interfaced with RIS. PACS comprises of various components such as acquisition modalities, workstations, network and storage.[1] The size of the storage, network bandwidth and number of workstations vary among institutions. Apart from the components of PACS, well trained information technology team having in-depth knowledge is also a requirement for smooth running of the department. But some basic aspects of PACS which the radiologists should know will be discussed here.

Acquisition

Image acquisition forms the entry point for PACS data, so any error at this point will affect the entire process. Digital modalities like CT, MRI and digital radiography (DR) can directly send the images to PACS. In computed radiography (CR) the existing conventional X-ray machine can be used along with photostimulable phosphor plates to generate digital images. Even in fully digital radiology departments, there is a requirement for digitization of films coming from outside hospitals for comparison. This is done by digitizers

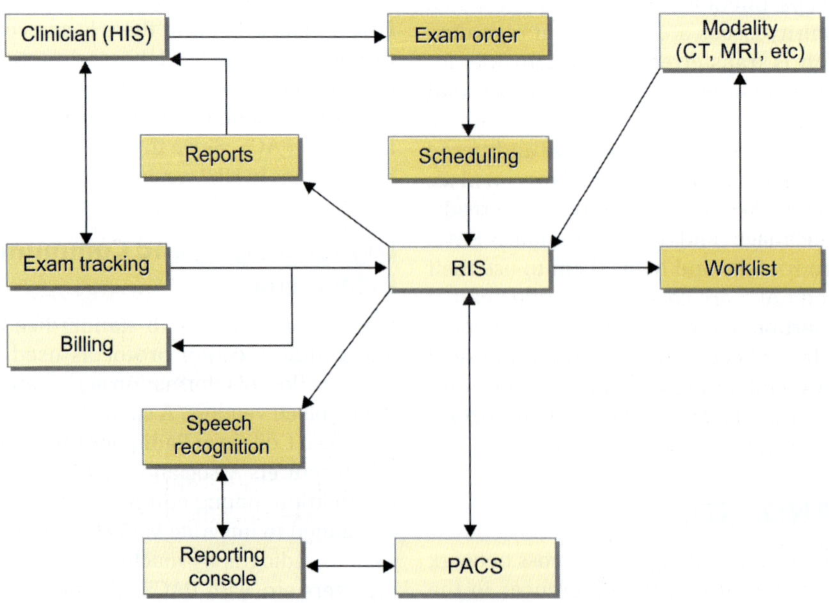

FIG.1: Typical workflow driven by radiology information system (RIS) in radiology department.

which scan the films using visible light or laser, converting them to digital format. Usually, the output of these digitizers is in DICOM format which can be stored in PACS.

Workstation

It is the interactive component of PACS where the radiologists interpret images and generate a report. It is the responsibility of the radiologist to ensure the image quality which, in turn, emphasizes their need to understand the basics of hardware. A typical workstation comprises of display monitors, computer and local storage. These workstations are connected by network cables. The computer should have enough computing power in the order of 3 MHz or above, and faster Random Access Memory (RAM) to do 3D rendering of large CT and MRI data sets.[6] In advanced workstation used for cardiac and vascular studies, dedicated video graphics card is usually required to improve the performance.

Display Monitors

Cathode ray tube (CRT) monitors utilize an older technology which has been used in televisions for decades and they are relatively cheaper. Liquid Crystal Display (LCD) is a newer technology and relatively expensive. However, the LCD technology has been improved to match the quality of best CRT monitors and is becoming cheaper. It is expected that in near future LCD monitors will replace CRT monitors. The advantages of LCD monitors over CRT are (a) Thin and light weight, (b) Less power consumption, (c) Brightness of display, (d) Flat surface, (e) Maintained aspect ratio.[7,8] One disadvantage of LCD monitor which is worth mentioning is that it has narrow viewing angle than CRT monitors.

Resolution

Spatial resolution of monitors is expressed in megapixels which is the number of pixels. Very high resolution monitors are expensive and slow to respond. So it is important to choose the resolution of monitors for the type of usage and workstation requirements.[1] Images of modalities having fixed matrix size such as US, CT and MRI, can be viewed optimally in 2 megapixel monitors. Radiographs pose a problem because they have very high resolution which is usually more than that of display monitors. One approach is to down sample the original image and displaying at a lower resolution in the monitor. Although finer details are lost in the process of down sampling, it has been shown that monitor resolution of more than 2–3 megapixels has no significant improvement in diagnostic accuracy.[9] Another approach with lower resolution monitors is zooming and panning the images so that the finer details are visualized. Visualization of microcalcification is very critical in mammography and demands for higher resolution monitors. Monitors with 5 megapixel resolution are recommended for mammography interpretation.[1]

Color and Grayscale Display

Most of the radiological images are in grey scale although certain modalities such as Doppler, PET, nuclear medicine images use colors. Color LCD monitors are superior in displaying color images. The quality of display of grayscale monitor is superior to that of color monitors of similar resolution because the images are blurred and less bright in color monitors. Expensiveness of the Color monitor over grayscale monitor is also a reason for increasing usage of grayscale monitors in many radiology departments. Usual recommendation is that lower resolution color monitors are used for viewing colored images whereas grayscale monitors are used for viewing high resolution images. Typically, one low resolution color monitor and two high resolution grayscale monitors are used in workstations.

The modern day browsers have become sophisticated and robust in such as way that the images can be streamed from the server to the browser without a need for a dedicated viewer. These zero footprint viewers need not have any high end hardware and because of this the users get a universal graphical user interface across all devices (PC, mobiles, etc.).

Network

Network is another important component which transmits data from one place to other. Four important factors to be considered while setting up a PACS network are (a) performance or the speed of the network, (b) reliability, (c) upgradability and (d) the cost involved. The workstations or computers used by radiologists to report are usually clients which are connected to a server. Clients get data from the server based on various queries. Typically there are many clients connected to a server by means of network cables which typically support multiple Gigabit data transfer. There are various equipment in a network such as router, switch which are used to manage the network and use the bandwidth efficiently. This kind of connections between computers within a hospital is called as Local Area network (LAN). This can be a wired network using cables or a wireless network. Usually wired network is preferred because of its performance, reliability and security. When multiple LANs are connected it is called as Wide Area Network (WAN). Performance and reliability of the network depend on how it is managed, which necessitates the requirement of trained personnel in the department. Network and error logs need to be checked on daily basis to ensure smooth running of network. Another technology called Virtual Private Network (VPN) which is commonly used nowadays to view the images from anywhere in the world using the internet infrastructure.[10] One of the problems in transmitting the images outside the hospital is lack of control and security over the transmitted data. Using this VPN protocol the internet infrastructure is tunnelled and used to reach the hospital LAN. This protocol ensures security of the transmitted data, though the data is transmitted across various public networks. This also enables the radiologists at a remote site to use all the facilities in the hospital LAN as if they are within the LAN. Users are given username and passwords and their privileges are set-up so that the data is secured in the network and avoiding their misuse. Also, numerous network and PACS configurations are possible such as access to certain sensitive information is based on user privileges.

It is very important to have a dedicated network for PACS and it should not be shared with other non-PACS network. This will ensure proper functioning and reduce congestion in the network. When many users are using the network simultaneously, it will cause congestion of even high bandwidth network. To avoid this problem to some extent, there are techniques to compress the image which will reduce the network load. There are two types of compression (a) lossy and (b) lossless. In lossy compression the decompression of the image will not result in the original image because of irreversible loss of image information during this process. Using the lossless compression technique which is a completely reversible process the original image can be obtained after decompression. This is the most preferred compression algorithm used in PACS.

The PACS and storage are usually located in the local site, however these days there are services available which run on cloud. Cloud based computing and services are becoming popular these days because of its low maintenance, high availability, relatively cheap and scalability. The computing resource, storage and the software run in a distant location and those hardware and software resources are availed by the user as a service. One important requisite for cloud based solutions is a reliable network as the entire operation is dependent on it.

Storage

Archiving can be online, near line or offline depending on the availability of data. Usually hard drive is used for online data storage which is readily available and accessed immediately. Tapes and optical media which are loaded automatically by juke-box are called as near-line storage.[11] In near-line storage, data is available in less than a minute. In offline storage, data is loaded manually and the loading time may vary. Some authors discourage the use of the term near-line.[1] This multi-tier system is used because of the high cost factor involved in online storage. As the cost of hard drives have been decreasing day by day, the use of offline storage should be reduced as far as possible because it involves manual intervention and the errors associated with it.

The amount of storage needed for a department should be calculated based on the number and types of imaging studies done and also the time duration for which they are kept in archive. Another consideration in choosing an appropriate storage is that it should be a robust, viable technology and should be upgradable in future. As any storage technology can fail, it is very important to have a failover mechanism especially in health care services. This is typically done by creating redundant copies so that even if a storage medium fails, data can still be recovered.

Redundant Array of Inexpensive Disks (RAID) is a popular technology employed in PACS. It provides high performance, availability and at the same time provides a copy of data in case any of the hard drive fails. RAID comprises of multiple hard drives which are functioning as a unit, which is controlled by a RAID controller. Since data is stored in multiple hard drives, recovery of data is possible in case of failure. Another method is to store the data in a Long Term Archive in addition to PACS. In this case the data is stored permanently and is available in long term archive even when the study is not available online. Availability of imaging data used in health care is very critical so it is recommended to store a copy of data in a different geographical location which is called as disaster recovery.

One of the challenges in traditional PACS system is that it is time consuming and hard to change over from one vendor to another. Every vendor use their own proprietary formats while storing the imaging data. Because of this the data migration is a challenge because it may lead to loss of crucial data during migration. Another limitation of traditional PACS is that it cannot handle non-DICOM images such as clinical photos, videos, pdfs etc. These non-DICOM modalities are on the rise in the recent past. A solution with open architecture called vendor neutral archive (VNA) has been developed to mitigate these issues. It can work across all the departments, can handle non-DICOM files, store them in a standard format and can work across vendors as well, overcoming the hassles of data migration. This new technology has shown wide acceptance and rapid adoption worldwide.

Related Applications

Apart from RIS and PACS, radiologists also commonly use various applications and software which make image interpretation easier, enable advanced post processing and generate reports in quicker and easier way. Some of the commonly used applications are discussed here.

Three-dimensional and Advanced Viewing

In the modern era of imaging, thin high resolution images are routinely acquired and they are utilised in three dimensional (3D) reconstructions. Many currently available commercial applications can provide a range of 3D reconstructions such as Maximum Intensity Projection (MIP), Surface Shaded Display (SSD) and Volume Rendering Technique (VRT) etc. These techniques help the radiologists to make use of the fullest potential of the modality. Curved reconstructions and VRT used to be a time consuming exercise but now these processes are automated by a click of a button. Other post processing techniques such as virtual bronchoscopy and colonoscopy can provide virtual endoluminal view. Modern workstations are also equipped with advanced post processing applications such as dual energy applications and computer aided detection (CAD).

With the emerging technology of dual energy CT, various post processing applications are available to decompose the image based on the material density. In this way it is possible to generate iodine only image and virtual non-contrast scans. Spectral imaging is also possible in which the keV can be changed by the user and image is processed by the workstation and displayed according to the selected keV. This processing can be useful in studying the material characteristics over a range of photon energies. Clinical application of this technique lies in differentiating hyperdensity because of bleed from contrast enhancement in post contrast scans.

The CAD is a technique in which the computer analyses the image set to show the region of interest based on predefined rules. Those areas will be again analyzed by the radiologist to come to a conclusion. This method has been applied in mammography, lung nodule detection and polyp detection. Advanced segmentation algorithms are available nowadays which can be useful in determining the volume of tumor or any solid organ which can be very useful in determining the response evaluation of tumors.

Speech Recognition

Report generation is a time consuming process if it involves typing of the report. Speech recognition software is aimed at reducing the time delay involved in typing a report. Various attempts were made since 1980s to device a robust speech recognition software.[11] But the earlier applications suffered many setbacks because of poor accuracy and inability to adapt to the accent of the radiologists. Various improvements have been made since then and the currently available speech recognition applications are robust enough to adapt itself to the accent of the user and it has in-built spelling check which includes words used in radiology. In addition, it has seamless integration with the PACS environment.

Natural Language Processing

Vast majority of radiology reports whether typed manually or using speech recognition softwares are unstructured, free narratives. Every person has their own way of describing a pathology. This introduces an obstacle when these data needs to be mined or when you are looking for a specific finding or diagnosis in a large number of radiology reports. Searching keywords may be a useful feature however they are not robust enough to yield the desired result. Keyword search will look for a specific word in the reports. But there may be many related terms for the same condition which could have been used by different radiologists. In this kind of situation keyword search will not help much. Natural language Processing (NLP) is a new technique which can automatically convert the unstructured, free narrative report to a structured one with an uniform radiology lexicon. In this way the salient findings in the reports are captured which can be used for various data mining methods, epidemiological research methods (especially retrospective studies), etc.

CONCLUSION

There has been a significant transformation in the way modern day radiology is practiced. Recent developments in information technology have been the key for this digital imaging revolution. These advancements will definitely improve the standard of radiology service and thereby the patient care. Management of large amount of data generated by radiology services is still a challenge but steady reduction in storage cost along with future advancements will negate these problems. Although RIS and PACS installations are steadily increasing in the country, complete digital radiology practice is still not practical in many centers. Analog practice is still the major component in day to day practice, but given the rapid growth in the technology, wide acceptance and its benefits, digital practice will eventually overrun the analog practice.

REFERENCES

1. Branstetter BF 4th. Basics of imaging informatics. Part 1. Radiology. 2007;243(3):656-67.
2. Hersh WR. Medical informatics. JAMA: the journal of the American Medical Association. 2002;288(16):1955-8.
3. Simborg DW. The case for the HL7 standard. Comput Healthc 1988;9(1):39-40, 42.
4. Mildenberger P, Eichelberg M, Martin E. Introduction to the DICOM standard. European Radiology. 2002;12(4):920-7.
5. Huang HK. PACS and imaging informatics: basic principles and applications. Wiley-Blackwell; 2011.
6. Indrajit I, Alam A. Computer hardware for radiologists: Part I. Indian J Radiol Imaging 2010;20(3):162 7.
7. Pärtan G, Mayrhofer R, Urban M, Wassipaul M, Pichler L, Hruby W. Diagnostic performance of liquid crystal and cathode-ray-tube monitors in brain computed tomography. Eur Radiol. 2003;13(10):2397-401.
8. Zuley ML, Willison KM, Bonaccio E, Miller DP, Leong DL, Seifert PJ, Somerville P, Destounis S. Full-Field Digital Mammography on LCD Versus CRT Monitors. AJR. 2006;187(6):1492-8.
9. Langer S, Bartholmai B, Fetterly K, Harmsen S, Ryan W, Erickson B, Andriole K, Carrino J. SCAR R&D Symposium 2003: comparing the efficacy of 5-MP CRT versus 3-MP LCD in the evaluation of interstitial lung disease. Journal of Digital Imaging. 2004;17(3):149-57.
10. Kumar S, Krupinski EA. Teleradiology. Springer; 2008.
11. Dreyer KJ, Mehta A, Thrall JH. PACS: a guide to the digital revolution [Internet]. Springer Verlag; 2002.

CHAPTER

47

Evidence-based Radiology and a Primer on Biostatistics

Sanjay Sharma, Ankur Goyal, Manisha Jana

INTRODUCTION

Evidence-based medicine (EBM) is defined as integrating the best research evidence with the available clinical expertise and expectations of the patient.[1-3] Dr Guyatt and Dr Sackett, from the Evidence-Based Medicine Working Group at McMaster University, Ontario, Canada, are the pioneers of EBM in modern clinical practice and first coined this term.[4] For proper understanding of EBM, all three of its basic constituents must be imbibed. Best research evidence means properly validated research in the field of diagnostic or therapeutic practice which is clinically relevant. Clinical expertise depends on the decision-making ability and expertise in treatment, based on one's clinical knowledge, experience and skill.

A basic understanding of biostatistics is very important for radiologists, not only to conduct the research themselves, but also to comprehend the existing literature (research evidence). Statistics is not only the analysis and interpretation of numerical data, but also includes collection and presentation of data. Application of statistics to biological and medical sciences is called *Biostatistics*.

This chapter includes an overview of evolution, types, components, strength and caveats of Evidence Based Practice (EBP) in our daily lives, illustrated with examples. A primer of various terms and concepts in biostatistics is also included.

BACKGROUND

The practice of medicine has hitherto remained 'eminence based', that is, based on individual experience and expertise.[3] According to Frieldland,[5] the traditional medical practice is based on the following assumptions:

1. The measure of authority is directly related to the weight of individual experience.
2. Understanding pathophysiology of a disease forms the foundation for clinical practice.
3. Conventional medical training and common sense enable one to evaluate new tests and treatments.
4. Clinical experience and expertise in a given subject are sufficient for the physician to develop clinical practice guidelines.

Traditional 'eminence-based practice' is more didactic, based on the individual expertise and does not always take into consideration the existing best research evidence. This is where the proponents of EBP differ from the traditional practice. The foundation of EBP rests upon the proper use of validated research evidence (e.g., meta-analysis, randomized controlled trials) to support one's clinical decision in diagnostic procedures, interventions and therapy. In no way it undermines the importance of individual knowledge or pathophysiology of disease.[6]

Why Evidence-based Practice?

The growing awareness and practice of EBM worldwide can be explained by a few basic needs in healthcare services. Firstly, with the ever-increasing number of newer disease entities, the physician needs to be constantly updating himself about the diagnosis, prognosis and treatment of the disease.[7] In this respect the conventional text books as a resource often prove inadequate.[8] Also searching for the desired data from the deluge of available medical journals is practically impossible for a busy medical practitioner, owing to the lack of time.[9,10] Secondly, the improved clinical skills in an experienced professional very often coexists with a declining up-to-date knowledge.[11] This forms an increasing 'knowledge gap' among the practitioners. In clinical practice, the knowledge of healthcare workers forms the backbone of the clinical decision making. The 'knowledge gaps' appear when the healthcare provider's knowledge is insufficient to meet the need of the patient.[3,12] The gap can be in 'background knowledge' i.e. general information regarding a disease or treatment; or 'foreground knowledge' which pertains to the latest information regarding the disease condition, any new diagnostic test or intervention.[3] The 'background knowledge' is usually obtained from books and well-established texts e.g., radiological anatomy and procedures for radiologists. 'Background knowledge' gaps can be encountered in rare diseases or an uncommonly performed procedure.[3] 'Foreground knowledge' gaps are more common. Sources of this type of knowledge lie in latest published literature. It becomes important for a practicing physician to identify the knowledge gap and be aware about where to search for the required evidence.[13]

The rising costs of healthcare make it imperative to justify the decision for any specific diagnostic test or treatment. Moreover, the freely available internet, effective search engines (MEDLINE, Pubmed, Google scholar etc.) and development of systematic reviews of the existing evidences in medicine and healthcare like the 'Cochrane Collaboration' have made tracking any evidence easier,[14] further supporting the evidence-based approach towards medical decisions. Archie Cochrane, a British epidemiologist, highlighted in 1972 that most treatment decisions were based on random selection of existing evidence or 'expert opinions' and not based on systematic review of the published research.[15] Cochrane collaboration is a non-profit organization consisting of volunteers all over the world who analyse the existing evidence and make the latest evidence-based information available.[14] Another reason for growing popularity of EBP is the development of evidence-based journals (e.g., *Evidence-based Medicine*) which contain systematic reviews, meta-analyses and evidence-based guidelines.[16]

Forms of Evidence-based Practice

There are two forms of evidence-based practice (EBP), the 'top-down' and the 'bottom-up'.[3,17] The 'top-down' practice is usually carried out by experts working for a government, large centralized resource like Cochrane Collaboration or a professional body like American College of Radiology. However, what practitioners (clinician or radiologist) are more concerned in daily life is with the 'bottom-up' approach. 'Bottom-up' EBP starts from the practitioner who encounters a problem, asks an answerable question regarding the problem, searches for the best available evidence and applies it in his practice after critical appraisal. These two forms of EBP are not mutually exclusive, but complimentary.[18] In the following sections of this chapter, we have elaborated the steps of 'bottom-up' EBP.

The 'Bottom-up' Evidence-based Practice

As described earlier, bottom-up EBP is the more relevant to daily practice of a busy clinician or radiologist. The concept was started by David Sackett in 1996. These steps are listed in **Table 1**.

Step 1: Ask

The first step of 'bottom-up EBP' is asking a question, arising from either the background or foreground knowledge gap.

TABLE 1: Steps of bottom-up evidence-based practice.[2,3]

Step	Summary	Explanation
1.	Ask	Asking an answerable question
2.	Search	Searching for the best available research evidence
3.	Appraise	Critical appraisal of the evidences for validity and impact assessment
4.	Apply	Application of the evidence in practice
5.	Evaluate	Evaluation of efficacy and effectiveness of first 4 steps

It is the foreground question that is usually needed to be answered to address the clinical problem. The foreground questions usually have four components, commonly abbreviated as PICO (patient, intervention, comparator and outcome) **(Table 2)**.[1,19]

The questions in clinical practice can relate either to the cause, predisposing factors, diagnosis or management of a certain entity. The radiologists in practice are more concerned with the diagnosis or management of a disease entity. While searching for the answers to a question, the practitioner should be aware of the kind of study to be looked for. For example, if a question relates to an etiology or risk factor, the ideal study design would be a randomized control trial (RCT), prospective cohort study or case control study. The questions related to disease frequency can be best answered by a prospective cohort study or a cross-sectional study. For questions related to diagnostic procedures, a cross-sectional study with consecutive or random sampling may be ideal. A cohort/survival study will be ideal to answer a question related to the disease prognosis; and therapy/intervention related questions can be better answered by an RCT or cohort study.[3]

While searching for evidence, one should be aware about the hierarchy of evidence.[20,21] The study designs are graded by the levels of evidence. On top of the hierarchy, are the systematic reviews of RCTs and cohort studies (level 1a) which are considered the least biased evidences. Level 1B includes RCTs and cohort studies with good validation and follow-up. Hitherto considered a superior evidence, an 'expert opinion' is downgraded at level 5. The levels of evidence are tabulated above **(Table 3)**.

In evidence-based radiology (EBR), when one searches for evidence, it must be valid and relevant. Since diagnostic

TABLE 2: Components of a question (PICO), illustrated by an example.[19]

Example: How effective is CT Pulmonary Angiography in the detection of pulmonary embolism compared to Ventilation-Perfusion scan, in suspected patients?

Component	Explanation	Example
Patient population/ clinical problem (P)	Patient's clinical situation or the problem of interest	Patients with suspected pulmonary embolism
Intervention (I)	Any exposure, including a diagnostic procedure or treatment in question	CT pulmonary angiography
Comparator (C)	Exposure, diagnostic test or treatment to which the main intervention is compared	Ventilation-perfusion scan
Outcome (O)	Result/outcome of interest	The accuracy in the diagnosis of pulmonary embolism

TABLE 3: Levels/hierarchy of evidence.[20,21]

Level of evidence	Description
1a	Systematic review (with homogeneity) of level 1 diagnostic studies or a clinical decision rule with 1b studies from different clinical centers
1b	Independent blind comparison of an appropriate spectrum of consecutive patients, all of whom have undergone both the diagnostic test and the reference standard
1c	Diagnostic finding for which specificity is so high that positive result rules in the diagnosis or for which sensitivity is so high that negative result rules out the diagnosis
2a	Systematic review (with homogeneity) of level 2 diagnostic studies
2b	Independent blind comparison but either in nonconsecutive patients or confined to a narrow spectrum of study patients (or both), all of whom have undergone both the diagnostic test and the reference standard; or a clinical decision rule not validated by means of a test set
3a	Systematic review (with homogeneity) of studies with a level of 3b and better
3b	Nonconsecutive study or independent blind comparison of an appropriate spectrum, but reference standard not applied to all study patients
4	Reference standard not applied independently or not applied blindly
5	Expert opinion without explicit critical appraisal or based on physiology, bench research, or "first principles"

imaging is not directly related to patient outcome and in view of the increasing cost of medical imaging, the technology assessment of an imaging tool has to be performed with assessment of some additional parameters.[22] The need for separate technology assessment also stems out from the concern regarding risk of increased radiation exposure in the imaging modalities.[22] A conceptual framework of the technologic assessment was described by Thornbury,[23] McNeil et al[24] and later Fryback.[25] In short, the hierarchy of technical assessment deals with the following:

1. Technical efficacy
2. Diagnostic accuracy (described by sensitivity, specificity, positive and negative predictive values, PPV and NPV respectively)
3. Diagnostic thinking efficacy (pre and post-test probability and likelihood ratios)
4. Therapeutic efficacy (whether the imaging modality can change the treatment decision)
5. Patient outcome efficacy (impact of the test on the patient)
6. Societal efficacy (the cost-effectiveness).

TABLE 4: Electronic resources for evidence-based practice.[13]

Name	Web link
McMaster University Health Information Research Unit: Evidence-based Health Informatics	http://hiru.mcmaster.ca/hiru
Pubmed: US National Library of Medicine and National Institutes of Health	http://www.ncbi.nlm.nih.gov/sites/entrez
Google scholar	http://scholar.google.com
MD consult	http://www.mdconsult.com
Cochrane collaboration	http://www.cochrane.org
SUM search	http://sumsearch.uthscsa.edu
American College of Physicians Journal Club	http://www.acpjc.org
British Medical Journal Evidence Based Medicine	http://ebm.bmj.com
BMJ Clinical Evidence	http://clinicalevidence.bmj.com/ceweb
National Library of Medicine	http://www.nlm.nih.gov
Centre for Evidence-based Medicine at Oxford	http://www.cebm.net
Centre for Evidence-based Radiology at the Brigham and Women's hospital	http://www.brighamandwomens.org/cebi/default.aspx

Step 2: Search

Once the question is formulated, the next step in EBP is searching for the best evidence. For this, the practitioner needs to be aware of how and where to look for. As already described, the textbooks are a good source of background knowledge, but the foreground knowledge gap need latest evidences, which cannot usually be found in textbooks, as they may be already outdated by the time they are published. The most up to date resources for the best evidences are the electronic resources (journals, search engines, information systems).[3] The common electronic resources are listed in **Table 4**.

Radiologic Electronic Resources

Unfortunately, there are limited available electronic resources providing information regarding diagnostic imaging modalities. Evidence-based radiology website (http://www.evidencebasedradiology.net) was developed by the St Vincent's University hospital in Ireland and provides proper 5-step process of EBM. Critical appraisal worksheets and excel spread sheets can be downloaded to create graph of conditional probabilities.[26,27]

Step 3: Critically Appraise

Once the proper evidences are available, one needs to assess them for validity and impact assessment. In routine practice, we tend to read an article without its proper critical appraisal. First step of critical appraisal of a primary research article (first-hand studies, such as RCT, experiments and survey) is the assessment of its validity, that is, whether the study is close to the truth and without bias.[28] The next step comprises of the impact assessment and applicability in one's own clinical practice.

Validity Assessment

The simple steps for validity assessment of a study are searching for answers to the following questions:[29]

1. What is the PICO of this study and whether they are relevant in one's own clinical scenario?
2. How well was the study performed?
3. Can the results be due to chance (bias)?

Assessment of validity of a study by asking the PICO questions is done by following the steps described by an acronym 'RAMMbo'. It also describes the processes to eliminate bias at each step. While critically appraising any study, the practitioner must try to get answers to all these questions, in order to decide if the results of the study are trustworthy **(Table 5)**.

Additionally, while appraising the internal validity of a study describing any new diagnostic test, the following questions are to be answered.[29]

1. Whether the test was evaluated on a group of patients similar to those on whom it is to be used in practice?
2. Whether there was an independent reference standard for proper blinded comparison?
3. Was the reference standard applied on all patients, independent of the test result?
4. Was the test validated on a separate, independent group of patients?

In an ideal study, answers to all of the above questions should be 'yes'. After the internal validity and methodology assessment, if study comes out to be a proper blinded randomized study without bias, the results are to be assessed for their relevance.

A statistically significant result is known by its *p-value*. It is a measure of the probability that the result is purely by chance.[28,30] A p value of less than 0.05 is considered statistically significant. Confidence intervals (CI) are an estimate of the range of values that are likely to include the real value. Usually they are described with 95% CI values.[28] Studies with larger sample tend to have narrower CI and are therefore more reliable.[31-33]

Impact Assessment

Impact assessment of diagnostic literature: After assessment for validity, the study should be evaluated for its impact or strength, usually found in the 'results' section. The important statistical parameters to be considered are sensitivity, specificity (with 95% CI), positive predictive value, negative predictive value, positive likelihood ratio, negative likelihood ratio and how these affect the pre and post-test probability.[34] For understanding these parameters, let us start with a contingency table **(Table 6)**.

True positive (TP) refers to the persons who are having the disease and are correctly detected positive by the test and true negative indicates people who do not have the disease and are correctly identified as negative. Sensitivity is a measure of how accurately a test can identify the persons having a disease. Specificity tells how correctly it can detect the persons not having a disease. Sensitivity and specificity, ideally, should be expressed with a 95% CI, which gives a better estimate of precision. For example, if a study states a range of sensitivity and specificity with 95% CI, it means that if the study is done100 times, the values of sensitivity and specificity will lie within the given range 95% of the times.[31-33]

Likelihood ratios (LR) reflect the discriminative power of a test.[35] Positive likelihood ratio (PLR) is the ratio of probability of a positive test result in a patient with disease to

TABLE 5: Assessment of validity of study in patient, intervention, comparator and outcome format.[29]

Questions	Assessment		Possible error/ bias	Ways to circumvent
Patient (P)- population in the study	Assessing for fair recruitment (**R**)	R	*Selection bias* (the subjects are not representative of the population of interest), or Small study sample leading to imprecise results	Randomization or Consecutive recruitment Increase the size of study population
Intervention (I)	How fairly were the subjects allocated (**A**) into groups? Whether equal management and follow-up were done (fair **M**aintenance) in both (except for the index test/ intervention)?	A M	*Allocation bias* (Lack of proper matching of subjects in the two groups e.g., age, sex etc.) *Treatment bias*	Randomization Equal management in both the groups apart from the index test or intervention
Comparator (C)	Same as above		Same as above	
Outcome (O)	Assessing for fair **M**easurement—valid and un**b**iased **o**utcome measurement	M b o	Measurement bias	Double-blinding

TABLE 6: A 2 x 2 contingency table describing outcome of a diagnostic test.[27]

Test outcome	Disease	
	Present	**Absent**
Positive	True positive (TP)	False positive (FP)
Negative	False negative (FN)	True negative (TN)

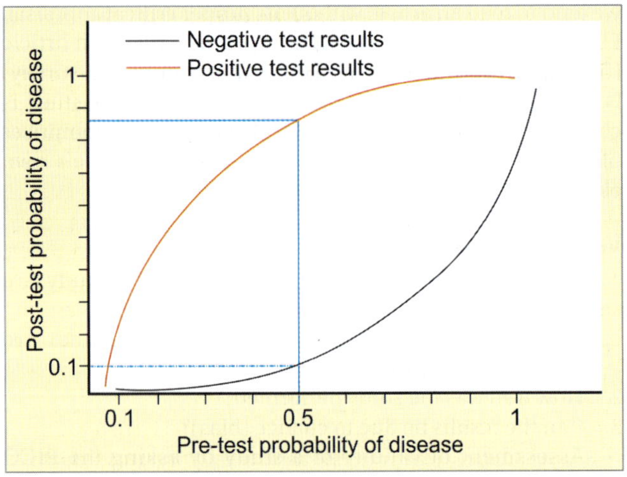

FIG. 1: Graph of conditional probability of a test showing high sensitivity and high specificity. Here, for a pre-test probability of 0.5, the post-test probability of a negative diagnostic test outcome is 0.1 and post-test probability of a positive test result is 0.85, which means the test can successfully 'rule out' the diagnosis as well as 'rule in' (confirm) the diagnosis.

the probability of a positive test in a person without disease. It is calculated by sensitivity divided by 1-specificity. Similarly, negative likelihood ratio (NLR) is the ratio of probability of a negative test in a person with disease to the probability of a negative test in a person without disease. NLR is calculated by 1- sensitivity divided by specificity. A PLR>10 and NLR <0.1 is considered significant. A PLR of >10 means strongly positive, 2 to 5 is moderately positive and 0.5 to 2 is weakly positive. Similarly, NLR of < 0.1 is considered strongly negative and 0.2 to 0.5 moderately or weakly negative.

Pre-test probability is the likelihood that the patient will have the disease in question even before the test is performed. It is usually decided by the prevalence of the disease and assessed by clinician without any mathematical analysis being involved. The pre-test probability is important for interpreting the results of a diagnostic test, comparing more than one test or deciding whether it is worth doing the test at all.[34,36] Once the pre-test probability and likelihood ratios are known, the post-test probability can be calculated. If LR>1, the post-test probability will be higher than the pre-test probability. It is the post-test probability that the practitioner is more concerned about while treating a patient. The concern is whether the test has altered the disease probability so that it now lies above the treatment threshold or below an exclusion threshold.[37] To calculate the post-test probability, one can multiply the pre-test odds by the LR, or refer to the graph of conditional probability or Fagan's nomogram **(Fig. 1)**.[38-40] Further details of these tools are beyond the scope of this chapter.

For better understanding, let us consider a situation relevant to a practicing radiologist. When a clinician questions whether it is prudent to perform a CT pulmonary angiography (CTPA) in a patient with suspected pulmonary thromboembolism (PTE), the radiologist needs to know the pre-test probability of PTE i.e., what according to the clinician is the risk of PTE in the given patient. Pre-test probability of 50% means that the clinician thinks there is a 50 % chance that the patient may have PTE. Now after proper literature search, we find that the PLR of CTPA is 10 and NLR is 0.02. Consulting the Fagan's nomogram, the positive post-test probability is around 90% and negative post-test probability is approximately 0.3%. This means the test can effectively rule in or rule out PTE, and, therefore, can be used.

Impact assessment of therapeutic literature: Critical appraisal of a therapeutic literature for internal validity should be performed in similar ways as described before. For impact assessment of a therapeutic literature, the important statistical parameters are relative risk (RR), absolute risk reduction (ARR), relative risk reduction (RRR), absolute risk increase (ARI) or relative risk increase (RRI), number needed to treat (NNT) or number needed to harm (NNH) and odds ratio.[41]

TABLE 7: A 2 x 2 contingency table describing the therapeutic test outcome.[41]

Exposure/ Treatment	Outcome of events		
	Yes	**No**	**Total**
Yes	Events in experimental group (a) EE	b	(a+b) Subjects in experimental group ES
No	Events in control group (c) CE	d	(c+d) Subjects in control group CS

For calculation of the above-mentioned parameters, let us consider another contingency **(Table 7)**.

Odd's ratio refers to ratio of odds of disease among exposed and odds of disease among unexposed. It is easier to calculate and straightforward, compared to RR. Relative risk means the risk of an event or developing a disease relative to exposure.[41] Mathematically, RR can be expressed as the ratio of risk in the treated/exposed group to the risk in the control group {[a/(a+b)]/[c/(c+d)]}. A relative risk >1 implies increased risk in the exposed group. Absolute risk reduction is the difference in the event rate between treatment and control groups {[a/(a+b)] – [c/(c+d)]}. Relative risk reduction is the difference in event rate between treatment and control groups, expressed as percentage (1-RR). Another important parameter is the number needed to treat (NNT) which is the inverse of ARR.[41-43] A lower NNT means that only few patients are needed to be treated to get a desirable benefit in at least some of them.[41-43]

Diagnostic systematic review and meta-analysis: A systematic review is a systematic collection, critical appraisal, and summary of all relevant studies on a specific topic.[44] Over the last few decades, as the number of available diagnostic and screening tests have increased significantly, the need of systematic analysis of all the available literature has also increased. Some of these studies may have inherent biases in their design whereas others may be well conducted. Since there is a plethora of evidence, a summary of all the available evidences should be deducted from them. Meta-analyses are statistical methods used to combine results from a number of different studies. Meta-analysis model aims at estimating: (a) the summary sensitivity and specificity and/or summary receiver operating characteristic (ROC) curves, and (b) common threats to the validity of the summary estimates.[45-48] Thus, meta-analysis is the quantitative counterpart of systematic review.

The steps involved in conducting a systematic review of a diagnostic test includes:

1. Finding the evidence
2. Assessing the study quality and applicability
3. Summarizing the evidence qualitatively or quantitatively (meta-analysis)
4. Clinical interpretation and application in developing a recommendation.[45]

Steps 1 and 2 have been discussed earlier. Discussion on the meta-analytical integration of evidence and the analysis is beyond the scope of this chapter. In the integration of diagnostic data, two or more paired statistics are taken into consideration viz., sensitivity and specificity, PPV and NPV etc. Summary estimate of sensitivity and specificity of various studies can be derived from various methods, summary ROC curves, Forrest Plot etc. ROC curve is a graph of test's sensitivity against 1-specificity and area under the curve (AUC) is a measure of the diagnostic accuracy.

While pooling data for meta-analysis, 'publication bias' should be kept in mind. It refers to the association of the publication probability of a study to its statistical significance. A study showing positive or good statistical significance is more likely to get published. There are several methods to estimate publication bias in a meta-analysis, e.g. Funnel plot. For the detailed understanding of Funnel plot the readers are requested to refer to more detailed treatise.[44]

In the clinical interpretation of evidence related to a diagnostic test, the important step is to determine the post-test probability, using the Fagan's nomogram or a graph of conditional probability, as described above.

Step 4: Apply

After proper critical appraisal of the available evidence, one should assess its applicability in the prevailing clinical context. This step can also be called 'external validation'.[49] Before applying the results in the individual patient, the following points should be considered.

1. Whether the diagnostic tests/treatment are feasible in your existing set-up?
2. Are there any other feasible alternatives?
3. Are the patients in existing clinical scenario sufficiently similar to the subjects of the study?
4. Whether the diagnostic test is changing the pre-test probability?
   (Here one needs to calculate the LR of a study, which can be calculated from sensitivity and specificity, vide supra. If the PLR of a study is >10 or NLR <0.1, the test can significantly alter the pre-test probability).
5. Consider the pros and cons of the diagnostic/or therapeutic test.
   (It is particularly important when the test or treatment under consideration has side effect or a risk, e.g., radiation exposure in diagnostic CT. In such cases, the risks associated with the test/treatment can be outweighed by the risk of the disease).[50]
6. Must take into consideration the patient's opinion.

Step 5: Evaluate

The last step is to evaluate your results in clinical practice, after going through all the four previous steps. This can be performed by evaluating the efficiency in executing all the four steps, and taking initiative to improve them.

How does Evidence-based Radiology (EBR) Differ from Evidence-based Medicine (EBM)?

Since Radiology is a technology-based subject, the practice of EBR differs from that of EBM in a few additional points under the step 'critical appraisal'. The additional five questions to be asked when assessing any imaging modality are as follows:[51]

1. Has the imaging methodology been described in sufficient detail to allow to reproduce the study in your own department?
2. Has the reference (gold standard) and the imaging test under evaluation been performed to the same standards of excellence?
3. Have technology development within the same modality been adequately considered in the study design and discussion?
4. Has the issue of radiation exposure been considered?
5. How were the MRI/CT images reviewed, on hard copy images or on a monitor?

Limitations of Evidence-based Practice

While the proposers of EBP see it as a tool of paradigm shift in the clinical decision-making, the critics suggest that it should be considered as an additional tool in the existing practice, giving importance to the other alternate forms of clinical practice also. They criticize the 'bottom-up EBP' for being time-consuming and not practically feasible in daily clinical practice. While EBP necessitates the convergence of various modalities and enhances multimodality practice, it is often seen as unhelpful. Some also believe that it is unproven, threatens professional autonomy and narrows the research agenda.[52,53]

How Can a Radiologist Practice EBR in His or Her Daily Life?

a. *In justifying a new diagnostic test.* When confronted to a question about performing a new diagnostic test in a patient, follow the previously stated five steps of EBP. It can help the radiologist in deciding whether the test is going to change the pre-test probability so as to establish or exclude the diagnosis.

b. *While studying an article, critically appraising it* (as described above) before applying its recommendations in your practice. Most radiology articles lack in proper statistical analysis and the information needed to assess validity is inadequate. Consolidated standards of reporting trials (CONSORT)[54] and the Standards for reporting of diagnostic accuracy (STARD)[55] are two initiatives to improve the reporting of clinical trials and studies of diagnostic accuracy. While studying any article, the radiologist should test them using the STARD or CONSORT criteria. One can use the proper format for critical appraisal of a diagnostic literature (available at http://www.srs-mcmaster.ca). In this manner, knowing the strength and weakness of the existing literature can help the radiologist to plan a proper study in a specific field.

c. *Applying principles of EBR in academic activities*: While presenting an article in a departmental Journal Club, a radiology resident could critically appraise it in the proper format, check for adequacy of the STARD criteria and summarize the strength and caveats of the article. This will help to spread the practice of EBR among the fellow colleagues.

BIOSTATISTICS PRIMER

Data refers to information regarding variables. Variables can be qualitative (categorical) or quantitative (numerical) and thus data can be of various types **(Table 8)**. Describing data using standard measures, tables and graphs is part of descriptive statistics.

Categorical data means data can be organized into groups which are summarized by proportions/rates/percentage. If there are only two groups, it is referred to as dichotomous data. If the groups can be arranged in a specific order, it is ordinal data. Categorical data can be depicted in frequency tables or bar charts. Mode is used for nominal data while ordinal data can be evaluated using median/mode.[56]

Numerical data can be continuous or discrete. Latter is also called count data and can have only integral values like number of lesions. Continuous data can be of interval or ratio type. Mean is used for continuous data and mode may be used for count data. The distribution of continuous data can be depicted using histograms.

TABLE 8: Types of data variables.

Types of data		Description	Examples
Nominal	Categorical	No specific order	Radiological modalities: USG, CT, MRI, etc.
Ordinal	Categorical	Groups can be arranged in meaningful order	Tumor staging, BIRADS
Interval	Numerical	Equal difference between units	Temperature in degree celsius
Ratio	Numerical	Equal difference between units with meaningful ratio and absolute zero	Height, weight, temperature in kelvin

Measures of Central Tendency and Variation

Normal distribution of data refers to symmetrical bell-shaped curve of frequency distribution of values with mean = median = mode. If asymmetric, it is called non-normal or skewed distribution.

Mean, median and mode are the measures of central tendency. Mean is the sum of all observations divided by the number of values. Median is the center value when observations are arranged in ascending order and corresponds to 50th percentile value. Median is less affected by outliers, compared to mean. Mode is the most frequently occurring observation and typically used in discrete variables.

Variability measures are range, variance and standard deviation. Range tells about the minimum and maximum values of the variable. Interquartile range denotes the difference between 25th and 75th percentile values, so tells about the central range, ignoring the outliers. Variance denotes the spread of values around the mean. Standard deviation is the square root of variance and is measured in the same unit as the variable, thus commonly used. For normal distribution, about 95% of the observations are expected to lie within two standard deviations from the mean.

Sample Size Calculation

Sample size depends on multiple factors, most important of which are:

- Acceptable *level of significance:* It refers to the p-value and is usually taken as 5%. This corresponds to the type I or α-error and is the probability of rejecting the null hypothesis when it is actually true
- *Power* of the study: It is usually kept as ~80%. Power = 1 - β. Type II or β error refers to the probability of not rejecting a false null hypothesis and is usually accepted up to 20%.
- Expected *effect size*: Sample size is inversely proportional to the square of effect size
- Underlying *event rate* in the population
- *Standard deviation* in the population

Thus, a larger sample is needed for common diseases, smaller effect size, stringent p-value, higher power and if there is high standard deviation of the variable in the population.

Measures of Effect

A 2 × 2 contingency table gives us sensitivity, specificity, positive and negative predictive values of a diagnostic test. The meaning of the effect variables is explained in **Table 9**. It may be noted that sensitivity is closely related to a type II error and specificity is closely related to the type I error.

Choice of Statistical Test

Statistical tests help us to derive the 'p' value. If latter is below our set threshold (usually ≤0.05), then the result is deemed statistically significant. This means that the difference is

TABLE 9: Statistical jargon explained.

Term	Mathematical expression/relationship	What does it imply for a diagnostic test
Sensitivity	TP/TP+FN	How well a test can identify patients with the disease
Specificity	TN/ TN+FP	How well a test can identify the persons without the disease
Positive predictive value	TP/TP+FP	
Negative predictive value	TN/TN+FN	
True positive rate	TP/TP+FN	Equivalent to sensitivity
True negative rate	TN/TN+FP	Equivalent to specificity
False positive rate	FP/FP+TN or 1-specificity	
False negative rate	FN/FN+TP or 1-sensitivity	
Power	1 – false negative rate (analogous to sensitivity of a diagnostic test)	Probability that the test will reject a false null hypothesis (i.e., it will not make a type II error)
Accuracy	TP+TN/TP+TN+FP+FN or True results/ total population or Sensitivity x prevalence + (Specificity)/ (1- prevalence), provided the prevalence is known	100% accuracy implies that the test will rightly detect all patients with or without the disease in a given population
Prevalence	TP+FN/ TP+FN+TN +FP	
Positive likelihood ratio (PLR)	Sensitivity/(1-specificity)	High PLR implies that if the test result is positive there is a high chance that the disease will be present
Negative likelihood ratio (NLR)	(1-sensitivity)/specificity	Low NLR implies that if the test result is negative there is a high chance that the disease will be absent
Pre-test odds	Prevalence/(1-prevalence)	
Pre-test probability	Patients with disease/ (patients with disease+ patients without the disease)	Represents the likelihood of a disease in subject, prior to investigation. Usually determined by clinicians based on the likelihood of the patient having a disease. Zero % pre-test probability indicates that the patient in all probability will not have disease
Post-test odds	Pre-test odds × likelihood ratio	Represents how confident a radiologist/ physician is that the patient will have the suspected disease, after performing the test in question. It increases if the pre-test probability is high
Post-test probability	Post-test odds/(post-test odds+1)	
p-value	Measurement of the probability that a result is purely by chance	Lower the p value, higher the probability that the observed result is statistically significant and not by chance

unlikely to be due to chance. The choice of a test depends upon the distribution of data, sample size, number of groups studied, type of variable and status of follow-up **(Table 10)**.

Kappa statistics assess the interobserver agreement in case of categorical variables. Intraclass correlation coefficient assesses the reliability of a test in case of continuous data. The tools for statistical analysis include MICROSOFT EXCEL, SPSS (IBM), STATA (Statacorp), MATLAB The Mathworks, R (Foundation for Statistical Computing), Open EPI, GraphPad Prism, etc. SPSS is one of the most popular tools used by

TABLE 10: Guidelines for choice of statistical test.

	Comparison				Association and regression	
	2 data sets		>2 sets			
	Paired	**Unpaired**	**Paired**	**Unpaired**	**Association**	**Regression**
Normally distributed continuous data (means)	*Paired t-test*	*Unpaired t-test*	Repeated measures Analysis Of Variance (ANOVA)	One-way ANOVA	*Pearson correlation* (Linear relationship)	Linear regression
Scores, ranks, non-normal continuous data (medians)	Wilcoxon signed rank test	Wilcoxon rank sum (Mann Whitney U test)	Friedman test	Kruskal-Wallis test	Spearman's rank correlation	Non-parametric regression
Dichotomous data (proportions)	McNemar's test	Fisher's exact (small sample)/ Chi square test (large sample)	Cochran's Q	Chi square	Contingency coefficients	Logistic regression

medical researchers. Newer versions of this package are released from time to time.

Majority of the radiological studies are cross-sectional observational studies with diagnostic tests done at one time point. If imaging findings are correlated with survival or development of complications by following up the study group, this becomes a cohort study. Case-control studies include imaging of healthy volunteers as well. Experimental studies assess the impact of a radiological interventions and randomized controlled clinical trials are the best way to assess advantages of procedures.

CONCLUSION

To conclude, evidence-based practice in radiology is a relatively new concept with its own advantages and limitations. Every radiologist should be aware of its concept and be able to apply it in their daily practice. All radiologists must have a basic understanding of the biostatistics to allow them to comprehend the latest research in proper perspective.

In practice, clinical decision making remains a combination of 'expert opinion', critical appraisal of the existing evidence and the judgment of the practitioner. A perfect balance between them can bring out the best patient care.

REFERENCES

1. Strauss SE, Rosenberg W, Glasziou P, et al. Introduction, in Evidence Based Medicine: How to Practice and Teach EBM 3rd ed. Churchill Livingstone, Edinburgh, Elsevier; 2005.pp.1-12.
2. Sackett DL, Rosenberg WM, Gray JA et al. Evidence based medicine: what it is and what it isn't. BMJ. 1996;312:71-2.
3. Kelly Am. Evidence based practice: an introduction and overview. Semin in Roentgenol. 2009;43:131-9.
4. Guyatt G, Cairns J, Churchill D, et al. Evidence-based medicine, a new approach to teaching the practice of medicine. J Am Med Assoc. 1992;268:2420-25.
5. Friedland D. Introduction, In evidence based medicine: a framework for clinical practice. Stamford, Conn, Appleton and Lange; 1998.pp.2-3.
6. Woods BP. What's the evidence? Radiology. 1999;213:635-37.
7. Currie LM, Graham M, Allen M et al. Clinical information needs in context: an observational study of clinicians while using a clinical information system. AMIA Annu Symo Proc; 2003.pp.190-4.
8. Antman EM, Lau J, Kupelnick B et al. A comparison of results of meta-analyses of randomized control trials and recommendations of clinical experts. Treatments for myocardial infarction. JAMA. 1992;268:240-8.
9. Haynes RB. Loose connections between peer-reviewed clinical journals and clinical practice. Ann Intern Med. 1990;113:724-8.
10. Sackett DL, Strauss SE. Finding and applying evidence during clinical rounds: the evidence cart. JAMA. 1998;280:1336-8.
11. Shuval K, Berkovits E, Netzer D et al. Evaluating the impact of an evidence-based medicine educational intervention on primary care doctors' attitudes, knowledge and clinical behavior: a controlled trial and before and after study. J Eval Clin Pract. 2007;13:581-98.
12. Strauss SE, Richardson WS, Haynes RB. Our reactions to knowing and not knowing, in Evidence Based Medicine: How to Practice and Teach EBM 3rd ed. Churchill Livingstone, Edinburgh, Elsevier; 2005.pp.18-9.
13. Kelly Am. Evidence based radiology: step 2- searching the literature (search). Semin Roentgenol. 2009;43:147-52.
14. Cochrane Collaboration Website: available at http://www.cochrane.org.
15. Cochrane AL. Critical review, with particular reference to the medical profession, in Medicines for the year 2000. London, Office of Health Economics; 1979.pp.1-11.
16. Evidence based medicine journal website. Available at http;//ebm.bmj.com.
17. Malone DE, Staunton M. Evidence-based practice in Radiology: step 5 (evaluate)- caveats and common questions. Radiology. 2007;243:319-28.

18. Van Beek EJ, Malone DE. Evidence-based practice in radiology education: why and how should we teach it? Radiology. 2007;243:633-40.
19. Glasziou P, Del Mar C, Salisbury J et al. Formulate an answerable question, in: Evidence based practice workbook (2nd ed). Boston, Blackwell Publishing; 2007.pp.21-34.
20. Levels of evidence. Oxford Centre for Evidence- Based Medicine Web site. http://www.cebm.net/levels_of_evidence.asp.
21. Dodd JD. Evidence-based practice in Radiology: steps 3 and 4- Appraise and apply diagnostic radiology literature. Am J Radiol. 2007;242:342-54.
22. Fryback DG, Thornbury JR. The efficacy of diagnostic imaging. Med Decis Mak. 1991;11:88-94.
23. Thornbury JR, Fryback DG. Technology assessment- an American view. Eur J Radiol. 1992;14:147-56.
24. McNeil BJ, Adelstein SJ. Determining the value of diagnostic and screening tests. J Nucl Med. 1976;17:439-48.
25. Finberg HV. Evaluation of computed tomography: achievement and challenge. Am J Roentgenol. 1978;131:1-4.
26. Centre for evidence based radiology in Ireland. Available at http//www.evidencebasedradiology.net/index.html.
27. Maceneaney PM, Malone DE. The meaning of diagnostic test results: a spreadsheet for swift data analysis. Clin Radiol. 200;55:227-35.
28. Cronin P. Evidence-based Radiology: step 3- primary literature validity (critical appraisal). Semin Roentgenol. 2009;43:153-7.
29. Sackett DL, Strauss SE, Richardson WS, et al. Evidence Based Medicine: How to Practice and Teach EBM 2nd ed. Churchill Livingstone,Edinburgh,Elsevier, 2000
30. Guyatt G, Jaeschke R, Heddle N et al. Basic Statistics for clinicians:1. Hypothesis testing. CMAJ. 1995;152:27-32.
31. Gardner MJ, Altman DG. Confidence intervals rather than p values: estimation rather than hypothesis testing. BMJ (Clin Res Ed). 1986;292:746-50.
32. Guyatt G, Jaeschke R, Heddle N et al. Basic Statistics for clinicians:2. Interpreting study results: confidence intervals. CMAJ. 1995;152:169-73.
33. Montori VM, Kleinbart J, Newman TB et al. Tips for learners of evidence based medicine: 2. Measures of precision (Confidence intervals). CMAJ 2004;171:611-615.
34. Cronin P. Evidence-based Radiology: step 3- critical appraisal of diagnostic literature. Semin Roentgenol. 2009;43:158-65.
35. Cronin P, Dwamena BA, Kelly AM, et al. Solitary pulmonary nodules and masses: A meta-analysis of the diagnostic utility of alternative diagnostic tests. Eur Radiol. 2008;18:1840-56.
36. McGinn T, Jervis R, Wisnivesky J, et al. Tips for teachers of evidence-based medicine. Clinical prediction rules (CPRs) and estimating pre-test probability. J Gen Intern Med. 2008;23:1261-8.
37. Chang PJ. Bayesian analysis revisited: A radiologist's survival guide. Am J Roentgenol. 1988;152:721-7.
38. Sackett DL, Haynes RB, Guyatt GH, et al. The interpretation of diagnostic data, in Clinical Epidemiology: A basic Science for clinical medicine (ed 2). Boston/ Toronto/London, Little, Brown. 1991;pp.92-3.
39. Fagan TJ. Nomogram for Bayes theorem. N Eng J Med. 1975;293:257.
40. Sackett DL, Richardson WS, Rosenberg W, et al. Is this evidence about a diagnostic test important? In Evidence based medicine, how to practice and teach EBM (ed 1), vol 127.Edinburgh, Churchill Livingstone,1998.
41. Cronin P. Evidence-based Radiology: step 3- critical appraisal of therapeutic literature. Semin Roentgenol. 2009;43:166-9.
42. Jaeschke R, Guyatt G, Shannon H et al. Basic statistics for clinicians. III. Assessing the effects of treatment: measures of association. Can Med Assoc J. 1995;152:351-7.
43. Barratt A, Wyer PC, Hatala R et al. Tips for learners of evidence based medicine. I. relative risk reduction, absolute risk reduction and number needed to treat. Can Med Assoc J. 2004;171: 353-8.
44. Jonathan A. C. Sterne and Roger M. Harbord. Funnel plots in meta-analysis.The Stata Journal. 2004;4(2):127-41.
45. Dwamena BA. Evidence-based radiology: step 3- diagnostic systematic review and meta-analysis (critical appraisal). Semin Roentgenol. 2009;43:170-9.
46. Whiting P, Rutjes AWS, Reitsma JB, et al. The development of QUADAS: a tool for the quality assessment of studies of diagnostic accuracy included in systematic reviews. BMC Med Res Methodol. 2003;3:25.
47. Lijmer JG, Bossuyt PM, Heisterkamp SH. Exploring sources of heterogeneity in systematic reviews of diagnostic tests. Stat Med. 2002;21:1525-37.
48. Deeks JJ, Macaskill P, Irwig L. The performance of tests of publication bias and other size effects in systematic reviews of diagnostic test accuracy was assessed. J Clin Epidemiol. 2005;58:882-93.
49. Cronin P. Evidence-based Radiology: step 4- Apply. Semin Roentgenol. 2009;43:180-1.
50. Del Mar C, Doust J, Glasziou P. Clinical Thinking: evidence, communication and decision making. London, BMJ Books. Blackwell Publishing Ltd. 2006
51. Dodd JD, MacEnenaey PM, Malone DE. Evidence based radiology: how to quickly assess the validity and strength of publication in the diagnostic radiology literature. Eur Radiol. 2004;14: 915-22.
52. Trinder L. A critical appraisal of evidence based practice. In: Trinder L, Reynolds S, eds. Evidence-based practice: a critical appraisal. Oxford, England: Blackwell Science. 2000;212-41.
53. Malone DE, Staunton M. Evidence based practice in radiology: step 5 (evaluate)- caveats and common questions. Radiology. 2007;243:319-28.
54. Moher D, Schulz KF, Altman D. The CONSORT statement: revised recommendations for improving the reports of parallel group randomized trials. JAMA. 2001;285:1987-91
55. Bossuyt PM, Teitsma JB, Bruns DE, et al. Towards complete and accurate reporting of studies of diagnostic accuracy: the STARD initiative. BMJ. 2003;326:41-4.
56. Anvari A, Halpern EF, Samir AE. Statistics 101 for Radiologists. Radiographics. 2015;35(6):1789-801. doi: 10.1148/rg.2015150112.

CHAPTER

48

Radiation Hazards and Radiation Units

Pratik Kumar, Anil Kumar Pandey

X-rays are so useful that it has become part of our life. X-ray examinations help in diagnosis. They fall under the category of ionizing radiation and hence, they are harmful too. Harmful effect of radiation on human body is called Radiation Hazards. In this chapter we discuss the harmful effect of radiation on human body (radiation hazards), how to protect the patient, staff, and public from radiation generated during the diagnostic and interventional procedures performed in radiology, and units associated with the measurement of radiation in these modalities.

THE BIOLOGICAL EFFECTS OF RADIATION

The ionizing radiations are those radiations which have enough energy to cause ionization of the atoms of the medium with which they interact. The ionization of atom means that the target atom (atom on which the radiation has been incident) looses one (or more) of its orbital electrons and hence bringing structural changes to the atom.

The ionizing radiation may be wave type (like X-rays and gamma rays) or particle type (particulate nature) like alpha, beta, protons, ions (Carbon ions) etc. Radioactive nuclei emit alpha, beta and gamma radiation. Alpha particles are heavy particles and may be considered as stream of helium nucleus. They are highly ionizing but lack penetrating capability. Hence, alpha particles usually can't penetrate sheets of papers or upper layer of our skin. It indicates that alpha sources outside our bodies don't pose much risk but may cause severe injuries if ingested inside the bodies. Beta particles which are stream of electrons are less ionizing than alpha particles but may penetrate some thickness of soft tissue, paper, wood etc. Beta particle is usually stopped by thin layer of metal. Gamma ray, which is electromagnetic waves, is least ionizing but possess very high penetration capabilities. In general, alpha particles contain about 20 times ionizing capability than that of gamma, 10 times than that of beta and about 2 times than that of neutrons.

All human beings are made of tiny structures called cells. The bigger a person is, the more number of cells he or she has. Children do not have as many cells as adults, but they have greater proportion of dividing cells. Chemical contents, physical shape and size of a living cell are continuously changing. A new cell is made when an existing cell grows and divides into two. The new cell is an exact copy of the old one. This change may be rapid or slow. In natural growth cycle of a cell, one step is linked with other as it is a continuous process, but for convenience these steps are named as different phase of growth cycle of the cell such as M phase, G1 phase, S phase and G2 phase. The cells are most sensitive to radiation during Mitosis (i.e. M phase) and G2 phase (i.e. Premitosis or RNA synthesis) and least sensitive during S phase (DNA synthesis).

First step of cell development is necessary to move on to the second step. In case of rapid development, the gap between the first step and second step is less, so the minimum time required to repair the damage created by the radiation, may not be available in case of rapid developing cells. In slow developing cell the time period to repair the break is available; therefore, slow developing cells are less sensitive to radiation in comparison to the fast/rapid developing cells. Similarly, any damage inflicted by radiation on the cell is expressed soon in case of rapidly developing cells as they progress fast through their cell-cycles.

The X-ray energy used in the diagnostic radiology varies from 25–125 kVp. They deposit their energy in a very small volume and are sufficient to produce ionization inside the human body. Radiation creates damage to the DNA by direct and indirect mechanism. In the direct mechanism, the X-ray hits the DNA molecules directly. DNA molecule gets ionized resulting in damage. In indirect mechanism, water molecules absorb the X-ray energy and dissociates into H^+ and OH^-. OH free radical contains an unpaired electron in the outer shell and is highly reactive. It reacts with DNA and creates the damage. It is estimated that 60–70% of radiation-caused DNA damage is due to OH free radical.

DAMAGE TO DNA BY THE RADIATION

THE EFFECT OF RADIATION

Chemical bonds hold DNA together. Loss of electrons causes chemical bond to change. Thymine one of the four bases of DNA, is supposed to bind with adenine on its opposing strand. However, loss of electrons caused by radiation makes thymine bind with another thymine on the same strand. When DNA is replicated to make new cells, coding errors occur and mutations result. Mutations result in damaged chromosomes. Cells then reproduce abnormally, causing both defects and cancer.

The types of damage that can occur to DNA molecules are:

- DNA single strand breaks
- DNA double strand breaks
- Sugar damage
- Base damage
- Local denaturation (separation of the two strands)
- DNA-DNA crosslinks
- DNA-Protein crosslinks.

These damages can lead to:

- Slow down in the cell synthesization (copies of its own DNA) so that there is a delay in cell dividing into two cells
- Delay in repair mechanism that will delay the cell cycle progression (as the cell progresses towards next cell division)
- Delays in cell proliferation (increase in cell number) of a population of cells
- Death of the cell
- Mutation of the cell
- Cell transformation (changes in the cell which will make them to behave as a cancer cell).

Cell death have been given special names also as cell necrosis (death of a contiguous fields of cell, the content of the cell leaks out into the surrounding tissue and blood supply), cell lysis (the cell simply bursts open and releases its contents into the surrounding), apoptosis (or programmed cell death) which is under genetic control (specific gene must be present active or inactive) and it requires energy and when the cells die, DNA fragments of specific sizes, and the content of the cells, are encapsulated in membranes as small vesicles. The damages incurred by different kinds of tissue vary with the type of radiation to which the person is exposed and the means of exposure. Direct exposure to radiation can affect the whole body. The body attempts to repair the damage caused by the radiation. However, at times the damage is so severe and widespread that repair is impossible. For example, thyroid gland is one of the most radiation-sensitive parts of the body, especially in babies and children. Absorption of too much radioactive iodine can cause thyroid cancer to develop several years after the exposure.

Different types of cell aberration can occur depending on the position of the cell cycles at the time of exposure to ionizing radiation. Most common is formation of dicentric and ring which can be visualized under microscope after the exposure above 10–25 cGy. Visualization of the ring or dicentric aberration means cell death has occurred. Certain types of aberration and/or mutation in gene can cause cancer. Mutation may occur even at low dose. There is no threshold of dose below which an ionizing radiation cannot induce mutation. However, at low doses and dose rates, the risk of mutation is very low, and it is lower for low dose rates at all doses. The relationship may be either linear or linear quadratic depending on type of radiation. X-rays follow linear-quadratic model, at low doses the relationship is linear with increase in dose, while at higher dose the relationship is square of the dose.

All cells and tissues are not equally sensitive to the radiation damages. The body cells which are actively cycling (reproducing) are more sensitive to the radiation damage. The reproducing cells replicate the DNA and any lasting damage to DNA leads to the loss of propagation of correct information in the reproduced cells (daughter cells). This may cause death or mutation of the daughter cells. Lymphocytes (white blood cells) and cells which form blood (bone-morrow) are constantly regenerating and thus are most sensitive to the radiation damage. Cells in gastrointestinal tract are also regenerating and hence are also sensitive to the radiation. On the other hand, the highlyl differentiated cells like neurons are very less cycling and are relatively radio-resistant. The law of Bergonie and Tribondeau sums up this that radio-sensitivity of a tissue is directly proportional to its growth rate and indirectly proportional to its degree of differentiation.

When living cells are irradiated the cells may be damaged. These damages may be repaired by the damaged (injured) cells and the tissue or organism remain normal i.e., no effect of radiation may be observed. If damages are too high to be repaired the cells may die. In fact millions of cells in our body die a natural death daily in our body and are replaced through normal biological process of cell cycle. If radiation exposure cause sudden death of a large number of cells the radiation effect will be visible in short span of time. If the irradiated cells are of one organ the organism may die. Sometimes, the cells which are damaged during irradiation repair the damage incorrectly, i.e. misrepair the damage leading to mutation or even malignancy (cancer).

Radiation exposure may be grouped into two types: Acute Exposure and Chronic Exposure. Acute exposure is defined as large radiation dose within short span of time while Chronic Exposure is low dose protracted during long period of time. In other words, acute exposure contains high dose and dose rate (exposure per unit time) and chronic exposure entails low dose and dose rate. Acute exposure to the skin may cause local radiation burn (erythema), hair loss (epilation), peeling of skin (desquamation, dry and wet) and blistering. Acute exposure to gonads may cause temporary or permanent sterility depending upon the doses. Acute exposure to eye lens may cause cataract. On the other hand chronic exposure does not show acute effects. It is to point-out here that acute exposure may also cause cancer and genetic effects in addition to acute effects. When a person or organism is exposed with large radiation doses in short duration the radiation effects appear immediately (acute or prompt effect). On the other hand, the chronic exposure leads to delayed effects which may take months and years to manifest. For example, the data from Hiroshima and Nagasaki Atom Bomb survivors show the peak incidence of leukemia at about 7 years after the exposure while other cancers peaked at about 38 years after the exposure. Cancer induction is a delayed effect of radiation exposure.

Oxygen Enhancement Ratio

The outcome of the irradiation of a living being is determined by many factors like the total dose delivered and the organ (part or whole body) involved in the exposure. Certain tissues (cells) may be more sensitive due to their high turn-around rate (fast growing or cycling cells). Similarly, well-oxygenated cells or cells with good supply of the blood are also vulnerable to the radiation effects since interaction of radiation with water and oxygen produces far more number of free radicals which damage the cells indirectly. This increased sensitivity of cells to radiation in the presence of oxygen may be measured by Oxygen Enhancement Ratio (OER) which is the ratio of radiation dose during the lack of oxygen (hypoxia) and the radiation dose in presence of oxygen for the same biological effect. Effect of oxygenation is more pronounced for low LET (Linear Energy Transfer) radiation or low ionising density radiation like X-rays, beta and gamma rays. The OER for most mammalian cells for low LET radiation is 2 to 4 while that for high LET (like alpha) it is 1. The cancer tumor is generally comprised of anoxic cells at the core and rapidly dividing and well-oxygenated cells at the outer-layer. The radiation treatment (radiotherapy) of the tumor kills the outer cells more effectively causing the tumor to shrink in size. If any massive dose to eliminate the whole tumor is given it might kill the patient. Instead, smaller daily doses are given to the cancer patients which kills the fast dividing tumor cells but provides healthy tissues a chance to recover. Again, hyperbaric oxygen can enhance the damage of hypoxic core of the tumor. Similarly, locally created hypoxia (like by using a tourniquet) may protect irradiated tissue.

Stochastic and Nonstochastic (Deterministic) Effects

The effect of radiation can be broadly classified as stochastic and deterministic effect. Stochastic effects are observed at low doses and these effects have no threshold. At low radiation dose the probability of occurrences of stochastic effect is low. As the dose increases the probability of occurrence of stochastic effect also increases. There is a linear relationship between absorbed dose and probability of effect. Examples of stochastic effects include hereditary effects and cancers. Cancer (which includes leukemia) and genetic effects follow linear nonthreshold dose response relationship.

Deterministic effects start after the absorption of certain amount of dose. It has a threshold, once the absorbed dose crosses the threshold these effects appear in all exposed subjects, and as the absorbed dose increases, the severity of the effect also increases. Examples of deterministic (also called nonstochastic) effects are various somatic effects including skin erythema, epilation, cataracts, impaired fertility etc. The threshold for skin effect is above 2 Gy.

Deterministic effects	Stochastic effects
Deterministic effects have a threshold of radiation dose below which no effect occurs	Stochastic effects have no threshold dose and hence may occur even at low loses
As the radiation dose increases over the threshold the severity of effects (worse outcome) increases	The probability of occurrence of effect increases with the radiation dose
All people who are exposed with the radiation dose exceeding the threshold dose would suffer with the deterministic effects	Only a portion of the exposed population (determined by the probability) will develop the effects. There is no severity linked with the radiation dose
Different effects, organs and population have different threshold doses	The value of probability for different stochastic effects and for different population may be different
All early effects and most normal tissue late effects are deterministic	Generally low doses carry the risk of stochastic effects only. Stochastic effects are delayed effects
Some examples of deterministic effects: • *Irradiation of Skin (acute) leads to*: - Transient Erythema at about 2 Gy - Fixed (main) Erythema at about 6 Gy - Temporary Epilation at about 3 Gy • Fixed epilation at about 7 Gy - Dry desquamation at about 14 Gy	*Examples of stochastic effects*: Cancer induction and hereditary effects of irradiation are stochastic effects. Hereditary effects are also celled
- Moist desquamation at about 18 Gy - Secondary ulceration at about 24 Gy • *Irradiation of gonads (male) leads to*: - Sterility (temporary) at about 2 Gy - Sterility (permanent) at about 4 Gy • *Irradiation of lens of the eye leads to*: - Cataract at about 2 Gy	genetic effects where mutations in the reproductive cells pass on to the off-spring (next generation) of the exposed individual
Deterministic effects are the result of the killing of a large number of cells by the radiation	Stochastic effects stem from the mutations and replication of the mutated cells. They may arise from single or small number of cells
Deterministic effects mostly occur at or after 500 mSv. For in-utero exposure, the deterministic effects occur only after 100 mSv	There is no such dose threshold for stochastic effects and may occur at low as well as high doses. However, low dose entail low probability and high dose has high probability for the incidence of stochastic effect

Dose and Dose-rate Effects

The biological effects of radiation dose and relationship between the radiation effects (consequences) and the corresponding radiation doses is called dose-response relationship. The reliable radiation dose-response is available only for larger radiation doses. However, it is the low dose and dose-rate which we encounter in our day-to-day life. Therefore, International Commission on Radiological Protection (ICRP) suggests to extrapolate the high radiation dose-response to the low dose by using Dose and Dose Rate Effectiveness Factor (DDREF). It is generally considered that if the effects are to be extrapolated from high dose and dose rate to the commonly encountered low dose and dose rate scenario it will lead to over-estimation of the effects (response). ICRP 103 (2007) recommends a DDREF of 2 for solid tumors for the exposures with photons and electrons which are sparsely ionising radiations. Therefore, ICRP 2007 stipulates that the risk coefficient has to be divided by 2 if the dose and dose-rate is low (with respect to the risk obtained at high dose and dose rate). Any dose of 100 mSv or below is taken as low dose and dose rate (may be 0.1 mGy/min) as stated by United Nations Scientific Committee on the Effects of Atomic Radiation (UNSCEAR 2012).

The radiation dose to human body and its effect can be summarized in a table as follows:

Radiation dose	Observable effects
0–50 mSv	None (irrespective of acute or protracted exposure)
50–100 mSv	None, might not be existing or too small to detect (irrespective of acute or protracted exposure)
100–500 mSv	Slightly increased cancer risk. Decrease in blood counts at around 500 mSv
500–1 Sv	Some observable effect may be visible in acute exposure
	Increased cancer risk over longer duration
	Above 500 mSv some changes in blood cells occur but recovers quickly
1–2 Sv	Nausea and fatigue in acute exposure
	Increased cancer risks over longer duration
2–3 Sv	Nausea and vomiting within 24–48 hours, medical attention is required
3–5 Sv	Nausea, vomiting, and diarrhea within hours, Loss of hair and appetite occurs within a week, medical attention is must, half of the population exposed will die if no medication attention is given
5–12 Sv	Death within a few days
Greater than 100 Sv	Death within few hours

Lethal Dose

The amounts of radiation dose (acute exposure) determine the outcome of the effects of the exposure. Larger doses are likely to cause larger number of causalities (killings) among their victims. For example, 1 Gy of whole body gamma dose (acute) may not result in any fatal outcome but not so for 2 Gy which may kill about 5% of exposed population. $LD_{50/60}$ indicates the Lethal Dose (LD) which may kill 50% of the exposed population within 60 days. For a healthy adult $LD_{50/60}$ is estimated between 4.5–5.4 Gy with medical support. $LD_{50/60}$ may be more than 5.4 Gy if autologous bone marrow or stem cell transplant is carried out.

Radiation Effect on Embryo

All human beings start life as a single cell that divides over and over again and grows into babies inside their mothers' bodies.

Embryo is composed of relatively few cells and has high rates of cell division and cell differentiation. Rapidly developing cells have found to be more sensitive to the radiation. Since Embryo/fetus has rapid developing cells, they are more sensitive to radiation than the adult.

Radiation produces no unique abnormalities. The effects vary with the amount of radiation dose, dose rate with which exposure has occurred and stage of development of the embryo/fetus (Table - given below). The radiation induced detriments seem to be more during organogenesis period and the early fetal period. The risk becomes comparatively less during second trimester and is considered least during third trimester. The malformations in organs in fetuses have a threshold value of 100–200 mGy during any stage of pregnancy. This 100 mGy has been suggested as the dose-limit for the decision about the medical termination of pregnancy during accidental (inadvertent) exposure of pregnancy.

Gestational age (week)	Effects of radiation exposure during pregnancy		
	Less than 50 mGy	50–100 mGy	More than 100 mGy
0–2	None	None	None
3–4	None	Probably none	Possible spontaneous abortion at very high dose
5–10	None	Uncertain	Possible malformation
11–17	None	Uncertain	Possible lowering of IQ (more than 15 points) depending upon dose. Incidence of mental retardation (more than 20%) possible depending upon dose
18–27	None	None	Reduction in IQ and mental retardation depending upon dose
>27	None	None	Neonatal death possible depending upon dose

A fetal dose of 1000 mGy is likely to kill 50% of embryos. 5000 mGy will kill 100% of human embryos or fetuses if they are less than 18 weeks of gestational age.

The risk of induction of cancer and hereditary diseases in the life later due to exposure in utero (i.e. irradiation during fetal stage) are stochastic in nature and probability for cancer and hereditary diseases increase with the radiation dose. The number of excess cancer cases (which includes leukemias and solid tumours) till 15 years of age following exposure in utero has been taken as 1 in 1700 per mGy of dose. A fetal dose of 25 mGy will make the risk of a fatal cancer double of the spontaneous risk of cancer if we consider these till the age of 15 years. 25 mGy fetal dose will increase the lifetime cancer risk by 0.5% **(Table 1)**.

In conclusion, there is not much significant increase of risk of induction of cancer in childhood among the children who may be exposed to diagnostic radiology examinations during gestation. Researchers have found about 14–40% increased risk of induction of cancer due to medical radiation but have cautioned against to take these data at face value due to limitations in the quality of the data (like small number of cases, wide confidence interval and indefinite radiation doses). However, care must be taken to prevent such accidental radiation exposure to the fetus during medical imaging.

Diagnostic Radiography in Women: Ten Day Rule to Twenty Eight Day Rule

International Commission on Radiological Protection (ICRP) recommended in 1966 that "whenever possible one should confine the radiological examination of the lower abdomen and pelvis to the ten days interval following the onset of menstruation." It was popularly named as ten days rule. The original proposal was for 14 days but was reduced to ten days to account for the variability of the human menstrual cycle. This ten days rule was devised to rule out any significant radiation dose to the fetus or embryo during radiological investigations. Later it was realized on the basis of growing evidences that the strict adherence to the ten days rule may be unnecessarily restrictive. Therefore, in 1984, ICRP recommended that radiological examinations may be carried out throughout the cycle until a period is missed. Therefore, the focus is shifted to the missed period or the possible pregnancy. When the number of cells in conceptus is small they are resistant to radiation effects and only very high dose (which are unlikely during medical imaging) may lead to failure to implant. Organogenesis starts 3–5 weeks post-conception and may have a threshold of radiation dose. Therefore, it was concluded that if there is missed period the woman should be considered pregnant unless proved otherwise and in such situation alternative method of imaging should be explored.

Radiation Dose to Eye Lens and Dose Limit

Irradiation of the lens of the eye may induce opacification or clouding of the lens resulting into the loss of vision several years after the radiation exposure. The radiation induced damages to lens depends upon the dose, type of the radiation, the way the radiation has been delivered, the genetic predisposition of the exposed individual and the location of the opacity in the lens. The opacity of the lens or clouding of lens of the eye which obstructs the passage of light is called cataract. Cataract may be mainly of three types depending upon its anatomical location in the lens. Cortical cataract is formed in the cortex of the lens which is the outside edge of the lens. Nuclear Cataract is found in the central portion of the lens. Posterior Subcapsular Cataract (PSC) is formed at the back of the lens and it is beneath the lens capsule (subcapsular). The lens capsule is a small sac (or membrane) which encloses the lens and holds it in its position. Radiation exposures have been found to induce cortical cataract and PSC. The earlier occupational dose limit of equivalent dose to the lens of eye was 150 mSv in a year and this limit was based on our understanding of the threshold dose for the induction of cataract at 5 Gy for single acute exposure and 8 Gy for the protracted exposure. The inadequacy of these observations which included insufficient follow-up, less accurate radiation dosimetry, not-so-perfect detection techniques and inadequate documentation of the radiation induced changes in lens became apparent in later years with the availability of the improved epidemiology and sensitivity to detect early changes in lens due to lower radiation doses. In April 2011, International Commission on Radiological Protection (ICRP) issued a statement revising the equivalent dose limit for eye lens to 20 mSv in a year averaged over defined period of 5 years with no single year exceeding 50 mSv in case of occupational workers. ICRP now considers 0.5 Gy as the threshold for the lens radiation injury leading to the cataract. This threshold dose is valid even for protracted or chronic exposure. ICRP defines the threshold dose as a dose resulting in a 1% incidence of the specified reaction in the tissue or organ **(Table 2)**.

International Atomic Energy Agency (IAEA) Technical Document No. 1731 entitled "Implications for occupational radiation protection of the new dose limit for the lens of the eye" published in 2013 chronicles a few typical eye lens doses encountered in various procedures.

TABLE 1: Probability of cancer and hereditary disease for fetal irradiation.

Fetal dose (mGy)	Probability of the disease: Fatal cancer till age of 15 years	Probability of the disease: Hereditary disease
1.1	1 in 30,000	1 in 38,000
1.4	1 in 24,000	1 in 30,000
1.7	1 in 20,000	1 in 24,000
2.4	1 in 14,000	1 in 24,000
3.3	1 in 10,000	1 in 13,000
6.8	1 in 5,000	1 in 6000
25	1 in 1300	1 in 1700

TABLE 2: ICRP dose limit for eye lens in planned exposure.

Occupational exposure in adult Workers (>18 yrs)		Occupational exposure in trainee (16–18 yrs)		Public exposure	
New (2011)	Old	New (2011)	Old	New (2011)	Old
20 mSv per year averaged over 5 consecutive years and 50 mSv in any single year	150 mSv in a year	20 mSv in a year	50 mSv in a year	15 mSv in a year	15 mSv in a year

Procedure	Unshielded eye lens dose (mSv)	Shielded eye lens dose (mSv) (lead glass/ goggle)
Hepatic chemoembolization	0.27–2.1	0.016–0.064
Iliac angiography	0.25–2.2	0.015–0.066
Neuroembolization (head, spine)	1.4 –11	0.083–0.34
Pulmonary angiography	0.19–1.5	0.011–0.045
TIPS creation	0.41–3.7	0.025–0.11
Cerebral angiography	0.046 (mean)	0.013–0.025
Endovascular aneurysm repair	0.010 (mean)	
Urology	0.026 (mean)	
Orthopedic	0.05	
Hysterosalpingography	0.14 (mean)	
Endoscopic retrograde Cholangiopancreatography (X-ray tube undercouch)	0.094 (mean)	
Endoscopic retrograde cholangiopancreatography (X-ray tube overcouch)	0.55 (mean) 2.8 (maximum)	

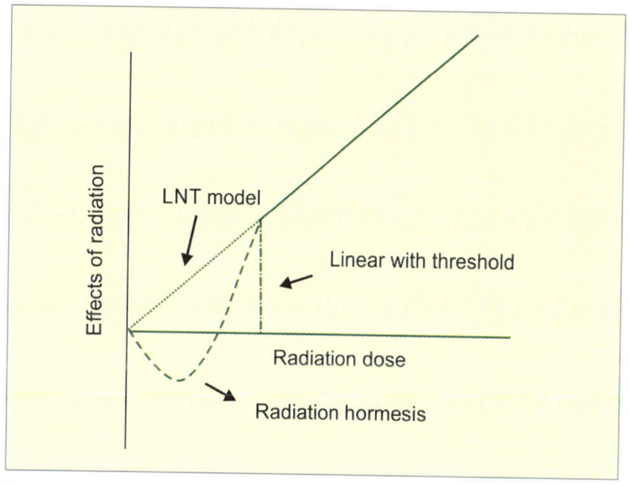

FIG. 1: Various hypotheses of low level radiation dose and its effect.

Protection of Patient, Staff, and Public from Radiation

Radiation Risk

Radiation risk calculation are based on the type of radiation, amount of energy absorbed, and which part of the body these energies is deposited. For example, certain amount of radiation energy deposited to the wrist has really no effect, however similar amount of energy deposited to blood forming organ may have an effect. One of worth-notable effect of low dose radiation which we come across in diagnostic and therapeutic radiological investigations is probability of cancer induction. The probability of cancer induction is low at low dose but never zero theoretically and therefore calls for the optimisation of radiation doses for all radiological investigations. One should keep in mind that it is not possible to differentiate or detect the cancer caused by diagnostic X-rays from cancer caused by other factors such as environmental, chemical or biological. The latency period of cancer induction may be in years or even in decade. This may be true for all carcinogens including radiation. This is especially true for low dose and low dose rate radiation. If the low level of radiation exposure has occurred today, its effect as a cancer may be expressed after few years of exposure.

Radiation Protection Guidelines and LNT Model

In 1950s, the scientific group created the radiation protection guidelines. At that time no one really knew the effect of low dose of radiation. It was decided to assume that the relation between the radiation dose and its effects are linear and proportional. It was also decided that any dose, no matter how small, could bring an effect. This is called a linear no threshold (LNT) model. Still this LNT model is in use to set radiation protection guidelines. Since this concept was easy to use and explain, most people presented this as a fact rather than saying that we do not know the effects of low doses of radiation or whether the low doses of radiation is safe. Effect of radiation at low doses is a controversial topic since it is difficult to get ideal epidemiological data. Cancer induction may be the only effect at low dose of radiation but there are also spontaneous incidences of cancer without radiation exposure (due to various other environmental carcinogens and biological factors). Such comparison demands similar control and study group in terms of life style, socioeconomic status, environment, age, sex, etc. except in radiation exposure history. Obviously it is hard to meet this ideal situation. Ubiquitous background radiation is another confounding factor which exposes all people living on this planet all the time with on an average 2–3 mSv (milli Sievert) annual dose. On the other hand there are researchers and their preliminary experimental results which may indicate about the existence of beneficial effect of low level radiation (called radiation hormesis) **(Fig. 1)**. At present it is thought prudent to consider low level radiation having linear relationship with risk (without having any threshold of a minimum dose) which signifies that even low level radiation entails some risk.

Every country has a regulatory authority to set the guidelines regarding radiation protection, make laws and to enforce them. These guidelines are based on LNT model and made in such a way that if followed properly, patient, staff and public all are protected. We must obey them. Atomic Energy Regulatory Board (AERB), Mumbai is the competent authority to enforce radiation safety in practice in India.

The first principle of radiation protection for the patient is justification.

Justification

X-ray examination should be undertaken only when there is medical question which need to be answered, the amount of benefit which patient is going to receive in comparison to the risk associated with this X-ray examination is high, and the information needed cannot be answered by any other investigation involving nonionizing radiation. In such condition, we say that X-ray examination is justified.

Some Facts that can help in Protecting Staff Patients and Public from Radiation

- X-rays are produced, emitted in isotropic direction; X-ray tube is shielded to protect patient and staff operating the machine.
- X-rays produced from the X-ray machine have a mixture of continuous spectrum starting from zero to maximum energy (equal to the kVp applied) and characteristic spectrum. If the spectrum is not filtered, the low energy X-rays (also called soft X-rays) will be absorbed completely on superficial organs of the patient body and contribute the patient dose; however these X-rays will not contribute in the image formation. X-rays are passed through the filter to remove these soft X-rays. Application of additional filter reduces the patient dose significantly.
- The X-rays emitted from the X-ray tube and directed towards the patient body are called primary X-rays. When these primary X-rays interact with the patient body, as a result of interaction scattered radiation are emitted in all direction.
- The energy of scattered radiation is almost equal to the primary radiation (a few keV less than the primary radiation). So it is most likely that the person standing in the room while X-rays are being energized will receive radiation exposure from the secondary radiation emitted from the patient body as a result of scattering.
- In case of overcouch X-ray tube, the radiologist will receive maximum exposure to the face, because scattered X-rays from the patients are directed towards the face. In under couch X-ray tube, the scattered radiations are directed towards the legs. Therefore, lead rubber flaps can be used to protect legs. Goggles must be used to protect the eyes.
- The lead apron of 0.25–0.50 mm Pb equivalent is worn by the radiologist to protect them from the secondary scattered radiation. In the interventional procedures they have to wear it for a longer duration. Due to prolonged time period of wearing the lead apron, some orthopedic problems of spinal injury have been reported in the literature for the interventional radiologist. Therefore, it is important (for both the radiologist and patient's viewpoint) that interventional radiological procedures or radiation related procedures will only be adopted when there is no other option available. Now a days, vest-skirt type lead aprons are available which shifts weight of the skirt apron at the waist.
- Lead free aprons incorporating Tungsten, Antimony and Bismuth or Barium, Aluminum, Tin, Titanium, Bismuth are available in the market. These aprons are environment friendly and recyclable as well. Lead is toxic and therefore, disposal of lead aprons needs proper care. It is desirable to check the protection/attenuation efficiency offered by these new lead-free protection aprons before it is put to use. Lead free aprons may offer the weight which is 20–40% lesser than that of conventional lead apron.
- Radiation burns (Radiation hazards) are different than the burn by the fire and hence requires specific expertise and experience to treat such cases. Radiation burns have been reported in the literature during the interventional fluoroscopic examinations. This needs to be prevented.

Since X-rays have high penetrating power, X-ray machines are needed to be installed in room having sufficient wall thickness such that outside the room the radiation penetrating through the wall must not exceed the limit set for public exposure. The entry of public or attendants is not allowed in the X-ray room while X-rays are being energized. There must be some warning signal displayed outside the X-ray room so that public must know that X-rays are being produced here. Public must know that X-rays beam is ON. The wooden door of the X-ray room must have sufficient lead shielding.

Cardinal principle of radiation protection is distance, time and shielding. The dose from the X-ray beam diminishes with the square of its distance from the source. This law is known as inverse square law. If the distance from the source is doubled, the dose reduces by one-fourth. So, one should maintain the maximum distance from the source to reduce dose. Radiation dose is directly proportional to the time duration spent with the source. It indicates to complete the job quickly (i.e. efficiency in job). By interposing shielding between the source and detector, the radiation dose decreases. One HVL (Half-value Layer) of a shielding material like lead, concrete or brick is the thickness of the material which when interspersed will attenuate the radiation to half.

General dose Reduction Measures that can be Adopted to Reduce Patient doses are:

- Increasing the distance between X-ray tube and patient helps to reduce dose. Doubling the distance will make the dose one-fourth.
- Collimation at the target/patient's body reduces dose and improves image quality also due to lesser scattering.
- Compression of the body reduces the thickness of the body and hence volume of irradiation. Amount of scattering is directly proportional to the volume of irradiated tissue. Therefore, compression of body reduces the amount of scattering and improves image contrast. With reduced thickness lower radiation dose is absorbed inside the body. That is why breast is compressed during mammography.
- Antiscatter grids are located between the patient and the image intensifier, or cassette or digital detector. Grids absorb most of the scatter radiation. Higher the grid ratio, better is the image quality but higher is the radiation dose to the patient. So, an optimum value of grid ratio needs to be selected. 8:1 for radiography and 5:1 for mammography is optimum. In radiography of children one may remove the grid since there is less scatter anyway due to smaller body volume of the children. Removing grid will enable the radiographer to reduce the radiographic parameters and hence reduce the dose to the pediatric cases.
- With increase in kVp, penetrating power of X-ray beam increases. It will deposit less amount of energy inside the patient body during radiography and hence the patient

dose will reduce. However, this will reduce the contrast in the image. In CT, higher kVp increases the patients' dose.

- X-ray beam contains both soft and hard X-rays. When X-ray beam is allowed to pass through the filter made of copper and aluminum the filter will attenuate the soft X-rays and allow the hard X-rays to pass through. Soft X-rays get absorbed on superficial organs and contribute to absorbed radiation dose and do not take part in the image formation. There is regulatory limit of minimum 2.5 mm aluminum total equivalent filtration to be present in X-ray beam in all radiography machines having 100 kVp or more.
- X-ray machines are available with automatic exposure timing control facility called automatic exposure control (AEC). These sensors monitors the transmitted X-ray from the patients, when amount of X-ray beam required for an optimum image quality is reached, it automatically turns off the X-ray beam falling on the patient body. In this way, it ensures the smallest amount of radiation have been administered to patient.
- Table top material should not absorb much radiation as the X-ray passes through it before reaching to patient/detector. However, it should be strong enough to carry the bulky patients. Carbon fiber has been proven to be the best material for X-ray system table top.
- Pulsed fluoroscopy reduces the dose to patients and staff significantly in interventional fluoroscopy. In pulse fluoroscopy the X-ray is emitted in pulses instead of continuous exposure. This effectively reduces the total time of emission of X-rays. Fifteen frames per second reduces radiation dose by about 25% while 7.5 frames per second may reduce the radiation dose to half. However, very low frame rate may lead to choppy image especially during imaging of a moving organ. Modern technology uses digital refresh memory to digitize the last image and showing it in the gap time of two consecutive X-ray pulses unless next pulse refreshes the image. This reduces the flickering of the image on monitor when very low frame rate pulse fluoroscopy is operated.

We need to quantify the damage created by the ionizing radiation. Following radiation units are used in radiology.

Radioactivity

Despite the strength of the forces that hold nucleons together to form an atomic nucleus, many nuclides are unstable and spontaneously change into other nuclides by radioactive decay. The phenomenon of radioactivity was discovered in 1896 by Antoine-Henri Becquerel. He demonstrated that uranium emits radiation without external source of energy. The emitted radiations had characteristics similar to X-rays, and were also deflected by a magnetic field. He was awarded the 1903 Nobel Prize for physics for his discovery, which he shared with Marie Curie and Pierre Curie. Marie Curie further investigated the phenomenon of radioactivity.

The activity of a sample of any radionuclide is the rate at which the nuclei of its constituent's atoms decay. If N is the number of nuclei present in the sample at a certain time, its activity R is given by

$$R = \frac{dN}{dt}$$

The minus sign is used to make R a positive quantity since dN/dt is intrinsically negative. The SI unit of activity is Becquerel.

$$1\ Becquerel = 1\ Bq = \frac{1\ decay}{Second}$$

The traditional unit of activity is the curie (Ci), which is defined as the activity of 1 gram of radium $^{226}_{88}Ra$.

$$1\ Ci = 3.7 \times 10^{10}\ decays\ per\ second = 3.7 \times 10^{10}\ dps$$

Question. Cabalt-60 (Co^{60}) has half life of 5.26 years. Let's suppose that we have 5 grams of Co^{60} in our radioisotope laboratory. Calculate its activity in Becquerel (Bq) and Curie (Ci).

$$\text{Activity} = \lambda N = \frac{0.693 \times N}{T_{½}} = \frac{0.693 \times 5\text{ gram}}{5.26\text{ years}}$$

$$= \frac{0.693 \times 5\text{ gram}}{5.26\text{ years}}$$

$$= \frac{0.693 \times 5\text{ gram}}{5.26 \times 365\text{ days}}$$

$$= \frac{0.693 \times 5\text{ gram}}{5.26 \times 365 \times 24\text{ hours}}$$

$$= \frac{0.693 \times 5\text{ gram}}{5.26 \times 365 \times 24 \times 60 \times 60\text{ seconds}}$$

$$= \frac{0.693 \times 5\text{ gram}}{5.26 \times 31536000\text{ sec}} \times \frac{1\text{ mol}}{59.9\text{ gram}} \times \frac{6.02 \times 10^{23}\text{ atoms}}{1\text{ mol}} \times \frac{1\text{ disintegration}}{1\text{ atom}}$$

$$= 2.10 \times 10^{14}\text{ disintegration per second (dps)}$$

$$= 2.10 \times 10^{14}\text{ Bq (since 1 Bq} = 1\text{ dps).}$$

$$= \frac{2.10 \times 10^{14}\text{ dps}}{3.7 \times 10^{11}\text{ dps}} \times 1\text{ Ci (Since 1 Ci} = 3.7 \times 10^{11}\text{ dps)}$$

$$= 5.7 \times 10^{2}\text{ Ci}$$

Radiation Units

When X-rays used in medical imaging interacts with any medium (human body or material like cassette, imaging plate, film, etc.), it transfers energy to the medium. This energy transfer is influenced by many factors. It is important to understand its nitty-gritty since risk to radiation has to be defined on the basis of the energy transfer pattern between interacting radiation and the medium it traverses through.

Fluence

X-ray may be thought of consisting of stream of energy packets (particles like) called X-ray photons. The stream of X-ray photons is called "X-ray fluence" which is defined as number of X-ray photons passing through per unit area when the area is perpendicular to the direction of photon stream.

$$\text{Hence, X-ray fluence} = \frac{\text{Number of photons}}{\text{Area of cross-section}}$$

Unit for fluence is cm^{-2}.

Flux

X-ray flux is defined as the X-ray fluence per unit time. In other words, number of X-ray photons passing through per unit area per unit time is called flux. It may be seen that flux is nothing but fluence rate which is fluence per unit time.

$$\text{X-ray flux} = \frac{\text{Number of photons}}{\text{Area}} \times \frac{1}{\text{Time}}$$

In fluoroscopy the concept of flux is important since radiation is "on" for longer time.

Energy Fluence

It is defined as amount of energy passing through unit area. If we know the energy of each X-ray photon the energy fluence may be defined as:

Energy fluence = Fluence × Energy of each X-ray photon

Since X-ray photons from X-ray tube are polyenergetic, therefore mean energy of X-ray photons have to be considered while calculating energy fluence.

$$\text{Mean energy of X-ray photons} = \frac{\text{Total energy of photons}}{\text{Number of photons}}$$

Energy fluence

$$= \frac{\text{Number of photons}}{\text{Area}} \times \frac{\text{Total energy of photons}}{\text{Number of photons}}$$

$$= \frac{\text{Energy}}{\text{Area}}$$

The energy of X-ray photon is in terms of keV.

(The maximum energy of X-rays photons is the maximum potential applied across cathode-anode in X-ray tube by selecting tube voltage at control console in terms of kVp).

Energy fluence has unit keV per Cm^2 which may be written as $keVCm^{-2}$.

Exposure

Exposure is defined as electrical charge produced by ionization created by the incident X-rays (radiation) in unit mass of air.

$$\text{Exposure} = \frac{\text{Amount of charge produced}}{\text{Irradiated mass of air}}$$

$$= \frac{\text{Charge}}{\text{Mass}}$$

$$= \frac{\text{Coulomb}}{\text{kg}} \text{ (SI unit)}$$

Traditional unit is Roentgen (R) which is defined as

$1 \text{ R} = 2.58 \times 10^{-4}$ Coulomb/kg of air

Or, 3876 R = 1 Coulomb/kg of air

The exposure rate is expressed in R/hr or mR/min.

R is valid for X-rays and gamma rays with energy up to 3 MeV. It is to note that the exposure and its unit R take care of the interaction of X-rays and gamma rays with air only.

Exposure is not applicable to electrons, beta or any charged particle. Exposure may be measured using ionization chamber. Since, there is not much difference between effective atomic number of air and soft tissue for the diagnostic range of energy, the absorbed dose to air or soft tissue may be regarded same. The concept of absorbed dose is for material.

Absorbed Dose

Absorbed dose indicates the amount of energy deposited by interacting ionization radiation (X-rays, gamma rays, electrons, beta, neutrons, alpha, protons, all radiation) with unit mass of matter.

$$\text{Absorbed dose} = \frac{\text{Amount of energy deposited}}{\text{Mass of matter}}$$

The unit of absorbed dose is Joule per kilogram ($J\ kg^{-1}$) and a special name has been given to this in SI unit is Gray.

1 Gray (Gy) = 1 Joule/kg

The traditional unit of absorbed dose is rad (Radiation absorbed dose)

1 Gy = 100 rad

1 rad = 0.01 Gy = 0.01 Joule/kg

The conversion factor between "Exposure" and "Absorbed dose" is called Roentgen to rad Conversion Factor (or F factor)

$$F = \frac{\text{Absorbed dose (rad)}}{\text{Roentgen (R)}}$$

F is defined as the absorbed dose in rad for a matter per Roentgen exposure for a given energy. For diagnostic energy range the F factor is about 1 for soft tissue and it signifies that for keV range R and rad is approximately same. However, value of 'F' for bone in keV range of X-rays is about 4 and this shows that bone absorbs about 4 times more dose than soft tissue due to predominant photoelectric effect at lower energy which increases with substance of high atomic number (like bone with respect to soft tissue).

The relation between absorbed dose to air and exposure is:

Dose to air (mGy) = 8.76 × Exposure (R)

1 R deposits 0.877 rad to dry air. This dose to air or air dose may also be equated with air kerma. The unit for air kerma is gray (Gy). Air kerma in air is the sum of kinetic energy of all charged particles generated when X-rays and gamma rays pass through unit mass of air.

Kerma

The ionizing radiation may be of two types, directly ionizing and indirectly ionizing. Directly ionizing radiations are those which carry charge with it (like alpha, electrons and beta). Directly ionizing radiation interacts with the electron of the atom of the medium through columbic forces. Indirectly ionizing radiation does not carry any charge and includes neutron, X-rays and gamma rays. The indirectly ionizing radiation deposits energy in the medium through two steps. In the first step, the interacting X-rays (or gamma and neutron) deliver/provides kinetic energy to the electrons of the medium through photoelectric, compton or pair production processes depending upon the energy of the incident X-rays. The electrons so produced are directly ionizing and in step two, they deposit their energy in the medium through the process of ionization and excitation. In some cases, where the range of such electrons is sufficiently high, some electrons may escape the medium.

The kerma stands for the kinetic energy released in the medium and is defined as total initial kinetic energy of all charge particles (electrons) relcased in the medium by the interacting X-ray (indirectly ionizing radiation) in a given mass. Kerma defines the above step one.

$$\text{Kerma (K)} = \frac{E_{tr}}{m}$$

E_{tr} = Sum of kinetic energy of electrons produced

m = Mass of the medium

Unit of kerma is joule/kg which is the unit for dose as well. SI unit for kerma is Gray (Gy) and traditional unit is rad. Kerma is defined for X-ray, gamma ray and neutrons only.

The kerma may be considered made of two parts, collision part and radiative part. When the electrons are liberated by the incident X-ray on the medium of low atomic number (air, water, soft tissue) the majority of these electrons expend their energy during interaction with the orbital electrons of the atoms of the medium. A very small part of liberated electrons may interact with the nuclei of the atoms of the medium giving off Bremsstrahlung X-rays (radiative part). If the energy transferred by the incident X-rays to the liberated electrons in the medium is deposited locally and Bremsstrahlung loses (radiative lose) is negligible, the absorbed dose equals to kerma. For diagnostic energy range absorbed dose equals to kerma. At higher energy of incident X-rays and gamma rays radiative loss is not negligible.

The quantity "Exposure" indicates the amount of ionization in air due to radiation interaction while radiation dose (or called radiation absorbed dose) refers the amount of radiation energy deposited to the medium (may be patient's body) with which the radiation (X-ray) has interacted. The term "Radiation Exposure" and "Radiation Dose" are many times used interchangeably especially in case of medical imaging where energy of X-rays used is in kilo-voltage range. Generally "Exposure" is measured using ionization chamber or any suitable measuring device while "Dose" is calculated from exposure and energy absorbed by X-rays per unit mass of the body.

Equivalent Dose

Equivalent dose may also be called radiation protection unit as it takes into account the potential of the radiation to cause biological damage. The ability to cause biological damage (effectiveness) varies with the type of radiation and is closely related with its ionizing capability. Various types of radiation has been assigned a "quality factor" which, though arbitrary chosen, may be linked with its relative biological effectiveness (RBE) related to linear energy transfer (LET) of radiation. The quality factor is called radiation weighing factor (W_R). W_R for X-rays, gamma rays, beta and electrons are 1, protons (>2 meV) has 5, neutrons (depending upon energy) has 5–20 and alpha particles W_R are 20.

Equivalent dose = Absorbed dose × W_R

The traditional unit for equivalent dose is Rem and the SI unit is Sievert (Sv). For X-rays W_R = 1 and hence, 1 mGy = 1 mSv.

Effective Dose

Radiosensitivity of various tissues is different. Therefore, radiation induced effect in different tissues are likely to be different even for similar equivalent dose for these tissues. Tissue have been assigned a tissue weighting factor (W_T) which represents the detriment (risk) of the radiation exposure to that tissue with respect to the uniform whole body radiation exposure. Bone marrow, colon, lung, breast, stomach each have been given W_T at 0.12, gonads at 0.08, bladder, liver esophagus and thyroid at 0.04, skin bone surface, brain and salivary glands have been given 0.01.

Effective dose = Σ Equivalent dose × W_T

Effective dose may be defined as sum of weighted radiation equivalent dose to various tissues/organs.

Effective dose has similar units as that of equivalent dose, i.e. traditional unit is Rem and SI unit is Sievert (Sv).

Radiation Dose Measurement in CT

The radiography is a projection imaging while CT scanner is a cross-sectional imaging. In the former, the radiation enters single body surface and maximum dose was delivered to the skin at the entrance. This measurement in case of radiography was called entrance skin dose (ESD). The ESD depends upon kV and mAs set on the control panel of the radiography machine. In contrast, radiation enters the body from all direction as X-ray tube revolves around the patient during exposure in CT scan. It makes the measurement of dose complex due to presence of significant amount of scatter dose and transmitted radiation when the X-ray tube is not directly over the point of measurement. Due to narrow collimation and requirement of good image, the mAs used in CT scanner are much higher than that in radiography. CT doses are measured in cylindrical phantom made of acrylic (or PMMA) with holes at center and periphery for placing ionization chambers **(Fig. 2)**. The body phantom has a diameter of 32 cm and head phantom has a diameter of 16 cm. Both phantoms have a length of 15 cm in Z-axis. The holes with diameter of 1 cm are made at 12, 3, 6, and 9 o'clock positions and are provided with well-fitted acrylic plug to fill the gap (hole) when not in use (by ionization chamber).

Computed Tomography Dose Index

Computed tomography dose index (CTDI) was originally planned as an index of dose and not a real patient dose. However, later CT dosimetry method for patient dosimetry was based upon CTDI. The $CTDI_{100}$ is a dose measured in a 100 mm

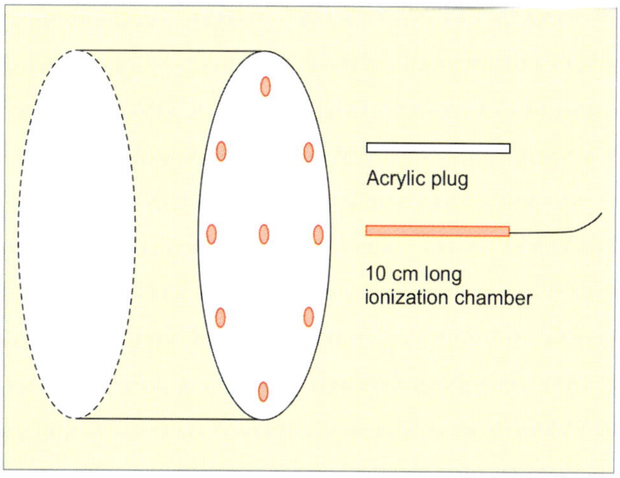

FIG. 2: CTDI phantom with chamber.

long cylindrical ionization chamber when the chamber is placed in CT scanner at its isocenter. The ionization chamber is aligned (its long axis) with the axis of the patient couch (i.e. Z-axis). One single axial scan is performed at the center of the ionization chamber without movement of the table.

$$CTDI_{100} = \frac{1}{\text{Beam width}} \times \int_{1=+50\text{ mm}}^{1=+50\text{ mm}} D(z).dz$$

D(z) = Radiation dose profile along Z-axis

The single axial scan at the center of the chamber with its beam width (i.e. in MDCT it is the product of number of channels and the size of the detector in channel) opened causes collection of charges created in ionization chamber, 50 mm on either side of its center due to scatter radiation along the Z-axis as well. Beam width may be denoted as NT where N is number of tomographic sections imaged or number of data channel used and T is the width of tomographic section along the Z-axis imaged by single data channel. For $CTDI_w$, the measurement of $CTDI_{100}$ is done at central and peripheral holes of the cylindrical acrylic (or PMMA) phantom.

$CTDI_w$ is a weighted measurement of $CTDI_{100}$

CTDI depends upon the field of view (FOV). Doses at the periphery and center of the phantom (i.e. $CTDI_{100,\ center}$ and $CTDI_{100,\ periphery}$) are not equal. CTDI at surface may be double of that at center. The average $CTDI_{100}$ which represents average dose to phantom has been termed as $CTDI_{weighted}$ or $CTDI_w$.

$CTDI_w = 1/3\ CTDI_{100,\ center} + 2/3\ CTDI_{100,\ periphery}$

In real work, we use CT scanner for series of slices or scans. These slices may be at gap, contiguous or overlapped. $CTDI_{volume}$ describes the dose to phantom in CT scan with series of slices and abbreviated as $CTDI_{vol}$.

$$CTDI_{vol} = \frac{1}{\text{Pitch}} \times CTDI_{100}$$

Pitch is defined in helical or spiral CT scanning as distance travelled by patient table in gantry (mm) during a full rotation of X-ray tube around the patient or phantom for unit beam width (NT) in mm.

$$\text{Pitch} = \frac{\text{Table moveme nt per axial scan (mm)}}{\text{Nominal beam width (NT) (mm)}}$$

$CTDI_{vol}$ represents the average radiation dose to phantom during scan and is reported on CT console for specific scan protocol. These values have been fed by the manufacturer after carrying out the measurement in phantom using specific scan protocol.

DLP is dose length product which is the product of $CTDI_{vol}$ and length of the CT scan.

$$DLP = CTDI_{vol} \times \text{Scan length}$$

The unit for $CTDI_{vol}$ is mGy. It should be noted that $CTDI_{vol}$ though represents average radiation dose to phantom but may be substantially different for a phantom which has different size from the phantom used in measurement. $CTDI_{vol}$ is independent of the length of the scan, i.e. coverage of scan. However, DLP takes length of scan into account. AAPM report 204 provides conversion factor for $CTDI_{vol}$ for different sizes of phantom which is called size specific dose estimates (SSDE). These factors may help us in arriving near the real doses involves in CT scan.

Size Specific Dose Estimate in CT Imaging

In recent time the use of CT imaging in patients has risen dramatically making it one of the most used imaging modalities. The CT imaging offers excellent images with cross-sectional slices which are quick and economical with respect to other advanced imaging modalities (like MRI). However, radiation dose delivered to the patient during the CT scan is an issue. In 2006 for US population, it was generally estimated that CT accounts for 12% of the imaging procedures using ionising radiation but contributed 46% of the collective dose. However, the method of dosimetry in CT scan is not straightforward and hence it is difficult to measure individual absorbed radiation dose and hence the health risk it poses. Even Effective Dose is not a proper parameter as this is derived in a phantom that adds relative weighting of radiosensitive organs. Effective dose represents the dose to the population and not the individual. Similarly Computed Tomography Dose Index (CTDI) and its derivative $CTDI_{vol}$ quantify the CT X-ray output and not the radiation dose to the patient in a CT scan. CTDI dose parameters have been defined for cylindrical phantoms of specified sizes (16 and 32 cm diameters) and made of PMMA (polymethyl methacrylate or acrylic). The radiation doses absorbed by the patient during CT scan does not depend upon the $CTDI_{vol}$ but on the size of the patient as well as on the attenuation of X-rays in the patients. Patients with different body size may absorb different radiation dose even if $CTDI_{vol}$ is same. For example, in a CT scanner if parameters selected remains same (e.g. 120 kVp and 200 mAs) the $CTDI_{vol}$ measured in a 32 cm phantom will remain same while in reality, the patient scanned at these parameters, if smaller than 32 cm diameter, will absorb more radiation dose than $CTDI_{vol}$ measured in the phantom (of diameter 32 cm). This may be checked by taking phantoms of 10 cm diameter, 16 cm diameter and 32 cm diameter and may be illustrated as below.

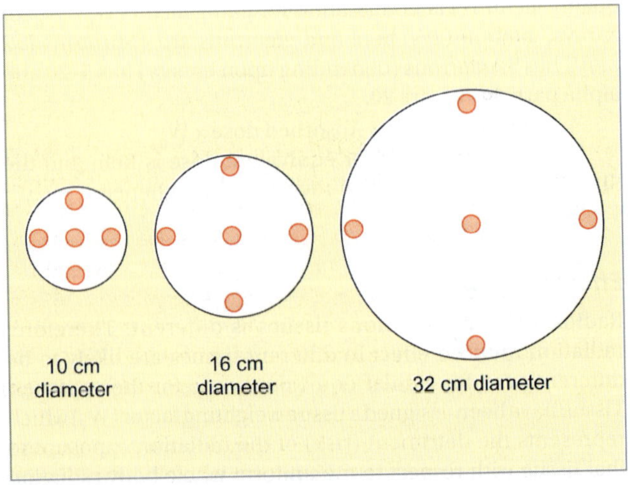

Cylindrical phantom diameter	Central hole dose	Peripheral hole dose	$CTDI_{vol}$
10 cm	47 mGy	47 mGy	47 mGy
16 cm	37 mGy	38 mGy	37 mGy
32 cm	10.8 mGy	21.6 mGy	18 mGy

The above sample table illustrates that if diameter of the phantom becomes half (from 32 cm to16 cm) $CTDI_{vol}$ increases by twice (from 18 mGy to 37 mGy). It is due to the fact that as the phantom becomes smaller the dose at central and peripheral holes become higher but dose at central hole increases much faster due to lesser attenuation of X-rays in the smaller phantom material. CT scanner always displays $CTDI_{vol}$ measured in 32 cm diameter cylindrical phantom whenever the operator chooses the scanning of the torso (body) irrespective of the real diameter of the patients. This may be even true for the torso of the pediatric cases as well.

To account this variation of patient dose with the variation in the size of the patient American Association of Physicists in Medicine (AAPM) came up with a Report No. 204 entitled "Size Specific Dose Estimates in Pediatric and Adult Body CT Examinations" in 2011 and suggested the conversion factors to translate $CTDI_{vol}$ measurements to the true measurements of the radiation dose on the basis of the thickness of the patient's body. In fact, AAPM Report 204 which is freely available in the internet, details the formation of four teams to investigate the question. Two teams used empirical methods of measurement of dose in cylindrical and orthomorphic phantom while other two teams attempted Monte Carlo simulations. Despite their varied techniques the coefficient arrived at by them were remarkably close. AAPM Report 204 proposed many descriptors for the patient's dimension including anterior-posterior (AP) dimension, lateral (LAT) dimension, combination of two AP+LAT and $(AP.LAT)^{1/2}$ (i.e. $\sqrt{AP}.\sqrt{LAT}$). The last parameter was called effective diameter. The effective diameter is the diameter of the patient which corresponds to a circle having an area equal to that of the patient at a given location. These dimensions may be measured at mid level either from CT topogram (or CT localizer radiography or scout view). They may also be measured by the physical calipers. AAPM Report No. 204 provides tables which gives a conversion factor F_{size}. When F_{size} is multiplied with $CTDI_{vol}$ it yields Size Specific Dose Estimate (SSDE) in terms of mGy.

$$SSDE\,(mGy) = F^{32X}_{size} \times CTDI^{32}_{vol}$$

Here, $CTDI^{32}_{vol}$ is the $CTDI_{vol}$ displayed in mGy by the CT scanner for the scan and given by the manufacturer for the body phantom of 32 cm diameter. F^{32X}_{size} is the conversion factor for 32 cm diameter reference phantom to that for a patient with known dimension. AAPM Report 204 gives conversion factor for AP, Lateral, A+P and effective diameter ($\sqrt{AP}.\sqrt{LAT}$). "x" in F^{32X}_{size} indicates that this factor should be taken from the appropriate table (out of four mentioned above). AAPM Report 204 suggests writing F^{32A}_{size} for AP, F^{32L}_{size} for lateral, F^{32S}_{size} for sum (A+P) and F^{32D}_{size} for effective diameter.

Similarly, AAPM Report 204 provides tables for F^{16X}_{size} as well which has to be used if CT scanner gives $CTDI_{vol}$ measured for 16 cm diameter phantom (i.e. $CTDI^{16}_{vol}$). The conversion factor, in general, will be more than unities (more than 1) if the effective diameters are smaller than the reference (32 cm and 16 cm respectively). AAPM Report 204 provides table for all four dimensions i.e., AP, LAT, AP+LAT and directly effective diameter $\sqrt{AP}.\sqrt{LAT}$. Depending upon the availability of the data one may use the suitable table.

One should keep in mind, however, that all tables in AAPM Report No. 204 are based upon the scan length (or phantom length) of 15–30 cm. The radiation dose to the patient during CT scan depends upon the scan length as well. Hence any scan length which is significantly different from this may lead to varied results.

Radiation Dose Measurement in Fluoroscopy

In fluoroscopy the users may use direct or indirect method of assessment of radiation dose to patient and staff. Direct method utilizes some measurement devices to be put at the point of measurement (patient's skin, at some reference point etc.) The measurement devices may be TLD, radiochromic film, MOSFET (metal-oxide-semiconductor field-effect transistor) dosimeter etc. Indirect method provides an estimate of radiation dose to patient by the direct measurement of some radiation-linked quantities (like, fluoroscopy time or dose area product i.e. DAP).

All fluoroscopy machines come equipped to measure the fluoroscopy X-ray "on" time. Fluoroscopy X-ray active time is also called "fluoroscopy time". This parameter is not good enough to provide the estimate of patient skin dose or staff dose.

Another indirect method to measure radiation dose to patient is dose area product (or kerma area product). DAP or KAP meter is a large area, flat, transparent, ionization chamber that is fitted into the collimator of X-ray tube. The X-ray passes through it and KAP meter intercepts the whole beam (X-ray field). It gives the measurement as the product of kerma and the area of the radiation beam in the unit $Gy.cm^2$ or any of its derivative like $mGy.cm^2$, $Gy.m^2$, $cGy.cm^2$ etc. This quantity is independent of distance and can be measured anywhere in the beam. This is true since as we go away from X-ray source the X-ray dose decreases with square of the distance from source (inverse square law) but area of the beam increases due to divergence, again, with square of the distance. This results in the product of radiation dose (kerma) and the X-ray field (area of the beam) to remain constant throughout the X-ray beam and hence KAP can be measured anywhere in the X-ray beam **(Fig. 3)**. KAP represents the total energy incident on the patient and hence is considered a good indicator of stochastic risk of the radiation exposure. KAP values may be used to arrive at effective dose as the conversion factor is available in literature.

The KAP takes non uniformity of the dose within the X-ray field into account like due to heel effect or due to utilization of any semitransparent shutter in any area of the field. It is easy to measure and all new fluoroscopy machines provide this data in real time. In some fluoroscopy machine, KAP may be calculated (rather measured) using generator and collimator settings. One should bear in mind that cumulative KAP reading does not indicate the risk of skin-exposure (skin burn) directly in the patient. Nonetheless, the scatter dose around the patient is largely proportional to KAP reading and hence may be a relative indicator of the radiation field around.

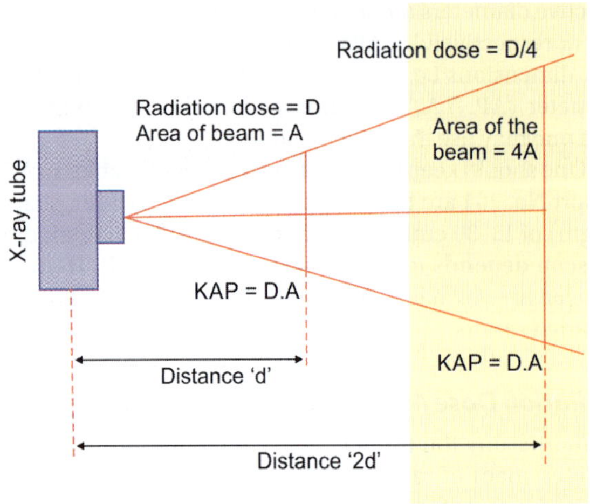

FIG. 3: Dose area product is independent of distance.

Nowadays, the fluoroscopic machines give cumulative doses at some reference point in terms of mGy which was designed to be an indicator of skin dose in the patient. The point of measurement of air kerma (calibrated free in air) has been defined at 15 cm from the isocenter of the isocentric machine (like c arm) towards the X-ray source. This point is intended to refer to the skin of the patient where radiation beam enters the patient. This reference point is called interventional reference point (IRP) and has been defined by International Electrotechnical Commission (IEC) standard 60601-2-43. However, one should keep in mind that cumulative dose at IEC reference point does not take into account back-scatter, table attenuation or in-field nonuniformity of dose. Also, actual skin may not be at IRP since the skin's position depends upon the position of the patient with respect to isocenter, patient thickness, angulations of beam, etc.

SUGGESTED READING

1. American Association of Physicists in Medicine (AAPM) Report No. 204, Size Specific Dose Estimates in Pediatric and Adult Body CT Examinations; 2011.
2. Faiz M Khan. The Physics of Radiation Therapy, Lippincott Williams and Wilkins; 2009.
3. IAEA. Radiation Protection of Patients. https://rpop.iaea.org/RPoP/RPoP/Content/index.htm.
4. International Atomic Energy Agency (IAEA) Technical Document No. 173. Implications for occupational radiation protection of the new dose limit for the lens of the eye; 2013.
5. JT Bushberg, JA Seibert, Leidholt EM Jr, JM Boone. The essential Physics of Medical Imaging. Lippincott Williams and Wilkins; 2002.

CHAPTER

49

Radiation Protection

Sapna Singh, Gaurav Shanker Pradhan, Swati Gupta

HISTORICAL PERSPECTIVE

Sir Wilhelm Roentgen discovered X-rays in the year 1895 and established the physical characteristics of these new found rays in a short period of time. However, the harmful effects of these rays were soon realized with severe dermatitis and eye complaints being reported within a few months of the discovery. Clarence E. Dally had been using his own left hand to check the output of X-ray tubes. In 1896, he developed an ulcerating carcinoma of his repeatedly exposed left hand. The delayed effects of radiation also started getting documented. In 1911 the death of Professor Benjamin Franklin drew a lot of attention to the delayed effects of radiation exposure. In 1896 he had used fluoroscopy on his abdomen for long periods leading to visceral degeneration and subsequent death. Muller won the Nobel Prize for documenting germline mutation as a delayed effect of ionizing radiation in 1927. Muller documented several cases of microcephaly and mental retardation in children of mothers who were exposed to pelvic radiotherapy early in pregnancy.[1]

Percy Brown was a radiologist historian who recorded case histories of the harmful effects of radiation in people exposed to radiation from 1911 onwards. The practice of using radiation to treat ankylosing spondylitis was stopped as soon as it was realized to be the cause of leukemia developing in these patients. Radiation induced leukemia in radiation workers was also reported around the same time by Duncan in 1942. In 1947, an Atom Bomb Casualty Commission (ABCC) was set up following the atomic bomb blasts on Hiroshima and Nagasaki cities of Japan. A very high incidence of mutations, leukemias and other malignancies, genetic effects in the form of microcephaly and mental retardation were reported in the population exposed in the blasts. In 1975, ABCC was renamed as Radiation Effects and Research Foundation (RERF) works on genetics, cancer induction and other delayed effects of ionizing radiation.[2]

REGULATORY BODIES FOR RADIATION PROTECTION

The various regulatory bodies lay down norms for radiation protection. In India the regulatory body is AERB or the Atomic Energy Regulatory Board. The NCRP or the National Commission for Radiation Protection is the regulatory body in United States of America while ICRP or International Commission on Radiological Protection is the name given to the regulatory body at the international level.

AERB: Atomic Energy Regulatory Board—India
NCRP: National Commission for Radiation Protection— USA
ICRP: International Commission on Radiological Protection—International level
ICRU: International Commission on Radiation Units and Measurements.

The ICRP was setup in 1928 and consists of a chairman, a secretary and 12 members from across the world. The AERB was set up on November 15 1983 by the President of India under section 27 of the Atomic Energy Act 1962. The purpose was to carry out certain safety and regulatory functions under the Act. The board has a full time chairman, a secretary, three part time members and an ex officio member.[3]

Functions of Atomic Energy Regulatory Board[4]

- *Registration of X-ray equipment:* For registration, the X-ray equipment must be approved from the point of view of radiation safety. Any person acquiring an X-ray machine either by purchase/transfer/gift/leasing or loan has to get it registered with the competent authority.
- *Commissioning/decommissioning of X-ray equipment:* Any commission/decommission of X-ray equipment requires registration with the competent authority.
- *Design certification:* There are design safety specifications in the AERB code which have to be met by the manufacturer/vendor.
- *No objection certificate:* Only NOC validated/type approved equipment can be marketed in the country. The manufacturer of the X-ray equipment should obtain a no objection certificate from the competent authority for equipment which are made indigenously.
- *Approval of the layout:* The layout of the stipulated X-ray installation should also be approved by the competent authority.

- *Inspection of X-ray installations:* The owner/employer should make available all X-ray installations for inspection at all reasonable times to the competent authority.
- *Certification of Radiation Safety Officer (RSO):* Any person who discharges the duties of a RSO should obtain a certificate from the competent authority. Certificate has to be granted on the basis of a person's educational qualifications, experience and testing and availability of dosimetry equipment.
- *Certification of service engineers:* Servicing of X-ray equipment can be undertaken only by a person holding a valid certificate from the competent authority. Certification would be granted on the basis of qualification, experience, training, availability of servicing facilities and safety record of such person.
- *Penalties:* Any person who contravenes the conditions of the registration/certification/licence granted to him or her by the competent authority or contravenes the provisions of the Radiation Protection Rules 1971 will be punishable under the Atomic Energy Act 1962 (sections 24, 25 and 26). The punishment may include fine or imprisonment or both. The quantum of punishment would depend on the severity of the offence.

Radiation Protection Survey and Program

It is the responsibility of the hospital administration to establish a radiation protection program. A Radiation Safety Committee (RSC) and a Radiation Safety Officer (RSO) should be appointed by the administration. Every department should have an RSO.[4] An RSO should be an officer who has undergone extensive training has knowledge of radiation physics, radiation biology, protection, instrumentation and dosimetry. Duties of an RSO include:

- Conducting radiation protection surveys on a regular periodic basis.
- Periodic quality assurance tests and maintaining a record of the same.
- Educating all radiation workers on relevant safety measures.
- Training new entrants.
- Implementing radiation surveillance measures.
- Maintaining a record of personal doses.
- Issuance of instructions about how to deal with radiation emergencies.
- Ensuring that all instruments in his/her custody are properly calibrated and maintained properly.
- Maintaining a record of all radiation surveys performed and the corrective measures taken in case of deficiencies.

The Radiation Safety Committee (RSC) comprises of a radiologist, a medical physicist, a senior nurse, internist and a nuclear medicine person. The duty of RSC is to perform a radiation protection survey which has five phases. The 5 phases include investigation, inspection, measurement, evaluation and recommendations regarding corrective measures.

PROTECTION AGAINST RADIATION HAZARD

The International Commission for Radiation Protection (ICRP) has advocated three general principles for radiation protection. These include:[5]

- *Justification:* This states that the practices adopted should produce a net positive benefit.
- *Optimization:* This states that all exposures should be kept as low as possible.
- *Dose limitation:* The dose should not exceed the limits that have been recommended for a particular practice.
- *Justification:* Every diagnostic practice should be justified, that is it should provide adequate benefit to the exposed individuals or to the society and outweigh the radiation risk involved, i.e. the benefit to risk ratio should be high. For example, the benefit to risk ratio is high when CT scan is performed for cerebrovascular hemorrhage and is low for screening mammography below 35 years of age.[6]
  There are three levels of justification of a radiological practice in medicine.[7]
  1. At the first and most general level, the proper use of radiation in medicine is accepted as doing more good than harm to society.
  2. At the second level is the justification of the procedure in improving the diagnosis or treatment and providing necessary information about the exposed individuals.
  3. At the third level, the application of the procedure to an individual should be justified.
- *Optimization:* The concept of ALARA states that radiation should be kept As Low As Reasonably Achievable.[8] In the United Kingdom this has been modified as As Low As Reasonably Practicable, i.e. ALARP, economic and societal factors being taken into account.[9] The optimization is applied at two levels for radiological protection in patients. The first level is in the appropriate selection, design and construction of the X-ray equipment and the second is in the day to day methods of working. The main aim of optimization is to adjust the protection measures in a manner which maximize the net benefit and keep the radiation doses as low as practicable.[10]
- *Dose limitation:* There is no defined threshold below which radiation damage would not occur. No radiation dose, however low its value, can be considered safe. Very low doses of radiation for example can produce radiation induced cancer and serious hereditary defects if the cells irradiated are the germ cells in the gonads.[11]
- *Maximum permissible dose (MPD):* It may be defined as the dose of ionizing radiation which an individual may accumulate over a long period of time with a negligible risk of significant body or genetic damage.
  MPD = 5 (N-1) R. Where N is age in years and R is the exposures in Roentgens. The unit of MPD is rem.
  The newer recommendation is MPD = age in years x 1 rem, i.e. the individual effective dose for a lifetime should not exceed the value of his/her age.

Tables 1 and 2 give the different dose limits as specified for the radiation workers and the general public.

TABLE 1: Recommended dose limits are specified for the radiation workers and the general public*.[4]

	Occupational workers		Public	
	Limit	**Annual equivalents**	**Limit**	**Annual equivalents**
ICRP	20 mSv/yr over 5 years	20 mSv	1 mSv/yr over 5 years	1 mSv
NCRP	Cumulative dose = Age in yrs × 10 mSv	50 mSv	5 mSv for 5 years period	1 mSv
AERB	100 mSv for 5 years period	30 mSv	1 mSv/yr for 5 years	1 mSv

(*According to the AERB safety code 2011)

TABLE 2: Recommendations for dose limits to eye and skin for occupational workers*.[4]

	Dose limits to skin, hands, feet (mSv/yr)	Dose limits to lens of eye (mSv/yr)
ICRP	500	150
NCRP	500	150
AERB	500	150

(*According to the AERB safety code 2011)

CARDINAL PRINCIPLES OF RADIATION PROTECTION

The cardinal principles of radiation protection are 'time distance shielding', i.e.

1. *Time:* The time of exposure should be kept as short as possible.

   Exposure = Exposure rate × Time

   Exposure is the product of the exposure rate and time. Hence for a smaller time of exposure, the resultant dose is smaller, for a larger time of exposure the dose is higher.[12]
2. *Distance:* The distance between the radiation and the exposed person should be kept as large as possible. The intensity (I) of radiation varies inversely with the square of the distance (d). This is known as the inverse square law.[13]

   $$I \propto 1/d^2$$

   If the distance is increased to twice the original, the radiation dose is reduced to one fourth.
3. *Shielding:* A shielding material should be inserted between the source of radiation and the exposed person.

Shielding means the attenuation of X-ray beam by certain materials like concrete, lead, etc. when placed between the source of radiation and the exposed individual. The shielding can be in the form of shielding of the X-ray tube, shielding of the room, personnel shielding or patient shielding.

The three types of radiation in radiation protection are:[14]

1. *Useful beam:* It is also called the primary beam. The useful or the primary beam is the radiation passing through the tube aperture.
2. *Leakage radiation:* This includes all radiation passing through the tube housing other than the useful radiation.
3. *Scattered radiation:* This includes all the radiation that has undergone a change in direction.

Source Shielding/Shielding of the X-ray Tube

The X-ray tube is lined with thin sheets of lead to prevent the X-rays produced in the tube from scattering in all directions. Shielding of the source protects both patients and radiation workers from leakage radiation. The leakage radiation exposure has to be limited to < 0.1 R per hour at 1 meter from the tube anode and hence the X-ray tube housing needs to be shielded. AERB recommends a maximum allowable leakage radiation from the tube housing of not greater than 1 mGy/hour/100 cm.

Room Shielding

A structural shielding of the X-ray room has to be done to ensure that the individuals outside these rooms are not exposed to unnecessary unwanted radiation.

There are two types of protective barriers.

1. *Primary barrier:* This is the one which is directly exposed to the useful beam. The atomic number and the thickness of the primary barrier should be such that it reduces the exposure rate of the useful beam to the permissible dose.
2. *Secondary barrier:* It is the one which is struck by radiation either by leakage from X-ray tube or by scattered radiation from the patient.

Room shielding can be done by 2 mm lead or 25 mm layer of high quality barium plaster, 225 mm of solid brick or 150 mm of concrete or 1/2 brick thickness and 1/2 inch plaster. The joints and holes must also be covered by similar protective barriers as the wall. The X-ray room shielding is influenced by the nature of occupancy of the adjoining area. Based on this various types of areas are identified:

A. *Control area:* It is defined as the area routinely occupied by radiation workers and exposed to an occupational dose. The shielding should be such that it reduces exposure in the control area <26 mC/kg/week.

B. *Uncontrolled area:* These areas are not occupied by occupational workers. The exposure rate in these areas should be reduced to <2.6 mC/kg/week.

Exposure Calculations

The exposure at any point is calculated on the basis of the following factors:

- *Workload:* It is the quantity of X rays (mAs) generated per week.

  Workload = mAs/week
- *Exposure (E):* This converts the workload into Roentgens.

- *Use factor (U):* It is defined as the time fraction for which the beam is directed at a particular barrier.
- *Distance (d):* The distance from the source of radiation is taken into consideration.
- *Occupancy factor (T):* This pertains to the time period for which the area will be occupied. T=1 means that the area will be occupied by the same individual for the entire day.[15]

Based on this, exposure at a given point will be calculated as:

$$E = E'WUT/d^2$$

The value obtained from this calculation can be used to determine the thickness of the primary barrier.

Half Value Layer (HVL)

It is defined as the thickness of a specific substance which when introduced into the path of a beam of radiation, reduces the exposure rate by 50% **(Table 3)**.

For example, if the calculated exposure at a point is 3.2 R/week and the permissible exposure is 0.1 R/week, the number of HVLs to achieve it would be 5. If the HVL of the beam is 0.25 mm of lead, the barrier thickness can be then calculated. It would be 0.25 x 5 = 1.25 mm.[12]

In general, the primary protective barrier should consist of 1/16 inch lead extending 7 feet from the floor when the X-ray tube is 5–7 feet from the wall. Primary protective barrier also takes care of leakage radiation.[12]

A secondary protective barrier should consist of 1/32 inch lead extending from the top of the primary barrier to the ceiling. The secondary barrier should overlap the primary barrier at least 0.5 inches at the seam.

Shielding of the X-ray Control Room

The control room of an X-ray equipment is a secondary protective barrier. It should never be located where the primary beam falls directly. The location of the control room should be such that the radiation should scatter twice before entering it. A lead equivalence of 1.5 mm is essential for the walls and the viewing window of the control booth.

For equipment operating at <125 kVp the control panel can be in the X-ray room while for equipments operating above 125 kVp the control panel should be in a separate room located outside the X-ray room. When located within the X-ray room, a distance of not less than 3 meters is recommended by the AERB between the control panel and the X-ray unit.

TABLE 3: Tube potential and the HVL*.[4]

Tube potential (kVp)	HVL	
	Lead (mm)	Concrete (inches)
40	0.03	0.13
80	0.19	0.42
100	0.24	0.6
125	0.27	0.76
150	0.28	0.86

(*According to the AERB safety code 2011)

When there is no fixed control booth as in mobile radiography it is recommended by the AERB that the technologist should remain at least 2 meters away from the X-ray tube and the primary beam. It is hence recommended that the length of the exposure cord on mobile radiographic units should be at least 2 meters.[16] The AERB also recommends that the size of the gantry room in the CT scanner should not be less than 25 m^2.

Shielding of the Personnel

Also follows the time-distance shielding principle.

Following steps should be taken to minimize radiation exposure to the occupational worker.[17]

- The workers should step behind the control booth or leave the room when possible, that is, should remain in the radiation area for as less time as possible.
- The distance between the radiation workers and the source of radiation, i.e. the X-ray tube should be maximized as the intensity of the radiation varies inversely as the square of the distance.
- Lead aprons, lead gloves, thyroid shields and eye glasses with side shields should be used to protect the personnel.
  - *Lead aprons:* Lead aprons are classified as secondary barriers as they provide protection only from scattered radiation and not the primary beam. Lead apron provides protection to the radiation workers and it is recommended that the minimum thickness of lead equivalence should be 0.5 mm for general purpose. The thickness of lead in the apron determines the protection it provides as 0.25 mm lead attenuates 66% of the beam at 75 kVp and thickness of 1 mm lead attenuates 99% of the beam at the same kVp.[17] For women radiation workers a customized lead apron that reaches below mid-thigh level and wraps completely around the pelvis is recommended to avoid any accidental exposure to a conceptus.[18] The lead aprons should be cared for properly. They should not be dropped on the floor, piled in a heap or draped over the back of a chair. When the apron is not being used, it should be hung on properly designed racks as improper care may lead to internal fracturing of the lead compromising its protective ability. The apron should be radiographed for defects such as internal tears and cracks at least once a year.
    Zero lead aprons: New aprons known as zero lead aprons or lead free aprons are available in the market which have a weight 20–40% less than the conventional lead aprons.[19] Lead is toxic and hence disposal needs proper care. The lead free aprons are made of tungsten, antimony and bismuth, tin, aluminium or barium. These are recyclable and hence disposal is not a problem.
  - Gonad shield, hand gloves and thyroid shields - These should have a minimum lead equivalence of 0.5 mm.

Shielding of the Patient

The various radiation protection measures involve choices of appropriate equipment and appropriate technique.

Equipment

The radiation protection features in the equipment include:

- *Beam filtration:* The function of the filters is to absorb low energy photons thereby increasing the mean energy penetrating power of the X-ray beam and hence reducing the patient dose. These beam filters absorb all rays below 10 kev. These low energy photons contribute to the patient dose without contributing to the image.
  The AERB has recommended the minimum total filtration for X-rays which depends on the kVp of the equipment **(Table 4)**.
  Total beam filtration should always be indicated on the tube housing and should not be less than 1.5 mm.
  For screen film mammography the total filtration in the useful beam should be at least 0.03 mm of molybdenum as per the AERB guidelines.
- *Beam collimation:* Collimators are used to reduce the area of exposure and limit it to the area of clinical interest. Tissues exposed directly to the primary beam receive much higher radiation dose then the tissues outside the primary beam. This unnecessary exposure of the tissues leads to higher radiation dosages. By using collimators to restrict exposure to only the area of clinical interest one can substantially reduce the radiation dose. The use of collimators also reduces the amount of scattered radiation reaching the image receptor with the resulting images having better contrast.
- *Table top for undercouch tubes* should be such that it allows a high beam transmission increasing the quantity of diagnostic photons reaching the film. A carbon filter material is generally used for high transmission tabletop.[20]
- *Image receptors:* Intensifying screens convert the absorbed X-ray energy into visible light acting as an image amplifiers and significantly reducing the patient absorbed dose. A fast screen (high speed) requires less exposure then a slow screen (low speed) to provide a given image density. Rare earth screen film combinations reduce patient dose without loss of diagnostic quality. Image intensifier tubes have efficient input phosphor that play a role in reducing dose to the patient.
- *Source to image receptor distance (SID):* An equipment with a large SID will result in a lower patient dose.[21]
- *Anti-scatter grids:* These reduce the scatter radiation reaching the film improving the quality of the resulting radiograph and hence reducing the chance of repeat exposure.[22]

Fluoroscopy X-ray Equipment

The AERB has recommended the following for fluoroscopy X-ray equipment.[4]

TABLE 4: Minimum total filtration for X-ray tubes*.[4]

Maximum rated tube potential (kVp)	Minimum total filtration (mm Al)
Less than 70	1.5
70 to and including 100	2.0
Above 100	2.5

(*According to the AERB safety code 2011)

- *Tube screen alignment:* The X-ray tube and fluoroscopic screen should be aligned and coupled in such a way that they move together in synchrony. Also, in all positions of the tube and screen the axis of the X-ray beam should pass through the centre of the screen.
- *Fluoroscopy tube housing and filtration:* Every housing for medical X-ray equipment shall be so constructed that leakage radiation through the tube housing shall not exceed an air kerma of 1 mGy in one hour at a distance of 1.0 m from the X-ray target.
- *Lead rubber flaps:* Protective flaps of lead equivalence 0.5 mm are suspended from the edge of the screen such that these flaps extend down to the table top in case of horizontal fluoroscopy and from the bottom of the screen in case of vertical fluoroscopy. The "bucky slot" is provided with a cover of 0.5 mm lead equivalence.[23]
- *Field limiting diaphragm:* Tube housing should be provided with a field limiting diaphragm even when the diaphragm is fully opened and the screen is at the maximum distance from the table, there is an unilluminated margin of at least 1 cm along the edges of the screen. The control knobs should be provided with local shielding of at least 0.25 mm lead equivalence.
- *Focus to table top distance:* This distance should not be less than 30 cm for fluoroscopy units.
- *Fluoroscopy timer:* There should be an audible signal after the preset site and the maximum range of the cumulative timer should not exceed 5 minutes. The built-in cumulative timer device and an audible warning system should ring after a preset fluoroscopy time to prevent excessive radiation exposure. If the screening time exceeds the preset time it can be reset but the radiologist must be aware of the dose implications of doing so.[23]
- *The fluoroscopy timer* is a means for monitoring the passage of exposure time.
- *Footswitch and visual indicator:* When the beam is on there is a visual indication on the control panel. For conducting the fluoroscopy examinations a foot operated pressure switch is provided.
- *Table top exposure:* The table top exposure should not be more than 5 Gy per minute.
- *Control panel:* This should indicate all exposure parameters like tube potential, exposure time and tube current. An indicator is provided on the control panel to show whether the X-ray beam is "ON or OFF"

Technique

Since repeat exposures give additional radiation dose, the importance of a good radiographic technique and optimum film processing cannot be overemphasized. Repeat images due to technical error must be minimised to reduce radiation dosages.[23]

- *Optimum film processing:* This helps to avoid repeat examinations.
- *Tube voltage and tube current:* A higher kVp leads to a lesser radiation dose because of the better penetration of the beam that leads to reduced scatter within the body. An attempt should be made to use the highest kVp possible without reducing the image contrast to an unacceptable level in order to reduce radiation dose to the patient.

It is recommended by the NCRP that the kVp and mA should be visible to the person performing the fluoroscopy procedure at all times.

- *Screening time and exposure factor:* Intermittent fluoroscopy rather than continuous fluoroscopy should be followed. The magnification mode should be avoided is it leads to an increase in the dose. The beam should be collimated to the smallest possible and the mA and kV should be kept as low as possible.

RADIATION PROTECTION IN INTERVENTIONAL RADIOLOGY

Lengthy fluoroscopy times and the acquisition of a large number of images during fluoroscopic procedures results in increased exposure of patients and operators.[24] Apart from the general radiation protection measures used in fluoroscopy some specific techniques applicable to Interventional radiology include:[25]

Pulsed Fluoroscopy

Conventional fluoroscopy produces a continuous radiation beam while pulsed fluoroscopy, as the name indicates, consists of pulsing the X-ray beam. In this the image is acquired only during a brief pulse of the X-ray beam say 10 millisecond. Dose is reduced in pulsed fluoroscopy by simply reducing the fraction of time the X-ray beam is on. Also, by using the lowest pulse rate possible, patient dose and fluoroscopy times can be reduced. At pulsed fluoroscopy with 15, 10 and 7.5 pulses/second, dose savings of 22%, 38% and 49% respectively, are achieved.[26]

Last Image Hold (LIH)

This enables the user to spend time interpreting the image without use of radiation. Last image hold combined with pulsed fluoroscopy reduces dose to the tune of 75%.

Road Mapping

A reference static image is displayed on a second monitor and is used as a mask for subtraction from the real time fluoroscopy display. The only objects left in the image are the vessel of interest and the catheter moving through it. Peak opacification is seen as maximum pixel values from a small bolus of contrast as it travels through the vessel of interest. Fluoroscopy is terminated by the operator when the whole vessel appears to be filled. Use of this technique shortens the procedure time thus decreasing patient and operator dose.

Dose Spreading Techniques

An alteration in the direction of the X-ray beam can reduce the maximum dose delivered to any one point on the patient's skin. This can be achieved by simply rotating the C-arm a few degrees. This is specially useful in prolonged procedures where entrance skin doses are high with a static X-ray beam. In these cases the beam can be moved by rotating the C-arm preventing erythema and epilation of the skin.[26]

Ultra Low Dose Fluoroscopy (ULD)

In ULD fluoroscopy, the system parameters are computer controlled and use the lowest optimal dose over a broad range of examinations and patient types while still producing quality images.

SAFETY OF RADIOGRAPHIC IMAGING DURING PREGNANCY

28 Day Rule

The 28 day rule states that any radiological examination, if justified can be carried out throughout the cycle unless a period is missed. If there is a missed period, a female should be considered pregnant unless proven otherwise. The 28 day rule has replaced the earlier 10 day rule which stated that any radiograph of in a female of reproductive age should be carried out within first days of menstrual cycle to avoid irradiating any possible pregnancy. The greatest risk to the fetus is between 8–15 weeks of pregnancy owing to the risk of chromosomal abnormalities and subsequent mental retardation and hence any radiation to the fetus should be avoided during this period **(Table 5)**. The effects may be both deterministic and stochastic. Various malformations that have been reported include microcephaly, exencephaly, malformations of the skull, mental retardation and hydrocephalus. Absence of eye, micropththalmia, absence of lens and cataract have also been reported. Skeletal malformations, cleft palate, clubfeet, spina bifida, have all been reported as radiation effects on the fetus.[27]

Table 6 gives recommendation for continuing pregnancy after radiation exposure as a function of gestational age and dose.

Another cause of concern is the radiation induced childhood cancer. The frequency of childhood cancer in an unexposed population is 1 in 1500 or 0.07% while the risk in a foetus exposed in utero to 1 rad (10 mGy) of radiation during the first trimester is 3.5 times more than an unexposed foetus. Hence multiplying the natural frequency with 3.5 gives us a value of 0.25% (3.5 x 0.07 = 0.25%) which is still low. Thus in 99.75% cases the child exposed in utero will not develop childhood cancer.[27]

According to the recommendations by the American College of Gynaecologists Committee on Obstetric Practice, radiation exposure through radiography, CT scan or nuclear imaging techniques results in a dose much lower than the dose associated with fetal harm. According to the recommendation if these techniques are necessary for the diagnosis to be made, they should not be withheld from a pregnant patient.

Recommended Dose Limits to Pregnant Women[3,4]

The recommendations of various authorities are as follows:

- *ICRP:* In pregnant females, a supplementary equivalent dose limit of 2 mSv applied to the surface of her lower

TABLE 5: Effects of prenatal exposure as a function of gestational age*.[28]

Gestational stage	Days after conception	Fetal dose		Observed effect
		Rad	mGy	
Perimplantation	0–14	5–10	50–100	Prenatal death
Major organogenesis	8–56	20–25	200–250	Most sensitive stage for growth retardation
	14–105			Small head size; most sensitive time for induction of childhood cancer
Rapid neuron development and migration	56–105	>10	>100	Small head size, seizures, decline in IQ points: 25 points/100 rad (1 Gy)
After organogenesis and rapid neuron development	105–term	>10	>100	Increased risk of childhood cancer
		>50	>500	Severe mental retardation observe at 16–25 wk

(*International Commission on Radiological Protection: Biological Effects After Prenatal Irradiation (Embryo and Fetus). Md:ICRP Publication 90;2003:1-200)

TABLE 6: Recommendation for continuing pregnancy after radiation exposure as a function of gestational age and dose*.[28]

Fetal absorbed dose			
Gestational age	**(<50 mGy)**	**(50–150 mGy)**	**(>150 mGy)**
< 2 wks	Recommended	Recommended	Recommended
2–8 wks	Recommended	May consider termination (in presence of other risk factors)	May consider termination (in presence of other risk factors)
8–15 wks	Recommended	May consider termination (in presence of other risk factors)	Higher risk conditions, but termination is not necessarily recommended
15 wks to term	Recommended	Recommended	Recommended

(*ICRP: Biological Effects After Prenatal Irradiation (Embryo and Fetus). Md:ICRP Publication 90;2003:1-200)

abdomen for the remainder of her pregnancy once pregnancy is established.

- *NCRP:* Recommends dose limit 0.5 mSv per month for the embryo/fetus for occupational pregnant workers.
- *AERB:* Recommends that once pregnancy is established the equivalent to surface of pregnant woman's abdomen should not exceed 2 mSv for the remainder of the pregnancy.

PERSONNEL DOSIMETRY

Persons who are exposed to radiation need to be monitored during the course of their work. The dosimeters should be properly worn, should receive proper care and be returned on time. The dosimeter should not be irradiated except during occupational exposure and proper environmental conditions should be ensured. Various dosimeters include pocket dosimeter, the film badge or thermoluminescent dosimeter. The dose is given as an estimate of the effective dose equivalent to the whole body in mSV for a 3 month period usually. The dosimeters have a dose measurement limit of 0.1-0.2 mSV.

The aim of personal monitoring is:

- To monitor and control individual doses.
- To be able to detect overexposures and suggest corrective measures.
- To maintain a record of the cumulative dose records.

Types of Dosimeter

- Immediate read
  - Pocket Ionization Chambers
  - Ionization detectors with dose accumulation function
- Delayed read/Personnel monitors
  - Film Badges
  - TLD
  - Optically Stimulated Light-emitting Dosimeters

Pocket Dosimeter

The pocket dosimeter consists of an ionization chamber and a movable quartz fibre. When X-rays enter the dosimeter, ionization causes the fibers to lose their charges giving a measure of the radiation dose. The pocket dosimeter however has several disadvantages in the form of low accuracy and being subject to human reading errors as reading is manual. Other disadvantages are its susceptibility to moisture and a limited range. The range of the pocket dosimeter is limited by the charge on the electrode which once gone, the device stops recording exposure.

Film Badge

A film badge uses a small double coated X-ray film sandwiched between several filters to help detect radiation. At least 6 pairs of filters are used to identify various components of incident radiation. The six types of windows are:

1. *Open window:* Alpha rays
2. *Plastic:* Gray—beta rays
3. *Cadmium:* Yellow—slow neutrons
4. *Thin copper:* Green-diagnostic X-rays
5. *Thick copper:* Pink-gamma and therapeutic rays
6. *Lead:* Black-fast neutrons and gamma rays

A different degree of blackening will be produced by the same quantity of radiation incident on the badge under each filter as various types of absorbers attenuate radiation of a given energy to a different extent. Film badges have been replaced by the thermoluminescent dosimeter (TLD) badges owing to several disadvantages[16] **(Table 7)**.

Thermoluminescent Dosimeter (TLD)

Certain materials known as phosphors have the tendency to emit light when heated. This property is known as thermoluminescence. Examples of such material include lithium fluoride (LiF), calcium fluoride (CaF_2), calcium sulphate ($CaSO_4$), lithium borate ($Li_2B_4O_7$) show thermoluminescence.

Principle

When a LiF crystal is exposed to radiation, few of the electrons get trapped at higher energy levels. When the crystal is heated, these electrons return to their stable energy levels.[12] The energy differences between the two orbital levels is emitted as light which is then measured by a photomultiplier tube. The amount of light emitted gives an estimate of the radiation dose as the two are proportional. The measurement of radiation from TLD is a two step procedure. First, the TLD is exposed to radiation. Then, the LiF crystal is heated in a TLD analyzer. On heating, light is emitted. A glow curve can be obtained by plotting the intensity of light as a function of the temperature. The highest peak and the area under the curve are proportional to the energy of the radiation and can be used to measure radiation dose. After the reading is obtained, the TLD can be annealed at a higher temperature which zeroes the TLD reading dose and is read for reuse.

Method to use TLD

The TLD card should be loaded in the cassette and should not be removed till the end of the service period. A TLD badge should always be worn by all persons working in the radiation and should not be shared by any other person. The TLD badge should always be stored in a radiation free place when not in use. While leaving the premises of the institution the badges should be submitted and not carried in a metro train where again these would be screened through the X-ray machine leading to erroneous readings. The badge should also not be left in radiation field or near ovens, hot plates, furnaces, burners, etc.

Where to Wear the TLD Badge

In radiography where no protective lead apron is being worn, a dosimeter can be worn either at the level of the waist or at the collar area. The trunk/waist level gives an estimate of the whole body exposure while the collar badge gives an estimate of the radiation received to the internal organs like thyroid. In fluoroscopy a protective lead apron is worn by the radiologist while performing the various fluoroscopic procedures. In such situations two TLD badges are to be worn ideally. One badge should be worn underneath the lead apron and the other needs to be worn at the level of the neck/collar region outside the lead apron. The one at the waist level gives an idea of the exposure received by the protected areas while the one at the collar level assesses the exposure to the unprotected organs. If it is not feasible to wear two and only one is to be worn, it should be worn in the neck region outside the lead apron as the neck receives about 10–20 times more exposure than the trunk which is protected by the lead apron.

TABLE 7: Comparison between film badges, TLD badges and electronic dosimeters.

Advantages	Disadvantages
Film badges	
• Relatively cheap • Permanent record of exposure • Wide dose ranges (0.2–2000 mSv) • Identifies type and energy of exposure • Easy to identify individual dosimeters	• Requires dark room and wet processing • Lower threshold for hard gamma radiation is 0.15 mSv • Cannot be used to assess finger dose. • Is affected by heat, humidity and chemicals [hence not suitable to monitor over periods > 1 month] • Accuracy ± 20 %
TLD badges	

• Chips can be reused
• Wide dose range (0.1–2000 mSv)
  - Direct reading of personal dose
  - Compact: Suitable for finger dosimetry
	• Requires high capital initially
	• No permanent record (other than glow curves)

Electronic personal dosimeter:	
• Direct reading and cumulative record storage (up to16Sv) • Can be 'zeroed' by user without deleting cumulative record • Measures personal dose at depth and at the skin directly to 1 micro Sv • Audible warning at high dose rates	• High cost • Battery should be renewed every year

How to Return the used TLD Cards

All the cards whether used or unused should be returned once the service period is over. This should be done along with the TLD/5 form. The TLD card should be arranged in the same order as listed in the TLD/5 forms and the nature of the radiation sources handled against the respective names in the TLD/5 form should be written. Sending of TLD by an air courier should be avoided to prevent screening of the package under X-ray machine at the airport. Plastic boxes should be used for returning the cards. If there is any damage to its filters (metallic pieces) or cassette holder, it should be immediately reported and a replacement be asked for. Personal numbers are allotted by Bhabha Atomic Research Centre, Mumbai to the radiation workers. These numbers are permanent and should not be changed. In case of any loss, a declaration stating the same duly signed by the RSO/Physicist should be immediately sent.

Overexposure

A dose exceeding 10 mSv is treated as overexposure and should be reported immediately to the institution and the concerned individual. The institution should arrange to investigate the cause of overexposure and report the findings to the appropriate authorities at BARC. A hematological examination including differential blood counts and chromosomal aberration test has to be carried out on the person receiving more than 10 mSv. All overexposure cases are reviewed by BARC and advice on necessary follow-up is given to the concerned institution.

Electronic Dosimeters

The sensitivity of the electronic dosimeters is 50–200 times that of TLD badges. These are based on single silicon diodes or Geiger Muller tubes. Electronic dosimeters provide the dose readings immediately and give out effective alarms when dose limits are exceeded.

COMPUTED TOMOGRAPHY (RADIATION EXPOSURE AND DOSE MODULATIONS)

Radiation Dose Measures: CT Specific

Because of its geometry and usage, CT is a unique modality and therefore has its own set of specific parameters for radiation dose. This modality is unique because the exposure is essentially continuous around the patient, rather than a projectional modality in which the exposure is taken from one or two source locations.[29]

Projectional radiographic exposures are taken from one source position and the entrance skin dose is much larger than the exit skin dose, creating a large radiation dose gradient across the patient. In contrast the tomographic exposure of CT scans with a full 360° rotation results in a radially symmetric radiation dose gradient within the patient.

Typical Dose Measurements

The radial dose gradient (the size of the difference from center to periphery) is affected by several factors, including the size of the object, the X-ray beam spectrum, and the attenuation of the material or tissue. In addition to the variations within the scan plane, there are variations along the length of the patient or phantom. These can be characterized by the z-axis dose distribution or radiation profile. The radiation profile is not limited to the primary area being imaged, and there are tails to this distribution from the nonideal collimation of the X-ray source and from scatter of photons within the object being exposed. These contributions can add up, creating additional absorbed dose in the primary area being imaged.

To account for the effects from multiple scans, several dose descriptors were developed.

- Multiple scan average dose (MSAD)
- Computed tomography dose index (CTDI)
- $CTDI_{100}$
- $CTDI_{W}$
- $CTDI_{vol}$
- Dose length product

Multiple Scan Average Dose

This is defined as the average dose resulting from a series of scans over an interval *I* in length[30]

$$\text{MSAD} = (1/\text{I}) \int_{-\pi 2}^{\pi 2} \text{D single (z) dz}$$

where 'I' is the interval of the scan length and 'D series(z)' is the dose at position z parallel to the z (rotational) axis resulting from the series of CT scans.

Computed Tomography Dose Index (CTDI)

It is defined as the radiation dose normalized to beam width measured from 14 contiguous sections.[31]

$$\text{CTDI} = (1/n\text{T}) \int_{-\pi}^{\pi} \text{D single (z) dz}$$

where n is the number of sections per scan, T is the width of the interval equal to the selected section thickness, and D single(z) is the dose at point z on any line parallel to the z (rotational) axis for a single axial scan.

$CTDI_{100}$

To overcome the limitations of CTDI with 14 sections, another radiation dose index—$CTDI_{100}$—was developed.

$$\text{CTDI}_{100} = (1/\text{NT}) \int_{-5\text{ cm}}^{5\text{ cm}} \text{D series (z) dz}$$

where 'N' is the number of acquired sections per scan (also referred to as the number of data channels used during acquisition) and 'T' is the nominal width of each acquired section. This index allowed measurement along the entire length of the pencil ionization chamber.

$CTDI_{W}$

$CTDI_{W}$ was created to represent a dose index that provides a weighted average of the center and peripheral contributions to dose within the scan plane. This index is used to overcome the limitations of $CTDI_{100}$ and its dependency on position within the scan plane.

$$\text{CTDI}_{W} = (1/3)(\text{CTDI}_{100})_{\text{center}} + (2/3)(\text{CTDI}_{100})_{\text{periphery}}$$

$CTDI_{vol}$

This parameter is an estimate of the average X-ray output from the acquired CT image series and takes into account the helical pitch and axial scan spacing.[32]

$$CTDI_{vol} = CTDI_{w} \times NT/I$$

where N is the number of acquired sections per scan and and T is the nominal width of each acquired section. The product of N x T is meant to reflect.

The total nominal width of the X-ray beam during acquisition and I is the table travel per rotation for a helical scan. Hence NT/I = 1/pitch

And $CTDI_{vol} = CTDI_{w}/pitch$.

Dose-length Product (DLP)

This value is simply the $CTDI_{vol}$ multiplied by the length of the scan (in centimeters) and is given in units of milligraycentimeters (mGycm):

$$DLP = CTDI_{vol} \times \text{scan length}$$ [33]

This descriptor is used to obtain an estimate of effective dose.

DLP values are easily converted to millisieverts by using conversion factors specific to the anatomic region imaged: The conversion factors listed by the American Association of Physicists in Medicine for the chest, abdomen, and pelvis are 0.014, 0.015, and 0.015[34] respectively. These conversion factors are periodically updated, so care should be taken to apply the most recent ones.

Effective radiation doses calculated from DLP values in a routine oncologic CT examination of the abdomen and pelvis **(Table 8)**.

FACTORS AFFECTING RADIATION DOSE AND QUALITY

Patient Factors

The patient's cross sectional area is a key factor in determining the radiation dose and image quality. Larger the patient, more is the radiation dose for the same image quality. Smaller patients require smaller doses. Hence children can and should be scanned at lower doses than that used for adults for the same clinical indication and body region. Radiation dose also varies according to the area being scanned, for example, air containing thorax should be scanned at lower radiation than the abdomen. This is because of the lower X-ray attenuation of the air containing regions as compared than those higher X-ray attenuation. The clinical indication is another key factor for radiation dose in CT. For example if the clinical indication involves inherently high contrast structures such as lung nodule or renal calculi the radiation doses are lower because image noise is less detrimental to the evaluation of these high contrast lesions.[36] On the contrary, low contrast lesions such as mediastinal lymph nodes, detection and characterization of tumors require higher radiation doses to minimize image noise and artefacts which increase at lower radiation doses.

Scanning Factors

Tube Current and Tube Current Time Product

There is a linear relationship between the tube current and radiation output from the X-ray tube. Smaller patients and lower X-ray attenuation regions like chest require lower tube current doses while larger patients and higher X-ray attenuating regions like shoulder and abdomen require higher tube currents. High contrast lesions like renal calculi and lung nodules require a lower tube current as these are less affected by image noise as compared to lesions with an inherent lower contrast. Most of the modern CT scanners have automatic exposure control (AEC) to modulate tube current but old CT scanners still operate with fixed tube currents and hence knowledge of the variation of tube current with the patient attenuation is necessary.

Tube Voltage

Alterations in tube voltage have a far greater effect on the radiation dose than tube current, e.g. a reduction of 15% in radiation dose can be achieved by a 15% reduction in tube current (linear relationship) while a reduction to the tune of 35% can be achieved in the radiation dose if the tube voltage is reduced by 15%. A decrease in voltage results in a change in CT numbers as well. Use of low voltages such as 100 kVp and 80 kVp results in higher attenuation than 120 kVp because the X-ray output energy at these low voltages is closer to the Iodine K-edge of 33 keV.

Hence the low kVp is beneficial for contrast-enhanced studies like angiography studies as iodine enhancement increases substantially with lower voltage.[36] Lower voltages also result in greater image contrast as the chances of scatter and scatter radiation which decrease contrast reduce with lower voltages. Thus lower voltages reduce radiation dose, improve contrast and improve iodine enhancement. Small children and smaller adults should always be scanned at lower voltages (<100 kV). The only disadvantage of low voltage is an increase in image noise. As a result newer techniques like iterative reconstruction are being used with scanners to enable usage of lower voltages.

TABLE 8: Effective doses calculated from DLP values.[35]

Region scanned	DLP (mGy·cm)	Conversion factor	Effective dose (mSv)
Abdomen and pelvis (portal venous phase)	681	0.015	10.2
Kidneys (delayed phase)	230	0.015	3.5
Bladder (delayed phase)	214	0.015	3.2

Detector Configuration

Detector configuration refers to the width of each detector row and the number of detector rows. If submillimeter sections are desired, thinner X-ray beam is needed which can increase the radiation dose. In wide area detectors (typically 74 cm) there is a problem of overranging, i.e. of the X-ray beam falling outside the desired anatomical regions of interest thereby increasing radiation doses. Modern scanners use adaptive shielding to improve radiation dose efficiency and reduce this overranging. Development of more efficient detector elements, more efficient integrated data assembly systems allow scanning at lower tube currents thereby reducing radiation dosages.

Gantry Rotation Time and Pitch

$$\text{Pitch} = \frac{\text{Table travel}}{\text{Collimated beam width}}$$

If the table travel, that is the movement of the CT table in mm per gantry rotation equals the width of the collimated beam the pitch is 1[36]. If the table travel is more than the beam width the pitch is more than 1 and sections are nonoverlapping while for a pitch <1 the sections are overlapping. Generally, the radiation dose is inversely proportional to the pitch. An increase in pitch results in decrease in radiation doses, increase in image noise, effective section thickness and decreased scanning time. The use of an appropriate pitch largely depends on the clinical indication.

TECHNIQUES FOR CONTROLLING RADIATION DOSE AT CT

Using Automated Exposure Control (AEC)

In automatic exposure control, the tube current is modulated according to the size of the patient.[37] For larger patients, the tube current in automatically increased while for the smaller patients, i.e. pediatric patients the tube current is automatically decreased. Thus by the AEC the tube current is dynamically altered to reduce radiation dose to the patient. Most modern scanners employ AEC techniques. The tube current gets modulated according to the regional X-ray attenuation measured from scout radiographs. There can be a transverse (x-y), longitudinal (z) or a combined (x-y-z) modulation. A combined modulation is usually preferred when available. A variation of the tube current during different portions of the cardiac cycle at ECG gated cardiac CT examination is also possible and is known as temporal resolution. With the use of AEC techniques, a close attention should be paid to the gantry isocentre. If there is off-centering it can increase the doses as the scanners use the patient width from the scout image to determine tube current for AEC.

Modifying the Acquisition Parameters

A reduction in radiation dosage can be achieved by altering the number of scanning phases and the scanning thickness. In CT angiography rather than using four phases (precontrast, postcontrast arterial, post-contrast venous and postcontrast delayed scanning) if two phases are used (arterial and venous phases) a reduction in the dosage to the tune of 50% can be achieved. The section thickness can also be altered to reduce radiation doses. If the noise index is kept constant at 15.3, the relative dose with 2.5 mm thick section would be around 2.3 times that with 5 mm thick sections.[38]

Optimum Tube Potential

Use of an optimum tube potential helps reduce radiation dose. Automatic voltage selection techniques have been developed by some vendors, e.g. Care kV by Siemens Healthcare, kV assist by GE Healthcare, etc.[39] Lower voltages are selected for contrast enhanced examinations and angiography as compared to the nonenhanced scans. A substantial reduction in chest and abdominal CT examination doses can be achieved by the use of automatic voltage selection techniques.

Iterative Reconstruction (IR)

Iterative reconstruction is an image reconstruction technique that reduces image noise. Lower levels of image noise result in lower levels of radiation dose. The various trade names for this technique are:

- Philips—i dose
- Siemens—IRIS (Iterative Reconstruction in Image Space)
- GE Healthcare ASIR
- AIDR—Tohsiba, Japan

In this a primary image is produced using the same filtered back projection, artificial raw data is created using a forward projection to the primary image and an updated image is generated by correlating the simulated data to the measured raw data. A final back projected image is produced as the output.

IR also results in effective reduction of various artifacts such as metal or streak artifacts.

KEY FEATURES OF PEDIATRIC CT PROTOCOLS

Adult CT protocols should not be followed in the pediatric patients and a size based adjustment of doses should be followed strictly.[39,40] The adjustment must be made based on the clinical indication. In order to avoid "missed" contrast boluses good scan timing is important. Fast scanning should be achieved by faster gantry rotation time and by using a higher nonoverlapping pitch. Multiphasic CT protocols should be avoided in the paediatric age group. When possible, ultrasound and MRI should be preferred over CT in children to avoid ionizing radiation.

STEPS TO ENSURE MINIMUM CT RADIATION

- The appropriateness or justification the CT scanning should be ensured.
- Clinical indication-specific CT protocols for different anatomic areas of the body should be created to help tailor CT dose.

- Automatic Exposure Control (AEC) should always be used in all CT examinations to reduce radiation dose
- The patient should be positioned correctly in the gantry. Off centering leads to incorrect tube current modulation by the AEC technique as the patient attenuation gets estimated incorrectly by off-centering.
- Voltage adjustment should be according to clinical indication and patient size.
- "Acquire thin and reconstruct thick" strategy helps decrease image noise and dose requirement.
- Overscanning beyond the anatomic area of interest should be avoided, e.g. for renal calculus CT can be initiated from the top of the kidneys to the pubic symphysis rather than from the dome of the diaphragm. Scanning of only the lung bases for lung nodule follow up rather than the entire lung parenchyma can be followed.
- Repetitive scanning increases radiation dose, hence multiphasic scanning should be undertaken only when clearly indicated for lesion detection and characterization. Split bolus technique can be adopted for CT urography rather than the multiphasic (CMP, parenchymal, excretory) CT technique.
- IR technique can be used to reduce image noise and artifacts seen at low radiation dose.[40]
- A periodic and frequent review of CT protocols should be undertaken for dose monitoring.

CONCLUSION

There are several technologic and scanning strategies available to image wisely without loss of diagnostic quality. A periodic review of the scanning protocols and dose tracking programs should be part of any dose management initiative. The goal should be to keep radiation dosages as low as reasonably achievable while preserving diagnostic information.

REFERENCES

1. Engel Hells P. Radiation protection in medical imaging. Radiography. 2006;12:153-60.
2. Millew RW. Delayed effects of external radiation exposure: a brief history. Radiation research. 1995;144:160-9.
3. Seeram E, Travis EC. Radiation protection. Philadelphia, New York: Lippincott; 1997.
4. AERB Safety Code (Code No AERB/RF-MED/SC) Mumbai 2011; 1-74
5. Shrimpton PC, Wall BF, Croft JR, Webb GAM. Medical exposure guidance on the 1990 recommendations of ICRP. Documents of NRPB. 1999;4(2):43-80.
6. Goldstone K, Yates SJ. Radiation issues governing radiation protection and patient doses in diagnostic imaging. Grainger and Allison's Diagnostic Radiology: a textbook of medical imaging 5th Edn. Adam A, Dixon AK, Grainger RG, Allison DJ, (Eds). New York Churchill Hill Livingstone; 2008. pp. 159-71.
7. Do KH. General principles of radiation protection in fields of diagnostic medical exposure. J Korean Med Sci; 2016.
8. National Council on Radiation Protection and Measurements. Implementation of the principle of As Low As Reasonably Achievable (ALARA) for medical and dental personnel. NCRP report no 107, Bethesda, Md: NCRP, 1990.
9. Webb GAM. The requirement to keep radiation exposures as low as reasonably practicable (ALARP). London HMSO, National Radiological Protection Board (NRPB/P/B); 1984.
10. Moores BM. A review of the fundamental principles of radiation protection when applied to the patient in diagnostic radiology. Radiation Protection Dosimetry 2016. pp. 1-9.
11. Wall BF, Fisher S, Shrimpton PC, Rae S. Current levels of gonadal irradiation from a selection of routine X-ray examination in Great Britain Harwell: National Radiological Protection Board (NRPB – R 105) 1980.
12. Christensen Radiation Protection. In Christensen's Physics of Diagnostic Radiology, 4th Edn. Curry TS, Dowdey JE, Murry RC (Eds). Philadelphia, London; 1990.
13. Shymko MJ. Minimizing occupational exposure. Radiologic Technology. 1998;70(1):89-90.
14. Selman Joseph. The fundamentals of X-ray and radium physics. 7th Edn. Charles Thomas Publisher. 1985. pp. 184-94.
15. Martin CJ. Radiation shielding for diagnostic radiology. Radiation Protection Dosimetry; 2015. pp. 1-6.
16. Grover SB, Kumar J, Gupta A, Khanna L. Protection against radiation hazards: regulatory bodies, safety norms, dose limits and protection devices. Indian J Radiol Imaging. 2002;12:157-67.
17. Simpkin DJ, Dixon RL. Secondary shielding barriers for diagnostic X-ray facilities: scatter and leakage revisited. Health Phys. 1998;74(3):350-65.
18. Brateman L. Radiation safety considerations for diagnostic radiology personnel. Radiographics. 1999;19:1037-55.
19. Çetin H, Yurt A, Yüksel SH. The absorption properties of lead-free garments for use in radiation protection. Radiation Protection Dosimetry. 2016;1-6.
20. National Council on Radiation Protection and Measurements. Medical X-ray, electron beam and gamma X-ray protection for energies upto 50 meV (equipment design, performance and use). Bethesda: NCRP publications (NCRP report no 102); 1989.
21. Sprawl P Jr. Physical principles of medical imaging 2nd Edn. Gaitherberg Md: Aspen; 1993. pp. 165-7.
22. Graham DT, Cloke P. Principles of radiological physics 4th Edn. Edinburg: Churchill Livingstone; 2003. pp. 325-38.
23. Meisinger QC, Stahl CM, Andre MP, et al. Radiation protection for the fluoroscopy operator and staff. AJR 2016;207:745-54
24. Bartal G, Vano E, Paulo G, et al. Management of patient and staff radiation dose in interventional radiology: current concepts. Cardiovasc Intervent Radiol. 2014;37:289-98.
25. Steele JR, Jones AK, Ninan EP. Establishing an interventional radiology patient radiation safety program. Radiographics. 2012;32:277-87.
26. Johnson DR, Kyriou J, Morton EJ, et al. Radiation protection in interventional radiology. Clinical Radiology. 2001;56:99-106
27. Parry RA, Glaze SA, Archer BR. Typical patient radiation doses in Diagnostic Radiology. Radiographics. 1999;19:1289-302.
28. ICRP: Biological Effects after Prenatal Irradiation (Embryo and Fetus) Md: ICRP Publication 90;2003:1-200.
29. McNitt Gray. Radiation dose in CT. Radiographics. 2002;22:1541-53.
30. Jucius RA, Kambic GX. Radiation dosimetry in computed tomography. Appl Opt Instrum Eng Med. 1977;127:286-95.
31. Shope TB, Gange RM, Johnson GC. A method for describing the doses delivered by transmission. X-ray Computed Tomography Med Phys. 1991;8:488-95.
32. McCollough CM, Schueler BA. Calculation of effective dose. Med Phys. 2000;27:838-44.

33. Shrimpton PC, Edyvean S. CT scanner dosimetry. Br J Radiol. 1998;71:1-3.
34. American Association of Physicists in Medicine. The measurement, reporting and management of radiation dose in CT. Report no 96, College park Md: American Association of Physicists in Medicine, 2008.
35. Tamm EP, Rong XJ, Coly D, et al. CT radiation dose reduction: how to implement change without sacrificing diagnostic quality. Radiographics. 2011;31:1823-32.
36. Kalra MK, Sodickson AD, Smith WM. CT radiation: key concepts for gentle and wise use. Radiographics. 2015; 35:1706-21.
37. Lee CH, Goo JM, Lee HJ, et al. Radiation dose modulation technique in multidetector CT era: from basics to practice. Radiographics. 2008;28:1451-9.
38. Kanal KM, Stewart BK, Kolokythas O, et al. Impact of operator selected image noise index and reconstruction slice thickness on patient radiation dose in 64 MDCT. AJR. 2007;189:219-25.
39. Yu L, Bruesewitz M, Thomas KB, et al. Optimal tube potential for radiation dose reduction in Pediatric CT: principles, clinical implementations and pitfalls. Radiographics. 2011;31:835-48.
40. Khawaja RD, Singh S, Otrakji A, et al. Dose reduction in pediatric abdominal CT: use of iterative reconstruction techniques across different CT platforms. Pediatric Radiol 2015;45:1046-55.

CHAPTER 50

Planning Modern Imaging Department with Regulatory Requirements in Radiology Practice

Ajay Gulati, Nidhi Prabhakar, Uma Debi

In the present modern era, diagnostic imaging has been increasing recognized to be an integral part of healthcare delivery services. Advancements in the sector of information technology complemented by development in digital information technology have resulted in a significant transformation of field of diagnostic imaging. This has resulted in providing more precise and timely diagnosis for various medical and surgical conditions.

Importance of recognizing the role of diagnostic imaging as a clinical service is essential by the healthcare professionals since it requires judicious clinical interpretation of imaging information available and further guidance to subsequent management decisions for better patient care. These is an ever increasing trend to include imaging in the early evaluation for patient management in order to improve the overall efficiency of health care delivery services.[1]

The diagnostic imaging is generally carried out by clinical radiology departments which may be within a multispecialty hospital or a stand-alone center.

Most modern radiology departments also provide interventional radiological services (minimally invasive treatments performed with imaging guidance) in addition to the diagnostic services. These interventional services may be a big source of revenue generation for the system in addition to providing necessary management support to other clinician colleagues.[2]

PLANNING AND ORGANIZATION

With increasing technological advancements, there is a continuous requirement of performing a comprehensive systematic planning and organization for launching any modern imaging department. It is imperative to understand that launching any new radiological center involves some important steps and roadmaps that have a direct influence on planning. The preliminary important step is to do a critical project analysis. Performing a cost benefit analysis will determine the financial viability of the project and ensure its operational success. Critical discussion with important staff members of the hospital and inputs from the supporting architects and engineers will help in ensuing successful launch of the center. Analyzing the requirements for imaging equipment, space and personnel are other key steps which have profound impact on physical planning. Subsequently scheduling and designing are other necessary requirements for successful project implementation.[3]

There are three horizontal levels of workflow (strategic, managerial and operational) in any institution, may it be a government hospital or corporate funded hospital. Planning must be centered on the strategic level of decision making. The second level is the managerial or administrative level which focuses on routine issues likely timely attendance and productivity, patient's waiting lists, staff scheduling and reassignments. The operational level is where the examinations and procedures are actually performed in any department **(Fig. 1)**.[4]

The major objectives of a radiology department include:

- To provide comprehensive high quality imaging service
- Establishment and confirmation of clinical diagnosis
- Providing high quality therapeutic/interventional radiology
- Commitment to training and research.

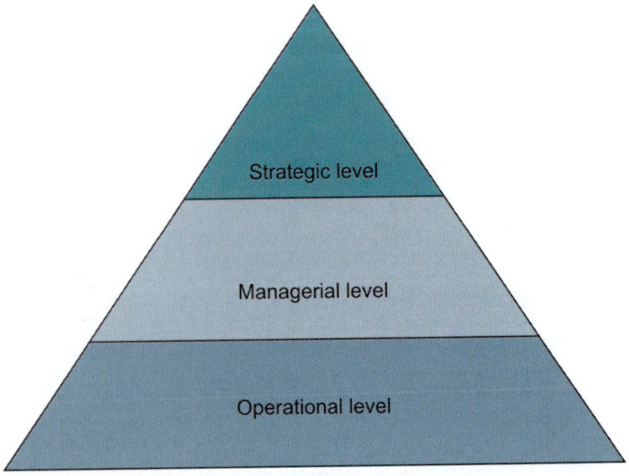

FIG. 1: Levels of radiological workflow.

DIVISIONS OF THE RADIOLOGY DEPARTMENT

The various sections of Radiology/Imaging services include:
- Radiography (X-ray machines/CR and DR System)
- Mammography
- Dual-energy X-ray absorptiometry (DEXA)
- Computed tomography (CT scan)
- Ultrasound with Doppler
- Magnetic resonance imaging (MRI)
- Digital subtraction angiography (DSA)
- Nuclear Imaging equipment.

To manage all these equipment with some producing rays/emissions which are harmful to health requires meticulous planning to ensure that radiation exposures to both patients and staff are optimized.[5]

LOCATION

The location of radiological department requires a very careful planning since it is one of the focal point of any hospital. The positions of different imaging facilities within the department is also important since it has a considerable impact upon the necessary requirements for radiation protection. Key aspects of planning should consider accessibility, workflow, patient comfort and traffic flow considerations, etc. Ease of access to patients from indoor wards, OPD and emergency department requires consideration. Central position on ground floor is generally preferred with some reserved space for further expansion to allow addition of equipment and services.[2] The location should be 10 meters away from the elevators due to their effect on the functioning of equipment in the department.[5]

A dedicated engineering approach is required to ensure a scientifically planned and optimally designed department with due importance paid to safety aspects thereby reducing risks associated with radiation to permissible levels. Strategic planning must be done with a clear understanding of the operational workflow in the department (staff movement, patient flow, material flow, technical procedures). Special attention to minor details related to operations can have significant impact on staff effectiveness and morale. Study of traffic patterns is an important prerequisite to the efficiency of any imaging department. This should be based on interactive discussions with the staff of the department and should consider the various activities like:[6]
- Movement of patients in and out of procedure rooms.
- Activity sequence within procedure rooms.
- Film processing and handling.
- Image interpretation and reporting.
- Filing.

LAYOUT

The layout of the department depends on the great extent the way the processes in the department are aligned and take place. Structural design and equipment layout plan should be carefully considered from a radiation protection perspective and should be in accordance with AERB guidelines. For ensuring operational efficiency and adequate radiation protection, it may be prudent to appropriately split the different functional areas to organize the workflow. These may be designed as:
- Public areas (reception and waiting lounge, preparation rooms, etc.)
- Staff areas (faculty offices, reporting chambers, etc.)
- Work areas (radiation rooms, console rooms, etc.).[2]

Corridors and doors leading to all patient areas and examination rooms should allow easy and safe movement of all patients, including handicapped or injured. Availability of toilet facilities is essential, particularly those suitable for handicapped patients. Also, the provision of safe storage facilities for patients' clothing and valuables during imaging is necessary.[6]

REGULATORY REQUIREMENTS

There are many regulatory bodies at the international and national level, which establish guidelines for radiation protection and recommend the permissible dose limits both for radiation personnel and the general public. The ICRP (International Commission for radiation protection) is the international body for regulation of radiation. Regulatory control for ensuring optimal safety of radiation in India is by Atomic Energy Regulatory Board (AERB).

AERB was constituted in 1983 and exercises powers of regulatory and legislative control envisaged under the Atomic Energy Act instituted by the Government of India in 1962. The main aim of the AERB is to ensure that use of ionizing radiation and nuclear energy in India does not cause undue risk to the health of people and the environment.

Main functions of AERB include:
- Safety review and assessment
- Licensing of various facilities
- Regulatory Inspections
- Regulatory enforcement
- Development of regulatory safety documents.

Safety standards and guidelines are an important aspect in early planning stages of a project since periodic safety review and assessment is one of integral component for exercising regulatory control. In order to ensure radiological safety, it is important to exercise strict administrative control over all facilities utilizing ionizing radiation in various equipment. Safety review ensures compliance to prescribed rules, safety requirements, obtaining operational licenses and other requirements of AERB. It is a continuous process throughout the lifetime of the facilities and ensures safety at all times. Safety review and assessment is required for generation of license for any equipment/facility and any noncompliance results in enforcement action like revocation or suspension of license.

AERB has an online portal for electronic licensing system for radiation applications termed E-LORA for facilitating users to file applications and necessary documents online.[7]

Regulatory Inspection (RI) is another key process of AERB through which it ensures that installation is compliant with the prescribed legal and regulatory licensing requirements.

AERB authorized inspectors perform both routine and special unannounced inspections to obtain realistic first hand information on the safety measures available at the facility and ensure regulatory compliance to safety requirements and relevant stipulations. The authorized inspectors have the power to take enforcement action at the site in consultation with the Competent Authority (Chairman, AERB), if required. This may be curtailment of activity or complete stoppage of function depending on the degree of noncompliance.

AERB formulates safety requirements and guidance for various radiation facilities in form of Regulatory Safety Documents. These are formulated as *Safety Codes and Standards* on the basis of internationally accepted safety standards and are periodically revised.[7]

Safety Code

Safety code elaborates various requirements to provide adequate assurance for radiation safety in aspects such as design, installation and operation of specific equipment and systems. Safety codes are for each practice elaborate requirements to be compiled by the licensee at all stages of activities. Safety assessment is based on satisfactory fulfillment of such requirements which are mandatory for the licensee in order to obtain the license by AERB. The safety code also covers roles and responsibilities of individuals involved in the manufacture, supply, servicing, operation and decommissioning of radiation facilities.[7]

Radiation Testing Facility for Demonstration of Type Approval

The dose limits for public and radiation workers are met by using shielding, protective devices and space requirements to the radiation testing facility should be in such manner as prescribed by the Competent Authority. Outside the radiation testing facility, the radiation warning placard should be displayed.

Radiation Protection Devices

Appropriate radiation protection devices **(Fig. 2A)** like barrier lead flaps, radiation shield, thyroid shield, lead apron, lead goggles and lead gloves, etc. should have appropriate lead equivalent as per AERB guidelines. These devices shall be verified periodically for its shielding adequacy. Further radiation warning signs **(Fig. 2B)** should be prominently displayed in front of the doors of all the radiation rooms in the radiology department.

Quality Assurance Program

The fundamental principles which govern the radiation protection include optimization, justification and the as-low-as-reasonably-achievable (ALARA) doses, which are to supplemented by sound quality control (QC) practices. A robust quality assurance program will ensure in maintaining optimal diagnostic performance of all equipment with minimum hazard and distress to patients. This professional approach will promote the due process of developing technical specifications, standards in accordance with the latest technical knowledge of the equipment.

Radiological Safety Officer

Every radiology department shall designate a Radiological Safety Officer (RSO) with written approval by the Competent Authority who should ensure compliance with the quality assurance program effectively in conformity with the prescribed regulatory requirements. RSO should possess adequate knowledge regarding radiation protection with the minimum qualifications and training as prescribed by the Competent Authority.

Quality Assurance Equipment

Supplier shall have appropriate quality assurance (QA) and radiation monitoring equipment for radiation testing of the

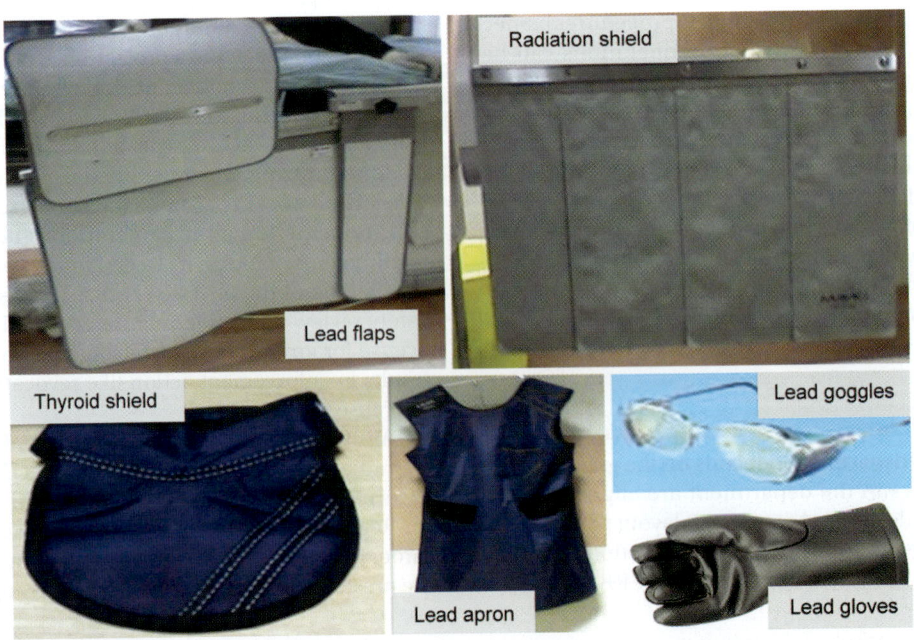

FIG. 2A: Radiation protection devices.

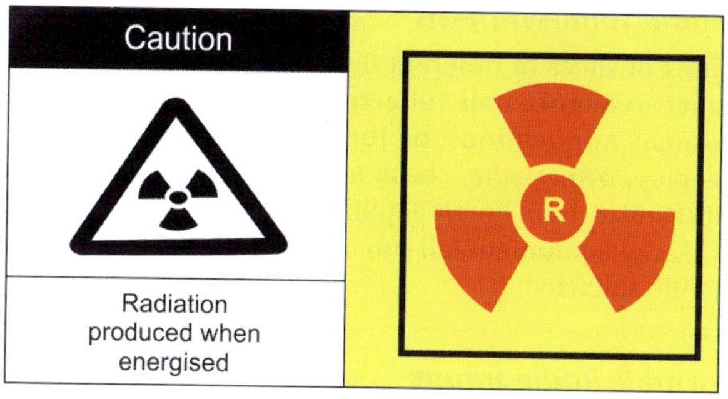

FIG. 2B: Radiation warning signs.

equipment producing ionizing radiation. There should be a valid calibration of the dosimeter equipment used to check the quality assurance to an acceptable standard.

EQUIPMENTS

The equipments used in this department are highly sophisticated and expensive. The major equipments and facilities are described here.

Conventional Radiography

The most important and easily performed imaging service in the front line of medical care is plain radiography. The X-ray unit must be able to perform all essential general radiographic examinations like chest, abdomen and extremities. In conventional radiography, majority of the radiographic examinations have been carried out by projecting the beam through the patient and allowing the transmitted beam to strike X-ray film or Intensifying screen to produce the latent image. The latent image can be made visible and permanent by processing the film with suitable chemicals **(Fig. 3)**.

Darkroom

When designing a darkroom, beside the operational considerations concerning the film development, the primary concern is the shielding of unexposed film from exposure to radiation (X-rays and daylight). The common location for a main darkroom is central in the imaging department. Dry and wet areas should be separate from each other and chemicals must be stored safely.[6]

Digital Radiography

Digital X-ray sensors are used in digital radiography in place of radiography film. Digital radiography systems are replacing films in the modern departments. It is a representation of continuous analog information into digital form by the use of computer which processes the digital data to form an image. The image quality of both digital image receptors and film screen image receptors remains almost same with lesser radiation dose in digital radiography. In the future, advanced processing techniques for example computer sided detection (CAD), temporal subtraction and dual energy subtraction will use to detect of subtle and focal lesions.[8] In digital radiography, a comprehensive quality assurance program should be implemented which included the quality control and continuous quality improvement.

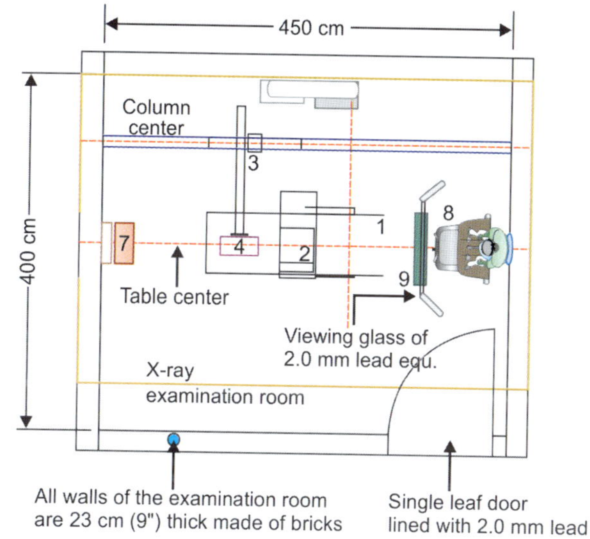

1. Examination table; 2. Spot film device; 3. Column stand; 4. X-ray tube head; 7. Chest stand; 8. Control unit; 9. MPB with lead glass viewing window of 1.7 mm lead equivalence

FIG. 3: Model Layout—X-ray installation.

Courtesy: e-Licensing of Radiation Applications (eLORA) System, July 2016.

Modulation transfer function (MTF) and detector quantum efficiency (DQE) are two objective performance measures to describe dose requirement and resolution.[9]

Three main digital detector technologies are commercially available which include:

Storage Phosphor Radiography (Computed Radiography, CR)

It uses storage-phosphor image plates having a detective layer of photostimulable crystals and separate image readout process.[10] This is advantageous and more cost effective as existing X-ray machines can be used to obtain digital images.

CR cassettes have storage phosphors which trap electrons during exposure which are subsequently extracted using a laser scanner.[11]

Dual-reading CR Systems

The detector material used by this system is transparent with light collection optics both in the front and the back side of the detector which improves quantum detection (DQE).[12]

Parallel Reading (Line Scanning)

Linear array of laser diodes are used in this system where all pixels work in one line simultaneously, thereby increasing the speed of processing with results that are comparable to most digital detectors for radiography.[11]

Needle-crystalline CR Detectors

A new detector material (CsBr: Eu2+) for storage phosphor systems facilitates producing thicker detector layer (improving DQE) without deteriorating spatial resolution (MTF).

Flat-panel Direct Detector Systems

There are two different detector systems (DS) technologies. Direct conversion systems or electro-direct systems use a photo conducting layer (amorphous selenium, a-Se), in which the absorbed X-ray energy is directly converted into charge on top of a TFT array. Indirect conversion systems or opto-direct systems use a scintillator (e.g., cesium iodide, CsI or gadolinium oxysulphide, GOS or Gadox) layered on top of an array with light-sensitive photodiodes with thin-film transistors (TFTs) **(Figs. 4 and 5)**.[13-15]

CCD Detector Technology

It is used to collimate the light emitted by a scintillator screen to the CCD, that can cause better image quality and decrease dose efficiency.[16] This optical coupling (demagnification) has made this technology more useful for chest X-ray.[17]

Slot-scanning CCD Technology

This technology is based on a CsI scintillator which is coupled to a linear array of CCDs that covers the whole slot that is used to scan the chest. The improved signal to noise produced by scatter reduction compensates for lower DQE of CCD technology, which can be translated to improve the quality or decrease the dose.[18]

Computer-aided Diagnosis

This system help radiologist in detection and differentiation of similar disease along with suggestion of abnormal region or lesion in the chest.

Dual-energy Subtraction

Two different X-ray energies are used to make exposure and remove bone or soft tissues by subtraction of the two images. It helps in detection of masses and nodules, improved detection of lesions of rib and to differentiate calcified and non-calcified lesions.[19,20]

Digital Tomosynthesis

Series of slices at different depths are produced using flat panel detectors and tube rotation in this technology.[21] Clinical applications of tomosynthesis include breast imaging, orthopedic, chest, and urinary applications with most advances in breast applications.[22]

X-ray equipment fall broadly into two groups portable/ mobile and fixed:

Portable Radiography

Equipment means the X-ray unit is capable of being taken to the destination to be used.It is very simple to use and can be packed into carrying cases and so transported. Portable sets relatively have low mA setting, can be dismantled for transfer. Mobile X-ray imaging is possible using these mobile X-ray units which are very helpful in digitalization in various emergency rooms.[23,24]

Wireless FPDs

Wireless portable DR system is now a reality. After exposure, it wirelessly transfer image data to the DR system. It has no cables and does not interfere with surrounding machines, so it is easy to handle as CR cassettes.[25] Typically a 17" × 14" image size is made available within 3s **(Fig. 6)**.

Mobile Image Intensifiers Units (C-Arm)

Mobile unit for fluoroscopy with an image intensifier is used during operation which reduces the number of X-rays during the procedure

Regulatory Requirements in the Use of X-ray Equipment

Authorization for X-ray Machine Supply

Authorization should be obtained by all suppliers for all models of X-ray equipment proposed to be supplied.

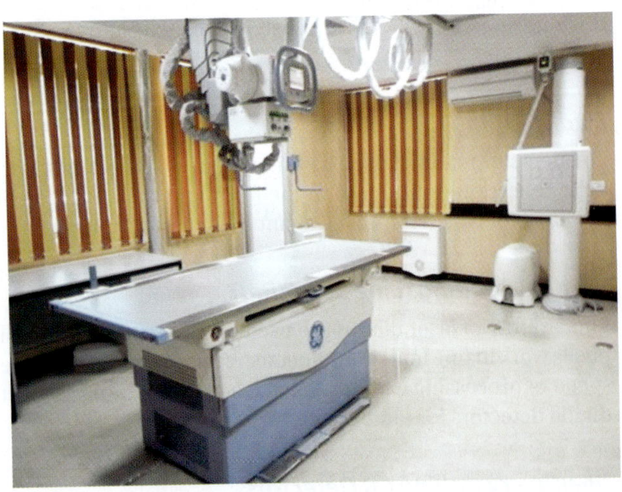

FIG. 4: DR flat panel X-ray unit.

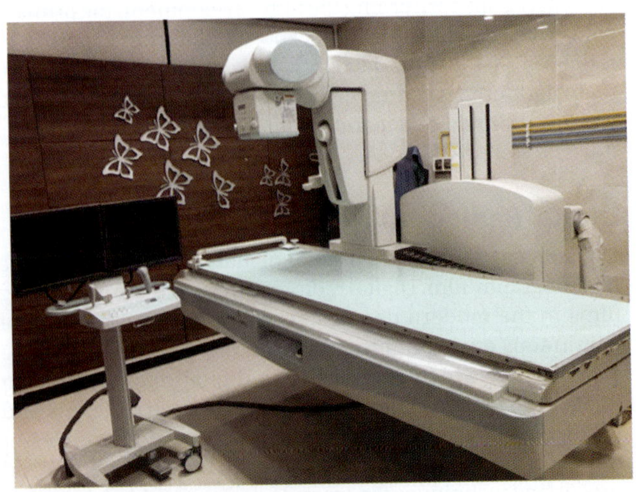

FIG. 5: DR and fluoroscopy unit (flat panel).

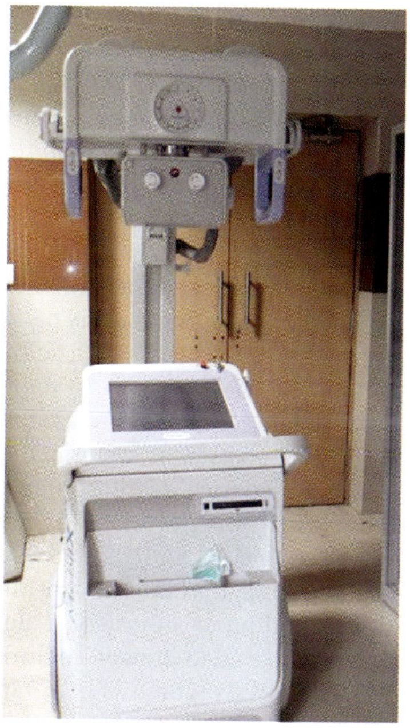

FIG. 6: Mobile digital radiography unit.

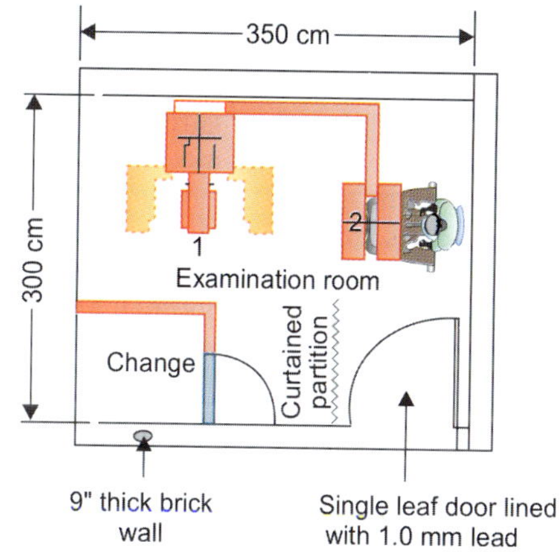

1. Mammography equipment; 2. Control unit with protective barrier of 1.5 mm lead equivalence

FIG. 7: Model layout—mammography installation.
Courtesy: e-Licensing of Radiation Applications (eLORA) System, July 2016.

Procurement of X-ray Equipment

The employer of X-ray facility shall procure NOC (No objection certificate) from authorized supplier for the approved X-ray equipment. Radiograph shall not be used for patient diagnosis unless license for operation is obtained from competent authority.

MAMMOGRAPHY

This radiography technique use high precision X-ray machine which gives reliable radiographic examinations of the breast along with reduced radiation dose which help in diagnosis of breast disease.[5]

Digital mammography is the alternative to Screen film mammography (SFM) which is being increasingly recognized **(Fig. 7)**. Solid-state detectors are used in digital mammography instead of the X-ray film. These convert the X-rays into electrical signals which are used to produce digital images.[26]

Various other advances in the field of mammography include:

Computer-aided Detection Systems

This system use software and digitized image to search for various findings of cancer like mass, abnormal density or calcification and mark these areas or lesions.

Breast tomosynthesis is also known as three dimensional (3-D) breast imaging and is based on flat panel detectors and tube rotation in an arc where series of slices of the breast are obtained. This allows better visualization of cancer and reduces the recall rates for additional imaging.[27]

Dual energy subtraction mammography and Contrast-enhanced digital mammography are also newer advanced techniques which help in improved lesion detection in difficult and indeterminate lesions.

Stereotactic biopsy from indeterminate lesions is also a recent advance.

DUAL-ENERGY X-RAY ABSORPTIOMETRY

Dual-energy X-ray absorptiometry (DEXA) is an imaging technique that is commonly used and most standard method to measure bone mineral density (BMD). DEXA provides an optimal combination of low cost, easy availability and accurate assessment which makes it the preferred option over other modalities.

The technique uses very small dose of ionizing radiation and relies on measurements of polychromatic spectra of X-rays for each image which is centered at variable energies to allow calcium, and therefore bone mineral density be assessed. The early-generation DEXA scanners used conventional pencil beam scanning; however recent technological advancements have resulted in equipment with fan beams, cone beams and c-arm technology allowing faster scans with improved image quality and better patient comfort **(Fig. 8)**.[28,29]

The DEXA scan is the most accurate and reliable way to diagnose and follow osteoporosis and predicts an individual's risk for developing fractures in future. It also aids as a useful tool in follow-up response to therapy and guides in taking treatment decisions. DEXA scans can also be used for assessment of soft tissue body mass composition with diagnostic accuracy that is nearly comparable to the hydrostatic weighing with certain caveats.[30,31]

Based on the site of examination, it may be categorized into:

Central DEXA-- Lumbar spine and hip

Peripheral DEXA-- forearm, hand, calcaneus.

The bone measures available from all DEXA scan modes include Bone mineral content (BMC), Bone area (BA) and Areal bone mineral density (aBMD).

Whole body DEXA also includes assessment of body composition measures which include objective measures of Fat Mass, Lean soft tissue mass (LSTM) and Fat free mass (FFM).[30]

COMPUTED TOMOGRAPHY

CT scan is a medical imaging modality which has become one of the most powerful tool for various diagnostic and therapeutic purposes in virtually all medical disciplines. The modern day CT systems generate volume of data that can be acquired by various techniques and protocols based on the clinical concern. CT is the workhorse diagnostic tool for imaging and evaluation of chest, abdomen and pelvis. CT is generally the initial approach in a time sensitive situation particularly in cases of trauma.

CT applications have greatly expanded because of increasing innovations in acquisition of image and reconstruction technologies. The modern day CT scanners (64 and 128 slice) can acquire sub-millimeter resolution images of the body parts in a few seconds. This allows depiction of the fine anatomical details of the body parts without any motion artifact **(Figs. 9A and B)**. The imaging data acquired can be post processed into various formats like volume rendered projections, multi planar and cine reformats, which allow the depiction of anatomical abnormalities with greater clarity. This also facilitates new applications such as Dynamic CT, CT angiography, cardiac CT, CT enterography, CT Colonography, CT urography and virtual endoluminal techniques like tracheobronchography. With recent advancements and availability of dual-energy CT, there is transition of CT from a solely morphological imaging technique to a more comprehensive imaging modality which can provide excellent anatomical information with insight to the functional and metabolic aspects of the pathology.[32]

CT angiography (CTA) allows the visualization of the entire vascular system after injection of contrast medium. Several imaging post-processing techniques are available enabling good display of the entire vascular system. The techniques which are most widely used include multi-planar and curved planar reformats (MPR), maximum intensity projection (MIP), Volume Rendering (VR) and Shaded Surface Display (3D-SSD). Sophisticated segmentation algorithms, removal of bone with thresh holding or subtraction algorithms and vessel analysis tools are also newer techniques which provide good vessel analysis which is comparable to DSA (Conventional angiography). The clinical applications for these various image postprocessing methods include steno-occlusive disease, aneurysms and vascular malformations.[33]

Virtual endoscopy (VE) is a recent development in post-processing technique that generates virtual endoscopic views. This technique obtains a perspective view of the display region and is used mainly for evaluation of anatomical cavities, which include the large vessels, colon, bronchial tree, and paranasal sinuses. VE is used to assess the areas, which are not directly accessible for conventional endoscopy. The perspective Volume Rendering Technique allows real-time fly through at high resolution mimicking the true endoscopy.

Installation of X-ray and CT scanner unit requires approval of AERB and need to conform to radiation protections measures **(Fig. 10)**. However, CT examination involves radiation exposure with potential risks and should be performed judiciously particularly in children who are more radio sensitive than adults.

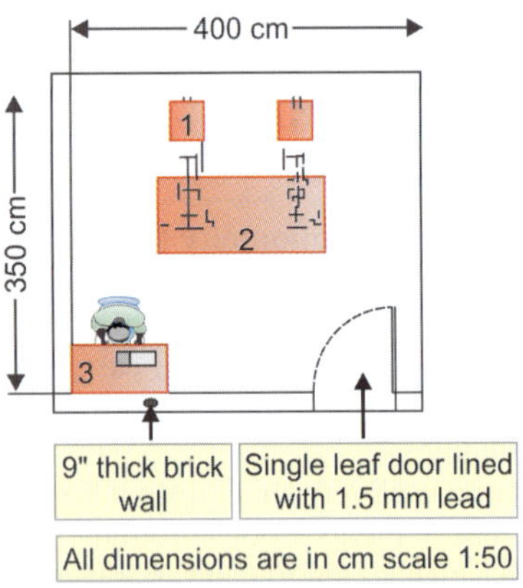

1. BMD equipment; 2. Examination table; 3. Evaluation unit

FIG. 8: Model layout—BMD installation.

Courtesy: e-Licensing of Radiation Applications (eLORA) System, July 2016.

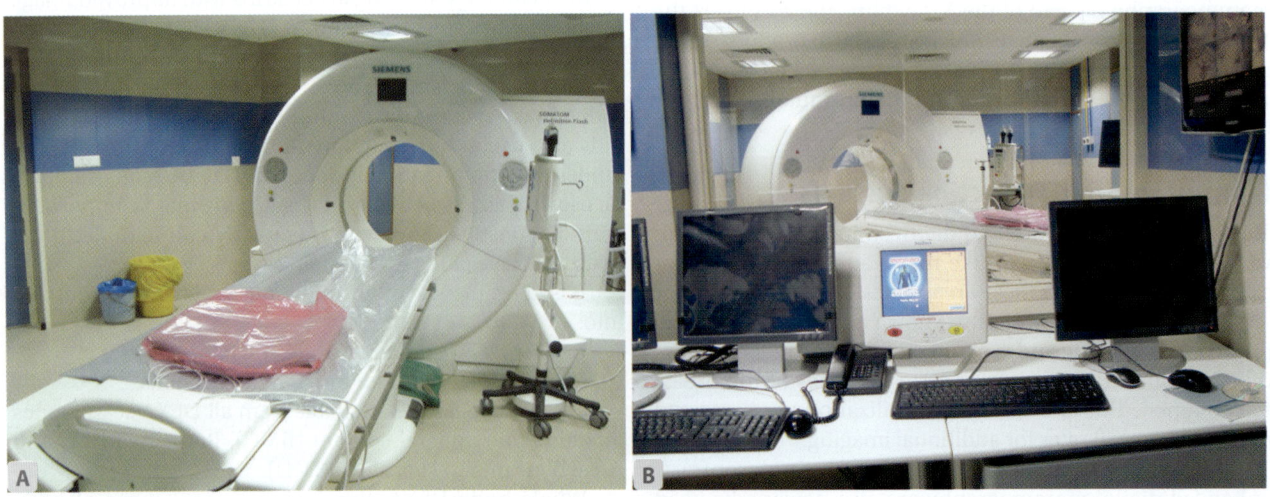

FIGS 9A AND B: 128 slice Dual source CT scanner.

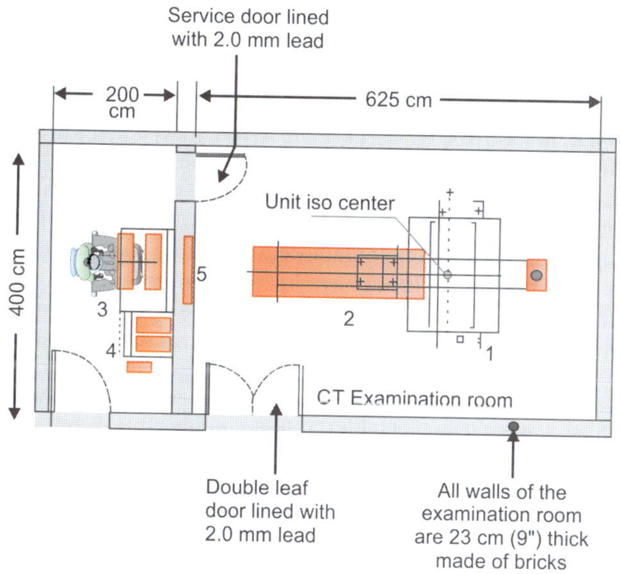

1. CT gantry; 2. Examination table; 3. Control unit; 4. Electronics; 5. Viewing glass 100 cm × 80 cm of 2.0 mm lead equivalence

FIG. 10: Model layout CT-scan installation.

Courtesy: e-Licensing of Radiation Applications (eLORA) System, July 2016.

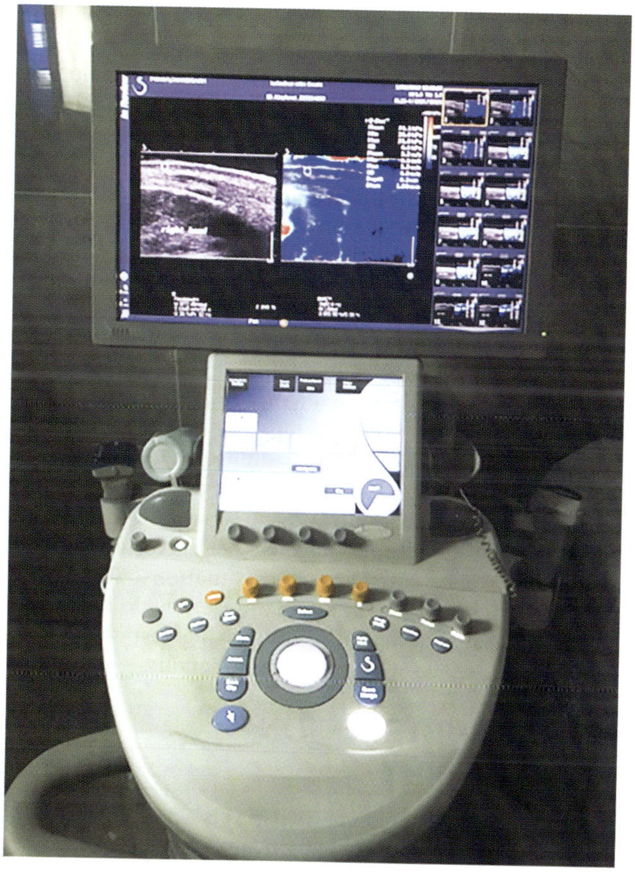

FIG. 11: Advanced ultrasound system.

ULTRASOUND

It is a non-invasive diagnostic modality that uses the transmission of high-frequency sound waves into the body to visualize the various internal organs of the body in real time. It has the important advantages of being widely available, low cost and does not use ionizing radiation. This modality has become one of the most preferred imaging for diagnostic, interventional, monitoring and follow-up of patients. It has a vital role in obstetrical imaging and is used both for assessing the fetal development and early diagnosis of many fetal anomalies.

Ultrasound is also useful for various guided interventions and can be performed on bedside in the triage of trauma patients. The quality of examination is however highly dependent on the experience of the sonographer in addition to the patient body habitus. The advanced ultrasound system include harmonic imaging, color and power Doppler and 3D and 4D reconstructions **(Fig. 11)**. Technical advances like elastography and computer aided diagnosis have expanded the clinical applications especially in breast sonography.[34] Recently therapeutic applications with high intensity focused ultrasound (HIFU) and micro-bubble assisted delivery of genes and drugs are showing promising results.[35] The rules and regulations for setting up an ultrasound machine are described under the PC-PNDT act section later in the chapter.

MAGNETIC RESONANCE IMAGING

Magnetic resonance imaging (MRI) is a noninvasive diagnostic modality which employs the physical properties of nuclear magnetic resonance (NMR) to image certain atomic nuclei within human body. MRI technically differs from CT scans and X-rays in that they do not use the damaging ionizing radiation. MRI uses high-strength magnetic fields that align the hydrogen nuclei within the body parts imaged and various radiofrequency pulses are put on and off repeatedly. The signals from human tissues are received by coils placed near the area of interest and fed to computer, which converts these signals into an image.

MRI can provide detailed structural information about of any region of the body, however in clinical practice its usefulness has been best explored and realized for neuroimaging and musculoskeletal imaging. It can detect or sometimes help in characterizing vital 'lesions' that might be missed or indeterminate on other imaging modalities.[36] MRI provides excellent white and gray matter differentiation of nervous tissues. An advantage of MRI is its ability to image directly in all three orthogonal planes which adds to its versatility and provides new insight to visualize and interpret pathologies. MRI scans provide exquisite soft tissue contrast far superior to that achievable by other imaging modalities. Advances in MR technologies have resulted in integrating perfusion, diffusion-weighted imaging, and spectroscopy which provide a new insight in the functional aspect of the pathologies and may improve the accuracy of diagnosis. With advances in computer hardware and post processing algorithms, MRI has become an indispensable medical imaging technique in the current medical practice.

There are however limitations which include long imaging times, lying in a narrow bore and continuous hammering noisy environment. Some susceptible patients experience anxiety and claustrophobia which may increase patient movement, causing motion artifacts thereby compromising the diagnostic quality. Advances in MR technology including availability of higher field strengths (3 Tesla), and newer wide-bore and open magnet designs have enabled faster scans, with better patient comfort and more simplified workflows **(Fig. 12)**. MRI is contraindicated in implanted electrical devices, cochlear implants, insulin pumps, ferromagnetic aneurysmal clips and metallic foreign bodies and implants.[37]

The planning and conceptual structural designing of MR Suite is critical for providing robust vibration restricted foundation with minimal disturbing electromagnetic interference that will comply with the technical requirements of the installation. Robust acoustical and electromagnetic shielding is mandatory for efficient and safe working. This requires careful and thorough planning for setting up of a Faraday cage or RF/EMI shielded room from the beginning of setting up any project. The quench vent is crucial for safety and must also be designed and installed as per the recommended layout to deal with any emergency situations. Since MRI systems do not emit ionizing radiations, they do not come under regulatory purview of AERB which is responsible for regulating safe usage of only ionizing radiations.

DIGITAL SUBTRACTION ANGIOGRAPHY

Digital subtraction angiography (DSA) is a specialized type of fluoroscopic technique which involves selective injection of contrast material into the vessels and acquires sequential images at rates which are technically not feasible with conventional film-changer and film-cassette technologies.

Diagnostic DSA is usually done at 2–3 frames per second (fps). Higher frame rates (e.g. 8–20) are more suited for imaging of high flow lesions e.g. arteriovenous malformations. DSA helps in evaluation of both the structural anatomy as well as hemodynamic status of the lesion. It even helps in the therapeutic management of various vascular disorders.

DSA has very high spatial and temporal resolution which exceeds both CT and MR Angiography. Single plane DSA has limitation in form of single plane demonstration of vasculature in one time frame. There have been advancements in DSA technology which have addressed this issue by development of biplane systems. Moreover, with 3D rotational ability in the same unit, it is possible to generate high quality 3 dimensional volume rendered images, even better than which can be achieved with CT angiography. This technique combines the anatomic resolution of DSA with simultaneous evaluation of 3D relationships which was previously feasible only with CT or MR angiography, and hence provides more comprehensive information than DSA alone. 3D DSA is being increasingly preferred in planning of procedures as it provides exquisite detailed anatomic information of complex vascular lesions and also guides in selecting the most suitable working projection while performing the procedure. It is therefore essential for both for the optimal diagnosis and interventional management of aneurysms/arteriovenous malformations at any location and can reduce the number of exposures.[38,39]

From regulatory requirements perspective, in addition to the layout requirements stated in **Figures 13 and 14**, the equipment used for interventional radiology procedures should have a duly calibrated Dose-Area-Product (DAP) Meter. Patient dose monitoring and recording facility should

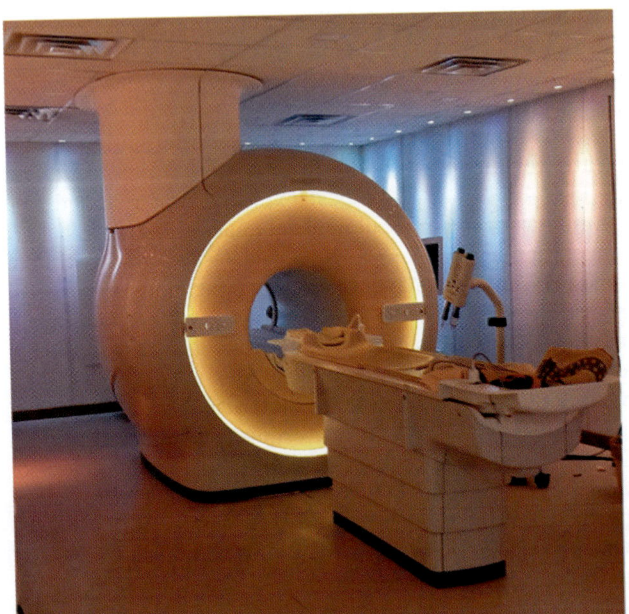

FIG. 12: 3 Tesla MRI system with coils

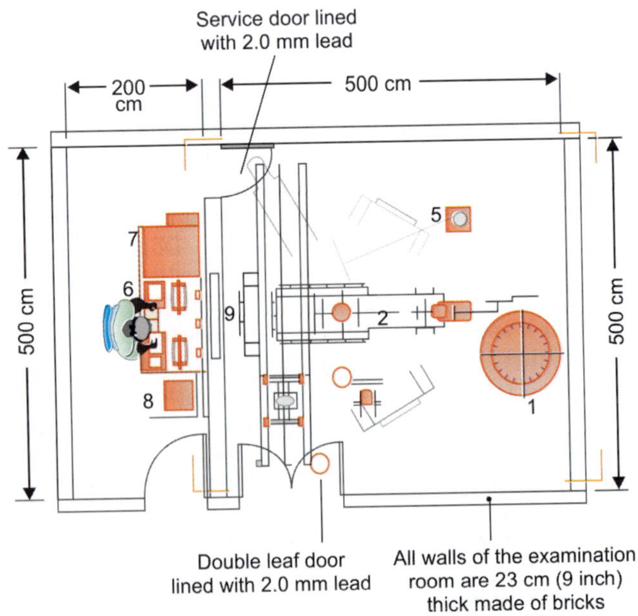

FIG. 13: Model layout—interventional radiology installation (1. C-arm; 2. Examination Table; 5. Fixed Radiation Shield; 6 to 8. Control Unit; 9. Viewing glass window of 120 cm x 100 cm of 2.0 mm lead equivalence).

Courtesy: e-Licensing of Radiation Applications (eLORA) System, July 2016.

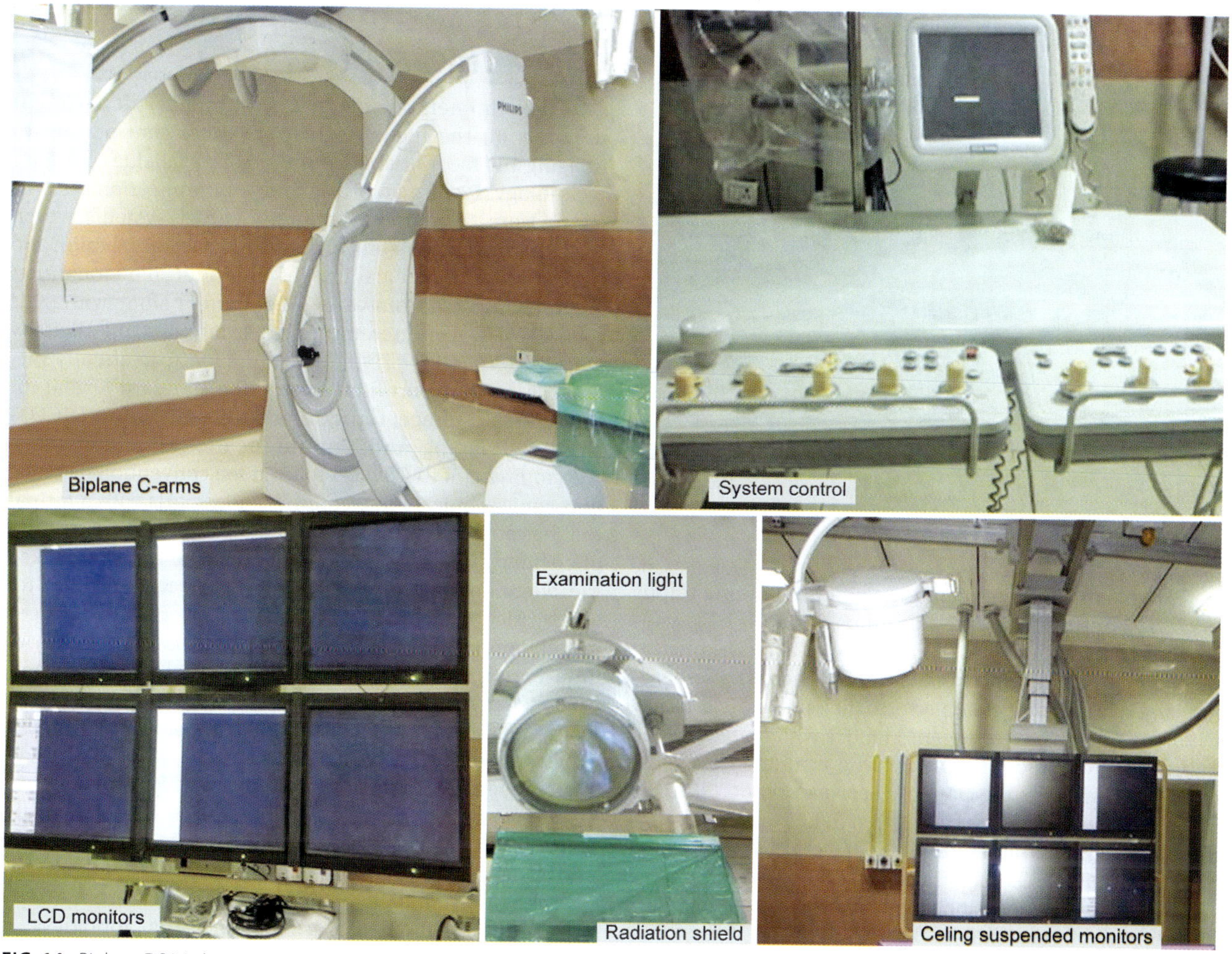

FIG. 14: Biplane DSA Lab.

be present which monitors dose related quantities i.e. total fluoroscopy time, number of cine runs, dose area product (mGy.cm^2), dose rate, cumulative Air Kerma and exposure parameters. Built-in Protective Device such as couch hanging protective flaps and ceiling suspended lead glass should be present. In addition Fluoroscopy timer with indicator alarm and foot switch and visual indicator are other important requirements.

Cone-beam computed tomography (CBCT) with digital flat panel detector has recently been incorporated for use in DSA systems. This allows the availability of performing fluoroscopy and subtraction angiography along with capability of obtaining soft-tissue information using computed tomography (CT) at the same working place during interventions. This can provide added information not apparent on conventional DSA which may result in alternate diagnosis, or revising the treatment plan. It aids in overall decision-making during interventions thereby helping in providing more standardized quality of care.[40]

Combined Angio-CT

Another newer advent is combination of angiography and sliding gantry CT system in a single suite. This allows fast and easy switching between CT and angio imaging without the need for patient transfer. This is helpful whenever treating patients requires the combination of both the modalities and the transfer from one modality to another includes risks and costs time e.g. trauma patients **(Fig. 15)**.

NUCLEAR IMAGING SYSTEMS

Nuclear medicine imaging is a type of medical imaging which provides unique insight into the functional information of changes occurring at cellular level that is unattainable with other imaging techniques. This involves administration of radiotracers (also called radiopharmaceuticals) which are detected by special types of cameras measuring their uptake and turnover. By providing information of the physiological processes, nuclear medicine offers a broad spectrum of applications for early and more accurate diagnosis and improved ability to determine the patient' response to treatment. Therapeutic applications of nuclear medicine are also adding another newer dimension to oncological management with promising results in treatment of thyroid cancer, neuroendocrine tumor, prostate cancer and palliation of bone pains where beta or alpha emitters are used.

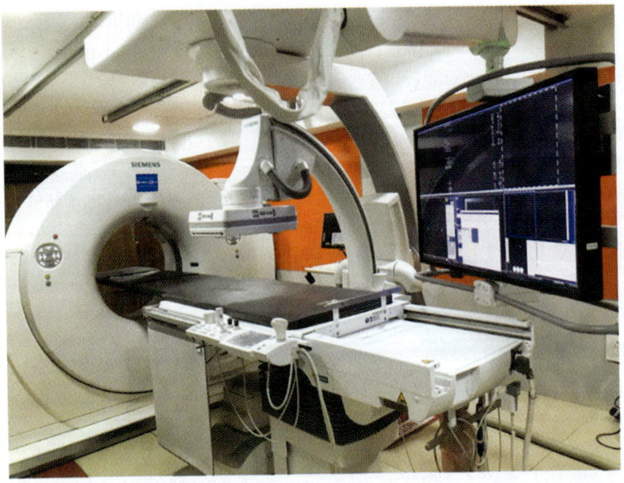

FIG. 15: Angio-CT Suite

Planar/single photon emission computed tomography (SPECT) and positron emission tomography (PET) scans are the most frequently used imaging modalities in nuclear medicine. The radiotracers must meet specified standards for safety and appropriate performance for clinical usage. Different tracers have different kinetics which are selected based on the clinical problem to be evaluated and that determine whether the patient receives a SPECT or PET scan. The primary difference between SPECT and PET scans is the type of radiotracers used. PET tracers commonly used include F18 FDG, Ga-68-DOTANOC, N-13 ammonia while the SPECT tracers routinely used include Tc-99m MDP, EC, Mebrofenin sestamibi, I-123, I-123 MIBG. The SPECT imagers have gamma camera detectors that can detect the gamma ray emissions, whereas the detectors in the PET scanner measure the photons and both equipment use this information to create three-dimensional images of internal organs. The major clinical application of PET scan is in the field of oncology for early and improved detection, staging, monitoring response to treatment, and to detect distant metastases.

With advent of hybrid imaging devices, combination of morphological information by computed tomography (CT) to the biological functional information by PET and SPECT has nearly transformed the conventional practice of cancer management. Integrated hybrid imaging has led to changing management paradigms which will continue to evolve in the future for delivering better patient care.[41]

The shielding requirements for a nuclear medicine facility include structural shielding for the various rooms and local shielding of the radionuclide sources used. Regulatory requirements are mentioned in AERB Safety Code for Nuclear Medicine Facilities, AERB/RF-SC/MED-2(Rev.2), 2011. Requisite regulatory consent from AERB should be obtained as per AERB Safety Guide for Consenting Process for Radiation Facilities.

PICTURE ARCHIVING AND COMMUNICATION SYSTEMS

The development of electronic (filmless) department depends on the technological advances that pertain to imaging and those arising from generally available computer technology. Picture archiving and communication systems (PACS) are computers, generally server systems which manage convenient storage, quick retrieval, distribution and transmission of medical images from multiple modalities. The imaging data from various equipment along with their reports are transmitted through a secure network digitally via PACS; thereby eliminating the need to manually file, retrieve, or transport film jackets. The standard format for PACS image storage, retrieval and transmission is DICOM (Digital Imaging and Communications in Medicine). Development of PACS has replaced the conventional analog film, paper clinical request forms and reports with a format that has completely computerized electronic display. PACS offers many advantages to radiologists with more organized radiology imaging data with access to various computer tools which can manipulate and post-process the images thereby enhancing the overall function and efficiency of data management. Capability of remotely viewing and interpreting images enables collaboration across provider teams thereby supporting primary and secondary health centers at point of care.

A modern PACS must possess capability for simultaneous display of new and preceding studies in a user-friendly manner for necessary review and comparison and access to prior radiology and clinical reports.[42]

The PACS architecture comprises of:

Centralized PACS—(hub and spoke, star topology) — single short-term storage unit to which every modality and every workstation is connected on a point to point basis.

Distributed PACS—composed of number of linked clusters, each with its own short term storage unit and one or more image acquisition modalities and several diagnostic/review workstations. Short-term storage is provided by one or more RAIDs (Random Array of Inexpensive Disks). RAID is composed of magnetic hard disks which are linked to a server which is connected directly to the PACS workstations. Connection can be made at various bandwidths, the highest generally being gigabit ethernet **(Figs. 16A and B)**.

The major benefits of PACS result from digitization of data which allows easy comparison, simultaneous multi location viewing, faster image retrieval, automatic chronological ordering and rapid database search.

Some of the disadvantages include the inherent costs and technological complexity which requires adequate trained hospital staff. A dedicated maintenance program and a carefully devised plan to provide essential clinical services in case of PACS failure.[43,44]

Hospital information system (HIS) is information management system which regulates all the information of

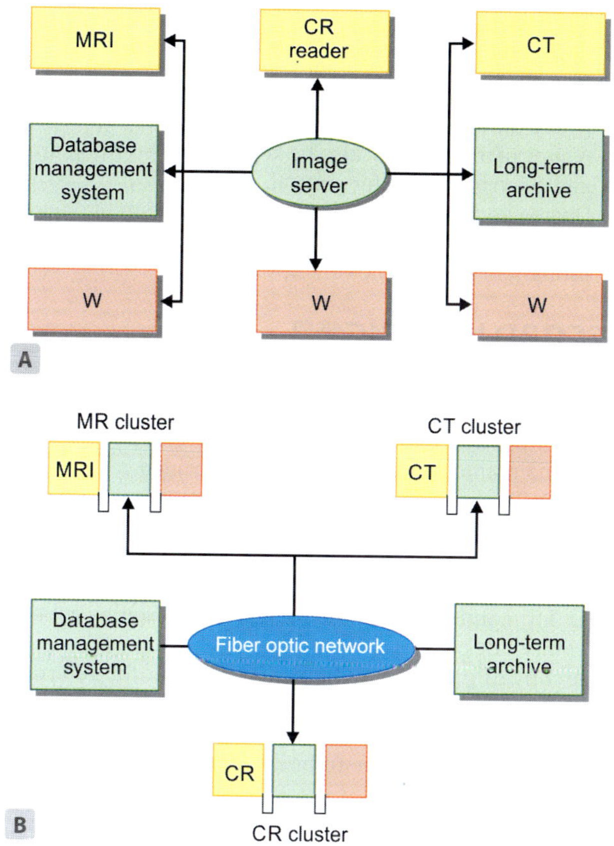

FIGS. 16A AND B: PACS architecture (A) with workstation; (B) with networking.

the patients to streamline processes within the hospital and reduce patient waiting time and ensures efficient workflow. They manage the data related to the various streams in the hospital like clinical information, pharmacy, nursing, radiology and laboratory/pathology departments, etc.

Radiology information system (RIS) can be a stand-alone computer platform, or may be a module of the HIS. It stores information specific to the radiology department including radiological reports .Modern RIS will incorporate some DICOM features such as modality work list, modality performed procedure step, interpretation work list, and structured reporting.

Health Level 7 is an internationally accepted standard for HIS and RIS systems.

HIS-RIS-PACS Integration should preferably be bidirectional. Input of demographic data is only once thereby minimizing human error. Any update to a patients demographic data or any scheduling is propagated to all systems HIS, RIS, or PACS automatically, hence providing advanced notice of events and allowing them to prepare.[45]

TELERADIOLOGY

Teleradiology is a growing practice of radiology which involves interpreting medical images while not physically present in the location where the images are generated.

It has proved to be a valuable tool in providing access to rapid and quality radiologic interpretations for studies performed in emergency room, ICU's and other examinations after routine working hours and on weekends. Teleradiology has facilitated a unique role of providing radiologists interpretation at distant remote and rural areas who do not have radiologists. There are however limitations and issues including lack of supervision of studies, gaps in the relevant medical history and clinical assessment of the patient which may compromise the quality and safety of patient care.

PRE-CONCEPTION AND PRE-NATAL DIAGNOSTIC TECHNIQUE (PC-PNDT) ACT

The Pre-natal Diagnostic Techniques (Regulation and prevention of misuse) Act was enacted on 20th September 1994. The Act came into existence after the government realized that the cause of skewed sex ratio, especially in parts of Northern India, was the prenatal termination of female fetuses. The easy availability of ultrasound was wrongly used for determining the sex of the unborn baby fetus as the girl child is unwelcome in many homes due to the cultural preference for a male heir, social stigmas in bringing up a girl child, economic burden of dowry and marriage expenses. There was a high preference for a boy child, and the indefensible choice of 'killing' the female child even before 'she' was born was often made. The act banned usage of diagnostic techniques for determining the sex of a fetus. The nomenclature of the Act was amended in 2002, and now it stands as Pre-conception and Pre-natal Diagnostic Techniques (Prohibition of Sex Selection) Act.[46]

Offenses under this act are *cognizable, non-compoundable and non-bailable.*[47] Implementing and prosecuting authorities under the Act are: Appropriate Authority (AA) at Union Territory, District and State levels; any officer authorized by AA, state or central governments; and any officer who has given notice of 15 days of the offence to the AA and his intent to make a complaint in the court.[47] Rules that have to be followed by medical professionals, who are using prenatal imaging equipment capable of sex determination, under this Act are listed below:

REGISTRATION[48,49]

1. All the nursing homes, ultrasound centers, and places where prenatal imaging equipment capable of sex determination, including ultrasound, has to be installed need to be registered. Registration needs to be done three months in advance. Any kind of ultrasound machine, including Doppler or not, needs to be registered even if the center does only pregnancy, only abdominal or cardiac scans. Registration is valid for five years since issue.
2. Two copies of Form 'A' should be submitted for registration along with all the documents pertaining to the ultrasound machine. In addition, an undertaking, which is notarized should be submitted that 'Sex selection and detection are not performed at the center and are punishable under

the law' message in the local language and English will be displayed at the center. An undertaking should also be submitted which states that 'sex selection and detection will not be done at the center.'

3. For registration renewal, an application has to be given at least one month before to the AA. The center is considered registered if authorities do not respond within 90 days.
4. If the application for registration renewal is not received on time, the center will be considered not registered, and the center will have to pay the penalty.
5. All the doctors including radiologists, gynecologists using ultrasound machine have to have their name registered. The doctors should be qualified as specified in the Act, to perform the ultrasound and registered in both the State medical council and office of the State Appropriate Authority.
6. No doctor, who is not registered in that particular center, can perform an ultrasound. If any doctor on a temporary basis (locum) has to perform an ultrasound, the appropriate authority should be notified and permission acquired after giving doctor's details: the doctor's medical council registration number and degree certificate, seven days in advance from the date of performance.
7. All ultrasound machines of a center, including the old machines, should be registered. The make and model and serial Number as well manufacturer's name is included in the PC-PNDT registration certificate.
8. When there is a change in the location of the radiology center or the ultrasound machine, it has to be informed to the appropriate authority 30 days prior to the change.
9. The certificate of registration has to be surrendered if there is a change in the ownership of the center, as the certificate is non-transferable. A fresh registration has to be applied by the new owner.
10. MRI and CT machines also need to be registered with the AA.

REQUIREMENTS AT THE ULTRASOUND CENTER[48,49]

1. Advertisements of pre-natal determination or pre-conception selection of sex are punishable under the Act.
2. The gender of a fetus cannot be disclosed to the referring doctor, patient, patient's relative, or anyone else, in word or sign language or any other means.
3. Persons who are working at an ultrasound center should display their name prominently on the overcoat worn by them or have an identity card.
4. The reception or waiting area and ultrasound room/rooms must display the center's registration certificate.
5. A board displaying 'sex selection and detection is not done at the center and is punishable under the PC-PNDT Act' in English, and the local language must be prominently exhibited in the reception/waiting area and the room where ultrasound is being performed.
6. A copy of the act must also be kept in the Reception area, and given to anyone for perusal.
7. Degree and State medical council registration of doctors who are performing procedures have to be displayed at a prominent place at the center.

RECORD KEEPING[48,49]

1. All antenatal ultrasound records are to be maintained for a duration of not less than two years, and if any case is pending, then the record of that particular patient must be maintained until the legal case is decided.
2. Form 'F' for maintenance of record for prenatal diagnostic test/procedure to be filled by ultrasound centers or genetic clinics for pregnant patients; Form 'E' for maintenance of records has to be filled by genetic laboratories; Form D' for maintenance of record has to be filled by genetic counseling centers.
3. A copy of patient's Aadhar, request from the referring doctor, a copy of the filled Form 'F', and the copy of ultrasound report or an electronic copy of ultrasound report and images are to be stored and made available when asked for.
4. Filling of Form 'F':
    a. The Form 'F's must be filled completely. There should not be any delay in filling up form. It should be completed as soon as the patient's ultrasound is done. No column should be left blank. Any blank area to be filled as not applicable.
    b. Two copies of Form 'F' have to be filled: One form has to be kept at the clinic, and the other submitted to the AA. In case of online submission: one form has to be submitted online, and the other copy must be retained at the clinic.
    c. Form 'F 'has to have details: the obstetric history of the patient, the number of children of the patient, the sex of each child, referring doctor, indication of ultrasound examination and the result of the ultrasound examination.
    d. Form 'F' has to be signed by the doctor who is performing the ultrasound examination. Doctor's name and designation should be written under his/her Full Signature.
    e. The patient must be given a receipt and a report with the doctor's signed declaration on sex determination.
    f. Monthly report has to given to AA by 5th of each month.

REFERENCES

1. Edwina H. The Future Delivery of Diagnostic Imaging Services in Wales December, 2009.
2. Aggarwal R, Planning an Imaging Department - Express Healthcare. (http://www.expresshealthcare.in)
3. Woodford DA. Project planning in the diagnostic imaging department. Radiol Manage. 1997;19(3):35-9.
4. Evan Leepson. Strategic Planning for Radiology: Opening an Outpatient Diagnostic Imaging Center. Radiology management March/April. 2003.
5. Singh H, Gayatri S. Radiology & Imaging Department. (http://www.drharisingh.com)
6. Salem D. Standard Specifications for Basic Diagnostic Radiology Departments. January 2011. (moh-gr.org/pdf/Standard%20 Specifications.pdf)
7. Regulatory requirements and model layout figures for various equipment and installations are courtesy (Amendment to AERB safety code on medical x-ray equipment and installations AERB/RF-MED/SC-3(Rev.2),2016 and (e-Licensing of Radiation Applications (eLORA) System (Medical Diagnostic Manual)-July 14, 2016.
8. Cornelia schaefor- Prokop, Uirich Neitzal, Henk W. Venema et al. Pigtail chest radiography: on and control of image quality update on modern technology dose containments. Eur Radio. 2008;18:1818-30.
9. Samei E. Performance of digital radiographic detectors: quantification and assessment methods. Advances in digital radiography: RSNA 2003: Categorical Course in diagnostic Radiology Physics; 2003.pp.37-47.
10. Korner M , Weber C H, Wirth S, Pfeifer K, Reiser MF, Treitl M. Advances in Digital Radiography: Physical Principles and System Overview. Radio Graphics. 2007;27:675-86.
11. Rivetti S, Lanconelli N, Bertolini M, Nitrosi A, Burani A, Acchiappati D. Comparison of different computed radiography systems: physical characterization and contrast detail analysis. Med Phys. 2010;37(2):440.
12. Arakawa S, Itoh W, Kohda K et al. Novel computed radiography system with improved image quality by detection of emissions from both sides of an imaging plate. SPIE Medical Imaging, poster presentation, 1999.
13. Samei E, Flynn MJ. An experimental comparison of detector performance for direct and indirect digital radiography systems. Med Phys. 2003;30:(4):608-22.
14. Metz S, Damoser P, Hollweck R et al. Chest radiography with a digital flat-panel detector: experimental receiver operating characteristic analysis. Radiology. 2005;234(3):776-84.
15. Bacher K, Smeets P, Vereecken L et al. Image quality and radiation dose in digital chest imaging: comparison of an amorphous silicon and an amorphous selenium flat-panel system. AJR. 2006;187:(3):630-7.
16. Bath M, Sund P, Mansson LG. Evaluation of the imaging properties of two generations of a CCD based system for digital chest radiography. Med Phys. 2002;29:2286-97.
17. Lawinski C, Mackenzie A, Cole H et al. Digital detectors for general radiography: a comparative technical report. National Health Service report 05078. K-CARE web site.http/www.kcare.co.uk/publkications/abstracts/ report05078.htm. 2005.
18. Samei E, Saunders RS, Lo JY et al. Fundamental imaging characteristics of a slot scan digital chest radiographic system. Med Phys. 2004;31(9):2687-98.
19. MacMahon H. Improvement in detection of pulmonary nodules: digital image processing and computer-aided diagnosis. Radiographics. 2000;20(4):1169-77.
20. Gilkeson RC, Sachs PB. Dual energy subtraction digital radiography: technical considerations, clinical applications, and imaging pitfalls (review). J Thorac Imag. 2006;21(4):303-13.
21. Dobbins JT, Godfrey DJ, McAdams HP. Chest tomosynthesis. Syllabus RSNA 2003, Advances in digital radiography: RSNA categorical course in diagnostic radiology physics. 2003;211-7.
22. Brice J. Will new DR technologies offer alternative to CT? Part2. http://www.auntminnie.com/index.aspx?Sec=sup&Sub=xra&Pag=dis&ItemId=90041. Updated March 25, 2010. Accessed October 28, 2010.
23. Heber MacMahon, NicholasJ. Yasillo, Michael Carlin Laser Alignment System for High Quality Portable Radiography RadioGraphIcs. 1992,12:111 20.
24. www.e-radiography.com
25. Lehnert T, Naguib NN, Ackermann H, Schomerus C, Jacobi V, Balzer JO, Vogl TJ. Novel, portable, cassette-sized, and wireless flat-panel digital radiography system: initial workflow results versus computed radiography. AJR Am J Roentgenol. 2011;196(6):1368-71.
26. http://www.radiologyinfo.org/en/info.cfm?pg=mammo
27. Katherine A. Leslie. Digital Mammography: Planning, Implementation, and Integration (Available at http://www.e-radimaging.com)
28. Larkin A. et al. Commissioning and Quality Assurance of Dual Energy X-ray Absorptiometry (DEXA) systems, Rad Prot Dosim 2008 (in press).
29. Sheahan N.F, Dowling A, O'reilly G, Malone J.F. Commissioning and quality assurance protocol for dual energy X-ray absorptiometry systems, Rad Prot Dosim. 2005;117:288-90.
30. Lohman TG, Harris M, Teixeira PJ, Weiss L. Assessing body composition and changes in body composition. Another look at dual-energy X-ray absorptiometry. Ann NY Acad Sci. 2000;904:45-54.
31. Lorente Ramos, R.M.; Azpeitia Armán, J.; Arévalo Galeano, N.; Muñoz Hernández, A.; García Gómez, J.M.; Gredilla Molinero J. Dual energy X-ray absorptimetry: Fundamentals, methodology, and clinical applications Radiologia. 2012;54:410-23.
32. Guillerman RP. Newer CT applications and their alternatives: what is appropriate in children? Pediatr Radiol. 2011;41(Suppl 2):534-48.
33. Lell MM et al. New Techniques in CT Angiography. Radio Graphics. 2006;26:S45-62.
34. Weinstein SP, Conant EF, Sehgal C. Technical advances in breast ultrasound imaging. Semin Ultrasound CT MR. 2006;27(4):273-83.
35. Harvey CJ, Pilcher JM, Eckersley RJ, Blomley MJ, Cosgrove DO. Advances in ultrasound. Clin Radiol. 2002;57(3):157-77.
36. Elsayes KM et al MRI characterization of 124 CT-indeterminate focal hepatic lesions: evaluation of clinical utility. HPB (Oxford). 2007;9(3):208-15.
37. http://www.frankshospitalworkshop.com/equipment/documents/X-ray/wikipedia/Radiology.pdf
38. Hochmuth A, Spetzger U, Schumacher M. Comparison of three-dimensional rotational angiography with digital subtraction angiography in the assessment of ruptured cerebral aneurysms. Am J Neuroradiol. 2002;23(7):1199-205.
39. JV Byrne, C Colominas, J Hipwell et al. Assessment of a technique for 2D–3D registration of cerebral intra-arterial angiography. The British Journal of Radiology. 2004;77:123-8.
40. Orth RC, Wallace MJ, Kuo MD. C-arm Cone-beam CT: General Principles and Technical Considerations for Use in Interventional Radiology Vasc Interv Radiol. 2008;19:814-21.

41. Nuclear Medicine Imaging in Diagnosis and Treatment. National Research Council (US) and Institute of Medicine (US) Committee on State of the Science of Nuclear Medicine. Advancing Nuclear Medicine through Innovation. Washington (DC): National Academies Press (US); 2007.
42. Ralston, Coleman R M, Beaulieu D M, Scrutchfield K, Perkins T. Progress toward Paperless Radiology in the Digital Environment: Planning, Implementation, and Benefits. J Digit Imaging. 2004;17(2):134-43. Epub 2004 Apr 19.
43. Ehsan Samei, J. Anthony Seibert, Katherine Andriole, Aldo Badano, Jay Crawford, Bruce Reiner, Michael J. Flynn, Paul Chang. AAPM/RSNA Tutorial on Equipment Selection: PACS Equipment Overview General Guidelines for Purchasing and Acceptance Testing of PACS Equipment. RadioGraphics. 2004;24:313-34.
44. Bryan S, Weatherburn GC, Watkins JR, Buxton MJ. "The benefits of hospital-wide picture archiving and communication systems: a survey of clinical users of radiology services". Br J Radiol 72. 1999;857:469-78.
45. Dundas DD. Installation of a PACS system The British Journal of Radiology. 2005;78:480-2.
46. Bhaktwani A. The PC-PNDT act in a nutshell. Indian J Radiol Imaging. 2012;22(2):133-4.
47. Patnaik AM, Kejriwal GS. A perspective on the PCPNDT Act. Indian J Radiol Imaging. 2012;22(2):137-40.
48. PCPNDT bare Act. Professional Book Publishers, 2011.
49. Mani S Guidelines for ultrasound owners and owners of clinics, diagnostic centers and owners of clinics, nursing homes and hospitals. Indian J Radiol Imaging. 2012;22(2):125-8.

CHAPTER

51

Recent Advances in PET/CT and PET/MR

Rakesh Kumar, Madhavi Tripathi

INTRODUCTION

The last decade has witnessed rapid advancements in the field of nuclear medicine. This can be attributed to the advancement in instrumentation and radiotracers for clinical use, and is evident with positron emission tomography/computed tomography (PET/CT) technology. In the present era of evidence-based medicine, the clinical indications for PET/CT have been increasing and expanding beyond oncological practice. Positron emission tomography/magnetic resonance (PET/MR) imaging is now available in advanced centers for specific clinical indications.

The authors would discuss the major advances in the applications of PET/CT and PET/MR in clinical nuclear medicine. It would be beyond the scope of this chapter to include the recent advances of instrumentation and radiotracers in the same.

POSITRON EMISSION TOMOGRAPHY/COMPUTED TOMOGRAPHY

Positron emission tomography (PET) is a diagnostic imaging technique, which can provide functional information of underlying metabolic processes that can be either physiological or pathological. There is a long list of PET radiotracers that can be used for imaging to provide information on glucose, amino acid and fatty acid metabolism, or target particular receptors on cells.

Standalone PET has now universally been replaced by PET/CT. Two important limitations of PET-only scanners were poor anatomical localization and limited resolution of abnormal radiotracer accumulation in the body. To overcome these combined PET/CT scanners were introduced into routine clinical practice after 2000. This widespread use of PET/CT was evidence based as PET/CT demonstrated higher specificity and sensitivity than either PET or CT alone for the management of various diseases especially in the field of oncology. PET/CT can provide the functional and morphological details of various pathological conditions in one procedure. Although many radiotracers are being used for PET-CT, ^{18}F-fluoro-2-deoxy-D-glucose (FDG) is the most commonly used radiotracer. FDG is an analogue of glucose and its uptake is proportional to the metabolism of glucose by physiological and pathological tissue. FDG is transported into the cell by GLUT transporters and most of the pathologies (tumors) usually demonstrate high FDG uptake based on the upregulation of GLUT transporters in comparison to the surrounding normal cells. After transport into tumor cell, FDG is phosphorylated by hexokinase into FDG-6-phosphate, which cannot continue through glycolysis because it is not a substrate for the enzyme glucose-6-phosphatase.[1,2] As a result, ^{18}F-FDG-6-phosphate is metabolically 'trapped' within the cell. ^{18}F-FDG-PET is now an established standard in the initial staging, restaging after treatment and monitoring the response to therapy of patients with various cancers. It also has a few applications in cardiology and neurology. In addition to qualitative image display, it is possible to semi-quantify the FDG uptake value normalized to the injected dose and body weight/surface area, which is known as "standardized uptake value" (SUV). The SUV provides an approximate indicator that correlates with FDG metabolism in the tissue. A lesion with an SUV greater than 2.5 is considered to have a high probability of malignancy. However, that is not always true and no particular cut-off for abnormality has been defined. Recently, a new quantitative parameter has been introduced which is described as tumor burden. This is a product of tumor volume and SUV. It has been reported to have higher accuracy than SUV alone in evaluating treatment response of solid tumors to chemotherapy.[3]

RECENT ADVANCES IN THE CLINICAL APPLICATIONS OF PET/CT

Oncology

PET/CT plays an important role in the management of cancer patients. It is primarily indicated for characterization of lesion equivocal on anatomical imaging, initial staging, treatment response evaluation, evaluation for recurrence, in detecting primary cancer in metastatic disease from unknown primary, and to provide prognostic information for various cancers.

Diagnosis

Computed tomography (CT) is the imaging modality of choice for detection and follow-up of lung nodules but has limited specificity especially in nodules less than 10 mm in size. PET/CT is increasing being used to characterize small solitary pulmonary nodule (SPN), which are difficult to evaluate on CT. PET/CT provides additional functional information and is useful in differentiating benign lesions from malignant ones **(Figs. 1A and B)**. Two systematic reviews of the literature with meta-analysis reported sensitivity ranging from 96 to 97% and specificity of 78–86% using PET for detection of malignant SPN.[4,5] It is important to note the limitations of PET-CT. FDG PET/CT has low sensitivity in detecting low grade tumors like bronchoalveolar carcinoma and bronchial carcinoid. Somatostatin receptor scintigraphy (SRS) with gallium-68 (Ga-68) tetra-azacyclododecane tetraacetic acid -D-Phe^1-Tyr^3-octreotide (DOTA-TOC) is useful for non-invasively characterizing intrabronchial tumors suspected to be carcinoids **(Figs. 2A and B)**. Sarcoidosis and active granulomatous infection like tuberculosis, and fungal infections (histoplasmosis or coccidioidomycosis) can be metabolically active and lead to false positive results.

Patients with cervical lymph node metastasis from an unknown primary tumor are a diagnostic dilemma from management perspective. FDG-PET can be a valuable tool in this subset of patients and can identify the primary tumor in approximately 30% patients.[6]

Mammography is the most widely used imaging tool for the screening for primary breast tumors but it has a lower sensitivity in women with radiographically dense breasts and in women with breast implants. PET/CT is useful in this subset of patients, it is also useful in detecting synchronous primary in the contralateral breast in known breast cancer patients **(Figs. 3A and B)**. However, MRI remains the gold standard for this purpose in selected cases. Recently positron emission mammography (PEM) has been introduced for

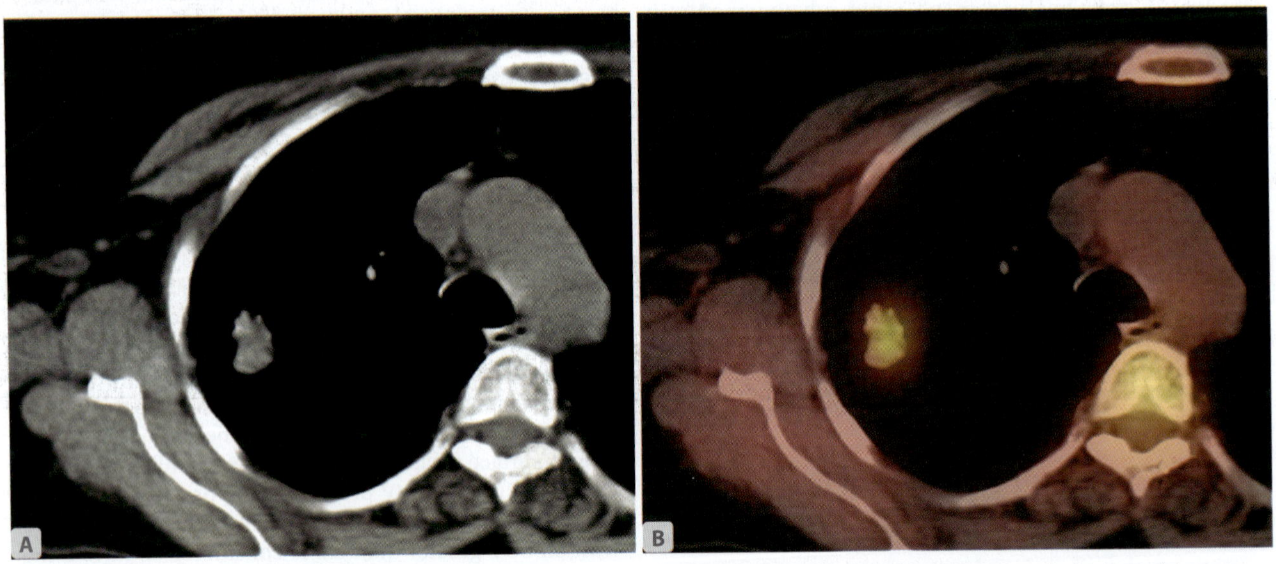

FIGS. 1A AND B: Chest CT of PET/CT shows solitary pulmonary nodule in right lung (A). PET/CT chest showing FDG uptake in the nodule suggestive of malignancy (B). FNAC of nodule confirmed the diagnosis of malignancy (adenocarcinoma).

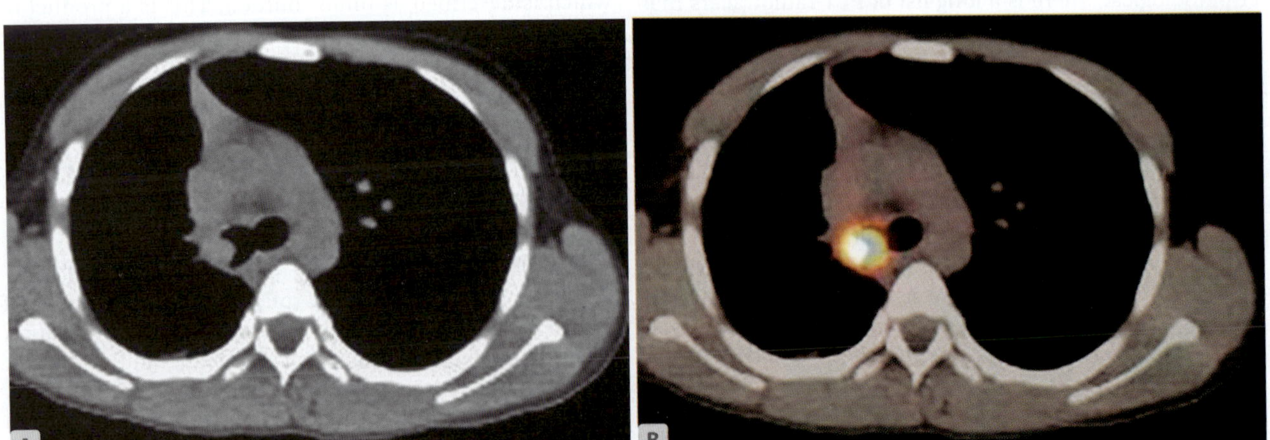

FIGS. 2A AND B: Transaxial CT of PET/CT shows a growth in the right main bronchus (A). transaxial fused PET/CT shows increased ^{68}Ga-DOTATOC uptake in the right intrabronchial mass (B) which was a synaptophysin positive carcinoid on histopathology.

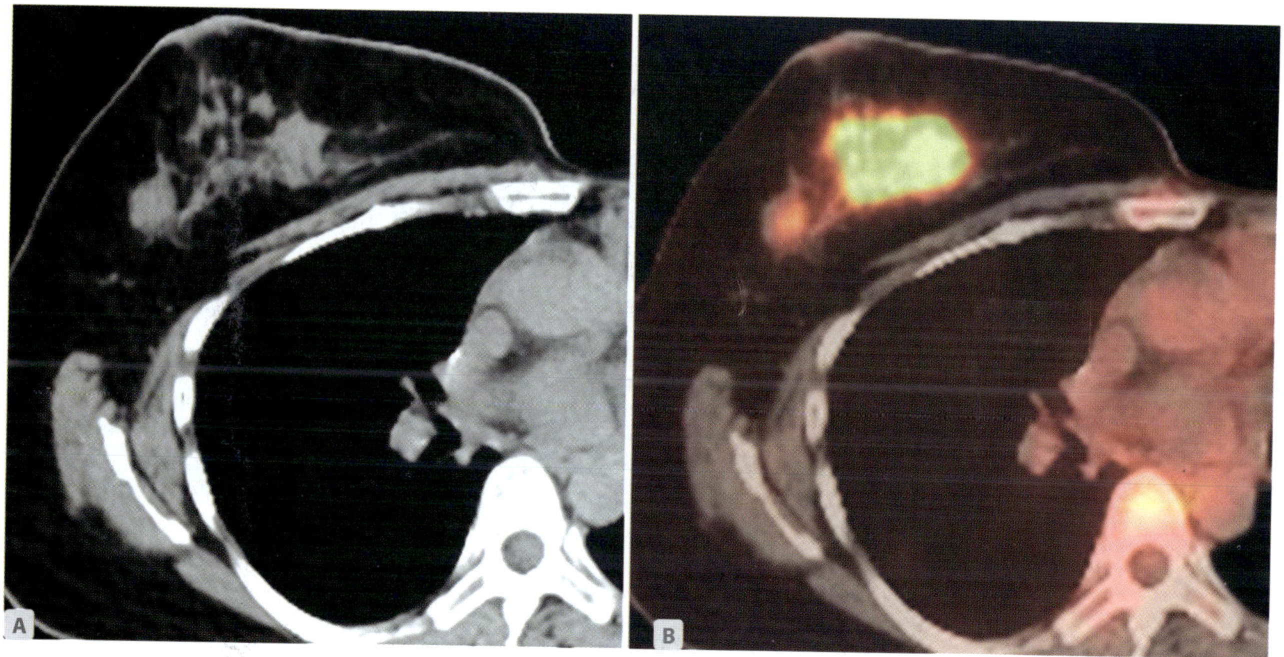

FIGS. 3A AND B: CT of PET/CT shows multiple nodules in right breast of patient who was treated for left breast cancer previously (A). PET/CT shows increased FDG uptake in all nodules suggestive of malignant nature of nodules (B) (additional primary in contralateral breast in known breast cancer patient).

characterization of breast lesions and has shown encouraging results.[7] Patients with carcinoma in situ, low-grade tumors, well-differentiated ductal and lobular breast cancer usually have significantly lower SUVs and can be misinterpreted as benign lesions.

Till recently, the role of FDG-PET in bladder cancer was very limited due to urinary excretion of FDG. The detection of primary tumor and local visceral tumor recurrence is limited due to the presence of excreted FDG in the urinary tract, which often masks the pelvic lesion. An intervention, thus, to reduce the urinary radioactivity without altering the tumor uptake seems needed. In a recent study, we used diuretic administration as an intervention, and demonstrated a sensitivity of 92% and specificity of 96% in patients with bladder carcinoma.[8] Diuretic administration significantly improved the detection of the primary tumor involving the bladder wall **(Figs. 4A to D)**.

Thymic tumors represent a broad spectrum of neoplastic pathologies with variable overlap in clinical and imaging presentation. PET/CT is useful in differentiating thymic hyperplasia from neoplasms, especially thymoma, carcinoma and lymphoma.[9] We have demonstrated a statistically significant difference in SUVmax for thymic hyperplasia, thymoma and thymic carcinomas **(Figs. 5A and B)**.[10]

FDG-PET/CT has lower sensitivity and specificity for neuroendocrine tumors (NET). In addition to FDG, other positron-emitting radiopharmaceuticals such as somatostatin analog (Ga-68 DOTA-TOC), ^{11}Carbon (^{11}C) -Hydroxyephedrine, ^{11}C-Epinephrine, ^{11}C-5-hydroxytryptophan and ^{18}F-Fluoro-dihydroxyphenylalanine (FDOPA) etc are also used. PET imaging with ^{68}Ga-DOTA-TOC is a valuable diagnostic tool in NETs as it targets the somatostatin receptors, which are variably expressed on these tumors. Our group demonstrated advantages of ^{68}Ga-DOTA-TOC over conventional FDG PET/CT in various NETs **(Figs. 6A to C)**.[11] ^{68}Ga-DOTATOC PET/CT emerged as a superior imaging technique with 100% sensitivity and positive predictive value (PPV) for detecting primary NET, as compared to CECT that had a sensitivity of 83%. 68Ga-DOTA-NOC PET/CT has been reported to be highly sensitive and specific for the detection of pheochromoctyomas and paragangliomas as reported by Naswa et al. in 35 patients.[12] It seems better than ^{131}I MIBG Scintigraphy for this purpose. Contrast-enhanced CT (CECT) is a standard investigative procedure in the localization of gastrinomas. Small tumors are often missed and metastatic lesions may remain occult on CT. Naswa et al. demonstrated usefulness of ^{68}Ga-DOTANOC PET/CT in patients with gastrinoma with negative or equivocal results on CECT.[13]

In brain tumors, FDG PET/CT has limited application due to inherent high glucose metabolism by brain parenchyma. FDG-PET CT may detect high-grade gliomas. FDG PET/CT has some role to play in patients with brain tumors treated by radiation therapy, where anatomical imaging modalities like CT and MRI can be limited in differentiating radiation necrosis from residual/recurrent tumor. New radiotracers like ^{11}C-methionine (^{11}C-MET), ^{11}C-tyrosine, ^{18}F-fluoro-tyrosine, ^{18}F-fluoroethyl-tyrosine (^{18}F-FET), 8-cyclopentyl-3-(3-^{18}F-fluoropropyl)-1-propylxanthine (^{18}F-CPFPX) and ^{18}F-fluoro-thymidine (^{18}F-FLT) and FDOPA have been evaluated due to their low brain uptake. The utility of ^{11}C-methionine, FDOPA and ^{18}F-FLT in the clinical setting has been suggested by a few studies.[14,15]

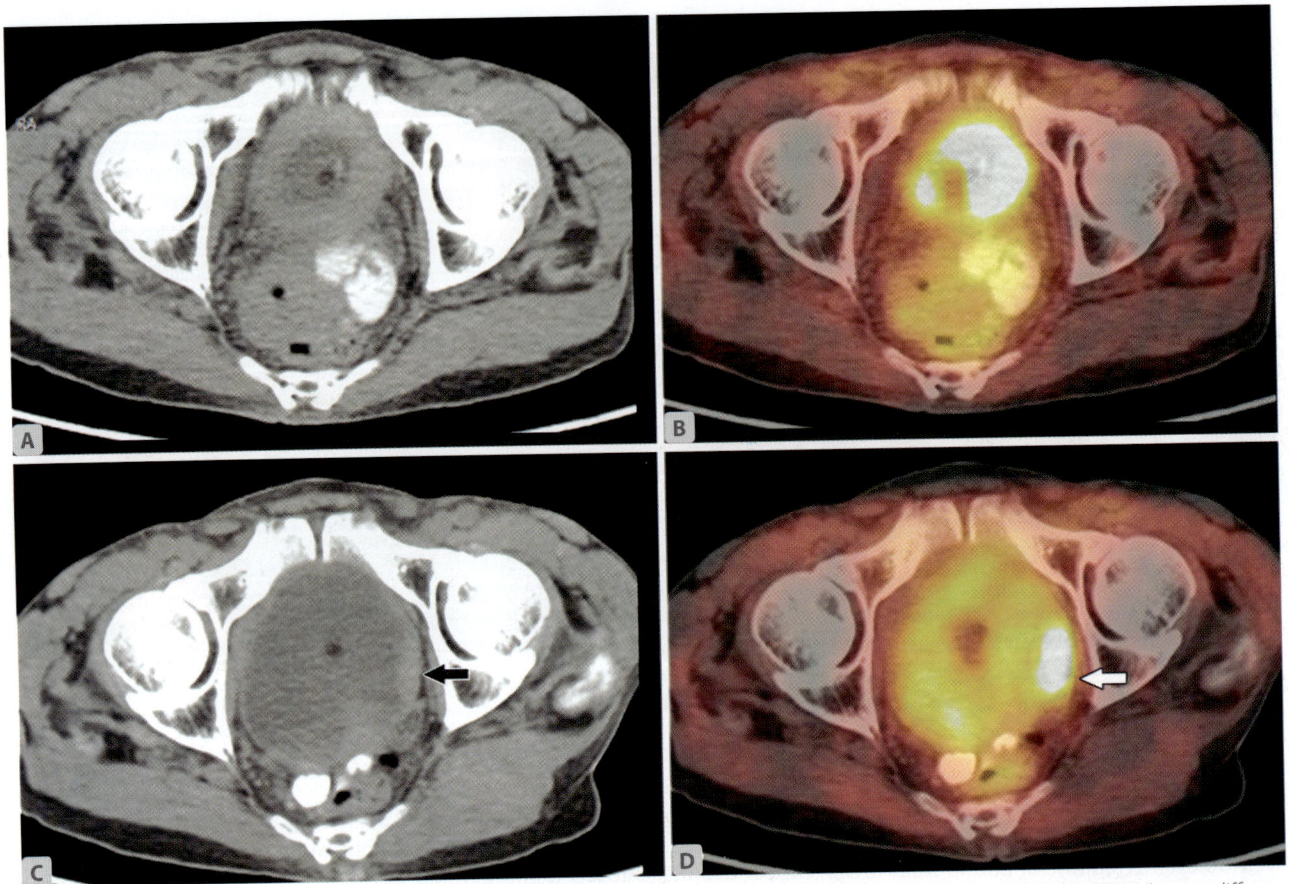

FIGS. 4A TO D: A 63-year-old man with carcinoma of the urinary bladder underwent staging PET/CT. Unenhanced axial CT image shows a diffuse thickening of urinary bladder wall with a catheter in situ (A). Corresponding axial PET/CT image shows a relative photon-deficient area in the region of the catheter bulb with urinary radioactivity occupying the remaining bladder cavity (B). Spot views of the urinary bladder were taken after diuretic administration which reveals the left lateral bladder wall thickening in a distended bladder on CT (C, bold arrow), which shows intense uptake on axial PET/CT (D, bold white arrow) with a high target to background ratio after the residual bladder activity has been cleared.

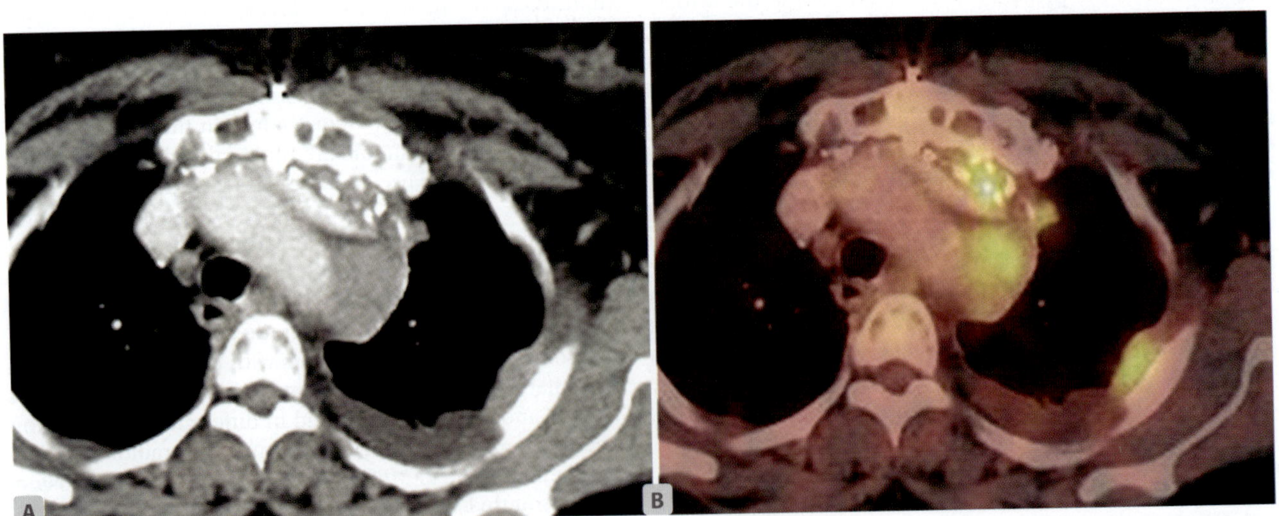

FIGS. 5A AND B: A 54-year-old man with thymic carcinoma underwent PET/CT. CECT axial image shows anterior mediastinal mass abutting arch of aorta with calcification. In addition, there is left pleural thickening (A). Corresponding axial PET/CT image shows an intense uptake in the anterior mediastinal mass seen on CT (B).

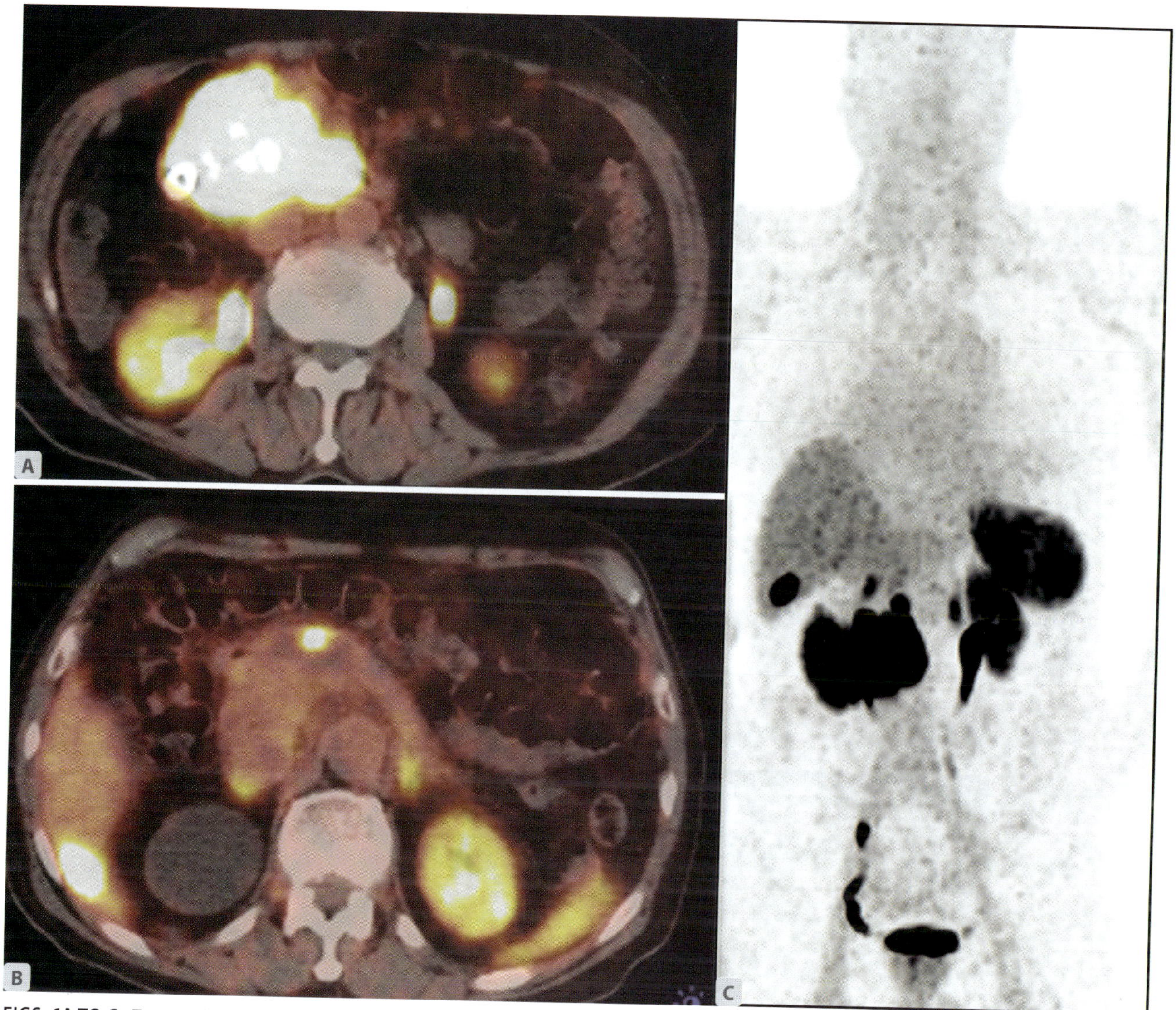

FIGS. 6A TO C: Transaxial ^{68}Ga-DOTATOC PET/CT images of abdomen (A) of a 42-year-old male patient presenting with pain abdomen showing intense tracer uptake in the pancreatic mass suggesting SSTR receptor expressing tumor. Also note a lesion in the liver showing increased ^{68}Ga-DOTATOC uptake suggesting metastasis (B). Projection image of whole body PET showing above described findings (C). A diagnosis of pancreatic NET was made. On histopathology, the mass turned out to be a well-differentiated NET.

Initial Staging

PET/CT has been found to play an important role in the initial staging of various tumors, which refers to assessing the local extent of disease, and in differentiating localized from disseminated disease.

For lung cancers, the FDG PET/CT has been primarily studied for non-small cell lung cancer (NSCLC) patients. In these patients regional and distant spread of the disease will change staging and guide the therapeutic approach **(Figs. 7A to E)**. PET/CT more accurately determines the T staging compared with either CT or PET alone. In one meta-analysis, PET/CT accurately predicted the T stage in patients with NSCLC in 82% of cases compared with 55% and 68% with PET alone and CT alone, respectively.[16] The additional advantages of PET/CT over CT are in differentiating central tumors from post obstructive atelectasis and detection of subtle areas of invasion.

In patients with Hodgkin's disease (HD) and non-Hodgkin's lymphoma (NHL), PET/CT detects more lesions, which change the stage of the disease in almost 15% of patients when compared to conventional imaging like CT.[17] For histopathological examination of the lesion in HD and NHL, PET-CT can guide the biopsy from suitable and easily accessible site.

In colorectal cancer (CRC) patients, regional nodal or distant metastasis is present in majority of them at initial presentation. CT is used as initial investigation for staging but PET/CT is superior in detecting unexpected hepatic and extrahepatic metastases **(Figs. 8A to D)**. In a recent meta-analysis on the value of FDG PET/CT in preoperative staging of colorectal cancer demonstrated a pooled sensitivity of 91%, and pooled specificity of 91%.[18] Mucinous adenocarcinoma is a subtype of CRC, which is less FDG avid and can produce false negative results in many cases.

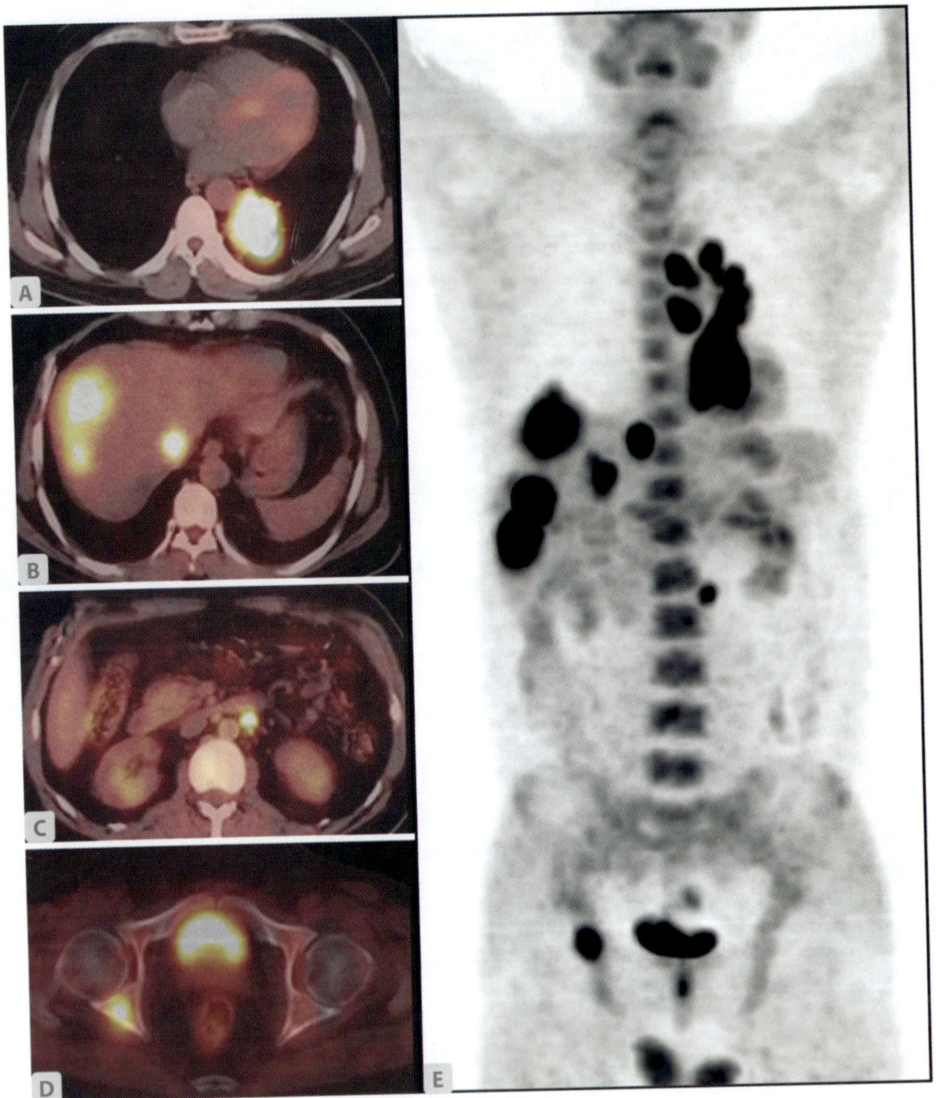

FIGS. 7A TO E: Transaxial [18]FDG- PET/CT images of chest, abdomen and pelvis (A to D) of a 62-year-old male patient presenting with chest pain and hemoptysis, showing intense tracer uptake in the left lower lung mass suggestive of malignant tumor (A). Also note multiple focal areas of increased FDG uptake in liver (B), left adrenal (C) and right acetabulum marrow (D) suggestive of metastatic disease. Projection image of whole body PET showing above described findings (E).

PET/CT can be useful in initial staging evaluation of breast cancer as it can detect axillary node involvement, however it is inferior in detecting lymph node metastasis when compared to sentinel lymph node biopsy. In selected patients who have high risk of nodal metastases, a clearly positive PET/CT carries a high positive predictive value for nodal metastases. The advantage of PET/CT in initial staging in breast cancer is detection of internal mammary lymph node and distant metastasis **(Figs. 9A and B)**. FDG PET/CT was found to be significantly more accurate for detecting axillary lymph node and distant metastases in 106 women in a recently published study.[19] Management of 15 patients (14%) was altered based on the FDG PET/CT findings, including 3 patients with axillary lymph node metastases, 5 patients with extra-axillary lymph node metastases, 4 patients with distant meta-stases and 3 patients with synchronous malignancies.

PET/CT differentiates resectable and unresectable disease in esophageal and gastric cancers and helps in avoiding futile surgeries; however, the detection of regional nodal metastases is limited due to the small volume of disease in some lymph nodes and small size of the metastatic lymph nodes **(Figs. 10A to G)**. In a recent study authors from Australia have shown that PET/CT changed the stage group in 56 (40%) patients and changed management in 47 (34%) of 139 patients.[20] The authors concluded that PET/CT provides incremental staging information compared with conventional imaging, changes management in one third of patients, and has powerful prognostic stratification in the primary staging of esophageal cancer. In a systematic review, Mazola et al. concluded that it appears reasonable to include FDG PET/CT in the diagnostic algorithm of patients with esophageal cancer in order to better define the optimal therapeutic approach.[21]

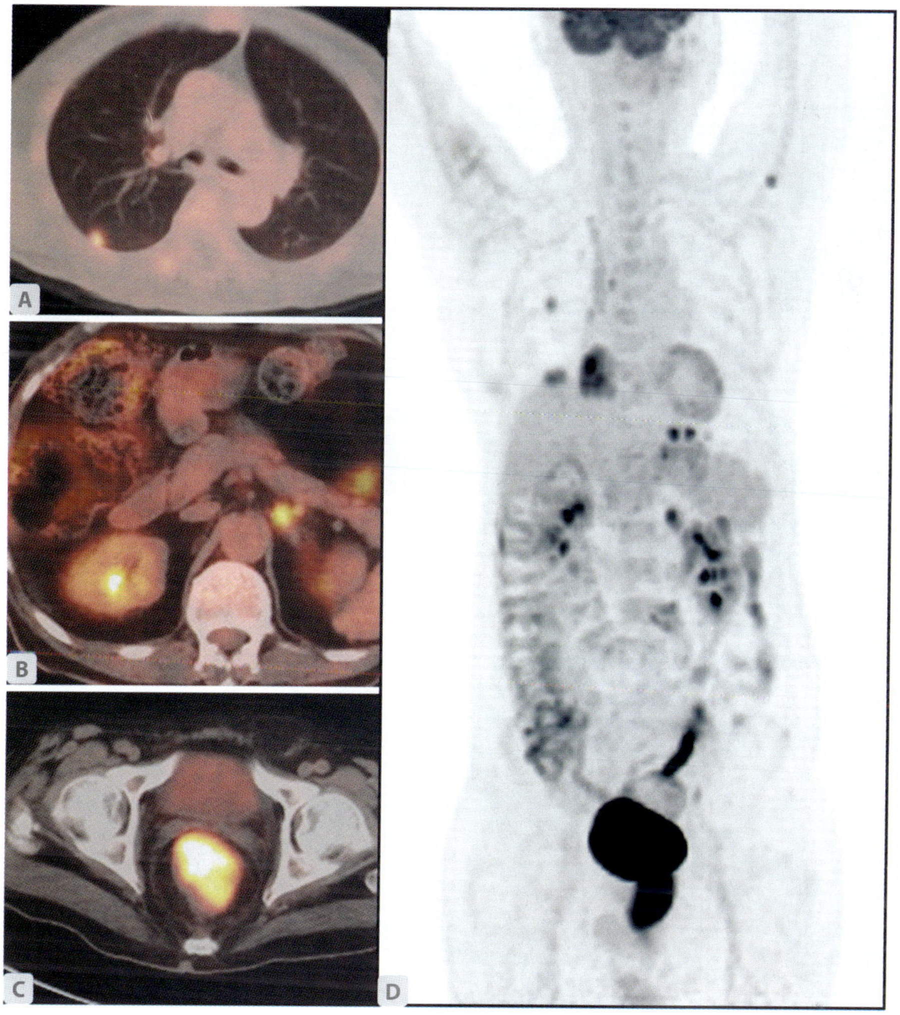

FIGS. 8A TO D: Transaxial 18FDG-PET/CT images of chest, abdomen and pelvis (A to C) of a 78-year-old male patient presenting with rectal mass, showing intense tracer uptake in the rectal mass suggestive of malignant primary tumor (C). Also note multiple focal areas of increased FDG uptake in the right lung (A) and left adrenal (B) suggestive of metastatic disease. Projection image of whole body PET showing above-described findings (D).

FDG PET/CT has a limited role in detecting soft-tissue metastasis to pelvic lymph nodes in patients with prostate cancer, owing to urinary excretion of FDG and low glucose uptake by tumor cells (usually a well-differentiated neoplasm) in these patients. ^{11}C-choline PET/CT is more accurate than FDG PET-CT in patients with prostate cancer. In a systemic review and meta-analysis of ^{18}F-choline and ^{11}C-choline PET/CT in the lymph node staging of prostate cancer prior to surgery involving 10 studies and 441 patients, Evangelista et al. demonstrated pooled sensitivity 49.2% and pooled specificity 95%.[22] A recent study highlighted the role of ^{68}Ga Glu-NH-CO-NH-Lys-(Ahx) [Ga-68(HBED-CC)] (Ga-68 PSMA 11) PET/CT for lymph node and metastases staging in high-risk prostate cancers.[23] This tracer has theranostic potential and can be labeled with ^{177}Lutetium for therapy in metastatic prostate cancer good results **Figure 11A to D.**[24] Another radiotracer ^{18}F-fluoro-5α-dihydrotestosterone (^{18}F-FDHT), a labeled analog of the major ligand for androgen receptor di-hydro-testosterone; has been used by few groups in limited number of patients. ^{18}F-Na-Fluoride PET/CT has high sensitivity for detecting bone metastases as compared to conventional bone scan due to high resolution of PET/CT scan.

The detection and staging of primary urothelial tumor and local visceral tumor recurrence is limited duc to the presence of excreted FDG in the urinary tract, which often masks the pelvic lesion and probably the adjacent lymph nodes. Diuretic administration significantly improved the detection of the primary tumor involving the bladder wall and regional lymph nodes metastasis.[8] In a recent study, Divgi et al. studied the utility of iodine-124 ^{124}I-girentuximab PET/CT in 195 patients with renal masses and demonstrated higher sensitivity and specificity as compared to CECT.[25]

In NET, ^{68}Ga-DOTA-TOC PET/CT is superior to conventional imaging and FDG PET/CT for detecting occult metastasis. In our experience, we have found that ^{68}Ga-DOTA-TOC PET/CT is the most sensitive and specific technique for initial staging of NET. CECT was found to have higher accuracy as compared to FDG PET/CT but lower accuracy than ^{68}Ga-DOTA-TOC PET/CT.[11,12]

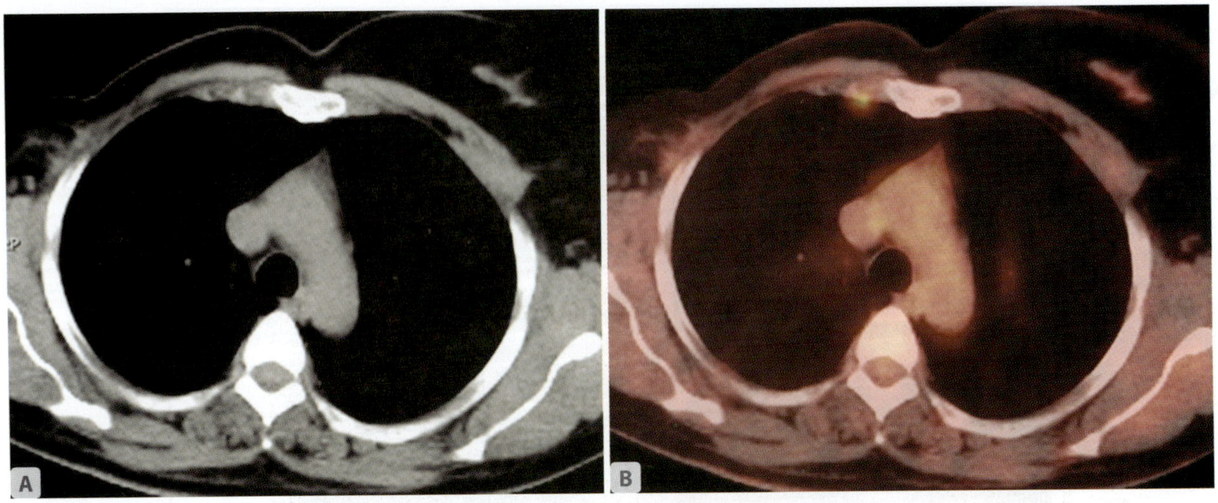

FIGS. 9A AND B: Chest CT of PET/CT shows no abnormality in a patient of right breast cancer (A). PET/CT chest showing FDG uptake in the subcentimeter right internal mammary suggestive of metastasis (B). Resolution of lymph node in postchemotherapy PET/CT confirmed the diagnosis of metastasis.

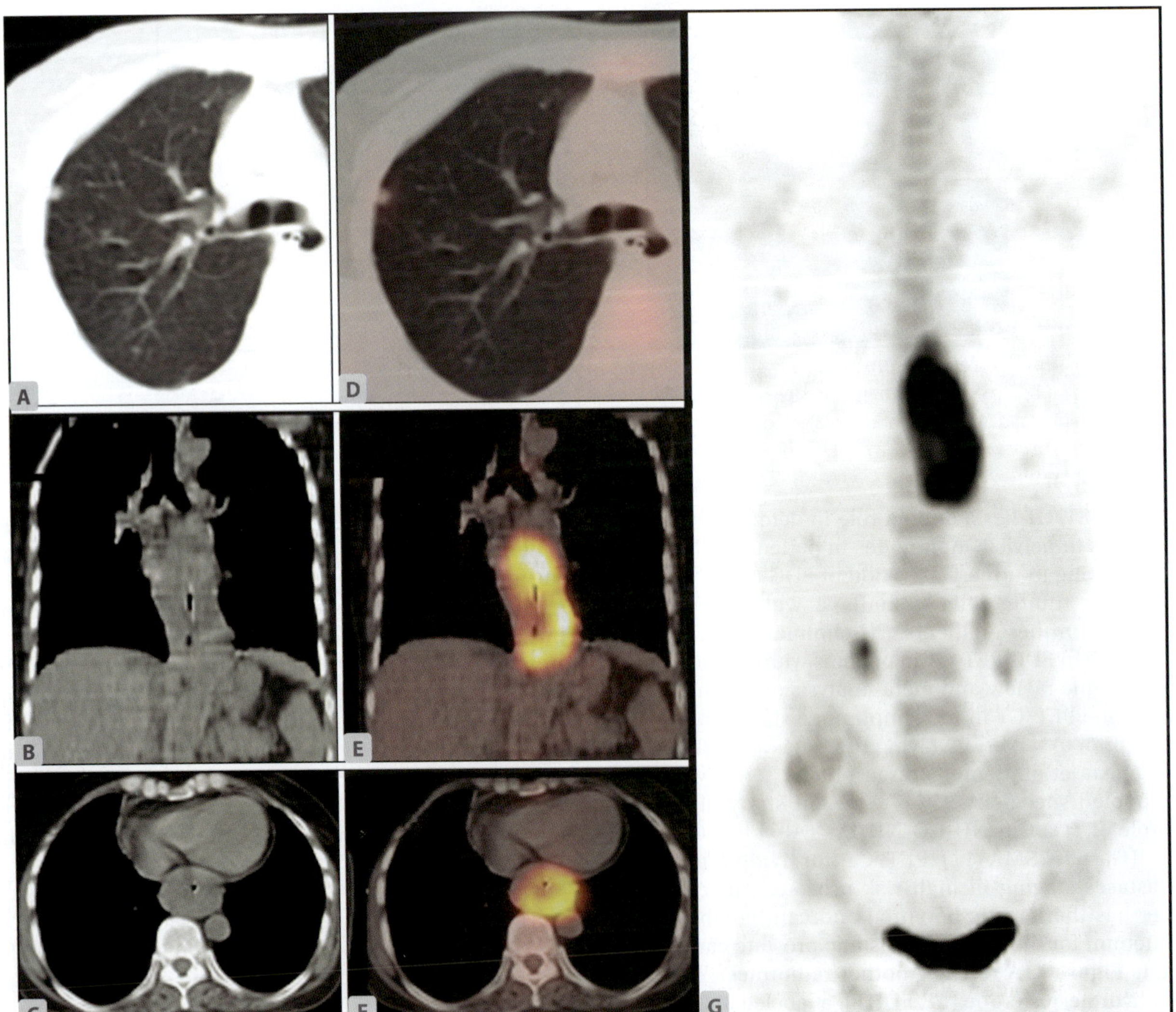

FIGS. 10A TO G: Chest CT of PET/CT shows diffuse thickening of lower half of esophagus and right pulmonary nodule (A to C). Corresponding ^{18}FDG-PET/CT images (D to F) show intense tracer uptake in the primary esophageal mass suggestive of malignant tumor and lung smetastasis. Projection image of whole body PET showing above-described findings (G).

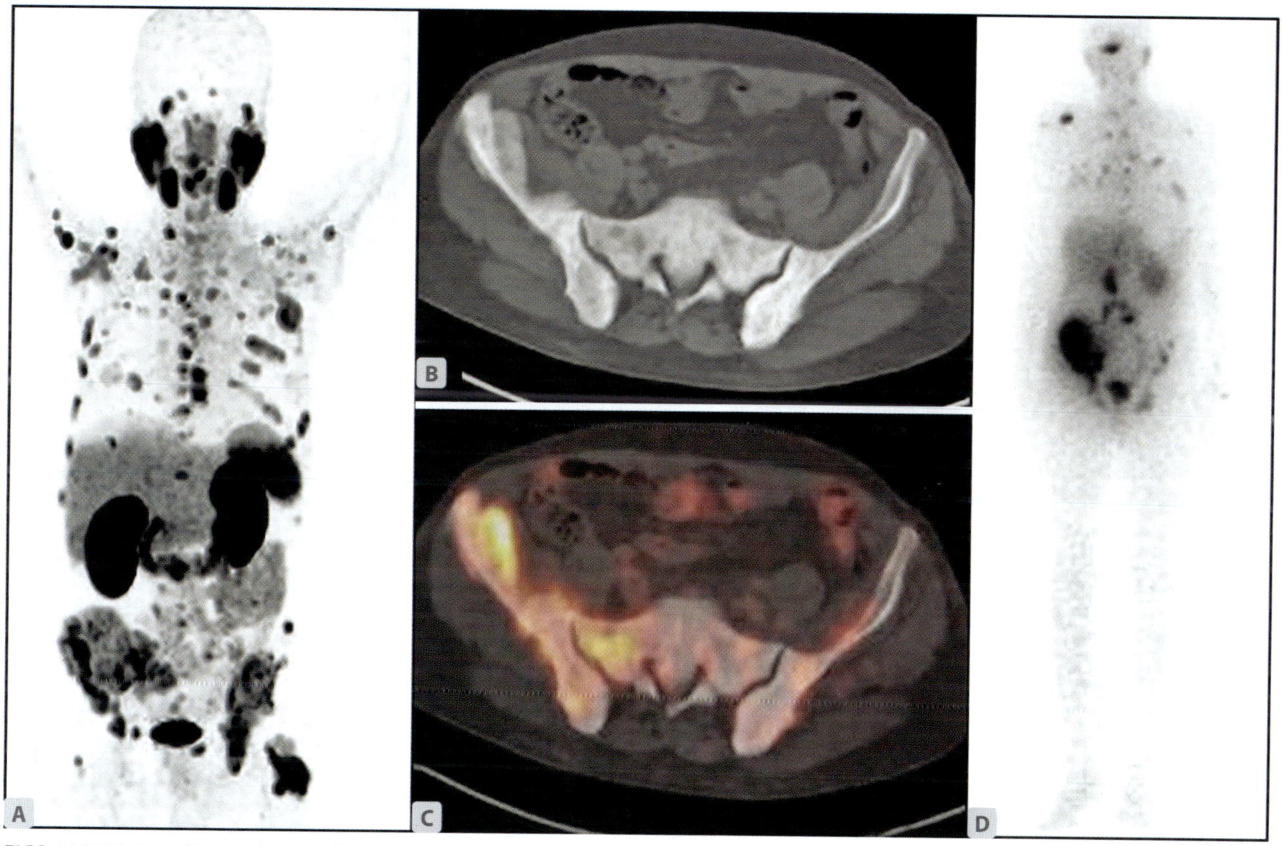

FIGS. 11A TO D: A 65-year-old male diagnosed and treated for metastatic prostate cancer showed progression and rise of PSA after docetaxel chemotherapy. ^{68}Ga-PSMA PET/CT study revealed PSMA expressing skeletal metastases (A to C). Patient was taken up for 177Lu-PSMA 617 therapy (D).

Treatment Response Evaluation

PET/CT has emerged as a useful imaging modality that can evaluate the therapy response and differentiate responders from non-responders during and after completion of treatment. Since many of the chemotherapeutic drugs used for targeted therapy are cytostatic and not cytocidal, conventional imaging like CT and MRI has limited value in evaluating the treatment response. PET/CT being a metabolic imaging modality, can demonstrate the treatment response earlier by determining the glucose uptake by tumor, which decreases earlier than the size in solid tumors. PET/CT performed after 1–2 cycles of chemotherapy in various malignancies can differentiate non-responsive disease from adequate response better than conventional imaging modalities and can guide the treatment plan accordingly.

PET-CT plays an important role in evaluation of treatment response after 1/2 cycles of chemotherapy in patients with lymphoma. It has been shown to have higher sensitivity, specificity and prognostic value when compared with CECT for mid-term therapy response **(Figs. 12A to J)**. PET-CT does not show any significant advantages over CECT when therapy evaluation is done after completion of treatment. In a recent study published by our group concluded though PET/CT depicts additional sites compared with contrast-enhanced CT and results in upstaging of disease. However, either PET/CT or contrast-enhanced CT may be used for response assessment and prognostication in stage III or IV nonlymphoblastic pediatric NHL.[26]

In breast cancer patients, PET/CT detects treatment-related metabolic changes much earlier than conventional imaging and clinical examination, once the chemotherapy has been initiated. There is strong correlation between the quantitative changes in SUV and overall clinical assessment of response of skeletal metastases to therapy and changes in tumor markers in breast cancer patients. We evaluated the role of FDG PET/CT for the assessment of response after two cycles of neo-adjuvant chemotherapy (NACT) for breast cancer and concluded that FDG PET/CT can differentiate responders from non-responders with high accuracy after two cycles of NACT in patients with locally advanced breast cancer (LABC).[27] ^{90}Y radioembolization [selective internal radiation therapy (SIRT)] has emerged as a valuable therapeutic option in unresectable, chemotherapy-refractory hepatic metastases from breast cancer. FDG PET/CT appears to be useful for predicting survival in these patients.[28]

Neoadjuvant chemoradiation therapy may result in significant tumor regression in patients with gastrointestinal malignancies. Delta SUVmax (Absolute SUVmax change) and response index (RI, percent SUVmax change) are best predictive parameters in response evaluation of neoadjuvant chemotherapy. Hendlisz et al, assessed the predictive value of FDG PET/CT metabolic response after a single course of

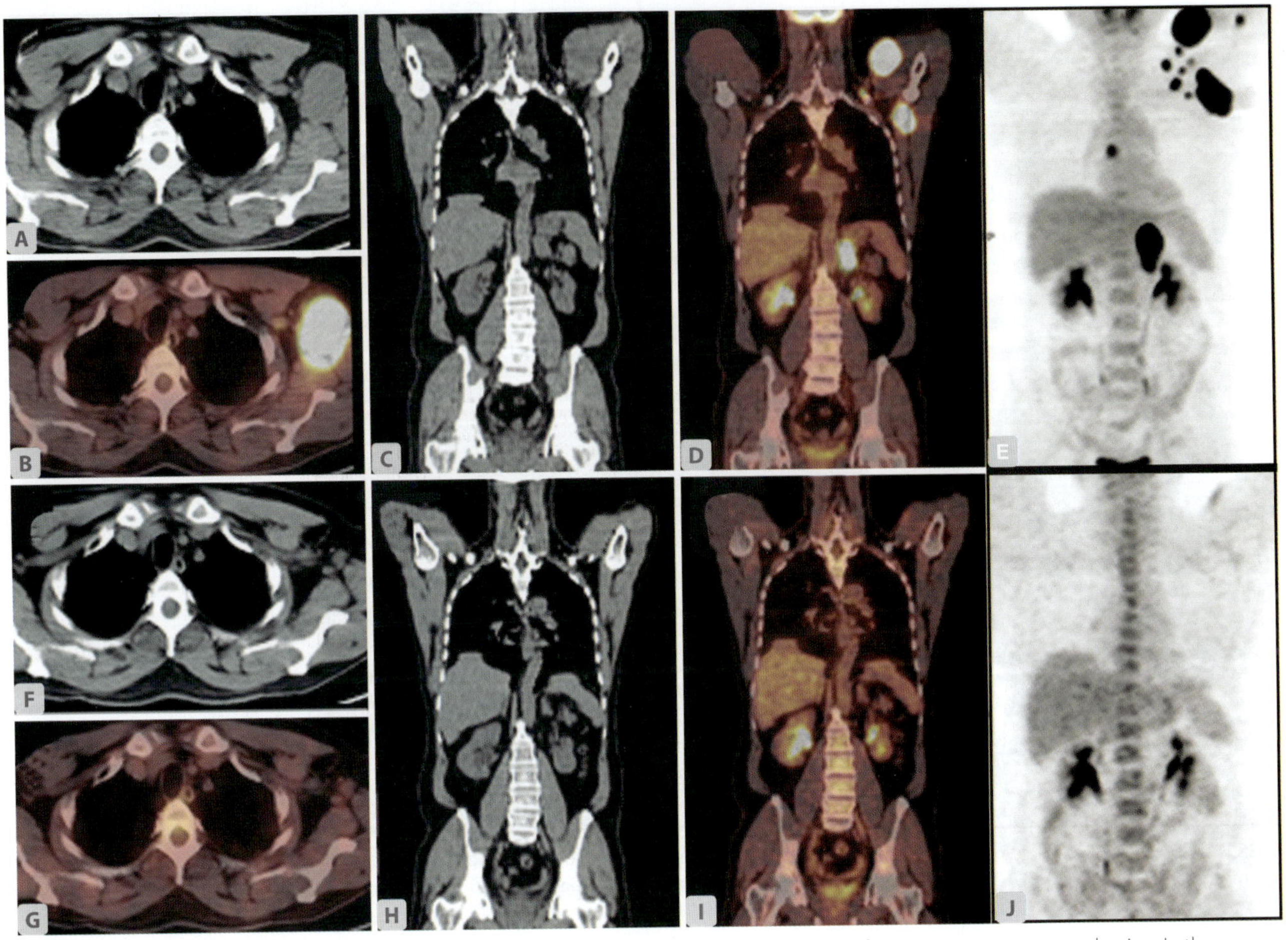

FIGS. 12A TO J: A 44-year-old man with NHL underwent baseline and postchemotherapy PET/CT for treatment response evaluation. In the baseline study (upper row), non-contrast CT of PET/CT shows enlarged left axillary lymph nodes, left deltoid muscle deposit and left adrenal lesions (A and C). Corresponding ^{18}FDG- PET/CT images (B and D) show intense tracer uptake in all lesion noted on CT. Projection image of whole body PET showing above-described findings (E). PET/CT done after 2 cycles of chemotherapy (lower row) demonstrated resolution of all lesions, suggestion of complete remission (F to J).

chemotherapy in patients with metastatic colorectal cancer and concluded that metabolic response measured by FDG-PET/CT after a single course of chemotherapy in metastatic CRC is able to identify patients who will not benefit from the treatment.[29] In patients with esophageal carcinoma, PET/CT is more specific than CT and endoscopic USG for loco-regional lymph node metastasis and response evaluation to neoadjuvant chemotherapy.

In bone tumors, PET/CT shows markedly reduced uptake early after the chemotherapy, while CT does not show definite change in tumor size. We studied 31 treatment naive osteosarcoma patients prospectively for treatment response by PET/CT scan after 3 cycles of neoadjuvant treatment and demonstrated that response can be predicted reliably by PET/CT scan early in disease course and PET/CT parameters correlate well with histologic necrosis.[30]

CT scanning is the imaging modality of choice in gastrointestinal stromal tumors (GIST), which can locate a mass lesion, contiguous organ invasion and distant metastases. Since the introduction of Imatinib mesylate, PET/CT is being used widely in GIST. PET/CT may show significant decrease in FDG uptake early after Imatinib therapy, while on conventional morphological imaging, tumor size may remain constant for a significant time and thereby, PET/CT accurately separates responders from non-responders in an early stage.

PET-CT has shown promising results for assessment of treatment response from newer anti-angiogenic agents (sunitinib and sorafenib) in patients with metastatic renal cell carcinoma, which might not show anatomical response such as decreasing size on conventional imaging.

Restaging/Recurrence/Prognosis

Many of the cancers recur even after the successful initial therapy. PET/CT is becoming standard of care in detecting the recurrence of various cancers and in determining the prognosis. This is one of the most acceptable clinical indications of PET/CT in oncology. PET/CT has proven role in assessing the prognosis of colorectal cancer, NSCLC, pancreatic cancer, lymphoma **(Figs. 13A to D)**, cervical cancer, melanoma, and other cancers.

In colorectal cancer, CT is frequently used to localize the site of possible recurrence, which has lower sensitivity and specificity. In a metaanalysis, comparing the diagnostic performance of PET, PET/CT, CT and MRI as whole-body imaging modalities for the detection of local and/or distant recurrent disease in CRC patients with high suspicion of recurrent disease, based on clinical findings or rise in carcinoembryonic antigen (CEA) level, whole-body PET and PET/CT were very accurate for the detection of local and/ or distant recurrent disease **(Figs. 14A to F)**.[31] In another meta analysis on colorectal liver metastases, FDG PET/CT had significantly higher sensitivity on a per-patient basis, compared with that of the CT, but not on a per-lesion basis. Sensitivity estimates for MR imaging with contrast were significantly superior to those for helical CT.[32]

PET/CT has higher sensitivity and specificity compared to PET alone and diagnostic CECT for lesion detection in suspected recurrence in patients of gall bladder cancer. We demonstrated a sensitivity of 97.6% and specificity of 90% in detecting gall bladder cancer recurrence in 62 PET/CT studies of 49 patients.[33]

In ovarian cancer, PET-CT has very important role in patients with rising tumor marker (CA-125) **(Figs. 15A to E)**. In a review by Son et al., PET/CT scan was found to be superior to CECT and MRI for detection of recurrent or residual ovarian cancer.[34] However, PET/CT may yield false-negative results in patients with small, necrotic, mucinous, cystic, or low-grade tumors. PET/CT may be false positive in the post-therapy setting, inflammatory and infectious processes. Despite these drawbacks, PET/CT is superior to CT and MR imaging for depiction of recurrent disease.

In NET, FDG-PET/CT has no definite role except in evaluation of prognosis. A positive FDG PET/CT in patients with NET is suggestive of undifferentiated NET (WHO grade III) and poor prognosis.

Total lesion glycolysis (TLG), which combines volumetric and metabolic information from FDG PET/CT can provide a better evaluation of the prognosis. In 105 consecutive patients with NSCLC who underwent staging FDG PET/CT before any therapy, the 1-year PFS was 0.0% for patients with high whole-body TLG (>655) and 50.0% for those with low whole-body TLG (≤655).[35]

Neurology

The availability of tracers imaging pathology in vivo is a step ahead of the use of FDG in neurodegenerative disorders. The amyloid tracers still have to find a place in the Indian markets but the availability of Tau tracers has enabled imaging Tau in vivo using PET/CT. We imaged Alzheimer's disease (AD) using Tau PET (18F-AD-ML-104) and could demonstrate an overlap of Tau pathology with areas of hypometabolism on FDG PET in the brains of AD patients. Tau deposition was found to have negative association with cognitive scores in these patients (unpublished data) **(Figs. 16A and B)**.

Miscellaneous

As stated previously the availability of new PET tracers has enabled improve the specificity for imaging pathology. ^{18}F fluorocholine PET enables improved localization of parathyroid adenomas in comparison of Tc-99m MIBI SPECT/CT **(Figs. 17A to G)**.

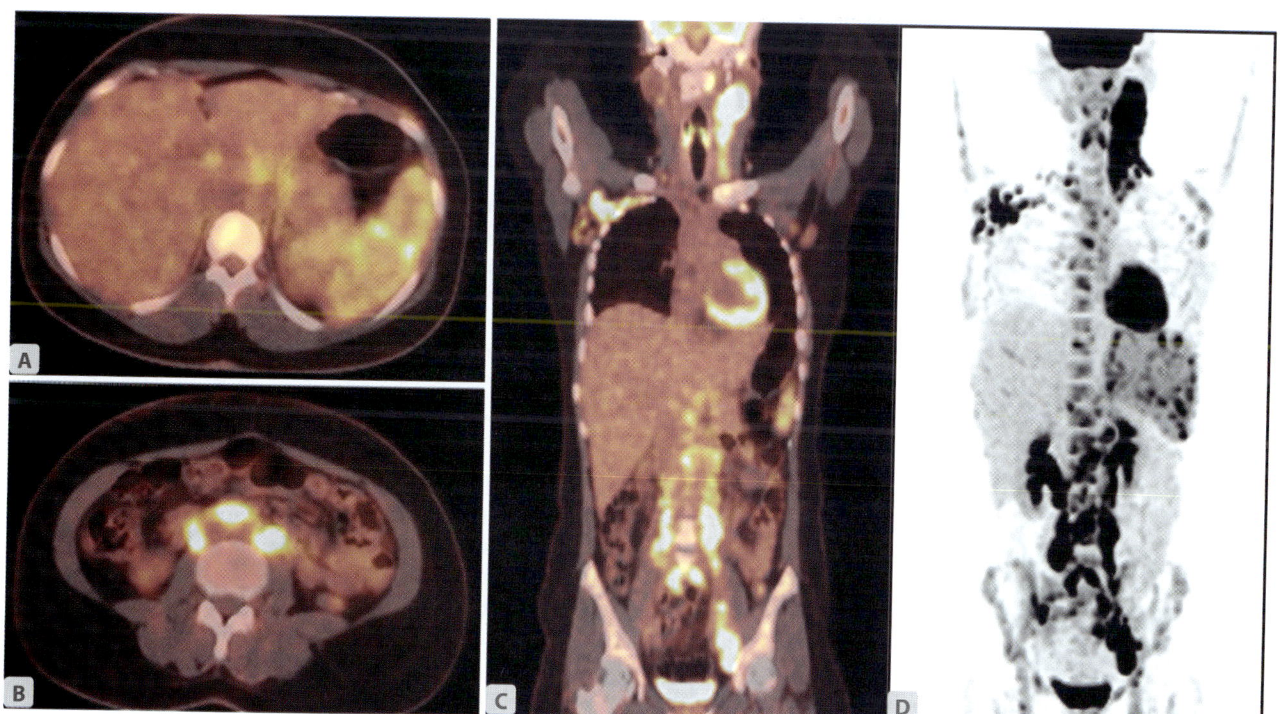

FIGS. 13A TO D: A 32-year-old man with NHL with complete remission after 6-cycles of chemotherapy presented with left cervical swelling and underwent PET/CT for restaging. Axial and coronal section of PET/CT shows splenic deposit, retroperitoneal, left pelvic, right axillary and left cervical lymph nodes (A to C). Projection image of whole body PET showing above-described findings (D). These findings were suggestive of recurrent disease.

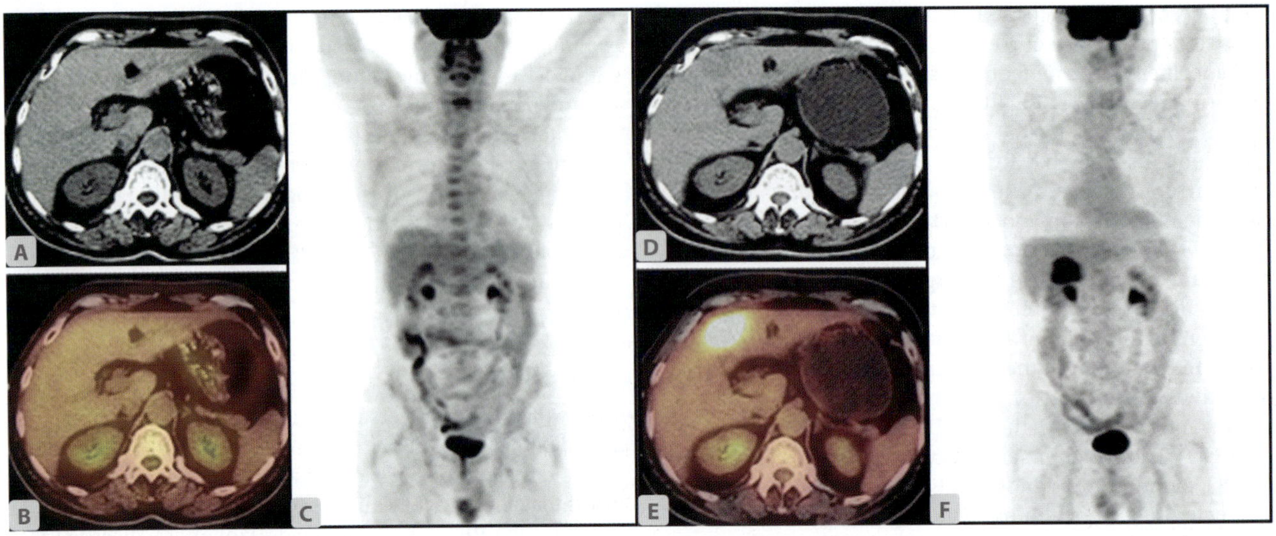

FIGS. 14A TO F: A 65-year-old man with a diagnosis of colorectal cancer who had normal PET/CT scan (right panel of images A to C) and CEA, 1-year back presented with recent rise in CEA levels, underwent PET/CT for restaging. CT of PET/CT shows hypodense liver lesion in segment IV (D). PET/CT shows increased FDG uptake in liver lesion suggestive of metastasis (E). Projection image of whole body PET showing above-described findings (F). These findings were suggestive of recurrent disease.

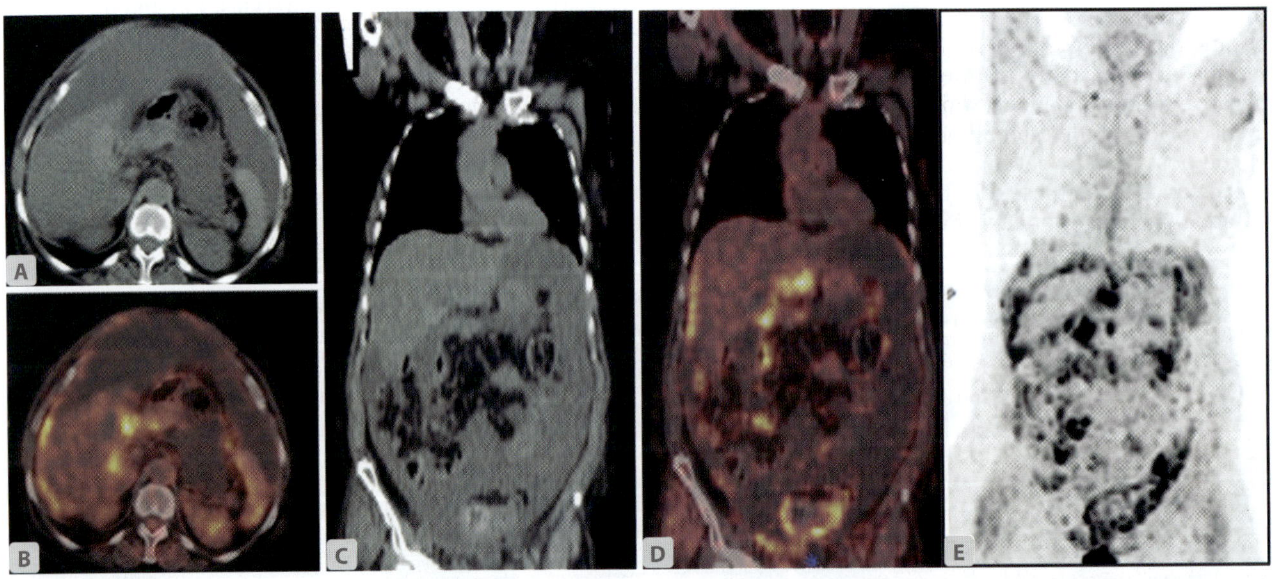

FIGS. 15A TO E: A 67-year-old woman with a diagnosis of ovarian cancer presented with recent rise in CA-125 levels and ascites, underwent PET/CT for restaging. CT of PET/CT shows ascites and peritoneal deposit (A to C). PET/CT shows increased FDG uptake in peritoneal deposit and ascites suggestive of metastasis (B and D). Projection image of whole body PET showing above-described findings (E). These findings were suggestive of recurrent disease.

The availability of ^{68}Ga Exendin enables specific binding to GLP-1 receptors targeting insulinomas in vivo which have poor somatostatin receptor expression **(Figs. 18A to C)**.

POSITRON EMISSION TOMOGRAPHY/ MAGNETIC RESONANCE

PET/CT has certain notable shortcomings, including the inability to perform simultaneous data acquisition leading to imaging artifacts and the significant radiation dose to the patient contributed by CT.[36,37] In addition, PET/CT has poor contrast among soft tissues and areas of complex anatomy, i.e. head and neck and pelvis. After 20 years of research, an integrated PET/MR scanner (Siemens) which enabled simultaneous acquisition of PET and MR was launched in 2010 in Munich, Germany.[38] There were many technical and practical hurdles before PET/MR was available for routine clinical imaging. Firstly, the photomultiplier (PMT)-based PET scanners do not work within or near the magnetic environment of an MR scanner. To overcome this, the developers used avalanche photodiode or silicon PMT-based PET detector systems.[39] Secondly, metallic objects such as surface coils used to get best MR image quality interfere with the gamma rays from PET, causing unwanted attenuation.

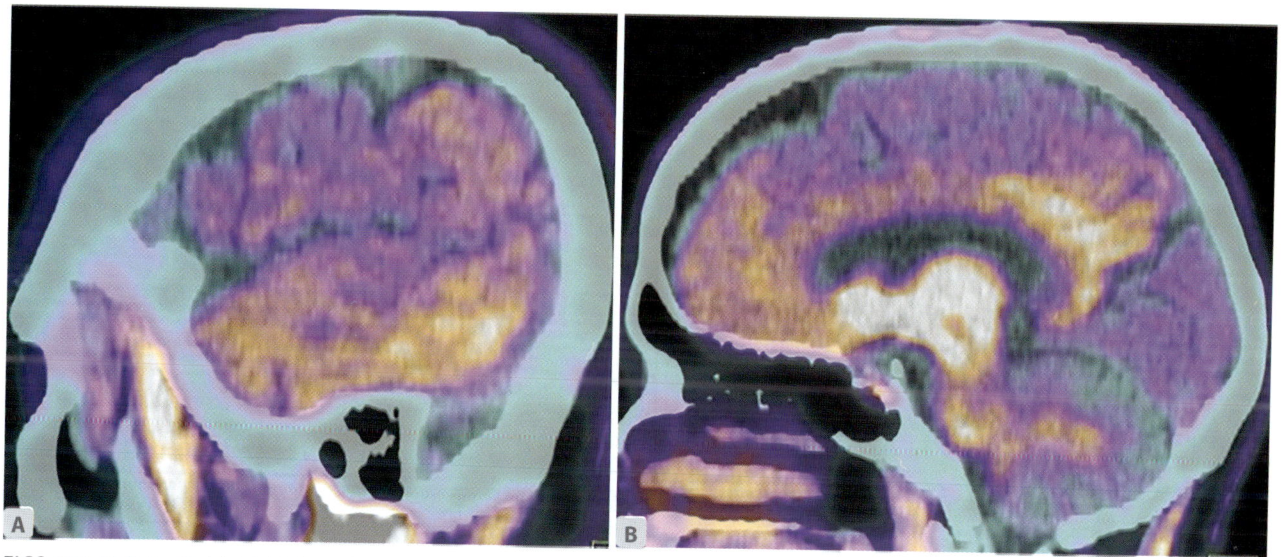

FIGS. 16A AND B: ^{18}F-AD-ML-104 Tau PET/CT fused sagittal images demonstrating abnormal tracer binding in the lateral temporal (A) and precuneal cortices (B).

This can be achieved by modification of surface coils to reduce their metal content. Thirdly, MR data are not readily usable for attenuation correction like PET/CT.[40] Therefore, quantification of PET data was not possible. Various approaches to overcome this problem[41] led to acceptable attenuation correction algorithms for PET/MRI.

CLINICAL APPLICATIONS OF PET/MR

Oncology

Staging

Correct staging is very important for management of various cancers. Combined PET/MR imaging obtains concerted information about anatomy, cellularity and biological activity of the tumor. The sensitivity and specificity in oncology staging can be significantly improved using PET/MR. There is relatively high physiological FDG-activity in liver in PET/CT leading to masking of focal liver lesions with only slightly elevated FDG activity. CT also has intrinsically lower soft-tissue contrast compared with MRI in the liver. Lesion conspicuity was significantly better on the MRI component when compared with the CECT component.[12] That is why the most common indication of PET/MR is the detection and characterization of liver lesions (primary and metastatic) **(Fig. 19)**. PET/MR is likely to be advantageous over PET/CT in the assessment of tumor invasion into adjacent structures in rectal, bladder, prostate and gynecological cancers.[43,44] Another indication requiring only regional extent imaging and expected advantages of PET/MRI is head and neck cancer due to its higher soft-tissue contrast. In these tumors, surrounding soft-tissue infiltration is important for local staging as well as surgical and radiotherapy planning.[45]

In addition, PET/MR will demonstrate improved accuracy in the assessment of spread to regional lymph nodes, especially in the pelvis, mediastinum and head- and-neck region **(Fig. 20)**.[44,45] It appears that combined PET/MR will enable a more thorough biological characterization of primary tumor and eventually metastases. Recently, Hirsch et al, reported PET/MR hybrid imaging in 15 children with multifocal malignant diseases and concluded that PET/MR is stable and reliable hybrid imaging modality, which generates a complementary diagnostic study of great additional value in pediatric cancer **(Figs. 21A to C)**.[46]

Overall, PET/MRI imaging has several advantages over PET/CT in many oncologic indications. Currently, the PET/CT-MRI approach offers the highest flexibility to provide complete staging concepts.

Response Evaluation

Accurate assessment of tumor response is essential in the management as well as in prognostication of cancer patients. Currently response is mainly evaluated by anatomical measures, known as the RECIST criteria (Response Evaluation Criteria in Solid Tumors). There are many limitations using these criteria in evaluating treatment response especially when patients are being treated with conventional cytotoxic therapy or molecularly targeted agents, which can provide therapeutic benefit without significantly reducing the tumor size. The use of PET/CT, combining metabolic and anatomical information for therapy evaluation, has a huge potential impact on the quality of patient treatment as well as on the evaluation of new therapy regimes. Standardized criteria for response evaluation in solid tumors by PET/CT–PERCIST was suggested in 2009,[47] and the impact of PET in response evaluation in e.g. lymphoma, is well established.[48] Similarly, diffusion-weighted MRI (DW-MRI) suggested that early changes in tumor diffusion values correlate with response to therapy. Additionally, dynamic contrast enhanced MRI can provide kinetics of tumor perfusion in pre and post-treatment setting to assess the response to therapy. Therefore, the PET/MR may provide unique advantages of both PET and MRI in exploring more specific changes in the tissue, making early therapy evaluation a safer endeavor.

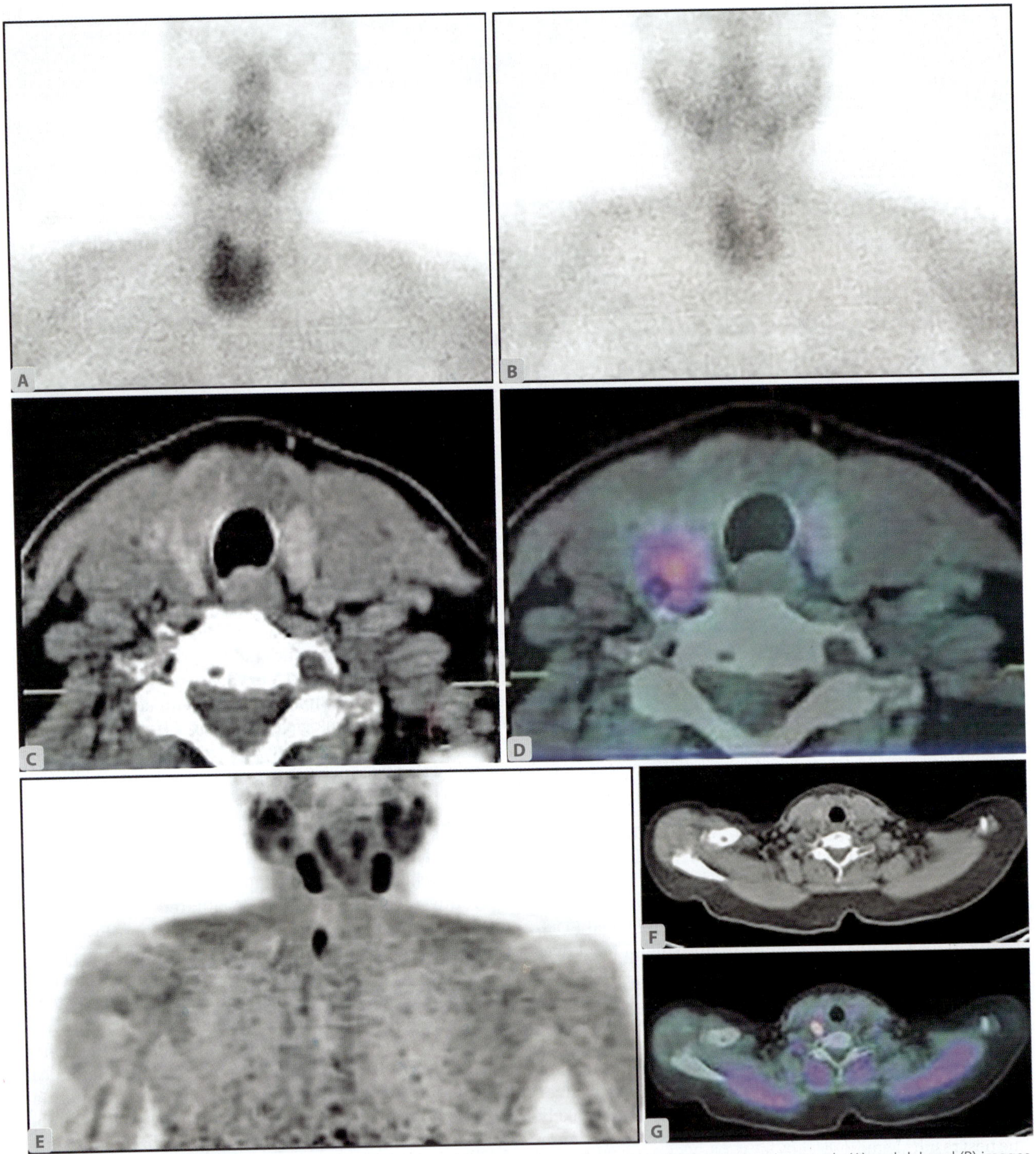

FIGS. 17A TO G: A 55-year-old female with primary hyperparathyroidism, ^{99}Tc MIBI parathyroid scintigraphy-planar early (A) and delayed (B) images showing a diffusely enlarged thyroid gland with washout and no focal tracer retention in relation to the poles of thyroid. Plain CT (C) and fused SPECT/CT transaxial (D) (neck-at level of thyroid) show a doubtful area of focal tracer accumulation in relation to the upper pole of right lobe of thyroid. ^{18}F-choline PET-MIP (E) clearly showing abnormal focal tracer accumulation in the right side of neck and plain CT (F) and fused PET/CT transaxial (G) confirming tracer accumulation in a right upper pole parathyroid adenoma.

Restaging

FDG-PET/CT can contribute in significant ways to the clinical management of patients particularly which have been previously treated by surgery or radiation and there is question of discrimination between post-treatment scar and recurrent tumor. However, in patients with brain tumors, metastatic liver disease and head neck cancer, PET/CT has limitations due to increased physiological FDG uptake and poor soft tissue contrast. In these patients PET/MR will demonstrate improved accuracy in detecting recurrence. It has been demonstrated that CECT has high sensitivity for liver lesions, but generally MRI is still considered superior. However, there

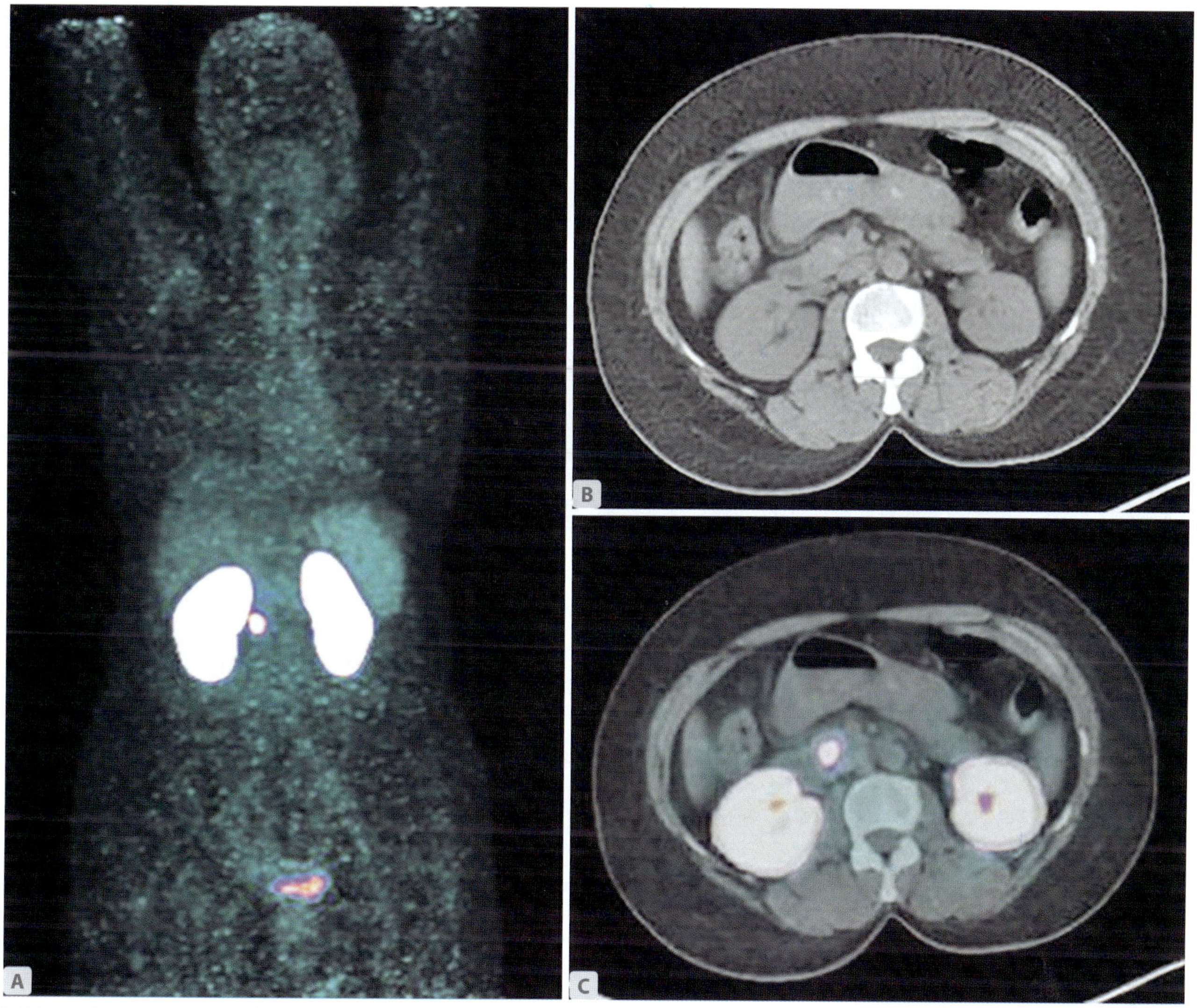

FIGS. 18A TO C: A 42-year-old female with recurrent hypoglycemia being worked up to localize an insulinoma. ^{68}Ga-Exendin PET/CT, MIP (A) showing focal tracer accumulation medial to the right kidney, localized to a small iso-to hyperdense lesion in the head of pancreas on plain CT (B) and fused PET/CT transaxial (C) at the level of pancreas.

are only few studies evaluating contrast enhanced PET/CT compared with MRI. A large meta-analysis did not find statistically significant differences in lesion detection.[49] Initial comparison of data acquired PET/CT-MRI system shows no difference in lesion detection when comparing CE PET/CT and non-CE MRI.[50]

Radiotherapy Treatment Planning

The best results of radiotherapy are obtained by the maximum radiation dose delivery to target tissue and reducing dose to minimum to surrounding normal tissue. This can be obtained by is the dose painting principle. Since PET/MR has advantages of better tumor delineation because of high resolution of MR and metabolic status of tumor by PET, it can be used for better defining targeted radiotherapy of tumor and avoiding normal tissues. Another issue in radiotherapy is tumor hypoxia, which is a key mechanism leading to radiotherapy resistance. Therefore, imaging technique for hypoxia mapping which can be integrated with radiotherapy planning systems is always warranted.[51] Thorwarth et al. demonstrated feasibility of dose painting using a dynamic 18F-MISO-PET scan.[52]

PET-based techniques using 64Cu-ATSM, 18F-MISO or 18F-FAZA can image hypoxia by binding to intracellular macromolecules when pO_2<10 mmHg.[53] Accumulation of most of PET tracers is flow-dependent while, MRI is thought to be most sensitive to perfusion related hypoxia. By simultaneous PET/MR it will be possible to describe tissue hypoxia by PET hypoxia tracer together with blood oxygen level dependent (BOLD) sequences, DW-MRI and/or DCE-MRI to distinguish between perfusion and diffusion as the most dominant cause of tumor hypoxia.[54,55]

Neurology

Anatomical imaging data is usually a prerequisite for processing and analysis of functional data in patients with neurological disorder. Till now this was achieved by

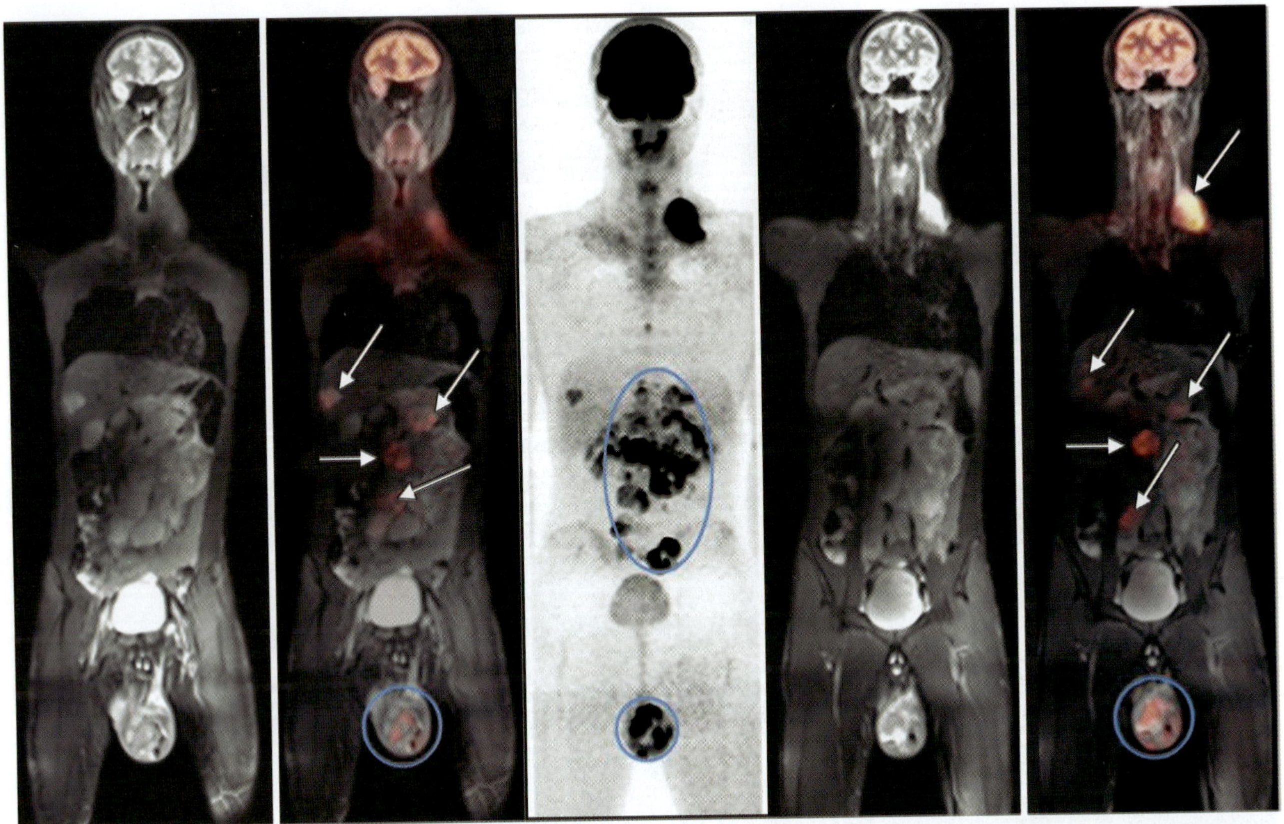

FIG. 19: A 15-year-old boy with left testicular tumor with left retroperitoneal, supraclavicular and hepatic metastases (arrows). The primary tumor in the left testicle and the retroperitoneal metastasis exhibit a very inhomogeneous enhancement of the glucose metabolism with larger metabolically inactive areas showing no enhancement. This can only be explained in part by tumor necrosis. The liver metastasis shows significantly enhanced glucose uptake.

Source: This figure is reproduced with permission from Franz Wolfgang Hirsch, Department of Paediatric Radiology, University of Leipzig, Liebigstr. 20a, 04103, Leipzig, Germany, hirw@medizin.uni-leipzig.de.[42]

software image fusion of structural and functional data. However, software image fusion has certain limitations, such as misregistration. Therefore, an integrated PET/MR will be helpful in patients with where visualized functional processes are time dependent in PET and MR. In functional neuropsychiatric examinations measuring task-induced changes of blood flow and oxygen consumption rate or the measurement of the arterial input function by MRI for its use in compartment modeling in quantitative PET studies.

In patients with Alzheimer's disease, PET/MR can be used for the early diagnosis, evaluation of disease progression and therapy response. In addition, morphologic images are essential to exclude other causes of dementia like multi-infarct dementia or normal-pressure hydrocephalus.[56,57]

Patients with refractory epilepsy despite medical treatment require surgery to resect the epileptogenic focus.[58] For success of surgical procedure structural and functional imaging data and concordance of modalities is of outmost importance. Therefore, these patients needs to undergo a battery of imaging and non-imaging tests like morphologic MRI, functional MRI, PET, and EEG for correct localization of epileptic focus. PET/MR will be useful in such patients and data can be obtained using single imaging test in one day rather than multiple imaging tests on different days causing immense loss of time and money.

Cardiology

Myocardial perfusion imaging (MPI) using SPECT and SPECT/CT is well established technique for the management of coronary artery disease (CAD). PET still plays a limited role in daily clinical routine for MPI as there is lack of solid data to support a superior accuracy of PET over SPECT. PET is the most reliable noninvasive tool for identification of myocardial viability in ischemic dysfunctional left ventricles and the only method validated in a prognostic interventional outcome study. However it has not been used as there are competing radiation-free methods in the hands of cardiologists, such as echocardiography and MRI, which allow identification of viability. PET/MR may be useful in evaluation of the vascular wall and the identification of plaques prone to rupture. It may help to explore evolving and investigational fields of cardiovascular imaging, such as vulnerable plaque characterization, in vivo stem cell tracking, and assessment of angiogenesis.

ACKNOWLEDGMENT

We are highly thankful to Franz Wolfgang Hirsch for providing PET/MR **(Figs. 19 to 21)**. These images were reproduced with permission from Franz Wolfgang Hirsch, Department of Paediatric Radiology, University of Leipzig, Liebigstr. 20a, 04103, Leipzig, Germany, hirw@medizin.uni-leipzig.de. Ref 42.

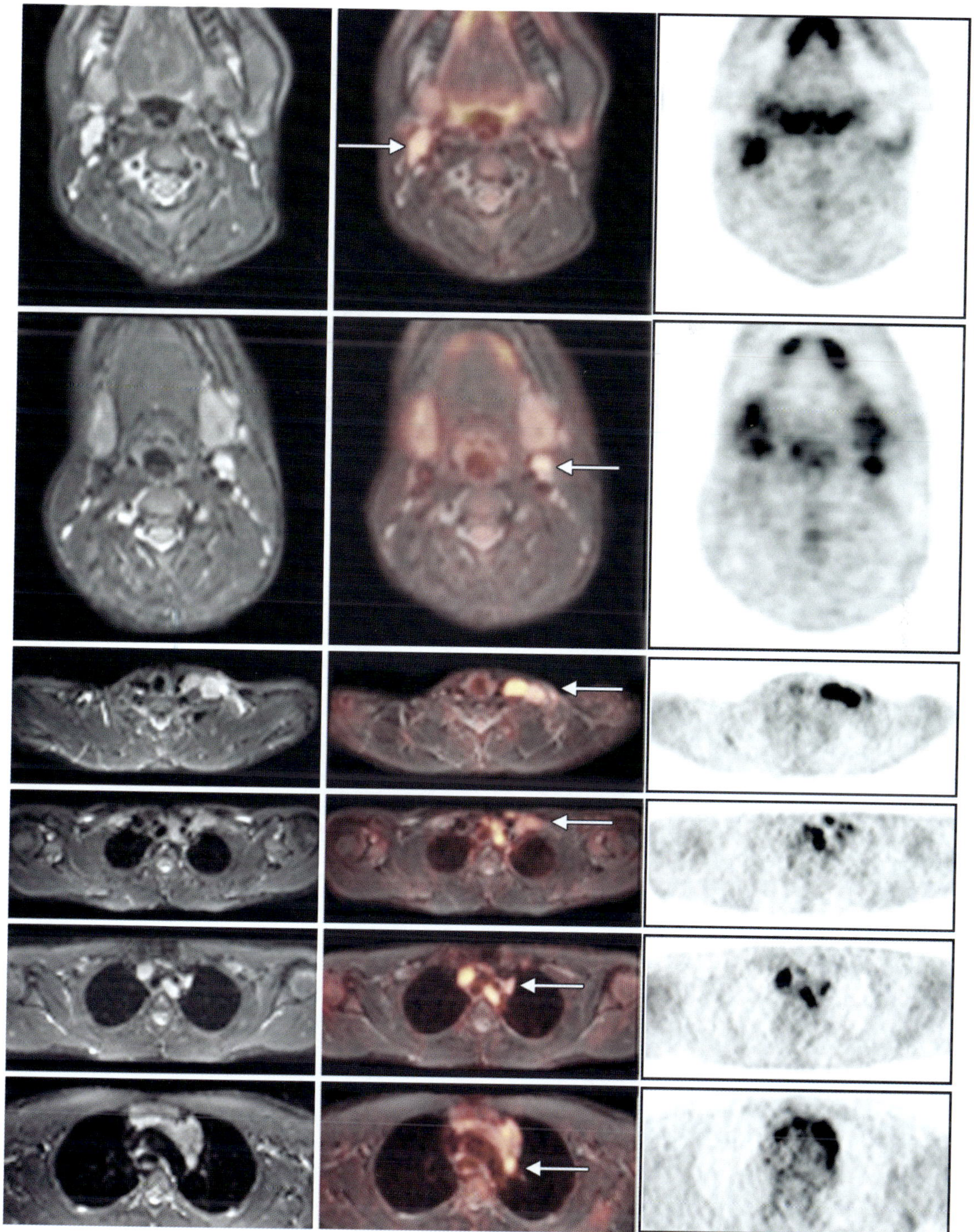

FIG. 20: A 13-year-old boy with Hodgkin disease stage II show involvement of both sides of the submandibular, cervical, and upper and middle mediastinum (arrows). Involvement of the submandibular lymph nodes (arrows) was not positively identified on MR criteria (size), but the PET image shows significantly enhanced FDG uptake. Arrows indicate positive PET/MR findings.

Source: This figure is reproduced with permission from Franz Wolfgang Hirsch, Department of Paediatric Radiology, University of Leipzig, Liebigstr. 20a, 04103, Leipzig, Germany, hirw@medizin.uni-leipzig.de.[42]

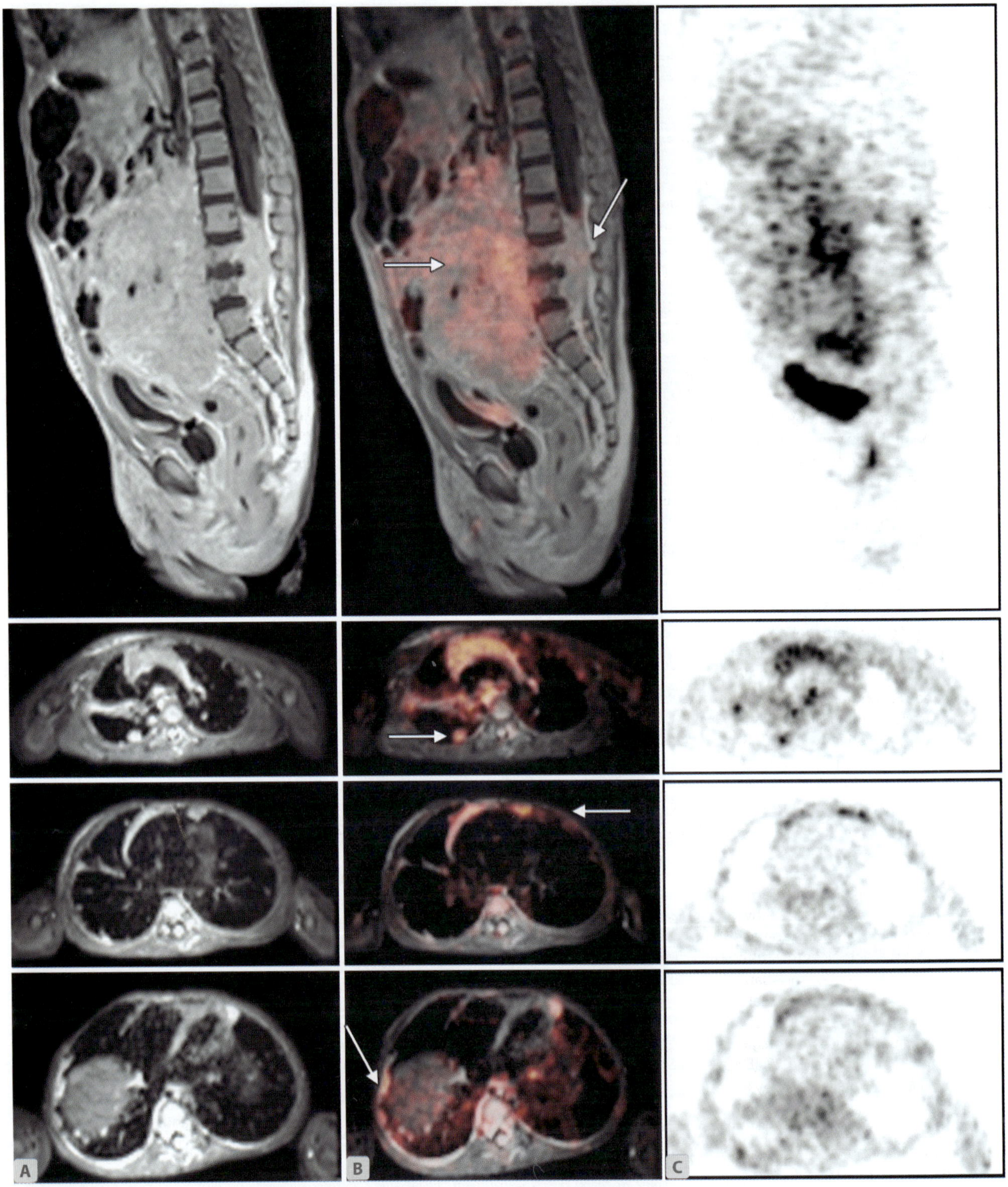

FIGS. 21A TO C: A 2-year-old boy with a large abdominal neuroblastoma that emanates from the sympathetic chain. Top row: The tumor (arrows) is growing into the spinal canal and involves the fourth and fifth lumbar vertebrae. The highly differentiated tumor shows only slightly intense inhomogeneous FDG uptake. Lower row: Transaxial slices show multiple (arrows) lung metastases and pleural metastases. The metastases are seen on the concordant respiratory-triggered T2-weighted TIRM images (A) and on the PET images (B and C); smaller metastases of 3–5 mm are clearly shown on the MR images. Arrows indicate positive PET/MR findings.

Source: This figure is reproduced with permission from Franz Wolfgang Hirsch, Department of Paediatric Radiology, University of Leipzig, Liebigstr. 20a, 04103, Leipzig, Germany, hirw@medizin.uni-leipzig.de.[42]

REFERENCES

1. Mochizuki T, Tsukamoto E, Kuge Y, et al. FDG uptake and glucose transporter subtype expressions in experimental tumor and inflammation models. J Nucl Med. 2001;42:1551-5.
2. McGowan KM, Long SD, Pekala PH. Glucose transporter gene expression: regulation of transcription and mRNA stability. Pharmacol Ther. 1995;66:465-505.
3. Sharma P, Gupta A, Patel C, Bakhshi S, Malhotra A, Kumar R.Pediatric lymphoma: metabolic tumor burden as a quantitative index for treatment response evaluation. Ann Nucl Med. 2012;26:58-66.
4. Gould MK, Maclean CC, Kuschner WG, Rydzak CE, Owens DK. Accuracy of positron emission tomography for diagnosis of pulmonary nodules and mass lesions: a meta-analysis. JAMA. 2001;285:914-24.
5. Fischer BM, Mortensen J, Hojgaad L. Positron emission tomography in the diagnosis and staging of lung cancer: a systematic, quantitative review. Lancet Oncol. 2001;2:659-66.
6. Miller FR, Hussey D, Beeram M, Eng T, McGuff HS, Otto RA. Positron emission tomography in the management of unknown primary head and neck carcinoma. Arch Otolaryngol Head Neck Surg. 2005;131:626-29.
7. Berg WA, Madsen KS, Schilling K, Tartar M, Pisano ED, Larsen LH, Narayanan D, Kalinyak JE. Comparative effectiveness of positron emission mammography and MRI in the contralateral breast of women with newly diagnosed breast cancer. Am J Roentgenol. 2012;198:219-32.
8. Nayak B, Dogra PN, Naswa N, Kumar R. Diuretic (18)F-FDG PET/CT imaging for detection and locoregional staging of urinary bladder cancer: prospective evaluation of a novel technique. Eur J Nucl Med Mol Imaging. 2012 Nov 24. [Epub ahead of print]
9. Gawande RS, Khurana A, Messing S, et al. Differentiation of normal thymus from anterior mediastinal lymphoma and lymphoma recurrence at pediatric PET/CT. Radiology. 2012;262:613-22.
10. Kumar A, Regmi SK, Dutta R, et al. Characterization of thymic masses using 18F-FDG PET-CT. Ann Nucl Med 2009;23:569-77.
11. Kumar R, Sharma P, Garg P, Karunanithi S, Naswa N, Sharma R, Thulkar S, Lata S, Malhotra A. Role of (68)Ga-DOTATOC PET-CT in the diagnosis and staging of pancreatic neuroendocrine tumors. Eur Radiol. 2011;21:2408-16.
12. Naswa N, Sharma P, Nazar AH, Agarwal KK, Kumar R, Ammini AC, Malhotra A, Bal C. Prospective evaluation of ^{68}Ga-DOTA-NOC PET-CT in phaeochromocytoma and paraganglioma: preliminary results from a single centre study. Eur Radiol. 2012;22:710-9.
13. Naswa N, Sharma P, Soundararajan R, Karunanithi S, Nazar AH, Kumar R, Malhotra A, Bal C. Diagnostic performance of somatostatin receptor PET/CT using (68) Ga-DOTANOC in gastrinoma patients with negative or equivocal CT findings. Abdom Imaging. 2012 Jun 29. [Epub ahead of print].
14. Tripathi M, Sharma R, Varshney R, et al. 'Comparison of F-18 FDG and C-11 Methionine PET/CT for the evaluation of recurrent primary brain tumors'. Clinical Nuclear Medicine. 2012;37:158-63.
15. Tripathi M, Sharma R, D'Souza M, et al. Comparative evaluation of F-18 fDOPA, F-18 FDG and F-18 FLT-PET/CT for metabolic imaging of low grade gliomas. Clinical Nuclear Medicine. 2009;34(12):878-83.
16. De Wever W, Stroobants S, Coolen J, Verschakelen JA. Integrated PET/CT in the staging of non–small cell lung cancer: technical aspects and clinical integration. Eur Respir J. 2009;33:201-12.
17. El-Galaly TC, d'Amore F, Mylam KJ, de Nully Brown P, Bøgsted M, Bukh A, Specht L, Loft A, Iyer V, Hjorthaug K, Nielsen AL, Christiansen I, Madsen C, Johnsen HE, Hutchings M. Routine bone marrow biopsy has little or no therapeutic consequence for positron emission tomography/computed tomography-staged treatment-naive patients with Hodgkin lymphoma. J Clin Oncol. 2012;30:4508-14.
18. Brush J, Boyd K, Chappell F, Crawford F, Dozier M, Fenwick E, Glanville J, McIntosh H, Renehan A, Weller D, Dunlop M. The value of FDG positron emission tomography/computerised tomography (PET/CT) in pre-operative staging of colorectal cancer: a systematic review and economic evaluation. Health Technol Assess. 2011;15:1-192.
19. Riegger C, Herrmann J, Nagarajah J, Hecktor J, Kuemmel S, Otterbach F, Hahn S, Bockisch A, Lauenstein T, Antoch G, Heusner TA. Whole-body FDG PET/CT is more accurate than conventional imaging for staging primary breast cancer patients. Eur J Nucl Med Mol Imaging. 2012;39:852-63.
20. Barber TW, Duong CP, Leong T, Bressel M, Drummond EG, Hicks RJ. 18F-FDG PET/CT has a high impact on patient management and provides powerful prognostic stratification in the primary staging of esophageal cancer: a prospective study with mature survival data. J Nucl Med. 2012;53:864-71.
21. Marzola MC, De Manzoni G, Grassetto G, Cordiano C, Al-Nahhas A, Alavi A, Rubello D. Extended staging of oesophageal cancer using FDG-PET - a critical appraisal. Eur J Radiol. 2012;81:21-30.
22. Evangelista L, Guttilla A, Zattoni F, Muzzio PC, Zattoni F. Utility of Choline Positron Emission Tomography/Computed Tomography for Lymph Node Involvement Identification in Intermediate- to High-risk Prostate Cancer: A Systematic Literature Review and Meta-analysis.Eur Urol. 2012 Sep 25. doi:pii: S0302-2838(12)01107-4.
23. Tulsyan S, Das CJ, Tripathi M, et al. Comparison of 68Ga-PSMA PET/CT and Multiparametric MRI for staging of high risk prostate cancer. Nuclear Medicine Communications. 2017;38:1094-102.
24. Yadav MP, Ballal S, Tripathi M, et al. 177Lu-DKFZ-PSMA-617 therapy in metastatic castration resistant prostate cancer: safety, efficacy and quality of life assessment. European Journal of Nuclear Medicine and Molecular Imaging. 2017;44:81-91.
25. Divgi CR, Uzzo RG, Gatsonis C, Bartz R, Treutner S, Yu JQ, Chen D, Carrasquillo JA, Larson S, Bevan P, Russo P. Positron Emission Tomography/Computed Tomography Identification of Clear Cell Renal Cell Carcinoma: Results From the REDECT Trial. J Clin Oncol. 2013;31:187-94.
26. Bakhshi S, Radhakrishnan V, Sharma P, Kumar R, Thulkar S, Vishnubhatla S, Dhawan D, Malhotra A. Pediatric non-lymphoblastic non-Hodgkin lymphoma: baseline, interim, and post-treatment PET/CT versus contrast-enhanced CT for evaluation-a prospective study. Radiology. 2012;262:956-68.
27. Kumar A, Kumar R, Seenu V, Gupta SD, Chawla M, Malhotra A, Mehta SN. The role of 18F-FDG PET/CT in evaluation of early response to neoadjuvant chemotherapy in patients with locally advanced breast cancer. Eur Radiol. 2009;19:1347-57.
28. Haug AR, Tiega Donfack BP, Trumm C, Zech CJ, Michl M, Laubender RP, Uebleis C, Bartenstein P, Heinemann V, Hacker M. 18F-FDG PET/CT predicts survival after radioembolization of hepatic metastases from breast cancer. J Nucl Med. 2012;53:371-7.
29. Hendlisz A, Golfinopoulos V, Garcia C, Covas A, Emonts P, Ameye L, Paesmans M, Deleporte A, Machiels G, Toussaint E, Vanderlinden B,

Awada A, Piccart M, Flamen P. Serial FDG-PET/CT for early outcome prediction in patients with metastatic colorectal cancer undergoing chemotherapy. Ann Oncol. 2012;23:1687-93.

30. Bajpai J, Kumar R, Sreenivas V, Sharma MC, Khan SA, Rastogi S, Malhotra A, Gamnagatti S, Kumar R, Safaya R, Bakhshi S. Prediction of chemotherapy response by PET-CT in osteosarcoma: correlation with histologic necrosis. J Pediatr Hematol Oncol. 2011;33:e271-8.
31. Maas M, Rutten IJ, Nelemans PJ, Lambregts DM, Cappendijk VC, Beets GL, Beets-Tan RG. What is the most accurate whole-body imaging modality for assessment of local and distant recurrent disease in colorectal cancer? A meta-analysis : imaging for recurrent colorectal cancer. Eur J Nucl Med Mol Imaging. 2011;38:1560-71.
32. Bipat S, van Leeuwen MS, Comans EF, Pijl ME, Bossuyt PM, Zwinderman AH, Stoker J. Colorectal liver metastases: CT, MR imaging, and PET for diagnosis—meta-analysis. Radiology. 2005;237:123-31.
33. Kumar R, Sharma P, Kumari A, Halanaik D, Malhotra A. Role of 18F-FDG PET/CT in detecting recurrent gallbladder carcinoma. Clin Nucl Med. 2012;37:431-5.
34. Son H, Khan SM, Rahaman J, Cameron KL, Prasad-Hayes M, Chuang L, Machac J, Heiba S, Kostakoglu L. Role of FDG PET/CT in staging of recurrent ovarian cancer. Radiographics. 2011;31:569-83.
35. Chen HH, Chiu NT, Su WC, Guo HR, Lee BF. Prognostic value of whole-body total lesion glycolysis at pretreatment FDG PET/CT in non-small cell lung cancer. Radiology. 2012;264:559-66.
36. Chawla SC, Federman N, Zhang D, Nagata K, Nuthakki S, McNitt-Gray M, et al. Estimated cumulative radiation dose from PET/CT in children with malignancies: a 5-year retrospective review. Pediatr Radiol. 2010;40:681-6.
37. Mattsson S, Söderberg M. Radiation dose management in CT, SPECT/CT and PET/CT techniques. Radiat Prot Dosimetry. 2011;147(1–2):13-21.
38. Delso G, Fürst S, Jakoby B, Ladebeck R, Ganter C, Nekolla SG, et al. Performance measurements of the Siemens mMR integrated whole-body PET/MR scanner. J Nucl Med. 2011;52:1914-22.
39. Pichler BJ, Judenhofer MS, Catana C, Walton JH, Kneilling M, Nutt RE, et al. Performance test of an LSO-APD detector in a 7-T MRI scanner for simultaneous PET/MRI. J Nucl Med. 2006;47:639-47.
40. Hofmann M, Pichler B, Schölkopf B, Beyer T. Towards quantitative PET/MRI: a review of MR-based attenuation correction techniques. Eur J Nucl Med Mol Imaging. 2009;36(Suppl 1):S93-104.
41. Zaidi H, Ojha N, Morich M, Griesmer J, Hu Z, Maniawski P, et al. Design and performance evaluation of a whole-body Ingenuity TF. PET-MRI system. Phys Med Biol. 2011;56:3091-106.
42. Assiri Y, Schmid D, Pietsch C, et al. Contrast-enhanced PET/CT vs. non-contrast enhanced PET/MRI in abdominal oncological lesions—Initial results. Annual Congress of the European Association of Nuclear Medicine, Milan, Italy, 2012.
43. Punwani S. Diffusion weighted imaging of female pelvis cancers: Concepts and clinical applications. Eur J Radiol. 2011;78:21-9.
44. Giannarini G, Petralia G, and Thoeney HC. Potential and limitations of diffusion-weighted magnetic resonance imaging in kidney, prostate, and bladder cancer including pelvic lymph node staging: A critical analysis of the literature. Eur Urol. 2012;61:326-40.
45. Jansen JFA, Schöder H, Lee NY, Stambuk HE, Wang Y, Fury MG, Patel SG, Pfister DG, Shah JP, Koutcher JA, and Shukla-Dave A. Tumor metabolism and perfusion in head and neck squamous cell carcinoma: pretreatment multimodality imaging with 1H magnetic resonance spectroscopy, dynamic contrast-enhanced MRI and [18F] FDG-PET. Int J Radiat Oncol Biol Phys. 2012;82:299-307.
46. Hirsch FW, Sattler B, Sorge I, Kurch L, Viehweger A, Ritter L, Werner P, Jochimsen T, Barthel H, Bierbach U, Till H, Sabri O, Kluge R.PET/MR in children. Initial clinical experience in paediatric oncology using an integrated PET/MR scanner. Pediatr Radiol. 2013 Jan 11. [Epub ahead of print].
47. Wahl RL, Jacene H, Kasamon Y, and Lodge MA. From RECIST to PERCIST: Evolving Considerations for PET Response Criteria in Solid Tumors. J Nucl Med. 2009;50:122S-150.
48. Hutchings M, Loft A, Hansen M, Pedersen LM, Buhl T, Jurlander J, Buus S, Keiding S, D'Amore F, Boesen AM, Berthelsen AK, and Specht L. FDG-PET after two cycles of chemotherapy predicts treatment failure and progression-free survival in Hodgkin Lymphoma. Blood. 2006;107:52-9.
49. Niekel MC, Bipat S, Stoker J. Diagnostic imaging of colorectal liver metastases with CT, MR imaging, FDG PET, and/or FDG PET/CT: A meta-analysis of prospective studies including patients who have not previously undergone treatment. Radiology. 2010;257:674-84.
50. Crook DW, Mader C, Kuhn FP, et al. Diagnostic performance of PET/MR versus PET/CT in the abdomen. Presented at: European Congress of Radiology, Vienna, 2012.
51. Bentzen SM and Gregoire V. Molecular imaging-based dose-painting: a novel paradigm for radiation therapy prescription. Semin Radiat Oncol. 2011;21:101-10.
52. Thorwarth D, Eschmann SM, Paulsen F, and Alber M. Hypoxia dose painting by numbers: a planning study. Int J Radiat Oncol Biol Phys. 2007;68:291-300.
53. Nehmeh SA, Lee NY, Schröder H, Squire OD, Zanzonizo PB, Erdi YE, Greco C, Mageras G, Pham HS, Larson SM, Ling CC, and Humm JL. Reproducibility of intratumor distribution of 18F-fluoromisonidazole in head and neck cancer. Int J Radiat Oncol Biol Phys. 2008;70:235-42.
54. Padhani AR, Krohn KA, Lewis JS, and Alber M. Imaging oxygenation of human tumors. Eur Radiol. 2007;17:861-72.
55. Dirix P, Vandecaveye V, De Keyzer F, Stroobants S, Hermans R, and Nuyts S. Dose painting in radiotherapy for head and neck squamous cell carcinoma: value of repeated functional imaging with 18F-FDG PET, 18F-Fluoromisonidazole PET, diffusion-weighted MRI, and dynam contrast-enhanced MRI. J Nucl Med. 2009;50:1020-7.
56. Ossenkoppele R, Tolboom N, Foster-Dingley JC, et al. Longitudinal imaging of Alzheimer pathology using [11C]PIB, [18F]FDDNP and [18F]FDG PET. Eur J Nucl Med Mol Imaging. 2012;39:990-1000.
57. Kenny ER, Blamire AM, Firbank MJ, et al. Functional connectivity in cortical regions in dementia with Lewy bodies and Alzheimer's disease. Brain. 2012;135:569-81.
58. Duncan J. The current status of neuroimaging for epilepsy. Curr Opin Neurol. 2009;22:179-84.

CHAPTER

52

Ethical and Legal Issues in Radiology

Chirag Kamal Ahuja, Mandeep Kang, Manavjit Singh Sandhu

"With great power (to heal people),
Comes great responsibility (to be ethical)"

What can be a more apt personification of this famous phrase, initially stated by Voltaire and lately by Uncle Ben (of Spiderman fame), than to medical profession.

The Hippocratic Oath makes us realize our duties and reiterates human expectations desired from us as medical professionals. As one interpretation of the original script rightly states,[1]

"I will follow that system of regimen which, according to my ability and judgment, I consider for the benefit of my patients, and abstain from whatever is deleterious and mischievous."

We, as true 'workers', try to achieve and maintain the greatest standards in treating 'OUR' patients. But being human, we falter at times, sometimes unknowingly and sometimes, though very rarely, knowingly. We have to realize the indubitable fact that in spite of doing the best we can as professionals, we are bound to be answerable for our actions even for the ones done for the betterment of patients. We cannot rest in the shade of the 'noble' medical profession. We have to be better equipped to prove at every step that the decisions we take are for the treatment of patient's infirmity. They say charity begins at home and the sooner we realize this, the better.

The two most significant changes in medicine in the past century have been the rapid evolution of scientific development and the rising belief among the general public that no mistake, inadequacy and failure should be accepted as a normal part of life. The latter understanding has created conflict between the seeker (patient) and the provider (doctor), so-much-so that one comes across many instances of violence between these two groups. Lately, the Indian physician has seen an upsurge in the incidence of manhandling at the hands of disgruntled patients. There have been many incidents of violence towards doctors, which have deeply dented their morale. As a response, many physicians are playing safe by not handling complex emergency cases and referring them to higher centres leading to compromise of immediate care that needs to be provided to such patients. The doctor-patient relationship appears to be at an all-time-low.

As we all live in a world governed by rules, laws and regulations which affect all citizens including doctors, we as radiologists, like all other doctors may be challenged legally on various grounds. Right from being accused by the police of committing a crime, facing claims of malpractice in a civil court to being charged with unprofessional conduct by medical boards and colleges, our community may be the subject of complaints registered by citizens through government agencies. In modern society the dictum 'If you provide a service, you may be sued' is very true. The increasing accountability of service providers including doctors has lead to cessation of many specialized examinations by them because of high rates of such examinations landing up in court. An example is that many radiologists in the west have given up interpreting mammograms because stricter laws there hold them responsible for even minutest of shortcomings, e.g. delay in personal communication of results to the referring physicians.

The radiologists, as other medical professionals, have to be equipped to safeguard their privileges and be vigilant towards their duties and responsibilities. They should have knowledge of the ethical and legal issues that are bound to crop up during their day-to-day practice and be able to handle them with courage and self-belief. The following chapter highlights the various aspects, apart from the clinical/patient-oriented work, which one has to experience as a doctor with some suggestions regarding how to handle them.

ETHICAL ISSUES

The Hippocratic oath teaches us to be ethically reasonable in our duties.[2] The basic principle has always been 'primum non-nocere'—first, do no harm. The moral principles or ethics, as they are called, are usually ingrained within us as individuals, however, there are circumstances when we may falter in the path to our duties and may inadvertently choose an unethical road, which may bring our profession to disrepute. More often than not, this occurs as a result of our lack of awareness to certain regulations to be followed during practice. Even if one rests aside the legal aspect, a clean consciousness in one's practice with respect to ethics is often emotionally rewarding. The various core principles, which govern good clinical and radiological practice, dwell on the principles of autonomy and individual dignity, beneficence, nonmaleficence, justice, prudence and accountability. The various ethical issues are briefly discussed below.

Doctor-patient Relationship

Since time immemorial the doctor-patient relationship is one of sacred trust. A patient usually approaches a doctor with complete trust and faith to seek a solution to his/her pain and ailment. He assumes that the doctor has the requisite knowledge, skills and competence to treat the illness and thus confides in him. It thus becomes an unwritten agreement once the doctor begins on his job. The doctor cannot promise or guarantee a cure but should be empathetic and truthful towards the patient and his own-self, be it in diagnosis or treatment. If the doctor feels that a certain case requires special attention in which he is not competent enough, he should rightfully transfer the patient to the appropriate specialist.

The medical community must realize that the patient confides in them and thus confidentiality of the patient's information regarding the illness and disease should not be disclosed to anyone unless absolutely necessary. The radiologist should hand over the report to either the patient or the referring physician. All the investigations and procedures that are advised should be in the patient's interest and not be guided by other gains. The patient should always be allowed to make informed decisions.

The doctor and all staff working under him/her should display utmost respect for the privacy and dignity of the patient. Their conduct and etiquette should be dignified and delicate. At the same time, the doctor must protect his own interests, e.g. performing a transvaginal ultrasound in the presence of a female attendant, to avoid embarrassing situations in case of any misunderstandings.

The doctor may be approached by patient's attendants at times who may try to influence him/her for any act of commission or omission that may not be in compliance with professional ethics or legal provisions, e.g. sex determination in a pregnant lady. In these cases, the doctor should remain vigilant, lest he/she may land in legal trouble. One should not easily succumb to any pressures or emotional blackmail and must not cross the ethical and legal boundaries.

Radiation Issues

The last decade has seen a tremendous surge in the incidence of radiation exposure due to the exponential rise in the number of radiological examinations being done for disease diagnosis. Radiology now accounts for over 98% of manmade human radiation exposure.[3] Although optimal dose limits are prescribed by various regulatory agencies for common man and professionals involved in radiation environments, they become nonfunctional when someone turns a patient and has to undergo repeated radiological examinations. Therefore it becomes the ethical duty of the radiologist performing the scans to comply with legislation with institution of appropriate measures to protect the health of patients and staff as he is the one who heads the gamut of various radiation-associated imaging procedures. He should ensure regular maintenance check of machines, adhere to badge monitoring requirements for staff and avoid excessive radiation exposure to patients in X-ray/CT examinations.[4] In all studies, he should adhere to the principles of justification of the investigation requested and optimization of the radiation dose [as low as reasonably achievable (ALARA) principle], especially in young patients who are most prone to the development of radiation-induced cancers in later life. Many workshops regularly conducted by radiation prevention societies reiterate approaches for effective implementation of justification, essential features of which are awareness (of radiation risks to patients, public, physicians and allied professionals), appropriateness (of radiological investigations to referred patients) and audit (of the effectiveness of the referral processes). These have been referred to as the three A's.[5] The radiologist heading a facility should ensure a detailed and documented procedure for protection of the patients and staff.

Patient Protection

The various measures that should be adopted for reducing the radiation exposures to the patient are avoidance of unnecessary investigations, use of radiation protection devices and minimizing the radiation exposure times. Many national and regional radiology societies have taken upon themselves to regulate the radiation dose to patients by sensitizing all those involved in the business. Image-wisely and image-gently are few of the many campaigns propagating the concept of low radiation exposure to patients.[6]

In case of contrast-induced reactions in patients undergoing any radiological investigation, quick action must be taken by a concerned specialist. More practically, the radiologist himself/herself should be trained in the same.

Staff Protection

Radiation protection measures in the form of lead aprons, protective gloves, use of screens, personalized radiation dose monitoring equipment should be adhered to. The pregnant staff should be relocated in the radiation free zones for work. There are various recommendations for preservation of radiation records of the department personnel with most agencies recommending to maintain till the entire tenure of one's employment and even uptil seventy-five years of age or at least 30 years after terminating work involving radiation exposure. It is also advisable to transfer the records to the next employer in case a worker changes jobs.

Public Protection

Appropriate signage should be displayed at appropriate places in the department which are under high radiation exposure. The attendants should not be asked to accompany the patients for radiological investigations unless required and if so, with full protection. Periodic surveillance of radiation levels should be carried out in and around rooms housing the radiation equipment. A radiation safety officer having necessary qualifications should be appointed for the overview of radiation zones.

Pregnancy, whether in staff or public, requires special consideration as all such personnel should not be allowed to enter the radiation fields. It becomes the responsibility of the radiologist to perform radiation free imaging in such patients. Inadvertent use of radiation may be harmful to the developing fetus and may lead to litigations at a later date. Thus, all the investigations requiring ionizing radiation should be withheld unless there is definite beneficial effect on the patient's condition.

Protection During Interventions

Interventional radiology (IR) has emerged as a therapeutic subspecialty of radiology and has picked up momentum over the last couple of decades as a minimally invasive treatment option. The risks involved in interventional procedures are more closely related to surgery than to diagnostic radiology. Thus, the duties of the radiologist performing interventions become stricter beginning right from when the patient comes for or is referred for some intervention till the time his/her condition improves for which he/she had been referred for initially.[7] Just like any surgical procedure, the nature of the disease process and treatment options needs to be explained to the patient after which he can make an informed decision regarding the option chosen by him. A written informed consent should subsequently be taken before embarking on the procedure. As all interventional procedures are image-guided, it becomes imperative that due care is taken with respect to radiation exposure as most of these procedures involve long fluoroscopy times. It is an interventional radiologist's duty to perform the procedure to the best of his/her capability in keeping with regional and international guidelines.[8,9]

IR is a completely clinical field and is governed by same principles, which hold true for physicians and surgeons. It is the senior's responsibility that the patient admitted under him/her receives most appropriate treatment. Any lack of care or complications at the hand of his subordinates will make him responsible for the consequences, following the principle of vicarious responsibility or 'respondeat superior'.

LEGAL ISSUES

The physician community falls under constant surveillance due to the consumer-provider relationship that it shares with the patients. A thorough awareness of our expected responsibilities and understanding of the legalities associated with our profession will help us to provide our best to the patients without undergoing the stress of any repercussions. The specific aspects, where radiologists should be strategic are:

Image Interpretation and Reporting

A radiologist is responsible for all aspects of a diagnostic examination. But it is his interpretation of the information obtained, embodied in the radiological report, that is the essential end product resulting from the contract between him and the patient. But the human eye and brain cannot match the extensive progress that radiology has seen in the recent past. In the words of Robinson:

The performance of the human eye and brain has failed to keep pace with the enormous technical progress in the first full century of radiology. Errors and variations in interpretation now represent the weakest aspect of clinical imaging.

Alleged misdiagnoses account for majority of malpractice lawsuits (60–70%) against radiologists. Thus interpreting the obtained images forms the major component of a radiologist's job. A uniform approach may prevent inadvertent error in studying the images of the necessary examination.

First Study the Images

The clinical information should be withheld until after the images have been read because it can generate a *framing bias* and alter a radiologist's independent opinion. Also try not to refer to previous reports until you have formulated your own opinion.

Know How the Examination was Performed

With such a wide range of imaging modalities available, the technical knowledge required has increased manifold. A radiologist should be well aware of the various technical aspects in various modalities like positioning, centering, etc in radiography, pulse sequences in MRI, pitch in helical CT, Doppler effects in ultrasound, the physiology of contrast media, digital image evaluation and various artifacts involved in different imaging modalities.

How to Look (Detect the Abnormalities)?

It is the most important task requiring skills and practice. One should be adept at detecting the normal range of appearances. Patient data should be checked along with the dates of examinations before interpreting any examination. A pattern approach should be followed so that no region of the image is missed. Tuddenham and McLaughlin studied the eye movements of experienced radiologists during film reporting and found an organized pattern of scanning, contrasting with the random scanning pattern of a beginner.[10] Many-a-times one needs to formulate an interventional treatment, which requires a precise judgment of the location of the pathology. It is very useful to create a 3 dimensional image of the lesion in one's mind. Thus, thinking three-dimensionally significantly simplifies treatment.

When an Abnormality is Found?

It is the knowledge and experience of the radiologist that determine the pathological differentials he/she generates foon viewing abnormal images. A detailed description of the abnormality is desirable for which following things should be kept in mind:

- Determine the anatomy of each abnormality
- Assess the radiopathology of each abnormality
- Check for any previous imaging investigations.

Reach a Conclusion

In reaching a conclusion to complete the interpretation, it is important to realize that 'common diseases occur commonly'. The chances of a common disease with atypical imaging manifestation is more than that of a common manifestation of an uncommon pathology which again is commoner than an atypical manifestation of an uncommon disease. A radiologist should be in a sound position to suggest the most appropriate further investigation, if further diagnostic specificity is required. In formulating the report, it is helpful to clearly separate the objective findings from the subjective conclusion.

Interpretation of the imaging findings is followed by a written radiology report which has come to be regarded as factual, rather than the radiologist's subjective opinion in legal circles. The essence of report writing is the ability to describe things and express opinions concisely and precisely. An ideal radiology report is 'most often right, though sometimes wrong, easy to read and not too long' as defined by a leading author.

When to Make the Report?

The report should not be recorded until after the processes of interpretation and conclusion have been thought through as a thorough understanding of the case is essential for an accurate and precise report.

Giving the Report a Title

The title of the imaging should precisely include the region covered in the examination, e.g. a frontal view of the chest radiograph should be specified lest the examination is assumed to include both the frontal and lateral projections and may have a bearing on the future medicolegal consequence. It is also important to indicate the techniques used, especially in specialized CT and MR examinations where a particular technique or sequence can miss a particular finding, e.g. subarachnoid hemorrhage may be missed on a routine T1 and T2 image while it can be exquisitely demonstrated on a FLAIR or DWI sequence.

Proofread the Report

Before issue, the reporting radiologist should check the report thoroughly, especially for typographical errors.

If an error is realized after dispatch of the report, a second report should be issued, replicating the first one with an addendum instead of an amended report.

General Format

The report can fall into two categories: those having a definite diagnosis and those in which a range of differential diagnoses are considered.

Definite Diagnosis

Clearly mentioned in the final impression with utmost precision when in no doubt.

Indefinite Diagnosis

When the diagnosis remains speculative, the format of the report should be divided into 'Findings' and 'Conclusion'. The findings section should record the objective data obtained from the images. Never try to give your subjective opinion in the findings. Conclude by giving what you think is the possible diagnosis. However, when in doubt, give the differentials along with an advice of appropriate further investigations.

Length of the Report

In general, brevity is a virtue. Lengthy reports are not recommended because they tax the patience of referring physicians. It has been suggested that clinicians judge the confidence of the radiologist to be inversely proportional to the length of the report.

Negative Reporting

It is conventionally accepted that radiology reports record abnormalities and things not mentioned can be taken to be normal. In cases where the clinical information suggests an abnormal finding but the images appear normal, the report should report normality. There are cases where the borderline between normal and abnormal is uncertain. In such cases, it is reasonable to state 'No definite abnormality seen...'

Internal Architecture

Sentence construction, use of descriptive phrases and the order in which things are set out are all part of the report architecture. Such skills accumulate with experience though some guidelines may be helpful. A good report should have 'brevity, relevance and clarity'. The main objectives of the report should be to:

- Focus the reader's attention early.
- Report the abnormalities as they are.
- Use phrases and adjectives to qualify nouns.
- Use familiar words.
- Get the anatomical terms right.
- Immediately communicate the findings to the referring physician when a life-threatening abnormality is detected.
- Recommend further diagnostic investigations, if diagnosis is inconclusive.

Appropriate image interpretation and report writing form the major roles of a radiologist and thus should be as precise and accurate as possible. In spite of that there are occasions when the radiologist's report is put under scanner by the patient[5] and his/her physician. Most of these pertain to specific investigations and body systems like mammography for breast cancer, chest radiograph for lung cancer, etc.

LAWS/LEGAL ACTS APPLICABLE TO MEDICINE

The Pre-natal Diagnostic Techniques (Regulation and Prevention of Misuse) Act (1994) and Pre-conception and Prenatal Diagnostic Techniques (Prohibition of Sex Selection) Rules, 1996

The PNDT [Pre-natal Diagnostic Techniques (Regulation and Prevention of Misuse)] Act came into existence in 1994[11] after the government realized that the cause of skewed sex ratio especially in parts of Northern India was the prenatal termination of female fetus. The advent and easy availability of ultrasound was being wrongly used for determining the sex of the fetus inside the mother's womb. As the girl child is unwelcome in many homes due to the traditional thinking, there was a high prevalence of 'killing' the female child even before 'she' was born. To check and curb this malpractice, strict rules were formulated which banned the communication regarding the gender of the fetus by the sonologist to the patient/attendants.

The Act has been a blessing as there has been a constant though gradual increase in the female sex ratio. However, many doctors including the radiologists and gynecologists believed that the paperwork involved was too much which was eating into their occupation time. The laws were so strict that not completing the required data would invite strict action against them even if they had followed all the legal rules. The details of the act have been discussed elsewhere in this book.

The Consumer Protection Act (1986)

This Act was formulated by the government of India in the year 1986 as an Act to provide for better protection of the interests of consumers and for that purpose to make provision for the establishment of consumer councils and other authorities for the settlement of consumers' disputes and for matters connected therewith. Of the various service providers included in the Act, doctor-patient relationship is also established as a consumer provider one. The doctor community is responsible for its actions and can be taken to task if an ill will can be proved against them. This may be harsh on us doctors as most of the times we try to alleviate the sufferings of 'our' patients with utmost care.

It is a general feeling among the doctors that they should not be equated with other service providers like shopkeepers, etc. because their jobs are vastly different. Yet malpractice by certain unscrupulous elements in our community has made our whole profession answerable. Medical negligence constitutes a wide portal in the present judiciary which has seen many doctors being tried for their negligent acts. Apart from the state judiciary which imposes sanctions on these individuals, the Medical Council of India also acts in coherence with the law agencies by debarring the practicing medical professionals from the state/national registers. These individuals, thereafter are not allowed to practice medicine until and unless their names have been cleared of misdeeds.

The radiologists may become a part of various lawsuits due to a number of reasons. The following discussion enumerates the various aspects of duty required of us and how to be careful in the provision of these duties once we are summoned by a legal agency for clarification of our practice. A radiologist's role may primarily be as a defendant or as a witness.

Radiologist as a Defendant

In a Malpractice Claim

On receiving a court notice regarding a malpractice claim, the radiologist should act calmly and not be intimidated by the notice. One should:

- Read the statement carefully to determine the exact nature of alleged malpractice.
- Assemble all of the available documents one has including radiology reports, request forms and diagnostic images, if in one's possession. Make copies and form a separate file.
- Contact one's insurer or medical defence lawyer without delay.

Duty of Care

A duty of care is intangible but generally accepted to be an obligation recognized by law to exercise diligence, care, knowledge, skill and caution in management. The duty may be different at different times for different patients. To further objectify the same, the Bolam principle is followed in many regions of the world and is most popular in Britain. It states that 'a doctor is not negligent if he acts in accordance with a practice accepted at the time as proper by a responsible body of medical opinion.' However, just as the medicine has evolved, the practice of law has also evolved. The 'Bolam' has now changed to 'Montgomery'[12] and the entire focus has shifted to 'patient oriented care' wherein it is expected that the interpreting and treating doctor should give all material evidence of any investigation or treatment modality to the patient before he/she decides on the treatment. It has transformed the concept of ethical medical practice to legal medical practice.

In spite of all linguistic endeavors regarding defining 'duty of care', it is ultimately, for the judge to determine the breach of care, which varies from case to case. Radiologists are required to provide the duty of care right from patient care to the interpretation of imaging findings.

Consent

The key elements of consent are that:

- It must be voluntary
- It must be informed—what is going to be done, why is it being done, what will be the result (including possible risks), what will happen if it is not done and what are the alternatives.
- It must be given in writing by a person who has capacity to give it and should be witnessed preferably by a person unrelated to both the parties.

We as radiologists should personally obtain consent before carrying out an investigation even if it has been previously taken by the referring physician, as he may not know precisely the risks involved in a particular investigation.

It is of more importance in case of invasive procedures like angiographies and radiological guided therapeutic procedures.[13] Any invasive procedure without informed consent is legally an assault—that is, the unlawful direct application of force to another individual. This is applicable in many countries across the world. No invasive procedure should be carried out without taking a written informed consent from the patient or nearest attendant. The primary consenter, if in sane mental health, should ideally be the patient himself/herself. If, for any reason, especially in a state where the patient is not in a position to understand the meaning or consequences of the investigation/procedure, the consent may be obtained from the immediate available relative. It should be a written comprehensive document.

Archiving and Ownership of Diagnostic Imaging Data

There are laws in many jurisdictions regarding retention of films in the public arena for a certain duration which may range from a minimum of 3 years till up to 25 years of patient's age after which they may be destroyed without seeking patient consent. Till this time, it is the responsibility of the concerned radiologist to preserve the imaging on which his/her reports are based. However, most patients and referring physicians opt to keep the films with them. The concept that the radiologist owns the images as 'tools of trade' is most important as the digital revolution portends a future of filmless radiology.[14] Until that is achieved, radiologists must record relevant hardcopy images on film, tape or disc. It is important that the images provided substantiate the dictated report.

Patient Referral

Although not a legal requirement, the importance of retaining referral information on each patient cannot be overstated from a medicolegal risk management point of view. Many a times the referral form by the physician is incomplete with respect to the clinical findings and provisional diagnosis. The information on the request form, often scanty, may be a telling factor in a radiologist's defence. There are instances when the patient is made to forego clinical examination in favor of imaging as well as duplicating examinations already undertaken. This 'defensive medicine' may at times lead to unnecessary imaging, the purpose of which is to protect the referring physician rather than benefit the patient. These examples have seen a steep rise in recent times when everyone wants to play safe in the era of ever-increasing law suits.

The second issue is whether a patient can self refer himself/herself to a radiologist or has to be referred by a treating physician.[15] The latter practice has seen reasonable growth in recent past where the physician has a financial interest in the imaging arrangements. The patient can do a self-referral till the time it is not seen to transgress into the ethical and legal responsibilities of the radiologist.

Radiologist as a Witness

As Expert Witness

Radiologists are the expert witnesses allowed to give an opinion, and the basis for it, within their recognized field of specialized knowledge and experience. A radiologist may be required to give evidence-testimony—in court for various reasons; as a defendant, or when the radiologist's report is relevant in other court actions. A summons is issued when a radiologist is required to provide evidence involving parties other than the radiologist. Refusal to attend court is not an option and failure to comply is a criminal offence.

Writing a Radiological Opinion

The document must show name, qualifications and address. The opinion should be honest, objective and based on the radiologist's experience and knowledge. Opinion should not be given on matters beyond one's limit of expertise.

Comments on Other Radiological Reports

As an expert, a radiologist may be required to be judgmental about reports by other professional colleagues. Without any bias, one should make his own opinion without belittling his fellow colleagues.

Appearing in Court

A good expert witness should understand his role and be well prepared, objective, independent, and credible. One should be able to use simple, nontechnical language, explain technical terms to lay people, answer questions directly and clearly, use consistent body language and should dress like a professional.

Personal Communication by the Radiologists

Malpractice lawsuits alleging failure of communication of radiologic results are prevalent and becoming more so in the western world. One analysis of court transcripts disclosed that communication problems were present in more than 70% of depositions while another claims it to be a causative factor in as many as 80% of malpractice lawsuits. A survey categorizing causes of malpractice litigation involving radiologists released in 1997 by the Physician Insurers Association of America and the American College of Radiology (ACR) found that the number of medical malpractice claims alleging communication failure had grown to become the fourth most frequent primary allegation against radiologists. This survey also disclosed that in nearly 60% of malpractice lawsuits involving radiologists, the referring physician had not been directly contacted regarding urgent or significant unexpected findings, even though in 75% of these cases, the medical record had shown that a radiology report was issued in a timely manner. Thus, approximately 75% of claims against radiologists stems from various sorts of errors in communication.[16]

Malpractice litigation involving radiologic communication is moving to center stage in the legal arena. Traditionally, radiologists have considered themselves to be consultants or "doctors' doctors," in the sense that they initiated radiologic examination only on the request of a referring physician and then rendered a radiographic interpretation and transmitted it to the same physician. Most radiologists believed that their duty to communicate interpretations was fulfilled with the sending of the radiology report from the radiology department, destined to be received by the referring physician without being concerned that the report might not be received or noticed by that physician. Nowadays due to easy and wide availability of radiologic techniques, we are receiving referrals for 'screening' for various disorders with no apparent symptoms. In the traditional referral, the referring physician suspected an abnormality, actively awaited the radiologic results, and was likely to follow-up with the radiologist if a written report was not forthcoming in a timely fashion. In the case of screening investigation, however, the patient would have no clinical sign or symptom; it was likely that both the physician and patient expected the radiology report to reveal normal findings, and, therefore, they might not actively seek the report—thus setting the stage for radiology reports to go astray without being noticed.

In the 1980s, the ACR issued its first Standard for Communication: Diagnostic Radiology. It stated: Some circumstances...may require direct communication of unusual, unexpected, or urgent findings to the referring physician in advance of a formal written report....The timeliness of direct communication should be based upon the immediacy of the clinical situation.

Issue of Self Referral

The medicolegal responsibility of the radiologist when reporting X-ray films is the same whether they were ordered by a registered medical practitioner, a physician or the patient himself. He has a duty of care to interpret the films correctly, accurately and having taken into account of all the information available. As radiological assessment nowadays involves complex imaging techniques, many of them being invasive involving considerable risks to the patient, the radiologist has to decide whether to agree to the request, having taken into consideration the source of the request, and whether the request is in the patient's best interest.[17] The radiologist would also have a duty to perform the test to the required standard, and without harm to the patient. If he agrees, he has a duty to ensure that the interpretation is correctly applied, having considered the individual patient and his clinical circumstances, even if the imaging has been done elsewhere.[18]

TELERADIOLOGY: WHO IS RESPONSIBLE?

Telemedicine has been defined by the World Medical Association as 'The practice of medicine over a distance, in which interventions, diagnostic and treatment decisions and recommendations are based on data, documents and other information transmitted through telecommunication systems.'

Teleradiology is a subset of telemedicine where the transmission of information across geographical boundaries is restricted to imaging data for interpretation and consultation. The teleradiology system has evolved in a huge way over the last couple of decades. Safeguards aimed at limiting access to only those authorized to have access, and to prevent breach of patient confidentiality need to be in place. It is arguable whether there is a doctor-patient relationship in teleradiology between the remote radiologist, who acts more like a consultant, and the patient. However, it may be argued that a duty of care exists once the radiologist accepts a request to provide medical services.[19] The radiologist responsible for the report may be in breach if it can be shown that he has not taken sufficient care when interpreting the films or in producing his report. Case law and legislation have yet to catch up with this rapidly developing area of healthcare. Some excellent reviews by Pattynama et al.[20] and Ross et al.[21] with relevance to the European system have generated apt questions and answers in this field of responsibility sharing. They have addressed some of these issues in their articles in the European Journal of Radiology.

CONCLUSION

The day we take the Hippocratic Oath on the completion of our medical graduation, we promise ourselves the care, hard work, truth and just treatment that we would provide to all our patients. Although most of us strive to attain this at all cost, there may be times when we may falter either due to the governing circumstances or our misjudgements. It is during this time that we are expected to stand for ourselves as practicing medical professionals and prove to the world our integrity. An awareness and knowledge of the medicolegal aspect of our practice is thus warranted. The brief review provided above may thus help in avoiding the legal hassles involved in providing appropriate care towards our patients. This review touches a few fronts where one can be challenged by patients, the duty that is often expected from us as professionals and some practical ways by which one can project one's work to the outer world without falling into legal conundrum in spite of giving our best for the community. Though a lot remains to be done in the Indian scenario with respect to the legal aspect of medicine, a thorough knowledge of medicine and laws is still essential for saving ourselves when the situation demands and to provide the best we can to our community and nation.

REFERENCES

1. https://www.britannica.com/topic/Hippocratic-oath accessed on February 07, 2019
2. Jhala CI, Jhala KN. The Hippocratic Oath: A comparative analysis of the ancient text's relevance to American and Indian modern medicine. Indian J Pathol Microbiol. 2012;55:279-82.
3. International Commission on Radiological Protection (ICRP). Radiological Protection in Medicine. Publication 105. Annals of the ICRP 2007a;37:1-63. Oxford: Pergamon Press.
4. Lau LS, Pérez MR, Applegate KE, Rehani MM, Ringertz HG, George R. Global quality imaging: Emerging issues. J Am Coll Radio. 2011;8:508-12.
5. Malone, J. New ethical issues for radiation protection in diagnostic radiology. Radiation Protection Dosimetry 2008;129:6-12.
6. https://www.imagewisely.org accessed on Feb 3, 2019
7. Zibners H. Legal Issues in Interventional Radiology: A Private Practitioner's Perspective. Semin Intervent Radiol. 2001;18:389-94.
8. Potchen EJ, JD, Hollstein BR. Information Management and the Legal Aspects of Interventional Radiology. Semin Intervent Radiol. 2001;18:367-74.
9. Capaccio E, Podestà A, Morcaldi D, Sormani MP, Derchi LE. How often do patients ask for the results of their radiological studies? Insights Imaging. 2010;1:83-5.
10. McLaughlin L, Bond R, Hughes C, McConnell J, McFadden S. Computing eye gaze metrics for the automatic assessment of radiographer performance during X-ray image interpretation. Int J Med Inform. 2017;105:11-21.
11. The Pre-Natal Diagnostic Techniques (Prohibition of Sex-Selection) Act, 1994. Act No. 57 of 1994 [20th September, 1994].
12. Lee A. 'Bolam' to 'Montgomery' is result of evolutionary change of medical practice towards 'patient-centred care'. Postgrad Med J. 2017;93:46-50.
13. Teoh MK. Medico-Legal Issues in Radiology. SMA News. 2005;37:7-9.

14. Berlin R. Storing Unread Radiologic Images in a PACs. Am J Roentgenol. 2011;196:W100.
15. Kilani RK, Paxton BE, Stinnett SS, Barnhart HX, Bindal V, Lungren MP. Self-referral in medical imaging: A meta-analysis of the literature. J Am Coll Radiol. 2011;8:469-76.
16. Berlin L. Communicating Findings of Radiologic Examinations: Whither Goest the Radiologist's Duty? Am J Roentgenol. 2002;178:809-15.
17. Hutchinson M, Rowe E. Yet another flawed study of self- referral? Am J Roentgenol. 2012;199:W414.
18. Berlin L. Malpractice and Ethical Issues in Radiology: Limiting Requests for Outside Radiographic Interpretations. Am J Roentgenol. 2013;200:W92.
19. Ross P, Sepper R, Pohjonen H. Cross-border teleradiology-experience from two international teleradiology projects. Eur J Radiol. 2010;73:20-5.
20. Pattynama PMT. Legal aspects of cross-border teleradiology. Eur J Radiol. 2012;73:26-30.
21. Ross P, Pohjonen H. Images crossing borders: Image and workflow sharing on multiple levels. Insights Imaging. 2011;2:141-8.

CHAPTER

53

Basics of Radiomics, Texture Analysis and Radiogenomics

Chandan J Das, Devasenathipathy Kandasamy, Ankur Goyal, Raju Sharma

INTRODUCTION

Recent advances in the field of Medicine have led to an ever-increasing volume of imaging data acquired using various radiological modalities. Traditionally, the imaging data is evaluated qualitatively by the radiologist to make a diagnosis. However, the images contain much more information than what the human eye can perceive. Each pixel in an image is data and this data can be used to derive useful information which is usually not apparent to the naked eye.

The process of extracting useful information from the images needs sophisticated algorithms and computational power. This process of extracting mineable quantitative information and its use to guide precision medicine for individual patients from radiological images is called *radiomics*.[1] It is based on the premise that the quantitative imaging analysis can yield information about pathophysiology and tumor biology. Its applications include additive role in the diagnosis and characterisation of lesions, predicting the grade and aggressiveness of tumors, prognostication, prediction and assessment of response to therapy. The radiomics data can be further collated with genomic data to generate clinically useful information and support for decision making which is called *radiogenomics*.[2] It is gaining popularity in onco-imaging for obvious reasons, but it can be useful in other areas as well. The step by step method of applying these tools will be discussed here.

BACKGROUND AND WORKFLOW IN RADIOMICS

Modalities like CT, MRI and PET-CT can be used for radiomics analysis.[1] The analysis of radiomics features is in a way similar to but more advanced than computer-aided detection/diagnosis (CAD/CADx). Both involve sophisticated computational and machine learning algorithms in bringing out features. The output of CAD is mainly targeted for a single outcome feature such as presence or absence of a lesion; whereas radiomics involves extraction of a large number of parameters from radiology images which can be stored in a database where data mining (search for patterns in data) can be performed to generate clinically relevant conclusions. These conclusions can be used to support decision making in the management of individual patients paving the way for precision medicine.

Radiomics involves the following steps:[1,2]

- Image Acquisition
- Segmentation of region of interest (ROI)
- Feature extraction
- Building radiomics classifiers and data sharing.

Image Acquisition

CT is the most commonly used modality for the radiomics analysis. Although it can be performed on any phase of CT scan regardless of the reconstruction algorithm, it is always important to keep the acquisition parameters and protocols uniform. Postcontrast scans provide better differentiation of solid versus necrotic areas compared to noncontrast CT. PET-CT is another modality which has been widely used for radiomics analysis which can provide insights into the relationships between the tumor biology and metabolic activity. MRI can provide multiple paradigms (different sequences) and better contrast resolution which can also be useful for feature extraction and classifier modeling. Dynamic contrast-enhanced scans can provide contrast kinetics information which can be used to correlate with specific gene expressions such as estrogen (ER) and progesterone receptors (PR). It can also be used to assess response to chemotherapeutic agents.

Segmentation of Region of Interest

Segmentation is one of the most critical aspects of radiomics analysis and at the same time, it is the weakest link in the entire process. For radiomics analysis of any lesion, it is necessary to segment the lesion out of the entire dataset so that the algorithms can analyze and extract data. Segmentation can be 2D or 3D depending on whether is it performed on a single slice or on the entire volume (multiple slices). Further, segmentation can be manual, semiautomatic or fully automatic and each of them has their own positives and downsides. Manual segmentation is performed manually on each slice by an experienced radiologist and it is usually considered as the gold standard.[3] Although there can be significant interobserver variability between radiologists and it is time-consuming. Hence it is not preferred in large volume data sets. There are several automatic segmentation methods available which can perform quick segmentation in large volume datasets. However, they are error-prone depending on the quality and type of images. To maintain a balance between accuracy and reproducibility, semiautomatic segmentation methods can provide the benefits of both automatic and manual methods. Here, the ROIs are manually curated after the preliminary automatic segmentation.

Feature Extraction

Feature extraction is the core of radiomics analysis after the images are prepared and curated by the previous steps. Typically, the features in the images are extracted automatically by feature extraction algorithms. The extracted features can be of many types as follows.[4]

- Semantic or shape features
- Agnostic features or texture analysis
    - First order statistic features
    - Second order statistic features
    - Higher order statistic features

Semantic features refer to the geometric features which are related to the shape of the lesion Segmentation of region of interest (ROI).[2] It includes volume, maximum dimension, sphericity, surface area, lesion compactness, necrotic areas, vascularity, etc. For instance, a spherical lesion will have the least surface area for a given volume which is an indicator of compactness. A lesion with spiculated margins will show a much larger surface area than a nonspiculated lesion of similar size. These features are those which radiologists are familiar with and used in standard lexicon.

Texture basically means surface variation; rough texture implies increased variation in the high and low points of the surface whereas smooth-texture implies little change.[5] Extrapolating to the field of radiology, this would mean the rate of change of grayscale values in the region of interest.

Agnostic features are purely quantitative features which can reflect the lesion heterogeneity.[2] These parameters enable accurate objective and detailed assessment of lesion heterogeneity, which may be associated with disease aggressiveness and patient prognosis.[6,7] The spatial and temporal relationship of the grayscale pixels/voxels is an indicator of the tumor phenotype which may correlate with the genetic variations.[8] There are different types of agnostic features depending on the level of complexity.

First order statistical texture metrics (Histogram analysis) describe the properties of a group of voxels in the ROI without any information on the spatial relationships of those voxels. They are histogram derived parameters such as mean, median, skewness, kurtosis, entropy (randomness), etc. These parameters are easy to understand and implement. Skewness is a indicator of the asymmetry of the histogram. Negative value means that the tail on the left side is longer **(Fig. 1A)**. Kurtosis is a measure of the flatness or peakedness of the histogram **(Fig. 1B)**. Negative values mean flatter curve and positive values indicate more peaked distribution.

Second order statistical texture metrics describe the location and arrangement of various voxels in the ROI. They also indicate the spatial heterogeneity of the voxels (the real texture analysis). There are numerous second order statistic features which are described and used in literature. Grey level co-occurrence matrix (GLCM) and Grey level run length matrix (GLRLM) are two of the commonly used parameters. GLCM describes the number of voxels with the same intensity in a particular distance and direction. GLRLM is a measure of the number of consecutive voxels with similar intensity in a particular direction. The descriptors of second order statistics include contrast, energy, correlation, inertia, cluster, prominence, cluster, shade, and others like Haralick metrics.

Higher order statistic features are those which are generated by statistical methods after transforming the image mathematically or after applying filters. These transformations can make the image fine/coarse, highlight the details, suppress the noise, etc. Transform analysis (Fourier, Law, wave spectrum) and Fractal structural analysis are higher-order methods.

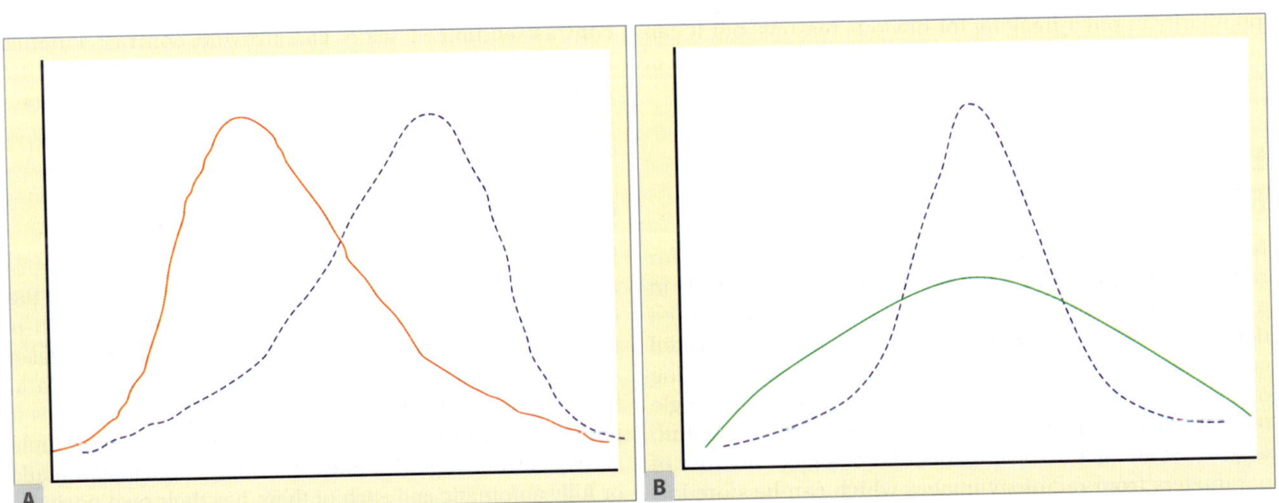

FIGS. 1A AND B: Skewness and Kurtosis. (A) Solid curve shows positively skewed data while dotted curve denotes negatively skewed data; (B) Dotted curve has higher kurtosis than the solid curve.

Building Radiomics Classifiers and Data Sharing

Most of the data obtained using feature extraction are redundant and may be meaningless. They may not be correlating with any of the desired endpoints. Hence, it is important to curate the data and make it more meaningful. This can be performed using various machine learning algorithms.[4]

- Unsupervised methods—dimensionality reduction and selection of features
  Example: Cluster analysis, principal component analysis
- Supervised methods—to check for any association with clinical outcomes
  Example: Random forests, regression analysis, neural networks

Once the association of radiomics features with clinical outcomes are available, it can be collated with data other than imaging such as serum biochemistry, genomic profile, histopathology, etc. These observations can be pooled in a shared archive among institutions to populate it and make it robust.

CLINICAL APPLICATIONS OF RADIOMICS AND TEXTURE ANALYSIS

Majority of the work on radiomics in CT has been done on kidneys, colon and lung while on MRI has been done in the brain, followed by breast and liver.[2,9,10]

Oncological Applications

The oncological applications of texture analysis include prognostication and predicting clinical outcomes in patients with esophageal and colorectal cancer, pancreatic neuroendocrine tumors, lung, liver and head and neck cancers. CT texture features also serve as an early marker of treatment response in metastatic renal cancer.

Random forest model has been used in characterization of hypervascular liver lesions. Mean of positive pixels (MPP) and entropy help in differentiating bland vs malignant portal vein thrombus. Characterization of colonic polyps and masses has also been achieved with high accuracy using features like gradient and curvature. In addition to characterization of lung nodules and mediastinal lymph nodes, texture features have been found useful in predicting response to chemotherapy in malignancies of lung (non small cell) and breast. Kurtosis has been found to be an independent predictor of patient survival in lung and colorectal cancers. Haralick texture analysis has been successfully used in distinguishing prostatic cancer from benign lesions and differentiating Gleason grades. Differentiating low and high-grade gliomas is another field where texture has found application. Lesion homogeneity and entropy have been utilized in differentiating benign and malignant renal lesions, lipopenic angiomyolipomas from renal cell carcinoma (RCC), clear-cell from non clear-cell RCC and low-grade from high-grade tumors.

Nononcological applications include quantification of liver and lung fibrosis and quantitative assessment of emphysema. Cardiac MRI texture features have been used for identifying scarred myocardium and classifying patients with low and high risk of arrhythmias. Other avenues include predicting risk of liver failure after resection and assessing abdominal aortic aneurysms for possibility of rupture.

Tools for Texture Analysis

The use of texture analysis can be facilitated by collaboration between Radiologists and experts in Mathematics. There are many mathematical tools and softwares available including open source and commercial products. They include freely available software packages like MaZda (Institute of Electronics, Technical University of Lodz, Lodz, Poland) and Image J, MATLAB (MathWorks Inc., Natick, MA) and TexRAD (TexRAD Ltd, www.texrad.com, Cambridge, UK part of Feedback Plc www.fbk.com), a proprictary commercial research software for texture analysis.

Radiogenomics

The term radiogenomics is a new direction in cancer research and refers to correlation of imaging data with genomic features (also known as imaging genomics). It is a correlation between imaging findings and gene expression mostly in case of cancer. However, this term has also been used to describe or study the genetic variations associated with radiation therapy. In this chapter, the term *"radiogenomics"* will only be used to describe the imaging of genomic features of cancer. Researchers say that radiogenomics will play a significant practical role in cancer research and will help to tailor the treatment to individual needs and in the long run will improve outcomes.

Evolution of Radiogenomics

Tissue imaging correlates with tissue pathology and radiological images have been used successfully to diagnose conditions affecting various organs of the body. The addition of genomic data in the last few years allows new correlations to be made between genomics and radiologic imaging.

Applications of Radiogenomics

Development of Imaging Biomarkers

In current clinical practice, radiogenomics has the potential to develop biomarkers of cancer without the use of invasive procedure like FNAC or biopsy. Various sophisticated techniques are used to find statistically significant correlations between imaging findings of MRI, CT, and PET-CT with the genomics of disease. As of now, the radiogenomics approach has proven successful in determining the correlation between MRI features with microRNA-mRNA of highly aggressive glioblastoma of brain. This approach has also been successfully applied in breast and liver cancer. Mazurowski et al. have shown that the contrast kinetics in MRI is associated with gene expression-based tumor molecular subtype in breast cancer patients.[11] More recently, Mu Zhou et al. have shown non-invasive diagnosis of molecular properties of non-small cell lung cancer using radiogenomic features.[12] Radiogenomics data can thus be mined meaningfully with the goal of developing robust imaging biomarkers which then can be used as noninvasive measurements of functional and pathological processes for treatment planning, prognosis, and therapy response. Combining phenotype and genetics may be an important strategy for advancing precision medicine.

Guiding Biopsy

The field of biomarker discovery and validation has been an exciting part of precision medicine which aims to tailor medical care to the individual by taking into account the variability in genes, tumor microenvironment and lifestyle. Biomarkers must accurately reflect the micro environment of the tumor.[13] Various assays or techniques have been used which might require assistance from surgical technique or biopsy. These techniques are invasive and samples are often obtained from only a portion of tissue which cannot completely represent the tumor's functional and pathological state. Radiogenomics may reliably identify important subregions noninvasively and can specify which part of the tumor to be sampled for a better diagnostic yield.

By combining various perfusion, diffusion and metabolic parameters derived from multiparametric MRI or PET/CT, important information can be obtained from discrete regions of the tumor.[13] These regions can subsequently be targeted for sampling and these samples can be sent for detailed histological, immunohistochemical, genetic, epigenetic, and proteomic analysis.

Improving Evaluation of Treatment Response and Patient Outcomes

Tumor heterogeneity has been described at the histological and genetic levels. Higher the intratumor genetic heterogeneity poorer is the clinical outcome. Radiogenomic analysis has been used to study tumor heterogeneity. Radiogenomic analysis can be used to evaluate therapy for individual tumors, assessment of treatment response, resistance and better prediction of patient outcome.[13] In a study of clear cell renal cell carcinoma patients, Jamshidi et al described radiogenomic risk score consisting of four CT imaging features (tumor necrosis pattern, transition zone, tumor-parenchyma interaction, and tumor-parenchyma interface) to predict disease-specific survival, independent of disease stage, disease grade, and performance status.[13,14]

Translation into Clinical Practice

Although many studies have shown early promise, Radiogenomics is still in its infancy and its full potential for clinical use is yet to be evaluated. For example, in cases of hepatocellular carcinoma, microscopic venous invasion (MVI) is a sign of poor prognosis and MVI was diagnosed by explanted tissue histology. Genomic pattern in the "venous invasion signature" were associated with presence of "internal arteries" and absence of "hypodense halos" with "tumor-liver difference," in CECT [13]. These CT findings were able to predict histological MVI with high precision and was associated with early disease recurrence as well as overall poor survival. Similarly, Radiogenomics analysis of clear cell RCC (ccRCC) revealed associations between CT features and underlying mutations. In ccRCC well-defined tumor margins, nodular tumor enhancement and intratumoral vascularity on CT have been linked to specific mutations of VHL gene whereas mutations of BAP1 and KDM5C were associated with an increased evidence of renal vein invasion. While mutations of VHL and PBRM1 were more common among solid ccRCC, mutations of SETD2, KDM5C and BAP1 were absent in multicystic ccRCC.[15] The ultimate clinical translation will happen once typical radiology reports are enhanced by incorporating the genomics data in addition to diagnostic radiological information to have an impact on patient management.[13]

Data Sharing

There should be provision of free open databases where images and the molecular features can be stored and which can be used and exchanged by various researchers to ensure studies of significant size for better statistical and meaningful analysis. Such databases may require large digital storage space and may incur a significant cost. Various online repositories such as the online CT image repository, the National Biomedical Image Archive (NBIA) hosted by NCI provide image data are currently available for reference.[13]

Radiogenomics offers imaging of various genomic features that may lead to improved decision making and thus improve patient outcomes in cancer patients. Radiogenomics has the potential to develop imaging biomarkers which may potentially aid cancer diagnosis, guide therapy, assessment of treatment response, and assessment of drug/therapy resistance and better predict patient outcome.[13] Finally, correlation of radiogenomic data may enable us to make a decision about where to biopsy, when necessary. Quantitative analysis of regionally distinct radiogenomic features has the potential to inform precisely about the best biopsy sites by identifying the locations within complex tumors that are most likely to contain important diagnostic, prognostic, or predictive information.[13] This is a field which is ideally suited to the application of artificial intelligence and deep learning and will expand in the future.

CHALLENGES

Apart from the benefits of radiomics and radiogenomics there are many challenges in their implementation. These fields are still in a nascent stage and will require further technological advancement and refinement to make them more user friendly in clinical practice.

The most important issues are highlighted below:

- *Reproducibility:* Almost all image acquisition parameters and reconstruction parameters have an effect on the radiomics parameters. It can vary between two different reconstruction kernels and even between two scanners. In MRI, the result is heavily dependent on the magnetic strength, slice thickness, FOV, etc. Similar issues can happen with PET-CT as well. Hence, to maintain uniformity, it is important to have a standard acquisition and reconstruction parameters. Differences in acquisition parameters are the main reason behind nonreproducibility of the radiomic metrics. The answer to this problem is the use of standardized acquisition protocols, reliable radiomic metrics which have low inter-scanner variation (reproducible), low intra-scanner variation (robust), and high test-retest performance (repeatable).

- There is no universal segmentation technique although automatic and semiautomatic segmentation algorithms have been developed. Computer-aided edge detection followed by manual adjustment has also been tried. Adequate reference standards in the form of histopathology and results of genomic testing will be necessary to explore the spatial relationship between imaging, genomics and histopathology.
- *Sample size:* Sometimes, the number of samples may not be enough to power the results. All patients may not have all the parameters (imaging, serology, etc). This highlights the importance of shared archive among various institutions.
- *Underlying correlation is abstract:* The correlation between the radiomics features and the underlying tumor biology is not straightforward. Hence, wherever there is a correlation with the underlying genomic profile or biochemical features, it may not be always explainable.
- *Redundancy of the quantitative parameters:* Using various types of texture analysis, multiple (hundreds) variables may be generated having a significant correlation with the clinical attributes. Thus, there is a need to eliminate redundancy and select the independent predictive parameters.
- Finally, most of these features are described from initial retrospective studies, with a small sample size, hence there is a need for well-designed prospective studies for prospective validation of the radiomics and radiogenomics data sets to ensure its reproducibility.

CONCLUSION

The field of Radiomics and Radiogenomics are in their infancy but are likely to see exponential growth in the coming years. Evidence based medicine with focus on objective quantifiable parameters will be the best way forward. Today when computational power has reached new heights, mineable imaging data has become a precious commodity which can help us find solutions to many complex and enigmatic clinical problems. It is imperative for radiologists to be aware of the basic concepts and understand the clinical applications of Radiomics. Radiology will play a pivotal role in curating and analysing robust mineable imaging data by prospectively using structured reporting with standardized lexicon and annotating images for the volume of interest which can then be subjected to radiomic analysis. The sharing of such data across institutions and national boundaries will allow high powered studies which will yield reliable metrics to improve diagnosis, prognostication and prediction of response to therapy. The application of artificial intelligence and deep learning will facilitate processing of large volumes of radiomic and radiogenomic data. This will enhance the field of Radiomics, make it more robust and eventually go a long way in deciding the right treatment, for the right patient, at the right time which will improve patient care and outcomes. The challenge will be to make this nascent field user friendly and incorporate it into the daily work flow of a busy Radiology department.

REFERENCES

1. Avanzo M, Stancanello J, El Naqa I. Beyond imaging: The promise of radiomics. Phys Medica PM Int J Devoted Appl Phys Med Biol Off J Ital Assoc Biomed Phys AIFB. 2017;38:122-39.
2. Gillies RJ, Kinahan PE, Hricak H. Radiomics: Images Are More than Pictures, They Are Data. Radiology. 2016; 278(2):563-77.
3. Vallières M, Freeman CR, Skamene SR, Naqa IE. A radiomics model from joint FDG-PET and MRI texture features for the prediction of lung metastases in soft-tissue sarcomas of the extremities. Phys Med Biol. 2015;60(14):5471-96.
4. Rizzo S, Botta F, Raimondi S, Origgi D, Fanciullo C, Morganti AG, et al. Radiomics: the facts and the challenges of image analysis. Eur Radiol Exp. 2018;2(1):36.
5. Varghese BA, Cen SY, Hwang DH, Duddalwar VA. Texture Analysis of Imaging: What Radiologists Need to Know. AJR Am J Roentgenol. 2019;212(3):520-8.
6. Balagurunathan Y, Gu Y, Wang H, Kumar V, Grove O, Hawkins S, et al. Reproducibility and Prognosis of Quantitative Features Extracted from CT Images. Transl Oncol. 2014;7(1):72-87.
7. Cyll K, Ersvær E, Vlatkovic L, Pradhan M, Kildal W, Avranden Kjær M, et al. Tumour heterogeneity poses a significant challenge to cancer biomarker research. Br J Cancer. 2017;117(3):367-75.
8. Aerts HJWL, Velazquez ER, Leijenaar RTH, Parmar C, Grossmann P, Carvalho S, et al. Decoding tumour phenotype by noninvasive imaging using a quantitative radiomics approach. Nat Commun. 2014;5:4006.
9. Larroza A, Bodí V, Moratal D. Texture Analysis in Magnetic Resonance Imaging: Review and Considerations for Future Applications. Assess Cell Organ Funct Dysfunct Using Direct Deriv MRI Methodol [Internet]. 2016 Oct 26 [cited 2019 Feb 23]; Available from: https://www.intechopen.com/books/assessment-of-cellular-and-organ-function-and-dysfunction-using-direct-and-derived-mri-methodologies/texture-analysis-in-magnetic-resonance-imaging-review-and-considerations-for-future-applications.
10. Lubner MG, Smith AD, Sandrasegaran K, Sahani DV, Pickhardt PJ. CT Texture Analysis: Definitions, Applications, Biologic Correlates, and Challenges. Radiogr Rev Publ Radiol Soc N Am Inc. 2017;37(5):1483-503.
11. Mazurowski MA, Grimm LJ, Zhang J, Marcom PK, Yoon SC, Kim C, et al. Recurrence-free survival in breast cancer is associated with MRI tumor enhancement dynamics quantified using computer algorithms. Eur J Radiol. 2015; 84(11):2117-22.
12. Zhou M, Leung A, Echegaray S, Gentles A, Shrager JB, Jensen KC, et al. Non-Small Cell Lung Cancer Radiogenomics Map Identifies Relationships between Molecular and Imaging Phenotypes with Prognostic Implications. Radiology. 2018;286(1):307-15.
13. Sala E, Mema E, Himoto Y, Veeraraghavan H, Brenton JD, Snyder A, et al. Unravelling tumour heterogeneity using next-generation imaging: radiomics, radiogenomics, and habitat imaging. Clin Radiol. 2017;72(1):3-10.
14. Jamshidi N, Jonasch E, Zapala M, Korn RL, Aganovic L, Zhao H, et al. The Radiogenomic Risk Score: Construction of a Prognostic Quantitative, Noninvasive Image-based Molecular Assay for Renal Cell Carcinoma. Radiology. 2015;277(1):114-23.
15. Karlo CA, Di Paolo PL, Chaim J, Hakimi AA, Ostrovnaya I, Russo P, et al. Radiogenomics of clear cell renal cell carcinoma: associations between CT imaging features and mutations. Radiology. 2014;270(2):464-71.

CHAPTER

54

Artificial Intelligence in Radiology

Chirag Kamal Ahuja, Kushaljit Singh Sodhi, Mandeep Garg, Mandeep Kang

INTRODUCTION

Artificial intelligence (AI) has taken the world by storm especially over the last few decades. Its application ranges from the healthcare sector to the automotive industry (driverless cars-Tesla, etc.), finance sector (Banking, Trading, etc.), military organizations, audit and advertising agencies, etc. The concept of AI can be understood by dissecting it into its two components, 'Artificial' and 'Intelligence'. According to the Cambridge dictionary, artificial refers to something 'made by people, often as a copy of something natural' while intelligence is 'the ability to learn, understand, and make judgments or have opinions that are based on reason'. Thus, AI is an attempt by mankind to replace/enhance the natural capabilities of humans to fulfill certain tasks which are based on high level understanding and reasoning. AI makes it possible for machines to learn from experience, adjust to new inputs and perform human-like tasks. In the words of John McCarthy,[1] who coined the term in 1955, AI is 'the science and engineering of making intelligent machines, especially intelligent computer programs.'

AI has evolved phenomenally over the last six decades and has transformed remarkably, from once being the staple of science fiction to presently, a close simulation of human cognition by computers. It has been helped by path-breaking technology in the form of exponential increase in the computational power and speed of systems, ever-rising storage capacity, ability of programmes to multi-task, availability of enhanced graphics processing units and affordability of all these factors. We, as medical personnel, are indeed at the dawn of a new era, which would transform the way we practice medicine. Personally speaking, radiology appears to be the earliest sub-specialty of medicine to be affected by the pace of AI as it is the one that is most avidly driven by technology and has seen considerable evolution over the last few decades. Would it significantly enhance the armamentarium of a radiologist and thereby, increase his value or attempt at replacing many of his capabilities and behaving as his competitor,[2] is a question that would have to be answered in near future. Time is probably ripe for us as radiologists to venture completely into the AI foray so that we become leaders in this field and guide our colleagues in optimal utilization of this potential weapon for the benefit of mankind against diseases.

Historical Perspective

The roots of AI can be traced back to the sixth decade of the nineteenth century when Alan Turing developed the "learning machine" and alongwith it, military applications of basic AI.[3] Simultaneously as Turing, Minsky and McCarthy launched the Artificial Intelligence project. Subsequently, the term was coined in 1955 by McCarthy. AI in its infancy explored topics like problem solving and symbolic methods. The US Defence showed interest and contributed to AI research. Algorithms of neural networks propelled the first two decades of its existence. This was followed by popularity of machine learning methods, which has been partly overtaken by deep learning mechanisms.

ARTIFICIAL INTELLIGENCE AND RADIOLOGY

Within medicine, most AI applications are directed to identification/detection (identifying abnormal findings or outliers), classification (categorizing patients to preformed groups), prognostication (predicting outcomes following diagnosis and treatment) and dimensionality reduction (reducing the number of redundant variables or highlighting the most informative variables). There has been a phenomenal rise in the publications related to artificial intelligence over the last half-a-century. **Figure 1** highlights the exponential increase in the published papers in the PubMed database ('Artificial Intelligence' used as a search word).

The seed of AI in radiology was laid many years ago with the introduction of digital picture archiving and communication system (PACS).[4] The enormous amount of data that PACS made available to the computers helped in evolution of AI through utilization of this data for machine learning purpose. In addition, image processing, retrieval, storage and communication between the referring physicians and radiologists became convenient, ultimately improving the patient care. At around the same time (1960s and 70s), computer-aided detection/diagnosis (CAD) systems

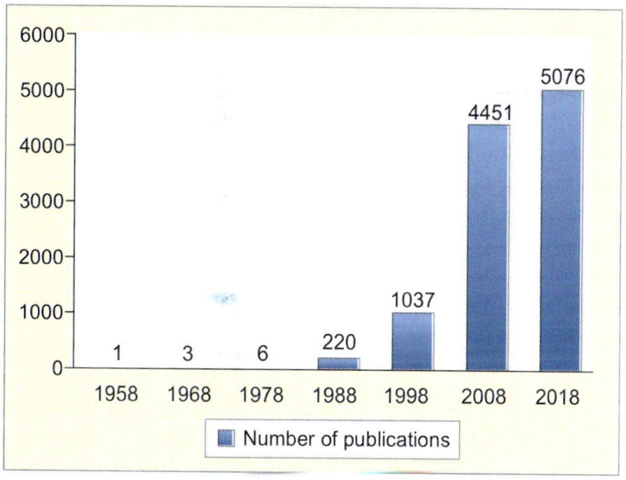

FIG. 1: Demonstrating the progressive increase in the number of publications on artificial intelligence over the last half-century. Note the exponential rise over the last two to three decades.

were developed which mimicked intelligent behavior of radiologists in the detection of lesions on chest X-ray and mammography.[5] This paved way for more experimentation with larger datasets and use of computed tomography (CT) and magnetic resonance (MR) images. In the last couple of years, CT and MRI have collectively accounted for more than 50% of articles in the field of AI research. Neuroradiology is the most involved subspecialty (accounting for about 30% of the publications), followed by breast, lung, musculoskeletal, cardiovascular, urogenital, and abdominal radiology, each representing between 6% and 9% of the total number of research papers. AI currently has an immense impact in radiology, with neuroradiology and particularly MRI as the major areas of impact.

It has had such a great impact that many radiology societies across the globe have dedicated a significant chunk of their attention and resources to AI. Radiological Society of North America (RSNA) and European Society of Radiology (ESR) had dedicated a significant proportion of their respective annual 2017 and 2018 meetings to AI. RSNA has infact floated a complete journal dedicated to AI research. Other societies like the Canadian Association of Radiologists (CAR) established an AI Working Group in 2017 with a mandate to discuss, deliberate and evolve the innovation, practice, policy and patient care issues related to the introduction and implementation of AI in imaging.[6] Time is therefore ripe for us as radiologists to harness the vast potential of AI and guide the other specialties to optimally utilize this resource in healthcare.

ARTIFICIAL INTELLIGENCE: CHARACTERISTICS AND IMPORTANCE

- **Automating repetitive learning and discovery through data**—AI adds automation to repetitive tasks with incredible quickness and without fatigue. In the process, it may discover new paradigms, which may have remained elusive from human eyes. However, human guidance is required at multiple points.
- **Adding intelligence to existing products**—AI invariably cannot exist individually. It adds to and improves the already existing solutions and devices.
- **Adaptation through progressive learning algorithms to let the data do the programming**—AI has an innate learning ability. The more data one feeds, the more robust it becomes. Through the back-projection and the feedback mechanisms, it progressively improves its own precision.
- **Analyzing more and deeper data using neural networks that have many hidden layers**—Specialized techniques of machine learning through neural networks have helped enhance the AI capabilities. AI has achieved incredible accuracy through deep neural networks.

Machine Learning: A Tool of Artificial Intelligence

Machine learning (ML) forms an important tool for development of algorithms for artificial intelligence. It is a method of computer based data science that provides them the ability to learn from existing data without being explicitly programmed.[7] It is, therefore, not a rule based methodology unlike its previous AI counterparts, e.g. Computer Aided Detection (CAD) algorithms. ML can broadly be divided into three categories **(Flowchart 1)**:[8]

1. *Supervised learning:* As the name suggests, the training of the machine requires supervision by a human expert, in this case a radiologist, by providing it with solved problems and assigning a *ground truth* as a solution to that problem in the 'learning phase'. Subsequently, the machine starts analyzing the data and predicts the outcome based on what it has been taught **(Fig. 2A)**. The classification techniques used in supervised learning methodology may be based on decision trees, K-nearest neighbours, support vector machine, random forests, Naïve Bayes classifier, etc and the regression techniques on linear/non-linear regression, local regression, ordinary least squares regression, neural networks, etc.
2. *Unsupervised learning:* In this form of learning, the algorithm is not instructed to produce certain results. Instead it tries to find correlations, identify latent patterns within data **(Fig. 2B)**. The output can be generated based on cluster analysis techniques (hierarchical clustering, K-means clustering) or dimension reduction techniques (linear discriminant analysis, principal component analysis).

   Supervised and unsupervised learning can be used in varying combinations to generate algorithms with 'semisupervised learning', which then can utilize the advantages of both these forms of learning mechanisms.
3. *Reinforcement learning:* This type of learning involves performing a certain task in a given environment by the machine for which it receives feedback as positive or negative reinforcements. Therefore, the learning achieved by the algorithm is as a result of its interactions with the environment without taking any previous training **(Fig. 2C)**.

   An example to illustrate these methodologies is identification of hemorrhage in noncontrast CT scan. Supervised learning involves training the algorithm to identify hemorrhage and the algorithm classifies the scans into those with bleed or not. In unsupervised learning, no such *ground truth* is given to the program, which tries to identify the pathology based on the perceived difference of contrast and brightness by the algorithm. In reinforced learning, the algorithm is appropriately *rewarded* once it generates the correct set of images it is required to, which it subsequently incorporates in its learning ability to better its accuracy in the same task. A machine-learning paradigm may use one or a combination of these methods namely supervised and unsupervised learning with a feedback loop in the reinforcement format.

FLOWCHART 1: The hierarchical correlation of the various techniques of artificial intelligence.

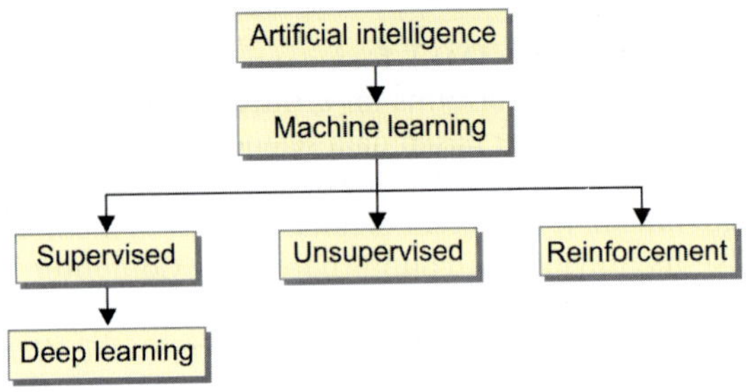

Deep Learning

Deep learning is a specialized form of supervised learning, which uses a specific architecture (neural network) to reach a conclusion. This has been a remarkable evolution in artificial intelligence, as the time, for example, to construct an image classification algorithm has tremendously reduced from years to days. These artificial neural networks (ANNs) are inspired and akin to actual biological nervous systems which are capable of processing large information datasets.[8] The processing elements that connect these networks are called neurons, cells or nodes. The basic structure of the ANNs consists of an input layer of neurons, few (one or more 'hidden') mid-level neuronal layers and one output layer **(Fig. 3)**. The middle-level 'hidden' layer is made up of a set of neurons, where each of these neurons is connected to all neurons in the previous layer. The strength of the network is governed by the individual strength of each connection, which is determined and quantified with its own weight. These weights are estimated through the training process of the network. The number of 'hidden layers' determines the 'depth' and the number of neurons per layer denotes the 'width' of the deep network, which constitutes its architecture. The processing pathway is governed by mathematical and statistical functions.

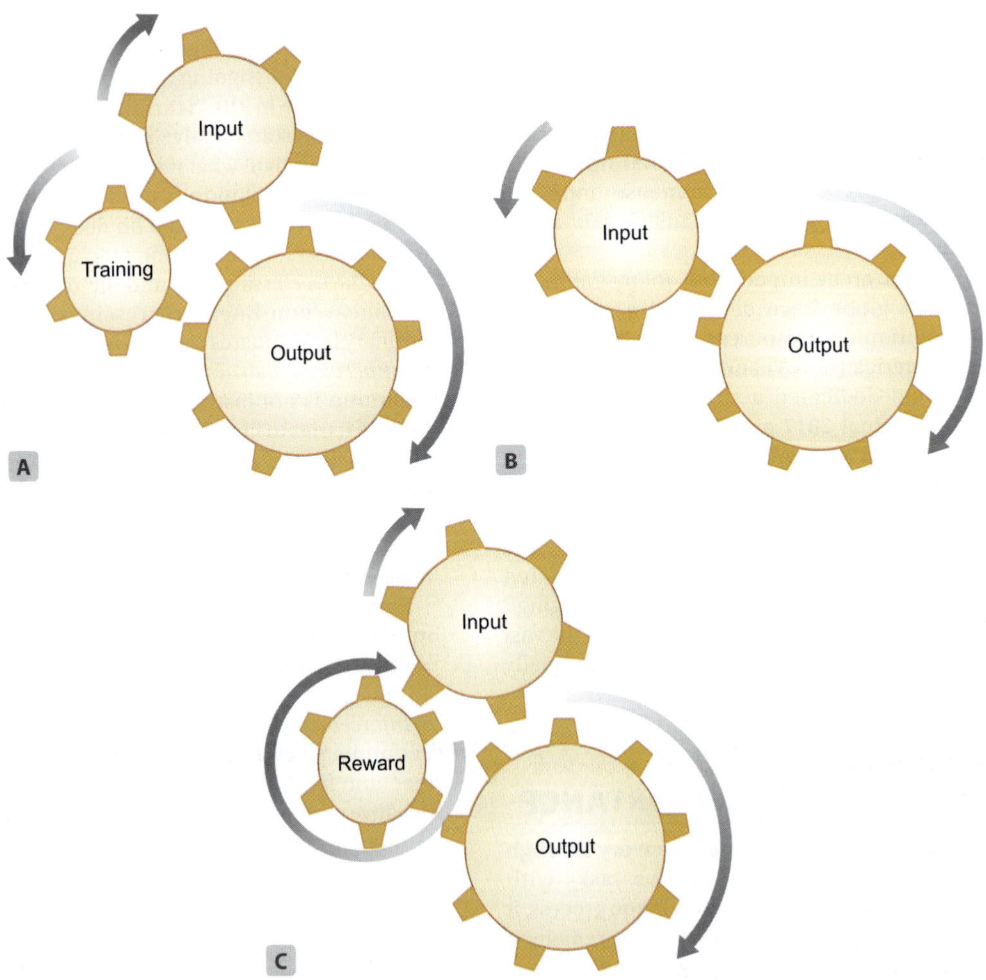

FIGS. 2A TO C: Various types of machine learning categories namely supervised (A), unsupervised (B) and reinforcement (C) learning.

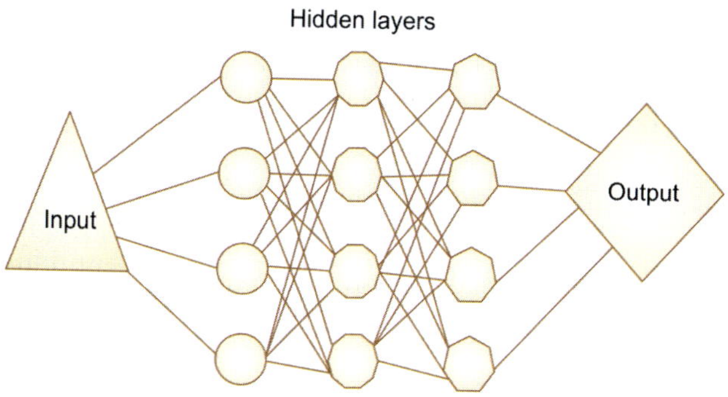

FIG. 3: The structure of an artificial neural network. Note that it resembles the brain neural network.

Training of the neural networks is done using a large number of cases. The major chunk of these cases (50–60%) is used for model training. The next step is validation (10–20%) followed by testing where 20–40% of the training data is used. All this data is walked through the network multiple times. The accuracy of predictions improve with the amount of training data as well the number of data incursions through the network. This training may be repeated using separate teaching models. The predictions are validated based on the ground truth. Once trained, the algorithm is tested on other datasets, which weren't used for training to assess its precision and robustness.

Deep learning can be classified into typical (normal) networks, which take nonstructured inputs and convolutional neural networks (CNNs), which take structured (two- or three-dimensional shaped) inputs. The latter is based on convolution, a mathematical operation and is commonly used in medical image analysis, especially for feature extraction from images. The difference from the typical or simple neural network is that instead of full connections, a small 'kernel' of weights is applied at each position, the purpose of which is to determine the value of the neuron of the next layer, akin to mathematical operation of convolution. Advantages of this system is that it reduces the number of weights and allows spatial invariance (identification of image features located in different locations).

Assessment Parameters of AI Algorithms

The effectiveness of AI algorithms in the interpretation of imaging findings and diagnosing pathologies becomes increasingly important as they gain wide acceptance in incorporation of modalities for disease diagnosis and classification. Various statistical parameters can be employed to detect their accuracy and predictive value. Statistically significant probability (*p* value) statistic is the most commonly used. 'Area under the curve ROC curve' (AUROC) is used for assessing the predictability of classification models (e.g. outcomes—good vs bad). Mean squared error (MSE), Mean absolute error (MAE) are used for models dealing with regression (e.g. predicting disease-progression free interval of glioma following surgery and radiotherapy on basis of MR features and patient general condition). Some variables are difficult to assess by these methods e.g. correctness of prediction of spatial localization of lesions on imaging by AI algorithms.

TABLE 1: Applications of artificial intelligence in radiology.

1.	Clinical requisition and scheduling the required exam (at the physician level)
2.	Patient screening for a particular exam
3.	Image acquisition
4.	Detection of pathology findings and features
5.	Automated interpretation of the findings
6.	Image management including display, archiving and retrieval
7.	Postprocessing, feature extraction, segmentation, registration, fusion, quantification, etc.
8.	Analysis of image quality
9.	Reporting and analytics (e.g. comparison with previous imaging)
10.	Automated dose estimation
11.	Scheduling appointments for follow-up exams/other radiology investigations and integration of current findings with other investigations

If an algorithm attempts at segmenting brain tumor and localizing to a particular area of the brain, the standard statistical methods of quantification of the predictive accuracy of that algorithm won't be useful.[9] Certain metrics like intersection over union, Dice coefficient, Jaccard index would be better suited to evaluate this algorithm. The segmented brain in this case can be compared with a 'ground truth' or the delineated tumor boundary by the radiologist. The degree of the overlap is taken as the representation of accuracy of this particular algorithm. This can further be combined with precision and recall rates i.e. correct identification of the pathology in addition to tumor segmentation accuracy. Mean average precision (MAP) can be used as a valid metric for the same. MAP is calculated by averaging the precision and recall rates at different thresholds of segmentation accuracy. Once appropriately validated, these imaging algorithms can then be used for clinical work in real environments.

APPLICATIONS OF AI IN IMAGING

AI is not solely restricted to imaging based diagnoses as is often understood by most professionals, probably because its entire idea originated with the introduction of computer-aided diagnosis (CAD) algorithms. It can be used at multiple levels in various radiology sections. Broadly, it has a role starting right from the stage of origin of the radiology investigation, i.e. at the clinician level, to giving appointments, performing examination, diagnosing the condition, dispatching the reports and further, in follow-up examinations. **Table 1** lists the areas of radiology where AI can play a significant role in radiology. We discuss subsequently these applications in detail.

Imaging Logistics

Automated scheduling of the exam right at the point where the physician orders it may be done on an integrated radiology platform. The suitable appointment dates and times may be decided by the automated software after detecting urgency of the exam asked for and the currently available imaging slots. Once the patient reports for the investigation, suitable screening methods can be applied to the patient to check for safety and other concerns, e.g. detecting metallic implants prior to MRI, allergy to iodine contrast before CT, etc. The machine learning algorithms based on the clinical input provided can subsequently do image protocolling. As a step further, the image review can be triaged in the order of suspected acuity. This would prevent delaying the reporting of a study, which has the potential to urgently change the management of the patient, and can have a bearing on his/her clinical outcome.

Image Acquisition and Optimization

AI-based algorithms could make imaging quick and relevant. Unnecessary imaging can be avoided and image characterization may improve. An automated program may recognize a lesion and suggest modifications in the imaging sequence, thus achieving optimal characterization of the lesion. Deep learning methods can also be used to improve image quality and can super-resolve imaging details based on inputs provided to them in the form of low-resolution images and corresponding paired high-resolution images. An example is the improvement in the quality of MR images obtained from 3T scanner. A study has shown reasonably good results in the attempt to enhance the image quality to create '7T-like' images.[10] Another potential use of AI can be in reducing the imaging times, e.g. increasing the no. of gradient directions in DTI increases the acquisition time. AI algorithms can reduce these times by predicting the final parameter maps (mean diffusivity, fractional anisotropy, etc.) from fewer angular directions.[11]

Image Transformation

This is an interesting use of AI. Images can actually be 'created' with different contrast or with features of different modalities. A study predicted T1 images from T2 images using deep network and vice versa[12] with reasonable accuracy. The development of synthetic images can prove a potential game-changer in MR imaging as this technology would have the capability to remarkably reduce scan times. There has also been an ongoing research to create MR images from CT images, though this is still in infancy. This, if it materializes, will prove to be a boon to patients who have a contraindication to MR imaging.

Pathology Detection, Feature Extraction and Postprocessing

Detecting subtle findings may sometimes be very difficult for the human eye. AI-based algorithms can aid in the detection of such lesions. Once identified, these lesions need to be further segmented or classified. Correctly delineating the lesion, especially with respect to its margins and edges is essential for following them up for progress after cytoreductive therapies, especially in cases of malignancies, etc.

CNS Imaging

Deep network algorithms can also be trained to detect specific image features of certain subtleties to be seen within a lesion like microhemorrhages, infarcts, etc. Dou et al.[13] attempted at identifying microhemorrhages from susceptibility-weighted images (SWI) by employing AI based algorithms. They achieved a sensitivity of >93% for the same. Another similar study detected established acute infarcts in the brain using a set of diffusion-weighted images with sensitivity of 94%.[14] A major area where this has a potential use is in the decision making for thrombolysis in cases of acute stroke. An assessment of diffusion perfusion mismatch needs to be made promptly in acute stroke patients to provide them the best therapy. Nielson et al.[15] have devised deep learning methods for the same with excellent results. There has been a lot of research in brain tumor segmentation and classification techniques. Various segmentation methodologies have been used alongwith a wide-variety of classifiers.[16,17] We, at our institute, in collaboration with dedicated imaging processing professionals, have worked on a number of algorithms for brain tumor segmentation and classification. The readers are directed to References[16,18,19] for the same.

Pulmonary Imaging

Wide interest has been shown in the detection, classification and management of pulmonary nodules. Deep learning algorithms have been devised with reasonably good pick-up rates.[20-22] Classifying them into benign and malignant nodules is quite challenging.

Breast Imaging

CAD algorithms have been used sincel long for lesion detection in breast. Many studies have shown the diagnostic value of machine learning techniques in different breast imaging modalities including mammography,[23] ultrasound,[24] MRI[25] and tomosynthesis.[26]

Other areas where ML algorithms are being developed are musculoskeletal imaging (bone age estimation using plain radiographs), prostate cancer detection, determination of coronary artery calcium score, etc.

Image Management (Display, Archiving and Retrieval)

The process of automated lesion detection needs to be error free. Prior to and following this task, i.e. from retrieving and viewing the images in the work-station to sending the output images too requires a lot of manual work. This can be easily ascribed to AI algorithms, which, using neural networks, can be trained for the same. Combining the imaging and textual data for comprehensive patient analysis also requires a lot of time, which too can be partially 'out-sourced' to machine learning algorithms. Various machine learning techniques like kernel methods, matrix factorization methods and network-based fusion methods may be applied for data integration and analysis.[27]

Image Quality Analytics

The evaluation of image quality is best performed by human eye. However, it requires a lot of attention and time. Therefore, with the passage of time, the human sensitivity regresses. Machine learning numerical observers have been developed as a surrogate for human observers.[28] For example, automated evaluation of image quality of liver MRI using deep learning architecture.[29]

Radiology Reporting and Analytics

AI techniques are capable of natural language processing. They can therefore be used for extracting information from the radiology reports and providing radiologic input data for other machine learning applications that process medical data. Extracting certain terms from the reports may help in quality control as well as track recommendations of the radiologist regarding follow-up of patients.

Automated Radiation Dose Estimation

AI algorithms could be used for organ radiation dose estimation from CT datasets. They could be trained to reduce dose on vulnerable organs during CT acquisition.

CHALLENGES/ETHICAL ISSUES OF AI IN MEDICINE AND RADIOLOGY

With the increasing use of AI algorithms in the detection, diagnosis, management, prognostication and follow-up of real clinical patients, many ethical dilemmas need to be addressed. There is concern that some of these algorithms may mimic human bias in decision-making. This may arise when these algorithms have been trained by datasets having ethnical homogeneity, whereby the results of these would not be extrapolable to other population groups. The intent behind the AI design may be unethical. A prominent example is the Volkswagen's algorithm, which allowed vehicles to pass emissions tests by reducing their nitrogen oxide emissions when they were being tested.[30] There is a real risk to the health care sector wherein the AI algorithms created by private sector designers could be used to guide patients towards certain drugs, tests, etc for their own profits. There is thus an urgent and real need to formulate guidelines, policies and regulations for the AI-healthcare sector so that the interests of patients are not compromised at any cost.

The current system of medicine dwells on the system of evidence based healthcare and hence, the medical knowledge has evolved into a combination of published literature and the data recorded in healthcare systems, as against physician's individual clinical experience. This shift, in fact, is presenting exciting opportunities to learn from compiled recorded data,[31] however, relying and becoming completely dependent on this form of data is unreasonable.

Ethical guidelines should be created to catch up with the age of machine learning and artificial intelligence that is staring deep at our profession. Physicians who use machine-learning systems should become more educated about their purpose, construction, the huge datasets they are built on and the limitations they come with. Living in darkness about the technology that is dawning upon our field would be like committing suicide knowingly and let others thrive. 'Survival of the fittest' has been a rule since life began, and it is applicable in all the spheres of life. Unless we become fit, we will lose the AI field to the ones that are fitter.

The introduction and creation of specialized algorithms in the provision of medical care widely opens a Pandora's box, especially the questions about the nature of the relationship that physicians will share with their respective patients. With the addition of AI to the scheme of things, it becomes increasingly unclear which parties are involved in a fiduciary compact, even if physicians are still the ones providing care. Will the success, or for that matter, the blame of treatment be shared by the physician, the AI algorithm formulator or the artificial intelligence programme is anybody's guess. The idea of confidentiality, once a cornerstone of Hippocratic ethics, described long ago, has now become near "decrepit".[32]

According to the Asilomar AI principles,[33] the prime concerns with proposed solutions are briefly listed below:

- *Safety:* Safety is of utmost importance in medical care. 'Primum non nocere' (first do no harm) has always been a tagline of medical care systems. AI systems should be self-sufficient in safety standards and should be secure throughout their operational lifetime, an essentiality that is required before they can be used on patients.
- *AI device failure, Responsibility and Judicial Transparency:* If an AI algorithm does the reverse of what it is meant to and causes harm in that process, it should be possible to ascertain why. The manufacturing team should be capable of identifying the reason of failure and should be answerable to the competent legal authority in unison with the medical professional/radiologist who has been assigned to take responsibility for the same. It would be worthwhile to incorporate a command wherein the AI program self-destructs if it envisions a threat to the patient whom it intends to benefit. Thus, the AI designers should be stakeholders in the moral implications of their use, misuse, and actions.
- *Privacy:* There would be a serious risk of patient privacy as the hefty data involved in AI programming needs to be freely available either on-site or in-cloud for the results to be utilizable to the patient community. Care should be taken not to disseminate the data to a third party, which may misutilized data for its own benefit. People should have the right to access, manage and control the data they generate. The application of AI to personal data must not unreasonably curtail people's real or perceived liberty.
- *Mutual and Shared Benefit:* AI technologies should benefit and empower, in addition to themselves, as many people as possible as part of the social responsibility to ones who cannot afford.
- *Loss of Human Control over AI technology:* This has been a perceived risk to many AI researchers since past times. A theoretical risk would be the AI technology taking decisions NOT to treat a patient whom it perceives will not benefit from treatment-akin to euthanasia. The 'intelligent' bots taking over the human decisions, in the current times, is

more of a fad than a near-future reality. Their current lack of 'emotional intelligence' would prevent them to behave adversely. At the same time, humans should choose how, whether and when to delegate decisions to AI systems, to human-chosen objectives. Also, AI systems designed to self-improve or self-replicate by feed-back/feed-forward mechanisms could lead to rapidly increasing quality or quantity. However, this must be subject to strict safety and control measures, so that they donot go beyond control.

ARTIFICIAL INTELLIGENCE: EXISTENTIAL DILEMMA FOR A RADIOLOGIST?

There was a lot of hue and cry when a piece of AI software 'ContaCT' was granted permission to diagnose cases of Acute Stroke on February 13, 2018 by the Food and Drug Administration (FDA). The allowance was granted based on the results of a trial named ALADIN, presented as a poster in 2018 International Stroke Conference accurately, which labeled middle cerebral artery M1 occlusion with a sensitivity of 97% and an overall accuracy of 78% as compared to an expert neuroradiologist. No publications, validation or other confirmations were subsequently done. The interesting thing was that the results obtained could be directly transmitted to a stroke neurologist without being read and approved by a radiologist. Does it mark the beginning of the end of 'OUR' existence? This was in fact preceded by a similar FDA approval of another software Arterys for cardiac segmentation (2017) and lately for liver and lung nodule detection.[34] However, what was not highlighted was the poor specificity. Aimed at possibly reducing the time to diagnose and at the same time earn from the concept, the lobbying by certain groups in making this technology legally acceptable has actually made a mockery of the general sensibility currently prevailing in medicine. It is akin to giving the control of one's (patient's) body to a piece of program, the latter determining what is wrong with it and what needs to be done to fix it, which is completely outrageous. As has been rightfully pointed out by one author group,[35] sole AI-based diagnosis would entail significant hurdles of patient acceptance of being treated and diagnosed by computers than human physicians. They believe that it would be better acceptable to patients to have algorithms that would aid physicians rather than those that eliminate and replace physicians. Another author[36] has remarked that radiologists would actually be in more demand after AI is established and has given the following reasons why they need not fear AI:

- AI lacks the power of communication and discussion, which the radiologists are capable of doing with the referring clinicians. Doctor-patient communication is also an important aspect, which the patients relish and this connection cannot be readily supplanted by machines.
- With the AI algorithms performing tasks such as image scanning, radiologists would have more time to focus on critical elements in imaging giving more direct attention to each review, focusing on precise problems and providing touch by interacting with patients and medical specialists.
- With too many complex variables and issues to be addressed in radiology, it would be impossible for AI to be comprehensive especially wherever a holistic approach is required. Machines distinctly lack critical and contextual thinking in reaching to their results.
- As AI becomes a part of the workflow, it would be possible to increase the productivity in terms of more studies being interpreted and channelizing human energies towards meeting accuracy and addressing complexities in imaging.

Apart from these, there are legal and regulatory hurdles in accepting machines to replace humans for disease treatments. All-in-all, AI is more of a blessing as it is adding armamentarium to the radiologist's repertoire than challenging his existence.

CONCLUSION

Artificial intelligence is here to stay. Of the entire field of medicine, the specialty of radiology is most to get impacted. It is supposed to potentially change radiology practice more than anything since Roentgen. Radiologists are used to facing technological challenges because, since the beginnings of its history, radiology has been the playfield of technological development.

An updated radiologist should be aware of the basic principles of AI, the methodology involved and its limitations. He need not essentially know the deepest details of these systems, but at the same time must learn the technical vocabulary used by data scientists to efficiently communicate with them. It would be best if AI serves the radiologist in giving more accurate reports, than to partly replace his jobs. Let the radiologist be the rider on the horse of artificial intelligence.

REFERENCES

1. John McCArthy. https://en.wikipedia.org/wiki/John_McCarthy_(computer_scientist): Accessed February 23, 2019.
2. G. Hinton, Machine learning and the market for intelligence, Mach. Learn. Mark. Intell. Conf. 2016, Machine Learning and the Market for Intelligence Conference 2016, Toronto, 2016.
3. Turing AM. Computing machinery and intelligence. Mind. 1950;59:433-60.
4. Hainc N, Federau C, Stieltjes B, et al. The bright, artificial intelligence-augmented future of neuroimaging reading. Front. Neurol. 2017;8:489.
5. Lee JG, Jun S, Cho YW et al. Deep learning in medical imaging: general overview. Korean J Radiol. 2017;18: 570-84.
6. Tang A, Tam R, Cadrin-Chênevert A, et al. Canadian Association of Radiologists (CAR) Artificial Intelligence Working Group. Canadian Association of Radiologists White Paper on Artificial Intelligence in Radiology. Can Assoc Radiol J. 2018;69(2):120-35.
7. Wang S, Summers RM. Machine learning and radiology. Med Image Anal. 2012;16(5):933-51.
8. Zaharchuk G, Gong E, Wintermark M, Rubin D, Langlotz CP. Deep learning in neuroradiology. Am J Neuroradiol. 2018;39(10):1776-84.

9. Handelman GS, Kok HK, Chandra RV, Razavi AH, Huang S, Brooks M, Lee MJ, Asadi H. Peering into the black box of artificial intelligence: evaluation metrics of machine learning methods. Am J Roentgenol. 2019;212(1):38-43.
10. Bahrami K, Shi F, Zong X, et al. Reconstruction of 7T-like images from 3T MRI. IEEE Trans Med Imaging. 2016;35:2085-97.
11. Golkov V, Dosovitskiy A, Sperl JI, et al. Q-space deep learning: twelve-fold shorter and model-free diffusion MRI scans. IEEE Trans Med Imaging. 2016;35:1344-51.
12. Vemulapalli R, Nguyen H, Zhou S. Deep networks and mutual information maximization for cross-modal medical image synthesis. In: Zhou S, Greenspan H, Shen D, eds. Deep Learning for Medical Image Analysis. London: Elsevier; 2017.
13. Dou Q, Chen H, Yu L, et al. Automatic detection of cerebral microbleeds from MR images via 3D convolutional neural networks. IEEE Trans Med Imaging. 2016;35:1182-95.
14. Chen L, Bentley P, Rueckert D. Fully automatic acute ischemic lesion segmentation in DWI using convolutional neural networks. Neuroimage Clin. 2017;15:633-43.
15. Nielsen A, Mouridsen K, Hansen M, et al. Deep learning: utilizing the potential in databases to predict individual outcome in acute stroke. In: Proceedings of the Annual Meeting of the International Society for Magnetic Resonance in Medicine, Honolulu, Hawaii. April 22–27. 2017;5665.
16. Sachdeva J, Kumar V, Gupta I, Khandelwal N, Ahuja CK. Segmentation, feature extraction, and multiclass brain tumor classification. J Digit Imaging. 2013;26(6):1141-50.
17. Korfiatis P, Kline TL, Erickson BJ. Automated segmentation of hyperintense regions in FLAIR MRI using deep learning. Tomography. 2016;2:334-40.
18. Sachdeva J, Kumar V, Gupta I, Khandelwal N, Ahuja CK. A dual neural network ensemble approach for multiclass brain tumor classification. Int J Numer Method Biomed Eng. 2012;28(11): 1107-20.
19. Sachdeva J, Kumar V, Gupta I, Khandelwal N, Ahuja CK. A novel content-based active contour model for brain tumor segmentation. Magn Reson Imaging. 2012;30(5): 694-715.
20. Liu Y, Balagurunathan Y, Atwater T, et al. Radiological image traits predictive of cancer status in pulmonary nodules. Clin Cancer Res. 2017;23(6):1442-9.
21. Ciompi F, Chung K, van Riel SJ, et al. Towards automatic pulmonary nodule management in lung cancer screening with deep learning. Sci Rep. 2017;7:46479.
22. Dhara AK, Mukhopadhyay S, Dutta A, Garg M, Khandelwal N. A Combination of Shape and Texture Features for Classification of Pulmonary Nodules in Lung CT Images. J Digit Imaging. 2016;29(4):466-75.
23. Huynh BQ, Li H, Giger ML. Digital mammographic tumor classification using transfer learning from deep convolutional neural networks. J Med Imaging (Bellingham). 2016;3(3): 034501.
24. Gu P, Lee WM, Roubidoux MA, Yuan J, Wang X, Carson PL. Automated 3D ultrasound image segmentation to aid breast cancer image interpretation. Ultrasonics. 2016;65:51-8.
25. Bickelhaupt S, Paech D, Kickingereder P, et al. Prediction of malignancy by a radiomic signature from contrast agent-free diffusion MRI in suspicious breast lesions found on screening mammography. J Magn Reson Imaging. 2017;46(2):604-16.
26. Samala RK, Chan HP, Hadjiiski L, Helvie MA, Wei J, Cha K. Mass detection in digital breast tomosynthesis: deep convolutional neural network with transfer learning from mammography. Med Phys. 2016;43(12):6654-66.
27. Li Y, Wu FX, Ngom A. A review on machine learning principles for multi-view biological data integration. Brief Bioinform. 2018;19(2):325-40.
28. Kalayeh MM, Marin T, Brankov JG. Generalization evaluation of machine learning numerical observers for image quality assessment. IEEE Trans Nucl Sci. 2013;60(3):1609-18.
29. Esses SJ, Lu X, Zhao T, Shanbhogue K, Dane B, Bruno M, Chandarana H. Automated image quality evaluation of T(2) -weighted liver MRI utilizing deep learning architecture. J Magn Reson Imaging. 2018;47(3):723-8.
30. Char DS, Shah NH, Magnus D. Implementing machine learning in health care—addressing ethical challenges. N Engl J Med. 2018;378:981-3.
31. Longhurst CA, Harrington RA, Shah NH. A 'green button' for using aggregate patient data at the point of care. Health Aff (Millwood). 2014;33:1229-35.
32. Siegler M. Confidentiality in medicine—a decrepit concept. N Engl J Med. 1982;307:1518-21.
33. AI Principles—Future of Life Institute, (n.d.). https://futureoflife.org/ai principles Accessed on February 23, 2019.
34. Bluemke DA. Radiology in 2018: Are you working with ai or being replaced by AI? Radiology. 2018;287:365-6.
35. Recht M, Bryan RN. Artificial Intelligence: Threat or Boon to Radiologists? J Am Coll Radiol. 2017;14(11):1476-80.
36. AI Will Not Replace Radiologists. https://insidebigdata.com/2018/08/08/ai-will-not-replace-radiologists. Accessed on February 23, 2019.

CHAPTER

55

Structured Reporting in Radiology

Ashu Seith Bhalla, Smita Manchanda, Manisha Jana

INTRODUCTION

A radiology report is a vital communication between the radiologist interpreting imaging studies, and treating clinician which significantly influences patient care. Although several clinicians do some level of interpretation of imaging studies themselves, there is an immense reliance on the formal radiology report to guide patient management. The report is accessible to, and hence read by patients too. Also, seldom is there any opportunity to correct one's own report, once it is already dispatched. The report will also be analysed in case of any subsequent conflict or negligence allegations.[1] Despite its importance, the subject of composing a good report is seldom taught as a formal subject during radiology residency, nor is external audit of reports performed in most departments.

STEPS OF RADIOLOGY REPORTING

The generation of radiology reports requires a systematic approach, which involves the interpretation of images in various windows, imaging planes and special reconstructions. The final opinion almost always requires the integration of clinical information. It is argued that the knowledge of clinical details add a bias to the report, as there is a pretest possibility to the diagnosis that is assigned by the radiologist without even looking at the images. On the other hand, ignoring the clinical information can lead to gross errors. It may thus be prudent to look at images first, note the findings and then assimilate the background information, to give the final opinion **(Flowchart 1)**.

TYPES OF REPORTS

There are two main forms of radiology reports:

1. *Nonstructured report*: Written as a narrative in free text.
2. *Structured report*: Written in predesigned templates in the form of checklists/bulleted texts.[2]

COMPONENTS OF A RADIOLOGY REPORT

Increasingly, the components of a radiology report are being formalized, and may soon become an essential parameter of quality assessment of an organization or an individual. In the United States, this is a part of merit based incentive payment system (MIPS), which is a component of Medicare access and CHIP reauthorization act.[3] A tier system is recommended for organizing a structured report, comprising of the following levels:

FLOWCHART 1: Steps of radiology reporting.

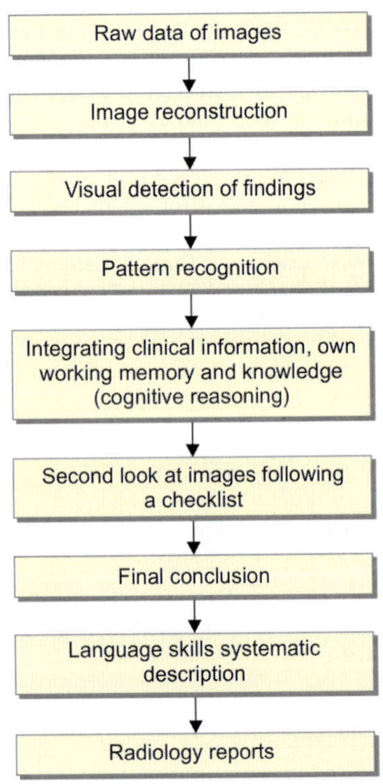

- *Tier 1*: Organization into headings—such as clinical evaluation, laboratory reports, imaging acquisition techniques, imaging findings and impression. These headings are frequently followed even in non-structured reporting formats. List of previous radiology investigations, especially those involving ionizing radiation is essential. The study type and protocols should also be detailed.
- *Tier 2*: Subheadings within the imaging findings section often based on organs/key anatomic structures imaged. Although several nonstructured reports will also have rough organs system headings, in a structured report these are in far more details often thus featuring as sub-subheadings and so on.
- *Tier 3*: A structured report often follows a standard lexicon in use for the concerned disease entity, e.g. Lung RADS or TNM staging, and the numerous headings in the imaging findings section are designed bearing in mind the criteria/components of the adopted lexicon. Follow up recommendations maybe given here.

COMPONENTS/CRITERIA OF A GOOD STRUCTURED REPORT

- The basic challenge of formulating any report is that it should convey all the relevant information, without being unduly lengthy or verbose. Long drawn descriptions, however vivid, do not often add to the scientific content of the report.
- The standard terminology/classification/staging being adopted must be in sync with that being used by the treating physician or surgeon. Hence, one must follow practise guidelines being adopted by the multidisciplinary team.[4] Adopt a standard set of evidence-based recommendations, and thus a standard lexicon. Use standard terminology to detail abnormalities.
- Incorporate all relevant key imaging features pertinent to the clinical condition.
- Whenever any measurements are reported, the screenshots of how the measurements were done must be saved into the picture archiving and communication system (PACS), or printed if films are being used. This ensures that when follow-up examinations are performed, re-measurements can be done at the same level and in the same plane. This is particularly important in oncology imaging, but also the benign diseases as mediastinal nodes. There is an initiative called AIM (Annotation and Image Mark-up) project, which aims to provide a tool for recording, storing and accessing quantitative measurement data.[5] This format will be machine-readable and hence allow more accurate comparison of quantitative data.

ERRORS IN RADIOLOGY REPORTS

Imaging forms a cornerstone of medical diagnosis today, and hence any error in radiological interpretation translates into an eventual error in diagnosis, resulting in patient mismanagement. It is however difficult to define an error, as the final histopathology diagnosis may not be available in majority of patients. Hence, a "peer review" system is used. Wherein, if the interpretation of a radiologist is substantially different from the consensus diagnosis of peers, it is taken as an error.[6]

Despite the development of advanced cross-sectional modalities, it is estimated that the prevalence of error in radiology reports is roughly the same as reported over 40 years back. In a 2010 study from Massachusetts General Hospital wherein experienced radiologists performed "second readings" reports of abdominal CTs earlier reported by themselves or others, discrepancy rates of 28–32% were reported.[7]

Types of Radiology Errors

There are two main types of errors in radiology reports:

1. Perceptual errors
2. Cognitive or interpretive errors.

Perceptual Errors

Perceptual error is essentially an error of detection i.e. a missed finding on initial interpretation, which is subsequently or retrospectively detected. This is the more frequent of the two types of errors, accounting for upto 80% of the mistakes.[6] This error is not deemed to have occurred in case the findings are subtle/minor. The causes of perceptual errors are multifactorial, and some of these are enlisted in **Table 1**.

Cognitive Errors (Interpretive Errors)

Cognitive errors are errors of interpretation, i.e. the finding is detected but its clinical significance/differential diagnosis are not clearly understood;[8,9] and hence the final conclusion is wrong. The causes and types of such interpretive errors are enlisted in **Table 2**.

Several classification systems of radiology errors exist, and the reader may refer to more detailed articles for the same. For example, Kim and Mansfield Categorization into 12 types of errors[10] or Classification Scheme by Provenzale et al.[11]

STRUCTURED VERSUS PROSE REPORTS

Pros of Structured Reporting

There are numerous advantages of adopting structured reporting formats:

- *Better clarity*: Use of consistent terminology makes the report more comprehensible to the treating clinician/surgeon. Since the report encompasses the criteria used in current guidelines or recommendations, clinician decision making is facilitated. In a study which compared structured vs non-structured reporting formats in pancreatic carcinoma, Brook et al. demonstrated that structured formats increased the surgeon's confidence regarding tumor resectability.[12]
- *Standard terminology across institutions*: If a patient chooses to change his hospital or clinician, or is referred

TABLE 1: Causes of perceptual errors.

- Lesion is not conspicuous
- Fatigue
- *Speed*: Interpreting too many examinations in a relatively short period of time
- *Distractions*: Phone calls, conversations
- *"Satisfaction search" phenomenon*: When one abnormality is picked up and the radiologist is satisfied, additional finding is missed

elsewhere; use of consistent terms makes it easier for the new team to assess the disease status. Hence, structured reports definitely have more clarity than free text ones in this scenario.

- *Reduction of diagnostic errors*: Following a checklist better ensures that no key site of involvement or imaging parameter is missed, hence reducing diagnostic errors. Although several factors contribute to diagnostic errors in radiology reports, missing findings in other organs when a dominant finding is detected is not infrequent. In a study on lumbar spine MRI reports by Quattrochi et al.,[13] it was shown that on use of structured reporting formats, additional relevant findings were reported in 28.5% patients which were missed in the initial unstructured reports.
- *Reduction of grammatical and typographical errors*: Since there is a decrease in the amount of free text to be composed in a structured format, the number of grammatical errors also reduce grammatical errors maybe related to meanings of words used (semantic errors), sentence construction or rules of grammar (syntactic errors) or spelling of words. Errors may also be inadvertent while typing (typographical error), or result from mistakes by digital speech recognition software. While grammatical errors may not alter the scientific content of the report, but these definitely leave a poor impression on the clinician or the patient reading the report. Structured formats reduce these errors, which can be seen in a significant number of nonstructured reports.[14,15]
- *Facilitates research*: The use of standard terms in description and final impression make it easier to retrieve data for any retrospective analysis.
- *Promotes evidence-based practices*: Since structured reporting formats are usually patterned on a standard guideline/recommendation for a particular disease entity, it promotes use of these evidence-based guidelines. Also, if the guidelines adopted are those that the treating clinician also follows, it enhances patient care and takes us closer to practice of precision medicine. A study by McKee et al on the impact of applying ACR Lung RADS reporting system in a lung cancer screening program, showed that the positive predictive value of study for the diagnosis of malignancy went up from 6.9 to 17.3% after applying Lung RADS.[16]
- *Complete documentation improves quality*: Overall reduction in diagnostic and grammatical errors improves the quality of reports. Also, the documentation is more complete with less errors of omission. These improvements should result in enhancement of referring clinician's satisfaction, decrease in complaints by patients or clinicians, and even reduction in liability suits. In a study of 336,062 abdominal USG reports it was shown that incomplete documentation by radiologists resulted in 2.5–5.5% loss of professional income.[17]

TABLE 2: Causes of cognitive errors.

Causes/types

- Lack of knowledge
- Clinical information is misleading resulting in cognitive bias—also called "framing bias"
- *Alliterative error/satisfaction of report*: When reporting in continuation or basis of previous report, one may make the same error of interpretation
- *Availability bias*: When one tends to be biased towards recently seen/made diagnosis
- *Anchoring bias:* When the radiologist tends to stick to the first finding or information that strikes them during interpretation, even though the subsequently detected findings may challenge it
- *Premature closure*: When a radiologist interprets the most obvious diagnosis, and "closes the case"; e.g. in case of known primary malignancies, interpreting every finding as metastases

Cons of Structured Reporting

The biggest challenge or obstacle to implementing structured reporting formats is the initial reluctance of reporting radiologists. This reluctance is based on several factors, which are the cons of structured reporting formats.

- Firstly, using a new system of reporting definitely involves a "learning curve" and slows down productivity and throughput.
- A structured report also curtails the individuality, and even expertise that a radiologist brings to a report. For instance, a radiology report by a first year resident in training or a subspecialist thoracic radiologist will read similar. The reporting format does not give much scope to the subspecialist to add additional points to the report on the basis of their knowledge.
- The strict adherence to the structured reporting format may also require change in the manner in which a radiologist interprets the images. For instance, most radiologists would tend to look at the primary imaging plane (axial in most instances), in one direction, often craniocaudal, and then view additional applicable windows as reconstructions.
- Structured formats often require "structure-wise" reporting, which will often necessitate one or multiple re-looks at the images to fill-in all the subheadings. While, the checklist ensures that all structures are seen individually, it is also argued that it slows the work flow without significantly altering the real content of the report.[2]
- There is higher chance of errors in reporting if "copy-paste" format is used either in structured reporting or even in free text reports versus reports that are dictated.

Reporting radiologists may omit to delete the "normal" statement in the report, despite having written abnormal findings. This creates conflicting statements within the report.

- Lastly, is the debate which of the two formats do the treating clinicians really prefer. Some studies have illustrated that structured reporting format does not enhance the comprehension of the report by the clinician.[18]
- A study of Italian radiologists and a similar one by United States academic radiologists showed that more than half of them have either never used structured reporting formats or not used them consistently.[19,20]

STEPS TO IMPLEMENTING STRUCTURED REPORTING FORMATS

- At local institutional levels, it is advocated that available or recommended reporting template should be modified according to institutional practices. This should be done by subspeciality radiologists in consultation with concerned physicians/surgeons.
- There are software solutions available which allow linking of the reporting template to specific imaging studies. On opening the examination, the reporting template also opens. Within the subheadings, drop down options of phrases can be provided which can be easily chosen.
- Typically, numerous disease specific protocols will be required. These may be adopted in phases.
- However, it is best that reporting radiologist is allowed to add additional free text content at the end, giving a degree of freedom to express complex situations/possibilities.
- Steps should also be taken to automate/reinforce standard operating procedures for notification of critical results to the treating physician/surgeon.

COMMON STRUCTURED REPORTING FORMATS IN USE/AVAILABLE RESOURCES

There are several resources providing standard reporting templates, some of these being:

- The Breast Imaging Reporting and Data System (BI-RADS), developed by the American College of Radiology[21]
- Lung Imaging Reporting and data System (Lung-RADS) by the American College of Radiology[16, 22, 23]
- Reporting templates by "RSNA Reporting Initiative"[24,25]
- Reporting templates of Society of Abdominal Radiology[26]
- Indian reporting formats (authors' experience) available for Chest and Head and Neck imaging.[27,28] A case of ameloblastoma is shown as an illustrative example in reporting format for jaw tumors **(Figs. 1A to E and Table 3)**.

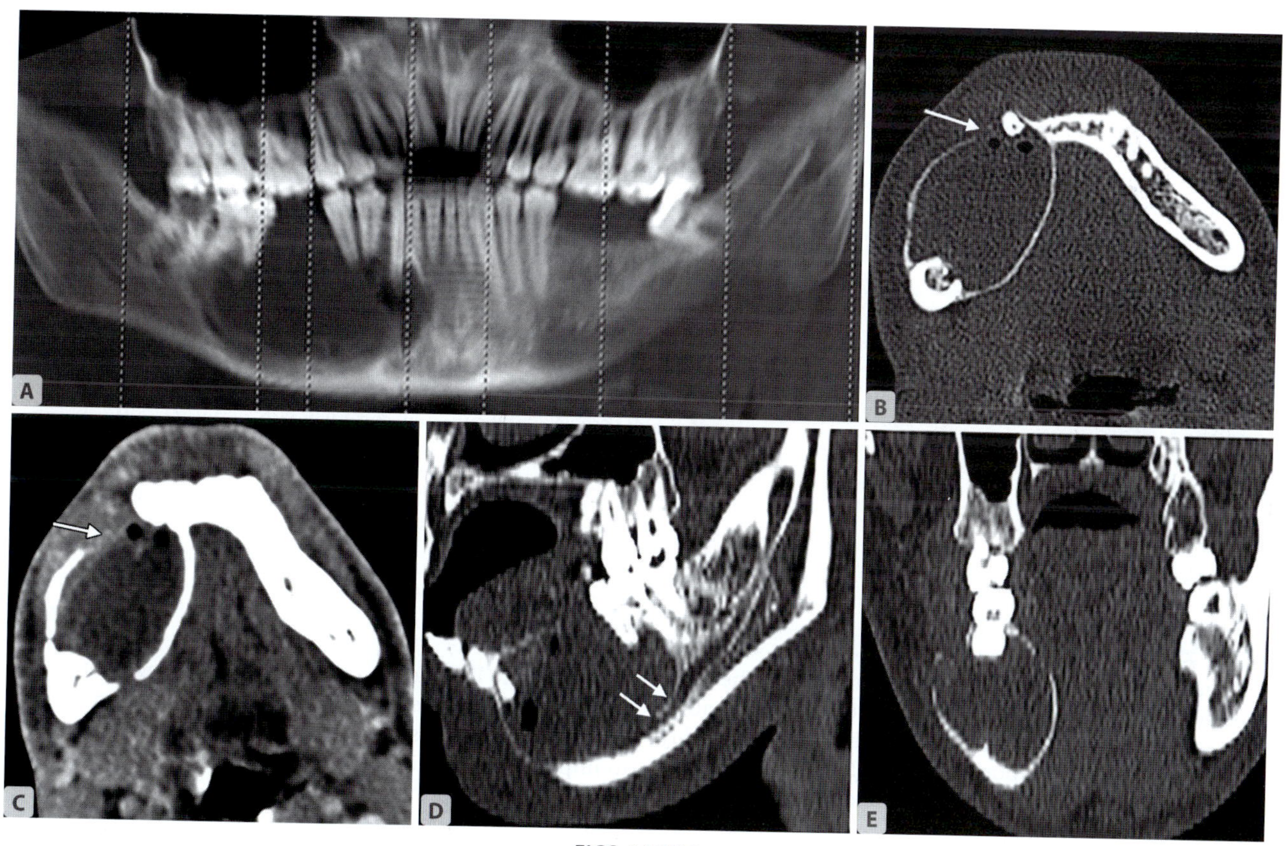

FIGS. 1A TO E

TABLE 3: Structured reporting format of a jaw tumor (ameloblastoma) shown in Figure 1.

Site of lesion	Mandible
Single/multiple	Single
Unilateral/bilateral (with side)	Unilateral, right side
Location (mandible/maxilla)	Mandible
Extent of lesion	Body of mandible (**Fig. 1A**)
Size of lesion	(CC × AP × TR) 3.5 = (3.9 × 3.1) cm
Character of lesion	Lytic, unilocular (**Fig. 1B**)
Buccolingual expansion (+/-)	+
Border: • Well defined/ill defined • Continuous/interrupted/eroded Bone destruction	 Well defined Interrupted Expansile with cortical breach (arrow in **Fig. 1B**)
Characteristic appearance	Nil
Tumor content: • Fluid/cystic • Solid • Mixed	 Mixed (**Fig. 1C**)
Density of lesion in comparison to adjacent soft tissue	Hypodense (**Fig. 1C**)
Calcification (+/-)	–
Adjacent bony changes (periosteal reaction/trabecular pattern)	–
Relationship to tooth: • Single/multiple • Pericoronal/periapical	 Multiple (**Fig. 1A**) Periapical
Overlying tooth: • Displacement • Resorption • Absent (secondary to extraction)	 – – Absent (canine to first molar) (**Fig. 1A**)
Involvement of adjacent vital structures *Mandible:* • Inferior alveolar nerve canal • Lower body continuity (mention thickness in mm) *Maxilla:* • Sinus • Ostiomeatal unit • Floor of orbit • Pterygoid plates	 Involved (arrows in **Fig. 1D**) Maintained (4.7 mm) (**Fig. 1E**) – – – –
Associated soft tissue Muscle/inflammation/fibrosis/lymph node	Soft tissue extending through cortical breach (arrow in **Fig. 1C**)
Imaging diagnosis	Ameloblastoma
Differential diagnosis	None

CONCLUSION

The importance of a radiology report cannot be over emphasized. It is often the only route of communication between a radiologist and the referring clinician. The quality and accuracy of the report, hence reflects the skill and knowledge base of the radiologist. Radiology reports are also susceptible to litigation in case of clinically significant errors. Hence, a periodic review and updating of one's radiology reporting formats or styles is essential. It is equally important to impart formal training to radiology residents on the 'art and science' of reports.

REFERENCES

1. Good practice for radiological reporting. Guidelines from the European Society of Radiology (ESR). Insights Imaging. 2011;2(2):93-6.
2. Ganeshan D, et al. Structured Reporting in Radiology. Academic Radiology 2018;25:66-73.
3. 60 of Ganeshan: 2016 radiology preferred specialty measure set. Available at: https://www.cms.gov/Medicare/Quality-Initiatives-Patient AssessmentInstruments/PQRS/downloads/Radiology_Specialty_Measure_Set.pdf. Accessed January 25, 2019.
4. Kahn CE, Heilbrun ME, Applegate KE. From guidelines to practice: How reporting templates promote the use of radiology practice guidelines. J Am Coll Radiol. 2013;10(4):268-73.
5. Rubin D, Mongkolwat P, Kleper V, Supekar K. Annotation and Image Mark-up: Accessing and Interoperating with the Semantic Content in Medical Imaging. Intelligent Systems, IEEE. 2009;24(1):57-65.
6. Bruno MA, Walker EA, Abujudeh HH. Understanding and Confronting Our Mistakes: The Epidemiology of Error in Radiology and Strategies for Error Reduction. RadioGraphics. 2015;35:1668-76.
7. Abujudeh HH, Boland GW, Kaewlai R, et al. Abdominal and pelvic computed tomography (CT) interpretation: discrepancy rates among experienced radiologists. Eur Radiol 2010;20(8): 1952-7.
8. Busby LP, Courtier JL, Glastonbury CM. Bias in Radiology: The How and Why of Misses and Misinterpretations. RadioGraphics 2018;38:236-47.
9. Lee CS, Nagy PG, Weaver SJ, Newman-Toker DE. Cognitive and System Factors Contributing to Diagnostic Errors in Radiology. AJR. 2013;201:611-17.
10. Kim YW, Mansfield LT. Fool me twice: delayed diagnoses in radiology with emphasis on perpetuated errors. Am J Roentgenol. 2014;202(3):465-70.
11. Provenzale JM, Kranz PG. Understanding errors in diagnostic radiology: proposal of a classification scheme and application to emergency radiology. Emerg Radiol 2011;18(5):403-8.
12. Brook OR, Brook A, Vollmer CM, et al. Structured reporting of multiphasic CT for pancreatic cancer: potential effect on staging and surgical planning. Radiology. 2015;274: 464-72.
13. Quattrocchi CC, Giona A, Di Martino AC, et al. Extra-spinal incidental findings at lumbar spine MRI in the general population: a large cohort study. Insights Imaging. 2013;4:301-8.
14. Hawkins CM, Hall S, Hardin J, et al. Prepopulated radiology report templates: a prospective analysis of error rate and turnaround time. J Digit Imaging. 2012;25:504-11.
15. Gunn AJ, Alabre CI, Bennett SE, et al. Structured feedback from referring physicians: a novel approach to quality improvement in radiology reporting. Am J Roentgenol. 2013;201:853-7.
16. McKee BJ, Regis SM, McKee AB, et al. Performance of ACR Lung-RADS in a clinical CT lung screening program. J Am Coll Radiol. 2015;12:273-6.
17. Duszak R, Jr, Nossal M, Schofield L, et al. Physician documentation deficiencies in abdominal ultrasound reports: frequency, characteristics, and financial impact. J Am Coll Radiol. 2012;9: 403-8.
18. Krupinski EA, Hall ET, Jaw S, et al. Influence of radiology report format on reading time and comprehension. J Digit Imaging. 2012;25:63-9.
19. Powell DK, Silberzweig JE. State of structured reporting in radiology, a survey. Acad Radiol. 2015;22: 226-33.
20. Bosmans JM, Weyler JJ, De Schepper AM, et al. The radiology report as seen by radiologists and referring clinicians: results of the COVER and ROVER surveys. Radiology. 2011;259:184-95.
21. American College of Radiology. The ACR breast imaging reporting and data system (BI-RADS) [web source]. November 11, 2003. https://www.acr.org/-/media/ACR/Files/RADS/BI-RADS/BIRADS-Atlas-Preface.pdf. Accessed January 28, 2019.
22. Lung Rads | American College of Radiology (Web Source). https://www.acr.org/Clinical-Resources/Reporting-and-Data-Systems/Lung-Rads. Accessed January 28, 2019.
23. Black WC. The Complementary Roles of the Vancouver Risk Calculator and Lung-RADS in Lung Cancer Screening. Radiology. 2019;22:18289. PMID: 30667334.
24. Radiology reporting initiative. Available at: https://www.rsna.org/Reporting_Initiative.aspx. Accessed January 25, 2019.
25. Morgan TA, Helibrun ME, Kahn CE, Jr. Reporting initiative of the Radiological Society of North America: progress and new directions. Radiology. 2014;273:642-5.
26. Al-Hawary MM, Francis IR, Chari ST, et al. Pancreatic ductal adenocarcinoma radiology reporting template: consensus statement of the Society of Abdominal Radiology and the American Pancreatic Association. Gastroenterology. 2014;146:291-304, e1.
27. Bhalla AS, Goyal A, Guleria R, Gupta AK. Chest tuberculosis: Radiological review and imaging recommendations. Indian J Radiol Imaging. 2015;25:213-25.
28. Manchanda S. Reporting template with illustrative cases (Inner ear, internal auditory canal and cochlear implant). In; Bhalla AS, Jana M (Eds). Temporal Bone Imaging. 2016, Jaypee Brothers Medical Publishers, 1st edn, 2016. pp.166-82.

AIIMS-MAMC-PGI's

Comprehensive Textbook of

DIAGNOSTIC RADIOLOGY

AIIMS-MAMC-PGI's

Comprehensive Textbook of DIAGNOSTIC RADIOLOGY

Third Edition

VOLUME 2

- Paediatric Imaging
- Gastrointestinal and Hepatobiliary Imaging

Editors

Arun Kumar Gupta MD FAMS
Professor and Head
Department of Radiodiagnosis
All India Institute of Medical Sciences
New Delhi, India

Anju Garg MD
Director Professor and Head
Department of Radiodiagnosis
Maulana Azad Medical College
New Delhi, India

Manavjit Singh Sandhu MD FICR
CCST (UK)
Professor and Head
Department of Radiodiagnosis
Postgraduate Institute of
Medical Education and Research
Chandigarh, India

JAYPEE

JAYPEE BROTHERS MEDICAL PUBLISHERS
The Health Sciences Publisher
New Delhi | London

Jaypee Brothers Medical Publishers (P) Ltd

Headquarter

Jaypee Brothers Medical Publishers (P) Ltd
4838/24, Ansari Road, Daryaganj
New Delhi 110 002, India
Phone: +91-11-43574357
Fax: +91-11-43574314
Email: jaypee@jaypeebrothers.com

Overseas Office

J.P. Medical Ltd
83 Victoria Street, London
SW1H 0HW (UK)
Phone: +44 20 3170 8910
Fax: +44 (0)20 3008 6180
Email: info@jpmedpub.com

Website: www.jaypeebrothers.com
Website: www.jaypeedigital.com

Inquiries for bulk sales may be solicited at: jaypee@jaypeebrothers.com

AIIMS-MAMC-PGI's Comprehensive Textbook of Diagnostic Radiology, ***Third Edition (Volumes 1 to 4)*** / *Arun Kumar Gupta, Anju Garg, Manavjit Singh Sandhu*

First Edition: 2016
Second Edition: 2019
Third Edition: 2021
Reprint: **2024**

ISBN: 978-93-90595-55-6

Printed at: Sanat Printers

ASSOCIATE EDITORS

VOLUME 1

Section 1: Genitourinary Imaging

Gaurav Shanker Pradhan DMRD DNB
Director Professor
Department of Radiodiagnosis
Maulana Azad Medical College
New Delhi, India

Alpana Manchanda MD
Director Professor
Department of Radiodiagnosis
Maulana Azad Medical College
New Delhi, India

Sapna Singh MD DNB MNAMS
Professor
Department of Radiodiagnosis
Maulana Azad Medical College
New Delhi, India

Section 2: Advances in Imaging Technology

Sanjay Sharma MD DNB MNAMS FRCR FICR
Professor
Department of Radiodiagnosis
(RP Center division)
All India Institute of Medical Sciences
New Delhi, India

Atin Kumar MD DNB MNAMS FICR
Professor
Department of Radiodiagnosis
(Trauma Centre Division)
All India Institute of Medical Sciences
New Delhi, India

Shivanand Gamanagatti MD MNAMS FICR
Professor
Department of Radiodiagnosis
(Trauma Centre Division)
All India Institute of Medical Sciences
New Delhi, India

VOLUME 2

Section 3: Paediatric Imaging

Ashu Seith Bhalla MD MAMS FICR
Professor
Department of Radiodiagnosis
All India Institute of Medical Sciences
New Delhi, India

Manisha Jana MD DNB FRCR
Additional Professor
Department of Radiodiagnosis
All India Institute of Medical Sciences
New Delhi, India

Devasenathipathy Kandasamy MD DNB FRCR
Additional Professor
Department of Radiodiagnosis
All India Institute of Medical Sciences
New Delhi, India

Priyanka Naranje MD DNB MNAMS
Associate Professor
Department of Radiodiagnosis
All India Institute of Medical Sciences
New Delhi, India

Section 4: Gastrointestinal and Hepatobiliary Imaging

Deep Narayan Srivastava MD MBA FAMS FICR
Professor
Department of Radiodiagnosis
All India Institute of Medical Sciences
New Delhi, India

Raju Sharma MD MAMS FICR
Professor
Department of Radiodiagnosis
All India Institute of Medical Sciences
New Delhi, India

VOLUME 3

Section 5: Chest and Cardiovascular Imaging

Sanjiv Sharma MD
Professor and Head
Department of Cardiovascular Radiology and Endovascular Interventions
CN Centre
All India Institute of Medical Sciences
New Delhi, India

Rashmi Dixit MD
Director Professor
Department of Radiodiagnosis
Maulana Azad Medical College
New Delhi, India

Section 6: Musculoskeletal and Breast Imaging

Mahesh Prakash MD MAMS FIACM FICR
Professor
Department of Radiodiagnosis
Postgraduate Institute of Medical Education and Research
Chandigarh, India

Anindita Sinha MD MAMS
Additional Professor
Department of Radiodiagnosis
Postgraduate Institute of Medical Education and Research
Chandigarh, India

VOLUME 4

Section 7: Neuroradiology Including Head and Neck Imaging

Paramjeet Singh MD FICR
Professor
Department of Radiodiagnosis
Postgraduate Institute of Medical Education and Research
Chandigarh, India

Shailesh B Gaikwad MD FNAMS CCST
Professor and Head
Department of Neuroimaging and Interventional Neuroradiology (CN Centre)
All India Institute of Medical Sciences
New Delhi, India

Vivek Gupta MD DM
Former Professor
Department of Radiodiagnosis
Postgraduate Institute of Medical Education and Research
Chandigarh, India

Ajay Garg MD
Professor
Department of Neuroimaging and Interventional Neuroradiology (CN Centre)
All India Institute of Medical Sciences
New Delhi, India

CONTRIBUTORS

Ajay Garg MD (Radiodiagnosis) Eur Dip in Neuroradiology (EDiNR) Eur Dip in Pediatric Neuroradiology (EDiPNR)
Professor, Department of Neuroimaging and Interventional Neuroradiology
CN Centre
All India Institute of Medical Sciences
New Delhi, India

Ajay Gulati MD MAMS
Additional Professor
Department of Radiodiagnosis
Postgraduate Institute of Medical Education and Research, Chandigarh, India

Ajay Kumar MD
Professor
Department of Radiodiagnosis
Postgraduate Institute of Medical Education and Research, Chandigarh, India

Akshay Kumar Saxena MD DNB FICR
Professor
Department of Radiodiagnosis
Postgraduate Institute of Medical Education and Research, Chandigarh, India

Alpana Manchanda MD
Director Professor
Department of Radiodiagnosis
Maulana Azad Medical College
New Delhi, India

Anil Kumar Pandey MSc PhD
Associate Professor (Medical Physics)
Department of Nuclear Medicine and PET
All India Institute of Medical Sciences
New Delhi, India

Anindita Sinha MD MAMS
Additional Professor
Department of Radiodiagnosis
Postgraduate Institute of Medical Education and Research
Chandigarh, India

Anjali Prakash DMRD DNB MNAMS
Director Professor
Department of Radiodiagnosis
Maulana Azad Medical College
New Delhi, India

Anju Garg MD
Director Professor and Head
Department of Radiodiagnosis
Maulana Azad Medical College
New Delhi, India

Ankur Goyal MD DNB MNAMS
Associate Professor
Department of Radiodiagnosis
All India Institute of Medical Sciences
New Delhi, India

Anmol Bhatia MD FPGI (Paediatric Radiology)
Assistant Professor
Department of Radiodiagnosis and Imaging
Postgraduate Institute of Medical Education and Research
Chandigarh, India

Anuj Prabhakar DNB DM (Neuroradiology)
Assistant Professor
Postgraduate Institute of Medical Education and Research
Chandigarh, India

Anupam Lal MD
Professor
Department of Radiodiagnosis
Postgraduate Institute of Medical Education and Research
Chandigarh, India

Arun Kumar Gupta MD FAMS
Professor and Head
Department of Radiodiagnosis
All India Institute of Medical Sciences
New Delhi, India

Ashu Seith Bhalla MD MAMS FICR
Professor
Department of Radiodiagnosis
All India Institute of Medical Sciences
New Delhi, India

Atin Kumar MD DNB MNAMS FICR
Professor
Department of Radiodiagnosis
(Trauma Center Division)
All India Institute of Medical Sciences
New Delhi, India

Chandan J Das MD DNB MAMS FICR FRCP
Additional Professor
Department of Radiodiagnosis
All India Institute of Medical Sciences
New Delhi, India

Chandrashekhara SH MD DNB MNAMS
Additional Professor
Department of Radiodiagnosis
Dr BRA Institute—Rotary Cancer Hospital
All India Institute of Medical Sciences
New Delhi, India

Chirag Kamal Ahuja MD DM (Neuroradiology)
Associate Professor
Department of Radiodiagnosis and Imaging
Postgraduate Institute of Medical Education and Research
Chandigarh, India

Deep Narayan Srivastava MD MBA FAMS FICR
Professor
Department of Radiodiagnosis
All India Institute of Medical Sciences
New Delhi, India

Devasenathipathy Kandasamy MD DNB FRCR
Additional Professor
Department of Radiodiagnosis
All India Institute of Medical Sciences
New Delhi, India

Ekta Dhamija MD
Associate Professor
Department of Radiodiagnosis
Dr BRA Institute—Rotary Cancer Hospital
All India Institute of Medical Sciences
New Delhi, India

Gaurav Shanker Pradhan DMRD DNB
Director Professor
Department of Radiodiagnosis
Maulana Azad Medical College
New Delhi, India

Gita Devi MD DNB
Assistant Professor
Department of Radiodiagnosis
Postgraduate Institute of Medical Education and Research
Chandigarh, India

Gurpreet Singh Gulati MD
Former Professor
Department of Cardiac Radiology
Cardio-Thoracic Sciences Centre
All India Institute of Medical Sciences
New Delhi, India

Harish Bhujade MD FVIR
Assistant Professor
Department of Radiodiagnosis
Postgraduate Institute of Medical Education and Research
Chandigarh, India

Jyoti Kumar MD DNB MNAMS FICR
Professor
Department of Radiodiagnosis
Maulana Azad Medical College
New Delhi, India

Kartik Ganga MD
Fellow
Department of Cardiovascular Radiology and Endovascular Interventions
All India Institute of Medical Sciences
New Delhi, India

Kirti Gupta MD, Neuropathology Fellowship (St Jude, USA)
Professor
Department of Histopathology
Postgraduate Institute of Medical Education and Research
Chandigarh, India

Kumble S Madhusudhan MD FRCR MAMS
Additional Professor
Department of Radiodiagnosis
All India Institute of Medical Sciences
New Delhi, India

Kushaljit Singh Sodhi MD PhD MAMS FICR
Professor
Department of Radiodiagnosis
Postgraduate Institute of Medical Education and Research
Chandigarh, India

Madhavi Tripathi MD DNB (Nuclear Medicine)
Additional Professor
Department of Nuclear Medicine and PET
All India Institute of Medical Sciences
New Delhi, India

Madhusudhan KS MD MAMS FRCR
Additional Professor
Department of Radiodiagnosis
All India Institute of Medical Sciences
New Delhi, India

Mahesh Prakash MD MAMS FIACM FICR
Professor
Department of Radiodiagnosis
Postgraduate Institute of Medical Education and Research
Chandigarh, India

Manavjit Singh Sandhu MD FICR CCST (UK)
Professor and Head
Department of Radiodiagnosis
Postgraduate Institute of Medical Education and Research
Chandigarh, India

Mandeep Garg MD FRCR
Professor
Department of Radiodiagnosis
Postgraduate Institute of Medical Education and Research
Chandigarh, India

Mandeep Kang MD MAMS FICR
Professor
Department of Radiodiagnosis
Postgraduate Institute of Medical Education and Research
Chandigarh, India

Manisha Jana MD DNB FRCR
Additional Professor
Department of Radiodiagnosis
All India Institute of Medical Sciences
New Delhi, India

Manish Modi MD DM
Professor
Department of Neurology
Postgraduate Institute of Medical Education and Research
Chandigarh, India

Manphool Singhal MD DNB MAMS FICR (India) FSCCT (USA) CMR-fellowship (London) CMR-Certification (SCMR USA and ESCVI France)
Additional Professor
Department of Radiodiagnosis
Postgraduate Institute of Medical Education and Research
Chandigarh, India

Mukesh Kumar Yadav (MD Radiodiagnosis)
Formerly Associate Professor
PGIMER, Chandigarh
Associate Professor
Department of Radiodiagnosis
All India Institute of Medical Sciences (IRCH)
New Delhi, India

Naveen Kalra MD FICR MAMS
Professor
Department of Radiodiagnosis
Postgraduate Institute of Medical Education and Research
Chandigarh, India

Nidhi Prabhakar MD DNB
Senior Research Associate
Department of Radiodiagnosis
Postgraduate Institute of Medical Education and Research
Chandigarh, India

Niraj N Pandey DM
Assistant Professor
Department of Cardiovascular Radiology and Endovascular Interventions
CN Centre
All India Institute of Medical Sciences
New Delhi, India

Niranjan Khandelwal MD Dip NBE FICR FAMS
Former Head
Department of Radiodiagnosis
Postgraduate Institute of Medical Education and Research
Chandigarh, India

Pankaj Gupta MD DNB
Assistant Professor
Department of Radiodiagnosis and Imaging
Postgraduate Institute of Medical Education and Research
Chandigarh, India

Paramjeet Singh MD FICR
Professor
Department of Radiodiagnosis
Postgraduate Institute of Medical Education and Research
Chandigarh, India

Pratik Kumar PhD (AIIMS) Dip RP (BARC)
Professor, Medical Physics Unit
BRA Institute Rotary Cancer Hospital
AIIMS, New Delhi, India

Priya Jagia MD DNB
Professor
Department of Cardiovascular Radiology and Endovascular Interventions
All India Institute of Medical Sciences
New Delhi, India

Priyanka Naranje MD DNB MNAMS
Associate Professor
Department of Radiodiagnosis
All India Institute of Medical Sciences
New Delhi, India

Punit Sharma MD
Former Senior Resident
Department of Nuclear Medicine
All India Institute of Medical Sciences
New Delhi, India

Radhika Batra MD DNB
Associate Professor
Department of Radiodiagnosis
Maulana Azad Medical College
New Delhi, India

Rajat Jain MD DNB FRCR FICR MNAMS
Assistant Professor
Department of Radiodiagnosis
Maulana Azad Medical College
New Delhi, India

Raju Sharma MD MAMS FICR
Professor
Department of Radiodiagnosis
All India Institute of Medical Sciences
New Delhi, India

Rakesh Kumar DRM DNB PhD
Professor and Head
Diagnostic Nuclear Medicine Division
Department of Nuclear Medicine and PET
All India Institute of Medical Sciences
New Delhi, India

Rakesh Kumar Vasishta MD FRCPath
Former Professor and Head
Department of Histopathology
Postgraduate Institute of Medical Education and Research
Chandigarh, India

Rashmi Dixit MD
Director Professor
Department of Radiodiagnosis
Maulana Azad Medical College
New Delhi, India

Sameer Vyas MD DM MAMS (Neuroradiology)
Additional Professor
Department of Radiodiagnosis
Postgraduate Institute of Medical Education and Research
Chandigarh, India

Sanjay Sharma MD DNB MNAMS FRCR FICR
Professor
Department of Radiodiagnosis
(Division at Rajendra Prasad Center for Ophthalmic Sciences)
All India Institute of Medical Sciences
New Delhi, India

Sanjeev Kumar MD
Associate Professor
Department of Cardiovascular Radiology and Endovascular Interventions
All India Institute of Medical Sciences
New Delhi, India

Sanjiv Sharma MD
Professor and Head
Department of Cardiovascular Radiology and Endovascular Interventions
CN Centre
All India Institute of Medical Sciences
New Delhi, India

Sapna Singh MD DNB MNAMS
Professor
Department of Radiodiagnosis
Maulana Azad Medical College
New Delhi, India

Satyam DNB MNAMS
Specialist
Department of Radiodiagnosis
Lok Nayak Hospital and Associated
Maulana Azad Medical College
New Delhi, India

Shailesh B Gaikwad MD FNAMS CCST
Professor and Head
Department of Neuroimaging and Interventional Neuroradiology
CN Centre
All India Institute of Medical Sciences
New Delhi, India

Shamim Ahmed Shamim MD (Nuclear Medicine)
Associate Professor
Department of Nuclear Medicine
All India Institute of Medical Sciences
New Delhi, India

Shashi Bala Paul PhD MAMS
Senior Scientist
Department of Radiodiagnosis
All India Institute of Medical Sciences
New Delhi, India

Shivanand Gamanagatti MD MNAMS FICR
Professor
Department of Radiodiagnosis
(Trauma Center Division)
All India Institute of Medical Sciences
New Delhi, India

Smita Manchanda MD DNB MNAMS
Associate Professor
Department of Radiodiagnosis
All India Institute of Medical Sciences
New Delhi, India

Smriti Hari MD MAMS
Professor
Department of Radiodiagnosis
All India Institute of Medical Sciences
New Delhi, India

Sreedhara BC MD FVIR
Assistant Professor
Department of Radiodiagnosis
Postgraduate Institute of Medical Education and Research
Chandigarh, India

Subrat Kumar Acharya DM FNASc
FASc FNA JC Bose Fellow
Former Professor and Head
Department of Gastroenterology
All India Institute of Medical Sciences
New Delhi, India

Sudesh Prabhakar MD DM
Former Professor and Head
Department of Neurology
Postgraduate Institute of Medical Education and Research
Chandigarh, India

Sudha Suri MD
Emeritus Professor
Department of Radiodiagnosis
Postgraduate Institute of Medical Education and Research
Chandigarh, India

Surabhi Vyas MD DNB MNAMS
Additional Professor
Department of Radiodiagnosis
All India Institute of Medical Sciences
New Delhi, India

Swati Gupta MD DNB FRCR
Associate Professor
Department of Radiodiagnosis
Maulana Azad Medical College
New Delhi, India

Tulika Singh MD
Additional Professor
Department of Radiodiagnosis
Postgraduate Institute of Medical Education and Research
Chandigarh, India

Ujjwal Gorsi (MD Radiodiagnosis)
Associate Professor
Department of Radiodiagnosis
Postgraduate Institute of Medical Education and Research
Chandigarh, India

Uma Debi MD
Associate Professor
Department of Radiodiagnosis
Postgraduate Institute of Medical Education and Research
Chandigarh, India

Veenu Singla MD
Professor
Department of Radiodiagnosis
Postgraduate Institute of Medical Education and Research
Chandigarh, India

Vikas Bhatia MD DNB
DM (Neuroradiology)
Assistant Professor
Department of Radiodiagnosis
Postgraduate Institute of Medical Education and Research
Chandigarh, India

Vineeta Ojha MD DNB
DM Senior Resident
Department of Cardiovascular Radiology and Endovascular Interventions
All India Institute of Medical Sciences
New Delhi, India

Virendra Jain MD FRCR
Former Senior Resident
Department of Radiodiagnosis
Maulana Azad Medical College
New Delhi, India

Vivek Gupta MD DM
Former Professor
Department of Radiodiagnosis
Postgraduate Institute of Medical Education and Research
Chandigarh, India

PREFACE TO THE THIRD EDITION

In 1996, a unique venture was jointly initiated by the faculty of Radiodiagnosis, All India Institute of Medical Sciences (AIIMS), New Delhi; Maulana Azad Medical College (MAMC), New Delhi; and Postgraduate Institute of Medical Education and Research (PGIMER), Chandigarh, India, to organize continuing medical education (CME) programs based on a series of imaging courses. An integral part of this endeavour was publishing books covering all organ systems. The aim was to provide state-of-the-art knowledge for postgraduate students as well as the practicing radiologists along with establishing a uniform pattern of teaching in radiology across the country.

The first series of seven imaging courses was successfully completed in the year 2000. A second series of these courses was then initiated in the year 2002 and was completed in 2004. This was also highly successful. The third series of seven extremely popular and successful courses covering all the organ systems and advances in physics was started in 2008 and was completed in 2013. The fourth series started in 2016 and was completed successfuly in 2020.

Every course in each of the series has resulted in publication of a book. These books have been very popular amongst residents as well as among practicing radiologists.

Considering the popularity of these books, the editors, along with publishers, M/s Jaypee Brothers Medical Publishers (P) Ltd, New Delhi, India, had decided to combine the individual course books into three volumes— *"AIIMS-MAMC-PGI's Comprehensive Textbook of Diagnostic Radiology"*. Its first edition was released in 2016.

In keeping pace with newer developments in the field of diagnostic radiology and in order to cater to the contemporary needs of users, the second edition of *"AIIMS-MAMC-PGI's Comprehensive Textbook of Diagnostic Radiology"* was presented in 2019 after a gap of three years. It was anticipated that with such a complete coverage of all the subjects, the users will not have to refer to any other book during their routine learning of diagnostic radiology.

However by the time fourth AIIMS MAMC PGI Imaging course series was near completion in early 2021, it was felt that there is a very strong need for updating of second edition along with addition of new chapters in view of rapid advancement of knowledge in the last few years. So third edition was planned. It was also agreed that in view of increasing size of individual course books and to keep the size of individual volumes of the Textbook handy and managable the whole textbook should be divided into four volumes from its current three volumes.

We are sure that residents and radiologists will find these comprehensive four volumes easy to handle and very useful in day-to-day practice.

We are once again grateful to all the contributors from the three apex academic institutions of India, i.e. AIIMS, New Delhi; MAMC, New Delhi; and PGIMER, Chandigarh, India.

We are thankful to M/s Jaypee Brothers Medical Publishers (P) Ltd, for helping us to make our dream come true.

Arun Kumar Gupta
Anju Garg
Manavjit Singh Sandhu

PREFACE TO THE FIRST EDITION

In 1996, a unique venture was jointly initiated by the faculty of radiodiagnosis at All India Institute of Medical Sciences, Maulana Azad Medical College, New Delhi, and Postgraduate Institute of Medical Education and Research, Chandigarh, India, to organize continuing medical education programs based on a series of imaging courses. An integral part of this endeavor was publishing books covering all organ systems. The aim was to provide state of the art knowledge for postgraduate students as well as the practicing radiologists along with establishing a uniform pattern of teaching in radiology across the country.

The first series of seven imaging courses was successfully completed in the year 2000. A second series of these courses was then initiated in the year 2002 and was completed in 2004. This was also highly successful.

With the great success of the second series, we, the current editors, decided to start a third series of these courses in 2008. Seven extremely popular and successful courses covering all the organ systems and advances in physics were completed in 2013.

Every course in each of the three series have resulted in publication of a book. These books have been very popular amongst residents as well as among practicing radiologists.

Considering the popularity of these books, we, the three current editors, along with publishers M/s Jaypee Brothers Medical Publishers (P) Ltd., decided to combine the individual books published so far into a *"AIIMS-MAMC-PGI's Comprehensive Textbook of Diagnostic Radiology"* with three volumes.

We are very happy to see the end result of this great effort.

We are sure that residents and radiologists will find these comprehensive three volumes easy to handle and very useful in day-to-day practice.

We are once again grateful to all the contributors from the three apex academic institutions of India, i.e. AIIMS, MAMC, New Delhi and PGIMER, Chandigarh, India.

We are thankful to M/s Jaypee Brothers Medical Publishers (P) Ltd., for helping us to make our dream come true.

Niranjan Khandelwal
Veena Chowdhury
Arun Kumar Gupta

ACKNOWLEDGMENTS

We would like to put on record our deep appreciation and gratitude:

To Professors Manorama Berry, Sudha Suri and Veena Chowdhury (Past Editors) the three pioneers who in 1996 took a bold initiative and started a unique teaching course now popularly known as AIIMS-MAMC-PGI's imaging course. By October 2020, four series, each series comprising of seven courses, have been completed. This course series has become extremely popular and every course is followed by the publication of a book which too is highly appreciated and popular.

To Professors Sima Mukhopadhyay, Sushma Vashisht and Niranjan Khandelwal who have been the Editors of past series and who contributed to organizing the earlier courses in their capacity as Heads of Departments.

To all the Associate Editors of the different course books who put in immense effort to bring the books out on time.

To all the Authors who contributed chapters without whom we could not have collected such an outstanding content of teaching and academic material.

To our respective hospitals for giving us the privilege and unique opportunity to work, which enabled us to amass data from patients and document images of diverse diseases that provide the reader with a wide spectrum of knowledge.

Our sincere and grateful thanks to Shri Jitendar P Vij (Group Chairman), Mr Ankit Vij (Managing Director), Mr MS Mani (Group President), Dr Richa Saxena (Associate Director-Professional Publishing), Ms Nedup Denka Bhutia (Development Editor) and Other staffs of M/s Jaypee Brothers Medical Publishers (P) Ltd, New Delhi, India, for their untiring coordination efforts in the production of this book.

We are very proud indeed at the culmination of two decades of these course series, to compile and present them together in the form of these four volumes of "*AIIMS-MAMC-PGI's Comprehensive Textbook of Diagnostic Radiology*".

Arun Kumar Gupta
Anju Garg
Manavjit Singh Sandhu

CONTENTS

VOLUME 1

Section 1: Genitourinary Imaging

VOLUME 2

Section 3: Paediatric Imaging

Section 4: Gastrointestinal and Hepatobiliary Imaging

VOLUME 3

Section 5: Chest and Cardiovascular Imaging

Section 6: Musculoskeletal and Breast Imaging

VOLUME 4

Section 7: Neuroradiology Including Head and Neck Imaging

SECTION

3

Pediatric Imaging

- Technical Considerations in Pediatric Imaging
- Recent Advances in Pediatric Radiology
- Frontiers in Research: Genomics, Radiogenomics, Texture Analysis, Safety of Gadolinium-based Contrast, etc.
- Vascular Interventions in Children
- Nonvascular Interventions in Children
- Imaging of Pediatric Trauma
- Neonatal Respiratory Distress
- Childhood Pulmonary Infections
- Imaging of Pediatric Chest Masses
- Pediatric Airway
- Pediatric Interstitial Lung Diseases
- Developmental Anomalies of Gastrointestinal Tract
- Imaging of Anorectal Anomalies
- Gastrointestinal Masses and Inflammatory Conditions of Gastrointestinal Tract in Children
- Hepatic and Pancreatic Masses in Children
- Imaging and Interventions in Pediatric Budd–Chiari Syndrome
- Childhood Biliopathies
- Congenital Anomalies of the Urinary Tract
- Urinary Tract Infections (Including Vesicoureteral Reflux and Neurogenic Bladder)
- Renal and Retroperitoneal Masses
- Evaluation of Female Pelvis and Testicular Abnormalities
- Imaging of Disorders of Sex Differentiation
- Skeletal Dysplasias
- Short Stature and Skeletal Maturity Assessment
- Spinal Dysraphism
- Imaging of Pediatric Joint Pathology
- Benign Bone and Soft-tissue Tumors and Conditions
- Pediatric Malignant Bone and Soft-tissue Tumors
- Congenital Brain Anomalies
- Hypoxic-ischemic Encephalopathy
- Craniospinal Sonography
- Infectious and Inflammatory Diseases of the Brain
- Pediatric Brain Tumors
- Metabolic Disorders of the Brain
- Pediatric Neck Lesions

CHAPTER

56

Technical Considerations in Pediatric Imaging

Surabhi Vyas, Ashu Seith Bhalla, Arun Kumar Gupta

INTRODUCTION

Technical factors such as the ability to position the patient and acquire images with the patient immobile, which are often taken for granted in adults, may appear as crippling problems in children. For this reason and because of the importance of minimizing radiation to the child, special attention must be paid to certain technical points. These will be discussed under the following six broadgroups:

1. Minimizing heatloss
2. Immobilization
3. Sedation
4. Reduction of radiation dosage
5. Reducing examination times [computed tomography/ magnetic resonance imaging (CT/MRI)]
6. Use of contrast media

MINIMIZING HEAT LOSS

Neonates and infants lose body heat rapidly, the risk of hypothermia being greatest in the premature baby with little subcutaneous fat. Local warmth may be obtained by special table-top heating cradles, but the most convenient way of avoiding heat loss is to maintain a room temperature of about 27°C. Room thermometer is an important piece of equipment. Enhanced humidity is not normally required for the duration of most of the diagnostic examination.[1]

IMMOBILIZATION

Atraumatic immobilization is essential in order to ensure proper positioning and to minimize patient motion. Commonly used immobilization devices are listed in **Box 1**. Desirable characteristics of immobilization device are: (1) It should result in minimum or no artifacts, (2) it does not disturb patient's sedation, and (3) it is easy to handle. Newborn babies and small infants need only soft sandbags and adhesive tape to stop movement. Towels and sheets can also be used to tightly wrap babies. Older and stronger children may require wrapping on immobilization boards in addition to tape and sandbags. **Figures 1A and B**. Cradle holding devices are available which enable the infant to be rotated in relation to the tabletop. It is, however, not possible to accommodate older children on such apparatus.[1-3]

BOX 1: List of immobilization devices available for pediatric imaging.

- Blanket
- Towels
- Vacuum cushion
- Tape with gauze pads
- Velcro® straps
- Body part supports and molds
- Polyurethane foam casts
- Thermoplastic mesh casts
- Sandbags
- Head clamps
- Grip rings
- Commercially available positioning apparatus (Pigg-O-stat, Pedia-poser Fuller chair)

SEDATION

A fundamental technical component for imaging is the need for the child to remain motionless during the duration of imaging. The aims of sedation/anesthesia during imaging or intervention, however, are to achieve not only control of motion but also to minimize discomfort and pain, safe completion of procedure, and control of anxiety. Generally, neonates and young infants can be managed with nonpharmacological methods detailed below; and do not require anesthesia/sedation. Similarly, intellectually age-appropriate children of >4–5 years can undergo imaging after careful explanation and information to the child. Nonpharmacological methods should be attempted to reduce need for sedation or anesthesia as far as possible.

Nonpharmacological Methods

Various nonpharmacological methods can be used to achieve a meaningful examination without sedating agents including the following:[4]

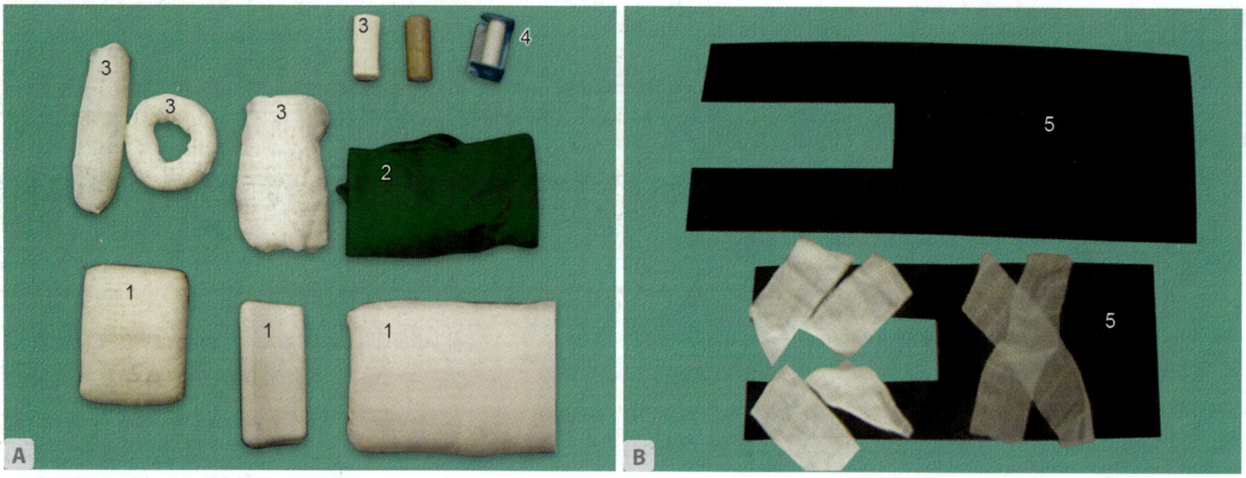

FIGS. 1A AND B: Examples of simple immobilization devices used in radiography. (A) Pads (1), folded sheet (2), gauze rollsfat content within. (3), and tape (4); and (B) Wooden boards of varying sizes (5) aided by gauze and tape serve as simple immobilization devices.

- Administration of sucrose, either alone or combined with a pacifierImmobilization devices such as swaddling the baby in a cozy blanket.
- Vacuum cushion or using sand bag or cushioned Velcro® straps.
- Feed and wrap; or feed and swaddle along with reduction in noise and illumination.
- *Sleep manipulation*: Mild sleep deprivation is employed before the examination so that the child may sleep during the examination. The commonly followed protocol is 1 hour delayed going to bed and 1 hour early rising.
- Hypnosis and distraction are known to decrease sedation time, need of sedation, and postprocedural pain.
- *Play therapy*: Toy models, video recordings, and pictures are used by a therapist to familiarize the child with the procedure to reduce anxiety and achieve cooperation.
- Parent involvement along with mock drill of the examination can be used to ensure cooperation.

Preanesthetic Evaluation

- All relevant risk factors must be taken into consideration before planning sedation.
- Knowledge of both the past and the present medical history is important.
- If the child's condition renders sedation to be a significant risk, precautionary measures such as securing the airway may be required before shifting the patient to radiology suite.[5]
- Documentation in the form of informed consent should be recorded according to institutional and local laws. Written instructions should also be provided to the parent or legal guardian regarding the sedative/anesthetic agents, route of administration, and possible adverse effects along with emergency contact details.

Nil per Orally (NPO) Status

- Aspiration is a significant concern in sedated children and, therefore, NPO guidelines should be adhered.[6]
- Allowance for oral intake include: clear liquids are allowable up to 2 hours before the procedure; breast milk: 4 hours; nonhuman milk including formula allowed till 6 hours; and light meal comprising clear fluid and toast till 6 hours.[7]
- Bowel obstruction or ileus is other factor that increases the risk of aspiration because it delays gastric emptying. In these patients, nasogastric suction of gastric contents should be performed and agents like metoclopramide to promote gastric emptying should be given.
- The actual risk of aspiration in children undergoing diagnostic imaging is unknown, but it is probably quite low. In one report, aspiration of gastric contrast was present in no >4% of children undergoing CT scan examination in a setting of trauma.[5,8,9]

Monitoring and Ensuring Safety

- Monitoring the patient in the radiology suite is not an easy task for the clinicians. Observing children from the CT or MRI control room through a glass window is much more difficult for the clinician than direct observation at the bedside and increases their reliance on monitoring devices. Hence, adequate monitoring devices should be available **(Fig. 2)**.
- Monitoring is further complicated during MRI because the scanner generates strong static, radiofrequency, and time-varied magnetic fields which interfere with the monitoring devices. Newer, nonferromagnetic monitors and cables have been devised which are safe and reliable within the scanning suite **(Fig. 3)**. Standard ferromagnetic monitors, if used, need to be placed outside the magnetic field or carefully shielded.[5,6]
- The radiology suite, especially MRI, presents a difficult environment for anesthesia to deal with complications such as respiratory arrest or cardiovascular collapse. Hence, the most important prerequisite to sedation is the availability of adequate equipment for resuscitation and personnel experienced in managing complications. If the radiology suite is not equipped with wall outlets for oxygen and suction, portable oxygen cylinders and suction apparatus should be available. Also, a cart with resuscitation drugs, defibrillator, and age- and size-appropriate

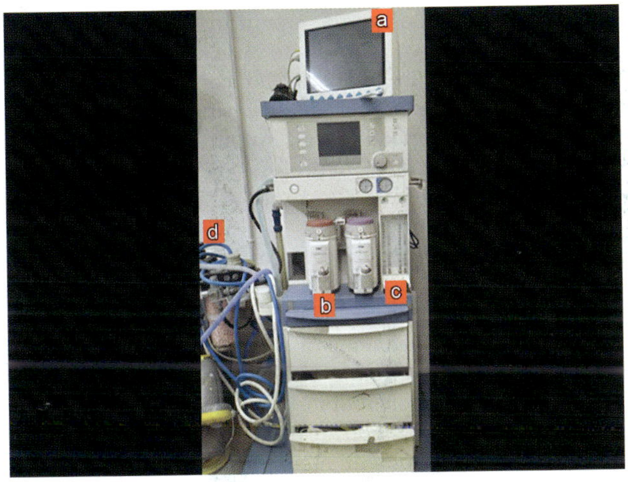

FIG. 2: Trolley mounted general anesthesia equipment comprising monitor (a), vaporizer for volatile anesthetic agents (b), glass flow tubes (c), and breathing system (d).

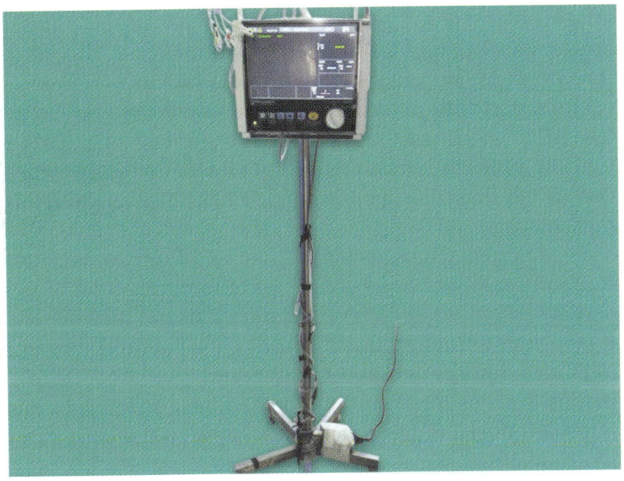

FIG. 3: Magnetic resonance imaging (MRI) compatible anesthesia monitor on a wheeled stand mount, for use in the MRI suite.

equipment for different age groups and body sizes for purpose of oxygen administration and intubation are absolutely essential.[5,6]

Sedative Agents

- The choice of the sedative agent depends on availability, local expertise and patient risk factors. The route of administration could be oral or parenteral. Intravenous route has the advantage of faster onset and reliable titration of dose. Other nonparenteral routes include the intranasal or rectal route. A detailed discussion of these agents is beyond the scope of this chapter.
- The commonly used sedative agents include barbiturates, benzodiazepines, and narcotics. Respiratory depression is the most important concern with barbiturates while vomiting is often seen with benzodiazepine such as midazolam. Narcotics are used as an adjunct to other sedative agents when where analgesia is desirable in addition to sedation.
- Besides these three groups of drugs, other commonly used agents include triclofos, chloral hydrate, propofol, and ketamine.
- Ketamine can be given by multiple routes and it seldom causes respiratory depression, unlike the opioids. Ketamine, however, may cause raised intracranial pressure and should not be used when this is an issue.

Risks of Anesthesia

The risks associated with the use of anesthesia are broadly categorized as immediate or short term and long term.

- *Immediate/short-term risks*:
  - These include hemodynamic instability, inadequate ventilation/organ perfusion, hypoglycemia, hypothermia, and allergic reactions.
  - The risk factors are presence of comorbidities such as significant cardiac disease, obesity, obstructive sleep apnea; younger age (like newborn and young infants) increases the risk.
  - Immediate risks are further categorized into major and minor risks:
    - Major risks occur in 1:10,000 patients and include fatality, cardiac arrest, and neurological injury.
    - Minor risks include laryngospasm and bronchospasm.
- *Long-term risks*:
  - These risks have been less well established with evidence of long-term neurocognitive effects of anesthetist/sedative agents obtained from animal studies. Similar studies in humans were nonconclusive as cognitive impairment and learning disability could be caused by the underlying illness(es).
  - A 2016 United States: Food and Drug Administration (US-FDA) report communicated caution regarding neurocognitive effects of these agents in children <3 years and pregnant patients in their third trimester of pregnancy.[10]
  - The United States: Food and Drug Administration now requires a warning of possible neurocognitive risk on the sedative/anesthetic agents labeling.
  - It is imperative for the requesting physician, anesthesiologist, and the radiologist to be aware of the possible risk factors associated with the use of anesthetic agents and take an informed decision regarding their benefit versus risk.
  - Broadly, though this incidence may not be clear, repeated use of anesthesia/sedation in children is discouraged.

Radiation versus Sedation (Computed Tomography versus Magnetic Resonance Imaging)

Magnetic resonance imaging is a radiation-free investigation modality; however, since it requires longer imaging time, it involves some form of sedation/anesthesia in pediatric patients, which may have long-term neurocognitive sequalae.[10,11] Moreover, there have been tremendous advancements in CT technology which has led to radiation dose reduction, and a shorter examination time. Therefore, the current debate stems from lowered radiation risk of CT examination without sedation/anesthesia versus radiation-free MRI which may require sedation/anesthesia. This is especially relevant as waiting period for MRI increases further due to requirement of anesthesia which may be limited in most centers.

Imaging may be possible without anesthesia or sedation in infants using nonpharmacological methods (elaborated earlier) and in older children who understand instructions. It is in young children that the need for sedation/anesthesia becomes imperative especially when the procedure is painful such as interventional procedures. A judicious and informed decision has to be made between the uses of the two modalities.

REDUCTION OF RADIATION DOSAGE

Conventionally, the concerns raised during pediatric imaging pertain to radiation exposure during CT examinations and there are various risk-predicting models which take into account the potential carcinogenic effects of radiation. Radiation can cause two types of changes: (1) *Deterministic,* which are predictable and are dose-dependent such as skin burns, hair loss; and (2) *Stochastic,* which are expressed as increased probability of genetic changes which may result in cancer. There are two main models of risk assessment:

- *Dose-related models*: These models predict the risks as a function of dose of radiation exposure. The *linear-no-threshold* hypothesis suggests that there is an increased risk of developing malignancy with every radiation exposure (even with a single CT examination). However, there is lack of evidence to suggest that the radiation exposure entailed during diagnostic CT examinations is associated with an increased malignancy risk in later life.[12]
- *Threshold models*: These models predict the risk of developing malignancy when the radiation dose is beyond a critical threshold for a particular patient group. It has been shown that a radiation dose of >100 mSv is associated with a significantly increased risk of developing cancer, which is significantly higher than the effective dose of a CT examination.[13] It has also been shown that risk of causation of cancers with exposures of <50 mSv is not statistically different from 0 radiation exposure.[14] Still, most physicians aim to minimize radiation exposure to pediatric patients, keeping in with the concerns of all, especially the parents.
- Regardless of the controversies in actual long-term risk of malignancy, it is essential to limit the dose of ionizing radiation to children as much as possible. Children are more sensitive than adults by a factor of 10 because, they have more time to express cancers than do adults and because they have more dividing cells. Also, girls are more sensitive than boys. Hence, applying the *ALARA (As Low As Reasonably Achievable) principle* in imaging becomes especially important in children.
- *Image gently*: The image gently campaign began in 2007, as an alliance of various organizations such as the Society of Pediatric Radiology, the American College of Radiology among others, with the aim to raise awareness regarding radiation exposure and dose readjustments when imaging children. In the last decade or so since its inception, the alliance has provided information to patients/parents, caregivers, and medical professions on various imaging modalities, dose reduction protocols with optimization of image quality.[15]

Reduction of dose during an examination can be done at several levels, i.e., rational use of referral criteria and modification of equipment and technique. The most important prerequisite is the evaluation of need for an examination and the choice of most suitable modality accordingly. Specific pediatric adaptation of equipment such as restriction devices and aids for immobilization are useful for dose saving. Besides modification of equipment, operator dependent factors, i.e., the technique is equally important.[16,17] Two major areas where reduction of radiation dose is critical are:

1. Radiography and fluoroscopy
2. Computed tomography

Radiography and Fluoroscopy

In procedures involving radiography and fluoroscopy, radiation dose reduction can be achieved at two broad levels:

1. Radiographic equipment related factors
2. Operator dependent techniques

Radiographic Equipment Related Factors

These include:

- Use of digital radiography
- Addition of filtration
- Use of carbon fiber materials
- In fluoroscopy:
  - Modern image intensifiers
  - Pulsed fluoroscopy
  - Last image hold-up system

Digital Radiography

Most modern computed radiography and digital radiography systems now effectively offer substantial patient dose reduction compared to screen-film radiography, repeated exposures are no longer necessary because the contrast resolution is sufficient over a wider range than with conventional screen-film combinations; in particular, fine catheters and tubes are clearly seen. Also, modern equipment has integrated "diagnostic reference dose levels". This is defined as dose levels for typical examinations for groups of standard sized patients. Using these presets, exposure can be adjusted as per the patient's size and hence dose may be reduced **(Figs. 4A to E)**. Despite these advantages, these may be counterbalanced by dose increases due to the radiographer's unawareness of possible overexposure, since the image quality can be manipulated by postprocessing. So, in order to reduce the radiation dose all guidelines, including appropriate collimation, appropriate, source-to-image distance (SID), focal spot size, and patient positioning should be practiced in digital techniques as well.[18,19] Collimation, particularly, is often neglected due to option of digitally cropping radiographs **(Figs. 5A and B)**.

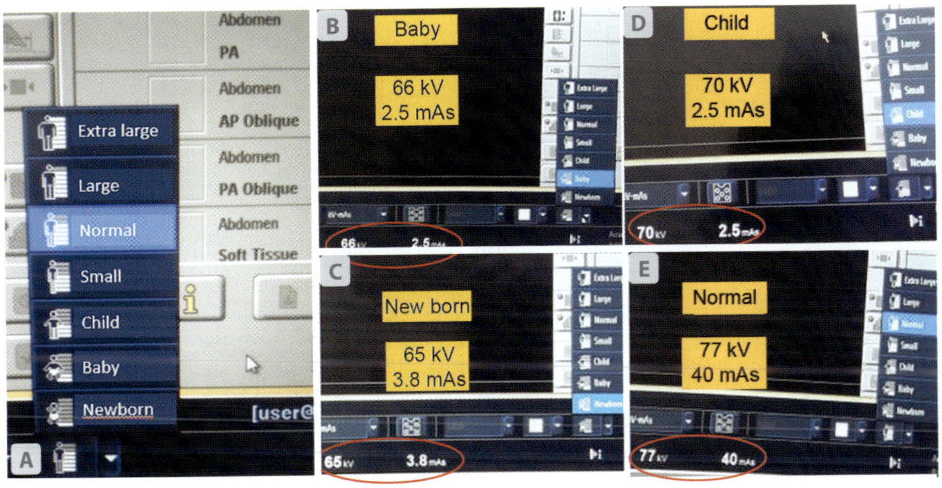

FIGS. 4A TO E: Various vendor-provided automated exposure control (AEC) presets for radiography (A). Note the difference in kV and mAs for different body habitus and age groups (B to E).

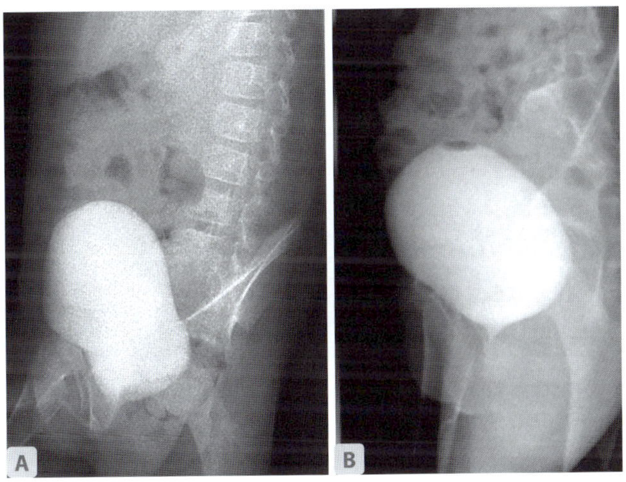

FIGS. 5A AND B: (A) Inappropriate and (B) appropriate collimation in a micturating cystourethrogram (MCU) in a child.

Additional Filtration

Additional filtration can reduce the entrance surface dose up to about 50% depending on the material used. Its use has the disadvantage that the image contrast is deteriorated and the tube load is increased.Adjustable additional filtration should be available for all X-ray tubes, which are used for pediatric exposures. The recommended materials for additional filtration are 1.0 mm aluminum and 0.1–0.2 mm copper. Steel filtration (0.7 mm) can also be used.[16,20,21]

Fluoroscopy

Image intensifiers: Over the years, as the use of image intensifiers has increased, digital fluoroscopy, especially with flat panel detectors, the patient dose has also reduced. Magnification during fluoroscopy should be restricted and instead digital zoom can be employed **(Figs. 6A to D)**.[16,17]

Pulsed fluoroscopy: Pulsed fluoroscopy reduces the effective screening time and hence, the dose can be dramatically reduced.[16,17]

Last image hold-up system: Saving of last image and cine loops results in substantial dose reductions. Exposures should only be obtained if higher resolution is desirable.[16,17]

Operator Dependent Techniques

These include:

- Use of appropriate field size
- Appropriate focal film distance and beam direction
- Avoiding use of anti-scatter grid
- Minimizing fluoroscopic time

Studies in the previous decade have shown that operator dependent changes could lead to dose reductions of about 30–50% with no increase in the cost.[22]

Field Size

This is the most important and most variable factor in the amount of radiation dose imparted to the patient and, hence, accurate field collimation should be meticulously followed. This is especially important in children because an increase in the field size in pediatric patients will cause a proportionally greater increase in individual exposure as compared to adults. This relatively higher increase is due to the smaller anatomical size of young patients. Compared to adults, a similar edge length increase in pediatric patients will lead to a larger percentage of the body surface area being irradiated. Also, because up to 40% of the red bone marrow of infants and toddlers is in the skull, and 25% in the femora of premature babies, correct patient positioning and collimation in the transverse axis is also important when chest and/or abdominal films are taken.[16,17] The actual field size also depends on a correctly functioning collimating system.[16,23]

Five frequent reasons for bad collimation in daily practice, and consequently for oversized field areas, are:

1. Lack of knowledge of age-dependent anatomy
2. No information on pathology
3. Difficulty in patient positioning
4. Difficulty in patient immobilization
5. Difficulty in handling of the radiographic and fluoroscopic equipment

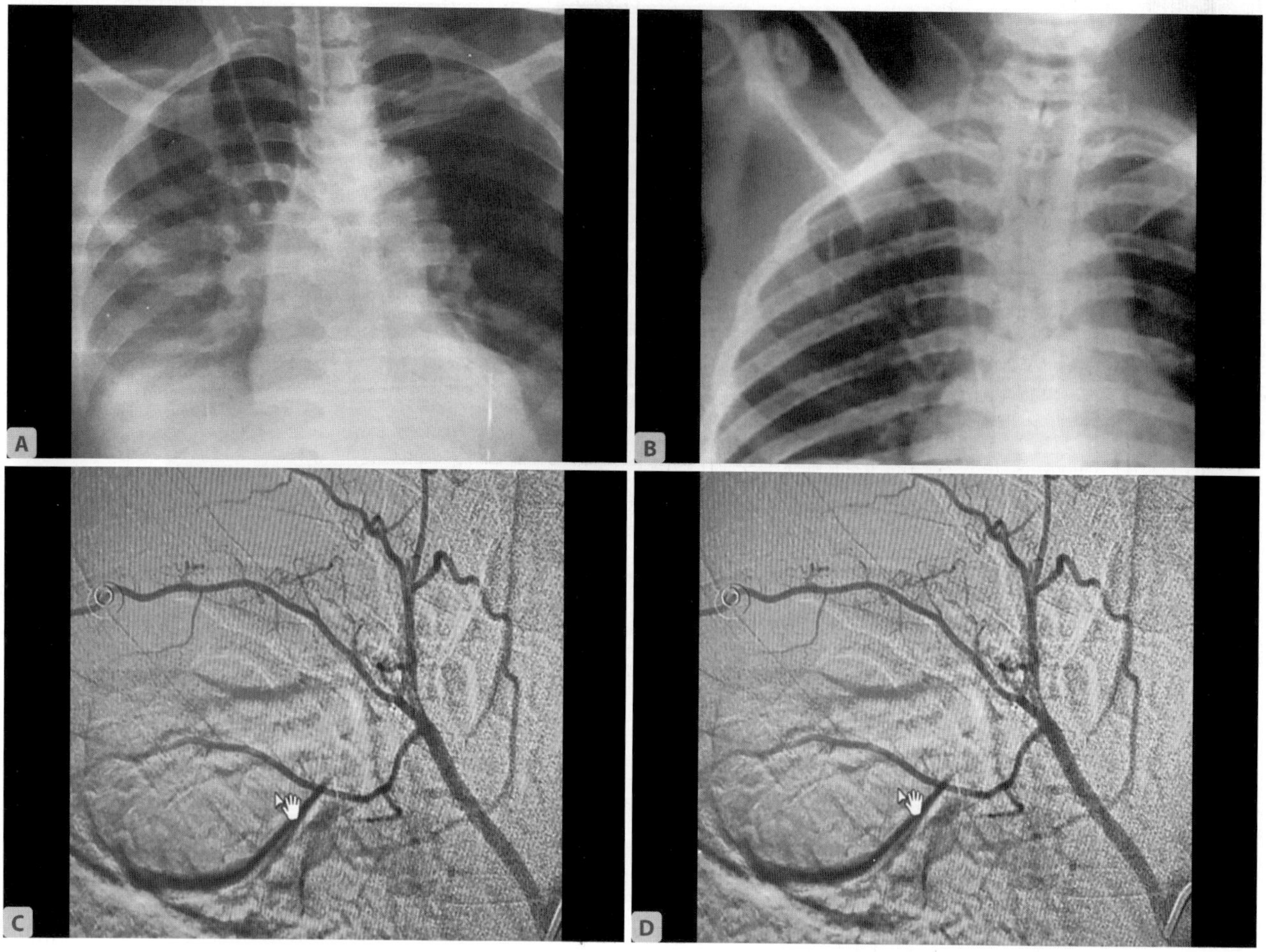

FIGS. 6A TO D: Use of digital zoom in fluoroscopy instead of magnification to reduce radiation exposure: (A and C) without and (B and D) with digital zoom.

Frequent training and supervision of the technicians and young radiologists is needed to optimize collimation, especially in neonates. In a European survey on neonatal chest radiography, only 15% of the films had an acceptable field size.[24] In chest radiograph, inadvertent exposure of both skull and abdomen; in abdominal radiograph inclusion of lower limbs increase the red marrow dose **(Figs. 7A and B)**.

Focus Film Distance

The radiographer should always try to select the largest possible focus-patient distance during radiography. For example, the longest distances are used for the upright anteroposterior spine for scoliosis (up to 300 cm). On the other hand, the focus-film distances (FFD) for radiographs performed with mobile units in neonatal wards (mainly chest and abdominal films) are often too short (<80 cm, sometimes even <60 cm). Ideally, the FFD should be at least 100 cm. Incorrect and varying FFD is important factor responsible for overexposure of patients in the intensive care units.[16,17]

Shielding of Sensitive Organs

The best gonadal protection is tight collimation to exclude the gonads from direct exposure. Gonadal shielding, which was commonly used till recently in pediatric imaging, is no longer recommended as its use is associated with a paradoxical increase in radiation exposure and reduction in the imaging quality.[25-27]

Beam Direction

Another important aspect for patient exposure is the beam direction [anteroposterior (AP)/posteroanterior (PA)]. The standard AP projection can be replaced by prone positions for a large number of examinations. For example, the gonadal and breast tissue dose in gastrointestinal or urographic examinations can greatly be decreased using PA instead of AP projection. In addition, patient thickness is decreased by compression of the belly in prone positioning, thereby decreasing the scattered dose.[16]

Anti-scatter Grid

Scattered radiation plays no major role in pediatric patients. Use of anti-scatter grid increases patient dose by a factor of 3–5. No grid is needed if the object thickness is <12 cm. No anti-scatter grid is needed for chest radiograph in most children, for the infant hip, and for abdominal films in infants or for most of the fluoroscopic examinations. However, a grid is needed for imaging of obese patients (diameter over 15 cm) and for high kV exposures (over 90 kV). A grid ratio of 8:1 is sufficient for all pediatric examinations.[16,17,28]

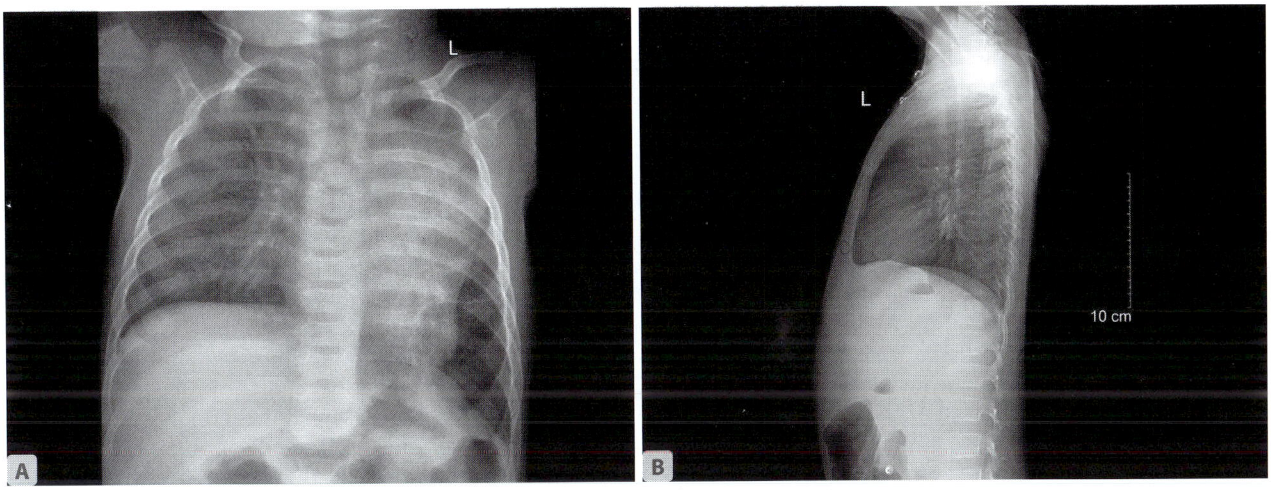

FIGS. 7A AND B: Chest radiograph frontal projection (A) showing **appropriate coverage**, lateral chest radiograph (B) showing inclusion of the abdominal area in the radiograph: inappropriate coverage.

Minimizing Fluoroscopic Time

The most important factor for dose reduction in fluoroscopy is the limitation of screening time. This depends mostly on the clear definition of the clinical questions, on the patient's disease, and on the radiologist's experience. Reduction of fluoroscopic time can be achieved by modifying some practices as a habit. Techniques such as collimating fluoroscopic field before placing the child on the table and use of fluoroscopy only after satisfactory positioning of the child are useful.[1,17,23]

Computed Tomography

Despite various recent developments in the CT technology, following facts should always be taken into account while performing a CT in pediatric cases. The skull contains nearly 30% marrow in a neonate, and it has been seen that CT brain leads to a higher absorbed dose than a CT of chest or abdomen in an older child of 6 years.[29] Therefore, it is imperative to use dose reduction measures in brain CT scans of children.[29,30] Chest is a naturally high-contrast area because of large attenuation differences that result from the presence of air in lungs and fat in mediastinum. As image noise affects the regions with lower contrast resolution more than higher contrast resolution, therefore, such regions such as lungs are less likely to be sensitive to image noise. So, low doses may be used.

Various manufacturers provide multiple protocols for different examination and as per the age of patient. Hence, when imaging for children, pediatric protocols should be followed. Ideally, all institutions must set their own scanning protocol, involving various parameters (tube voltage, tube current, slice thickness, collimation, and pitch) optimized as per the use. The important point to remember is that different manufacturers use different techniques for dose modulation so the user should know about the system's characteristics before trying to attempt any change in scanning parameters.[31] Any changes should be performed using appropriate (weight range) phantoms.

BOX 2: Dose reduction techniques employed in computed tomography (CT).

Strategies for dose reduction employed in CT:
- Tube current modulation
- Tube voltage reduction (low kV techniques)
- Use of dual-energy CT
- Iterative reconstruction

The various dose reduction techniques employed in CT are enumerated in **Box 2**.

Tube Current Modulation

Newer multidetector CT (MDCT) scanners are equipped with automatic exposure control system (AEC) under different names (Care dose 4D, Dose right, AutomA, etc.). These dose modulation systems work in various ways, so as to adjust the radiation dose according to the patient's body size and attenuation. AEC reduces the patient's dose without compromising image quality.[29]

The radiation dose is essentially reduced by controlling the tube current which is performed by three methods. These methods are based on (a) patient size, (b) z axis, and (c) angular or rotational AEC. Most of the scanners use combination of all these methods.[29] The scanner uses the projection radiograph data (topogram/scanogram) to assess size and attenuation of patient and accordingly dose is modulated using patient size and z axis. In angular AEC, the dose is modulated so as to equalize the photon flux to the detector while the tube is rotating. This is needed because the human body is noncircular and hence the attenuation of the beam varies at different projections. Generally, lateral projections are more attenuating than anteroposterior projections. By using AEC there is considerable reduction in the magnitude exposure dose in the range of 35–60%.[29] AEC, thus, is helpful in reducing the patient's dose, especially in pediatric cases.

Tube Voltage Reduction

The effects of reducing the tube voltage kV on image quality are summarized in **Box 3**. As the **Box 3** shows, the enhanced conspicuity of contrast comes with the trade-off of increased noise; this trade-off is eminently suitable for pediatric patients due to their small size and thickness.

Reduction in tube voltage to 80 kV has been shown acceptable for patients of weight <67 kg and linear dimension <32 cm (using a 64-row scanner).[32] In fact, a further reduction to 70 kV is possible with recent scanners (for body weight <40 kg).[33]

Applications of low KV technique include:
- CT angiography (allows use of less contrast and lower injection rate)
- CT urography
- CT enterography
- Any examination of hyperenhancing lesions, for example, in solid organs such as liver/kidney.
- CT chest

Several vendors provide automatic tools for kV selection, which the scanner can do based on size of the patient and the type of examination entered. These include:
- Care kV (Siemens)
- kV Assist (GE)
- Sure kV (Canon)

These tools result in substantial dose reduction; up to 68% in chest CT angiography and 26% in contrast-enhanced computed tomography (CECT) chest/abdomen.[34] Low kV technique, however, is not useful/only minimally useful in larger size patients or in noncontrast computed tomography (NCCT) examinations. Also, in those with metallic implants, the technique worsens the streak artifacts.

Dual Energy Computed Tomography

Recently dual energy CT scanners have been introduced which are faster and have ability to provide greater information about tissue composition than obtained by single energy scanners.
- It allows lower contrast volumes to be used for low kV CT angiography studies.
- Noncontrast CT can be omitted in pediatric imaging by creating virtual noncontrast images. Contrast media can be subtracted, and the patient is spared from the radiation **(Figs. 8A to F)**.

Detailed discussion of the DECT applications is beyond the scope of the chapter.

Iterative Reconstruction

Refer to Chapter 2 for details.

BOX 3: Effects of low kV technique.
- Lower radiation dose (roughly related to square of the voltage)
- Increase in image noise
- Increase in iodine contrast-to-noise ratio (CNR)

REDUCING EXAMINATION TIMES IN COMPUTED TOMOGRAPHY AND MAGNETIC RESONANCE IMAGING

Reducing Computed Tomography Scan Time

Scanning in young children and infants is complicated by motion artifacts, prevention of which requires some form of sedation. The faster scanning capabilities of the modern scanners allow scanning to be competed without sedation in babies <6 months of age after feeding. However, in older infants and children, some form of sedation is commonly required to obtain diagnostic quality images. With the increasing awareness regarding long-term cognitive adverse effects of general anesthesia medications, rapid CT scan techniques become relevant in awake-free breathing imaging without motion artifacts.

Advantages of using rapid scanning techniques are:
- May obviate need for sedation/GA. Hence, it is useful in children <5 years of age where "awake" CT can be performed.
- Allows "free breathing" CT without significant degradation of image quality due to motion artifacts.
- Reduction of radiation dose (if wide area detector CT used), or combined with low kV technique (for example, ultrahigh pitch CT with low kV technique).
- Reduction of intravenous contrast volume is at times possible.

Strategies for rapid scanning in MDCT scanners: With the increasing number of detectors and rapid rotation times, the acquisition time in modern MDCT scanners has substantially reduced over the years. However, the following recent advances aim at decreasing the acquisition times even further:
- Ultra high pitch CT: Pitch of >3
- Wide area detectors

Ultrahigh-pitch Computed Tomography

It uses a pitch of >3 by using a dual source scanner in comparison to the usual pitch of 0.5–1.5 used in routine CT for adults. However, this feature is exclusively available on Siemens Healthineers Dual source CT scanners (e.g., Somatom Definition Flash and Somatom Force). Use of higher pitch results in sampling gaps, causing artifacts; and hence is not achievable with single source scanners. Use of two X-ray sources helps to fill in the sampling gaps, reducing/eliminating these artifacts. There is a concern, however, that "over-ranging" is required to fill in the gaps, resulting in increased radiation dose. This limitation has been overcome in the newer generation dual source CT scanners through the use of "adaptive beam collimation".

Applications of ultrahigh-pitch CT include body CT particularly chest CT, wherein, dynamic airway imaging can be performed due to better temporal resolution. This can be achieved even when the child is awake and free breathing. In CT angiography, it helps in reducing contrast volume requirement.[35,36]

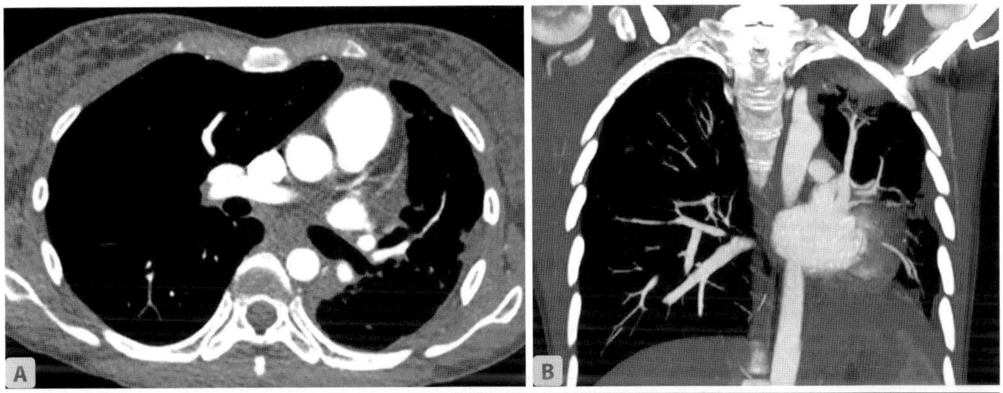

Total mAs 2109 Total DLP 110 mGycm

	Scan	KV	mAs / ref.	CTDIvol* mGy	DLP mGycm	TI s	cSL mm
Patient Position F-SP							
Topogram	1	120	35 mA	0.14 L	5	3.7	0.6
PreMonitoring	2	120	20	1.23 L	1	0.28	10.0
Contrast							
Monitoring	3	120	20	8.61 L	9	0.28	10.0
DE_CTPA	10A	80	65 / 179				
	10B	Sn140	32 / 76	2.82 L	95	0.28	0.6

C

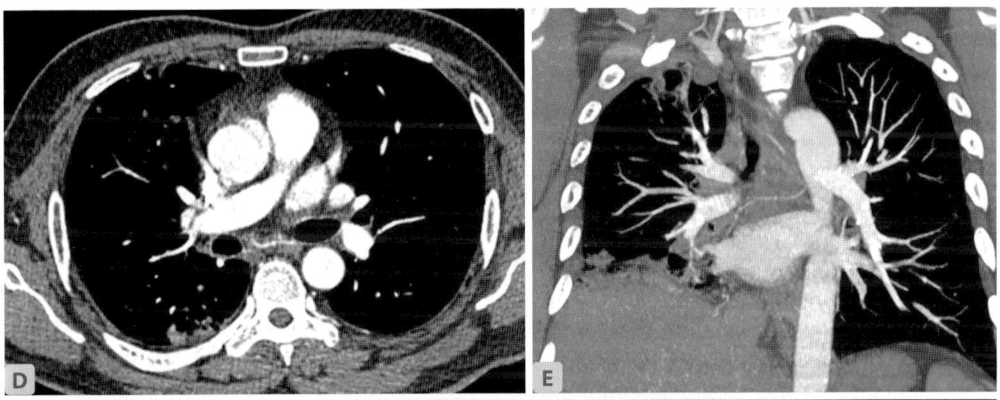

Total mAs 3175 Total DLP 438 mGycm

	Scan	KV	mAs / ref.	CTDIvol* mGy	DLP mGycm	TI s	cSL mm
Patient Position F-SP							
Topogram	1	120	35 mA	0.14 L	5	3.7	0.6
PreMonitoring	2	120	20	1.20 L	1	0.5	10.0
Contrast							
Monitoring	3	120	20	2.40 L	2	0.5	10.0
Thorax	5	100	148 / 148	6.13 L	215	0.5	0.6
Thorax	6	100	148 / 148	6.13 L	215	0.5	0.6

F

FIGS. 8A TO F: CT bronchial angiography using dual energy computed tomography (DECT) mode (A to C) with mA of 270 and kV of 80 shows a total. CT bronchial angiography using single energy mode (D to F) with mA of 245 and kV of 100.

Wide Area Detector Computed Tomography

Certain newer scanners (currently two models) have an ultrawide detector array (16 cm). This allows coverage of field of view (FOV) of 16 cm in a single country rotation. This is referred to as axial scanning (versus helical scanning). A single rotation is completed in 0.28–0.35 seconds, and there is no z-axis motion. Axial scanning has mainly found applications in cardiac imaging. In pediatrics, axial technique is useful for the following:[37]

- Cardiac CT

- Body CT in infants or young children (body weight <10 kg)
- Airway dynamic imaging (acquired through limited area of interest)
- Head and neck imaging
- Imaging single extremity or joint

The two scanners with this feature are:
1. GE revolution (256 detector rows)
2. Canon Aquilion One^{TM}/Genesis (320 detector rows)

Estimates of comparison of timings and doses among various scanners are available online.[38]

Reducing Magnetic Resonance Scan Time

Various MRI techniques have been developed to minimize scanning times.[39] These include:
- Automated protocol selection software
- Parallel imaging
- Simultaneous multisection (SMS) imaging
- Radial k-space sampling
- Compressed sensing reconstruction

Automated Protocol Selection Techniques

The automated protocol selection softwares help to improve the quality and efficiency of an examination by guiding the user with optimum imaging parameters, FOV, and contrast administration protocols. These may achieve a reduction of scan time by up to 20%.[39]

The commercially available products include:
- SmartExam (Philips Healthcare)
- READY Brain (GE Healthcare)
- Dot (Siemens Healthineers)

Applications include automated vertebral labeling, liver segmentation, and liver fat estimation among others.

Parallel Imaging

Parallel imaging techniques involve under-sampling of the k-space and as the length of the MRI scan depends on the number of phase encoding lines, it reduces sampling time. However, it leads to wrap around or aliasing artifacts and reduction of signal-to-noise ratio (SNR) due to reduced signal acquired. The loss of SNR is lesser in 3 T scanner compared to 1.5 T scanner. The reduction in time duration depends on the acceleration factor, so that an acceleration factor of 2 would halve the scan time. In practice, the acceleration factor ranges from 1.5 to 4. Multichannel phased array coils are used in parallel imaging.

The two *reconstruction strategies* used in parallel imaging are:
1. *Image domain reconstruction*: Correction of aliasing is performed after Fourier transformation. For example, SENSE (sensitivity encoding, Philips), mSENSE (modified sensitivity encoding, Siemens), AS-SET (Array spatial sensitivity encoding, GE).
2. *K-space domain reconstruction*: Correction is done before image reconstruction. For example, GRAPPA (generalized autocalibrating partial parallel acquisitions, Siemens) and ARC (autocalibrating reconstruction for Cartesian imaging, GE). Another technique is two-dimensional (2D) controlled aliasing in parallel imaging (CAIPIRINHA, Siemens) which accelerates both phase encoding and partition encoding directions.

Applications of parallel imaging include:
- Whole body imaging
- Magnetic resonance angiography
- Cardiac imaging
- Pharyngeal dynamic imaging
- Breathhold three-dimensional (3D) abdominal imaging especially in nonsedated pediatric patients

Simultaneous Multisection Imaging

Simultaneous multisection imaging is a technique wherein multiband radiofrequency (RF) pulse is employed in multiple sections. These are, however, applied in a single repetition time and read out is also single reducing the acquisition time. It is used in combination with parallel imaging (for coil encoding).

The term "section acceleration factor" refers to number of images acquired at a time (of multiple sections). More the section acceleration factor, less the imaging time; and it typically varies from 2 to 8. The technique is better suited to 1.5 T scanners (versus 3.0 T) scanners.[39]

Commercially available products include:
- Simultaneous Multi-Slice (Siemens)
- Hyperband (GE)
- Multi-Band SENSE (Philips)

Applications of SMS imaging include:
- Neuroimaging along with echo-planar imaging (EPI), diffusion-weighted images (DWI), and functional MRI [blood oxygen level dependent (BOLD) imaging]
- Diffusion-weighted images in abdominal imaging
- Fast-spin-echo (FSE) sequence in musculoskeletal imaging
- Spine imaging along with parallel imaging

Radial K-space Sampling

Radial k-space sampling (unlike Cartesian sampling) involves sampling in radial direction (blades) passing through the center of k-space. This results in reduced acquisition times and reduced motion artifacts. The technique is better suited to 1.5 T scanners (versus 3.0 T) scanners. The disadvantages are that contrast-to-noise ratio (CNR) and SNR are not good at the periphery (versus central k-space) causing blurring. Also, radial k-space technique works best for axial images and not so for coronal/sagittal planes.

Commercially available products include:
- PROPELLER (periodically rotated overlapping parallel lines with enhanced reconstruction, GE Healthcare)
- MultiVane Philips **(Figs. 9A to D)**
- BLADE (Siemens Healthineers)

Applications include:
- Abdominal imaging with and without respiratory triggered T2-weighted (T2W) imaging.

- Brain imaging, using fluid-attenuated inversion recovery (FLAIR) images to reduce motion artifacts and improving SNR and CNR.
- Volumetric interpolated breath-hold examination (VIBE) for contrast-enhanced abdominal MRI.
- Central nervous system (CNS) and orbital imaging in nonsedated pediatric patients.

Compressed Sensing Magnetic Resonance Imaging Reconstruction

Compressed sensing MRI reconstruction is a technique under evaluation, which relies on under-sampling of the k-space to reduce scan time; with an improved temporal resolution. It can be used with both 1.5 and 3 T scanners; however, the SNR is relatively lower in 1.5 T scanner. It is often used in tandem with parallel imaging. Disadvantage includes a long (>30 min) reconstruction times, which is especially relevant in pediatric patients undergoing imaging under anesthesia.

The commercially available products include:

- Golden-angle radial sparse parallel (GRASP)-VIBE (GRASP-VIBE; Siemens Healthineers)
- HyperSENSE (GE Healthcare)
- Compressed SENSE (Philips Healthcare)

Applications include:

- Abdominal imaging especially contrast-enhanced multiphase scans.
- Three-dimensional GRE CEMRI especially free-breathing pediatric imaging.
- Free-breathing 3D MRCP
- Time-of-flight (TOF) angiography of head and neck vessels
- Cardiac imaging (cine)
- Musculoskeletal imaging

USE OF CONTRAST MEDIA

Intravenous Contrast Use

Most principles and recommendations of contrast usage in children are similar to those in adults with a few pertinent exceptions which are discussed here.

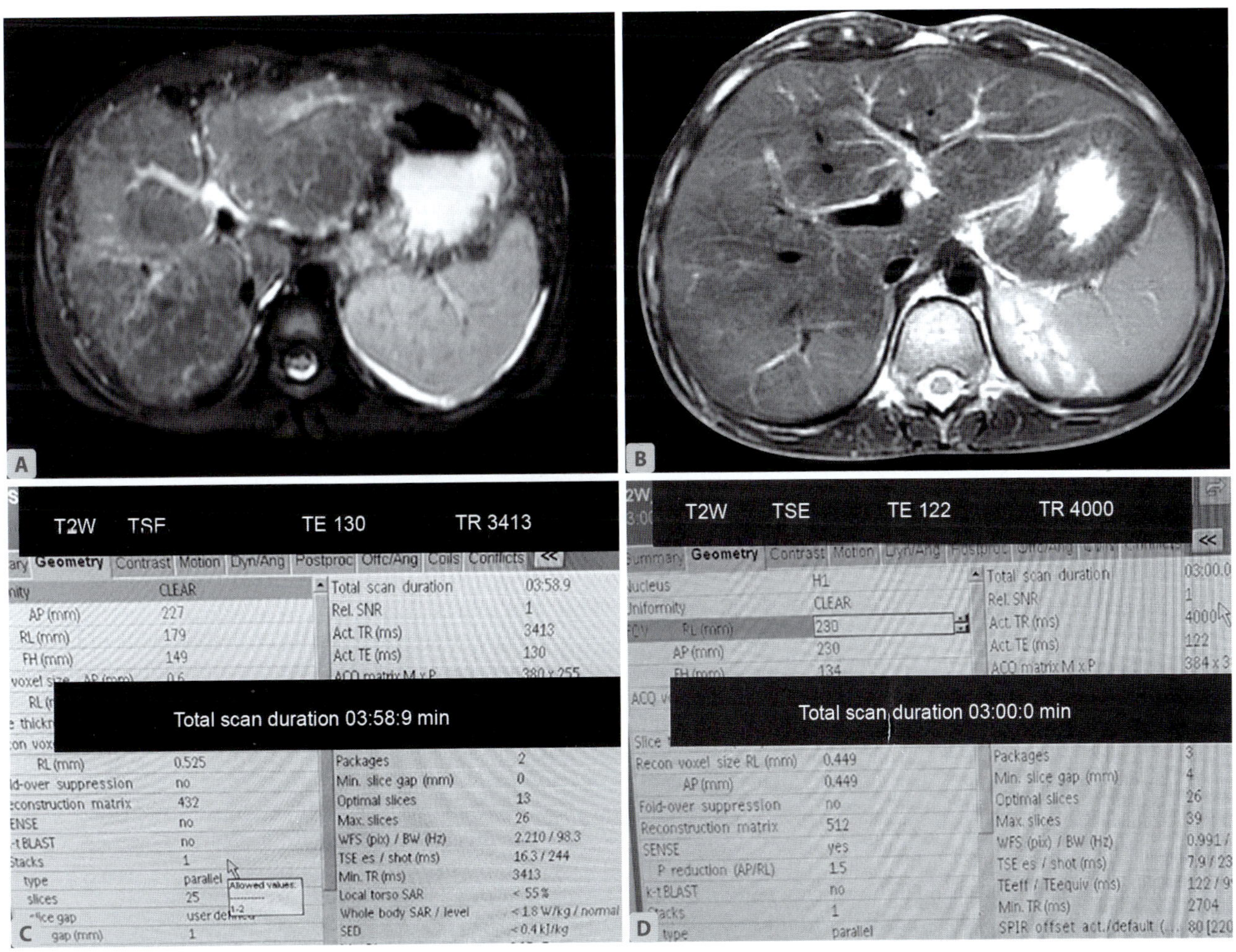

FIGS. 9A TO D: (A) Axial T2-weighted (T2W) SPAIR; and (B) Axial T2 MultiVane of different patients; (C) The duration of the acquisition of former is 3 minutes 58 seconds; and (D) Compared to 3 minutes for the latter. (TSE: turbo spin-echo)

TABLE 1: Cannula size, color coding, and maximum flow rates.

Cannula size (gauge)	Color	Maximum flow rate (mL/s)
24	Yellow	1.5
22	Blue	2.5
20	Pink	4.0
18	Green	5.0

Source: Courtesy Dr Smita Manchanda, AIIMS, New Delhi.

- *Venous access* should be preceded by topical anesthetic gel application by half an hour. This renders the procedure tolerable for a child. Two possible areas can be prepared to take into account a potentially failed application site. Small gauge needles are used, often 22–25 gauge. The cannula size and maximum flow rates are illustrated in **Table 1**.
- *Warming of contrast medium* makes injection through fine needles easier and less painful.[5,6]
- *Contrast osmolality* consideration is important; especially in neonates, infants, and young children. The use of hyperosmolar contrast agents causes fluid shift from extravascular to intravascular compartment, causing increased blood volume for which children have lower tolerance than adults. If this intravascular volume expansion is large, it can cause pulmonary edema and cardiac failure, more so in those with pre-existent cardiac dysfunction.
- *Contrast medium viscosity* has a bearing on contrast flow rate, especially while using a pressure injector. It is important to check the venous catheter for maximum permissible flow rates, especially in CT angiography studies. It has been shown that higher viscosity agents when warmed to body temperature resulted in fewer contrast extravasations.[40]
- *Iodine-based compounds:*
  - Nonionic agents to be used
  - Low osmolar monomers (osmolality 600–800 mOsm/kg water) are preferred over iso-osmolar dimer to reduce the risk of renal injury (osmolality 290 mOsm/kg water).[41]
  - Dose up to 2 mL/kg, iodine concentration: 300–320 mg/L.
- *Contrast reactions*:
  - Contrast reactions may be anaphylactic/allergic or dose dependent. A complete discussion of those is beyond the scope of this chapter.
  - Particular caution is required for avoidance of contrast extravasation in children; as the resultant local reaction can be severe.
  - *Allergic-like reactions* to contrast media are rare in children. Mechanism of reaction appears to be anaphylactoid, with no prior exposure necessary; and rarely anaphylactic. The reaction appears to be independent to dose and contrast concentration and range from mild to severe, similar to those in adults. Children <10 years of age and elderly have been found to have the lowest adverse reaction rates.[42] It is, however, important to keep children and infants under close observation both during and after contrast administration as they may not be able to convey the discomfort faced by them.
  - *Treatment of allergic-like reactions* is similar to that of adults; however, dose calculation is done based on the weight of the patient. A chart may be used for ready reference. Supplemental oxygen with appropriately sized face masks and emergency resuscitation equipment should also be available. The treatment includes:
    - Diphenhydramine is the commonly used agent in case of severe cutaneous reactions in dose of 1–2 mg/kg of body weight by intravenous (IV) or intramuscular (IM) route. Side effect includes hypotension.
    - Albuterol as inhaled bronchodilator (2 puffs MDI) for bronchospasm and wheeze
    - Epinephrine is used in severe reactions with laryngeal edema, bronchospasm, hypotension/tachycardia in dose of 0.01 mg/kg IV slow push over 2–5 minutes (1:10,000 concentration—10 mL vial); maximum up to 0.3 mg (3 mL) per dose OR 0.15 mg (EpiPen Jr)/0.3 mg (EpiPen) IM (1:1,000 concentration)
  - In those with previous history of allergic-like reactions, *premedication* with corticosteroid and antihistaminic agent may be used similar to adults, even though there is lack of conclusive evidence of benefit of their use in children.

Oral Use of Contrast Media

Enteric Contrast Media for Fluoroscopic Examination

Barium Sulfate

It is an inorganic barium containing white crystalline radiopaque compound. As it is poorly soluble in water, it is used in suspension form administered via oral, rectal route or via stomy openings (gastrostomy, jejunostomy, colostomy, cecostomy, and colonic mucous fistula) for opacification of hollow viscus in various fluoroscopic studies. Some institutes, however, do not use it per rectally.[43] The density of barium sulfate in suspension is described as a ratio of either weight of barium sulfate per 100 g weight (w/w) or weight of barium sulfate per 100 mL volume (w/v) **(Figs. 10A and B)**.

Various commercially available preparations of barium sulfate in suspension and powder forms are available. The concentration of barium sulfate used for various investigations are:

- Barium swallow, upper gastrointestinal (UGI), single contrast: 90–100%
- Barium swallow, UGI, double contrast: 200–250%
- Barium meal follow through: 50–60%
- Barium enema, single contrast: 30%
- Barium enema double contrast: 70–100%

Advantages of barium sulfate suspension include:

- It is an inexpensive contrast medium compared to most iodinated contrast media.

- It is palatable and well tolerated orally, especially when mixed with a flavoring medium.
- It can be diluted and administered by syringe or transesophageal catheter.
- As it is not metabolized or absorbed in the gut, it is excreted unchanged per rectally.

Disadvantages include:
- If used in perforated viscus, it can extravasate into the peritoneum where it is retained indefinitely and may cause inflammatory reaction.
- Aspirated barium in the bronchial tree can rarely cause respiratory distress.

Iodinated Water-soluble Contrast Media

Iodinated contrast agents are also commonly used enteric contrast agents. Most of these have a bitter taste and thus have to be used with a carrier agent or with a syringe or transesophageal catheter. High osmolality contrast medium (HOCM) such as gastrografin® (diatrizoate meglumine diatrizoate sodium) which is approved for enteric administration in adults may be unsuitable for young children and infants due to risk of aspiration leading to pneumonia and the possible fluid shifts.[44] All low osmolar contrast media (LOCM) for intravenous route can be used for oral/per rectal administration.[44]

Enteric Contrast Media for Computed Tomography

As children and infants have no significant retroperitoneal and intraperitoneal fat, the demarcation between solid organs and bowel loops is facilitated by enteric contrast agents. Enteric contrast media can be positive (increased attenuation), negative (reduced attenuation), or neutral (similar attenuation as that of water). Even though use of positive contrast medium can potentially increase the radiation dose, its judicious use can facilitate diagnostic imaging. Rectal administration of enteric contrast is reduced due to multiplanar reconstructions and use of MDCT.

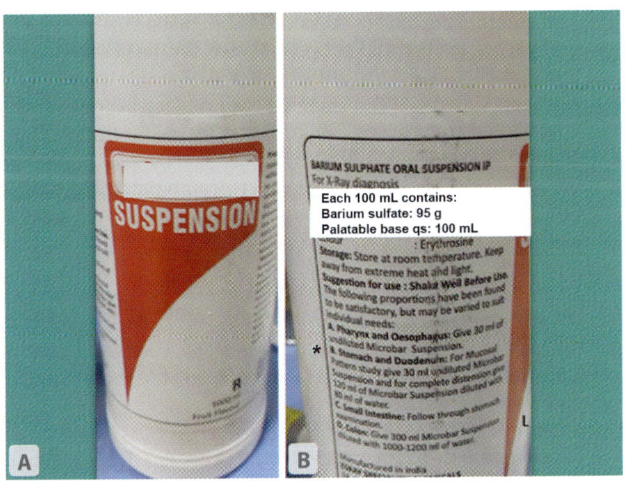

FIGS. 10A AND B: Commercially available barium sulfate suspension (95% w/v) used for barium swallow and meal UGI studies. The container provides usage and dilution instructions (*). (UGI: upper gastrointestinal)

Positive oral contrast: Positive oral contrasts include:
- *Barium sulfate suspension*: Dilute barium sulfate suspension (2%) can be used without causing streak artifacts on CT. However, in case of suspected bowel perforation, iodine-based compounds are indicated.
- *Water soluble iodine-based contrast agents*: Enterically administered water soluble contrast media are associated with low risk of anaphylactoid reaction.[45] Two types of iodine-based oral contrast used are:
  i. *Diluted HOCM, for example, diatrizoate meglumine*: Due to its high osmolality and possible risk of aspiration pneumonia, these are rarely used.
  ii. *Diluted low osmolar contrast medium (LOCM)*: The risk of aspiration pneumonia and pulmonary edema are low; however, these agents are also hyperosmolar to serum and require caution during administration.

Dose and administration: *Dilution of LOCM*: 1 mL of LOCM to 30 mL of carrier fluid. The dose is dependent on the age of the patient such that for infants <1 month, 45 mL of prepared solution, for 1 month to 1 year 90 mL, 1–6 years 120 mL, 6–12 years 180 mL, 12–16 years 240 mL and for >16 years 300 mL of prepared solution is administered.[46] The amount of solution is divided in three doses; first dose is given 90 minutes before CT examination, second dose 30 minutes prior, and the third just before the examination. The contrast can be given orally or via transesophageal catheter.

Negative and neutral oral contrast:
- Water is the safest and inexpensive neutral contrast; however, it is absorbed by the bowel and thus limits distension of the more distal loops.
- Up to 0.1% barium sulfate suspension containing sorbitol is used as a neutral CT enteric contrast. Sorbitol reduces water absorption and thus helps in optimum distension of the bowel loops.
- Milk is another inexpensive enteric contrast, which has an added advantage of slowing peristalsis due to the fat content.
- For CT enterography, water mixed with polyethylene glycol 3,350 (PEG) can be used similar to MR enterography.[46]

Magnetic Resonance Contrast Agents

Magnetic resonance contrast agents are covered in the next chapter.

CONCLUSION

In conclusion, the aim of all those who are dealing with pediatric imaging should be to achieve a diagnostically adequate examination with minimum radiation exposure and discomfort to the child, requiring minimum time, with due diligence for anesthesia and sedation. This goal can only be achieved if the radiologists and technicians in-charge are committed to quality control programs, and are aware of the issues pertaining to radiation protection in children.

REFERENCES

1. Levick RK, Spriqq A. In: Whitehouse GH, Worthington BS (Eds): Pediatric Radiology in Techniques in Diagnostic Imaging (3rd edn). 1996;389-404.
2. Tani S, Mizuno N, Abe S. Availability and improvement of a vacuum-type immobilization device in pediatric CT. Abstract in English on pubmed. Nippon Hoshasen Gijutsu Gakkai Zasshi. 2002;58(8):1073-9.
3. Bontrager KL. Pediatric Radiography in Textbook of Radiographic Positioning and Related Anatomy (5th edition). St Louis: Mosby; 2001. pp. 629-64.
4. Edwards AD, Arthurs OJ. Paediatric MRI under sedation: Is it necessary? What is the evidence for the alternatives? Pediatr Radiol. 2011;41:1353-64.
5. Frush DP, Bisset GS. Sedation of children for emergency imaging. RCNA. 1997;35(4):789-97.
6. Chudnofsky C, Krauss B, Brustowic Z (Eds). Sedation for Radiologic Imaging in Pediatric Procedural Sedation and Analgesia. Maryland, USA: Lippincott Williams and Wilkins; 2001. pp. 169-78.
7. American Society of Anesthesiologists Committee. Practice guidelines for preoperative fasting and the use of pharmacologic agents to reduce the risk of pulmonary aspiration: application to healthy patients undergoing elective procedures: an updated report by the American Society of Anesthesiologists Committee on Standards and Practice Parameters. Anesthesiology. 2011;114(3):495-511.
8. Lim-Dunham JE, Narra J, Benya EC, Donaldson JS. Aspiration after administration of oral contrast material in children undergoing abdominal CT for trauma. AJR Am J Roentgenol. 1997;169(4): 1015-8.
9. Ferris EJ. The Radiological Society of North America 82nd Scientific Assembly and Annual Meeting Chicago, Illinois: Radiological Society of North America; 1996.
10. FDA Drug Safety Communication. (2017). FDA review results in new warnings about using general anaesthetics and sedation drugs in young children and pregnant women. [online] Available from http://www.fda.gov/Drugs/DrugSafety/ucm532356.htm. [Last accessed September, 2020].
11. Davidson AJ, Disma N, de Graaff JC. Neurodevelopmental outcome at 2 years of age after general anaesthesia and awake regional anaesthesia in infancy (GAS): an international multicentre, randomised controlled trial. Lancet. 2016;387:239-50.
12. American Association of Physicists in Medicine. (2011). Position statement. Radiation risks from medical imaging procedures. [online] Available from http://www.aapm.org/org/policies/details.asp?id=318&type=PP. [Last accessed September, 2020].
13. Committee to Assess Health Risks from Exposure to Low Levels of Ionizing Radiation, National Research Council. Health Risks from Exposure to Low Levels of Ionizing Radiation: BEIR VII Phase 2. Washington, DC: The National Academies Press; 2006. [online] Available from http://www.nap.edu/openbook.php?isbn=030909156X [Last accessed September, 2020].
14. Hendee WR, O'Connor MK. Radiation risks of medical imaging: separating fact from fantasy. Radiology. 2012;264:312-321.
15. The Image Gently Alliance. (2014). Translation of Image Gently Resources—Posters and Brochures. [online] Available from https://www.imagegently.org/Global-Resources [Last accessed September, 2020].
16. Schneider K. Radiation Protection in pediatric radiology: How important is what? In syllabus of 20th Postgraduate Course European Society of Pediatric Radiology. 1997. pp. 95-101.
17. Protection of the patient in diagnostic radiology: Summary of the current ICRP principles, by Atomic Energy Regulatory Board: Mumbai; 1987. pp. 3-16.
18. Uffmann M, Schaefer-Prokop C. Digital radiography: The balance between image quality and required radiation dose. Eur J Radiol. 2009;72(2):202-8.
19. Willis CE. Optimizing digital radiography of children. Eur J Radiol. 2009;72(2):266-73.
20. Fearon T, Vucich J. Normalized pediatric organ absorbed doses from CT examinations. AJR Am J Roentgenol. 1987;148:171-4.
21. Nicholson RA, Thornton A, Akpan M. Radiation dose reduction in pediatric fluoroscopy using added filtration. Br J Radiol. 1995;68(807):296-300.
22. Ruiz MJ, Vañó E, González L, Fernández JM. Dose–area product values in frequently performed complex paediatric radiology examinations. Br J Radiol. 1996;69(818):160-4.
23. Shah R, Gupta AK, Rehani M. Evaluation of radiation dose to children undergoing radiological examinations and reduction of dose by protective methods. (Unpublished data) Deptt. of Radiodiagnosis, AIIMS, 2002.
24. Schneider K. Evolution of Quality assurance in pediatric radiology. Radiation Protection Dosimetry. 1995;57:119-23.
25. Jeukens CRLPN, Kütterer G, Kicken PJ, Frantzen MJ, van Engelshoven JMA, Wildberger JE, et al. Gonad shielding in pelvic radiography: modern optimised X-ray systems might allow its discontinuation. Insights Imaging. 2020;11:15.
26. Marsh RM, Silosky M. Patient shielding in diagnostic imaging: discontinuing a legacy practice. AJR Am J Roentgenol. 2019;212:755-7.
27. AAPM. (2019). AAPM Position Statement on the Use of Patient Gonadal and Fetal Shielding PP32A. [online] Available from https://www.aapm.org/org/policies/details.asp?id=468&type=PP. [Last accessed September, 2020].
28. Drury P, Robinson A. Fluoroscopy without the grid: A method of reducing the radiation dose. Br J Radiol. 1980;53(626):93-9.
29. Söderberg M, Gunnarsson M. Automatic exposure control in computed tomography—an evaluation of systems from different manufacturers. Acta Radiol. 2010;51(6):625-34.
30. Chan CY, Wong YC, Chau LF, Yu SK, Lau PC. Radiation dose reduction in paediatric cranial CT. Pediatr Radiol. 1999.
31. Gudjónsdóttir J, Ween B, Olsen DR. Optimal use of AEC in CT: A literature review. Radiol Technol. 2010;81(4):309-17.
32. Guimarães LS, Fletcher JG, Harmsen WS, Yu L, Siddiki H, Melton Z, et al. Appropriate patient selection at abdominal dual-energy CT using 80 kV: relationship between patient size, image noise, and image quality. Radiology. 2010;257(3):732-42.
33. Niemann T, Henry S, Duhamel A, Faivre JB, Deschildre A, Colas L, et al. Pediatric chest CT at 70 kVp: a feasibility study in 129 children. Pediatr Radiol. 2014;44(11):1347-57.
34. Siegel MJ, Hildebolt C, Bradley D. Effects of automated kilovoltage selection technology on contrast-enhanced pediatric CT and CT angiography. Radiology. 2013;268(2):538-47.
35. Strauss KJ, Goske MJ, Towbin AJ, Sengupta D, Callahan MJ, Darge K, et al. Pediatric chest CT diagnostic reference ranges: development and application. Radiology. 2017;284(1):219-27.
36. Goske MJ, Strauss KJ, Coombs LP, Mandel KE, Towbin AJ, Larson DB, et al. Diagnostic reference ranges for pediatric abdominal CT. Radiology. 2013;268(1):208-18.
37. Sorantin E, Riccabona M, Stücklschweiger G, Guss H, Fotter R. Experience with volumetric (320 rows) pediatric CT. Eur J Radiol. 2013;82(7):1091-7.
38. Imaging Technology News. (2019). Comparison charts: computed tomography systems. Imaging Technology News website. [online] Available from https://www.itnonline.com/content/computed-tomographysystems. Updated January 4, 2019. [Last accessed September, 2020].

39. Kozak BM, Jaimes C, Kirsch J, Gee MS. MRI techniques to decrease imaging times in children. RadioGraphics.2020;40(2):485-502.
40. Davenport MS, Wang CL, Bashir MR, Neville AM, Paulson EK. Rate of contrast material extravasations and allergic-like reactions: effect of extrinsic warming of low-osmolality iodinated CT contrast material to 37 degrees C. Radiology. 2012;262(22106356):475-84.
41. Thomsen HS. Guidelines for contrast media from the European Society of Urogenital Radiology. AJR Am J Roentgenol. 2003;181:1463-71.
42. Cohen MD, Herman E, Herron D, White SJ, Smith JA. Comparison of intravenous contrast agents for CT studies in children. Acta Radiol. 1992;33(1449887):592-5.
43. Callahan MJ, Talmadge JM, MacDougall RD, Kleinman PL, Taylor GA, Buonomo C. Selecting appropriate gastroenteric contrast media for diagnostic fluoroscopic imaging in infants and children: a practical approach. Pediatr Radiol. 2017;47(4):372-81.
44. American College of Radiology. (2020). ACR Committee on Drugs and Contrast Media: ACR Manual on Contrast Media. [online] Available from https://www.acr.org/-/media/ACR/Files/Clinical-Resources/Contrast_Media.pdf [Last accessed September, 2020].
45. Davis PL. Anaphylactoid reactions to the nonvascular administration of water-soluble iodinated contrast media. AJR Am J Roentgenol. 2015;204:1140-5.
46. Callahan MJ, Talmadge JM, MacDougall R, Buonomo C, Taylor GA. The use of enteric contrast media for diagnostic CT, MRI, and ultrasound in infants and children: a practical approach. AJR Am J Roentgenol. 2016;206:973-9.

CHAPTER

57

Recent Advances in Pediatric Radiology

Akshay Kumar Saxena, Kushaljit Singh Sodhi, Anmol Bhatia

INTRODUCTION

Medical professionals learn about the recent advances through the research work published in the medical journals. In the modern era, such journals are available in both print and electronic format. The articles dwelling upon pediatric radiology are published not only in the radiology journals, but also in journals in the fields of allied specialties like pediatrics and pediatric surgery. There is no strict definition of recent advances. For an avid reader, recent advances mean the literature published in last few months (say 1 year); for a research worker dedicated to a particular topic, only the articles published in that context would constitute recent advances while for a general radiologist, changing trends over last few years would qualify for recent advances. Given the plethora of articles available in medical literature and differing needs of the radiologists, it is impossible to cater to the need of all. This chapter dwells upon only some of the recent advances in the subspeciality of pediatric radiology in various imaging modalities. Readers are encouraged to enhance their knowledge by reading the recent journals and the referred articles in this chapter.

ULTRASOUND

Contrast-enhanced Ultrasound

Conventional gray-scale ultrasound (US) along with color and spectral Doppler is the most commonly used diagnostic tools in imaging various body organs. Color Doppler imaging provides information about presence/absence and direction of flow. However, its role is limited to evaluating predominantly large blood vessels having fast flow of blood within them. Accordingly, it is mainly used in assessing large vessels of limbs, main abdominal vessels (predominantly hepatoportal axis), and carotids. Its role is limited if we consider detection of perfusion level flow.[1] This limitation can be overcome by adding microbubble contrast agents along with specialized US techniques. The role of microbubbles is to enhance signal from blood within the vessels and specialized US techniques are then used to suppress intrinsic tissue signal by various means, thus making this almost as effective as magnetic resonance imaging (MRI) to evaluate different organs of the body and masses/lesions arising from them.[1]

Contrast Agents used in Ultrasound[1]

Contrast agents being used in contrast-enhanced ultrasound (CEUS) are gas-filled microbubbles with phospholipid shell covering on outside to stabilize them. The diameter is kept <7 μm, so that they can pass through the capillaries. US contrast agents are divided into two generations based on the type of gas used within the microbubble shells. First-generation contrast agents have air which is covered by galactose microparticle shell. These types of microbubbles undergo early destruction during the scanning because of which only intermittent scanning is possible. Second-generation contrast agents contain agents such as sulfur hexafluoride or perfluoro gas-containing agents. These second-generation contrast agents can be used for continuous real-time scanning using a low mechanical index (MI) technique. These agents are injected intravenously and act like "blood-pool contrast agents". They are excreted from the body through breathing and liver and do not undergo renal excretion. Hence, they can be safely administered in children with renal disorders.[1]

Physical Principles of Contrast-enhanced Ultrasound

There is significant difference between tissue and microbubble compressibility and this property is utilized in CEUS, the tissue being nearly incompressible and gases in microbubble being compressible. The US beam makes microbubble oscillate and makes it undergo compression and rarefaction leading to change in size. The change in size of the microbubbles varies with the acoustic power of the US beam. At quite low acoustic power (MI <0.2), microbubbles behave linearly. At higher power, they undergo relatively greater expansion during rarefaction phase than size reduction during compression. Microbubbles, thus, show asymmetrical oscillations characterized by tendency to expand more than compress. By increasing the power even more, microbubbles get shattered and destroyed and this produces very intense, though transient, signal. By utilizing all these properties of microbubbles, US signal is enhanced thereby increasing US yield.[1]

Mechanical Index

Mechanical index is calculated as peak rarefactional pressure/square root of US frequency. It is considered to give an indication of the propensity of sound to cause cavitation in medium, i.e., it expresses microbubble disruption probability during US scan. In the past, few techniques such as destructive contrast-specific techniques with relatively high MI have exploited signal produced by microbubbles rupture after application of high-intensity US beams.

Now-a-days, another technique is in use which utilizes the nonlinear oscillation property of microbubbles being used at a low MI ($0.2 < MI < 0.5$) in non-destructive type contrast-specific techniques. In such technique, persistent signal is achieved rather than intermittent signal thus enabling real-time scanning. This leads to better detection of focal lesions, their perfusion changes as well as perfusion defects, and improves the overall diagnostic confidence.[1]

Applications in Pediatric Imaging

Box 1 summarizes the European Society of Pediatric Radiology (ESPR) Uroradiology Task Force and European Society of Urogenital Radiology (ESUR) Pediatric Working Group—imaging recommendations in pediatric uroradiology for CEUS in children.[2]

Various studies have been published describing the utility of CEUS in varied indications in children. They are enlisted below:

- *Evaluation of parenchymal injuries following blunt abdominal trauma*: Valentino et al.[3] in their study of 27 children with blunt abdominal trauma, with contrast-enhanced CT scan as the gold standard, showed the performance of CEUS to be better than B-mode US. CEUS had a high sensitivity (92.2%), specificity (100%), negative predictive value (NPV) (100%), and positive predictive value (PPV) (93.8%) for the detection of solid organ injury. In comparison, B-mode US performed less well and had a sensitivity of 57.1%, specificity of 86.7%, NPV of 86.4%, and PPV of 80%. The authors argued that CEUS may be considered for triage of children with abdominal trauma who are hemodynamically stable in order to reduce the number of CT scans and radiation exposure to the children. Similarly, Menichini et al.[4] in their study of 73 children with abdominal trauma and CT as the gold standard showed that CEUS was superior to gray-scale US in detecting parenchymal injuries. They showed a sensitivity, specificity, PPV, NPV, and accuracy of 100%, 100%, 100%, 100%, and 100%, respectively for CEUS for the detection of parenchymal injuries as compared to 38.8%, 100%, 100%, 12.8%, and 44%, respectively for gray-scale US. Hence, CEUS has a potential of superseding contrast-enhanced computed tomography (CECT) scan in the children as the initial as well as the main imaging modality with minor or moderate severity abdominal trauma.[5]
- *Identification and characterization of focal liver lesions*: The most common focal hepatic lesions which have been evaluated using intravenous CEUS include hemangioma, focal nodular hyperplasia (FNH), focal fat, adenomas, and regenerative nodules.[6,7] In a study by Jacob et al.[8] in 44 children with focal hepatic lesions, the diagnostic accuracy of CEUS was compared with either CECT or MRI or both. They detected an agreement between the CEUS and the reference imaging in 29 of 34 cases (85.4%). Further, CEUS showed a specificity of 98% for identification of benign lesions and NPV of 100% which suggest that CEUS is comparable in its performance to CECT and MRI.
- *Acute appendicitis*: CEUS has been shown to be a promising imaging investigation for diagnosing acute appendicitis as well as identification of the inflammation stage. In the study of 50 patients by Incesu et al.,[9] a statistically significant difference was seen between mean resistance index (RI) values of the normal appendix, suppurative appendicitis, and gangrenous appendicitis. Contrast-enhanced power Doppler (CEPD) US was shown to have an accuracy of 98% and sensitivity of 100% in the diagnosis of acute appendicitis. Further, CEPD US helped in identification of 100% of suppurative appendicitis and gangrenous appendicitis preoperatively. This study, however, enrolled both adult and pediatric patients with only 9/50 being <16 years of age.
- *Detection of vesicoureteral reflux*:[10-15] This has been covered in detail in the Chapter number 19 entitled "Urinary Tract Infections (including VUR and Neurogenic Bladder)".
- *Pediatric oncology in solid malignancies*: CEUS use has been evaluated in pediatric abdominal as well as pelvic tumors and is technically feasible.[16] It leads to slight improvement in inter-reviewer agreement for detecting tumor margins, local tumor invasion, and lymphadenopathy.[16]
- *Ultrasound-guided percutaneous transhepatic cholecysto-cholangiography (PTCC)*: Zhou LY et al.[17] conducted a study to ascertain the feasibility of US-guided PTCC with microbubbles for evaluation of infants with ambiguous

BOX 1: Box summarizing the potential indications for contrast-enhanced ultrasound (CEUS) in infants and children.[2]

Intracavitary

- Contrast-enhanced voiding urosonography (CEVUS) for vesicoureteral reflux (VUR) or bladder rupture
- Sonogenitography for evaluation of genital malformations, intersex, and cloacal malformations
- Sonourethrography for urethra
- Punctures and drainages in percutaneous nephrostomy, abscess drainage—Leakage? Fistulae? Drain position?

Intravenous

- Transcranial imaging mainly for vascular problems
- Imaging of parenchymal organs for detection and characterization of focal lesions (tumors, infections, and trauma)
- Assessment of vessels patency
- Assessment of organ perfusion in cases of trauma, post-transplantation, and central lines
- Utility for bowel, testis, and joints

features of extrahepatic biliary atresia (EHBA). The study included nine infants with conjugated hyperbilirubinemia and gallbladder length of >15 mm. US findings were equivocal for EHBA. US-guided PTCC was successful in all nine infants. EHBA was diagnosed in four infants, with diagnosis further confirmed at surgery and liver biopsies. The authors concluded that infants with unspecified type of EHBA or showing indeterminate findings on US can benefit from US-guided PTCC. They concluded that US-guided PTCC with microbubbles is safe and effective procedure to rule out EHBA in infants with equivocal findings on ultrasonography (USG).

Shear Wave Elastography

There has been a significant development in the recent years regarding the development of different techniques for measurement of elasticity of the various tissues. Elasticity measurement methods involve two common factors: (1) applying a force or stress and (2) then measuring the mechanical response. The most common types of external sources for application of force/stress are external vibrators, compression devices, or acoustic radiation force. The measurement of the mechanical response can be performed using X-ray, US imaging, optical and acoustic signals, or MRI.[18]

The techniques for imaging elasticity of the tissues using US can be divided into two groups mainly: (1) strain imaging and (2) shear wave elasticity or velocity measurement. In strain imaging techniques, compression is given to the tissue which results in strain, which leads to the linear deformation along the line of the force application and the strain is measured from the degree by which the distortion in the tissue is there. Strain imaging techniques are based on the fact that tissues which are stiffer demonstrate low strains. An image using a gray-scale or color-coded map is generated which shows the pattern of relative tissue stiffness and is assessed subjectively. Elasticity coefficient (Young's modulus) is not directly calculated by the strain imaging. However, region of interests (ROIs) can be drawn in the target area as well as in the adjacent region (which acts as a reference considering it to be a normal tissue) and the strain ratios can be calculated providing a semiquantitative measure.[19]

Shear wave techniques demonstrate the pattern of the shear wave velocity propagation which is induced using a mechanical vibrator or a focused US beam (acoustic radiation force). These shear waves induce mechanical waves in the direction of the force applied. The tissue's elasticity is directly deduced by measuring the speed of this shear wave propagation. Shear wave elastography (SWE) is based on the fact that stiffer tissues induce a higher shear wave propagation speed. The main advantage of shear wave techniques is that the shear wave generation and shear wave velocity measurement are operator independent and hence it provides a numerical value that can be related to the degree of the tissue stiffness.[19]

When a broadband pulse with a central frequency of 50–200 Hz is applied to the tissue periphery or along a line within the tissue, it results in generation of two different types of waves. The first wave displaces the tissue parallel to the direction of wave propagation. This wave is relatively fast and is known as the compression wave. The compression wave travels at approximately 1,500 m/s. The second wave displaces tissue perpendicular to the direction of wave propagation. This wave is called as shear wave which is very slow (as compared to the compression wave) and travels at speed of approximately 3 m/s. These shear waves are then tracked by the same transducer which also measures the speed of the wave. The speed of the shear wave increases with increase in the stiffness of the tissues.[19] Shear wave speed may be converted to Young's modulus with the help of the following formula:

$$SWS\,(m/s) = \sqrt{\frac{\mu}{p}} = \sqrt{\frac{E}{3p}}$$

where μ is the shear modulus in units of Pa, ρ is the density of the medium, and E is the Young's modulus in units of Pa [note $\mu = E/[2(1+v)] \approx E/3$, as v is the Poisson's ratio, which is assumed to be 0.5 to account for tissue incompressibility].[20]

Several studies have been published describing the utility of SWE in varied indications in children in different organs. They are enlisted below:

- *Determining the degree of liver fibrosis* **(Figs. 1A and B)** *in chronic parenchymal diseases and other systemic disorders affecting the liver*: Kim et al.[21] in their meta-analysis of 12 studies in children and adolescents showed that SWE has a summary sensitivity of 81% and a specificity of 91% for the prediction of significant liver fibrosis. Further subgroup analysis demonstrated SWE to have an excellent performance which was correlating well with each degree of liver fibrosis. Bailey et al.[22] evaluated SWE velocities of the liver in children with normal weight and with obesity and showed that SWE velocity is statistically more in children showing increased echogenicity of the liver than in those children with livers having normal echogenicity (1.53 ± 0.38 m/s vs. 1.17 ± 0.27 m/s) on US. They concluded that SWE is useful for evaluating liver stiffness in children and has a potential of being a quantitative biomarker for assessing liver stiffness.
- *For diagnosis and monitoring of muscle stiffness in children with cerebral palsy (CP) as well as for grading and for response assessment to treatment*: Vola et al.[23] evaluated the role of SWE to measure muscle stiffness in children having CP and compared the values in normal children. They showed that children having CP had greater SWE values as compared to the healthy children ($p < 0.001$). They showed a significant correlation (Spearman correlation coefficient being 0.74) between the SWE values and clinical assessment score using Modified Ashworth Scale (MAS) in children with CP. They concluded that SWE may be a useful investigative tool for diagnosis as well as longitudinal monitoring of the stiffness of muscles as well as useful for grading and response assessment to treatment.
- *Diagnosing and monitoring the children with proven or suspected increased intracranial pressure (ICP)*: Dirrichs et al.[24] evaluated the technical feasibility of obtaining SWE values in brain of infants and compared the SWE values of healthy infants with those having hydrocephalus with suspected or proven increased ICP. A direct correlation

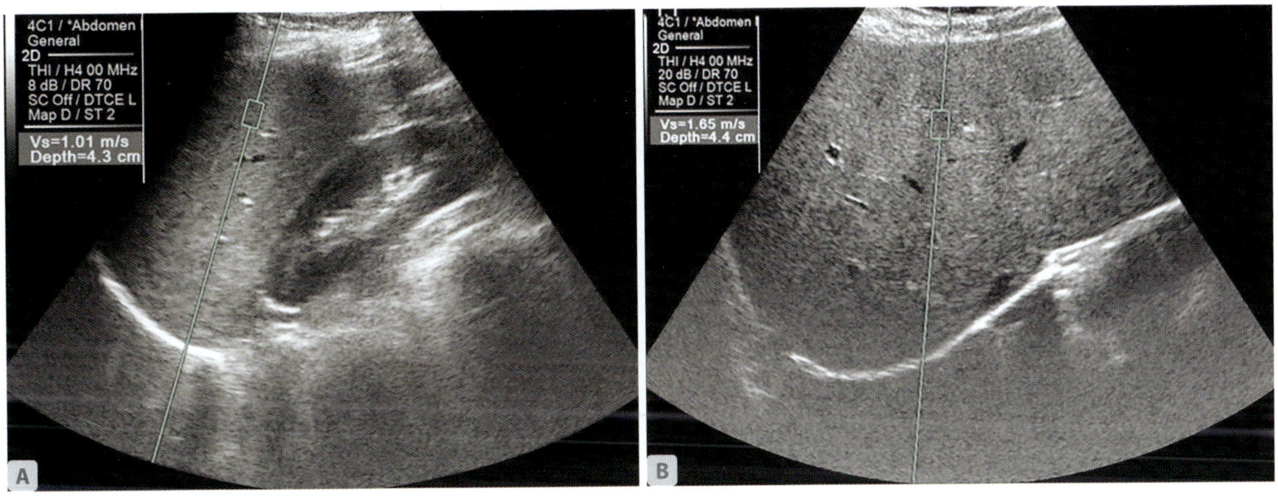

FIGS. 1A AND B: Shear wave elastography images of liver in children with obesity with normal liver (A) and fatty liver (B). The shear wave speed in child with normal liver (A) is 1.01 m/s, while in the child with fatty liver (B) is increased and is 1.65 m/s.

was found between raised ICP and raised SWE values ($r = 0.69$, $p < 0.001$). In infants with increased ICP, mean SWE value was 30.8 kPa as compared to 16.2 kPa in infants with nonincreased ICP. They concluded that SWE may be used as a noninvasive surrogate marker for raised ICP in children.

- *Differentiating biliary atresia (BA)* ***(Fig. 2)*** *from other causes of neonatal/infantile liver diseases*: Leschied et al.[25] conducted a study to determine whether SWE can differentiate BA from other causes of neonatal/infantile liver diseases depending on the liver stiffness values. Mean SWE using Virtual Touch Quantification (VTQ) and Virtual Touch IQ (VTIQ) software were found to be significantly higher in children with BA as compared to children without BA ($p < 0.05$). They concluded that SWE values are significantly increased in neonates and infants with BA. Dillman et al.[26] similarly conducted a study to evaluate the diagnostic performance of SWE for differentiating BA from other causes of neonatal cholestasis. They also compared shear wave speed and laboratory values between patients with and without BA. They showed that SWE had a sensitivity of 92.3% and specificity of 78.6% in making a diagnosis of BA and concluded that SWE can help in distinguishing BA from other causes of neonatal cholestasis. Wang et al.[27] evaluated the utility of SWE for making a diagnosis of BA and for differentiating BA from infantile hepatitis syndrome by measuring liver stiffness. In this study, the mean SWE value of liver in children with BA was higher than that seen in controls and children with infantile hepatitis. SWE showed a sensitivity of 97.4%, specificity of 100%, PPV of 100%, and NPV of 96.9% in diagnosis of BA. They concluded that SWE can help in distinguishing BA from infantile hepatitis syndrome. Zhou et al.[28] evaluated the utility of supersonic shear wave elastography (SSWE) for making a diagnosis of BA in infants with conjugated hyperbilirubinemia. The authors reported that although SSWE is feasible and is useful in differentiating patients with BA from non-BA, its diagnostic performance was not higher as compared to gray-scale US. Duan et al.[29] conducted a study to evaluate the role of SWE in measuring liver stiffness for diagnosing BA and distinguishing it from infantile hepatitis. SWE showed a sensitivity of 84.3% and a specificity of 89.7% for diagnosis of BA. SWE combined with finding of abnormal gallbladder showed the best diagnostic performance with sensitivity and specificity of 80.4% and 100%, respectively. They concluded that SWE helps in differentiating BA from other cholestatic hepatic diseases as well as increases the diagnostic specificity of gray-scale US.

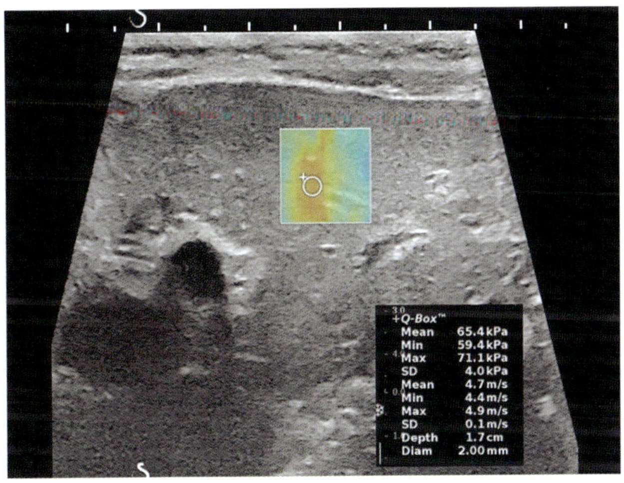

FIG. 2: Shear wave elastography image of liver in an infant with biliary atresia showing increased stiffness with a mean value of 65.4 kPa.

- *Evaluating the spleen stiffness* ***(Figs. 3A and B)*** *for predicting esophagogastric varices in children with chronic liver diseases like BA*: Yokoyama et al.[30] evaluated the role of SWE of the spleen in predicting esophageal varices in 34 children with BA. The highest area under the receiver operating characteristic (AUROC) curve was found for the splenic stiffness (0.900) for the detection of esophagogastric varices and the cutoff value of 4.12 m/s showed a sensitivity of 92.9% and specificity of 90%.

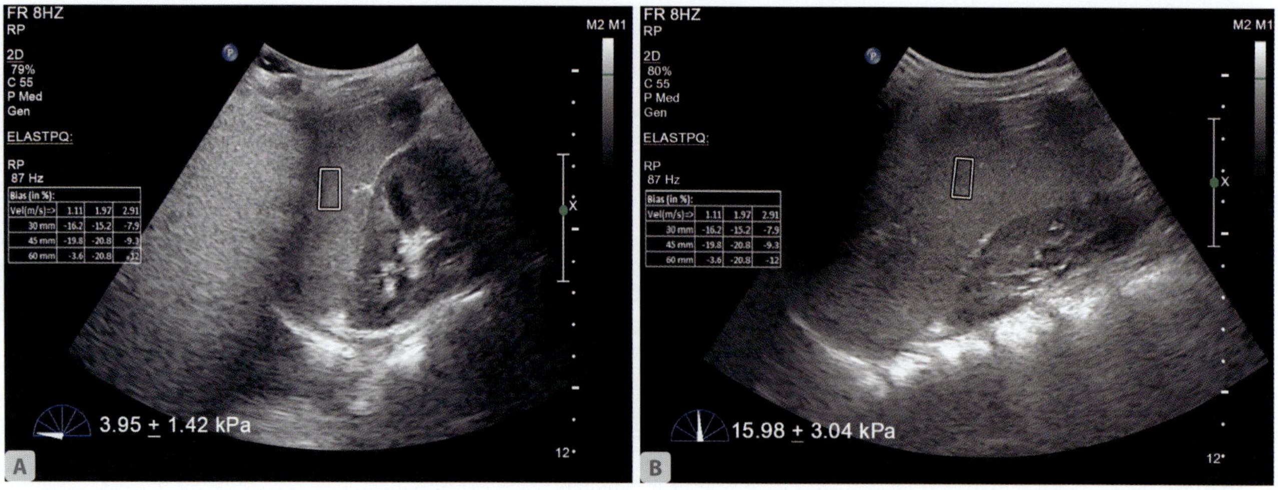

FIGS. 3A AND B: Shear wave elastography images of spleen in children with normal spleen (A) and enlarged spleen (B) in portal hypertension. The shear wave value in child with normal spleen (A) is 3.95 kPa, while in the child with enlarged spleen in portal hypertension (B) is increased to 15.98 kPa.

They concluded that SWE of spleen is the most accurate predictor of esophageal varices in children with BA.

- *Thyroid disorders*: Palabıyık et al.[31] evaluated role of SWE in measuring the elasticity of normal thyroid gland in children and adolescents and evaluate its role for making a diagnosis of autoimmune thyroiditis in children. They found that average SWE value of thyroid in children with autoimmune thyroiditis was 3.7 ± 1.2 m/s which was significantly greater than in healthy children (1.82 ± 0.3 m/s). They concluded that SWE is a useful investigative tool which may be used in addition to routine US in evaluation of the thyroid disorders in children.

COMPUTED TOMOGRAPHY

Dual-energy Computed Tomography

Dual-energy CT (DECT) is a technique that uses two separate X-ray photon energy spectra and allows the interrogation of materials that are having different attenuation properties at different energy levels. DECT uses image acquisition at both high (120 kVp) and low (80 kVp) kVp values and can be used as a supplement to the information that is gained from conventional CT. Low kVp at 80 kV imaging improves the conspicuity of otherwise difficult to visualize subtle contrast enhancement. Quantitative analysis of the degree of enhancement can be done by using iodine selective images and measuring iodine concentration in designated region of interest.[32] Imaging is based on the principle that iodine, with its k edge present close to the mean energy of the low kVp X-ray spectrum, demonstrates a higher dual energy ratio (steeper slope of increase with increasing concentration) than calcium.[33] Additionally, postprocessing techniques allow the creation of iodine maps displaying the iodine content or virtual nonenhanced images that subtract the iodine content. Both of these image sets can then be superimposed to create iodine overlay maps that juxtapose the gray-scale images of virtual nonenhanced set with the colored iodine maps.[33]

Dual-energy CT maximizes the information gained from a single acquisition with no increase in radiation exposure or acquisition times. The radiation dose is divided between the low- and high-energy acquisitions such that total dose may even be less than single energy scans as the virtual nonenhanced images can replace the nonenhanced images.[34] Main potential clinical applications of DECT in children are listed below:

- *Vascular imaging*: Common clinical indications include coarctation of aorta, Takayasu arteritis, and noninflammatory aortitis like midaortic dysplastic syndrome.[35] The software for the automated bone removal in DECT angiography studies separates bone from iodine based on atomic number differences of calcium and iodine. DECT has the advantage of less error in segmentation of bone as compared to the threshold attenuation-based technique which is used in single-energy acquisitions. It has been shown that segmentation errors occur in 1.5% cases of dual-energy acquisitions as against 12.4% cases of single-energy CT acquisitions.[35]
- *Assessment of perfused lung blood volume and lung vessels*: Clinical indications include pulmonary thromboembolism, pulmonary atresia, pulmonary arterial hypertension (PAH), and arteriovenous malformations (AVMs).[35] DECT provides anatomic information as well as lung perfusion status. The perfused blood volume image shows the distribution of iodine in the parenchyma, which helps in visualizing and quantifying the perfusion defects. Areas with perfusion defects demonstrate decreased or absent iodine content and the pulmonary vasculature with absent or slow flow is coded red. Zhang et al.[36] in their study of 32 children with nephrotic syndrome compared a combined 120 kVp image and blood-pool images. Up to 28.1% emboli were seen only on perfusion images. The perfusion defects were typically peripheral in location, wedge-shaped, and were segmental or lobar in distribution. They concluded that DECT pulmonary angiography

improves the detection of pulmonary emboli in the pediatric population.

- *Masses (in chest as well as abdomen)*: DECT is particularly valuable in the evaluation of abdominal masses in children where single-phase contrast-enhanced examinations are preferred over multiphase imaging to minimize radiation exposure. A single-phase DECT examination generates both iodine and virtual nonenhanced images, which may be helpful for lesion characterization. It also may reduce radiation exposure by obviating a true nonenhanced image acquisition.[35]
- *Bowel imaging in evaluation of disorders such as infections, Crohn's disease, ulcerative colitis, and graft-versus-host disease (GVHD)*: The findings in infectious and inflammatory bowel disease are wall thickening and associated hyperemia showing an increased iodine content. The findings in poorly perfused bowel include decreased or absent iodine content.[35]
- *Composition of renal calculi*: Common renal stones in children in decreasing order of frequency include calcium oxalate, calcium phosphate, struvite, cysteine, and uric acid.[35] It is clinically important to distinguish between uric and nonuric acid stones because uric acid stones are medically managed with urine alkalization, while calcium, cysteine, and struvite stones need to be removed mechanically (using extracorporeal shock wave lithotripsy) or fragmented using ureteroscopic techniques if they fail to pass spontaneously.[35]
- *Evaluation of tumor response to treatment*: Residual or viable tumor shows iodine enhancement and high iodine concentrations, while decreased iodine content is seen in the lesions which have been treated successfully.[35]

FLUOROSCOPY

Percutaneous Transhepatic Cholecystocholangiography

Percutaneous transhepatic cholecystocholangiography involves transhepatic puncture of gallbladder under US guidance followed by injecting iodinated contrast medium under fluoroscopy guidance to assess the patency of the biliary tree. It is used for differentiating BA from other causes of infantile cholestasis. This technique was first introduced by Treem WR et al.[37] and a few subsequent studies[38-40] endorsed its role in evaluation of infantile cholestatic jaundice. More recently, Lee et al.[41] reported their experience regarding effectiveness of sonography-guided PTCC in early diagnosis and determination of type of BA. The study population included 22 infants with neonatal cholestasis. The age range was 1–138 days with mean age of 49.7 days. Among the 18 patients who underwent PTCC successfully, EHBA was ruled out in 13 patients while five patients were diagnosed with EHBA. The diagnosis of EHBA was subsequently confirmed at surgery. In four patients where PTCC could not be performed, EHBA was diagnosed in two patients. No complications, attributable to PTCC, were observed. They concluded that PTCC is a safe and useful technique and can help in exclusion when BA cannot be ruled out using the routine screening investigations. It may also be useful in determining type of BA preoperatively.

Jensen et al.[42] reported their experience in ascertaining whether a combination of PTCC and liver biopsy can lead to reduction in unnecessary laparotomy. The study population for this retrospective study consisted of 128 infants with cholestasis. About 46 of these infants had undergone PTCC while 41 infants, in addition, had simultaneous liver biopsy. The technical success rate for PTCC was reported to be 83% (19/23) in the subset of population where the gallbladder was small or absent on initial US. The authors reported negative laparotomy rate of 17% (1/6 patients) when PTCC and liver biopsy were used together to diagnose EHBA. The complications were reported in four patients which included bleeding in two patients, fever with raised transaminases in one patient, and oxygen desaturation in one patient. The authors concluded that PTCC, when coupled with simultaneous liver biopsy, leads to lowest negative laparotomy rate. In another recent study, Sujka JA et al.[43] reported avoidance of surgery in three critically ill infants by demonstrating normal opacification of gallbladder, biliary system, and duodenum at PTCC.

MAGNETIC RESONANCE IMAGING

Lung Magnetic Resonance Imaging

The use of lung MRI in the children evolved mainly to reduce high radiation exposure which occurs during CT scan. One CT scan is equal to 100–200 chest radiographs in terms of radiation dose.[44] It is said that around 80–90% of all CT chest may be replaced by MRI having good diagnostic value.[44] In fact, in few individual cases, MRI may even be superior to the CT scan. The utility of lung MRI has been explored in pediatric population for evaluating the pulmonary as well as mediastinal abnormalities **(Figs. 4 and 5)**.[45-51]

Plus Pathologies of the Lung at Magnetic Resonance Imaging in Children

Plus pathologies are the disorders where the findings are easy to be picked up on MRI and with a proper examination technique and protocol, MRI is at par with CT in these disorders. The list includes all disorders having alveolar exudates and infiltration by infections,[45-51] primary tumors or metastases,[52] and airway disorders such as cystic fibrosis and allergic bronchopulmonary aspergillosis (ABPA).[46]

Minus Pathologies of the Lung at Magnetic Resonance Imaging in Children

Minus pathologies are the disorders which have a questionable benefit on MRI. For example, if cysts **(Figs. 6A and B)**, congenital pulmonary airway malformation (types I and II), etc., are suspected, CT would still be indicated as first-line cross-sectional imaging modality in children.[53]

Ultrashort Echo Time Sequences

The use of T1-weighted (T1W) ultrashort echo time (UTE) sequences for imaging of the lung was first described by Togao et al. in 2007.[54] But in the recent years only is this idea being explored up again and is being implemented technically, after the manufacturers realized the use of extremely short echo times. The T1W UTE sequences are available as

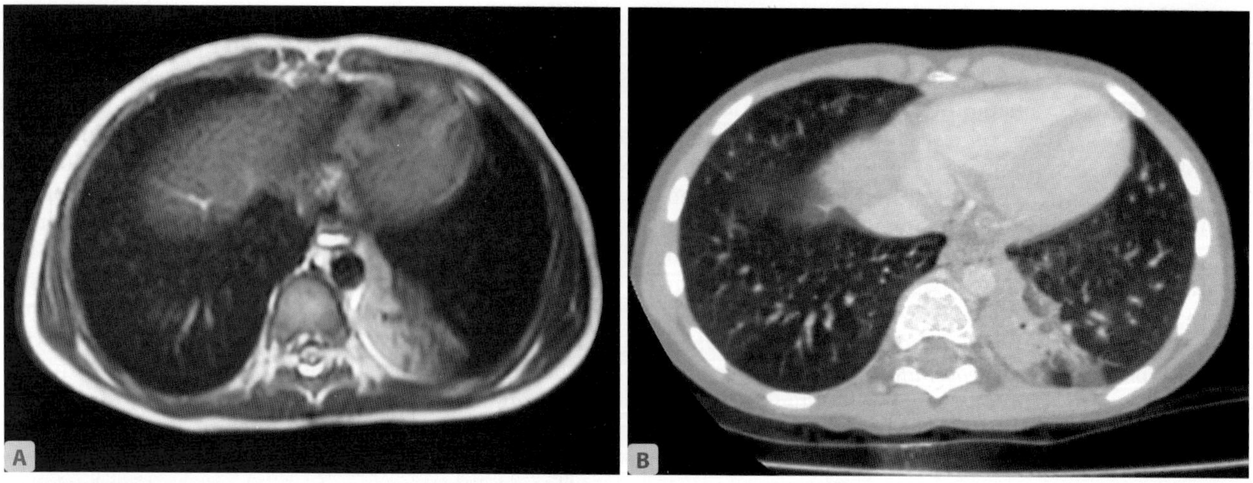

FIGS. 4A AND B: (A) Axial T2-weighted (T2W) MR image showing consolidation in the left lower lobe; and (B) Axial CT image at the corresponding level shows similar consolidation.

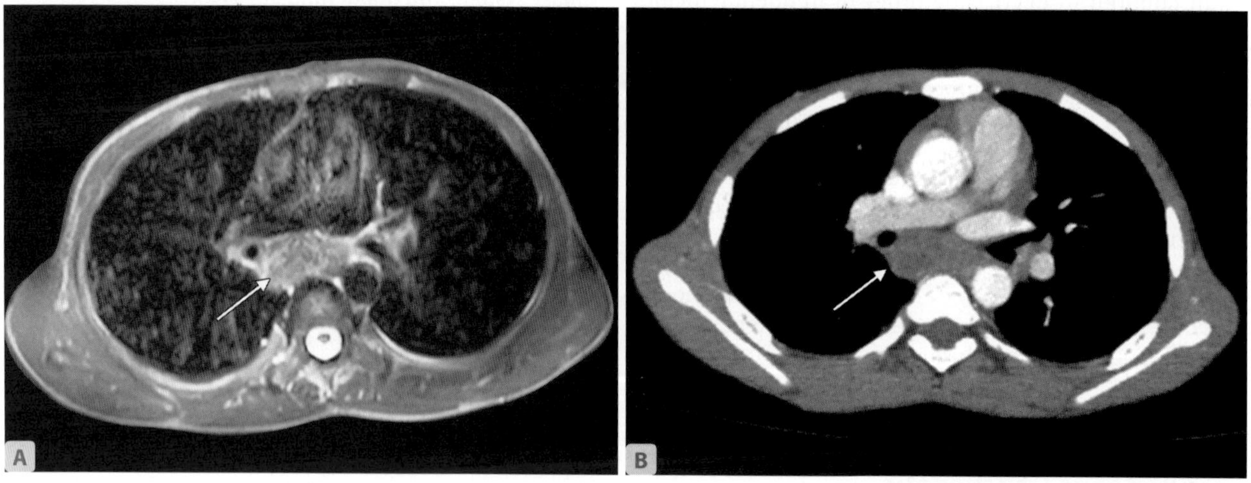

FIGS. 5A AND B: (A) Axial T2W MR image showing lymph node in subcarinal location (white arrow); and (B) Axial CECT image at the corresponding level showing lymph node (white arrow) similar to MRI. (CECT: contrast-enhanced computed tomography; T2W: T2-weighted; MRI: magnetic resonance imaging)

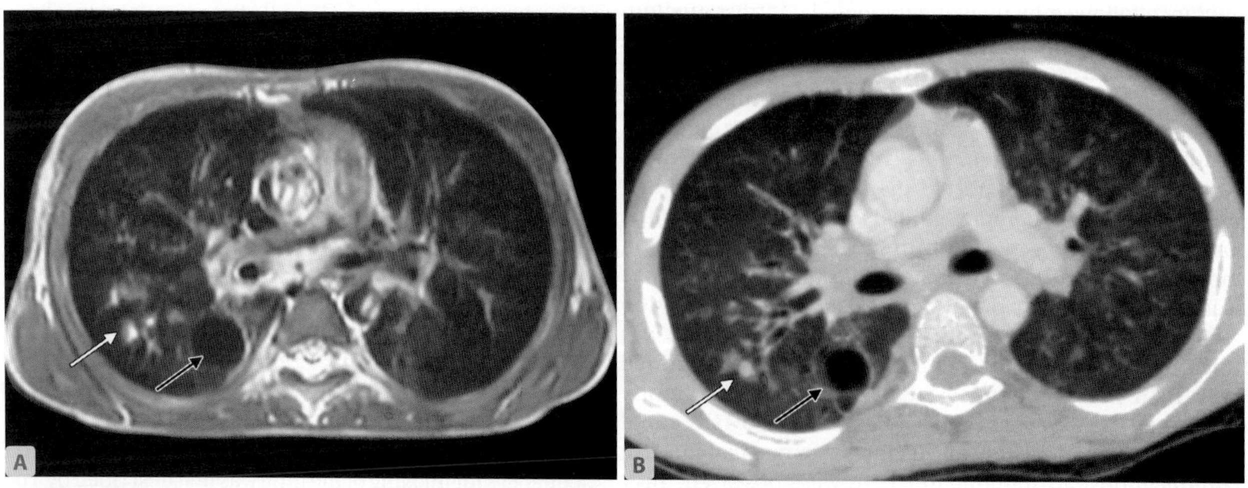

FIGS. 6A AND B: (A) Axial T2-weighted (T2W) MR image showing nodules (white arrow) and air-filled cyst (black arrow) in right lower lobe; and (B) Axial CT image at the corresponding level showing nodules (white arrow) and air-filled cyst (black arrow) in the right lower lobe similar to magnetic resonance imaging (MRI).

three-dimensional (3D) sequences which are reconstructible in isovoxel geometry or as two-dimensional (2D) sequences, having an execution time of 13 seconds (having a slice width of 2.5 mm) or as zero echo time sequences. The technical background of these three sequences has been published recently.[55]

The sequences appropriate for T1W 3D imaging have a high spatial resolution which is in the submillimeter range and can be reconstructed in all three planes due to the isovoxel geometry of around 0.86 mm. No contrast is used in this sequence. Further, it is a respiratory gated sequence and is performed additionally with K-space readout in a special spiral fashion. This helps in further reduction of motion artifacts.[55-57]

Functional Magnetic Resonance Imaging

Phase-resolved functional lung (PREFUL) MRI imaging, which is a further development of Fourier decomposition MRI,[44] has shown very encouraging results of dynamic regional ventilation and perfusion mapping.[41] It holds a potential to transform into a patient-friendly MRI spirometry test providing novel clinically relevant information which can help in guiding clinical decision-making.[44] PREFUL MRI is based on a gradient echo fast low-angle shot (FLASH) sequence. PREFUL is advantageous in pediatric population as it is a free-breathing technique with a relatively short examination time and there is no need for administration of intravenous contrast agent. It helps in creating the perfusion, ventilation, and dynamic flow-volume loop maps after the acquisition of the images through the use of complicated registration and postprocessing algorithms.[44]

Whole-body Magnetic Resonance Imaging

Recent advances in MRI technology have made it possible to image the entire body—from vertex to toes through MRI in short duration. It has the added advantages of better soft-tissue resolution as compared to nuclear scans and is free of ionizing radiation. These images are acquired at multiple stations in the same sitting, which are later reconstructed by a software algorithm so that the single stitched image of the entire scanned area can be visualized. There occurs a signal loss at the periphery which is compensated by allowing an overlap of around 3–5 cm between the adjacent stations which results in seamless images.[58] The selection of the imaging protocols and sequences depends on the disease under evaluation. The sagittal and coronal planes are commonly used, with axial plane least commonly used due to long acquisition time. Short tau inversion recovery (STIR) sequence is the most commonly used sequence in whole-body MRI (WBMRI) of children as it allows visualization of signal changes even in the hypercellular marrow of the pediatric population **(Figs. 7A and B)**. It also provides more uniform suppression of fat compared with T2 fat saturation (fat-sat) images.[58] Disadvantage of STIR sequence includes increased acquisition times and lack of visibility of calcified lesions.

The major role of WBMRI in pediatrics has been in its use in the initial staging and treatment response of pediatric malignancies.[59,60] In this group of patients, lack of ionizing radiation with WBMRI is an undisputable advantage. It provides excellent soft-tissue contrast and hence is ideal for evaluation of brain, liver, and bone marrow while positron emission tomography with CT scan outscores it in evaluation of lungs and lymph node involvement.[59,60] Studies have demonstrated comparable diagnostic performance of WBMRI and nuclear studies in evaluation of lymphoma, Ewing's sarcoma, neuroblastoma, and rhabdomyosarcoma.[59,60] Diagnostic accuracy of WBMRI for detecting the tumor spread into the abdominal organs, lymph nodes, and the central nervous system has been shown to increase when diffusion-weighted sequences are also added to the routine imaging protocol. Regacini et al.[61] conducted a study to see whether diffusion-weighted WBMRI has a potential to replace CECT for initial staging of Hodgkin lymphoma in pediatric population. They found an excellent sensitivity of WBMRI for Hodgkin lymphoma staging in pediatric population and concluded that WBMRI may be considered an alternative to CECT, particularly since it free

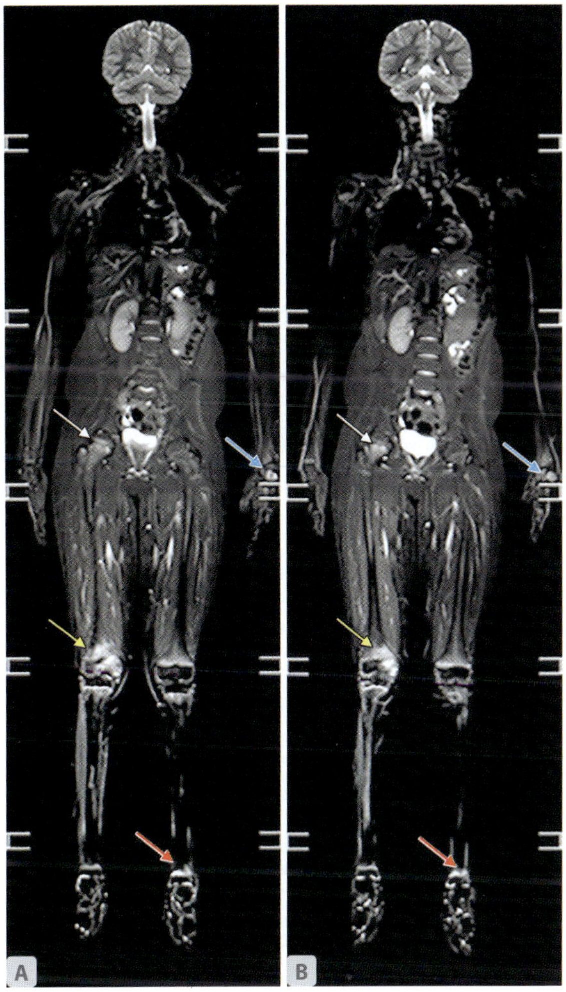

FIGS. 7A AND B: Whole-body coronal short tau inversion recovery (STIR) images in a case of chronic recurrent multifocal osteomyelitis showing abnormally increased signal in the right femoral neck (white arrows), distal epiphysis and metaphysis of the right femur (yellow arrows), distal metaphysis of left tibia (red arrows), and carpal bones on the left side (blue arrows).

of ionizing radiation exposure. Evaluation of tumor burden in case of neurofibromatosis and detection of tumors in cancer predisposition syndromes such as Li-Fraumeni, Von Hippel-Lindau, and Beckwith-Wiedemann syndromes have also been demonstrated.[62] Nononcologic applications include evaluation of subclinical edema as occurs in chronic recurrent osteomyelitis and diseases with multiple sites of skeletal and muscular involvement such as McCune-Albright syndrome, hypophosphatasia, and suspected child abuse.[63] Role of WBMRI in the evaluation of disease status in inflammatory myopathies in children has also been explored in recent years. WBMRI has been shown to be useful in detecting clinically uninvolved areas of muscle inflammation, which may prove to be better accessible for biopsy.[64]

CONCLUSION

Several good articles have been published in recent years contributing to improved patient care. The current trends stress on the need of keeping the radiation dose to the minimum possible level when investigating the pediatric patients. Readers are encouraged to stay in touch with recent developments. The task forces of the pediatric radiology societies across the world regularly publish guidelines and recommendations related to different areas of pediatric imaging which help to optimize the workflow and increase the diagnostic performance. Use of electronic resources is recommended as quick and inexpensive means for maintaining up to date knowledge.

REFERENCES

1. Cosgrove D. Ultrasound contrast agents: an overview. Eur J Radiol. 2006;60:324-30.
2. Riccabona M, Avni FE, Damasio MB, Ording-Müller LS, Blickman JG, Darge K, et al. ESPR Uroradiology Task Force and ESUR Paediatric Working Group—Imaging recommendations in paediatric uroradiology, part V: childhood cystic kidney disease, childhood renal transplantation and contrast-enhanced ultra-sonography in children. Pediatr Radiol. 2012;42:1275-83.
3. Valentino M, Serra C, Pavlica P, Labate AM, Lima M, Baroncini S, et al. Blunt abdominal trauma: diagnostic performance of contrast-enhanced US in children—initial experience. Radiology. 2008;246:903-9.
4. Menichini G, Sessa B, Trinci M, Galluzzo M, Miele V. Accuracy of contrast-enhanced ultrasound (CEUS) in the identification and characterization of traumatic solid organ lesions in children: a retrospective comparison with baseline US and CE-MDCT. Radiol Med. 2015;120:989-1001.
5. Laugesen NG, Nolsoe CP, Rosenberg J. Clinical Applications of Contrast-Enhanced Ultrasound in the Pediatric Work-Up of Focal Liver Lesions and Blunt Abdominal Trauma: A Systematic Review. Ultrasound Int Open. 2017;3:E2-7.
6. Anupindi SA, Biko DM, Ntoulia A, Poznick L, Morgan TA, Darge K, et al. Contrast-enhanced US Assessment of Focal Liver Lesions in Children. Radiographics. 2017;37:1632-47.
7. El-Ali AM, Davis JC, Cickelli JM, Squires JH. Contrast-enhanced ultrasound of liver lesions in children. Pediatr Radiol. 2019;49:1422-32.
8. Jacob J, Deganello A, Sellars ME, Hadzic N, Sidhu PS. Contrast-enhanced ultrasound (CEUS) characterization of grey-scale sonographic indeterminate focal liver lesions in pediatric practice. Ultraschall Med. 2013;34:529-40.
9. Incesu L, Yazicioglu AK, Selcuk MB, Ozen N. Contrast-enhanced power Doppler US in the diagnosis of acute appendicitis. Eur J Radiol. 2004;50:201-9.
10. Darge K, Moeller RT, Trusen A, Butter F, Gordjani N, Riedmiller H. Diagnosis of vesicoureteric reflux with low-dose contrast-enhanced harmonic ultrasound imaging. Pediatr Radiol. 2005;35:73-8.
11. Darge K, Riedmiller H. Current status of vesicoureteral reflux diagnosis. World J Urol. 2004;22:88-95.
12. Darge K, Trusen A, Gordjani N, Riedmiller H. Intrarenal reflux: diagnosis with contrast-enhanced harmonic US. Pediatr Radiol. 2003;33:729-31.
13. Darge K, Bruchelt W, Roessling G, Troeger J. Interaction of normal saline solution with ultrasound contrast medium: significant implication for sonographic diagnosis of vesicoureteral reflux. Eur Radiol. 2003;13:213-8.
14. Darge K, Troeger J. Vesicoureteral reflux grading in contrast-enhanced voiding urosonography. Eur J Radiol. 2002;43:122-8.
15. Darge K. Diagnosis of vesicoureteral reflux with ultrasonography. Pediatr Nephrol. 2002;17:52-60.
16. McCarville MB, Kaste SC, Hoffer FA, Khan RB, Walton RC, Alpert BS, et al. Contrast-enhanced sonography of malignant pediatric abdominal and pelvic solid tumors: preliminary safety and feasibility data. Pediatr Radiol. 2012;42:824-33.
17. Zhou LY, Chen SL, Chen HD, Huang Y, Qiu YX, Zhong W, et al. Percutaneous US-guided Cholecystocholangiography with Microbubbles for Assessment of Infants with US Findings Equivocal for Biliary Atresia and Gallbladder Longer than 1.5 cm: A Pilot Study. Radiology. 2017;286:1033-9.
18. Dietrich CF, Cantisani V. Current status and perspectives of elastography. Eur J Radiol. 2014;83:403-4.
19. Bercoff J, Tanter M, Fink M. Supersonic shear imaging: a new technique for soft tissue elasticity mapping. IEEE Trans Ultrason Ferroelectr Freq Control. 2004;51:396-409.
20. Nightingale K. Acoustic radiation force impulse (ARFI) imaging: a review. Curr Med Imaging Rev. 2011;7:328-39.
21. Kim JR, Suh CH, Yoon HM, Lee JS, Cho YA, Jung AY. The diagnostic performance of shear-wave elastography for liver fibrosis in children and adolescents: A systematic review and diagnostic meta-analysis. Eur Radiol. 2018;28:1175-86.
22. Bailey SS, Youssfi M, Patel M, Hu HH, Shaibi GQ, Towbin RB. Shear-wave ultrasound elastography of the liver in normal-weight and obese children. Acta Radiol. 2017;58:1511-8.
23. Vola EA, Albano M, Di Luise C, Servodidio V, Russo S, Corrado B, et al. Use of ultrasound shear wave to measure muscle stiffness in children with cerebral palsy. J Ultrasound. 2018;21:241-7.
24. Dirrichs T, Meiser N, Panek A, Trepels-Kottek S, Orlikowsky T, Kuhl CK, et al. Transcranial Shear Wave Elastography of Neonatal and Infant Brains for Quantitative Evaluation of Increased Intracranial Pressure. Invest Radiol. 2019;54:719-27.
25. Leschied JR, Dillman JR, Bilhartz J, Heider A, Smith EA, Lopez MJ. Shear wave elastography helps differentiate biliary atresia from other neonatal/infantile liver diseases. Pediatr Radiol. 2015;45:366-75.
26. Dillman JR, DiPaola FW, Smith SJ, Barth RA, Asai A, Lam S, et al. Prospective Assessment of Ultrasound Shear Wave Elastography for Discriminating Biliary Atresia from other Causes of Neonatal Cholestasis. J Pediatr. 2019;212:60-5.
27. Wang X, Qian L, Jia L, Bellah R, Wang N, Xin Y, et al. Utility of Shear Wave Elastography for Differentiating Biliary Atresia From Infantile Hepatitis Syndrome. J Ultrasound Med. 2016;35:1475-9.
28. Zhou LY, Jiang H, Shan QY, Chen D, Lin XN, Liu BX, et al. Liver stiffness measurements with supersonic shear wave elastography

in the diagnosis of biliary atresia: a comparative study with grey-scale US. Eur Radiol. 2017;27:3474-84.
29. Duan X, Peng Y, Liu W, Yang L, Zhang J. Does Supersonic Shear Wave Elastography Help Differentiate Biliary Atresia from Other Causes of Cholestatic Hepatitis in Infants Less than 90 Days Old? Compared with Grey-Scale US. Biomed Res Int. 2019;2019:9036362.
30. Yokoyama S, Ishigami M, Honda T, Kuzuya T, Ishizu Y, Ito T, et al. Spleen stiffness by 2-D shear wave elastography is the most accurate predictor of high-risk esophagogastric varices in children with biliary atresia. Hepatol Res. 2019;49:1162-8.
31. Palabıyık FB, İnci E, Çakır ED, Hocaoğlu E. Evaluation of Normal Thyroid Tissue and Autoimmune Thyroiditis in Children Using Shear Wave Elastography. J Clin Res Pediatr Endocrinol. 2019;11:132-9.
32. Tulwadhva UP, Wortman JR, Sodickson AD. Use of dual-energy CT and iodine maps in evaluation of bowel disease. Radiographics. 2016;36:393-406.
33. Patino M, Prochowski A, Agrawal MD, Simeone FJ, Gupta R, Hahn PF, et al. Material separation using dual-energy CT: current and emerging applications. Radiographics. 2016;36:1087-105.
34. Graser A, Johnson TR, Chandarana H, Macari M. Dual energy CT: preliminary observations and potential clinical applications in the abdomen. Eur Radiol. 2009;19:13-23.
35. Siegel MJ, Ramirez-Giraldo JC. Dual-Energy CT in Children: Imaging Algorithms and Clinical Applications. Radiology. 2019;291: 286-97.
36. Zhang LJ, Wang ZJ, Zhou CS, Lu L, Luo S, Lu GM. Evaluation of pulmonary embolism in pediatric patients with nephrotic syndrome with dual energy CT pulmonary angiography. Acad Radiol. 2012;19:341-8.
37. Treem WR, Grant EE, Barth KH, Kremers PW. Ultrasound-guided percutaneous cholecystocholangiography for early differentiation of cholestatic liver disease in infants. J Pediatr Gastroenterol Nutr. 1988;7:347-52.
38. Meyers RL, Book LS, O'Gorman MA, White KW, Jaffe RB, Feola PG, et al. Percutaneous cholecysto-cholangiography in the diagnosis of obstructive jaundice in infants. J Pediatr Surg. 2004;39:16-8.
39. Shin KM, Ryeom HK, Choe BH, Kim KC, Kim JY, Lee JM, et al. Ultrasound-guided Percutaneous Cholecysto-Cholangiography for the Exclusion of Biliary Atresia in Infants. J Korean Radiol Soc. 2006;55:177-82.
40. Nwomeh BC, Caniano DA, Hogan M. Definitive exclusion of biliary atresia in infants with cholestatic jaundice: the role of percutaneous cholecysto-cholangiography. Pediatr Surg Int. 2007;23:845-9.
41. Lee SY, Kim GC, Choe BH, Ryeom HK, Jang YJ, Kim HJ, et al. Efficacy of US-guided percutaneous cholecystocholangiography for the early exclusion and type determination of biliary atresia. Radiology. 2011;261:916-22.
42. Jensen MK, Biank VF, Moe DC, Simpson PM, Li SH, Telega GW. HIDA, percutaneous transhepatic cholecysto-cholangiography and liver biopsy in infants with persistent jaundice: can a combination of PTCC and liver biopsy reduce unnecessary laparotomy? Pediatr Radiol. 2012;42:32-9.
43. Sujka J, Weaver KL, Poola AS, Rivard DC, Hendrickson RJ. Percutaneous transhepatic cholecysto-cholangiography (PTCC): An alternative to intraoperative cholangiography in high risk infants suspect for biliary atresia. J Pediatr Surg Case Rep. 2018;38:61-3.
44. Hirsch FW, Sorge I, Vogel-Claussen J, Roth C, Gräfe D, Päts A, et al. The current status and further prospects for lung magnetic resonance imaging in pediatric radiology. Pediatr Radiol. 2020;50:734-49.
45. Sodhi KS, Sharma M, Lee EY, Saxena AK, Mathew JL, Singh M, et al. Diagnostic Utility of 3T Lung MRI in Children with Interstitial Lung Disease: A Prospective Pilot Study. Acad Radiol. 2018;25:380-6.
46. Sodhi KS, Gupta P, Shrivastav A, Saxena AK, Mathew JL, Singh M, et al. Evaluation of 3T lung magnetic resonance imaging in children with allergic bronchopulmonary aspergillosis: Pilot study. Eur J Radiol. 2019;111:88-92.
47. Sodhi KS, Khandelwal N, Saxena AK, Bhatia A, Bansal D, Trehan A, et al. Rapid lung MRI—paradigm shift in evaluation of febrile neutropenia in children with leukemia: a pilot study. Leuk Lymphoma. 2016;57:70-5.
48. Sodhi KS, Khandelwal N, Saxena AK, Singh M, Agarwal R, Bhatia A, et al. Rapid lung MRI in children with pulmonary infections: Time to change our diagnostic algorithms. J Magn Reson Imaging. 2016;43:1196-206.
49. Sodhi KS, Sharma M, Saxena AK, Mathew JL, Singh M, Khandelwal N. MRI in Thoracic Tuberculosis of Children. Indian J Pediatr. 2017;84:670-6.
50. Sodhi KS, Bhatia A, Samujh R, Mathew JL, Lee EY. Prospective Comparison of MRI and Contrast-Enhanced MDCT for Evaluation of Pediatric Pulmonary Hydatid Disease: Added Diagnostic Value of MRI. AJR Am J Roentgenol. 2019;19:1-6.
51. Rana P, Sodhi KS, Bhatia A, Saxena AK, Suri D, Singh S. Diagnostic accuracy of 3-T lung magnetic resonance imaging in human immunodeficiency virus-positive children. Pediatr Radiol. 2020;50: 38-45.
52. Liszewski MC, Görkem S, Sodhi KS, Lee EY. Lung magnetic resonance imaging for pneumonia in children. Pediatr Radiol. 2017;47:1420-30.
53. Mon RA, Johnson KN, Ladino-Torres M, Heider A, Mychaliska GB, Treadwell MC, et al. Diagnostic accuracy of imaging studies in congenital lung malformations. Arch Dis Child Fetal Neonatal Ed. 2019;104:F372-7.
54. Togao O, Tsuji R, Ohno Y, Dimitrov I, Takahashi M. Ultrashort echo time (UTE) MRI of the lung: assessment of tissue density in the lung parenchyma. Magn Reson Med. 2019;64:1491-8.
55. Wielpütz MO, Triphan SMF, Ohno Y, Jobst BJ, Kauczor HU. Outracing lung signal decay—potential of ultrashort echo time MRI. Rofo. 2019;191:415-23.
56. Ohno Y, Koyama H, Yoshikawa T, Seki S, Takenaka D, Yui M, et al. Pulmonary high-resolution ultrashort TE MR imaging: Comparison with thin-section standard- and low-dose computed tomography for the assessment of pulmonary parenchyma diseases. J Magn Reson Imaging. 2016;43:512-32.
57. Hahn AD, Higano NS, Walkup LL, Thomen RP, Cao X, Merhar SL, et al. Pulmonary MRI of neonates in the intensive care unit using 3D ultrashort echo time and a small footprint MRI system. J Magn Reson Imaging. 2017;45:463-71.
58. Goo HW. Whole Body MRI in children: Current imaging techniques and clinical applications. Korean J Radiol. 2015;16:973-85.
59. Atkin KL, Ditchfield MR. The role of whole-body MRI in pediatric oncology. J Pediatr Hematol Oncol. 2014;36:342-52.
60. Littooij AS, Kwee TC, Barber I, Granata C, Vermoolen MA, Enríquez G, et al. Whole-body MRI for initial staging of paediatric lymphoma: prospective comparison to an FDG-PET/CT-based reference standard. Eur Radiol. 2014;24:1153-65.
61. Regacini R, Puchnick A, Luisi FAV, Lederman HM. Can diffusion-weighted whole-body MRI replace contrast-enhanced CT for initial staging of Hodgkin lymphoma in children and adolescents? Pediatr Radiol. 2018;48:638-47.
62. Monsalve J, Kapur J, Malkin D, Babyn PS. Imaging of cancer predisposition syndromes in children. Radiographics. 2011;31:263-80.
63. Axelsen MB, Eshed I, Duer-Jensen A, Møller JM, Pedersen SJ, Østergaard M. Whole-body MRI assessment of disease activity and structural damage in rheumatoid arthritis: first step towards an MRI joint count. Rheumatology (Oxford). 2014;53: 845-53.
64. Huang ZG, Gao BX, Chen H, Yang MX, Chen XL, Yan R, et al. An efficacy analysis of whole-body magnetic resonance imaging in the diagnosis and follow-up of polymyositis and dermatomyositis. PLoS One. 2017;12:e0181069.

CHAPTER

58

Frontiers in Research: Genomics, Radiogenomics, Texture Analysis, Safety of Gadolinium-based Contrast, etc.

Devasenathipathy Kandasamy, Atin Kumar, Manisha Jana, Raju Sharma

INTRODUCTION

Over a period of time, imaging has evolved from just a diagnostic tool which can give information on the location and morphology of lesions to a versatile tool which can provide functional as well as structural information and in certain cases even the molecular composition. Pediatric imaging like other subspecialties of imaging has also gained a lot from the ongoing revolution in imaging technology. Technological improvement has happened in the scanner hardware, acquisition techniques, postprocessing algorithms, etc. As a pediatric radiologist, it is important to keep ourselves aware and updated with all the latest developments in this field. In this chapter, we discuss the latest developments in the field of imaging with a special emphasis on pediatric imaging.

BASICS OF GENOMICS

Genomics is a discipline which deals with structure, functioning, evolution, mapping, and editing of genomes. Molecular genetics has a very important role in the diagnosis, characterization, assessment of treatment response, and follow-up of various disease entities especially tumors.[1] Currently, the vast majority of genetic testing is related to tumors. It is also used in characterization of other diseases which are related to genetic mutations and gene inheritance. It is considered that cancer is a disease of genes, which occurs because of genetic alterations related to cell growth and division. There can be numerous mutations happening in the cell but the vast majority of them will not have any effect on the survival of the cell. These large numbers of mutations which do not have any neoplastic potential (preneoplastic) are generally called passenger mutations.[2] Only very few of those mutations may gain the potential to grow selectively and invade which are called driver mutations.[2] A typical cancer needs 1–8 such driver mutations to occur **(Fig. 1)**. The entire genome can be classified into two parts namely exon and intron **(Flowchart 1)**. *Exon* is the part of the genome which codes for and expresses itself as proteins and *introns* are segments which do not really code for any protein or structure. Their function is not fully understood. Together all the exons in the genome are referred to as *exome* and the method of sequencing them is called "whole exome sequencing." Few common pediatric malignancies or syndromes with recognized genetic associations are namely "Wilms tumor (WT-1)," "retinoblastoma (RB-1)," "neuroblastoma (NSD-1)," and "neurofibromatosis (NF-1, NF-2)," etc.[3] Most of the pediatric malignancies are because of the mutations in the tumor suppressor genes which are otherwise responsible for keeping a check on tumor genesis. There are few genes such as *ALK, KIT,* and *MET* which encode for various kinases and can also get mutated leading to tumor genesis.[3] Currently, most of the driver mutations are recognized in the exon part of the genome and the genetic testing is also focused on the exon which only forms 1.5% of the entire genome. The remaining part of the genome is formed by introns which do not code for any protein, but they play an important role in gene expression. The mutations involving the introns and epigenes can also be often responsible for carcinogenesis. These mutations are not fully understood and

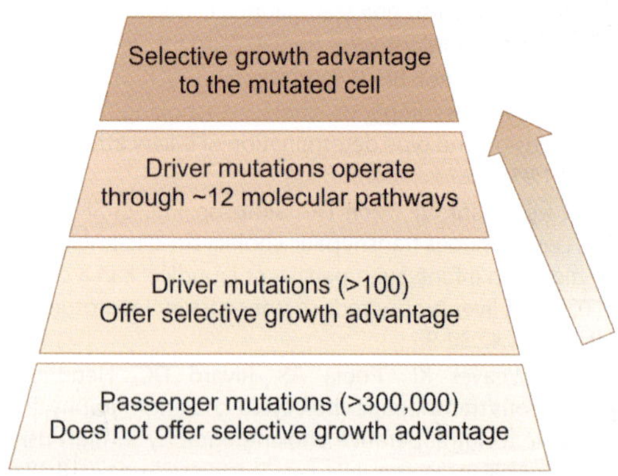

FIG. 1: Typical cancer genesis.

FLOWCHART 1: Whole genome.

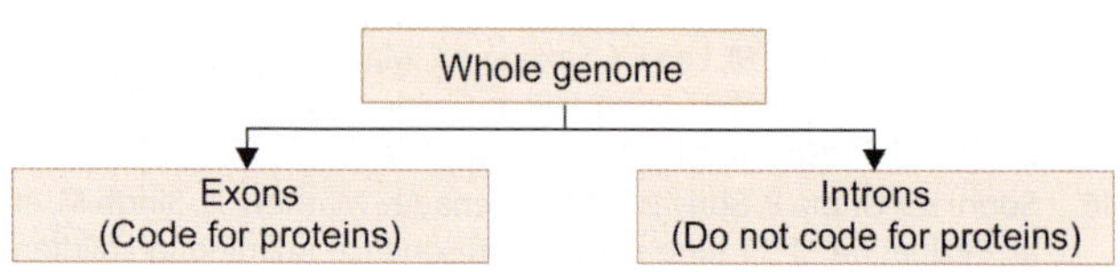

TABLE 1: Conventional radiomics pipeline.

Acquisition	Segmentation	Feature extraction	Feature selection and data building	Data mining and prediction models
• Data acquisition using a uniform protocol • Any change in parameters can affect the output	• Segmentation is an error-prone step but critical • Choice of segmentation ○ Manual ○ Auto ○ Semi	• Heart of radiomics • >600 features can be extracted • Semantic, agnostic, etc.	• Too much data and redundancy • Selection of most important features using statistical methods • Populate with clinical, HPE, genetic information • Handle missing data	• Using ML, DL, or statistics—find the pattern and association • Usually supervised • Create a predictive model—validate

(DL: deep learning; HPE: histopathology; ML: machine learning)

hence they are not recognized. The driver mutations act via various molecular signaling pathways to eventually affect cell fate, survival, and genome maintenance.[4] When the tumor grows, more and more mutations happen which can provide enhanced capabilities such as invasiveness and metastatic potential to the tumor. This is one of the reasons why the tumors can be heterogeneous and can be quite different in morphology from its metastasis.

There are various ways to sequence the genome based on our needs. We can just sequence the exon part of the genome which is most commonly performed because it is less expensive or the entire genome including exons and introns can be sequenced. There are also methods to sequence a single or a set of genes which are known to be associated with a disease. Similarly, there are various techniques to sequence the genome. The traditional method called "Sanger sequencing" is a slow process because it sequences a single DNA fragment at a time whereas newer techniques called "next generation sequencing (NGS)" can perform a simultaneous massive parallel processing of millions of fragments. Hence, it is much faster than the traditional method. NGS is actually an umbrella terminology which includes a variety of modern high throughput sequencing technologies. NGS can do both short-read sequencing and long-read sequencing. Short-read methods are less expensive and commonly used in clinical practice.[1]

TEXTURE ANALYSIS, RADIOMICS, AND RADIOGENOMICS

Radiological images have a large number of qualitative as well as quantitative (macro) features which are usually interpreted by the radiologists to come to a diagnosis. However, like any digital image radiological images are also made of multiple pixels. The pattern of arrangement of those pixels and their gray-scale relations are not visible to the human eye. There is a lot of information hidden in those pixel and gray-scale arrangements which are not apparent to our naked eye. The process of decoding this pattern and mining numerous quantitative features using computer algorithms from digital radiological images is called "texture analysis" or "radiomics."[1,4,5] These features can be correlated with various outcome variables of the disease process. When these radiomics features are correlated with the underlying genetic profile of the tumors it is called as "radiogenomics."[1,4,5] This entire process right from image acquisition till the correlation of quantitative parameters with genetic profiling is referred to as "radiomics pipeline"[6] **(Table 1)**. Radiogenomics is an evolving field and currently the radiomic features are also being correlated with proteomics and metabolomics as well.[6] Study of sensitivity of tumors to radiation therapy and correlation with the genetic profile is also known as "radiogenomics"; however, its usage in the radiotherapy realm has been overtaken by the radiology realm in recent times and will not be discussed in this chapter. With the evolution in NGS and other technological advancements in genetic profiling, the role of radiogenomics is also becoming more and more important. There are various reasons why radiogenomics has carved out an important role in the management of patients with cancer. In some situations, radiogenomics has many advantages compared to even genetic profiling. Once the radiogenomics is correlated with a particular tumor's genetic profile, it can be used to predict the genetic profile without even performing genetic testing. Imaging is a high throughput technique producing huge amounts of data which can be easily mined and correlated with genetic profile. The process of radiogenomics can be almost completely automatic and cheap compared to genetic profiling. Radiogenomics can be performed over the entire tumor, peritumoral areas and even the metastasis whereas biopsy and genetic testing can only be performed on a small piece of tissue which may not be representative of the entire tumor. Radiogenomics has the advantage of being noninvasive and can be performed at multiple time points and even in the follow-up of these tumors. The tumor tissues including their metastases are spatially heterogeneous and radiogenomics has the ability to profile all the areas in all time points of imaging. Hence, with the current potential of radiogenomics the role of imaging has progressed form radiology-histology diagnosis to molecular diagnosis and risk stratification.[7]

Radiomics can be applied to any cross-sectional modalities such as computed tomography (CT), magnetic resonance imaging (MRI), and positron emission tomography (PET-CT). Any radiomics pipeline will involve the following steps:

- Image acquisition
- Segmentation of region of interest (ROI)
- Feature extraction
- Building radiomics classifiers and data sharing (Machine learning methods or statistical methods)

Broadly, there are two approaches to the radiomics pipeline; conventional or traditional radiomics and deep learning radiomics. In *conventional radiomics*, the lesion delineation is done automatically or manually and feature extraction is done based on manual selection. Once these handcrafted features are extracted, they will be processed using statistical methods (univariate or multivariate analysis) or machine learning methods (Bayesian networks, Support vector machines, random forests, etc.). Machine learning algorithms are generally considered superior and require less human involvement. In *deep learning radiomics* the entire radiomics pipeline is performed by a deep learning process such as convolutional neural networks (CNN). Here, feature extraction, selection, and classification are performed by CNN without any human input.[8]

Image Acquisition

Computed tomography is the most commonly used modality in the radiomics pipeline. Since the choice of acquisition parameters can influence the radiomics output it is important to keep the acquisition parameters uniform. Postcontrast images are widely used compared to noncontrast images because of their better contrast resolution. MRI and PET-CT can also be used as an input for radiomics pipeline. MRI can provide multiple paradigms in morphological (T1W, T2W, etc.) and functional imaging (diffusion-weighted imaging and dynamic contrast-enhanced imaging).

Segmentation

Segmentation is one of the critical steps in the conventional radiomics pipeline because it is error-prone and time consuming. The errors created in this step will be propagated to the rest of the pipeline. This issue is largely offset in deep learning radiomics because of less human involvement. There are three types of segmentations: (1) Manual, (2) Semi-automatic, and (3) Automatic. Manual segmentation is performed by an experienced radiologist, which is time consuming. However, this type has the advantage of being accurate. Automatic segmentation does not involve human input but it is error-prone. Semi-automatic method provides a balance between the other two types in which the radiologist curates the segmentation performed by automated algorithms.

Feature Extraction

Feature extraction is the heart of radiomics and this step is performed largely by the computer algorithms (handcrafted or by deep learning). The features extracted can be of many types as follows:[9]

- Semantic or shape features
- Agnostic features or texture analysis
  - First-order statistic features
  - Second-order statistic features
  - Higher-order statistic features

Semantic features are the ones usually recognized by radiologists such as shape, size, necrosis, vascularity, sphericity, spiculations, calcifications, etc., which forms the usual radiologists' lexicon.[10] *Agnostic features* are quantitative features which do not have any subjectiveness to them. These depend on the type and number of gray scales and their locations in the segmented tumor. These agnostic features are also known as texture features which can be of different types depending on the level of complexity. *First-order* statistical metrics simply describe the histogram analysis of the segmented grayscale pixels. These include mean, median, skewness, entropy, kurtosis, etc. These values just depend on the values of grayscale pixels but not on the location of those pixels. *Second-order* statistical metrics, on the other hand, depend on and describe the location and arrangement of those pixels. These metrics bring out the microscopic heterogeneity of the tumor. The commonly used second-order metrics are gray level co-occurrence matrix (GLCM) and gray level run length matrix (GLRLM).[5] However, there are numerous others which are described in the literature. For instance, group pixels arranged in two different ways will have similar first-order metrics whereas they will have different second-order metrics. *Higher-order* statistical features are those which are obtained after subjecting the images to filter and mathematical transformations. These include methods such as highlighting the features by applying coarse/fine filters, transform analysis, and fractal analysis.

Building Radiomics Classifiers and Data Sharing

This is the step where the selected features are mined and correlated with outcome variables. Redundant features are removed and correlating variables are selected and classified. There can be many features which are correlating with the outcome but they may be similar to each other which need selection of features having the strongest association. This step can be either supervised or unsupervised. Sometimes there may be missing data which is especially true when you are handling clinical data. There are various methods described in the literature to handle missing data. Once patterns and associations are recognized between the features and variables such as serum biochemistry, genomic profile, histopathology, etc., a predictive model is created and validated. A shared database can be developed to allow participation from various institutions and also across countries and make it more robust.

The applications of radiogenomics include development of imaging biomarkers, guiding biopsy, and improved assessment of treatment response and patient outcomes. There are various challenges and limitations in the implementation and utility of radiomics; some of which are discussed below. Reproducibility is a major challenge in radiomics because almost all features are dependent on the acquisition parameters which are bound to be nonuniform among institutions. Efforts should be made to keep them uniform to make it robust and reproducible. Errors introduced by the segmentation process, paucity of robust reference standards, missing data, and less number of samples are the few other challenges.

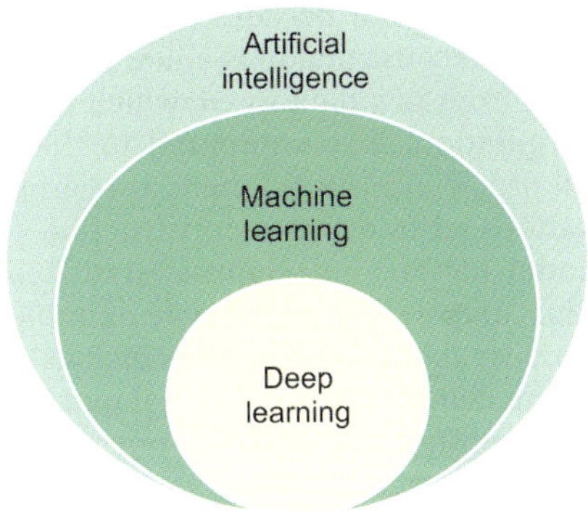

FIG. 2: Artificial intelligence is an umbrella terminology. Deep learning is a subset of machine learning which in turn is a subset of artificial intelligence.

ARTIFICIAL INTELLIGENCE

Artificial intelligence (AI) is a concept which has been there in the computer science field for many decades. Over decades the technology has evolved and has become sophisticated. It has become a part of our day-to-day life. In the last few years because of few developments in AI, diagnostic imaging is becoming the hot field for AI. It is an umbrella term which includes various technologies and algorithms enabling the computers to perform tasks which are otherwise considered too complex for computers **(Fig. 2)**. Machine learning (ML) is a type of AI in which the computers can learn to do a task from the input data fed to them without explicit coding. This is the area which has exciting prospects in the field of diagnostic imaging. Recently, ML has evolved rapidly and has the potential to compete with human intelligence. This was made possible by deep learning methods such as convolutional neural network (CNN) or deep neural network (DNN).[11,12] The architecture of CNN and DNN is inspired by the neuronal architecture of the human brain. CNN has multiple layers of nodes which are connected with each other in a complex way. There is an input layer through which data (images in radiology) is fed. The input layer analyzes the input data, extracts numerous features and they are, in turn, fed into deeper layers where further analyses happen. Based on the analysis, classification and decisions are made and presented in the output layer. The algorithms which are doing the analyses are quite flexible and they can correct themselves based on the reference standard by altering the weighting factor for a given feature to come to a decision (**Flowchart 2**). This kind of inherent flexibility in making decisions by learning is akin to human brain learning based on experiences. This sophistication in the software domain is also paralleled by hardware improvements making these complex computations possible.

There are three broad types of learning in ML namely supervised, unsupervised, and semi-supervised learning.[11] Each of them has their own advantages, disadvantages, and use case scenarios. The most common type of learning used in medical imaging is supervised learning in which a labeled data set (learning data set) is used to teach the algorithm. In this learning phase the algorithm learns from the labeled data (lesion or no lesion, malignant or benign). The knowledge

FLOWCHART 2: Schematic flow diagram of a typical supervised deep learning process.

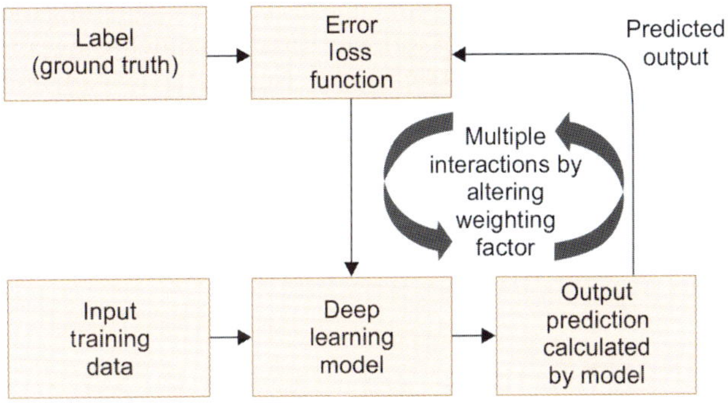

gained from the training data set will be used to make predictions in the test data set. Usually, the percentage of samples in the training data set is 70% and in the test data set is 30%. Although supervised learning enables us to train the algorithm to perform a desired task, it needs accurate labeling of images by experts which can be a tedious job. In unsupervised learning, input data without any labeling is fed to the algorithm and it tries to find an underlying pattern in the input data and classifies them (MRI vs. CT, organ systems, etc.). Since there is no manual labeling of data sets required in unsupervised learning, large data sets can be used. However, it is challenging to teach a desired task in this approach. There is a third approach called semi-supervised learning which is gaining popularity.[12] In this a smaller labeled data and a larger unlabeled data set are used to train the algorithm.

Machine learning has a variety of uses in medical imaging such as classification of images (abnormal, normal, etc.), detection of lesions or abnormality (lung, bone metastases, etc.), segmentation (marking out the abnormal area in images for various quantification purposes) or optimizing imaging data acquisition and workflow (triaging critical cases against less critical ones rather than chronological reporting list). There are few limitations in the currently available ML methods which will be overcome in the future. Currently, ML methods need a large number of samples which are not always available. This can be partly overcome by the usage of transfer learning which involves transfer of knowledge in related domains to medical imaging so as to reduce the number of samples required to train the algorithm. Another limitation is the requirement of accurate labeling of training data sets which needs huge man-hours from radiologists. There are few methods to offset this such as using semi-supervised learning and natural language processing (NLP) to extract labels directly from radiology reports. AI is currently a black box where the logic behind the decision made is not apparent to humans. This makes it difficult to adopt these decisions blindly without knowing the basis. Currently, there are various approaches available to make this black box "AI" a more interpretable AI which will make AI even more reliable and attractive to users.[13] Besides the above, there are issues in the regulatory domains such as how to validate a model, who will be responsible (radiologist or AI vendor) for the consequences if an error occurs in deciding the management. These issues will be ironed out in due course of time as the entry of AI in clinical practice seems inevitable.

Perceptions on the future of AI in radiology are variable. Some may think that it can never replace radiologists and it can only be used to perform mundane tasks such as counting the lesions, report transcription, etc., (assistive intelligence).[14] Others may think that eventually AI will be able to learn and become robust enough to replace radiologists (autonomous intelligence).[15] It is hard to predict the future of AI, but it is quite likely that the role will be somewhere in between these two extremes where both radiologists and AI will have a fruitful coexistence (augmented intelligence).

RECENT ADVANCES IN COMPUTED TOMOGRAPHY AND MAGNETIC RESONANCE IMAGING

Computed tomography also had its share of recent advances such as dual-energy CT (DECT) and iterative reconstruction. DECT is a revolutionary technology in which CT data is acquired at two different kVps almost simultaneously. The principle behind this technology was conceived many decades ago, but the hardware technology was not robust enough till the last decade. Body tissues behave in a nonlinear way when they interact with X-rays of different kVps. This gives rise to a characteristic dual energy ratio (attenuation at lower kVp/attenuation at higher kVp) for different body tissues. Using this principle the composition of the body tissues can be identified. In a conventional single energy CT, calcification, blood clot, and even contrast can appear similar to each other depending on the concentration. However, with DECT all these materials can be differentiated which opens up many possibilities. There are different methods used by different vendors to collect dual energy data. It can be achieved by using two tubes working on two different kVps (Siemens Healthineers), single tube with fast kVp switching (GE Healthcare), single tube with sandwich detector selectively collecting high and lower energy photons (Philips medical systems) or single tube with twin beam technology (Siemens Healthineers). Each method has its own advantages and disadvantages although a discussion of that is beyond the scope of this chapter.

Although images are acquired using two kVps, because of the adoption of iterative reconstruction and other dose saving technologies the radiation dose in DECT is comparable to single energy CT.[16] In fact, it will be less if virtual noncontrast (VNC) CT images are used instead of true acquired noncontrast images. VNC images are generated from the dual energy data set without actually acquiring them. They are comparable to true noncontrast CT, however, their attenuation values may not be equal and very fine calcifications can be missed on VNC. Other applications of DECT are iodine mapping which would highlight the enhancing areas, fat decomposition, and its quantification in conditions such as fatty liver in children and virtual monoenergetic images which can be used to remove artifacts and improve contrast resolution in images.[17]

Radiation dose is an important consideration while performing CT scan and there have been various hardware and protocol improvements such as automatic tube current modulation in the last few decades to reduce the radiation burden. Iterative reconstruction is a new method of image reconstruction from raw data in CT which can drastically reduce the radiation dose compared to the traditional filtered back projection (FBP). There are various types of implementations of iterative reconstruction techniques such as model based and adaptive statistical iterative reconstruction. Depending on the type of implementation the radiation dose reduction can be as high as 80–90% and it would require complex computational requirements and longer image reconstruction time.[18] In practical terms, up to 50–60% of dose reduction can be achieved by using iterative reconstruction without compromising on the reconstruction speed.[18,19]

One of the main drawbacks of MRI compared to other modalities in pediatric imaging is the time taken to acquire images. Over the period of many decades the MRI technology has evolved and the time taken to acquire images has decreased significantly. Even with the current technology, MR acquisition is time consuming which necessitates sedation, anesthesia, etc., which have their own issues. In this section, we will discuss few of the latest sequence acceleration technologies which can significantly reduce image acquisition time.

Parallel imaging is a technology which has been there for some time now and it is worth mentioning here for its capability in bringing down the acquisition time significantly. The length of sequence is directly proportional to the number of phase encoding steps. Normally, if the number of phase encoding steps is decreased significantly, it will lead to aliasing artifacts in the final image. Parallel imaging does it without artifacts by utilizing the ability of phased array coils. By decreasing the number of phase encoding steps (related to acceleration factor) parallel imaging decreases the acquisition time. An acceleration factor of 2 reduces the image acquisition time by half.[20] The acceleration factor depends on the number of individual receiving elements in phased array coils. By leveraging the unique location and sensitivity profile of coils, the images from multiple receivers can be composed to form a single image without aliasing artifacts. There are two most common methods of forming the final image using parallel imaging. SENSitivity Encoding (SENSE) utilizes the image domain and GeneRalized Autocalibrating Partially Parallel Acquisitions (GRAPPA) utilizes the k-space domain. Parallel imaging can be implemented in almost any sequence. There are few limitations of parallel imaging such as one cannot increase the acceleration factor beyond a limit and low signal-to-noise ratio (SNR) in the image.

Simultaneous multisection (SMS) imaging is a novel technique using multiband radiofrequency (RF) transmission to acquire multiple slices simultaneously. Because of the multiple frequencies used in the RF, protons in multiple slices are activated and signals are read. This approach is quite different from parallel imaging because there is no reduction in the number of phase encoding steps. Hence, there is no aliasing or loss of SNR. It can be implemented in conjunction with parallel imaging which would further reduce the sequence time.[21] The reduction in time is proportional to the number of simultaneously acquired slices which is called the section acceleration factor (range from 2 to 8).[22]

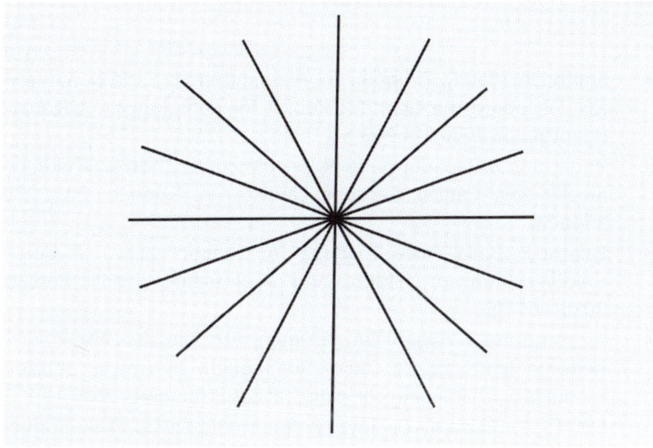

FIGS. 3A AND B: "Cartesian" and "Radial" k-space filling.

Radial k-space sampling is a type of non-Cartesian k-space filling in which each line will be arranged in radial fashion overlapping each other in the center of the k-space **(Figs. 3A and B)**. In conventional Cartesian method the k-space is filled line by line which is why it is prone to motion artifacts. By filling the k-space in a radial manner (like a stack of stars) there are two benefits.[23] Firstly, because of repeated sampling of central k-space the motion gets eliminated and there is an increase in contrast resolution. Secondly, the peripheral k-space is undersampled leading to sequence acceleration. In addition, because of less chance of motion there is less need to repeat a sequence and there is a potential to obviate the need for the time-consuming respiratory triggering of sequences.

Compressed sensing is another revolutionary technology which is based on the premise that the current MRI acquisition has a lot of data redundancy. With appropriate methods images can be generated from much less number of data points eventually reducing the acquisition time. Compressed sensing has three important components: (1) Pseudorandom sampling, (2) Sparse transformation, and (3) Iterative reconstruction.[24] Pseudorandom sampling of k-space distributes the aliasing artifacts randomly so that they are not apparent on images, sparse transformation generates images from an undersampled data and iterative reconstruction is used to remove artifacts. There are various commercial products available for compressed sensing nowadays. One limitation with compressed sensing is that it is computation intensive and takes time for reconstruction. However, better algorithms and hardware computational ability will overcome these limitations in future.

Apart from the above there are techniques involving automated sequence planning and AI driven workflow and image reconstructions are available which have the potential to reduce MR imaging time.

MAGNETIC RESONANCE IMAGING CONTRAST SAFETY

Compared to iodinated contrast agents, gadolinium (Gd)-based contrast agents have an excellent safety profile. Gd-ion is paramagnetic and it causes T1 shortening which is the basis of its contrast property. Gd-ion is toxic and that is why proper chelation is necessary. Once they are chelated their toxicity is drastically reduced and they are excreted without any Gd deposition. However, in situations where the excretion is delayed there is a possibility that the Gd-ions can get dislodged and deposited in tissues. Deposition of Gd in body tissues can lead to issues such as nephrogenic systemic fibrosis (NSF) which is a fatal disorder causing extensive fibrosis of skin and internal solid organs. This is the reason why Gd-based contrasts are contraindicated in patients with chronic kidney disease stage 4 and 5. Even in children with normal renal function there is evidence of Gd deposition in the metaphysis of bones and in globus pallidus and dentate nuclei in the brain who had multiple Gd-based contrast administration.[25,26] It is also found that the deposition is linearly related to the cumulative dose of contrast. Also, the risk of deposition seems to be higher with linear and nonionic contrast compared to cyclical and ionic compounds.[27,28] The mechanism and the long-term ill effects of these Gd deposits in bones and brain are not fully understood. This leads to concerns in neonates where the glomerular filtration rate (GFR) tends to be <30 mL/min/1.73 m^2 because of immature renal function. Children are at increased risk of developing long-term contrast-related complications because of their longer life expectancy. Since there is a risk of developing NSF in neonates in future, the risks and benefits of administration of Gd-based contrast should be thought of by the radiologists.

CONCLUSION

The domain of pediatric radiology and radiology in general has evolved over a period of decades. Improvements have happened in areas such as hardware, software algorithms, and allied domains such as genetics which have the potential to completely transform the way we have practiced pediatric radiology. In the years to come, imaging is going to evolve in the same direction at a much faster rate. It is important as a pediatric radiologist to be aware of the developments in these domains to keep ourselves in the business in future.

REFERENCES

1. Smith DA, Pfau D, Tirumani SH, Alessandrino F, Sadri N, Ramaiya NH. Decoding the Genomic Report for Radiologists. AJR Am J Roentgenol. 2020;214:949-61.
2. Vogelstein B, Papadopoulos N, Velculescu VE, Zhou S, Diaz Jr. LA, Kinzler KW. Cancer Genome Landscapes. Science. 2013;339: 1546-58.
3. Saletta F, Dalla Pozza L, Byrne JA. Genetic causes of cancer predisposition in children and adolescents. Transl Pediatr. 2015;4:67-75.
4. Alessandrino F, Smith DA, Tirumani SH, Ramaiya NH. Cancer genome landscape: a radiologist's guide to cancer genome medicine with imaging correlates. Insights Imaging. 2019;10:111.
5. Das CJ, Kandasamy D, Goyal A, Sharma R. Basics of Radiomics, Texture Analysis and Radiogenomics. In: Gupta AK, Garg A, Sandhu MS, eds. Diagnostic Radiology: Advances in Imaging Technology. New Delhi: JP Medical Ltd.; 2019.
6. Bodalal Z, Trebeschi S, Nguyen-Kim TDL, Schats W, Beets-Tan R. Radiogenomics: bridging imaging and genomics. Abdom Radiol NY. 2019;44:1960-84.
7. Bai HX, Lee AM, Yang L, Zhang P, Davatzikos C, Maris JM, et al. Imaging genomics in cancer research: limitations and promises. Br J Radiol. 2016;89:20151030.
8. Berger MF, Mardis ER. The emerging clinical relevance of genomics in cancer medicine. Nat Rev Clin Oncol. 2018;15:353-65.
9. Rizzo S, Botta F, Raimondi S, Origgi D, Fanciullo C, Morganti AG, et al. Radiomics: the facts and the challenges of image analysis. Eur Radiol Exp. 2018;2:36.
10. Lubner MG, Smith AD, Sandrasegaran K, Sahani DV, Pickhardt PJ. CT Texture Analysis: Definitions, Applications, Biologic Correlates, and Challenges. RadioGraphics. 2017;37:1483-503.
11. Moore MM, Slonimsky E, Long AD, Sze RW, Iyer RS. Machine learning concepts, concerns and opportunities for a pediatric radiologist. Pediatr Radiol. 2019;49:509-16.
12. Neri E, de Souza N, Brady A, Alberich Bayarri A, Becker CD, Coppola F, et al. What the radiologist should know about artificial intelligence—an ESR white paper. Insights Imaging. 2019;10:44.
13. Ghosh A, Kandasamy D. Interpretable Artificial Intelligence: Why and When. Am J Roentgenol. 2020;214:1137-8.
14. Cabitza F, Rasoini R, Gensini GF. Unintended Consequences of Machine Learning in Medicine. JAMA. 2017;318:517-8.
15. Kruskal JB, Berkowitz S, Geis JR, Kim W, Nagy P, Dreyer K. Big Data and Machine Learning—Strategies for Driving This Bus: A Summary of the 2016 Intersociety Summer Conference. J Am Coll Radiol. 2017;14:811-7.
16. Uhrig M, Simons D, Kachelrieß M, Pisana F, Kuchenbecker S, Schlemmer HP. Advanced abdominal imaging with dual energy CT is feasible without increasing radiation dose. Cancer Imaging Off Publ Int Cancer Imaging Soc. 2016;16:15.
17. Kamps SE, Otjen JP, Stanescu AL, Mileto A, Lee EY, Phillips GS. Dual-Energy CT of Pediatric Abdominal Oncology Imaging: Private Tour of New Applications of CT Technology. AJR Am J Roentgenol. 2020;214:967-75.
18. Image Wisely. (2018). Iterative Reconstruction in CT. https://www.imagewisely.org/Imaging-Modalities/Computed-Tomography/Iterative-Reconstruction-in-CT. Iterative Reconstruction in CT: What Does It Do? How Can I Use It? [online] Available from https://www.imagewisely.org/imaging-modalities/computed-tomography/imaging-physicians/articles/adaptive-iterative-reconstruction-in-ct [Last accessed August, 2020].
19. Sulieman A, Adam H, Elnour A, Tamam N, Alhaili A, Alkhorayef M, et al. Patient radiation dose reduction using a commercial iterative reconstruction technique package. Radiat Phys Chem. 2020;108996.
20. Deshmane A, Gulani V, Griswold MA, Seiberlich N. Parallel MR imaging. J Magn Reson Imaging JMRI. 2012;36:55-72.
21. Fritz J, Fritz B, Zhang J, Thawait GK, Joshi DH, Pan L, et al. Simultaneous Multislice Accelerated Turbo Spin Echo Magnetic Resonance Imaging: Comparison and Combination With In-Plane Parallel Imaging Acceleration for High-Resolution Magnetic Resonance Imaging of the Knee. Invest Radiol. 2017;52:529-37.
22. Todd N, Josephs O, Zeidman P, Flandin G, Moeller S, Weiskopf N. Functional Sensitivity of 2D Simultaneous Multi-Slice Echo-Planar Imaging: Effects of Acceleration on g-factor and Physiological Noise. Front Neurosci. 2017;11.
23. Pipe JG. Motion correction with PROPELLER MRI: application to head motion and free-breathing cardiac imaging. Magn Reson Med. 1999;42:963-9.
24. Yang ACY, Kretzler M, Sudarski S, Gulani V, Seiberlich N. Sparse Reconstruction Techniques in MRI: Methods, Applications, and Challenges to Clinical Adoption. Invest Radiol. 2016;51:349-64.
25. Kanda T, Ishii K, Kawaguchi H, Kitajima K, Takenaka D. High signal intensity in the dentate nucleus and globus pallidus on unenhanced T1-weighted MR images: relationship with increasing cumulative dose of a gadolinium-based contrast material. Radiology. 2014;270:834-41.
26. Darrah TH, Prutsman-Pfeiffer JJ, Poreda RJ, Ellen Campbell M, Hauschkac PV, Hannigan RE. Incorporation of excess gadolinium into human bone from medical contrast agents. Met Integr Biometal Sci. 2009;1:479-88.
27. Kanda T, Osawa M, Oba H, Toyoda K, Kotoku J, Haruyama T, et al. High Signal Intensity in Dentate Nucleus on Unenhanced T1-weighted MR Images: Association with Linear versus Macrocyclic Gadolinium Chelate Administration. Radiology. 2015;275:803-9.
28. Radbruch A, Weberling LD, Kieslich PJ, Eidel O, Burth S, Kickingereder P, et al. Gadolinium retention in the dentate nucleus and globus pallidus is dependent on the class of contrast agent. Radiology. 2015;275:783-91.

CHAPTER

59

Vascular Interventions in Children

Sanjeev Kumar, Niraj N Pandey, Sanjiv Sharma

INTRODUCTION

The spectrum of pediatric vascular pathology differs from the adult population and it varies greatly to include congenital and acquired disorders. Although catheter-directed angiography remains the gold standard for diagnosis of vascular pathology, most vascular pathologies in the child can be adequately diagnosed with noninvasive imaging techniques (magnetic resonance angiography, computed tomographic angiography, or Doppler ultrasonography) with only a few exceptions, such as intrarenal arterial stenosis, small vessel vasculitis, and visceral vascular malformations. Catheter-directed vascular procedures are mainly reserved for therapeutic purposes. Vascular interventional procedures in the pediatric age group have come a long way since the earliest cardiovascular intervention of balloon atrial septostomy in patient of congenital heart disease. The advancement of catheter and wire technology has made it increasingly possible for complex vascular interventions to be performed in children, including embolization, angioplasty with stent insertion, thrombolysis, and endovascular neurological procedures. Children are not merely "little adults" nor are the diseases to which they are particularly susceptible, variants of diseases in adult life. Excessive crying, unwillingness for examination, and their inability to describe complaints make a child the most difficult patient. Vascular access route and techniques are also vastly different as compared to adult patients considering the small size of these vessels. Special considerations in children include the use of appropriate equipment and adequate dosing of contrast and of the various medications used during angiography, particularly in patients <15 kg in weight. However, it is a challenge to the pediatric interventionist to master the art of "talking" and achieve a successful examination. A friendly environment, affectionate attitude of the medical staff, and a carefully and rapidly performed study go a long way in conducting a successful procedure.

SPECIAL CONSIDERATIONS FOR THE PEDIATRIC PATIENT

A discussion between the interventional radiologist and referring physician ensures that the appropriate procedure is performed, the risks for the particular patient are appreciated, and the likely benefit to accrue to the patient is understood. It is particularly imperative to pay special attention to the following details while conducting a pediatric angiography or intervention. These are:

- Vascular access
- Choice of sedation or anesthesia
- Maintenance of temperature control
- Fluid balance
- Radiation safety
- Equipment selection

A dedicated team consisting of the operating radiologist, the radiation and hemodynamic technologists, and the nursing attendant are needed to prepare the catheterization laboratory, prepare and handle the patient, and assist during the procedure. A high-resolution digital angiography system is required to obtain reliable diagnostic images quickly and to monitor the interventional procedure.

Patient Preparation

History and Physical Examination

A detailed discussion on the patient's history taking and examination relevant to general as well as specific angiographic interventional procedures is outside the scope of this chapter. **Box 1** lists the several components that need to be assessed while evaluating the patient.

Informed Consent

The parent or guardian of a minor child, and when possible, the patient himself, should understand the reasons for undergoing the procedure, the risks and benefits, the consequences of refusing the procedure, and the alternative therapies available. He or she should then give consent for the procedure.

Coagulation

Whenever there is a bleeding diathesis, risk of hemorrhage, or a plan to perform systemic thrombolysis, coagulation studies are obtained. Blood is sent for grouping and cross-matching whenever there is ongoing or expected blood loss. Heparin is administered for arterial catheterization procedures in a dose

BOX 1: Preprocedure clinical evaluation of the patient.

- History of the current problem
- Pertinent medical and surgical history
- *Review of the organ systems:*
  - Cardiac
  - Pulmonary
  - Renal
  - Hepatic
  - Hematologic (e.g., coagulopathy, hypercoagulable state)
  - Endocrine (diabetes)
- History of allergies
- Current medications
- Directed physical examination

of 50 U/kg for diagnostic and 100 U/kg for revascularization procedures.

Anesthesia

Most diagnostic studies are carried out with intravenous (IV) sedation. Difficult interventions such as device implantation or particularly painful procedures are conducted under general anesthesia.

In most children, conscious sedation is used, in which the child is conscious, drowsy, and may even close his eyes, but is responsive to verbal commands and able to protect his reflexes and airway. Midazolam is a commonly used, short-acting benzodiazepine that is metabolized by the liver. Its dose is 0.2–1 mg/kg body weight (KBW) IV. The onset of action is 3–5 minutes and the duration of action is 60 minutes. The major side effects are respiratory depression and apnea. A combination of three drugs namely, (1) demerol (50 mg), (2) promethazine (12.5 mg), and (3) triclofos (12.5 mg), known as DPT, are the other agent used for conscious sedation. A mixture of the three is made into a 2-mL solution to be given in a dose of 0.06–0.1 mL/KBW intramuscular (IM). For deeper sedation, a combination of diazepam (0.1 mg/KBW) and morphine (0.1 mg/KBW) may be given IV. Respiratory depression may occur with higher doses.

Patient Immobilization and Appropriate Positioning

An extremely important aspect of obtaining vascular access relates to taking the time and effort to position the baby. This can be particularly challenging when procedure is undertaken using conscious sedation without general anesthesia. For femoral access, it helps greatly to elevate the pelvis and hips of the child using a small roll. The limbs should be abducted slightly and laterally rotated. Smaller children are immobilized on a restraining board. Older children will have hand and leg restraints but, if uncooperative, will need to be anesthetized.

Temperature Control

Neonates and especially premature babies may become hypothermic if a warm operating environment is not maintained. The room temperature should be increased, radiation heaters are required, and the child should be covered quickly while preparing the groin and draping.

TABLE 1: Ratio of radiation dose to the skin in relation to age.

Age (in years)	1	5	10	15
Angiography—20 films	1.4	3.0	4.8	7.5
Fluoroscopy—4 minutes	3.2	4.8	6.8	8.8

Diet and Medications

Small children need not to be kept fasting for >3–4 hours prior to the procedure. Routine antibiotics are not prescribed except for high-risk procedures, e.g., splenic embolization.

Dose of Radiation and Fluids

Gordon I et al.[1] calculated and published the ratio of radiation dose to the skin (in rads) for various procedures that is given in **Table 1**.

One must try and minimize the radiation exposure to children who are believed to be more sensitive to the effects of radiation and likely to live for many years with these effects. Digital systems probably do not reduce radiation exposure. However, several precautions may be taken by the operator to reduce the dose. Fluoroscopy at the lowest dose possible (reduce the mAS), pulsed fluoroscopy, removing the scatter grids, and addition of rare earth filters in the X-ray tubes help to reduce radiation doses to the patient.

All fluids and medication must be scaled to the patient size. One may easily administer excessive amounts of fluids and contrast without realizing it. Digital systems (more so with biplane angiography systems) help to bring down the volume of contrast material and speeding up procedures. Most infants can tolerate 4 mL/kg of contrast whereas children over 6 months can tolerate 6 mL/kg, if it is delivered as several injections spread over a period of time. It is important to maintain patient hydration if such large doses are employed.

TECHNIQUES

Vascular procedures in pediatric patients require a substantially different approach than that used in the adult population. Many considerations must be taken into account when treating the pediatric population, including the small caliber vessel size, anticipation of spasm, the risk for infection, the propensity for children to rapidly form collateral circulation, the inevitability of growth, and the strong tendency for restenosis and growth arrest to occur.

Access

Introducer sheaths should be used to preserve vascular access, since multiple catheters/guidewire insertions or exchanges may be needed. Micropuncture access set and special pediatric access sheaths are available in 4–6 F sizes. These are usually introduced by using a cannula (18–21 G) and a 0.021" guidewire. The angle of entry of the needle should be less perpendicular to the skin and a small nick in the skin with the blade should be given before introducing the sheath to prevent pain and a possible vasovagal reaction. Care should be taken to prevent an inadvertent incision in the anterior vessel wall while using the blade.

PROCEDURES

The major vascular interventional procedures performed in children can be grouped into:

- Embolization
- Angioplasty
- Thrombolysis
- Foreign body removal

Embolization

Percutaneous transcatheter embolization has replaced surgery for many pediatric vascular problems and is a treatment alternative in patients where surgery has little to offer. Microcatheter systems, which were initially developed for adult neurovascular interventions, are ideal for pediatric applications. They permit access to small vessels and territories that were previously inaccessible. Hydrophilic-coated steerable guidewires permit negotiation of complex vascular loops without provoking spasm or causing dissection.

Embolization procedures should only be performed by experienced physicians familiar with the equipment and technical aspects of the procedure. Discussion with the pediatric physicians or surgeons, their support, and backup is essential for a safe and successful procedure.

The various pediatric vascular conditions treated by using embolotherapy can be grouped as follows:

- Vascular anomalies, e.g., arteriovenous malformation (AVM), arteriovenous fistula (AVF), venous malformation (VM), lymphatic malformation (LM), and hemangioma
- Hemorrhage from bleeding vessels (due to pseudo-aneurysms or vascular involvement in trauma, tumor, or inflammation) in various organ systems
- Other conditions, e.g., tumors and organ ablation

Goals of embolotherapy include: (i) An adjunctive goal, e.g., preoperative, adjunct to chemotherapy, or radiation therapy, (ii) A curative goal, e.g., definitive treatment such as that performed in cases of aneurysms, AVFs, AVMs, and traumatic bleeding, and (iii) A palliative goal, e.g., relieving symptoms, such as of a large AVM, which cannot be cured by using embolotherapy alone.

Embolization Materials and Substances

Materials used in embolization include coils, ethanol, sodium tetradecyl sulfate, n-butyl cyanoacrylate (NBCA) glue, polyvinyl alcohol (PVA) particles, microspheres, and gelatin sponge (Gelfoam).

Vascular Anomalies

Vascular anomalies are grouped into two categories: (1) Hemangiomas and (2) Vascular malformations. Vascular malformations are categorized further as high-flow lesions (AVM, AVF), low-flow lesions (capillary malformation, VM, and LM), or combined vascular malformations. Embolotherapy with a variety of embolic materials is commonly used in the treatment of vascular anomalies.

Hemangioma

Hemangiomas are benign tumors that require no treatment in most patients. Most of the uncomplicated hemangioma undergoes spontaneous involution with a small proportion of cases requiring intervention. These are children with lesions in life-threatening locations, local complications like hemorrhage, ulceration and necrosis, and functional or cosmetic disfigurements. Systemic corticosteroids have been the first line of treatment for many years. Recently, nonselective beta-blockers, such as oral propranolol and topical timolol, have emerged as promising and safer therapies.[2] In rare cases, embolization may be necessary (particularly in patients in whom therapy is needed urgently) because of spontaneous hemorrhage or functional abnormality caused by the extreme size of the lesion or the particular anatomic location or because of significant congestive heart failure.[3] In addition, embolotherapy is considered useful prior to surgical resection in selected patients and in patients in whom a hemangioendothelioma causes Kasabach–Merritt phenomenon (platelet trapping).[3] Embolotherapy of a hemangioma or hemangioendothelioma can be performed with the use of PVA particles. Coils are infrequently used since they cause more proximal occlusion with potential for recruitment of supply from other arteries and they block future access to the lesion if needed.

The goal of embolotherapy is to block a large percentage of the tumoral vessels, thereby preventing further trapping and destruction of the platelets and hastening involution of the lesion. Some tumors may require several sessions of embolotherapy because of revascularization of the tumor or to prevent exceeding the limits of radiation and contrast burden in one session. Infantile hepatic hemangioendotheliomas, a variant of infantile hemangioma, usually are multiple and frequently are complicated by congestive heart failure. In the clinical setting, the goal of embolotherapy is to reduce hepatic arterial flow, which sufficiently relieves high-output cardiac failure. A variety of embolic materials have been used. In some patients, embolization of other nearby arteries (e.g., intercostals) may also be necessary.[4] Arterial portography should be performed to exclude the possibility of feeders from the portal system.

A rare entity called noninvoluting hemangioma, which is found in the adult population, may also respond to transcatheter embolization (usually with particles such as PVA or microspheres). This procedure is usually performed to improve the cosmetic appearance.

Arteriovenous Malformation

Arteriovenous malformations are typically characterized by a nidus of abnormal vessels in which shunting of arterial blood to veins occurs. These vascular anomalies are usually present during childhood, but often demonstrate a sudden increase in size in response to trauma, hormones, or other stimuli. Although a clinical grading system has been used among surgeons, no grading system has been developed for imaging. Most AVMs can be managed by transcatheter embolization and/or sclerotherapy. Some focal AVMs can be treated by surgical excision. Proximal embolization or ligation of the feeding arteries usually worsen matters because of subsequent recruitment of collaterals and transluminal embolization of the nidus cannot be performed afterward. The collaterals that develop are more problematic in terms of transcatheter treatment; however, proximal embolization of the feeding arteries may be performed if indicated prior to surgical excision.

Whenever possible during primary embolotherapy, the nidus should be embolized.[3] Absolute alcohol is the most effective agent in the treatment of AVMs. If the nidus cannot be reached through the feeding arteries, direct percutaneous cannulation of the nidus can be attempted. In selected patients with AVMs, another therapeutic approach is embolic occlusion of the venous outflow.

Cervicofacial Arteriovenous Malformations

For dental arcade AVMs, spontaneous or catastrophic hemorrhage during tooth extraction is a common presentation. Embolization of an AVM in this region requires superselective catheterization of the involved branches of external carotid artery and other regional arterial branches (e.g., thyrocervical trunk) using microcatheters and the coaxial technique.[5]

Embolotherapy can be performed with NBCA, alcohol, particles, and/or microcoils, depending on the nature and extent of the malformation. Gelfoam can also be used for preoperative embolization. Patients with dental AVMs associated with acute bleeding and loose teeth should undergo embolization immediately prior to tooth extraction. Possible complications of embolotherapy of cervicofacial AVMs include stroke, nerve paralysis, skin necrosis, infection, blindness, and pulmonary embolism.

Extremity Arteriovenous Malformations

In the extremities, AVMs can be diffuse and may involve the entire extremity (Parkes-Weber syndrome). Extremity AVMs typically present with extremity-length discrepancy, high cardiac output, pain, and ulceration. Extremity lesions can be treated with multiple embolizations[5] and/or surgical resections or amputation of the extremity **(Figs. 1A and B)**.

A detailed pre-embolization angiographic examination is important for mapping the feeders and draining veins. During the injection of contrast material, the injection rate and duration should be adjusted so that arteriovenous connections can be identified accurately. A high injection rate in a short period is appropriate for AVMs.

Selective catheterization with microcatheters is required to reach the nidus of the AVM. Significant complications of embolotherapy possibly include skin necrosis (blisters), nontarget embolization (which also includes pulmonary emboli), and systemic sclerosant toxicity if a liquid agent (e.g., alcohol) is used.

Pulmonary Arteriovenous Malformations

Pulmonary AVMs are also called pulmonary AVFs. They have a high association with Osler-Weber-Rendu syndrome (also called hereditary hemorrhagic telangiectasia syndrome). Symptoms may include dyspnea, cyanosis, and clubbing. Paradoxical embolization may cause stroke or brain abscess. This anomaly can be classified as simple or complex on the basis of the number of feeders and draining veins. In simple lesions, a single artery and vein are involved; in complex lesions, two or more supplying arteries and one or more draining veins are involved.

Most pulmonary AVMs (80%) are simple. Although a surgical approach (thoracotomy and resection) is the traditional mode of therapy, transcatheter embolization is currently a preferred alternative.[6] Transcatheter embolization offers significantly reduced morbidity and mortality rates, particularly in hereditary hemorrhagic telangiectasia syndrome.

Embolotherapy for AVMs can be performed with coils, vascular plugs, or detachable balloons. Possible complications of embolotherapy include nontarget embolization in the systemic circulation (through the AVM shunt) or in other noninvolved pulmonary arteries. Therefore, properly sizing the coil to the feeding (afferent) artery is essential. A preliminary detailed angiography is essential for mapping the feeders and draining veins, paying particular attention to the size of the feeders. Basically, a successful embolization is accomplished by nesting one or more coils in the feeding artery, which occludes flow through the AVM shunt **(Figs. 2A and B)**.

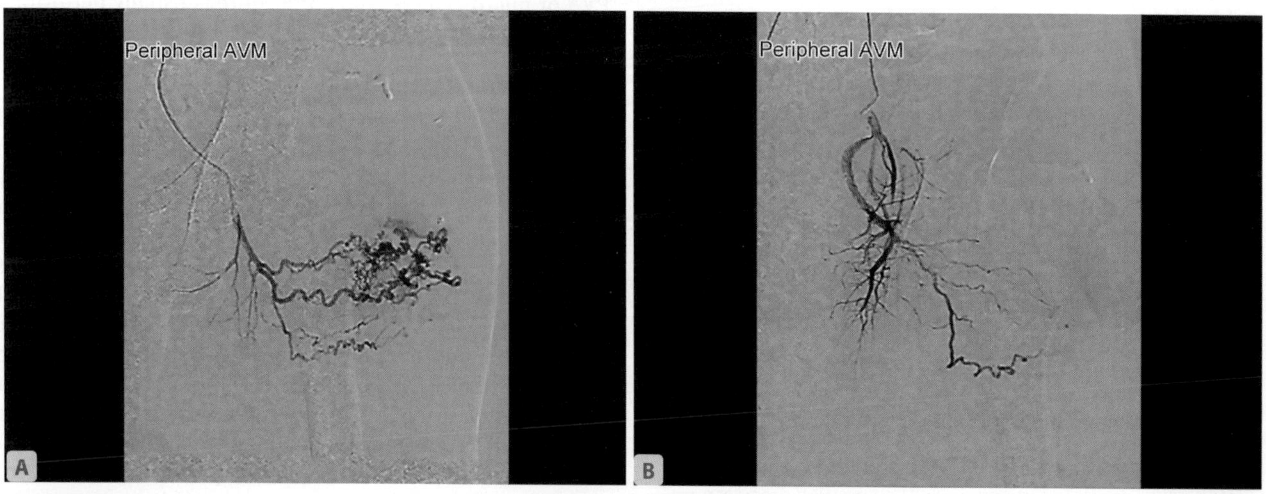

FIGS. 1A AND B: An arteriovenous malformation (AVM) of the left gluteal region, with feeders from the superior gluteal branch (left internal iliac artery, posterior branch): (A) Pre- and (B) postembolization [using n-butyl cyanoacrylate (NBCA)] angiograms.

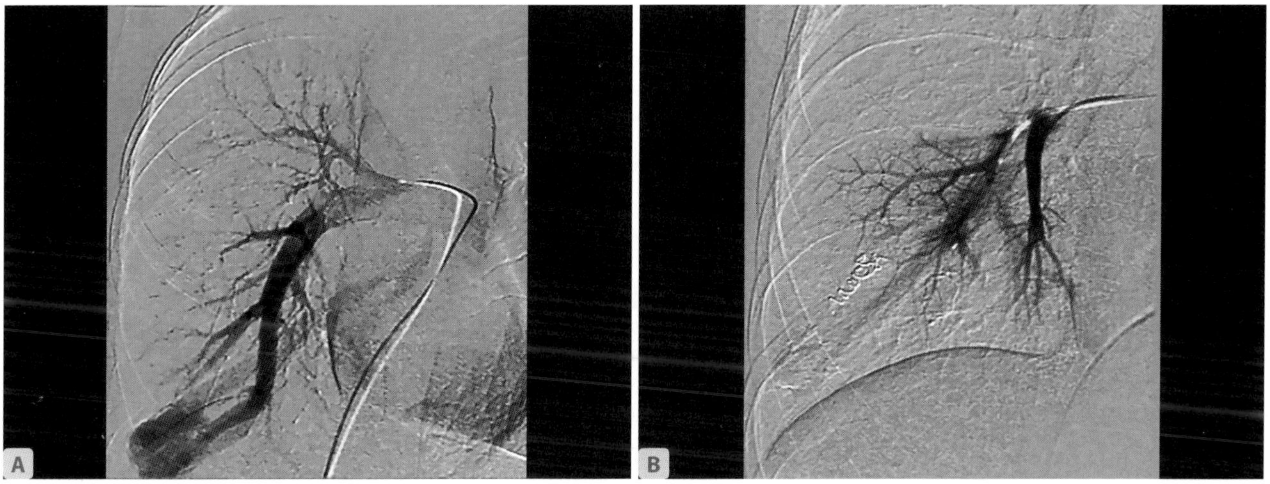

FIGS. 2A AND B: Right lower lobe pulmonary arteriovenous malformation. (A) Pre- and (B) postembolization (fibered platinum coils for smaller feeder and vascular plug for large feeder) angiograms.

Generally, feeding arteries >3 mm should be embolized. Feeders <3 mm have low risk of paradoxical embolization and should be left alone unless they are simple and straightforward technically. A coil that is 2–3 mm larger than the feeding artery is usually selected. For vascular plug, a 30–50% oversizing is recommended. If the feeding artery is large in caliber (>12 mm), a balloon occlusion of the proximal artery via a second groin puncture can be used for a more controlled coil deployment. Postembolization syndrome can occur and is characterized by pleuritic chest pain, pleural fluid, atelectasis, fever, and leukocytosis.

Arteriovenous Fistula

Arteriovenous fistulas are relatively large arteriovenous connections and may be congenital or secondary to trauma, surgery, or underlying vascular abnormality (e.g., neurofibromatosis). AVFs may be seen in any part of the body. A patient may present with cardiac failure, localized growth disturbances, neurologic deficits, and ischemic changes. Unlike AVMs, AVFs can be cured with embolotherapy. The embolotherapy technique used depends on the size, location, and hemodynamics of individual lesions. The goal of embolotherapy is to occlude the fistula and the immediate draining vein.

Embolization can be achieved by using detachable coils or balloons or tissue adhesives (glue or Onyx). Gelfoam or particles are not appropriate for use in AVF embolization. Detachable coils[7] or balloons are ideal because these embolic materials can be positioned optimally before they are detached. Balloons also have the advantage of conforming to the size and shape of the abnormal vessels. Microcoils can be dislodged; however, this complication can be minimized by performing flow-control techniques [e.g., balloon occlusion, tourniquet, or blood pressure (BP) cuff control]. The other disadvantage of coil embolization is that the clot that forms around the coil may dissolve, resulting in recanalization. Appropriate nesting of several coils (packing) can minimize recanalization. Also, thrombosis can be augmented by soaking the coils in thrombin before deployment or by injecting sclerosants around the coils. If adequate coil packing cannot be accomplished, tissue adhesive can be effectively used in combination with coils. Covered stents can also be particularly useful for acquired AVFs (single communications). They have the advantage of maintaining patency of the parent artery. Often, a combined strategy using different techniques is necessary.

Venous Malformation

Venous malformations are the most common type of vascular malformations and can vary significantly in size and clinical presentation. These lesions (usually distinguished by a bluish discoloration with swelling and pain) may also be associated with systemic syndromes such as blue rubber bleb nevus syndrome or Maffucci syndrome. Sinus pericranii (communication between intracranial and extracranial venous drainage) is also commonly associated with craniofacial VMs. These lesions can be treated with embolotherapy (sclerotherapy) and/or surgical excision.[8,9] The type of treatment used depends on the morphology, size, and location of the malformation.

A preliminary venogram is usually obtained to evaluate the deep venous system and to determine if any communication exists between the VM and the extremity veins. In particular, a venogram is performed on extremity VMs. The lesion is localized by using ultrasonography and the largest-appearing cystic portion of the lesion is selected. Then, the lesion is accessed by using real-time ultrasonographic guidance and a small angiocatheter needle (typically, 20–22 G). The lesion is studied with contrast agent injections under fluoroscopy as well as digital subtraction angiography (DSA). Subsequently, sclerotherapy is performed by using ethanol (absolute alcohol) or sodium tetradecyl sulfate mixed with a contrast medium (ethiodol or iodinated contrast) under real-time fluoroscopic control **(Figs. 3A and B)**. Foam sclerotherapy is a technique where a mixture of room air and sclerosant is injected and potentially results in greater agent-malformation contact and lowers volume of sclerosant required.

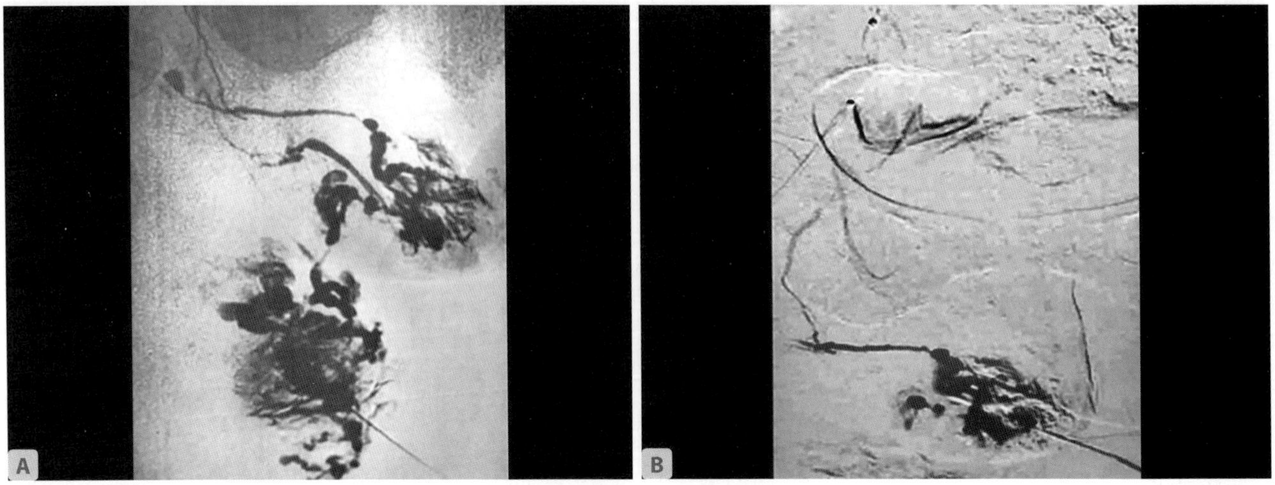

FIGS. 3A AND B: A diffuse venous malformation in the right thigh. (A) Direct puncture venogram showed minimal flow into deep veins; and (B) Sodium tetradecyl sulfate was slowly injected under fluoroscopic control. Successful occlusion of the malformation was achieved.

If draining veins are present (as they commonly are), manual compression or a tourniquet should be used to reduce washout of the sclerosant material from the malformation. If large draining veins are present, these veins can be embolized with coils via a percutaneous approach before sclerotherapy. For large head and neck VMs, airway involvement can be a challenging component of the condition in terms of treating the patients. Because alcohol and sodium tetradecyl sulfate cause significant edema after sclerotherapy, airway patency should be carefully monitored during and after the sclerotherapy procedure. In patients with large head and neck VMs requiring surgical debulking, presurgical sclerotherapy with NBCA glue can be performed because NBCA causes no significant edema.

Two common problems associated with sclerotherapy include skin necrosis (blisters) and/or nerve damage or paralysis. Nerve damage or paralysis can result from the direct toxic effect of the sclerosant agent and/or compression of the nerve by focal compartmental tissue edema (compartment syndrome). In addition, hemoglobinuria is a relatively common complication; this is treated by aggressive hydration and alkalinization. A less common but more severe complication is cardiac toxicity resulting from the systemic effect of absolute alcohol.

Lymphatic Malformation

Lymphatic malformations can be grouped as microcystic, macrocystic, and mixed. The mixed form of anomaly is probably the most common form of LM. Lymphatic cysts contain lymphatic fluid. When a single cystic mass (previously termed cystic hygroma when found in the neck) or a conglomerate mass containing a few macrocysts is encountered, surgical excision is considered the most effective treatment. However, some lesions respond really well to sclerotherapy without any complications after one or several sclerotherapy sessions.

When a mixed form of LM is encountered, the best therapeutic approach may be sclerotherapy for cystic masses, followed by surgical debulking. The microcystic LM or the microcystic component of the mixed form does not contain cystic spaces on radiologic studies (including MRI). It demonstrates a characteristic contrast-enhanced pattern of rings and arcs. The sclerosant agents most commonly used are antibiotics (doxycycline), ethanol, sodium tetradecyl sulfate and, most recently, OK-432 (a derivative of group A streptococci). For patients older than 8 years, doxycycline is the most commonly used sclerosant agent. If the patient is younger than 8 years, the options are alcohol, sodium tetradecyl sulfate, or OK-432. The amount of alcohol used depends on the patient's weight, which is a limiting factor in most procedures involving alcohol.

The interventional therapeutic approach used for LMs is similar to the sclerotherapy technique used for VMs; however, an initial venogram is usually unnecessary.

Hemorrhage

Several types of hemorrhage can be treated with embolization. Examples include hemoptysis, epistaxis, and gastrointestinal (GI) tract, post-traumatic, and iatrogenic hemorrhage (e.g., postbiopsy or nephrostomy tube insertion).

Gastrointestinal Hemorrhage

Major causes of upper GI tract hemorrhage are ulcer disease, gastritis and varices. The most common causes of a lower GI tract hemorrhage are vascular malformations and bleeding after endoscopic biopsy. If the bleeding source is identified on arterial angiogram, the patient is treated by using either intra-arterial vasopressin infusion (Pitressin) or embolization of the bleeding mesenteric artery. Embolization is usually the first line of treatment in patients with upper GI tract bleeding and is used as the second line of treatment in patients with lower GI tract bleeding (usually used if vasopressin treatment fails).[10]

Embolization in the arcades proximal to the bleeding vasa recta is recommended to minimize the risk of bowel necrosis. The most commonly used embolic agents are coils (macrocoils or microcoils) and Gelfoam pieces (torpedoes).

Coil embolization is particularly helpful if the bleeding is caused by focal vascular abnormalities such as a false aneurysm. Some interventional radiologists have also used PVA, although the use of PVA or other particles should be avoided because of the risk of bowel infarction. After embolization, control angiography is performed to determine if bleeding (contrast material extravasation) continues via any collaterals. The primary advantage of embolotherapy is the immediate cessation of bleeding without need for prolonged catheterization (unlike vasopressin infusion therapy).

Pelvic Hemorrhage

Intractable pelvic hemorrhage, usually post-traumatic, should be approached in a similar interventional fashion. A surgical approach to control active bleeding in acute trauma setting is usually not favored. Detailed angiographic examination with superselective injections in the branches of the internal iliac artery is mandatory. Embolization can be performed by using an autologous blood clot, Gelfoam torpedoes, PVA particles, NBCA, coils, or detachable balloons.[11] At the capillary level, embolization with small particles or Gelfoam powder is contraindicated (because of the elimination of collateral flow, which results in massive tissue necrosis).

A specific anatomic relationship between the fracture site and the affected vessel often allows embolization of the branch (frequently the obturator artery) even when no obvious bleeding site is detected.[12] In particular, liquid or particle embolization of the inferior gluteal branch of the anterior division should be avoided to minimize the possibility of sciatic nerve injury (this branch supplies muscles of the thigh and buttocks and the sciatic nerve). In addition, embolization of the posterior division of the internal iliac artery should be avoided because of the risk of gluteal necrosis.

Hemoptysis

Hemoptysis is considered massive when at least 300 mL of blood is lost in <24 hours and it may be life-threatening. Common causes of massive hemoptysis are cystic fibrosis, bronchiectasis, tuberculosis, and aspergillosis. Malignancy is rarely a cause. Surgical intervention is usually not feasible because of severe pulmonary disease; therefore, embolization of the bleeding bronchial arteries can be lifesaving.[13]

Bronchial arteries are variable. They usually arise from the descending thoracic aorta between thoracic vertebrae T4 and T7. The right bronchial artery arises from the intercostobronchial trunk in most patients (>90%). The left bronchial artery usually arises directly from the aorta and is multiple in most patients. Occasionally, the right and left bronchial arteries arise from a common trunk.

Although some bronchial branches may supply the spinal cord, the most important of these branches is the artery of Adamkiewicz. This artery usually arises from an intercostal or lumbar artery on the left. Other spinal branches from the right intercostobronchial artery, thyrocervical, or costocervical arteries may be identified. A preliminary thoracic aortogram may be performed, which usually shows abnormal bronchial arteries. An aortogram helps in outlining the bronchial anatomy.

Because of potential source of collaterals, a subclavian arteriogram also is obtained, particularly if the upper lung field is involved. Then, the bronchial arteries are catheterized and studied with selective injections. The most common appearance of the abnormal bronchial artery (the bleeding source) is increased caliber of the bronchial artery with some hypervascularity over the lung field. Contrast agent extravasation, shunting from bronchial to pulmonary arteries, or aneurysmal changes in the involved bronchial artery rarely are identified.

Embolotherapy is usually performed with particles (PVA or embospheres) and Gelfoam pledgets **(Figs. 4A and B)**. When the decision is made to use particles, appropriately-sized particles should be used. Sizes are usually 500–710 μm for PVA and 500–800 μm for embospheres. Use of coils is inappropriate and absolute alcohol or cyanoacrylate is no longer used for bronchial artery embolization because of the risk of tissue necrosis (bronchial and/or esophageal).

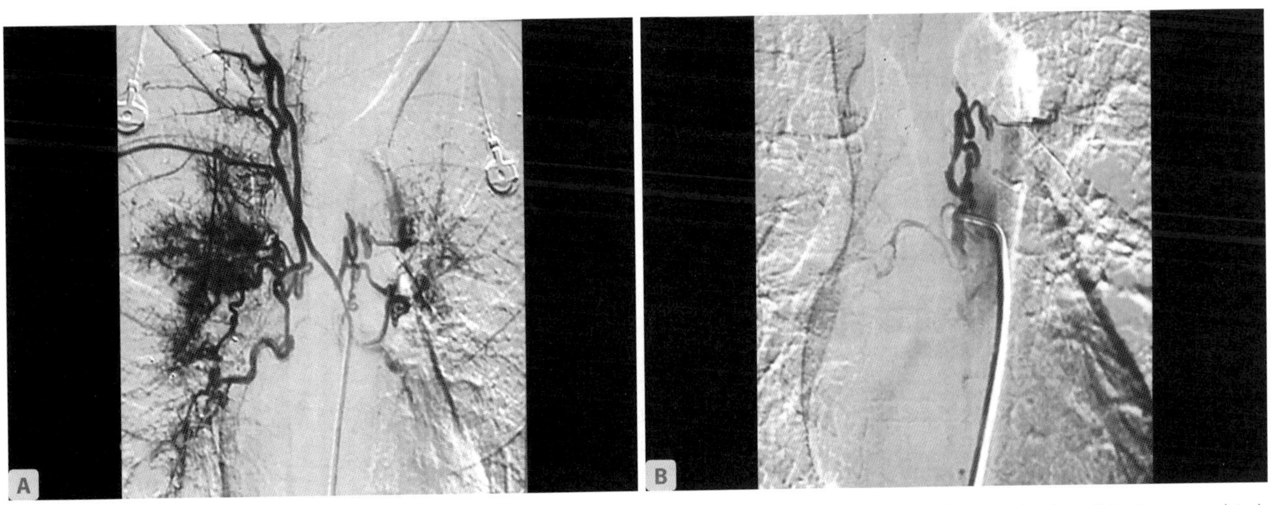

FIGS. 4A AND B: A patient with hemoptysis due to bronchiectasis in the right upper and middle lobe. (A) Selective injection of the hypertrophied right intercostobronchial trunk revealed multiple feeders with parenchymal blush; and (B) After embolization with polyvinyl alcohol (PVA) particles and Gelfoam, the culprit vessel is completely occluded.

Embolization is performed as selectively as possible (when necessary, by using a microcatheter and coaxial technique) to minimize tissue necrosis and nontarget embolization (e.g., spinal artery). Special care should be taken to prevent reflux by injecting the embolic material slowly under continuous fluoroscopic control. Gelfoam pledgets/torpedoes usually are used to occlude the abnormal artery more proximally after particle embolization.

Epistaxis

Intractable epistaxis is a nosebleed that does not respond to conservative treatment (nasal spraying of vasoconstrictors, nasal packing, and blood transfusion). Etiologies include uncontrolled hypertension with or without superficial mucosal abnormality (e.g., Osler-Weber-Rendu syndrome).

Epistaxis can be treated by either surgical means (e.g., cautery, vascular ligation) or endovascular embolotherapy. Internal carotid arteriograms are obtained to exclude aneurysms. Then, the external carotid artery is catheterized and control angiography is performed initially to map the vascular anatomy and to check for the presence of a collateral supply to the intracranial circulation.

During catheterization of the external carotid artery and its branches, vasospasm is a common problem. Nitroglycerin can be used to treat this. The target branch is usually the pterygopalatine division of the internal maxillary artery, which is distal to the origin of the meningeal and temporal arteries. By using a microcatheter, the pterygopalatine division is catheterized and embolized with particles (most commonly PVA). If bleeding is not caused by a neoplastic entity, embolotherapy can be performed in the 250–500 μm range. If a neoplastic entity is the cause, the capillary bed needs to be embolized. This embolization can be accomplished by using smaller particles (150–250 μm).

Although the procedure is considered safe if performed by an experienced physician, possible complications can occur. These include ischemia, pain, cranial nerve damage, blindness, and stroke.

Post-traumatic Hemorrhage

Post-traumatic hemorrhage can be due to either a blunt or penetrating injury to a vessel, typically arteries in the extremities with penetrating injuries or associated fractures or arteries to the organs (e.g., renal arteries, after blunt trauma). Some patients may present after an orthopedic procedure, such as total hip replacement. An angiographic study is mandatory, not only to aid selecting in the appropriate subsequent embolization procedure but also in planning for possible future surgical interventions.

Coil embolization is appropriate in extremity branch arteries responsible for the bleeding because it offers a fast and permanent occlusion of the vessel. The bleeding vessel should be embolized proximal and distal to the site of arterial injury. Avoid embolization of arteries that endangers limb viability. Hemorrhage or AVF formation after organ biopsy (particularly renal biopsy), or iatrogenic traumatic hemorrhage, is a common complication (i.e., iatrogenic traumatic hemorrhage) that can be treated with embolization **(Figs. 5A and B)**.

Pseudoaneurysm

Pseudoaneurysms occur secondary to trauma or infection and consist of leakage of blood into the confined perivascular space at the site of a vessel wall disruption. Embolization is a good alternative to surgical repair and is often the treatment of choice, especially when pseudoaneurysms are not accessible or when the patient is not a surgical candidate because of sepsis or other medical conditions.[14,15]

Embolic materials used for pseudoaneurysms include coils, detachable balloons, thrombin, Gelfoam, and NBCA **(Figs. 6A to C)**. In large-neck pseudoaneurysms, a stent placement combined with coil embolization has been described. If the involved vessel cannot be catheterized or if a pseudoaneurysm is close to the skin surface (typically a pseudoaneurysm in the groin after cardiac catheterization), the pseudoaneurysm can be directly punctured with a fine needle (e.g., 22 G) and thrombin or NBCA can be injected.

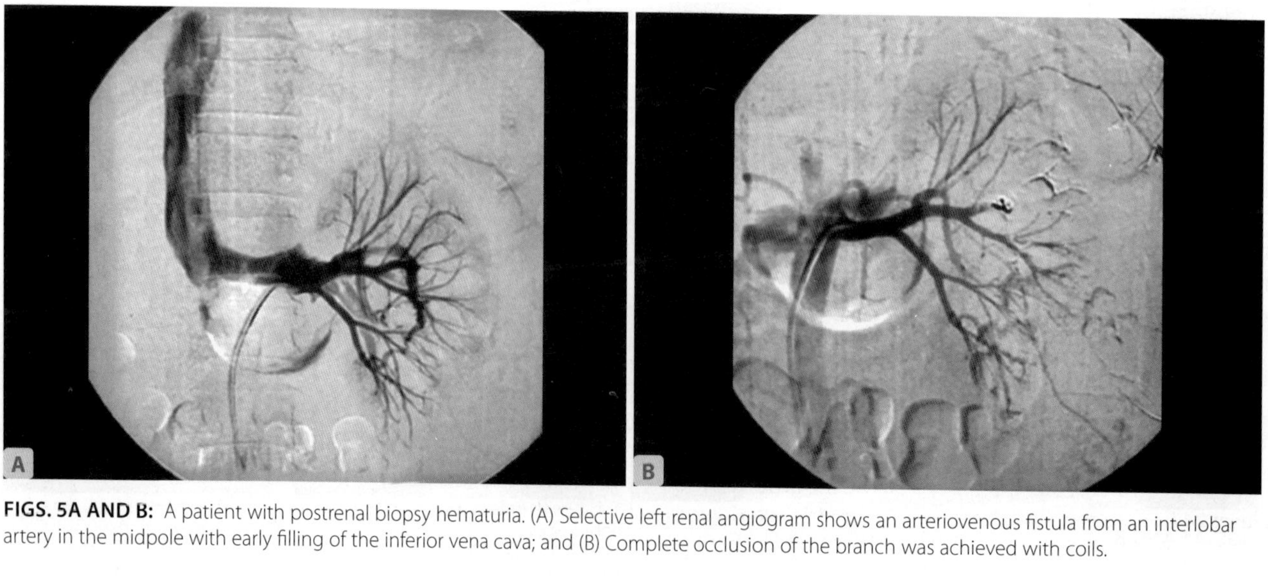

FIGS. 5A AND B: A patient with postrenal biopsy hematuria. (A) Selective left renal angiogram shows an arteriovenous fistula from an interlobar artery in the midpole with early filling of the inferior vena cava; and (B) Complete occlusion of the branch was achieved with coils.

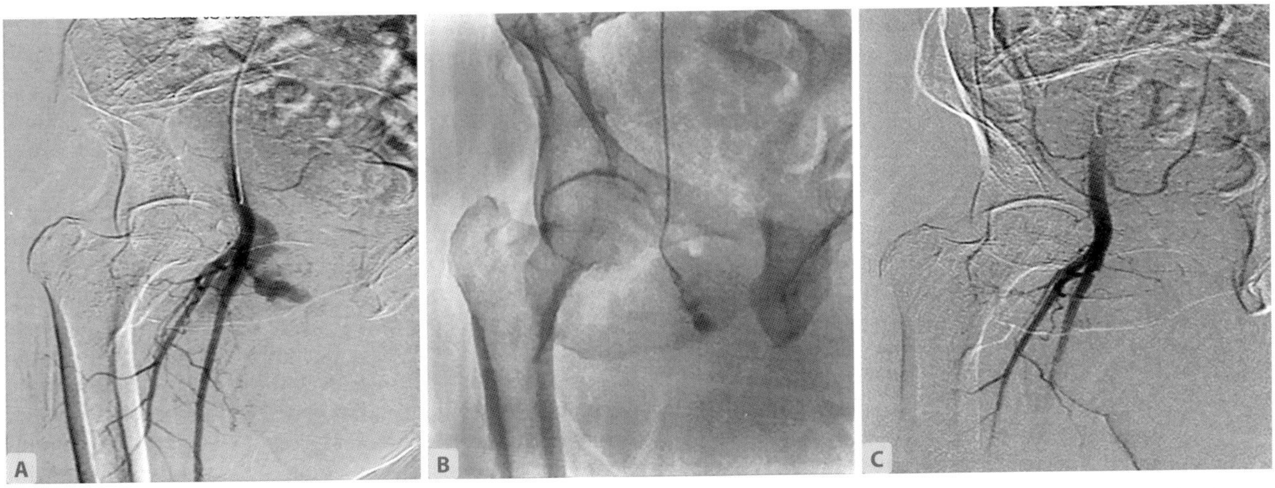

FIGS. 6A TO C: A postcatheterization pseudoaneurysm in the right groin. (A) Selective injections into the right common femoral artery showing pseudoaneurysm from proximal superficial femoral artery with small neck; (B) The neck was selectively cannulated and Gelfoam pledget was injected into neck; and (C) Postembolization angiogram—no filling of pseudoaneurysm.

When the involved artery is embolized with coils, the artery also should be embolized distal to the origin of the pseudoaneurysm so that collaterals do not fill the aneurysm.

Malignant Tumors

Indications for embolotherapy in neoplastic conditions include preoperative embolization and palliative embolization. Embolization helps alleviate symptoms, reduces further dissemination, and increases the response to other treatment modalities (e.g., radiation therapy). Embolotherapy can be used for many types of malignant tumors.[16] Renal malignancy is the most common type of tumor treated with embolotherapy. In particular, tumors extending into the hilum or other adjacent structures for which surgical removal is difficult are treated by using embolotherapy. In these patients, prior embolization of the tumor shrinks the mass and minimizes blood loss during surgical removal.

Unresectable tumors can be made operable by means of embolotherapy. If the entity is in its end-stage (disseminated metastatic deposits), the technique can be used for palliation to control pain and hematuria. Other reported malignancies in which embolotherapy has been used include pelvic malignancies and bone tumors. Hemorrhage resulting from malignancy or radiotherapy (e.g., due to radiation cystitis) can be controlled by using embolotherapy.

Chemoembolization

Chemoembolization is commonly performed in hepatic malignancies.[17] The technique is used in patients with unresectable liver tumors and metastatic liver disease. An essential prerequisite for chemoinfusion/chemoembolization is the presence of a patent portal vein with hepatopetal flow. The bilirubin level should be <3 mg/dL to perform chemoinfusion/chemoembolization safely.

Vigorous IV hydration is required before the procedure for at least 24 hours. Initially, a superior mesenteric arteriogram is usually obtained to demonstrate a variant origin of hepatic artery (accessory or replaced, originating from the superior mesenteric artery) and to demonstrate patency of the portal vein. Then, the celiac trunk and, subsequently, the common hepatic artery are catheterized and studied to outline the vascular anatomy.

The involved lobar hepatic artery or, more commonly, the first- or second-order branches of this artery is subsequently catheterized by using a microcatheter and the chemoinfusion material is injected under fluoroscopic guidance. The tip of the catheter must be placed distal to the cystic and gastroduodenal arteries. The most commonly used chemoinfusion mixture consists of 10 mL of iopamidol (Isovue), 20 mL of ethiodol, and 60 mg of doxorubicin. The chemoinfusion is usually followed by embolization with a slurry of gelatin sponge powder (Gelfoam).

Lidocaine is intra-arterially administered to reduce pain after the chemoinfusion/chemoembolization treatment.

Organ Ablation

Splenic embolization can be used as a preoperative therapy or as an alternative to surgical removal of the spleen. Indications include post-traumatic bleeding, variceal bleeding secondary to portal hypertension or splenic vein thrombosis, hypersplenism, thalassemia major, thrombocytopenia, idiopathic thrombocytopenic purpura, Gaucher's disease, and Hodgkin's disease. Embolotherapy is performed with superselective catheterization/embolization of the splenic artery by using embolic particles while the tip of the catheter is beyond the caudal pancreatic artery. Careful fluoroscopic control of the splenic area is required to limit the total infarction to approximately 60% of the spleen.

Renal embolization is an alternative to surgical removal of the kidney and indications include end-stage renal disease or renovascular hypertension (RVH) requiring unilateral or bilateral nephrectomy and renal transplant with native kidneys in situ. The procedure requires selective catheterization of the renal artery with further advancement of the catheter, so that the catheter is wedged or with the use of a balloon occlusion catheter to minimize the possibility of embolic material spillage into the aorta. The preferred embolic agents are particles (e.g., PVA) and/or liquid agents such as ethanol or NBCA. Postinfarction syndrome is relatively common and characterized by pain, which can be managed with narcotics. This pain usually subsides within 48–72 hours.

Angioplasty

The techniques for balloon dilatation of vascular stenosis are the same for children as for adults. Balloon dilatation can be carried out safely even in small children and can permit access to peripheral stenoses. Small balloon catheters (2 mm) and small shaft catheters (3.8 F) can be used with 4 F delivery systems. Small steerable guidewires [e.g., 0.018" or 0.014" percutaneous transluminal coronary angioplasty (PTCA) wires] can be used to cross small distal stenosis. For the renal arteries, low profile balloons in diameters of 3–4 mm are employed. Larger balloons up to 20 mm in size are used to treat recurrent coarctation or peripheral pulmonary stenosis. High pressure balloons (up to 17 atm burst pressure) are available with smaller sizes for fibrous stenosis or restenotic lesions.

The major indications for angioplasty in children are:

- Renal artery stenosis (RAS)
- Aortic stenosis
- Coarctation of aorta
- Transplant renal artery stenosis
- Peripheral pulmonary stenosis
- Systemic-to-pulmonary artery shunt stenosis
- Budd-Chiari syndrome due to hepatic vein/inferior vena cava (IVC) stenosis.

Percutaneous transluminal renal angioplasty (PTRA) is the treatment of choice for RAS. Nonspecific aortoarteritis (NSAA) is responsible for 61% of RAS in our country. Other causes include fibromuscular dysplasia (28%), atherosclerosis (8%), polyarteritis nodosa (2.5%), and renal artery aneurysm of indeterminate etiology (0.5%). NSAA is a chronic and progressive panarteritis of unknown cause that commonly affects the aorta, its major branches, and the pulmonary arteries and results in stenosis, occlusion, dilatation, or formation of aneurysms in the involved blood vessels.[18,19] Stenosis or obstruction is the most common angiographic abnormality, frequently involving the aorta and the renal arteries, and resulting in systemic hypertension. The complexity of pathological changes in the wall of the aorta and widespread nature of involvement make surgical revascularization a very difficult option. There is also a high prevalence of graft occlusion. Due to these reasons, nonsurgical revascularization techniques have been increasingly used in the treatment of this group of patients.[20-22]

The goals of therapy in RVH include control of BP and restoration of renal blood flow. We accept the patients for treatment by nonsurgical revascularization if they have hypertension uncontrolled by single-drug therapy, angiographic evidence of at least 70% stenosis in the renal artery or the aorta with a pressure gradient of >20 mm Hg, and a normal erythrocyte sedimentation rate (ESR). Patients with an elevated ESR and/or a positive C-reactive protein test are considered to have an active arteritis and are not generally accepted for this treatment, except in certain situations (uncontrolled hypertension, severe ventricular dysfunction, flash pulmonary edema, and deteriorating renal function).

Antihypertensive medication is stopped 24 hours before angioplasty, except for sublingual administration of 5–10 mg nifedipine if the BP is >170/110 mm Hg. The patients are treated with aspirin (175–330 mg) daily for 3 days before angioplasty and this treatment is continued for 6 months after treatment. Heparin (100 IU/KBW) is given IV during the procedure and is not reversed afterward. BP medication is withheld for 24 hours after the procedure, except for sublingual administration of nifedipine (5–10 mg) if the BP is >160/100 mm Hg. If there is severe, uncontrolled hypertension before renal angioplasty, the BP is controlled with nitroprusside drip infusion.

For renal angioplasty, a pigtail catheter is positioned in the abdominal aorta above the origin of renal arteries for continuous pressure measurement and diagnostic DSA. The diseased renal artery is selectively catheterized through another arterial sheath in the opposite groin and trans-stenotic pressure gradient is measured. The angiographic catheter is replaced by a commercially available,

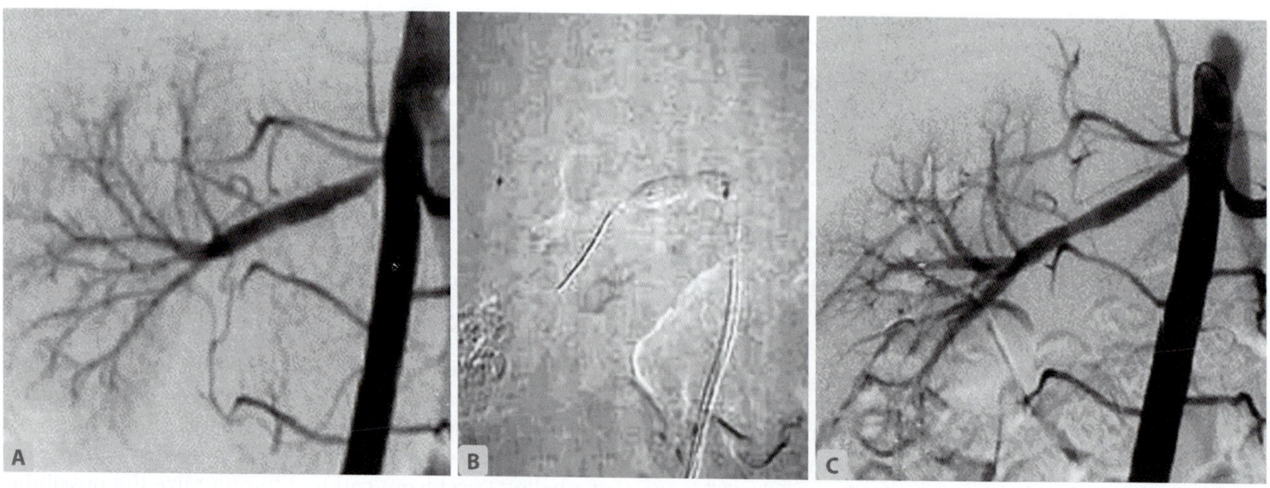

FIGS. 7A TO C: (A) A 12-year-old female with hypertension: Tight ostial stenosis of right renal artery due to aortoarteritis; (B) The right stenosis was treated with balloon angioplasty with a mild residual waist; and (C) The lesion opened up well with mild residual disease.

appropriate-sized balloon catheter by using standard exchange technique. The diameter of the involved vessel is measured and a balloon catheter of same size is used for angioplasty. Three to five inflations, for up to 45 seconds each, are performed until the balloon "waist" is no longer present or has decreased substantially **(Figs. 7A to C)**. We do not use oversized balloon catheters in patients with mild residual stenosis or trans-stenotic pressure gradients in order to avoid the risk of arterial rupture. Immediately after the procedure, trans-stenotic pressure is measured and an angiogram is obtained to assess the adequacy of angioplasty.

Alternatively, the procedure can be completed through a single groin approach too. After crossing the stenosis with the angiographic catheter, an 0.014" or 0.018" exchange guidewire is placed in a distal intrarenal branch and a 6 F or 7 F (depending upon the patient size) guiding (right coronary or renal double curve configuration) catheter is placed at the ostium of the diseased artery. The appropriately compatible balloon catheters (sometimes, PTCA balloons in monorail configuration may also be used) are then used to dilate the lesion. The advantage of this approach is the avoidance of a second puncture, although the cost of hardware increases.

If there is an obstructive dissection or a recurrent ostial stenosis, renal artery stent placement is considered. Pretreatment with ticlopidine (250 mg twice daily) beginning 3 days before angioplasty is then advisable. This should be continued for at least 6 weeks after the procedure. A preshaped renal guiding catheter is positioned at the ostium of the diseased renal artery over an exchange guidewire positioned in a secure distal location in the artery. The selection of the diameter and length of the stent is based on the angiographic morphology of the involved artery. It is advisable to give sublingual nifedipine (5–10 mg) or an intra-arterial bolus of trinitroglycerin (100–200 mg) in the renal artery before stent placement. The stent is positioned across the lesion and released by inflating the balloon at the desired inflation pressure for up to 30 seconds. Various stent designs are available for use in this location. Balloon-mounted stents are generally preferred for an ostial stenosis. A check angiogram is obtained at the end of the procedure to assess the adequacy of stent release. Intravascular ultrasound is a useful technique to define the endpoint of intervention. Angioplasty or stent placement in the aorta is performed by a similar technique.

Angioplasty is considered technically successful if: (i) The aortic or renal artery lumen after angioplasty has <30% residual stenosis, (ii) The arterial lumen is at least 50% larger than its pretreatment diameter, and (iii) The pressure gradient is <20 mm Hg and has decreased at least 15 mm Hg from the pretreatment gradient.

The clinical results of the angioplasty are judged as follows: (i) Cure (normal BP after the procedure without antihypertensive drug therapy), (ii) Improved (at least 15% reduction in diastolic pressure or a diastolic pressure <90 mm Hg with the patient taking less antihypertensive medication than before the procedure), and (iii) Failed (no change in BP after the procedure). All patients cured or improved are considered to have benefited from angioplasty. Follow-up is performed by BP and medication evaluation 1 day, 1 week, and 4–6 weeks after treatment and then at 6-month intervals. Follow-up angiograms are performed in patients with recurrence of hypertension, in whom contralateral nephrectomy of poorly or nonfunctioning kidney for residual hypertension is planned and in those patients who consent for the procedure. Angioplasty is repeated if restenosis is detected.

Percutaneous transluminal angioplasty (PTA) of the aortic stenosis in NSAA can also be carried out by a similar technique **(Figs. 8A to D)**. The angiographic features, including eccentricity of the stenosis and presence of diffuse adjacent

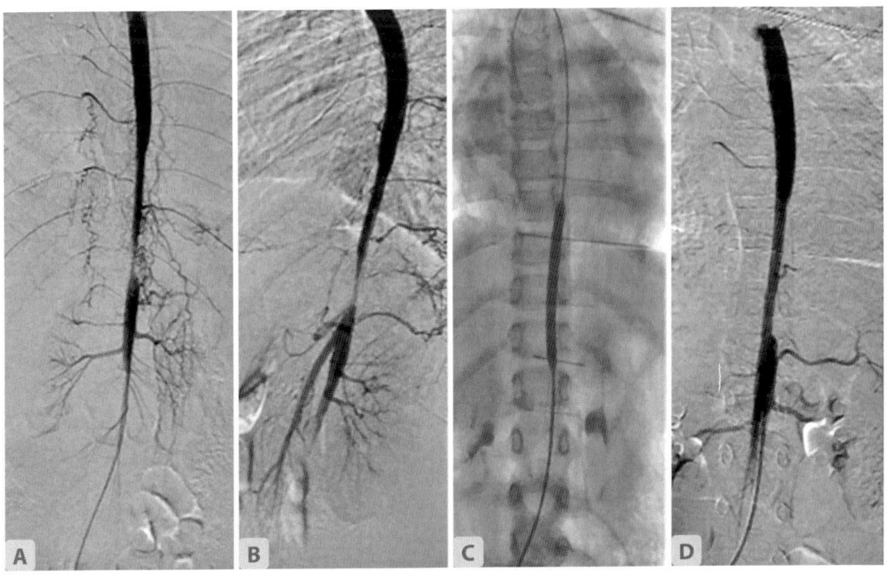

FIGS. 8A TO D: Supraceliac aortic stenosis (due to aortoarteritis) in a 12-year-old girl with severe left ventricular dysfunction. (A) Anteroposterior (AP) view; (B) Lateral view aortogram showing long segment tight stenosis of the supraceliac aorta; (C) Balloon angioplasty of the stenosed segment; and (D) Postangioplasty aortogram showing significant reduction of degree of stenosis with reduction of the trans-stenotic pressure gradient. The patient did well on clinical follow-up.

disease, location of the stenosis in juxtadiaphragmatic segment of the aorta, and presence of calcification, adversely affect the outcome of PTA, most of whom develop large intimal flaps. Stents have been occasionally used as a "bail-out" measure in salvaging an obstructive dissection in such situations and rarely electively in the treatment of native stenosis. Stents provide an immediate relief of symptomatic obstructive dissection and are also useful in the treatment of recurrent stenosis after successful angioplasty. We do not advocate elective use of stents due to young age of the patients, the cost involved, and lack of knowledge about the long-term behavior of stents in the aorta at a growing age. Until recently, it was felt that this disease is characterized by skip areas of involvement. The findings of recent studies, using cross-sectional imaging techniques, suggest that nonspecific aortitis involves a continuous length of the aorta, producing mural and luminal changes in some areas, and only mural changes in the intervening segments. This observation has therapeutic implications. The site of surgical reconstruction or balloon positioning in PTA is based on the demonstration of angiographically normal adjacent segments. The results of cross-sectional imaging suggest that there are extensive wall changes even in angiographically normal areas. The unpredictable outcome of PTA and surgical revascularization in nonspecific aortitis, in our opinion, is caused by the placement of a bypass graft or the balloon catheter within the diseased segments and not from normal to normal aortic segment. In this regard, intravascular ultrasound may be useful in guiding the interventional procedures. Overall, aortic PTA has specific technical problems but has a high technical and clinical success rate. The complication rate is low. Late remodeling occurs in most patients and is responsible for delayed clinical benefit, despite poor technical success in some patients.

Arterial stenosis associated with renal transplantation can often be improved. These obstructions may be at or beyond the suture line. It is important to evaluate the hemodynamic significance of proximal stenosis because in some of these patients, extensive peripheral disease due to rejection nullifies the benefit of dilating the proximal lesions.

Peripheral pulmonary artery stenosis can sometimes be treated effectively but at moderate risk. Because of the elasticity of pulmonary arteries, these lesions require large balloons for small increase in artery size. Arterial rupture can occur, resulting in death. Because there are no surgical options to treat these lesions, balloon dilatation is the procedure of choice when treatment is clinically indicated. Stenting is a safer and more effective approach to these lesions.

After the modified Blalock–Taussig (BT) shunt is placed, stenosis can develop in the subclavian artery, the proximal or distal anastomosis, the graft, or the pulmonary artery. All of these may be treated except the graft stenosis. The best results are obtained in those patients with a traditional BT shunt where the subclavian artery has been directly connected to the pulmonary artery, but this surgery is rarely performed nowadays. Most BT shunts are performed with Gore-Tex grafts, which limit the amount of stretching of the stenosis. Narrowing within the graft is probably caused by kinking, thrombosis, or fibrointimal proliferation.

Complications of Angioplasty Procedures

Vascular spasm can occur, particularly in PTRA, and may in turn provoke thrombosis and segmental infarction. About 100 U/kg of heparin is usually given to prevent this and more may be required for prolonged procedures. Monitoring of heparinization with measurements of activated clotting time (ACT) should be done. Spasm may be treated with direct intra-arterial injection of nitroglycerin (0.25–1.00 µg/kg/min).

Thrombosis may occur at the PTA site or at the groin. If it does, then thrombolytic therapy is indicated. Intimal dissection is part of any PTA procedure and usually does not cause flow obstruction. If an obstructive dissection develops, stents may be used. Vascular rupture is always a concern, but can be avoided by appropriate balloon selection.[23]

Thrombolysis

Experience with thrombolysis in children is limited but has increased because of the need to treat complications of cardiac or peripheral angiography or intervention. Procedures requiring insertion of devices mounted on large shafts are more likely to result in femoral artery thrombosis. The other indications include thrombosis of BT shunts, dialysis fistula, pulmonary artery thrombosis, iliofemoral thrombophlebitis, aortic thrombosis in neonates, and brachial artery occlusion after supracondylar fracture. Contraindications for the procedure include recent surgery or trauma (within the past 6 weeks), any intracranial or GI bleed within the past 3 months, renal failure, gangrene, or significant pregangrenous changes in the affected organ system or extremity.

Thrombolytic agents include streptokinase, urokinase, or recombinant tissue plasminogen activator (rtPA). Urokinase is the most commonly employed agent. Local low-dose therapy is unlikely to produce systemic changes in coagulation whereas systemic therapy may cause undesirable bleeding. The dose of urokinase for local low-dose infusion is 300–500 IU/kg/h. High dose, short duration treatment given locally often produces clearing of thrombus. Treatment failures usually relate to delays in implementing therapy, resulting in maturation of thrombus. The fibrinogen level, thrombin time, prothrombin time, and activated partial thromboplastin time are monitored at regular intervals and the children are observed in an intensive care unit or neonatal nursery. In patients with relatively high-risk of bleeding, combined pharmacomechanical thrombolysis may be considered as it significantly reduce the overall dose of thrombolytic agents and also reduce overall procedural time **(Figs. 9A and B)**.

Complications of intra-arterial thrombolysis include systemic bleeding (<5% cases), compartment syndrome due to extremity edema, tissue breakdown products entering systemic circulation causing renal shutdown, hyperkalemia causing cardiac arrhythmias, etc. Appropriate patient selection and preprocedure evaluation may help prevent these complications.[24]

Foreign Body Removal

Intravascular foreign bodies may result from the complex interventional hardware, monitoring systems, and indwelling

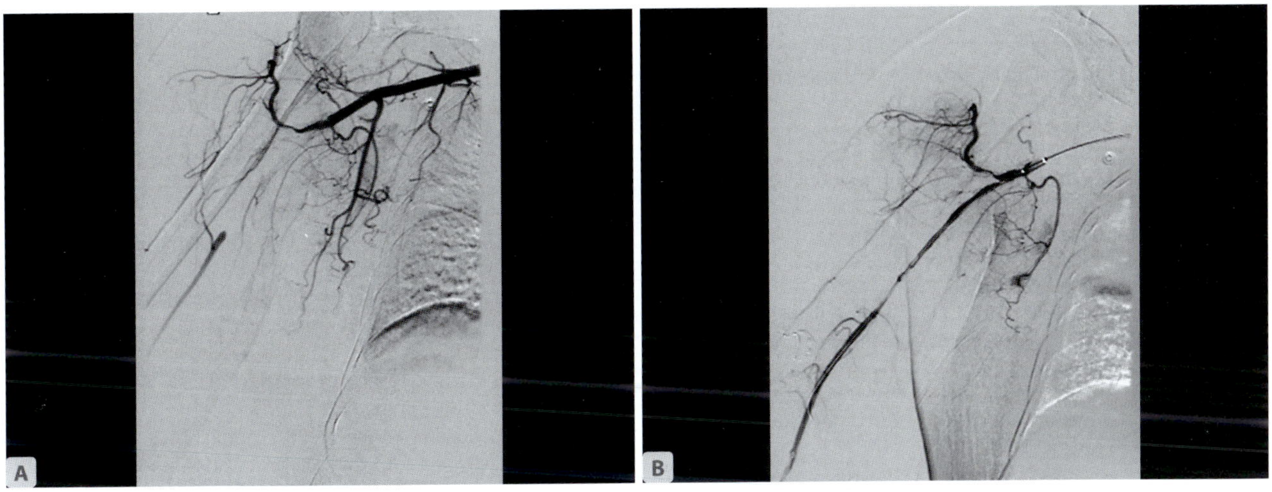

FIGS. 9A AND B: Acute thrombosis of right brachial artery (due to vasculitis) in an 11-year-old boy, presented with acute upper limb ischemia. (A) Right arm angiogram showing complete thrombotic occlusion of brachial artery in proximal part with reformation in distal part; and (B) Post pharmacomechanical thrombolysis, significant reduction in thrombus burden, with establishment of antegrade flow in brachial artery. Patient had significant clinical improvement of ischemic symptoms.

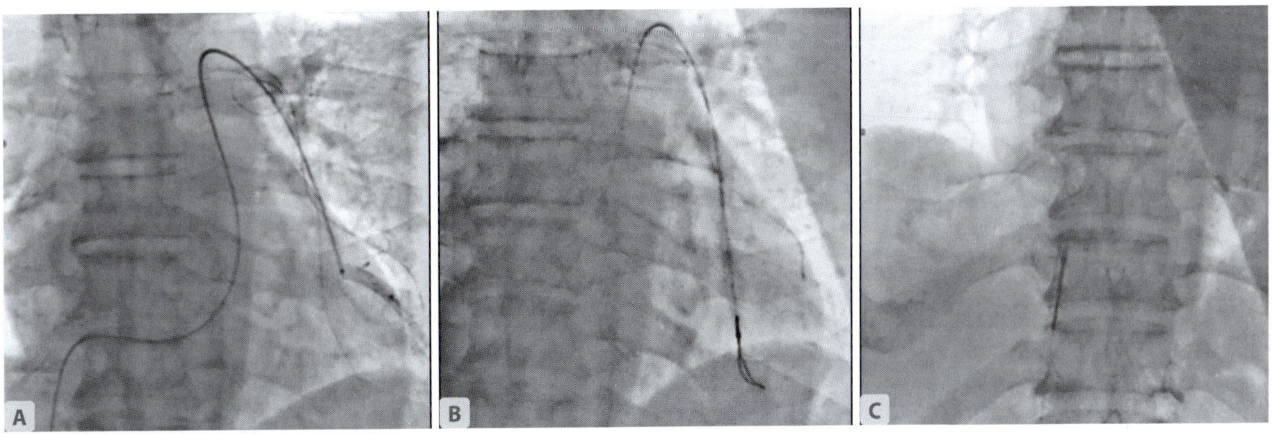

FIGS. 10A TO C: Inadvertent peripherally inserted central catheter (PICC) line migration in left pulmonary artery (LPA) during placement, in 10-year-old boy, planned for chemotherapy for lymphoma. (A) Fluoroscopic image showing PICC line curled in LPA with snare catheter advanced from right femoral vein approach in LPA; (B) One end of PICC line being caught with snare; and (C) Catheter snare PICC line assembly being retrieved.

catheters that are increasingly being used these days. These may be catheter fragments, pieces of guidewires, metallic coils, stents, electrodes, or ventriculoatrial shunt tubing. Large fragments are believed to pose a risk of thrombosis, spasm, hemorrhage, and arrhythmia.[25] Snares, deflectable guidewires, wire baskets, and intravascular forceps (bioptomes) may be used to retrieve these objects **(Figs. 10A to C)**.

CONCLUSION

Pediatric vascular intervention has come a long way and has shown safety and efficacy with ever-expanding indication. As more and more of the procedures that are currently being performed in adults get gradually adapted for use in the pediatric population, it may be possible to perform safe and successful interventions in many of the pediatric vascular lesions that are otherwise being referred for surgery. These include use of atherectomy devices or lasers that may be used for fibrointimal proliferation that develops in bypass grafts or stents or in cases of coarctation and recoarctation of the aorta once the vessel wall structure is better understood. Endovascular stenting of the neonatal ductus may replace the surgical creation of aortopulmonary shunts. Percutaneous insertion of central lines and creation of portacaval anastomosis may increasingly get applied to the pediatric patients as well.

One of the important points to remember is the risk of radiation damage and the long-lasting impact of its after effects may be a serious problem in this age group, particularly in interventional procedures that require increased fluoroscopic times or multiple sessions. Newer devices or materials or those with uncertain safety should be used with caution in children and only in situations where other more suitable and safer alternatives do not exist. Finally, it should be remembered that pediatric vascular intervention is not only a science, but a fine art and knowledge of minute details of craftsmanship are important for successful outcome.

REFERENCES

1. Gordon I, Evans K, Peters AM, Kelly J. Diagnostic Imaging in Pediatrics. Pediatrics. 1987;21:661-70.
2. Haggstrom AN, Drolet BA, Baselga E, Chamlin SL, Garzon MC, Horii KA, et al. Prospective study of infantile hemangiomas: clinical characteristics predicting complications and treatment. Pediatrics. 2006;118:882-7.
3. Castaneda-Zuniga WR. Vascular embolotherapy. In: Castaneda-Zuniga WR (Ed). Interventional Radiology. Philadelphia: Lippincott Williams and Wilkins; 1997.
4. Mavrogenis AF, Rossi G, Calabrò T, Altimari G, Rimondi E, Ruggieri P. The role of embolization for hemangiomas. Musculoskelet Surg. 2012;96:125-35.
5. Rosen RJ, Nassiri N, Drury JE. Interventional management of high-flow vascular malformations. Tech Vasc Interv Radiol. 2013;16: 22-38.
6. Chamarthy MR, Park H, Sutphin P, Kumar G, Lamus D, Saboo S, et al. Pulmonary arteriovenous malformations: endovascular therapy. Cardiovasc Diagn Ther. 2018;8:338-49.
7. Vaidya S, Tozer KR, Chen J. An overview of embolic agents. Semin Interv Radiol. 2008;25:204-15.
8. Burrows PE. Endovascular treatment of slow-flow vascular malformations. Tech Vasc Interv Radiol. 2013;16:12-21.
9. Qiu Y, Chen H, Lin X, Hu X, Jin Y, Ma G. Outcomes and complications of sclerotherapy for venous malformations. Vasc Endovasc Surg. 2013;47:454-61.
10. Orron DE, Bloom AI, Neeman Z. The role of transcatheter arterial embolization in the management of nonvariceal upper gastrointestinal bleeding. Gastrointest Endosc Clin North Am. 2018;28:331-49.
11. Moore HM, List A, Holden A, Osborne TM. Therapeutic embolization for acute haemorrhage in the abdomen and pelvis. Australas Radiol. 2000;44(2):161-8.
12. Hoffer EK. Transcatheter embolization in the treatment of hemorrhage in pelvic trauma. Semin Interv Radiol. 2008;25: 281-92.
13. Martin LN, Higgins L, Mohabir P, Sze DY, Hofmann LV. Bronchial Artery Embolization for Hemoptysis in Cystic Fibrosis Patients: A 17-Year Review. J Vasc Interv Radiol. 2020;31:331-5.
14. Mazer MJ, Baltaxe HA, Wolf GL. Therapeutic embolization of the renal artery with Gianturco coils: limitations and technical pitfalls. Radiology. 1981;138:37-46.
15. Khattak YJ, Alam T, Shoaib RH, Sayani R, Haq TU, Awais M. Endovascular embolisation of visceral artery pseudoaneurysms. Radiol Res Pract. 2014;2014:258954.
16. Chuang VP, Soo CS, Wallace S. Ivalon embolization in abdominal neoplasms. AJR Am J Roentgenol. 1981;136:729-33.
17. Poliektov N, Johnson DT. Treatment of liver tumors with transarterial chemoembolization. Semin Interv Radiol. 2018;35:350-5.
18. Liu YQ. Radiology of aortoarteritis. Radiol Clin North Am. 1985;23:671-88.
19. Sharma S, Rajani M, Talwar KK. Angiographic morphology in nonspecific aortoarteritis (Takayasu's arteritis): a study of 126 patients from North India. Cardiovasc Interv Radiol. 1992;15: 160-5.
20. Sharma S, Saxena A, Talwar KK, Kaul U, Mehta SN, Rajani M. Renal artery stenosis caused by nonspecific arteritis (Takayasu disease): results of treatment with percutaneous transluminal angioplasty. AJR Am J Roentgenol. 1992;157:417-22.
21. Sharma S, Bahl VK, Saxena A, Kothari SS, Talwar KK, Rajani M. Stenosis in the aorta caused by non-specific aortitis: results of treatment by percutaneous stent placement. Clin Radiol. 1999;54:46-50.
22. Sharma S, Gupta H, Saxena A, Kothari SS, Taneja K, Guleria S, et al. Results of renal angioplasty in nonspecific aortoarteritis (Takayasu disease). J Vasc Interv Radiol. 1998;9:429-35.
23. Ge BH, Copelan A, Scola D, Watts MM. Iatrogenic percutaneous vascular injuries: clinical presentation, imaging, and management. Semin Interv Radiol. 2015;32:108-22.
24. Obara H, Matsubara K, Kitagawa Y. Acute limb ischemia. Ann Vasc Dis. 2018;11:443-8.
25. da Motta Leal Filho JM, Carnevale FC, Nasser F, Santos ACB, de Oliveira Sousa W, Zurstrassen CE, et al. Endovascular techniques and procedures, methods for removal of intravascular foreign bodies. Rev Bras Cir Cardiovasc. 2010;25:202-8.

CHAPTER

60

Nonvascular Interventions in Children

Priyanka Naranje, Devasenathipathy Kandasamy, Shivanand Gamanagatti

INTRODUCTION

Pediatric interventional radiology (IR) has emerged as an essential adjunct to management of various surgical and medical conditions of children. Performing an image-guided intervention in children is challenging.

The interventional procedure may be categorized into: (a) Vascular interventions and (b) Nonvascular interventions. Vascular interventions have been described elsewhere in this book and in this chapter nonvascular procedures will be discussed. Prior to any intervention, the most important step consists of patient evaluation and preprocedure care. Every intervention should have a proper and valid referral. If necessary, a direct discussion with the referring physician is appropriate.

PATIENT EVALUATION AND PREPROCEDURE CARE

This includes reviewing the medical records as well as the available imaging. If required any specific specialty consultation or reimaging should be organized. Evaluation of the imaging is important in order to plan the technical feasibility of performing the procedure such as biopsy or collection drainage. It also helps to plan the choice of modality for performing the IR procedure thereby enables scheduling the case under most suitable equipment (e.g., lung nodule biopsy under CT guidance). Many nonvascular interventions are performed using ultrasonography (USG) and fluoroscopy; preprocedure screening with USG helps to assess the feasibility and also improves the procedure accuracy. Moreover, it gives an opportunity for parents and children to meet the IR team when a proper explanation about the procedure should be done and this time can be used to obtain informed written consent for the procedure.

Another prerequisite prior to the procedure is evaluation of the various necessary laboratory reports. The coagulation parameters should be within normal limits or else these should be rectified prior to intervention. Renal function parameters should be evaluated prior to any intervention needing administration of intravenous (IV) contrast media; however, IV contrast is seldom needed in nonvascular procedures.

SEDATION AND ANESTHESIA

Sedation is one of the most important factors determining the technical success of a procedure and it also decreases the actual time of procedure. Children may be unable to cooperate for the procedure and crying and body movements can significantly impair the procedure. Hence, anesthetic agents are required to perform a successful intervention. Choice of anesthetic agent depends upon the estimated duration and the degree of pain associated with the procedure. Longer and painful procedures may need general anesthesia (GA) while shorter and less painful procedures may be performed under conscious sedation. Moreover, all procedures should be done in a room well equipped with pulse oximeter monitor, resuscitation devices and emergency drugs are needed to handle any adverse situation.

BASIC PROCEDURES

Fine-needle Aspiration/Biopsy

The most common image-guided nonvascular procedures requested are fine-needle aspiration (FNA) and biopsy. Common indications for these procedures are diagnosis of underlying inflammatory/malignant pathology, metastatic disease, and tumor staging. Few contraindications, although relative, include—uncorrectable coagulation abnormalities and nonavailability of a safe percutaneous pathway to reach the desired lesion. For abdominal biopsies, ascites is also considered as a contraindication.

The basic prerequisite for FNA and biopsies are the same as described earlier. Special care should be taken for correcting the coagulopathies, if any, prior to the procedure. A 22–23-gauge (G) spinal lumbar puncture (LP) needle is the most preferred needle for FNA. For deep-seated lesions 22-G Chiba needle may be needed. Most of the FNAs may be performed under sedation and local anesthesia (LA).

Image-guided biopsies although safe still carry a risk of bleeding and hence, these should always be performed with all precautions. Nowadays most of the procedures are performed using either automated or semi-automated biopsy guns. In certain situations, a coaxial system may prove to be very helpful in cases where multiple passes are required such as FNAs and biopsies from lung lesions. Generally, 18–20 G biopsy gun suffices for most of the true cut biopsies but the throw length of the cutting needle should be chosen depending upon the size of the lesion. US guidance is preferred over CT guidance for most of the pediatric FNAs and biopsies barring few procedures related to lung lesions, where CT may be needed.[1] Also US guidance prevents the child from unnecessary radiation.

Sampling Technique

Patient should be kept in a comfortable position preferably supine for most of the procedures, but other positions such as prone, oblique, and even sitting position may be opted for, if deemed necessary. For all FNAs and biopsies, the shortest and safest path should be chosen and any vital structure lying in the path between the target and skin should be avoided **(Fig. 1)**. Lesions situated on the surface of the liver should be approached by a path having a sizable amount of normal liver parenchyma between the lesion and site of capsular puncture to reduce hemorrhagic complications. FNAs and biopsies should not be attempted if the child is crying or restless as patient movement may cause inadvertent needle movement resulting in organ injury and bleeding. Also, the needle tip should always be monitored throughout the procedure.

For FNA, once the needle tip reaches the target organ the stylet should be removed and small to and fro as well as rotating movement should be done with the tip placed in the lesion. Sample for FNA may be obtained using either slight suction technique with a 10-mL syringe or nonsuction technique to prevent contamination of sample by red blood cells.

Various needles and biopsy guns are commercially available and prior to any biopsy proper knowledge of the device is mandatory. The performing radiologist should know about the functioning of device (automated or semi-automated gun) and throw length of the cutting needle **(Figs. 2A and B)**. While performing biopsy special care is to be taken (more than FNA) to avoid any vital structure as slight negligence leading to vital structure injury may be catastrophic.

Abscess Drainage

Percutaneous drainage is the preferred treatment for various abdominal/pleural collections and abscesses. This may be performed using either of the two basic techniques. For large and superficial collections one-step procedure (*Trocar technique*) may be used; whereas relatively small and deeper collections or collections adjoining vital structures are suitable for *Seldinger technique*. In trocar technique, the catheter is mounted over a stiff cannula with a stylet; and this assembly is directly inserted into the collection under image guidance as a one-step procedure. In Seldinger technique, 18/17.5-G needle is used for the initial puncture and a guidewire is introduced into the collection via this needle. Further serial dilatation of the track is done and then a catheter is placed. Choice of catheter depends upon the consistency of the collection. For thick collections wide bore catheters (10–14 F) with large holes such as Malecot catheter may be required whereas for clear or less viscous collections 8–10 F pigtail catheter may suffice.

THORACIC INTERVENTIONS

Guided aspiration of pleural fluid is the most commonly requested nonvascular intervention of the thorax. Other interventions include guided insertion of percutaneous drainage catheters for large/thick/septated pleural/mediastinal collections and FNA/biopsy of lung/mediastinal lesions.

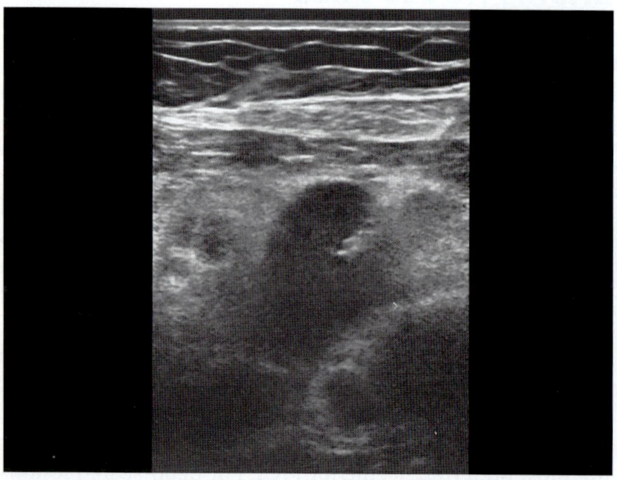

FIG. 1: Ultrasonographic (USG) image showing fine-needle aspiration (FNA) being performed with needle tip in mesenteric lymph node in a child.

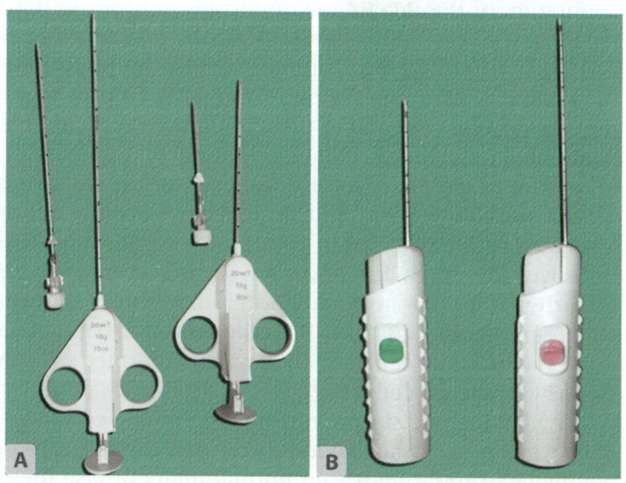

FIGS. 2A AND B: Biopsy devices. (A) Semi-automated biopsy gun and (B) Automated biopsy gun.

Pleural fluid aspiration may be requested either for diagnostic purposes or sometimes it may be a therapeutic tap. Single time aspiration using a small-gauge needle is performed for small and clear pleural effusions; however, thick/septated and nonresolving effusions require continuous drainage via a percutaneous drainage catheter. For large collections trocar technique may be used **(Figs. 3A to E)** but for smaller collections Seldinger technique is preferable. Special care should be taken to prevent pneumothorax while attempting these procedures, for instance, in single time aspiration a three-way stop cock along with tubing should be attached to the hub of the needle to prevent entry of air into the pleural cavity. Similarly, if a drainage catheter is placed it should be connected to an underwater seal bag rather than a routine urobag. Fibrinolytic therapy may be needed for thick and septated collections and various agents such as streptokinase, urokinase, and tissue type plasminogen activator (tPA) are available. Studies have shown urokinase and tPA to be safer options.[2,3]

Thoracic lesions in contact with the chest wall and, hence, visible on US should be sampled under US guidance; however, lung/mediastinal lesions not visible on US will require CT guidance **(Fig. 4A and B)**. The basic technique remains the same as described above except for few modifications and precautions. Multiple pleural punctures should be avoided to prevent pneumothorax and for this purpose coaxial devices are useful. Facility for oxygen administration, suction, and chest tube insertion should be available.

GASTROINTESTINAL INTERVENTIONS

Salivary Gland Interventions

These include US-guided injection of botulinum toxin in submandibular and sometimes parotid glands. Botulinum injection is performed for treatment of drooling in children with neurological impairment.[4] While injecting botulinum, care should be taken so as to provide uniform distribution of drug throughout the gland. This may be achieved by placing the needle at a deeper level and withdrawing it while the drug is being injected. FNAs and biopsy of salivary gland lesions may be safely done under US guidance; however, the risk of needle track seeding exists in cases of epithelial malignancy.

Esophageal Interventions

One of the most common childhood problems is *esophageal stricture*, which may be secondary to corrosive ingestion or surgical anastomosis.[5,6] Balloon dilatation for esophageal strictures is a well-recognized interventional treatment **(Figs. 5A to D)**.[5,6] It should be done under sedation/GA and fluoroscopic guidance. Curved/straight-tip angiographic catheter with (0.035 in) hydrophilic, floppy J-tip guidewire may be used to cross the stricture. Size of the balloon depends upon the size of the patient and ranges from 8- to 18 mm. A rough guide may be obtained from the width of the thumb of the child, which should be the upper limit of the size of the balloon to be used.[5] Complete dilatation should be attempted

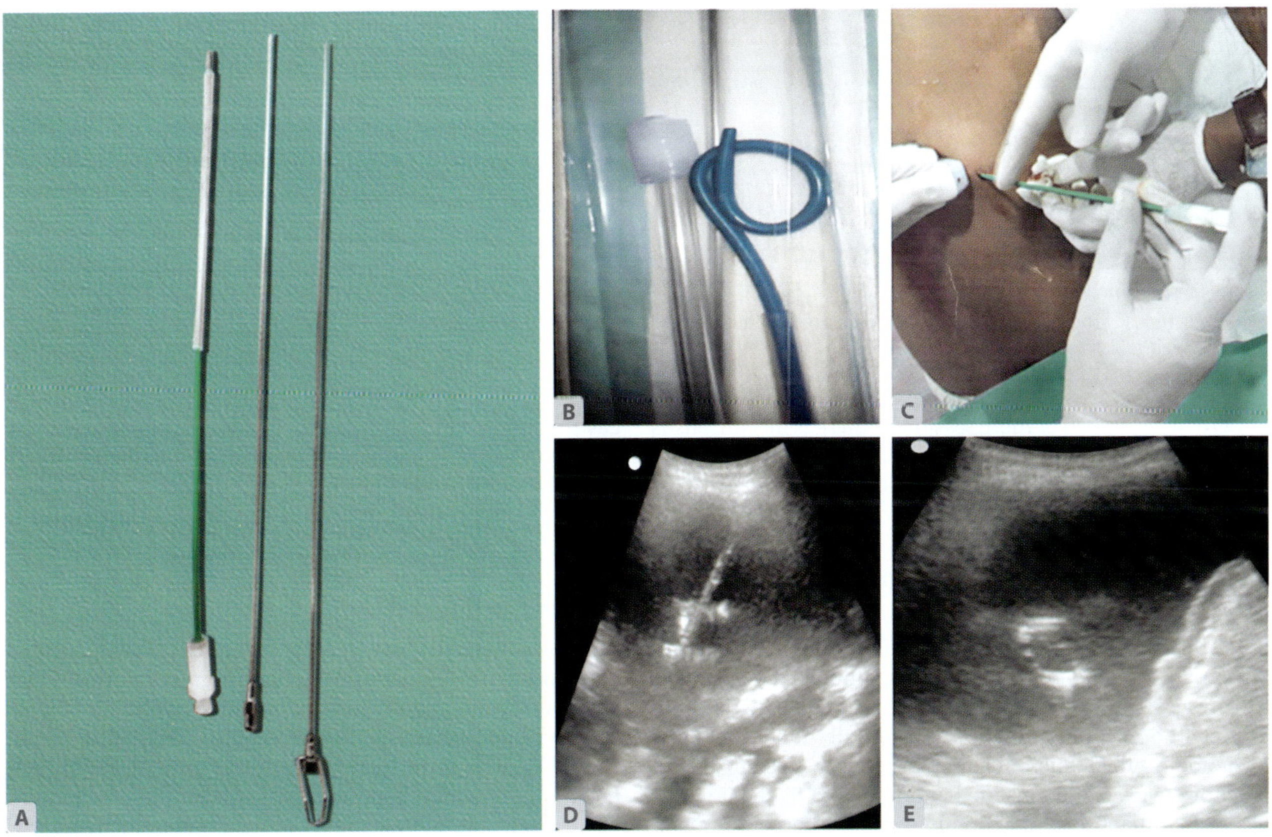

FIGS. 3A TO E: Trocar technique for drainage of large pleural collections. (A and B) Pigtail catheter with trocar. (C) Insertion being done by pushing the trocar and catheter until reaching the pleural cavity. (D) ultrasonography (USG) showing trocar catheter in collection. (E) Final position of pigtail catheter after removing trocar.

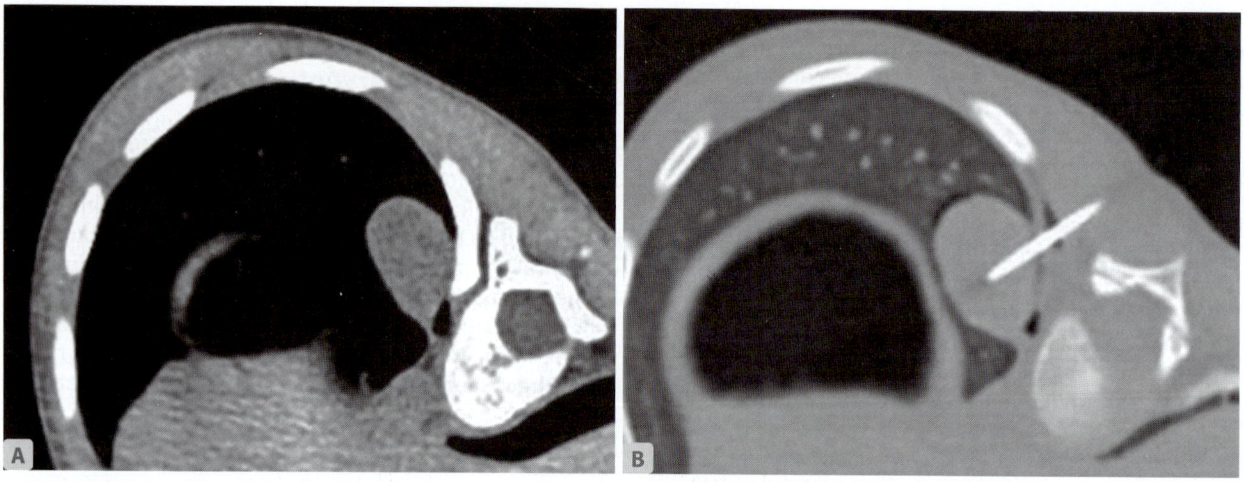

FIGS. 4A AND B: A 5-year-old patient with osteosarcoma of right femur and single lung nodule; biopsy being performed under CT guidance.

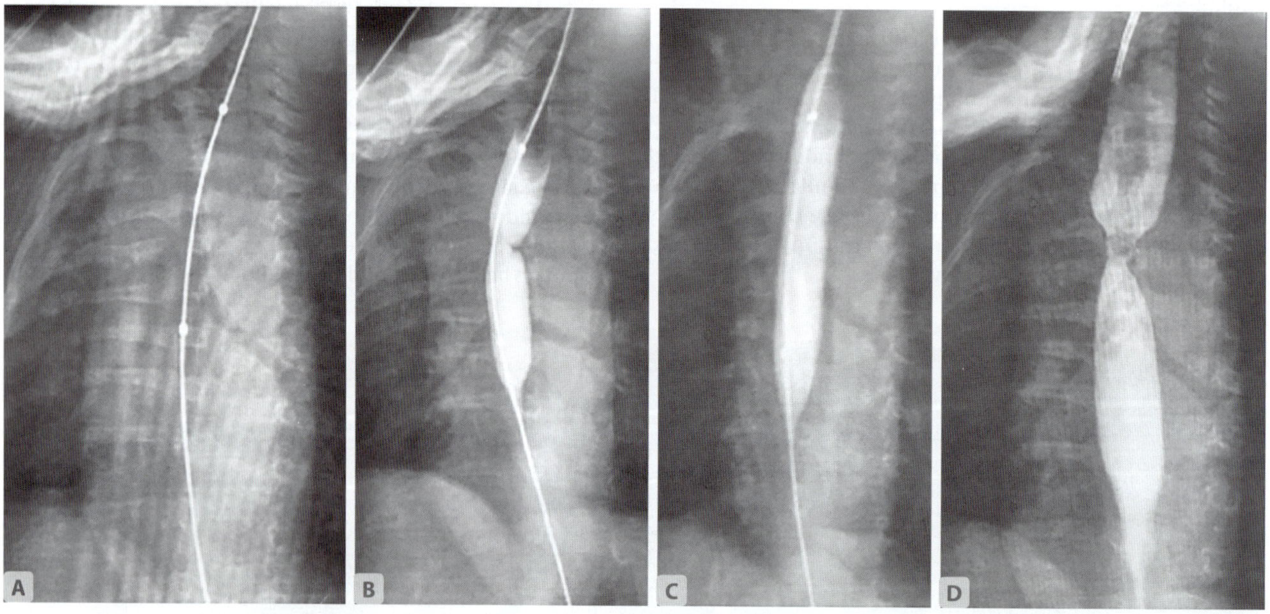

FIGS. 5A TO D: (A) Image showing balloon catheter placed across the stricture. (B) Balloon catheter being inflated with formation of waist at the site of stricture. (C) The waist within the balloon was removed; and (D) Postdilatation contrast study showing free flow of contrast, however, residual stricture seen, which requires another session.

progressively in two or more sessions.[7] There is no consensus regarding the time to keep balloon inflated; however, authors have suggested balloon inflation for 10–30 seconds.[8]

Gastric Interventions

Percutaneous gastrostomy is one of the radiological interventions which may be requested in patients requiring long-term (>6 weeks) nutritional supplementation such as patients having neurodisability, craniofacial anomalies, severe gastroesophageal reflux disease, etc. This is done under fluoroscopic guidance and initially the stomach is distended with air and punctured by a thin-gauge needle. An anchor device is then inserted and pulled to fix the anterior wall of stomach to the abdominal wall.[9] Thereafter, again the stomach is punctured and the tract is dilated in order to insert a pigtail catheter. This may be further converted to gastrojejunostomy by passing the guidewire into the jejunum through the same track and inserting the catheter over it **(Fig. 6)**. Care should be taken during the procedure to prevent colonic puncture/injury, which may lead to formation of gastrocolic fistula.

Hepatic Interventions

Common hepatic interventions requested in pediatric patients are percutaneous FNA, biopsy, and drainage of liver abscess. The technique remains the same for FNA and biopsy as described previously. However, the coagulation profile should be within normal limits for any patient undergoing hepatic intervention, especially biopsy. Also, the lesion should be approached via substantial normal liver parenchyma.

Percutaneous insertion of the drainage catheter may be required in selected cases of liver abscess.[10,11]

Depending upon the size and location of the abscess either trocar or Seldinger technique may be used.

Biliary Intervention

Percutaneous biliary drainage may be required in children having malignant obstructive jaundice as in patients with metastatic lymph nodes encasing the common bile duct, primary pancreatic tumors, or metastatic involvement of pancreas.[12] Prior to the procedure, status of biliary confluence (patent/blocked) should be ascertained and accordingly procedure should be performed. In case of a patent primary confluence the catheter may either be placed in the right or the left ductal system. Left-sided drainage is generally better tolerated by the children because of less inconvenience caused; and also, it is easy to perform under US guidance. In case of a blocked primary confluence, the duct which is draining the maximum part of liver should be targeted and at least one-third of liver should be drained.

Sedation is a must with coagulation profile under normal limits. For patients with a deranged prothrombin time fresh frozen plasma (FFP) may be required. Ideally, the puncture should be performed using a micropuncture set containing a 21-G needle and 018" guidewire which can be further dilated to accommodate 035" guidewire. After initial puncture performed under US guidance the procedure should be carried under fluoroscopic guidance and efforts should be made to cross the strictured segment and place an internal-external drainage catheter across the stricture reaching up to the duodenum **(Fig. 7A)**. However, at times, it may not be possible to negotiate the stricture in the first attempt when the system is grossly dilated. In these cases, patient may be scheduled for a second session to attempt internalization while the external drain is left in place (**Fig. 7B**). Once the system collapses, the internalization of the biliary drainage becomes easier. If internalization fails and the patient is on an external drainage then adequate care should be taken to maintain hydration and electrolyte balance caused by bile loss.

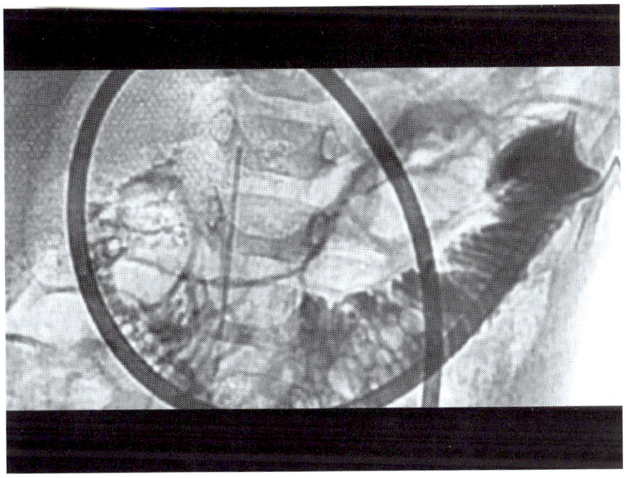

FIG. 6: Gastrojejunostomy image with tip of malecots in proximal jejunum.

Pancreatic Interventions

Pancreatic interventions include FNA/biopsy of pancreatic mass and drainage of peripancreatic collections. While attempting pancreatic FNA/biopsy, care should be taken to avoid traversing through spleen, colon, and normal pancreatic parenchyma.

Pancreatitis is relatively rare in children and is generally seen secondary to trauma. Sometimes, a pseudocyst may form and drainage may be required. While planning drainage the smallest and safest pathway without any intervening abdominal viscera should be chosen for catheter placement; however, if no safe pathway is available transgastric approach may be taken.[13] US guidance is preferred for drainage of various abdominal collections; however, if proper acoustic window is not available then the drainage should be performed under CT guidance.

GENITOURINARY INTERVENTIONS

Common interventions of the genitourinary system include renal biopsies, drainage procedures, percutaneous nephrostomy and ureteric dilatation and stenting.

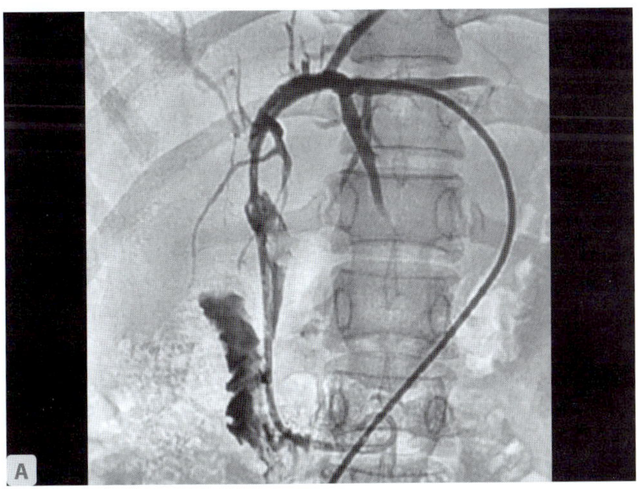

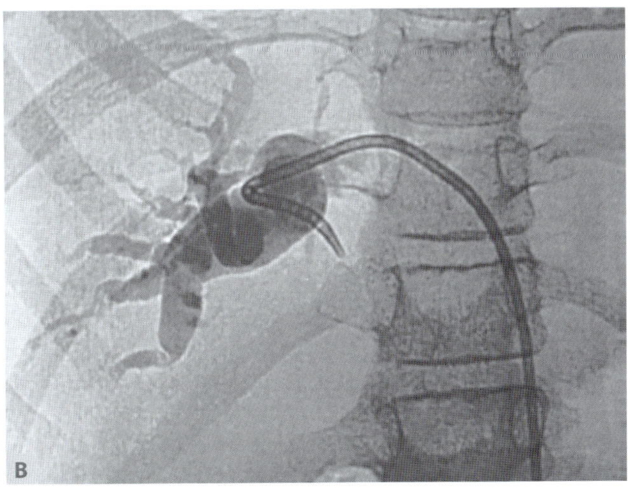

FIGS. 7A AND B: (A) Image showing internal–external drainage catheter (Ring biliary catheter) placed across the stricture with collapsed biliary system; and (B) Grossly dilated biliary system with external drainage catheter *in situ*.

Renal Biopsy

Renal biopsy is required for the diagnosis of renal parenchymal disease or renal masses for tissue diagnosis. Being a painful procedure sedation/GA may be needed for a successful biopsy. All renal biopsies are done under US guidance and retroperitoneal approach is preferred especially in cases with renal masses to prevent intraperitoneal seeding **(Fig. 8)**. While sampling renal masses a coaxial technique is preferred.[14] Sampling of renal capsule should be avoided as it may increase the chances of bleeding/hematoma. Postbiopsy hematuria though common is minimal and self-limiting. In cases of continuous significant hematuria, patient should be worked up to rule out pseudoaneurysm/arteriovenous fistula, which if present, may need angiographic embolization for treatment.

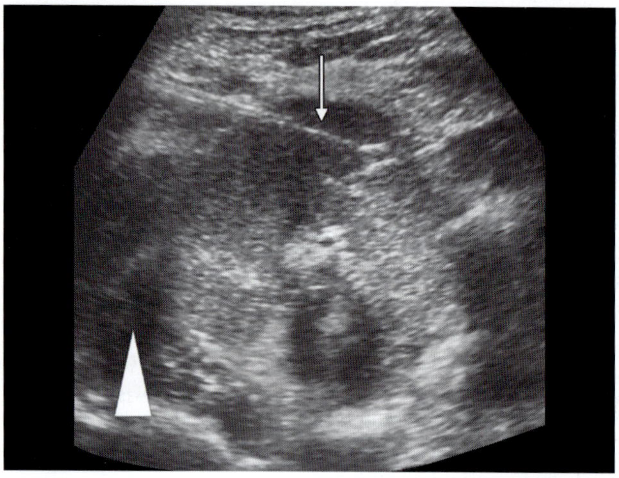

FIG. 8: Ultrasonography (USG) guided renal biopsy. The sampling notch of the biopsy gun is placed in cortex through retroperitoneal approach (arrow). Small perinephric hematoma is also noted (arrowhead).

Percutaneous Nephrostomy

Common indications for percutaneous nephrostomy (PCN) are obstructive renal disease, urinary diversion, and for removal of renal stones or placement of antegrade ureteric stent. In cases of obstructive disease or when simply urinary diversion is needed lower polar calyx puncture is preferred. However, if PCN is performed as an initial step for ureteric stenting or percutaneous nephrolithotomy then upper/interpolar calyx should be punctured **(Figs. 9A and B)**. Intercostal approach may be needed to access the upper pole calyx.[15]

Commonly, the patient is placed in a prone or semiprone position. The initial puncture of selected calyx (upper or lower) is done under USG guidance. It is preferable to puncture the selected calyx via an oblique posterolateral approach (at 25° from the median plane, with the hub toward patient's flank) to avoid renal hilar vessels.[16] Once the needle tip is inside the calyceal system, urine is seen coming out of the needle as soon as the stylet is removed. At this point, a small amount of diluted contrast may be injected to map the anatomy of pelvicalyceal system and ureter. Further, a floppy tip wire is inserted and directed toward the ureter and using Seldinger technique drainage catheter is positioned in the renal pelvis. The catheter should be properly secured by using various commercially available devices or may be sutured to the skin and dressing should be applied.

Ureteric Dilatation and Stenting

Common indication of ureteric dilatation and stenting in pediatric patients is post-transplant ureteral stricture. Upper pole calyx or interpolar calyx puncture is required for all ureteric interventions (**Fig. 10A**). Dilatation and stenting may be done via a pre-existing PCN catheter or through a new antegrade puncture. Initially, a 0.035" hydrophilic floppy J-tip guidewire is placed in the ureter (**Fig. 10B**). Then an angled 5-F angiographic catheter is advanced over it to reach the

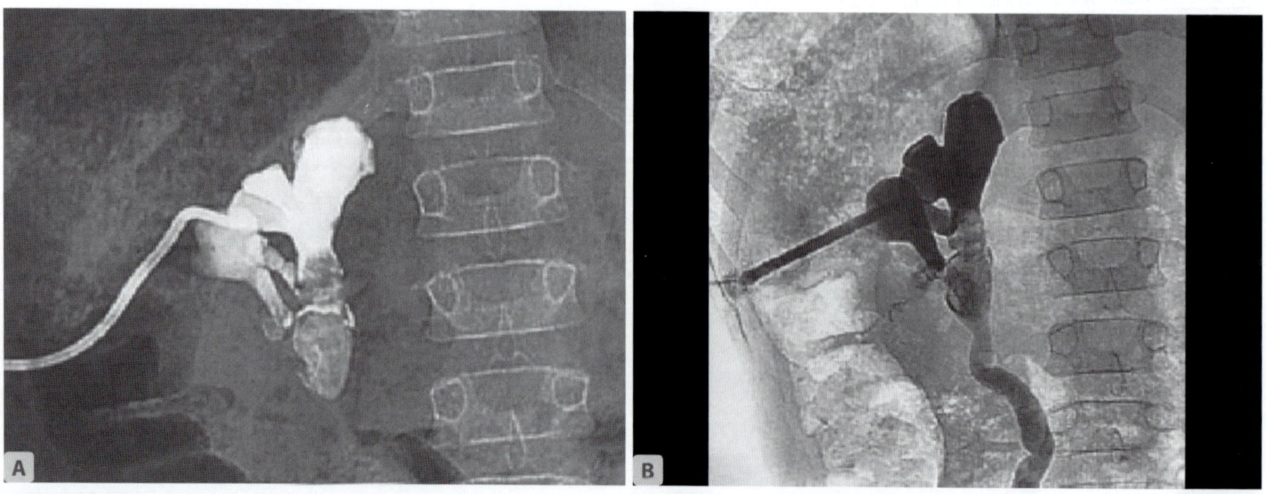

FIGS. 9A AND B: (A) Percutaneous nephrostomy (PCN) pigtail drainage catheter through upper pole calyx, as patient planned for percutaneous nephrolithotomy (PCNL); and (B) Pigtail catheter replaced with a 12-F sheath in upper pole calyx for PCNL.

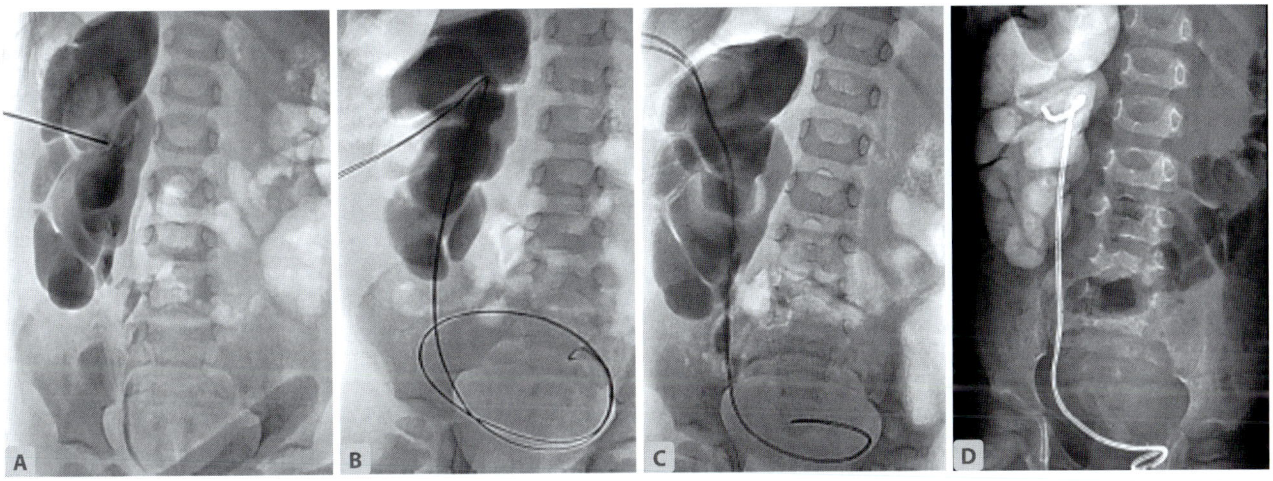

FIGS. 10A TO D: (A) Contrast study following interpolar calyx puncture. (B) Guidewire was negotiated across the stricture with tip lying within the urinary bladder lumen. (C) Further catheter was advanced into the bladder; and (D) Double J-stent was placed over the stiff metallic guidewire.

stricture site and using the combination of guidewire and catheter the stricture is negotiated (**Fig. 10C**). Sometimes, floppy straight tip guidewire may be needed to cross the stricture. After crossing the stricture hydrophilic floppy guidewire is exchanged for a stiff metallic (0.035" Amplatz extra stiff) guidewire, over which the balloon dilatation of stricture is done. Thereafter, a double J-ureteric stent is inserted over the same guidewire using the stent pusher (**Fig. 10D**). The proximal end of the stent may be secured using a suture anchored in one of the side holes so as to position the proximal end of the stent in the renal pelvis while the wire is being withdrawn. A PCN tube should also be placed in the renal pelvis with external end capped for next 24 hours so as to perform antegrade nephrostogram to ensure proper functioning of the stent. Later these stents are removed cystoscopically.

MUSCULOSKELETAL INTERVENTIONS

Common interventions of bone and soft tissues in children include FNA/biopsies, aspiration procedures (detailed in initial part of this chapter), and ablation procedures for osteoid osteoma and aneurysmal bone cyst (ABC).

Radiofrequency ablation of osteoid osteoma is one of the standards of care treatment options, in addition to long-term analgesia and surgical excision. Clinical success rates of the procedure have been reported in the range of 85% to 92% in various studies.[17-19] The procedure is performed under CT guidance and general anesthesia. After initial localization of the lesion, entry point, and approach are planned (**Figs. 11A** to **D**). Bone biopsy needle (11G) is kept perpendicular to the proximal cortex at the entry point. The shortest distance to the nidus is chosen for access in general; however, if neurovascular bundle is in the path then a steep oblique approach may have to be selected. Since procedure is done in GA, prone position is generally avoided and rotating the limb according to the approach required can be done. After entering the nidus, the stylet is removed and RF probe is introduced through the cannula. Both monopolar and bipolar RF systems may be used; using bipolar negates the need for grounding pads. Complete ablation of the nidus should be achieved. Postprocedure care includes adequate analgesia. Infections, neurovascular damage, growth plate disturbance, or articular bone damage are reported complications of the procedure. Follow-up for assessment of pain should be done 1 month and 6 months after the procedure and follow-up imaging can also be done at 6 months. In case of residual/recurrent disease, a second thermal ablation can also be done with good success rates.

CONCLUSION

Barring a few, most of the interventions performed in children are similar to adults; but, interventions in children are more challenging due to their small size and uncooperative nature due to the associated pain. It is thus essential to have an experienced team consisting of interventional radiologists, anesthetists and nurses for successful pediatric interventions. Also critical is the availability of size-appropriate hardware. Concern regarding radiation may be addressed by performing most of the interventions under US guidance, with judicious use of fluoroscopy/CT.

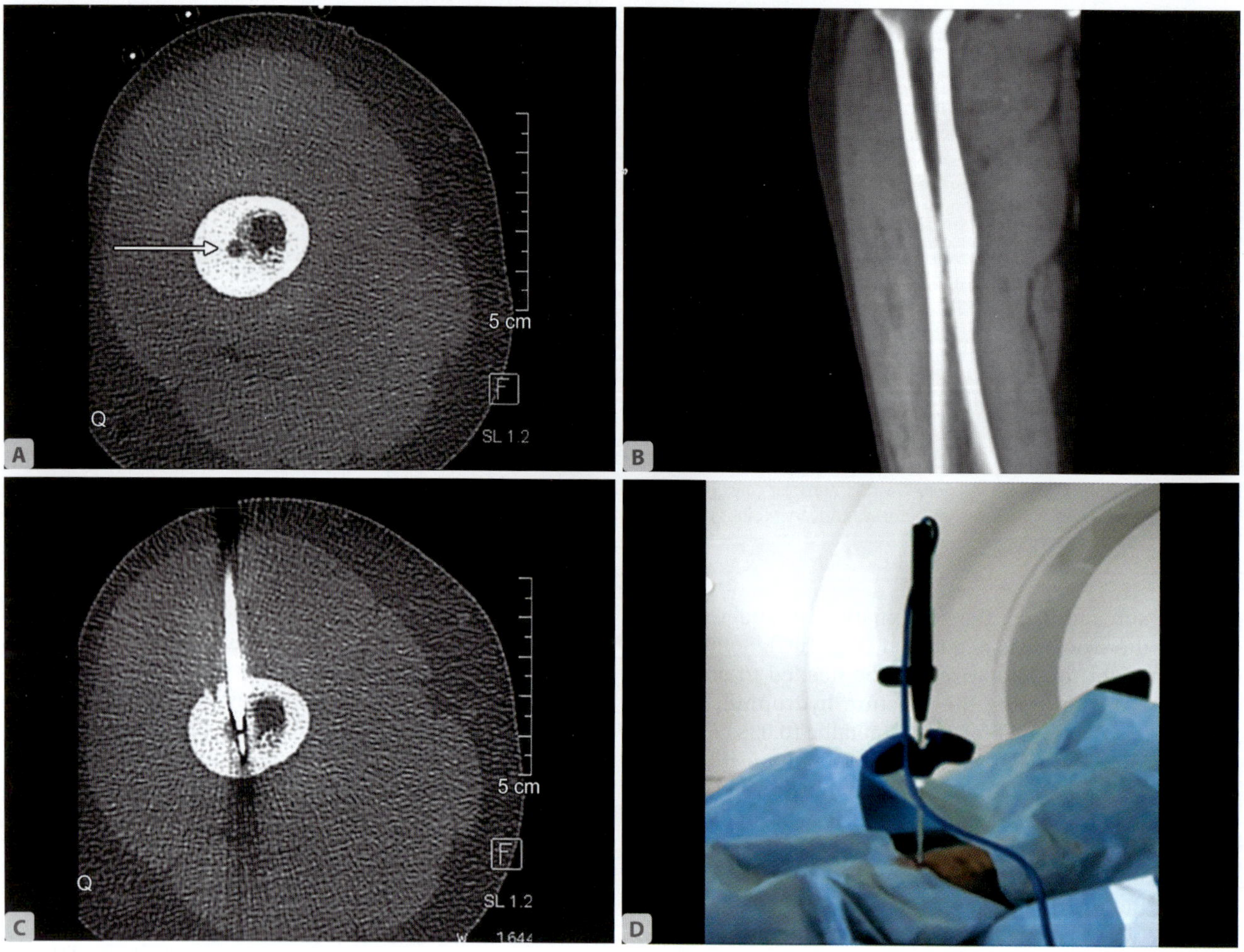

FIGS. 11A TO D: Radiofrequency ablation (RFA) of osteoid osteoma. (A and B) Femur shaft osteoid osteoma in diaphysis of femur (arrow). (C) Electrode tip in nidus; and (D) RFA probe position.

REFERENCES

1. Roebuck DJ. Pediatric interventional radiology. Imaging. 2001;13:302-20.
2. Haaga JR, Nakamoto D, Stellato T, Novak RD, Gavant ML, Silverman SG, et al. Intracavitary urokinase for enhancement of percutaneous abscess drainage: Phase II trial. AJR Am J Roentgenol. 2000;174(6):1681-5.
3. Beland MD, Gervais DA, Levis DA, Hahn PF, Arellano RS, Mueller PR. Complex abdominal and pelvic abscesses: Efficacy of adjunctive tissue-type plasminogen activator for drainage. Radiology. 2008;247(2):567-73.
4. Pena AH, Cahill AM, Gonzalez L, Baskin KM, Kim H, Towbin RB. Botulinum toxin A injection of salivary glands in children with drooling and chronic aspiration. J Vasc Interv Radiol. 2009;20:368-73.
5. Hamza AF, Abdelhay S, Sherif H, Hasan T, Soliman H, Kabesh A, et al. Caustic esophageal strictures in children: 30 years' experience. J Pediatr Surg. 2003;38:828-33.
6. Ko HK, Shin JH, Song HY, Kim YJ, Ko GY, Yoon HK, et al. Balloon dilation of anastomotic strictures secondary to surgical repair of esophageal atresia in a pediatric population: Long-term results. J Vasc Interv Radiol. 2006;17:1327-33.
7. Gercek A, Ay B, Dogan V, Kiyan G, Dagli T, Gogus Y. Esophageal balloon dilation in children: Prospective analysis of hemodynamic changes and complications during general anesthesia. J Clin Anesth. 2007;19:286-9.
8. Roebuck DJ, McLaren CA. Gastrointestinal intervention in children. Pediatr Radiol. 2010;41(1):27-41.
9. Amaral J, Connolly B. Pediatric interventional radiology. In: Geary DF, Schefer F (Eds). Comprehensive pediatric nephrology. Philadelphia: Elsevier; 2008. pp. 1053-78.
10. Simeunovic E, Arnold M, Sidler D, Moore SW. Liver abscess in neonates. Pediatr Surg Int. 2009;25:153-6.
11. Lee SH, Tomlinson C, Temple M, Amaral J, Connolly BL. Imaging-guided percutaneous needle aspiration or catheter drainage of neonatal liver abscesses: 14-year experience. AJR Am J Roentgenol. 2008;190:616-22.
12. Roebuck DJ, Stanley P. External and internal-external biliary drainage in children with malignant obstructive jaundice. Pediatr Radiol. 2000;30:659-64.

13. Curry L, Sookur P, Low D, Bhattacharya S, Fotheringham T. Percutaneous cystgastrostomy as a single-step procedure. Cardiovasc Intervent Radiol. 2009;32:289-95.
14. Roebuck D, Michalski AJ. Core biopsy of renal tumors in childhood [abstract]. Med Pediatr Oncol. 2003;41:283.
15. El-Nahas AR, Shokeir AA, El-Kenawy MR, Shoma AM, Eraky I, El-Assmy AM, et al. Safety and efficacy of supracostal percutaneous nephrolithotomy in pediatric patients. J Urol. 2008;180:676-80. [Epub: J Urol. 2009;182(2):802-3].
16. Roebuck D. Pediatric interventional radiology: An overview. In: Spitz L, Coran A (Eds). Operative pediatric surgery. London: Hodder Arnold; 2006. pp. 1025-37.
17. Chahal A, Rajalakshmi P, Khan SA, Rastogi S, Srivastava DN, Gamanagatti S. CT-guided percutaneous radiofrequency ablation of osteoid osteoma: Our experience in 87 patients. Indian J Radiol Imaging. 2017;27(2):207-15.
18. Mahnken AH, Tacke JA, Wildberger JE, Günther RW. Radiofrequency ablation of osteoid osteoma: initial results with a bipolar ablation device. J Vasc Interv Radiol. 2006;17(9): 1465-70.
19. Rosenthal DI, Hornicek FJ, Torriani M, Gebhardt MC, Mankin HJ. Osteoid osteoma: percutaneous treatment with radiofrequency energy. Radiology. 2003;229(1):171-5.

CHAPTER

61 Imaging of Pediatric Trauma

Shivanand Gamanagatti, Atin Kumar

INTRODUCTION

Trauma accounts for nearly 50% of all the mortalities in children.[1] In children, most of the fatalities occur before the arrival to the hospital, whereas death rates in hospitalized children are uniformly low across the world.[1,2]

The most common single organ system injury, which is associated with the highest mortality in pediatric age group, is head trauma and nearly 80% of patients with head injuries have been associated with other organ injuries such as thoracoabdominal injuries. Children are not simple mini adults. Pediatric patients have many anatomical, physiological, and imaging differences in contrast to adult patients. Radiologists and physicians should be aware of these differences in the assessment and management of pediatric trauma patient.

ANATOMIC DIFFERENCES IN CHILDREN FROM ADULTS: EFFECT ON PEDIATRIC TRAUMA MANAGEMENT[3] (TABLE 1)

- Smaller body size leads to greater distribution of traumatic injuries with resultant multiple injuries.
- Relatively greater body surface area of children contributes to greater heat loss.

TABLE 1: Anatomic differences in children.

Head-to-body ratio is greater	• More serious head injury • Cervical spine injury patterns differ
Liver and spleen	• Less protected by ST, muscle
Kidneys	• Less protected • More mobile
Smaller body size	• Multiple organ injuries common • Greater distribution of injury
Bones	• Have more elasticity and plasticity • Reversible deformities, without manifesting a typical fracture

- Liver and spleen are more anteriorly located and less protected by rib cage, and musculature and subcutaneous tissues make them more susceptible to injury.
- Relatively large size of the kidneys compared to their body size, and more mobility and less protection from rib cage make them very susceptible to deceleration injury.
- Unfused growth plates make them susceptible to physeal injuries leading to limb-length discrepancies and deformities following healing.
- Children have larger head-to-body ratio and thinner cranial bones (less than age of 4 years, the calvarium is unilaminar and lacks dipole) due to which injuries to the head are more serious.
- Young growing bones have increased plasticity and elasticity, hence they are more likely to bend or buckle than developing complete fracture. The periosteum is thicker, more elastic, and less firmly adherent to underlying bone, usually remains intact over an underlying fracture helping in early healing of fractures.
- Due to increased elasticity and plasticity of bones, rib fractures are less common than adults and also major internal injuries can occur without rib fractures.
- In newborn, bony cortex is thin and porous, later transforms into dense lamellar bone beginning in the diaphysis. There is transitional zone (metaphysis) between thin porous and dense lamellar bone, which is the most weak part of the bone leading to typical metaphyseal (toddler) fractures.
- Growth plate (physis) is a cartilaginous flat disk between epiphysis and metaphysis, becomes progressively undulated after puberty when closes. The physis is a weak part and more prone to injury.

PHYSIOLOGICAL DIFFERENCES IN CHILDREN FROM ADULTS[3-5]

- In pediatric age group, circulation may remain steady for prolonged time but can deteriorate dramatically at any time.
- Children are more susceptible to hypothermia.
- After initial assessment, efficient continuous observation and preventive measures should be taken to safeguard

quick response in case of sudden deterioration, particularly essential in the era of nonoperative management.

Imaging differences in children are based on following aspects:

- Children have small body, higher respiratory and heart rates, less subcutaneous tissue fat, and unossified bones, hence their imaging demands a higher spatial and temporal resolution.
- Some traumatic conditions can be evaluated by ultrasound (US) in infants and young children than in adults could only be evaluated by computed tomography (CT) scan, such as solid organ injuries/intracranial bleed.
- They are more sensitive to radiation and estimated risk of developing radiation-induced cancer is quite high in young children as compared to adults **(Fig. 1)**. Therefore, utmost radiation protection is compulsory, one should use dedicated imaging algorithms, alternative imaging modality, and radiation reducing protocols [e.g., as low as reasonably achievable (ALARA) principle and pediatric dedicated CT protocols].

IMAGING METHODS[6]

The primary assessment of any child with trauma should be emphasized on the following questions **(Flowchart 1)**.

- *Radiographs*: During primary survey, chest and pelvic radiographs are obtained to look for source of bleed. During secondary survey, radiographs are obtained based on findings of physical examination. In majority of the cases, radiographs are obtained for medico-legal purpose rather than clinical necessity; however, radiographs play important role in skeletal trauma. Imaging of skeletal trauma begins with radiographs and very few patients require imaging beyond plain film, at least two perpendicular/oblique views should be obtained. In a suspected case of nonaccidental injury, one should obtain good quality skeletal survey.[7]
- *Ultrasound*: State of the art US with high frequency transducers (7–5 MHz) having color Doppler facility is necessary for a thorough imaging, particularly neonates and young children. However, in the emergency bay area portable US equipment with 3–5 MHz transducer is used for detecting presence of free fluid, which is termed as "focused abdominal sonography for trauma (FAST)." FAST has 90% sensitivity and 95% specificity for detecting intraperitoneal fluid which represents hemorrhage in trauma setting. The FAST has very low sensitivity for detecting specific organ injuries.

Potential Benefits of the Focused Abdominal Sonography for Trauma Examination[8]

- Quickly recognize the source of bleed in a hemodynamically unstable patient.
- Appraises a stable and conscious trauma patient with negative physical findings, who are usually not subjected to routine imaging.
- Helps to prioritize imaging studies in the polytrauma patient (e.g., stable FAST positive patient should undergo torso CT rather than extremity fracture imaging).
- Helps to avoid CT imaging in a child with FAST negative, who are less likely to have intra-abdominal injury.

CT scan: CT is the modality of choice for a fast, consistent, and complete assessment of any polytrauma child. The current generation multidetector CT (MDCT) scanners are very fast, have extremely short rotation time, improved Z-axis resolution and multiplanar reconstruction capabilities. Contrast media is necessary to identify the solid organ injuries and vascular injuries; hence, one should use weight-adapted contrast media dose and age-adapted delay protocols. The modern CT scanners have automated radiation dose reduction techniques such as *automatic tube current modulation* that can substantially reduce patient dose. Currently, there are two methods used in the CT systems: (1) z-axis modulation; and (2) angular (x- and y-axis) modulation. In pediatric patients, however, a more critical approach should be adopted with the CT examination being

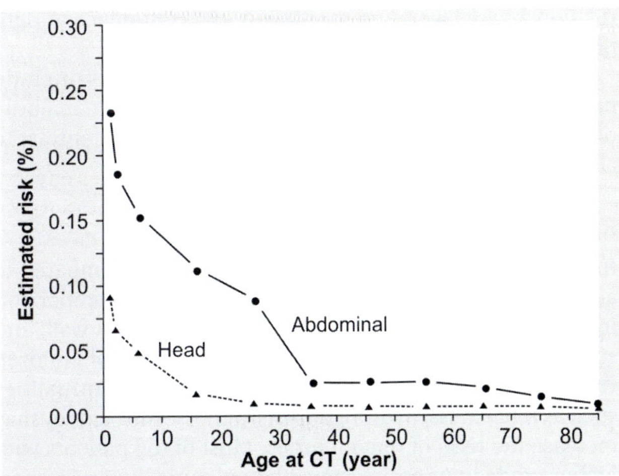

FIG. 1: Diagram showing estimated risk of cancer versus CT performed at different age group.

FLOWCHART 1: Primary assessment of any child with trauma.

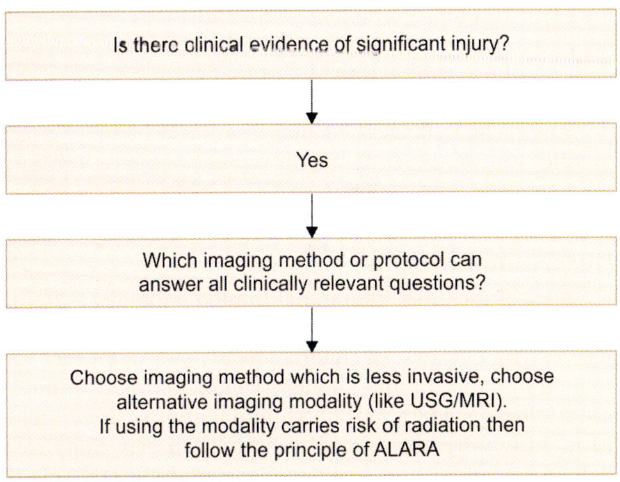

(ALARA: as low as reasonably achievable; MRI: magnetic resonance imaging; USG: ultrasonography)

tailored to the specific clinical question being asked, to avoid unnecessary radiation dose.[9]

The indications for torso CT are directed by the mechanism of injury, findings of initial physical examination, observations of chest and pelvic radiographs, and status of FAST.

Some of the common indications for torso CT include:
- Fractures of the upper ribs and sternum to look for vascular injuries.
- Persistent hemorrhagic output from intercostal tubes or pneumomediastinum to look for bronchial or vascular injury.
- Abnormal widening of mediastinum on chest radiograph to look for thoracic aortic injury.
- Thoracolumbar spinal fractures.
- Lap-belt ecchymosis, gross hematuria, positive FAST scans, all patients with penetrating injury and signs of peritonitis to look for bowel injury.

Controversies in use of Whole-body CT in Pediatric Trauma Patients[9]

- An important issue is radiation and is well-established that children are very sensitive to radiation.
- With available collective evidence suggests the limited efficacy of whole-body CT on reducing trauma related deaths in children and also it incurs expensive imaging resources.
- Also, there is risk of demonstrating clinically insignificant findings by overinterpretation of CT findings.

Due to these controversies:
- There is desperate need for policy makers to develop appropriateness criteria for the whole-body CT in pediatric trauma patients.
- The primary survey of pediatric trauma should consist of the conventional trauma series (lateral radiograph of the cervical spine, AP radiograph of the pelvis, and chest radiograph) and FAST. This methodology will control the need for additional imaging with CT.

Magnetic resonance imaging (MRI): MRI is rarely used in acute trauma setting except in situations such as suspected case of diffuse axonal injury or spinal cord injury without radiographic abnormality (SCIWORA), also to detect occult musculoskeletal injuries.[10] Major drawbacks include longer imaging times, dependence on patient cooperation, and frequent need for sedation.

Abdominal Trauma[11-13]

Majority of the blunt abdominal trauma patients are being managed by nonoperative management (NOPM) over the past several decades. In children, nearly 90% of injuries are related to blunt trauma, though skeletal and head injuries are clinically evident, intra-abdominal injuries are difficult to identify only on physical examination especially in a comatose child. Thus, imaging plays an important role in diagnosis and management.

Currently, contrast-enhanced CT is the modality of choice that helps in exact characterization and defining the exact extent of injury for deciding need of urgent surgery, angioembolization or NOPM.[14]

CT evaluation of torso does not require use of oral contrast. Single phase of CT with use of nonionic contrast media at dosage of 2 mL/kg and scan delay of 60–70 seconds is essential to identify intrathoracic and abdominal injuries. Delayed imaging through kidneys is performed to look for pelvicalyceal injuries and CT cystogram is performed in patients suspected with bladder injuries by injecting diluted contrast media through infant feeding catheter or Foley's catheter.

In children, following blunt abdominal trauma, solid-organ injuries predominate, with the spleen being the most commonly injured organ, followed by the liver and the kidney.

Spleen and Liver

Spleen is the most commonly affected organ followed by liver; occur in 6–10% children with blunt abdominal trauma. Typical imaging patterns of liver and splenic injury include contusion, laceration, intraparenchymal and subcapsular hematomas, and vascular injuries such as active extravasation and pseudoaneurysms **(Figs. 2A to D and 3A to D)**. Delayed complications include pseudoaneurysm, biloma, and infarction.

Pancreas

Pancreatic injuries are rare, may occur in isolation, and may be associated with other organ injuries and seen in 1–2% of children with blunt abdominal trauma. The most common mechanisms associated with pancreatic injury include handle bar injuries of bicycle riding. Typical patterns of pancreatic injury include laceration, transection, and contusion **(Figs. 4A to D)**.

Few indirect signs such as peripancreatic fat stranding/ fluid without any other solid organ injury and fluid between the splenic vein and pancreas may give clue to search for underlying pancreatic injury. Two important imaging information should be conveyed to the surgeon, first is thickness of pancreatic parenchyma involved ≥50%, secondly relationship of laceration to splenoportal confluence to right or left.

Delayed complications of pancreatic injury include pancreatitis and pseudocyst formation. In children, majority of pancreatic injuries are managed by NOPM in contrast to adults in whom surgery is preferred.

Kidney

In children renal injuries are more common as compared to adults, because of their relatively large size in comparison to body size, more mobile, less protected by chest wall, and surrounding fat. Renal injuries occur in 4–14% of children with blunt abdominal trauma. Pre-existing abnormalities such as renal mass, hydronephrosis, or horseshoe kidney may increase the risks of renal injuries. Most of the patients with higher-grade injuries present with hematuria, however, most of the injuries are of mild degree (grade 1–2) **(Figs. 5A to D)**.

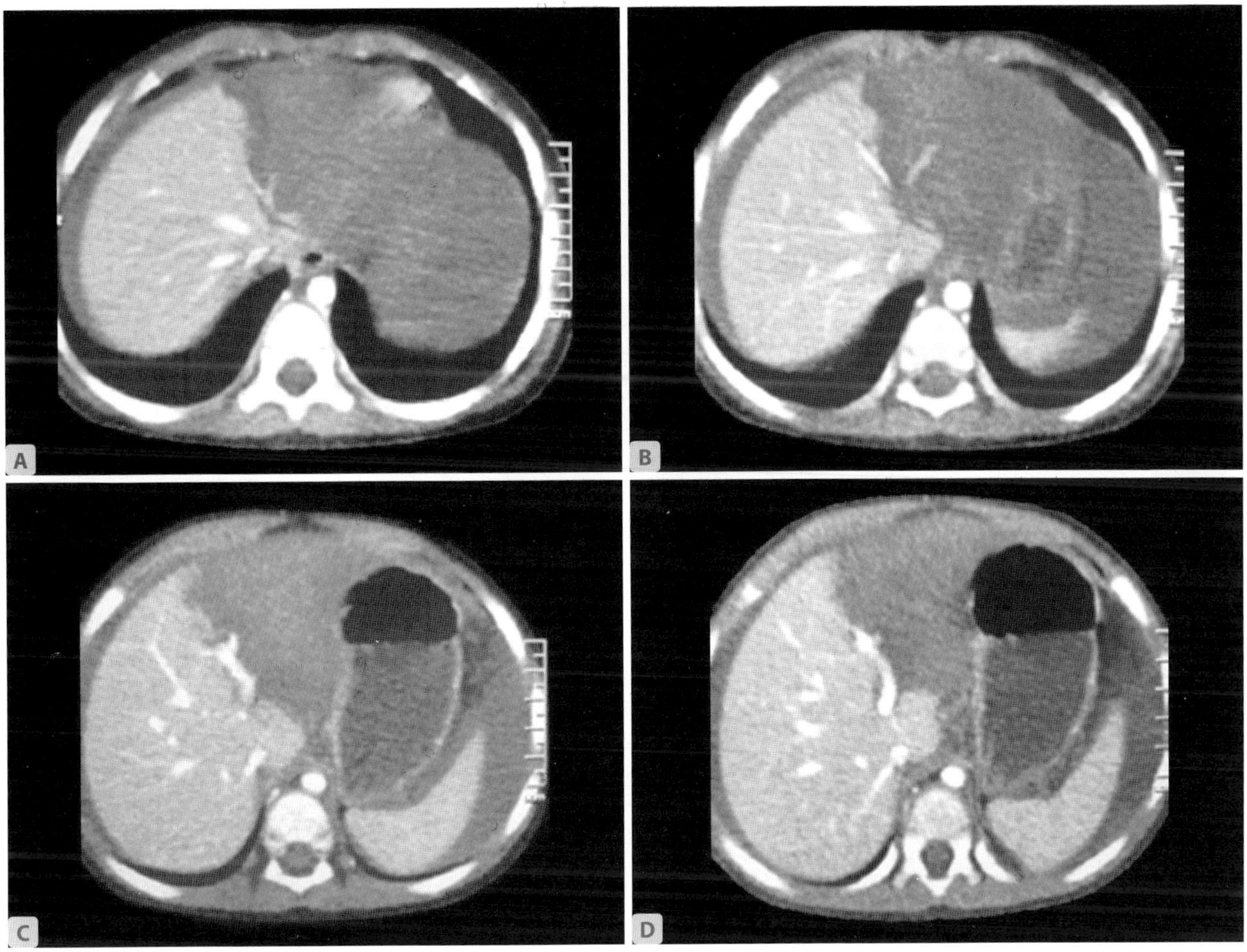

FIGS. 2A TO D: Axial CT sections of liver showing large contusion involving lateral segment of left lobe of liver with hemoperitoneum.

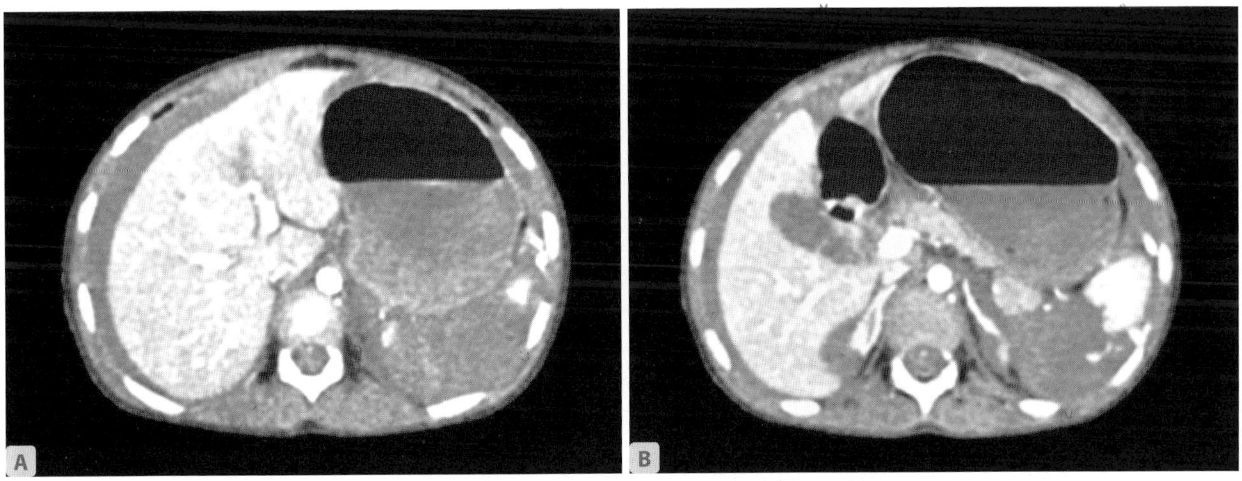

FIGS. 3A TO D: *Continued*

Continued

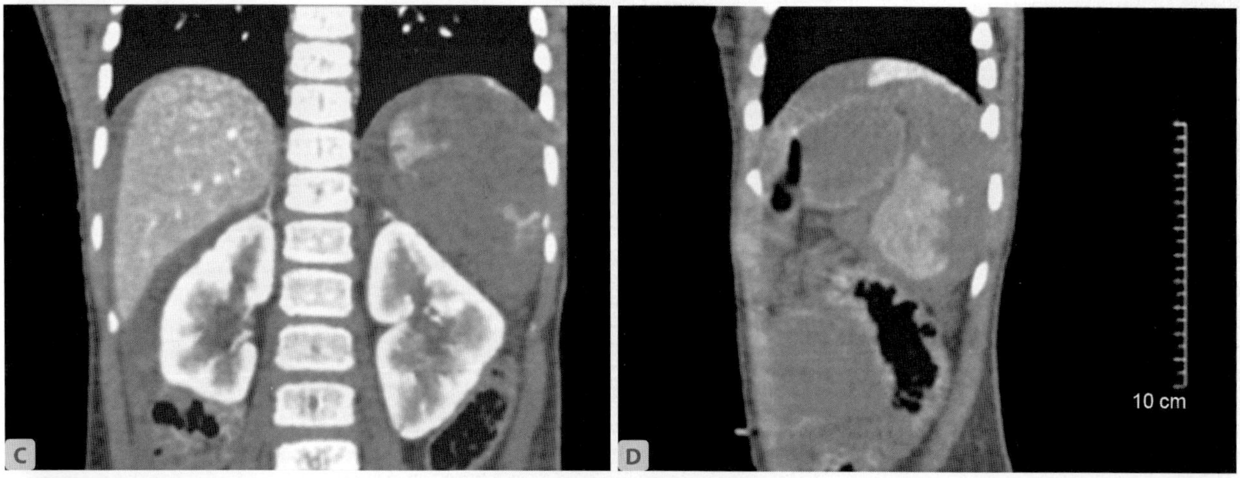

FIGS. 3A TO D: Axial CT: (A and B) and coronal (C) and sagittal MPR (D) images of upper abdomen showing large contusion involving >50% of splenic parenchyma suggsting Grade 3 lesion with hemoperitoneum.

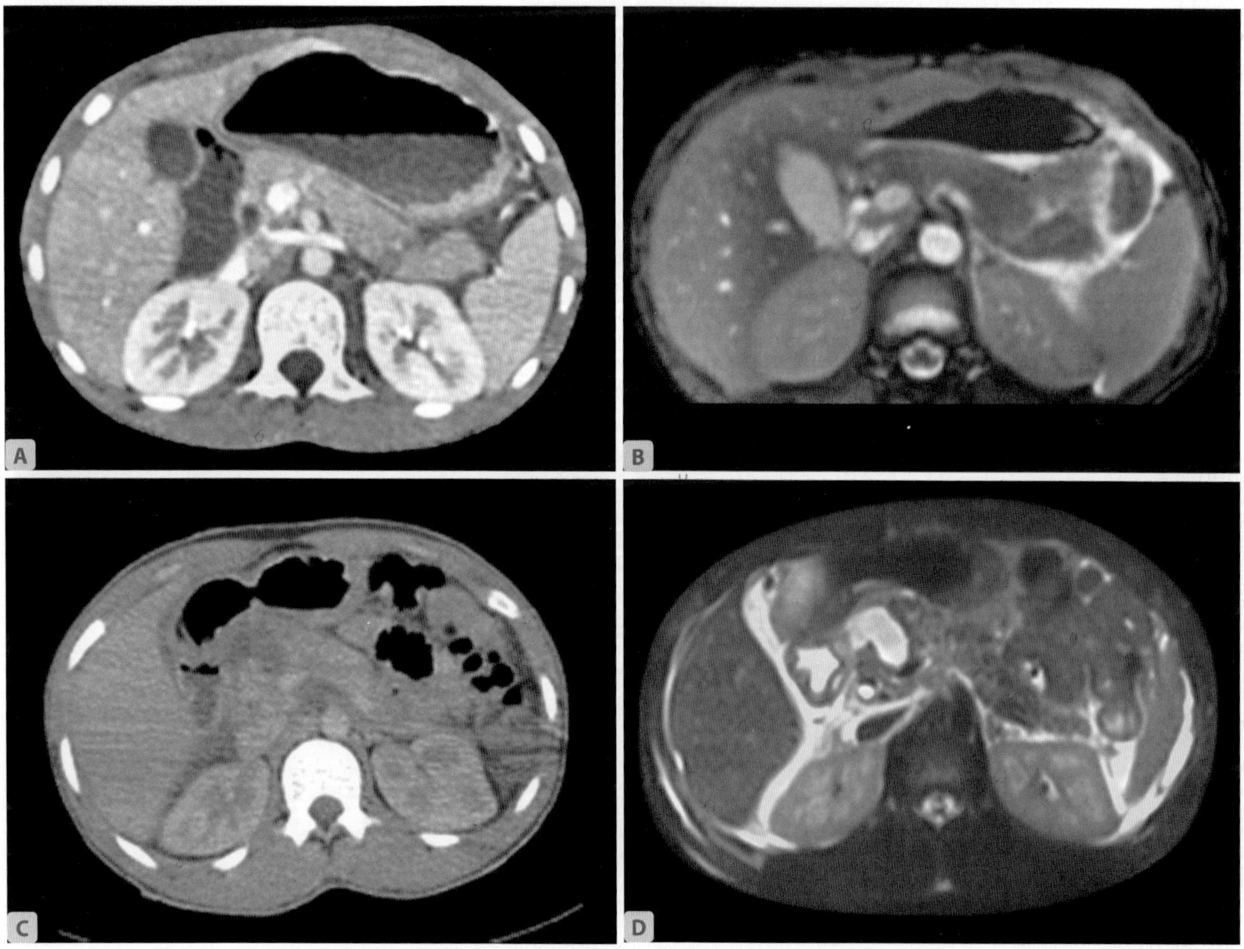

FIGS. 4A TO D: Axial CT and fast imaging with steady-state precession (True-FISP): MR images showing linear complete laceration involving tail of pancreas with peripancreatic minimal free fluid collection (A and B). Axial CT and T2-weighted fat saturated (T2W-FS) image showing complete laceration with fluid collection in the region of head of pancreas (C and D).

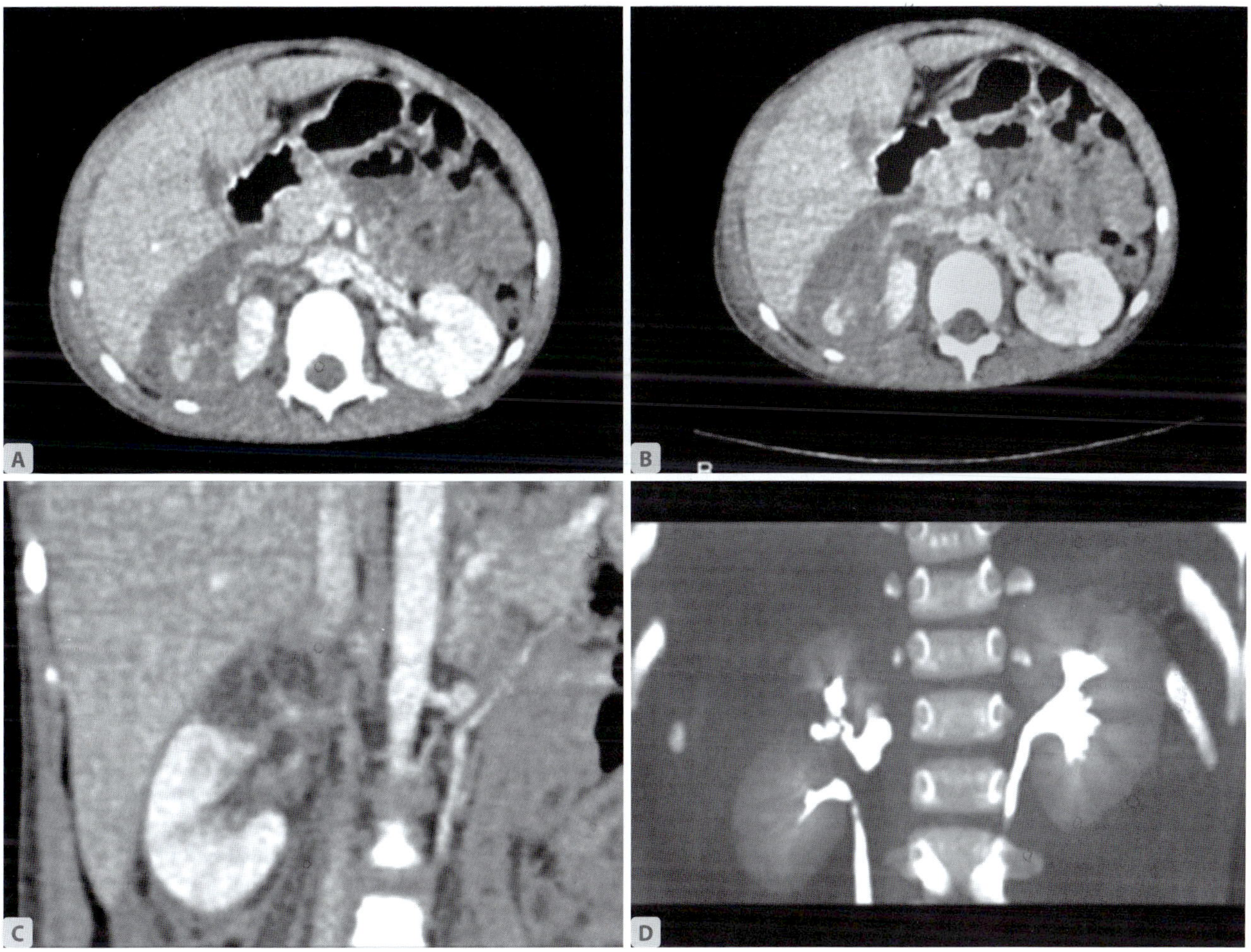

FIGS. 5A TO D: Axial CT: (A and B) and coronal multiplanar reconstruction (MPR) (C) images of upper abdomen showing laceration involving upper pole of right kidney with perinephric hematoma and there is evidence of contrast leakage from the upper pole calyx in delayed scan (D).

Majority of renal injuries are managed by NOPM assisted by urinary diversion either by double-J (DJ) stent or percutaneous nephrostomy in case of pelvicalyceal or ureteric injuries.

Delayed complications of NOPM include delayed hemorrhage due to pseudoaneurysm or arteriovenous fistula, renal scarring, and persistent urinoma.

Bowel and Mesentery

These injuries are very serious if they go undetected or missed, since bowel and mesenteric injuries are one of the indications for emergent surgery. In children with lap belt or handle bar injury, one should suspect these injuries, can occur in 1–8% of children with blunt abdominal trauma. It has become very challenging for the attending radiologist to differentiate perforating from nonperforating bowel injury. Definitive CT findings of bowel injury include bowel wall defect, free extraluminal gas, and abnormal bowel wall enhancement **(Figs. 6A and B)**. Extraluminal air is very specific for bowel injury but not sensitive enough since many full thickness bowel injuries may not show free air. Other causes of extraluminal air include mechanical ventilation, pulmonary barotrauma, intraperitoneal bladder rupture, and pneumomediastinum.

Unexplained peritoneal fluid without any obvious solid organ injury or pelvic fracture, or hypoperfusion complex, one should suspect mesenteric injury.

Definitive CT signs of mesenteric injury include mesenteric hematoma, mesenteric extravasation of contrast, vascular beading, and abrupt termination of mesenteric vessels.

Duodenal injuries are very rare, may occur in isolation or may be associated with pancreatic injuries. Presence of retroperitoneal air should rise the suspicion of duodenal perforation. Identification of duodenal perforation is very critical since it requires urgent surgery.

Delayed complications of bowel and mesenteric injuries include collections of enterocutaneous fistula, obstruction, and pseudoaneurysms.

Chest Trauma

Blunt Trauma Chest[9]

After the head injuries, chest injuries are leading cause of death in children following trauma. Blunt injuries are more

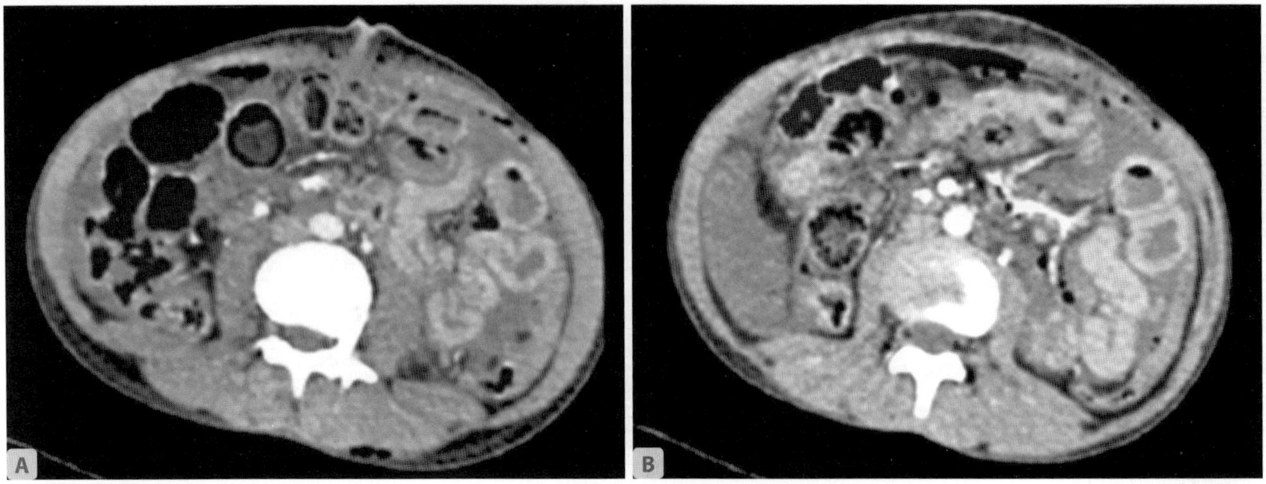

FIGS. 6A AND B: Axial CT sections: (A and B) of mid abdomen showing presence of pneumoperitoneum and abnormal enhancement of walls of small bowel loops with hemoperitoneum suggestive of bowel injury.

common than penetrating injury. Portable chest radiograph in emergency bay area remains important means to detect tension pneumothorax and hemothorax.

Extended FAST helps in detecting hemothorax and hemopericardium, which requires urgent intervention. Pneumoscan using high-frequency linear probe helps in detecting pneumothorax.

Once a severely injured child is stabilized hemodynamically, further imaging using CT scan is performed to identify internal injuries such as contusion, laceration, pneumothorax, hemothorax, pericardial effusion or any vascular injury.

Currently, CT is the modality of choice to assess chest injury in polytrauma pediatric patients.

Chest wall injuries: In children, rib fractures are less common than in adults because of the plasticity and elasticity of bones; however, internal injuries can occur without overlying rib fractures.

- Fractures of the upper ribs and clavicle may be associated with either vascular or tracheobronchial injuries.
- Lower rib fractures are often associated with injuries to either liver or spleen.

Fracture of the trachea or of a bronchus gives following radiological findings:

- Misplaced endotracheal tube, but a deformed bronchial contour can also be helpful in the diagnosis.
- In the most advanced cases fallen lung sign with collapse of the lung not to the hilum but toward the diaphragm can be seen.

Pleura

Pneumothorax usually results from alveolar rupture, other mechanisms include air leakage into pleural space from penetrating injury, from lung laceration or in association with air leak from the tracheobronchial tree (pneumomediastinum).

Diagnosis of pneumothorax is simple on upright chest radiographs, but on supine radiographs, pneumothorax is more difficult to appreciate and is suspected by indirect signs such as deep sulcus sign and double diaphragm sign.

CT is very sensitive to detect small pneumothorax **(Fig. 7A)**, but it is of no clinical significance unless the patient is receiving positive-pressure ventilation support.

Presence of a tension pneumothorax **(Fig. 7B)**, as evidenced by midline shift on chest radiograph, requires urgent chest tube insertion and therefore this information should be communicated to the treatment team.

Hemothorax: May result either from venous or arterial source into the pleural cavity. Extended FAST is used to detect hemothorax in emergency bay area. On supine radiograph, small hemothorax goes undetected unless the fluid quantity is very large, seen as veil-like opacity over the hemithorax.

CT is very sensitive for detecting small effusions/hemothorax; however, Hounsfield values are not helpful in defining the nature of fluid **(Figs. 8A and B)**. CT is also helpful for accurate assessment of chest tube placement and its complications.

Pulmonary parenchyma: CT is the ideal modality to look and define the extent of parenchymal injuries. Pulmonary contusion is usually seen as patch of ground glass attenuation or consolidation without air bronchogram adjacent to the site of impact or rib fracture. They usually clear over 3–10 days. If the opacities do not clear or increase over a period of this time frame, one should suspect development of acute respiratory distress syndrome (ARDS) or infection.

Lung laceration is seen as air-filled/fluid cavity surrounded by an area of consolidation due to contusion **(Figs. 9A to D)**. Peripherally located lacerations may involve the pleural surface, a bronchopleural fistula may develop. Lung laceration may take 3 weeks to months to resolve.

Pneumomediastinum: The most common source is terminal airspaces, other sources include tracheobronchial tree,

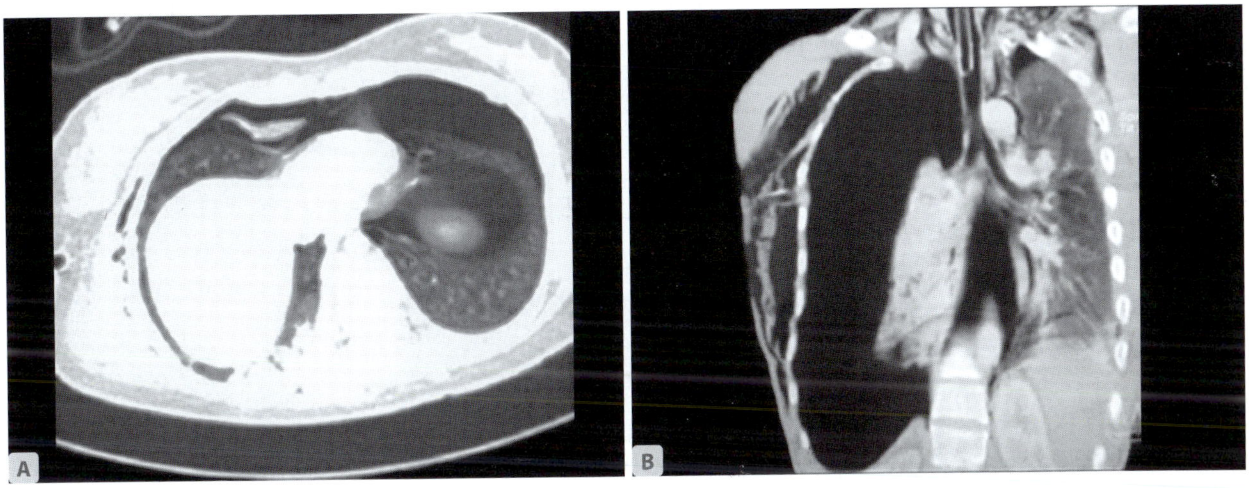

FIGS. 7A AND B: Axial and coronal multiplanar reconstruction (MPR) images of lungs showing bilateral minimal pneumothorax (A) and tension pneumothorax on right side with collapse of underlying lung (B).

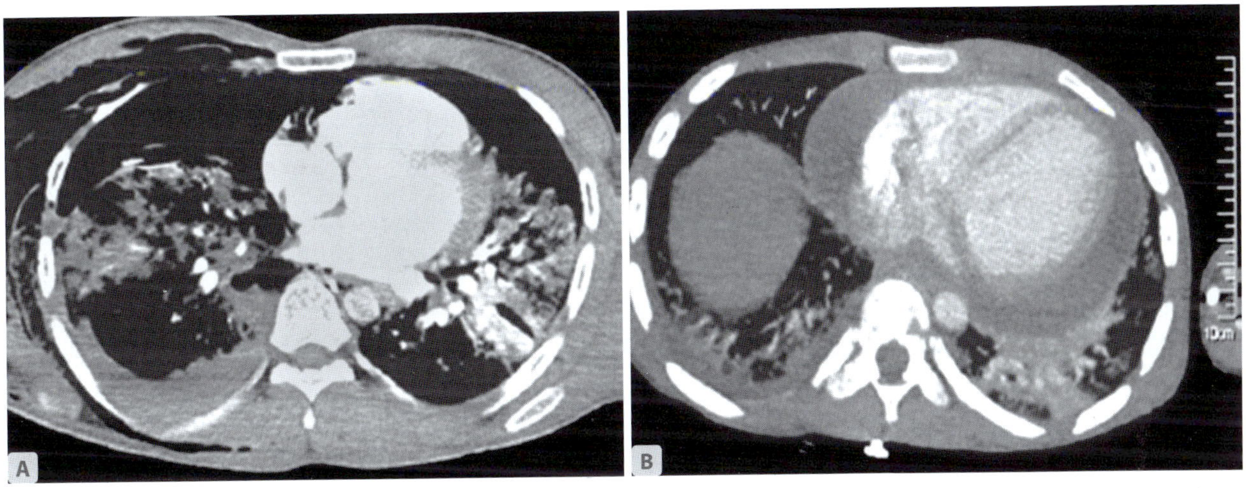

FIGS. 8A AND B: Axial CT section of thorax showing right-side hemothorax with contusion in bilateral lungs (A) and hemopericardium with minimal right-side hemothorax (B).

esophagus, and head and neck injuries. Pneumomediastinum may sometimes extending inthe neck, chest wall, and retroperitoneum. Pneumomediastinum is recognized by streaky air collections outlining mediastinal structures such as thymus and peribronchial sheath. Another sign of pneumomediastinum is the so-called "continuous diaphragm sign" which is due to air beneath the heart.

Rupture of the esophagus is very rare in pediatric trauma. Whenever source of pneumomediastinum is not explained, CT esophagogram should be performed, with water-soluble contrast material, to look for esophageal injury **(Figs. 10A and B)**.

Identification of mediastinal *hematoma* is very important, since it may be an indirect sign of underlying major vascular injury such as aortic or aortic arch branches injury, which may be clinically occult. Mediastinal widening criterion on chest radiograph used for adult patients is not applicable to pediatric patients. CT angiography is the modality of choice to rule out aortic injury; however, aortic injuries are very rare in pediatric patients as compared to adults.[9]

Cardiac injuries are rare but may include both myocardial laceration with ventricular shunting or pericardial hemorrhage **(Figs. 8A and B)** and possibly present with a cardiac tamponade. Chest radiograph may show enlargement of cardiac silhouette, however, more precisely evaluated by CT angiography.

Diaphragmatic injuries are rare in children, however, usually seen on the left side.

Penetrating Chest Trauma

Penetrating chest injuries may occur either due to gunshot wounds or due to sharp metallic objects (stab injuries). Unlike blunt chest trauma (associated with injury to chest wall, pleura, and lung) penetrating injuries are associated with injuries to vital structures including heart, great vessels, esophagus, and trachea, and are usually fatal.

Musculoskeletal Injuries[7,10]

Many unique features of the growing skeleton pose specific challenges in imaging skeletal trauma (vide supra). Differences in the composition and development of the pediatric skeleton (as compared with adults) result in

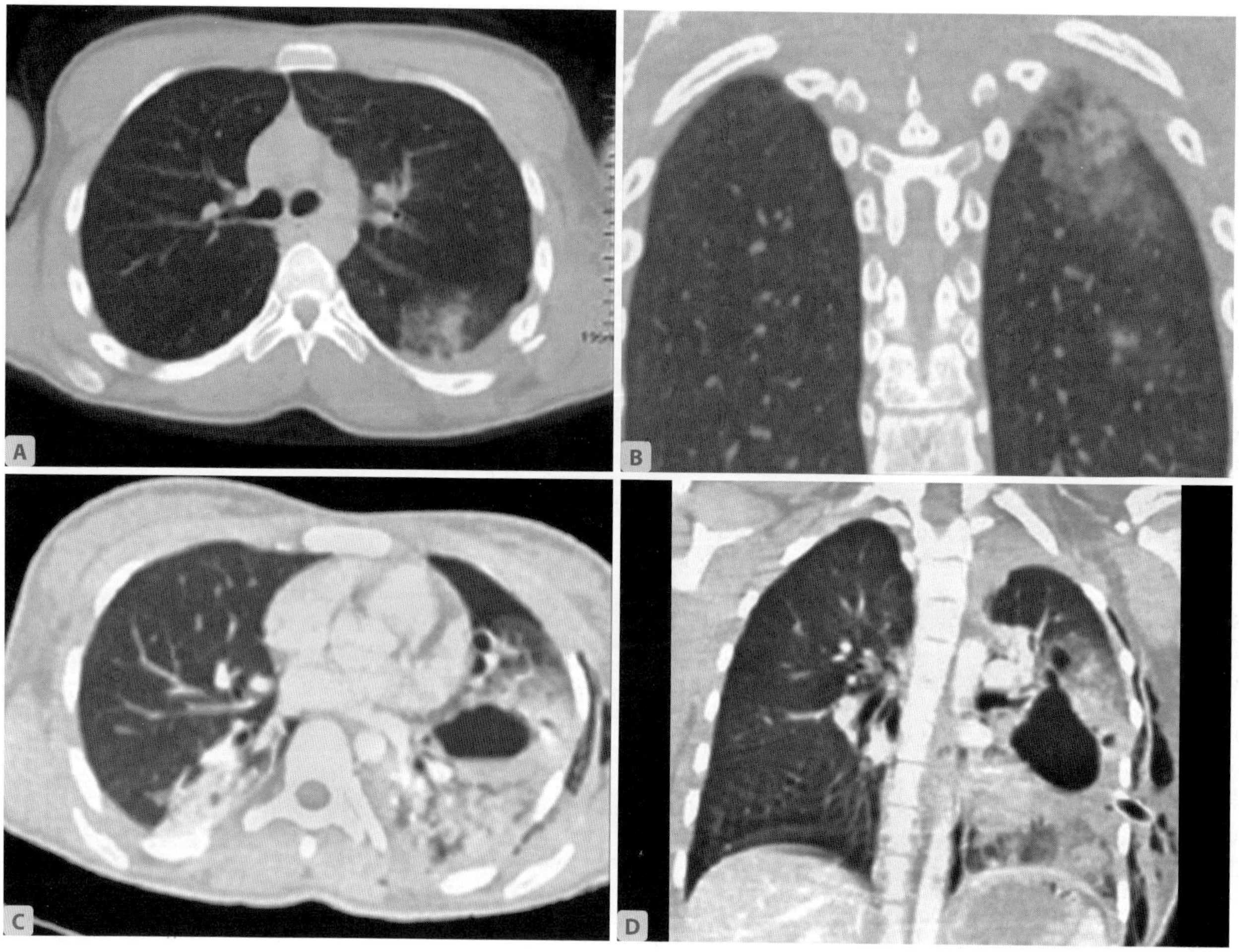

FIGS. 9A TO D: Axial and coronal maximum intensity projection (MIP) images: (A and B) of lung showing ground glass attenuation lesion in left upper lobe close to the chest wall suggestive of lung contusion. Axial and coronal MIP (C and D) images of lung showing large air-filled cavity in left upper lobe with surrounding consolidation suggestive of laceration with surrounding contusion. Note minimal pneumothorax on left side.

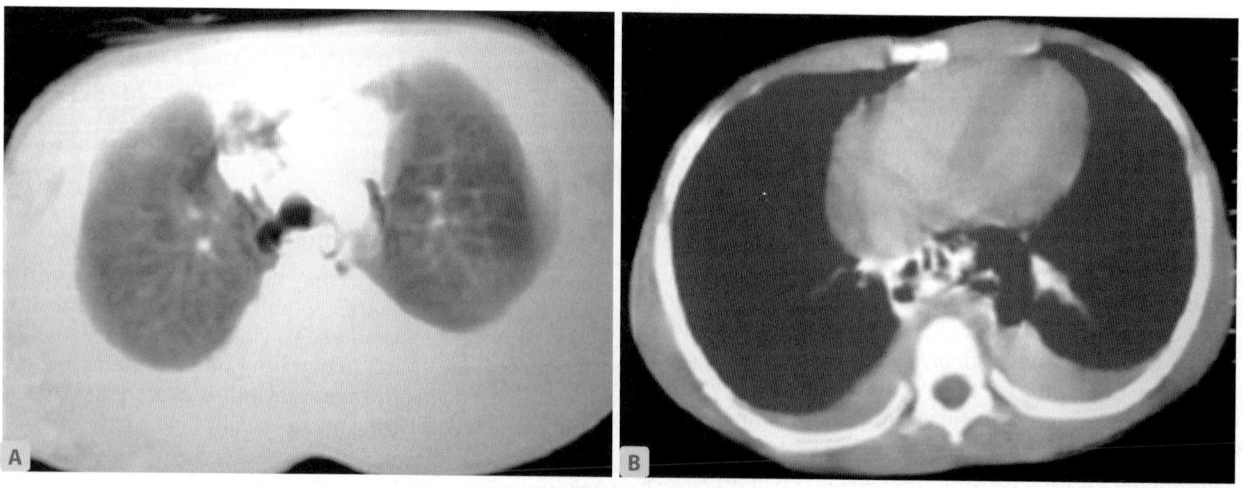

FIGS. 10A AND B: Axial CT sections of thorax showing pneumomediastinum (A) and contrast leakage from the esophagus (B) given orally suggestive of esophageal rupture.

characteristic injuries and fractures. Imaging of these injuries typically begin with plain films, and in the majority no further radiologic evaluation is required. However, CT and MRI are used as supplementary imaging studies in pediatric patients with suspected skeletal trauma.

Imaging[15]

Plain Radiographs

In most cases, imaging of pediatric skeletal trauma begins with radiographs and very few patients require imaging beyond plain films, this is particularly true in cases of common fractures.

At least two perpendicular views should be obtained. Occasionally, oblique or other views may be required to identify subtle fracture.

CT Scan

Fractures involving complex anatomical areas such as pelvis, tibia, spine, scapula, foot and ankle require evaluation with CT scan. MDCT with three-dimensional (3D) reconstruction and volume rendered techniques (VRT) help in defining the exact extent and classifying the fractures. CT is also used to assess fracture nonunion, chronic osteomyelitis, and bony bar secondary to physeal injury.

Magnetic Resonance Imaging

With acute pediatric trauma, although plain radiography is still the primary imaging tool, MR imaging has evolved into an essential adjunct diagnostic tool for the prompt identification of occult musculoskeletal injuries, growth plate injuries and their complications, osteochondritis dissecans **(Figs. 11A to C)**, avulsion fractures, stress fractures, and soft-tissue injuries can be diagnosed early and confidently with MR imaging when other imaging modalities are equivocal. Drawbacks of MRI include longer imaging times, dependence on patient co-operation, and frequent need for sedation.

Types of Injuries

Account for 10–12% of children coming to emergency and trauma center. Young growing bones have increased plasticity and elasticity, hence, they are more likely to bend or buckle than developing complete fracture.

Because of unique anatomical differences, children present with unique kind of fractures such as plastic deformity (bend), torus, and greenstick fractures.[7,10] Other special types of fractures seen in children include growth plate injuries and metaphyseal (toddler) fractures.

Types of Pediatric Fractures (Fig. 12)

- Plastic deformity (bowing fracture)
- Torus fracture
- Greenstick fracture
- Complete diaphyseal fractures
- Toddler fracture

Plastic deformation (bowing fracture) results from angulation and compressive force producing a gradual curve across the length of whole bone. It occurs most frequently in distal radius and ulna.

Torus fractures are also known as "buckle fractures" and are incomplete fractures occurring on the concave side of the bone with outward buckling of the cortical margin. These fractures occur most commonly in the metaphyseal regions of long bones **(Fig. 13)**.

Greenstick fracture shows complete break of the cortex on the tension side and plastic deformation of the opposite cortical border **(Fig. 14)**.

Complete fracture occurs when the fracture line extends completely through the both cortices and the most commonly seen in diaphyseal region.

Toddler fracture, its type of spiral (oblique nondisplaced) fracture due to torsion usually occurs in the lower limbs. Toddler's fracture, if it occurs in first year of life, one should suspect child abuse, and when the child begins to walk, these are usually due to trauma **(Figs. 15A and B)**.

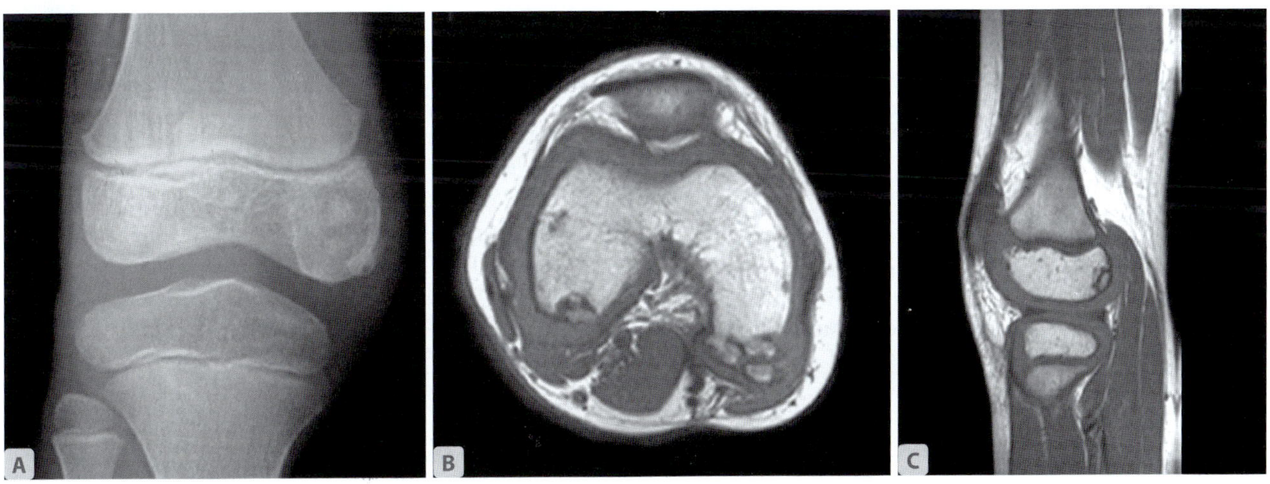

FIGS. 11A TO C: Anteroposterior (AP) radiograph of left knee: (A) showing multiple loose bodies overlying the medial condyle of left femur. Axial and sagittal magnetic resonance (MR) (B and C) images showing osteochondral lesions involving both condyles of left femur with multiple loose bodies in relation to medial condyle.

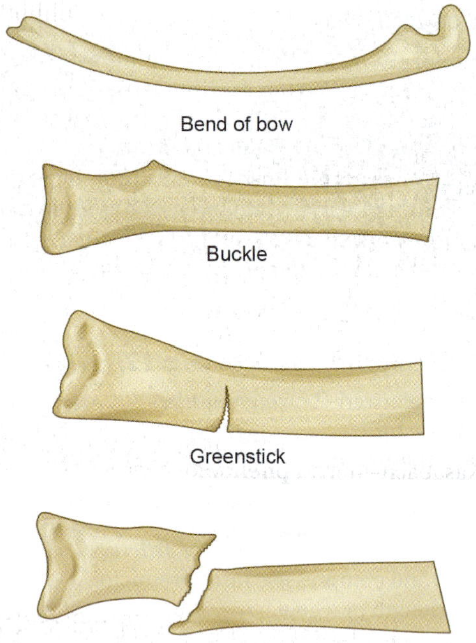

FIG. 12: Diagram showing various types of pediatric fractures.

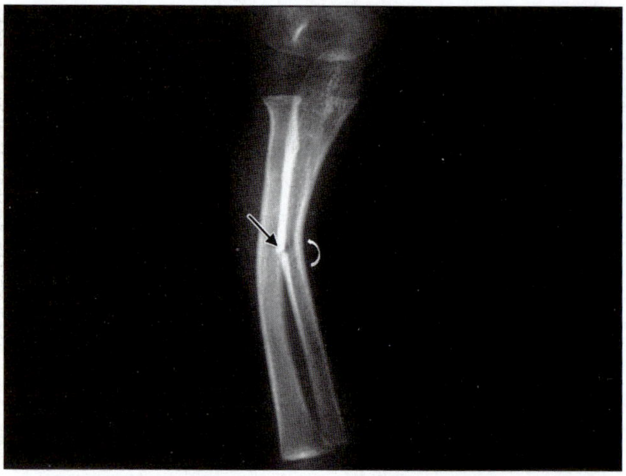

FIG. 14: Typical example of green stick fracture showing complete break of the cortex on the tension side (arrow) and plastic deformation of the opposite cortical border (curved arrow).

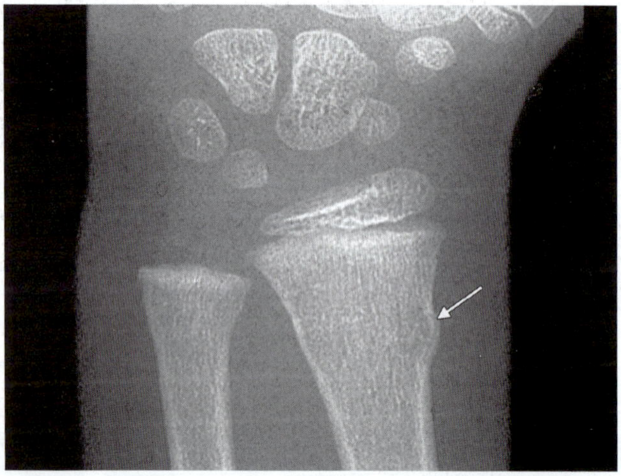

FIG. 13: Anteroposterior (AP) radiograph of wrist showing torus fracture with outward buckling of the cortical margin of lower end of radius in the metaphyseal region (arrow)

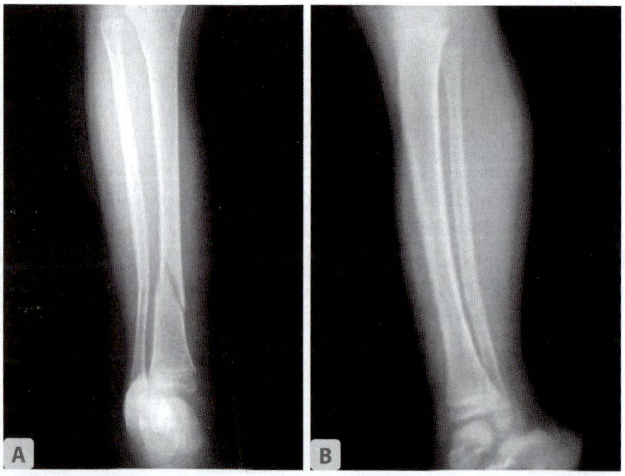

FIGS. 15A AND B: (A) Anteroposterior (AP) and (B) lateral radiographs of right leg showing a greenstick fracture of fibula and oblique (toddler) fracture of tibia.

Physeal Fractures

Salter–Harris classification is a well-recognized classification system for defining the physeal injuries in children and it relates the radiological appearance of physeal fractures with treatment and long-term complications.

Salter–Harris classification

- Transverse through physis
- Through physis but with a metaphyseal fragment
- Through physis and epiphysis and therefore intra-articular
- Through epiphysis, across physis, and through metaphysis (II and III)
- Physeal crush injury **(Figs. 16A to C)**

A practical rule of thumb is: "Higher the grades of physeal injury, the greater chances of growth plate are getting affected". Types I, II, and III injuries have a reasonably better prognosis, than type V injury, which has a worse prognosis because of damage to the growth plate. Complications of physeal injuries include malunion, premature fusion of growth plate (bony bar) resulting in growth impairment and deformity **(Figs. 17A to D)**.

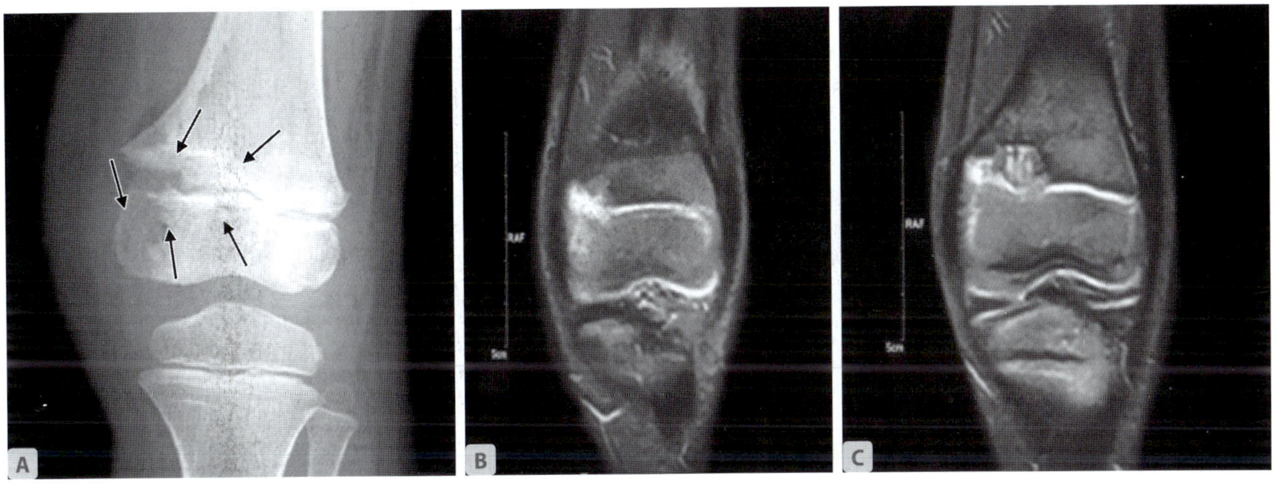

FIGS. 16A TO C: Anteroposterior (AP) radiograph (A) and coronal short inversion time inversion-recovery magnetic resonance (STIR MR) images (B and C) of right knee showing type V fracture of Salter–Harris classification involving the medial aspect of growth plate.

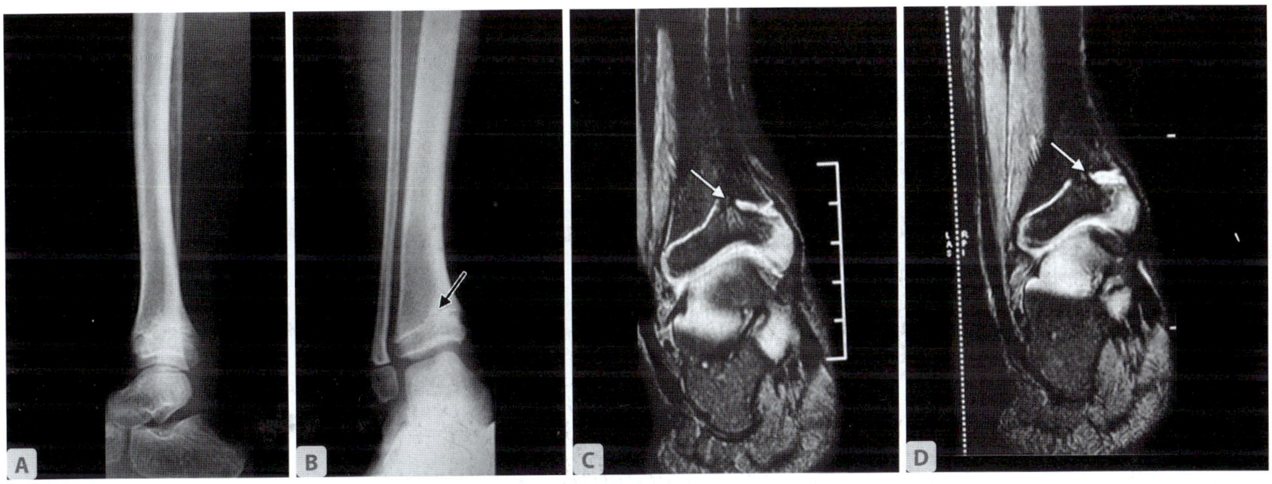

FIGS. 17A TO D: Anteroposterior (AP) and lateral radiographs: (A and B) of tibia including ankle joint showing bony bar (arrows) across the growth plate confirmed on MR images (C and D).

Head Trauma[16]

Head injury in children is major cause of mortality and morbidity following trauma in childhood. Imaging plays vital role in identification and defining the extent of injury.

The mechanism of injury in children varies depending on age, in younger children, accidental falls are frequent cause, whereas in older children, bicycle injuries and motor vehicle accidents are more common.

Children have larger head-to-body ratio and thinner cranial bones (less than age of 4 years, the calvarium is unilaminar and lacks dipole) due to which injuries to the head are more serious.

Broad Classification

- *Primary lesions:* Primary lesions are the direct result of trauma (already occurred at the time of presentation).
- *Secondary lesions:* As complications of primary lesions (preventable)
    - *Acute and subacute:* Include cerebral edema, ischemia, and brain herniation.
    - *Chronic:* Hydrocephalus, the cerebrospinal fluid (CSF) leak, leptomeningeal cyst, and encephalomalacia.

According to Location of Lesions

- *Intra-axial:* Cortical contusions, intracerebral hematoma, axonal shearing injuries, gray matter injury, and vascular injury.
- *Extra-axial:* Epidural, subdural, subarachnoid, and intraventricular hemorrhage.

Skull Fractures[17]

Types of skull fractures seen in children following trauma include: Linear, diastatic, depressed, and compound fractures. Depressed skull fractures are associated with underlying cerebral contusion and dural tears.

Imaging appearances of skull fractures are similar to those seen in adults. However, there are few differences as compared to adults.[18]

- In children <2 years, skull fractures may result from minor trauma because calvarium is softer and thinner than in adults.
- Calvarium is unilaminar without diploe till the age of 4 years. Thus, skull offers less protection to the underlying brain parenchyma.

Extra-axial Injury

- Epidural hematoma (EDH) **(Figs. 18A and B)**
- Subdural hematoma (SDH) **(Figs. 19A and B)**
- Subarachnoid hemorrhage
- Intraventricular hemorrhage

Imaging findings of these abnormalities in children are similar to those in adults.

However, there are few differences as compared to adults:

- In children, SDH is more common than EDH, because dura is more firmly adherent to inner table.
- Subdural hematoma is bilateral in 80% of cases and more extensive (due to less adhesive subdural space).
- Epidural hematoma is less common, and when it does occur, is more often from venous origin than arterial.
- Epidural hematoma or SDH is often venous in origin and evolves slowly, and hence close monitoring is very critical, since the clinical presentation is less dramatic initially as compared to adults.

Intra-axial injuries include contusions **(Fig. 20)**, diffuse axonal injury (DAI) **(Figs. 21A to D and 22)** and intracerebral hematomas. The imaging appearances of these abnormalities are similar to those in adults. However, inner aspect of skull is relatively smooth as compared to adults, hence, contusions are less common in children.

Secondary Head Injury

Diffuse cerebral swelling (edema) results from:

- Increase in cerebral blood volume (hyperemia)
- Vasogenic edema, or
- An increase in tissue fluid (cytotoxic edema).

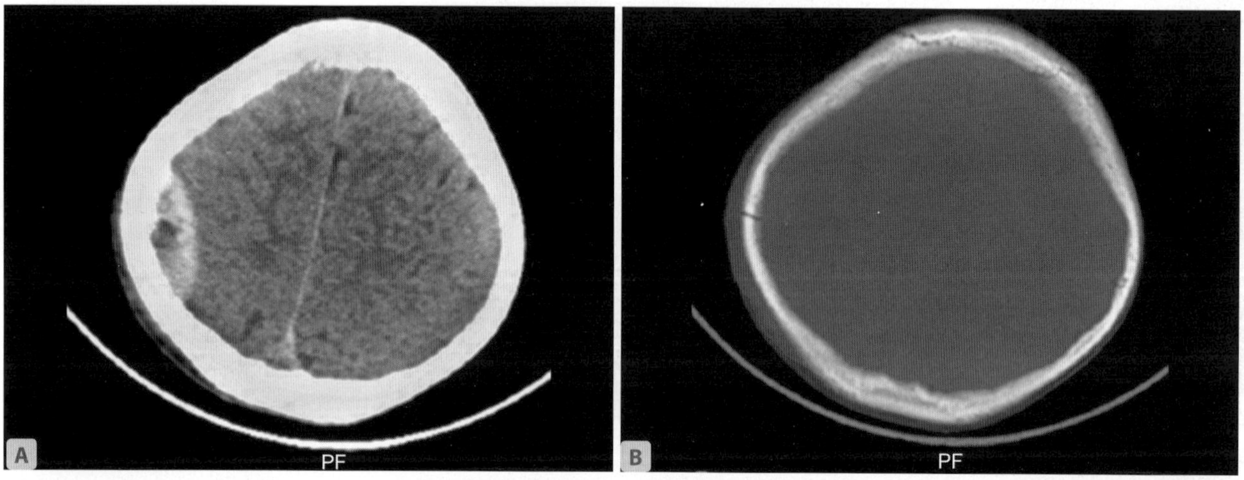

FIGS. 18A AND B: Axial CT sections in brain window (A) and bone window (B) showing small biconvex epidural hematoma in parietal region with linear nondepressed fracture of overlying parietal bone.

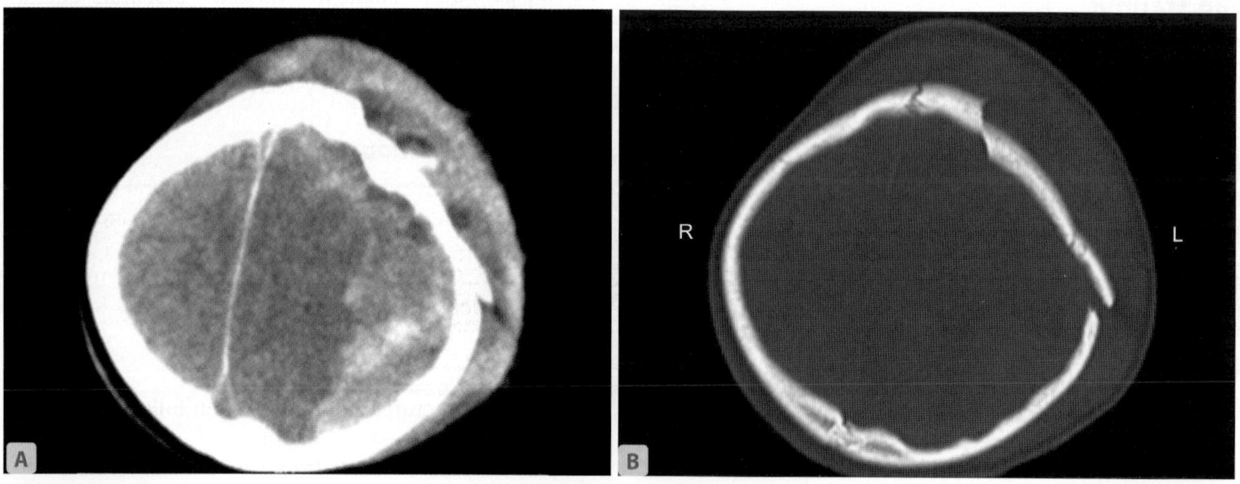

FIGS. 19A AND B: Axial CT sections in bone window (A) and brain window (B) showing subdural hematoma along left cerebral convexity with depressed fracture of overlying frontal bone.

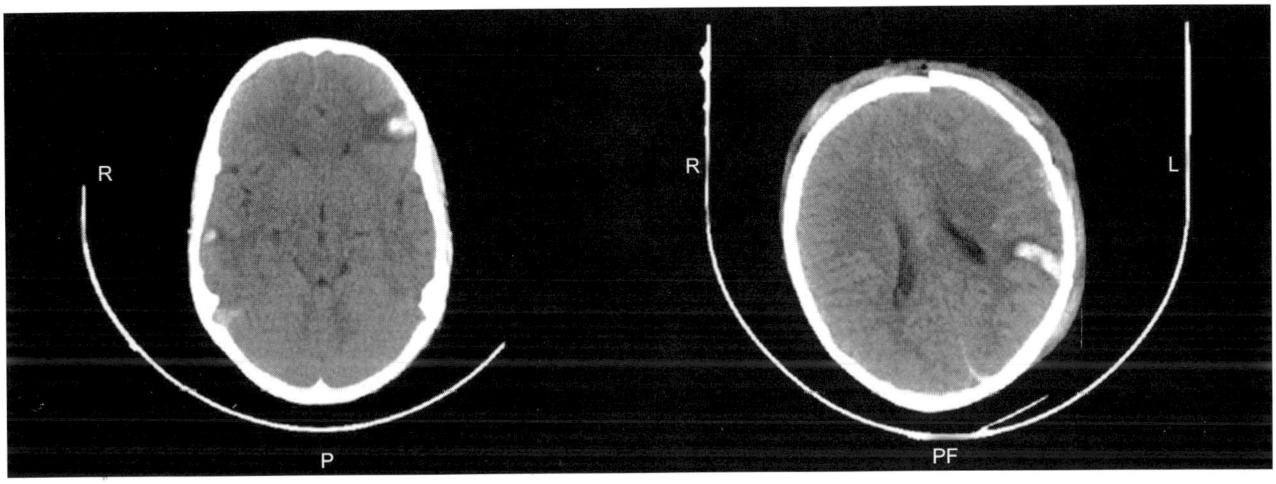

FIG. 20: Axial CT sections of brain showing multiple contusions in left frontal, parietal, and right temporal lobes associated with mild perilesional edema. Note depressed fracture of frontal bone.

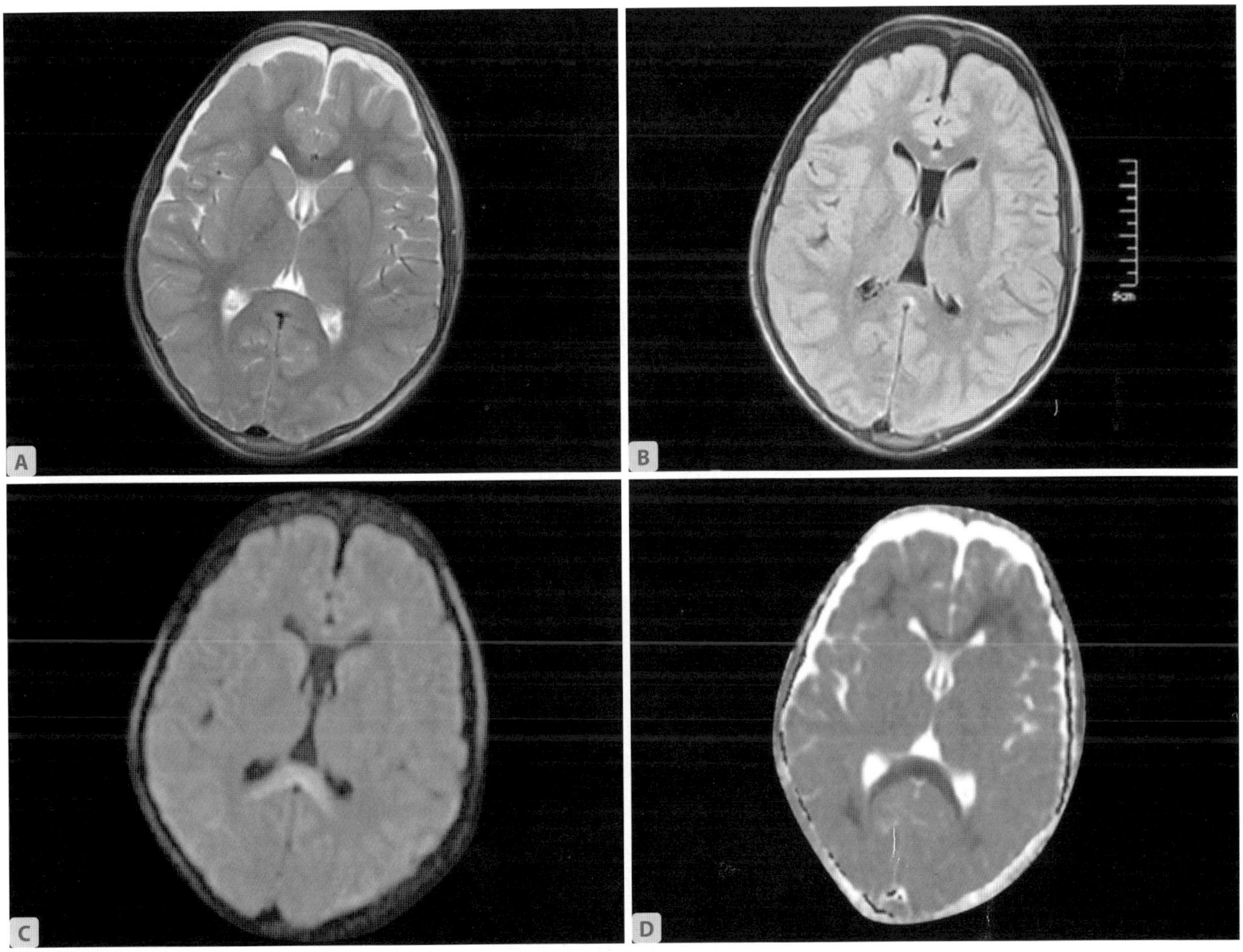

FIGS. 21A TO D: Axial T2 weighted (T2W) (A), fluid-attenuated inversion recovery (FLAIR) (B), diffusion-weighted imaging (DWI) (C), and apparent diffusion coefficient (ADC) map (D) showing diffuse axonal injury involving the splenium of corpus callosum.

Imaging features of cerebral edema include effacement of the cerebral sulci and cisterns, compression of the ventricles and loss of gray-white differentiation. The cerebellum and brainstem are usually spared in cerebral edema and may appear hyperdense (on CT) relative to the affected cerebral hemispheres.

Brain herniation occurs secondary to mass effect produced by cerebral edema.

Types of herniation include:

- Subfalcine
- Uncal
- Transtentorial
  - Descending
  - Ascending
- Transcalvarial through skull defect

All types of herniations are serious signs of cerebral injury, will ultimately lead permanent vascular complications.

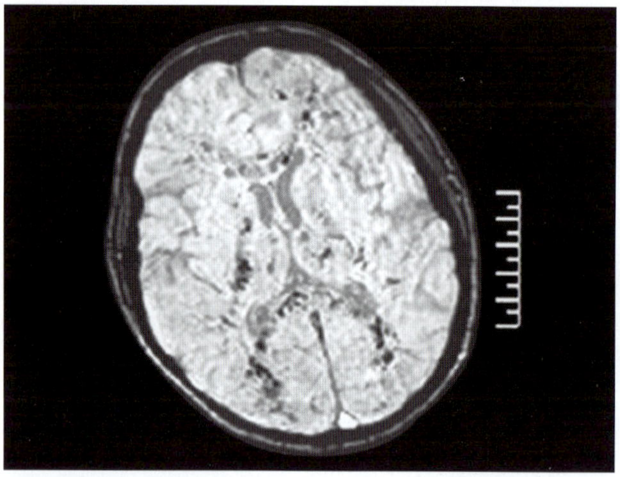

FIG. 22: Fast low angle shot magnetic resonance imaging (FLASH MR) image showing multiple foci of hemorrhages involving gray-white matter junctions and corpus callosum with blooming effect suggestive of diffuse axonal injury.

Traumatic Ischemia–Infarction

Infarctions usually result from cerebral herniations due to cerebral edema. Transfalcine or transtentorial herniation compresses the anterior or posterior cerebral arteries respectively. Cerebral ischemia can also occur due to regional or global cerebral blood flow changes, that will lead to gliosis as a long-term sequel **(Figs. 23A and B)**.

"Growing fracture" refers to interval widening of the space between the fracture margins on successive skull radiographs. Usually seen in children and delayed complications of skull fractures and are accompanied by dural tear in association with a calvarial defect. CSF pulsations eventually widen the dural defect and expand the fracture margins **(Figs. 24A to G)**.

Spinal Injuries

In children, spinal injuries are rare because of greater mobility and elasticity of spinal column, account for <5% all traumatic injuries because of anatomical and biomechanical properties of the growing spine, and there is difference in the pattern of injuries and also the outcomes of spinal injuries in children as compared to adults **(Box 1)**.[16]

Of all the spinal injuries, thoracic spine is affected in nearly 50–60% of cases, 10–15% involve lumbar spine and <5% involve cervical spine and multisegmental in 20–25% cases. Types of cervical spine injuries are mentioned in **Box 2**.

Indications for Imaging Cervical Spine Include (When to Image)[19,20]

Clinical examination can confidently exclude C-spine injuries:

- National Emergency X-Radiography Utilization Study (NEXUS) or Canadian C-spine rule should be adopted, used, and taught.
- Advanced trauma life support (ATLS) practice: NEXUS + Movement test.

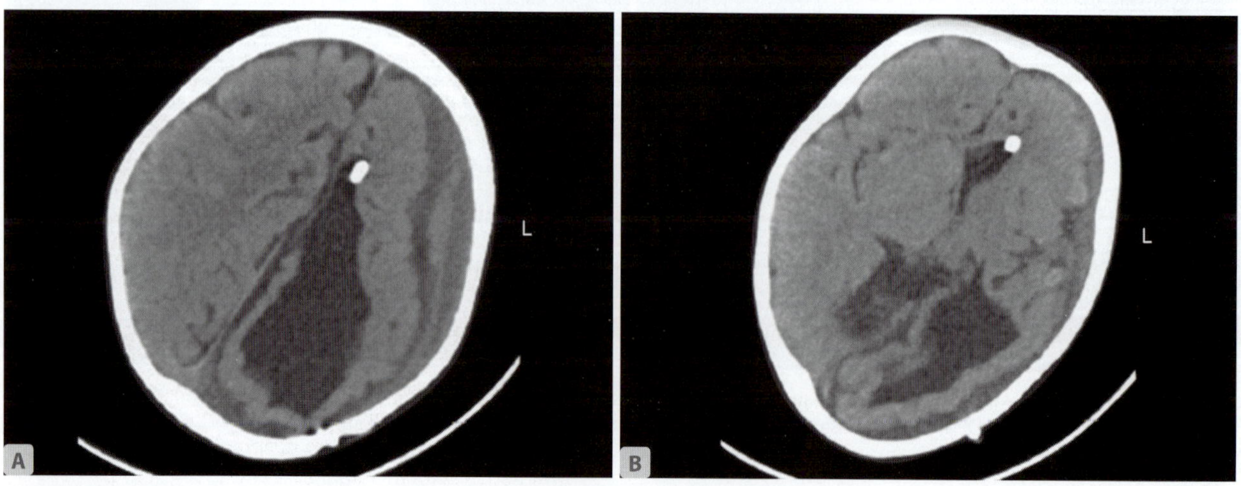

FIGS. 23A AND B: Axial CT sections of brain showing atrophic changes in left cerebral hemisphere with ex-vacuo ventriculomegaly with ventriculoperitoneal (VP) shunt in situ and subdural hygroma, sequelae of post-traumatic brain injury.

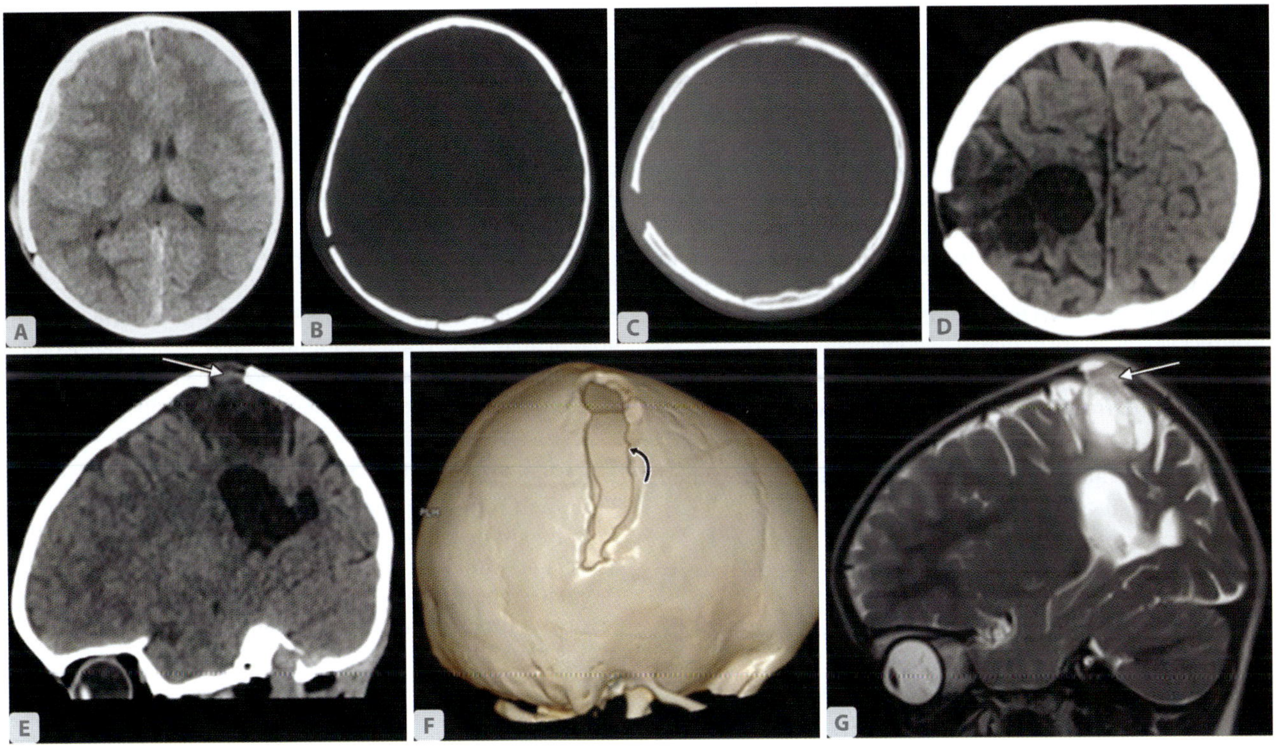

FIGS. 24A TO G: Growing fracture: Initial CT images (A and B) showing linear fracture involving parietal bone without any underlying brain injury. Follow up CT scan (C and D) at 6 months showed widening of the fracture line with gliosis of underlying brain parenchyma. Scans at 1.5 years (E to G) showed irregular widening of fracture line (curved arrow) and herniation of brain parenchyma through the calvarial defect (arrows).

BOX 1: Anatomic differences in the pediatric cervical spine.[3]

- Relatively larger head size: Flexion injuries >> extension injuries
- Smaller neck muscle mass: Ligamentous injuries more common than fractures
- Infantile bony column can lengthen significantly: SCIWORA
- Facet joints with a more horizontal orientation offer less resistance to the forces
- Incomplete ossification makes interpretation of bony alignment difficult
- Increased preodontoid space up to 4–5 mm (3 mm in an adult)
- Pseudosubluxation of C2 on C3 seen in 40% of children
- Prevertebral space size may change because of variations with respiration

BOX 2: Types of cervical spine injuries.[16]

- Spinal cord injury without radiographic abnormality (SCIWORA), **(Figs. 25A and B)**
- Occiput–C1 injury **(Figs. 26A and B)**
- Atlantoaxial injuries **(Figs. 27A and B)**
- Atlantoaxial rotatory subluxation **(Fig. 28)**
- Traumatic spondylolisthesis of C2 (Hangman fracture)
- Subaxial injuries (C3–C7)
- Posterior ligamentous injuries
- Wedge compression fractures
- Facet dislocations

How to Image Pediatric Spine

- >9 years old = Same rule as adults
  - NEXUS supports this strategy
- <9 years old = No solid data on how to image exists
  - No solid data on CT versus radiography
  - Children are more sensitive to radiation
  - Start with radiographs
  - If head CT is done in young children: Extend it through C2.

Indications for Thoracolumbar CT[20]

- Motor vehicle crash at >35 mph
- Falls of >15 feet
- Automobile hitting pedestrian with pedestrian thrown >10 feet
- Assaulted with a depressed level of consciousness
- Known cervical injury
- Rigid spine disease

When indicated in young children <9 years, radiographic evaluation consisting of a cross-table lateral view, an anteroposterior view, and an open-mouth view has the sensitivity of 89% and the negative predictive value of nearly 100 in detecting cervical spine injuries.

However, in older children (<9 years), CT is the modality of choice for imaging any form of spinal injury.

Magnetic resonance imaging is indicated in presence of neurological deficit to know the status of posterior ligamentous complex, status of the spinal cord and the disk injury.

Spinal cord injury without radiographic abnormality (SCIWORA) is almost unique to the pediatric population and occurs as a consequence of a stretch or distraction injury to the relatively flexible spinal column that exceeds the tensile limits of the spinal cord. Because of increased musculoskeletal elasticity, which serves to dissipate the kinetic energy transferred to the child's body during trauma thus preventing fracture or dislocation is not shared by the spinal cord, which may lead to the occurrence of spinal cord injury without radiological abnormality **(Figs. 25A and B)**. Another theory, SCIWORA results either from ischemia due to direct vessel injury or due to hypoperfusion.[16]

Atlantoaxial Rotatory Fixation/Subluxation

Atlantoaxial rotatory fixation is one of the causes of a torticollis in children. Rotation is the primary movement at atlantoaxial joint. This normal rotation becomes limited or fixed in rotatory atlantoaxial subluxation. The etiology of this condition unknown may be related to increased laxity ligaments and capsular structures secondary to trauma.

It is very important to recognize this entity because it indicates a compromised atlantoaxial joint and may potentially cause neural damage or even death. Imaging evaluation of this condition is difficult because child head is being in rotated position during CT scan, hence one may falsely interpret it as rotatory subluxation. Imaging trick to make the diagnosis of this condition is to see the anterior arch of atlas, which always follows the chin or nasal septum. If the anterior arch of C1 does not follow either chin or nasal septum, then one should suspect this condition[21] **(Fig. 28)**.

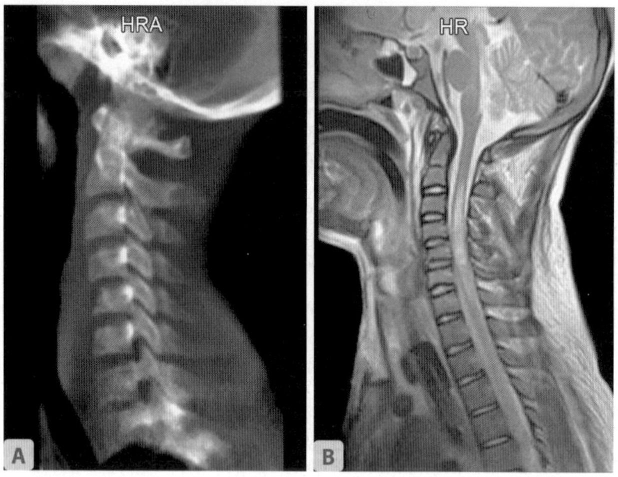

FIGS. 25A AND B: Lateral radiograph of cervical spine (A) and sagittal T2-weighted magnetic resonance imaging (T2W MR) image (B) showing evidence of cord contusion without any obvious visible radiographic abnormality suggestive of spinal cord injury without radiological abnormality (SCIWORA).

Thoracic and Lumbar Spine Trauma

Thoracolumbar injuries are seen either following fall from height or following road traffic injury and are usually associated with other organ injuries. Of all the spinal injuries, thoracic spine is affected in nearly 50–60% of cases, 10–15% involve lumbar spine and <5% involve cervical spine and multisegmental in 20–25% cases. The most common type of fracture in the thoracolumbar region is compression fracture **(Figs. 29A and B)**. CT is the modality of choice to demonstrate the fracture extent.[16]

Nonaccidental Injury

Nonaccidental injury (NAI) can be defined as any violent act or series of acts of commission or omission by child's parent or caregiver that results in harm or potential harm to the child.

Investigation of the suspected NAI is a sensitive multidisciplinary task where imaging plays an important role. A correct diagnosis is very crucial for the safety of the child; however, cases are missed due to misinterpretation of images.

As a radiologist, we need to be aware of possible symptoms, presentations, and imaging spectrum of NAI and also we have to cooperate with clinicians in thorough medical investigation.

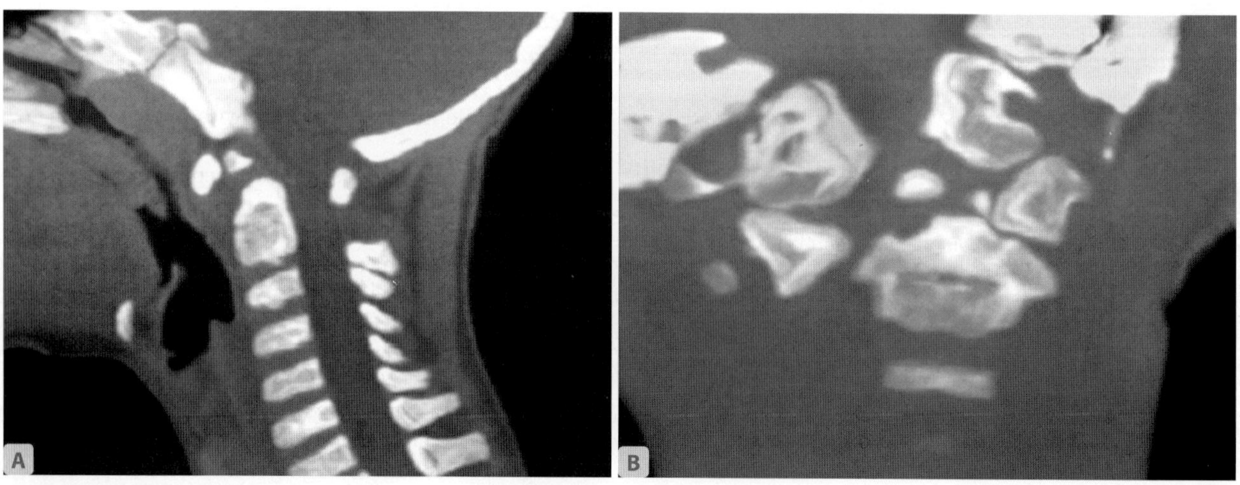

FIGS. 26A AND B: Sagittal multiplanar reconstruction (MPR) (A) and coronal thick maximum intensity projection (MIP) (B) images showing type 1 fracture of dense of C2 vertebra and atlanto-occipital subluxation.

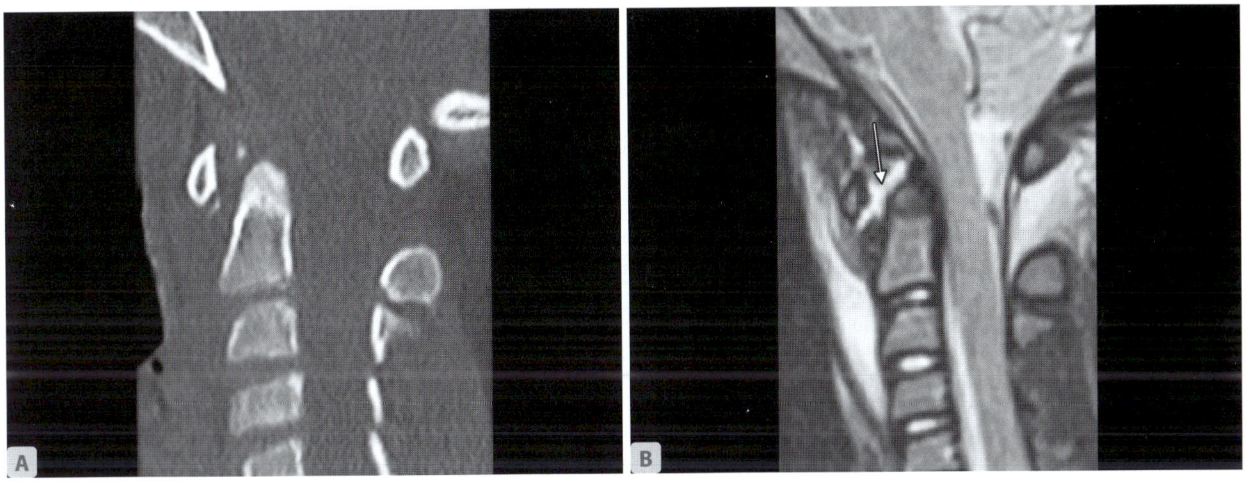

FIGS. 27A AND B: Sagittal computed tomography (CT) (A) and sagittal T2 weighted (T2W) MR (B) images showing widening of atlanto-dental interval (arrows) suggesting atlantoaxial dislocation.

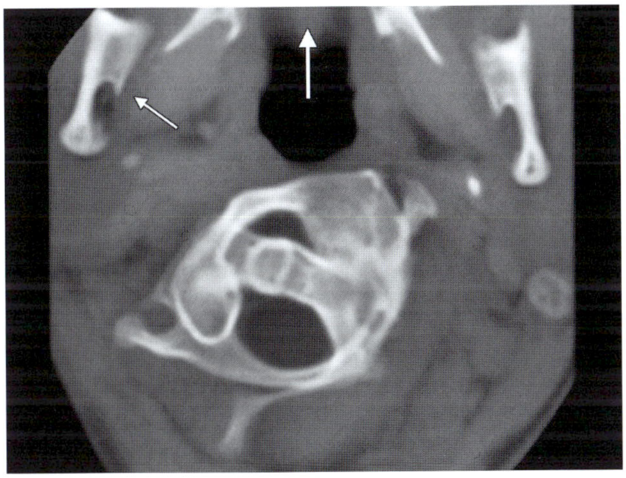

FIG. 28: Atlantoaxial rotatory fixation showing anterior arch of C1 is directed toward right side (thin arrow) rather than directing toward nasal septum/chin (block arrow).

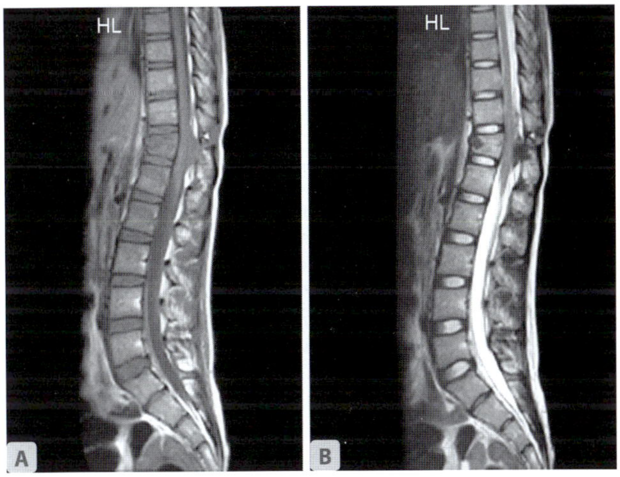

FIGS. 29A AND B: Sagittal T1 weighted (T1W) (A) and T2 weighted (T2W) MR (B) images showing wedge compression fracture of D12 vertebral body with epidural hematoma. Cord shows normal signal intensity.

Imaging Findings of Nonaccidental Injury (Table 2)

Any type of injury/fracture may occur in NAI. Some of the imaging features are highly specific, some are moderately specific and some are very common but carry low specificity. A complete skeletal survey is almost always mandatory in suspected NAI for patients under 2 years of age; its utility diminishes and provides little value after the age of 5 years. Between the ages of 2 and 5 years, imaging is guided by specific clinical indicators of abuse and should be individually prescribed as per the recommendation of American Academy of Pediatrics.[22]

Skeletal survey consists of both appendicular skeleton and axial skeletal imaging (ACR 2006).[23]

Appendicular skeletal survey consists of:

- Arms AP
- Forearms AP
- Hands PA
- Thighs AP
- Legs AP
- Feet AP or PA

TABLE 2: Imaging findings of nonaccidental injury.

High specificity	Moderate specificity	Common but low specificity
CMLs*	Multiple Fractures especially bilateral	SPNBF**
Rib fractures, especially posternomeddial	Fractures of different ages	Clavicular fractures
Scapular fractures	Epiphyseal separations	Long bone shaft fractures
Spinous process fractures	Vertebral body fractures and subluxation	Linear skull fractures
Sternal fractures	Digital fractures	
	Complex skull fractures	
	Pelvic fractures	

*CML: classic metaphyseal lesion

**SPNBF: subperiosteal new bone formation

Axial skeletal survey consists of:

- Chest frontal AP and lateral including ribs and thoracic spine
- Pelvis AP to include mid-lumbar spine
- Lumbosacral spine (lateral)
- Cervical spine (frontal and lateral)
- Skull (frontal and lateral) (in addition to CT scanner)

CONCLUSION

Imaging in pediatric trauma must use specific techniques with adapted protocols and algorithms taking the child's specific conditions into consideration. These differ from standard adult imaging strategies and protocols.

REFERENCES

1. Jaffe D. Emergency management of blunt trauma in children. N Engl J Med. 1991;324:1477-82.
2. Miniño A, Heron M, Smith B, Kochanek KD, Centers for Disease Control and Prevention, National Center for Health Statistics, et al. Deaths: final data for 2004. Natl Vital Stat Rep. 2007;55(19):1-119.
3. Marx JA, Holberger RS. Rosen's emergency medicine: concepts and clinical practice, 5th edition. United States: Mosby; 2002. pp. 267-81.
4. Kao SC, Smith WL. Skeletal injuries in the pediatric patient. Radiol Clin North Am. 1997;35:727-46.
5. Resnik CS. Diagnostic imaging of pediatric skeletal trauma. Radiol Clin North Am. 1989;27:1013-22.
6. Kellenberger CJ. Imaging children—what is special? Ther Umsch. 2009;66(1):55-9.
7. Johnson KJ, Bache E, Baert AL. Imaging in Pediatric Skeletal Trauma: Techniques and Applications, 1st edition. Berlin, Germany: Springer; 2008. pp. 1-11.
8. Soudack M, Epelman M, Maor R, Hayari L, Shoshani G, Heyman-Reiss A, et al. Experience with Focused Abdominal Sonography for Trauma (FAST) in 313 pediatric patients. J Clin Ultrasound. 2004;32:53-61.
9. Westra SJ, Wallace EC. Imaging evaluation of pediatric chest trauma. Radiol Clin North Am. 2005;43(2):267-81.
10. Sanchez TR, Jadhav SP, Swischuk LE. MR imaging of pediatric trauma. Magn Reson Imaging Clin N Am. 2009;17(3):439-50.
11. Stanescu LA, Gross JA, Bittle M, Mann FA. Imaging of blunt abdominal trauma. Semin Roentgenol. 2006;41(3):196-208.
12. Saladino RA, Lund DP. Abdominal trauma. In: Fleisher GR, Ludwig S, Henretig FM (Eds). Textbook of Pediatric Emergency Medicine, 5th edition. Philadelphia: Lippincott Williams & Wilkins; 2006. pp. 1339-48.
13. Rose JS. Ultrasound in abdominal trauma. Emerg Med Clin North Am. 2004;22(3):581-9.
14. Bixby SD, Callahan MJ, Taylor GA. Imaging in pediatric blunt abdominal trauma. Semin Roentgenol. 2008;43(1):72-82.
15. Barnes H. Pediatric Skeletal Trauma—Plain Film to MRI: Imaging Techniques. Appl Radiol. 2007;36(8):24-33.
16. Cakmakci H. Essentials of trauma: Head and spine. Pediatr Radiol. 2009;39(Suppl 3):391-405.
17. Zimmerman RA, Bilaniuk LT. Pediatric head trauma. Neuroimaging Clin N Am. 1994;4:349-66.
18. Schutzman SA, Greenes DS. Pediatric minor head trauma. Ann Emerg Med. 2001;37:65-74.
19. Daffner RH. Controversies in cervical spine imaging in trauma patients. Semin Musculoskelet Radiol. 2005;9(2):105-15.
20. Daffner RH, Hackney DB. ACR Appropriateness Criteria on suspected spine trauma. J Am Coll Radiol. 2007;4(11):762-75.
21. Rajagopal KV, Lakhkar BN, Banavali S. CT demonstration of rotatory atlantoaxial subluxation. Indian J Radiol Imaging. 2000;10:175-6.
22. Christian CW, Committee on Child Abuse and Neglect, American Academy of Pediatrics. The evaluation of suspected child physical abuse. Pediatrics. 2015;135(5):e1337-54.
23. American College of Radiology. (2006). ACR practice guideline for skeletal surveys in children. [online] Available from http://www.acr.org/SecondaryMainMenuCategories/quality_safety/guidelines/pediatric/skeletal_ surveys.aspx. [Last accessed July, 2020].

CHAPTER

62

Neonatal Respiratory Distress

Akshay Kumar Saxena, Kushaljit Singh Sodhi, Anmol Bhatia

INTRODUCTION

A newborn is called a neonate till the age of 28 days of postnatal life. Respiratory distress is the most common morbidity necessitating the admission of a neonate in an intensive care unit (ICU). Respiratory distress is said to be present with at least two of the following three features:[1]

1. Tachypnea (respiratory rate >60 breaths/min)
2. Retractions (intercostal, subcostal, sternal, or suprasternal)
3. Noisy respiration (grunt, stridor, or wheeze)

Respiratory distress occurs in 11–14% of all live births.[2] Gestational age has pronounced effect on incidence of neonatal respiratory distress with incidence of respiratory distress on 1st day of life being higher in babies born at lesser gestation. Kumar and colleagues reported 60% incidence of respiratory distress in babies <30 weeks of gestational age which reduced to 5–6% in babies with gestational age >34 weeks.[2] There are several causes which can give rise to respiratory distress during the neonatal period. They can broadly be classified as follows:[3]

- *Causes affecting respiration at alveolar level*: Hyaline membrane disease (HMD), meconium aspiration syndrome (MAS), pneumonia, pneumothorax, pulmonary hemorrhage, transient tachypnea of the newborn (TTNB), primary pulmonary hypertension, etc.
- *Structural anomalies of the respiratory tract*: Congenital lobar overinflation (CLO), congenital pulmonary airway malformation (CPAM), congenital diaphragmatic hernia (CDH), choanal atresia, tracheoesophageal fistula, etc.
- *Extrapulmonary causes*: Chest wall abnormalities, congenital heart disease, metabolic acidosis, etc.

The management of neonatal respiratory distress depends upon clinical history, examination, radiology, and laboratory data. The radiology of important causes of respiratory distress in neonates is discussed below.

MEDICAL CAUSES OF NEONATAL RESPIRATORY DISTRESS

Hyaline Membrane Disease

Hyaline membrane disease (HMD), also known as respiratory distress syndrome (RDS), is the most common cause of respiratory distress in preterm babies accounting for up to 60% incidence in babies born at or before 29 weeks of gestation.[4] It is a manifestation of pulmonary immaturity and results from impaired surfactant production by type 2 pneumocytes leading to formation of hyaline membranes within alveoli and terminal airways, hence the name. Oxygen therapy along with surfactant supplementation currently forms the cornerstone of treatment for HMD. Persistent barotraumas and oxygen toxicity in these neonates, due to intensive oxygen and ventilation therapy, can lead to bronchopulmonary dysplasia (BPD).[5]

The radiological evaluation of HMD has traditionally relied upon chest radiography. The chest X-ray (CXR) findings in untreated HMD reflect the generalized acinar collapse which occurs due to surfactant deficiency. CXR demonstrates decreased expansion of lungs, symmetric generalized consolidation depending upon the severity, nonvisualization of normal pulmonary vessels, and air bronchograms **(Figs. 1A and B)**.[6] The commonly seen "reticulogranular" pattern of opacities in HMD represents the collapsed alveoli, seepage of fluid into the interstitium from capillary leak, and distension by air of innumerable bronchioles that are more compliant when compared to the surfactant-deficient lung. These radiographic findings reach to maximum severity around 12–24 hours of life. In severe cases, there may be complete bilateral "whiteout" of lungs due to extensive consolidation.[7]

The CXR findings of HMD are also affected by the timing of the surfactant administration. Early on, despite prevention

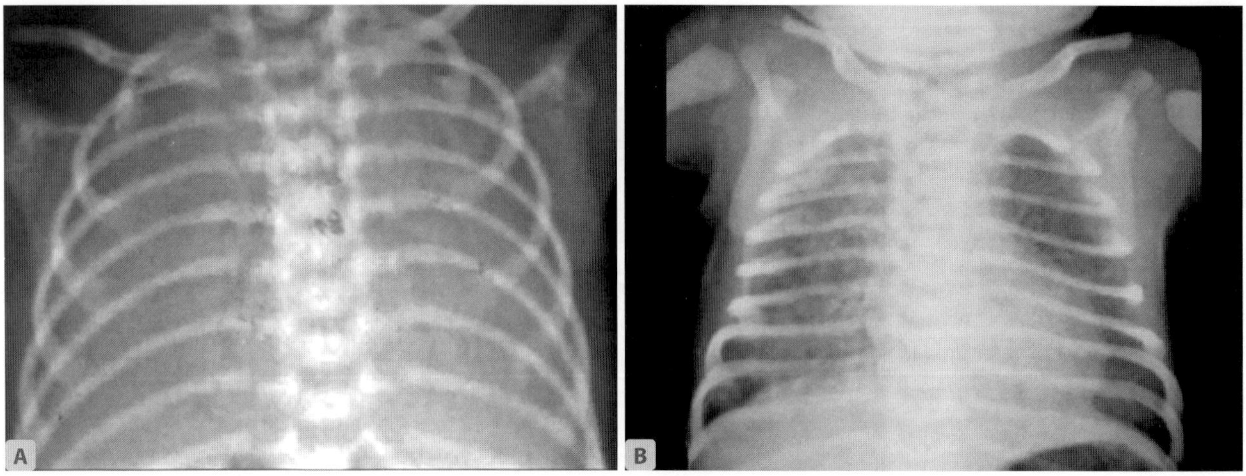

FIGS. 1A AND B: (A) Chest X-ray AP view of a preterm neonate with respiratory distress soon after birth reveals low volume lungs with bilateral consolidation with "whiteout" of lungs suggestive of HMD; and (B) In another preterm neonate with respiratory distress soon after birth, consolidation is less extensive. (AP: anteroposterior; HMD: hyaline membrane disease)

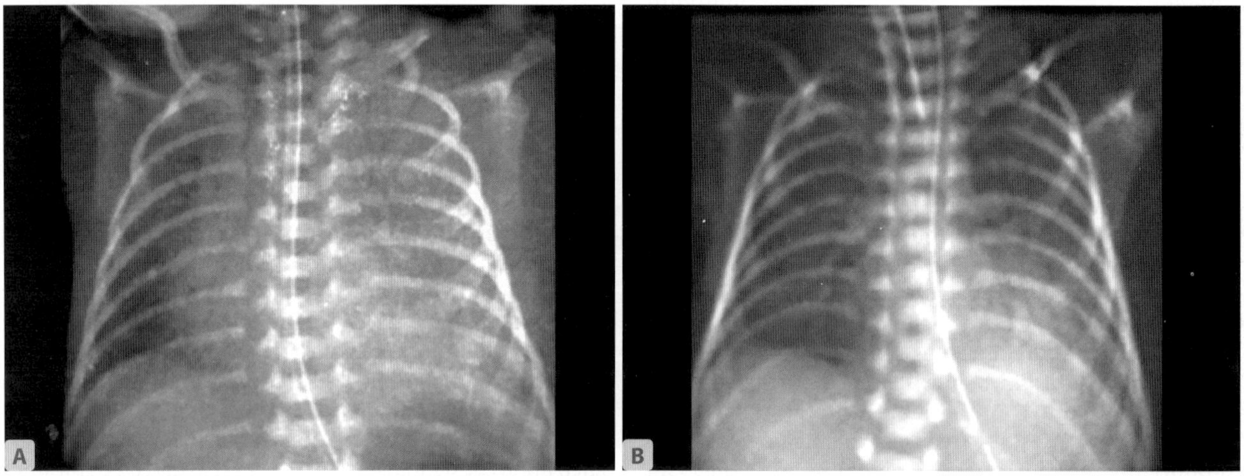

FIGS. 2A AND B: (A) Chest X-ray AP view of a preterm neonate with respiratory distress soon after birth reveals low volume lungs with bilateral consolidation with "whiteout" of lungs suggestive of HMD; and (B) 18 hours after surfactant administration, there is asymmetric clearing of upper zones. (AP: anteroposterior; HMD: hyaline membrane disease)

with surfactant, the lungs are hypoaerated and have a reticulogranular pattern due to fluid in the interstitium and atelectatic alveoli. The surfactant administration usually results in some clearing **(Figs. 2A and B)**, which may be symmetrical or asymmetrical. Since the surfactant does not gets distributed evenly throughout the lungs, it is common to seen areas of lung showing improvement which alternate with the areas of unchanged RDS.[8]

With positive-pressure ventilation usually given in these infants, there is decrease in the lung opacity suggesting a radiological improvement. However, the positive pressure which is required for lung aeration may disrupt the epithelial lining resulting in interstitial and alveolar edema. It can further lead to dissection of air into the peribronchovascular interstitium, resulting in pulmonary interstitial emphysema (PIE) **(Fig. 3)**. Radiographically, PIE is seen as 1–4 mm linear lucent areas that are relatively of uniform size radiating outward from the pulmonary hilum and extend up to the periphery of the lungs.[9] This can result in formation of subpleural blebs which may rupture into pleural cavity resulting in pneumothorax or can also extend toward the mediastinum leading to pneumomediastinum or pneumopericardium.

Since, portable chest radiography imparts ionizing radiation and involves delay in availability of information to the clinician, alternative strategies in evaluation of HMD are desirable. Ultrasound has recently emerged as an alternative to chest radiography for the diagnosis and follow-up of HMD. The advantages of ultrasound include lack of ionizing radiation and portability. Two different types of techniques—transabdominal and transthoracic—have been utilized for diagnosis and follow-up of HMD. The transabdominal approach was the earlier method for evaluation of HMD. Using this approach, a few studies[10-12] have described a typical pattern of increased retrodiaphragmatic (retrohepatic and retrosplenic hyperechogenicity) which has high sensitivity and specificity for the diagnosis of HMD. Incomplete clearance of this retrodiaphragmatic hyperechogenicity **(Figs. 4A and B)** on serial transabdominal lung sonography has been reported to predict the future occurrence of BPD.[12-14] However, these studies differed in the exact postnatal day on which follow-up transabdominal lung sonography can be performed for prediction of BPD. The transthoracic lung sonography for RDS was described by Copetti et al.[15] They evaluated 40 preterm newborn infants with respiratory distress and reported that the ultrasound consistently showed echographic "white lung" or generalized alveolar-interstitial syndrome **(Fig. 5)**, abnormalities of pleural line (small subpleural consolidations, thickening, irregularity, and coarse appearance), and an absence of areas with a normal pattern ("spared areas"). Simultaneous presence of these findings could identify RDS with a sensitivity and specificity of 100%. Utility of transthoracic sonography has been corroborated by subsequent studies.[16-19] A recent systematic review[20] has reported that transthoracic technique appears to be superior to the transabdominal approach for diagnosis of neonatal RDS as the subgroup analysis demonstrated transthoracic technique to have marginally better sensitivity (99%, 97%, respectively) as well as better specificity (98%, 82%, respectively). Lung ultrasonography, using a combination of transabdominal and transthoracic approach, has also been reported to be highly reliable for diagnosing pulmonary complications of RDS.[21]

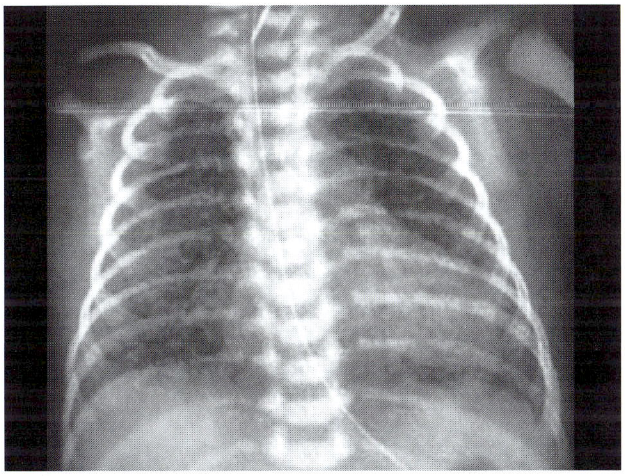

FIG. 3: Follow-up chest X-ray of a patient of HMD reveals lucent lesions suggestive of PIE. (HMD: hyaline membrane disease; PIE: pulmonary interstitial emphysema)

Transient Tachypnea of the Newborn (TTNB)

Whereas HMD is a disease of premature neonates, TTNB affects term babies. In the fetal life, the lungs are distended with fluid. This fluid is cleared from the lungs during the squeeze through the birth canal, while additional fluid is cleared by capillaries and lymphatics within the lungs. The delay in clearance of pulmonary fluid leads to TTNB which is also known as "wet lung disease." The neonates present with mild or moderate respiratory distress soon after birth.[22] Typically, the disease is self-limiting with resolution of symptoms in 6–24 hours. Uncommonly, the symptoms may last 2–5 days when it becomes necessary to exclude alternative causes of respiratory distress.[3]

The radiographic features of TTNB include mild hyper-inflation, mild cardiomegaly, small pulmonary effusion, and prominent interstitial markings in perihilar region **(Fig. 6)**. TTNB may mimic reticulogranular pattern of HMD, but lacks the underaeration seen in HMD. The radiographic features may occasionally look similar to pulmonary edema or MAS.[22]

Copetti and Cattarossi[23] evaluated the lung sonographic findings in TTNB and its clinical relevance. They reported that in neonates with TTNB, lung sonography showed a difference in echogenicity between the upper and lower areas of the lung. This was due to the presence of compact

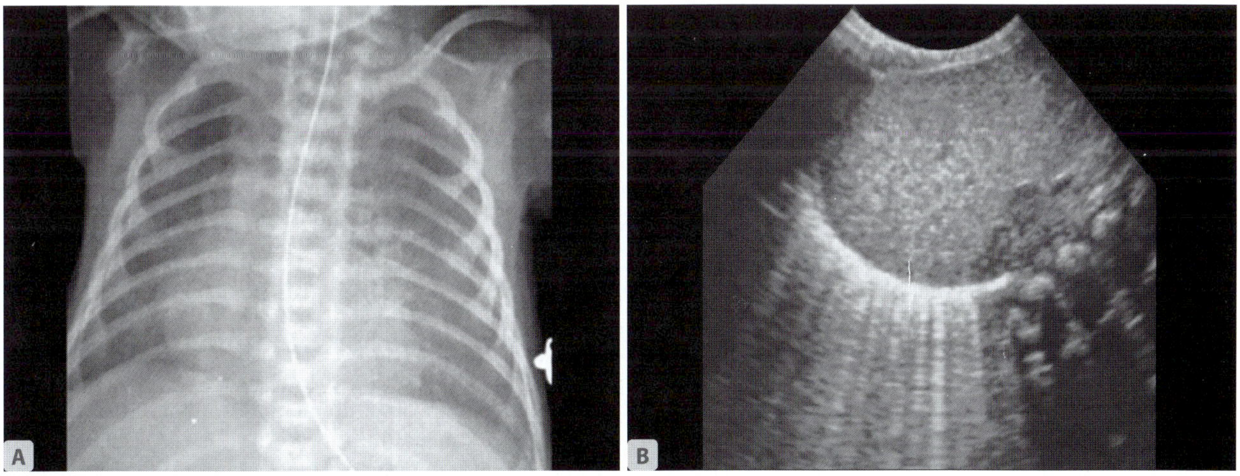

FIGS. 4A AND B: (A) Chest X-ray AP view of a preterm neonate with respiratory distress soon after birth reveals low volume lungs with bilateral consolidation with "whiteout" of lungs suggestive of HMD; and (B) Coronal transabdominal sonography reveals diffuse retrodiaphragmatic hyperechogenicity suggestive of HMD. (AP: anteroposterior; HMD: hyaline membrane disease)

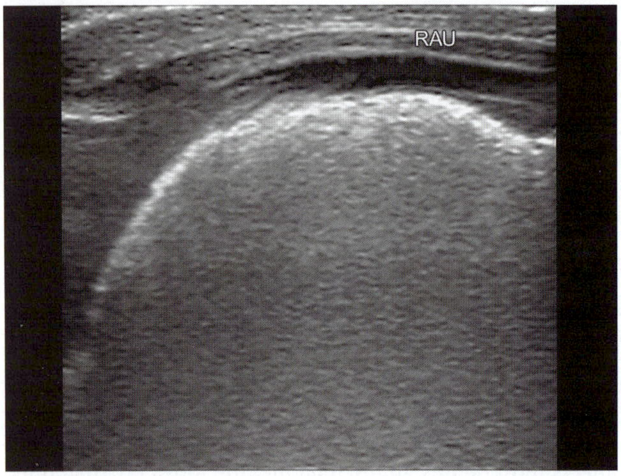

FIG. 5: Transthoracic ultrasound image of a preterm neonate with hyaline membrane disease (HMD) showing whiteout of lung due to confluent B-lines.

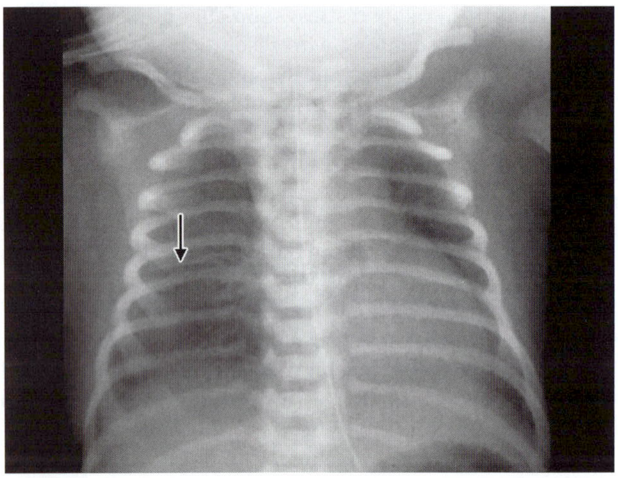

FIG. 6: Transient tachypnea of the newborn (TTNB): Chest X-ray of a term neonate born by cesarean section and respiratory distress soon after birth reveals normal volume lungs with perihilar infiltrate, prominent cardiac silhouette, and pleural fluid in minor fissure (black arrow).

comet-tail artifacts (B-lines) in the inferior lung fields, which were sparsely seen in the superior lung fields. They named this finding as the "double lung point". In this study, "double lung point" was not seen in healthy neonates, neonates with HMD, pneumonia, atelectasis, pneumothorax, or pulmonary hemorrhage. Thus, the specificity and sensitivity of the "double lung point" was 100% for the diagnosis of TTNB. Another recent study by Ibrahim and colleagues[24] have reported the sensitivity, specificity, positive predictive value, and negative predictive value of "double lung point" to be 69.6%, 100%, 100%, and 39.1%, respectively for the diagnosis of TTNB. However, "double lung point" cannot be considered pathognomonic of TTNB as it has also been reported in pneumothorax.[25]

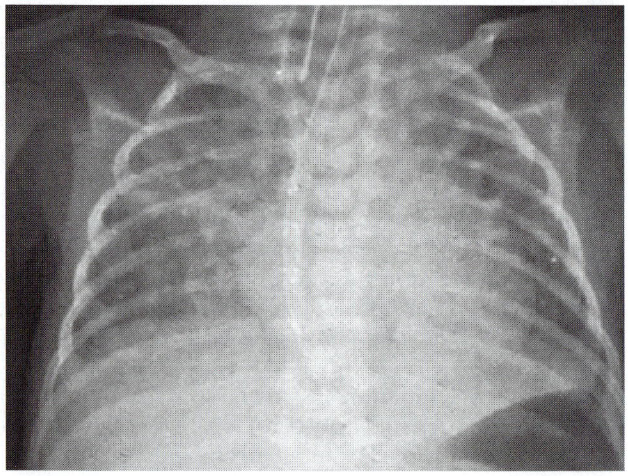

FIG. 7: Chest X-ray anteroposterior (AP) view of a neonate on ventilator with respiratory distress reveals patchy consolidation in right lung suggestive of pneumonia.

Neonatal Pneumonia

Pneumonia is an important cause of neonatal respiratory distress in India with all cases of neonatal respiratory distress being treated as pneumonia at the first referral unit.[18] In a study which evaluated the causes of respiratory distress in outborn neonates brought to a referral unit, Mathur et al.[26] reported pneumonia as a cause of respiratory distress in more than two-thirds of cases. However, this study did not include patients having surgical causes of respiratory distress. The pneumonia may set in due to transplacental spread, lack of asepsis during delivery, aspiration of amniotic fluid, or be acquired during hospital stay for other ailments. Ventilator-associated pneumonia (VAP) is the second most common hospital-acquired infection (HAI) among pediatric and neonatal ICU patients[27,28] and is responsible for a very high mortality in neonatal ICU patients. The majority of cases are of bacterial etiology.

Radiographically, pneumonia is characterized by pulmonary opacities **(Fig. 7)**. However, similar appearance may be seen in RDS, TTNB, and MAS. Presence of pleural effusion is a helpful pointer toward pneumonia. Furthermore, some of these conditions may coexist with pneumonia.[22] The patients with positive radiograph who do not grow causative organism from blood culture are considered "probable pneumonia".[29] It is important to note that in some of the patients with pneumonia, CXR may be normal and diagnosis is made on isolation of organism from blood culture.[26] Rarely, pneumonia may mimic mass lesion.

Meconium Aspiration Syndrome

Meconium aspiration syndrome (MAS) is predominantly seen in term and postmature neonates. While, 10–15% of the neonates pass meconium in utero, it is rarely seen before 37 weeks of gestational age.[29] Fetus manifests normal shallow regular respiratory movements during intrauterine life. Fetal hypoxia stimulates deep gasping respirations. In addition,

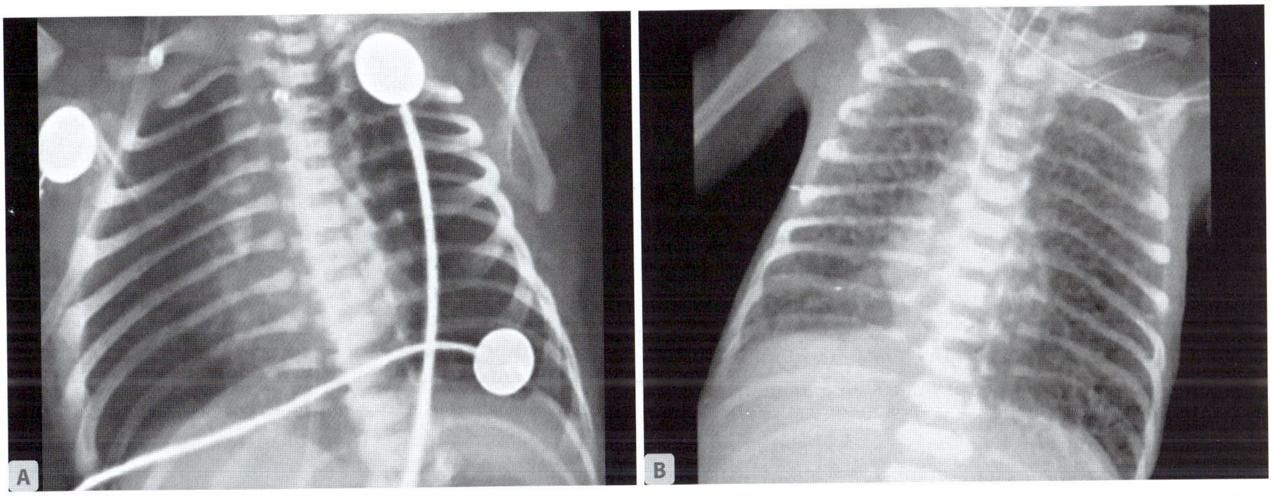

FIGS. 8A AND B: Term neonate with meconium aspiration. (A) Chest X-ray (CXR) anteroposterior (AP) view reveals bilateral hyperinflation; and (B) In another neonate with respiratory distress and suspected meconium aspiration, CXR AP view reveals bilateral pulmonary opacities. Pulmonary opacities in meconium aspiration may be due to atelectasis, chemical pneumonitis, or superadded pneumonia.

it also leads to premature passage of meconium in utero. Meconium is sterile, but locally irritant. It can cause obstruction of medium and small airways. In addition, it is a good medium for bacterial growth. The severity of MAS depends on several factors including consistency of meconium, adequacy of oropharyngeal suction, associated asphyxia, resuscitative measures, etc.

The radiographic appearance in meconium aspiration is variable **(Figs. 8A and B)**. Incomplete bronchial obstruction leads to generalized hyperinflation along with patchy areas of atelectasis secondary to complete bronchial obstruction. There may be subsequent development of pneumothorax and pneumomediastinum. The radiographic appearance may be further complicated by pulmonary edema (because of cerebral, myocardial, or renal dysfunction secondary to ischemia), pulmonary hemorrhage, RDS, or pneumonia.[22] Some of the babies with meconium aspiration may eventually develop persistent pulmonary hypertension of newborn.[3]

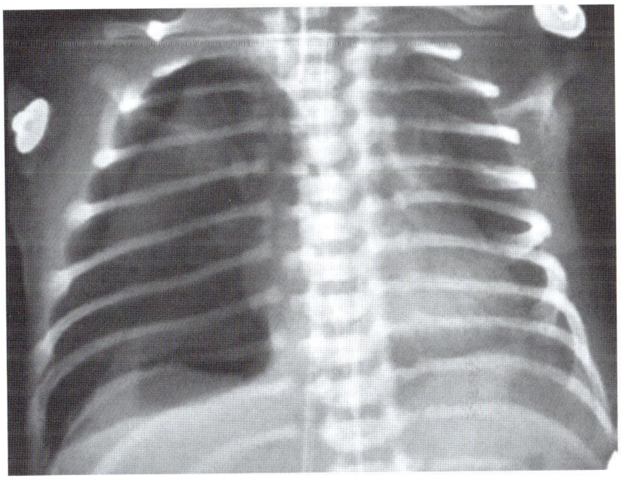

FIG. 9: Neonate on ventilator developed respiratory distress. Chest X-ray anteroposterior (AP) view revealed gross right pneumothorax.

Pneumothorax

Pneumothorax is defined as presence of air within the pleural cavity and is an uncommon but significant cause of neonatal respiratory distress.[26,30] Timely identification can be lifesaving. It can occur spontaneously or be secondary to infection, meconium aspiration, ventilation barotraumas **(Fig. 9)**, or lung deformity. Spontaneous pneumothorax is more commonly seen in premature babies (about 6%) as compared to term babies (1–2%). The radiographic diagnosis of pneumothorax, although of great clinical significance, can be missed on the X-rays as apicolateral accumulation of air is rather uncommon in the supine films. In the supine position, air preferentially accumulates in anteromedial and subpulmonic recesses.[31] The position of air collection is also modified by underlying lung disease. Subpulmonic pneumothorax presents as a relatively lucent region in the left or right upper abdominal quadrant. Sometimes, the only radiographic sign of subpulmonic pneumothorax is deep lateral costophrenic angle (deep sulcus sign).[32] Recent studies have found chest ultrasound to be as reliable as CXR[33,34] and better than clinical evaluation[35] for diagnosis of pneumothorax.

SURGICAL CAUSES OF NEONATAL RESPIRATORY DISTRESS

Several conditions in neonates causing respiratory distress require surgical intervention for management. Although listed as the causes of respiratory distress in neonates, it is to be remembered that the following disorders may present beyond the neonatal period. In addition, even if discovered during neonatal period, they may be managed conservatively initially. Some of these conditions, like diaphragmatic hernia, can be diagnosed antenatally. Conversely, some of these pathologies may be discovered accidentally in later life and pose dilemma regarding the need for surgery.

Congenital Lobar Overinflation

Congenital lobar overinflation (CLO) is a disease of multifactorial origin characterized by focal abnormality of a large airway. Unfortunately, the exact abnormality of large airway frequently remains a mystery as it is left inside the body of the child proximal to the ligated bronchial stump. However, potential culprits include bronchomalacia, webs, kinks, and anomalous crossing vessels. Whatever the etiology may be, the result is impairment of bronchial function and hyperinflation of a pulmonary lobe.[36] Left upper lobe is the most common site of involvement (42.2%), followed by right middle lobe (35.3%), and right upper lobe (20.7%).[37] The hyperinflated lobe causes mediastinal shift and atelectasis of the adjacent lobes.

Prenatal diagnosis is unusual in CLO. Postnatally, the age of onset of symptoms and degree of respiratory distress may be variable. However, >50% become symptomatic within 1st week. Not all the symptomatic patients may require immediate surgery.[36,38] The postnatal chest radiograph, if acquired early in life, may reveal overdistended fluid-filled lobe. Later on, the radiograph shows characteristic hyperinflation of a lobe with splayed pulmonary vessels, atelectasis of adjacent lobes, and contralateral mediastinal shift **(Fig. 10)**. The differential diagnosis is pneumothorax wherein the hyperlucent region will be devoid of pulmonary vascular markings. In case the diagnosis is uncertain on CXR, computed tomography (CT) scan can be performed to resolve the diagnosis. CT will show the reduced attenuation of the involved lobe/segment (s) with attenuated pulmonary vascular markings **(Figs. 11A and B)** in patients of CLO. CT can also reveal treatable extrinsic and intrinsic treatable cause of partial bronchial obstruction.[37]

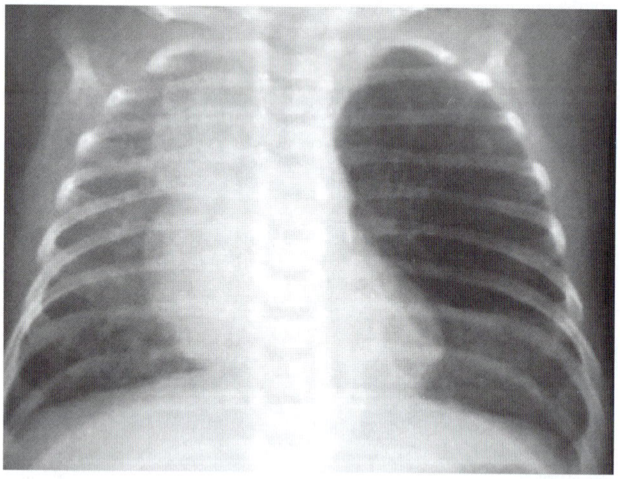

FIG. 10: Chest X-ray anteroposterior (AP) view of a neonate with respiratory distress reveals emphysematous left upper lobe with contralateral mediastinal shift suggestive of congenital lobar overinflation. Presence of vascular markings differentiates congenital lobar overinflation from pneumothorax.

Uncommonly, the CLO may affect two lobes **(Fig. 12)**. Either the lobes may be affected simultaneously or the second hyperinflated lobe may be detected after first thoracotomy. The bilobectomy procedure may be performed as one-stage or two-stage procedure.[38]

Congenital Pulmonary Airway Malformation

Congenital pulmonary airway malformation (CPAM) is a hamartomatous lesion believed to occur because of the failure of pulmonary mesenchyme into normal bronchoalveolar tissue.[22,37] On the basis of pathological findings, Stocker[39] classified the CPAM into five types. However, radiological classification consists of four types:[37]

1. *Type I*: It constitutes 50% of CPAM patients and shows multiple or single large cysts which communicate with the bronchial tree of the affected lobe.
2. *Type II*: It constitutes 40% of CPAM and shows multiple cysts that rarely exceed 1.2 cm in diameter and communicate with the bronchial tree of the affected lobe.
   About one-third of these patients have associated congenital anomalies.
3. *Type III*: It is less common type (<10% of patients). It consists of multiple small (<0.5 cm) cysts and may appear solid on imaging. It usually causes mass effect on mediastinum.

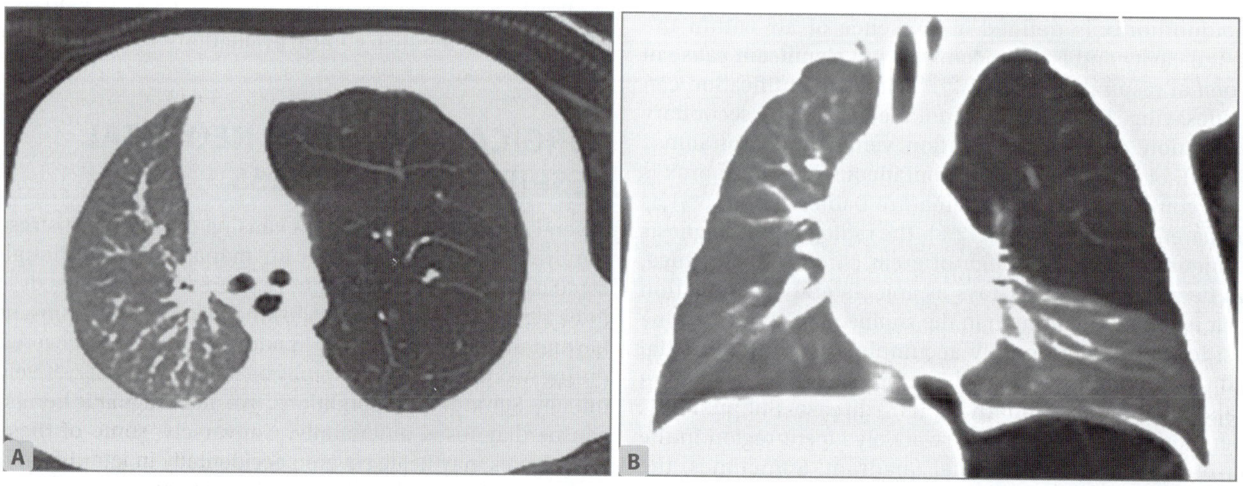

FIGS. 11A AND B: Axial (A) and coronal (B) CT scan images in a case of congenital lobar overinflation (CLO) involving the left upper lobe showing reduced attenuation of the involved lobe with attenuated vasculature.

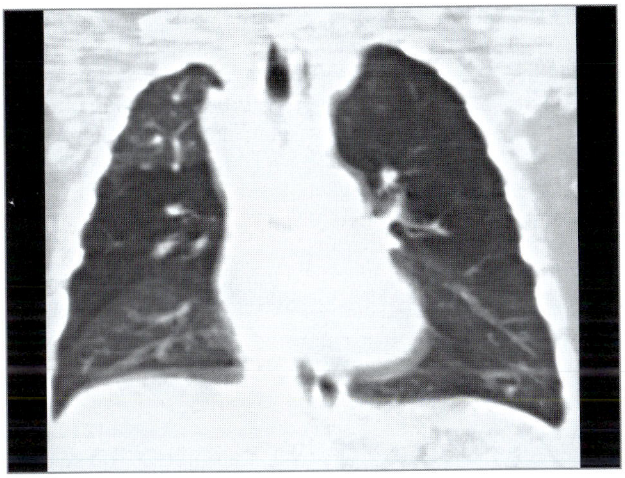

FIG. 12: Coronal CT scan images in a case of bilateral congenital lobar overinflation (CLO) involving the left upper lobe and right middle lobe showing reduced attenuation of the involved lobes with attenuated vasculature.

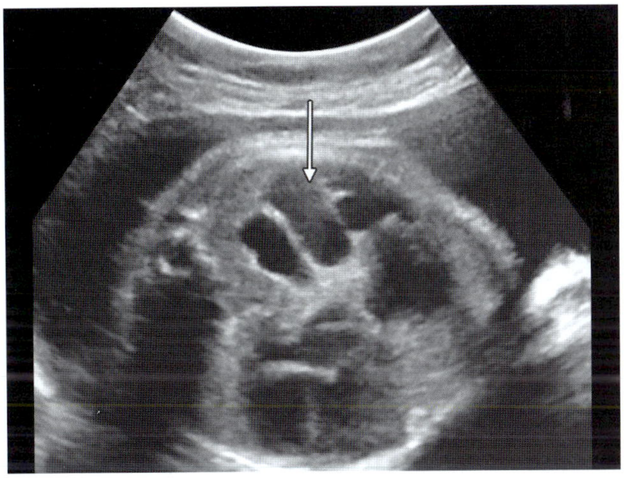

FIG. 13: Antenatal USG image showing cystic lesions in the lung (white arrow) suggestive of CPAM. (CPAM: congenital pulmonary airway malformation; USG: ultrasonography)

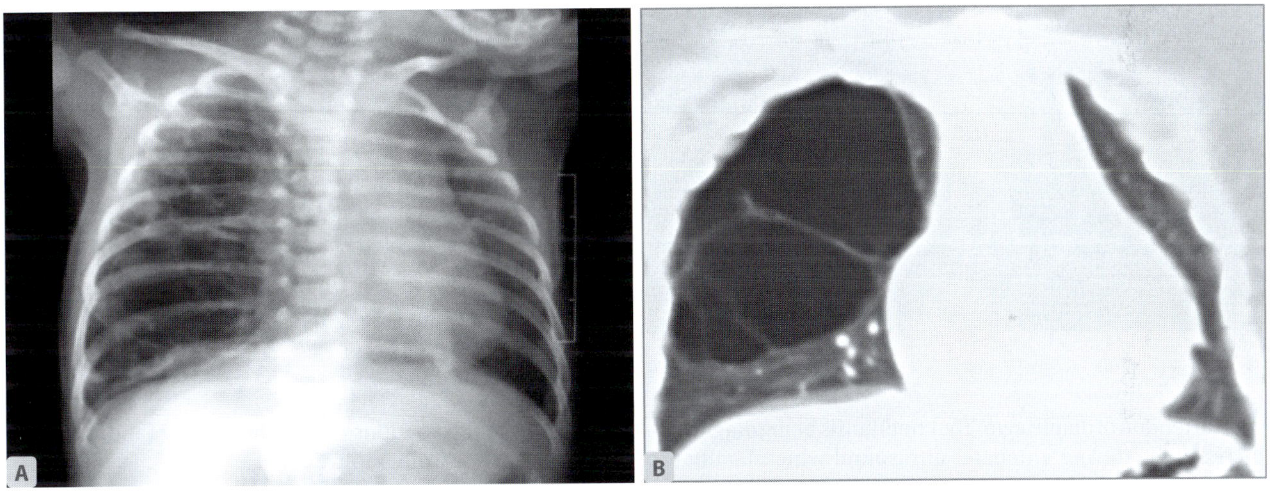

FIGS. 14A AND B: (A) CXR of a neonate showing increased lucency on the right side with mediastinal shift to the left side. The differentials include CLO, CPAM, and loculated pneumothorax; and (B) This needs to be further evaluated on CT which shows multiple cystic lesions in the right lung suggestive of type 1 CPAM. (CLO: congenital lobar overinflation; CPAM: congenital pulmonary airway malformation; CXR: chest X-ray; CT: computerized tomography)

4. *Type IV*: It is the rarest type of CPAM (<1%) in which large cystic lesions are seen and is indistinguishable from the cyst predominant type 1 pleuropulmonary blastoma.

Antenatal ultrasound may depict CPAM as a pulmonary mass **(Fig. 13)** with associated polyhydramnios or fetal anasarca. The disease is usually unilateral with single lobe involvement seen in 95% of patients. Bilateral disease is rare (2%). Neonatal respiratory distress occurs if the CPAM is large and causes mediastinal shift. The cysts may be detected radiographically in 90% of patients and better characterized with CT **(Figs. 14A and B)** which also helps in excluding CLO as differential diagnosis. It is to be noted that radiological classification of CPAM may not corroborate with pathological classification.[40] When the lesion abuts diaphragm, CDH needs to be excluded. This can be done through contrast study of the gastrointestinal tract. CPAM also needs to be differentiated from pneumatoceles. The diagnosis of pneumatoceles can be made if an earlier normal chest radiograph is available or when subsequent radiographs (or CT scan) show complete resolution of disease. Mesenchymal cystic hamartoma can mimic CPAM radiographically. Malignant masses may occasionally be seen within CPAM.[41,42]

Congenital Diaphragmatic Hernia

Congenital diaphragmatic hernia signifies intrathoracic herniation of abdominal organs through a defect in the diaphragm. Its incidence varies from 1:2,000 to 1:5,000 in live births. Many fetuses with the diaphragmatic hernia are stillborn. Among the live-born, 28–50% may have associated anomalies. The diaphragmatic defect may be located anteromedially (Morgagni hernia) **(Figs. 15A to C)**, posterolaterally (Bochdalek hernia) **(Figs. 16A to C)**, or in the

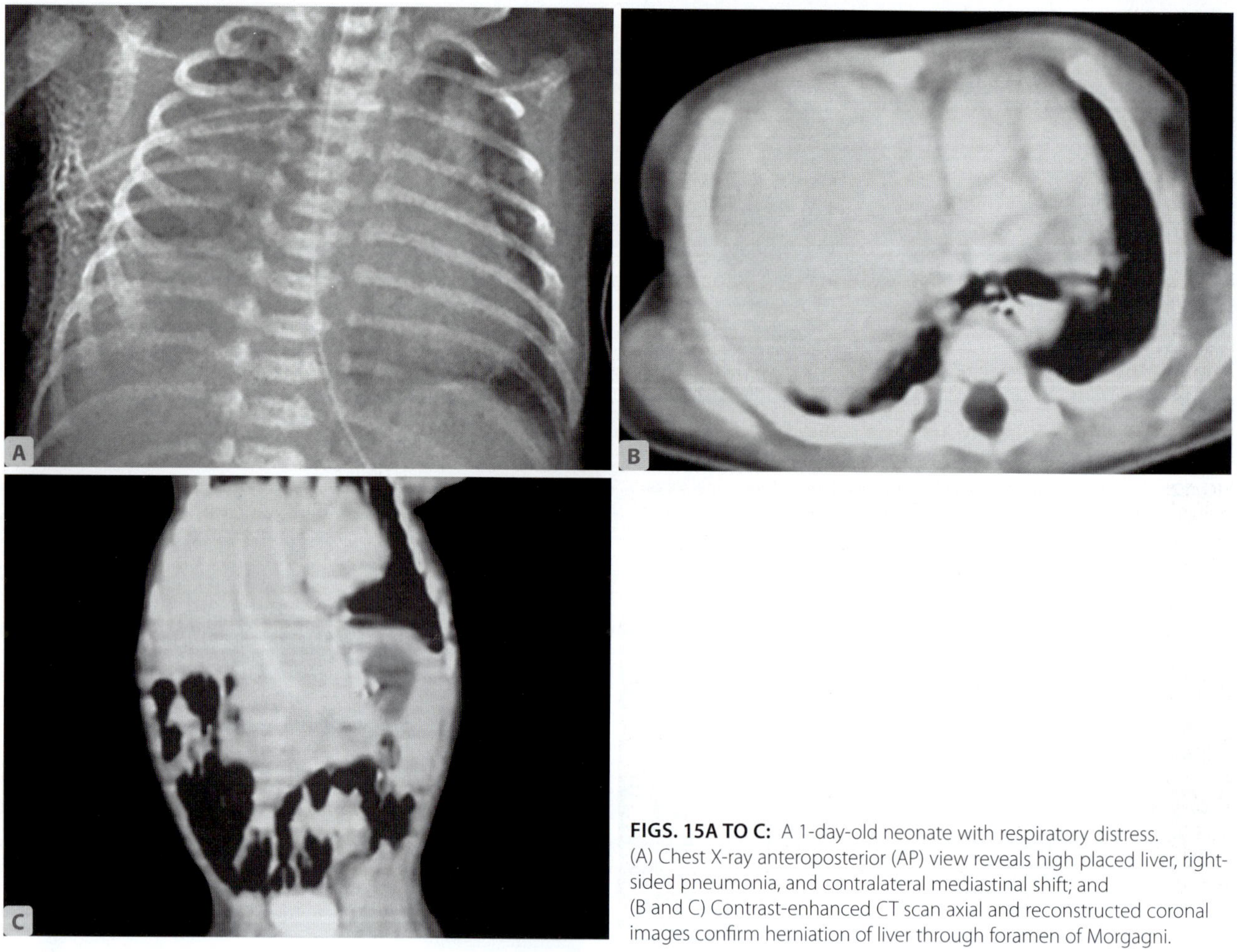

FIGS. 15A TO C: A 1-day-old neonate with respiratory distress. (A) Chest X-ray anteroposterior (AP) view reveals high placed liver, right-sided pneumonia, and contralateral mediastinal shift; and (B and C) Contrast-enhanced CT scan axial and reconstructed coronal images confirm herniation of liver through foramen of Morgagni.

central tendon of diaphragm. The condition is being diagnosed increasingly during antenatal ultrasound which facilitates supervised institutional delivery. Bag and mask therapy during neonatal resuscitation may worsen the respiratory distress. Diaphragmatic hernia is accompanied by pulmonary hypoplasia, pulmonary immaturity, hypoplastic left heart, and persistent pulmonary artery hypertension of the newborn.[43]

The radiographic appearance depends on the contents of hernia sac and distension of bowel. If radiograph is acquired early, the bowel may be fluid-filled or collapse resulting in opacity of variable size in lower hemithorax with contralateral mediastinal shift. Subsequently, air can be identified in the herniated bowel loops making the diagnosis straightforward. However, in some cases, it may need to be differentiated from congenital cystic adenomatoid malformation. This may require a contrast study of the gastrointestinal tract to establish the diagnosis. After the diagnosis of diaphragmatic hernia is established, search should be made for associated congenital malformations using sonography (abdomen and head) and echocardiography.

Esophageal Atresia with Tracheoesophageal Fistula

Although Western literature does not consider esophageal atresia with tracheoesophageal fistula a common cause of neonatal respiratory distress,[30] it has been shown to be the most common cause of neonatal respiratory distress which required admission in neonatal surgical ICU.[44] Esophageal atresia can be diagnosed at birth with the baby pouring out oral secretions. The baby can develop respiratory distress due to aspiration pneumonia as also due to distended stomach. Antenatal sonography may reveal polyhydramnios. Postnatal diagnosis can be made by localizing the "gastric" tube coiled in the upper esophageal pouch **(Fig. 17)**. Small volume of nonionic contrast can be injected through the tube before acquiring the radiograph for better localization.[3] However, spillage of contrast may make the situation worse.[44]

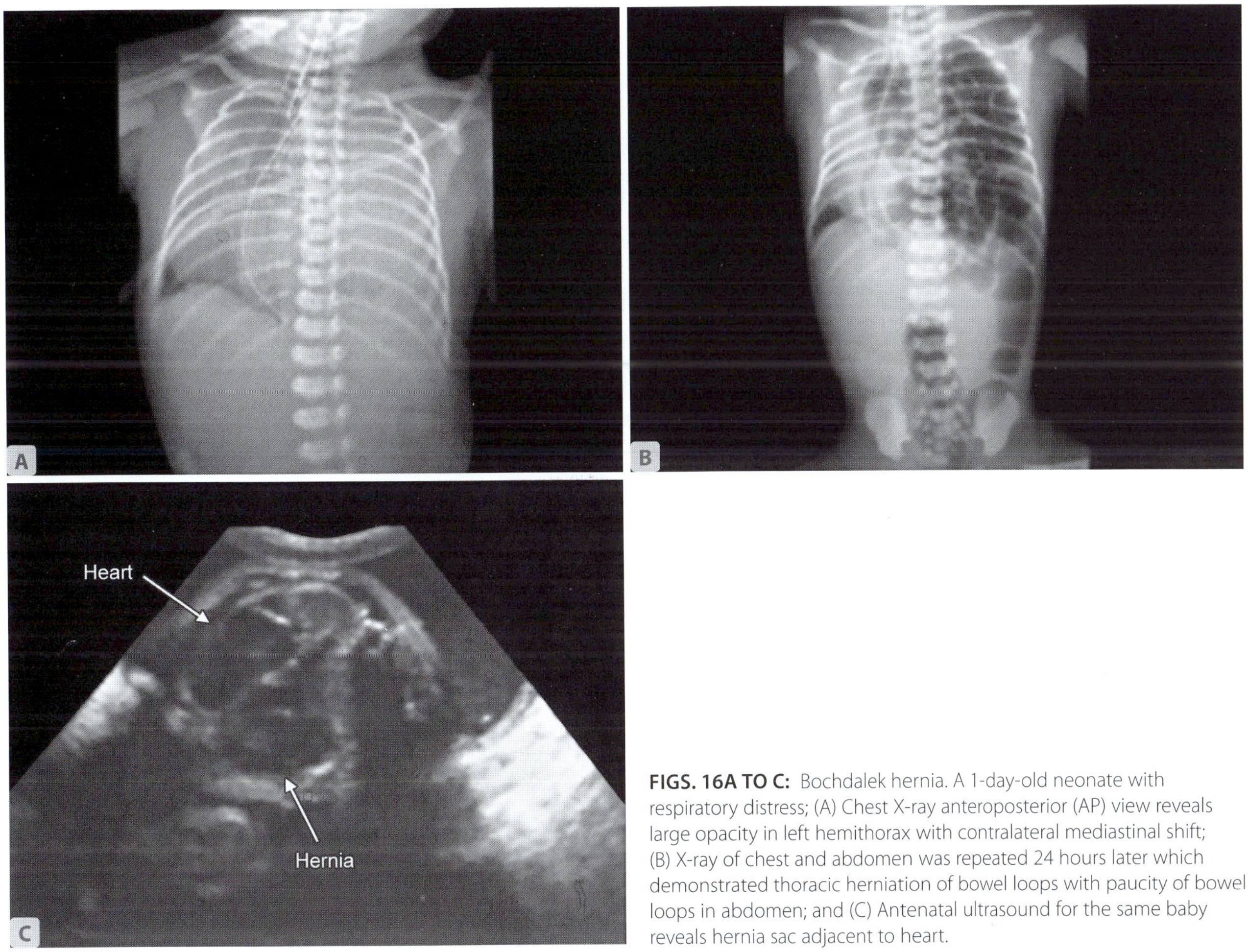

FIGS. 16A TO C: Bochdalek hernia. A 1-day-old neonate with respiratory distress; (A) Chest X-ray anteroposterior (AP) view reveals large opacity in left hemithorax with contralateral mediastinal shift; (B) X-ray of chest and abdomen was repeated 24 hours later which demonstrated thoracic herniation of bowel loops with paucity of bowel loops in abdomen; and (C) Antenatal ultrasound for the same baby reveals hernia sac adjacent to heart.

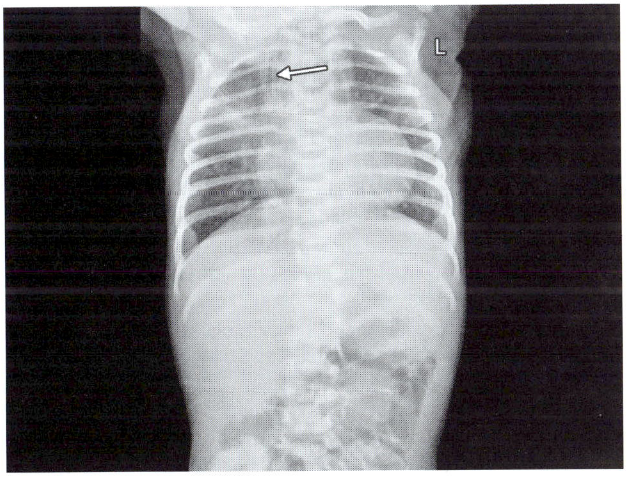

FIG. 17: A 1-day-old neonate with respiratory distress and pooling of saliva. Chest X-ray anteroposterior (AP) view reveals coiling of nasogastric tube in upper esophageal pouch (white arrow) suggestive of esophageal atresia. Presence of air in abdomen confirms the presence of tracheoesophageal fistula.

MISCELLANEOUS CAUSES

Bronchogenic and esophageal duplication cysts[45] **(Figs. 18A to C)** are congenital lesions which can cause neonatal respiratory distress by virtue of mass effect on surrounding structures or because of superadded pneumonia. If located in mediastinum, CT is required to characterize the lesion and demarcate its size and extent. Careful evaluation is required to exclude intraspinal communication to exclude neuroenteric cyst. Intrapulmonary bronchogenic cyst is difficult to differentiate radiologically from other congenital cystic lesions.

Some of the congenital cardiac anomalies (e.g., transposition of the great arteries) can cause neonatal respiratory distress. Echocardiography and catheter angiography are the mainstay of diagnostic workup.

Several other conditions can cause respiratory distress in neonates. These include bony defects of the chest wall, metabolic acidosis, anemia, polycythemia, primary pulmonary arterial hypertension, hyperthermia, choanal atresia, etc.[3,26,30]

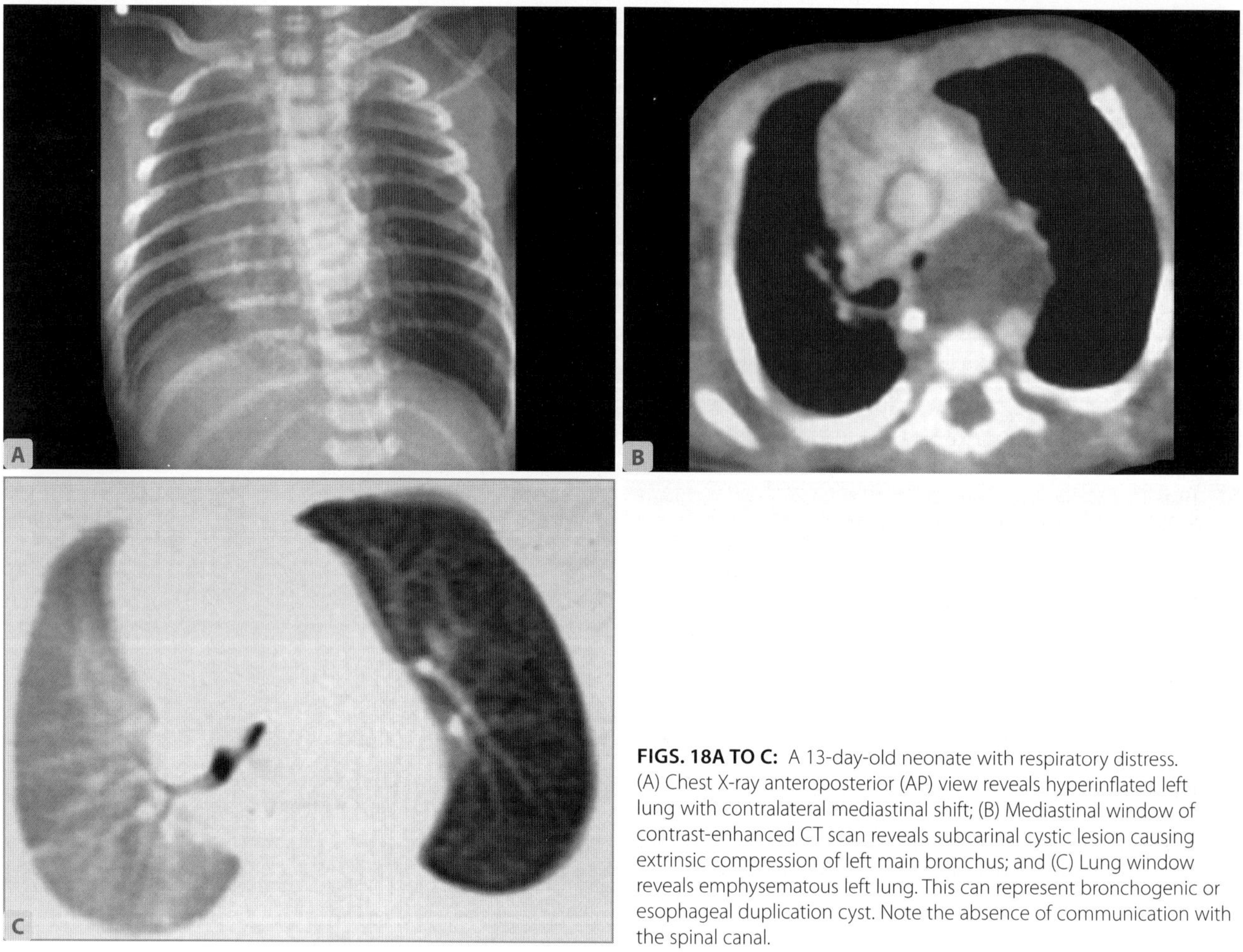

FIGS. 18A TO C: A 13-day-old neonate with respiratory distress. (A) Chest X-ray anteroposterior (AP) view reveals hyperinflated left lung with contralateral mediastinal shift; (B) Mediastinal window of contrast-enhanced CT scan reveals subcarinal cystic lesion causing extrinsic compression of left main bronchus; and (C) Lung window reveals emphysematous left lung. This can represent bronchogenic or esophageal duplication cyst. Note the absence of communication with the spinal canal.

REFERENCES

1. Guha DK. NNF recommended basic perinatal-neonatal nomenclature. In: Guha DK (Ed). Neonatology—Principles and Practice, 1st edition. New Delhi: Jaypee Brothers Medical Publishers (P) Ltd; 1998. pp. 131-2.
2. Kumar P, Kumar R, Narang A. Spectrum of neonatal respiratory distress at PGI. Bull NNF. 2000;14:8-12.
3. Diwakar KK. Clinical approach to respiratory distress in newborn. Indian J Pediatr. 2003;70:S53-9.
4. Guyer B, Hoyert DL, Martin JA, Ventura SJ, MacDorman MF, Strobino DM. Annual summary of vital statistics—1998. Pediatrics. 1999;104:1229-46.
5. Northway WH, Rosan RC, Porter DY. Pulmonary disease following respirator therapy of hyaline-membrane disease. Bronchopulmonary dysplasia. N Engl J Med. 1967;276:357-68.
6. Marini C, Bulleri A, Cambi L, Marinari A, Bernardini M, Bartalena L, et al. The neonatal respiratory insufficiency syndrome: the role of the chest radiogram. Radiol Med. 1997;94:463-7.
7. Kurl S, Heinonen KM, Kiekara O. The first chest radiograph in neonates exhibiting respiratory distress at birth. Clin Pediatr. 1997;36:285-9.
8. Dinger J, Schwarze R, Rupprecht E. Radiological changes after therapeutic use of surfactant in infants with respiratory distress syndrome. Pediatr Radiol. 1997;27:26-31.
9. Helbich TH, Popow C, Dobner M, Wunderbaldinger P, Zekert M, Herold CJ. New-born infants with severe hyaline membrane disease: radiological evaluation during high frequency oscillatory versus conventional ventilation. Eur J Radiol. 1998;28:243-9.
10. Avni EF, Braude P, Pardou A, Matos C. Hyaline membrane disease in the newborn: diagnosis by ultrasound. Pediatr Radiol. 1990;20:143-6.
11. Bober K, Swietliński J. Diagnostic utility of ultra USG for respiratory distress syndrome in neonates. Med Sci Monit. 2006;12:440-6
12. Ahuja CK, Saxena AK, Sodhi KS, Kumar P, Khandelwal N. Role of transabdominal ultrasound of lung bases and follow-up in premature neonates with respiratory distress soon after birth. Indian J Radiol Imaging. 2012;22:279-83.
13. Avni EF, Cassart M, de Maertelaer V, Rypens F, Vermeylen D, Gevenois PA. Sonographic prediction of chronic lung disease in the premature undergoing mechanical ventilation. Pediatr Radiol. 1996;26:463-9.

14. Pieper CH, Smith J, Brand EJ. The value of ultrasound examination of the lungs in predicting BPD. Pediatr Radiol. 2004;34:227-3.
15. Copetti R, Cattarossi L, Macagno F, Violino M, Furlan R. Lung ultrasound in respiratory distress syndrome: a useful tool for early diagnosis. Neonatology. 2008;94:52-9.
16. Liu J, Cao HY, Liu Y. Lung ultrasonography for the diagnosis of neonatal respiratory distress syndrome: a pilot study. Zhonghua Er Ke Za Zhi. 2013;51:205-10.
17. Vergine M, Copetti R, Brusa G, Cattarossi L. Lung ultrasound accuracy in respiratory distress syndrome and transient tachypnea of the newborn. Neonatology. 2014;106:87-93.
18. Sawires HK, Abdel-Ghany EA, Hussein NF, Seif HM. Use of lung ultrasound in detection of complications of respiratory distress syndrome. Ultrasound Med Biol. 2015;41:2319-25.
19. Rachuri H, Oleti TP, Murki S, Subramanian S, Nethagani J. Diagnostic Performance of Point of Care Ultrasonography in Identifying the Etiology of Respiratory Distress in Neonates. Indian J Pediatr. 2017;84:267-70.
20. Hiles M, Culpan AM, Watts C, Munyombwe T, Wolstenhulme S. Neonatal respiratory distress syndrome: chest X-ray or lung ultrasound? A systematic review. Ultrasound. 2017;25:80-91.
21. Lovrenski J. Lung ultrasonography of pulmonary complications in preterm infants with respiratory distress syndrome. Ups J Med Sci. 2012;117:10-7.
22. Newman B. Imaging of medical disease of the newborn lung. Radiol Clin North Am. 1999;37:1049-65.
23. Copetti R, Cattarossi L. The "double lung point": an ultrasound sign diagnostic of transient tachypnea of the newborn. Neonatology. 2007;91:203-9.
24. Ibrahim M, Omran A, AbdAllah NB, Ibrahim M, El-Sharkawy S. Lung ultrasound in early diagnosis of neonatal transient tachypnea and its differentiation from other causes of neonatal respiratory distress. J Neonatal Perinatal Med. 2018;11:281-7.
25. Volpicelli G, Audino B. The double lung point: an unusual sonographic sign of juvenile spontaneous pneumothorax. Am J Emerg Med. 2011;29:355.e1-2.
26. Mathur NB, Garg K, Kumar S. Respiratory distress in neonates with special reference to pneumonia. Indian Pediatr. 2002;39:529-37.
27. Garner JS, Jarvis WR, Emori TG, Horan TC, Hughes JM. CDC definitions for nosocomial infections. In: Olmsted RN (Ed). APIC Infection Control and Applied Epidemiology: Principles and Practice. St. Louis: Mosby; 1996. pp. 1-19.
28. Gaynes RP, Edwards JR, Jarvis WR, Culver DH, Tolson JS, Martone JW, et al. Nosocomial infections among neonates in high-risk nurseries in the United States. Pediatrics. 1996;98:357-61.
29. Wiswell TE, Bent RC. Meconium staining and meconium aspiration syndrome. Pediatr Clin North Am. 1993;40:955-81.
30. Hermansen CL, Lorah KN. Respiratory distress in the newborn. Am Fam Physician. 2007;76:987-94.
31. Tocino IM, Miller MH, Fairfax WR. Distribution of pneumothorax in the supine and semirecumbent critically ill adult. Am J Roentgenol. 1985;144:901-5.
32. Gordon R. The deep sulcus sign. Radiology. 1980;136:25-7.
33. Cattarossi L, Copetti R, Brusa G, Pintaldi S. Lung Ultrasound Diagnostic Accuracy in Neonatal Pneumothorax. Can Respir J. 2016;2016:6515069.
34. Liu J, Chi JH, Ren XL, Li J, Chen YJ, Lu ZL, et al. Lung ultrasonography to diagnose pneumothorax of the newborn. Am J Emerg Med. 2017;35:1298-302.
35. Raimondi F, Fanjul JR, Aversa S, Chirico G, Yousef N, de Luca D, et al. Lung Ultrasound for Diagnosing Pneumothorax in the Critically Ill Neonate. J Pediatr. 2016;175:74-8.e1.
36. Schwartz DS, Reyes-Mugica M, Keller MS. Imaging of surgical diseases of the newborn chest. Intrapleural mass lesions. Radiol Clin North Am. 1999;37:1067-78.
37. Biyyam DR, Chapman T, Ferguson MR, Deutsch G, Dighe MK. Congenital lung abnormalities: embryologic features, prenatal diagnosis, and postnatal radiologic-pathologic correlation. Radiographics. 2010;30:1721-38.
38. Ghribi A, Mekki M, Krichene I, Jouini R, Maazoun K, Sahnoun L, et al. Congenital bilobar emphysema. J Pediatr Surg. 2008;43: e5 7.
39. Stocker JT. Congenital and developmental diseases. In: Dail OH, Hammar SP (Eds). Pulmonary Pathology, 2nd edition. Heidelberg: Springer-Verlag; 1994. pp. 155-90.
40. Shimohira M, Hara M, Kitase M, Takeuchi M, Shibamoto Y, Kurono K, et al. Congenital pulmonary airway malformation: CT-pathologic correlation. J Thorac Imaging. 2007;22:149-53.
41. d'Agostino S, Bonoldi E, Dante S, Meli S, Cappellari F, Musi L. Embryonal rhabdomyosarcoma of the lung arising in cystic adenomatoid malformation: case report and review of the literature. J Pediatr Surg. 1997;32:1381-3.
42. West D, Nicholson AG, Colquhoun I, Pollock J. Bronchioloalveolar carcinoma in congenital cystic adenomatoid malformation of lung. Ann Thorac Surg. 2007;83:687-9.
43. Thébaud B, Mercier JC, Dinh-Xuan AT. Congenital diaphragmatic hernia: a cause of persistent pulmonary hypertension of the newborn which lacks an effective therapy. Biol Neonate. 1998;74:323-36.
44. Kumar A, Bhatnagar V. Respiratory distress in neonates. Indian J Pediatr. 2005;72:425-8.
45. Sodhi KS, Saxena AK, Narasimha Rao KL, Singh M, Suri S. Esophageal duplication cyst: an unusual cause of respiratory distress in infants. Pediatr Emerg Care. 2005;21:854-6.

CHAPTER

63

Childhood Pulmonary Infections

Jyoti Kumar, Anjali Prakash, Alpana Manchanda

INTRODUCTION

Respiratory tract infections are the most common cause of illness in children and one of the most common indications for imaging. It should be remembered that children are not small adults and the spectrum of disorders that affects the pediatric population can be quite different from that seen in adults. Clinical evaluation is difficult and the history is inevitably difficult to elicit, no matter how observant the parents are. There is extra emotional concern when children fall sick and all together; these issues are of great importance to a radiologist, especially in thoracic disorders where imaging of the chest is frequently one of the first tools after clinical assessment.[1]

PNEUMONIA

Epidemiology

The various pathogens that can cause pneumonia in children include viruses, bacteria, mycobacterium, mycoplasma, fungi, protozoa, and helminths. In neonates, bacterial pneumonia is more common than viral pneumonia. While bacterial pneumonia results from pathogens acquired during delivery, neonates are protected from viral pathogens owing to maternal antibody transfer. Between 2 months and 2 years of age group, viruses cause 95% of all respiratory infections. The incidence of bacterial infection increases after 2 years of age. *Mycoplasma pneumoniae* (MP) is the cause in approximately 30% of pulmonary infections in school-going children and young adults >6 years of age.[2]

The factors that increase the risk for childhood pneumonia are large families, siblings of school-aged children, congenital heart disease, congenital immune disorders, and neuromuscular disorders that depress the patient's ability to clear infected secretions or to suppress aspiration.[3]

Infections reach the lower respiratory tract via three routes: (1) The airways, (2) The blood vessels, and (3) By direct spread from extrapulmonary sites. Inhalation or aspiration of airborne organisms or infected secretions are the most common route for infection. Infection via pulmonary vasculature may be a result of diffuse sepsis or septic emboli as in cases of endocarditis. Direct spread of infection from mediastinum, chest wall, abdomen, or neck is an uncommon occurrence.[3]

Imaging

Although clinical symptoms and signs are helpful indicators of the presence of disease, radiographic investigation is often required to confirm the clinical diagnosis and to help decide whether or not antibiotics or more extensive workup is necessary.[4] The various roles of imaging in children with pneumonia are: evaluation of possible pneumonia, determination of specific etiologic agent, exclusion of other pathology, evaluation of the child with failure of pneumonia to clear, and evaluation of complications related to pneumonia.[5]

In infants and young children, the signs and symptoms of pneumonia may be more nonspecific than in adults. Although fever and respiratory symptoms like cough, wheezing, tachypnea, or retractions are the presenting symptoms in most cases, nonrespiratory symptoms like malaise and irritability, headaches, chest pain, or abdominal pain are also a common mode of presentation in children. Lower lobe pneumonia may be recognized on the superior aspect of abdominal radiographs being obtained for abdominal pain as pleuritic chest pain from lower lobe may get referred to upper abdomen. Physical examination may be less reliable in children. Also, laboratory tests including elevated erythrocyte sedimentation rate, C-reactive protein, and leukocytosis are neither sensitive nor specific. Chest radiography is a technique which is heavily relied upon to determine the likelihood of underlying bacterial illness in children and has been shown to alter the management decisions in children with pneumonia.[5]

Most chest infection imaging is carried out using *radiographs.* It is generally agreed that chest radiographs should be obtained when fever is present in conjunction with respiratory symptoms. Although cost, radiation dose, and procedure time increase, when both frontal and lateral radiographs are used, certain radiographic findings like hyperinflation are better evaluated on a lateral radiograph, especially in infants.

The etiological agent cannot be characterized from radiographs alone.[4] The main objective of imaging in pneumonia is whether the patient is likely to have viral or bacterial pneumonia. The specific bacterial agent is usually not the clinical question expected to be resolved by radiography alone as there is considerable overlap between the imaging findings resulting from various infectious agents. Underlying lung conditions can alter the appearance of radiographic findings. Various noninfectious processes can also simulate infection on radiography.

Ultrasound (US) plays an important role in the evaluation of parapneumonic effusion (PPE), guiding drainage procedures, and follow-up of effusion/empyema.

Computed tomography (CT) has a very limited role in primary assessment of uncomplicated pneumonia. In pediatric lower respiratory infection, CT is indicated:[6,7]

- When complications of bacterial pneumonia are suspected. One of the goals of CT in cases of persistent illness is to separate suppurative pleural from parenchymal pathology as most of the former require interventional procedures while lung parenchymal complications are managed conservatively;
- To exclude underlying abnormality in recurrent infection;
- To evaluate immunocompromised children with normal radiographs but with clinical suspicion of respiratory infection;
- To guide the type and site of tissue sampling;
- To assess the sequelae of respiratory infection (e.g., postviral bronchiolitis obliterans).

Magnetic resonance (MR) is a promising technique for evaluation of children with chronic lung conditions who require repeated CT examinations.[2]

Viral Pneumonia

Viral infection predominantly affects the mucosa of the airways resulting in bronchiolitis, typically seen in children <2 years of age. The process may remain confined to the medium and small airways or may extend into the adjacent lung tissue resulting in peribronchiolar opacities. Respiratory syncytial virus (RSV) is the most common cause, others being rhinovirus, parainfluenza, and adenovirus.[4] Most of these are acquired by inhalational route. Edema, increased mucosal secretions, and necrotic debris in the lumen result in blockade of airways, more marked at the level of the bronchioles and cause air trapping. Children are more predisposed to air trapping and collapse in viral infection than adults due to the following reasons: (1) Bronchi and bronchioles are smaller in diameter, (2) Collateral pathways of ventilation, including pores of Kohn and channels of Lambert are not well-developed. These do not mature until about 8 years of age, and (3) Mucus secretion is more in children.

Radiographic Signs

Radiographic signs of diffuse hyperinflation are hyperlucency, depression of the hemidiaphragm to >6 anterior or 10 posterior ribs, flattening of the diaphragms, widening of intercostal spaces, and increased retrosternal space. On the lateral view, findings of flattening of the hemidiaphragms and increased anteroposterior diameter, which often becomes more than the superior to inferior diameter, are often better evaluated **(Figs. 1 and 2A and B)**. When thick mucus inspissates resulting in complete plugging of the airway, there is segmental atelectasis. This is seen as wedge-shaped areas of density, more common in the middle and lower lung **(Fig. 3)**. Inflammation extending into the adjacent lung tissue can cause peribronchial edema and result in bronchopneumonia which manifests as bilateral, usually symmetrical peribronchial cuffing and thickening in the central perihilar location. On the lateral view, increased hilar size and density may be used as a marker for perihilar peribronchial thickening. Doughnut-like appearance owing to central lucency on cross-section and tram-track line appearance of bronchi are seen radiating from the hilum. Pleural effusion and lymph node enlargement are atypical.[2,4,5]

Pitfalls

Although the central peribronchial thickening, hyperinflation, and areas of segmental atelectasis are typical of viral infection in infants and small children, there are various pitfalls. Expiratory films may give the erroneous impression of peribronchial thickening. Sometimes, bacterial pneumonia like pertussis pneumonia (rare due to widespread immunization) mimics the appearance of viral pneumonia. Segmental atelectasis in viral pneumonia may be overinterpreted as consolidation in bacterial pneumonia. Secondary bacterial infection may develop in few cases of viral infection, related to altered immunity and ubiquitous pathogen, confounding the radiological picture.[4] Also, if bronchial wall thickening is present between bouts of acute illness, it suggests chronic airway disease such as asthma or cystic fibrosis, immunodeficiency, or chronic aspiration. Reactive airway disease may appear very similar to viral bronchiolitis and need clinical differentiation.[3]

Complications

Although most infants recover uneventfully, viral pneumonias may result in long-standing complications of bronchiolitis

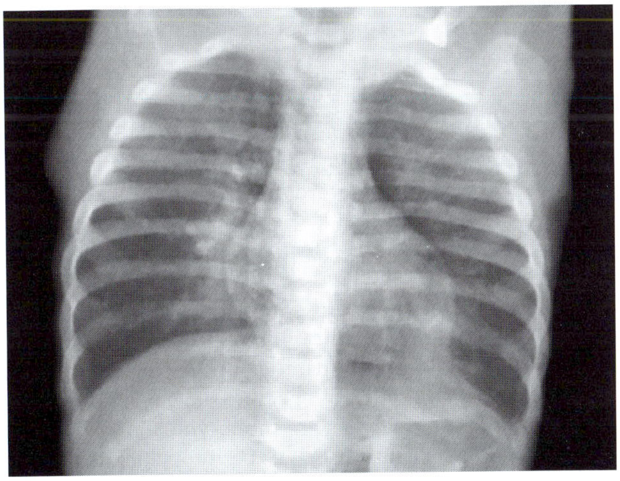

FIG. 1: Viral pneumonia: Frontal radiograph in a 4-month-old boy shows hyperinflation with increased peribronchial markings.

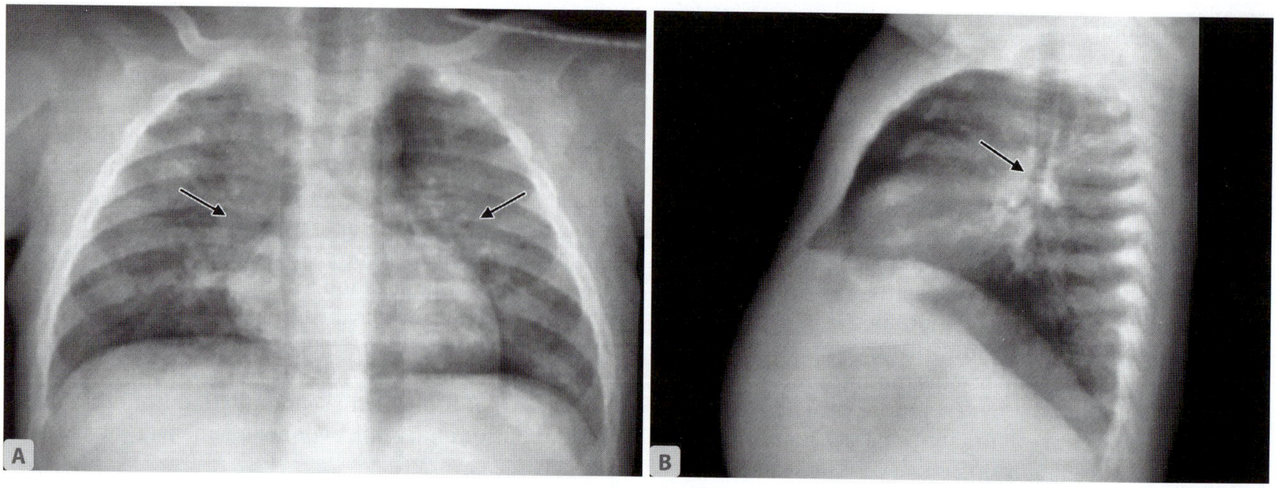

FIGS. 2A AND B: Viral pneumonia. (A) Frontal radiograph in a 5-month-old child shows increased peribronchial markings (black arrows); and (B) Lateral radiograph shows prominent density and size of the hila, a supportive finding of increased peribronchial markings (black arrow).

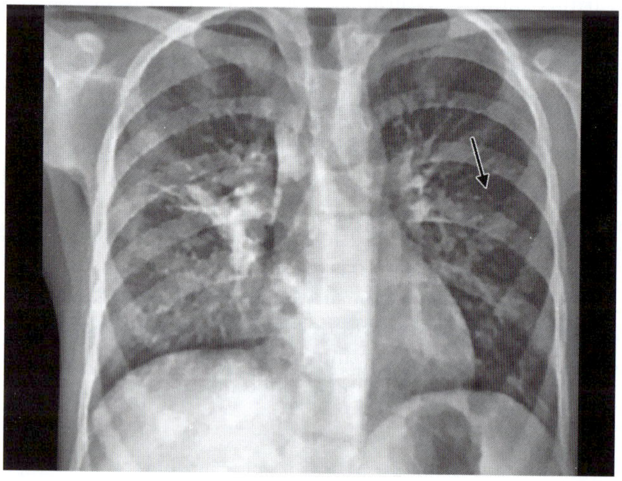

FIG. 3: Viral pneumonia: Frontal radiograph in a 4-year-old girl depicts prominent bronchovascular markings with triangular right perihilar area of atelectasis (black arrow).

obliterans and Swyer–James syndrome (unilateral hyperlucent lung) discussed later.[4]

Coronavirus Disease 2019 Pneumonia

This is a new highly contagious viral pneumonia caused by a novel coronavirus [severe acute respiratory syndrome coronavirus 2 (SARS-CoV-2)] of unclear origin. Overall symptoms in children are relatively mild as compared to adults.[8]

Typical chest X-ray findings in coronavirus disease 2019 (COVID-19) patients include bilateral peripheral and/or subpleural ground-glass opacities and/or consolidation. Both unilateral and bilateral opacities have been observed, although bilateral opacities are more typical of COVID-19 **(Figs. 4A and B)**. Features such as peribronchial thickening and/or peribronchial distribution of lung opacities are more commonly seen in pediatric population. Atypical features like unilateral segmental or lobar consolidation, central distribution of opacities, single round consolidation, lymphadenopathy, and pleural effusion can be seen.[9]

Chest CT may be done when there are features of severe pneumonia, suspected bacterial superinfection, or immunocompromised state. CT features include bilateral peripheral and/or subpleural ground-glass opacities and/or consolidation predominantly in the lower lobes **(Fig. 4C)**.

Other features include peribronchial thickening, fine reticulations, and "crazy paving" pattern and reverse halo sign seen as central ground-glass haze surrounded by parenchymal consolidation. Pleural effusion and lymphadenopathy are atypical findings.[9]

Peribronchial distribution of the lung opacities and bronchial wall thickening are relatively more frequent in the pediatric population.[10] However, the disease course is generally milder with overall better prognosis.

Bacterial Pneumonia

Bacterial pneumonia is usually a result of *Streptococcus pneumoniae (S. pneumoniae)*, other common agents being *Haemophilus influenzae* (*H. influenzae*) and *Staphylococcus pneumoniae*. The usual route of spread is via inhalational route. On imaging, bacterial pneumonia can present as air-space pneumonia or bronchopneumonia.

Air-space pneumonia is classically the result of *S. pneumoniae* and *Klebsiella pneumoniae* (*K. pneumoniae*). Inflammatory exudates and edema within the acini result in segmental or lobar consolidation **(Fig. 5)**. This is usually unilateral in contrast to viral pneumonias. Air bronchograms, when seen, are typical. There is usually little or no volume loss as the airways are not primarily affected.

Bronchopneumonia is usually seen with infection by *Staphylococcus aureus (S. aureus)*, gram-negative bacteria, and MP. Infection begins in terminal and respiratory bronchioles rather than alveoli. The disease then spreads to peribronchiolar alveoli that produce acinar filling and lobular consolidations. This results in patchy consolidation, loss of

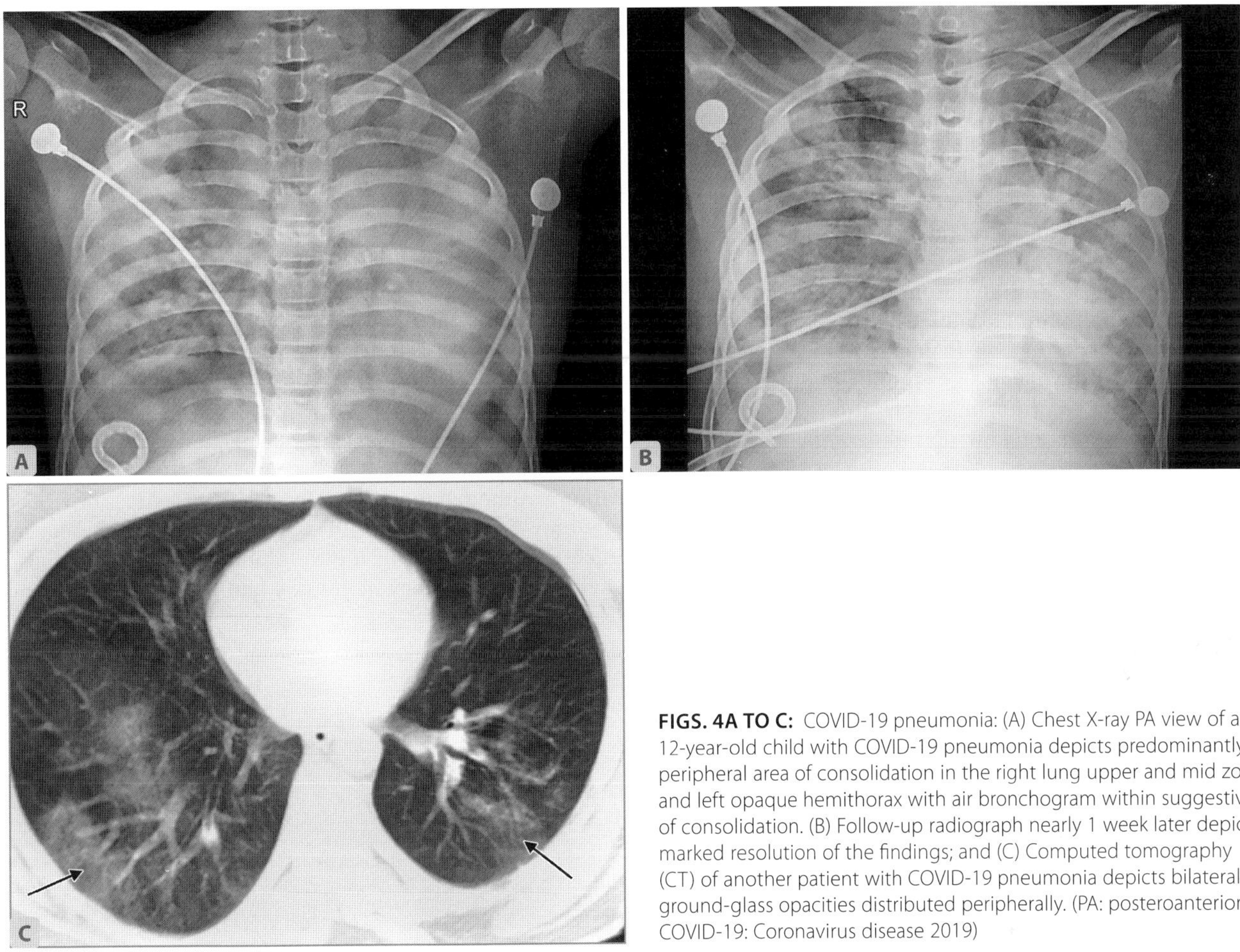

FIGS. 4A TO C: COVID-19 pneumonia: (A) Chest X-ray PA view of a 12-year-old child with COVID-19 pneumonia depicts predominantly peripheral area of consolidation in the right lung upper and mid zone and left opaque hemithorax with air bronchogram within suggestive of consolidation. (B) Follow-up radiograph nearly 1 week later depicts marked resolution of the findings; and (C) Computed tomography (CT) of another patient with COVID-19 pneumonia depicts bilateral ground-glass opacities distributed peripherally. (PA: posteroanterior; COVID-19: Coronavirus disease 2019)

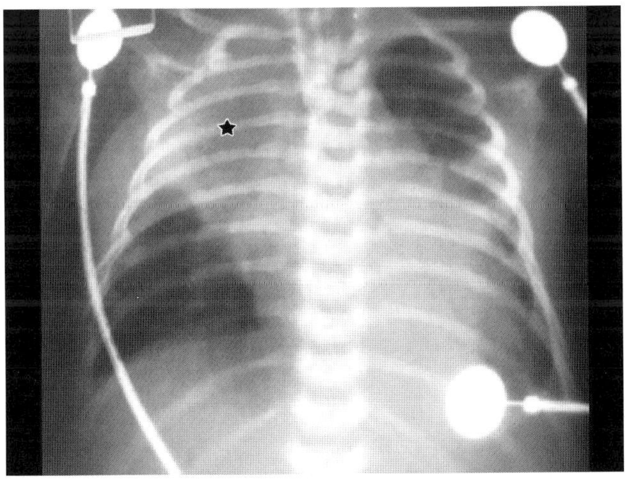

FIG. 5: Lobar pneumonia: Frontal radiograph in a 3-month-old infant shows consolidation of the right upper lobe suggesting a bacterial pneumonia.

volume with absence of air bronchograms. When affected areas coalesce, the shadowing may become more uniform and resemble lobar pneumonia.

There may be accompanying pleural effusions, which are rarely associated with viral disease.

Sometimes, lobar consolidation may be difficult to distinguish from atelectasis seen in viral pneumonias (in fact, these may coexist as superadded infection that is common secondary to obstructed airway). It may be remembered that accompanying signs of volume loss like fissural distortion, mediastinal shift, and compensatory hyperinflation, seen with atelectasis, are unusual in consolidated lung.[4]

Although more gradual, the pneumonia generally resolves completely. Radiological improvement may lag behind clinical improvement by days or weeks, usually taking 1–2 weeks **(Figs. 6A and B)**. However, severity of the disease agent and underlying host factors may result in complications like cavitary necrosis, empyema, and abscess formation.[4,5] Increase in antibiotic usage has led to increase in the incidence of complications.[4]

In a study by Bettenay et al.,[11] it was suggested that both clinical and radiographic criteria overestimate the number of children with bacterial pneumonia by a significant proportion, owing to low positive predictive value. However, it was the high negative predictive value in the range of 80–90% that was useful in excluding bacterial pneumonia and affected the management decisions.

Round Pneumonia

Round pneumonia is also common in young children, <8 years of age. This is due to paucity of collateral channels of ventilation as described earlier. This is most often due to *S. pneumoniae* and simulates a mass lesion.[2,5] These often involve the posterior and lower lobes, as the exudates moves into the dependent portions of the lung. In a child with fever, diagnosis of round pneumonia should always be considered when a round mass-like lesion is encountered **(Figs. 7A and B)**. Round pneumonia may contain air bronchograms and show ill-defined margins in at least a part of the border, suggesting the diagnosis. A lateral radiograph can help to make the diagnosis as round pneumonia is often less mass-like on an orthogonal view. This is one of the few clinical settings where follow-up radiography 2 weeks after antibiotic therapy is essential in children to rule out an underlying mass lesion, like bronchogenic cyst.[2] Apart from round pneumonia, nonresolving and recurrent pneumonia are the other indications for follow-up radiographs. These may also be done in children who have an underlying condition such as immunodeficiency, cystic fibrosis, or sickle cell anemia.

In most children with pulmonary infections, the specific etiological agent is never documented. Invasive diagnostic procedures are usually not warranted and even when done, specific etiological agent is still not identifiable because of ongoing treatment with antibiotics.[5]

Few specific appearances pertaining to different bacterial agents may be mentioned here. Staphylococcal pneumonia presents with lobar or multilobar consolidation. Complications are most common with this organism. Pleural effusion is common which may develop into empyema. A frequent feature of staphylococcal pneumonia is pneumatocele formation, which is otherwise rare. It is seen as a round thin-walled lucency due to collection of air in the interstitium. This may result in pneumothorax secondary to rupture. Although they generally disappear in days or weeks, few may persist for months.[6] Septicemic staphylococcal infection may result in multiple nodules which may also cavitate. Nodules may be miliary and diffuse or fewer and

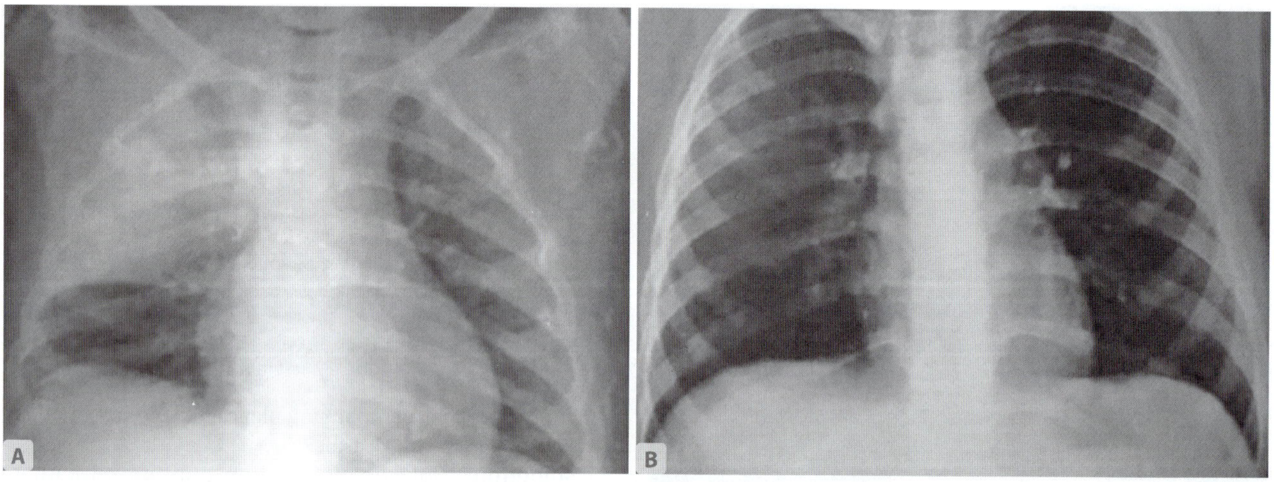

FIGS. 6A AND B: Lobar pneumonia. (A) Frontal radiograph in a 2-year-old child shows consolidation of the right upper lobe; and (B) Patient was put on antibiotics and radiograph obtained 2 weeks later shows complete radiological clearance.

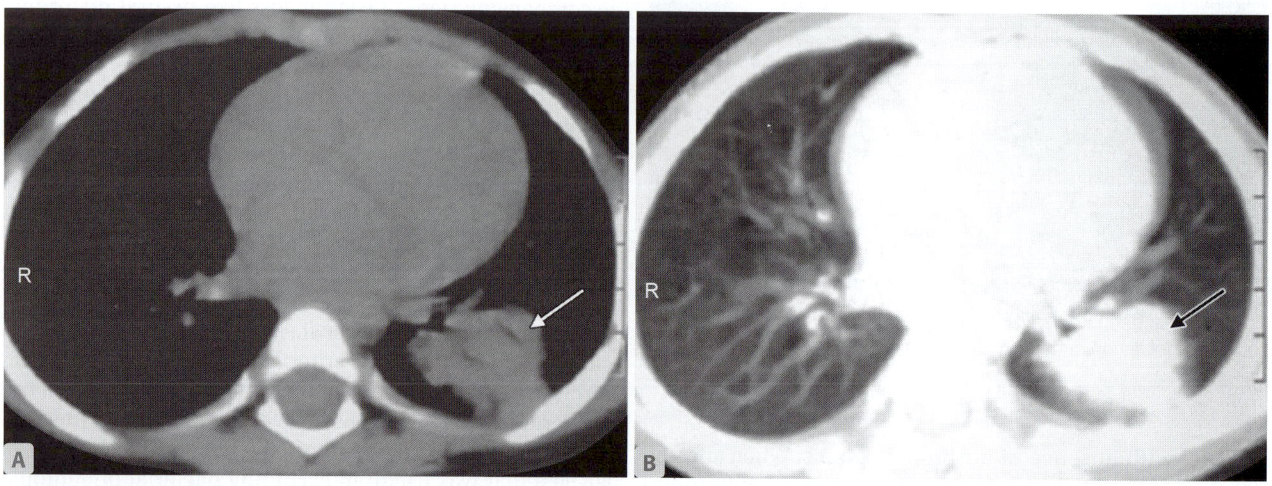

FIGS. 7A AND B: Round pneumonia: Axial CT images in a 2-year-old child with fever shows a round mass-like lesion with air bronchogram (white arrows). This was a case of round pneumonia.

random in distribution. Vessels may be seen reaching up to the nodules **(Figs. 8A and B)**.

In cases of infection with *K. pneumoniae*, a gram-negative bacillus, there is homogeneous opacification with copious inflammatory exudate which may result in an increase in the lung volume resulting in expansile pneumonia **(Fig. 9)**. Empyema and abscess are common complications.[6]

Mycoplasma pneumoniae is a significant cause of community-acquired pneumonia in school-aged children. MP usually affects older children and young adults >6 years of age with a mean age of 8–9 years. It is uncommon in children <3 years of age. These children may present with indolent symptoms unlike viral and round pneumonia. Extrapulmonary manifestations of gastrointestinal/skin/joint/central nervous system (CNS) may also be seen. On imaging, it can have a broad spectrum of appearances which may simulate viral or bacterial pneumonia. The varied radiographic appearance could be focal, unilateral reticular opacities, focal unilateral ground-glass opacities, or bilateral perihilar peribronchial thickening akin to viral bronchiolitis. Dense consolidation is usually not seen. The radiographic changes are more severe than the clinical symptoms. Hilar lymph nodes and pleural effusions can be associated.[6]

Exclusion of Other Pathologies

Since the clinical symptoms of pneumonia in children are fairly nonspecific, other pathologies that may simulate pneumonia must be excluded. It is essential to look at the ribs and the airways to exclude other potential causes of respiratory distress in children. For example, rib erosions in cases of neuroblastoma **(Figs. 10A and B)** and fractures in cases of child abuse are pointers to the correct diagnosis. Also, stridor due to vascular rings around the airway is common in children, compared to adults and warrants a careful look at the airways. Evaluation of the diameter of the airways should be stressed as a routine part of evaluation of pediatric chest radiographs. Other mimics of pneumonia pattern include pulmonary vasculitis, adult respiratory distress syndrome, hemorrhage from pulmonary embolism, and neoplasms/lymphoproliferative disorders. Sometimes, a normal but prominent thymus may also mimic pneumonia.[12]

Progressive or Fulminant Pneumonia

Progressive pneumonia is pneumonia that worsens both clinically/radiologically despite adequate antibiotic therapy. Pneumonia is called fulminant when there is marked clinical/radiological worsening after clinical presentation over 24–48 hours. In this setting, nonbacterial infections and other mimics of pneumonia may need to be considered.[2]

Nonresolving or Recurrent Pneumonia

Nonresolving or chronic pneumonia is a pneumonia that does not improve within 1 month. Recurrent pneumonia is defined as >1 episode in 12 months or >3 episodes in a lifetime.

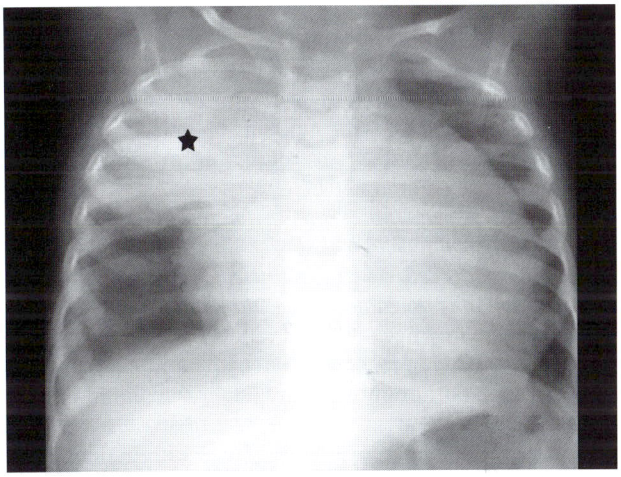

FIG. 9: Expansile pneumonia: Frontal radiograph in a 4-month-old infant shows lobar consolidation with bulging of the fissure suggesting expansile pneumonia (star).

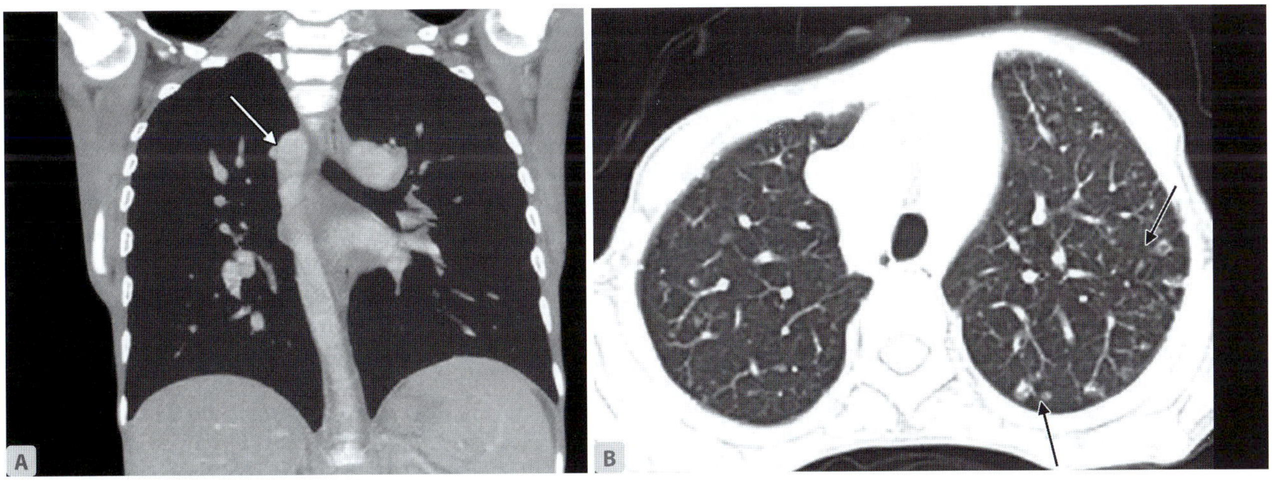

FIGS. 8A AND B: Infective endocarditis with septic emboli. (A) Coronal reformatted CT image on mediastinal window settings shows right-sided aortic arch in a case of ventricular septal defect with infective endocarditis (white arrow); and (B) Multiple nodular lesions, few showing feeding vessel sign, are seen on axial contrast-enhanced computed tomography (CECT) at lung window settings (black arrows).

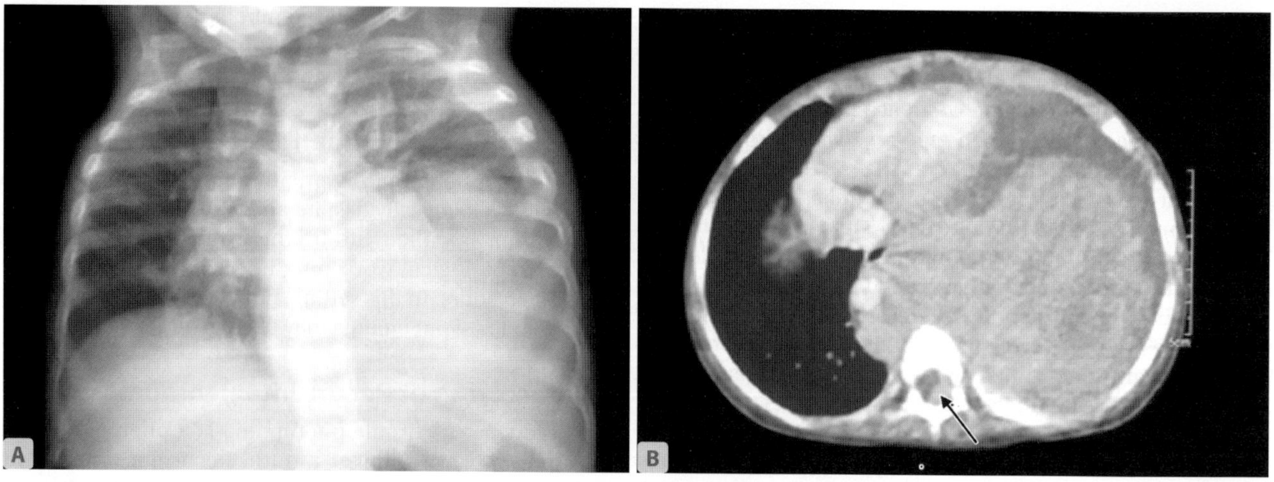

FIGS. 10A AND B: Neuroblastoma. (A) Chest radiograph in a 2-year-old girl shows opacity in the left mid and lower zone with accompanying left pleural effusion. Note erosion and splaying of the left posterior 7–10th ribs differentiating neuroblastoma from pneumonia; and (B) CT scan shows a posterior mediastinal mass displacing heart and aorta with extension into spinal canal (black arrow).

In patients with nonresolving pneumonia on antibiotic and other therapy, with noncontributory chest radiograph, contrast-enhanced CT is the modality of choice.

The various causes of recurrent or nonresolving pneumonia are enumerated below:[2,5]

- *Aspiration syndrome—owing to swallowing disorders due to neuromuscular disorders or immaturity, gastroesophageal reflux, H-type fistula, and esophageal obstruction (foreign body, vascular ring)*: For assessment of swallowing mechanism, swallow examination should be done using solid food coated with barium, followed by thickened barium mixture and finally thin liquid barium. In case H-type tracheoesophageal fistula is suspected, tube esophagogram should be done, with patient in the prone position and using a horizontal beam. Combined bronchoscopy and endoscopy are the investigation of choice.[6]

  Aspiration pneumonia cannot only result from entry of fluid/particulate material, but also results from endogenous secretion in distal airways. Aspiration typically affects the lower dependent lobes. Posterior upper lobes become dependent in the supine position. While chronic lung aspiration results from swallowing dysfunction, gastroesophageal reflux, inability to protect the airway from oral secretions, or a combination of above factors, acute aspiration may occur as a complication of anesthesia.

  Hydrocarbon pneumonia and lipoid pneumonia are two examples of named aspiration pneumonias. Hydrocarbon pneumonia results from aspiration of volatile hydrocarbons and usually presents acutely. On chest radiographs, bilateral scattered opacities can be seen in middle/lower zones, which may progress to acute respiratory distress syndrome (ARDS). Obstructive empyema, atelectasis, and pneumatoceles can be the sequelae.[2]

  Lipoid pneumonia results from aspiration of fatty substance, e.g., as a result of ingestion of oils as a part of cultural practice. The clinical presentation is subacute to chronic, but with marked changes on radiographs. The findings on chest radiographs range from bilateral central ill-defined air-space opacities, ground-glass opacification, and septal thickening with ground-glass opacities giving crazy paving pattern to dense consolidation. Low density consolidation although typical is not a common finding. The consolidation slowly improves after ingestion of oils is stopped. However, scarring/fibrosis may be permanent sequelae.[2]

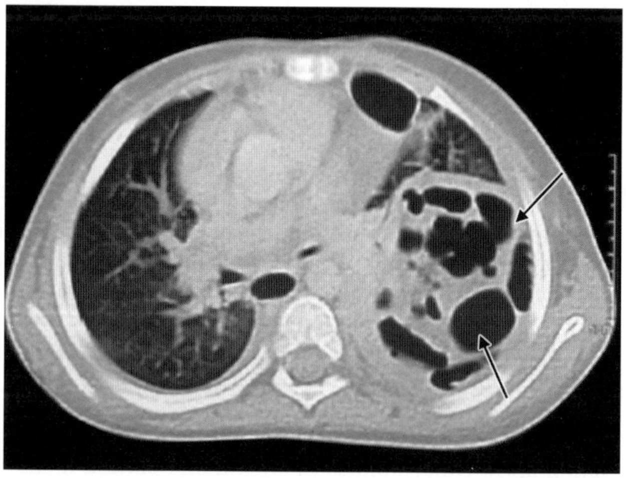

FIG. 11: Congenital pulmonary airway malformation: Computed tomography (CT) in a 3-year-old child with recurrent pneumonia shows multiseptated cystic mass with thickened walls in the left lower lobe (black arrows). The diagnosis of congenital cystic adenomatoid malformation (CCAM) was confirmed at surgery.

- *Underlying developmental lesions—like congenital pulmonary airway malformation* ***(Fig. 11)****, bronchogenic cyst, sequestration, and tracheal bronchus*: Differentiating an infected from a noninfected lung malformation may be extremely difficult or even impossible. Comparison with previous radiographs can be a great help in determining whether there is a new air-fluid level within a pre-existing lesion/perilesional consolidation to suggest infection of an underlying lesion.

- *Bronchial obstruction—foreign body, mucoid impaction, lymph nodes, neoplasm, and cardiovascular anomaly*: Foreign bodies usually lodge in the bronchial tree and affect the lower lobes or the right middle lobe. Only large ones may lodge in the trachea. Foreign body aspiration may occur while eating and present acutely with cough and choking. However, many a times, children do not remember the episode or are too young to do so and hence present with chronic pneumonia. Very small foreign bodies such as grass may migrate to the peripheral bronchi. Inorganic foreign bodies are usually inert and only result in mechanical obstruction whereas organic foreign bodies such as peanuts also incite an inflammatory reaction in addition to mechanical obstruction. Organic foreign bodies may also get fragmented and then spread into peripheral bronchi or bronchi of other lobes.

  Up to 85% of foreign bodies are nonopaque on chest radiographs. When a foreign body is suspected, radiographic assessment should start with paired inspiratory and expiratory films or fluoroscopy. Bilateral decubitus film may be obtained if fluoroscopy is not available and expiratory film is difficult to obtain. Fluoroscopy can depict mediastinal shift to affected side on inspiration and features of air trapping with reduced diaphragmatic movement on the affected side. In selected cases, CT may also be done. Distal atelectasis, especially in the lower lobes, pulmonary abscess, bronchiectasis, and bronchiolitis obliterans are the complications that may be encountered. Stenosis of the bronchus can result which predisposes to further infections.[2,6]
- Underlying systemic disorders—immunodeficiency (congenital and acquired), asthma, cystic fibrosis, and immotile cilia disease.

Evaluation of Associated Complications

Suppurative complications of pneumonia may involve the pleura, lung parenchyma, and rarely the pericardium.

Pleural Complications

A parapneumonic effusion is a pleural fluid collection adjacent to infected lung. It may be simple or complicated depending on whether the infective organism is present or not within the collection. The term empyema is used when there is frank pus within the collection.[13]

Empyema in children is a different condition from that in adults. Although associated with significant morbidity, it is almost never fatal in contrast to adults, where mortality is nearly 20%, probably due to the higher incidence of premorbid conditions.[13]

The most common agents involved are *S. pneumoniae*, *S. aureus*, other streptococci (including *Streptococcus pyogenes*), *H. influenzae*, *MP*, *Pseudomonas* species, and *Mycobacterium tuberculosis (M. tuberculosis)*.[13]

Initially, there is pleural inflammation secondary to involvement of the subpleural lung. This leads to increase in pleural fluid production with influx of inflammatory cells resulting in simple PPE. There is consequent fibrin production, resulting in fibrinous septations, resulting in complicated PPE when fluid is thickened. Later, there is pus formation, resulting in frank empyema. Eventually, a thick fibrous peel may trap the lung and may result in long-term restriction of lung function.[13] The infection may also spread from the pleura and lungs to the soft tissues and bones of the chest wall. This is most frequently seen with *Actinomyces*, *Aspergillus*, and *M. tuberculosis* infections.[2]

Chest radiography and US are the imaging modalities of choice to detect effusions and guide drainage of complicated effusions. Chest radiography is usually the first investigation. The signs vary from obliteration of the costophrenic angle, meniscus of fluid tracking along the lateral chest wall in small effusions to complete opacification of the hemithorax with contralateral mediastinal shift in larger effusions **(Figs. 12 and 13)**. Pleural cap may be visualized. Loculated effusions tend to have a lenticular shape **(Fig. 14)**. In cases of empyema, there may be scoliosis concave to the side of the collection, due to pain. On supine films, there may be homogeneous haze of the affected hemithorax. Subpulmonic effusion may be better seen on a decubitus film.

Ultrasound is used to confirm the presence of effusion, characterize it, and guide drainage. Effusions may be anechoic or show fine internal echoes and fibrinous septations **(Figs. 15A to C)**. US may also be used to characterize nonshifting nature of loculated fluid by scanning the patient in supine and sitting position. In cases of fibrous rind formation, pleural thickening is seen with lack of mobility of the underlying lung, suggesting entrapment. When a very organized collection is difficult to distinguish from the underlying consolidated lung, color Doppler may be used to demonstrate vessels in the consolidated lung in contrast to the avascular pleural collection.[13]

Computed tomography is reserved for special circumstances, e.g., failing tube drainage and in immunocompromised individuals to detect associated parenchymal and mediastinal abnormalities. On CT, features of empyema include pleural thickening and enhancement, increased

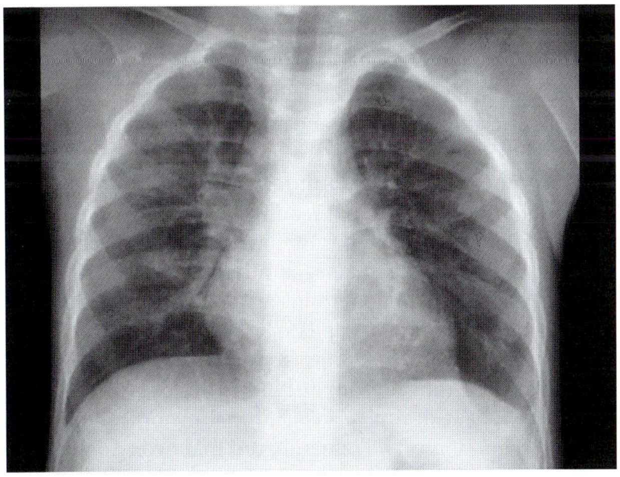

FIG. 12: Pleural effusion: Frontal radiograph of a child shows blunting of the left costophrenic angle suggesting effusion. This was confirmed on ultrasound.

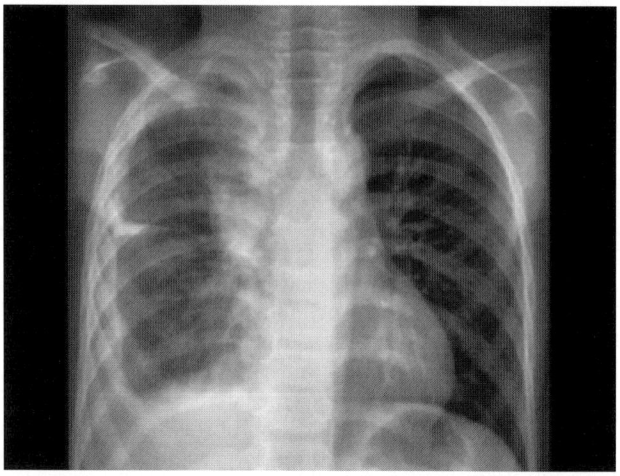

FIG. 13: Pleural effusion: Frontal radiograph of a 10-year-old child shows blunting of the right costophrenic angle with fluid tracking along the lateral chest wall and the horizontal fissure in addition to the opacities in the right lung.

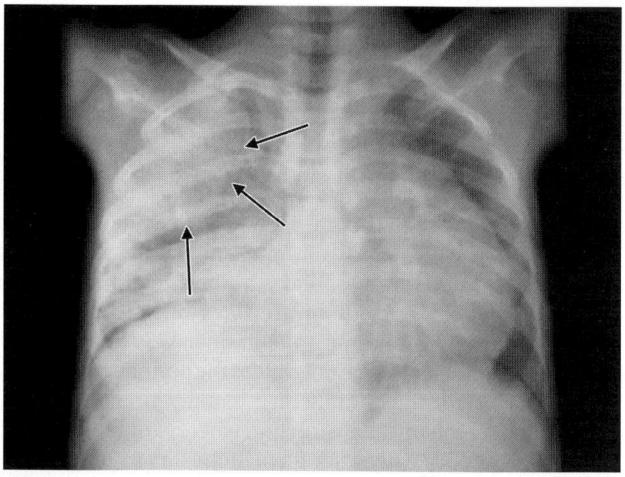

FIG. 14: Loculated pleural effusion; Frontal radiograph of a 10-year-old child shows lenticular-shaped soft-tissue opacity along the right upper lateral chest wall suggesting loculated pleural effusion (black arrows). The underlying lung shows areas of consolidation and atelectasis.

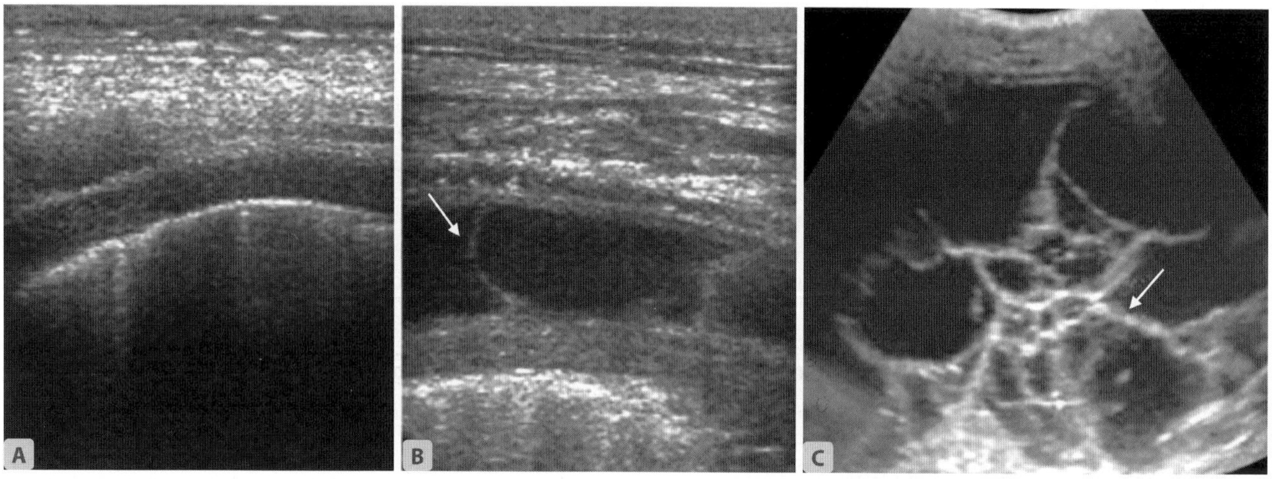

FIGS. 15A TO C: Ultrasound in cases of pleural effusion may depict the (A) clear nature of fluid or (B and C) show fine fibrinous septations (white arrows in B and C).

density and thickening of extrapleural fat, increased density of extrathoracic fat, and lenticular shape suggesting loculation. Pleural thickening and enhancement are better appreciated in the parietal pleura, as the visceral pleura is difficult to differentiate from the underlying consolidated lung. Although septations are not readily appreciable on CT, their presence may be inferred from air loculi within the pleural collection. This is due to air separating into tiny bubbles due to septations rather than forming an air-fluid level **(Fig. 16)**.[13] CT can also be helpful in depicting malpositioned chest tubes **(Figs. 17A and B)**.

Treatment ranges from antibiotic therapy, simple tube drainage, chest drainage insertion with fibrinolytics, and even surgery. It must be remembered that even an anechoic collection may contain frank pus. Therefore, imaging is not the basis for deciding whether the patient requires drainage. This decision is dependent on whether the collection is increasing in size or the patient is having respiratory embarrassment due to the collection.[13]

Another clinical problem which may arise is differentiation between empyema and a lung abscess. This is important because the treatment of abscess is primarily medical and insertion of drainage tube increases the risk for bronchopleural fistula (BPF) formation. While irregular thick wall and acute angle with chest wall favor the diagnosis of lung abscess, split pleura sign and compression of the adjacent lung favor the diagnosis of empyema.[13]

Lung Parenchymal Complications

The various complications include cavitary necrosis, pulmonary abscess, pulmonary gangrene, pneumatocele, and BPF. These names depend on the severity and distribution of the complication, status of the adjacent lung parenchyma, and its temporal relationship with resolution of infection.[2,5,14-16]

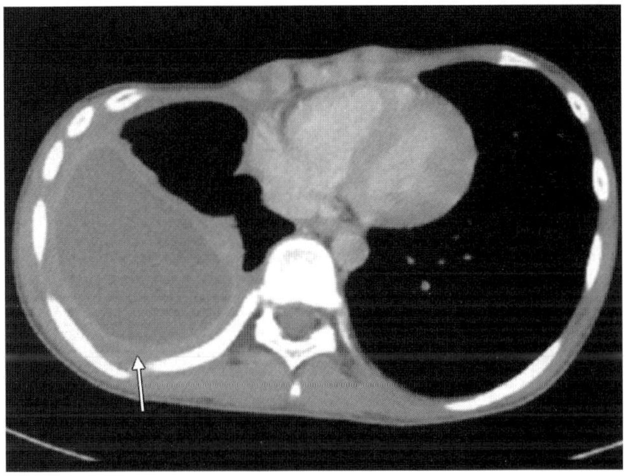

FIG. 16: Empyema: Axial contrast-enhanced computed tomography (CECT) shows lenticular shape of the collection with pleural thickening and enhancement with increased thickness and density of extrapleural fat (white arrow).

Cavitary necrosis is the most common complication encountered in children. *S. pneumoniae* and *S. aureus* are the frequent associated organisms. It is defined as a dominant area of necrosis with associated variable number of thin-walled cysts. On CT, it appears as decreased contrast enhancement, lack of normal lung architecture, loss of lung pleura margin, and multiple thin-walled cavities filled with air or fluid with no peripheral enhancement **(Figs. 18A and B)**. The finding of decreased enhancement is indicative of pulmonary parenchymal ischemia or impending cavitary necrosis **(Figs. 19A and B)**. Cavitary necrosis is visualized on chest radiographs when air enters the cavities due to bronchial communication. Although associated with a protracted course, most patients are managed conservatively in contrast to adults. To distinguish between underlying cystic malformation of the lung with secondary infection and cavitary necrosis of the lung, it may not be possible on a single radiograph. Comparison with previous chest radiographs or follow-up may be necessary for differentiation.[5,16]

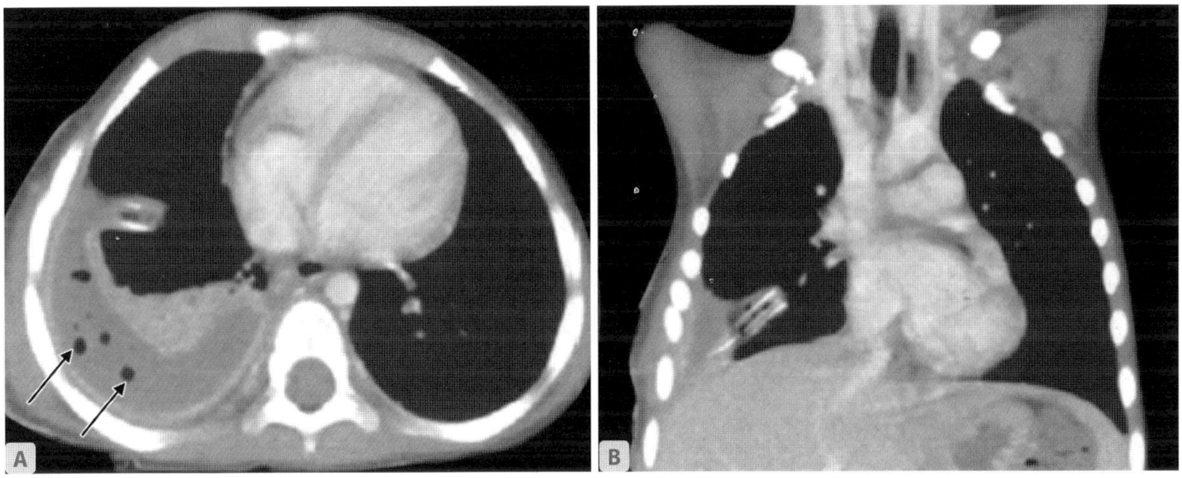

FIGS. 17A AND B: Empyema: Axial and coronal reformatted contrast-enhanced computed tomography (CECT) images depict the loculated right pleural collection with foci of air within (black arrows). Note is made of split pleura sign and underlying atelectasis. It is important to note the position of the chest tube which appears malpositioned.

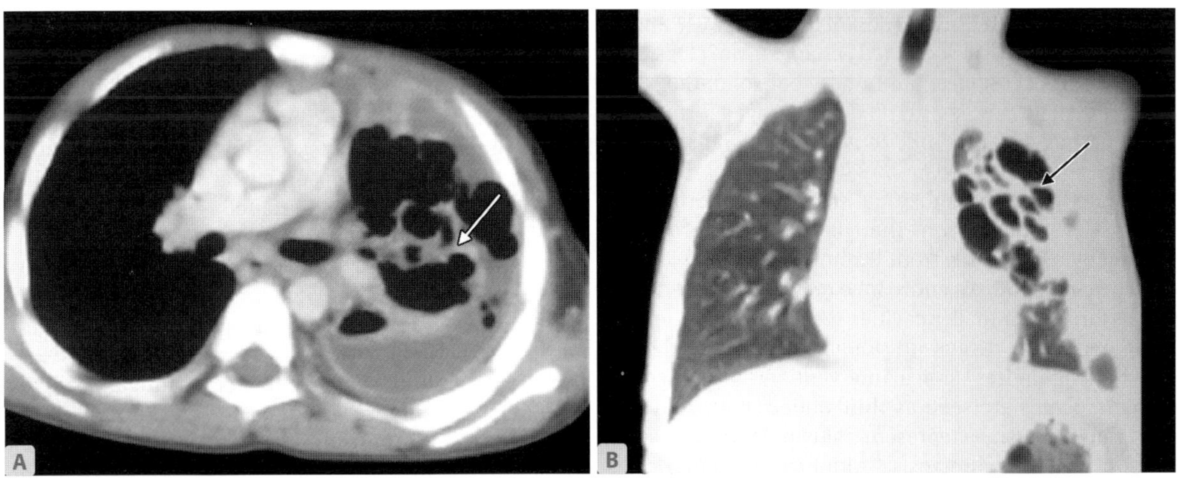

FIGS. 18A AND B: Cavitary necrosis: Computed tomography (CT) findings in a 7-year-old boy shows multiloculated cavity within consolidated lung (white and black arrows).

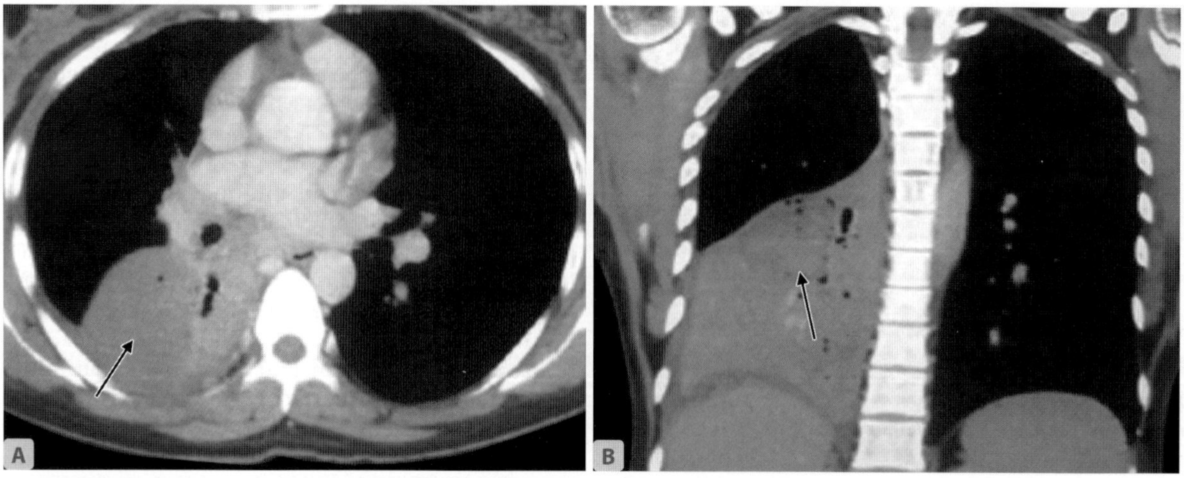

FIGS. 19A AND B: (A and B) Axial and coronal reformatted CT images of an adolescent with severe pneumonia shows consolidation of the right lower lobe with bulging of the lobe and areas of decreased parenchymal enhancement within (black arrows), probably reflecting areas of ischemia and impending gangrene.

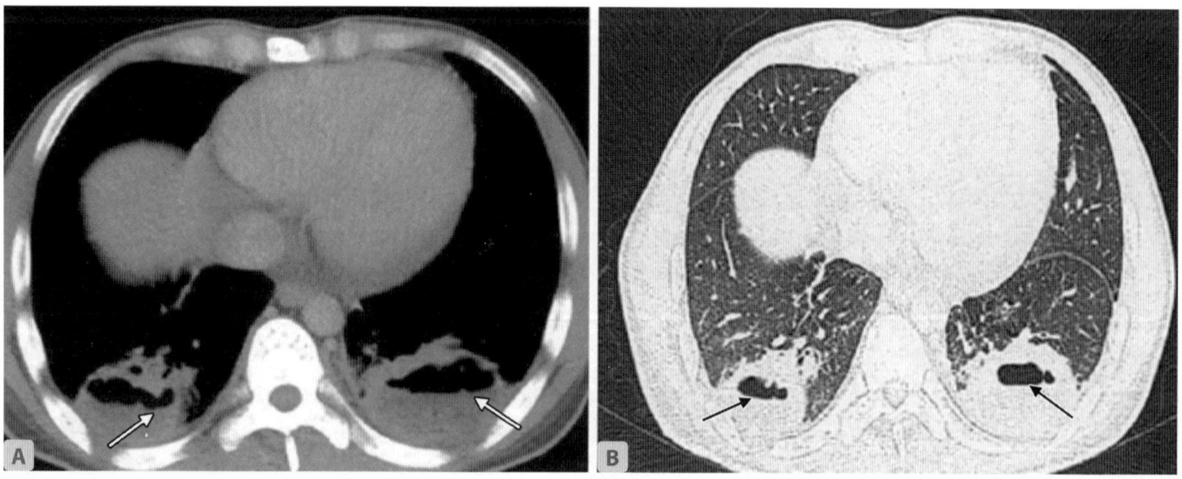

FIGS. 20A AND B: Lung abscesses: Axial contrast-enhanced computed tomography (CECT) images show abscesses with air-fluid levels in bilateral posterior-dependent lungs suggesting aspiration as the probable cause (white and black arrows).

Lung abscess is fairly uncommon in immunocompetent children and is defined as collection of fluid or air within the lung parenchyma with a well-defined enhancing rim **(Figs. 20A and B)**.[5,14-16] In early stages, pulmonary consolidation may show a low density center with no definite cavity formation. Common pathogens are *S. pneumoniae, S. aureus*, and *K. pneumoniae*.[7]

Pulmonary gangrene is the final stage of a continuum of pulmonary devascularization. There is extensive necrosis of lung parenchyma resulting from thrombosis of large vessels secondary to infection. An entire lobe may get necrosed with bulging fissures and smaller cavities may coalesce to form a single large irregular cavity with sloughed lung parenchyma. This most often requires surgical intervention.

Pneumatoceles are seen as thin-walled air-containing cysts on imaging and may represent a later or less severe stage of resolving or healing necrosis.[2] Although pneumatoceles are most characteristic of *S. aureus* infection, other causes are *Pneumococcus, H. influenzae, Streptococcus, M. tuberculosis,* and *Escherichia coli (E. coli)*. They are also known after hydrocarbon ingestion. These do not show any rim enhancement and surrounding lung parenchyma is normal. When pneumatoceles develop in infected areas, inflammatory exudate may seep into them and produce air-fluid levels that simulate lung abscesses. However, true lung abscesses have a thicker and often somewhat shaggy wall. While most pneumatoceles resolve spontaneously with time, those with air-fluid levels may require drainage.

Bronchopleural fistula is a communication between a bronchus/lung parenchyma and the pleural cavity. Central BPF commonly results from trauma and postpneumonectomy. Peripheral BPF manifests as a result of infection [lung abscess, tuberculosis (TB), bacterial, fungal], malignancy, trauma, and surgery. Diagnosis is based upon increasing amount of sputum production and air in the pleural cavity which may be loculated.[6] Air within the pleural cavity prior to intervention/drainage can either result from infection with gas-forming organisms or BPF. CT may demonstrate direct communication between the pleural space and the bronchial tree in cases of BPF.

Purulent Pericarditis

Pericardial fluid is not uncommonly encountered during US and CT of children with pneumonia. This may also result in cardiac tamponade when there is rapid accumulation. When the clinical features go unrecognized, the radiologist may be the first one to suggest the diagnosis **(Figs. 21A and B)**.[13]

Chronic Effects of Pneumonia

Most cases of pneumonia resolve completely. However, a few children may develop chronic complications. Chronic complications include bronchiectasis, predisposition to asthma, constrictive bronchiolitis, fibrothorax, constrictive pericarditis, and fibrosing mediastinitis.

- Bronchiectasis may occur in cases of infection with persistent collapse or foreign body aspiration **(Fig. 22)**. It usually affects the medium-sized bronchi, as the proximal bronchi have more cartilage in their walls. Only allergic bronchopulmonary aspergillosis shows a tendency to attack the proximal bronchi. Diffuse bronchiectasis may also occur due to chronic recurrent pulmonary infection (including pneumonia, TB, pertussis), particularly in cases of cystic fibrosis and primary ciliary dyskinesia syndromes.[3]
- Constrictive bronchiolitis (bronchiolitis obliterans) occurs owing to fibrosis resulting in concentric narrowing/obliteration of bronchioles. It can occur as a result of infection, collagen vascular diseases, toxins, and drugs.
    - *Swyer-James-MacLeod syndrome* is a form of post-infectious obliterative bronchiolitis that occurs following an insult to the developing lung (before the age of 8 years). It is most frequent after a viral infection, in particular adenoviral infection and also post-mycoplasma infection. The lung served by the

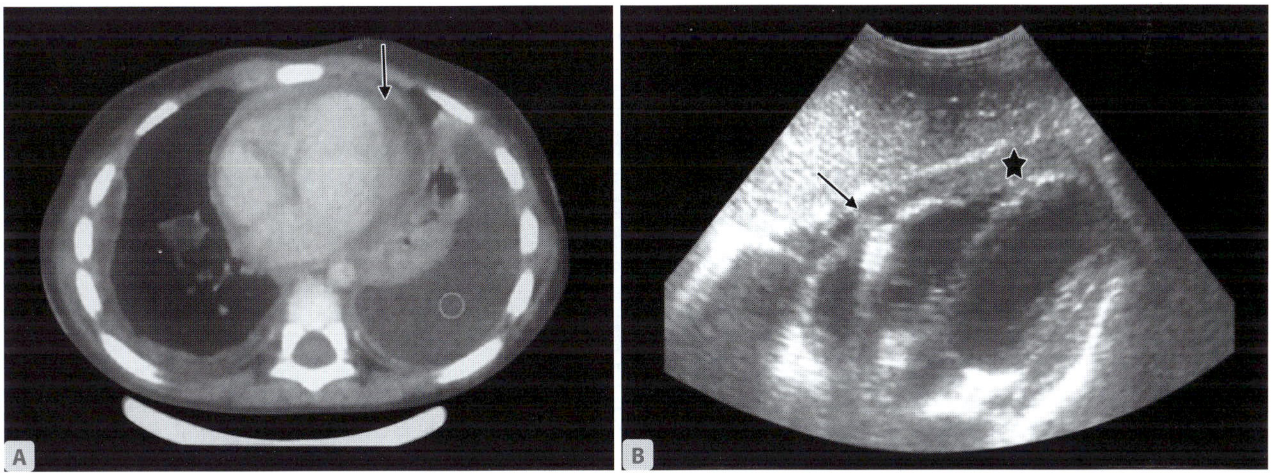

FIGS. 21A AND B: Purulent pericarditis. (A) Axial contrast-enhanced computed tomography (CECT) image shows pericardial (black arrow) as well as pleural fluid in a case of pneumonia; and (B) Correlative ultrasound image shows thick pericardial fluid (star) with septations (black arrow).

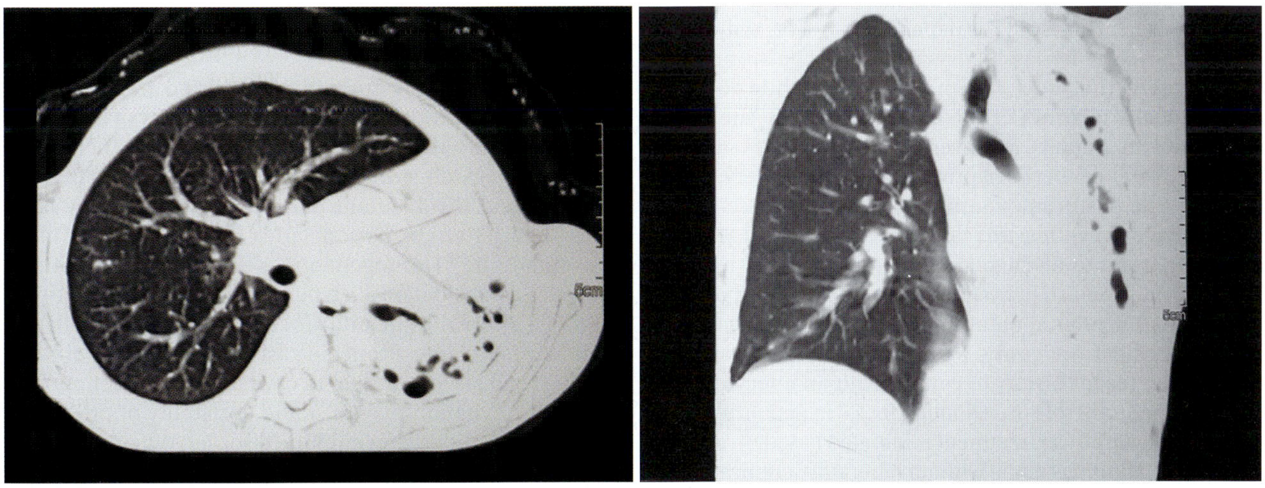

FIG. 22: There is complete collapse of the left lung with bronchiectatic changes in a 8-year-old child consequent to chronic pneumonia.

affected bronchi and bronchioles remains inflated due to collateral air drift. Pulmonary tissue as well as pulmonary artery and its branches are hypoplastic. Patients are typically asymptomatic and may present in adulthood with progressive exertional dyspnea or repeated respiratory infections. Disease on chest radiography is predominantly unilateral, giving rise to the key finding of unilateral transradiancy. This reflects hypoplasia of pulmonary vasculature as well as obliterative bronchiolitis. Ipsilateral air trapping is the key finding. The hilum of the affected lung is small. The affected lung is small or normal in volume in contrast to congenital lobar emphysema. CT changes are more complex than chest radiographs. It more commonly shows areas of bilateral abnormalities depicting areas of decreased attenuation. Air trapping can be confirmed on expiratory scans. Areas of cylindrical bronchiectasis may also be seen. There may be areas of collapse and scarring.[17]

- Fibrothorax results from extreme fibrosis involving both visceral and parietal pleura which may fuse together. This results in reduced volume of the hemithorax and reduced mobility of lungs. The mediastinum shifts to the affected side. Treatment of fibrothorax is decortication.

  When the lung cannot expand due to pleural fibrosis, it results in a trapped lung. This results in negative pressure within the pleura leading to accumulation of pleural fluid. The treatment is again decortication and not drainage of pleural fluid which has accumulated only due to mechanical reasons. It is important to ensure that the underlying lung is healthy prior to decortication as desired improvement will not occur after decortication if the lung is fibrosed or diseased.[2]
- Fibrosing mediastinitis results from fibrosis within the mediastinum. The most common infectious agents are *M. tuberculosis* and *Histoplasma capsulatum*. This condition can produce symptoms owing to compression of central airways, pulmonary artery and veins, superior vena cava, and esophagus.[2]

TUBERCULOSIS

The pathological form of TB is dependent on sensitivity of the infected host and is classified as primary or postprimary.[18] Primary TB, the most common form in childhood, is radiologically distinct from postprimary TB the most common form in adults. However, recent literature[19] suggests that the differences between primary and postprimary TB are blurring. The postprimary form of TB is being increasingly seen in children with significant destructive sequelae. It is more important to distinguish between active and inactive TB than to distinguish between primary and postprimary TB.

Due to difficulty in obtaining suitable sputum samples and low sensitivity of gastric washings, chest radiography in a child with recent history of contact with an infected adult plays an important role in evaluation for TB in pediatric cases. Many times, empirical treatment is initiated based on clinical and imaging findings alone without laboratory confirmation. Positive culture from an infected adult contact may also guide treatment.[20]

Primary Pulmonary Tuberculosis

Primary TB represents the reaction to first exposure and is often a subclinical condition. Incubation period varies from 2 to 10 weeks and ends when the patient becomes sensitized (i.e., has a positive skin test). As the infecting bacteria are inhaled, it incites a local inflammatory reaction in the bronchiole/alveolus, usually peripherally in a subpleural focus, called the Ghon focus. From this focus, lymphatic spread to the local hilar or mediastinal lymph nodes may occur.[17] The combination of a peripheral granuloma, involved lymphatics, and lymph nodes is known as Ghon complex. In most cases, the immune response is usually enough to limit the infection, which heals with calcification and is then called Ranke complex. Primary focus is usually quite small as compared to the large lymph nodes. In young infants or in cases with underlying illness or impaired nutrition resulting in impaired defenses, progressive primary disease may occur. Enlarging pulmonary focus of consolidation and caseation followed by liquefaction occurs. This leads to cavitation and rupture into a bronchus that may result in acute tuberculous bronchopneumonia.[20] These children are usually quite ill with weight loss and failure to thrive.

Primary TB may be asymptomatic when the child is well and the disease is detected during a routine skin test. It may otherwise present in four major ways in childhood, in addition to a normal chest radiograph:

1. Lymphadenopathy
2. Lobar or segmental parenchymal disease
3. Pleural effusion
4. Miliary involvement

Lymphadenopathy

Lymph node enlargement with or without parenchymal abnormality is the radiological hallmark of primary TB in childhood. The favored lymph nodal sites are right paratracheal, hilar, subcarinal, and aortopulmonary window region. Lymphadenopathy is seen in 83–96% of pediatric cases of TB compared to 10–45% of adult TB population.[20-22] Contrast-enhanced CT may depict characteristic low attenuation nodes with rim enhancement **(Figs. 23A and B)**.

Parenchymal Disease

There is a tendency toward right-sided parenchymal involvement, likely due to increased probability of inhalation of particles into the straighter right bronchus. There is no consensus regarding zonal predilection in primary TB.[20] The parenchymal involvement patterns described vary from ill-defined parenchymal opacities to segmental or lobar consolidation.[20] Homogeneous, dense, and well-defined air-space consolidation is a typical appearance of primary TB **(Fig. 24)**. There may be multifocal air-space consolidation or diffuse nodularity. Bronchiectasis may be seen in areas of previous collapse. Evolution to cavitary TB is uncommon in children. Cavitation may raise the possibility of previously unsuspected underlying immune disorder. When cavitation occurs, it is known as progressive primary TB. Calcification occurs after caseation of the primary lesion and is seen earlier in infants (6 months after infection) than in older children

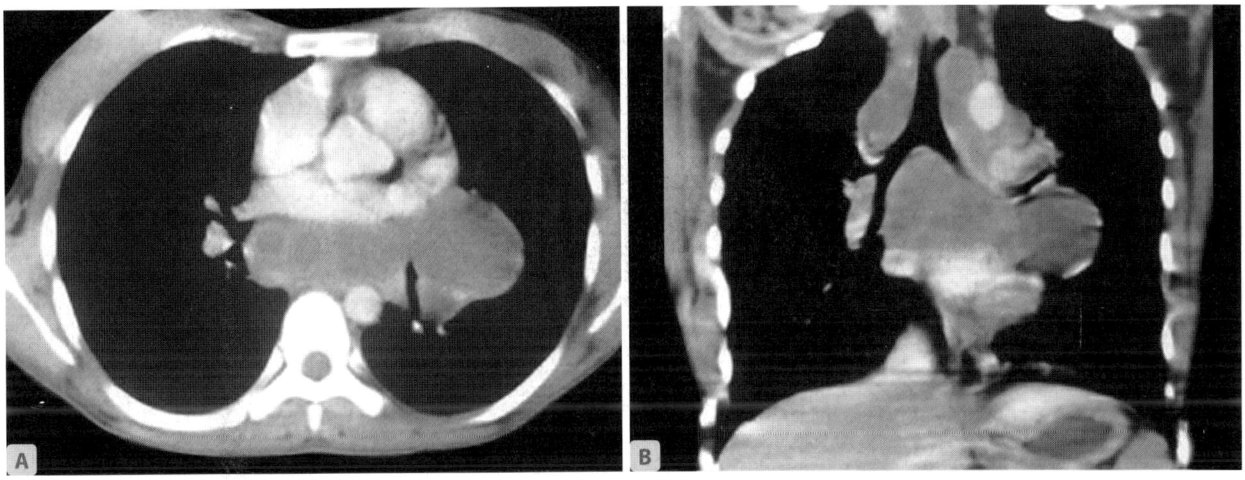

FIGS. 23A AND B: Tuberculosis: Axial and coronal reformatted contrast-enhanced computed tomography (CECT) images at mediastinal window settings depict large necrotic rim-enhancing lymph nodes in a case of tuberculosis in a 5-year-old girl.

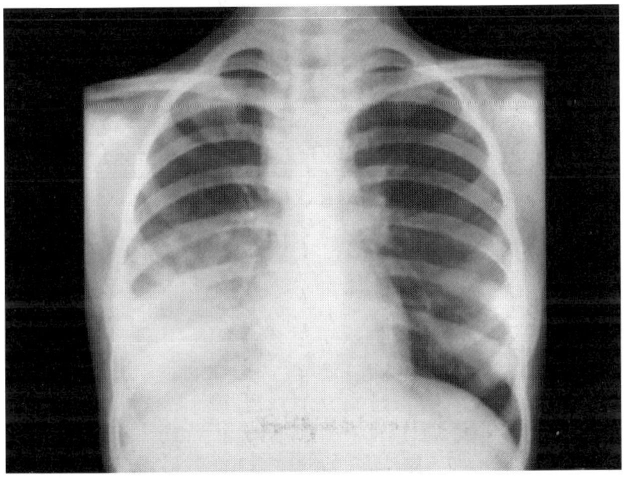

FIG. 24: Tuberculosis: Frontal radiograph in an 8-year-old child with proven tuberculosis shows right paratracheal lymphadenopathy with homogeneous consolidation in the right lower lobe.

(2–3 years after infection) **(Figs. 25A and B)** Fibrotic and calcified lesions may persist.[3,7]

Bronchial stenosis may result from lymph nodal compression but more commonly from direct extension into the bronchi. Bronchial wall involvement is more commonly seen in primary TB than postprimary TB. On chest radiograph, obstructive hyperinflation, atelectasis, mucoid impaction, and postobstructive pneumonia can be seen **(Figs. 26A to C)**. CT shows long segment narrowing and irregularity of the bronchi and extrinsic compression.

Direct extension of lymph nodes into bronchi can result in bronchopneumonia.

Parenchymal consolidation may simulate bacterial pneumonia, but presence of lymph nodes points toward the diagnosis of TB.

Pleural Effusion

Pleural effusions usually occur due to hypersensitivity to tubercular protein rather than direct extension from the

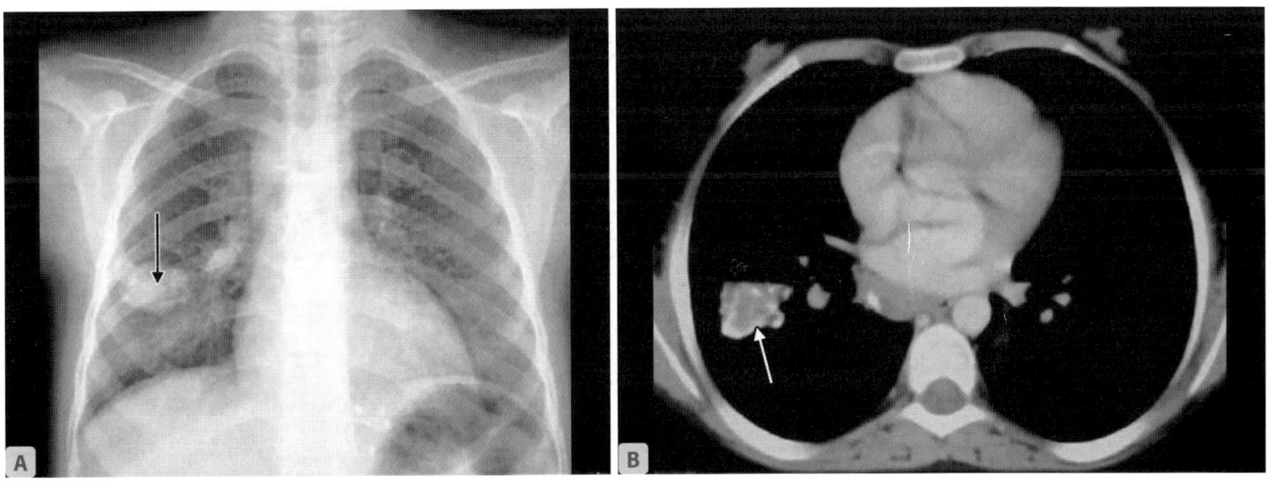

FIGS. 25A AND B: Tuberculosis in an 11-year-old child. (A) Frontal radiograph of an 11-year-old child reveals prominence of the right paratracheal stripe and hilum with nodule in the right lung field (black arrow); and (B) Axial contrast-enhanced computed tomography (CECT) image shows the calcified lymph nodes with granuloma in the right lung with foci of calcification (white arrow).

parenchymal focus in cases of primary TB. Effusions are not a common feature of primary TB in young children and are more commonly encountered in adolescents and adults.[20]

Miliary Tuberculosis

Hematogenous spread occurs as a rule but is self-limited in primary TB. However, when an overwhelming number of mycobacteria are discharged into the bloodstream, it can cause miliary infection of the lungs.[6,18] Infants are more susceptible to miliary TB, possibly due to low immunity at this age. CT can detect miliary disease earlier than chest radiographs **(Figs. 27A to C)**. Most often, miliary TB presents as an acute disease but sometimes more insidiously as pyrexia of unknown origin. However, in both cases, the mortality remains high.[20]

Postprimary Tuberculosis

It is usually seen in older children and adolescents. It results from reactivation of dormant residual foci or by second infection from a different strain.[22]

Postprimary TB is characterized by parenchymal disease with an anatomic bias for the upper lung zones. Typically, the lesions are located in the apical and posterior segments of the upper lobes and superior segments of the lower lobes, probably due to relatively higher oxygen tension and impaired lymphatic drainage.[20] However, no portion of the lungs has immunity. Bilateral and multilobar involvement is fairly frequent **(Fig. 28)**.

Cavitation is a characteristic radiographic finding. Cavitation is usually seen within an area of consolidation. The wall of the cavities may be thick and irregular. Cavitation correlates with bacterial load, drug resistance, infectivity, and prognosis. Thin-walled cavities may persist after treatment, which can result in secondary infection, mycetoma formation, and hemoptysis from vascular erosions. Air-fluid level in the cavity can be a result of TB itself or by bacterial superinfection. Heavy seeding of the bronchial tree is likely, particularly in the presence of cavitation and widespread bronchopneumonia may result resulting in centrilobular nodule formation **(Figs. 29 and 30)**. Centrilobular nodules may be seen away from the cavities with no lobar predilection.

Cicatrization atelectasis is a common finding after postprimary TB. Bronchiectasis may be seen, either as a result of cicatricial bronchostenosis after local infection or more commonly due to fibrosis of lung parenchyma with secondary bronchial dilatation **(Figs. 31A to C)**. Calcification is often seen coincident with increasing fibrosis.[6,18] Airway and pleural involvement is less common in postprimary than primary TB. Necrotic rim enhancing or calcified lymph nodes may be encountered.

Miliary TB due to hematogenous spread can be seen with postprimary TB as well. The findings are similar to those in

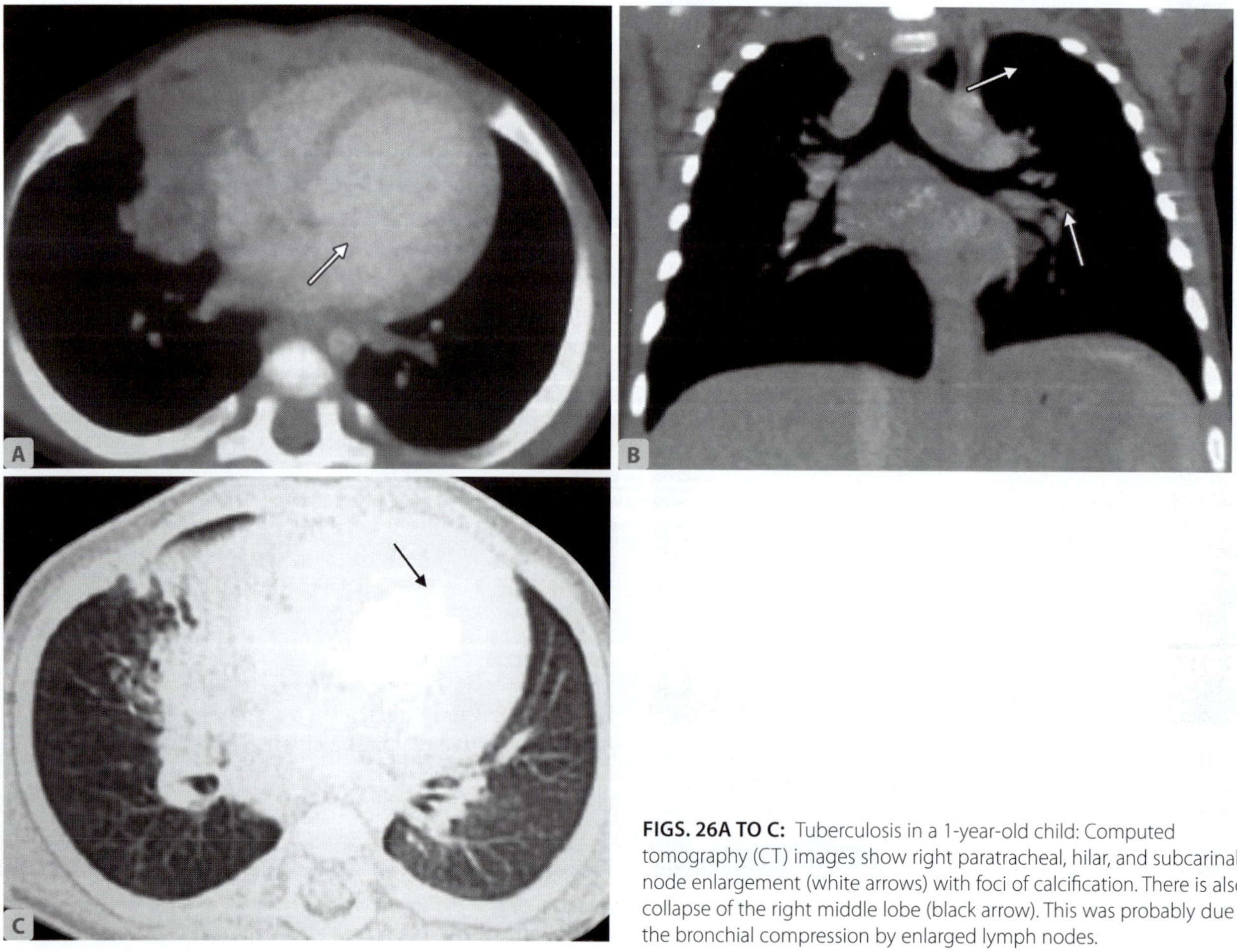

FIGS. 26A TO C: Tuberculosis in a 1-year-old child: Computed tomography (CT) images show right paratracheal, hilar, and subcarinal node enlargement (white arrows) with foci of calcification. There is also collapse of the right middle lobe (black arrow). This was probably due to the bronchial compression by enlarged lymph nodes.

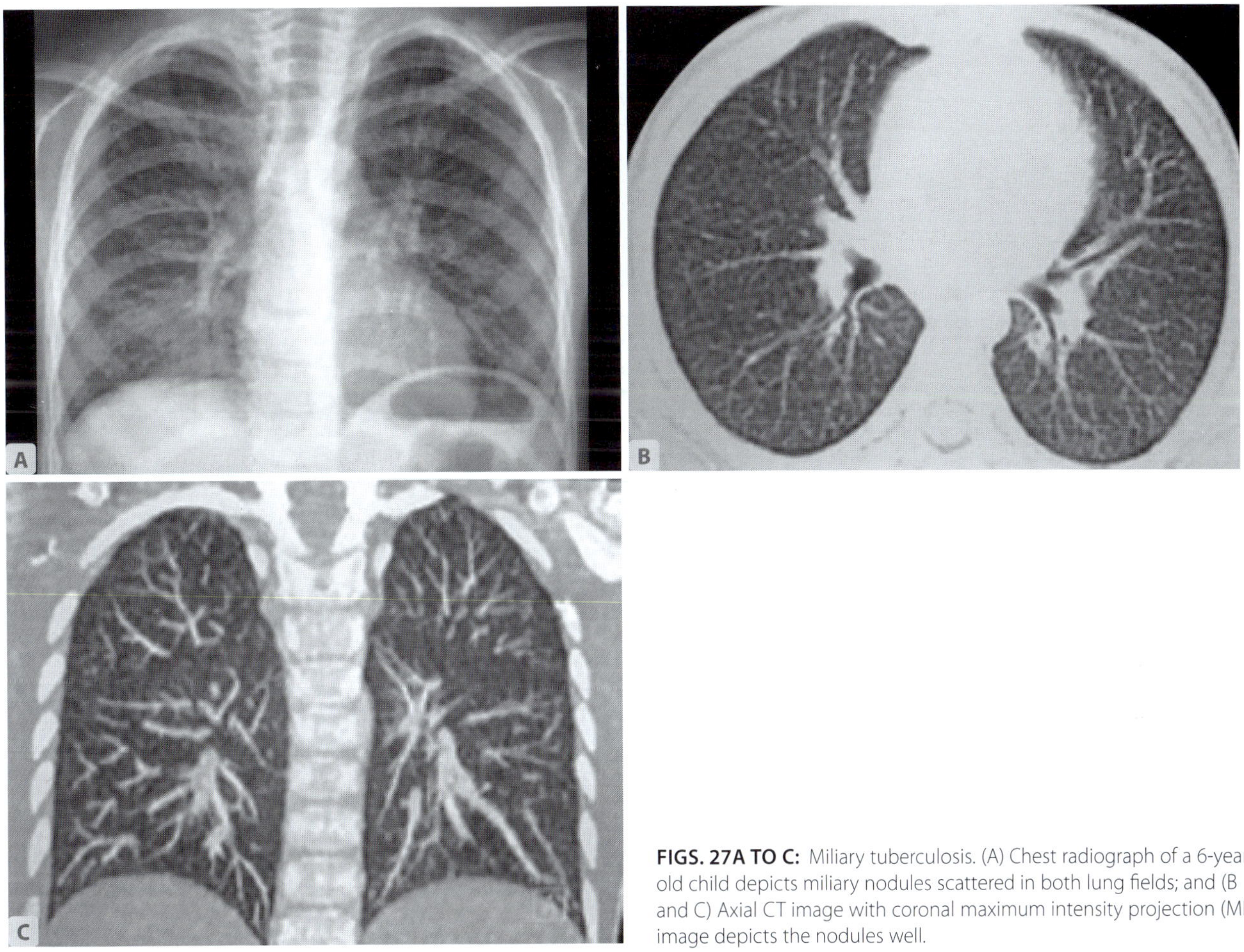

FIGS. 27A TO C: Miliary tuberculosis. (A) Chest radiograph of a 6-year-old child depicts miliary nodules scattered in both lung fields; and (B and C) Axial CT image with coronal maximum intensity projection (MIP) image depicts the nodules well.

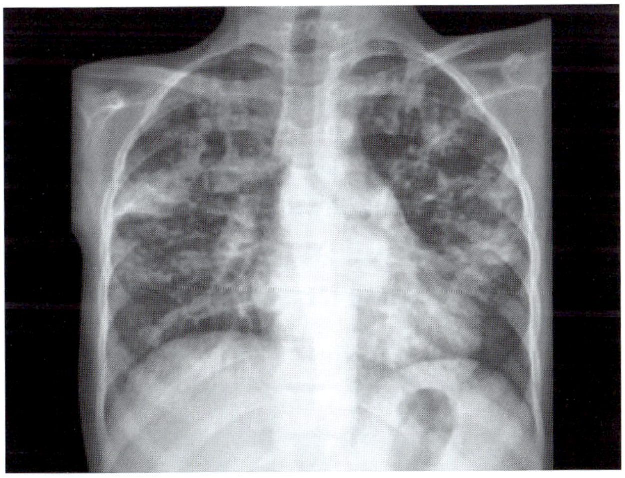

FIG. 28: Tuberculosis: In an adolescent with tuberculosis, frontal radiograph depicts multifocal areas of consolidation in both lungs with an area of cavitation in the right upper lobe.

primary TB. Both well-defined and poorly-defined nodular opacities, 2–3 mm in size are seen scattered randomly in both lungs. Coalescence of small nodules may form larger nodules or even consolidation. There may be reticulonodular opacities with thickening of the interlobular septa. Ground-glass opacities may also be seen on high-resolution computed tomography (HRCT) when small granulomas below the resolution of the scan are superimposed on exudative changes of the lung.[6,18]

Role of Computed Tomography

Computed tomography may be done when TB is suspected in children, but the radiographic findings are inconclusive or when complications are suspected or disease activity needs characterization.

Signs of Disease Inactivity in Tuberculosis

Findings that may persist on imaging even when disease becomes inactive include calcified granulomas and calcified lymph nodes. These carry an extremely low risk of reactivation **(Fig. 31)**. Other findings include fibronodular disease and thin-walled cavities. These carry a higher risk of reactivation. If fibronodular disease is stable for last 6 months as compared with previous radiographs, then it can be considered inactive.[22]

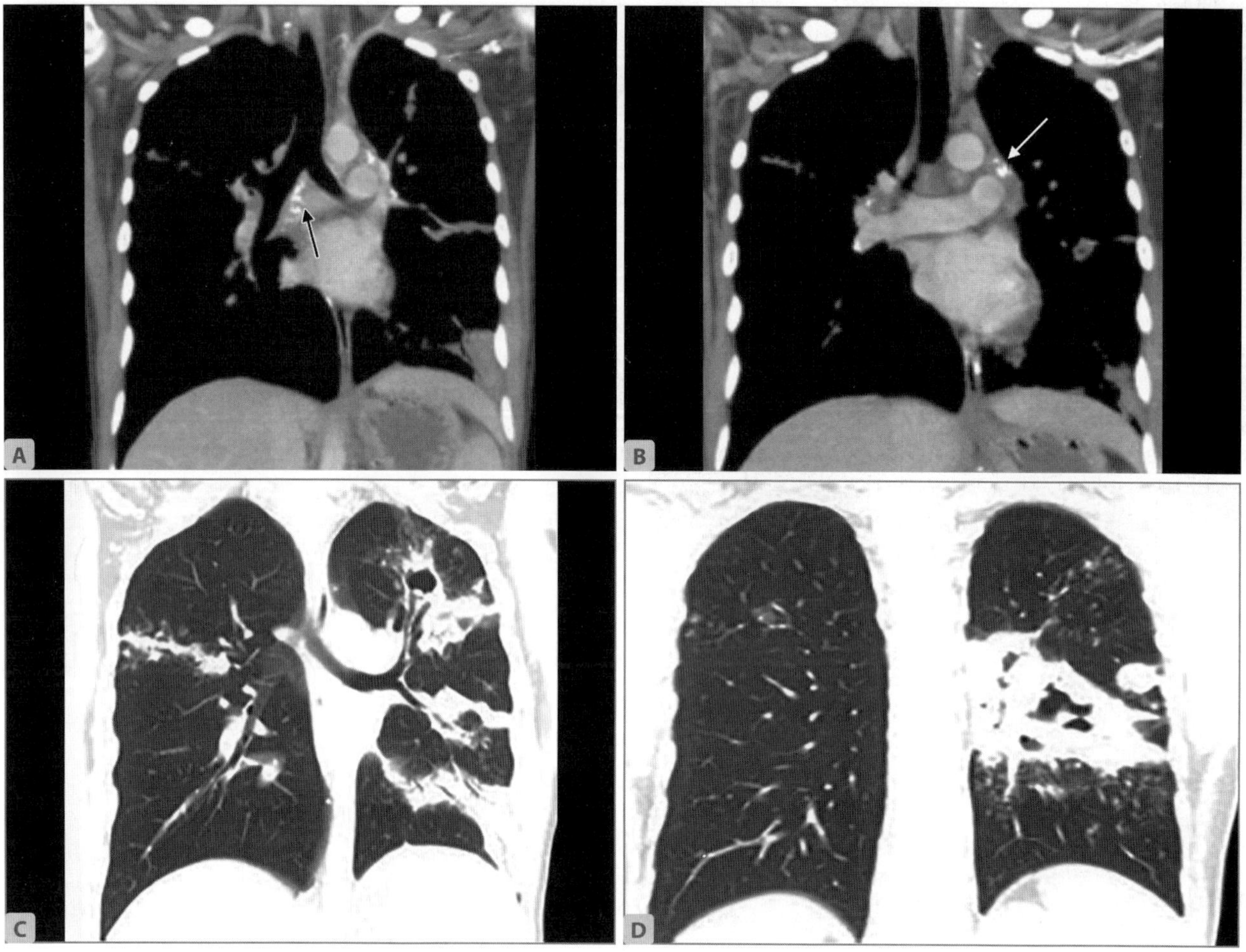

FIGS. 29A TO D: Tuberculosis: In a 12-year-old girl, coronal reformatted CT images at mediastinal (A and B) and lung window (C and D) settings show mediastinal nodes with foci of calcification (arrows) and multifocal patches of consolidation bilaterally with areas of cavitation and other centrilobular nodules.

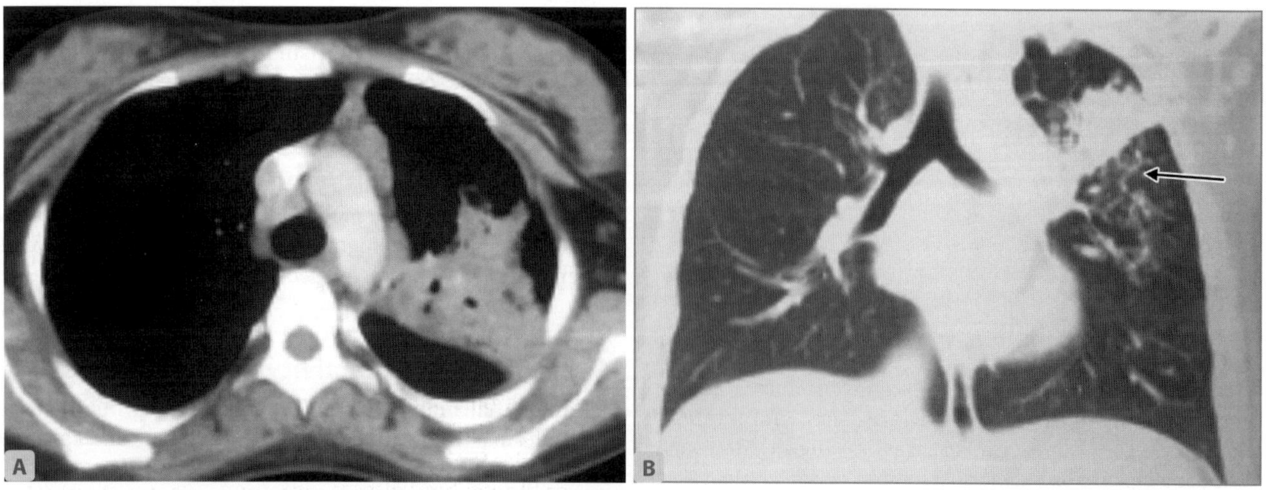

FIGS. 30A AND B: Tuberculosis. (A) In an adolescent, axial contrast-enhanced computed tomography (CECT) image at mediastinal window shows evidence of mediastinal lymph nodes with left upper lobe consolidation; and (B) Coronal reformatted CT image at lung window depicts consolidation in the left upper lobe with few adjacent centrilobular nodules (black arrow).

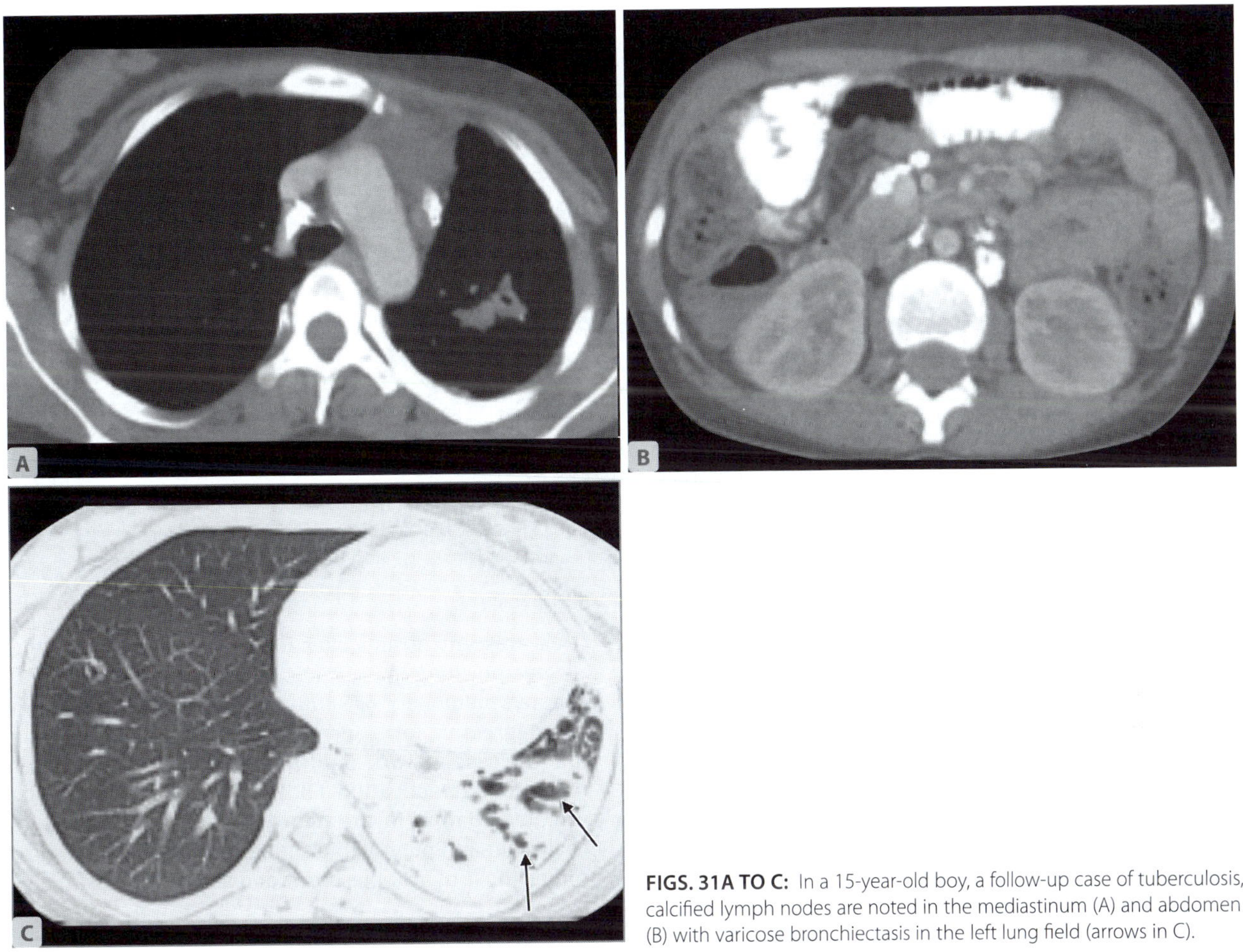

FIGS. 31A TO C: In a 15-year-old boy, a follow-up case of tuberculosis, calcified lymph nodes are noted in the mediastinum (A) and abdomen (B) with varicose bronchiectasis in the left lung field (arrows in C).

However, if prior imaging is not available, then clinical and laboratory evaluation is required. Chest CT may also aid in better characterization of disease activity.

FUNGAL INFECTIONS

Fungi that can cause pneumonia can be either pathogenic (affecting immunocompetent host) or saprophytic (affecting immunocompromised host). The fungi that can infect the immunocompetent host include coccidioidomycosis, blastomycosis, and histoplasmosis and that usually infect the immunocompromised host include *Pneumocystis, Candida, Aspergillus*, and Mucormycosis. Necrosis, cavitation, calcification, chronic inflammatory reaction, and pleural disease may all occur. These resemble tuberculous lesions. There are no conclusive radiographic criteria that can distinguish mycosis from TB or one mycosis from another. Few common radiographic patterns are enumerated in **Table 1**. Other important features are highlighted in the following discussion.

TABLE 1: Radiographic characteristics of fungal and actinomyces infection.[3]

Infection	Common radiographic patterns
Blastomycosis	Consolidation, cavitation
Cryptococcosis	Consolidation, nodules
Invasive aspergillosis	Bronchocentric or angiocentric lesions, halo and air crescent signs
Coccidioidomycosis	Simulates tuberculosis, thin-walled cavities
Histoplasmosis	Simulates tuberculosis

Aspergillosis

Aspergillus can produce four distinct patterns in children depending on the immune status and patient's pre-existing disease—(1) simple aspergilloma (fungal ball), (2) allergic bronchopulmonary aspergillosis (ABPA), (3) invasive pulmonary aspergillosis (airway invasive or angioinvasive), and (4) chronic pulmonary aspergillosis.[23]

1. Fungal ball (aspergilloma) can form in preexisting cavities formed by tuberculous infection, bronchiectasis, or fibrotic lung disease and is unusual in children. It is usually seen in the upper lobes or apical segments of lower lobes because most of the cavities are caused by previous TB **(Fig. 32)**. Mobility can be demonstrated in most cases, except when it nearly completely fills the cavity with no

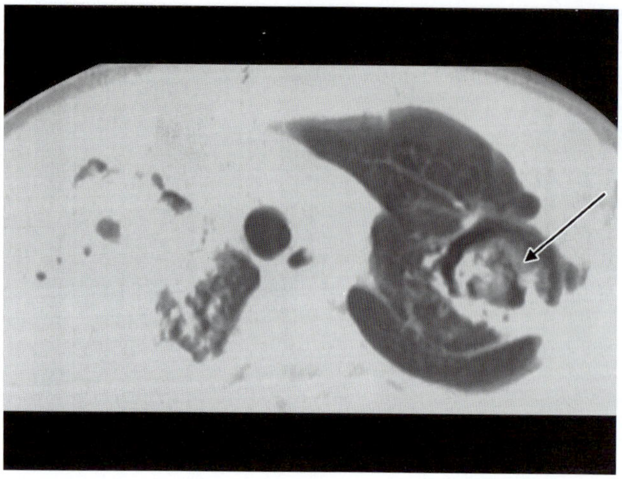

FIG. 32: Aspergilloma: A well-defined rounded opacity with a meniscus sign is seen in a thin-walled cavity in the left upper lobe in the background of fibrocavitatory disease.

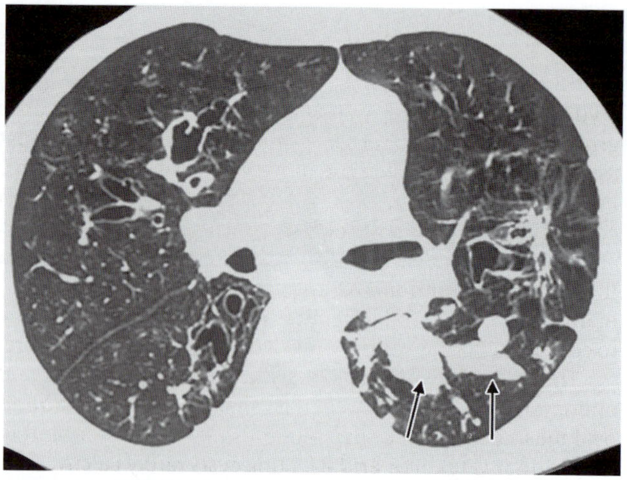

FIG. 33: Allergic bronchopulmonary aspergillosis: There are features of central bronchiectasis with finger-in-glove appearance in left lung (black arrows) due to mucin-filled bronchi in a child with asthma.

space to move around. In contrast, the air crescent sign of invasive aspergillosis usually does not have a background of fibrocavitatory disease. Pronounced-associated inflammatory reaction may result in hemoptysis.[17]

2. Allergic bronchopulmonary aspergillosis is a hypersensitivity reaction to the presence of *Aspergillus fumigatus*. It is most commonly seen in association with asthma and cystic fibrosis. The immune reaction results in thick mucin plugging the bronchi. Imaging may show gloved finger appearance due to mucin-filled bronchi outlined because of collateral air drift **(Fig. 33)**. Mucin may show high density likely due to mineral deposition within. There may be patchy areas of atelectasis and emphysema. Central bronchiectasis may be seen. *Aspergillus* infection may be suggested in children with cystic fibrosis, when there are large patches of consolidation, often disproportionate to the magnitude of disease.
3. Invasive aspergillosis is invariably noted in immunocompromised neutropenic patients with leukemia or after bone marrow or solid organ transplantation. It may be airway invasive or angioinvasive. The two forms may coexist and it is not always possible to distinguish between the two types.
   i. Airway invasive form—multifocal bronchocentric or angiocentric air-space opacities may be seen. Peribronchiolar nodules, centrilobular micronodules (<5 mm), ground-glass opacities, and consolidation may be seen.
   ii. Angioinvasive form—wedge-shaped opacities can result from infarction as a consequence of hyphal invasion of blood vessels. They are typically seen in subpleural areas. Few nonspecific but distinctive features are halo sign and air crescent sign. The halo sign represents hemorrhage surrounding the nodule due to vascular invasion. It is seen earlier and with greater frequency than the air crescent sign. The air crescent sign is seen in the recovery phase when neutrophilic count rises; retraction of the necrotic lung from the viable lung parenchyma results in a crescent of air collection, partially outlining the necrotic lung.[17]
4. Chronic pulmonary or semi-invasive aspergillosis is a less aggressive form seen in patients with underlying lung disease or with mild immunosuppression.[3] This may mimic reactivation TB. It usually starts as a focus of consolidation in the upper lobes, which may have cavitation and pleural thickening. The findings may also mimic those of histoplasmosis and actinomycosis.

Histoplasmosis

This is endemic in many parts of the United States, especially in Ohio and Mississippi river valleys. The initial exudative phase simulates primary complex of TB; only the pulmonary foci are mostly multifocal. About 95% of patients are asymptomatic in the initial phase. The disease resembles TB in all phases. Hilar and mediastinal lymph nodes may be enlarged. The chronic form shows fibrobronchiectatic changes and calcific nodules similar to postprimary TB.

Disseminated histoplasmosis may occur in an infant or in the immunocompromised and resembles miliary TB. Massive hepatosplenomegaly may be seen with granulomatous or calcific foci.

A rare but serious complication is fibrosing mediastinitis, which may result in compression of the pulmonary artery, superior vena cava, airway, and esophagus. In the west, chronic histoplasmosis is a frequent cause of mediastinal fibrosis in children while TB remains a common cause in the Indian community.[3]

Coccidioidomycosis

Coccidioidomycosis, caused by *Coccidioides immitis*, is endemic in Southwestern deserts of USA. The radiographic manifestations are similar to TB in all phases, including consolidation, lymph nodes, and pleural effusions. The primary complex lasts only a few weeks—duration being shorter than in TB. Residual calcifications may occur. Small thin-walled cavities, commonly seen in adults, are less common in children.[3]

PARASITIC INFESTATIONS

Hydatid Disease of the Lung

Hydatidosis, caused by larval stage of *Echinococcus granulosus* and *Echinococcus multilocularis*, is the most frequently encountered type of hydatid disease in humans. Humans are accidental hosts when they acquire ova through contaminated water or direct contact with sheep, dogs, and cats. While in adults, hepatic involvement is more common than lungs; in children, the lungs are the most common site of involvement. The lung facilitates the growth of the cyst due to compressible nature and the presence of negative pressure.

The wall of hydatid cyst consists of pericyst, ectocyst, and endocyst. Intact cysts are seen as sharply defined round to oval masses of variable size seen most commonly in mid to lower zones **(Figs. 34A and B)**. Lung cysts rarely calcify.

Rupture or superimposed infection may result in varied appearances giving rise to air crescent sign, water lily sign, onion peel sign, and dry cyst sign among others. When the hydatid ruptures into an adjacent bronchiole, air enters the cyst between the layers of the cyst giving rise to "air crescent" sign. In addition to the "crescent" or the "meniscus" sign, when there is air within the endocyst as well, it results in the "Cumbo" or "onion peel" sign. The "water lily" sign refers to the floating membranes at the surface of the air-fluid level in the cyst. If the contents get expectorated out, it results in the formation of "empty" or "dry" cyst. Rupture of the cyst can also lead to superinfection with abscess formation giving rise to rim enhancement of the lesion **(Fig. 35)**.[23,24]

Others

Few parasites including *Ascaris lumbricoides*, *Necator americanus*, *Ancylostoma duodenale*, and *Strongyloides stercoralis* may pass through lungs as a part of their life cycle. They enter the pulmonary vessels and can cause edema and hemorrhage. These may result in unilateral or bilateral transient migratory pulmonary opacities with no segmental distribution. Blood and sputum eosinophilia may be present along with pulmonary opacities (Loeffler's syndrome).[17]

Paragonimiasis is endemic in the Orient and is a common cause of necrosis and calcification in lungs and is difficult to distinguish from TB radiologically.

PULMONARY INFECTIONS IN IMMUNOCOMPROMISED CHILDREN

Pneumonia is common in the immunocompromised host. Immunocompromised status may be a result of congenital immunodeficiency states, acquired as in human immunodeficiency virus (HIV)/acquired immunodeficiency syndrome (AIDS), poor nutritional status, immunotherapy for cancer, and posttransplant state.

The agents that cause pneumonia include the pathogens that cause infection in the normal host as well as other opportunistic pathogens acquired from resident mucosal flora/nosocomially, depending on how severe the immunodeficiency is or how much time has elapsed after chemotherapy or transplant.[2]

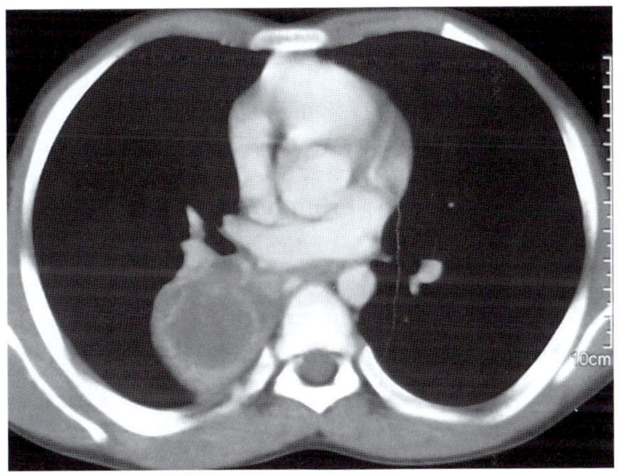

FIG. 35: Infected hydatid: There is a rim enhancing fluid containing well-defined lesion in the right lower lobe. This was confirmed to be an infected hydatid on surgery.

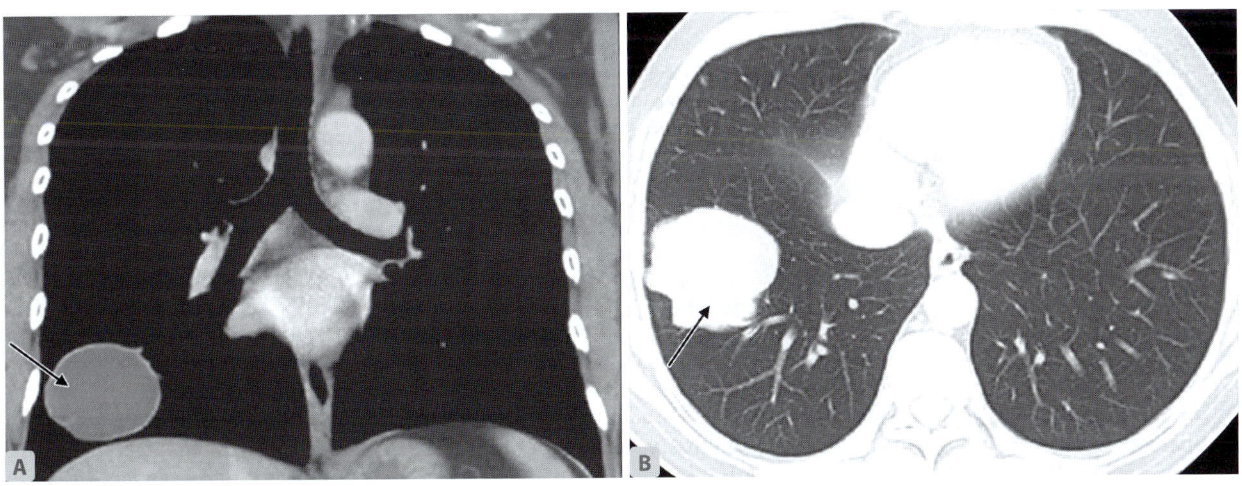

FIGS. 34A AND B: Hydatid cyst: Homogeneous well-defined rounded fluid attenuation mass lesion is noted in the right lower lobe.

The radiographic appearance of pulmonary infections in the immunocompromised is not specific. Hence, the aim of imaging is to narrow the differential diagnosis based upon pattern recognition, clinical presentation, level of immune compromise, and current drug therapy. When chest radiograph findings are noncontributory, chest CT is often done if clinical suspicion of lung infection is high. CT shows increased sensitivity for detection, characterization and delineation of the extent of lung abnormality, picking up more than one pattern of opacity, planning a diagnostic procedure, and assessing response to treatment.[24,25]

Bacterial Pneumonias

Typical pneumonias (*S. pneumoniae, S. aureus*) occur as in immunocompetent children, but with increased frequency and severity. The radiological appearance is that of bronchopneumonia and lobar pneumonia as in immunocompetent children but with an increased incidence of empyema and lung abscess. Other uncommon pathogens include *Salmonella* species, *Klebsiella* species, *Pseudomonas* species, *E. coli*, and other atypical organisms such as *Mycoplasma*. These can produce a wide variety of appearances, including bilateral patchy reticulonodular infiltrates and patchy or confluent air-space opacification. Also common are polymicrobial infections.[25]

Pyogenic infectious airway disease has been increasingly recognized in recent years in immunocompromised population, including bronchitis, bronchiolitis, and bronchiectasis.

Mycobacterial Pneumonias

The risk of TB increases in HIV, malnutrition, diabetes, and malignancy. Tuberculin test is less useful and treatment response is poorer in this subset of patients. Primary TB usually manifests as massive adenopathy and pattern of consolidation is similar to that in primary TB in immunocompetent children. Miliary pattern may also be encountered. Subcarinal group of lymph nodes are the most common. On MRI, lymph nodes have a strikingly low signal on T2 and short tau inversion recovery (STIR) images. Pleural effusion is uncommon.[25]

The nontuberculous mycobacteria, *M. avium-intracellulare* or *M. kansasii*, have also been observed as cause of infection in pediatric patients with immunocompromise. Children tend to be older in age and have nonspecific features of air-space opacification, nodular opacities, cavitation, bronchiectasis, and mediastinal nodes. Compared with *M. tuberculosis* infection, nontubercular mycobacteria show less surrounding infiltration, less bronchogenic spread, more contiguous involvement, cavities with thinner walls, and greater involvement of bilateral middle and lower lung lobes.[23,25]

Fungal Pneumonias

Pneumocystis jirovecii (*P. jirovecii*) is a common pulmonary pathogen in immunocompromised children, particularly with AIDS, although the incidence has decreased because of prophylactic treatment.[25] Children with *P. jirovecii* pneumonia (PJP) are usually younger than those with other pulmonary conditions, with a peak age incidence at 4–5 months. PJP can be fulminant, with a mortality rate as high as 40–50%. Most patients have a CD4+ count <100 cells/mm^3. Radiographic findings include a normal radiograph, hyperinflation with prominent perihilar bronchovascular markings, or air-space opacities. PJP needs to be included in the differential diagnosis of any infant with rapidly progressive pneumonia, even in those not known to have HIV infection as approximately 45% of children with PJP are not known to have HIV at the time of presentation. The use of PJP prophylaxis does not exclude the diagnosis. CT is the imaging modality of choice. CT features include patchy areas of ground-glass haze, especially in the perihilar location **(Figs. 36A and B)**. Interlobular septal thickening may be present. Other findings include lymphadenopathy, nodules, and mass lesions. Pulmonary air cysts may be seen. Pneumothorax and pneumomediastinum may occur. Pleural effusion is uncommon and suggests other pathology.[25]

Infection with *Cryptococcus neoformans*, histoplasmosis, mucormycosis, and invasive aspergillosis are the other fungal infections that may be encountered. Typically, fungal infections in immunocompromised state present as peripheral ill-defined nodules with surrounding ground-glass haze (CT halo sign) that represents surrounding hemorrhage. Apart from fungal nodules, viral pneumonia and organizing pneumonia are other causes of this sign.

Viral Pneumonias

Viral pathogens include RSV, parainfluenza, influenza, adenovirus, cytomegalovirus (CMV), measles, varicella, and herpes simplex virus.

Transmission of RSV is primarily via the hands contaminated with secretions from the mouth or nose. The radiographic findings are diffuse, patchy, or nodular air-space opacities rather than interstitial infiltrates. Secondary bacterial infections are more common.[25]

Cytomegalovirus pneumonia is another common infection in immunocompromised state. In HIV infection, it usually presents when the CD4+ counts fall below the level of 50 cells/mm^3. Chest radiographs may be normal, may show reticulonodular or air-space pattern of disease. CT features include ground-glass attenuation, nodules, consolidation, and masses. Other features may be cavitation, bronchiectasis, lymphadenopathy, and pleural effusions.

Lymphocytic Interstitial Pneumonitis

Lymphocytic interstitial pneumonitis (LIP) is seen in severe immunocompromise, especially with HIV infection. It is believed to be a response of the lymphoid system to circulating antigens of infectious agents (Epstein–Barr virus) or to HIV itself. It is most frequently diagnosed in children over 2 years of age. The course of the disease is relatively indolent compared to PJP. It presents with insidious development of respiratory distress and mild cough. Associated findings include generalized lymphadenopathy, salivary gland enlargement, hepatosplenomegaly, and clubbing of fingers.[26]

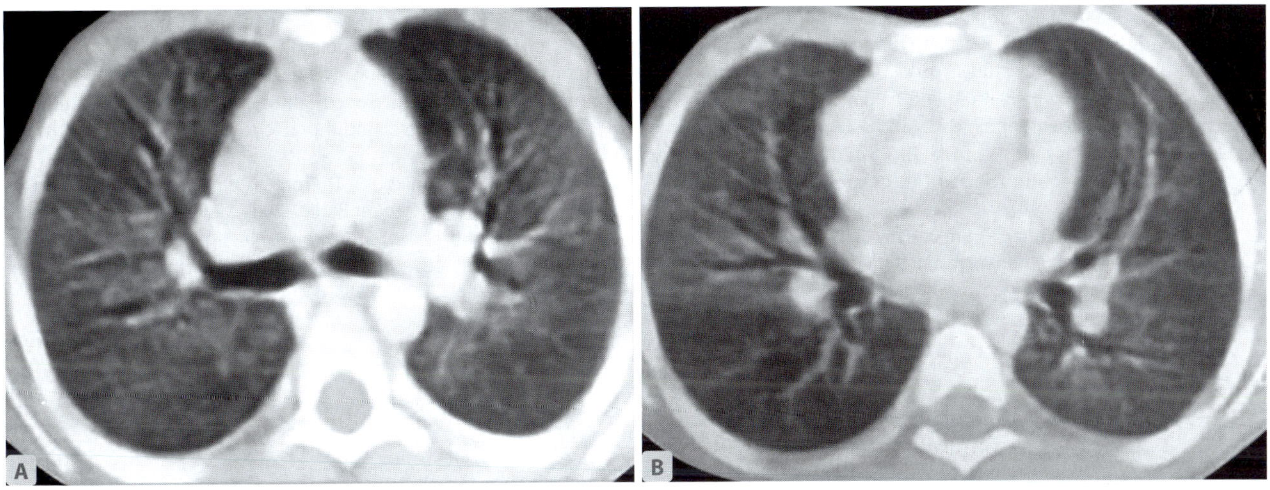

FIGS. 36A AND B: *Pneumocystis jirovecii* pneumonia (PJP): Areas of ground-glass opacification are seen in bilateral lungs in a proven case of PJP in a 6-year-old HIV-positive boy. (HIV: human immunodeficiency virus)

Clinical features and radiographic appearance are usually sufficient to make the diagnosis. Chest radiographs range from mild prominence of bronchovascular markings to the more classical description of adenopathy and reticulonodular markings. Nodules may measure up to 2–3 mm in diameter. Lymphadenopathy may be massive but with no airway compression, in contradiction to tuberculous adenopathy. On CT, diffuse ground-glass opacity, poorly defined centrilobular nodules, interlobular septal thickening, and thickening of the bronchovascular interstitium may be seen. Bronchiectasis and cyst formation may complicate the disease. LIP responds successfully to steroid treatment.[16]

CONCLUSION

It is important to be familiar with the role of imaging in the diagnosis and management of various pediatric pulmonary infections as these remain a major cause of infant and child morbidity and mortality worldwide.

REFERENCES

1. Frush DP. Pediatric chest imaging. Radiol Clin North Am. 2005;43:11-12.
2. Eslamy HK, Newman B. Pneumonia in normal and immunocompromised children: an overview and update. Radiol Clin North Am. 2011;49:895-920.
3. Adler B, Effmann EL. Pneumonia and pulmonary infection. In: Slovis TL (Ed). Caffey's Diagnostic Imaging, 11th edition. Amsterdam: Mosby-Elsevier; 2008. pp. 1184-7.
4. Markowitz RI, Ruchelli E. Pneumonia in infants and children: radiological-pathological correlation. Semin Roentgenol. 1998;2:151-62.
5. Donnelly LF. Imaging in immunocompetent children who have pneumonia. Radiol Clin North Am. 2005;43:253-65.
6. McPhillips M. Infection. In: Carty H, Brunelle F, Stringer DA, Kao S (Eds). Imaging in Children, 2nd edition. Amsterdam: Elsevier Churchill Livingstone; 2005. pp.1075-118.
7. Copley SJ. Application of computed tomography in childhood respiratory infections. Br Med Bull. 2002;61:263-79.
8. Xia W, Shao J, Guo Y, Peng X, Li Z, Hu D. Clinical and CT features in pediatric patients with COVID-19 infection: different points from adults. Pediatr Pulmonol. 2020;55:1169-74.
9. Foust AM, Phillips GS, Chu WC, Daltro P, Das KM, Garcia P, et al. International expert consensus statement on chest imaging in pediatric COVID-19 patient management: imaging findings, imaging study reporting and imaging study recommendations. Radiol Cardiothorac Imaging. 2020;2:e200214.
10. Chen A, Huang J, Liao Y, Liu Z, Chen D, Yang C, et al. Differences in clinical and imaging presentation of pediatric patients with COVID-19 in comparison with adults. Radiol Cardiothorac Imaging. 2020. [Online ahead of print].
11. Bettenay FAL, de Campo JF, McCrossin DB. Differentiating bacterial from viral pneumonias in children. Pediatr Radiol. 1988;18:453-4.
12. Winant AJ, Schooler GR, Concepcion ND, Lee EY. Current Updates on Pediatric Pulmonary Infections. Semin Roentgenol. 2017;52:35-42.
13. Calder A, Owens CM. Imaging of pleural effusions and empyema in children. Pediatr Radiol. 2009;39:527-37.
14. Donnelly LF, Klosterman LA. Pneumonia in children: Decreased parenchymal contrast enhancement—CT sign of intense illness and impending cavitary necrosis. Radiology. 1997;205:817-20.
15. Donnelly LF, Klosterman LA. The yield of CT of children who have complicated pneumonia and noncontributory chest radiography. AJR Am J Roentgenol. 1998;170:1627-31.
16. Donnelly LF, Klosterman LA. Cavitary necrosis complicating pneumonia in children: sequential findings on chest radiography. AJR Am J Roentgenol. 1998;171:253-6.
17. Hansell DM, Armstrong P. Infections of the lungs and pleura. In: Hansell DM, Armstrong P, Lynch DA, McAdams HP (Eds). Imaging of Diseases of the Chest, 4th edition. Amsterdam: Mosby-Elsevier; 2005. pp. 183-276.
18. Santos JF. Tuberculosis in children. EJR. 2005;55:202-8.

19. Veedu PT, Bhalla AS, Vishnubhatla S, Kabra SK, Arora A, Singh D, et al. Pediatric vs adult pulmonary tuberculosis: a retrospective computed tomography study. World J Clin Pediatr. 2013;2:70.
20. Agrons GA, Markowitz RI, Kramer SS. Pulmonary tuberculosis in children. Semin Roentgenol. 1993;28:158-72.
21. Leung AN, Muller NL, Pineda PR, Fitzgerald JM. Primary tuberculosis in childhood: radiographic manifestations. Radiology. 1992;182:187-91.
22. Nachiappan AC, Rahbar K, Shi X, Guy ES, Mortani-Barbosa EJ, Shroff GS, et al. Pulmonary tuberculosis: role of radiology in diagnosis and management. Radiographics. 2017;37:52-72.
23. Garg M, Prabhakar N, Gulati A, Agarwal R, Dhooria S. Spectrum of imaging findings in pulmonary infections. Part 2: Fungal, mycobacterial, and parasitic. Pol J Radiol. 2019;84:e214.
24. Turgut AT, Altinok T, Topcu S, Kosar U. Local complications of hydatid disease involving thoracic cavity: imaging findings. EJR. 2009;70:49-56.
25. George R, Andronikou S, Theron S. Pulmonary infection in HIV-positive children. Pediatr Radiol. 2009;39:545-54.
26. Theron S, Andronikou S, George R, Plessis J, Goussard P, Hayes M, et al. Non-infective pulmonary disease in HIV-positive children. Pediatr Radiol. 2009;39:555-64.

CHAPTER

64

Imaging of Pediatric Chest Masses

Devasenathipathy Kandasamy, Smita Manchanda, Arun Kumar Gupta

INTRODUCTION

Thoracic masses in children may be located in the mediastinum, lung, or the chest wall. Majority of these are surgical conditions. The spectrum ranges from incidentally detected developmental lesions to aggressive malignant tumors. Chest radiography is the initial modality for their detection and ultrasonography (USG) can aid in characterization. However, these lesions require further evaluation with computed tomography (CT) or magnetic resonance imaging (MRI). While obtaining the CT, special attention must be given to radiation issues in children and dedicated pediatric CT protocols should be followed. Although MRI has the limitations of long imaging time often requiring general anesthesia, it should be substituted for CT whenever possible.

LUNG MASSES

These can be classified as:

- *Congenital*:
  - Abnormal lung bud development—congenital lobar emphysema, unilateral pulmonary agenesis/aplasia, pulmonary hypoplasia, and hypogenetic lung syndrome (the conditions are described separately in this book)
  - *Hamartomatous lesions*: Congenital pulmonary airway malformation (CPAM), lung cysts, and hamartoma
  - *Abnormality of separation of lung bud*: Sequestration
  - *Vascular anomalies*: Congenital arteriovenous malformation (AVM).
- *Inflammatory*: Lung abscess, hydatid cyst
- *Neoplastic*: Metastases, benign [recurrent respiratory papillomatosis (RRP), fibroleiomyomatous hamartoma, hemangioma], malignant (inflammatory myofibroblastic tumor, pleuropulmonary blastoma, mucoepidermoid carcinoma, carcinoid, anaplastic lymphoma, rhabdomyosarcoma).

Congenital Pulmonary Airway Malformation

This was previously known as congenital cystic adenomatoid malformation (CCAM). This relatively rare entity is considered a focal pulmonary dysplasia and is defined as "a multicystic mass of pulmonary tissue in which there is proliferation of immature bronchial structures at the expense of alveolar development". Pathologically, the affected lobe is increased in volume and weight. The cysts are lined by cuboidal or columnar epithelium and the walls contain smooth muscle and elastic tissue.

- Type I is most common and contains 1–4, varying sized air-filled large cysts over 2.0 cm in diameter. It may resemble congenital lobar emphysema, especially if unilocular.
- Type II is characterized by numerous small- to medium-sized thin-walled cysts of up to 2 cm in diameter and prognosis is bad when associated with other congenital malformations.
- Type III is the least common. It is seen as a large solid lesion with multiple tiny fluid-filled cysts.[1]

Congenital pulmonary airway malformation may be seen in stillborn infants, with a classical triad of hydramnios, fetal ascites, and cystic or solid mass in the fetal chest. The intrathoracic mass causes venous obstruction, which in turn is responsible for fetal ascites. On antenatal ultrasound, CPAM is seen as an echogenic intrathoracic mass, which may or may not have cysts. After birth, it presents with neonatal respiratory distress. In the older infant, it may cause pulmonary infection. The lesion is usually unilateral and occurs with equal frequency in both lungs with slight predilection for the upper lobes. CPAM usually involves an entire lobe or lung and produces mediastinal shift. The prognosis is usually poor due to large size and early in utero cardiovascular compromise.

Type I appears as a multicystic lesion with a tendency for recurrent infection in older children. Types II and III are usually associated with respiratory distress in the newborn, often with other congenital anomalies. Radiographically, types I and II demonstrate a multilocular air-filled bubbly mass. At this stage, the differential diagnosis includes congenital diaphragmatic hernia (in which the abdomen will be gasless) and staphylococcal pneumatoceles (uncommon in the neonatal period). If one of the cysts becomes extremely large with very thin walls, it may resemble a pneumothorax or congenital lobar emphysema. Prenatal diagnosis may be made on ultrasound. Ultrasound is also helpful in the evaluation of fluid-filled or solid-appearing lesions. The solid lesions demonstrate highly reflective interfaces within due to the walls of the minute cysts. In uninfected CPAM, CT shows multilocular cystic mass with thin walls **(Figs. 1A and B)** while in infected lesion, CT shows a complex mass with a mixture of solid and cystic lesions with variable definition and thick walls. The treatment is surgical excision even if the patient is asymptomatic. Type III lesion is seen as a solid pulmonary mass and may be seen in the neonatal period.[2]

The venous and arterial connections to the pulmonary circulation are normal in pure CPAM. However, *hybrid lesions* (CPAM with sequestration) may exist with abnormal vascular connections feeding or draining the lung lesions **(Figs. 2A to C)**. CT angiography is essential to map out the systemic feeding artery and venous drainage.

Pulmonary Sequestration

A bronchopulmonary sequestration is defined as a congenital mass of nonfunctioning lung tissue which contains both bronchial and alveolar elements but which lacks communication with tracheobronchial tree and receives blood supply from an anomalous systemic artery. Its venous drainage may be via the pulmonary veins, inferior vena cava, or the azygos system. Sequestration occurs when a supernumerary lung bud develops caudal to the normal lung bud. If arrest occurs early in development, its communication with the foregut remains, sharing its blood supply. If arrest occurs later, the sequestrated segment is connected with foregut through a fibrous band. This malformation has been further classified as intralobar in which the abnormal tissue is contained within the normal lung and its pleural covering and extralobar in which the sequestration is separate from the lung parenchyma and has its own pleural covering.

Intralobar sequestration predominantly occurs in lower lobes, usually on the left side. It tends to present later in life as an incidental finding on chest radiograph or because of recurrent infections. Patients may also present with hemoptysis if there is communication with bronchial tree. The sequestrated segment may communicate with the adjacent lung as a result of infection or occasionally cystic spaces in the lesion may communicate directly with bronchial tree.

On a chest radiograph and CT, the lesion appears as an oval, spherical, or triangular basal opacity **(Figs. 2A to C)**. It is ill-defined and often contains multiple cysts of variable sizes, simulating CPAM. Indeed pulmonary sequestration may coexist with CPAM and then it is called a hybrid lesion of the lung. Other differential diagnosis includes pneumonia, bronchogenic cyst, or pulmonary neoplasm. Most often, the abnormal vascular supply is a large vessel arising from the aorta either above or below the diaphragm. It is important to demonstrate the abnormal vascular channel on CT or MR angiography not only for diagnosis, but also to avoid potential hemorrhage if surgery is contemplated.[3]

Extralobar sequestration occurs in contiguity with the left hemidiaphragm in 90% of the patients and is often seen incidentally as a basal soft-tissue mass at or below the diaphragm with associated diaphragmatic hernia in almost 30% of patients. These masses enhance on contrast-enhanced computed tomography (CECT). Sometimes, aeration may occur in this opacity. As it is completely separated from the lung, there is less chance of secondary infection.

Bronchogenic Cyst

This congenital lesion presents after the newborn period. It arises as a result of anomalous supernumerary budding of the tracheal diverticulum of the ventral foregut. The cyst has a fibrous wall containing cartilage and is lined by respiratory epithelium and may be filled with air, mucoid, or serous fluid or combination of this. The location of the cyst may be central (near hilum or mediastinum) or peripheral in the lung. Mediastinal bronchogenic cysts are more common and the usual locations are subcarinal, paratracheal, and along the bronchi. Intrapulmonary cysts can be perihilar or peripheral. The central cyst is usually solitary and asymptomatic until infection occurs that produces hemoptysis, fever, cough, or purulent expectoration. There is no direct communication of mediastinal bronchogenic cysts with the tracheobronchial

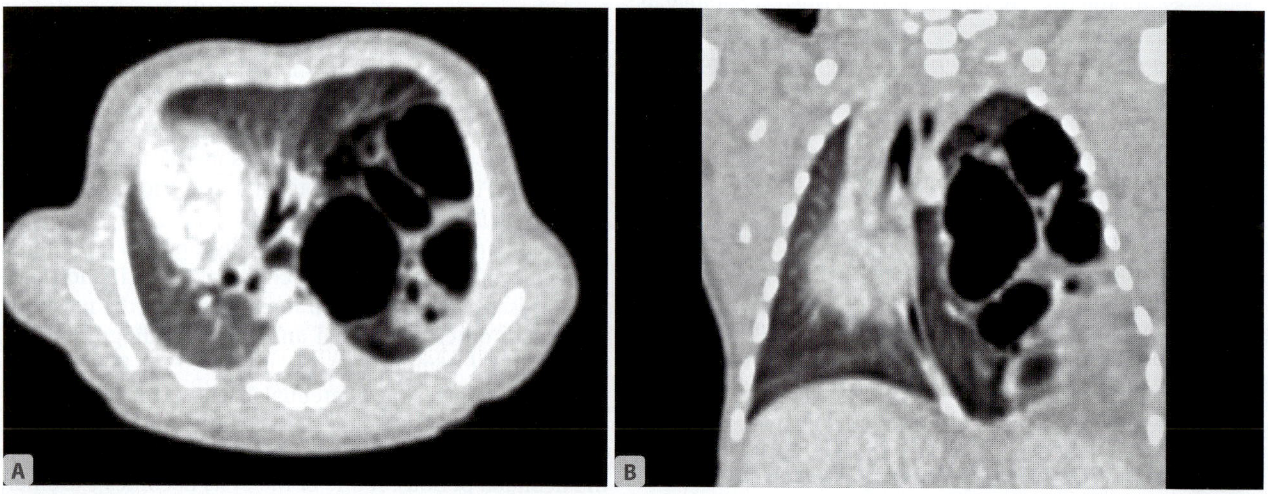

FIGS. 1A AND B: Congenital pulmonary airway malformation (CPAM). (A and B) Computed tomography (CT) of chest (axial and coronal sections) shows a thin-walled multicystic left lung mass with mediastinal shift.

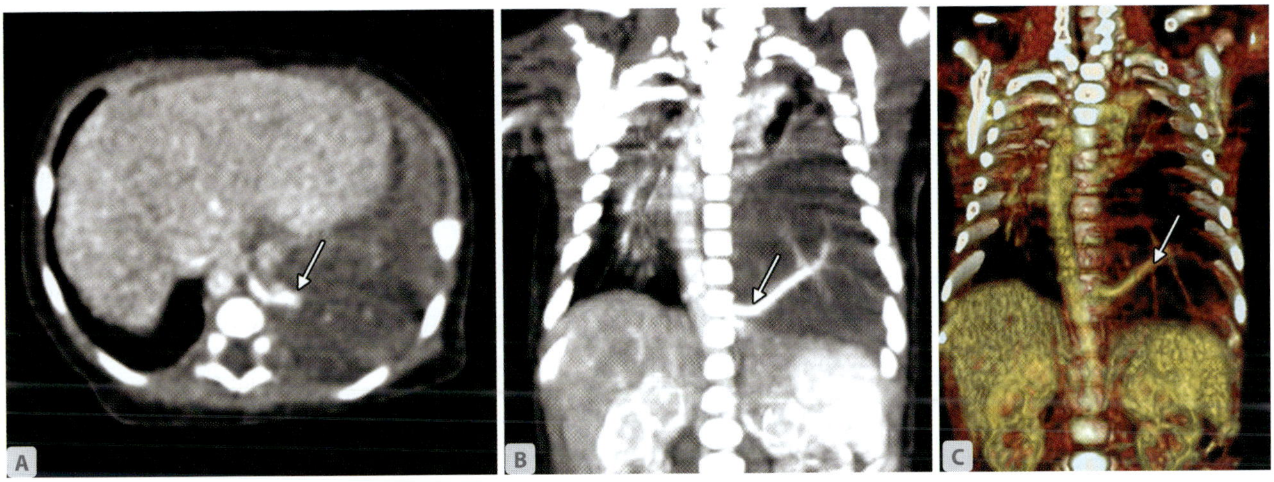

FIGS. 2A TO C: Hybrid lesion. (A) Axial CECT showing a mass lesion in the left lower lobe with a hypertrophied arterial feeder (arrow); and (B and C) Thin MIP and VRT showing the mass supplied by dominant arterial feeder arising from thoracic aorta (arrows). The lesion was surgically removed and proven as hybrid lesion (CPAM and sequestration). (CECT: contrast-enhanced computed tomography; CPAM: congenital pulmonary airway malformation; MIP: maximum intensity projection; VRT: volume rendering technique)

tree. However, the mediastinal bronchogenic cysts may be attached to major airways through a stalk. Rapid enlargement may be seen in infected cysts and respiratory distress may be profound. When peripheral, the cysts may be multiple and extensive. With multiple cysts, respiratory distress and even death may occur shortly after birth. Bronchial communication is common with peripheral cysts with air-fluid levels and more rapid development of infection.

Chest radiograph shows round or oval, smooth, sharply marginated, thin-walled, homogeneous water density mass, or air-filled cyst in the mediastinal or perihilar location. Mass effect over the adjacent trachea, bronchus, or esophagus may be demonstrable. An air-fluid level and thick wall may be seen in infected cysts. On CT, a hypodense, isodense, or hyperdense mass lesion may be seen depending on the nature of fluid contents[4] **(Figs. 3A to C)**. The differential diagnosis on chest radiograph of a fluid-filled intrapulmonary bronchogenic cyst includes round pneumonia **(Figs. 4A and B)**, primary or metastatic pulmonary neoplasm, and interlobar effusion. Air or fluid-filled cyst should be differentiated from small congenital cystic adenomatoid malformation, pneumatocele, and pulmonary abscess. Complications of bronchogenic cysts include infection, hemorrhage, spontaneous pneumothorax, and rarely development of malignancy.[5]

Vascular Lesions

Vascular malformations may be isolated or part of a congenital syndrome like hereditary telangiectasia. When multiple or large, they may cause high output cardiac failure and cyanosis from right-to-left shunting. A pulmonary AVM or varix may be seen on a radiograph as a well-defined, serpiginous, or lobulated opacity. Calcification is rare.[6] Associated linear density representing a feeding vessel may be seen. If the feeding vessel is not apparent, the lesion may simulate a granuloma or metastasis. A thin-section CT pulmonary angiogram would demonstrate an arterial malformation to best advantage. Pulmonary angiography with and embolization is the treatment of choice.[7]

Lung Abscess

A lung abscess develops when necrosis, suppuration, and cavitation occur in a localized infection of lung parenchyma. The necrotic cavity filled with purulent material may develop an air-fluid level, if erosion into the airway has occurred. Staphylococci, alpha- and beta-hemolytic streptococci, *Pseudomonas*, *Klebsiella*, and aspirated anaerobic mouth flora are the common organisms for the lung abscesses. With the advent of antibiotics and prompt therapy, incidence of primary lung abscess has markedly reduced. However, secondary abscess in an immunocompromised and severely ill patient has become more frequent.

The radiological appearance depends on the relative amount of necrosis, consolidation, and presence of gas in the necrosis. In early stages, discrete pneumonic consolidation is seen on chest radiograph. CT at this stage may show a low density center in the area of consolidation. There is absence of air bronchogram within the abscess **(Figs. 5A and B)**. When the cavity attains sufficient size and is filled with air after a bronchial communication, an air-fluid level will be seen. The abscess wall is enhancing, thick, and shaggy. Ultrasound is also useful to demonstrate lung abscess and to perform ultrasound-guided aspiration.[8]

Cavitary necrosis is a more common complication of chest infection in children. It is seen as a well-demarcated area of necrosis filled with multiple small irregular cysts **(Fig. 6)**. Affected part of the lung parenchyma does not enhance.[9] Round pneumonia is a localized infective pneumonia which appears as a rounded lung mass. This occurs in young children in whom collateral air circulation through pores of Kohn is not well-developed. The consolidation remains localized and forms a mass-like round opacity on chest radiographs. In children with clinical features of chest infection, round

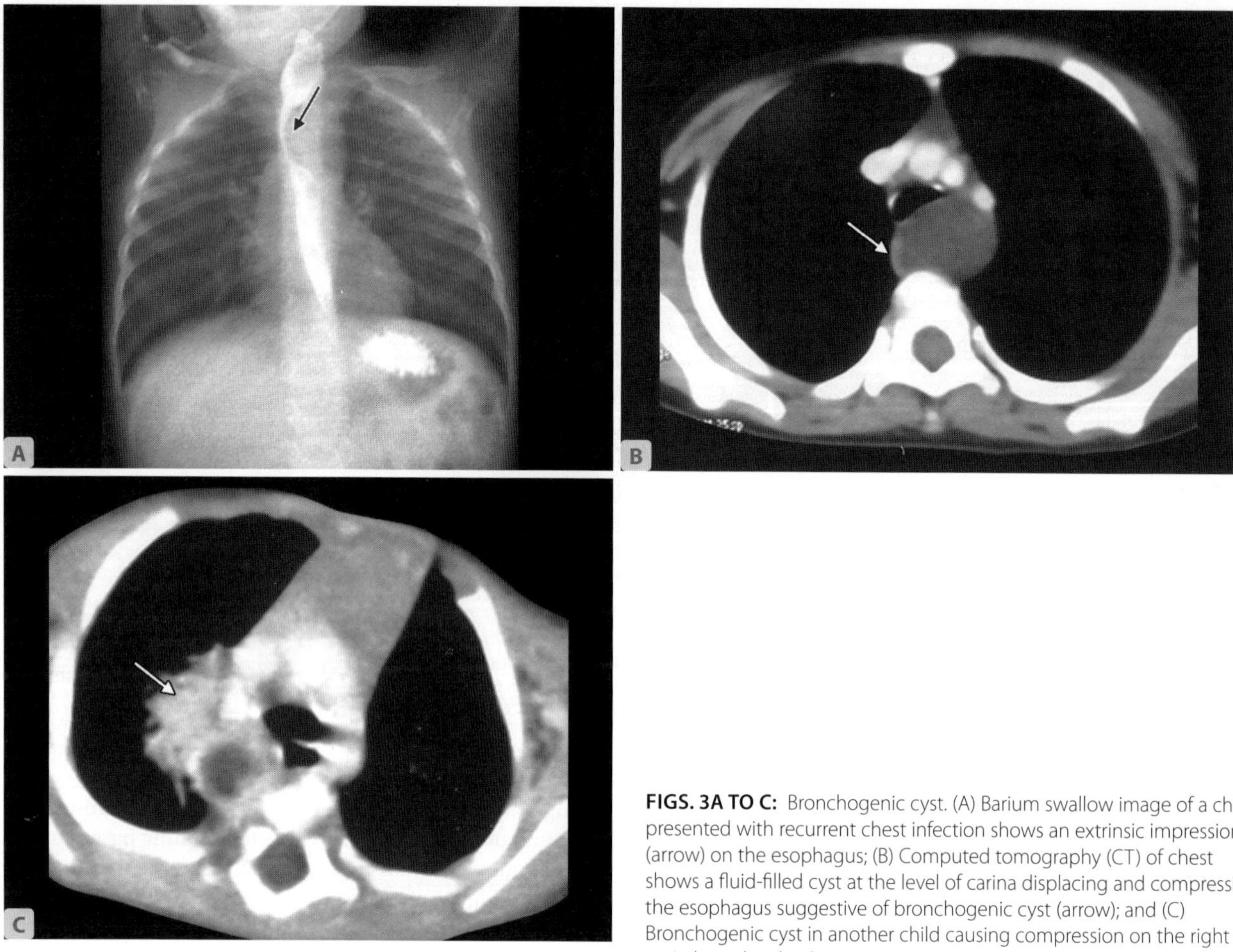

FIGS. 3A TO C: Bronchogenic cyst. (A) Barium swallow image of a child presented with recurrent chest infection shows an extrinsic impression (arrow) on the esophagus; (B) Computed tomography (CT) of chest shows a fluid-filled cyst at the level of carina displacing and compressing the esophagus suggestive of bronchogenic cyst (arrow); and (C) Bronchogenic cyst in another child causing compression on the right main bronchus leading to consolidation of right upper lobe (arrow).

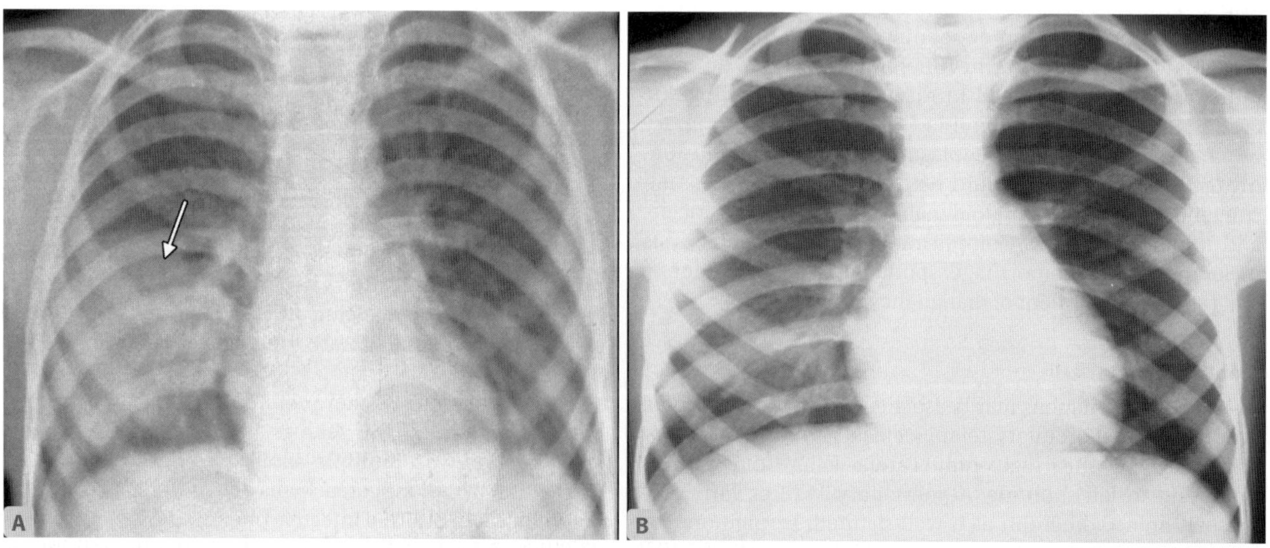

FIGS. 4A AND B: Round pneumonia. (A and B) Chest radiograph shows a round opacity in the right lower zone (arrow) which has completely disappeared in the follow-up radiograph typical for a round pneumonia.

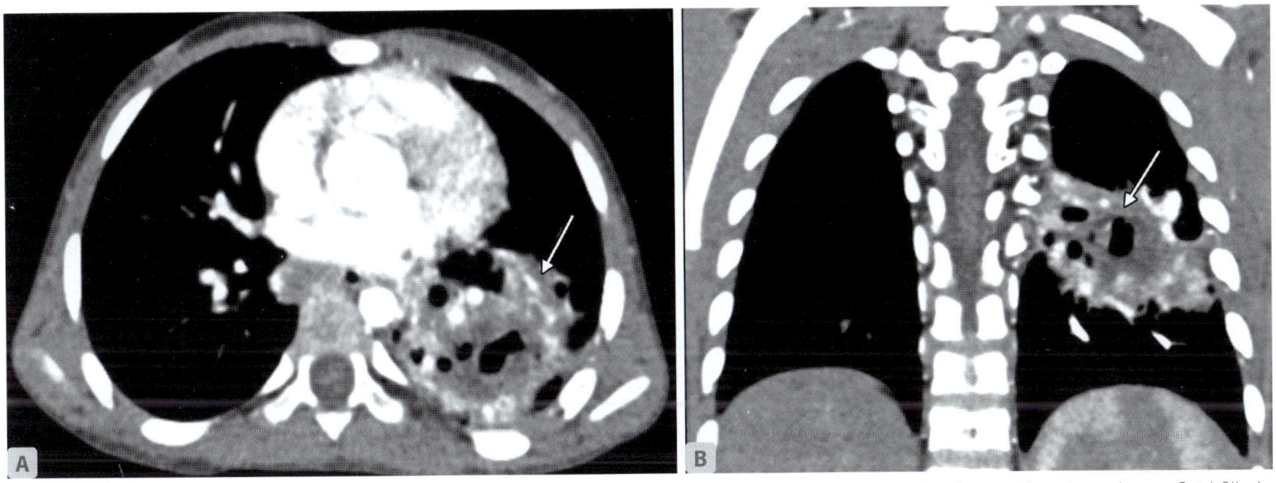

FIGS. 5A AND B: Evolving lung abscess. (A and B) Contrast-enhanced computed tomography (CECT) axial and coronal sections show a fluid-filled rounded lesion with air lucencies within left lower lobe with ill-defined wall (arrows).

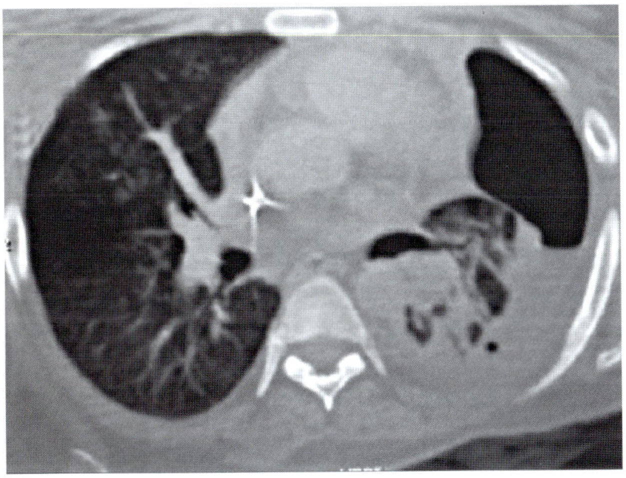

FIG. 6: Cavitary necrosis: Contrast-enhanced computed tomography (CECT) of chest of a leukemic child shows left lung consolidation with irregular cavities within. Variable sizes of the cavities help to distinguish it from air bronchogram. Associated hydropneumothorax is also seen.

pneumonia is the most likely cause of lung mass on chest radiographs.[10]

Hydatid Cysts

This is caused by infestation with *Echinococcus granulosus* and *Echinococcus multilocularis*. As hydatid cyst grows, it compresses the adjacent lung tissue into a fibrotic capsule known as pericyst. The cyst itself has a thin smooth wall, consisting of two adherent layers, the laminated ectocyst and thin lining endocyst. It grows rapidly and nearly two-thirds may rupture either in the surrounding lung, bronchial tree, or pleura.

Chest radiograph shows spherical or oval well-defined homogeneous opacity **(Figs. 7A and B)**. It may be single, multiple, unilateral, or bilateral. Lung hydatids rarely calcify. When the pericyst ruptures into an airway and air dissects between pericyst and ectocyst, this gives rise to the characteristic meniscus or crescent sign. When the cyst ruptures into an airway, an air-fluid level results. Sometimes, the cyst wall is seen crumpled up and floating in fluid which lies within the noncollapsed pericyst. This is described as a water-lily sign or camalote sign. Fluid content is demonstrated on CT or MRI. With secondary infection, the membranes may disintegrate, walls thicken, and the appearance is indistinguishable from bacterial lung abscess on chest radiograph. Sometimes, all contents of the cyst may be expelled through the bronchial tree and resultant dry cyst is seen as air-filled cavity.[11] Lesions abutting the chest wall or diaphragm can also be diagnosed on ultrasound which shows the characteristic cystic mass with floating membranes.

Pulmonary Metastasis

Metastases are the most common malignant lesion of the lung in children. The common primary tumors that metastasize to the lung include Wilms' tumor, osteosarcoma, Ewing's sarcoma, rhabdomyosarcoma, lymphoma, leukemia, germ cell tumors, and neuroblastoma. The metastasis may be single or multiple, vary in size from a small nodule to large mass, or a lymphangitis pattern may be seen. With a known primary malignancy, chest radiograph is always necessary to look for metastasis, and if present, further imaging studies may not be indicated. However, CT is routinely indicated in patients with normal chest radiographs in cancers with high incidence of lung metastases and whom the management would alter. Such cancers include most sarcomas, choriocarcinoma, and germ cell tumors. CT is also required if metastasectomy is considered. On CT, the metastases are seen as a round sharply defined nodules or masses with homogeneous attenuation. Deposits from Wilms' tumor, Hodgkin's disease, and osteosarcoma may cavitate and when peripheral, these may cause a pneumothorax. Osteosarcoma is the most common cause of calcified metastases; it may also be associated with calcified mediastinal lymph nodes and calcified pleural deposits[12] **(Figs. 8A to C)**. Thyroid carcinoma causes miliary deposits with 2–5 mm nodules. Lymphoma and leukemia may also cause lung deposits. An air bronchogram within a lung nodule is a characteristic feature of the lymphomatous nodule.[21] Hilar adenopathy and interstitial disease may be

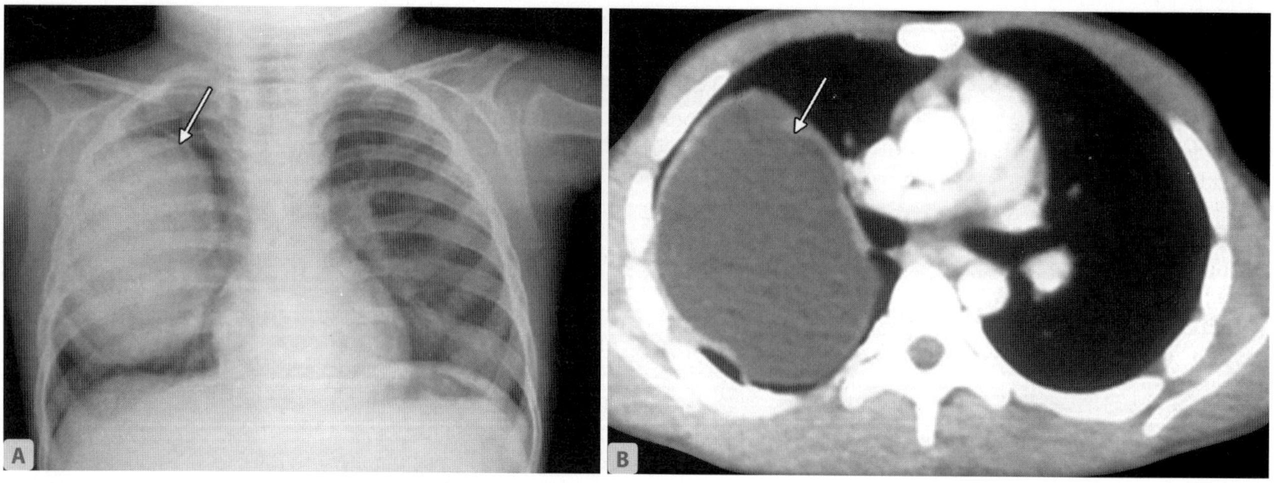

FIGS. 7A AND B: Hydatid cyst. (A and B) Chest radiograph and contrast-enhanced computed tomography (CECT) of chest shows a well-defined homogeneous oval mass (arrows) in right lung. The lesion shows fluid attenuation on computed tomography (CT).

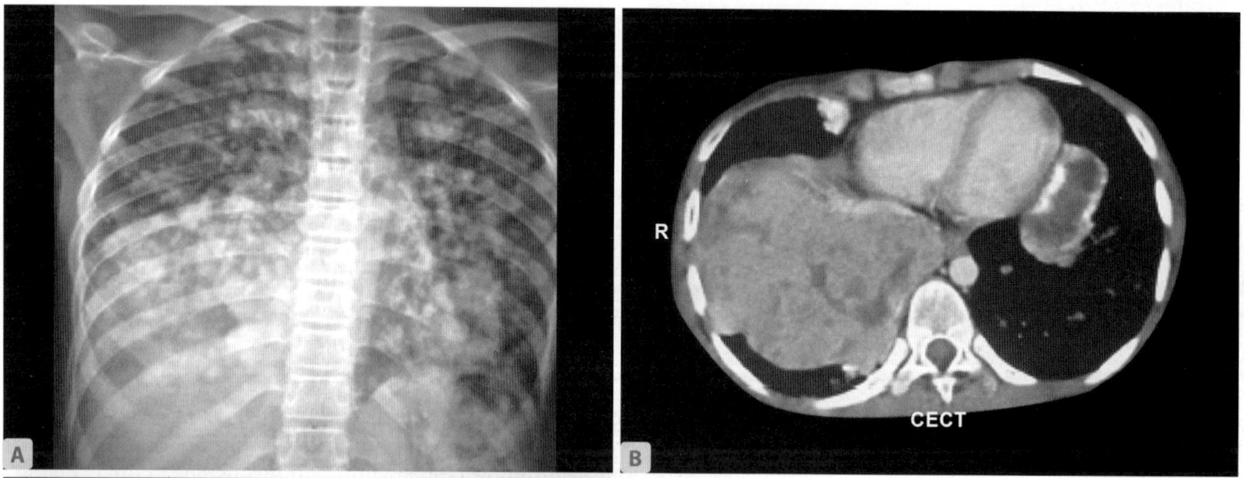

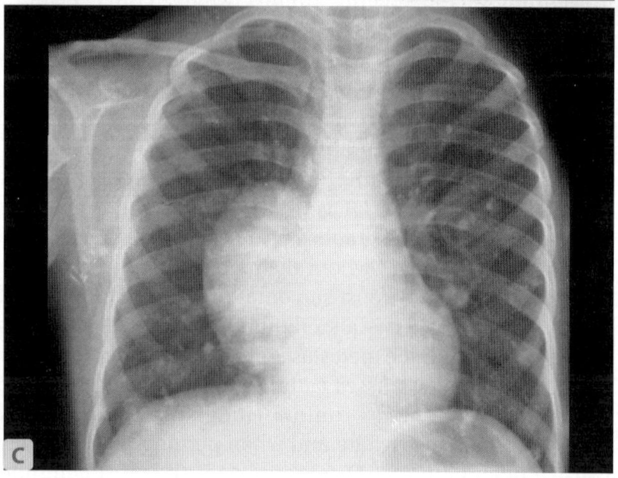

FIGS. 8A TO C: Lung metastases from osteosarcoma. (A) Chest radiograph shows bilateral extensive nodules and masses; (B) Computed tomography (CT) shows a right lower lobe mass with multiple small bilateral nodules and masses with calcifications; and (C) Chest radiograph of another child with history of left upper limb amputation for osteosarcoma shows multiple calcified lung metastases.

associated. Lymphangitic spread on chest radiograph is seen as reticular or reticulonodular pattern. On high-resolution computed tomography (HRCT), nodules are seen in continuity with a vessel. Also, there is beading and thickening of interlobular and interlobar septa and irregular thickening of bronchovascular bundles. It is important to note that in patients with known extrathoracic malignancies, large number of the lung nodules detected on CT as metastases are actually benign and may represent granulomas.[13] This is especially common in areas with high incidence of tuberculosis or histoplasmosis.

Primary Lung Tumors

Primary pulmonary neoplasms in children are uncommon. The largest group of malignant tumors in childhood is grouped under the name *pleuropulmonary blastoma*. These occur in children as well as in adults; however, both are considered as distinct entities. Pleuropulmonary blastoma of the childhood arises from primitive blastomatous tissues and develops in pre-existing congenital lung lesions like cystic adenomatoid malformation, sequestration, or bronchogenic cysts.[14]

This tumor may be small and present as a solitary pulmonary nodule or large and occupy the entire thorax. The lesion may be multicystic, cystic solid, or entirely solid, with malignancy rate increasing in that order. The chest radiograph shows a large mass which may have features of local invasion **(Figs. 9A to C)**. CT and MR features are variable and range from fluid-filled cysts with solid nodule, solid mass causing mediastinal shift and lung collapse, shows areas of necrosis within a heterogeneously enhancing mass. Pleural effusion may be present; however, chest wall invasion is uncommon.[15] Metastases may occur in the liver and central nervous system. Prognosis is poor.

Mesenchymal sarcomas of childhood may be associated with developmental cystic lesions like bronchogenic cyst, cystic adenomatoid malformation, or congenital pulmonary cyst. These include leiomyosarcoma, rhabdomyosarcoma, and fibrosarcoma.

Bronchogenic carcinoma is extremely rare but can occur in older children. Carcinoid tumor and salivary gland tumors may also be seen. Carcinoid is typically an intensely enhancing, endobronchial mass with usually no extraluminal component **(Figs. 10A to C)**.

Initial clinical diagnostic consideration in primary lung tumors is usually pneumonia resulting in delayed diagnosis.[16] Other rare primary lung tumors include hemangiopericytoma and Askin tumor.

Inflammatory myofibroblastic tumor, previously called inflammatory pseudotumor, is a proliferation of plasma cells, histiocytes, and granulocytes and could represent a reparative response to infection. It is classified as a neoplasm of borderline behavior as there are aggressive features (local invasion, distant metastases). The typical imaging feature is of a large mass with coarse calcification **(Figs. 11A and B)**. On CECT, the mass shows heterogeneous enhancement with no cavitation and adjacent organ invasion.[17]

The most common benign neoplasm is squamous papilloma.[17] Airway and pulmonary papillomas are usually coexistent in papillomatosis. This condition typically affects

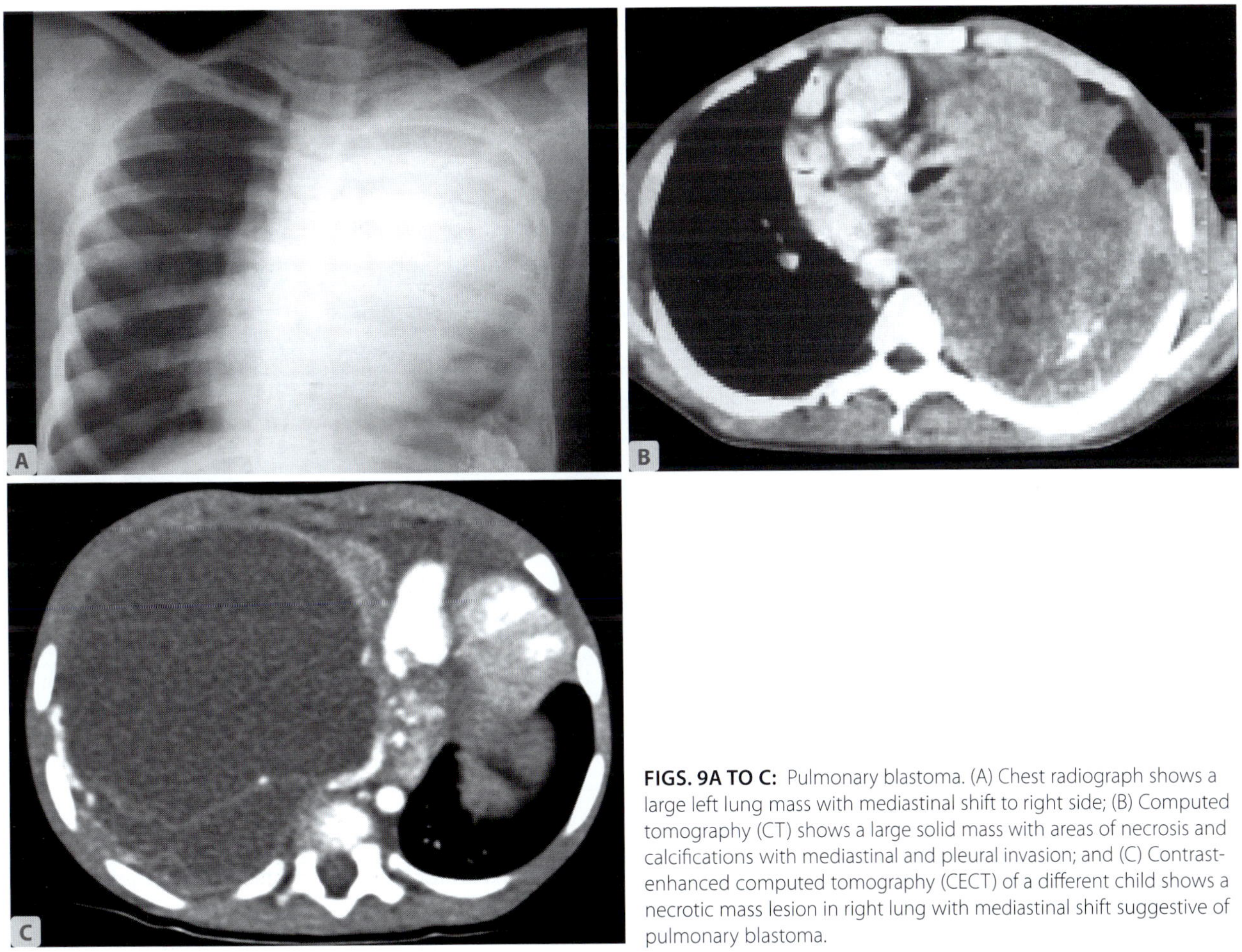

FIGS. 9A TO C: Pulmonary blastoma. (A) Chest radiograph shows a large left lung mass with mediastinal shift to right side; (B) Computed tomography (CT) shows a large solid mass with areas of necrosis and calcifications with mediastinal and pleural invasion; and (C) Contrast-enhanced computed tomography (CECT) of a different child shows a necrotic mass lesion in right lung with mediastinal shift suggestive of pulmonary blastoma.

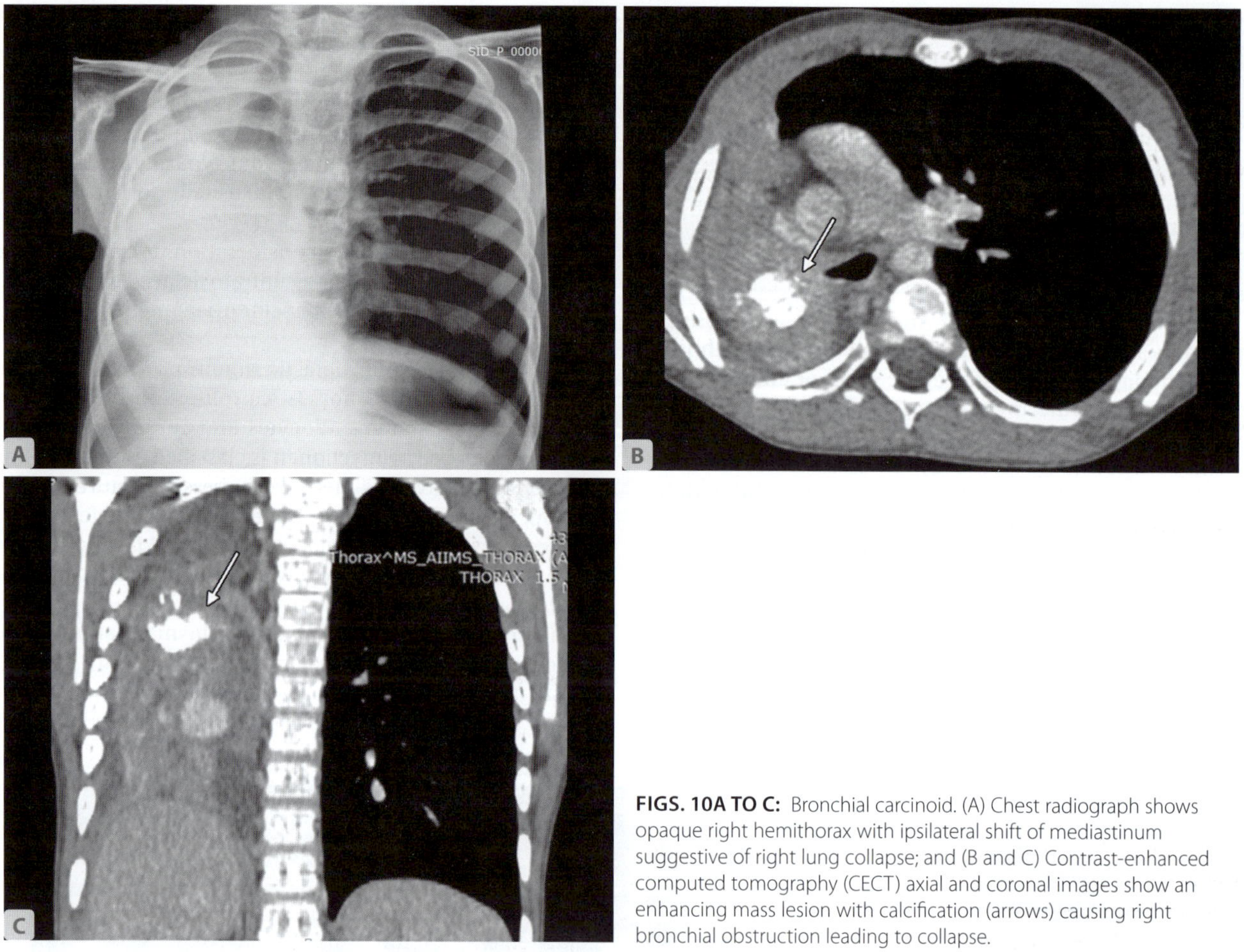

FIGS. 10A TO C: Bronchial carcinoid. (A) Chest radiograph shows opaque right hemithorax with ipsilateral shift of mediastinum suggestive of right lung collapse; and (B and C) Contrast-enhanced computed tomography (CECT) axial and coronal images show an enhancing mass lesion with calcification (arrows) causing right bronchial obstruction leading to collapse.

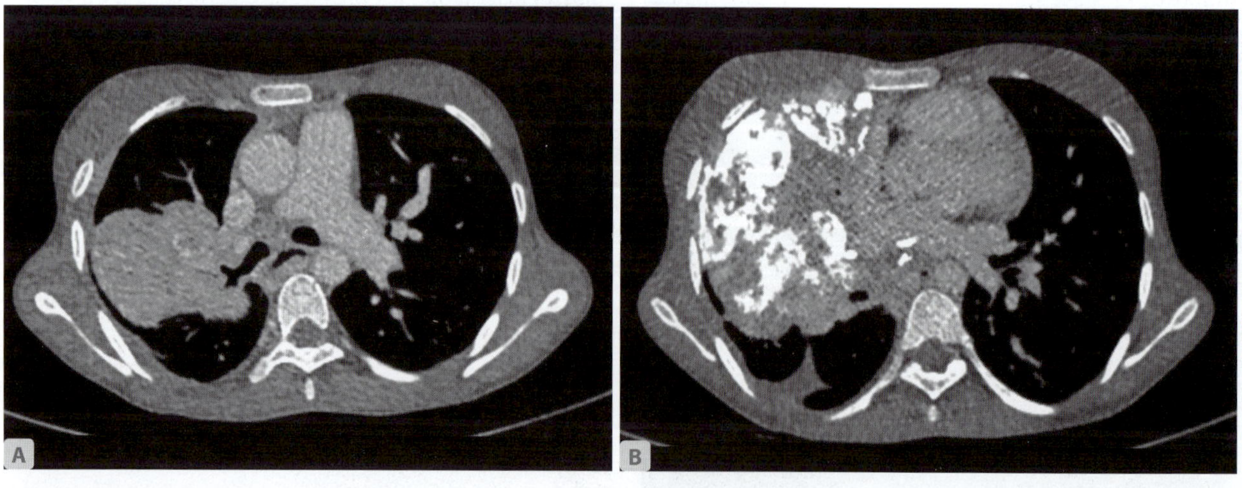

FIGS. 11A AND B: Inflammatory myofibroblastic tumor. (A and B) Contrast-enhanced computed tomography (CECT) shows a large mass lesion involving the right middle and lower lobes with extensive calcifications.

children and young adults and is often limited to the larynx. It may involve the intrathoracic airways and also present with cavitating lung nodules and is referred to as RRP. These lesions have a high propensity for recurrence and even malignant transformation.

MEDIASTINAL MASSES

The primary thoracic masses in children are most commonly located in the mediastinum. The mediastinal masses represent a wide variety of congenital anomalies and cysts in addition to neoplasms. Children with mediastinal masses are frequently asymptomatic and most often chest X-ray is done for nonspecific symptoms like fever, malaise, and cough. Airway compression, particularly before the age of 1 year, is an important presentation. Respiratory distress results from easily compressible rings of the infant's trachea and bronchi. The risk of airway compression and high incidence of malignancy require prompt diagnosis and treatment for a child with mediastinal tumor.

Mediastinal masses can be classified as per their location into anterior, middle, and posterior mediastinal masses. Since these compartments are not anatomical spaces, masses may often involve more than one compartment. In this situation, location of the center of the mass direction of displacement of adjacent structures, such as trachea and great vessels, is useful to suggest the likely region of origin.

Anterior Mediastinal Masses

Approximately 30% of mediastinal masses occur in anterior mediastinum. These include the four "Ts": (1) Teratoma (and other germ cell tumors), (2) Thymic tumor, (3) Thyroid tumor or cysts, and (4) "Terrible" lymphoma/leukemia. As thymus or thyroid tumors are rare in the pediatric age group, important differential diagnosis of anterior mediastinal mass consists of germ cell tumor and lymphoma.

Germ Cell Tumors

These include dermoid, teratoma, teratocarcinoma, choriocarcinoma, embryonal carcinoma, seminoma, endodermal sinus tumors, and mixed germ cell tumors. Most germ cell tumors arise in anterior mediastinum near thymus and few arise in other mediastinal compartments.

Teratomas may be benign (mature) or malignant (immature). Mature teratomas usually attain a large size before they present with symptoms. Both mature and immature teratomas are seen as lobulated anterior mediastinal soft-tissue masses. Calcifications are common. On CT, teratomas are seen as complex solid or cystic solid masses with variable wall thickness. Calcification, teeth, and fat densities are more readily visualized on CT[18] **(Fig. 12A)**. However, macroscopically demonstrable fat is unusual in malignant teratoma.

Seminoma arising in mediastinum is rare and metastatic seminoma in the mediastinum from occult gonadal lesion should always be excluded with USG of scrotum. Seminoma is seen as a bulky, homogeneous anterior mediastinal mass on CT and may simulate lymphoma. Rarely, calcifications may be present. Involvement of adjacent structures is uncommon; however, metastases to lymph nodes, lung, or bone may be present. Endodermal sinus tumor (yolk sac tumor) is a poorly differentiated embryonal carcinoma, occurs often in males, and patients usually have systemic symptoms and elevated serum alpha-fetoprotein. These tumors as well as most other nonseminomatous malignant germ cell tumors have nonspecific imaging features. On CT, these are seen as large irregular, heterogeneous mediastinal masses with areas of necrosis, cystic degeneration, and hemorrhages **(Fig. 12B)**.[19]

Lymphoma

Lymphomas are the most common cause of mediastinal masses in children. Both Hodgkin's and non-Hodgkin's lymphoma (NHL) (especially lymphoblastic lymphoma) can present with large anterior mediastinal masses. However, lymphadenopathy may be present anywhere in the mediastinum or the hila. CT is the modality of choice for evaluation and staging of lymphoma. On CT, mediastinal lymphadenopathy in lymphoma may be discrete; however, more often it produces conglomerate homogeneous lymph node masses **(Figs. 13A and B)**. Mass effect such as vascular displacement, compression of trachea, or obstruction of superior vena cava (SVC) is common with large masses.[20] Necrosis and hemorrhages are rare, but it may be seen in large masses of lymphoma. Calcification is also rare in lymphoma.

In Hodgkin's lymphoma, if the transverse diameter of mediastinal lymph nodal mass measured on chest radiograph at T4–T5 level exceeds transverse thoracic diameter, it is called bulky disease.

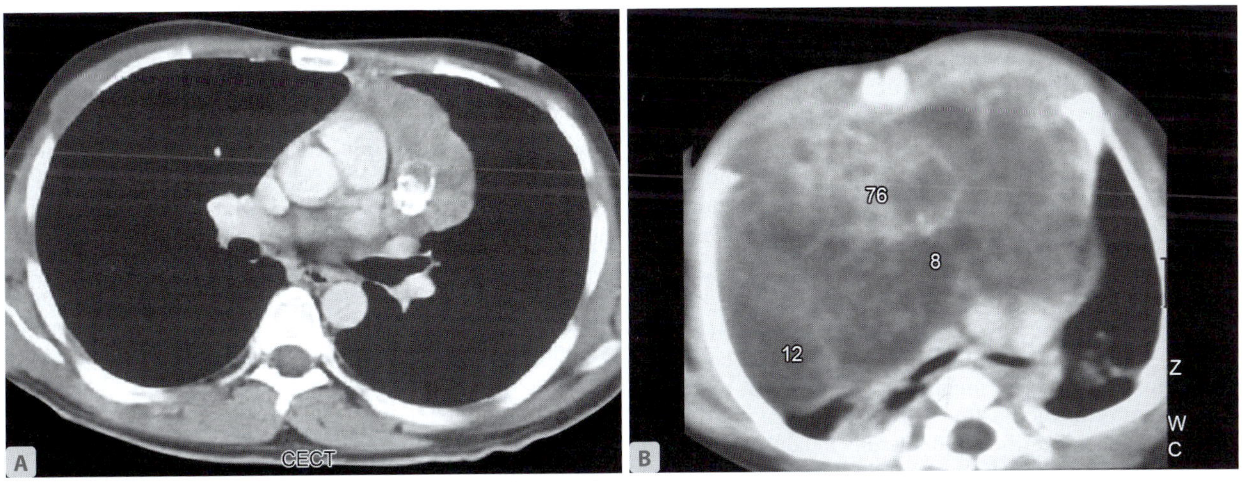

FIGS. 12A AND B: Mediastinal germ cell tumor. (A) CT shows an anterior mediastinal mass containing coarse calcification; and (B) Contrast-enhanced computed tomography (CECT) of another child shows a large heterogeneous mass in the anterior mediastinum suggestive of malignant germ cell tumor.

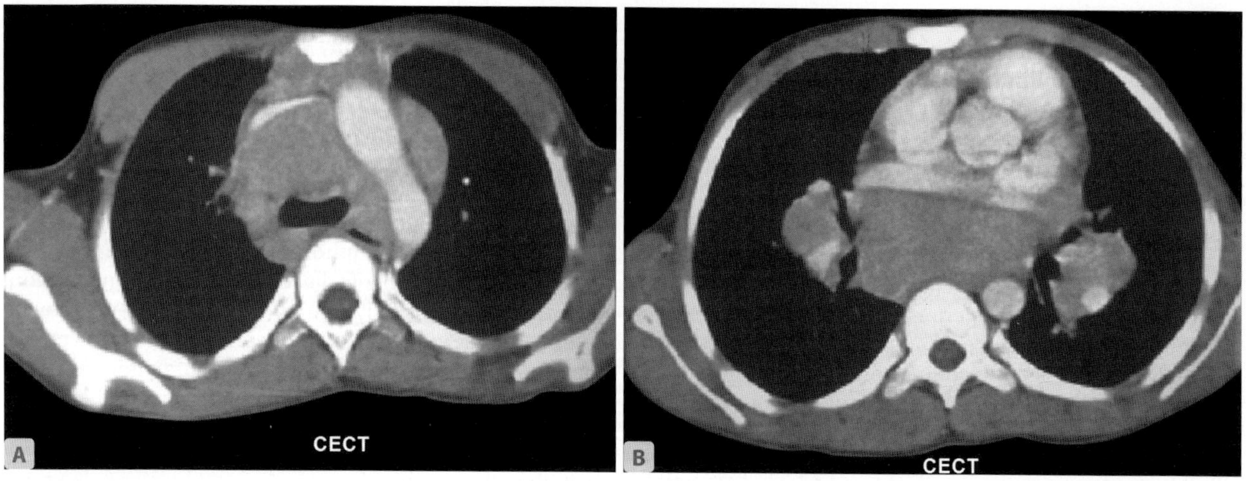

FIGS. 13A AND B: Hodgkin's lymphoma (HL). (A and B) Computed tomography (CT) images at carinal and subcarinal levels show bilateral conglomerate homogeneous lymph node enlargement.

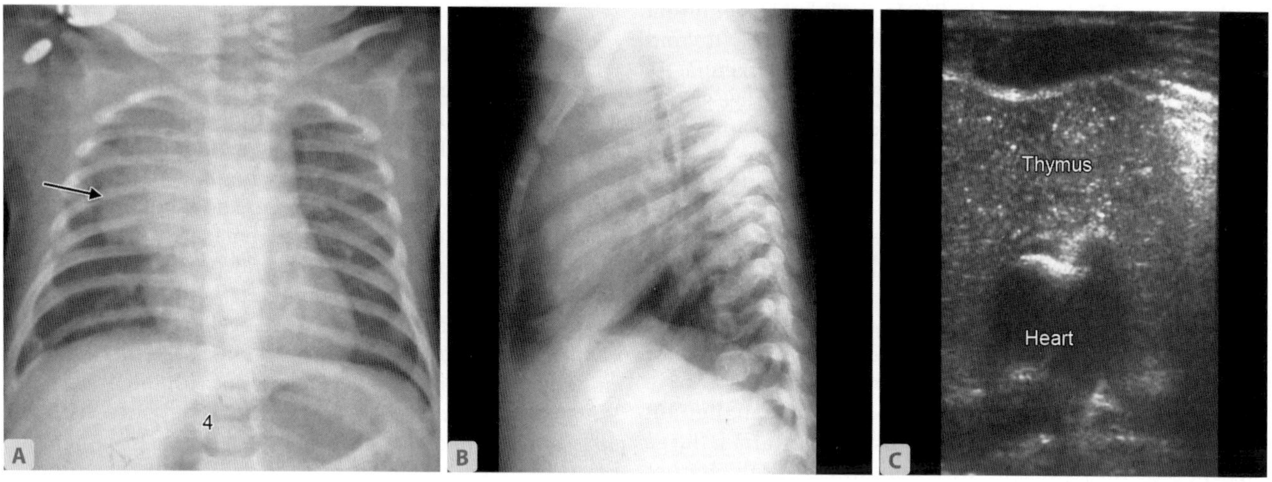

FIGS. 14A TO C: Normal thymus. (A and B) Chest radiograph AP and lateral view show an anterior mediastinal soft tissue showing sail sign (black arrow in A); and (C) USG of the child shows the "starry sky" appearance of normal thymus. (AP: anteroposterior; USG: ultrasonography)

It is denoted as suffix X to the stage and associated with inferior prognosis. It is uncommon for NHL to be limited to mediastinum only at the presentation. However, some NHL primarily involves anterior mediastinum. These include primary mediastinal large B-cell lymphoma and lymphoblastic lymphoma, the later is a T-cell NHL. Both these aggressive lymphomas are seen in children and young adults. Patients usually present with dyspnea, stridor, and SVC syndrome.[21] On imaging, large, often heterogeneous and infiltrative, anterior mediastinal mass is seen.

Thymic Masses

Prominent but normal thymus is the most common pseudotumor of anterior mediastinum **(Figs. 14A to C)**. On imaging, anterior mediastinal tumors displace the trachea and esophagus posteriorly and laterally in contradistinction to a normal enlarged thymus which does not displace adjacent structures.

Hyperplasia of thymus is uncommon and may occur in Graves' disease, lymphoma, leukemia, and Langerhans cell histiocytosis. It may also occur as a rebound thymic enlargement after chemotherapy.

Thymic cyst is of developmental origin, representing persistent tubular remnants of the third pharyngeal pouch. The cyst is usually asymptomatic and incidentally seen on chest radiograph. It is unilocular or multilocular and varies in size. CT is helpful in diagnosis.

Thymoma is rare in childhood. The association of thymoma and myasthenia gravis is also much less in children than in adults. In radiographs, thymoma is seen as a variable-sized lobulated soft-tissue mass in anterior mediastinum. On CT, thymomas are generally seen as lobulated, homogeneously enhancing masses with smooth contour. They tend to grow asymmetrically to one side of the mediastinum. Calcifications may be present and this helps to differentiate thymoma from lymphoma. Rarely, thymoma may have pleural effusion with nodular pleural deposits or diffuse pleural thickening mimicking mesothelioma or pleural metastases.[22] On MRI, thymoma is homogeneously isointense on T1-weighted images and heterogeneously hyperintense on T2-weighted images.[23]

Lymphangioma

Lymphangioma, also known as cystic hygroma, results from failure of primary lymphatic sac to establish drainage into the venous system. It is an uncommon cause of mediastinal masses in children. Most are caused by extension form other sites, such as neck or axilla, into the mediastinum.[24] Most are located in anterior or middle mediastinum, but few may be seen in posterior mediastinum. It often presents as a large soft consistency mass and rarely causes airway obstruction. Pathologically, these are lymphatic malformations macrocystic, microcystic, or combined morphology. Chest radiograph shows well-demarcated mass which may have a lobulated outline. On USG, macrocystic components are seen as cystic masses with internal echoes and septations. Mild vascularity may be seen on color Doppler. Microcystic component is highly echogenic. MRI is required to assess the entire extent of lymphangioma. CT and MRI demonstrate a well-circumscribed avascular cystic mass with septations and mild wall enhancement **(Fig. 15)**. Areas of fat density may be demonstrated. Fluid-fluid levels may also be seen due to hemorrhages or protein contents. The septations show enhancement on contrast-enhanced MRI (CEMRI). The mass tends to envelop or mold to adjacent structures. The microcystic type may be seen as highly enhancing soft-tissue mass on CEMRI.[25]

Pericardial Cysts

These are rare benign unilocular anterior mediastinal cyst containing clear fluid. Most are developmental in origin. On radiographs, these are seen as well-defined, rounded, or teardrop-shaped mass in cardiophrenic angles abutting the heart. Most are seen on the right side. On CT or MRI, these are seen as well-demarcated nonenhancing cysts.

Middle and Posterior Mediastinal Masses

Common masses in middle mediastinum are enlarged lymph nodes or bronchogenic cyst. Lymph node enlargement may be in the paratracheal or hilar locations that are mostly due to viral, tubercular, or fungal infections, leukemia, lymphoma, and histiocytosis. Massive adenopathy is seen in lymphoma and leukemia in which the nodes are confluent. Aneurysms of aorta, pulmonary artery, or coronary artery are also rare causes of middle mediastinal masses. Bronchogenic cyst is discussed under congenital lung conditions. Almost 40% of mediastinal masses in children are located in the posterior mediastinum and majority of these are neurogenic tumors or cystic duplications.[26] Rare causes of posterior mediastinal tumors include hemangiomas and vascular malformations, extramedullary hematopoiesis, germ cell tumors, Ewing's sarcoma, and rhabdomyosarcoma.

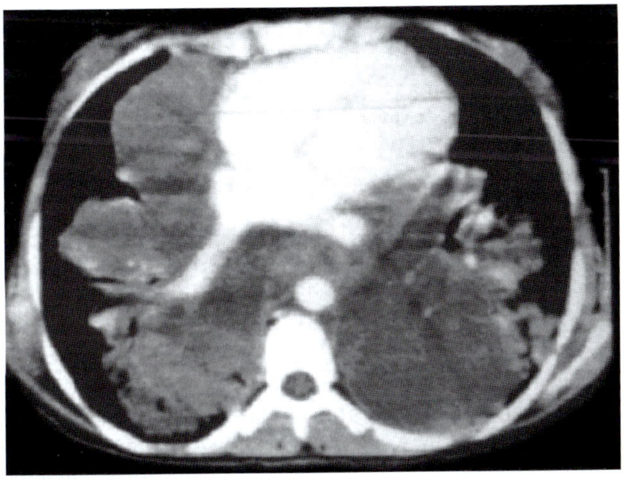

FIG. 15: Mediastinal lymphangioma: Computed tomography (CT) shows a multiseptated, lobulated bilateral cystic mediastinal mass.

Neurogenic Tumors

These include ganglion tumors (ganglioneuroma, ganglio-neuroblastoma, and neuroblastoma), nerve sheath tumors (neurofibroma and schwannoma), and paraganglioma.

Neuroblastoma and Other Ganglion Tumors

Ganglion tumors are derived from the sympathetic ganglia and include neuroblastoma (malignant), ganglioneuroma (benign), and ganglioneuroblastoma (having both components). They usually occur in the superior half of the posterior mediastinum and cannot be differentiated on the basis of imaging alone.

Neuroblastoma is the second most common solid tumor in children after brain tumors and represents 10% of all childhood cancers.[27] Thorax is the second most common site for neuroblastoma after the abdomen. It usually occurs in children <2 years of age, but may rarely occur up to the age of 10 years. These may also be diagnosed on prenatal USG. Neuroblastoma is malignant, but has a better prognosis in mediastinum when diagnosed under 1 year of age.

Patients with thoracic neuroblastoma have symptoms due to primary mass or the metastases. They present with respiratory distress or cord compression. Those with metastatic disease have pain, fever, and weight loss. Rarely, neuroblastoma may be detected as an asymptomatic mass on chest radiograph. Usual appearance of neuroblastoma on chest radiograph is of a smooth elongated paraspinal mass with rib or vertebral erosion and characteristic splaying of ribs. Calcifications are seen in up to 30% of cases.[28] On CT, a soft-tissue mass with speckled, irregular, and granular calcification is seen in the posterior mediastinum **(Figs. 16A and B)**. It shows mild contrast enhancement, occasionally with areas of necrosis and hemorrhages. Rib erosion and widened intervertebral foramina may be seen. Other bony changes include pedicular flattening, spinal canal enlargement, posterior vertebral scalloping, and localized kyphoscoliosis. Intraspinal extension is frequent even in absence of neurologic signs and symptoms. Vascular encasement and mediastinal lymphadenopathy may also be seen, though uncommonly. MRI is the modality of choice for staging because the intraspinal spread and spread along nerves and bone marrow involvement are better demonstrated by MRI. As bone metastases are common, radiographic skeletal survey and a bone scan using technetium 99m-methylene diphosphonate (^{99m}Tc-MDP) or ^{123}I-meta-iodobenzylguanidine (MIBG) are usually obtained as a part of

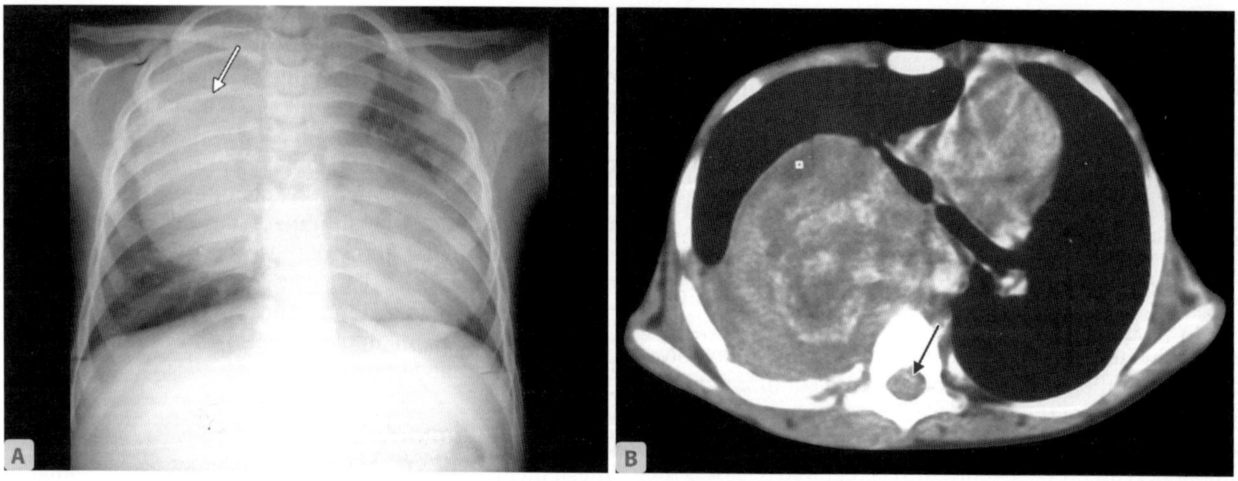

FIGS. 16A AND B: Thoracic neuroblastoma. (A) Chest radiograph shows a large posterior mediastinal mass lesion in the right side crossing the midline. There are erosions seen in the posterior ends of multiple contiguous ribs (white arrow) on right side with increased intercostal spaces; and (B) Computed tomography (CT) shows a large mass in the right paravertebral location with areas of necrosis and calcification. There is evidence of intraspinal extension (black arrow) as well.

imaging workup. Bony metastases are lytic or lytic sclerotic and have characteristic appearances.[29]

Median age for the diagnosis of ganglioneuroblastoma is 5 years and that for the ganglioneuroma is 10 years.[27] Ganglioneuroblastoma is more differentiated malignancy and has a good prognosis. These tumors are usually asymptomatic until they invade or compress adjacent structures, metastasize to distant sites, or produce unusual paraneoplastic syndromes. Nonspecific symptoms include fever, malaise, back pain, or anemia. Lower limb weakness is present in lesions involving the spinal canal. The imaging features of ganglioneuroblastoma are similar to neuroblastoma. About 20% of ganglioneuroblastomas have calcification and show low homogeneous attenuation with minimal contrast enhancement **(Figs. 17A to C)**. Ganglioneuroma is a benign tumor which occurs in older children and is seen as a large smooth spherical mass or small elongated sausage-shaped mass which shows low homogeneous attenuation with minimal contrast enhancement. Differential diagnosis of neurogenic tumors includes malignant sarcoma arising from chest wall or inflammatory lesion such as actinomycosis.

Neurofibroma and Schwannoma

Neurofibroma and schwannomas are nerve sheath tumors. Schwannoma is encapsulated and does not contain nerve fibers while neurofibroma is unencapsulated and hence has nerve fiber within it. In thorax, these tumors arise from intercostals or sympathetic nerves. These tumors are mostly benign, asymptomatic, and seen under 20 years of age. On imaging, neurofibroma and schwannoma are similar in appearance and seen as solid, well-defined round or oval masses.[30] Neurofibroma usually occurs in patients with systemic neurofibromatosis rather than a solitary lesion. It is more often bilaterally located in posterior mediastinum. Chest radiograph in addition to this lesion shows "ribbon-like" rib deformities or scoliosis. On CT, the soft-tissue mass is homogeneous with low attenuation and mildly enhances with contrast. It may extend to spinal canal, showing characteristic dumb-bell shape. In the plexiform variety, the mass may be confluent.

Paraganglioma

These are rare neurogenic tumors of the posterior mediastinum and actually represent extra-adrenal pheochromocytoma. These are derived from chromaffin cells of the sympathetic nervous system. Imaging features are nonspecific, but the diagnosis is usually established on the basis of excessive catecholamine secretions.

Duplication Cysts

Abnormal closure of ventral foregut results in formation of bronchogenic cyst. These are described above in congenital lung conditions. Abnormal closure of dorsal foregut results in enterogenic duplication cysts and these include esophageal duplication cyst and neurenteric cyst. Esophageal duplication cyst constitutes almost 10–15% of all duplications of the gastrointestinal tract. In contrast to bronchogenic cyst which occurs in early age, the majority of children with esophageal duplications are over 10 years of age at the onset of symptoms. The lesion is smooth in outline, varies in size, and usually impinges on a barium-filled esophagus, but rarely communicates with esophageal lumen. CT and MRI demonstrate the cystic and avascular nature of the lesion. These modalities clearly demonstrate precise size, location, its relation to adjacent organs, and transdiaphragmatic extension. Technetium 99m-pertechnetate scintigraphy demonstrates gastric mucosa in the cyst, thereby confirms the preoperative diagnosis.

The neurenteric cyst results from incomplete separation of the foregut from notochord. These have a vertebral body cleft communicating with the spinal canal. It contains both neural and gastrointestinal elements. It may be limited to the chest as a blind sac or may extend below the diaphragm where it either ends blindly or communicates with the intestinal tract. Most neurenteric cysts are discovered in infancy because of esophageal and tracheobronchial compression.[31]

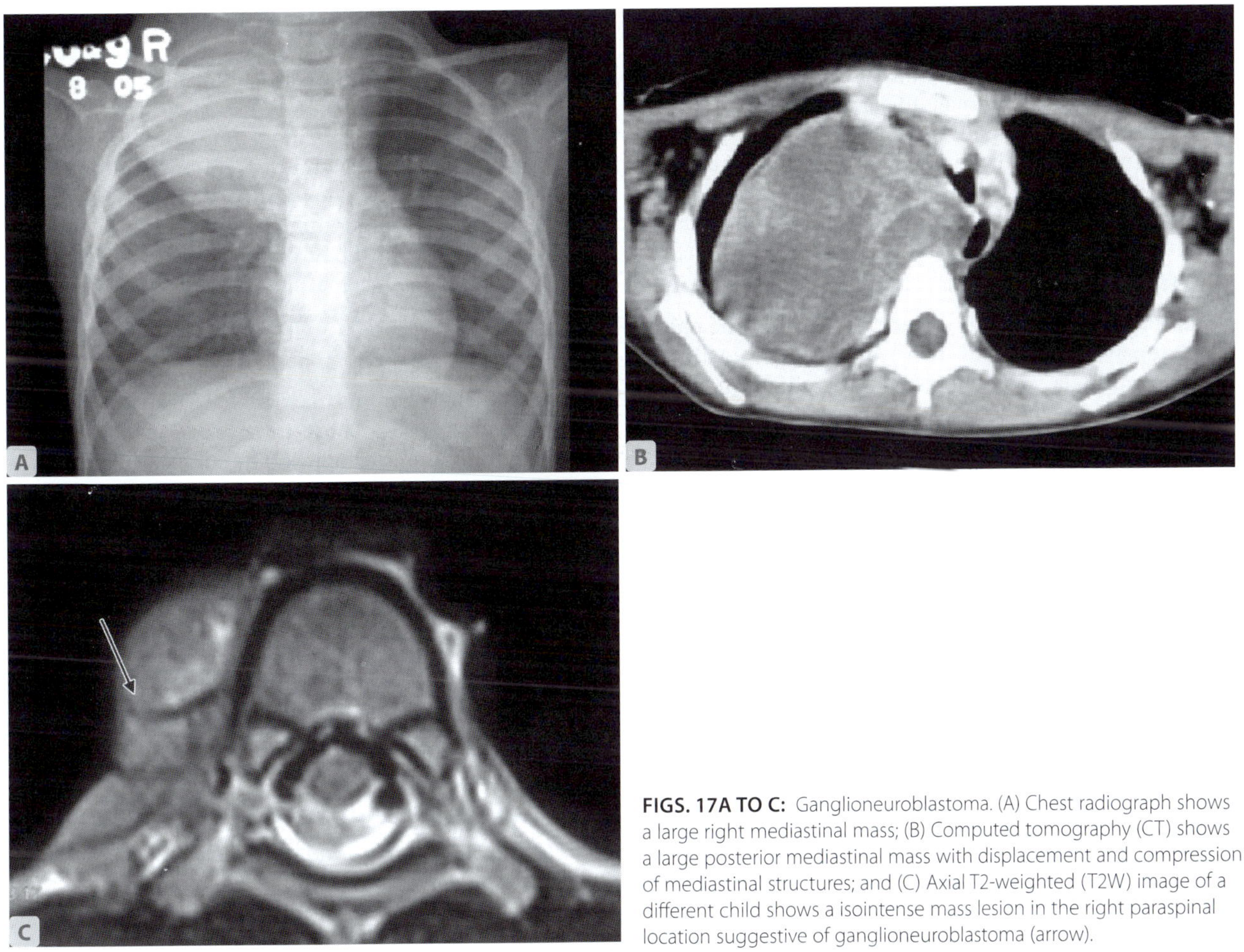

FIGS. 17A TO C: Ganglioneuroblastoma. (A) Chest radiograph shows a large right mediastinal mass; (B) Computed tomography (CT) shows a large posterior mediastinal mass with displacement and compression of mediastinal structures; and (C) Axial T2-weighted (T2W) image of a different child shows a isointense mass lesion in the right paraspinal location suggestive of ganglioneuroblastoma (arrow).

Anterior Thoracic Meningocele

Though rare, this entity is to be considered in the differential diagnosis of posterior mediastinal masses. It occurs due to spinal canal anomalies in which the leptomeninges herniate through the neural foramina. It is seen usually in patients of neurofibromatosis with kyphoscoliosis where the meningocele is at the apex of the convexity. MRI confirms the diagnosis.

Extramedullary Hematopoiesis

It is rarely seen in hematological disorders, most commonly in thalassemia. It is usually asymptomatic, but may rarely cause cord compression. On imaging, it is seen as bilaterally symmetrical, well-defined, and lobulated lower thoracic paraspinal soft-tissue mass.

CHEST WALL MASSES

Chest Wall Infections

Chest wall is the uncommon site for infections and abscesses as compared to the lungs. These are easily diagnosed clinically; however, imaging is required to assess the deeper extent. Ultrasound is useful to detect and localize chest wall abscess. It is seen as cystic mass with debris. On CT, the abscess is seen as a cystic area with wall enhancement. CT is especially useful to detect associated osteomyelitis of the rib and deeper extent of the abscess. Chest wall infection without the well-formed abscess is seen as a heterogeneous, ill-defined mass on CT.

Lymphangioma

These are focal or diffuse masses that tend to involve subcutaneous tissues of the neck, chest wall, or axilla. These may extend into mediastinum. Imaging features are similar to those described above for mediastinal lymphangiomas.

Hemangioma

Hemangiomas are the most common soft-tissue tumors in children. The usual sites are head and neck, chest, and extremities. These are usually present at birth; however, after initial proliferation, the majority of these disappear spontaneously. Small superficial hemangiomas have characteristic appearance and of no clinical significance. Large and extensive lesions may have mass effect. On color Doppler USG, large vascular channels with both arterial as well as venous flow are seen.[32] On MRI, hemangiomas are seen as lobulated masses iso and high signal intensity on T1- and T2-weighted images, respectively, with areas of flow voids representing vascular channels and diffuse enhancement following contrast administration. During involution, high T1 signal intensity is seen due to fatty replacement.

Venous malformations may have similar appearance; however, unlike hemangiomas, these are not tumors. On imaging, venous malformations tend to be solid without dilated vascular channels and on color Doppler, there is minimal or no detectable flow at all. Phleboliths are frequently seen as calcified focal lesions within the mass.

Neurofibroma

Neurofibroma and schwannoma may also involve the chest wall. Extensive chest wall involvement by plexiform neurofibromatosis may be seen in children with neurofibromatosis type 1 (NF1). These tumors may cause secondary bony abnormalities in the form of ribbon appearance of the ribs, scalloping of the vertebral bodies, and kyphoscoliosis.

Benign Osseous Masses

Fibrous dysplasia of the rib is the most common osseous lesion of the chest wall. These are frequently seen as incidental findings on imaging. Radiographically, it is seen as a focal, well-defined, and expansile lytic lesion of the rib. Alternatively, there may be diffuse fusiform enlargement of the rib with ground-glass matrix. Osteochondromas (or exostosis) are benign bony outgrowths with cartilage cap on the surface. These usually occur in long bones; however, ribs, sternum, scapula, clavicle, or spine may also be involved. Most are asymptomatic and detected incidentally while others may be symptomatic due to mass effect on adjacent structures. Malignant transformation is rare. In radiography, osteochondroma is seen as a bony outgrowth with both cortex and medulla that are continuous with the host bone. CT and MRI show similar features and cartilage cap is better evaluated on these modalities. Irregularity or thickening of the cartilage cap >2 cm is suspicious for malignant transformation into chondrosarcoma.[33] Enchondroma of the rib usually occurs in adults and uncommon in children. It is seen as a well-defined, expansile lytic lesion of the rib with endosteal scalloping. Calcifications may also be present.

Mesenchymal hamartoma of the chest wall is a rare benign tumor of infancy. It is a mature mesenchymal tumor containing bone, cartilages, fat, and fibrous tissues. On imaging, it is seen as a large complex cystic solid soft-tissue mass along with destruction of one or several contiguous ribs. Intense enhancement is seen in solid parts of the mass.[34]

Primitive Neuroectodermal Tumor

These include Ewing's sarcoma of the bone and primitive neuroectodermal tumor (PNET) of the chest wall (Askin tumor). Clinically, these present a large painful soft-tissue mass, often associated with cough and dyspnea. The current terminology for these tumors is Ewing's sarcoma family of tumors (ESFTs). On chest radiographs, large thoracic soft-tissue mass with or without associated rib destruction is seen **(Figs. 18A to C)**.

Computed tomography demonstrates large extrapleural mass with heterogeneous contrast enhancement and rib destruction. The extraosseous soft-tissue mass component is disproportionately larger than the bone lesion. Very large tumors may occupy most part of the hemithorax and cause lung collapse and mediastinal shift to the contralateral side. Pleural effusion may be present, but it is usually not massive. Incidence of lung metastases is high and hence, careful lung evaluation should also be done on CT. MRI appearance is similar to CT. These tumors may also have skip lesions along the intercostal nerves. These tumors are usually treated with chemoradiotherapy followed by surgery; however, the prognosis is poor.[35]

Rhabdomyosarcoma

It is the second most common malignancy of the chest wall in children.[36] Chest wall rhabdomyosarcomas are more aggressive than those occurring in the head and neck or genitourinary tract. On radiographs, soft-tissue mass is seen with or without rib destruction **(Figs. 19A and B)**. CT and MR features are nonspecific and similar to those of ESFT.

Miscellaneous Malignant Chest Wall Masses

Both HL and NHL may secondarily involve the chest wall by direct extension from mediastinal or pleural disease. Most common pattern is of homogeneous parasternal chest wall mass contiguous with anterior mediastinal lymphadenopathy. Rib or sternum may be eroded or appears normal in spite of large chest wall mass. Uncommonly, discrete and isolated chest wall may also be seen with lymphoma. Neuroblastoma may involve the chest wall as a direct extension from posterior mediastinal tumor.[37] MRI is most useful to evaluate the extent of chest wall as well as spinal involvement by neuroblastoma. Osteosarcoma of the rib is uncommon in children. It is seen as a destructive lesion of the rib with new bone formation. Associated soft-tissue components are also present, although not as massive as PNET.

Other rare malignant chest wall tumors in children include congenital fibrosarcoma, mesenchymal chondrosarcoma, and malignant peripheral nerve sheath tumor (MPNST). Their imaging features are nonspecific.

CONCLUSION

Pediatric chest masses form a heterogeneous group of disorders involving chest wall, mediastinum and lung. The pathologies affecting children are quite different than in adults. It is important for the radiologists to be aware of the different types of chest masses.

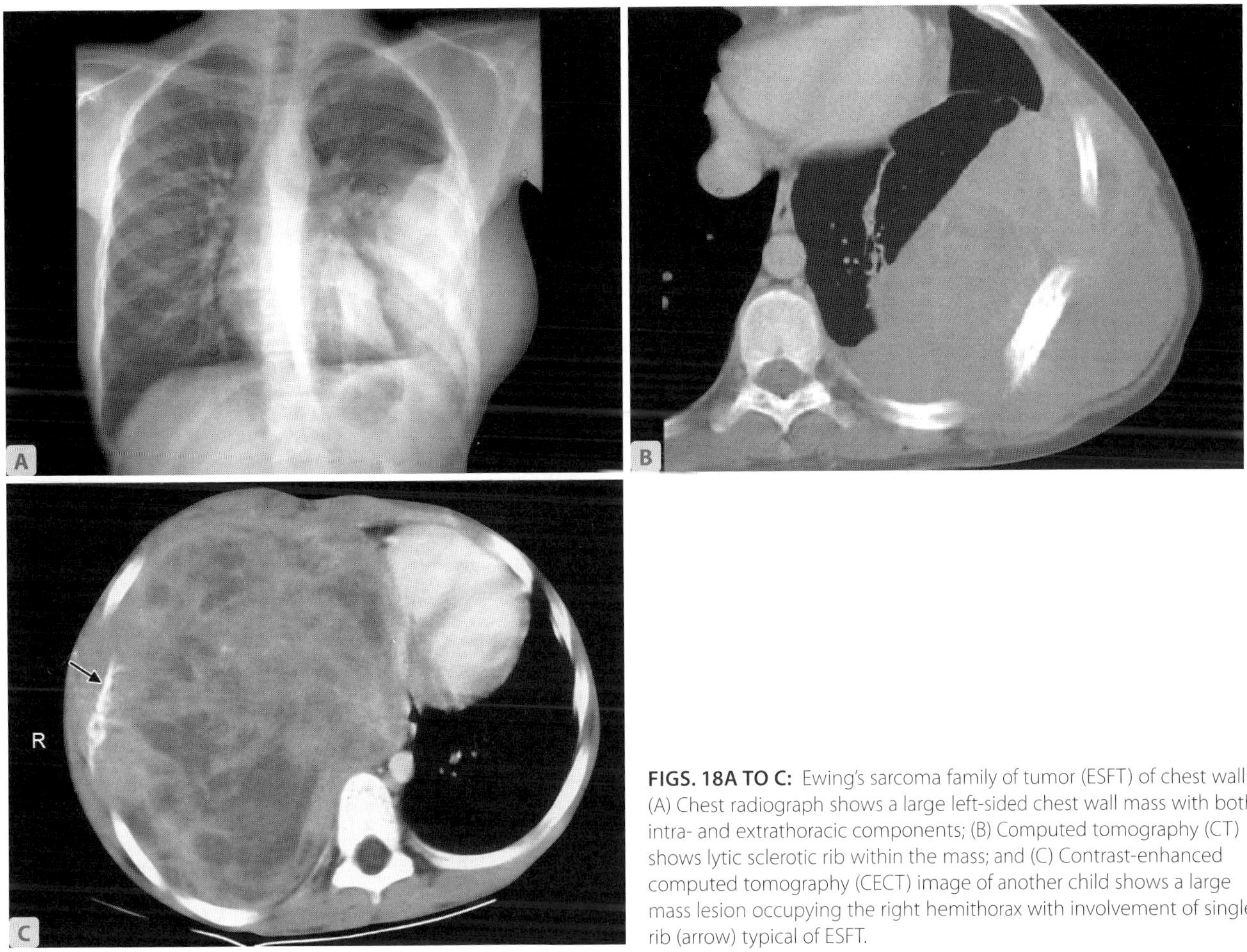

FIGS. 18A TO C: Ewing's sarcoma family of tumor (ESFT) of chest wall: (A) Chest radiograph shows a large left-sided chest wall mass with both intra- and extrathoracic components; (B) Computed tomography (CT) shows lytic sclerotic rib within the mass; and (C) Contrast-enhanced computed tomography (CECT) image of another child shows a large mass lesion occupying the right hemithorax with involvement of single rib (arrow) typical of ESFT.

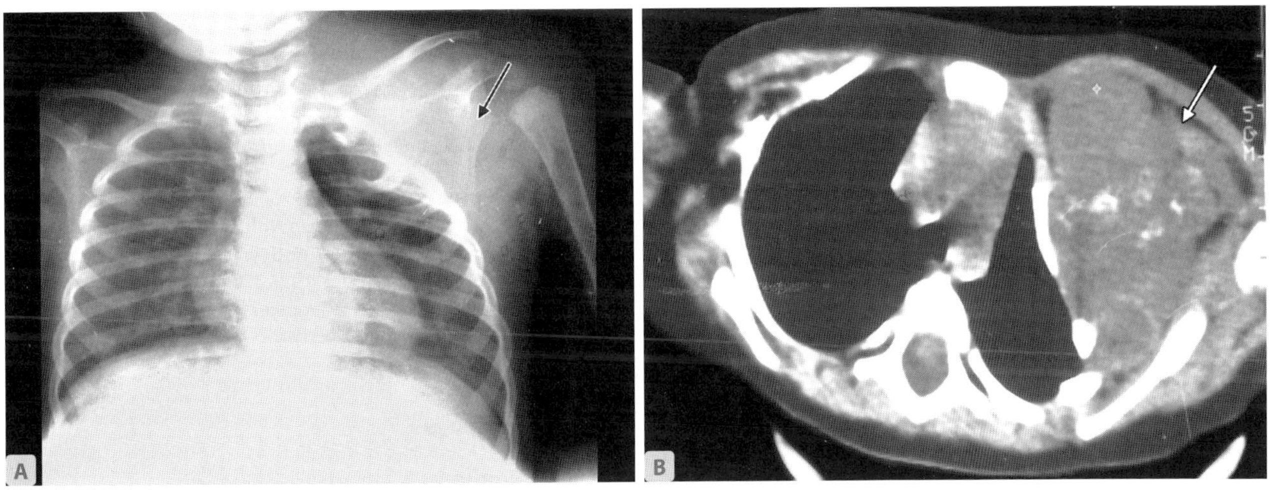

FIGS. 19A AND B: Rhabdomyosarcoma. (A) Chest radiograph shows a soft-tissue opacity (arrow) in the left axillary region; and (B) Computed tomography (CT) scan of the child shows a soft-tissue mass lesion (arrow) in the left axilla with multiple areas of calcification leading to deformation of left-sided ribs.

REFERENCES

1. Stocker JT, Madewell JE, Drake RM. Congenital cystic adenomatoid malformation of the lung: classification and morphologic spectrum. Hum Pathol. 1977;8:155-71.
2. Winters WD, Effaman EL. Congenital masses of the lung: prenatal and postnatal imaging evaluation. J Thorac Imaging. 2001;16:196-206.
3. Lee EY, Siegel MJ, Sierra LM, Foglia RP. Evaluation of angio-architecture of pulmonary sequestration in pediatric patients using 3D MDCT angiography. AJR Am J Roentgenol. 2004;183: 183-8.
4. Reed JC, Sobonya RE. Morphologic analysis of foregut cysts in the thorax. AJR Am J Roentgenol. 1974;120:851-60.
5. McAdams HP, Kitejczyk WM, Rosado-de-Christensen ML, Matsumoto S. Bronchogenic cyst: imaging features with clinical and histopathologic correlation. Radiology. 2000;217:441-6.
6. Paterson A. Imaging evaluation of congenital lung abnormalities in infant and children. Radiol Clin North Am. 2005;43:303-23.
7. Abushaban L, Uthaman B, Endrys J. Transcatheter coil closure of pulmonary arteriovenous malformations in children. J Interven Cardiol. 2004;17:23-6.
8. Yang PC, Luh KT, Lee YC, Chang DB, Yu CJ, Wu HD, et al. Lung abscesses: US examination and US-guided transthoracic aspiration. Radiology. 1991;180:171-5.
9. Donnely LF. Practical issues concerning imaging of pulmonary infections in children. J Thorac Imaging. 2001;16:238-50.
10. Rose RE, Ward BH. Spherical pneumonias in children simulating pulmonary and mediastinal masses. Radiology. 1973;106: 179-82.
11. Erdem CZ, Erdem LO. Radiological characteristics of pulmonary hydatid disease in children: less common radiological appearances. Eur Radiol. 2003;45:123-8.
12. Rastogi R, Garg R, Thulkar S, Bakhshi S, Gupta A. Unusual thoracic CT manifestations of osteosarcoma: review of 16 cases. Pediatr Radiol. 2008;38:551-8.
13. Aquino SL. Imaging of metastatic disease to the thorax. Radiol Clin North Am. 2005;43:481-95.
14. Manivel JC, Priest JR, Watterson J, Steiner M, Woods WG, Wick MR, et al. Pleuropulmonary blastoma. The so-called pulmonary blastoma of childhood. Cancer. 1988;62:1516-26.
15. Orazi C, Inserra A, Schingo PM, De Sio L, Cutrera R, Boldrini R, et al. Pleuropulmonary blastoma, a distinct neoplasm of childhood: report of three cases. Pediatr Radiol. 2007;37: 337-44.
16. Lal DR, Clark I, Shalkow J, Downey RJ, Shorter NA, Klimstra DS, et al. Primary epithelial lung malignancies in the pediatric population. Pediatr Blood Cancer. 2005;45:683-6.
17. Dawani A, Bhalla AS, Jana M, Agarwala S, Naranje P. Primary pulmonary tumors in pediatric population: imaging markers for predicting histology. J Indian Assoc Pediatr Surg. 2020. [Epub ahead of print].
18. Brown LR, Muhm JR, Aughenbaugh GL, Lewis BD, Hurt RD. Computed tomography of benign mature teratomas of the mediastinum. J Thorac Imaging. 1987;2:66-71.
19. Lee KS, IM JG, Han CH. Malignant primary germ cell tumors of the mediastinum: CT features. AJR Am J Roentgenol. 1989;153: 947-51.
20. Arya LS, Narain S, Tomar S, Thavaraj V, Dawar R, Bhargawa M. Superior vena cava syndrome. Indian J Pediatr. 2001;69:293-7.
21. Shukla NN, Trippett TM. Non-Hodgkin lymphoma in children and adolescents. Curr Oncol Rep. 2006;8:387-94.
22. Thomas CR, Wright CD, Loeherer PJ. Thymoma: state of art. J Clin Oncol. 1999;17:2280-9.
23. Santana L, Givica A, Camacho C. Best cases from AFIP: thymoma. Radiographics. 2002;22:95-102.
24. Sumner TE, Volberg FM, Kiser PE, de Shaffner LS. Mediastinal cystic hygroma in children. Pediatr Radiol. 1981;11:160-2.
25. Konez O, Borrows PE. Magnetic resonance of vascular anomalies. Magn Reson Imaging Clin North Am. 2002;10:363-88.
26. Mea MP, Benson M, Slovis TL. Imaging of mediastinal masses in children. Radiol Clin North Am. 1993;31:583-604.
27. Lonergan GJ, Schwab CM, Suarez ES, Carlson CL. Neuroblastoma, ganglioneuroblastoma, and ganglioneuroma: radiologic-pathologic correlation. Radiographics. 2002;22:911-34.
28. Softka CM, Semelka RC, Kelekis NL, Worawattanakul S, Chung CJ, Gold S, et al. Magnetic resonance imaging of neuroblastoma using current techniques. Magn Reson Imaging. 1999;17:193-8.
29. Hiorns MP, Owens CM. Radiology of neuroblastoma in children. Eur Radiol. 2001;11:2071-81.
30. Laurent F, Latrabe V, Lecesne R, Zennaro H, Airaud JY, Rauturier JF, et al. Mediastinal masses: diagnostic approach. Eur Radiol. 1998;8:1149-59.
31. Strollo DC, Rosado-de-Christenson ML, Jett JR. Primary mediastinal tumours. Part II: tumors of the middle and posterior mediastinum. Chest. 1997;112:1344-57.
32. Paltiel HJ, Burrows PE, Kozakewich HP, Zurakowski D, Mulliken JB. Soft-tissue vascular anomalies: utility of US for diagnosis. Radiology. 2000;214:747-54.
33. Lee KC, Davis AM, Cassar-Pullicino VN. Imaging the complications of osteochondromas. Clin Radiol. 2001;57:18-28.
34. Groom KR, Murphy MD, Howard LM. Mesenchymal hamartoma of the chest wall: radiologic manifestations with emphasis on cross-sectional imaging and histopathological comparison. Radiology. 2002;222:205-11.
35. Fefferman NR, Pinkney LP. Imaging evaluation of chest wall disorders in children. Radiol Clin North Am. 2005;43:355-70.
36. Shamberger RC, Grier HE. Chest wall tumors in infants and children. Semin Pediatr Surg. 1994;3:267-76.
37. Wyttenbach R, Vock P, Tschappeler H. Cross-sectional imaging with CT and/or MRI of pediatric chest tumors. Eur Radiol. 1998;8:1040-9.

CHAPTER

65

Pediatric Airway

Ashu Seith Bhalla, Surabhi Vyas, Priyanka Naranje

INTRODUCTION

Diseases affecting the airway, extrinsic or intrinsic, are frequent in children compared to adults. Also, these are more often symptomatic as children have smaller airways that are more prone to collapse. Hence, even mild edema can result in symptoms. Clinically, the presentation of these disorders may be acute or chronic. In their acute form, the airway disorders can be life-threatening. "Always look at the airway" is a lesson that must be emphasized in pediatric radiology.[1-4]

The airway is referred to as the *upper airway* (above the thoracic inlet) or *lower airway* being below it. While the predominant presentation of upper airway obstruction is inspiratory stridor, that of lower airway obstruction is expiratory wheeze.[2,3] Other clinical presentations include feeding difficulty, respiratory distress, tachypnea, nasal flaring, chest wall retractions, hemoptysis, fever, failure to thrive, and even no symptoms.[2] Diseases affecting the pediatric airway are broadly classified in **Table 1**.

TABLE 1: Diseases affecting the pediatric airway.

Upper airway obstruction	Lower airway obstruction

Acute:
• Croup
• Epiglottitis
• Retropharyngeal cellulitis and abscess
• Exudative tracheitis
• Foreign body
Chronic:
• Space-occupying lesions:
  – Adenoidal enlargement
  – Enlarged pharyngeal tonsils
  – Juvenile nasopharyngeal angiofibroma
• *Fixed airway narrowing:*
  – Stenosis/stricture
• *Congenital:*
  – Micrognathia
  – Macroglossia
  – Laryngeal malacia
  – Laryngeal cysts
	Central airway:
	• *Extrinsic causes:*
	  – *Congenital:*
	    ▪ Vascular compression, vascular malformations
	    ▪ Bronchopulmonary foregut malformations—bronchogenic cyst
	    ▪ Thoracic deformity
	  – *Inflammatory:*
	    ▪ Lymph nodes
	    ▪ Mediastinal abscess/cellulitis
	  – *Masses:*
	    ▪ Hemangioma
	    ▪ Lymphoma
	    ▪ Germ cell tumor
	• *Intrinsic causes:*
	  – *Wall abnormalities:*
	    ▪ Congenital:
	      ♦ Tracheobronchomalacia
	      ♦ Tracheal stenosis
	      ♦ Bronchopulmonary foregut malformations
	      ♦ Bronchial atresia
	      ♦ Tracheoesophageal fistula
	      ♦ Tracheobronchial branching anomalies
	    ▪ *Inflammatory:*
	      ♦ Exudative tracheitis
	      ♦ Tuberculosis
	      ♦ Fibrotic stricture
	      ♦ Postintubation stricture
	    ▪ *Intraluminal:*
	      ♦ Foreign body
	      ♦ Masses: Hemangioma, carcinoid
	Peripheral airway:
	• Asthma
	• Bronchiectasis
	• Bronchiolitis/small airway disease

IMAGING MODALITIES

The goals of imaging are to delineate:

- Location of the abnormality
- Whether the involvement is diffuse or focal
- Whether the involvement is extrinsic or intrinsic. If the lesion is an intrinsic process, it is mural or intraluminal and is the obstruction fixed or dynamic.[2]

Challenges of Imaging

- The radiographic evaluation of airways in infants and young children is challenging due to inability to obtain motionless end-inspiratory and end-expiratory images.
- The resultant artifacts are especially noticeable in high-resolution computed tomography (HRCT) images.
- Also, the caliber of airways of young children is small and difficult to detail in infants and small children.

Plain Radiographs

Plain radiographs are the primary and often only imaging modality used in evaluation of children with airway obstruction. The evaluation should include frontal and lateral high kV radiographs of the upper airways [also referred to as soft-tissue neck (STN)] and frontal and lateral views of the chest. When an endobronchial foreign body (FB) is suspected, decubitus chest views have been reported to be useful. Expiratory radiographs aid in demonstrating air trapping. However, in times of multidetector computed tomography (MDCT), these are seldom used and have been replaced by CT.

Fluoroscopy

Fluoroscopy of the airway demonstrates dynamic airway collapse during expiration in children with tracheobronchomalacia.[2] Decubitus fluoroscopy may be performed in cases of suspected FB in infants and young children, lying on the affected side, demonstrating the relative immobility of lung on respiration. With advances in MDCT, fluoroscopy is seldom employed.

Barium Swallow

A barium swallow may be useful for demonstrating gastroesophageal reflux in patients with chronic aspiration simulating asthma. This study is also helpful for establishing the diagnosis of vascular rings and slings, although cross-sectional imaging is eventually required for better anatomic delineation.

Multidetector Computed Tomography

Relative to MRI, CT has the advantage of rapid scan times enabling performance of the examination without sedation; it has the disadvantage of radiation exposure and need for using contrast. *Dynamic CT* can be obtained as a paired inspiratory-expiratory scan in older cooperative children.

In uncooperative children, cine-CT can be used. *Cine-CT* involves rapid acquisition of images of the airway throughout the respiratory cycle during free breathing. Once the site of suspected airway stenosis or malacia is localized, CT images are rapidly and sequentially acquired at the same axial level. Cine-CT technique can provide multiple images of the airway during inspiration and expiration, even in tachypneic patients.

Multiplanar and three-dimensional (3D) volume-rendered image reconstructions including virtual bronchoscopy further enhance the accuracy of MDCT in delineating the level of narrowing, degree of obstruction, segment length, and distal airway.[5]

Techniques of Dynamic Airway Imaging[6-8]

- *Paired inspiratory-expiratory*: Older, cooperative child, and larger field of view (FOV) are possible.
- *Ultra-high pitch CT*: Pitch >3, available on Siemens health scammer dual-source CT (DSCT scanners), e.g., Somatom Definition Flash or Somatom Force (limitation—craniocaudal coverage 4–6 cm only achievable depending on width of the detector and hence not useful in older children).
- Dynamic helical scanning, e.g., adaptive four-dimensional (4D) spiral, Siemens Healthineers—wide area detector.

Magnetic Resonance Imaging

MRI can demonstrate abnormal airway motion in addition to anatomic causes of obstruction. The protocol includes axial and sagittal T1-weighted (T1W) as well as short tau inversion recovery (STIR) images.

Dynamic (cine) MRI studies can be used to evaluate airway motion in real time. Sagittal midline MR cine (fast gradient echo imaging) is performed. Axial MR cine images are obtained craniocaudally at the level of mid-tongue in those with obstructive sleep apnea.[9] The use of cine MR imaging during coughing for evaluation of tracheal collapsibility in patients with suspected tracheomalacia has been described.[10,11]

Ultrashort echo time MRI (UTE-MRI) has been reported to be useful in assessing the tracheal dynamics in neonates without the need for sedation or any increased risk.[12]

UPPER AIRWAY OBSTRUCTION

Plain radiographs STN [anteroposterior (AP)/lateral] are frequently employed in upper airway obstruction. It is, hence, essential to be familiar with the normal anatomy.

Normal Anatomy (Figs. 1A to C)

Epiglottis

The normal epiglottis has very thin borders. Epiglottis may appear artifactually thickened if imaged obliquely—this is due to both the left and right sides being imaged next to each other. This is referred to as the "omega"appearance.[1,2]

Aryepiglottic Folds

Aryepiglottic folds are mucosal folds which extend from the epiglottis superiorly to the arytenoid cartilages, posteroinferiorly. On a lateral radiograph, these appear thin and convex inferiorly.

Subglottic Trachea

On frontal views, subglottic trachea appears rounded with lateral convexities or "shoulders". On the lateral view, it should not be narrower than the airway above or below it.

Retropharyngeal Soft Tissues

Normally, the soft tissues between the posterior aspect of the aerated pharynx and anterior aspect of the vertebral column should not be more than the anteroposterior diameter of the vertebral bodies. However, "pseudothickening" of the retropharyngeal soft tissues may be seen if the radiographs are obtained in a flexed position of the neck, especially in infants with short necks. The radiographs should, hence, be performed with adequate neck extension. The thickness of soft tissues is measured transversely somewhere between the level of adenoids superiorly to base of epiglottis inferiorly, below which these are normally thicker due to the presence of esophagus.

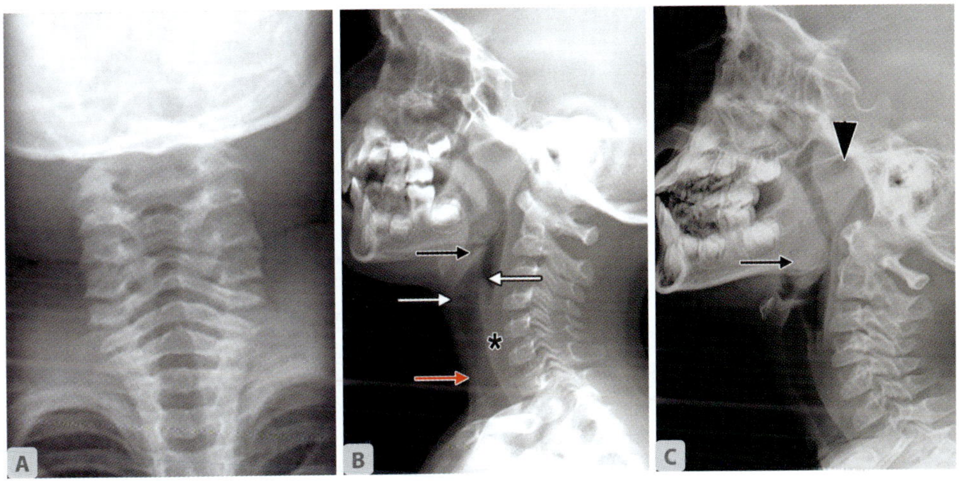

FIGS. 1A TO C: Normal frontal (A) and lateral (B) radiographs neck of a 5-year-old child; and (C) Lateral radiograph of a 9-year-old boy showing enlarged tonsils (white arrow), adenoids (arrowhead), epiglottis (black arrow), glottis (white arrow), aryepiglottic folds (small white arrow), subglottic trachea (red arrow), and retropharyngeal soft tissues (asterisk).

Tonsils/Adenoids

At <6 months of age, the adenoids are rarely visible on radiography. There is rapid proliferation during infancy with peak size reaching between 2 and 10 years. A size up to 12 mm is considered normal. Subsequently, during the second decade, there is reduction in size.

Acute Obstruction

The most common causes of acute upper airway obstruction are inflammatory, followed by FB. Ingestion of corrosive/caustic substances is another cause.

Croup (Acute Laryngotracheobronchitis)

Croup is a benign, self-limiting acute inflammatory condition of the upper airways. It results from viral infection and is the most common cause of upper airway obstruction in young children and infants (6 months to 3 years of age). Affected children present with "croupy" (barky) cough and inspiratory stridor.

The purpose of obtaining radiographs in a suspected case of croup is to exclude secondary causes such as FB. It, however, has characteristic findings—on frontal radiographs, there is loss of the normal shoulders (lateral convexities) of the subglottic trachea due to subglottic edema. The subglottic trachea becomes elongated, extending below the level of the pyriform sinuses. The appearance is referred to as a "church steeple" or "inverted V" appearance. Lateral radiographs may reveal similar narrowing of the subglottic trachea with loss of its wall definition.

Epiglottitis

Unlike croup, epiglottitis is a life-threatening condition requiring emergency intubation. The most common organism responsible is *Haemophilus influenzae*. Affected children present with abrupt onset of fever, dysphagia, stridor, and worsening of respiratory distress in recumbent position. The classic mean age of presentation is 3–5 years (older than croup). Now with availability of vaccination, the incidence of this entity has significantly declined and patients may present at a later age (13–14 years).

Diagnosis is made on basis of presentation and physical examination. If not, a single lateral radiograph of neck may be obtained. This reveals markedly thickened epiglottis ("thumb" appearance). The pathological thickening of epiglottis can be differentiated from "omega" appearance, due to associated thickening of aryepiglottic folds in the former. The thickened aryepiglottic folds appear convex superiorly.

Retropharyngeal Cellulitis and Abscess

Retropharyngeal space inflammation is usually of pyogenic origin, following upper respiratory tract infection. Patients present with fever, dysphagia, a stiff neck, and occasional stridor. It is most common between 6 and 12 months of age.

Lateral radiographs reveal thickening of the retropharyngeal soft tissues. On radiographs, the only conclusive finding differentiating cellulitis from abscess is the presence of gas within the latter. Contrast-enhanced CT scans can aid in the distinction of cellulitis from a drainable fluid collection. An abscess appears as a well-defined, low-attenuation area with an enhancing rim **(Figs. 2A and B)**.

Exudative Tracheitis

Exudative tracheitis is also referred to as membranous laryngotracheobronchitis or membranous croup. It is a purulent infection of the trachea characterized by formation of exudative plaques along the tracheal walls. Patients are older than croup, typically 6–10 years of age, and are also more ill. The causative organism may be *Staphylococcus aureus* or the infections may be multimicrobial.

The characteristic finding on radiographs is a linear soft tissue-filling defect (membrane) seen within the airway. A plaque-like irregularity of the tracheal wall is also suggestive. Other findings include narrowing of subglottic trachea

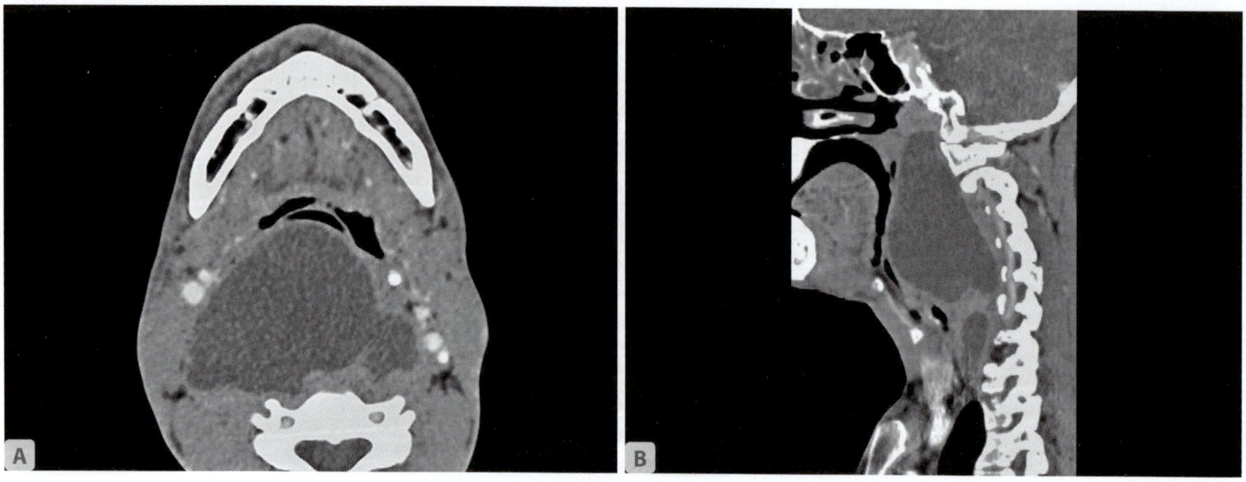

FIGS. 2A AND B: Retropharyngeal abscess: Contrast-enhanced CT neck in a patient with low-grade fever, respiratory distress, and dysphagia shows a large peripherally enhancing, prevertebral abscess compressing airway.

(symmetric or asymmetric) with loss of its wall definition. The older age of the patient (>3 years) aids in distinction from croup.

Foreign Body

Postaspiration, most FBs lodge in the lower airway. Foreign bodies in the larynx or trachea are much less common and the patients present with sudden onset stridor and respiratory distress. Foreign bodies, if lodged in the esophagus, may also present with respiratory symptoms. Radiographs reveal either a radiopaque FB or soft-tissue density within the airway or loss of definition of the airway wall **(Figs. 3A to C)**.

Chronic Obstruction

The clinical presentation in children with chronic upper airway obstruction differs from that of acute obstruction. While these children may present with stridor, symptoms of sleep apnea or snoring are more common.

Obstructive Sleep Apnea

Sleep apnea may be seen in 1–6% of children.[1,13] The various causes include any space-occupying lesion or fixed narrowing, which may be congenital, inflammatory, or neoplastic in etiology.

At various levels, the causes are:

- *Nasal cavity/Nasopharynx*: Adenoidal enlargement, choanal atresia, and juvenile angiofibroma.
- *Oropharynx*: Micrognathia or retrognathia with posterior displacement of tongue **(Fig. 4)**, macroglossia, and glossoptosis.
- *Hypopharynx*: Hypopharyngeal collapse.
- *Larynx*: Laryngomalacia, congenital cysts.

Large hemangiomas/vascular malformations can cause airway obstruction at any level.

MRI is useful in evaluation of patients with obstructive sleep apnea (OSA). Indications for dynamic MR sleep imaging include persistence of OSA despite tonsillectomy and adenoidectomy, OSA with predisposition to obstruction at multiple sites (craniofacial anomalies, Down syndrome), and evaluation of OSA before any complex airway surgery and obesity.

Enlarged Tonsils/Adenoids

The most common cause of chronic upper airway obstruction is enlargement of adenoids and palatine tonsils. Enlargement of lingual tonsils results in OSA only uncommonly. On a lateral radiograph, enlarged adenoids appear as convex soft-tissue mass (>2 cm) in the posterior nasopharynx narrowing or obliterating the nasopharyngeal air lucency. CT also demonstrates tonsillar adenoidal enlargements as well **(Figs. 5A to C)**. Enlarged palatine tonsils appear as soft-tissue mass projecting on the posterior aspect of soft palate.[1] On T2-weighted (T2W) and STIR images, adenoids and tonsils appear hyperintense.

Glossoptosis

Glossoptosis means abnormal posterior motion of the tongue during sleep and is associated with underlying hypotonia, macroglossia, or micrognathia. Macroglossia and micrognathia may be diagnosed on lateral radiograph. However, glossoptosis can be demonstrated on dynamic sleep fluoroscopy or cine MRI.

Hypopharyngeal Collapse

Congenital hypopharyngeal collapse refers to cylindrical collapse of the hypopharynx, with its anterior, posterior, and lateral walls all moving centrally. It is associated with disorders of decreased muscular tone. This can be diagnosed on cine fluoroscopy or MRI.

Osseous Causes

Children with mandibular hypoplasia (micrognathia) or retrognathia have OSA consequent to posterior tongue.

Subglottic Obstruction

Subglottis is a common site of obstruction in children.

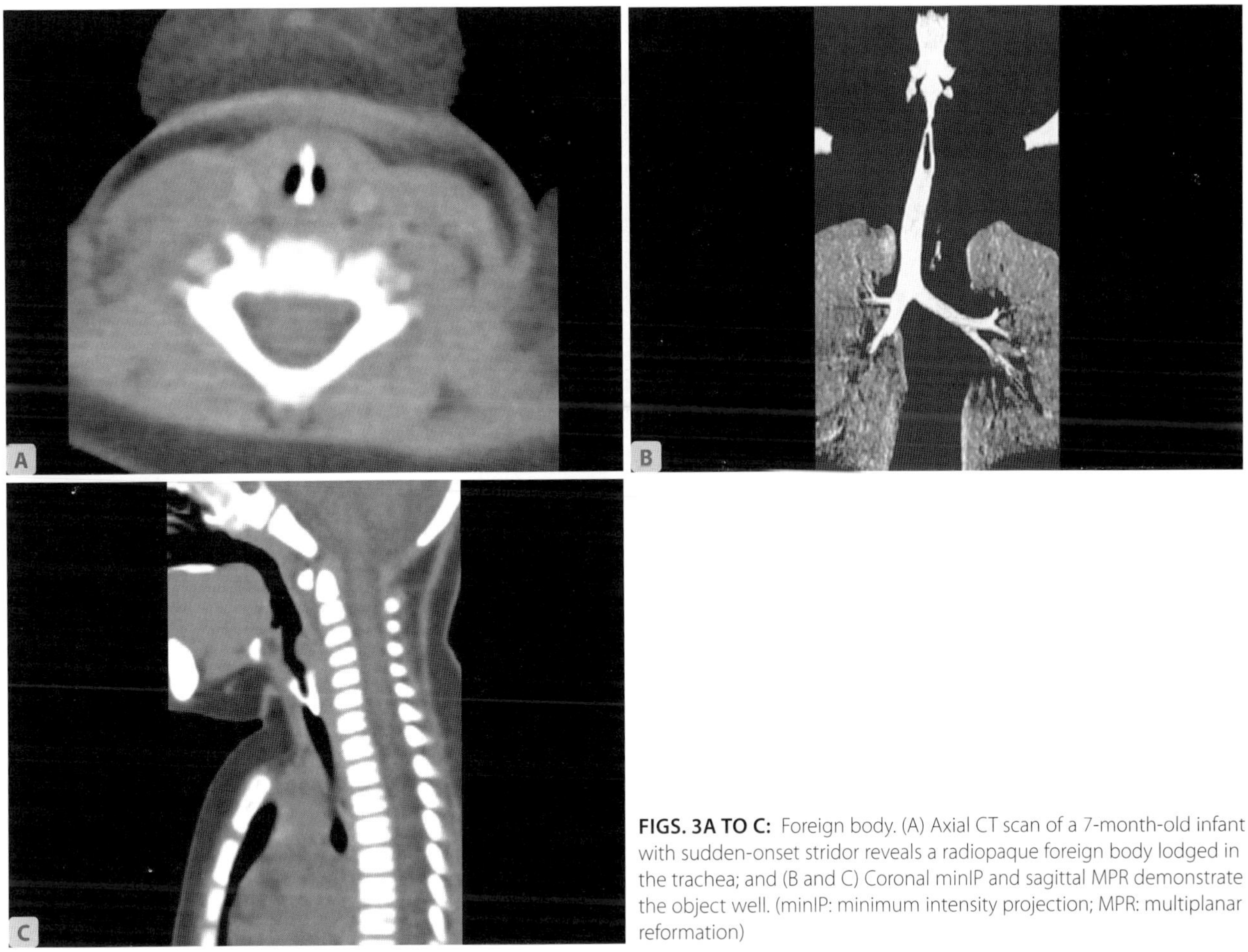

FIGS. 3A TO C: Foreign body. (A) Axial CT scan of a 7-month-old infant with sudden-onset stridor reveals a radiopaque foreign body lodged in the trachea; and (B and C) Coronal minIP and sagittal MPR demonstrate the object well. (minIP: minimum intensity projection; MPR: multiplanar reformation)

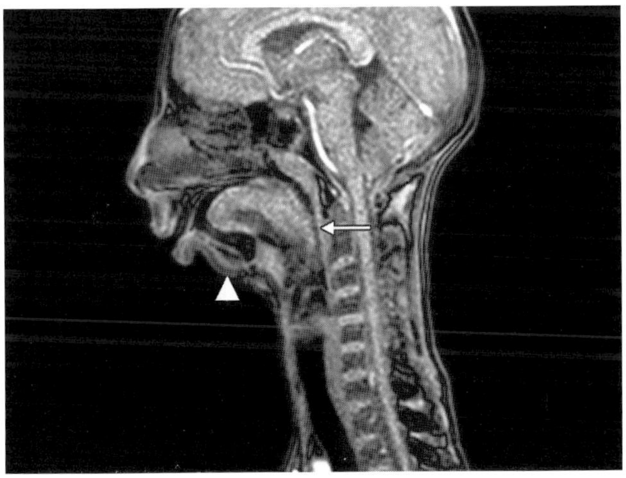

FIG. 4: Micrognathia with posterior displacement of tongue. Still image from cine MRI shows the retrognathia (arrowhead) and displaced tongue narrowing the oropharyngeal airway (white arrow).

Subglottic Stenosis

Short segment subglottic stenosis is often congenital in origin **(Figs. 6A and B)**.

Postintubation Stenosis

Prolonged intubation can lead to either tracheomalacia or airway stenosis, particularly with oversized endotracheal tubes or balloon cuffs. Airway stenosis consequent to prolonged intubation usually occurs at the level of cricoid cartilage, which is the narrowest part of the upper airway **(Figs. 7A to C)**.[14]

Subglottic Hemangioma

Hemangiomas located in the soft tissues of the neck may extend into the subglottic airway. Large hemangiomas or vascular malformations can cause obstruction at any level **(Figs. 8 and 9)**. These present in infancy, often at <6 months of age and may be associated with hemangiomas of the face or trunk.

Plain radiographs reveal asymmetric subglottic narrowing with associated soft tissue. Ultrasonography

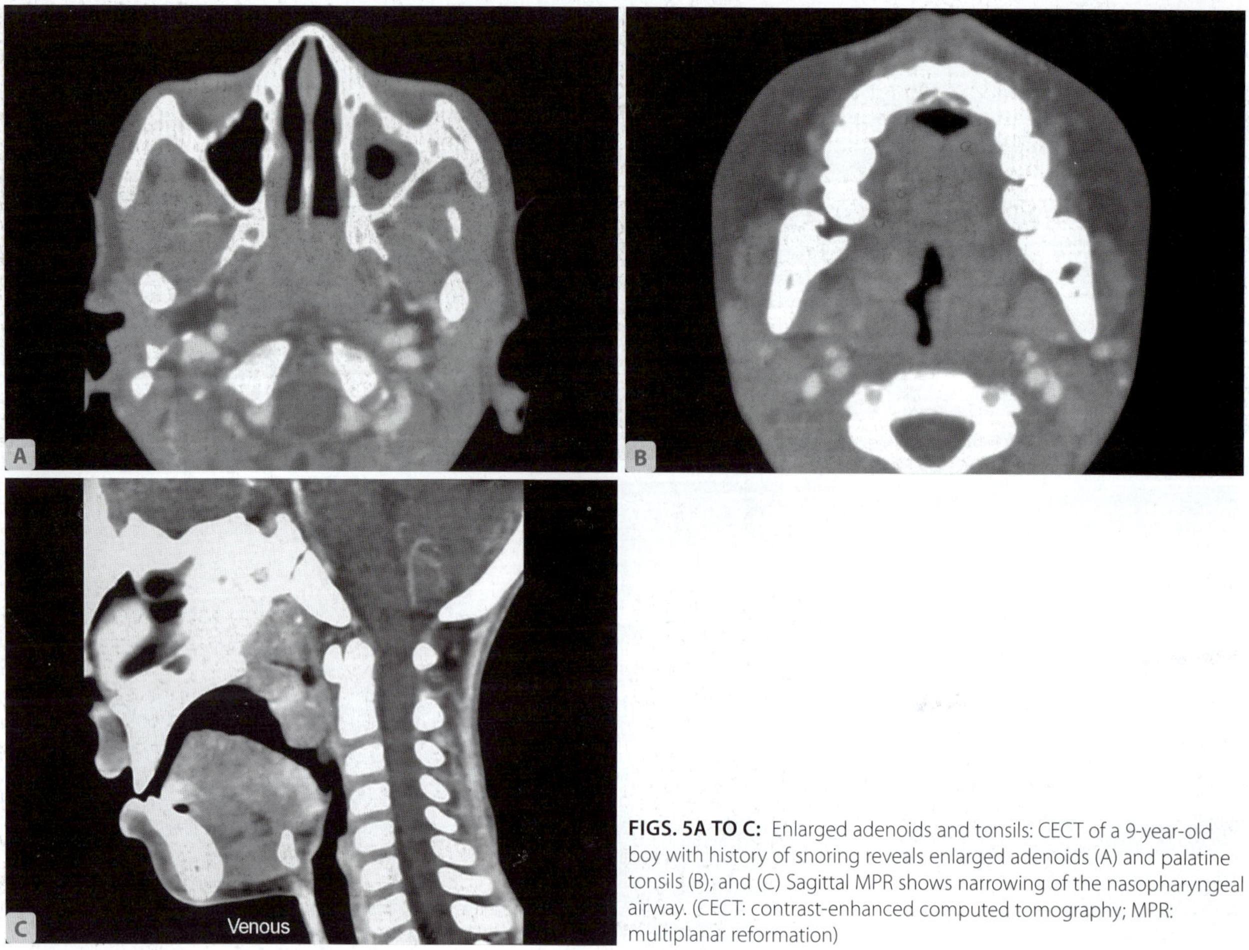

FIGS. 5A TO C: Enlarged adenoids and tonsils: CECT of a 9-year-old boy with history of snoring reveals enlarged adenoids (A) and palatine tonsils (B); and (C) Sagittal MPR shows narrowing of the nasopharyngeal airway. (CECT: contrast-enhanced computed tomography; MPR: multiplanar reformation)

(USG) of upper airway region is useful in identifying the lesion and assessment on color Doppler provides diagnostic information **(Fig. 8C)**. On cross-sectional imaging, the lesions show intense contrast enhancement which may be nodular. These lesions are unilateral or bilateral, but often asymmetric and occasionally circumferential. On T2W images, as elsewhere, hemangiomas appear hyperintense. Although a benign lesion with a natural history of proliferation and involution, complications of bleeding and airway obstruction can be life-threatening. Spontaneous regression is typical. Endoscopy confirms the diagnosis. When the presentation demands active management, as in patients with symptomatic airway compromise, treatment options include systemic or intralesional corticosteroids, laser ablation, interferon therapy, or surgical excision.[15]

LOWER AIRWAY OBSTRUCTION

Central Airways

The central causes of airway obstruction may be extrinsic or intrinsic (involving either the wall or lumen).

Investigations include frontal and lateral radiographs of the airway and chest. The neck radiographs help to exclude upper airway obstruction. Chest radiographs should be evaluated for tracheal caliber, cardiac size, position of the aortic arch, mediastinal widening, asymmetric lung aeration, lung collapse or consolidation, and radiopaque FB. The length of tracheal narrowing and involvement of anterior/posterior walls should be noted. If the radiographs are suggestive of an intrinsic cause of obstruction, then one can proceed with fiberoptic bronchoscopy. If the suspected cause is extrinsic, then further cross-sectional imaging is indicated.

The choice between CT and MRI is not clearly defined. While MRI has the advantage of being radiation free and not dependent on intravenous contrast, its main drawback is the long scanning times. The need for sedation especially in a child with airway compromise often negates the advantages of MRI, making CT the preferred modality. Both modalities offer good contrast between the central airway and surrounding structures, while the lungs are better visualized on CT.

Extrinsic Causes

Any mass lesion of the mediastinum such as nodes and cysts includes the nonvascular causes of airway compression. Chest wall deformities may similarly result in airway compromise.

The classical vascular causes include double aortic arch, anomalous left pulmonary artery (pulmonary sling), and innominate artery compression syndrome. However, several other vascular causes such as dilatation of pulmonary artery,

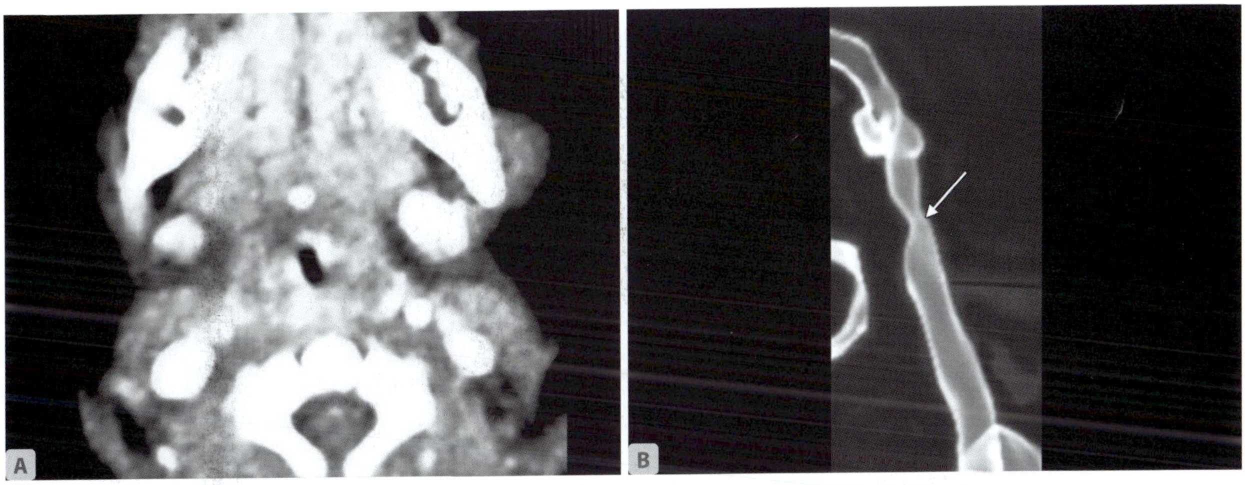

FIGS. 6A AND B: Subglottic stenosis: CECT of a newborn with stridor. Axial (A) and sagittal VRT (B) images show a short segment, smooth subglottic stenosis (arrow). (CECT: contrast-enhanced computed tomography; VRT: volume rendering technique)

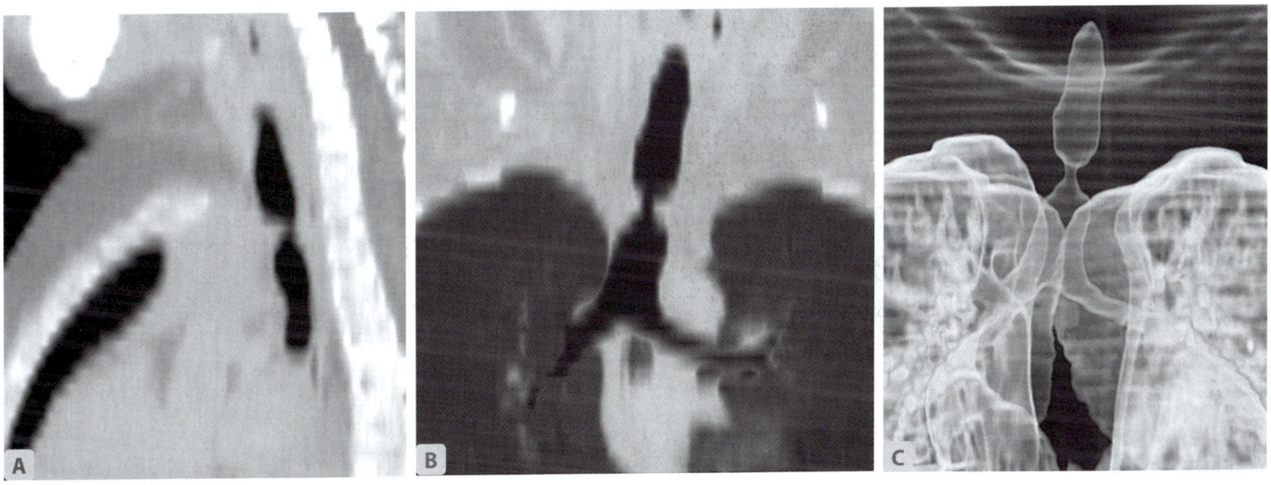

FIGS. 7A TO C: Postintubation stenosis: A short segment, smooth stenosis is seen in upper trachea on sagittal MPR (A), coronal minIP (B), and VB (C) CT images of a child with history of prolonged intubation. (minIP: minimum intensity projection; MPR: multiplanar reformation)

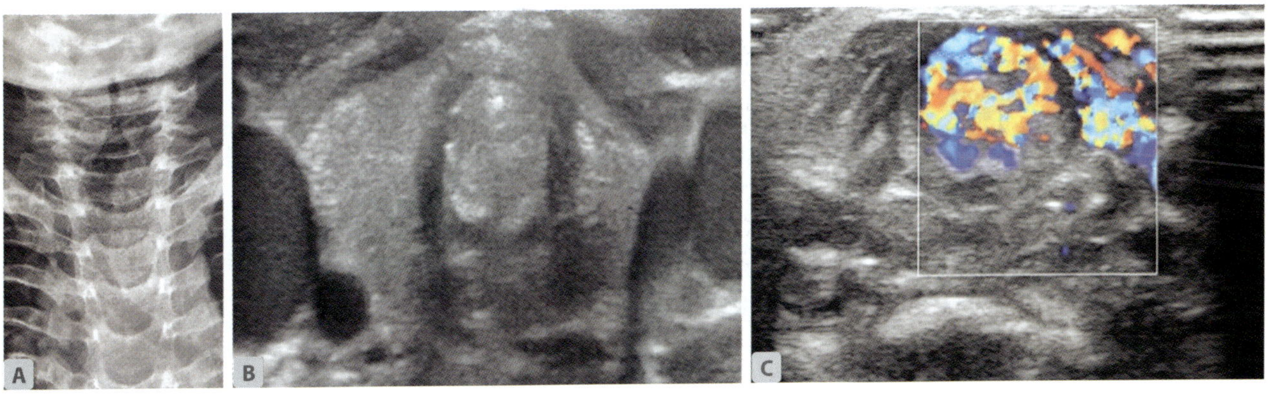

FIGS. 8A TO C: Subglottic hemangioma. (A) Frontal radiograph shows narrowing in the subglottic region; and (B and C) Ultrasonography (USG) of upper airway shows echogenic mass in subglottic region showing intense vascularity on color Doppler.

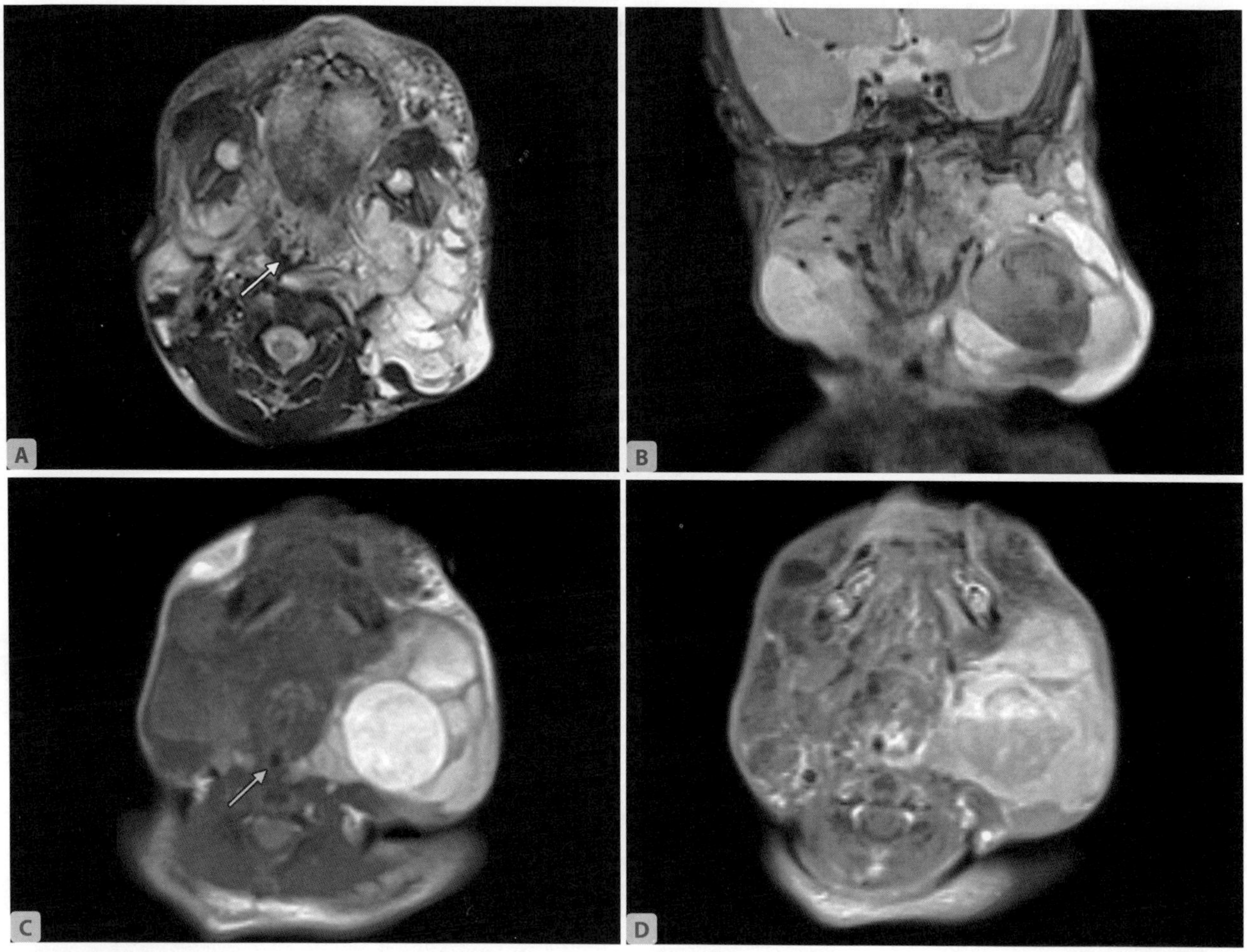

FIGS. 9A TO D: Venolymphatic malformation with airway compression. (A and B) T2WI showing hyperintense multicystic mass in left parotid and submandibular regions extending in parapharyngeal space causing airway narrowing (white arrow); (C) T1WI shows hyperintense contents within (suggestive of hemorrhage) (white arrow); and (D) Fluid levels are also noted within the lesion. (T1WI: T1-weighted image; T2WI: T2-weighted image)

enlargement of ascending aorta, midline descending aorta, and right arch with aberrant left subclavian artery can also result in airway compression. A vascular ring encircling the airway occurs as a result of the failure of primitive vascular structures to fuse and regress normally during the development of the aortic arch, pulmonary arteries, and/or ductus arteriosus. Patients with vascular rings may have wheezing, stridor, feeding difficulties, choking episodes, or even aspiration pneumonia, depending on the degree of tracheal and esophageal narrowing. Plain radiographs and barium swallow cannot reliably distinguish among the types of vascular ring. Cross-sectional imaging, either with CT or MR, is helpful in delineating the anatomy and aiding in presurgical planning and postsurgical assessment.[16]

Vascular Causes

Vascular rings (Tables 2 and 3):

- *Double aortic arch*: It is a congenital arch anomaly and is the most common vascular ring to cause airway compression. It is usually an isolated anomaly. Both right and left arches are seen to arise from the ascending aorta and join to form the descending aorta. Right arch is commonly larger and posterosuperior.

The two arches surround and compress the trachea anteriorly and esophagus posteriorly **(Figs. 10A and B)**. The level of compression is mid to lower thirds of intrathoracic trachea.[17] **(Table 2)**. On radiography, lateral tracheal indentations are seen. On cross-sectional imaging, it is important to determine the dominant arch (side), as the surgical approach differs accordingly **(Figs. 10A and B)**.

Right arch with aberrant left subclavian artery: This is an arch anomaly wherein the aortic arch is located to the right of trachea. The left subclavian artery (LSA) originates from the proximal descending aorta and courses to the left behind the esophagus. In 60% cases, there is dilatation of origin of the LSA (aortic diverticulum of Kommerell).[18] It is commonly an asymptomatic finding with only 5% patients having symptoms. However, this anomaly may be associated with a constricting left ligamentum arteriosum, forming a vascular ring and causing airway compression. If the ligamentum arteriosum connects to LSA, it forms a loose vascular ring,

TABLE 2: Vascular rings.

Aortic abnormalities	Incidence	Embryology	Associations	Age of presentation/symptoms
Double aortic arch	Most common	Persistent bilateral fourth branchial arches	Mostly isolated	• Symptomatic • Infancy
Right aortic arch with aberrant left subclavian artery (SCA)	Second most common	Interrupted hypothetical left arch [between left common carotid artery (CCA) and left SCA]	Mostly isolated	• Often asymptomatic • "Loose ring" between left SCA and persistent left ligamentous arteriosum
Left aortic arch with aberrant right SCA	–	–	–	Ring formed between right SCA and intact right ligamentum arteriosum

TABLE 3: Imaging features of vascular rings.

	CXR	Barium swallow	CTA/MRA
Double aortic arch	• Right-sided/bilateral aortic knuckles • Trachea midline (abnormal) • Narrowing—supracarinal • Lateral—anterior bowing, narrowing • Air trapping—infrequent	• Right/bilateral indentations on esophagus • Lateral view posterior indentation • Level aortic arch	• Right arch dominant—classical variant (majority 70%) • Higher, larger • Left—smaller/atretic band may cause traction on left SCA • Important to identify dominant arch • Nondominant side operated • Aortic diverticulum (in case of atretic segment) • Square (trapezoid) symmetric appearance of major arch branches • "Four artery sign" • Lower trachea/carina narrowing
Right aortic arch with aberrant left subclavian artery (SCA)	• Right-sided aortic knuckle • Lateral—rounded mass like opacity retrotracheal, just above arch of aorta (space is called Raider triangle)	• Right lateral and posterior indentation • Oblique angled to left shoulder • Normal left aortic arch indentation absent	• Right-sided aortic arch • Four brachiocephalic branch vessels (instead of three) • Lateral SCA last branch • Aortic diverticulum at origin, retroesophageal • Airway narrowing—variable, lower trachea • Ligamentum arteriosum is not directly visualized

(CTA: computed tomography angiography; CXR: chest X-ray; MRA: magnetic resonance angiography)

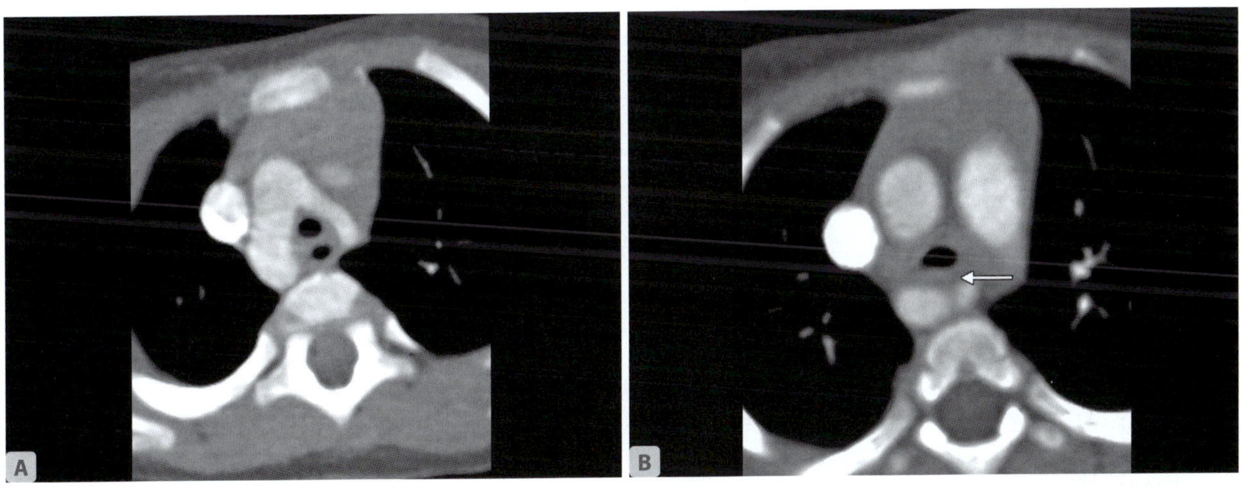

FIGS. 10A AND B: Double aortic arch. (A and B) Axial computed tomography angiography (CTA) images show right-sided dominant arch with mild extrinsic anterior compression on lower trachea and posterior compression on esophagus (white arrow).

while if it extends to the aortic diverticulum of Kommerell, a tight vascular ring is formed.

On frontal radiograph, there is aortic arch indentation on the right wall of the trachea with tracheal deviation to the left **(Figs. 11A to C)**. Right-sided descending aorta may also be seen. Lateral view reveals indentation on the posterior aspect of trachea. On barium swallow, frontal views show a filling defect coursing from right inferior to left superior. On lateral view, there is posterior esophageal indentation. Cross-sectional imaging is indicated when there is clinical or radiographic evidence of airway compression.

There are several other aortic arch anomalies which can result in airway compression; these are uncommon. Some of these are associated with cervical position of aortic arch. Computed tomography angiography (CTA)/ magnetic resonance angiography (MRA) can demonstrate the location of the arch, its major branches, and associated airway narrowing. A patent ductus arteriosus (PDA) is also well-delineated. Ligamentum arteriosum is not directly seen on CTA/MRA; although some indirect signs can point to its presence, i.e., presence of aortic diverticulum, tracheal narrowing/distortion. Also, these are mostly opposite to aortic arch side. It is to be noted that incidence of aortic arch anomalies may be different form associated airway narrowing, as not all anomalies will result in airway compression. Also, congenital heart diseases should be looked for even in nongated CTA/MRA and reported as far as possible.

Midline descending aorta: In this anomaly, the descending aorta is positioned immediately anterior to the vertebral body, instead of the normal left paravertebral location. It may be an isolated lesion or be associated with hypoplastic right lung and hence mediastinal shift or aortic arch anomalies. Malposition may result in airway compression due to crowding of structures. Radiographs are often normal and cross-sectional imaging reveals the diagnosis.

Pulmonary sling: Pulmonary sling refers to a pulmonary artery anomaly wherein the left pulmonary artery arises from the proximal right pulmonary artery, forming a "sling" around the trachea. It subsequently passes between the trachea and esophagus as it courses toward the left lung.[19] **(Fig. 12A)**. It may be associated with congenital heart disease and complete tracheal rings, worsening the airway compromise **(Fig. 12A and B)**. Frontal radiograph reveals asymmetric lung inflation. On lateral radiograph, there is posterior compression of the trachea with anterior esophageal impression. It is the only vascular ring to course between the trachea and esophagus, to be associated with asymmetric lung inflation and also the only one to cause anterior indentation on the esophagus.

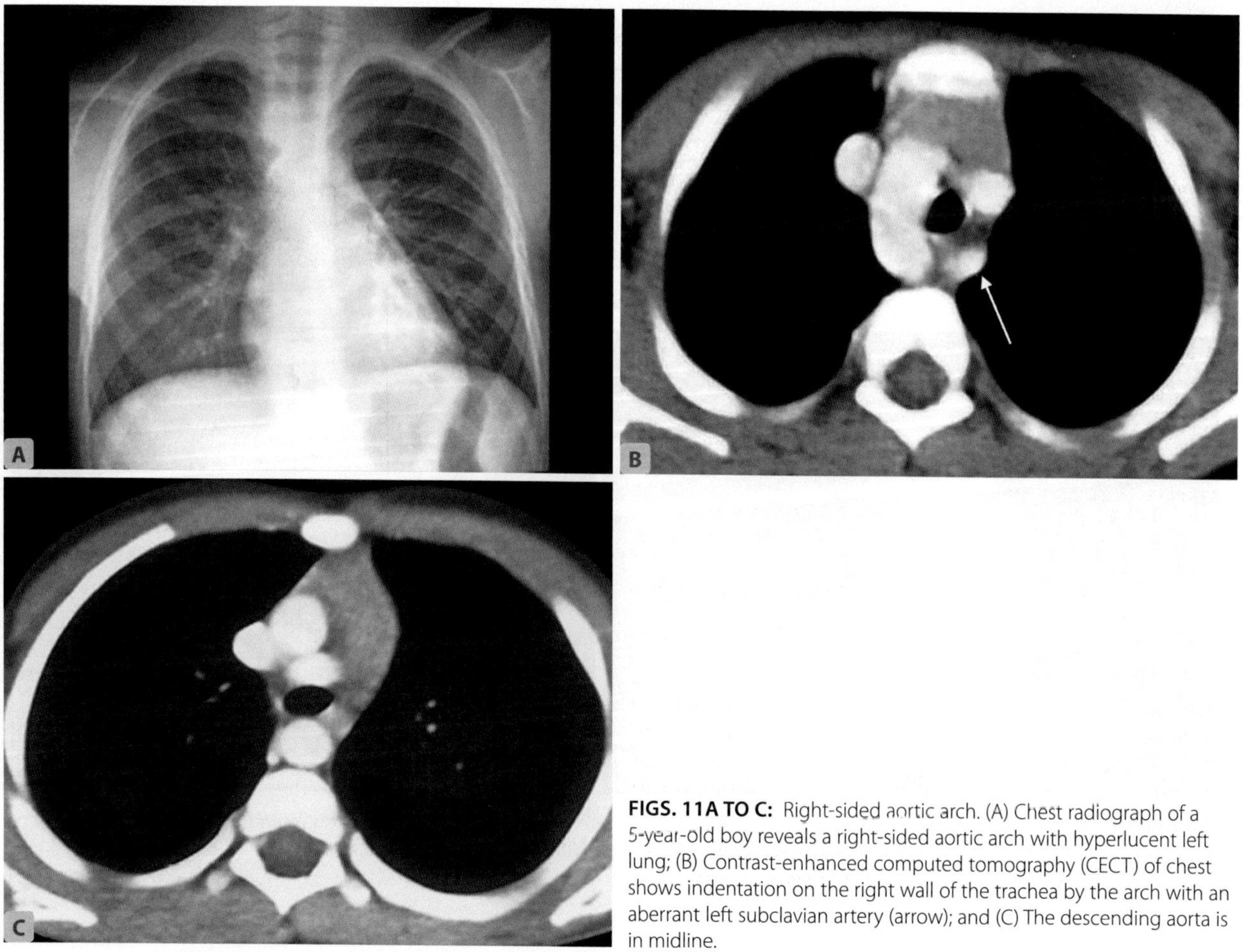

FIGS. 11A TO C: Right-sided aortic arch. (A) Chest radiograph of a 5-year-old boy reveals a right-sided aortic arch with hyperlucent left lung; (B) Contrast-enhanced computed tomography (CECT) of chest shows indentation on the right wall of the trachea by the arch with an aberrant left subclavian artery (arrow); and (C) The descending aorta is in midline.

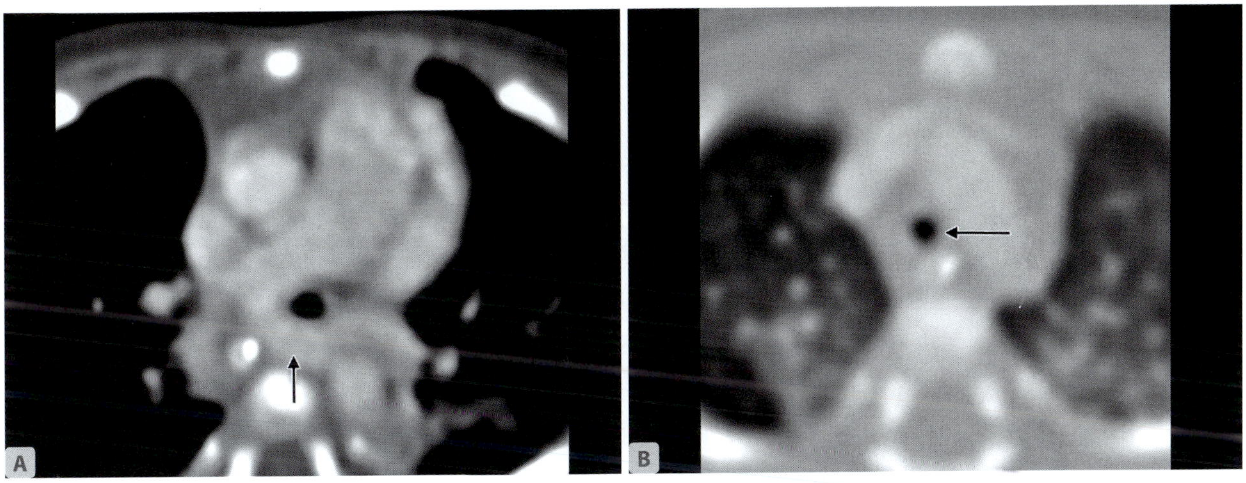

FIGS. 12A AND B: Pulmonary sling type II. (A) Axial contrast-enhanced computed tomography (CECT) image showing the left pulmonary artery (black arrow) coursing posterior to lower trachea; and (B) Associated complete cartilage ring giving a rounded appearance to trachea (black arrow).

FLOWCHART 1: Types of pulmonary slings.

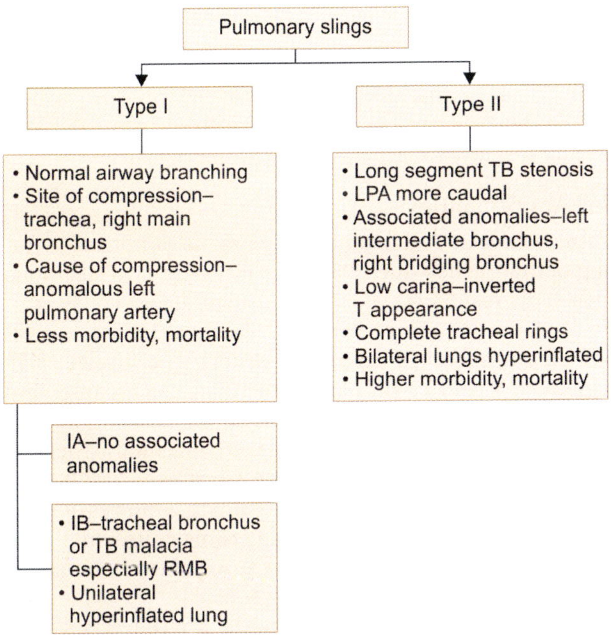

(RMB: right main bronchus; TB: tuberculosis; LPA: left pulmonary artery)

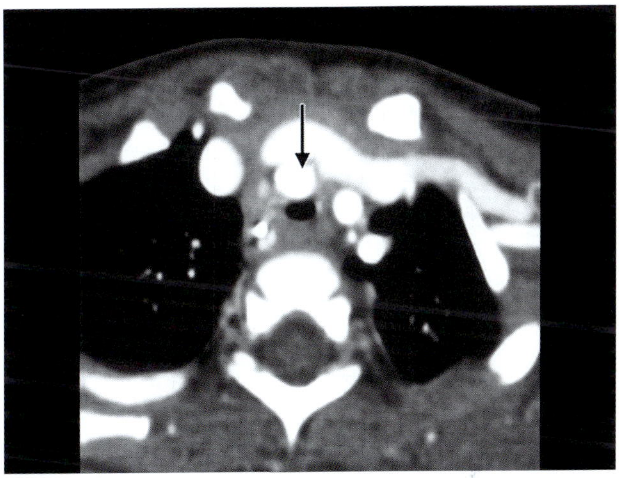

FIG. 13: Innominate artery compression syndrome: Computed tomography angiography (CTA) axial image shows the right brachiocephalic artery compressing the anterior tracheal wall (black arrow).

Types of pulmonary slings: There are two types on basis of associated airway anomalies[17] **(Flowchart 1)**.

Innominate artery compression syndrome: Innominate artery (brachiocephalic) crosses the trachea anteriorly, just below the thoracic inlet. In infants, it arises more to the left than adults.[20] In addition, the presence of a large thymus in the mediastinum and lack of rigidity of infantile trachea result in tracheal compression. The range of symptoms varies from none to stridor and dyspnea resulting from severe compression. Most children outgrow the disease and surgery is reserved only for those with severe compression. Lateral radiographs reveal focal anterior indentation of the trachea. CT and MRI detail the severity of the compression and exclude other causes **(Fig. 13)**.

Vascular Malformations

Vascular malformations may be venous, lymphatic, or mixed venolymphatic. Although these lesions are usually soft and compressible, giant malformations of the neck and/or chest can compress airway.

Bronchopulmonary foregut malformations: Bronchogenic cysts are among most common cystic lesions in the pediatric chest. The most common location is around the carina. Hence, when large, these result in compression of the proximal bronchi **(Figs. 14A to C)**. They can occur anywhere along the respiratory tract. The dilated proximal esophageal pouch in patients of esophageal atresia can also exert a mass effect on the adjoining airway **(Fig. 15)**.

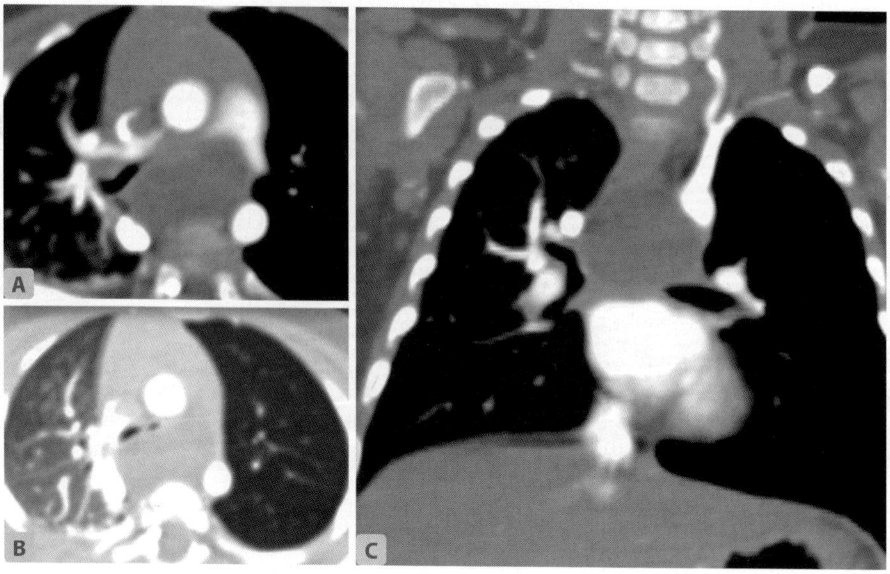

FIGS. 14A TO C: Bronchogenic cyst: Subcarinal cystic lesion causing severe compression of left main bronchus with resultant hyperinflation and lucency of left lung.

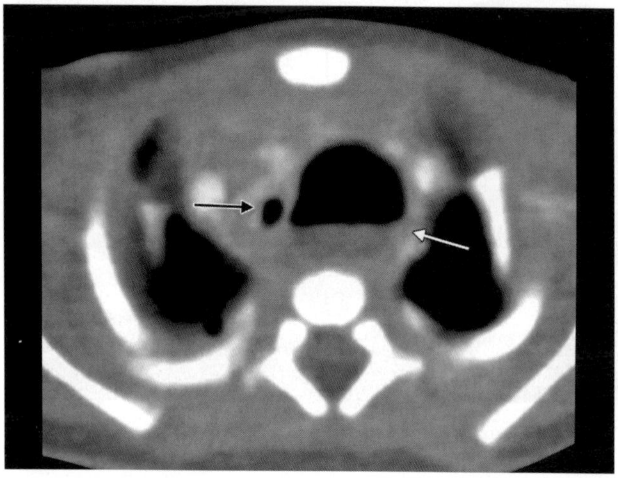

FIG. 15: Esophageal atresia: Contrast-enhanced computed tomography (CECT) of a neonate with esophageal atresia, performed to evaluate respiratory distress shows the dilated proximal esophageal pouch (white arrow) causing significant compression of the trachea (black arrow).

Inflammatory causes: Deep neck space infections, when they spread into the mediastinum, can compress the airway **(Figs. 16A to C)**. Large paravertebral abscesses, even tubercular, may result in significant airway compression. Mediastinal lymphadenopathy, tubercular, or fungal infections can also narrow the airway by mass effect **(Figs. 17A to D)**.

Masses: Lymphoma is the most common childhood neoplasm to cause symptomatic airway compromise in children. Other neoplasms that tend to narrow the airway by extrinsic mass effect include infantile hemangiomas, germ cell tumors, rhabdomyosarcomas, and neurogenic tumors **(Figs. 18A and B)**.

Intrinsic Causes

Intrinsic causes include those involving the wall, which may be dynamic (tracheomalacia) or fixed (stenosis) and intraluminal lesions.

Wall Abnormalities

Tracheomalacia: Tracheomalacia refers to abnormal softening of the trachea due to abnormality of the cartilaginous rings. This results in intermittent (expiratory) collapse of the trachea. The narrowing of the tracheal lumen is most marked during forced expiration, coughing, or the Valsalva maneuver. It may be primary or secondary to compression by masses or vascular structures. Similar condition may involve the proximal bronchi. It may be congenital associated with syndromes such as cystic fibrosis or even result from chronic inflammation, chronic extrinsic compression, or prior intubation.[21] The characteristic clinical presentation is of an expiratory wheeze. Various causes of tracheomalacia are shown in **Table 4**.

The diagnosis cannot be made on the basis of a single radiograph. Fluoroscopy and typically fiberoptic bronchoscopy can demonstrate the characteristic dynamic collapse of the trachea. Airway fluoroscopy done in a lateral projection is the traditional radiographic method of diagnosing tracheomalacia. However, bronchomalacia is difficult to diagnose on fluoroscopy and dynamic/multiphasic CT/MR imaging are preferred methods for this entity. On a single-phase inspiratory CT, the diagnosis is difficult, although the trachea may demonstrate an abnormal shape being flattened slightly posteriorly in the membranous part **(Figs. 19A to D)**. The diagnostic criteria on imaging are >50% reduction in tracheal/bronchial caliber on expiratory scans. Paired inspiratory-expiratory MDCT/cine MDCT is more sensitive to demonstrate the expiratory collapse and requires the measurement of the area of trachea in both the phases.[22]

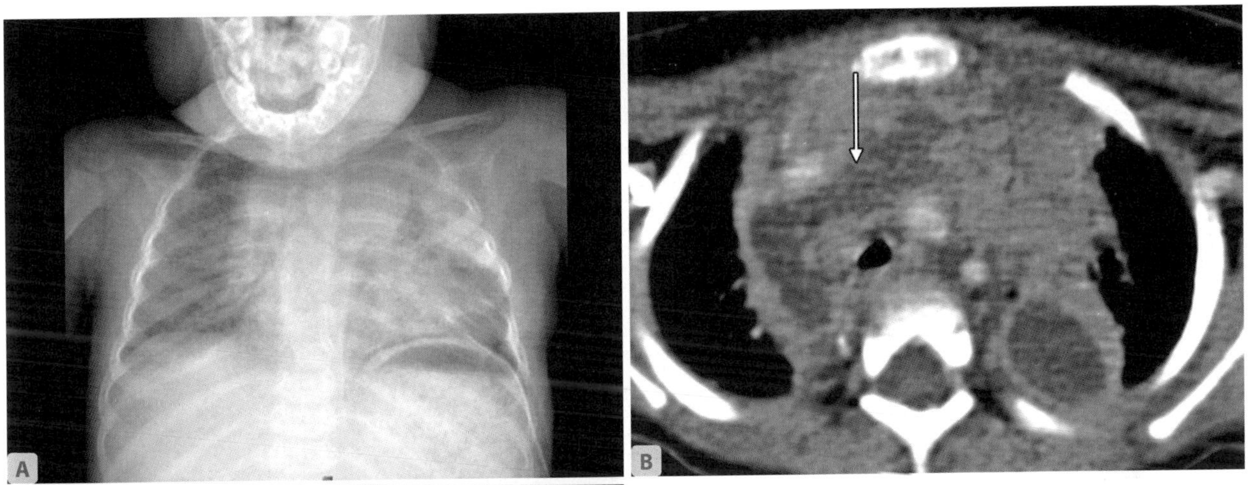

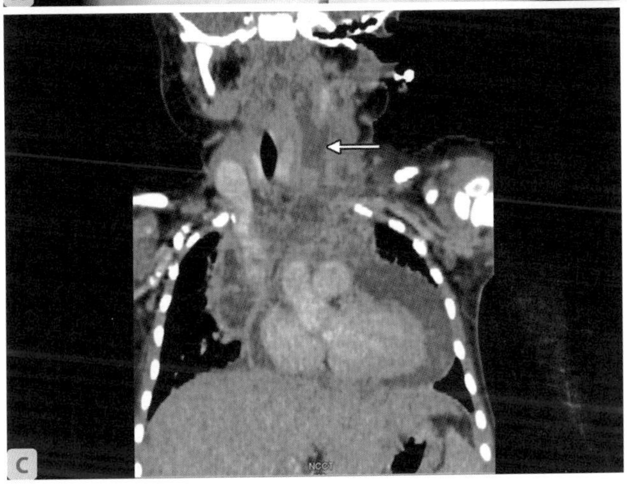

FIGS. 16A TO C: Descending necrotizing mediastinitis: The deep neck space collections extending into the mediastinum causing mild compression on intrathoracic trachea (white arrows).

Stenosis: Fixed tracheal stenosis may be congenital or acquired. Congenital tracheal stenosis results from absence of the membranous portion of the trachea resulting in complete or near complete cartilaginous tracheal rings. The various patterns of tracheal stenosis include generalized stenosis, carrot- or funnel-shaped segmental stenosis, and focal stenosis. Focal stenosis usually involves the lower trachea. A tight focal stenosis causes more severe symptoms than a long, mild stenosis. It may be associated with congenital heart disease, pulmonary sling, tracheoesophageal fistula (TEF), or skeletal abnormalities. On axial imaging, trachea appears as a round or complete circle (O-shaped). Other findings include circumferential narrowing of the entire length of the trachea and fusion of the cartilaginous tracheal rings posteriorly.[23]

Congenital tracheal web is a rare entity. The web is usually not associated with deformity of the tracheal cartilage or the tracheal wall. CT reveals a web-like structure traversing and narrowing the tracheal lumen,[24] which is well-demonstrated on coronal reformatted images and virtual bronchoscopy.

Bronchopulmonary foregut malformations: Bronchopulmonary foregut malformations include a wide spectrum of disorders such as: tracheal agenesis, tracheal stenosis, tracheal fistula, branching anomalies, bronchial stenosis, or lung agenesis and hypoplasia as well as bronchogenic cysts are also included in this group. These anomalies may present with respiratory distress in the newborn, recurrent pulmonary infections, or mass lesions later in life. This chapter deals with anomalies affecting the major bronchi.

Bronchial atresia and sequestration: Bronchial atresia most often involves the left upper lobe. On CT, a mucocele is identified as a hypo- or fluid-attenuating branching structure distal to the atretic bronchus near the hilum. The pulmonary parenchyma distal to the atretic segment is often lucent and demonstrates air trapping. The affected region may even be outlined by pseudo-fissures.

Bronchial atresia may be isolated or associated with a retained systemic vascular connection, when it is referred to as intralobar sequestration. The imaging appearance is virtually identical to that of isolated bronchial atresia, except that the atretic bronchus is ectopically located at the margin of the lung. Rarely, such ectopic bronchi may not be atretic but have a connection with the gastrointestinal tract, usually the esophagus. Such cases are usually accompanied by bronchiectasis and accumulated secretions from impaired clearance of lung parenchyma. It is hence important to look for airway abnormalities, pulmonary parenchymal abnormalities, retained systemic vascular connections, anomalous pulmonary venous drainage, and airway communication with the gastrointestinal tract in patients with suspected bronchopulmonary foregut malformations.[25,26]

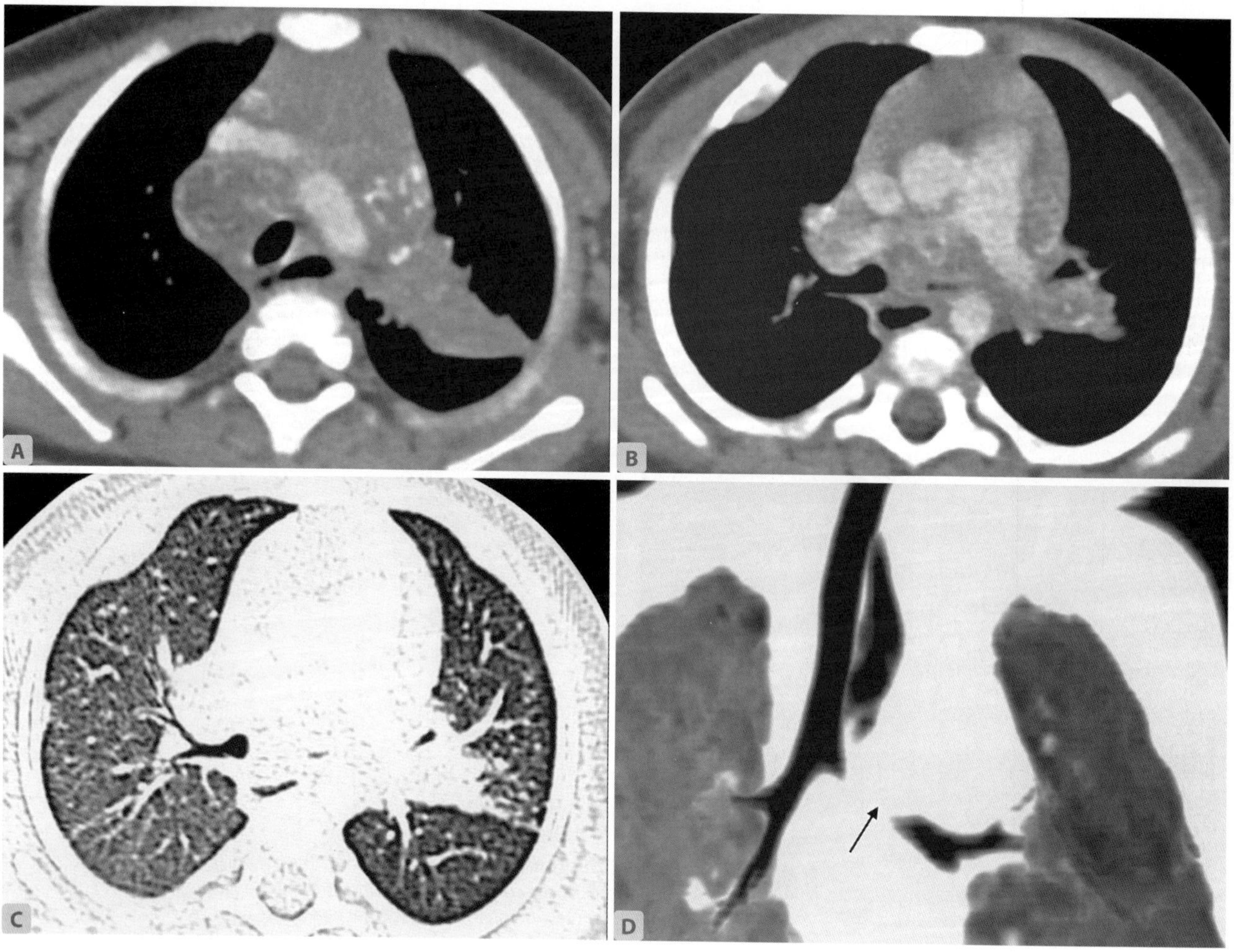

FIGS. 17A TO D: Tubercular lymphadenopathy. (A) CECT of a 6-year-old boy reveals conglomerate, necrotic, and calcific mediastinal lymphadenopathy with left upper lobe consolidation; (B to D) A more caudal section of mediastinal window and lung window and minIP show narrowing of the left main (arrow) and upper lobe bronchi. (CECT: contrast-enhanced computed tomography; minIP: minimium intensity projection)

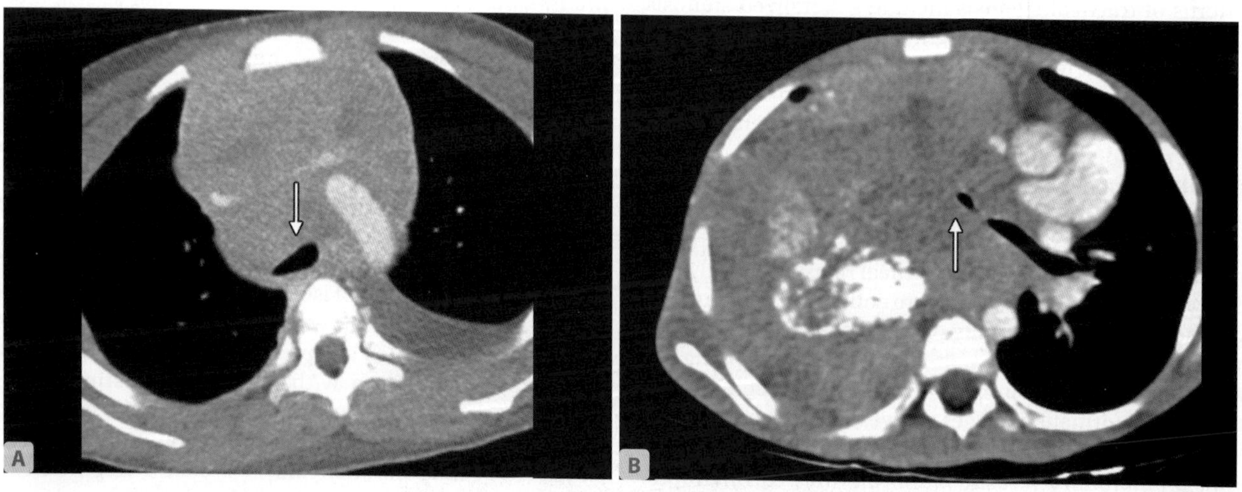

FIGS. 18A AND B: Masses causing airway compromise. (A) Lymphoma: Anterior and middle mediastinal mass causing tracheal compression (white arrow); and (B) Thoracic Neuroblastoma: Contrast-enhanced computed tomography (CECT) showing a large posterior mediastinal mass lesion with calcifications causing displacement and compression of the major bronchi, especially the right main bronchus (white arrow).

Tracheoesophageal fistula: Esophageal atresia with or without TEF is believed to result from a faulty separation of the embryonic trachea and esophageal remnants. The most common type of these is proximal esophageal atresia with distal TEF (up to 80–90%). H-shaped TEFs with no atresia constitute up to 5–8%. Typical clinical presentation includes failure to pass a feeding tube in a newborn with a history of polyhydramnios at prenatal ultrasound, excessive secretions from the mouth, and respiratory distress. Chest radiograph demonstrates the feeding tube catheter ending/coiling in the proximal thoracic esophagus. The presence of air in the distal gastrointestinal tract confirms the presence of a distal TEF. In such patients, it is important to observe the airway as there is frequently associated tracheomalacia.[17] Also, a dilated proximal esophageal pouch can result in airway compression. Patients with H-type fistula may present with recurrent aspiration or small airway disease (SAD). While contrast esophagogram is the investigation of choice, CT scan may demonstrate the fistula **(Figs. 20A and B)**.

TABLE 4: Etiologies of tracheomalacia.

Congenital	Acquired
• Defective cartilage maturation • Most common central airway anomaly	• Degeneration of cartilage • Intubation • Infection • Trauma

Tracheobronchial branching anomalies: Tracheobronchial branching anomalies may be seen as an isolated finding or accompanying heterotaxy syndromes, pulmonary sling, and conditions associated with pulmonary underdevelopment (agenesis, aplasia, or hypoplasia). The most common among these is the tracheal bronchus or "pig bronchus" **(Figs. 21A and B)**. A tracheal bronchus arises from the trachea or mainstem bronchus and aerates either the entire upper lobe or a segment.[27] An accessory cardiac bronchus or tracheal diverticulum is also relatively common anomalies. An accessory cardiac bronchus arises from the medial wall of the right mainstem bronchus or bronchus intermedius, grows toward the pericardium terminating as a blind-ending stump or branching further **(Figs. 21C and D)**. Tracheal diverticula are seen arising with an arrow stalk from

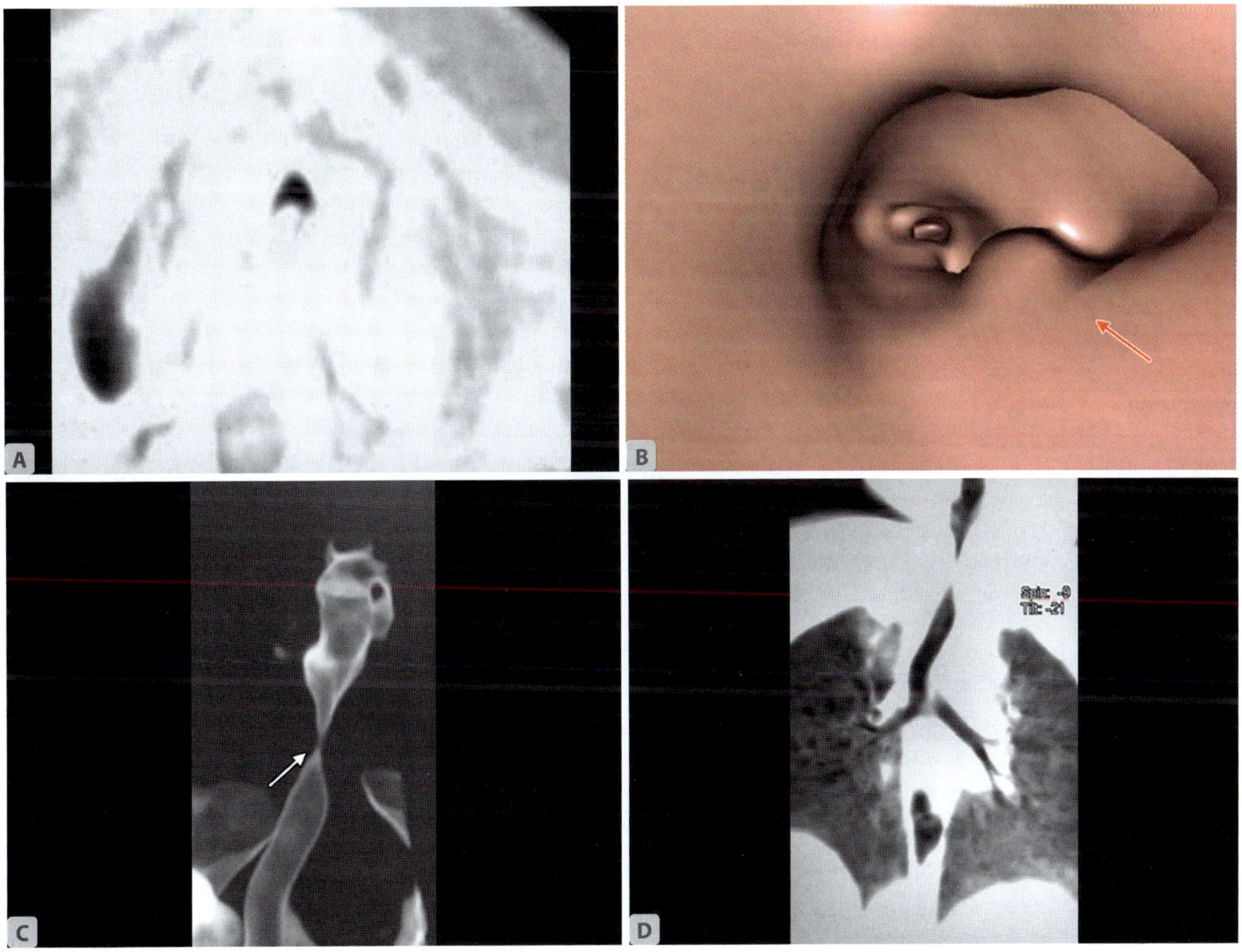

FIGS. 19A TO D: Tracheomalacia: Axial CT (A) and virtual bronchoscopy image (B) of a neonate with stridor showing slight posterior bowing of the trachea. minIP (C) and VRT images (D) show narrowing of subglottic trachea. On bronchoscopy, this narrowing was found to be dynamic. (minIP: minimum intensity projection; VRT: volume rendering technique)

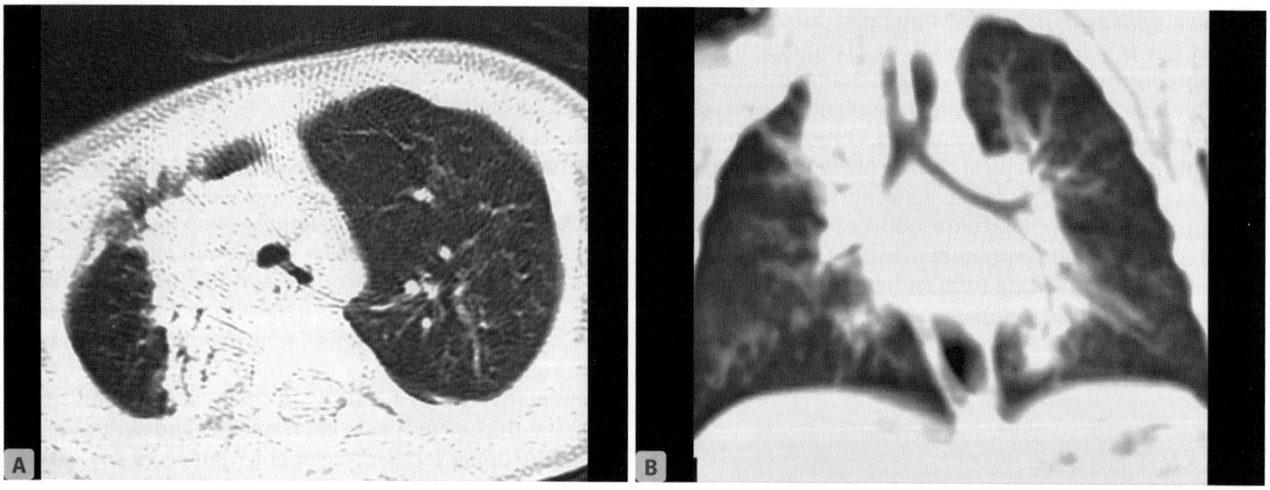

FIGS. 20A AND B: Tracheoesophageal fistula (TEF). (A) Axial CT of an infant reveals a communication between the trachea and esophagus with right upper lobe consolidation; and (B) Coronal multiplanar reformation (MPR) also demonstrates the fistula.

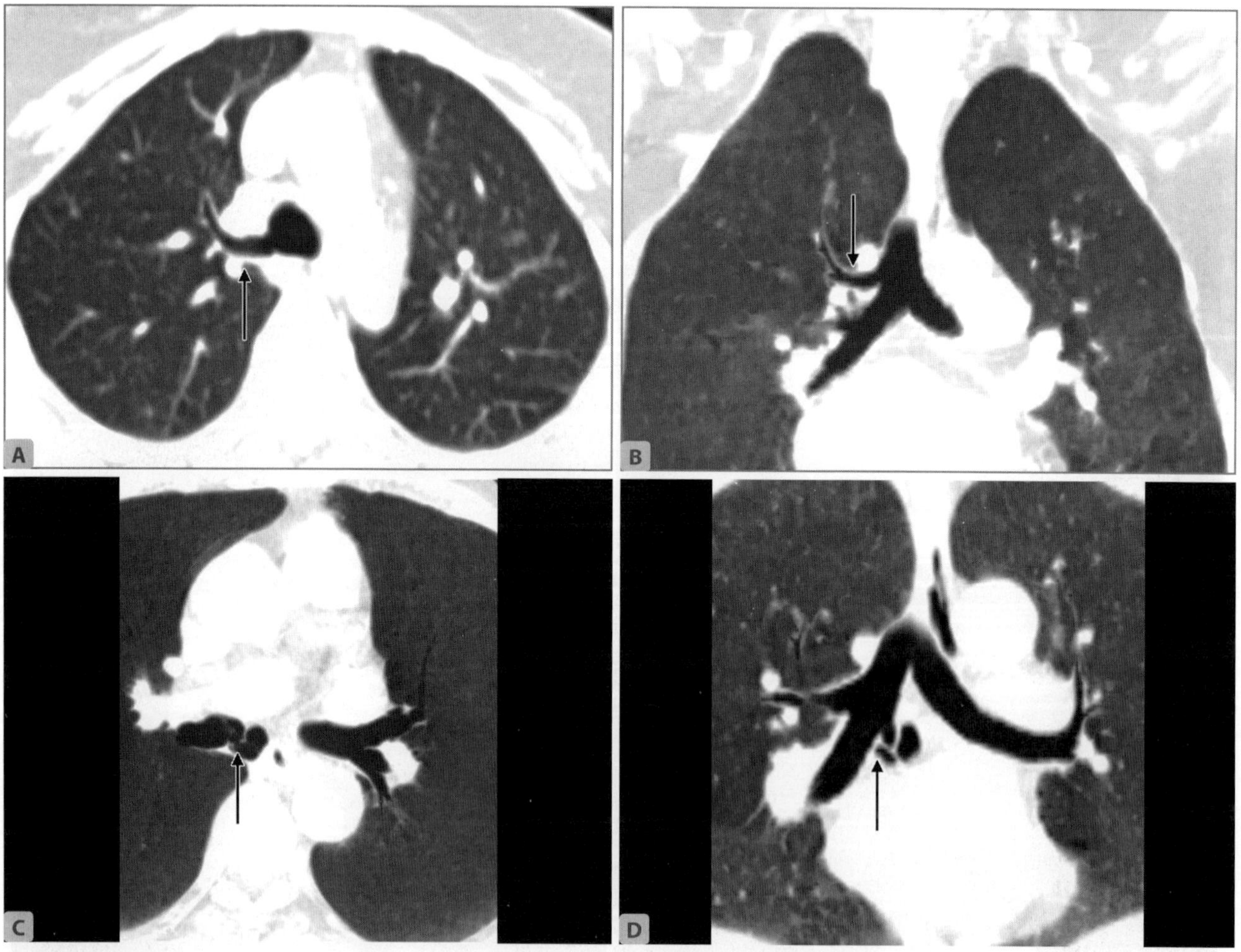

FIGS. 21A TO D: Tracheal bronchus: Axial lung window (A) and coronal minimum intensity projection (minIP) (B) reveal an accessory bronchus arising from the trachea and aerating the posterior segment of right upper lobe (black arrows); and (C and D) Cardiac bronchus: Accessory bronchus arising from the medial wall of the right mainstem bronchus, grows toward the pericardium terminating as a blind-ending stump (black arrows).

the right posterolateral wall of the trachea near the thoracic inlet.[4] Other abnormal branching patterns include tracheal trifurcation, bilateral right-sided isomerism, or bilateral left-sided isomerism. A detailed classification of tracheobronchial branching anomalies has been given in "Imaging of the tracheobronchial tree" in AIIMS-MAMC-PGI Imaging Course Series, Diagnostic Radiology-Chest and Cardiovascular Imaging, 3rd edition.[20] Lobe-based tracheobronchial classification is shown in **Table 5**.[28]

Metabolic conditions: Hunter syndrome (a mucopolysaccharidosis) may cause the deposition of mucopolysaccharides in the walls of the major airways that result in progressive airway narrowing due to wall thickening and anteroposterior collapse.[29]

Acquired: Acquired tracheal or bronchial strictures usually result from chronic inflammation, often tubercular **(Figs. 22A to E)**. Another cause of acquired airway strictures is post-traumatic sequelae.

Intraluminal Causes

The FB is the most common cause of bronchial obstruction. Soft-tissue masses of the trachea and bronchi are rare.

Foreign body: FB aspiration is most often seen in infants and toddlers (8 months–3 years). The bronchi are the most common site of lodgment (76%) while laryngeal (6%) or tracheal

TABLE 5: Lobe-based tracheobronchial classification.

Categories of tuberculosis (TB) anomaly	Entities
Bronchial situs anomalies/ anomalies of entire lung	• Right isomerism • Left isomerism • Situs inversus
Upper lobe	• Tracheal bronchus • Right preeparterial bronchus • Right posteparterial bronchus • Left eparterial bronchus • Left prehyparterial bronchus
Middle lobe	Gross upward displacement of middle lobe bronchus
Lower lobes	Suprasuperior bronchus
Others	• Accessory cardiac bronchus • Types 1 and 2 bridging bronchus

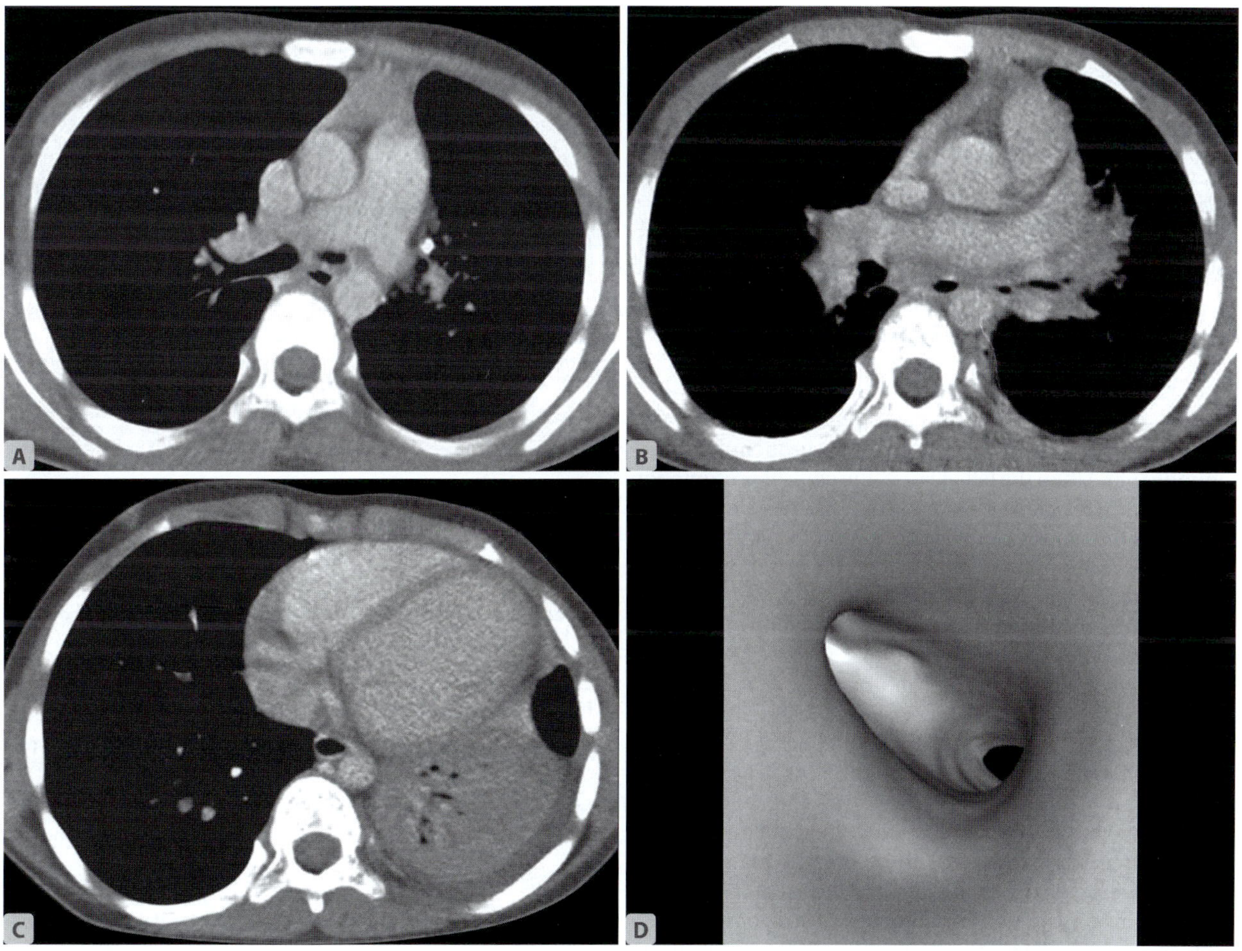

FIGS. 22A TO E: *Continued...*

Continued...

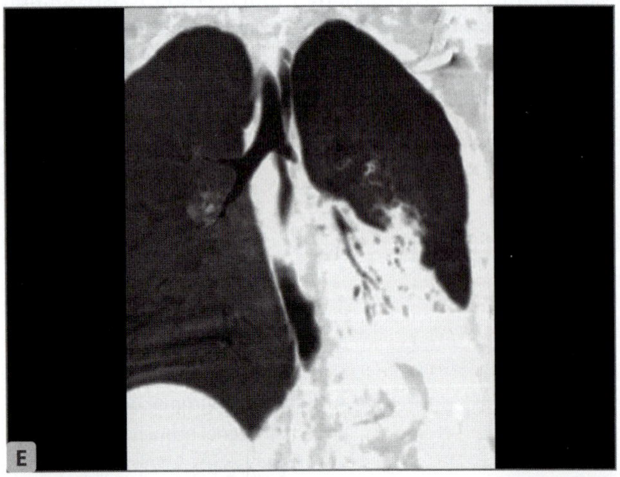

FIGS. 22A TO E: Inflammatory stricture: (A to C) Cranial to caudal CECT sections reveal narrowing of the left main and lower lobe bronchi with ill-defined surrounding soft tissue and collapse of left lower lobe; (D) VB images also confirm the main bronchus stricture with nonvisualization of the distal airway; and (E) Coronal minIP shows a long segment involvement. (CECT: contrast-enhanced computed tomography; minIP: minimum intensity projection)

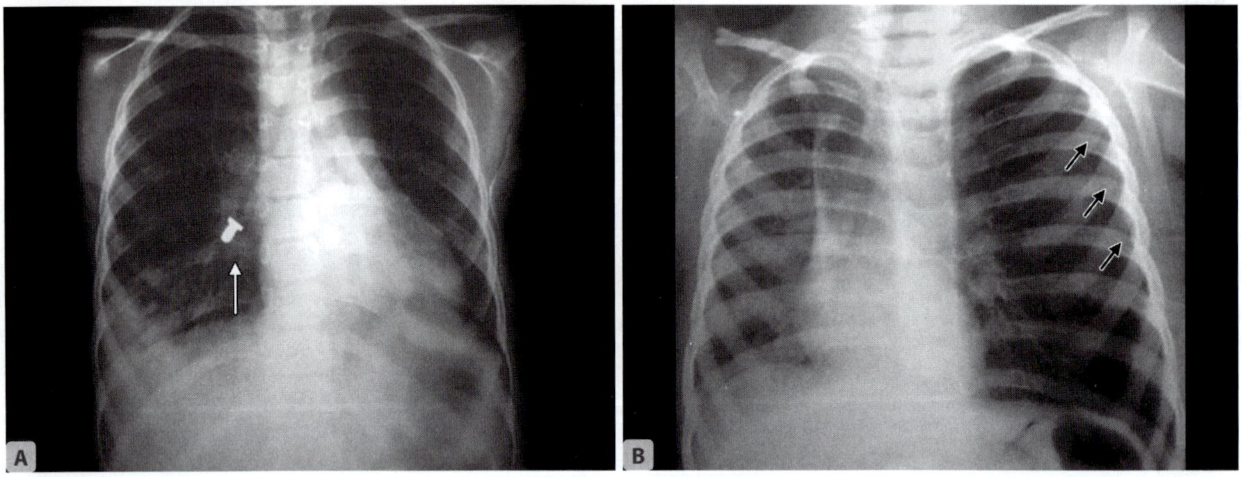

FIGS. 23A AND B: Foreign body. (A) Chest radiograph demonstrates a radiopaque foreign body in the right lower lobe bronchus with consolidation in the distal lung (white arrow); and (B) Chest radiograph of a 2-year-old boy with history of foreign body aspiration and sudden-onset respiratory distress reveals a hyperinflated left lung with spontaneous pneumothorax (short black arrows) and extensive subcutaneous emphysema.

(4%) lodgment is far less common. Right bronchus is more common (58%) than the left (42%).[30] The clinical presentation may be acute while more often the symptoms remain indolent. The symptoms and signs can mimic asthma, upper respiratory infection, or pneumonia. The history of aspiration is often not elicited. FB may lead to partial ("ball-valve" effect) or complete obstruction, resulting in hyperinflation or collapse, respectively. Chest radiograph findings include asymmetric lung aeration, lung consolidation or atelectasis, and even pneumothorax or pneumomediastinum **(Figs. 23A and B)**. Metallic FBs can be identified on plain radiographs (**Fig. 23A** and **Flowchart 2**). However, commonly aspirated airway FBs are food products, particularly nuts and seeds, which are not radiopaque enough to be identified at conventional radiography **(Figs. 24A to D)**. These organic materials can swell following absorption of water and then rapidly change a partial airway obstruction to a complete obstruction.

Inspiratory radiographs alone may be normal in up to a third of patients (14–35%) with FBs. The lung volume of

FLOWCHART 2: Types of foreign body (FB).

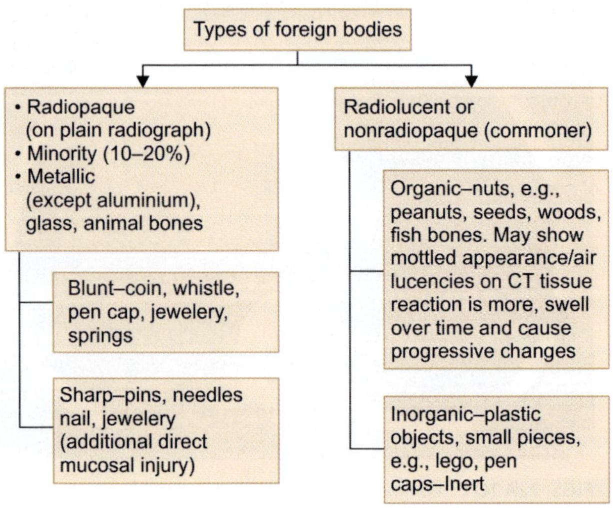

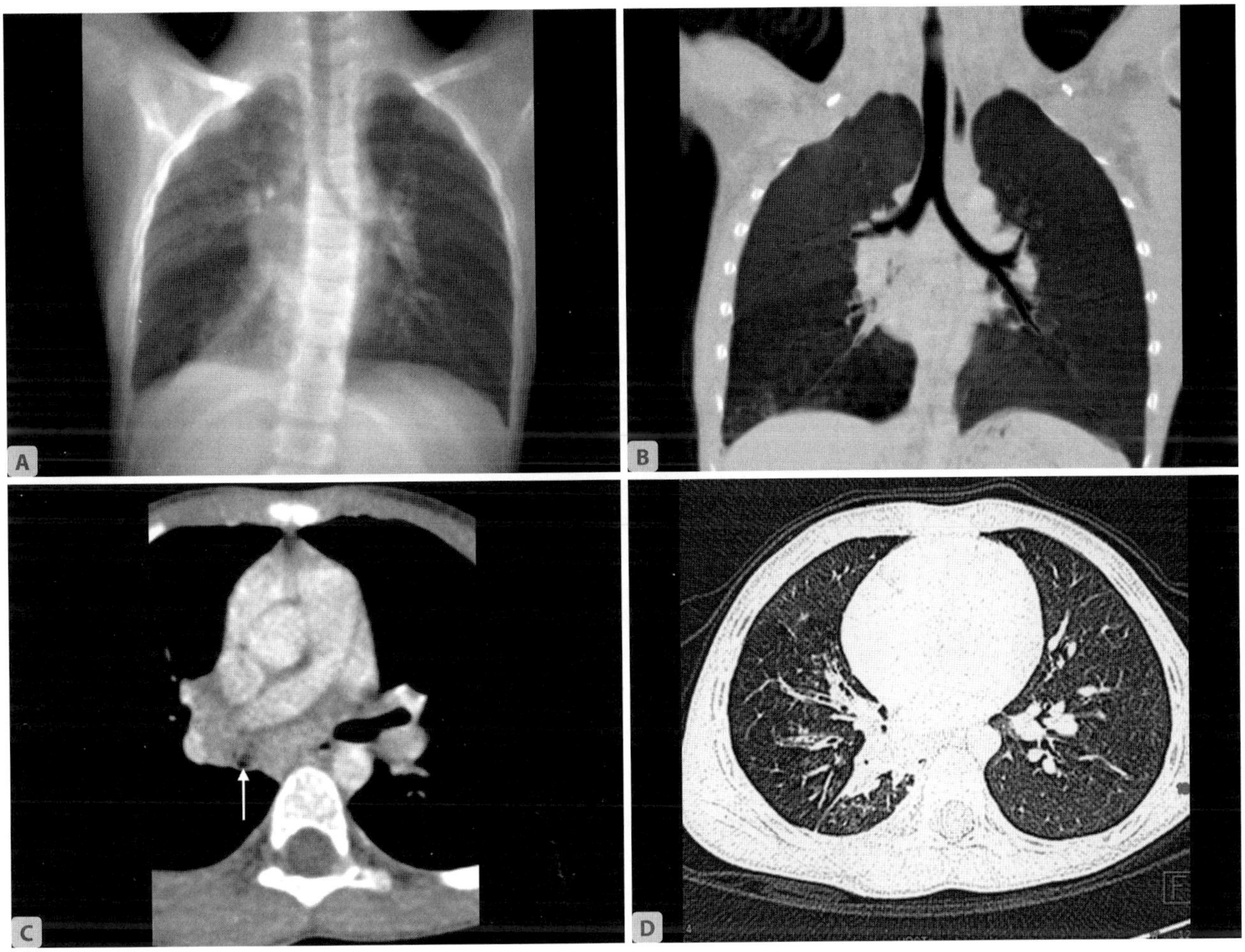

FIGS. 24A TO D: Foreign body. (A) Chest radiograph of a 6-year-old boy with history of recurrent high-grade fever reveals right paracardiac opacities with tram-track lesions; and (B to D) CT scan reveals abrupt cutoff of the right bronchus intermedius with intraluminal contents (white arrow) and distal bronchiectasis. A peanut was removed on bronchoscopy.

the affected lung/segment may be normal, increased, or decreased. Majority (up to 97%) of the FBs are nonradiopaque. The characteristic radiographic finding is that the lung volume remains static with no change in different phases of respiration. This can be demonstrated by obtaining paired inspiratory-expiratory radiographs in cooperative children. In infants and uncooperative children, bilateral decubitus radiographs of the chest or fluoroscopy can demonstrate the same finding. The differential diagnosis of an asymmetric, lucent lung includes Swyer–James syndrome and pulmonary hypoplasia. However, air trapping may be seen in partial obstruction.

Computed tomography is not routinely advocated in evaluation of a bronchial FB. It may, however, be performed as workup for nonresolving pneumonia or collapse or even stridor **(Figs. 24A to D)**.[31] CT is also a good option when the clinical setting does not strongly warrant bronchoscopy or if bronchoscopy is not readily available. On CT, FBs are well-demonstrated as filling defects in the bronchus, besides detailing the changes in the distal lung. It can identify both opaque and nonopaque FBs. Kosucu et al. reported a 100% sensitivity and specificity of CT in the evaluation of endobronchial FBs.[32] Applegate et al. while evaluating low-dose helical CT found a sensitivity of 83% and specificity of 89% for visualizing plastic pieces in the airway. Peanuts, however, were not well-visualized in the same study.[33] Indirect findings of FB in TB tree are described in **Table 6**. Even esophageal FBs can present acutely with symptoms related to airway compression or with complications consequent to perforation and neck and/or mediastinal infection **(Flowchart 3)**.

Mucous plugs: Mucous plugs are another cause of intraluminal airway obstruction and result from inspissation of bronchial secretion. Compared to adults, these are infrequent in children, but can be encountered in those with impaired cough reflex, cystic fibrosis, primary ciliary dyskinesia, or asthma. The most common site of impaction is the major bronchi and an acute presentation is more common than chronic one.

On imaging, mucous plugs appear very similar to an organic FB, i.e., both have low attenuation and may display trapped air foci or a strand-like linear pattern. The secondary causes of obstruction are also seen; however, atelectasis

TABLE 6: Indirect findings of FB in TB tree.

Complications	Imaging findings
• Hyperinflation/air trapping (due to ball-valve mechanism of obstruction) • Most common	• Seen in both acute/chronic FB aspiration • Unilateral/segmental/bilateral (in tracheal FB) • Involved lung increased in volume • Fixity of volume on dynamic or multiphasic imaging (fluoroscopy, inspiratory-expiratory, or decubitus imaging) • Limited diaphragmatic excursion • Hyperlucent lung (due to air and resultant oligemia) • Mediastinal shift ±
• Atelectasis • Postobstructive pneumonia • Seen in about one-fourth of cases	• More frequent in chronic or delayed presentation • Increase lung density with volume loss • Air bronchogram may be present in early cases or partial obstruction • "Shifting atelectasis" if FB migrates
Combination of hyperinflation and atelectasis in same hemithorax	• As lung adjacent to atelectasis will hyperinflate • Nonspecific, seen in any airway obstruction
Bronchiectasis	In delayed/chronic presentation
Air leaks: • Pneumothorax • Pneumomediastinum • Subcutaneous emphysema • Epidural emphysema (pneumorrhachis)—very rare	• Rare • Due to rupture of alveoli as intrathoracic pressure increases • ven more rarely due to direct perforation of TB tree (sharp objects)

(FB: foreign body; TB: tuberculosis)

FLOWCHART 3: Imaging algorithm for suspected foreign body (FB) in airway.

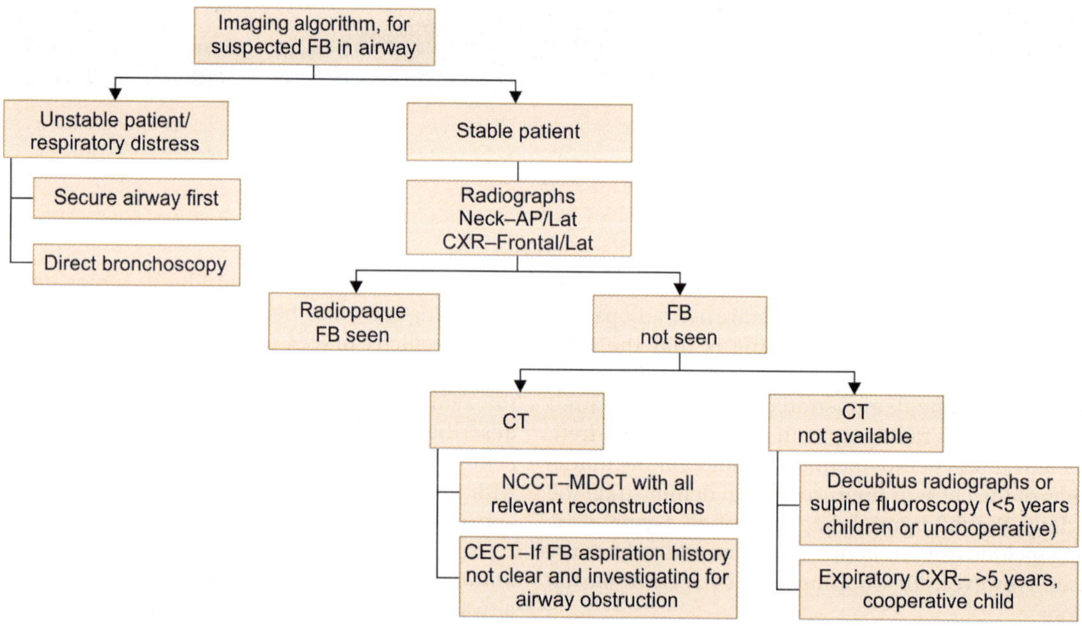

(AP: anteroposterior; CECT: contrast-enhanced computed tomography; CXR: chest X-ray; MDCT: multidetector computed tomography; NCCT: noncontrast-enhanced computed tomography)

and postobstructive pneumonia are far more common with mucous plugs; unlike air trapping is more frequent in FB.[34]

Inflammatory

Tuberculosis: Occasionally, enlarged lymph nodes erode into the bronchus and result in endobronchial fibrosis or luminal occlusion. Intraluminal granulomas may occur in the trachea or bronchi. Airway involvement in tuberculosis may be seen in up to 30% of cases.[35,36]

Tumors: Tracheal soft-tissue masses include tracheal papilloma while bronchial masses may be carcinoid tumors. Carcinoid tumor is the most common among these. Rare lesions include adenoid cystic carcinoma, mucoepidermoid carcinoma, inflammatory myofibroblastic tumor, juvenile xanthogranuloma, and metastasis.[37,38]

Carcinoid tumors comprise about 80% of endobronchial neoplasms in children and adolescents. These present in children or young adults and may be associated with neuroendocrine secretion. Most carcinoid tumors occur in the mainstem or lobar bronchi and patients present with dyspnea, wheezing, cough, or hemoptysis. CT reveals typically intensely enhancing, ovoid lesions with a long axis parallel to the bronchovascular bundle. These lesions may have intraluminal, mural, and extrabronchial components. Associated collapse, consolidation, or air trapping is often seen **(Figs. 25A to C)**. They are relatively slow growing masses and complete surgical resection offers the best chance of cure.

Peripheral Airways

Small airway diseases such as asthma and bronchiolitis are more common than central causes of obstruction.

Small Airway Disease/Bronchiolitis

Small airway diseases refer to term for disorders affecting peripheral airways with no wall cartilage, typically including terminal and respiratory bronchioles.[39]

Acute

Acute inflammation of the bronchi and bronchioles is common in children and is most often infective in etiology. Plain radiographs reveal hyperinflation with increased perihilar markings. This entity is covered in detail in the chapter on Pulmonary Infections.

Chronic

The causes of chronic, SAD in children include: constrictive bronchiolitis, extrinsic allergic bronchiolitis, diffuse panbronchiolitis, follicular bronchiolitis, and lung disease of prematurity. The chest radiograph and even CT findings are often nonspecific, though the underlying etiologies may be quite variable. CT scan reveals ground-glass opacities with mosaic attenuation and air trapping. Mild bronchiectasis with bronchial wall thickening may be seen.

Constrictive Bronchiolitis

Although constrictive bronchiolitis may present as a unilateral hyperlucent lung (Swyer-James syndrome), it is more often bilateral. There are several causes of this entity including infection (viral or mycoplasma), toxic and fume exposure, collagen vascular diseases such as rheumatoid arthritis, and complication of bone marrow or heart-lung transplant.[40]

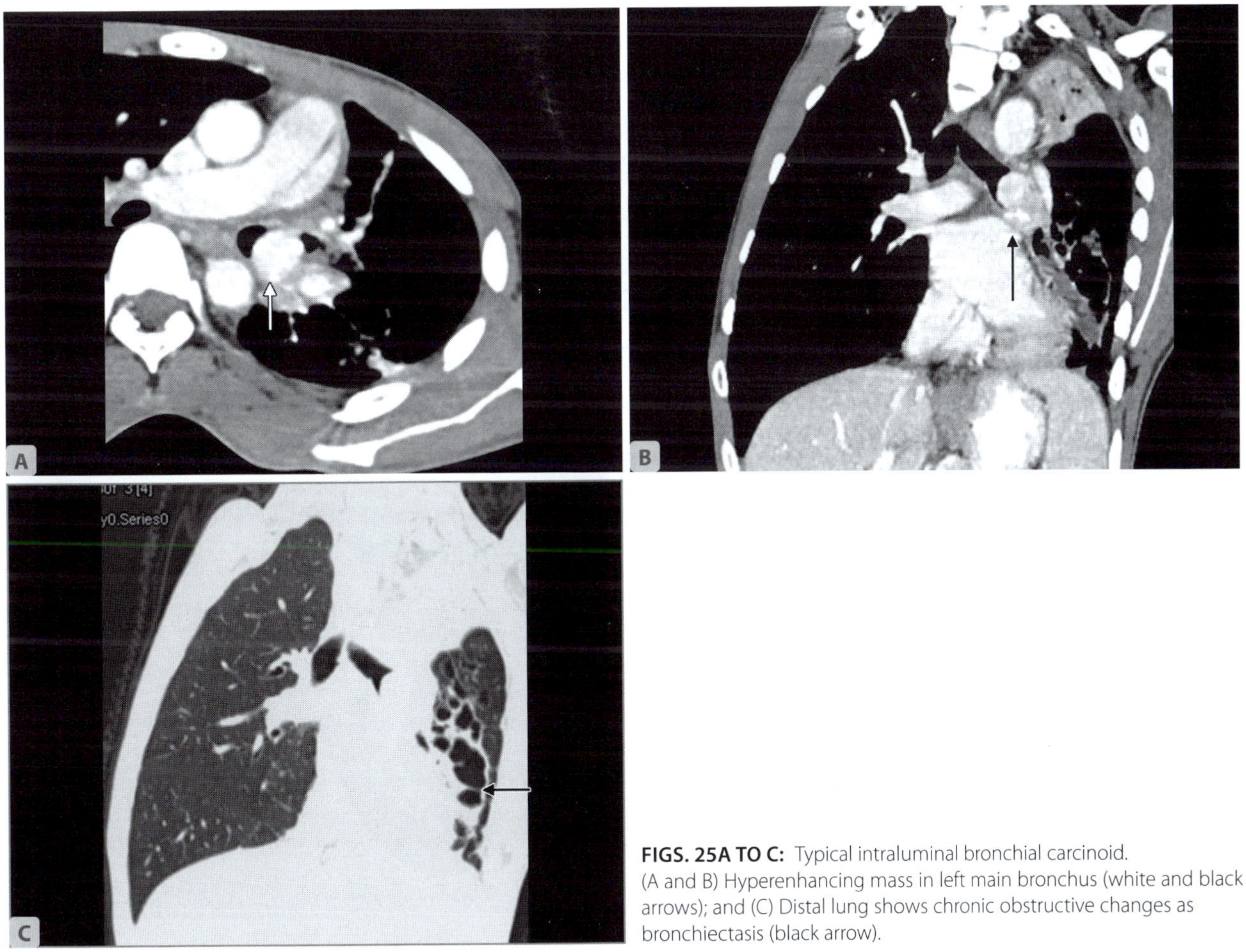

FIGS. 25A TO C: Typical intraluminal bronchial carcinoid. (A and B) Hyperenhancing mass in left main bronchus (white and black arrows); and (C) Distal lung shows chronic obstructive changes as bronchiectasis (black arrow).

HRCT reveals a prominent mosaic attenuation with bronchial abnormalities including bronchiectasis and air trapping (**Figs. 26A** and **B**). The pattern is similar to severe asthma or cystic fibrosis.

Hypersensitivity Pneumonitis

Hypersensitivity pneumonitis is characterized by peribronchial cellular infiltration, developed in response to an antigen exposure. In the acute stage, CT reveals multiple, ill-defined centrilobular nodules while in the subacute or chronic stage, mosaic alternation with expiratory air trapping is seen **(Figs. 27A and B)**. Areas of fibrosis may also be present.

Follicular Bronchiolitis

Follicular bronchiolitis is the second major form of SAD characterized by centrilobular nodules and a bronchial wall thickening. It is a lymphoproliferative disorder with multiple etiologies, e.g., immunodeficiencies and connective tissue diseases.

Diffuse Panbronchiolitis

Diffuse panbronchiolitis is an exudative form of bronchiolitis seen in Eastern and Southeastern Asia. CT reveals multiple small centrilobular nodules and linear opacities diffusely distributed in both the lungs.

Lung Disease of Prematurity

This is a unique form of airway disease seen in premature infants with bronchopulmonary dysplasia. It is a destructive diffuse lung disease occurring in a background of rapid alveolar growth. CT helps in excluding other causes of chronic respiratory distress such as central airway lesions.

Bronchiectasis

Bronchiectasis is a common cause of respiratory symptoms in children. It is often the result of chronic inflammation causing damage to the supporting structure of the airways. Also,

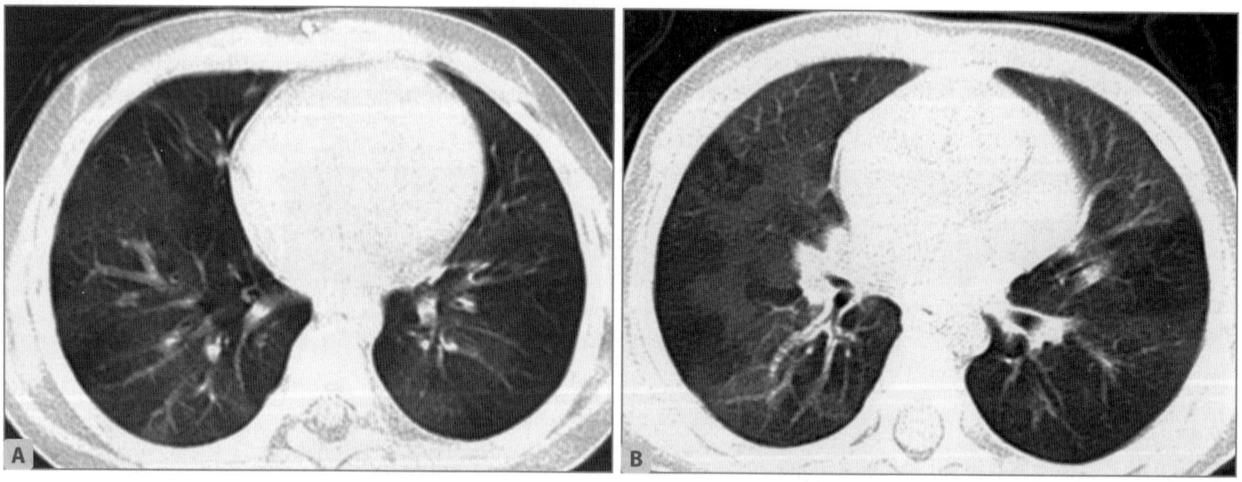

FIGS. 26A AND B: Constrictive bronchiolitis. (A and B) Axial CT lung window of a 4-year-old boy with history of dyspnea reveals prominent mosaic attenuation with air trapping in both lungs.

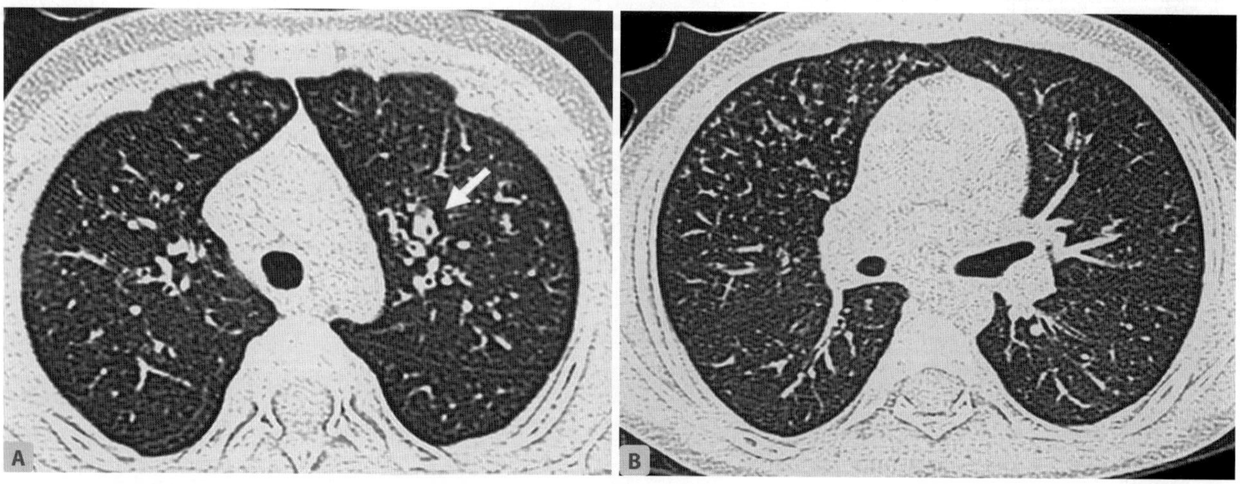

FIGS. 27A AND B: Chronic bronchiolitis. (A and B) High-resolution computed tomography (HRCT) of an 8-year-old child reveals multiple, ill-defined centrilobular nodules and bronchial wall thickening (arrow).

chronic or recurrent inflammation due to immunodeficiency states may cause bronchiectasis. Other etiologies include abnormal mucus as in cystic fibrosis and abnormal mucociliary clearance in children with ciliary dyskinesias **(Figs. 28A and B)**.[41] Proximal bronchial obstruction due to an intrinsic or extrinsic cause may also lead to bronchiectasis in the distal lung. Aspiration secondary to gastroesophageal reflux due to its chronic, recurrent nature has also been postulated as a cause of bronchiectasis.

Patients typically present with recurrent infections. Chest radiographs are relatively insensitive in detecting early changes, with HRCT being the imaging modality of choice. Chest radiographs reveal multiple cystic, ring or tram-track lucencies with bronchial wall thickening. In case of secondary infection, mucous plugging, air-fluid levels, bronchial wall thickening, and even enlarged draining nodes may be seen[42] **(Figs. 28 and 29)**.

Asthma/Reactive Airway Disease

The terms are used for reversible recurrent airway obstruction resulting from hyperresponsive airways with triggers being environmental or even emotional. The term reactive airway disease is employed in younger children (2–6 years age typically). The peak age of prevalence of asthma in children is 6–11 years, with a male predominance. Up to 30% of these persist into adulthood. Chest radiographs are usually normal and are indicated in case of poor response to therapy, suspected complications, or suspicion of an alternate diagnosis. Radiographs reveal hyperlucency of lungs or foci of atelectasis. The differential diagnosis includes viral bronchiolitis. CT is seldom indicated in asthma and reveals nonspecific findings of SAD **(Figs. 30A and B)**.[43] Findings of secondary allergic bronchopulmonary aspergillosis (ABPA) may be seen **(Fig. 31)**.

Complications are more frequent in younger children as their bronchi are smaller and more easily occluded in an exacerbation. Complications include: lobar collapse, segmental or subsegmental atelectasis, pneumonia, and air leaks [pneumomediastinum, subcutaneous emphysema, and rarely pneumothorax or pulmonary interstitial emphysema (PIE)].

In conclusion, it is critical to evaluate the airway in all children presenting with acute, chronic, or recurrent respiratory symptoms. Multiphasic imaging is essential. Plain radiographs and fluoroscopy form the initial methods of evaluation, with CT being required often for a complete diagnosis.

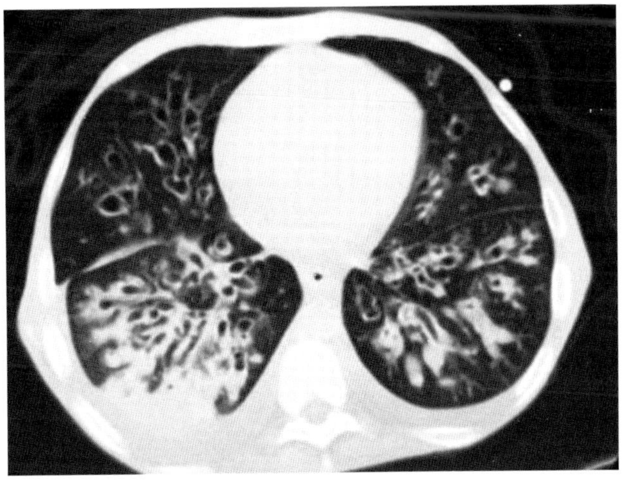

FIG. 29: Bronchiectasis: CT shows tubular bronchiectasis in bilateral lungs with bronchial wall thickening and mucus plugging in a child with secondary infection.

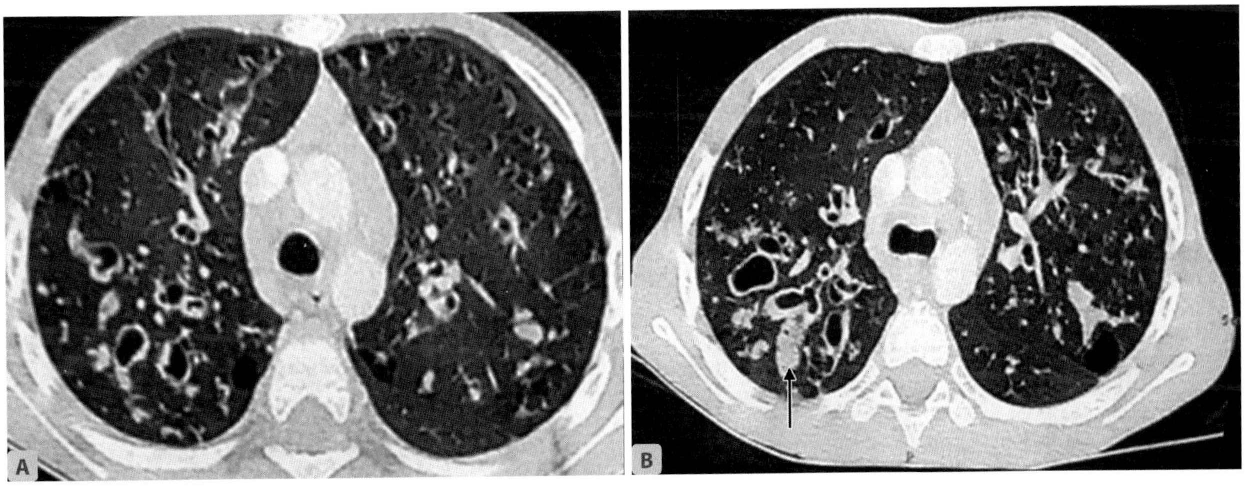

FIGS. 28A AND B: Cystic fibrosis: CT reveals areas of bronchiectasis, bronchial wall thickening, air trapping, and mucus plugging (black arrow).

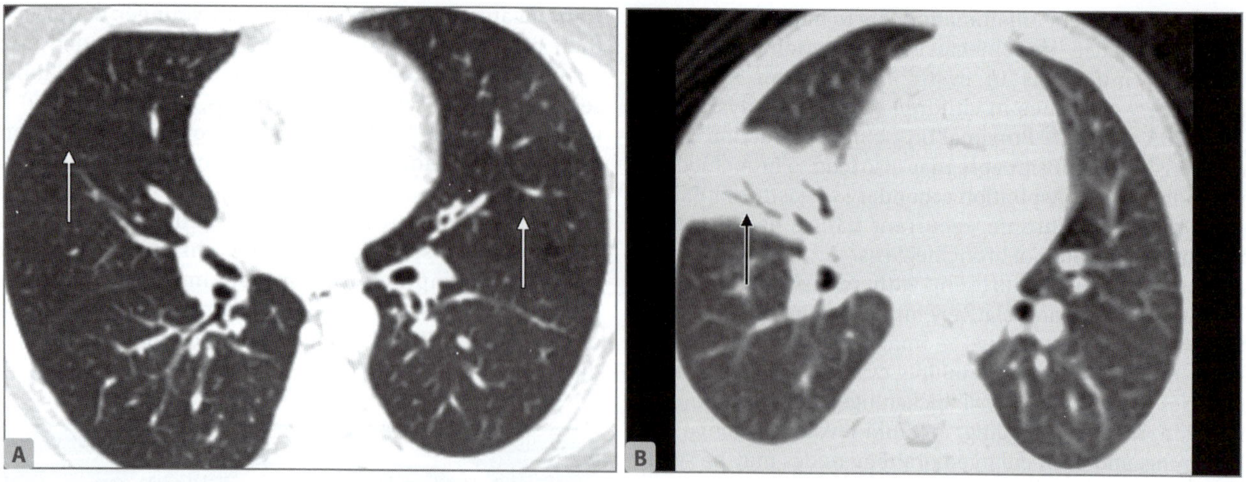

FIGS. 30A AND B: Asthma in two different patients: (A) CT showing multiple subtle areas of air trapping in both lungs (white arrows); and (B) Another child with asthma showing right middle lobe collapse (common site of atelectasis in asthmatics) (black arrow).

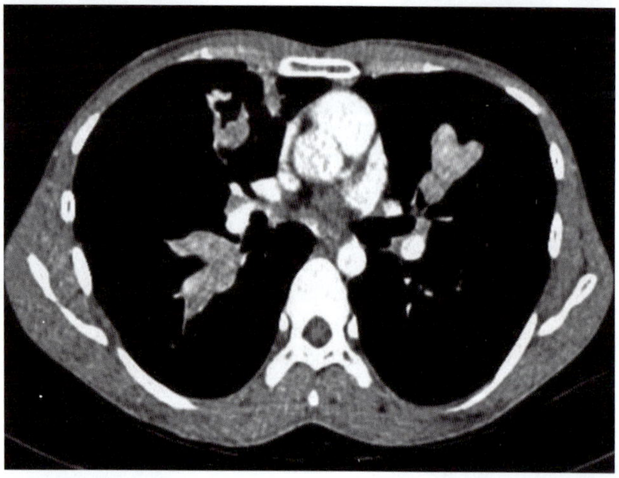

FIG. 31: Allergic bronchopulmonary aspergillosis (ABPA): A 16-year-old asthmatic boy showing multiple bilateral tubular bronchiectasis with bronchoceles giving a "finger-in-glove" appearance.

REFERENCES

1. Long FR. Imaging evolution of airway disorders in children. Radiol Clin North Am. 2005;43(2):371-89.
2. Yedururi S, Guillerman RP, Chung T, Braverman RM, Dishop MK, Giannoni CM, et al. Multimodality imaging of tracheobronchial disorders in children. Radiographics. 2008;28(3):e29.
3. Donnelly LF. Airway. In: Donnelly LF (Ed). Diagnostic Imaging Pediatrics. USA: Amirsys; 2005.
4. Donnelly LF. Airway. In: Donnelly LF (Ed). Fundamentals of Pediatric Radiology. Philadelphia: Saunders; 2001.
5. Sundarakumar DK, Bhalla AS, Sharma R, Hari S, Guleria R, Khilnani GC. Multidetector CT evaluation of central airways stenoses: Comparison of virtual bronchoscopy, minimal-intensity projection, and multiplanar reformatted images. Indian J Radiol Imaging. 2011;21(3):191-4.
6. Westra SJ. High-pitch CT, decreasing need for sedation and its potential side effects: some practical considerations and future directions. Pediatr Radiol. 2019;49(1):297-300.
7. Andronikou S, Chopra M, Langton-Hewer S, Maier P, Green J, Norbury E, et al. Technique, pitfalls, quality, radiation dose and findings of dynamic 4-dimensional computed tomography for airway imaging in infants and children. Pediatr Radiol. 2019;49(5):678-86.
8. Gottumukkala RV, Kalra MK, Tabari A, Otrakji A, Gee MS. Advanced CT Techniques for Decreasing Radiation Dose, Reducing Sedation Requirements, and Optimizing Image Quality in Children. Radiographics. 2019;39(3):709-26.
9. Donnelly LF. Obstructive sleep apnea in pediatric patients: evaluation with cine MR sleep studies. Radiology. 2005;236(3):768-78.
10. Suto Y, Tanabe Y. Evaluation of tracheal collapsibility in patients with tracheomalacia using dynamic MR imaging during coughing. AJR Am J Roentgenol. 1998;171(2):393-4.
11. Faust RA, Remley KB, Rimell FL. Real-time, cine magnetic resonance imaging for evaluation of the pediatric airway. Laryngoscope. 2001;111(12):2187-90.

12. Bates AJ, Higano NS, Hysinger EB, Fleck RJ, Hahn AD, Fain SB, et al. Quantitative Assessment of Regional Dynamic Airway Collapse in Neonates via Retrospectively Respiratory-Gated (1) H Ultrashort Echo Time MRI. J Magn Reson Imaging. 2019;49(3):659-67.
13. Andersen IG, Holm JC, Homøe P. Obstructive sleep apnea in obese children and adolescents, treatment methods and outcome of treatment—a systematic review. Int J Pediatr Otorhinolaryngol. 2016;87(2):190-7.
14. John SD, Swischuk LE. Stridor and upper airway obstruction in infants and children. Radiographics. 1992;12(4):625-43.
15. Bitar MA, Moukarbel RV, Zalzal GH. Management of congenital subglottic hemangioma: trends and success over the past 17 years. Otolaryngol Head Neck Surg. 2005;132(2):226-31.
16. Choo KS, Lee HD, Ban JE, Sung SC, Chang YH, Kim CW, et al. Evaluation of obstructive airway lesions in complex congenital heart disease using composite volume-rendered images from multislice CT. Pediatr Radiol. 2006;36(3):219-23.
17. Dillman JR, Attili AK, Agarwal PP, Dorfman AL, Hernandez RJ, Strouse PJ. Common and uncommon vascular rings and slings: a multi-modality review. Pediatr Radiol. 2011;41(11):1440-54.
18. Kellenberger CJ. Aortic arch malformations. Pediatr Radiol. 2010;40(6):876-84.
19. Lee KH, Yoon CS, Choe KO, Kim MJ, Lee HM, Yoon HK, et al. Use of imaging for assessing anatomical relationships of tracheobronchial anomalies associated with left pulmonary artery sling. Pediatr Radiol. 2001;31(4):269-78.
20. Backer CL, Mongé MC, Popescu AR, Eltayeb OM, Rastatter JC, Rigsby CK. Vascular rings. Semin Pediatr Surg. 2016;25(3):165-75.
21. Fraga JC, Jennings RW, Kim PC. Pediatric tracheomalacia. Semin Pediatr Surg. 2016;25(3):156-64.
22. Douros K, Kremmydas G, Grammeniatis V, Papadopoulos M, Priftis KN, Alexopoulou E. Helical multi-detector CT scan as a tool for diagnosing tracheomalacia in children. Pediatr Pulmonol. 2019;54(1):47-52.
23. Berrocal T, Madrid C, Novo S, Gutiérrez J, Arjonilla A, Gómez-León N. Congenital anomalies of the tracheobronchial tree, lung, and mediastinum: embryology, radiology, and pathology. Radiographics. 2004;24(1):e17.
24. Legasto AC, Haller JO, Giusti RJ. Tracheal web. Pediatr Radiol. 2004;34(3):256-8.
25. Newman B. Congenital bronchopulmonary foregut malformations: concepts and controversies. Pediatr Radiol. 2006;36(8):773-91.
26. Yang G, Chen L, Xu C, Yuan M, Li Y. Congenital bronchopulmonary foregut malformation: systematic review of the literature. BMC Pediatr. 2019;19(1):305.
27. Ghaye B, Szapiro D, Fanchamps JM, Dondelinger RF. Congenital bronchial abnormalities revisited. Radiographics. 2001;21(1): 105-19.
28. Chassagnon G, Morel B, Carpentier E, Ducou Le Pointe H, Sirinelli D. Tracheobronchial Branching Abnormalities: Lobe-based Classification Scheme. Radiographics. 2016;36(2):358-73.
29. Davitt SM, Hatrick A, Sabharwal T, Pearce A, Gleeson M, Adam A. Tracheobronchial stent insertions in the management of major airway obstruction in a patient with Hunter syndrome (type-II mucopolysaccharidosis). Eur Radiol. 2002;12(2):458-62.
30. Hegde SV, Hui PK, Lee EY. Tracheobronchial foreign bodies in children: imaging assessment. Semin Ultrasound CT MR. 2015;36(1):8-20.
31. Laya BF, Restrepo R, Lee EY. Practical Imaging Evaluation of Foreign Bodies in Children: An Update. Radiol Clin North Am. 2017;55(4):845-67.
32. Koşucu P, Ahmetoğlu A, Koramaz I, Orhan F, Ozdemir O, Dinç H, et al. Low-dose MDCT and virtual bronchoscopy in pediatric patients with foreign body aspiration. AJR Am J Roentgenol. 2004;183(6):1771-7.
33. Applegate KE, Dardinger JT, Lieber ML, Herts BR, Davros WJ, Obuchowski NA, et al. Spiral CT scanning technique in the detection of aspiration of LEGO foreign bodies. Pediatr Radiol. 2001;31(12):836-40.
34. Hong WS, Im SA, Kim HL, Yoon JS. CT evaluation of airway foreign bodies in children: emphasis on the delayed diagnosis and differentiation from airway mucus plugs. Jpn J Radiol. 2013;31(1):31-8.
35. Goussard P, Gie R. Airway involvement in pulmonary tuberculosis. Paediatr Respir Rev. 2007;8(2):118-23.
36. Goussard P, Gie RP, Kling S, Andronikou S, Lucas S, Janson J, et al. Bronchoscopic assessment of airway involvement in children presenting with clinically significant airway obstruction due to tuberculosis. Pediatr Pulmonol. 2013;48(10):1000-7.
37. Curtis JM, Lacey D, Smyth R, Carty H. Endobronchial tumours in childhood. Eur J Radiol. 1998;29(1):11-20.
38. Eyssartier E, Ang P, Bonnemaison E, Gibertini I, Diot P, Carpentier E, et al. Characteristics of endobronchial primitive tumors in children. Pediatr Pulmonol. 2014;49(6):E121-5.
39. Kothari NA, Kramer SS. Bronchial diseases and lung aeration in children. J Thorac Imaging. 2001;16(4):207-23.
40. Yu J. Postinfectious bronchiolitis obliterans in children: lessons from bronchiolitis obliterans after lung transplantation and hematopoietic stem cell transplantation. Korean J Pediatr. 2015;58(12):459-65.
41. Chang AB, Bush A, Grimwood K. Bronchiectasis in children: diagnosis and treatment. Lancet. 2018;392(10150):866-79.
42. Singh A, Bhalla AS, Jana M. Bronchiectasis Revisited: Imaging-Based Pattern Approach to Diagnosis. Curr Probl Diagn Radiol. 2019;48(1):53-60.
43. Richards JC, Lynch D, Koelsch T, Dyer D. Imaging of Asthma. Immunol Allergy Clin North Am. 2016;36(3):529-45.

CHAPTER 66

Pediatric Interstitial Lung Diseases

Priyanka Naranje, Ashu Seith Bhalla, Manisha Jana

TERMINOLOGY AND BACKGROUND

Pediatric interstitial lung diseases (ILD) are not only less frequently encountered compared to adults; but also are less understood and reported. An understanding of the basic forms is required before embarking on discussion of the individual causes.

Interstitial lung diseases is a broad term referring to disorders that affect the pulmonary interstitium and affect the distal airspaces resulting in impairment of gas exchange.[1]

Diffuse lung diseases (DLDs): Since all disorders categorized as ILD do not necessarily involve only interstitium but also predominantly affect airspaces, the term DLD is often preferred. No term is perfect as all ILDs are not diffuse in distribution.[1]

Childhood interstitial lung disease (ChILD) syndrome: This term refers to a clinical syndrome, employed when an infant <2 years of age, meets two of the four following criteria.[1]

1. Respiratory symptom such as cough and breathing difficulty.
2. Respiratory signs such as tachypnea, retractions, or adventitious sounds.
3. Hypoxemia
4. Diffuse lung diseases on chest X-ray (CXR) or computed tomography (CT).

The term is used after excluding common disorders **(Flowchart 1)**.

CLASSIFICATION[1]

The classification of chILD was given by the American Thoracic Society (Kurland G et al.[1] and essentially divides it into two major groups).

I. Diseases More Prevalent in Infancy

These can be divided into four major subgroups.

A. Diffuse developmental disorders
B. Lung growth abnormalities
C. Specific conditions of undefined etiology
D. Surfactant mutation and associated disorders

FLOWCHART 1: Terminologies in pediatric diffuse lung diseases (DLDs).

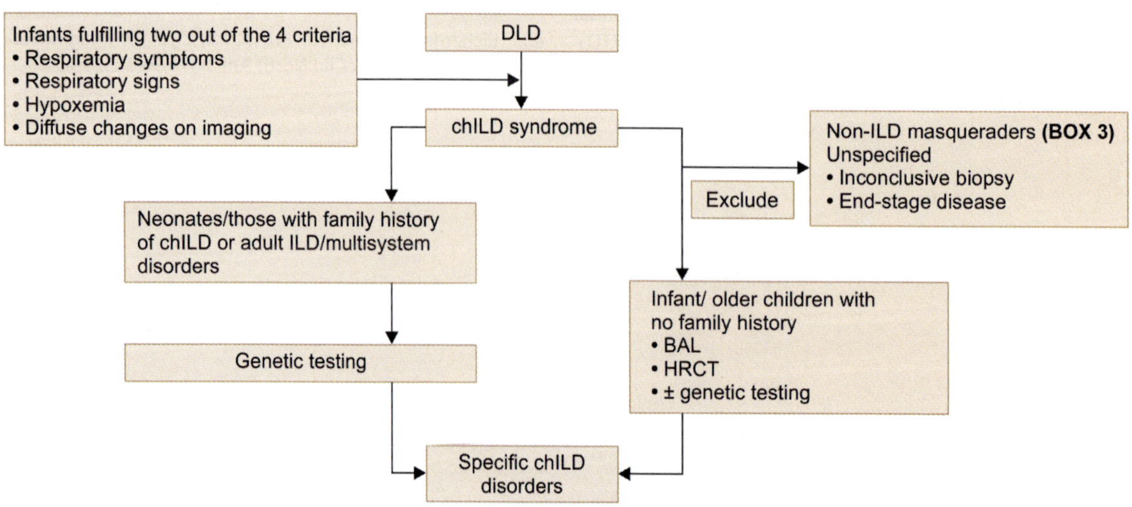

(BAL: bronchoalveolar lavage; chILD: childhood interstitial lung disease; HRCT: high-resolution computed tomography; ILD: interstitial lung disease)

A and B: Diffuse Developmental Disorders and Lung Growth Abnormalities

As the name indicates, the disorders in this group are growth/development associated. These are discussed in **Table 1**.[1-6]

C: Specific Conditions of Undefined Etiology

Pulmonary Interstitial Glycogenosis

Pulmonary interstitial glycogenosis (PIG) is a DLD wherein the mesenchymal cells located in the walls of alveoli increase in number.[1,7] This proliferation is mostly reactive and, hence, is mostly a consequence or association of an underlying disorder. Its associations include:

- Pulmonary hypoplasia
- Chronic lung disease of prematurity
- Pulmonary cysts, e.g., congenital pulmonary airway malformation
- Pulmonary arterial hypertension

Imaging findings are nonspecific and include:

- Areas of interstitial thickening/fibrosis with architectural distortion **(Figs. 5A and B)**
- Areas which are hyperinflated
- Cystic lucencies
- Ground glass opacities (GGO)
- Often adjoining/associated with primary abnormalities listed above

Neuroendocrine Cell Hyperplasia of Infancy (NEHI)

Neuroendocrine hyperplasia of infancy is a disorder affecting the peripheral airways and results from proliferation of the neuroendocrine cells located within the mucosa (epithelial layer) lining the airways. Affected infants present with dyspnea and tachypnea. On examination, chest retractions are present and patient has hypoxemia. CT reveals characteristic GGO particularly involving the right middle lobe and lingula. Rest of the lungs show area of air trapping, thus appear hyperlucent

TABLE 1: Diffuse developmental disorders and lung growth abnormalities and their salient features.[1-6]

Category	Entities	Pathology	Imaging	Prognosis
Diffuse developmental disorders[1-3]	Acinar dysplasia	• Developmental arrest in pseudoglandular stage • Poorly formed alveoli	• Diffuse airspace opacification (GGO, consolidation) • Pneumothorax Pneumomediastinum	Poor
	Congenital alveolar dysplasia	Developmental arrest at a later stage (late canalicular/saccular). Simplified alveolar pattern, lymphangiectasia, abnormal capillaries	Same as above; with additional findings of septal thickening due to dilated lymphatics	Poor
	Alveolar capillary dysplasia with misalignment of pulmonary veins	Alveolar capillaries do not have contact with airspace epithelium. Pulmonary veins run along the bronchovascular interstitium (rather than in the interlobular septae), lymphatics are dilated	Variable; may be normal or GGO/septal thickening	Poor, associated with pulmonary lymphangiectasia,[3] other GI and GU abnormalities
Lung growth abnormalities	Pulmonary hypoplasia	Restriction of lung development (either primary or secondary)	Small hyperlucent lung. May be complicated by secondary infections **(Figs. 1A to C)**	Variable, depends on associated factors as well, e.g., autosomal recessive polycystic kidney disease, Jeune's asphyxiating thoracic dystrophy
	Chronic neonatal lung disease (e.g., bronchopulmonary dysplasia)	• Secondary to insult to a premature lung after birth • HPE shows peribronchial fibrosis, obliterative bronchiolitis, arterial hypertension	• *Chest radiograph*: Reticular opacities, hyperinflation, atelectatic bands **(Figs. 2A and B)** • *CT*: Bronchial wall thickening, air trapping, interstitial thickening, subpleural opacities	Variable
	Associated with chromosomal anomalies[4-6]	Reduced alveolar number, cysts/overinflation, interstitial septal thickening	• Subpleural cysts[4] (in trisomy 21) **(Figs. 3A to C)** • Overinflation of upper and middle lobes (filamin A mutation), associated with CNS gray matter heterotopia[5,6]	Depends on the primary pathology
	Associated with congenital heart diseases	Vascular abnormality (arterial and venous hypertension)	PAH, mosaic attenuation, septal thickening **(Figs. 4A to C)**	Depends on the primary cardiac anomaly

(CNS: central nervous system; GGO: ground glass opacity; GI: gastrointestinal; GU: genitourinary; HPE: histopathological examination; PAH: pulmonary arterial hypertension)

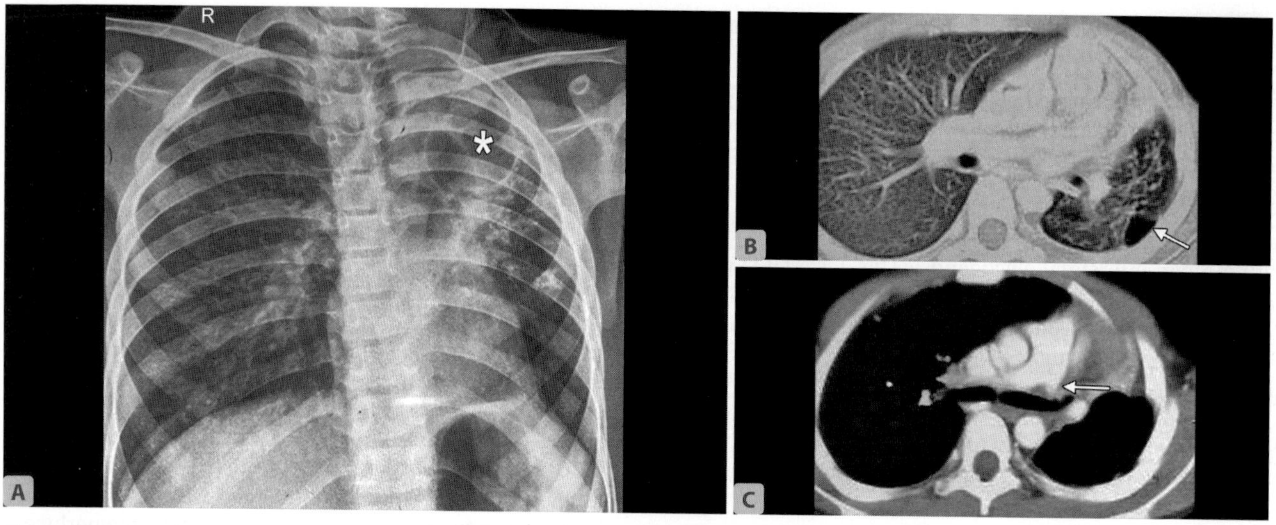

FIGS. 1A TO C: Lung growth abnormality. Left pulmonary hypoplasia complicated by recurrent infection. (A) Small volume left lung with fibrosis and a thin-walled cavity (asterisk). (B) Small volume left lung with fibrosis and cavity (arrow). (C) Small left pulmonary artery (arrow).

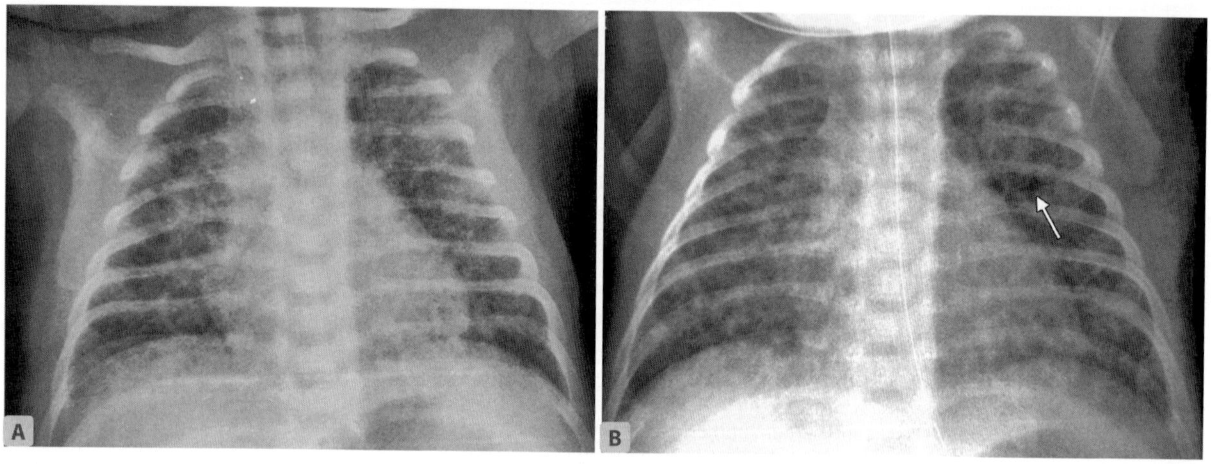

FIGS. 2A AND B: Bronchopulmonary dysplasia. Serial radiographs of a newborn on prolonged oxygen treatment. (A) Radiograph at day 18 and (B) day 27 show increasing reticular markings and hyperinflation on the later radiograph. Cystic changes (arrow in B) develop later during the course of the disease.

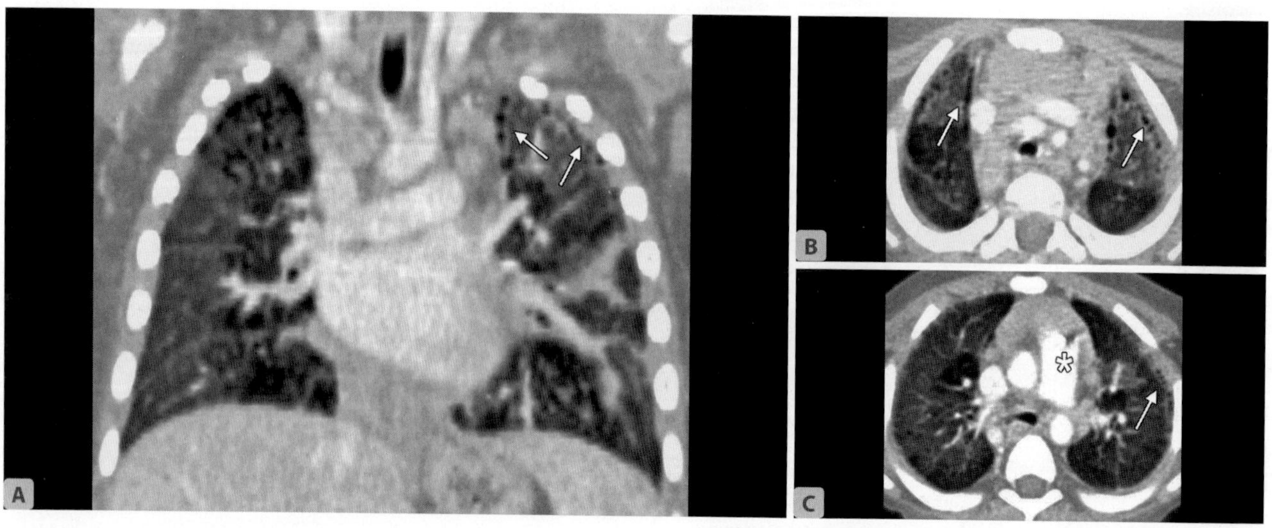

FIGS. 3A TO C: Diffuse lung disease in *Down's syndrome* and ASD: Single layer of subpleural cysts (arrows in A to C) is a characteristic appearance seen in Down's syndrome. The mosaic attenuation seen in bilateral lungs is due to the associated atrial septal defect (ASD) and pulmonary arterial hypertension. Main pulmonary artery is dilated (asterisk in C).

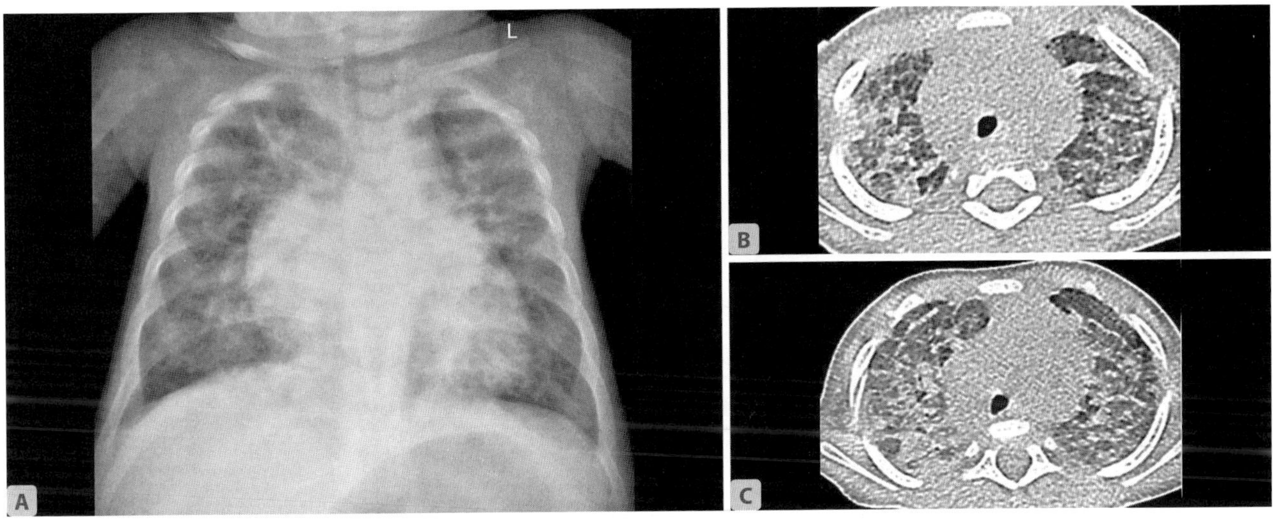

FIGS. 4A TO C: Diffuse lung disease in atrioventricular septal defect (AVSD) and pulmonary artery hypertension. (A) Chest X-ray (CXR): Cardiomegaly and prominent vascular markings in central lung. (B and C) CT: Scattered GGOs with mosaic attenuation in both lungs.

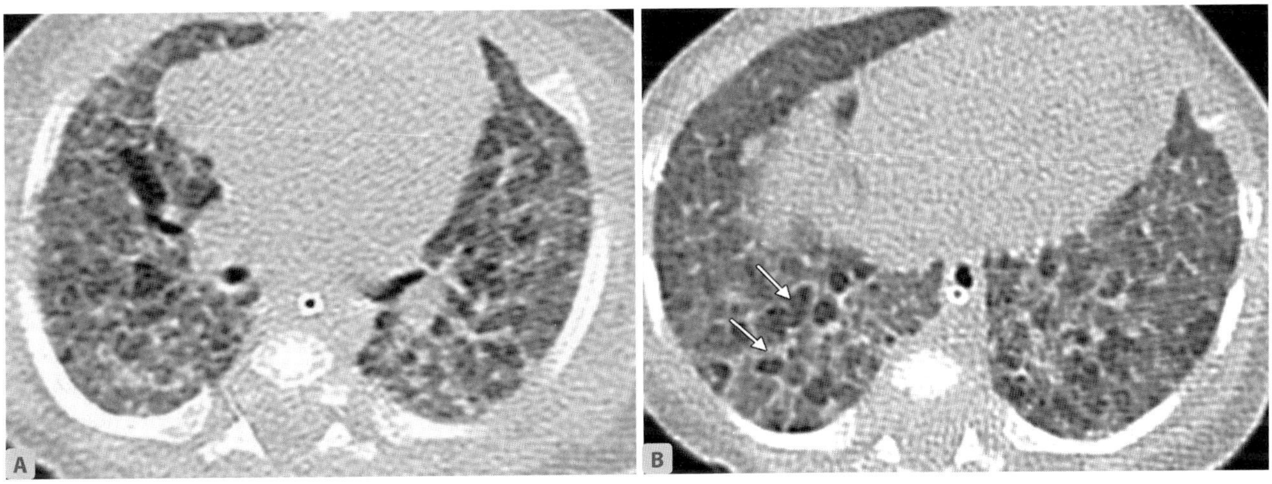

FIGS. 5A AND B: Pulmonary interstitial glycogenosis: A 34-week-preterm neonate at 28 days after birth had increased respiratory rate and persistent oxygen requirement. She had associated pulmonary artery hypertension. CT images reveal diffuse ground glass opacity (GGO) with smooth inter- and intralobular septal thickening. Foci of air trapping (arrows) and cystic changes also noted, preferentially at basal segments.

(Figs. 6A to C).[0] The overall management strategy is mostly supportive, as these patients improve over time.

D. Surfactant Mutation and Associated Disorders

Pulmonary surfactant is essentially a lipoprotein complex that lines the alveolar mucosa, preventing its collapse, besides other secondary functions. It is produced within the type II pneumocytes of the alveolar epithelium **(Flowchart 2)**.[9,10] There are four types of proteins related to surfactant production; surfactant proteins A, B, C, and D; of which B and C are the most clinically significant. Alveolar macrophages are involved in the clearance and degradation of the surfactant **(Flowchart 3)**.

Surfactant mutation related disorders are one of the most significant chILD disorders. Depending on the inheritance and mutation, the age of presentation is variable and ranges from neonatal to adolescents, or even adults [in the granulocyte-macrophage colony-stimulating factor (GM-CSF) receptor gene disorders]. Several radiological patterns have been described with bilateral GGO being a dominant imaging feature.

Table 2 describes the major disease entities in this subgroup.[9,10]

Chronic Pneumonitis of Infancy

This term refers to a characteristic histopathological pattern of interstitial edema and inflammatory exudate; along with diffuse uniform type II pneumocyte hyperplasia; seen in infants. The alveoli are filled with exudates containing macrophages and eosinophilic debris. This pattern was found to be unique among the infants and was strikingly different from adult DLDs. CPI is a histopathological pattern which is

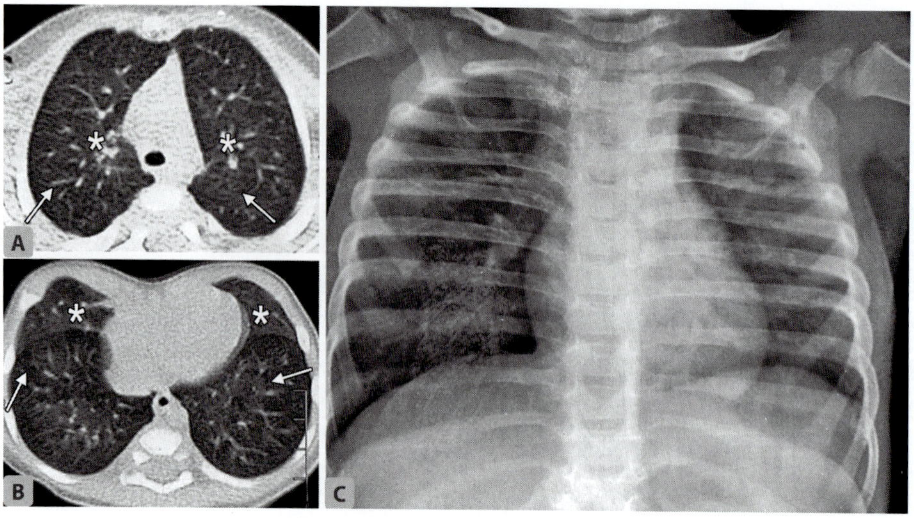

FIGS. 6A TO C: Neuroendocrine cell hyperplasia of infancy. A 40-days-old neonate with increased respiratory rate. (A and B) CT reveals central ground glass opacity (GGO) (asterisk) and peripheral air trapping (arrows). (C) Follow-up radiograph revealed mild residual hyperinflation in right lung. The child also had symptomatic improvement.

FLOWCHART 2: Mechanism of surfactant production.

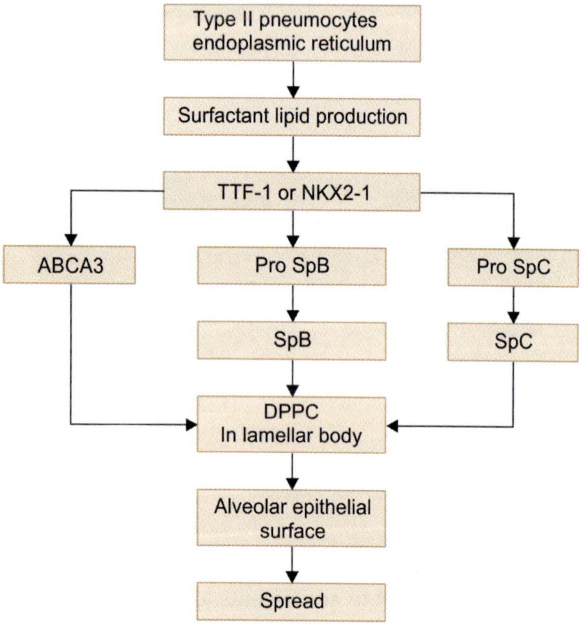

[ABCA3: ATP-binding cassette transporter; ATP: adenosine triphosphate; DPPC: dipalmitoylphosphatidylcholine. Phospholipid (lecithin) which is the main constituent of surfactant; SpB: surfactant protein B encoded by *SFTPB* gene; SpC: surfactant protein C encoded by *SFTPC* gene; TTF-1: thyroid transcription factor 1; NKX2-1- NKX homeobox 2-1, encodes TTF-1 (TTF-1, NKX2-1 regulate the gene transcription within these cells)]

most commonly associated with surfactant protein mutation disorders especially SpC mutations. *ABCA3* mutation can also give rise to this pattern; although there may be slight difference under electron microscopic examination.

II. Disorders not Specific to Infancy

A. Disorders of the normal host
B. Disorders related to systemic diseases
C. Disorders of immunocompromised host
D. Diseases masquerading as ILD

A. Disorders of Normal Host

This group includes the following disorders:

- Infectious and postinfectious diseases
- Environmental agents related
- Aspiration syndrome
- Eosinophilic pneumonia

Infectious or Postinfectious Disorders

The most significant among these is postinfective bronchiolitis; or constrictive bronchiolitis (CB) or constrictive obliterative bronchiolitis (COB). COB is the result of infection occurring in infants/young children (<3 years of age). It is most commonly reported with adenovirus infections; but has also been seen following other infections such as measles or respiratory syncytial virus (RSV). It has several synonyms, such as Swyer–James–MacLeod syndrome and postinfective bronchiolitis obliterans (PIBO). Constrictive bronchiolitis can also occur in other clinical settings such as post-transplant (hematopoietic stem cell transplant or lung transplant) when it is referred to as bronchiolitis obliterans (BO).

Imaging is characterized by hyperinflation/air trapping resulting in mosaic attenuation **(Fig. 8A and B)**. Mild bronchiectasis may also be seen. Reflex vasoconstriction eventually results in decrease in pulmonary artery diameter. The classical description of the entity on CXR is of a unilateral small hyperlucent lung with small hilum. However, COB is more often bilateral.

Environmental Agents Related Disorders

Since occupational exposure to metal dust is not a significant factor in children; this group of disorders is uncommon in children. Among these, hypersensitivity pneumonitis (HP) is the most frequently encountered entity. The imaging features

FLOWCHART 3: Mechanism of surfactant degradation.

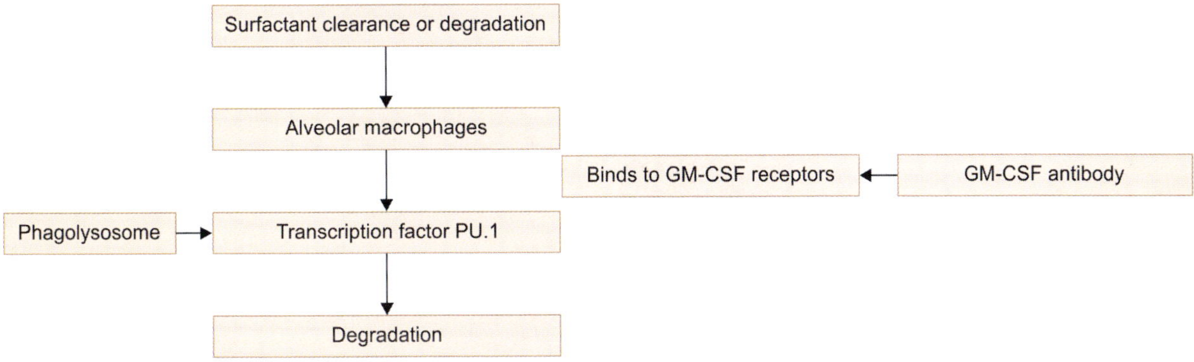

(CSF-2: colony-stimulating factor 2; GM-CSF: granulocyte-macrophage colony-stimulating factor)

TABLE 2: Surfactant mutation disorders.[9,10]

Mutation	Inheritance	Age of presentation	Radiopathological pattern	Course
SpB	Recessive	Infants, term neonates (vs. RDS)	Pulmonary alveolar proteinosis (PAP), GGO, crazy-paving	• Often fatal • Partial deficiency has better survival
SpC	Autosomal dominant/ arises de novo	Variable postnatal	• CPI • DIP • NSIP • GGO ± cysts	Variable
ABCA3	Autosomal recessive	Late onset	• PAP • CPI, DIP, NSIP (less common)	• Less severe • Better prognosis
NKX2-1 deletion/ loss of function	Autosomal dominant	• Multisystem (brain-thyroid-lung syndrome) • Choreoathetosis, atonia, congenital hypothyroidism	RDS-like or other patterns as above	Variable
GM-CSF receptor genes	Autosomal recessive	Variable, infants to adults	PAP, nonspecific **(Figs. 7A to C)**	Suspect if *SpC* or *ABCA3* mutation absent and serum GM-CSF levels increased

(*ABCA3*: ATP-binding cassette transporter 3; CPI: chronic pneumonitis of infancy; DIP: desquamative interstitial pneumonia; GGO: ground glass opacity; GM-CSF: granulocyte-macrophage colony-stimulating factor; NKX2-1: NKX homeobox 2-1, encodes TTF-1; NSIP: nonspecific interstitial pneumonitis; PAP: pulmonary alveolar proteinosis; RDS: respiratory distress syndrome; SpB: surfactant protein B encoded by *SFTPB* gene; SpC: surfactant protein C encoded by *SFTPC* gene)

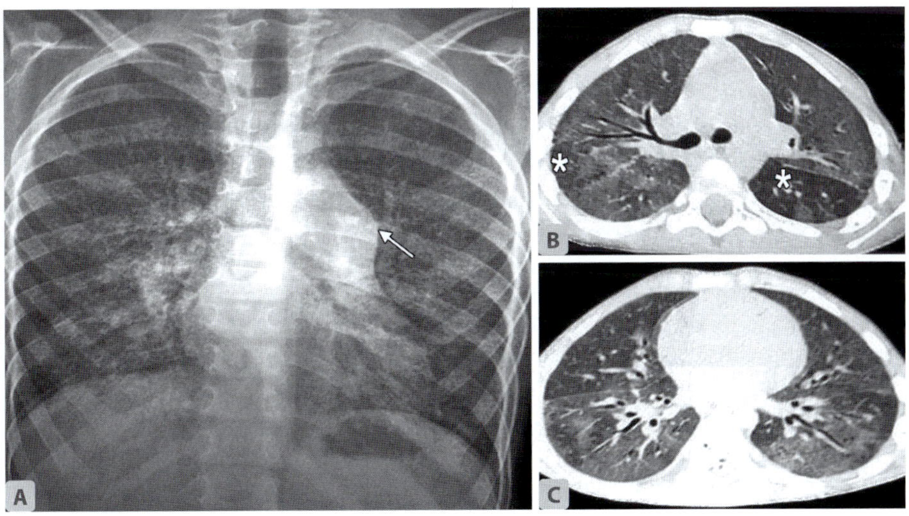

FIGS. 7A TO C: DLD in GM-CSF mutation in a 7-year-old boy with chronic respiratory distress. (A) Chest X-ray: Central GGO with prominence of pulmonary artery (arrow). (B and C) CT: Diffuse GGO with scattered areas of air trapping (asterisk). (CT: computed tomography; DLD: diffuse lung disease; GGO: ground glass opacities; GM-CSF: granulocyte-macrophage colony-stimulating factor)

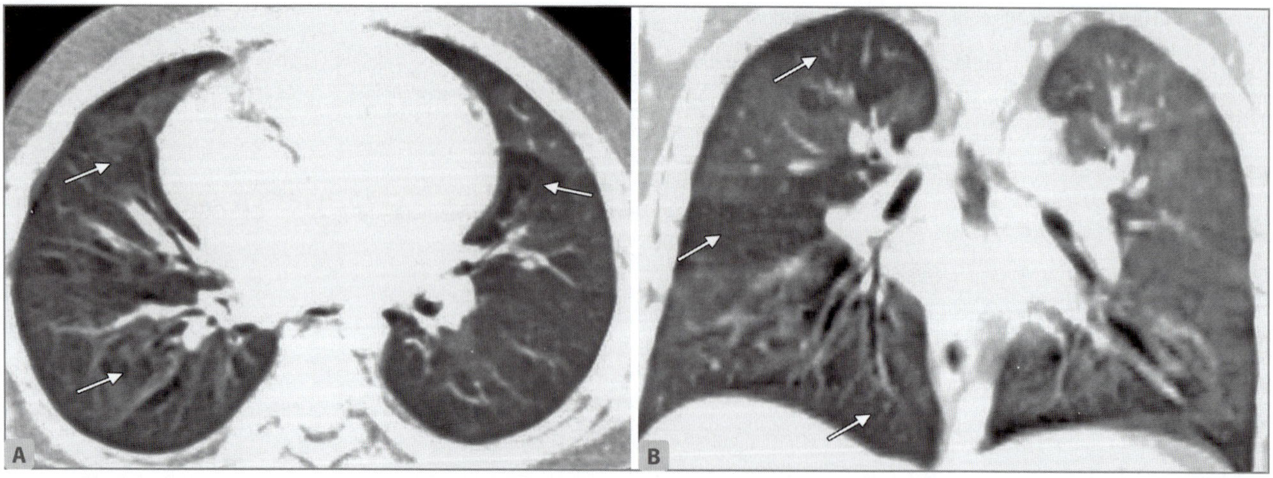

FIGS. 8A AND B: Constrictive obliterative bronchiolitis in a 10-year-old boy with wheezing and respiratory distress. CT images show patchy areas of air trapping, seen as lucent areas (arrows), leading to an appearance simulating "mosaic attenuation".

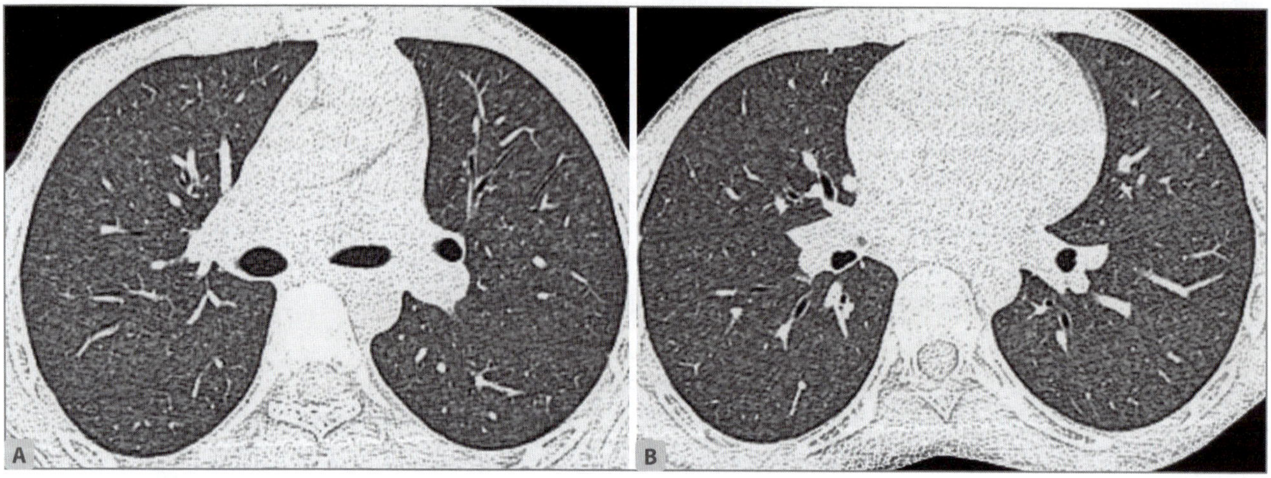

FIGS. 9A AND B: Hypersensitivity pneumonitis in a 16-year-old boy with history of exposure to pigeon droppings. CT shows classical ground glass centrilobular nodules uniformly spread throughout both lungs.

are similar to those encountered in adults **(Figs. 9A and B)**. Lung disease consequent to toxic inhalation of noxious fumes is another entity which may be seen.

Aspiration Syndromes

Aspiration is common in children and a frequent cause of recurrent pneumonia and postinfective fibrosis. It has also been reported in up to half the chILD cases, although a clear cause-effect relationship is not established. Consolidation and volume loss with bronchiectasis are seen in bilateral lower lobes followed by right upper lobe **(Figs. 10A and B)**. In cases of exogenous lipoid pneumonia due to mineral oil ingestion or inhalation, low density foci may be seen within the consolidation **(Figs. 11A to C)**.

Eosinophilic Pneumonia

Eosinophilic lung disorders display similar imaging to adults **(Figs. 12A and B)**. These are rare and include eosinophilic pneumonias, allergic bronchopulmonary aspergillosis (ABPA), and drug reactions.

B. Disorders related to Systemic Diseases

Systemic disorders associated with ILD in children are listed in **Box 1**.

Immune-related Disorders

This group of disorders includes connective tissue diseases (CTDs) and vasculitides. Among the CTDs progressive systemic sclerosis (PSS) and juvenile dermatomyositis most frequently result in pulmonary involvement. Pulmonary involvement is encountered mostly in adolescents. Similar to adults, nonspecific interstitial pneumonia (NSIP) **(Figs. 13A and B)** is the most common imaging pattern; followed by organizing pneumonia (OP). Patients of Sjögren syndrome may have lymphocytic interstitial pneumonia (LIP), although it is more frequent in adults. Similarly follicular bronchiolitis (FB) may also be seen.

In those with vasculitis including systemic lupus erythematosus (SLE) or anti-GBM disease (previously known as GoodPasture syndrome); diffuse alveolar hemorrhage (DAH) results in bilateral GGO. DAH (synonym: diffuse

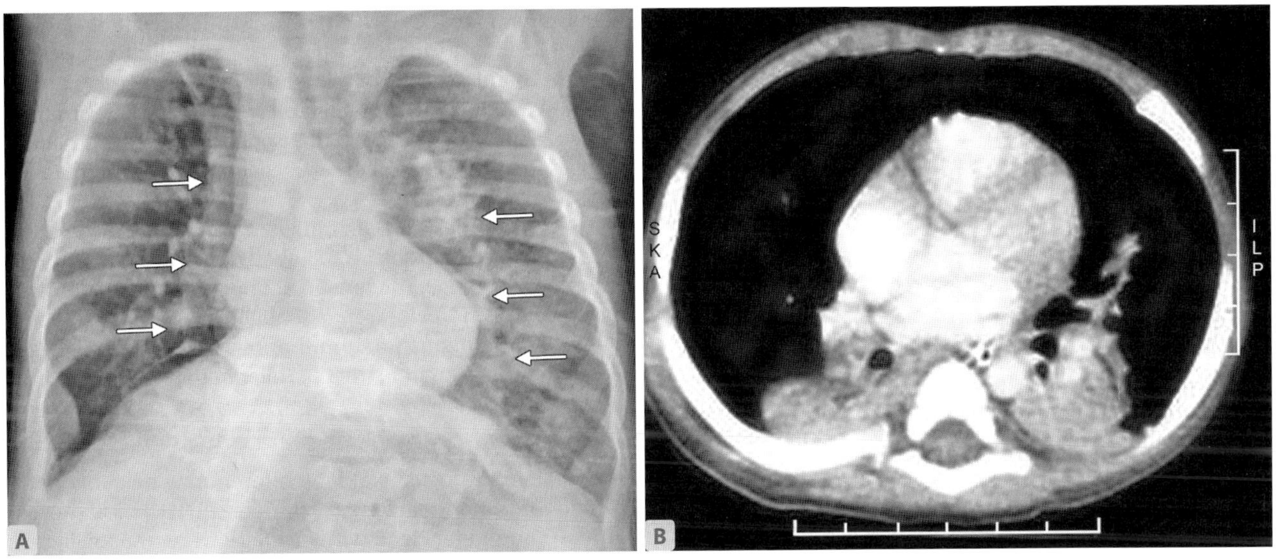

FIGS. 10A AND B: Aspiration pneumonia in a child with gastroesophageal reflux. (A) Chest X-ray (CXR): Central paraspinal consolidation (arrows) and distal compensatory hyperinflation, as evidenced by flattening of domes of both diaphragms. (B) CT: Paravertebral dense consolidation in the lower lobes.

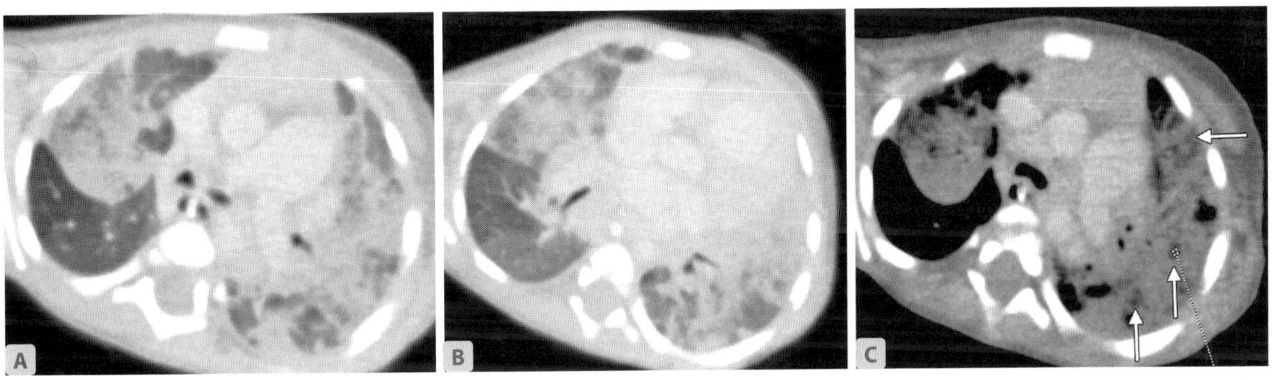

FIGS. 11A TO C: Endogenous lipoid pneumonia in a 2-year-old child with primary immunodeficiency. Bilateral dense areas of ground glass opacity (GGO)/consolidation are seen with internal low-attenuation areas (arrows in C) showing an attenuation of -105.

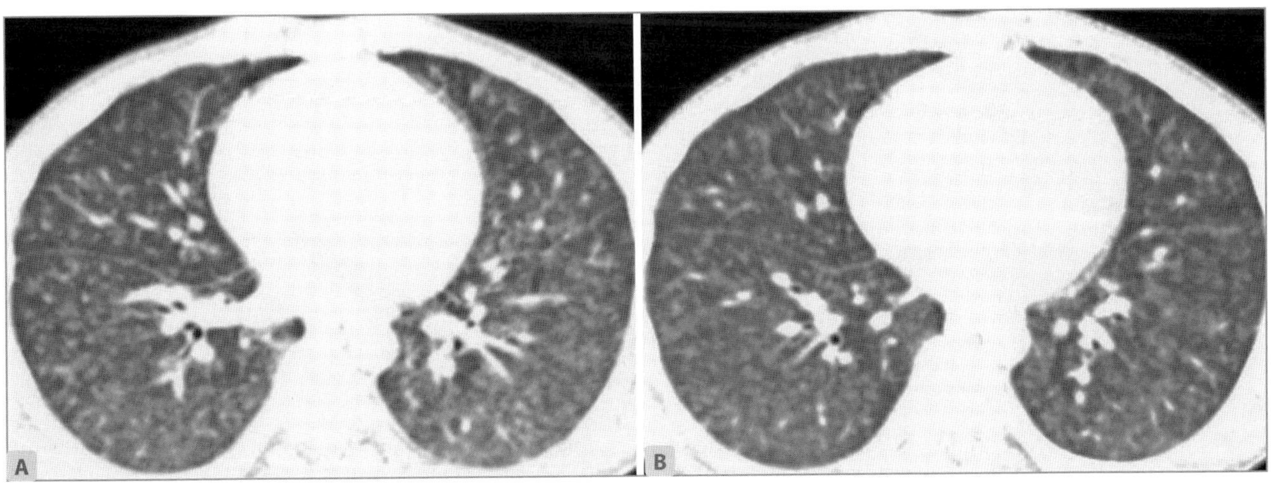

FIGS. 12A AND B: Acute eosinophilic pneumonia in a boy. CT reveals diffuse ground glass and solid centrilobular nodules diffusely scattered over both lungs. The child has peripheral eosinophilia. The imaging appearance is similar to hypersensitivity pneumonitis **(Fig. 9)**.

pulmonary hemorrhage/DPH) results in diffuse GGO, lobular GGO, and ill-defined or GG centrilobular nodules with sparing of lung apices and costophrenic (CP) angles. On CT perivenular region also appears spared. Causes of DAH in children are listed in **Table 3**. While DAH **(Figs. 14A and B)** is characteristically associated with rapid clearing/resolution on imaging, repeated hemorrhages can result in septal thickening (intra- and interlobular) **(Figs. 15A and B)**.

Storage Disorders

Storage disorders are an important cause of diffuse lung abnormalities encountered in children. The child is often a known patient of storage disorder, but may also be first suspected on imaging if a "crazy paving" CT appearance is seen alongside hepatosplenomegaly.[11-15]

Lysosomal disorders are the most common group resulting in ILD **(Table 4)**[11-16] and frequent pattern of GGO **(Figs. 16A to D)** with superimposed septal thickening (PAP like). Bronchial wall thickening and reticulonodular pattern is also reported. This is because Gaucher cells deposit in the peribronchovascular tissues.

Sarcoidosis

Pulmonary involvement in sarcoidosis is infrequent in young children (<5 years); and mostly seen in older children and adolescents, wherein the imaging pattern is similar to adults.

Langerhan's Cell Histiocytosis

Langerhan's cell histiocytosis (LCH) is a cause of cystic pattern of ILD in both children and adults. However, in adults, pulmonary LCH (PLCH) is mostly limited to the lungs and is encountered in young smokers, particularly males. On the other hand, in children, the lung involvement is part of the multisystemic involvement and it has a reported variable incidence of 20–50%.[16] However, isolated/predominant lung changes in the absence of other sites (bone, liver, spleen, and skin) are distinctly rare.

On CT, nodules are seen initially which are subsequently replaced by irregular, bizarre-shaped cysts **(Figs. 17A to D)**. Unlike adults, the characteristic of upper lobar involvement may not be seen in children; although CP angles are mostly spared. Spontaneous pneumothorax often occurs. Calcific specks may be present in thymus/hilar nodes.

BOX 1: Systemic disorders associated with ILDs in children.

- Immune-related disorders
- Storage disorders
- Sarcoidosis
- Langerhans cell histiocytosis

C. Disorders of Immunocompromised Host

Immunocompromised state in children may be congenital [primary immunodeficiency disorders (PIDD)] or acquired human immunodeficiency virus-acquired immunodeficiency syndrome (HIV-AIDS). DLDs related to these are listed in **Box 2**.

Lymphocytic Interstitial Pneumonia

Lymphocytic interstitial pneumonia (LIP) has been described in children with HIV infection and less frequently with

TABLE 3: Causes of diffuse alveolar hemorrhage (DAH) in children.

Vasculitis	Systemic lupus erythematosus (SLE)
	GPA (formerly Wegener's granulomatosis)
	EGPA (formerly Churg–Strauss syndrome)
	Anti-GBM disease (formerly Goodpasture syndrome)
Heiner syndrome	DAH with cow milk allergy
Idiopathic	

(GPA: granulomatosis with polyangiitis; EGPA: eosinophilic granulomatosis with polyangiitis; GBM: glomerular basement membrane)

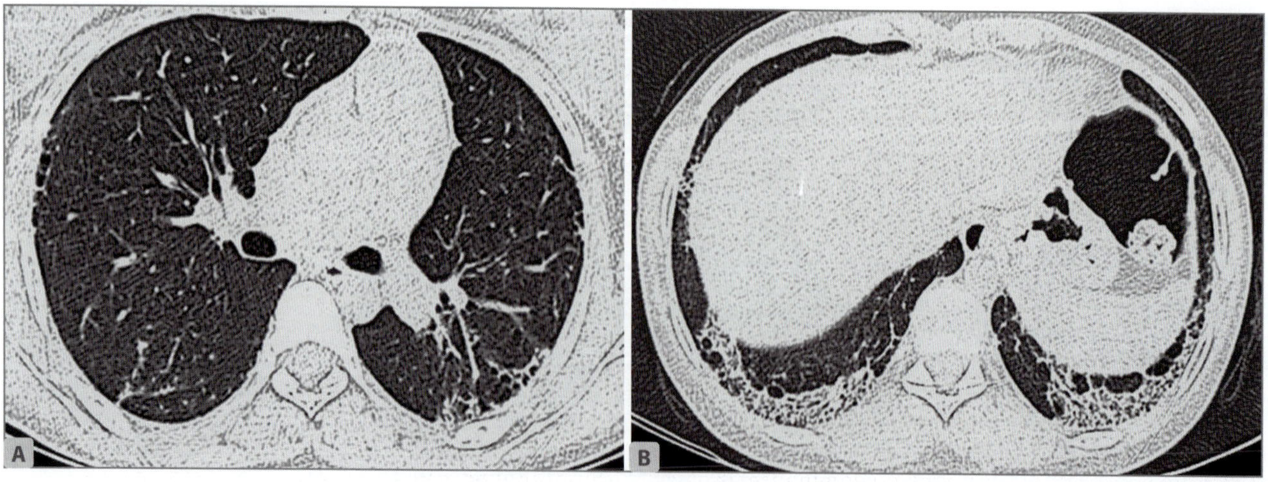

FIGS. 13A AND B: CT of a 14-year-old girl with SLE showing fibrotic NSIP pattern. (NSIP: nonspecific interstitial pneumonia; SLE: systemic lupus erythematosus)

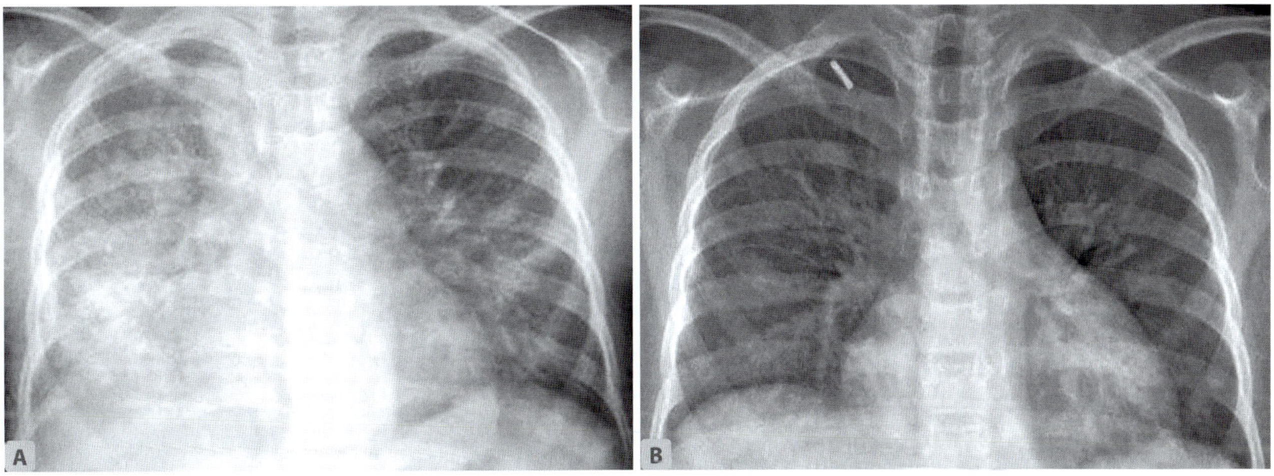

FIGS. 14A AND B: DAH in a child with SLE: Serial radiographs taken at an interval of 7 days. (A) Radiograph at presentation: Right opaque hemithorax and left central perihilar consolidation. (B) Radiograph 7 days after steroids: Complete clearance of radiographic abnormality. (DAH: diffuse alveolar hemorrhage; SLE: systemic lupus erythematosus)

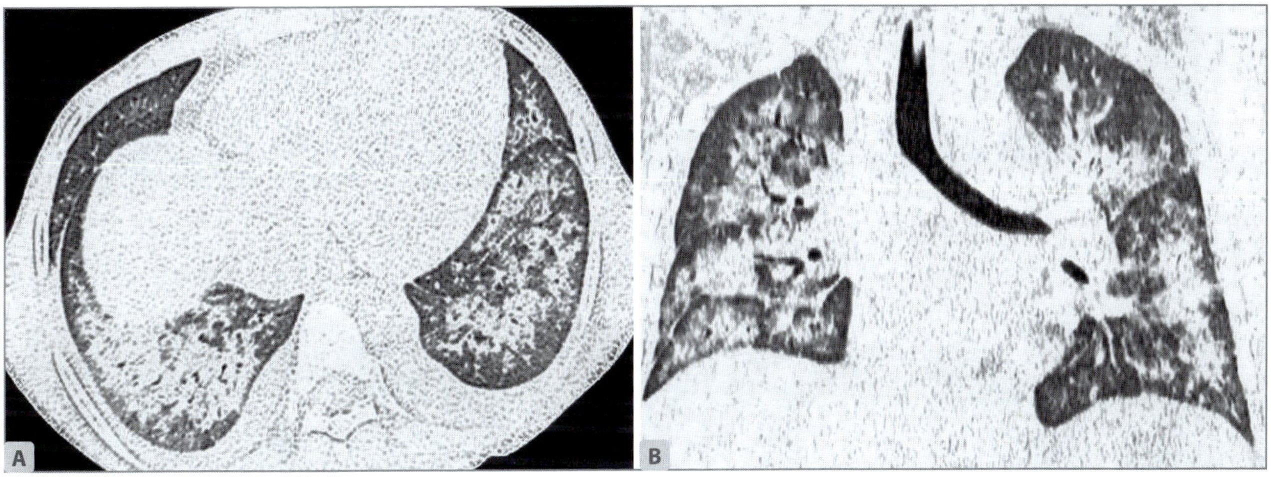

FIGS. 15A AND B: Classical CT appearance of diffuse alveolar hemorrhage (DAH). Same patient as in **Figure 14**. Note the sparing of the apical and basal zones, and the peripheral part of lungs.

TABLE 4: Lysosomal storage disorders associated with childhood interstitial lung disease (ChILD).

Name	Pathology	Imaging features
Niemann–Pick disease • Types A and B most commonly associated, type C rare	Deposition of lipid laden macrophages and characteristic NP cells	Upper lobe GGO, septal thickening at the bases[11,12]
Gaucher disease[13] • Type 3 and 1 (after splenectomy)	Deposition of lipid laden macrophages and characteristic gaucher cells	GGO, PAP, pulmonary arterial hypertension, hepatopulmonary syndrome[14,15]

(GGO: ground glass opacity; NP: Niemann–Pick; PAP: pulmonary alveolar proteinosis)

common variable immunodeficiency (CVID).[17] LIP associated with AIDS is far more frequent in children (20–40%); while it is encountered less commonly in adults (30%).[17]

Imaging features described include nodules (subpleural or centrilobular) with a lower lobe predominance. Bronchi may also show wall thickening or dilation. Cysts are frequent **(Figs. 18A and B)**.[17] Another pattern observed in PIDD, especially CVID is small airway disease (follicular bronchiolitis, FB).

Opportunistic infections such as *Pneumocystis carinii (jirovecii)* pneumonia (PCP) or viral pneumonia are a well-described cause of DLD in immunocompromised hosts. Extensive bacterial or fungal infections can result in extensive bilateral consolidations in PIDD such as chronic

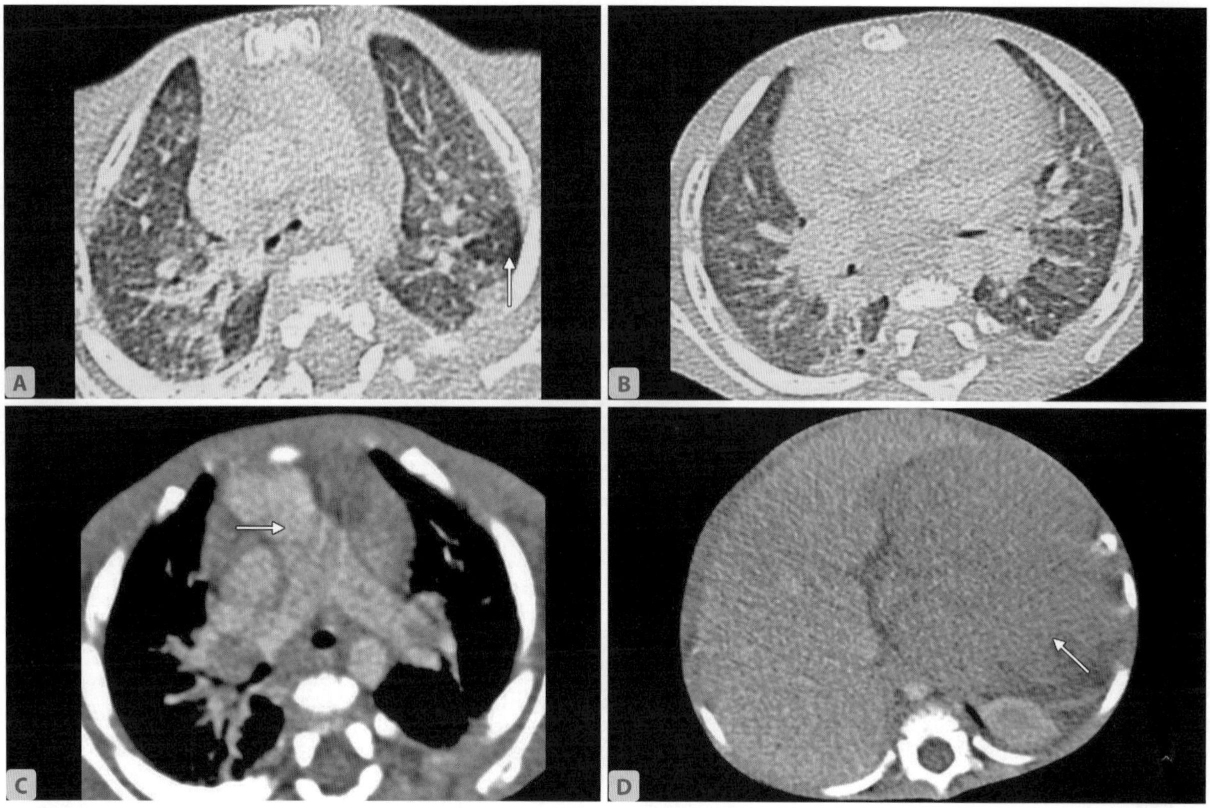

FIGS. 16A TO D: Pulmonary involvement in Type I Gaucher's disease in a 4-year-old boy. Diffuse ground glass opacity in both lungs with patchy areas of sparing (arrow in A); pulmonary artery hypertension (arrow in C); splenomegaly (arrow in D).

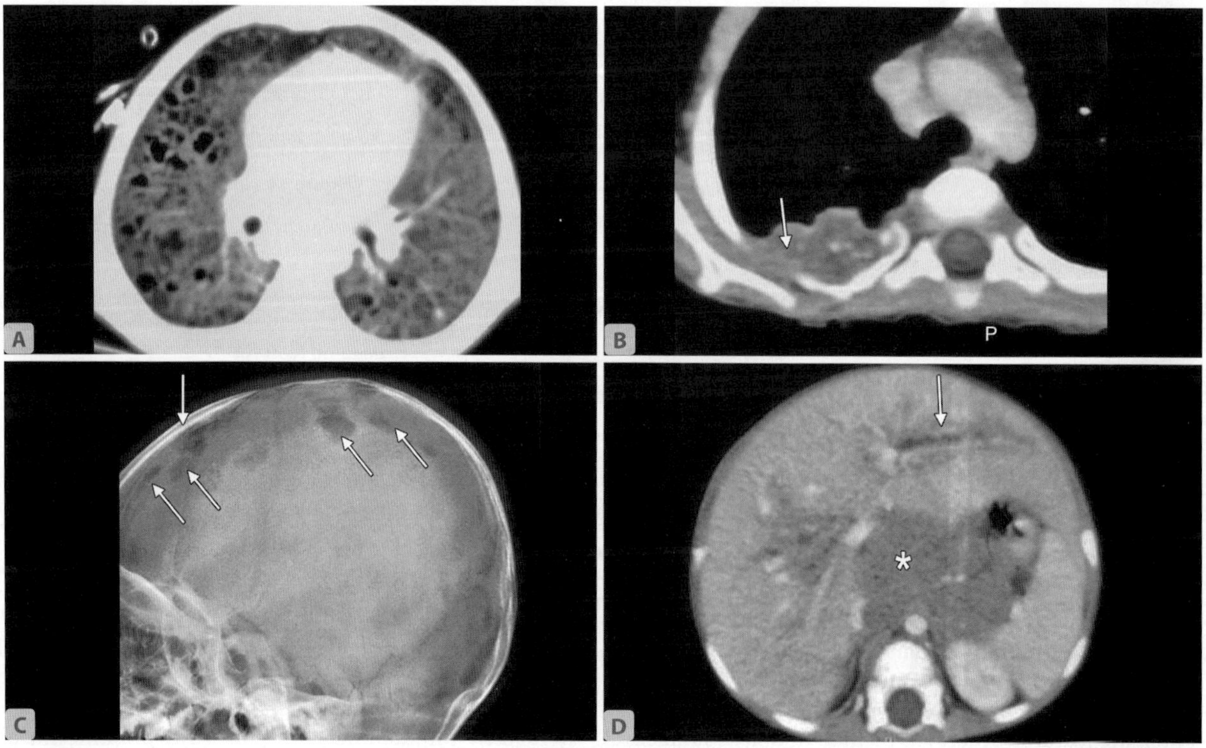

FIGS. 17A TO D: Multisystem Langerhans cell histiocytosis (LCH) in a 4-year-old boy. Random nodules and thin-walled cysts in both lungs (A). Expansile lytic lesion of right-sided 5th rib (arrow in B). Typical calvarial geographic lytic lesions (arrows in C). Periportal hypodensity (arrow in D) with retroperitoneal lymphadenopathy (asterisk in D).

granulomatous disease (CGD). A complete discussion of these is beyond the scope of this chapter.

Related to Transplantation and Rejection

Small airway disease (obliterative bronchiolitis form) can develop in patients with chronic graft-versus-host disease (GVHD) in hematopoietic stem cell transplant (HSCT) and less frequently in solid organ transplants (SOT) recipients. This entity in transplant setting is referred to as bronchiolitis obliterans syndrome (BOS). CT reveals air trapping with or without bronchial wall thickening and mild bronchiectasis. Centrilobular nodules are less frequent (vs. FB).

Another entity encountered in post-HSCT setting is transplant-associated thrombotic microangiopathy (TA-TMA). The entity mainly involves the kidneys, pulmonary involvement is extremely rare, and is in the form of pulmonary arterial hypertension (PAH). Lung parenchyma appears normal on imaging.

Pleuroparenchymal Fibroelastosis

Pleuroparenchymal fibroelastosis (PPFE) is a rare form of idiopathic interstitial pneumonia recently described in adults. A rare idiopathic form has also been described in children which has a more fulminant course and worse prognosis than the adult form. It has been reported with HSCT, SOT, high-dose chemotherapy, and with dyskeratosis congenital.[18]

BOX 2: Disorders of immunocompromised host.

- Infections
- Related to therapeutic interventions
- Related to transplantation and rejection syndrome
- Diffuse alveolar damage (unknown etiology)

Computed tomography features are of apical pleural thickening associated with subpleural consolidation and subsequent fibrosis. Associated bronchiectasis and subpleural cysts are also reported, which can rupture causing spontaneous pneumothorax.

D. Disorders Masquerading as Interstitial Lung Diseases (Box 3)

Several disorders lead to diffuse lung changes which can mimic chILD disorders (**Box 3**).

Congestive Changes due to Cardiac Cause

Congestive changes occur due to pulmonary venous hypertension (PVH) in those with a cardiac cause (dysfunction or valvular disease or septal defect), with back pressure changes. Lung parenchyma shows smooth interlobular septal thickening with GGO, with or without pleural effusion.

Congestive Vasculopathy

Pulmonary veno-occlusive disease (PVOD) is a cause of precapillary pulmonary hypertension. PVOD is characterized by intimal fibrosis and hence narrowing/occlusion of peripheral pulmonary veins. On CT, there is thickening of interlobular septae (mostly smooth, but may be nodular). Hilar/mediastinal nodes and pulmonary artery dilation (due to PAH) are seen in addition.

Lymphatic Disorders

Since lymphatics also run in the walls of the secondary pulmonary lobule, their dilatation gives rise to smooth thickening of the septae **(Figs. 19A to D)** and GGO (similar to PVH or PVOD). In addition chylous pleural effusion and/or ill-defined mediastinal soft tissue may be seen. Lymphatic disorders include:

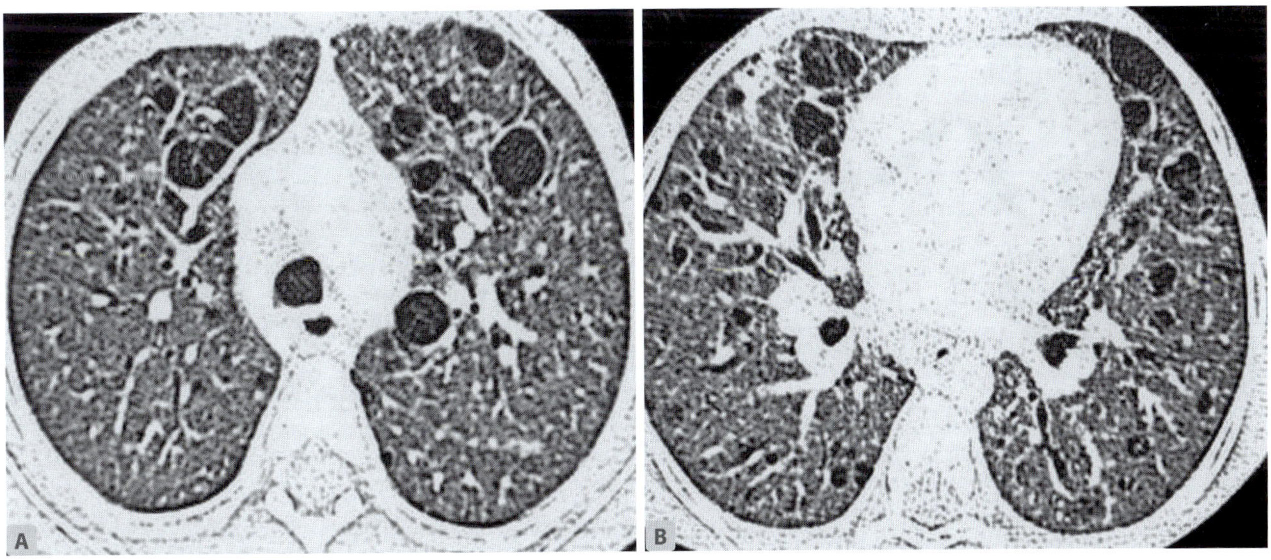

FIGS. 18A AND B: Lymphocytic interstitial pneumonia (LIP) in a retropositive 5-year-old boy. CT reveals perilymphatic distribution of thin-walled cysts. The child had palpable cervical lymphadenopathy.

- Lymphangiectasia (dilated lymphatics)
  - Primary (associations: Noonan syndrome, Turner syndrome)
  - Secondary (any cause of obstruction to drainage)
- Lymphangiomatosis (proliferation of lymphatics)

Arterial Hypertensive Vasculopathy

Pulmonary capillary hemangiomatosis (PCH) is an entity that is associated with capillary proliferation occurring in the walls of alveoli. It is also a cause of postcapillary pulmonary hypertension, similar to PVOD. However, these patients often present with hemoptysis and the condition is extremely rare in children. On CT, extensive bilateral centrilobular nodules (ill-defined), along with PAH is the hallmark of PCH.

BOX 3: Disorders masquerading as interstitial lung diseases.

- Congestive changes (due to cardiac cause)
- Congestive vasculopathy, PVOD
- Lymphatic disorders
- Arterial hypertensive vasculopathy

(PVOD: pulmonary veno-occlusive disease)

III. Unclassified Disorders

This group includes:

- End-stage diseases wherein the cause could not be ascertained **(Figs. 20A to C)**.
- The second situation is if the lung biopsy is nondiagnostic.

PATTERN APPROACH (TABLE 5)

As in adult DLDs, most patients will report for imaging with a clinical diagnosis of chILD without a definite underlying cause. In these situations, the pattern-based approach is immensely useful to narrow down the differential diagnoses and guide further investigations.

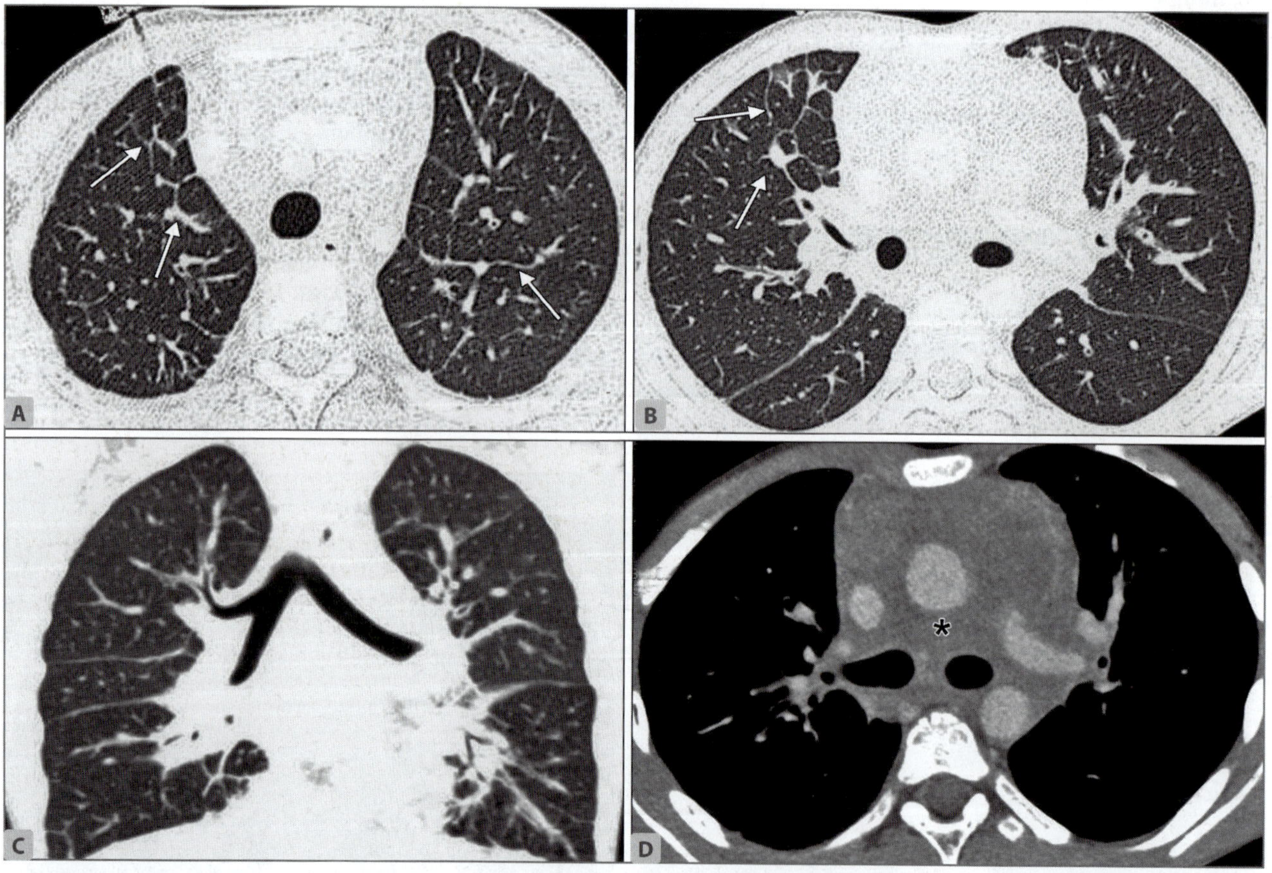

FIGS. 19A TO D: Mediastinal fibrosis causing *pulmonary lymphatic dilatation* masquerading as interstitial lung disease (ILD): Smooth septal thickening of both lungs, predominantly central, perihilar and bilateral apical distribution (arrows in A to C). Sheet-like hypodense soft tissue (asterisk in D) in the mediastinum encircling the mediastinal vascular structures and carina (D).

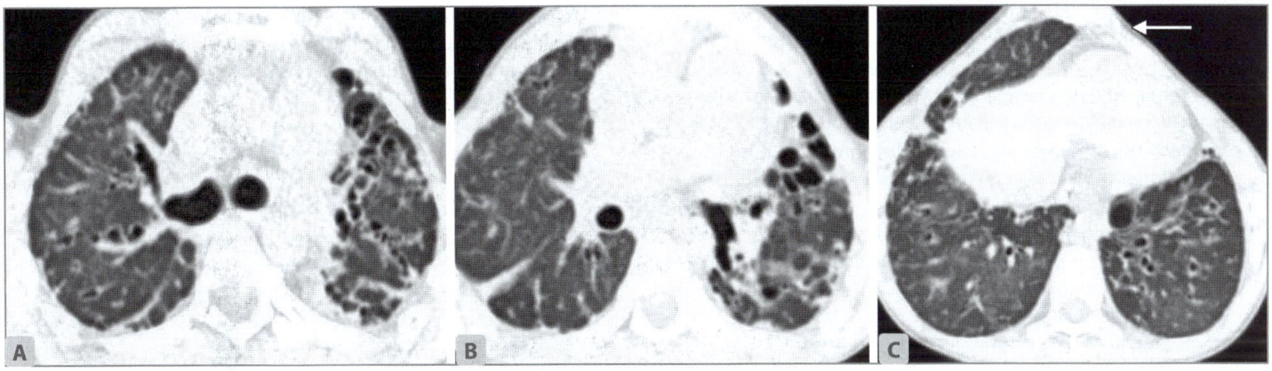

FIGS. 20A TO C: End-stage interstitial lung disease (ILD) in a 10-year-old girl. CT reveals bilateral upper lobe predominant fibrosis and traction bronchiectasis; and pectus carinatum deformity (arrow in C) due to reduced volume of the hemithoraces.

TABLE 5: Pattern approach toward differential diagnosis of childhood diffuse lung diseases (DLDs) on high-resolution computed tomography (HRCT).

Pattern	Additional information	Differential diagnosis (DDs) in infancy (<2 years)	DDs in older children
GGO	Acute/subacute presentation	Infections (viral)	Infections, pulmonary edema/ARDS, hypersensitivity pneumonitis, DAH
	Chronic presentation	NEHI, errors of surfactant metabolism, storage disorders	Errors of surfactant metabolism, storage disorders, NSIP
Septal thickening/ reticular pattern	NSIP/UIP pattern	Errors of surfactant metabolism, storage disorders	Connective tissue diseases, errors of surfactant metabolism
	Interlobular septal thickening	Lung growth abnormalities (e.g., BPD), PIG, PVOD, lymphatic disorders, congestive changes secondary to cardiac dysfunction	Venous/lymphatic edema
	Upper lobe fibrosis		• Sarcoidosis • Chronic hypersensitivity pneumonitis
Nodules	Random		• Miliary-infective • High-density-alveolar microlithiasis
	Centrilobular		Infective (TB), bronchiolitis
	Perilymphatic		Sarcoidosis, LIP
Cysts	Peribronchovascular/perilymphatic		LIP
	Random		LCH, sequel of infection (PJP)
	Subpleural/basal	Trisomy 21	Fibrotic ILD/NSIP

(ARDS: acute respiratory distress syndrome; BPD: bronchopulmonary dysplasia; DAH: diffuse alveolar hemorrhage; GGO: ground glass opacities; ILD: interstitial lung diseases; LCH: Langerhans cell histiocytosis; LIP: lymphocytic interstitial pneumonia; NEHI: neuroendocrine cell hyperplasia of infancy; NSIP: nonspecific interstitial pneumonia; PAP: pulmonary alveolar proteinosis; PJP: *Pneumocystis jirovecii* pneumonia; PIG: pulmonary interstitial glycogenosis; PVOD: pulmonary veno-occlusive disease; UIP: usual interstitial pneumonia)

REFERENCES

1. Kurland G, Deterding RR, Hagood JS, Young LR, Brody AS, Castile RG, et al. An Official American Thoracic Society Clinical Practice Guideline: Classification, Evaluation, and Management of Childhood Interstitial Lung Disease in Infancy. Am J Respir Crit Care Med. 2013;188:376-94.
2. Guillerman RP, Brody AS. Contemporary perspectives on pediatric diffuse lung disease. Radiol Clin North Am. 2011;49(5):847-68.
3. Dishop MK. Diagnostic pathology of diffuse lung disease in children. Pediatr Allergy Immunol Pulmonol. 2010;23(1):69-85.
4. Gonzalez OR, Gomez IG, Recalde AL, Landing BH. Postnatal development of the cystic lung lesion of Down syndrome: suggestion that the cause is reduced formation of peripheral air spaces. Pediatr Pathol. 1991;11(4):623-33.
5. Taylor PA, Dishop MK, Lotze TE, Mallory GB, Guillerman RP. Congenital multilobar emphysema: a characteristic lung growth disorder attributable to filamin A gene mutations. Pediatr Radiol. 2009;39(suppl 3):S516.
6. Robertson SP. Filamin A: phenotypic diversity. Curr Opin Genet Dev. 2005;15(3):301-7.

7. Guillerman RP. Imaging of childhood interstitial lung disease. Pediatr Allergy Immunol Pulmonol. 2010;23(1):43-68.
8. Brody AS, Guillerman RP, Hay TC, Wagner BD, Young LR, Deutsch GH, et al. Neuroendocrine cell hyperplasia of infancy: diagnosis with high-resolution CT. AJR Am J Roentgenol. 2010;194(1):238-44.
9. Semple TR, Ashworth MT, Owens CM. Interstitial Lung Disease in Children Made Easier…Well, Almost. Radiographics. 2017;37: 1679-703.
10. Suzuki T, Sakagami T, Young LR, Carey BC, Wood RE, Luisetti M, et al. Hereditary pulmonary alveolar proteinosis: pathogenesis, presentation, diagnosis, and therapy. Am J Respir Crit Care Med. 2010;182(10):1292-304.
11. Nicholson AG, Florio R, Hansell DM, Bois RM, Wells AU, Hughes P, et al. Pulmonary involvement by Niemann-Pick disease. A report of six cases. Histopathology. 2006;48(5):596-603.
12. Sévin M, Lesca G, Baumann N, Millat G, Lyon-Caen O, Vanier MT, et al. The adult form of Niemann-Pick disease type C. Brain. 2017;130 (Pt 1):120-33.
13. Nagral A. Gaucher disease. J Clin Exp Hepatol. 2014;4(1):37-50.
14. Hill SC, Damaska BM, Tsokos M, Kreps C, Brady RO, Barton NW. Radiographic findings in type 3b Gaucher disease. Pediatr Radiol. 1996;26(12):852-60.
15. Kim JH, Park CH, Pai MS, Hahn MH, Kim HJ. Hepatopulmonary syndrome in Gaucher disease with right-to-left shunt: evaluation and measurement using Tc-99m MAA. Clin Nucl Med. 1999;24(3):164-6.
16. Sharma S, Dey P. Childhood pulmonary Langerhans cell histiocytosis in bronchoalveolar lavage: a case report along with review of literature. Diagn Cytopathol. 2016;44(12): 1102-6.
17. Becciolini V, Gudinchet F, Cheseaux JJ, Schnyder P. Lymphocytic interstitial pneumonia in children with AIDS: high-resolution CT findings. Eur Radiol. 2001;11(6):1015-20.
18. von der Thüsen JH. Pleuroparenchymal fibroelastosis: its pathological characteristics. Curr Respir Med Rev. 2013;9(4): 238-47.

CHAPTER

67

Developmental Anomalies of Gastrointestinal Tract

Alpana Manchanda, Anju Garg, Radhika Batra

INTRODUCTION

Derangement of embryological development can lead to malformations at any point along the gastrointestinal tract (GIT) from the oropharynx to the anorectum. Most of these abnormalities manifest clinically with GIT obstruction and present with vomiting and abdominal distention. Bile-stained vomiting occurs when the obstruction is below the ampulla of Vater, whereas vomiting of clear gastric contents indicates obstruction above the second part of the duodenum. Abdominal distention indicates a low level of obstruction. However, one must remember that patients may present with overlapping features. Also, both vomiting and abdominal distention may occur in conditions where there is absence of anatomic abnormality of the GIT.[1] Developmental lesions of the neonatal GIT can be grouped as follows:[1]

ANATOMICAL

Attributed to embryological maldevelopment:

- Esophageal atresia with or without fistula
- Antropyloric atresia
- Antral diaphragm
- Duodenal atresia
- Duodenal stenosis
    - Intrinsic
    - Extrinsic
    - Midgut malrotation with peritoneal bands
- Anorectal atresia

Attributed to in utero catastrophic (ischemic) complication:

- Jejunoileal atresia
- Colonic atresia or stenosis
- Complicated meconium ileus

FUNCTIONAL

- Meconium plug syndrome and its variants
- Megacystis-microcolon-intestinal hypoperistalsis

COMBINED ANATOMICAL-FUNCTIONAL

- Hypertrophic pyloric stenosis (HPS)
- Midgut volvulus (complicating midgut malrotation)
- Uncomplicated meconium ileus
- Colonic aganglionosis (Hirschsprung's disease)

IMAGING MODALITIES

The imaging methods available to investigate the GIT in the neonate include plain film radiography, contrast studies of the GIT and ultrasonography. Nuclear scintigraphy, computed tomography (CT), and magnetic resonance imaging (MRI) are uncommonly required in infants.

Plain Film Radiography

It is simple, inexpensive, widely available, and usually the first and sometimes the only examination performed. The plain radiograph of the abdomen in supine position is the most commonly performed projection in children for abdominal evaluation. Air is an inherent contrast and the morphology and distribution of gas enables plain film diagnosis. Recognition of bowel gas features/patterns on a plain radiograph guides a radiologist in diagnosing intestinal obstruction, pneumoperitoneum, duodenal, and jejunal atresias. In the above conditions, a plain X-ray of the abdomen can be diagnostic in the appropriate clinical setting. Compared to a CT scan, a plain radiograph entails less radiation and the temporal evolution of the disease can be assessed on serial/follow-up X-rays. However, lack of contrast resolution and difficulty in interpretation due to overlapping structures are some of its limitations.[2] An anteroposterior supine radiograph may be sufficient only if the purpose is to evaluate a palpable mass or the presence of calcification. If obstruction is suspected, additional films are required. A cross-table lateral projection with the infant in supine position is best in terms of leaving the patient virtually undisturbed. However, a left-lateral decubitus view with a horizontal beam has the advantage of better identification of free gas over the liver and better anatomical definition of bowel loops than in a frontal projection. If only one film is desired, a prone radiograph will give the most information regarding free gas as well as defining the level of obstruction. Occasionally, a prone lateral film is valuable for detection of gas in the rectum.[1]

The various abdominal radiographic projections routinely performed and the features evaluated in them are given in **Table 1**.[3,4]

Gas Pattern in Neonates

The normal bowel gas pattern in neonates is quite different from that seen in older children and adults. Within seconds after birth, air enters the GIT and it can be seen radiographically in the stomach. Air is seen in the small bowel within the first hour, it reaches the cecum within 3–4 hours, and appears in the sigmoid colon by 11 hours. Gas fluid levels are generally absent except in the stomach and occasionally in the right colon. It is characterized by gas throughout the small and large bowel and little fluid with respect to air so that bowel-air interfaces are thin and sharp, with few if any loops identified; rather, the gas distribution is one of multiple, closely apposed, rounded, or polyhedral structures. Small and large bowel cannot be distinguished on a plain radiograph due to nondevelopment of haustrae.[5]

A gasless abdomen after the first few hours of life is occasionally seen in normal infants as well as in those with uncontrollable vomiting, continuous gastric aspiration, severe dehydration, esophageal atresia without a fistula, and deficient air swallowing secondary to central nervous system (CNS) depression. Obstruction is manifested by distention of portion of the GIT proximal to the obstruction with little or no gas below. By observing the number and distribution of distended bowel loops and air-fluid levels, one can estimate the approximate level of obstruction **(Figs. 1A and B)**.

TABLE 1: Bowel gas features evaluated on abdominal radiographs.

Radiographic projections of abdomen X-rays	Features evaluated
Abdomen supine	Soft-tissue mass or calcification, position, caliber of bowel loops (gas pattern)
Abdomen erect	Free intraperitoneal air (pneumoperitoneum), distribution, and number of air-fluid levels
Abdomen left lateral decubitus view (in suspected perforation, ischemia, and obstruction)	Small pockets of extraintestinal air, portal venous gas, and differential air-fluid levels
Abdomen in prone position	Is best for assessment of rectal gas, to rule out bowel obstruction
Prone cross table lateral view (X-ray abdomen in prone position with horizontal beam)	Helps to differentiate mechanical from functional obstruction. Rectal gas suggests ileus while absence of air in rectum is indicative of mechanical obstruction

Contrast Studies

Air is the cheapest, easiest, and most commonly available contrast medium. The presence of gas within the bowel can be very useful in delineating abnormalities, particularly a proximal high atresia. Occasionally, one may require to inject air to delineate the bowel better and it can be instilled by nasogastric tube or per rectum.[6]

Contrast studies of the GIT such as the contrast swallow, upper gastrointestinal (UGI) study or contrast enema is performed under fluoroscopic guidance. Radiation exposure to the patient can be reduced by adhering to the ALARA (as low as reasonably achievable) principle. The practices which help in reducing the radiation dose include use of: (a) Intermittent pulsed fluoroscopy; (b) Last image capture; (c) Appropriate collimation; (d) Removing antiscatter grid;

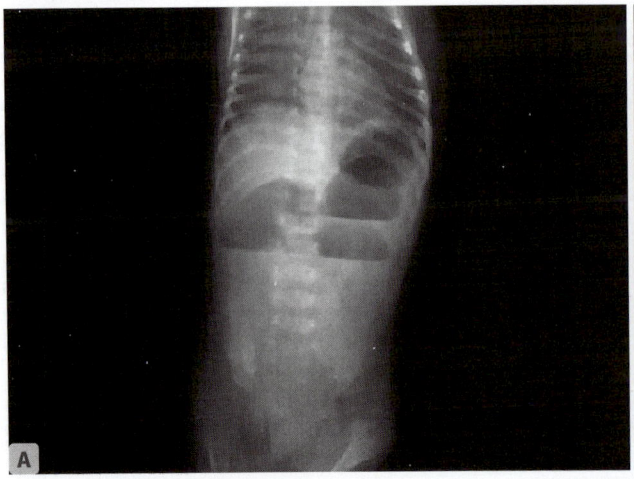

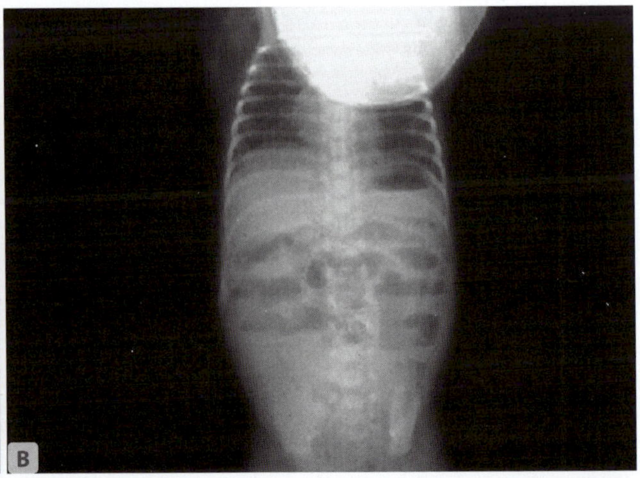

FIGS. 1A AND B: Plain X-ray abdomen erect view reveals (A) few (three) air-fluid levels in proximal small bowel with absence of distal air diagnostic of a (high small bowel jejunal) obstruction in a newborn presenting with bilious vomiting; (B) In contrast, multiple air-fluid levels seen in another neonate with abdominal distention are indicative of a low small bowel (ileal) obstruction.

(e) Avoiding digital magnification; and (f) Reducing the distance between the patient and image intensifier.[7]

Barium in the form of barium sulfate is the primary contrast medium used to demonstrate the GIT. Barium is not used in the following circumstances: (i) Suspected perforation of hollow viscus, where preferably a low osmolar nonionic water soluble iodinated contrast medium should be used, e.g., iohexol (omnipaque); (ii) Instances of lower small-bowel obstruction when retained fluid proximally is likely to cause oral barium suspension to precipitate and degrade the images; (iii) When a cleansing effect is also desired, as in attempted reduction of meconium ileus or meconium plug; and (iv) In contrast studies in neonates due to increased risk of bowel perforation and leak.

Ionic water-soluble contrast media are used rectally for therapeutic purposes in case of uncomplicated meconium ileus for stimulating evacuation of retained thick tenacious intestinal contents by virtue of their high osmolarity, which increases the intraluminal fluid and bulk. This, however, may cause water and electrolyte imbalance and appropriate patient hydration and electrolyte homeostasis should be carefully maintained. High osmolal and ionic contrast media (meglumine and sodium diatrizoate) are contraindicated when investigating esophageal problems because of risk of aspiration and consequent pulmonary edema.

Nonionic contrast media are ideal for most of the circumstances. Nevertheless, utmost care and close fluoroscopic monitoring should be done in all patients who are at a risk of aspiration. In suspected Hirschsprung's disease, in which the rate of evacuation has some potential diagnostic value, barium should be preferred. The radiologist should modify the routine use of contrast as needed in a particular case.

Ultrasonography

The role of ultrasound has increased in recent years, especially for neonatal bowel disorders. Ultrasonography has been found to be highly accurate in the diagnosis of HPS. It is useful in the diagnosis of gastric and duodenal duplications and in the detection of duodenal dilatation accompanying intrinsic or extrinsic duodenal obstruction, such as duodenal atresia and stenosis. Ultrasound is valuable in the investigation of abdominal distention or palpable mass lesions because of easy and accurate detection of ascites as well as meconium peritonitis and intraperitoneal cystic lesions such as intestinal duplications and mesenteric or omental cysts.[1]

Computed Tomography

CT is not the first line of investigation in the evaluation of pediatric bowel pathology. However it can be used as a second-line modality which can provide valuable information regarding the location of pathology and to characterize it whenever conventional investigations do not provide adequate information.

ESOPHAGUS

Esophageal Atresia and Tracheoesophageal Fistula

Esophageal atresia with or without tracheoesophageal fistula (TEF) is the most common congenital abnormality of the esophagus, manifesting itself during the neonatal period, occurring in about 1 in 2,500–4,000 live births.[8] It is usually sporadic and its etiology is uncertain.[6] No definite familial tendency has been documented in esophageal atresia, but more than one case in the same family has been noted.

Embryology

The trachea and esophagus develop from the common foregut during the early first trimester. During the 5th and 6th weeks of gestation, the common foregut divides into trachea and esophagus. Incomplete separation results in esophageal atresia with or without associated TEF. Because separation of the trachea and esophagus occurs cranial to tracheal branching of the carina, TEFs generally present above the carina.[9]

Clinical Presentation

The presentation is usually in the first few hours of life with the newborn having excessive oral secretions, choking, and sometimes even cyanosis. Typically, symptoms become more pronounced during the first feed. The abdomen may be distended due to air passing through the distal fistula into the stomach or may be scaphoid or gasless in patients who have atresia without a fistula or atresia with a proximal fistula. Patients with an H-fistula usually present later with history of choking while feeding, cough, cyanosis, recurrent or chronic pneumonias, and a distended abdomen from tracheal gas passing through the fistula into the esophagus and stomach.[9]

Esophageal atresia may be diagnosed by antenatal ultrasound. It is suspected on the basis of maternal polyhydramnios with an absent fluid-filled stomach, the proximal esophageal pouch seen as a central anechoic area in the fetal neck or upper chest. The presence and size of the TEF determines the amount of fluid in the stomach and GIT. Associated anomalies in the other systems may be identified. The atresias may be multiple and involve the esophagus, duodenum, and anus.

Classification

Esophageal atresia and TEF have been classified based on their anatomical and radiographic appearance, i.e., on the basis of presence (and location) or absence of a TEF **(Figs. 2A to E)**. They have been variously designated as types A to E according to the gross classification (or 1–5) as follows:[6]

- Type A—esophageal atresia without fistula (7.8%)
- Type B—esophageal atresia with proximal fistula (0.8%)
- Type C—esophageal atresia with distal fistula (85.8%)
- Type D—esophageal atresia with fistula in both the pouches (1.4%)
- Type E—H-type fistula without atresia (4.2%)

In the majority of patients, the atresia occurs between the proximal and middle thirds of the esophagus with a gap of varying length between the atretic pouches.[6]

Most commonly, there is a proximal esophageal atresia with a distal TEF (Type C). This occurs in approximately 85.8% of cases. Next most common, occurring approximately in 7.8% cases, is isolated esophageal atresia. H-type fistula occurs in approximately 4.2% of cases. Esophageal atresia with proximal TEF or with both proximal and distal TEFs are quite rare.[10]

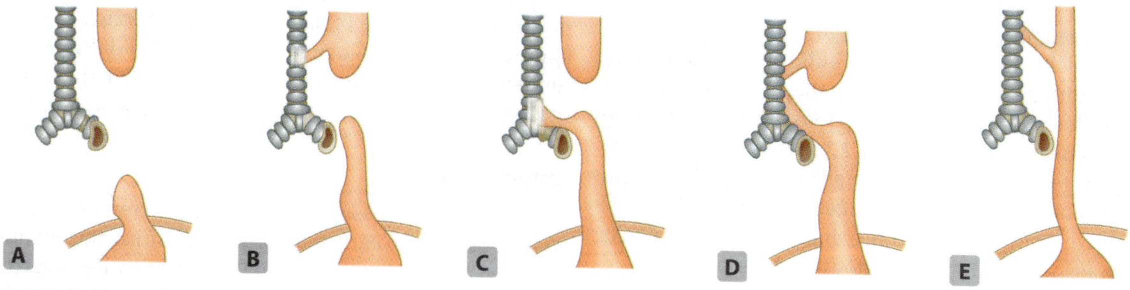

FIGS. 2A TO E: Types of esophageal atresia/tracheoesophageal fistula (TEF). Type C fistula is the most common while type E is a TEF without atresia (H-type fistula).

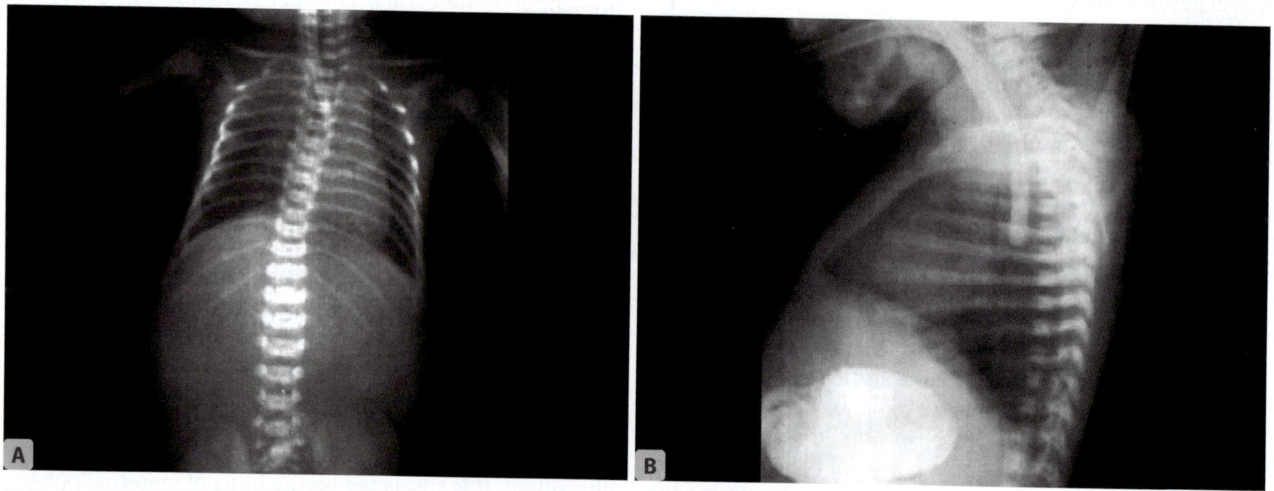

FIGS. 3A AND B: Type A esophageal atresia. (A) Frontal radiograph of chest and abdomen showing a catheter in the proximal pouch. The abdomen is gasless; (B) Lateral film shows the tip of the tube at the level of 4th dorsal vertebra.

Approximately 50–70% of patients with esophageal atresia have additional anomalies. The VACTERL syndrome is seen in 15–30% of patients. "V" is for vertebral and vascular abnormalities. Of these, a right-sided aortic arch is seen in 5% cases. "A" is for anal and auricular malformations. "C" is for cardiac abnormalities such as ventricular septal defects, patent ductus arteriosus, and complex cyanotic heart disease. "TE" is for TEF and esophageal atresia. "R" represents renal abnormalities and "L" is for limb malformations.[11] A person is designated to have VACTERL abnormality if there are three or more anomalies of the vertebral, anorectal, cardiac, tracheal, esophageal, renal, and limb system without any chromosomal aberration.[7] Other syndromes such as CHARGE syndrome (coloboma, heart malformation, choanal atresia, mental retardation, genitourinary, and ear malformations) and Down syndrome can also be associated.

Imaging Features

A plain radiograph of the chest taken soon after birth reveals a proximal esophageal pouch distended with air, thereby indicating the diagnosis on plain radiographs. In equivocal cases, a thin soft rubber nasogastric tube is passed into the proximal pouch and about 5 cc of air is injected. A frontal radiograph of the chest showing a dilated proximal esophageal pouch with round distal margin and coiled nasogastric tube within is diagnostic. The distended air-filled proximal esophageal pouch may make visualization of the lower cervical and upper dorsal spine more clear. A lateral radiograph though not routinely indicated shows considerable anterior bowing and narrowing of the trachea by the dilated blind esophageal pouch.[6] Plain radiograph of the chest should include the abdomen to evaluate the presence of air in the GIT. The presence of air in the stomach and the small bowel indicates esophageal atresia with a distal TEF which is seen on plain radiographs in both types C and D tracheoesophageal fistulae. Absence of air in the stomach eliminates the possibility of a distal fistula as is seen in types A and B tracheoesophageal fistulae. The possibility of proximal TEF, however, cannot be eliminated **(Figs. 3A and B and 4)**.

Air confined to the stomach raises the possibility of associated duodenal atresia and necessitates a follow-up plain film examination.

Routine contrast examination is generally contraindicated in the neonate with esophageal atresia and TEF because of risk of aspiration.[7] Hence, use of radiopaque contrast in the proximal pouch should be avoided. Swallowed air or air through nasogastric tube is usually adequate for the diagnosis and to demonstrate the extent of the proximal pouch. If positive contrast examination is needed then isotonic nonionic contrast medium should be used in minimal

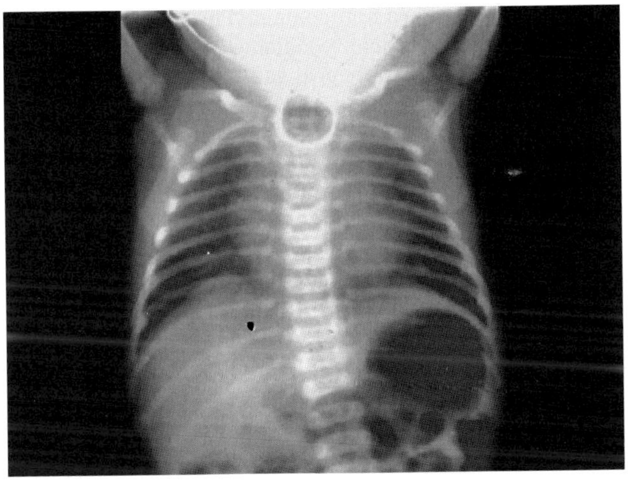

FIG. 4: Esophageal atresia with distal tracheoesophageal fistula (type C): Coiled nasogastric tube is seen in the proximal esophageal pouch. Air is seen in the stomach and bowel.

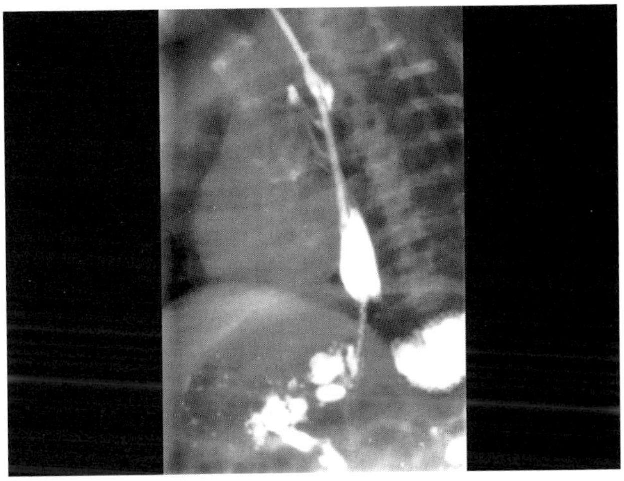

FIG. 5: Contrast esophagogram demonstrating an oblique tract of an H-type tracheoesophageal fistula arising from the anterior wall of the esophagus and passing cephalad to the posterior tracheal wall with contrast filling the tracheobronchial tree.

amount under fluoroscopic monitoring. Immediately after the study, contrast should be aspirated. The study should be done with the infant in the lateral position and to facilitate demonstration of associated fistula, if any, the infant can be turned prone. The infant should not be put in supine position because of the risk of aspiration.[12]

Congenital, isolated TEF without atresia (type E in **Fig. 2**) also termed as "H-type fistula", differs from other types of TEF in its presenting features and appearance. Patients typically present with episodes of choking or coughing. The children with H-type of fistula may present late with symptoms of recurrent lung infection due to aspiration.[2] The pattern of pneumonia is usually more widespread, resulting in difficulty in delineation of fistula.[12]

Large fistulae generally present early in life and are easily picked up on a contrast swallow study. H-type fistulae are more commonly small, inconstantly patent, and may need repeated examination before they are diagnosed. Though H-type fistulas can be at any level, most are at the thoracic inlet, between C7 and T2 vertebral bodies. The connection is angulated superiorly from the esophagus to the trachea, thus accounting for the more precise but less popular appellation of the N-type fistula **(Fig. 5)**. The best way to demonstrate H-type TEF is with careful injection of contrast medium via a nasogastric tube, first placed at gastroesophageal (GE) junction and then gradually withdrawing the nasogastric tube with simultaneous injection of contrast under fluoroscopic guidance at various levels of the esophagus. The main reason that the H-type TEF is inconstantly patent is that the normal esophageal mucosa is quite redundant and usually occludes the esophageal side of the fistula. Normal active swallowing may not distend the esophagus sufficiently to allow passage of contrast into the fistula.[13] The patient should be viewed in the lateral or steep prone oblique projection with the right side down. Care should be taken to separate tracheal and esophageal lumens during the study so that fistula is readily identified between them. If the contrast appears in the trachea or lungs, it is very important to be certain if the contrast went through a fistula or was aspirated. If in doubt, then the investigation must be repeated once the trachea is cleared of the contrast.

H-type fistulas are commonly demonstrated by contrast studies.[6] However, bronchoscopy and endoscopy are more sensitive methods and may be indicated to confirm the diagnosis, especially in a symptomatic older child where the contrast esophagogram is normal.

Computed tomography is occasionally used in the preoperative evaluation of neonates with TEF and has proved to be a noninvasive and quick investigation. As compared with conventional bronchoscopy or catheterization, CT does not require any general anesthesia. The improved spatial and temporal resolution of new generation of scanners facilitates assessment of small defects such as TEF. Either direct sagittal acquisition or axial acquisition with multiplanar reconstruction may help in demonstrating the precise location of fistula and the length of the gap between esophageal segments. Alternatively, length of the atretic segment can be assessed by passing a feeding tube from above and a metal bougie from below, via a gastrostomy.

The knowledge of the origin of the fistula is helpful to the surgeon not only in deciding the side of the thoracotomy (right or left), but also in anticipating the gap to be bridged. The most important advantage of CT is that both esophagus and trachea are seen in their natural (unstretched) positions, and the interpouch gap can be measured accurately.[14]

High resolution CT scan on a 64-slice CT scanner has shown to provide definitive diagnosis and help in surgical planning in critically ill neonates with H-Type TEF by distending the esophagus with air (by means of nasogastric feeding tube) during CT acquisition. Such a maneuver has proved to be very useful in optimizing the visualization of the fistula which may be totally or partially closed by a valve-like mucosal flap or by a spasm of the muscular layer of the esophagus.[15]

Treatment

Surgical correction of the fistula is the treatment of choice which can be done by endoscopic, thoracoscopic or as standard open repair. The side of the aortic arch should always be determined and reported on the plain radiograph. This information is important to the surgeon because the surgical approach to the mediastinum for repair of esophageal atresia with a distal TEF is from the side opposite to the aortic arch. When plain radiograph fails to indicate the side of the arch, CT or a cardiac ultrasound can localize the arch.

In esophageal atresia with a distal fistula, primary repair is possible as the length of the gap between the esophageal segments is usually short. When there is atresia with no distal fistula, there is usually a long gap (of the order of about five vertebral bodies) between the proximal and distal esophageal segments. The growth of the esophageal segments during the first few months of life tends to lessen the gap, thereby making a delayed primary repair feasible. A gastrostomy is established for feeding in the meantime.

Radiological Evaluation of Postoperative Complications

Most patients of isolated esophageal atresia and TEF do well following surgical repair which is performed early in life between 1 and 7 days. Nevertheless, complications following surgery do occur and can be grouped under early and late complications. The **early complications** include: (i) Leakage at the anastomotic site (14–16%); (ii) Esophageal stricture; and (iii) Recurrent fistula. Oral feeding is not started for 1–2 weeks following surgery, till the edema subsides. A contrast study of the esophagus should be performed prior to the institution of oral feeds. A low-osmolar nonionic contrast should be used as leakage at the anastomotic site is the most commonly identified early complication of surgical repair.

Postoperative leak has been found to be more common in patients who have undergone a primary surgical repair than those who have had a thoracoscopic repair. The leakage can be a contained leak or a noncontained leak. Around 75% of patients who develop a non-contained leak after surgery are known to develop a stricture. Patients with long gap atresia, which is defined as esophageal gap >2.5 cm, are known to develop postoperative leak more frequently compared to patients with short gap atresia (i.e., esophageal gap <2.5 cm).

Stricture is another common complication which can occur following esophageal atresia repair. Most often, the stricture or narrowing is slight at the site of anastomotic repair and may persist for years, even though the patient has no functional problem **(Figs. 6A and B)**. Those with true stricture at anastomotic site are symptomatic and generally respond to bougie dilatation with reoperation generally not required. However, if a stricture is associated with GE reflux (GER), the stricture may not respond to dilatation if it continues to be exposed to the acidic gastric contents. Hence, patients with postoperative strictures should be evaluated for reflux by UGI series or pH monitoring.

A *TEF can recur* (3–14% cases) again at the anastomotic site following surgery and is believed to be related to anastomotic leakage with erosion into trachea caused by local inflammation.

The ***late complications*** which can occur following repair of an esophageal atresia are long-term dysphagia, dysmotility, GER, tracheomalacia, rib fusion, and scoliosis. Dysmotility is present in nearly all patients who have had esophageal atresia and along with dysphagia have been known to persist till adulthood.

Gastroesophageal reflux is also commonly associated and has been reported in 40–70% of cases. Reflux is thought to be related to the shortening of the intra-abdominal portion of the esophagus, or occur secondary to the surgical repair. Reflux may lead to peptic esophagitis and is likely to be the cause of more distal strictures in those who have had a history of repaired esophageal atresia. Other known complications of GE reflux Disease (GERD) which are known to occur are aspiration, bronchial hyperactivity, and airway damage. Around 50% of GERD patients respond to medical treatment while around 15% of post-TEF repair patients with GERD are known to require an anti-reflux surgical procedure.

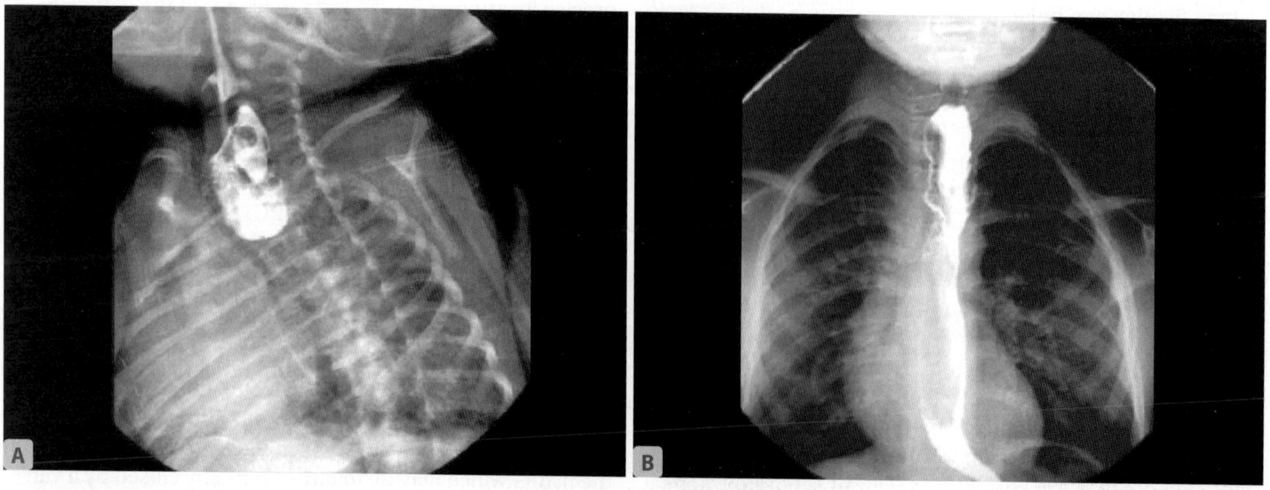

FIGS. 6A AND B: (A) Esophageal atresia with distal tracheoesophageal fistula (TEF) in a neonate. Lateral radiograph shows contrast-filled dilated proximal esophageal pouch bowing the trachea anteriorly; (B) Barium swallow following primary anastomosis of esophageal atresia demonstrates slight narrowing at the anastomotic site (D4 vertebral level). The child had mild respiratory distress with dysphagia.

Tracheomalacia is thought to occur due to chronic intrauterine compression of trachea by a distended upper esophageal pouch.

STOMACH

Microgastria

Congenital microgastria is an extremely rare anomaly in which fetal rotation of the stomach fails to occur. The stomach is small and underdeveloped. There is no differentiation into fundus, body, antrum and pyloric canal, and the lesser and greater curvatures also do not develop.[13] It is believed to occur as a result of atresia of normal foregut development in the 5th week of embryonal development.

Microgastria is often accompanied by other congenital anomalies such as malrotation, asplenia, renal, limb, and vertebral and cardiac anomalies (VACTERL syndrome).[8] The common association between microgastria and upper extremity limb reduction defects has led to the term microgastria-limb reduction complex.[13]

Clinical Presentation

The clinical presentation of microgastria depends on the stage at which gastric development has been arrested. On prenatal ultrasound, it may mimic esophageal atresia due to failure to visualize a distended stomach. Postnatally, microgastria presents with postprandial vomiting, failure to thrive, developmental delay, growth retardation, malnutrition, and aspiration pneumonia. Most of the symptoms are due to secondary GER.[8]

Imaging Features

On plain radiograph, microgastria results in the absence of the normal gastric bubble. An upper GI study shows a small tubular stomach in the midline (<25% of normal size). The esophagus (megaesophagus) appears to take over the storage function of the small capacity stomach. The GE junction is incompetent and GE reflux is present. It results in associated esophageal dysmotility, secondary to its massive dilatation.[8]

Treatment

The treatment of microgastria depends on its severity. The less severe forms may be treated conservatively, with surgery reserved as the first line of treatment in severe cases. The surgical treatment consists of creation of a Hunt–Lawrence pouch (a double lumen roux-en-Y jejunal pouch) as a gastric reservoir, which allows for the secondary esophageal changes to resolve.[8]

DEVELOPMENTAL OBSTRUCTIVE DEFECTS

Gastric Atresia

Isolated gastric atresia is very rare and accounts for <1% of all congenital obstructions and presents with complete gastric outlet obstruction.[16] Almost all gastric atresias occur at the pylorus or antrum. They are thought to be due to localized vascular occlusion in fetal life and not due to failure of recanalization of the intestinal tract.[6] Gastric atresia is classified into three types **(Fig. 7)**.[12]

1. Type A: Complete atresia with no connection between the stomach and duodenum
2. Type B: Complete atresia with a fibrous band connecting the stomach and duodenum, and
3. Type C: A gastric membrane or diaphragm producing atresia

Gastric atresia may be familial or associated with multiple atresias and with epidermolysis bullosa. The newborn presents mainly with nonbilious vomiting within the first few hours after birth. As obstruction is complete, a plain radiograph of the abdomen reveals a "**single bubble appearance**" with marked dilatation of the stomach, proximal to the obstruction, and absence of gas in the small bowel and colon **(Figs. 8A and B)**. This appearance is diagnostic and most patients are taken directly to surgery without any contrast imaging.[11] Surgical intervention involves bypassing the obstruction and creation of patent lumen.

Prepyloric Membrane or Antral Web/Diaphragm

A prepyloric membrane or antral web is a rare cause of symptomatic gastric obstruction in the newborn.[5] Patients with webs or stenosis of the pylorus, rather than complete atresia may present later in life or even in adulthood because the obstruction is incomplete.[13] The most common presenting symptom is cyclic postprandial vomiting and

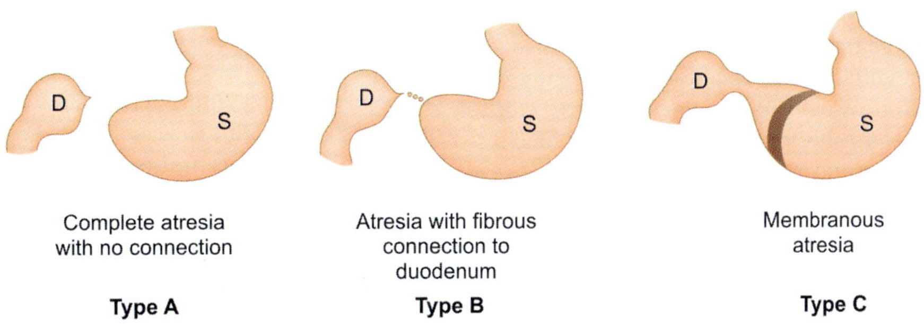

FIG. 7: Schematic representation of types of gastric atresia: (A) Complete atresia; (B) Atresia with fibrous connection; and (C) Membranous atresia. (S: stomach, D: duodenum).

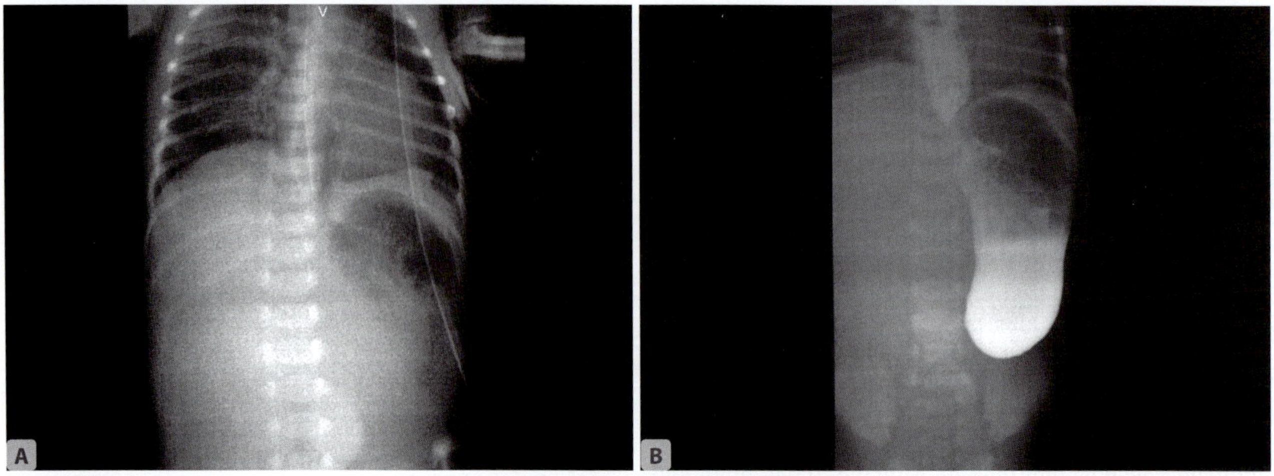

FIGS. 8A AND B: Gastric atresia. (A) Plain radiograph shows a distended stomach with nonvisualization of air distally; (B) Barium upper gastrointestinal (UGI) study reveals complete gastric outlet obstruction with no passage of contrast into duodenum consistent with complete atresia.

episodes of transient vomiting.[14] Radiographically, the stomach is dilated with varying degrees of distal air, the extent of which depends on the degree of obstruction. In patients with incomplete obstruction, webs are more common than stenosis.[8] Incomplete obstruction due to web or diaphragm is more commonly encountered than complete atresia which is very rare.

It is difficult to diagnose an antral web on imaging studies. On UGI barium studies, a web is seen as a thin, 2–3 mm, linear circumferential filling defect traversing the barium column producing a reduction in the antral lumen, typically located 1–2 cm from the pylorus with a normal pyloric canal.[11] On ultrasound, the membrane may be visible if the stomach is filled with clear fluid and appears as echogenic band extending centrally from the lesser and greater curvatures in the prepyloric region. A mucous strand may be mistaken for an antral membrane. On the basis of clinical and radiographic findings, the definitive diagnosis of antral web can be confirmed endoscopically.[2]

Hypertrophic Pyloric Stenosis

Hypertrophic pyloric stenosis is a common developmental surgical condition affecting young infants in the first few months of life. It is characterized by hypertrophy of pyloric circular muscle and redundancy of the pyloric mucosa. Its etiology is unknown. Possible causes include hypersecretion with resulting duodenal irritation and pylorospasm. There is constant association with hyperplasia of the antral mucosa. Abnormal innervation of pylorus and lack of nitric oxide synthetase may be responsible for the pylorospasm that leads to muscular hypertrophy and gastric outlet obstruction.[9]

Clinical Presentation

The incidence of HPS is approximately 3 in 1,000 live births and boys are affected 4-5 times more commonly than girls. There is a familial disposition typically seen in first born male infants. Affected patients usually present between 2 and 6 weeks of age with a classical history of projectile nonbilious vomiting which may be intermittent or occur with every feed. It needs to be differentiated from other conditions that can manifest with nonbilious vomiting **(Box 1)**.[17] HPS is never seen beyond 3 months of age, except reported in premature infants, in whom, enteral feeding has been started late.[18]

BOX 1: Differential diagnosis of nonbilious vomiting in an infant.

- Hypertrophic pyloric stenosis
- Pylorospasm
- Preampullary duodenal stenosis

Diagnosis can be made on appropriate history. Late clinical presentation results in palpation of an "olive" mass in the subhepatic region of an infant which represents the thickened pylorus. Antral peristaltic waves can also be observed.[6]

In most cases, a clinical diagnosis can be confidently made. If not diagnosed promptly, protracted vomiting may lead to dehydration and development of hypochloremic metabolic alkalosis. However, most patients usually do not have metabolic abnormalities due to early diagnosis on imaging.

Imaging Features

Ultrasonography

Ultrasonography is the imaging modality of choice in an infant suspected of having pyloric stenosis with a reported accuracy approaching 100%.[17] By virtue of being noninvasive, it is able to visualize the pyloric muscle directly and obtain measurements of muscle thickness and has replaced barium evaluation.[19,20] Ultrasound examination is typically performed with a high frequency linear transducer as the stomach, pylorus, and duodenum are very superficial in an infant.[21] A 6–10 MHz probe provides the depth to visualize the pylorus. The gallbladder, which is adjacent to the pylorus, serves as a good landmark.[6] Longitudinal and transverse images through the pylorus are obtained with the infant in the right posterior oblique position while scanning the right upper quadrant just off the midline. In this position, any fluid in the fundus of the stomach moves into the antrum and pyloric region, distending these regions. The stomach should not be emptied prior to the examination as this makes identification of antropyloric area difficult. If there is inadequate distention of the antrum, the infant may be given a glucose solution or water, orally or via a nasogastric tube. If fluid is administered, it should be removed at the end of the examination to prevent further vomiting and the risk of aspiration. In addition, if there is a lot of gas, scanning the baby in the prone position may help in visualization of the pyloric region.[21] Ultrasound is a dynamic study which allows direct visualization of both morphological and quantitative features of the pyloric canal.

The **classic findings** are of a **thickened echo-poor pyloric muscle** and an **elongated pyloric canal**.[19,20,22] The thickened muscle is seen as two curved bundles of mixed but generally low reflectivity bulging into the base of the duodenal cap and gastric antrum. The mucosal echoes are seen as one or two central bright lines. On transverse images, the hypertrophic pylorus has a doughnut appearance representing the reflective central mucosa and submucosa surrounded by echo-poor muscle. The hypertrophic muscle may look nonuniform on transverse scanning of the pylorus.[23] This is related to the sonographic artifact of anisotropic effect because of the orientation of the muscle fibers.[6] Other signs include exaggerated peristaltic waves that terminate at the pylorus, esophageal reflux and little if any gastric emptying.

An experienced examiner can frequently make the diagnosis just by qualitative assessment of the thickness of the pyloric wall. The exact measurements that separate a normal pylorus from a hypertrophic one are controversial.[20,22,24] However, as a general guide, a **pyloric canal length >15 mm, muscle thickness >3.0 mm, and transverse serosa-to-serosa diameter >15 mm is consistent with HPS (Figs. 9A and B).** At least two values should be positive. A muscle thickness <2.0 mm is unequivocally normal. A muscle thickness between 2 and 2.9 mm is abnormal but nonspecific, and can be seen in gastritis and pylorospasm as well as in HPS. Though pylorospasm may mimic HPS on sonography as there is some pyloric muscle thickening and/or slight elongation of the pyloric canal, pylorospasm is transient and generally resolves in 30 minutes. An important pointer for diagnosing pylorospasm is that there is considerable variation in measurement or image appearance with time during the study.[25] Borderline muscle thickness measurements are more likely to occur in premature than in term infants.

During sonography, the dynamic passage of gastric contents through the antropyloric region is important. A wide-open pylorus through which there is normal passage of gastric contents excludes HPS.

A number of ancillary sonographic signs of HPS have been described[21] **(Fig. 10)**.

- *"Shoulder sign"*—refers to an indentation upon the gastric antrum produced by hypertrophy of the pyloric muscle.
- *"Double tract sign"*—this refers to fluid, trapped in the mucosal folds in the center of an elongated pyloric canal seen as two sonolucent streaks in the center.
- *"Nipple sign"* is produced due to the evagination of redundant pyloric mucosa into the distended portion of the antrum.

Color Doppler evaluation of the pylorus may reveal hyperemia within the muscle and mucosal layers.

False negative diagnosis may be made if the stomach is overdistended, because it can displace the pylorus posteriorly, making it difficult to visualize the pyloric canal. If the scan is not in the midline, or is tangential to the antrum, the antral wall can simulate a thickened pyloric muscle, leading to a false positive diagnosis. **Box 2** depicts the key imaging features of HPS.

Barium Study

A barium study should be performed if ultrasound is inconclusive or GER is suspected.[25] If gastric distention is severe, a nasogastric tube should be passed and the stomach emptied. With the patient in the prone oblique position,

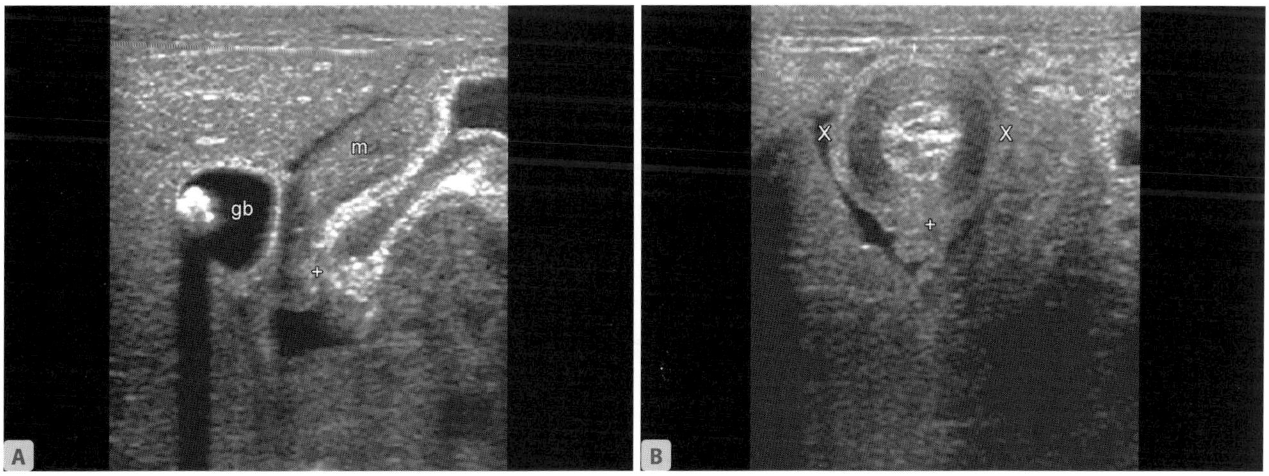

FIGS. 9A AND B: (A) Hypertrophic pyloric stenosis: Longitudinal ultrasound image showing an elongated thickened pylorus seen as two curved bundles of low reflectivity (m). The mucosal echoes are seen as central bright lines. Gallbladder (gb) shows sludge within. Minimal fluid is present around the stomach; (B) Transverse section shows the muscle thickness as an echo poor rim—"Bull's eye" sign. Serosa-to-serosa measures 15 mm (cursors).

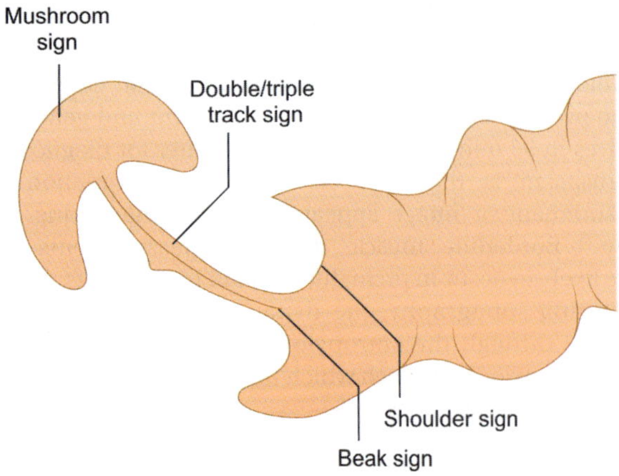

FIG. 10: Schematic representation of signs of hypertrophic pyloric stenosis.

BOX 2: Key imaging findings of hypertrophic pyloric stenosis.

On high resolution US

- Muscle thickness >3.0 mm
- Pyloric canal length >15 mm
- Transverse serosa-to-serosa diameter >15 mm

On barium UGI study

- "String sign": Passage of thin streak of barium into narrow elongated pyloric canal
- "Double string sign": Barium caught between mucosal folds in pyloric canal
- "Beak sign": Seen at the entrance of pyloric canal when the thick muscle narrows the canal

(UGI: upper gastrointestinal; US: ultrasonography)

the tube is placed in the antrum and adequate barium is injected via the tube under fluoroscopic control and spot films are taken.

Most of the infants, with and without HPS, show some degree of pylorospasm. In HPS, generally barium will pass through the antropyloric region within 1–10 minutes, but may be delayed as long as 20–25 minutes. The **pyloric canal** is narrowed (the "string sign") and elongated and almost always curved upward posteriorly **(Fig. 11)**. **Combination of narrowing and elongation** is the **hallmark** of HPS **on barium study**. Barium may be caught between folds overlying the hypertrophied muscle and parallel lines (the "double-string sign") may be seen **(Fig. 12)**. The enlarged muscle mass looks much like an "apple-core lesion", with undercutting of the distal antrum and proximal duodenal bulb. The "beak sign" is noted as the thick muscle narrows the barium column as it enters the pyloric canal. Virtually, all of the above signs can be seen transiently in infants especially those with some degree of spasm. The study should be continued sufficiently long to document the persistence of the findings in order to assure the diagnosis of pyloric stenosis. Occasionally, an associated antral web or diaphragm may be identified.

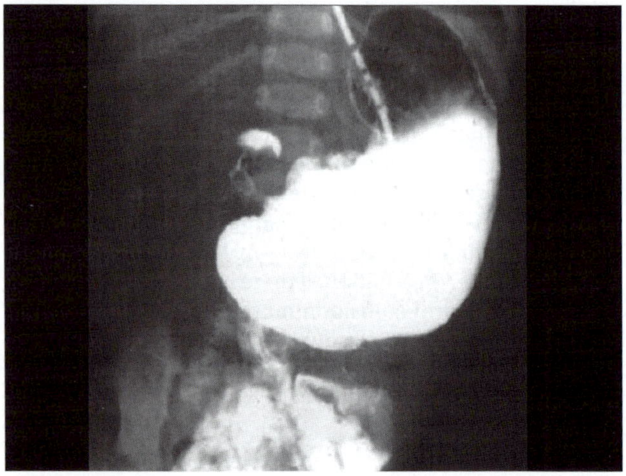

FIG. 11: Upper gastrointestinal (UGI) barium study in a child with pyloric stenosis. The markedly narrowed pylorus curves upward and posteriorly to the duodenal bulb which shows an impression of the hypertrophied muscle in the base.

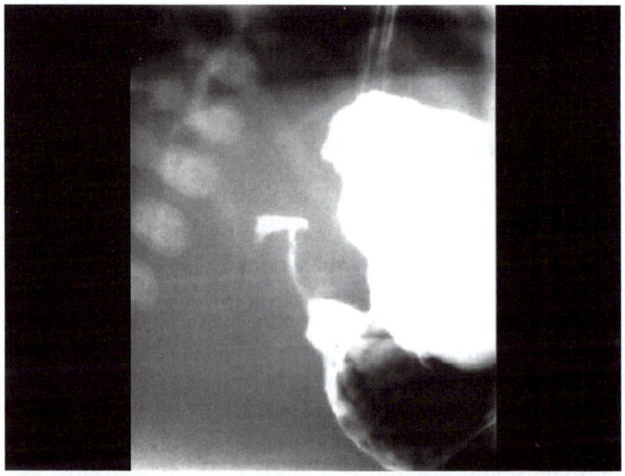

FIG. 12: Characteristic findings of hypertrophic pyloric stenosis in a 6-week-old boy with history of vomiting: The pyloric canal is narrowed and elongated and the base of the duodenal bulb is stretched by the pyloric mass.

Adult Idiopathic Hypertrophic Pyloric Stenosis (AIHPS)

It is a mild form of HPS which may rarely present later in adult life. Its exact incidence is not known, as majority of these patients are asymptomatic for years. Around 80% of patients with the adult form of the disease are men which is in concordance with the male preponderance of congenital HPS. The primary form of AIHPS should be differentiated from the secondary form which is caused by diseases such as peptic ulcer disease, hypertrophic gastritis, or malignancy.[26]

In AIHPS, the pylorus is bulbous or fusiform with its thickest portion at the pyloroduodenal junction. Patients present with symptoms of delayed gastric emptying not associated with any pain.

The radiologic and endoscopic studies may be nonspecific. However, the diagnosis should be suspected if there is elongation of the pyloric canal and is accompanied by marked dilatation of the stomach.

In AIHPS, the "string sign" may be seen as an extremely thin line of barium on an UGI study. A marked thickening of the pyloric muscle may produce a convex indentation at the base of the duodenal bulb, causing a mushroom-like deformity (Kirklin's sign). The presence of a barium-filled cleft between the hypertrophied muscle and the fibers of the pylorus can project into either one or both sides of the pylorus, proximal to the base of the bulb (Twining's sign). However, none of these signs are pathognomonic and presence of two or more of them strengthens the radiologic diagnosis. Endoscopy may be useful and the classic finding that has been described is the "donut" or the cervix sign which consists of a fixed narrow pylorus with a smooth border.

Treatment

Surgery is the treatment of choice of both the pediatric and adult forms of HPS. In the congenital type of HPS, surgical pyloromyotomy is the preferred treatment. It involves division of the thickened outer muscle while the inner layer of the pylorus is left intact. This opens a wider channel to allow the contents of the stomach to pass easily. Normal emptying of the stomach occurs within 2–3 days after the procedure. However, muscle thickness gradually regresses to normal and may even take 5 months to return to normal after successful surgery. In the 1st week after surgery, the pyloric muscle can be of the same thickness or even thicker than before surgery. The dimensions gradually return to normal with anterior muscle normalizing before the posterior part (3 mm by 3 months as against 5 months for the posterior muscle wall).[27] In contrast, in AIHPS, pyloroplasty and laparoscopic pyloromyotomy have been tried with successful results.[28]

An increased incidence of renal anomalies such as pelviureteric junction obstruction, primary megaureter, duplex kidney, renal agenesis or ectopia, and horseshoe kidney have been reported in patients with HPS.[26]

Ectopic Pancreas

It is defined as the presence of pancreatic tissue outside its normal location with lack of any anatomic or vascular connection with the pancreas. Ectopic pancreas is mainly seen to occur in the proximal GIT in the stomach (26%), duodenum (28%), and proximal jejunum (16%).[29]

Clinical Presentation

Ectopic pancreas is most often detected incidentally. It can present in children or adults with chronic and nonspecific symptoms. The patient may present with symptoms related to the location of ectopic pancreatic tissue, i.e., abdominal pain, obstruction or gastrointestinal bleeding. If it prolapses into the pylorus, it can produce symptoms of intermittent obstruction.[16]

The embryologic basis of ectopic or heterotopic pancreas is not known, but the most likely theory is abnormal migration, wherein deposits of pancreatic tissue are "dropped" in to the developing gastrointestinal system, anatomically separate from the main body of pancreas.

Histologically, it mimics the orthotopic pancreas and appears most often as a solid intramural mass <3 cm size. The heterotopic pancreatic tissue may be present in the submucosal, muscularis, or subserosal layers in the GIT.

Imaging Features

This congenital anomaly is rarely diagnosed at imaging with most cases identified at surgery or autopsy. On barium meal UGI study, ectopic pancreas appears typically as a 1–3 cm intramural mass with a broad base and smooth surface along the greater curvature of the gastric antrum within 6 cm of the pylorus. The mass has a small central barium-filled pit or umbilication which is characteristic and helps it to differentiate from other intramural masses.

At endoscopy, it appears as a submucosal mass with the central umbilication more often seen endoscopically than at imaging. On endoscopic US, the location and morphology of the mass is delineated and most commonly appears as a solid submucosal mass which is hypoechoic relative to the hyperechoic submucosa.

On CT, the ectopic pancreatic mass is described as usually small, oval or flat shape and has an endoluminal growth pattern with ill-defined microlobulated margins.

In contrast, gastrointestinal stromal tumor (GIST) which is most commonly seen in the stomach followed by the small intestine is a submucosal lesion which grows extraluminally.

The attenuation and enhancement characteristics of the lesion reflect its microscopic composition. Heterotopic tissue which has predominantly acini shows enhancement which is homogeneous and greater than or equal to the orthotopic pancreas. Lesions which are hypoattenuating are found to have more of ductal structures.

On MRI, ectopic/heterotopic pancreas can be differentiated from other lesions by its characteristic high signal intensity on T1-weighted sequences similar to that of the pancreas. The ectopic tissue shows intense enhancement in the arterial phase similar to that of the native pancreatic tissue. On T2-weighted images and magnetic resonance cholangiopancreatography (MRCP), a dilated duct in the heterotopic pancreas has been described which is also referred to as the "ectopic duct" sign and is pathognomonic of ectopic pancreas.[29]

The complications associated with ectopic pancreas include pancreatitis, pseudocyst formation, malignant degeneration, GI bleeding, bowel obstruction, and intussusceptions.

Treatment

Ectopic pancreas diagnosed incidentally does not require any treatment. In a symptomatic patient surgical resection of the involved segment is done where there is suspicion of malignancy.

SMALL BOWEL

Duodenum

Duodenal obstruction is a relatively common form of intestinal obstruction in the newborn. It has an incidence of 1 in 5,000 to 1 in 10,000 live births with congenital duodenal obstruction occurring for half of all cases of bowel obstruction.[30] It may be complete (duodenal atresia) or incomplete. Complete duodenal obstruction is seen more frequently than congenital gastric obstruction.[16] Incomplete obstruction may be intrinsic, such as duodenal stenosis caused by a web or "windsock" membrane; or more often, extrinsic, e.g., duodenal compression from bands, annular pancreas, etc. Intrinsic and extrinsic obstructions may coexist **(Table 2)**.

Duodenal Atresia and Stenosis

Duodenal atresia and stenosis represent a spectrum of duodenal obstruction ranging from complete to partial obstruction, presenting from prenatal life to later childhood or even adulthood.[3]

Atresia is much more common than stenosis, but the etiology is the same. Atresia or stenosis occurs when the duodenum, which is a solid tube till about 3–6 weeks' gestation, fails to recanalize partially or completely. Unlike jejunal and ileal atresia, it does not appear to be related to intrauterine ischemia.[16] Atresia and stenosis almost always occur in the region of the ampulla of Vater (about 80% are just distal to the ampulla); thus, they are frequently accompanied by abnormalities of the bile duct and pancreas. Annular pancreas occurs in 20% of patients with duodenal atresia or stenosis. It may contribute to the duodenal obstruction but is seldom or never found without intrinsic obstruction of the duodenum.

Duodenal atresia and stenosis may be associated with other congenital anomalies, such as intestinal atresia, esophageal atresia with or without fistula, and congenital heart disease and may be part of VACTERL association. About 30% of the patients have Down syndrome.[31-33] Biliary anomalies such as bifid common duct, choledochal cyst, and gallbladder agenesis are also known to occur with duodenal atresia/stenosis.[34]

Clinical Presentation

Duodenal atresia is the congenital UGI obstruction which presents at the earliest and can be even diagnosed on prenatal ultrasound. Findings on prenatal ultrasound consist of polyhydramnios which occurs in 30–50% cases with premature birth seen in nearly half of the patients.

Duodenal atresia and stenosis occur with equal frequency in boys and girls. **Bilious vomiting in the first few hours of life** is the **cardinal symptom** but those with duodenal stenosis can present at variable times, because the clinical findings depend on the degree of stenosis. Bilious vomiting is a feature **in 80% of neonates with duodenal atresia as the atresia is present distal to the ampulla of Vater**. In the remaining 20%, the vomitus is nonbilious[6] and can simulate HPS.

TABLE 2: Causes of duodenal obstruction in the newborn.

Intrinsic	Extrinsic
Duodenal atresia	Ladd's bands in malrotation
Duodenal stenosis	Midgut volvulus with malrotation
Duodenal web or diaphragm	Annular pancreas
	Intestinal duplication/duplication cyst
	Preduodenal portal vein

Imaging Features

In newborns with duodenal atresia, the **abdominal radiograph** is usually **diagnostic**. Air is present in the stomach and proximal duodenum, but there is no air distally in the GIT. Erect film shows two gas-fluid levels in which the higher, larger bubble to the left is the stomach and the other bubble is the dilated proximal duodenum which is seen above the region of obstruction.[11] Thus, the typical appearance of a "**double-bubble sign**" represents air, or air and fluid-filled distended stomach and duodenal bulb **(Fig. 13)**. As the obstruction has been present in utero, i.e., long-standing, the obstructed duodenum is typically large, appearing around 33–50% of the size of the stomach. At times, if the pylorus remains wide open, it may not be possible to distinctly separate the two bubbles.[3] **In duodenal stenosis, the stomach and duodenal bulb are usually distended, but air is present in the distal bowel.**

In newborns with evidence of complete duodenal obstruction on abdominal radiograph, there is mostly no need for further radiologic investigation and the patient can be directly taken up for surgery. In certain instances such as vomiting or recent feeding in the new born, the stomach or duodenal bulb may not distend, then the specific double-bubble appearance may not be seen even when duodenal atresia exists.

Malrotation is known to occur in half the patients of duodenal atresia, but it has been seen that these patients do not suffer from midgut volvulus. The decreased risk of midgut volvulus is thought to be due to lack of peristalsis as there is no bowel gas distal to the duodenal obstruction.[30] However, if clinically a suspicion of malrotation exists, an UGI contrast study should be performed.

Treatment

The newborn with congenital duodenal obstruction, complete or partial, requires surgery and is frequently taken

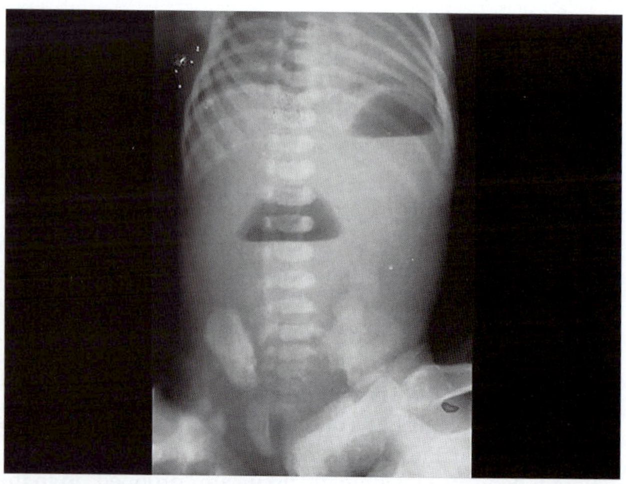

FIG. 13: Duodenal atresia: Erect film of the abdomen demonstrating the classical "double bubble" sign.

to surgery without any more radiological investigation other than the plain film. However, further radiological study is required for making a preoperative diagnosis, specifically to distinguish between a cause of partial obstruction for which operation may be delayed, such as duodenal stenosis, from midgut volvulus, which requires emergent surgery. In these cases, when the infant is clinically stable, an UGI series may be very useful. On UGI study, duodenal stenosis appears as dilatation of the duodenum proximal to the point of obstruction with abrupt caliber change.[6]

Duodenal Web/Intraluminal Duodenal Diaphragm

Duodenal web or diaphragm is a thin membrane partially obstructing the duodenum, accounting for 10–31% of congenital duodenal obstruction.[34] It is usually located in the second part of the duodenum at the level of ampulla of Vater, attached to the wall. It occurs due to the failure of recanalization in the primitive foregut between 9th and 11th week of gestation. A duodenal web is associated with malrotation, annular pancreas, and preduodenal portal vein.[7]

The following types of duodenal web have been described:

- Duodenal atresia/complete imperforate web.
- Windsock web or imperforate intraluminal duodenal diverticulum.
- Perforated duodenal web which is an intraduodenal diverticulum with central/eccentric opening.

Clinical Presentation

The presentation is little later in the neonatal period or infancy as compared to duodenal atresia. Patients may present with features of obstruction such as abdominal distention or vomiting. The symptoms and age of presentation of a perforated duodenal web depends on the size of the perforation. A perforated duodenal web contains central or eccentric openings which result in varying degree of partial duodenal obstruction. The smaller the size of the perforation or opening of the web, earlier is the age of presentation with partial duodenal obstruction in the neonate, while a larger fenestration can present later in childhood with nonspecific abdominal distention or vomiting due to its less obstructive nature.[34]

Imaging Features

In patients with duodenal webs, the findings on UGI study vary. In some, the appearance is of complete obstruction, in others there is narrowing of the duodenum. In the latter, a web is indistinguishable from simple duodenal stenosis. The most diagnostic appearance of a web is that of a thin, convex, curvilinear defect extending for a variable distance across the lumen of the duodenum. Sometimes, due to propulsion of peristalsis the duodenal web or membrane elongates and presents like an intraduodenal diverticulum, mimicking a wind sock[2] **(Fig. 14)**. The "windsock" appearance is seen in an adult or older child and is not seen in newborns. This appearance is probably due to stretching and redundancy of the web caused by years of peristalsis, proximal to an incomplete obstruction.[35] At UGI examination, a windsock deformity is seen when contrast distends the dilated proximal duodenum and outlines a thin web that bulges into the nondilated distal segment **(Fig. 15)**.

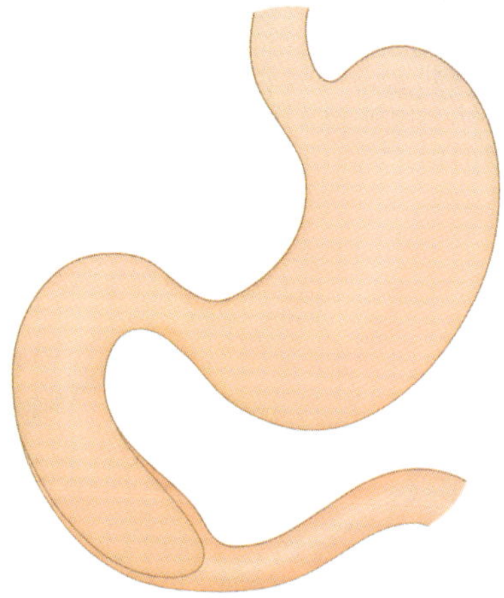

FIG. 14: Schematic representation of "windsock appearance" of intraluminal duodenal web presenting like an intraduodenal diverticulum.

Duodenal webs are known to occur with other lesions such as duodenal bands, midgut volvulus, duodenal atresia, and with obstructing diaphragms in other parts of the GIT. So, during surgery, even if obstruction is due to one lesion, a search for coexisting diaphragm/s should be made on surgical exploration. Also, when a duodenal diaphragm is found during surgery, other developmental lesions should be excluded at exploration.

Annular Pancreas

Annular pancreas is a developmental malformation which may lead to UGI obstruction (UGIO) due to anomalous pancreatic tissue encircling the second part of duodenum. It results from incomplete rotation of the ventral pancreatic bud during the 7th week of gestation. The encircling pancreatic ring may be partial or complete and known to include the major pancreatic duct **(Fig. 16)**. It produces a fixed stenosis of the underlying duodenum which is not relieved by removing the pancreatic ring.[34]

Clinical Presentation

Annular pancreas may present at any age and presentation depends on the degree of narrowing of duodenum and the severity of the resulting symptoms. It can remain asymptomatic or can present in children or adults with chronic nonspecific symptoms. It typically presents in an adult from 3rd to 6th decade with pancreatitis, obstruction, and jaundice. Rarely, it can present with symptoms of duodenal obstruction in a neonate.[34] The duct of the pancreatic annulus is often a separate duct entering the duodenum opposite the ampulla of Vater. Duodenal contents may reflux through this resulting in pancreatitis.

Imaging Features

Plain radiographs are usually normal. In a patient presenting with obstruction, plain radiograph may show duodenal

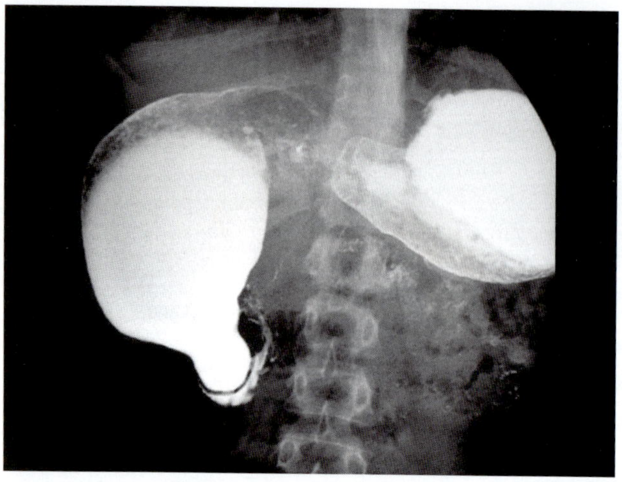

FIG. 15: Barium upper gastrointestinal study in a 10-year-old girl with recurrent vomiting reveals typical "windsock appearance" of duodenal web obstructing second part of duodenum with proximal dilatation.

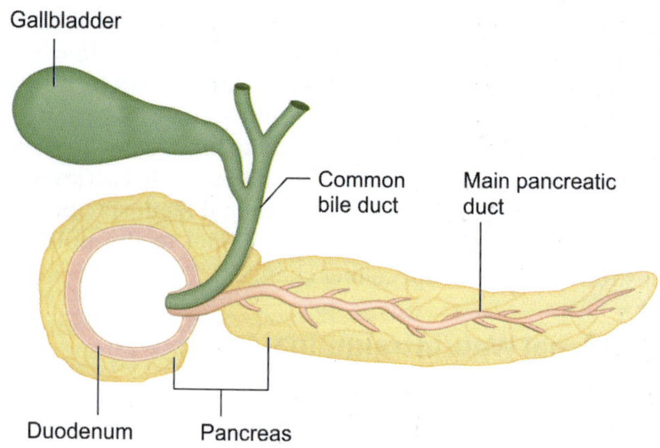

FIG. 16: Schematic representation of pancreatic tissue completely encircling the second part of duodenum: Annular pancreas.

dilatation. Partial or complete obstruction at the second part of duodenum may be seen on UGI contrast study. Diagnosis on ultrasound may be difficult, but pancreatic tissue may be seen adjacent to the descending duodenum and it may resemble a mass.

Multidetector CT (MDCT) and MRI provide a more definitive diagnosis, especially MRCP which delineates the pancreatic duct and its circumferential course to the duodenum. The diagnosis of complete annular pancreas is more straight forward with complete rim of pancreatic tissue enveloping second part of duodenum. Findings of incomplete annular pancreas may be more subtle. Three types of incomplete annular pancreas have been described—anterolateral extension, posterolateral extension, and both anterior and posterior extension, depending on the extension of pancreatic tissue in relation to duodenum. Of these, the type with anterior and posterior extension is highly specific of incomplete annular pancreas.

Treatment

Treatment of annular pancreas is by bypassing the duodenal obstruction by duodenoduodenostomy or gastrojejunostomy.

Preduodenal Portal Vein

Preduodenal portal vein is a rare anomaly which occurs due to an abnormal development of the portal vein. It is rarely the sole cause of duodenal obstruction and is rarely diagnosed preoperatively. The obstruction which is seen is due to a primary and obstructing duodenal lesion such as intraluminal membrane or web and such a lesion should be suspected in these patients if duodenal obstruction is present.[21] It is thus important for the surgeon to be aware of the association of this anomaly with the other congenital lesions causing duodenal obstruction.[6]

A preduodenal portal vein (persistent left vitelline vein) results from normal situs asymmetry and is commonly seen in patients with heterotaxy. The resultant portal vein courses anterior to the pancreas and duodenum and in doing so can produce indentation and compression of the duodenum.

Clinical Presentation

Preduodenal portal vein in symptomatic children is usually seen with manifestations of other malformations such as malrotation with duodenal Ladd bands, duodenal atresia, biliary atresia, and cardiac defects.[34]

Imaging Features

The condition is diagnosed by identifying the prepancreatic course of the portal vein on sonography, CT, and MRI. It is now believed that in most cases of duodenal obstruction associated with a preduodenal portal vein, the preduodenal portal vein is usually an incidental finding.

When malrotation with duodenal bands is associated, the vein may be contained within the band, but it is not transected during surgery.[12]

Anomalies of Rotation and Fixation

Intestinal rotation anomalies or "malrotation" are a spectrum of anomalies in which there is a congenitally abnormal position of small and large bowel within the peritoneal cavity occurring as a result of abnormal rotation of the midgut and mesenteric fixation.

Embryology

The midgut is the portion of the bowel that extends from the distal second part of the duodenum to the distal transverse colon and is supplied by the superior mesenteric artery (SMA). The embryonic midgut achieves its final position in the peritoneal cavity by undergoing 270° counterclockwise rotation through a series of steps.

Three steps of rotation of the gut occur in utero. The gut is initially in the form of a straight tube with the duodenojejunal junction (DJ) and cecum lying along a straight line. During its growth, the gut forms a primary loop along the axis of the SMA. The first rotation is the 90° counterclockwise rotation of the duodenum and cecum, which results in the DJ junction to lie in the right upper quadrant and the cecum in the left lower quadrant. At around 6th week of gestation, the growth of the intestine results in its herniation into the umbilical cord and a second counterclockwise rotation of 90° occurs at the DJ junction. By the 10th week of gestation, the herniated bowel starts returning into the abdominal cavity and the duodenum undergoes its final 90° of rotation to lie in the left upper quadrant and also undergoes fixation at the ligament of Treitz. The cecum undergoes its final 180° of rotation and terminates in the right lower quadrant and undergoes fixation to the posterior peritoneum **(Figs. 17A to D)**.

Thus, the bowel is suspended from a mesentery that is attached to the posterior abdominal wall and extends from the left upper quadrant to the right lower quadrant. The duodenal C-loop configuration resembles the 270° rotation which it has undergone. During the final process of bowel rotation and fixation, the dorsal mesenteries of the ascending and descending colon are resorbed and there is elongation of the ascending colon with descent of cecum in the right lower quadrant with a broad-based mesentery. These processes continue postnatally for several months.

When all or part of physiological rotation of bowel is arrested, a wide variety of anomalies of intestinal rotation and mesenteric fixation occur which consist of nonrotation, true malrotation, or reversed rotation.

- *Nonrotation*: It is the most common positional anomaly of the GIT wherein the normal process of rotation is arrested after the initial 90° of counterclockwise rotation. Thus, the DJ junction and the small bowel come to lie entirely on the right of the abdomen, and the cecum and the rest of the colon are all located on the left side of the abdomen **(Figs. 18A and B, Fig. 19B)**. It is an asymptomatic condition demonstrated incidentally on barium studies in older children or adults. The small and large bowel share a common mesentery with the mesenteric root being broad, hence there is a low risk of midgut volvulus.
- *True malrotation*: This occurs when the arrest of rotation occurs beyond the stage of nonrotation, i.e., two 90° rotation occur in the counterclockwise direction which brings the DJ junction and cecum nearer to each other. It results in a shorter mesenteric root which is not fixed with a narrow base from which the bowel is suspended which has a tendency to twist on its axis. The horizontal part of the duodenum rotates and lies posterior to the mesenteric vessels. This twist leads to extrinsic compression of the bowel causing bowel obstruction, and if the twist persists, it may lead to occlusion of the mesenteric vessels. This twist of malfixed intestines around the short mesentery is called a midgut volvulus **(Figs. 19A to D)**. In patients with malfixation of the bowel, in addition to the absence of a normal mesentery, frequently there are aberrant peritoneal bands (Ladd's bands). These bands extend from the malpositioned cecum across the duodenum and attach to the hilum of the liver, posterior peritoneum

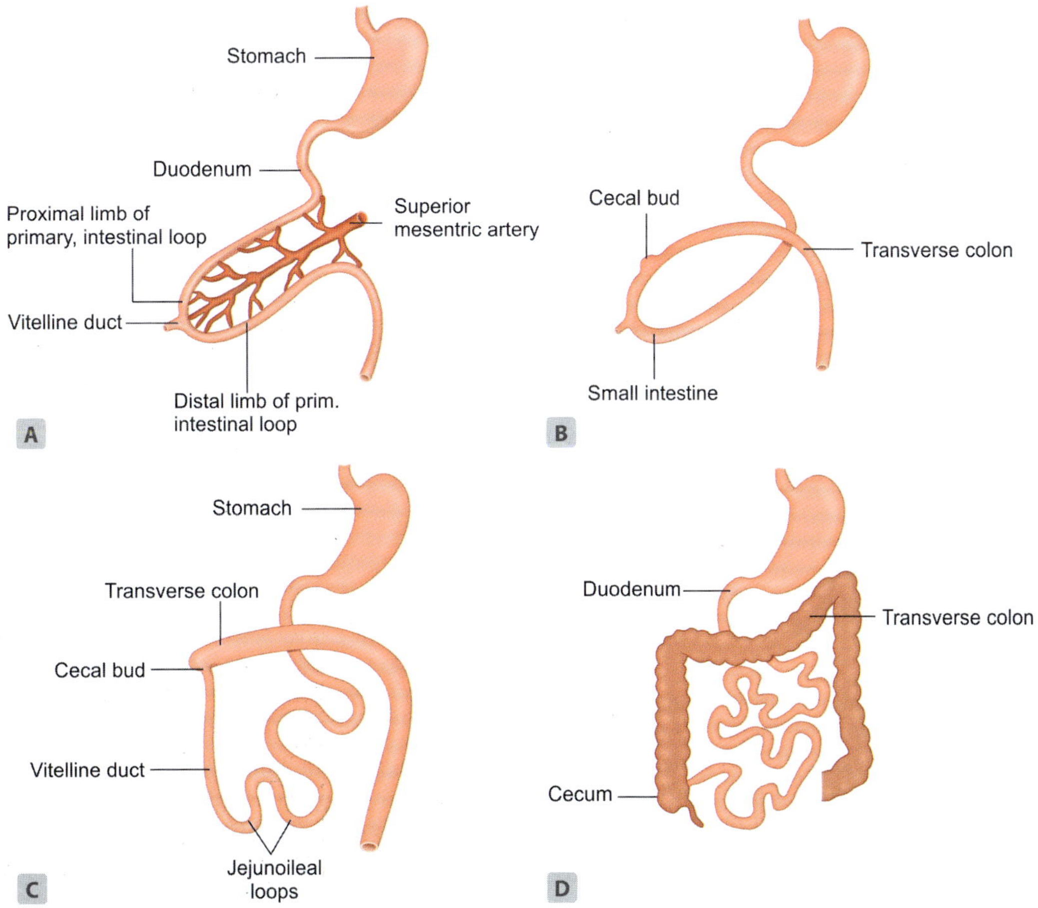

FIGS. 17A TO D: Diagrammatic representation of physiological midgut rotation.

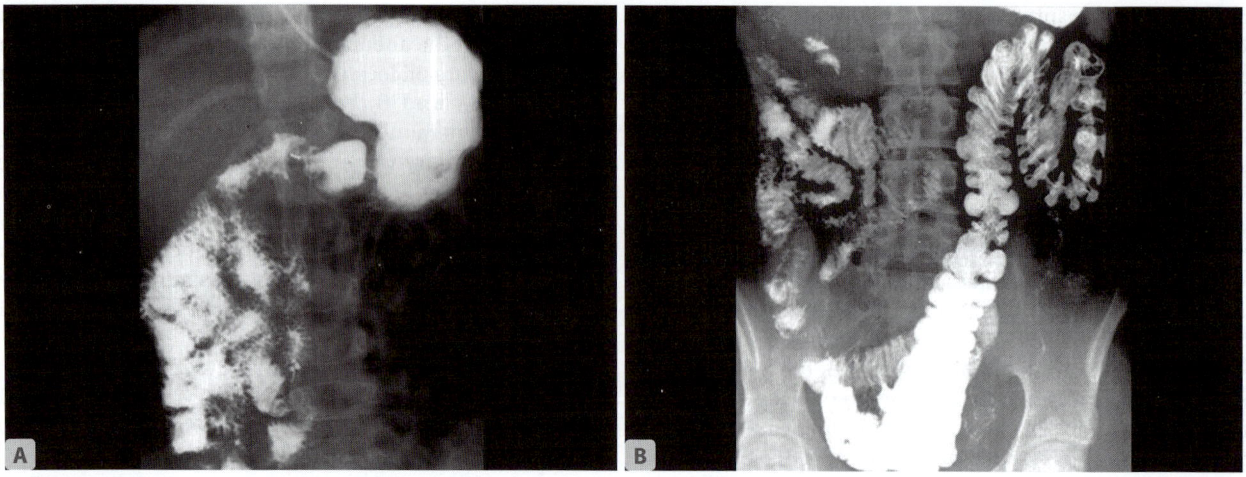

FIGS. 18A AND B: Barium meal follow through study shows (A) jejunal loops on the right side of the abdomen; and (B) colon and cecum on the left side with the ileum seen crossing the midline from right to left—nonrotation.

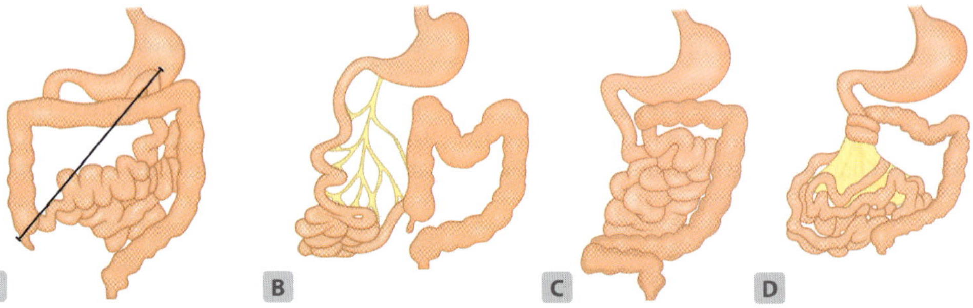

FIGS. 19A TO D: Illustration of anomalies of rotation and fixation. (A) Normal; (B) Nonrotation; (C) Intestinal malrotation without volvulus; and (D) Malrotation with midgut volvulus.

or abdominal wall and can cause extrinsic duodenal obstruction[31] **(Figs. 20A and B and 21)**.

- *Reversed intestinal rotation*: It is a rare rotational anomaly in which there is a change in rotational direction. A normal 90° rotation is followed by a 90° or 180° inverse rotation. This results in the DJ junction in the left upper quadrant and the cecum is malrotated and medially placed. In this anomaly, the duodenum lies anterior to the SMA and the cecum and transverse colon lie behind the pedicle of mesenteric attachment (i.e., located posteriorly between the aorta and SMA instead of the duodenum).

The true incidence of malrotation is not known as many patients may remain clinically silent. Its estimated prevalence is high, around 1 in 500 live births.[7]

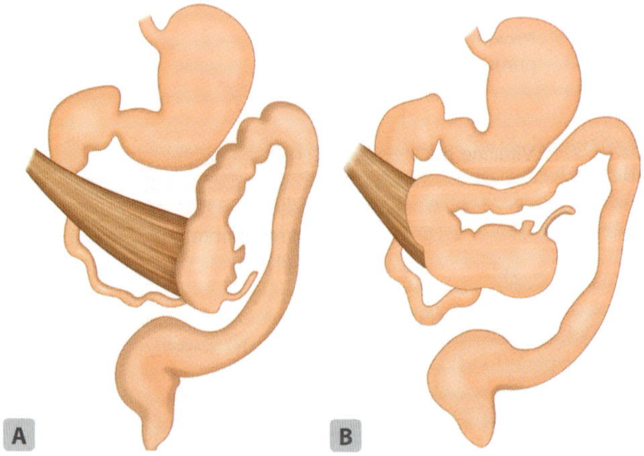

FIGS. 20A AND B: Diagrammatic representation of Ladd's bands causing duodenal compression in patients with malrotation. The cecum is left sided (A) and midline (B) in position and has dense peritoneal bands crossing over the duodenum.

Clinical Presentation

The typical presentation of malrotation with midgut volvulus is early in life, with 75% cases occurring in newborns and up to 90% of cases within 1st year of life.[30,36] Patients present with bilious vomiting and symptoms of intestinal obstruction. The bowel obstruction may be caused by the volvulus, by Ladd's bands, or both. Signs and symptoms of sudden onset of bilious vomiting in a newborn who has been normal for the first few days of life should be considered to be due to a midgut volvulus until proved otherwise.

Malrotation in adults has an insidious onset, may manifest in them with symptoms ranging from acute abdominal pain and vomiting to mild intermittent episodes of abdominal pain and malabsorption. It may also be an incidental finding on imaging especially in adults.[36]

Malrotation is associated with numerous other anomalies such as jejunal or duodenal stenosis or atresia, annular

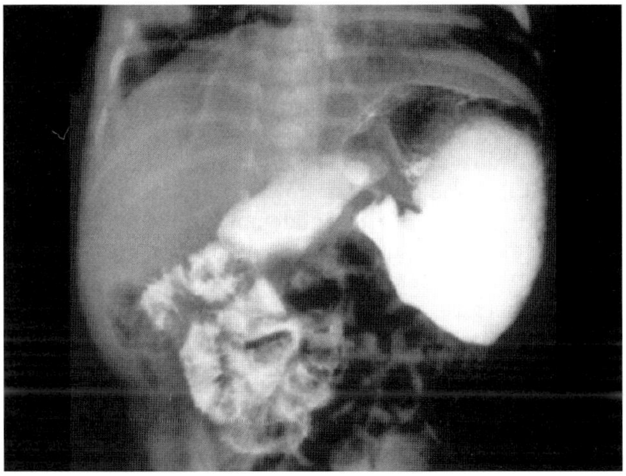

FIG. 21: Midgut malrotation with Ladd's bands: Barium study shows distended proximal duodenum with tapering at the level of obstruction indicative of extrinsic compression. The small intestine, distal to the usual site of the ligament of Treitz, lies below the duodenum and to the right.

pancreas, and Hirschsprung's disease. It has been found to occur in children when the normal embryologic position of the developing gut was disrupted as in omphalocele, gastroschisis or congenital diaphragmatic hernia. Malrotation is also very common in children with heterotaxy syndrome.[36]

Imaging Features

Plain radiographs may show features of duodenal obstruction due to partially obstructing Ladd's bands. The duodenal bulb dilatation is less than that seen with duodenal atresia. Plain abdominal radiographs may not be diagnostic of malrotation and may show stomach and proximal duodenum distended with air and with little bowel gas beyond. When there is a volvulus, the plain films may show features of distal bowel obstruction. Bowel wall-thickening and pneumatosis may be present due to volvulus-induced ischemia. The fluid-filled bowel loops associated with volvulus can simulate an abdominal mass. The abdomen may be gasless, which may be due either to proximal obstruction or to diffuse bowel necrosis in midgut volvulus. Of all the congenital anomalies that result in bilious emesis, only malrotation is likely to produce a normal abdominal film.[31]

Suspected malrotation requires an emergent contrast study. **Barium meal UGI study** is the **examination of choice** for the **diagnosis of malrotation** with **midgut volvulus**. Meticulous technique is required to document the duodenal course and location of DJ junction (Ligament of Treitz) and to evaluate for duodenal obstruction. Normally, the DJ junction lies to the left of the body or the left of the left-sided pedicles of the first or second lumbar vertebra at the level of the duodenal bulb. In malrotation, it is located lower and to the right of normal location described above. It is important to remember that the DJ junction is mobile due to relative laxity of peritoneal ligaments in children younger than 4 years of age[36] and may lie in the right upper abdomen without any evidence of malrotation. The DJ junction may be pushed inferomedially by an overdistended stomach, chronic bowel dilatation, and enlarged spleen or in the presence of a nasojejunal tube.[6] This inferior displacement of DJ junction is more common in premature children seen on frontal view of UGI study. A lateral view of the contrast-filled duodenum is an important additional view in the UGI study when evaluating for malrotation. Normal duodenum, being a retroperitoneal structure, is seen to lie posterior to the stomach on lateral views with the fourth part of the duodenum superimposed on the second part of duodenum. This superimposed relationship is lost in case of malrotation of duodenum as it is seen to course anteriorly. An abnormal position of the DJ flexure may be the only indication of malrotation, as in 16% of cases cecum occupies its normal position.

In up to 15% of the UGI studies, there may be a false positive diagnosis of malrotation which may be due anatomical variance such as:

- *Duodenum inversum*: It is a rare, usually asymptomatic congenital condition wherein the third part of the duodenum tracks superiorly and posteriorly before crossing the midline at a high level above the pancreas toward the ligament of Treitz which is usually in normal position.
- *Duodenal redundancy or wandering duodenum*: This appears as longer and more meandering course of the duodenum to the right of the spine, instead of the typical C-shaped course. But, it crosses the midline at the normal level with the normal position of the ligament of Treitz.

Hence, to improve the diagnostic accuracy of identification of malrotation on the UGI study, the following has been recommended.

- The duodenal course and the DJ junction should be noted on fluoroscopy.
- Both frontal and lateral projections should be acquired to demonstrate the position of DJ junction.
- Care must be taken not to overfill the stomach as with overdistention, the position of duodenum and normal DJ junction may be obscured. Also, an overdistended stomach may displace the normal DJ junction inferiorly.
- Manual palpation during the UGI study should be performed by the radiologist to determine the mobility of the duodenum.
- Other imaging studies should be reviewed, if available.
- If diagnosis is in doubt or equivocal, delayed abdominal radiographs should be obtained to identify the position of the cecum as 80% of individuals with malrotation have an abnormal position of the cecum.
- If the clinical manifestations do not correspond to the findings of the UGI study, then the UGI contrast may be repeated on the following day.

Steps performed for a repeat UGI study in an infant which aid in visualization of the DJ junction are:

- Barium to be administered via a nasogastric tube.
- Only small/limited amount of barium to be given.
- The patient should be in the right lateral position at the beginning of the study so as to promote early emptying of the barium from the stomach to the duodenum.
- Air can be injected through the NG tube to push the small amount of barium into the duodenum.

The proper technique of performing an UGI study as described above for documentation of normally rotated C-loop should be followed. This is possible when on fluoroscopy the first bolus of contrast is tracked as it leaves the stomach.

Appearance of Midgut Volvulus

When volvulus occurs, there may be **complete or partial duodenal obstruction**. With complete obstruction, the contrast column may terminate in tapered or in a beak-like configuration. In patients with acute duodenal obstruction from Ladd's bands, the duodenum may show a kinked configuration that may resemble a Z-shape instead of a normal C-loop. More commonly, the volvulus is intermittent with incomplete bowel obstruction with contrast filling the proximal small bowel. Occasionally, the **pathognomonic "corkscrew pattern"** of the twisted duodenum and jejunum is seen in the **barium meal UGI study** due to their clockwise spiraling around the SMA **(Figs. 22A and B)**. This may lead to ischemia of the bowel if the SMA is compromised. In malrotation, the cecum and right colon may have abnormal mobility. The cecum is in the right upper quadrant or in midline in malrotation. A colonic beak may be present in the right colon on barium enema in the presence of volvulus.[31] In the past, a contrast enema was the first investigation performed to evaluate for malrotation.[6] This has been replaced by an UGI study due to its greater sensitivity and specificity for malrotation. The cecum may be mobile in neonates and may be seen in the right upper quadrant in the absence of malrotation.

Ultrasound may be useful in the early detection of midgut malrotation as well as complicating midgut volvulus **(Figs. 23A to D)**. A distended proximal duodenum with a tapered end in front of the spine is consistent with malrotation in the proper clinical setting. If, in addition, one finds peritoneal fluid and edematous bowel loops on the right, the diagnosis of volvulus can be made. An UGI series is mandatory if this diagnosis must be confirmed or excluded prior to surgery.

On ultrasound and CT, the diagnosis of malrotation with volvulus is given when in the clinical context of acute duodenal obstruction an abnormal SMA or superior mesenteric vein (SMV) anatomy is seen. The SMV normally rests to the right and anterior to the SMA. When the SMV is to the left of the SMA, this is highly suggestive of volvulus. When the SMV is anterior to the SMA, this is suggestive of malrotation with possible volvulus. **Color Doppler US** demonstrates the **"whirlpool"** ***sign*** which is **diagnostic** of midgut volvulus due to clockwise spiraling of the mesentery, SMV and its tributaries, fat, bowel, and branches of SMA around the SMA. A dilated duodenum can be followed as it enters into the volvulus. Inversion of the mesenteric vessels or the SMV rotation sign is not a specific finding of midgut volvulus, because it may be present in normal population, patients with situs inversus and patients with abdominal masses. **Box 3** depicts the key imaging features of malrotation with midgut volvulus.

CT is not the procedure of choice for evaluation of malrotation. But if performed, the normal retroperitoneal course of the duodenum should be followed, and if visualized, indicates that normal rotation of the bowel has occurred. CT features of malrotation consist of (a) nonvisualization of the third part of duodenum across the midline from right to left, (b) position of small bowel loops in right upper abdomen, (c) colonic loops located on the left side, and (d) reversal of normal position of SMA and SMV.[37]

The CT findings of midgut malrotation complicated by midgut volvulus are: (1) The "whirl" sign of small-bowel loops and SMV spiraling around the SMA **(Figs. 24A and B)**; (2) A dilated, fluid-filled, obstructed stomach and proximal duodenum; (3) Thick-walled loops of ischemic right-sided small bowel with potential pneumatosis intestinalis and mesenteric edema; and (4) Free intraperitoneal fluid.

Treatment

The treatment of midgut volvulus is emergent, necessitating immediate surgery with correction of existing metabolic and electrolyte derangements. Prompt diagnosis of malrotation with midgut volvulus is important, as a mortality of 3% is reported due to it. Around 15% of midgut volvulus cases demonstrate bowel strangulation at the time of surgery due to arterial and venous compromise of the bowel segment which has undergone volvulus.

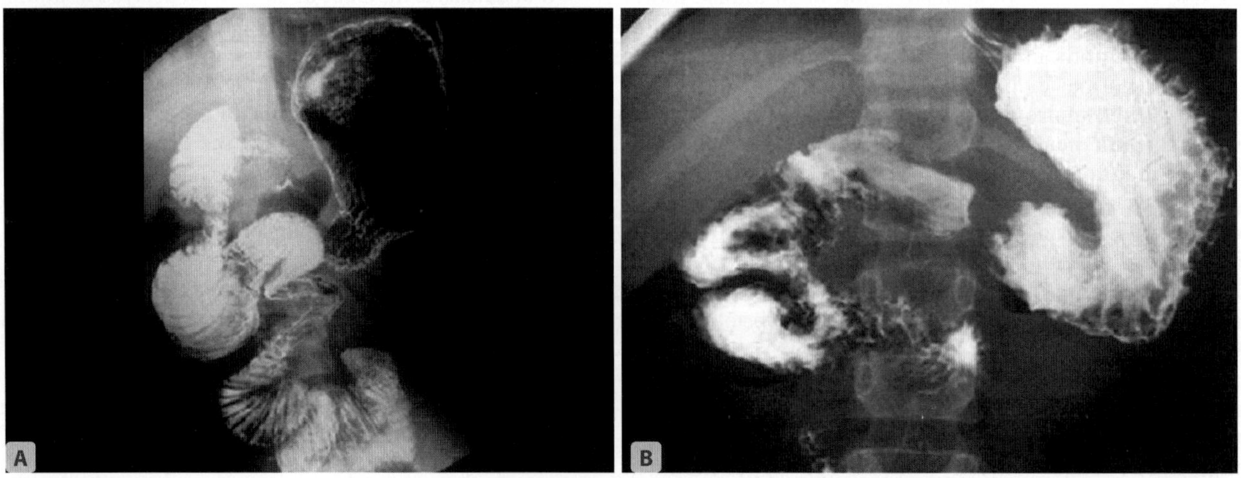

FIGS. 22A AND B: Upper gastrointestinal (UGI) barium study in two different patients showing classic "corkscrew" appearance of the duodenum in midgut volvulus.

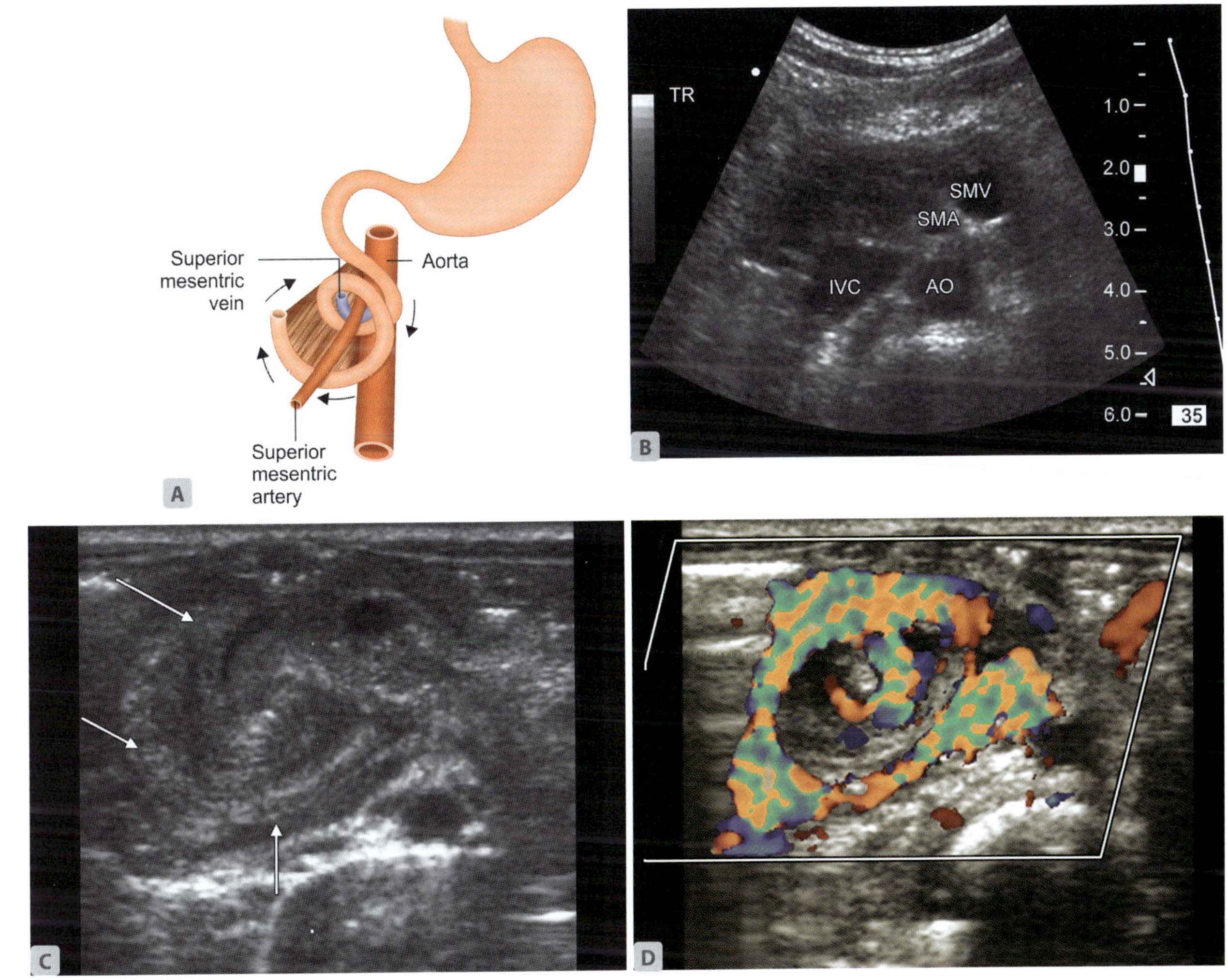

FIGS. 23A TO D: Malrotation with midgut volvulus. (A) Schematic representation of midgut volvulus; (B) Gray-scale ultrasound depicting loss of normal SMA/SMV relationship with SMV lying anterior and to the left of SMA in a patient with malrotation; (C) with clockwise twist of SMV, bowel, and mesentery around SMA (arrows); and (D) giving characteristic "whirlpool sign" on Color Doppler imaging.

BOX 3: Diagnostic imaging features of malrotation with midgut volvulus.

- **On upper gastrointestinal contrast study**
  - "Corkscrew appearance" of duodenum—pathognomonic
  - Beaked tapering of obstructed duodenum in complete obstruction
  - Malposition of duodenojejunal junction
- **On US and color Doppler**
  - "Whirlpool" or "swirl" sign of clockwise twist of dilated duodenum, mesentery, SMV, and tributaries around SMA

(SMA: superior mesenteric artery; SMV: superior mesenteric vein)

The standard surgical procedure for malrotation with volvulus is Ladd's procedure which consists of—surgical detorsion, identification and lysis of Ladd's band, straightening of duodenum along the right abdomen with cecum placed in the left lower quadrant, thereby broadening the base of the mesentery and creating a space/separation between the DJ junction and cecum resembling nonrotation. An incidental appendectomy is performed.[3]

Jejunoileal Atresia and Stenosis

The incidence of small bowel atresias (i.e., jejunal, jejunoileal or ileal) is 1:400–1500 and is more common than duodenal or colonic atresia. In decreasing frequency the sites of involvement of small bowel atresia are distal ileum, proximal jejunum, distal jejunum, and proximal ileum.[2] Jejunal atresia comprises around 50% of small bowel atresias and may be associated with other jejunal and ileal atresias.[5]

As compared to atresia, stenosis of bowel is less common.

Etiopathogenesis

Most jejunal and ileal atresias and stenoses, except those that are familial, are thought to be **secondary to ischemic injury** to the developing gut. The ischemia may be due to primary vascular accident, usually in the mid-second trimester or secondarily to a mechanical obstruction, as may occur in case of an in utero volvulus.[31] There is no solid core phase in the development of jejunum and ileum, so recanalization is not thought to be involved. Jejunoileal atresia may involve the bowel anywhere from the ligament of Treitz to the ileocecal

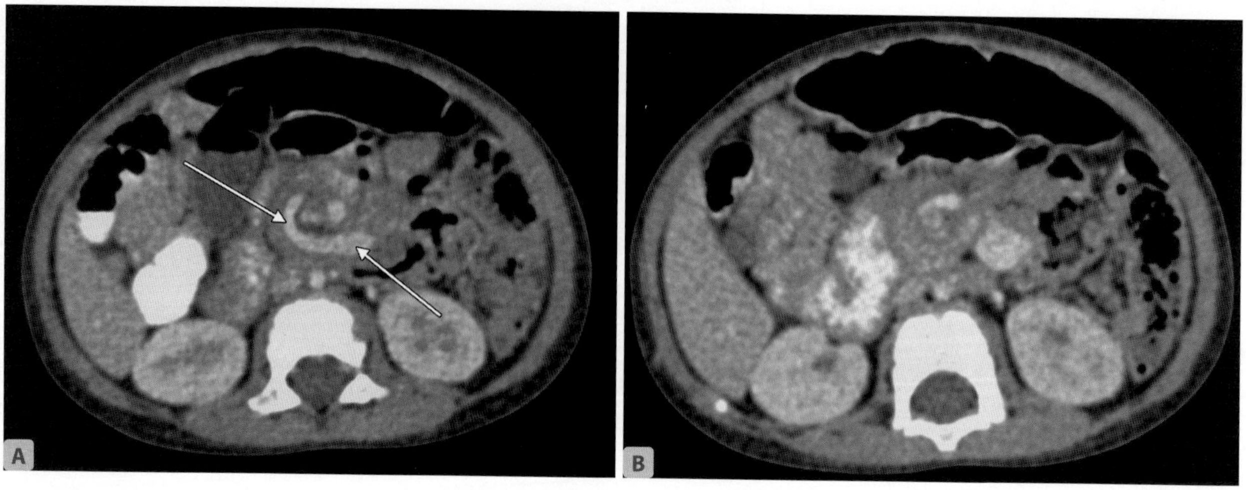

FIGS. 24A AND B: Axial contrast-enhanced computed tomography (CECT) of the abdomen showing characteristic "whirlpool" sign—clockwise twisting of the superior mesenteric vein (arrows) and mesentery around the superior mesenteric artery.

valve with the **majority** of cases of **atresia** occurring at the **extremes of the small bowel**. The devascularized bowel becomes necrotic and is resorbed leaving an atretic area of varying length with its attached mesentery. Atresias have been found in patients where prenatal gut ischemia or compression of bowel segments such as gastroschisis and intrauterine volvulus has occurred.

Clinical Presentation

It usually manifests in the first day or two of life with signs of bowel obstruction. Proximal atresia may present with bilious vomiting; whereas more distal atresias present with abdominal distention. There may be failure to pass meconium. Meconium may pass if atresia is located in the jejunum or occurred late in intrauterine life.

Classification

Small bowel atresia usually occurs as an isolated anomaly of the GIT. Several forms of atresia have been described surgically, but it is not possible to differentiate them by imaging studies.[4]

There are **four types** of small bowel atresia[3] **(Figs. 25A to D)**.

1. *Type I:* Membranous or web-like occlusion composed of mucosal and submucosal elements with no interruption of the muscularis.
2. *Type II:* Atresia with a solid fibrous cord connecting the atretic bowel ends, but the mesentery is intact. All the three layers of the intestinal wall are interrupted.
3. *Type III:* Complete absence of a segment of bowel (total atresia) as well as a portion of the mesentery (V-shaped defect in the mesentery). It is the most common form accounting for around 45% cases.
4. *Type IV:* The familial form of multiple atresias.

There are two unusual forms of atresia that are inherited.[24] They are:

i. "Apple peel" or "Christmas tree" atresia.
ii. A syndrome of multiple intestinal atresias.

"Apple peel" or "Christmas tree" atresia is a rare variant of Type III atresia which consists of proximal jejunal atresia with absence of the distal SMA, shortening of the small bowel distal to the atresia and absence of the dorsal mesentery. This type of atresia is probably caused by prenatal occlusion of the SMA, distal to the origin of the right colic and ileocolic arteries. The distal small intestine spirals around its vascular supply giving the characteristic apple peel appearance **(Fig. 25D)**. The result is a very short intestine with a propensity toward necrotizing enterocolitis.[38]

The syndrome of multiple intestinal atresias with intraluminal calcification is transmitted as an autosomal recessive pattern. There are multiple atresias from stomach to rectum. The radiological hallmark of this syndrome is extensive calcification of intraluminal contents between the areas of atresia. Nonhereditary bowel atresias may also demonstrate intraluminal calcification.[31]

Imaging Features

Plain radiograph of the abdomen demonstrates typical findings of small-bowel obstruction. The site (jejunal or distal ileal) of the atresia can be suspected by the number and location of gas-filled loops of bowel[6] **(Fig. 26)**. Proximal jejunal atresia may have a few markedly dilated loops, the so-called triple bubble sign. More distal atresia typically has a more uniform dilatation of multiple small bowel loops with associated air-fluid levels. The loop just proximal to the site of atresia is frequently disproportionately distended with a bulbous end.

If the ischemic event that produced the atresia caused a perforation, there may be evidence of meconium peritonitis which is a chemical peritonitis occurring as a result of extruded bowel contents producing an intense peritoneal inflammatory reaction. It leads to the formation of dense fibrotic tissue which often calcifies, resulting in characteristic intraperitoneal calcifications. Peritoneal calcifications may be identified on plain films as a consequence of meconium peritonitis, wherein they are seen as linear or flocculent areas

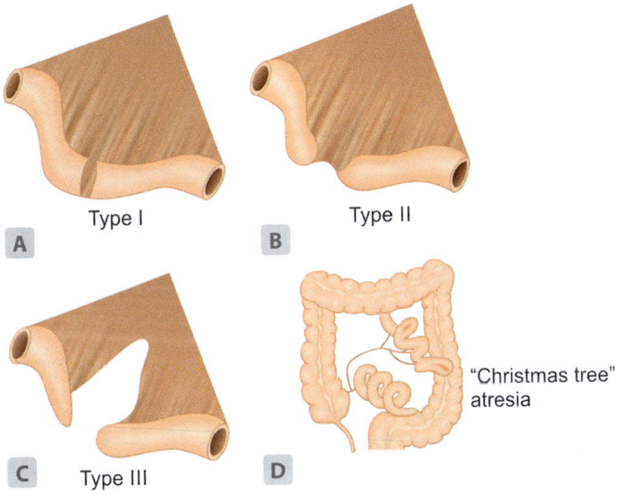

FIGS. 25A TO D: Types of small bowel atresia.

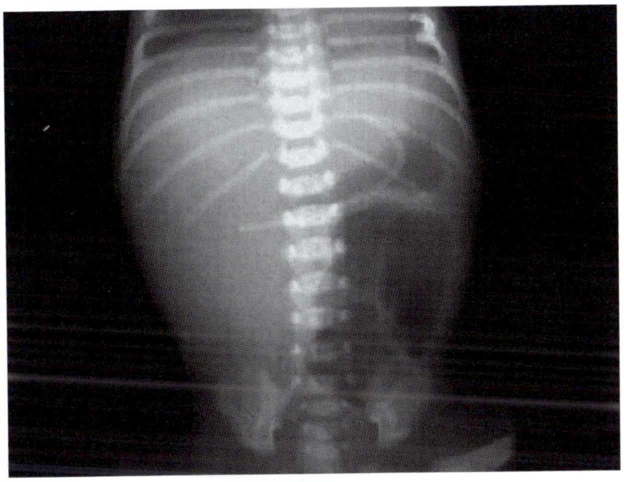

FIG. 26: Small bowel atresia: Air is seen in the stomach and dilated part of the jejunum proximal to the atresia.

of calcification within the peritoneal cavity **(Fig. 27)**. The most frequent finding is a linear calcification under the free edge of the liver, though any or all portions of the peritoneum may be involved.[8] The calcification may extend into the scrotum through a patent vaginal process to produce a calcified mass in the scrotum.[38] The association of **meconium peritonitis** with **small bowel obstruction** is virtually diagnostic of **small bowel atresia**.[8] The peritoneal calcifications are seen regardless of the site of small bowel atresia, secondary to in utero perforation and meconium peritonitis.[7]

Ultrasound depicts the **calcifications** of **meconium peritonitis** as highly echogenic linear or clumped foci in the abdomen or pelvis. The appearance of meconium peritonitis on US may be either generalized or cystic **(Fig. 28)**. In the generalized condition, highly echogenic material spreads throughout the abdomen and around the bowel loops to produce a **characteristic "snowstorm" appearance**. Encysted collections of meconium show a variable appearance from homogeneous to heterogeneous echogenicity and may be ill-defined or well-defined.

Sonography may also be useful in differentiating ileal atresia from meconium ileus. In ileal atresia, the bowel contents are echopoor while in meconium ileus, the dilated bowel loops are filled with echogenic material.[25]

Additional imaging is not required in the presence of a high intestinal obstruction. A contrast enema is required for further evaluation for low bowel obstruction to distinguish between a large and distal small bowel obstruction as the differentiation of the two on plain radiographs may be difficult or impossible.

Contrast enema should be performed with water soluble low osmolar contrast media introduced via a soft rectal catheter. Care must be taken to perform the enema as the distal blind pouch is prone to perforation. The one diagnostic finding to be looked for in the contrast enema performed in a setting of low bowel obstruction is the presence or absence of a microcolon **(Fig. 29)**. A microcolon is defined as a diffuse and small caliber (usually <1 cm diameter) colon which is normal in length with involvement of the entire colon. The colon is small owing to lack of use rather than anatomic or functional abnormality. The more distal the small bowel obstruction, the smaller the colon. A **microcolon** or unused colon occurs when no or little intestinal juices (succus entericus) reaches the colon and is **highly suggestive** of a **distal small bowel obstruction** (meconium ileus or ileal atresia). A normal sized colon almost always excludes these diagnoses.[31]

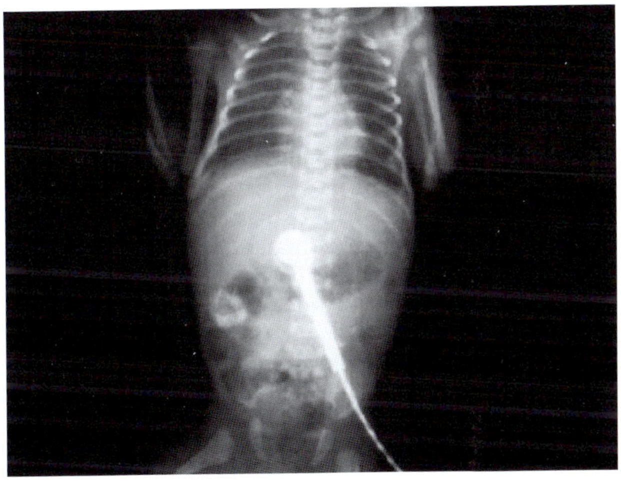

FIG. 27: Plain radiograph of the abdomen in a case of meconium peritonitis shows coarse clumped calcification in the right flank.

Differential Diagnosis

Meconium ileus is a differential of distal ileal atresia and can be differentiated from the latter on the basis of appearance of microcolon on contrast enema which shows filling defects typical of meconium pellets.

Complications

The complications which can occur in small bowel atresia are: (1) Meconium peritonitis, which occurs secondary to perforation (2% cases); (2) Postoperative short bowel

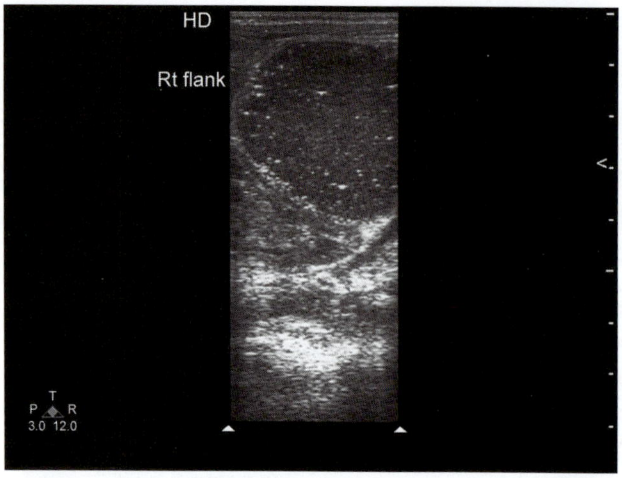

FIG. 28: High resolution ultrasound abdomen in a 4-day-old neonate presenting with abdominal distention reveals well-defined cystic mass with echoes within in the right flank: Meconium cyst.

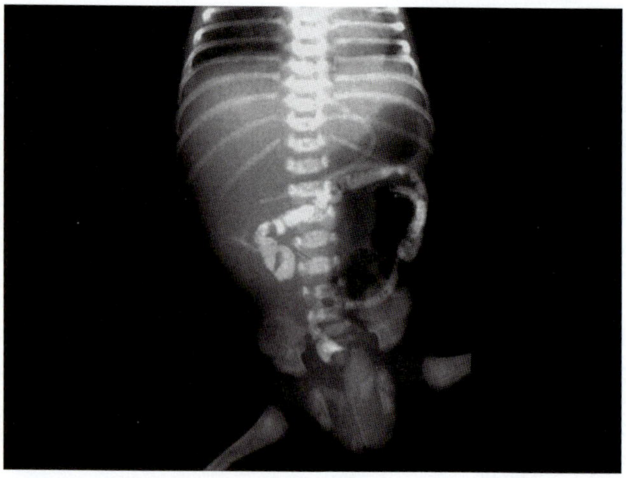

FIG. 29: Small bowel atresia: Contrast enema demonstrates a microcolon (same patient as in **Fig. 26**).

syndrome with disruption of intestinal motility; (3) Strangulation; and (4) Anastomotic stenosis.

Treatment

The treatment of patients of jejunal and ileal atresia or stenosis is surgical. Surgical treatment involves resection of the atretic portion of the intestine with reanastomosis. The proximal dilated bowel may remain dilated for some time in the postoperative period showing delayed motility with delayed passage of contrast across a widely patent anastomosis.

Meconium Ileus

Meconium ileus is a low intestinal obstruction caused by impaction of abnormal thick and tenacious meconium in the distal ileum in a neonate.[31] It is usually associated with cystic fibrosis with up to 90% of full-term neonates with meconium ileus known to have cystic fibrosis.[7] It is a presenting feature of cystic fibrosis in 5–10% of these patients.[31] The lack of normal pancreatic enzymes leads to thick, tenacious meconium that collects in the distal ileum and cecum, occluding its lumen and resulting in high-grade distal small bowel obstruction **(Fig. 30)**. Neonates generally present with failure to pass meconium.

Meconium ileus can be complicated or uncomplicated, with complicated meconium ileus being seen in up to half of the patients which include intestinal atresia, volvulus of the distal intestinal loop, and perforation with meconium or pseudocyst formation.[6]

Imaging Features

Meconium ileus is the most common mimic of small bowel atresia clinically and on plain films.[8] Plain radiograph may demonstrate a distal bowel obstructive pattern with air-fluid levels. Bowel loops may vary in size, a finding seen less often in atresia. The dilated small-bowel loops that contain air can mimic colon loops in size and course. In addition, some air mixes with the viscid meconium and results in a bubbly appearance in the right lower quadrant. This "soap bubble

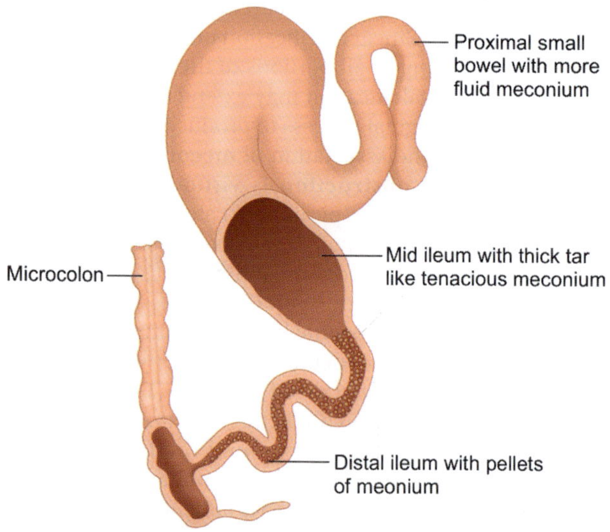

FIG. 30: Diagrammatic representation of meconium ileus with meconium pellets inspissated in collapsed distal ileum leading to proximal small bowel obstruction.

appearance" is not specific and a similar fecal pattern can be seen with any cause of distal intestinal obstruction such as ileal atresia, colonic atresia, aganglionosis of the terminal ileum and meconium plug syndrome.[38] Patients with meconium ileus have fewer air-fluid levels than patients with small-bowel atresias. Meconium peritonitis may occur and may be associated with peritoneal calcifications. A localized perforation forms a meconium pseudocyst which may have peripheral curvilinear calcifications seen on plain radiographs. The term pseudocyst is also used to refer for a mass of necrotic and fluid-filled bowel loops with a fibrous wall which may be seen as a mass on radiographs.[6]

Ultrasound can detect abnormal bowel dilatation and echogenic bowel contents in infants with meconium ileus. On ultrasound, complications of meconium peritonitis or pseudocyst are seen as echogenic material lying outside the bowel loops with or without associated calcification.

The colon of babies with meconium ileus is often said to be the smallest of all colons and is empty except for a few occasional pellets of meconium. The distal 10–30 cm of ileum appears dilated due to meconium within and may even displace the right colon to the left.[31]

Definitive diagnosis is made with a **low osmolality water-soluble contrast enema** which demonstrates a **microcolon with inspissated meconium pellets** identified in the collapsed distal ileum with dilated small bowel proximal to the obstruction **(Fig. 31)**.

Contrast enema, apart from diagnosing the condition, is used as a therapeutic procedure. Water-soluble contrast agents which are hyperosmolar to plasma are preferred for therapeutic effect as it will draw water into the lumen of the bowel and soften the meconium plugs. Diatrizoate meglumine and diatrizoate sodium (gastrografin) are preferred as a hypertonic contrast and are highly hyperosmotic as compared to other water-soluble agents.[3]

Uncomplicated cases of meconium ileus may be treated with multiple contrast enemas, i.e., one or two enemas per day. The aim is to introduce the contrast into the dilated small bowel proximal to the obstructing inspissated meconium. The patient should be well hydrated if high-osmolarity agents are used because of fluid shifts it causes with careful fluid and electrolyte monitoring. Success rates between 50 and 65% have been reported with therapeutic enema for complete resolution of the obstruction.

Patients diagnosed with complicated meconium ileus clinically, or on plain radiographs with presence of calcification or free intraperitoneal air, are candidates for surgery with no role of enema procedure in such patients. Surgery is also indicated for those patients in whom therapeutic enema is unsuccessful in relieving the obstruction.

Megacystis-microcolon-intestinal Hypoperistalsis Syndrome (Berdon Syndrome)

Megacystis-microcolon-intestinal hypoperistalsis syndrome (MMIHS) is a pseudoatresia. There is a functional small bowel obstruction with a microcolon, malrotation, and a large unobstructed bladder. There is a 2:1 female predominance with associated genitourinary and congenital heart malformation in up to 14% cases. This syndrome is considered one of the severest forms of functional intestinal obstruction in the newborn.

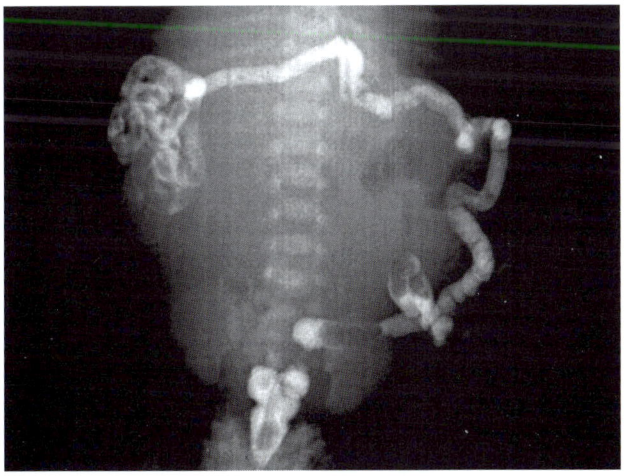

FIG. 31: Meconium ileus: Water soluble contrast enema showing a microcolon. Filling defects due to meconium are seen in colon and distal ileum.

Upper GI contrast study shows hypomotility of small bowel with retrograde peristalsis. On contrast enema there is microcolon and malrotation is seen in >50% cases. Ultrasound reveals a dilated bladder with bilateral hydroureteronephrosis.[25] The prognosis is poor for long-term survival with most patients dying without treatment within first 6 months of life.

Meckel's Diverticulum

Meckel's diverticulum is a **congenital blind pouch** in the small bowel which results from an **incomplete obliteration of the proximal part of the vitelline duct** (omphalomesenteric duct) between the 5th and 7th week of gestation. It results in a true diverticulum (wall layers identical to small bowel) arising from the antimesenteric border of the distal ileum.[39] It has its own blood supply. The *"rule of 2's"* is commonly associated with Meckel's diverticulum, i.e., it is found in 2% of the population, twice as common in males, most frequently found in those <2 years of age and usually 2 feet from the ileocecal valve. It may contain ectopic gastric mucosa (15%) which predisposes to adjacent ulceration and bleeding. Rarely, a giant Meckel's diverticulum may be seen with a diameter >5 cm.

Clinical Presentation

Meckel's diverticulum is usually clinically occult and presents secondary to complications. It occurs equally in both sexes, but symptoms from complications are more common in males. The incidence of complications varies from 4 to 40%, mostly in the younger age group. GI hemorrhage in the form of **painless rectal bleeding** is the most common complication in children reported in over 90% of cases. It occurs due to ectopic gastric or pancreatic mucosa in the diverticulum. Bleeding is usually minor resulting in chronic anemia.[28] It may also be profuse. It may present with melena due to ulceration of ectopic gastric mucosa in its wall. In 20–30% of patients, it may give rise to symptoms such as inflammation and/or perforation which may often be indistinguishable from acute appendicitis. Small bowel obstruction may occur due to inflammatory adhesions, volvulus or intussusception, when the diverticulum inverts and acts as a lead point. The obstructed the diverticulum may result in diverticulitis. In adults, it can also present as a neoplastic mass.

Imaging Features

Preoperative evaluation of a Meckel's diverticulum is difficult and **radiological studies** such as plain abdominal radiograph, barium meal follow through, and ultrasound are **often nondiagnostic** and often of limited diagnostic value. The diverticulum appears as any other intestinal loop on a small bowel follow-through study due to its small ostium, peristalsis, and rapid emptying. On meticulous fluoroscopic examination on barium meal follow through study, or when enteroclysis is performed, a diverticulum may be seen as a **saccular outpouching** from the **distal ileum** along the **antimesenteric border**.[3]

On ultrasound, a Meckel's diverticulum is not easy to identify when it is collapsed and may appear as any other intestinal loop. However, when inflammed, the appearance of a blind ending loop of bowel resembles that of acute appendicitis. CT also has low sensitivity for detection of uncomplicated Meckel's diverticulum, wherein it is seen as a blind-ending fluid or gas-filled structure in continuity with the small bowel. CT can show enteroliths, intussusception, diverticulitis, and small bowel obstruction. Extravasation of contrast material into the lumen of the diverticulum has been reported when active bleeding occurs at the time of CT scanning.[40] On CT, heterotropic tissue or neoplasm within the diverticulum appears as a nodular or polypoid intraluminal mass.

In suspected symptomatic Meckel's diverticulum, preoperative evaluation includes technetium-99m (^{99m}Tc)-pertechnetate scanning. ^{99m}Tc is injected intravenously, and over time it accumulates in the mucin-secreting cells of the gastric tissue and ectopic gastric mucosa. As symptoms such as bleeding is caused by the ectopic gastric issue, **^{99m}Tc scanning** is **most reliable** in the **diagnosis** in **symptomatic cases**. In children, the scan has a sensitivity of 85% and specificity of 95% while in adults the sensitivity is only around 60%. However, there is little or no uptake of the isotope when there is scant or no gastric mucosa present.

Treatment

The treatment of complicated Meckel's diverticulum is surgical resection. With the development of minimally invasive surgery, laparoscopic diagnosis with resection of symptomatic diverticulum is advocated.[3]

Enteric Duplication

Gastrointestinal duplications are uncommon congenital abnormalities that may occur anywhere in the GIT. The most common locations are the distal ileum followed by esophagus, colon, jejunum, stomach, and duodenum.[37] Colonic and rectal duplications are rare. Multiple duplications may be present in 15–20% cases.[25] Typically, a duplication contains all muscle layers of the GIT and may possess a common wall with the bowel or hang-free on its own mesentery.[41]

Embryology

The etiology of alimentary tract duplication is uncertain and many hypotheses have been proposed to explain its embryogenesis such as (a) abnormal recanalization, (b) attempt of incomplete/abortive twinning, (c) diverticula formation during recanalization stage of bowel, and (d) environmental factors such as trauma or hypoxia.[3]

Gastrointestinal tract duplications are of two types—(1) cystic and (2) tubular. Cystic duplications account for approximately 80% of cases are spherical in shape and have no communication with the bowel lumen. In contrast, tubular duplications account for around 20% of the cases and are more likely to communicate with the adjacent bowel lumen and are often ulcerated. They typically occur along the mesenteric border of the intestine and share a common blood supply. Thus, the tubular type of duplication may complicate bowel-sparing surgery because of difficulty in preserving the enteric blood supply. The cystic variety usually contains a clear mucoid substance which is secreted from the mucosa itself. It may at times be hemorrhagic due to ulceration of the ectopic gastric mucosa. Unlike neurenteric cysts, duplication cysts are usually not associated with vertebral segmental anomalies.[39]

Enteric duplication occurs in the late first or early second trimester. The duplication has smooth muscle in its wall with gastrointestinal mucosal lining. The wall thickness is 3–5 mm as seen in normal bowel. It is usually adjacent to and in most instances does not communicate with the GIT. In most cases of hemorrhage or ulceration, gastric mucosa is present. Esophageal duplications are located at the posterior aspect of the esophagus. Gastric duplication is found along the greater curvature of the stomach interposed between the stomach and the transverse colon.

Malrotation, genitourinary anomalies, and jejunal or ileal atresias are also seen with duplication cysts.

Clinical Presentation

Most GI duplications manifest during the 1st year of life. In adults, they are rarely symptomatic and are usually detected incidentally or at endoscopy.[37] Duplications are more common in boys except for gastric ones, which occur without gender predominance.

Duplications can present with a variety of symptoms and signs depending on the site and size of duplication. Upper esophageal duplications present with symptoms due to tracheal compression. Other symptoms include abdominal pain, nausea, and vomiting. In the presence of heterotopic gastric mucosa, patients may present with gastrointestinal hemorrhage or even perforation. Duodenal duplication cysts can lead to pancreatitis. Patients may also present with distention, ulceration, volvulus, infection, and an abdominal mass lesion with obstruction or intussusception, particularly when the duplication is in the region of the ileocecal valve or duodenum.

Imaging Features

Plain radiographs may demonstrate a mass lesion, especially in the chest in the case of esophageal duplication **(Figs. 32A to C)**. The bowel gas pattern may suggest an obstruction, particularly with duodenal or ileal duplications. Enteric duplication cysts may reveal mural calcifications.

On barium studies, duplications are usually not seen as they do not communicate with the GIT. They may rarely get filled with barium during contrast examinations. **Barium study** reveals **extrinsic compression (Figs. 33A to C)** of the **bowel or an obstruction.**

On ultrasonography, a duplication cyst appears as a well-defined, unilocular anechoic mass with good through transmission **(Fig. 34)**. Rarely, the contents are reflective or contain septations secondary to hemorrhage or inspissated material within the lumen. A highly reflective mucosa and a surrounding echo poor muscular wall may be seen as the duplication is of gastrointestinal origin.[42,43] This is most easily identified in the dependent portion of the cyst.[25] The presence

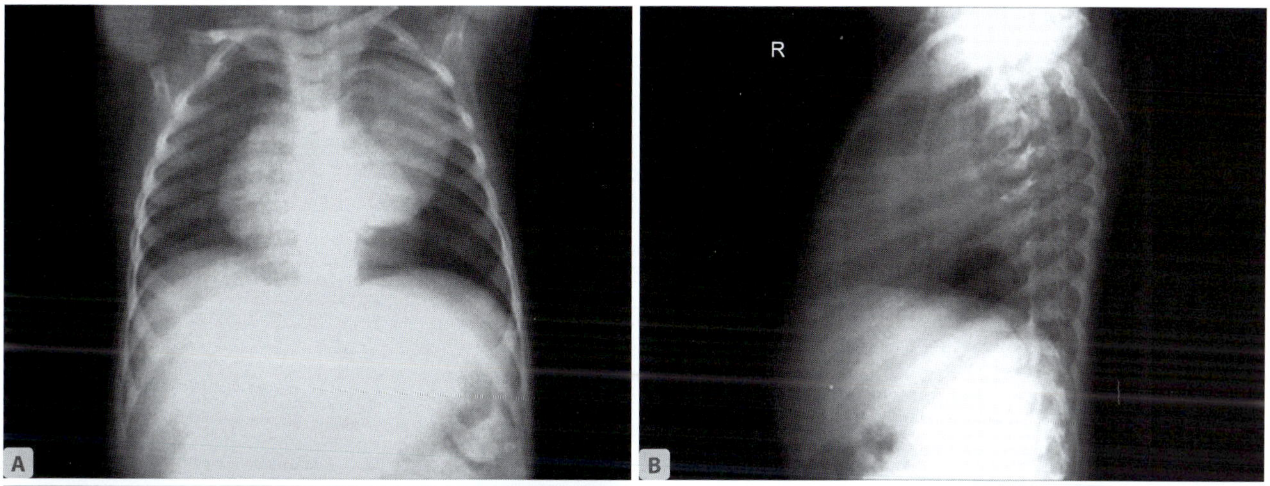

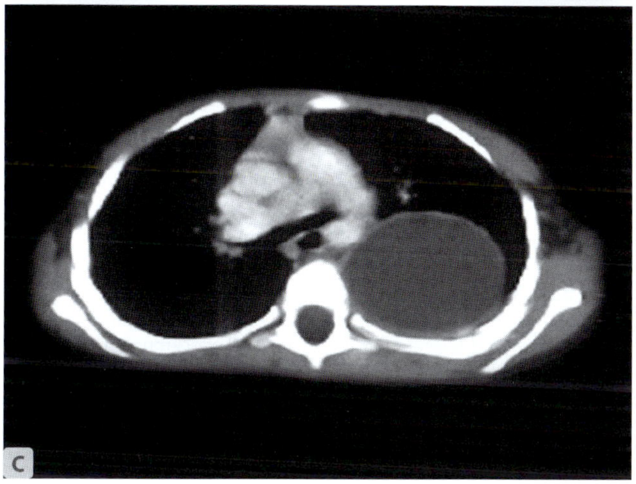

FIGS. 32A TO C: Esophageal duplication: Chest PA showing a well-defined soft-tissue mass in the left hemithorax (A) lying posteriorly in the lateral film (B). There is associated hyperinflation of the left lung. The vertebral bodies appear normal. CT chest shows a well-defined oval homogeneous nonenhancing mass of fluid attenuation in the posterior mediastinum (C).

of this double-layered appearance, i.e., "gut wall signature" is relatively specific for the diagnosis of duplication cyst. The inner layer is the hyperechoic mucosa and the outer layer is the hypoechoic muscle. This feature was considered useful to exclude other cystic masses, such as mesenteric or omental cyst, choledochal cyst, ovarian cyst, pancreatic pseudocyst or abscess. However, it has been seen that some cystic lesions such as Meckel's diverticula, mesenteric cysts, and ovarian cysts may show a layered wall that simulates this sign. In spite of this, a **cystic mass** having a **bi-layer wall**, located adjacent to the bowel, should suggest a strong possibility of a **duplication cyst**. Sometimes, the reflective lining may be absent as a result of extensive mucosal ulceration by gastric enzymes. Also, in some instances with inflammation the layers may be obscured.[41]

Radionuclide studies may be useful in 30% of patients where the enteric duplications have gastric mucosa. Free pertechnetate is taken up and secreted by gastric mucosa, thus, localizing the enteric duplication.[9]

CT or MRI may be useful in further characterizing the nature of enteric duplication cysts when the diagnosis is unclear by depicting the location, extent of the cyst as well as complications and other associated anomalies. On CECT/CEMR, the duplication cyst appears as a well-marginated, smooth-walled mass of fluid attenuation/signal with mild enhancement of the wall and arises from or is extrinsic to the gastrointestinal wall **(Figs. 32C and 33C)**. An area of high attenuation in the cyst may be seen due to hemorrhage or proteinaceous material. A duplication cyst complicated by infection appears as a cystic mass with a thick-enhancing wall or septa and surrounding inflammation.

LARGE BOWEL

Colonic Obstruction

Obstruction of the colon in the newborn may be either anatomical or functional. The first type includes atresia of the colon and with a functional element, aganglionosis or Hirschsprung's disease. A group of poorly understood disorders such as meconium plug, neonatal small left colon syndrome, etc., cause transient self-limited functional obstruction.

Colonic Atresia

Colonic atresia is quite rare as compared to atresias of the small bowel.[31] It is thought to be **secondary to a vascular insult**. Multiple atresia syndromes may involve the colon in addition to small bowel. Proximal location is more common than distal with atresias beyond the splenic flexure being unusual. If atresia is located in the ascending colon, it may

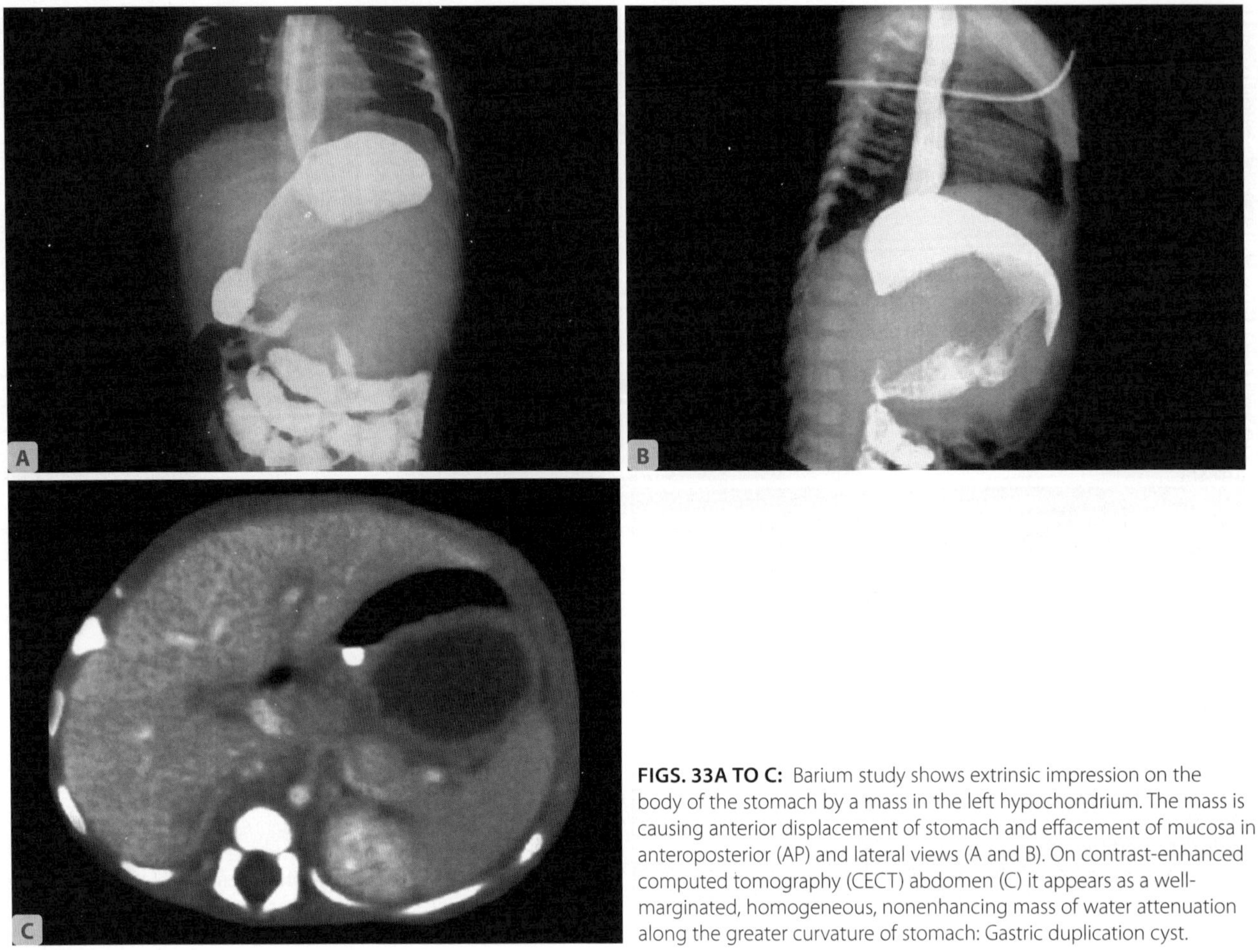

FIGS. 33A TO C: Barium study shows extrinsic impression on the body of the stomach by a mass in the left hypochondrium. The mass is causing anterior displacement of stomach and effacement of mucosa in anteroposterior (AP) and lateral views (A and B). On contrast-enhanced computed tomography (CECT) abdomen (C) it appears as a well-marginated, homogeneous, nonenhancing mass of water attenuation along the greater curvature of stomach: Gastric duplication cyst.

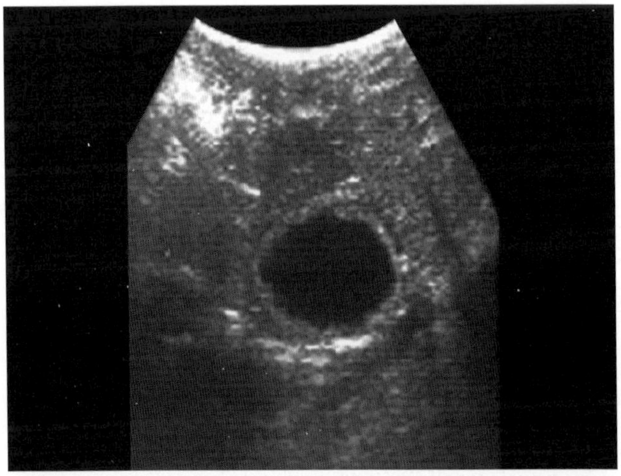

FIG. 34: Ultrasound abdomen reveals a well-defined, smooth-rounded cystic lesion with inner echogenic mucosal stripe and outer hypoechoic muscle layer: Enteric duplication cyst.

often be indistinguishable from obstruction of the distal ileum.[38] The classification system based on the anatomic appearance is same as with jejunoileal atresia. Type I represents a diaphragmatic occlusion, type II represents a complete atresia with a blind, solid cord extending between the two ends of atretic segment; and type III represents a complete atresia with complete separation and an associated V-shaped mesenteric defect.

Clinical Presentation

Patients present with abdominal distention, vomiting, and failure to pass meconium. Presentation may be delayed up to 48 hours, if the atresia is proximal.

Imaging Features

Prenatal sonography may demonstrate dilatation of the colon proximal to the atresia. Polyhydramnios is uncommon as the atresia is distal and thus allows resorption of swallowed amniotic fluid.[3]

Plain radiograph may demonstrate a distal obstruction with multiple air-fluid levels and may be nonspecific. Occasionally, a hugely and disproportionately dilated loop of bowel may be present and render the plain film evaluation highly suggestive of the diagnosis.[5] There is dilatation of the proximal colon up to the level of the atresia, unless multiple atresias are present. Air-fluid levels are seen on horizontal beam radiographs with no gas in rectum on prone film.

Contrast enema shows a microcolon distal to the atresia that terminates blindly, and is devoid of filling defects of meconium ileus. There is obstruction to the retrograde flow of barium at the site of atresia. The colon may have a hook or question-mark appearance at the site of atresia and is often nonfixed or malpositioned in the midline. The distal colon segment may perforate into the peritoneal cavity during a contrast enema because often the blind end is covered with only mucosa.

Treatment

The treatment of colonic atresia is surgical. The proximal bowel should be evaluated at the time of surgery as associated proximal atresia is seen in 15–20% of patients of colonic atresia.[3]

Hirschsprung's Disease/Aganglionosis of the Colon/Congenital Megacolon

Hirschsprung's disease is a condition caused by absence of normal ganglion cells in a segment of the effected colon leading to a form of low intestinal obstruction. It accounts for around 15–20% of cases of neonatal bowel obstruction.[38]

Embryology

In normal intrauterine development, neuroenteric cells migrate from the neural crest to the upper end of the GIT by 5 weeks and then proceed in a caudal direction. These cells reach the rectum by 12 weeks and commence the intramural migration from Auerbach's (myenteric) plexus to the submucosal plexus. Hirschsprung's disease is caused by **abnormal neural crest cell migration** resulting in arrested distal migration of these cells.[6] As the normal migration is continuous from proximal to distal, the part of the GIT distal to the site of arrest is aganglionic.[13]

Hirschsprung's disease can be classified into short, ultrashort, long segment (up to splenic flexure) and total colonic aganglionosis. In the **majority of cases** (80%), the **aganglionic segment** is **limited to the rectosigmoid region** (short segment aganglionosis). The aganglionosis always involves the anus and internal sphincter and extends proximally for a variable distance. The transition from innervated to aganglionic bowel is found in the rectosigmoid region in 73% of patients, the descending colon in 14%, and more proximal colon in 10%, according to Swenson et al.[8] Total colonic aganglionosis involves the entire colon and part of the terminal ileum. It can very rarely involve the large as well as whole of the small bowel, which is incompatible with life. At the other end of the spectrum is ultrashort segment Hirschsprung's disease which is also rare. In this type, the aganglionosis is limited to the region of the internal anal sphincter.[6] The ultrashort segment is one in which the involved aganglionosis is a very short distal rectal segment <2 cm. Though the ganglion cells are absent, the transition zone is not a feature. It can only be diagnosed by manometry and is usually not diagnosed in the neonatal period.[8]

Skip lesions in Hirschsprung's disease are believed to be unlikely to exist if one accepts the concept of neuronal migration down the GIT. It is likely that such areas represent areas of intrauterine ischemic insult leading to destruction of ganglion cells.[12]

However, according to published literature, skip lesions or zonal aganglionosis, though a controversial condition, is known to occur in Hirschsprung's disease with 29 cases reported till date. It is defined as presence of single or multiple segments of ganglionated bowel in between segments of aganglionosis. Skip lesions have been found to occur predominantly in patients with total colonic aganglionosis or long segment Hirschsprung's disease. The diagnosis of skip segment should be considered when there is treatment failure, recurrent enterocolitis, or refractory constipation postoperatively in a known patient of Hirschsprung's disease. The presence of a skip area of normally innervated colon in total colonic aganglionosis may influence the surgical management enabling the surgeons to preserve and use the ganglionated skip area during pull through operations.[44]

Hirschsprung's disease may be associated with certain congenital anomalies such as intestinal atresia and malrotation. Down syndrome is present in 2–3% cases.

Clinical Presentation

The absence of ganglion cells interrupts the normal propagation of colonic peristalsis. Neonates with Hirschsprung's disease typically present with delayed passage of meconium beyond the first 48 hours of life. They may present with abdominal distention, bilious vomiting, or enterocolitis. Over 80% of patients present within the first 6 weeks in life. It is more common in term infants and almost all present before 5 years of age. Hirschsprung's disease is about 3-4 times as common in boys than in girls. Older children may present with chronic constipation. Hirschsprung's disease can be complicated by life-threatening enterocolitis which presents with diarrhea, abdominal distention, and fever and may progress to perforation with peritonitis.[6]

Imaging Features

Plain films may demonstrate features of distal bowel obstruction. However, a dilated colon proximal to the distal and smaller aganglionic segment is the more typical finding **(Fig. 35)**. A small gas-filled rectum can be seen, especially on prone films, and may help in the diagnosis. The absence of rectal gas is not specific for Hirschsprung's disease as it is commonly seen in infants with sepsis and necrotizing enterocolitis.[25] At times, the bowel pattern may appear normal. Less commonly (4%), pneumoperitoneum may be seen in patients with long segment or total colonic disease secondary to colonic perforation.

The **radiographic diagnosis** is made by **contrast enema** and is directed toward identifying the **transition zone** which is the most specific sign of **Hirschsprung's disease (Fig. 36)**. This is where the normal-sized distal aganglionic bowel changes in caliber to join the proximal ganglionic bowel.[6] This finding may not be obvious in the newborn, hence, careful attention should be given to the technique of performing barium enema.

Technique of Contrast Enema

Water soluble iso-osmolar contrast agents are preferred in neonates as hyperosmolal contrast will lead to increased

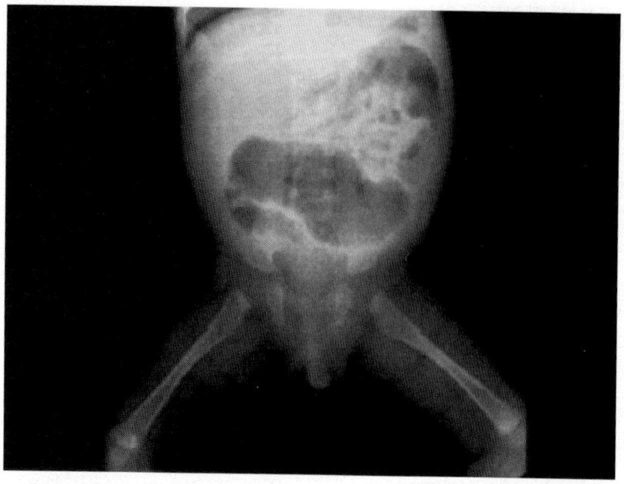

FIG. 35: Plain X-ray abdomen showing a dilated proximal sigmoid colon with a smaller distal sigmoid with relatively little rectal gas in a neonate with Hirschsprung's disease.

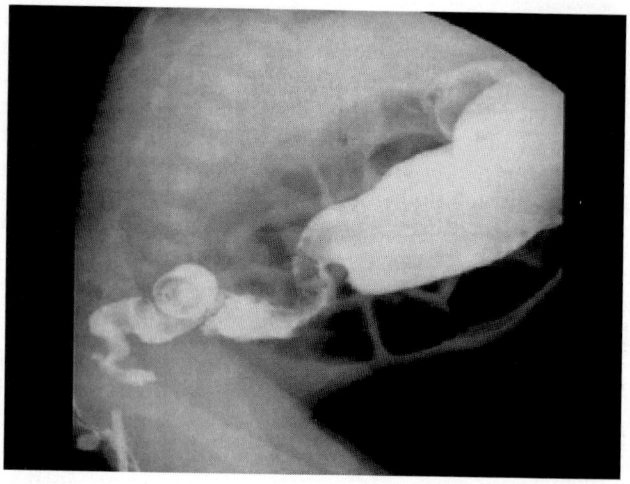

FIG. 36: Hirschsprung's disease: Barium enema shows an abrupt transition from the narrow caliber rectosigmoid (aganglionic) to the larger caliber more proximal sigmoid colon.

bowel distention. Barium is not used if there is another cause of obstruction suspected such as meconium ileus or in case of a perforation. In an older child being evaluated for constipation, barium is the contrast-agent preferred.[13] Barium enema is performed on an unprepared patient by inserting a straight-tipped catheter to a point just beyond the anal sphincter. Balloon catheters are not used to avoid expanding a narrow segment of aganglionic colon and may, thus, obscure the diagnosis. There is also risk of perforation of the stiff aganglionic rectum.[31] Barium contrast should be prepared with normal saline to avoid possibility of water absorption from the large surface area of dilated colon.[39] With the patient in the lateral position, barium suspension is introduced slowly by gravity drip infusion under fluoroscopic monitoring. The infusion is stopped and restarted as serial spot radiographs are obtained. As filling progresses into the descending colon, the patient is rolled into the supine position. If the examination is positive, the diagnosis in most cases is made by the time the barium fills the proximal descending colon. Rapid infusion of barium suspension can distend and mask the transition zone. When the transition zone is observed, the examination should be discontinued because filling of the more proximal dilated bowel beyond the transition zone may lead to impaction. However, distention of the bowel proximal to the aganglionic segment is gradual, and a transition zone is seen in only 50% of neonates during the 1st week of life.[38]

The **transition zone** generally is **funnel-shaped** and it is an **important diagnostic feature**. In some instances, the transformation from dilated bowel to narrowed bowel is abrupt **(Figs. 37A and B)**. In other cases, the funneling of the bowel occurs incrementally over a long segment of bowel to appear almost imperceptible because of the gradual change in caliber. In long segment Hirschsprung's disease, a variable portion of the colon proximal to the sigmoid colon is aganglionic **(Fig. 38)**. The pathological transition zone is usually somewhat more proximal than the radiological one. Under fluoroscopic visualization, **irregular saw-toothed mucosal pattern** may be seen due to disordered contractions in the aganglionic colon **(Fig. 39)**. Another radiographic appearance of Hirschsprung's disease that has been described in neonates and young infants in whom the rectosigmoid region appears normal is the presence of straight transverse bands in the involved segment of colon. These bands are thought to represent areas of persistent spasm.[12]

The **rectosigmoid index** can be used in the diagnosis of Hirschsprung's disease confined to the rectum. This compares the ratio of the rectal diameter to the sigmoid diameter and is considered abnormal if the sigmoid colon is more dilated than the rectum (R/S index <1).[6]

The immediate postevacuation film may be useful in identifying the collapsed distal aganglionic segment. Delayed radiographs taken after 24 hours may show prolonged retention of barium, which is a strong indicator of Hirschsprung's disease when enema findings have been inconclusive **(Figs. 40A and B and Box 4)**. Other signs observed on delayed films is contrast media mixed with stool or a more obvious transition zone than seen on immediate films.[6]

In total colonic Hirschsprung's disease, barium enema may be nondiagnostic with no discordant sizes in the distal large bowel. A useful sign is a colon that is shortened with flexures pulled down and rounded in appearance (question mark colon). A true microcolon appearance similar to that seen in distal ileal atresia is rare.[9]

Diagnostic Investigations

Patients with a high index of suspicion for Hirschsprung's disease should undergo a methodical evaluation. Two **screening tests** for the diagnostic work-up are contrast study and anorectal manometry. Manometric study is noninvasive, nonionizing, and does not require much patient preparation, and if positive, should be confirmed by a rectal biopsy.[45]

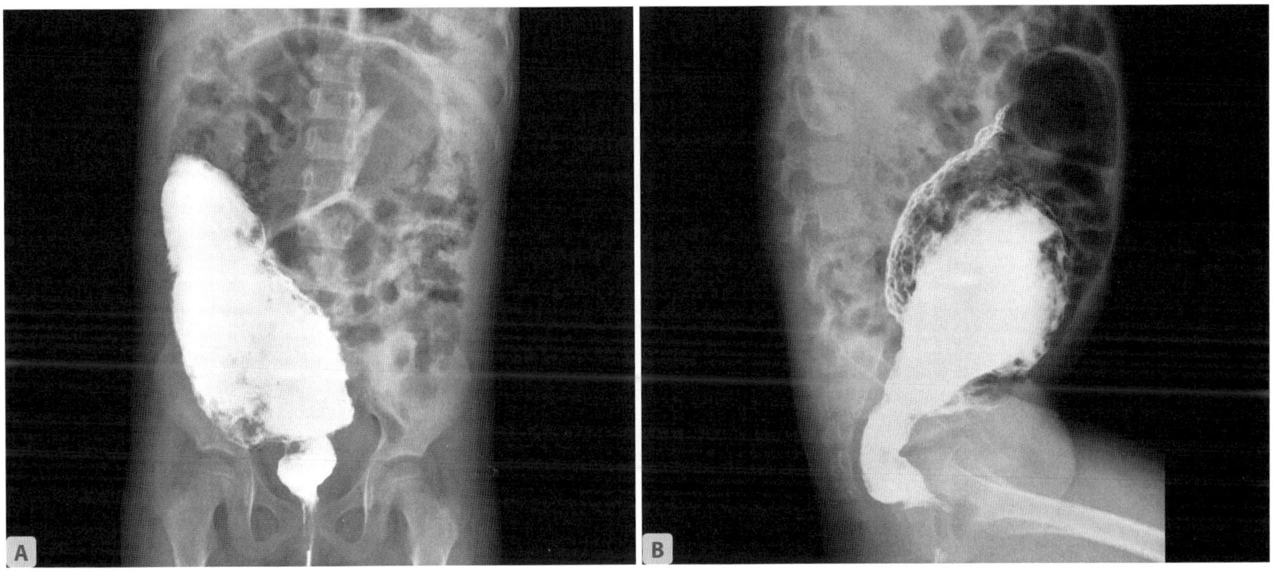

FIGS. 37A AND B: Anteroposterior (AP) and lateral views of barium enema reveal pronounced dilatation of the descending colon and proximal sigmoid colon with abrupt change in caliber in the rectosigmoid region: Hirschsprung's disease.

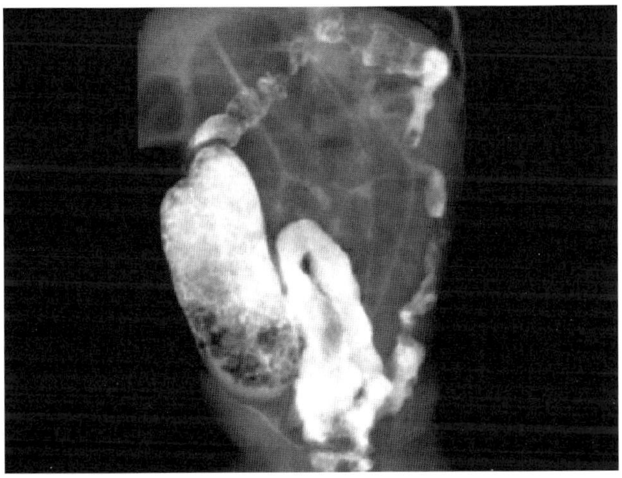

FIG. 38: Barium enema reveals a colon of reduced caliber from rectum to hepatic flexure with markedly dilated colon (cecum and ascending colon) proximal to it—long segment aganglionosis.

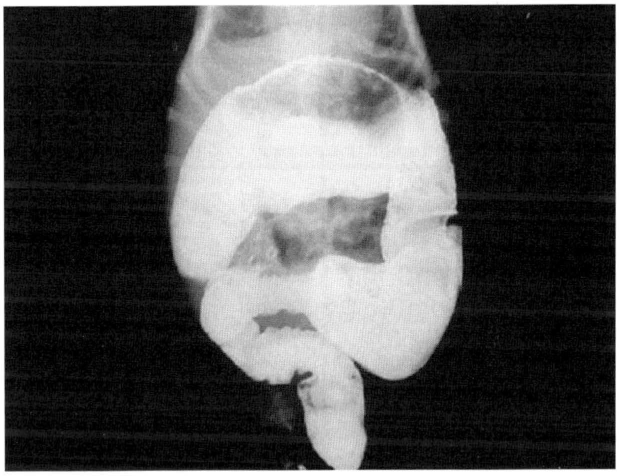

FIG. 39: Colonic aganglionosis with transition zone in sigmoid colon showing irregular mucosal outline/contractions.

This relies on anal sphincter reflex relaxation in response to distention of the rectum and is absent in patients with Hirschsprung's disease.

Confirmation of Hirschsprung's disease is by means of a rectal suction biopsy in patients <6 months of age as an OPD procedure. Contrast enema can be safely performed 24 hours after a suction biopsy, though ideally the enema should precede a biopsy.[6] While in a child who is >12 months old, a full thickness rectal biopsy is the procedure of choice and is performed under general anesthesia. For rectal biopsy, adequate sample of mucosa and submucosa is obtained at three levels around 2 cm, 3 cm, and 4 cm above the anal verge, as below this line the normal anus shows relative hypoganglionosis.[45] Histopathologic findings in patients with Hirschsprung's disease consist of absent ganglion cells, hypertrophied nerve fibers and increased acetylcholinesterase staining.

Treatment

Surgical treatment of Hirschsprung's disease consists of resection of the aganglionic segment, confirmation of ganglia in the proximal bowel and pull through of the normal innervated bowel through the sphincteric mechanism. This is known by the name of Duhamel and Soave procedures. Leaks, strictures, and residual obstruction, or delayed bowel control are some of the postoperative complications known to occur.

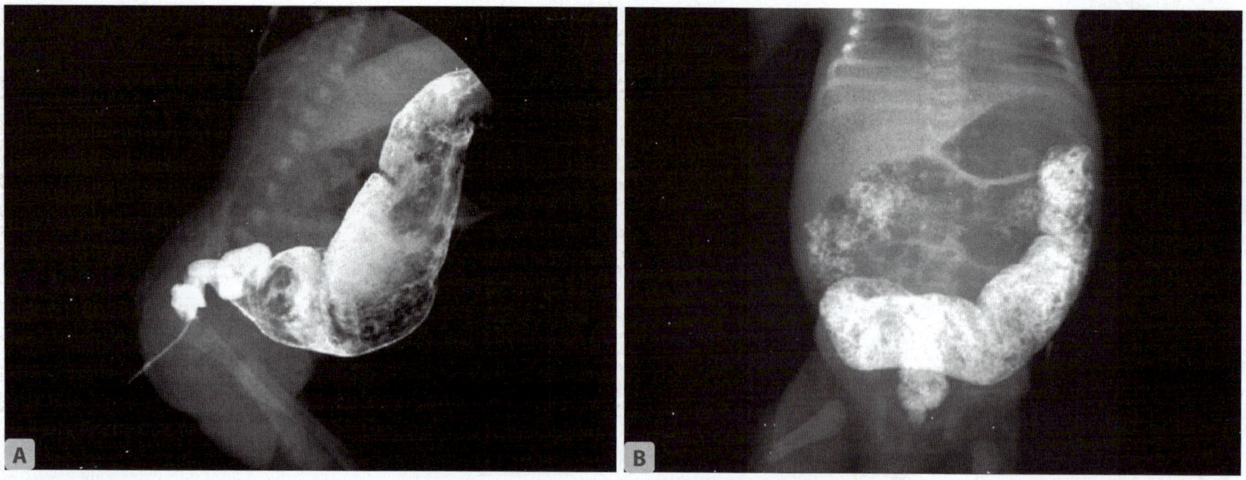

FIGS. 40A AND B: (A) Short segment Hirschsprung's disease with aganglionosis of rectum and distal sigmoid and marked dilatation proximal to it; (B) 24 hour film showing significant retention of barium.

BOX 4: Key radiological features of Hirschsprung's disease on contrast enema.

- Zone of transition between aganglionic segment and dilated proximal bowel
- Serrated appearance of aganglionic segment (due to irregular colonic contractions)
- Rectosigmoid ratio <1.0
- Retention of contrast on postevacuation film

Functional Immaturity of the Colon/Neonatal Functional Colonic Obstruction

Functional immaturity of the colon is a common cause of neonatal obstruction, especially in premature babies. It comprises of several entities, most common being small left colon syndrome and meconium plug syndrome.[38] They are both conditions of colonic dysmotility which present as distal bowel obstruction in neonates. Both conditions overlap with each other and also with Hirschsprung's disease. The exact etiology is not known and is thought to be associated with functional immaturity of the ganglion cells of the colon. The babies are frequently infants of diabetic mothers or mothers who have received magnesium sulfate for eclampsia.

Clinical Presentation

In general, babies with functional immaturity of the colon are not sick as compared to other babies presenting with low intestinal obstruction.[31]

Most infants present within the first 24–36 hours of life with abdominal distention, biliary emesis and failure to initiate the normal passage of meconium. This is due to transient colonic inertia with failure of normal peristalsis in a normally innervated colon.[12]

Plain radiography findings are nonspecific showing distal bowel obstruction with no gas seen in the distal colon or rectum.[6]

Small Left Colon Syndrome

The contrast enema demonstrates a distended right and transverse colon with transition to a very small caliber descending and rectosigmoid colon, occurring near the splenic flexure, with the rectum being of normal caliber, i.e., a variable part of left colon is small in caliber, resembling a microcolon. Typically, there is improvement in the clinical and radiological finding over the next few hours or days. The condition may mimic Hirschsprung's disease, but there are several findings which help in differentiating the two **(Table 3)**.[2] Also, the rectosigmoid ratio is normal against an abnormal rectosigmoid ratio in Hirschsprung's disease.[7]

It is important to follow the patients closely because if they have Hirschsprung's disease, they will return with intestinal problems such as constipation or diarrhea.

Meconium Plug Syndrome

This is the most frequent cause of delayed passage of meconium in infants. In this condition, meconium is in the colon but is not the underlying cause of obstruction, which is a result of the functional obstruction. Contrast enema performed is both diagnostic and therapeutic in such infants. Low osmolal contrast should be used with careful attention to hydration of the neonate.

In meconium plug syndrome, the colon is usually of normal caliber with a long-filling defect due to meconium plug. The meconium plug occupies the rectosigmoid region, but may extend throughout the colon. A normal evacuation pattern is established following stimulation of rectum by enema or occasionally digital examination.[6]

Meconium plug syndrome needs to be differentiated from meconium ileus. The term meconium ileus is reserved for bowel obstruction secondary to inspissated meconium in the distal small bowel and proximal colon, most often seen in patients of cystic fibrosis.[6]

In both meconium plug syndrome and left colon syndrome, patients appear symptomatically better after enema examination. Prognosis is good and patients usually resolve in a few days with supportive care. At times,

TABLE 3: Differentiating features between small left colon syndrome and Hirschsprung's disease.

Points of difference	Small left colon syndrome	Hirschsprung's disease
Change in caliber/transition	Usually at splenic flexure with proximal distended right colon and transverse colon	Transition usually more distal, most commonly at rectosigmoid
Type of transition	Abrupt change in caliber	Cone-shaped and gradual change
Caliber of involved segment	Left colon is usually smaller in caliber than normal colon	Near normal caliber of aganglionic colon
Rectum	In most patients rectum is quite distensible	The aganglionic colon is of uniform caliber to the anus

distinction from Hirschsprung's disease is not possible and a rectal biopsy should be performed in those children in whom the symptoms do not resolve.[31]

CONCLUSION

Imaging plays an important role in most neonatal as well as childhood developmental lesions of the GIT, which usually presents with obstruction. The role of imaging may vary from establishment of diagnosis, evaluation of associated abnormalities, surgical planning or therapy for some conditions. Plain radiographs and contrast examinations serve as primary imaging modalities. CT and MRI help in more complex cases as they provide excellent anatomical detail.

Plain radiographs are often diagnostic in neonates with complete gastric and duodenal atresia and generally do not require any further radiological investigation. An upper GI contrast study should be performed in all patients presenting with incomplete intestinal obstruction. Ultrasound is useful in evaluating developmental lesions such as HPS, enteric duplication cysts, midgut malrotation, meconium ileus, and meconium peritonitis.[25]

It is important to be familiar with the role and usefulness of various imaging modalities so that they can be used judiciously. The aim of every radiological study is to obtain maximum possible information while avoiding unnecessary radiation exposure and minimizing patient discomfort.

ACKNOWLEDGEMENTS

I would like to thank Dr Prince and Mohit for the illustrations.

REFERENCES

1. Silverman FN, Kuhn (Eds). The gastrointestinal tract. Caffey's Pediatric X-ray Diagnosis: An Integrated Imaging Approach. United States: Mosby; 1993.
2. Kandasamy D, Sharma R, Gupta AK. Bowel Imaging in Children: Part 1. Ind Jr Pediatr. 2019; 86:805-16.
3. Hernanz-Schulman M, Bowel S. Congenital and neonatal abnormalities. Caffey's pediatric diagnostic imaging, 12th edition. Philadelphia: Elsevier Saunders; 2013.
4. Prasad GR, Aziz A. Abdominal Plain Radiograph in Neonatal Intestinal Obstruction. J Neonat Surg. 2017;6(1):6.
5. Hernanz-Schulman M. Imaging of neonatal gastrointestinal obstruction. Radiol Clin North Am. 1999;37:1163-86.
6. Donohue V, Twomey EL. The neonatal and non-neonatal gastro-intestinal tract. In: Carty H, Brunelle F, Stringer DA Kazo Simon CS (Eds). Imaging children, Volume 2, Second edition. London: Elsevier Churchill Livingstone; 2005. pp. 1305-528.
7. Ngo AV, Stanescu AL, Phillips GS. Neonatal Bowel Disorders Practical Imaging Algorithm for Trainees and General Radiologists. AJR. 2018;210:976-88.
8. Leonidas JC, Singh SP, slovis TL. Congenital Anomalies of the Gastrointestinal tract. In: Kuhn Jerald P, Slovis Thomas L, Haller Jack O (Eds). Caffey's Pediatric Diagnostic Imaging, Volume 1, 10th Edition. United States: Mosby; 2004. pp. 113-62.
9. McAlister WH, Kronemer KA. Emergency gastrointestinal radiology of the newborn. Radiol Clin North Am. 1996;34:819-44.
10. Ein SH, Shandling B. Pure esophageal atresia: A 50-year review. J Pediatr Surg. 1994;29:1208-11.
11. Iuchtman M, Brereton RJ, Spitz L, Kiely EM, Drake D. Morbidity and mortality in 46 patients with the VACTERL association. Isr J Med Sci. 1992;28:281-4.
12. Swischuk LE. Alimentary tract. In: Swischurk LE (Ed). Imaging of the Newborn, Infant and Young child, 5th edition. Philadelphia: Lippincott Williams and Wilkins; 2004. pp. 341-482.
13. Schlesinger AE, Parker BR. Abdomen and gastrointestinal tract. In: Kuhn JP Slovis TL, Haller JO (Eds). Caffey's Pediatric Diagnostic Imaging, volume 2, Section VI, 10th Edition. United States: Mosby; 2004. pp. 1421-690.
14. Ratan SK, Varshney A, Mullick S, Saxena NC. Evaluation of neonates with esophageal atresia using chest CT Scan. Pediatr Surg Int. 2004;20:757-61.
15. Ou P, Seror E, Layouss W, Revillon Y, Brunelle F. Definitive diagnosis and surgical planning of H-type tracheoesophageal fistula in a critically ill neonate: First experience using air distension of the esophagus during high-resolution computed tomography acquisition. J Thorac Cardiovasc Surg. 2007;133: 1116 7.
16. Berrocal T, Torres I, Gutierrez J, Prietio C, del Hoyo ML, Lamas M. Congential Anomalies of the upper gastrointestinal tract. Radiographics. 1999;19(4):855-72.
17. Schulman MH. Infantile hypertrophic pyloric stenosis. Radiology. 2003;227:319-31.
18. Chung E. Infantile hypertrophic pylotic stenosis: genes and environment. Arch Dis Child. 2008;93:1003-4.
19. Haller JO, Cohen HL. Hypertrophic pyloric stenosis: Diagnosis using ultrasound. Radiology. 1986;161:335-9.
20. Hayden CK Jr, Swischuk LE, Lobe TE, Schwartz MZ, Boulden T. Ultrasound: The definitive imaging modality in pyloric stenosis. Radiographics. 1984;4:517-30.
21. Amodio J, Fefferman N. Ultrasound of pediatric abdominal and scrotal emergencies. App Radiol. 2007;36(12):22-9.

22. Blumhagen JD, Maclin L, Krauter D, Rosenbaum DM, Weinberger E. Sonographic diagnosis of hypertrophic pyloric stenosis. Am J Roentgenol. 1988;150:1367-70.
23. Hernanz-Schulman M, Sells LL, Ambrosino MM, Heller RM, Stein SM, Neblett WW, 3rd. Hypertrophic pyloric stenosis in the infant without a palpable olive: Accuracy of sonographic diagnosis. Radiology 1994;193:771.
24. O'Keeffe FN, Stansberry SD, Swischuk LE, Hayden CK, Jr. Antropyloric muscle thickness at US in infants: what is normal? Radiology. 1991;178:827-30.
25. Gupta AK, Guglani B. Imaging of Congenital Anomalies of the Gastrointestinal Tract. Indian J Pediatr. 2005;72(5):403-14.
26. Atwell JD, Levick P. Congenital hypertrophic pyloric stenosis and associated anomalies in the genitourinary tract. J Pediatr Surg. 1981;16:1029-35.
27. Dias SC, Swinson S, Torrão H, Gonçalves L, Kurochka S, Vaz CP, et al. Hypertrophic pyloric stenosis tips and tricks for ultrasound diagnosis. Insights Imaging. 2012;3:247-50.
28. Vaos G, Misiakos EP. Congenital Anomalies of the Gastrointestinal Tract Diagnosed in Adulthood—Diagnosis and Management. J Gastrointest Surg. 2010;14:916-25.
29. Rezwani M, Menias C, Sandrasegaran K, Olpin JD, Elsayes KM, Shaaban AM. Heterotopic Pancreas Histopathologic Features, Imaging Findings, and Complications. Radiographics. 2017;37:484-99.
30. Tantillo K, Dym RJ, Chernyak V, Scheinfeld MH, Taragin BH. No way out: Causes of duodenal and gastric outlet obstruction. Clin Imaging. 2020;65:37-46.
31. Buonomo C. Neonatal gastrointestinal emergencies. Radiol Clin North Am. 1997;35:845-64.
32. Bailey PV, Tracy TF, Connors RH, Mooney DP, Lewis JE, Weber TR. Congenital duodenal obstruction: A 32-year review. J Pediatr Surg. 1993;28:92-5.
33. Fonkalsrud E, de Lorimier A, Hays D. Congenital atresia and stenosis of the duodenum: A review compiled from the members of the surgical section of the American Academy of Pediatrics. Pediatrics. 1969;43:79-83.
34. Brinkley MF, Tracy ET, Maxfield CM. Congenital duodenal obstruction: causes and imaging approach. Pediatr Radiol. 2016;46:1084-95.
35. Pratt A. Current concepts of the obstructing duodenal diaphragm. Radiology. 1971;100:637-43.
36. Applegate KE, Anderson JM, Klatte EC. Intestinal malrotation in children: a problem-solving approach to the upper gastrointestinal series. Radiographics. 2006;26(5):1485-500.
37. Lee NK, Kim S, Jeon TY, Kim HS, Kim DH, Seo HI, et al. Complications of congenital and developmental abnormalities of the gastrointestinal tract in adolescents and adults: evaluation with multimodality imaging. Radiographics. 2010;30(6):1489-507.
38. Berrocal T, Lamas M, Gutierrez J, Torres I, Prieto C, del Hoyo ML. Congenital Anomalies of the small Intestine, Colon and Rectum. Radiographics. 1999;19(5):1219-36.
39. Thomas KE, Owens CM. The Pediatric Abdomen. In: Sutton D (Ed). Textbook of Radiology and Imaging, Volume 1, 7th Edition. London: Churchill Livingstone; 2002. pp. 849-84.
40. Macari M, Balthazar EJ. The acute right lower quadrant: CT evaluation. Radiol Clin North Am. 2003;41:1117-36.
41. Di Serafino M, Mercogliano C, Vallone G. Ultrasound evaluation of the enteric duplication cyst: the gut signature. J ultrasound. 2016;19(2):131-3.
42. Macpherson RI. Gastrointestinal tract duplications: Clinical, pathologic, etiologic and radiologic considerations. Radiographics. 1993;13:1063-80.
43. Barr LL, Hayden CK Jr, Stansberry SD, Swischuk LE. Enteric duplication cysts in children: Are their ultrasonographic wall characteristics diagnostic? Pediatr Radiol. 1990;20:326-8.
44. O' Donnell AM, Puri P. Skip segment Hirschsprung's disease: a systematic review. Pediatr Surg Int. 2010;26(11):1065-9.
45. Ambartsumyan L, Smith C, Kapur RP. Diagnosis of Hirschsprung's disease. Pediatr Develop Pathol. 2020;23(1):8-22.

CHAPTER

68

Imaging of Anorectal Anomalies

Arun Kumar Gupta, Manisha Jana, Devasenathipathy Kandasamy

INTRODUCTION

Anorectal anomalies (ARAs) are rare with an incidence of approximately 1 in 5,000 births.[1] They have a slight male preponderance.[2] Quite often they are associated with other anomalies and the presence and severity of the associated anomalies decide the clinical course in a vast majority.[2-4]

EMBRYOLOGY OF THE CLOACA RELATED TO ANORECTAL ANOMALIES

Embryology of the cloaca can be described under internal and external cloaca.

Internal Cloaca

It is an endodermal reservoir which is in contact with the surface ectoderm at the cloacal membrane. At present, there is a general agreement that the division of internal cloaca occurs in two stages (Tourneux's method), i.e., a combination of craniocaudal extension of the urorectal septum and lateral ingrowths of the mesenchyma.[5] Most of the ARAs can be explained by this mechanism of combined division. This process of division of primitive hindgut into a ventral urogenital sinus and a dorsal cloaca is completed by 7th week of gestation.[6]

External Cloaca

On the other hand, external cloaca refers to the partitioning of the proctodeal pit, the perineum, and the genital folds. By the end of 7th week and early 8th week, after the cloacal membrane ruptures; the distal end of hindgut is occluded by epithelial growth at the distal end. This part again recanalizes at the end of 8th week in order to form distal anal canal.[5,6]

Essentially, the rectal group of ARAs consists of those abnormalities which are intrinsic in the partitioning of the internal cloaca, whereas aberrations in the external cloacal division result in the anal group of malformations.

CLASSIFICATION

Three major classifications of ARAs exist, and are the following:

1. International classification, 1970 **(Table 1)**
2. Wingspread classification, 1984 **(Table 2)**
3. Krickenbeck classification, 2005 **(Table 3)**

International classification was considered by some to be too detailed and too complex. A simplified version of it was, therefore, considered and is known by the name of Wingspread classification[7] (so called because the meeting to decide it was held at the Wingspread convention center in Racine, Wisconsin). More recently, another classification was proposed in the Krickenbeck conference on anorectal malformations in 2005.[8] All the classifications primarily depend on the location of the blind ending rectal pouch; and the presence/absence, and type of fistula.

In the author's experience, if one is dealing with a large number of ARAs in a major hospital, then use of international classification is essential. On the other hand, for general teaching and occasional encounter with these patients, Wingspread classification should be adequate.

INFORMATION REQUIRED IN A PATIENT OF ANORECTAL ANOMALY

Four major answers, one is looking for, are the following:

1. Level of the blind terminal bowel and of any fistula, if present
2. Levator muscle mass status
3. Associated congenital anomalies
4. Nerve supply status to the levator muscle group

The last one is assessed by clinical tests while the rest are evaluated by imaging.

CLINICAL CLUES

Males

Perineum should be carefully scrutinized for any orifice. Visible orifice suggests an anal translevator anomaly

TABLE 1: Anorectal anomalies: International classification (1970).

Level	Male	Female
High anomalies	• Anorectal agenesis: – Without fistula – With fistula: ▪ Rectovesical ▪ Rectoprostatic urethral fistula ▪ H or N type fistula (*not described in original classification*) • Rectal atresia	• Anorectal agenesis: – Without fistula – With fistula: ▪ Rectovesical ▪ Cloacal anomalies ▪ Rectovaginal (high) • Rectal atresia • H or N type fistula *(not described in original classification)*
Intermediate anomalies	• Anal agenesis: – Without fistula – With fistula: ▪ Rectobulbar • Anorectal stenosis	• Anal agenesis: – Without fistula – With fistula: ▪ Rectovaginal (low) ▪ Rectovestibular • Anorectal stenosis
Low anomalies	• At normal anal site: – Covered anus, complete – Anal stenosis • At perineal site: – Anterior perineal anus – Anocutaneous fistula	• At normal anal site: – Covered anus, complete – Anal stenosis • At perineal site: – Anterior perineal anus – Anocutaneous fistula • At vulvar site: – Anovestibular fistula – Vulvar anus – Anovulvar anus

(exception—rectal atresia). External orifice may be located anywhere from the normal anal site to the tip of penis.

In the absence of a perineal orifice, level of the anomaly is difficult to predict although the majority will be rectal lesions. In these patients, urine may be examined next (after collection and not catheterization) for meconium or squamous epithelial cells. In the absence of meconium, an invertogram should be done while presence of meconium in urine requires a defunctioning colostomy.

Females

Noncommunicating anomalies occur rarely in females. Careful examination for the site and number of orifices must be made.

If only one orifice is present, then it indicates a cloacal anomaly with a common cloaca for the urethra, vagina, and rectum. Colostomy is required.

If two orifices are visible in the vulva with no anal orifice, then one of them is of the urethral, while the other one is of

TABLE 2: Anorectal anomalies: Wingspread classification[7] (1984).

Level	Male	Female
High anomalies	• Anorectal agenesis: – Without fistula – With rectoprostatic urethral fistula • Rectal atresia	• Anorectal agenesis: – Without fistula – With rectovaginal fistula • Rectal atresia
Intermediate anomalies	• Anal agenesis without fistula • Rectobulbar urethral fistula	• Anal agenesis without fistula • Rectovaginal fistula • Rectovestibular fistula
Low anomalies	• Anocutaneous fistula • Anal stenosis	• Anovestibular fistula • Anocutaneous fistula • Anal stenosis
Cloacal malformations	Rare	Rare

the vaginal orifice. Meconium would come from the latter due to the associated rectovaginal fistula. Colostomy is again indicated.

If three orifices are visible, then two of them are respectively of the urethra and the vagina, both at their normal site, while the third one is the bowel which could be at the normal anal site, or it might open as a fistulous track anteriorly at an abnormal site—either in the perineum or in the vestibule.

IMAGING WORKUP

During the imaging of a case with ARA, one or more of a number of investigations can be carried out—invertography; contrast opacification of the urinary tract, fistula or colon; ultrasound; computed tomography (CT) and magnetic resonance imaging (MRI) scan. All these investigations are complementary, providing information regarding different facets of the complex problem of ARA.

Invertography

Invertography was first described by Wangensteen and Rice in 1930.[9]

Technique: Six to eight hours after the birth, a newborn baby with ARA should be held upside down for at least 3 minutes, and then a strict lateral view (in this upside down position) is taken with the thighs of the baby flexed at hip, and beam accurately centered on the greater trochanter. Anal dimple and the natal cleft should be outlined by barium paste. In a correctly taken radiograph: (1) Both the ischial bones would accurately superimpose; and (2) The terminal blind bowel will be rounded and well-distended. Interpretation of an invertogram should be attempted only; if both these features are present otherwise it may be fallacious.

Interpretation: Basic purpose of invertography is to identify the relationship of the gas bubble in the blind pouch to

TABLE 3: Anorectal anomalies: Krickenbeck classification[8] (2005).

Type	Any gender	Male	Female
Low	• Anal stenosis • Imperforate anus without fistula • Anal agenesis with rectoperineal fistula		• Anal agenesis with rectovestibular fistula
Intermediate/ High	• Anal or anorectal agenesis without fistula • Rectal atresia	• Anal or anorectal agenesis: - Rectourethral bulbar fistula - Rectourethral prostatic fistula - Rectovesical fistula	• Rectal atresia • Cloacal anomalies: - Short canal (<3 cm) - Long canal (>3 cm)

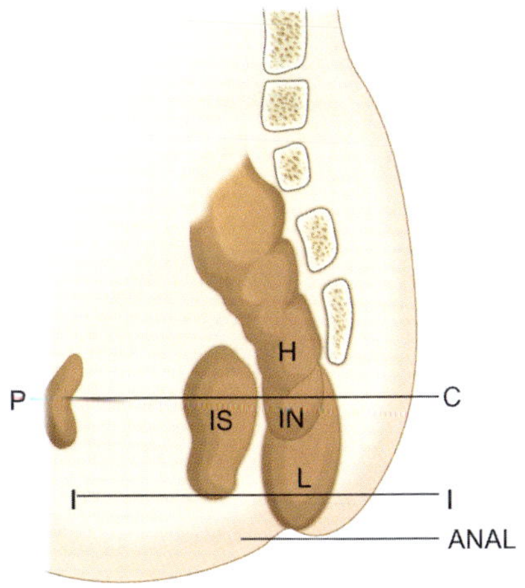

FIG. 1: Line drawing showing high (H), intermediate (IN), and low (L) anomalies and their relationship to pubococcygeal (PC) and ischial (I) lines.

the bony pelvis, which in turn indicates the relation to the levator ani muscle complex. Information contained in an invertogram can be interpreted in two ways.

1. By using three lines, a concept which was first put forward by Stephens and Smith (1971).[10] The three lines are: (i) Pubococcygeal (PC) line, (ii) The ischial (I) line or I point, and (iii) The anal pit line **(Fig. 1)**. A gas bubble situated above the PC line is designated "high" anomaly, one located between the PC and I line or point "intermediate" anomaly, and if it extends below the I line (point), then it is called "low" anomaly **(Figs. 2A to C)**.
2. However, Cremin (1971)[11] did not find PC line very accurate. He proposed an "M line" or "M point", which is located at the junction of upper two-thirds and lower one-third of the ischium **(Figs. 2A to C)**. Anomalies are then divided into "high" and "low" types with no intermediate category.

Accuracy of invertography to differentiate supralevator (gas bubble above the I line or point) and infralevator lesions (gas bubble below the I line or point) has been reported to range from 60 to 87%. One must be aware of the potential pitfalls of this technique in order to avoid misdiagnosis. Some of the common reasons are listed here:

- Insufficient time for the gas to reach the terminal bowel.
- Meconium blocking the terminal segment.
- In a crying child, puborectalis sling may move significantly up or down giving erroneous results.
- Gas may escape through a fistula.
- Improper technique—in positioning, centering or marker placement.

Besides the conventional upside down invertography described above, two more methods have been described to obtain the same information. They are as follows:

1. Prone cross-table lateral view (Narasimharao et al., 1983).[12]
2. CT invertography (Leighton and de Campo, 1989).[13]

During the reading of an invertogram, besides evaluating the level of bowel gas, one should also look for the following:

- *Spine*: Congenital anomalies of the spine are common.
- Presence of gas in the region of urinary bladder and vagina, which would indicate an underlying fistula.

Contrast Studies

Purpose of any contrast study is:

- To confirm the level of blind bowel pouch, and
- To document the presence (or absence) and level of the fistula between the gastrointestinal (GI) and the genitourinary (GU) system.

Contrast Studies in Males

- *Retrograde urethrography (RGU)/micturating cysto-urethrography (MCU)*: Prior to or even after the colostomy, RGU is a good technique to demonstrate the fistula. If negative, then RGU is followed by MCU in the same sitting to demonstrate the possible fistula.
- *Distal cologram*: Once colostomy has already been done, then distal cologram, in the author's experience, is a reliable technique to demonstrate the fistula. Fluoroscopy with image intensifier, use of water-soluble contrast media, and raising the intraluminal pressure in the distal colon[14,15] to fill the fistula more consistently are some of the prerequisites in this technique. In a case with colostomy, distal cologram should be done first, and only if it is negative in demonstrating the fistula, then RGU/MCU should be done in the same sitting.
  Sometimes the fistula is not documented in spite of all the efforts but on RGU, an acute backward angulation of the posterior urethra and on colography an anteroinferior "beaking" of the blind rectal pouch is seen **(Figs. 3A and B)**—these findings suggest the presence of fistula or adhesion.
- *Direct catheterization*: If a patient has a cutaneous fistula, then direct catheterization and retrograde injection of

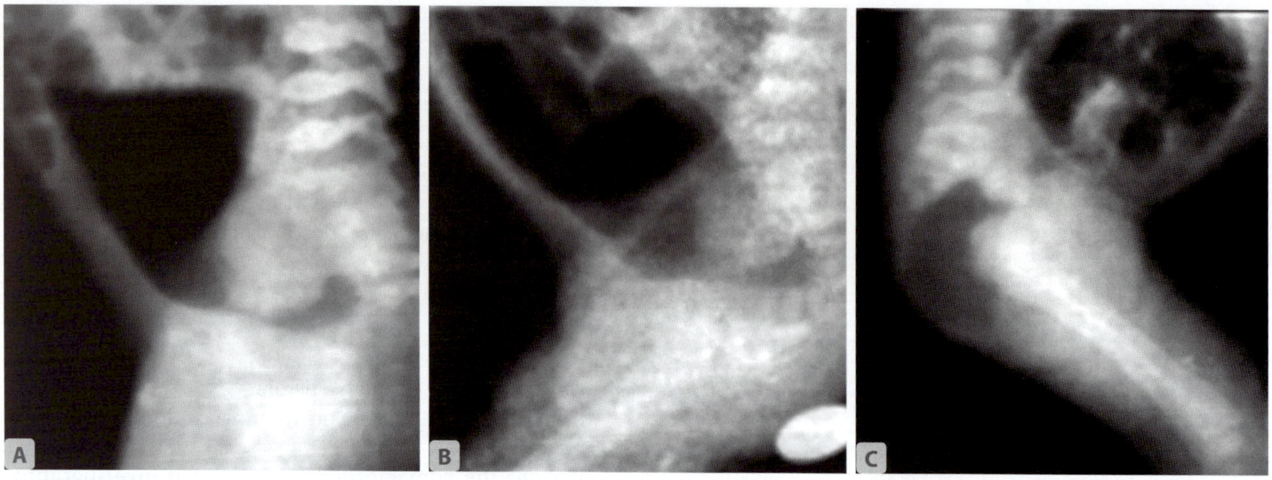

FIGS. 2A TO C: Examples of: (A) high, (B) intermediate, and (C) low anomalies on invertography.

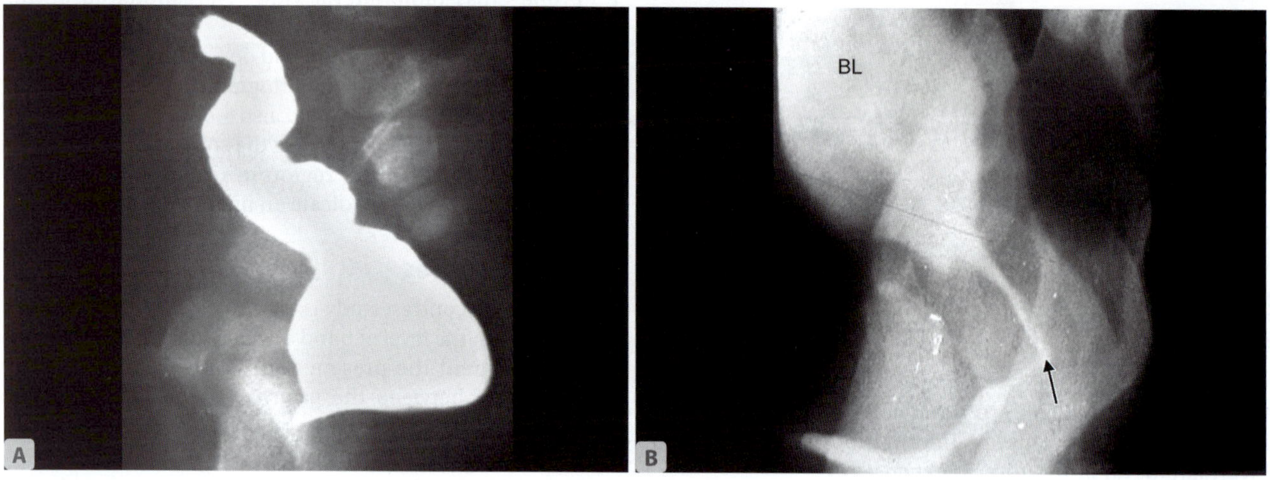

FIGS. 3A AND B: Pointers to fistula. (A) "Beaking" from anteroinferior angle of blind rectal pouch on colography and (B) "acute backward angulation" (arrow) of posterior urethra on retrograde urethrography (RGU) without actually filling the fistula, indicating presence of underlying fistula or adhesion. (BL: bladder)

contrast into the fistula should be carried out. However, urethra and bladder should be first outlined with a catheter (filled with radiopaque contrast) in situ.

ANORECTAL ANOMALY IN MALES

These are discussed under high, intermediate, and low anomalies.

High Anomalies

In these patients, the imperforate bowel or its fistulous connection lies above the puborectalis sling of the levator ani muscle. Various types described under this group are the following:

Anorectal Agenesis without Fistula

Anorectal agenesis without fistula is uncommon. Invertography and contrast studies would show the blind rectal pouch lying at or cranial to the PC line with no suggestion or demonstration of a fistula.

Anorectal Agenesis with Rectoprostatic Urethral Fistula

Anorectal agenesis with rectoprostatic urethral fistula is the most common type in this group. Most common site of fistulous opening is at the level of the verumontanum, but rarely it may open either more cranially closer to the bladder neck or more distally just above the bulb **(Figs. 4A and B)**.

H or N Type of Rectoprostatic Urethral Fistula

H or N type of rectoprostatic urethral fistula is extremely rare. This entity was not even described in the original International classification. There is an H- or N shaped fistulous connection between the prostatic urethra and the anterior wall of the rectum just cranial to the valves. Characteristically, urethra distal to the site of fistula is usually stenotic **(Figs. 5A and B)**.

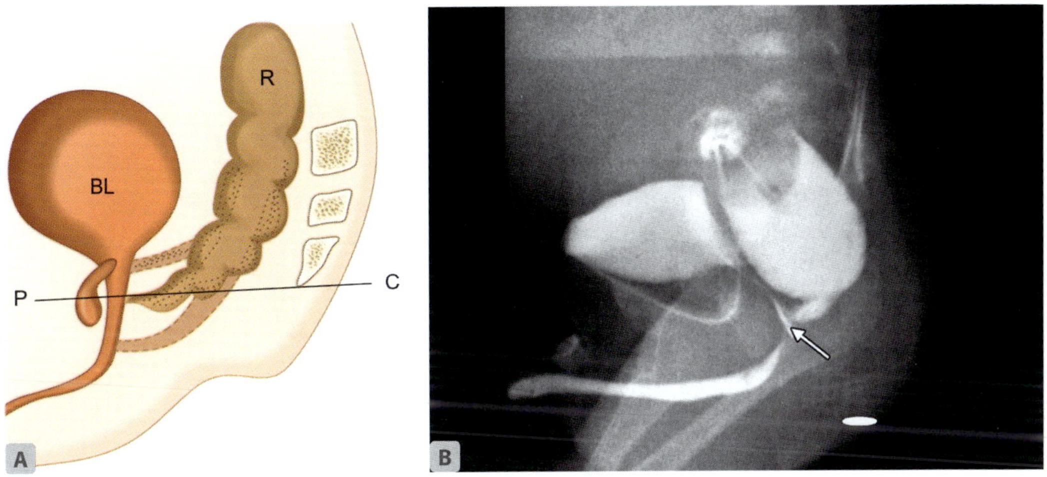

FIGS. 4A AND B: Rectoprostatic urethral fistula: (A) schematic drawing and (B) a case. As indicated by dotted lines, fistula may enter either more cranial or distal to verumontanum (arrow—fistula). (BL: bladder; R: rectum)

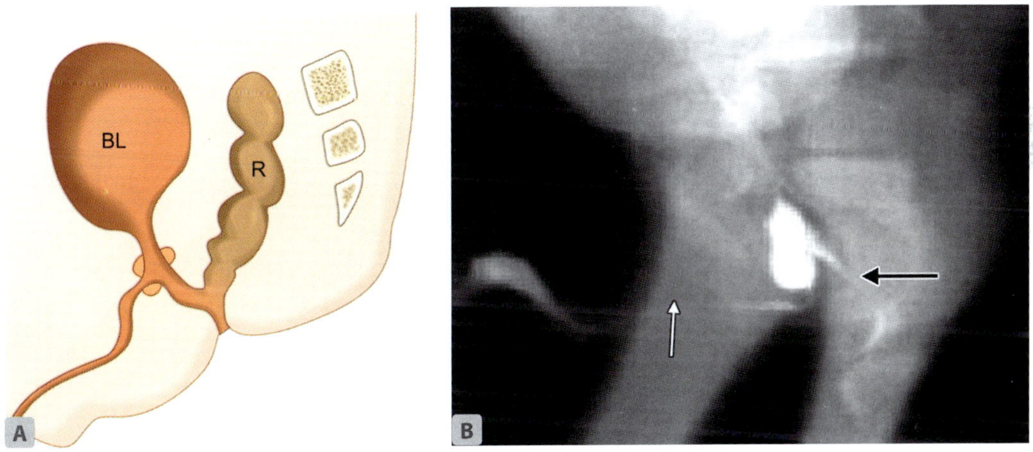

FIGS. 5A AND B: H or N fistula is extremely rare: (A) Diagrammatic representation shows the patent anal canal and the small caliber of the penile urethra. (B) Retrograde urethrogram in a patient showing a fistula (block arrow— fistula, arrow—narrow penile urethra). (BL: bladder; R: rectum)

Rectovesical Fistula

Rectovesical fistula is also rare. Fistulous tract usually enters close to the bladder base. During contrast injection into the distal colon via colostomy site, urinary bladder would fill first **(Figs. 6A and B)** without opacifying the urethra, thereby, excluding a urethral fistula. This sequence of events must be carefully monitored and specifically looked for real time on the image intensifier. It is very important to differentiate this type of fistula from the rare more cranially located rectoprostatic urethral fistula by the observations described above.

Rectal Atresia

It is a rare and an unusual condition. In these patients, the terminal bowel ends blindly at varying levels. Anus and the anal canal are normal and the bowel in between these two segments is deficient (either a short membranous or a long, string-like) **(Figs. 7A to D)**. Its etiopathogenesis is believed to be a vascular insult after the formation of a normal rectum. Complete documentation in such cases requires contrast injection from both ends (i.e., distal cologram + anal canal opacification) simultaneously. Rectal atresia, though a high lesion, has good prognosis as the anus and associated sphincter complex is unaffected.[5]

Intermediate Anomalies

Intermediate anomalies are termed so due to a complex relationship to puborectalis muscle. Thus, the blind terminal bowel is lying on (i.e., above) the puborectalis sling muscle, a feature of "high" anomalies, but the fistulous track when present is within or through the sling, a criterion for diagnosing "low" anomalies. Thus, features of both the "high" and the "low" anomalies are present in this group of anomalies.

Anal Agenesis without Fistula

Invertography and distal cologram would reveal the blind bowel pouch to lie between the PC line and the I point without demonstrating a fistula.

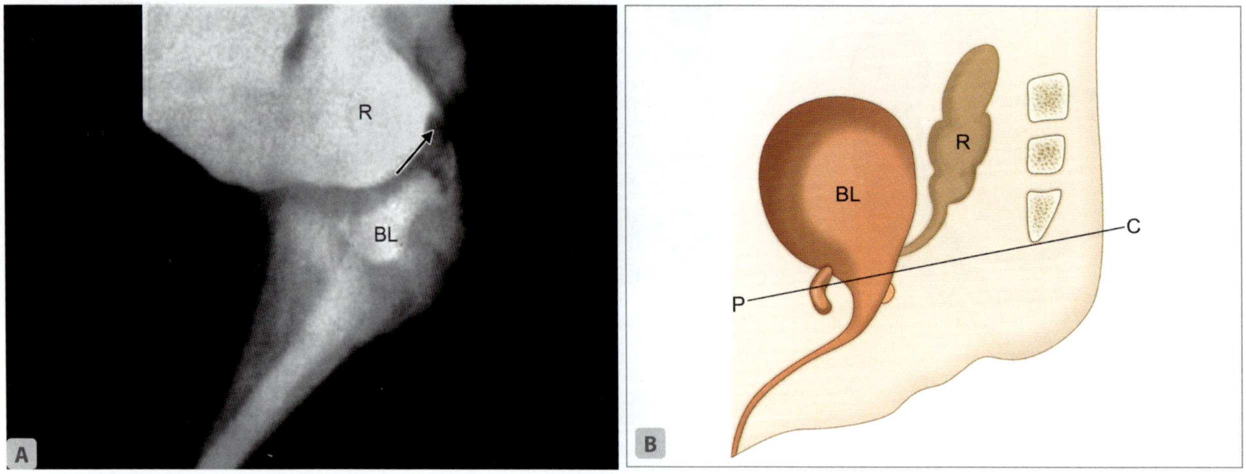

FIGS. 6A AND B: Rectovesical fistula—another rare type filling on distal colography—note the filling of urinary bladder immediately after opacification of the rectum (arrow—fistula). (BL: bladder; R: rectum)

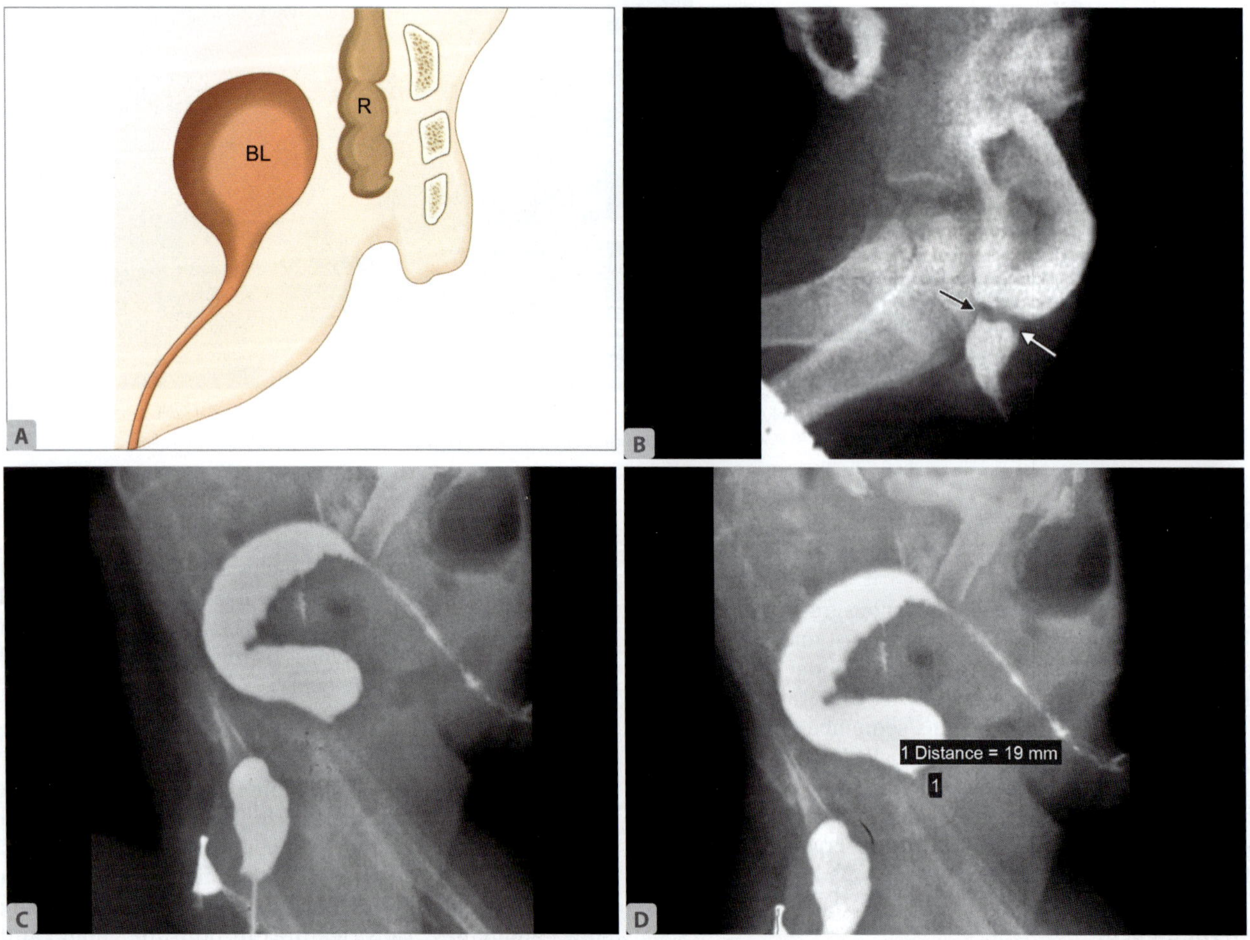

FIGS. 7A TO D: Rectal atresia: (A) Diagrammatic representation. (B to D) Contrast study in two different patients. Opacification was done from both ends of the site of atresia. On a conventional film, 1 cm metallic scale helps in accurately measuring the distance of atretic bowel (arrows—atretic segment in B). (C and D) Digital fluoroscopy of a patient with long segment atresia: measurement has to be done at the console using electronic calipers. (BL: bladder; R: rectum)

Anal Agenesis with Rectobulbar Urethral Fistula[16]

Two types are described **(Figs. 8A to D)**—either the fistula is short, wide and enters the posterior surface of the bulb directly **(Fig. 8B)**, or it is long, thin, passing distally within the cavernous tissues of the penis in midline to enter the undersurface of the urethra **(Figs. 8C and D)**.

Anorectal Stenosis

Anorectal stenosis is rare. It is generally agreed that "anal stenosis" should be classified under the low anomalies while stenosis occurring up to 4 cm within the anus are more appropriate to be termed "anorectal stenosis". Mechanism of its formation is postulated to be ischemic and is thus similar to rectal atresia described earlier.

Low Anomalies

These are essentially "anal deformities". Various types are listed here:

1. Anocutaneous fistula (covered anus, incomplete)
2. Anterior perineal anus
3. Covered anal stenosis
4. Anal membrane stenosis
5. Covered anus, complete
6. Imperforate anal membrane

The entire group of low anomalies can be readily appreciated on the clinical examination itself, and imaging is usually not indicated. First two subtypes are briefly described here.

Anocutaneous Fistula

In this condition, the anal canal is of normal caliber till the level of anal valves beyond which it is suddenly reduced to a tube of small caliber and runs forward covered by skin to open anywhere from the ventral surface of the penile shaft to an area adjacent to the anal site **(Figs. 9A to C)**. Although fistulogram is not necessary, but if required it can be readily carried out.

Anterior Perineal Anus

In this condition, anus is normal in appearance but is located more anteriorly than the normal site close to the posterior or membranous urethra. This is an important differential in

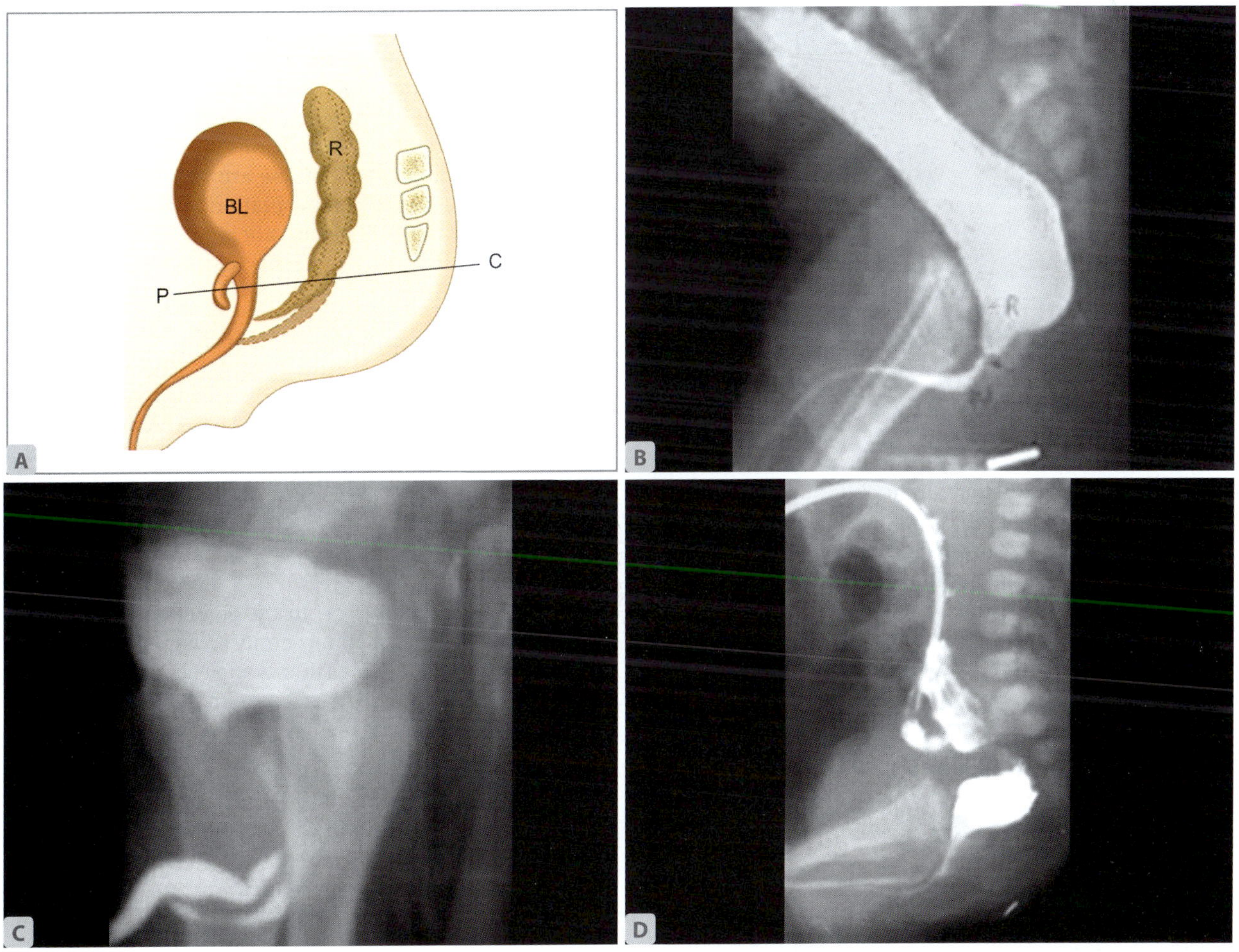

FIGS. 8A TO D: Rectobulbar urethral fistulae: (A) Diagrammatic representation. (B) Proximal type and (C and D) distal type, two cases. Note that the fistula is long and narrow which enters the undersurface of penile urethra in (C) and (D) compared to (B). (BL: bladder; R: rectum)

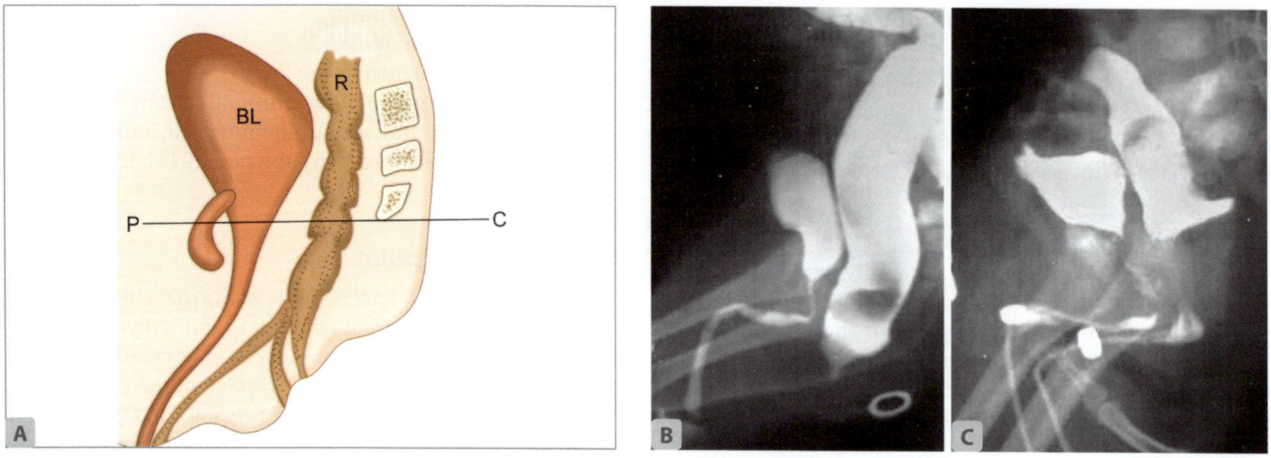

FIGS. 9A TO C: Anocutaneous fistula: (A) Diagrammatic representation shows that the fistula can open anywhere from near the anal opening to the tip of penis. (B and C) Two different cases showing (B) opening near anal opening and (C) near tip of penis. (BL: bladder; R: rectum)

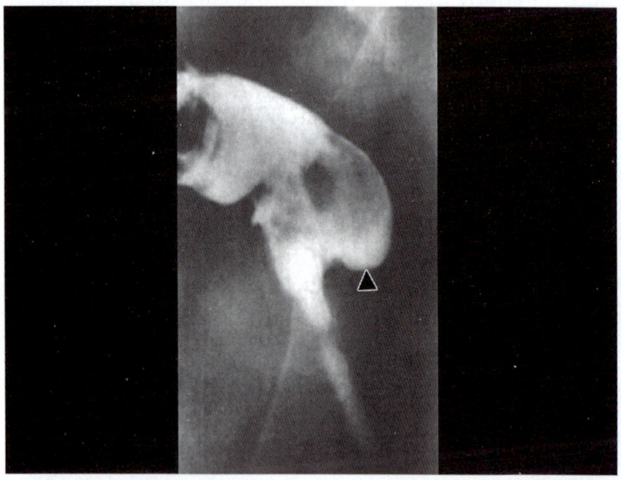

FIG. 10: Anterior perineal anus demonstrated on barium enema—note removal of cannula and posterior shelf (arrowhead).

the list of causes of constipation in children. On per rectal examination, "posterior shelf"—a characteristic finding of this condition might be felt which can also be demonstrated on barium enema examination **(Fig. 10)**. Cannula may distort the anal anatomy due to sheer mechanical pressure. Therefore, the catheter/cannula should be removed before the film is taken in strict lateral view at the time of barium defecation.

ANORECTAL ANOMALY IN FEMALES

Anorectal anomalies are divided into high, intermediate, and low types.

High Anomalies

Anorectal Agenesis with High Rectovaginal Fistula (Without a Urogenital Sinus Defect)

The vagina, urinary bladder, and urethra are normal. Rectal fistula enters the posterior (dorsal) wall of the vagina **(Figs. 11A to C)**. Rectovaginal fistulae have been classified as "high" or "low" depending on the level of the terminal bowel, and these terms do not refer to the level of entry of fistula into the vagina.

Vaginogram or distal cologram following colostomy would readily demonstrate these fistulae.

The recent change in concept about the rectovaginal fistulae is based on the very high association of rectovaginal fistulae and cloacal malformations. It is conceptualized that isolated rectovaginal fistulae are very rare and almost always a part of cloacal malformation.[6,8] This explains the change in the Krickenbeck classification from Wingspread classification; where the term rectovaginal fistula is omitted.[6,8]

Rectal Atresia

Rectal atresia is similar to the lesions seen in males. It may be associated with rectovaginal fistula **(Figs. 12A and B)**. This is an extremely rare condition and has not been described in the various classifications published in the literature so far. However, it should be placed under high-type anomalies.

Rectovesical Fistula

Rectovesical fistula must be an extremely rare condition in females. We have not seen this entity so far. Probable reason for its rarity is anatomy since uterus and vagina are interposed between GI and GU tract. On documentation, the appearance should be similar to that seen in males.

H or N Type of Fistula

H or N type fistula is another extremely rare condition in females, and is similar to that seen in males **(Fig. 13)**. This entity has also not been described in the various classifications published in the literature so far.

Cloacal Anomalies

This is a very large and one of the most complex groups of anomalies which is beyond the scope of this text. In these

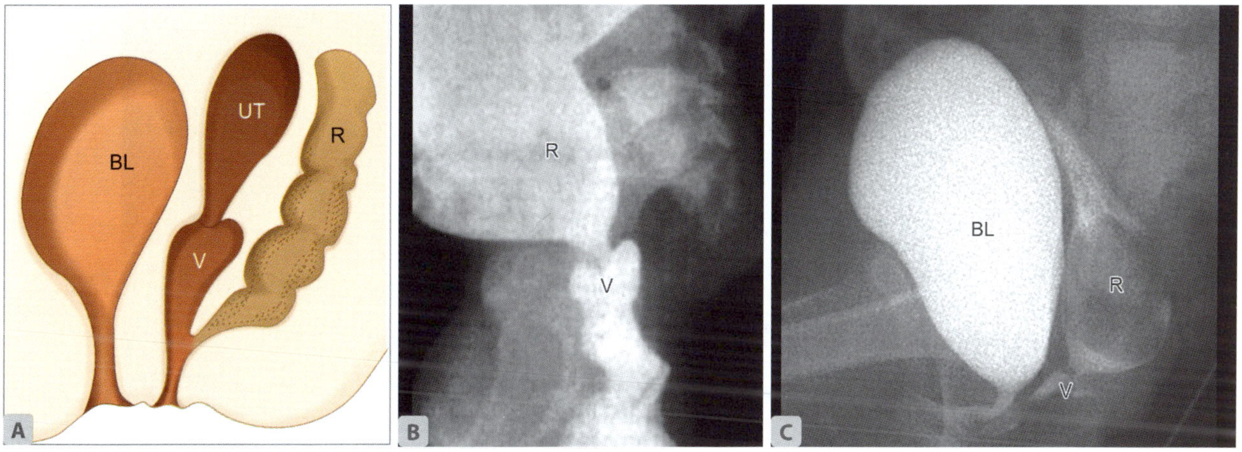

FIGS. 11A TO C: Rectovaginal fistula: (A) Diagrammatic representation. (B) High rectovaginal fistula demonstrated on vaginogram. (C) A low rectovaginal fistula demonstrated on simultaneous distal cologram and micturating cystourethrography (MCU). Difference in "high" and "low" rectovaginal fistulae lies in the level of blind bowel pouch and not on the site of entry of fistula into the vagina. (R: rectum; V: vagina; BL: bladder; UT: uterus)

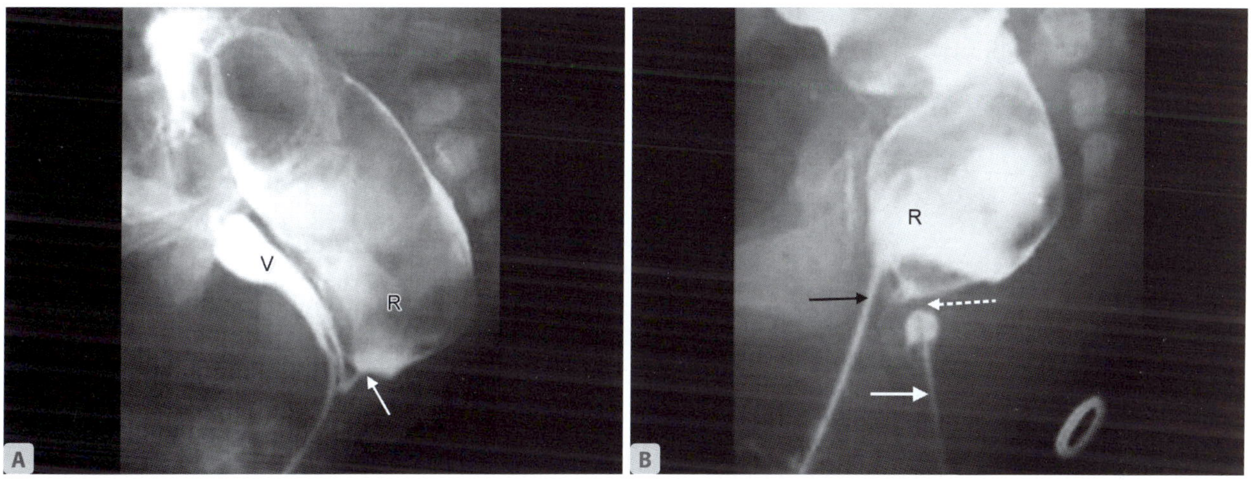

FIGS. 12A AND B: Rectal atresia with rectovaginal fistula. Retrograde contrast study demonstrates the rectovaginal fistula (arrow in A). When one catheter is inserted into the rectum through the fistula (arrow in B); and another through the anal orifice into the blind distal segment (block arrow in B); the small shelf-like atretic segment (dotted arrow in B) is visualized. (R: rectum; V: vagina)

anomalies, there is only a single orifice for the urethra, vagina, and rectum. A large number of subtypes based on the internal anatomy have been described. Retrograde injection of contrast through the external orifice as well as colography would delineate the internal anatomy **(Fig. 14)**. Some of the most severe forms may present immediately after birth with acute respiratory distress due to a hugely dilated vagina. It can be associated with other urogenital anomalies **(Fig. 15)**.

In the recent classification, cloaca is classified as intermediate/high ARA in females; and further divided in two types: (1) Short common canal (<3 cm); and (2) Long common canal (>3 cm). It is very important to differentiate these two as the long common canal cloacal malformations have higher risk of associate anomalies and a poorer prognosis. Usually, pelvic floor and external sphincter muscles are poorly developed in these children.[6]

Intermediate Anomalies

Anal Agenesis without Fistula

Anal agenesis without fistula is easy to diagnose by inverted plain films of the abdomen especially taken in lateral views.

Rectovestibular Fistula

From the anterior wall of the rectum arises a fistula which opens externally in the vestibule. Usually, it is narrow and long (>1 cm) **(Fig. 16A)**. Diagnosis is evident on clinical examination by noting three orifices in the vestibule (urethra, vagina, and fistula) and combining it with a gentle probe test. Retrograde injection of contrast through the fistulous opening would readily opacify the fistula and the rectum **(Fig. 16B)**.

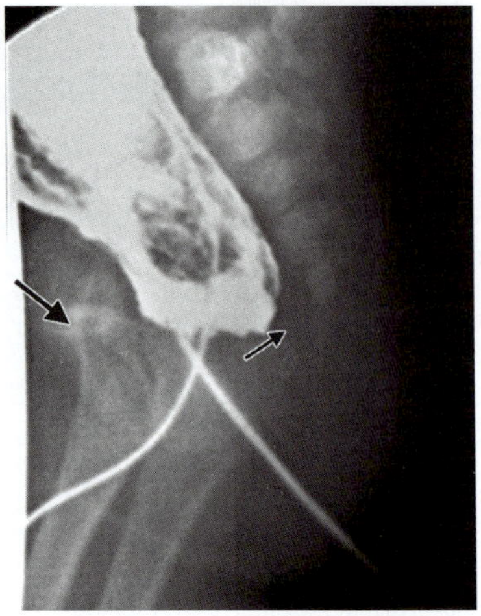

FIG. 13: H or N type fistula in a girl child. Cutaneous fistula (arrow) and urethral communication (bigger arrow).

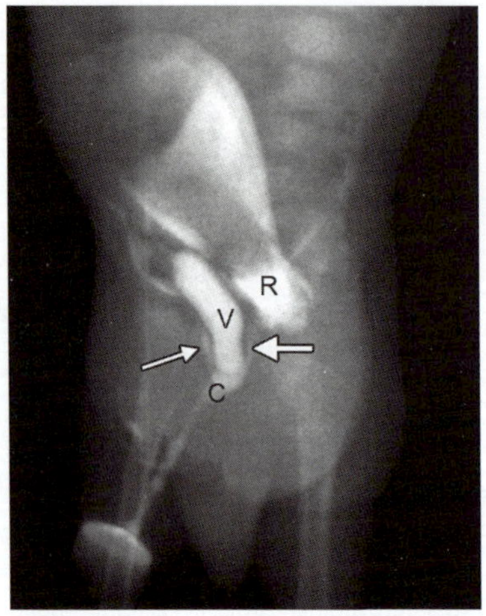

FIG. 14: Cloaca: The common channel (C) leading into urethra (arrow) and vagina (V); while rectum (R) opening into the vagina (block arrow).

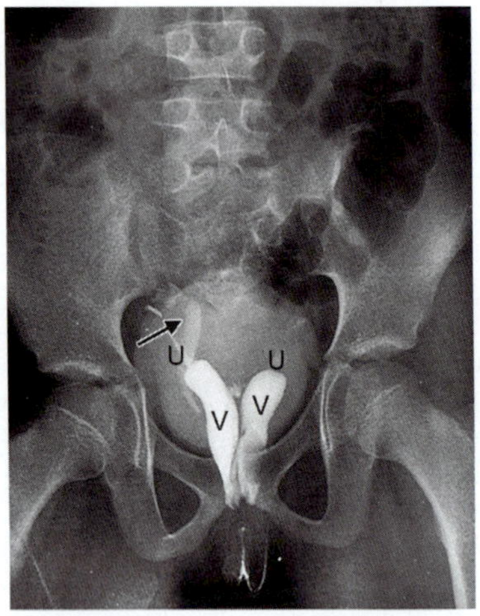

FIG. 15: Uterine didelphys in a case of cloaca. Note two vaginae (V), uterine cavities (U), and right-sided vesicoureteral reflux (VUR) (arrow).

Low Rectovaginal Fistula

Low rectovaginal fistula is very rare. Its difference from the high type has already been discussed earlier.

Low Anomalies

These are again designated as "anal deformities".

Anovestibular Fistula

Like rectovestibular fistula, it opens in the vestibule. However, its length is very short (<1 cm) and well-formed anal canal extends quite low down close to the skin at the anal site **(Figs. 17A and B)**. A probe would pass not only upward parallel to the vagina, but to some extent, it can be turned posteriorly just beneath the perineum. The latter maneuver cannot be achieved in rectovestibular fistula. Contrast study, if at all done, demonstrates the anatomy clearly.

Anocutaneous Fistula/Anterior Perineal Anus

Anocutaneous fistula/anterior perineal anus is similar to those observed in males.

Anal Stenosis

Anal stenosis is similar to the lesions in males.

Anorectal Agenesis without Fistula

Anorectal agenesis without fistula is uncommon and can be seen in both males and females. There is a blind terminal bowel without any fistula. Invertography and contrast studies would show variable length of the blind rectal pouch with no suggestion or demonstration of a fistula **(Figs. 18A and B)**.

UNCOMMON ANORECTAL ANOMALY: POUCH COLON

This is a rare form of high ARA where either entire colon or a part of it is replaced by a "pouch" like dilated structure. The dilation is variable and can even range till 15 cm. This is commonly associated with a fistula. Four types have been described.[17] Type 1 is the most severe form **(Figs. 19A and B)**, where the entire colon is replaced by a pouch and there is a rectovesical fistula. Type 4 is the least severe one, where almost entire colon except the terminal part is abnormal. Etiology of this anomaly is controversial; although early in utero vascular insult to the segment of bowel has been proposed as a possibility. In all of the types, the length of the colon is short (variable; depending on the types); and the abnormal part has thick wall and sharp demarcation from the normal bowel wall.[17]

INVESTIGATIONS

As the first step, a careful and detailed clinical examination is absolutely essential. This may provide a number of clues

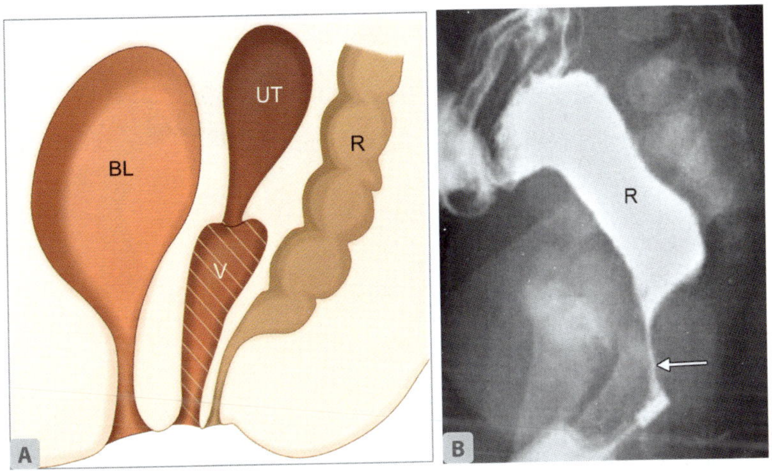

FIGS. 16A AND B: Rectovestibular fistula—demonstrated on retrograde contrast injection—note the long, narrow fistulous track (arrow). (R: rectum; V: vagina; BL: bladder; UT: uterus)

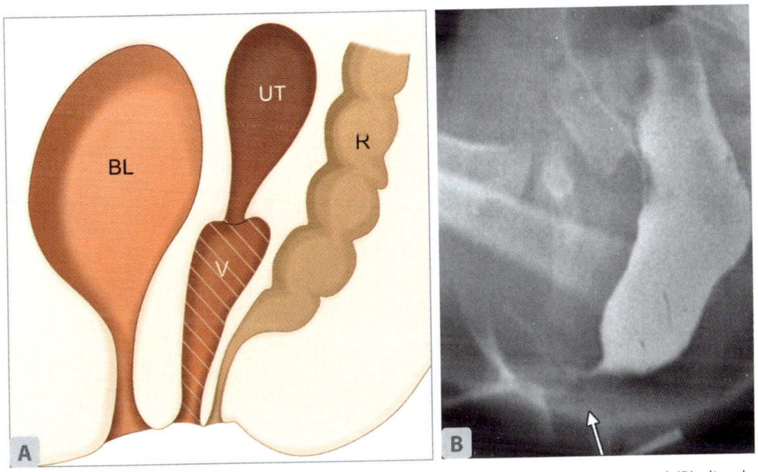

FIGS. 17A AND B: Anovestibular fistula: (A) Diagrammatic representation and (B) distal cologram showing fistula (arrow). (R: rectum; V: vagina; BL: bladder; UT: uterus)

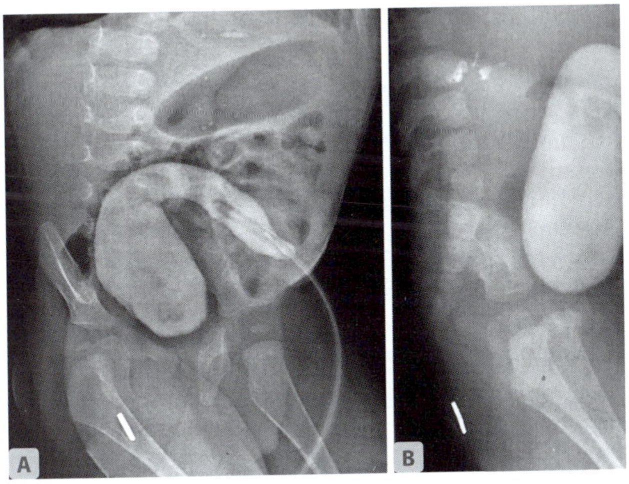

FIGS. 18A AND B: Anorectal agenesis without fistula in a female neonate with a flat perineum and no anal opening. Note the high ending of the blind ending rectal pouch. The smooth ending and absence of any anterior "beak" (compared to Fig. 3) points against the presence of fistula.

pointing to a specific type of the anomaly. This has been discussed earlier.

Invertography: Its role is similar to that described earlier in males.

Contrast studies: Noncommunicating anomalies are rare in females. Communication of the bowel may be either to the exterior and, therefore, visible as an abnormal orifice or internally into one of the pelvic viscera. Contrast studies can be carried out to demonstrate both the types.

OTHER INVESTIGATIONS (BOTH FOR MALE AND FEMALE ANORECTAL ANOMALIES)

Besides the invertography and the conventional contrast studies, other newer imaging modalities have also an important role to play prior to as well as after the surgery.

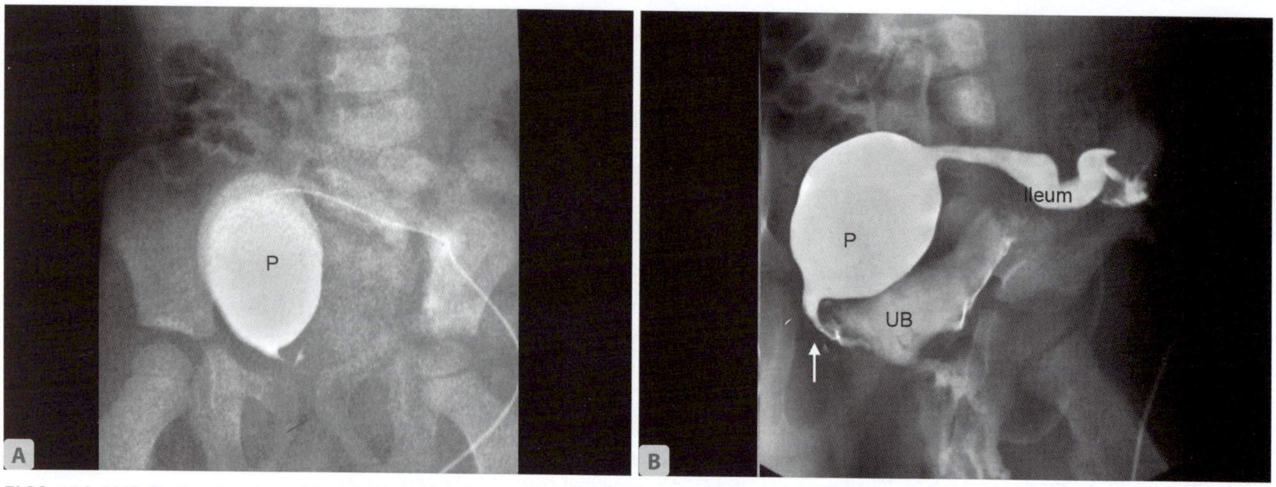

FIGS. 19A AND B: Pouch colon with colovesical fistula. Distal loopogram performed from ileostomy stoma reveals entire colon to be replaced by a globular " pouch" (P) and a fistula with the urinary bladder (UB) (arrow). Note associated sacral dysgenesis.

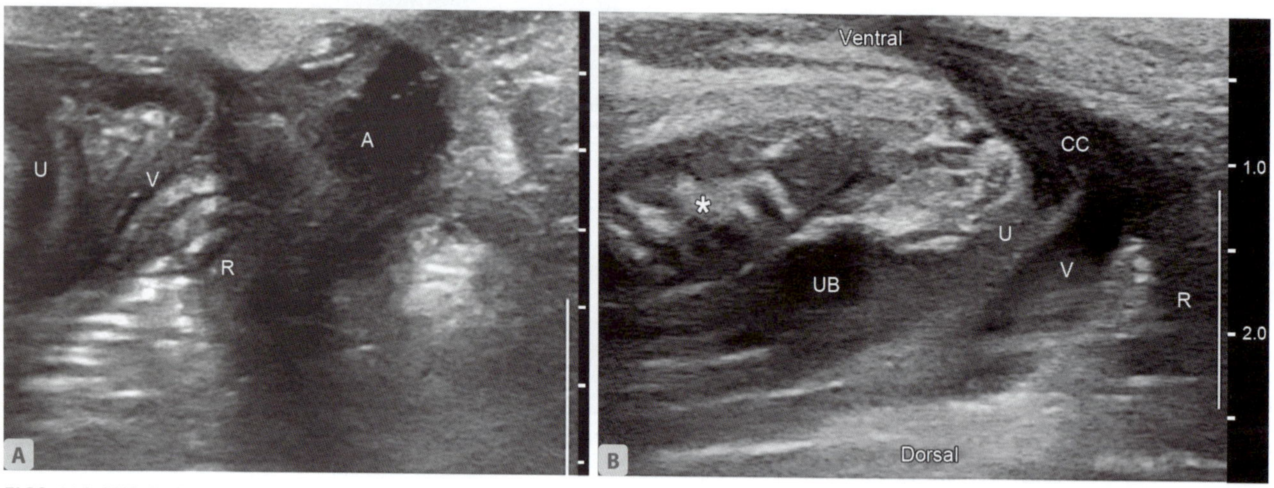

FIGS. 20A AND B: Transperineal ultrasonography (USG). (A) Normal midsagittal image in a girl showing urethra (U), vagina (V), rectum (R), and anal canal (A). Cloacal malformation in a 2-year girl. (B) Midsagittal image shows a common canal (CC) communicating with rectum (R), vagina (V), and urethra (U). Normal symphysis pubis has an irregular serrated appearance (asterisk). Note the small length of the common canal, which has a better prognosis.

Ultrasound

The usual advantages of ultrasound in pediatric age group include easy availability, quick and reliable imaging technique without the risk of ionizing radiation. The utility of ultrasound in ARAs is multifactorial. First, it can be used as a screening tool of the abdomen and pelvis for other associated anomalies.[18] Secondly, a quick screening of the spine using a high-frequency linear transducer is recommended in order to rule out occult spinal dysraphism in these children.[19,20] Thirdly, transperineal ultrasound using high-frequency linear transducer has additional advantage in assessing the anal sphincter complex, the location of the blind ending rectal pouch and, less commonly, evaluation of abnormal fistulous tracts.[21-23]

Transperineal ultrasonography (USG) should be performed with the child supine, the legs and the hips elevated. Transducer should be placed in the midsagittal plane and the distance from the blind-ending rectal pouch to skin should be measured. A few studies have suggested that if the distance is >15 mm; it should be called a high ARA; and a distance <15 mm as low type ARA. A fistula is seen as a hypoechoic tract between urethra/rectum/vagina **(Figs. 20A and B)**. The major disadvantages of this technique include a long learning curve and operator dependence. Also, in a crying or straining child, this distance might decrease because of increased intra-abdominal pressure.

Computed Tomography Scan

Computed tomography can be used preoperatively to demonstrate the thickness of muscles [puborectalis sling and external anal sphincter (EAS)]. In the postoperative period,[24,25] it demonstrates the relationship of the pulled-through bowel (neorectum) to the above muscles (i.e., whether neorectum is central, eccentric or even outside the sling) and any evidence of fat drawn into the sling **(Fig. 21)**—all of these may be the reason for the incontinence in the

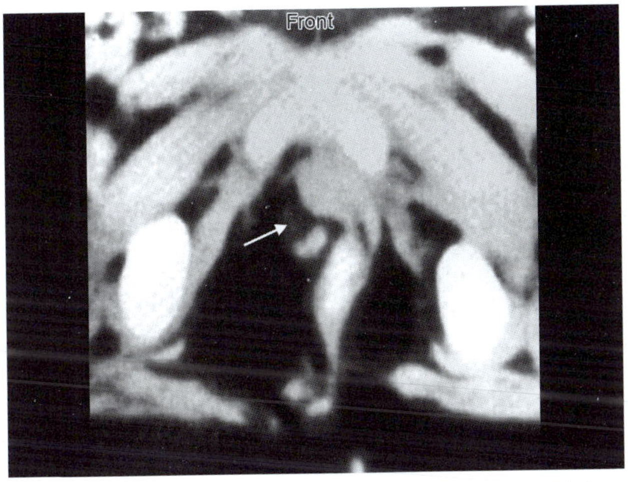

FIG. 21: Pelvic CT, postoperative—fat has been drawn along with the neorectum (arrow) which was the cause of incontinence.

postoperative period.[26] However, with the advances in MRI; CT has mostly been replaced by MRI in preoperative as well as postoperative evaluation in ARAs.

Magnetic Resonance Imaging Scan

With the recent advances in MRI resulting in faster sequence acquisitions, superior spatial and contrast resolution of the images; it plays a crucial role in preoperative evaluation of ARAs. The utility is manifold; it demonstrates the sphincter complex and levator ani muscle with great details; detects associated abdominopelvic anomalies; and can even detect associated occult spinal dysraphism in the same study. Although genitography is superior in assessing the fistulous tract in most cases; complete assessment of the urogenital tract and associated anomalies often require a detailed MRI of abdomen and pelvis.[6] The suggested MRI protocol in ARAs is given in **Table 4**.

The acquisition of images should be done using specified imaging planes. Axial sections should be acquired along a pubococcygeal plane extending from superior margin of pubic bone to the coccyx bone (on a sagittal image).[7] Coronal sections should be acquired perpendicular to this line.

On an MRI, either qualitative/quantitative estimate of the EAS should be done **(Figs. 22A to D)**. Structural integrity of the levator ani and EAS should be carefully evaluated.[27-29] Presence of fistula is better appreciated on a fat-suppressed T2-weighted (T2W) image, and can be either hyperintense/hypointense in appearance **(Figs. 23A and B)**.

Postoperative MRI: Postoperative incontinence is not uncommon in ARAs. Careful evaluation should be done for the location of the neoanus, any fat interposition and the integrity and bulk of the EAS.[30] **(Figs. 24A to C)**. Sometimes, residual fistula tract may persist and even give rise to a posterior urethral diverticulum.[31] Also, presacral/pelvic masses may be left behind during surgery if a careful preoperative evaluation is not done.[32]

TABLE 4: Suggested MRI protocol for anorectal anomalies.

Region	Sequence	Plane	Useful for evaluation of
Pelvis	T1-weighted spin-echo (T1W SE)	Axial	• External anal sphincter (EAS) • Pubococcygeus, iliococcygeus, puborectalis
Pelvis	T1W SE	Coronal	Levator hammock
Pelvis	T2-weighted turbo-spin-echo (T2W TSE)	Axial	• External anal sphincter • Pubococcygeus, iliococcygeus, puborectalis, fistula tract
Pelvis	T2W TSE	Coronal	Levator hammock
Pelvis	T2W TSE fat-suppressed	Sagittal	Fistula tract
Spine	T1W SE	Axial and sagittal	Spinal dysraphism
Spine	T2W TSE	Axial and sagittal	Spinal dysraphism/associated anomalies such as Currarino's triad
Abdomen	T2W TSE	Axial and coronal	• Kidneys and ureters • Other associated anomalies

RELATIONSHIP OF SACRAL DEVELOPMENT AND LEVATOR MUSCLE DEVELOPMENT

In order to determine the levator muscle mass prior to surgery, CT and MRI are routinely used. However, if these modalities are not available, then a good indicator is the development of the sacrum as seen on plain radiographs. It has been observed that:

- If sacrum is normal then muscle mass and innervation are also normal;
- If S4, S5 are absent then muscle and innervation are usually still normal;
- If S3–S5 are absent then there is variable degree of deficiency of the muscle mass, and patient is usually incontinent;
- If S1–S5 are absent then muscles are markedly hypoplastic, and all the patients are incontinent.

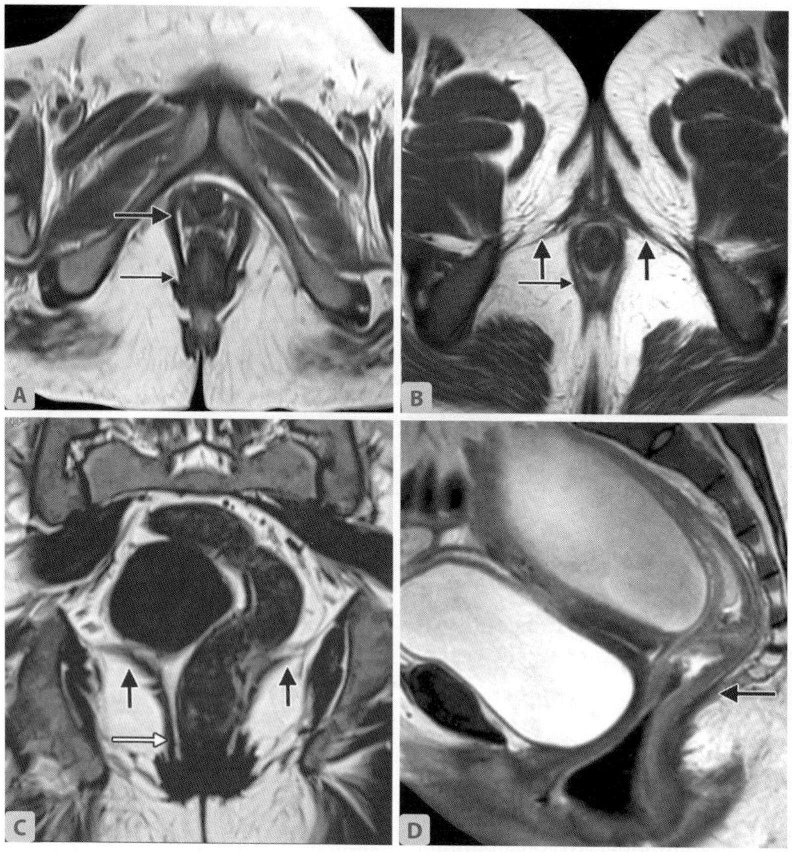

FIGS. 22A TO D: Normal pelvic MRI. (A and B) Axial sections showing puborectalis (arrow in A), sphincter vaginae (block arrow in A). External anal sphincter (EAS) (arrows in B and C), superficial transversus perinei muscle (block arrows in B). Levator hammock (block arrows in C and D).

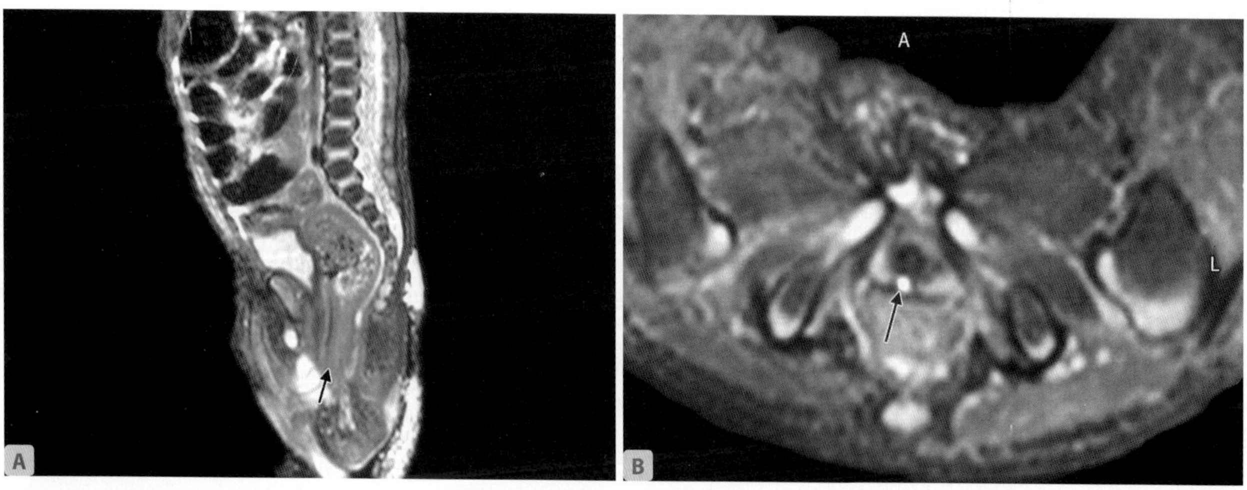

FIGS. 23A AND B: Rectourethral fistula on magnetic resonance imaging (MRI) (arrows).

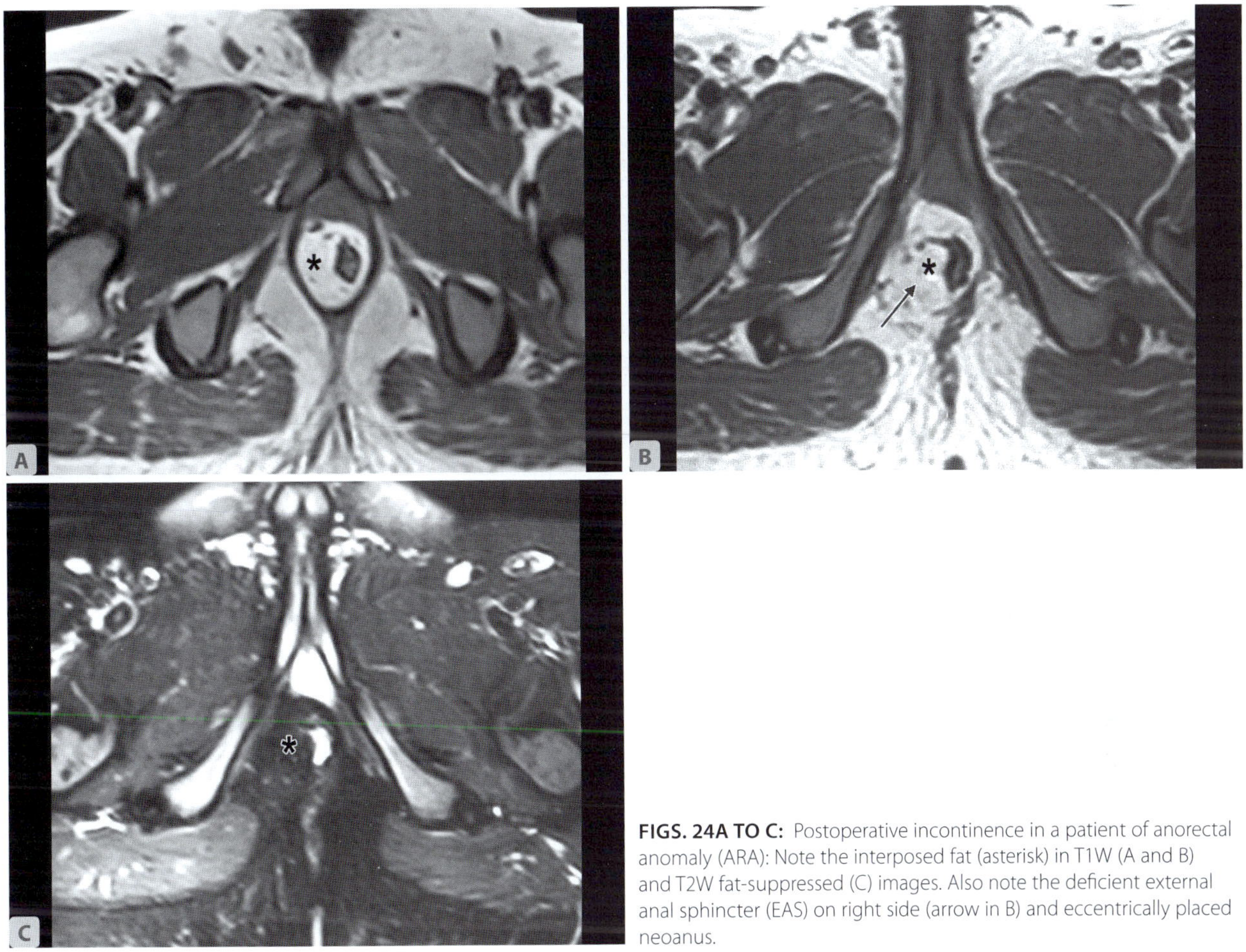

FIGS. 24A TO C: Postoperative incontinence in a patient of anorectal anomaly (ARA): Note the interposed fat (asterisk) in T1W (A and B) and T2W fat-suppressed (C) images. Also note the deficient external anal sphincter (EAS) on right side (arrow in B) and eccentrically placed neoanus.

ASSOCIATED ANOMALIES

Anorectal anomalies are frequently associated with other congenital anomalies. Its incidence varies from 20 to 70% depending upon the efforts put in to find the anomalies. Almost any system may be affected, but the spine, GU, GI, and the cardiac systems are more frequently affected **(Fig. 25A)**. Supralevator, i.e., high and intermediate anomalies are much more likely to have the associated anomalies than the infralevator lesions.

Syndromic associations of ARAs include caudal regression syndrome **(Figs. 25B and 26)**, Currarino's triad, Down's syndrome **(Figs. 27A and B)**, fetal alcohol syndrome, Walker-Warburg syndrome, and many more[6,33] which are beyond the scope of this chapter.

DIAGNOSTIC ALGORITHM

Diagnostic algorithms in a new case of ARA are shown in **Flowcharts 1 and 2** for male and female, respectively. A combination of the clinical findings and the information provided by invertography are used to make the crucial decision on day 1.

Anorectal anomalies are rare complex congenital malformations which need a teamwork between the pediatrician, pediatric surgeon, and the pediatric radiologist with an aim to deliver the best possible management, utilizing the available investigations and resources in a planned and judicious manner.

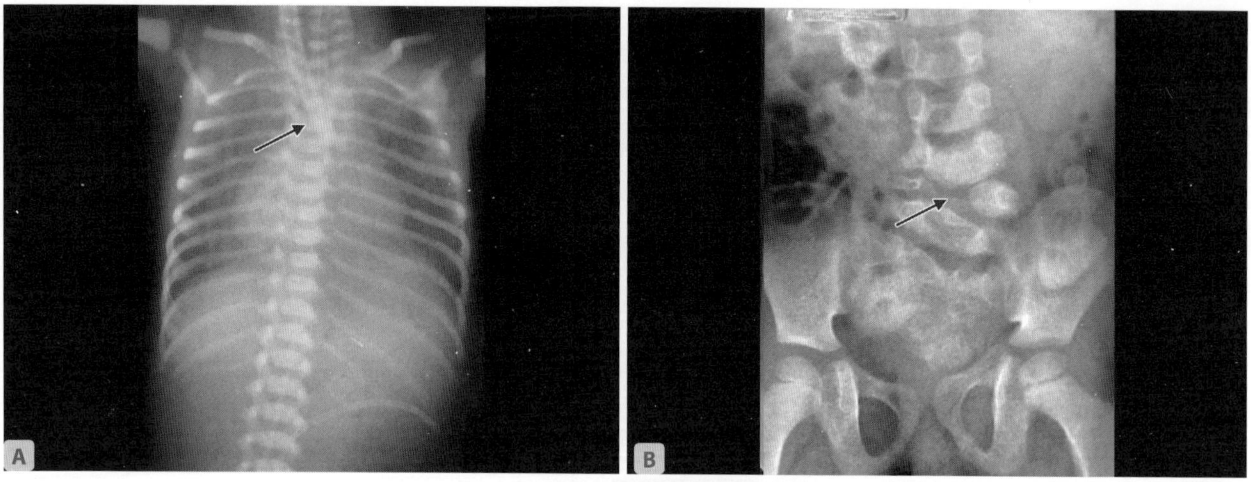

FIGS. 25A AND B: Associated anomalies: Esophageal atresia (A) blind ending proximal pouch (arrow). Partial sacral agenesis (arrow in B).

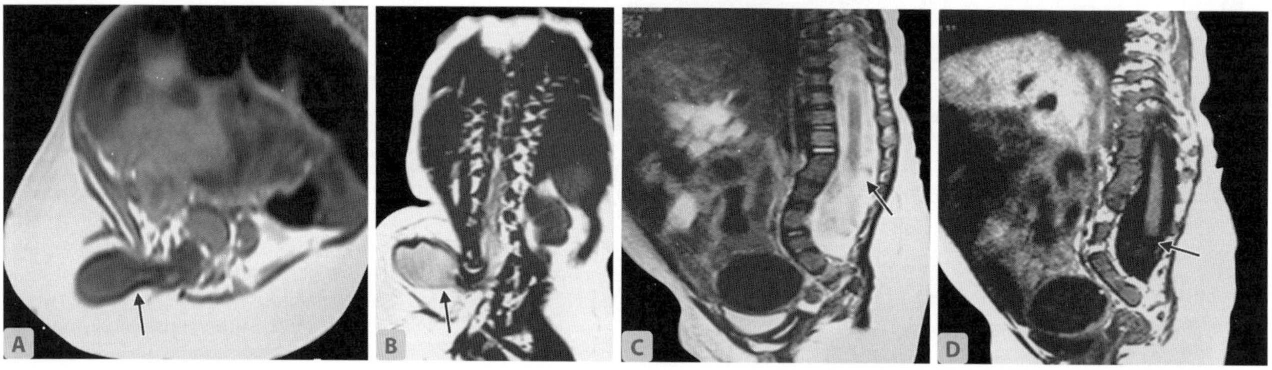

FIGS. 26A TO D: Associated anomalies: Closed spinal dysraphism with caudal regression. Skin-covered back mass containing cerebrospinal fluid (CSF) and fatty component (arrow in A and B). Sacral dysgenesis with club-shaped high-ending spinal cord (arrow in C and D) as a part of caudal regression syndrome.

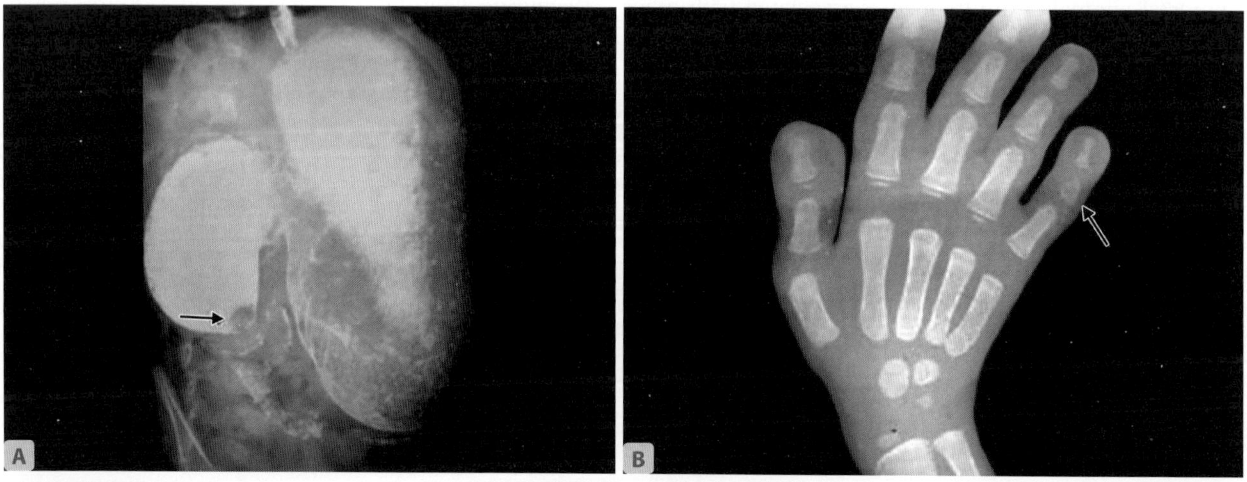

FIGS. 27A AND B: Anorectal anomaly (ARA) can be associated with Down's syndrome. (A) Barium meal study reveals grossly dilated stomach and first part of duodenum; and narrowing at second part of duodenum: duodenal atresia (arrow). (B) Hand radiograph reveals characteristic finding of clinodactyly (arrow).

FLOWCHART 1: Diagnostic algorithm in a male anorectal anomaly.

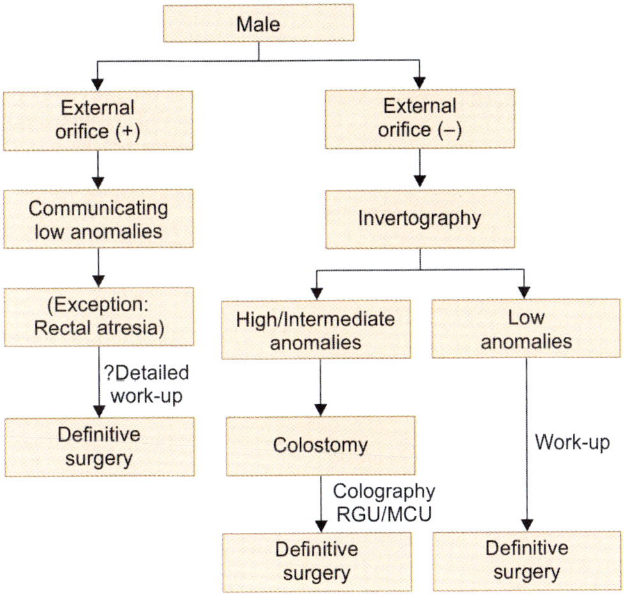

FLOWCHART 2: Diagnostic algorithm in a female anorectal anomaly.

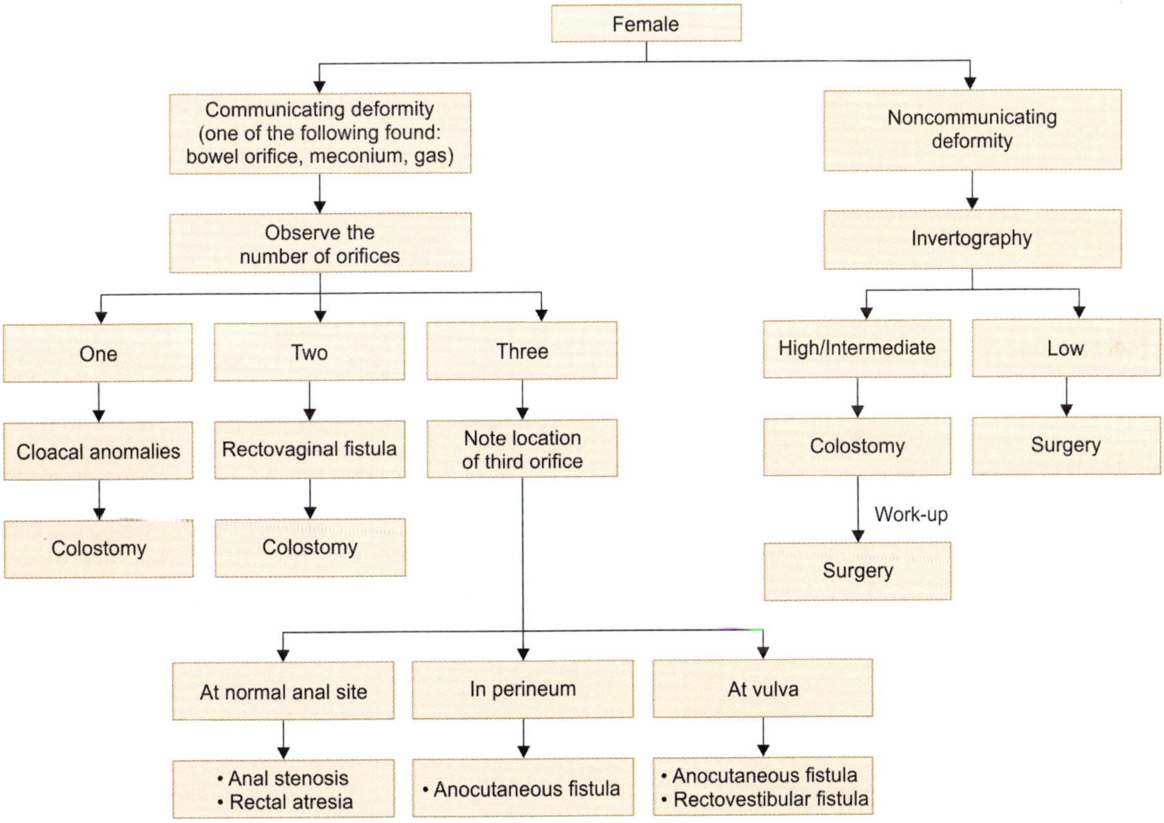

REFERENCES

1. Levitt MA, Peña A. Anorectal malformations. Orphanet J Rare Dis. 2007;2:33.
2. Berrocal T, Lamas M, Gutiérrez J, Torres I, Prieto C, del Hoyo ML. Congenital anomalies of the small intestine, colon, and rectum. Radiographics. 1999;19(5):1219-36.
3. Ratan SK, Rattan KN, Pandey RM, Mittal A, Magu S, Sodhi PK. Associated congenital anomalies in patients with anorectal malformations: a need for developing a uniform practical approach. J Pediatr Surg. 2004;39(11):1706-11.
4. Kumar A, Agarwala S, Srinivas M, Bajpai M, Bhatnagar V, Gupta DK, et al. Anorectal malformations and their impact on survival. Indian J Pediatr. 2005;72(12):1039-42.
5. Nievelstein RA, van der Werff JF, Verbeek FJ, Valk J, Vermeij-Keers C. Normal and abnormal embryonic development of the anorectum in human embryos. Teratology. 1998;57(2): 70-8.
6. Alamo L, Meyrat BF, Meuwly JY, Meuli RA, Gudinchet F. Anorectal malformations: finding the pathway out of the labyrinth. Radiographics. 2013;33:491-512.
7. Stephens FD, Smith ED, Paul NW. Anorectal Malformations in Children: Update 1988. New York, NY: Alan R Liss; 1988.
8. Holschneider A, Hutson J, Peña A, Beket E, Chatterjee S, Coran A, et al. Preliminary report on the International conference for the development of standards for the treatment of anorectal malformations. J Pediatr Surg. 2005;40(10):1521-6.
9. Wangensteen OH, Rice CO. Imperforate anus: a method of determining the surgical approach. Ann Surg. 1930;92:77-81.
10. Stephens FD, Smith ED. Anorectal Malformations in Children. Chicago: Year Book Medical Publishers; 1971.
11. Cremin BJ. The radiological assessment of anorectal anomalies. Clin Radiol. 1971;22:239-50.
12. Narasimharao K, Prasad G, Katariya S, Yadav K, Mitra S, Pathak I. Prone cross-table lateral view: an alternative to the invertogram in imperforate anus. AJR Am J Roentgenol. 1983;140:227-9.
13. Leighton DM, de Campo M. CT invertograms. Pediatr Radiol. 1989;19:176-8.
14. Niedzielski JK. Invertography versus ultrasonography and distal colostography for the determination of bowel-skin distance in children with anorectal malformations. Eur J Pediatr Surg. 2005;15(4):262-7.
15. Peña A, Hong A. Advances in the management of anorectal malformations. Am J Surg. 2000;180(5):370-6.
16. Gupta AK, Bhargava S, Rohtagi M. Anal agenesis with recto-bulbar fistula. Pediatr Radiol. 1986;16:222-4.
17. Narsimha Rao KL, Yadav K, Mitra SK, Pathak IG. Congenital short colon with imperforate anus (pouch colon syndrome). Ann Pediatr Surg. 1984;1:59.
18. Boemers TM, Beek FJ, Bax NM. Guidelines for the urological screening and initial management of lower urinary tract dysfunction in children with anorectal malformations: the ARGUS protocol. BJU Int. 1999;83(6):662-71.
19. Kim SM, Chang HK, Lee MJ, Shim KW, Oh JT, Kim DS, et al. Spinal dysraphism with anorectal malformation: lumbosacral magnetic resonance imaging evaluation of 120 patients. J Pediatr Surg. 2010;45(4):769-76.
20. Unsinn KM, Geley T, Freund MC, Gassner I. US of the spinal cord in newborns: spectrum of normal findings, variants, congenital anomalies, and acquired diseases. Radiographics. 2000;20(4): 923-38.
21. Haber HP. Ultrasonography of imperforate anus in neonate: an approach correlated with current surgical concepts. Ultraschall Med. 2009;30(2):189-95.
22. Haber HP, Seitz G, Warmann SW, Fuchs J. Transperineal sonography for determination of the type of imperforate anus. AJR Am J Roentgenol. 2007;189(6):1525-9.
23. Le Bayon AG, Carpentier E, Boscq M, Lardy H, Sirinelli D. Imaging of anorectal malformations in the neonatal period. J Radiol. 2010;91(4):475-83.
24. Ikawa H, Yokoyama J, Sanbonmatsu T, Hagane K, Endo M, Katsumata K, et al. The use of computerized tomography to evaluate anorectal anomalies. J Pediatr Surg. 1985;20:640-4.
25. Kohda E, Fujioka M, Ikawa H, Yokoyama J. Congenital anorectal anomaly: CT evaluation. Radiology. 1985;157:349-52.
26. Taccone A, Martucciello G, Fondelli P, Dodero P, Ghiorzi M. CT of anorectal malformation—a postoperative evaluation. Pediatr Radiol. 1989;19:375-8.
27. Paramasivam S, Proietto A, Puvaneswary M. Pelvic anatomy and MRI. Best Pract Res Clin Obstet Gynaecol. 2006;20(1):3-22.
28. Fröhlich B, Hötzinger H, Fritsch H. Tomographical anatomy of the pelvis, pelvic floor, and related structures. Clin Anat. 1997;10(4):223-30.
29. Tang S, Tong Q, Mao Y, Wang Y, Li S, Cao Z, et al. Magnetic resonance imaging measurement of the anorectal striated muscle complex in normal children. J Pediatr Surg. 2006;41(9):1549-55.
30. Raman VS, Agarwala S, Bhatnagar V, Gupta AK. Correlation between functional outcomes and postoperative pelvic magnetic resonance imaging in children with anorectal malformation. J Indian Assoc Peditar Surg. 2015;20(3):116-20.
31. Pena A, Grasshoff S, Levitt M. Reoperations in anorectal malformations. J Pediatr Surg. 2007;42:318-25.
32. Eltomey MA, Donnelly LF, Emery KH, Levitt MA, Peña A. Postoperative pelvic MRI of anorectal malformations. AJR Am J Roentgenol. 2008;191:1469-76.
33. Kumar A, Gupta AK, Bhatnagar V. Low anorectal malformation associated with sacrococcygeal teratoma. Trop Gastroenterol. 2004;25:101-2.

CHAPTER

69

Gastrointestinal Masses and Inflammatory Conditions of Gastrointestinal Tract in Children

Arun Kumar Gupta, Devasenathipathy Kandasamy, Raju Sharma, Manisha Jana

PART A: CONGENITAL AND NEOPLASTIC LESIONS

INTRODUCTION

The diagnostic evaluation of a gastrointestinal tract (GIT) mass in an infant or child is a challenging problem. The role of diagnostic imaging is to identify the precise location, the organ of origin and the extent of pathologic process with a minimal number of imaging procedures.

Gastrointestinal tract masses in children include:

- Masses arising from the GIT, i.e., esophagus to rectum
- Mesenteric and omental masses

Clinically, the patient may present with either a palpable abdominal lump as in hypertrophic pyloric stenosis (HPS), large GIT tumors, mesenteric masses or the mass may be clinically nonpalpable, e.g., gastrointestinal polyps and these latter group of patients may present with other abdominal symptoms such as abdominal pain, distention, bleeding or occasionally with the symptoms related to the mass effect on other organs.

Imaging modalities available for the evaluation of GIT masses in children are:

- Plain radiographs
- Contrast studies
- Ultrasonography (US)
- Computed tomography (CT)
- Magnetic resonance imaging (MRI)
- Angiography

The presenting symptoms of a patient govern to a large extent, the type of initial investigation performed. Thus, in a child with an abdominal lump, the US is the initial investigation of choice whereas in patients presenting with nonspecific abdominal symptoms without a palpable abdominal mass, an abdominal radiograph or contrast study may be done initially.

PLAIN RADIOGRAPHS

Plain radiographs do not have any significant role in the diagnostic evaluation of patients with GIT masses. However, in certain clinical situations, where a patient presents with atypical features, plain radiographs may be obtained to exclude an acute process such as small bowel obstruction and bowel perforation. Also in masses with calcification, e.g., teratoma, plain radiographs are diagnostic.[1]

CONTRAST STUDIES

Clinical circumstances of the patient determine which contrast study to be performed and in what fashion. Over the years, with advancements in the imaging technology and increasing experience with newer modalities, the diagnostic algorithms have changed dramatically in most diseases. The role of barium studies in the evaluation of GIT masses in children has declined significantly in most situations except for conditions such as polyposis where they continue to be the initial investigation of choice.

ULTRASONOGRAPHY

The US is the screening modality of choice in a child suspected to have an intra-abdominal mass.[2] It is quick, easy to perform, rarely requires sedation, requires no patient preparation, and is free of ionizing radiation. Lack of intra-abdominal fat in infants and children allows better visualization of intra-abdominal structures when compared with adults. It can yield information about intraperitoneal fluid, presence and location of mass, nature of mass, i.e., whether cystic or solid, presence or absence of adenopathy, etc.

COMPUTED TOMOGRAPHY

The CT is an extremely accurate and fast imaging modality and is playing an increasing role in the radiological evaluation of GIT masses in children. It can provide information about the bowel wall, mesentery, lymph node status, peritoneum, omentum, and solid organs. It is useful in assessing the extent of mass lesion. Optimal and uniform opacification of bowel loops is required along with intravenous contrast in a dose of 2 mL/kg. Short sedation may be required especially in children between 4 months and 4 years of age. Relative disadvantage of CT is the radiation exposure. Spiral CT further decreases the scan time and allows the use of three-dimensional (3D) reconstruction algorithms.

MAGNETIC RESONANCE IMAGING

MR imaging offers exquisite soft-tissue resolution, excellent delineation of vascular structures, multiplanar ability and absence of ionizing radiation but because of expense, limited availability, motion artifacts from bowel peristalsis and frequent need for sedation, it is usually reserved only for equivocal cases. Also, the total scan time is considerably longer than in CT and claustrophobia is a real issue in pediatric patients. MR compatible anesthesia equipment is another important requirement.

ESOPHAGEAL MASSES IN CHILDREN

In general, the appearance of the normal esophagus in infants and children is similar to that in adults, except for the following variations:

- Air is more often noted in the esophagus in neonates and children than in adults and is a normal finding due to aerophagia from feeding or crying.
- In children <5 years of age, thoracic esophagus may lie slightly to the right of the spine. This variation must be borne in mind in these young patients so that the esophagus is not mistaken for adenopathy.

Masses arising from the esophagus are very rare in children. They can be broadly classified into:

- Congenital
- Neoplastic

Congenital Masses

Esophageal duplication cysts (DCs) occur most commonly in the distal third of esophagus.[3] DC is a spherical/tubular structure that is lined by alimentary tract epithelium, has smooth muscle in its wall, and is usually attached to the GIT. They share a common muscular wall and blood supply with the adjacent bowel. Ectopic gastric mucosa can be seen in all locations of enteric DCs but is most common in esophageal duplications where autodigestion of pulmonary tissue can lead to massive hemoptysis.

Clinical Presentation

- Patient may be asymptomatic and DC is diagnosed incidentally on a chest radiograph.
- Dysphagia or dyspnea may be present due to compression of the esophagus or tracheobronchial tree, respectively, especially if located in upper two-thirds of esophagus.
- Rarely, pain from peptic ulceration or hemoptysis, if the cyst ruptures into the tracheobronchial tree, may be the presenting features.

Associated anomalies include gastric duplication and partial pericardial absence.

Imaging Features

Plain radiograph: A well-defined posterior mediastinal mass with displacement of the trachea/bronchus may be seen depending upon the site and size of mass.

Barium swallow: Extrinsic compression of the esophagus by the mass may be appreciated.

US: Using a high frequency transducer through posterior chest wall an esophageal DC located in the posterior mediastinum and abutting the posterior chest wall can be diagnosed based on the wall characteristics.

The cyst is typically anechoic, but the presence of echogenic contents represents either hemorrhage or inspissated secretions.

CT and MRI are helpful in demonstrating the relationship of the cyst to the surrounding structures. DC appears as a homogeneous, round, sharply outlined, fluid-filled mass located adjacent to the esophagus. If mucoid material or calcium is present within, then higher attenuation values of the fluid will be noted.

Technetium-99m (^{99m}Tc)-pertechnetate scan confirms the presence of ectopic gastric mucosa within the DC.

Neurenteric cysts arise due to incomplete separation of foregut from the notochord. They can have residual communication with the spinal canal either via a sinus tract or a fibrous band. They contain both the GI and neural elements in the wall. Radiographic appearance is similar to that of enteric DC except for the presence of associated vertebral anomalies.

Presence of dorsal vertebral anomalies in association with a posterior mediastinal mass on a frontal chest radiograph **(Figs. 1A to D)** in a child suggests the diagnosis of neurenteric cyst.[3] MRI can help to delineate the associated intraspinal anomalies.

Neoplasms

Primary esophageal tumors are extremely rare in children. Most of those that do occur are benign tumors such as leiomyoma, neurofibroma, fibroma, hemangiomas, and polyps. Of the malignant esophageal tumors, secondary tumors, especially lymphomas and rarely metastasis are more likely to affect children than a primary neoplasm. Esophageal lymphomas account for <1% of total GIT lymphomas in children.

GASTRIC MASSES IN CHILDREN

Gastric masses can be broadly classified into:

- *Congenital:* Duplication cyst
- *Acquired outlet obstruction of stomach:* Hypertrophic pyloric stenosis
- *Neoplasms:* Both benign and malignant
- *Miscellaneous:* Bezoars

Significant differences occur in the radiographic appearance and investigation of gastric masses in younger children as compared with adults:

- Distended and air-filled stomach is commonly seen in normal infants because they swallow a large amount of air while crying/feeding.
- Because ulcers and mucosal diseases are relatively rare in children, single-contrast barium studies are usually more helpful than double-contrast studies.
- In single-contrast studies, gastric emptying may normally be slow in infancy, and this should not be confused as indicative of HPS.

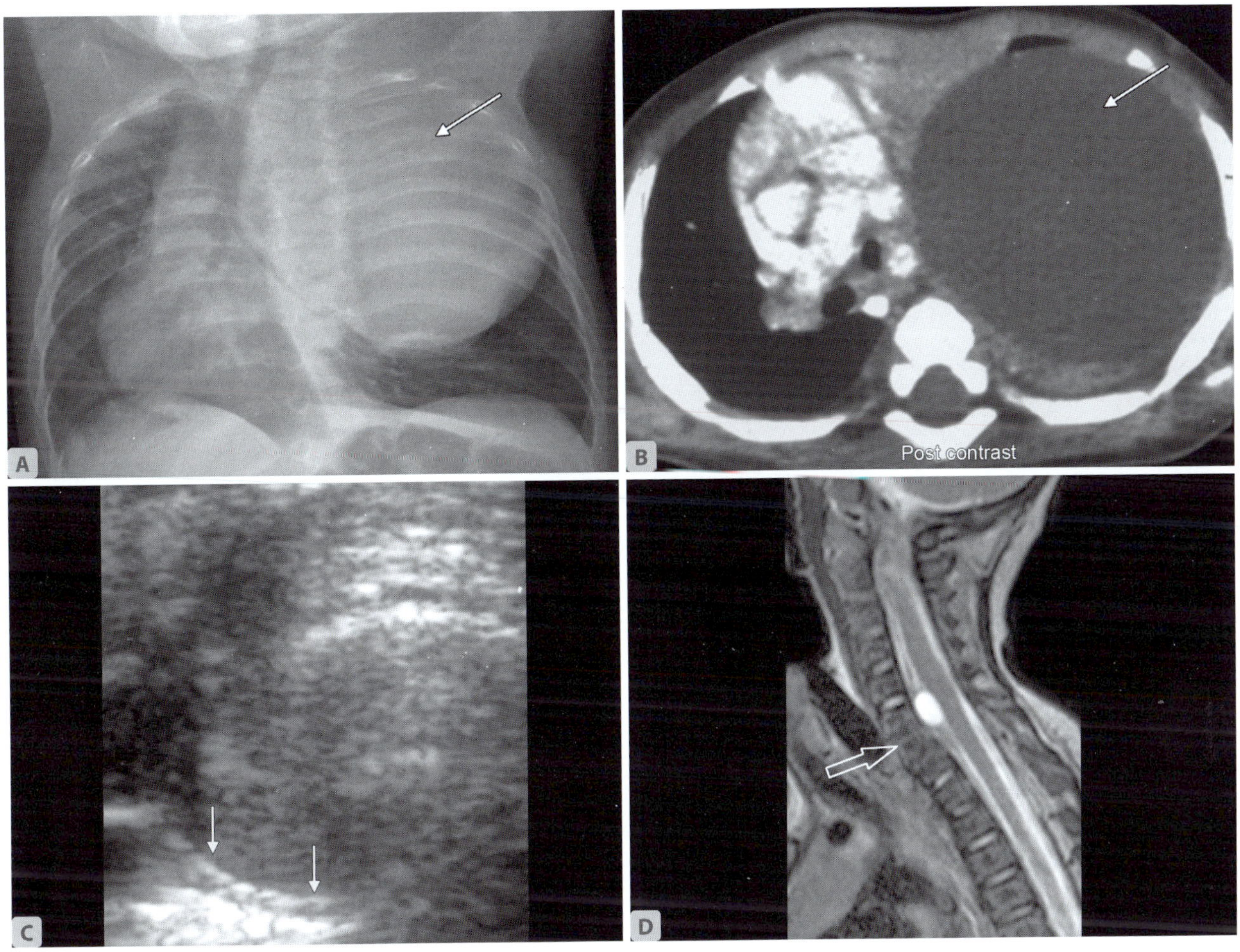

FIGS. 1A TO D: Neurenteric cyst: Chest radiograph (A) showing a large mediastinal mass seen in the left hemithorax (arrow). Contrast-enhanced computed tomography (CECT) (B) also showing the fluid attenuation mass causing shift of mediastinum toward left side (arrow). USG image (C) showing the cystic nature of the lesion with thick wall (small arrows) consistent with duplication cyst. Patient also underwent MRI to look for intraspinal extension. It (D) showed congenital block vertebra at the cervicothoracic junction (outlined arrow) and intraspinal extension of the cyst.

Congenital

Gastric duplication cysts are rare accounting for only 3.8% of all gastrointestinal duplications. A female preponderance has been noted. DCs usually occur in the antral region along its greater curvature.[4] Gastric DCs may have associated multiple duplications in the bowel.

Clinical Presentation

Gastric duplication cyst usually presents in early infancy with one or more of the following:

- Vomiting, fever, pain, and anemia. Vomiting may be related to partial or complete small bowel or pyloric obstruction. Larger cysts may also be palpable clinically.
- Complications such as perforation, hemorrhage, and fistula from ulceration due to aberrant pancreatic or gastric tissue may be present.

Imaging Features

Barium studies: In its typical location along the greater curvature of gastric DC impinges on the stomach causing its upward displacement while in the late films of the same follow through study transverse colon is displaced downward **(Figs. 2A to C)**. This combination of gastric and colonic displacements in the same study is reported to be a specific finding in an appropriate clinical setting.

Ultrasonography: Gastric DCs are typically anechoic on US but the presence of echogenic contents represents either hemorrhage or inspissated secretions.

Due to its location, gastric DC may simulate pseudo-pancreatic cyst on US but a more specific diagnosis can usually be made using a high frequency, usually linear, transducer probe by observing the characteristic appearance of bowel wall, i.e., echogenic mucosal stripe surrounded by hypoechoic line of muscle wall. US is usually more than sufficient to diagnose cystic duplication.

Computed tomography: On CT scan, DC is seen as a fluid-filled mass with an enhancing well-defined rim or wall.

Acquired Outlet Obstruction of Stomach

Hypertrophic pyloric stenosis is the most common cause of gastric outlet obstruction in infants. There is hypertrophy and hyperplasia of the circular muscle of pylorus with thickening

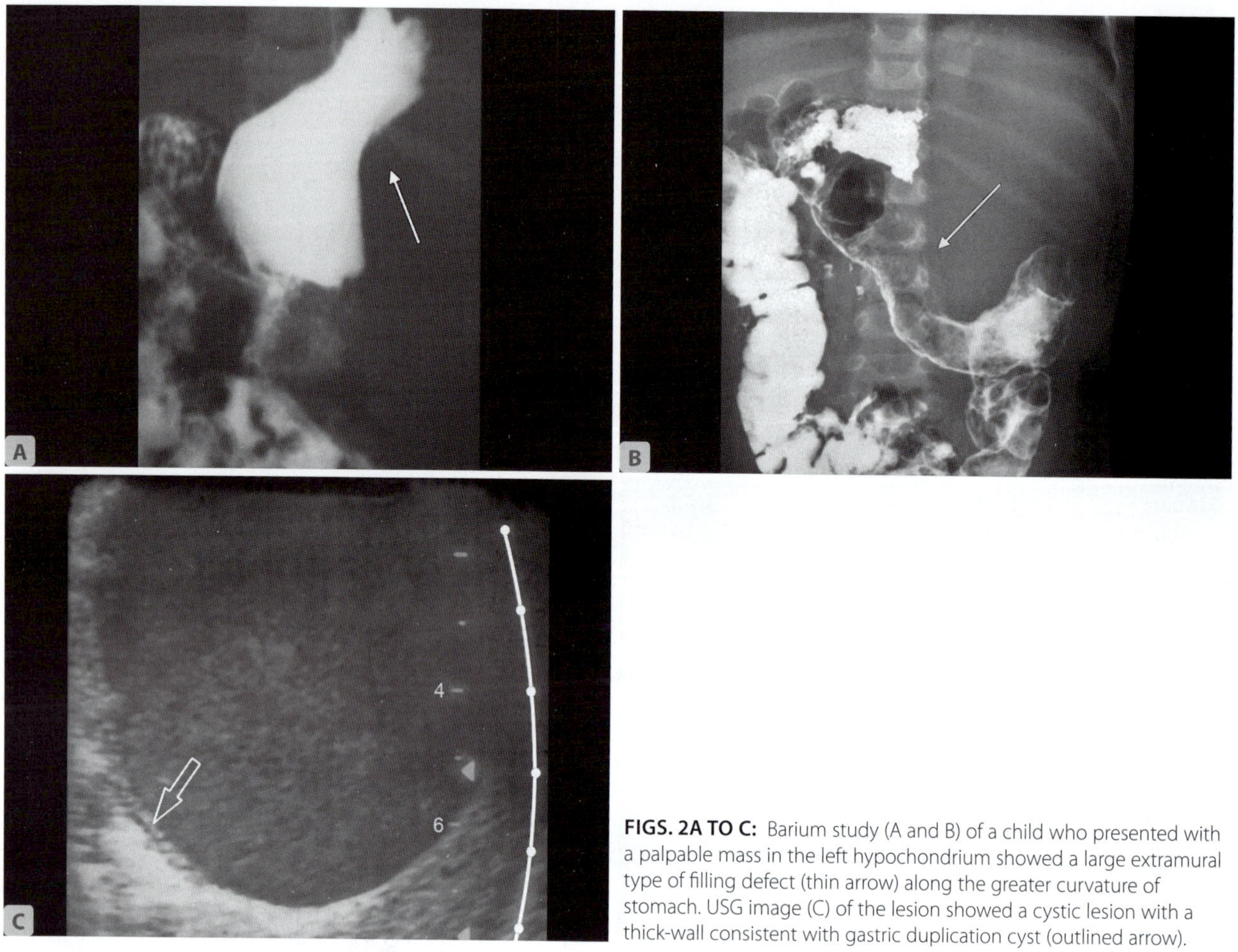

FIGS. 2A TO C: Barium study (A and B) of a child who presented with a palpable mass in the left hypochondrium showed a large extramural type of filling defect (thin arrow) along the greater curvature of stomach. USG image (C) of the lesion showed a cystic lesion with a thick-wall consistent with gastric duplication cyst (outlined arrow).

and lengthening of pylorus gradually progressing to gastric outlet obstruction.

Etiology

Etiology is unknown but several mechanisms have been postulated, two important ones are:

1. Abnormal nerve cells of myenteric plexus. Electron microscope studies have disproved this hypothesis.
2. Hyperacidity causing prolonged pylorospasm leading to muscle hypertrophy.

Clinical Presentation

Typically, the child presents at 3 weeks of age with nonbilious and projectile vomiting. There is a male predominance with a ratio of 4:1. Usually, the baby is well at birth and vomiting begins at 2nd to 3rd week of life with progression from regurgitation to projectile vomiting after every feed. On clinical examination, a lump (olive) may be palpable in the epigastrium in about 80% of cases. Exaggerated peristaltic wave may be seen traveling from left upper quadrant (LUQ) across the epigastrium. Presentation before 1st week and after 3 months of age is rare.

Diagnosis of classical HPS is based on clinical history and finding of a mass on abdominal palpation.

For confirmation of clinical findings nowadays US is the modality of choice. Only in equivocal cases barium study should be done.

Imaging Features

Plain radiograph, if done, may show increased gastric distention with air and little amount of small bowel or colonic air.

Ultrasonography[5-10]

Technique

- A high frequency linear transducer probe (7–10 MHz) should be used.
- Child is positioned in supine or right posterior oblique (RPO) position.
- Adequate amount of gastric fluid is essential to provide the ultrasonic window and identification of anatomical structures. By placing a nasogastric tube and filling of saline through it keeps the whole procedure under control.
- On transverse section, the upper pole of right kidney is identified and the transducer is moved toward the xiphoid process. When pyloric canal is located, the transducer is angled to align it to the long axis of pyloric canal. The

lumen of pylorus is always a straight line in HPS in the longitudinal plane. This is important because scanning in tangential plane can produce false positive results.

Findings on US[11]

- Thickness of muscle is the most sensitive and specific measurement. It is measured from the outer edge of echogenic mucosa to the outer edge of muscle on both longitudinal and transverse scan and these measurements should be in close agreement. Normal wall thickness of pyloric canal is <2 mm. Earlier workers had proposed that thickness >4 mm is abnormal but recently it has been agreed that the critical value should be decreased and presently if pyloric wall thickness is >3 mm then it is considered abnormal **(Fig. 3A)**.
- Total pyloric canal length (TPL) is more variable than muscle thickness. Length >17 mm is considered abnormal, whereas <14 mm is felt to be unequivocally normal. However, diagnosis should not be made on pyloric canal length alone.
- Increase in wall thickness and TPL are the two main diagnostic features.
- Other findings which may be present are:
  - "Empty cervix sign": Hypertrophic muscle mass indents the duodenal bulb and bulges into the antrum, an appearance resembling that of empty cervix.
  - "Mucosal nipple sign": Redundant pyloric mucosa may protrude into the antrum.
  - Hyperperistalsis of stomach with failure of gastric contents to pass into the duodenum.
  - Overdistended, fluid-filled stomach, and also the squared off rather than rounded configuration of the end of stomach can provide indirect clues to the diagnosis of HPS.

Barium Study

It is always advisable to put a nasogastric tube so that gastric filling with barium is better. Findings could be:

- Delayed gastric emptying
- Elongated and narrowed pyloric canal—"string sign". This is one of the most important finding for diagnosis of HPS on barium study **(Fig. 3B)**.
- "Double track" of barium may be seen if the hypertrophied muscle squeezes the lumen into separate compartments.
- Indentation of the gastric antrum and duodenal bulb producing "shoulder sign".
- "Beak sign" is produced as the barium column enters the narrowed pylorus.
- Hyperperistaltic waves seen stopping at the pylorus.

Diagnosis of HPS cannot be based only on delayed gastric emptying because delay could be due to pylorospasm and gastritis as well.

After the completion of the barium study, residual barium should be drained via the nasogastric tube before tube removal in order to prevent aspiration of barium into the lungs.

Treatment

HPS is treated with Ramstedt pyloromyotomy. Postoperatively the normal gastric emptying is usually resumed within 2–3 days. Muscle thickness may remain abnormal on US for up to 6 weeks. Most important is to assess the gastric emptying in postoperative period preferably with barium.

Hypertrophic pyloric stenosis is not an emergency. False positive diagnosis must be avoided. Since HPS is a progressive disease borderline cases must be re-examined in a day or two to avoid unnecessary surgeries.

NEOPLASTIC MASSES

These could be benign or malignant.

Benign Masses[12]

Polyps may be present in isolation or may be associated with several polyposis syndromes such as Peutz-Jeghers, juvenile polyposis syndromes as well as familial polyposis

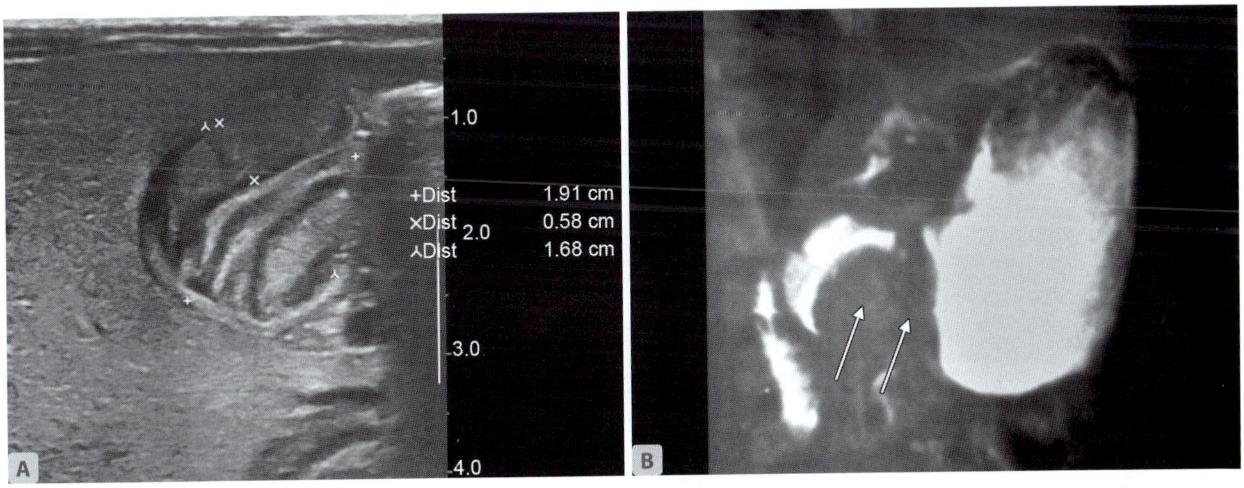

FIGS. 3A AND B: USG image using a high resolution linear probe showed severe thickening and lengthening of the pyloric muscle (marked in calipers) typical for hypertrophic pyloric stenosis (HPS). In another patient with HPS, barium swallow showed the elongated and narrowed pyloric canal (arrow).

coli. They are commonly hamartomatous polyps. Barium upper gastrointestinal study readily detects these as well-circumscribed filling defects that interrupt the normal mucosal pattern.

Benign gastric tumors are rare in children. They are usually derived from mesenchymal tissue. Two relatively common masses are teratoma and leiomyoma.

Gastric Teratoma[1,13,14]

Stomach is a rare site for development of teratoma. They have a benign clinical course. These usually occur in infants <1 year of age. A strong male preponderance is observed. Most common site is along the greater curvature.

Clinical presentation: They are often large in size and presents as a palpable abdominal mass. GI bleeding and proximal GIT obstruction may be the other presenting features.

Imaging features: On both US and CT a large solid mass with areas of cystic component is seen in the epigastric region, usually along the greater curvature. Calcification is seen in nearly half the cases **(Figs. 4A to C)**. Abdominal radiographs would show an epigastric soft-tissue mass with areas of calcification.

Gastrointestinal Stromal Tumor[15-18]

Gastrointestinal stromal tumor (GIST) is extremely rare in children. The histology and natural course are quite different from the adult counterpart. In contrast to the adult type, most of GISTs occurring in pediatric age group are negative for c-kit mutation. They can be sporadic or can be a part of syndromes such as carneys triad or neurofibromatosis type 1. About 60–70% of all GISTs occur in the stomach. Histologically, and on imaging they resemble leiomyoma. About 10–30% are malignant but majority are benign. Factors indicating higher probability of malignancy are: Extraintestinal location, size >5 cm, central necrosis, extension into adjacent organs and presence of metastases

Imaging features: Barium may show a smooth, rounded, and well-circumscribed filling defect in the stomach with or without central ulceration.

CT: A homogeneous soft-tissue mass with uniform contrast enhancement is seen on CT. Large lesions may contain necrotic areas **(Figs. 5A to D)**. CT provides excellent delineation of exophytic component of the mass which is otherwise difficult to assess on barium studies. Lymph nodal metastasis is extremely rare and it can be used to differentiate

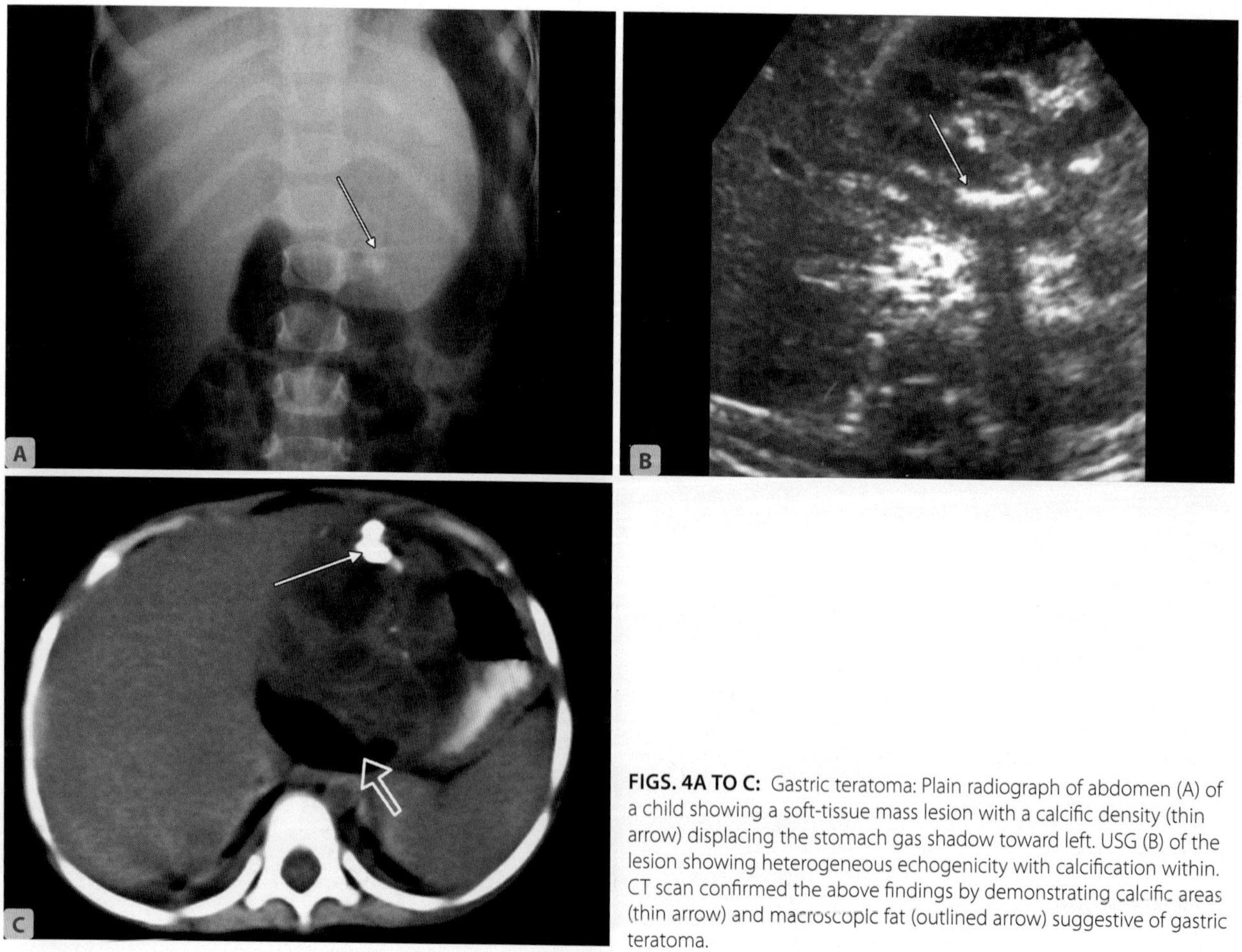

FIGS. 4A TO C: Gastric teratoma: Plain radiograph of abdomen (A) of a child showing a soft-tissue mass lesion with a calcific density (thin arrow) displacing the stomach gas shadow toward left. USG (B) of the lesion showing heterogeneous echogenicity with calcification within. CT scan confirmed the above findings by demonstrating calcific areas (thin arrow) and macroscopic fat (outlined arrow) suggestive of gastric teratoma.

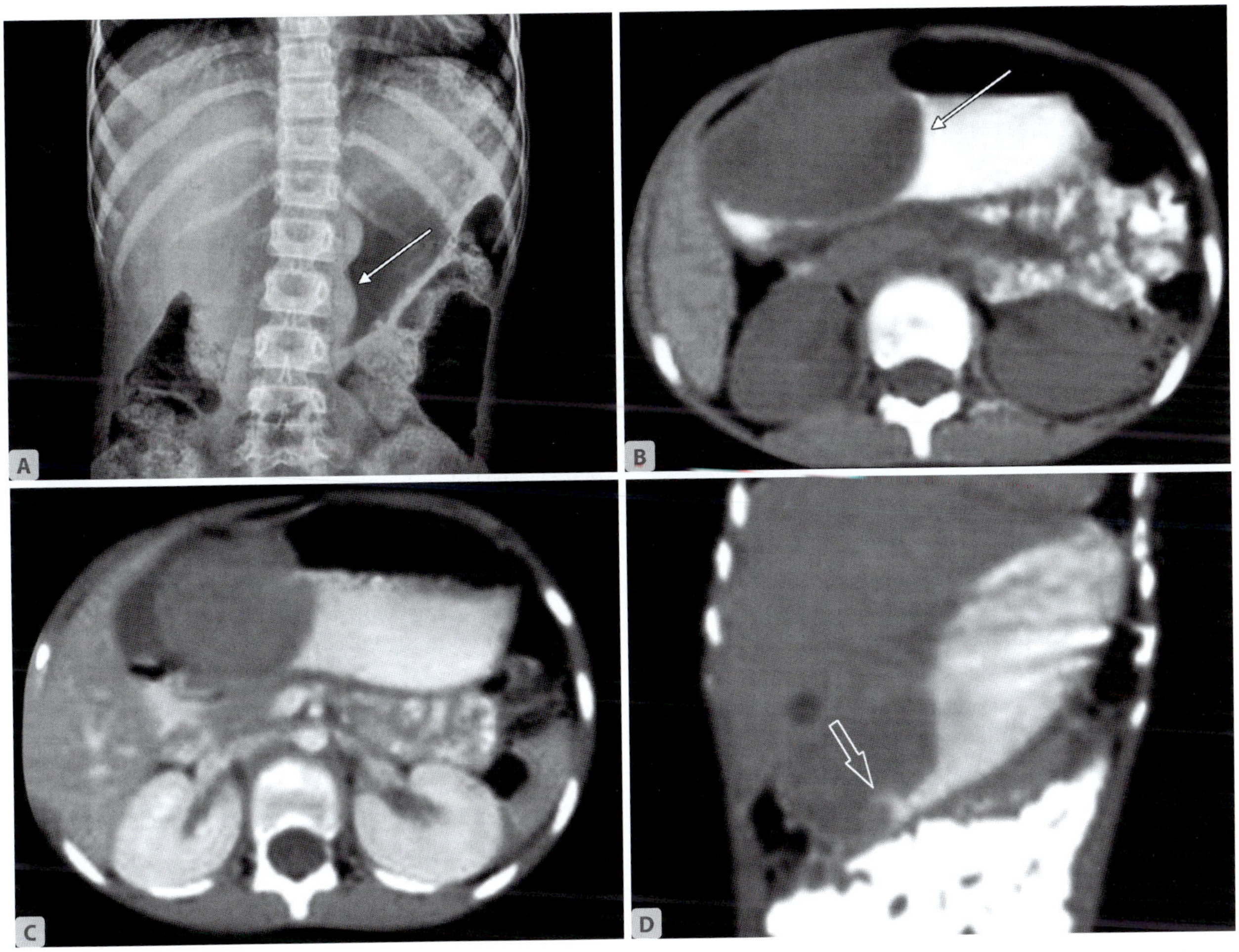

FIGS. 5A TO D: GIST: Abdominal radiograph showing a soft-tissue opacity (arrow) seen in within the expected gas-filled outline of stomach. Contrast-enhanced computed tomography (CECT) with positive oral contrast showing soft-tissue mass (arrow) seen within the stomach arising from the lesser curvature and anterior wall of antrum of stomach. Coronal MPR showed a focus of ulceration in the mass lesion (outlined arrow) which is typical for this entity. (GIST: gastrointestinal stromal tumor; MPR: multiplanar reformation or reconstruction)

GIST from lymphoma. Calcification is uncommon. A rare case of ossified GIST **(Fig. 6)** has also been reported.[15]

Other benign tumors are lipoma, fibroma, neurogenic tumor, and hemangiomas.[19]

Malignant Gastric Tumors

Adenocarcinoma of Stomach

Adenocarcinoma of stomach is a disease of adults but cases have occasionally been reported in children.[20] Clinical presentation is as a chronic gastric ulcer. Detection is usually late **(Fig. 7)** and is associated with a poor prognosis. Endoscopy should therefore be undertaken in any patient with persistent chronic gastric ulcer symptoms.

Gastric Lymphoma

Gastric lymphoma is the most common malignancy of stomach in children.[21-23] Stomach is the second most common site of primary GIT lymphomas in children after ileum. This is in contrast with adults where stomach is the

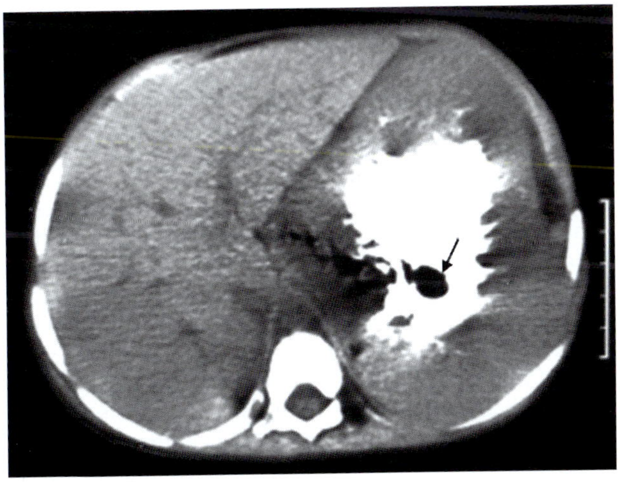

FIG. 6: Ossified gastric GIST: NCCT abdomen shows a densely ossified mass in the epigastrium. Note extension of gas into the center of the mass (arrow) from its medial side suggesting communication with the gastric lumen. (GIST: gastrointestinal stromal tumor; NCCT: noncontrast computed tomography)

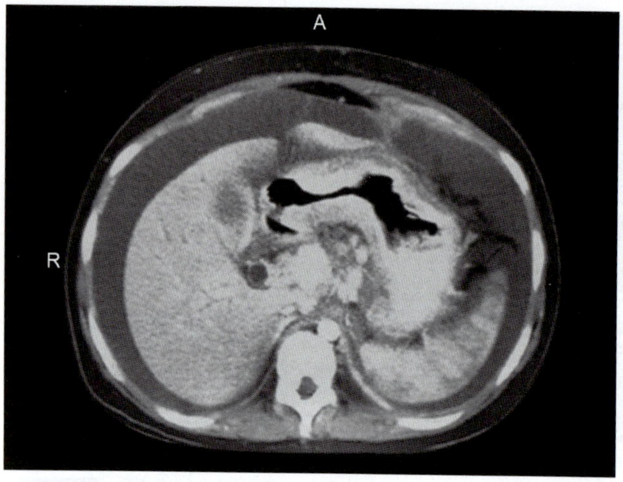

FIG. 7: Gastric adenocarcinoma: CT shows significant thickening of gastric walls with luminal narrowing and ascites.

most common site of primary GIT lymphomas and accounts for approximately 80% of all cases.

Clinical presentation: Patient may present with abdominal pain, abdominal mass, and weight loss.

Imaging features: Barium studies may show an intraluminal mass with ulceration, fold thickening, or narrowing of lumen.

CT usually demonstrates gastric wall-thickening with smoothly lobulated outer border. CT is particularly valuable in the diagnosis of gastric lymphoma since the disease originates in the submucosa and endoscopic biopsy may yield limited information especially in early stages.

Gastric Leiomyosarcoma

Gastric leiomyosarcoma is an exceedingly rare condition.[16] It is usually seen in children <1 year of age but can occur at any age. *Carneys triad* has been described, i.e., gastric leiomyosarcoma, pulmonary chondromas, and extra-adrenal paraganglioma. It usually affects young females with an average age of 19 years. Mortality rate is almost 20% mostly due to paraganglioma.

Bezoars[24]

A bezoar is a mass of ingested, non radiopaque foreign material in the stomach. At one time they were mainly a problem of older children and for most part were trichobezoars (hair) and phytobezoars (vegetable matter). Recently, lactobezoars have become common especially in premature infants due to the formation of dense milk coagulum when powdered milk is mixed with inadequate quantities of water.

Trichobezoar is the most common and is due to chronic hair swallowing by mentally disturbed children especially young females. Over a period of time an intraluminal mass develops representing matted hair, trapped food particles, and air taking the shape of stomach. It may extend into the duodenum and even small bowel.

Clinical Presentation

Patient may present with a mass or with history of gastric outlet obstruction. A palpable mass in the LUQ or epigastrium is common. Limited mobility is typically seen in smaller masses. Complications such as gastric outlet obstruction, perforation, hemorrhage, and ulceration may also be the cause for presentation.

Imaging Features

Plain abdominal radiograph may show a mottled epigastric mass often rimmed by gas. This can mimic food residue. Therefore, it is important to know when the child ate last and a delayed fasting film can sort out problem cases.

Barium studies: Bezoar produces a filling defect. After the barium has been expelled from the stomach, barium that has adhered to the surface of the bezoar forms a mottled shadow of increased density. Delayed films may show extension of the bezoar into the duodenum or jejunum.

On US, a curved broad band of increased echogenicity is seen with distal acoustic shadowing produced by air inside and around the bezoar. No details of the mass can be appreciated.

On CT, an intragastric mass with entrapped air, debris, and contrast is seen **(Figs. 8A to C)**.

Lactobezoars usually disappear after formula adjustment and increased water intake.

Tricho and phytobezoars require surgical removal to prevent complications.

SMALL BOWEL MASSES IN CHILDREN

Masses can be classified into:

- *Congenital:* Enteric duplication cysts
- *Infectious:* Abdominal Koch's
- *Neoplastic:* Both benign and malignant
- *Miscellaneous:* Intussusception and intramural hematoma

Congenital

Enteric Duplication Cyst[25-28]

Embryologically, DCs arise from abnormalities of development, separation, and recanalization of primitive foregut during the late first or early second trimester. Spherical duplications usually do not communicate with the GIT while the much less common tubular type frequently does communicate. Although they can occur anywhere in the GIT, the most common site is the distal ileum followed by esophagus. Approximately 40% of the patients present by 1st month of age while 85% present during the 1st year of life.

Duodenal DCs are rare. They may present with gastric outlet obstruction and on imaging can mimic pseudopancreatic cyst. Ileal DCs lie on the mesenteric border of normal small bowel and their muscular wall is often intimately attached to the muscular wall of the normal bowel. Therefore, surgical removal is often impossible without resecting the adjacent loop of bowel. Very rarely, persistent fibrous connection to the spinal cord can exist.

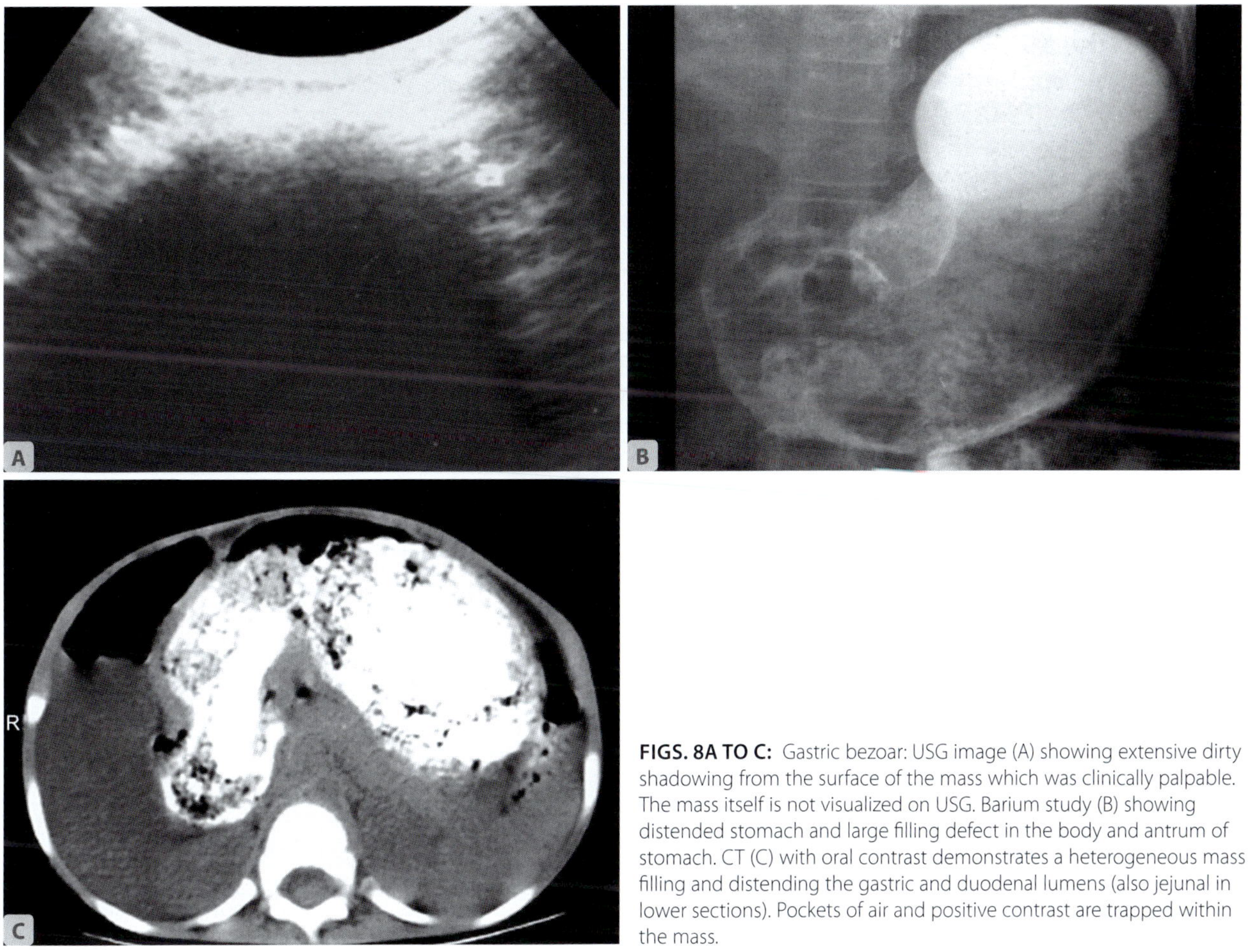

FIGS. 8A TO C: Gastric bezoar: USG image (A) showing extensive dirty shadowing from the surface of the mass which was clinically palpable. The mass itself is not visualized on USG. Barium study (B) showing distended stomach and large filling defect in the body and antrum of stomach. CT (C) with oral contrast demonstrates a heterogeneous mass filling and distending the gastric and duodenal lumens (also jejunal in lower sections). Pockets of air and positive contrast are trapped within the mass.

In such cases, anterior vertebral body segmentation anomalies can be seen. Most are solitary, but they can be multiple. Transdiaphragmatic extension into chest has been reported.

Clinical presentation: Patient may present with abdominal pain, abdominal mass, and vomiting or abdominal distention secondary to intestinal obstruction. Presence of ectopic gastric or pancreatic mucosa may result in complications such as bleeding or perforation.

Imaging features: US is the modality of choice in the initial examination of any child suspected to have DC. It shows a well-defined, usually unilocular, cystic anechoic mass. The characteristic appearance of bowel wall showing "rim-sign" with echogenic inner-rim of mucosa surrounded by a relatively hypoechoic layer representing gut muscle is diagnostic **(Figs. 9A to C)**. Unfortunately, not all DCs have this sign either because the mucosal layer has been enzymatically destroyed or the duplication is tubular and communicating type and so is not always fluid-filled. Also, rimming may be seen in any cyst where bleeding occurs and fibrin is deposited along the cyst wall, most often in the ovarian cyst. ^{99m}Tc-pertechnetate scan then becomes useful since ectopic gut mucosa usually takes up ^{99m}Tc-pertechnetate. Another interesting finding of DC is the presence of peristalsis in the cyst wall which may be appreciated in real time scanning. CT would show a cystic mass with sharp and enhancing wall. Differential diagnosis includes mesenteric cyst, omental cyst, ovarian cyst, choledochal cyst, and pancreatic pseudocyst.

NEOPLASTIC MASSES

Neoplastic masses could be benign or malignant.

Benign

Benign small bowel tumors, which include hemangiomas, lipomas, GIST **(Fig. 10)**, neurofibromas, and fibromas are rare in children.[29,30]

Polyps of small bowel are usually seen in association with polyposis syndromes especially Peutz-Jeghers and juvenile gastrointestinal polyposis.

Clinical presentation: Patient may be asymptomatic and detection is incidental. Most common clinical presentation is crampy abdominal pain and bloody stools due to recurrent enteroenteric intussusception.

Imaging features: If the presentation is not acute, the polypoidal mass or masses are readily identified in most cases as filling defects on barium meal follow through. If the

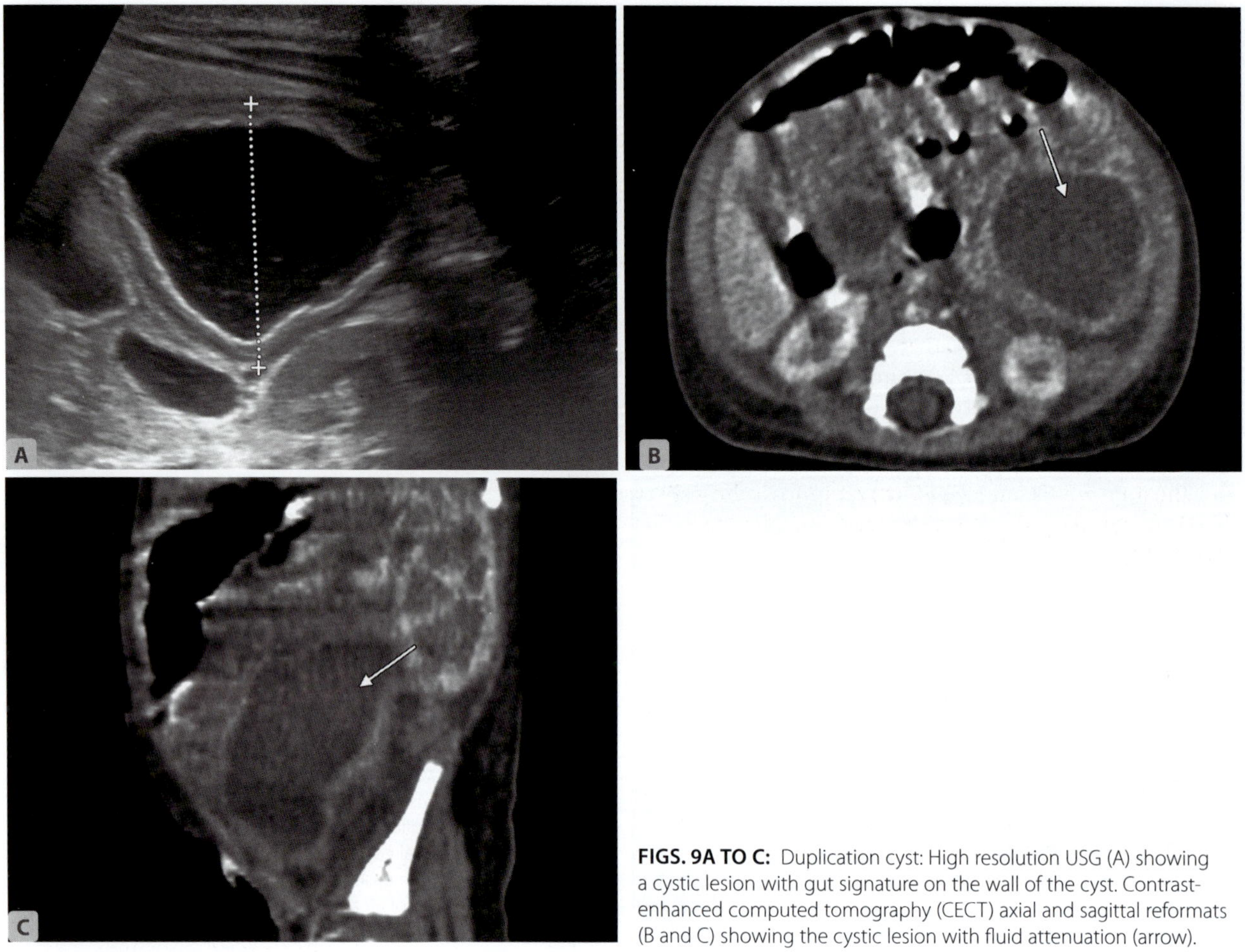

FIGS. 9A TO C: Duplication cyst: High resolution USG (A) showing a cystic lesion with gut signature on the wall of the cyst. Contrast-enhanced computed tomography (CECT) axial and sagittal reformats (B and C) showing the cystic lesion with fluid attenuation (arrow).

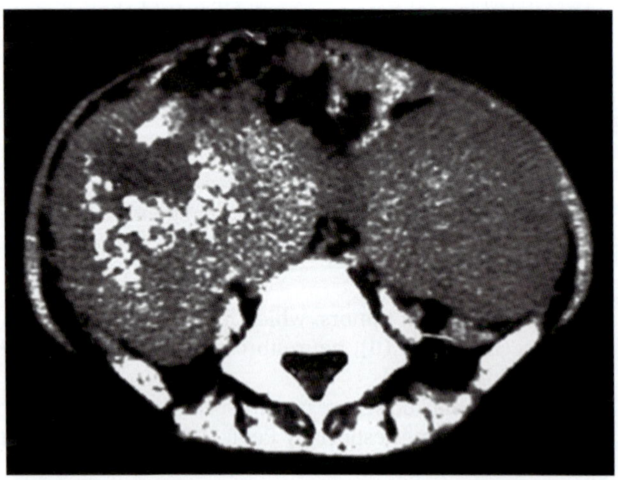

FIG. 10: Small bowel GIST: NCCT abdomen shows a large bilobed soft-tissue mass with areas of calcification. (GIST: gastrointestinal stromal tumor; NCCT: noncontrast computed tomography)

condition presents as intussusception, the lead point may be seen as a polypoidal mass on barium meal follow through (BaMFT) studies.

Malignant Small Bowel Masses

Malignant masses of the small bowel include lymphoma, adenocarcinoma, leiomyosarcomas, and carcinoid. Of these, lymphoma is the most common tumor. All the benign tumors have their malignant counterparts. Also patients with polyposis syndromes can develop GI malignancies.

Small Bowel Lymphoma (Figs. 11A to F)[16,18,22,24]

Although relatively rare, childhood lymphomas constitute the most common small bowel malignancy in children. Those under 8 years of age are at the greatest risk. Burkitt lymphoma, which has a strong male predominance, is the most common type of lymphoma.

In children, GI lymphomas account for 19% of total lymphomas and majority occur in ileum followed by stomach and jejunum. This is in contrast with adults in whom primary GI lymphomas occur in only 4–12% cases and the most common site is stomach.

Clinical presentation: Nausea, vomiting, abdominal pain, altered bowel habits, GI bleeding, small bowel obstruction, and a palpable abdominal mass or features of intussusception are some of the features with which a patient may present. Approximately 25% patients present with intussusception.

Burkitt lymphoma is the most common leading point in children of >4 years of age presenting with ileocolic intussusception.

Imaging features: The investigations performed would depend upon the clinical presentation. Plain abdominal radiograph is usually nonspecific and may be normal, show a soft-tissue mass, or may show features of intussusception with small bowel obstruction.

Barium meal follow through may be the initial investigation performed if the patient presents with unusual abdominal pain or features of subacute intestinal obstruction. BaMFT may demonstrate a stricture, mass or features of intussusception **(Fig. 11A)**. Findings are similar to that seen in adult lymphomas and six radiological patterns have been described on barium: Aneurysmal, nodular, ulcerative, constrictive, mesenteric, and sprue patterns.

The appearance on BaMFT may mimic Crohn's disease (CD) or tuberculosis and differentiation may be difficult based only on imaging.

If there is a suspicion of an abdominal mass, then US is the most appropriate initial imaging study. On USG, an atypical target is seen, i.e., a hypoechoic mass due to bowel wall-thickening, usually in the right iliac fossa (RIF), with a central irregular echogenic area due to the bowel lumen **(Figs. 11D to F)**. Also, enlarged nodes and ascites may be frequently seen.

CT is crucial to demonstrate the full extent of the mass and any associated lesions. CT findings **(Figs. 11B and C)** include one or more of the following:

- Marked bowel wall-thickening
- Luminal narrowing
- Aneurysmal dilatation
- Bulky mesenteric and RP nodal masses with loop separation
- Intussusception
- Small bowel obstruction
- Omental, mesenteric, and peritoneal dissemination
- Ascites and pleural effusion
- Renal, hepatic, splenic, and pancreatic lesions
- Calcification is uncommon in untreated cases

Leiomyosarcomas[29]

Leiomyosarcomas can also rarely occur in small bowel especially in <1 year age group. Most commonly they present with small bowel obstruction, perforation, intussusception, bleeding, and anemia. Obstruction in a newborn can cause meconium peritonitis. On CT, they resemble leiomyomas, i.e., soft-tissue mass with areas of necrosis **(Figs. 12A to C)**, and may be even calcification. Intestinal leiomyosarcomas in children are smaller at diagnosis than in adults and majority are resectable and have a slightly better prognosis. Metastases have been reported in regional lymph nodes, lung, liver, and bone.

Gastrointestinal Stromal Tumors

These tumors are similar to those in stomach. Small bowel GISTs account for 20–30% of total cases. Large masses with areas of necrosis are common CT findings.

Adenocarcinoma

Adenocarcinoma of the small bowel is extremely rare in children. Most cases occur in the second decade.

Clinical presentation may be nonspecific and includes nausea, vomiting, and small bowel obstruction. On *barium meal follow through* study, tumor is seen as a short segment narrowing **(Fig. 13A)**, an appearance which may simulate tubercular stricture of small bowel.

Generally, the prognosis is poorer than in adults because of late diagnosis since symptoms are nonspecific and there is a low index of suspicion.

Intussusception (Fig. 13B)

Intussusception is the prolapse of one portion of bowel into the other. The segment of intestine that prolapses is called the intussusceptum while the receiving segment is the intussuscipiens. Ileocolic intussusception is most commonly seen (90%) in children. Ileo-ileocolic, colocolic, and ileoileal intussusceptions are rarer. It commonly affects children <2 years of age and is more frequent in boys.

Unlike in adults where majority of intussusception are due to pedunculated polypoidal tumor (80%, mostly lipoma), in children only 5% cases are due to identifiable lead points such as Meckel's diverticulum, DCs, lymphoma, polyps, and hematoma. Lead points are more frequent in children <1 month or >4 years of age where approximately 50% of cases may be caused by lead points.

Clinical Presentation

The classical triad of abdominal pain, red currant jelly stools, and palpable abdominal mass is seen in <50% cases. Diagnosis may be difficult and delay may be life-threatening due to bowel necrosis and complications. Therefore, imaging modalities play a vital role in diagnosing or excluding intussusception.

Imaging Features

Although US is the initial investigation of choice, plain abdominal radiograph and barium enema may be done in equivocal cases during the course of evaluation.[31]

Ultrasound features are:[32-35]

- A mass with either an atypical target or a concentric ring appearance in transverse section **(Figs. 14A to C)** and sandwich/pseudokidney appearance in sagittal plane.
- Since any condition causing bowel wall-thickening, e.g., inflammation, edema, hematoma, etc., may mimic intussusception on US, an extremely useful differentiating sonographic feature is the characteristic appearance of eccentric, semilunar, and echogenic mesenteric fat on transverse section that is pulled along with the vessels and lymph nodes into the intussusception.
- US may be able to depict lead point and detect other intra-abdominal lesions unrelated to intussusception.
- On color Doppler imaging absence of blood flow might indicate the presence of ischemia or necrosis and vigorous attempts at reduction in such patients should be avoided.

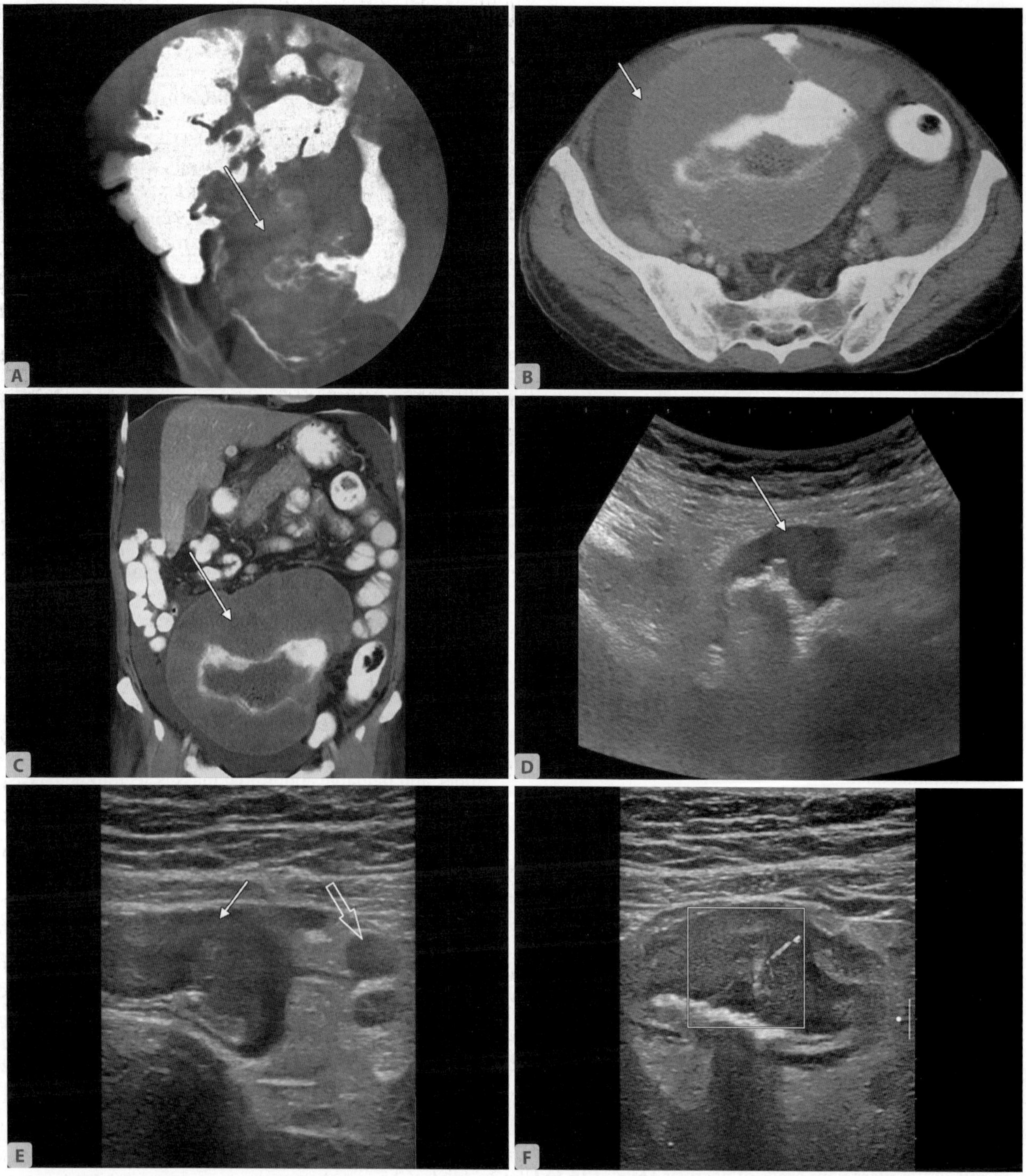

FIGS. 11A TO F: Small bowel lymphoma: BaMFT (A) shows dilated bowel with irregular outline, narrow lumen and significant wall-thickening (arrow). CT with oral contrast (arrow) (B) showing a large soft-tissue mass with a contrast containing bowel (C) within it (arrow). USG images (D to F) in a different child with small bowel lymphoma showing irregular mass like thickening of wall (arrow) with associated lymphadenopathy (outlined arrow) and internal vascularity. (BaMFT: barium meal follow through)

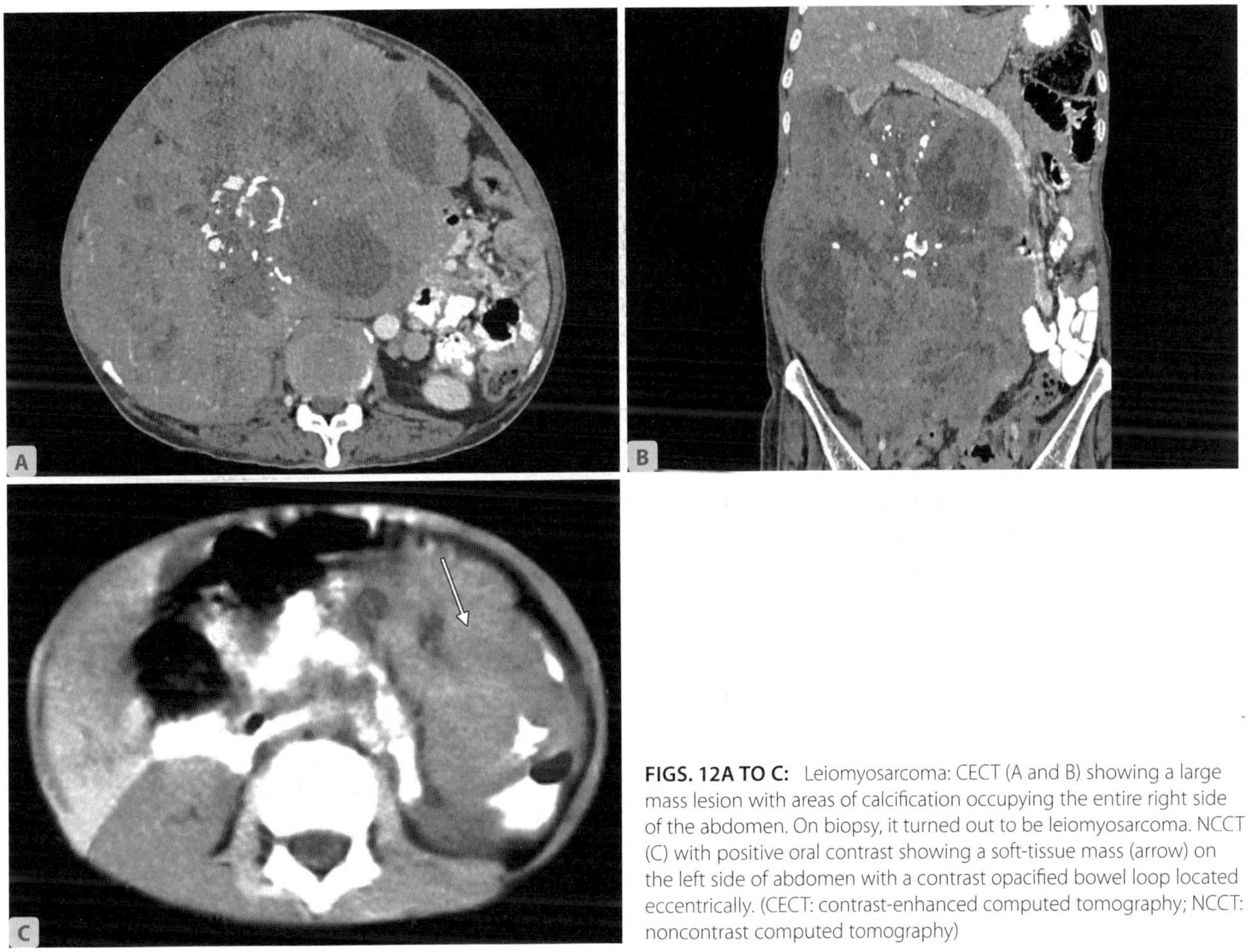

FIGS. 12A TO C: Leiomyosarcoma: CECT (A and B) showing a large mass lesion with areas of calcification occupying the entire right side of the abdomen. On biopsy, it turned out to be leiomyosarcoma. NCCT (C) with positive oral contrast showing a soft-tissue mass (arrow) on the left side of abdomen with a contrast opacified bowel loop located eccentrically. (CECT: contrast-enhanced computed tomography; NCCT: noncontrast computed tomography)

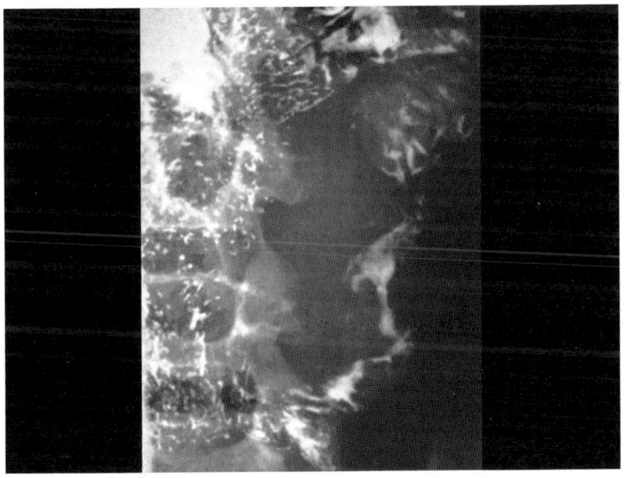

FIG. 13A: Small bowel adenocarcinoma: BaMFT shows marked degree of narrowing, irregularity, and loss of normal fold pattern in a segment of small bowel. (BaMFT: barium meal follow through)

Plain radiographs: If done might show:[31]

- Soft-tissue mass in the region of cecum or transverse colon with meniscus sign (due to the presence of rim of gas around the intussusceptum)
- Absence of cecal gas or stool
- Features of small bowel obstruction

The sensitivity of plain abdominal radiographs in diagnosing intussusception is low. The best positive predictor is the presence of a soft-tissue mass in the abdomen and the absence of cecal gas even in prone position. The only way to exclude intussusception is the presence of cecal gas. However, misidentification of air can lead to false negative results.

Diagnostic barium enema had been the gold standard for the diagnosis till mid-80s when it was realized that sonography could be highly accurate in the diagnosis of intussusception. Since about 50% of patients with clinical suspicion of intussusception turn out to be normal on barium enema, US rather than barium enema should be done initially in all patients with suspected intussusception. When used appropriately, a negative US obviates unnecessary diagnostic enemas and the use of enema can be limited to therapeutic purpose only. On a diagnostic barium enema study, an intussusception is seen as a convex intraluminal filling defect **(Fig. 13B)**. Coiled spring appearance may be produced as the contrast insinuates between the intussusceptum and the intussuscipiens.

Reduction can be attempted using either dilute barium/water soluble contrast (hydrostatic) or more recently using air (pneumatic) each under either fluoroscopic or US guidance.[36-38]

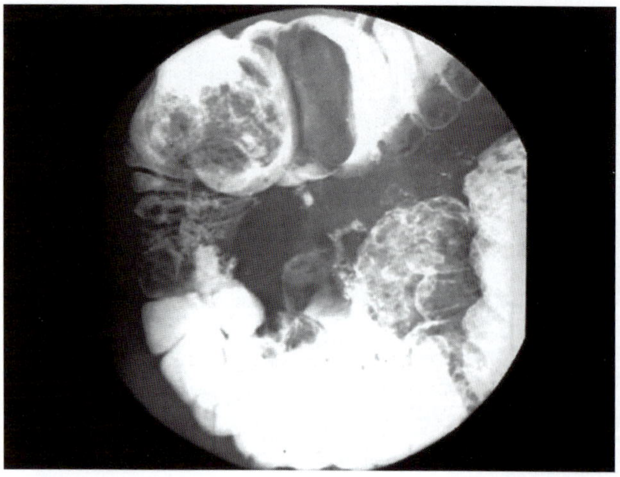

FIG. 13B: Intussusception: Barium enema shows a filling defect due to intussusceptum head in the proximal transverse colon.

Procedures for reduction using barium enema **(Figs. 14D and E)**:

- Hydration status and vitals should be checked, an intravenous line should be established, procedure is explained to the parents and their written consent is obtained.
- Anal opening is occluded using an appropriate sized Foley's catheter.
- About 25% weight/volume (w/v) barium or a diluted (1:3 or 1:4) water soluble contrast is used; latter is preferred in young infants with long duration of symptoms.
- Rule of 3's is followed, that is:
    - Reservoir is kept at 3 feet high from the table (5 ft in case of water soluble contrast)
    - Reduction attempt is maintained for 3 minutes.
    - A maximum of 3 attempts are made.

For air enema reduction pressure between 85 and 120 mm Hg is safe.

Successful reduction is marked by free flow of contrast into the terminal ileum with disappearance of soft-tissue mass.

Some workers prefer air enema under fluoroscopy than barium reduction because it is quicker, easy, less messy, and exposes patient to lower amount of radiation. Recent studies have shown that US with saline reduction is safe with comparable results. Pneumatic reduction under US guidance has been tried and might have fewer complications but is much more cumbersome.

The only contraindications to enema reduction are clinical features of peritonitis, shock, and radiological features of perforation.

Relatively lower rates of successful reduction are obtained in the following situations:

- Symptoms for >24 hours
- Presence of associated small bowel obstruction or rectal bleeding
- Presence of lead points
- Position of intussusceptum, e.g., those located distally, is more difficult to reduce.
- Ileoileal and ileoileocolic types are more difficult to reduce.
- US appearance of an atypical target indicating more tight intussusception is less likely to be reduced than one with concentric ring appearance suggesting a more loose type of intussusception, though this criteria is not considered reliable now.

Major complication of enema reduction is perforation. Perforation rates in both hydrostatic and pneumatic reduction are comparable and is <1%, provided air pressures are not exceeded and proper technique is followed.

Increased risk of perforation is noted in infants <6 months of age, >36 hours duration of onset, and absent flow on color Doppler imaging.

There is 5–10% recurrence rate after successful hydrostatic or pneumatic reduction. Most recur within 72 hours. Children with recurrent intussusception appear to be more likely to have a lead point than those with single episode.

MESENTERIC MASSES IN CHILDREN

Mesenteric masses may be classified as:[39-41]

- Cystic
- Neoplastic

Mesenteric cysts, omental cysts, and lymphangiomas are believed to be different manifestations of a common problem, i.e., malformation of lymphatic system in which the lymphatic vessels of the mesentery fail to establish communication with the central lymphatic system resulting in the formation of large masses with dilated fluid-filled lymphatic spaces. They may adhere to the adjacent organs but do not invade them. Rarely, they may be associated with lymphatic malformation elsewhere.

Clinical Presentation

Most of these patients present in the first few years of life but rarely in the newborn period. Presenting features include:

- Abdominal distention, pain, and abdominal mass or features of small bowel obstruction
- Rarely, diffuse lymphangiomas may extend via patent processus vaginalis and present as an inguinal hernia.
- Diffuse lymphangiomas can produce protein losing enteropathy.

Imaging Features

Plain radiograph may show a soft-tissue mass displacing the gas-filled bowel loops. Mesenteric mass would displace the bowel loops around it while an omental mass would displace the bowel loops posteriorly **(Figs. 15A and B)**. Features of small bowel obstruction may also be seen.

US features include:

- Cystic anechoic mass which is usually unilocular but may show fine septations. Presence of echoes within suggests blood, chyle, or purulent material.
- Mesenteric and omental cysts are solitary and occasionally multiloculated, whereas abdominal lymphangiomas are more widespread and multicystic.
- Mesenteric cysts are usually mobile and changes shape.

CT: On CT, a large and thin-walled cystic, sometimes multiseptate, mass is seen which displaces the bowel loops posteriorly **(Fig. 15B)**. Mural calcification is rare.

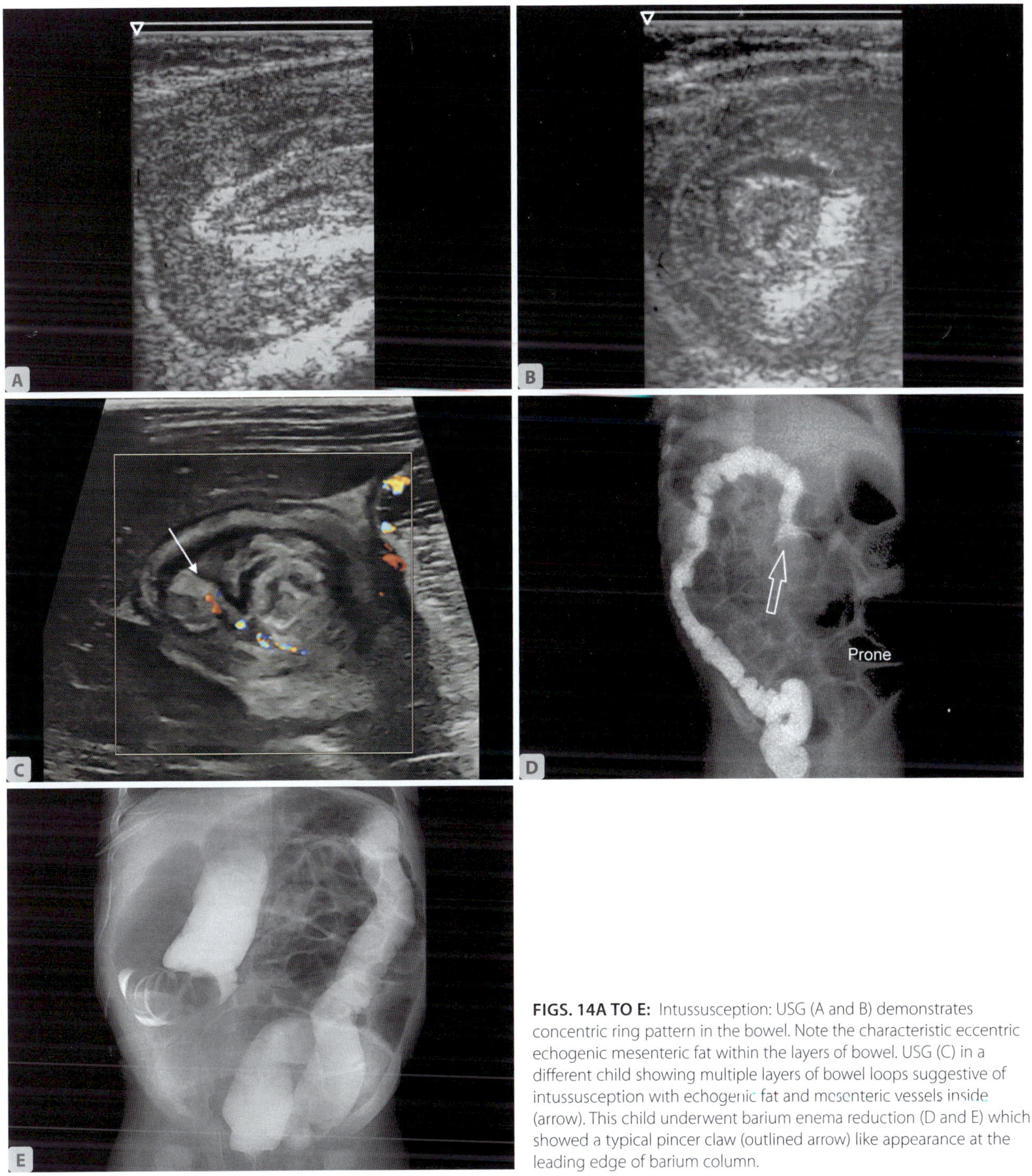

FIGS. 14A TO E: Intussusception: USG (A and B) demonstrates concentric ring pattern in the bowel. Note the characteristic eccentric echogenic mesenteric fat within the layers of bowel. USG (C) in a different child showing multiple layers of bowel loops suggestive of intussusception with echogenic fat and mesenteric vessels inside (arrow). This child underwent barium enema reduction (D and E) which showed a typical pincer claw (outlined arrow) like appearance at the leading edge of barium column.

MRI: Cyst may have signal intensity ranging from fluid (low on T1W and high on T2W) to fat (high on T1W) depending upon the content of fluid.

Differential Diagnosis

Differential diagnosis includes loculated ascites, fluid-filled viscus (pseudoascites), ovarian cyst, cystic teratoma, and DC.

Mesenteric and Omental Tumors

Most common neoplasms involving the mesentery are lymphomas (usually in the disseminated form) and metastasis.

Lymphoma: Non-Hodgkin's lymphoma (NHL) is more common than Hodgkin's disease. It is usually associated with retroperitoneal lymphadenopathy.

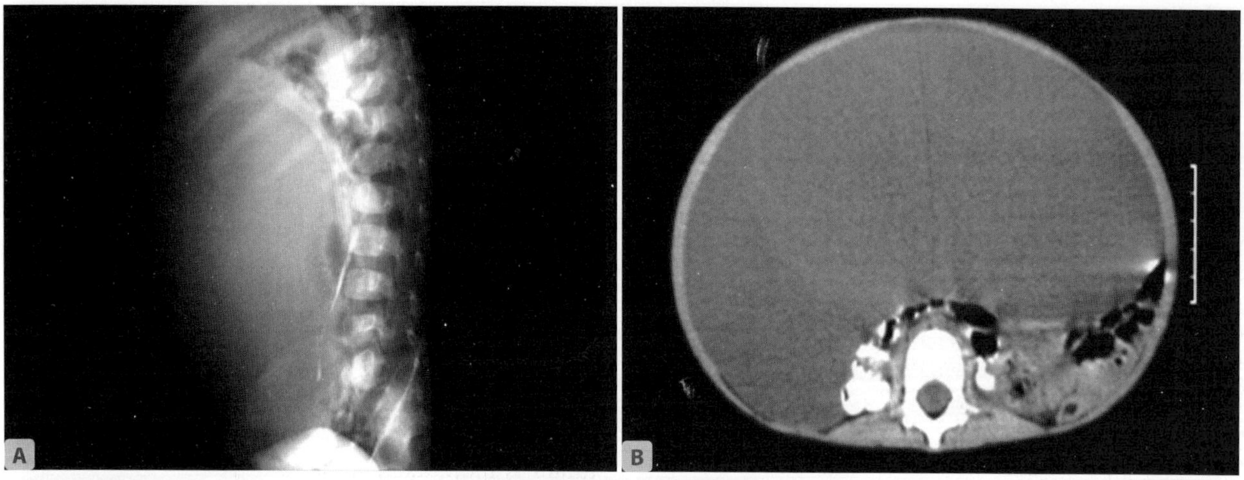

FIGS. 15A AND B: Lateral view of an excretory urography (A) shows a large omental mass displacing the bowel loops posteriorly. CT scan (B) confirms the lesion as omental cyst displacing the bowel loops posteriorly around the spine.

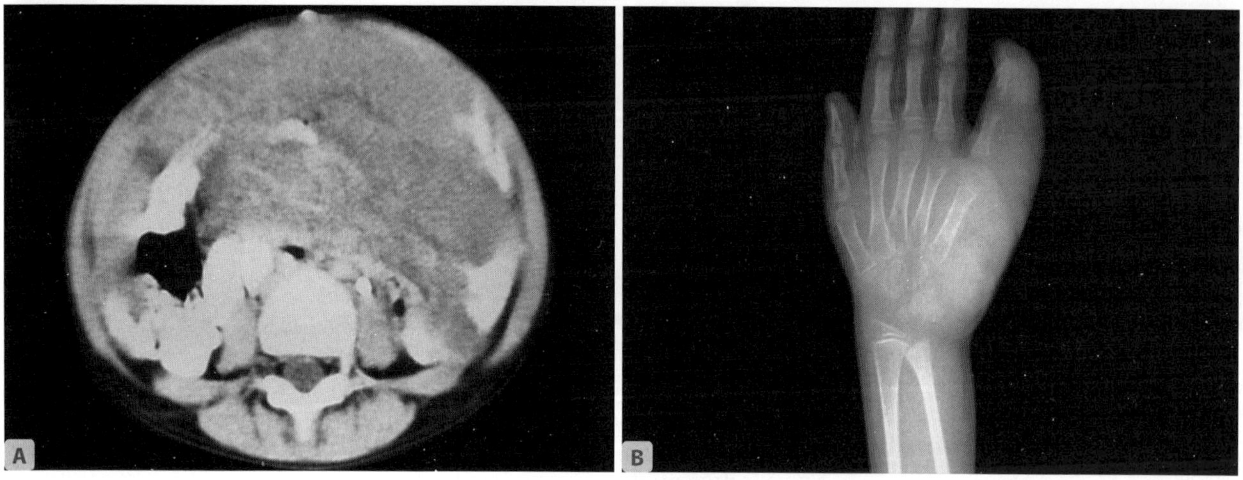

FIGS. 16A AND B: Mesenteric neurofibroma: CT shows a diffuse relatively homogeneous soft-tissue mass in the mesentery. Right hand radiograph of the same child showed a large neurofibroma on the ulnar side of upper limb.

Metastasis may appear on CT as discrete rounded or cake-like masses, ill-defined masses, or simply as mesenteric fat streakiness.

Primary omental and mesenteric neoplasms are rare and include fibromas, neurofibromas **(Figs. 16A and B)**, lipomas, lipoblastomas, desmoid, and yolk-sac tumor.

Fibroma: It is the most common primary mesenteric neoplasm. It appears solid and homogeneous on CT.

Lipomas are well-defined homogeneous mass of fat attenuation **(Fig. 17)**.

Lipoblastoma is a heterogeneous mass with soft tissue attenuation areas within a focal fatty mass.

Desmoid tumor occurs typically in post colectomy patients with Gardener syndrome.

Yolk-sac tumor is highly malignant. It is the most common gonadal tumor occurring in childhood. Occasionally, however, they can arise in mesentery and can appear on CT as well-defined heterogeneous solid mass with low-attenuation areas within.

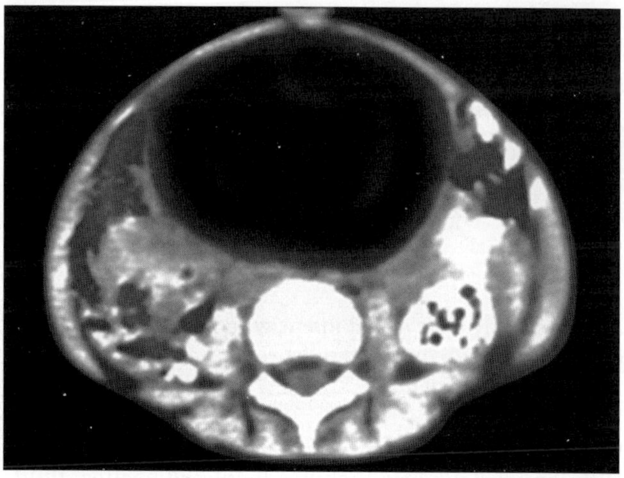

FIG. 17: Mesenteric lipoma: On CT a large fat attenuating mesenteric mass is seen.

Intraperitoneal teratoma is usually cystic. Identification of multi-tissue origin, especially when fat and calcification are seen, can lead to the correct diagnosis.

Cystic mesothelioma is a rare primary neoplasm of peritoneal cavity, seen most commonly in adult females, but may occasionally be seen in children. It has a predilection for surface of pelvic viscera.

COLONIC MASSES IN CHILDREN

Colonic masses can also be classified as:

- Congenital
- Inflammatory
- Neoplastic

Congenital

Duplication Cysts[42,43]

Colonic duplication cysts are much less frequent than in small bowel but if they are large then they can produce mass effect or obstruction of the bowel. Urinary tract obstruction due to pressure on the urinary bladder by rectal DC has been observed **(Figs. 18A and B)**. Ectopic gastric or pancreatic mucosa can cause ulceration, bleeding, and perforation. They may be spherical but in about 50% of cases it is tubular.

Neoplasms

Most large bowel tumors in children are benign, i.e., juvenile polyps. Less common causes include hereditary polyposis syndrome and primary colonic malignancy.

Benign Colonic Neoplasms

Isolated juvenile polyp: This is the most common tumor of colon in children between 4 and 6 years of age. Some consider it inflammatory, others describe them as hamartomatous. These are not true neoplasms. They can be single or multiple and are most commonly (75–85%) located in the rectum or sigmoid region but they can occur anywhere in the colon. They are rarely seen in neonates.

They usually present with bleeding per rectum. Occasionally, there may be anemia, mucoid diarrhea, or colocolic intussusception.

Polyposis syndromes: A number of syndromes have been described with multiple colonic polyps **(Figs. 19A to D)**. Peutz-Jeghers syndrome, Gardner's syndrome, generalized juvenile polyposis syndrome, familial adenomatous colonic polyposis syndrome, and Turcot syndrome.

Malignant Colonic Neoplasm[44,45]

Adenocarcinoma of colon is uncommon in childhood. Most occur in the colon and rectum, usually in the second decade. No sex predilection is observed. In young infants, a colonic tumor is more likely to be leiomyoma, leiomyosarcoma, and other sarcomas than adenocarcinoma. Predisposing conditions are seen in only about 9–12% of cases and includes familial adenomatous polyposis (FAP), Gardner's syndrome, ulcerative colitis, and cystic fibrosis.

Clinical features include abdominal pain, nausea, vomiting, diarrhea, weight loss, GI bleed, and obstructive symptoms. In children, the diagnosis of colorectal carcinoma has a much poorer prognosis than in adults for several reasons:

- Because of nonspecific clinical features and a low index of suspicion patients usually present at an advanced stage. About 70–90% already have local, nodal, or metastatic spread at the time of diagnosis compared with 40% in adults.
- *Aggressive histological subtype*: Approximately 50% are aggressive mucinous adenocarcinomas as compared to 5% in adults.

Imaging: Appearance is similar to that in adults **(Figs. 20 and 21)**.

Plain films are either normal or show features of intestinal obstruction. Mucinous tumors may show areas of punctate calcification at the primary site and also in the metastatic deposits.

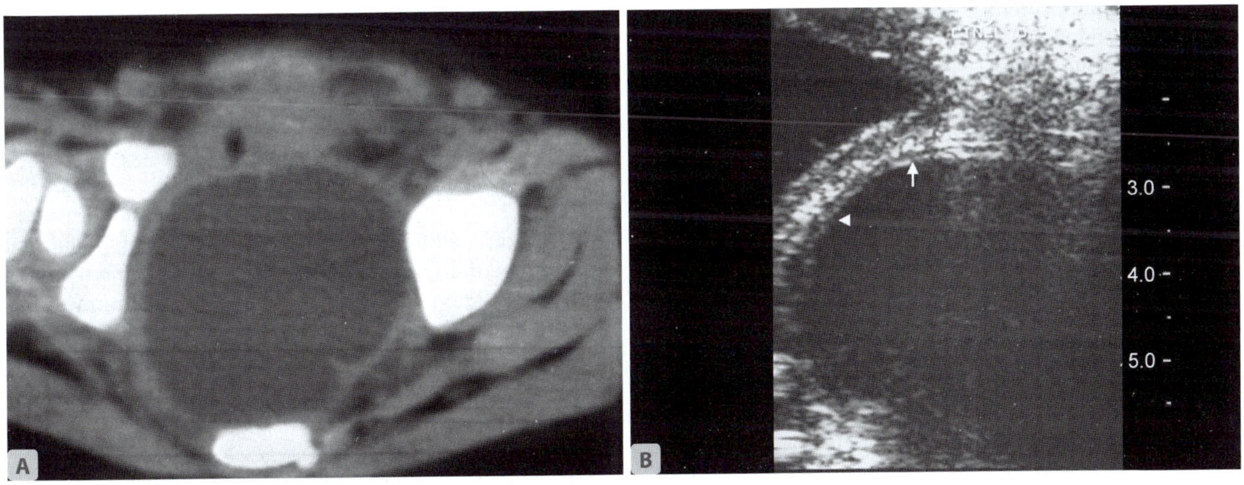

FIGS. 18A AND B: Rectal duplication cyst: On CECT (A), a fluid attenuating cystic lesion is seen in pelvis posterior to posterior urethra and compressing rectum. USG (B) confirmed the cystic nature of the lesion with thick wall. (CECT: contrast-enhanced computed tomography)

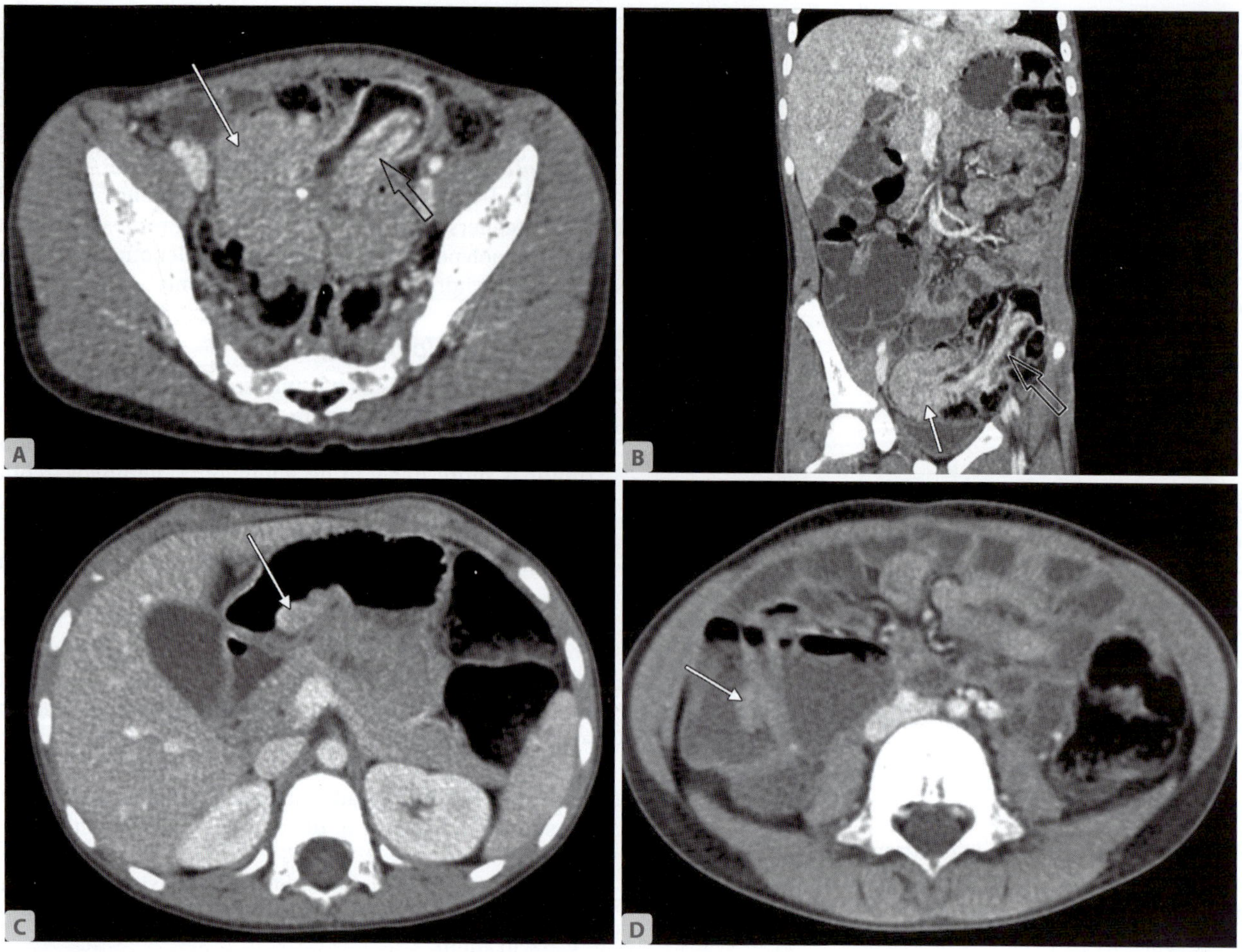

FIGS. 19A TO D: CTE images (A to D) of a child with Peutz–Jegher syndrome showing a large polyp (thin arrow) in large bowel causing intussusception (outlined arrow). There are multiple other polyps in stomach (thin arrow in C) and ascending colon (thin arrow in D). (CTE: CT enterography)

Barium enema is used as a screening modality. Intraluminal filling defect or apple-core lesion may be seen.

US is not performed for suspected colorectal carcinoma, but when used for evaluation of nonspecific abdominal pain, may demonstrate a mass lesion involving the bowel.

CT is valuable for diagnosis and staging of disease. The bowel wall thickness, relation of mass to surrounding structures, adenopathy, and distant metastasis can be evaluated.

MRI has better soft-tissue contrast, but because of expense, low availability, and motion artifacts and need for sedation CT is preferred.

Gastric gastrointestinal stromal tumors: Colonic GIST accounts for only about 5% of cases. Features are similar to GIST anywhere in the intestine.[46]

Colon is a much less frequent site for the development of lymphoma than the small bowel.

CONCLUSION

- Gastrointestinal masses in children are significantly different when compared with GI masses in adults. In children, primary malignant tumors of GIT are very rare. Masses in intestinal tract are much more likely to be benign developmental lesions such as DCs. Benign neoplastic processes are also more common than malignant lesions.
- Successful management of these masses depend on coordinated efforts of pediatric radiologist, pediatrician, and pediatric surgeon. The age of patient and the clinical presentation guide the initial imaging technique. Precise diagnostic evaluation allows selection of the proper surgical and medical treatment.

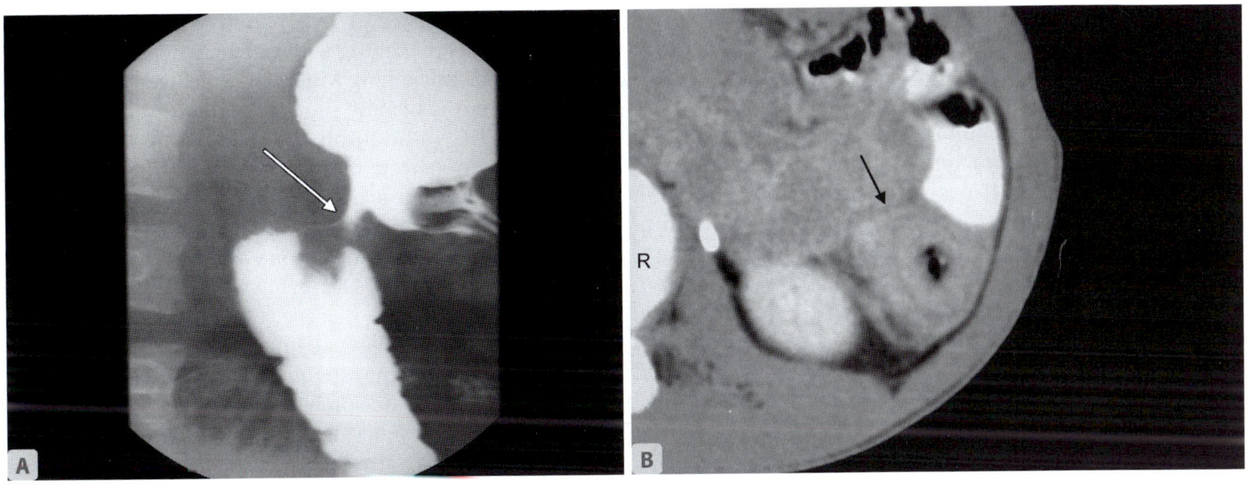

FIGS. 20A AND B: Adenocarcinoma of colon: Barium enema (A) of a child showing short segment narrowing (thin arrow) in descending colon with mucosal irregularity. The lesion on CT scan (B) is seen as luminal narrowing with associated soft tissue (thin black arrow). The lesion was resected and proven to be adenocarcinoma of descending colon.

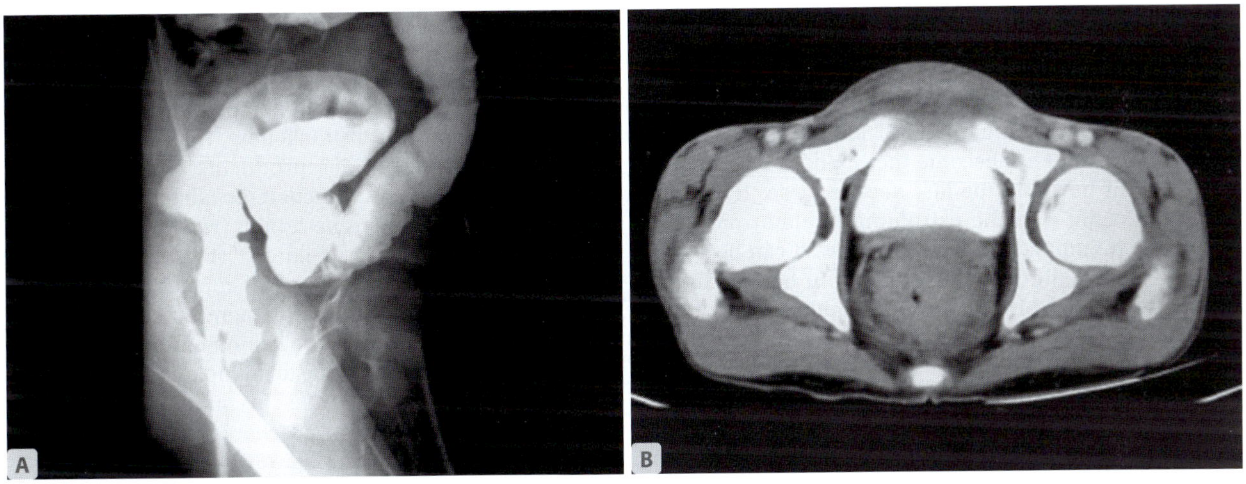

FIGS. 21A AND B: Carcinoma rectum: Barium enema (A) showing marked narrowing and irregularity of the rectum. CT pelvis (B) showed diffuse thickening of rectal wall with early infiltration of adjacent tissues.

PART B: BOWEL IMAGING IN CHILDREN: INFLAMMATORY AND INFECTIVE LESIONS

INTRODUCTION

Bowel is one of the most dynamic organs in our body which is difficult to evaluate on imaging modalities. Bowel imaging in children is even more challenging because they are less cooperative, organs are small to image and the spectrum of pathologies are quite different from the adult counterpart. This part of chapter will deal with inflammatory and infective pathologies of gastrointestinal tract (GIT) in children and also the advantages and disadvantages of various imaging modalities.

INFECTIVE DISEASES

Tuberculosis

Tuberculosis (TB) is one of the leading causes of deaths worldwide and India has the largest number of TB patients in the world according to the World Health Organization.[47] India alone constitutes roughly around 25% of all TB cases in the world.[18] Apart from pulmonary involvement, nodal, and abdominal involvement by TB are the most common sites. In bowel, ileocecal (IC) involvement is the most common site of involvement.[48] Other less common sites of bowel involvement are colon, jejunum, duodenum, etc. Depending on the immune response by the host there can be three forms of TB involvement in bowel namely ulcerative, ulcerohypertrophic, and hypertrophic type.[48,49] If the host response is good it usually leads to hypertrophic type and if the host immune response is poor it leads to ulcerative type. Of the above types, ulcerohypertrophic type poses a diagnosis dilemma because it can mimic malignant masses. Until the last decade, barium meal follow through (BaMFT) used to be the choice of imaging modality to evaluate bowel TB. Although BMFT is excellent for the evaluation of mucosal involvement, it is poor for the evaluation of extraluminal features which is critical for the management of these patients. Barium may demonstrate contracted, coned, irregular cecum; gaping, incontinent IC valve; narrowed, rigid terminal ileum; matted and fixed bowel loops with or without strictures. Some of the signs described on BMFT for the diagnosis of IC TB which are of historical importance are Fleischner's sign, Stierlin sign, gooseneck deformity, purse string stenosis, etc., **(Figs. 22A to C)**. USG is also a good modality to evaluate bowel loops especially the IC junction which can show wall-thickening, increased vascularity, surrounding enlarged nodes, and mesenteric changes. It can be coupled with USG contrast which will increase the accuracy and usefulness of USG significantly. However, the expertise of performing bowel USG with contrast in our country is quite limited. Another downside of USG is that it cannot evaluate the proximal bowel loops optimally. Enterography is a relatively new technique which can be coupled with either CT (CT enterography) or MRI (MR enterography) has become the standard of care in the evaluation of bowel in the last decade or so. It provides excellent insight into the extraluminal abnormalities of infective or inflammatory bowel diseases. It can be used to diagnose and to differentiate active from healed disease. Although CTE and MRE have comparable sensitivity and specificity in bowel evaluation, MRE is generally preferred over CTE in children because of radiation concerns. On enterography, TB involvement of bowel will be seen as wall-thickening and abnormal enhancement with associated enlarged or necrotic lymph nodes, peritoneal thickening, and ascites **(Figs. 23A to E)**. Active disease is seen as stratified wall-thickening with mucosal hyperenhancement whereas wall-thickening with poor or delayed homogeneous enhancement is usually seen in healed disease **(Figs. 24A and B)**. MRE, in addition to the above features, has the ability to demonstrate multiple other paradigms which can reliably differentiate active disease from healed disease. Wall hyperintensity on T2-weighted images, diffusion restriction of bowel wall, mesenteric edema and increased vascularity are the signs of active disease. However, all the above features can be seen in Crohn's disease (CD) as well.[3] TB can mimic CD on clinical, biochemical, imaging, and histopathological features. Long segment involvement, skip lesions, and left colon involvement are some features which would favor CD rather than TB. Presence of necrotic nodes is quite specific to TB and its presence should point toward the diagnosis of TB regardless of other imaging features.[3] Involvement of other parts of small bowel such as jejunum and duodenum by TB can have a nonspecific appearance on imaging and usually needs sampling to diagnose them **(Figs. 25A to C)**.

Tuberculosis involving the IC region and peritoneum can present as an abdominal mass in children. In IC TB, the IC valve may be so thick that it mimics a mass in the RIF. The patient may present with nonspecific complaints with a RIF mass. Both CT and US would demonstrate adherent bowel loops, gross bowel wall-thickening, thickened mesentery, and large regional nodes producing a soft-tissue mass centered around the IC junction. Loculated ascites, as may be seen with tuberculous peritonitis (wet form), may present as an abdominal mass in children[50] **(Figs. 26A to C)**. It may contain septations and debris. US appearance of loculated ascites can mimic mesenteric or omental cyst. In the dry form of tuberculous peritonitis, bowel, omentum, or mesentery may be clumped together due to multiple caseous nodules on the surface and adhesions, often becoming palpable and may present as a mass. On US, a very characteristic "Swiss-cheese" appearance may be noted **(Fig. 26B)**.

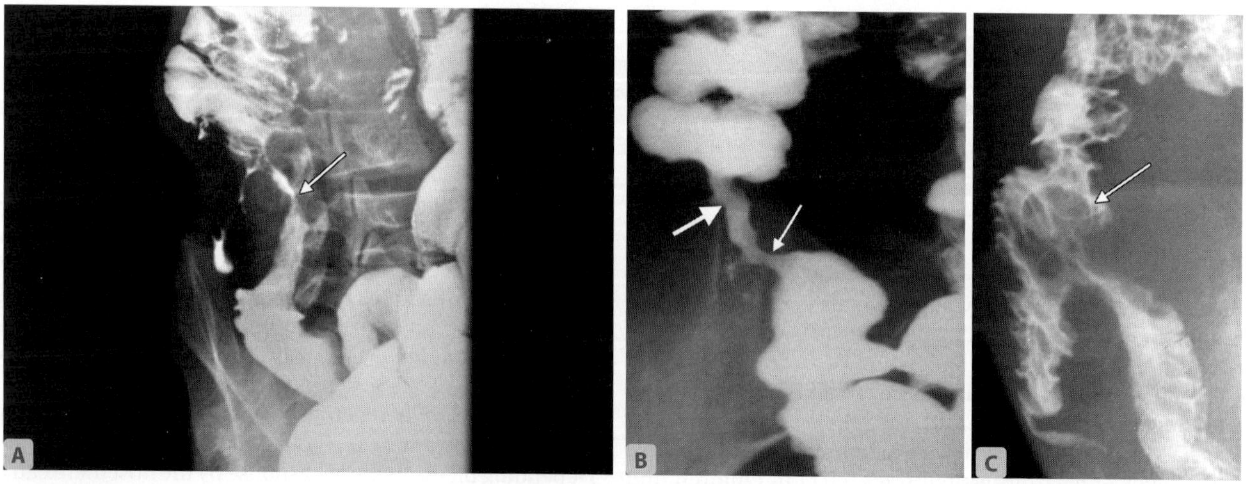

FIGS. 22A TO C: Signs of ileocecal (IC) tuberculosis (TB) on BMFT: Image (A) showing narrowing of terminal ileum and IC junction (arrow) suggestive of string sign. Also the cecum is contracted. In image (B) the terminal ileum is dilated, both cecum and proximal ascending colon are contracted (thick arrow) with patent IC valve (thin arrow) suggestive of Stierlin sign. On fluoroscopy the barium was seen to rapidly emptying into colon due to the irritable cecum. Image (C) showing edematous IC valve leading to mushroom-like filling defect (thin arrow) suggestive of Fleischner sign. (BMFT: barium meal follow through)

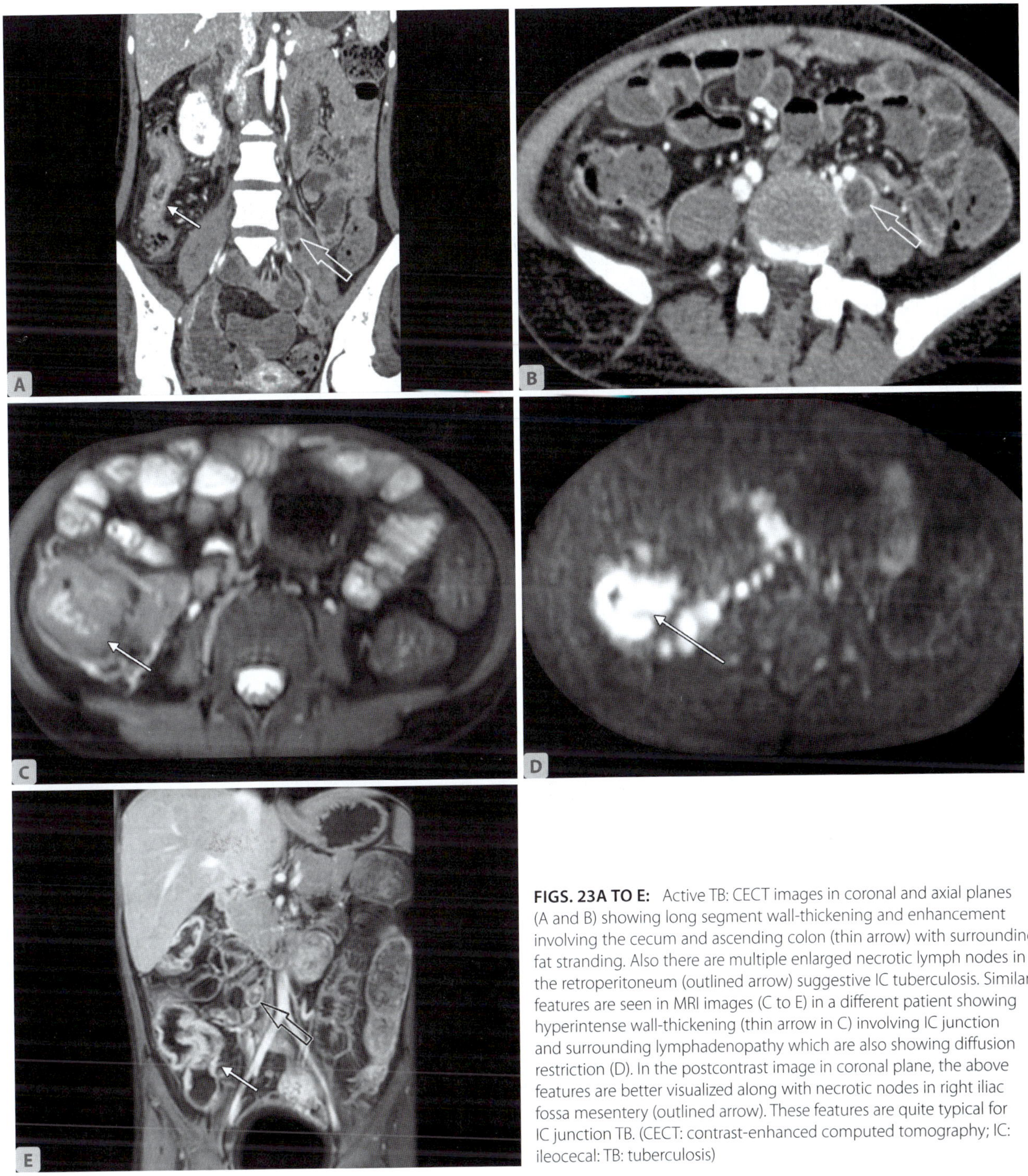

FIGS. 23A TO E: Active TB: CECT images in coronal and axial planes (A and B) showing long segment wall-thickening and enhancement involving the cecum and ascending colon (thin arrow) with surrounding fat stranding. Also there are multiple enlarged necrotic lymph nodes in the retroperitoneum (outlined arrow) suggestive IC tuberculosis. Similar features are seen in MRI images (C to E) in a different patient showing hyperintense wall-thickening (thin arrow in C) involving IC junction and surrounding lymphadenopathy which are also showing diffusion restriction (D). In the postcontrast image in coronal plane, the above features are better visualized along with necrotic nodes in right iliac fossa mesentery (outlined arrow). These features are quite typical for IC junction TB. (CECT: contrast-enhanced computed tomography; IC: ileocecal: TB: tuberculosis)

Acute Appendicitis

Acute appendicitis is one of the common diagnoses in children presenting to emergency with abdominal pain and is the most common cause of abdominal surgery in children.[18] It is caused by acute inflammation of appendix. The classical clinical presentation is periumbilical pain, tenderness in the McBurney's point, fever, and leukocytosis. The exact site of tenderness may vary depending on the position of appendix. The most common position is retrocecal followed by subcecal position.[51] Most of the times the diagnosis is made on clinical grounds; however, imaging is necessary to confirm the diagnosis and to rule out the other mimickers such as mesenteric adenitis, ileitis, and adnexal inflammation. Perforation with generalized peritonitis is unusual because

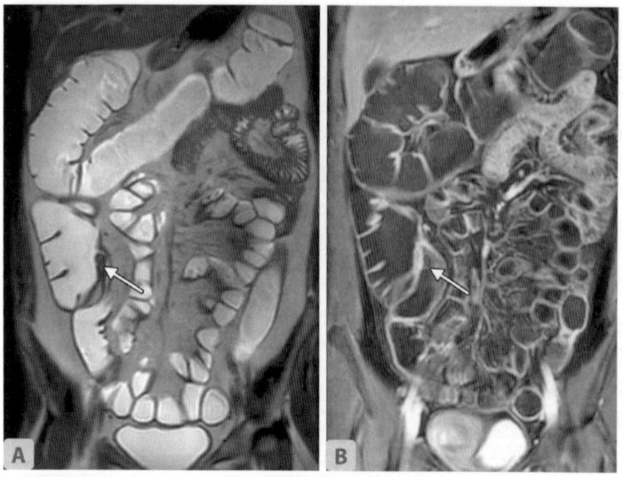

FIGS. 24A AND B: Healed TB: MRE images in coronal plane in a patient treated with antitubercular therapy showing mild wall-thickening (arrow on A) which is T2 hypointense suggestive of fibrosis along with homogeneous enhancement (arrow on B) on postcontrast image. The above features are suggestive of healed TB. (MRE: magnetic resonance enterography; TB: tuberculosis)

omentum effectively contains the perforation. USG is the initial investigation of choice to evaluate a child with suspected acute appendicitis.[52] Radiographs are often noncontributory. CT is usually avoided in this scenario because of ionizing radiation although it is also accurate in diagnosing the condition. USG may show an aperistaltic, noncompressible, and dilated blind-ending appendix. There can be edematous echogenic fat and fluid collection around it **(Figs. 27A to C)**. Sometimes appendix may not be visible and can be replaced by an appendicular mass or even abscess **(Figs. 28A to C)**. Appendicolith within the lumen may cause shadowing on USG **(Fig. 28)**. Wall-thickening of 3 mm or more and outer diameter of appendix >6 mm are quite diagnostic for acute appendicitis. Graded compression technique on USG is found to increase the likelihood of visualizing appendix which involves application of gradual increasing pressure of probe at the site of tenderness. By employing this technique the overlying bowel loops can be displaced without causing much pain to the child. When the USG findings are equivocal, CT or MRI can be used as a problem solving tool.[52] MRI because of its safe nature and high accuracy of over 90% is coming up as an alternative

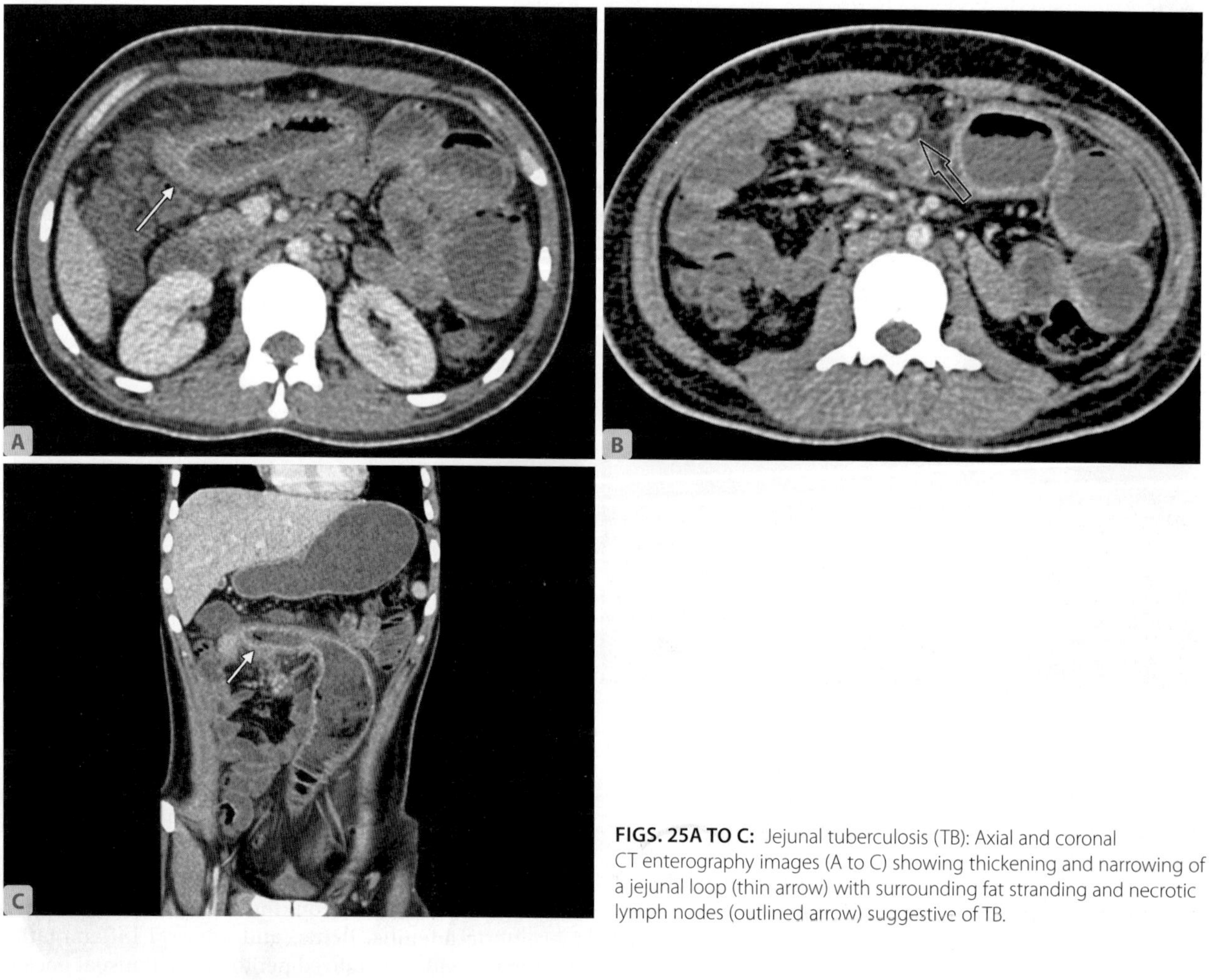

FIGS. 25A TO C: Jejunal tuberculosis (TB): Axial and coronal CT enterography images (A to C) showing thickening and narrowing of a jejunal loop (thin arrow) with surrounding fat stranding and necrotic lymph nodes (outlined arrow) suggestive of TB.

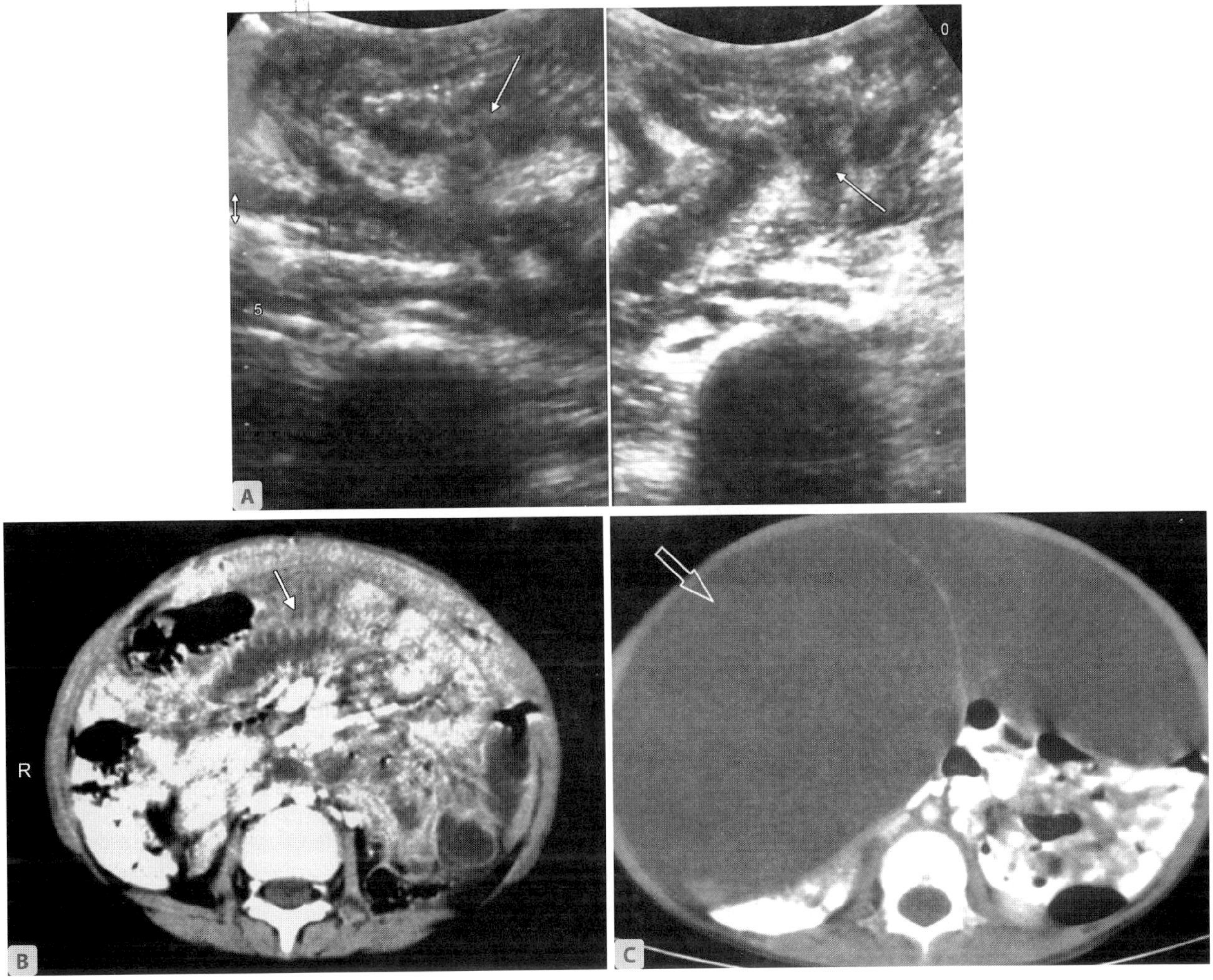

FIGS. 26A TO C: Peritoneal tuberculosis (TB): USG (A) and CECT axial images (B) showing clumping of bowel loops (arrow) and increased echogenicity of mesenteric fat giving a Swiss-cheese appearance in a child diagnosed with abdominal TB. In another child who presented with abdominal mass, CECT (C) showed a loculated collection (outlined arrow) in the peritoneal cavity displacing the bowel loops suggestive of loculated ascites. (CECT: contrast-enhanced computed tomography)

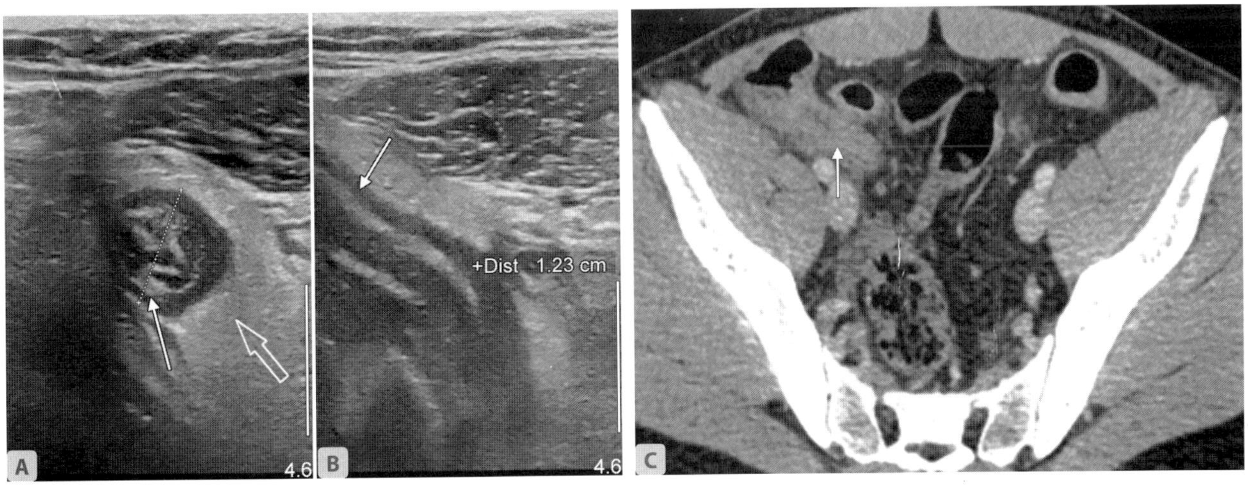

FIGS. 27A TO C: Acute appendicitis: High resolution USG images (A and B) of a young patient who presented with periumbilical pain showing thickening of appendix (thin arrow) with surrounding inflamed (hyperechoic) fat (outlined arrow). Contrast-enhanced computed tomography (C) also showed inflamed and thickened appendix suggestive of acute appendicitis.

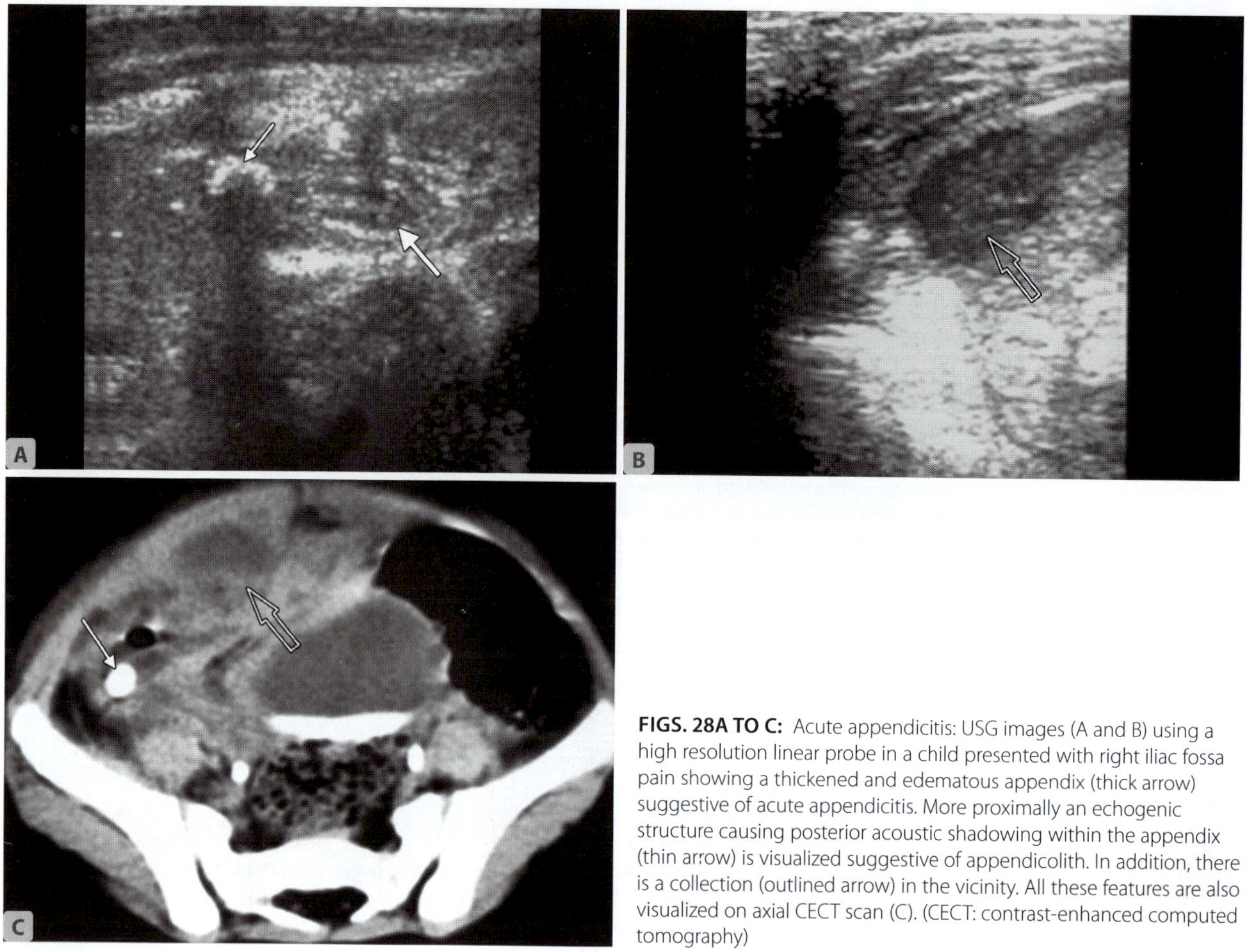

FIGS. 28A TO C: Acute appendicitis: USG images (A and B) using a high resolution linear probe in a child presented with right iliac fossa pain showing a thickened and edematous appendix (thick arrow) suggestive of acute appendicitis. More proximally an echogenic structure causing posterior acoustic shadowing within the appendix (thin arrow) is visualized suggestive of appendicolith. In addition, there is a collection (outlined arrow) in the vicinity. All these features are also visualized on axial CECT scan (C). (CECT: contrast-enhanced computed tomography)

modality to screening USG.[53-56] MRI and CT findings are essentially similar to what is seen on USG such as thickening of appendix and adjacent structures, periappendiceal inflammation or collection **(Fig. 28)**. T2 fat suppressed and not fat suppressed images are the important sequences used in the evaluation of acute appendicitis on MRI.

Neutropenic Enterocolitis

Neutropenic enterocolitis or typhlitis is a life-threatening condition predominantly affecting neutropenic children with leukemia/lymphoma on immunosuppressive therapy or any other cause of immunosuppression.[57] The exact underlying pathogenesis is not clear although it seems to be a combination of ischemia, infection, and inflammation leading to bacterial invasion into the cecal wall. Cecum is the most common site of involvement; however, it can also extend to other parts of colon. Commonly associated organisms are cytomegalovirus and pseudomonas.[58] This entity is usually associated with less inflammation due to the blunted host immune response which also leads to faster spread of infection. CT is the modality of choice for this entity which can show wall-thickening of cecum with or without surrounding collection or signs of perforation. Pneumatosis can also be seen in few cases. CT can be used in the follow-up of these patients to evaluate treatment response. USG can also be used as an alternative investigation in certain clinical situations and it can also show similar findings that of CT. However, these findings on CT as well as USG are nonspecific in nature and it has to be interpreted in the light of clinical features to arrive at a correct diagnosis.

Meckel Diverticulitis

Meckel diverticulum is the most common congenital structural abnormality of GIT which can be present in up to 2% of individuals.[18] It is an embryological remnant of omphalomesenteric duct which is located in the antimesenteric border of terminal ileum. Up to 60% of them can have heterotopic mucosa (mostly gastric mucosa).[59] Most of these are asymptomatic and they become symptomatic when they get complicated. Common complications are GI bleed, diverticulitis, small bowel obstruction and perforation. Rarely, it can present with malignancy as well. In uncomplicated diverticulum, it is difficult to detect them on USG or CT scan. On both, the imaging they may look similar to the surrounding bowel loops and, hence, easily missed. Nuclear scintigraphy using pertechnetate can be useful in up to 60% of cases in detecting them due to the tracer uptake by the ectopic gastric mucosa.[60]

INFLAMMATORY DISEASES

Necrotizing Enterocolitis

Necrotizing enterocolitis (NEC) is the most common bowel condition affecting the premature babies. It is a severe form of enterocolitis which can be potentially life-threatening and can be associated with significant morbidity. The factors which predispose to NEC are low birth weight, prematurity (90%), hypoxia, sepsis, and any other condition requiring intensive care.[61] Most of the children are <10 days old. The presenting symptoms are usually bilious vomiting, abdominal distention, and poor feeding. Precise pathogenesis of NEC is not yet clear; however, most accepted theory is that a combination of ischemia and inflammation affecting the bowel wall leading to increased permeability to intestinal microbes and eventually spread of infection. The most common site of NEC is distal ileum. Supine abdominal radiograph is the investigation of choice and it can be combined with lateral decubitus or cross-table lateral view to demonstrate free peritoneal air. Most common appearance on radiograph is dilated bowel loop which is a nonspecific finding. However, if the position of the dilated bowel loops is persistent over a period of 24–36 hours (persistent loop sign), it is considered as a specific sign of NEC.[62] Presence of pneumatosis intestinalis (bubbly appearance) with or without portal venous air is also a specific sign[63] **(Figs. 29A and B)**. Sometimes thumbprinting sign suggestive of wall edema of the dilated loop can also be seen. The role of bedside USG is coming up in the management of NEC which can show bowel wall-thickening, free fluid, collection and pneumatosis in the bowel wall **(Fig. 29C)**. USG may also show tiny bright echoes suggestive of air bubbles moving within the mesenteric veins and portal vein.

Eosinophilic Gastroenteritis

Eosinophilic gastroenteritis is a relatively uncommon entity which is characterized by diffuse infiltration of bowel wall by eosinophils.[64] It is a chronic inflammatory pathology and it is usually self-limiting and most of these patients have peripheral eosinophilia. It can involve any part of the GIT but gastric antrum is almost always involved. CT and USG are the commonly performed investigations which may show nonspecific features such as bowel wall-thickening **(Figs. 30A to D)**. Hence, sampling is necessary to make the diagnosis.

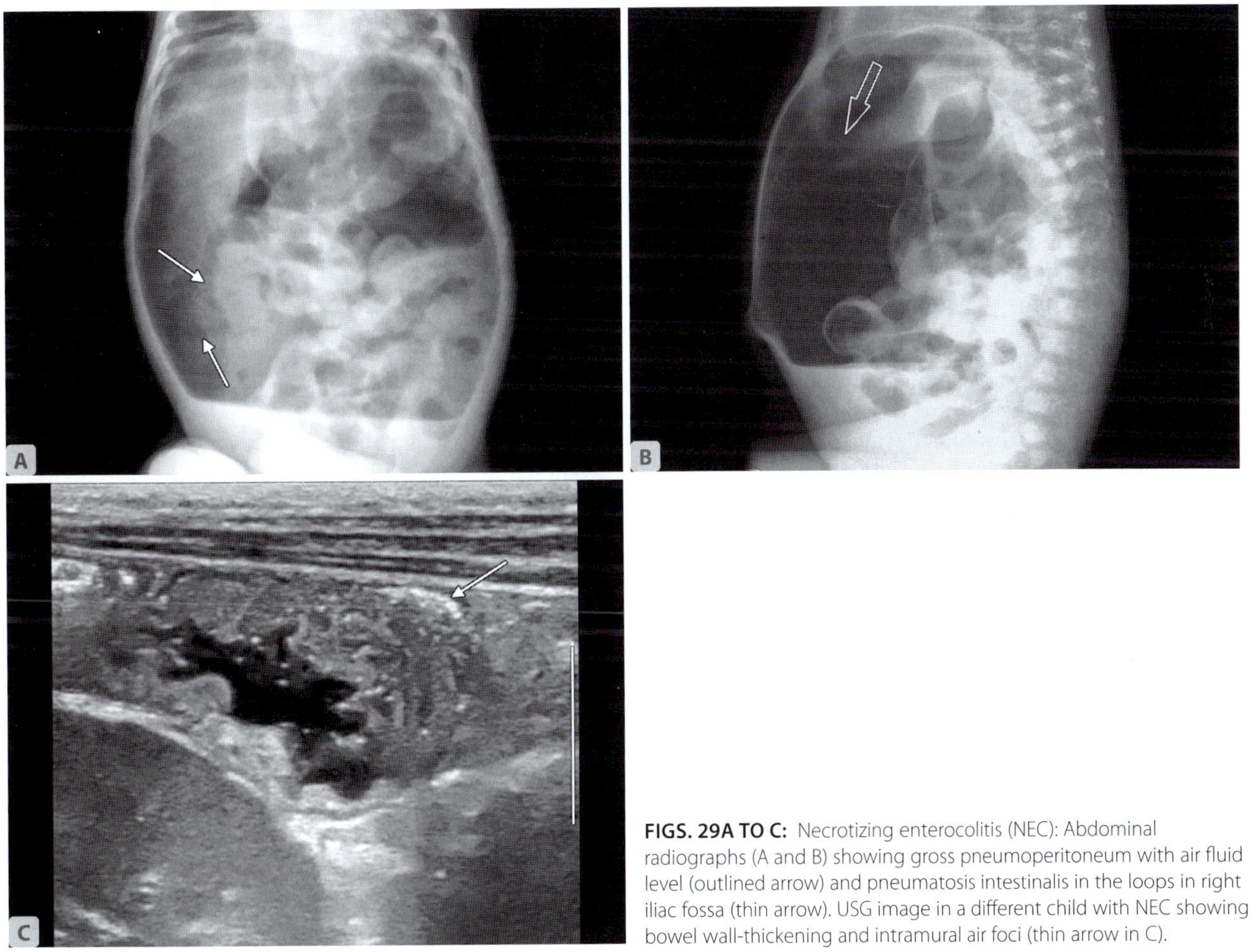

FIGS. 29A TO C: Necrotizing enterocolitis (NEC): Abdominal radiographs (A and B) showing gross pneumoperitoneum with air fluid level (outlined arrow) and pneumatosis intestinalis in the loops in right iliac fossa (thin arrow). USG image in a different child with NEC showing bowel wall-thickening and intramural air foci (thin arrow in C).

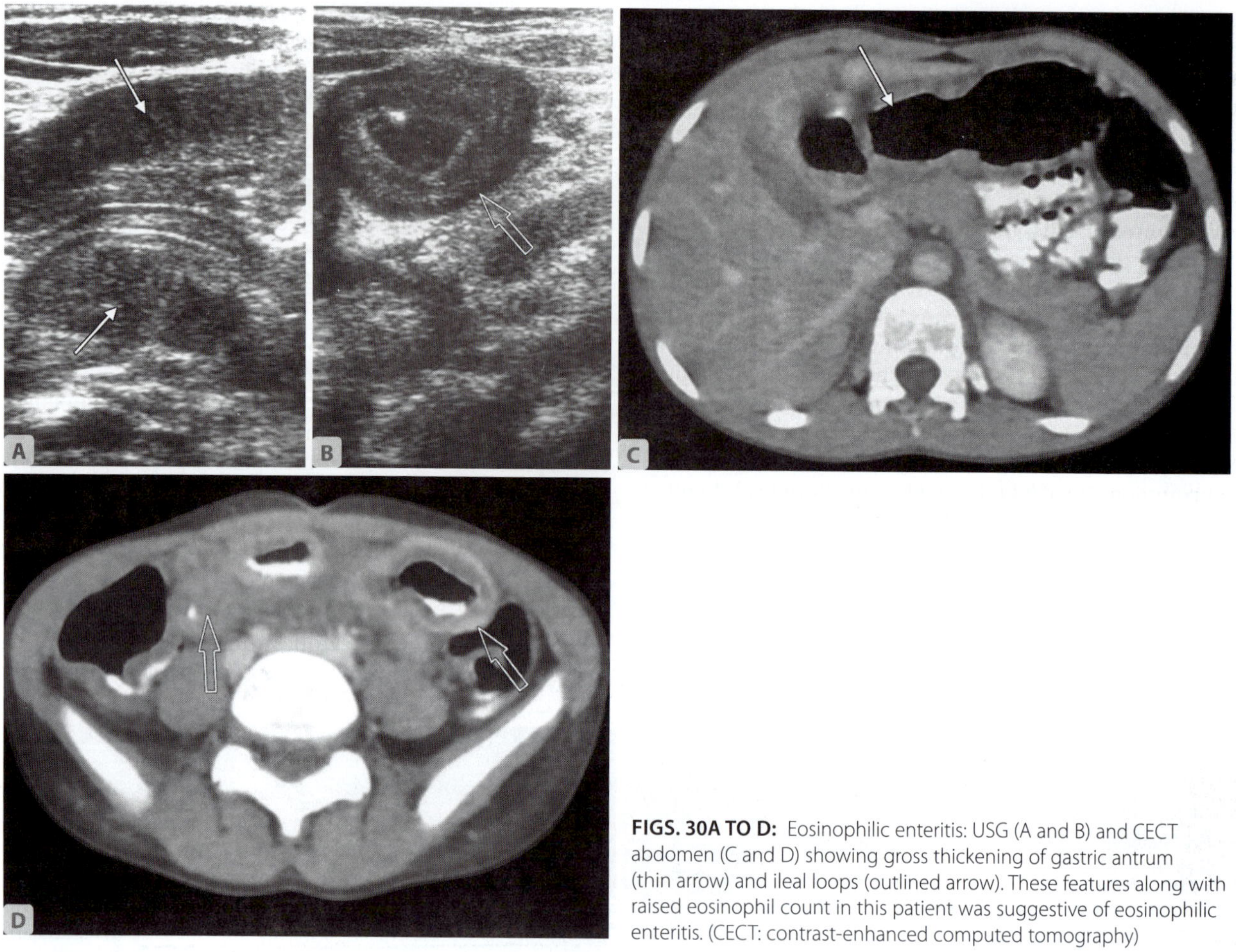

FIGS. 30A TO D: Eosinophilic enteritis: USG (A and B) and CECT abdomen (C and D) showing gross thickening of gastric antrum (thin arrow) and ileal loops (outlined arrow). These features along with raised eosinophil count in this patient was suggestive of eosinophilic enteritis. (CECT: contrast-enhanced computed tomography)

Crohn's Disease

Crohn's disease is a chronic idiopathic granulomatous inflammatory process affecting the GIT. It was considered to be the disease of the west till a decade or so ago. However, there is steady increase in the number of patients with CD in India as well.[65-67] Although less in number compared to adults the incidence of CD in children is increasing because of increased awareness among the pediatricians. Apart from GI involvement CD can present with a variety of extraintestinal manifestations such as hepatitis, cholangitis, arthritis, etc. CD is a transmural inflammatory pathology which can affect any part of GIT. Terminal ileum is the most commonly affected region in GI (about 70%) and, hence, it mimics TB a lot on imaging.[68] Colon is the second most common site of involvement. As discussed above there are features on imaging which can be used to differentiate CD from TB. Some of those features are quite nonspecific and, hence, it needs a systematic multidisciplinary approach to manage these patients. Imaging forms an integral part of this multidisciplinary team. Imaging modality of choice to evaluate these patients is enterography which can be performed either on CT or MRI. Enterography is a technique in which child is made to drink a large quantity (up to 900 mL or as much as possible) of diluted mannitol (or other osmotic solutions such as Peglec or Volumen®) over a period of 45 minutes which will distend the bowel loops during the examination.[69] Bowel distention facilitates better visualization of wall-thickening and enhancement on imaging. In children, MRE is the preferred modality over CTE both in baseline and follow-up. MRE has the advantage of better characterization of active versus fibrotic disease and lack of ionizing radiation. In contrast to adults performing enterography in children is a tedious task. It has to be tailored according to the age of the child and the local expertise available. In children over 7 years or so there is no need for sedation or anesthesia and procedure can be performed with their co-operation. In children of aged 4–7 years, decision should be based on whether the child can drink orally or not. Contrast can be administered through a nasogastric tube if the child is not able to drink the required amount of contrast. For children <4 years, the study needs to be performed under anesthesia with endotracheal intubation to prevent aspiartion.[69] After intubation, oral contrast can be administered using a nasogastric tube. Once the study is complete the stomach contents have to be emptied before extubating the child. The primary role of imaging in CD is to diagnose the disease, classify the phenotype, differentiating active from fibrotic disease, look for complications and assess response to treatment. Imaging features of active disease are wall-thickening with wall stratification and mucosal hyperenhancement, engorged and prominent vasa recta (comb sign), mesenteric edema, abnormal bowel motility and presence of abscess, sinuses, and fistulae **(Figs. 31 and 32)**. MRE is better than CTE in characterizing the activity by showing submucosal edema better on T2W images, changes in bowel motility, magnetization transfer property, and restriction of diffusion **(Figs. 33A and B)**. Imaging signs of healed disease are late progressive homogeneous enhancement of bowel wall, submucosal fatty infiltration, and pseudodiverticulum formation in the antimesenteric border and surrounding fibrofatty proliferation **(Figs. 34A to D)**. Bowel wall-thickening, reactive adenopathy, and stricture are nonspecific features which can be present in both active and healed disease. USG is an upcoming technique which when combined with contrast medium [contrast-enhanced ultrasound (CEUS)] has shown comparable accuracy to MRE for terminal ileal and IC junction disease. CEUS is not as effective as MRE/CTE for the evaluation of jejunal loop involvement. Imaging plays a critical role in the management of these patients by differentiating active from fibrotic disease because the management approach is quite different from one another. Strictures with activity will undergo medical therapy whereas those with fibrosis will undergo operative management.

Ulcerative Colitis

Ulcerative colitis (UC) is characterized by superficial inflammation of colonic mucosa almost always involving rectum. In contrast to CD, UC shows mucosal inflammation starting from rectum without any skip areas.[70] Since UC is primarily a mucosal disease and colorectal region is well evaluated by colonoscopy, imaging has a limited role in their management. Imaging is needed when colonoscopy

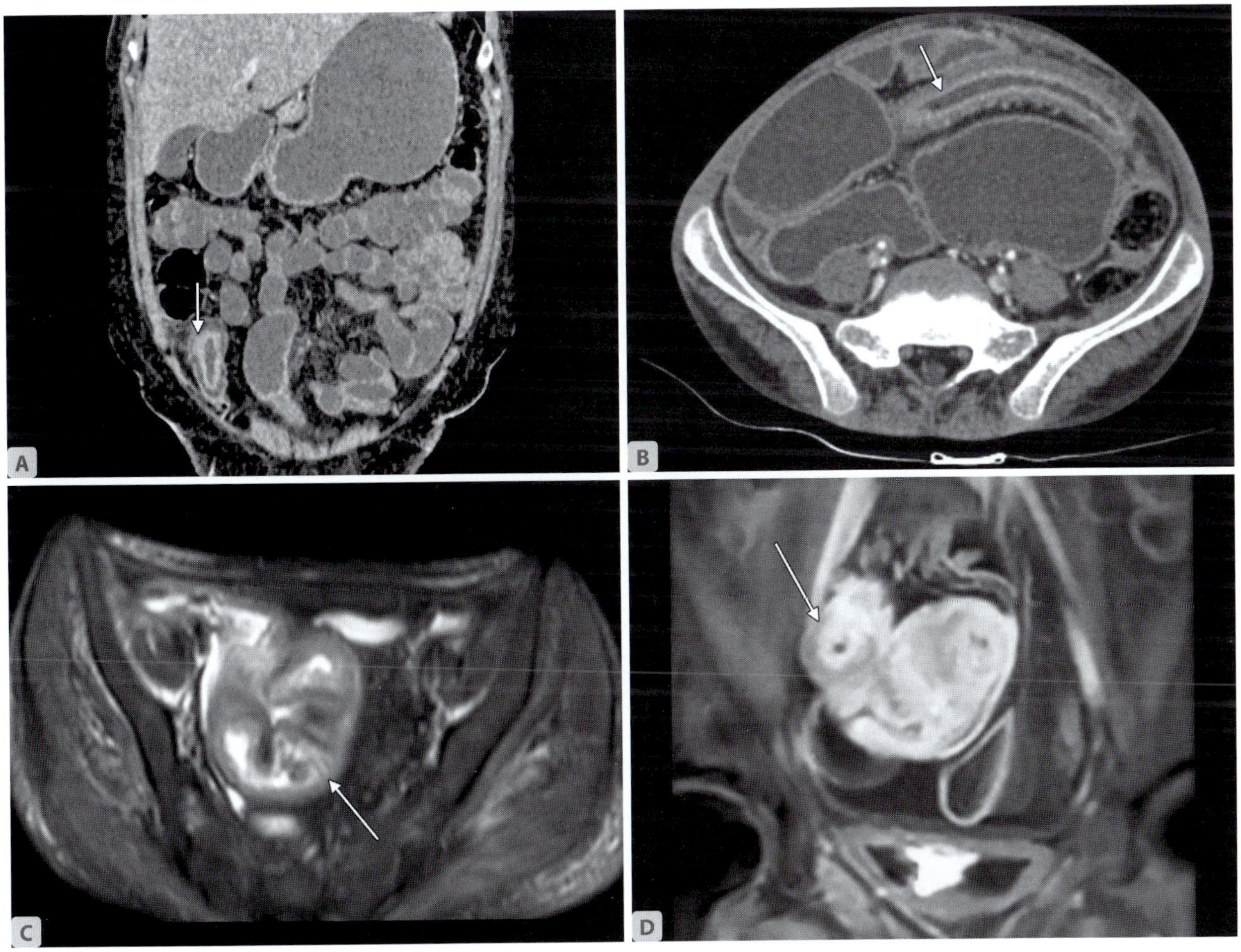

FIGS. 31A TO D: Active Crohn's disease (CD): Coronal and axial images of CT enterography (CTE) (A and B) showing wall-thickening with mural stratification (thin arrow) in the distal ileal loop. In another patient, magnetic resonance enterography (MRE) showing thickening and T2 hyperintensity (C) of distal ileal loops (thick arrow) which showed stratified mural enhancement (thin arrow) on postcontrast image (D). These changes are quite typical for active phase of CD.

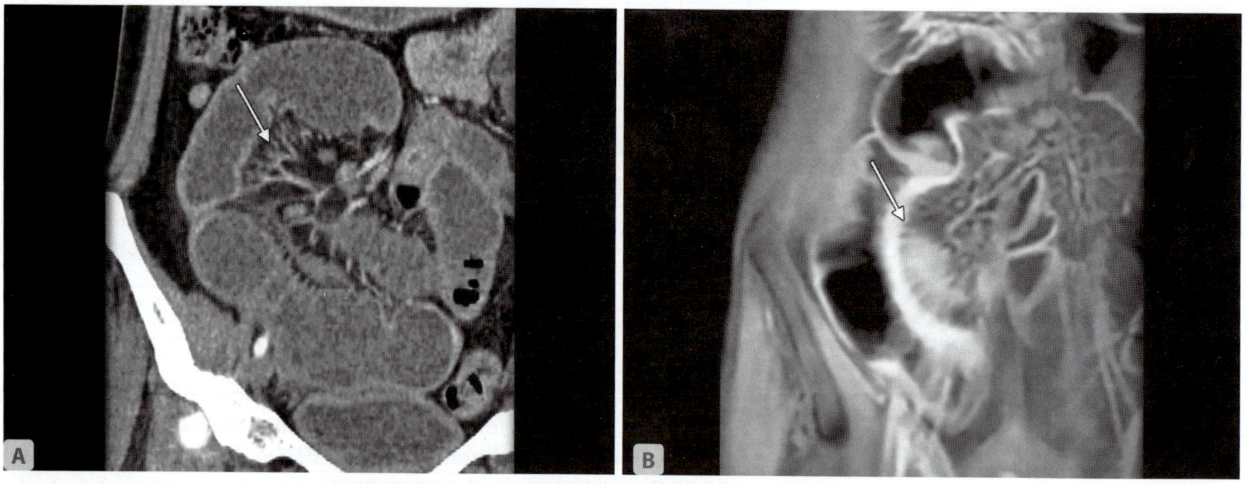

FIGS. 32A AND B: Comb sign: Coronal images of CT enterography (CTE) (A) and magnetic resonance enterography (MRE) (B) in separate patients showing prominent and engorged vasa recta (thin arrow) suggestive of comb sign. Also in image B there is asymmetrical thickening involving the mesenteric border of the ileal loop.

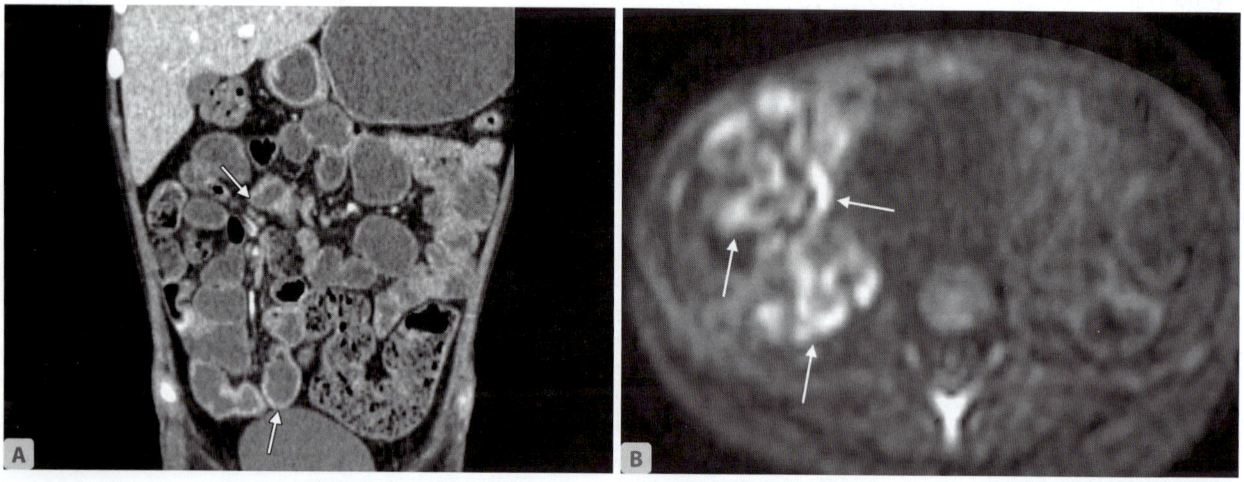

FIGS. 33A AND B: Crohn's Disease: Coronal reformat of CT enterography (CTE) (A) showing multiple short segment bowel wall-thickening (thin arrow) which are much better depicted on diffusion-weighted (DW) MR images (hyperintensities in image B) (thin arrow). This case demonstrates the utility of DWI in the detection of inflamed bowel segments in Crohn's disease.

is not feasible in situations such as fulminant colitis and toxic megacolon. Barium enema is rarely performed for this purpose nowadays which may show granular appearance of mucosa in acute phase and lead pipe appearance in chronic phase **(Fig. 35)**. USG and CT can also show features of wall-thickening and submucosal edema in the involved part of colon.

Celiac Disease

Celiac disease or nontropical sprue is the most common gluten-related disease which is characterized by atrophy of villi in proximal bowel and malabsorption.[71] Common presentation in children includes constipation, abdominal pain, iron deficiency anemia, and failure to thrive. It is considered as a T-cell mediated autoimmune disease with a recognized genetic predisposition. Biopsy obtained by endoscopy is the gold standard for the diagnosis which can be supported by high serum level of anti-tissue transglutaminase.[72] Imaging features are quite nonspecific and not accurate enough to make a diagnosis of celiac disease. Barium studies can show mild dilatation of small bowel loops due to excess fluid, diluted barium, loss of folds

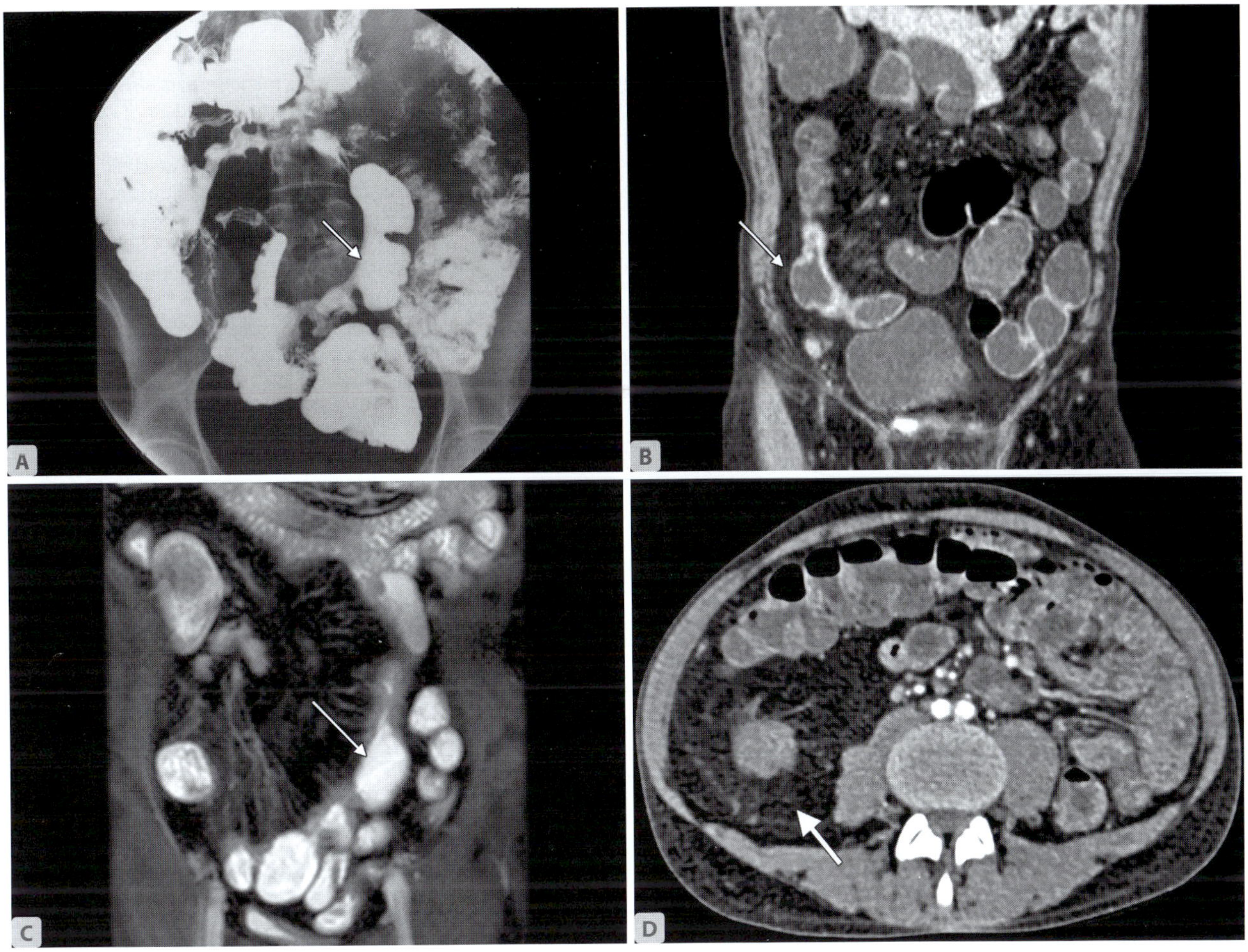

FIGS. 34A TO D: Fibrotic Crohn's disease (CD): BaMFT (A), CTE (B), and MRE (C) images of three different patients showing pseudodiverticulum (thin arrow) formation in the antimesenteric border of ileal loops. CTE image in axial plane (D) showing wall-thickening of ascending colon with poor enhancement and surrounding fibrofatty proliferation (thick arrow). These features are typical for fibrotic type of CD. (BaMFT: barium meal follow through; CTE: CT enterography; MRE: magnetic resonance enterography)

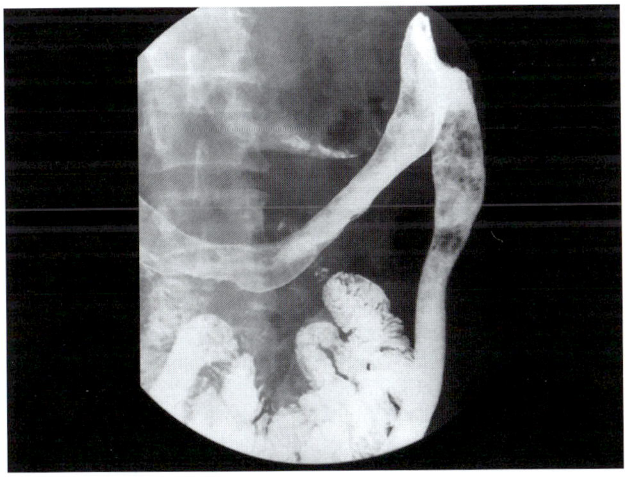

FIG. 35: Ulcerative colitis: Barium study of a patient with a long-standing history of ulcerative colitis showing featureless appearance of colon with associated mild narrowing and shortening suggestive of lead pipe colon.

in jejunum and increased folds in ileum, segmentation, and flocculation of barium.[18] Cross-sectional modalities are usually not useful for the diagnosis, however, they can show enlarged mesenteric nodes with fat-fluid level. These modalities are useful when patients develop complications such as lymphoma (usually T cell) and adenocarcinoma.

CONCLUSION

Imaging of GIT is a challenging problem especially in children. It is imperative for the radiologists to be aware of the spectrum of disorders affecting this age group and the choice of imaging modalities for a given clinical situation. USG still plays an important role as a screening modality in the evaluation of abdominal pathologies. When USG findings are inadequate or equivocal, CT or MRI can be used depending on the clinical suspicion and availability.

REFERENCES

1. Cairo MS, Grosfeld JL, Weetman RM. Gastric teratoma: unusual cause for bleeding of the upper gastrointestinal tract in the newborn. Pediatrics. 1981;67:721-4.
2. Golden CB, Feusner JH. Malignant abdominal masses in children: quick guide to evaluation and diagnosis. Pediatr Clin North Am. 2002;49:1369-92, viii.
3. Superina RA, Ein SH, Humphreys RP. Cystic duplications of the esophagus and neurenteric cysts. J Pediatr Surg. 1984;19:527-30.
4. Gupta AK, Berry M, Mitra DK. Gastric duplication cyst in children: report of two cases. Pediatr Radiol. 1994;24:346-7.
5. Teele RL, Smith EH. Ultrasound in the diagnosis of idiopathic hypertrophic pyloric stenosis. N Engl J Med. 1977;296:1149-50.
6. Hayden CK, Swischuk LE, Lobe TE, Schwartz MZ, Boulden T. Ultrasound: The definitive imaging modality in pyloric stenosis. Radiographics. 1984;4:517-30.
7. Hallam D, Hansen B, Bødker B, Klintorp S, Pedersen JF. Pyloric size in normal infants and in infants suspected of having hypertrophic pyloric stenosis. Acta Radiol Stockh Swed. 1987;36:261-4.
8. Neilson D, Hollman AS. The ultrasonic diagnosis of infantile hypertrophic pyloric stenosis: technique and accuracy. Clin Radiol. 1994;49:246-7.
9. Hernanz-Schulman M, Sells LL, Ambrosino MM, Heller RM, Stein SM, Neblett WW 3rd. Hypertrophic pyloric stenosis in the infant without a palpable olive: accuracy of sonographic diagnosis. Radiology. 1994;193:771-6.
10. Blumhagen JD, Noble HG. Muscle thickness in hypertrophic pyloric stenosis: sonographic determination. AJR Am J Roentgenol. 1983;140:221-3.
11. Kandasamy D, Sharma R, Gupta AK. Bowel Imaging in Children: Part 1. Indian J Pediatr. 2019;86:805-16.
12. Murphy S, Shaw K, Blanchard H. Report of three gastric tumors in children. J Pediatr Surg. 1994;29:1202-4.
13. Mathew M, Gupta A, Narula MK, Anand R, Jain AK, Chandha R. Gastric teratoma: a report of B cases. Indian J Radiol Imaging. 2002;12:507-10.
14. Sugandhi N, Gupta AK, Bhatnagar V. Gastric teratoma: unusual location and difficulties in diagnosis. Trop Gastroenterol. 2012;33:75-7.
15. Gupta AK, Berry M, Mitra DK. Ossified gastric leiomyoma in a child: a case report. Pediatr Radiol. 1995;25:48-9.
16. Navarro O, Dugougeat F, Daneman A. Sonographic signs that characterize the gastrointestinal origin of abdominal neoplasms in children: 4 case reports. Can Assoc Radiol J. 2000;51;250-3.
17. Bluth EI, Merritt CRB, Sullivan MA. Ultrasonic Evaluation of the Stomach, Small Bowel, and Colon. Radiology. 1979;133:677-80.
18. Kandasamy D, Sharma R, Gupta AK. Bowel Imaging in Children: Part 2. Indian J Pediatr. 2019;86:817-29.
19. Thompson WM, Kende AI, Levy AD. Imaging characteristics of gastric lipomas in 16 adult and pediatric patients. AJR Am J Roentgenol. 2003;181:981-5.
20. Dixon WL, Fazzari PJ. Carcinoma of the stomach in a child. JAMA. 1976;235:2414-5.
21. Dunnick NR, Harell GS, Parker BR. Multiple 'bull's-eye' lesions in gastric lymphoma. AJR Am J Roentgenol. 1976;126:965-9.
22. Ng YY, Healy JC, Vincent JM, Kingston JE, Armstrong P, Reznek RH. The radiology of non-Hodgkin's lymphoma in childhood: a review of 80 cases. Clin Radiol. 1994;49:594-600.
23. Kurugoglu S, Mihmanli I, Celkan T, Aki H, Aksoy H, Korman U . Radiological features in paediatric primary gastric MALT lymphoma and association with Helicobacter pylori. Pediatr Radiol. 200;32:82-7.
24. Newman B, Girdany BR. Gastric trichobezoars—sonographic and computed tomographic appearance. Pediatr Radiol. 1990;20: 526-7.
25. Barr LL, Hayden CK, Stansberry SD, Swischuk LE. Enteric duplication cysts in children: are their ultrasonographic wall characteristics diagnostic? Pediatr Radiol. 1990;20:326-8.
26. Macpherson RI. Gastrointestinal tract duplications: clinical, pathologic, etiologic, and radiologic considerations. Radiographics. 1993;13:1063-80.
27. Spottswood SE. Peristalsis in duplication cyst: a new diagnostic sonographic finding. Pediatr Radiol. 1994;24:344-5.
28. Bhat NA, Agarwala S, Wadhwa S, Gupta AK, Bhatnagar V. Thoracoabdominal intestinal duplication with absent inferior vena cava. Pediatr Surg Int. 2001;17:540-2.
29. Gupta AK, Berry M, Mitra DK. Gastrointestinal smooth muscle tumors in children: report of three cases. Pediatr Radiol. 1994;24:498-9.
30. Chattopadhyay A, Kumar V, Maruliah M, Rao PLNG. Duodeno-jejunal obstruction by a hemangioma. Pediatr Surg Int. 2002;18:501-2.
31. Sargent MA, Babyn P, Alton DJ. Plain abdominal radiography in suspected intussusception: a reassessment. Pediatr Radiol. 1994;24:17-20.
32. Bowerman RA, Silver TM, Jaffe MH. Real-time ultrasound diagnosis of intussusception in children. Radiology. 1982;143:527-9.
33. Harrington L, Connolly B, Hu X, Wesson DE, Babyn P, Schuh S. Ultrasonographic and clinical predictors of intussusception. J Pediatr. 1998;132:836-9.
34. Gupta AK, Berry M, Bhargava PS. Atypical Target Pattern: Sonography in GIT lesions. Australas Radiol. 1987;31:281-6.
35. Gupta AK, Berry M, Bhargava S. Sonographic double target in a case of type Ia cecal duplication cyst. J Clin Ultrasound JCU. 1987;15:273-5.
36. del-Pozo G, Albillos JC, Tejedor D, Calero R, Rasero M, de-la-Calle U, et al. Intussusception in children: current concepts in diagnosis and enema reduction. Radiogr Rev Publ Radiol Soc N Am Inc. 1999;19:299-319.
37. Chan KL, Saing H, Peh WC, Mya GH, Cheng W, Khong PL, et al. Childhood intussusception: ultrasound-guided Hartmann's solution hydrostatic reduction or barium enema reduction? J Pediatr Surg. 1997;32:3-6.
38. Swischuk LE. The current radiologic management of intussusception: a survey and review. Pediatr Radiol. 1992;22:317.
39. Haney PJ, Whitley NO. CT of benign cystic abdominal masses in children. AJR Am J Roentgenol. 1984;142:1279-81.
40. Konen O, Rathaus V, Dlugy E, Freud E, Kessler A, Shapiro M, et al. Childhood abdominal cystic lymphangioma. Pediatr Radiol. 2002;32:88-94.
41. Zarewych ZM, Donnelly LF, Frush DP, Bisset GS. Imaging of pediatric mesenteric abnormalities. Pediatr Radiol. 1999;29:711-9.
42. Jewell CT, Miller ID, Ehrlich FE. Rectal duplication: an unusual cause for an abdominal mass. Surgery. 1973;74:783-5.
43. Bhadoo D, Chand K, Jana M, Gupta AK, Bhatnagar V. Colonic duplication: Treatment by limited division of common wall. J Indian Assoc Pediatr Surg. 2015;20:146-7.
44. Karnak I, Ciftci AO, Senocak ME, Büyükpamukçu N. Colorectal carcinoma in children. J Pediatr Surg. 1999;34:1499-504.
45. Radhakrishnan CN, Bruce J. Colorectal cancers in children without any predisposing factors. A report of eight cases and review of the literature. Eur J Pediatr Surg.2003;13:66-8.

46. Karnak I, Kale G, Tanyel FC, Büyükpamukçu N. Malignant stromal tumor of the colon in an infant: diagnostic difficulties and differential diagnosis. J Pediatr Surg. 2003;38:245-7.
47. World Health Organization. (2020). Tuberculosis (TB). [online] Available from https://www.who.int/news-room/fact-sheets/detail/tuberculosis. [Last accessed September, 2020].
48. Sharma R, Madhusudhan KS, Ahuja V. Intestinal tuberculosis versus crohn's disease: Clinical and radiological recommendations. Indian J Radiol Imaging. 2016;26:161-72.
49. Debi U, Ravisankar V, Prasad KK, Sinha SK, Sharma AK. Abdominal tuberculosis of the gastrointestinal tract: Revisited. World J Gastroenterol WJG. 2014;20:14831-40.
50. da Rocha EL, Pedrassa BC, Bormann RL, Kierszenbaum ML, Torres LR, D'Ippolito G. Abdominal tuberculosis: a radiological review with emphasis on computed tomography and magnetic resonance imaging findings. Radiol Bras. 2015;48:181-91.
51. de Souza SC, da Costa SRMR, de Souza IGS. Vermiform appendix: positions and length—a study of 377 cases and literature review. J Coloproctology. 2015;35;212-6.
52. Swenson DW, Ayyala RS, Sams C, Lee EY. Practical Imaging Strategies for Acute Appendicitis in Children. Am J Roentgenol. 2018;211:901-9.
53. Thieme ME, Leeuwenburgh MM, Valdehueza ZD, Bouman DE, de Bruin IG, Schreurs WH, et al. Diagnostic accuracy and patient acceptance of MRI in children with suspected appendicitis. Eur Radiol. 2014;24:630-7.
54. Dibble EH, Swenson DW, Cartagena C, Baird GL, Herliczek TW. Effectiveness of a Staged US and Unenhanced MR Imaging Algorithm in the Diagnosis of Pediatric Appendicitis. Radiology. 2018;286:1022-9.
55. Dillman JR, Gadepalli S, Sroufe NS, Davenport MS, Smith EA, Chong ST, et al. Equivocal Pediatric Appendicitis: Unenhanced MR Imaging Protocol for Nonsedated Children—A Clinical Effectiveness Study. Radiology. 2015;279:216-25.
56. Mushtaq R, Desoky SM, Morello F, Gilbertson-Dahdal D, Gopalakrishnan G, Leetch A, et al. First-line Diagnostic Evaluation with MRI of Children Suspected of Having Acute Appendicitis. Radiology. 2019;291:170-7.
57. Rodrigues FG, Dasilva G, Wexner SD. Neutropenic enterocolitis. World J Gastroenterol. 2017;23:42-7.
58. Machado NO. Neutropenic enterocolitis: A continuing medical and surgical challenge. North Am J Med Sci. 2010;2:293-300.
59. Dillon PA, Warner BW. Chapter 89: Gastrointestinal Bleeding. in: Coran AG (Ed). Pediatric Surgery (Seventh Edition). United States: Mosby; 2012. pp. 1147-54.
60. Swaniker F, Soldes O, Hirschl RB. The utility of technetium 99m pertechnetate scintigraphy in the evaluation of patients with Meckel's diverticulum. J Pediatr Surg. 1999;34:760-4; discussion 765.
61. Gephart SM, McGrath JM, Effken JA, Halpern MD. Necrotizing Enterocolitis Risk. Adv Neonatal Care. 2012;12:77-89.
62. Caplan M. Chapter 73: Necrotizing Enterocolitis and Short Bowel Syndrome. in: Gleason CA, Devaskar SU (Eds). Avery's Diseases of the Newborn (Ninth Edition). Philadelphia: WB Saunders; 2012. pp. 1022-9.
63. Epelman M, Daneman A, Navarro OM, Morag I, Moore AM, Kim JH, et al. Necrotizing enterocolitis: review of state-of-the-art imaging findings with pathologic correlation. Radiographics. 2007;27:285-305.
64. Sunkara T, Rawla P, Yarlagadda KS, Gaduputi V. Eosinophilic gastroenteritis: diagnosis and clinical perspectives. Clin Exp Gastroenterol. 2019;12:239-53.
65. Makharia GK. Rising incidence and prevalence of Crohn's disease in Asia: Is it apparent or real? J Gastroenterol Hepatol. 2006;21:929-31.
66. Makharia GK, Ramakrishna BS, Abraham P, Choudhuri G, Misra SP, Ahuja V, et al. Survey of inflammatory bowel diseases in India. Indian J Gastroenterol. 2012;31:299-306.
67. Ray G. Inflammatory bowel disease in India—Past, present, and future. World J Gastroenterol. 2016;22:8123-36.
68. Caprilli R. Why does Crohn's disease usually occur in terminal ileum? J Crohns Colitis. 2008;2:352-6.
69. Mollard BJ, Smith EA, Dillman JR. Pediatric MR Enterography: Technique and Approach to Interpretation—How We Do It. Radiology. 2014;274:29-43.
70. Jung SA. Differential Diagnosis of Inflammatory Bowel Disease: What Is the Role of Colonoscopy? Clin Endosc. 2012;45:254-62.
71. Dickson BC, Streutker CJ, Chetty R. Coeliac disease: an update for pathologists. J Clin Pathol. 2006;59:1008-16.
72. Webb C, Norström F, Myléus A, Ivarsson A, Halvarsson B, Högberg L, et al. Celiac disease can be predicted by high levels of anti-tissue transglutaminase antibodies in population-based screening. J Pediatr Gastroenterol Nutr. 2015;60:787-91.

CHAPTER

70

Hepatic and Pancreatic Masses in Children

Kushaljit Singh Sodhi, Akshay Kumar Saxena, Anmol Bhatia

INTRODUCTION

Focal hepatic masses in children include benign lesions such as cysts (congenital, i.e., simple or acquired like hydatid cysts), abscesses, granulomas, and neoplasms (benign and malignant tumors, primary, and metastatic lesions). Malignant neoplasms and abscesses are more common than simple cysts and benign tumors.

Pancreatic tumors are rare in infants and children. They can be cystic or solid, benign or malignant, and endocrine or exocrine in origin. Pancreatoblastoma, islet cell tumors, and solid and papillary epithelial neoplasms (SPEN) are the most important tumors of childhood. Pseudocysts of pancreas secondary to pancreatitis are more common than cystic tumors of the pancreas.

IMAGING

Plain radiography is of limited diagnostic value in the evaluation of pediatric masses. Calcification in tumors such as hepatoblastoma and pancreatoblastoma may be detected on abdominal radiographs. Pulmonary complications such as basal pneumonitis, pleural effusions in hepatic abscesses, and pulmonary metastasis may be seen on chest radiographs.

Ultrasonography (US) and computed tomography (CT) remain the primary imaging modalities for investigating hepatic and pancreatic masses. Majority of the lesions, particularly tumors, require more than one modality to reach at a definitive diagnosis. US is the initial investigation of choice as the location, nature of the lesion (cystic or solid), relationship to adjacent organs, associated lymphadenopathy, and invasion of the vascular structures by the mass can all be well seen on US. In children, US has the ability to visualize the entire pancreas well because of the relatively large left lobe of liver as an acoustic window during scanning. Color Doppler flow imaging and intraoperative US further help in the diagnosis and patient's management.[1]

Once a mass is suspected to be a tumor, contrast-enhanced CT scan should be performed as it is more accurate than US in distinguishing various neoplastic lesions and it has the best capability to assess extrahepatic spread of the disease such as lymphadenopathy and omental or peritoneal spread.[1] However, it is important to note a few technical considerations while performing the CT scan. Many of the patients require sedation for performing a technically satisfactory study. Generally, the sedation is provided by the anesthetists. The radiologist should ensure that the patient undergoes preanesthetic checkup prior to the date of appointment. In addition, need for keeping the child nil orally on the day of appointment should be carefully impressed upon. Failure to adhere to these precautions may lead to postponement of study. The nil per oral guidelines are less stringent for smaller children and for clear fluids **(Table 1)**.[2]

With the advent of multidetector spiral CT, it is now possible to image the abdomen during the arterial and portal venous phases. Lu et al.,[3] however, have advocated that imaging of the pancreas should be done in the "pancreatic phase" only. This phase occurs in the interval between the arterial and portal venous phase at 40–70 seconds after the bolus injection of contrast at a rate of 3 mL/sec. During this phase there is maximum pancreatic parenchymal enhancement with accentuation of the lesion-to-pancreas contrast. The use of this phase alone has the benefit of reducing the radiation exposure to the patient. Single phase evaluation of focal hepatic lesions is also recommended by "image gently" campaign.[4] Apart from doing the single phase studies, it is important to carefully adjust the kV and mAs according to the weight of the child.[2] This will avoid unnecessary high radiation to these children. Most of the vendors now provide for children-specific scanning protocols and radiologists should ensure that technologists are adhering to these protocols.

TABLE 1: Nil per oral guidelines for computed tomography (CT) scan.[2]

Age	Solids and milk/formula	Clear liquids
>3 years	Stop 6–8 h before sedation	Stop 2–3 h before sedation
6 months to 3 years	Stop 6 h before sedation	Stop 2–3 h before sedation
<6 months	Stop 4–6 h before sedatio	Stop 2 h before sedation

Magnetic resonance imaging (MRI) is superior to both US and CT in characterizing the lesion and showing its extent, particularly vascular invasion,[5,6] but it is reserved as a problem-solving modality because of its inherent limitations namely high cost, lack of easy availability and compulsory sedation in nearly all infants and children which makes its routine use impractical. However, due to the lack of ionizing radiation and multiplanar imaging capabilities, MR and magnetic resonance cholangiopancreatography (MRCP) are especially useful in the pediatric population.

Radionuclide scanning of the liver using ^{99m}Tc-sulfur colloid has a sensitivity and specificity of 80–85% each. It can be supplemented with single photon emission computed tomography (SPECT) which can detect lesions as small as 1 cm diameter (sensitivity and specificity of 90–95% each). Regarding characterization of a known hepatic mass, ^{99m}Tc-labelled red blood cell (RBC) scanning has the greatest utility in diagnosing cavernous hemangiomas by achieving a specificity of nearly 100% (barring occasional false positives due to small hepatocellular carcinomas (HCC) or hypervascular metastasis).[7]

Angiography has limited role except for the vascular road-mapping of tumors when surgery or therapeutic embolization is considered.

Imaging, usually US, may also be required for providing guidance for interventional procedures such as fine-needle aspiration cytology (FNAC).

HEPATIC MASSES

Table 2 summarizes the salient features of common malignant and benign hepatic lesions in children across the different age groups. Of note, one should remember that although the lesions usually are seen in a particular age group, at times, they may have an atypical age of presentation.

Malignant Hepatic Tumors

Primary malignant hepatic tumors constitute nearly 1.5% of all pediatric tumors and 15% of all abdominal masses in children.[8] About two-thirds of these are malignant, of which hepatoblastoma, HCC, and rarely sarcomas constitute the majority.[5,9]

Hepatoblastoma

The term "hepatoblastoma" was coined by Willis in 1962 for hepatic tumors of embryonal origin which were histologically different from HCC.[10] Hepatoblastoma is the most frequent malignancy of liver in children and is seen at <5 years of age.[2,11] The peak incidence occurs between 18 and 24 months of age. The patient usually presents with an abdominal mass but less frequently anorexia, weight loss, jaundice, and pain due to hemorrhage or rupture may be the presenting features. A number of conditions such as Beckwith-Wiedemann syndrome, hemihypertrophy, familial adenomatous polyposis (FAP), Gardner syndrome, Wilms' tumor, sexual precocity, and osteopenia can be associated with hepatoblastoma. Serum alpha-fetoprotein (AFP) is elevated in about 80% of these patients.[9]

Pathologically, hepatoblastoma contains small and primitive epithelial cells resembling those in fetal liver tissue. When mesenchymal elements such as osteoids are also present in addition to epithelial elements, the hepatoblastoma is classified as mixed variant. There is no significant survival difference between the epithelial and mixed forms of hepatoblastoma. Vascular invasion is less frequent compared to HCC. Calcification may be present. The tumor metastasizes most commonly to the lungs followed by lymph nodes, brain, peritoneum, and diaphragm.

Several methods are available for staging of hepatoblastoma.[12] The most commonly used is PRETEXT (PRE-Treatment EXTent of tumor) system which was introduced in 1992 and has become the primary method of risk stratification for hepatoblastoma in numerous multicenter trials across the world. The PRETEXT system is made of two components: (1) The PRETEXT group and (2) The annotation factors. The liver, in this system, is divided by the hepatic veins and portal veins into its four sections: (1) Left lateral (Couinaud segments 2 and 3), (2) Left medial (segments 4a and 4b), (3) Right anterior (segments 5 and 8), and (4) Right posterior (segments 6 and 7). The PRETEXT group number reflects the maximum number of contiguous liver sections that are free of tumor **(Table 3)**.[12] The annotation factors include V (hepatic venous/inferior vena cava involvement), P (portal venous involvement), E (extrahepatic disease contiguous with the main liver tumor), F (multifocality), R (tumor rupture), C (caudate lobe involvement), N (lymph node metastases), and M (distant metastases). The PRETEXT annotation factors are summarized in **Table 4**.[13]

On imaging, hepatoblastoma is generally seen as a single, well-defined lesion with lobulated outline, mostly located in the right lobe. Less commonly, the lesion may involve the left lobe or even be multicentric. On US, the lesion has generally inhomogeneous echotexture, may be hyperechoic[14] with anechoic areas corresponding to necrosis or hemorrhage. Calcifications in the lesion appear as echogenic foci with distal shadowing. A rare cystic form of hepatoblastoma has also been described which is completely anechoic on US but may reveal mural nodule.[11] Hepatoblastoma may also appear as diffuse parenchymal inhomogeneity with multiple cystic lesions.[15] In case of vascular invasion, portal vein may show intraluminal thrombus. On Doppler studies, peak systolic Doppler frequency shifts in the hepatic artery are usually >4 KHz.[9] If available, noncontrast CT **(Fig. 1A)** scan generally reveals hypodense or isodense and calcification may be detected in as many as 50% of cases.[16] Calcification is typically coarse and dense. On CECT, hepatoblastoma appears as low attenuating mass which may show inhomogeneous enhancement **(Fig. 1B)**. In the early phase of dynamic CT, the tumor may appear hyperdense and show rim enhancement indicating increased vascularity. The septations within the tumor are best seen after contrast enhancement **(Fig. 2)**.

On MRI, hepatoblastoma appears as a low-intensity mass on T1-weighted image (T1WI) and increased signal intensity mass on T2-weighted image (T2WI) **(Figs. 3A and B)**. It shows heterogenous postcontrast enhancement **(Fig. 3C)**. Hypointense bands (corresponding to fibrotic areas) may be seen on both T1W and T2W images. Tumor thrombus in the

TABLE 2: Summarizing the salient features of common hepatic lesions in children.

Lesion	Salient clinical and laboratory features	Salient radiological features
Age group: Up to 5 years		
Hepatoblastoma	AFP elevated	Coarse and chunky calcifications, solid mass, may show invasion of veins, enhancement is usually less than adjacent liver
Embryonal rhabdomyosarcoma	AFP normal	Intraductal growth pattern
Hemangioma	AFP normal, child may present with cardiac heart failure/coagulopathy/ hypothyroidism	Shows fine granular pattern of calcification, enhances more than the adjacent liver, early peripheral nodular enhancement with gradual central filling in small lesions while larger lesions usually show incomplete filling with central hypodense areas representing fibrosis and thrombus
Mesenchymal hamartoma	AFP normal	Cystic lesion showing enhancement of septa and solid portion No foci of calcification
Metastases	Present or past history of primary malignant lesion	Usually multifocal
Age group: 6–10 years		
Undifferentiated embryonal sarcoma	AFP normal	Solid on ultrasound, cystic appearance on CT and MRI, shows enhancement of the solid portion and septa
Metastases	Present or past history of primary malignant lesion	Usually multifocal
Hydatid cyst	Endemicity or history of travel to endemic area	Cystic lesion with varied appearances, focus of calcification
Simple cyst	Incidental	Cystic lesion with no enhancement
Age group: >10 years		
Hepatocellular carcinoma	AFP elevated, underlying predisposing liver disease (like biliary atresia, hereditary tyrosinemia, glycogen storage disorder, etc.)	Solid, focal or multifocal, heterogeneous with areas of hemorrhage and necrosis, may show invasion of veins
Fibrolamellar carcinoma	AFP normal	No underlying liver disease, solitary mass, homogeneous, nonenhancing central fibrous scar which is hypointense on T2WI
Focal nodular hyperplasia	AFP normal, strong predilection for girls	Homogeneous enhancement, central vascular and myxoid scar which is hyperintense on T2WI and shows delayed enhancement
Adenoma	AFP normal, history of use of oral contraceptive or androgenic steroid use or presence of glycogen storage disease	No central scar, heterogeneous in appearance with areas of fat/ hemorrhage, areas of fat suppression seen suggesting presence of fat and glycogen
Metastases	Present or past history of primary malignant lesion	Usually multifocal
Hydatid cyst	Endemicity or history of travel to endemic area	Cystic lesion with varied appearances, focus of calcification
Simple cyst	Incidental	Cystic lesion with no enhancement

(AFP: alpha-fetoprotein; T2WI: T2-weighted images)

TABLE 3: PRETEXT staging of hepatic tumors.[12]

PRETEXT-I	One section is involved and three adjoining sections are free
PRETEXT-II	One or two sections are involved, but two adjoining sections are free
PRETEXT-III	Two or three sections are involved and no two adjoining sections are free
PRETEXT-IV	All four sections are involved

(PRETEXT: PRE-Treatment EXTent of tumor)

hepatic or portal vein appears as an area of increased signal intensity in the normal flow of vessels. MRI is better than CT and US for demonstration of tumor margins and vascular invasion. However, CT is superior for detecting calcification.

Hepatocellular Carcinoma

This tumor generally occurs in children older than 5 years. There are two age peaks in childhood, the first is between 2 and 4 years and the second one occurs between 12 and 14 years.[17] Childhood HCC (hepatocellular carcinoma) is

TABLE 4: Summarizing the PRETEXT annotation factors.[13]

Factor	Annotation	Positive definition
Hepatic venous/inferior vena cava involvement	V	Any of the following is met: • The tumor is obliterating all the three first-order hepatic veins or the intrahepatic IVC • The tumor is encasing (>50% or 180°) all three first-order hepatic veins or the intrahepatic IVC • Tumor thrombus seen in any one (or more) of the first-order hepatic vein or the intrahepatic IVC
Portal venous involvement	P	Any of the following is met: • The tumor is obliterating either both first-order portal veins or the main portal vein (MPV) • The tumor is encasing (>50% or 180°) either both first-order portal veins or the MPV • Tumor thrombus seen in either or both the right and left portal veins, or the MPV
Extrahepatic disease contiguous with the main liver tumor	E	Any of the following is met: • Tumor crosses boundaries/tissue planes • Tumor is surrounded by normal tissue >180° • Peritoneal nodules (not lymph nodes) are present so that there is at least 1 nodule measuring 10 mm or larger or at least 2 nodules measuring 5 mm or larger
Multifocality	F	Two or more discrete hepatic tumors with normal intervening liver tissue
Tumor rupture	R	Free fluid in the abdomen or pelvis with one or more of the following findings of hemorrhage: • Internal complexity/septations within fluid • High-density fluid on CT (>25 HU) • Imaging characteristics of blood or blood degradation products on MRI • Heterogeneous fluid on ultrasound with echogenic debris • Visible defect in tumor capsule or Tumor cells are present within the peritoneal fluid or Rupture diagnosed pathologically in patients who have received an upfront resection
Caudate lobe involvement	C	Tumor involving the caudate
Lymph node metastases	N	Any one of the following criteria is met: • Lymph node with short-axis diameter of >1 cm • Portocaval lymph node with short-axis diameter >1.5 cm • Spherical lymph node shape with loss of fatty hilum
Distant metastases	M	Any one of the following criteria is met: • One noncalcified pulmonary nodule ≥5 mm in diameter • Two or more noncalcified pulmonary nodules, each ≥3 mm in diameter • Pathologically proven metastatic disease

(IVC: inferior vena cava; PRETEXT: PRE-Treatment EXTent of tumor)

associated with diseases such as glycogen storage disease (Type I), cystinosis, hereditary tyrosinemia, Wilson disease, alpha-1-antitrypsin deficiency, extrahepatic biliary atresia, and giant-cell hepatitis. Association with cirrhosis is less common than in adults. Serum AFP is elevated in 40–50% of patients.[6]

Hepatocellular carcinoma can appear as focal, multinodular or diffuse form with variable and nonspecific appearances. When solitary, the lesion is common in the right lobe. On sonography, HCC is characterized by variable echogenicity pattern with predominantly hypo-, iso-, or hyperechoic echotexture. Calcification may be seen in 10% of patients but is less common than in hepatoblastoma. US appearances may be indistinguishable from hepatoblastoma.

On noncontrast CT scan, lesion is of low attenuation and generally reveals inhomogeneous enhancement after contrast. On dynamic CT, majority are hypervascular and may reveal areas of peripheral enhancement in the early vascular phase and later become hypodense to liver parenchyma **(Figs. 4A and B)**. On MRI, these tumors are usually hypointense on T1WI and hyperintense on T2WI. The vascular invasion is demonstrated as loss of normal flow void in the vessels.

Fibrolamellar Hepatocellular Carcinoma

It is a rare subtype of HCC but it has a better prognosis if resected. This tumor is usually seen in young females (mean age 23 years); but it can occur in children. AFP level is usually not elevated.[18] CT reveals a well-defined hypodense mass which shows variable enhancement after contrast injection. A central fibrotic scar and calcification are more commonly seen (30% and 50% of cases respectively)[19] in

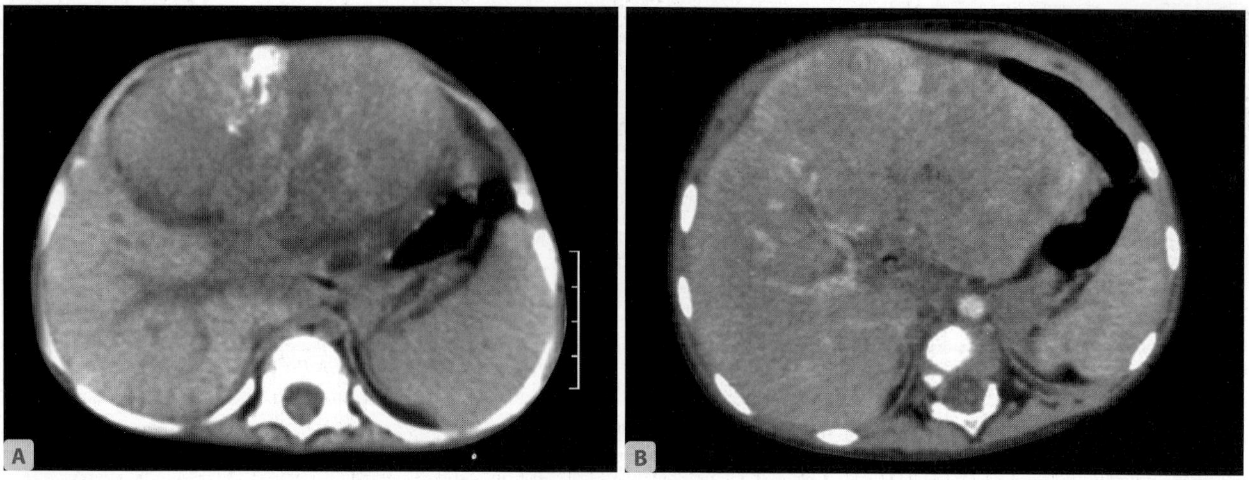

FIGS. 1A AND B: NCCT scan. (A) in a 14-month-old male patient with hepatoblastoma shows a large well-defined hypodense mass replacing the left lobe of liver. Coarse calcification is seen within the mass; CECT (B) image in another patient shows heterogeneously enhancing mass lesion in left lobe. (CECT: contrast-enhanced computed tomography; NCCT: noncontrast computed tomography)

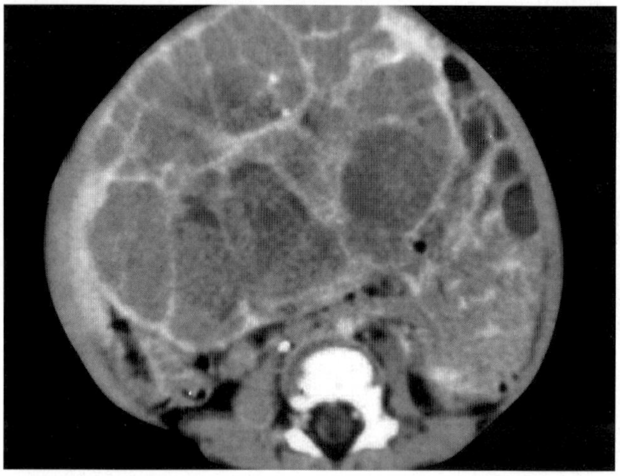

FIG. 2: CT in a case of hepatoblastoma shows inhomogeneous enhancement and multiple enhancing septae.

fibrolamellar subtype of HCC **(Figs. 5A and B)**. MRI can be used to distinguish fibrolamellar HCC from focal nodular hyperplasia (FNH). The fibrous central scar of fibrolamellar HCC is hypointense on both T1WI and T2WI. On the other hand, the central scar of FNH is hyperintense on T2WI.[20]

Undifferentiated Embryonal Sarcoma

Undifferentiated embryonal sarcoma (UES) is a rare, aggressive tumor of mesenchymal origin, and commonly affects children between 6 and 10 years of age with a slight male predominance.[21] It is said to be malignant counterpart of mesenchymal hamartoma and is believed to arise in the background of pre-existing mesenchymal hamartoma.[22] On histopathology, it shows primitive spindle-shaped, sarcomatous satellite cells which are closely packed in sheets or whorls in a background of loose myxoid tissue, containing hematopoiesis foci in up to 50% of cases.[21]

Children usually present with an abdominal mass, pain, and discomfort. UES is usually large at presentation, is solitary involving the right lobe of the liver (in up to 75% of cases), and is predominantly solid with occasional cystic, necrotic, or hemorrhagic areas.[21] AFP levels are not raised.[23]

Plain radiographs show a large and soft-tissue opacity without calcification. On ultrasound, the tumor is solid and isoechoic to hyperechoic **(Figs. 6A and B)** relative to normal liver, along with small anechoic areas that may represent necrosis, hemorrhage, or cystic degeneration.[21] The tumor is predominantly water attenuation on CT **(Fig. 6C)** which correlates with a large component of myxoid stroma seen on histology. A densely enhancing peripheral rim can be seen in relation to the pseudocapsule. Sometimes, hyperattenuating areas/foci can be seen which represent hemorrhage and calcifications.[21,24,25] On MRI, the tumor shows low signal intensity on T1WI and increased signal intensity on T2WI. Pseudocapsule is seen as a hypointense rim on T1WI and T2WI. Increased signal intensity areas on T1WI correspond to hemorrhagic areas. Internal debris, fluid levels, and septa may be seen on T2WI.[21,24,25] Heterogeneous enhancement of the tumor is seen after contrast administration. Metastases in UES usually occur to the lungs and bone.

Treatment consists of complete resection of the tumor. Multimodal treatment has shown improved survival rates in the recent years. Patients having unresectable masses and are not responsive to chemotherapy can be treated with liver transplantation.

Rhabdomyosarcoma

This is the most common tumor of the biliary tree in children and accounts for 0.04% of all cancers in children. It occurs at a median age of 3 years and is rare after the first decade.[26] There is a male preponderance. The tumor may arise in the liver, intrahepatic ducts, intrahepatic cyst, gallbladder, cystic duct, extrahepatic duct, and ampulla or choledochal cyst. Patient usually presents with jaundice and abdominal distention.

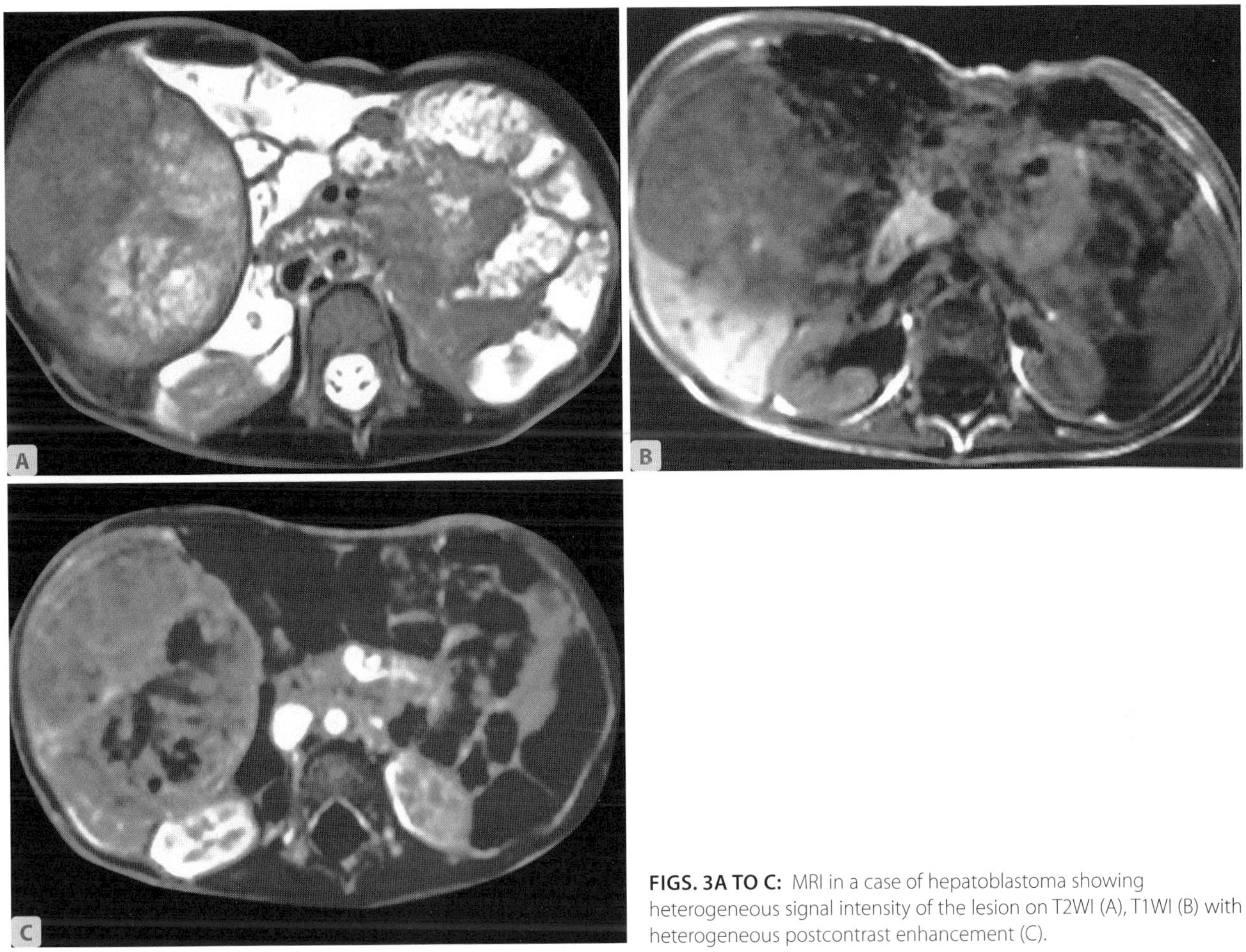

FIGS. 3A TO C: MRI in a case of hepatoblastoma showing heterogeneous signal intensity of the lesion on T2WI (A), T1WI (B) with heterogeneous postcontrast enhancement (C).

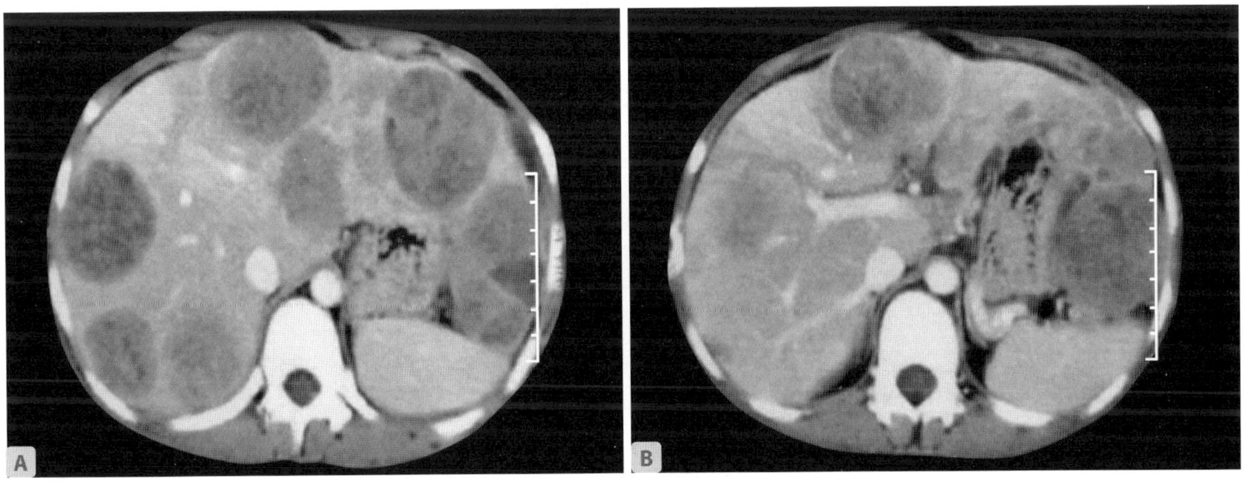

FIGS. 4A AND B: CT scan in an 11-year-old male patient with multicentric hepatocellular carcinomas (HCC). There are multiple lesions seen in both lobes of liver which show peripheral enhancement. The left branch of portal vein is not opacified suggestive of invasion.

Ultrasonography **(Fig. 7A)** shows biliary dilatation with a hyperechoic intraductal mass. The portal vein may be displaced but is not thrombosed. Larger lesions have areas of necrosis. CT **(Figs. 7B and C)** shows an intraductal mass with or without biliary dilatation. The mass is heterogeneous in attenuation with variable contrast enhancement. On MRI, the mass is of low-signal intensity on T1W images and hyperintense on T2W images. MRCP shows dilated ducts and the entire extent of the lesion **(Fig. 8)**.

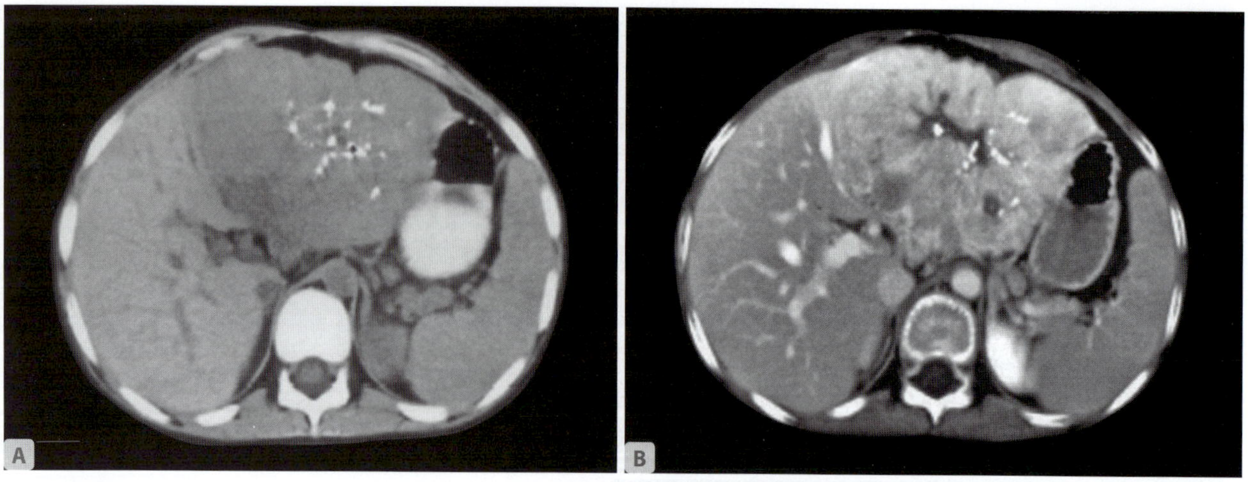

FIGS. 5A AND B: CT scan in a 16-year-old female patient with fibrolamellar HCC. NCCT (A) shows a well-defined hypodense mass in the left lobe of liver with central calcification and lobulated border; CECT (B) shows inhomogeneous enhancement with central hypodense scar. (CECT: contrast-enhanced computed tomography; HCC: hepatocellular carcinomas; NCCT: noncontrast computed tomography)

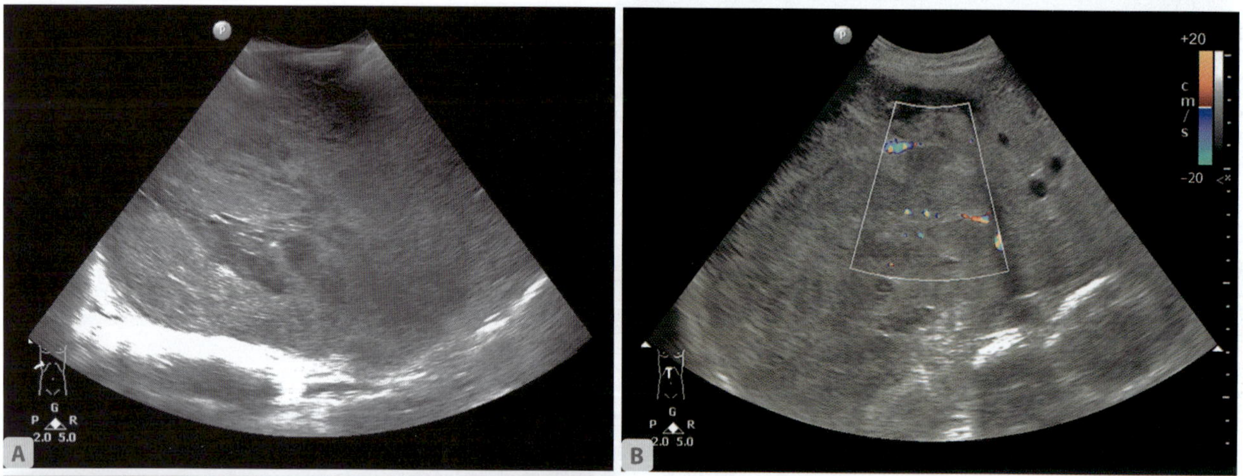

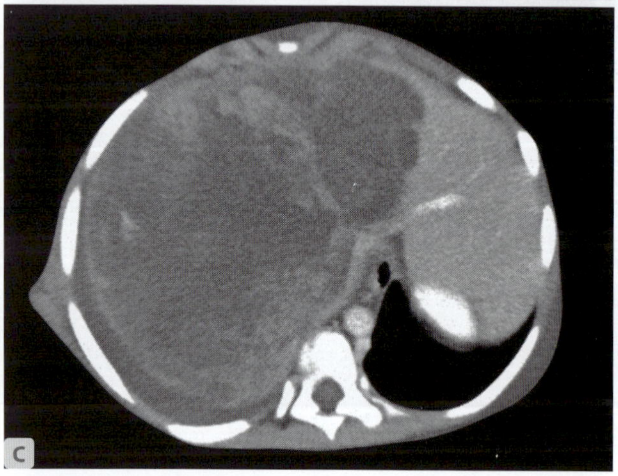

FIGS. 6A TO C: Gray-scale ultrasound image of the liver in a 10-year-old girl showing heterogeneous solid lesion in the right lobe of the liver (A); On doppler image (B), the lesion is showing small focal areas of vascularity; CECT image shows a predominantly hypodense lesion (C) with solid enhancing areas. FNA showed undifferentiated embryonal sarcoma. (CECT: contrast-enhanced computed tomography; FNA: fine-needle aspiration)

Hepatic Metastases

The common primary malignancy to metastasize to liver in children are neuroblastoma, Wilms' tumor, GI tumors, Ewing's sarcoma, rhabdomyosarcoma, lymphomas, and leukemias.[2,11] The metastases may be single or multiple **(Figs. 9 and 10)**. These are usually nonspecific lesions appearing hypoechoic on US, hypodense on contrast-enhanced CT scan, hypointense on T1 and hyperintense on T2W MR images. If required, diagnosis can be clinched by fine-needle aspiration cytology under sonographic guidance.

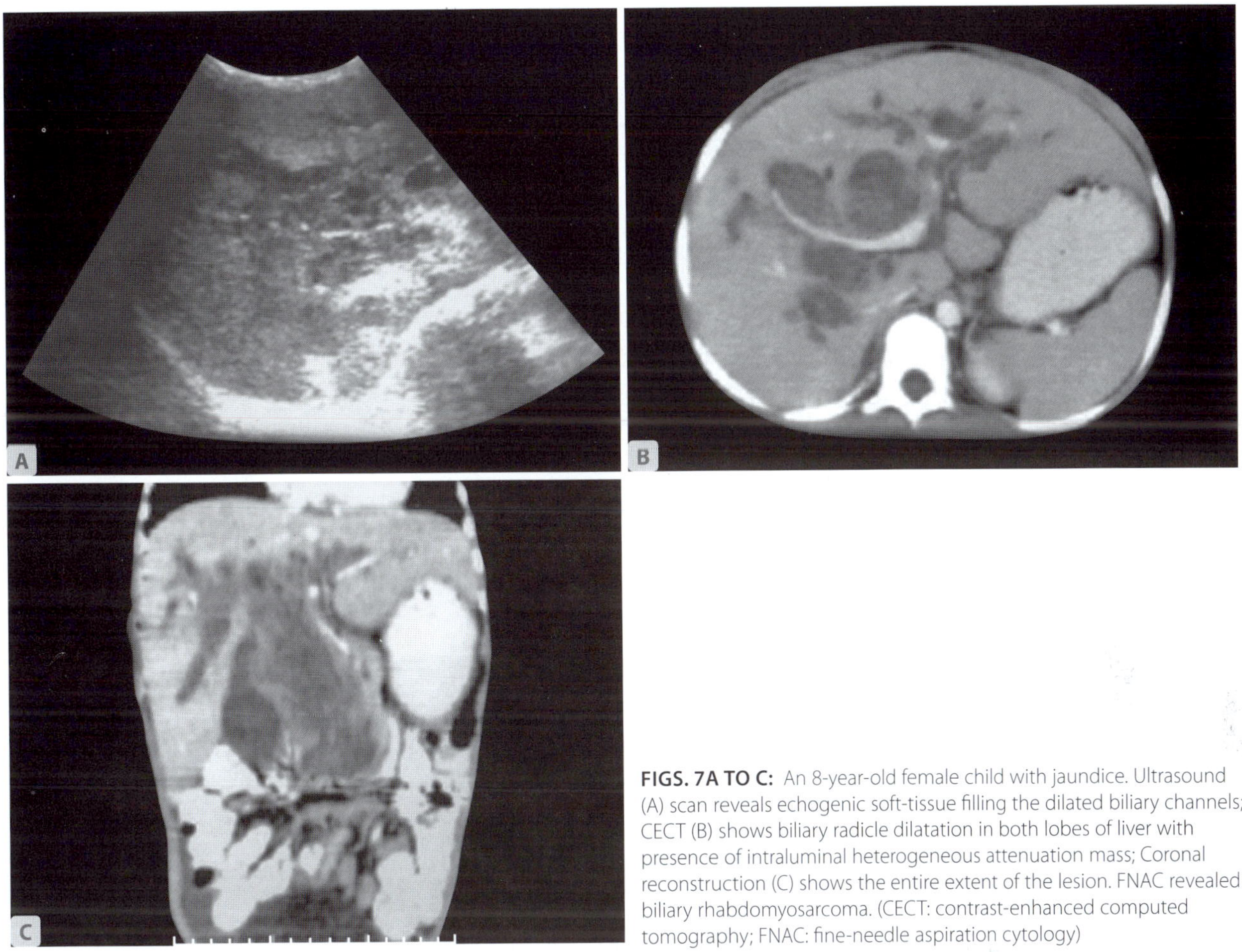

FIGS. 7A TO C: An 8-year-old female child with jaundice. Ultrasound (A) scan reveals echogenic soft-tissue filling the dilated biliary channels; CECT (B) shows biliary radicle dilatation in both lobes of liver with presence of intraluminal heterogeneous attenuation mass; Coronal reconstruction (C) shows the entire extent of the lesion. FNAC revealed biliary rhabdomyosarcoma. (CECT: contrast-enhanced computed tomography; FNAC: fine-needle aspiration cytology)

Epithelioid Hemangioendothelioma

Epithelioid Hemagioendothelioma (EHE) is a tumor of intermediate malignant potential. It is seen usually in young to middle-aged patient population, with only a few cases reported in pediatric population.[27,28] There is a relative female predominance (male:female::3:2). AFP levels are in normal range.[29]

On gross examination, EHE are usually seen as multifocal, ill-defined nodules and masses distributed throughout the both lobes (in up to 82% cases) predominantly along the periphery, but may occur as a solitary mass. These nodules vary in size from a few millimeters to up to 15 cm, and larger nodules can be seen to form confluent masses. Calcifications can be seen in up to 23% of cases. On microscopic examination, they show a mixture of dendritic and epithelioid cells having evidence of vascular differentiation.[29]

Two patterns have been described at imaging, which include multifocal and solitary pattern. The multifocal form presents with multiple nodules along the periphery, which tend to coalesce to form larger masses. Solitary masses demonstrate a target like appearance. There is associated capsular flattening or retraction as a result fibrosis, which may be detected at imaging.

At ultrasound, EHE nodules are hypoechoic because of myxoid stroma in the central part, but they may be hyperechoic with a hypoechoic rim or isoechoic with a hypoechoic halo. Dynamic CECT imaging in larger lesions shows peripheral and progressive centripetal enhancement with incomplete fill-in even on. Smaller lesions can show enhancement in the central with centrifugal progression at dynamic imaging.[30] On MRI, the lesions are generally hypointense on T1WI with a more hypointense signal in central portion, representing necrosis, hemorrhage, or calcification. The lesions are heterogeneously hyperintense on T2WI with a more hyperintense signal in central portion. A dark halo may be seen on T1WI or T2WI; which may sometimes be hyperintense on T1WI. After the administration of contrast, peripheral enhancement is seen typically, however heterogeneous enhancement may be seen in large lesions.[31-33] The peripheral halo is usually non-enhancing.

Benign Hepatic Neoplasms

These account for one-third of all primary hepatic tumors. Most of these tumors are of vascular origin, viz., hemangioma.[9] Less common tumors are mesenchymal hamartoma, FNH, and hepatic adenoma.

Hemangioma

Liver hemangiomas are one of the vascular tumors of liver in children according to the International Society for the Study

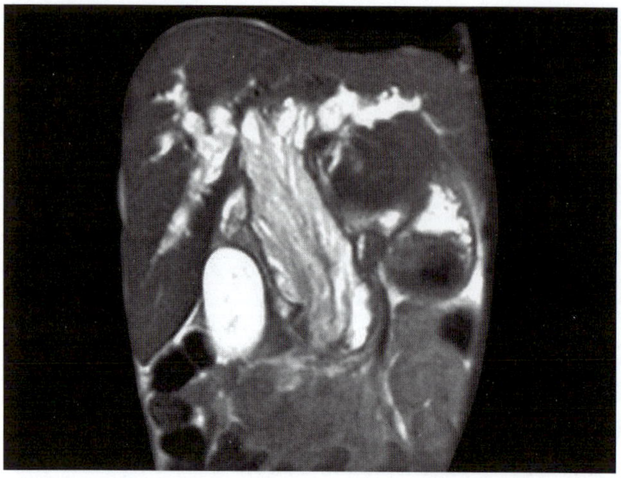

FIG. 8: T2-weighted (T2W) coronal image in a case of biliary rhabdomyosarcoma shows the dilatation of the biliary tree with heterogeneous hyperintensity of the intraductal tumor.

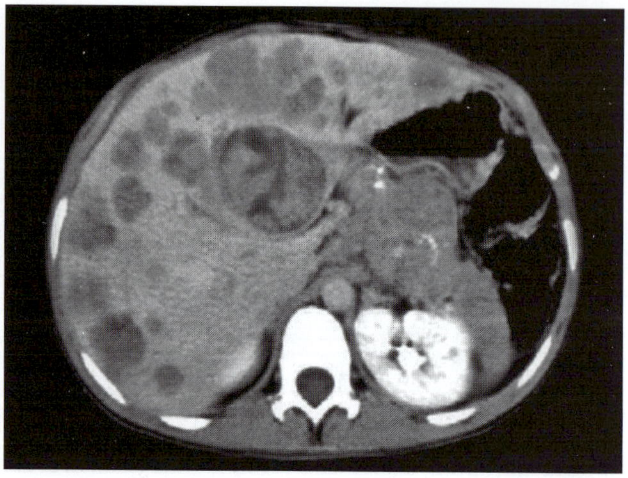

FIG. 10: Multiple well-defined hypodense lesions are seen in liver on contrast-enhanced computed tomography (CECT) in a case of pancreatoblastoma metastasizing to liver.

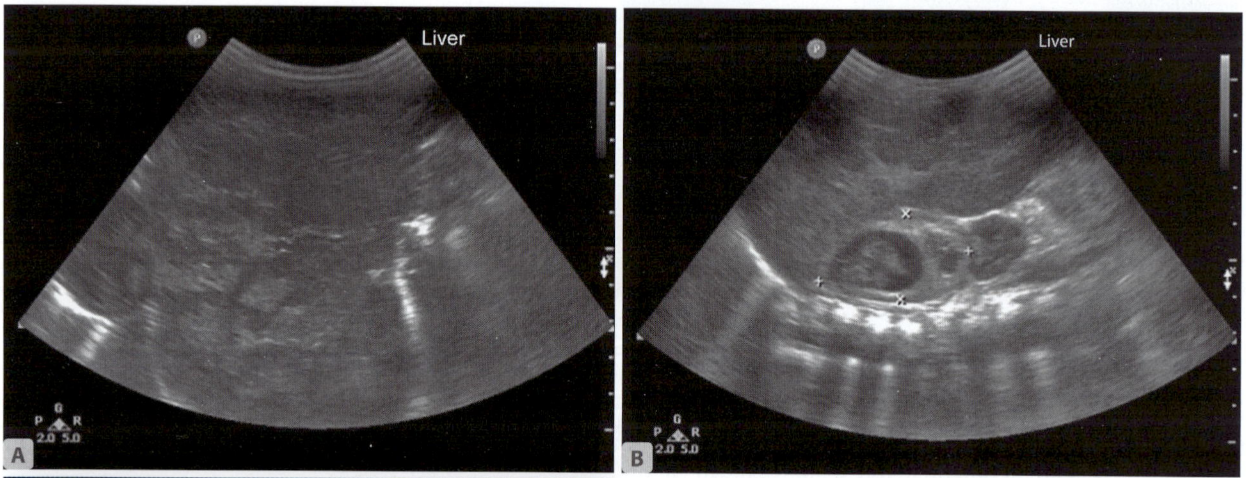

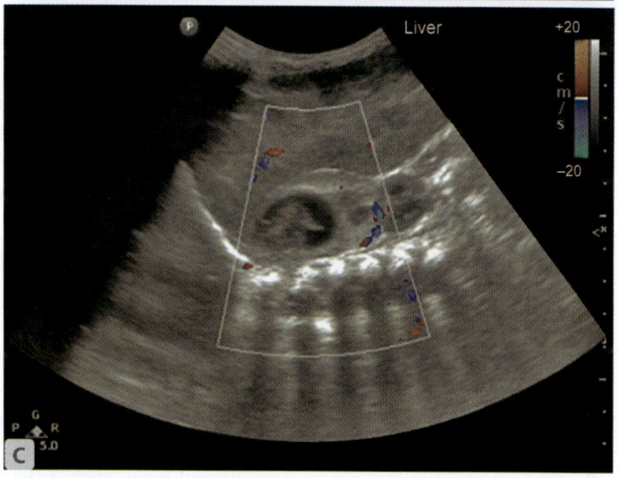

FIGS. 9A TO C: Ultrasound images in a 1-month-old infant showing multiple hyperechoic and hypoechoic lesions scattered in the liver along with a suprarenal mass suggestive of adrenal neuroblastoma with liver metastases.

of Vascular Anomalies (ISSVA) classification of vascular anomalies. They are classified as infantile and congenital. Infantile hemangiomas are seen to occur more frequently, usually begin to grow after birth typically during the 1st year of life, followed by and involuting phase between 1 and 7 years, and lastly an involuted phase between 8 and 12 years.[34] Infantile hemangiomas are positive for glucose transporter-1 protein (Glut-1) that facilitates the transport of glucose across RBC membranes. Congenital hemangiomas are seen to be fully developed at birth and are Glut-1 negative. Congenital hemangiomas are divided into a rapidly involuting group, which involute usually within 12–14 months of age,[35] and a noninvoluting group.[34,35] The differentiation among these tumors may be impossible at initial diagnosis. The development of liver hemangiomas is related to the upregulation of angiogenic factors and downregulation of the inhibitors of angiogenesis, and the trigger is related to viral insult or somatic mutation.[34]

Infantile hemangiomas occur more commonly in girls, with a female to male ratio of 3–5:1, and they are more common in fair-skinned individuals. Most liver hemangiomas are clinically silent and remain undetected. Others are discovered on prenatal ultrasound or postnatal imaging that is performed for various reasons. Even though most liver hemangiomas are asymptomatic, life-threatening complications may occur, especially in the setting of multifocal lesions or congestive heart failure related to an intralesional shunt, hypothyroidism resulting from overproduction of type III iodothyronine deiodinase, fulminant hepatic failure, and/or abdominal compartment syndrome. In some patients with liver hemangioma, consumptive coagulopathy may develop as a result of intralesional thrombosis, hemorrhage, and hemolysis.[36,37]

On sonography, hemangiomas are typically small (<3 cm in diameter), homogeneous, well-defined, and hyperechoic with distal acoustic enhancement. Larger lesion can be heterogeneous.[38] On noncontrast CT, it is hypo- to isodense and well-defined. On dynamic contrast studies, early, peripheral, dense nodular enhancement with later centripetal fill-in is noted **(Figs. 11 and 12)**. Complete isodense filling occurs in not <3 minutes and not >30 minutes after injection in two-thirds of these lesions. When above features can be demonstrated, no further investigation is required. But the lesion can show variable contrast enhancement and variable fill-in. In this equivocal state, MRI and scintigraphy are helpful.

On MRI, hemangioma appears hypo- or isointense to liver on T1WI. On T2WI, it shows marked hyperintensity with centripetal fill-in on post-contrast imaging similar to that on CECT.

On Tc-labeled RBC scanning, it shows increased activity in blood pool phase and on delayed scanning. This study has 100% specificity for the diagnosis of hemangioma. For lesion larger than 2 cm, both MRI and ^{99m}Tc RBC imaging have similar accuracy (95%) but for lesion smaller than 2 cm, MRI is more sensitive. However, SPECT ^{99m}Tc RBC imaging is more specific than MRI.

Hepatic angiography is rarely required in establishing the diagnosis of hemangioma. Rarely when surgery is contemplated in symptomatic hemangioma, angiography can be helpful in defining the vascular anatomy.

Mesenchymal Hamartoma

Mesenchymal hamartoma is the second most common benign hepatic tumor next to vascular lesions.[39] This tumor usually presents as an asymptomatic abdominal mass in children <2 years of age and is twice as common in boys than girls. Rarely children may present with cardiac failure due to presence of large shunt in the lesion.

Pathologically, this tumor is seen as a well-circumscribed mass with multiple cystic areas.[39] On sonography,[40] the tumor appears as a well-defined, multilocular mass with anechoic spaces separated by echogenic septae **(Fig. 13)**. This has been described as "swiss cheese" appearance.[39] On CT scanning, the tumor is seen as a complex mass containing areas of low attenuation separated by solid septae and stroma which enhance with intravenous contrast administration[41] **(Figs. 14A and B)**. On MRI, the cystic spaces show high signal on T2WI and low signal on T1WI. The signal intensity, however, depends on the protein content and presence of hemorrhage within the cysts.

Focal Nodular Hyperplasia and Hepatic Adenoma

This benign lesion is uncommon and constitutes <2% of pediatric hepatic tumors.[7] Childhood hepatic adenoma is associated with glycogen storage disease, Fanconi anemia and galactosemia. Both these tumors are well-circumscribed masses with variable echogenicity and enhancement patterns. However, presence of a central low attenuation scar favors the diagnosis of FNH. When the distinction based on these imaging modalities is uncertain, radionuclide sulfur colloid scintigraphic study is very helpful. As high as 60% of FNH accumulate colloid while hepatic adenoma appears as focal defects.[7,9,42] Focal hepatic mass which is seen as hot area on sulfur colloid scan is diagnostic of FNH.

PELIOSIS HEPATIS

This is a rare entity characterized by small blood-filled spaces in the liver. It is found in association with type I glycogen storage disease, HIV infection and intake of androgens.[10,17] On US, there are scattered areas of heterogeneous echogenicity of liver along with cystic lesions. CT demonstrates areas of low attenuation which show variable contrast enhancement. MRI shows increased signal intensity on T2WI and variable signal on T1WI depending upon the contents of the cysts.[11]

INFLAMMATORY LESIONS

Pyogenic Hepatic Abscess

These are usually associated with various predisposing conditions such as systemic sepsis, appendicitis, inflammatory bowel disease, omphalitis, and trauma or chronic granulomatous disease of childhood.[43] In neonates, gram-negative and in older children *Staphylococcus aureus* are the most common organisms. When the abscesses are multiple, they usually are the result of ascending biliary infection. When solitary, right lobe is affected more often. Children often present with fever, upper abdominal pain, tender hepatomegaly and leukocytosis.

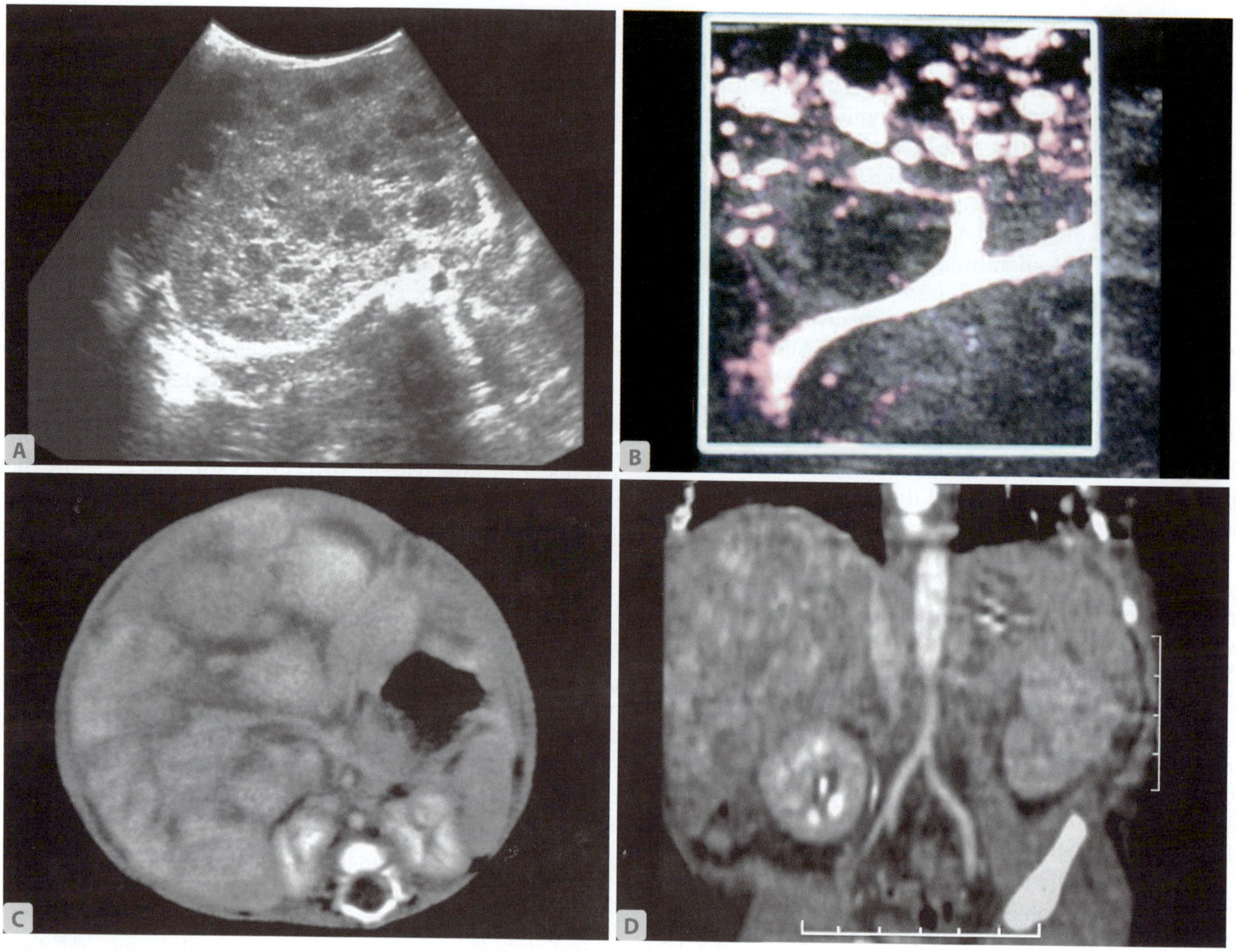

FIGS. 11A TO D: Imaging finding in diffuse infantile hemangioma. (A) Gray-scale ultrasound reveals multiple well-defined hypo- to anechoic lesions in both lobes of liver; Power Doppler (B) revealed markedly increased vascularity in these lesions. (C) In another patient axial contrast-enhanced computed tomography (CECT) scan demonstrates multiple enhancing hypervascular lesions diffusedly distributed in both lobes of liver while coronal reformatted image; (D) shows sudden change in aortic caliber, distal to celiac artery.

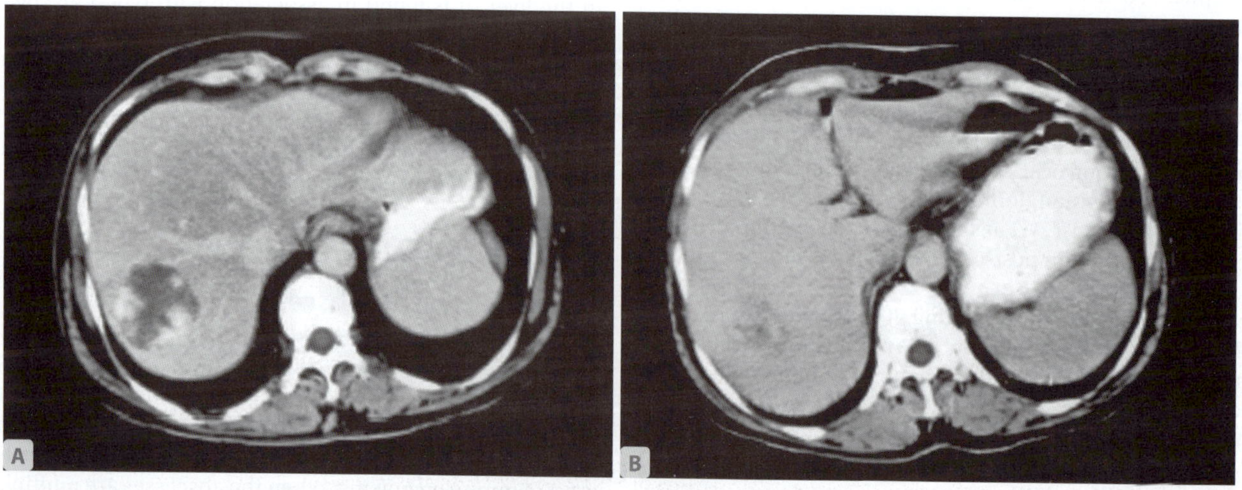

FIGS. 12A AND B: (A) Venous phase contrast-enhanced computed tomography (CECT) image in a case of hemangioma showing dense nodular enhancement in a peripherally located hepatic mass. (B) Delayed phase reveals lesion to be almost isodense to liver.

The abscesses pass through three stages, viz., the stage of suppuration, the stage of liquefaction, and the stage of resolution including fibrosis, cystic residual lesion, and calcification. These stages influence imaging appearance of the abscesses.

Ultrasonography is the initial and usually the only investigation required in patients suspected to have hepatic abscesses. Abscess may appear anechoic, hypoechoic, hyperechoic or as a complex mass with thick irregular walls and through-transmission **(Fig. 15)**. Early lesions tend to be echogenic and ill-defined. If gas is detected, it clinches the diagnosis. Occasionally septations, fluid-fluid levels, and echogenic debris may be noted.[44]

On CT, most abscesses are sharply defined, hypodense masses which may show rim enhancement on contrast administration.[9] Intralesional gas, although highly suggestive of the diagnosis, is seen in only 20% of patients. Double-target sign consisting of a low-density central area surrounded by hyperdense zone and then a peripheral hypodense zone may also be noted **(Figs. 16 and 17)**.

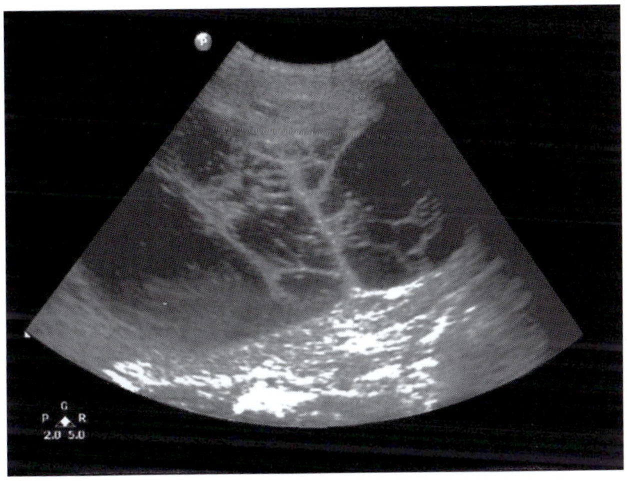

FIG. 13: Ultrasound image of liver in a 7-month-old boy reveals a large multilocular cystic mass with septae in the right lobe of liver in a case of mesenchymal hamartoma.

On scintigraphy examination using either Ga-67 or In-111, the lesions are "hot". In-111 scanning provides increased specificity because it is not taken up by benign or malignant lesions. Chest radiographs show elevated hemidiaphragm, pleural effusion, and basal atelectasis or infiltrates.

When the diagnosis cannot be established based on clinical or CT findings, percutaneous needle aspiration performed under sonographic or CT guidance can be helpful in diagnosis and also for providing percutaneous aspiration or catheter drainage.[45,46]

Amebic Hepatic Abscess

It is caused by *E. histolytica* and approximately 3–9% of cases of intestinal amebiasis are complicated by hepatic abscesses. Liver is invaded by one of the three routes, viz., (i) portal vein (most common), (ii) lymphatics, or (iii) via direct extension through colonic wall.

Amebic abscess is most often solitary (85%) and affects the right lobe more (72%) than left lobe (13%). Chest radiograph is abnormal in approximately 50–78% of cases which includes elevation of right hemidiaphragm, basal pulmonary infiltrates, or pleural effusion. On sulfur-colloid scans and gallium scans, the abscess appears as cold center with a hot rim. On ultrasound, the lesion is usually round or oval, hypoechoic mass with homogeneous low-level internal echoes and distal acoustic enhancement **(Fig. 18)**. Compared to pyogenic abscess, amebic abscess is more likely to be round or oval in shape (82% vs. 60%), sonographically hypoechoic with fine low-level echoes (58% vs. 36%) and shows absence of a definite wall.[47]

CT appearance of amebic abscess is variable and nonspecific. Lesion is usually low attenuating (10–20 HU) with an enhancing rim **(Fig. 19)**. It may appear uni- or multiocular and may demonstrate nodularity of the margin. On MRI, amebic abscess appears as a round or oval area showing low signal intensity on T1WI and hyperintensity on T2WI.

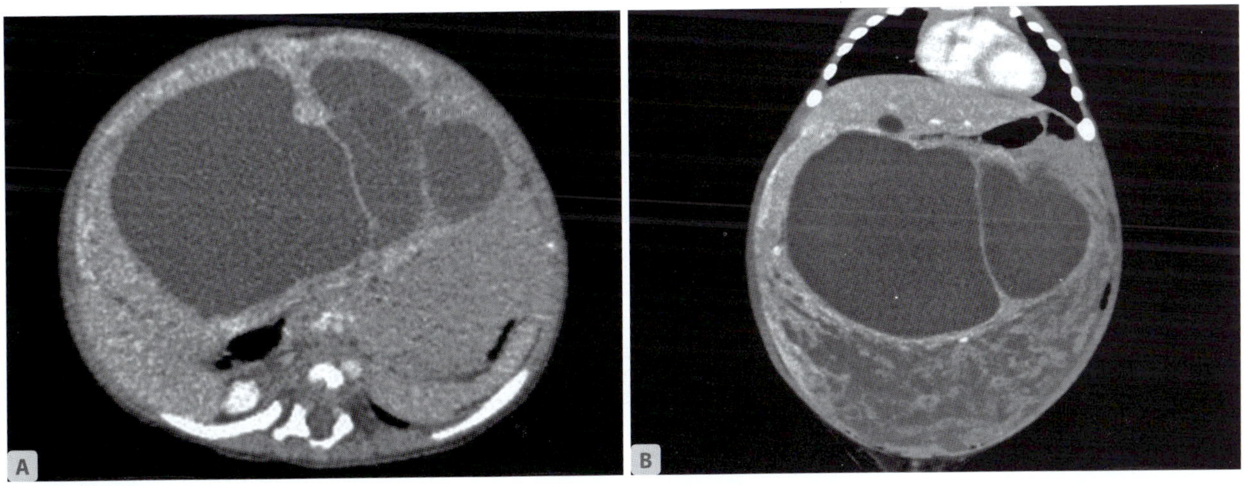

FIGS. 14A AND B: Axial (A) and coronal (B) reformatted images of a 7-month-old infant with mesenchymal hamartoma reveals a multiloculated cystic mass with enhancing septae.

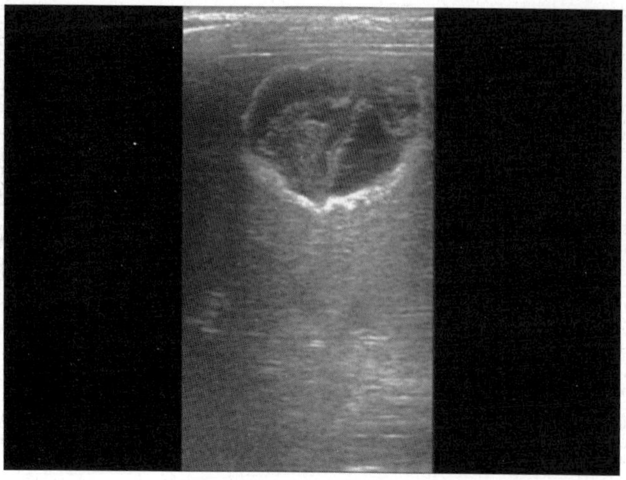

FIG. 15: Ultrasound image showing a pyogenic liver abscess with central anechoic area with internal echoes and thick irregular shaggy wall. Increased through-transmission is seen.

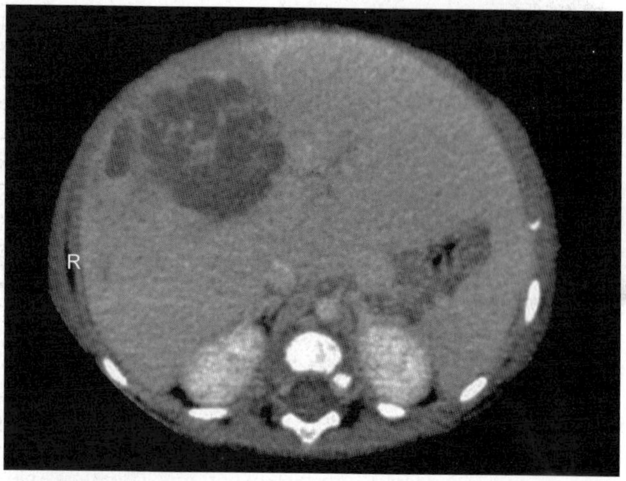

FIG. 16: Axial contrast-enhanced computed tomography (CECT) image showing a pyogenic liver abscess with central hypodense area with irregular walls and enhancing septae.

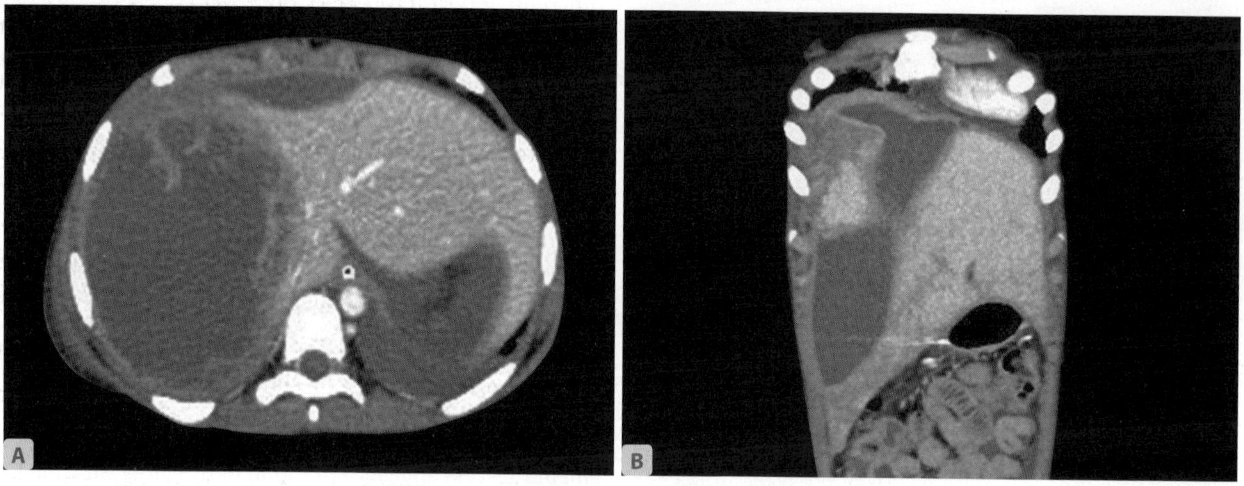

FIGS. 17A AND B: Axial (A) and coronal (B) contrast-enhanced computed tomography (CECT) images showing a pyogenic liver abscess with central hypodense area with irregular walls and enhancing septae which was communicating with the perihepatic collection suggestive of rupture.

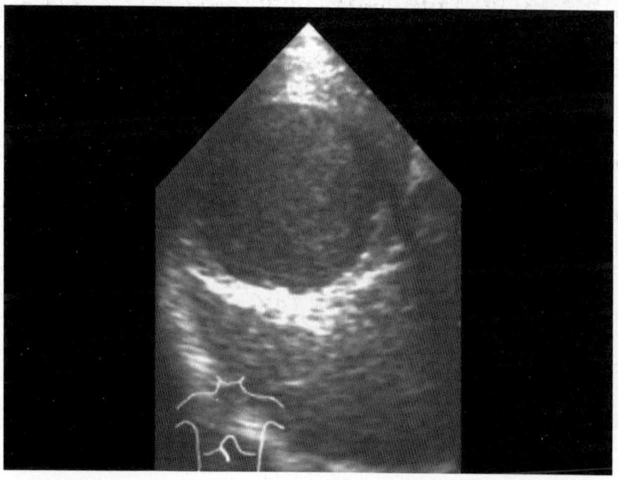

FIG. 18: Ultrasound (US) of liver in a case of amebic liver abscess shows a well-defined rounded hypoechoic lesion with fine low level internal echoes and an almost imperceptible wall.

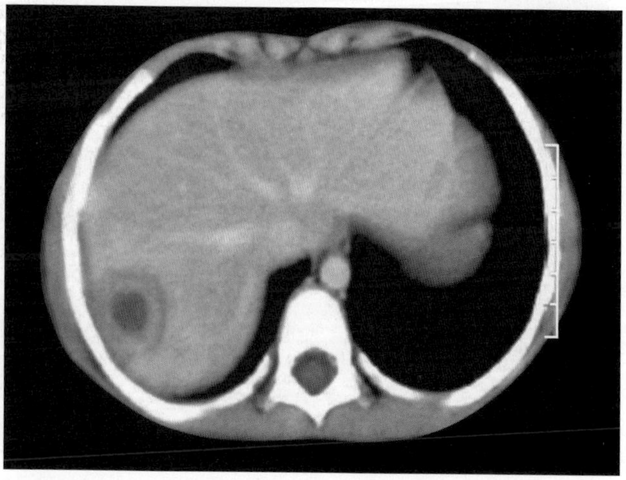

FIG. 19: CT scan in a case of liver abscess shows a hypodense lesion with thick wall in the right lobe of liver. A thin rim of perilesional fluid is seen.

Fungal Abscess

This is more commonly seen in immunocompromised patients such as those receiving chemotherapy, acquired immunodeficiency syndrome (AIDS), lymphoma or acute leukemia. Liver is frequently involved secondary to hematogenous spread of mycotic infection from other organs, most commonly the lungs. Of the various fungi, *Candida* is the most common agent.[48]

Sonographically, four major types are seen: (i) "Wheel within a wheel" appearance where a peripheral hypoechoic zone surrounds an inner echogenic wheel which, in turn, surrounds a central hypoechoic nidus, (ii) "Bull's eye" lesion where a hyperechoic center is surrounded by hypoechoic rim, (iii) "Uniformly hypoechoic"—the most common appearance **(Fig. 20)**, and (iv) "Echogenic" lesion, caused by scar formation.

On CT scan, the most common pattern is multiple, small, and rounded lesions of low attenuation. The lesion may show calcification. MR shows increased signal intensity on T1WI and STIR (short T1 inversion recovery) sequences.

Granulomatous Lesions

Various granulomatous diseases which may affect liver include tuberculosis, histiocytosis, and sarcoidosis.

Tuberculosis of the liver usually occurs in miliary form with nodules ranging in size from 0.5 to 2 mm which are too small to be seen on US or CT. The most common finding in such cases is hepatomegaly without focal lesions. A diffusely heterogeneous echotexture on US has also been reported. Macronodular involvement is uncommon[39] and usually manifests as single or multiple focal lesions of varying sizes which are hypoechoic on US and hypodense on CT **(Fig. 21)**. These lesions may show peripheral rim enhancement and a central hypodensity due to caseation.[49,50]

Echinococcal Disease (Hydatid Cyst)

The disease is worldwide and is most often caused by *Echinococcus granulosus. E. multilocularis* is less common but is more aggressive pathogen and rarely encountered in our country.

Hydatid cyst has three layers. The outer pericyst is formed by the compressed, modified host tissue which is a rigid protective zone. The two inner layers (ectocyst and endocyst) are parasitic in origin. The ectocyst is approximately 1 mm thick and may calcify. The innermost germinal layer (endocyst) is the living parasite which produces laminated membrane and scolices. Up to 60% of the cysts are multiple.

Plain radiograph shows calcification of the cyst wall in 20–30% of cases. Calcification, however, does not indicate death of the parasite.[51] On sulfur-colloid scans, they are cold and may show a rim of increased activity on gallium scans.

Sonographic appearance depends on the maturity of the cyst **(Figs. 22A and B)**. It can be (i) completely anechoic, well-encapsulated cyst, (ii) anechoic cyst with hydatid sand, (iii) multiseptated cyst, with daughter cysts and echogenic material within cysts—the characteristic "Water-lily" sign, and (iv) a densely-calcified mass. When infected, the hydatid cysts lose their characteristic appearance and are indistinguishable from liver abscess.

On CT **(Figs. 23A to D)**, hydatid cyst is usually uni- or multilocular, well-defined with either thick or thin wall. Daughter cysts are usually located at the periphery and can be floating freely and altering the patient's position may change the position of these cysts thereby confirming the diagnosis. Curvilinear wall calcification may be seen.

On MR, hydatid cyst has low intensity on T1WI and high signal intensity on T2WI **(Figs. 24A and B)**. Pericyst usually has low intensity signal on both T1WI and T2WI. Calcification is not detected on MR, although MR better

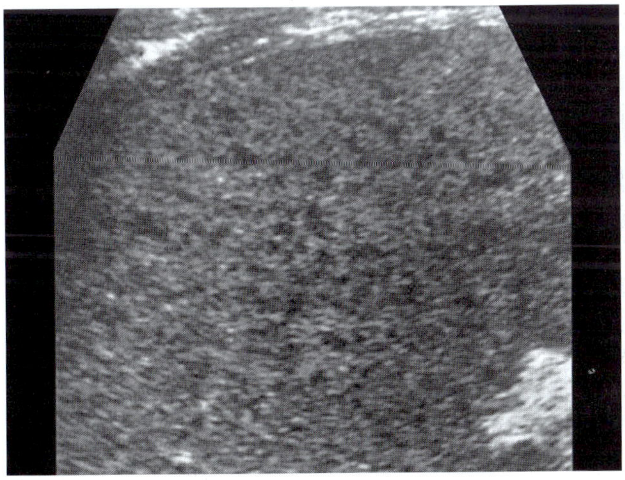

FIG. 20: Ultrasound reveals multiple tiny hypoechoic lesions diffusedly scattered in both lobes of liver in a case of candidiasis.

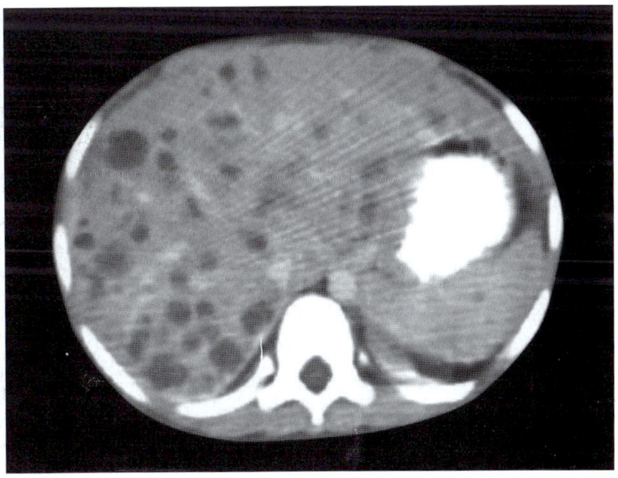

FIG. 21: Contrast-enhanced computed tomography (CECT) abdomen shows multiple well-defined hypodense lesions in both lobes of liver and spleen. Fine-needle aspiration cytology (FNAC) confirmed tuberculosis.

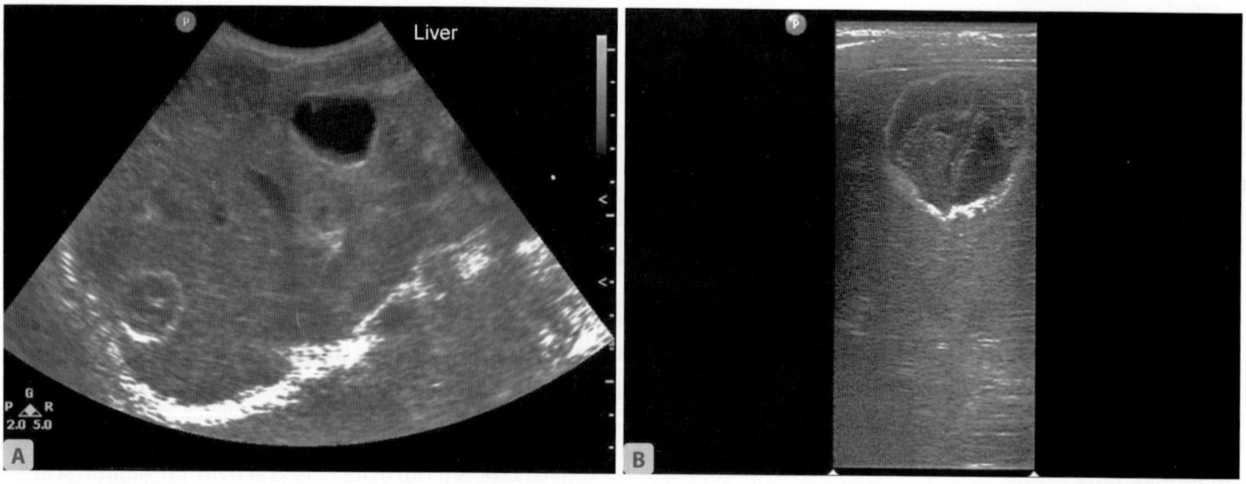

FIGS. 22A AND B: Ultrasound image. (A) Showing multiple small size cystic lesions with varied appearance (anechoic as well as with central echogenic components). In addition, one of the lesions (B) is also showing curvilinear echogenic membranes inside.

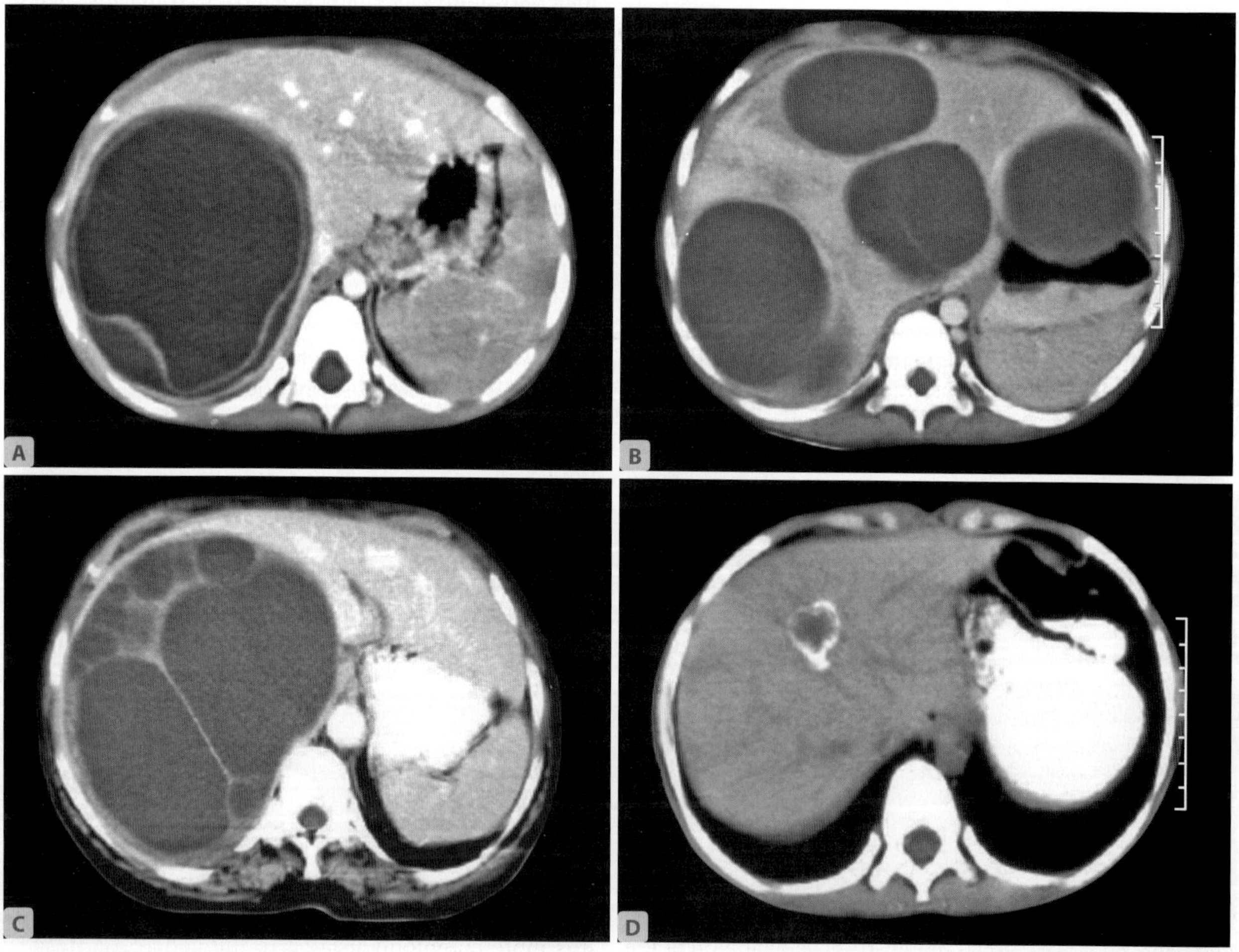

FIGS. 23A TO D: CT scan findings in hydatid cysts. (A) Unilocular cyst with undulating membrane. (B) Multiple cysts with one of them showing septation. (C) Multiseptated cyst in right lobe of liver with multiple peripheral daughter cysts. (D) Partially calcified cyst.

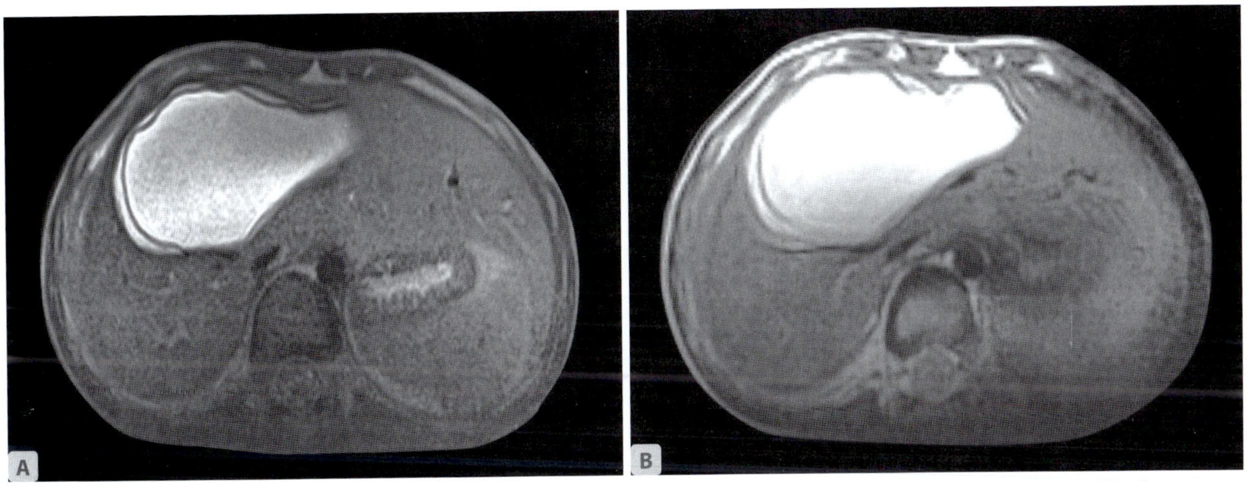

FIGS. 24A AND B: MRI in liver hydatid: T2 axial (A) and MultiVane-XD axial (B) showing hyperintense cystic lesion in liver with undulating membranes inside.

demonstrates the membranes inside the lesions when compared to CT.

Hydatid cyst may rupture into the biliary tree, and pleural, pericardial or the peritoneal cavity, thereby increasing the mortality to 50%.[52,53] Presence of undulating membrane on either US or CT suggests contained rupture.

SIMPLE HEPATIC CYST

This arises from bile duct epithelium and is seen in about 5–14% of the general population. It is usually asymptomatic and rarely causes pain, biliary obstruction or hepatomegaly.

On sonography **(Fig. 25)**, this lesion is usually solitary, well-defined, and anechoic and reveals enhanced through-transmission. CT features of simple cyst include low attenuating (0–15 HU) lesion with imperceptible or thin smooth walls, homogeneous appearance and total lack of contrast enhancement. On MR, they are sharply demarcated hypointense lesion on T1WI and hyperintense on T2WI.[9]

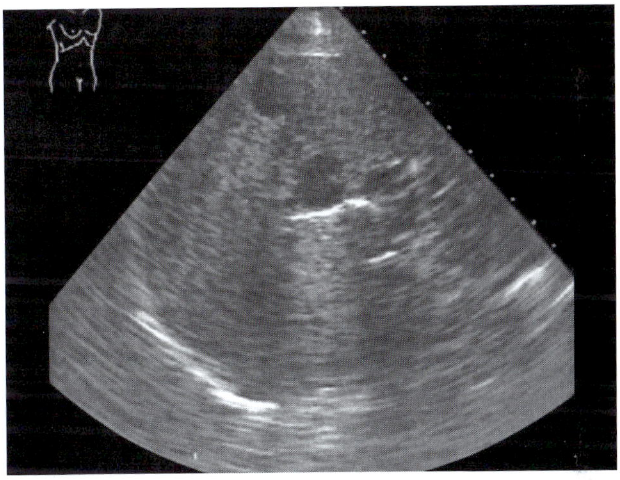

FIG. 25: Ultrasound of liver in a 4-year-old child reveals two anechoic lesions with imperceptible wall and distal acoustic enhancement suggestive of simple cysts.

POLYCYSTIC LIVER DISEASE

This is characterized by multiple liver cysts of varying sizes. Approximately, 57–74% of patients with adult polycystic kidney disease will show liver cysts. Extent of liver involvement is not proportional to the renal disease. In typical congenital hepatic fibrosis, cysts are not grossly visible. However, in the polycystic variant, numerous large and small cysts coexist with hepatic fibrosis.[54]

CAROLI'S DISEASE

This represents type V (Todani) choledochal cyst and is characterized by segmental nonobstructive dilatation of the intrahepatic bile ducts. It is associated with hepatic fibrosis, medullary sponge kidney, and infantile polycystic renal disease. Patient presents with abdominal pain secondary to cholangitis or to biliary calculi. US typically shows ectatic ducts surrounding portal vein radicles (intraluminal portal vein sign).[55] The counterpart of this intraluminal portal vein sign is the "central dot" sign seen on CT. The common duct and gallbladder are dilated. MRCP is indicated to define the anatomy of the biliary tree in Caroli's disease.

PANCREATIC MASSES

Pancreatoblastoma

The term "pancreatoblastoma" was first coined by Horie et al. for infantile tumors of the pancreas.[56] This tumor is located in the body or tail region of pancreas. According to some authors, it is more commonly located in the pancreatic head.[56,57] It usually occurs in newborns and children <8 years of age. The mean age at presentation is 6 years. The congenital form is associated with Beckwith–Wiedemann syndrome.[55] Patient presents with an abdominal mass, weight loss, pain, nausea, and diarrhea. These tumors secrete AFP, alpha-1-antitrypsin, and lactate dehydrogenase. These tumors are usually large at presentation (7–12 cm) and show areas of necrosis.

Microscopically, pancreatoblastoma consists of acinar cells. Small areas of squamous differentiation (squamoid corpuscles) are typically present.[58] The tumor is well-encapsulated and has a good prognosis after surgery. If metastases are seen at the time of diagnosis, the prognosis is poor.

Barium studies may reveal features of mass effect **(Fig. 26A)**. Ultrasound shows a heterogeneous or predominantly hypoechoic mass. Sometimes cystic areas and foci of calcification are seen within the mass **(Fig. 26B)**. Even when these tumors are present in the head of pancreas they do not cause biliary obstruction despite their large size **(Fig. 26C)**. This is due to the soft and gelatinous consistency of these tumors.[59] The tumor may directly spread into the portal vein.[60] Vascular encasement commonly involves the mesenteric vessels and inferior vena cava. Aortic encasement, however, has not been described.

On CT, the tumor is hypodense and shows mild enhancement. Sometimes it is seen as a multiloculated mass with enhancing septae. Central necrosis may be seen **(Figs. 27A and B)**. The most common metastases seen in pancreatoblastoma are to the liver. Metastatic spread may also occur to lymph nodes, peritoneal cavity, and the lungs. Bony metastases are very rare.

Magnetic resonance shows these tumors as hypointense on T1W images and iso- or hyperintense on T2W images. Contrast enhancement is variable.

Imaging in pancreatoblastoma is required to localize the organ of origin of the mass and to determine the extent of spread. It is important to distinguish pancreatoblastoma from other pediatric masses such as neuroblastoma, lymphoma, or Wilms' tumor.

Islet Cell Tumors

Islet cell tumors are rare pancreatic neoplasms that produce and secrete hormones to a variable degree. Insulinoma, glucagonoma, gastrinoma, vasoactive intestinal polypeptide producing tumor, and somatostatinoma have been reported in childhood.[11] Insulinomas are the most common islet cell tumors. The majority of these lesions are solitary (80%) and benign (90%). The usual age of presentation is over 4 years of age although islet cell adenomas have been reported to occur in the neonatal period.

Functional tumors are diagnosed due to the hormonal activity and imaging is needed for preoperative localization. Insulinomas lead to hypoglycemia and the affected children show seizure activity and erratic behavior which is relieved by the administration of glucose. The diagnosis is confirmed

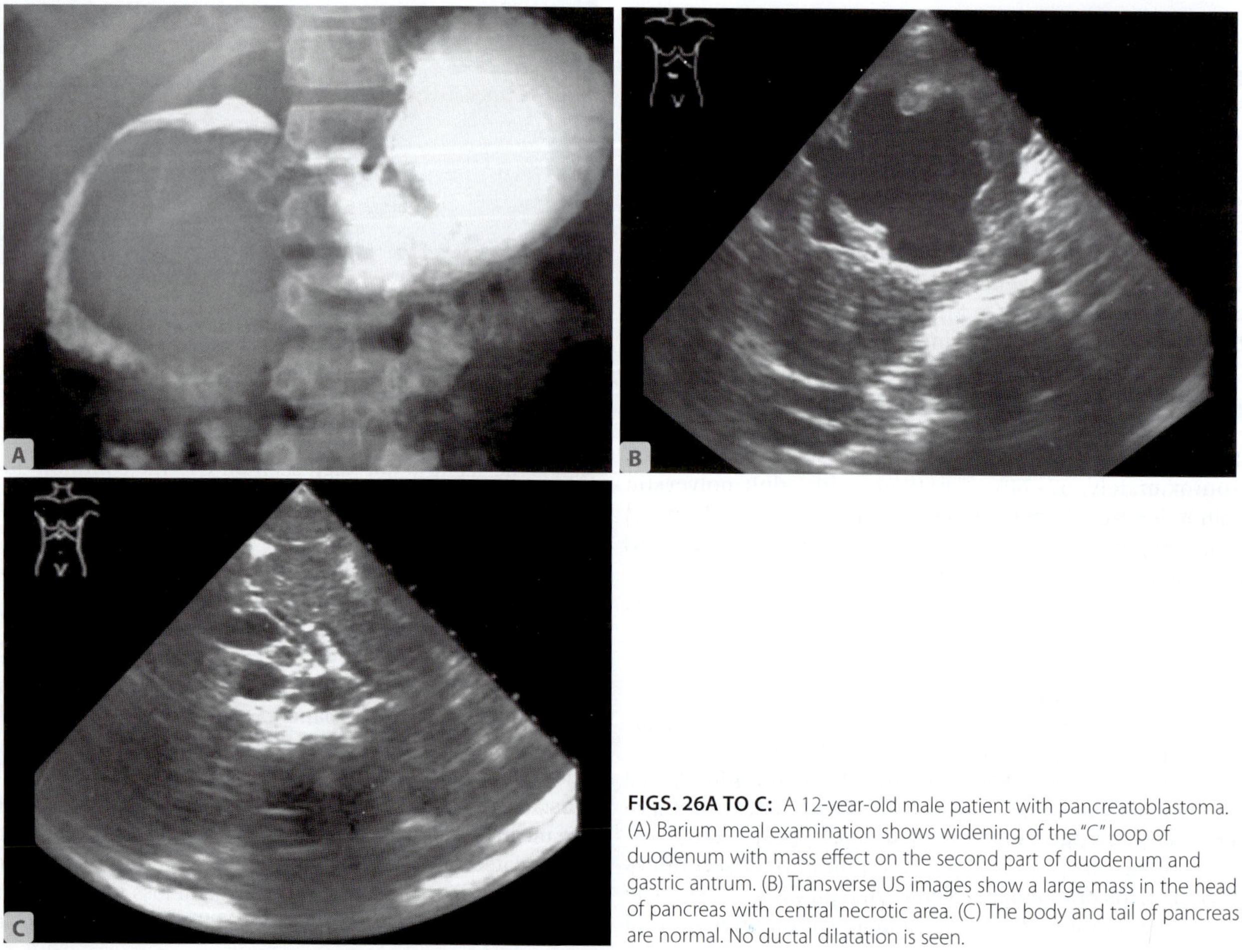

FIGS. 26A TO C: A 12-year-old male patient with pancreatoblastoma. (A) Barium meal examination shows widening of the "C" loop of duodenum with mass effect on the second part of duodenum and gastric antrum. (B) Transverse US images show a large mass in the head of pancreas with central necrotic area. (C) The body and tail of pancreas are normal. No ductal dilatation is seen.

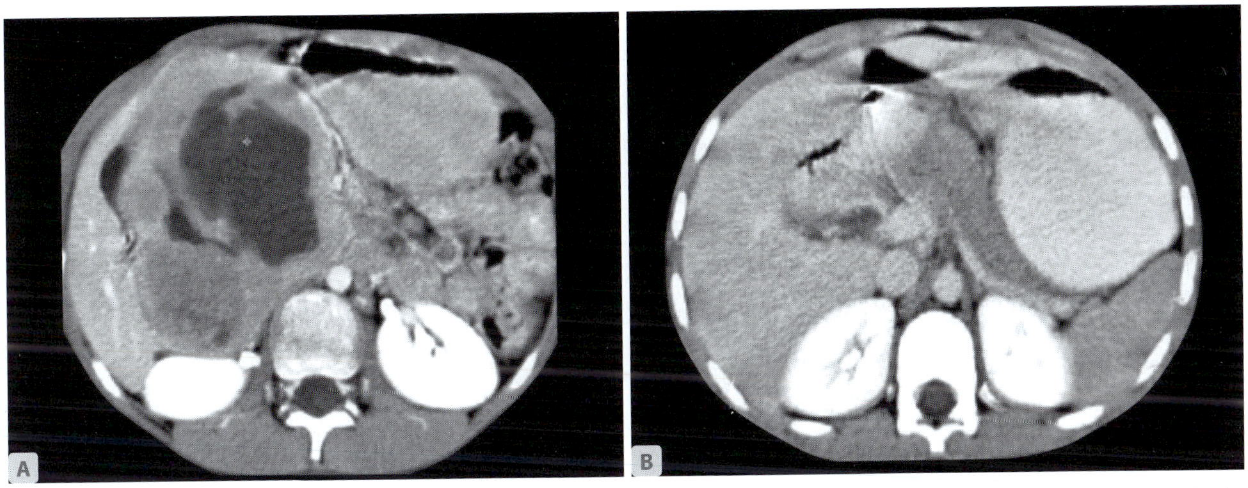

FIGS. 27A AND B: Contrast-enhanced computed tomography (CECT) in the case of pancreatoblastoma shows a large heterogeneous mass in the head of pancreas with central necrosis. There is no dilatation of biliary radicles (A) or pancreatic duct in visualized body and tail of pancreas (B).

by reproducible hypoglycemia in a controlled environment (fasting) and by showing concomitant hyperinsulinemia. **Table 5** shows the clinical and laboratory features of patients with functional islet cell tumors.

Nonfunctioning tumors are usually large at the time of presentation and contain necrotic and calcified areas. They are easily detected due to the mass effect that they produce.

With the availability of helical CT and MRI, invasive imaging techniques such as selective celiac and mesenteric angiography and venography with venous sampling are rarely being used for the diagnosis of islet cell tumors. Selective arteriography is diagnostic in 60–70% of cases while transhepatic portal venous sampling has been reported to have an 86% success rate for tumor localization.[61]

Endoscopic ultrasound is an excellent imaging technique with sensitivity and specificity of 93% and 95%, respectively.[62] On US, these tumors are usually seen as well-defined hypoechoic lesions. A hyperechoic rim may sometimes be seen. Isoechoic and hyperechoic lesions have also been described.

On dual phase helical CT, small islet cell tumors are seen as homogeneous hyperattenuating lesions on the arterial as well as portal venous phase. However, these tumors are hypervascular and the attenuation difference between the lesion and the normal pancreatic parenchyma is more in the arterial phase than in the portal venous phase. Nonfunctioning islet cell tumors also have similar characteristics. Larger lesions show heterogeneous enhancement **(Figs. 28A and B)**. There is no precise data about the sensitivity of biphasic CT for islet cell tumor diagnosis because of the rarity of such studies. The reported sensitivity of CT for localizing functional islet cell tumors is 71–82%.[63]

Fat suppressed T1WI shows islet cell tumors as low signal intensity lesions compared to the normal pancreas. These lesions are hyperintense on T2WI. Some islet cell tumors may be hypointense on T2WI also due to the presence of fibrous tissue. The sensitivity of MR imaging ranges from 24 to 100%.[64] This conflicting data is due to the small reported patient series and the variations in the imaging sequences used.

TABLE 5: Clinical and laboratory features of islet cell tumors.

Functioning islet cell tumor	Clinical presentation	Laboratory findings
Insulinoma	Hypoglycemic attacks, atypical seizures	Low fasting plasma glucose, hyperinsulinemia
Gastrinoma	Peptic ulcers, diarrhea, malabsorption	Elevated serum gastrin
Glucagonoma	Necrolytic migratory erythema	Hyperglycemia
VIPoma	Watery diarrhea, flushing	Hypokalemia, achlorhydria, elevated plasma peptide

Solid and Papillary Epithelial Neoplasm (Frantz Tumor)

This tumor was first described by Frantz in 1959. Solid and papillary epithelial neoplasm (SPEN) is an uncommon low-grade malignant pancreatic tumor which occurs in young women. The usual age of presentation ranges from 10 to 74 years with the mean age at diagnosis being 25 years.[65] However, it also occurs in the pediatric population. It is common in blacks and East Asian patients.

Patients present with an abdominal mass, pain, nausea, and early satiety. The tumor is usually large at presentation and shows areas of necrosis and hemorrhage resulting in cystic cavities. Peripheral calcification is seen in one-third of cases.

Microscopically SPEN has characteristic histological features. The solid areas in the lesion are traversed by numerous delicate blood vessels. The disruption of this delicate vascular network leads to intralesional hemorrhage. Acellular spaces form subsequently, which fill with myxoid connective tissue.

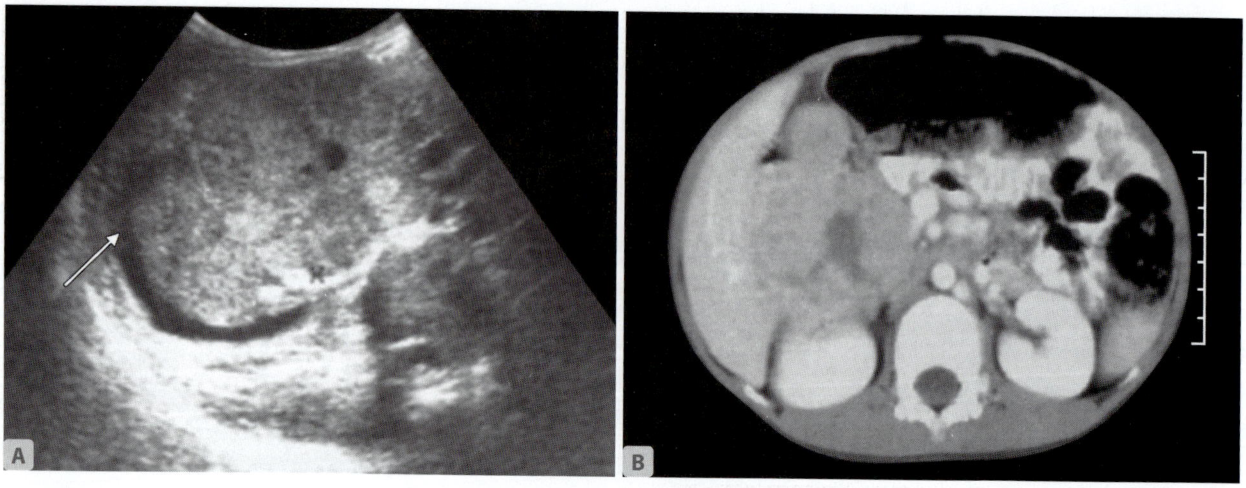

FIGS. 28A AND B: An 8-year-old boy with abdominal mass. (A) US reveals a solid mass lesion with duodenum (arrow) draped around it. (B) Contrast-enhanced computed tomography (CECT) confirms a large heterogeneous mass with central necrosis in the head of pancreas. Histopathological examination of surgical specimen revealed nonfunctioning neuroendocrine tumor of the pancreas.

On US, the tumor shows variable echotexture. Hyperechoic areas are seen due to hemorrhage. The tumor shows heterogeneous attenuation on CT. On MRI **(Figs. 29A to C)**, areas of high signal intensity may be seen on T1WI due to presence of hemorrhagic debris within the tumor. A fluid-debris level may be seen on imaging.

Solid and papillary epithelial neoplasm needs to be distinguished from other cystic lesions of the pancreas such as microcystic adenoma, mucinous cystadenoma, and cystadenocarcinoma, nonfunctioning islet cell tumor, and hemorrhagic pseudocysts. Microcystic adenoma is well-circumscribed lesion with microscopic cystic spaces. This lesion is seen in older women and has no malignant potential. Mucinous cystadenoma may have large cystic spaces and shows fluid-debris levels such as SPEN. This can be differentiated from SPEN due to the presence of multiple loculi and septations. Mucinous cystadenoma is a premalignant lesion and can transform into cystadenocarcinoma.

Mesenchymal Tumors

These account for 1–2% of all pancreatic tumors.[59] These include lymphangioma, lipoma, teratoma, schwannoma, and lymphoma. Their exact prevalence in the pediatric population is unknown.

Lymphangioma is a multicystic lesion with cysts of varying sizes separated by thin septa. CT shows a uni- or multilocular cystic mass with enhancing septa. Calcification is rarely seen within the lesion. Pancreatic lymphangioma may be intraglandular or may be connected to the gland by a pedicle. These lymphangiomas are liable to undergo torsion.

Lipoma is seen as homogeneous well-defined nonenhancing lesion with attenuation value of –30 to –120 HU.

Pancreatic teratoma originates from pluripotential cells and contains both cystic and solid elements such as hair, teeth, cartilage, and dermal appendages. On CT, a complex solid cystic mass with calcifications and fatty component is seen.

Pancreas is an unusual site for visceral schwannomas. In tumors with Antoni type A tissue (organized cellular component), a solid enhancing mass with central necrosis or an inhomogeneous hypodense lesion is seen on CT. In tumors with Antoni type B tissue (loose hypocellular component), CT shows a homogeneous fluid attenuation lesion without any significant contrast enhancement.

Less than 1% of non-Hodgkin's lymphoma (NHL) can be seen in the pancreas. AIDS-related NHL may also involve the pancreas. Pancreatic lymphoma can present as diffuse infiltrating lesion in the pancreas **(Figs. 30A and B)** or as focal well-defined mass.

Primary pancreatic sarcoma accounts for 0.6% of pancreatic malignancies. CT shows a heterogeneous solid mass with inhomogeneous enhancement.[66] Imaging findings cannot distinguish sarcoma from adenocarcinoma.

Pancreatic desmoids are relatively rare tumors with limited cases in the literature. It is difficult to distinguish these tumors radiologically from other malignant soft-tissue tumors **(Figs. 31A to D)**.[66]

Pancreatic Adenocarcinoma

It is the most common pancreatic malignancy occurring in the sixth decade of life but is relatively rare in children. The incidence of pancreatic carcinoma in children is not known. Welch[67] reviewed 38 patients of pancreatic carcinoma in children and found that the age at the time of diagnosis ranged from 3 months to 18 years with a mean age of 9.2 years. Abdominal pain and epigastric mass were the common presentations. Unlike in adult patient, jaundice was found to be less common presenting symptom in children.

The imaging features are similar to those seen in adults. Ultrasound shows a poorly defined, homogeneous or inhomogeneous hypoechoic mass in the pancreas. CT assesses the local extension of the tumor and determines the resectability of the lesion.

Pseudocysts

These are frequent complications of pancreatitis regardless of its etiology. An overall incidence of 10–12% has been reported in pancreatitis with a 30% incidence in case of

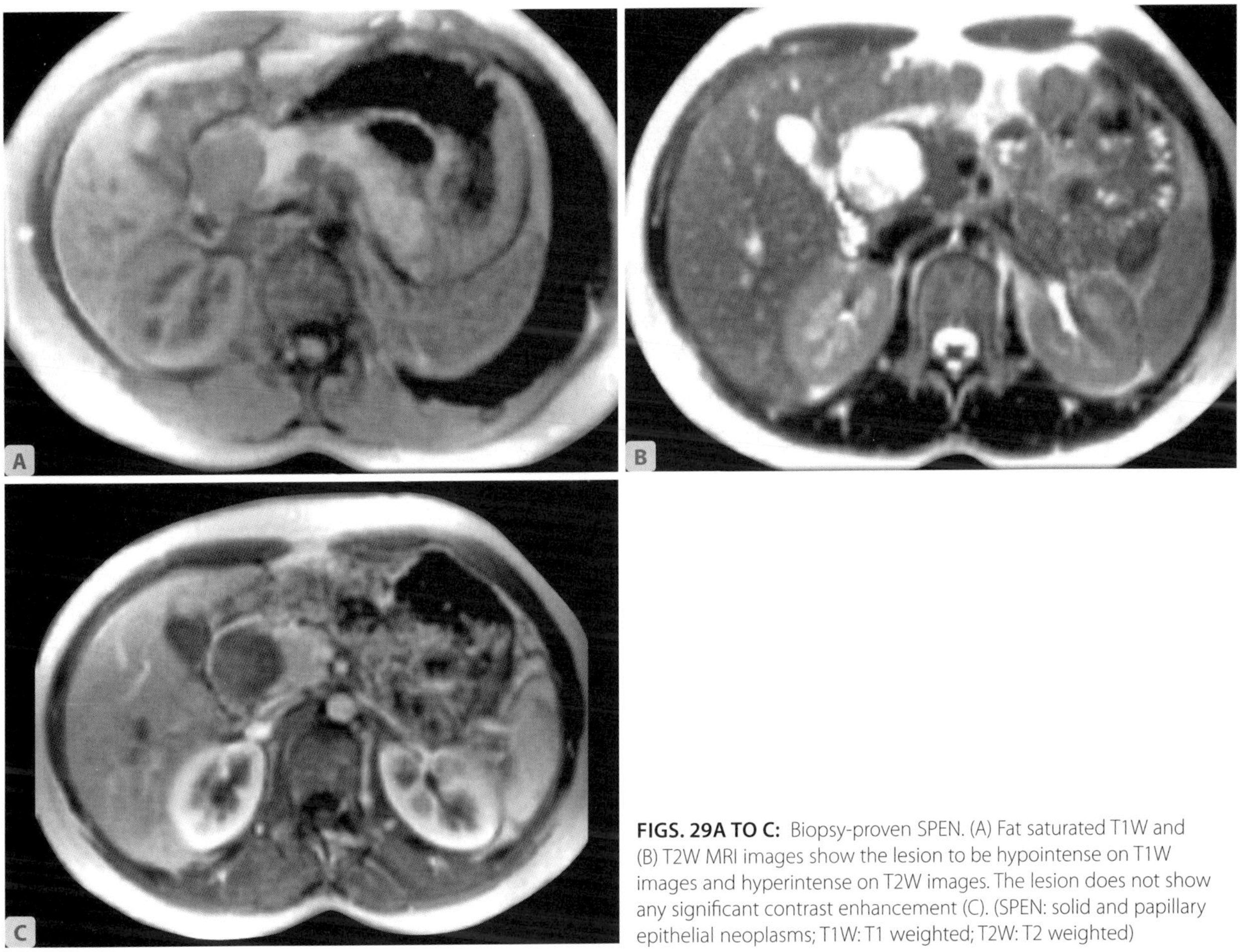

FIGS. 29A TO C: Biopsy-proven SPEN. (A) Fat saturated T1W and (B) T2W MRI images show the lesion to be hypointense on T1W images and hyperintense on T2W images. The lesion does not show any significant contrast enhancement (C). (SPEN: solid and papillary epithelial neoplasms; T1W: T1 weighted; T2W: T2 weighted)

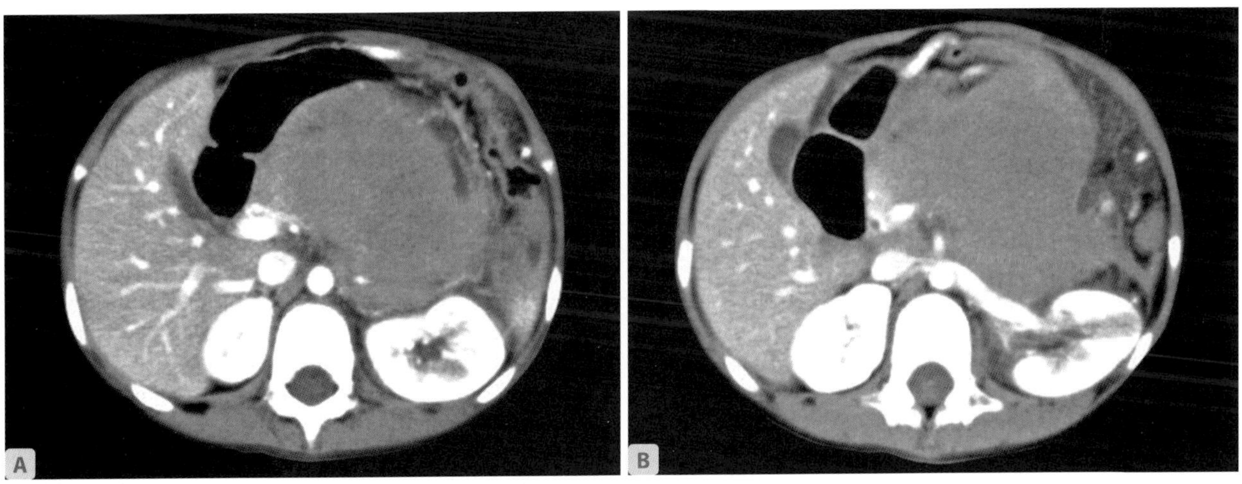

FIGS. 30A AND B: Biopsy-proven non-Hodgkin's lymphoma (NHL) in a 6-year-old boy: Axial contrast-enhanced computed tomography (CECT) images (A and B) show a large homogeneously enhancing mass lesion replacing the entire pancreas.

traumatic pancreatitis.[68] Thus, pseudocysts occur more often in children with traumatic pancreatitis compared with those with nontraumatic pancreatitis.

Acute pancreatitis is uncommon in childhood. The most common etiology is multisystem disease (Reye's syndrome, sepsis, shock, viral infections, and hemolytic uremic syndrome).[69] Other common causes include blunt trauma, congenital anatomic abnormalities, drug toxicity, and metabolic diseases. Children with pancreatitis present with abdominal pain, nausea, and vomiting.

Ultrasonography is the initial imaging modality for detecting pseudocysts in children with pancreatitis.

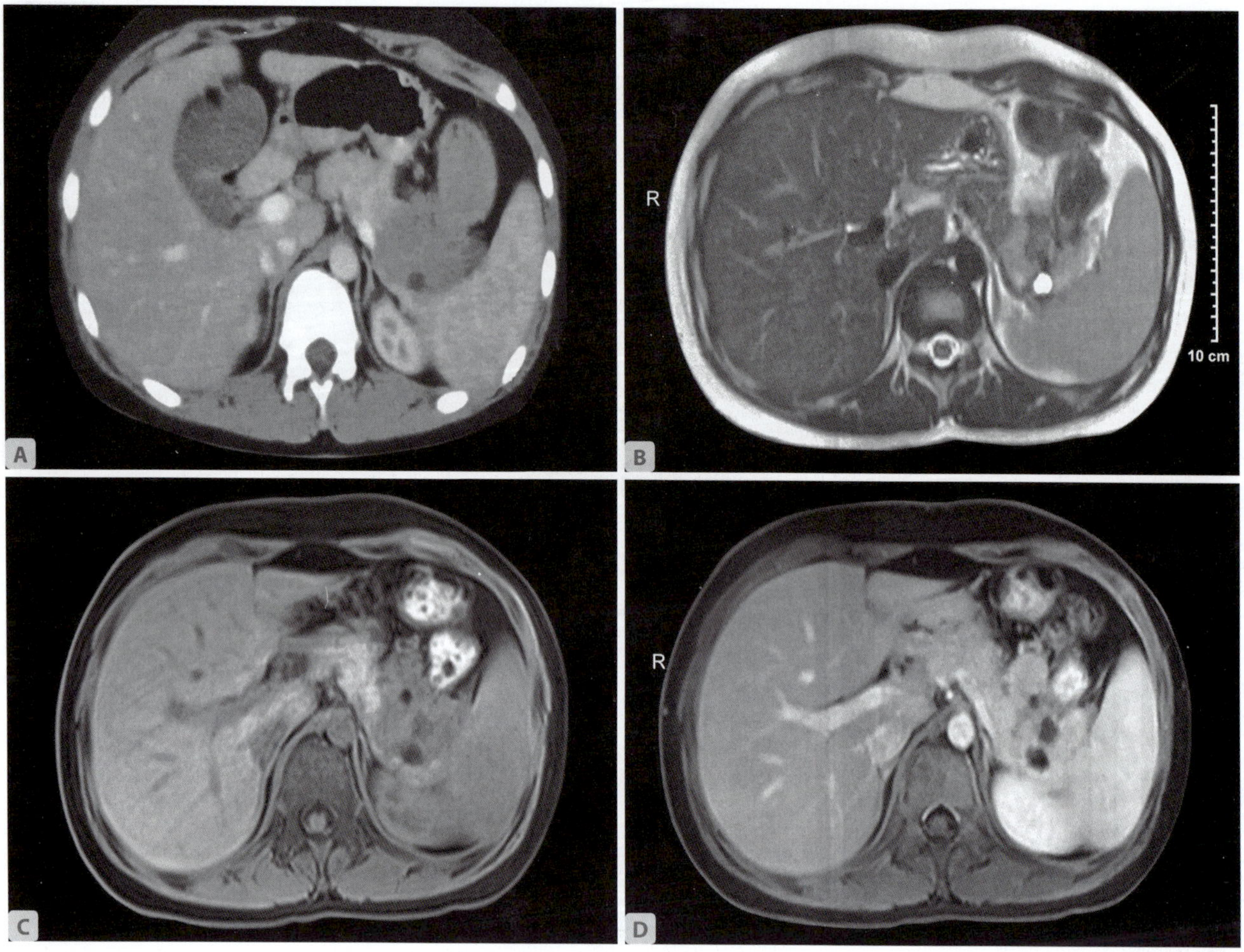

FIGS. 31A TO D: Biopsy-proven desmoid tumor in a 14-year-old boy: Axial contrast-enhanced computed tomography (CECT) image (A) shows a soft-tissue mass in the pancreatic tail region. The mass is heterogeneously hyperintense on T2WI (B), isointense on T1WI (C) and shows postcontrast enhancement (D). Few nonenhancing cystic areas are also seen in it.

Pseudocyst is seen as a well-defined anechoic lesion with or without debris. CT is indicated when the pancreas is not well-visualized on US. On CT, pseudocyst is seen as a low-attenuating lesion with enhancing walls **(Figs. 32A and B)**. High attenuation in the pseudocyst occurs due to hemorrhage or infection.

Magnetic resonance imaging and MRCP provide an increased contrast, thereby helps in better characterization of fluid collections. MRI is superior to CT in demonstrating debris within fluid collections and pseudocysts. A fluid-filled pseudocyst will show a high-signal intensity on T2WI and low signal intensity on T1WI **(Figs. 33A and B)**. In case of complicated or recurrent pancreatitis, MRCP is done to evaluate the pancreatic ductal system for congenital ductal anomalies, delineate the site of disruption and communication of the pseudocyst with the ductal system **(Fig. 33C)**.[70] The knowledge of the status of pancreatic duct is important as it helps in deciding the further plan of management. Nealon and Walser in 2002 proposed a classification of pseudocysts based on pancreatic duct anatomy in which seven different types of pseudocysts were described depending on whether there is communication between the cyst and duct, presence or absence of stricture in the pancreatic duct, and presence or absence of features of chronic pancreatitis.[71]

In the recent years, endoscopic ultrasound (EUS) has emerged as a highly useful diagnostic as well as therapeutic investigation in children. It has a high accuracy and high sensitivity and offers high quality images especially for the subtle abnormalities. It has been found better than MRI and/or CT scan. EUS is being utilized in recurrent pancreatitis, congenital anomalies, microlithiasis, pancreatic pseudocysts, as well as pancreatic masses. It is a safe and cost-effective having both diagnostic and therapeutic roles in pseudocysts.[72]

Pancreatic pseudocysts may resolve spontaneously. In the past nonresolving or infected pseudocyst was drained surgically. Percutaneous drainage is an alternative mode of treatment. Its advantages over surgical drainage include early treatment prior to cyst wall maturation and reduction of length and cost of hospital stay.[73]

Pancreatic Tuberculosis

Abdominal tuberculosis is uncommon in children with a reported incidence of 10% under the age of 10 years.[74]

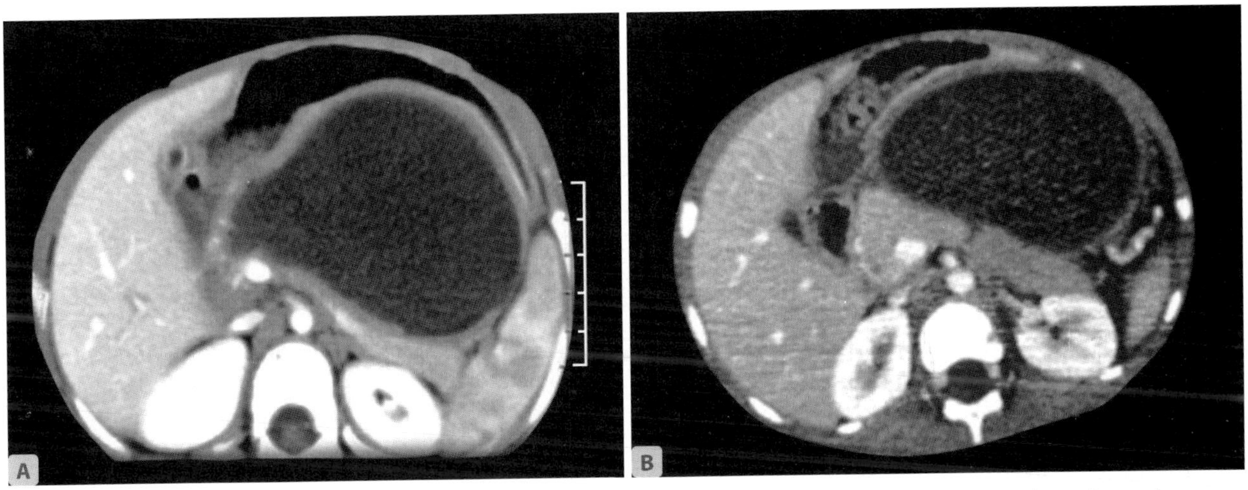

FIGS. 32A AND B: (A) Contrast-enhanced computed tomography (CECT) in a 3-year-old girl patient with pancreatitis and pseudocyst shows a large well-defined fluid attenuation lesion with enhancing wall in the lesser sac. (B) CECT section in another patient with traumatic pancreatitis shows laceration of the pancreas with a fluid collection in the lesser sac.

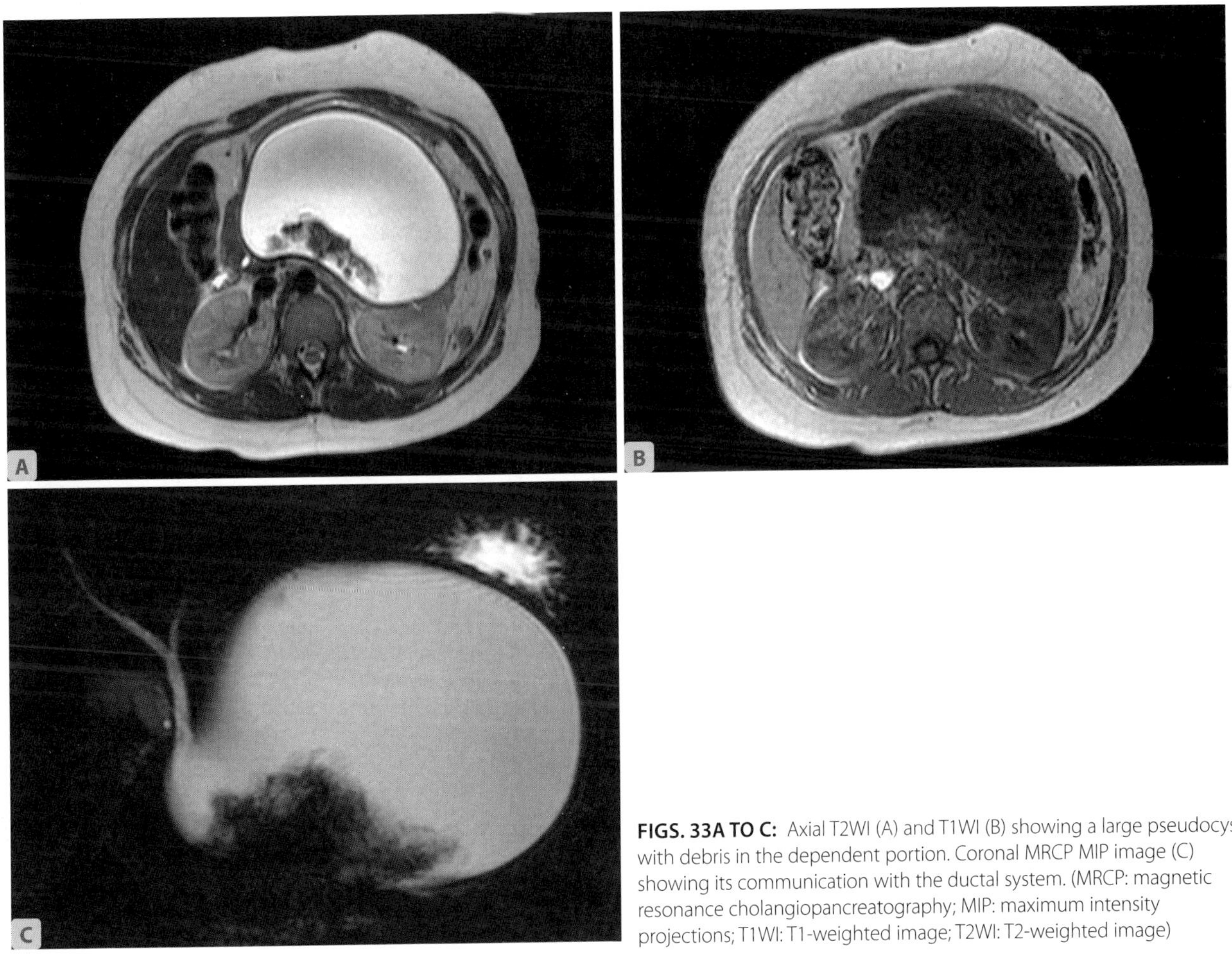

FIGS. 33A TO C: Axial T2WI (A) and T1WI (B) showing a large pseudocyst with debris in the dependent portion. Coronal MRCP MIP image (C) showing its communication with the ductal system. (MRCP: magnetic resonance cholangiopancreatography; MIP: maximum intensity projections; T1WI: T1-weighted image; T2WI: T2-weighted image)

Only 1–5% of cases of pulmonary tuberculosis are complicated by abdominal tuberculosis. Tuberculosis infrequently involves the pancreas. Pancreatic involvement in children was first reported by Andronikou et al. in 2002.[75]

The common presenting features are pain, fever, anorexia, and weight loss. Obstructive jaundice, vomiting, and anemia are less common symptoms.

Ultrasound shows an enlarged pancreas with focal hypoechoic lesions especially in the head region. A cystic lesion may sometimes be seen. CT shows multiple hypodense lesions. The imaging findings are nonspecific and may be mimicked by pancreatic carcinoma or focal pancreatitis. Associated ancillary findings such as hypodense peripancreatic or mesenteric lymph nodes, ascites, mural thickening of the ileocecal region can help in prospectively diagnosing tuberculosis.[76] The diagnosis should, however, be confirmed on US- or CT-guided biopsy.

SUMMARY

Hepatic and pancreatic masses in children are a common clinical problem in pediatric population. Judicious use of various imaging modalities can help to reach at a correct preoperative diagnosis in the majority. Awareness of the imaging characteristics, advantages, and limitations of different imaging techniques is crucial for diagnosis and management.

REFERENCES

1. Kane RA. Liver imaging update. Seminars in ultrasound, CT and MRI. 1992;13:311-2.
2. Takano H, Smith WL. Gastrointestinal tumors of childhood. Radiol Clin North Am. 1997;35:1367-89.
3. Lu DS, Vedantham S, Krasny RM, Kadell B, Berger WL, Reber HA. Two-phase helical CT for pancreatic tumors: Pancreatic versus hepatic phase enhancement of tumor, pancreas, and vascular structures. Radiology. 1996;199:697-701.
4. Image Gently. (2020). Image Gently Mission Statement Update. [online] Available from www.imagegently.org [last accessed June, 2020].
5. Boechat MI, Kangarloo H, Ortega J, Feig S, Stanley P, Gilsanz V, et al. Primary liver tumors in children: Comparison of CT and MR imaging. Radiology. 1988;169:727-32.
6. Weinreb JC, Cohen JM, Armstrong E, Smith T. Imaging the pediatric liver: MRI and CT. AJR Am J Roentgenol. 1986;147: 785-90.
7. Drane WE. Nuclear medicine techniques for the liver and biliary system. Update for the 1990s. Radiol Clin North Am. 1991;29:1129-50.
8. Weinberg AG, Finegold MJ. Primary hepatic tumors of childhood. Hum Pathol. 1983;14:512-37.
9. Siegel MJ. Pediatric liver and biliary tract. In: Margulis AR, Burhennes HJ, (Eds): Alimentary Tract Radiology, 5th edition. USA: Mosby-Year Book Inc.; 1994.
10. Willis RA. The pathology of the tumors of children. In: Cameron R, Wright GP, (Eds). Pathological Monographs. London: Oliver and Boyd; 1962. pp. 57-61.
11. Miller JH, Greenspan BS. Integrated imaging of hepatic tumors in childhood. Part I: Malignant lesions (primary and metastatic). Radiology. 1985;154:83-90.
12. Roebuck DJ, Olsen Ø, Pariente D. Radiological staging in children with hepatoblastoma. Pediatr Radiol. 2006;36:176-82.
13. Towbin AJ, Meyers RL, Woodley H, Miyazaki O, Weldon CB, Morland B, et al. 2017 PRETEXT: radiologic staging system for primary hepatic malignancies of childhood revised for the Paediatric Hepatic International Tumour Trial (PHITT). Pediatr Radiol. 2018;48:536-54.
14. Dachman AH, Pakter RL, Ros PR, Fishman EK, Goodman ZD, Lichtenstein JE. Hepatoblastoma: Radiologic-pathologic correlation in 50 cases. Radiology. 1987;164:15-9.
15. Men S, Hekimoðlu B, Tüzün M, Arda IS, Pinar A. Unusual US and CT findings in hepatoblastoma: A case report. Pediatr Radiol. 1995;25:507-8.
16. Amendola MA, Blane CE, Amendola BE, Glazer GM. CT findings in hepatoblastoma. J Comput Assist Tomogr. 1984;8:1105-9.
17. Schlesinger AE, Parker BR. Tumors and tumor-like conditions. In: Kuhn JP, Slovis TL, Haller JO (Eds). Caffey's Pediatric Diagnostic imaging, 10th edition. USA: Mosby; 2004. pp. 1493-508.
18. Blickman JG, Connolly SA. Pediatric imaging: Liver, biliary tree, and pancreas. In: Gazelle GS, Saini S, Mueller PR (Eds). Hepatobiliary and Pancreatic Radiology, Imaging and Intervention, 1st edition. Germany: Thieme Medical Publishers; 1998. pp. 240-70.
19. Brandt DJ, Johnson CD, Stephens DH, Weiland LH. Imaging of fibrolamellar hepatocellular carcinoma. AJR Am J Roentgenol. 1988;151:295-9.
20. Horton KM, Bluemke DA, Hruban RH, Soyer P, Fishman EK. CT and MR imaging of benign hepatic and biliary tumors. Radiographics. 1999;19:431-51.
21. Buetow PC, Buck JL, Pantongrag-Brown L, Marshall WH, Ros PR, Levine MS, et al. Undifferentiated (embryonal) sarcoma of the liver: pathologic basis of imaging findings in 28 cases. Radiology. 1997;203:779-83.
22. Rakheja D, Margraf LR, Tomlinson GE, Schneider NR. Hepatic mesenchymal hamartoma with translocation involving chromosome band 19q13.4: a recurrent abnormality. Cancer Genet Cytogenet. 2004;153:60-3.
23. Siegel MJ, Chung EM, Conran RM. Pediatric liver: focal masses. Magn Reson Imaging Clin North Am. 2008;16:437-52.
24. Ros PR, Olmsted WW, Dachman HH, Goodman ZD, Ishak KG, Hartman DS. Undifferentiated (embryonal) sarcoma of the liver: radiologic-pathologic correlation. Radiology. 1986;161:141-5
25. Chung EM, Lattin Jr GE, Cube R, Lewis RB, Marichal-Hernández C, Shawhan R, et al. From the archives of the AFIP: pediatric liver masses: radiologic-pathologic correlation. Part 2. Malignant tumors. Radiographics. 2011;31:483-507.
26. Ruymann FB, Raney RB Jr, Crist WM, Lawrence W Jr, Lindberg RD, Soule EH. Rhabdomyosarcoma of the biliary tree in childhood. A report from the Intergroup Rhabdomyosarcoma Study. Cancer. 1985;56:575-81.
27. Adler B, Naheedy J,Yeager N, Nicol K, KlamarJ. Multifocal epithelioid hemangioendothelioma in a 16-year-old boy. Pediatr Radiol. 2005;35:1014-8.
28. Da Ines D, Petitcolin V, Joubert-Zakeyh J, Demeocq F, Garcier JM. Epithelioid hemangioendothelioma of the liver with metastatic coeliac lymph nodes in an 11-year-old boy. Pediatr Radiol. 2010;40:1293-6.
29. Makhlouf HR, Ishak KG, Goodman ZD. Epithelioid hemangioendothelioma of the liver: a clinico- pathologic study of 137 cases. Cancer. 1999;85:562-82.
30. Miller WJ, Dodd GD 3rd, Federle MP, Baron RL. Epithelioid hemangioendothelioma of the liver: imaging findings with pathologic correlation. AJR Am J Roentgenol. 1992;159:5-7.

31. Leonardou P, Semelka RC, Mastropasqua M, Kanematsu M, Woosley JT. Epithelioid hemangioen. dothelioma of the liver: MR imaging findings. Magn Reson Imaging. 2002;20:631-3.
32. Ros LH, Fernández L, Villacampa VM, Ros PR. Epithelioid hemangioendothelioma of the liver: characteristics on magnetic resonance imaging—case report. Can Assoc Radiol J. 1999;50:387-9.
33. Lyburn ID, Torreggiani WC, Harris AC, et al. Hepatic epithelioid hemangioendothelioma: sono- graphic, CT, and MR imaging appearances. AJR Am J Roentgenol. 2003;180:1359-64.
34. Mulliken JB, Fishman SJ, Burrows PE. Vascular anomalies. Curr Probl Surg. 2000;37:517-84.
35. Berenguer B, Mulliken JB, Enjolras O, Boon LM, Wassef M. Rapidly involuting congenital hemangioma: clinical and histopathologic features. Pediatr Dev Pathol. 2003;6:495-510.
36. Christison-Lagay ER, Burrows PE, Alomari A, Dubois J, Kozakewich HP, Lane TS, et al. Hepatic hemangiomas: subtype classification and development of a clinical practice algorithm and registry. J Pediatr Surg. 2007;42(1):62-7.
37. Huang SA, Tu HM, Harney JW, Venihaki M, Butte AJ, Kozakewich HP, et al. Severe hypothyroidism caused by type 3 iodothyronine deiodinase in infantile hemangiomas. N Engl J Med. 2000;343: 185-9.
38. Abramson SJ, Lack EE, Teele RL. Benign vascular tumors of the liver in infants: Sonographic appearance. AJR Am J Roentgenol. 1982;138:629-32.
39. Ros PR, Goodman ZD, Ishak KG, Dachman AH, Olmsted WW, Hartman DS, et al. Mesenchymal hamartoma of the liver: Radiologic-pathologic correlation. Radiology. 1986;158: 619-24.
40. Narasimharao KL, Narasimhan KL, Katariya S, Suri S, Kaushik S, Mitra SK. Giant hamartoma of liver mimicking malignancy. Postgrad Med J. 1988;64:398-400.
41. Stanley P, Hall TR, Woolley MM, Diament MJ, Gilsanz V, Miller JH. Mesenchymal hamartomas of the liver in childhood: Sonographic and CT findings. AJR Am J Roentgenol. 1986;147:1035-9.
42. Rogers JV, Mack LA, Freeny PC, Johnson ML, Sones PJ. Hepatic focal nodular hyperplasia: Angiography, CT, sonography, and scintigraphy. AJR Am J Roentgenol. 1981;137:983-90.
43. Chusid MJ. Pyogenic hepatic abscess in infancy and childhood. Pediatrics. 1978;62:554-9.
44. Newlin N, Silver TM, Stuck KJ, Sandler MA. Ultrasonic features of pyogenic liver abscesses. Radiology. 1981;139:155-9.
45. Towbin RB, Strife JL. Percutaneous aspiration, drainage, and biopsies in children. Radiology. 1985;157:81-5.
46. Rajak CL, Gupta S, Jain S, Chawla Y, Gulati M, Suri S. Percutaneous treatment of liver abscesses: Needle aspiration versus catheter drainage. AJR Am J Roentgenol. 1998;170:1035-9.
47. Ralls PW, Colletti PM, Quinn MF, Halls J. Sonographic findings in hepatic amebic abscess. Radiology. 1982;145:123-6.
48. Miller JH, Greenfield LD, Wald BR. Candidiasis of the liver and spleen in childhood. Radiology. 1982;142:375-80.
49. Brauner M, Buffard MD, Jeantils V, Legrand I, Gotheil C. Sonography and computed tomography of macroscopic tuberculosis of the liver. J Clin Ultrasound. 1989;17:563-8.
50. Denton T, Hossain J. A radiological study of abdominal tuberculosis in a Saudi population, with special reference to ultrasound and computed tomography. Clin Radiol. 1993;47:409-14.
51. Beggs I. The radiology of hydatid disease. AJR Am J Roentgenol. 1985;145:639-48.
52. Lewall DB, McCorkell SJ. Rupture of echinococcal cysts: Diagnosis, classification, and clinical implications. AJR Am J Roentgenol. 1986;146:391-4.
53. Jain R, Sawhney S, Berry M. Hydatid disease: CT demonstration and follow-up of a cystogastric fistula. AJR Am J Roentgenol. 1992;158:212.
54. Wan SK, Cochlin DL. Sonographic and computed tomographic features of polycystic disease of the liver. Gastrointest Radiol. 1990;15:310-2.
55. Tomà P, Lucigrai G, Pelizza A. Sonographic patterns of Caroli's disease: Report of 5 new cases. J Clin Ultrasound. 1991;19:155-61.
56. Horie A, Yano Y, Kotoo Y, Miwa A. Morphogenesis of pancreatoblastoma, infantile carcinoma of the pancreas: Report of two cases. Cancer. 1977;39:247-54.
57. Willnow U, Willberg B, Schwamborn D, Körholz D, Göbel U. Pancreatoblastoma in children. Case report and review of the literature. Eur J Pediatr Surg. 1996;6:369-72.
58. Drut R, Jones MC. Congenital pancreatoblastoma in Beckwith-Wiedemann syndrome: An emerging association. Pediatr Pathol. 1988;8:331-9.
59. Klöppel G, Maillet B. Classification and staging of pancreatic nonendocrine tumors. Radiol Clin North Am. 1989;27:105-19.
60. Gupta AK, Mitra DK, Berry M, Dinda AK, Bhatnagar V. Sonography and CT of pancreatoblastoma in children. AJR Am J Roentgenol. 2000;174:1639-41.
61. Grosfeld JL, Vane DW, Rescorla FJ, McGuire W, West KW. Pancreatic tumors in childhood: Analysis of 13 cases. J Pediatr Surg. 1990;25:1057-62.
62. Anderson MA, Carpenter S, Thompson NW, Nostrant TT, Elta GH, Scheiman JM. Endoscopic ultrasound is highly accurate and directs management in patients with neuroendocrine tumors of the pancreas. Am J Gastroenterol. 2000;95:2271-7.
63. Sheth S, Fishman EK. Imaging of uncommon tumors of the pancreas. Radiol Clin North Am. 2002;40:1273-87.
64. Ichikawa T, Peterson MS, Federle MP, Baron RL, Haradome H, Kawamori Y, et al. Islet cell tumor of the pancreas: Biphasic CT versus MR imaging in tumor detection. Radiology. 2000;216: 163-71.
65. Buetow PC, Buck JL, Pantongrag-Brown L, Beck KG, Ros PR, Adair CF. Solid and papillary epithelial neoplasm of the pancreas: Imaging-pathologic correlation on 56 cases. Radiology. 1996;199:707-11.
66. Ferrozzi F, Zuccoli G, Bova D, Calculli L. Mesenchymal tumors of the pancreas: CT findings. J Comput Assist Tomogr. 2000;24:622-7.
67. Welch KJ. The pancreas. In: Ravitch MM, Randolph JG, Rowe MI, (Eds). Pediatric Surgery, 3rd edition. Chicago, IL: Year book; 1984. pp. 1090-6.
68. Eichelberger MR, Hoelzer DJ, Koop CE. Acute pancreatitis: The difficulties of diagnosis and therapy. J Pediatr Surg. 1982;17:244-54.
69. Weizman Z, Durie PR. Acute pancreatitis in childhood. J Pediatr. 1988;113:24-9.
70. Habashi S, Draganov PV. Pancreatic pseudocyst. World J Gastroenterol. 2009;15:38-47.
71. Nealon WH, Walser E. Main pancreatic ductal anatomy can direct choice of modality for treating pancreatic pseudocysts (surgery versus percutaneous drainage). Ann Surg. 2002;235:751-8.
72. Lal SB, Venkatesh V, Rana SS, Anushree N, Bhatia A, Saxena A. Paediatric acute pancreatitis: Clinical profile and natural history of collections. Pancreatology. 2020;S1424-3903(20)30098-3.
73. Amundson GM, Towbin RB, Mueller DL, Seagram CG. Percutaneous transgastric drainage of the lesser sac in children. Pediatr Radiol. 1990;20:590-3.
74. Aston NO. Abdominal tuberculosis. World J Surg. 1997;21:492-9.
75. Andronikou S, Welman CJ, Kader E. The CT features of abdominal tuberculosis in children. Pediatr Radiol. 2002;32:75-81.
76. Takhtani D, Gupta S, Suman K, Kakkar N, Challa S, Wig JD, et al. Radiology of pancreatic tuberculosis: A report of three cases. Am J Gastroenterol. 1996;91:1832-4.

CHAPTER

71

Imaging and Interventions in Pediatric Budd–Chiari Syndrome

Kumble S Madhusudhan, Sanjay Sharma

INTRODUCTION

Budd–Chiari syndrome (BCS) is a rare vascular disease of the liver in which there is obstruction to the venous drainage of blood out of the liver. Therefore, it is also called as *hepatic venous outflow tract obstruction* (HVOTO). The obstruction may occur at the level of hepatic veins (HVs), inferior vena cava (IVC), or both. The IVC can get obstructed at its intrahepatic segment or suprahepatic course. Since the term "HVOTO" also includes cardiac conditions which lead to congestive hepatopathy and the veno-occlusive disease, the term BCS is more widely accepted.[1]

While BCS more commonly affects adult population, the true incidence in children is not clearly known. Indian data has shown that the pediatric patients account for approximately 5–10% of all BCS cases.[2,3] In view of lack of awareness of this disease and the nonspecific presenting symptoms, the diagnosis is often delayed. Imaging plays an important role in the diagnosis of pediatric BCS. Ultrasonography (USG) is the most valuable imaging modality as it not only plays a role in the diagnosis, but also in guiding radiological interventions.[4] Percutaneous radiological intervention, which is aimed at recanalization of the occluded venous channel and/or relieving the symptoms of portal hypertension, is the treatment of choice. The aims of imaging are to detect the disease, demonstrate the anatomical location and length of occlusion, and identify the hepatic parenchymal changes and signs of portal hypertension.

PATHOPHYSIOLOGY

The pathophysiology of pediatric BCS relates to the spectrum of the changes seen on imaging **(Fig. 1)**.[5] Presumably, the inciting event is the thrombosis of HV and/or IVC that occurs spontaneously or secondary to various underlying etiologies described below.[1] The liver has three hepatic veins draining into the IVC **(Figs. 2A to C)**. Involvement of one or two hepatic veins is usually without any consequence. Generally, it is the occlusion of all three hepatic veins that are needed for appearance of clinical symptoms.[6] Subsequently, the thrombosis either recanalizes or more commonly organizes to result in the formation of discrete "membranous webs," fibrotic stenosis, or occlusions. The occluded segment of HV and/or IVC may be short (<5 mm) or long (5–20 mm) segment or fibrotic and cord like.[4] There is sequential involvement of the HV and IVC. One may, therefore, note various stages of involvement of the three HVs and IVC.

As a result of occlusion of one HV, the other patent HV dilates and venovenous collateral channels develop to divert the blood from the occluded HV to the patent HV. However, as the disease progresses, the patent HVs may also get occluded. In an attempt to drain blood out of the liver, several other collaterals develop from the occluded HV to hepatic capsular veins and suprahepatic IVC. These collaterals are inadequate to satisfactorily drain the liver of its venous blood. Thus, there is progressive increase in the hepatic sinusoidal pressure leading to portal venous hypertension.[7] Long-standing portal hypertension subsequently results in complications like esophageal varices, splenomegaly, and ascites.[1] Due to constantly elevated sinusoidal pressure, there is ischemic necrosis in the perisinusoidal compartment and deposition of fibrosis in the liver parenchyma. If it is left untreated, cirrhosis ensues. Since the caudate lobe drains directly into the IVC through multiple veins, it may often remain uninvolved by the disease and undergoes compensatory hypertrophy along with the dilatation of the caudate vein(s).

ETIOLOGY AND CLINICAL PRESENTATION

The pediatric BCS may be primary or secondary **(Table 1)**. Various underlying coagulopathies have been identified as a cause of primary BCS in children. Approximately 50–80% of children with primary BCS have an underlying etiology.[8] In the remaining, no cause is identified. The etiologies causing primary pediatric BCS include systemic conditions which result in hypercoagulability. These include thrombophilia, protein C and protein S deficiency, antithrombin III deficiency, antiphospholipid antibody syndrome, factor V Leiden mutation, Janus kinase 2 (JAK2) mutation, homocysteinemia, etc. Poor hygiene and low standards of living have also been found to be associated with pediatric BCS.[9] Secondary BCS is caused by tumors and infective/

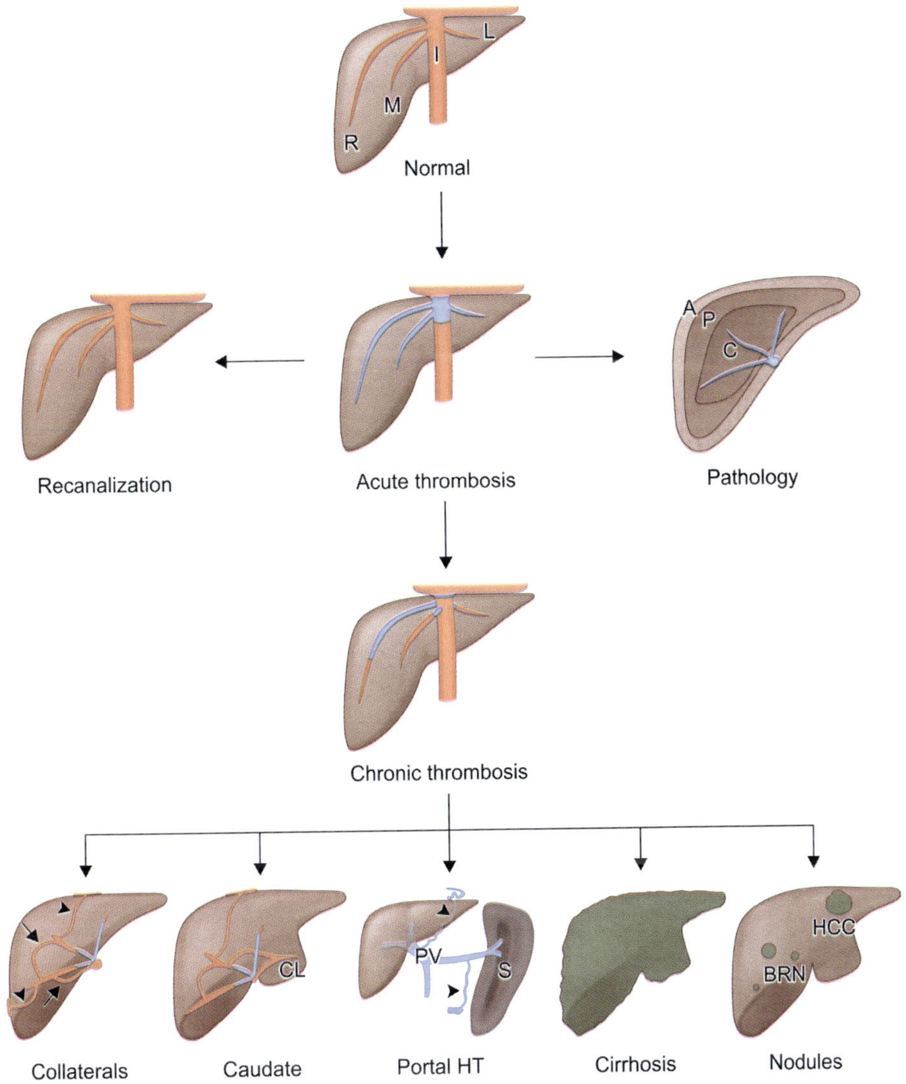

FIG. 1: Schematic diagram of the pathophysiology of Budd–Chiari syndrome. Arrows indicate venovenous collaterals and arrowheads indicate portosystemic collaterals. (a: ascites; brn: benign regenerative nodules; c: central liver; cl: caudate lobe; hcc: hepatocellular carcinoma; HT: hypertension; I: inferior vena cava; L: left hepatic vein; M: middle hepatic vein; p: peripheral liver; pv: portal vein; R: right hepatic vein; s: spleen)

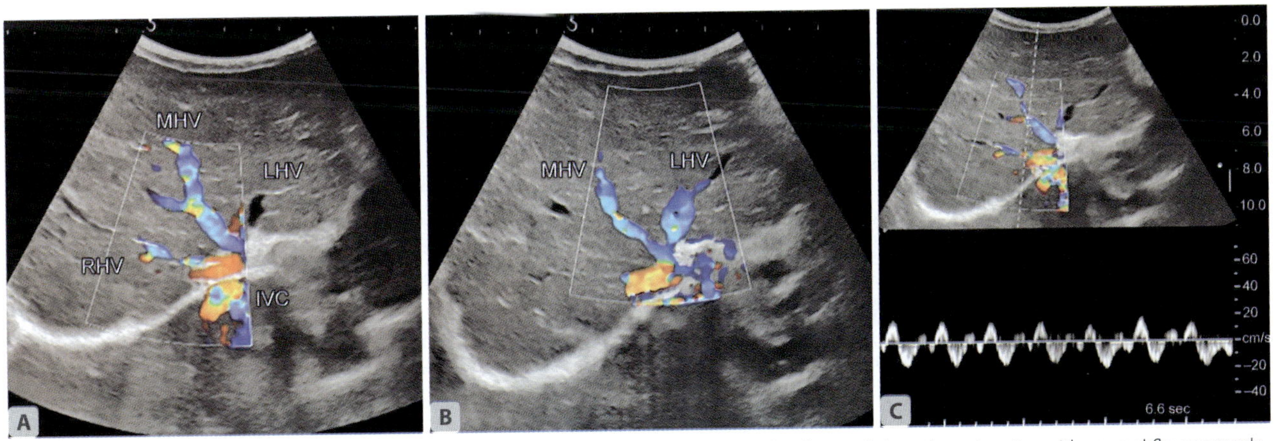

FIGS. 2A TO C: Normal hepatic venous anatomy: (A and B) Color Doppler ultrasonography shows all three hepatic veins with normal flow towards the IVC. (C) Normal pulsatile spectral waveform is seen within the middle hepatic vein. (IVC: inferior vena cava; LHV: left hepatic vein; MHV: middle hepatic vein; RHV: right hepatic vein)

TABLE 1: Etiology of pediatric Budd–Chiari syndrome (BCS).

Types	Causes
Primary BCS	• Thrombophilia • Protein C and protein S deficiency • Antithrombin III deficiency • Antiphospholipid antibody syndrome • Factor V Leiden mutation • Janus kinase 2 (JAK2) mutation • Homocysteinemia • Paroxysmal nocturnal hemoglobinuria • Myeloproliferative disorders
Secondary BCS	• Infections like abscesses • Hepatic tumors • Retroperitoneal tumors (renal, adrenal) • Behcet's syndrome • Trauma
Idiopathic	—

BOX 1: Forms of clinical presentation of pediatric Budd–Chiari syndrome.

- Asymptomatic
- Fulminant
- Acute
- Subacute
- Chronic (most common)

TABLE 2: Morphological classification of pediatric Budd–Chiari syndrome.

Based on type of vein involved	
Type I	Inferior vena cava
Type II	Hepatic vein
Type III	Mixed (inferior vena cava and hepatic vein)
Based on length of venous involvement	
Web or membranous	Thin web
Short segment	<5 mm long
Long segment	5–20 mm long
Near complete or complete	>20 mm long

TABLE 3: Imaging signs of pediatric Budd–Chiari syndrome.

Direct signs	• Thrombosis of hepatic vein (HV) or inferior vena cava (IVC) • Occlusion or nonvisualization of HV or IVC
Indirect signs	• Venovenous collaterals • Dilated caudate vein • Enlarged caudate lobe • Hepatic atrophy-hypertrophy complex • Dilated accessory HVs • Hepatic parenchymal perfusion changes • Benign regenerative nodules • Ascites • Features of portal hypertension

inflammatory diseases developing around the HV and IVC and causing their occlusion by compression or invasion.[1]

The clinical presentation of pediatric BCS has been classified into five types **(Box 1)**.[1,10] These include asymptomatic, fulminant, acute, subacute, and chronic forms. Patients may be *asymptomatic* when there are large collaterals which sufficiently drain the liver preserving liver function. The rarer *fulminant* form occurs when all the three hepatic veins are rapidly occluded by thrombosis. The patients present with features of hepatic encephalopathy, renal failure and coagulopathy, and have tender hepatomegaly. In *acute* form, there is a few weeks history of abdominal pain and distension due to ascites, jaundice, and liver dysfunction.[10] The patients with *subacute* form of the disease have symptoms like abdominal discomfort, lump due to splenomegaly, and mild jaundice for few months before presentation. The *chronic* form, which is the most common type (60%), has symptoms lasting over 6 months and may present with variceal bleeding, hepatic encephalopathy, and gross ascites.[1]

MORPHOLOGICAL CLASSIFICATION

Depending on the type of the venous channel involved, pediatric BCS has been classified into three types **(Table 2)**.[11] Type I involves IVC, type II involves HV, and type III is mixed type, involving both HV and IVC. Type II is the most common type (72%), followed by type III (24%) and type I (4%).[12] This classification helps in planning radiological interventions. Classification can also be made based on the length of venous obstruction into web or membranous, short segment, long segment, and near-complete or complete occlusion **(Table 2)**.

IMAGING MODALITIES

The various imaging modalities used in the evaluation of pediatric BCS include USG, computed tomography (CT) scan, magnetic resonance imaging (MRI), and venography.[13] Among these, USG is the most accurate diagnostic modality with sensitivity and accuracy of 90% and 95%, respectively.[5] It is a simple modality that requires no sedation and involves no ionizing radiation. Therefore, it is the diagnostic modality of first choice. It also plays a major role in guiding the radiological interventions. CT scan and MRI are performed when the USG diagnosis is equivocal and for evaluation of complications like hepatic nodules and portal vein thrombosis. Uncommonly, the disease may be incidentally detected when imaging is done for an unrelated indication. Contrast venography of HV or IVC may be occasionally necessary to evaluate the equivocal findings on USG. The findings seen on imaging depend on the stage of the disease and are divided into direct and indirect signs **(Table 3)**.

IMAGING DIAGNOSIS OF PEDIATRIC BUDD–CHIARI SYNDROME

Ultrasonography

As mentioned previously, USG is the imaging modality of first choice for evaluation of patients with a clinical suspicion of BCS. The findings on USG are divided into two categories: (1) Direct and (2) Indirect signs.[4,14]

Direct signs are seen involving the HV or IVC itself. In acute BCS, the HV contains echogenic material in the lumen suggestive of acute thrombus **(Figs. 3A and B)**. No flow is seen within the vein on color Doppler USG (CDUSG). The vein itself may not be dilated and shows thin smooth walls. This thrombus may either resolve spontaneously or with treatment or may evolve into a chronic thrombus.[15] In subacute and chronic cases, the HV and IVC show partial or complete occlusion by an organized thrombus **(Figs. 4A to C)**. The pathology may be either complete occlusion or varying degrees of stenosis. On the B-mode image, the occluded segment may show three different morphologies. In membranous occlusion, there is a thin web-like echogenic lesion causing occlusion **(Figs. 5A and B)**.[16] In short segment occlusion, the length of HV or IVC involvement is <5 mm and the segment appears as an echogenic area with no flow on CDUSG **(Figs. 4A to C)**.[17] The occlusion may be a long segment (5–20 mm) or involve entire HV and may appear as an echogenic cord with no flow **(Figs. 6A and B)**. The segment of the HV or IVC proximal to the occlusion is usually dilated and may show either smooth or irregular outline, the latter finding being due to recanalization of a thrombosed segment. The segment shows slow forward or reversed flow on CDUSG.[5] The atrial transmitted pulsations are absent and the vein shows monophasic flow **(Figs. 7A to C)**. Uncommonly, the flow within the HV or IVC may be too slow to be detected by CDUSG. At the site of occlusion, there is aliasing due to eddy currents in flow and in cases of stenosis, the segment shows high peak systolic velocity (PSV), often >100 cm/s.[17] The three HVs are often involved with variable severity which can be demonstrated on USG **(Figs. 8A to C)**. Multiple segments may be involved in the same vein.

There are various indirect signs which assist in making the diagnosis of BCS.[4] These include venovenous collaterals, enlarged caudate and accessory veins, hepatic atrophy-

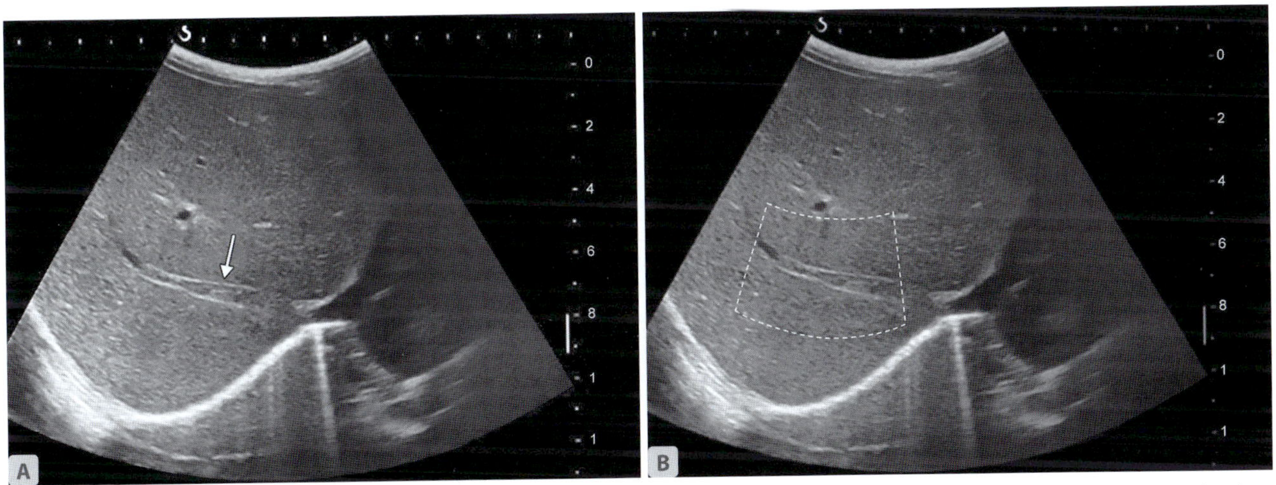

FIGS. 3A AND B: Ultrasonography of acute hepatic vein thrombosis: (A and B) B-mode and color Doppler images show echogenic material in the right hepatic vein (arrow) with no flow suggestive of acute thrombosis.

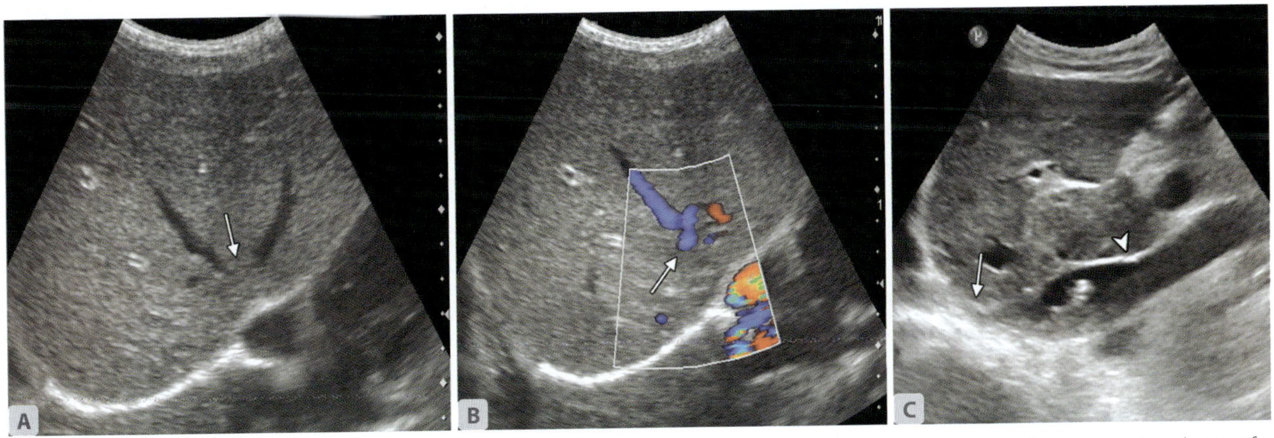

FIGS. 4A TO C: Ultrasonography of chronic Budd–Chiari syndrome: (A and B) B-mode and color Doppler images show long segment occlusion of ostia of middle and left hepatic veins (arrow in A) with collaterals near the occlusion (arrow in B). (C) B-mode image shows short segment occlusion of suprahepatic inferior vena cava (arrow) with its dilatation (arrowhead).

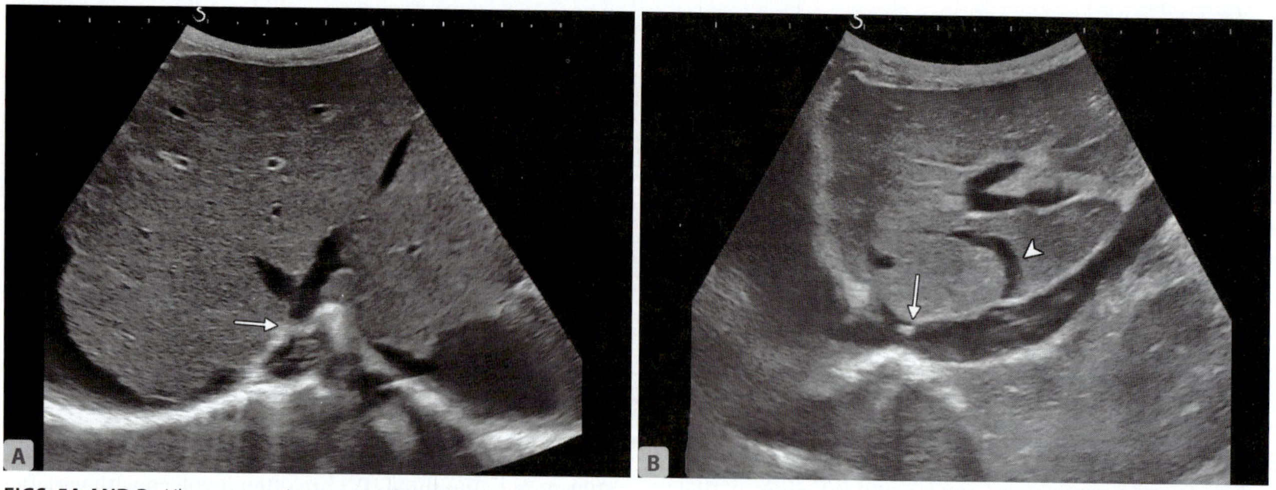

FIGS. 5A AND B: Ultrasonographic images of membranous occlusion: (A) B-mode image shows membrane-like web occluding the common ostium of middle and left hepatic veins (arrow). (B) B-mode image shows a discrete echogenic web (arrow) in the suprahepatic inferior vena cava, likely due to calcification. Prominent caudate vein is noted (arrowhead).

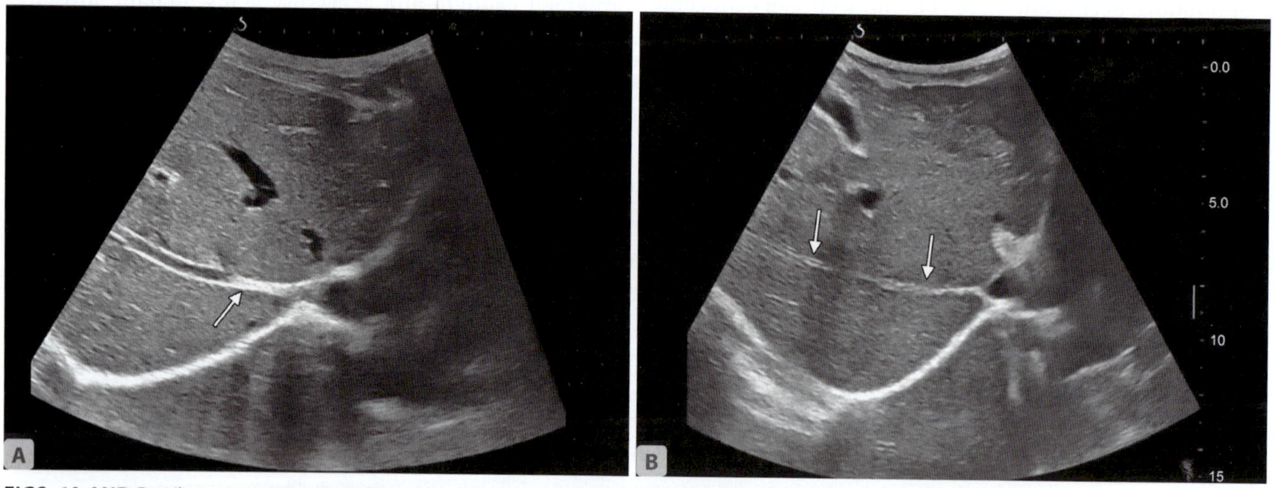

FIGS. 6A AND B: Ultrasonography of cord-like veins: B-mode images of two children with Budd–Chiari syndrome show long segment cord-like appearance of right hepatic vein (arrows) due to chronic organized thrombosis and fibrosis.

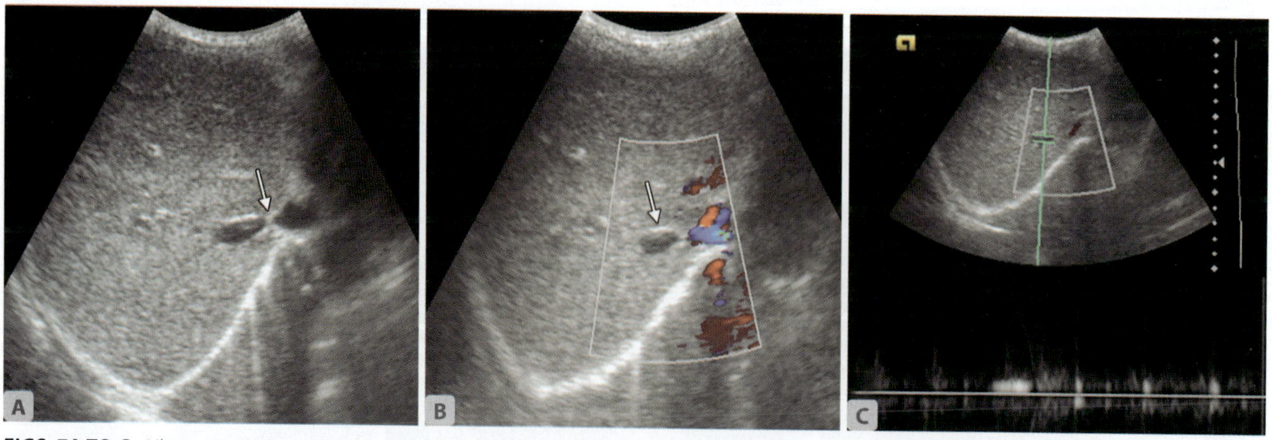

FIGS. 7A TO C: Ultrasonography with color Doppler in Budd–Chiari syndrome: (A) B-mode image shows membranous occlusion of the right hepatic vein (arrow). (B) Color Doppler image shows no color filling in the right hepatic vein (arrow). (C) Doppler image shows mild monophasic flow in the right hepatic vein.

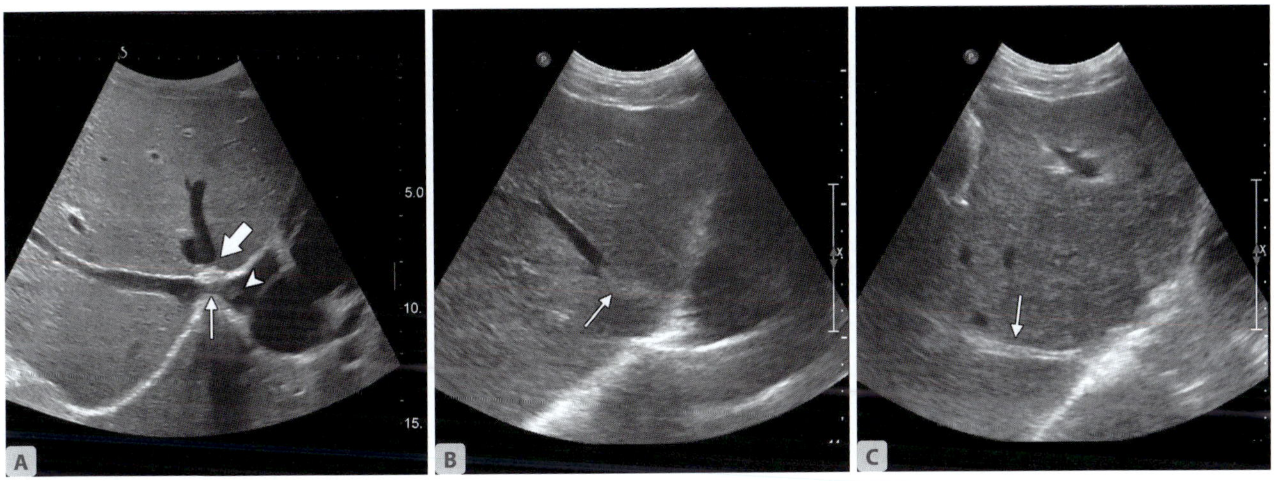

FIGS. 8A TO C: Ultrasonography of variable hepatic vein involvement: (A) B-mode image shows short segment occlusion of middle hepatic vein (block arrow) with stenosis of the ostium of right hepatic vein (arrow) and surrounding acute thrombus extending into the inferior vena cava (arrowhead). (B and C) B-mode images in another patient show absent left hepatic vein, long segment occlusion of middle hepatic vein (arrow in B), and cord-like right hepatic vein (arrow in C).

hypertrophy complex, focal liver lesions, and alterations secondary to portal hypertension.

Venovenous collaterals run either between two HVs or between HV and systemic veins like hepatic capsular veins or suprahepatic IVC **(Figs. 9A to D)**.[5] These develop in an attempt to bypass obstruction and reduce hepatic congestion. These collateral channels are classically described as "comma" shaped and are seen within the liver parenchyma. The flow direction is from more obstructed to less obstructed HV and from HV to systemic veins. They are seen in about 60% of cases.[18] The caudate vein drains directly into the IVC and is usually not affected. Hence, this vein dilates and becomes one of the major drainage pathways for the liver **(Figs. 10A to C)**.[19] A caudate vein caliber of >3 mm has a diagnostic specificity of 94% for BCS.[19] In addition, accessory hepatic veins (e.g., right inferior accessory hepatic vein), when present, are also uninvolved and may dilate to drain the liver parenchyma.[18] The segments of the liver which drain the blood like, the caudate lobe, undergo hypertrophy and the peripheral segments, which suffer more congestion, undergo atrophy **(Figs. 10A to C)**.[2,20] The caudate lobe enlarges both in anteroposterior and longitudinal dimensions unlike cirrhosis. Findings which are seen secondary to portal hypertension include dilated portal vein, hepatofugal flow in the portal vein, ascites, splenomegaly, and portosystemic collaterals like paraumbilical collaterals **(Figs. 11A to C)**.

As the disease progresses, the liver shows features of cirrhosis like coarsening of echotexture, widening of fissures, and nodular outline. An uncommon, but well-known, complication of chronic BCS is development of benign hepatic nodules. These are variably called as nodular regenerative hyperplasia, benign hyperplastic nodules, and focal nodular hyperplasia (FNH) like nodules.[21] Although found in adults, they are very rare in children. They vary from 0.5 to 4 cm in size and are either single or multiple **(Figs. 12A and B)**. They appear hypoechoic or hyperechoic on B-mode images and may show internal vascularity.

Contrast-enhanced USG (CEUS) involves performing USG after administration of USG contrast agents.[4,21] This technique has been used in the evaluation of pediatric BCS. It has been shown to add diagnostic value to USG in equivocal cases. Where the visibility near the HV ostium is obscured due to cardiac pulsations, CEUS helps in improving the visualization and thus the diagnosis. Additional use of CEUS is in the characterization of hepatic nodules found in pediatric BCS.[4,22] Thus, it may avoid the use of CT scan or MRI. On CEUS, these nodules show enhancement in the early phase after injection of the contrast agent and do not show washout **(Figs. 13A to D)**. In the later phase, the lesion appears isoechoic with the surrounding liver parenchyma.

Sonoelastography is another technique which is being increasingly used in patients of BCS.[4,23] Liver stiffness (LS) is an important measure of fibrosis in the parenchyma. However, in BCS, both congestion of liver parenchyma and parenchymal fibrosis adds to the stiffness. Hence, LS is usually very high in these patients and does not correlate with the histological stage of fibrosis. Although routine measurement may not be important, it has role in the follow-up of patients after radiological intervention **(Figs. 14A and B)**. After recanalization of the occluded vessel, the LS significantly reduces within 24 hours.[24] Thus, this could be an additional parameter to assess the success of the procedure.

An important role of USG is in guiding radiological interventions.[4,25,26] The transfemoral, transjugular, and transhepatic routes, used for performing interventions, all require USG guidance for puncturing the common femoral, internal jugular, or the hepatic veins, respectively. Once the access is gained, USG guidance helps in adjusting the direction of the needle to optimally perforate the occluded segment **(Figs. 15A and B)**. Further, USG helps in the accurate positioning of the stent prior to deployment and in assessing the patency of the vein or stent immediately after the procedure **(Figs. 15A and B)**.

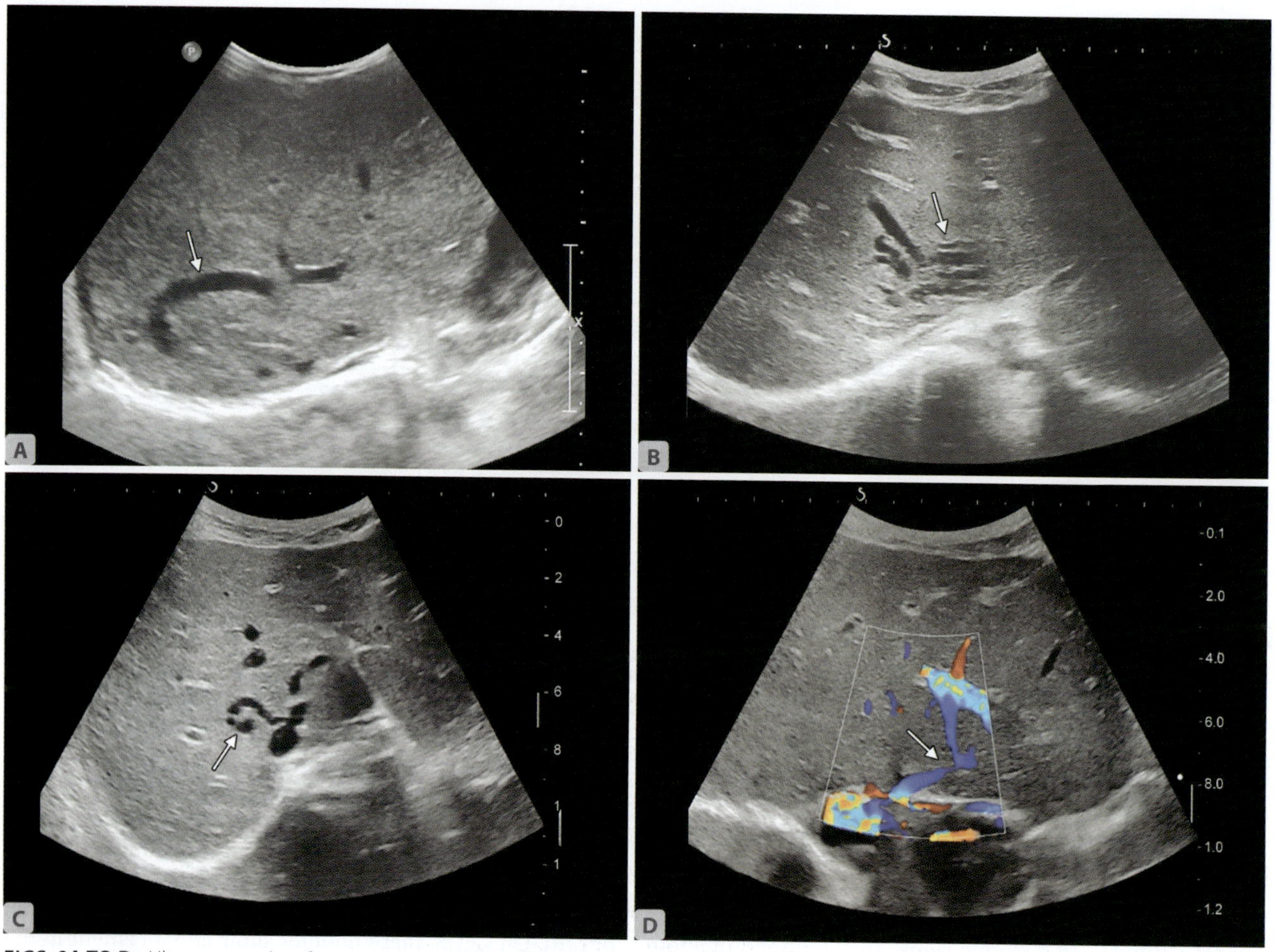

FIGS. 9A TO D: Ultrasonography of venovenous collaterals. (A to C) B-mode images show comma-shaped (arrow in A) and multiple other venovenous anechoic tortuous vascular channels around the occluded hepatic veins (arrows in B and C); and (D) Color Doppler image shows flow in a venovenous collateral channel (arrow).

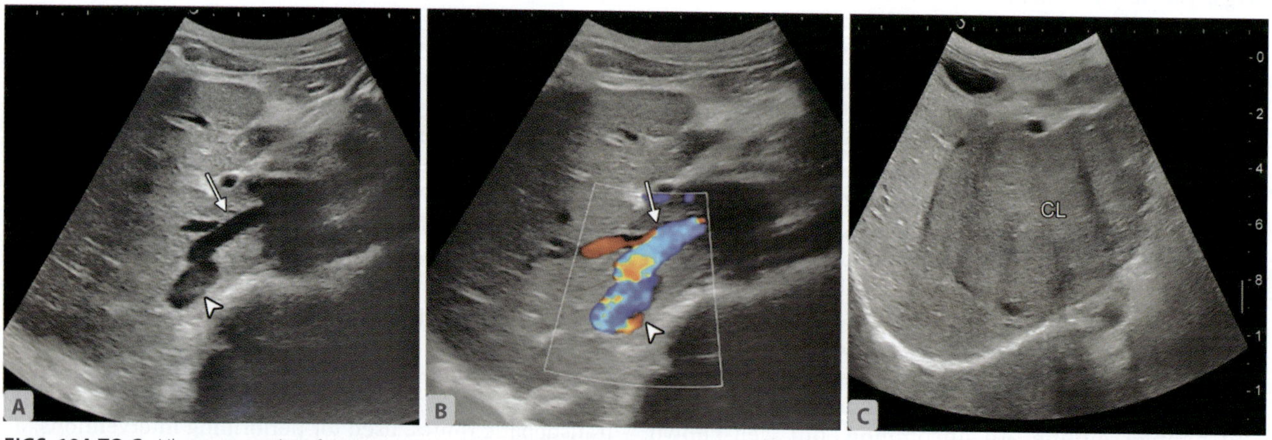

FIGS. 10A TO C: Ultrasonography of caudate lobe and its draining vein. (A and B) B-mode and color Doppler images show dilated caudate vein (arrow) with flow toward the inferior vena cava (arrowhead); and (C) B-mode image, of another patient, shows a large caudate lobe (CL).

Computed Tomography

Computed tomography scan is less preferred in the evaluation of pediatric BCS owing to the radiation risk that it exposes. However, it may still be done in situations when MRI is not available, the diagnosis is missed on USG or CT is done for other causes. The HV and IVC are better seen in the venous phase. The scan shows hypodense nonenhancing thrombus in (acute) or nonvisualization (subacute or chronic) of a segment or the entire length of the HV or IVC **(Figs. 16A and B)**. Calcification may be

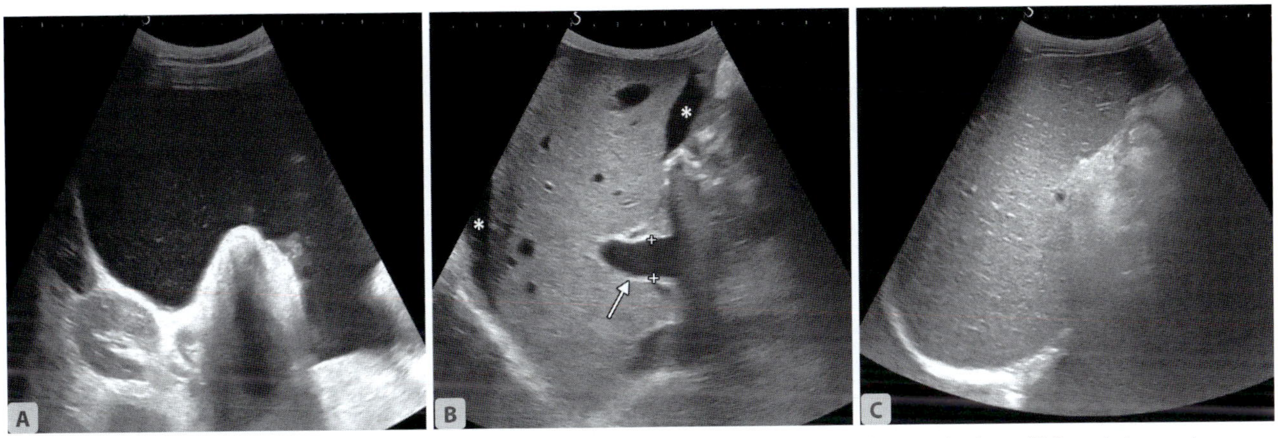

FIGS. 11A TO C: Ultrasonography of portal hypertension. (A) B-mode image shows gross ascites with internal echoes. (B) B-mode image shows dilated main portal vein (arrow) and ascites (asterisk); and (C) B-mode image shows splenomegaly.

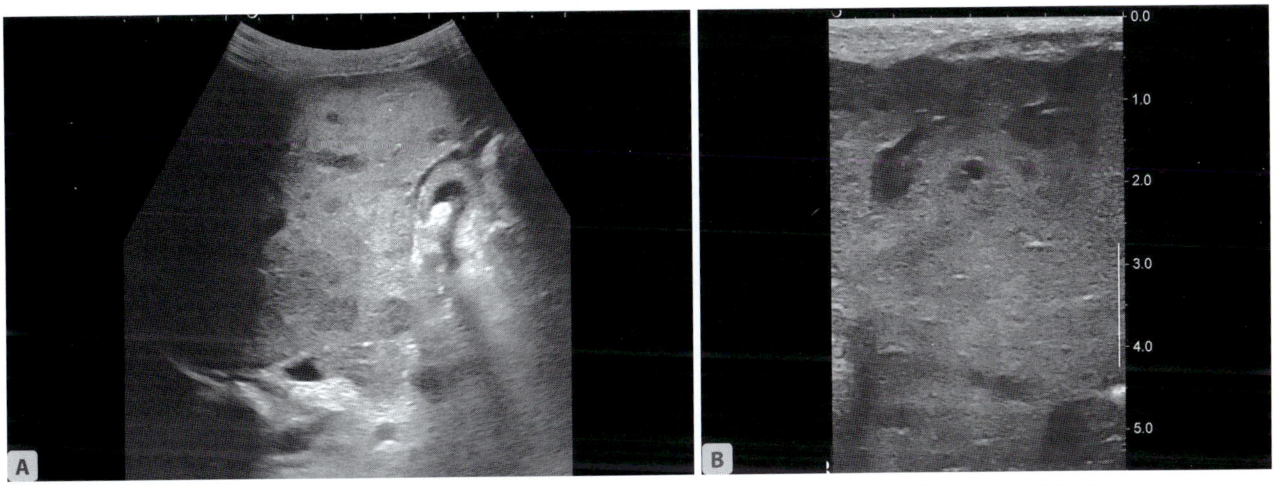

FIGS. 12A AND B: Ultrasonography of benign regenerative nodules. (A and B) B-mode images using low frequency and high frequency transducers show multiple hypoechoic nodules in the liver parenchyma in a 5-year-old child with Budd–Chiari syndrome.

seen in chronic thrombus. Multiplanar reconstructions are useful for better visualization of the occluded segments, in oblique planes for HV and in sagittal plane for IVC **(Figs. 17A and B)**.[13]

In acute BCS, the liver parenchyma typically shows higher contrast enhancement of the central portions and decreased enhancement of the peripheral portions.[5] If a delayed scan is acquired, the peripheral portions show enhancement giving the "flip-flop" pattern of enhancement **(Figs. 18A to C)**.[27] In addition, ascites and splenomegaly are frequently seen. Sometimes, the caudate lobe shows strong and variable contrast enhancement, giving a fan-shaped appearance **(Figs. 19A to C)**.[28]

In subacute or chronic BCS, the liver shows diffuse hypoperfusion. The "spider web" collaterals may be occasionally seen **(Figs. 20A to C)**.[29] In addition, venovenous collaterals bypassing the occluded HV may be visible **(Figs. 21A to C)**.[30] Occlusion of the IVC is associated with dilated infrahepatic IVC and enlarged azygous and hemiazygous veins. The caudate lobe is enlarged as is the caudate vein **(Figs. 22A to C)**. Portosystemic collaterals may be seen due to portal hypertension and are located in the peripancreatic, splenic hilar, retroperitoneal, and periumbilical regions. Sometimes, there is dilatation of the hepatic artery due to reduced portal flow.[27]

Benign regenerative nodules are better characterized on a multiphase contrast-enhanced CT scan.[31] These nodules, 0.5–4 cm in size, show intense and homogeneous enhancement in the arterial phase and become isodense or mildly hyperdense in the portal venous and delayed phases **(Figs. 23A to D)**. Sometimes, the nodules may be hyperdense in the plain scans. These features help in its differentiation from hepatocellular carcinoma (HCC) which shows arterial phase hyperenhancement and washout in the venous and delayed phases **(Figs. 24A to C)**.

Magnetic Resonance Imaging

Magnetic resonance imaging is not commonly performed in the evaluation of pediatric BCS due to the requirement of general anesthesia, long scan times, motion artifacts due to breath-hold difficulties, and higher cost. However, it may occasionally be necessary in cases where the diagnosis is unclear and in the characterization of hepatic nodules.

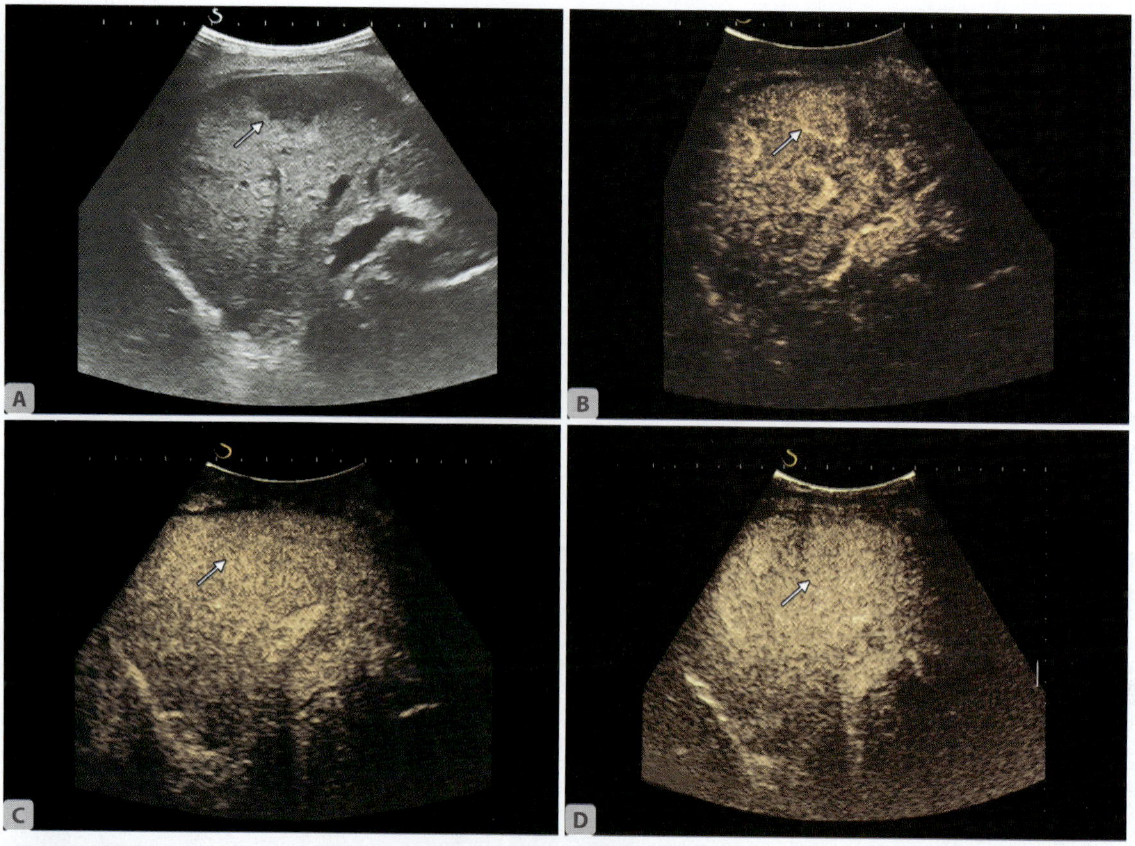

FIGS. 13A TO D: Contrast-enhanced ultrasound of benign liver nodules in Budd–Chiari syndrome. (A) B-mode image shows a hypoechoic nodule (arrow) in liver; and (B to D) arterial, venous, and delayed phase images after contrast administration show enhancement of the lesion in the arterial phase with no washout (arrows).

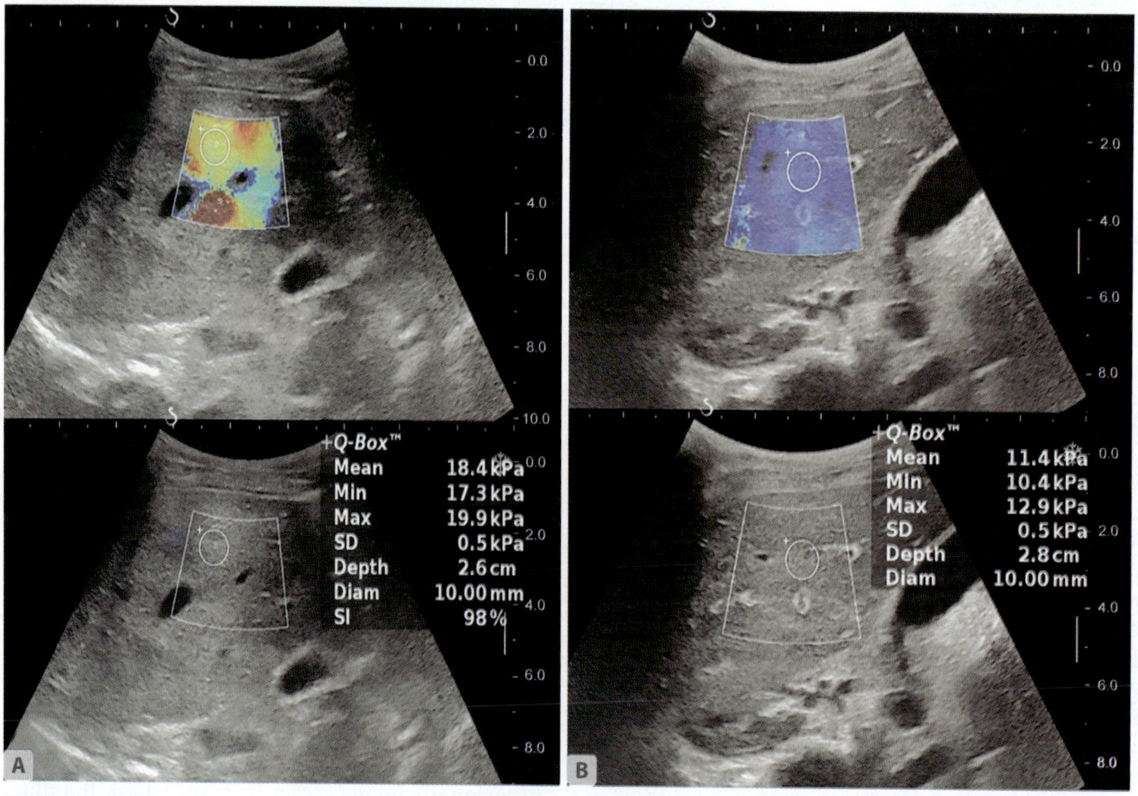

FIGS. 14A AND B: Shear wave elastography in Budd–Chiari syndrome. (A) Elastography image before radiological intervention shows a mean liver stiffness of 18.4 kPa; and (B) Elastography image 24 hours after angioplasty of right hepatic vein shows reduction of mean liver stiffness to 11.4 kPa.

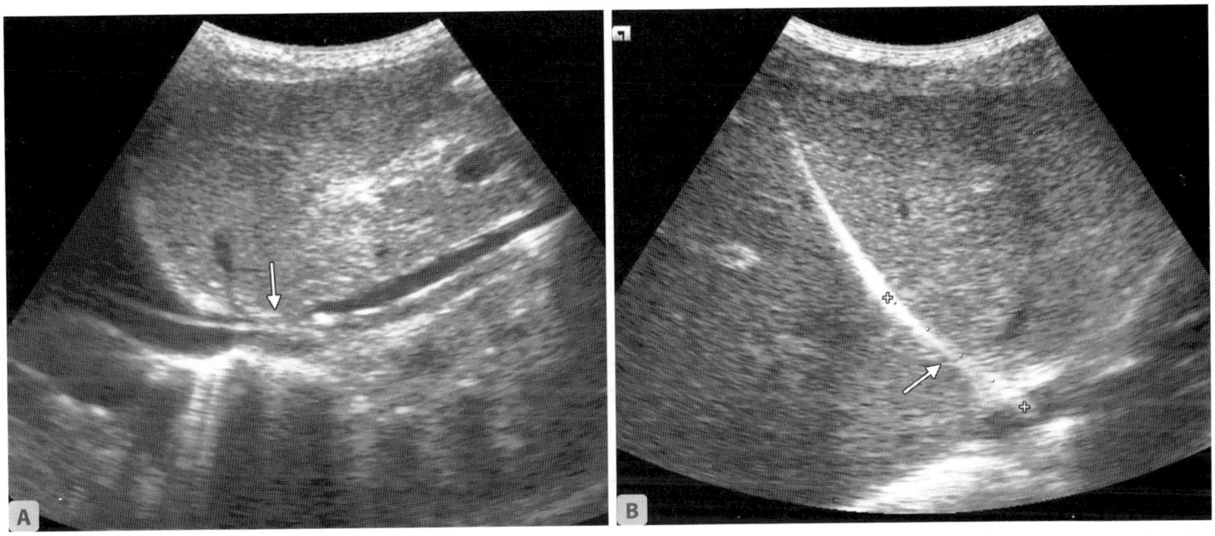

FIGS. 15A AND B: Ultrasonography (USG) in radiological intervention. (A) B-mode image shows perforation of inferior vena cava web and passage of guidewire under USG guidance (arrow); and (B) B-mode image in a case of transhepatic middle hepatic vein stenting, in another patient, shows the perforation of the obstructed ostium under ultrasound guidance (arrow).

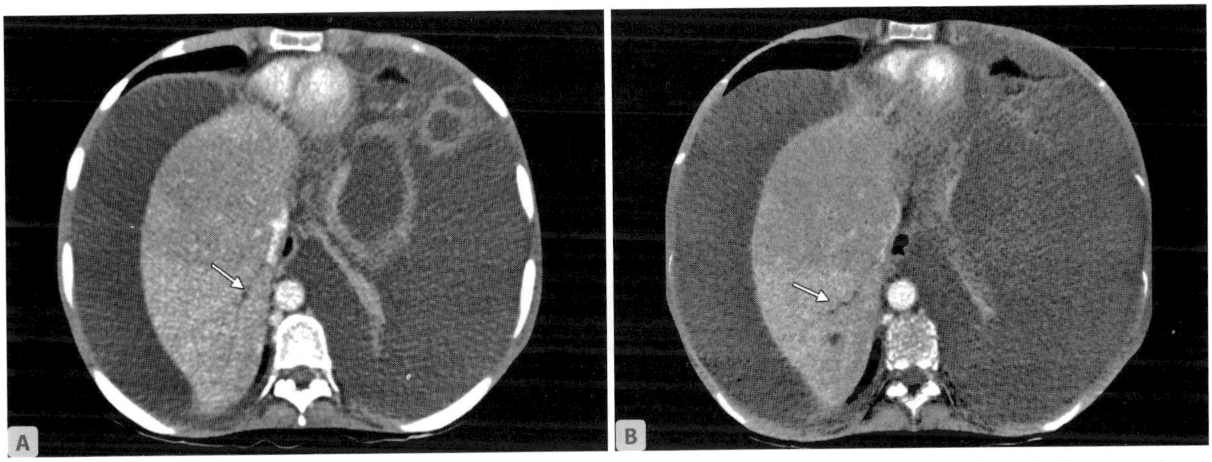

FIGS. 16A AND B: Computed tomography (CT) scan in acute Budd–Chiari syndrome. (A and B) Axial contrast-enhanced CT image and minimum intensity projection show hypodense thrombus in the right hepatic vein (arrows) with perfusion abnormalities in the liver parenchyma. Gross ascites is noted.

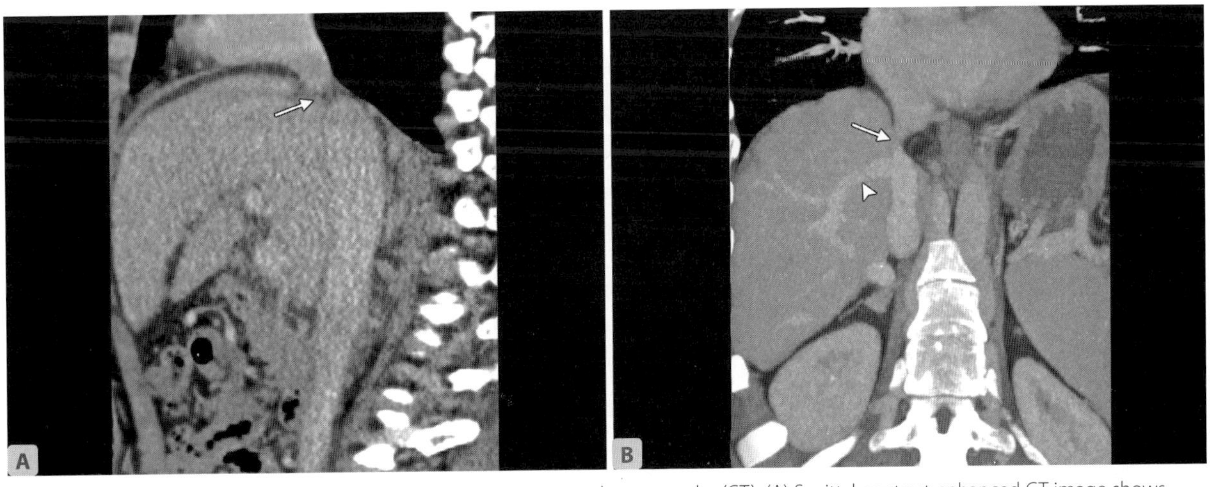

FIGS. 17A AND B: Role of multiplanar reconstructions on computed tomography (CT). (A) Sagittal contrast-enhanced CT image shows short segment occlusion of the suprahepatic inferior vena cava (IVC) (arrow); and (B) Oblique coronal maximum intensity projection image shows short segment stenosis of the suprahepatic IVC (arrow) with a large collateral (arrowhead).

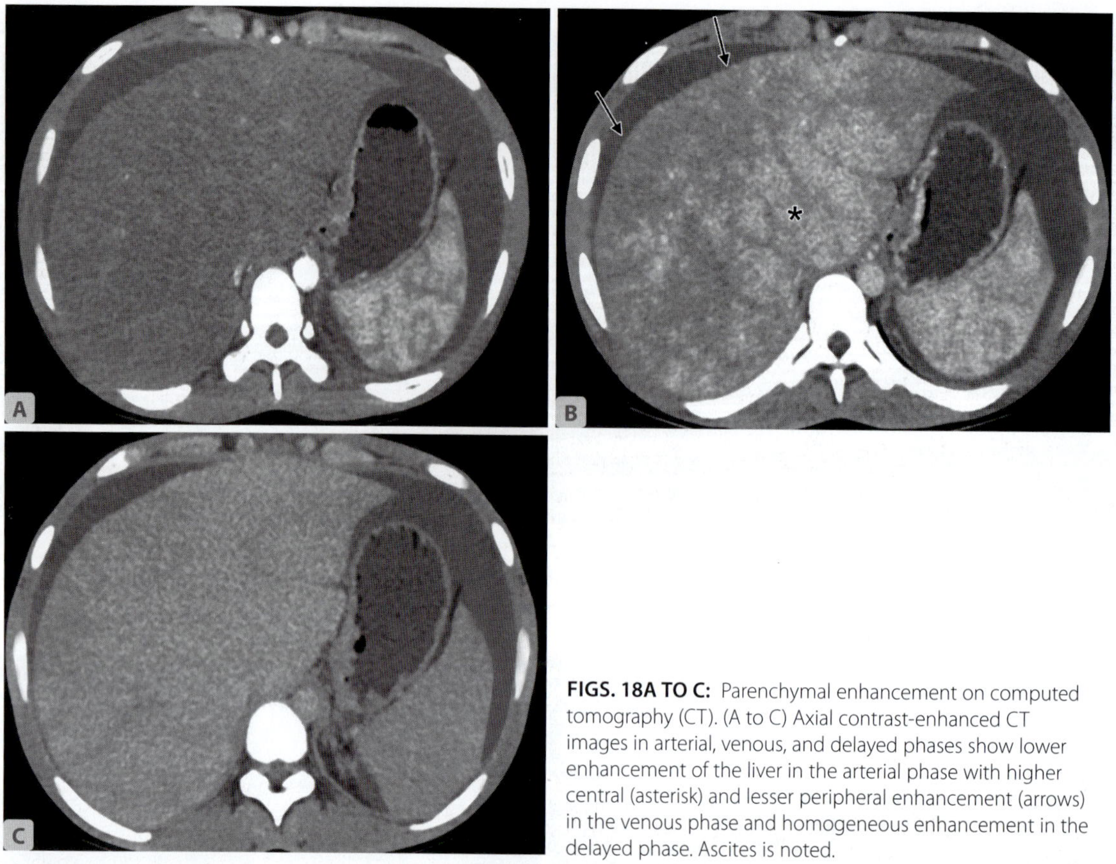

FIGS. 18A TO C: Parenchymal enhancement on computed tomography (CT). (A to C) Axial contrast-enhanced CT images in arterial, venous, and delayed phases show lower enhancement of the liver in the arterial phase with higher central (asterisk) and lesser peripheral enhancement (arrows) in the venous phase and homogeneous enhancement in the delayed phase. Ascites is noted.

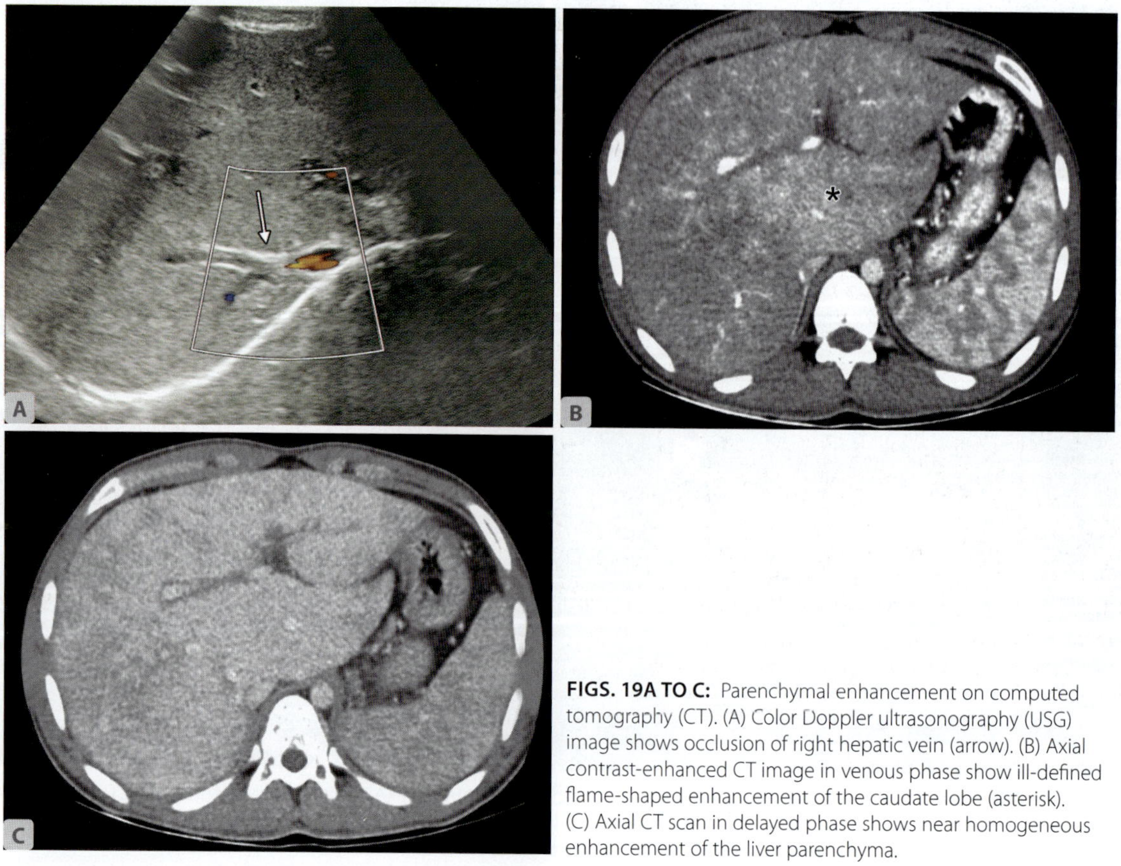

FIGS. 19A TO C: Parenchymal enhancement on computed tomography (CT). (A) Color Doppler ultrasonography (USG) image shows occlusion of right hepatic vein (arrow). (B) Axial contrast-enhanced CT image in venous phase show ill-defined flame-shaped enhancement of the caudate lobe (asterisk). (C) Axial CT scan in delayed phase shows near homogeneous enhancement of the liver parenchyma.

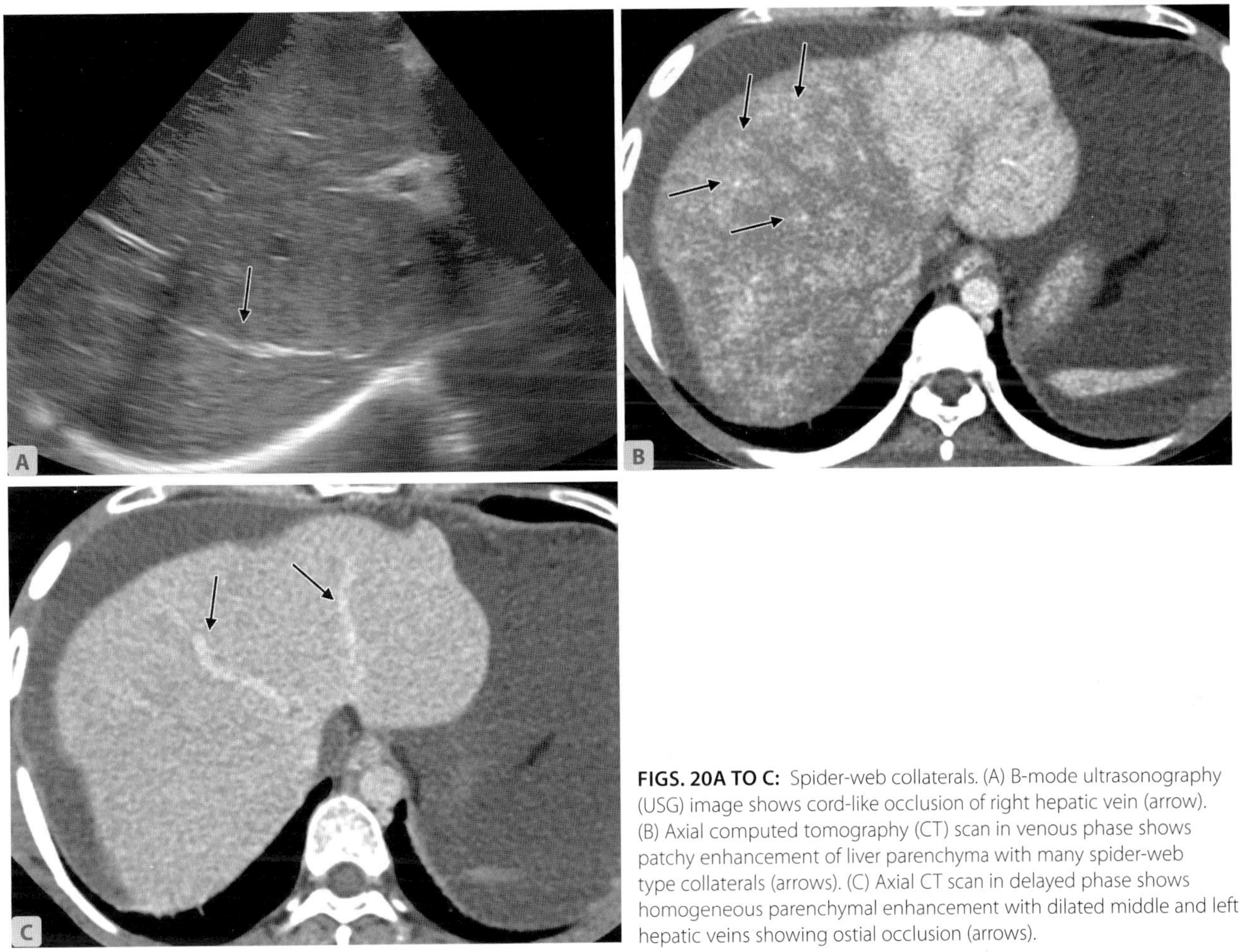

FIGS. 20A TO C: Spider-web collaterals. (A) B-mode ultrasonography (USG) image shows cord-like occlusion of right hepatic vein (arrow). (B) Axial computed tomography (CT) scan in venous phase shows patchy enhancement of liver parenchyma with many spider-web type collaterals (arrows). (C) Axial CT scan in delayed phase shows homogeneous parenchymal enhancement with dilated middle and left hepatic veins showing ostial occlusion (arrows).

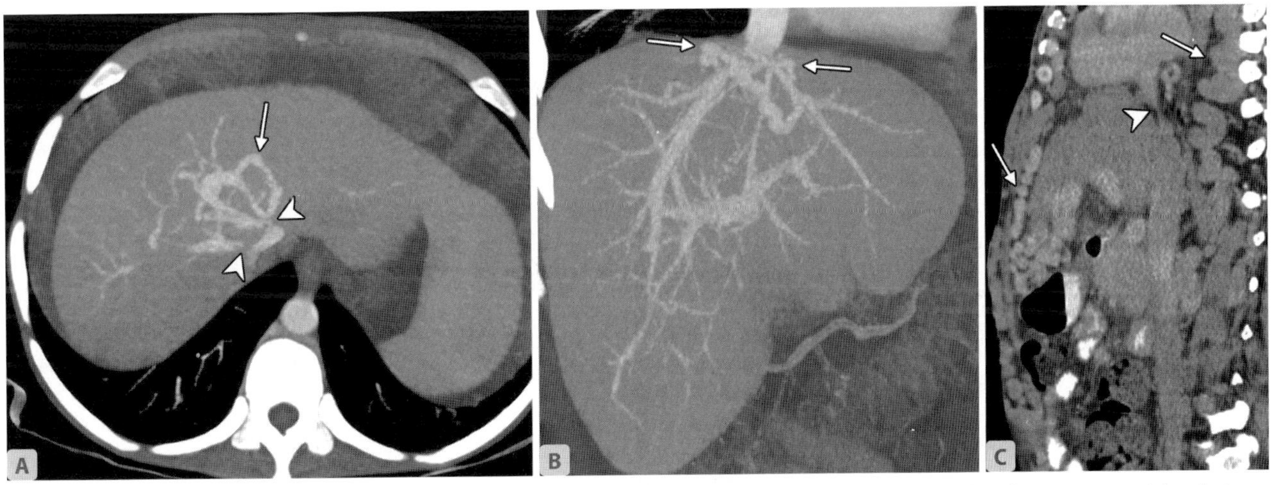

FIGS. 21A TO C: Venovenous collaterals on CT scan. (A and B) Axial and coronal maximum intensity projection show hepatic vein ostial occlusion (arrowheads) with multiple venovenous collaterals (arrows); and (C) Sagittal image shows short segment occlusion of suprahepatic inferior vena cava (arrowhead) with multiple paravertebral and abdominal wall collaterals (arrows).

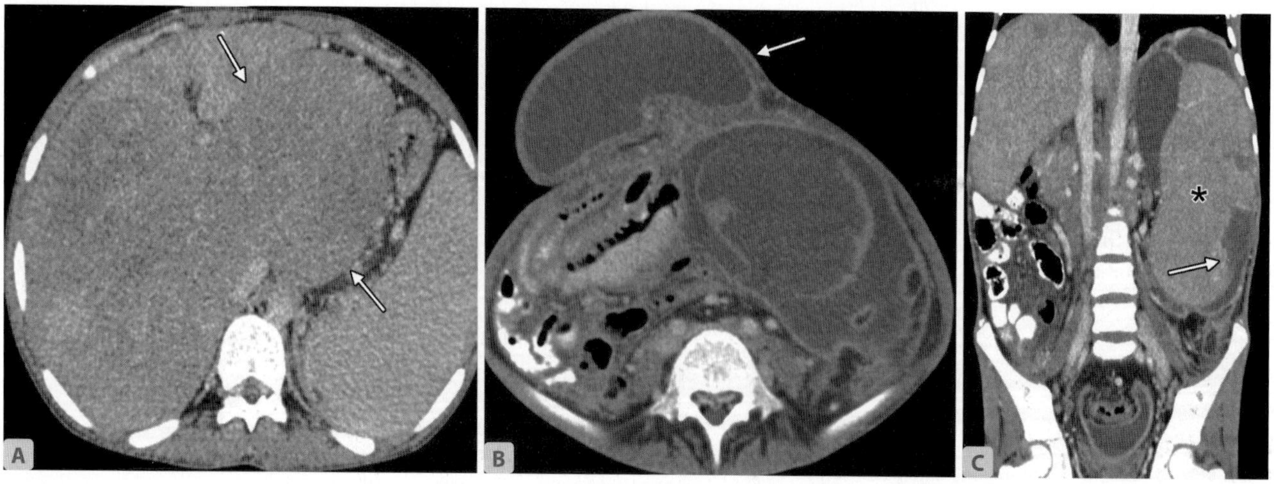

FIGS. 22A TO C: Other changes on CT scan. (A) Axial contrast-enhanced CT image shows grossly enlarged caudate lobe (arrows). (B) Axial contrast-enhanced CT image shows ascites with loculations and umbilical hernia (arrow); and (C) Coronal contrast-enhanced CT image shows splenomegaly (asterisk) with peripheral wedge-shaped hypodensities suggesting infarcts (arrow).

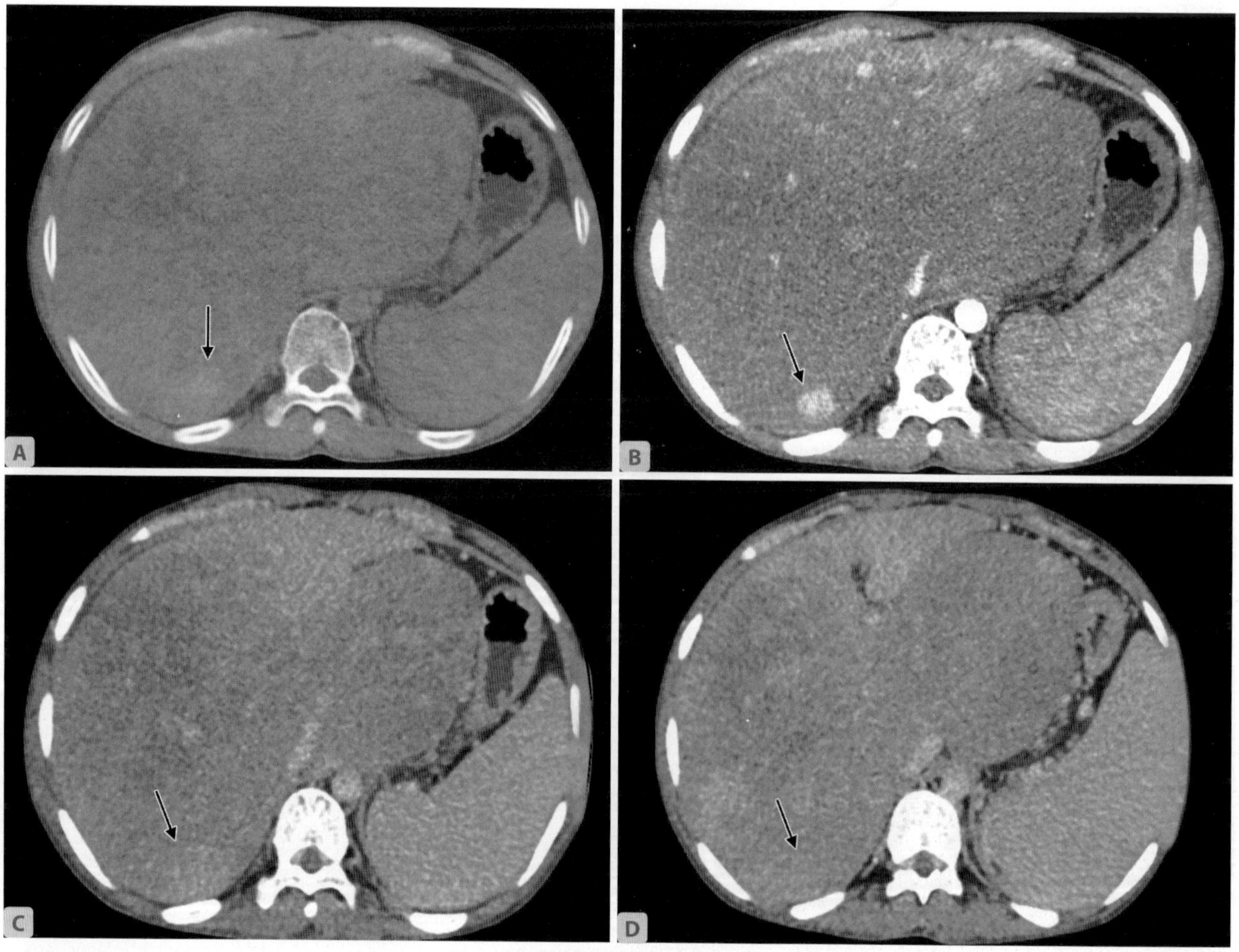

FIGS. 23A TO D: CT scan of benign regenerative liver nodule. (A) Noncontrast CT scan shows subtle hyperdensity within the nodule (arrow). (B) Arterial phase image shows homogeneous enhancement of the nodule (arrow). Other multiple enhancing smaller nodules are also seen. (C and D) Venous and delayed phases show that the lesion is isodense without any washout (arrows).

Balanced steady state sequences provide information on the status of veins without the need of contrast agent **(Figs. 25A to F)**. However, contrast-enhanced MRI should be performed whenever necessary for more accurate evaluation.

The HV and the IVC show occlusion and dilatation proximal to the occluded segment.[5,28] On T2-weighted sequences, the peripheral parts of the liver show hyperintense signal as they are more congested with higher water content **(Figs. 25A to F)**.[5] The same areas appear hypointense on T1-weighted sequences.

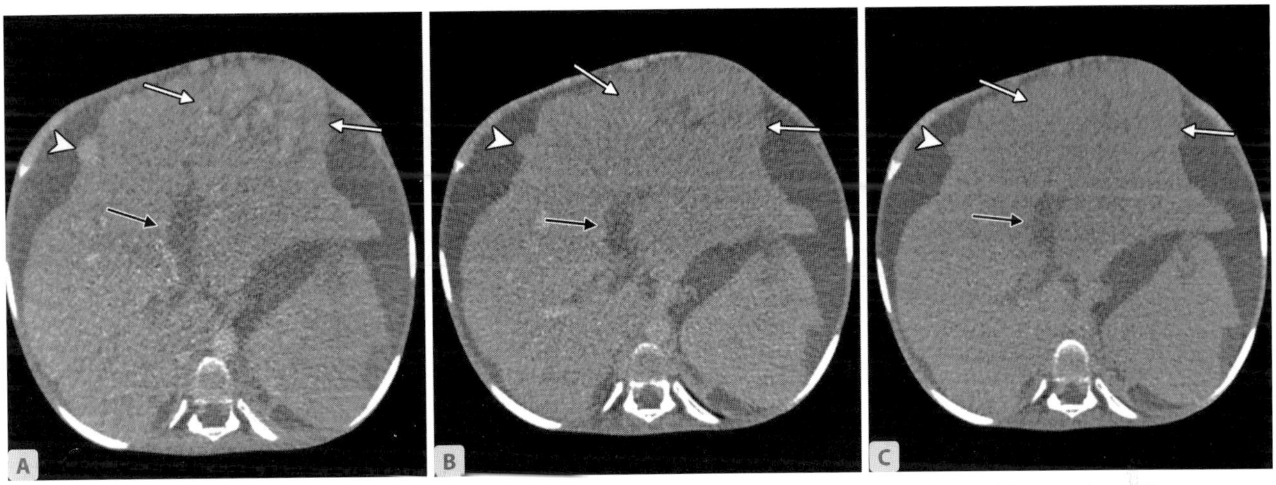

FIGS. 24A TO C: CT scan of hepatocellular carcinoma (HCC) in Budd–Chiari syndrome. (A to C) Arterial, venous, and delayed phase CT images show an ill-defined arterial phase heterogeneously hyperenhancing lesion (white arrows) in the left lobe which shows mild washout in venous and delayed phases, with portal vein thrombosis (black arrows), suggestive of infiltrative HCC. Another arterial enhancing nodule (arrowhead) is also seen in left lobe showing mild washout suggestive of HCC.

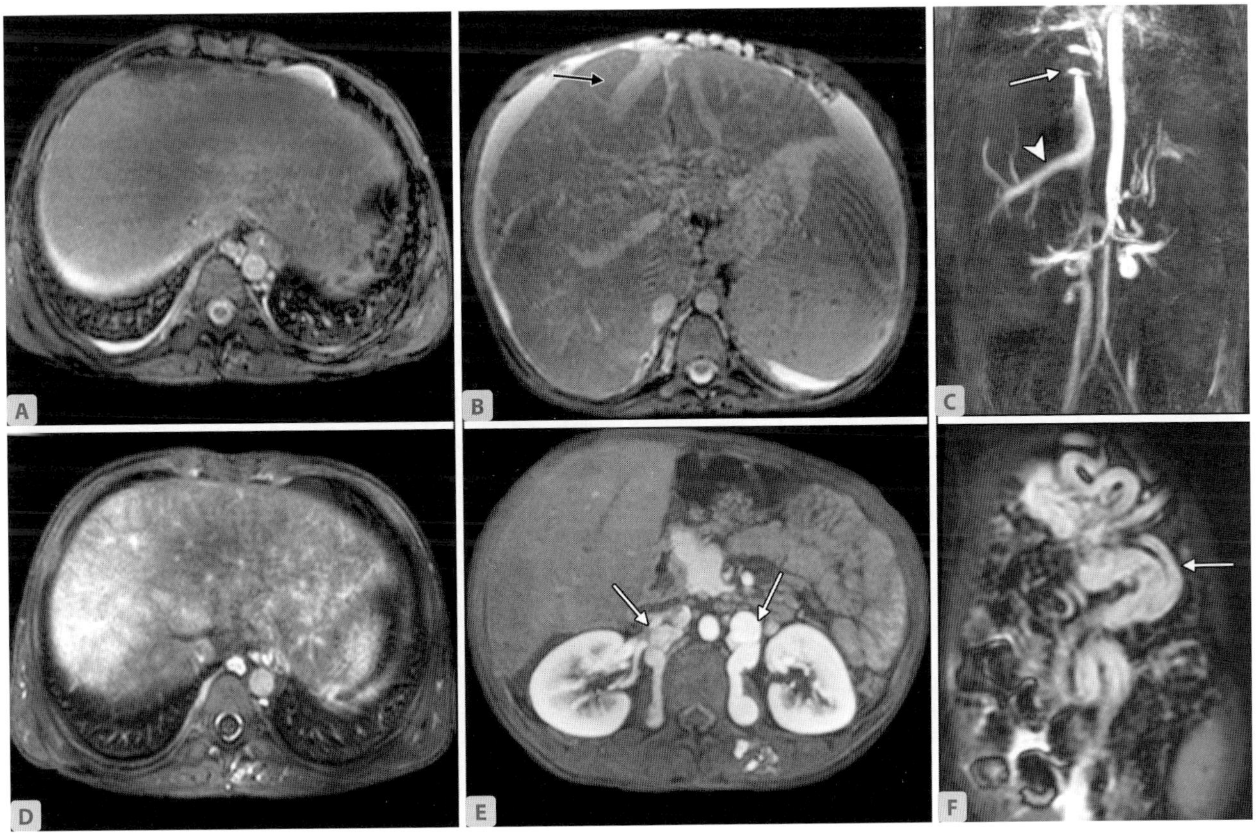

FIGS. 25A TO F: Magnetic resonance imaging in chronic Budd–Chiari syndrome. (A and B) Axial balanced steady-state sequences show absence of hepatic veins with a large paraumbilical collateral (black arrow in B) and ascites. (C) Coronal maximum intensity projection of angiography images show complete occlusion of suprahepatic inferior vena cava (arrow) with dilated right inferior accessory hepatic vein (arrowhead). (D and E) Contrast-enhanced axial T1-weighted images show heterogeneous parenchymal enhancement and large paravertebral collaterals (arrows in E). (F) Coronal balanced steady-state sequence shows large abdominal wall collaterals (arrow).

The contrast enhancement of the liver parenchyma is similar to that described under CT scan.[32] In acute BCS, the central portion of the liver shows more contrast enhancement than the periphery. In subacute or chronic BCS, the parenchymal enhancement is more heterogeneous **(Figs. 26A to D)**.

The benign regenerative nodules typically appear hyperintense on T1 and isointense or hypointense on T2-weighted images **(Figs. 27A to H)**.[31] There is no restriction of diffusion. They show hyperenhancement in the arterial phase with no washout in the venous and delayed phases. On the hepatobiliary phase of liver-specific contrast agent (like gadobenate dimeglumine), these lesions appear hyperintense or isointense. Unlike these, HCC appears hypointense on T1, hyperintense on T2, shows diffusion restriction frequently, arterial phase hyperenhancement, and washout in the venous and delayed phases. Usually, they are hypointense in the hepatobiliary phase.

Venography

Occasionally, when the diagnosis is uncertain, venography of HV or IVC may be performed to clarify the diagnosis. Typically, this is seen with intrahepatic segment of IVC, which may be compressed by the enlarged caudate lobe and appears falsely occluded on USG.[13]

Here, either the IVC or the HV may be punctured under the guidance of USG and venogram is obtained under fluoroscopy after injecting iodinated contrast agent. When a cavogram is obtained, both anteroposterior and lateral views are obtained for accurate diagnosis **(Figs. 28A to C)**. Presence of obstruction to the flow of contrast at the level of HV ostium or the IVC confirms the diagnosis of BCS. Membranous occlusion may be seen as a rounded cutoff or may show a fine jet of contrast through the pinhole orifice in the occluding web. Other types of occlusion may be seen as a beak or irregular cutoff. The study also shows the collateral veins which could be spider web collaterals or venovenous collaterals which bypass the obstruction **(Figs. 28A to C)**.[13] Additional advantage is the ability to measure intravascular pressures.[28] Although invasive venography is considered to be the gold standard for diagnosis of BCS, it alone cannot clearly define the length of the occlusion required for planning radiological interventions.[28]

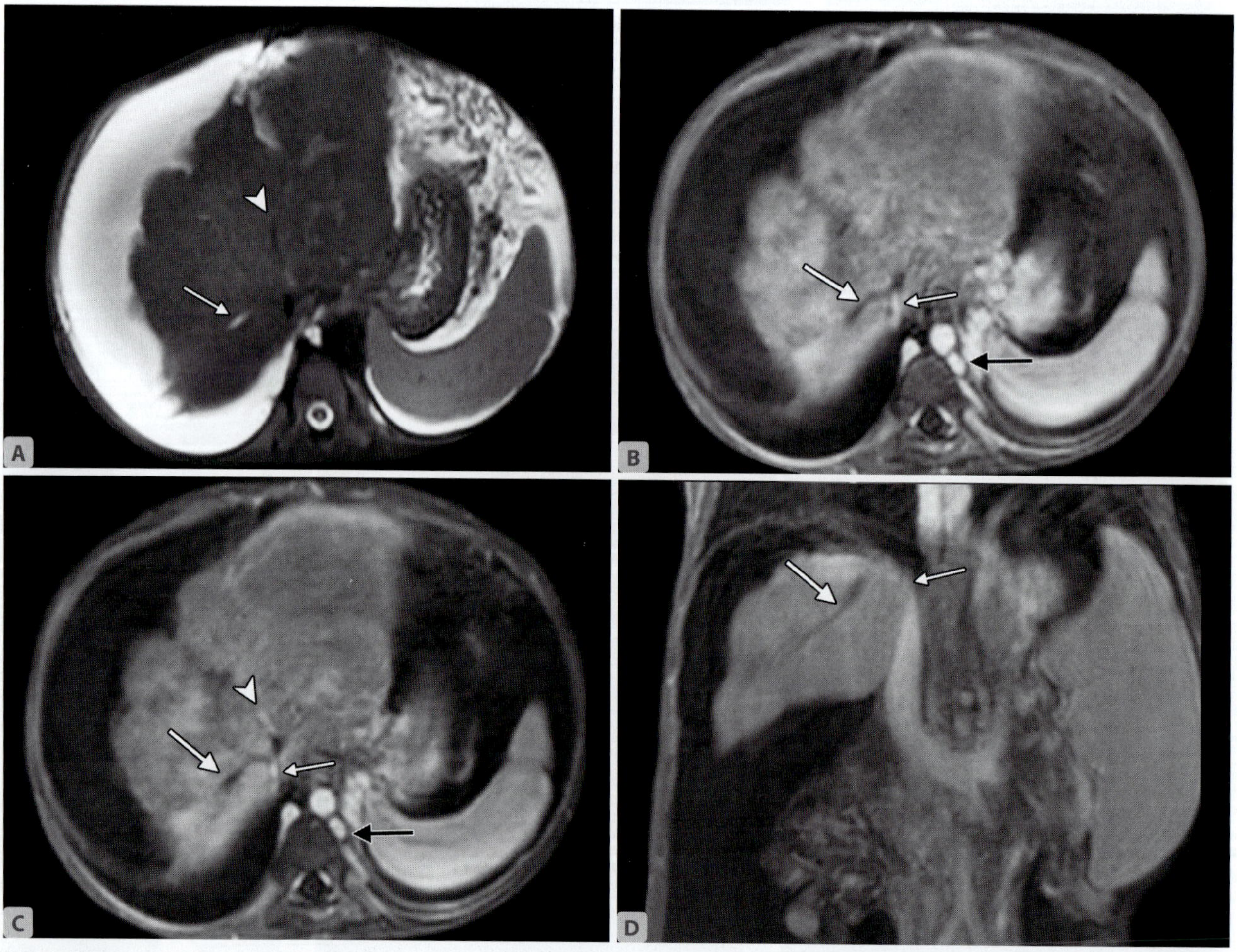

FIGS. 26A TO D: Magnetic resonance imaging in chronic Budd–Chiari syndrome. (A) Axial T2-weighted image shows cirrhotic liver with partially visualized right (arrow) and middle (arrowhead) hepatic veins and gross ascites. (B to D) Axial, delayed, and coronal venous phase images show nonenhancement of right hepatic vein (white thick arrows) and partial delayed enhancement of middle hepatic vein (arrowhead in C) with severe stenosis of inferior vena cava (long thin arrow). Paravertebral collaterals are noted (black arrow).

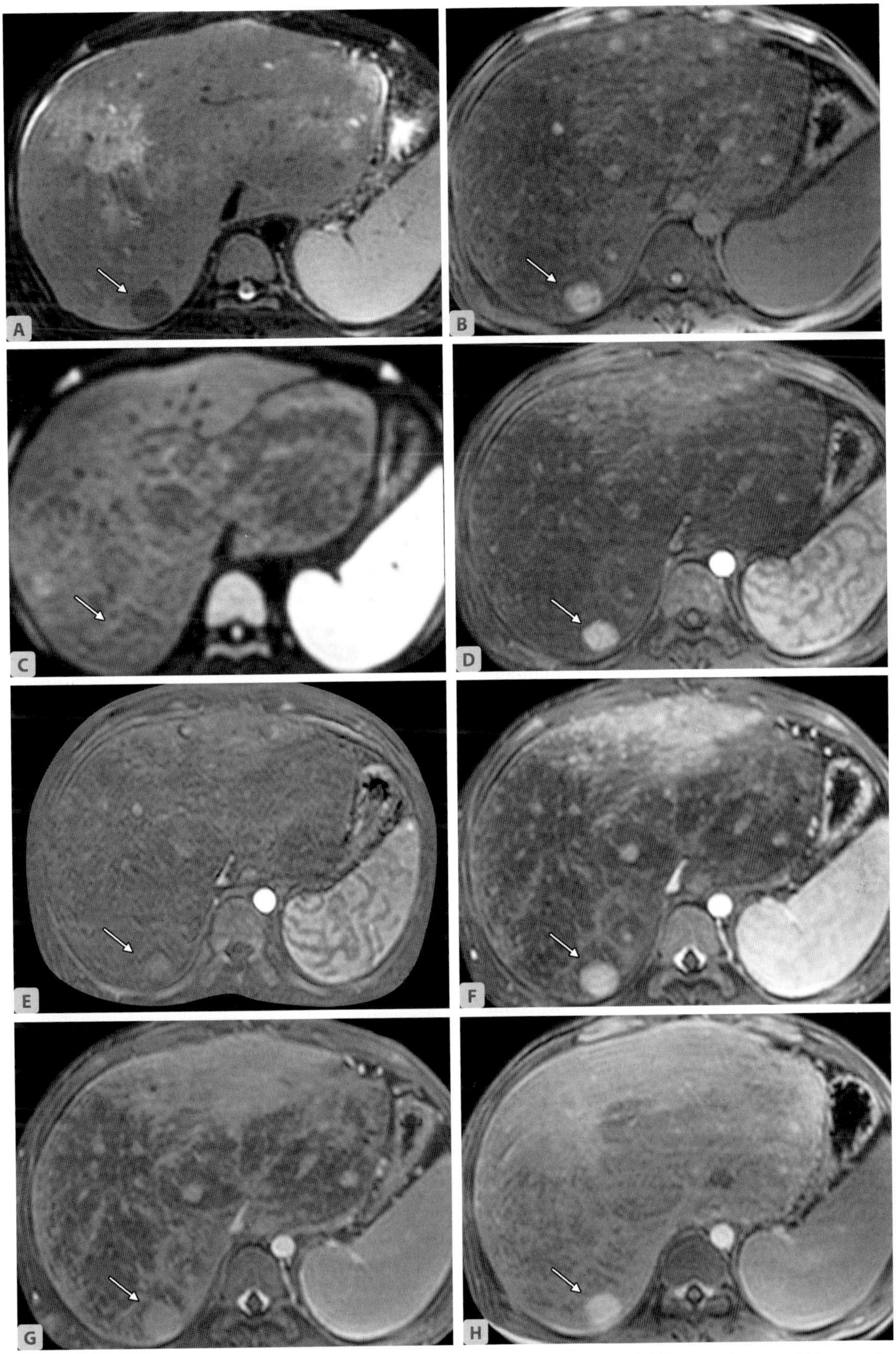

FIGS. 27A TO H: Magnetic resonance imaging of benign regenerative nodules. (A to C) T2, T1, and diffusion-weighted axial images show enlarged liver with a T2 hypointense and T1 hyperintense nodule without diffusion restriction (arrows) in segment 7. Multiple similar smaller nodules are also seen. (D to H) Arterial, arterial subtracted, venous, delayed, and hepatobiliary phase axial contrast-enhanced T1-weighted images show the nodule with mild arterial phase enhancement and persistence of enhancement in the venous, delayed, and hepatobiliary phase, suggestive of benign regenerative nodule (arrows). Similar other enhancing smaller nodules are also seen. Liver shows heterogeneous contrast enhancement consistent with Budd–Chiari syndrome.

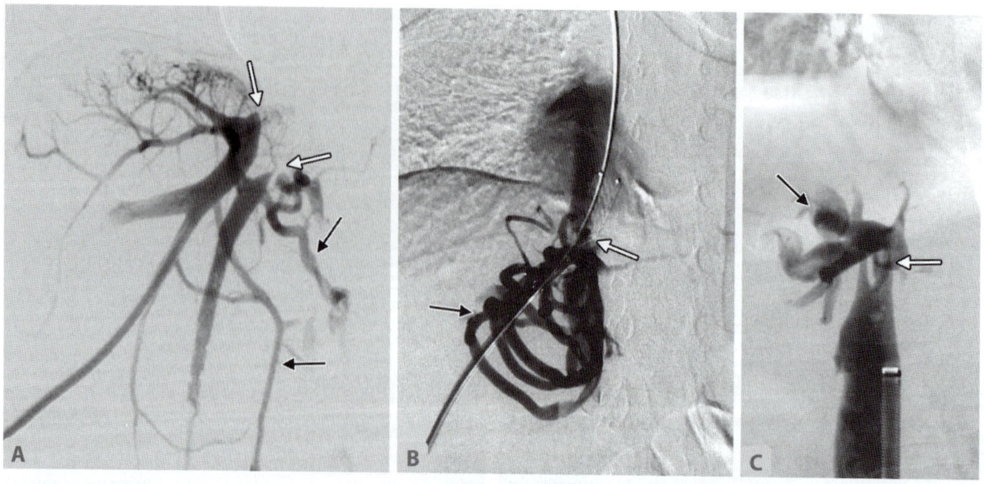

FIGS. 28A TO C: Digital subtraction angiography in Budd–Chiari syndrome. (A) Right hepatic venogram shows ostial occlusion of right and middle hepatic veins (white arrows) with multiple collaterals (black arrows). (B) Middle hepatic venogram shows occlusion of a previously placed stent (white arrow) with multiple collaterals (black arrow) draining into the inferior vena cava (IVC). (C) Inferior vena cavogram shows occlusion of intrahepatic IVC segment (white arrow) with adjacent collaterals (black arrow).

MANAGEMENT OF PEDIATRIC BUDD–CHIARI SYNDROME

Management of pediatric BCS requires multidisciplinary team approach involving pediatric gastroenterologist, pediatric interventional radiologist, pediatric hematologist, and pediatric surgeon. The type of treatment depends on the stage of the disease at presentation.

In acute stage, the children may be managed by anti-coagulation and intravascular thrombolysis, wherever possible.[7] Ascites is managed by diuretics and paracentesis. In subacute or chronic stages, which form the most common types of presentation, radiological interventions are the mainstay of treatment.

Radiological Interventions

Percutaneous radiological interventions have become the established treatment of choice in the management of subacute and chronic pediatric BCS.[12,18] These procedures have shown to be safe with excellent long-term outcomes. These are performed under general anesthesia.

Hepatic Vein Thrombolysis

Thrombolysis of the HV can be performed when the child presents with acute thrombosis of the HVs. Once the diagnosis of the thrombus is made on USG and color Doppler, thrombolysis may be planned.[33] Recanalization of at least one HV should be the aim of the procedure.

Under USG guidance, the right internal jugular vein (IJV) is punctured and an 8–10F-sized vascular sheath is placed, with the tip in IVC. The HV which is to be thrombolyzed is subsequently catheterized. When all three veins show acute thrombosis, then thrombolysis of right HV (RHV) is preferred, as it drains blood of a larger portion of the liver. Once the HV is catheterized, an infusion catheter (5F) is positioned with all its side holes in the thrombosed vein. Usually, a combination of mechanical and chemical thrombolysis gives better results.[33]

In mechanical thrombolysis, a 4–6 mm-sized balloon catheter is inflated in the thrombosed vein to macerate the thrombus. This is then followed by chemical thrombolysis, with either urokinase or recombinant tissue plasminogen activator (rtPA). The procedure involves giving a bolus dose of the thrombolytic agent followed by continuous infusion over 24–48 hours, with assessment by check venogram every 8–12 hours. The bolus dose of urokinase is 4,400 U/kg and maintenance dose is 4,400 U/kg/h, respectively. Similarly, the bolus and maintenance doses of rtPA are 0.1–0.3 mg/kg and 0.01–0.03 mg/kg/h, respectively.[34] During infusion, regular (every 6–12 h) monitoring of coagulation profile with international normalized ratio (INR) and activated partial thromboplastin time (aPTT) is highly desirable.

Once venogram establishes the patency of the HV, proper anticoagulation should be maintained and continued till the cause of the thrombosis is identified and treated. If an anatomical lesion is found, it should be treated during thrombolysis by either angioplasty or stenting.[33] If the procedure is not successful, collaterals may gradually develop and a definitive treatment in the form of direct intrahepatic portosystemic shunt (DIPS) may done at a later date.

Angioplasty

Angioplasty or venoplasty is the procedure where a balloon catheter is used to dilate and recanalize the occluded segment of the HV or IVC.[12,35] This procedure is preferred for membranous occlusions and occlusions which are <5 mm in length on USG. Size of the balloon catheter depends on the caliber of the HV or IVC proximal to the occlusion and it is preferable to use a balloon catheter 2–4 mm larger than the caliber of the vessel. Usually, for HV, 6–10 mm and for IVC, 12–18 mm-sized balloon catheters are used.

For HV angioplasty, both transhepatic and transjugular routes can be used. For IVC, usually transfemoral route is used. If the transfemoral route fails, then a combined transfemoral and transjugular route may be used for angioplasty. Once the level of obstruction is reached using a catheter or a sheathed stiff cannula, a guidewire or sheathed puncture needle is used to probe and cross the obstructive lesion **(Figs. 29 and 30)**. Subsequently, an extra-stiff or ultra-stiff guidewire is placed and balloon catheter is inserted over it. Once the balloon is in position at the site of occlusion, it is inflated completely to break the fibrous structure responsible for the obstruction. Following this, a venogram is performed to check for any residual stenosis. If present, repeat angioplasty with the same or slightly larger (by 2 mm) balloon may be performed. The procedure is usually successful in a majority of the children. If it still fails, then stent should be placed.

Stent Placement

Placement of stents should be deferred wherever possible in children as they have a long growing period ahead and the stent may become a limiting point for growth. However, in cases with short segment occlusions (5–20 mm), angioplasty is known to fail and hence primary stenting is desirable.[12,35] Stenting is also the treatment of choice in children after failed angioplasty. The balloon-mounted stents are preferred over the self-expandable stents as they can be deployed more precisely. The size of the stent, similar to balloon catheter, depends on the caliber of the venous channel and should be slightly larger (by about 1–2 mm) than the venous lumen.

The steps of the stent placement procedure are mostly similar to the balloon angioplasty. Once the occlusion is crossed and a stiff guidewire is placed across it, the stent device is inserted over the wire **(Figs. 31A to C)**. Once the stent is accurately positioned, using fluoroscopic landmarks and USG, the balloon holding the stent is inflated and stent is deployed. The catheter is removed after deflation of the balloon. A venogram is obtained to check for the patency. If there is residual waist, repeat balloon dilatation is necessary to remove the waist. Overdilatation with a larger caliber balloon should be avoided as it may fracture the struts of the stent. Predilatation of the occluded segment is usually not necessary prior to stent placement.

Direct Intrahepatic Portosystemic Shunt

In children with BCS, attempt should always be made to recanalize the HV or IVC as it re-establishes the physiological flow and relieves hepatic congestion. However, in cases where all the HV show nonrecanalizable long segment occlusions, angioplasty or stenting is not possible. The only option is to perform a DIPS to reduce liver congestion and treat portal hypertension like hematemesis and ascites.[12,35] This procedure diverts major part of the blood in the portal vein to the suprahepatic IVC, thereby reducing hepatic congestion, portosystemic pressure gradient, and portal hypertension. Since the blood flow to the liver is bypassed, it may result in liver dysfunction and encephalopathy. Hence, preprocedure liver function tests should be normal or near-normal to avoid post-DIPS complications like liver failure and hepatic encephalopathy.

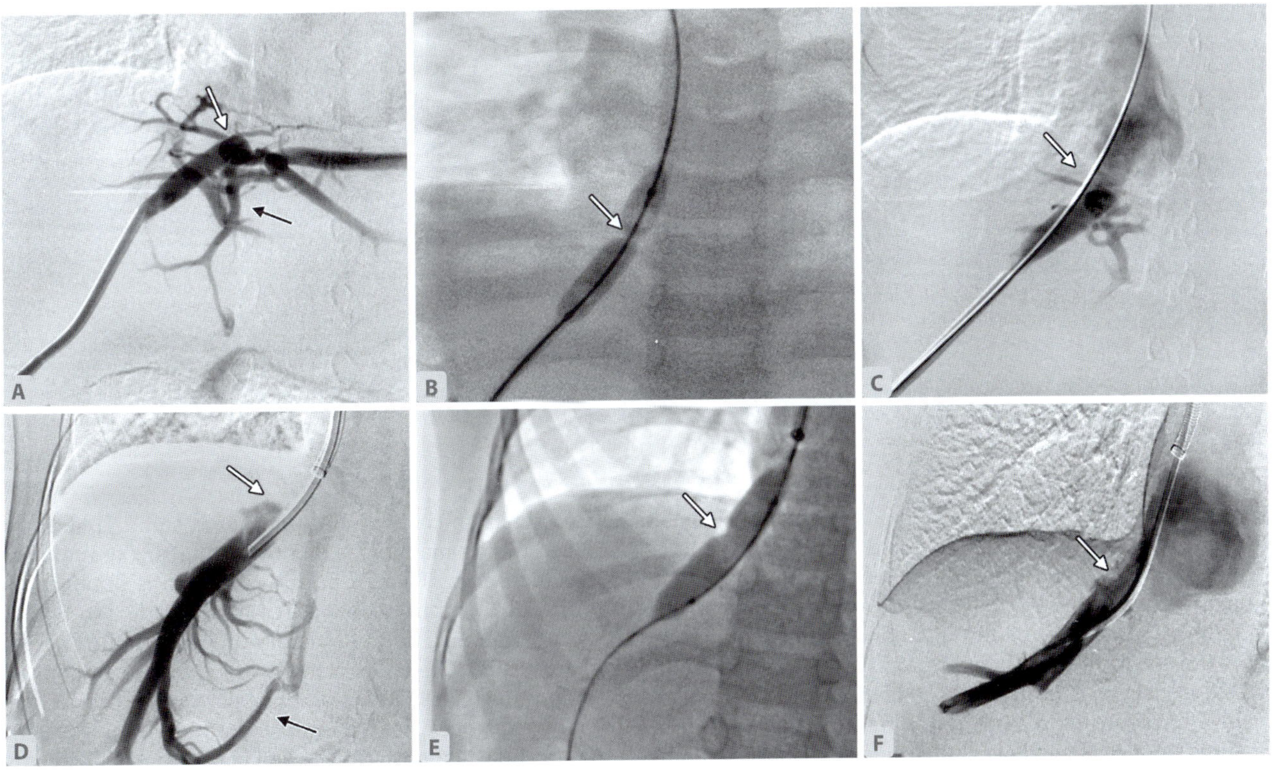

FIGS. 29A TO F: Hepatic vein angioplasty procedure: Angioplasty of middle hepatic vein through transhepatic route. (A) Middle hepatic venogram shows ostial occlusion of the vein (white arrow) with surrounding collaterals (black arrow). (B) Balloon angioplasty (8 × 40 mm) shows a waist (white arrow). (C) Venogram after angioplasty shows opening of the occlusion (white arrow) with marked reduction in the collaterals. Angioplasty of right hepatic vein (in another patient) through transjugular route. (D) Right hepatic venogram shows ostial occlusion of the vein (white arrow) with collaterals (black arrow) draining to inferior vena cava. (E) Balloon angioplasty (10 × 40 mm) shows waist (white arrow); (F) Venogram after angioplasty shows opening of the occlusion (white arrow) with disappearance of collaterals.

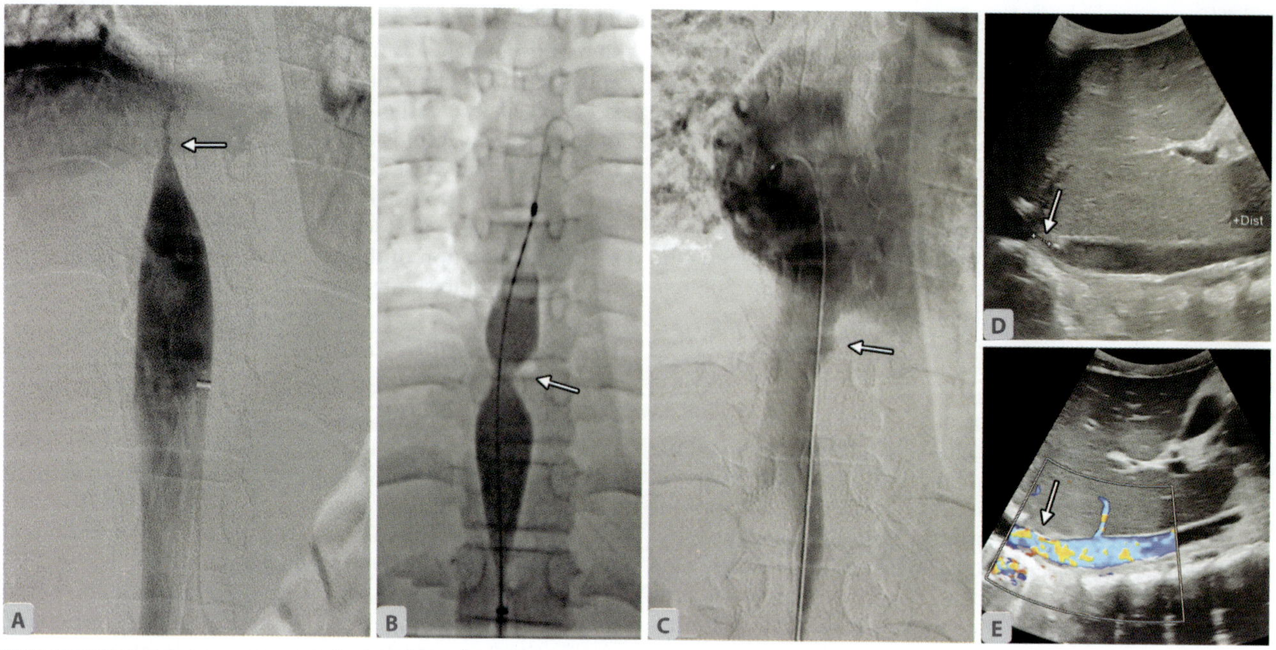

FIGS. 30A TO E: Inferior vena cava angioplasty through transfemoral route. (A) Inferior vena cavogram shows beak-like occlusion of suprahepatic segment (white arrow). (B) Balloon angioplasty (14 × 40 mm) shows a waist (white arrow). (C) Cavogram after angioplasty shows opening of the occlusion (white arrow). (D and E) Ultrasonography before and after angioplasty shows the opening of the occlusion (white arrows).

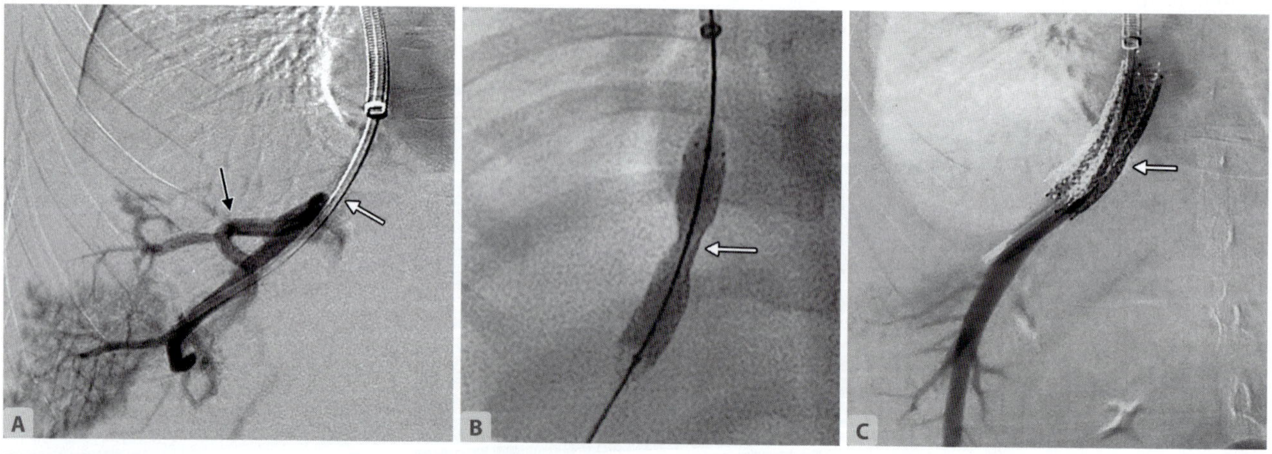

FIGS. 31A TO C: Hepatic vein stenting through transjugular route. (A) Right hepatic venogram shows ostial occlusion of the vein (white arrow) with surrounding collaterals (black arrow). (B) Balloon mounted stent placement (8 × 37 mm) shows a waist (white arrow). (C) Venogram after stenting shows opening of the occlusion (white arrow) with disappearance of the collaterals.

This procedure is usually performed through transjugular route **(Figs. 32A to F)**. The sheathed metallic cannula is positioned at the level of suprahepatic or intrahepatic IVC and directed to the right. Then, a catheter/trocar stylet assembly (5F) is inserted through the cannula and pushed onto the liver with a jab. Then with help of USG, the direction of the trocar stylet is adjusted so as to hit the right portal vein 1 cm from its bifurcation. Once the portal vein is entered, an exchange length stiff guidewire is inserted into the superior mesenteric vein through the right portal vein. Subsequently, the track is dilated using an 8-mm balloon catheter, followed by a venogram study using a sizing catheter to determine the length of the stent to be used. Then, a hybrid stent with both covered and uncovered portions or two separate covered and uncovered stents (placed in an overlapping manner) is deployed. The size of the stent is usually 8 mm. Then, a portal venogram is obtained to confirm flow within the stent. It would be ideal to obtain pressure gradients between the portal vein and IVC before and after DIPS. The target is to attain a pressure gradient of 5–10 mm of Hg. A higher gradient will result in persistence of symptoms of portal hypertension and too low gradient (<5 mm Hg) will increase the risk of hepatic encephalopathy and liver dysfunction.

The principle of stent placement is that for the track in the liver parenchyma covered stent (stent graft) should be used to prevent its occlusion by bile leak and hepatocytes ingrowth. The part of the stent in the right and main portal

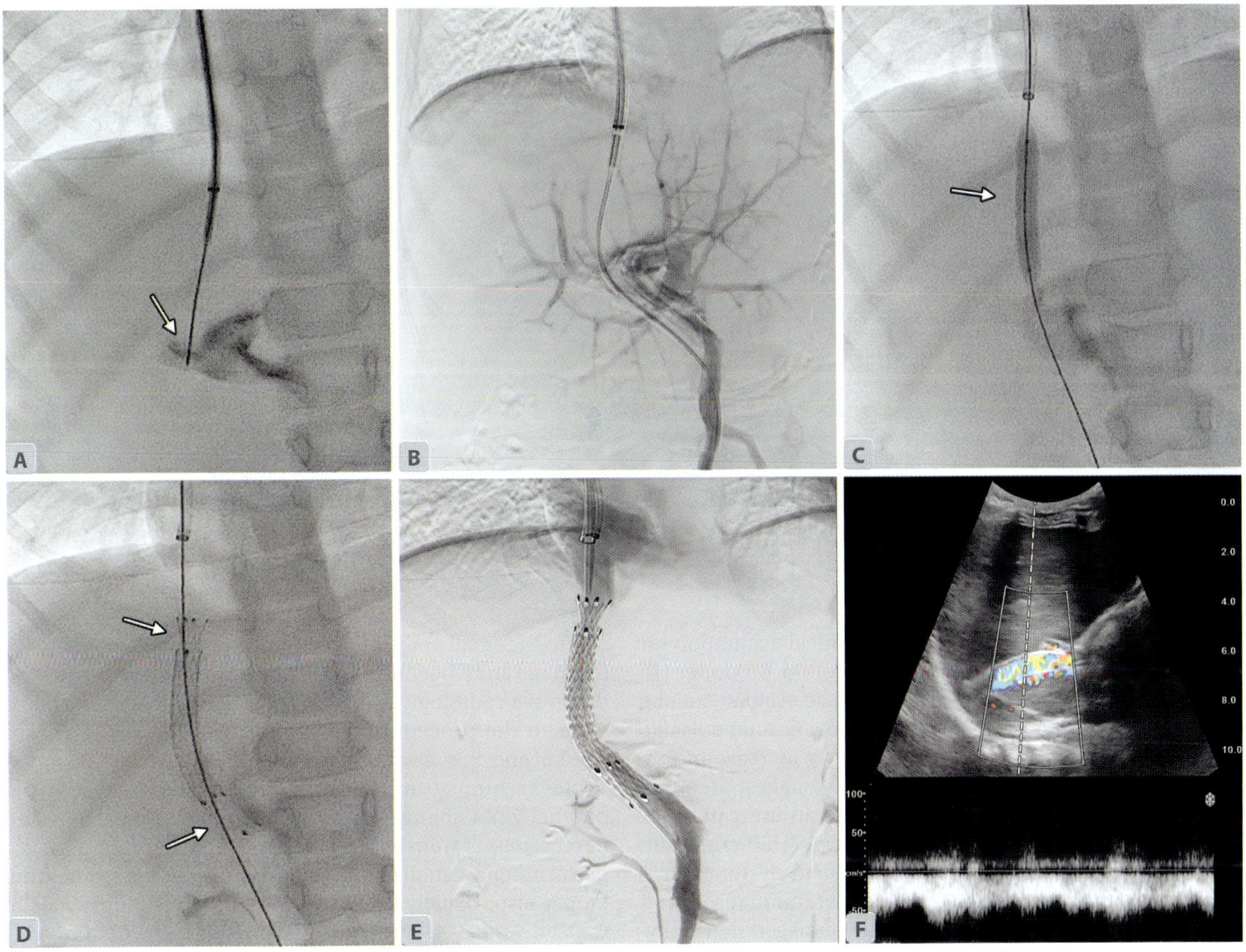

FIGS. 32A TO F: Direct intrahepatic portocaval shunt (DIPS) placement. (A) Puncture of the right portal vein through transjugular route (white arrow). (B) Mesenteric venogram shows portal vein and its branches. (C) Balloon angioplasty of the track (white arrow). (D) Placement of two overlapping stents (uncovered distally and covered proximally; white arrows). (E) Venogram after DIPS shows good opacification of the stent. (F) Color Doppler ultrasonography after 72 hours shows good flow within the stent.

vein should be uncovered (self-expandable metallic stent), so that it does not occlude the flow into the branches of the right and left portal veins. Further, the positioning of the ends of the stent is also critical. The proximal end should not project too much into the suprahepatic IVC and the distal end should be at the level of portal vein bifurcation or slightly projecting into the main portal vein. This is important to allow future liver transplantation. The adequate lengths of unstented IVC and main portal vein are necessary for performing surgical anastomosis to the liver allograft.

Complications and Management

Various complications can occur during and after the percutaneous interventions performed for pediatric BCS. The incidence of complications is in the range of 5–7%.[36] The most serious complication is hemorrhage which may occur from the HV or IVC rupture, puncture of pericardium resulting in cardiac tamponade, or peritoneal bleed due to portal vein rupture during DIPS. Temporary balloon occlusion or immediate placement of covered stent helps in controlling the bleeding. Pericardial hematoma causing cardiac tamponade may require surgery. Hemoperitoneum may occur if a transhepatic route is used. This can be prevented by embolization of the liver parenchymal tract with coils or gelfoam.

Other less serious complications include puncture site hematoma, pneumothorax, liver laceration, thrombosis of the stent, hepatic encephalopathy, restenosis, and liver failure. Many of these can be managed conservatively. Thrombosis of the stent and restenosis require repeat interventional procedure.

Follow-up and Outcomes of Interventions

After the therapeutic interventions, all children should be put on oral anticoagulants to maintain the INR between 2 and 3.[35] If the patient has an underlying genetic hypercoagulable state as an etiology, the anticoagulation should be continued for life. In the absence of any identifiable cause, it may be stopped after a period of 5 years.

All children must be regularly followed-up clinically and by USG. The standard protocol is to evaluate them first at 1 month and then every 3 months in the first year followed

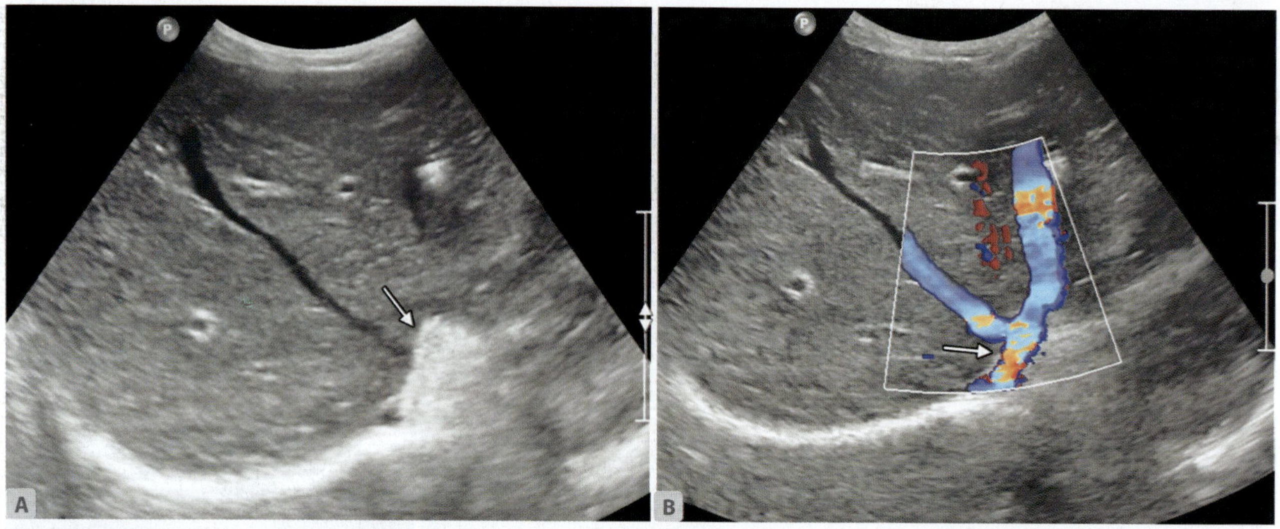

FIGS. 33A AND B: Ultrasonography (USG) during follow-up after radiological intervention. (A and B) B-mode and color Doppler USG images show stented left hepatic vein (arrow in A) having good flow (arrow in B).

by every 6 months thereafter.[37] After clinical evaluation for symptoms, USG with color Doppler should be done. On USG, patency of the vein or stent should be evaluated along with spectral waveform which should show normal pulsatile flow **(Figs. 33A and B)**. Any turbulence or increase in PSV of above 100 cm/s in the HV stent may suggest stenosis. Any stenosis of >30% of the diameter is an indication for reintervention.[38] Peak systolic velocities of <50 cm/s and >250 cm/s within a DIPS stent suggest stent dysfunction.[39] The former may be associated with hyperammonemia and hepatic encephalopathy and is usually managed medically, but occasionally DIPS stent reduction may be needed. A PSV of >250 cm/s indicates stenosis of the stent and balloon angioplasty or restenting may become necessary. Additional findings to evaluate are the presence of ascites, morphological changes in the liver, and development of liver nodules.

Studies have shown excellent (about 90%) long-term patency after angioplasty and stenting of HV and IVC in pediatric BCS.[40,41] Reintervention rate is in the range of 10–20%. Survival rates are above 90% at 5 years.

Other Percutaneous Procedures

In addition to the major recanalization procedures performed for pediatric BCS, few other interventions are also performed.[42]

Ascites drainage is an important procedure. Although it can be performed without guidance in most cases due to the large volume, there are two problems. One, it refills quickly and second, not >500–700 mL can be drained at a single time due to the small body habitus. Hence, percutaneous catheter drainage may become necessary immediately before the definitive radiological intervention. Further, this drainage prior to the procedure also helps the child recover from general anesthesia without respiratory problems.

Liver biopsy may also be performed to assess the parenchymal changes and for prognostication. The same percutaneous transhepatic or transjugular route used for performing recanalization procedure is used for obtaining biopsy also. Usually, an 18G semi-automatic biopsy needle is used and 3–4 cores (1.5–2 cm long) are obtained. If transhepatic route is used, the tract is then embolized with coils or gelfoam pledgets.

CONCLUSION

Pediatric BCS is an uncommon vascular disease of the liver. The clinical presentation is nonspecific and the diagnosis is often delayed. Imaging, particularly USG, plays a significant role not only in the diagnosis of the disease, but also in guiding radiological interventions. CT scan and MRI are only required for problem solving. The radiological interventions depend on the disease morphology and include thrombolysis, angioplasty, stent placement, or DIPS. Following these interventions, a regular follow-up is necessary to ensure continued venous patency, prevent complications, and detect disease recurrence. A complete knowledge of the diagnostic findings and standard percutaneous radiological interventions helps in judicious management of children with BCS.

REFERENCES

1. Bayraktar UD, Seren S, Bayraktar Y. Hepatic venous outflow obstruction: three similar syndromes. World J Gastroenterol. 2007;13:1912-27.
2. Dilawari JB, Bambrey P, Chawla Y, Kaur U, Bhusnurmath SR, Malhotra HS, et al. Hepatic outflow obstruction (Budd–Chiari syndrome). Experience with 177 patients and a review of the literature. Medicine (Baltimore). 1994;73:21-36.
3. Shukla A, Bhatt P, Gupta DK, Modi T, Patel J, Gupte A, et al. Budd–Chiari syndrome has different presentations and disease severity during adolescence. Hepatol Int. 2018;12:560-6.
4. Madhusudhan KS, Sharma S. Ultrasonography in pediatric Budd–Chiari syndrome. Pediatr Radiol. 2020. [Epub ahead of print].
5. Faraoun SA, Boudjella MA, Debzi N, Benidir N, Afredj N, Guerrache Y, et al. Budd–Chiari syndrome: an update on imaging features. Clin Imaging. 2016;40:637-46.
6. Aydinli M, Bayraktar Y. Budd–Chiari syndrome: etiology, pathogenesis and diagnosis. World J Gastroenterol. 2007;13: 2693-6.
7. Menon KV, Shah V, Kamath PS. The Budd–Chiari syndrome. N Engl J Med. 2004;350:578-85.
8. Valla DC. Hepatic vein thrombosis (Budd–Chiari syndrome). Semin Liver Dis. 2002;22:5-14.
9. Shrestha SM, Okuda K, Uchida T, Maharjan KG, Shrestha S, Joshi BL, et al. Endemicity and clinical picture of liver disease due to obstruction of the hepatic portion of the inferior vena cava in Nepal. J Gastroenterol Hepatol. 1996;11:170-9.
10. Hadengue A, Poliquin M, Vilgrain V, Belghiti J, Degott C, Erlinger S, et al. The changing scene of hepatic vein thrombosis: recognition of asymptomatic cases. Gastroenterology. 1994;106:1042-7.
11. Patil P, Deshmukh H, Popat B, Rathod K. Spectrum of imaging in Budd–Chiari syndrome. J Med Imaging Radiat Oncol. 2012;56: 75-83.
12. Kathuria R, Srivastava A, Yachha SK, Poddar U, Baijal SS. Budd–Chiari syndrome in children: clinical features, percutaneous radiological intervention, and outcome. Eur J Gastroenterol Hepatol. 2014;26:1030-8.
13. Brancatelli G, Vilgrain V, Federle MP, Hakime A, Lagalla R, Iannaccone I, et al. Budd–Chiari syndrome: spectrum of imaging findings. AJR Am J Roentgenol. 2007;188:W168-76.
14. Trivedi CR, Thakkar H, Sannananja B, Shah HU. Ultrasound and Doppler features of Budd–Chiari syndrome in pediatric population. Ultrasound Q. 2015;31:45-54.
15. Chaubal N, Dighe M, Hanchate V, Thakkar H, Deshmukh H, Rathod K. Sonography in Budd–Chiari syndrome. J Ultrasound Med. 2006;25:373-9.
16. Lim JH, Park JH, Auh YH. Membranous obstruction of the inferior vena cava: comparison of findings at sonography, CT, and venography. AJR Am J Roentgenol. 1992;159:515-20.
17. Faraoun SA, Boudjella MA, Debzi N, Afredj N, Guerrache Y, Benidir N, et al. Budd–Chiari syndrome: a prospective analysis of hepatic vein obstruction on ultrasonography, multidetector-row computed tomography and MR imaging. Abdom Imaging. 2015;40:1500-9.
18. Cheng DL, Xu H, Li CL, Lv WF, Li CT, Mukhiya G, et al. Interventional treatment strategy for primary Budd–Chiari syndrome with both inferior vena cava and hepatic vein involvement: patients from two centers in China. Cardiovasc Intervent Radiol. 2019;42: 1311-21.
19. Bargallo X, Gilabert R, Nicolau C, Garcia-Pagan JC, Bosch J, Bru C. Sonography of the caudate vein: value in diagnosing Budd–Chiari syndrome. AJR Am J Roentgenol. 2003;181:1641-5.
20. Bargalló X, Gilabert R, Nicolau C, García-Pagán JC, Ayuso JR, Brú C. Sonography of Budd–Chiari syndrome. AJR Am J Roentgenol. 2006;187:W33-41.
21. Zhang R, Qin S, Zhou Y, Song Y, Sun L. Comparison of imaging characteristics between hepatic benign regenerative nodules and hepatocellular carcinomas associated with Budd–Chiari syndrome by contrast enhanced ultrasound. Eur J Radiol. 2012;81:2984-9.
22. El Ali AM, Davis JC, Cickelli JM, Squires JH. Contrast-enhanced ultrasound of liver lesions in children. Pediatr Radiol. 2019;49:1422-32.
23. Wang HW, Shi HN, Cheng J, Xie F, Luo YK, Tang J. Real-time shear wave elastography (SWE) assessment of short- and long-term treatment outcome in Budd–Chiari syndrome: A pilot study. PLoS One. 2018;13:e0197550.
24. Mukund A, Pargewar SS, Desai SN, Rajesh S, Sarin SK. Changes in liver congestion in patients with Budd–Chiari syndrome following endovascular interventions: assessment with transient elastography. J Vasc Interv Radiol. 2017;28:683-7.
25. Zhang C, Fu L, Zhang G, Xu L, Shun H, Wang Z, et al. Ultrasonically-guided inferior vena cava stent placement: experience in 83 cases. J Vasc Interv Radiol. 1999;10:85-91.
26. Gipson MG, Smith MT, Durham JD, Brown A, Johnson T, Ray CE, et al. Intravascular US-guided portal vein access: improved procedural metrics during TIPS creation. J Vasc Interv Radiol. 2016;27:1140-7.
27. Cazals-Hatem D, Vilgrain V, Genin P, Denninger MH, Durand F, Belghiti J, et al. Arterial and portal circulation and parenchymal changes in Budd–Chiari syndrome: a study in 17 explanted livers. Hepatology. 2003;37:510-9.
28. Erden A. Budd–Chiari syndrome: a review of imaging findings. Eur J Radiol. 2007;61:44-56.
29. Xiang H, Han J, Ridley WE, Ridley LJ. Spider's web sign: Budd–Chiari syndrome. J Med Imaging Radiat Oncol. 2018;62:110.
30. Cho OK, Koo JH, Kim YS, Rhim HC, Koh BH, Seo HS. Collateral pathways in Budd–Chiari syndrome: CT and venographic correlation. Am J Roentgenol. 1996;167:1163-7.
31. Brancatelli G, Federle MP, Grazioli L, Golfieri R, Lencioni R. Large regenerative nodules in Budd–Chiari syndrome and other vascular disorders of the liver: CT and MR imaging findings with clinicopathologic correlation. AJR Am J Roentgenol. 2002;178:877-83.
32. Erden A, Erden I, Yurdaydin C, Karayalcin S. Hepatic outflow obstruction: enhancement patterns of the liver on MR angiography. Eur J Radiol. 2003;48:203-8.
33. Sharma S, Texeira A, Texeira P, Elias E, Wilde J, Olliff SP. Pharmacological thrombolysis in Budd–Chiari syndrome: a single centre experience and review of the literature. J Hepatol. 2004;40:172-80.
34. Raffini L. Thrombolysis for intravascular thrombosis in neonates and children. Curr Opin Pediatr. 2009;21:9-14.
35. Sharma VK, Ranade PR, Marar S, Nabi F, Nagral A. Long-term clinical outcome of Budd–Chiari syndrome in children after radiological intervention. Eur J Gastroenterol Hepatol. 2016;28:567-75.

36. Wei X, Hao X, Da-Hai Y, Mao-Heng Z, Qing-Qiao Z, Yu-Ming G. Analysis of interventional treatments of Budd–Chiari syndrome and the related complications: a study of 1006 cases. Panminerva Med. 2013;55:371-6.
37. Ding PX, Zhang SJ, Li Z, Fu MT, Hua ZH, Zhang WG. Long-term safety and outcome of percutaneous transhepatic venous balloon angioplasty for Budd–Chiari syndrome. J Gastroenterol Hepatol. 2016;31:222-8.
38. Han G, Qi X, Zhang W, He C, Yin Z, Wang J, et al. Percutaneous recanalization for Budd–Chiari syndrome: an 11-year retrospective study on patency and survival in 177 Chinese patients from a single center. Radiology. 2013;266:657-67.
39. Hayek G, Ronot M, Plessier A, Sibert A, Abdel-Rehim M, Zappa M, et al. Long-term outcome and analysis of dysfunction of transjugular intrahepatic portosystemic shunt placement in chronic primary Budd–Chiari syndrome. Radiology. 2017;283:280-92.
40. Rathod K, Deshmukh H, Shukla A, Popat B, Pandey A, Gupte A, et al. Endovascular treatment of Budd–Chiari syndrome: Single center experience. J Gastroenterol Hepatol. 2017;32:237-43.
41. Chen ZK, Fan J, Cao C, Li Y. Endovascular treatment for hepatic vein-type Budd–Chiari syndrome: effectiveness and long-term outcome. Radiol Med. 2018;123:799-807.
42. Cura M, Haskal Z, Lopera J. Diagnostic and interventional radiology for Budd–Chiari syndrome. Radiographics. 2009;29:669-81.

CHAPTER

72

Childhood Biliopathies

Rashmi Dixit, Sapna Singh, Anju Garg

INTRODUCTION

A wide range of disease processes involve the pediatric gallbladder and bile ducts varying from congenital, developmental, and inflammatory to neoplastic in nature. Clinical presentation is often with jaundice or nonspecific symptoms which overlap in various disease processes, hence imaging plays a vital role in establishing the diagnosis and guiding management decisions.

IMAGING MODALITIES[1-8]

Ultrasound (US) is generally the first imaging modality: It is noninvasive, inexpensive, and does not require sedation or exposure to radiation. US should be performed after a 4–6 hours fast to ensure optimal distention of the biliary system. It is especially useful to differentiate obstructive from nonobstructive jaundice.

Magnetic resonance imaging (MRI) can evaluate the biliary system, the surrounding liver parenchyma, and other abdominal viscera usually without need for administration of contrast and does not involve ionizing radiation. MRI in children has to be planned to optimize signal to noise ratio (SNR) and answer the clinical question at hand. Heavily T2-weighted sequences are used to generate magnetic resonance cholangiopancreatography (MRCP) images that allow visualization of gallbladder, bile ducts, and the pancreatic duct without contrast. Breath-hold techniques can be used in older children who can co-operate, while respiratory gating can be used in younger children. Like ultrasound, the child should be fasting for 4–6 hours to ensure optimal distention of the biliary tree and so that a full stomach does not obscure the ducts. MRCP protocols should include a thick slab single-section acquisition (for the entire biliary tree) and thin (1–5 mm) contiguous sections. A three-dimensional (3D) sequence should be performed whenever breathing is regular. It provides better SNR and spatial resolution than two-dimensional (2D) imaging. Moreover, anomalies can be better understood on 3D images. However, MRCP is limited in neonates and infants, as biliary ducts <1 mm in diameter are difficult to visualize. MR contrast agents have a role in evaluation of periductal inflammation and tumors of the biliary system. Hepatobiliary contrast agents may help to distinguish true biliary obstruction from dilated ducts without obstruction and visualize bile leaks in postoperative patients. However, due to equivocal utility and concerns regarding CNS deposition their use is best avoided.

Although ***computed tomography (CT)*** is inferior to MR for evaluation of the biliary tree, it is often used after ultrasonography (US) due to its wider availability and faster aquisition times. CT exposes the child to ionizing radiation and does require sedation. It is mainly indicated in the evaluation of tumors and complications of biliary disease such as cirrhosis and portal hypertension. Contrast-enhanced examination is usually done with acquisition in the portal venous phase. Multiplanar reformats (MPR) and minimum intensity projections (minIP) allow better evaluation of the biliary tree.

Hepatobiliary scintigraphy is used to provide physiologic information, particularly regarding patency of the biliary system.

Invasive investigations include percutaneous transhepatic cholangiography, percutaneous cholecystocholangiography, intraoperative cholangiography, and endoscopic retrograde cholangiopancreatography (ERCP). However, they are technically challenging and expose the child to radiation. In the pediatric population, ERCP has a complication rate of nearly 33% which is higher than the complication rate for adults. These investigations are, therefore, reserved for cases where noninvasive investigations are inconclusive, especially for surgical candidates.

NORMAL ANATOMY[9-12]

Normal Bile Ducts

The normal common hepatic and common bile duct (CBD) are generally identified in most cases on US. The normal CBD increases in diameter with age. Measuring from inner wall to inner wall, the CBD diameter should be <1.6 mm up to 1 year of age, <4 mm in childhood and <7 mm in adolescents and adults. The normal left and right hepatic ducts can often be seen on US in older children. The cystic duct is visualized only when dilated, usually only the most distal portion being seen. The normal peripheral intrahepatic biliary radicles are not well visualized with US, CT, or MRI and are seen only when dilated.

Magnetic resonance cholangiopancreatography reliably delineates the right and left hepatic ducts, common hepatic duct, and CBD in most children and adolescents. The neonatal biliary tree is challenging to visualize and extrahepatic biliary ducts may be the only ducts visible.

Normal Gallbladder

The normal gallbladder is well visualized on US and its size is proportional to the age of the child and/or body surface area. The gallbladder in neonates is approximately 1.3 cm in length increasing to 3.4 cm in infancy, being <1 cm in width in both. By 16 years of age, the average length of the gallbladder is 8 cm and the average width is <3.5 cm. The wall is well-defined with hyperechoic mucosa and measures <3 mm in thickness when the gallbladder is well distended. The gallbladder wall may appear fallaciously thickened if it is not optimally distended as in a nonfasting state or due a halo effect caused by fluid between gallbladder and liver. Folds or kinks can be normally seen in the gallbladder and can simulate pathology.

CHOLESTATIC PROCESSES[13-17]

Jaundice is the most common problem in the neonatal period, occurring in approximately 60% of term infants and 80% of preterm infants. Since jaundice in neonates is commonly physiological, not all jaundiced neonates need to be investigated. Physiologic jaundice, a normal finding that occurs during the first 2 weeks of life in term and preterm infants, is transient and consists of unconjugated hyperbilirubinemia. It occurs as the metabolism of bilirubin in the neonate is in transition from the fetal stage, when the placenta eliminates bilirubin, to the adult stage when bilirubin is excreted via the hepatocytes into the biliary system and then into the gastrointestinal tract. Jaundice persisting beyond 2 weeks in nonbreastfed neonates warrants prompt evaluation as per the Cholestasis Guideline Committee. In breastfed infants, physiologic jaundice may persist up to 3 weeks. This is due to substances in the breast milk of some mothers that impair conjugation of bilirubin. Even so, abnormally dark urine or acholic stool should raise concern for underlying cholestasis (or conjugated hyperbilirubinemia). Serum bilirubin levels can help to confirm the diagnosis of cholestasis. The biochemical criteria for the diagnosis of cholestasis are: conjugated bilirubin >1.0 mg/dL if total bilirubin <5.0 mg/dL or conjugated bilirubin >20% if total bilirubin >5.0 mg/dL.

Several conditions may produce neonatal jaundice that is not physiologic which may be transient or persistent. The important conditions responsible for transient neonatal jaundice include adrenal hemorrhage, bile-plug syndrome, hemolysis, infective hepatitis, drugs, metabolic diseases, sepsis, and total parenteral nutrition (TPN). Biliary atresia, neonatal hepatitis, and choledochal cysts are the important conditions responsible for persistent neonatal jaundice. Of these, biliary atresia and hepatitis are responsible for 70–80% of cases and imaging evaluation is often directed at distinguishing between the two. Persistent jaundice can less often be due to Alagille syndrome, Caroli's disease, and spontaneous bile duct perforation. The causes of jaundice in neonates are summarized in **Table 1**.

Biliary Atresia[18-21]

Biliary atresia accounts for approximately one-third cases of neonatal cholestasis and is the most common cause of persistent neonatal jaundice that requires surgical management. The incidence of biliary atresia is reported to be 1 in 8,000–16,700 live births with a higher incidence for Asian populations.

Biliary atresia is characterized by an inflammatory and fibrosing obstruction of extrahepatic and intrahepatic bile ducts. The exact cause is not known but several factors have been implicated. An immune-mediated inflammatory obstruction of the biliary tree due to a viral infection is one common theory for pathogenesis of biliary atresia. Other possible causes include ductal plate malformation, abnormal fetal circulation, genetic factors, and environmental toxins. The underlying pathologic process is progressive fibrosis of the biliary tree with consequent cholestasis. This ultimately results in hepatic fibrosis and cirrhosis.

Affected children typically present in the neonatal period, although the pathologic process may begin in the antenatal period. Patients usually have severe, persistent cholestatic jaundice, acholic or white stools and high-colored urine. If the diagnosis is delayed, features of cirrhosis and vitamin K coagulopathy may be seen.

Classification[22,23]

Several classification systems for biliary atresia have been developed. The classification system given by Kasai, based on the level of atresia, is commonly used. It classifies biliary atresia into three types of which type III is the most common and only type I is considered truly surgically correctable. The Kasai classification is summarized in **Table 2** and **Figure 1**.

Anomalies and Malformations Associated with Biliary Atresia[24-29]

In 70–85% of patients, there are no associated anomalies or malformation, the so-called *nonsyndromic* or *perinatal biliary atresia*. Classically, these children do not have jaundice at birth, but jaundice develops progressively within the first 2

TABLE 1: Causes of neonatal jaundice.

Transient causes	Persistent causes
• Adrenal hemorrhage	• Biliary atresia*
• Infective hepatitis	• Neonatal hepatitis*
• Sepsis	• Alagille syndrome/bile duct paucity
• Hemolysis	• Progressive familial intrahepatic cholestasis
• Metabolic diseases	Gestational alloimmune liver disease
• Bile plug syndrome	Choledochal cyst*
• Drug related	Spontaneous perforation of the CBD

*common causes of persistent jaundice.
(CBD: common bile duct)

TABLE 2: Kasai classification of biliary atresia.

Type	Characteristic
Type I	Obliteration of the common bile duct, but proximal ducts are patent
Type II	Common hepatic duct is obliterated, but bile ducts are found at porta hepatis
Type IIa	Common hepatic duct is obliterated, but both cystic and common bile ducts are patent
Type IIb	Obliteration of both cystic common hepatic and common bile duct
Type III	No patent hepatic or hilar ducts

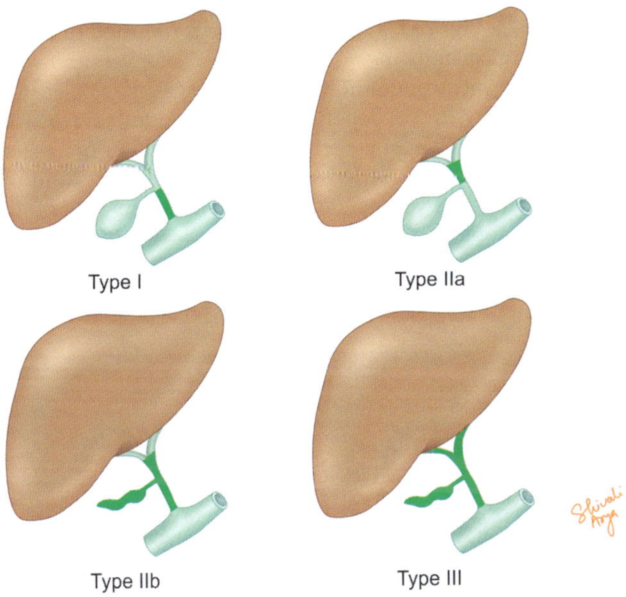

FIG. 1: Line diagram depicting the Kasai classification of biliary atresia.

months. Approximately 15–30% cases of biliary atresia have associated congenital anomalies. Laterality defects are seen in 10–15% of infants with biliary atresia which is known as biliary atresia splenic malformation (BASM) or embryonal biliary atresia also referred to as syndromic, congenital/fetal or prenatal biliary atresia. Associated extrahepatic anomalies seen in these patients include asplenia or polysplenia, situs inversus, and symmetric bilobed liver. Also seen are malrotation of gut, interruption or absence of inferior vena cava, preduodenal portal vein, aberrant hepatic artery, and cardiac anomalies. *Importantly, biliary atresia is almost always present if polysplenia or situs inversus is demonstrated in a jaundiced infant.* The complex anatomy in these patients makes surgical treatment of biliary atresia more difficult. The residual 5–10% cases of biliary atresia are associated with congenital anomalies such as intestinal atresia, imperforate anus, renal anomalies, and cardiac abnormalities.

Imaging

Ultrasound, hepatobiliary scintigraphy, and MRI are the main imaging modalities used in the evaluation of biliary atresia.

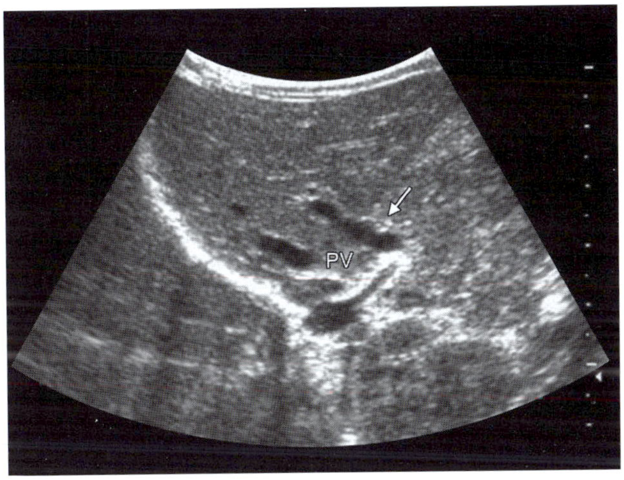

FIG. 2: Ultrasound (US) of a neonate with biliary atresia showing an echogenic triangular cord anterior to the portal vein—"Triangular cord" sign.

Ultrasound[1,12,30-43] is the initial imaging modality for infants with cholestatic jaundice and suspected biliary atresia. It is best performed after a 4-hour fast using an appropriate high-frequency transducer. It can exclude other anatomic causes of cholestasis, such as a choledochal cyst and may be able to confirm the diagnosis of biliary atresia. US can, however, not be used to rule out the diagnosis of biliary atresia. The most helpful US features of biliary atresia include the *triangular cord sign, abnormal gallbladder, absence of the CBD, and hypertrophied hepatic artery.* These can be seen when correctly searched for with a high-frequency transducer.

The *"triangular cord sign"* is a triangular or cord like hyperechoic structure seen just anterior to the bifurcation of the main portal vein (MPV). It is thought to represent the fibrous ductal remnant of the bile duct at the porta hepatis. A thickness of the echogenic cord of >4 mm on longitudinal US images has sensitivity varying from 73–80% and specificity of 98–100% for biliary atresia **(Fig. 2)**. Another measurement that has been suggested is echogenic anterior wall of the right portal vein (EARPV): this is measured just proximal to the right portal vein bifurcation (rather than MPV bifurcation), a measurement of >4 mm on a longitudinal scan is abnormal. A modified triangular cord thickness has also been described to improve accuracy, requiring a cord thickness of >2 mm at the anterior branch of the right branch of portal vein on longitudinal sections. False negative findings may occur due to several reasons. The triangular cord sign may not be evident early on in the disease, or it may be obscured by diffuse increase in periportal echogenicity due to inflammation or cirrhosis. An enlarged right hepatic artery may also mask the sign. The sign is better appreciated on longitudinal images and may not be apparent on transverse images due to the tapering nature of echogenicity.

The gallbladder is usually *absent* in neonates with biliary atresia (BA). When the gallbladder is visualized it is often abnormal. A combination of three features, i.e., (i) Length of the gallbladder <15–19 mm, (ii) An irregular or lobular contour of the wall, and (iii) Thin mucosa or absence of complete and smooth echogenic mucosal lining—the so-called "*gallbladder ghost triad*" is highly suggestive of biliary atresia. Another finding described is a length-to-width ratio of >5.2. A meta-analysis of US studies has shown 95% sensitivity (95% CI 70–99) and 89% specificity (95% CI 79–94) using the triangular cord sign and abnormality of gallbladder taken together **(Figs. 3A to C)**. Visualization of a normal gallbladder, however, does not exclude the diagnosis of biliary atresia. A normal gallbladder may be seen when the atresia is distal to the insertion of the cystic duct. Repeat examination after an oral feed may help to differentiate biliary atresia from neonatal hepatitis in these cases. Change in gallbladder size after a milk feed suggests patency of the common hepatic and CBDs and is seen in infants with neonatal hepatitis. In biliary atresia, the gallbladder length is not affected by oral feeding. A small gallbladder may be seen without biliary atresia in neonatal hepatitis with severe hepatocellular dysfunction or in preterm jaundiced infants on TPN. Gallbladder wall-thickening is not a feature of biliary atresia and this finding should prompt evaluation for other causes of neonatal jaundice.

The common bile duct is not seen in cases of biliary atresia but is difficult to visualize even in normal neonates being less than a millimeter in diameter **(Figs. 4A to D)**. Hepatic artery diameter is significantly larger in infants with biliary atresia than in hepatitis or normal controls. Color Doppler should be used to avoid misdiagnosing the hepatic artery for a normal CBD. Studies have reported that a hepatic artery diameter >1.5 mm is 92% sensitive, 87% specific, and 89% accurate and hepatic artery diameter-to-portal vein diameter ratio of >0.45 is 76% sensitive, 79% specific, and 78% accurate for diagnosis of biliary atresia **(Figs. 5A and B)**. Another finding reported on color Doppler US is increased hepatic subcapsular flow defined as arterial flow extending to the hepatic surface. This finding has a sensitivity of 100% and specificity of 86% for the diagnosis of biliary atresia.

Cystic lesions 5 mm to 4 cm in size may be visualized in 8–11% of cases at the porta hepatis, the so-called "*cystic form of biliary atresia*". Some authors have also reported the presence of small round or tubular cystic lesions smaller than 5 mm or *microcysts* at the porta as a useful sign of biliary atresia (see **Fig. 7A**). The cystic vairety is reported to have a better surgical outcome.

A wide spectrum of nonspecific changes may be seen in cases of biliary atresia, depending on the type and severity. The liver size and the echogenicity may be normal or increased. There may be decreased visualization of bile ducts and the peripheral portal venous radicles producing an abnormally homogeneous appearance of liver. Typically, intrahepatic bile duct dilatation is not seen in biliary atresia. Cirrhosis and

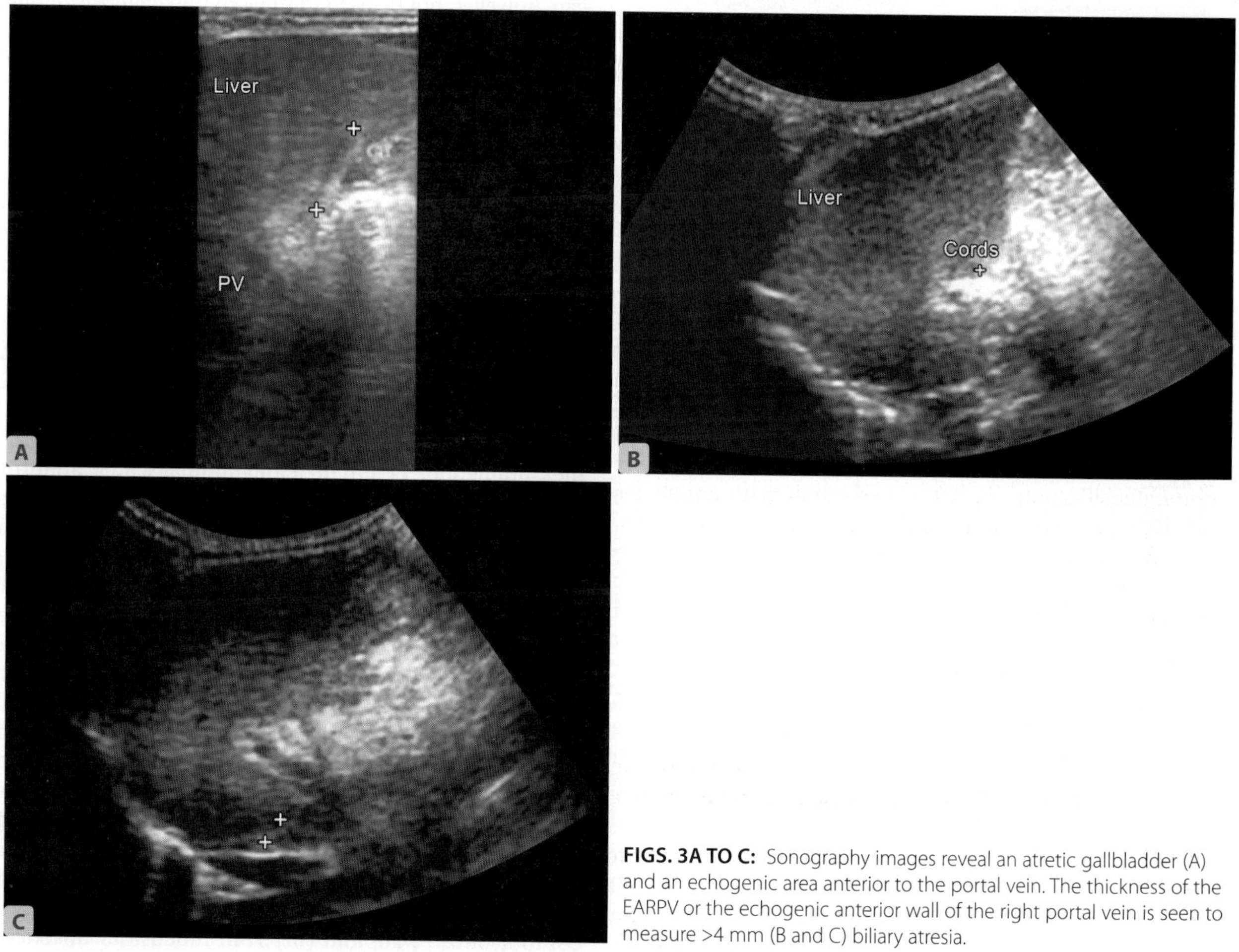

FIGS. 3A TO C: Sonography images reveal an atretic gallbladder (A) and an echogenic area anterior to the portal vein. The thickness of the EARPV or the echogenic anterior wall of the right portal vein is seen to measure >4 mm (B and C) biliary atresia.

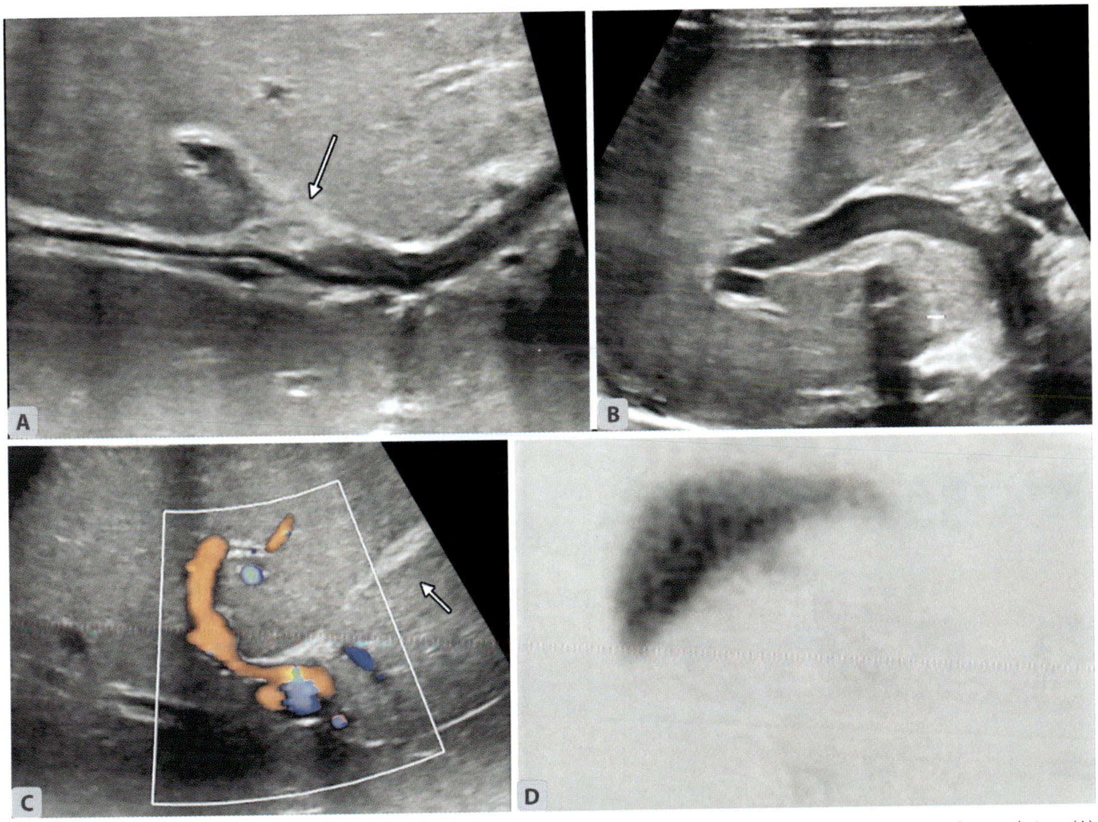

FIGS. 4A TO D: High resolution USG images (A to C) of a 1.5-month-old child with persistent jaundice shows the triangular cord sign. (A) CBD is not seen anterior to the portal vein (B and C). A small linear echogenicity is seen in the GB fossa with nonvisualization of GB (arrow in C). HIDA scan of same patient shows no gut activity on 24-hours delayed scan; (D) Biliary atresia. (CBD: common bile duct; GB: gallbladder; HIDA: hepatobiliary iminodiacetic acid; USG: ultrasonography)

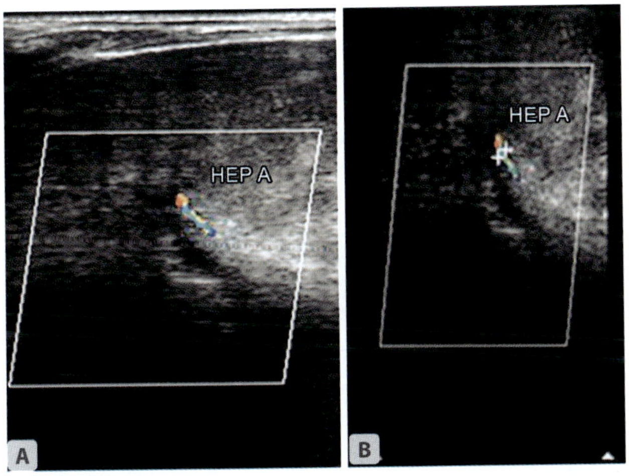

FIGS. 5A AND B: Color Doppler showing color fill in of the hepatic artery which is enlarged. The diameter of the artery is >1.5 mm in a case of biliary atresia.

features of portal hypertension may be apparent in the late stages. Associated malformations must be searched for in all cases.

Recently US elastography, especially shear wave elastography (SWE), has revealed higher values in infants with biliary atresia compared with those having other liver diseases. Its diagnostic performance has, however, not been reported to be more than that of gray-scale US. Another technique that has been found to be useful in some recent studies is US percutaneous cholangiocystography with microbubble based contrast. This can be helpful in equivocal cases. Visualization of microbubbles entering into the duodenum rules out BA.

A follow-up US may be useful if the initial US is either normal or suggests neonatal hepatitis but the cholestatic jaundice does not improve or worsens.

An inconclusive US examination is followed up by hepatobiliary scintigraphy[44-48] commonly referred to as hepatobiliary iminodiacetic acid (HIDA) or di-isopropyl iminodiacetic acid (DISIDA) scan. The iminodiacetic acid derivative generally used is mebrofenin because of its higher hepatic excretion. Oral phenobarbital is given for 5 days prior to the study to increase the biliary excretion of the isotope and the child should be fasting for 2 hours prior to the examination. The study is considered normal when the hepatic parenchyma is visualized almost immediately after administering the isotope with activity being seen subsequently in the intrahepatic biliary ducts, the extrahepatic biliary ducts, and the gallbladder and finally the small bowel (usually within 1 h). Neonatal hepatitis is the likely diagnosis when the hepatocyte clearance is delayed but activity is visualized in the small intestine within 24 hours. The presence of radioisotope in the gastrointestinal tract by 24 hours essentially excludes biliary atresia. No activity in the intestine by 24-hours, however, is not specific to biliary atresia. Severe hepatocellular dysfunction in neonatal hepatitis also results in inability to excrete detectable amounts of radiotracer into the gastrointestinal tract. The reported sensitivity of scintigraphy varies between 91.7 and 100% and specificity between 35 and 76.9% **(Fig. 6)**.

Magnetic resonance imaging especially MRCP[3-5,43,49-51] is being increasingly used to evaluate biliary atresia. It may obviate the need for more invasive imaging such as percutaneous transhepatic cholangiography or biopsy if normal biliary tract anatomy is demonstrated. In infants with cholestatic jaundice, MRCP findings of biliary atresia are nonvisualization of the extrahepatic bile duct, absent or a small, abnormal gallbladder, and periportal fibrosis. Gallbladder can be considered abnormal when its length is <15 mm; it has an abnormal elongated tubular shape even when length ≥15 mm or presence wall irregularity. On MR periportal fibrosis is seen as a triangular area of high signal on T2-weighted (T2W) images anterior to the porta and as a hypointense area running parallel to the portal vein branches on T1-weighted (T1W) images. On contrast administration this becomes isointense with liver. Some authors have measured the maximum thickness of the periportal signal and referred to this as the *MR triangular cord thickness (MR-TCT)*. In contrast to the triangular cord sign on US, that is, measured along the anterior aspect of the portal vein, the authors measured the MR-TCT on any side of the portal vein where its thickness was the greatest and suggested a cut-off value of 5.1 mm for the diagnosis of biliary atresia. At times a focal area of fluid signal/cyst may be seen on T2W images within the high signal intensity periportal fibrosis **(Figs. 7A and B)**. The authors reported that three MRI features—nonvisualization of CBD, abnormal gallbladder morphology and MR-TCT >5.1 mm when selected as discriminators of biliary atresia demonstrated high diagnostic performance with 97.3% sensitivity, 94.8% specificity, and 96.2% accuracy—comparable to US. Diffusion-weighted images (DWI) and other advanced MR techniques have also been evaluated in biliary atresia. On DWI, patients of biliary atresia showed lower liver apparent diffusion coefficient (ADC) values than control group. The ADC values also show a negative correlation with the degree of liver fibrosis in postoperative patients. On intravoxel incoherent motion (IVIM) evaluation, hepatic D* values have been reported to be lower than those in normal children. The more the liver stiffness lower the D*values (pseudo diffusion coefficient).

Magnetic resonance imaging, however, has a number of limitations. Since MRCP sequences are basically fluid-sensitive sequences they depend on production and excretion of bile for visualization of the biliary system. When the hepatic function is abnormal such as in hepatitis and sclerosing cholangitis (SC), the CBD may not be visualized resulting in a false positive diagnosis of biliary atresia. In addition, the normal biliary tree is not consistently visualized

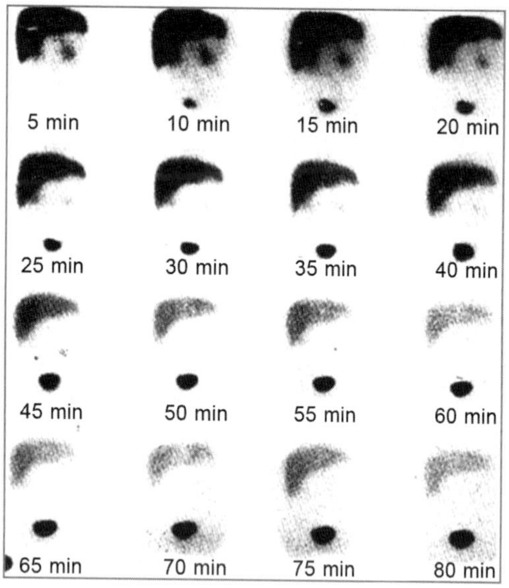

FIG. 6: Scintigraphy using ^{99m}TC-IDA scan in a neonate with cholestasis shows good hepatocyte extraction of the radiotracer but no bowel opacification due to biliary atresia. (IDA: iminodiacetic acid)

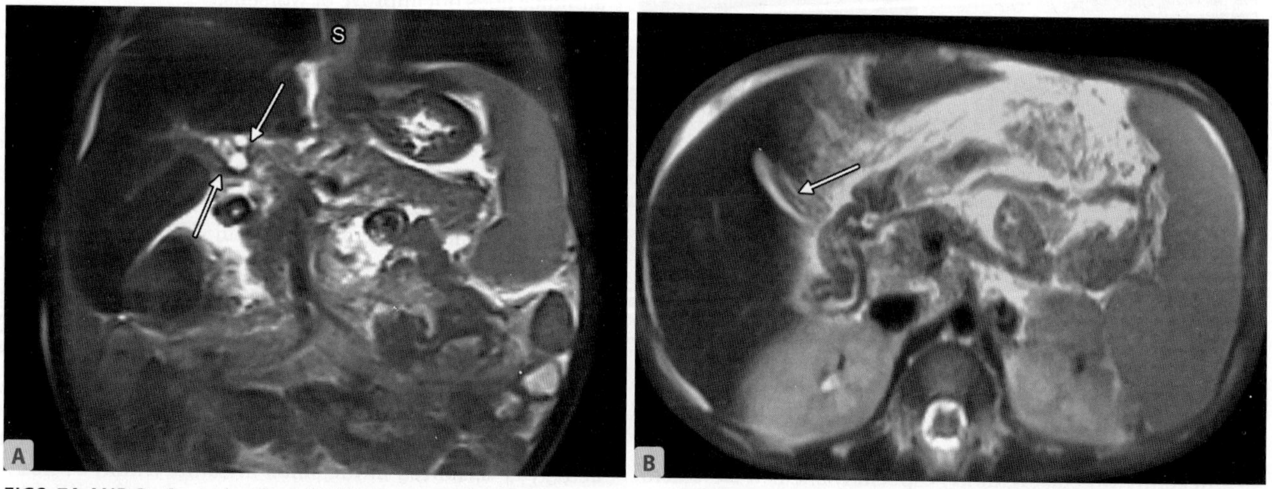

FIGS. 7A AND B: Coronal and axial T2W MR images of a 4-month-old child with persistent obstructive jaundice reveal small cysts at the porta (arrows in A). The CBD is not visualized either within the pancreatic head or in the suprapancreatic region. (A and B) A small atretic gallbladder is visualized in the GB fossa (arrow in B)—consistent with biliary atresia. Note is also made of splenomegaly and free fluid in abdomen. (CBD: common bile duct; GB: gallbladder; T2W MR: T2-weighted magnetic resonance)

under 3 months of age. Use of hepatobiliary contrast agents has been suggested in addition to conventional MRCP images. Absence of excretion into the bowel is expected in biliary atresia but like HIDA this is not specific to biliary atresia, in addition there are concerns regarding gadolinium administration in children.

Liver biopsy[14,48] can help to confirm the diagnosis of biliary atresia. A liver biopsy using an 18-gauge needle has sensitivity of 90% and specificity of 96% for diagnosis of biliary atresia in children with cholestasis. Histopathological findings of biliary atresia are proliferation of intralobular bile ductules, loss of ductular microvilli, bile plugging, and periductal inflammatory fibrosis. However, early in the disease process (within the first month) these findings may be absent, resulting in a false-negative liver biopsy and misinterpretation as neonatal hepatitis. When ultrasound, nuclear scintigraphy, MRCP, and liver biopsy are inconclusive intraoperative, transhepatic or endoscopic cholangiography may be necessary. Even when the diagnosis of biliary atresia is made on imaging, surgeons at many institutes go ahead with an intraoperative cholangiogram, which is regarded as the gold standard, before proceeding to surgical correction.

Neonatal hepatitis as discussed is the major differential of biliary atresia. In addition, the cystic variety of biliary atresia must not be confused with a choledochal cyst.[42] Clinically, cholestasis is less severe in a choledochal cyst. The cyst of biliary atresia is smaller and not associated with intrahepatic ductal dilatation, unlike choledochal cyst. Absence of sludge or calculi in the cyst favors the diagnosis of biliary atresia over choledochal cyst. Besides other features of biliary atresia such as the "*triangular cord sign*" and atretic gallbladder can be seen in cases of biliary atresia. The cyst of biliary atresia may show morphologically abnormal/obliterated intrahepatic ducts on cholangiography but no evidence of communication with the intestine is seen.

Management[12,37,52]

The mean survival in biliary atresia when left untreated is around 18 months. Kasai procedure or hepatico-enterostomy is the most common surgical treatment for biliary atresia, best performed before the infant reaches 2 months of age. This involves excision of the atretic bile ducts along with a Roux-en-Y hepaticojejunostomy. The proximal common hepatic duct should be patent (type I biliary atresia) in order for this to be a definitive treatment. This is true only in 10–15% cases, in the rest Kasai procedure is used as a palliative measure until a liver transplant is needed. The criterion for adequate drainage is total bilirubin concentration of <2.0 mg/dL within 3 months of surgery.

On imaging fluid-filled bowel loops, may be seen in the region of the porta hepatis on postoperative US scans, and should not be mistaken for a collection. Biliary scintigraphy can be used to evaluate the patency of the porto-enterostomy. Isotopic activity should appear in the bowel by 1 hour after administration. The most common complication of Kasai procedure is ascending cholangitis. There can be subsequent cystic dilatation of the intrahepatic bile ducts and the so-called "*bile lake*" formation secondary to stasis. These accumulations of bile are easily seen on US, CT, and MRI and can be drained percutaneously with variable results. Following Kasai procedure, percutaneous biliary drainage and balloon dilatation of bilio-digestive anastomosis can be performed in cases of biliary sepsis and anastomotic stricture respectively.

Neonatal Hepatitis[1,53,54]

Neonatal hepatitis represents a morphologic alteration of the liver that occurs as a nonspecific reaction to various insults. The disease may be idiopathic (55%), familial (10%), infectious (20%), or metabolic (15%) in etiology.[12] Idiopathic neonatal hepatitis is the most common cause of neonatal cholestasis accounting for one-third to two-thirds of cases.

The incidence ranges from 1 in 4,800 to 1 in 9,000 live births. Male preterm infants are more commonly affected. More than half of neonates with this disorder have jaundice of varying degree within the first week of life, about one-third show failure to thrive and have a fulminant course leading to extensive hepatocellular damage. On clinical examination, hepatosplenomegaly is found and a bleeding diathesis may be present. Laboratory tests reveal abnormal elevation of liver enzyme levels.

Imaging

Ultrasonography and radionuclide scintigraphy are the most widely used imaging modalities. US findings, however, are nonspecific. US may show a normal or enlarged liver with increased parenchymal echogenicity and poor visualization of intrahepatic biliary radicles. The biliary tree and gallbladder are usually normal in neonatal hepatitis **(Figs. 8A and B)**. At times, a small gallbladder may be seen in neonatal hepatitis due to decreased bile volume. As stated earlier, a change in gallbladder size after milk feeding is seen in neonatal hepatitis. Hepatic artery enlargement is not a feature of neonatal hepatitis. On MR imaging, T2W images may reveal to periportal edema; however, this finding is nonspecific. Visualization of the normal CBD and gallbladder are useful to rule out biliary atresia **(Figs. 9A to E)**. On scintigraphy excretion of radiotracer into the bowel is used to exclude the diagnosis of biliary atresia. Finally, liver biopsy or intraoperative cholangiography may be required to differentiate between biliary atresia and neonatal hepatitis. The differences between biliary atresia and neonatal hepatitis are summarized in **Table 3**.

Bile Duct Paucity[12,37]

Another rare cause of neonatal or delayed pediatric cholestatic jaundice is paucity of bile ducts. Bile duct paucity is said to be present when histologic examination demonstrates that the ratio of intralobular ducts to portal tracts[55] is <0.9. Disorders with bile duct paucity have been divided into two major groups: Nonsyndromic and syndromic bile duct paucity (SBDP) or Alagille's syndrome. The nonsyndromic variety may occur due to metabolic (α-1 antitrypsin deficiency, hypopituitarism, and cystic fibrosis), infectious [rubella, congenital syphilis, cytomegalovirus (CMV), and hepatitis B], immunologic, chromosomal (Down syndrome) and miscellaneous disorders (Zellweger's syndrome and Ivemark's syndrome).

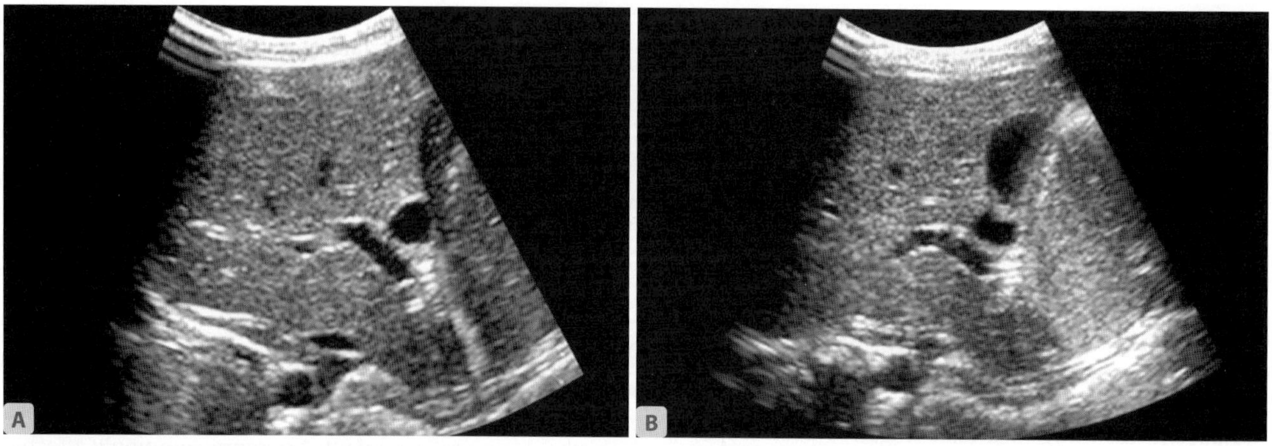

FIGS. 8A AND B: Gray scale sonograms of a jaundiced neonate showing increased hepatic echogenicity with a normal sized gallbladder—neonatal hepatitis.

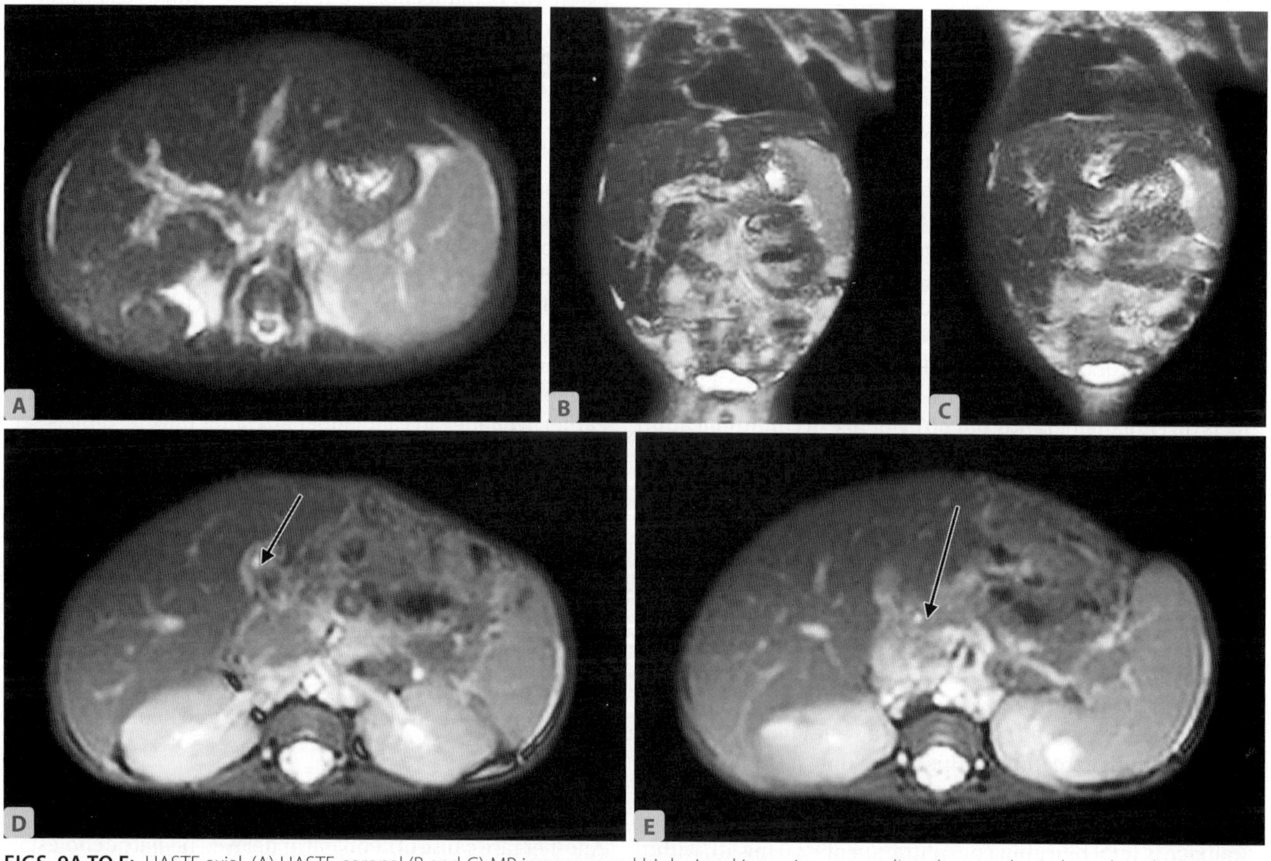

FIGS. 9A TO E: HASTE axial. (A) HASTE coronal (B and C) MR images reveal high signal intensity surrounding the portal vein branches due to periportal edema. The CBD is seen anterior to portal vein in (A). TRUFISP axial (D and E) MR images reveal a near normal gallbladder arrow in (D) and the intrapancreatic CBD arrow in (E) - neonatal hepatitis. (CBD: common bile duct; MR: magnetic resonance)

Alagille Syndrome[12,54]

Alagille syndrome is also called "arteriohepatic dysplasia". It occurs due to mutations in the *JAG1* and *NOTCH2* genes and inheritance is autosomal dominant. Alagille syndrome is an uncommon cause of chronic cholestasis, characterized by the presence of intrahepatic bile duct paucity on liver biopsy. In addition to the biopsy findings the diagnosis of Alagille syndrome requires of three of the following five features: characteristic peculiar facies, cholestasis, congenital cardiac defects (usually hypoplasia/stenosis of peripheral branches pulmonary arteries or Tetralogy of Fallot), ocular abnormalities, and vertebral anomalies (butterfly vertebra).

TABLE 3: Differentiating features of biliary atresia and neonatal hepatitis.

Ultrasound and Doppler finding	Biliary atresia	Neonatal hepatitis
Triangular cord sign	Present	Absent
Hepatic artery	Enlarged >1.5 mm	Normal
Hepatic artery/ Portal vein ratio	>0.45	
Hepatic subcapsular flow	Present	Absent
Gallbladder	• Usually absent • GB ghost triad • No response to milk feed • Never thick-walled	• Normal GB usually • Response to milk feed +
Common bile duct	• Not seen • Cysts at porta (10%)	• Normal • No cyst
Associated findings	Laterality malformation present in 10–15%	Absent
Scintigraphy	No accumulation in GIT in 24 h	Accumulation in GIT may or may not be seen depending on liver function

(GB: gallbladder; GIT: gastrointestinal tract)

The abnormal facies include a large forehead, small-pointed chin, hypertelorism and a poorly developed nasal bridge. Ocular abnormalities are most typically posterior embryotoxon and pigmentary retinopathy. Other vascular abnormalities seen include aneurysms of intracranial vessels, Moyamoya syndrome, anomalies of internal carotid artery and intra-abdominal arterial stenosis or aneurysms. Renal dysplasia, renal tubular acidosis and renovascular hypertension may also be seen. Clinical presentation is with jaundice, xanthomas, mental retardation, and growth failure consequent to fat malabsorption. These patients have a higher risk for hepatocellular carcinoma in childhood and adolescence; hence, regular abdominal imaging and α-fetoprotein (AFP) screening are recommended. It is important to distinguish Alagille syndrome from biliary atresia, as management of Alagille syndrome is essentially medical and infants with Alagille syndrome who undergo the Kasai procedure have a worse prognosis with higher morbidity and progression of liver disease. Around 15% of patients of Alagille syndrome may require liver transplantation due to development of liver failure consequent to cirrhosis and or severe clinical symptoms not responsive to medical management.

Ultrasound findings may be similar to neonatal hepatitis or biliary atresia. Hence, radiographs are invaluable to demonstrate bony findings such as butterfly vertebrae. An abnormal gallbladder morphology on US may be seen in both Alagille syndrome and biliary atresia, but the triangular cord sign is not seen in the former. Hepatic artery enlargement is less commonly seen in Alagille syndrome than in biliary atresia. It is hypothesized that on MRCP the extrahepatic biliary tree should be seen.

On hepatobiliary scintigraphy, absence of isotope excretion into the bowel may be seen in some patients leading to a wrong diagnosis of biliary atresia. Cholangiography reveals a hypoplastic or small CBD and hypoplasia or absence of opacification of intrahepatic ducts. The diagnosis of Alagille syndrome is mainly clinical, and based on liver biopsy and genetic testing.

Progressive Familial Intrahepatic Cholestasis[19,54,56]

Progressive familial intrahepatic cholestasis (PFIC) is a constellation of three slightly different and rare autosomal recessive disorders of bile production. These disorders are caused by mutations which afflict hepatocellular transport genes responsible for canalicular export and bile formation. The mean age at presentation is 3 months, but some patients may not be symptomatic till much later, even adolescence depending on the specific type. PFIC1 and PFIC2 present in neonates, and have low normal serum gamma-glutamyl transferase (GGT). PFIC1 was first reported in Amish people and referred to as Byler's disease, later it was reported from Greenland as well. PFIC2 is a similar disease but occurs mainly in the Middle East and Europe. PFIC3, on the other hand, generally presents later varying from late infancy to adulthood. These patients have impaired biliary phospholipid secretion resulting in elevated serum GGT. A few cases of PFIC have been reported from India as well.

Clinical presentation is with jaundice, intense pruritus, pancreatitis, and failure to thrive. Initially, the jaundice and pruritus may be intermittent but ultimately become persistent. The disease progresses to liver failure if left untreated. PFIC2 is associated with increased risk of malignancy. Imaging of PFIC shows a normal liver in neonatal period. However, the US and the MRCP are useful in excluding other causes of extrahepatic cholestasis. Later, findings of cirrhosis may be seen.

Treatment is a combination of medical and surgical management. Choleretics and nutritional management of fat malabsorption and pruritus is done. Some patients may require surgical management such as partial external biliary diversion (such as cholecystostomy), and finally liver transplantation.

Gestational Alloimmune Liver Disease and Neonatal Hemochromatosis[54,57-59]

Gestational alloimmune liver disease, or GALD, occurs due the production of maternal immunoglobulin G (IgG) antibodies against fetal hepatocytes. Neonatal hemochromatosis is the consequence of severe liver disease in the new born manifesting as extrahepatic siderosis. Although neonatal hemochromatosis may occur as a result of neonatal liver failure from any cause but GALD is the most common etiology. It is a rare cause of neonatal cholestasis presenting as liver failure in neonates. Antenatally, there is intrauterine growth retardation and oligohydramnios, and multiorgan dysfunction is evident soon after birth. US examination of neonates is usually normal, but a patent ductus venosus is said to be typical.

MR imaging can demonstrate iron deposition in the liver, pancreas, and heart with sparing of the reticuloendothelial system. Diagnosis can be established by showing presence of extrahepatic siderosis by MR imaging or buccal/minor salivary gland biopsy. It has been reported that neonatal hemochromatosis due to GALD shows good response to intravenous immunoglobulin and exchange transfusion; but, liver transplantation may be required.

Inspissated Bile Syndrome[12,37,54]

Inspissated bile syndrome or bile-plug syndrome refers to bile duct obstruction as a result of impaction of viscous bile or sludge within the ducts. Inspissated bile is a common cause of prolonged neonatal jaundice. Predisposing conditions for formation of sludge include TPN, drugs such as diuretics, and cephalosporins, prematurity, congenital heart disease, hemolytic conditions, and disturbance of the enterohepatic circulation, which may be due to intestinal resection. On US scans, CBD is dilated with a normal gallbladder. Sludge, seen as low level echoes, can be visualized in the bile duct and gallbladder. When isoechoic sludge fills the gallbladder lumen, the gallbladder is difficult to visualize. The occluding bile plug tends to be slightly hyperechoic with no posterior acoustic shadowing. It is seen in nearly one-third cases. The condition may resolve spontaneously or on treatment with ursodeoxycholic acid. Sometimes ERCP or percutaneous saline lavage or drainage may be needed.

Spontaneous Perforation of Common Bile Duct

Perforation usually occurs at the junction of the cystic and common hepatic duct and, rarely, it occurs in the common hepatic or CBD or the gallbladder. The etiology is uncertain but several causes have been postulated including developmental weakness of the bile duct wall, weakness resulting from the reflux of pancreatic secretions, calculi or inspissated bile. It is seen in infants within the first 3 months of life who present with jaundice and ascites. The liver function tests are essentially normal. Diagnosis is established based on clinical, sonographic, and scintigraphic findings.

Sonography reveals normal ducts with fluid in the peritoneal cavity. The fluid may be septated and is located in subhepatic region. Aspiration may reveal bile-stained fluid. Hepatobiliary scintigraphy depicts the leak.

Choledochal Cyst[12,37,60-66]

Choledochal cysts are uncommon anomalies of the biliary system with dilatation of the extrahepatic and/or the intrahepatic bile ducts. Their incidence in Western countries is approximately 1 in 15,000 live births. They are more common in East Asian populations with an incidence of approximately 1 in 13,000 in Japan. About 80% of cases are diagnosed before the age of 10 years and they are sometimes seen even on antenatal US examinations. Nearly 20% of patients remain asymptomatic until adulthood. There is a definite female preponderance with 75% cases occurring in females.

The etiopathogenesis of choledochal cysts is not well understood and several factors have been implicated. According to some authors choledochal cyst occurs as a result congenital malformation of the ductal plate (Further discussed with Caroli's disease). A more commonly accepted, hypothesis is that choledochal malformations which occur as a result of an *anomalous pancreaticobiliary junction (APBJ)*. APBJ implies an early union of the CBD and pancreatic duct. This results in a long suprasphincteric common channel allowing reflux of pancreatic enzymes into the bile ducts due to higher pressure in the pancreatic duct and the absence of a sphincteric mechanism. This damages the bile duct epithelium resulting in dilatation. It is believed that arrest in migration of the CBD—pancreatic duct junction into the duodenal wall, during development, is the embryological basis of a long common channel. A long common channel is defined as the union of the pancreatic duct and the CBD >15 mm from the ampulla of Vater. Depending on the morphology APBJ has been classified into various types by Komi et al.[63] depicted in **Table 4** and **Figure 10**.

APBJ is noted in as many as 57–96% patients with a choledochal cyst; however, it may also occur without an

TABLE 4: Classification of anomalous pancreaticobiliary ductal junction by Komi et al.

Type	Description
Type I	Right-angled union without an accessory pancreatic duct
Type II	Acute-angled union without an accessory pancreatic duct
Type III	Right- or acute-angled union with an accessory pancreatic duct

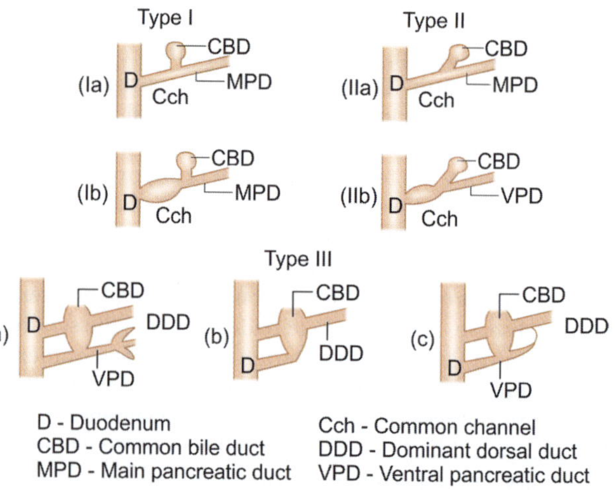

FIG. 10: Line diagram depicting APBJ as per Komi's classification. Type I—right-angled union without an accessory pancreatic duct. Ia—common channel is not dilated, Ib—dilated common channel. Type II—acute-angled union without an accessory pancreatic duct. IIa—common channel is not dilated, IIb—dilated common channel. Type III—a right-angled or acute-angled union with an accessory pancreatic duct. (APBJ: anomalous pancreaticobiliary junction)

associated cyst. It has also been suggested that primary strictures of the common bile duct also have a role to play in formation of choledochal cyst. The location and severity of the CBD stricture probably influences the morphology of the cyst. For instance, a long or tight stricture may result in cystic changes; on the other hand, fusiform dilatation is likely due to a low grade or short stricture. Preoperative identification of these strictures is important as treating the choledochal cyst alone without treating the stricture could result in recurrent episodes of cholangitis.

Classification[67-70]

The classification of choledochal malformations is challenging due to lack of common etiopathogenic basis. The initial classification given by Alonso-Lej in 1959 consisted only of the three extrahepatic cyst types. It was subsequently revised by Todani et al.[68] in 1977 to include intrahepatic biliary cysts and is widely used. This is summarized in **Table 5** and **Figure 11**. This classification was later modified to accommodate for the presence of APBJ. Besides the types I–V in the revised Todani classification, two additional types have been proposed: Type "ID" to describe dilation of the central portion of the cystic duct along with diffuse dilatation of the CBD and Type VI as an isolated cystic duct dilation with normal CBD. This classification is summarized in **Table 6**. Type I cysts are the most common representing around 50–90% of all choledochal cysts, while type IV cysts are the second most common type occurring in 30–40% of cases.

Some authors have suggested that Todani classification groups together diseases with different etiopathogenesis and that the division between type I and IVA is subjective. Only a morphological description should hence be used instead of a numerical classification. However, at present Todani classification remains the most widely used classification system.

Clinical presentation in infants is generally with a triad of abdominal pain, jaundice, and a palpable right upper quadrant mass. In older children, the presentation is more

TABLE 5: Todani classification of choledochal cyst.

Type	Description
Type IA	Cystic dilatation of extrahepatic ducts
Type IB	Focal dilatation of extrahepatic ducts
Type IC	Fusiform dilatation of extrahepatic ducts
Type II	CBD diverticulum
Type III	Focal dilatation of the intraduodenal portion of CBD—choledochocele
Type IVA	Multiple intrahepatic and extrahepatic cysts
Type IVB	Multiple extrahepatic cysts
Type V	Multiple dilatations of the intrahepatic ducts (Caroli's disease)

(CBD: common bile duct)

TABLE 6: Modified Todani classification of choledochal cysts.

Type	Description
Type IA	Cystic dilation of the extrahepatic ducts associated with APBJ
Type IB	Segmental dilation of the extrahepatic ducts without APBJ
Type IC	Fusiform dilation of extrahepatic ducts associated with APBJ
Type ID*	Dilation of the central part of the cystic duct*
Type II	One or more diverticula of the extrahepatic ducts
Type IIII	Choledochocele (dilation of the intraduodenal portion of the duct)
Type IVA	Multiple cystic intra- and extrahepatic ducts with APBJ
Type IVB	Multiple extrahepatic ductal cysts
Type V (or Caroli's disease)	Saccular dilation of the intrahepatic ducts
Type VI*	Isolated cystic duct dilatation*

*Proposed additional types not officially a part of modified Todani classificartions.

(APBJ: anomalous pancreaticobiliary junction)

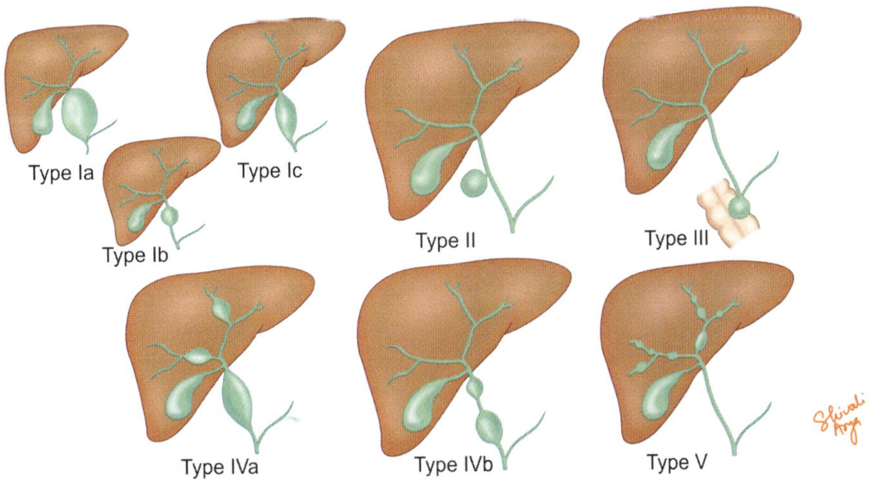

FIG. 11: Line diagram depicting Todani's classification of choledochal cysts.

variable and nonspecific. Complications include cholangitis, cystolithiasis, cholelithiasis, pancreatitis, cirrhosis, portal hypertension, and rarely, even malignant transformation. Incidence of malignancy is reported to be around 4% arising within the cyst or adjacent biliary or pancreatic ducts. It is most commonly seen with type I and type IVA choledochal cysts.

Imaging[12,37,66,69-74]

Ultrasound is the initial imaging modality to diagnose a choledochal cyst **(Figs. 12A to C)**. *CT* is helpful in ruling out other causes of biliary dilation and evaluating for complications. MRCP is extremely useful not only to diagnose a choledochal cyst but also to characterize it according to the Todani classification. It is generally the only imaging required after an US. Cyst size, extent of intrahepatic/extrahepatic bile duct involvement, and relationship to the cystic duct and even APBJ can be evaluated. MRCP can also detect intraductal filling defects due to sludge, calculi, or neoplasms, stenosis and anomalies of intrahepatic ducts. It reduces the need for invasive imaging such as ERCP or intraoperative cholangiography and the attendant complications. The major drawback is that a large choledochal cyst obscures the common channel of APBJ **(Figs. 13A and B)**. Some authors advocate the use of liver-specific contrast agents in difficult cases in order to delineate subtle dilatations and strictures of the biliary ducts and to define APBJ when it is not well visualized on conventional MRCP images. However, in general, contrast agents are best avoided in children due to concerns regarding tissue deposition. ERCP is regarded as the most definitive and reliable diagnostic method of revealing choledochal cysts and anomalous pancreaticobiliary ductal union **(Figs. 14A and B)**. Hepatobiliary scintigraphy can confirm excretion of radiotracer into the choledochal cyst, but yields limited anatomic information and is insufficient for determining cyst type or planning surgical reconstruction. At times the choledochal cyst does not fill with the radionuclide and the diagnosis can be missed.

On imaging, type I choledochal cyst is seen as a large right upper quadrant cystic structure that extends to porta, communicates with the biliary tree, and is separate from the gallbladder. The intrahepatic ducts are usually not dilated but may, at times, be dilated to varying degrees in type IC choledochal cyst **(Figs. 15 to 18)**.

Type IV cysts, most of which are IVA are visualized as multiple fusiform or cystic dilatations of intra and extrahepatic bile ducts. A stricture or narrowing at the level of the hepatic hilum may be seen in type IVA cysts which

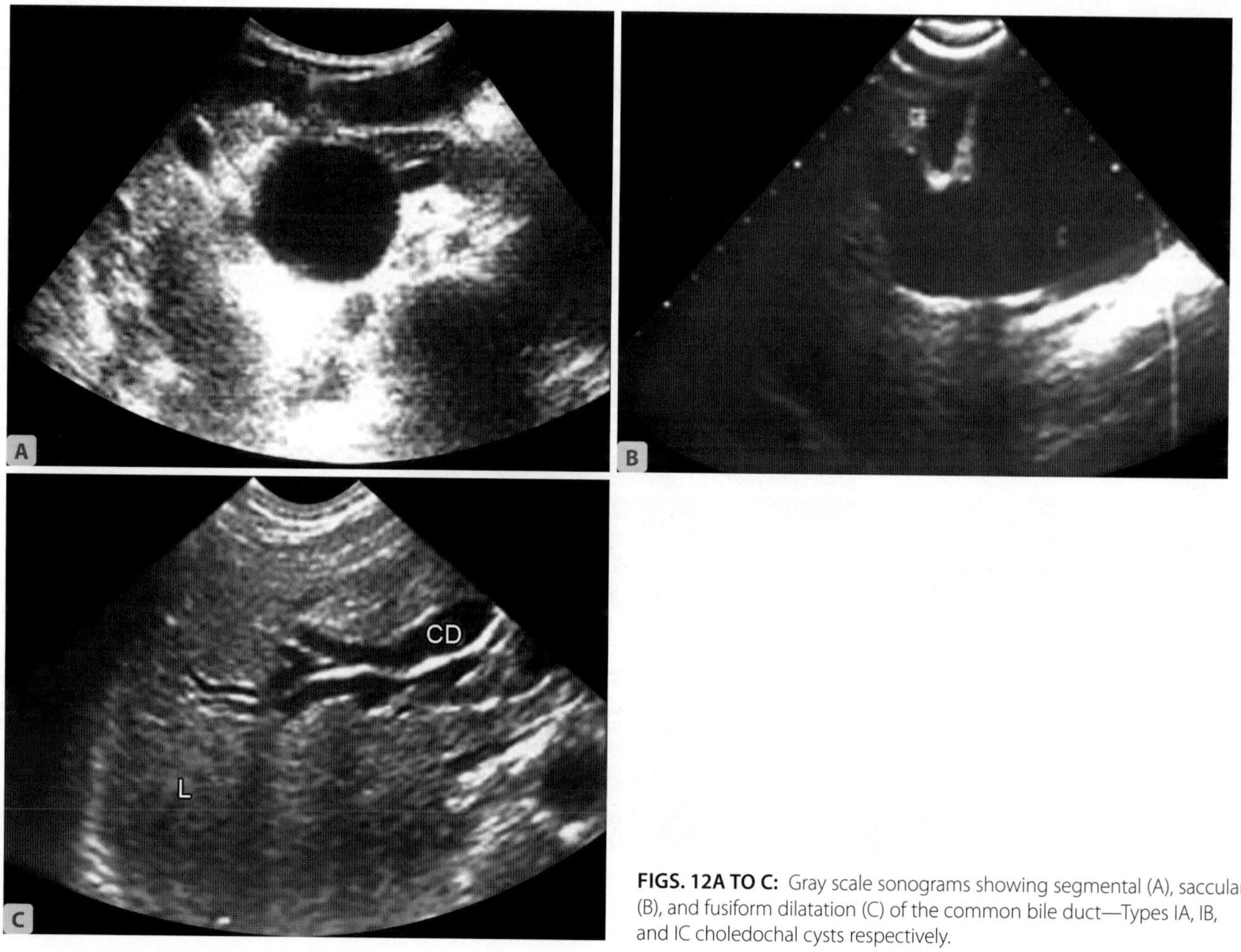

FIGS. 12A TO C: Gray scale sonograms showing segmental (A), saccular (B), and fusiform dilatation (C) of the common bile duct—Types IA, IB, and IC choledochal cysts respectively.

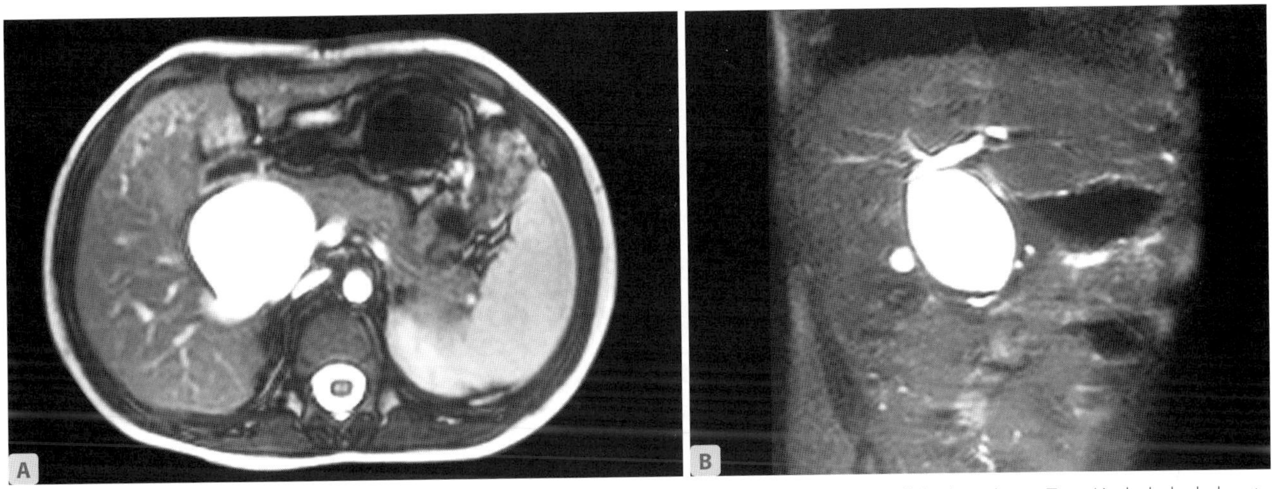

FIGS. 13A AND B: True FISP axial and HASTE coronal MR images showing a cystically dilated common bile duct due to Type IA choledochal cyst.

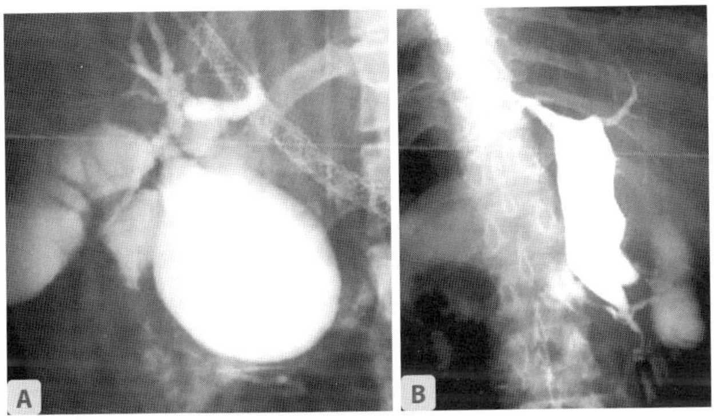

FIGS. 14A AND B: ERCP images illustrating saccular and fusiform dilatation of common duct with nondilated intrahepatic biliary radicles—Type IA and IC choledochal cysts respectively. An anomalous pancreatobiliary junction is noted in B with the CD joining the pancreatic duct at right angles.The long common channel is not dilated. (ERCP: endoscopic retrograde cholangiopancreatography)

may be responsible for the intrahepatic dilatation. This stricture at the hilum may help in distinguishing fusiform type IVA cysts from type IC cysts. In type IC, the intrahepatic ducts are involved in a continuous fashion without any hilar stricture **(Figs. 19A and B)**.

Both types I and IVA cysts may undergo malignant transformation. Malignancies include cholangiocarcinoma, squamous cell carcinoma, sarcoma, and gallbladder cancer; cholangiocarcinoma being the most common **(Figs. 20A and B)**. Irregular wall-thickening in the cyst with or without an enhancing mass should raise the suspicion for cholangiocarcinoma. Papillary adenocarcinoma may be visualized as solitary or multiple enhancing papillary lesions. Irregular heterogeneously enhancing, gallbladder wall-thickening suggests gallbladder malignancy.

Type IVB cysts are rare with multiple extrahepatic dilatations only.

Type II cysts account for only 2–3% of all choledochal cysts. They are seen as diverticulae arising from any part of

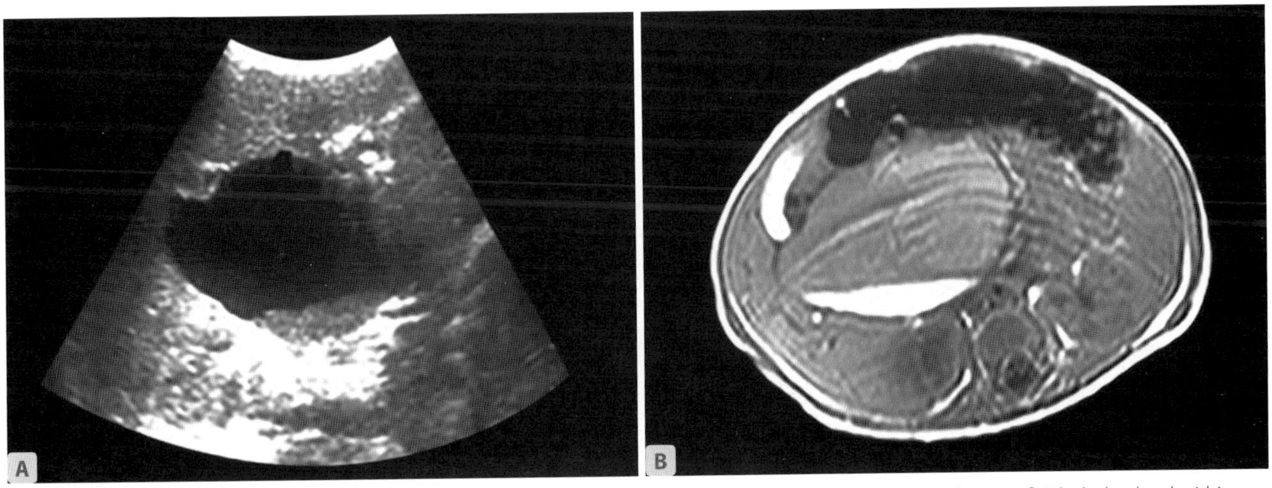

FIGS. 15A AND B: Ultasonography (US) (A) and T1-weighted (T1W) axial (B) magnetic resonance (MR) image showing fluid–sludge level within a huge Type I choledochal cyst.

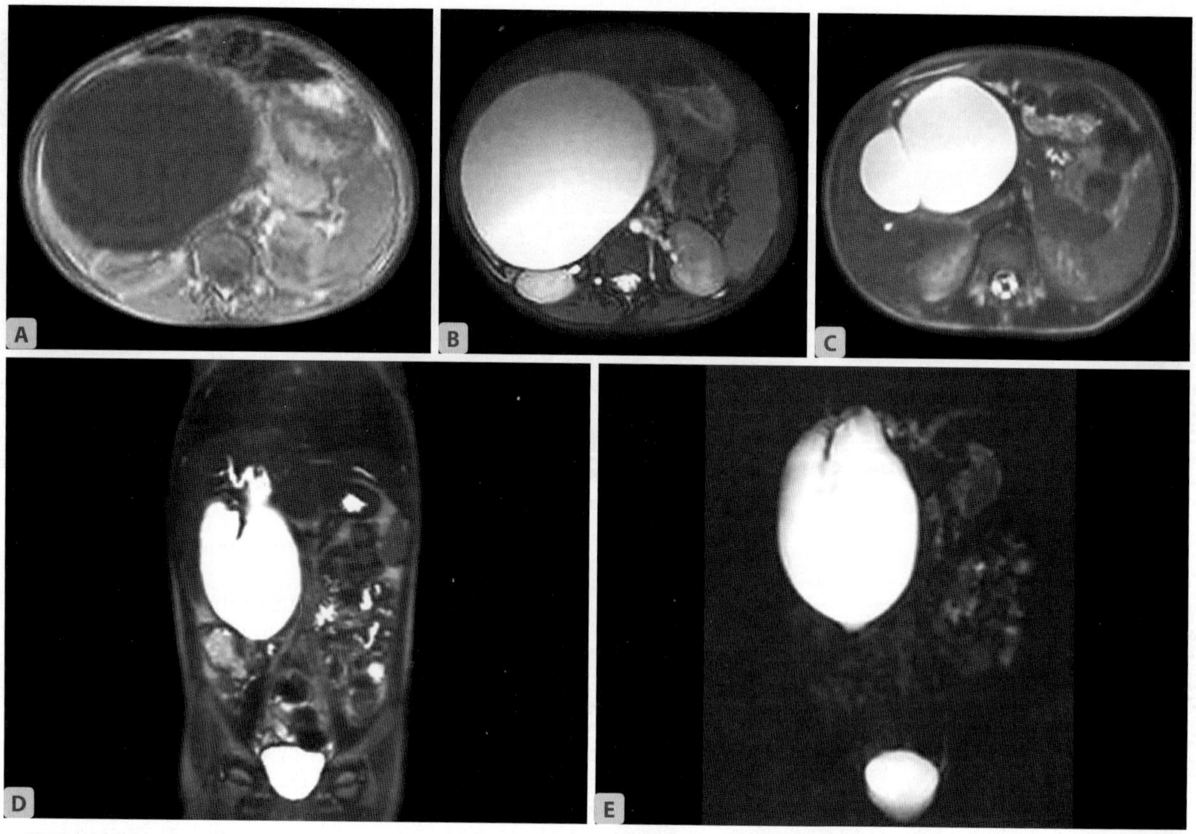

FIGS. 16A TO E: Axial, T1-weighted (T1W) (A); Axial T2-weighted (T2W) (B and C) and HASTE coronal (D) images revealing the cystic nature of choledochal cyst seen as hypointense signal on T1 and hyperintense on T2W magnetic resonance (MR) images. RARE sequence (E) showing the cyst to a saccular dilatation of the common bile duct Type I choledochal cyst.

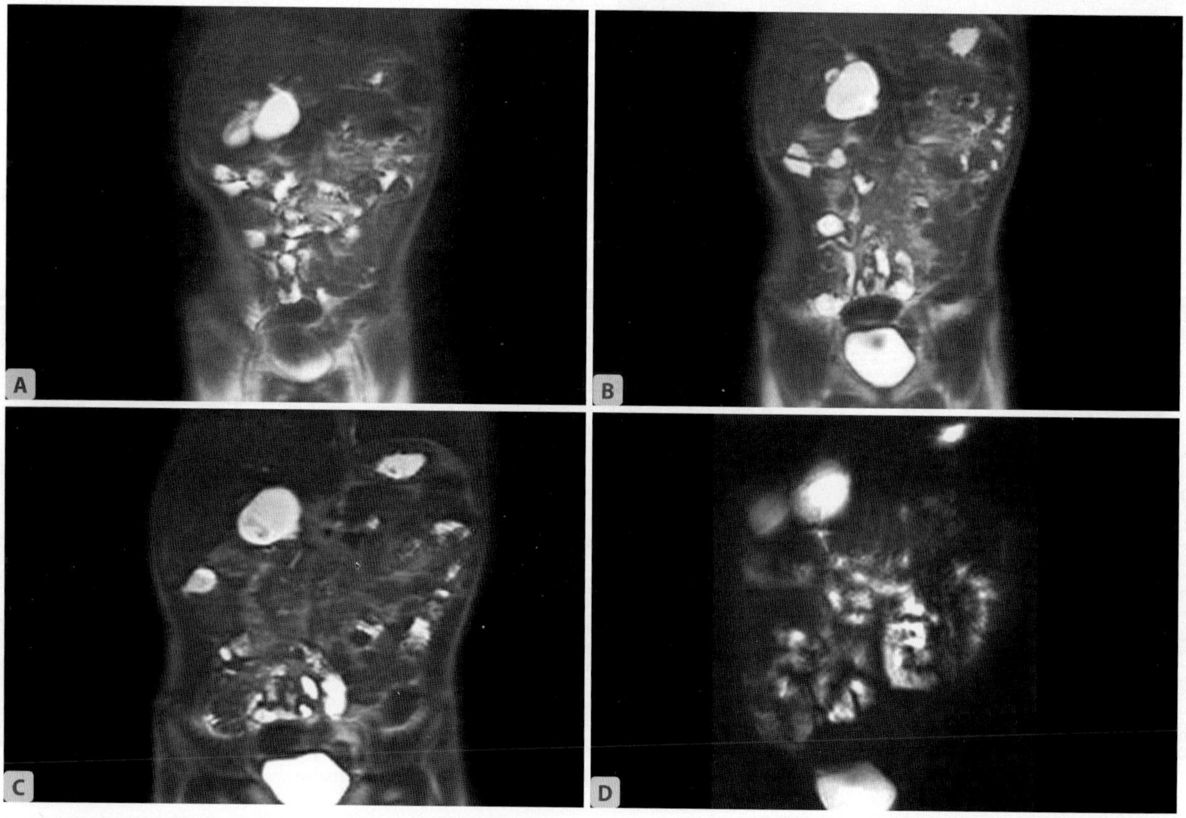

FIGS. 17A TO D: HASTE coronal (A to C) and RARE sequence (D) magnetic resonance (MR) images showing a focal segmental dilatation of the common bile duct. The normal caliber duct proximal to the dilatation is visualized—Type IB choledochal cyst.

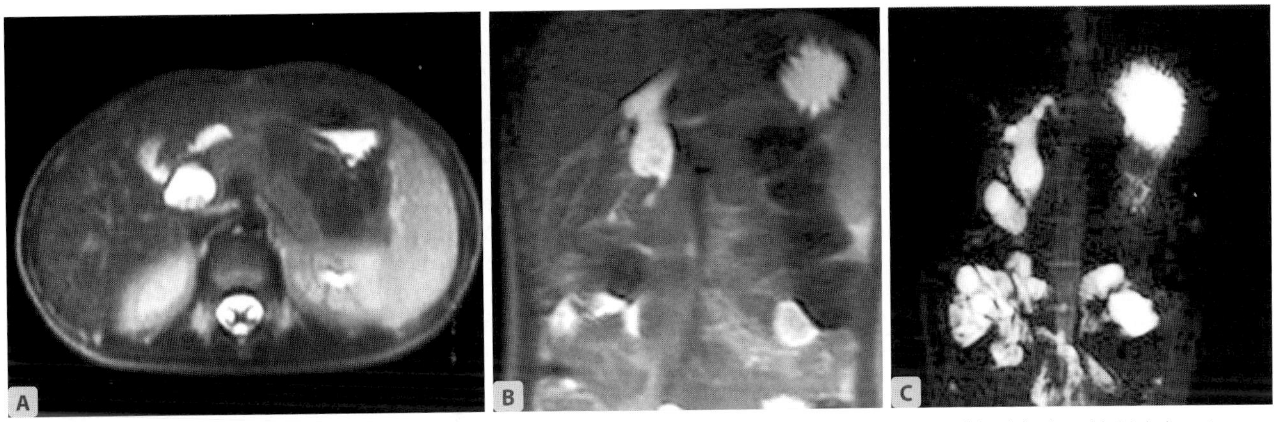

FIGS. 18A TO C: HASTE axial (A) and coronal (B) magnetic resonance (MR) images reveal a fusiform dilatation of the bile duct. Multiple hypointense foci suggestive of calculi seen within (A) —Type IC choledochal cyst with calculi.

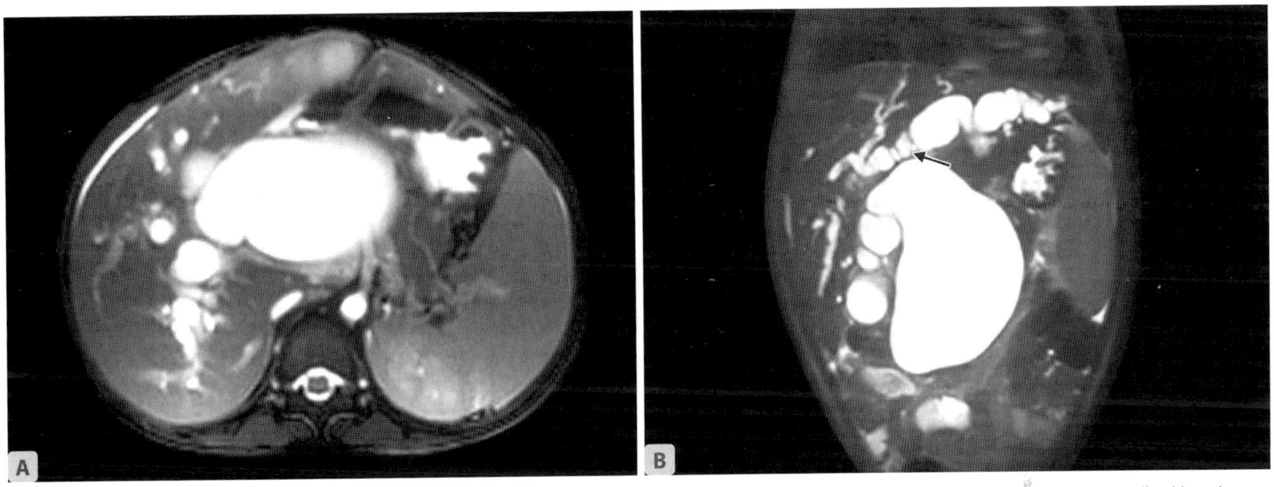

FIGS. 19A AND B: Type IVA choledochal cyst seen on True FISP axial and HASTE coronal magnetic resonance (MR) images as cystically dilated extrahepatic bile duct and multiple fusiform dilatations of intrahepatic ducts. Note the stricture at the level of hepatic hilum (arrow).

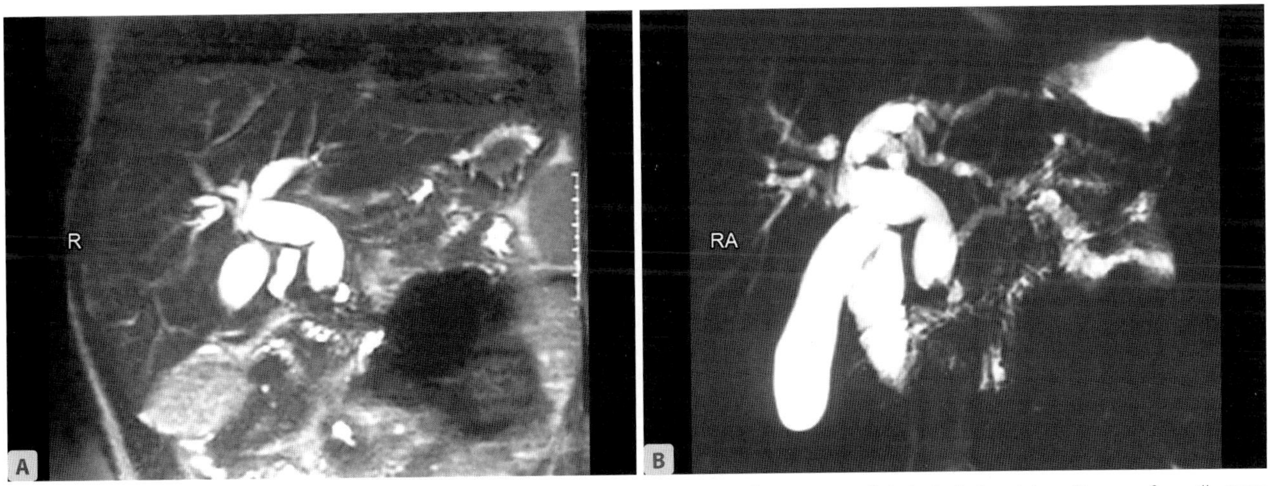

FIGS. 20A AND B: HASTE coronal and SSFSE or MRCP images in a 20 year old **patient** known case of choledochal cyst since 8 years of age illustrate fusiform dilatation of common duct with an irregular polypoid filling defect at its lower end MPD is also dilated (B)—malignant transformation in a Type I choledochal cyst.

the extrahepatic bile duct and may be visualized on MR or cholangiography. US may show an anechoic cyst adjacent to a normal the CBD with a normal gallbladder.

Type III choledochal cysts, also called choledochoceles, represent only 1–5% of all choledochal cysts. These are seen as dilatation of the intraduodenal portion of the CBD, without APBJ. Ziegler et al.[74] reported that choledochoceles were found in an older age group of males presenting with acute pancreatitis and should be classified separate from the revised Todani classification due to differences in clinical presentation and demography. These are generally difficult to visualize on noninvasive imaging. Location of a cyst near the pancreaticobiliary junction on US should raise the suspicion of type III choledochal cyst. It has been reported that MRCP may not be sensitive for detection of a small choledochocele which may only be visualized after contrast medium is injected under pressure during an ERCP.

Type V choledochal cyst or Caroli's disease is discussed separately.

The differential diagnosis of choledochal cyst includes several other cystic lesions including hepatic cyst, enteric duplication cyst, pancreatic pseudocyst, hepatic artery aneurysm, and spontaneous perforation of the CBD. Careful US imaging to show biliary communication, attention to wall characteristics combined with color Doppler flow imaging (CDFI)/MRI can help to differentiate these conditions.

Management[12,37]

Type I and IV choledochal cysts are treated by early excision with bilioenteric reconstruction. Surgeons need an exact anatomic map of the pancreaticobiliary ductal union because it is essential that the choledochal cyst must be completely resected without pancreatic ductal injury. Surgical excision with Roux-en-Y anastomosis gives excellent results and reduces bile stasis, risk of cholangitis, and malignancy, although the risk for malignancy may remain elevated for >15 years after surgery. When the anatomy is more complicated, a simple drainage is carried out but these patients have risk of recurrent cholangitis, lithiasis, pancreatitis, and cancer. Type II and III choledochal cyst have a very low risk of malignancy and are generally treated by diverticulectomy and endoscopic sphincterotomy, respectively. For large choledochoceles transduodenal excision may be done.

Radiological interventions that may be done in a choledochal cyst include preoperative percutaneous biliary drainage in the presence of sepsis and management of calculi prior to definitive surgical treatment.

Caroli's Disease and Caroli's Syndrome[12,37,69,75-78]

Caroli's disease or type V choledochal cyst is also known as communicating cavernous ectasia of intrahepatic bile ducts. It is a rare congenital disorder with segmental, saccular, nonobstructive dilatation of the intrahepatic bile ducts. Although, congenital cystic dilatation of the intrahepatic bile ducts was first described by Vachell and Stevens in 1906, Caroli first clearly defined this disease entity in 1958. Caroli's disease more often involves the left lobe of the liver but may affect the right or both lobes of the liver. Isolated ectasia of the intrahepatic biliary radicles without other hepatic abnormalities is referred to as Caroli's disease. On the other hand, when ectasia of small and large bile ducts is associated with congenital hepatic fibrosis it is referred to as Caroli's syndrome. The latter is more common than Caroli's disease. Fibrosis can ultimately lead to liver cirrhosis and portal hypertension in this group of patients.

Caroli's disease is uncommon, accounting for <10% of choledochal cysts, occurring more frequently in women and is considered to be a congenital ductal plate malformation. Ductal plate refers to a sleeve or cylinder of hepatoblasts or hepatic precursor cells surrounding the developing portal vein branches. This remodels around the 12th week of gestation to form the bile ducts and ductules. Depending upon the level of the biliary tree affected various disease entities can be seen. Involvement of small interlobular bile ducts results in biliary hamartoma (von Meyenburg complexes) or congenital hepatic fibrosis. When medium-size intrahepatic ducts are involved the result is autosomal dominant polycystic liver disease. Caroli's disease is the consequence of ductal plate malformation involving the large intrahepatic bile ducts. In "Caroli's syndrome" all levels of the biliary tree are involved resulting in features of both congenital hepatic fibrosis and Caroli's disease. Abnormal growth rate of the biliary epithelium and lack of the normal involution of the ductal plates surrounding the portal tracts lead to biliary cysts surrounding the portal tracts.

Caroli's disease usually occurs sporadically with no family history of the disease. Rarely, Caroli's disease has been described in families with autosomal dominant polycystic kidney disease appearing to follow an autosomal dominant pattern of inheritance. On the contrary, Caroli's syndrome shows an autosomal recessive pattern of inheritance. It is often seen in association with autosomal recessive polycystic kidney disease. Other associated renal cystic diseases include renal tubular ectasia, medullary sponge kidney, and nephronophthisis with cysts in the renal medulla and corticomedullary junction.

Clinical Features

Most patients with Caroli's disease present with fever, recurrent, crampy abdominal pain, and jaundice during childhood or early adulthood. These symptoms are the result of bile stasis and stone formation. Other symptoms and signs include pruritus, pale stools, intermittent jaundice, and hepatomegaly.

Complications include cholangitis, lithiasis, biliary cirrhosis, and malignant transformation **(Figs. 21A and B)**. Cholangiocarcinoma has been reported in up to 7% of people with congenital cystic dilation of the intrahepatic bile ducts, which is >100 times greater than in the general population.

Imaging

Ultrasound findings include segmental or diffuse saccular outpouchings or fusiform dilatation of the intrahepatic bile ducts with complete or incomplete echogenic septa that cross the dilated ducts. These dilated ducts may give the appearance of surrounding the portal vein radicles—*"the*

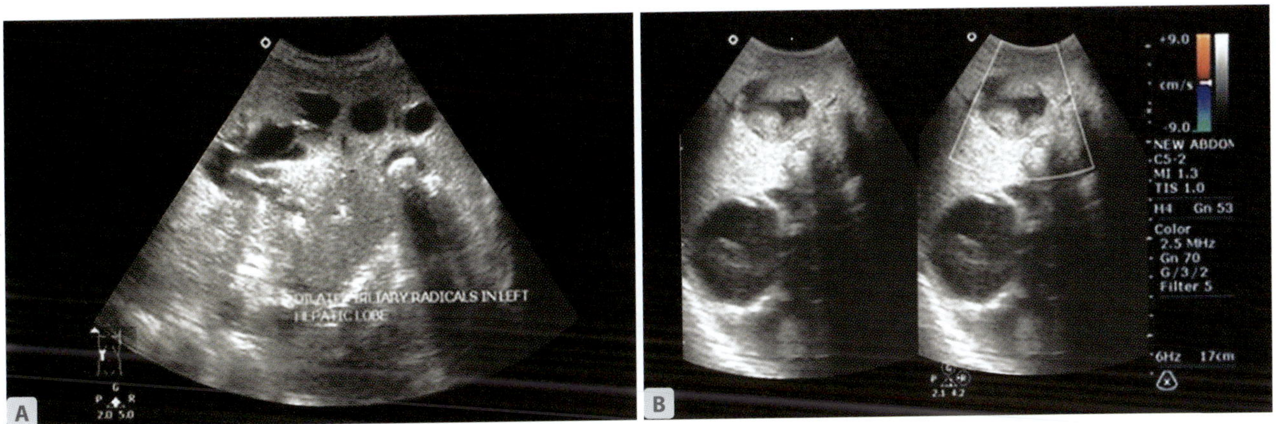

FIGS. 21A AND B: Ultrasound images in an adolescent male showing multiple saccular areas of biliary dilatation within the liver parenchyma. Echogenic foci with distal acoustic shadowing are seen in one of the cysts s/o intraductal calculi. One of the larger cysts shows presence of soft tissue along the walls with vascularity-cholangiocarcinoma developing in Caroli's disease.

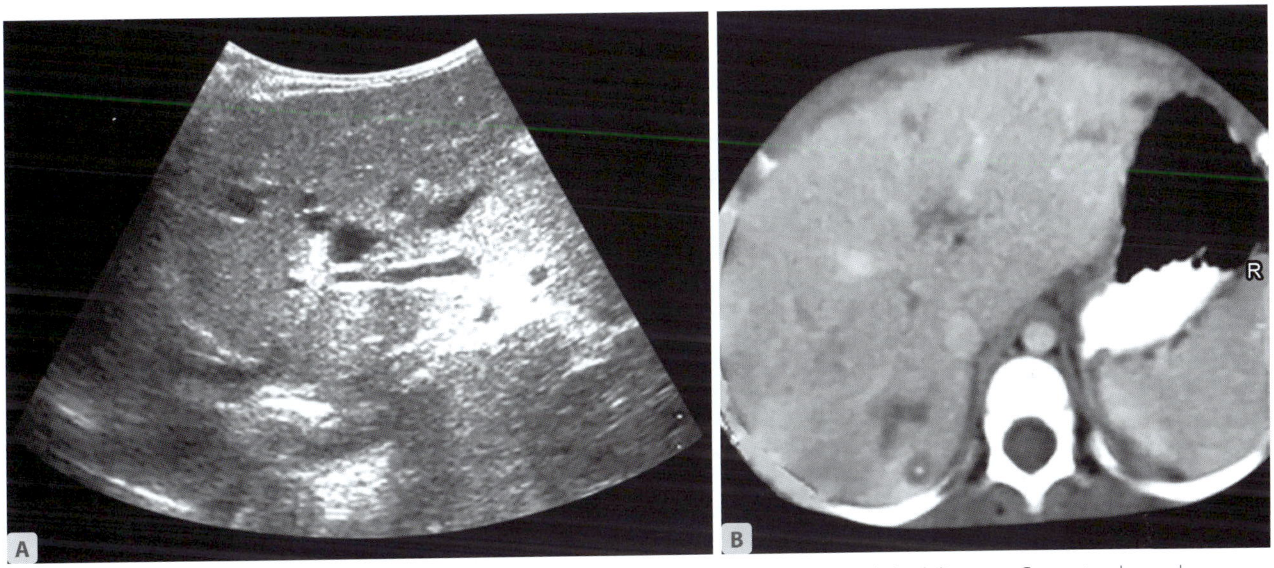

FIGS. 22A AND B: Transverse sonogram (A) showing multiple intrahepatic cysts communicating with the biliary tree. Contrast-enhanced computed tomography (CECT) (B) in another patient showing segmental intrahepatic duct dilatation with the "central dot" sign—Caroli's disease.

intra-aluminal portal vein sign". On color Doppler, no color fill in is seen in the dilated ducts while color flow can be seen in portal vein branches. The dilated channels are visualized as multiple low (near water) attenuation fusiform or cystic lesions on CT and as T2-hyperintense structures on MR and should not be confused with hepatic cysts or hamartomas. The "*central dot sign,*" produced by enhancement of the portal vein branches and adjacent hepatic artery engulfed by dilated intrahepatic bile ducts is highly suggestive of Caroli's disease and can be easily seen on contrast-enhanced CT or MRI **(Figs. 22A and B)**. MRCP is particularly useful to demonstrate the connection between these cystic structures and the biliary tree thus differentiating Caroli's disease from polycystic liver disease. At times extrahepatic ductal dilatation may be associated. Enhancing soft tissue within the cystic spaces or ducts should raise the suspicion for malignancy **(Figs. 23A to D)**.

In patients with Caroli's syndrome besides cysts, associated findings of congenital hepatic fibrosis are seen in the form of a dysmorphic liver with enlargement of the lateral segment of left lobe, normal or enlarged medial segment of left lobe and an atrophic right lobe. A small medial segment is distinctly uncommon in congenital hepatic fibrosis unlike alcoholic or viral hepatitis. Regenerative nodules, enlargement of hepatic artery, associated findings of portal hypertension and renal anomalies may also be seen in this subgroup of patients.

The differential diagnosis of Caroli's disease includes polycystic liver disease, SC, recurrent pyogenic cholangitis (RPC), choledochal cyst, biliary papillomatosis, and (occasionally) obstructive biliary dilatation. In SC, the ductal dilatation is more isolated and elongated and not cystic as in Caroli's disease, and associated with wall-thickening. Also, these patients often have associated inflammatory

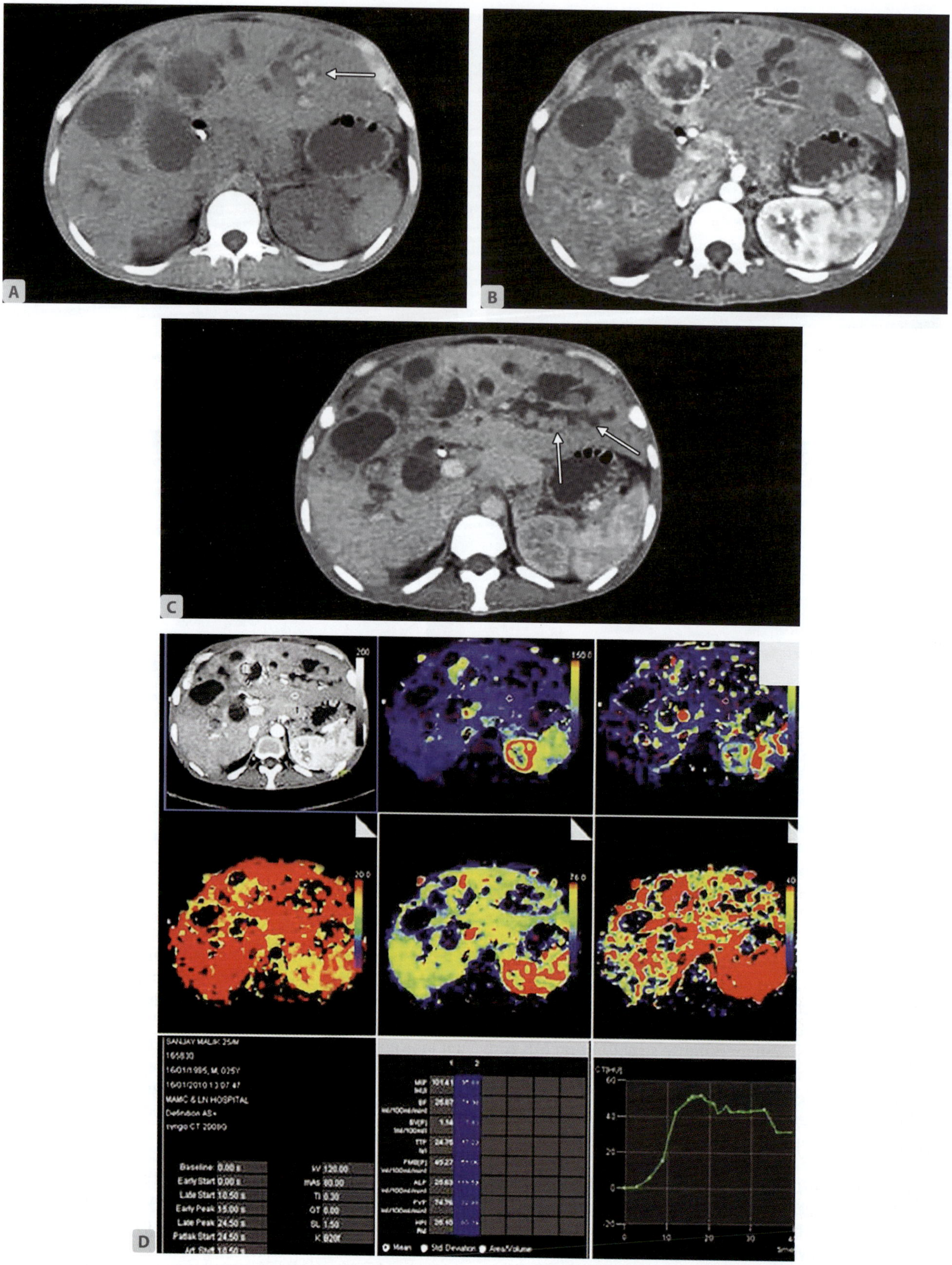

FIGS. 23A TO D: Triphasic CT showing multiple saccular dilatations of the biliary tree (A). Hepatic arterial phase showing intense rim and polypoidal enhancement of the mass (B) washout is seen in the portal venous phase (C). Nonenhancing intraductal calculi are also seen (arrows)—Caroli's disease with a mitotic polypoidal mass. (D) Perfusion study with ROI placed over the intraductal lesion and normal liver reveals increased HPI values 80.79% for the lesion. Higher BF, BV, PMB, and HPI are observed. Biopsy revealed it to be a intraductal cholangiocarcinoma.

bowel disease. RPC is more challenging to exclude, however, saccular dilatation favors Caroli's disease and is unusual in RPC. However, Caroli's disease with diffuse fusiform dilatation can be difficult to distinguish.

Management

Management of Caroli's disease is difficult and a conservative nonoperative approach is used initially, especially in bilobar disease. This may be in the form of cyst drainage, stone removal, and antibiotics. Regular surveillance for potential malignant transformation is essential. Definitive treatment is surgical. Segmental or unilobar Caroli's disease is managed by resection, while complicated disease with involvement of both lobes is best managed by orthotopic liver transplantation.

BILIARY CHANGES ASSOCIATED WITH SYSTEMIC DISEASES

Biliary Changes in Cystic Fibrosis[12,37,79]

Pulmonary disease is classical of cystic fibrosis. In addition, many patients have associated abnormalities of the pancreas, spleen, liver, and biliary system. Symptomatic liver disease is seen in 2–18% patients of cystic fibrosis and can be the presenting feature of this disorder. Rarely, the patient may present in the neonatal period with cholestatic jaundice. Inspissated bile in cystic fibrosis may be a cause of prolonged neonatal jaundice.

Ultrasound in cystic fibrosis may depict a small gallbladder with thick walls often containing sludge and/or stones. The gallbladder function is usually normal. The bile ducts, both intra- and extrahepatic, demonstrate a "beaded" appearance consequent to areas of ductal strictures with intervening dilatation. Duct wall irregularity and intraductal calculi and debris can also be seen **(Fig. 24)**. MRCP demonstrates these changes to advantage.

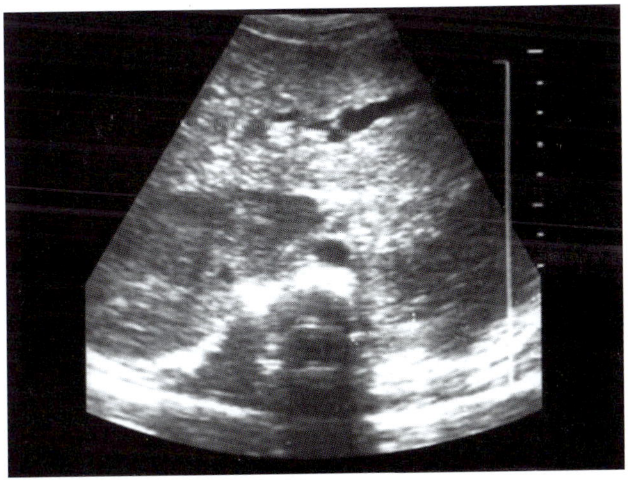

FIG. 24: Ultrasonography (USG) of a child with cystic fibrosis reveals irregular left hepatic duct dilatation with nonshadowing intraluminal echogenic foci.

Sclerosing Cholangitis[12,37]

Sclerosing cholangitis is a chronic progressive disease in which there is inflammation and obliterative fibrosis of the medium and large intrahepatic and/or extrahepatic bile ducts. SC may occur in psoriasis, cystic fibrosis, systemic malignancies, Langerhans cell histiocytosis, and sickle-cell anemia. Many children with SC may show an overlap syndrome with autoimmune hepatitis. In addition, there are some inherited forms of SC including a neonatal form and those associated with mutations in the *ABCB4 (MDR3)* gene. About 60–80% cases have associated inflammatory bowel disease, mostly ulcerative colitis. The incidence is estimated to be 0.2 per 100,000 with a male predominance.

Clinical presentation is with abdominal pain, fatigue, jaundice, splenomegaly, hepatomegaly, ascites, fever, and weight loss, and abnormal liver function tests.

Imaging

On US irregular, multisegmental intrahepatic biliary dilatation may be seen. Thickening of intrahepatic and extrahepatic ducts is depicted as brightly echogenic tissue surrounding the portal venules and common duct. Intraluminal debris consisting of nonshadowing, mobile echoes may be present due to biliary sludge or desquamated bile duct epithelium or pus. There may be signs of cirrhosis or portal hypertension.

Computed tomography, though not the preferred investigation, may show multifocal discontinuous areas of minimal intrahepatic biliary dilatation without a mass **(Figs. 25A and B)**. Benign reactive lymphadenopathy may occasionally occur and it should not be taken as a strong indicator of malignancy without other supportive signs. Cholangiocarcinoma has rarely been reported in children with primary sclerosing cholangitis (PSC).

Magnetic resonance cholangiopancreatography is the preferred modality for noninvasive diagnosis of SC. MRCP demonstrates an irregular/beaded appearance of the biliary tree, and peripheral "floating" bile ducts in the liver. These are due to intrahepatic biliary strictures with intervening normal caliber or dilated ducts **(Figs. 26A to C)**. Less often extrahepatic biliary strictures can be seen. Associated changes in liver parenchyma on MRI include increased periportal intensity and peripheral wedge-shaped or "triangular" T2 hyperintensity in association with dilated ducts. Sensitivity of MRCP is nearly 84–86% for the detection of SC in children, which is roughly similar to ERCP. In the presence of active inflammation, periductal enhancement can be visualized with intravenous gadolinium.

Cholangiography has been considered the gold standard for diagnosis of PSC and ERCP is preferable to PTC for demonstrating the intrahepatic and extrahepatic ductal narrowing and dilatations with "skip" lesions.

The treatment and prognosis depend on the associated pathology. Medical treatment includes ursodeoxycholic acid based on a reported beneficial effect in adults with PSC. Liver transplantation may be required in 20–30% of pediatric patients with SC who develop end-stage liver disease.

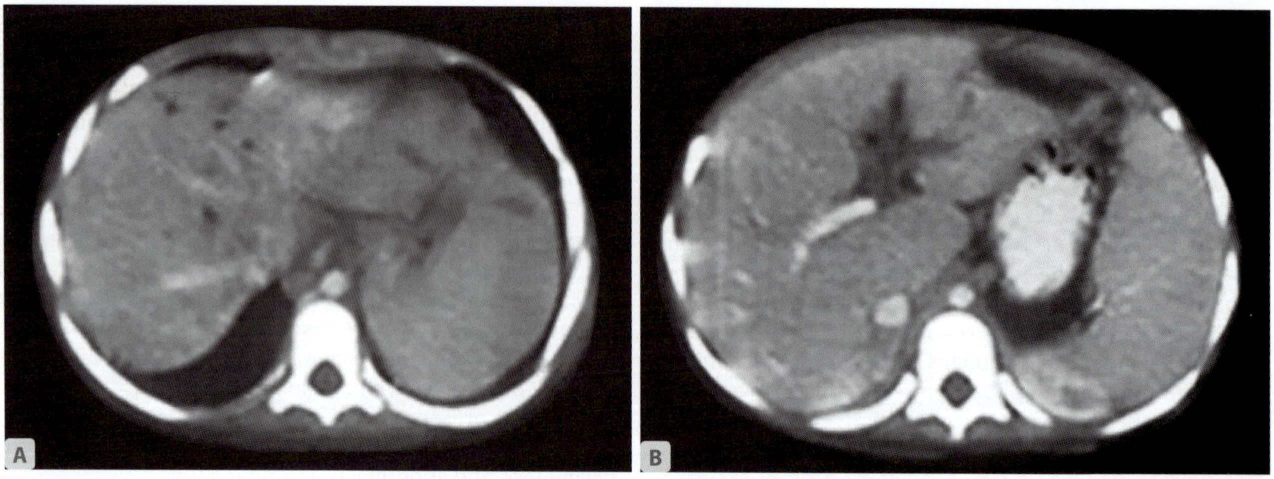

FIGS. 25A AND B: Contrast-enhanced computed tomography (CECT) scans of an adolescent with sclerosing cholangitis show tubular structures in left lobe with "skip" areas of biliary dilatation.

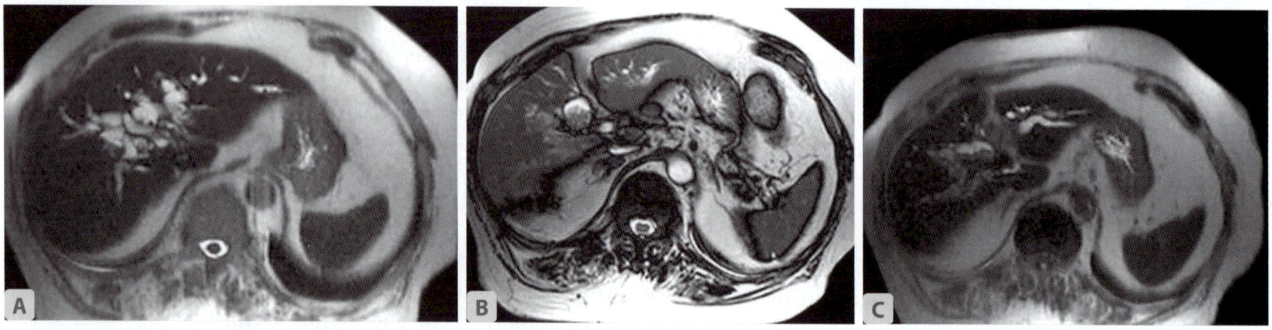

FIGS. 26A TO C: HASTE axial (A and C) TRUFISP axial (B) MR images revealing irregular multisegmental intrahepatic biliary dilatation with evidence of pruning and skip dilatation. Intraluminal debris is seen as a hypointense material filling the common duct and the biliary radicles—sclerosing cholangitis.

Immunoglobulin G4-related Disease[12,80]

Immunoglobulin G4-related disease (IgG4-RD) is very rare in children, but an important entity to distinguish from SC. It is a group of inflammatory diseases in which there is lymphoplasmacytic infiltration of tissues with a preponderance of IgG4-positive plasma cells. This is accompanied with fibrosis. IgG4-related biliary diseases can be difficult to distinguish from SC, however, the wall-thickening tends to be more marked in the former. Since the imaging findings of these entities may be similar differentiation depends on histopathology, elevated serum IgG4 levels, associated findings (such as IgG4-related pancreatitis), and response to steroids. It can also present with mass-like hepatic lesions called "inflammatory pseudotumors".

Portal Hypertensive Biliopathy[81-83]

It is a rare cause of childhood cholestasis. Portal hypertensive biliopathy (PHB) is defined as abnormal biliary changes that take place most often secondary to extrahepatic portal vein obstruction (EHPVO) with portal cavernoma formation and portal hypertension.[84] Portal cavernous transformation is seen as many dilated pericholedochal and periportal collaterals that bypass the portal vein obstruction. These may rarely lead to biliary obstruction. This condition may be asymptomatic or could lead to a cholestatic state which is rare in children. The term "portal biliopathy" actually describes an intra- or extrahepatic biliary stricture in patients with portal cavernoma. Extrinsic compression of the common duct by dilated venous collaterals together with pericholedochal fibrosis from the inflammatory process causing portal thrombosis may lead to biliary stricture and dilatation of the proximal biliary tree. This condition sometimes causes the formation of secondary biliary stones and cholangitis. There are two types of clinical features in portal biliopathy: (i) Those related to chronic cholestasis, probably explained by strictures caused by either compression of the biliary lumen by enlarged collaterals or by ischemia and (ii) Those related to biliary stones, which are probably responsible for biliary pain and cholangitis.

Imaging

US and color Doppler can show varices around the bile duct and gallbladder wall with dilatation of the duct **(Figs. 27A and B)**. MRCP is an excellent technique to demonstrate the full spectrum of findings. It reveals biliary stenosis, a wavy appearance of the bile ducts with smooth tapering strictures or an angulated appearance of the ducts.

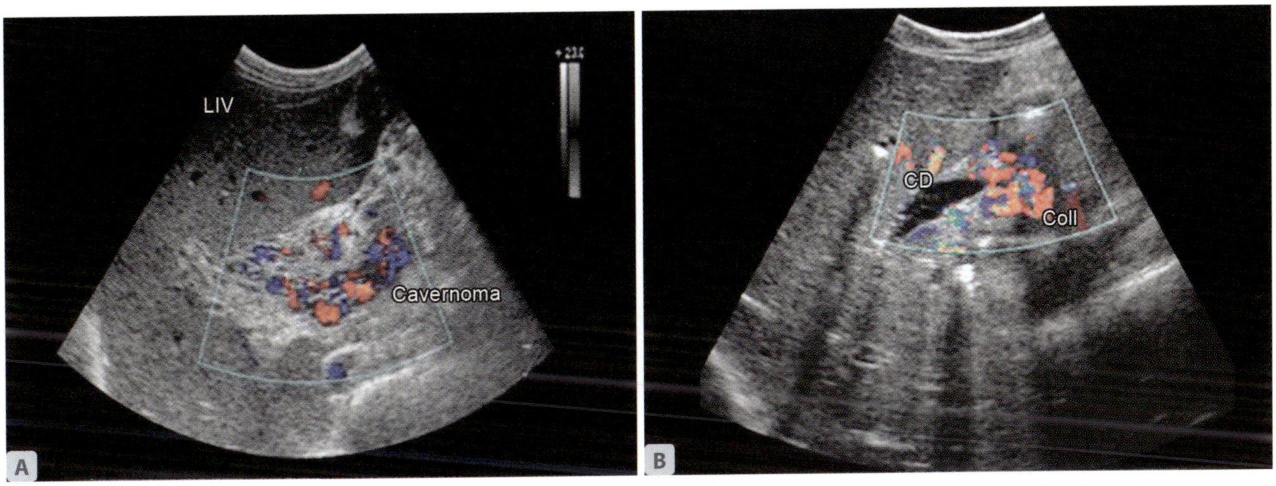

FIGS. 27A AND B: Doppler images revealing multiple anechoic tubular structures replacing the portal vein with color fill in s/o portal cavernoma formation. There is extrinsic compression with resultant dilatation of the common bile duct—portal hypertensive biliopathy.

There is associated upstream dilatation of the bile ducts. It can distinguish between calculi and varices. Biliary findings on MRCP have been classified into three types by Shin et al.[83] (1) Varicoid, (2) Fibrotic, and (3) Mixed. Varicoid irregularities are seen as smooth indentations due to cavernous transformation. Smooth localized strictures with wall-thickening are seen in the fibrotic type. The thickened-wall shows delayed increased enhancement on dynamic imaging suggesting an ischemic etiology. The mixed type shows irregular wall contour and thickening with no delayed enhancement, suggesting a nonischemic or inflammatory cause.

On ERCP, the typical changes are irregularities in the CBD and hepatic ducts (smooth tapering strictures) and localized saccular dilatations. Filling defects suggestive of CBD stones may be seen.

Treatment is focused on the management of portal hypertension and relief of obstructive jaundice due to the portal cavernoma is managed endoscopically. Stenting with or without balloon dilatation of CBD is recommended and the stent needs to be replaced regularly. Endoscopic management, however, needs to done with care due to the risk of bleeding from varices. Portosystemic shunt surgery can be done in cases which cannot be managed endoscopically and is considered the first line of treatment by some surgeons.

CHOLELITHIASIS AND CHOLEDOCHOLITHIASIS[12,54,84-86]

Gallstones may be seen in children of any age and have been described on third-trimester antenatal US scans. Gallstones that occur in the early in neonates and are of unknown etiology. Gallstones that develop after birth are associated with risk factors similar to those for development of biliary sludge such as cephalosporins usage, frusemide, prematurity, congenital heart disease, hemolytic conditions, and TPN. Most of the neonatal gallstones resolve spontaneously by 1 year of age after removal of precipitating factors but occasionally cholecystitis and choledocholithiasis have been reported. Neonatal cholelithiasis is generally visualized as small echogenic foci in the gallbladder lumen. Posterior acoustic shadowing may not be evident unless the calculi are larger than 3 mm **(Fig. 28)**.

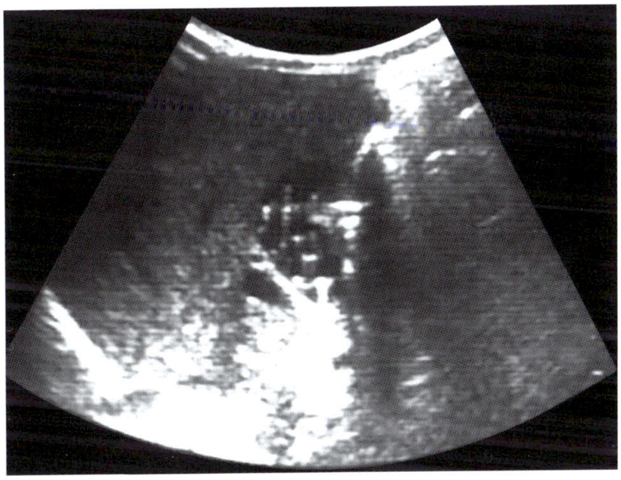

FIG. 28: Ultrasonography (USG) showing multiple echogenic foci within the gallbladder lumen with no distal shadowing—gallstones in a neonate.

The etiological factors for gallstone disease in older children and adolescents include cystic fibrosis, hemolytic anemia, sickle-cell disease, TPN, obesity, oral contraceptives, and pregnancy.

The prevalence of cholelithiasis in children below 16 years of age is low but an increasing number of cases are being reported. While infants and younger children are usually asymptomatic, older children and adolescents may present with "adult" symptoms of colicky right upper quadrant pain, abdominal distension, nausea, and vomiting. Like adults, US is the modality of choice and often the only imaging required. The US findings of gallbladder calculi in children are the similar to adults: Echogenic foci with posterior acoustic shadowing, which are mobile. A contracted gallbladder, bladder with calculi, may also produce the typical wall-echo-shadow complex. A thickened hyperemic gallbladder

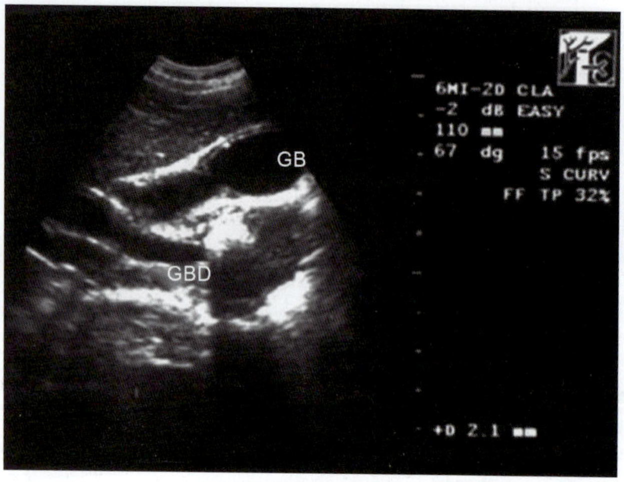

FIG. 29: Gray scale sonogram of a 9-year-old child showing choledocholithiasis with proximal common bile duct (CBD) dilatation.

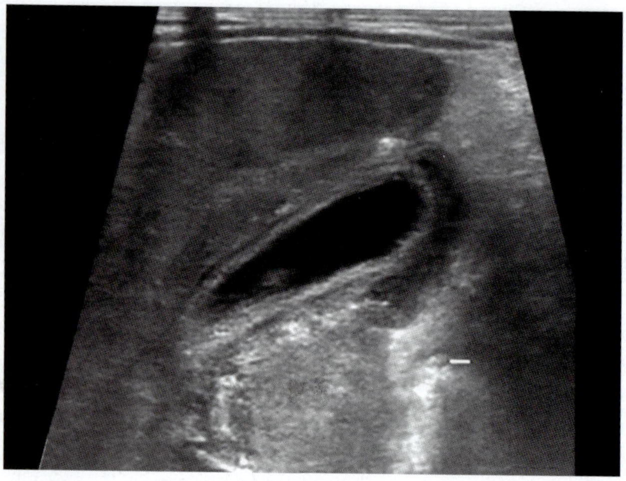

FIG. 30: USG of a child with Salmonella sepsis and right upper quadrant tenderness shows a marked GB wall thickening, but no calculi due to acalculus cholecystitis. (GB: gallbladder; USG: ultrasonography)

wall with surrounding fluid is seen in gallstone associated cholecystitis. At times calcified gallstones may also be seen on abdominal X-rays.

Up to 13% of pediatric patients undergoing cholecystectomy for cholelithiasis show CBD calculi. Most are passed out spontaneously. US features of CBD calculi are similar to gallbladder calculi though it is much less sensitive for CBD calculi. Extrahepatic bile duct dilatation is also seen, but may be absent in up to 33% of cases **(Fig. 29)**. MRCP demonstrates CBD calculi as hypointense intraluminal filling defects with a sensitivity of 97%.

An interesting entity is ceftriaxone-associated biliary pseudolithiasis. Ceftriaxone, a third-generation cephalosporin, is known to result in biliary sludge or biliary calculi. Since this lithiasis is reversible and disappears on stoppage of therapy it is called "pseudolithiasis." The incidence of pseudolithiasis varies between 15 and 46% usually appearing after 6th day of therapy and disappearing by 15 days after stoppage of therapy but may take longer. Most children are asymptomatic and detected incidentally on US and in these cases cessation of therapy is not required.

MISCELLANEOUS GALLBLADDER PATHOLOGY

Acalculous Cholecystitis[87,88]

Acalculous cholecystitis refers to gallbladder inflammation without calculi. it is thought to be the consequence of biliary stasis or ischemia. The condition may be acute (symptomatic for less than a month) or chronic (symptoms persisting for over 3 months). Clinical features include fever, jaundice, abdominal pain, and vomiting. Laboratory investigations reveal leukocytosis and deranged liver function test. Acute acalculous cholecystitis (AAC) most often occurs in the immediate postoperative period. Other predisposing conditions include systemic medical illnesses, severe trauma, burns, multiple transfusions, metabolic diseases, intravenous narcotics, salmonella sepsis or hyperalimentation. Bacterial and viral infections have also been implicated in some cases. AAC is associated with high morbidity and mortality.

On ultrasound, the gallbladder is thick-walled (>3.5–4 mm) but shows no calculi though sludge may be seen. Pericholecystic fluid and mucosal membrane sludge can be seen. The presence of two of these features, in addition to the absence of gallstones, is used to establish the diagnosis of AAC. In the appropriate clinical setting, isolated gallbladder wall-thickening may be used to suggest the diagnosis **(Fig. 30)**. Chronic acalculus cholecystitis is not usually seen in children. Treatment of the acute variety can be medical or with cholecystectomy.

Gallbladder Dyskinesia[86]

Gallbladder dyskinesia is said to be present when there is poor gallbladder contractility. Children present with chronic abdominal pain. Hepatobiliary scintigraphy, followed by cholecystokinin injection which causes gallbladder contraction, may be diagnostic. If the ejection fraction is <35% it is abnormal.

Gallbladder Hydrops[88-90]

Hydrops of the gallbladder refers to abnormal distention of the gallbladder with no wall-thickening or inflammation. It could be due to intrinsic obstruction of cystic duct due to abnormally thick bile. The obstruction may also be extrinsic, such as due to periportal lymph nodes. Vasculitis has also been implicated as a cause. Serous fluid secreted by the gallbladder mucosa causes distention in the presence of obstruction. Importantly "*transient gallbladder dilation*" should not be called hydrops and the term should be used for cases in which there is prolonged cystic duct obstruction so that bile is replaced by clear, thin, and colorless liquid. Predisposing conditions include conditions causing bile stasis such as dehydration or prolonged fasting, infection or hyperalimentation and Kawasaki's syndrome. Clinical features include jaundice, abdominal distention, and a right upper quadrant lump. However, cases may be completely asymptomatic. In acute hydrops, gallbladder is >3 cm in length in infants and >7 cm in older children on US. The wall is not thickened and sludge may be seen. In general, there is no dilatation of the rest of the biliary tract.

BILIARY NEOPLASMS[12,37]

Rhabdomyosarcoma is only primary tumor of the pediatric biliary tract. It is usually of the embryonal subtype, and may arise from the ampulla, CBD, hepatic ducts and even in a choledochal cyst. The median age at presentation is 3 years, being slightly more common in males. Jaundice, acholic stools, and abdominal distention are the usual presenting features. Other clinical features include abdominal pain, vomiting, and intermittent fever. On US examination, a mass at the porta hepatis is the most common finding. A dilated CBD with intraluminal contents may be apparent. Presence of arterial waveforms within the intraductal mass can be seen on Doppler, and this is useful to differentiate between biliary rhabdomyosarcoma and a sludge-filled choledochal cyst. CT may demonstrate a soft-tissue mass filling the common duct and expanding it. Liver invasion and intrahepatic bile duct dilatation may be seen. In up to 30% cases, metastatic disease of the regional lymph nodes, peritoneum, and omentum may be present.

Magnetic resonance imaging and MRCP are excellent techniques to confirm that the mass originates within the biliary system. The tumor is isointense to muscle on T1, hyperintense on T2WI. Asymmetric mural thickening of the CBD may be seen. Central tumor necrosis may be marked when it may be difficult to distinguish it from a choledochal cyst. The solid portion of the tumor enhances heterogeneously helping to distinguish the two. The current treatment modalities include of surgery, radiation, and chemotherapy in varying combination.

Rarely tumors arising in close proximity to the common duct may involve it.

Biliary dilatation may be seen with extrahepatic tumors, such as large pancreaticobiliary masses and lymphoma.

BILIARY COMPLICATIONS OF PEDIATRIC LIVER TRANSPLANTATION[37]

Some of the most common complications following liver transplantation involve the biliary tree. They are seen in 5–34% of pediatric liver transplant recipients, affecting function and consequently prognosis. Bile duct leakage usually occurs early, within the first 3 months after the surgery. US and MR provide indirect evidence of leak although hepatocyte specific contrast agents may help to demonstrate the leak. HIDA scans with delayed imaging are helpful to confirm bile leaks. Delayed complications, such as lithiasis and stenosis, are seen months or years after transplantation and may be treated by interventions via endoscopic or percutaneous route.

CONCLUSION

Cholestasis in childhood is both a diagnostic and therapeutic challenge. US remains the first-line investigation, but multimodality imaging approach is generally needed before an appropriate treatment strategy can be worked out. Improvements in imaging techniques and understanding of the molecular mechanisms underlying childhood biliary pathology can contribute to early diagnosis with improved management and better outcome for these children.

ACKNOWLEDGEMENT

The authors are grateful to Dr Shivali Arya for her illustration of **Figures 1 and 11**.

REFERENCES

1. Gubernick JA, Rosenberg HK, Ilaslan H, Kessler A. US approach to jaundice in infants and children. Radiographics. 2000;20:173-95.
2. Lam WW, Lam TP, Saing H, Chan FL, Chan KL. MR cholangiography and CT cholangiography of pediatric patients with choledochal cysts. AJR Am J Roentgenol. 1999;173:401-5.
3. Egbert ND, Bloom DA, Dillman JR. Magnetic resonance imaging of the pediatric pancreaticobiliary system. Magn Reson Imaging Clin N Am. 2013;21:681-96.
4. Kim MJ, Park YN, Han SJ, Yoon CS, Yoo HS, Hwang EH, et al. Biliary atresia in neonates and infants: Triangular area of high signal intensity in the porta hepatis at T2-weighted MR cholangiography with US and histopathologic correlation. Radiology. 2000;215:395-401.
5. Saito T, Terui K, Mitsunaga T, Nakata M, Kuriyama Y, Higashimoto Y, et al. Role of pediatric endoscopic retrograde cholangiopancreatography in an era stressing less-invasive modalities. J Pediatr Gastroenterol Nutr. 2014;59:204-9.
6. Blumfield E, Moore MM, Drake MK, Goodman TR, Lewis KN, Meyer LT, et al. Survey of gadolinium-based contrast agent utilization among the members of the Society for Pediatric Radiology: a Quality and Safety Committee report. Pediatr Radiol. 2017;47(6):665-73.
7. Griffin N, Charles-Edwards G, Grant LA. Magnetic resonance cholangiopancreatography: The ABC of MRCP. Insights Imaging. 2012;3(1):11-21.
8. Yeh BM, Liu PS, Soto JA, Corvera CA, Hussain HK. MR imaging and CT of the biliary tract. Radiographics. 2009;29(6):1669-88.
9. Gwal K, Bedoya MA, Patel N, Rambhatla SJ, Darge K, Sreedharan RR, et al. Reference values of MRI measurements of the common bile duct and pancreatic duct in children. Pediatr Radiol. 2015;45(8):1153-9.
10. Siegel MJ. Pediatric Sonography, 4th edition. Philadelphia: Wolters Kluwer/Lippincott Williams & Wilkins; 2011.
11. McGahan JP, Phillips HE, Cox KL. Sonography of the normal pediatric gallbladder and biliary tract. Radiology. 1982;144:873-5.
12. Sharafinski ME Jr, Meyers AB, Vorona G. Pediatric cholangiopathies: diseases of the gallbladder and biliary tract. Abdom Radiol (NY). 2017;42(1):69-85.
13. Moyer V, Freese DK, Whitington PF, Olson AD, Brewer F, Colletti RB, et al. Guideline for the evaluation of cholestatic jaundice in infants: Recommendations of the North American Society for

Pediatric Gastroenterology, Hepatology and Nutrition. J Pediatr Gastroenterol Nutr. 2004;39(2):115-28.
14. Nicholas J. Diseases of the Pediatric Gallbladder and Biliary Tract. In: Richard MSL, Gore M (eds). Textbook of Gastrointestinal Radiology. Philadelphia: Elsevier, Saunders; 2015. pp. 2180-99.
15. Balestreri W. Neonatal cholestasis. J Pediatr Gastroenterol Nutr. 1985;106:171-84.
16. Maisels MG. Neonatal jaundice. In: Avery GB (Ed). Neonatology, Pathophysiology, and Management of the Newborn. Philadelphia: JB Lippincott; 1987.
17. Kliegman RM, Behrman RE. Jaundice and hyperbilirubinemia in the newborn. In: Behrman RE, Vaughan VC III (Eds). Nelson Textbook of Pediatrics, 13th edition. Philadelphia: WB Saunders; 1987.
18. Lilly JR. Biliary atresia: The jaundiced infant. In: Welch KJ, Randolph JG, Ravitch MM (Eds). Pediatric Surgery. Chicago: YearBook, l; 1985.
19. Verkade HJ, Bezerra JA, Davenport M, Schreiber RA, Mieli-Vergani G, Hulscher JB, et al. Biliary atresia and other cholestatic childhood diseases: advances and future challenges. J Hepatol. 2016;65(3):631-42.
20. Mack CL, Sokol RJ. Unraveling the pathogenesis and etiology of biliary atresia. Pediatr Res. 2005;57(5 Pt 2):87R-94R.
21. Hartley JL, Davenport M, Kelly DA. Biliary atresia. Lancet. 2009;374(9702):1704-13.
22. Miyano T, Fujimoto T, Ohya T. Current concept of treatment of biliary atresia. World J Surg. 1993;17:332-6.
23. Kasai M. Treatment of biliary atresia with special reference to hepatic portoenterostomy and its modifications. Prog Pediatr Surg. 1974;6:5-52.
24. McIlhenny J, Campbell SE, Raible RJ, Antaki GM. Pediatric case of the day: Biliary atresia and polysplenia syndrome. AJR Am J Roentgenol. 1996;167:269, 271-3.
25. Haber BA, Russo P. Biliary atresia. Gastroenterol Clin North Am. 2003;32:891-911.
26. Schwarz KB, Haber BH, Rosenthal P, Mack CL, Moore J, Bove K, et al. Extrahepatic anomalies in infants with biliary atresia: Results of a large prospective North American multicenter study. Hepatology. 2013;58:1724-31.
27. Shneider BL, Brown MB, Haber B, Whitington PF, Schwarz K, Squires R, et al. A multicenter study of the outcome of biliary atresia in the United States, 1997 to 2000. J Pediatr. 2006;148:467-74.
28. Davenport M, Savage M, Mowat AP, Howard ER. Biliary atresia splenic malformation syndrome: An etiologic and prognostic subgroup. Surgery. 1993;113:662-8.
29. Mirza B, Iqbal S, Sheikh A. Biliary atresia associated with polysplenia syndrome, situs inversus abdominus, and reverse rotation of intestine. APSP J Case Rep. 2012;3:14.
30. Baumann U, Ure B. Biliary atresia. Clin Res Hepatol Gastroenterol. 2012;36:257-9.
31. Humphrey TM, Stringer MD. Biliary atresia: US diagnosis. Radiology. 2007;244(3):845-51.
32. Choi SO, Park WH, Lee HJ, Woo SK. 'Triangular cord': a sonographic finding applicable in the diagnosis of biliary atresia. J Pediatr Surg. 1996;31(3):363-6.
33. Zhou LY, Wang W, Shan QY, Liu BX, Zheng YL, Xu ZF, et al. Optimizing the US diagnosis of biliary atresia with a modified triangular cord thickness and gallbladder classification. Radiology 2015;277(1):181-91.
34. Lee HJ, Lee SM, Park WH, Choi SO. Objective criteria of Triangular cord sign in biliary atresia on US scans. Radiology. 2003;229:395-400.
35. Kanegawa K, Akasaka Y, Kitamura E, Nishiyama S, Muraji T, Nishijima E, et al. Sonographic diagnosis of biliary atresia in pediatric patients using the 'triangular cord' sign versus gallbladder length and contraction. AJR Am J Roentgenol. 2003;181(5):1387-90.
36. Zhou L, Shan Q, Tian W, Wang Z, Liang J, Xie X. Ultrasound for the Diagnosis of Biliary Atresia: A Meta-Analysis. AJR Am J Roentgenol. 2016;206:W73-W82.
37. Rozel C, Garel L, Rypens F, Viremouneix L, Lapierre C, Décarie JC, et al. Dubois Imaging of biliary disorders in children. Pediatr Radiol. 2011;41(2):208-20.
38. Tan Kendrick AP, Phua OB, Ooi Bc, Tan CE. Biliary atresia making the diagnosis by gallbladder ghost triad. Pediatr Radiol. 2003;33:311-5.
39. Kim WS, Cheon JE, Youn BJ, Yoo SY, Kim WY, Kim IO, et al. Hepatic arterial diameter measured with US: Adjunct for US diagnosis of biliary atresia. Radiology. 2007;245(2):549-55.
40. Redkar R, Davenport M, Howard ER. Antenatal diagnosis of congenital anomalies of the biliary tract. J Pediatr Surg. 1998;33:700-4.
41. De Matos V, Erlichman J, Russo PA, Haber BA. Does "cystic" biliary atresia represent a distinct clinical and etiological subgroup? A series of three cases. Pediatr Dev Pathol. 2005;8:725-31.
42. Koob M, Pariente D, Habes D, Ducot B, Adamsbaum C, Franchi-Abella S. The porta hepatis microcyst: an additional sonographic sign for the diagnosis of biliary atresia. Eur Radiol. 2017;27:1812-21.
43. Yoon H, Shin HJ, Kim MJ, Lee MJ. Quantitative Imaging in Pediatric Hepatobiliary Disease. Korean J Radiol. 2019;20(9):1342-57.
44. Tulchinsky M. The SNM practice guideline on hepatobiliary scintigraphy. J Nucl Med. 2010;51:1825.
45. Poddar U, Bhattacharya A, Thapa BR, Mittal BR, Singh K. Ursodeoxycholic acid–augmented hepatobiliary scintigraphy in the evaluation of neonatal jaundice. J Nucl Med. 2004;45:1488-92.
46. Treves ST. Pediatric Nuclear Medicine/PET, 3rd Edition. New York: Springer; 2007.
47. Dolgin SE. Answered and unanswered controversies in the surgical management of extrahepatic biliary atresia. Pediatr Transplant. 2004;8:628-31.
48. Park WH, Choi SO, Lee HJ, Kim SP, Zeon SK, Lee SL. A new diagnostic approach to biliary atresia with emphasis on the ultrasonographic triangular cord sign: Comparison of ultrasonography, hepatobiliary scintigraphy, and liver needle biopsy in the evaluation of infantile cholestasis. J Pediatr Surg. 1997;32:1555-9.
49. Norton KI, Glass RB, Kogan D, Lee JS, Emre S, Shneider BL. MR cholangiography in the evaluation of neonatal cholestasis: Initial results. Radiology. 2002;222:687-91.
50. Kim YH, Kim MJ, Shin HJ, Yoon H, Han SJ, Koh H, et al. MRI-based decision tree model for diagnosis of biliary atresia. Eur Radiol. 2018;28(8):3422-31.
51. Siles P, Aschero A, Gorincour G, Bourliere-Najean B, Roquelaure B, Delarue A, et al. A prospective pilot study: can the biliary tree be visualized in children younger than 3 months on magnetic resonance cholangiopancreatography? Pediatr Radiol. 2014;44:1077-84.
52. Takahashi A. Tsuchida Y, Suzuki N, Kuroiwa M, Ikeda H, Hirato J, et al. Incidence of intrahepatic biliary cysts in biliary atresia after hepatis portoenterostomy and histopathologic findings in the liver and porta hepatic at diagnosis. J Paediatr Surg. 1999;34:1364-8.

53. Moyer MS, Balistreri WF. Prolonged neonatal obstructive jaundice. In: Walker WA, Durie PR, Hamilton JR, Walker-Smith JA, Watkins JB (Eds). Pediatric Gastrointestinal Disease. Philadelphia: BC Decker; 1991.
54. Shamir SB, Kurian J, Kogan-Liberman D, Taragin BH. Hepatic Imaging in Neonates and Young Infants: State of the Art. Radiology. 2017;285(3):763-77.
55. Levy AD, Rohrmann CA, Murakata LA, Lonergan GJ. Caroli's disease: Radiologic spectrum with pathologic correlation. AJR Am J Roentgenol. 2002;179:1053-7.
56. Srivastava A. Progressive familial intrahepatic cholestasis. J Clin Exp Hepatol. 2014;4(1):25-36.
57. Whitington PF. Gestational alloimmune liver disease and neonatal hemochromatosis. Semin Liver Dis. 2012;32(4): 325-32.
58. Tsai A, Paltiel HJ, Sena LM, Kim HB, Fishman SJ, Alomari AI. Neonatal hemochromatosis and patent ductus venosus: clinical course and diagnostic pitfalls. Pediatr Radiol. 2009;39(8):823-7.
59. Hayes AM, Jaramillo D, Levy HL, Knisely AS. Neonatal hemochromatosis: diagnosis with MR imaging. AJR Am J Roentgenol. 1992;159(3):623-5.
60. Sela-Herman S, Scharschmidt BF. Choledochal cyst, a disease for all ages. Lancet. 1996;347:779.
61. Soares KC, Arnaoutakis DJ, Kamel I, Rastegar N, Anders R, Maithel S, et al. Choledochal cysts: Presentation, clinical differentiation, and management. J Am Coll Surg. 2014;219(6):1167-80.
62. Shi LB, Peng SY, Meng XK, Peng CH, Liu YB, Chen XP, et al. Diagnosis and treatment of congenital choledochal cyst: 20 years' experience in China. World J Gastroenterol. 2001;7(5):732-4.
63. Komi N, Udaka H, Ikeda N, Kashiwagi Y. Congenital dilatation of the biliary tract; new classification and study with particular reference to anomalous arrangement of the pancreaticobiliary ducts. Gastroenterol Jpn. 1977;12(4):293-304.
64. Nagi B, Kochhar R, Bhasin D, Singh K. Endoscopic retrograde cholangiopancreatography in the evaluation of anomalous junction of the pancreaticobiliary duct and related disorders. Abdom Imaging. 2003;28(6):847-52.
65. Iwai N, Yanagihara J, Tokiwa K, Shimotake T, Nakamura K. Congenital choledochal dilatation with emphasis on pathophysiology of the biliary tract. Ann Surg. 1992;215(1):27-30.
66. Todani T, Watanabe Y, Toki A, Morotomi Y. Classification of congenital biliary cystic disease: Special reference to type Ic and IVA cysts with primary ductal stricture. J Hepatobiliary Pancreat Surg. 2003;10(5):340-4.
67. Alonso-Lej F, Rever WB Jr, Pessagno DJ. Congenital choledochal cyst, with a report of 2, and an analysis of 94, cases. Int Abstr Surg. 1959;108(1):1-30.
68. Todani T, Watanabe Y, Narusue M, Tabuchi K, Okajima K. Congenital bile duct cysts: Classification, operative procedures, and review of thirty-seven cases including cancer arising from choledochal cyst. Am J Surg. 1977;134:263-9.
69. Lewis VA, Adam SZ, Nikolaidis P, Wood C, Wu JG, Yaghmai V, et al. Imaging of choledochal cysts. Abdom Imaging. 2015;40(6): 1567-80.
70. Michaelides M, Dimarelos V, Kostantinou D, Bintoudi A, Tzikos F, Kyriakou V, et al. A new variant of Todani type I choledochal cyst. Imaging evaluation. Hippokratia. 2011;15(2):174-7.
71. Courtier JL, Perito ER, Rhee S, Tsai P, Heyman MB, MacKenzie JD. Targeted MRI contrast agents for pediatric hepatobiliary disease. J Pediatr Gastroenterol Nutr. 2012;54(4):454-62.
72. Komi N. New classification of anomalous arrangement of the pancreaticobiliary ductal (APBD) in choledochal cyst: A proposal of new Komi classification of APBD. J Jpn Pancr Soc. 1991;6: 234-43.
73. Misra SP, Gulati P, Thorat VK, Vij JC, Anand BS. Pancreaticobiliary ductal union in biliary diseases. An endoscopic retrograde cholangiopancreatographic study. Gastroenterology. 1989;96:907-12.
74. Ziegler KM, Pitt HA, Zyromski NJ, Chauhan A, Sherman S, Moffatt D, et al. Choledochoceles: Are they choledochal cysts? Ann Surg. 2010;252(4):683-90.
75. Torra R, Badenas C, Darnell A, Brú C, Escorsell A, Estivill X. Autosomal dominant polycystic kidney disease with anticipation and Caroli's disease associated with a PKD1 mutation. Kidney Int. 1997;52(1):33-8.
76. Brancatelli G, Federle MP, Vilgrain V, Vullierme MP, Marin D, Lagalla R. Fibropolycystic Liver Disease: CT and MR Imaging Findings. Radiographics. 2005;25(3):659-70.
77. Caroli J, Soupault R, Kossakowsky J. La Dilatation Polycystique congenitale des voies biliairis intrahepatiques. Sem Hôp Paris. 1958;14:128-35.
78. Toma P, Lucigraj G, Pelizza A. Sonographic patterns of Caroli's disease report of 5 new cases. J Clin Ultrasound. 1991;19:155-8.
79. Oppenheimer EH, Esterly JR. Hepatic changes in young infants with cystic fibrosis. Possible relation to focal biliary cirrhosis. J Pediatr. 1975;86:683-9.
80. Pieringer H, Parzer I, Wöhrer A, Reis P, Oppl B, Zwerina J. IgG4-related disease: an orphan disease with many faces. Orphanet J Rare Dis. 2014;9:110.
81. Perego P, Cozzi G, Bertolini A. Portal biliopathy. Surg Endosc. 2003;17:351-2.
82. Malkan GH, Bathia SJ, Bashir K. Cholangiopathy associated with portal hypertension. Gastroint Endos. 1999;49:344-8.
83. Shin SM, Kim S, Lee JW, Kim CW, Lee TH, Lee SH, et al. Biliary abnormalities associated with portal biliopathy: evaluation on portal hypertensive biliopathy evaluation on MR cholangiography. AJR Am J Roentgenol. 2007;188:W341-7.
84. Poddar U. Gallstone Disease in Children. Indian Pediatr. 2010;47:945-53.
85. Triunfo S, Rosati P, Ferrara P, Gatto A, Scambia G. Fetal cholelithiasis: a diagnostic update and a literature review. Clin Med Insights Case Rep. 2013;6:153-8.
86. Svensson J, Makin E. Gallstone disease in children. Semin Pediatr Surg. 2012;21:255-65.
87. Tsakayannis DE, Kozakewich HP, Lillehei CW. Acalculous cholecystitis in children. J Pediatr Surg. 1996;31:127-30; discussion 130-1.
88. Garel L, Lucaya J, Piqueras J. Acute acalculous cholecystitis owing to salmonella sepsis. Pediatr Radiol. 2003;33:905-6.
89. Appleby GA, Forestier E, Starck CJ. Hydrops of the gallbladder in the neonatal period. Acta Paediatr Scand. 1981;70:117-20.
90. Bowen A. Acute gallbladder dilatation in a neonate: Emphasis on ultrasonography. J Pediatr Gastroenterol Nutr. 1984;3: 304-8.

CHAPTER

73

Congenital Anomalies of the Urinary Tract

Arun Kumar Gupta, Chandan J Das, Smriti Hari

INTRODUCTION

Anomalies of the urogenital tract are among the most common organ system anomalies found in the children. Approximately, 3.2% of infants had an abnormality of the genitourinary tract and one-half of these patients required surgical intervention.[1] Prompt and accurate imaging diagnosis of these anomalies is important so that correctible abnormalities can be treated in a timely manner and a genetic workup may be performed that may aid in future pregnancy planning.

IMAGING MODALITIES

The backbone of pediatric urologic imaging has been ultrasound (USG), voiding cystourethrography (VCUG), radionuclide scintigraphy, and magnetic resonance imaging (MRI). The small physical habitus of pediatric patients and absence of ionizing radiation make USG an ideal imaging method. The results of USG usually determine what further examination is required. The role of intravenous urography (IVU) is to answer specific questions (e.g., to show the calyceal anatomy which may be helpful in establishing the cause of a small kidney) and to differentiate some unusual causes of ureteral obstruction (ureteral valve, ureteral polyp, and retrocaval ureter) from the usual pelviureteric junction (PUJ) obstruction.[2] VCUG is essential for the evaluation of the bladder, urethra, and to rule out reflux. Diuretic renography is used to differentiate obstructive from nonobstructive hydronephrosis or hydroureter. Diuretic renography gives quantitative functional information, such as differential renal function.

Antenatal Sonography

It is estimated that a structural fetal anomaly is detected by antenatal sonography in 1% of all screened pregnancies. Of these anomalies, one-fifth is believed to be manifestations of genitourinary origin.[3] Fetal sonography allows for early detection of hydronephrosis. Because it has been shown that renal growth and development are affected adversely by prenatal urinary tract obstruction, antenatal hydronephrosis has become a common indication for postnatal radiologic workup to exclude vesicoureteral reflux (VUR) and posterior urethral valve (PUV) and to determine whether the hydronephrosis is obstructive or nonobstructive. The most common causes of nonobstructive hydronephrosis are VUR and nonobstructive primary megaureter. Obstructive causes include PUJ obstruction, ureterovesical junction (UVJ) obstruction, ureteral ectopia with or without ureterocele, and PUV (in boys).[4]

Magnetic Resonance Urography

Magnetic resonance urography (MRU) has become a useful adjuvant in evaluating urogenital anomalies.[5] MRU is free of radiation and has the distinct advantage of providing both anatomic and functional information in one go. MRU allows a one-stop-shop evaluation of the renal parenchyma, collecting system, vasculature, bladder, and surrounding structures. A comprehensive MRU protocol is a two-part imaging technique composed of precontrast sequences (static MRU) and postcontrast sequences (dynamic or excretory MRU).

Static MRU uses heavily T2-weighted fluid-sensitive sequences in which urine-containing structures are bright. Three-dimensional (3D) respiratory triggered T2 sequences can be reconstructed to create maximum intensity projections (MIPs). MRU has been shown to be superior to US both in the detection of occult upper pole moieties and in demonstrating ureteral ectopy without depending on excretory function of the kidney.[6] This is also true for the detection of dysplastic ectopic kidneys that are very difficult to see with other imaging modalities **(Figs. 1A and B)**.

Dynamic MRU uses the excretory function of kidney and can provide both anatomic and functional information. Intravenous gadolinium is administered, and sequential 3D dynamic sequences are acquired till excretory phase. The dynamic sequences are the basis of the functional calculation, assessment of renal perfusion, evaluation of renal transit, and excretion.[7] MRU has been shown to be superior to renal scintigraphy in demonstration of precise anatomic information and in distinguishing between pyelonephritis and scar.[8-10]

Although MRU is a powerful study with numerous advantages, few limitations do exist. MRU can have relatively

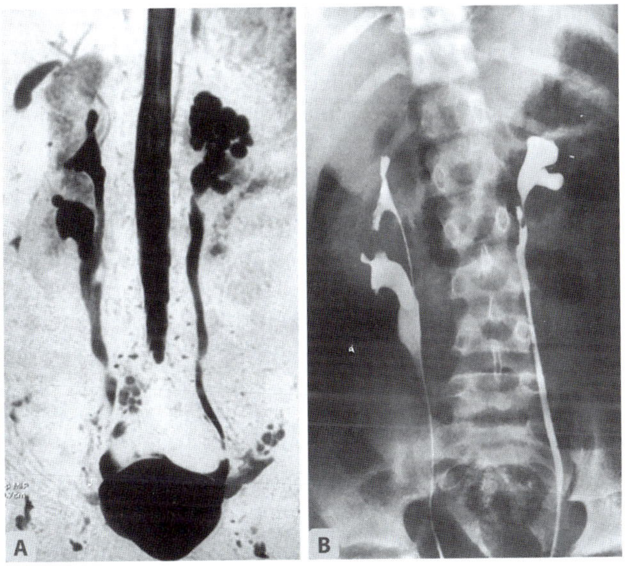

FIGS. 1A AND B: (A) MR urogram (coronal HASTE image) shows complete duplication of pelvicalyceal system on right side joining to form a single ureter and left hydronephrosis in a 4-year-old child; (B) Corresponding IVU image of the same patient showing almost complete correlation with the MR urogram image. Note cystic changes of segmental dysplastic kidney in left upper pole seen only in MRU (A) but not visualized in IVU (B). (IVU: intravenous urography; MRU: magnetic resonance urography)

long imaging times and is sensitive to motion artifact, which necessitates sedation for young children. An important limitation of the dynamic MRU is that it is contraindicated in patients with moderate renal insufficiency (GFR < 30 mL/min) although a non-contrast static MRU can be performed.[9]

Voiding Ultrasonography

Voiding ultrasonography (VUS) is another modality for the detection of VUR in children. Although VCUG and radionuclide cystography are currently the two most commonly used techniques to evaluate VUR, recent developments of commercially available echoenhancing agents have significantly improved the sonographic detection of fluid movement within the urinary tract. SonoVue (Bracco, Milan, Italy) can be used as contrast agent for VUS. VUS can be used in workup of urinary tract infections, follow-up of known VUR, and in the evaluation of reflux in renal transplant patients. In our experience, this has very high sensitivity and specificity to diagnose vesicoureteric reflux.

CT Angiography and CT Urography

Pediatric CT angiography (CTA) and CT urography (CTU) are considered only after USG and MRI have been exhausted or when CT is considered superior for clinical imaging objectives. Using a 64-channel multidetector computed tomography (MDCT) scanner for abdominal CTA and abdominopelvic CTU in neonates to adolescent patients, average radiation exposures are approximately 1–2 mSv with scan times of 1.5–4.0 seconds.[10] This radiation dose is equivalent to that of approximately 50–100 chest radiographs. CTA applications for the pediatric urology patient include

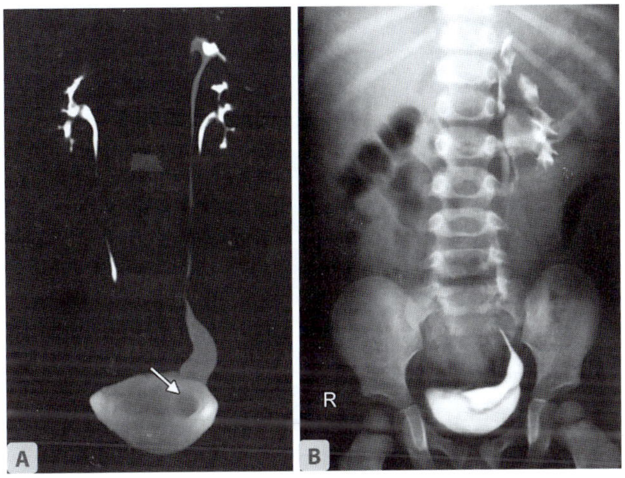

FIGS. 2A AND B: CT urography. (A) CT urogram showing the ureterocele as filling defect (arrow) with left-sided duplex system; (B) A delayed image of IVU of the same patient showing a similar finding. (IVU: intravenous urography)

evaluation of vascular anatomy, vascular morphology, and traumatic vascular injury. CTU common applications include the evaluation of suspected or known congenital anomalies **(Figs. 2A and B)**, obstructive uropathy, and trauma. Acquisitions may be performed as a single dedicated urographic 8–10 minutes delay acquisition.

Neonatal Kidney

The normal US appearance of the neonatal kidney **(Fig. 3)** is markedly different from that of an older child or an adult, i.e., the cortex is thinner, often lobulated in outline and more reflective than the liver, the pyramids are large and relatively hypoechoic compared with the cortex, the capsule is not well-defined and the sinus fat is much less noticeable.[11] The age of transition from the neonatal to an adult pattern is very variable and may occur at 2–3 months after birth, but can persist for up to 6 months of age.

Dynamic radionuclide scans are generally best obtained after 4 weeks of age when some renal maturity has occurred. The neonatal diethylenetriamine penta-acetic acid (DTPA) scan is characterized by poor visualization of the kidneys. Relatively poor function as seen on nuclear scanning does not imply irreversible damage, and no long-term management decisions should be taken on the basis of these results; rather the scan should be repeated either when the infant is older (around 3 months) or following a drainage procedure.[12]

There is generally no place for an IVU in the first 2–3 days of life. USG is the imaging modality of choice. If an IVU is undertaken, delayed images at 6, 12, and 18 hours may be necessary to visualize the kidneys. IVU should be done with a nonionic contrast medium at a concentration of 30% iodine up to a maximum dose of 3 mL/kg.

Embryologic Development of the Urinary Tract

A brief review of the embryologic development of the urinary tract is very helpful in understanding these congenital genitourinary malformations. The renal parenchyma is derived from the primitive metanephros.[13] As the primitive

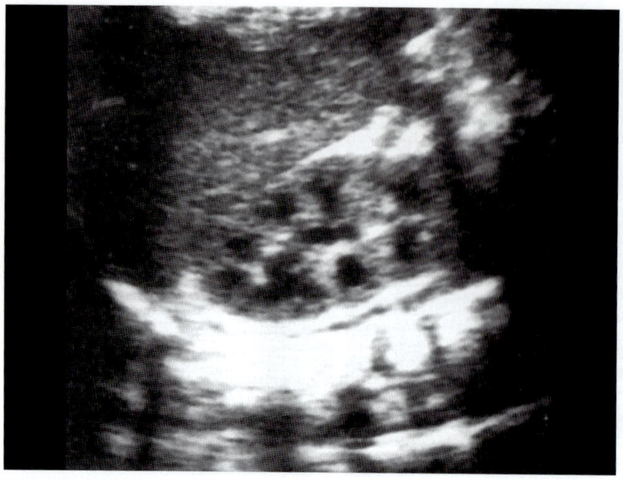

FIG. 3: Normal neonatal kidney: The cortex is relatively thin and echogenic, the medullary pyramids appear large and relatively hypoechoic and minimal sinus structures are seen.

metanephros migrates upward and matures, it takes the form of normal kidney. A specific rotation also occurs so that when the renal pelvis originally points anteriorly, a gradual inward and medial rotation takes place so that the anteriorly facing pelvis is finally facing anteromedially.

The ureteric bud develops as an outpouching from the metanephric or Wolffian duct. The ureteric bud grows upward and eventually meets the primitive renal parenchymal tissue. The cloaca forms the larger portion of the bladder and urethra. The Wolffian duct descends and forms the epididymis, ejaculatory duct, and vas deferens in the male. In the female, the Wolffian duct disappears and the Müllerian ducts give rise to the female internal genitalia.

ABNORMALITIES OF KIDNEY

Renal Agenesis

Renal agenesis, the complete congenital absence of renal tissue results from the failure of the ipsilateral ureteric bud to contact the nephrogenic blastema. The ipsilateral renal artery is absent.

Bilateral renal agenesis is the most severe anomaly of the genitourinary system and occurs in 1-3 per 10,000 live births. It is noted predominantly in males and is incompatible with life. On prenatal USG, severe oligohydramnios, absence of fetal bladder, and both kidneys are highly suggestive of bilateral renal agenesis.

Unilateral agenesis occurs in about 1 in 1,000 of the general population, predominantly in males and on the left side. The most common associated genitourinary anomalies include uterovaginal atresia (or duplication) in females and absent seminal vesicle or seminal vesicle cyst in males.[14] A number of syndromes are associated with unilateral renal agenesis, such as the VACTERL (vertebral defects, anal atresia, cardiac defects, tracheo-esophageal fistula, renal anomalies, and limb abnormalities) association, Fanconi pancytopenia, and Kallmann syndrome. The present kidney may show VUR, ectopic location, malrotation, PUJ obstruction, and multicystic dysplasia.

Imaging Features

In clinical practice, it is quite difficult to be certain whether one is dealing with true unilateral agenesis or a very small nonfunctioning kidney. USG might show that a nonexcreting kidney that is actually present but may be nonfunctional. Conversely, ^{99m}TC dimercaptosuccinic acid (DMSA) scintigraphy might reveal a small unilateral dysplastic/ hypoplastic kidney that was difficult to be evaluated on USG, but which is nonetheless present with some function. If the USG and nuclear studies fail to show a small kidney, then contrast-enhanced computed tomography (CECT) should be done which may confirm the absence along with absent ipsilateral renal artery.

Rotational Anomalies

As the kidney ascends to its final position opposite the second lumbar vertebra, it undergoes rotation so that finally the renal hilum is directed medially and slightly forward. In incomplete rotation, or nonrotation, the hilum continues to face anteriorly, the calices project out from either side of the pelvis on a standard frontal radiograph, and the proximal ureter is displaced laterally. Nonrotation and incomplete rotations are most common rotational anomalies. They may be unilateral or bilateral and often accompany ectopia **(Figs. 4A and B)**, or fusion anomalies. In an IVU, oblique views are of great help in establishing that the malrotated kidney is otherwise normal.[15]

Anomalies of Renal Position

Normally, the kidneys are located opposite first to third lumbar vertebrae. Anomalies of renal position range from minor degrees of unilateral malposition to totally abnormal positioning of both kidneys. The clinical significance of this finding lies in the fact that these ectopic kidneys are more susceptible to trauma, iatrogenic injury, obstruction, calculi, reflux, and infection. There is a high incidence of aberrant and multiple renal arteries and veins.

Ipsilateral/Uncrossed Ectopia

In this anomaly, the ectopic kidney is on the same side as the vesical opening of its ureter. It can be further divided into cranial or caudal ectopias according to whether they are above or below the normal position. In cranial renal ectopia, the affected kidney, usually the left, is within the lower thorax.[16] In caudal renal ectopia the abnormal kidney lies below normal position; it may be abdominal (above iliac crest, below L3), iliac (iliac fossa) or pelvic (true pelvis).

Imaging Features

A thoracic kidney appears as a well-defined, posteroinferior mediastinal mass on chest radiograph. IVU confirms the thoraciclocationofthekidney.CTmayshowthethoracickidney with diaphragmatic defect and the adrenal gland is seen lying above, behind or below it. Blood supply is from an elongated renal artery from aorta at normal level **(Figs. 5A and B)**, or occasionally from an accessory renal artery from thoracic aorta. In cases of caudal renal ectopia, renal outline is not visible in expected position on an abdominal X-ray. IVU shows the malrotated, ectopic kidney draining into the

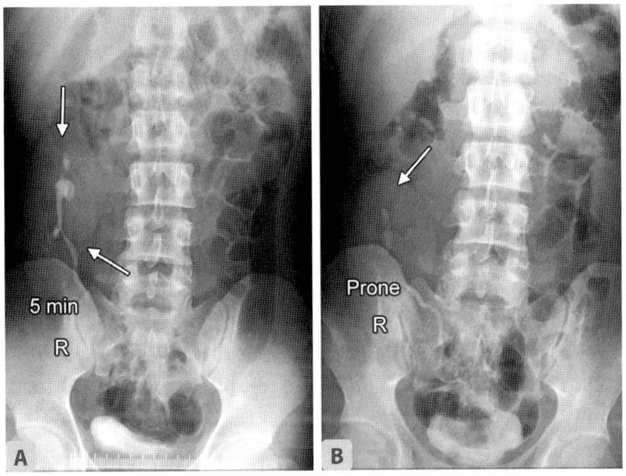

FIGS. 4A AND B: Malrotation: IVU supine (A) and prone (B) showing caudal ectopic right kidney with malrotation of PCS. (IVU: intravenous urography; PCS: pelvicalyceal system)

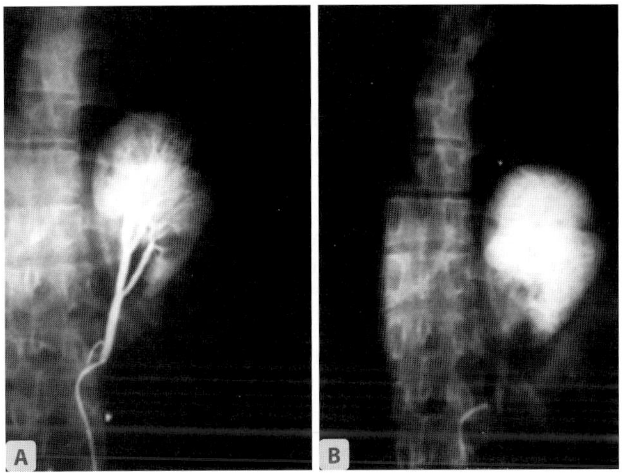

FIGS. 5A AND B: Thoracic kidney: Conventional angiogram (A) showing intrathoracic left kidney being supplied by an abnormally long renal artery; (B) Delayed image showing complete nephrostogram.

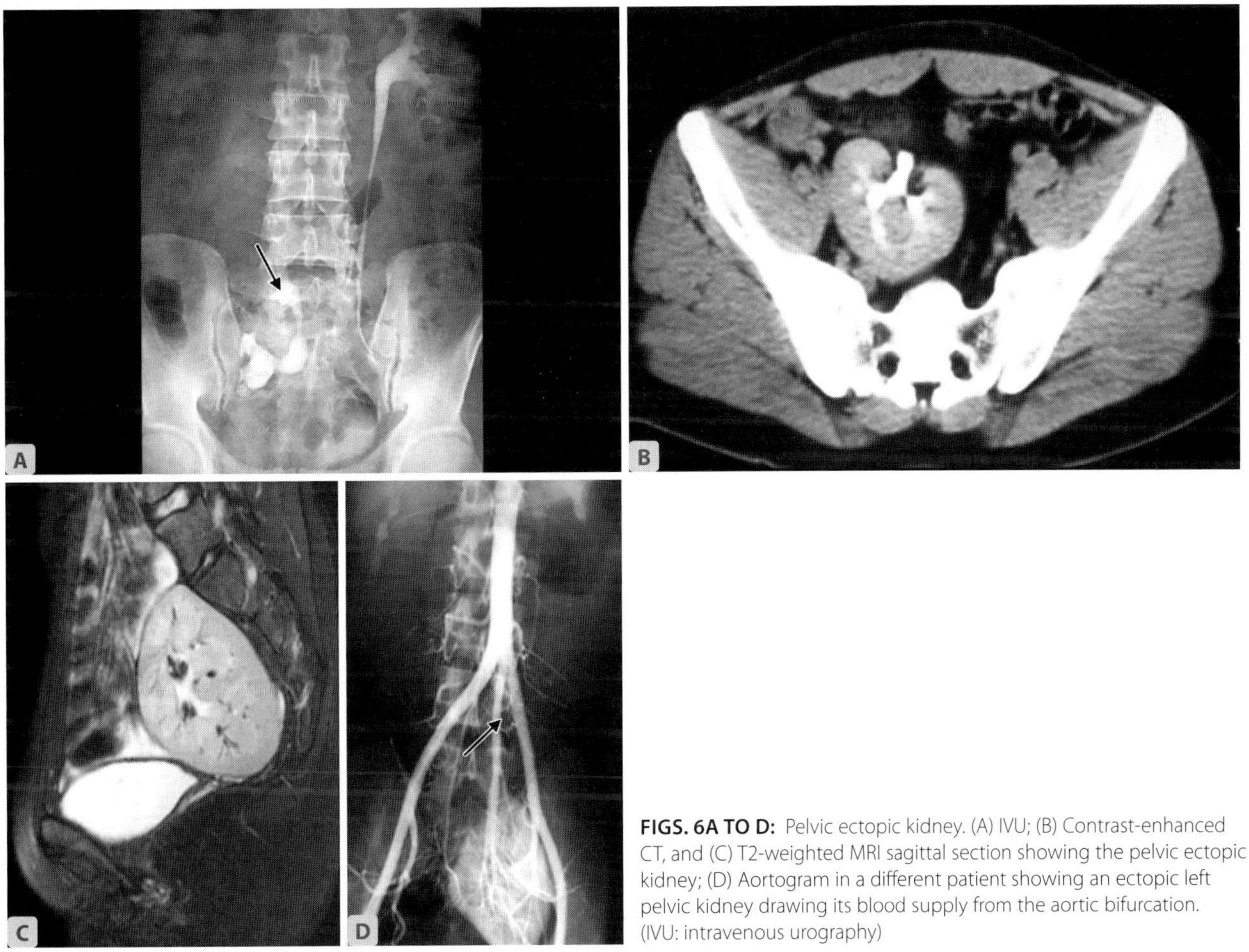

FIGS. 6A TO D: Pelvic ectopic kidney. (A) IVU; (B) Contrast-enhanced CT, and (C) T2-weighted MRI sagittal section showing the pelvic ectopic kidney; (D) Aortogram in a different patient showing an ectopic left pelvic kidney drawing its blood supply from the aortic bifurcation. (IVU: intravenous urography)

bladder via a short ureter **(Fig. 6A)**. CT can easily distinguish the ectopic kidney from various abdominal and pelvic masses **(Fig. 6B)**. CTU is helpful in hydronephrosis and to delineate distal ureters. MRI can also depict the ectopic kidney nicely **(Fig. 6C)**. When the kidney is pelvic, the arterial supply usually arises from the aortic bifurcation **(Fig. 6D)**. These aberrant arteries may cross and obstruct the ureter. It is important to recognize these vessels prior to surgery.[17]

Crossed Renal Ectopia

In crossed renal ectopia, the kidney is in opposite side of midline from its ureteral orifice. It may occur with fusion (most common), without fusion (15%), or in a solitary kidney (least common).[18] In fused crossed ectopia (unilateral fused kidney), the kidney crosses the midline to the opposite side of the body and fuses with the kidney on that side. Crossed, fused renal ectopia is more common in males and on the right side. The anomalous kidney usually lies below the orthotopic kidney and the fusion is between the lower pole of the orthotopic kidney and the upper pole of the ectopic kidney. Malrotation, particularly in the ectopic kidney, is the rule.[19] The importance of these conditions is that it may present as an abdominal mass or PUJ obstruction or with VUR.

Imaging Features

The USG reveals an unusually large kidney on the affected side with an absent kidney on the opposite side. In cases of fused ectopia, the renal sinuses lie in different planes, run in different directions and the fused kidneys are inseparable. The diagnosis of renal ectopia is generally established from the IVU or CTU. IVU delineates the morphology of the crossed kidneys and shows the insertion of ureter into their respective trigone on the side of origin **(Fig. 7)**.

Horseshoe Kidney

The horseshoe kidney is the most frequent renal fusion anomaly, occurring in 1 in 400 people. It is characterized by fusion of the lower poles across the midline through an isthmus of tissue anterior to the aorta and inferior vena cava. The usual position of the isthmus is at the junction of the aorta with the inferior mesenteric artery. The ureters exit from the anteriorly positioned renal pelvises to descend inferiorly. Most (90%) cases are asymptomatic but may be associated with PUJ obstruction, VUR, infection, urolithiasis, and malignancy. Carcinoma and Wilms' tumor can occur in the horseshoe kidney.[20] The abnormal position also leaves the kidney more susceptible to trauma. Horseshoe kidney may be associated with Turner syndrome, trisomy 18, Fanconi anemia, and Laurence-Moon-Biedl syndrome, or as a part of VACTERL association.

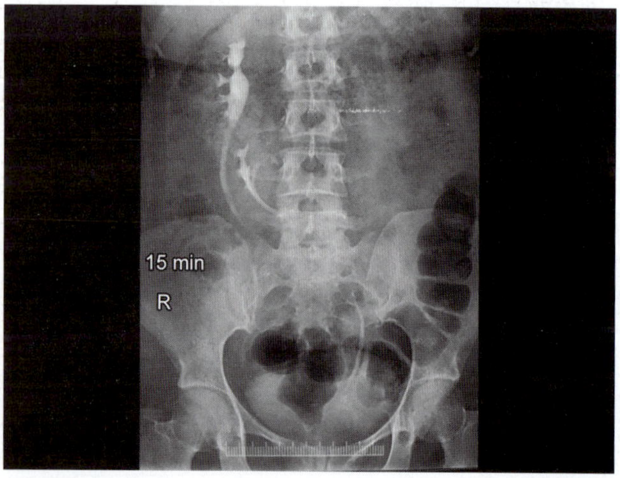

FIG. 7: Crossed fused ectopia: IVU showing the left kidney crossing over and fusing with the lower pole of right kidney. Note that the ureters always drain into their corresponding site, i.e., right to right VUJ and left to left VUJ. (IVU: intravenous urography; VUJ: vesicoureteric junction)

Imaging Features

On X-ray the lower poles of the kidneys are seen to lie too close to the spine **(Fig. 8A)**. USG shows the curved configuration of the horseshoe kidney with elongated, poorly defined lower poles.[21] IVU reveals U-shaped nephrogram and the lower calyces descend toward the midline near the isthmus, resulting in the "hand-holding calyces" appearance **(Fig. 8B)**. The lower calyces are often medial to the ureter on the same side. As each ureter crosses the isthmus, it curves laterally and then assumes a normal medial course giving rise to the "flower-vase" appearance. CT is especially useful in showing the degree and site of fusion, and nature of the isthmus **(Fig. 8C)**. Renal parenchymal and collecting system abnormalities (duplex system, hydronephrosis, and calculi) are also picked up on CTU **(Fig. 8D)**.[22]

Ureteropelvic Duplication (Duplex Kidney)

A duplex kidney shows two separate pelvicalyceal systems. The two draining ureters may join before emptying into the bladder (partial duplication/bifid ureters) or insert separately into the bladder (complete duplication). 85% of completely duplicated ureters follow the Weigert-Meyer rule according to which the upper ureter inserts into the bladder in a position more inferior and medial to the orifice of the lower moiety ureter. In these cases, the ectopic ureter draining the upper pole moiety frequently ends in a ureterocele and is obstructed, whereas reflux typically occurs into the lower moiety.

Imaging Features

The USG shows two distinct echo complexes with intervening renal parenchyma **(Fig. 9A)**. On IVU or CT urography, duplex kidney is well seen with double ureters **(Fig. 9B)**. There may be poor or no excretion by the upper pole moiety. Nonfilling of the obstructed upper pole moiety results in the downward displacement of the lower pole calyces, called the "drooping lily" sign. VCUG may demonstrate reflux into the lower pole ureter. Saddle reflux or yo-yo reflux is unique to partial duplications which have a single distal ureter. Occasionally, nuclear scan is the first to suggest a renal duplication. MRI coupled with MR urography is often the best modality **(Figs. 9C and D)**.[23]

Renal Hypoplasia

In simple renal hypoplasia, also called miniature or dwarf kidney, the affected kidney is significantly smaller than normal, but is otherwise well formed both grossly and histologically, and functions normally in proportion to its mass. The main renal artery and its branches are uniformly small. The opposite kidney is generally large owing to compensatory hypertrophy. It does not affect total kidney function unless the opposite kidney is diseased or absent.[24]

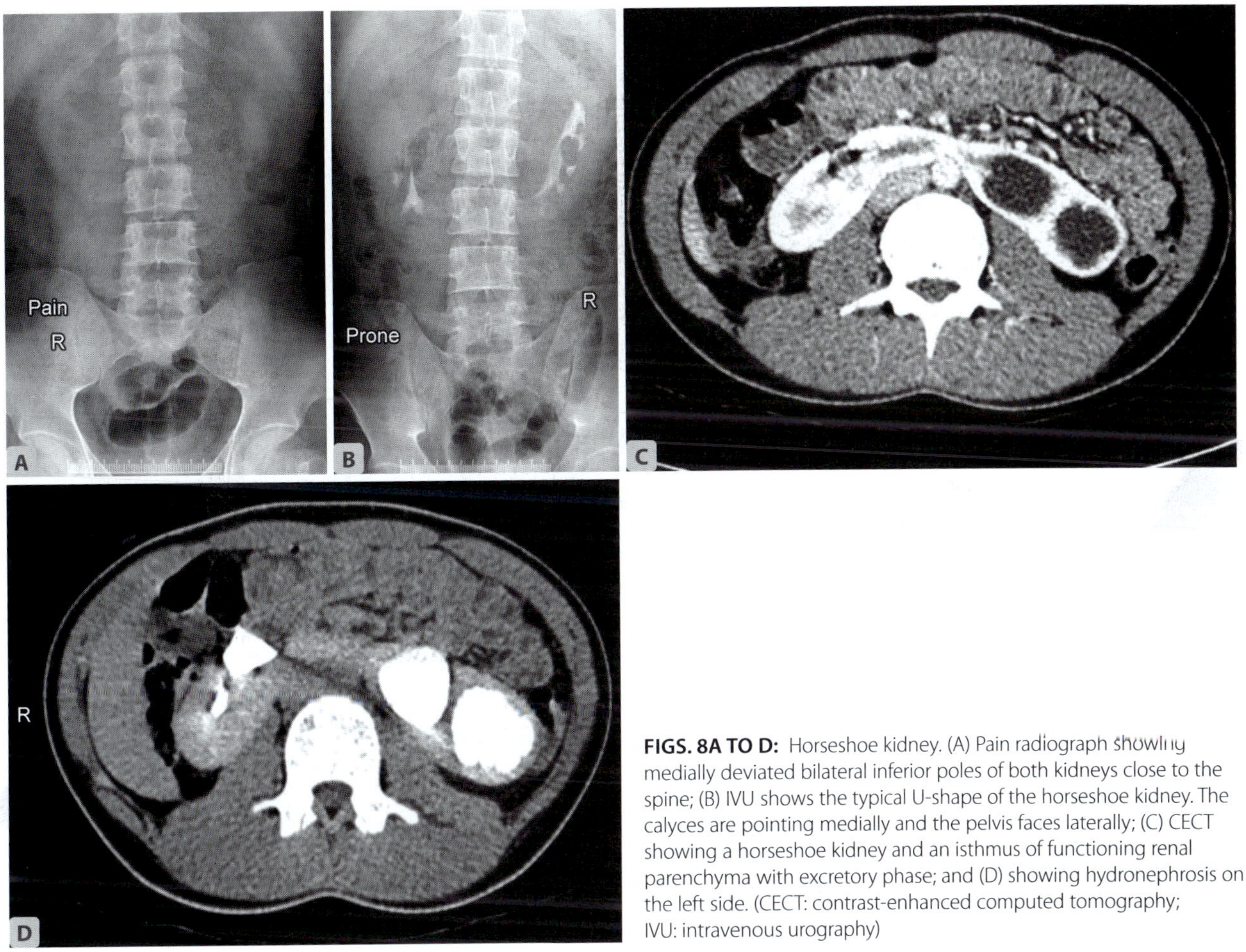

FIGS. 8A TO D: Horseshoe kidney. (A) Pain radiograph showing medially deviated bilateral inferior poles of both kidneys close to the spine; (B) IVU shows the typical U-shape of the horseshoe kidney. The calyces are pointing medially and the pelvis faces laterally; (C) CECT showing a horseshoe kidney and an isthmus of functioning renal parenchyma with excretory phase; and (D) showing hydronephrosis on the left side. (CECT: contrast-enhanced computed tomography; IVU: intravenous urography)

Cystic Renal Dysplasia

Renal dysplasia is a congenital renal parenchymal malformation occurs in 2–4 in every 1,000 births. Cystic renal dysplasia has been classified by Potter into four types.[25] Type I is infantile or autosomal recessive polycystic kidney disease (ARPKD); type II, multicystic dysplastic kidney disease (MDK); type III, autosomal dominant (adult type) polycystic kidney disease (ADPKD); and type IV, partial or intermittent urinary outflow obstruction (obstructive dysplasia).[25,26]

Autosomal Recessive Polycystic Kidney Disease

Autosomal recessive polycystic kidney disease is characterized by bilateral, symmetrical renal cystic disease. There is 25% likelihood of recurrence in a future pregnancy. Pathologically, there is saccular dilatation of renal collecting tubules. In ARPKD, the liver is always involved by hepatic cysts, bile duct ectasia and periportal fibrosis. Clinically, it is characterized by a variable mixture of renal failure and portal hypertension.[26]

Imaging Features

Ultrasound is the most common imaging modality used for diagnosis. The numerous acoustic interfaces provided by the cyst walls lead to solid and homogeneously hyperechoic kidney on USG **(Fig. 10A)**. The enlarged kidneys maintain their reniform shape and show absent or poor corticomedullary differentiation.[27] A characteristic perirenal halo may be seen, representing the peripherally compressed hypoechoic normal cortex around the hyperechoic medulla. Tiny, punctate, echogenic foci develop with time due to calcium deposition and correlate with renal failure. These foci do not show posterior acoustic shadowing but may cause ring-down artifacts.

Noncontrast computed tomography (NCCT) shows bilateral symmetrically enlarged kidneys with multiple punctate calcific foci **(Fig. 10B)**. Contrast-enhanced CT shows a prolonged striated nephrogram **(Fig. 10C)** due to trapping of contrast in the medulla. There is minimal excretion of contrast. MRI is a useful modality which can evaluate the kidneys and liver together especially the biliary abnormality **(Figs. 10D and E)**.

Antenatal USG diagnosis can be made when oligohydramnios with markedly enlarged, echogenic kidneys is noted. These infants are at risk for pulmonary hypoplasia and often die in the neonatal period.

Multicystic Dysplastic Kidney

Multicystic dysplastic kidney is the second most common abdominal mass in a neonate after hydronephrosis with an incidence of 1 in 4,300 live births. The affected kidney is

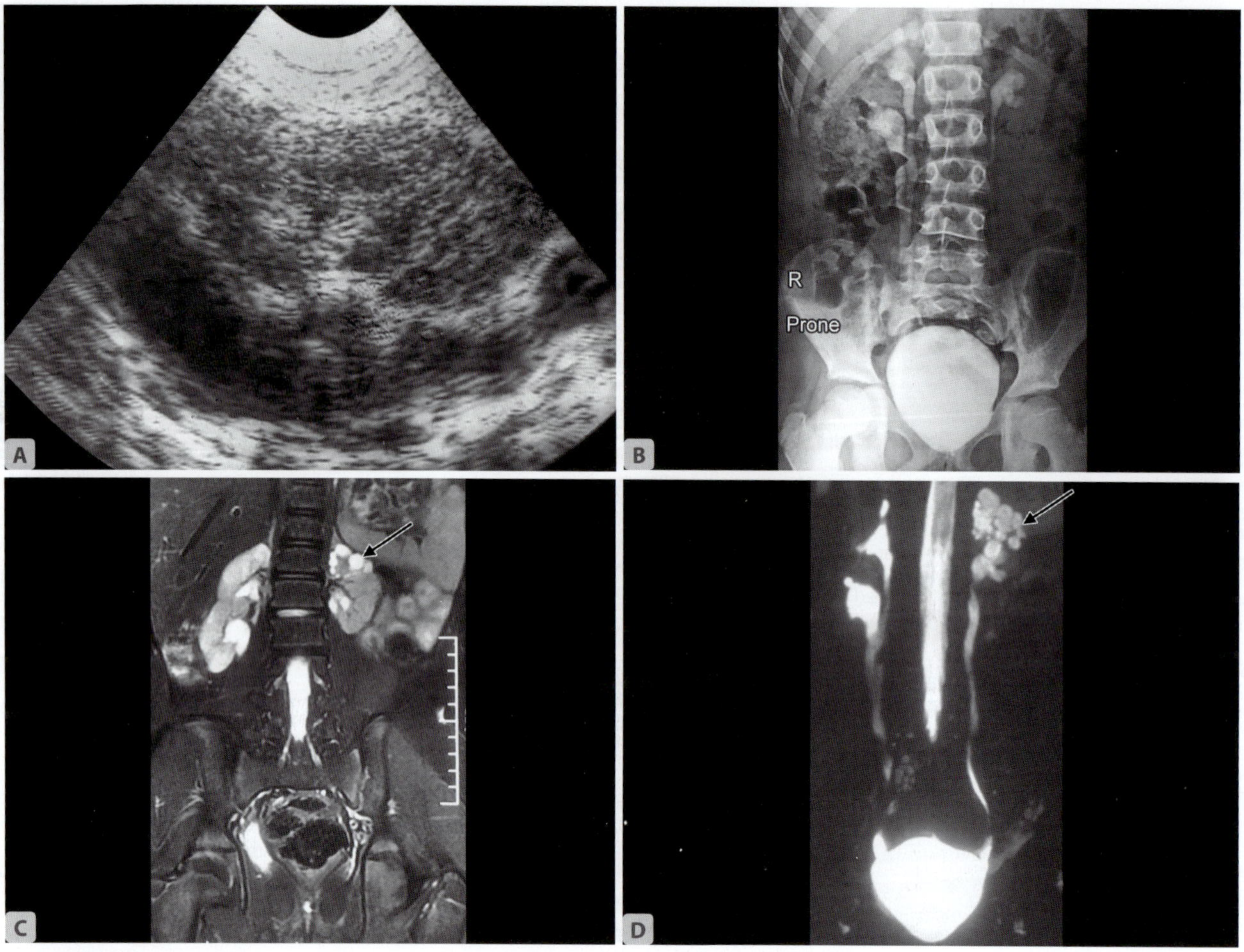

FIGS. 9A TO D: Duplex right kidney. (A) Ultrasonography showing duplex system with dilated upper system including its ureter; (B) IVU shows two separate PCS and the two ureters joining inferiorly to become one; (C) T2 coronal MRI image showing two separate PCS; and (D) MRU showing exactly similar findings with the IVU. Note is made of cystic dysplasia (arrow) in upper pole of left kidney (C,D). (IVU: intravenous urography; MRU: magnetic resonance urography; PCS: pelvicalyceal system)

nonfunctioning, replaced by numerous cysts and dysplastic tissue. It varies in size from 10–15 cm to only 1–2 cm. Classically, it can be of two forms: (1) *pelvi-infundibular* (more common) and (2) *hydronephrotic* MDK (less frequent) type.

The abnormality is usually unilateral with a normal contralateral kidney allowing for a good prognosis. There is a 3–5% familial recurrence of the disease suggesting a genetic influence.[28] The contralateral renal abnormalities include VUR, PUJ obstruction, and UVJ obstruction.[29]

Imaging Features (Figs. 11A and B)

Ultrasonography findings include the presence of variably sized noncommunicating cysts separated by echogenic areas without any normal renal parenchyma **(Fig. 11A)**.[30] USG allows a definitive diagnosis to be made, however, in a small percentage of cases in the neonate, it may be difficult to distinguish it from large PUJ obstruction. In MDK, there is usually one "cyst" which is larger than the others and lies laterally, whereas in PUJ obstruction the dilated renal pelvis is centrally located and the peripheral calyces are seen to extend from it **(Figs. 12A and B)**. In such situations dynamic nuclear imaging may be useful since the demonstration of function indicates PUJ obstruction. CT can show multiple low attenuation cysts replacing normal renal parenchyma with minimal or no contrast enhancement and excretion. T2-weighted (T2W) MRI can also show the cysts nicely due to fluid in the cyst **(Fig. 11B)**.

Autosomal Dominant (Adult Type) Polycystic Kidney Disease

Autosomal dominant (adult type) polycystic kidney disease is an autosomal dominant hereditary disease characterized by the presence of multiple bilateral renal macrocysts. There is cystic involvement of liver (50%) and pancreas (9%). This disorder most frequently manifests after the third decade of life but now is frequently being diagnosed in infants and children. Children with ADPKD may have hypertension, proteinuria, or hyperlipidemia.

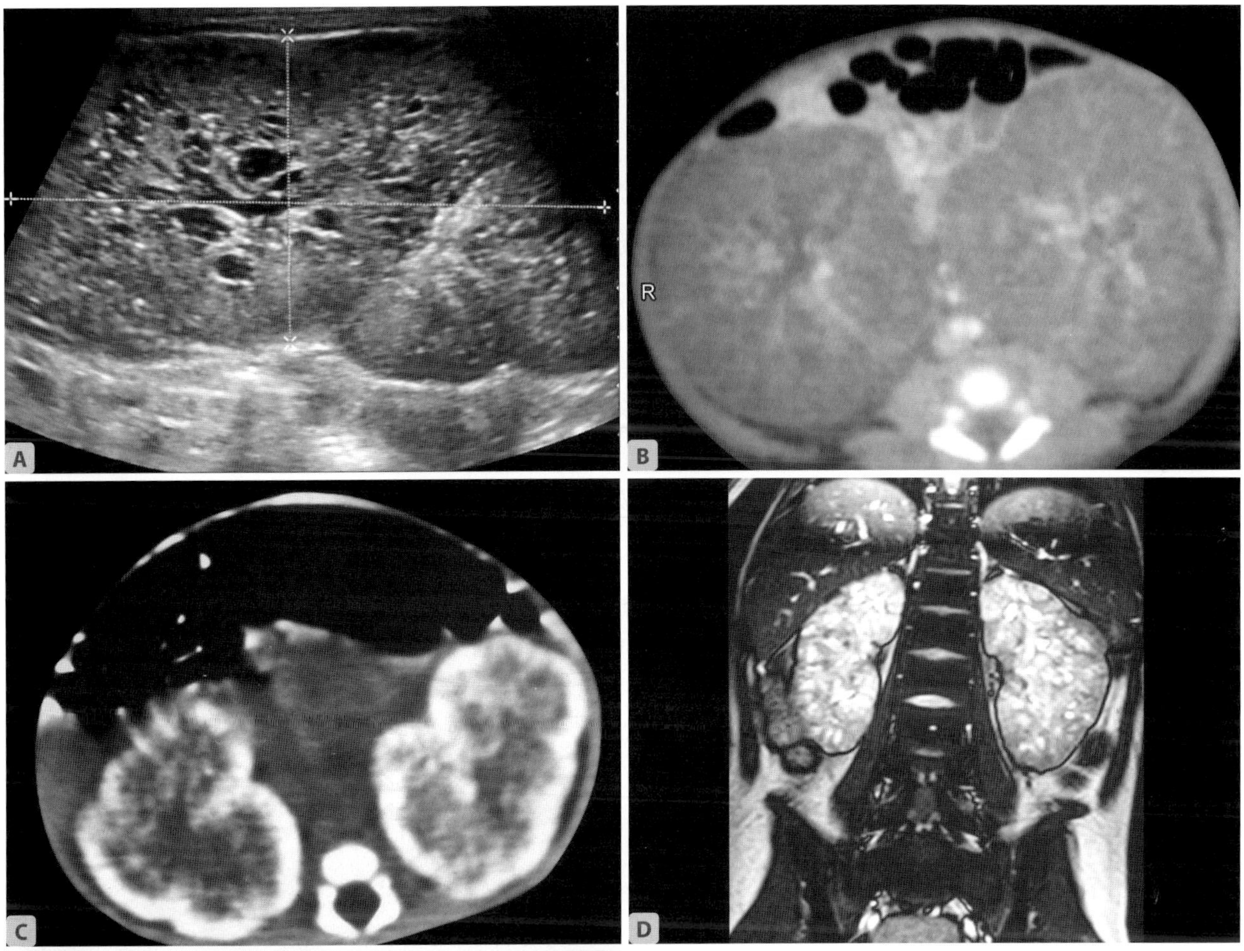

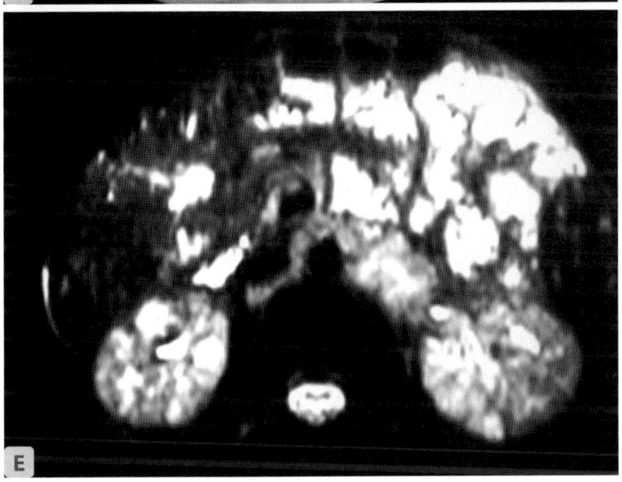

FIGS. 10A TO E: Autosomal recessive polycystic kidney. (A) Ultrasonography (USG) shows markedly enlarged, homogeneously hyperechoic, kidney with few tiny medullary cysts and absent corticomedullary differentiation; (B) Noncontrast CT showing bilateral enlarged kidneys with radiating hyperdensities from medulla; and (C) Contrast-enhanced CT of a different patient shows bilateral symmetrically enlarged kidneys showing a prolonged striated nephrogram due to trapping of contrast in the medulla; (D) T2-weighted (T2W) MRI coronal and (E) axial images showing enlarged both kidneys with multiple focal areas of T2 hyperintensities with loss of corticomedullary differentiation. Note that associated abnormal signal intensity of liver due to hepatic fibrosis.

Imaging Features

Ultrasonography shows multiple cysts with normal renal size and echotexture **(Fig. 13A)** with sensitivity of 100%. Renal contour is typically normal early in life, becoming bosselated as more cysts develop.[31]

Intravenous urography shows smoothly marginated rounded, radiolucent defects in the nephrographic phase, leading to a "Swiss-cheese" pattern.

Contrast-enhanced computed tomography can readily show the nonenhancing hypodense cysts with intervening normally enhancing renal parenchyma and the associated cysts in the liver and pancreas **(Fig. 13B)**. Cysts can be complicated by hemorrhage, infection, calcification, and secondary calculi formation. MRI is useful in equivocal cases as it can reliably demonstrate hemorrhage within the cysts.

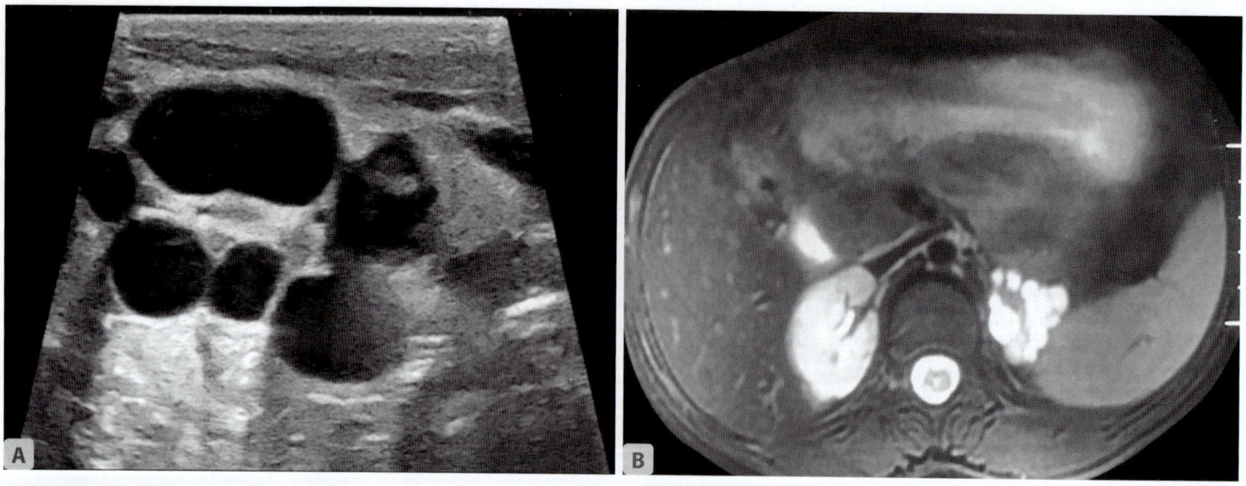

FIGS. 11A AND B: Multicystic dysplastic kidney. (A) USG shows variably sized, noncommunicating cysts separated by echogenic areas throughout the kidney; (B) T2W MRI axial image showing the multiple cysts replacing left kidney.

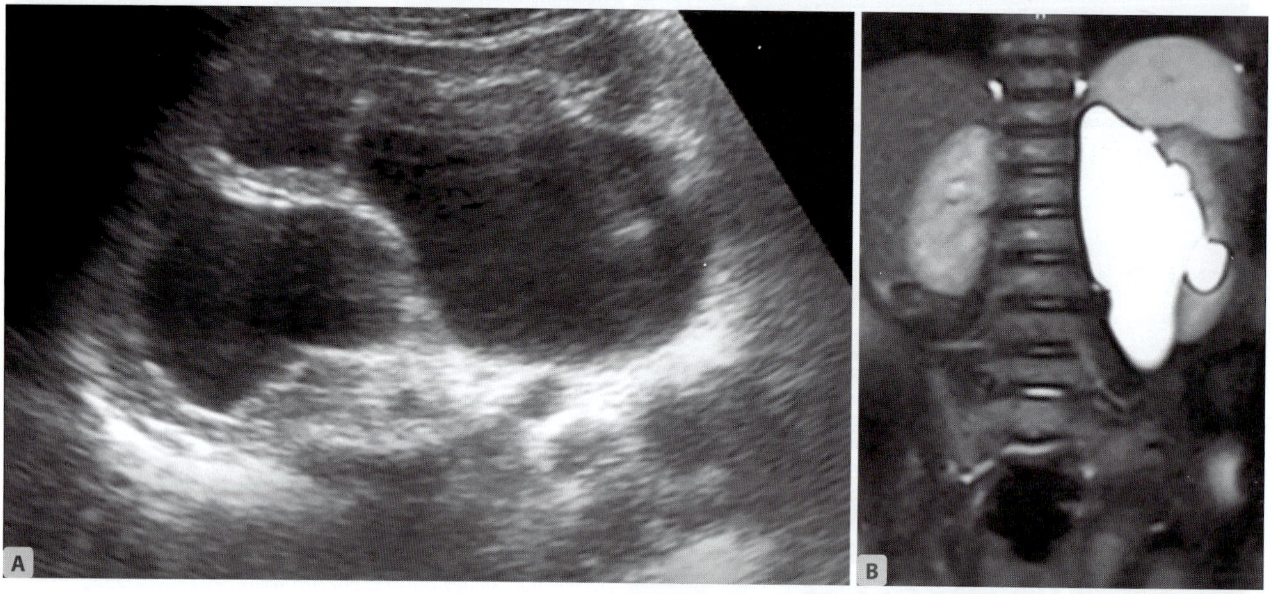

FIGS. 12A AND B: PUJ obstruction. (A) Longitudinal US scan of the kidney showing a central distended pelvis with rounded caudal margin which is connected to dilated calyces; (B) T2W MRI coronal image showing grossly dilated left renal pelvis out of proportion to the calyces and the calyces placed peripherally. Note absence of dilatation of ureter. (PUJ: pelviureteric junction; T2W: T2 weighted)

Pelviureteric Junction Obstruction

Idiopathic obstruction at the PUJ is the most common cause of neonatal hydronephrosis.[32] In more than half the cases obstruction is functional rather than anatomical.[33] Obstruction may also be due to an intrinsic stenosis of the PUJ.[34] PUJ obstruction may occur in a duplex system (almost always lower moiety), malrotated, horseshoe, and ectopic kidneys. In unilateral PUJ obstruction, the opposite kidney is sometimes absent, duplicated or dysplastic.[35]

Pelviureteric junction obstruction occurs more commonly in males than females and on the left side. There can be bilateral involvement in 10–30% of patients. Infants present with a palpable abdominal lump. Older children may present with intermittent abdominal pain with vomiting, hematuria, or urinary tract infection.

Imaging Features

On USG, the hydronephrotic kidney is often enlarged and contains dilated renal pelvis in the center, around which multiple cystic areas corresponding to the dilated calyces can be seen **(Fig. 12A)**. Ureter is not visualized.

Duplex Doppler can be used to differentiate obstructive from nonobstructive dilatation of the renal collecting system. A resistive index (RI) of >0.7 in the peripheral intrarenal arteries indicates obstructive dilatation. However, the RI value is age-dependent and in children <4 years of age the RI

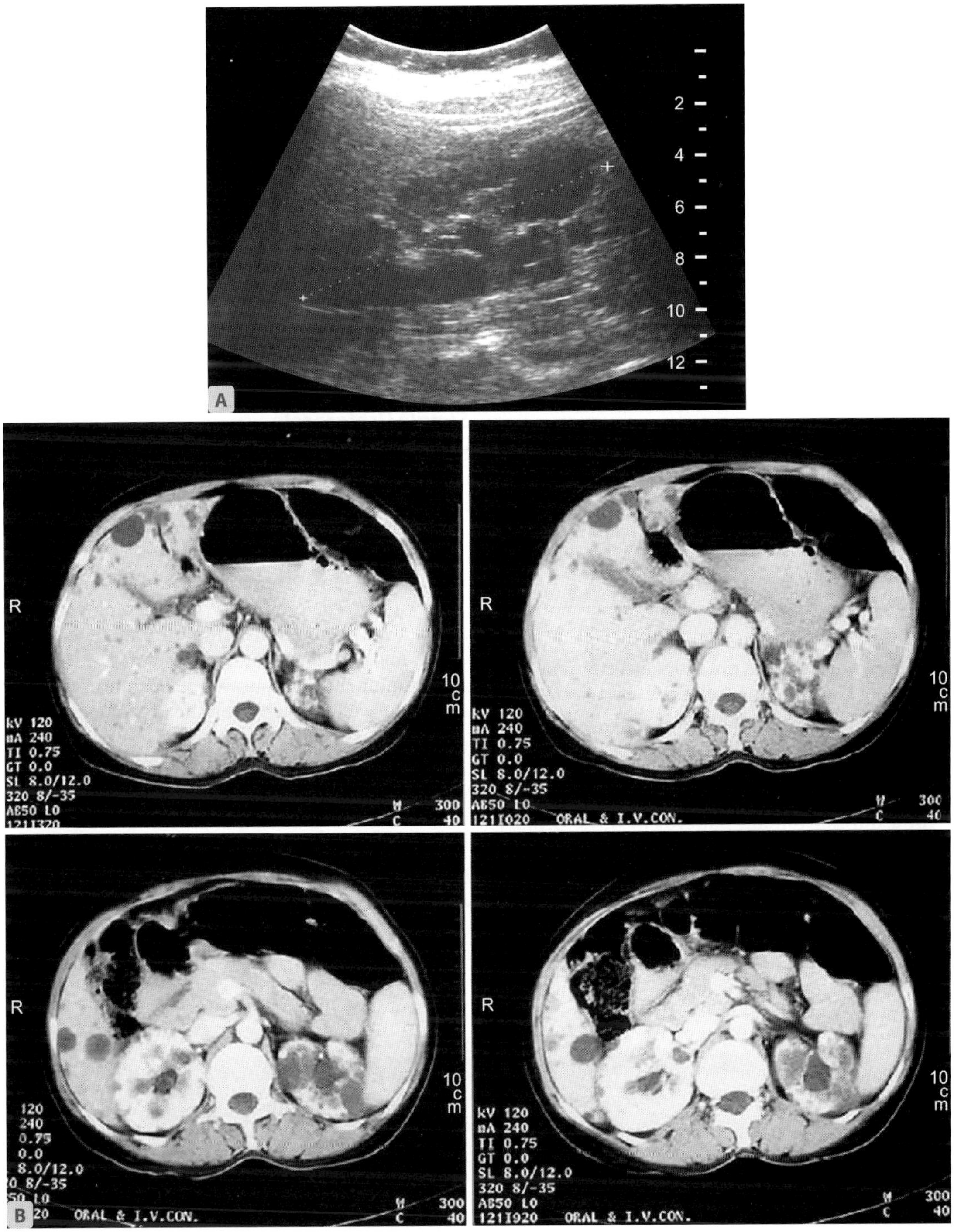

FIGS. 13A AND B: Autosomal dominant polycystic kidney. (A) USG shows multiple noncommunicating cysts; (B) Contrast-enhanced CT showing bilateral renal cysts and multiple cysts in liver. (USG: ultrasonography)

is normally >0.7. In these cases, the RI of the affected system can be compared with the opposite side.[36] Measurements of the resting RI and 10 minutes following intravenous frusemide can give better results. The postfrusemide study shows an increase in RI in both the obstructed and nonobstructed kidneys, but the obstructed kidney shows a significant increase of >0.1.[37]

On IVU, the classical PUJ obstruction presents with delayed opacification of the collecting system, marked pyelocaliectasis, narrowing at PUJ, incomplete visualization of ureter, and retention of contrast material in the collecting system on delayed films.[38,39]

The urographic appearance of PUJ obstruction varies depending upon the cause.[40,41] In most PUJ obstructions the extrarenal pelvis enlarges out of proportion to the degree of caliectasis.

Voiding cystourethrography is done in infants with PUJ obstruction to exclude coincidental reflux.[42] CT is needed in very few circumstances. CTU is the best method for assessing isthmus anatomy when PUJ obstruction involves a horseshoe kidney **(Figs. 8C and D)**. MRI can also be used to delineate the PUJ obstruction **(Fig. 12B)**.

Imaging has a role in postsurgical evaluation of PUJ obstruction. Edema at the PUJ anastomosis site frequently causes partial obstruction in the early postoperative period and gradual resolution takes place over days to weeks. Serial diuretic radionuclide renography is probably the most informative way to monitor urodynamics as long as renal function is satisfactory.[43]

Pelviureteric junction obstruction can be mimicked by prominent extrarenal pelvis and pathological obstruction at PUJ especially by calculus. Although the extrarenal pelvis appears distended, it tapers smoothly into the ureter with no evidence of hold-up of contrast **(Fig. 14)**. Calculus can be seen on CT scan obscured on IVU causing PUJ obstruction **(Fig. 15)**.

ANOMALIES OF THE URETER

Ectopic Ureter

An ectopic ureter is one that does not insert at its normal VUJ. Intravesical ectopia is not so common. Extravesical ectopia is more common and clinically important. It is more common in girls and is associated with a duplicated system in at least 85% of cases. It is the upper pole ureter that opens ectopically. In girls, the ectopic ureter presents with continuous leakage of urine with a normal voiding pattern. In boys, urinary incontinence is not a problem as the ectopic opening is above the strongly developed external sphincter of urethra.

Imaging Features

The pelvicalyceal system and ureter draining ectopically may be visualized on delayed films of an IVU. In female, it can open into the vagina or urethra **(Fig. 16A)**. USG is helpful if the anomalous ureter is dilated, in which case it can be followed down to and beyond the bladder **(Fig. 16B)**. In male, the ectopic opening can be seen in posterior urethra **(Fig. 16C)**. Recently, MRU has proved capable of displaying dilated collecting systems, ectopic ureters, and ureteroceles demonstrating ectopic extravesical ureteric insertions, thereby providing a global view of the malformation **(Figs. 17A to C)**.

Ureterocele

Ureterocele is a cystic dilatation of the intravesical segment of the ureter. It is of two types—(1) simple ureterocele and (2) ectopic ureterocele.

Simple Ureterocele

Simple ureterocele presents as a rounded cystic mass in the normal VUJ. It is more commonly bilateral and is seen in nonduplicated systems.

Imaging Features

The findings on IVU are characteristic. In the early films, the ureterocele is seen as a round, radiolucent defect at the trigone with well-defined smooth wall. As contrast collects within the bladder and in the ureterocele a radiolucent halo representing the nonopacified wall of the ureterocele is seen. This is the well-known "cobra head" appearance **(Fig. 18A)**. On USG, ureterocele may be seen as a cystic mass projecting into the lumen of the bladder and may show distension and collapse **(Fig. 18B)**.

Ectopic Ureterocele (Figs. 19 and 20)

Ectopic ureterocele is more common than the simple type and is unilateral in 90% of patients.[44] Ectopic ureterocele commonly occurs in a duplicated system and is almost always connected with the upper moiety ureter. The ectopic ureterocele represents the dilatation and protrusion of the

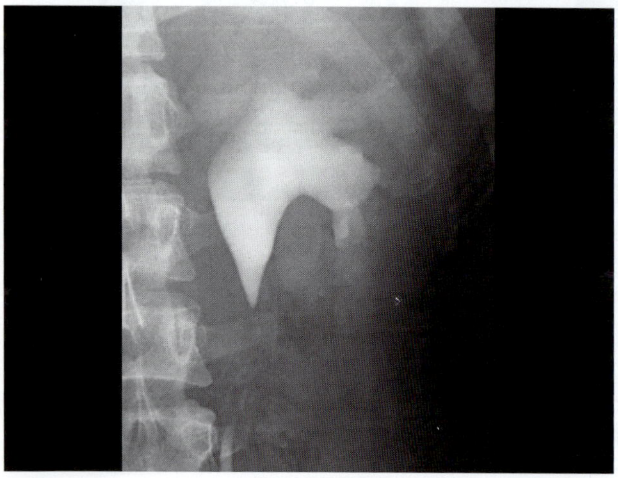

FIG. 14: Left extrarenal pelvis without obstruction. Though the pelvis appears distended, it tapers smoothly into the ureter with no evidence of hold-up of contrast.

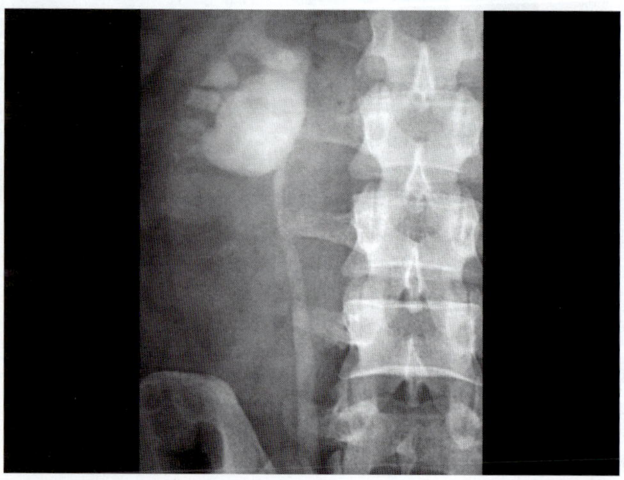

FIG. 15: PUJ obstruction mimic: IVU showing dilatation of right renal pelvis. The obstruction was due to a lucent PUJ calculus. (IVU: intravenous urography; PUJ: pelviureteric junction)

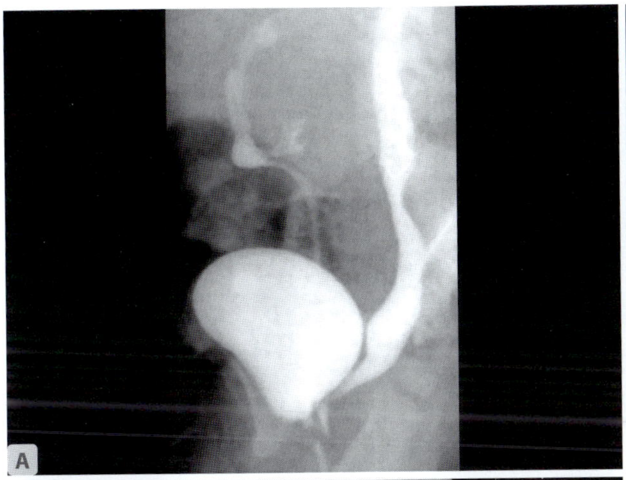

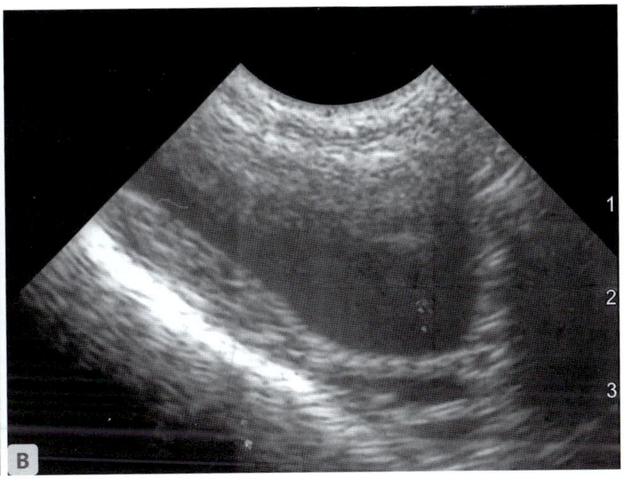

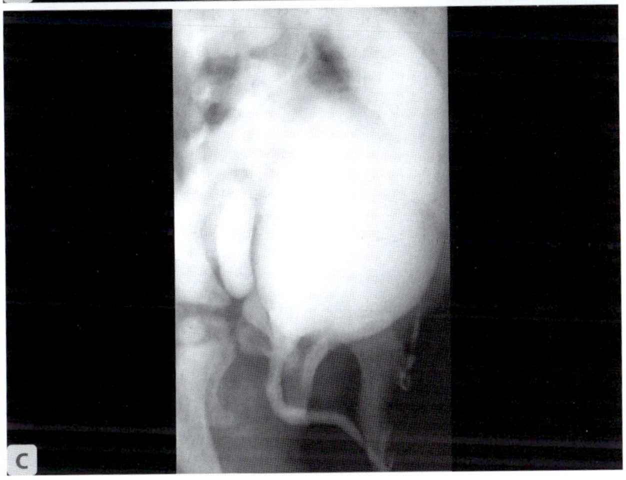

FIGS. 16A TO C: Ectopic ureter. (A) IVU in a female with history of urinary dribbling showing left dilated ureter opening below the location of VUJ into vagina; (B) Ultrasonography of the same patient showing the fluid (urine)-filled vagina posterior to the urinary bladder into which ureter could be traced; (C) IVU in a male showing right ureter opening ectopically into the prostatic urethra. (IVU: intravenous urography; VUJ: vesicoureteric junction)

entire submucosal segment of the ureter into the lumen of the bladder and at the bladder neck.

Imaging Features

On USG, the ureterocele is seen as an intravesical cystic lesion (cyst within cyst). Ipsilateral kidney may reveal "duplex system" **(Fig. 19A)**. On IVU, ureterocele is usually seen as a rounded and eccentric filling defect at the base of the urinary bladder **(Fig. 19B)**. The outline of the ureterocele is usually clearly defined by the contrast material except for its lower margin which is confluent with the bladder base and bladder neck **(Figs. 19C and D)**. This is in contrast to the simple ureterocele which is intravesical and therefore completely outlined. Cecoureterocele is an ectopic ureterocele which has a broad base and is located more inferiorly in the bladder and extends into the bladder neck area or urethra **(Figs. 20A and B)**.

Primary Megaureter

Primary megaureter is an uncommon, nonhereditary lesion caused by an adynamic distal segment that prevents normal and caudal progression of ureteral peristalsis.

On IVU, the dilated ureter tapers smoothly but abruptly just above the ureterovesical junction. Even when the entire ureter is affected, the lower third shows greatest dilatation **(Fig. 21A)**.

Real-time USG shows disproportionately greater dilatation of the lower ureter, hyperperistalsis with to and fro movement of urine, and the relatively narrowed adynamic distal segment **(Fig. 21B)**. VCUG should always be performed to make sure VUR is not the major cause of a wide ureter.[45]

Magnetic resonance urography is also useful to delineate the dilated ureters and MR fluoroscopy can be used to demonstrate the adynamic distal segment **(Fig. 21C)**.

ANOMALIES OF THE URINARY BLADDER

Complete Duplication

Complete duplication of the urinary bladder is extremely rare.[46] Two bladders lie side by side with separate urethra **(Figs. 22A and B)**. Bladder may be compartmentalized into two parts by a septum in the sagittal or coronal plane. In female, bladder duplication may be associated with

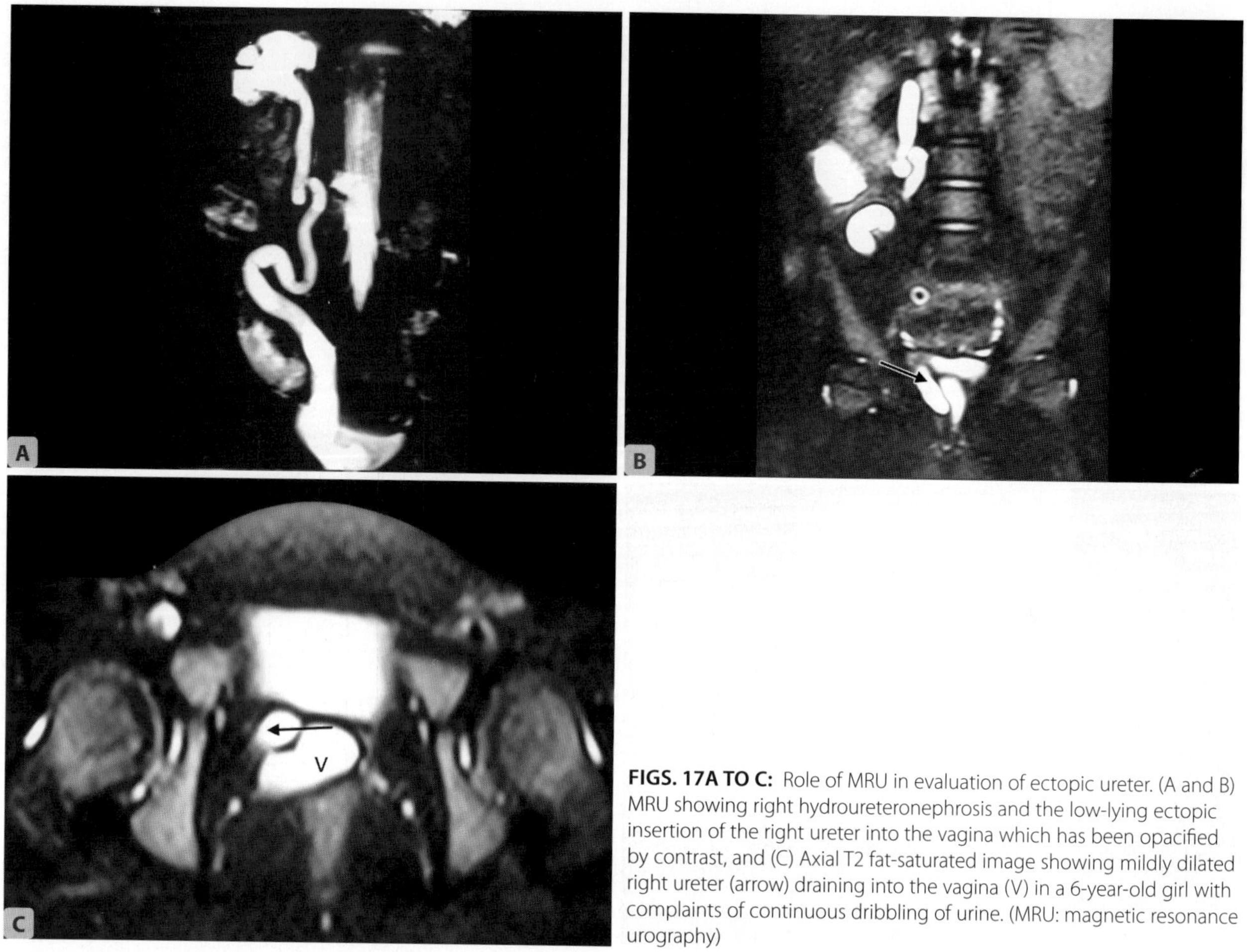

FIGS. 17A TO C: Role of MRU in evaluation of ectopic ureter. (A and B) MRU showing right hydroureteronephrosis and the low-lying ectopic insertion of the right ureter into the vagina which has been opacified by contrast, and (C) Axial T2 fat-saturated image showing mildly dilated right ureter (arrow) draining into the vagina (V) in a 6-year-old girl with complaints of continuous dribbling of urine. (MRU: magnetic resonance urography)

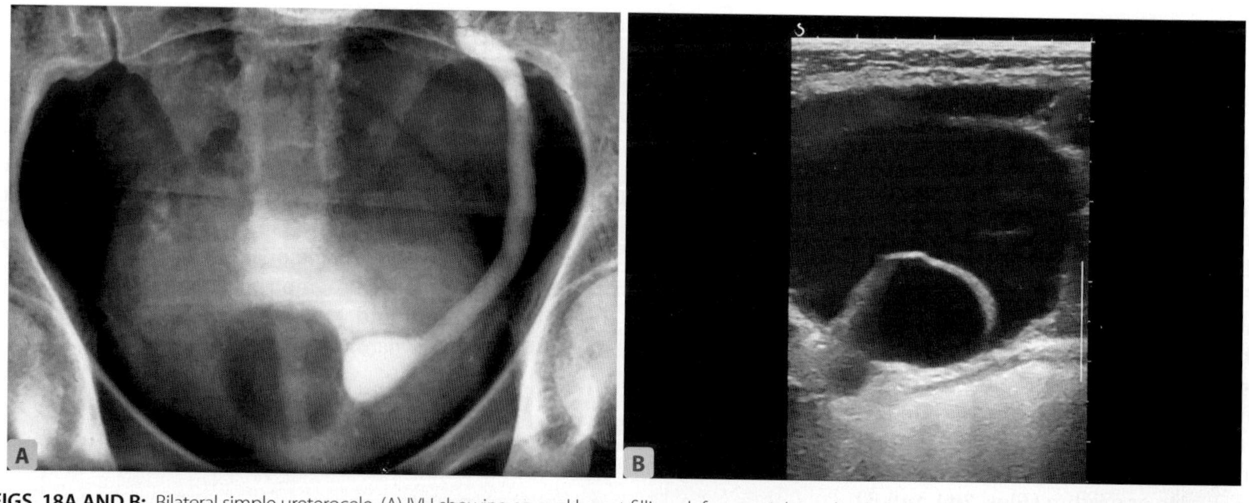

FIGS. 18A AND B: Bilateral simple ureterocele. (A) IVU showing an oval lucent filling defect on right and radiolucent halo around contrast-filled dilated lower end left ureter, representing nonopacified ureterocele on right and classical "cobra head" appearance on the left side; (B) Ultrasonography of urinary bladder showing ureterocele as cystic lesion with thin wall at the UVJ. Ureterocele shows contraction and expansion on real-time USG. Corresponding ureter can be traced into it. (IVU: intravenous urography; USG: ultrasonography; UVJ: ureterovesical junction)

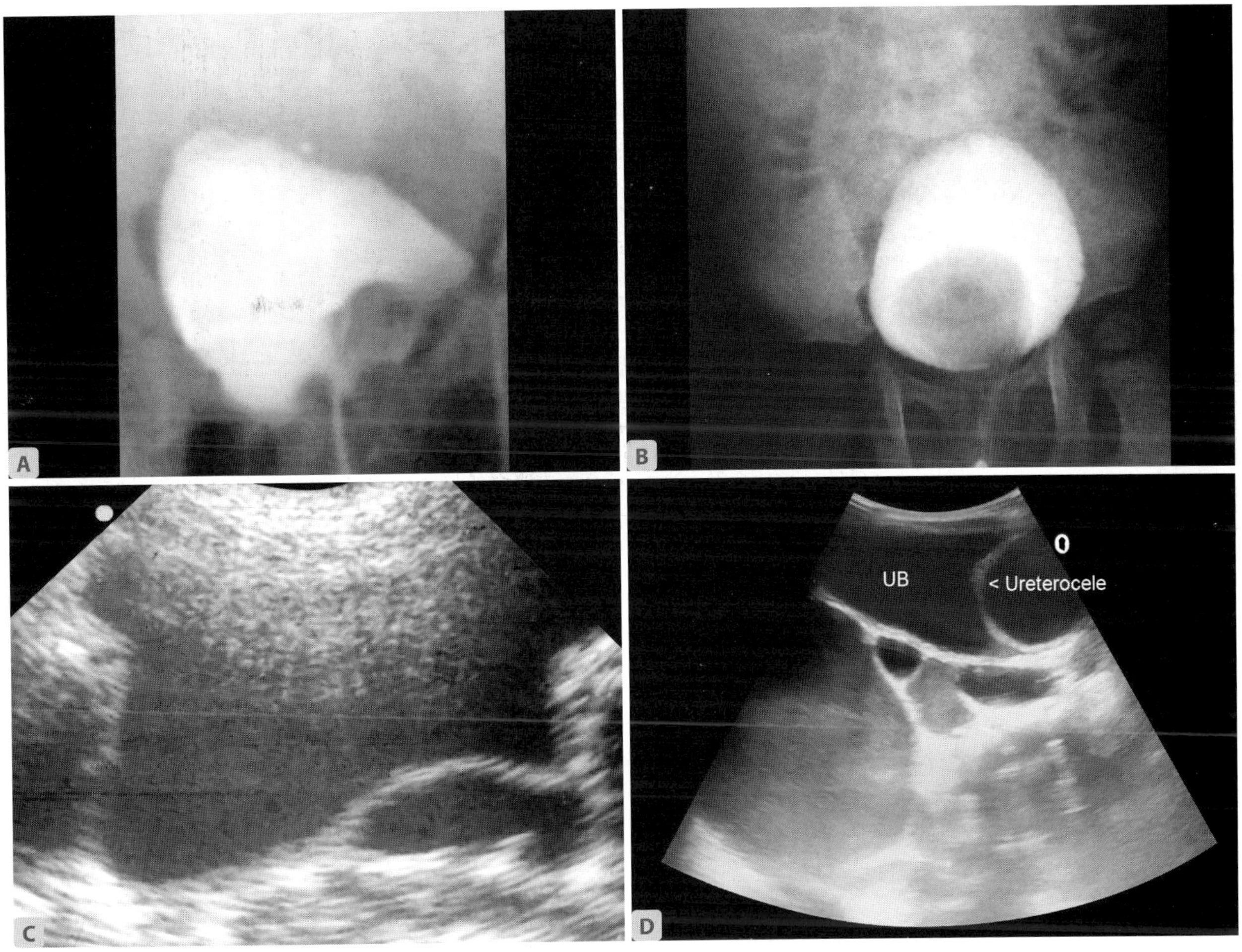

FIGS. 19A TO D: Ectopic ureterocele. (A and B) Contrast-filled bladder in two cases shows the ureterocele as a well-defined filling defect confluent with and reaching up to the bladder base. Note the ill-defined border inferolaterally in (A). Ultrasonography (C) and (D) showing a cystic structure close to urinary bladder marked as "ureterocele" in (D) cyst within cyst appearance.

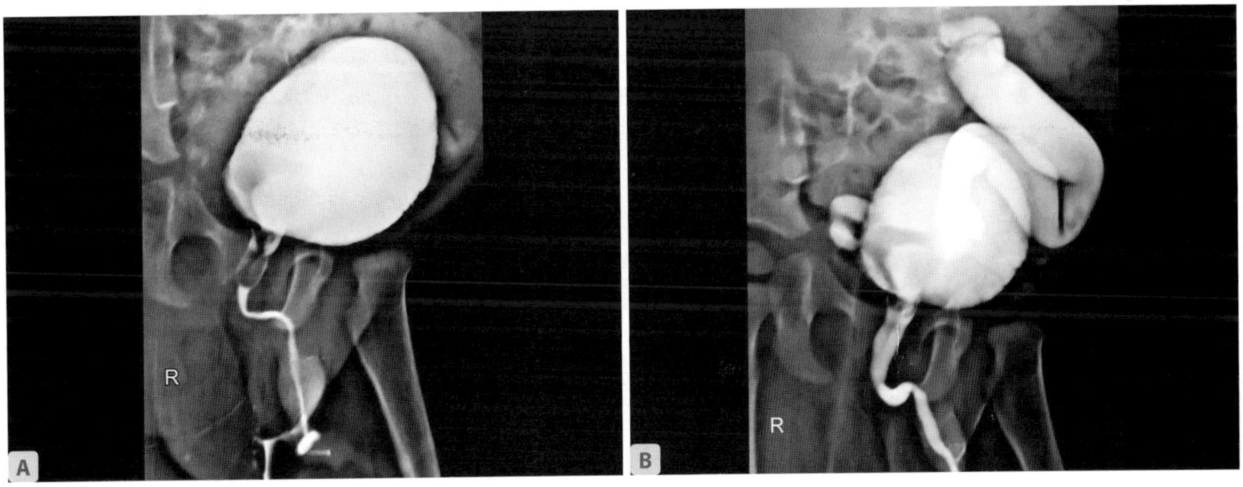

FIGS. 20A AND B: Ectopic ureterocele: Cecoureterocele. (A) Micturating film showing the relation of the filling defect-like structure with the posterior urethra; (B) Dilated left ureter associated with the ectopic ureterocele is also seen. This is a form of vesicourethral ureterocele known as "Cecoureterocele".

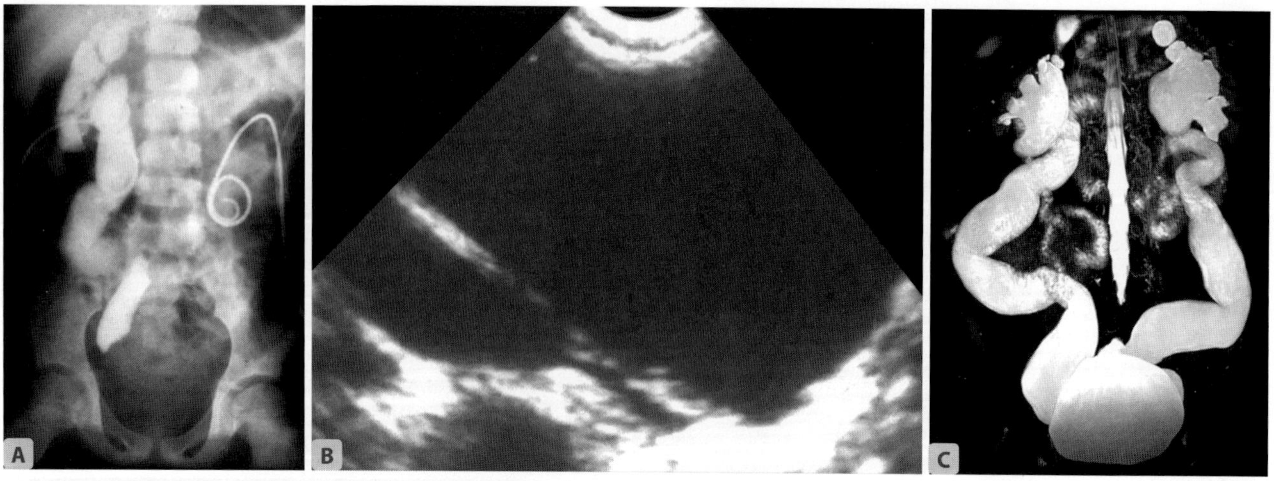

FIGS. 21A TO C: Primary megaureter. (A) Antegrade contrast study right side showing hydroureteronephrosis till the lower end which is tapered. Note that contrast has not entered urinary bladder; (B) Ultrasonography showing the dilated right ureter with narrow distal segment which did not show peristalsis on real-time USG, features consistent with primary megaureter; (C) MRU in a different patient showing grossly dilated aperistaltic (confirmed on MR fluoroscopy) ureters suggestive of primary megaureter. (MRU: magnetic resonance urography; USG: ultrasonography)

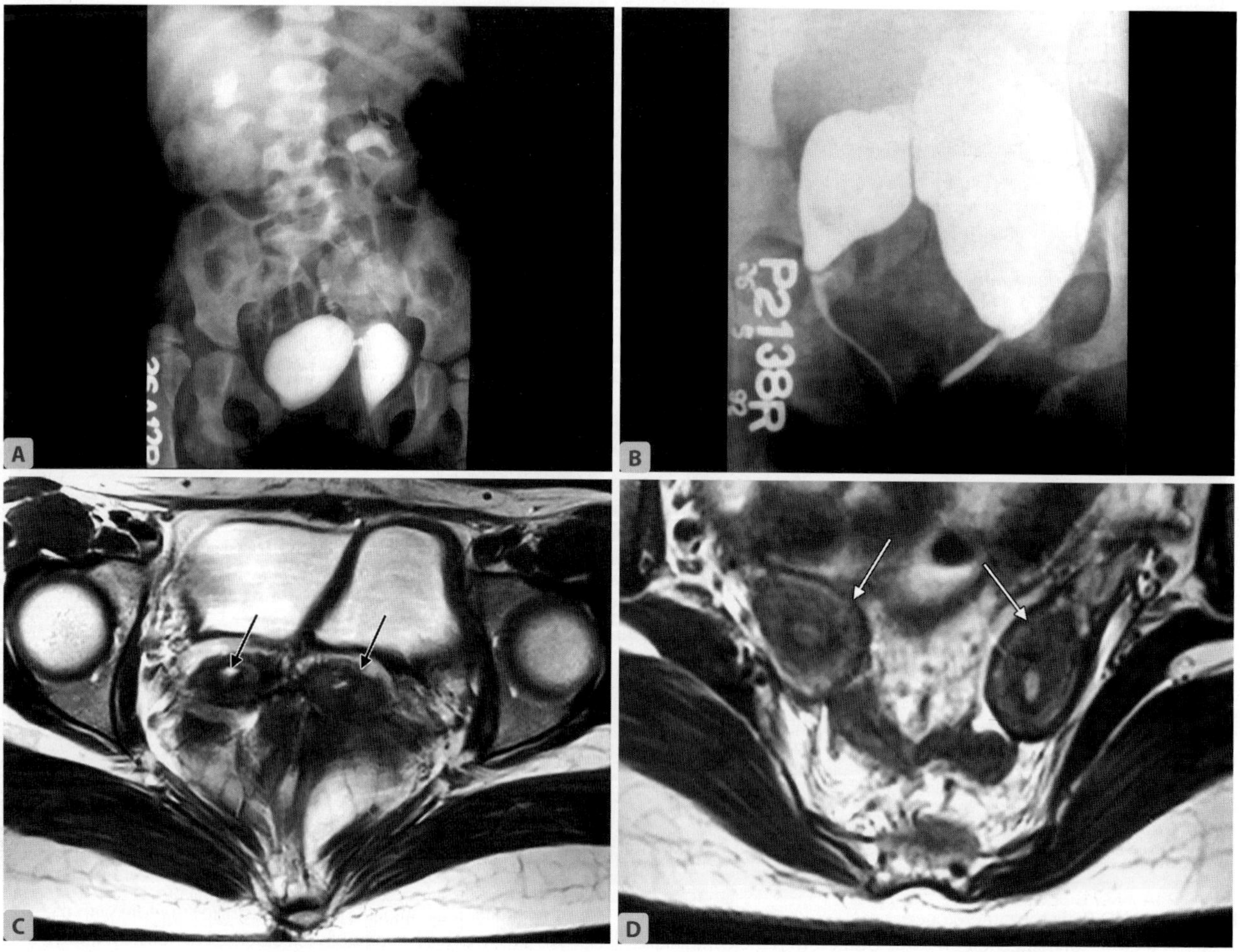

FIGS. 22A TO D: Bladder duplication. (A) IVU in a male showing complete duplication of the urinary bladder in the sagittal plane; (B) MCU showing both the bladders having separate urethrae. MRI of a female patient (C and D) showing duplication of urinary bladder along with complete duplication of uterus (arrow). (IVU: intravenous urography; MCU: micturating cystourethrography)

duplication of uterus and both these anomalies can be seen nicely on MRI **(Figs. 22C and D)**.

Bladder Exstrophy

Exstrophy is the most common anomaly of the urinary bladder.[47] In its most severe manifestation, the rectus abdominus muscle is widely separated and bladder lies open and everted on the anterior abdominal wall. With an associated epispadias, the urethral mucosa covers the dorsum of a short penis and the urethra opens on the dorsal surface of the penis. Plain radiograph of abdomen and pelvis demonstrates diastasis of the symphysis pubis **(Fig. 23A)**. On micturating cystourethrography (MCU), there is associated VUR **(Fig. 23B)**.

Bladder Diverticulae

Most bladder diverticulae are localized outpouchings of the bladder mucosa between fibers of the detrussor muscles (pseudo-diverticulae). Bladder diverticulae may be primary (idiopathic) or secondary.

Primary or idiopathic diverticulae are the most common, can occur anywhere but most frequently in the trigonal areas. A common type of bladder diverticulum, referred to as paraureteral diverticulum or "Hutch diverticulum", is located laterally and cephalad to the ureteral orifice **(Fig. 24)**. In male infants, bladder diverticulum must be distinguished from bilateral protrusion of the urinary bladder into the inguinal rings anteriorly. These outpouchings also called "bladder ears" are transient and disappear with growth. Secondary diverticulae develop as a result of chronically increased intravesical pressure and are seen mostly in patients with posterior urethral valves.

Bladder diverticulae are best imaged by contrast cystography, USG, and CT.

Neurogenic Bladder

Neurogenic bladder is most often seen with myelomeningocele or a related myelodysplastic anomaly (occult spinal dysraphism, sacral agenesis). The radiographs of the affected area may show spina bifida and widened interpedicular distance with defective pedicles.[48]

On VCUG, bladder is usually elongated pointing upward (Christmas tree shape) with varying degrees of trabeculation and sacculation **(Fig. 25A)**. On USG, the bladder shows multiple diverticuli and sacculations of the wall **(Fig. 25B)**. During voiding, bladder neck is wide (in contrast to PUV) with dilatation of proximal posterior urethra, forming a funnel shape. Distal urinary stream is usually poor with significant postvoid residual urine. Associated VUR is common.

Prune Belly Syndrome

Prune belly syndrome is a rare congenital syndrome usually affecting the males characterized by lax, wrinkled abdominal wall, which is frequently associated with undescended testis and urinary tract anomalies.[49] On VCUG, bladder is enlarged and elongated but lacks trabeculations and dilated high placed posterior urethra is a characteristic finding **(Figs. 26A to C)**.

Urachal Anomalies

Failure of the urachus to regress may result in congenital anomalies, viz., patent urachus, urachal cyst, urachal sinus, and urachal diverticulum.[50] The diagnosis of patent urachus can be made either by catheterization of the bladder through the umbilicus or by VCUG with films taken in lateral projection. Diagnosis of urachal sinus is made by catheterization and opacification of the umbilical fistula. Urachal diverticulum is demonstrated by VCUG with films in lateral projection

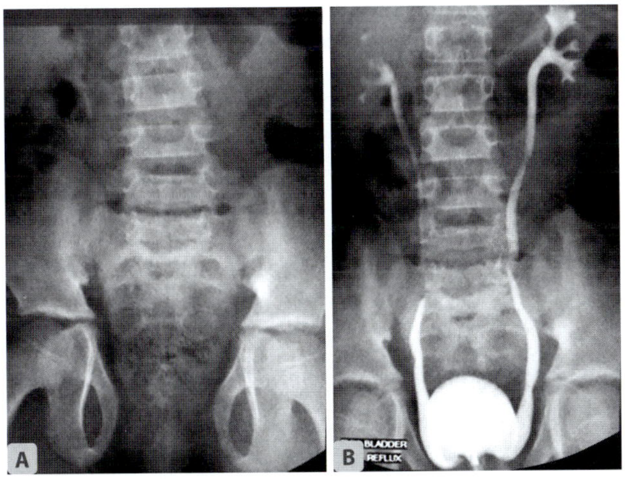

FIGS. 23A AND B: Exstrophy of the bladder. (A) Plain radiograph showing classical diastasis of symphysis pubis; (B) MCU showing small capacity postoperative bladder with bilateral VUR. (MCU: micturating cystourethrography; VUR: vesicoureteral reflux)

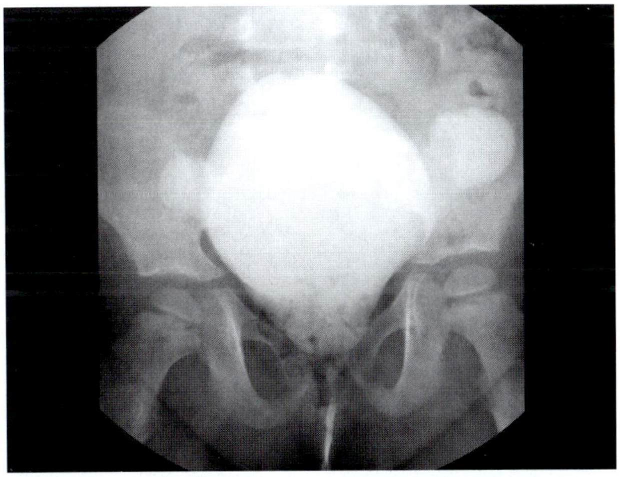

FIG. 24: Hutch diverticulum: MCU showing bilateral ear-like contrast-filled paraureteric (Hutch) diverticulae. (MCU: micturating cystourethrography)

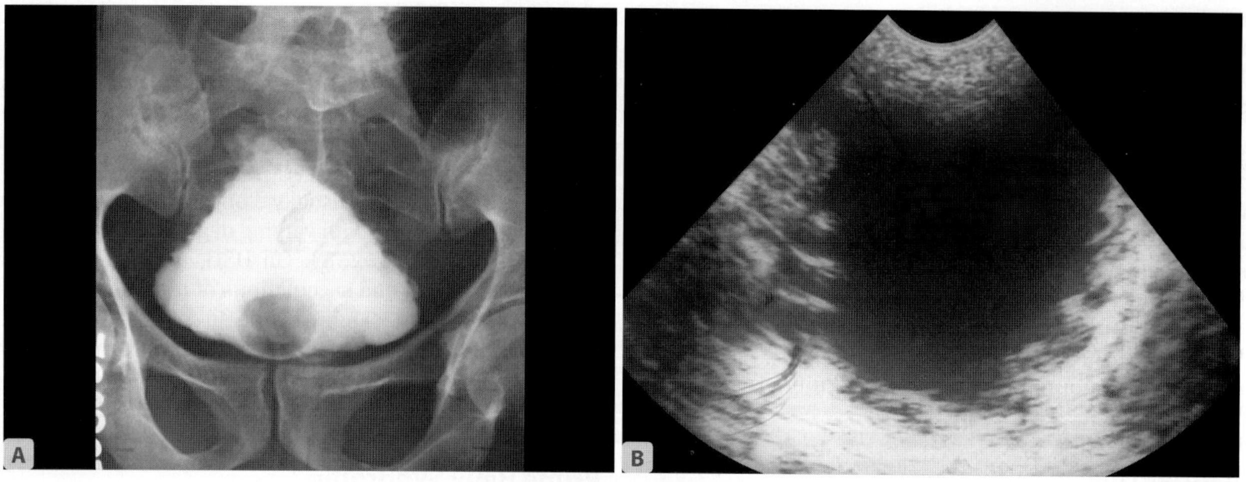

FIGS. 25A AND B: Neurogenic bladder. (A) VCUG showing small capacity urinary bladder which is elongated upward with trabeculations and sacculations (Christmas tree or pinecone shape). Note is made of spina bifida at L5 vertebra; (B) USG showing multiple diverticuli and sacculations of the bladder wall. (VCUG: voiding cystourethrography)

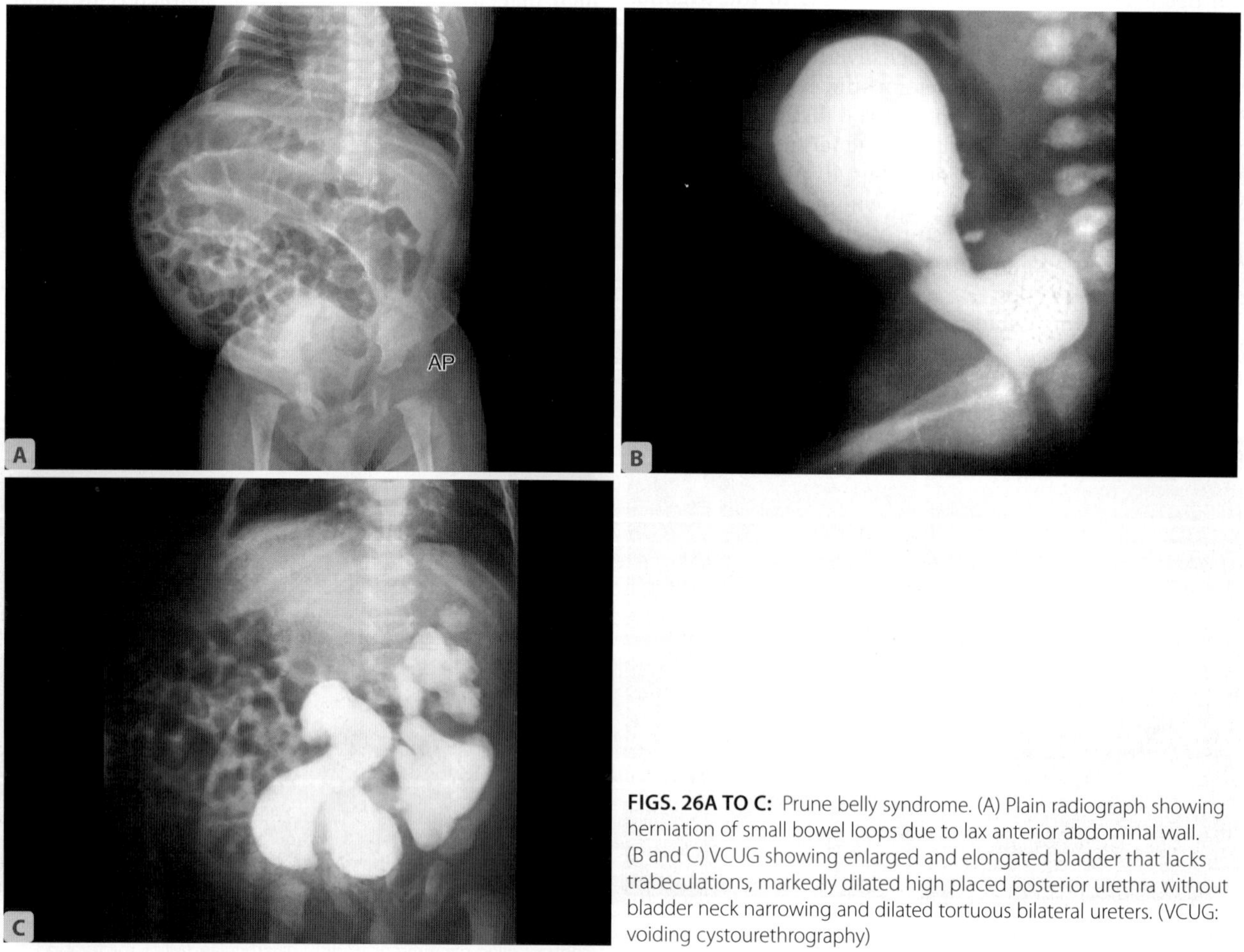

FIGS. 26A TO C: Prune belly syndrome. (A) Plain radiograph showing herniation of small bowel loops due to lax anterior abdominal wall. (B and C) VCUG showing enlarged and elongated bladder that lacks trabeculations, markedly dilated high placed posterior urethra without bladder neck narrowing and dilated tortuous bilateral ureters. (VCUG: voiding cystourethrography)

(Fig. 27). Diagnosis of urachal cysts is more difficult. The cystogram may show only an extrinsic compression on the dome of the bladder in the midline or slightly to one side. US, CT, or MRI may demonstrate the lesion better.

ABNORMALITIES OF THE URETHRA

Posterior Urethral Valve

Posterior urethral valve is the most common congenital obstructive lesion of the urethra leading to end-stage renal disease in boys. Three types of PUVs have been recognized based on urethroscopic findings.[51]

The most common form of PUV is *Type I characterized by* two fibroepithelial valve-like folds which originate from the lower pole of the verumontanum and course obliquely to the most distal portion of the prostatic urethra. The 2-folds fuse anteriorly, leaving a cleft as the only passage for urine. *Type II and III are rare.*

Imaging Features

Voiding cystourethrography is the gold standard for imaging PUV. On voiding films, the posterior urethra is markedly dilated and elongated down to the level of PUV. The transition between the dilated posterior and anterior normal urethra is abrupt with a thin stream **(Fig. 28A)**. Urethral polyp can mimic PUV. The valves may be seen as two radiolucent lines. Classic PUV is not visible on a retrograde urethrogram since the valves are displaced and flattened against the urethral wall by the retrograde flow of contrast.

Secondary obstructive changes of varying severity develop in the bladder, ureters, and kidneys. The bladder becomes hypertrophied and trabeculated and develops saccules and diverticulae. There is bladder neck hypertrophy seen as narrowing on VCUG. In approximately 50% of patients, VUR **(Fig. 28B)** may be present.[52]

Ultrasonography is a valuable modality for evaluation of PUV. Mid-line sagittal scans of the base of the bladder through suprapubic approach or through perineum may show dilatation of the proximal posterior urethra.[53] Upper tract changes are better seen on USG. The prenatal USG may reveal bilateral hydroureteronephrosis, thickened bladder wall, and a dilated posterior urethra in sagittal scans (Keyhole sign).[54] Fetal MRI is the best imaging test for antenatal diagnosis in late gestation.[55]

Male Hypospadias/Epispadias

Hypospadias is a condition in which the urethral meatus opens on the ventral surface of the penis at a point proximal to the glans. In epispadias, the urethral orifice is located on the dorsal aspect of the penis. Epispadias is usually seen in association with various forms of exstrophy. In either, hypospadias or epispadias, VCUG demonstrates a foreshortened urethra. MRI may be useful as it can evaluate the status of the phallus.

Anterior Urethral Diverticulum and Anterior Urethral Valve

Anterior urethral diverticulum is a saccular outpouching of the ventral aspect of the anterior urethra commonly near penoscrotal junction. The diverticulum has a well-defined valve such as anterior lip and a less well-defined posterior lip. On VCUG, the typical saccular diverticulum of the anterior urethra fills with contrast material and appears as an oval-shaped structure on the ventral aspect of anterior urethra **(Figs. 29A and B)**. At times, RGU may be required to demonstrate the neck of the diverticulum.

Anterior urethral valve is a semilunar fold similar to anterior lip of a urethral diverticulum with absence of posterior lip. VCUG is the diagnostic modality of choice

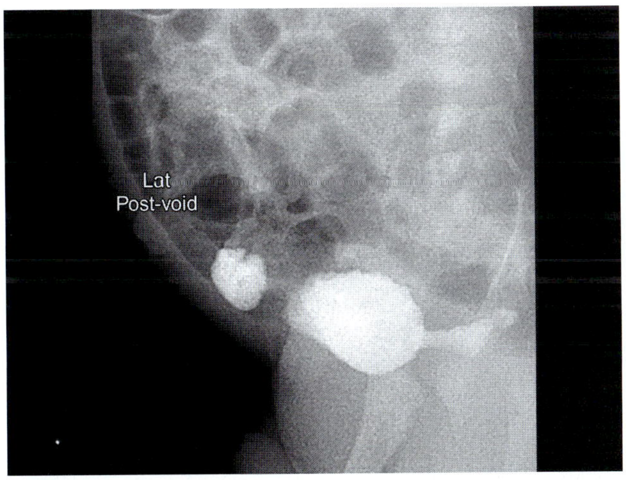

FIG. 27: Urachal diverticulum: Blind-ending dilated urachus seen at the anterior superior aspect of the bladder.

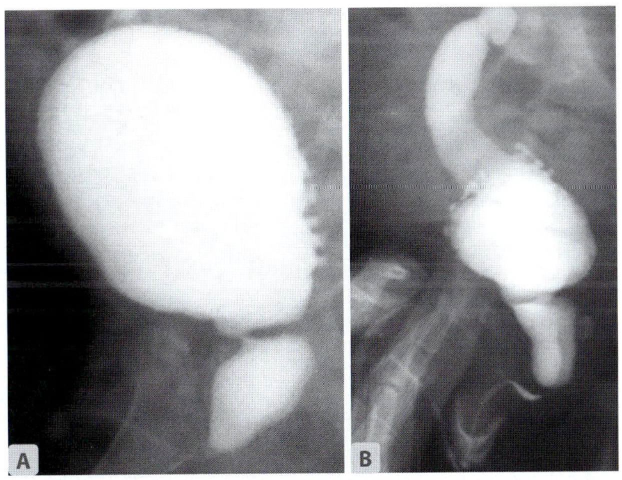

FIGS. 28A AND B: Posterior urethral valve. (A) MCU showing markedly dilated posterior urethra with bladder neck hypertrophy (seen as narrowing) and thin stream of contrast in anterior urethra. Bladder shows back pressure changes of multiple saccules and diverticulae; (B) Another patient with similar changes along with reflux into dilated right ureter. (MCU: micturating cystourethrography)

for anterior urethral valves. Typically, the urethra appears dilated proximal to the valve and narrowed distal to it. A valve may appear as a linear filling defect along the ventral wall, or it may be indicated by an abrupt change in the caliber of the dilated urethra.

Urethral Duplication

Urethral duplication may be complete or incomplete and may take several forms.[56] Two separate structures may originate from the bladder and persist with separate external drainage; a common urethra may originate from the bladder and duplicate distally; or a duplicated origin may unite distally into a single external orifice.[56,57] The diagnosis is made by VCUG or catheterization and opacification of both the urethras. The phallus could be one containing two urethras or duplicated with one urethra in each phallus **(Figs. 30A and B)**.

Megalourethra

Megalourethra is a rare anomaly in which abnormal development of the corpus spongiosum and corpus cavernosum results in congenital dilatation of penile urethra without obstruction. The penile urethra is seen markedly dilated and fusiform, with tapering both distally and proximally into a relatively normal urethra. Scaphoid megalourethra is more common than fusiform type. On US, scaphoid type appears as a localized saccular dilatation of the penile urethra caused by a localized absence of the corpus spongiosum **(Fig. 31A)**. On VCUG, the affected part of urethra balloons markedly causing a large smooth bulge on the ventral surface of the urethra assuming a scaphoid configuration **(Fig. 31B)**.[58]

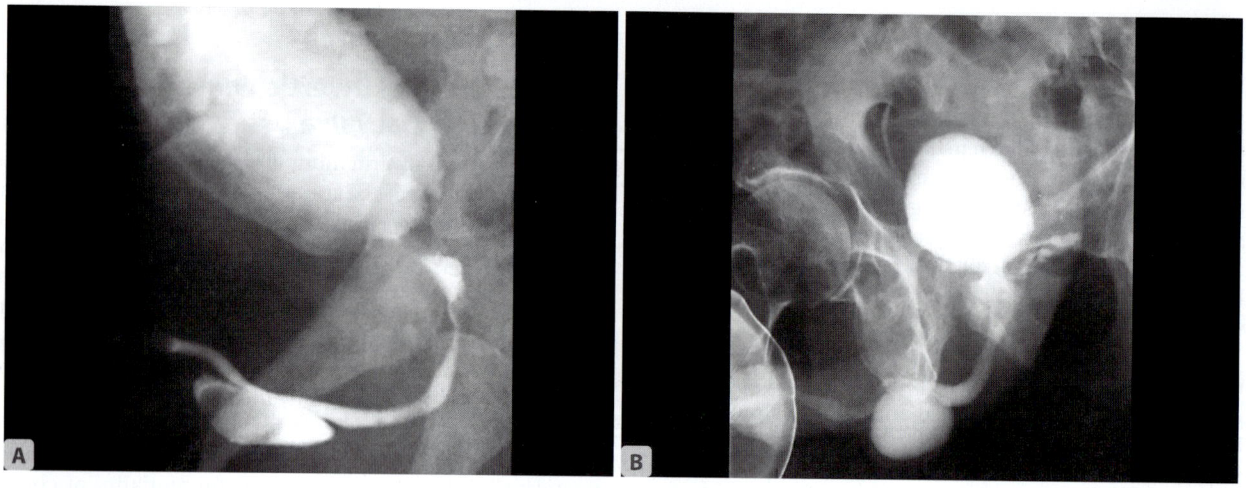

FIGS. 29A AND B: Anterior urethral diverticulum. (A and B) VCUG in two different patients showing relatively narrow neck diverticulum on the ventral aspect of the anterior urethrae. (VCUG: voiding cystourethrography)

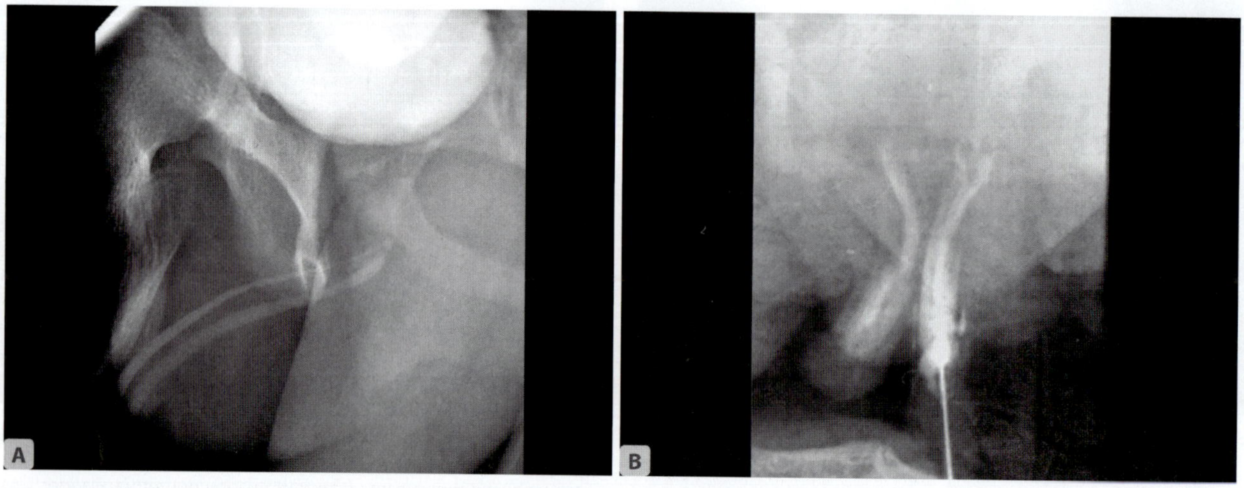

FIGS. 30A AND B: Urethral duplication. (A) MCU showing duplication of urethra within a single phallus; (B) Another patient showing complete duplication of phallus and urethra. (MCU: micturating cystourethrography)

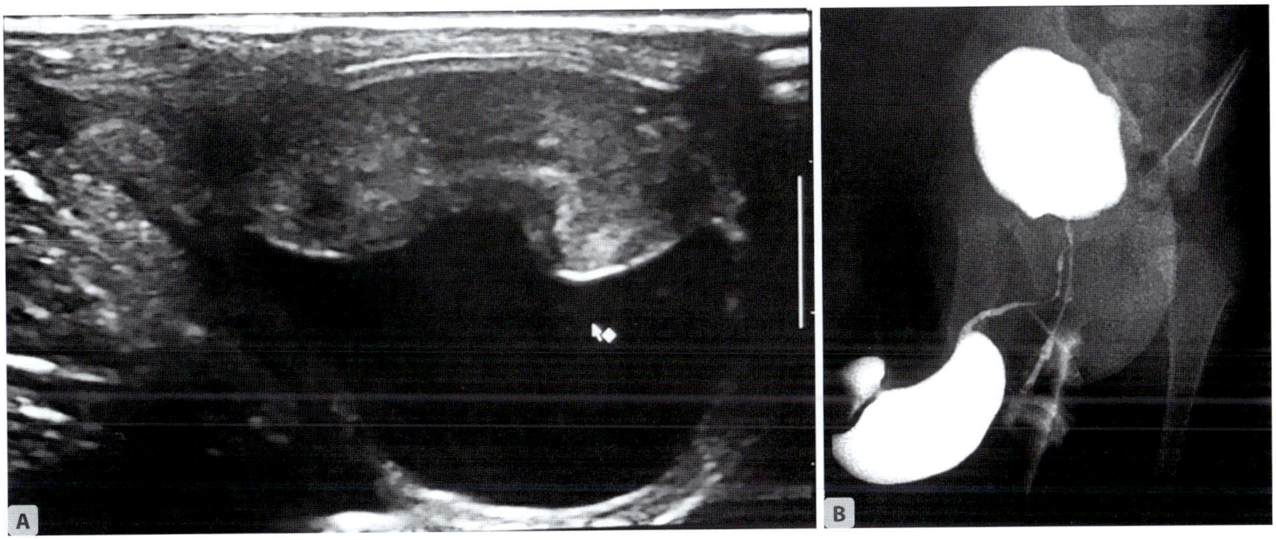

FIGS. 31A AND B: Megalourethra. (A) USG showing a cystic lesion in penile shaft with defect in spongiosa; (B) VCUG showing a broad-based contrast-filled dilated structure in relation to penile urethra suggestive of scaphoid type of megalourethra. The broad base differentiates it from diverticulum which has a narrow neck. (VCUG: voiding cystourethrography)

REFERENCES

1. Steinhardt JM, Kuhn LP, Eisenberg B. Ultrasound screening of healthy infants for urinary tract abnormalities. Pediatrics. 1988;82:609-12.
2. Kraus SJ. Genitourinary Imaging in Children in Pediatric Urology. Pediatr Clin North Am. 2001;48:1381-424.
3. Johnson CE, Elder JS, Judge NE, Adeeb FN, Grisoni ER, Fattlar DC. The accuracy of antenatal ultrasonography in identifying renal abnormalities. Am J Dis Child. 1992;186(10):1181-4.
4. Harvie S, McLeod L, Acott P, Walsh E, Abdolell M, Macken MB. Abnormal antenatal sonogram: An indicator of disease severity in children with posterior urethral valves. Can Assoc Radiol J. 2009;60(4):185-9.
5. Payabvash S, Kajbafzadeh AM, Saeedi P, Sadeghi Z, Elmi A, Mehdizadeh M. Application of magnetic resonance urography in diagnosis of congenital urogenital anomalies in children. Pediatr Surg Int. 2008;24(9):979-86.
6. Staatz G, Rohrmann D, Nolte-Ernsting CC, Stollbrink C, Haage P, Schmidt T, et al. Magnetic resonance urography in children: Evaluation of suspected ureteral ectopia in duplex systems. J Urol. 2001;166:2346-50.
7. Perez-Brayfield MR, Kirsch AJ, Jones RA, Grattan-Smith JD. A prospective study comparing ultrasound, nuclear scintigraphy and dynamic contrast enhanced magnetic resonance imaging in the evaluation of hydronephrosis. J Urol. 2003;170:1330-4.
8. Grattan-Smith JD, Jones RA. MR urography in children. Pediatr Radiol. 2006;36:1119-32.
9. Grobner T. Gadolinium—a specific trigger for the development of nephrogenic fibrosing dermopathy and nephrogenic systemic fibrosis? Nephrol Dial Transplant. 2006;21:1104-8.
10. Brody AS, Frush DP, Huda W, Brent RL, American Academy of Pediatrics Section on Radiology. Radiation risk to children from computed tomography. Pediatrics. 2007;120:677-82.
11. Han BK, Babcock DS. Sonographic measurements and appearances of normal kidneys in children. AJR Am J Roentgenol. 1985;185:611-6.
12. De Brugn R, Gordon I, Mc Hugh K. Pediatric Uroradiology. In: Grainger RG, Allison D (Eds). Diagnostic Radiology: A Textbook of Medical Imaging. New York: Churchill Livingstone; 2001. pp. 1717-64.
13. Sadler TW (Ed). Langman's Medical Embryology, 9th edition. Philadelphia, PA: Lippincott Williams and Wilkins; 2004.
14. Trigaux JP, Van Beers B, Delchambre F. Male genital tract malformations associated with ipsilateral renal agenesis: Sonographic findings: J Clin Ultrasound. 1991;19:3-10.
15. Shalaby-Rana E, Lowe LH, Blask AN, Majd M. Imaging in pediatric urology. Pediatr Clin North Am. 1997;44:1065-89.
16. Jefferson KP, Persad RA. Thoracic kidney: a rare form of renal ectopia. J Urol. 2001;165(2):504.
17. Pennington DJ, Zerin JM. Imaging of the urinary tract in children. Pediatr Ann. 1999;28:678-86.
18. Glodny B, Petersen J, Hofmann KJ, Schenk C, Herwig R, Trieb T, et al. Kidney fusion anomalies revisited: Clinical and radiological analysis of 209 cases of crossed fused ectopia and horseshoe kidney. BJU Int. 2009;103(2):224-35.
19. Solanki S, Bhatnagar V, Gupta AK, Kumar R. Crossed fused renal ectopia: Challenges in diagnosis and management. J Indian Assoc Pediatr Surg. 2013;18:7-10.
20. Bégin LR, Guy L, Jacobson SA, Aprikian AG. Renal carcinoid and horseshoe kidney: A frequent association of the two rare entities—a case report and review of the literature. J Surg Oncol. 1998;68:113-9.
21. Strauss S. Sonographic features of horseshoe kidney. J Ultrasound Med. 2000;19(1):27-31.
22. Pozniak MA, Nakada SY. Three-dimensional computed tomographic angiography of a horseshoe kidney with ureteropelvic junction obstruction. Urology. 1997;49(2):267-8.
23. El-Nahas AR, Abou El-Ghar ME, Refae HF, Gad HM, El-Diasty TA. Magnetic resonance imaging in the evaluation of pelvi-ureteric junction obstruction: An all-in-one approach. BJU Int. 2007;99(3):641-5.

24. Tokunaka S, Osanai H, Hashimoto H, Takamura T, Yachiku S, Mori Y. Severe hypertension in infant with unilateral hypoplastic kidney. Urology. 1987;29:618-20.
25. Osathanondh V, Potter EL. Pathogenesis of polycystic kidneys. Survey of results of microdissection. Arch Pathol. 1964;77:510-2.
26. Avni FE, Garel C, Cassart M, D'Haene N, Hall M, Riccabona M. Imaging and classification of congenital cystic renal diseases. AJR Am J Roentgenol. 2012;198(5):1004-13.
27. Gupta AK, Berry M. Recessive polycystic kidney disease and congenital hypertrophic pyloric stenosis. Pediatric Radiol. 1991;21:160.
28. Srivastava T, Garola RE, Hellerstein S. Autosomal dominant inheritance of multicystic dysplastic kidney. Pediatr Nephrol. 1999;13(6):481-3.
29. Kaneyama K, Yamataka A, Satake S, Yanai T, Lane GJ, Kaneko K, et al. Associated urologic anomalies in children with solitary kidney. J Pediatr Surg. 2004;39(1):85-7.
30. Eckoldt F, Woderich R, Smith RD, Heling KS. Antenatal diagnostic aspects of unilateral multicystic kidney dysplasia—sensitivity, specificity, predictive values, differential diagnoses, associated malformations and consequences. Fetal Diagn Ther. 2004;19(2):163-9.
31. Avni FE, Guissard G, Hall M, Janssen F, DeMaertelaer V, Rypens F. Hereditary polycystic kidney diseases in children: Changing sonographic patterns through childhood. Pediatr Radiol. 2002;32(3):169-74.
32. Talner LB. Specific causes of obstruction. In: Pollack HM (Ed). Clinical Urography. Philadelphia: WB Saunders Co.; 1990. pp. 1629-751.
33. Park JM, Bloom DA. The pathophysiology of UPJ obstruction. Current concepts. Urol Clin North Am. 1998;25(2):161-9.
34. Rohtagi M, Bajpai M, Gupta DK, Gupta AK. Role of ultrasound-guided percutaneous antegrade pyelography in the diagnosis of obstructive uropathy. Indian Pediatrics. 1992;29:425-31.
35. Alladi A, Aggarwal S, Gupta AK, Bal CS, Mitra DK, Bhatnagar V. Postnatal outcome and natural history of antenatally detected hydronephrosis. Pediatric Surg Int. 2000;16:569-72 .
36. Platt JF, Rubin JM, Ellis JH, Dipietro MA. Duplex Doppler US of the kidney-differentiation of obstructive from non-obstructive dilatation. Radiology. 1989;171:515-7.
37. Mallek R, Bankier AA, Etele-Hainz A, Kletter K, Mostbeck GH. Distinction between obstructive and non-obstructive hydronephrosis: Value of diuresis duplex Doppler sonography. AJR Am J Roentgenol. 1996;166:113-7.
38. Ramsey PG. Opacification of the renal parenchyma in obstruction and reflux. Paediatr Radiol. 1976;4:226-32.
39. Dunbar JS, Nogardy MB. The calyceal crescent—a roentgenographic sign of obstructive hydronephrosis. Am J Roentgenol Radium Ther Nucl Med. 1970;110:520-8.
40. Stephens FD. Ureterovascular hydronephrosis and the "aberrant" renal vessels. J Urol. 1982;128:984-7.
41. Whitfield HN, Britton KE, Hendry WF, Wickham JE. Furosemide intravenous urography in the diagnosis of PUJ obstruction. Br J Urol. 1985;57:351.
42. Lebowitz RL, Blickman JG. The coexistence of ureteropelvic junction obstruction and reflux. AJR Am J Roentgenol. 1983;180:231-8.
43. Chandrasekharan VV, Srinivas M, Bal CS, Gupta AK, Agarwal S, Mitra DK, et al. Functional outcome after pyeloplasty for unilateral symptomatic hydronephrosis Pediatr Surg Int. 2001;17:524-7.
44. Nussbaum AR, Dort JP, Jeffs RD, Gearhart JP, Sanders RC. Ectopic ureter and ureterocoele: Their varied radiographic manifestations. Radiology. 1986;159:227-35.
45. Ramaswamy S, Bhatnagar V, Mitra DK, Gupta AK. Congenital Segmental giant megaureter. J Pediatr Surg. 1995;30:123-4.
46. Dunetz GN, Bauer SB. Complete duplication of bladder and urethra. Urology. 1985;25:179-82.
47. Cohen HL, Kravets F, Zucconi W, Ratani R, Shah S, Dougherty D. Congenital abnormalities of the genitourinary system. Semin Roentgenol. 2004;39(2):282-303.
48. Bauer SB. Neurogenic bladder dysfunction. Pediatr Clin North Am. 1987;34:1121-40.
49. Jennings RW. Prune Belly syndrome. Semin Pediatr Surg. 2000;9:115-20.
50. Suita S, Nagasaki A. Urachal remnants. Semin Paediat Surg. 1996;5:107-15.
51. Wendelin SH. The urinary bladder. In: Davidson AJ, Hartman DS (Eds). Radiology of the Kidney and Urinary Tract. Philadelphia: WB Saunders Co.; 1994. pp. 607-48.
52. Chatterjee SK, Banerjee S, Basak D, Basu AK, Chakravarti AK, Chatterjee US, et al. Posterior urethral valves: The scenario in a developing center. Pediatr Surg Int. 2001;17:2-7.
53. Cohen HL, Susman M, Haller JO, Glassberg KI, Shapiro MA, Zinn DL. Posterior urethral valve: Transperineal US for imaging and diagnosis in male infants. Radiology. 1994;192:261-4.
54. Mandelia A, Bajpai M, Agarwala S, Gupta AK, Kumar R, Ali A. The role of urinary TGF-β_1, TNF-α, IL-6 and microalbuminuria for monitoring therapy in posterior urethral valves. Pediatr Nephrol. 2013;28(10):1991-2001.
55. Goenka A, Jain V, Sharma R, Gupta AK, Bajpai M. MR diagnosis of penile agenesis: is it just absence of a phallus? Pediatr Radiol. 2008;38:1109-12.
56. Jana M, Gupta AK, Prasad KR, Goel S, Tambade VD, Sinha U. Pictorial essay: congenital anomalies of male urethra in children. Indian J Radiol Imaging. 2011;21:38-45.
57. Effman EL, Lebowitz RL, Colodny AH. Duplication of urethra. Radiology. 1976;119:179-85.
58. Kester RR, Woopan UM, Ohm HK. Congenital megalourethra. J Urol. 1990;4:1213-5.

CHAPTER

74

Urinary Tract Infections (Including Vesicoureteral Reflux and Neurogenic Bladder)

Anmol Bhatia, Kushaljit Singh Sodhi, Akshay Kumar Saxena

INTRODUCTION

Urinary tract infection (UTI) is a common cause of fever in pediatric population. Although many of the children with UTI recover with an excellent long-term outcome, few of the children have long term complications and/or sequelae like hypertension, chronic kidney disease (CKD), and end-stage renal disease (ESRD). These complications necessitate early investigations, prompt treatment, and close follow-up.[1,2] Various interventions, including follow-up radiological investigations, adequate prophylactic antibiotics, and surgical management, are also required for reducing the incidence of the long-term chronic morbidities.[3-5]

The urine culture is an important component of the workup of a child with presumed UTI. The culture helps in identification of the organism which is causing the infection and thereby helping regarding the initiation of appropriate antibiotics. UTI is considered as clinically significant when the culture shows >100,000 colony-forming unit (CFU)/mL.[3,4] However, reduced CFU can also be seen in UTI due to presence of confounding factors (e.g., dilution due to hydration and increased voiding frequency).[3,4]

INCIDENCE

It is said that 7% girls and 2% boys will have a UTI episode before 6 years of age.[3,6] During infancy, boys are more at-risk, with 10-fold greater risk in uncircumcised boys as compared to boys who are circumcised.[3,6] However, beyond the infancy, more girls are seen to develop UTI.

Of the children who have UTI, up to 25–40% are shown to have vesicoureteral reflux (VUR).[5,7] Among the children with febrile UTI, 50–91% will show photopenic areas on renal nuclear scan, suggesting acute pyelonephritis (APN).[5,8] When VUR and APN coexist, abnormalities are seen on nuclear scan in 79–86% of children.[8,9] Although, VUR and APN are also seen independently of one another.[9,10]

About 38–57% of the children who are diagnosed with APN diagnosed by scintigraphy are known to develop permanent renal scars.[5,11-13] However, the possibility of APN leading to renal scars is not always dependent on the grade of VUR.[13]

RADIOLOGICAL MODALITIES FOR IMAGING OF URINARY TRACT INFECTION

Imaging includes renal ultrasound (US) which helps in detection of congenital anomalies, hydronephrosis, and renal scars; micturating cystourethrogram (MCUG) for detecting VUR; and ^{99m}Tc-labeled dimercaptosuccinic acid (DMSA) scan to look for renal scars.

Role of Ultrasound in First-time Urinary Tract Infection

Ultrasound is very useful in picking up structural anomalies including anomalies in renal size, hydronephrosis, and duplicated collecting systems. Furthermore, US is a noninvasive, radiation-free modality, and requires no sedation. However, due to its low yield for additional important clinical information, its role has been questioned in many studies.[14]

Although, studies[15] have also shown that US picks up renal abnormalities which correlate with a higher prevalence and severity of VUR and hence US in children with UTI should be performed routinely.

VESICOURETERAL REFLUX

Vesicoureteral reflux is the retrograde passage of urine from the bladder into the ureters and kidneys. It can occur due to one of the following causes:[16,17]

- Abnormality of ureterovesical junction (UVJ)
- Marginally competent UVJ becoming incompetent due to UTI
- Lateral ureteral ectopia
- Abnormal bladder wall, e.g., prune belly syndrome
- Bladder outlet obstruction and neurogenic bladder
- Reflux following interference of UVJ (iatrogenic)

As it is generally believed that VUR correlates to risk of renal scar development, pediatric patients with UTI undergo various radiological investigations to detect VUR.

Pathophysiology of Vesicoureteral Reflux and Pyelonephritis

The distal most part of ureter traverses in an oblique fashion through the wall of the bladder ending into the ureteral orifice. Over a period of time, as the urine distends the bladder, compression on the submucosal and intramural portions of ureter helps in preventing the retrograde flow of the urine. A shorter intramural-submucosal length is associated with an increased risk of VUR.[5] The intramural-submucosal length changes with age and in children, it ranges between 7 mm and 12 mm.[18] In the surgeries involving ureteral reimplantation, the aim is to increase the ureteral course running obliquely within the wall of the urinary bladder resulting in lengthening of intramural-submucosal portion.[5]

Vesicoureteral reflux and urinary stasis predispose to infection resulting in entry of the bacteria in the renal parenchyma, which leads to edema and inflammation. The parenchymal microvasculature then gets compressed, which leads to ischemia, necrosis, and abscess formation,[5] which if not resolved leads to renal scars. ^{99m}Tc-DMSA scan is considered to be the imaging of choice to diagnose APN and renal scars as it has a very high sensitivity.[5,19] Both of these appear as photopenic areas and one has to rely on the temporal course to distinguish between them.

Imaging Findings in Acute Pyelonephritis

Urographic [intravenous urography (IVU)] findings consist of diffuse renal enlargement, decreased patchy or striated nephrogram, delayed calyceal opacification, and attenuation or effacement of the pelvicalyceal system (PCS). Renal US may be entirely normal or may show generalized or patchy decrease (rarely increase) in parenchymal echogenicity with decreased vascularity **(Fig. 1)**. US is mainly performed for detection of associated abnormalities, e.g., calculi, obstructive uropathy, or nephrocalcinosis.[20]

Renal scintigraphy with ^{99m}Tc-glucoheptonate (GH) or DMSA with a 91% sensitivity and 99.9% is the imaging modality of choice for acute pyelonephritis.[21] Cortical scintigraphy demonstrates focally reduced or absent accumulation of the tracer in the cortex without any evidence of volume loss; the defects can be solitary, multiple, or may involve the entire kidney giving rise to a mottled tracer distribution **(Figs. 2 and 3)**. On contrast-enhanced computed tomography (CECT) and contrast-enhanced magnetic resonance (CEMR), the affected kidney may show a striated nephrogram with multiple, poorly enhancing wedge-shaped (rarely round and irregular) areas fanning out from the calyces and reaching up to the cortex of the kidney **(Fig. 4)**.

All children having APN require US and DMSA scans in the acute stage; if the US is normal but the isotope scan is abnormal, follow-up scanning 3–6 months later is suggested, to detect whether the kidney has healed or scarred.[20,22]

Acute Focal Bacterial Nephritis

In this form of APN, which is also called acute lobar nephronia, the inflammatory process is localized or segmental, often affecting a renal pole or one moiety of a duplex kidney. On renal US, the swollen part of the kidney appears as a hypoechoic poorly marginated mass with low-level echoes scattered throughout **(Fig. 5)**. Acute infection produces wedge-shaped areas with decreased perfusion on Doppler US,[23] which is better seen on power Doppler.[20] However, power Doppler US is not as sensitive for pyelonephritis as DMSA scan. The CECT shows ill-defined areas of poor enhancement which may be seen as wedge-shaped hypodense zones. In general, the renal mass is not sharply defined from adjacent parenchyma and lacks a well-defined enhancing wall **(Fig. 6)** in contrast to a renal abscess where relatively well-defined enhancing wall is seen **(Fig. 7)**. A decreased uptake of the tracer is seen in the affected area on renal scintigraphy.

Grading of Vesicoureteral Reflux

The accepted classification for the grading of VUR is the International Reflux Study Committee's classification, which helps in generating a standardized reporting format.[24]

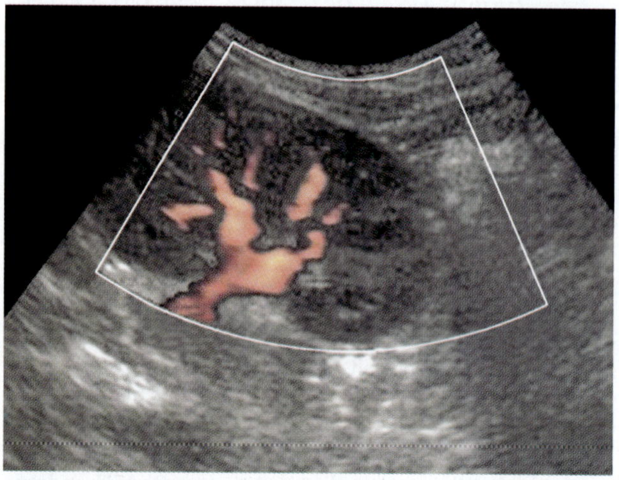

FIG. 1: Power Doppler ultrasound of kidney reveals a well-defined area of altered echogenicity at lower pole, which demonstrates decreased flow and perfusion, corresponding to acute pyelonephritis.

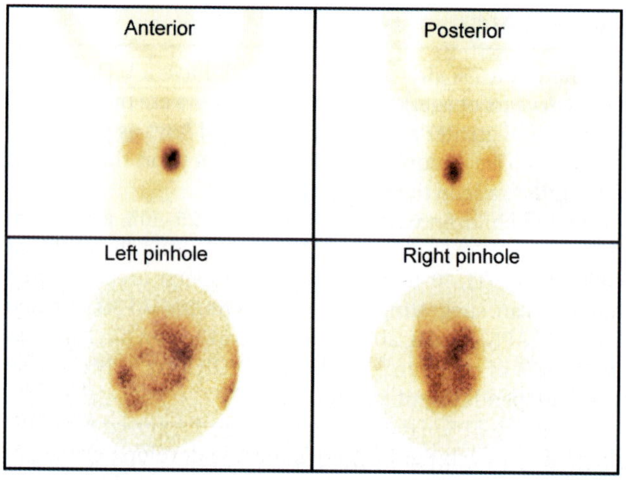

FIG. 2: ^{99m}Tc-labeled-dimercaptosuccinic acid scan showing multiple photopenic areas in both kidneys, suggestive of pyelonephritis.

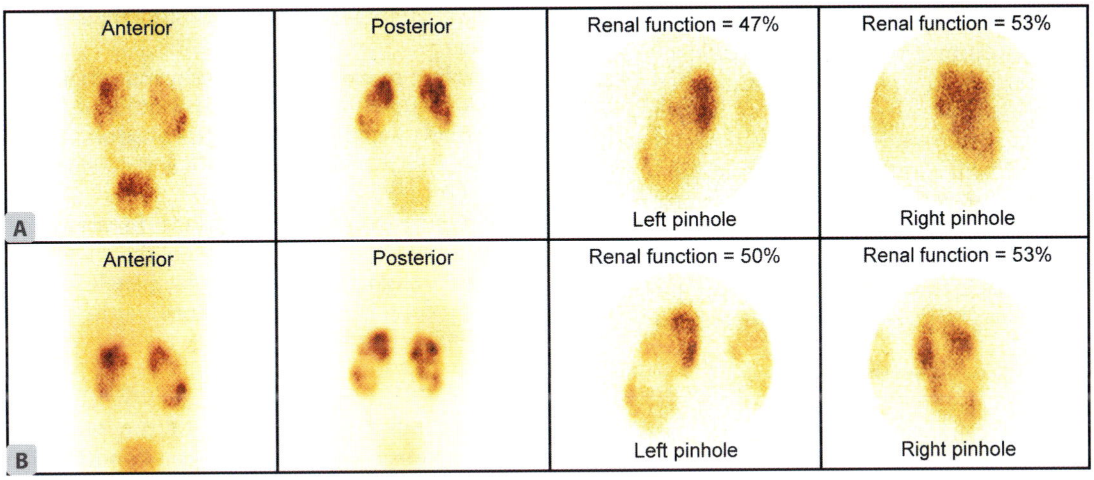

FIGS. 3A AND B: Consecutive ^{99m}Tc-labeled-dimercaptosuccinic acid scans in (A) 2008 and (B) 2010 showing persistent photopenic defects in both kidney cortices, indicative of renal scarring.

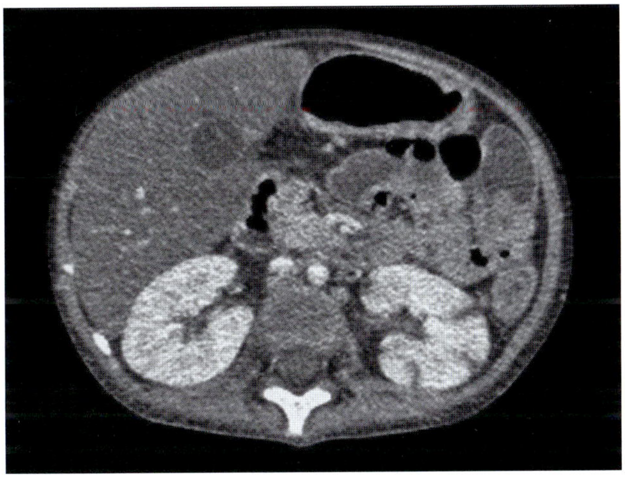

FIG. 4: Contrast-enhanced computed tomography of abdomen demonstrates well-defined poorly enhancing areas of acute pyelonephritis in left kidney.

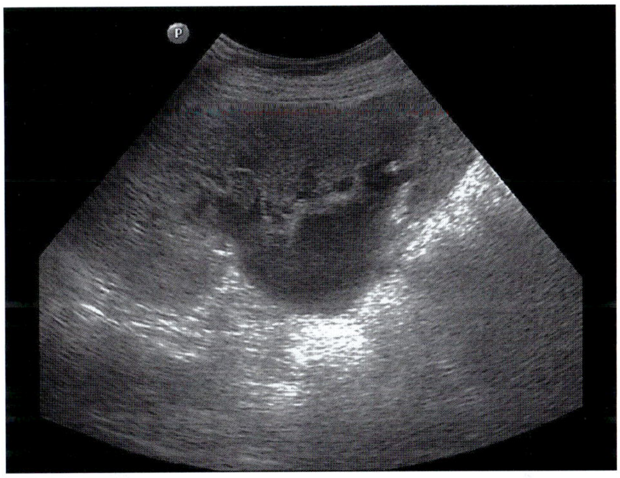

FIG. 5: Ultrasound image showing ill-defined hypoechoic lesion in the midpole of the left kidney with internal echoes and septations suggestive of an abscess.

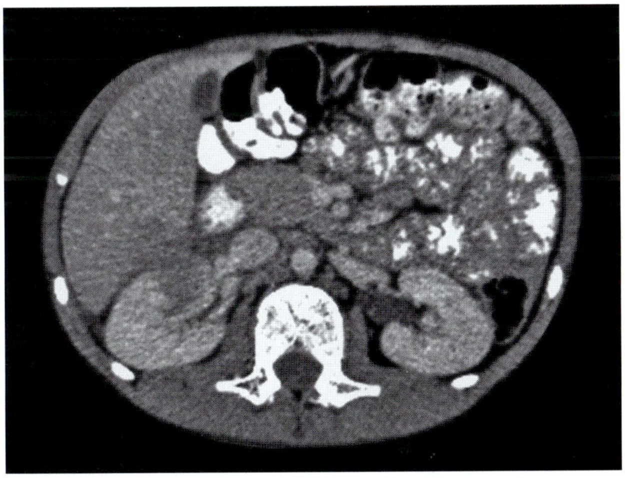

FIG. 6: Contrast-enhanced computed tomography of abdomen demonstrates ill-defined poorly enhancing in right kidney suggestive of acute focal nephritis.

- *Grade I*: Reflux to the ureter only
- *Grade II*: Reflux to the ureter and PCS without dilatation
- *Grade III*: Reflux to the PCS with mild dilatation or tortuosity of the ureter, mild dilatation of PCS, with normal or slightly blunted calyceal fornices
- *Grade IV*: Reflux to moderately dilated ureter and PCS with blunting of the forniceal angles; however, there is preservation of papillary impressions in majority of the calyces
- *Grade V*: Reflux into grossly dilated ureter and PCS with loss of papillary impressions in majority of the calyces.

Imaging of Vesicoureteral Reflux

- Micturating cystourethrogram (MCUG)
- Radionuclide cystography (RNC)
- Contrast-enhanced voiding urosonography (ceVUS)
- Magnetic resonance imaging (MRI)

Micturating Cystourethrogram

Micturating cystourethrogram, also known as voiding cystourethrogram (VCUG), is one of the most commonly performed fluoroscopic investigations in children.[25] It is the primary diagnostic procedure for evaluation of VUR in children. MCUG helps in documentation of the presence of VUR, grading of reflux, and whether reflux occurs during micturition or bladder filling phase **(Figs. 8 and 9)**.

A proper technique is essential for performing MCUG. Catheterization should be done with strict aseptic precautions and contrast should be injected using the gravity drip or by hand injection.[26]

Recommended views for MCUG study[25] are:

- Early filling phase of bladder
- *Full bladder phase*: The expected bladder capacity (in milliliters) is calculated using the formulae: Weight in kg × 7 for infants, [2 × age (years) + 2] × 30 for children <2 years of age, and [age (years)/2 + 6] × 30 for those 2 years of age or older.[25,27]
- *Voiding phase to demonstrate urethra*: This should be obtained in the right and left anterior oblique positions. For girls, supine position is also to be obtained.
- *Renal view after voiding*: To look for contrast in PCS due to VUR.
- *Bladder view after voiding*: It helps in assessing the degree of emptying of bladder. Most of the children <1 year of age fail to empty the bladder completely during MCUG,[28] but a complete emptying of bladder helps in excluding bladder neuropathy.

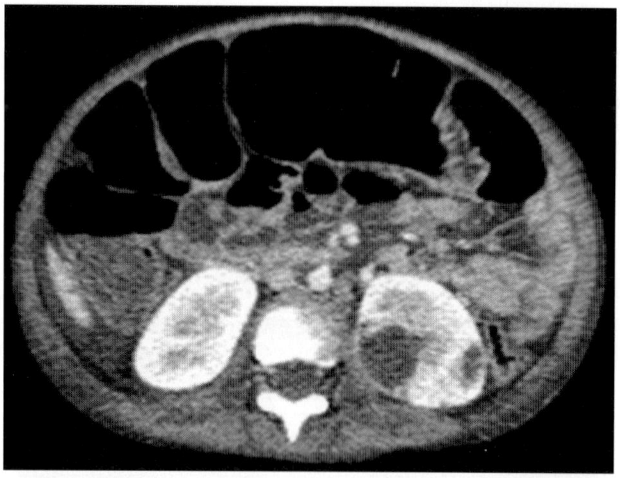

FIG. 7: Contrast-enhanced computed tomography of abdomen showing peripherally enhancing hypodense lesions in the left kidney suggestive of abscesses.

Practice and Concept of Cyclical Voiding

Cyclical voiding is recommended during MCUG to increase the detection rate of VUR. A second voiding phase helps increase the VUR detection significantly,[25,29,30] which is as high as 19.5%.[29] There is also a probability of detecting an increased grade of reflux compared to that seen on the first void.[29,30] This is significant as surgical intervention is required only in high grades of reflux.

With recent advances in fluoroscopy, dose reduction can be easily achieved without any perceived loss of image quality.[31-34] Using high-quality image-capture technology, it can also reduce radiation dose.[35,36]

In a comparison between spot films and image-capture acquisition, the latter provided diagnostically comparable images with a 57% reduction in skin radiation dose.[25] Per se, low magnification, low-pulse-per-second fluoroscopy, and image-grab acquisition should be used as much as possible within locally formulated MCUG protocols.

Radionuclide Cystography

Reflux can also be graded with RNC **(Fig. 10)**. There are two types of RNC: (1) Direct and (2) Indirect.

Indirect RNC is done by injecting ^{99m}Tc-mercapto-acetyltriglycine (^{99m}Tc-MAG3) or ^{99m}Tc-diethylenetriamine-

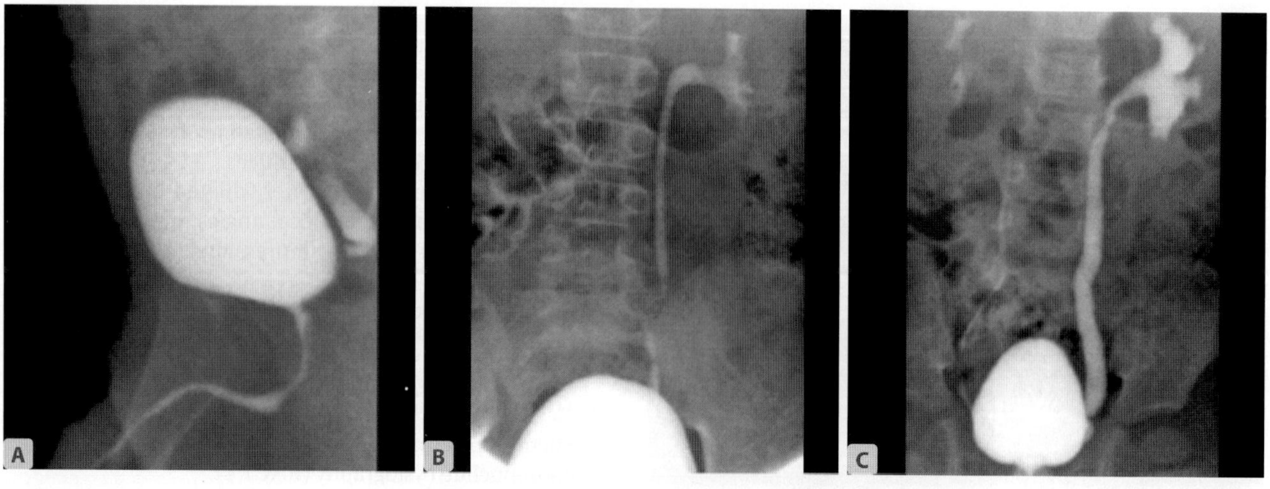

FIGS. 8A TO C: Grades I–III vesicoureteral reflux: Micturating cystourethrogram reveals left-sided (A) Grade I reflux; (B) Grade II reflux; (C) Grade III reflux.

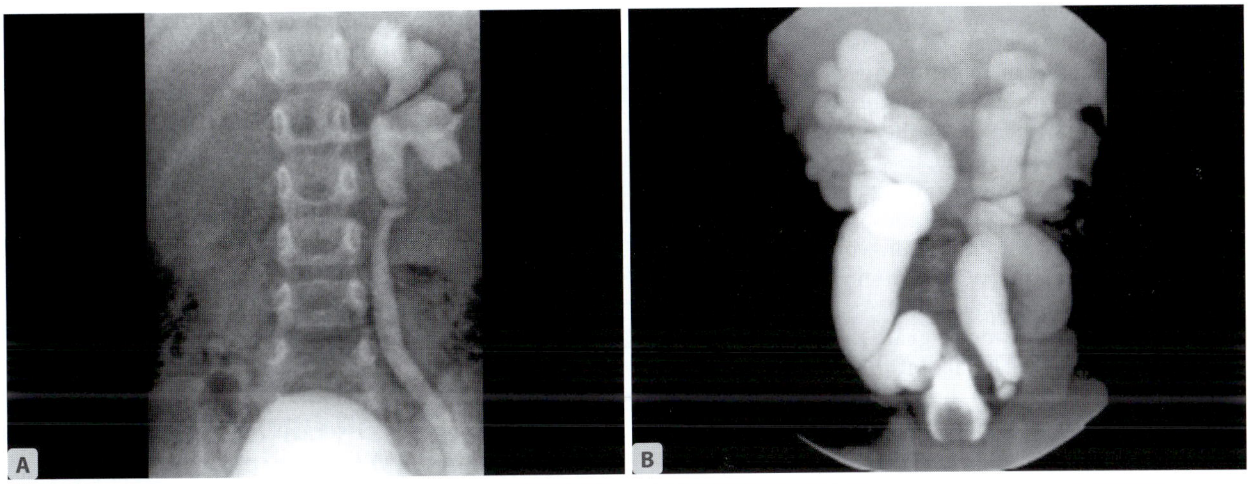

FIGS. 9A AND B: (A) Left grade IV and (B) bilateral grade V reflux are seen on micturating cystourethrogram.

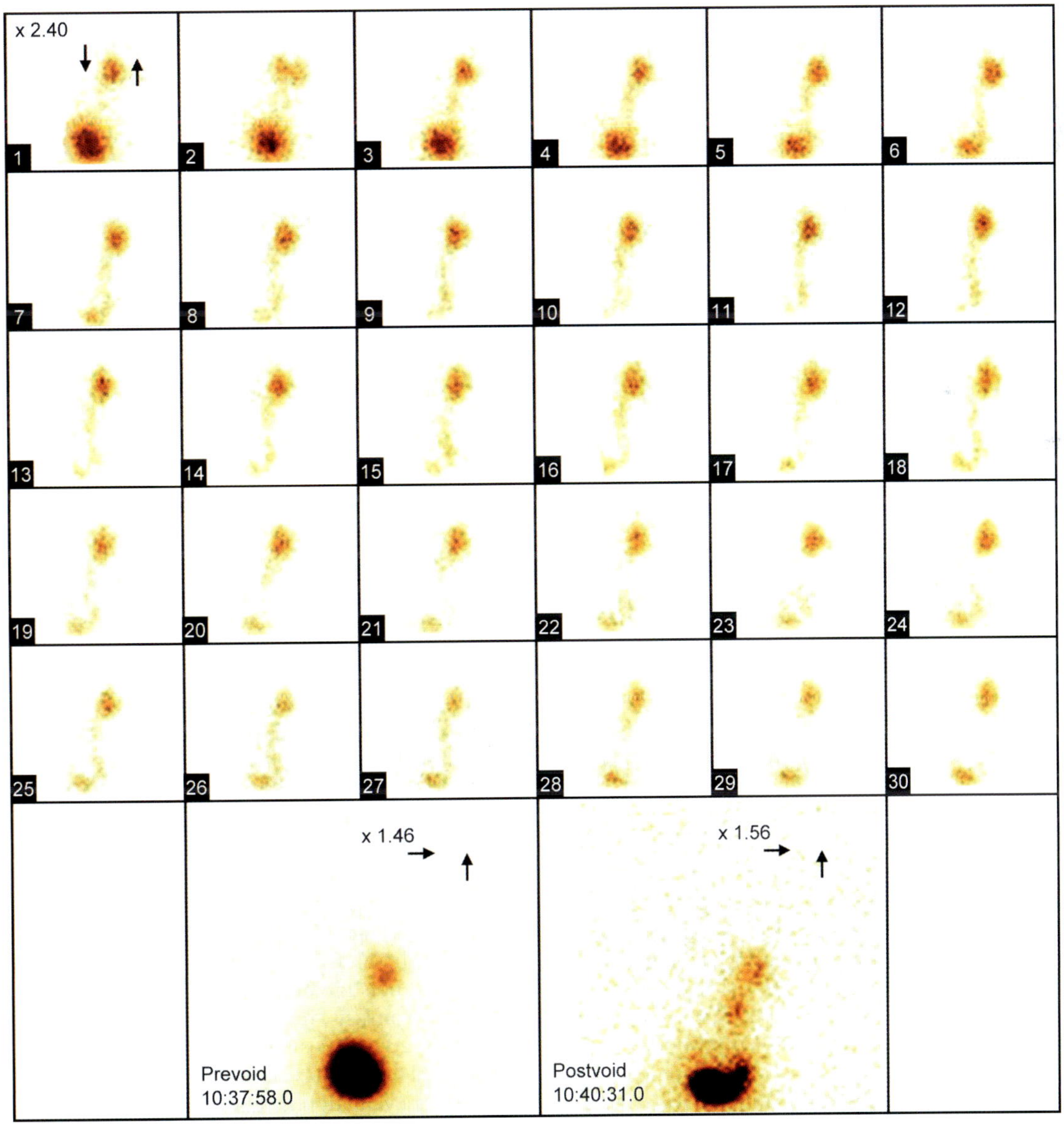

FIG. 10: ^{99m}Tc-sulfur colloid direct radionuclide cystography; Retrograde movement of tracer is seen from the right kidney into the upper ureter, indicative of high-grade right-sided vesicoureteral reflux.

pentaacetic acid (^{99m}Tc-DTPA) and this is followed by imaging of the kidneys in a dynamic fashion.[5] A time-activity curve shows an abrupt increase in activity in the PCS, if VUR is there. The main advantage of indirect technique is that there is no need for bladder catheterization, although an intravenous cannula is required.

The reported sensitivity of indirect RNC is less than direct RNC and ranges between 22% and 51%.[5,31] Indirect RNC should be limited for the patients in whom catheterization of bladder is not possible. Children should be toilet-trained to maximize its sensitivity.

The radionuclide cystogram has 1/100th of the radiation exposure of a standard MCUG.[3] Further, as the child is continuously imaged in a direct RNC (versus intermittent with fluoroscopy), it is, therefore, more sensitive in picking up VUR than MCUG.[3,32-36] Fluoroscopic MCUG is more accurate at grading of VUR and can also show associated anomalies in spine, anatomy of bladder and urethra, and other anatomic details in the upper urinary tract that cannot be identified with RNC.[3,4]

The radiation dose to gonads in RNC is around 10–20 µGy.[5,37] Use of "last-frame grabber" technology, which is a low-dose fluoroscopy technique, can potentially help in reducing the VCUG gonadal dose to 17–52 µGy.[5,38] Hence, even with the use of modern fluoroscopy machines, the effective dose of VCUG is still higher than that of RNC.[39]

Contrast-enhanced Voiding Urosonography

It is a dynamic radiological investigation that allows the morphologic and functional assessment of the entire genitourinary tract. It by done by instilling an ultrasonographic contrast agent (USCA) within the bladder.[40-42] Compared to MCUG, it is more sensitive and picks up higher grades of VUR.[41-43] The main advantage of ceVUS, as against VCUG, is that ceVUS is a radiation-free modality. VUR is demonstrated on ceVUS by the presence of contrast in the ureters and/or PCS.[44] Darge and Troeger[45] proposed a classification of VUR based on US. However, due to depiction of the ureters on ceVUS, it is easy to use the international classification for reflux while performing ceVUS.[46]

However, the inability to obtain a single image showing the entire urinary tract may cause difficulty in the interpretation of the ceVUS. This can be overcome in small children by using a lateral approach using a convex transducer, thereby obtaining an image in the coronal plane depicting the entire ureters, PCS, and the bladder. Furthermore, we can also generate compound ceVUS images.[47]

The basic procedural steps of ceVUS are:

- Ultrasound of the kidneys and bladder
- Catheterization of bladder followed by intravesical administration of normal saline and contrast.
- Repeat scan of the bladder and kidneys during and after filling of the bladder and later on during voiding.[40,42]

The most commonly used USCAs are first-generation ultrasound contrast agent Levovist (Bayer Schering Pharma, Berlin, Germany) and second-generation ultrasound contrast agent SonoVue (Bracco, Milan, Italy).[40,42] Harmonic imaging (HI) improves the detection of microbubbles and increases the sensitivity of VUS.[41]

Role of Magnetic Resonance Imaging in Diagnosing Urinary Tract Infection

Magnetic resonance imaging can help in detection of pyelonephritis and renal scars. It is a radiation-free modality and can provide structural detail even in children with poor renal function. However, it is not routinely used due to its limited availability, high cost, longer scan times, and need for long sedation/anesthesia support. Technical feasibility of direct and indirect MR cystography techniques has been discussed in a few studies;[48,49] however, there have been no studies comparing it with VCUG.

GUIDELINES FOR UROLOGIC IMAGING IN URINARY TRACT INFECTION: FROM HISTORY TO CURRENT PERSPECTIVE

First set of guidelines were published by the Royal College of Physicians (RCP) in 1991 for imaging of UTI in children.[50] It was recommended that every child between 0 year and 7 years of age with first UTI should have an US and DMSA scan. Children up to 1 year of age should also have a MCUG.

Subsequently, in 1999, practice parameters were given by the American Academy of Pediatrics (AAP) and their recommendations for imaging workup were wide, supporting US and MCUG or RNC in all children with UTI who are <2 years old.[51] The American Academy of Family Physicians recommended to perform DMSA after UTI treatment to look for renal scars.[52] This has been described as the "bottom-up" approach as the initial aim is to detect VUR. Once VUR is seen, the child is assumed to be at increased risk for development of renal scars and DMSA is then to be done several months later to look for renal scars.

In recent years, there has been development of several imaging algorithms which differ among various clinicians and vary across various hospitals worldwide.[53] Another evolution in practice guidelines was seen in 2007 European Society of Pediatric Radiology recommendations.[54] Their guidelines suggest US of all children with UTI and if it is normal but there is suspicion of APN, early DMSA scan is recommended. If APN is detected on DMSA scan, then VCUG or RNC is recommended later to look for VUR.[5] Normal DMSA scan obviates the need for VCUG or RNC.[55,56] This is called as the "top-down" approach because now the initial diagnostic concern is of APN and not VUR.[5]

In 2011, a revision of the practice guidelines was released by the AAP.[57] The biggest change from the 1999 guideline was in the section on urologic imaging. The main action statements related to imaging are:

- Febrile infants and young children with UTI should undergo renal and bladder US.
- Although MCUG should not be routinely performed after the first episode of febrile UTI, it is indicated if there is hydronephrosis, renal scar, or other findings suggesting high-grade VUR or obstructive uropathy and in other atypical or complex clinical circumstances.
- Further evaluation is required, if there is a recurrence of febrile UTI.

TREATMENT GUIDELINES FOR REFLUX

The significance of reflux deals with the issue of recurrent APN and development of renal scars. A common dilemma is whether to treat or not to treat a particular child. Traditional therapy includes long-term antibiotic prophylaxis to prevent infections along with observation, in anticipation of the child outgrowing the reflux.[3]

High spontaneous resolution rates have been seen, especially for lower grades of reflux, but this adds to the cost of long-term use of antibiotics and repeated MCUG. Surgical intervention is usually reserved for those children showing noncompliance with medical treatment or nonresolving VUR, febrile breakthrough UTIs, and renal scar progression, after prolonged follow-up.[3]

The American Urological Association convened the Pediatric VUR Guidelines Panel for making guidelines to determine whether to treat VUR medically or surgically.[58] They recommended surgery for higher grades of reflux. The standard surgical care is open surgical repair (e.g., ureteral reimplantation). To reduce the morbidity, extravesical approach has also been proposed. Success rates for surgical techniques are 98% for treating VUR. The surgical developments, combined with a tendency to avoid antibiotics overuse, resulted in a shift toward earlier surgery. This has been stressed upon even more with the use of laparoscopic techniques in many centers.[59] In endoscopic treatment of VUR, however, success rates of 70–90% have been reported for curing VUR. It is important to know that all VUR does not require an intervention and treatment does not always reduce the incidence of complications.[60]

In the meta-analysis, which was conducted by the American Urological Association 2010, emphasis has been put on the management of bladder and bowel dysfunction (BBD). It was shown that children with BBD had higher incidence of UTI even on antibiotic prophylaxis, lower rates of resolution of VUR, and decreased success rates of endoscopic treatment of VUR. Results have shown a higher risk of developing UTI in children with both VUR and BBD, as against the children having VUR or BBD alone. The incorporation of diagnosis and treatment of BBD into the initial evaluation of the children resulted in better overall outcomes. Children with VUR and coexisting BBD should undergo timely intervention in form of biofeedback, timed voiding, anticholinergic drugs, or alpha blockers to avoid the lower urinary tract symptoms or voiding patterns have been shown to have a downgrading of their reflux by two or more grades on an average.[61]

NEUROGENIC BLADDER

Neurogenic bladder is defined as malfunctioned urinary bladder which can be seen in any kind of neurologic disorder. The age of presentation may vary from neonates to adolescence. The children usually present with failure to empty bladder, frequency, nocturia, urgency, retention, incontinence, UTI, and vesical stones. In contrast to adult patient in whom neurogenic bladder is most often due to an acquired, usually traumatic spinal cord lesion, the vast majority of children affected with this disorder have a myelomeningocele or a related myelodysplastic anomaly (occult spinal dysraphism, sacral agenesis).

Myelomeningocele can occur at any level of the spine, but is most often located in the lumbosacral area. The radiographs of the affected area show widening of the neural canal, defect in the posterior neural arches in the form of absence of the posterior spinous processes, and widened interpedicular distance involving several segments, with elongated and flattened or defective pedicles.[16]

Occult myelodysplasia is a group of congenital anomalies of the spinal cord in which the overlying skin is intact, although cutaneous stigmata of the disorder may be present such as local hair overgrowth, hyperpigmentation, hemangioma, a skin dimple, or an ill-defined soft-tissue mass due to a lipoma. These anomalies include tethered cord, diastematomyelia, intraspinal lipoma, dermoid cyst, and hamartoma. Radiographs of the spine may show osseous changes similar to those seen in myelomeningocele and sometimes scoliosis or broad vertebral bodies.

Children with this disorder commonly have inappropriate detrusor muscle contraction and external sphincter relaxation, resulting in uncontrolled voiding pattern with incomplete bladder emptying.[16,62,63] Initially, the upper tracts are normal but due to poor bladder emptying, secondary changes of reflux and infection result. Complete evaluation of patients suspected of having neurogenic bladder requires MCUG for assessment of lower urinary tract, US, and one of the functional studies of IVU or scintigraphy for upper tract. However, for the diagnosis of primary cause, examination with plain radiographs and MRI is essential.

Ultrasound shows a small contracted/large atonic bladder, with or without wall thickening, increased postvoid residual urine, diverticula/pseudodiverticula, and hydroureteronephrosis.

Best imaging tool is MCUG which typically shows an elongated towering bladder **(Figs. 11A and B)**. MCUG can help in identifying three types of bladder dysfunction:

1. Contractile bladders
2. Intermediate bladders
3. Acontractile bladders

The findings in the different kinds of neurogenic bladder are summarized in **Table 1**.

Further, associated varying degrees of VUR may be seen. Urodynamic techniques have assumed a major role in the evaluation of neurogenic bladder and contributed significantly to the management.

ACKNOWLEDGMENTS

We wish to thank Dr Anish Bhattacharya, Professor and Dr BR Mittal, Professor and Head, Department of Nuclear Medicine for their kind help and support in providing images of ^{99m}Tc-DMSA scans and ^{99m}Tc-sulfur colloid direct radionuclide cystography scans.

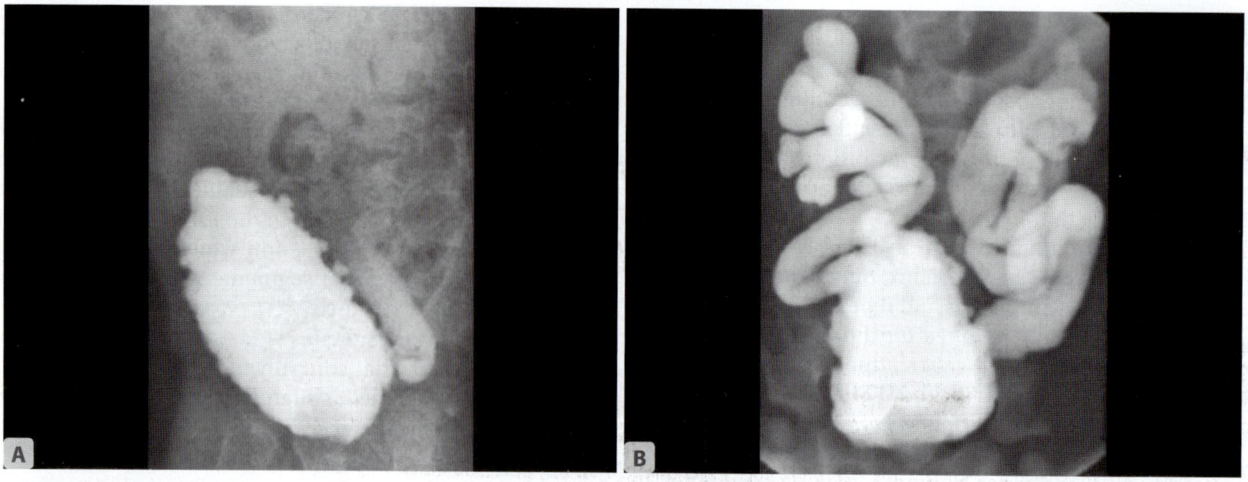

FIGS. 11A AND B: Neurogenic bladder. (A) Micturating cystourethrogram (MCUG) shows an elongated bladder with trabeculations and sacculations with grade I vesicoureteral reflux (VUR); (B) MCUG in another patient showing neurogenic bladder with grade V VUR.

TABLE 1: A summary on the features of different types of neurogenic bladder.

Types of bladder	Findings
Contractile bladder	Trabeculated thick-walled bladder, bulging posterior urethra up to the contracted urethral sphincter suggestive of detrusor sphincter dyssynergia
Intermediate bladder	Bladder neck closes at early filling, bladder neck opens with increasing volume and pressure, and no bulging of posterior urethra as seen in contractile bladders
Acontractile bladder	Opened up bladder neck during the entire filling phase suggestive of incontinence, pericatheter leakage of the contrast suggesting sphincter weakness

REFERENCES

1. Luk WH, Woo YH, Au-Yeung AWS, Chan JCS. Imaging in pediatric urinary tract infection: a 9-year local experience. AJR Am J Roentgenol. 2009;192:1253-60.
2. Larcombe J. Urinary tract infection in children: clinical evidence. BMJ. 1999;319:1173-5.
3. Bauer R, Kogan BA. New Developments in the Diagnosis and Management of Pediatric UTIs. Urol Clin North Am. 2008;35:47-58.
4. Linda S. Urinary tract infections in infants and children. In: Walsh P (Ed). Campbell's Urology, 8th edition. Baltimore: Saunders; 2002. pp. 1846-84.
5. Lim R. Vesicoureteral reflux and urinary tract infection: evolving practices and current controversies in pediatric imaging. AJR Am J Roentgenol. 2009;192:1197-208.
6. Marild S, Jodal U. Incidence rate of first-time symptomatic urinary tract infection in children under 6 years of age. Acta Pediatr. 1998;87:549-52.
7. Cleper R, Krause I, Eisenstein B, Davidovits M. Prevalence of vesicoureteral reflux in neonatal urinary tract infection. Clin Pediatr (Phila). 2004;43:619-25.
8. Rushton HG, Majd M. Dimercaptosuccinic acid renal scintigraphy for the evaluation of pyelonephritis and scarring: a review of experimental and clinical studies. J Urol. 1992;148:1726-32.
9. Ditchfield MR, De Campo JF, Cook DJ, Nolan TM, Powell HR, Sloane R, et al. Vesicoureteral reflux: an accurate predictor of acute pyelonephritis in childhood urinary tract infection? Radiology. 1994;190:413-5.
10. Sastre JB, Aparicio AR, Cotallo GD, Colomer BF, Hernandez MC. Urinary tract infection in the newborn: clinical and radioimaging studies. Pediatr Nephrol. 2007;22:1735-41.
11. Lin KY, Chiu NT, Chen MJ, Lai CH, Huang JJ, Wang YT, et al. Acute pyelonephritis and sequelae of renal scar in pediatric first febrile urinary tract infection. Pediatr Nephrol. 2003;18:362-5.
12. Zaki M, Badawi M, Al Mutari G, Ramadan D, Rahman MA. Acute pyelonephritis and renal scarring in Kuwaiti children: a follow-up study using 99mTc DMSA renal scintigraphy. Pediatr Nephrol. 2005;20:1116-9.
13. Oh MM, Jin MH, Bae JH, Park HS, Lee JG. Moon DG. The role of vesicoureteral reflux in acute renal cortical scintigraphic lesion and ultimate scar formation. J Urol. 2008;180:2167-70.
14. Zamir G, Sakran W, Horowitz Y, Koren A, Miron D. Urinary tract infection: Is there a need for routine renal ultrasonography? Arch Dis Child. 2004;89:466-8.
15. Huang HP, Lai YC, Tsai IJ, Chen SY, Tsau YK. Renal ultrasonography should be done routinely in children with first urinary tract infections. Urology. 2008;71:439-43.
16. Vashist S. Radiology of lower urinary tract. In: Donnelly LF (Ed). Diagnostic Radiology: Pediatric Imaging, 2nd edition. New Delhi: Jaypee Brothers Medical Publishers (P) Ltd; 2004. pp. 208-22.
17. Alon U, Berant M, Pery M. Intravenous pyelography in children with urinary tract infection and vesicoureteral reflux. Pediatrics. 1989;83:332-7.
18. Cussen LJ. Dimensions of the normal ureter in infancy and childhood. Invest Urol. 1967;5:164-78.
19. Ataei N, Madani A, Habibi R, Khorasani M. Evaluation of acute pyelonephritis with DMSA scans in children presenting after the age of 5 years. Pediatr Nephrol. 2005;20:1439-44.
20. Sandhu MS, Lal A. Pediatric kidney: medical conditions. In: Donnelly LF (Ed). Diagnostic Radiology: Pediatric Imaging, 2nd

edition. New Delhi: Jaypee Brothers Medical Publishers (P) Ltd; 2004. pp. 160-81.

21. Jakobson B, Soderlungh S, Berg U. Diagnostic significance of 99mTc-DMSA scintigraphy in urinary tract infection. Arch Dis Child. 1992;67:1338-42.
22. Lebowitz RL, Mandell J. Urinary tract infection in children: putting radiology in its place. Radiology. 1987;165:1-9.
23. Dubbins PA. The kidney. In: Allen PL, Dubbins PA, Pozniak MA, McDicken WN (Eds). Clinical Doppler Ultrasound. New York. Churchill Livingstone; 2000. pp. 169-90.
24. International Reflux Study Committee. Medical versus surgical treatment of primary vesicoureteral reflux: a prospective international reflux study in children. J Urol. 1981;125:277-83.
25. Agrawalla S, Pearce R, Goodman TR. How to perform the perfect voiding cystourethrogram? Pediatr Radiol. 2004;34:114-9.
26. Weese DL, Greenberg HM, Zimmern PE. Contrast media reactions during voiding cystourethrography or retrograde pyelography. Urology. 1993;41:81-3.
27. Kaefer M, Zurakowski D, Bauer SB, Retik AB, Peters CA, Atala A, et al. Estimating normal bladder capacity in children. J Urol. 1997;158:2261-4.
28. Sillen U. Bladder function in healthy neonates and its development during infancy. Urology. 2001;166:2376-81.
29. Papadopoulou F, Efremidis SC, Oiconomou A, Badouraki M, Panteleli M, Papachristou F, et al. Cyclic voiding cystourethrography: is vesicoureteral reflux missed with standard voiding cystourethrography? Eur Radiol. 2002;12:666-70.
30. Paltiel HJ, Rupich RC, Kiruluta HC. Enhanced detection of vesicoureteral reflux in infants and children with use of cyclic voiding cystourethrography. Radiology. 1992;184:753-5.
31. De Sadeleer C, De Boe V, Keuppens F, Desprechins B, Verboven M, Piepsz A. How good is technetium-99m mercaptoacetyltriglycine indirect cystography? Eur J Nucl Med. 1994;21:223-7.
32. Unver T, Alpay H, Biyikli NK, Ones T. Comparison of direct radionuclide cystography and voiding cystourethrography in detecting vesicoureteral reflux. Pediatr Int. 2006;48:287-91.
33. McLaren CJ, Simpson ET. Direct comparison of radiology and nuclear medicine cystograms in young infants with vesicoureteric reflux. BJU Int. 2001;87:93-7.
34. Lebowitz RL. The detection and characterization of vesicoureteral reflux in the child. J Urol. 1992;148:1640-2.
35. Sükan A, Bayazit AK, Kibar M, Noyan A, Soyupak S, Yapar Z, et al. Comparison of direct radionuclide cystography and voiding direct cystography in the detection of vesicoureteral reflux. Ann Nucl Med. 2003;17:549-53.
36. Saraga M, Stanicic A, Markovic V. The role of direct radionuclide cystography in evaluation of vesicoureteral reflux. Scand J Urol Nephrol. 1996;30:367-71.
37. Van den Abbeele AD, Treves ST, Lebowitz RL, Bauer S, Davis RT, Retik A, et al. Vesicoureteral reflux in asymptomatic siblings of patients with known reflux: radionuclide cystography. Pediatrics. 1987;79:147-53.
38. Kleinman PK, Diamond DA, Karellas A, Spevak MR, Nimkin K, Belanger P. Tailored low-dose fluoroscopic voiding cystourethrography for the reevaluation of vesicoureteral reflux in girls. AJR Am J Roentgenol. 1994;162:1151-4.
39. Ward VL, Strauss KJ, Barnewolt CE, Zurakowski D, Venkatakrishnan V, Fahey FH, et al. Pediatric radiation exposure and effective dose reduction during voiding cystourethrography. Radiology. 2008;249:1002-9.
40. Darge K. Voiding urosonography with ultrasound contrast agents for the diagnosis of vesicoureteric reflux in children. I. Procedure. Pediatr Radiol. 2008;38:40-53.
41. Darge K. Voiding urosonography with US contrast agents for the diagnosis of vesicoureteric reflux in children. II. Comparison with radiological examinations. Pediatr Radiol. 2008;38:54-63.
42. Darge K. Voiding urosonography with US contrast agent for the diagnosis of vesicoureteric reflux in children: an update. Pediatr Radiol. 2010;40:956-62.
43. Papadopoulou F, Anthopoulou A, Siomou E, Efremidis S, Tsamboulas C, Darge K. Harmonic voiding urosonography with a second-generation contrast agent for the diagnosis of vesicoureteral reflux. Pediatr Radiol. 2009;39:239-44.
44. Darge K, Trusen A, Gordjani N, Riedmiller H. Intrarenal reflux: diagnosis with contrast-enhanced harmonic US. Pediatr Radiol. 2003;33:729-31.
45. Darge K, Troeger J. Vesicoureteral reflux grading in contrast-enhanced voiding urosonography. Eur J Radiol. 2002;43:122-8.
46. Lebowitz RL, Olbing H, Parkkulainen KV, Smellie JM, Tamminen-Möbius TE. International system of radiographic grading of vesicoureteric reflux: international reflux study in children. Pediatr Radiol. 1985;15:105-9.
47. Duran C, Beltrán VP, González A, Gómez C, Riego JD. Contrast-enhanced Voiding Urosonography for Vesicoureteral Reflux Diagnosis in Children. Radiographics. 2017;37:1854-69.
48. Teh HS, Gan JS, Ng FC. Magnetic resonance cystography: novel imaging technique for evaluation of vesicoureteral reflux. Urology. 2005;65:793-4.
49. Takazakura R, Johnin K, Furukawa A, Nitta N, Takahashi M, Okada Y, et al. Magnetic resonance voiding cystourethrography for vesicoureteral reflux. J Magn Reson Imaging. 2007;25:170-4.
50. Guidelines for the management of acute urinary tract infection in childhood. Report of a Working Group of the Royal College of Physicians. J R Coll Physicians Lond. 1991;25:36-42.
51. Biassoni L, Chippington S. Imaging in Urinary tract Infections: Current Strategies and New Trends. Sem Nucl Med. 2008;38:56-66.
52. Practice parameter: the diagnosis, treatment, and evaluation of the initial urinary tract infection in febrile infants and young children. American Academy of Pediatrics. Committee on Quality Improvement. Subcommittee on Urinary Tract Infection. Pediatrics. 1999;103:843-52.
53. Ross JH, Kay R. Pediatric urinary tract infection and reflux. Am Fam Physician. 1999;59:1472-8.
54. Shah L, Mandlik N, Kumar P, Andaya S, Patamasucon P. Adherence to AAP practice guidelines for urinary tract infections at our teaching institution. Clin Pediatr (Phila). 2008;47:861-4.
55. Riccabona M, Avni FE, Blickman JG, Dacher JN, Darge K, Lobo ML, et al. Imaging recommendations in paediatric uroradiology: minutes of the ESPR workgroup session on urinary tract infection, fetal hydronephrosis, urinary tract ultrasonography and voiding cystourethrography, Barcelona, Spain, June 2007. Pediatr Radiol. 2008;38:138-45.
56. Preda I, Jodal U, Sixt R, Stokland E, Hansson S. Normal dimercaptosuccinic acid scintigraphy makes voiding cystourethrography unnecessary after urinary tract infection. J Pediatr. 2007;151:581-4.
57. Roberts KB. Revised AAP Guideline on UTI in Febrile Infants and Young Children. Am Fam Physician. 2012;86:940-6.
58. Agras K, Ortapamuk H, Naldoken S, Tuncel A, Atan A. Resolution of cortical lesions on serial renal scans in children with acute pyelonephritis. Pediatr Radiol. 2007;37:153-8.
59. Elder JS, Peters CA, Arant BS, Ewalt DH, Hawtrey CE, Hurwitz RS, et al. Pediatric vesicoureteral reflux guidelines panel summary report on the management of primary vesicoureteral reflux in children. J Urol. 1997;157:1846-51.
60. Yeung CK, Sihoe JD, Tam YH, Lee KH. Laparoscopic excision of prostatic utricles in children. BJU Int. 2001;87:505-8.
61. Edwards A, Peters CA. Managing vesicoureteral reflux in children: making sense of all the data. F1000Res. 2019;8:F1000.
62. Lorenzo AJ, Khoury AE. Endoscopic treatment of reflux: management pros and cons. Curr Opin Urol. 2006;16:299-304.
63. Bauer SB. Neurogenic bladder dysfunction. Paediatr Clin North Am. 1987;34:1121-40.

CHAPTER

75

Renal and Retroperitoneal Masses

Anju Garg, Alpana Manchanda, Radhika Batra

INTRODUCTION

The retroperitoneum is a potential space that extends along the posterior most aspect of the abdominal cavity from the level of the diaphragm to the pelvic brim. Masses in this space can arise from the kidneys, adrenal glands, lymph nodes, lymphatic channels, sympathetic ganglia or other neural tissue, and iliopsoas muscle. As symptoms of retroperitoneal disease are nonspecific and physical examination is difficult, retroperitoneal masses grow quite large before they are detected.

IMAGING

The multitude of diagnostic imaging modalities available for evaluation of abdominal masses in infants and children requires a logical and analytical approach to avoid unnecessary expense, radiation, and potential morbidity. Ultrasound (US) is the most frequently selected first imaging modality on the basis of availability, ease of performance (as there is no need for intravenous contrast or patient sedation), low cost and absence of radiation exposure. The highest possible frequency probes should be used to maximize resolution. Color Doppler enables characterization of tumor vascularization and assessment of vascular invasion. US has a high diagnostic efficacy for common pediatric abdominal masses and in many cases it may give a complete diagnosis obviating the need for any further investigation. If the US examination is technically limited because of excessive bowel gas or body habitus, or if the mass is incompletely evaluated by US or thought to be neoplastic, computed tomography (CT) or magnetic resonance imaging (MRI) can be done. In the case of a suspected neoplasm, these modalities further refine the differential diagnosis, define the local and regional extent of the mass and detect metastases.

Computed tomography is an extremely accurate and fast imaging modality, displaying high quality cross-sectional images. Multidetector CT allows excellent reconstructions in planes other than the original scanning plane. Isotropic multiplanar reconstructions (MPRs) of thin overlapping slices in the coronal and sagittal plane provide excellent delineation of the location and extent of retroperitoneal masses. The use of pre- and postcontrast scanning should be minimized in children; the use of oral contrast is helpful in distinguishing bowel from nodal disease. Short sedation may be required, especially in younger children. A relative disadvantage of CT is the radiation exposure. Chest CT may be required in cases of suspected neoplasms to evaluate presence of lung metastases.

The advantages of MRI include its unique ability to directly acquire multiplanar images, superior contrast resolution, and lack of ionizing radiation. Its major disadvantages are cost, limited availability, and need for sedation. Faster scanners and newer imaging sequences currently allow accurate lesion characterization in a reasonably short scanning time. Typical sequences used are precontrast T1- and T2-weighted (T2W) gradient echo sequences and postcontrast fat suppressed T1W images. Images should be obtained in at least two orthogonal planes to permit direct evaluation of extent of retroperitoneal disease.

Functional MRI like diffusion-weighted imaging (DWI) can act as a problem-solving tool in evaluation of some of the renal and retroperitoneal mass lesions. DWI along with apparent diffusion coefficient (ADC) values can yield significant qualitative and quantitative functional information about tumors that can be used to improve tumor detection, characterization of tumor, and monitoring the response to therapy.[1] DWI can help guiding biopsy in solid tumors away from necrotic areas. With the introduction of new generation MR scanners and advent of free breathing DWI, diffusion-weighted whole body (WB) imaging with background body signal suppression (DWIBS) has now become feasible, which has promising application in primary tumor detection as well as metastatic work-up in various pediatric tumors.[2]

Conventional abdominal radiographs infrequently provide a definite diagnosis for a suspected abdominal mass but can suggest a mimicking process such as constipation and fecal retention or a distended urinary bladder. The nature of an abdominal mass can sometimes be inferred on abdominal radiographs by the presence or absence of calcification in the mass and the location of the mass as indicated by the pattern of bowel displacement and other signs of mass effect.

With the availability of cross-sectional imaging modalities like US, CT, and MRI, intravenous urography (IVU) has a very limited role to play in the evaluation of suspected cases of retroperitoneal or even renal masses as it provides only indirect evidence of the mass.

Radionuclide imaging offers functional information that is not attainable with traditional radiographic imaging. Technetium-99m-dimercaptosuccinic acid (^{99m}Tc-DMSA) renal cortical scintigraphy has a role in preoperative assessment of functional renal parenchyma in cases of bilateral renal tumors, selected for nephron sparing surgery (NSS). Iodine-123-metaiodobenzylguanidine (123I-MIBG) scintigraphy is a sensitive and specific radionuclide imaging modality routinely used for the detection of neuroblastoma (NBL) involvement. ^{99m}Tc-methylene diphosphonate (^{99m}Tc-MDP) bone scan may be useful for detection of bony metastases in some malignant renal and retroperitoneal tumors in children. ^{18}F-labeled fluoro-2-deoxyglucose positron emission tomography (^{18}F-FDG-PET) is a functional imaging modality based upon the metabolic activity of viable tumor tissue and can be incorporated into CT or MRI. FDG-PET CT/MR has well-established role in primary staging and response assessment of pediatric lymphoma. This can also be useful in detection of synchronous tumor, distant metastases, and post-treatment evaluation of residual tumor in various malignant renal and retroperitoneal mass lesions.

The first step in evaluating these masses is to decide whether the mass is located in the retroperitoneal space. Anterior displacement of retroperitoneal organs and major abdominal vessels strongly suggest that the mass arises in the retroperitoneum. After confirming the retroperitoneal location, the next step is to decide whether it is arising from a retroperitoneal organ or is a primary retroperitoneal tumor arising outside the major retroperitoneal organs. Certain radiologic signs have been described to determine the origin of a mass.[3] When a tumor arises from an organ, the organ appears to be embedded in the tumor. This is called the positive embedded organ sign. When a tumor compresses an adjacent pliable organ [such as the hollow viscera or inferior vena cava (IVC)], it deforms the organ into a crescent shape. This is the negative embedded organ sign and is seen in primary retroperitoneal tumors. When the edge of an adjacent organ is distorted into a "beak", it indicates that the tumor probably arises from the organ. This is called the "positive beak sign". On the other hand, when an adjacent organ has rounded edges, it indicates that the retroperitoneal mass does not arise from that organ, this finding is called a negative beak sign **(Figs. 1A to D)**. When a large mass arises from a small organ, the organ sometimes becomes undetectable—the phantom (invisible) organ sign.

RENAL MASSES

Renal masses can be congenital, infective, inflammatory or neoplastic in nature. Non-neoplastic masses have been discussed elsewhere in the book and this chapter will deal with the renal neoplasms in children.

An abdominal mass in a child in the 1st year of life is usually of renal origin. Benign renal masses (mainly developmental, only 20% being true neoplasms)[4] predominate in early infancy, but beyond the 1st year of life and during the first decade, primary tumors of the kidney become more common. The various pediatric renal neoplasms, their frequency, and age of presentation are given in **Table 1**.[5]

WILMS' TUMOR (NEPHROBLASTOMA)

Wilms' tumor was first described by a German surgeon named Max Wilms in 1899. It is the most common renal malignancy in childhood accounting for 80–90% of pediatric renal tumors and 12% of childhood cancers.[6] It is rare during the 1st year of life and is commonly seen between 1 and 5 years of age with a peak at 3 years.[6] Occasionally, Wilms' tumor has been described in teenagers and adults.

Etiopathogenesis

Wilms' tumors can arise sporadically, can develop in association with genetic syndromes, or can be familial. Up to 12% of children with Wilms' tumor have associated congenital anomalies. The incidence of co-existent genitourinary anomalies—cryptorchidism, hypospadias, ambiguous genitalia, horseshoe kidney—is the highest (5%) followed by hemihypertrophy (2.5%), and aniridia (1%).[7] About 33% of children with sporadic aniridia develop Wilms' tumor and these tumors are frequently bilateral. Certain syndromes have a predisposition to Wilms' tumor. These include the Beckwith-Wiedemann syndrome (macroglossia, exomphalos, and gigantism), Denys-Drash (pseudohermaphroditism and glomerulonephritis), Sotos (cerebral gigantism), Bloom (immunodeficiency and facial telangiectasia) and Perlman syndromes.[4] Wilms' tumor has also been reported in children with neurofibromatosis, with imperforate anus, and rectourethral fistula.

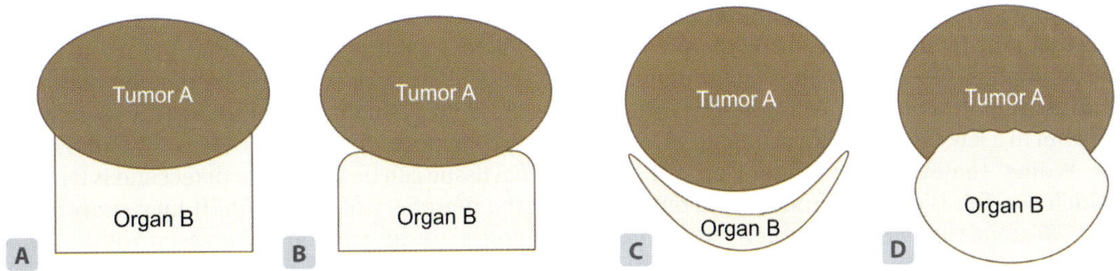

FIGS. 1A TO D: Schematic diagram showing possible relationships of retroperitoneal masses to retroperitoneal organs,[3] (A and B) Beak sign. Drawings illustrate the pos itive beak sign (A), in which Tumor A arises from Organ B, and the negative beak sign (B), in which Tumor A does not arise from Organ B, (C and D) Embedded organ sign. Drawings illustrate the negative embedded organ sign (C), in which Tumor A simply compresses Organ B, and the positive embedded organ sign (D), in which Tumor A arises from Organ B so that the organ appears to be embedded in the tumor.

TABLE 1: Most common age of presentation for renal neoplasms.[5]

Renal neoplasm (prevalence)	Age range	Peak age
Wilms' tumor (80%)		
Unilateral form	1–11 years	3½ years
Bilateral form	2 months to 2 years	15 months
Mesoblastic nephroma (3%)	0–1 years	1–3 months
Clear cell sarcoma (4–5%)	1–4 years	2 years
Rhabdoid tumor (2%)	6 months to 9 years	6–12 months
Miscellaneous tumors (7%)		
Renal cell carcinoma	6 months to 60 years	10–20 years*
Multilocular cystic nephroma	3 months to 4 years	1–2 years
Angiomyolipoma	6–41 years	10 years†
Ossifying renal tumor of infancy	6 days to 14 months	1–3 months
Metanephric adenoma	15 months to 83 years	None
Renal medullary carcinoma	10–39 years	20 years
Lymphoma		
Hodgkins	>10 years	Late teens
Non-Hodgkins	Any age child	<10 years

* von Hippel–Lindau syndrome.

† Tuberous sclerosis, neurofibromatosis, von Hippel–Lindau syndrome.

Two loci on chromosome 11 have been implicated in the genesis of a minority of Wilms' tumors. Locus 11p13 is known as the *WT1* gene, and locus 11p15 is known as the *WT2* gene. An abnormal *WT1* gene is present in patients with Wilms' tumor, aniridia, genitourinary abnormalities, and mental retardation (WAGR) syndrome or Drash syndrome; an abnormal *WT2* gene is present in patients with Beckwith-Wiedemann syndrome or hemihypertrophy. However, the genetics of Wilms' tumor appear to be multifactorial, and abnormalities at other sites, including chromosomes 1, 12, and 8, are also recognized. Familial Wilms' tumor is rare, occurring in approximately 1% of cases, and is not associated with mutations in chromosome 11.[8]

Clinical Features

Most children present with a painless abdominal mass often discovered accidentally by the parents or by the physician on a routine examination. The mass is hard rather than firm, nontender, and commonly unilateral. Wilms' tumor is almost always solitary, but in a few cases multifocal unilateral lesions may be seen. Wilms' tumor can be bilateral in 4–13% of children of which two-thirds are synchronous and one-third metachronous.[9] Bilateral tumors occur earlier, have a higher incidence of associated congenital anomalies, and a higher incidence of nephroblastomatosis than seen in unilateral tumors.

If the tumor ruptures or if hemorrhage occurs, there may be rapid enlargement of the mass with development of acute symptoms. Fever, leukocytosis, malaise, anorexia, and gross or microscopic hematuria may occur. Hypertension can occur due to disruption of blood flow to and from the kidney, compression of renal tissues by tumor, or rarely production of renin by the tumor itself. Rarely, some tumors may become hormonally active and can cause Cushing's syndrome or hypoglycemia.

Pathology

Wilms' tumor is characterized by an abnormal proliferation of the metanephric blastema cells, which are believed to be primitive embryologic cells of the kidney. The gross appearance of a Wilms' tumor is that of a large, bulky, solid mass with a well-defined pseudocapsule of compressed renal parenchyma that separates it from the rest of the kidney with distortion of the renal parenchyma and collecting system. The tumor typically spreads by direct extension and displaces adjacent structures but does not usually encase or elevate the aorta. Foci of hemorrhage, necrosis, and cyst formation are commonly found, especially if the tumor is large or has previously been treated with radiation or chemotherapy. There may be vascular invasion of the renal vein and IVC with occasional extension into the right atrium. Metastases are most commonly found in the lungs (85% of cases), liver, and regional lymph nodes.

Histologically, the classic Wilms' tumor is "triphasic": It contains epithelial (tubular and glomerular), blastemal (small round cells), and stromal (spindle and myxoid) cell lines. Not all tumors, however, contain all cell lines and the proportion as well of degree of differentiation of cell lines is highly variable from one tumor to the next.[7] Apart from the predominant cell lines, the prognosis of children with Wilms' tumor is heavily dependent on the presence of anaplasia. Its presence has been found to be more significant than tumor staging when assigning prognosis. A "favorable" histology lacks anaplastic changes, whereas one with "unfavorable" histology demonstrates extreme nuclear and mitotic atypia characteristic of anaplasia. Approximately 90% of Wilms' tumors are of "favorable" histology.

Imaging

Plain abdominal radiographs show evidence of a large flank mass. Calcification is seen in <10% of cases.[4] Chest radiographs are routinely done in all cases to look for evidence of lung metastases which indicate advanced stage disease **(Fig. 2)**.

On US, the tumor is visualized as a predominantly solid and slightly hyperechoic mass causing gross renal enlargement. A clear margination of the tumor from the rest of the kidney is often possible due to the pseudocapsule which may be hypo- or hyperechoic **(Figs. 3A and B)**. Normal native renal tissue can be difficult to detect and is typically stretched at the periphery of the lesion. It may show hydronephrotic changes. Cystic areas are often seen within the mass which correlate with presence of hemorrhage or cystic degeneration. Invasion of the IVC and extension into the right atrium can be readily detected on US **(Figs. 4A and B)**. Intrahepatic IVC can be assessed relatively easily but differentiation of invasion from displacement and compression may be difficult. A clue

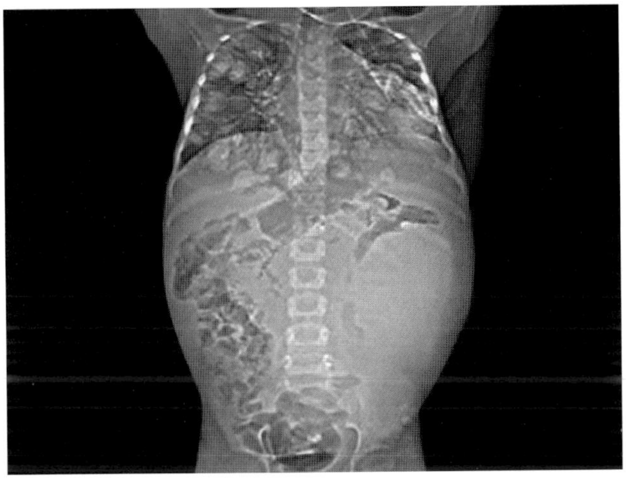

FIG. 2: Plain radiograph of the chest and abdomen shows evidence of a soft-tissue mass in the left lumbar and iliac fossa with displaced bowel loops. Multiple rounded opacities seen scattered through both lung fields consistent with pulmonary metastases.

to the presence of obstruction is the dilatation of the hepatic veins. Doppler can also confirm the presence of a thrombus and show its extent. Thrombus confined to the renal vein is less easy to detect because of distortion. Invasion into neighboring organs such as the liver can be evaluated by the real-time US. If the mass is seen to move freely from the organ, then invasion or adherence to the organ can be ruled out.[10] US is excellent for detecting the tumor itself and its vascular extension but is limited in its ability to assess extracapsular extension of tumor, lymph node involvement, and small contralateral tumors.

Abdominal CT scan is more sensitive than ultrasound in identifying tumor extent, nodal, liver, and contralateral kidney involvement. CT has the advantage of detecting the precursor condition, nephroblastomatosis. On CT, Wilms' tumor is seen as a large, well-defined mass of heterogeneous attenuation, which enhances to a lesser degree than the normal renal parenchyma **(Figs. 5A to C)**. The normal renal parenchyma can be seen stretched and splayed at the periphery of the mass—the "positive beak sign" **(Figs. 3C and 6A and B)**. Areas of low attenuation coincide with tumor necrosis and/or fat deposition. Calcification may be seen in a few cases. Capsular invasion may be suggested by a pattern of exophytic growth and contour irregularity. Contrast-enhanced CT scan allows evaluation of the renal veins and IVC for tumor thrombus though sensitivity is less than sonography **(Figs. 7A and B)**. CT scan may identify regional adenopathy, although it cannot differentiate tumor replacement from reactive adenopathy. Nodal involvement differentiates between stage II and III, but neither CT nor surgical exploration is accurate and its distinction remains histological at present. Peritoneal, omental, and mesenteric involvement of Wilms' tumor can be depicted accurately by CT.

MRI of the abdomen is the first choice complementary imaging procedure after US evaluation as it does not use any ionizing radiation.[11] MRI is also the preferred imaging modality in children with known bilateral Wilms' tumors or known bilateral tumor predisposition.[12] On MRI, the tumor appears as a well-defined mass with signal intensity similar to that of the spleen and slightly lower than that of the normal renal cortex on T1W images. On T2W images, the tumor appears isointense to normal renal cortex. Areas of high signal intensity correspond to the presence of hemorrhage or necrosis. The pseudocapsule is seen as a hypointense rim surrounding the tumor on both T1 and T2 pulse sequences **(Figs. 3D and E)**. On contrast administration, the tumor enhances heterogeneously and characteristically less than the normal renal parenchyma.

MRI can accurately assess tumor size, gross composition, and regional spread, although, as with all other imaging modalities, it cannot define subtle capsular invasion.[2] It can also accurately identify the presence of liver metastases and caval thrombus. Advantages over US and CT scan include the use of specific flow sequences in the search for tumor thrombus and multiplanar imaging in evaluating caval displacement by tumor.

The solid components of the Wilms' tumor typically show restricted diffusion on DW images.[13,14] DWI can differentiate between viable and necrotic areas within the tumor, which is useful in selecting the optimal site for biopsy. It helps in assessing the response to neoadjuvant chemotherapy showing a reduction in tumor size and an increase in ADC values seen in tumors responding to chemotherapy, whereas nonresponding lesions tend to have persistent low ADC values.[11] ADC values of residual viable tumor obtained from DWI have also been found to be useful in postchemotherapy stratification of histological subtypes of Wilms' tumor (lower ADC values in the high-risk blastemal type compared with various subtypes of the intermediate risk).[15] Besides this, DWI can aid in detection of small synchronous tumors in the same or contralateral kidneys.[1]

With the diagnostic information provided by US, CT/MRI, the role of IVU has significantly reduced in the present day imaging work-up of Wilms' tumor. On IVU, both frontal and lateral views are required for a proper three-dimensional concept of the mass. The appearance of the tumor on the IVU depends on the location of the tumor within the kidney. An intrarenal mass can be seen to cause splaying and distortion of the calyces. Tumors in the upper pole and posterior location cause more calyceal distortion than lower pole or anterior tumors, which can readily grow exophytically. A centrally located tumor may cause a hydronephrotic appearance associated with calyceal distortion.

Role of FDG-PET-CT in Wilms' tumor is still being elucidated.[16] Although primary and metastatic Wilms' tumors have been shown to be FDG-avid, currently, FDG-PET does not have a role in the initial diagnostic staging of Wilms' tumor due to the concerns of additional radiation exposure.[13,17] However, it has an important role in: (1) Evaluating the response to neoadjuvant chemotherapy with higher maximum standardized uptake value (SUV_{max}) being found in poor responders compared with good responders to chemotherapy;[17,18] (2) Directing biopsy from areas of active tumor activity, if it is deemed necessary;[19] (3) Providing additional information about active residual or recurrent disease over anatomic cross-sectional imaging studies;[18] and (4) Accurate staging and detection of the full extent of metastatic disease in children with relapse.[13]

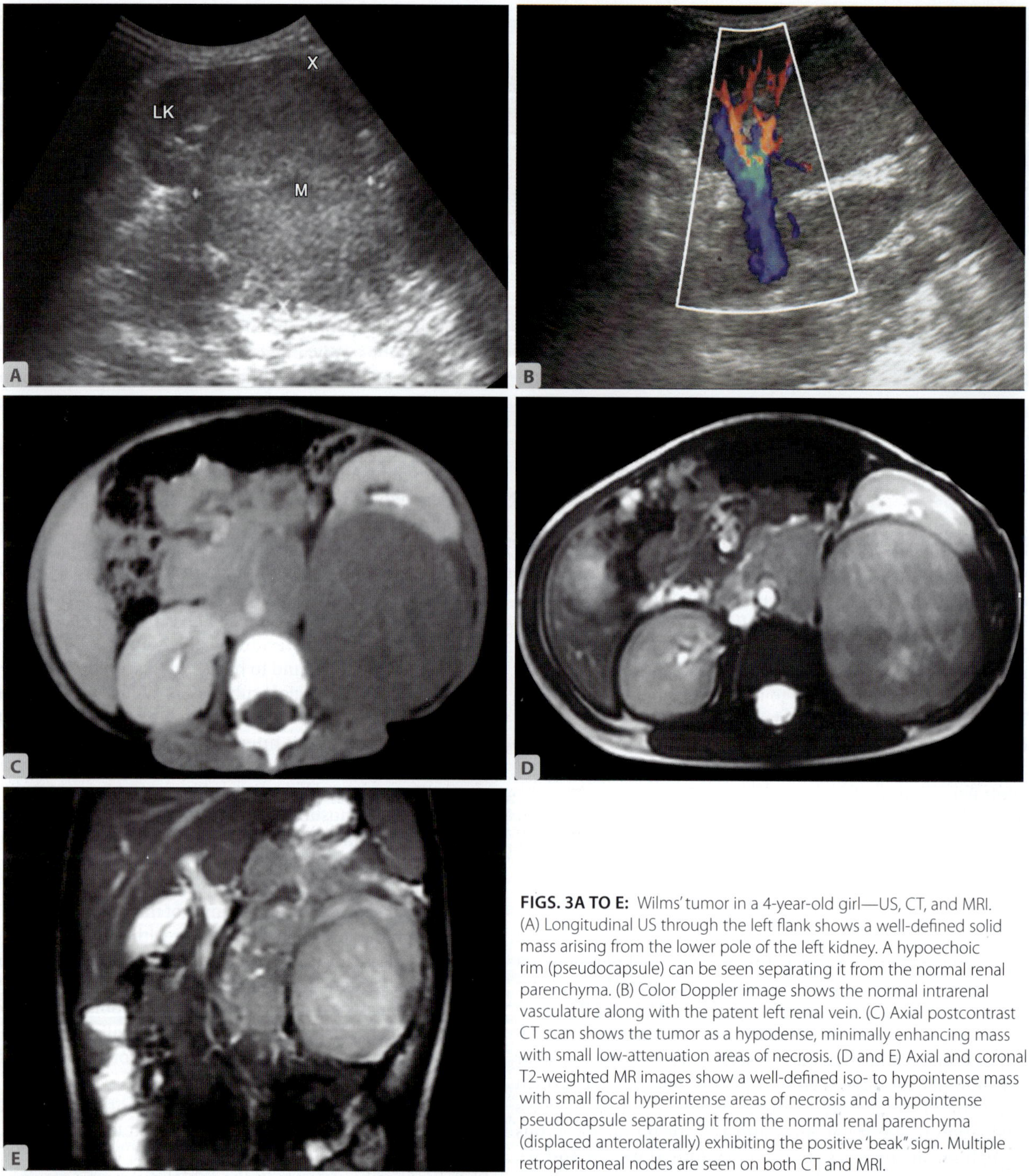

FIGS. 3A TO E: Wilms' tumor in a 4-year-old girl—US, CT, and MRI. (A) Longitudinal US through the left flank shows a well-defined solid mass arising from the lower pole of the left kidney. A hypoechoic rim (pseudocapsule) can be seen separating it from the normal renal parenchyma. (B) Color Doppler image shows the normal intrarenal vasculature along with the patent left renal vein. (C) Axial postcontrast CT scan shows the tumor as a hypodense, minimally enhancing mass with small low-attenuation areas of necrosis. (D and E) Axial and coronal T2-weighted MR images show a well-defined iso- to hypointense mass with small focal hyperintense areas of necrosis and a hypointense pseudocapsule separating it from the normal renal parenchyma (displaced anterolaterally) exhibiting the positive 'beak" sign. Multiple retroperitoneal nodes are seen on both CT and MRI.

Tumor Staging

Staging of Wilms' tumor initially developed by North American National Wilms' Tumor Study Group (NWTSG) has been adopted by Children's Oncology Group (COG). A similar staging system is used by European International Society of Pediatric Oncology (SIOP) group, but after a course of preoperative neoadjuvant chemotherapy, rather than upfront surgery as in COG studies. The current staging system utilized by COG and SIOP is described in **Table 2.**[12,13] Both of them are postoperative staging systems, essentially based on surgical and pathological findings. However, imaging plays a role in (1) defining the preoperative local extent of tumor mass as this can guide surgeons while operating, and (2) assessing the distant metastases to establish the overall disease stage. CT and MRI are considered to have similar accuracy in loco-regional staging of Wilms' tumor.[20] Different institutions opt for either CT or MRI depending upon the availability of the imaging modality and other patient-related

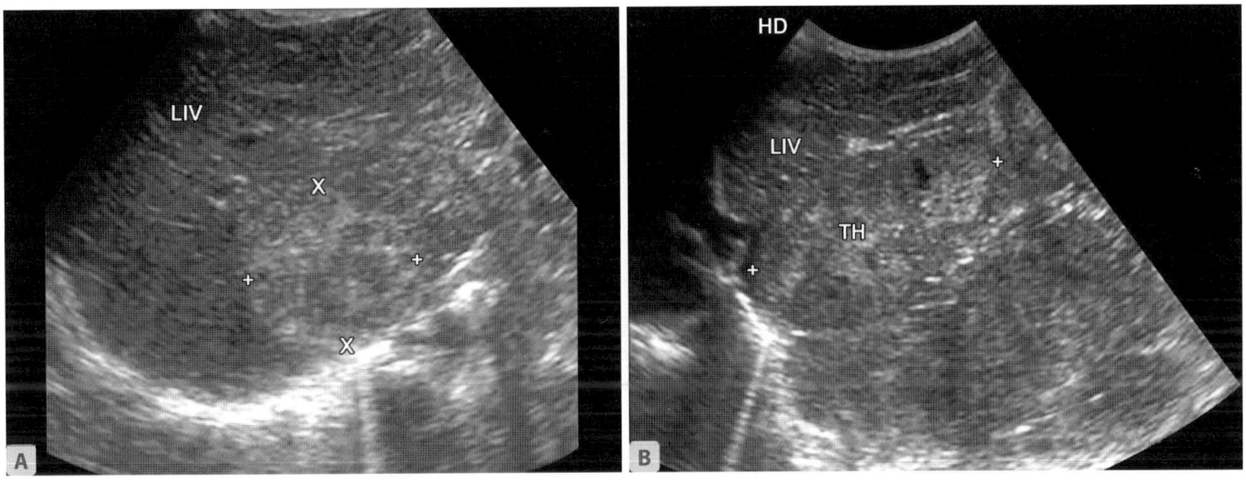

FIGS. 4A AND B: Transverse and longitudinal US image in a case of Wilms' tumor showing an isoechoic thrombus (TH) filling the inferior vena cava (IVC).

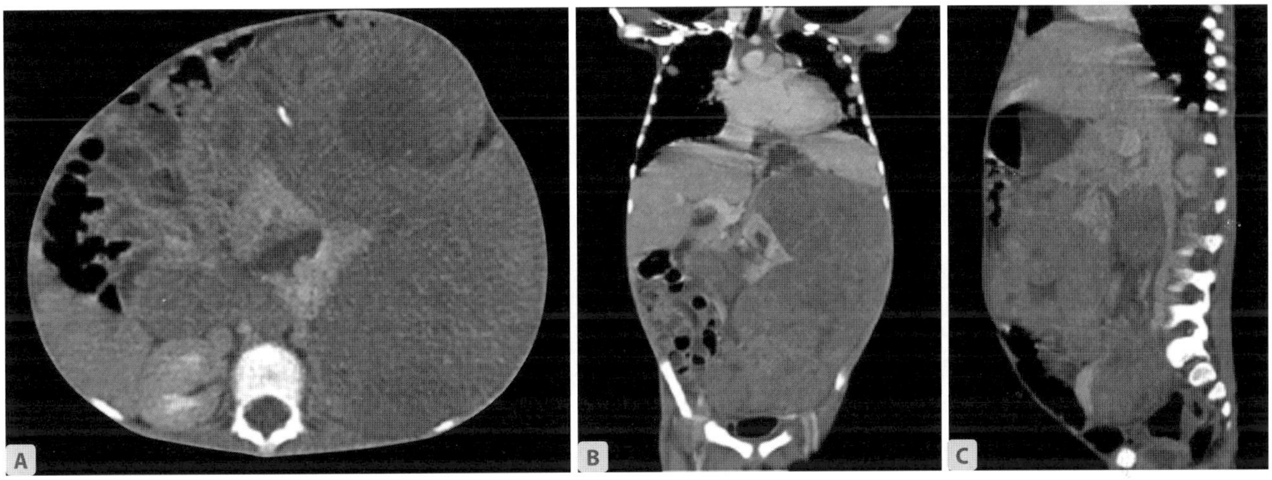

FIGS. 5A TO C: Multidetector computed tomography (MDCT) of a large left Wilms' tumor. (A and B) Axial CT and coronal multiplanar reconstruction (MPR) show a large heterogeneous left renal mass with areas of low attenuation due to necrosis. Small focus of calcification is also seen. Residual renal parenchyma is displaced anteromedially by the mass and shows the positive "embedded organ" sign. The mass enhances less than the normal renal parenchyma. Note the ill-defined nodular hypoattenuating area anterior to the right kidney, aorta, and inferior vena cava (IVC) representing adenopathy. Vessels are not encased or elevated. Multiple metastases can be seen in the lung fields. (C) Parasagittal MPR image shows the entire IVC which is compressed by the mass but there is no invasion or thrombus formation.

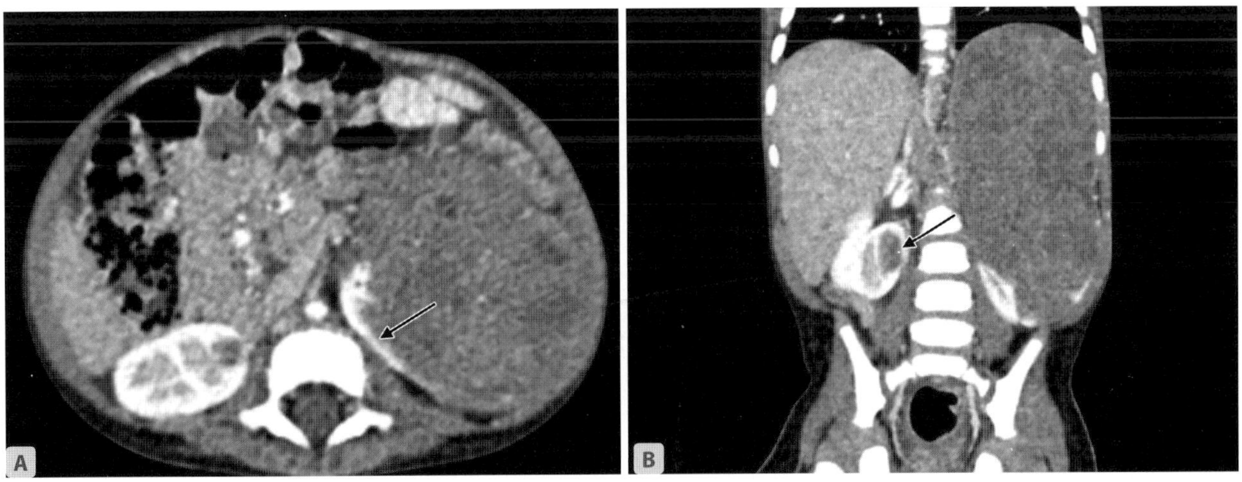

FIGS. 6A AND B: Wilms' tumor in a 2-year-old girl: Contrast-enhanced axial (A) and coronal (B) CT images show a large relatively well-defined poorly enhancing heterogeneous mass lesion arising from the left kidney which demonstrates "positive beak/claw sign" with the residual enhancing renal parenchyma (arrow in A). A small, oval, hypodense, nonenhancing lesion seen in the right kidney was a nephrogenic rest (arrow in B).

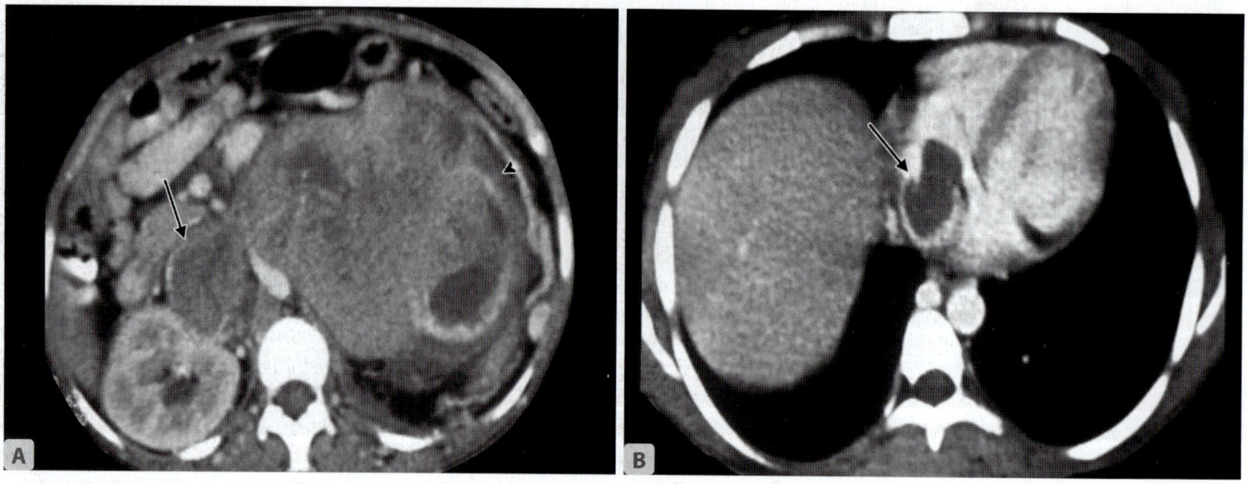

FIGS. 7A AND B: Wilms' tumor showing vascular invasion: Contrast-enhanced axial CT images (A and B) in a 6-year-old boy with a large Wilms' tumor arising from left kidney show tumor thrombus extension into left renal vein (black arrow head in A) and inferior vena cava (IVC) (black arrow in A), which are distended by thrombus. There is extension of tumor thrombus into the right atrium (black arrow in B).

TABLE 2: Staging system of Wilms' tumors (WT) utilized by the National Wilms' Tumor Study Group (NWTSG)/COG and SIOP.[12,13,16]

Stage	Children's Oncology Group (COG)	International Society of Pediatric Oncology (SIOP)
I	The tumor is limited to the kidney with intact capsule and is excised completely	• The tumor limited to kidney or surrounded by fibrous pseudocapsule and completely resected • Necrotic tumors or chemothearapy changes in perirenal fat or renal sinus do not upstage if completely resected
II	• The tumor extends beyond the kidney but is excised completely • Capsular penetration, renal vein involvement, and renal sinus involvement may also be found • No residual tumor apparent at or beyond margins of excision	• The tumor extends beyond kidney • Or, penetrates renal capsule or pseudocapsule into perirenal fat • Or, infiltrates renal sinus and/or vessels • Or, invades adjacent organs or vena cava • And is completely resected
III	• Residual intra-abdominal tumor (nonhematogenous) exists after the completion of surgery. Lymph node findings are positive • Tumor extends beyond surgical margins either microscopically or macroscopically • Diffuse peritoneal contamination by growth or spillage • Tumor is removed in more than one piece • Contiguous tumor extension into adjacent organs resulting in incomplete resection • Preoperative tumor rupture into retroperitoneum or peritoneal cavity • Preoperative tumor biopsy	• Incomplete excision of tumor (gross or microscopic residual tumor) • Or, any abdominal lymph nodes involved • Or, peritoneal implants or penetrates peritoneal surface • Or, tumor thrombi at resection margin • Or, tumor has ruptured • Or, tumor has had surgical (not needle) biopsy
IV	• Distant hematogenous metastasis (lungs, liver, bone, and brain) • Lymph node metastases outside the abdomen/pelvis	• Hematogenous metastasis • Or, lymph node metastases outside the abdomen/pelvis
V	• Synchronous bilateral involvement has occurred • Each side is assigned a stage from I to III, and histology is based on biopsy findings	• Bilateral renal tumors at diagnosis • Each side should be staged separately

factors. MRI is more sensitive for detection of contralateral synchronous lesions.[20]

- *Local extent*: The key imaging findings that should be carefully evaluated in the abdomen include:
  - Infiltration of tumor into adjacent structures
  - Intravascular extension of tumor into the renal vein, IVC, and right atrium **(Figs. 7A and B)**
  - Detection of tumor extension to proximal ureter
  - Involvement of regional lymph nodes although size and morphology based imaging criteria are not always accurate in differentiating benign and malignant lymph node; therefore, surgical lymph node sampling is imperative for accurate staging.[21]

- *Signs of tumor rupture (intraperitoneal and retroperitoneal)*: It is important to detect tumor rupture for staging and therapy planning, as it is a major risk factor for abdominal recurrence. CT detection of preoperative tumor rupture may aid the surgeon in preoperative planning before laparotomy.[22] Some of the imaging findings which suggest tumor rupture are poorly defined tumor margins, fat stranding around the tumor, presence of retroperitoneal fluid, ipsilateral pleural effusion, and peritoneal fluid extending beyond the cul-de-sac (irrespective of Hounsfield units).[12,16,22] Intratumoral hemorrhage, subcapsular fluid collection, or presence of a small amount of peritoneal fluid does not necessarily indicate tumor rupture.[22]
- *Tumor spread to peritoneum*: Peritoneal spread is often associated with intraperitoneal tumor rupture. This is seen as irregular peritoneal thickening, peritoneal nodularity, and ascites, along with mesenteric and omental solid masses on US, CT, and MRI.[23]

- *Size of the tumor*: Size of the tumor can be accurately measured on both CT and MRI. The volume of the tumor is determined from the largest diameter in the three planes (L × B × H × 0.523) by MRI or CT. If the tumor is large and cannot be differentiated from the kidney, then the tumor and kidney should be measured as a single unit.[11]
- *Distant metastases*: Hematogenous spread of the tumor with distant metastases is seen in approximately 20% of children with Wilms' tumor at time of initial diagnosis.[12] Lungs are the most common site for distant metastases accounting for 80–85% cases followed by liver.[12,16]

Chest CT and pulmonary metastases **(Figs. 8A to D)**: The role of CT scan of the chest in the evaluation and subsequent management of pulmonary lesions found only on CT is controversial and its prognostic importance is equivocal.[13,16,24] Chest CT is now mandatory for a complete staging protocol. It is a highly sensitive technique in the evaluation of parenchymal lung disease and enables the identification of lesions not visible on chest radiographs **(Fig. 8D)**. It is also more sensitive in the detection of calcified

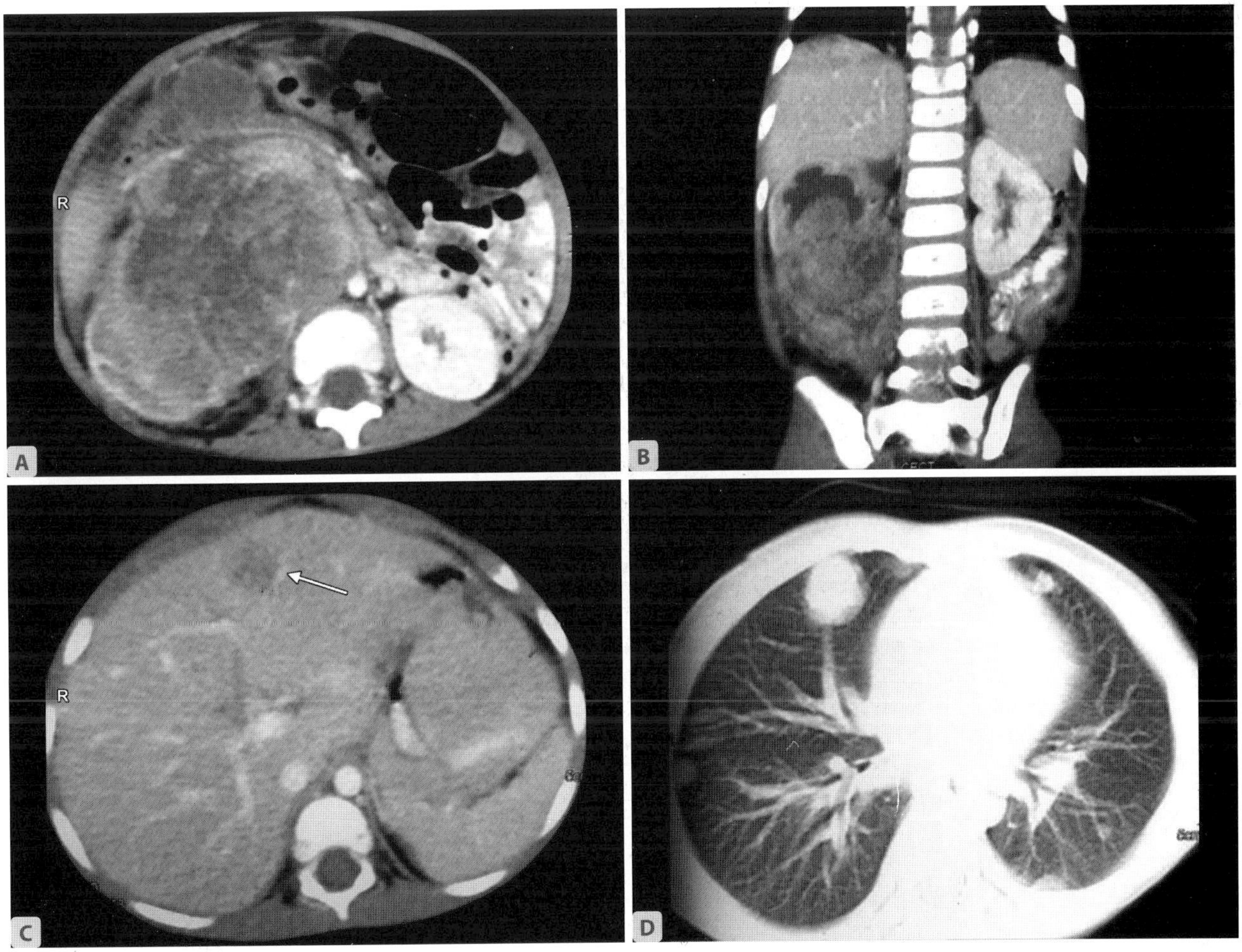

FIGS. 8A TO D: Wilms' tumor in a 4-year-old boy with pulmonary and hepatic metastases: Axial (A) and coronal (B) contrast-enhanced CT images show a large, irregular, heterogeneously enhancing mass lesion arising from the mid and lower pole of right kidney and showing nonenhancing necrotic areas within. The mass is infiltrating into the renal pelvis with resultant obstruction and dilatation of the residual upper pole calyces. Postcontrast axial CT scan through liver (C) shows hepatic metastasis as a well-defined round hypodense lesion (white arrow) in segment IV of liver. Axial sections through the chest in lung window (D) reveal multiple, bilateral, and rounded metastatic lesions predominantly in basal and subpleural location.

nodules. Controversy arises in staging the disease when chest CT identifies lesions not seen on chest radiographs (CT-only lesions). The results of many studies have shown that treating according to chest CT findings does not change the final outcome of children with Wilms' tumor.[25] Also, it has been shown that CT-only lesions are not invariably tumor, demonstrating the need for histopathological confirmation.[26]

USG, CT, and MRI can reliably detect hepatic metastases, which appear as solitary or multiple variable sized focal lesions within the hepatic parenchyma. On USG, they are usually hyperechoic compared to rest of liver. Smaller lesions can be easily detected on contrast-enhanced CT/MRI of abdomen done for evaluation of primary tumor and typically appear as hypoenhancing focal lesions **(Fig. 8C)**.

Management

The treatment strategy of Wilms' tumors has become a model for the successful multidisciplinary approach to pediatric solid tumors as the overall survival has now approached 90%.[12] There are two schools of management strategies as followed by American COG and European SIOP. The American practice is initial surgical removal of tumor followed by adjuvant chemotherapy dictated by the staging found at surgery. European oncologists favor initial neoadjuvant chemotherapy before proceeding to surgery. As the management of Wilms' tumor is fundamentally different in both the regimens (COG and SIOP), the imaging protocol also varies. In both the cases, a base line imaging is performed at time of diagnosis, which determines the renal origin of the lesion and its locoregional extent as well as detects distant metastases. As the patients in SIOP guidelines receive neoadjuvant chemotherapy, a repeat imaging is performed after completion of chemotherapy before going to the surgery **(Figs. 9A to C)**. CT chest for distant pulmonary metastasis is repeated only if pretreatment imaging shows positive findings.[11] The prognosis for Wilms' tumor patients is excellent and there is little evidence to suggest that the overall relapse-free survival is adversely affected by either approach.

The optimal surgery includes a transperitoneal approach with nephrectomy and biopsy of adjacent regional lymph nodes, whether enlarged or not. NSS is the primary management of choice in children presenting with bilateral Wilms' tumor at diagnosis.[16] Partial nephrectomy and other forms of NSS are also considered alternative to total nephrectomy in the management of unilateral Wilms' tumor in children with tumor involving a solitary or horseshoe kidney, in the cases of genitourinary abnormalities of the other kidney and in children with syndromic predisposition to develop metachronous Wilms' tumor in the contralateral kidney.[7,16] Preoperative imaging using CT with multiplanar reconstructions or multiplanar MRI plays an important

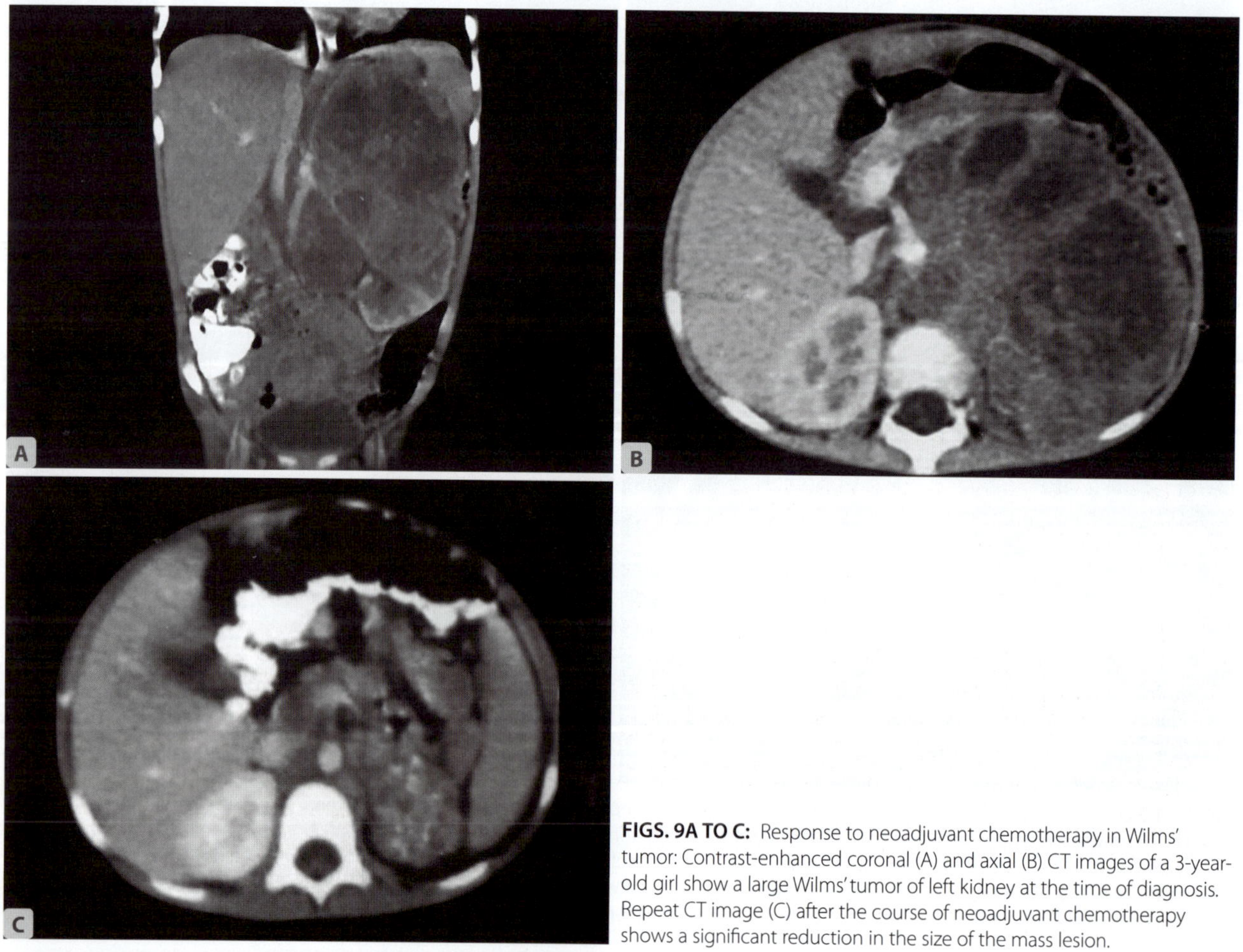

FIGS. 9A TO C: Response to neoadjuvant chemotherapy in Wilms' tumor: Contrast-enhanced coronal (A) and axial (B) CT images of a 3-year-old girl show a large Wilms' tumor of left kidney at the time of diagnosis. Repeat CT image (C) after the course of neoadjuvant chemotherapy shows a significant reduction in the size of the mass lesion.

role in identifying candidates for NSS and determining the resectability of the lesion by the accurate delineation of tumor margin and its extent.[11,16] Features on imaging which suggest the feasibility of an NSS are described in **Table 3**. Besides this, preoperative angiographic studies preferably magnetic resonance angiography (MRA) is useful in accurate demonstration of vascular supply and venous drainage in cases with bilateral Wilms' tumor. ^{99m}Tc-DMSA renal scintigraphy is used for assessment of functioning renal tissue in children with bilateral Wilms' tumor, where renal conservative surgery is being contemplated.

Pretreatment Biopsy

The latest SIOP-UMBRELLA management protocol recommends neoadjuvant chemotherapy to be started without biopsy confirmation, thereby increasing the importance of imaging studies in suggesting an accurate presumptive diagnosis of Wilms' tumor. However, to reduce the chances of a non-Wilms' histology receiving inappropriate chemotherapy regimen, a percutaneous core needle biopsy is indicated in the presence of unusual features.[11,27] Besides unusual clinical presentation, i.e., age >10 years, urinary infection, septicemia, or presence of hypercalcemia, and certain imaging features warrant a biopsy to confirm the histological diagnosis.[27] These imaging features have been described in **Table 4**.

Differential Diagnosis

The most important differential diagnosis of a Wilms' tumor is *neuroblastoma*. Although Wilms' tumor characteristically arises from the kidney whereas a NBL displaces the kidney, differentiation may be difficult in the presence of a large exophytic Wilms' tumor or with renal invasion of NBL. Features favoring Wilms' tumor are nonhomogeneous internal structure of tumor with hemorrhage and necrosis, round or oval shape with regular margins, and absence of calcification. Classical features of an abdominal NBL are ill-defined margins, tumor calcifications, tumor extension across midline, and displacement and encasement of vascular structures. Encasement of aorta, paravertebral extension, and invasion of spinal canal, if seen, are highly predictive of NBL whereas tumor invasion of IVC suggests Wilms' tumor.

Other differentials are mesoblastic nephroma (seen in children younger than 6 months), renal cell carcinoma (RCC) (peak age 10–20 years), clear cell sarcoma, and rhabdoid tumor of the kidney (RTK). In cases with bilateral Wilms' tumor, differential of lymphoma should also be considered.

TABLE 3: Imaging criteria suitable for nephron sparing surgery (NSS).

I	Tumor restricted to one pole of kidney or peripheral at mid-kidney
II	Volume <300 mL at the time of diagnosis
III	Unifocal tumor
IV	Adequate adjacent normal renal parenchyma to achieve oncological safe margin after excision of the tumor
V	Tumor involving <1/3 of the kidney with at least 66% of remnant renal tissue spared for normal renal function
VI	No signs of preoperative rupture
VII	Absence of involvement of renal pelvis and calyces
VIII	Absence of invasion of surrounding organs
IX	Absence of thrombus in the renal vein or IVC
X	Absence of lymph nodal involvement

(IVC: inferior vena cava)

Follow-up and Screening

Follow-up care after treatment must be long (if possible, lifelong) because Wilms' tumor may recur after several years. Most relapses occur within the chest and abdomen, and usually occur within the first 2 years following diagnosis. The latest SIOP-UMBRELLA protocol recommends chest X-ray and abdominal ultrasound every 3 months for all patients for a period of 2 years after completion of the treatment. Shorter intervals should be considered for subgroups of patients at high risk of early relapse (high-risk histology in stages III to V and intermediate risk histology in stage IV). These patients should have abdominal ultrasound/Chest X-ray every 2 months during the 1st year.[11] Chest CT should be performed after the end of treatment, if there is persistent disease after neoadjuvant chemotherapy.

Screening for Wilms' tumor in patients with associated syndromes should begin at 6 months of age with initial CT followed by serial ultrasonography (US) every 3 months up to 7 years of age. After the age of 7 years, screening can be discontinued because the risk of developing Wilms' tumor decreases significantly.[9,28]

NEPHROBLASTOMATOSIS

The nephrons of the kidney develop from the metanephric blastema. This development is normally complete by the 36th week of intrauterine life. The term "nephrogenic rests (NRs)" implies persistence of the metanephric blastema beyond 36 weeks of gestation. Nephroblastomatosis is the presence of multiple NRs, which may be multifocal or diffuse. These abnormal foci of persistent nephrogenic cells are regarded as precursor lesions and have the potential for malignant transformation into Wilms' tumor. They are found incidentally in 1% of infants. It is currently believed that NRs give rise to approximately 30–40% of unilateral Wilms' tumors,[9] and they are found in up to 99% of bilateral Wilms' tumors.[5]

TABLE 4: Unusual imaging features that warrant a pretreatment biopsy.

I	Presence of large lymphadenopathy
II	Presence of significant intratumoral calcifications
III	Inflammation/infiltration of psoas
IV	Nonvisibility of renal parenchyma
V	Almost totally extrarenal process
VI	Pulmonary metastasis in children younger than 2 years
VII	Extrahepatic and extrapulmonary metastases

Pathology

Nephrogenic rests are classified histologically as dormant, sclerosing, hyperplastic, or neoplastic. Dormant and sclerosing rests are usually microscopic and not considered to have malignant potential. Hyperplastic and neoplastic rests are grossly visible as small nodules surrounded by normal parenchyma. NRs can also be classified into perilobar and intralobar on the basis of location and the syndromes with which they are associated. Perilobar rests lie in the peripheral cortex or columns of Bertin. They are associated with Beckwith–Wiedemann syndrome and hemihypertrophy, Perlman syndrome, and trisomy 18. Malignant degeneration into Wilms' tumor is most common in patients with Beckwith–Wiedemann syndrome and hemihypertrophy, occurring in 3% of cases.[9] Intralobar rests are considerably less common than the perilobar type but have a higher association with Wilms' tumor development. These rests are found in 78% of patients with Drash syndrome and nearly 100% of patients with sporadic aniridia and are also seen in patients with WAGR syndrome.[5]

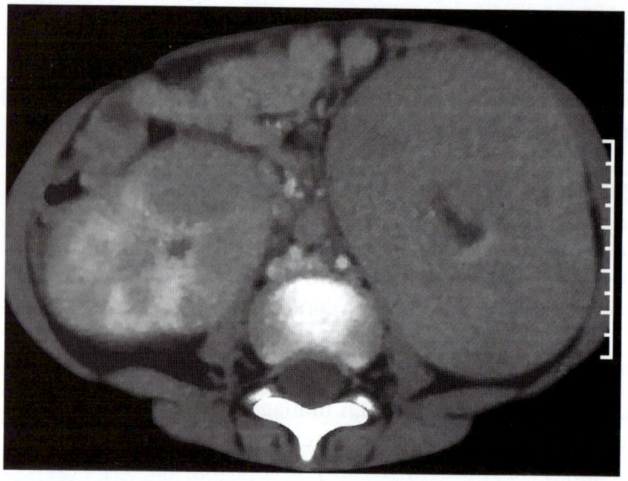

FIG. 10: Nephroblastomatosis in a 1-year-old child: Contrast-enhanced axial CT scan shows large nonenhancing hypodense masses in both the kidneys, larger on the left. Histological examination showed Wilms' tumor on the left side.

Imaging Features

Nephroblastomatosis may either be diffuse or multifocal. In the more common multifocal type, the NRs resemble normal renal cortex on all modalities and can be scattered throughout the kidneys; US shows large and irregularly lobulated kidneys with hypoechoic to isoechoic homogeneous mass-like regions within the renal parenchyma. These masses are often asymmetric and peripheral and the corticomedullary differentiation is poor. They are better defined on contrast-enhanced CT and MRI as focal nonenhancing masses **(Fig. 6)**.[29] In general, these nodules appear fairly homogeneous in contrast to a Wilms' tumor which is always heterogeneous in appearance.

The diffuse form typically manifests as reniform enlargement with a thick hypoechoic rim on US. This abnormal tissue surrounds the renal periphery and compresses the centrally located residual parenchyma. At CT, the peripheral rim of nephroblastomatosis is homogenously hypodense and nonenhancing, and causes distortion of the pelvicalyceal system **(Fig. 10)**. The remaining functional parenchyma may characteristically exhibit a pattern resembling stag's antlers. On MRI, the nephroblastomatosis is homogeneously hypointense on T1W images and varies from iso- to hyperintensity on T2W images. It is best seen after contrast administration becoming sharply demarcated from the highly enhancing normal renal parenchyma.

MRI may be able to distinguish a sclerotic from a hyperplastic nephrogenic rest.[19,30] Sclerotic rests typically appear dark on T2W images, while hyperplastic rests are usually hyperintense, similar to Wilms' tumor. In the setting of bilateral nephroblastomatosis or bilateral Wilms' tumors on treatment, it is thought that hypointense lesions on T2W images (sclerotic rests) may simply be observed, whereas hyperintense lesions may require further chemotherapy or local resection.[30] CT is unable to make this distinction.[30]

Differentiating NRs from a small Wilms' tumor can be difficult on imaging in some cases.[12] Increasing size on follow-up imaging, spherical shape of the lesion and heterogeneous enhancement are findings suspicious of neoplastic transformation.[5] At present, DWI cannot distinguish with certainty small Wilms' tumor from NRs or NBL, based on mean ADC values.[12,23,31] However, DWI allows better visualization of small NR/NBL foci and can also detect additional NBL lesions not seen on the classical MRI sequences both at presentation and after neoadjuvant chemotherapy.[23,31]

The differential diagnosis of nephroblastomatosis includes renal lymphoma, leukemia, or even polycystic kidneys.

MESOBLASTIC NEPHROMA (BOLANDE'S TUMOR)

Mesoblastic nephroma is the most common solid renal tumor identified in the first 3–6 months of life. It is a nonfamilial and benign tumor arising from the renal connective tissue. Originally thought to represent congenital Wilms' tumor, it was first described as a separate entity by Bolande et al. in 1967.

Clinical Presentation

A large and palpable abdominal mass in a neonate is the most common presentation. The peak age at presentation is approximately 3 months. Additional signs and symptoms include hematuria, hypertension, vomiting, and hypercalcemia seen in a minority of cases. Increased renin levels are often present. Some cases are detected at prenatal sonography and may be associated with polyhydramnios, hydrops, and premature delivery.

Pathology

Grossly, mesoblastic nephroma has a yellow, homogeneous, rubbery appearance likened to a uterine leiomyoma with no capsule and poorly defined margins. Unlike Wilms' tumor, foci of hemorrhage and necrosis are uncommon in this entity. The tumor has two morphologic variants—

namely, the classic and cellular type. Microscopically, the classic type shows sheets of benign connective tissue and mature spindle cells arranged in bundles and fascicles with entrapped dysplastic tubules and glomeruli. The cellular variant is highly cellular with immature mesenchymal cells and a high number of active mitotic figures, but no significant pleomorphism. Tumor necrosis and hemorrhage are more frequently seen with the cellular variant. These tend to have a poorer prognosis and are mainly seen in infants and children older than 3 months.[29]

Imaging

On US imaging, a mesoblastic nephroma typically appears as a well-defined, solid, and homogeneous lesion **(Figs. 11A and 12C)**. A distinctive "ring sign" may be seen in typical intrarenal congenital mesoblastic nephroma (CMN). This vascular ring sign, as described by Chan et al.,[32] is an anechoic or hypoechoic vascular ring surrounding the tumor on ultrasound and is considered a feature of the typical or nonaggressive mesoblastic nephroma. On color Doppler examination, this vascular ring demonstrates significant vascularity, and on spectral Doppler examination, it demonstrates both arterial and venous waveforms **(Fig. 12D)**.

CT and MRI demonstrate the presence of a large solid, mostly homogeneous intrarenal mass typically involving the renal sinus without invasion of the vessels.[33] On contrast administration, the tumor shows no or minimal enhancement **(Fig. 11B)**. Entrapment of urine or collecting system may lead to the excretion of contrast material within the mass. On MRI, the mass shows intermediate signal intensity, similar to the renal cortex and the skeletal muscle on the T1W and increased signal on the T2W images. The benign or the classic mesoblastic nephroma may demonstrate a peripheral, markedly enhancing ring on the postcontrast T1W images, corresponding to the vascular ring seen on US. DWI shows restricted diffusion in solid portions of the tumor, likely related to increased cellularity.[34]

Cellular or aggressive CMN appears more heterogeneous and shows hemorrhagic, necrosis, and cystic areas, which are uncommon in classic tumors.[35] Postcontrast CT images show variable focal enhancement of only the solid components. Noncontrast CT and T1W images may show high attenuation/high-signal-intensity foci of hemorrhage in the cellular subtype.[35] Due to aggressive growth pattern, this subtype often grows to large size, frequently crossing the midline and occasionally encasing the vessels and invading the adjacent organs.

On prenatal sonography, a mesoblastic nephroma may be first diagnosed when the detailed fetal anomaly scan is performed at 18–20 weeks' gestation, as a unilateral and solid paravertebral mass with low level echoes **(Figs. 12A and B)**. Differentiation between a solid and a cystic mass can easily be made on ultrasound to differentiate between a mass and hydronephrosis. Associated polyhydramnios is common and is thought to occur due to increased renal blood flow and impaired renal concentrating ability leading to fetal polyuria and subsequent polyhydramnios. If the mass is very large, it may be difficult to determine the organ of origin in some cases. Fetal MRI may be helpful in determining the organ of origin.

Differential Diagnosis

Imaging cannot definitively differentiate a mesoblastic nephroma from a congenital Wilms' tumor. Histologic examination is the only definitive test. The younger age of presentation, lack of well-defined margins, absence of tumor capsule, and central intrarenal location with involvement of renal sinus favor the diagnosis of mesoblastic nephroma. Other differential diagnoses include multicystic dysplastic kidney and congenital adrenal NBL.

Treatment and Prognosis

Mesoblastic nephroma generally exhibits benign behavior and is successfully treated with nephrectomy alone. Rarely,

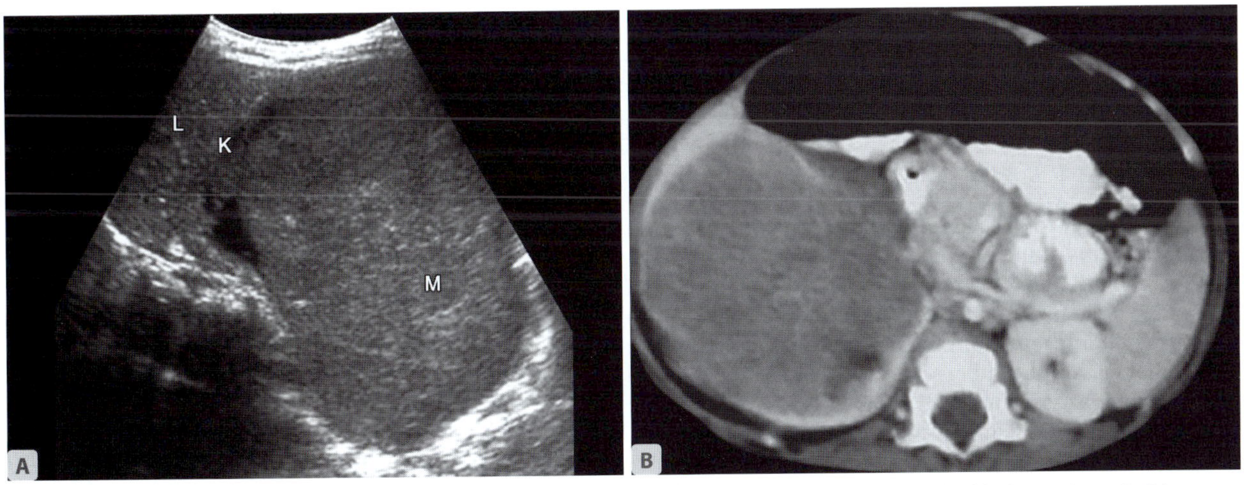

FIGS. 11A AND B: Mesoblastic nephroma: (A) Longitudinal US and (B) contrast-enhanced axial CT in a 6-month-old infant with a palpable abdominal mass shows a large, central, solid homogeneous mass arising from the right kidney. The enhancing normal renal tissue is seen along the periphery in B. (M: mass; K: hydronephrotic kidney; L: liver)

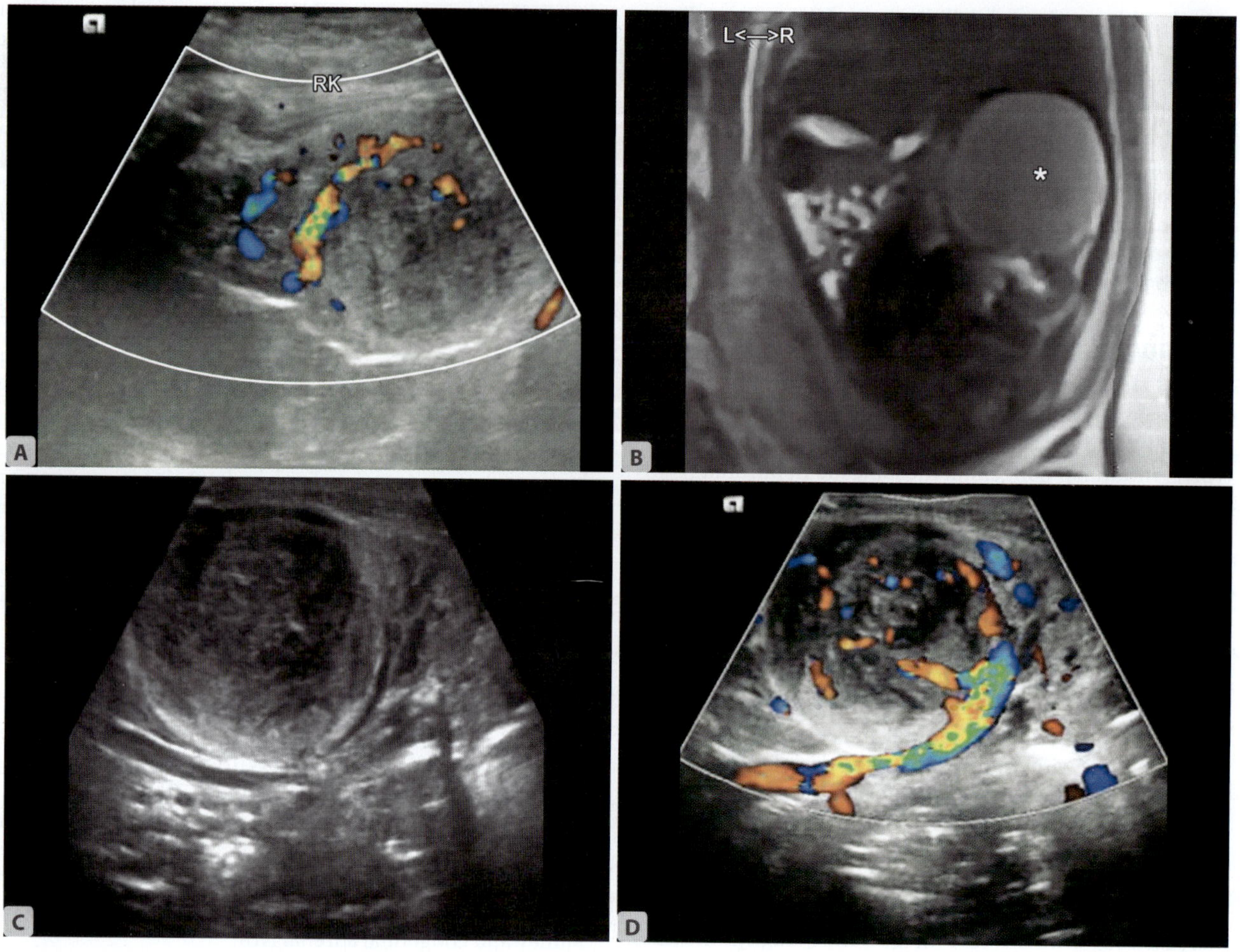

FIGS. 12A TO D: Congenital mesoblastic nephroma: Antenatal USG at 37 weeks (A) shows a large solid hyperechoic mass in upper pole of right kidney with internal vascularity. Prenatal MRI at 37 weeks' (B) shows well-circumscribed T2 iso- to hyperintense mass (asterisk) in upper pole of right kidney showing positive beak sign. Postnatal USG of right kidney (C and D) shows a well-defined solid heterogeneously hyperechoic mass in the upper pole showing marked internal vascularity. The vascular "ring sign" is absent. Right nephrectomy was done. Histopathology revealed mesoblastic nephroma-cellular type.

the lesion may recur locally if incompletely resected or metastasize to the lungs, brain, or bones. Therefore, it is currently recommended that patients be closely followed-up for 1 year after surgical resection.[3] The prognosis is best if the tumor is diagnosed and resected before 6 months of age.

CLEAR CELL SARCOMA

Clear cell sarcoma of the kidney (CSSK) once thought to be a variant of Wilms' tumor accounts for 4–5% of primary renal tumors in childhood.[4] The peak incidence is at 1–4 years of age and a male predominance has been reported.[5] It has a nonspecific presentation, most often manifesting as an abdominal mass. The tumor is characterized by its aggressive behavior and is associated with a higher rate of relapse and mortality than Wilms' tumor. It may metastasize to the bones, lymph nodes, brain, liver, and lungs; in some cases long after nephrectomy.

Pathology

At gross analysis, the tumor is soft and well-circumscribed. At histologic analysis, small cells with inconspicuous nucleoli and ill-defined cell membranes and a prominent capillary network commonly characterize this tumor. However, there is a spectrum of appearances, in which only 20% have clear cells.[5]

Imaging

Imaging studies do not allow differentiation of clear cell sarcoma from Wilms' tumor **(Figs. 13A and B)**. A sharply demarcated, predominantly solid, heterogenous, intrarenal mass without intravascular extension is seen on all modalities. At CT, the tumor enhances heterogeneously and less than adjacent kidney and shows nonenhancing foci, which correspond to hemorrhage and necrosis.[36] However, calcifications are infrequent.[36] At MRI, the tumor has low to intermediate signal intensity on T1W images and high signal intensity on T2W images with cystic areas.[33,37] Bone is the most common site of metastasis; hence, this was historically known as bone metastasizing tumor of infancy.[33] Bone metastases may be osteolytic, osteoblastic, or mixed. The discovery of a metastatic lesion in the skeleton in a child with a presumed diagnosis of Wilms' tumor should suggest that the tumor is likely to be a clear cell sarcoma. Once a CCSK

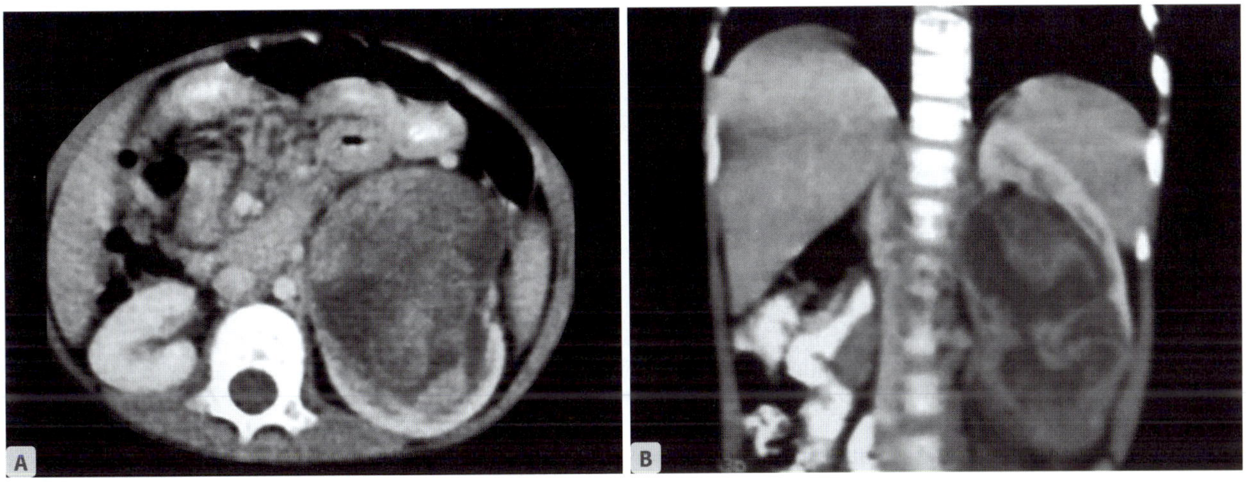

FIGS. 13A AND B: Clear cell sarcoma of kidney: Contrast-enhanced CT images of a 4-year-old boy showing a large well-defined mass lesion arising from left kidney. The lesions shows heterogeneous enhancement with nonenhancing necrotic areas within. Preoperative presumptive diagnosis was Wilms' tumor. Postoperative histopathological examination proved to be clear cell sarcoma.

is diagnosed, a WB FDG-PET (sensitivity ± 90%), WB MRI (sensitivity ± 82%), or ^{99m}Tc bone scan (sensitivity ± 71%) to detect bone metastases, and a brain MRI for cerebral metastase are recommended for staging purposes.[38]

Treatment

Treatment consists of nephrectomy and chemotherapy with current survival rates of 60–70%.[5] WB MRI, bone scan, or FDG-PET scan is advised in addition to standard follow-up examinations if bone relapse is suspected and for patients with a relapse detected elsewhere. Brain MRI is also advised if any suspicion of a cerebral relapse exists and if a relapse is detected at another site.

RHABDOID TUMOR

Rhabdoid tumor of the kidney is a rare and highly aggressive malignancy of early childhood comprising 2% of all pediatric renal malignancies.[3] Rhabdoid tumor is seen early in life; 80% of cases occur in patients <2 years and 60% before 1 year of age.[8] The median age at presentation is 11 months with a slight male predominance.[39]

Clinical Presentation

Most patients present with advanced stage disease and symptoms may be related to metastatic disease. Concomitant brain tumor or other soft tissue-tumors are distinctive features of this entity.

Pathology

The macroscopic appearance of rhabdoid tumor is nonspecific. It arises centrally (unlike Wilms' tumor) and has an infiltrative growth pattern. Local invasion of renal parenchyma and renal vein are common. Distant metastases to the lung and liver are also common and association with synchronous and metachronous brain metastases is a distinctive feature. Association with synchronous primary brain tumors has been reported in 10–15% of patients. Primitive neuroectodermal tumor (PNET), ependymoma, and cerebellar and brainstem astrocytoma have all been documented.[39] Soft-tissue and thymic tumors may also occur in association with malignant rhabdoid tumor.

At histologic analysis, the tumor is characterized by monomorphic cells with prominent eosinophilic nucleoli and characteristic filamentous intracytoplasmic inclusions.[5] Some areas of the tumor may superficially resemble the blastemal pattern of Wilms' tumor.

Imaging

In most instances, RTK cannot be differentiated from Wilms' tumor based on imaging alone. US, CT, and MRI show a large heterogenous mass with indistinct margination, characteristically involving the renal hilum with associated vascular invasion.[33] If present, a number of features may suggest the diagnosis of RTK: Subcapsular fluid collections, soft-tissue tumor lobules interspersed by areas of necrosis or hemorrhage, and curvilinear calcifications outlining tumor lobules.[5,40] Subcapsular fluid collection represents either subcapsular hemorrhage or a crescentic area of necrosis.[40] This appears hypoattenuating on CT, and may appear hyperintense on T1W MRI, and does not show enhancement on postcontrast study. The crescentic subcapsular fluid collection, although seen in more than half of patients with RTK, it is not specific for rhabdoid tumor, and has been reported in other childhood renal tumors.[33] In fact, given the rarity of rhabdoid tumor, a renal mass with a subcapsular fluid collection is more likely to represent Wilms' tumor.[16] Similar to Wilms' tumor, vascular invasion of the renal vein and IVC may be seen.[16] Radiological investigation should also include cross-sectional imaging for the common sites of metastases (lung, liver, and brain) and bone scintigraphy, WB MRI or FDG-PET (bone metastases).

Treatment and Prognosis

Of all the pediatric renal tumors, the prognosis of children with RTK is the poorest. Despite aggressive surgery and chemotherapy, RTK has the poorest prognosis among all pediatric renal tumors. There is a high rate of local tumor recurrence following surgical resection. Survival is poor, with an 18-month survival rate of only 20%.[40]

RENAL CELL CARCINOMA

Renal cell carcinoma is primarily a tumor of the adult population and <2% of all cases occur in the pediatric age range.[5] The mean age of presentation is 9–10 years.[33] RCC is the second most common renal malignancy of childhood after Wilms' tumor. Although Wilms' tumor is much more common than any other malignancy in the first decade of life, RCC is more common than Wilms' tumor in the second decade of life.[41]

Renal cell carcinoma is associated with von Hippel-Lindau syndrome, in which the tumors tend to be multiple and manifest at a younger age. This syndrome must be ruled out in pediatric patients diagnosed with RCC, especially when the tumor is bilateral.[3]

Clinical Presentation

Clinical manifestations are similar to those in adults. Gross painless hematuria, flank pain, and a palpable mass are the most common presenting symptoms. Hematuria is more frequent in patients with RCC than in patients with Wilms' tumor.

Pathology

The pediatric RCC is different from adult RCC. The most frequent type of RCC in children is translocation associated carcinoma accounting for 20–47% of cases in contrast to clear cell carcinoma commonly seen in adults.[42] However, RCCs associated with VHL are usually clear cell type. Translocation of RCC is associated with Xp11.2 translocation, that involves gene fusion and subsequent overexpression of transcription factor E3 (TFE3).[41] The tumor forms an infiltrative solid mass with variable necrosis, hemorrhage, calcification, and cystic degeneration. There is distortion of the normal renal architecture and formation of a pseudocapsule. The tumor invades locally with spread to adjacent retroperitoneal lymph nodes. In contrast to adults, the retroperitoneal lymph node involvement is more commonly seen at the time of diagnosis, even with small tumors.[43] Metastases to the lungs, bones, liver, or brain are found in 20% of patients at diagnosis.[5] Compared with Wilms' tumor, RCC is more likely to manifest bilaterally and more likely to metastasize to bone.[4]

Imaging

At imaging, translocation of RCCs generally has a heterogeneous appearance owing to solid and cystic components with hemorrhage, necrosis, and calcifications. The tumors are typically centered in the medulla and contained within the kidney with unusual exophytic component.[43] Translocation of RCC typically appears hyperdense (45–60 HU) as compared to the adjacent cortex.[44] Focal or rim-like calcifications are commonly seen. At contrast-enhanced CT, this shows heterogeneous enhancement with both solid and nonenhancing cystic components that represent old hemorrhage and/or necrosis.[43,44] The solid portions typically show mild to moderate enhancement and enhance less intensely compared with the adjacent cortex during all three phases of enhancement.[51] Prolonged enhancement at delayed phase CT is also typically seen.[43] The tumor margins are well-defined, and a progressively enhancing peripheral rim, corresponding to the pathologically observed capsule, is best seen on delayed phase CT images.[43,44]

On MRI, translocation of RCC is usually hypointense on T2W images and isointense to hyperintense on T1W images, often with a heterogeneous T1W and T2W signal due to cystic and solid components with hemorrhage, necrosis, and calcification.[41] A fibrotic, low T1W and T2W capsule is often present. On gadolinium-enhanced imaging, the mass demonstrates heterogeneous enhancement, usually less than that of the adjacent renal parenchyma. Diffusion-weighted sequences may demonstrate areas of restriction within the tumor owing to the hypercellularity.

Differential Diagnosis

Renal cell carcinoma and Wilms' tumor may be indistinguishable based on imaging features alone. RCC tends to be smaller and exhibits calcifications more frequently (25% of RCC vs. 9% of Wilms' tumor).[9] Both Wilms' tumor and RCC tend to spread to adjacent lymph nodes and metastasize to the lung and liver; however, RCC is more likely to involve bone.[5]

MULTILOCULAR CYSTIC RENAL TUMOR

The term multilocular cystic renal tumor (MCRT) refers to two distinct entities: Cystic nephroma (CN) and cystic partially differentiated nephroblastoma (CPDN). Both are benign renal tumors that have well-defined margins and consist entirely of cystic lesions with multiple thin walled septations. In CN, the septa are composed entirely of differentiated tissues. If immature or blastemal cells are present in the septa, the lesion is termed CPDN.[29]

Multilocular cystic renal tumors have a biphasic age and sex distribution—two-thirds occur in a predominately male pediatric population between 3 months and 2-years-old; approximately one-third occur in a mostly female population, with a peak in the fifth and sixth decades of life. There is no association with cysts in other organs and only sporadic association with other congenital anomalies.

Clinical Presentation

Presenting symptoms vary with patient age. Children typically present with a painless, progressively enlarging, and palpable abdominal or flank mass that has a variable growth rate and may be discovered incidentally. Adults can present with a variety of nonspecific signs and symptoms including abdominal and flank pain, urinary tract infection, and hypertension.

Pathology

Cystic nephroma and CPDN are indistinguishable from each other on gross examination and consist of a well-defined multiloculated mass of noncommunicating cysts that is surrounded by a thick fibrous capsule and compressed renal parenchyma. The mass is typically large and commonly arises from the lower pole of the kidney. Calcification is rare. Necrosis and hemorrhage are uncommon but are usually seen in association with herniation of the tumor into the renal pelvis or ureter, which damages the thin layer of transitional epithelium.

At microscopic examination, however, CN is clearly distinct from CPDN. In CN, the septa consist of fibrous tissue, which may contain well-differentiated epithelial cells. The presence of poorly differentiated tissues or blastemal cells in the septa characterize CPDN. It is essential to distinguish between CN and CPDN because the blastemal component theoretically portends the risk of Wilms' tumor development.

Imaging

Cystic nephroma and CPDN cannot be distinguished at imaging. Abdominal radiographs may demonstrate a soft-tissue mass with curvilinear and peripheral calcification. On US, CT, and MRI, a MCRT typically appears as a well-circumscribed encapsulated intrarenal multiseptated cystic mass with no solid or nodular elements **(Figs. 14A and B)**. The loculi can range in size from microscopic to 4 cm in diameter and very small loculi may mimic solid components because of their innumerable, closely packed acoustic interfaces.[45] On CT, the cystic spaces have an attenuation value similar to or slightly greater than water. Herniation of the tumor into the collecting system is a characteristic feature.[41] On MR T1W images, the cyst contents show variable signal intensities depending on the concentration of old hemorrhage or protein and a high signal intensity on T2W images. The fibrous capsule and septa are hypointense on both T1W and T2W images. Capsular and septal enhancement is seen on contrast administration on both CT and MRI. Associated urinary tract obstruction may be evident.

Differential Diagnosis

The main differential diagnosis is cystic Wilms' tumor. Identification of solid nodular elements in the septa should suggest the diagnosis of Wilms' tumor and not MCRT. Other lesions that may mimic MCRT include multicystic dysplastic kidney, cellular variety of mesoblastic nephroma, clear cell carcinoma, and RCC.[29]

Treatment and Follow-up

As neither the clinical nor the imaging features of MCRT can predict its histologic characteristics, surgery—either nephrectomy or NSS—is required for both diagnosis and treatment. If pathologic analysis proves that the tumor is a CPDN, regular noninvasive monitoring is suggested because the presence of blastemal cells in the septa of a CPDN implies the potential for more aggressive behavior despite the usually benign course of the tumor.

ANGIOMYOLIPOMA

Angiomyolipomas (AMLs) are benign hamartomatous masses in the kidney containing fat, smooth muscle, and blood vessels in varying proportions. Up to 80% of all patients with tuberous sclerosis (both adults and children) have AML.[4] When associated with tuberous sclerosis, these tumors are more likely to be multifocal, bilateral, and of greater size. Association with neurofibromatosis and von Hippel-Lindau syndrome has also been described.

Clinical Presentation

Most commonly AMLs are found incidentally in asymptomatic children. Clinical symptoms are related to the occurrence of tumor bleeding which correlates with the size of tumor. AMLs smaller than 4 cm are usually asymptomatic. Those larger than 4 cm are more likely to bleed spontaneously and manifest clinically as pain and hematuria or even severe life-threatening hemorrhage.[4]

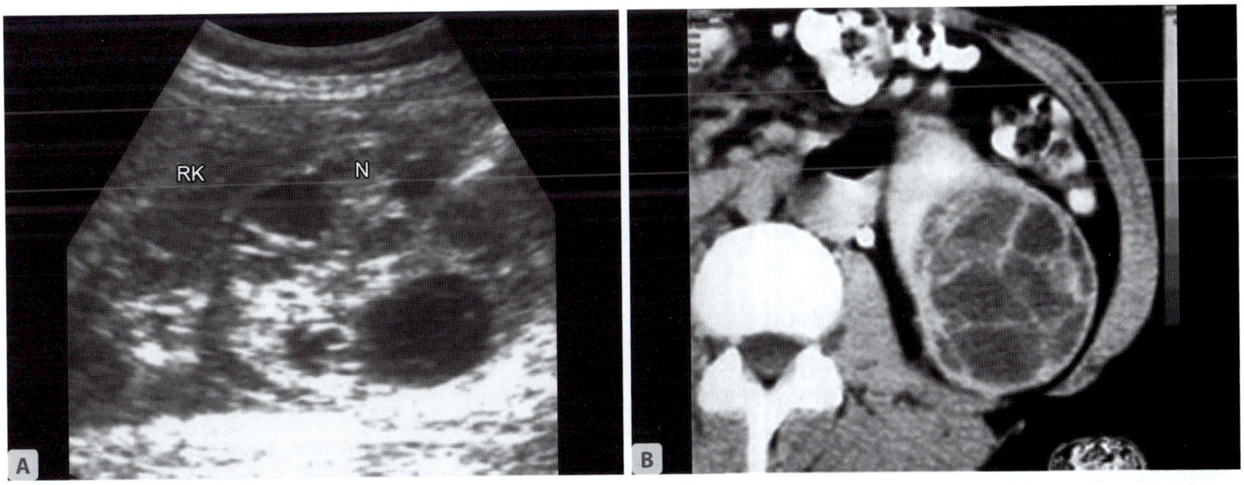

FIGS. 14A AND B: Multilocular cystic nephroma. (A) Longitudinal US and (B) contrast-enhanced (CE) axial CT demonstrates an intrarenal sharply circumscribed and multiloculated mass with enhancing septae on CECT.

Pathology

On gross examination, AML appears as an intrarenal mass varying in diameter from 3 to 20 cm. It is well-demarcated from surrounding compressed renal parenchyma but it has no capsule. Rarely, it may behave aggressively and invade the collecting system, renal vein, IVC, and retroperitoneal lymph nodes. Microscopically, a mixture of lipomatous tissue, blood vessels, and smooth muscle characterizes AML.

Imaging

Imaging studies are diagnostic if a characteristic fatty component is identified. On US, AML is seen as a heterogeneous mass, predominantly echogenic, without through transmission **(Fig. 15A)**. CT is the most reliable imaging modality and shows the presence of a renal mass with significant fat attenuation within it **(Figs. 15B and C)**. However, in the case of small lesions thin sections and single voxel measurements may be needed to confirm the diagnosis.[46] MRI can also detect fat within an AML which gives high-signal intensity signal on both T1W and T2W images with suppression of signal on fat-saturated pulse sequences. T1W gradient-recalled-echo MR sequences are useful for depicting diffuse signal loss on opposed-phase images of lipid-poor AML, which may not have bulk-fat signal intensity on standard T1W and T2W MRI. Also, the India-ink appearance at the border between the fat-containing mass and renal parenchyma is particularly helpful for identifying small lesions.[33,47] Angiography, which may be performed for embolization of a focal lesion prior to surgery, shows a hypervascular lesion with tortuous, somewhat aneurysmal arteries, venous puddling, but no vascular encasement or arteriovenous shunting.[48]

Screening, Follow-up, and Treatment

Conservative management is recommended for patients with known masses smaller than 4 cm. In children with tuberous sclerosis, it is expected that by 10 years of age, 80% will have developed AML, if monitored. The intensity of monitoring varies between centers. Serial US examinations every 2–3 years before 10 years of age and every 8–12 months thereafter are recommended with the aim of identifying and monitoring growing lesions.[5] Lesions that have bled or lesions larger than 4 cm may require renal-sparing surgery or selective transcatheter embolization in an attempt to spare as much renal parenchyma as possible.[4]

OSSIFYING RENAL TUMOR OF INFANCY

Ossifying renal tumor of infancy is a rare benign renal mass and is reported only in young children ranging from 6 days

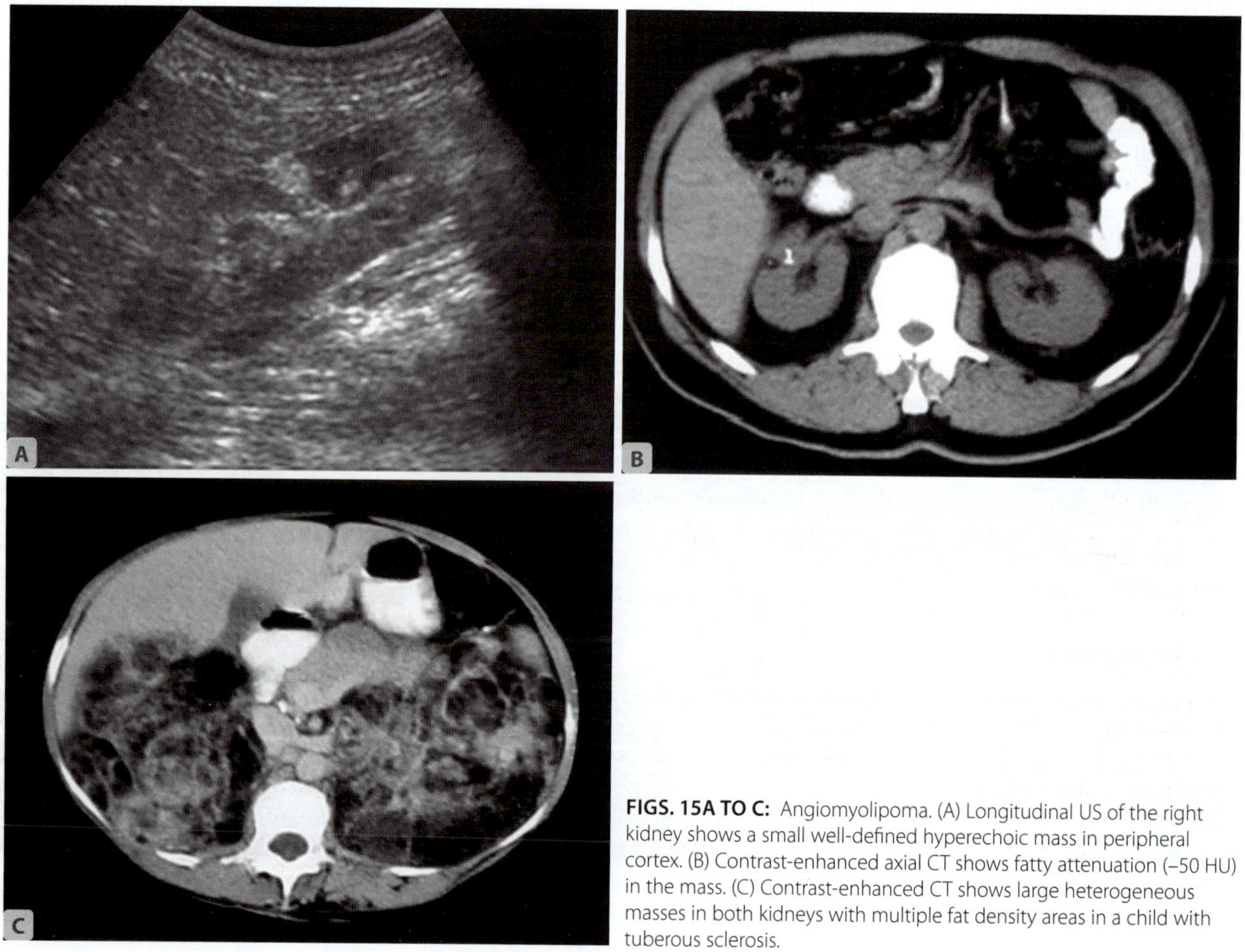

FIGS. 15A TO C: Angiomyolipoma. (A) Longitudinal US of the right kidney shows a small well-defined hyperechoic mass in peripheral cortex. (B) Contrast-enhanced axial CT shows fatty attenuation (–50 HU) in the mass. (C) Contrast-enhanced CT shows large heterogeneous masses in both kidneys with multiple fat density areas in a child with tuberous sclerosis.

to 14 months. Boys are more commonly affected than girls.[49] The tumor is relatively small (2–3 cm) and resembles renal calculi, except that it is attached to the renal parenchyma. The mass is centrally located at or near the renal papilla from where it extends in a polypoid fashion into the collecting system. Microscopically, ossifying tumors are composed of an osteoid core, osteoblasts, and proliferating spindle cells.

Imaging

The renal outline is usually maintained; however, filling defects with partial obstruction of the collecting system are often seen. Because of its location within the collecting system and its characteristic ossification, ossifying renal tumor of infancy may mimic a staghorn calculus, which would be exceedingly rare in the age group in which this lesion occurs. At US, the mass is echogenic with shadowing, and hydronephrosis may be present. Intratumoral flow may be seen with color Doppler imaging.[50] CT shows a well-defined mass, often calcified, with variable contrast enhancement, which distinguishes the tumor from a calculus.[50] MRI of ossifying renal tumor describes low signal intensity on T2W images due to calcification and possibly to dense cellularity.[50]

METANEPHRIC ADENOMA (NEPHROGENIC ADENOFIBROMA AND EMBRYONAL ADENOMA)

Metanephric adenoma is a benign renal tumor that can occur at any age and has been reported in patients as young as 15 months and as old as 83 years. It is more common in female patients.[5] Presenting features include pain, hypertension, hematuria, a flank mass, hypercalcemia, and polycythemia.

Imaging

On imaging, metanephric adenomas are typically well-circumscribed and hypovascular. On ultrasound, they may appear hypoechoic, isoechoic, or hyperechoic relative to renal parenchyma or even cystic with a mural nodule.[51] Doppler evaluation shows the lesion to be hypovascular. They are characteristically hyperdense to renal parenchyma on unenhanced CT and enhance to a lesser extent than renal parenchyma on contrast-enhanced CT.[51] Small calcifications may be present within the tumor. On MR, metanephric adenoma is usually hypointense on T1W and T2W imaging with reduced enhancement as compared to renal parenchyma.

LYMPHOMA

Lymphoma either involves the kidney secondarily from direct retroperitoneal extension or by hematogenous metastases. In children, non-Hodgkin lymphoma—especially Burkitt lymphoma–is more likely to involve the kidney. As many as 62% of patients with lymphoma have renal involvement at autopsy although only 3–8% of these patients demonstrate renal involvement at CT.[5] The existence of primary renal lymphoma without evidence of systemic disease is still debatable.

Clinical Presentation

Lymphomatous involvement of the kidney typically does not produce symptoms until late in the disease. Flank or abdominal pain, hematuria, anemia, weight loss, and a palpable mass are the most common clinical findings. Hypertension is rare. Of importance, similar to the central nervous system and testes, the kidneys represent a common sanctuary site for lymphoma where recurrences may occur.[52]

Imaging

Imaging findings are variable and include solitary or multiple renal masses or nodules, diffuse infiltration, direct invasion from contiguous retroperitoneal extension, and least commonly isolated perinephric disease. The most common radiologic pattern is multiple parenchymal masses or nodules that occasionally distort the renal contour and displace the collecting system. Lymphomatous masses have a nonspecific CT appearance. They are usually homogeneous, hypodense on nonenhanced and contrast-enhanced images, and may mimic multiple renal cysts. At US, they are hypoechoic and may demonstrate increased through transmission **(Figs. 16A to C)**. On MRI, lymphomatous nodules are hypointense or isointense on T1W imaging, hypointense on T2W imaging, and enhance to a lesser extent than adjacent renal parenchyma.[47,53]

Diffuse infiltration of the kidney may result in reniform enlargement. Retroperitoneal disease occasionally leads to vascular and ureteric encasement. Perinephric involvement can arise from retroperitoneal disease (most commonly) or transcapsular spread of parenchymal involvement. The CT findings of perinephric disease are variable and include small curvilinear areas of high attenuation, soft-tissue attenuation nodules, thickening of the Gerota fascia, or a mass contiguous with retroperitoneal disease. Lymphomatous masses often exhibit restricted diffusion on DW MRI and demonstrate increased ^{18}F-FDG avidity on PET.[33]

LEUKEMIA

Renal involvement by leukemia is rare at presentation but may occur at relapse. Leukemic involvement of the kidneys in children most often arises from acute lymphoblastic leukemia (ALL), which is the most common childhood malignancy.[54] Renal involvement generally occurs along with involvement of other extramedullary sites such as mediastinum, liver, pancreas, lymph nodes, etc. Renal symptoms such as hypertension or renal failure are rare. Leukemic infiltration of the kidneys most commonly causes bilateral and diffuse renal enlargement with distortion of the calyceal system. Solitary or multiple focal nodular deposits may be seen in the renal parenchyma. On imaging, the kidneys are enlarged but maintain their shape. There is loss of corticomedullary differentiation on US with a heterogeneous echotexture. CT and MRI show the same findings, i.e., bilaterally enlarged kidneys with loss of corticomedullary differentiation, altered parenchymal attenuation and decreased cortical enhancement.[4] Nodular deposits are seen as hypoechoic on US which are nonenhancing on CT and MRI **(Fig. 17)**. The differential diagnosis includes nephroblastomatosis, lymphomatous deposits, and simple cysts.

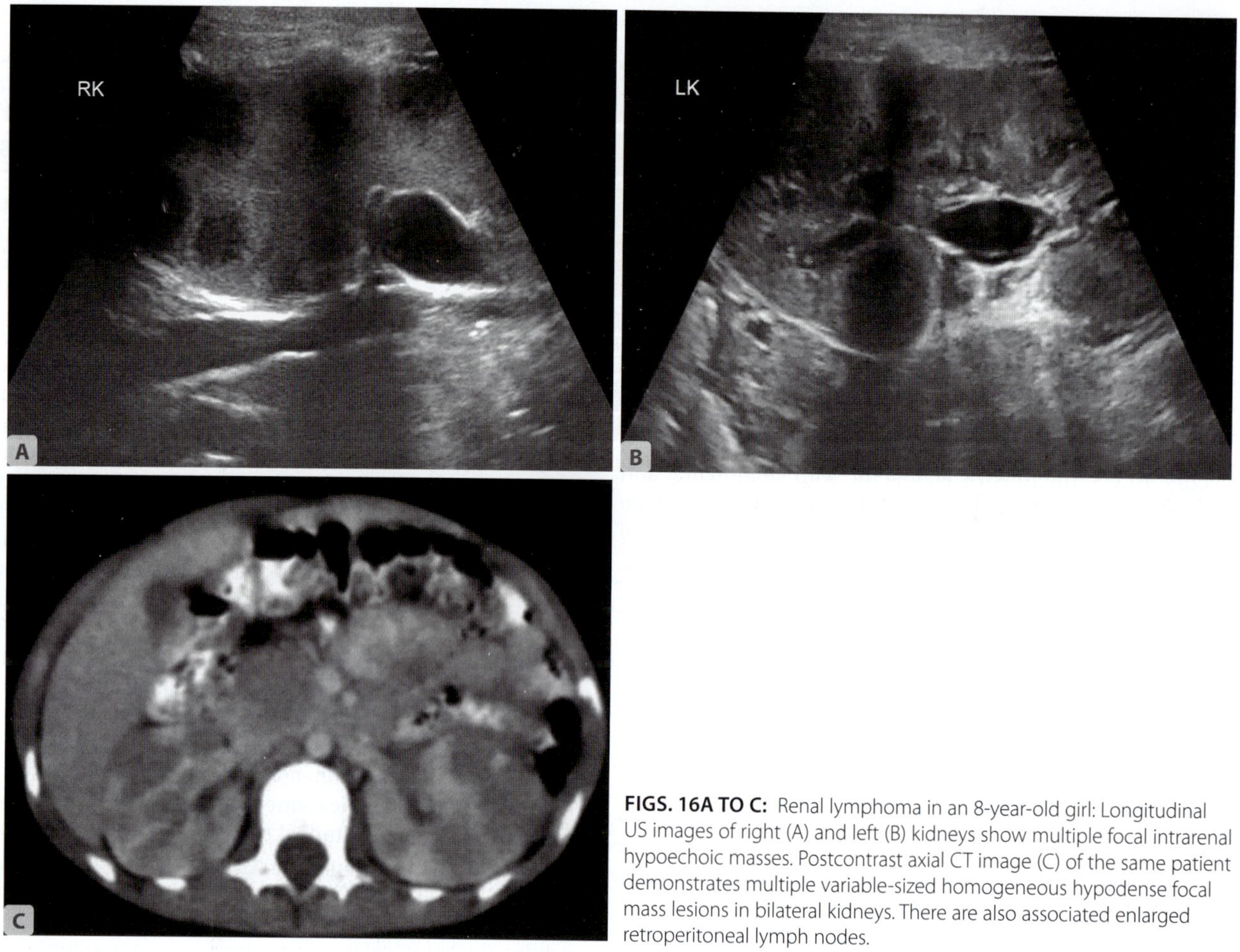

FIGS. 16A TO C: Renal lymphoma in an 8-year-old girl: Longitudinal US images of right (A) and left (B) kidneys show multiple focal intrarenal hypoechoic masses. Postcontrast axial CT image (C) of the same patient demonstrates multiple variable-sized homogeneous hypodense focal mass lesions in bilateral kidneys. There are also associated enlarged retroperitoneal lymph nodes.

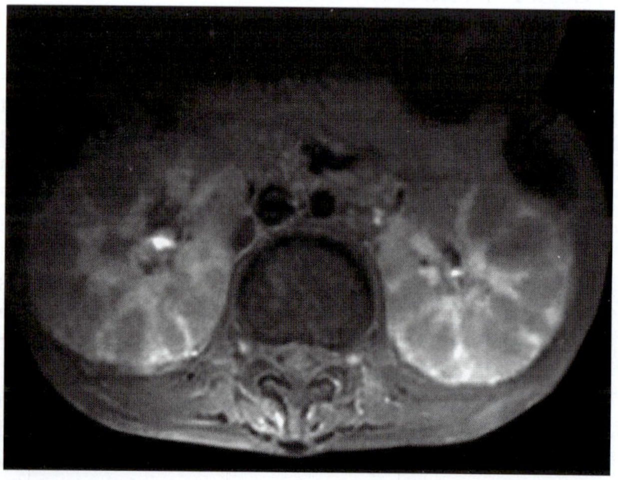

FIG. 17: Renal leukemia: Postcontrast T1-weighted axial image shows leukemic infiltration of the kidneys in a 12-year-old boy as multiple nonenhancing nodular lesions in the renal parenchyma. This appearance is indistinguishable from that of lymphoma.

PRIMARY NEUROGENIC TUMORS OF THE KIDNEY

Primitive Neuroectodermal Tumor

Primitive neuroectodermal tumors are rare malignant lesions most commonly occurring in the chest and extremities but have been reported to occur in the kidney. At histological examination, the tumor features small round cells and areas of extensive necrosis. On imaging, these lesions resemble Wilms' tumors. A large poorly defined heterogeneous mass with areas of necrosis and minimal or no enhancement are found. Calcifications may be present.[29]

Neuroblastoma

Primary renal NBLs have been reported but are rare. Imaging appearances resemble those of Wilms' tumor. Secondary renal involvement from contiguous adrenal and retroperitoneal NBL is more common and an incidence of 20% of cases has been reported.[55] Renal invasion occurs more frequently in undifferentiated histology and high stage (3 or 4) tumors. Extension may occur by tumor spread along vessels or by direct infiltration of the renal capsule, especially the upper pole contiguous with the adrenal gland.

Other rare primary tumors of the kidney are renal medullary carcinoma, metanephric stromal tumor, hemangiopericytoma or reninoma.[4,5] Desmoplastic small round cell tumor (DSRCT) and synovial cell sarcoma can rarely affect the kidneys in children.[41] Metastases to the kidney are extremely rare in children. Osteosarcoma metastases have been reported.[56]

CYSTIC DISEASES OF THE KIDNEY

Although simple cysts of the kidneys are more common in adults, they are more frequent in childhood than was previously appreciated and may even be seen in utero. The routine use of US nowadays and its high sensitivity in the diagnosis of cystic lesions account for the increased number of cysts reported.

It is believed that if a cyst is small, asymptomatic, and meets all the standard US criteria for a simple cyst (no internal echoes or septations, good through transmission, and smooth wall) then no further evaluation is required. Follow-up sonography is recommended to detect changes in the size or appearance of the cyst that might indicate the need for surgical treatment. If a cyst is symptomatic (producing hypertension or dangerously attenuating the overlying cortex), surgery may be indicated despite a benign appearance at US.

For unifocal cysts, some authors have proposed adapting the Bosniak classification for application in pediatric patients.[57-59] Wallis et al. proposed a modification of the Bosniak criteria for US, as children are most often studied with this modality rather than CT.[57] Early retrospective studies show good interobserver agreement in classifying tumors and suggest an ability to separate benign cysts from tumors.[57-59] Karmazyn et al. made a further modification to include the Bosniak IIF criteria [slight septal thickening (>1 mm), thin calcification, or septal Doppler flow] in modified class III.[58] No further imaging is required for modified Bosniak I and II cysts.

Bosniak III and IV (complex) cysts at US should be further evaluated with CT or MRI, and if the findings of complex cyst are confirmed, surgical resection should be under-taken. According to this system, MCRT would be classified as grade III (wall thickness and septa ≥1 mm with Doppler flow and possible calcifications).[58] Cystic Wilms' tumor and other predominantly cystic renal tumors would be classified as grade IV (wall or septal nodules or soft-tissue component). This modified Bosniak classification system and associated management guidelines need to be validated with prospective studies.

ADRENAL MASSES

Adrenal masses in children may be due to neoplasms, hemorrhage, abscess, and cysts. Neoplasms of the adrenal gland may arise from the medulla or the cortex. Medullary neoplasms are of neural crest origin and so may arise not only from the adrenal medulla but also from the sympathetic chain and include NBL, ganglioneuroblastoma, ganglioneuroma, and pheochromocytoma. Adrenal cortical neoplasms are the carcinoma and adenoma. Rarely, other neoplasms such as smooth muscle tumors can occur in children.

NEUROBLASTOMA

Neuroblastoma is by far the most frequent adrenal neoplasm, being the third most common pediatric malignancy, after leukemia and central nervous system tumors. It is also the most common malignancy encountered in the first month of life. The median age of diagnosis is 2 years and 90% of the diagnoses are made in children under the age of 5 years.[60] The tumor is congenital and cases have been identified on in utero ultrasound examination. There is a genetic predisposition to NBL and the tumor has occurred in siblings and in identical twins.

Site

Neuroblastomas arise from primordial neural crest cells, which are the precursors of the sympathetic nervous system. As a result they can be found anywhere along the sympathetic chain or in the adrenal medulla. Two-thirds of NBLs are located in the abdomen and of these approximately two-thirds arise in the adrenal gland and the rest from the retroperitoneal sympathetic ganglia, followed by the posterior mediastinum (20%).[61] Less common sites are the pelvis (2–3%) and the neck (1–5%). Occasionally, in the presence of metastatic disease, no definite primary tumor can be found.

Clinical Features

Neuroblastoma has a wide spectrum of clinical symptoms which depend on the site, extent, and the biological features of the primary tumor, and the presence of distant metastatic disease. The majority of children with NBL present with a palpable abdominal mass. This may be an incidental finding in an otherwise healthy child or in a child clearly unwell with lethargy, anemia, weight loss, and failure to thrive from widespread dissemination of tumor. In half of the patients with intraspinal tumor extension, peripheral neurologic deficits, and neurological symptoms from compression of the nerve roots or the cord may be present.[42] Metastatic involvement of the periorbital bones and soft tissues results in ecchymosed orbital proptosis, which is also described as "raccoon eyes" and may be misinterpreted as nonaccidental injury. Compression of the optic nerves by metastases may cause blindness. Massive hepatic metastases can cause increased intra-abdominal pressure and death from respiratory insufficiency. Encephalopathic symptoms may be encountered. In <2% of cases, NBLs can present with paraneoplastic syndromes: Opsoclonus-myoclonus-ataxia syndrome or watery diarrhea.[62] NBLs may also be discovered incidentally during scanning for other reasons, e.g., antenatal ultrasound, chest radiograph for pneumonia, or screening protocols.

Urinary excretion of high levels of catecholamine metabolites occurs in 85–90% of patients.[60] These metabolites are identified as vanillylmandelic acid (VMA) and homovanillic acid (HVA). The VMA/HVA ratio in patients with disseminated disease correlates with prognosis. Vanillacetic acid (VLA) in urine indicates a poor prognosis.

Pathology

The tumors arise from the primitive neuroectodermal cells. Histologically, NBLs are composed of small round and rosette forming cells which may be difficult to distinguish from similar round cells seen in Ewing's sarcoma, rhabdomyosarcoma (RMS), and even leukemia. Classically three different types of neural crest tumors are described based on the degree of differentiation of these primitive cells and subsequent variable malignancy. NBL is considered the most malignant, ganglioneuroma a benign and ganglioneuroblastoma with a mixed mature and undifferentiated histology as a "semi-malignant" or intermediate manifestation of this neoplastic disease. Within a given tumor the state of maturation may change, specially in an infant, the degree of malignancy may decrease and the neoplastic process may disappear.

Imaging

Imaging of NBL requires evaluation of the primary tumor and the metastatic extent of disease.

Plain radiographs: Abdominal radiographs may show the presence of an abdominal mass. One of the characteristic findings in NBL is calcification, which can be demonstrated in about one half of abdominal NBLs (compared with only <10% in Wilms' tumor). The calcification is usually finely stippled but may also be linear or ring-shaped and can sometimes be seen in areas of metastases such as lymph nodes or liver. Evidence of erosion of vertebral body or widened interpedicular distance suggests intraspinal extension.

Ultrasound: The mass is seen as a predominantly solid, poorly defined, heterogeneous, echogenic mass with few echopoor areas **(Fig. 18A)**. Calcification is commonly seen **(Fig. 19A)**. The displaced kidney can be identified, most often inferolateral to the mass, with a well-defined plane between the mass and the kidney. In rare cases, a NBL may invade

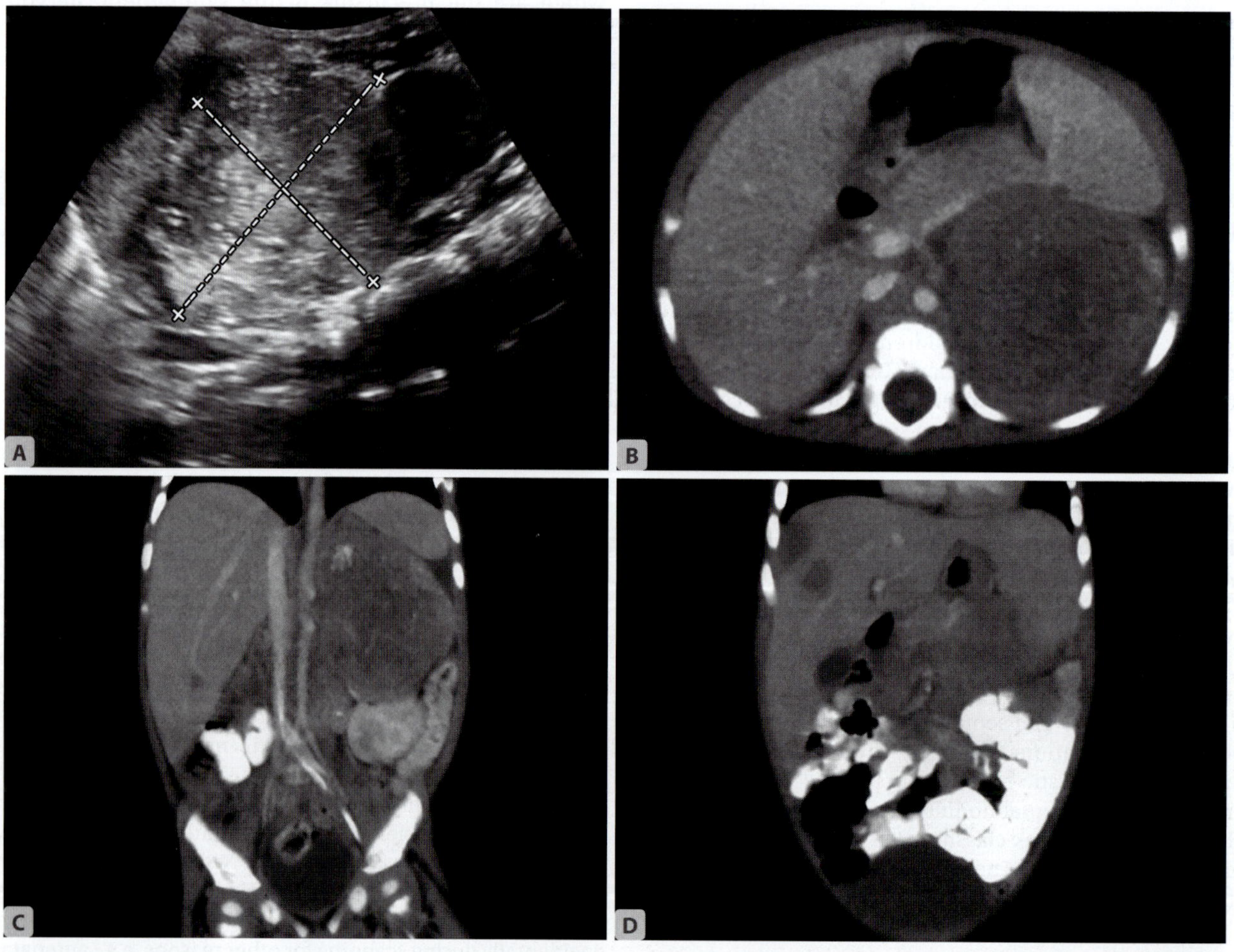

FIGS. 18A TO D: Neuroblastoma in a 10-month-old boy. (A) US image shows a large well-defined solid hyperechoic mass lesion in left supra renal location. Contrast-enhanced axial (B) and coronal (C and D) CT images show a large heterogeneously enhancing solid, left adrenal mass with inferior displacement of left kidney and anterior displacement of pancreas and spleen. There is an area of calcification (arrow in C) noted within the tumor. *Note*: made of multiple hypodense nodular metastatic lesions in liver.

the kidney and then it is impossible to differentiate from Wilms' tumor. The tumor often extends across the midline and can be seen to encase and anteriorly displace the aorta, IVC, and other vascular structures rather than invade them. The opposite kidney may also be displaced by large masses. US is useful in detecting differential movements of the tumor relative to the adjacent organs, i.e., liver and ipsilateral kidney. If there is no differential movement, involvement is likely. Nodal and focal hepatic metastases can be identified.

Antenatal and perinatal US examination has resulted in an apparent increase in the incidence of fetal or congenital NBL. The US appearance is variable and ranges from cystic through solid to mixed with foci of calcification. The differential diagnosis of this appearance is adrenal hemorrhage, extralobar pulmonary sequestration, and CMN.

CT and MRI: Further axial imaging for staging of a newly discovered NBL can be performed with either CT or MRI of the primary site. Both modalities can accurately assess the location and the size of the primary tumor, the vascular encasement and tumor resectability, but may sometimes be equivocal in the evaluation of invasive growth and lymphadenopathy. MRI is superior to CT in determining marrow infiltration and intraspinal extension of tumor.

On CT, a NBL is seen as a large, heterogeneous, lobulated soft-tissue mass that shows mild heterogeneous enhancement **(Fig. 18)**. Coarse, finely stippled or curvilinear calcifications are seen in >90% of the abdominal **(Figs. 18 and 19)** and 50% of the thoracic NBLs on CT.[62] Low-attenuation areas seen within the tumor represent necrosis or hemorrhage. NBL typically encases and displaces vascular structures but does not invade them **(Fig. 20)**. On MRI, the tumor is typically heterogeneous, with low signal on T1W and high-signal intensity on T2W images and shows little or no enhancement **(Figs. 21A and B)**. Cystic and hemorrhagic areas within the tumor can be well-identified but not calcification. On DWIs, NBLs show increased tumor signal which is attributed to restricted diffusion of water protons within the dense tumor matrix.[63]

The tumor is usually lobulated and lacks an identifiable capsule. Involved nodes at the renal hila, porta, and in the retroperitoneum are often large. Distinguishing between the primary tumor and the adjacent nodal disease is often difficult. Adrenal tumors frequently displace the ipsilateral kidney inferiorly while paravertebral tumors may push the kidney anteriorly. NBL can invade the ipsilateral kidney in about 20% cases and these tumors have to be carefully differentiated from Wilms' tumor on imaging **(Figs. 22A and B)**.

Both CT and MRI can demonstrate retrocrural and paravertebral extension and encasement and compression of the major abdominal vessels. Spinal canal extension is more common with thoracic than with abdominal tumors and the extent of extension, spinal cord displacement, and compression are better seen on MRI.

Hepatic metastases have two distinct patterns—either diffuse infiltration seen in 4S infants, which may be indiscernible on CT, but is clearly seen on MRI as

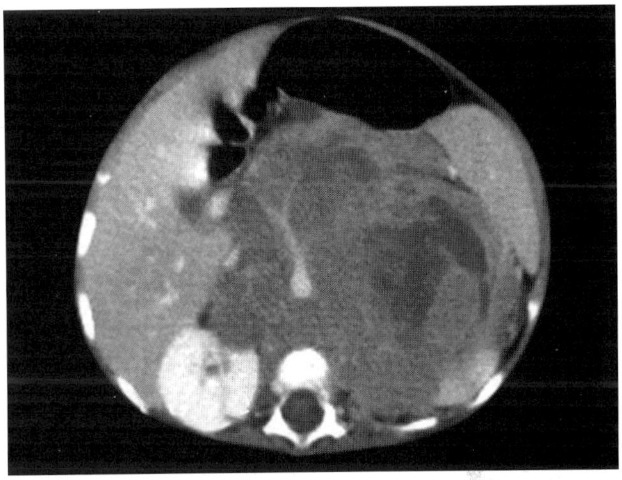

FIG. 20: Neuroblastoma: Contrast-enhanced computed tomography (CECT) axial image in a 2-year-old child shows a large lobulated left abdominal mass with few hypodense necrotic areas within. The mass elevates and encases the aorta and its branches. The inferior vena cava (IVC) is displaced anteriorly and to the right. The left kidney is displaced inferolaterally.

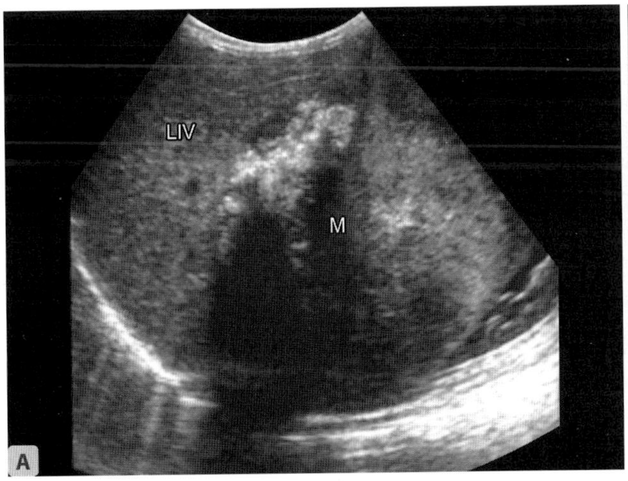

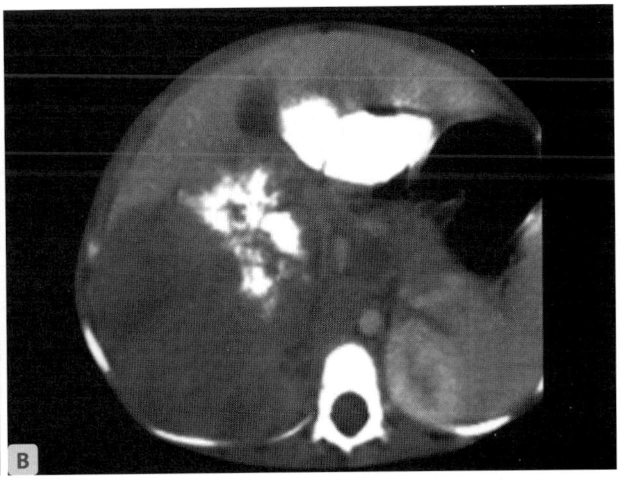

FIGS. 19A AND B: Neuroblastoma. (A) US and (B) contrast-enhanced axial CT shows a solid, right adrenal mass with a large area of calcification within. Multiple retroperitoneal nodes are also seen on CT.

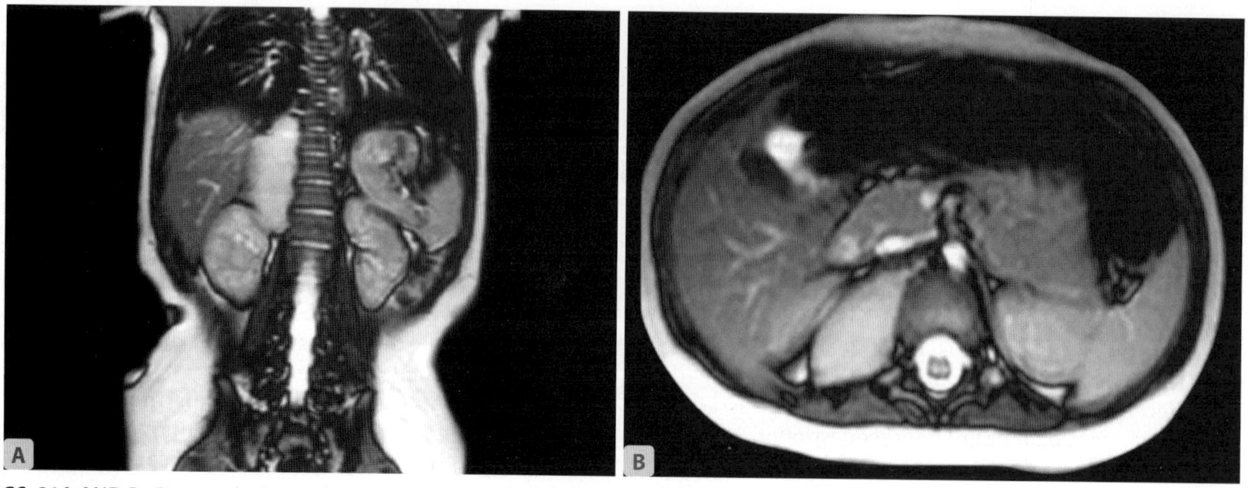

FIGS. 21A AND B: Paravertebral neuroblastoma. (A) Coronal and (B) axial T2-weighted MR images in a child presenting with opsoclonus-myoclonus syndrome show a well-defined hyperintense solid mass seen in the right paravertebral region superior to the right kidney. There is no evidence of intraspinal extension of the tumor.

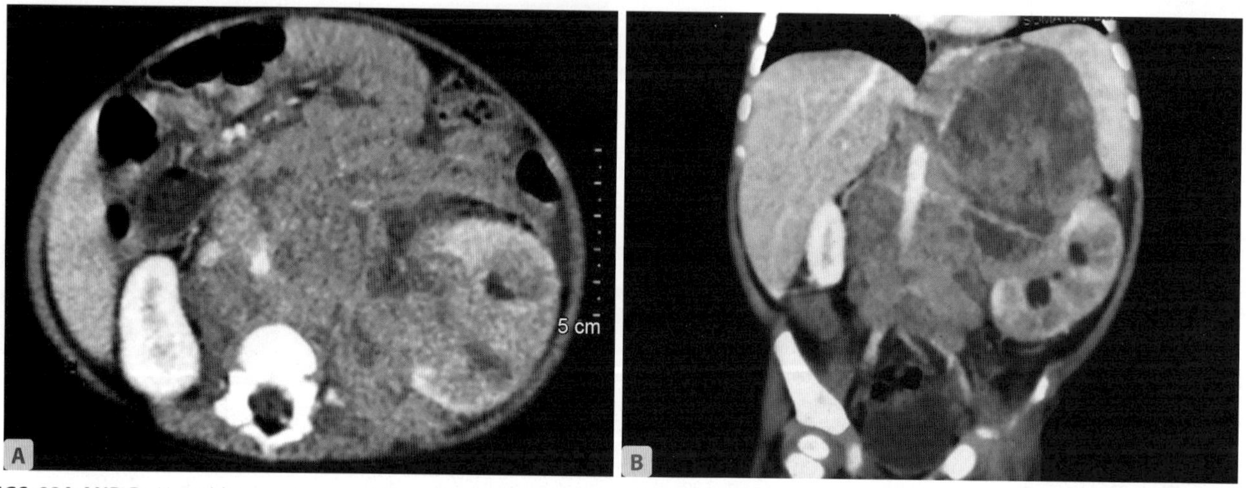

FIGS. 22A AND B: Neuroblastoma invading kidney: Contrast-enhanced axial (A) and coronal (B) CT images of a 1-year-old boy show a large heterogeneously enhancing mass lesion in the retroperitoneum in the left side and extending across midline. The mass is displacing the left kidney inferolaterally with negative beak sign suggesting an extra-renal origin. The lesion shows areas of internal necrosis and characteristically encases and displaces aorta, inferior vena cava (IVC), and bilateral renal artery. Important point to note that the lesion is secondarily invading the left kidney at places, which can be seen in some cases of abdominal neuroblastoma.

characteristically bright signal on T2W images; or focal nodular lesions seen in older children with stage 4 disease which can be readily identified on both CT and MRI. Lung metastases are rare, occurring in approximately 3% cases.[64]

If the child has presented with bone pain, it is likely that initial imaging will include skeletal radiographs. Discrete lytic areas or metaphyseal lucencies are typical of metastatic involvement and plain film appearances can simulate leukemic infiltration. However, the bones may appear normal even in the presence of metastases. Skull radiographs may also show lytic areas or sutural widening due to underlying dural involvement **(Figs. 23A to C)**. MRI plays an important role in assessing disseminated disease in the bone marrow. Bone marrow disease is usually seen as diffuse infiltration, but it may also present a nodular pattern with areas of low- and high-signal intensity on T1W and T2W images, respectively. Both CT and MRI may be needed for detection and follow-up of cranial disease particularly with recurrent disease. Bony erosion is identified on CT **(Figs. 24A and B)**, both CT and MRI can demonstrate soft-tissue deposits and focal dural involvement whereas diffuse leptomeningeal disease is best seen on contrast-enhanced MRI.

Some studies suggest that MRI with whole body short tau inversion recovery (STIR) imaging can replace the combination of CT and bone scintigraphy for overall assessment of stage 4 disease in children with NBL reducing the radiation exposure and the number of sedation procedures required.[65]

Nuclear scanning: Two-thirds of patients with NBL have metastatic bone disease at diagnosis. ^{99m}Tc -MDP *whole-body* bone scintigraphy should be performed on all patients at diagnosis. It is more sensitive than a radiographic skeletal

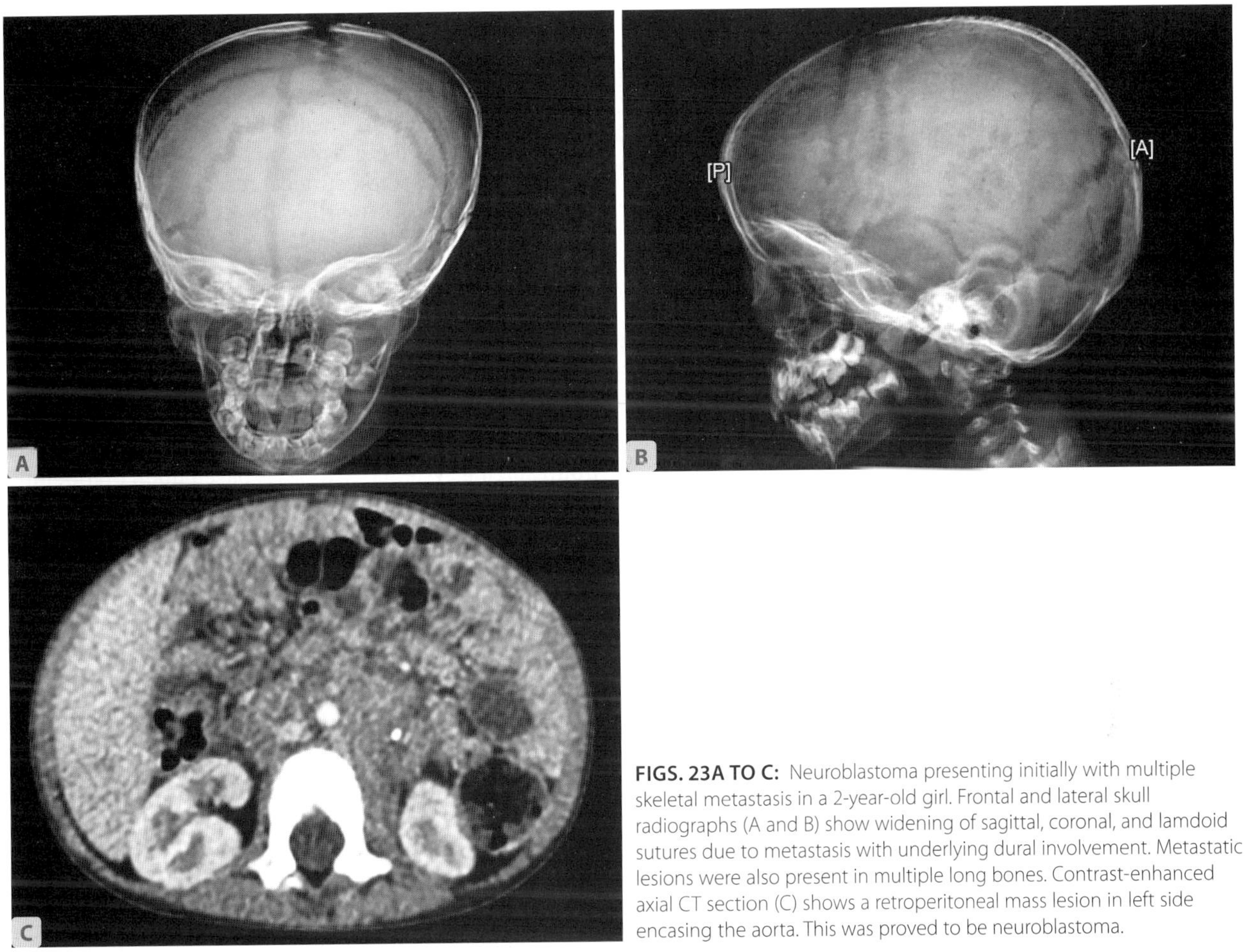

FIGS. 23A TO C: Neuroblastoma presenting initially with multiple skeletal metastasis in a 2-year-old girl. Frontal and lateral skull radiographs (A and B) show widening of sagittal, coronal, and lamdoid sutures due to metastasis with underlying dural involvement. Metastatic lesions were also present in multiple long bones. Contrast-enhanced axial CT section (C) shows a retroperitoneal mass lesion in left side encasing the aorta. This was proved to be neuroblastoma.

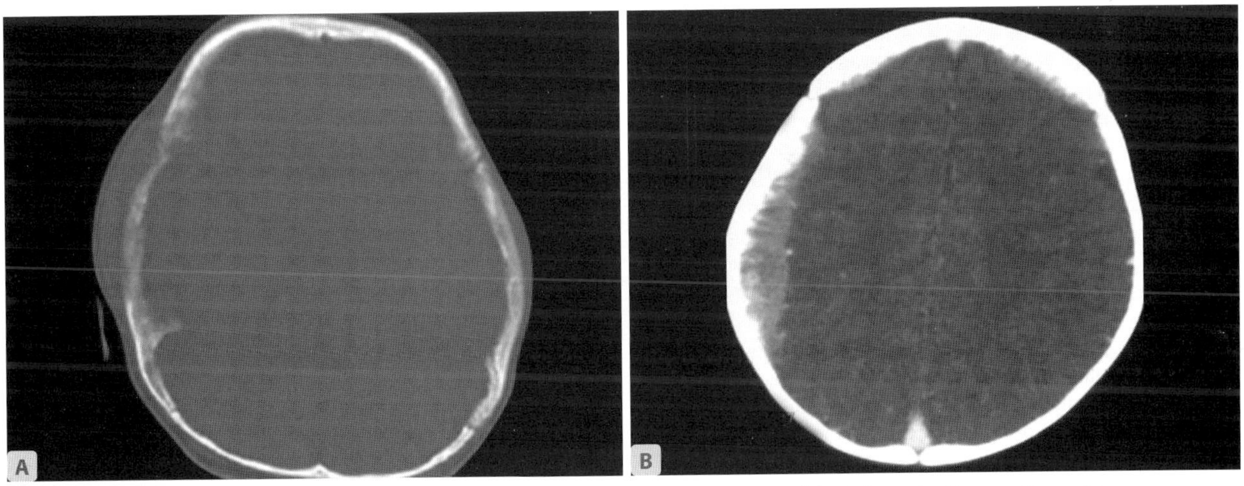

FIGS. 24A AND B: Cranial metastasis in neuroblastoma. (A) CT cranium shows bony erosion of the right parietal bone with overlying soft-tissue thickening. (B) Contrast-enhanced CT image of the brain in another child shows bony metastasis in frontal and right parietal bone with underlying enhancing dural soft-tissue mass.

survey. Plain radiographs should be performed on suspicious areas of abnormal increased tracer uptake. The primary tumor frequently takes up ^{99m}Tc-MDP and is consequently seen on bone data acquisition.

Metaiodobenzylguanidine imaging plays an important role in diagnosis and follow-up of patients with NBL. MIBG labeled with either I^{123} or I^{131} should be done in all patients. MIBG is an analog of catecholamine precursors and is taken up by catecholamine-producing cells and although other neuroendocrine tumors such as pheochromocytoma, medullary carcinoma of thyroid, and carcinoid tumors also take up MIBG, these are extremely rare in the pediatric population. Therefore, uptake of MIBG is considered specific for NBL.

Metaiodobenzylguanidine is taken up by both—the primary tumor and metastases and shows high sensitivity (88%) and specificity (99%) in detecting primary tumor and metastatic involvement (cortical bone, bone marrow, and lymph nodes) in >90% of patients.[64] MIBG scanning is less sensitive than MDP at detecting bone involvement and using only MIBG may result in an underestimate of bone metastases. False negative MIBG scans do occur and therefore many centers combine MIBG and MDP in the diagnostic work-up of children with NBL to minimize the incidence of false-positive or false-negative results.

Positron emission tomography has emerged as a promising modality for revealing NBL in both soft-tissue and skeleton. FDG uptake is directly proportional to tumor burden and to tumor-cell proliferation. Primary tumor and metastatic spread concentrate FDG avidly before therapy, whereas after therapy variable patterns of accumulation have been observed. PET scanning can be useful in MIBG-negative cases and during follow-up when assessing response to treatment.[13,66] An emerging PET/CT compound is Ga-68 DOTATATE, which utilizes somatostatin receptor expression in NBLs. The peptide binds to somatostatin receptors and can, therefore, be used for diagnosis and follow-up.[67]

TABLE 5: International Neuroblastoma Staging System.[68]

Tumor stage	Description
Stage 1	Localized tumor confined to the area of origin; complete gross resection with or without microscopic residual disease; identifiable ipsilateral and contralateral lymph nodes negative macroscopically
Stage 2A	Localized tumor with incomplete gross excision, identifiable ipsilateral and contralateral lymph nodes negative microscopically
Stage 2B	Unilateral tumor with complete or incomplete gross resection with positive ipsilateral regional lymph nodes contralateral lymph nodes negative microscopically
Stage 3	Tumor infiltrating across the midline with or without regional lymph node involvement; unilateral tumor with contralateral regional lymph node involvement; or midline tumor with bilateral regional lymph node involvement
Stage 4	Dissemination of tumor to distant lymph nodes, bone, bone marrow, liver, or other organs (except as defined in stage 4S)
Stage 4S	Localized primary tumor (as defined for stage 1 or 2) with dissemination limited to skin, liver, or bone marrow (<10% tumor cells, and MIBG scan negative in the marrow) limited to infants <1 year of age

(MIBG: metaiodobenzylguanidine)

Staging

The age of the patient and the stage of disease at diagnosis are the two most important predictors of survival in NBL. Two systems are used for the staging of NBLs. The International Neuroblastoma Staging System (INSS)[68] is a postsurgical staging system based on surgical resectability, lymph node involvement, and bone marrow involvement (**Table 5**).

A more recently introduced recognized variant of NBL, stage 4N (N = nodes) has been described which is not included in the INSS classification. This has been added for children with distant nodal spread, but no bony cortical involvement on account of better prognosis.[62]

International Neuroblastoma Risk Group (INRG) proposed a more comprehensive staging system for assessing the presurgical risk.[69] This International Neuroblastoma Risk Group Staging System (INRGSS) is based upon preoperative imaging findings and it supplements the postsurgical INSS rather than replacing it. Consequently both are used in the management of NBL patients.[70,71] INRGSS is summarized in **Table 6**. Various image-defined risk factors (IDRFs) have been defined by the INRG to describe the relationship between the tumor and adjacent vascular, major airway, or nervous system structures that ideally should not be injured at surgery. The IDRFs are imaging features that predict the risk of tumor resection.[70] With the INRGSS, the focus has shifted from surgicopathologic staging to imaging. The IDRFs relevant to retroperitoneal NBLs are summarized in **Table 7**. Vessel encasement is defined as 50% or greater encirclement of the vessel with the exception of the renal vasculature where any tumor abutting the renal vessels is regarded as an IDRF.[72] Absence of any of these IDRFs results in more complete surgical resection, whereas the presence of IDRFs is associated with significant postoperative morbidity.[73]

Imaging Strategy

According to the guidelines established by INRG, there are certain mandatory and optional imaging examinations to be performed at the time of diagnosis for patients with NBL for assessing both locoregional disease and distant metastases.[72] The imaging strategy has been described in **Box 1**.

TABLE 6: International Neuroblastoma Risk Group Staging System (INRGSS).[69,70]

Tumor stage	Description
L1	Localized tumor not involving vital structures, as defined by the list of IDRFs, and confined to one body compartment
L2	Local-regional tumor with presence of one or more IDRFs
M	Distant metastatic disease (except stage MS tumor)
MS	Metastatic disease in children younger than 18 months with metastases confined to skin, liver, and/or bone marrow (<10% involvement)

(IDRFs: image-defined risk factors)

TABLE 7: Description of image-defined risk factors (IDRFs) as relevant to retroperitoneal neuroblastoma.[72]

Anatomic region	Descriptions
Multiple body compartments	Ipsilateral tumor extension within two body compartments (i.e., neck and chest, chest and abdomen, or abdomen and pelvis)
Abdomen and pelvis	• Tumor infiltrating porta hepatis and/or hepatoduodenal ligament • Tumor encasing branches of superior mesenteric artery at mesenteric root • Tumor encasing origin of celiac axis and/or origin of superior mesenteric artery • Tumor invading one or both renal pedicles • Tumor encasing aorta and/or vena cava • Tumor encasing iliac vessels • Pelvic tumor crossing sciatic notch
Intraspinal tumor extension	Intraspinal tumor extension (whatever the location) provided that more than one-third of spinal canal in axial plane is invaded, the perimedullary leptomeningeal spaces are not visible, or the spinal cord signal intensity is abnormal
Infiltration of adjacent organs and structures	Pericardium, diaphragm, kidney, liver, duodenopancreatic block, and mesentery

BOX 1: Imaging strategy in neuroblastoma.[72]

- *Mandatory imaging examinations:*
  - MRI or CT of primary tumor compartment
  - MRI preferred modality
  - IV contrast agent optional for MRI
  - IV contrast agent mandatory for CT
  - Chest X-ray
  - I^{123}-MIBG scintigraphy (SPECT or SPECT-CT)
- *Optional imaging examinations:*
  - ^{99m}Tc-MDP bone scintigraphy (when primary tumor is MIBG negative)
  - Plain X-ray of abnormal skeletal region (when single equivocal skeletal uptake on MIBG or bone scan)
  - Abdominal imaging for hepatic metastases (when primary tumor is outside the abdomen)
    - USG or MRI abdomen generally preferred over CT abdomen
  - Contrast-enhanced CT chest (when pleuropulmonary abnormalities are suspected on clinical examination or chest X-ray)
  - Brain imaging (in presence of neurological symptoms other than spinal cord compression or MIBG/bone scan uptake of skull base or orbits)
    - MRI is recommended over CT

(MIBG: metaiodobenzylguanidine)

TABLE 8: Key differentiating features between neuroblastoma and Wilms' tumor.[13]

Features	Neuroblastoma	Wilms' tumor
Age group	Commonly seen in <2 years of age	Slightly older age group with peak in 3–5 years
Tumor composition	Predominantly solid mass lesion and cystic components are uncommon	More heterogeneous mass and more commonly shows cystic components
Tumor origin and margin	Poorly marginated retroperitoneal mass, commonly arising from adrenal gland and displaces the kidney	Well-circumscribed mass arising from kidney and demonstrates claw sign at the interface with renal parenchyma
Pattern of vascular involvement	Encases and displaces vascular structures but does not invade them	Invades the vascular structures with extension into renal vein and inferior vena cava
Pattern of extension	Commonly crosses across midline and can extend through neural foramina into spinal canal	No such patterns are seen
Calcification	Very common (seen in 80–90%)	Uncommon (seen in 10–15%)
Common sites of metastases	Bone/bone marrow	Lung

Differential Diagnosis

The differential diagnosis encompasses all pediatric abdominal masses, particularly Wilms' tumor, teratoma, lymphoma, metastatic retroperitoneal lymhadenopathy, and rhabdoid tumor. The key differentiating points between NBL and Wilms' tumor have been summarized in **Table 8**. A congenital NBL diagnosed in the neonatal period needs to be differentiated from neonatal adrenal hemorrhage. The diagnosis of adrenal hemorrhage is usually made by US, which identifies the mass and shows, in sequential examinations, decreasing size and cystic evolution. Color Doppler is useful to show avascularity of adrenal hemorrhage. MRI may show the classic signal intensity pattern of aging blood products, but diagnostic difficulties can occur because of bleeds of different ages. Other pediatric adrenal tumors, such as pheochromocytoma and adrenal carcinoma, are much less common.

Management and Follow-up

Treatment depends on several factors including stage of the disease at the time of presentation and response to initial therapy. Surgery, chemotherapy, and radiation therapy all have a role to play. Primary surgical resection is done for localized tumors and initial chemotherapy for those that are unresectable, followed by delayed surgery once they decrease in size. Imaging is helpful in assessing the response to preoperative therapy **(Figs. 25A and B)**.

The imaging strategy in the follow-up period depends largely on the imaging protocols followed by various pediatric oncology set-ups. Regular follow-up is required after surgery to assess the tumor bed for local recurrence. Follow-up is also essential in nonoperable tumors to assess response to chemotherapy and to determine the most appropriate time for delayed surgery. Imaging includes chest radiographs, abdominal US, and CT/MRI of the primary site. ^{99m}Tc-MDP and I^{123}-MIBG scanning are performed until they have returned to normal or until the end of treatment. PET/CT or single photon emission computed tomography (SPECT)/CT may be more sensitive than MIBG in detecting recurrence, as the initial MIBG-positive tumor can become MIBG-negative when it recurs.

GANGLIONEUROBLASTOMA

A ganglioneuroblastoma is intermediate in aggressiveness in the spectrum of neural crest tumors between the frankly malignant NBL and the benign ganglioneuroma. Most occur in the abdomen and thorax. Clinically, they present with effects of a mass lesion, hormonal manifestations being rare. Occasionally, they can be discovered incidentally on imaging performed for some other purpose.

Imaging and investigation are the same as described for NBLs **(Figs. 26A to C)**. Catecholamine excretion is usually increased. Biopsy is required for diagnosis but sampling errors may occur due to variable tumor composition. DW-MRI can help in differentiation between NBL and ganglioneuroblastoma as NBLs generally have lower ADC values than ganglioneuroblastomas.

GANGLIONEUROMA

This tumor is benign and is formed of nerve fibers and mature ganglion cells. Most ganglioneuromas occur in the posterior mediastinum. Only one-third occur in the abdomen, and most are paravertebral, rarely from adrenal medulla. It may be associated with neurofibromatosis type 1. These tumors generally occur in older children or adolescents, who are often asymptomatic. Hormonally, active lesions are rare. They may be discovered incidentally on radiographs or present with mass effect. The imaging appearances are similar to those of NBL but unlike NBLs, they are well-encapsulated masses. The abdominal lesions may even encase the aorta and the IVC and their branches or invade the spinal canal. The definitive diagnosis depends on histological examination of tumor tissue. Surgical removal may be difficult particularly when the mass is encasing vital structures or with intraspinal extension. In these cases, conservative management is advocated with regular clinical and imaging follow-up.

PHEOCHROMOCYTOMA

Pheochromocytoma is an uncommon neoplasm in children.[42] Like neuroblastoma, pheochromocytoma is of neural crest origin, secretes catecholamines, and may be located in the adrenal medulla or anywhere along the sympathetic chain. In children, 70% of pheochromocytomas occur in the adrenal gland and 20% have bilateral involvement. About 30% have extra-adrenal involvement and most of these occur in the upper abdomen. Other less common extra-adrenal sites include the sympathetic chain anywhere from base of skull to pelvis, urinary bladder, spermatic cord, and vagina. Multiple lesions are present in 30–70% of children. Malignancy occurs in <10%.[74]

Pheochromocytoma usually presents in older children and a familial occurrence is well-documented. It has been seen as a part of multiple endocrine neoplasia (MEN-2) syndrome. It has also been associated with a number of diseases including neurofibromatosis, von Hippel–Lindau disease and Sturge–Weber syndrome.

Clinical Presentation

Clinical presentation is usually related to the secretion of catecholamines. Patients may present with hypertension,

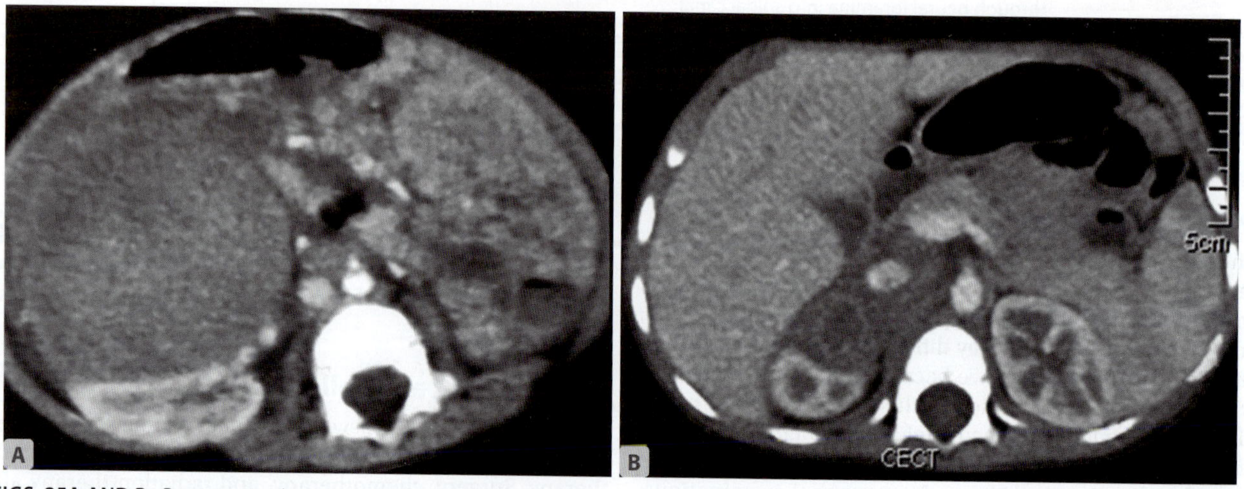

FIGS. 25A AND B: Response to chemotherapy in neuroblastoma: Contrast-enhanced axial (A) CT image of an 18-month-old boy shows a large retroperitoneal neuroblastoma displacing the right kidney at the time of diagnosis. Repeat axial contrast-enhanced computed tomography (CECT) image (B) after course of chemotherapy shows significant reduction in the size with central necrosis of the neuroblastoma.

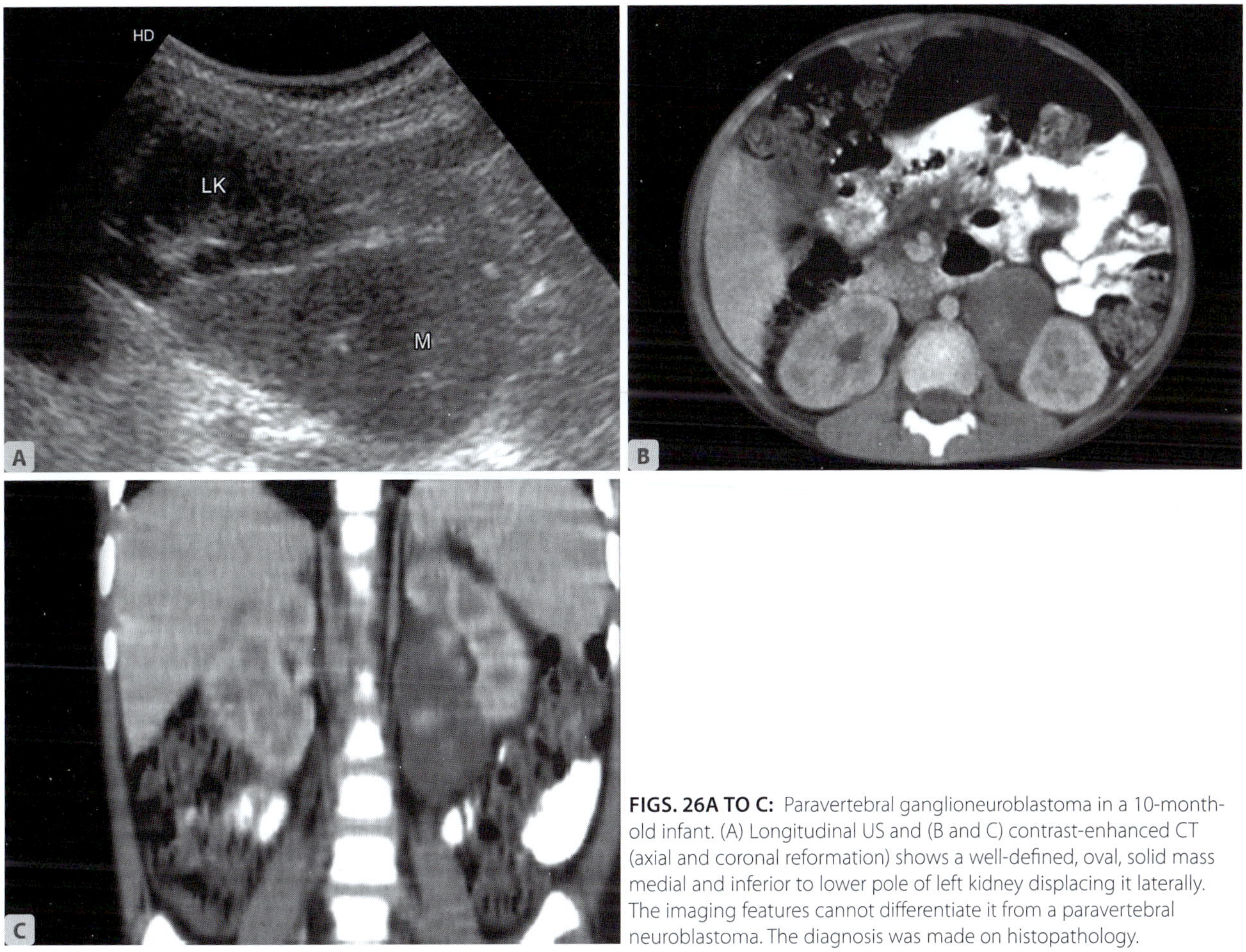

FIGS. 26A TO C: Paravertebral ganglioneuroblastoma in a 10-month-old infant. (A) Longitudinal US and (B and C) contrast-enhanced CT (axial and coronal reformation) shows a well-defined, oval, solid mass medial and inferior to lower pole of left kidney displacing it laterally. The imaging features cannot differentiate it from a paravertebral neuroblastoma. The diagnosis was made on histopathology.

sweating, headaches, visual blurring, flushing, tachycardia, hypertensive encephalopathy, weight loss, and diarrhea. Urinary catecholamines are usually markedly elevated, much more so than with NBL.

Imaging

On ultrasound, a pheochromocytoma may be seen as a well-defined hypoechoic mass which may be homogenous or heterogenous due to hemorrhage and necrosis **(Fig. 27A)**. Calcification is uncommon. Sonography easily detects lesions in and adjacent to adrenal glands but is less sensitive than CT and MRI for lesions in mid and lower abdomen. On CT, the lesions have a soft-tissue attenuation with diffuse, mottled, or rim-like enhancement **(Figs. 27B and C)**. Adrenergic blockade, to prevent a hypertensive crisis, is not required prior to nonionic contrast administration during CT scanning.[6] On MRI, pheochromocytomas have a low signal on T1W images and high signal on T2W images with intense enhancement and slow washout after contrast administration **(Figs. 28A and B)**. Malignancy is best determined by identifying distant metastases to nonchromaffin tissues such as lung, liver, bone, and lymph nodes.[74] I^{131}-MIBG can accurately localize a pheochromocytoma, but does not show the anatomy as well as CT or MRI. It is particularly helpful in detecting nonadrenal tumors (paragangliomas). MIBG may be positive in the abdomen even when a US is negative and MIBG should always be done prior to surgery to detect or exclude multiple sites of disease.

ADRENAL CORTICAL TUMORS

Adrenocortical tumors (ACT) are very rare in children with a worldwide annual incidence of 0.3 per million children below the age of 15 years.[75] 75% of children who develop ACT are <5 years old at the time of diagnosis. The incidence is higher in young girls with a female/male ratio of 2:1, whereas in adolescence the sex ratio is equal. Two syndromes have a clear association with this tumor: Li-Fraumeni syndrome is associated with mutations of the *p53* gene, and Beckwith-Wiedemann syndrome which has mutations in the 11p15 region.

Clinical Features

More than 75% of ACT are functional, secreting one or more hormones (androgens, cortisol, aldosterone, or estrogens). Virilization, with early onset of pubic hair, hypertrophy of the clitoris or penis, accelerated growth, gynecomastia or acne, is the most common presentation. The second most common manifestation is with hypercortisolism (Cushing's syndrome), while presentation with a palpable

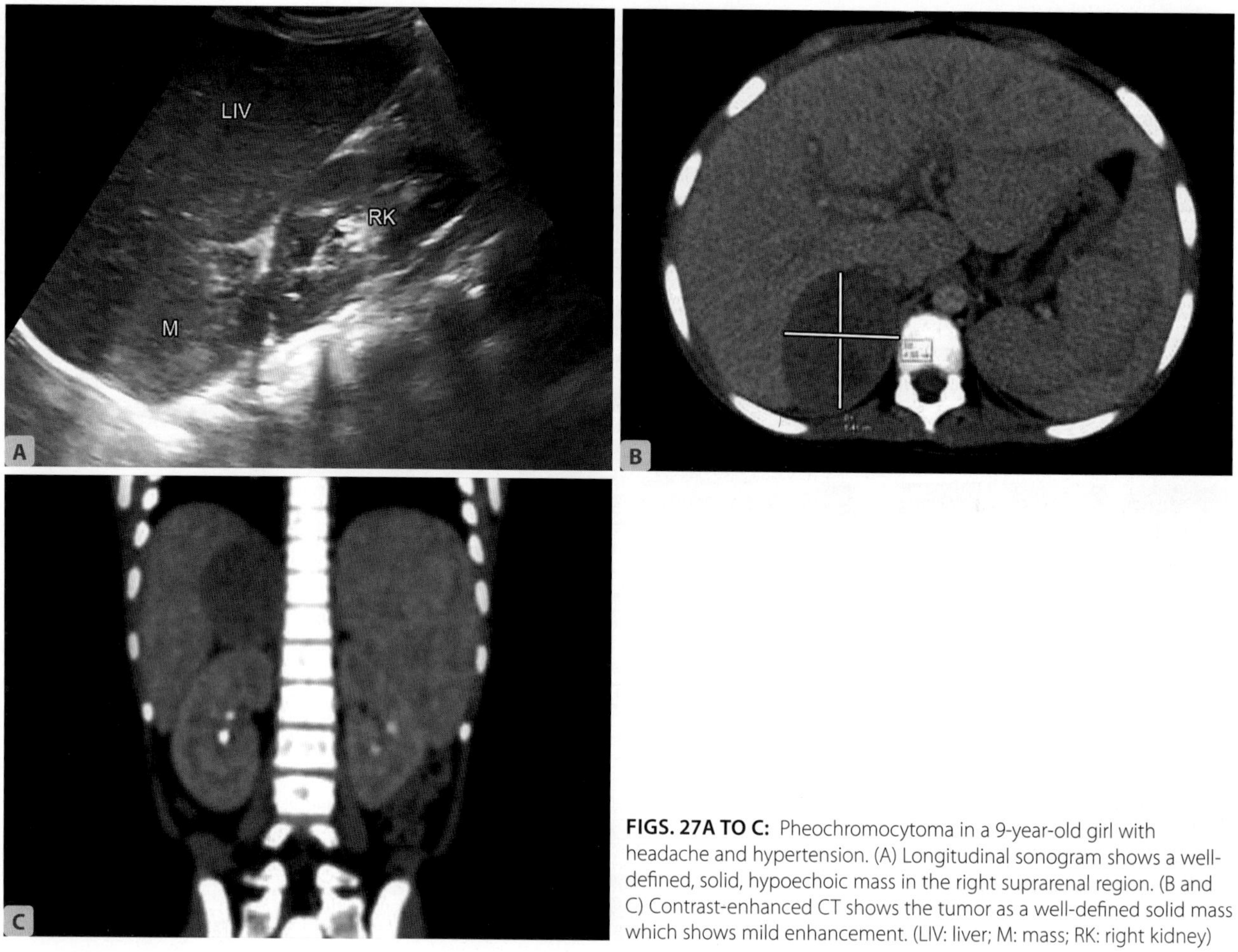

FIGS. 27A TO C: Pheochromocytoma in a 9-year-old girl with headache and hypertension. (A) Longitudinal sonogram shows a well-defined, solid, hypoechoic mass in the right suprarenal region. (B and C) Contrast-enhanced CT shows the tumor as a well-defined solid mass which shows mild enhancement. (LIV: liver; M: mass; RK: right kidney)

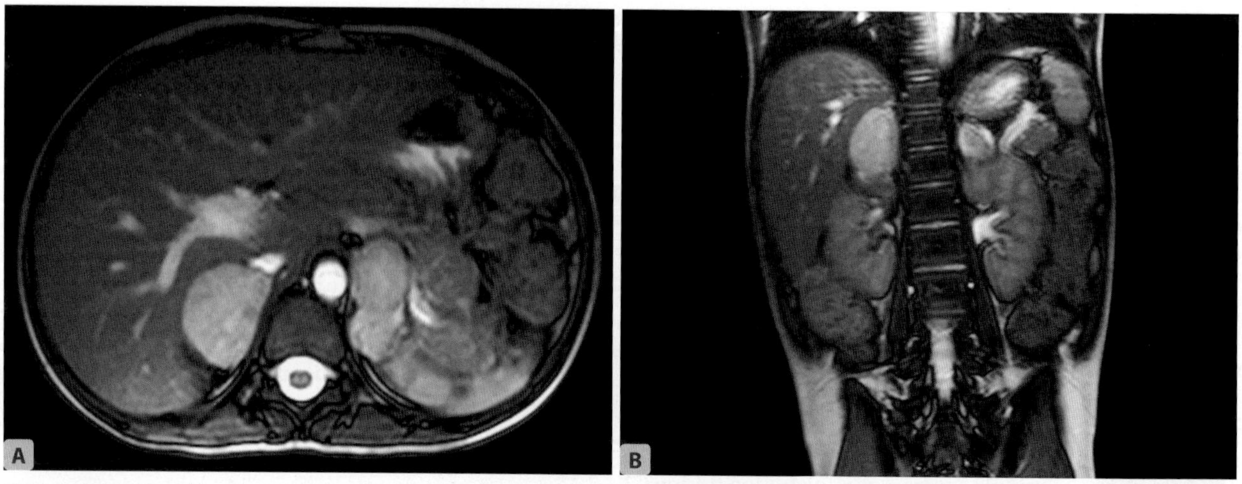

FIGS. 28A AND B: Bilateral pheochromocytoma in a 13-year-old girl: T2-weighted axial (A) and coronal (B) MR images show well-defined hyperintense focal mass lesions involving bilateral adrenal glands (right larger than left).

abdominal mass is unusual. Hypertension may be seen in up to 43% at diagnosis.[75] This may be due to either mineralocorticoid or glucocorticoid excess, increased aldosterone production or simply renal artery compression by the tumor, and the hypertension usually resolves after tumor resection. Diagnosis of an ACT is supported by raised levels of androstenedione, dehydroepiandrosterone-sulphate (DHEA-S), testosterone, and urinary steroids. These hormones are also useful markers for the detection of tumor recurrence during follow-up. The combination of hormone production and adrenal mass is diagnostic of an adrenocortical tumor.

Imaging Features

On all three modalities (US, CT, and MRI), the smaller lesions tend to have a fairly homogeneous appearance **(Figs. 29A and B)** and areas of hemorrhage, necrosis, and calcification are seen in the larger lesions. A characteristic central scar with radiating linear bands representing areas of necrosis and calcification is often seen in the large lesion.[74] Adrenal adenoma usually contain intracellular lipid and are typically hypodense (<10 HU) on noncontrast CT scan. Microscopic fat present within these lesions can be easily detected on chemical shift MRI **(Figs. 30A to D)**.

The tumor tends to be locally aggressive and frequently invades the IVC and may extend into the right atrium.[76] The tumor may also metastasize to lung, nodes, bone, and liver. MRI is the modality of choice and demonstrates the primary tumor, caval extension, and liver metastases. Chest CT to exclude or detect pulmonary metastases should be performed at first diagnosis.

The classification of benign from malignant ACTs is not clear cut and is the subject of much debate.[6] Even established histopathological criteria and algorithms adapted from tumors in adults do not allow a clear classification in children. Differentiation between adenoma and carcinoma is in practice somewhat arbitrary, and all patients (even those with a seemingly benign adenoma completely resected) require close follow-up initially. The majority of ACTs in children are interpreted pathologically as malignant in most studies. Factors favoring malignancy include size over 5–10 cm, weight over 200 g, invasion into the periadrenal soft tissues or IVC.[6]

Surgical resection is the mainstay of treatment. Younger children, particularly those <5 years, with pathologically malignant ACTs have a significantly better prognosis than older children and adolescents.[6]

ADRENAL HEMORRHAGE

Adrenal hemorrhage occurs almost exclusively in newborns in association with perinatal asphyxia, trauma, or bacterial (typically meningococcal) septicemia. The precise cause is unknown but is thought to be stress related or due to birth trauma, as there is an increased frequency in larger babies or babies of diabetic mothers. The hemorrhagic process may involve the whole gland or part of one, or both adrenal glands in about 10% of cases.

Clinical Features

In a moderate or massive degree of adrenal hemorrhage, there is clinically a palpable flank mass due to the caudal displacement of the ipsilateral kidney from the hemorrhagic mass. The mass is usually not palpable at birth and develops over the following 24 hours. The child will often become jaundiced and present with vomiting. The mass typically regresses within days to a few weeks with resorption of the clot. Acute or late adrenal insufficiency is uncommon even in bilateral adrenal hemorrhage.

Imaging Features

US demonstrates a suprarenal mass that is variable in echogenicity. In the acute phase, the hemorrhage is usually echogenic representing clot formation **(Fig. 31)**. Over several weeks, the hemorrhage becomes echofree as the clot lyses and becomes liquified. The hemorrhage gradually decreases in size and may result in adrenal calcification. If there is no evidence of ultrasonographic resolution after several days, other diagnoses including NBL and its variants, but also benign conditions such as an adrenal cyst or extra-adrenal abnormality from a surrounding structure including an enteric duplication cyst need to be considered.

In older children, post-traumatic adrenal hemorrhage has been described to occur in some 3% of blunt abdominal injury and often associated with ipsilateral lesions of the liver, kidney or spleen. It seems more likely to occur on the right side is usually asymptomatic and, also, without evidence of subsequent adrenal insufficiency.

ADRENAL CYSTS

Large adrenal cysts may be found in older children. These are usually endothelial lined and found incidentally. Their importance lies in their being mistaken for adrenal neoplasms.

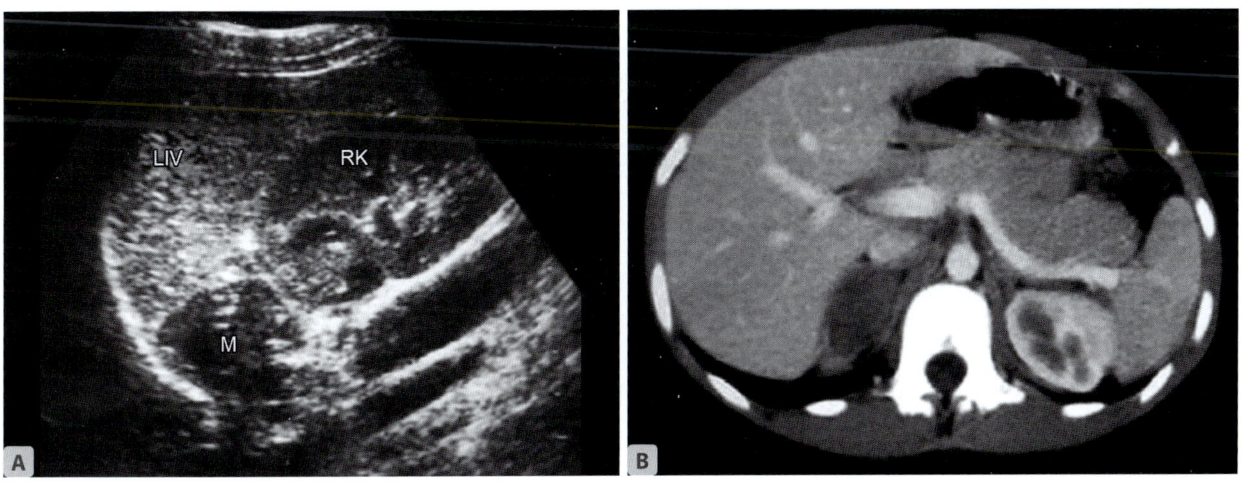

FIGS. 29A AND B: Adrenal adenoma: (A and B) US and contrast-enhanced axial CT scans show a small well-defined mass in the right suprarenal region in a 12-year-old boy, hypodense on CT with no evidence of calcification.

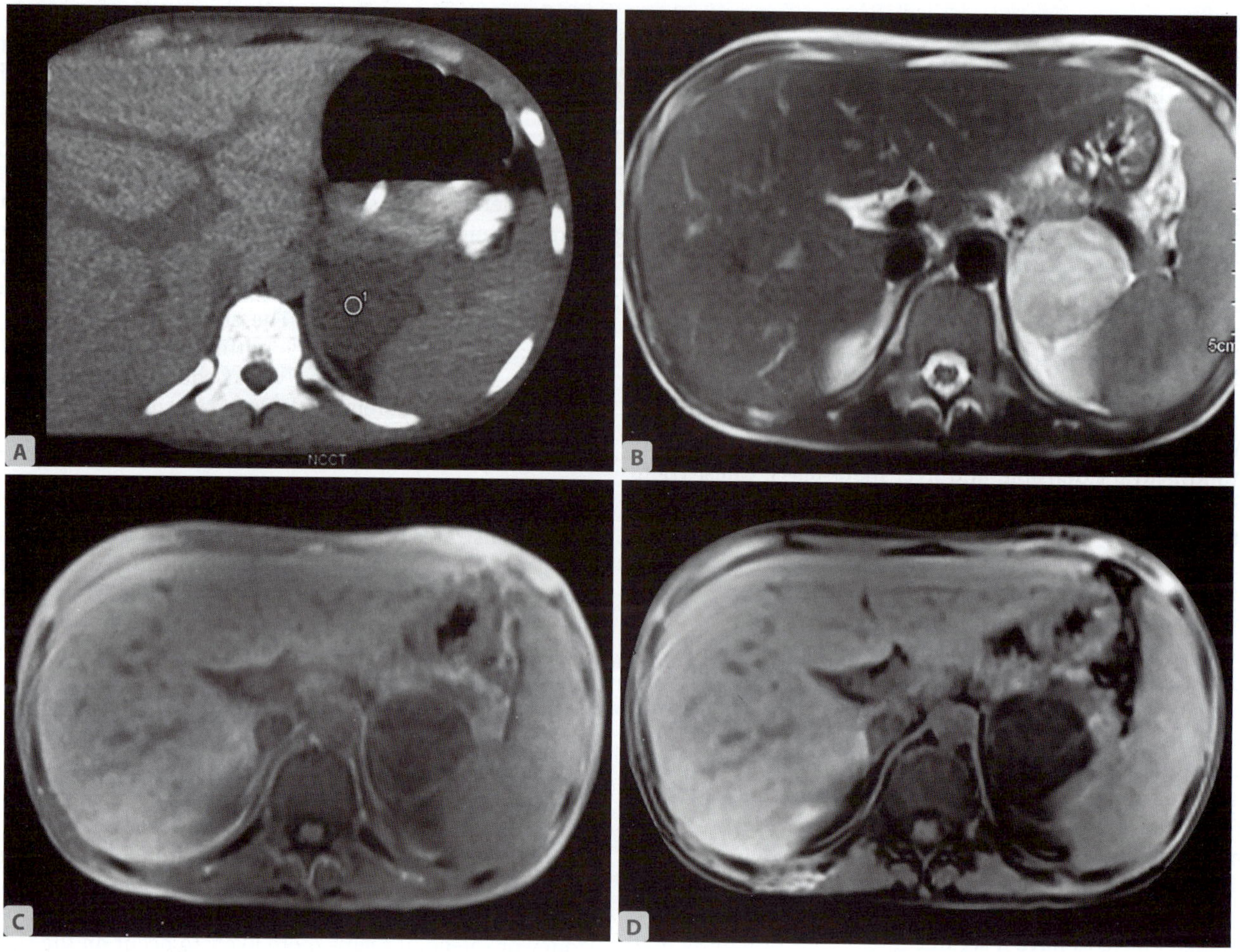

FIGS. 30A TO D: Adrenal adenoma in a 13-year-old boy. (A) Noncontrast axial CT image showing a well-defined hypodense mass lesion in left suprarenal location with average Hounsfield unit (HU) value of the lesion being 7.5 (<10 HU). (B) On T2-weighted MR image, the lesion shows iso- to slightly hyperintense signal. In-phase (C) and opposed-phase (D) MR images demonstrate significant signal suppression on opposed phase image as compared to in phase image suggestive of presence of microscopic fat within the lesion. CT and MR imaging features consistent with lipid rich adrenal adenoma.

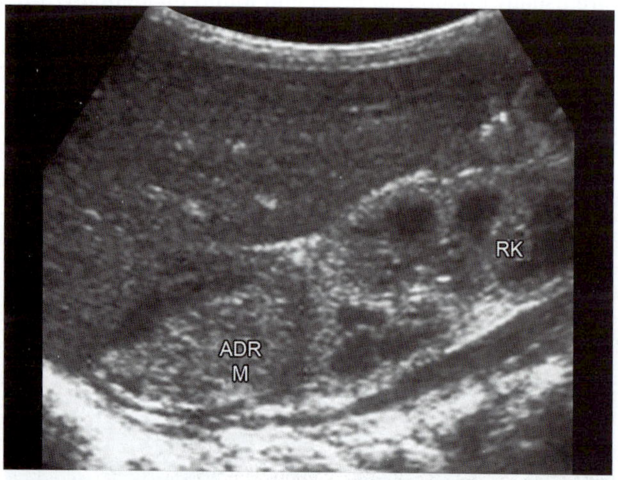

FIG. 31: Adrenal hemorrhage: Longitudinal US scan through the right flank in a 9-day-old infant shows a well-defined cystic mass in the right suprarenal regional with a fluid-fluid level.

If cross-sectional imaging shows a smooth thin-walled cyst without any evidence of solid components, and there is no endocrine dysfunction, hypertension, infection or metastatic disease, they can be managed conservatively because adrenal neoplasms seldom have large cystic components and never present as thin smooth-walled cystic structures without solid components.

PRIMARY RETROPERITONEAL TUMORS

Primary tumors of retroperitoneum are rare tumors that originate in the retroperitoneal space but outside the major organs in that space. These neoplasms are generally derived from neurogenic cells, embryonic rests, or mesenchymal cells and may be benign or malignant.

NEUROGENIC TUMORS

Neurogenic tumors may arise from tissue of the sympathetic (autonomic) nervous system and include extra-adrenal NBL

(**Fig. 23**), ganglioneuroblastoma (**Fig. 26**) and ganglioneuroma, or from neuroectoderm as in the case of a primitive peripheral neuroectodermal tumor. Extra-adrenal pheochromocytoma also arises in the retroperitoneum. The site of origin of all these tumors is in the paravertebral gutter with resultant anterior and lateral displacement of other retroperitoneal structures including kidneys, ureters, and the IVC. Their imaging and investigations are similar to that of their adrenal counterparts and have been discussed above. Uncommon neuroectodermal tumors are paraganglioma, neurofibroma, neurofibrosarcoma, neurolemmoma, or schwannoma. Although occasionally isolated tumors, they are often seen as multiple tumors in patients with neurofibromatosis.

GERM-CELL TUMORS

Germ-cell tumors are derived from the primordial germinal epithelial layer cells and two-thirds of these tumors are extragonadal in location. These include germinomas, embryonal carcinoma, endodermal sinus tumor, choriocarcinoma, gonadoblastoma, and teratoma. Teratomas, the most common of germ-cell tumor, account for 3.5–4% of all germ-cell tumors in children.[77] They contain all three embryonal layers—ectoderm, mesoderm, and endoderm. They are the third most common tumors of the retroperitoneum in children following NBL and Wilms' tumor. The ratio of girls to boys is 2:1. Malignancy is seen in 10–15% cases. Increase in abdominal girth is the most common presenting symptom, frequently accompanied by pain, nausea, vomiting, and weight loss. The presence of a palpable abdominal mass is an almost universal finding. Occasionally, the tumor is present antenatally and diagnosed at birth, these neonatal teratomas have a higher incidence of malignancy than those in older children. Malignant teratomas can produce alpha-fetoprotein and its serum levels can be used to monitor response to therapy/recurrence.[78]

Imaging

Plain radiographs may demonstrate calcification or formed bony components such as teeth and phalanges, which are pathognomonic.

The tumor may be cystic, solid, or mixed. Although US demonstrates the solid or cystic nature of the tumor, CT defines the true location and character of the mass better and is useful to delineate the extent of the disease in retroperitoneum and its relationship to major vessels (**Figs. 32A and B**). Fat may be identified in about half the cases and fat-fluid levels may sometimes be seen. Internal homogeneity, fat density, cyst formation, and calcification are important predictors of a benign retroperitoneal tumor on CT.[79]

MESENCHYMAL TUMORS

Lipomatous Tumors

These are often quite large at the time of diagnosis and are usually benign. They include lipoma, lipoblastoma, and liposarcoma-like lipoblastomatosis. These tumors are best visualized on CT and MRI showing homogeneous fatty attenuation at CT and homogeneous signal identical to that of fat on all MRI sequences. The boundaries of the mass are clearly delineated because of marked contrast in signal intensity with surrounding structures. Lipoblastoma is extensive and locally invasive and difficult or impossible to remove completely. Its appearance on imaging studies may be similar to lipoma but some cases have shown areas of relatively increased attenuation on CT, which on pathologic examination have been shown to be regions of myxoid material. Liposarcoma is extremely rare in children, but is locally invasive and also metastatic to distant sites.

Rhabdomyosarcoma and Undifferentiated Sarcomas

Rhabdomyosarcoma accounts for 5–8% of childhood cancer and presents in a wide variety of histologic types and patterns of spread of tumor. Retroperitoneal RMSs are rare tumors. The tumors infiltrate locally, invade lymphatics and blood vessels, and frequently present with distant hematogenous metastases to the lungs, bone marrow, and bone. Retroperitoneal lymph nodes, bone marrow metastases, and distant hematogenous metastases to the lungs are common at presentation. Other sarcomas occasionally seen in children and adolescents

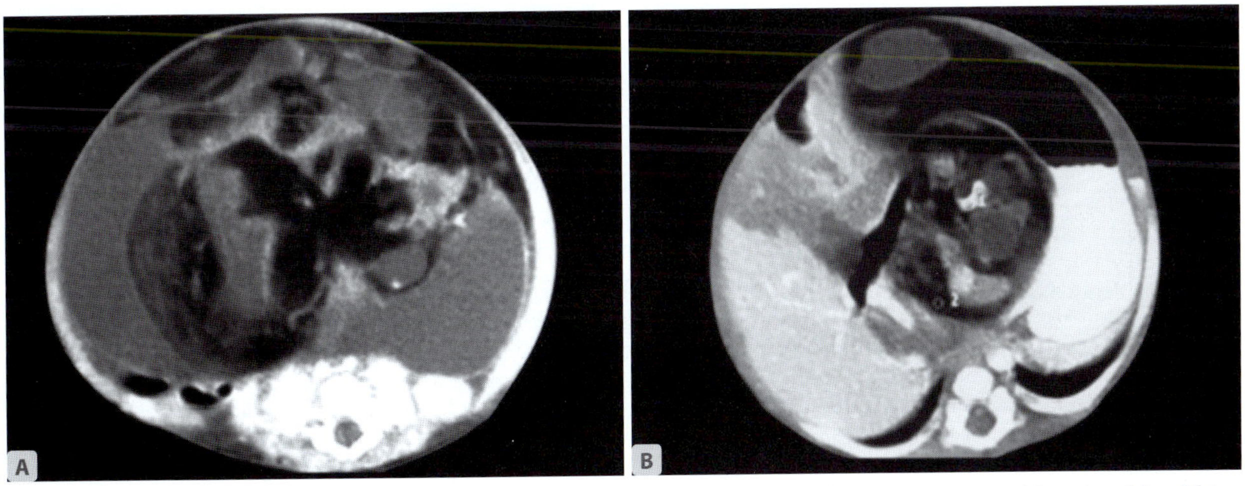

FIGS. 32A AND B: Teratoma: (A) Contrast-enhanced axial CT section shows a large well-defined heterogeneous mass with cystic, solid, and fat attenuation components in a 3-month-old child. (B) A higher section shows the presence of a tooth within the mass, clinching the diagnosis.

include fibrosarcoma, neurofibrosarcoma, malignant fibrous histiocytoma, hemangiopericytoma, and leiomyosarcoma.

RETROPERITONEAL LYMPHATIC MALFORMATION

A lymphatic malformation (LM) is a benign tumor of congenital lymphatic origin. LMs can be of two types—macrocystic and microcystic. Macrocystic LM consists of multiple dilated and poorly developed lymphatic channels. The cystic spaces are lined with endothelium and contain multiple thin septa and chylous fluid while a microcystic LM has multiple very small cysts, appearing almost solid in consistency. Although it may present early as a palpable abdominal mass, the soft nature of this lesion, makes it difficult to identify on physical examination. The mass may compress adjacent structures, particularly displacing and obstructing the ureters. On US, a LM is seen as a cystic mass with multiple, apparently noncommunicating, fluid-containing cystic regions, separated by thin septae **(Fig. 33)**. Internal echoes representing blood, pus, or chyle may be present and form fluid-fluid levels.

On MRI, a macrocystic LM is seen as multiloculated cystic mass which insinuates along tissue planes or displaces adjacent structures. It is hypointense on T1W and hyperintense on T2W images. The presence of internal contents can give a heterogenous appearance. Fluid-fluid levels may be seen. A retracted clot can mimic a mural nodule (nonenhancing) or solid component. CT findings of LMs are similar to MRI findings, although septae may not be well seen **(Fig. 34)**. Faint linear calcifications may be seen in the septa on CT. On contrast administration, no or faint peripheral capsular and septal enhancement can occur.

LYMPH NODE MASSES

Isolated retroperitoneal lymph node enlargement in children is unusual and associated findings help to clarify the diagnosis. Retroperitoneal lymphadenopathy can be benign, most often infective—tubercular, or it can occur with a variety of malignant processes including metastatic lymph node enlargement or lymphoma.

Metastasis to retroperitoneal nodes in children occurs by spread from primary retroperitoneal malignancies such as Wilms' tumor, NBL, or spread from testicular or ovarian malignancies **(Fig. 35)**. Intra-abdominal lymphoma in children is nearly always non-Hodgkin's lymphoma, most commonly Burkitt's lymphoma. Retroperitoneal lymphadenopathy generally occurs along with bowel, hepatic, or spleen involvement. Initial presentation with retroperitoneal masses is uncommon and more likely to be associated with lymphomas related to pharmacologic immunosuppression.

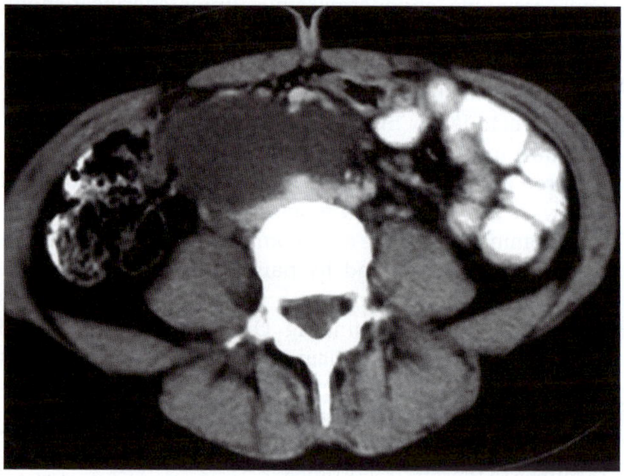

FIG. 34: Lymphatic malformation: Contrast-enhanced axial CT shows a cystic mass in midline with thin imperceptible walls, just anterior to the major abdominal vessels, displacing the mesenteric vessels anteriorly.

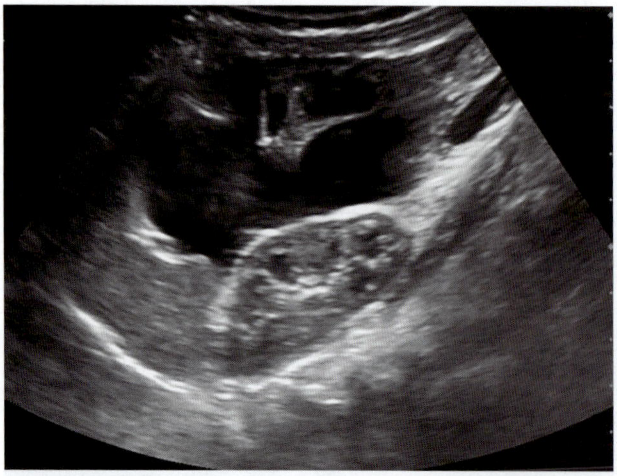

FIG. 33: Lymphatic malformation: US of right flank in a 6-month-old child shows a macrocystic lymphatic malformation (LM) lying anteroinferior to the right kidney. It is seen as a multiloculated cystic lesion, insinuating along tissue planes.

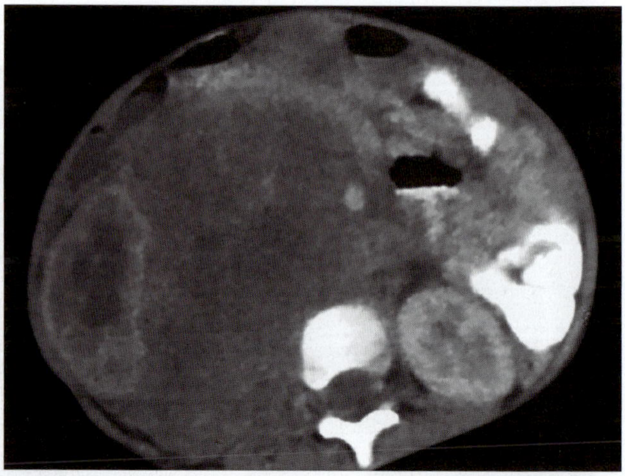

FIG. 35: Metastatic testicular germ-cell tumor: Contrast-enhanced CT shows massive, low attenuation retroperitoneal lymphadenopathy displacing the right kidney laterally (negative beak sign seen) in a diagnosed case of testicular germ-cell tumor in a 2-year-old boy.

CT is the most frequently used modality for evaluation of enlarged nodes. However, MRIs, especially fat-suppressed T2W images, are very sensitive for the detection of lymph nodes and perform better than CT particularly in children who have a paucity of fat. CT and MRI use nonspecific criterion of size and are limited in their ability to differentiate benign from malignant nodes. Contrast-enhanced MR lymphography using ultrasmall supermagnetic iron oxide (USPIO) particles is a promising technique in differentiating benign from metastatic nodes and providing information on lymph node morphology and function.[80] FDG-PET may be more sensitive and specific for evaluation of lymphomas and certain retroperitoneal metastases depending on the primary.

RETROPERITONEAL ABSCESS AND HEMATOMA

Tuberculous spondylitis is the most common cause of an iliopsoas abscess in our country. The inflammatory mass shows a variety of appearances ranging from diffuse homogeneous enlargement of the iliopsoas muscle to discrete masses containing central areas of low CT attenuation or high-signal intensity on T2W MRI **(Figs. 36A to C)**. Postcontrast images show abscesses as expansile lesions with nonenhancing necrotic centers, intense peripheral enhancement and enhancement of the surrounding tissue. Calcification may occasionally be seen on CT and plain radiographs. Although vertebral involvement can be well-appreciated on both CT and MRI, MRI scores over CT in detecting intraspinal extension of the inflammatory granulation tissue/abscess and cord compression. US can detect the psoas abscess as a sonolucent region within the psoas muscle with associated fluid along the margins of the psoas and can serve as a guide for diagnostic and therapeutic drainage of these abscesses.

Hematomas of the retroperitoneum are most commonly the result of severe blunt trauma or a surgical procedure. Spontaneous retroperitoneal hematomas, usually within the iliopsoas muscle, can be seen in patients with hemophilia or other bleeding diathesis. On US, CT, and MRI, the muscle is seen to be enlarged with characteristic changing pattern of an evolving hemorrhage within it.

CONCLUSION

Seventy to eighty percent of abdominal masses in infants and children are retroperitoneal in origin, renal being the most common. Imaging aims to diagnose the site, nature, extent, and stage of the disease, so as to determine the appropriate management. The various imaging modalities available need to be used in a logical sequence as governed by the findings in an individual case and availability of facilities.

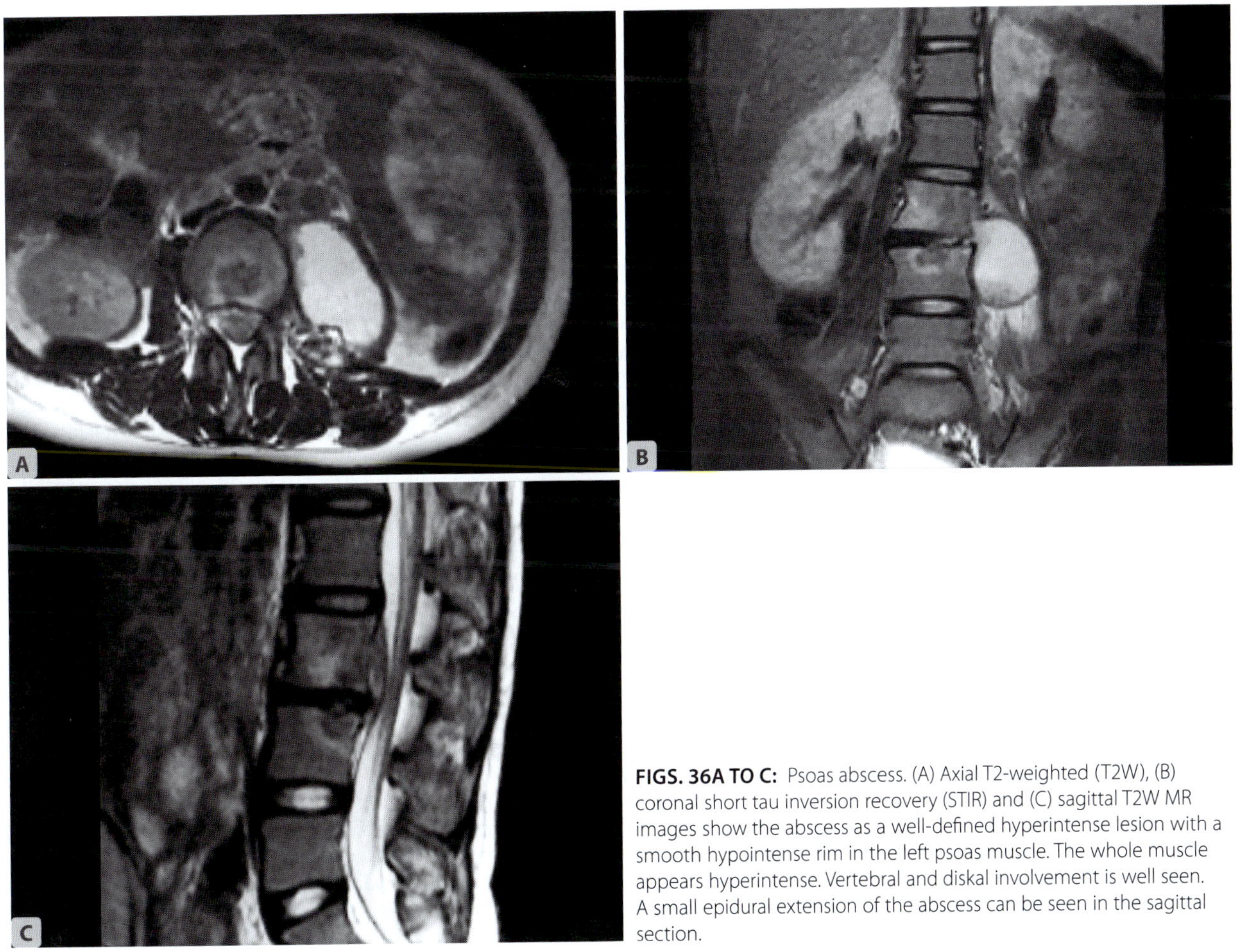

FIGS. 36A TO C: Psoas abscess. (A) Axial T2-weighted (T2W), (B) coronal short tau inversion recovery (STIR) and (C) sagittal T2W MR images show the abscess as a well-defined hyperintense lesion with a smooth hypointense rim in the left psoas muscle. The whole muscle appears hyperintense. Vertebral and diskal involvement is well seen. A small epidural extension of the abscess can be seen in the sagittal section.

REFERENCES

1. Gawande RS, Gonzalez G, Messing S, Khurana A, Daldrup-Link HE. Role of diffusion-weighted imaging in differentiating benign and malignant pediatric abdominal tumors. Pediatr Radiol. 2013;43(7):836-45.
2. de Oliveira Schiavon JL, Pioner GG, Lederman HM. MRI in Pediatric Oncology, Abdominal Tumors: Diffusion. Curr Radiol Rep. 2014;2:75.
3. Nishino M, Hayakawa K, Minami M, Yamamoto A, Ueda H, Takasu K. Primary Retroperitoneal Neoplasms: CT and MR Imaging Findings with Anatomic and Pathologic Diagnostic Clues. Radiographics. 2003;23:45-57.
4. Geller E, Smergel EM, Lowry PA. Renal neoplasms of childhood. Radiol Clin North Am. 1997;35(6):1391-413.
5. Lowe HL, Isuani BH, Heller RM, Stein SM, Johnson JE, Navarro OM, et al. Paediatric renal masses: Wilms' tumor and beyond. Radiographics. 2000;20(6):1585-603.
6. McHugh K. Renal and adrenal tumours in children. Cancer Imaging. 2007;7(1):41-51.
7. White KS, Grossman H. Wilms' and associated renal tumors of childhood. Pediatr Radiol. 1991;21:81-8.
8. Charles AK, Vujanic GM, Berry PJ. Renal tumors of childhood. Histopathology. 1998;32:293-309.
9. Lonergan GJ, Martinez-Leon MI, Agrons GA, Montemarano H, Suarez ES. Nephrogenic rests, nephroblastomatosis, and associated lesions of the kidney. Radiographics. 1998;18:947-68.
10. Smets AM, de Kraker J. Malignant tumours of the kidney: Imaging strategy. Pediatr Radiol. 2010;40:1010-8.
11. Brillantino C, Rossi E, Minelli R, Bignardi E, Coppola M, Zeccolini R, et al. Current role of imaging in the management of children with Wilms tumor according to the new UMBRELLA protocol. Trans Med. 2019;9(1):206.
12. Servaes SE, Hoffer FA, Smith EA, Khanna G. Imaging of Wilms tumor: an update. Pediatr Radiol. 2019;49:1441-52.
13. Dumba M, Jawad N, McHugh K. Neuroblastoma and nephroblastoma: a radiological review. Cancer Imaging. 2015;15:5.
14. Stanescu AL, Acharya PT, Lee EY, Phillips GS. Pediatric Renal Neoplasms: MR Imaging-Based Practical Diagnostic Approach. Magn Reson Imaging Clin N Am. 2019;27(2):279-90.
15. Littooij AS, Nikkels PG, Hulsbergen-van de Kaa CA, van de Ven CP, van den Heuvel-Eibrink MM, Olsen ØE. Apparent diffusion coefficient as it relates to histopathology findings in post-chemotherapy nephroblastoma: A feasibility study. Pediatr Radiol. 2017;47(12):1608-14.
16. Chung EM, Graeber AR, Conran RM. Renal Tumors of Childhood: Radiologic-Pathologic Correlation Part 1. The 1st Decade: From the Radiologic Pathology Archives. Radiographics. 2016;36: 499-522.
17. Begent J, Sebire NJ, Levitt G, Brock P, Jones KP, Ell P, et al. Pilot study of F(18)-Fluorodeoxyglucose positron emission tomography/ computerised tomography in Wilms' tumour: correlation with conventional imaging, pathology and immunohistochemistry. Eur J Cancer. 2011;47(3):389-96.
18. Qin Z, Tang Y, Wang H, Cai W, Fu H, Li J, et al. Use of 18F-FDG-PET-CT for assessment of response to neoadjuvant chemotherapy in children with Wilms tumor. J Pediatr Hematol Oncol. 2015;37(5):396-401.
19. Grundy P, Perlman E, Rosen NS, Warwick AB, Glade Bender J, et al. Current issues in Wilms' tumor management. Curr Probl Cancer. 2005;29:221-60.
20. Servaes S, Khanna G, Naranjo A, Geller JI, Ehrlich PF, Gow KW, et al. Comparison of diagnostic performance of CT and MRI for abdominal staging of pediatric renal tumors: a report from the Children's Oncology Group. Pediatr Radiol. 2015;45(2):166-72.
21. Gow KW, Roberts IF, Jamieson DH, Bray H, Magee JF, Murphy JJ. Local staging of Wilms' tumor—computerized tomography correlation with histological findings. J Pediatr Surg. 2000;35:677-9.
22. Khanna G, Naranjo A, Hoffer F, Mullen E, Geller J, Gratias EJ, et al. Detection of preoperative Wilms tumor rupture with CT: a report from the Children's Oncology Group. Radiology. 2013;266(2):610-7.
23. Brisse HJ, Smets AM, Kaste SC, Owens CM. Imaging in unilateral Wilms tumour. Pediatr Radiol. 2008;38(1):18-29.
24. Owens CM, Veys PA, Pritchard J, Levitt G, Imeson J, Dicks-Mireaux C. Role of chest computed tomography at diagnosis in the management of Wilms' tumor: A study by the United Kingdom Children's Cancer Study Group. J Clin Oncol. 2002;20:2768-73.
25. Tongaonkar HB, Qureshi SS, Kurkure PA, Muckaden MA, Arora B, Yuvaraja TB. Wilms' tumor: An update. Indian J Urol. 2007;23:458-66.
26. Ehrlich PF, Hamilton TE, Grundy P, Ritchey M, Haase G, Shamberger RC, et al. The value of surgery in directing therapy for patients with Wilms' tumor with pulmonary disease. A report from the National Wilms' Tumor Study Group (National Wilms' Tumor Study 5). J Pediatr Surg. 2006;41:162-7.
27. de la Monneraye Y, Michon J, Pacquement H, Aerts I, Orbach D, Doz F, et al. Indications and results of diagnostic biopsy in pediatric renal tumors: A retrospective analysis of 317 patients with critical review of SIOP guidelines. Pediatr Blood Cancer. 2019;66(6):e27641.
28. Beckwith JB. Children at increased risk for Wilms' tumor: monitoring issues. J Pediatr. 1998;132:377-9.
29. Carneiro RC, Fordham LA. Tumors of the Urinary Tract. In: Carty H, Brunelle F, Stringer DA, Kao S (Eds). Imaging Children (2nd Edition). London: Churchill Livingstone Publications; 2005. pp. 777-804.
30. Rohrschneider WK, Weirich A, Rieden K, Darge K, Troger J, Graf N. US, CT and MR imaging characteristics of nephroblastomatosis. Pediatr Radiol. 1998;28:435-43.
31. Platzer I, Li M, Winkler B, Schweinfurth P, Pabst T, Bley T, et al. Detection and differentiation of paediatric renal tumours using diffusion-weighted imaging: an explorative retrospective study. Cancer Res Front. 2015;1:178-90.
32. Chan HS, Cheng MY, Mancer K, Payton D, Weitzman SS, Kotecha P, et al. Congenital mesoblastic nephroma: Clinicoradiological study of 17 cases representing the pathological spectrum of the disease. J. Paediatr. 1987;111(1):64-70.
33. Gee MS, Bittman M, Epelman M, Vargas SO, Lee EY. Magnetic resonance imaging of the pediatric kidney: benign and malignant masses. Magn Reson Imaging Clin N Am. 2013;21(4):697-715.
34. Ko SM, Kim MJ, Im YJ, Park KI, Lee MJ. Cellular mesoblastic nephroma with liver metastasis in a neonate: prenatal and postnatal diffusion-weighted MR imaging. Korean J Radiol. 2013;14(2):361-5.
35. Chaudry G, Perez-Atayde AR, Ngan BY, Gundogan M, Daneman A. Imaging of congenital mesoblastic nephroma with pathological correlation. Pediatr Radiol. 2009;39(10):1080-6.
36. Glass RB, Davidson AJ, Fernbach SK. Clear cell sarcoma of the kidney: CT, sonographic, and pathologic correlation. Radiology. 1991;180(3):715-7.
37. Siegel MJ, Chung EM. Wilms' tumor and other pediatric renal masses. Magn Reson Imaging Clin N Am. 2008;16(3):479-97.
38. Gooskens SL, Graf N, Furtwängler R, Spreafico F, Bergeron C, Ramírez-Villar GL, et al. Position paper: Rationale for the treatment of children with CCSK in the UMBRELLA SIOP-RTSG 2016 protocol. Nat Rev Urol. 2018;15(5):309-19.
39. Agrons GA, Kingsman KD, Wagner BJ, Sotelo-Avila C. Rhabdoid tumor of the kidney in children: A comparative study. AJR Am J Roentgenol. 1997;168:447-51.

40. Chung CJ, Lorenzo R, Rayder S, Sotelo-Avila C. Rhabdoid tumors of the kidney in children: CT findings. AJR Am J Roentgenol. 1995;164:697-700.
41. Chung EM, Lattin GE Jr, Fagen KE, Kim AM, Pavio MA, Fehringer AJ, et al. Renal Tumors of Childhood: Radiologic-Pathologic Correlation Part 2. The 2nd Decade: From the Radiologic Pathology Archives. Radiographics. 2017;37(5):1538-58.
42. Geller JI, Ehrlich PF, Cost NG, Khanna G, Mullen EA, Gratias EJ, et al. Characterization of adolescent and pediatric renal cell carcinoma: a report from the Children's Oncology Group study AREN03B2. Cancer. 2015;121(14):2457-64.
43. Wang W, Ding J, Li Y, Wang C, Zhou L, Zhu H, et al. Magnetic resonance imaging and computed tomography characteristics of renal cell carcinoma associated with Xp11.2 translocation/TFE3 gene fusion. PLoS One. 2014;9(6):e99990.
44. Koo HJ, Choi HJ, Kim MH, Cho KS. Radiologic-pathologic correlation of renal cell carcinoma associated with Xp11.2 translocation. Acta Radiol. 2013;54(7):827-34.
45. Agrons GA, Wagner BJ, Davidson AJ, Suarez ES. Multilocular cystic renal tumor in children: Radiologic-pathologic correlation. Radiographics. 1995;15:653-69.
46. Kurosaki Y, Tanaka Y, Kuramoto K, Itai Y. Improved CT fat detection in small kidney angiomyolipomas using thin sections and single voxel measurements. J Comput Assist Tomogr. 1993;17:745-8.
47. Pedrosa I, Sun MR, Spencer M, Genega EM, Olumi AF, Dewolf WC, et al. MR imaging of renal masses: correlation with findings at surgery and pathologic analysis. Radiographics. 2008;28(4):985-1003.
48. Strouse PJ. Paediatric Renal Neoplasms. Radiol Clin North Am. 1996;34(6):1081-100.
49. Vazquez JL, Barnewolt CE, Shamberger RC, Chung T, Perez-Atayde AR. Ossifying renal tumor of infancy presenting as a palpable abdominal mass. Pediatr Radiol. 1998;28:454-7.
50. Lee SH, Choi YH, Kim WS, Cheon JE, Moon KC. Ossifying renal tumor of infancy: findings at ultrasound, CT and MRI. Pediatr Radiol. 2014;44(5):625-8.
51. Bastide C, Rambeaud JJ, Bach AM, Russo P. Metanephric adenoma of the kidney: clinical and radiological study of nine cases. BJU Int. 2009;103(11):1544-8.
52. Averill LW, Acikgoz G, Miller RE, Kandula VV, Epelman M. Update on pediatric leukemia and lymphoma imaging. Semin Ultrasound CT MR. 2013;34(6):578-99.
53. Sheth S, Ali S, Fishman E. Imaging of renal lymphoma: patterns of disease with pathologic correlation. Radiographics. 2006;26(4):1151-68.
54. Hilmes MA, Dillman JR, Mody RJ, Strouse PJ. Pediatric renal leukemia: spectrum of CT imaging findings. Pediatr Radiol. 2008;38:424-30.
55. Albregts AE, Cohen MD, Gallani CA. Neuroblastoma Invading the kidney. J Paediatr Surg. 1994;29:930-3.
56. Raby WN, Kopplin P, Weitzman S. Metastatic osteosarcoma of the kidney presenting as renal haemorrhage. J Paediatr Haematol/Oncol. 1996;18:321-2.
57. Wallis MC, Lorenzo AJ, Farhat WA, Bägli DJ, Khoury AE, Pippi Salle JL. Risk assessment of incidentally detected complex renal cysts in children: potential role for a modification of the Bosniak classification. J Urol. 2008;180(1):317-21.
58. Karmazyn B, Tawadros A, Delaney LR, Marine MB, Cain MP, Rink RC, et al. Ultrasound classification of solitary renal cysts in children. J Pediatr Urol. 2015;11(3):149.e1-6.
59. Peng Y, Jia L, Sun N, Li J, Fu L, Zeng J, et al. Assessment of cystic renal masses in children: comparison of multislice computed tomography and ultrasound imaging using the Bosniak classification system. Eur J Radiol. 2010;75(3):287-92.
60. Kushner B, Cheung NK. Neuroblastoma: An overview. Haem/Onc Ann. 1993;1:189-201.
61. Rha SE, Byun JY, Jung SE, Chun HJ, Lee HG, Lee JM. Neurogenic tumors in the abdomen: Tumor types and imaging characteristics. Radiographics. 2003;23:29-43.
62. Hirons MP, Owens CM. Radiology of neuroblastoma in children. Eur Radiol. 2001;11:2071-81.
63. Uhl M, Altehoefer C, Kontny U, Il'yasov K, Büchert M, Langer M. MRI-diffusion imaging of neuroblastomas: First results and correlation to histology. Eur Radiol. 2002;12:2335-8.
64. Lonergan GJ, Schwab CM, Suarez ES, Carlson CL. Neuroblastoma, ganglioneuroblastoma, and ganglioneuroma: radiologic-pathologic correlation. Radiograhics. 2002;22:911-34.
65. Laffan EE, O' Connor R, Ryan SP, Donoghue VB. Whole body magnetic resonance imaging: A useful additional sequence in paediatric imaging. Pediatr Radiol. 2004;34:472-80.
66. Sharp SE, Shulkin BL, Gelfand MJ, Salisbury S, Furman WL. 123I-MIBG Scintigraphy and 18 F-FDG PET in Neuroblastoma. J Nucl Med. 2009;50(8):1237-43.
67. Mittal BR, Agrawal K, Shukla J, Bhattacharya A, Singh B, Sood A. Ga-68 DOTATATE PET/CT in neuroendocrine tumours: Initial Experience. J Postgrad Med Edu Res. 2013;47(1):1-6.
68. Brodeur GM, Pritchard J, Berthold F, Carlsen NL, Castel V, Castelberry RP, et al. Revisions of the international criteria for neuroblastoma diagnosis, staging, and response to treatment. J Clin Oncol. 1993;11:1466-77.
69. Cohn SL, Pearson ADJ, London WB, Monclair T, Ambros PF, Brodeur GM. The International Neuroblastoma Risk Group (INRG) Classification System: An INRG Task Force Report. J Clin Oncol. 2009;27:289-97.
70. McCarville MB. Imaging neuroblastoma: what the radiologist needs to know. Cancer Imaging. 2011;11(1A):S44-7.
71. Monclair T, Brodeur GM, Ambros PF, Brisse HJ, Cecchetto G, Holmes K. The International Neuroblastoma Risk Group (INRG) Staging System: An INRG Task Force Report. J Clin Oncol. 2009;27(2):298-303.
72. Brisse HJ, McCarville MB, Granata C, Krug KB, Wootton-Gorges SL, Kanegawa K. International Neuroblastoma Risk Group Project. Guidelines for imaging and staging of neuroblastic tumors: consensus report from the International Neuroblastoma Risk Group Project. Radiology. 2011;261(1):243-57.
73. Simon T, Häberle B, Hero B, von Schweinitz D, Berthold F. Role of surgery in the treatment of patients with stage 4 neuroblastoma age 18 months or older at diagnosis. J Clin Oncol. 2013;31(6):752-8.
74. Daneman A. Adrenal Gland. In: Kuhn JP, Slovis TL, Haller JO (Eds). Caffey's Pediatric Diagnostic Imaging Vol. 2, 10th Edition. United States: Mosby Publications; 2004. pp. 1894-908.
75. Bonfig W, Bittman I, Bechtold S, Kammer B, Noelle V, Arleth S, et al. Virilizing adrenocortical tumors in children. Eur J Paedtiatr. 2003;162:623-8.
76. Michalkiewicz E, Sandrini R, Figueiredo B, Miranda EC, Caran E, Oliveira-Filho AG, et al. Clinical and outcome characteristics of children with adrenocortical tumors: A report from the International Pediatric Adrenocortical Tumor Registry. J Clin Oncol. 2004;22:838-45.
77. Nguyen CT, Kratovil T, Edwards MJ. Retroperitoneal teratoma presenting as an abscess in childhood. J Pediatr Surg. 2007;42:21-3.
78. Rattan KN, Kadian YS, Nair VJ, Kaushal V, Duhan N, Aggarwal S. Primary retroperitoneal tumors in children: A single institution experience: African J Paediatr Surg. 2010;7(1):5-8.
79. Hayasaka K, Yamada T, Saitoh Y, Yoshikawa D, Aburano T, Hashimoto H, et al. CT evaluation of primary benign retroperitoneal tumor. Radiat Med. 1994;12:115-20.
80. Bellin MF, Lebleu L, Meric JB. Evaluation of retroperitoneal and Pelvic node metastases with MRI lymphangiography. Abdom Imaging. 2003;28:155-63.

CHAPTER

76

Evaluation of Female Pelvis and Testicular Abnormalities

Anmol Bhatia, Kushaljit Singh Sodhi, Akshay Kumar Saxena

FEMALE PELVIS

Ultrasonography (USG) is the most useful modality for imaging genital organs in infants and children because it is a noninvasive and painless study which does not require sedation for the baby [in contrast to computed tomography (CT) and magnetic resonance (MR) examinations]. The lack of ionizing radiation makes ultrasound (US) very attractive as a pediatric imaging modality.[1,2]

Knowledge of simple embryology and basic physiology is required to evaluate the children presenting with precocious puberty, amenorrhea, lower abdominal pain, suspected pelvic masses, or ambiguous genitalia, which are key reasons for imaging of female pelvis in children.

Computed tomography remains useful for tumor staging, follow-up, and in acute abdomen. Magnetic resonance imaging (MRI) provides exact demonstration of findings in different planes especially in cases of complex anomalies, when US findings are inconclusive.[3]

NORMAL ULTRASOUND ANATOMY OF GENITAL ORGANS IN INFANTS AND CHILDREN

The size and shape of the ovaries and of uterus vary during childhood, are age dependent, and under hormonal influence. The maternal and placental hormones produce a relatively larger size of the neonatal uterus and ovaries. The uterus has a prominent, echogenic endometrial lining.[1,2]

During infancy, the size, shape, and echotexture of the uterus and ovaries remain relatively stable. However, the ovaries are never dormant and follicles or cysts can be seen at every age. About 2–3 years before the onset of puberty, the uterine volume gradually increases with accelerated growth occurring during puberty.[2]

Uterus

Uterine anatomy changes with age of the child **(Figs. 1A to C)**. The uterus in neonates is prominent due to effects of maternal and placental hormones.[4,5] The cervix is larger than the fundus (fundus-to-cervix ratio 1/2 <1), the length of uterus is approximately 3.5 cm, and the maximum thickness is approximately 1.4 cm. Echogenic endometrial lining is often seen. Fluid can also be seen sometimes within the endometrial cavity. During infancy, the proportion of cervix to uterine body changes to 1:1. This tubular shape is stable until 2–3 years before the onset of puberty.[2]

The prepubertal uterus is tubular in configuration (anteroposterior dimension of cervix equal to anteroposterior dimension of fundus) or is of a spade shape (anteroposterior dimension of cervix is larger than anteroposterior dimension of fundus).[6-9] The endometrium is normally not well-seen; however, central lining can be seen in some cases using high-frequency transducers. The length varies between 2.5 and 4 cm and the thickness is not >10 mm.

During puberty, the greatest growth occurs in the fundus and corpus, altering to a pear-shaped uterus (~25 mL). The pubertal uterus is pear shape in configuration (fundus larger than cervix) (fundus-to-cervix ratio = 2/1 to 3/1)[6-9] **(Fig. 1C)** which is similar to that seen in adults and is 5–8 cm long, 3 cm wide, and 1.5 cm thick. The endometrial lining is visualized which varies with the different phases in the menstrual cycle. The endometrial canal is seen as a thin echogenic interface and the endometrium demonstrates cyclical changes every cycle. The measurement of the endometrial thickness includes both endometrial lines.

Doppler US of the uterine artery can be used to confirm the onset of puberty. In prepubertal girls, the pulsed Doppler demonstrates a narrow systolic waveform without positive diastolic flow. In postpubertal girls, a broad systolic waveform is seen with positive diastolic flow.[6]

Ovaries

The size of ovaries is usually described by estimating their volume: Neonatal ovaries measure 1–3.6 mL.[2,6] In infants, measurements are average of slightly >1 cm^3 during infancy and 0.67 cm^3 for the 2nd year of life.[10,11]

Multiple follicles in the ovaries are normal in a neonatal ovary. After birth, follicle-stimulating hormone (FSH) rises in the newborn period due to the abrupt lack of the placental and maternal hormones. During the 2nd year of life, the FSH level decreases, but a pulsatile secretion of FSH persists at a

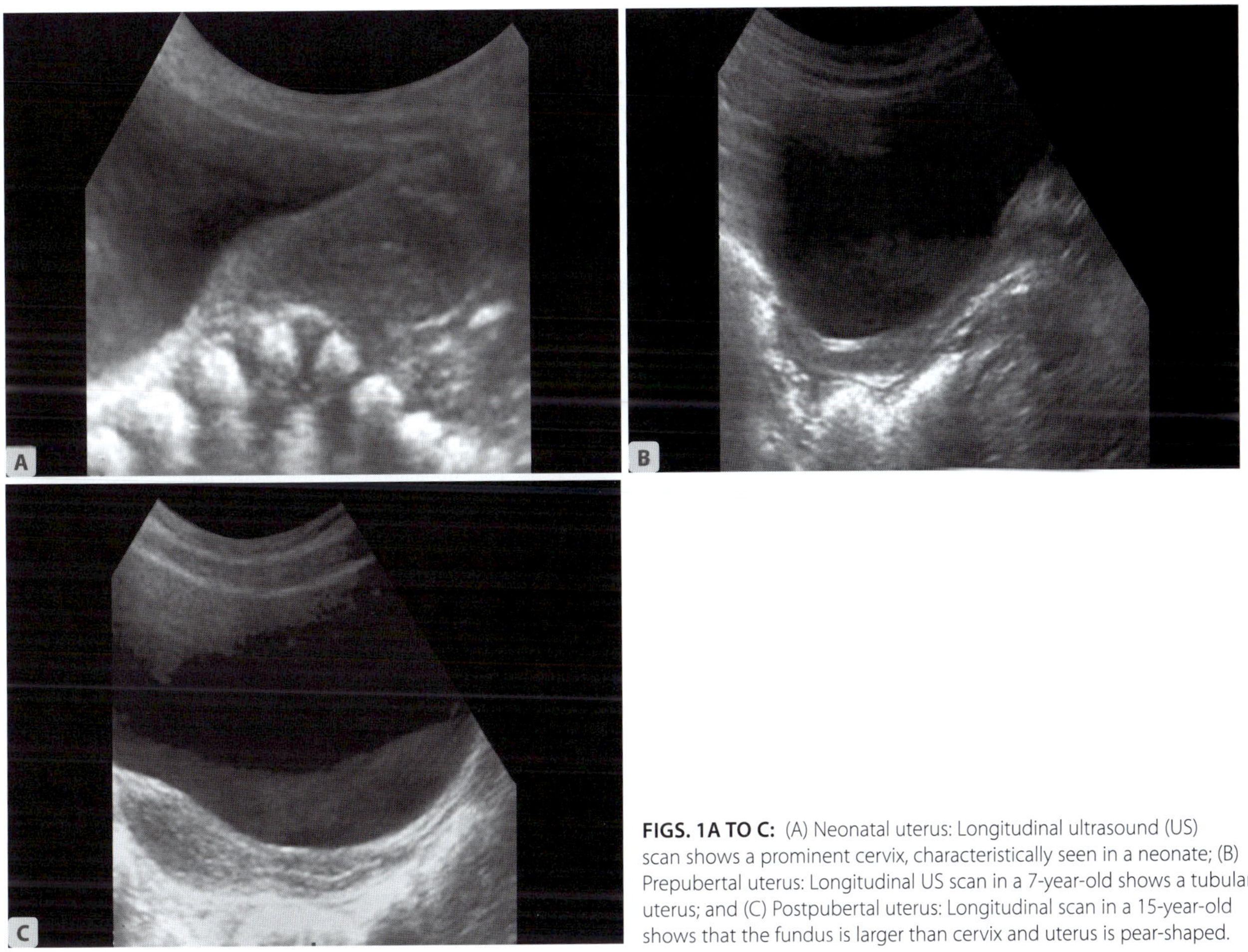

FIGS. 1A TO C: (A) Neonatal uterus: Longitudinal ultrasound (US) scan shows a prominent cervix, characteristically seen in a neonate; (B) Prepubertal uterus: Longitudinal US scan in a 7-year-old shows a tubular uterus; and (C) Postpubertal uterus: Longitudinal scan in a 15-year-old shows that the fundus is larger than cervix and uterus is pear-shaped.

low level. The ovary thus contains mature follicles at all ages. Antral follicles (tertiary follicles) are fluid-filled follicles, which are round in shape and usually <9 mm in size in the prepubertal girl.[1,2]

The mean ovarian volume in girls <6 years of age is ≤1 cm^3. The increase in ovarian volume starts after 6 years of age.

In prepubertal girls (6–10 years of age), ovarian volume ranges between 1.2 and 2.3 cm^3. In premenarchal girls (11–12 years of age), ovarian volume ranges between 2 and 4 cm^3 **(Table 1)**. In postmenarchal girls, the ovarian volume averages around 8 cm^3.

Microcystic follicles are routinely imaged (in up to 84% of normal girls) from birth to 24 months of age and in 68% of girls between 2 and 12 years of age).[12] The following measurements can be considered as upper normal values for prepubertal girls: Uterine length of 4.5 cm, uterine thickness of 1 cm (the single most useful criteria), and ovarian volume of 4–5 cm^3.[1,2]

TABLE 1: Pediatric ovarian volumes.

Age (year)	Mean volume (cm^3)	Standard deviation
1	1.05	0.7
2	0.67	0.35
3	0.7	0.2
4	0.8	0.4
5	0.9	0.02
6	1.2	0.4
7	1.3	0.6
8	1.1	0.5
9	2.0	0.8
10	2.2	0.7
11	2.5	1.3
12	3.8	1.4
13	4.2	2.3

Source: Cohen HL, Shapiro MA, Mandel FS, Shapiro ML. Normal ovaries in neonates and infants: a sonographic study of 77 patients 1 day to 24 months old. AJR Am J Roentgenol. 1993;160:583-6; Orsini LF, Salardi S, Pilu G, Bovicelli L, Cacciari E. Pelvic organs in premenarcheal girls: real-time ultrasonography. Radiology. 1984;153:113-6.

Ovarian Cysts

Ovarian cysts can be classified as physiological, functional, or neoplastic.[13] When a normal mature follicle fails to involute and continues to enlarge, secondary to hormonal imbalance, a functional or retention cyst results. These cysts may develop from preovulatory follicles (follicular cysts) or from postovulatory follicles (corpus luteum cysts) and usually range from 4 to 10 cm in size.[13-15]

Cysts up to 2 cm are usually follicles. Larger cysts (>2 cm) may be pathologic, particularly if persistent.[2] Follow-up US of ovarian cysts is recommended to ensure resolution after 6 weeks or after one and a half menstrual cycles.[16-18] Maternal hormones may cause large neonatal ovarian cysts.[19] Although retention cysts are usually asymptomatic and detected incidentally on sonograms, they may cause pain related to pressure or hemorrhage.

Follicular and corpus luteum retention cysts cannot be differentiated with imaging studies. However, corpus luteum cysts tend to be more symptomatic. Diagnosis requires correlation with the date of the last menstrual period or tissue sampling. Serial sonography is suggested, since the majority of functional cysts demonstrate cyclic changes or regress spontaneously.

On sonograms, a nonhemorrhagic functional cyst appears as a smooth, unilocular cystic mass. The sonographic features that suggest hemorrhage within a simple cyst are variable and depend on the age of the blood. Most hemorrhagic ovarian cysts are seen as complex masses with septations, low-level echoes, a fluid-debris level, or coagulated blood. Hemorrhagic cysts are avascular on Doppler sonography. Clot lysis and resolution are an important diagnostic feature. With time, the cyst becomes more sonolucent or anechoic.[2,13]

ANOMALIES OF THE FEMALE PELVIS

Müllerian Duct Anomalies

According to anatomic findings, Müllerian duct anomalies (MDAs) have been classified by the American Society for Reproductive Medicine as summarized in **Table 2**. However, this classification does not include vaginal anomalies, for which an alternative classification system has been described which is summarized in **Table 3**.

As can be seen in the classifications, the anomalies can be obstructive or nonobstructive in nature. Because of the frequent association between anomalies of lateral fusion and anomalies of vertical fusion, it is helpful to consider these anomalies according to the presence or absence of obstruction.

TABLE 2: Summarizing the MDAs proposed by the American Society for Reproductive Medicine.

Classes	Description
I	Müllerian agenesis/hypoplasia
I-A	Agenesis/hypoplasia of vagina (uterus: Normal/have one or more malformations)
I-B	Agenesis/hypoplasia of cervix
I-C	Agenesis/hypoplasia of fundus
I-D	Agenesis/hypoplasia of fallopian tube
I-E	Combined agenesis or hypoplasia (≥2 findings from classes I-A to I-D)
II	Unicornuate uterus
II-A	Rudimentary horn with an endometrial cavity communicating with the (single-horned) uterus
II-B	Rudimentary horn with an endometrial cavity not communicating with the uterus
II-C	Rudimentary horn having no endometrial cavity
II-D	No rudimentary horn
III	Uterus didelphys
IV	Bicornuate uterus
IV-A	Complete bicornuate: Septum is extending to the internal os or external os
IV-B	Partial bicornuate: Septum is confined to the fundus
V	Septate uterus
V-A	Complete septate: Septum extends to the internal os
V-B	Partial septate: Septum does not reach the internal os
VI	Arcuate uterus
VII	DES-related anomalies of uterus
VII-A	T-shaped uterus
VII-B	T-shaped uterus with dilated horns
VII-C	Hypoplasia of uterus

(DES: diethylstilbestrol; MDAs: Müllerian duct anomalies)

TABLE 3: Classification of vaginal anomalies.

Classes	Description
I	Transverse vaginal septum: May be obstructing or nonobstructing
II	Longitudinal vaginal septum: May be obstructing or nonobstructing
III	Stenosis or iatrogenic injury

Müllerian Agenesis/Mayer–Rokitansky–Küster–Hauser Syndrome

Second most common cause of primary amenorrhea and primary infertility, the most common being the gonadal dysgenesis.[20,21] It is characterized by atresia of vagina with an absent or a rudimentary uterus (which may be a unicornuate or bicornuate ion configuration) and normal ovaries. The child's karyotype is normal (46,XX). Renal anomalies (agenesis, ectopia) can be seen in up to 50% of cases; skeletal or spinal anomalies occur in 12% of cases. In 6–10% of cases, functioning endometrium may be seen within the rudimentary uterus, which results in unilateral hematometra. Mayer-Rokitansky-Küster-Hauser (MRKH) syndrome is subdivided in two types: (1) Type I (isolated) or Rokitansky; and (2) Type II **(Figs. 2A to C)** or Müllerian duct aplasia, renal dysplasia, and cervical somite anomalies (MURCS) association.

Obstructive Müllerian Anomalies

Failure of vertical fusion or canalization of the urogenital sinus or the Müllerian duct system may result in cervical stenosis or atresia, vaginal atresia, or transverse vaginal septa. A transverse vaginal septum can occur at many levels of the vagina and creates a blockage of the vagina and uterus. In

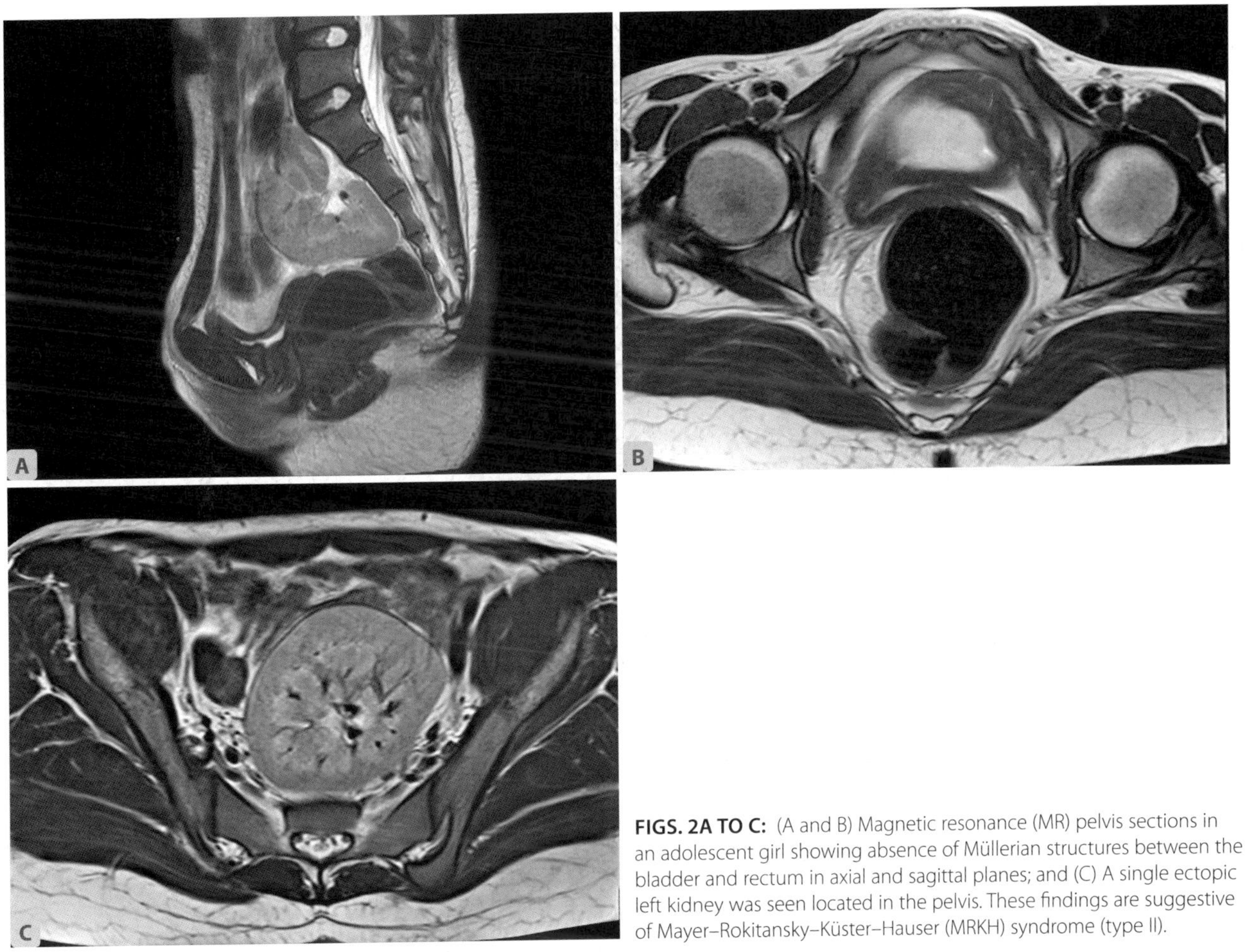

FIGS. 2A TO C: (A and B) Magnetic resonance (MR) pelvis sections in an adolescent girl showing absence of Müllerian structures between the bladder and rectum in axial and sagittal planes; and (C) A single ectopic left kidney was seen located in the pelvis. These findings are suggestive of Mayer–Rokitansky–Küster–Hauser (MRKH) syndrome (type II).

addition, hymenal tissue may be imperforate. Imperforate hymen is the most common genital outflow tract anomaly.

Most of the cases of hydrometrocolpos in the neonatal group coexist with a urogenital sinus or cloaca.[22,23] Hematometrocolpos presenting in adolescent girls is secondary to vaginal obstruction by an imperforate hymen. The patient presents at puberty with primary amenorrhea and cyclic lower abdominal or pelvic pain.[24] US typically shows a fluid-filled mass posterior to the bladder, which represents the dilated vagina **(Figs. 3A and B and 4A and B)**. The uterus may also be dilated. The dilated uterus can be differentiated from the vagina by the cervical margin and thicker wall. Not infrequently, hematometrocolpos is present with duplication anomalies.[25] In the newborn period, a bulging mass (hydrocolpos) may be noted at the introitus.

Hematometrocolpos is cured by addressing the obstruction whereas hematometra needs a hysterectomy.

Nonobstructive Müllerian Anomalies

The unicornuate uterus appears as a curved, elongated uterus with tapering of the fundal segment off midline (the "banana-like" configuration) on T2-weighted MR images.

Normal uterine zonal anatomy is maintained. The rudimentary horn, when present, usually demonstrates lower signal intensity on T2-weighted images. Communication with rudimentary horn can be easily demonstrated on MRI.

Partial fusion of the Müllerian ducts results in the bicornuate uterus. MRI shows uterine horns separated by an intervening cleft in the external fundal myometrium of longer than 1 cm. Normal zonal anatomy is seen in each horn and there is a dividing septum which is composed of myometrium.

The uterus didelphys results from nonfusion of the two Müllerian ducts. Two separate normal-sized uterine horns and cervices are demonstrated on T2-weighted MR images **(Figs. 5A to C)**.

A longitudinal vaginal septum is present in 75% of cases, occasionally complicated by transverse septa causing obstruction. The two uterine horns are usually widely separated, with preservation of the endometrial and myometrial widths.

A septate uterus is seen when there is incomplete resorption of the final fibrous septum between the two uterine horns. The septum may be partial or it may be complete and extends to the external cervical os. The differentiation between the septate and the bicornuate uterus is clinically important as the septate uterus is associated with a higher rate of reproductive complications. T2-weighted MR images taken parallel to the long axis of the uterus demonstrate a

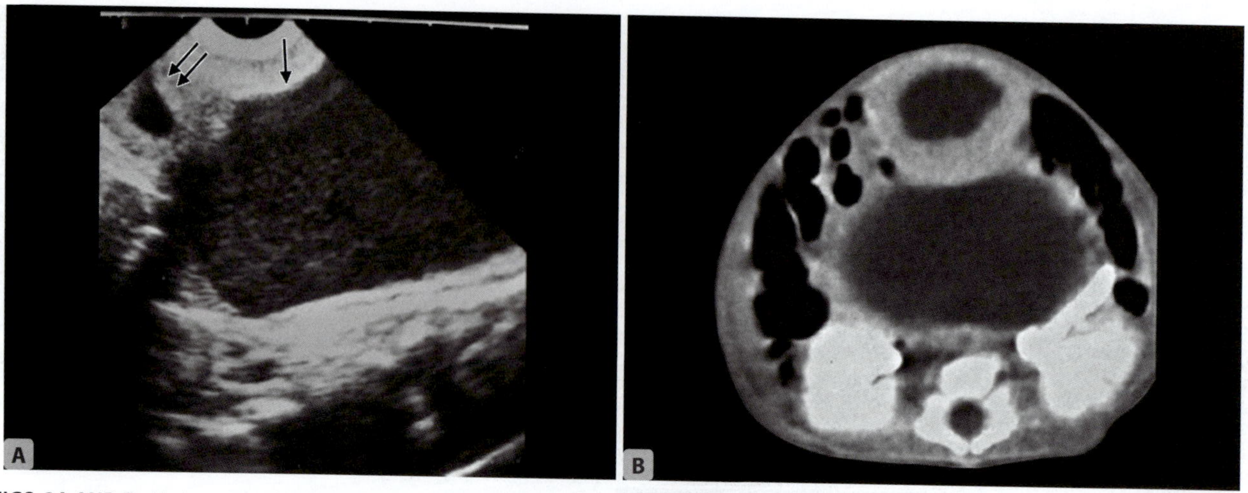

FIGS. 3A AND B: Hydrometrocolpos in a 1-year-old female child with palpable midline pelvic lump. (A) Ultrasound shows a fluid-filled distended vagina (arrow) and the uterine cavity with its thick myometrium (double arrows); and (B) CT scan reveals two fluid-filled structures separate from the displaced small urinary bladder, consistent with distended uterine cavity and vagina.

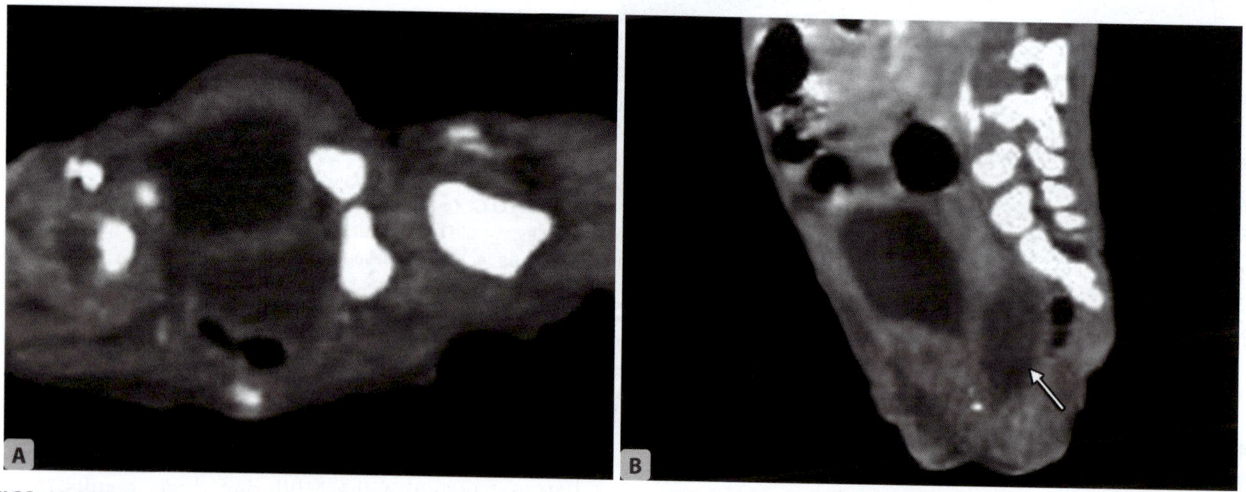

FIGS. 4A AND B: CT scan. (A and B) Axial and sagittal images of hydrocolpos in a 4-month-old intrauterine growth restriction (IUGR) child showing cystic structure (arrow) behind urinary bladder, anterior to rectum, and inferior to uterus, consistent with hydrocolpos.

convex, flat, or concave (<1 cm) external uterine contour and the presence of the fibrous septa.[26]

Primary Amenorrhea

Primary amenorrhea is defined as:

- No menarche by 16 years of age.
- No thelarche or adrenarche by 14 years of age
- No menarche >3 years after adrenarche and thelarche[1]

The presence or absence of secondary sexual development at clinical examination and visualization of Müllerian structures at US is the basis for further laboratory tests. Common causes for primary amenorrhea include gonadal dysgenesis (Turner syndrome) (33% cases), Müllerian (uterovaginal) anomalies (20% cases), central hypothalamic-pituitary causes (15% cases), constitutional delay (often familial) (10% cases), and other causes like systemic, psychiatric issues (22% cases).

Multiple syndromes result in primary amenorrhea including Turner syndrome, MRKH syndrome, Kallmann syndrome, Prader–Willi syndrome, androgen insensitivity syndrome, and Swyer syndrome.[27-29]

In Swyer syndrome (XY gonadal dysgenesis), no functional gonads are present to induce puberty, in an otherwise normal girl whose karyotype is found to be XY. The gonads are found to be nonfunctional streaks. Estrogen and progesterone therapy is commenced. The nonfunctioning gonads are removed because of their risk of developing gonadoblastoma.[2]

Turner Syndrome

Patients with XO karyotype (approximately 70% of cases with Turner syndrome) have a prepubertal uterus and nonvisualized or streaky gonads (ovaries).[30] In rare instances, especially in mosaic karyotypes, the gonads can be normal in

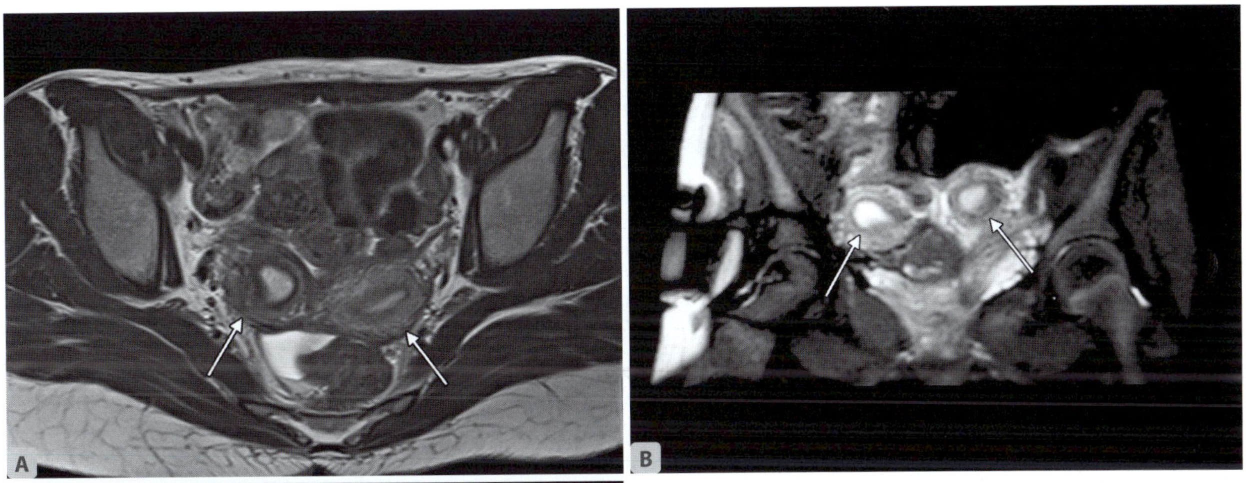

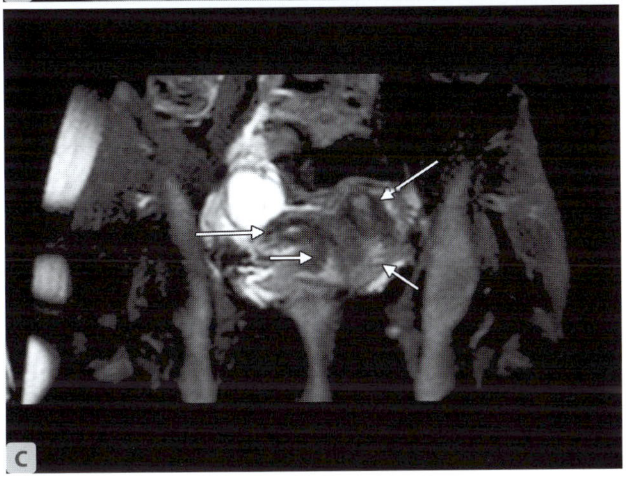

FIGS. 5A TO C: Magnetic resonance (MR) pelvis sections showing two uterine cavities (long white arrows in A to C) and two separate cervixes (short white arrows in C). The findings are suggestive of uterus didelphys.

appearance.[30] Spontaneous puberty occurs in 5–15% of cases with Turner syndrome.[31]

Polycystic Ovary Syndrome

Polycystic ovary syndrome (PCOS) is an endocrine disorder resulting in chronic anovulation. PCOS is a common cause of infertility and amenorrhea. It is associated with Stein–Leventhal syndrome, which includes obesity and hirsutism. On US, multiple, small follicles (over 10) may be noted with increased echogenicity of the stroma. The ovaries are often 1.5–3 times larger than normal; however, the ovarian volume may be normal in 30% of cases.[2] The diagnosis of PCOS is confirmed biochemically.

PELVIC MASSES IN CHILDREN

Benign Ovarian Neoplasms

Ovarian teratomas are the most common benign ovarian neoplasm in pediatric patients.[2] Mature teratomas or dermoid cysts constitute for two-thirds of pediatric ovarian tumors.[13]

Typically, they are found in adolescents. Dermoids contains two cell layers: (1) mesoderm and (2) ectoderm. Teratomas are made up of elements from all three layers, including the endoderm. Two-thirds of patients present with an abdominal mass and the rest with pain due to torsion or hemorrhage. About 25% of teratomas are bilateral. Malignancy is found in 2–10%. Teratomas may have cystic, solid, or mixed appearance on US due to its contents. They appear echogenic due to contained fat, hair, sebum, or calcium (teeth, bone). Anechoic components are due to serous fluid or sebum.[32] Approximately, 10–15% of benign teratomas are purely anechoic masses at sonography. Another 10–15% of teratomas are predominantly echogenic.

Peripheral nodules and shadowing each occur in 70% of teratomas in postpubertal girls. In contrast, mural nodules occur in only 40% of prepubertal girls and shadowing in only 15%.[13] Other features of teratomas include fat- or hair-fluid levels and central soft-tissue masses.[32,33]

CT and MR imaging are useful in further characterization. The most characteristic CT appearance of a benign teratoma is that of a predominantly fluid-filled lesion containing a mixture of fat, hair, debris, and calcifications **(Figs. 6A to C)**. Calcifications (either teeth or bone) often are localized to the solid globular protuberance (i.e., mural nodule or dermoid plug) arising from the cyst wall. Rarely, a teratoma appears on CT scans as a primarily fatty mass without calcification. If fat or a combination of fat and calcium is identified within a cystic mass, a specific

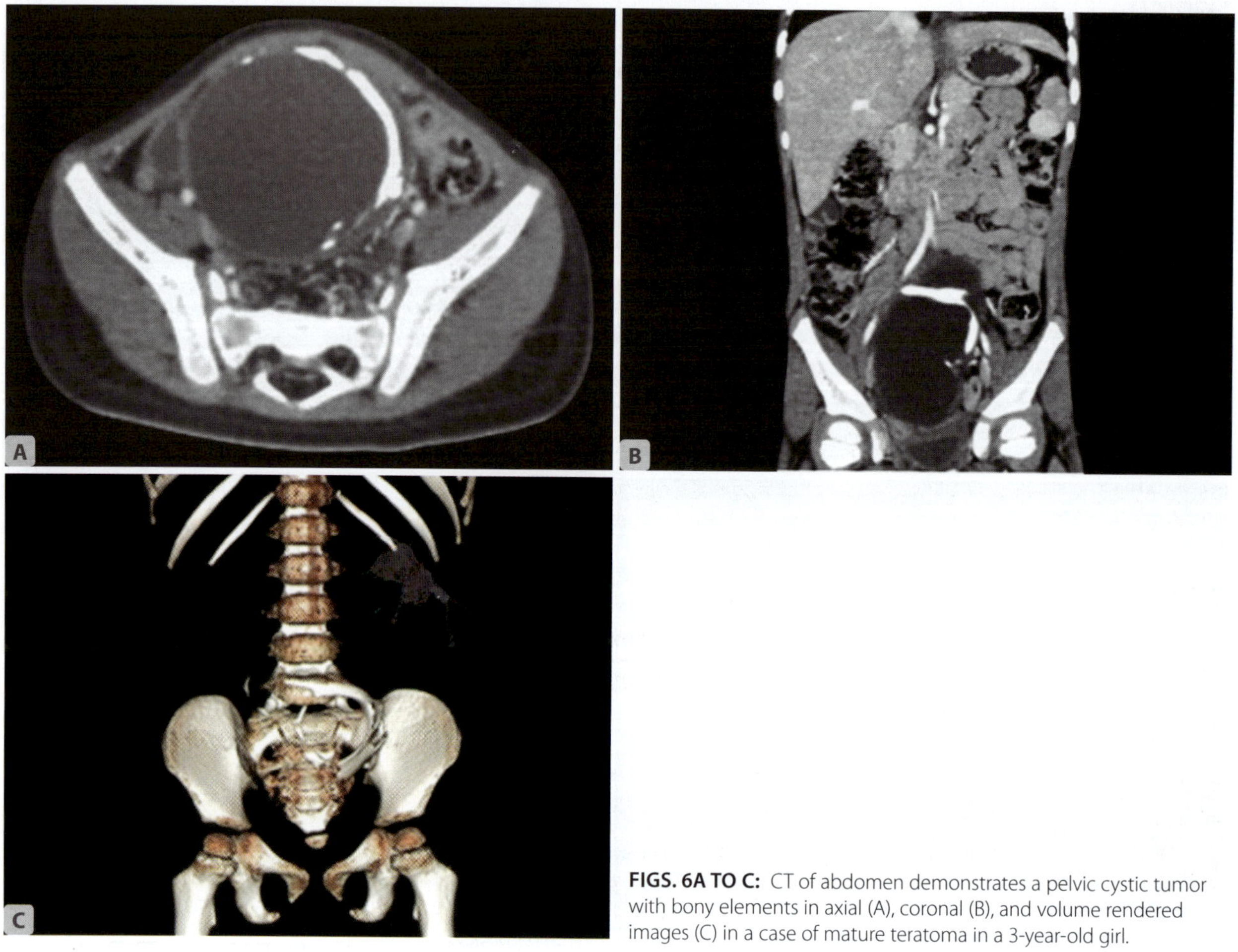

FIGS. 6A TO C: CT of abdomen demonstrates a pelvic cystic tumor with bony elements in axial (A), coronal (B), and volume rendered images (C) in a case of mature teratoma in a 3-year-old girl.

diagnosis of teratoma can be made. In general, two-thirds of teratomas display characteristic CT features. On MR images also, cystic teratomas vary in signal intensity depending on their tissue composition.[19] On T1-weighted images, fat appears as an area of high signal intensity, while serous fluid has low signal intensity. On T2-weighted images, fat and serous fluid have high signal intensity. Calcifications, bone, and hair have low signal intensity on MR images.[13]

Malignant Neoplasms

Malignant pelvic lesions in the female pelvis are rare and can arise from bone (Ewing's sarcoma, coccygeal teratomas), soft tissue of muscles, uterus, or bladder (rhabdomyosarcoma) or have neurogenic origin (neuroblastoma). Some cystic and solid masses have particular diagnostic features (teratomas), but often additional imaging modalities (MR/CT) and/or histology are necessary to confirm a specific diagnosis.

Sacrococcygeal teratoma is one of the most common presacral tumors which contain derivates of three germinal layers. These tumors occur more frequently in girls and are classified into four types, according to the location. Type I is predominantly external, while type IV is presacral with no external component in it. CT and MRI are useful for depiction of location, its differentiation, and extent of this tumor **(Figs. 7A and B and 8A and B)**.

Rhabdomyosarcoma is the most common soft-tissue sarcoma in children. Peak incidence is between 2 and 6 years. The genitourinary tract is a common site of origin.

In girls, rhabdomyosarcoma can arise from the bladder or vagina and surrounding tissues. About 6% are sarcoma botryoides, which is an embryonal rhabdomyosarcoma originating from the vagina, cervix, or bladder of young girls. The tumor characteristically resembles a bunch of grapes.

Malignant Ovarian Neoplasms

Malignant pelvic neoplasms with gynecologic origin are rare in children and include sex cord stromal tumors (granulosa cell, theca cell, fibroblast, Leydig and Sertoli cells) and germ cell tumors (dysgerminoma, malignant teratoma, endodermal sinus tumor, embryonal carcinoma, and choriocarcinoma) **(Figs. 9 and 10)**. Sex cord stromal tumors represent 8% of ovarian neoplasm and affect all age groups. The more common type is granulosa cell tumors. Due to the estrogenic effects of these tumors, females present with pseudoprecocious puberty, endometrial bleeding, and sonographic findings of enlargement of the

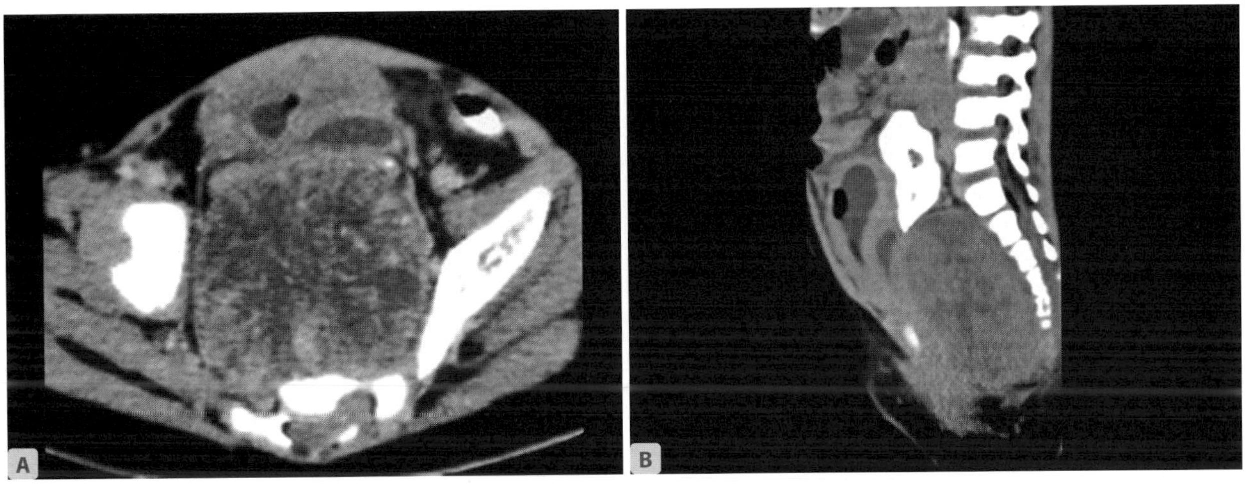

FIGS. 7A AND B: CT scan. (A and B) Axial and sagittal images of malignant sacrococcygeal teratoma in a 2-year-old female child which also demonstrated bony involvement along with markedly raised alpha-fetoprotein (AFP) levels.

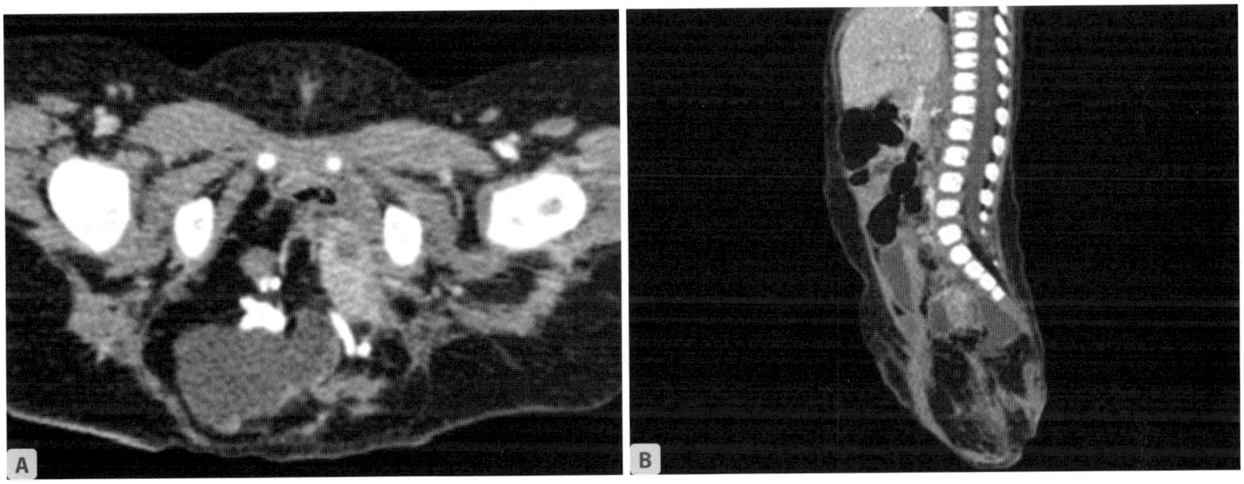

FIGS. 8A AND B: Axial and sagittal CT scan in another patient of sacrococcygeal teratoma which demonstrates areas of fat, calcification, and cystic components within this tumor.

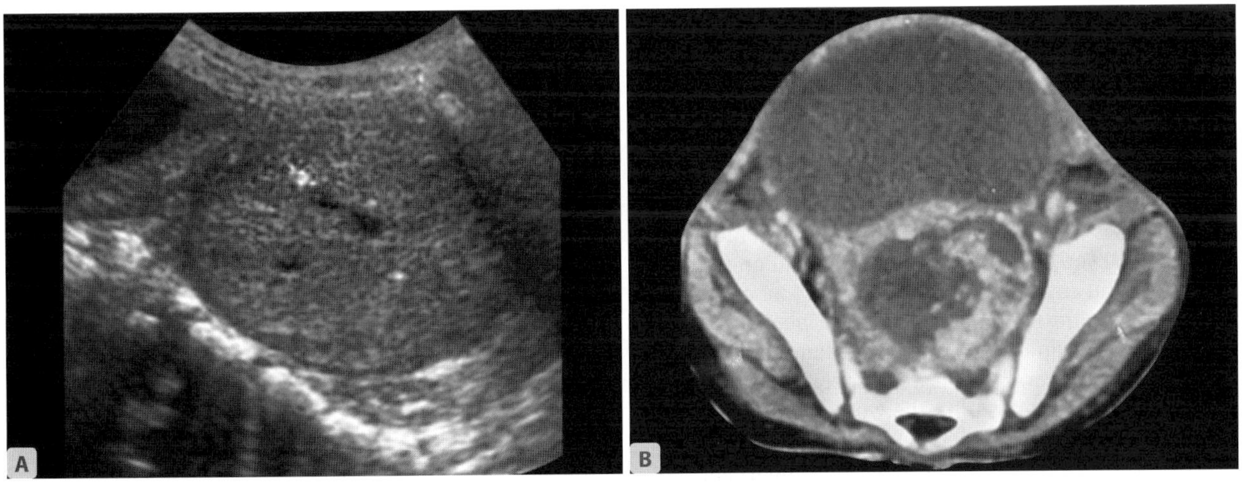

FIGS. 9A AND B: (A) Ultrasound shows a well-encapsulated predominantly solid adnexal mass with calcific foci and few cystic areas. Biopsy revealed malignant germ cell tumor; and (B) CT scan reveals a large heterogeneous solid cystic pelvic mass with a calcific foci.

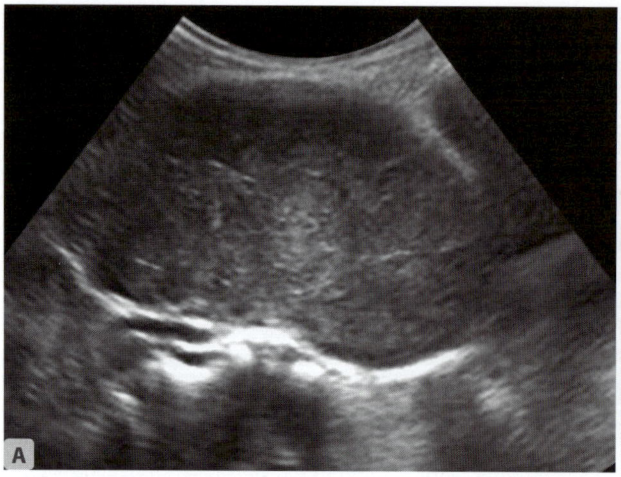

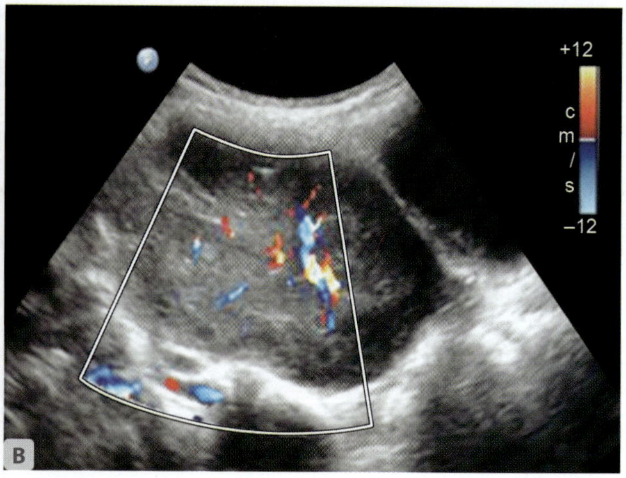

FIGS. 10 AND B: Dysgerminoma right ovary. (A and B) Ultrasound pelvis reveals a solid pelvic mass in the right adnexa, which on color Doppler demonstrates mild increased central vascularity.

uterus and thickening of the endometrium. The appearance of sex cord tumors vary and range from large multicystic masses to small solid masses.[34]

Children with germ cell tumors present often with asymptomatic pelvic or abdominal masses. With imaging, solid masses are found, which are echogenic on US and have soft-tissue attenuation on CT **(Figs. 9A and B)**. Other findings include calcifications, central necrosis, irregular walls, thick septations, papillary projections, and free abdominal and pelvic fluid. Metastasis occurs in lungs, liver, and peritoneum. Yolk sac tumor is a germ cell tumor and is a rare, malignant tumor composed of cells that line the yolk sac of the embryo. The tumor is most often found in children before the age of 2 years. As with most other pelvic masses, ovarian yolk sac tumors grow very large before being noticed clinically.[2]

Ovarian Torsion

Ovarian torsion is the twisting of an ovary on its ligamentous supports, which may lead to reduction of the blood supply.[23]

Symptoms of ovarian torsion are nonspecific, making it difficult to differentiate from other causes of acute abdomen. Ovarian torsion is commonly associated with a cyst or tumor, which is typically benign; the most common being mature cystic teratoma.

Ultrasound is the primary imaging modality which is used in a case of suspected ovarian torsion. The most constant finding on US is a large ovary (>4 cm).[35] US may demonstrate multiple small (up to 25 mm) uniform cysts aligned in the periphery of the engorged ovary in up to 74% of cases. This appearance is due to follicles that have been displaced to the periphery due to the marked edema and venous congestion.[36,37] However, this is a nonspecific sign and may be seen in normal ovaries of fertile women and in patients with PCOS and are not solely diagnostic of ovarian torsion. However, in the setting of acute pain, multiple peripheral cysts in a unilaterally enlarged ovary are helpful in diagnosing ovarian torsion.[35]

The typical color Doppler sonographic finding in ovarian torsion is the absence of arterial flow. However, the most frequent finding is either decrease or absence of venous flow (93%).[35] The diagnostic findings incorporating both grayscale and color Doppler study include a twisted vascular pedicle and the whirlpool sign.[38,39] A twisted vascular pedicle is known to be detected in 88% of cases of ovarian torsion.[39]

Although CT is not advocated to diagnose a case of ovarian torsion, it may be incidentally detected on CT as it is increasingly being used in evaluation of patients with abdominal pain. Moreover, when CT or USG reveals an indeterminate pelvic of adnexal mass, MRI is the next step for further characterization. Features of ovarian torsion on cross-sectional imaging include an enlarged ovary, deviation of the uterus to the twisted side, smooth wall thickening of the twisted adnexal cystic mass, thickening of the fallopian tube, peripheral cystic structures, ovarian hemorrhage, abnormal ovarian enhancement, and fluid in the pelvis.[1,2,23]

Tubo-ovarian Abscess

Pelvic inflammatory disease more commonly affects postpubertal girls. The inflammatory process usually begins in the cervix, ascending to the endometrium, fallopian tubes, and, rarely, to the ovaries, parametrium, and peritoneal cavity. The diagnosis is made clinically, based on symptoms of pain, vaginal discharge, and fever. US, CT, or MRI is useful for detecting complications such as pyosalpinx, tubo-ovarian abscess.[13]

Pyosalpinx appears as a hypoechoic tubular mass with internal debris whereas tubo-ovarian abscess is seen as a complex mass, often with debris, septations, and irregular thick walls. After antibiotics, pelvic inflammatory disease may resolve completely or lead to sequelae such as hydrosalpinx or adhesions. CT can complement US. At CT, a tubo-ovarian abscess often appears as a soft-tissue mass with central areas of lower attenuation and thick walls. Occasionally, air or an air-fluid level may be seen.

Ectopic Pregnancy

Ectopic pregnancy is a known but infrequent cause of pelvic mass in postpubertal girls.

The most specific US finding for diagnosing an ectopic pregnancy is the visualization of an extrauterine embryo. More often, ectopic pregnancy is manifested as a nonspecific echogenic or complex adnexal mass, often associated with cul-de-sac fluid and an enlarged uterus with a pseudogestational sac.[40,41] A pseudogestational sac has only a single echogenic ring representing parietal decidua whereas an early intrauterine pregnancy has a double-ring appearance resulting from visualization of the inner decidua capsularis and outer parietal decidua. Because of the nonspecificity of the adnexal masses, it is vital to correlate the US appearance with the level of the β subunit of human chorionic gonadotropin (hCG).

NONGYNECOLOGIC PELVIC MASSES

Pelvic masses of nongynecologic origin include appendiceal abscesses, fluid collections, and fluid-filled bowel, which can be confounded with primary adnexal lesions.[13]

On sonograms, periappendiceal abscess appears as a complex mass in the right lower quadrant. If an appendicolith or gas is present, bright echoes with shadowing may be noted. Positive US findings of appendicitis are diameter over 6 mm, lack of compressibility, increased vascularity of the appendical wall, appendicolith, adjacent abdominal free fluid, increased echogenicity of adjacent mesenteric fat, and enlarged lymph nodes.

Cerebrospinal fluid pseudocysts are infrequent complications of ventriculoperitoneal shunting, resulting from loculation of draining cerebrospinal fluid. On sonograms, uninfected pseudocysts appear as hypoechoic masses. When infected, pseudocysts become more complex, containing internal echoes or septations. Fluid-filled bowel may potentially be confused with an adnexal cyst at US. In most cases, bowel can be identified due to peristalsis detected with real-time imaging. In addition, complicated fluid collections resulting from bleeding or ascites due to peritoneal metastases may be confused with ovarian masses. These collections may change with changes in patient position.

Other nongynecological cystic masses which can be seen in the pelvis include mesenteric cysts, duplication cysts, urachal remnants, Meckel's diverticulum, ureteroceles, dilated ureters, hydronephrosis in ectopic kidneys, vascular and lymphatic malformations, abscess, and hematoma. The larger the size of the lesion, the more difficult it is to determine its origin.

IMAGING OF TESTICULAR ABNORMALITIES

The clinical manifestations in testicular abnormalities include pain, swelling, redness, or a palpable mass. These include undescended testes, hydrocoele, varicocele, acute scrotum, scrotal tumors, benign testicular cysts, testicular microlithiasis, scrotal trauma, scrotal hernia, and systemic diseases with testicular involvement.

Gray-scale USG in combination with color or power Doppler imaging is a well-accepted technique for assessing testicular abnormalities.[42] US permits differentiation between lesions that require urgent surgery (testicular torsion, malignant tumors, and traumatic rupture) and those that can be managed conservatively (e.g., epididymo-orchitis, torsion of the testicular appendages).

Undescended Testes

Various terms such as maldescended, undescended, retractile, and ectopic testes have been used in the literature. Hormann M has illustrated the entity of "undescended testes" in their review on scrotal imaging in children.[43] "Undescended testes" includes the following:[44]

- *Maldescended testis*: Testis is not descended into the normal position, which is 4 cm below the inguinal ligament.
- *Cryptorchidism*: Abdominally positioned testis.
- *Incompletely descended testis*: Testis lying in the region of inguinal canal **(Figs. 11A and B)** anywhere between the external and internal inguinal ring.[45]
- *Obstructed testis*: Testis which is seen lying in the superficial pouch.
- *Prescrotal retention*: Testis is located within the scrotal sac, but is at a higher position (<4 cm below the inguinal ligament).
- *Retractile testis*: Testis which is located in the normal position but retracts at times in cases of patent processus vaginalis and cremasteric muscle contraction.
- *Ectopic testis*: Testis which is located outside the normal path of descent and can be seen anywhere in groin, perineum, penile root, femoral triangle, and opposite scrotum (crossed ectopia).
- *Absent testis*: No viable testicular tissue is present.
- Approximately, 3.5% of all male term infants, 20% of preterm, and 100% of infants with a birth weight of <800 g have undescended testis. In 80% of these male infants, the testes get descended by the age of 1 year.[43] After 1 year of age, the descent of the undescended testis usually does not occurs. Hence, one should wait and re-evaluate the child with undescended testis at age of 9–12 months.

Untreated undescended testes may lead to infertility, especially when it is lying in the abdominal cavity. Also, a significantly higher risk for development of malignancy is seen in undescended testes.[45,46] Intra-abdominal testes has a four times greater risk for tumor development than an inguinal testis.[47] The most frequent tumors in undescended testes include seminoma followed by embryonal cell carcinoma. The majority of undescended testes can be detected with US, as 75–80% are found to be located in the inguinal canal between the internal and external inguinal ring.[45]

Higher intra-abdominal locations make detection with US more difficult. MR imaging is recommended in such cases. MR imaging offers excellent images of the testes, but it is associated with a high cost and the need for sedation or anesthesia in small children due to long duration of the sequence protocols.[43]

Inguinal-scrotal Hernia

Inguinal-scrotal hernia is defined as the passage of intestinal loops and/or omentum into the scrotum.[42] The prevalence of inguinal hernia is higher in preterm neonates. The hernia is more frequently located on the right side, as the right

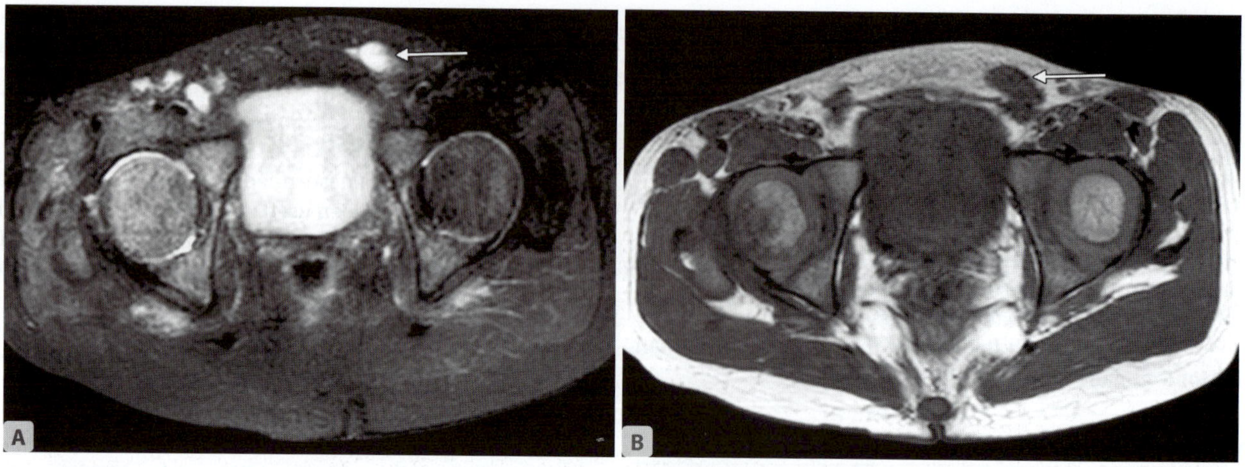

FIGS. 11A AND B: T2W and T1W MR axial sections showing undescended testis (arrows in A and B) on left side which is hyperintense on T2 and isointense on T1. Faint hypointense line of rete testis is seen in the testis on T2W images. (T1W: T1-weighted; T2W: T2-weighted; MR: magnetic resonance)

processus vaginalis closes later than the left.[48] Physical examination is usually sufficient to allow diagnosis in most cases. US examination is indicated in patients with inconclusive physical findings, in patients with acute scrotum, and also to investigate contralateral involvement in patients in whom only a unilateral hernia is clinically evident.[49]

The diagnosis of hernia is achieved by visualization of air bubble movement and/or intestinal peristalsis during the real-time examination. The herniated omentum is seen as a highly echogenic structure on US. Inguinal rings >4 mm are an indication for prophylactic herniorrhaphy.[49] Color or power Doppler imaging is useful in inguinal-scrotal hernia to investigate intestinal and testicular perfusion. Urgent surgery is indicated in patients with an aperistaltic akinetic dilated bowel loop (a sign of strangulation).[50]

Hydrocele

Hydrocele is collection of fluid between the visceral and parietal layers of the tunica vaginalis and/or along the spermatic cord. It is one of the most common causes of painless scrotal swelling in children. In the normal scrotum, 1–2 mL of serous fluid may be observed in the potential tunica vaginalis cavity and should not be mistaken for hydrocele. Virtually all hydroceles are congenital in neonates and infants and associated with a patent processus vaginalis, which allows peritoneal fluid to enter the scrotal sac.[42,51] In older children and adolescents, hydroceles are usually acquired and are often result of an inflammatory process, testicular torsion, trauma, or a tumor.

At USG, congenital hydrocele appears as an anechoic fluid collection surrounding the anterolateral aspects of the testis, which may sometimes extend to the inguinal canal or as a fluid collection with low-level swirling echoes[51] **(Fig. 12)**.

Spermatic cord cyst is a less common type of hydrocele, which more commonly appears as a fluid collection in the spermatic cord and results from closure of the processus vaginalis above the testis and below the internal inguinal ring **(Figs. 13A and B)**. Two types of spermatic cord hydrocele are known. The first type is encysted hydrocele of the cord,

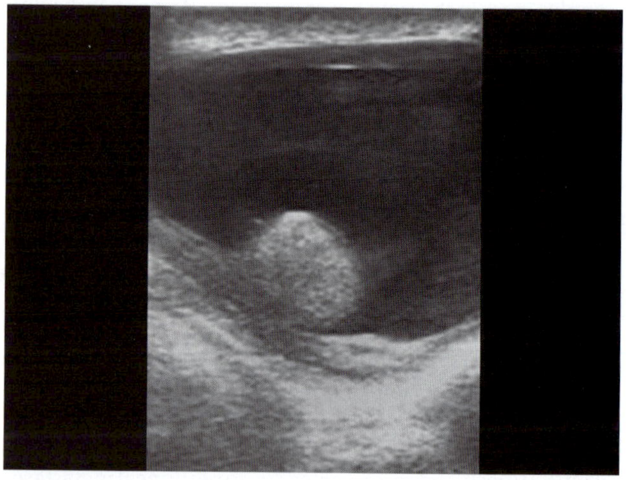

FIG. 12: Hydrocele; Longitudinal ultrasound of the right hemiscrotum shows a fluid collection surrounding the testes.

where the fluid collection does not communicate with the peritoneum or the tunica vaginalis. The second type is the funicular hydrocele, where there is a fluid collection along the cord, communicating with the peritoneum at the internal ring.

Most congenital hydroceles (80%) resolve spontaneously before the age of 2 years. However, surgical treatment is usually applied in spermatic cord and abdominoscrotal hydroceles.[42]

Cystic Dysplasia of the Testis

Cystic dysplasia of the testis is detected incidentally while evaluating children with renal dysplasia. It involves cystic dilatation of the rete testes. It is usually associated with dysplasia or absence of the ipsilateral kidney.[43]

Testicular Calcification (Microcalcification)

Testicular microcalcification is usually an incidental finding. Testicular microlithiasis is defined as multiple calcifications

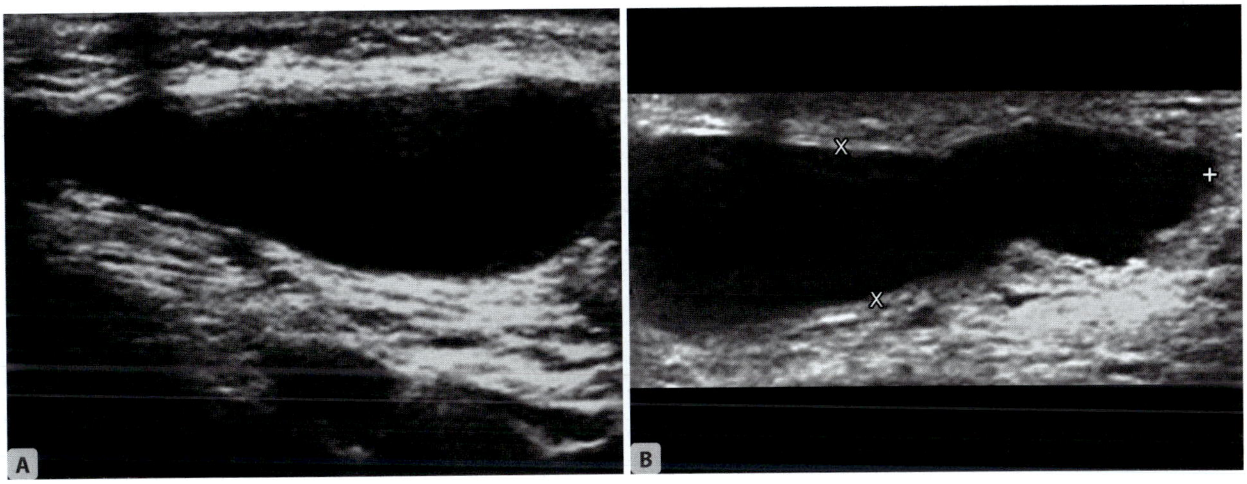

FIGS. 13A AND B: Spermatic cord hydrocele (funicular hydrocele). (A) Longitudinal scan of the right spermatic cord of a 2-year-old child, shows a fluid collection along the cord, communicating with the peritoneum at the internal ring; and (B) Ultrasound in another patient with spermatic cord hydrocele.

that are <2 mm and seen as hyperechoic foci.[43] They usually have a syndromic association (Klinefelter syndrome, pseudohermaphroditism) or are associated with congenital anomalies (undescended testes) or they could be idiopathic; they are also seen in tumors and are of unknown cause.

The calcifications are seen as fine, bright, and non-shadowing hyperechoic foci (five or more on any single view) that are uniform in size and are distributed in a diffuse pattern or in peripheral clusters.[43] As testicular microlithiasis is considered to be a premalignant condition thus, serial scrotal US monitoring (once per year) is recommended.[52]

Acute Scrotum

Acute scrotum refers to a clinical setting of sudden-onset scrotal pain, redness, and swelling, which is most frequently caused by acute epididymo-orchitis, torsion of the testicular appendages, or testicular torsion.[42] Since scrotal involvement is usually unilateral, one should start the examination on the asymptomatic side first to have a basis for comparison. Color Doppler imaging or power Doppler imaging should be added to gray-scale US.

Epididymo-orchitis

Epididymo-orchitis is a common cause of acute scrotum in children.[42] It is mainly of infectious origin. The infection usually originates in the bladder or prostate gland, spreads through the vas deferens and the lymphatics of the spermatic cord to the epididymis, and finally reaches the testis, causing epididymo-orchitis. Isolated orchitis can also occur, but is rare.

There are two reported peaks of prevalence: Under 2 years of age and over 6 years of age. Many conditions predispose to epididymo-orchitis, which include imperforate anus, ureteral ectopia to the seminal vesicle, bladder exstrophy, neurogenic bladder, posterior urethral valves, and dysfunctional voiding. Chronic mild trauma may also result in mild noninfective epididymo-orchitis.[43] Children usually come with pain of acute onset, which is not as rapid onset as in torsion, along with skin reddening and edema. It is difficult to do a clinical examination due to pain and uplifting the scrotum beyond the symphysis pubis relieves pain (Prehn's sign).[43]

The epididymal head is the most affected region and reactive hydrocele and wall thickening are also frequently present. Increased size and decreased, increased, or heterogeneous echogenicity of the affected organ are usually observed. On color Doppler imaging, there is increased blood flow within the epididymis, testis, or both[43] **(Figs. 14A and B and 15A and B)**. Occasionally, the entire epididymis is affected. Malignancies such as leukemia and lymphoma, that diffusely infiltrate the testicular parenchyma, may have a US appearance similar to that of diffuse orchitis. In such cases, the clinical history is extremely important.

In cases of coexisting orchitis, the testis is enlarged and on US will show a heterogeneous echotexture.[53] Color Doppler shows hyperemia in the affected regions, which helps to distinguish it from torsion. This hyperemia is seen to disappear rapidly with improvement of symptoms after initiation of treatment.[54] On spectral Doppler analysis, a low-resistance waveform pattern with decreased resistance index (RI) <0.5 is seen.[55]

Granulomatous epididymo-orchitis is a chronic inflammation occurring in postpubertal boys.[42] The affected part of the epididymis, mainly the tail, is enlarged with heterogeneous echogenicity.[56] At color Doppler imaging, chronic epididymo-orchitis does not demonstrate the increased blood flow, typical of acute epididymitis. The sonographic features can be similar to those of epididymal adenomatoid tumor; however, patients with chronic epididymitis present with a painful mass whereas the tumor is usually painless.

Torsion of the Testicular Appendages

The appendages are sessile structures, which thus predisposes them to torsion and the appendix testis is most often affected.[42] Torsion of the appendix testis occurs mainly in prepubertal boys (aged 7–14 years), is more frequent on the left side, and is a common cause of acute scrotum in this age group.[57]

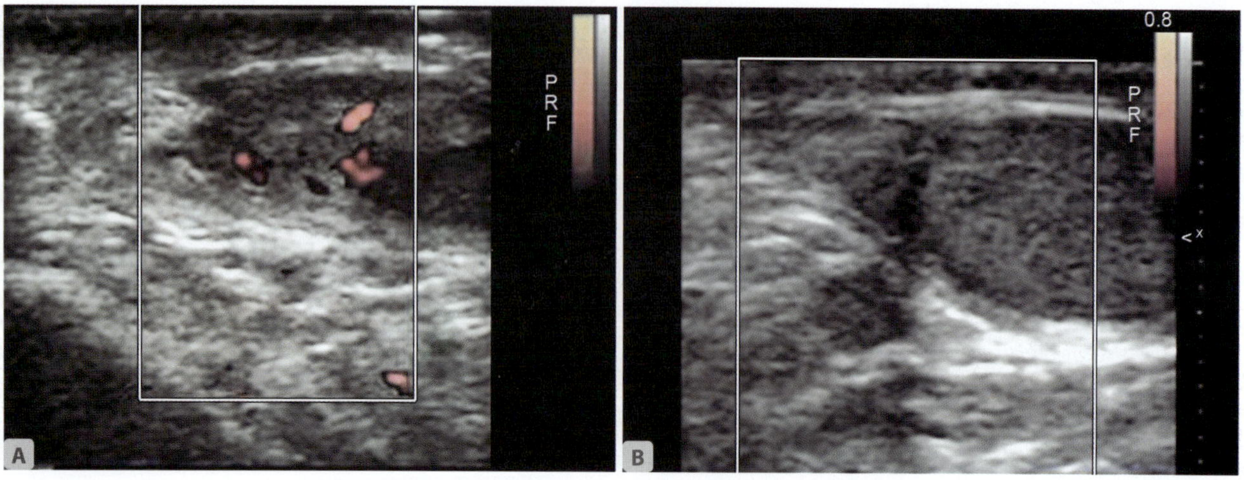

FIGS. 14A AND B: Epididymitis. (A) Epididymis is enlarged, heterogeneous, and demonstrates increased flow on color Doppler; and (B) Normal opposite epididymis is shown for comparison.

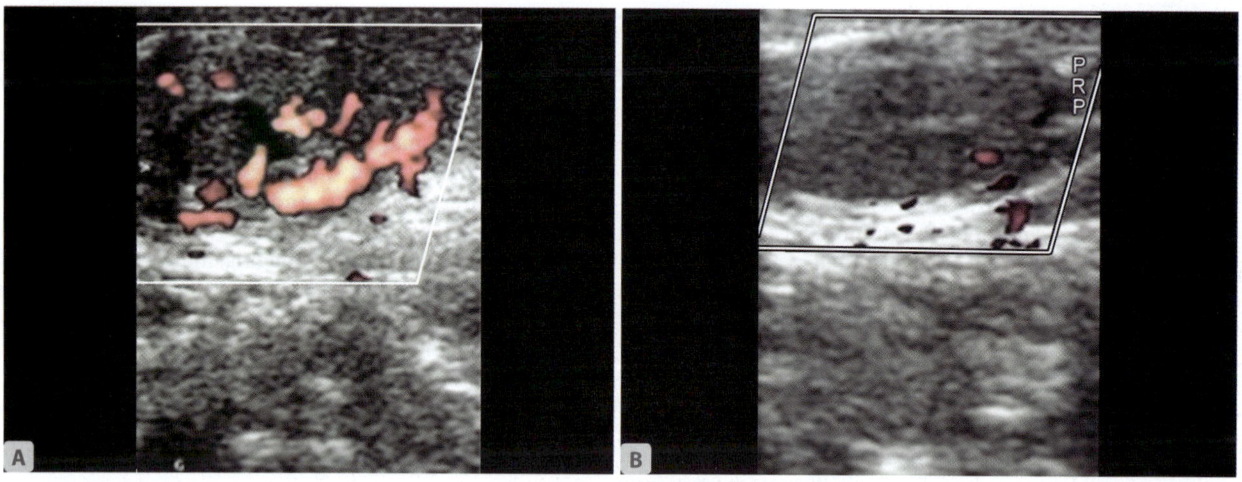

FIGS. 15A AND B: Epididymo-orchitis in a 9-year-old boy. (A) Ultrasound revealed enlarged epididymal head with heterogeneous echotexture of epididymis and testes, which demonstrated increased vascularity on power Doppler; and (B) Opposite normal left testis is shown for comparison.

Affected patients typically present with gradual or sudden intense pain, usually localized in the upper pole of the testis. At physical examination, the classic finding in these children is a small nodule which is palpable along the superior aspect of the testis, which is called the "blue dot" sign. This is seen in nearly one-third of patients and this is a pathognomonic feature of this entity.

At US, the twisted appendage is seen as a round extra-testicular mass with high or mixed echogenicity depending on the evolution time.[58] Associated findings include an enlarged epididymal head, reactive hydrocele, and scrotal skin thickening. There is no Doppler signal in the twisted appendage and the epididymis and scrotal tunics are hypervascularized. Management is conservative, in contrast to torsion of the spermatic cord, and the pain resolves after 2–3 days. The appendix gets atrophic and finally calcifies.

Testicular Torsion

Testicular torsion entails first venous and later arterial flow obstruction. The extent of testicular ischemia in these patients depends on the degree of twisting (180–720°) and the duration of the torsion. Testicular salvage is more likely in patients treated within 6 hours after the onset of torsion, hence the need for an urgent, immediate diagnosis.[42]

Testicular torsion is of two types: (1) Extravaginal; and (2) Intravaginal.

Extravaginal torsion or supravaginal torsion occurs before the tunica vaginalis and the gubernaculum get fixed to the scrotal wall and therefore is seen only in the perinatal period.[59] At birth itself, the testis is infarcted and necrotic and clinical presentation is of a painless mass, swelling, and discoloration of the scrotum. US will show an enlarged testis with heterogeneous echotexture, hydrocele, thickening, and loss of color flow in the spermatic cord and testis.

Intravaginal torsion can occur at any age, but is more common in adolescents. A known predisposing factor is the "bell clapper" deformity, in which the tunica vaginalis joins high on the spermatic cord, leaving the testis free to rotate.[43]

Differentiation between testicular torsion and epididymo-orchitis is important, since scrotal pain, swelling, and redness are clinical symptoms common to these two entities. Generally, pain in testicular torsion has a sudden onset whereas in orchitis, it is more gradual. However, 5% of children with orchitis have sudden onset of pain and only 50% of patients with testicular torsion have an acute attack.

The pain is typically constant with no increase in the intensity seen on palpation or movement and is not relieved when the scrotum is elevated above the pubic symphysis in contrast to inflammatory conditions.

In the early phases of torsion (1–3 h), testicular echogenicity appears normal. With progression, enlargement of the affected testis and increased or heterogeneous echogenicity are common findings. Sonographic evaluation of the spermatic cord is an essential part of the examination. The point of cord twisting can be identified at the external inguinal orifice. About 24 hours after the onset of symptoms, there is reversal to normal echogenicity and 10 days later, the testis gets atrophic.[43] A definitive diagnosis of complete testicular torsion is made when blood flow is visualized on the normal side but is absent on the affected side.[41]

Two kinds of torsion are known to occur: (1) Complete (>360°); and (2) Incomplete (<360°) torsion.[43] In complete torsion, epididymis is the initial organ to show absent flow, but 6 hours later a collateral arterial supply develops from the inferior epigastric artery, misleading the examiner and resulting in a false-negative diagnosis. Incomplete torsion refers to cord twisting of <360°, in which some arterial flow persists in the affected testis (seen in 20% of cases in one series). The venous flow is obstructed. Therefore, one should always examine the testicular perforating arteries to avoid false-negative results on Doppler study.[43]

Additional information can be obtained from pulsed-wave Doppler imaging, with which decreased or reversed diastolic flow may be evident on the affected side and from scintigraphy and MR imaging.[60,61]

Normal echogenicity with mild testicular enlargement has been reported as a good sign of viability whereas marked enlargement, heterogeneous echotexture, and scrotal wall hypervascularity are signs of testicular infarction and necrosis.

Acute Idiopathic Scrotal Edema

Acute idiopathic scrotal edema is a self-limiting disease which is characterized by edema and erythema of the scrotum.[62] It is the fourth most common cause of acute scrotum in patients aged below 20 years, following epididymitis, testicular torsion, and torsion of appendages.[62,63] Since clinically it manifests similar to those of other surgically correctable acute scrotal disease, it is important to confirm diagnosis, using US and Doppler to avoid unnecessary surgery.

Exact etiology of this entity remains unclear however, it is considered as a variant of angioneurotic edema.[63] Patients with idiopathic scrotal edema may also show eosinophilia, which may be the result of allergic reaction. In most reported cases, all source of infection was excluded from surrounding structures. It is also known that as mostly unilateral, perineal or inguinal erythema is coexistent in half of the cases.[63-65] However, bilateral involvement was more common in one study by Lee et al. (75%) compared with previous studies.[62] The most common characteristic of it is scrotal wall edema **(Fig. 16)**, which is easily visualized on US, which has also been confirmed by surgical findings.[65]

Several studies have described the following US and Doppler findings:

- Marked thickening of the scrotal wall, with heterogeneous striated and edematous appearance, with increased flow.
- Increased peritesticular blood flow.
- Mildly reactive hydrocele.[64,65]
- The testes and epididymis are normal in appearance and do not show increased vascularity.[66]
- Enlargement and increased vascularity of the inguinal lymph nodes.

As it is a self-limiting disease, surgical intervention should be avoided. US examination along with Doppler is very useful to differentiate between other acute scrotal diseases and acute idiopathic scrotal edema.

Scrotal Tumors

The incidence of scrotal tumors is estimated at 0.5–2.0 cases per 100,000 boys.[67] Scrotal tumors typically manifest as painless scrotal swelling. Owing to its excellent spatial resolution, US is highly sensitive for identifying scrotal masses.[68] This technique allows differentiation between cystic and solid tumors and classification as intra- or extratesticular. The term paratesticular refers to a group of extratesticular lesions that are not easily identified as originating from a particular tissue. CT is reserved for detecting spread in malignant tumors while MR imaging is useful for characterizing the tumor content or better delineation of extratesticular solid masses.[69] Certain tumor markers (α-fetoprotein and hCG) also help to make a more precise diagnosis.

Testicular Tumors

Testicular tumors account for 1% of all pediatric solid tumors.[42] They have two peaks of prevalence, first before 3 years of age and secondly in the postpubertal period. They usually manifest as a painless scrotal mass. However, in approximately 10% of patients, testicular tumor is associated

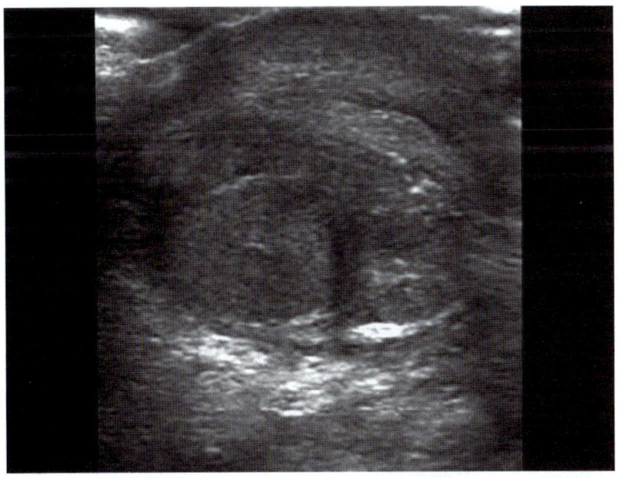

FIG. 16: Acute idiopathic scrotal edema. Transverse ultrasound scan of both hemiscrota shows marked thickening of scrotal walls.

with pain due to hemorrhage or infarction, mimicking torsion, or epididymitis. Testicular tumors are subdivided into two groups: (1) Germ cell tumors; and (2) Nongerm cell tumors.

Germ Cell Tumors

Germ cell tumors result from the transformation of primitive germ cells. These pluripotent cells can remain non-differentiated (seminomas), become slightly differentiated (embryonal carcinoma), or transform into differentiated embryonal (mature or immature teratomas) or extraembryonal (choriocarcinoma) structures.[70]

For clinical purposes, germ cell tumors are also divided into two groups: (1) Seminomatous; and (2) Nonseminomatous germ cell tumors.[71]

Seminomas

In comparison with nonseminomatous tumors, occur in older population, with an average patient age of 40.5 years. Seminoma is extremely radiosensitive and radiotherapy for low-stage tumors is very effective, resulting in a 5-year survival rate of 95%.[71]

Nonseminomatous Germ Cell Tumors

Yolk sac tumor, also known as endodermal sinus tumor, is the most common germ cell tumor, accounts for 80% of childhood testicular tumors, with most cases occurring before the age of 2 years. In its pure form, yolk sac tumor is rare in adults; however, it is present in 44% of adult cases of mixed germ cell tumor.[72]

Alpha-fetoprotein is normally produced by the embryonic yolk sac and thus serum α-fetoprotein levels are elevated in >90% of patients with yolk sac tumor.[71] These markers are also useful in follow-up to check for regression or recurrence of the tumor.

The US findings are nonspecific, usually showing a solid mass replacing the entire testis. The presence of hypoechoic areas within the tumor, which indicates areas of necrosis, is a frequent finding **(Figs. 17A to C)**. As with all germ cell tumors, spread is predominantly via the lymphatic system; hence, the lymphatic pathway should be included in the initial workup.

The second most common germ cell tumor is teratoma, which is classified as mature, immature, and those with malignant areas. Generally, teratomas occur in children <4 years of age.[71]

The sonographic appearance depends on the components of the three germinal layers (endodermal, mesodermal, and ectodermal). Cysts are a common feature and may be an echoic or complex, depending on the cyst contents (i.e., serous, mucoid, or keratinous fluid). Teratoma may appear as a complex mass with cystic components or a cystic lesion with

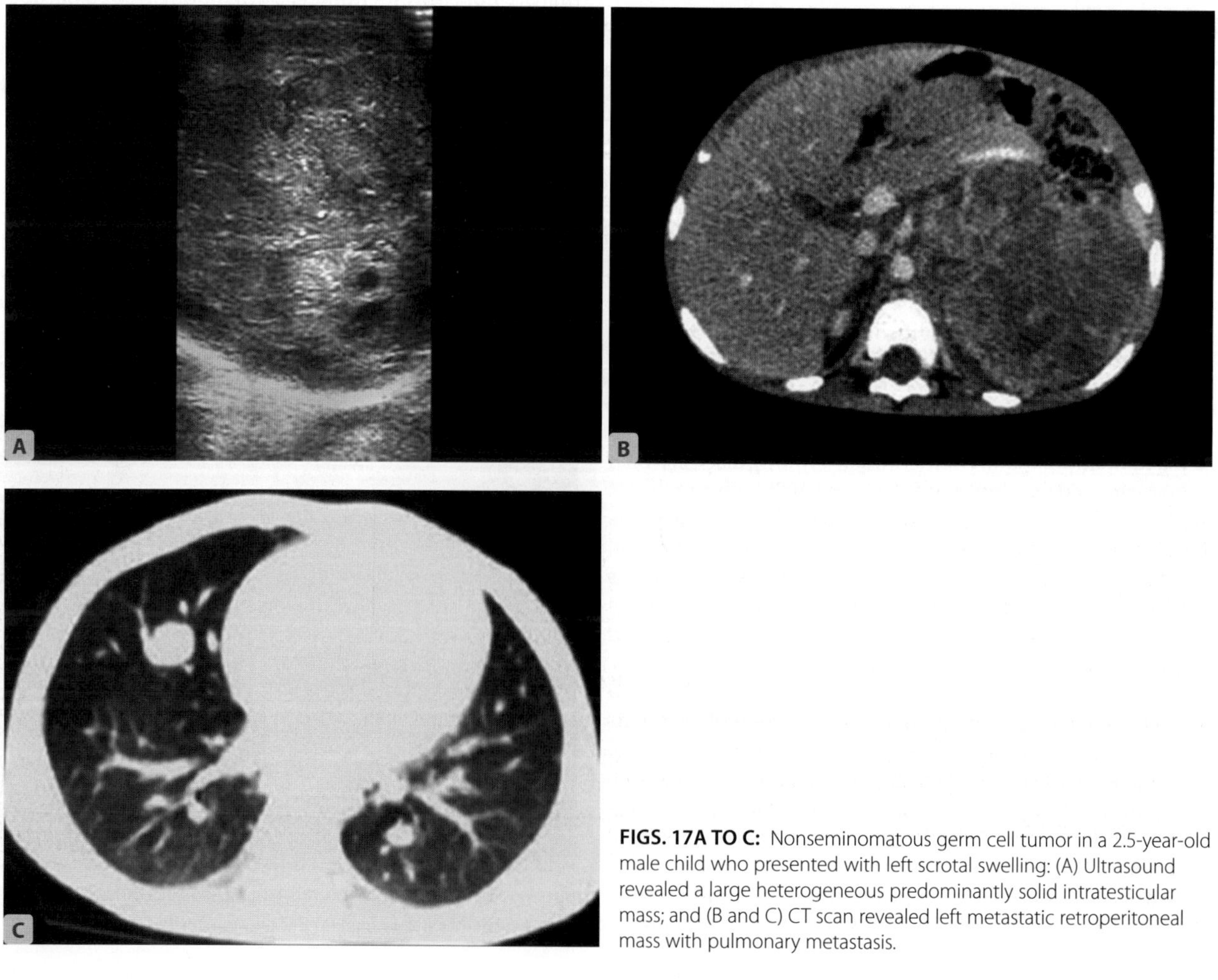

FIGS. 17A TO C: Nonseminomatous germ cell tumor in a 2.5-year-old male child who presented with left scrotal swelling: (A) Ultrasound revealed a large heterogeneous predominantly solid intratesticular mass; and (B and C) CT scan revealed left metastatic retroperitoneal mass with pulmonary metastasis.

peripheral solid components or calcifications and echogenic intratumor fat **(Figs. 18A and B)**.[71] These tumors are usually benign in prepubertal children, so tissue-sparing surgery may be possible; however, in adolescents, they are often malignant and require orchidectomy.

Testicular epidermoid *cyst* is the most common benign testicular tumor with no malignant potential. Epidermoid cysts are composed of keratinizing, stratified, and squamous epithelium with a well-defined fibrous wall. The cyst contains cheesy material and may resemble a solid tumor at US. Several sonographic patterns have been described: An echogenic lesion surrounded by a hypoechoic or echogenic rim, a target appearance, and an "onion ring" configuration with alternating echogenic and anechoic areas within the lesion.[73] The presence of well-delineated borders and a vascularity at color Doppler imaging favor the diagnosis. In inconclusive cases, MR imaging can aid in identification. On contrast-enhanced images, they are seen as sharply demarcated, low signal-intensity, and nonenhancing lesions.[74]

Although the radiologic appearance of epidermoid cyst is quite characteristic, it is not, however, pathognomonic. Teratomas and other malignant tumors may also have a similar appearance and mass should be carefully evaluated for any irregular borders, which might suggest a malignant lesion. Because carcinoma cannot be completely excluded, orchiectomy is usually performed. However, if the lesion has been thoroughly evaluated and if there is a strong possibility that it is an epidermoid cyst, it is recommended to perform a testis-sparing enucleation rather than orchiectomy.[71]

Nongerm Cell Tumors

Nongerm cell tumors are less frequent than germ cell tumors and can develop from the gonadal stroma (Leydig cell tumor), sex cord cells (Sertoli cell tumor), or sex cord cells plus stroma (gonadoblastoma).[42]

These account for nearly 4% of all testicular tumors.[71] The prevalence is higher in the pediatric age group, for which nongerm cell tumors constitute 10–30% of all testicular neoplasms.[71] About 90% of all nongerm cell tumors are benign. Unfortunately, no radiologic criteria allow definite differentiation of benign from malignant disease and orchiectomy is usually performed in all cases. Even with histologic analysis, it is difficult at times to determine the biologic behavior of these tumors.

Leydig cell tumors are the most common in this group, accounting for 1–3% of all testicular tumors. They can be seen in any age group, with 20% of cases reported to occur in patients younger than 10 years, 25% in patients aged 10–30 years, 30% in patients aged 30–50 years, and 25% in patients older than 50 years.[75] Nearly 30% of patients will have an endocrinopathy secondary to secretion of androgens or estrogens by the tumor. Leydig cell tumors are generally small solid masses, but they may show cystic areas, hemorrhage, or necrosis **(Fig. 19)**.[75] Their sonographic appearance is also variable and is indistinguishable from that of germ cell tumors.

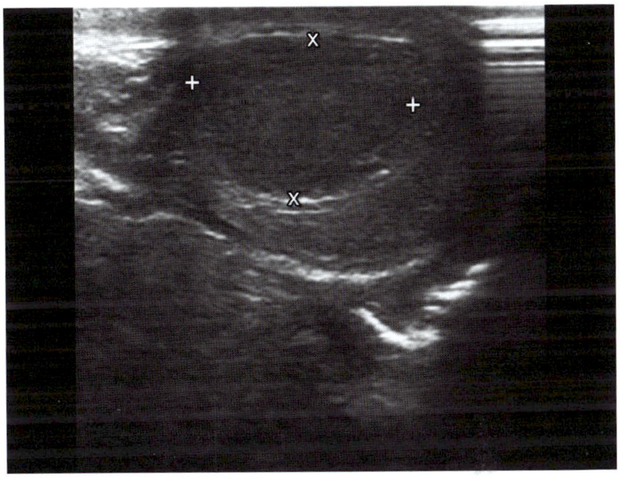

FIG. 19: Testicular ultrasound showing a hypoechoic intratesticular lesion in a child with Leydig cell tumor of testes.

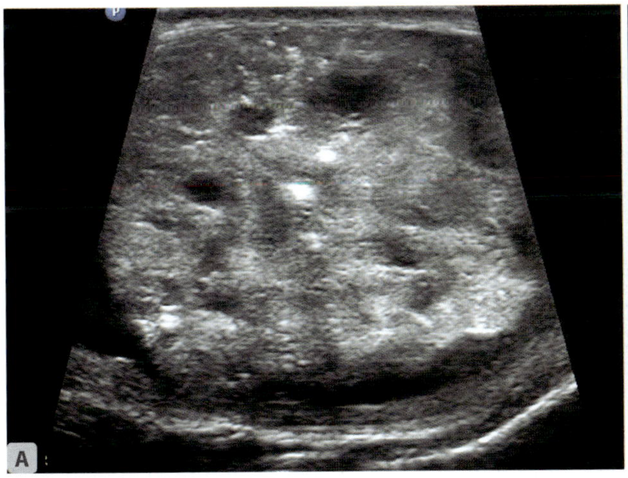

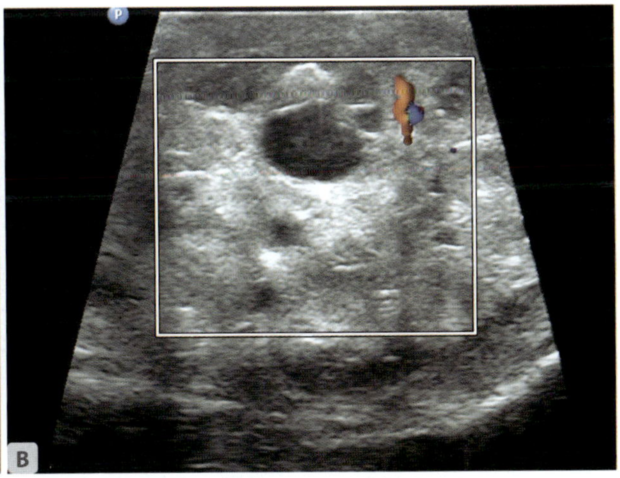

FIGS. 18A AND B: (A) Ultrasound images of a malignant teratoma of testis in a 6-month-old infant showing testis replaced by a large heterogeneous mass showing foci of calcifications, solid areas, and well as cystic areas; and (B) Focal vascularity is seen in solid area on color Doppler.

Sertoli cell tumors are less common than Leydig cell tumors and constitute <1% of testicular tumors. They are less hormonally active, but gynecomastia can occur.[75] Sertoli cell tumors are typically well-circumscribed, unilateral, and round to lobulated masses. A subtype is the large-cell calcifying Sertoli cell tumor, which is most often seen in the pediatric age group. This subtype commonly manifests as multiple and bilateral masses, which, as the name implies, are distinguished by large areas of calcification that are readily seen with US.[76] This subgroup has been associated with Peutz–Jeghers syndrome and Carney syndrome (pituitary adenomas, mucocutaneous pigmentation, and myxomas of the heart, skin, eyelids, and breast).[71,76]

Gonadoblastoma is a dysgenetic lesion occurring in the setting of gonadal dysgenesis and intersex syndromes. Approximately, 80% of the patients are phenotypically female.[75,76]

Other Testicular Tumors

Primary follicular lymphoma of the testes is an infrequent tumor, with only few reported cases.[77] However, secondary involvement is common in patients with acute lymphoblastic leukemia and non-Hodgkin B-cell lymphoma.[78] At US, there are two relatively more common patterns of involvement, which are seen in both leukemia and lymphoma: The more common diffuse type, in which the testis is enlarged and hypoechoic and the focal type, which demonstrates multiple hypoechoic nodules. Increased blood flow may be seen on color Doppler images, which may simulate an inflammatory lesion.

Primary leukemia of the testis is rare. However, the testis is a common site of leukemia recurrence in children, with 80% of patients being in bone marrow remission.[79,80] It is believed that the blood–testis barrier allows leukemic cells to be "hidden" during chemotherapy. The clinical characteristics and sonographic appearance of leukemia of the testis can be quite varied, as the tumors may be unilateral or bilateral, diffuse or focal, and hypoechoic or hyperechoic[79,80] **(Figs. 20A and B)**.

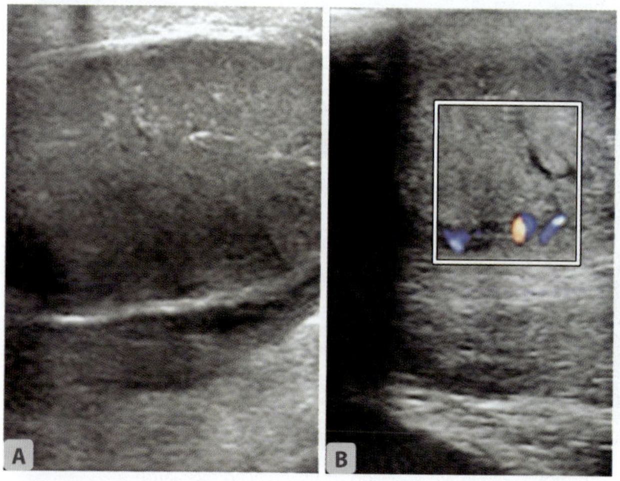

FIGS. 20A AND B: (A and B) Ultrasound reveals diffuse leukemic infiltration of testes in a child with lymphoblastic leukemia.

Metastasis of other solid tumors, such as Wilms' tumor, neuroblastoma, and retinoblastoma, that may affect the testis, have also been reported.[42]

Benign testicular cysts can be located either within the tunica albuginea or the parenchyma.[71] Tunica albuginea cysts are typically peripherally located and may be single or multiple. Recognition of their classic location and appearance usually helps in making this diagnosis. Careful analysis must be done to differentiate these lesions from cystic neoplasms, typically teratomas. If the cystic lesion has any solid components, it should be considered malignant.

EXTRATESTICULAR TUMORS

Paratesticular Rhabdomyosarcoma

The most common extratesticular tumor is paratesticular rhabdomyosarcoma, which originates in the spermatic cord or scrotal tunics.[42] The majority of these tumors occur in the first 2 decades of life and belong to the embryonal histopathologic subtype. At US, paratesticular rhabdomyosarcoma is seen as a hypo- or hyperechoic solid mass that may envelop or invade the epididymis and testis, which demonstrates hypervascularity at color Doppler imaging.[81]

Computed tomography is often recommended in the initial workup to determine tumor spread and MR imaging can be performed, if required, to delimit the borders of the mass relative to the epididymis and testis.[82] Long-term survival is expected in patients under 10 years of age with disease confined to the scrotum.

Adenomatoid Tumor

Adenomatoid tumors are benign, solid extratesticular lesions that can originate from the epididymis, tunica vaginalis, or spermatic cord. They are the most common tumor of the epididymis and occur more often in the lower pole than in the upper pole by a ratio of 4:1.[83] Usually, an incidental finding, adenomatoid tumors manifest as a painless scrotal mass, with the majority diagnosed in patients aged 20–50 years.[84] They are typically unilateral and occur more frequently on the left side. When they grow noninvasively into the testicular parenchyma, they can simulate intratesticular disease.

At US, they appear as a solid extratesticular mass with variable echogenicity.[84,85] Commonly, MR imaging demonstrates low signal intensity relative to the testicular parenchyma on T2-weighted images. However, the appearance is not specific and should be differentiated from granulomatous epididymitis, a chronic form of epididymitis that manifests as a painful palpable mass. At color Doppler imaging, vessels are observed within the adenomatous tumor whereas usually no vessels are seen in granulomatous epididymitis.[42]

Epididymal cysts, although not true tumors, typically manifest as a palpable mass and are of lymphatic origin. Because they contain clear serous fluid, they are seen as an anechoic, well-defined mass with increased through transmission. Epididymal cysts cannot be differentiated from spermatoceles, which are secondary to obstruction and dilatation of the efferent ductal system. However, the latter occur exclusively in postpubertal boys.[84]

Primary malignant tumors of the epididymis are rare in children; epididymal involvement is largely due to metastatic spread from B-cell acute lymphoblastic leukemia and B-cell non-Hodgkin lymphoma.[84]

Epididymal Cystadenoma

Papillary cystadenoma of the epididymis is a benign epithelial neoplasm. It is seen in up to 60% of men with von Hippel–Lindau disease.[84] Although the sporadic variety is usually seen in middle-aged men, it is seen earlier in patients with von Hippel–Lindau disease. The sonographic appearance is variable. It can appear as a solid appearance with few cystic spaces or can appear as multiloculated cystic lesion with small papillary projections.[83-85] In patients with von Hippel–Lindau disease, sonographic criteria for diagnosis of epididymal cystadenoma consist of: (a) A predominantly solid epididymal mass >10 × 14 mm; and (b) Slow growth. At MR imaging, a cystic mass with septations or mural nodules can be seen.

Lipoma

Lipoma is the most common benign tumor of the spermatic cord and can occur at any age.[84] At US, it is a well-defined, homogeneous, and hyperechoic paratesticular lesion.[85,86] At MR imaging, lipoma appears uniform and follows fat signal intensity with all sequences, including fat-suppressed sequences, which confirms the diagnosis.[87]

Fibrous Pseudotumor

Fibrous pseudotumor is considered as a benign, reactive fibrous paratesticular tissue. As it can grow up to large sizes, therefore, it can mimic a neoplasm. It commonly arises from the tunica vaginalis. The sonographic appearance is nonspecific[83,85] and calcification is commonly seen. The lesion can dislodge and become freely mobile within the scrotal sac; such a lesion is known as a "scrotal pearl". At MR imaging, owing to the presence of fibrosis, the lesion has low-signal intensity on both T1- and T2-weighted images with variable enhancement.

ADRENAL RESTS

These are a rare cause of testicular masses, which can be seen in patients with congenital adrenal hyperplasia (CAH) and rarely in those with Cushing syndrome. These rests are usually <5 mm and can be found in the testis and surrounding tissues in 7.5–15% of newborns and 1.6% of adults.[87] If these

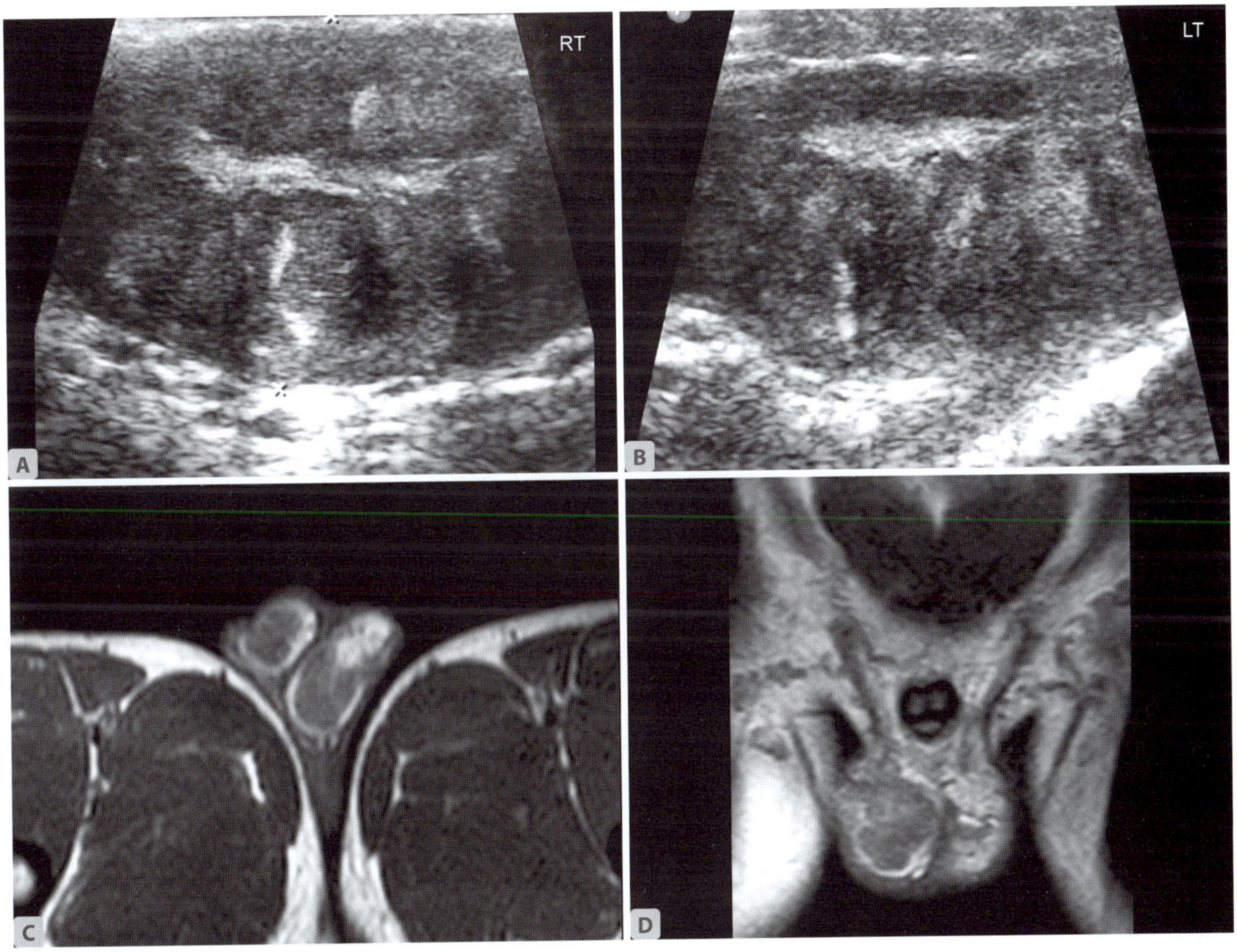

FIGS. 21A TO D: A 12-year-old boy with precocious puberty. (A and B) Ultrasound images showing right and left testis replaced by heterogeneous solid lesions; and (C and D) T2-weighted (T2W) axial and coronal images showing bilateral testis replaced by isointense lesions having lobulated margins. The findings are typical of adrenal rest tumors.

cells are exposed to elevated levels of adrenocorticotropic hormone, they can enlarge to form masses.

These were present in 11 of 20 patients (55%) with CAH, in one series reported by Aso C et al.[42] As potential malignancy is extremely rare, testicular biopsy is not required, even when the mass increases in size.

The sonographic appearance of adrenal rests is variable, with some series describing predominantly hypoechoic masses and others reporting heterogeneously hyperechoic masses with shadowing **(Figs. 21A and B)**.[87,88] On MR imaging, these have been reported to have low-signal intensity on both T1- and T2-weighted images **(Figs. 21C and D)**.[89] It is important to recognize these as benign lesions to avoid unnecessary orchiectomy.

Sarcoidosis is a multisystem, chronic granulomatous disease that rarely affects the genital tract. Although, it more commonly affects the epididymis but can, in some cases, also involve the testis. Testicular lesions can be solitary, but they are more commonly multiple, small, and bilateral masses.[90] Testicular sarcoidosis is more common in African-Americans than in other racial groups.

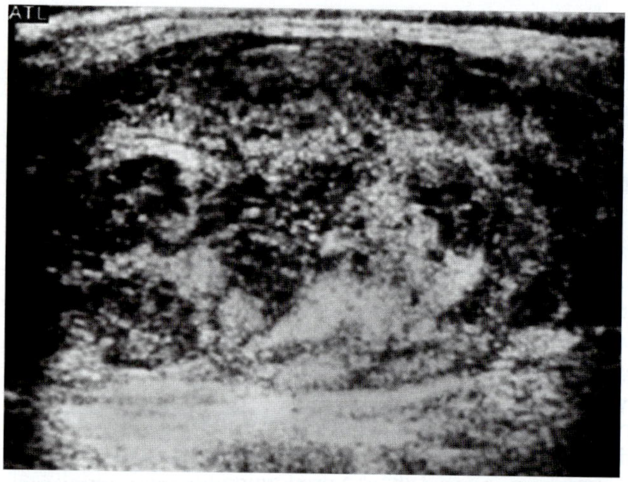

FIG. 22: Longitudinal ultrasonogram in a 12-year-old child (with history of scrotal injury while playing football) shows a large heterogeneous soft-tissue mass in the left scrotal sac, suggestive of testicular hematoma.

SCROTAL INVOLVEMENT IN SYSTEMIC DISEASES

Scrotal involvement can be seen in many systemic diseases.[42] The testes are affected in 15–37% of patients with Henoch-Schönlein purpura.[91,92] In this disease, scrotal symptoms may even precede other manifestations. US findings include scrotal wall thickening, epididymal enlargement, and reactive hydrocele. Involvement is bilateral in the majority of cases; hence, this entity should be considered when bilateral US findings similar to those of inflammatory epididymitis are visualized.

Scrotal Trauma

Scrotal trauma, in children, can result from a trivial fall, sports, or motor vehicle and straddle accidents. Since physical examination is limited by swelling and pain, US is a good modality for its detection. Lesions range from extratesticular hematoma to testicular rupture. Extratesticular hematomas may be quite large and their echogenicity changes over time, being echogenic in the acute state and anechoic during follow-up **(Fig. 22)**. Conservative treatment is recommended except in cases of impaired testicular flow and testicular rupture that are rare, but should be suspected when the margins of the testis are poorly defined or disruption of the capsular blood flow is observed.[42] MR imaging increases the diagnostic confidence and is useful in preoperative workup of testicular rupture.[93] MRI is extremely helpful for evaluation of scrotal blunt trauma owing to its high tissue contrast, multiplanar imaging, and ability to depict hemorrhage at different stages. The low signal from the albuginea is a remarkable sign, ensuring testicular integrity.

REFERENCES

1. Gare L, Dubois J, Grignon A, Filiatrault D, Vliet GV. US of the pediatric female pelvis: a clinical perspective. Radiographics. 2001;21:1393-407.
2. Stranzinger E, Strouse PJ. Ultrasound of the pediatric female pelvis. Semin Ultrasound CT MR. 2008;29:98-113.
3. Lang IM, Babyn P, Oliver GD. MR imaging of pediatric uterovaginal anomalies. Pediatr Radiol. 1999;29:163-70.
4. Nussbaum AR, Sanders RC, Jones MD. Neonatal uterine morphology as seen on real-time US. Radiology. 1986;160:641-3.
5. Hata K, Nishigaki A, Makihara K, Takamiya O, Hata T, Kitao M. Ultrasonic evaluation of the normal uterus in the neonate. J Perinat Med. 1989;17:313-7.
6. Haber HP, Mayer EI. Ultrasound evaluation of uterine and ovarian size from birth to puberty. Pediatr Radiol. 1994;24:11-3.
7. Holm K, Laursen EM, Brocks V, Muller J. Pubertal maturation of the internal genitalia: an ultrasound evaluation of 166 healthy girls. Ultrasound Obstet Gynecol. 1995;6:175-81.
8. Buzi F, Pilotta A, Dordoni D, Lombardi A, Zaglio S, Adlard P. Pelvic ultrasonography in normal girls and in girls with pubertal precocity. Acta Paediatr. 1998;87:1138-45.
9. Orbak Z, Sagsoz N, Alp H, Tan H, Yildirim H, Kaya D. Pelvic ultrasound measurements in normal girls: relation to puberty and sex hormone concentration. J Pediatr Endocrinol Metab. 1998;11:525-30.
10. Cohen HL, Shapiro MA, Mandel FS, Shapiro ML. Normal ovaries in neonates and infants: a sonographic study of 77 patients 1 day to 24 months old. AJR Am J Roentgenol. 1993;160:583-6.
11. Orsini LF, Salardi S, Pilu G, Bovicelli L, Cacciari E. Pelvic organs in premenarcheal girls: real-time ultrasonography. Radiology. 1984;153:113-6.
12. Cohen HL, Eisenberg P, Mandel F, Haller JO. Ovarian cysts are common in premenarchal girls: a sonographic study of 101 children 2–12 years old. AJR Am J Roentgenol. 1992;159:89-91.
13. Surratt, JT, Siegel MJ. Imaging of pediatric ovarian masses. Radiographics. 1991;11:533-48.
14. Fleischer AC, Daniell JF, Rodier J, Lindsay AM, James AE. Sonographic monitoring of ovarian follicular development. J Clin Ultrasound. 1981;9:275-80.
15. Ritchie WGM. Sonographic evaluation of normal and induced ovulation. Radiology. 1986;161:1-10.

16. Templeman C, Fallat ME, Blinchevsky A, Hertweck SP. Noninflammatory ovarian masses in girls and young women. Obstet Gynecol. 2000;96:229-33.
17. de Silva KS, Kanumakala S, Grover SR, Chow CW, Warne GL. Ovarian lesions in children and adolescents–an 11-year review. J Pediatr Endocrinol Metab. 2004;17:951-7.
18. Brandt ML, Helmrath MA. Ovarian cysts in infants and children. Semin Pediatr Surg. 2005;14:78-85.
19. Nussbaum AR, Sanders RC, Hartman DS, Dudgeon DL, Parmley TH. Neonatal ovarian cysts: sonographic-pathologic correlation. Radiology. 1988;168:817-21.
20. Rosenberg HK, Sherman NH, Tarry WF, Duckett JW, Snyder HM. Mayer-Rokitansky-Kuster-Hauser syndrome: US AID to diagnosis. Radiology. 1986;161:815-9.
21. Carranza-Lira S, Forbin K, Martinez-Chequer JC. Rokitansky syndrome and MURCS association: clinical features and basis for diagnosis. Int J Fertil Womens Med. 1999;44:250-5.
22. Blask AR, Sanders RC, Gearhart JP. Obstructed uterovaginal anomalies: demonstration with sonography. I. Neonates and infants. Radiology. 1991;179:79-83.
23. Banerjee AK, Clarke O, MacDonald LM. Sonographic detection of neonatal hydrometrocolpos. Br J Radiol. 1992;65:268-71.
24. Sugar NF, Graham EA. Common gynecologic problems in prepubertal girls. Pediatr Rev. 2006;27:213-23.
25. Strouse PJ. Sonographic evaluation of the child with lower abdominal or pelvic pain. Radiol Clin North Am. 2006;44:911-23.
26. Sala E. Magnetic resonance imaging of the female pelvis. Semin Roentgenol. 2008;43:290-302.
27. Ziereisen F, Guissard G, Damry N, Avni F. Sonographic imaging of the pediatric female pelvis. Eur Radiol. 2005;15:1296-309.
28. Robert Y, Mestdagh P, Ziereisen F, Launay S, Avni F. Imaging of the female pelvis in adolescence. J Radiol. 2001;82:1765-80.
29. Haber HP, Ranke MB. Pelvic ultrasonography in Turner syndrome: standards for uterine and ovarian volume. J Ultrasound Med. 1999;18:271-6.
30. Mazzanti L, Nizzoli G, Tassinari D, Bergamaschi R, Magnani C, Chiumello G, et al. Spontaneous growth and pubertal development in Turner's syndrome with different karyotypes. Acta Paediatr. 1994;83:299-304.
31. Matarazzo P, Lala R, Artesani L, Franceshini PG, de Sanctis C. Sonographic appearance of ovaries and gonadotropin secretions as prognostic tools of spontaneous puberty in girls with Turner's syndrome. J Pediatr Endocrinol Metab. 1995;8:267-74.
32. Sheth S, Fishman EK, Buck JL, Hamper UM, Sanders RC. The variable sonographic appearances of ovarian teratomas: correlation with CT. AJR Am J Roentgenol. 1988;151:331-4.
33. Sisler CL, Siegel MJ. Ovarian teratomas: a comparison of the sonographic appearance in prepubertal and postpubertal girls. AJR Am J Roentgenol. 1990;154:139-14.
34. Outwater EK, Wagner BJ, Mannion C, McLarney JK, Kim B. Sex cord-stromal and steroid cell tumors of the ovary. Radiographics. 1998;18:1523-46.
35. Albayram F, Hamper UM. Ovarian and adnexal torsion: spectrum of sonographic findings with pathologic correlation. J Ultrasound Med. 2001;20:1083-9.
36. Breech LL, Hillard PJ. Adnexal torsion in pediatric and adolescent girls. Curr Opin Obstet Gynecol. 2005;17:483-9.
37. Graif M, Itzchak Y. Sonographic evaluation of ovarian torsion in childhood and adolescence. AJR Am J Roentgenol. 1988;150: 647-9.
38. Vijayaraghavan SB. Sonographic whirlpool sign in ovarian torsion. J Ultrasound Med. 2004;23:1643-9.
39. Lee EJ, Kwon HC, Joo HJ, Suh JH, Fleischer AC. Diagnosis of ovarian torsion with color Doppler sonography: depiction of twisted vascular pedicle. J Ultrasound Med. 1998;17:83-9.
40. Dashefsky SM, Lyons EA, Levi CS, Lindsay DJ. Suspected ectopic pregnancy: endovaginal and transvesical US. Radiology. 1988;169:181-4.
41. Filly RA. Ectopic pregnancy: the role of sonography. Radiology. 1987;162:661-8.
42. Aso C, Enríquez G, Fité M, Torán N, Piró C, Piqueras J, et al. Gray-scale and color Doppler sonography of scrotal disorders in children: an update. Radiographics. 2005;25:1197-214.
43. Hormann M, Balassy C, Marcel O, Philipp MO, Pumberger W. Imaging of the scrotum in children. Eur Radiol. 2004;14:974-83.
44. Whitaker RH. Undescended testes: the need for a standard classification. Br J Urol. 1992;70:1-6.
45. Oyen RH. Scrotal ultrasound. Eur Radiol. 2002;12:19-34.
46. Nguyen HT, Coakely F, Hricak H. Cryptorchidism: strategies in detection. Eur Radiol. 1999;9:336-43.
47. Campbell HE. The incidence of malignant growth in the undescended testicle: a reply and reevaluation. J Urol. 1959;81:663-8.
48. Siegel MJ. The acute scrotum. Radiol Clin North Am. 1997;35:959-76.
49. Chou TY, Chu CC, Diau GY, Wu CJ, Gueng MK. Inguinal hernia in children: US versus exploratory surgery and intraoperative contralateral laparoscopy. Radiology. 1996;201:385-8.
50. Ogata M, Imai S, Hosotani R, Aoyama H, Hayashi M, Ishikawa T. Abdominal ultrasonography for the diagnosis of strangulation in small bowel obstruction. Br J Surg. 1994;81:421-4.
51. Gooding GA, Leonhardt WC, Marshall G, Seltzer MA, Presti JC. Cholesterol crystals in hydroceles: sonographic detection and possible significance. AJR Am J Roentgenol. 1997;169:527-9.
52. Drut R. Yolk sac tumor and testicular microlithiasis. Pediatr Pathol Mol Med. 2003;22:343-7.
53. Dogra VS, Gottlieb RH, Mayumi O, Rubens DJ. Sonography of the scrotum. Radiology. 2003;227:18-36.
54. Rifkin MD, Cochlin DLl. Scrotal masses (and scrotal enlargement). In: Rifkin MD, Cochlin DLI (Eds). Imaging of the Scrotum and Penis. London: Martin Dunitz Ltd.; 2002. pp. 33-95.
55. Jee WH, Choe BY, Byun JY, Shinn KS, Hwang TK. Resistive index of the intrascrotal artery in scrotal inflammatory disease. Acta Radiol. 1997;38:1026-30.
56. Salmeron I, Ramirez-Escobar M, Puertas F, Marcos R, Garcia-Marcos F, Sanchez R. Granulomatous epididymo-orchitis: sonographic features and clinical outcome in brucellosis, tuberculosis and idiopathic granulomatous epididymo-orchitis. J Urol. 1998;159:1954-7.
57. Monga M, Scarpero HM, Ortenberg J. Metachronous bilateral torsion of the testicular appendices. Int J Urol. 1999;6:589-91.
58. Hesser U, Rosenborg M, Gierup J, Karpe B, Nystrom A, Hedenborg L. Gray-scale sonography in torsion of the testicular appendages. Pediatr Radiol. 1993;23:529-32.
59. Brown-Casillas VJ, Montalvo AM, Albores-Saavedra J. Intrauterine spermatic cord torsion in the newborn: sonographic and pathologic correlation. Radiology. 1990;177:755-7.
60. Paltiel HJ, Connolly LP, Atala A, Paltiel AD, Zurakowski D, Treves ST. Acute scrotal symptoms in boys with an indeterminate clinical presentation: comparison of color Doppler sonography and scintigraphy. Radiology. 1998;207:223-31.
61. Watanabe Y, Dohke M, Ohkubo K, Ishimori T, Amoh Y, Okumura A, et al. Scrotal disorders: evaluation of testicular enhancement patterns at dynamic contrast-enhanced subtraction MR imaging. Radiology. 2000;217:219-27.
62. Lee A, Park SJ, Lee HK, Hong HS, Lee BH, Kim DH. Acute idiopathic scrotal edema: ultrasonographic findings at an emergency unit. Eur Radiol. 2009;19:2075-80.
63. Klin B, Lotan G, Efrati Y, Zlotkevich L, Strauss S. Acute idiopathic scrotal edema in children—revisited. J Pediatr Surg. 2002;37:1200-2.

64. Van Langen AM, Gal S, Hulsmann AR, De Nef JJ. Acute idiopathic scrotal edema: four cases and a short review. Eur J Pediatr. 2001;160:455-6.
65. Kaplan GW. Acute idiopathic scrotal edema. J Pediatr Surg. 1977;12:647-9.
66. Varga J, Zivkovic D, Grebeldinger S, Somer D. Acute scrotal pain in children—ten years' experience. Urol Int. 2007;78:73-7.
67. Kay R. Prepubertal testicular tumor registry. J Urol. 1993;150:671-4.
68. Woodward PJ, Schwab CM, Sesterhenn IA. Extratesticular scrotal masses: radiologic-pathologic correlation. Radiographics. 2003;23:215-40.
69. Cramer BM, Schlegel EA, Thueroff JW. MR imaging in the differential diagnosis of scrotal and testicular disease. Radiographics. 1991;11:9-21.
70. Martelli H, Patte C. Gonadal tumors in children. Arch Pediatr. 2003;10:246-50.
71. Paula J, Woodward PJ, Sohaey R, O'Donoghue MJ, Green DE. Tumors and tumor-like lesions of the testis: radiologic-pathologic correlation. Radiographics. 2002;22:189-216.
72. Frush DP, Sheldon CA. Diagnostic imaging for pediatric scrotal disorders. Radiographics. 1998;18:969-85.
73. Schwerk WB, Schwerk WN, Rodeck G. Testicular tumors: prospective analysis of real-time US patterns and abdominal staging. Radiology. 1987;164:369-74.
74. Cho JH, Chang JC, Park BH, Lee JG, Son CH. Sonographic and MR imaging findings of testicular epidermoid cysts. AJR Am J Roentgenol. 2002;178:743-8.
75. Ulbright TM, Amin MB, Young RH. Tumors of the testis, adnexa, spermatic cord, and scrotum. In: Ulbright TM, Amin MB, Young RH (Eds). Atlas of Tumor Pathology. Washington: Armed Forces Institute of Pathology; 1999. pp. 1-290.
76. Chang B, Borer JG, Tan PE, Diamond DA. Large-cell calcifying Sertoli cell tumor of the testis: case report and review of the literature. Urology. 1998;52:520-2.
77. Pileri SA, Sabattini E, Rosito P, Zinzani PL, Ascani S, Fraternali-Orcioni G, et al. Primary follicular lymphoma of the testis in childhood: an entity with peculiar clinical and molecular characteristics. J Clin Pathol. 2002;55:684-8.
78. Dalle JH, Mechinaud F, Michon J, Gentet JC, de Lumley L, Rubie H, et al. Testicular disease in childhood B-cell non-Hodgkin's lymphoma: the French Society of Pediatric Oncology experience. J Clin Oncol. 2001;19:2397-403.
79. Mazzu D, Jeffrey RB, Ralls PW. Lymphoma and leukemia involving the testicles: findings on gray-scale and color Doppler sonography. AJR Am J Roentgenol. 1995;164:645-7.
80. Heaney JA, Klauber GT, Conley GR. Acute leukemia: diagnosis and management of testicular involvement. Urology. 1983;21:573-7.
81. Mak CW, Chou CK, Su CC, Huan SK, Chang JM. Ultrasound diagnosis of paratesticular rhabdomyosarcoma. Br J Radiol. 2004;77:250-2.
82. Mason BJ, Kier R. Sonographic and MR imaging appearances of paratesticular rhabdomyosarcoma. AJR Am J Roentgenol. 1998;171:523-4.
83. Kim W, Rosen MA, Langer JE, Banner MP, Siegelman ES, Ramchandani P. US–MR imaging correlation in pathologic conditions of the scrotum. Radiographics. 2007;27:1239-53.
84. Yang DM, Kim SH, Kim HN, Kang JH, Seo TS, Hwang HY, et al. Differential diagnosis of focal epididymal lesions with gray scale sonographic, color Doppler sonographic, and clinical features. J Ultrasound Med. 2003;22:135-42.
85. Akbar SA, Sayyed TA, Jafri SZ, Hasteh F, Neill JS. Multimodality imaging of paratesticular neoplasms and their rare mimics. Radiographics. 2003;23:1461-76.
86. Pretorius E. MRI of the male pelvis and bladder. In: Siegelman ES (Ed). Body MRI. Philadelphia: Elsevier Saunders; 2005. pp. 372-86.
87. Vanzulli A, DelMaschio A, Paesano P, Braggion F, Livieri C, Angeli E, et al. Testicular masses in association with adrenogenital syndrome: US findings. Radiology. 1992;183:425-9.
88. Seidenwurm D, Smathers RL, Kan P, Hoffman A. Intratesticular adrenal rests diagnosed by ultrasound. Radiology. 1985;155:479-81.
89. Berg NB, Schenkman NS, Skoog SJ, Davis CJ. Testicular masses associated with congenital adrenal hyperplasia: MRI findings. Urology. 1996;47:252-3.
90. Burke BJ, Parker SH, Parker KD, Pienkos EJ. The ultrasonographic appearance of coexistent epididymal and testicular sarcoidosis. J Clin Ultrasound. 1990;18:522-6.
91. Ben-Sira L, Laor T. Severe scrotal pain in boys with Henoch-Schönlein purpura: incidence and sonography. Pediatr Radiol. 2000;30:125-8.
92. Laor T, Atala A, Teele RL. Scrotal ultrasonography in Henoch-Schönlein purpura. Pediatr Radiol. 1992;22:505-6.
93. Muglia V, Tucci S, Elias J, Trad CVS, Bilbey J, Cooperberg PL. Magnetic resonance imaging of scrotal diseases: When it makes the difference. Urology. 2002;59:419-23.

CHAPTER

77

Imaging of Disorders of Sex Differentiation

Manisha Jana, Arun Kumar Gupta, Sanjay Sharma

INTRODUCTION

Disorders of sex differentiation (DSD), formerly known as intersex disorders, are complex and uncommon conditions where a definite sexual identity cannot be assigned to an individual; and the external sexual characteristics do not follow the usual male or female pattern. The incidence is approximately 1 per 1,000 live births. This condition is associated with immense psychological and social impact to the children as well as the family. Early diagnosis is very essential in order to ensure an early treatment and proper gender assignment. Knowledge of internal genital anatomy is crucial in the overall management of these patients. The role of a radiologist is to demonstrate this anatomy using different imaging techniques. An understanding of the normal sexual differentiation is essential before interpreting the pathological state.

NORMAL SEXUAL DIFFERENTIATION[1,2]

Genital primordia of a fetus are intrinsically programed to differentiate into female sex. However, in the presence of a Y chromosome the undifferentiated gonads differentiate into testes. Anti-Müllerian hormone (AMH), which is secreted by the Sertoli cells of the testes, inhibits the development of Müllerian ducts (i.e., female structures) while testosterone secreted from Leydig cells of the testes maintain and differentiate Wolffian ducts (i.e., male structures). Thus, presence of Y chromosome differentiates the genital primordia into a male. On the other hand, in the absence of Y chromosome, testicular tissue and its two hormones are absent due to which there is no inhibition of Müllerian ducts by AMH. Wolffian ducts regress because of lack of testosterone. End result is a normal female child.

IMAGING OF A CHILD WITH DISORDERS OF SEX DIFFERENTIATION[3-7]

Disorders of sex differentiation presenting with ambiguous genitalia form a challenging clinical problem. Biochemical and chromosomal assays, besides the radiological evaluation, are required in order to completely address its different aspects. Genitography, ultrasound, and magnetic resonance imaging (MRI) are routinely employed. Judicious use of minimum investigations to obtain maximum information should be the goal.

Genitography[3,8]

As most of these children have a urogenital sinus (UGS) the anatomy displayed using genitography becomes essential in treatment planning as regard the corrective surgery for gender assignment. In this technique, water-soluble contrast is injected retrogradely, via the external genital opening so as to outline the genital anatomy. Contrast is injected, either by placing the nozzle of a syringe (flush technique) or the tip of an end-hole catheter (catheter technique), within the external genital opening **(Figs. 1A and B)**. It aims to address the following:

- Degree of masculinization of the UGS and the urethra.
- Vaginal status, i.e., its presence, size, and any cervical indentation by the uterus.
- Junctional site of vagina with the urethra, i.e., whether low, middle, or high junction **(Figs. 2A to C)**. Low, middle, or high vaginal insertion determines the morphological female, indeterminate, or the male urethral type, respectively.
- Presence of uterus/fallopian tubes, either by their direct opacification or indirectly by visualization of cervical indentation at the cranial end of the contrast-filled vagina.

It must be realized that no genitographic appearance is specific for one particular type of DSD. It only depicts the degree of virilization of genitalia. Genitography only provides information about the status of the derivatives of Müllerian and Wolffian ducts. Gonadal evaluation is not possible. The technique is "invasive" and it uses ionizing radiation.

Other Imaging Modalities

Ultrasound and MRI are two noninvasive cross-sectional imaging techniques available for examination of the pelvic structures. Addition of pelvic ultrasonography has been a

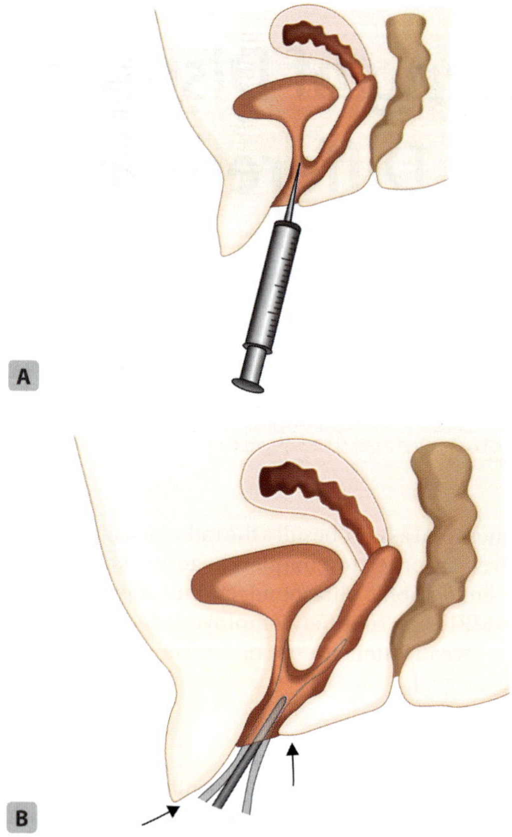

FIGS. 1A AND B: Techniques of genitography, flush technique (A) and catheter technique (B). In former, tip of the syringe nozzle is within the external opening and barrel is pressed against the perineum. In latter, single hole catheter should be used and its tip should be in the common urogenital sinus. Dotted lines show the potential pitfall if the tip enters either channel selectively. Arrows in (B) indicate compression of perineal skin around the catheter to prevent reflux of contrast.

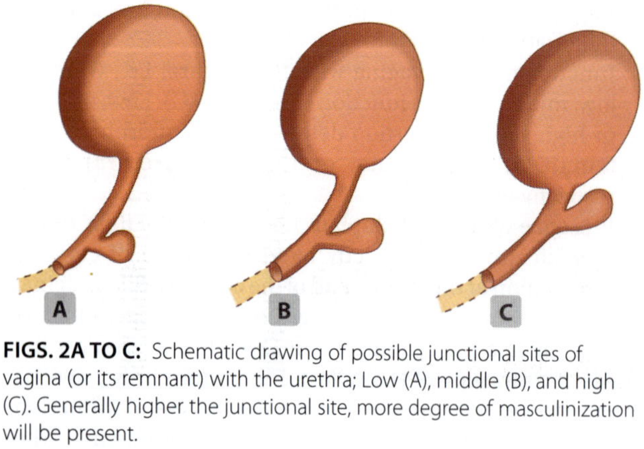

FIGS. 2A TO C: Schematic drawing of possible junctional sites of vagina (or its remnant) with the urethra; Low (A), middle (B), and high (C). Generally higher the junctional site, more degree of masculinization will be present.

valuable supplement to genitography and karyotyping in the work-up of a child with DSD for assessing not only gonads but also the presence of uterus and cervix, but has its usual limitations of small field of view, observer dependence, and inability to keep the child's urinary bladder adequately distended to provide a sonographic window. In cases of complex congenital anomalies, USG alone may not be sufficient and MRI is required.

Transperineal ultrasonography (TPUS) is another useful modality for evaluation of lower genital tract anatomy.[9-12] Using a high-frequency linear transducer directly placed over the perineum; it is possible to visualize the lower genital tract anatomy with great detail **(Figs. 3A to C)**. UGS length can also be measured by TPUS,[11] although the main disadvantage of this technique is operator dependence. As of now, there is no specific imaging guideline regarding its utility in DSD.

A complete ultrasonography in a child would include an abdominal, pelvic evaluation, and evaluation of inguinal canal **(Figs. 4A and B)** and scrotum (in males). The utility of ultrasound is listed in **Box 1**.

MRI has several advantages over ultrasonography in the evaluation of internal genital tract anatomy and gonads.[6,13-15] Owing to its superior soft-tissue contrast resolution and large field of view; it comes handy as a problem solving tool in complex developmental anomalies in order to delineate the genital anatomy in detail. Image analysis should include the assessment of uterus, vagina, ovaries, testes, penis, and clitoris. In the neonatal period, the ovaries and uterus are physiologically prominent due to maternal hormonal influence. Diffusion-weighted MRI, especially at high b values, is more helpful than routine sequences for the detection of gonads (ovaries as well as testes).[16,17] CT now has a very limited role to play due to the widespread use of MRI **(Figs. 5A to F)**. A suggested MRI protocol is listed in **Box 2**.

The visualization of internal genital structures in patients of DSD on MRI is variable. At AIIMS, genitography, ultrasound, and MRI were performed in 33 children of intersex disorder (13 days to 17 years of age) after appropriate clinical work-up, karyotyping, and hormonal analysis.[18] The ability to detect common UGS, vagina, and gonads by each modality was assessed. Surgical follow-up was available in 17 cases whereas karyotype, hormonal assay, and biochemical profile were taken as a proof of diagnosis in the remaining 16 cases. Common UGS was properly evaluated in 48% cases by genitography, and none by ultrasound or MRI. Vagina was detected by genitography, US, and MRI in 100%, 39.4%, and 78%, respectively. Uterus was detected by genitography, US, and MRI in 69%, 75%, and 100% cases, respectively. US detected 21 inguinal and 8 intra-abdominal gonads (total 44%), whereas MRI detected 40 inguinal and 11 intra-abdominal gonads (total 77.3%).[18] Relatively hypointense (even hyperintense) gonad on T2-weighted (T2W) images could be atrophic or dysgenetic gonads and requires histological analysis.

Another additional advantage of MRI over other imaging modalities is that it can differentiate hypertrophied phallus from normal penis. Supporting muscles of phallus, viz., bulbospongiosus (BS), ischiocavernosus (IC), and superficial transverse perinei (STP) have been stated to help to differentiate enlarged clitoris from penis on MRI **(Fig. 6)**. In the study at AIIMS,[19] it was found that well-developed BS and IC muscles are a better indicator of chromosomal (karyotype) than hormonal (urethral type) sex. Well-developed supporting muscles suggest a likely male karyotype. However, when these muscles are indeterminate or nonvisualized, it cannot predict

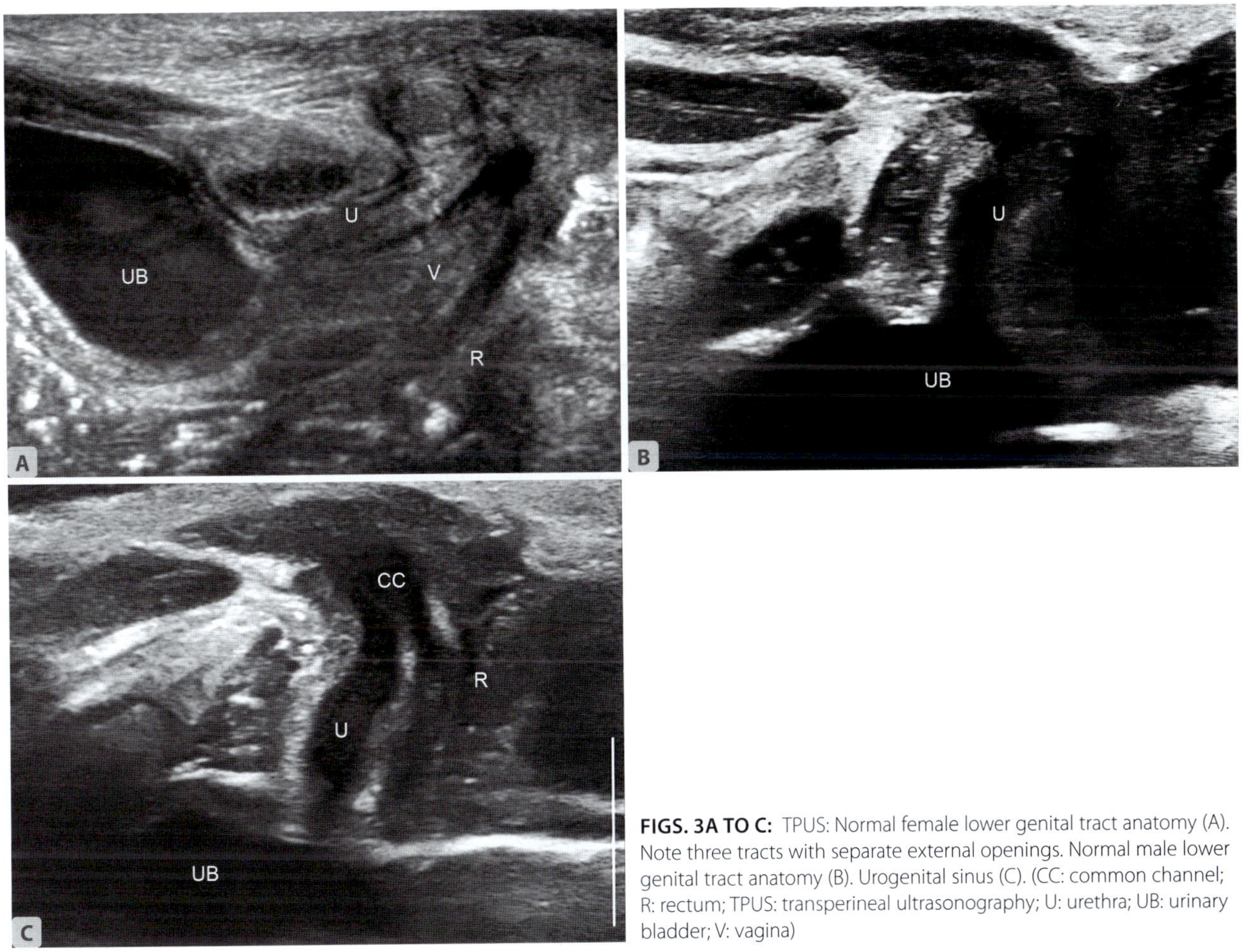

FIGS. 3A TO C: TPUS: Normal female lower genital tract anatomy (A). Note three tracts with separate external openings. Normal male lower genital tract anatomy (B). Urogenital sinus (C). (CC: common channel; R: rectum; TPUS: transperineal ultrasonography; U: urethra; UB: urinary bladder; V: vagina)

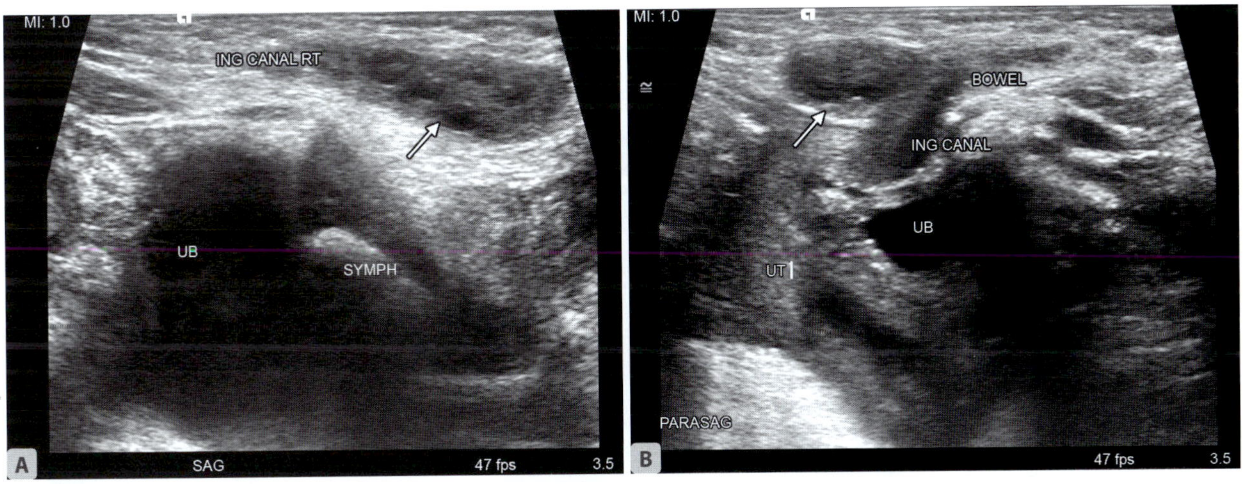

FIGS. 4A AND B: Inguinal hernia containing ovary (arrows) in a girl child with DSD: Midline sagittal (A) and parasagittal (B) ultrasound. (DSD: disorders of sex differentiation; ING: inguinal; UB: urinary bladder)

the chromosomal (karyotype) sex, but may suggest a female or indeterminate urethral type. STP muscle is not visualized in a large majority but when seen, it suggests a likely male karyotype. Poor or nonvisualization of this muscle gives no clue about the chromosomal sex or urethral type.[19] Literature is silent on MRI findings of these muscles in different types of intersex patients.

Magnetic Resonance Appearance of Genital Structures

T2-weighted turbo spin echo (T2W TSE) sequence is the most useful sequence for delineation of internal genital tract anatomy. Fat suppression improves the detection of the gonads (testes and ovaries).

BOX 1: Uses of ultrasound in disorders of sex differentiation (DSD).

- Identification and characterization of gonads
- Localization of undescended/ectopic testes
- Demonstration and characterization of Müllerian structures/Wolffian duct derivatives
- Adrenal gland evaluation [in congenital adrenal hyperplasia (CAH)]
- Detection of inguinal hernia, especially in female DSD (may have ovaries as content)
- Visualization of common channel/UGS in TPUS
- Detection of complications (e.g., malignancy in streak gonads, testicular adrenal rest tumors in CAH)

(TPUS: transperineal ultrasound; UGS: urogenital sinus)

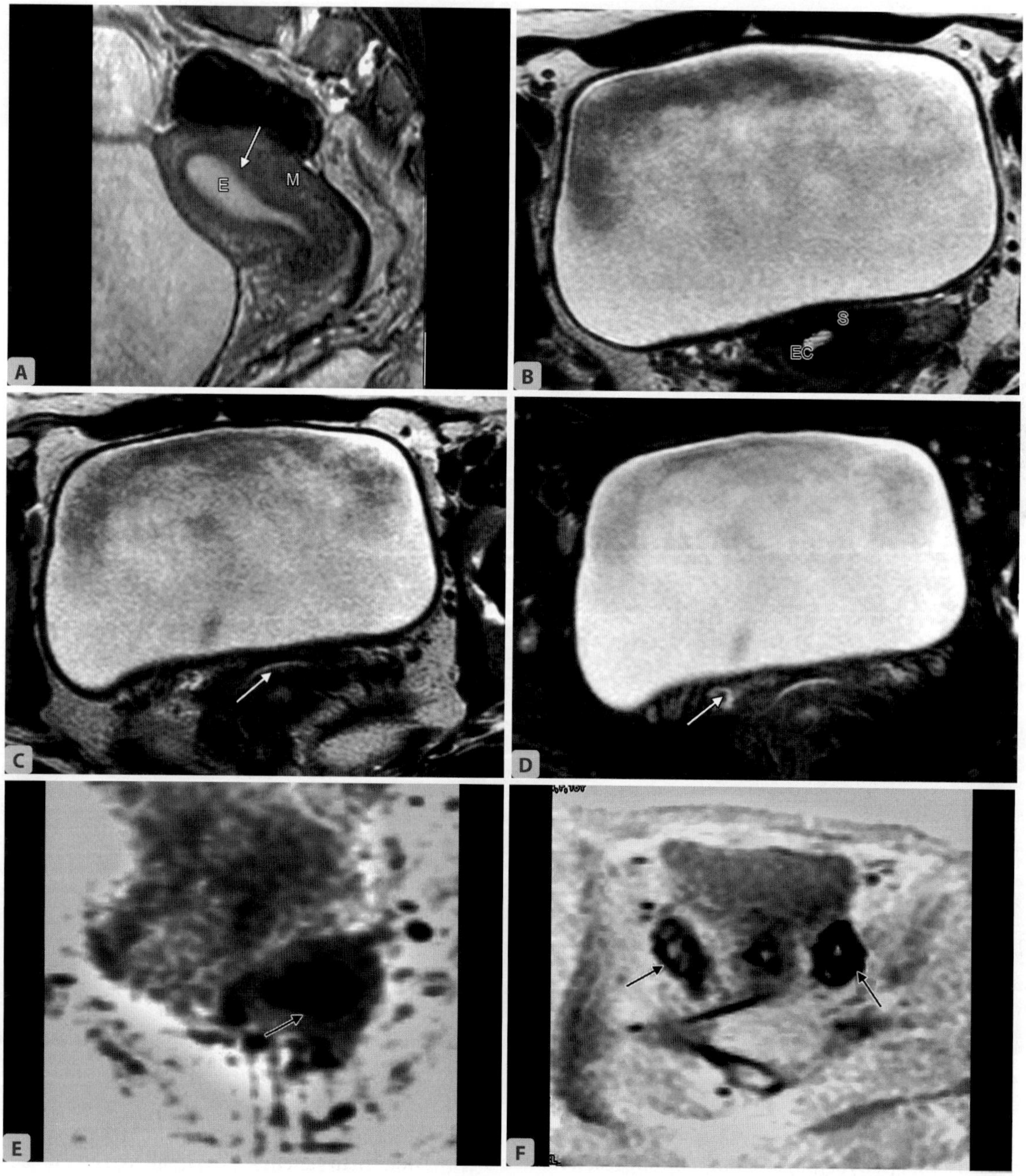

FIGS. 5A TO F: Normal appearances on MRI: T2W sagittal MRI (A) showing endometrium (E), junctional zone (arrow), and outer myometrium (M). T2W axial images (B and C) showing normal cervix (B) with inner hyperintense endocervical canal (EC) and outer hypointense stroma (S). Normal vagina seen as hyperintense flattened structure (arrow in C). Surrounding venous plexus is better appreciated on T2W fat suppressed image (arrow in D). Normal endometrium showing restricted diffusion on high b-value diffusion weighted images (arrow in E). Normal ovarian stroma showing restricted diffusion (arrows in F). (MRI: magnetic resonance imaging; T2W: T2 weighted)

BOX 2: Magnetic resonance (MR) imaging protocol in disorders of sex differentiation (DSD).

Pelvis:
- T2W TSE axial
- T2W TSE fat suppressed axial
- T2W TSE sagittal
- T2W TSE coronal
- T1W SE axial
- DWI (b values 0, 400, and 800)

Abdomen:
- T2W TSE axial

(DWI: diffusion-weighted imaging; T1W: T1-weighted; T2W: T2-weighted; SE: spin echo; TSE: turbo spin echo)

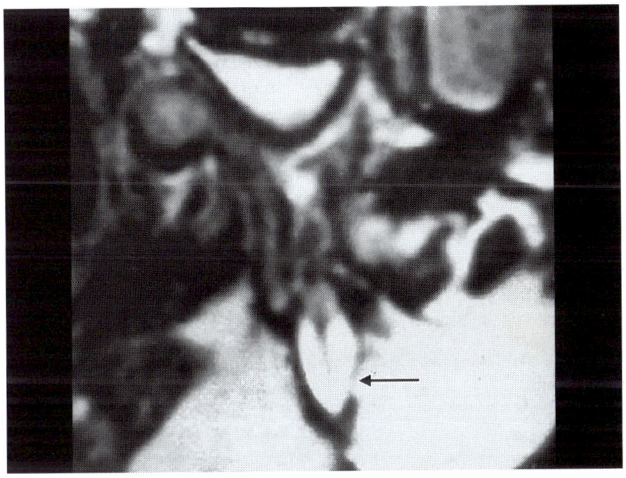

FIG. 6: Coronal T2W MRI shows the normal clitoral appearance. Compare this with **Figure 14.** (T2W MRI: T2-weighted magnetic resonance imaging)

The normal appearances of the genital structures are given in **Table 1, Figures 5 and 6.**

CLASSIFICATION OF DISORDERS OF SEX DIFFERENTIATION

Over the years, a number of workers have put forth contradictory views regarding classification of DSD. Paquin et al.,[20] based on a study of 7 patients, concluded that presence and appearance of urogenital sinus on imaging itself is not diagnostic of any specific type of DSD. Shopfner[21] studied 66 children of DSD and classified them into six types, demonstrating progressive masculinization from type I to type VI. He believed that each genitographic type represented a specific type of DSD, an observation in direct contradiction to Paquin et al.[20] and other subsequent workers. A French team of endocrinologists and radiologists[1,22] carried out studies in >120 patients and concluded, unlike Shopfner,[21] that no genitographic pattern is specific for any particular type of DSD. At AIIMS, our conclusion is similar to that of Paquin et al.[20] and the French team.[1]

More recently, a new classification system was proposed by European Society for Pediatric Endocrinology and the Lawson Wilkins Pediatric Endocrine Society in 2006.[23] In this classification, the term "intersex" was replaced by DSD and various types were also renamed **(Table 2)**. There are three broad categories; although there are overlaps among these groups **(Fig. 7)**.

1. *46,XX DSD [earlier known as "female pseudohermaphroditism"(FPH)]*: Occuring due to gonadal/ovarian developmental abnormality or androgen excess.
2. *46, XY DSD (earlier known as male pseudohermaphroditism)*: Resulting due to testicular developmental abnormality or androgen insufficiency/poor function.
3. Sex chromosome DSD (abnormal number of chromosomes such as 47XXY, 45X).

46,XX DSD (Earlier Known as Female Pseudohermaphroditism)[1,3,24-27]

Children of this group usually have a female karyotype 46,XX with presence of virilized external genitalia (of variable degrees). 46,XX DSD [earlier known as female pseudohermaphroditism (FPH)] comprises two broad groups:

1. *Disorders of androgen excess:*
   - Congenital [congenital adrenal hyperplasia (CAH) is the most common one]
   - Exogenous androgen excess (maternal anabolic steroid use)
2. Gonadal developmental disorder: This includes a subset of ovotesticular DSD and XX testicular DSD.

In group (1), normal ovaries, uterus, and tubes are present. Disorders of group (2) are discussed later along with ovotesticular DSD.

Etiopathogenesis: These disorders result from the action of an extragonadal testosterone on a normal female fetus resulting in virilization of genitalia to varying degrees. A number of mechanisms may be responsible but the most common one is CAH, resulting from an enzymatic defect (21-hydroxylase deficiency being the most common) in adrenal steroidogenesis.[25] Other uncommon causes include maternal exposure to anabolic steroids and progesterone; or placental aromatase deficiency.[26]

Phenotypic changes: Degree of virilization of the urogenital sinus and the external genitalia vary,[27,28] depending upon the time of onset of the insult and the amount of androgen. Based on the degree of virilization it can be classified either as complete or incomplete.

- *Complete virilization* is equivalent to Prader type V and results from massive amounts of androgens in the early phase of embryonic development. Clinically the external genitalia, i.e., the penis and the scrotum are like that of a normal male except that the scrotum is empty. Genitography reveals a male type urethra **(Fig. 8A)**, which at times may be associated with an underdeveloped vagina opening high on the vertical portion (high junction). Cervical impression is absent or difficult to appreciate. MRI or pelvic sonography would demonstrate presence of uterus and gonads **(Fig. 8B)**. MRI or CT shows bilateral adrenal hyperplasia **(Fig. 8C)**. Bone age is accelerated **(Fig. 8D)**. It is advisable to rear these children as male.

TABLE 1: Appearances of genital structures (normal as well as dysgenetic).

Structure	T1WI	T2WI	DWI	Best seen in
Uterus • *Endometrium* • *Myometrium*	 Hypointense Intermediate	 Hyperintense Divided in two areas: (1) Inner hypointense junctional zone, and (2) Outer intermediate myometrium	 Restricted diffusion No restriction	 T2W sagittal
Vagina	Hypointense	Central hyperintensity, peripheral hypointense wall, surrounded by hyperintense venous plexus	No restricted diffusion	T2W axial
Hypoplastic uterus	Intermediate	Similar to normal uterus, but signal intensity may be reduced	Variable	T2W sagittal
Ovaries	Hypointense	Hyperintense with even brighter follicles	Restricted diffusion	Axial T2W fat suppressed, axial high b value DWI
Testes	Hypointense	Hyperintense; with central hypointense structure (attachment of gubernaculum)	Restricted diffusion	Axial T2W fat suppressed, axial high b value DWI
Streak gonads	Hypointense	Intermediate to hypointense	Variable	Axial T2W fat suppressed, axial high b value DWI
Penis	Hypointense	Hyperintense, with three distinct divisions into corpora cavernosa and corpus spongiosum. Supporting muscles (bulbocavernosus, ischiocavernosus, and transverse perineal muscles) appear intermediate signal intensity		Coronal and sagittal T2W fat suppressed images
Clitoris	Hypointense	Hyperintense, but without the differentiation of corpora and the muscles		Sagittal T2W (considered hypertrophied if length >1 cm beyond the pubic rami)

(DWI: diffusion-weighted imaging; T1WI: T1-weighted imaging; T2WI: T2-weighted imaging)

TABLE 2: Classification of disorders of sex differentiation (DSD).[23]

New nomenclature	Earlier known as	Karyotype	External genitalia	Gonads and internal genitalia
46,XX DSD	Female pseudohermaphroditism (FPH)	46,XX	Variable virilization	Uterus and ovaries (commonly)
46,XY DSD	Male pseudohermaphroditism (MPH)	46,XY	Ambiguous, undermasculinized	Testes
Ovotesticular DSD	True hermaphroditism	46,XX (the most common), 46,XX/XY mosaicism, 46,XY	Ambiguous	Variable combination of testes/ovary/ovotestes
46,XY complete gonadal dysgenesis	XY female sex (XY sex reversal)	46,XY	Female	Streak gonads, müllerian structures
46,XX testicular DSD	XX male sex (XX sex reversal)	46,XX	Male	Testes, male internal genitalia

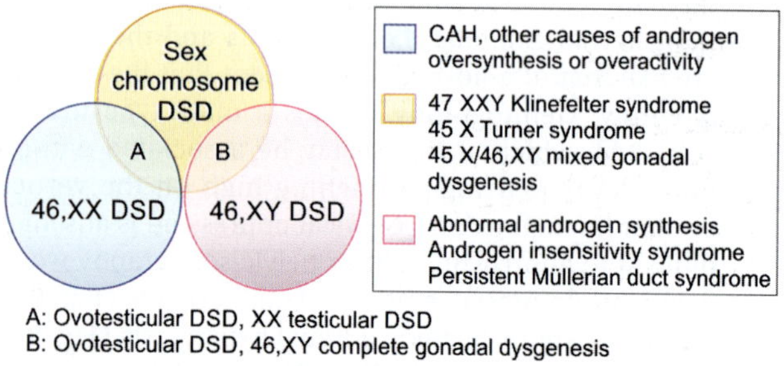

FIG. 7: Three broad categories of disorders of sex differentiation (DSD). (CAH: congenital adrenal hyperplasia)

- *Incomplete virilization* type **(Figs. 9 and 10)** is equivalent to Prader types I to IV and occurs as a result of exposure to lesser amounts of androgens later during the embryonic development. Clinically, external genital appearance varies from simple clitoral hypertrophy (Prader type I) to perineal hypospadias (Prader type IV). Genitography reveals a well-developed vagina with cervical impression **(Figs. 9A, 10A and B)**, uterus and tubes **(Figs. 10C and D)**. These patients should be reared as female.

Magnetic resonance images demonstrate masculinized external genitalia with normal ovaries **(Fig. 11A)** and uterus **(Fig. 11B)**. It may show enlarged adrenal glands due to

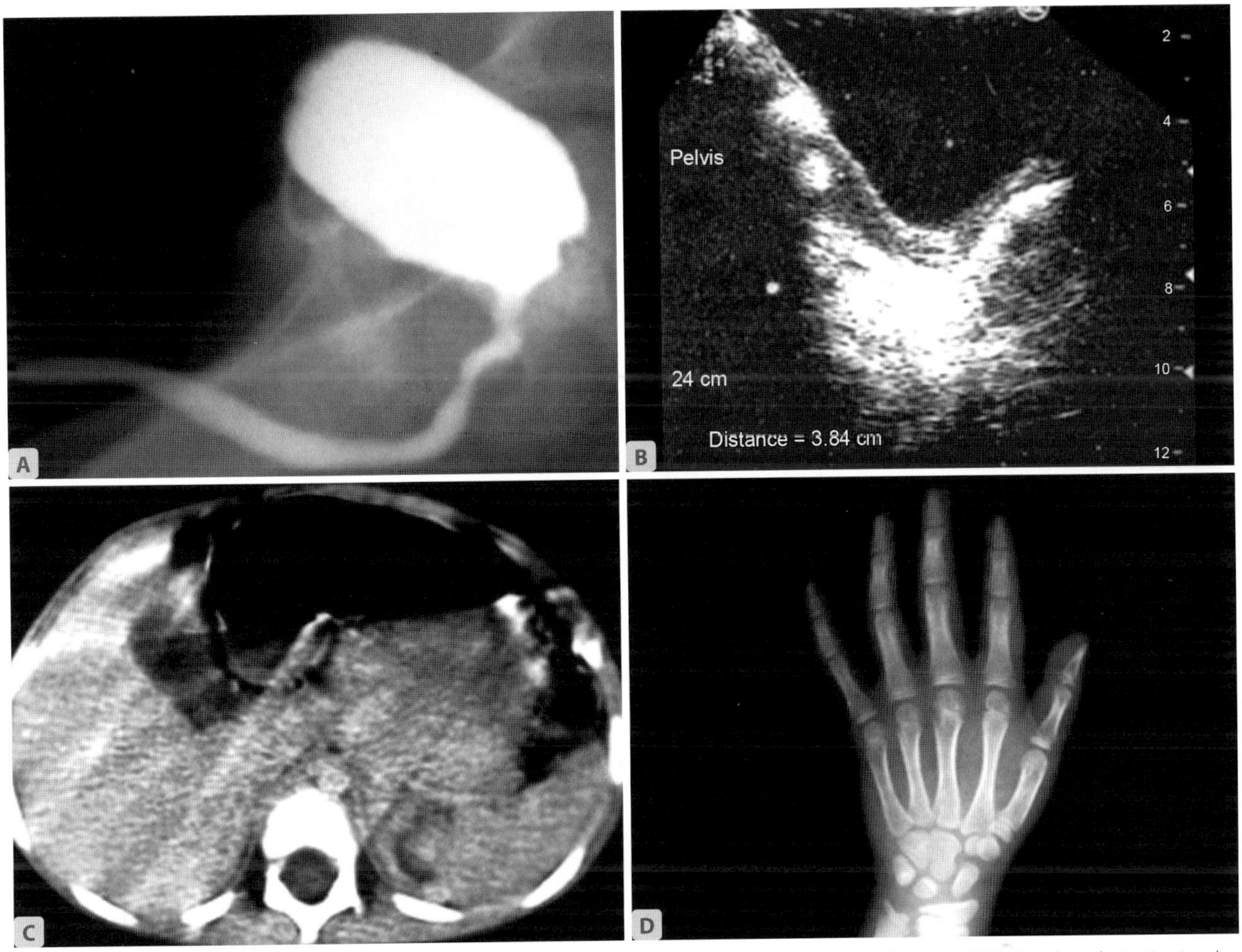

FIGS. 8A TO D: A 4-year-old child with 46, XX DSD, complete virilization type; Genitography (A) did not show any Müllerian duct derivative in a boy with normal external genitalia with cryptorchidism. Pelvic sonography, (B) revealed presence of a well-formed uterus. CT (C) demonstrated bilateral adrenal hyperplasia, (D) bone age is accelerated.

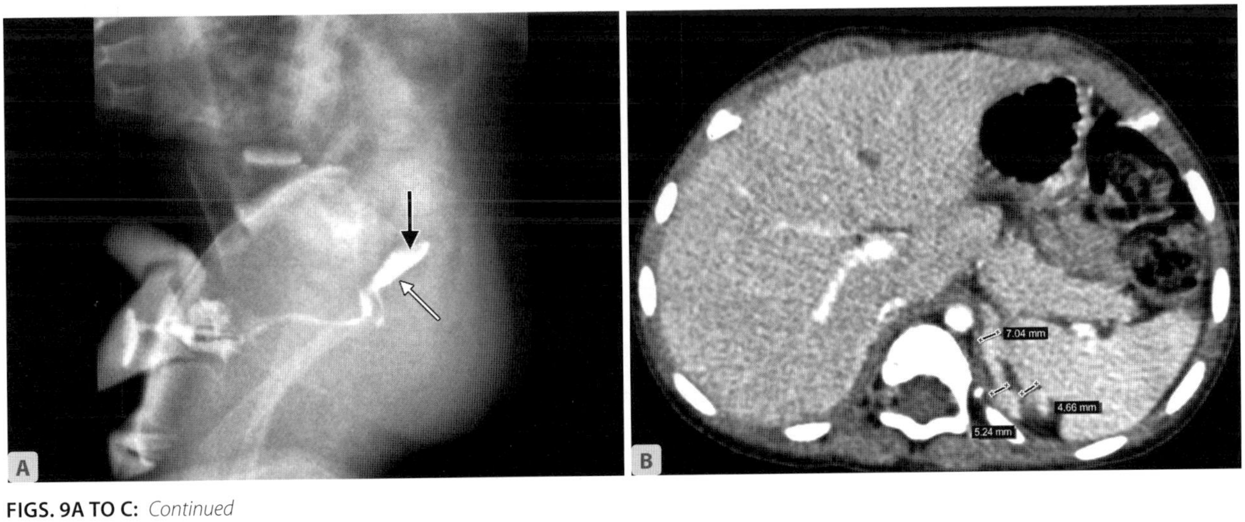

FIGS. 9A TO C: *Continued*

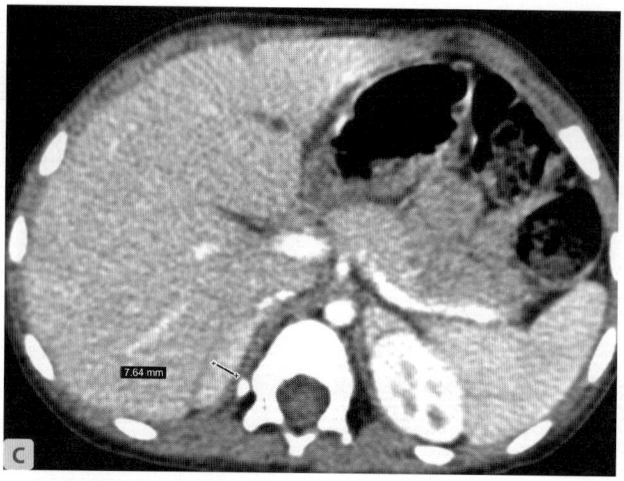

FIGS. 9A TO C: A 6-year-old child with 46,XX DSD, complete virilization type; Genitography (A) shows male type urethra with presence of well-formed vagina (arrow) and a cervical indentation (block arrow). CT (B and C) revealed bilateral adrenal hyperplasia. (DSD: disorders of sex differentiation)

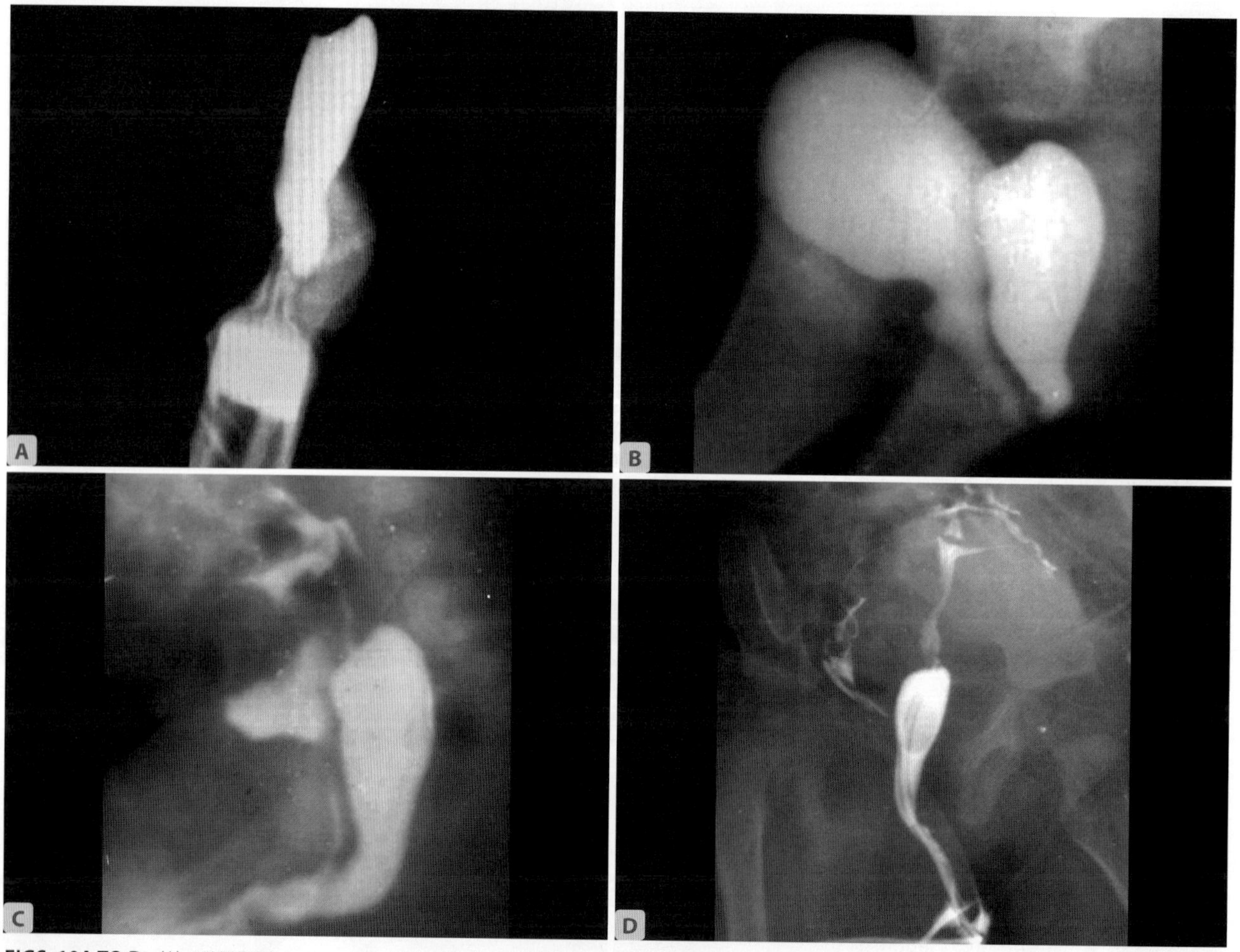

FIGS. 10A TO D: (A) 46,XX DSD, incomplete virilization types (different cases): Flush technique genitography filled only a well-formed vagina. Note a concave upward filling defect on top of the vagina, the cervical identification, presence of which indirectly denotes a well-formed uterus; (B) 46,XX DSD, incomplete virilization types: Both urethra and vagina, open together very low, close to the surface of perineum. Again note negative filling defect, the cervical indentation. Uterus and tubes are not opacified in both (A) and (B); (C and D) 46,XX DSD, incomplete virilization types: Picture is similar to (B) except that contrast has entered the uterine cavity and tubes with spill over into the peritoneal cavity. (DSD: disorders of sex differentiation)

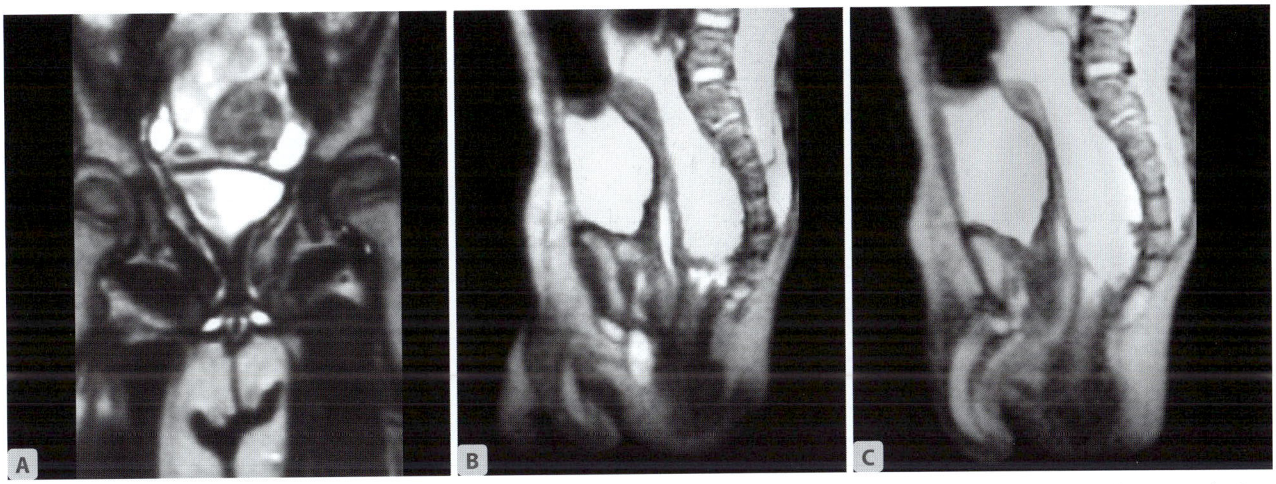

FIGS. 11A TO C: MRI in 46,XX DSD due to CAH. (A) Coronal T2WI shows bilateral normal ovaries with high signal intensity; (B) Midline sagittal MRI: Normal uterus well seen; (C) Externally, hypertrophied clitoris seen. (CAH: congenital adrenal hyperplasia; DSD: disorders of sex differentiation; MRI: magnetic resonance imaging; T2WI: T2-weighted imaging)

adrenal hyperplasia. Although external genitalia of complete virilization type of FPH are similar to those of males, there are no testes at any site. In patients of incomplete virilization type of FPH, the hypertrophied clitoris mimics penis due to prominent corpora cavernosa and corpus spongiosum **(Fig. 11C)**. The uterus and the vagina may be filled with clear urine due to reflux into them through the urogenital sinus.

46,XY DSD (Earlier Known as Male Pseudohermaphroditism)[1,3,24-26,29-32]

Patients of this group of disorder have a variable external phenotype—either ambiguous genitalia, normal male or normal female); and the chromosomal sex is 46,XY. It can be divided into two broad groups:

1. *Defect in androgen synthesis or function:*
   - Defect in androgen synthesis:
     - Luteinizing hormone (LH) receptor mutation
     - 17-β hydroxysteroid dehydrogenase deficiency
     - 5-α reductase deficiency
     - Male CAH
   - Defect in androgen function:
     - Androgen insensitivity syndrome (AIS) (complete, partial or mild)
     - Persistent Müllerian duct syndrome (AMH deficiency) (in this entity, the external appearance is like a male).
2. *Gonadal development disorder:*
   - Ovotesticular DSD
   - Complete gonadal dysgenesis
   - Partial gonadal dysgenesis

Final definitive diagnosis would require sophisticated laboratory facilities for estimation of these hormones.

Phenotype: The external phenotype in this group of disorders is variable among the subtypes. In complete AIS, the external genitalia are that of a female. In persistent Müllerian duct syndrome (PMDS, AMH deficiency), the external genitalia are that of a male. In all the other disorders of the subgroup (a), there is variable genital ambiguity and hypospadias **(Figs. 12A to C)**.

Imaging Appearances

In complete AIS (previously called "complete testicular feminization syndrome"), genitography would demonstrate a short, blind-ending vagina without any evidence of cervix and a separate urethral opening **(Figs. 13 and 14A to C)**. Testes can be identified on MRI. On MRI, uterus and ovaries are not seen; instead there is a short blind-ending vagina.

Persistent Müllerian duct syndrome (PMDS) or AMH deficiency syndrome: This is also called "male with uterus" because on clinical examination of the external genitalia, these patients appear as normal male with the urethra opening at the tip of a normally formed penis. They also have cryptorchidism (or inguinal hernia) and internally fully developed Müllerian duct derivatives, i.e., well-formed vagina and uterus **(Figs. 15A and B)** are present.

In all the other subtypes of 46,XY DSD group externally there is an ambiguous genitalia; and internally a variable-sized urogenital sinus with a small-sized vagina without cervical impression are seen **(Figs. 16A to D)**. MRI is invaluable in identifying the undescended testes and the penile structure **(Figs. 17A to C)**.

46,XY pure/complete gonadal dysgenesis (earlier known as "XY female") is also known as "Swyer syndrome":[33] In this disorder, the individual is genotypically male (46,XY) but the testes are dysgenetic/streak-like **(Figs. 18A to F)**. The dysgenetic gonads do not produce testosterone and hence the result is an external female genitalia. These children are reared as girls, who later on present with primary amenorrhea. The streak gonads do not show usual hyperintense signal on T2WI MRI and are often difficult to identify on imaging. It is very important to remove these testicular tissues, as they are prone to development of malignancy.[33]

If a newborn has perineal hypospadias and 46,XY karyotype, it is important to assume that the child is a male with congenital urogenital malformation. Detailed radiological

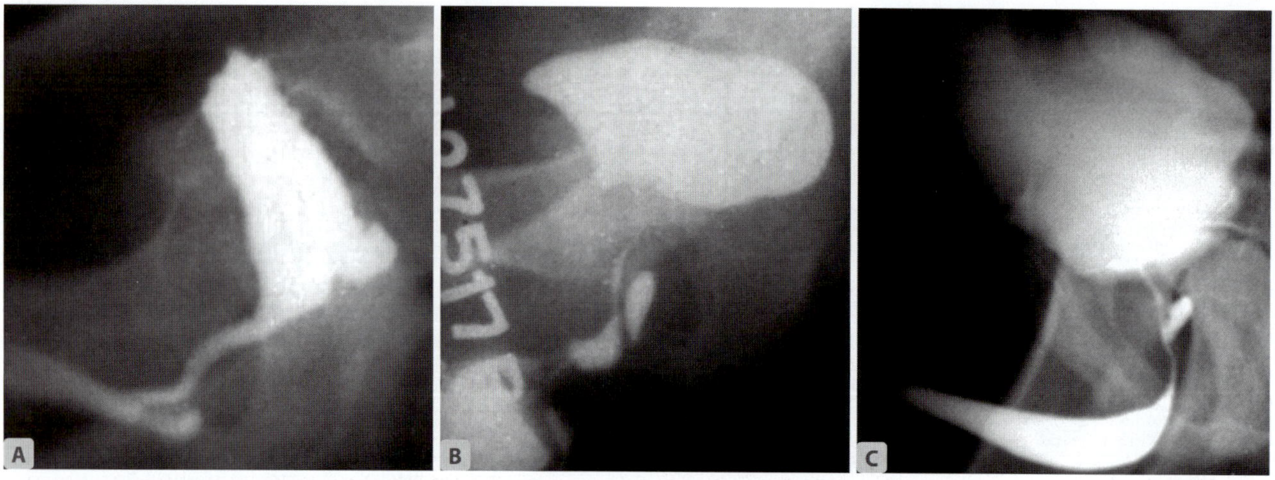

FIGS. 12A TO C: 46,XY DSD (different cases): Note that the junctional site is low (A), middle (B), and high (C). As the junctional site moves up, the degree of masculinization also increases which is evident by longer, male type urethra. In (C), small vaginal remnant, also called utriculus is arising from the vertical portion of the urethra. Also note absence of cervical indentation and the top of the vaginal remnants remaining round. (DSD: disorders of sex differentiation)

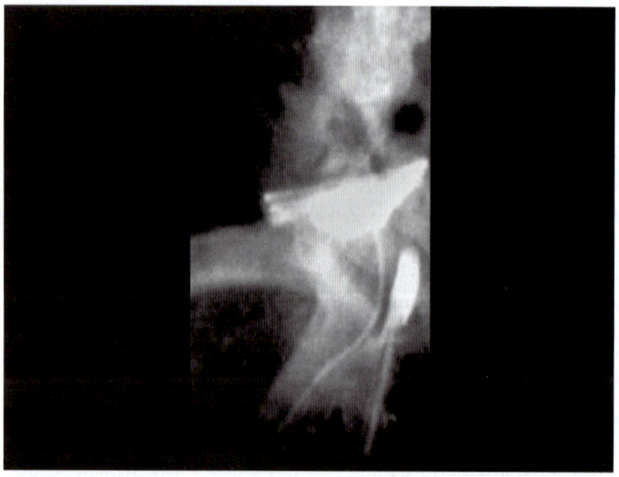

FIG. 13: 46,XY DSD, complete testicular feminization syndrome type: Clinically, no ambiguity in the external genitalia which was female type, i.e., two separate openings, one each for urethra and vagina present. Simultaneous, separate catheterization of both the openings with retrograde contrast injection demonstrates a small, hypoplastic, blind-ending vagina with rounded top and absence of cervical indentation. Sonography or MRI would show absence of uterus or cervix. (DSD: disorders of sex differentiation; MRI: magnetic resonance imaging)

and laboratory investigations are essential to reach the final diagnosis. A comparison of clinical and imaging findings in 46,XY DSD subgroups is given in **Table 3**.

Ovotesticular Disorders of Sex Differentiation (Earlier Known as True Hermaphroditism)[1,8,26]

Majority (50–80%) of ovotesticular DSD patients have a 46,XX karyotype with both the ovary and the testicular tissue present in the same patient or even same gonad. Various possible combinations in which these tissues may occur in ovotesticular DSD and are shown in **Figure 19**.

Other possible karyotypes in this group include 46,XX/XY mosaicism or even more rarely, 46,XY. Clinically, before puberty, these patients present with an ambiguous external genitalia but later presentation may be varying such as cryptorchidism, breast development in a patient reared up as a male, hematuria (actually menstruation through the urogenital sinus opening) in those reared up as a male, amenorrhea in those reared up as female, inguinal hernia, etc.

Genitography shows a urogenital sinus of variable size with a relatively well-developed vagina which may open at varying level into the urethra. Contrast might also enter into the uterus and tubes **(Fig. 20)**.

MRI demonstrates both an ovary and a testis (one or both of which may be replaced by an ovotestis) and variable internal and external genitalia.

Final diagnosis is made only after laparotomy, identification of the Müllerian and Wolffian duct derivatives and gonadal biopsy and histopathological examination of the gonads.

Surgical management consists of excision of inappropriate gonadal tissues followed by appropriate genitoplasty of external genitalia.

CLUES TO THE DIAGNOSIS

At most centers especially in India, laboratory facilities for a detailed investigation of a case of DSD are lacking. Under these circumstances, by combining the information of karyotyping genitographic anatomy and MRI, one can reach at a reasonably correct "working diagnosis" within a short period of time and thus the sex of rearing can be assigned to the child at an early age. The diagnostic approach is shown in **Table 4**. MRI is now more widely used. With increasing experience in interpreting the complex anatomy of DSDs, it is necessary that MRI should form an essential component in the diagnostic work-up of these patients for reaching definitive diagnosis.

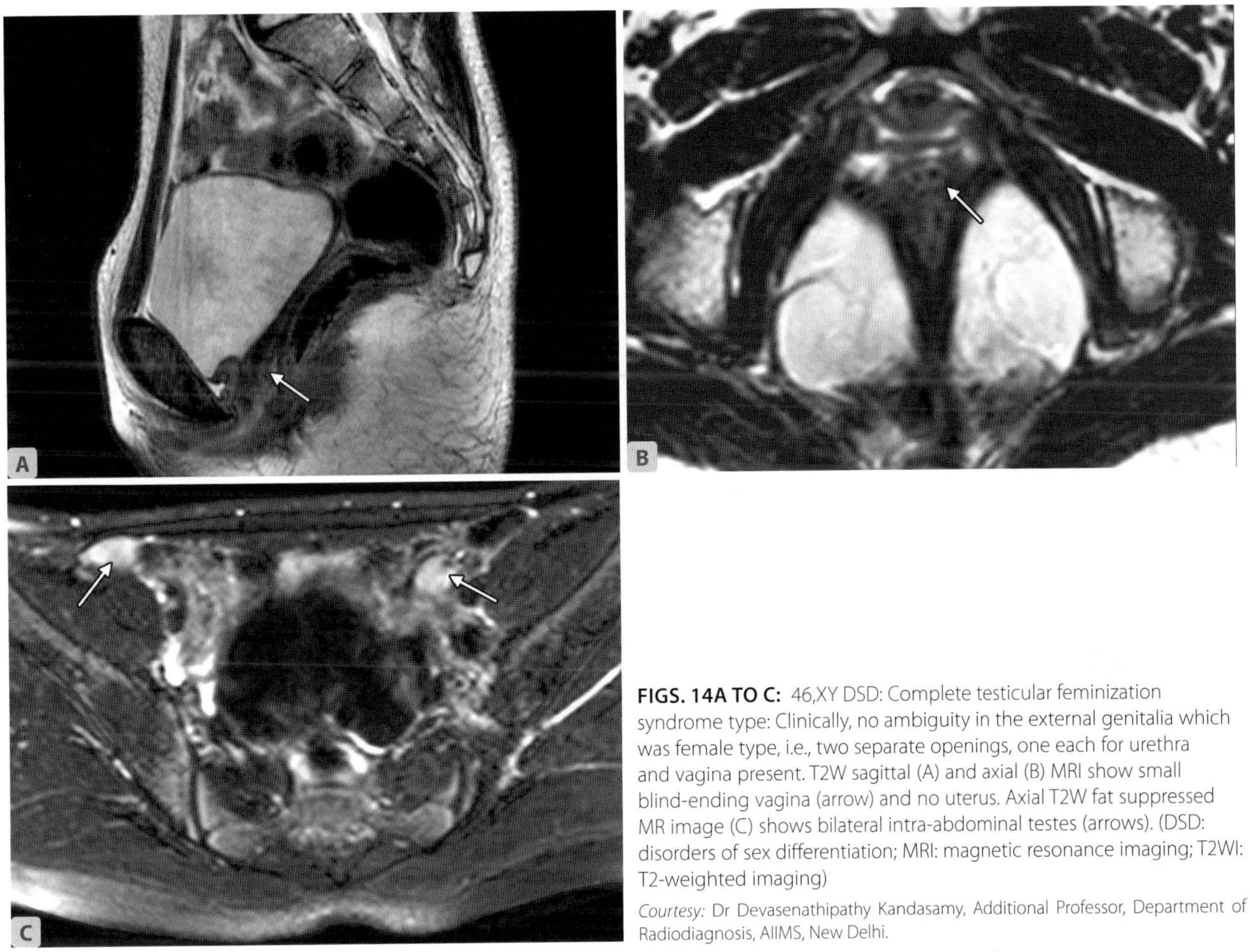

FIGS. 14A TO C: 46,XY DSD: Complete testicular feminization syndrome type: Clinically, no ambiguity in the external genitalia which was female type, i.e., two separate openings, one each for urethra and vagina present. T2W sagittal (A) and axial (B) MRI show small blind-ending vagina (arrow) and no uterus. Axial T2W fat suppressed MR image (C) shows bilateral intra-abdominal testes (arrows). (DSD: disorders of sex differentiation; MRI: magnetic resonance imaging; T2WI: T2-weighted imaging)

Courtesy: Dr Devasenathipathy Kandasamy, Additional Professor, Department of Radiodiagnosis, AIIMS, New Delhi.

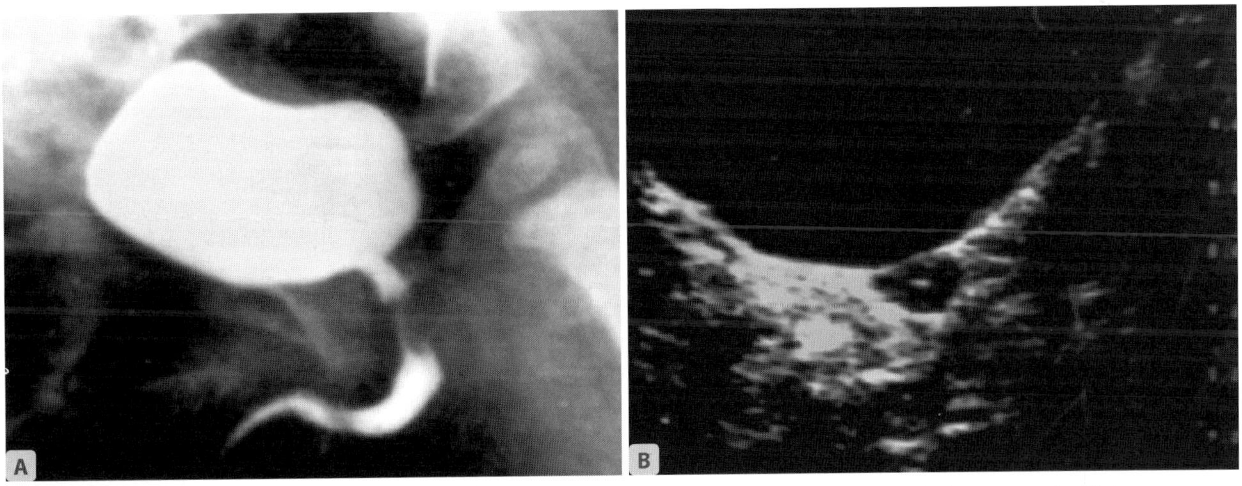

FIGS. 15A AND B: 46,XY DSD, PMDS (AMH deficiency): Genitography (A) documents a male type urethra only. On sonography (B), however, a good-sized uterus and cervix was detected. Example of "male with uterus". (AMH: anti-Müllerian hormone; DSD: disorders of sex differentiation; PMDS: persistent Müllerian duct syndrome)

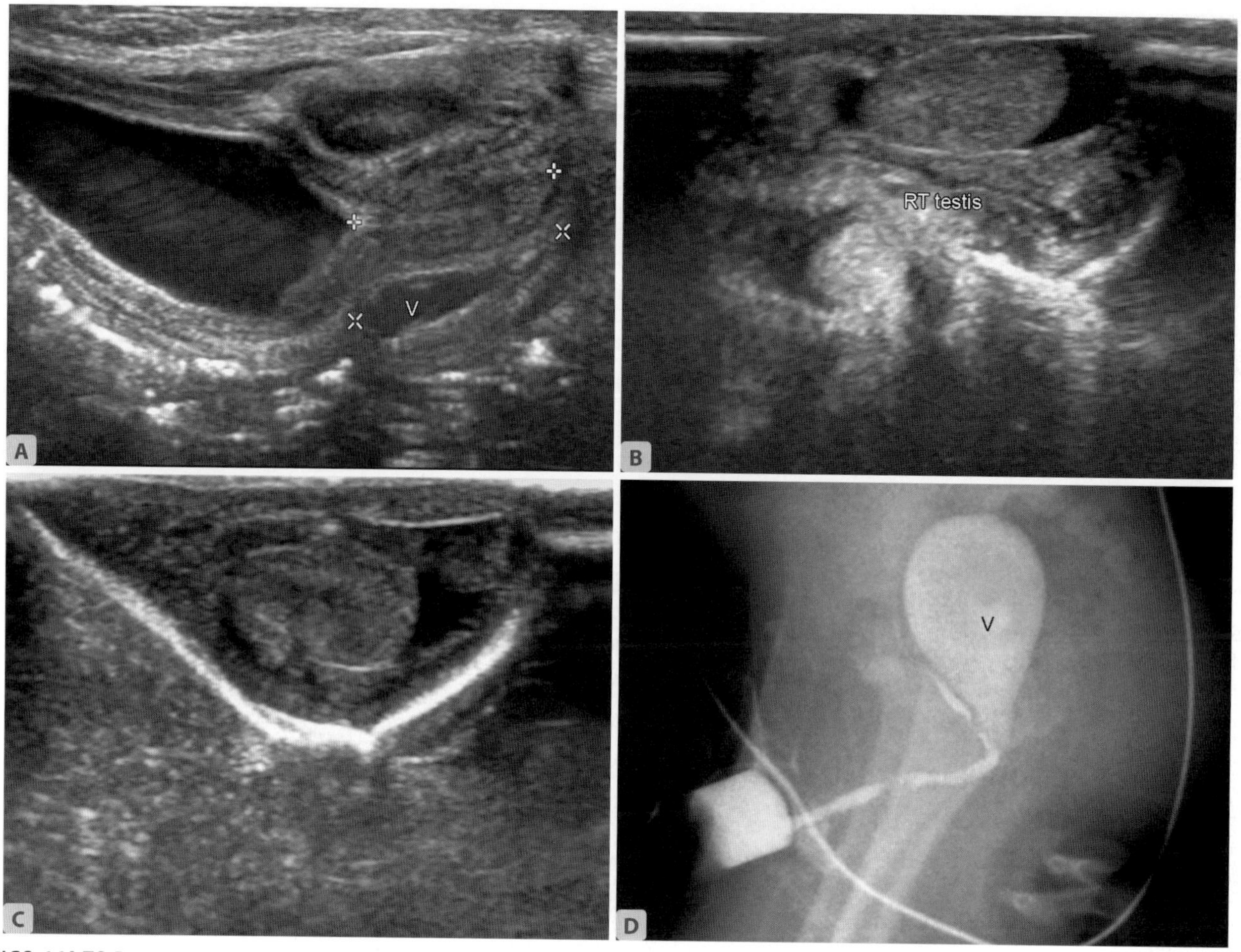

FIGS. 16A TO D: 46,XY DSD, partial androgen insensitivity type: A newborn girl child presented with ambiguous genitalia; Sagittal TPUS image (A) showed presence of blind-ending vagina (V) without uterus. Both testes seen in bilateral labial folds (B and C) genitography (D) showed a well-formed vagina (V) without cervical indentation. (DSD: disorders of sex differentiation; TPUS: transperineal ultrasonography)

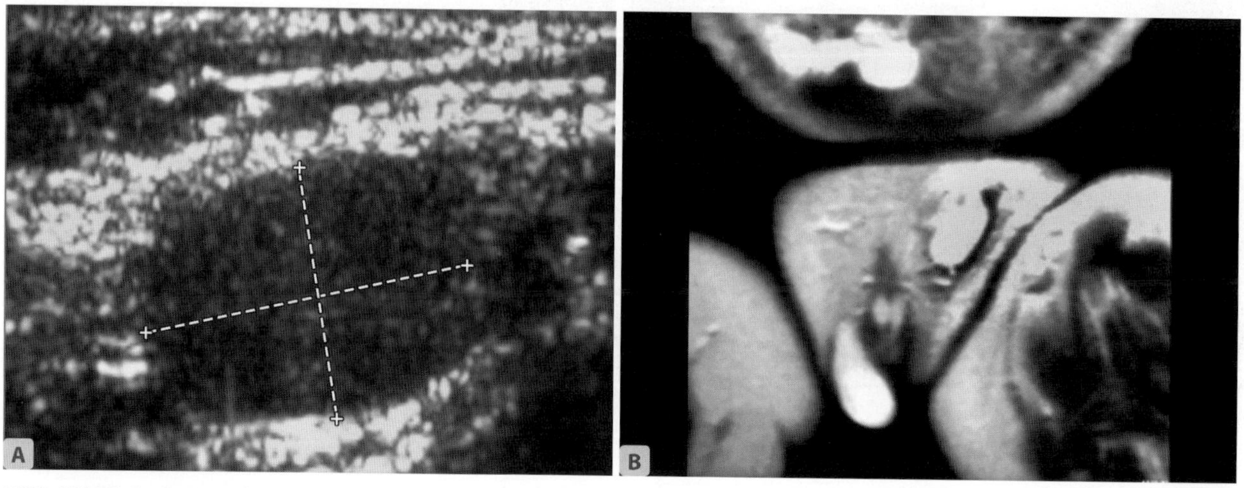

FIGS. 17A TO C: *Continued*

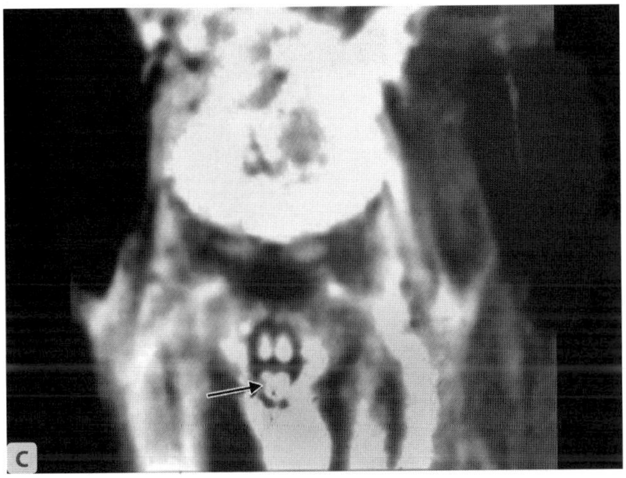

FIGS. 17A TO C: MRI in 46 XY DSD: Undescended testes.
(A) Ultrasonography detects a gonad at inguinal canal; (B) T2W coronal MRI demonstrates bilateral undescended testes as high signal masses; (C) Corpora cavernosa and spongiosum are well-demonstrated, presence of these suggests male type of anatomy. (DSD: disorders of sex differentiation; MRI: magnetic resonance imaging; T2WI: T2-weighted imaging)

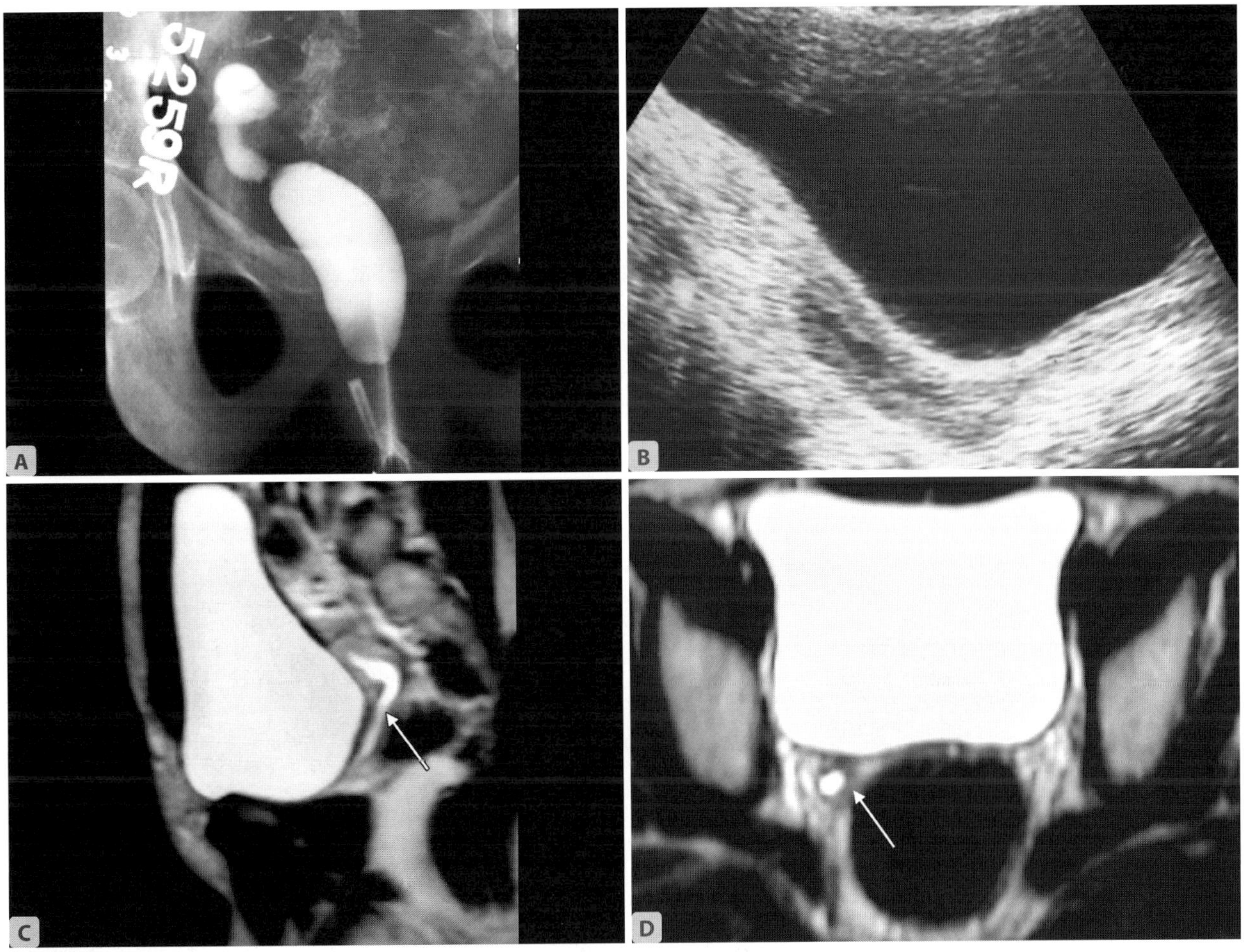

FIGS. 18A TO F: *Continued*

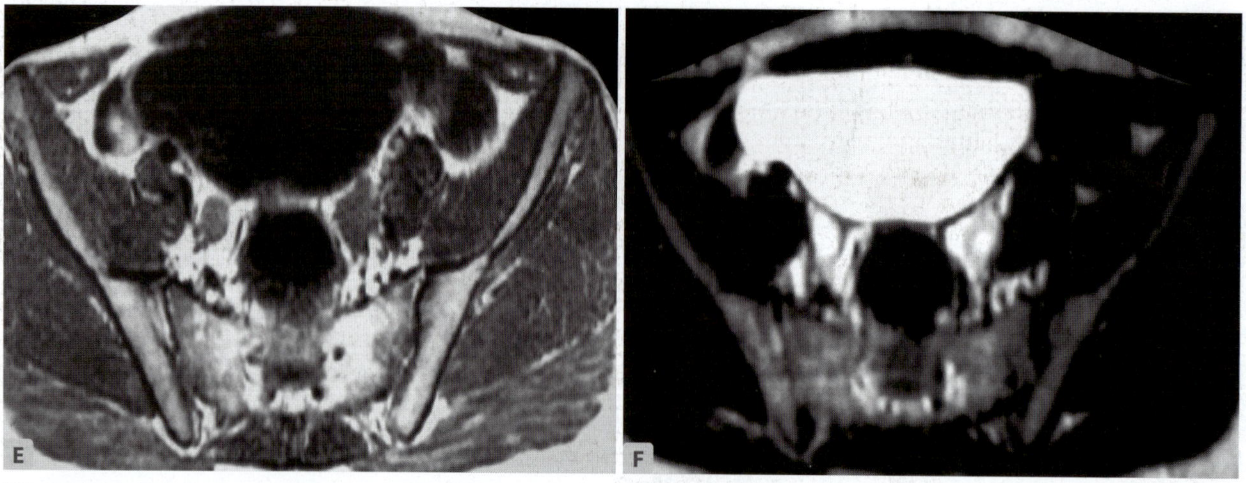

FIGS. 18A TO F: 46,XY pure gonadal dysgenesis: Genitography documents right-sided Müllerian duct structures (A). On ultrasound sagittal image uterus is seen (B). Sagittal T2W MRI demonstrates well-formed uterus (arrow in C). Axial T2W MRI localizes the uterus to right side only (arrow in D). Axial T1W (E) and T2W MRI (F) demonstrate bilateral gonads. Histologically both were dysgenetic. (MGD: mixed gonadal dysgenesis; MRI: magnetic resonance imaging; T1W: T1-weighted; T2W: T2-weighted; US: ultrasound)

TABLE 3: Clinicoradiological features of 46,XY disorders of sex differentiation (DSD).

	Clinical presentation	External genitalia	Internal genitalia	Gonads
Complete AIS	Primary amenorrhea	Female	Blind-ending vagina, no uterus	Testes (usually undescended)
Partial AIS	Ambiguous genitalia	Ambiguous/hypospadias	Urogenital sinus, vagina without any uterus	Undescended testes
5-α reductase deficiency	Ambiguous genitalia	Ambiguous/hypospadias	Urogenital sinus, vagina without any uterus	Undescended or ectopic testes
PMDS (AMH deficiency)	Cryptorchidism/inguinal hernia	Male	Well-developed vagina and uterus	Testes
46,XY pure gonadal dysgenesis	Primary amenorrhea	Female	Uterus (small), vagina, and Fallopian tubes	Streak gonads

(AIS: androgen insensitivity syndrome; AMH: anti-Müllerian hormone; PMDS: persistent Müllerian duct syndrome)

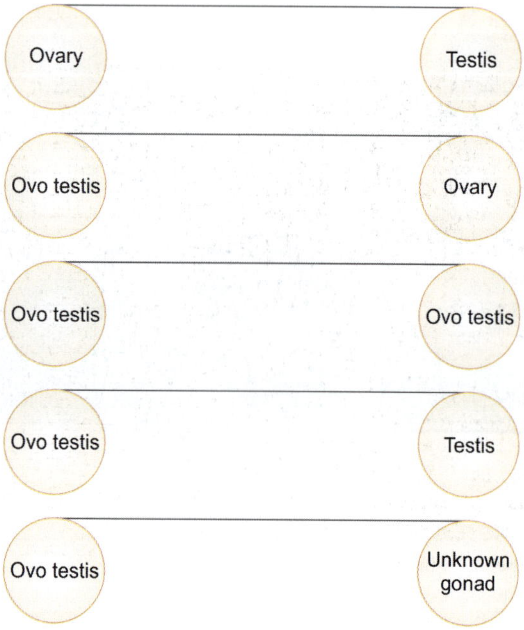

FIG. 19: Ovotesticular DSD. Schematic drawing to show all possible combinations of testicular and an ovarian tissue, on the two sides.

(DSD: disorders of sex differentiation)

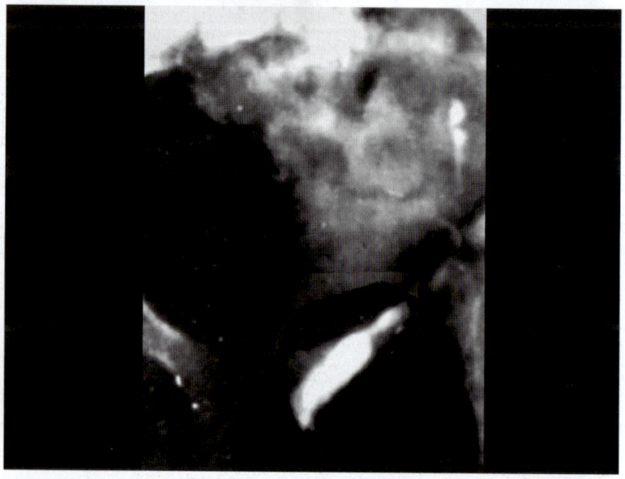

FIG. 20: Ovotesticular DSD, genitography: demonstrates presence of Müllerian duct derivative only on the left side. Due to the presence of testicular tissue on the contralateral side, Müllerian duct structures do not differentiate on that side. (DSD: disorders of sex differentiation)

NEOPLASMS IN DISORDERS OF SEX DIFFERENTIATION

The streak gonads in DSD (especially with a Y chromosome) are prone to development of gonadoblastoma. Gonadoblastoma itself is a benign tumor but has a propensity to transform into malignancies such as dysgerminoma, yolk-sac tumor, embryonal carcinoma, seminoma, and immature teratoma.[34,35] Gonadoblastomas **(Figs. 21A to C)** may present as masses with foci of calcification within a dysgenetic gonad. Henceforth, it is advisable to surgically remove the streak gonads.

CONCLUSION

Disorders of sex differentiation are disorders with complex clinical problems. Radiology is a key component of the multidisciplinary team approach involved in patient care; alongside clinical examination, biochemical, and genetic studies. Genitography, ultrasonography, and MRI are important imaging tools. Except perhaps for the evaluation of urogenital sinus, most of the other information required in DSD can be obtained reliably by MRI. Role of the radiologist is not to arrive at a diagnosis, but to accurately demonstrate the genital anatomy. This is often difficult as the conditions encountered are diverse in etiology and often incompletely expressed. The final diagnosis is established by putting clinical findings with a combination of cytogenetic, biochemical, and radiological studies. An early decision regarding the phenotypic sex lessens the psychological impact on the child, and is crucial in parent counseling.

TABLE 4: Diagnostic algorithm in a child with DSD. Criteria used: Karyotyping + genitographic anatomy.

Genitographic anatomy → / Karyotyping ↓	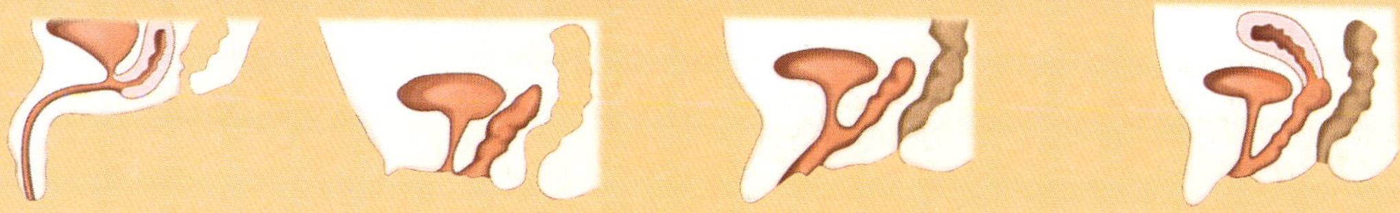			
Chromatin Positive (XX)	46,XX DSD (Total virilization type)	—	—	• 46,XX DSD (Partial virilization type) • Ovotesticular DSD
Chromatin Negative (XY)	46,XY DSD (AMH deficiency only)	46,XY DSD (Androgen receptor insensitivity type: complete testicular feminization syndrome)	46,XY DSD Causes: • Deficiency of 5-α reductase • Defective biosynthesis of testosterone • Incomplete testicular feminization syndrome	• 46,XY complete gonadal dysgenesis • 46,XY DSD with combined AMH and testosterone deficiency

(AMH: anti-Müllerian hormone; DSD: disorders of sex differentiation)

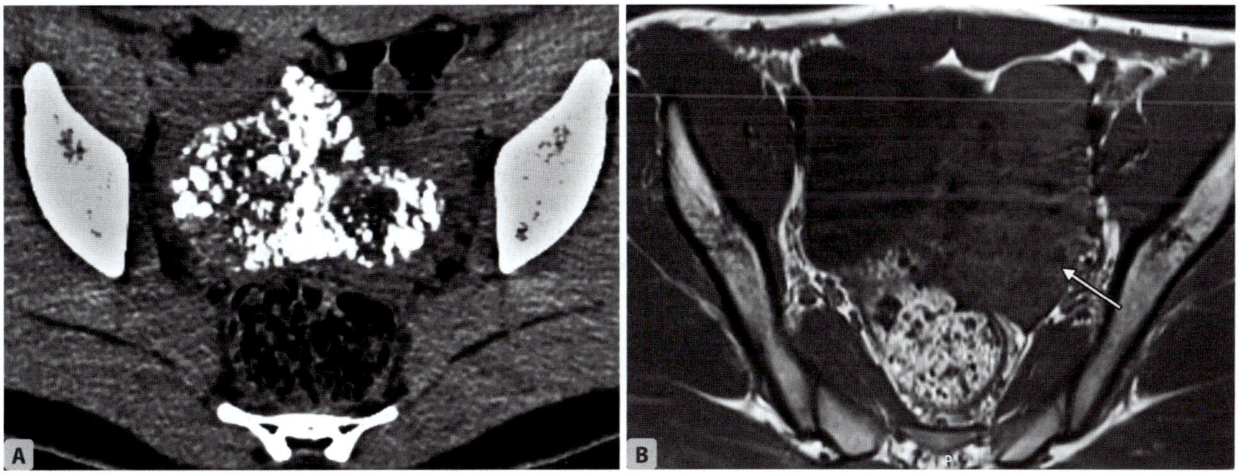

FIGS. 21A TO C: *Continued*

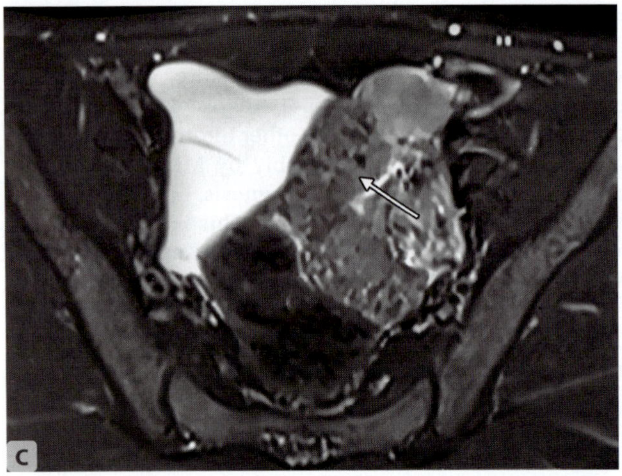

FIGS. 21A TO C: Gonadoblastoma in a streak gonad in an 18-year-old girl. The large pelvic mass showed multiple foci of dense calcification (A). On T1W MRI (B) the mass was predominantly hypointense. On T2WI (C) it was hyperintense; with the calcified area appearing hypointense (arrow).

Courtesy: Dr Devasenathipathy Kandasamy, Additional Professor, Department of Radiodiagnosis, AIIMS, New Delhi.

REFERENCES

1. Josso N, Karger S, Basel (Eds). The Intersex Child of Pediatric and Adolescent Endocrinology. 1981;8:240-60.
2. Chavhan GB, Parra DA, Oudjhane K, Miller SF, Babyn PS, Pippi Salle FL. Imaging of ambiguous genitalia: classification and diagnostic approach. Radiographics. 2008;28(7):1891-904.
3. Silverman F (Ed). Caffey's Pediatric X-ray Diagnosis (9th edition). Chicago: Yearbook Medical Publishers Inc.; 1993. p. 2.
4. Cohen HL, Bober SE. Imaging the pediatric pelvis: The normal and abnormal genital tract and simulators in its diseases. Urol Radiol. 1992;14:273-83.
5. Cremin BJ. Intersex states in young children: The importance of radiology in making a correct diagnosis. Clin Radiol. 1974;25: 63-73.
6. Gambino J, Coldwell B, Dietrich R, Walot I, Kangarloo H. Congenital disorders of sexual differentiation: MR findings. Pictorial Essay. AJR Am J Roentgenol. 1992;158:363-7.
7. Horowity M, Glassberg KI. Ambiguous genitalia: Diagnosis, evaluation, and treatment. Urol Radiol. 1992;14:306-18.
8. Gupta AK. Imaging of intersex. In: Subbarao K, Banerjee S, Aggarwal SK (Eds). Diagnostic Radiology and Imaging. 1997;1:860-9.
9. Garel L. Abnormal sex differentiation: who, how and when to image. Pediatr Radiol. 2008;38(suppl 3):S508-11.
10. Scanlan KA, Pozniak MA, Fagerholm M, Shapiro S. Value of transperineal sonography in the assessment of vaginal atresia. AJR Am J Roentgenol. 1990;154:545-8.
11. Lindert J, Niort O, Tushaus L, Tafazzoli-Lari K, Wunsch L. Perineal ultrasound offers useful information in girls with congenital adrenal hyperplasia. 2016;12:427.e1-6
12. de Jesus LE, Fazecas T, Ribeiro BG, Dekermacher S. Transperineal Ultrasound as a Tool to Plan Surgical Strategies in Pediatric Urology: Back to the Future?. Urology. 2017;104:175-8.
13. Kanemoto K, Hayashi Y, Kojima Y, Maruyama T, Ito M, Kohri K. Accuracy of ultrasonography and magnetic resonance imaging in the diagnosis of non-palpable testis. Int J Urol. 2005;12(7): 668-72.
14. Secaf E, Hricak H, Gooding CA, Ho VW, Gorczyca DP, Ringertz H, et al. Role of MRI in the evaluation of ambiguous genitalia. Pediatr Radiol. 1994;24:231-5.
15. Wright NB, Smith C, Rickwood AMK, Carty HML. Review: Imaging children with ambiguous genitalia and intersex states. Clin Radiol. 1995;50:823-9.
16. Umeoka S, Koyama T, Saga T, Fujiwara T, Kido A, Fukuhara K, et al. Ectopically located gonads in a patient with mixed gonadal dysgenesis: detection by diffusion-weighted MRI. Abdomen Imaging. 2005;30:637-40.
17. Krishnaswami S, Fonnesbeck C, Penson D, McPheeters ML. Magnetic resonance imaging for locating nonpalpable undescended testicles: a meta-analysis. Pediatrics. 2013;131:e1908-16.
18. Haloi AK, Gupta AK, Sharma S. Radiological evaluation of children with intersex disorders with ambiguous genitalia using genitography, ultrasonography and MR imaging. AJR Am J Roentgenol. 2001;178:50.
19. Sharma S, Gupta AK, Haloi AK. MR imaging of muscles supporting the phallus: A clue to the true sex in an intersex child. Radiology. 2002;225:669.
20. Paquin AJ, Baker DH, Finby N, Evans JA.. The urogenital sinus: Its demonstration and significance. J Urol. 1957;78:796-807.
21. Shopfner CE. Genitography in Intersex Problems. In: Kaufmann HJ, Karger S, Basel, (Eds). Progress in Pediatric Radiology. New York: München; 1970. pp. 97-115.
22. Josso N, Fortier B, Faure C. Genitography in intersexual states: A review of 86 cases with new criteria for the study of the urogenital sinus. Acuta Endocrinologica. 1969;62:165-80.
23. Hughes IA, Houk C, Ahmed SF, Lee PA; LWPES Consensus Group; ESPE Consensus Group. Consensus statement on management of intersex disorders. Arch Dis Child. 2006;91(7):554-63.
24. Moshiri M, Chapman T, Fechner PY, Dubinsky TJ, Shnorhavorian M, Osman S, et al. Evaluation and Management of Disorders of Sex Development: Multidisciplinary Approach to a Complex Diagnosis. Radiographics. 2012;32:1599-618.
25. Auchus RJ, Chang AY. 46,XX DSD: the masculinised female. Best Pract Res Clin Endocrinol Metab. 2010;24(2):219-42.
26. Eapen A, Chandramohan A, Simon B, Putta T, John R, Kekre A. Imaging Evaluation of Disorders of Sex Development. J Gastrointestinal Abdominal Radiol. 2019. [online] Available from https://www.thieme-connect.com/products/ejournals/pdf/10.1055/s-0039-3402101.pdf [Last accessed June, 2020].
27. Prader A. Der Genitalbefund beim Pseudohermaphroditismus feminus der kongenitalen adrenogenitalen Syndroms. Helv Paediatr Acta. 1954;9:231-48.
28. Ogilvy-Stuart AL, Brain CE. Early assessment of ambiguous genitalia. Arch Dis Child. 2004;89(5):401-7.
29. Michala L, Creighton SM. The XY female. Best Pract Res Clin Obstet Gynaecol. 2010;24(2):139-48.

30. Grasso D, Borreggine C, Campanale C, Longo A, Grilli G, Macarini L. Usefulness and role of magnetic resonance imaging in a case of complete androgen insensitivity syndrome. Radiol Case Rep. 2016;10(2):1119.
31. Nezzo M, De Visschere P, T'sjoen G, Weyers S, Villeirs G. Role of imaging in the diagnosis and management of complete androgen insensitivity syndrome in adults. Case Rep Radiol. 2013;2013:158484.
32. Nakhal RS, Hall-Craggs M, Freeman A, Kirkham A, Conway GS, Arora R, et al. Evaluation of retained testes in adolescent girls and women with complete androgen insensitivity syndrome. Radiology. 2013;268(1):153-60.
33. Da Silva Rios S, Monteiro IC, Braz Dos Santos LG, Garcia Caldas N, Rios Chen AC, Rios Chen J, et al. A case of Swyer syndrome associated with advanced gonadal dysgerminoma involving long survival. Case Rep Oncol. 2015;8(1):179-84.
34. McCann-Crosby B, Mansouri R, Dietrich JE, McCullough LB, Sutton VR, Austin EG, et al. State of the art review in gonadal dysgenesis: challenges in diagnosis and management. Int J Pediatr Endocrinol. 2014;2014(1):4.
35. Kim KS, Kim J. Disorders of sex development. Korean J Urol. 2012;53(1):1-8.

CHAPTER

78

Skeletal Dysplasias

Gaurav Shanker Pradhan, Radhika Batra, Sapna Singh

INTRODUCTION

The skeletal dysplasias (SD) are a large heterogeneous group of disorders with dysplastic bony growth and usually an underlying genetic basis characterized by abnormal growth, shape, number, texture, or integrity of bones. SD may be subdivided into osteochondrodysplasia and dysostoses. Osteochondrodysplasias occur due to genetic mutation and have progressive changes in the bone/cartilage throughout life due to changing phenotype while dysostoses occur due to abnormal blastogenesis and remain static throughout life. The osteochondrodysplasias are further subdivided into osteodysplasia and chondrodysplasia depending on whether the dysplasias are due to disturbance in osteoid production or chondroid formation respectively. Osteodysplasias are characterized by osteopenia or osteosclerosis, whereas chondrodysplasias manifest as a short stature as they affect the cartilage and thus affect the linear growth of bones. Depending on the part of the skeleton involved, disproportionate short stature due to chondrodysplasia can be either short limb dwarfism or short trunk dwarfism. The dysplasias may manifest as:

- Abnormal growth—affecting shape, contour, and size of involved bones.
- An abnormal number of bones—less or more in number.
- Abnormal texture—reduced or increased remodeling and mineral deposition leading to an abnormal bony matrix (also known as osteodystrophy).

In the neonatal period, the prevalence of SD has been estimated to be 2.4/10,000 births.[1] There was a lack of understanding of the etiology of SD. So, various classifications emerged based on techniques that were used to identify these abnormalities or on a clinical basis. Some classifications have recently come up, highlighting genetic basis of these dysplasias with increased detection of underlying chromosomal aberrations.[2,3]

Radiographs are often the first imaging modality used in arriving at the diagnosis. The radiologist is unaware of the detailed genetic studies, which are both time consuming and usually unavailable immediately. So, any abnormality has to be picked on standard radiographs based on the abnormality affecting growth, number, or texture of bones. Therefore, we need to use classifications based on radiological findings.[4-6]

NOSOLOGY AND CLASSIFICATION OF SKELETAL DYSPLASIA

The first-ever classification of skeletal dysplasia which was based on clinical findings and description of radiographs was done by the "*International Nomenclature of Constitutional Diseases of Bones*" group in 1970. Since then, the nomenclature of skeletal dysplasia is confusing. Advances in medical knowledge and research involving genetics of SD led to a new nomenclature not only based on clinical and radiological findings but also on molecular phenotypes which made it more extensive and confusing. According to the latest 10th edition of the International Skeletal Dysplasia Society (ISDS) Nosology and Classification of Genetic Skeletal Disorders which was published in 2019, skeletal dysplasia includes 461 different diseases that are classified into 42 groups based on their clinical, radiographic, and/or molecular phenotypes.[7] Out of these large number of dysplasias, only six entities constitute around 40% of all SD namely achondroplasia, pseudoachondroplasia, osteogenesis imperfecta, multiple epiphyseal dysplasia (MED), spondyloepiphyseal dysplasia, and metaphyseal chondrodysplasia.

Despite the addition of molecular tests in recent classifications, it is important to remember that detailed clinical and radiographic evaluation still plays a pivotal role in the diagnosis of SD.

The various groups and important examples of dysplasias in each group in ISDS Nosology and Classification (10th edition) are summarized in **Table 1**.

CLINICAL PRESENTATION OF SKELETAL DYSPLASIAS

Skeletal dysplasia is suspected in children with unexplained short stature, particularly if it is disproportionate, and in children with facial dysmorphism such as cleft palate, micrognathia, midface hypoplasia and depressed nasal bridge. Dysplasia should be differentiated from other causes of short statures, such as familial short stature, endocrine disorders, and metabolic disorders. Clinical evaluation includes complete history especially birth and family history with pedigree analysis, various anthropometric

TABLE 1: List of 42 groups of skeletal dysplasias with associated examples in each group.

Group number	Group name	Examples of important disorders of the group
1.	*FGFR-3* chondrodysplasia group	Thanatophoric dysplasia, achondroplasia, hypochondroplasia
2.	Type II collagen group	Achondrogenesis type 2, spondyloepiphyseal dysplasia congenita (SEDC), Kniest dysplasia, spondyloepiphyseal dysplasia with marked metaphyseal changes (SEMD), Stickler syndrome type 1
3.	Type II collagen group	Stickler syndrome type 2 and 3
4.	Sulfation disorders group	Achondrogenesis type IB, diastrophic dysplasia (DTD), Ehlers–Danlos syndrome
5.	Perlecan group	Silverman–Handmaker and Rolland–Desbuquois syndrome, Schwartz–Jampel syndrome
6.	Aggrecan group	Spondyloepiphyseal dysplasia, (Kimberley type), spondyloepimetaphyseal dysplasia, aggrecan type
7.	Flamin group and related disorders	Frontometaphyseal dysplasia, Larsen syndrome
8.	*TRPV4* group	Metatropic dysplasia, SMD (Kozlowski type), SEMD Maroteaux type (pseudo-Morquio syndrome type 2)
9.	Ciliopathies with major skeletal involvement	Chondroectodermal dysplasia (Ellis–van Creveld syndrome), short rib-polydactyly syndrome type 1/3, asphyxiating thoracic dysplasia (Jeune syndrome)
10.	Multiple epiphyseal dysplasias and pseudoachondroplasia group	Multiple epiphyseal dysplasias (MED), pseudoachondroplasia, Stickler syndrome, recessive type
11.	Metaphyseal dysplasia	Metaphyseal dysplasia, Schmid type, and Jansen type
12.	Spondylometaphyseal dysplasia (SMD)	SMD, Sutcliffe type or corner fracture types
13.	Spondylo-epi-(meta)-physeal dysplasias [SE(M)D]	Dyggve–Melchior–Clausen (DMC) dysplasia
14.	Severe spondylodysplastic dysplasias	Achondrogenesis type 1, spondylometaphyseal dysplasia, Sedaghatian type
15.	Acromelic dysplasias	Trichorhinophalangeal dysplasias, acrodysostosis
16.	Acromesomelic dysplasias	Acromesomelic dysplasias, Maroteaux type, and Osebold–Remondini type
17.	Mesomelic and rhizomelic dysplasias	Mesomelic dysplasias, dyschondrosteosis
18.	Bent bone dysplasias	Campomelic dysplasia
19.	Primordial dwarfism and slender bones groups	Multiple epiphyseal dysplasias with microcephaly and nystagmus (Lowry–Wood syndrome)
20.	Dysplasias with multiple joint dislocations	Multiple epiphyseal dysplasias (recessive type), Desbuquois dysplasia, Ehlers–Danlos syndrome
21.	Chondrodysplasia punctate (CDP) group	CDP, X-linked dominant (Conradi–Hünermann type), CDP X-linked recessive, brachytelephalangic type and rhizomelic CDP
22.	Neonatal osteosclerotic dysplasias	Caffey disease
23.	Osteopetrosis and related disorders	Osteopetrosis, pycnodysostosis
24.	Other sclerosing bone disorders	Osteopoikilosis, melorheostosis, osteopathia striata, craniometaphyseal dysplasia, Pyle disease
25.	Osteogenesis imperfecta and decrease bone density group	Osteogenesis imperfecta and Bruck syndrome
26.	Abnormal mineralization group	Hypophosphatasia, vitamin D resistant rickets, Familial hyperparathyroidism
27.	Lysosomal storage diseases with skeletal involvement (dysostosis multiplex)	Mucopolysaccharidosis and mucolipidosis
28.	Osteolysis group	Familial expansile osteolysis, Progeria, Hajdu–Cheney syndrome
29.	Disorganized development of skeletal components	Multiple cartilaginous exostoses (osteochondromas), Fibrous dysplasia, fibrodysplasia ossificans progressiva (FOP), Ollier's and Maffucci disease, osteofibrous dysplasia

Continued

Continued

Group number	Group name	Examples of important disorders of the group
30.	Overgrowth (tall stature) syndrome with skeletal involvement	Weaver syndrome, Sotos syndrome
31.	Genetic inflammatory/rheumatoid like osteoarthropathy	Progressive pseudorheumatoid dysplasia, chronic infantile neurologic cutaneous articular syndrome
32.	Cleidocranial dysplasia and related disorders	Cleidocranial dysplasia, Yunis–Varon syndrome
33.	Craniosynostosis syndromes	Pfeiffer syndrome, Apert syndrome, Crouzon syndrome, and Carpenter syndrome
34.	Dysostoses with predominant craniofacial involvement	Mandibulofacial dysostoses, acrofacial dysostoses, frontonasal dysplasia
35.	Dysostoses with predominant vertebral and without costal involvement	Currarino syndrome, Klippel–Feil syndrome
36.	Patellar dysostoses	Nail–patella syndrome
37.	Brachydactyly (without extraskeletal manifestations)	Brachydactyly type A1, A2, B, B2, C, D, E, and Cooks syndrome (Brachydactyly with anonychia)
38.	Brachydactyly with extraskeletal manifestations	Rubinstein–Taybi syndrome
39.	Limb hypoplasia-reduction defects groups	TAR, Holt–Oram syndrome, Fanconi anemia, Poland syndrome
40.	Ectrodactyly with/without other manifestations	Split hand foot malformations, Hartsfield syndrome
41.	Polydactyly–Syndactyly–Triphalangism group	Various syndromes associated with polydactyly and syndactyly
42.	Defect in joint formation and synostoses	Radioulnar synostosis with amegakaryocytic thrombocytopenia, multiple synostoses syndrome

(FGFR: fibroblast growth factor receptor; TAR: thrombocytopenia-absent radius; TRPV4: transient receptor potential vanilloid 4)

Source: Adapted from International Skeletal Dysplasia Society (ISDS) Nosology and classification of the skeletal dysplasia, 10th edition, published in 2019.[7]

measurements, description of the limb involvement, hair quality, cleft palate, eye abnormalities, immunological/hematological data, and even internal organ abnormalities such as cystic kidney, or hepatosplenomegaly seen during abdominal ultrasonography.

Disproportionate short stature is the most common presentation of skeletal dysplasia, systemic causes of short stature are usually proportionate. Exceptions include few forms of osteogenesis imperfecta and hypophosphatasia (HPP) which may present with proportionate short stature.

Another important consideration in dealing with skeletal dysplasia is the concept of lethality. About 50 disorders are included in the group of lethal dysplasias. By far the most common lethal dysplasia, at or before birth, is thanatophoric dysplasia. Other relatively common lethal SD include homozygous achondroplasia, achondrogenesis type I, osteogenesis imperfecta type II, etc.

Usually, these conditions are lethal because the infant possesses a small rib cage as a direct result of having short ribs, leading to respiratory insufficiency and death in most cases. The chest/abdominal circumference ratio in these cases is usually <0.85 and reflects the reduction of chest size. No children of asphyxiating thoracic dysplasia (ATD) who have managed to live beyond 2 years and have been reported to die of respiratory insufficiency. The reason for this appears to be the growth of the thoracic cage, resulting in adequate respiratory function. It is therefore very critical when dealing with a newborn with skeletal dysplasia to establish the diagnosis quickly and then to decide if the child should receive ventilator care.[8,9]

The nonlethal SD are a much larger group. Some dysplasias may present at birth or even prenatally such as achondroplasia. Many others may not manifest until a failure of growth is noted, hence the age of presentation is highly variable. They are considered according to the time of appearance, at birth or early infancy, or others after 2 years of age. The nonlethal dysplasia commonly presenting at the time of birth is heterozygous achondroplasia. The radiographic findings are quite specific to this disorder, which is differentiated from pseudoachondroplasia where the head is normal-sized.

Most patients of nonlethal dysplasias, if managed properly, can live relatively normal and productive lives.

RADIOLOGICAL EVALUATION

Skeletal Survey

The skeletal survey for the diagnosis of skeletal dysplasia includes the following radiographs according to the American College of Radiology (ACR) and the Society for Pediatric Radiology (SPR) guidelines.[10]

Axial Skeleton

- Skull—anteroposterior (AP) and lateral (also assess cervical spine on lateral skull radiograph)
- Chest—Frontal view (also assess thoracic spine)

- Pelvis—AP view (also assess lumbar spine)
- Lateral radiograph of the thoracolumbar spine

Appendicular Skeleton

- One upper limb
- One lower limb
- Left hand—for bone age

As most SD are symmetric in nature, therefore, we acquire radiographs of the appendicular skeleton on one side only, however, in cases with epiphyseal irregularity or stippling, it is recommended to obtain radiographs of both sides upper and lower limbs because Conradi-Hünermann type chondrodysplasia punctata (CDP) often causes asymmetric epiphyseal stippling.

Special views may be included according to suspicion for particular dysplasia, for example, lateral radiograph of the knee to demonstrate patellar cartilage stippling in Zellweger syndrome and for "double patella sign" in MED.

As dysplasias continue to evolve phenotypically throughout life, serial radiographs are recommended and comparison should always be made with previous radiographs to assess the evolution of disease and complications. Repeat survey is usually recommended after a period of about 1 year so that to reduce radiation exposure to the child and to allow for new skeletal changes to manifest. For example, metaphoric dysplasia manifests as a short limb disorder at infancy but gradually changes to short trunk dwarfism in children and adults due to progressive kyphoscoliosis.

After obtaining the above radiographs, they need to be analyzed systematically. Offiah and Hall have described a very useful systematic approach for the evaluation of the skeletal survey given by mnemonic ABCD.[11]

- *A*—Anatomical localization
- *B*—Bones
- *C*—Complications
- *D*—Dead/alive

A—Anatomical Localization

Skeletal dysplasias can involve either the axial skeleton (skull and spine, ribcage, and pelvis) or the appendicular skeleton (long bones). Various prefixes are used for skeletal dysplasia depending on the part involved. For example, when the spine or any of its parts are shortened, the prefix "spondylo" is used and it causes short trunk dwarfism, cranio/cranial for the skull, facio/facial for facial bones, mandibulo for mandible, cleido for clavicle, costo for ribs, and ischio/ilio/pubic for pelvis. Involvement of the long bones causes short limb dwarfism and is subclassified into rhizomelia (proximal segment shortening involving the humerus and/or femur), mesomelia when, there is a shortening of the middle segment of limb (radius and tibia), acromelia when there is a shortening of the distal segment of the limbs (hands and feet) and micromelia when there is a shortening of all segments of the limbs.

These definitions are important because the terminologies of many disorders were created based on radiologic findings, although they may be confusing at times. The SD are often classified according to whether the epiphysis, the metaphysis or the diaphysis is involved. Thus, the tubular bones must be viewed before the closure of the epiphyseal plate. Epiphyseal involvement leads to premature osteoarthritis. Metaphyseal involvement manifests as short bones and diaphyseal involvement leads to deformities of bones.

B—Bones

The following mnemonic of five ''S's'' is very helpful for analysis of bones:

1. *Structure*
2. *Shape*
3. *Size*
4. *Sum*
5. *Soft tissues*

Structure

Assessment of the structure of bone includes the general appearance of the bones, bone density, and the presence of wormian bones, tumorous lesions such as exostoses, and enchondromas. After identifying a particular abnormality, its distribution further helps to narrow the diagnosis. For example, osteosclerosis may diffusely affect all bones or may be limited to certain bones, or appear as bone islands as seen in osteopoikilosis, or metaphyseal striations as seen in osteopathia striata.

Shape

Certain alterations in shape can suggest a specific diagnosis and these alterations in shape may diffusely involve the whole bone or may be localized to a part of a bone, for example, in the limbs, alteration may be seen in metaphyses, which may be flared, or the epiphyses may be stippled or cone-shaped. Various alterations can occur in the shape of vertebral bodies of the spine that include severe platyspondyly giving the wafer-thin appearance of vertebral bodies are seen in the thanatophoric dysplasias, hooked vertebral bodies (mucopolysaccharidoses), and posterior scalloping of the vertebral bodies in achondroplasia. In the pelvis, sloping acetabular roofs of the mucopolysaccharidoses and horizontal trident roofs are seen in achondroplasia.

Size

Bones can be short/long, large, broad, or hypoplastic, e.g., the fibula is relatively long in comparison to the tibia in hypochondroplasia, but relatively short in campomelic dysplasia.

Sum

Analyzing the radiographs for the number of bones that can be multiple in number, very few in number, or maybe fused, can provide a clue to a particular dysplasia. For example, chondroectodermal dysplasia has supernumerary teeth, diastrophic dysplasia may have multiple epiphyseal centers in the patella in some forms, while multiple centers in the calcaneum are almost pathognomonic of Larsen's syndrome. Certain dysplasias have absent bones such as patella in Nail-patella syndrome, absent radius in Holt-Oram syndrome or TAR (thrombocytopenia absent radius) syndrome. Fused carpal bones may be seen in Ellis-van Creveld syndrome. Polydactyly is seen in many dysplasias; it is classified as being preaxial if it occurs on the side of the thumb or big toe, and postaxial on the side of the little finger or toe.

Soft Tissues

Associated soft-tissue abnormalities such as wasting, excessive soft tissues, contractures, and calcification may change not only the diagnosis but also the patient's prognosis. For example, the simultaneous presence of multiple enchondromas and phleboliths changes the diagnosis to Maffucci's syndrome from Ollier's disease and it has prognostic significance as there is a greater risk of malignancy of up to about 30% in the latter.

C—Complications

After a certain diagnosis is made, careful assessment for associated complications is important from a management point of view. For example, fractures are common complications in both osteoporotic (e.g., osteogenesis imperfecta) and osteosclerotic (e.g., osteopetrosis) conditions. Mucopolysaccharidosis (MPS) can have atlantoaxial instability which can cause cervical myelopathy. Apart from the complications of the disease itself, we should not forget to look for complications of therapy, such as increasing angular deformity, excessive rate of the distraction of a leg length osteotomy site or infection, which may be local or distant (e.g., following bone marrow transplantation for osteopetrosis).

D—Dead or Alive

Knowing the status of the patient being dead or alive points to the lethality of the dysplasia and also the appropriate genetic counseling of the parents.

CROSS-SECTIONAL IMAGING MODALITIES

Computed tomography (CT) and magnetic resonance imaging (MRI) are helpful ancillary modalities to assess intracranial and spinal cord anomalies in SD. They are also helpful in assessing not only bony abnormalities of the cranium and the spinal canal, but also permit detailed evaluation of internal soft-tissue structures **(Figs. 1A and B)**. Bony craniofacial anomalies can be well assessed by three-dimensional CT. Detailed imaging of the spine using MR helps in preoperative workup before reconstructive surgery.[8,12] Thus, these modalities help in planning management and help in improving the prognosis.

PRENATAL DIAGNOSIS OF SKELETAL DYSPLASIA

It is difficult to diagnose SD in utero during a routine ultrasound. This is because of the global involvement of multiple anatomic regions simultaneously in skeletal dysplasia as compared to anomalies of other systems which are usually regional in nature. Therefore, evaluation of skeletal dysplasia needs a meticulous step-by-step approach for assessment of long bones, spine and thorax, fetal head, mineralization of bones, and for any joint contractures/dislocations. The bones should be evaluated for number, absence or deficiency, (absent, delayed or supernumerary) ossification centers, contour abnormality, mineralized content, and fractures. If there is disproportionate limb shortening, then the segment (rhizo, meso, or acromelic) involved should be assessed. The dysplasia may be suspected during a routine ultrasound if an abnormal or short bone or

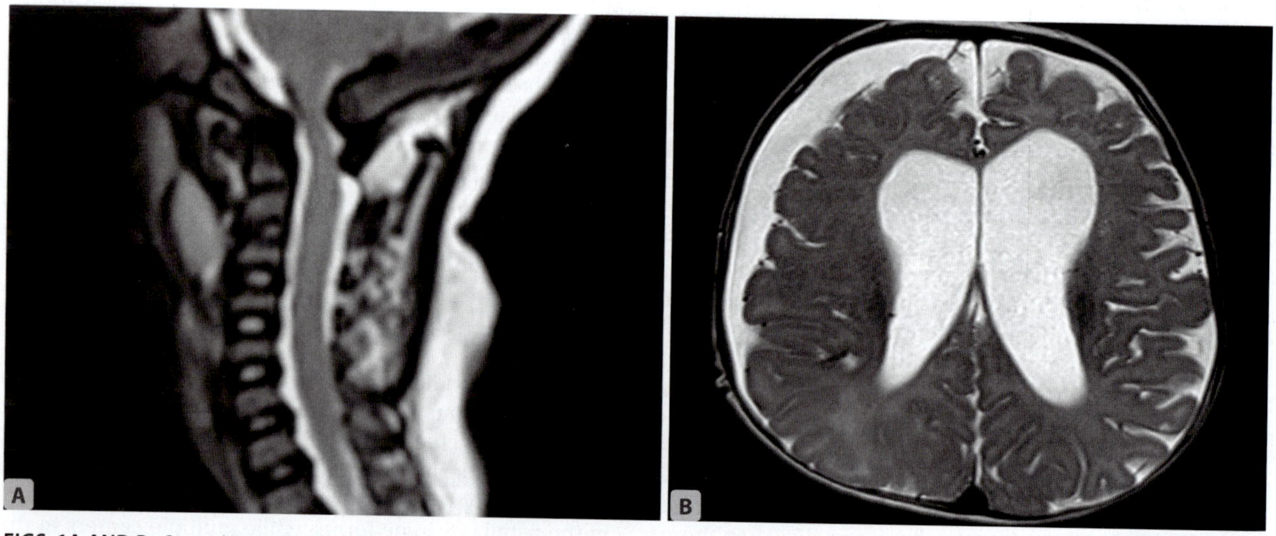

FIGS. 1A AND B: Sagittal T2W (A) and axial T2W (B) MRI images of a 1-year-old patient of proven case of achondroplasia with positive FGFR mutation demonstrate the narrowing of foramen magnum at CV junction with obliteration of anterior and posterior subarachnoid spaces and upstream obstructive hydrocephalous. (CV: craniovertebral; FGFR: fibroblast growth factor receptor; MRI: magnetic resonance imaging; T2W: T2 weighted)

Source: Case courtesy by Dr Mohammad Shoaib, Maulana Azad Medical College, New Delhi.

some other abnormal skeletal finding is detected. It is also important to evaluate chest circumference, femur length-abdominal circumference ratio to assess the possibility of lethality, besides evaluating for other craniofacial and skeletal anomalies.[13,14]

Practical Approach to Skeletal Dysplasia

As the SD often have diverse and overlapping radiological findings and there are around 461 diseases arranged into 42 groups, a discussion of all the groups is beyond the scope of this book. Also, apart from a few common entities, rest are all so rare that even the experienced clinical or radiologist may find it difficult to accurately diagnose them. Therefore, after analyzing a skeletal survey of the patient, it is practically very useful to approach the dysplasias according to the pattern of involvement in terms of predominant anatomic location (as epiphyseal, metaphyseal, diaphyseal, and dysplasias with predominant spine involvement), altered bone density as sclerosing or osteopenic dysplasias, a common constellation of findings such as dysostosis multiplex, dysplasias with a single site or segment, etc.

Various important lethal and nonlethal skeletal dysplasia are discussed under the following groups as follows:[15]

- Epiphyseal dysplasia
- Metaphyseal dysplasia
- Diaphyseal dysplasia
- Dysplasia with predominant involvement of the spine
- Dysostoses multiplex
- Sclerosing or osteopenic dysplasias
- Dysplasias with a single site or segment involvement
- Dysplasias with multiple joint dislocations
- Entities with disorganized development of skeletal components
- Dysostoses

Epiphyseal Dysplasias

All heterogeneously diverse dysplasias belonging to this broad group share common radiological findings of abnormal epiphyses and epiphyseal irregularity which can lead to early osteoarthritis and deformities such as coxa vara and genu valgum.

Chondrodysplasia Punctata Group

It can be divided into rhizomelic chondrodysplasia punctata (RCDP) which is autosomal recessive and Conradi-Hünermann type which has both autosomal dominant and X-linked dominant forms.

Rhizomelic Chondrodysplasia Punctate

Clinicopathological findings: It is transmitted as an autosomal recessive trait with a female preponderance. Most of the cases manifest clinically before 2 years of age. There is craniofacial dysmorphism (flat face with depressed nasal bridge and hypertelorism), ocular abnormalities (cataracts and optic atrophy), severe mental retardation, spastic tetraplegia and joint contractures with symmetric limb shortening (usually maximal in upper arms). Skin changes may include ichthyosis. Mucoid degeneration in the epiphyseal center has been seen histologically which leads to fragmentation of the epiphyses. This becomes a nidus for calcareous deposits or punctate ossification. Stillbirth or early death is usual, usually within the first year of life because of respiratory complications.[16] Tracheal stenosis or spinal cord compression is often the cause of death in the rhizomelic group.

Radiological Findings

Limbs: Findings in the limbs include stippled calcification **(Fig. 2A)** of the cartilage at the end of the epiphyses of long bones at birth which disappears by 1 year of age in survivors of the disease and epiphyses become irregular. There is symmetric rhizomelic or mesomelic limb shortening with metaphyseal splaying.[14] There can be delayed ossification of carpal bones.

Spine: Lumbar and thoracic regions show coronal clefts (unossified cartilage between anterior and posterior ossification centers of vertebral bodies which ossify with time, **Fig. 2B**). Stippling may occur but it is not always as prominent as seen in nonrhizomelic CDP.

Nonrhizomelic Chondrodysplasia Punctate (Conradi–Hünermann Type)

This is a benign nonrhizomelic group with a good prognosis having similar craniofacial and dermal changes such as the rhizomelic form of chondrodysplasia punctata. However, the limb-shortening is less severe and is often asymmetric. Intelligence is normal. Additionally, there is a presence of structural abnormalities of the vertebral bodies which may cause spinal deformity.

Imaging Features

Limbs: In mild cases, punctate calcification may be present only in the tarsus and carpus with no limb-shortening. In severe cases, there is widespread involvement with stippling seen in ankles, feet, patellae, hands, and wrists (pelvis, vertebrae, intervertebral disks, sternum, scapulae, rib cartilages, and mandible may also be involved). The stippling may be periarticular and extended into the tissues outside the normal epiphyses.

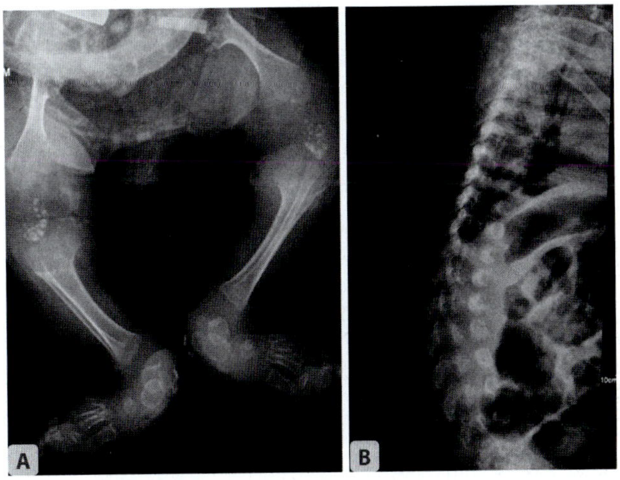

FIGS. 2A AND B: In a case of rhizomelic chondrodysplasia punctata (CDP), anteroposterior (AP) radiograph of bilateral lower extremities (A) demonstrate rhizomelic shortening with epiphyseal stippling. The lateral radiograph (B) of thoracolumbar spine shows coronal clefts.

Thorax and pelvis: No special features apart from epiphyseal stippling.

Spine: Marked stippling is seen in the vertebral and paravertebral regions.

Other areas: Calcification of the larynx and tracheal ring cartilage is sometimes found and tracheal stenosis is an important cause of mortality in these children.

The radiologic appearance is characteristic and should not be confused with other conditions **(Fig. 2)**. Rhizomelia, coronal clefts, and mental retardation help to differentiate RCDP from other forms of CDP. Zellweger syndrome involves stippled calcification in the patellar bone and usually does not have coronal clefts. In cretins, there can be epiphyseal fragmentation which is however larger and conforms to the expected shadow of theepiphysis.

Multiple Epiphyseal Dysplasia

Clinical features: It is transmitted in an autosomal dominant manner in most of the cases. Mild dwarfism with flexion deformities and degenerative arthritis is frequentlypresent.

Imaging features: Radiographic findings are especially prominent in the hip, knee, wrist, and ankles.

The ossification centers appear late, show delayed mineralization, and are fragmented. They ossify from multiple centers and can have a *"mulberry appearance"*. The secondary centers are small and flattened. The fusion of ossification centers is also delayed, and a fragmented piece of the center may result in the formation of a loose body. In older patients, slipped epiphyses may occur with resultant deformities of joint, such as tibiotalar slant, genu valgum, and premature osteoarthritis **(Fig. 3)**. The metaphyseal changes are especially noticeable in metacarpal and metatarsal bones. There are short broad phalanges with the irregularity of epiphyseal ends of bones. The spine is affected in two-thirds of patients and changes include mild anterior wedging with the mild irregularity of the anterior aspect of endplates associated with scoliosis and multiple Schmorl's nodes typically in mid-thoracic spine. It can mimic Scheuermann's disease. Double patella sign in lateral radiograph of the knee is considered highly pathognomic, but it is also uncommonly seen in pseudochondrodysplasia.[17]

The involvement of multiple epiphyses with relative lack of metaphyseal change helps in differentiating this condition from Perthes' disease. In cretins, the bone age is severely retarded, which is a helpful differentiating feature.

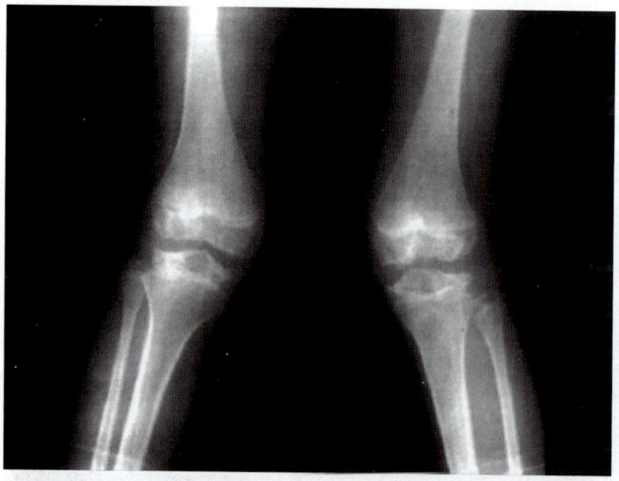

FIG. 3: X-ray of both knees anteroposterior (AP) view showing epiphyseal flattening with irregularity of both distal femora and proximal tibia with mild fibular flattening and resultant genu-valgum, in a case of multiple epiphyseal dysplasia.

Pseudoachondroplasia

Clinical features: Pseudoachondroplasia is an autosomal dominant dysplasia caused due to mutation affecting the *COMP* gene similar to MED. Since both pseudoachondroplasia and MED share a common gene mutation, there is considerable overlap in the age of presentation and radiographic appearance in both entities except for the fact that pseudoachondroplasia is more severe in clinical and radiographic involvement as compared to MED.

Imaging findings: Vertebral bodies show the presence of anterior tongue-like projection which disappears with age and is replaced by platyspondyly giving rise to the short limb-short trunk dwarfism. This is known as central tongue appearance and is highly pathognomic of the disease. The main differential diagnoses of pseudoachondroplasia include MED and achondroplasia. MED and pseudoachondroplasia may be differentiated based on the clinical history and certain almost pathognomic radiologic findings. Clinically, pseudoachondroplasia has joint and ligamentous laxity with the presence of central anterior tongue and platyspondyly whereas MED shows restricted and painful movements with double-layered patella on lateral knee radiograph. Secondly, in pseudoachondroplasia, the dwarfism and shortening of the extremities are severe as compared to MED as it is considered a more severe manifestation of mutation on the same gene.[17]

Metaphyseal Dysplasia

This group of dysplasias has a widening of metaphysis or metaphyseal irregularity and eventual limb shortening, which can be rhizomelic typically seen in thanatophoric dysplasia, achondroplasia, metaphyseal chondrodysplasia and mesomelic/acromelic as in Ellis-van Creveld syndrome and ATD.

Thanatophoric Dysplasia

Clinical features: As the name implies, thanatophoric dysplasia meaning "death bearing", is the most common lethal bony dysplasia. Clinically, the disease is so severe that it may be recognized in utero, with a family history of polyhydramnios and spontaneous abortions. The neonate has markedly shortened limbs with a normal size of the trunk, however, the thorax is markedly narrow in contrast to protruding abdomen with the resultant inability of the infant to inflate the lung.

Imaging Features

Limbs: Markedly shortened rhizomelic tubular bones along with bowing, bony widening, and presence of flaring of the metaphyses. Bowed femora are characteristic and appear like telephone receivers **(Fig. 4A)**.

Skull: Findings in the skull include frontal bossing, macrocephaly, cloverleaf skull with a small skull base, and foramen magnum **(Fig. 4B)**.

Thorax and pelvis: Thoracic capacity is reduced along with short ribs with flaring of their anterior ends **(Fig. 4C)**. Changes in pelvis include small, squared innominate bones, and sacrosciatic notches. The pubic and ischial bones are also wide and short **(Fig. 4A)**.

Spine: Vertebral bodies are flattened with a reduced height of their middle portions and consequently prominent intervertebral disk spaces, while posterior neural arches are normally formed. This gives a typical H-shaped appearance of vertebrae on the AP view. Narrowing of the spinal canal is the most marked in the lumbar region. The features distinguishing this dysplasia from achondroplasia are severe universal vertebra plana in the spine and short tubular bowed bones of limbs.

Prenatal diagnosis by sonography is possible. Polyhydramnios, poor fetal activity, and the presence of extra ossification pelvic centers can help in the diagnosis of the dysplasia in utero.[18]

Achondroplasia

Clinicopathological features: Achondroplasia is the most common type of nonlethal dysplasia presenting with rhizomelic dwarfism. It is a hereditary condition with an autosomal dominant mode of transmission, though now most cases may be due to spontaneous mutation of the *FGFR3* gene associated with increased paternal age, in 85% of cases. The disorder shows a generalized defect in enchondral bone formation. It presents at birth and is characterized clinically by a large head with brachycephaly, prominent frontal bones with a depressed nasal bridge, rhizomelic dwarfism, constricted thorax, and trident hands due to separation of third and fourth digits. The apophyseal growth is deficient toward the metaphysis, resulting in a V-shaped defect in which the epiphysis is incorporated. A fibrous band growing from periosteum can interpose between the epiphysis and the ossifying cartilage with resultant stunting of longitudinal growth.

Imaging Features

Skull: Defective growth of the base of the skull and facial bones giving a pinched appearance with compensatory overexpansion of vault of skull and frontal regions. The foramen magnum is small and funnel-shaped. CT and MRI of the craniocervical region show associated **(Fig. 5A)** abnormalities of the cervicomedullary junction. Due to the narrowing of the foramen magnum, associated upstream obstructive hydrocephalus can be seen.

Thorax and pelvis: Anteroposterior diameter of chest is decreased due to short ribs. Changes in pelvis include square

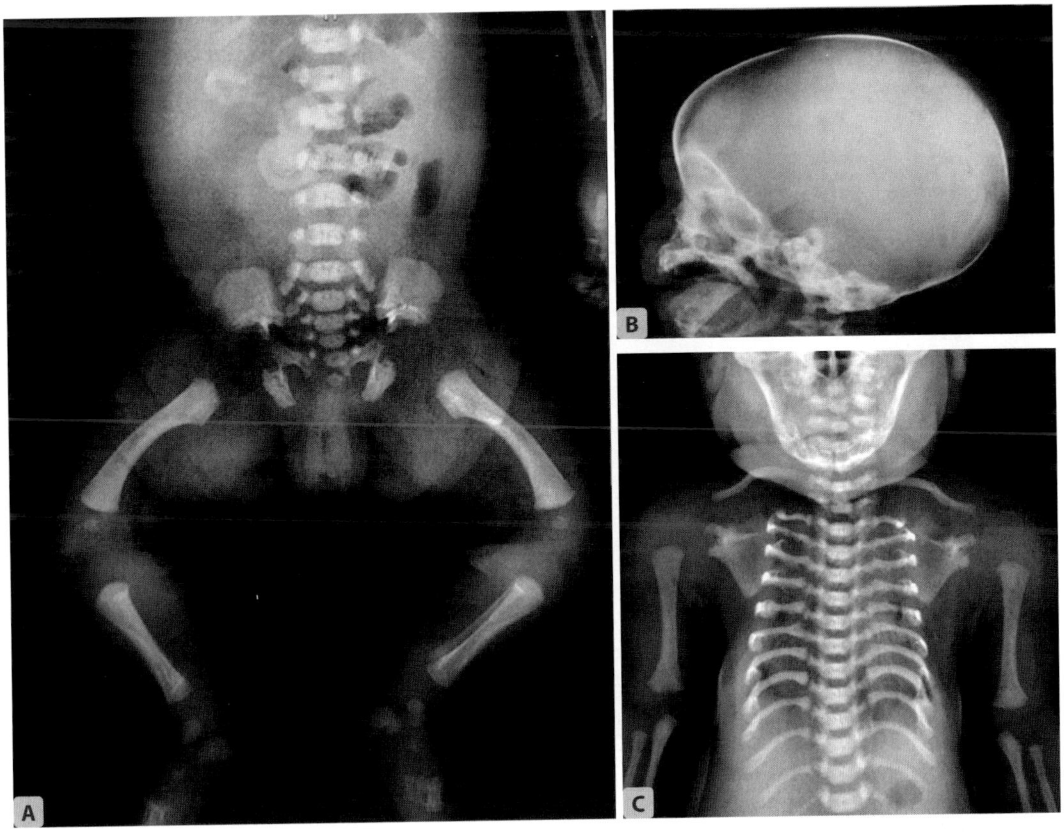

FIGS. 4A TO C: In a 1-day-old newborn child of thanatophoric dysplasia: Anteroposterior (AP) radiograph (A) of pelvis with both lower extremities demonstrate small-squared iliac, small pubic bones with widening of pubic symphysis. Bilateral femurs are shortened and bowed giving telephone handle appearance. Lateral radiograph of skull (B) shows macrocephaly with frontal bossing and small skull base. AP radiograph of thorax (C) shows small-sized thoracic cavity with shortened ribs with flared anterior ends.

iliac bones with posteriorly set horizontal acetabular roof and small sacrosciatic notches giving classical *"tombstone appearance"* **(Fig. 5B)**.

Spine: Vertebral bodies are either normal or mildly reduced in height with other spinal abnormalities including a reduction in interpedicular distances in the lumbar region with short and thick pedicles with resultant narrowing of the spinal canal and posterior vertebral scalloping **(Figs. 5C and D)**. With advancing age, severe spinal cord compromise and disk protrusions become especially important and are best evaluated by MRI.

Limbs: Rhizomelic shortening of proximal bones, with deep-seated epiphyses in flared metaphyses, gives a V-shaped appearance (Chevron deformity), mostly seen at the lower end of the femur and disappears with age **(Fig. 5E)**. Shortening and widening of tubular bones of hand and feet, with typical involvement of proximal and middle phalanges, can also be seen. Space between 3rd and 4th digits is widened giving rise to the characteristic "trident hand".

There is rarely any difficulty in diagnosing achondroplasia, however, it must be differentiated mainly from thanatotropic dysplasia in children and hypochondroplasia in adults. In hypochondroplasia, the radiologic findings are quite similar but less severe than achondroplasia and the skull is never affected.

Hypochondroplasia

Clinical features: This dysplasia is transmitted in an autosomal dominant mode and affects the same *FGFR* gene receptor as achondroplasia. The clinical features include short stature and disproportionate short limbs. The head is normal, which distinguishes it from achondroplasia. It usually manifests after 2–4 years of life.

Imaging Features

Limbs: Show rhizomelia with metaphyseal flaring. Mild symmetric brachydactyly is seen involving all the metacarpals and phalanges, unlike achondroplasia in which 2nd to 5th metacarpals and proximal phalanges are more affected. Trident hand is not seen in hypochondroplasia.

Spine: Similar to achondroplasia-like reduced interpedicular distances, however, other vertebral changes are mild, and spinal canal stenosis is less. In contrast to achondroplasia, the skull, pelvis, and hands are essentially normal.

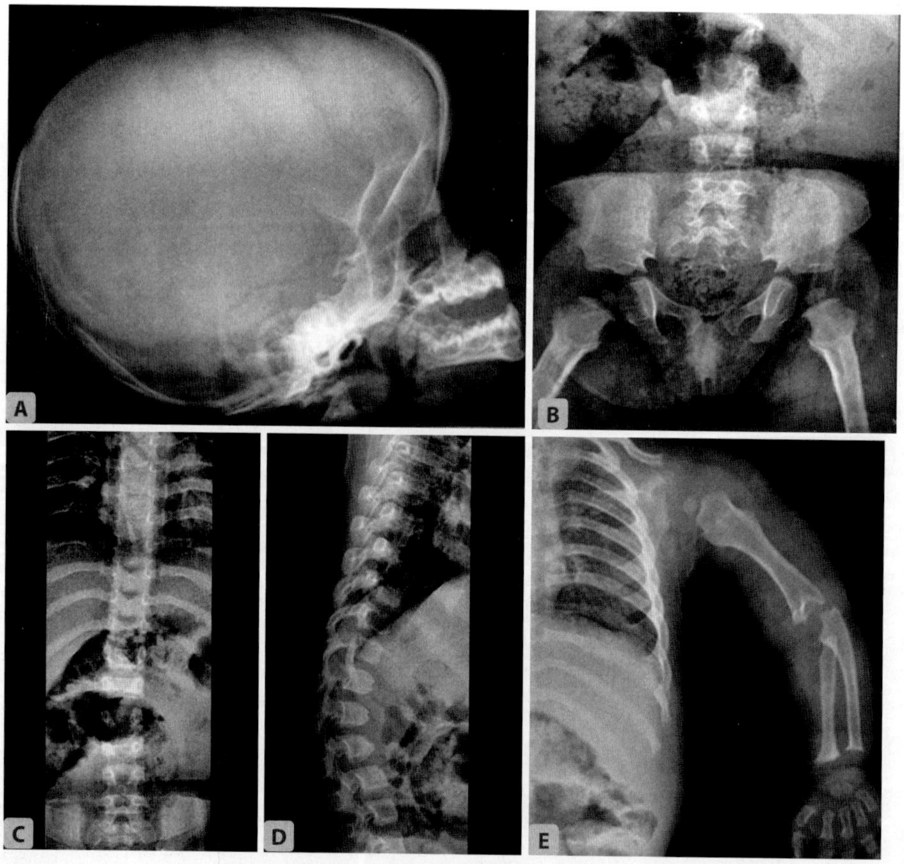

FIGS. 5A TO E: In a 2-year-old child of achondroplasia: lateral radiograph of skull (A) shows depressed nasal bridge with hypoplasia of facial bones giving pinched appearance, small size of base of skull with macrocephaly and frontal bossing. Anteroposterior (AP) radiograph of pelvis (B) shows presence of small pelvis with squaring of iliac wings with horizontal acetabular roof giving tombstone appearance. AP (C) and lateral (D) radiographs of DL spine shows decreasing interpedicular distance and posterior vertebral scalloping. AP radiograph of upper extremities (E) showing rhizomelic shortening of humerus with V-shaped defect of the distal humeral metaphysis.

Asphyxiating Thoracic Dysplasia (ATD, Jeune Syndrome)

Clinical features: This is an autosomal recessive condition, which is evident at birth. The infants have characteristically constricted chests with shortening of the extremities. There is also a marked pulmonary hypoplasia. Most infants die due to respiratory distress while renal failure is frequent in those that survive.

Imaging Features

Thorax and pelvis: Features include "high handlebar" appearance of clavicles along with narrow thorax, short horizontal ribs, and wide irregular costochondral junctions. Changes in pelvis include short ilia with flat acetabular roof and downward spike-like projections giving "trident appearance" to the acetabulum.

Limbs: Premature ossification of the capital femoral epiphysis is fairly common with the presence of metaphyseal irregularity. Shortening of middle and distal phalanges can occur due to premature fusion of cone-shaped epiphyses.

Skull and spine: These are normal.

It is not associated with congenital heart disease.[19] It can be differentiated from chondroectodermal dysplasia by the presence of short ribs, hepatic fibrosis, and a higher incidence of progressive renal disease. Besides, there are less frequent polydactyly and less frequent nail changes.

Chondroectodermal Dysplasia (Ellis–van Creveld syndrome)

Clinical features: This is short-limbed dwarfism and presents at birth, as the mode of inheritance is autosomal recessive. It is characterized by dysplasia of ectodermal elements (including hair, teeth, and nails), congenital cardiac defects, and polydactyly. There is a distal shortening of limbs, absent or hypoplastic nails, abnormal hair, dysplastic teeth, and upper lip abnormalities. Death is common in childhood due to cardiac and pulmonary complications.

Imaging Features

In addition to changes in ATD, there is the presence of carpal fusion, postaxial poly, and syndactyly. Drumstick appearance due to bulbous enlargement of proximal end of ulna and distal end of radius along with dislocation of radial heads anteriorly is also a characteristic finding. Medial tibial exostoses, wide but hypoplastic lateral aspect of proximal tibia, genu valgum, and fibular shortening are other typical features. Atrial septal defect is a commonly associated cardiac abnormality. The spine and skull are normal.

Metaphyseal Chondrodysplasia

Metaphyseal chondrodysplasias are a large heterogeneous group of disorders.

Jansen Type

Clinical features: This is a rare severe dysplasia due to excessive proliferating hypertrophic cartilage in the metaphyses. There is swelling of joints, bowed forearms and legs, and dwarfism detectable at birth.

Imaging features: In infancy, there is marked irregularity of the metaphyses, widened growth plate, and bowing of tubular bones with diffuse osteopenia. Subperiosteal resorption of bones and fractures also occur in childhood. There is cupping of the metaphyses with a wide zone of irregular calcification. There is resultant dwarfism with metaphyseal flaring and bowed bones. Spine shows minimal platyspondyly. There is basilar and supraorbital ridge sclerosis with osteopenia of the skull vault.

In the early cases, the differential diagnosis includes renal osteodystrophy and HPP, however, the radiological features are diagnostic.

Schmid Type

Clinical features: Presents in early childhood and this is often misdiagnosed as rickets because of metaphyseal changes. It is transmitted as an autosomal dominant trait and manifests as mild dwarfism.

Imaging features: The skeletal abnormalities are not evident at birth but appear in the third and fourth year of life. Radiological findings include growth plate widening, metaphyseal irregularity, and flaring especially in the knee and hip joints. Coxa-vara is common due to the involvement of the metaphyses of proximal femora. The spine and hands are not involved.

Mckusick Type

It is also known as cartilage hair hypoplasia. Patients also show irregular metaphyses with bowing and dwarfism, but the brittle and short hair accompanying the syndrome help in differentiation.

Hypophosphatasia

Hypophosphatasia is a rare metabolic systemic disorder that occurs due to mutation in the gene encoding tissue nonspecific alkaline phosphatase (TNSALP) leading to the low activity of alkaline phosphatase (ALP) in the body. Low levels of ALP lead to impaired metabolism and accumulation of inorganic pyrophosphates which interfere with the growth of hydroxyapatite crystals and thus causing defective mineralization and skeletal abnormalities.

Clinical features: Four clinical groups are recognized according to the age of onset, although the distinction between them is not always possible due to the variability in presentation due to variable deficiency of ALP. These include the perinatal (in utero or at birth), infantile (<6 months), childhood (>6 months to <18 years) and adult (>18 years) form. Earlier the onset of the disease, more the severity of disease which can range from death in the perinatal form to bone fragility and dental abnormalities in the adult form of HPP.

Imaging Features

Perinatal form: The radiological features in the perinatal form include diffuse profound defective ossification with broad, irregular metaphyses, seen prominently at the wrists, knee, and costochondral junctions. The cranial sutures also appear wide due to defective ossification. Fractures are common.

Infantile form: It is characterized by the widening of the cartilaginous growth plate and frayed and cupped metaphyses with the epiphyses showing spotty demineralization. Mild irregularity of the diaphysis can also be evident due to defective mineralization. The skull shows premature fusion with subsequent craniosynostosis, often with a brachycephalic configuration.[18]

Childhood form: The characteristic features in childhood form include bowed legs or knock knees, mild rachitic changes, premature loss of deciduous teeth, and dental caries. Craniosynostosis is usually not present.

Adult form: The adult form is characterized by the presence of osteopenia, Looser's zones, and actual fractures.

The perinatal form of HPP was considered lethal, but with the availability of enzyme replacement therapy, the mortality has gone down. The differential diagnosis of the perinatal form includes other fatal short limb dwarfisms, osteogenesis imperfecta, and severe rickets. Osteogenesis imperfecta can be ruled out by the presence of wormian bones and fractures and the absence of metaphyseal punched out defects. In rickets, there are no punched out metaphyseal defects and elevated serum ALP. Metaphyseal chondrodysplasia can be differentiated by normal bone structure and no punched out metaphyseal defects.

Dysplasia with Predominant Involvement of Diaphyses

Oto-palato-digital Spectrum Disorders

It is a group of related diseases including Melnick–Needles syndrome, Otopalatodigital syndrome type 1 and 2, and frontometaphyseal dysplasia and collectively referred to as oto-palato-digital spectrum disorders. As the name suggests, these disorders involve the malformations in-ear ossicles causing hearing problems, developmental defects of mouth (palate), and skeletal anomalies involving the digits (fingers/toes).

Melnick–Needles syndrome is at the most severe end of the spectrum and is usually seen in females as it is fatal in utero in males because it is an X-linked dominant disorder. Clinically, they present with a typical craniofacial and skeletal abnormalities with typical facial appearance (prominent supraorbital ridge, depressed nasal bridge, down-slanted palpebral fissure and hyperteleroism). Radiological features include micrognathia, sclerosis of skull bones, scoliotic/kyphotic deformity of the spine with the anterior concavity of vertebrae, multiple constrictions of ribs giving rise to ribbon-shaped ribs, dysplastic pelvis and bowed limbs with metaphyseal flaring and distorted diaphyseal contour with irregular thickened cortices.

Frontometaphyseal Dysplasia

Clinical manifestations include childhood-onset, short trunk with long extremities, prominent supraorbital ridges, micrognathia, and joint contractures. The radiologic features of this dysplasia include calvarial hyperostosis, prominent supraorbital ridge, absent frontal sinuses, hypoplasia of angle, and condylar processes of the mandible, antegonial notching of the body of mandible, flaring of the iliac wings with the widening of ischial bones. Changes in tubular bones include fibular waviness and bowing, tibia recurvatum, elongation of metacarpal bones and phalanges with erosion and fusion of carpal and tarsalbones.

Otopalatodigital syndrome (OPD) type 1 and 2: Type 1 OPD syndrome is the mildest of the OPD spectrum disorders and is fully manifest in males only, while females having only mild expression. It is characterized by the presence of supraorbital hyperostosis, abnormalities of thumb and digits such as short and spatulate thumb, broad distal phalanges, and clinodactyly which is the most prominent in 5th digit. Type 2 OPD syndrome is more severe than type 1 with more prominent skull base sclerosis, prominent anomalies of thumb and digits, and thoracic hypoplasia.

Dysplasia with Major Involvement of the Spine

This group includes dysplasias having epiphyseal involvement with platyspondyly and include disorders such as spondyloepiphyseal dysplasia congenita (SEDC) and tarda, Kniest dysplasia and achondrogenesis type 2.

Spondyloepiphyseal Dysplasia Congenita

As the name suggests, SEDC affects the spine and proximal epiphyses of long bones at birth and is an autosomal dominant disease due to mutation of mutation in *COL2A1* gene on chromosome locus 12q13.1 which codes for type II collagen protein. The hallmark of the disease is delayed ossification of epiphyses at birth.

Clinical features: This short limb dwarfism is characterized by mild shortening of the limbs, cleft palate, flat face, short neck, and increased anteroposterior chest diameter. Progressive kyphoscoliosis occurs as the child grows. Knock-knees and bowleg deformities are common. The hands and feet are normal.

Imaging Features

Spine: The height of vertebral bodies is decreased with pear-shaped vertebrae seen in infancy due to a lack of development of the posterior portion of vertebral bodies. Later on, in childhood, it progresses to anterior wedging, irregularity, and generalized flattening with reduced intervertebral disks and eventual development of kyphoscoliosis and lumbar lordosis. The interpedicular distances are narrowed in the lumbar region. Atlanto-axial dislocation due to hypoplasia of dens can also be present and poses a risk for cervical myelopathy.

Thorax and pelvis: The chest is broad and bell-shaped and of decreased height. There are, in addition, short-squared scapulae with flared anterior ends of ribs, delay in sternal ossification, and pectus-carinatum. There is a marked delay in ossification of the pubic bones and the proximal portion of femora. The femoral heads often ossify from multiple centers and progressive coxa vara develops with premature osteoarthritis. Prominent shortening of the neck of femora with small femoral heads well below the level of greater trochanter can be seen.

Limbs: The epiphyses are irregular and the metaphyses show flaring secondary to abnormal epiphyses and irregularity in long tubular bones. The ossification may be delayed. Bones of hands and feet are typically not involved **(Fig. 6)**.

Spondyloepiphyseal dysplasia congenita needs to be differentiated from spondyloepiphyseal dysplasia tarda (SEDT), Morquio's disease, diastrophic dwarfism, metatrophic dwarfism, and MEDs. Moriquo's disease can be differentiated from SEDC as Moriquo's disease has a central beaking of the spine with increased or maintained intervertebral disk spaces. Also, unlike SEDC hands and feet are abnormal in Moriquo's disease.

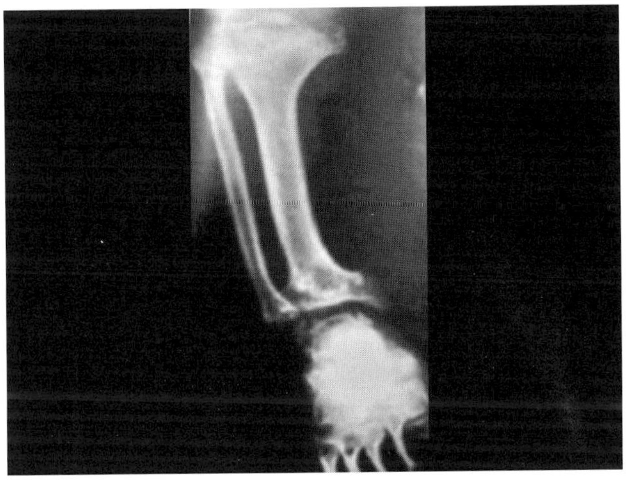

FIG. 6: Epiphyseal and metaphyseal irregularities with metaphyseal widening involving both tibia and fibula with angular deformity at the ankle joint in a case of spondyloepiphyseal dysplasia congenita.

X-linked Spondyloepiphyseal Dysplasia Tarda

Clinical features: This condition is seen exclusively in males as it is transmitted as a sex-linked trait. It becomes evident after 5 years of age due to impaired growth of the spine. The dwarfism is of the short limb type. Premature hip osteoarthritis with pain and limited motion is noticed around puberty.

Imaging Features

Spine: Platyspondyly is prominently present in the spine **(Figs. 7A and B)**. Other features include dense bone on the central and posterior portion of the endplates giving rise to a heaped up or hump-shaped appearance. The disk spaces consequently appear wide anteriorly and narrow posteriorly. The odontoid process may be deformed. The thoracic spine may have disk protrusions. Degenerative changes in the spine develop in early adult life.

Thorax and pelvis: There is a relative increase in the anteroposterior diameter of the chest. Pelvic bones and femoral necks may be small with the presence of coxa vara. Osteoarthritis involving hip can be disabling **(Fig. 7C)**.

Spondyloepiphyseal dysplasia tarda can be differentiated from SEDC as SEDT manifests in young boys compared to SEDC which is apparent at birth with the spine, hip, and joint changes more severe with progressive deformities in SEDC than SEDT. Other differentials include MED/pseudoachondroplasia which can be differentiated by looking for evidence of involvement of hands and feet in both MED and pseudoachondroplasia, hands, and feet are typically normal in SEDC/SEDT. Furthermore, platyspondyly is either absent as MED or moderate in pseudoachondroplasia, whereas both SEDC/SEDT has prominent platyspondyly. Morquio's disease can be excluded by the absence of severe platyspondyly and severe dysplasia of the peripheral epiphyses.

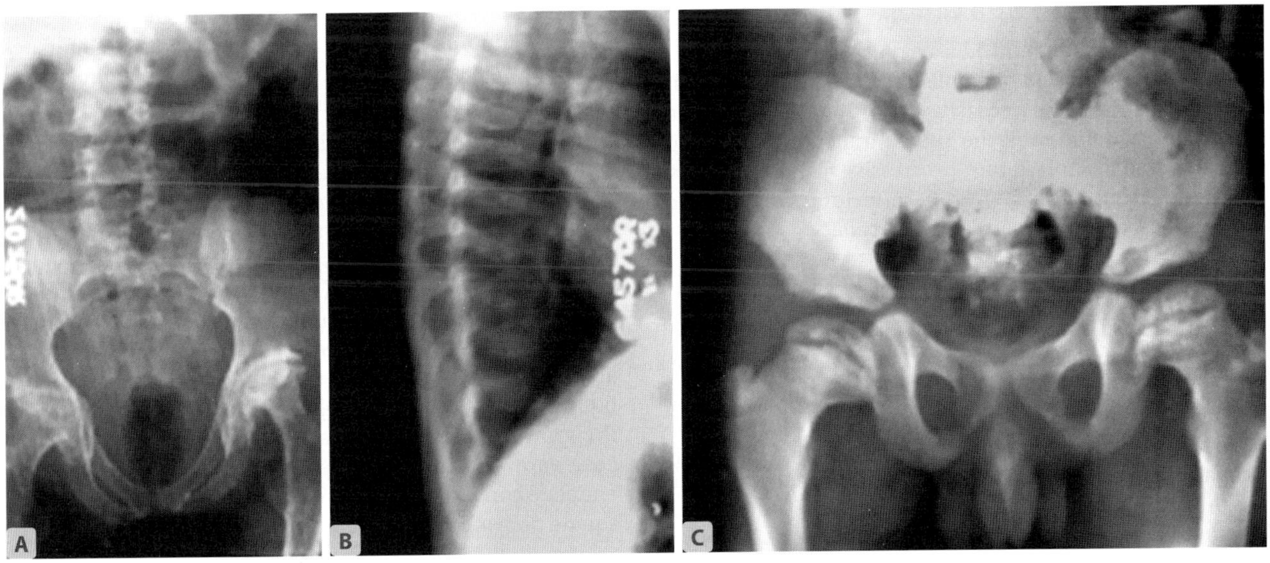

FIGS. 7A TO C: (A) X-ray spine anteroposterior (AP) and (B) lateral views showing generalized platyspondyly; (C) X-ray pelvis AP view-rounded flared ilia with distal tapering and bilateral symmetrical capital femoral epiphyseal flattening, sclerosis, and fissuring in a case of spondyloepiphyseal dysplasia tarda.

Kniest Dysplasia

Kniest dysplasia, also an autosomal dominant type II collagenopathy like SEDC affecting the same gene locus with similar clinical presentation in the form of short limb dwarfism with delayed ossification at birth and in infancy. However, dumbbell-shaped femora and coronal clefting of the spine are also noted at birth. Other findings include megaepiphyses with cloud-like calcifications, flattening of epiphyses of metacarpals, and enlargement at ends of metacarpals and proximal phalanges giving rise to bulbous metacarpophalangeal and proximal interphalangeal joints.

Achondrogenesis

Clinicopathologic features: Achondrogenesis is a phenotypically diverse group of chondrodysplasias characterized by a short trunk and micromelia. Achondrogenesis is classified into two types, type I and type II. In achondrogenesis I, the child is usually stillborn or dies soon after birth. Achondrogenesis II is not lethal and usually appears in children of consanguineous parents.

Imaging features: The radiologic findings in achondrogenesis I include hypoplastic and deformed iliac bones, extremely deficient ossification of vertebral bodies, pubic and ischial bones. There is severe micromelia involving the tubular bones, which are deformed and short with wide cupped ends. The ribs are also short and show cupped, flared ends. Rib fractures are present in some patients. The skull and other membranous bones are involved.

Imaging features in achondrogenesis II include shortening of bones in distal extremities. The bones are curved and distal segments may be absent. The ossification of bones of hand and feet is delayed. Polydactyly of the hands and feet is common. The skull and other membranous bones are not involved, distinguishing it from type I.

Diastrophic Dysplasia Group

Clinical features: The term "diastrophic" meaning twisted or crooked has been used to highlight the phenotype resulting from this autosomal recessive disorder. This dysplasia group has a mutation in the sulfate transporter gene. It is characterized by short stature, progressive scoliosis, kyphosis, clubfeet, Hitchhiker's thumb, multiple contractures, dislocations, deformed ears, and cleft palate.

Imaging Features

Limbs: There is micromelic dwarfism with markedly shortened tubular bones with a widening of metaphyses. The radiologic features include cortical thickening and diaphyseal sclerosis. The endosteal involvement is more than the periosteal involvement **(Fig. 8)**. The first metacarpal is oval and usually hypoplastic. There is delayed appearance of the epiphyses with flattening and deformity, seen characteristically in proximal and distal femora. Epiphyses in hand and foot bones may be irregular, distorted, and deformed. A disproportionate shortening of ulna and fibula can be present. Narrowing of joint spaces especially of hip and elbows can be seen. Short and broad femoral necks are also frequently seen.

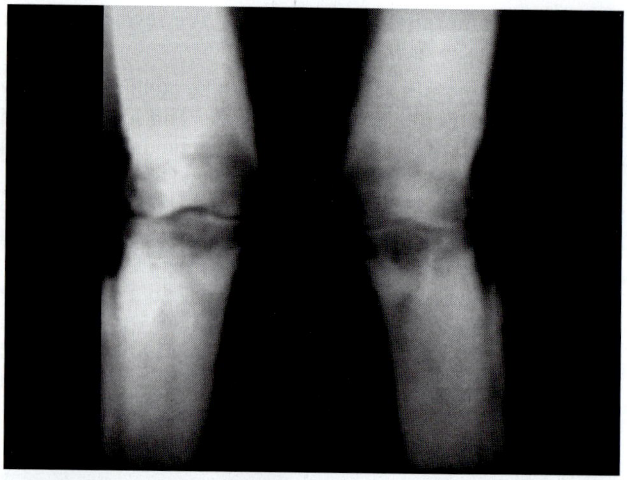

FIG. 8: Symmetrical (both periosteal and endosteal) new bone formation, obliterating the medullary cavity, sparing only the ends of the bones in a case of diastrophic dysplasia.

Spine: Scoliosis is progressive leading to spinal abnormalities, instability, cord compression, and death.

Diastrophic dysplasia needs to be differentiated from achondroplasia and Morquio's syndrome. The oval metacarpal of diastrophic dwarfism is the most distinguishing feature. The presence of a basal segment of innominate bone and the lack of reduction of the interpedicular distances in the lumbar region distinguish it from achondroplasia. The characteristic spinal changes in form of anterior beaking of lumbar vertebrae and "simian shaped" pelvis in Morquio's syndrome help in differentiating it from diastrophic dysplasia.

Spondylometaphyseal Dysplasias

Clinical features: This dysplasia is characterized by abnormalities in the vertebrae and metaphyses of tubular bones. Currently, there are around 10 described subtypes of SMD. The most important subtypes are Kozlowski and Sutcliffe types. In Kozlowski type, there is short stature, kyphosis and scoliosis, diminutive hands, and feet with bowing of bones.

Imaging features: Radiological findings include markedly retarded skeletal maturation with degenerative changes in joints. There is a flattening of vertebral bodies with pedicles located medially and altered spinal curvatures **(Figs. 9A and B)**. Metaphyseal irregularity is most evident at the ends of long bones **(Fig. 9C)**. Proximal femora are commonly involved with resultant coxa-vara. The iliac bones are shortened with small sacrosciatic notches and horizontal acetabular roof. In Sutcliffe type, there are small triangular bony fragments at the periphery of metaphyses adjacent to the growth plate (corner fracture appearance) and severe coxa vara. In the spine, the findings include exaggerated endplate convexity, anterior wedging of vertebral bodies and square or ovoid vertebral bodies.[19]

Metaphoric Dysplasia

Clinical features: Metaphoric means changing body proportions as the patient age as there are short extremities and normal trunk at birth but as age progresses there is

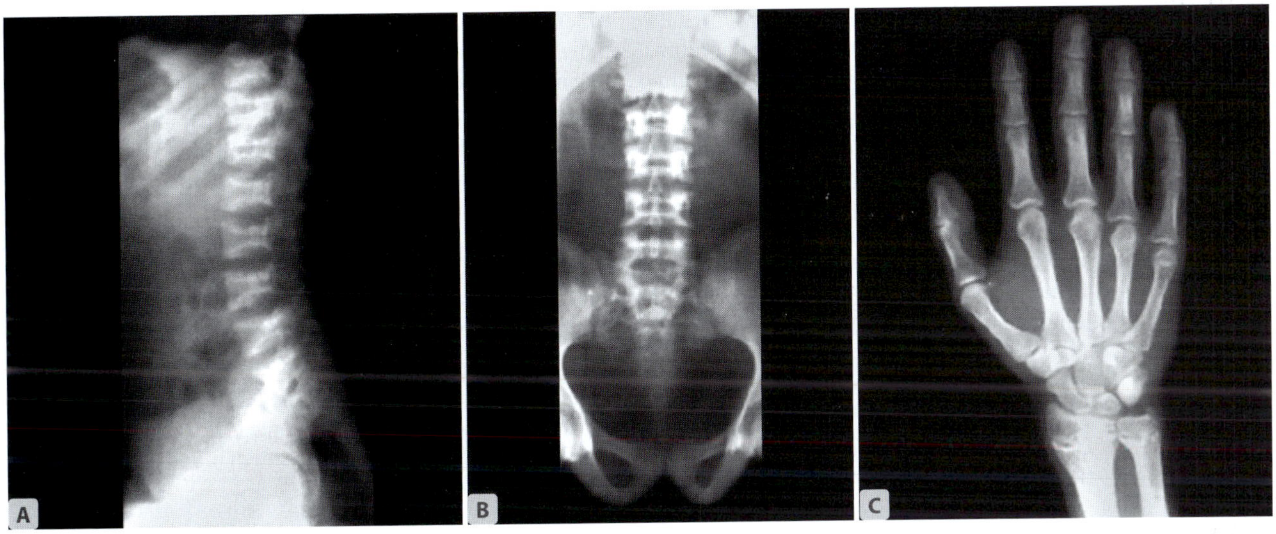

FIGS. 9A TO C: Lateral (A) and anteroposterior (AP) (B) radiographs of lumbar spine showing platyspondyly with endplate irregularity and sclerosis. Posteroanterior (PA) radiograph of left hand (C) showing metaphyseal cupping and irregularity involving distal metaphysis of radius and ulna in a case of spondylometaphyseal dysplasia.

spinal kyphoscoliosis with resultant short trunk relative to extremities, hence, the name "metatrophic dysplasia."

Imaging Features

Limbs: The limb bones are short with characteristic trumpet-like flaring of their metaphyses. The appearance of ossification centers may be delayed. With growth, the proximal ends of the femora (typically the lesser trochanter) develop a "battle-axe" configuration. The epiphyses show delayed appearance and are small and deformed.

Thorax and pelvis: The thorax is elongated with decreased AP diameter due to short ribs in infancy. There is severe anterior bowing of sternum with the development of kyphoscoliosis in childhood. Changes in pelvis include short ilia with curved lateral margins, flat acetabular roof, wide Y-shaped triradiate cartilage, and small sacrosciatic notches.

Spine: In the spine, vertebral bodies are markedly reduced in height (severe generalized platyspondyly) and appear rectangular or diamond-shaped and can show anterior wedging. The intervertebral disk spaces consequently appear large. The neural arches are well developed. In later childhood, the vertebrae become wedge-shaped with humped-up central and dorsal portions. Progressive spinal malalignment and secondary distortion of the thorax occurs. There may be hypoplasia of the dens with resultant atlantoaxial instability.

Since this dysplasia presents as rhizomelic shortening with a normal trunk at birth such as achondroplasia and later on changes into short trunk dysplasia similar to spondyloepiphyseal dysplasia congenita. Hence, its differential diagnoses include both achondroplasia and SEDC.

Dysostosis Multiplex

Mucopolysaccharidoses and Mucolipidoses

These are complex carbohydrate metabolism abnormalities associated with the absence of lysosomal enzymes needed for degradation of glycosaminoglycans (GAGs) or mucopolysaccharides which get deposited in various tissues causing coarse facies, mental retardation, and organomegaly. They can be diagnosed through specific metabolic tests such as fibroblast culture and assay. The role of radiologists in this group of disorders is limited but important especially in the evaluation of multiple skeletal abnormalities seen associated with them. As these disorders have multiple common skeletal abnormalities, they are also known as dysostoses multiplex. The common skeletal features in this group include epiphyseal abnormalities, proximal pointed metacarpals, and beaking in the spine. The two representative entities in this group namely Hurler's and Morquio's syndrome are described.

Mucopolysaccharidosis-I (Hurler's syndrome)

Clinical features: It is a rare disorder of mucopolysaccharide metabolism due to deficiency of alpha-L-iduronidase enzyme and is transmitted as an autosomal recessive trait. Clinical features manifest in early infancy and include a large head with eyes wide apart, shrunken bridge of the nose, everted lips, protruding tongue, poorly formed teeth, hepatosplenomegaly, and dorsolumbar kyphosis. Progressive mental retardation and corneal opacities are invariably present with death occurring at a younger age compared to other mucopolysaccharidoses.

Imaging Features

Skull: Macrocephaly and J-shaped sella which occur due to deposition of GAGs in the pituitary gland causing its enlargement.

Spine: Odontoid hypoplasia, atlantoaxial subluxation, anteroinferior beaking of vertebral bodies, hypoplasia of vertebra around the thoracolumbar region resulting in kyphosis and gibbus deformity with platyspondyly.

Thorax and pelvis: Paddle or oar-shaped ribs (thin posteriorly and broad anteriorly). Hypoplasia of lateral ends of the clavicle, small scapulae, and cardiomegaly. The changes in pelvis include hypoplasia of base of ilia, poor development of acetabulum, and medial portions of the femoral head leading to arthropathy.

Limbs: In the hands, changes include pointing of proximal ends of metacarpal bones and shortening and widening of short tubular bones. Other features include short and wide diaphyses, notching of the proximal humerus and long and narrow femoral neck, hypoplasia of lateral tibia resulting in genu valgum.

Hurler's syndrome may be confused with Morquio's syndrome, but changes in the spine, skull, and long bones help in differentiating between the two conditions.

Mucopolysaccharidosis-IV (Morquio's syndrome)

Clinical features: Clinical features include dwarfism with low dorsal kyphosis, flexion deformities of both hips and knees, knock knees, and flat feet. The head is thrust forward and appears shrunken between high shoulders. Deformities become noticeable after 1 year of age.

Imaging findings: MPS-IV shows similarities to MPS-I such as an enlarged skull, dorsolumbar kyphosis in the spine, and atlantoaxial instability. Findings specific to MPS-IV include normal sized sella (unlike MPS-I), central beaking of vertebrae, and platyspondyly with maintained/increased intervertebral disk spaces **(Figs. 10 and 11)**.

Mucolipidoses

These are inherited as an autosomal recessive trait and this group exhibits clinical features depending on the deficiency of the enzyme involved. The radiologic features resemble those of MPS except that urinary excretion of mucopolysaccharides is not increased.

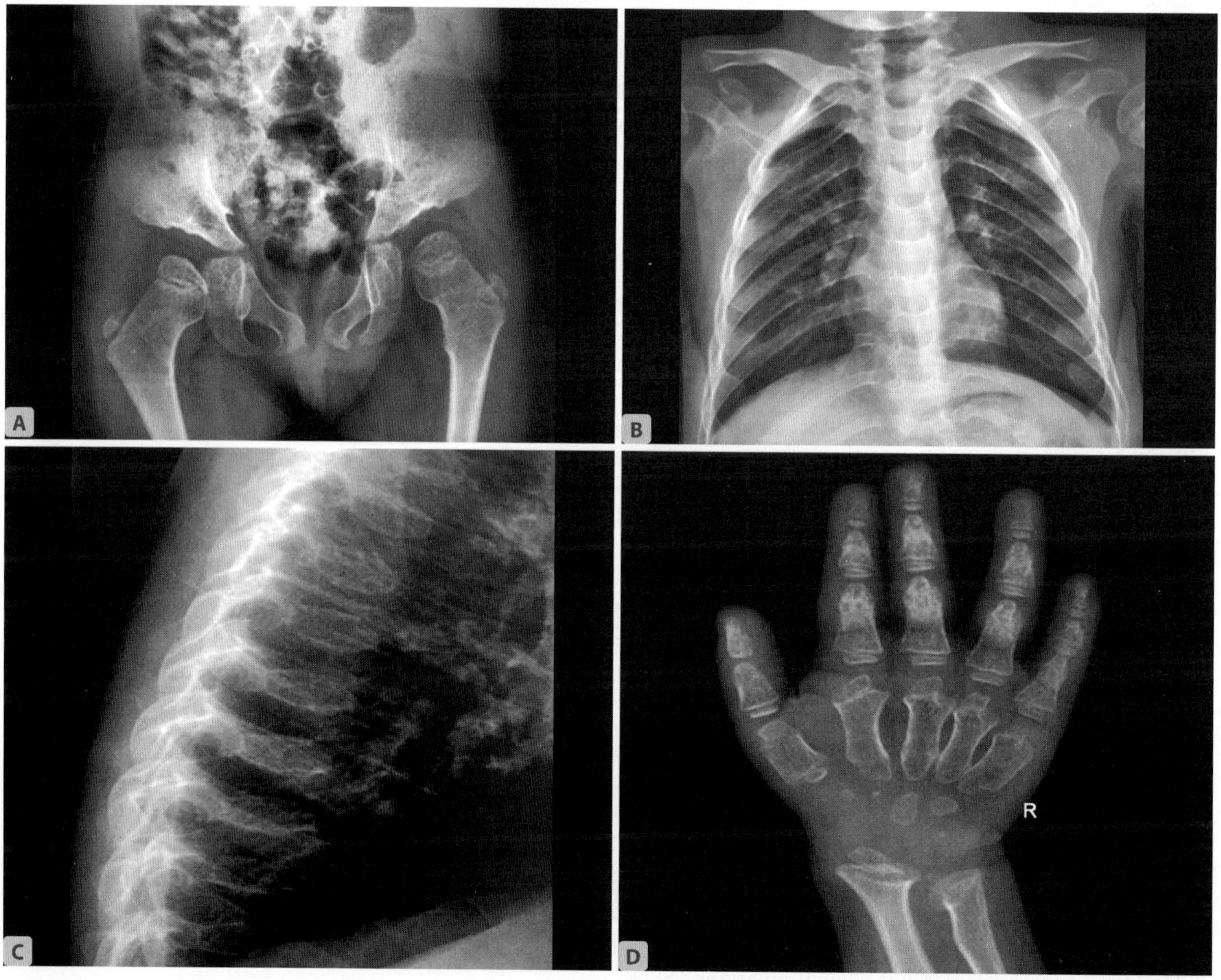

FIGS. 10A TO D: In a 3-year-old case of mucopolysaccharidosis-IV, anteroposterior (AP) radiograph of pelvis (A) shows inferior tapering of bilateral iliac bones with poorly developed acetabulum and femoral heads. AP radiograph (B) of thorax show oar-shaped ribs which are tapered posteriorly and wide anteriorly. Lateral radiograph of DL spine (C) shows platyspondyly with central beaking of vertebrae. AP radiograph (D) of left hand show proximally pointed metacarpal bones and bullet-shaped phalanges.

Source: Case courtesy by Dr Mohammad Shoaib, Maulana Azad Medical College, New Delhi.

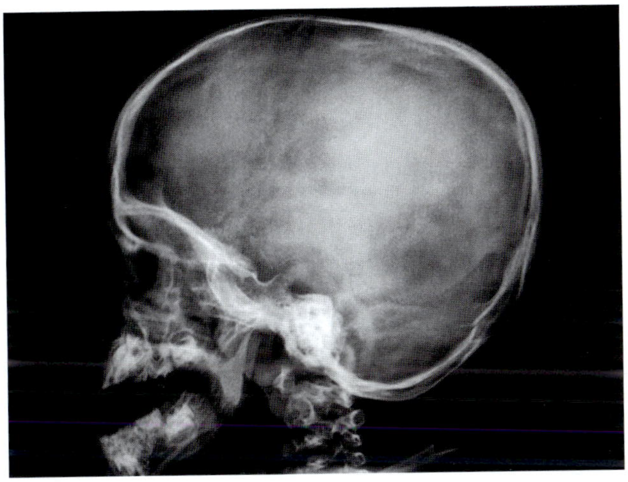

FIG. 11: Another patient of MPS-IV in which lateral radiograph of skull shows the presence of odontoid hypoplasia which is responsible for atlantoaxial instability and compressive myelopathy in these patients.

Source: Case courtesy by Dr Mohammad Shoaib, Maulana Azad Medical College, New Delhi.

DYSPLASIA WITH ALTERED BONE DENSITY: OSTEOPENIC OR SCLEROSING DYSPLASIAS

Dysplasias with Decreased Bone Density (Osteopenic Dysplasia)

Osteogenesis Imperfecta

Clinical features: The dysplasia is seen to result from both quantitative and qualitative abnormalities of type I collagen leading to increased bone fragility and low bone density, hence, it is also known as "brittle bone disease". Clinically, there is thin skin with ligamentous laxity and easy bruising, blue sclerae, dentinogenesis imperfecta (abnormal dentition), premature otosclerosis, with the presence of hydrocephalus. Osteogenesis imperfecta congenita occurs early in life while osteogenesis imperfecta tarda is less severe and occurs later in life. Clinical features in osteogenesis imperfecta congenita include a paper-thin soft skull with short broad extremities with deformities due to multiple fractures.

Imaging features: Osteogenesis imperfecta is characterized by diffuse osteopenia in both axial and appendicular skeleton, pencil-thin cortices, and multiple fractures.

Limbs: Based on the radiographic appearance of the extremities, Fairbank classified osteogenesis imperfecta into three groups. The first group includes patients with thin gracile bones **(Fig. 12A)**. This is the most common expression of the disease. The bone cortices and shafts are thin with poorly defined trabeculae. The second group includes those patients with short thick limbs. The term "thick-bone type" is a misnomer, as the cortices are thin with reduced bony density. In this group, there is severe micromelia with an increase in the width of the bones **(Fig. 12B)**. This group has a poor prognosis. The third and least common is a group of cases with cystic changes in the extremities with altered modeling of the bone. These occur in severely affected patients and other features include flared hyperlucent metaphyses traversed by coarse trabeculae giving a honeycomb appearance. Patients who survive infancy often undergo a change from the thick limb type to the cystic or gracile type.[19]

Fractures in osteogenesis imperfecta occur most commonly in the lower limbs. Microfractures can occur at the junction of metaphyses and epiphyses. These fractures are asymmetrical and are seen as dense lines due to repeated trauma. Avulsion injury due to normal muscle pull can occur. Multiple telescoping fractures, which begin to occur in utero, lead to micromelia and bowing deformities. Fracture healing is usually normal, but tumoral callus and pseudoarthroses can occur. Hyperplastic callus usually occurs after a trauma or surgical intervention. Multiple radiolucent scalloped areas with sclerotic margins referred to as popcorn calcifications can occur in metaphysis or epiphysis in severely affected patients. This is thought to result from the traumatic fragmentation of the cartilage growth plate. Laxity, tendon ruptures, fractures deformities, and premature degenerative processes all contribute to wide-scale deformities.

Skull: In the skull, changes include enlargement of mastoid and frontal sinuses. Wormian bones are commonly seen, arranged in a mosaic pattern, along the lambdoid suture. Platybasia with or without basilar impression is a frequent deformity. A basilar impression with platybasia is referred to as the *"Tam-o-Shanter"* skull. Premature otosclerosis can also result due to the thickening of stapes footplate, stapedial crural fractures, obliteration of oval window, and flattening of the cochlea, which can be well depicted by CT. Dental abnormalities include teeth with absent pulp chambers and root canals, deformed and twisted roots, and absence of enamel. Jaw fractures with excessive callus can follow dental extraction.

Spine: Spinal changes include flattened vertebral bodies, which can be biconcave or wedged anteriorly, with severe kyphoscoliosis, which is progressive **(Fig. 12C)**.

Thorax and pelvis: Findings in the chest include thinning of ribs, multiple rib fractures with callus formation. The pelvis is frequently triradiate with the presence of compression fractures and protrusio acetabulae. Shepherd's crook deformity of the femur can also be present.

Sonographic detection of disease is possible in utero by using three diagnostic criteria described by Münoz and associates:

1. Detection of crumpled or wrinkled appearance due to fractures of long bones
2. Detection of severe demineralization of the calvaria, which is associated with excellent visualization of intracranial contents, and
3. Shortening of the femur to more than three standard deviations below mean value. Other features can also be detected which include platyspondyly, beaded ribs, small thoracic circumference, and wormian bones. Serial scans are important, as they can help in determining prognosis and in planning type of delivery.[20]

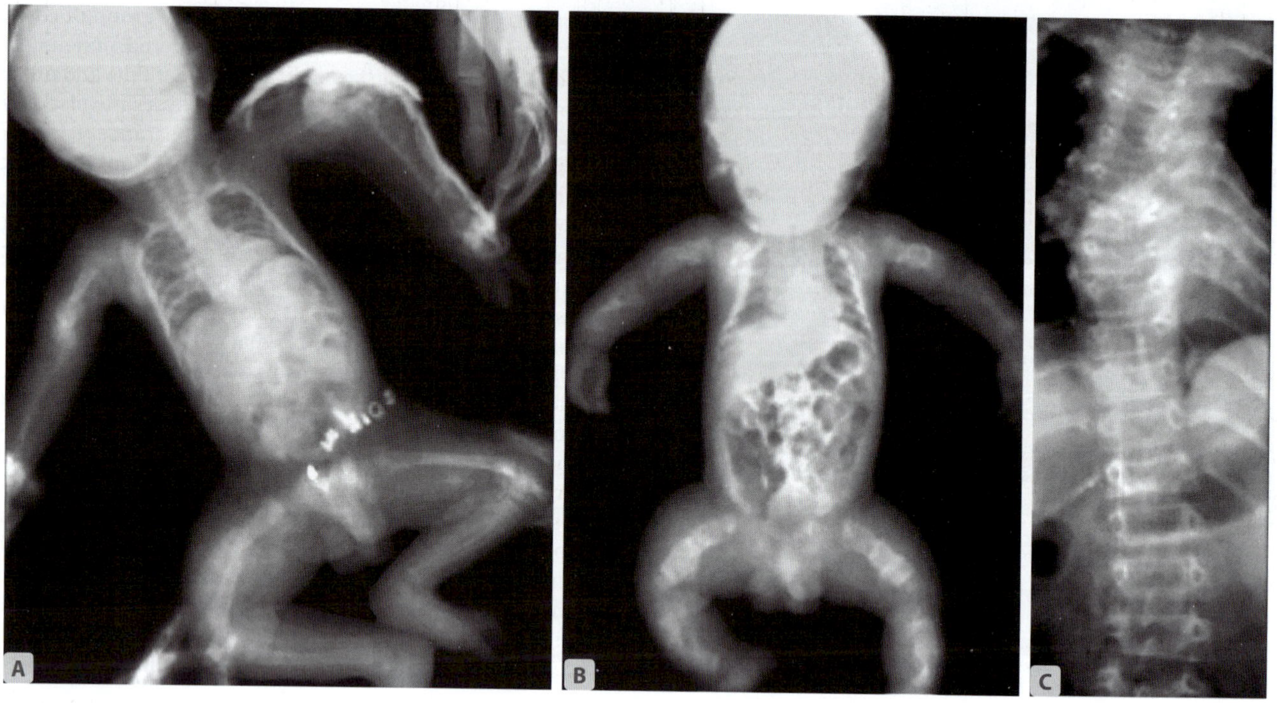

FIGS. 12A TO C: (A) Infantogram showing a case of osteogenesis imperfecta congenita (thin bone type) with bone with thin cortices and decreased bone density with presence of fractures in diaphysis of both humeri and right femora with exuberant callus formation; (B) Infantogram showing a classical case of osteogenesis imperfecta congenita (thick bone type) with short and broad bones and decreased bony density, platyspondyly, multiple diaphyseal fractures in all the long bones of the extremities and ribs with callus formation; (C) Radiograph of the lumbar spine (AP view) showing generalized decrease in bone density with platyspondyly in a case of osteogenesis imperfecta tarda.

Dysplasias with Increased Bone Density (Sclerosing or Osteosclerotic Dysplasia)

Increased bone density on radiographs can be due to sclerosis or hyperostosis.

These dysplasias can be further classified into:[17]

- Dysplasia due to disturbance in endochondral bone formation: Osteopetrosis, pyknodysostosis, bone islands and osteopoikilosis, and osteopathia striata.
- Dysplasia due to disturbance in intramembranous bone formation: Progressive diaphyseal dysplasia.
- Mixed (disturbance in both endochondral and membranous ossification sclerosing dysplasias: Melorheostosis and overlap syndromes).

Osteopetrosis

Clinicopathological features: The primary defect is the failure of normal osteoclastic activity, which causes failure of normal bone remodeling with resultant obliteration of medullary canal of bones leading to bone marrow failure causing anemia and extramedullary hematopoiesis leading to hepatosplenomegaly. There can be various modes of inheritance, both autosomal recessive and dominant types have been described.

Four different types can be commonly recognized, which include the precocious type, the delayed-type, the intermediate type, and the tubular acidosis type.

Imaging features: The radiological findings in *precocious type* include generalized osteosclerosis, failure of corticomedullary differentiation, and defective modeling of bones.

Limbs: Defective modeling of distal femora leads to the metaphyseal flaring called "Erlenmeyer flask deformity."[21] A club-like appearance due to defective modeling frequently results with the presence of transverse striations **(Fig. 13A)**. Alternating areas of mature bone and sclerotic osseous tissue can give a "bone within bone" appearance.

Skull: While the entire calvaria is involved, the cartilaginous portion of the base is more severely involved. Calvaria is thick with dense inner and outer tables, broad diploic spaces with the hair-on-end appearance, and small cranial foramina. The skull base shows appreciable marrow activity, well shown by MR imaging.

Spine: The changes in the spine include radiodense vertebral bodies with endplate sclerosis known as sandwich vertebrae.

In the *delayed-type*, the findings are less severe compared to the precocious type. Osteosclerosis, defective undertubulation with a thick cortex and a bone within the bone appearance, characterize this type of osteopetrosis **(Figs. 13B and C)**.

In *intermediate type*, there is bone sclerosis, primarily of the skull base with the involvement of facial bones. Interference with normal bone modeling, bone within the bone appearance, and ischemic necrosis of the femoral head can also be present.

In the *tubular acidosis type*, there is osteopetrosis with renal tubular acidosis and intracerebral calcifications, primarily in basal ganglia and periventricular region. Other radiologic findings include the obliteration of the medullary cavity and pathologic fractures. Progressive improvement of the abnormalities is also seen.

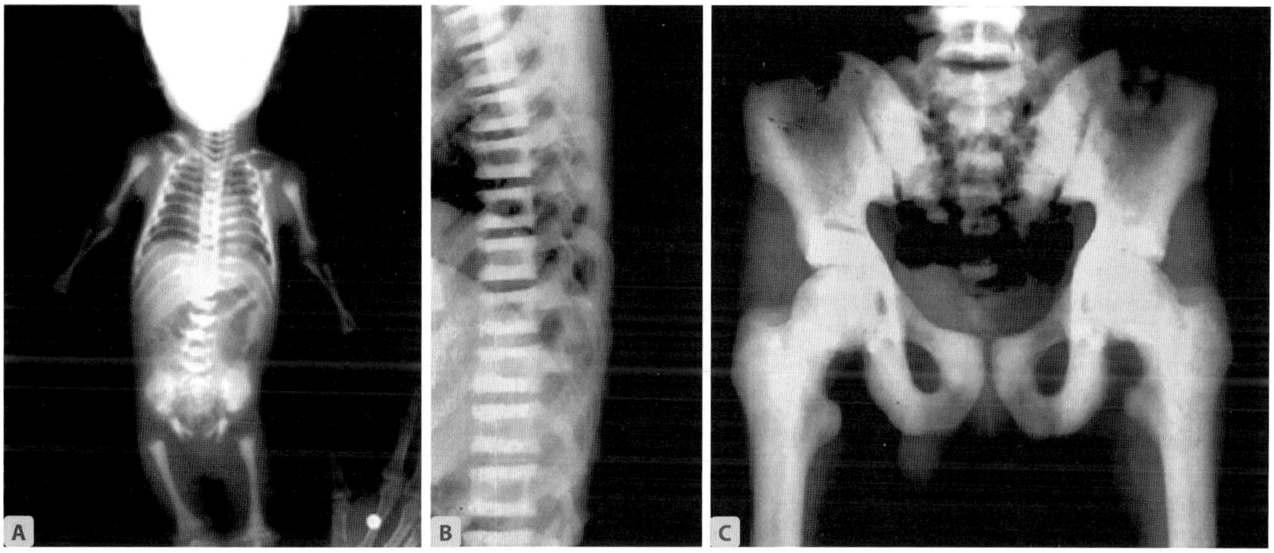

FIGS. 13A TO C: (A) Generalized increase of bone density involving vertebrae, pelvic bones, and extremities with transverse metaphyseal lucencies in a case of osteopetrosis, infantile type; (B) Generalized increase of bone density involving axial skeleton evident as endplate sclerosis in multiple dorsal and lumbar vertebrae; (C) X-ray pelvis of the same patient showing generalized increase of bone density in a case of osteopetrosis, adolescent type.

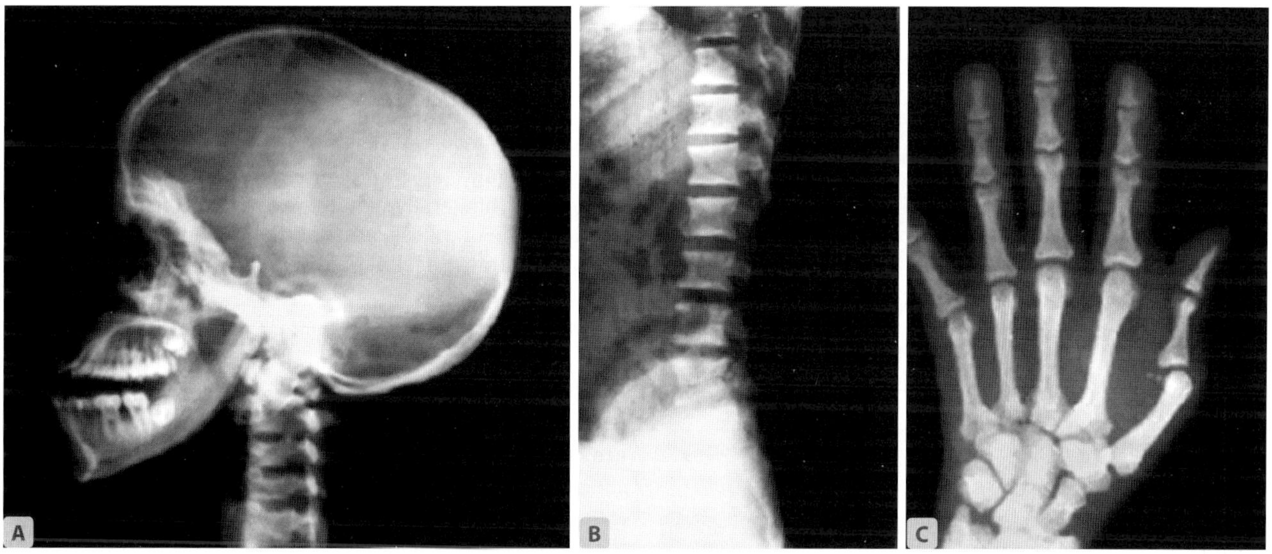

FIGS. 14A TO C: (A) Skull lateral view showing widely open sutures, open anterior and posterior fontanels with absent angle of mandible in a case of pyknodysostosis; (B) Increased bone density with spool-shaped lumbar vertebral bodies along with fractures involving pars interarticularis at multiple levels; (C) Increased bone density with acro-osteolysis in a case of pyknodysostosis.

Pycnodysostosis

Clinical features: It is transmitted as an autosomal recessive trait. Clinically, there are short limbs with a tendency to fracture, irregular dentition, and respiratory problems. Patients are usually short and <150 cm inheight.

Imaging Features

Skull: The radiologic findings include generalized osteosclerosis with thick sclerotic skull base, vault, and orbital rims. There is a marked delay in the closure of sutures with the presence of wormian bones. The mandible is frequently hypoplastic with loss of normal angulation (become obtuse) **(Fig. 14A)**.

Spine: Changes in the spine include sclerosis of vertebral bodies, segmentation anomalies, and spondylolisthesis **(Fig. 14B)**.

Limbs: The bones of the hand are short with hypoplasia or osteolysis of the distal phalanges (acro-osteolysis) **(Fig. 14C)**. The medullary cavity of tubular bones may be maintained or mildly narrow.

Pyknodysostosis can be differentiated from osteopetrosis by its typical appearance of skull, mandible, and hands.

Osteopoikilosis

Clinical features: This condition is asymptomatic and does not produce physical deformity. Male preponderance is seen. The condition is associated with linear scleroderma. The disease is of little clinical concern.

Imaging features: Punctate, rounded, and sometimes linear sclerotic densities of 1–10 mm are seen in medullary cavities of compact bone. These densities predominate toward ends of long bones. The pelvis is affected frequently **(Fig. 15)**. The skull, ribs, and spine are usually spared in this condition.

Osteopathia Striata

Clinical features: The condition is usually asymptomatic, although sometimes it may be associated with vague joint pains.

Imaging features: There are multiple linear densities of varying width having an axial distribution, prominently seen in the ends of long bones. They usually extend into the epiphysis, where punctate and confluent opacities can occur **(Fig. 16)**.

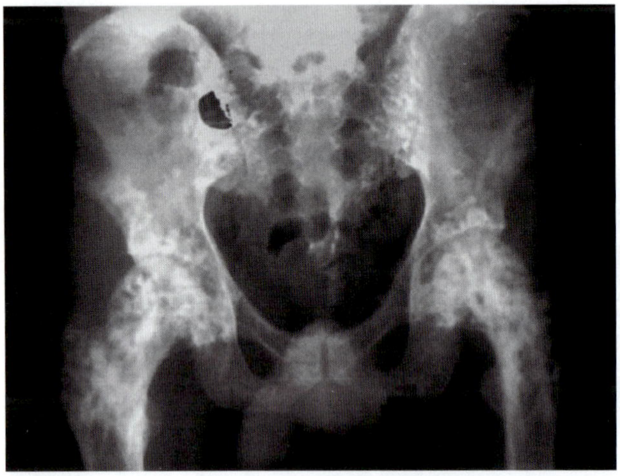

FIG. 15: Numerous small dense rounded opacities symmetrically involving the pubic bones and both femora in a case of osteopoikilosis.

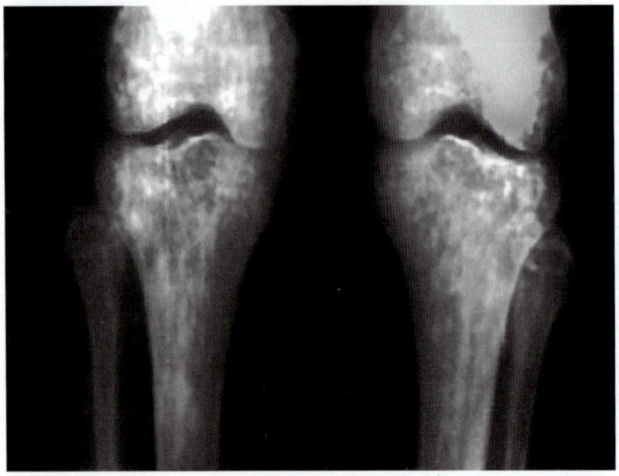

FIG. 16: Multiple linear opacities running vertically through the metadiaphysis and epiphysis with punctate opacities in a case of osteopathia striata.

Except for skull and clavicles, the remaining skeleton can all be involved. It is a disease of little clinical consequence.

Melorheostosis

Clinical features: It is also called Leri's disease. It is a rare sclerosing dysplasia of unknown etiology and is often seen in association with osteopoikilosis. It is characterized by the involvement of long bones and adjacent soft tissues is usually observed after 3 years of age. Severe pain is often the presenting symptom. Thickness and fibrosis of overlying skin are present. Tumors or malformations of blood vessels and lymphatics can be other cutaneous associations.

Imaging features: Multiple areas of dense hyperostosis are observed with a linear and segmental distribution corresponding to one or more sclerotomes in this condition.

Superficial cortical deposits are the rule, though the disease may also encroach the medullary cavity **(Fig. 17)**. The resulting contour has been likened to candle wax flowing down the margin of the bone. The disease is usually monomelic and involves bones in one limb. Bony overgrowth can occur. Soft-tissue ossification commonly occurs in the periarticular region between two affected bones of a limb.

Progressive Diaphyseal Dysplasia (Camurati–Engelmann Disease)

Clinical features: It is an autosomal dominant disorder with the variability of expression with symptoms usually occurring in or after the second decade, such as bone enlargement, abnormal gait, leg pain, and muscle weakness. It is a generalized, bilaterally symmetric dysplasia of bone primarily involving the diaphysis and sparing the epiphysis. It is also called Camurati-Engelmann disease.

Imaging Features

The radiologic features include cortical thickening and diaphyseal sclerosis. The endosteal involvement is more than periosteal involvement. Tibia, femur, and humerus are commonly involved in decreasing order of frequency,

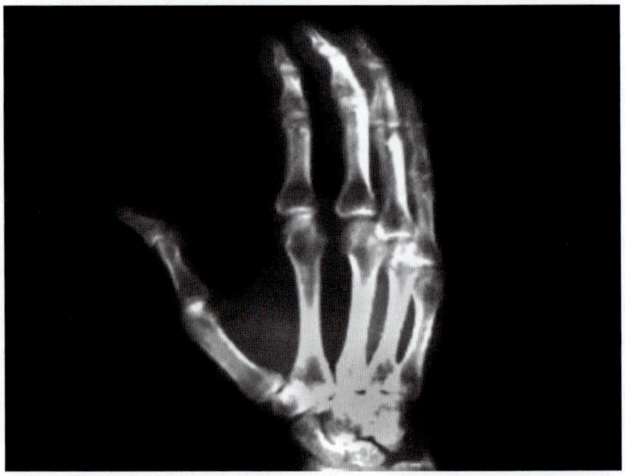

FIG. 17: Hyperostosis encroaching on the medulla of the proximal phalanges of the ring and middle fingers in a case of melorheostosis.

while any bone can be involved. Sclerosis of the skull base is common with the encroachment of cranial nerves with associated complications. Changes in the spine include vertebral sclerosis especially in the posterior parts of vertebral bodies and neural arches.

Craniodiaphyseal Dysplasia

Clinical features: It is an autosomal recessive disorder characterized by deformity of face, nasal and lacrimal obstruction, and cranial nerve palsies.

Imaging features: The radiologic features include massive and progressive hyperostosis of the skull and facial bones with obliteration of the paranasal sinuses. The involvement of the long bones varies in severity, although cortical thickening and lack of normal modeling are typical. The ribs, clavicles, and ilia are wide and sclerotic, whereas the changes in the spine are mild and preferentially located in the vertebral arches.

Craniometaphyseal Dysplasia

Clinical features: It is clinically characterized by facial deformity, broad mass at the base of the nose, hypertelorism, nasal obstruction, deafness, and malocclusion of teeth.

Imaging features: There is progressive sclerosis around the sutures with sclerosis of the skull base. Besides, there is an obliteration of paranasal sinuses and loss of lamina dura of teeth. Osteosclerosis in the diaphyses of tubular bones is noted in infancy, which later disappears and is replaced by modeling defects. There are an additional metaphyseal expansion and club-shaped epiphysis. Ribs and medial part of clavicles can be widened. The spine is rarely affected.

Dysplasia with Single Site or Segment Involvement

There are many dysplasias which involve either a single segment of limb (e.g., mesomelic dysplasias involving bones of forearms and lower legs, acrodysplasia which involves bones of hand and feet), single-site of involvement such as the involvement of membranous bones in cleidocranial dysplasia.

Mesomelic Dysplasias

Dyschondrosteosis: It is the most common mesomelic dysplasia which is transmitted as an autosomal dominant trait with a female predominance. It is also called as "Léri-Weill syndrome".

Clinical features: It is characterized by the presence of reducible dorsal dislocation of distal ulna known as "Madelung deformity and mesomelic short stature".

Radiological features: There is a shortening of bones of the forearm (radius is more affected than ulna). There is a shortening of the radius with bowing appearance and the triangular shape of the distal end of the radius. The distal end of the ulna is subluxated giving rise to bayonet-shaped deformity called "Madelung deformity". The radial head can also dislocate. Similar changes in the lower leg can result in deformity of ankle mortice. Madelung deformity is characteristic of dyschondrosteosis and not seen in other mesomelic dysplasias.

Nievergelt type: It is the most severe type of mesomelic dysplasia, which is characterized by marked shortening and deformity in the bones of the lower leg as compared to forearms. It is often accompanied by visible bony prominences in the lower legs. Hypoplasia of bones of forearm and leg is common **(Fig. 18)**. Dysplasia of tibia may result in atriangular or rhomboid configuration of tibia and slanting of the growth plate of the tibia. Proximal radioulnar synostosis is seen with restricted mobility. A fusion of tarsal and carpal bones is also seen.

Acrodysplasia—Trichorhinophalangeal Dysplasia

Clinical features: It is transmitted as an autosomal dominant trait and characterized by sparse scalp hair, pear-shaped nose, and deformity of proximal interphalangeal joints. Three types of dysplasia have been described.

Imaging features: The characteristic radiologic findings in type I dysplasia include cone-shaped epiphysis in hands producing a U-shaped pattern with osseous shortening, especially in middle phalanges of second and third digit with ivory epiphysis being common in the distal phalanges. The proximal femoral epiphyses are small and often demonstrate changes resembling Perthes' disease. Pectus carinatum, scoliosis, and kyphosis can also be seen. In type II dysplasia, there are cone-shaped epiphyses in the thumb and other digits with the presence of multiple exostoses, which distort and expand the bone.[22] There is asymmetric limb growth, tibiofibular synostosis, short fibula, wide femoral neck, and changes similar to Perthes' disease. Segmentation errors in the spine and macrocephaly may occasionally be present. In type III dysplasia, there is a severe generalized shortening of tubular bones of the hand without the presence of exostosis.

Cleidocranial Dysplasia

Clinical features: This dysplasia has an autosomal dominant mode of inheritance. There is delayed or deficient ossification

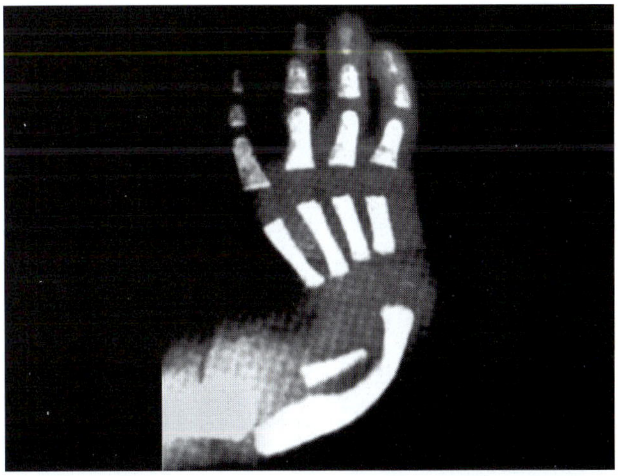

FIG. 18: Newborn infant with hypoplastic radius, curved ulna with absent thumb in a case of mesomelic dysplasia.

of membranous bones such as skull and clavicles. Midline structures are primarily affected in this dysplasia and the disease manifests in infancy.

Imaging Features

Skull: Consequent to deficient ossification, there is markedly delayed ossification of skull bones, more so in the region of the parietal bone, with resultant wide sutures. Basilar invagination may occur as a consequence of large foramen magnum. Wormian bones are frequently seen.

Thorax and pelvis: The clavicle may be absent in its outer or middle parts or rarely may be absent in its entire extent **(Fig. 19A)**. The thorax is small-sized with a small hypoplastic scapula.[18,23] Pelvis is severely affected with severe under mineralization of its constituent bones, giving a "see-through" appearance **(Fig. 19B)**. The increased angle between the femoral neck with shaft can give rise to coxa valga.

Spine: Spinal changes include failure of fusion of neural arches, vertebral bodies wedging with scoliosis, supernumerary ossification centers in thoracic region, pars interarticularis defects frequently seen in lumbar spine and spina bifida occulta.[16]

Limbs: In the hand, there can be delayed carpal bone ossification, pseudoepiphysis in metacarpal bones, long 2nd and 5th metacarpals with supernumerary ossification centers, short 2nd and 5th phalanges and acro-osteolysis **(Fig. 19C)**. In the lower extremities, tibiotalar slant and short fibulae may also be present.

Yunis–Varon syndrome encompasses findings of cleidocranial dysplasia, small mandible, absence of thumbs, and first metatarsals and absence of distal phalanges.

SKELETAL DYSPLASIAS WITH MULTIPLE DISLOCATIONS

Two rare but important SD that can present as multiple joint dislocations are Larsen syndrome and Desbuquois syndrome. Typical radiological findings reported in Larsen syndrome include multiple joint dislocations involving hips, knees, and elbows, spinal curvature abnormalities, extra ossification centers of the calcaneum, and supernumerary carpal bones. On the other hand, Desbuquois syndrome has a typical radiological appearance involving iliac bones and medial femoral necks, in which iliac bones are hypoplastic with short femoral neck and there is beaking of the medial metaphysis of femur giving rise to "monkey wrench" appearance. Other findings include accelerated ossification of carpal and tarsal bones and extra ossicles between metacarpals/metatarsals and phalanges of 1st and 2nd digits/toes.

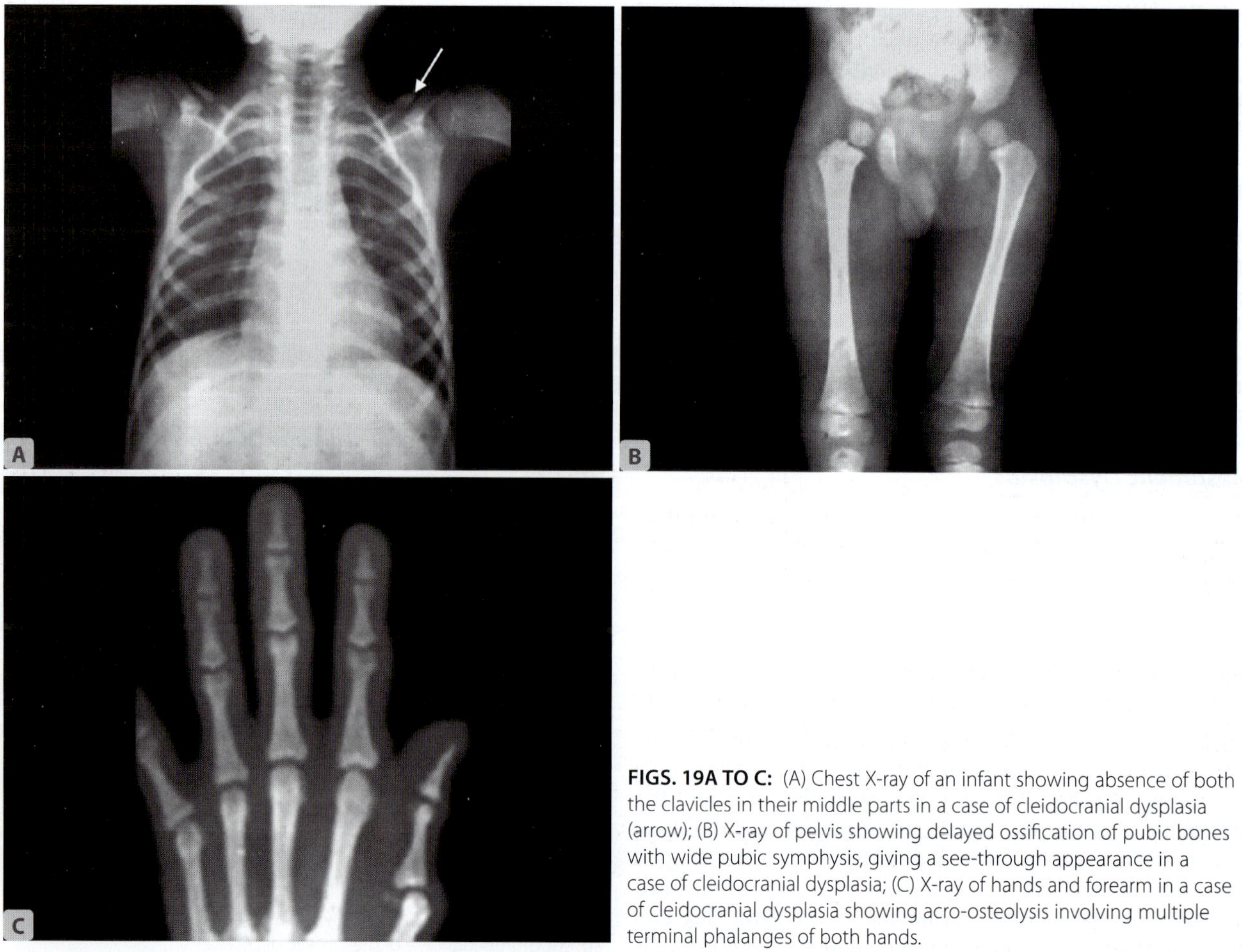

FIGS. 19A TO C: (A) Chest X-ray of an infant showing absence of both the clavicles in their middle parts in a case of cleidocranial dysplasia (arrow); (B) X-ray of pelvis showing delayed ossification of pubic bones with wide pubic symphysis, giving a see-through appearance in a case of cleidocranial dysplasia; (C) X-ray of hands and forearm in a case of cleidocranial dysplasia showing acro-osteolysis involving multiple terminal phalanges of both hands.

Disorganized Development of Cartilage and Fibrous Components of the Skeleton

Dysplasia Epiphysealis Hemimelica

Clinical features: The clinical features consist of pain, deformity, and restricted motion of affected joints.

Imaging features: The radiological features of this dysplasia include early appearance and excessive growth of epiphysis with irregularly calcified mass projecting from the epiphysis.

The irregular mass may initially appear distinct from the surrounding bone, though eventually, it fuses with the adjacent epiphysis. The distal femur and distal tibia are among the common sites of involvement. Epiphyseal involvement on one side of the body may be associated with hemihypertrophy. Spinal abnormalities including scoliosis can occur.

Multiple Cartilaginous Exostoses

Clinical features: This condition, also called diaphyseal aclasis, is characterized by cartilage capped exostosis. It occurs more commonly in boys, who develop painless lumps near ends of long bones. They have mild shortness of stature.

Imaging features: The radiological appearance and size of exostoses are variable. They arise on the metaphyseal side of the growth plate and point away from the epiphyses with associated metaphyseal expansion and deformity **(Fig. 20)**. In hands, however, the origin can be in the epiphysis. The forearms are frequently deformed as a consequence of bowing of radius, dislocation of the radial head, ulnar angulation of distal end of radius, and shortening of the ulna. The long tubular bones are frequently involved; however, ribs, scapula, and pelvis can also be affected. Vertebral involvement though uncommon can lead to compression of spinal cord or nerve roots. Complications related to osteochondroma include interference with growth, compression of adjacent structures, and malignant transformation. Malignant transformation may be indicated by the continued growth of osteochondroma even after cessation of normal growth, changing the appearance of calcification in cartilage cap and irregular outline or bony destruction of exostosis.

Enchondromatosis (Ollier's Disease)

Clinical features: Clinically, there is asymmetrical limb shortening with an expansion of affected bone and occasionally pathological fracture.

Imaging features: The radiological features include radiolucent masses, which may be round or triangular in the tubular bones of the hand, which may show considerable expansion and pathological fracture. Focal area of calcification can be present in the mass **(Fig. 21)**. Cartilaginous areas extending from physis lead to interference with growth and resultant shortening and deformity. The femur and tibia are most commonly involved. In pelvis V-shaped radiolucent areas are seen in iliac bones. The enchondromas may stop growing or even regress in adulthood. Chondrosarcoma can occur in one-fourth of patients.

Enchondromatosis with Hemangiomas (Maffucci's Syndrome)

The radiological features are akin to Ollier's disease with soft-tissue masses due to hemangiomas and phleboliths in hands and feet **(Fig. 22)**. The hemangiomas can disappear and they need not overlie the bone lesions. A higher incidence of malignant transformation is seen compared to Ollier's disease.

Fibrous Dysplasia

Clinical features: This dysplasia is seen in the first three decades with a female preponderance. There is deformity and pain related to involved bones with a pathological fracture at times. The lesions tend to be unilateral. Histologically, medullary bone is seen to be replaced by fibrous tissue and cysts. This dysplasia can be monostotic or polyostotic. The association of polyostotic fibrous dysplasia, sexual precocity,

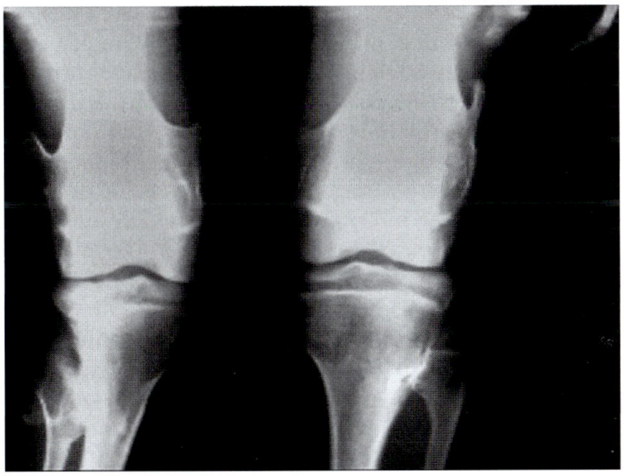

FIG. 20: Multiple bony exostosis seen involving both lower femora and upper ends of tibia and fibulae with metaphyseal modeling deformity.

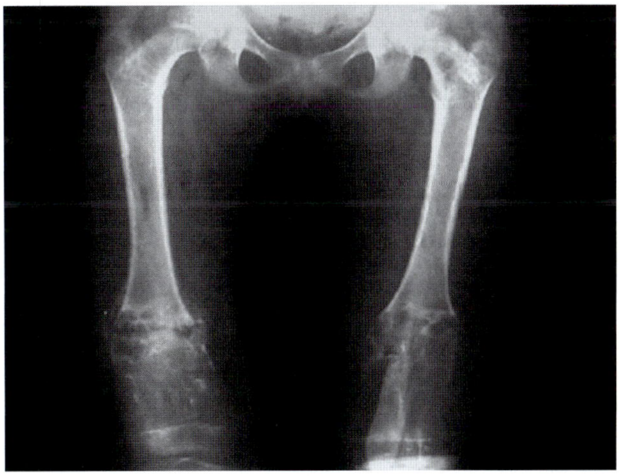

FIG. 21: X-ray of both knees AP view showing marked bony expansion with loss of cortical integrity of the distal femoral metaphysis with intramedullary calcification and lucencies in a case of Ollier's disease.

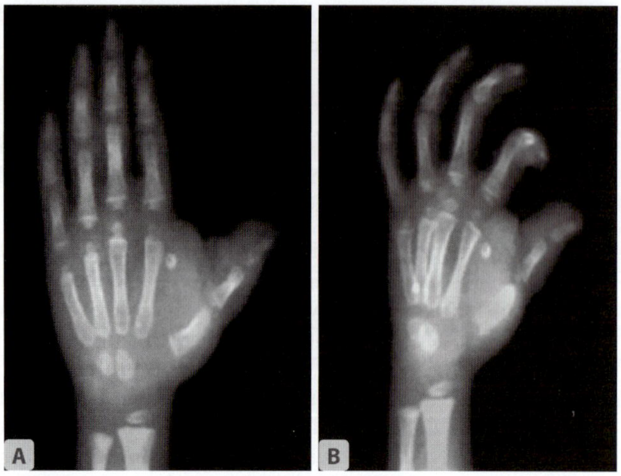

FIGS. 22 A AND B: X-ray of right hand AP view showing soft-tissue swelling with presence of calcified phleboliths suggestive of hemangioma between the metacarpal bones in a case of Maffucci syndrome. Enchondromatosis may not be present in the region of hemangioma as in this case.

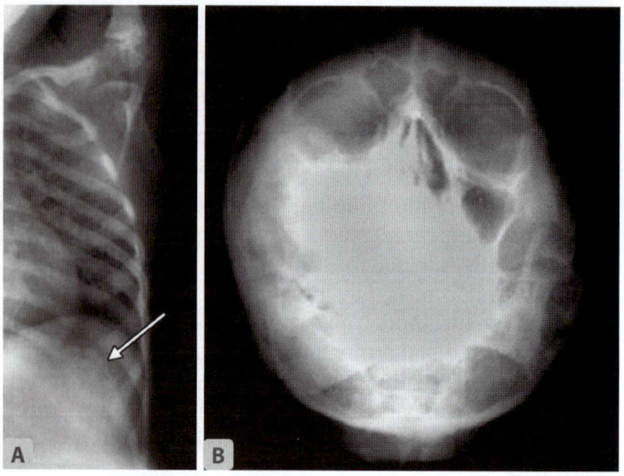

FIGS. 23A AND B: (A) Bony expansion with lysis and ground-glass haze in a case of fibrous dysplasia involving the 10th rib posteriorly (arrow); (B) Bony expansion with ground glass haze and uniformly increased density seen involving the right maxillary sinus, right zygoma, and right hemimandible on Water's view.

café-au-lait pigmentation in females, constitutes the McCune Albright syndrome. Sarcomatous degeneration can occur in about 1% of cases.

Imaging features: The radiological features include "ground glass" appearance or radiolucent areas of altered trabeculae in the ribs and long bones with associated patchy sclerosis and expansion **(Fig. 23A)**. There is endosteal scalloping and cortical thinning. Localized or asymmetrical overgrowth of bones may be seen. Pathological fractures and deformities due to bone softening such as "shepherd's crook deformity" can occur. The skull shows asymmetrical thickening of the vault with sclerosis of the base with obliteration of the paranasal sinuses **(Fig. 23B)** and marked facial deformity giving a "leontiasis ossea" appearance.[24,25]

DYSOSTOSES

Dysostoses with Cranial and Facial Involvement

Craniosynostosis

Clinical features: There is a local cessation of growth and distortion of calvarial configuration due to premature fusion of one or more cranial sutures.

Imaging features: Isolated closure of sagittal suture is encountered most frequently. Unilateral closure of lambdoid suture leads to flattening of the back of the head or plagiocephaly. Cloverleaf skull is associated with premature synostosis of multiple sutures.

Craniofacial Synostosis

Clinicoradiological features: Crouzon's syndrome is characterized by craniosynostosis, exophthalmos, and midface recession. The disorder is caused by a mutation in the gene for fibroblast growth factor. The skull is brachycephalic with the fusion of coronal, sagittal, and lambdoid sutures, usually seen by 3 years of age. Hypertelorism, hypoplastic maxilla, hydrocephalus, and spinal anomalies can also occur.

Dysostoses with Predominant Axial Involvement

Vertebral segmentation defects and Sprengel's deformity: Various vertebral segmentation defects can occur. Multiple block vertebrae are seen in cervico-oculo-acoustic syndrome or Wildervanck syndrome. Sprengel's deformity can occur as an isolated abnormality of the scapula, which is small, triangular, elevated, and rotated so that its medial border faces the spine, or as a part of Klippel-Feil syndrome.

Dysostosis with Predominant Involvement of Extremities

Dysostosis with predominant involvement of extremities can occur alone or as a part of a widespread dysplasia. There can be various deformities affecting the limbs, for example, there can be a partial or complete absence of limbs or fingers, radioulnar synostosis, polysyndactyly, and clinodactyly.

Certain neonatal anomalies in hand, foot, and arm can be a pointer to the presence of skeletal dysplasia. For instance, clinodactyly (finger curvature in medial or lateral plane) can be seen in Cornelia de Lange syndrome, Down syndrome, Nail-patella syndrome, radial hypoplasia or aplasia can be seen in Cornelia de Lange syndrome, Trisomy 18 **(Figs. 24A and B)**, metacarpal hypoplasia can be seen in chondrodystrophia calcificans congenita, polydactyly in chondrodystrophia calcificans congenita, Ellis-van Creveld syndrome, syndactyly in acrocephalosyndactyly (Apert's syndrome), chondrodystrophia calcificans congenita, Cornelia de Lange syndrome, broad thumb in acrocephalosyndactyly camptodactyly (permanent finger flexion at the proximal interphalangeal joint due to contractures or fascial abnormality) in Morquio's syndrome and Nail-patella syndrome.

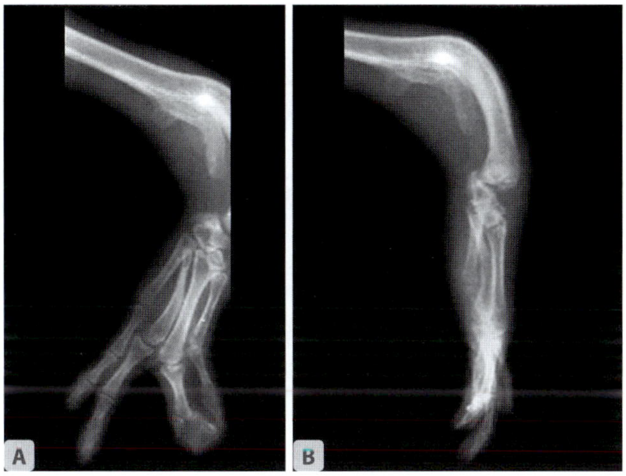

FIGS. 24A AND B: Radial aplasia with curved ulna and absent thumb in a case of Trisomy 18.

Bone Abnormalities Secondary to Disturbances of Extraskeleton Systems

Bone abnormalities can result secondary to endocrine, hematologic, neurologic, renal, gastrointestinal, and cardiopulmonary diseases. These diseases of bone classified under "constitutional diseases of bone" are secondary abnormalities and not classified under SD.

CONCLUSION

Systematic evaluation of skeletal survey and knowledge of salient features of commonly seen skeletal dysplasia can lead to a specific diagnosis of skeletal dysplasia.

The establishment of diagnosis is important for reasons such as genetic counseling and assessing recurrence risk, prenatal diagnosis in future pregnancies, prediction of adult height, and most importantly, clinical management including prevention of complications and disabilities.

REFERENCES

1. Camera G, Mastroiacovo P. Birth prevalence of skeletal dysplasias in the Italian multi-centric monitoring system for birth defects. In: Papadatos CJ, Bartsocas CS (Eds). Skeletal Dysplasias. New York: Alan R. Liss; 1982. pp. 441-9.
2. Spranger J. International classification of osteochondrodysplasias. Eur Pediatr. 1992;151:407-15.
3. Lachman Ralph S. International nomenclature and classification of the osteochondrodysplasias. Pediatr Radiol. 1998;28:737-44.
4. Jean F, Le Merrer M, Chauvet ML. Osteochondrodysplasias, dysostosis, disorders of calcium metabolism, congenital malformations syndromes and other disorders. Pediatr Radiol. 1997;27:366-87.
5. Horton W. Advances in the genetics of human chondrodysplasias. Pediatr Radiol. 1997;27:422-7.
6. Superti-Furga A, Bonafé L, Rimoin DL. Molecular pathogenetic classification of genetic disorders of the skeleton. Am J Med Gene (Semin Med Genet). 2001;106:282-93.
7. Mortier GR, Cohn DH, Cormier-Daire V, Hall C, Krakow D, Mundlos S, et al. Nosology and classification of genetic skeletal disorders: 2019 revision. Am J Med Genet Part A. 2019;179:2393-419.
8. Kirks Donald R, Thorne Griscom N. Practical Pediatric Imaging Diagnostic Radiology of Infants and Children (3rd edition). Philadelphia, New York: Lippincott-Raven Publishers; 1999.
9. Krakow D, Alanay Y, Rimoin LP, Lin V, Wilcox WR, Lachman RS, et al. Evaluation of prenatal onset osteochondrodysplasias by ultrasonography: A retrospective and prospective analysis. Am J Med Genet A. 2008;1;146A(15):1917-24.
10. Watson SG, Calder AD, Offiah AC, Negus S. A review of imaging protocols for suspected skeletal dysplasia and a proposal for standardisation. Pediatr radiol. 2015;45:1733-7.
11. Offiah AC, Hall CM. Radiological diagnosis of the constitutional disorders of bone. As easy as A, B, C? Pediatr radiol. 2003;33: 153-61.
12. Behrman Richard E, Kliegman Robert M, Jenson Hal B. Nelson Textbook of Pediatrics (16th edition) India reprint. Noida, Uttar Pradesh: Harcourt Asia Pte Ltd, Thompson press(I) Ltd: 2000. pp. 2113-36.
13. Kitoh H, Lachman RS, Brodie SG, Mekikian PB, Rimoin DL, Wilcox WR. Extrapelvic ossification centers in thanatophoric dysplasia and platyspondylic lethal skeletal dysplasia. Pediatr Radiol. 1998;28:759-63.
14. Pozanski AK. Punctate epiphysis: A radiological sign not a disease. Pediatr Radiol. 1994;24:418-24.
15. Spranger JW, Brill PW, Hall C, Superti-Furga A, Unger S. Bone dysplasias: an atlas of genetic disorders of skeletal development. USA: Oxford University Press; 2018.
16. Lachman Ralph S. The cervical spine in the skeletal dysplasias and associated disorders. Pediatr Radiol. 1997;27:402-8.
17. Panda A, Gamanagatti S, Jana M, Gupta AK. Skeletal dysplasias: a radiographic approach and review of common non-lethal skeletal dysplasias. World j radiol. 2014;6:808.
18. Taybi H, Lachman RS. Radiology of syndromes, metabolic disorders and skeletal dysplasias. St Louis: Mosby Year Book Publications; 1996.
19. Donald R. Diagnosis of Bone and Joint Disorders (4th edition). Philadelphia, United States: WB Saunders Company: An imprint of Elsevier Science; 2002. p. 5.
20. Murray Ronald O, Jacobson Harold G, Stoker Dennis J. The Radiology of Skeletal Disorders, Exercises in Diagnosis (3rd edition). London, United Kingdom: Churchill Livingstone; 1990. p. 2.
21. Faden MA, Krakow D, Ezgu F, Rimoin DL, Lachman RS. Erlenmeyer Flask bone deformity in the skeletal dysplasias. Am J Med Genet A. 2009;149A (6):1334-45.
22. Andres G. Phalangeal cone shaped epiphyses of the hand: Their history, diagnostic sensitivity and specificity in cartilage hair dysplasia and the trichorhinophalangeal syndrome I and II. Pediatr Radiol. 1998;28:751-8.
23. David S. Textbook of Radiology and Imaging (7th edition). London, United Kingdom: Churchill Livingstone; 2003. p. 2.
24. Leet AI, Collins MT. Current approach to Fibrous Dysplasia and McCune Albright syndrome. J Child Orthop; 2007;1(1):3-17.
25. Grainger Ronald G, David A. Grainger and Allison's Diagnostic Radiology: A Textbook of Medical Imaging (3rd edition). London, United Kingdom: Churchill Livingstone; 1997.

CHAPTER 79

Short Stature and Skeletal Maturity Assessment

Manisha Jana, Arun Kumar Gupta, Priyanka Naranje

INTRODUCTION

From the moment one is born until the time one has grown up, the bones go through a set of characteristic changes—the skeletal maturity or sometimes also referred to as "bone age." Therefore, skeletal maturity is the only indicator of development that is available from birth to full maturity.[1] Skeletal maturity, in pathological terms, denotes consolidation of new tissues by calcification of the fibrous and cartilaginous elements. It is distinct from growth. In clinical terms, one may describe each individual passing from a stage of "wholly immature" to a stage of "wholly mature" through a normal growth process. At any particular stage, one individual might be more or less mature than another individual.

"Short stature" can be defined as a height that is two or more standard deviations below the expected mean gender-specified age. Short stature can happen because of a wide range of diseases; which can be nutritional deficiency, metabolic or endocrine disorders, genetic disorders, and skeletal dysplasia among many. Short stature can even be familial or constitutional, when no other causes are found. Nevertheless, short stature raises parental concern and often requires a detailed approach involving multiple specialties.

Estimation of skeletal maturity is an integral component of evaluation for short stature. Hence, in this chapter, both will be discussed in an integrated manner.

MEASUREMENT OF MATURITY

Maturity can be measured by observing certain events which occur in all individuals along the "road to full maturity". These are called "developmental milestones"[2] which could be dental, skeletal, or pubertal development (secondary sexual characters, i.e., pubic hair, breast development, and penis development).

In an ideal situation, the developmental milestones should occur in all the individuals, invariably in the same order and should cover the entire developmental span evenly and completely. Only skeletal maturity provides developmental milestones closest to such an ideal situation. It is, therefore, the most commonly used parameter of maturity in clinical practice.

In addition, the method employed to assess "skeletal maturity" is noninvasive, inexpensive and independent of body size, weight, and chronological age. All these advantages make assessment of maturity by "skeletal maturity" method an ideal clinical tool.

SKELETAL MATURITY ASSESSMENT: WHY IS IT NECESSARY?

Skeletal maturity assessment is required in clinical practice for two major reasons:

1. In pediatric endocrinological problems and growth disorders
2. For medicolegal reasons.

1. In the field of pediatric endocrinology, skeletal maturity assessment is not only essential but highly crucial for a number of reasons:[2]
   - For diagnosing underlying cause in children with short stature and growth delay **(Fig. 1)**.
   - For reassuring young people with nonpathological but unusual growth delay.
   - Monitoring growth hormone and anabolic steroid therapy.
   - Monitoring treatment in various endocrinopathies, e.g., hypothyroidism, congenital adrenal hyperplasia.
   - In the differential diagnosis of sexual precocity.
   - For prediction of adult height.
   - For selection of children in sports.

   Public health reasons—Comparison of environmental, dietary, and other factors between different populations.
2. For medicolegal reasons, estimation of age of an individual is important both for the medical jurist and lawyers. The gravity of offence is dependent upon particular age and also certain rights are given to the persons only at certain age.[3] Estimation of age is, therefore, of considerable importance from the point of view of administration of justice. This is important in a number of situations: Identification, employment, criminal responsibility, judicial punishment, consent for marriage, rape, criminal abortion, prostitution, etc.[3]

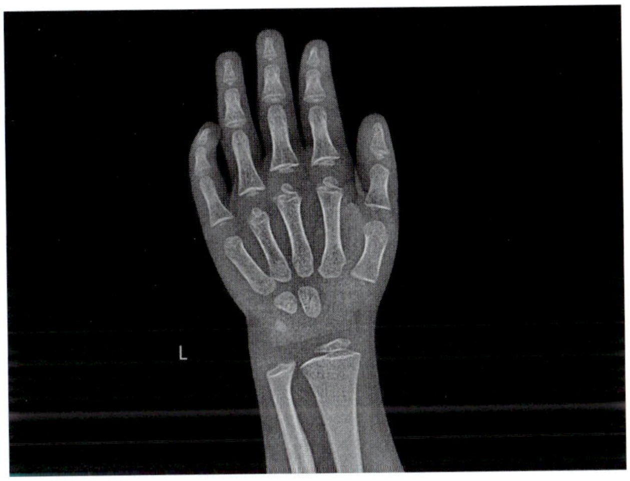

FIG. 1: Radiograph of left hand and wrist of a girl. Chronological age: 11 months. Bone age, TW2 method: RUS-2.9 years, CS-2.3 years, 20 bone–bone age-2.7 years. (CS: Carpal score; RUS: radius, ulna, and short bones; TW2: Tanner and Whitehouse II method)

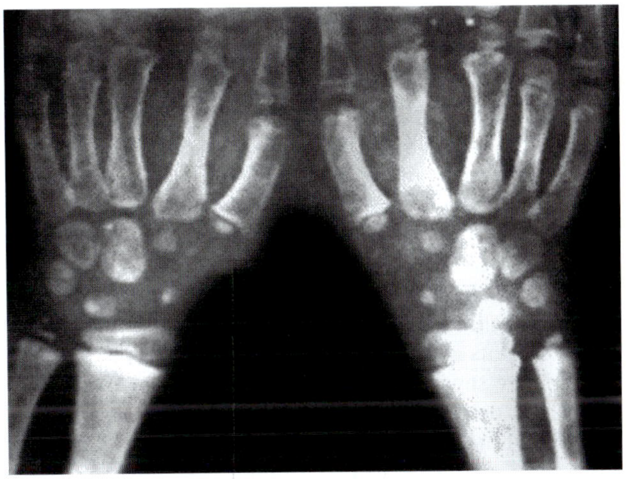

FIG. 2: Posteroanterior radiograph of both wrists of a 14-year-old male. Note asymmetrical appearance of carpal centers on the two sides, a major drawback of the technique using "appearance-fusion" of centers as the basis.

Most difficult problem arises in estimation of age of adolescent girls. Period of adolescence extends from puberty to full maturity.

Factors to be taken into consideration for estimation of age are:[3]

- Dentition, i.e., number of teeth in each jaw
- Pubarche
- Thelarche
- Menarche
- Height, weight, general configuration, and development of body
- Radiological examination of joints

METHODS TO ASSESS SKELETAL MATURITY

Skeletal maturity in an individual child is assessed by comparing his or her state of bone development with the standards that have already been evolved from examination of radiographs of normal children.[2-4] Different methods use different standards for determining skeletal maturity. The three important methods are:

1. Appearance and fusion of ossification centers
2. Greulich and Pyle atlas method (GP method)
3. Tanner and Whitehouse II method (TW2 method)

Appearance and Fusion of Ossification Centers

The earliest method for assessing skeletal maturity was by observing the time of appearance and fusion of various ossification centers.

Although this method has the advantage of being simple, quick, and easy to calculate, it has significant drawbacks[5-7] and the two major ones are: Ossification centers especially those of carpal bones may have extremely variable appearance and fusion time **(Fig. 2)** even on the two sides of the same individual, and secondly the bone age calculated by this method usually has a wide range, thereby, diminishing its clinical usefulness in pediatric endocrine diseases.

For these reasons, it became apparent that this method was neither valid nor reliable and hence inadequate and unsatisfactory for estimating skeletal maturity in children with pediatric endocrine diseases where crucial decisions for treatment are based to a large extent on this information.[7]

However, this method still has its utility in medicolegal cases.[3,8] This is more so in adolescent girls involved in rape, kidnapping, and prostitution where courts directive will change depending on age. Also, whether to try a boy or girl involved in some offence under juvenile act or not will depend on his/her age.

Radiology plays a crucial role in all these cases.[3] However, it is important to remember that radiological bone age must be interpreted along with other clinical parameters of growth before final decision.

For Indian children, standards have been established by a number of workers.[3,7-11] Using prepared charts the degree of skeletal development or "bone age" can be calculated readily. Different sets of radiographs are required for bone age estimation depending upon the chronological age, e.g.,

- Posteroanterior (PA) radiograph of wrist and hand.
- Elbow, knee, shoulder—either one or both ends depending upon expected age.
- Pelvis anteroposterior (AP) for iliac crest appearance and fusion.

At AIIMS two published data for children from Delhi are followed[8,9] for calculating bone age by this method.

Table 1 enlists the age ranges covered in different radiographs (based on appearance and fusion of epiphyses). It is to be kept in mind that at each of these sites, there may be wide variation in appearance and fusion of epiphyses;[12-15] but often a combination of radiographs can be of help in controversial cases. By and large, hand radiographs are the most reliable and most commonly performed one for bone age estimation.

Greulich and Pyle Method

In 1940, Greulich and Pyle published an atlas **(Fig. 3)** of standards of skeletal maturity based on longitudinal studies in 1930s of a relatively small number of Euro-American children living in Cleveland who were above average in economic and educational status.[16] This atlas was the turning point in establishing scientific standards of skeletal maturity. It is still the most widely used method in the Western countries due to its relative simplicity to use.

The atlas consists of a set of standard (typical) radiographs of the wrist and hand representing a particular bone age at some 30 points along the maturity scale. Standards for boys and girls are separate since girls mature earlier than boys. In order to determine the skeletal maturity of a child, the user should match the radiograph under question "as close as possible" to one of the plates in the atlas and the closest match represents that child's bone age. Thus a bone age of "12" means the child is as mature as the "average 12 years old".

Although the atlas for GP method is most commonly used as described above but the same atlas also describes "maturity indicators" for individual bones which form the basis for the Tanner and Whitehouse method.

Popularity of GP method is due to its simple methodology providing accurate information and similar reproducibility.[17] However, two important drawbacks are:[2] Subjectivity of matching process and the scale used for expressing maturity, i.e., maturity is expressed by "most likely" chronological age after the matching process and this "most likely" age is then designated as "bone age". Some studies found GP method to be inaccurate.[14]

TABLE 1: Age ranges covered in different radiographs (based on appearance and fusion of epiphyses).

Hand radiograph	Up to 18 years
Elbow	Up to 14 years
Humerus upper end	Up to 16 years
Medial end of clavicle	18–22 years
Knee joint	10–20 years
Ischial tuberosity	14–16 years
Iliac crest	15–22 years
Hip joint	14–17 years

Tanner and Whitehouse II Method

Tanner et al. in 1962, revolutionized skeletal maturity assessment by introducing the bone specific scoring system.[2] The study was carried out in an average socioeconomic level British (Scottish) children in 1950s. It was later modified to TW2 method in 1975. The conclusion drawn from the greatest drawback of GP method was that the maturity scale should be defined in a manner which does not refer directly to age. In TW2 method this disadvantage was eliminated.[2] Till date this is the most accurate and reliable method for skeletal maturity assessment.

Tanner and Whitehouse II method **(Fig. 4)** is based on the principle that each bone develops to a reasonable, constant final shape, and a sequence of recognizable state can be defined right from the appearance to the final shape all along the developmental journey. Each bone is thus classified into eight or nine stages (A to H or I) to which weighted scores are assigned. Boys and girls have different scores for the same stage of a bone. Each stage differs from the next by "maturity indicators," i.e., slight change in shape which is presented both in visual form as well as written descriptions by the side of each stage in the atlas. While calculating skeletal maturity, both the visual and the descriptive information are used for assigning the stage but in case of any doubt, latter, i.e., descriptive information is used for making the final decision.

In 2001, an updated version of the "Tanner-Whitehouse method", the TW3 method was published. Unlike TW2, it took into account various secular trends and their relationship with total bone maturity.[18]

Technique

For TW2 and TW3 methods a PA radiograph of the left hand and wrist is used. During positioning it is important to keep

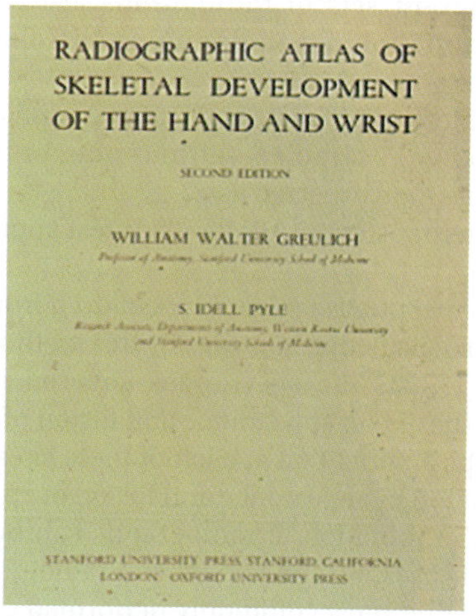

FIG. 3: Greulich and Pyle (GP) method bone age atlas.

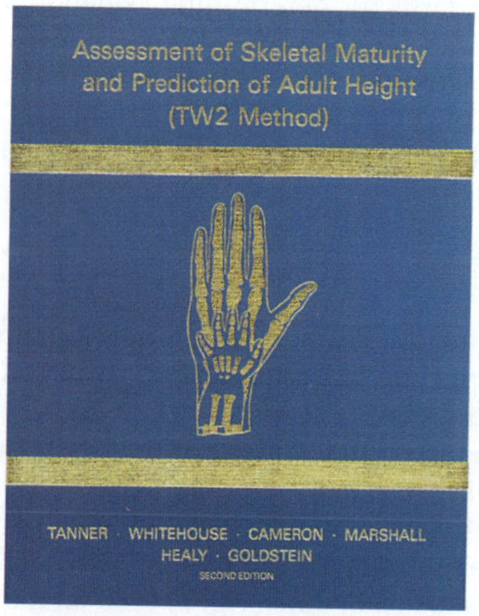

FIG. 4: Tanner and Whitehouse II (TW2) method bone age atlas.

the long axis of the middle finger, forearm, and arm in direct line and also upper arm and forearm in the same horizontal plane. Centering is done on the third metacarpal head at a film focus distance of 30 inches (75 cm).

X-ray film is viewed with fingers pointing upward and thumb on the right side of the viewer **(Fig. 5)**.

In this method 20 bones are assessed based on the TW2 atlas **(Fig. 4)** and score is assigned to them. The scores are summed up. Three separate maturity scoring systems are derived, i.e., carpal score (CS) for the seven carpals (out of the eight carpals pisiform is not considered for calculations), the "radius-ulna-short" bone (RUS) score for 13 bones comprising the radius, ulna, and short bones of hand (I, III, and V fingers only) and finally the TW2-20 bone score which combines both the carpal and the RUS components. For each of these three scoring systems, different "weighted scores" are assigned. At the end of the atlas a series of tables as well as centile standard curves are given for each of these three bone age scores from which "bone age" can be directly read for a given total score.

Finally three bone ages are thus obtained:

1. Radius-ulna-short bone age
2. Carpal bone age
3. 20 bone–bone age

Tanner and Whitehouse II and TW3 methods are useful till the age of 18 years (RUS and 20 bone–bone age) in boys and till 16 years in girls (RUS and 20 bone–bone age). However, upper limit for carpal bone age is 15 years in boys and 13 years in girls.

Comparison of Greulich and Pyle and Tanner and Whitehouse II Methods

A number of studies have compared the two standard methods. GP method is easy and faster to do while TW2 is a more laborious, time-consuming technique, and requires more training. Bone age was found to be closer to chronological age by TW2 method.[19] However, TW2 was less reproducible between observers in this study.[19] The conclusion of most studies[19-22] is to use one method, preferably TW2 method, when performing serial measurements on an individual patient.

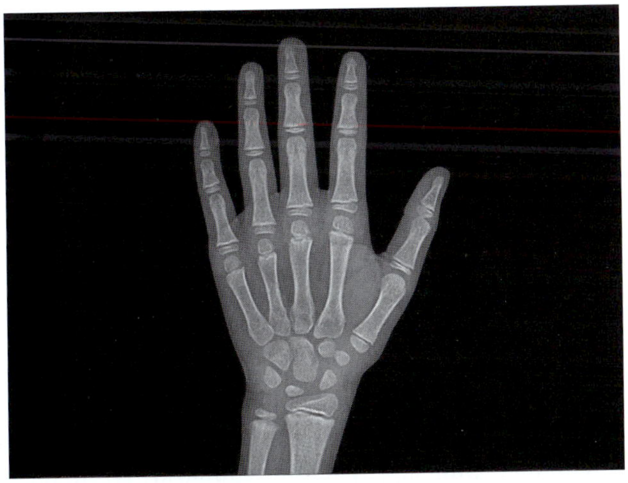

FIG. 5: While reviewing the radiograph of left hand and wrist by TW2 method, X-ray film should be put up with fingers pointing upwards and thumb directed to viewer's right side. (TW2: Tanner and Whitehouse II method)

Automated Bone Age Estimation

To eliminate the various sources of inter- and intraobserver errors associated with TW2 method (as well as for GP method and even for carpal bone maturation), a number of studies[23-27] have reported use of computer systems. Almost all of them found computer-aided systems to be reliable with results close to that with expert's interpretation. With time, TW2 method may become easy and a routine procedure with the help of these computer programs.

BoneXpert (Visiana, Denmark) is a commercially available automated bone-age calculation software, developed on Danish population. This offers a server-based automated calculation of bone age. The bone-age calculation is done on left hand radiograph using all three available methods (GP, TW2, and TW3). In this software, the user has to upload a digital image of the left hand radiograph; following which an automated outline marking of the 1st, 3rd, and 5th complete digital rows and calculation of bone take place **(Figs. 6A and B)**. The whole process is server-based. The report can be optimized to give bone age in all three methods (GP, TW2, and TW3). On adding the parent's height in the given proforma; it even provides a predicted adult height of the child. One unique feature in the calculation by BoneXpert is that it does not take into account the carpal bones at all. It has been found to be fairly reproducible, quick and easy to use and lacks the interobserver variation that can happen in atlas-based calculations.[28,29] It can estimate bone age for 2.5–17 years for boys and 2–15 for girls.

Ultrasound-based Bone Age Calculation

In November 2003, a German company called "Sunlight" introduced an ultrasound-based device to test skeletal age in children and adolescents.[30] In this method of bone-age estimation the child need not be referred to some specialized center but can be performed at the pediatrician's clinic with results in years and months available on the spot. Results are reported to be closely related to those produced by traditional method of GP atlas.

But this needs larger studies at various centers by independent workers before finally it can be accepted as a routine technique.

Magnetic Resonance-based Bone Age Assessment

A magnetic resonance (MR)-based bone-age assessment method was devised by Tereda et al.[31,32] on an open MR scanner. Bone age was estimated on hand and wrist images. Although they found this method to be correlating well with hand radiographs; the main drawback was the long imaging time. As of now, this is not widely used in clinical practice.

Indian Scene

Skeletal maturation is dependent not only on intrinsic factors such as genetic, racial, familial, and hormonal but also on

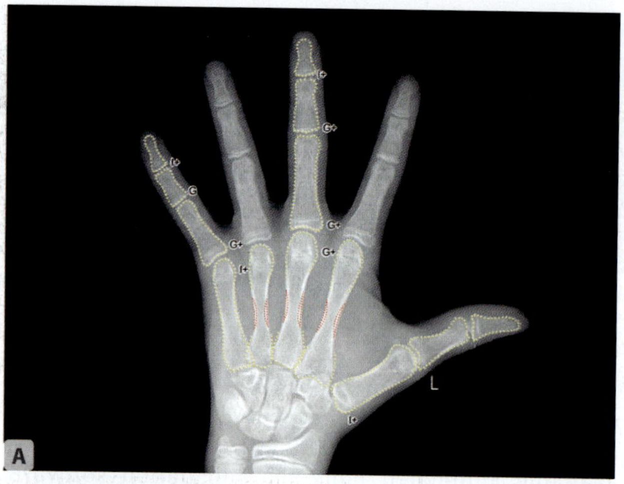

B

			X-ray date
Birth date	16/01/2010	Height	
		Father's height	
Ethnicity	Asian Chinese	Mother's height	
Age	7.03 years		
Bone age (GP)	8.40 years	Pred. adult height	
Bone age SDS			
Bone age (TW2)	8.89 years	Report date	
		Image file	
Bone health index	3.84	Hand	Left
BHI SDS		Physician	

FIGS. 6A AND B: Automated bone-age estimation software. (A) The marking of the first, 3rd and 5th rows; (B) Automated bone-age calculation format. Chronological age: 7.03 years; bone age (TW2): 8.89 years; bone age (GP): 8.4 years; bone age (TW3): 7.97 years. (GP: Greulich and Pyle method; SDS: standard deviation scores; TW2: Tanner and Whitehouse II method)

extrinsic factors such as socioeconomic status, nutrition, chronic illness, and climate. When there is interplay of so many factors then the standards for one population may not be applicable to another population. Ideally each country, even within different regions of each country, should establish their own standards through longitudinal (or at least cross-sectional) studies of normal children. However, due to an ethical issue of exposing normal children to radiation hazard such studies have not been carried out in large numbers. The next best thing is to apply well-established methods to our own population and compare the results. From India few studies[7,33] have been carried out using both GP and TW2 methods to assess skeletal maturity. Maniar[7] assessed Indian children with GP method but found progressively increasing delay after 2nd year of life. This method was therefore, not found applicable to Indian children by the author.[7]

On the other hand Maniar[7] applied the same set of radiographs as above to TW2 method. At any age between 1 and 7 years, the difference was found to be <0.8 years. Hence, TW2 method was found to be by far the best method applicable to Indian children. Our experience at AIIMS[34] in 100 normal healthy children is similar (unpublished data) and we concluded that TW2 method can be directly applied to Indian children. TW2 has been a standard method used in all pediatric endocrinology OPD patients at AIIMS for >3 decades.

To conclude, despite the difficulties of assessing bone age, and the assumptions on which various methods are based, skeletal maturity assessment is clinically relevant in that it provides the only means of assessing rates of maturational change throughout the growing period.[1] Of the various methods available, TW2 is the most accurate method and it can be applied directly to Indian population. However, this method requires correct positioning, precise radiographic technique, and skilled interpretation. Awareness among the pediatricians and radiologists of India about TW2 method and its advantages is essential before it can become part of routine workup in every department all over the country. For medicolegal purposes, however, method of appearance and fusion of ossification centers continues to be in use because age groups covered under MLC problems cannot be evaluated by other two methods.

ACCELERATED AND DELAYED BONE AGE

Skeletal maturity is the result of complex interplay of many factors, including nutrition and several hormones including growth hormone, corticosteroids, and sex hormones. In **Figure 7**, interplay of various hormones influencing bone age is shown. While growth hormone (GH), thyroid hormones, estrogen and androgen promote bone growth and maturation; glucocorticoids hamper bone maturation.[35,36] Hence, an excess of glucocorticoid as well as lack of GH and thyroid hormones will result in a delayed bone age **(Figs. 8A and B)** and short stature. An accelerated bone age **(Fig. 9)** and tall stature can result from an excess of growth hormone.

CAUSES OF SHORT STATURE

"Short stature" can be defined as a height that is two or more standard deviations below the expected mean gender-specified age. Short stature can happen because of a wide range of diseases, which includes nutritional deficiency, metabolic or endocrine disorders, genetic disorders, skeletal dysplasia among many. Short stature can even be familial or constitutional, when no other causes are found.

Dysmorphism and disproportionate short stature can be seen in various skeletal dysplasias. Causes of proportionate short stature include syndrome such as Down syndrome, Turner syndrome, endocrinologic (hypothyroidism, hypopituitarism, isolated GH deficiency, hypogonadism, precocious puberty, pseudohypoparathyroidism), gastrointestinal (GI) (celiac disease, malabsorption), chronic infections, chronic renal, and pulmonary diseases.

IMAGING EVALUATION IN SHORT STATURE

The imaging evaluation should be tailored according to the clinical details. In most cases, the radiological evaluation begins with bone-age assessment. Interpretation of the bone age, along with other imaging/clinical/laboratory findings, can provide complete diagnosis.

Other radiologic investigations pertinent to the evaluation of short stature include:

- *Skeletal survey*: In suspected skeletal dysplasia
- *Magnetic resonance imaging (MRI) brain*: Suspected hypopituitarism, Cushing syndrome, central precocious puberty
- *Ultrasound (US) neck*: Suspected congenital/Juvenile hypothyroidism
- *US and CT/MRI abdomen*: Precocious puberty, Cushing syndrome (congenital adrenal hyperplasia will require testicular ultrasound also)

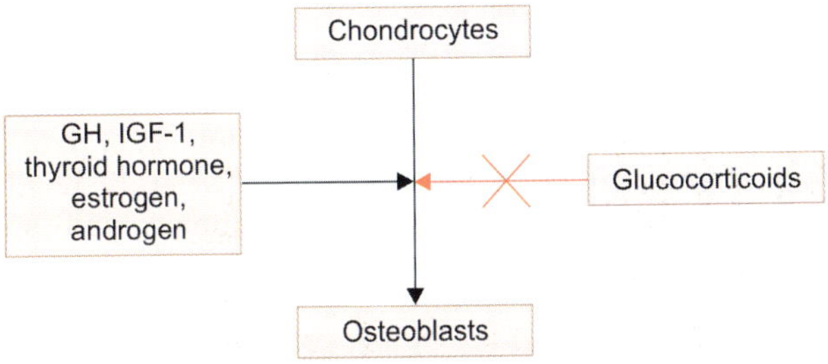

(GH: growth hormone; IGF-1: insulin-like growth factor-1)

FIG. 7: Influence of various hormones in proliferation of chondrocytes and their differentiation into osteoblasts.

IMAGING FINDINGS IN SPECIFIC DISEASE ENTITIES

Hypopituitarism[37-44]

Hypopituitarism can be congenital or acquired. Congenital hypopituitarism can result from hypoplastic anterior pituitary, pituitary stalk interruption syndrome. MRI of sella is the ideal imaging modality.

Acquired causes include Langerhan's cell histiocytosis (LCH), craniopharyngioma, hypothalamic hamartoma/glioma, germinoma, etc.

Usually during the evaluation of congenital pituitary hypoplasia, intravenous contrast administration is not

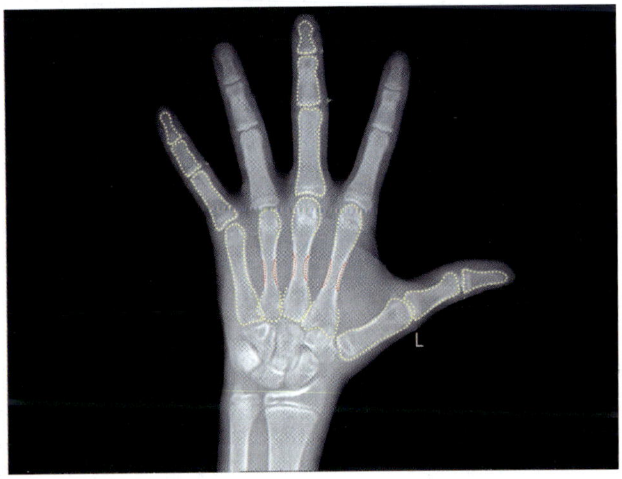

FIG. 9: Advanced bone age in a boy; Chronological age: 11.75 years; bone age (TW2): 15.66 years; bone age (GP): 14.74 years. (GP: Greulich and Pyle method; TW2: Tanner and Whitehouse II method)

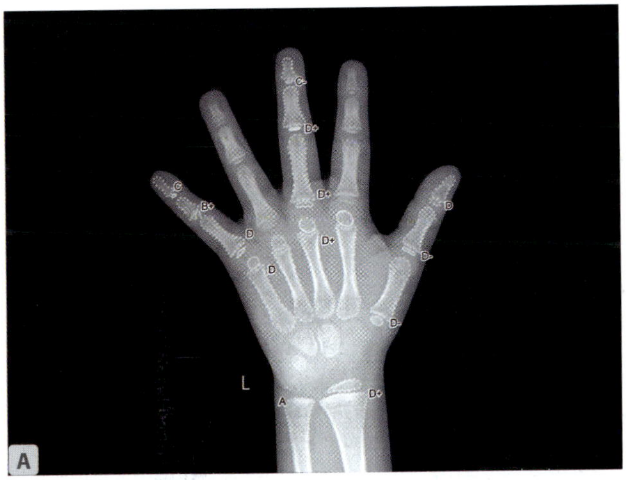

A

			X-ray date 16/02/2017
Birth date	11/02/2011	Height	
		Father's height	
Ethnicity	Asian American	Mother's height	
Age	6.02 years		
Bone age (GP)	2.69 years	Pred. adult height	
Bone age SDS	–3.64		
Bone age (TW3)	3.08 years		
Bone health index (BHI)	3.73		
BHI SDS			

B

FIGS. 8A AND B: Delayed bone age in a girl; Chronological age: 6.02 years; bone age (GP): 2.69 years; bone age (TW3): 3.08 years (GP: Greulich and Pyle method; SDS: standard deviation scores; TW3: Tanner and Whitehouse III method)

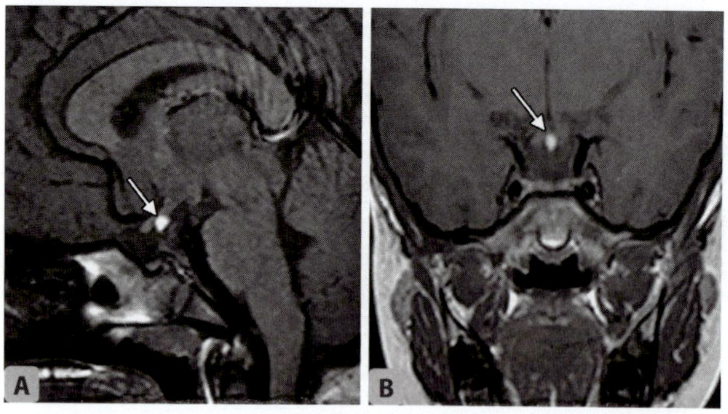

FIGS. 10A AND B: Pituitary stalk transection syndrome with ectopic posterior pituitary bright spot and hypoplastic pituitary. T1W sagittal (A) and coronal (B) MR images reveal a small sella, small anterior pituitary and an ectopic posterior pituitary bright spot (arrows). The stalk is not visualized. (MR: magnetic resonance; T1W: T1 weighted)

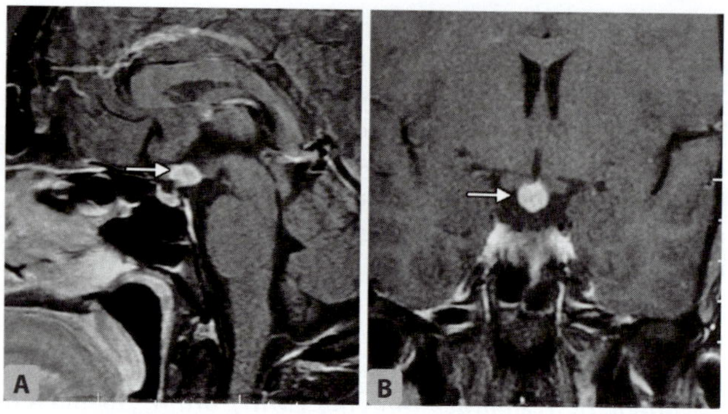

FIGS. 11A AND B: LCH involving the stalk and hypothalamus: T1W sagittal (A) and coronal (B) postcontrast MR images show thickening of stalk, globular lesion and hyperenhancement involving hypothalamus. (LCH: Langerhan's cell histiocytosis; MR: magnetic resonance; T1W: T1 weighted)

essential. However, evaluation of the acquired causes requires intravenous contrast administration.

Pituitary hypoplasia:[37,38] The anterior pituitary tissue is compressed along the sellar floor. On MRI, the height of the anterior pituitary is <2 mm. Herniation of cerebrospinal fluid (CSF) in the sella results in a partial empty sella.

Ectopic posterior pituitary/stalk interruption syndrome ***(Figs. 10A and B)***: Normal posterior pituitary is hyperintense on T1-weighted (T1W) MR images. In this condition, the hyperintense bright spot is absent in its usual location. Instead, it is found in ectopic locations such as near the infundibulum or hypothalamus along with an absent or fibrotic stalk.[39-41] The anterior pituitary is also small.

Langerhan's cell histiocytosis ***(Figs. 11A and B)***: This is a rare entity. It can be seen as part of multisystem affection by LCH. Hypothalamo-pituitary axis is the most common site of intracranial involvement.[42-44] Involvement of the pituitary stalk is manifested on imaging as a thickening and enhancement of the stalk. Absence of posterior pituitary bright spot is an imaging finding seen in central diabetes insipidus caused by LCH.

Craniopharyngioma ***(Figs. 12A to D)***: This tumor of the sella commonly manifests as a complex solid-cystic suprasellar mass, with variable sellar component as well. The cystic component is hyperintense on T1W with only minimal enhancement of the cyst wall. No solid component is usually present. A less common variant (papillary type) of this tumor is seen as solid enhancing suprasellar tumor.

Hypothalamic hamartoma/glioma ***(Figs. 13A to C)***: Hypothalamic hamartomas are seen as well-defined suprasellar mass. The signal intensity is similar to the gray matter signal intensity on all MR sequences and no enhancement is seen on postcontrast images.

Hypothyroidism

Congenital or juvenile hypothyroidism can result in a marked short stature, usually associated with intellectual disability. Structurally, the thyroid gland can be hypoplastic, absent or ectopic. Ultrasound neck is useful in diagnosing absence of thyroid gland in its normal location. However, ruling out an ectopic thyroid gland will require nuclear scans such as ^{99m}Tc pertechnetate or I-123 scan **(Figs. 14A to C)**.[45]

There are various well-described skeletal changes in long-standing hypothyroidism; including osteopenia, markedly delayed bone age, metaphyseal sclerotic bands at the end of long bones, and irregular stippled epiphyses **(Figs. 15A to C)**.

Congenital hypothyroidism can rarely be associated with incomplete isosexual precocious puberty (Van Wyk Grumbach syndrome).[46] Clinically there is menarche, occasionally breast development, but absence of pubic hair development. This results due to the structural similarities among thyroid-stimulating hormone (TSH), follicle-stimulating hormone (FSH), and their receptors. In congenital hypothyroidism, very high levels of TSH can bind to FSH receptors and lead to activation of follicular cells, and ovarian stimulation leading to estrogen production. Ovaries are enlarged with multiple cysts **(Figs. 16A to C)**. However, the luteinizing hormone (LH) level and LH/FSH ratio is usually low (in comparison, LH/FSH ratio is high in normal puberty). On imaging, features of incomplete precocious puberty with a delayed bone age should alarm one for this disorder.

Cushing Syndrome

Cushing syndrome can be due to endogenous or exogenous glucocorticoid excess. Endogenous glucocorticoid excess can be due to adrenal adenoma; or due to excess of adrenocorticotropic hormone (ACTH) secretion. Excess of ACTH secretion can be seen in either pituitary microadenoma or ectopic tumors (e.g., thymic carcinoid).

Usual imaging workup includes dynamic contrast-enhanced MRI brain, MRI/adrenal protocol CT abdomen. Ectopic ACTH secreting lesions are difficult to find on imaging; and often CT/MRI chest and abdomen are performed for the same.

Adrenocorticotropic hormone secreting pituitary microadenoma is usually a small lesion, T1W and T2W

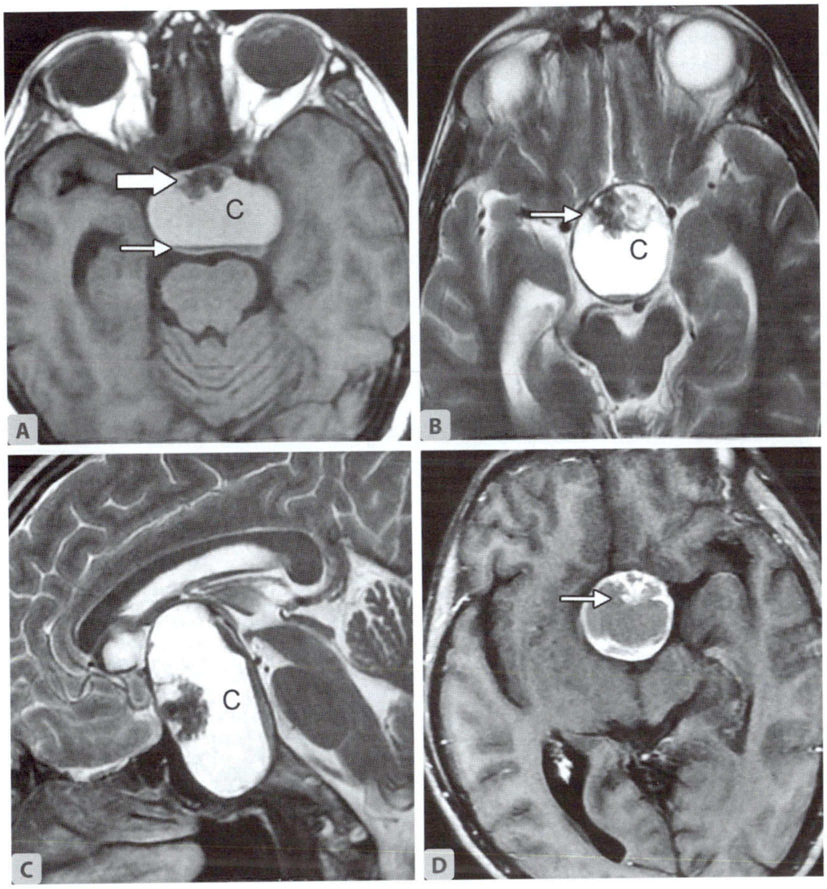

FIGS. 12A TO D: Craniopharyngioma: T1W axial MR image (A) shows hyperintense internal content of the cyst (C), with layering (arrow) and solid hypointense component anteriorly (block arrow). Axial T2W image (B) shows the cyst content as hyperintense. Sagittal T2W image showing sellar as well as suprasellar extension of the lesion with solid component anteriorly (arrow). Contrast-enhanced image (D) showing thin cyst wall enhancement as well as enhancement of the solid component (arrow). (MR: magnetic resonance; T1W: T1 weighted; T2W: T2 weighted)

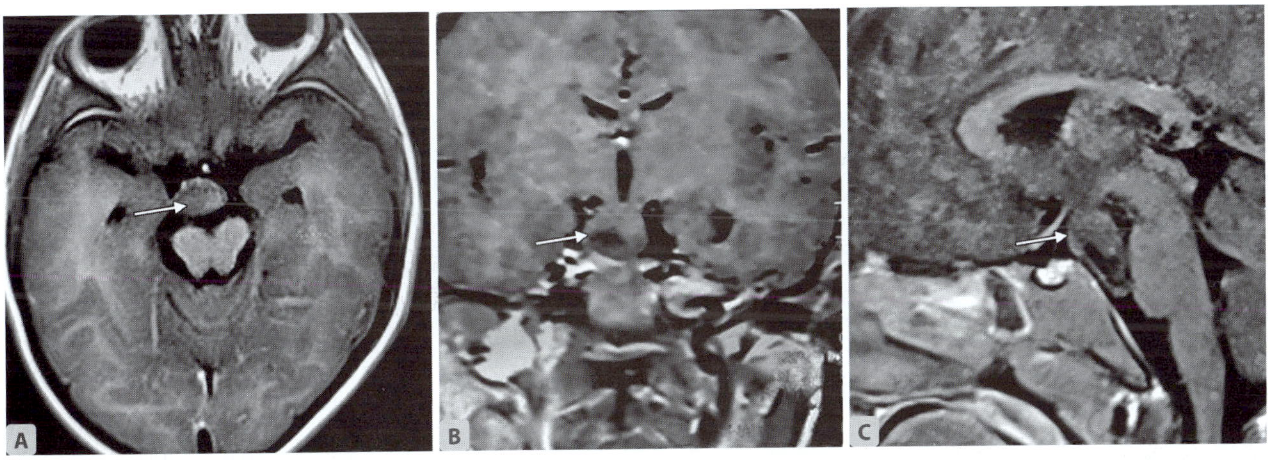

FIGS. 13A TO C: Hypothalamic hamartoma: Axial (A), coronal (B), and sagittal (C). T1W contrast enhanced MR images reveal a solid nonenhancing hypothalamic mass (arrow) isointense to gray matter.

hypointense hypoenhancing focal lesion. However, on a 30-minutes delayed scan, it shows increased signal intensity compared to the rest of the anterior pituitary **(Figs. 17A to D)**.

The bone age is usually normal and can even be advanced. Other skeletal manifestations include osteopenia, multiple vertebral collapses, and fractures with hypertrophied callus formation **(Fig. 18)**.

Precocious Puberty

Precocious puberty is defined as the onset of puberty before 8 years in girls and 9 years in boys.[47-50] Primarily precocious

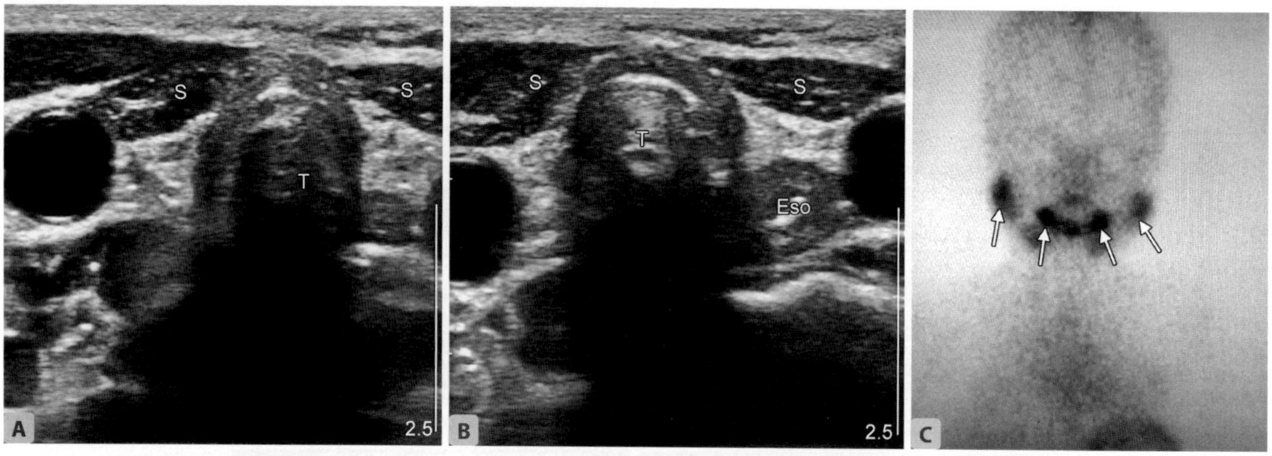

FIGS. 14A TO C: Congenital hypothyroidism: Ultrasound neck (A and B) shows no thyroid gland anterior to trachea (T). Note the strap muscles (S) of the neck are apposed to the anterior wall of trachea. Tc-99m pertechnetate scan (C) reveals absence of thyroid uptake. Note normal salivary gland uptake (arrows).

Courtesy: Dr Devasenathipathy Kandasamy.

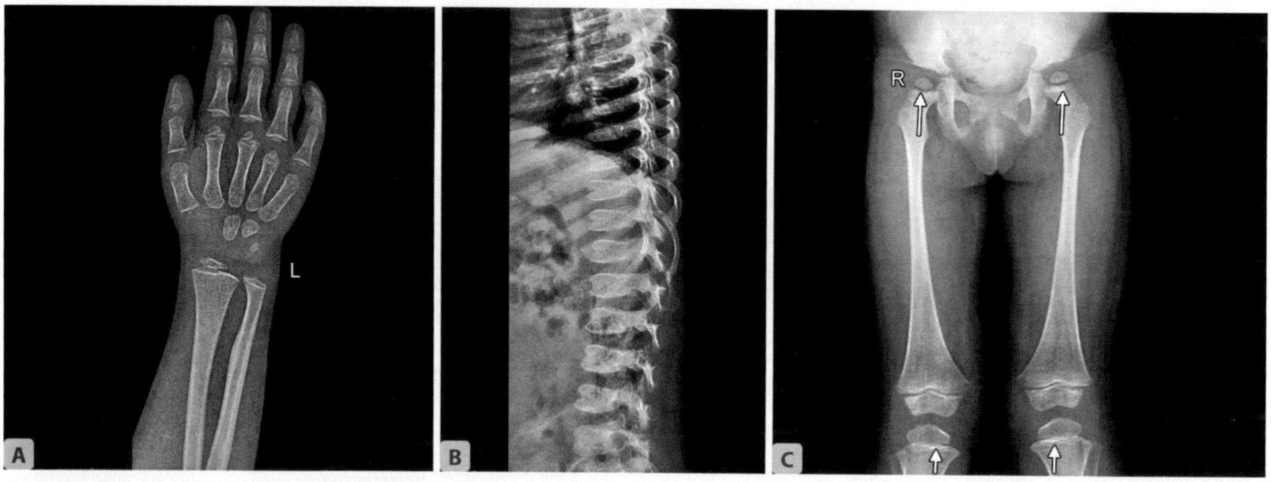

FIGS. 15A TO C: Skeletal changes in long-standing untreated hypothyroidism. Delayed bone age in an 11-year-old girl (A). Osteopenia with flattening of vertebral bodies (B). Metaphyseal sclerotic bands (arrows in C).

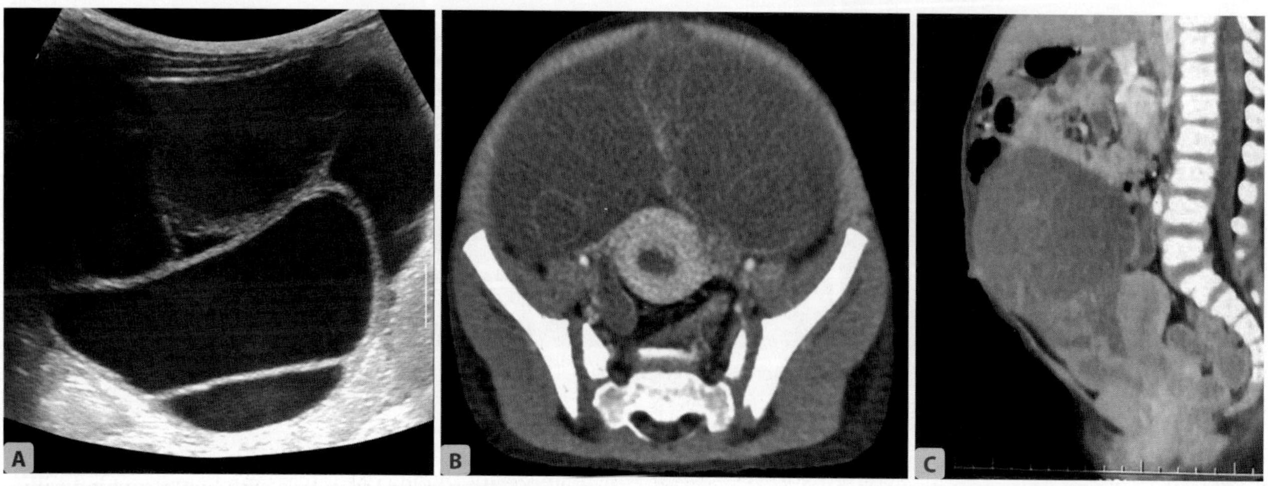

FIGS. 16A TO C: Van Wyk-Grumbach syndrome, patient same as in previous image. She presented with pain and swelling in abdomen, precocious puberty (premature menarche) and short stature; although there was no development of pubic hair. Ultrasound pelvis (A) reveals bilateral enlarged cystic ovaries. Axial (B) and sagittal (C) CECT images reveal enlarged pubertal uterus and bilateral enlarged cystic ovaries. Incomplete isosexual precocity along with a delayed bone age should raise a suspicion of this disorder. (CECT: contrast-enhanced computed tomography)

Courtesy: Dr Devasenathipathy Kandasamy.

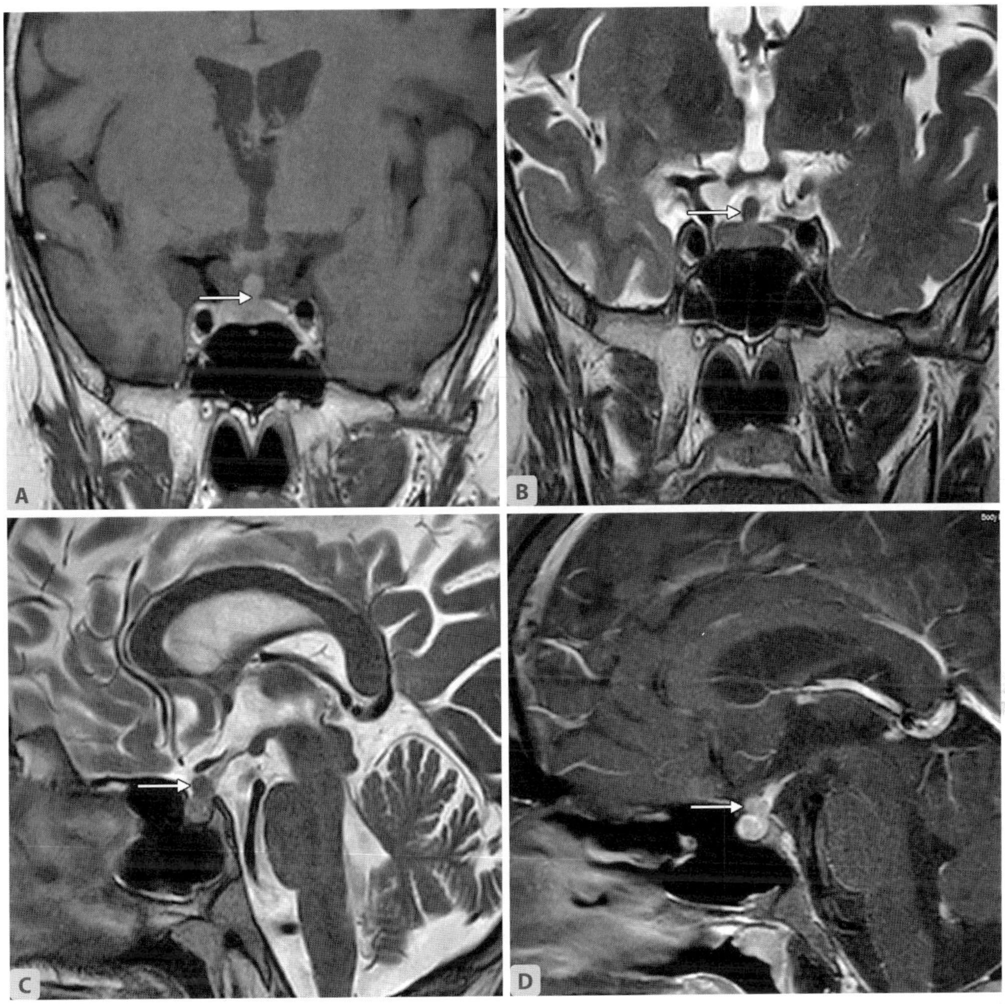

FIGS. 17A TO D: Cushing syndrome due to pituitary microadenoma in a child. Coronal T1W (A), T2W (B), sagittal T2W (C), and sagittal T1W postcontrast (D) images show the microadenoma (arrow) near the stalk. (T1W: T1 weighted; T2W: T2 weighted)

Courtesy: Dr Devasenathipathy Kandasamy.

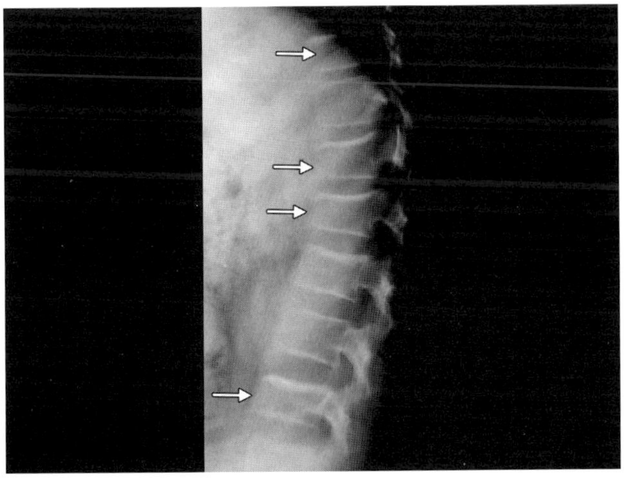

FIG. 18: Spinal radiograph in a child with Cushing syndrome reveals osteopenia and multiple vertebral collapses (arrows).

puberty can be of two types: (1) central and (2) peripheral. Central precocity results from oversecretion of gonadotropin-releasing hormone (GnRH) and hyperstimulation of the gonads. It may result from various causes such as infections, hydrocephalus, central nervous system (CNS) tumors, etc.

When the increased secretion of sex hormones (estrogen and androgen) is a result of any lesion in the gonad itself (or secondary to adrenal pathology such as congenital adrenal hyperplasia); it is called peripheral precocious puberty. In males, congenital adrenal hyperplasia can result in precocious puberty and a short stature. Testicular ultrasound should also be done along with adrenal USG/CT in these children as testicular adrenal rests are not uncommon **(Figs. 19A to E)**.

In girls, causes of peripheral precocious puberty include ovarian cyst or tumors (e.g., juvenile granulosa cell tumor). Hence, along with abdominal ultrasound, a detailed pelvic ultrasound should also be done. It is essential to be well-

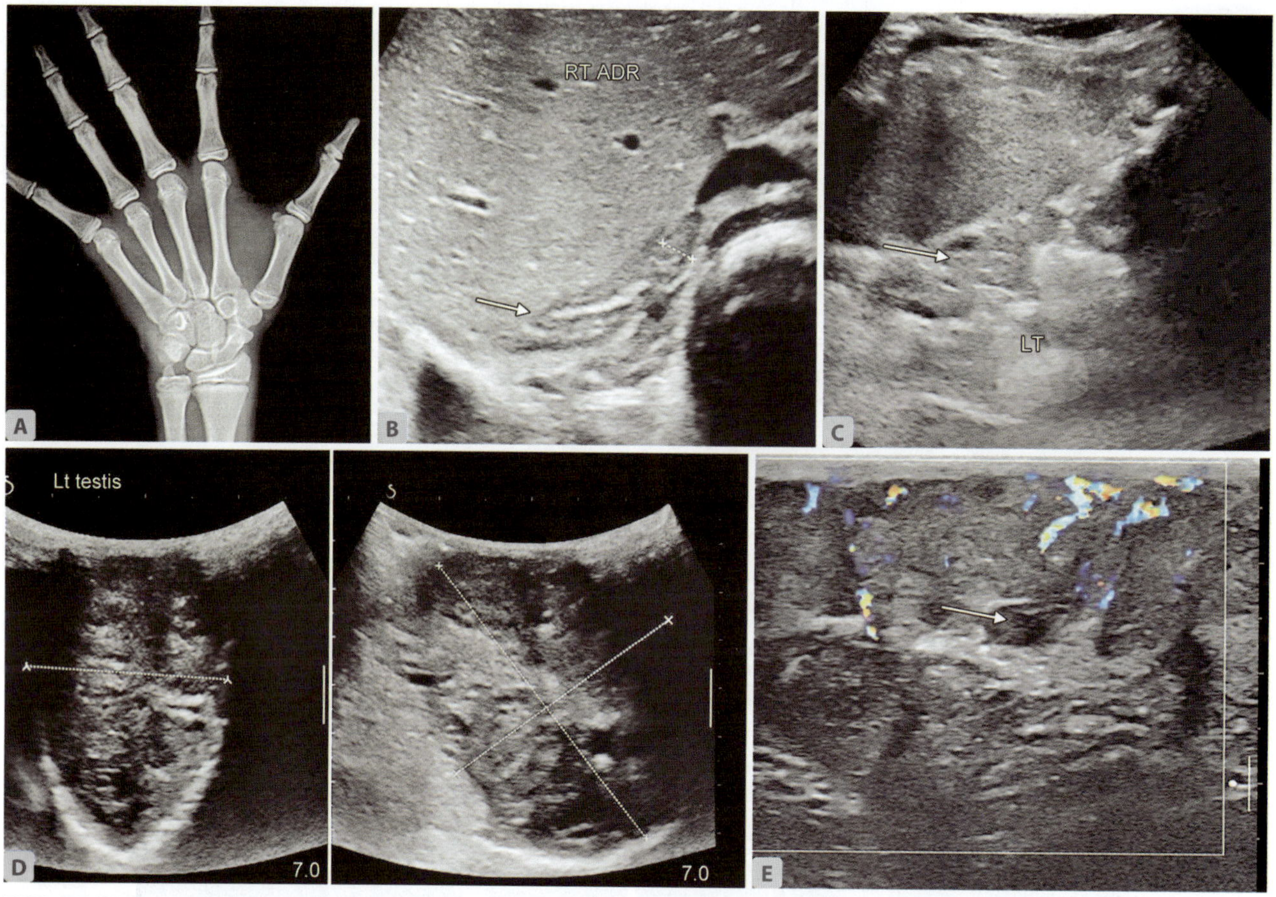

FIGS. 19A TO E: Congenital adrenal hyperplasia with testicular adrenal rest. Hand radiograph of a 6-year-old boy showing advanced bone age (A). Ultrasound abdomen (B and C) shows bilateral adrenal enlargement (arrows). Scrotal ultrasound (D) reveals heterogeneously enlarged bilateral testes. High-resolution ultrasound (E) of testis reveals hypoechoic focal lesions (arrow).

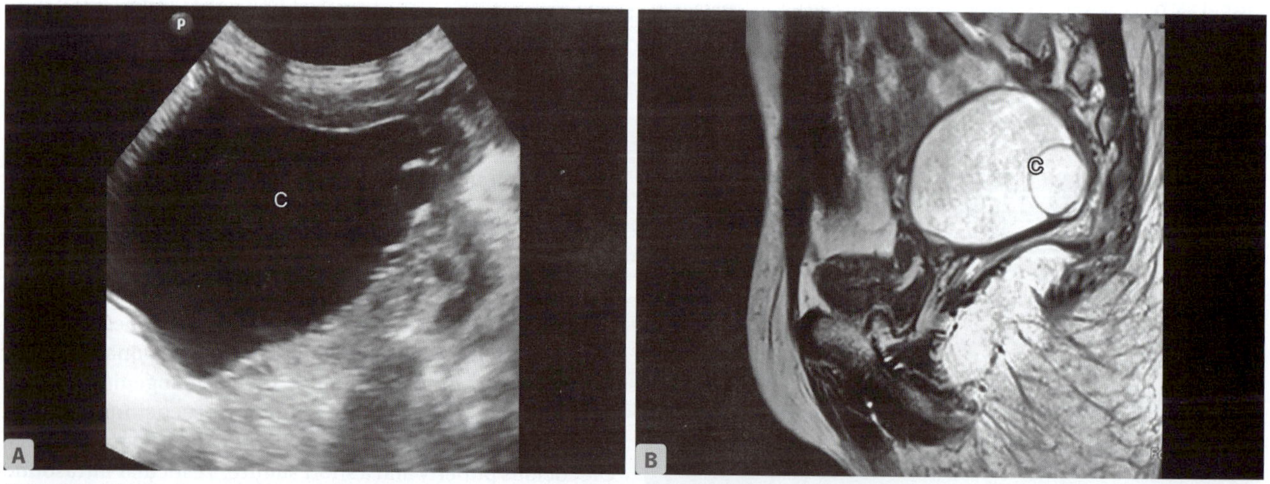

FIGS. 20A AND B: Functioning ovarian cyst causing precocious puberty and short stature in a 6-year-old girl. Ultrasound abdomen (A) and T2W sagittal MRI (B) show ovarian cyst (C) with "cyst within cyst" appearance. (MRI: magnetic resonance imaging; T2W: T2 weighted)

versed with the normal appearance of a prepubertal ovary; as even a functional ovarian cyst itself **(Figs. 20A and B)** can cause precocious puberty.

Juvenile granulosa cell tumors usually present as a heterogeneous solid-cystic mass **(Figs. 21A to C)**.

Hepatic tumors such as hepatoblastoma, teratoma, or hepatocellular carcinoma can sometimes secrete LH or human chorionic gonadotropin (hCG) and cause precocious puberty.

Table 2 enlists some of the important causes of short stature in children and the diagnostic clues.

A simplified approach toward a child with short stature is given in **Flowchart 1**.

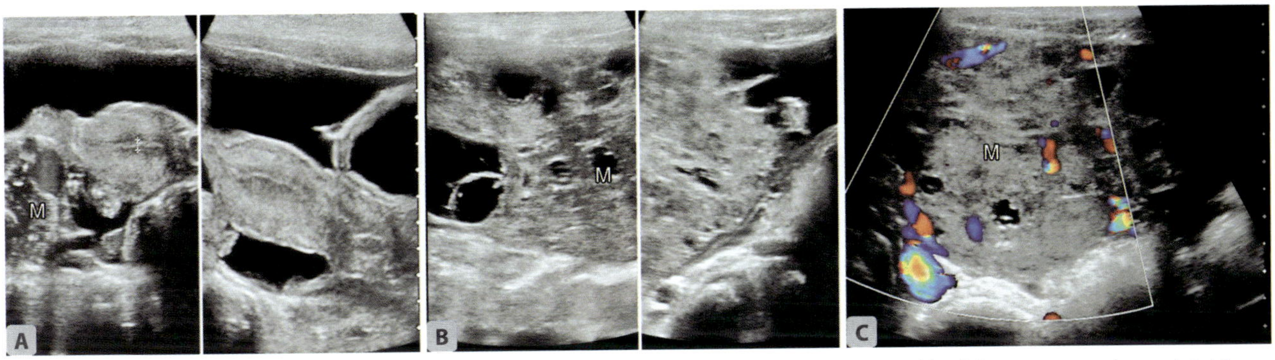

FIGS. 21A TO C: Juvenile granulosa cell tumor causing precocious puberty and short stature in a 3-year-old girl. Bone age was advanced. Pelvic US shows an uterus having pubertal shape and proportions, with well-identified thin endometrium (A). A large solid cystic right adnexal mass (M) is seen, having scattered color flow (B and C). (US: ultrasound)

TABLE 2: Clinic-radiological diagnosis in causes of short stature.

Disease	*Bone age*	*Other imaging findings/clinical clue*
Hypothyroidism	Delayed	Skeletal: Osteopenia, metaphyseal sclerotic band, epiphyseal irregularity, and stippling Others: Mental retardation, absence/hypoplastic/ectopic thyroid gland
Hypopituitarism	Significantly delayed	Imaging will vary and depend on the cause (detailed above)
Isolated GH deficiency	Delayed	Acquired: Recent head trauma/CNS infection/radiation treatment Congenital: Midline craniofacial anomalies, hypoglycemia, bone age, and height becomes progressively delayed with age after a normal length at birth
Precocious puberty	Advanced	Imaging findings depend on the cause (detailed above)
Cushing syndrome	Delayed	Skeletal: Osteopenia, fracture with hypertrophic callus, platyspondyly Adrenal adenoma/pituitary microadenoma/ectopic ACTH secreting tumor
Turner syndrome	Delayed	Hypoplastic uterus, streak ovaries, short 4th metacarpals
Familial short stature	Normal	Midparental height analysis
Constitutional delay	Delayed	Delayed onset of puberty, resulting in a normal adult height
Idiopathic	Normal	After exclusion of pathologies

(ACTH: adrenocorticotropic hormone; CNS: central nervous system)

FLOWCHART 1: Simplified algorithm of approach toward short stature.

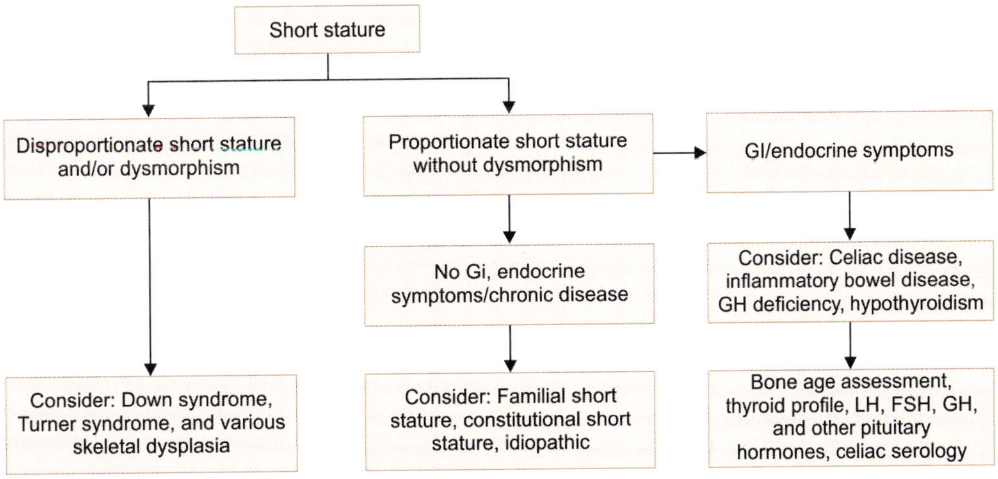

(FSH: follicle-stimulating hormone; LH: luteinizing hormone; GH: growth hormone; GI: gastrointestinal)

REFERENCES

1. Cox LA. The biology of bone maturation and ageing. Acta Paediatr Suppl. 1997;423:107-8.
2. Tanner JM, Whitehouse RH, Cameron N, Marshall WA, Healy MJR, Goldstein H. Assessment of Skeletal Maturity and Prediction of Adult Height (TW2 method), 2nd edition. London: Academic Press; 1983.
3. Kangne RN, Sami SA, Deshpande VL. Age estimation of adolescent girls by radiography. JFMT. 1999;16(1):20-6.
4. Gupta AK. Chapter 20: Skeletal Maturity Assessment. How is skeletal age measured? [online] Available from http://vms.cc.wmich. edu/~Anemone/anth354/tsld091.htm. [Last accessed June, 2020].
5. Kovi R, Körner A, Varkony J, Kis É. Bone age discrepancy on hand radiographs. Pediatr Radiol. 2000;30(7):500.
6. Marshall WA. Individual variations in rate of skeletal maturation. Nature. 1969;221(195):91.
7. Maniar B. Skeletal maturity in Indian children. Indian J Pediatr. 1987;54:295-302.
8. Modi's Medical Jurisprudence and Toxicology, 1999.
9. Jain S. Estimation of age from 13 to 21 years. JFMT. 1999;16(1):27-30.
10. Bajaj ID, Bhardwaj OP, Bhardwaj S. Appearance and fusion of important ossification centers. A study in Delhi population. Indian J Med Res. 1967;55:1064-7.
11. Sharat S, Khanduja PC, Agarwal KN, Saha MM, Gupta S, Bhardwaj OP. Skeletal growth in school children. Indian Pediatr. 1970;7:98-108.
12. Mughal AM, Hassan N, Ahmed A. Bone Age Assessment Methods: A Critical Review. Pak J Med Sci. 2014;30(1):211-5.
13. Paterson RS. A radiological investigation of the epiphyses of the long bones. J Anat. 1929;64:28-46.
14. Flecker H. Roentgenographic observations of the times of appearance of epiphyses and their fusion with the diaphyses. J Anat. 1932;67:118-64.
15. Pillai MJS. The study of epiphyseal union for determination of age of South Indians. Ind J Med Res. 1936;23:1015-7.
16. Greulich WW, Pyle SI. Radiographic atlas of skeletal development of hand and wrist. Stanford: Stanford University Press; 1950.
17. King DG, Steventon DM, O'Sullivan MP, Cook AM, Hornsby VP, Jefferson IG, et al. Reproducibility of bone ages when performed by radiology registrars: An audit of Tanner and Whitehouse II versus Greulich and Pyle methods. BJR. 1994;801(67):848-51.
18. Tanner JM, Healy M, Goldstein H, Cameron N. Assessment of skeletal maturity and prediction of adult height (TW3 method), 3rd edition. London: WB Saunders, Harcourt Publishers Ltd; 2001.
19. Benso L, Vannelli S, Pastorin L, Angius P, Milani S. Main problems associated with bone age and maturity evaluation. Horm Res. 1996;45(2):42-8.
20. Gilli G. The assessment of skeletal maturation. Horm Res. 1996;45(2):49-52.
21. Cole AJ, Webb L, Cole TJ. Bone age estimation: A comparison of methods. BJR. 1988;728(61):683-6.
22. Bull RK, Edwards PD, Kemp PM, Fry S, Hughes I. Bone age assessment: A large scale comparison of the Greulich and Pyle, and Tanner and Whitehouse (TW2) methods. Arch Dis Child. 1999;81:172-3.
23. Canovas F, Banegas C, Cyteval M, Jaeger M, DiMéglio A, Bonnel F, et al. Carpal bone maturation assessment by image analysis from computed tomography scans. Horm Res. 2000;54:6-13.
24. Drayer NM, Cox LA. Assessment of bone age by Tanner and Whitehouse method using a computer-aided system. Acta Paediatr Suppl. 1994;406:77-80.
25. Frisch H, Riedl S, Wadhor T. Computer-aided estimation of skeletal age and comparison with bone age evaluation by the method of Greulich-Pyle and Tanner-Whitehouse. Pediatr Radiol. 1996;26(3):226-31.
26. Sato A, Ashizawa K, Anzo M, Otsuki F, Kaneko S, Tanaka T, et al. Setting up an automated system for evaluation of bone age. Endocr J. 1999;46:S97-100.
27. Tanner JM, Gibbons RD. A computerized image analysis system for estimating Tanner–Whitehouse 2 bone age. Horm Res. 1994;42(6):282-7.
28. van Rijn RR, Lequin MH, Thodberg HH. Automatic determination of Greulich and Pyle bone age in healthy Dutch children. Pediatr Radiol. 2009;39:591-7.
29. Thodberg HH, Kreiborg S, Juul A, Pedersen KD. The BoneXpert method for automated determination of skeletal maturity. IEEE Trans Med Imaging. 2009;28:52-66.
30. Sunlight introduces Ultrasound-based bone age testing. [online] Available from http://www9.medica.de/cgi-bin/md/content.cgi?lang=2 and ticket=g_u_e_s_t and oid=11275 and print=1/1/99 [Last accessed June, 2020].
31. Terada Y, Kono S, Tamada D, Uchiumi T, Kose K, Miyagi R, et al. Skeletal age assessment in children using an open compact MRI system. Magn Reson Med. 2013;69:1697-702.
32. Terada Y, Kono S, Uchiumi T, Kose K, Miyagi R, Yamabe E, et al. Improved reliability in skeletal age assessment using a pediatric hand MR scanner with a 0.3T permanent magnet. Magn Reson Med Sci. 2014;13:215-9.
33. Prakash S, Cameron N. Skeletal maturity of well-off children in Chandigarh, North India. Ann Hum Biol. 1981;8:175-80.
34. Gupta AK, Menon PSN, Seth V. Skeletal maturity by TW2 method in normal, healthy children at AIIMS (unpublished data).
35. Bajpai A, Kabra M, Gupta AK, Menon PS. Growth pattern and skeletal maturation following growth hormone therapy in growth hormone deficiency: factors influencing outcome. India Pediatr. 2006;43(7):593-9.
36. Satoh M. Bone age: assessment methods and clinical applications. Clin Pediatr Endocrinol. 2015;24(4):143-52.
37. Chaudhary V, Bano S. Imaging of pediatric pituitary endocrinopathies. Indian J Endocrinol Metab. 2012;16(5):682-91.
38. Delman BN. Imaging of Pediatric Pituitary Abnormalities. Endocrinol Metab Clin North Am. 2009;38:673-98.
39. Kulkarni C, Moorthy S, Pullara SK, Rajeshkannan R, Unnikrishnan AG, et al. Pituitary stalk transection syndrome: Comparison of clinico-radiological features in adults and children with review of literature. Indian J Radiol Imaging. 2012;22(3):182-5.
40. Ioachimescu AG, Hamrahian AH, Stevens M, Zimmerman RS. The pituitary transaction syndrome: Multifaceted presentation in adulthood. Pituitary. 2012;15:405-11.
41. Argyropoulou M, Perigram F, Brauner R, Brunelle F. Magnetic resonance imaging in diagnosis of growth hormone deficiency. J Pediatr. 1992;12:886-91.
42. D'Ambrosio N, Soohoo S, Warshall C, Johnson A, Karimi S. Craniofacial and Intracranial Manifestations of Langerhans Cell Histiocytosis: Report of Findings in 100 Patients. AJR Am J Roentgenol. 2008;191:589-97.
43. Prayer D, Grois N, Prosch H, Gadner H, Barkovich AJ. MR Imaging Presentation of Intracranial Disease Associated with Langerhans Cell Histiocytosis. Am J Neuroradiol. 2004;25:880-91.
44. Hamilton BE, Salzman KL, Osborn AG. Anatomic and Pathologic Spectrum of Pituitary Infundibulum Lesions. AJR. 2007;188:W223-32.

45. Chang YW, Lee DH, Hong YH, Hong HS, Choi DL, Seo DY. Congenital Hypothyroidism: Analysis of Discordant US and Scintigraphic Findings. Radiology. 2011;258:872-9.
46. Rastogi A, Bhadada SK, Bhansali A. An unusual presentation of a usual disorder: Van Wyk-Grumback syndrome. Indian J Endocrinol Metab. 2011;15(Suppl 2):S141-3.
47. Jakubowska A, Grajewska-Ferens M, Brzewski M, Sopyło B. Usefulness of imaging techniques in the diagnostics of precocious puberty in boys. Pol J Radiol. 2011;76(4):21-7.
48. Pectasides D, Pectasides E, Psyrri A. Granulosa cell tumor of the ovary. Cancer Treat Rev. 2008;34(1):1-12.
49. Gittleman AM, Price AP, Coren C, Akhtar M, Donovan V, Katz DS. Radiology-Pathology Conference: Juvenile granulosa cell tumor. J Clin Imaging. 2003;27(4):221-4.
50. Gupta AK, Jana M, Kumar A. Imaging in short stature and bone age estimation. Indian J Pediatr. 2019;86(10):939-51.

CHAPTER

80

Spinal Dysraphism

Raju Sharma, Ankur Goyal, Devasenathipathy Kandasamy

INTRODUCTION

Spinal dysraphism is one of the most common congenital disorders associated with significant morbidity and mortality with estimated incidence of approximately 0.05–0.25 per 1,000 births.[1] It can be defined as an incomplete fusion of midline mesenchymal, bony, and neural structures.[2]

Spinal dysraphism is broadly classified into open and closed type. Most of the open spinal dysraphic states can be detected prenatally using ultrasound or fetal magnetic resonance imaging (MRI). Postnatal imaging is usually performed to look for associated central nervous system (CNS) anomalies (hydrocephalus, Chiari malformation) and in postoperative patients presenting with progressive neurological deficit to look for any treatable cause. Most of the closed spinal dysraphic states remain asymptomatic at birth and are suspected in the presence of high-risk cutaneous markers or when these children present with neurological deficit later in life.[3]

Magnetic resonance imaging is the modality of choice for evaluating spinal dysraphism.[4-6] It is helpful in the classification, diagnosis, and treatment planning of these disorders.

CLASSIFICATION

Most of the dysraphic spinal states can be explained on the basis of specific abnormality in early embryonic development which spans over the period of 3rd to 8th week of intrauterine life and classification based on embryology has been proposed **(Box 1)**. Since our understanding of human embryology is likely to evolve, this classification is also likely to change over a period of time. Recently, Tortori-Donati P et al.[5,6] proposed a classification system based on clinicoradiological features **(Flowchart 1)**, which is now widely accepted and followed. Spinal dysraphism is classified into two categories: (1) Open spinal dysraphism (OSD); and (2) Closed spinal dysraphism (CSD). Neural tissue is exposed to the environment in OSDs whereas CSDs are covered by skin, with cutaneous markers present in up to 50% of cases.

First step in the evaluation of patients with dysraphism is thorough clinical assessment **(Figs. 1A to C)**. The child's back should be evaluated to look for presence/absence of skin covering, back mass, and cutaneous stigmata of dysraphism **(Box 2)**.[3,5,6]

BOX 1: Embryological classification of spinal dysraphism.

Anomalies of gastrulation:

- Disorders of notochordal integration:
  - Dorsal enteric fistula
  - Neurenteric cysts
  - Split cord malformations (diastematomyelia)
  - Dermal sinus
- Disorders of notochord formation:
  - Caudal regression syndrome
  - Segmental spinal dysgenesis

Anomalies of primary neurulation:

- Myelomeningocele
- Myeloschisis
- Lipomas with dural defect:
  - Lipomyelomeningocele
  - Lipomyeloschisis
- Intradural lipoma

Anomalies of secondary neurulation and retrogressive differentiation:

- Filar lipoma
- Tight filum terminale
- Abnormally elongated spinal cord
- Persistent terminal ventricle
- Terminal myelocystocele

Anomalies of unknown origin:

- Cervical myelocystocele
- Meningocele

EMBRYOLOGY

It is vital to know the development of the spinal cord to understand the different types of spinal dysraphism. The development of the bony spine and intraspinal contents begins in the 1st month of gestation.[7,8] The spinal cord

FLOWCHART 1: Clinicoradiological classification proposed by Tortori-Donati P et al.

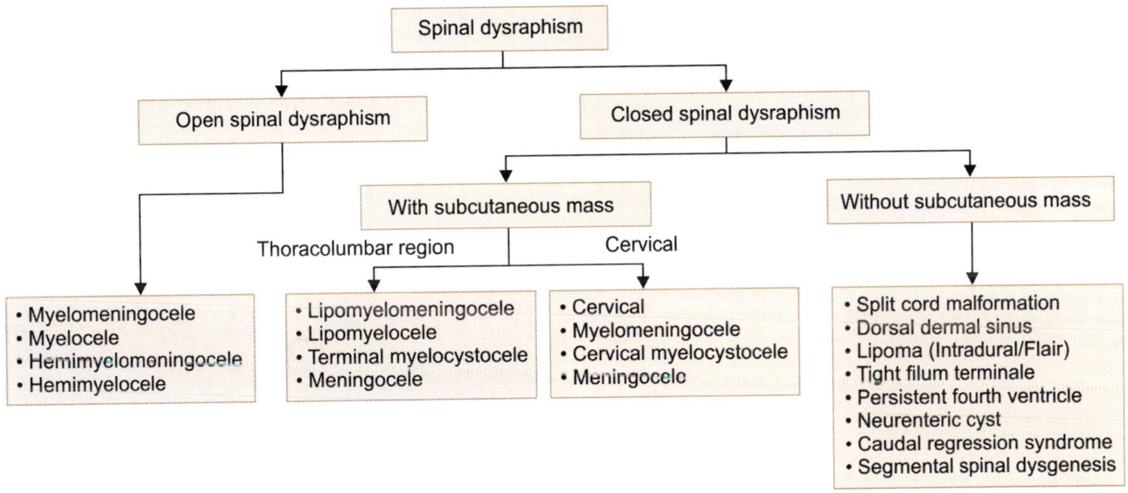

develops from ectoderm and the development occurs during three stages: (1) Neurulation, (2) Canalization, and (3) Retrogressive differentiation. During the 1st week of gestation, there is a proliferation of ectodermal cells along the surface of the embryo to form the primitive streak. This is the neural plate which forms a groove in the midline and during the 3rd week of gestation, it begins to fold laterally. The folds begin to approach each other dorsally near the midline at the neural groove and the neural plate, thus closes to form the neural tube. This is referred to as the stage of neurulation.

Simultaneous with the stage of neurulation, the overlying ectoderm of the skin separates from the neural tube and fuses in the midline. The perineural mesenchyme grows around the neural tube to form the meninges, bone, and muscle. Majority of the dysraphic states including myelomeningocele, myelocele, and lipomyelomeningocele are thought to occur at this stage of development of the spine and spinal cord.

During the next stage called canalization, the caudal end of the neural tube elongates into a caudal cell mass and ependyma lines a central tubular structure. It is believed that persistence of portions or abnormal development of the caudal cell mass may give rise to intradural lipoma, sacral teratoma, and tethered low-lying spinal cord.

Finally, during the stage of retrogressive differentiation (between 5 and 6 weeks), there is a decrease in the size of the central lumen and in the caudal cell mass and formation of the spinal cord, conus medullaris, and filum terminale. The underlying cause for different types of spinal dysraphism is thought to be an insult—either genetic or acquired that interferes with the normal process of neurulation, canalization, or retrogressive differentiation.

IMAGING MODALITIES

Magnetic resonance imaging is the imaging modality of choice for the diagnosis and characterization of spinal dysraphism. Other modalities play a supplemental role.

Plain radiographs (anteroposterior and lateral views) are mandatory for evaluation of the vertebral column.[5,9] The findings seen on plain radiographs include focal spina bifida, widened spinal canal, scoliosis, segmentation anomalies like block vertebrae, butterfly vertebrae, and other congenital abnormalities. Bony spur may be seen in cases of diastematomyelia. Radiographs are used as preliminary screening examination that can help to guide further imaging workup.

Ultrasonography (USG) is primarily useful in the antenatal diagnosis of spinal dysraphism **(Figs. 2 to 4)** and is also of use in the neonate and infant.[4] It becomes progressively less useful as ossification of posterior elements proceeds during the 1st year of life. Prenatal sonography can detect the open widened neural arch with flared laminae, can show the meningomyelocele sac, and detect hydrocephalus and other associated cranial anomalies. Direct sonography of the sac in children using high frequency transducers can provide information regarding the contents of the sac. However, for complete and more detailed information, an MR scan is usually required.

Computed tomography (CT) is useful in demonstration of the bony spur in cases of split cord malformation (SCM). Myelography and postmyelogram CT were used prior to the advent of MRI.

Magnetic resonance imaging provides an accurate and noninvasive method for evaluating spinal dysraphism, making it the modality of choice. The excellent contrast resolution, wide field of view, and multiplanar images allow evaluation of the entire spinal cord, contents of the back mass, detect cord tethering, associated syringomyelia, Chiari malformation, and other associated abnormalities. T1-weighted (T1W) images (sagittal, axial, and coronal plane) demonstrate the malformation in the majority of the cases. T2-weighted (T2W) images are helpful in the demonstration of syrinx and associated pathologies like dermoid and epidermoid cyst.[6,9] **Box 3** delineates the MRI protocol for imaging these children. Patients with spinal dysraphism may have multiple spinal anomalies. For instance, a patient with myelomeningocele may have associated syringohydromyelia and Chiari malformation. Therefore, it cannot be overemphasized that the entire spine needs to be imaged if a cutaneous or vertebral anomaly suggests the presence of a malformation. Fetal MRI

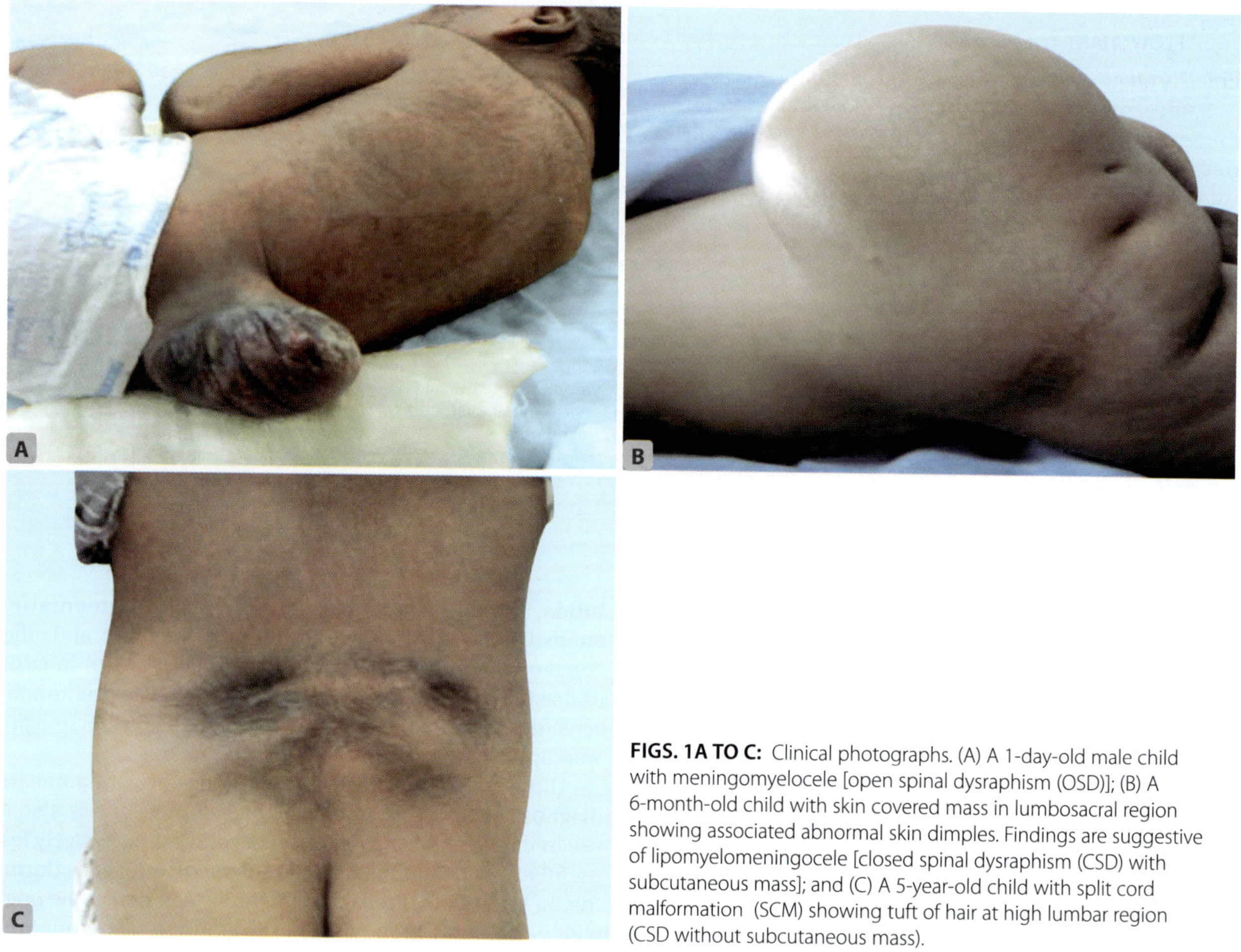

FIGS. 1A TO C: Clinical photographs. (A) A 1-day-old male child with meningomyelocele [open spinal dysraphism (OSD)]; (B) A 6-month-old child with skin covered mass in lumbosacral region showing associated abnormal skin dimples. Findings are suggestive of lipomyelomeningocele [closed spinal dysraphism (CSD) with subcutaneous mass]; and (C) A 5-year-old child with split cord malformation (SCM) showing tuft of hair at high lumbar region (CSD without subcutaneous mass).

BOX 2: Cutaneous lesions associated with spinal dysraphism.

High index of suspicion:
- Hypertrichosis
- Atypical dimples
- Acrochordons/pseudotails/true tails
- Lipomas
- Hemangiomas
- Aplasia cutis or scar
- Dermoid cyst or sinus

Low index of suspicion:
- Telangiectasia
- Capillary malformation (port-wine stain)
- Hyperpigmentation
- Melanocytic nevi
- Teratomas

is used as complementary modality to USG **(Figs. 2 to 4)** for the antenatal diagnosis of spinal anomalies and associated hydrocephalus.[10,11]

OPEN SPINAL DYSRAPHISM

Open spinal dysraphism implies exposure of neural tissue or its covering meninges to the external environment without any cutaneous covering. The nonneurulated embryonic neural tissue is called placode and is exposed in this category of dysraphism.[5] This category includes myelomeningocele, myelocele, hemimeningocele, and hemimyelomeningocele. Myelomeningocele accounts for approximately 99% cases of OSD while myelocele, hemimeningocele, and hemimyelomeningocele are distinctively rare.

Myelocele and Myelomeningocele

Myelomeningocele and myelocele are the most common form of OSD, occurring in up to 2 per 1,000 live births and females are affected slightly more than males.[5] The incidence has decreased in the last two decades because of the use of folate supplementation in pregnant mothers in the period before conception to 6 weeks after conception.[4,12] The mechanism of preventive action of folate is not fully understood.

Superficial ectoderm does not disjoin from the neuroectoderm, thereby producing a midline defect. The neural tube remains open and the neural folds remain in continuity with the cutaneous ectoderm at the skin surface.[5,6] The affected newborn is identified by the presence of a placode of reddish neural tissue in the middle of the back that is exposed to air because of the absence of overlying skin. Most common location of OSDs is the lumbosacral region (44%) followed by thoracolumbar region (32%). In contrast to lumbar meningomyelocele, cervical meningomyelocele is classified as a CSD. Imaging is usually not done as the diagnosis is clinically obvious and is a neurosurgical emergency.

Some authors suggest that MRI should be performed whenever possible as it can characterize the various components of the malformation, evaluate associated abnormalities (hydromyelia, Chiari II malformation, and hydrocephalus), and identify hemimyelomeningocele and hemimyeloceles.[13] Imaging of untreated OSDs demonstrates dehiscence of skin, subcutaneous fat, muscle, and bone at the level of spina bifida **(Figs. 5 and 6)**. In a meningomyelocele, the ventral subarachnoid space is distended displacing the neural placode posteriorly **(Fig. 5)** while myelocele lies flush with the skin surface without cerebrospinal fluid (CSF) space expansion **(Figs. 6A to C)**.

After surgery, the infants have a neurological defect that is stable. Imaging is indicated if the patient deteriorates neurologically despite adequate treatment of associated hydrocephalus or if the neurological examination findings are unusual.[14,15] MRI done in the postoperative setting may show the cord to be low lying and covered by skin graft; the stretched spinal cord may be tethered at this level **(Figs. 7 and 8)**. The spinal cord may be thinned out and may show cavitation at any level **(Fig. 7)**. Intraspinal mass (epidermoid or dermoid cyst) may be associated.[15] Dermoid differs from epidermoid by the presence of appendages of skin. On imaging, both conditions appear similar. These lesions usually appear hypointense on T1W images and hyperintense on T2W images similar to CSF **(Fig. 9)**. They may have complex signal intensity when there is hemorrhage or when the cyst becomes infected.

Causes of postoperative neurological deterioration include retethering **(Figs. 7 and 8)**, cord ischemia, spinal cord cysts and cavitation **(Figs. 7A and B)**, diastematomyelia,

BOX 3: Magnetic resonance imaging (MRI) protocol for imaging in spinal dysraphism.

- Sagittal (whole spine), axial, and coronal T2-weighted (T2W) or 3D-isovoxel T2W SPACE/CUBE/VISTA
- Sagittal (whole spine), axial, and coronal T1-weighted (T1W) spine
- T1W FS in axial or sagittal plane
- Sagittal and axial T2W brain screening
- Optional sequences
- Single-shot or 3D myelogram
- MRI may be performed in prone position for assessment of occult cord tethering to look for CSF dorsal to conus

(CSF: cerebrospinal fluid; 3D: three-dimensional; FS: fat-suppressed)

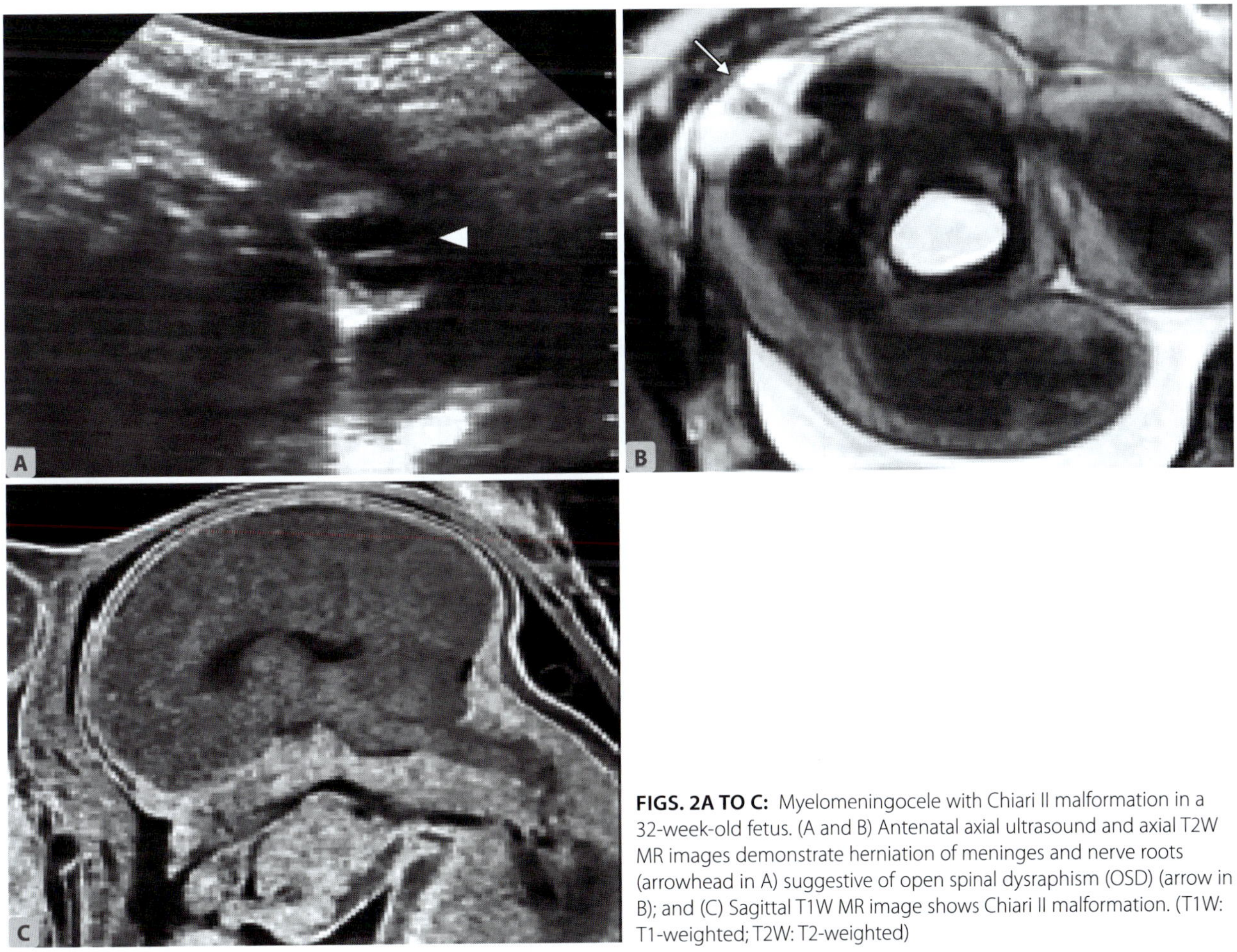

FIGS. 2A TO C: Myelomeningocele with Chiari II malformation in a 32-week-old fetus. (A and B) Antenatal axial ultrasound and axial T2W MR images demonstrate herniation of meninges and nerve roots (arrowhead in A) suggestive of open spinal dysraphism (OSD) (arrow in B); and (C) Sagittal T1W MR image shows Chiari II malformation. (T1W: T1-weighted; T2W: T2-weighted)

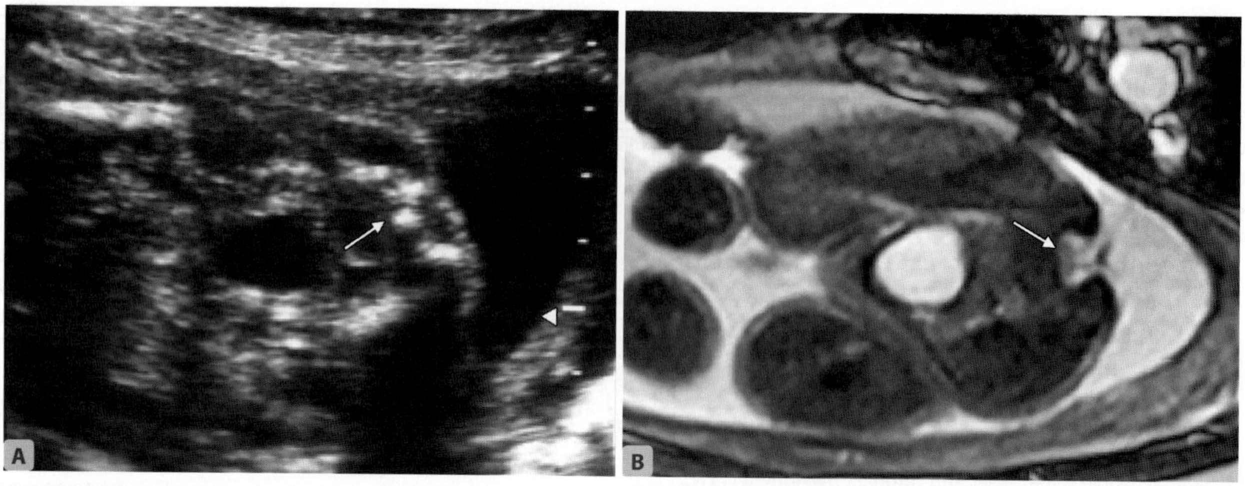

FIGS. 3A AND B: Myelocele with Chiari II malformation in a 26-week-old fetus. (A and B) Antenatal axial ultrasound and axial T2-weighted (T2W) images demonstrate widening of the spinal canal with absence of posterior elements. Neural placode is flush with the skin surface (arrows).

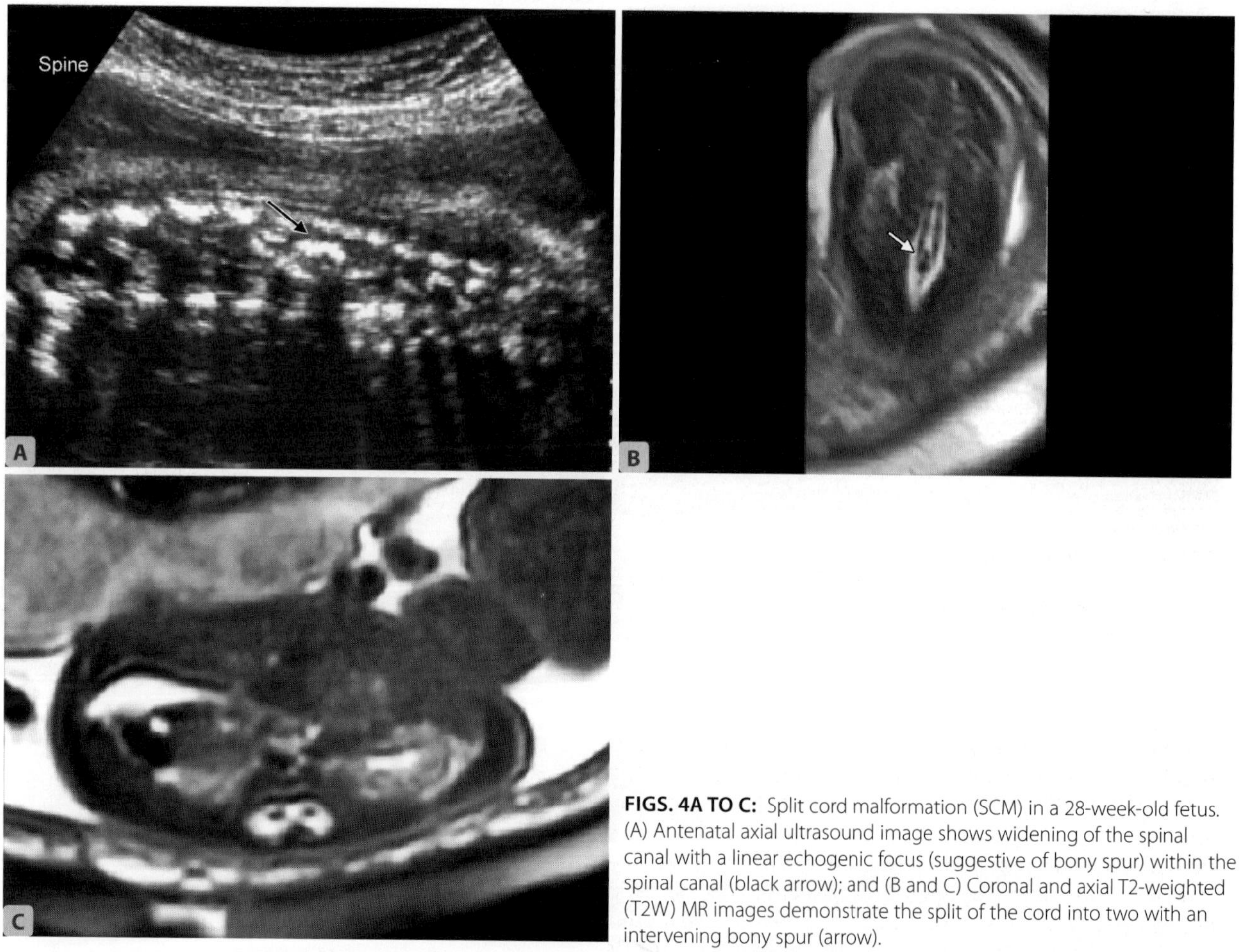

FIGS. 4A TO C: Split cord malformation (SCM) in a 28-week-old fetus. (A) Antenatal axial ultrasound image shows widening of the spinal canal with a linear echogenic focus (suggestive of bony spur) within the spinal canal (black arrow); and (B and C) Coronal and axial T2-weighted (T2W) MR images demonstrate the split of the cord into two with an intervening bony spur (arrow).

and hydrocephalus. All these are easily amenable to detection by MR.[14] Surgical release of the adherent cord is effective and leads to improved motor function in almost 80% of patients. Up to 85% of OSD patients have a concurrent hydrocephalus and nearly all patients have an associated Chiari II malformation.[5,16]

Chiari II Malformation

Various theories have been put forward to explain this entity, but the recent theory by McLone and Knepper[17] best explains this association which is shown in **Figure 10** and it has also been shown that most of these CNS anomalies

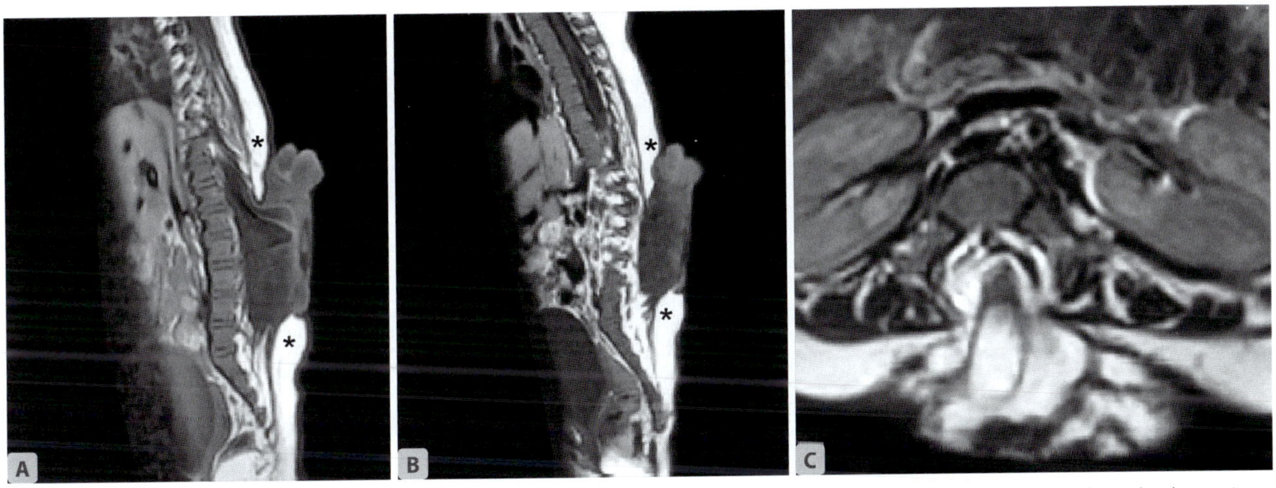

FIGS. 5A TO C: Lumbosacral meningomyelocele in a 2-day-old female. (A and B) Sagittal T1W images show a large mass in the lower lumbar region without skin covering; and (C) Axial T2W image shows exposed neural placode with traversing dorsal and ventral nerve roots. Notice dehiscent subcutaneous fat (asterisks in A and B). Ventral subarachnoid space is distended in contrast to myelocele which lies flush with the skin surface without CSF space expansion. Also note small syrinx in the cord at thoracic level. (CSF: cerebrospinal fluid; T1W: T1-weighted; T2W: T2-weighted)

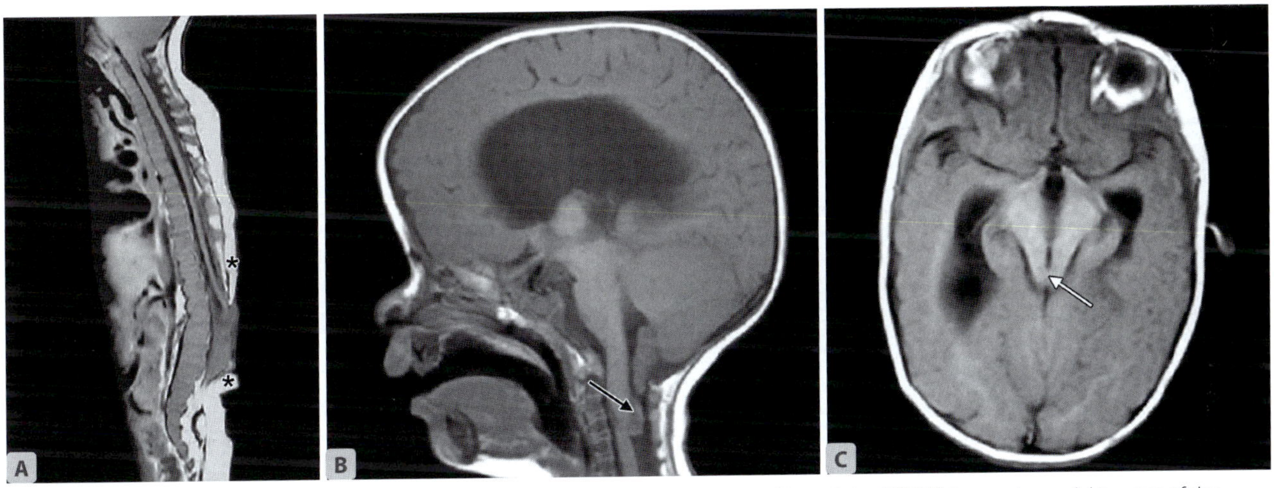

FIGS. 6A TO C: Myelocele with Chiari II malformation in a 1-day-old newborn. (A) Sagittal T1-weighted (T1W) image shows dehiscence of the subcutaneous fat (asterisks). Neural placode is exposed and flush with the skin surface without expansion of the subarachnoid space; (B) Sagittal T1W image of the brain shows small posterior fossa with herniation of cerebellar tonsil behind cervical cord (black arrow); and (C) Axial T1W image at midbrain level shows abnormal posterior tectal beaking (white arrow) with dilated temporal horns.

can be reversed or even prevented by early intrauterine repair of the defect which highlights the importance of early diagnosis of this condition.[18,19] As against less pronounced tonsillar herniation seen with Chiari I, in Chiari II, there is marked tonsillar herniation **(Figs. 3 and 6)**. Tectal beaking, low-lying torcular herophili, and hydrocephalus are usual associations with this malformation. Tonsillar herniation should be assessed on midsagittal nonfat-suppressed T1W image. Anatomical landmark followed is a line connecting basion with opisthion.[20] While drawing the line signal intensity of bone, marrow should not be used. Since there is gradual ascent of cerebellar tonsil with age, criteria for tonsillar ectopia changes with age (≥6 mm—0–10 years, ≥5 mm—10–30 years, ≥4 mm—30–80 years, and ≥3 mm—>80 years).

Hemimyelocele/Hemimyelomeningocele

This is the rarest form of OSD and results when SCM is associated with defective primary neurulation of one of the hemicord which forms part of myelomeningocele. Hemimyelocele/myelomeningocele **(Figs. 11 and 12)** also has associated Chiari II malformation in up to 40% of cases.[21,22] Clinical clues to the diagnosis include asymmetrical neurological deficit and presence of hirsutism along one side of the exposed neural defect.[23] **Table 1** reviews the entities discussed under OSD.

CLOSED SPINAL DYSRAPHISM

Closed spinal dysraphism is a heterogeneous group of disorders. In patients with CSD, early diagnosis may be

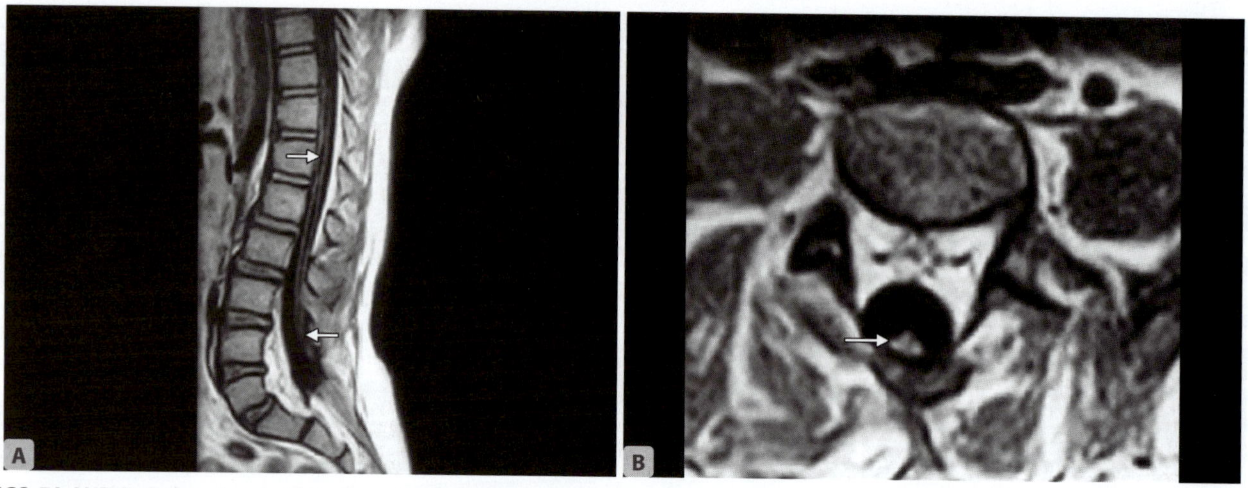

FIGS. 7A AND B: Tethered cord with hydromyelia in a 2-year-old male after surgery for lumbosacral meningocele. (A and B) Sagittal T1-weighted (T1W) and axial T1W images show low-lying tethered cord reaching up to L4-L5 disk level with thinning (arrow in B) and hydromyelia (short arrows in A) with abnormal eccentric location of cord indicating adhesion.

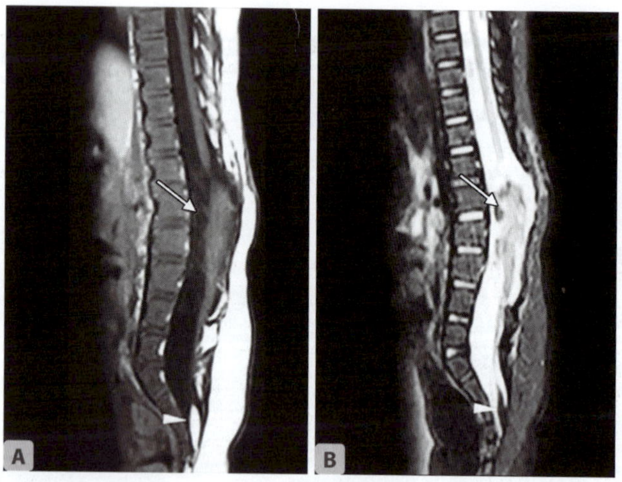

FIGS. 8A AND B: Postoperative fibrosis following meningomyelocele closure in a 5-year-old female. (A and B) Sagittal T1W and T2W images demonstrate low-lying cord tethered by fibrotic tissue, hypointense on T1W and T2W images (arrows). Also note the presence of filar lipoma (arrowheads) showing hyperintensity on T1W and hypointensity on T2W fat-suppressed images. (T1W: T1-weighted; T2W: T2-weighted)

useful, as spinal dysraphism may lead to distortion of the nerve roots with growth, resulting in neurological sequelae in the lower extremities. Early diagnosis is necessary to prevent neurological sequelae by performing early surgical procedures.

Closed Spinal Dysraphism with Subcutaneous Mass

Closed spinal dysraphisms with subcutaneous mass at the lumbosacral region include lipomyelocele, lipomeningomyelocele, meningocele, and myelocystocele. Among these, lipomyelocele and lipomyelomeningocele are common entities and lipomyelocele is twice as common as lipomyelomeningocele. At cervical level, differential diagnosis of CSD with subcutaneous mass includes cervical meningomyelocele, meningocele, and myelocystocele.[5,6]

Lipoma with Dural Defect (Lipomyelocele and Lipomyelomeningocele)

The lipoma extends from the subcutaneous region up to/into the spinal canal (through the vertebral and dural defect). Lipomyelomeningocele consists of a large subcutaneous skin covered mass in lumbosacral region that contains fat, neural tissue, CSF, and meninges.[24] This results from premature separation of surface ectoderm from neural ectoderm prior to formation of proper neural tube which allows ingress of intervening mesoderm into neural tube which in turn prevents further neurulation.[8] These mesodermal components specifically differentiate toward adipose tissue and form fatty component of these disorders. Clinically, there is a midline soft nontender mass above level of the intergluteal crease which extends asymmetrically into one buttock. Associated cutaneous malformation is seen in 50% of cases. Differentiation of lipomyelocele from lipomyelomeningocele is by position of lipoma-placode interface. In lipomyelomeningocele, the lipoma-placode interface is outside the confines of spinal canal **(Figs. 13A to C)** whereas in lipomyelocele, interface is either inside or at the edge of spinal canal **(Figs. 14A to C)**. In lipomyelocele, size of the subarachnoid space ventral to the cord is normal; however, the size of the canal may be increased depending on size of the lipoma. On the other hand, in the lipomyelomeningocele, there is ballooning of subarachnoid space ventral to the cord. This condition is associated with tethered cord, hydromyelia, and Chiari I malformation.[9] Some researchers have suggested that instead of lipoma-placode interface, presence of fluid component in the mass should be the deciding factor for differentiating between these two.[25] In lipomyelomeningocele, the expanded CSF space herniates through the dural and bony defect into the subcutaneous region. Though this is usually accompanied

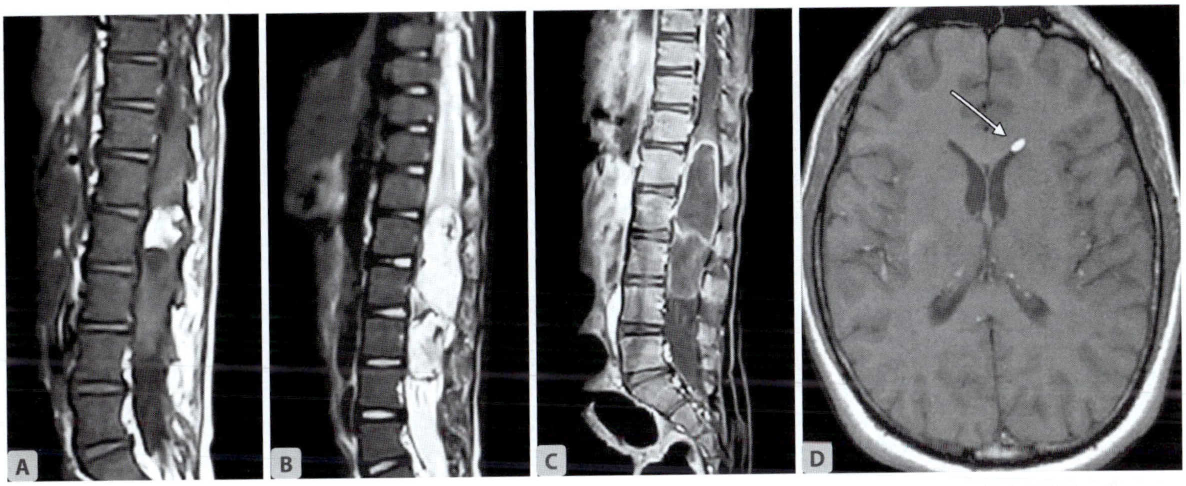

FIGS. 9A TO D: Infected dermoid cyst in a 12-year-old child with a history of meningomyelocele repair. (A to C) Sagittal T1W, T2W, and postgadolinium images show focal expansion of spinal cord at level of conus by a hyperintense (on T2W) mass with foci of T1 hyperintensity suggesting fat. Note peripheral rim enhancement following gadolinium indicating infected cyst; and (D) Axial T1W image of brain demonstrates a hyperintense focus in the left frontal horn (arrow). Findings are suggestive of infected dermoid cyst with rupture. (T1W: T1-weighted; T2W: T2-weighted)

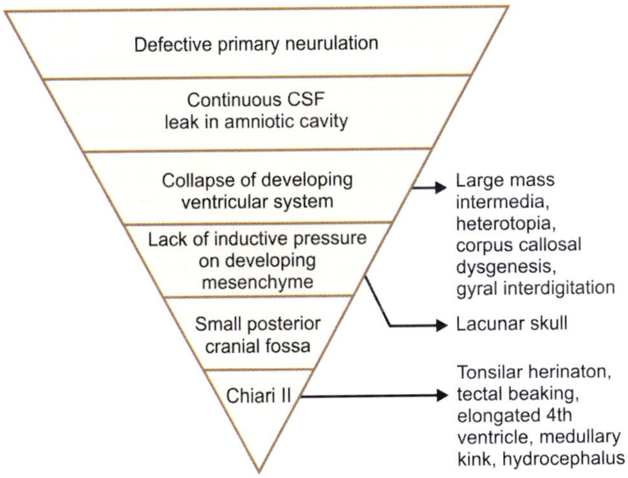

FIG. 10: McLone and Knepper theory explaining the pathogenesis of Chiari II malformation. (CSF: cerebrospinal fluid)

by the herniation of neural placode as well, but in cases the lipoma is asymmetric, then the lipoma-placode interface may lie within the spinal canal.

Meningocele

Meningocele is characterized by herniation of meninges through bony defect covered externally by the skin. The embryological basis remains unexplained.[8] As per definition, the mass should not contain any of spinal cord segments or nerve root as content **(Figs. 15A and B)**. Rarely, filum terminale may remain tethered at the neck of the sac. On imaging, CSF-filled dural outpouching is seen to herniate via the spina bifida, intervertebral foramen, or sacral foramen. More than 80% meningoceles are located in the lumbosacral spine. The bony defect may involve the posterior elements, anterior aspect of sacrum, lateral aspect of spine, or distal sacrum (intrasacral meningocele).

Anterior Sacral Meningocele

Anterior sacral meningocele is characterized by herniation of meninges through anterior sacral defect, forming a cyst-like structure filled with CSF continuous with subarachnoid space of spinal cord. When this condition is associated with anorectal anomaly, it is called Currarino triad. Majority of cases remain asymptomatic and are detected incidentally either on pelvic examination or imaging. Differential diagnosis includes cystic sacrococcygeal teratoma, large ovarian cyst, and neurenteric cyst. Demonstration of continuity of cyst with thecal sac ensures diagnosis of anterior sacral meningocele **(Figs. 16A to C)**.

Myelocystocele

This rare entity constitutes about 5% cases of CSD and its embryological basis is not fully understood.[5,8] It could represent severe disruptive form of terminal ventricle, a defect in secondary neurulation. It has three components: (1) Skin covered posterior meningocele, (2) Hydromelic terminal cord into meningocele, and (3) Posterior spina bifida. Myelocystocele may be terminal or segmental (cervical). Differential diagnosis includes simple dorsal meningocele and myelomeningocele. Continuity of the dilated central canal with the caudal cyst is diagnostic of myelocystocele and helps to differentiate it from other entities.[26] The hydromyelic cyst and meningocele do not communicate with each other.[24] **Table 2** revisits the conditions included in CSD with subcutaneous mass.

Closed Spinal Dysraphism without Subcutaneous Mass

This group includes a wide variety of abnormalities in which imaging plays a crucial role in making the diagnosis.

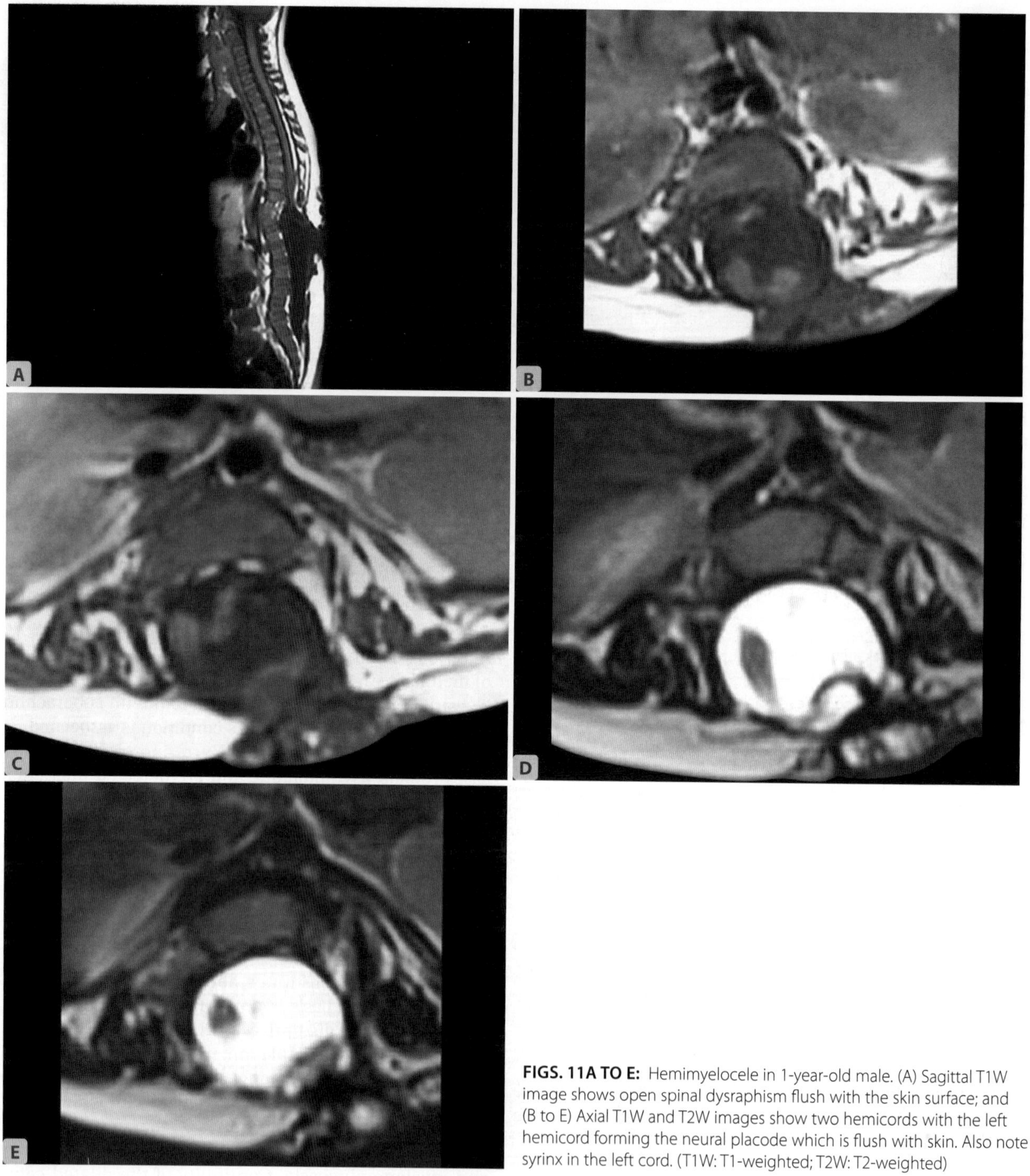

FIGS. 11A TO E: Hemimyelocele in 1-year-old male. (A) Sagittal T1W image shows open spinal dysraphism flush with the skin surface; and (B to E) Axial T1W and T2W images show two hemicords with the left hemicord forming the neural placode which is flush with skin. Also note syrinx in the left cord. (T1W: T1-weighted; T2W: T2-weighted)

Posterior Bony Spina Bifida

This is the simplest form of CSD and is characterized by defective fusion of the posterior bony element. Isolated posterior spina bifida is seen in up to 5% of the general population. Usually, insignificant, further imaging is not indicated unless there is neurological deficit or high-risk cutaneous markers are present **(Box 2)**. Defect is commonly seen at L5-S1 level **(Fig. 17)**. Care should be taken not to diagnose this entity in children <6 years on radiographs since it is physiological to see unfused posterior elements in lumbosacral region up to 6 years of age.[9]

Lipoma (Intradural and Intramedullary)

Lipoma results from early disjunction between neuroectoderm and ectoderm.[8] Lipoma is most commonly seen at lumbosacral level and is usually subpial in location.

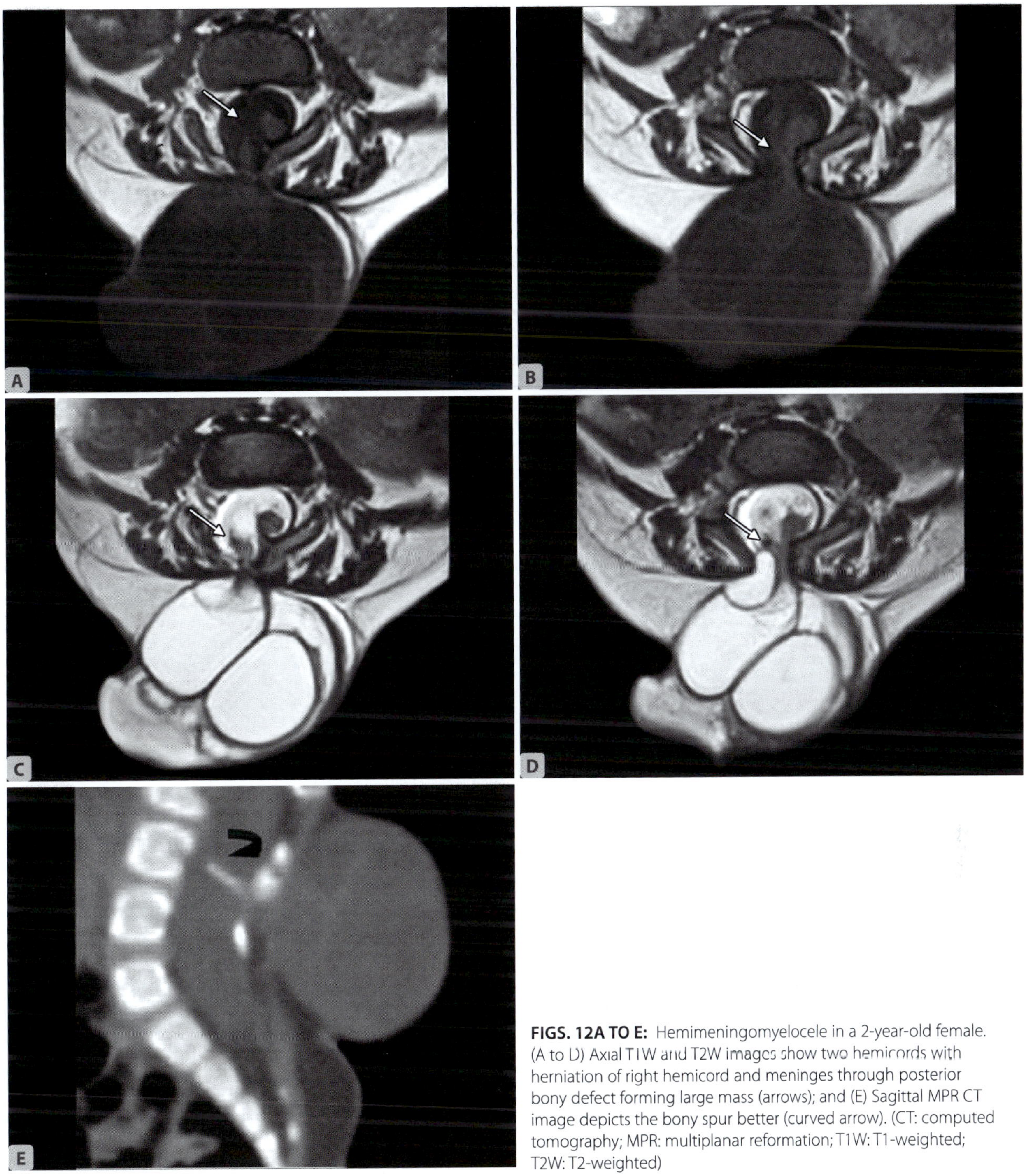

FIGS. 12A TO E: Hemimeningomyelocele in a 2-year-old female. (A to D) Axial T1W and T2W images show two hemicords with herniation of right hemicord and meninges through posterior bony defect forming large mass (arrows); and (E) Sagittal MPR CT image depicts the bony spur better (curved arrow). (CT: computed tomography; MPR: multiplanar reformation; T1W: T1-weighted; T2W: T2-weighted)

TABLE 1: Summary of entities covered under open spinal dysraphism (OSD).

Myelomeningocele (99% cases of OSD)	Neural placode protrudes above skin surface due to expansion of ventral subarachnoid space
Myelocele	• Neural placode flush with skin surface • Normal thickness of ventral subarachnoid space
Hemimyelocele/Hemimyelomeningocele	Myelocele/Myelomeningocele involving one hemicord in diastematomyelia

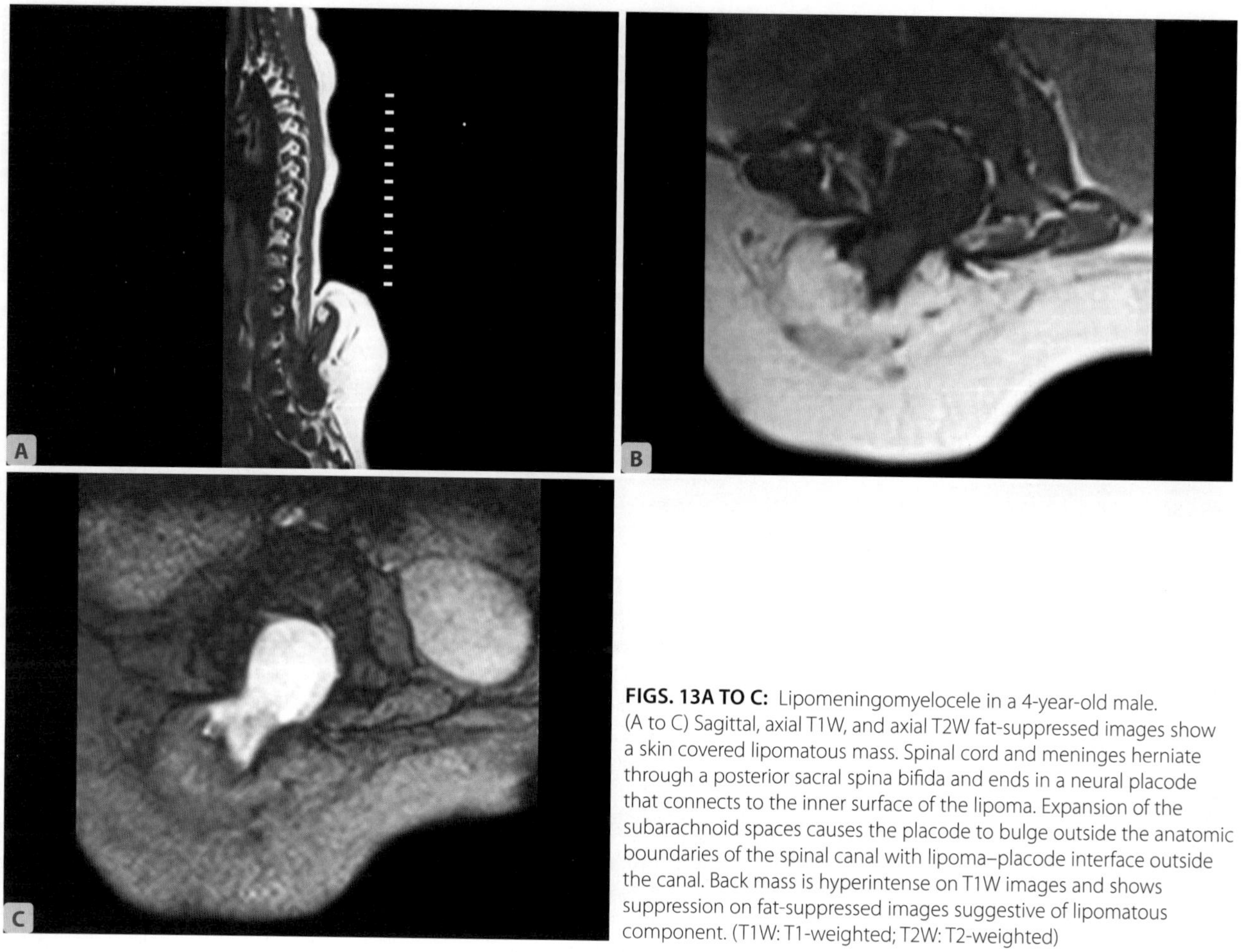

FIGS. 13A TO C: Lipomeningomyelocele in a 4-year-old male. (A to C) Sagittal, axial T1W, and axial T2W fat-suppressed images show a skin covered lipomatous mass. Spinal cord and meninges herniate through a posterior sacral spina bifida and ends in a neural placode that connects to the inner surface of the lipoma. Expansion of the subarachnoid spaces causes the placode to bulge outside the anatomic boundaries of the spinal canal with lipoma–placode interface outside the canal. Back mass is hyperintense on T1W images and shows suppression on fat-suppressed images suggestive of lipomatous component. (T1W: T1-weighted; T2W: T2-weighted)

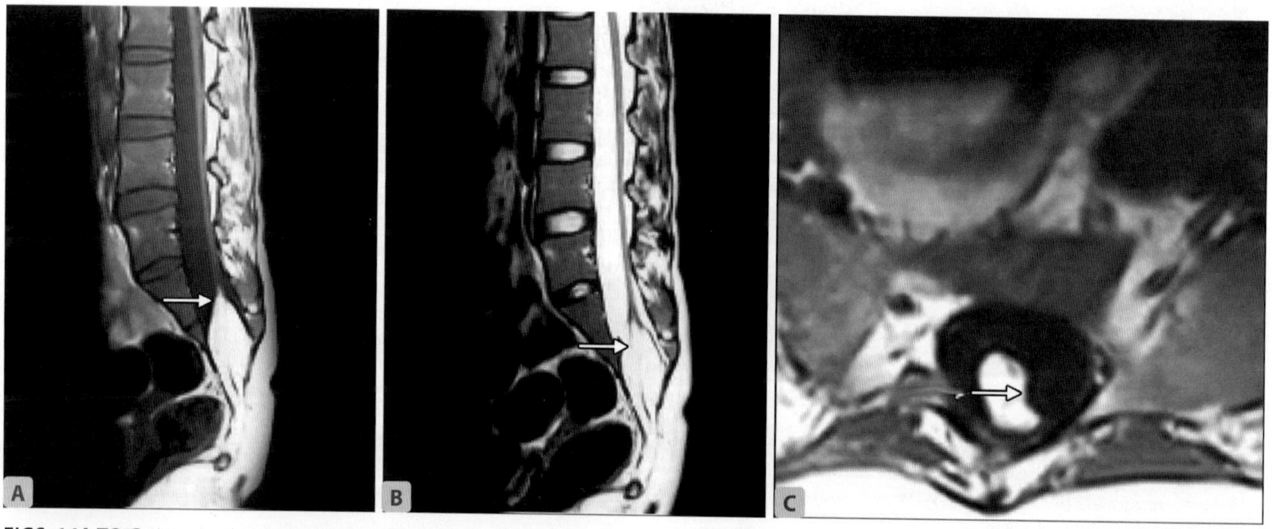

FIGS. 14A TO C: Lipomyelocele in a 2-year-old male. (A and B) Sagittal T1W and T2W images show T1 hyperintense intraspinal mass adherent to cord continuous with subcutaneous fat through wide spina bifida (arrow); and (C) Axial T1W image better depicts intraspinal fatty component. Note lipoma–placode interface within the confines of the spinal canal (arrow). (T1W: T1-weighted; T2W: T2-weighted)

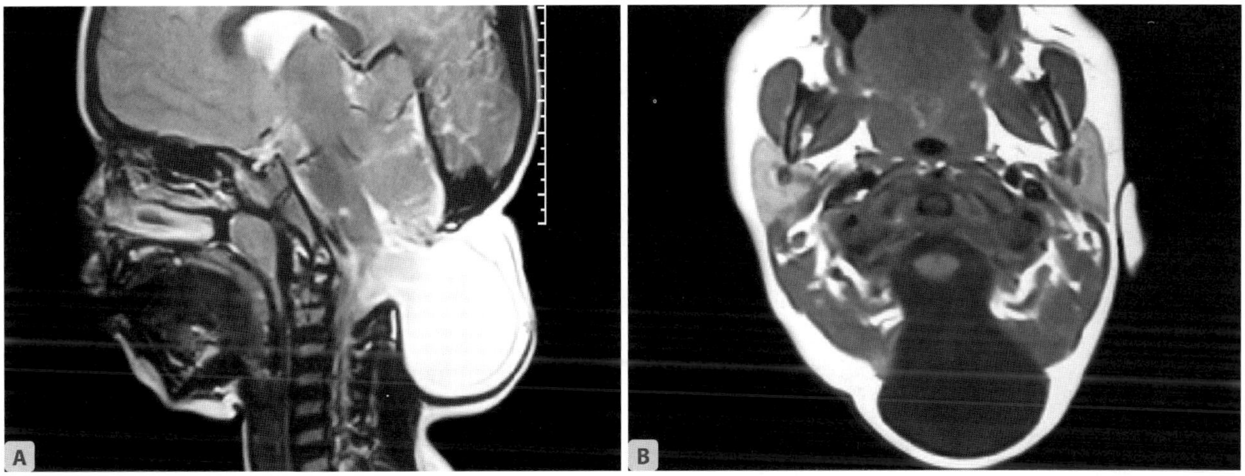

FIGS. 15A AND B: Posterior cervical meningocele in a 6-month-old-male. (A and B) Sagittal T2W and axial T1W images show herniation of the meninges in the upper cervical region. Note associated skin covering and lack of herniation of neural elements. (T1W: T1-weighted; T2W: T2-weighted)

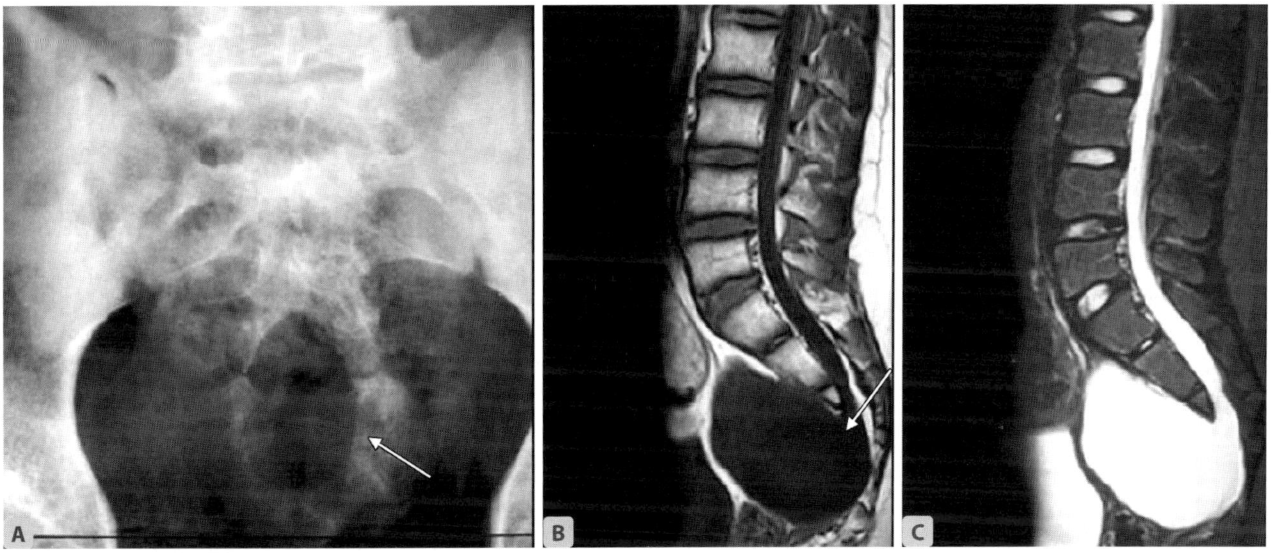

FIGS. 16A TO C: Anterior sacral meningocele in a 15-year-old female. (A) Radiograph sacrum AP view shows scimitar sacrum (arrow); and (B and C) Sagittal T1W and T2W images show a large presacral cyst contiguous with the spinal canal (arrow). Also note the sacral defect. (AP: anteroposterior; T1W; T1-weighted; T2W: T2-weighted)

They occur more commonly in females, peak in the first 5 years of life, and usually present with tethered cord syndrome. Lipomas are contained within intact dural sac and are located in midline dorsally. On MR, lipoma appears as a mass which follows signal intensity of subcutaneous fat on all pulse sequences [high signal intensity on T1W and fast spin echo (FSE) T2W images, hypointense on fat-saturated images].

Filum Terminale Lipoma

Filum terminale lipoma probably results from defective secondary neurulation which leads to persistence of mesodermal elements within filum terminale which later differentiate toward adipose tissue.[5,8] Incidental detection of fatty signal (hyperintense on T1W) in the filum is a normal finding seen in up to 5% of general population and is referred as fatty filum.[27] Diagnosis of filum terminale lipoma should be made when the fatty filum measures >2 mm **(Figs. 8 and 18)**. This condition may or may not be associated with cord tethering.

Tight Filum Terminale Syndrome

Tight filum terminale syndrome occurs due to defective retrogressive differentiation of neural tube formed by the process of secondary neurulation resulting in short and thick filum terminale (>2 mm) which causes abnormal stretching of spinal cord with secondary neurological deficit.[5,6,9] Associated anomalies include posterior spina bifida, scoliosis, and kyphoscoliosis. According to some authors, tight filum terminale is a clinical syndrome and not an imaging diagnosis. It can be seen with anomalous filum

TABLE 2: Summary of entities covered under closed spinal dysraphism (CSD) with subcutaneous mass.		
Lipoma with dural defect	Lipomyelomeningocele	Lipoma–placode interface outside the spinal canal due to expansion of ventral subarachnoid space
	Lipomyelocele	• Lipoma–placode interface within the spinal canal • Normal thickness of ventral subarachnoid space
Meningocele		• Herniation of meninges [cerebrospinal fluid-filled sac lined by dura and arachnoid] through bony defect, either anteriorly or posteriorly and covered with skin • No nerve root/cord within
Myelocystocele: Terminal/Segmental		Dilated central canal (large hydromyelia) herniating into posterior meningocele

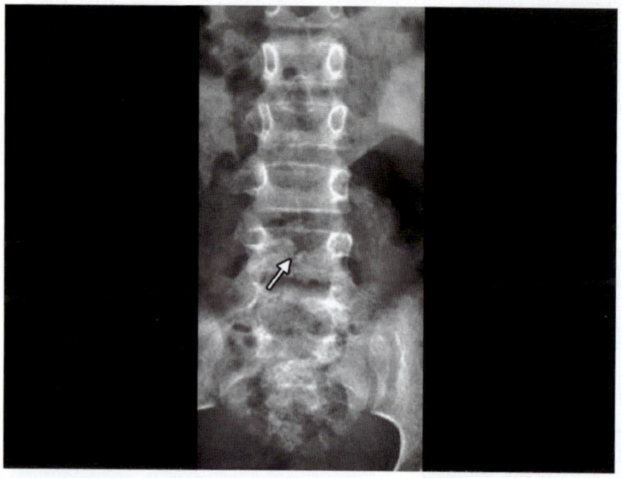

FIG. 17: Isolated spina bifida in an 8-year-old male. Radiograph lumbosacral spine anteroposterior (AP) view shows absence of fusion of posterior elements of L4 and L5 (arrow).

terminale, SCM, and in postoperative period after surgery for OSD **(Figs. 19A and B)**. The treatment is surgical section of the filum terminale.

Persistent Terminal Ventricle

Persistent terminal ventricle results from defect in the process of secondary neurulation, resulting in the formation of small ependymal lined cavity within conus medullaris. Usually, asymptomatic but may present with low backache and bladder dysfunction. There is dilatation of the ependymal canal immediately above the filum terminale with slight expansion of conus. This condition needs to be differentiated from intramedullary tumor which can be done by its central location, CSF isointense signal intensity, and by noting lack of contrast enhancement following gadolinium and on follow-up imaging.[6,9] Other differentials include focal syrinx and intraspinal arachnoid cyst; however, this distinction is not clinically relevant and they can be differentiated only on histology.[27]

Neurenteric Cyst

Neurenteric cyst results from incomplete regression of neuroenteric canal. Complete failure of regression manifests as dorsal enteric fistula which is very rare.[8] They are enteric-lined cysts that present within the spinal canal and exhibit a definite connection with the spinal cord and/or vertebra. They may communicate with an extraspinal component of cyst in the mediastinum or mesentery through a dysraphic vertebra or they may attach by a fibrous stalk to the vertebra or gut.[5,28] The peak incidence is during the first two decades of life and the most common location is thoracic spine followed by cervical spine. Vertebral anomalies are common though not invariable. Most cysts lie in the cervicothoracic junction or close to the conus medullaris.

Typically, neurenteric cysts are located ventral to the cervicothoracic cord. Diagnosis should be thought of whenever a posterior mediastinal mass is seen along with congenital vertebral anomalies **(Figs. 20A to C)**. Neurenteric cysts are isointense to CSF on T1W images and hyperintense on T2W images.[28] No enhancement occurs after contrast administration. Usually, the child is asymptomatic, but can present with symptoms related to compression of airways, esophagus, or atrium. Neurological deficit occurs secondary to intraspinal component of cyst and demonstration of this component and associated vertebral segmentation anomaly is critical in establishing the diagnosis.

Table 3 reviews the disease entities covered under CSD without subcutaneous mass.

Split Cord Malformation

In SCM, the spinal cord is partially or completely split into two hemicords by either an osteocartilaginous septum or by a fibrous septum. Usually, these hemicord unite distally after splitting into two. Each segment has a central canal and dorsal and ventral nerve roots. Over 90% of the cases occur in female patients. SCM most commonly occurs in the thoracolumbar region (between D9 and S1 vertebral levels) and approximately 50–75% of patients have cutaneous stigmata at the site of cord split.[4-6]

Split cord malformation is classified as type 1 and type 2 based on state of the dural tube and nature of the medial septum.[21] In Pang type 1 **(Figs. 21A to F)**, each hemicord has a separate dural and arachnoid covering separated by a bony spur or septum (osteocartilaginous). In type 2 **(Figs. 22A to F)**, the hemicords are contained in a single dural sac and arachnoid covering without a rigid median septum (60% cases). Medial septum may be complete or incomplete and may course obliquely dividing the cord asymmetrically. Cleft is located at the caudal end of splitting in the majority of cases. SCM may be difficult to appreciate on sagittal MR images. Axial and coronal images show cord splitting as well as septum. However, fibrous septum may be very thin and is best demonstrated using thin axial/coronal T2W images.[9] SCM is suspected clinically in the presence of asymmetric

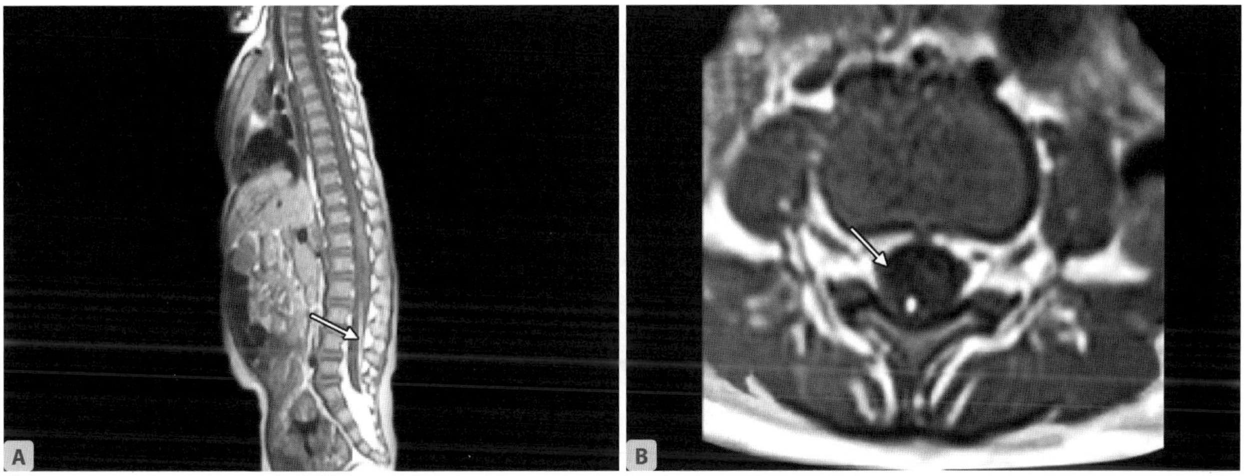

FIGS. 18A AND B: Filum terminale lipoma in a 10-month-old female. (A and B) Sagittal T1W and axial T2W images show thickened filum terminale with T1 hyperintensity indicating fatty filum terminale (arrows). (T1W: T1-weighted; T2W: T2-weighted)

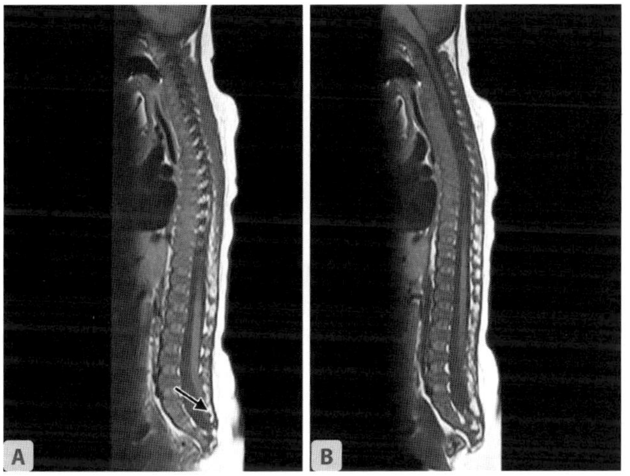

FIGS. 19A AND B: Tight filum terminale (tethered cord syndrome) in an 8-month-old female. (A and B) Sagittal T1-weighted (T1W) images show thickened filum terminale with tethered, low conus medullaris (arrow).

neurological deficit and in presence of hairy tuft high along the back. It is important to look for this abnormality in all cases of dysraphic spine because of its frequent association. If not recognized prior to repair, it may be responsible for neurological deficit secondary to cord tethering. Commonly associated anomalies include: Cord tethering seen in around 75% of patients and syringohydromyelia (50% of patients). It may affect the normal cord above or below the cleft and extend into one or both hemicords. Intramedullary tumors **(Figs. 23A to C)** have also been reported in the hemicord.[29] Vertebral anomalies are a rule and include spina bifida, widened interpedicular distance, hemivertebrae, and fused vertebrae.

Dorsal Dermal Sinus

Dorsal dermal sinus (DDS) is an epithelium-lined tract beginning at the skin surface which can communicate with the CNS and its meningeal coating. This results from defective disjunction of surface ectoderm from developing neural tube which leads to persistence of ectodermal connection between spinal cord and external skin.[8] Sinus tract usually ends at a level above the external opening because of the ascent of the spinal cord. The points of attachment of skin and spinal cord remain segmental or metameric, so the dermatome of involvement predicts the site of neural abnormality. Males and females are affected equally. The sinus ostium is typically midline and small hemangiomas may surround the ostium. The sinus tract extends deeply through the subcutaneous layer and between the bifid laminae toward the dura. It may end superficial to the dura, at the dura, or deep to the dura.

Clinically dimples below top of the intergluteal crease end blindly whereas dimples above the level of intergluteal crease are highly suspicious. Patients become symptomatic either by infection or due to associated dermoid and epidermoid tumors.[30] DDS will be seen as hypointense tract in both T1W and T2W images extending from skin surface to spinal canal **(Figs. 24A to C)**.[31] Sagittal and axial MR sequences are good to demonstrate the extraspinal portion of the dermal sinus tract, though the intraspinal portion is hard to identify. In such cases, three-dimensional (3D) MR myelography can better delineate the tract and its intraspinal component. The differential diagnosis of DDS includes low sacrococcygeal midline dimple and pilonidal sinus, both of which do not enter the spinal canal.

Two other similar-appearing entities need to be considered while evaluating linear tracts in this region.[25] Both are characterized by a cigarette burn-like mark on the overlying skin. One is limited dorsal myeloschisis or pseudodermal sinus.[25] It consists of a solid fibroneural tract linking the skin to the cord. Since there is no lumen, the risk of infection is less but may present with cord tethering. The intraspinal tract can usually be clearly identified attaching to the cord. The second entity is meningocele manqué (missed or atretic meningocele).[25] It consists of a linear band extending from the dorsal surface of the cord to the dura and does not have any extraspinal component. The band

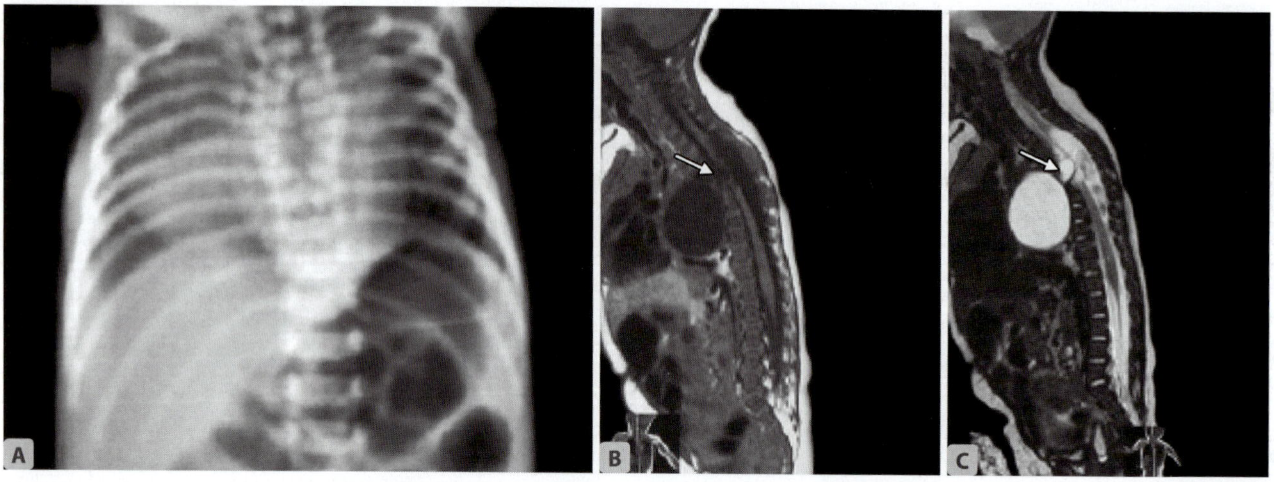

FIGS. 20A TO C: Neurenteric cyst in a 1-month-old male. (A) Chest radiograph AP view shows vertebral segmentation anomalies with large posterior mediastinal mass; and (B and C) Sagittal T1W and T2W images demonstrate a dumbbell-shaped mass extending from mediastinum into the spinal canal (arrows). Posterior subarachnoid space is dilated. (AP: anteroposterior; T1W: T1-weighted; T2W: T2-weighted)

TABLE 3: Summary of entities covered under closed spinal dysraphism (CSD) without subcutaneous mass.

Simple	Spina bifida	Defective fusion of posterior bony elements, usually at L5-S1
	Lipoma	Intradural/intramedullary midline fatty lesion or fatty filum terminale (>2 mm) and may present with tethered cord. No dural defect
	Tight filum terminale syndrome	Short and thick (>2 mm) filum. This causes cord tethering and low-lying conus
	Persistent terminal ventricle	Small central cerebrospinal fluid cavity in mildly expanded conus, immediately above filum terminale
	Dorsal dermal sinus	• Epithelium-lined tract from skin (inferiorly) to cord/meninges (superiorly) in the midline • Often associated with spinal dermoid at cauda equina/conus
Complex	Neurenteric cyst	• Enteric-lined cysts within spinal canal with definite connection with cord and vertebra; extraspinal component of cyst lies in posterior mediastinum or mesentery • Associated vertebral anomalies are common
	Split cord malformation	• Cord is partially or completely split into two • Associations: Scoliosis, cord tethering, and syrinx
	Caudal regression syndrome	Partial agenesis of lumbosacral spine with imperforate anus, malformed external genitalia, renal aplasia, and bladder exstrophy
	Segmental spinal dysgenesis	Segmental cord and vertebral dysgenesis

may contain nerve roots, fibrous tissue, or mixture. It is very difficult to visualize and one may diligently search for this entity in case of unexplained tethered cord syndrome. Focal cord deformity may be seen. About 20% cases of type 2 SCM may have meningocele manqué.[25]

Caudal Agenesis (Caudal Regression Syndrome)

This is an uncommon malformation seen in 0.1–0.25:10,000 of normal pregnancies. However, it occurs in about one in 350 infants of diabetic mothers, representing an increase of about 200 times.[32] This syndrome is characterized by partial agenesis of lumbosacral spine, imperforate anus, malformed external genitalia, renal aplasia, bladder exstrophy, etc. Plain films are adequate for demonstrating bony hypogenesis, but do not show associated cord abnormalities. Sagittal T1W MR images are excellent for evaluating caudal vertebral agenesis, level and shape of conus, and cord tethering.[6,32]

The anatomy and position of the conus defines two distinct types of abnormalities.[33] In type I **(Fig. 25)**, the conus ends above the level of L1, is typically deformed, and terminates abruptly at D11 or D12, as if the normal distal tip was absent (nearly always club or wedge shaped). In this type, with high conus, the sacral deficit is typically large and the sacrum typically ends at or above S1. More severe the malformation, greater the number of absent vertebra and more cephalic is cord termination. In type II **(Fig. 26)**, the conus ends lower (below L1) and is elongated, stretched caudally, and tethered by a thick filum or transitional lipoma. In these patients, the sacrum tends to be relatively well-preserved, with identifiable portions of S2 or lower vertebral segments. Type 1 is associated with significant neurological deficit when compared to type 2 caudal agenesis. **Box 4** enlists the various

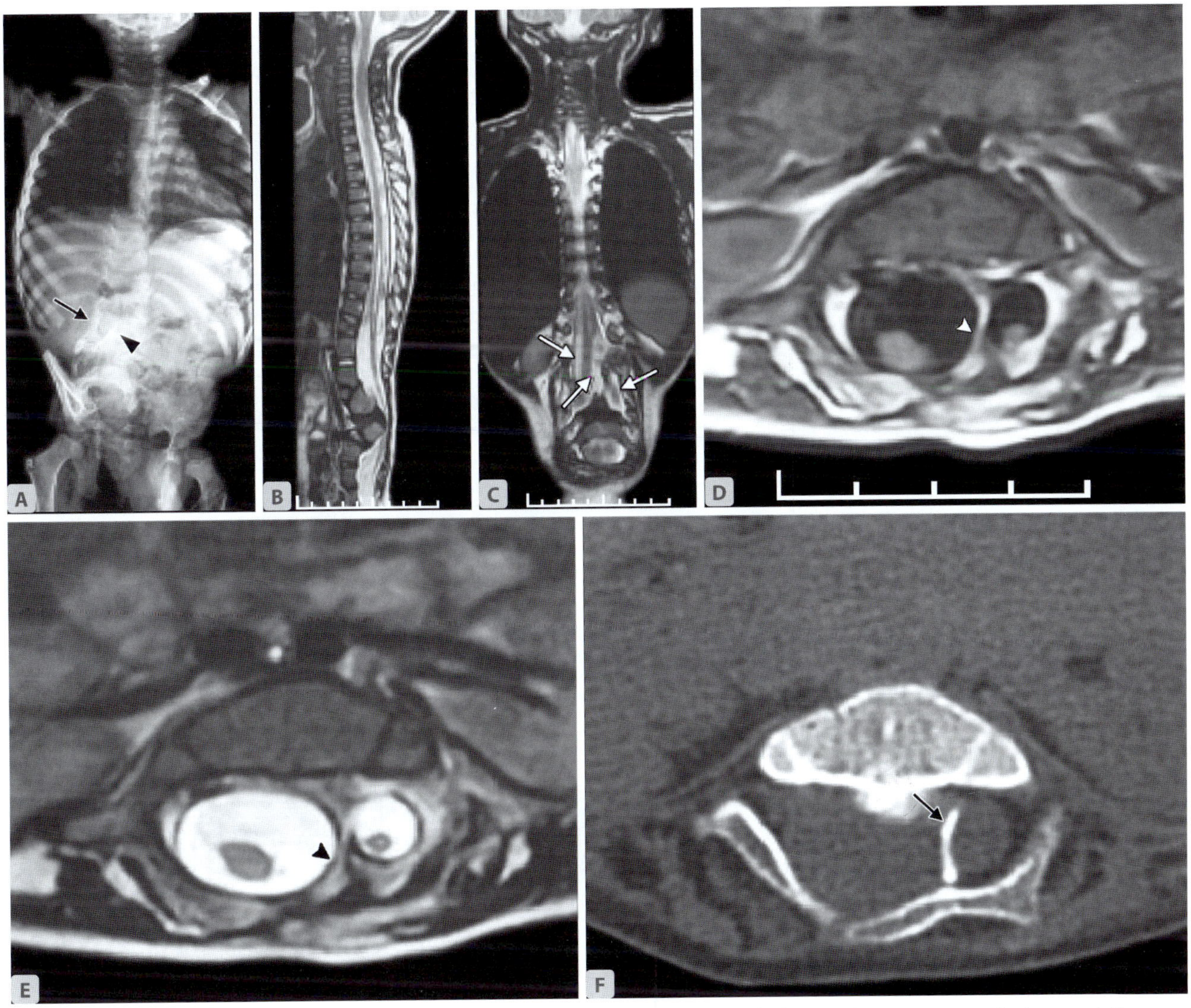

FIGS. 21A TO F: Type 1 split cord malformation (SCM) in an 8-year-old boy. (A) Radiograph whole spine demonstrates vertebral segmentation anomalies with intersegmental bar (arrow). Presence of vertical intersegmental bar strongly suggests SCM. Also, note the presence of bony spur (arrowhead); (B) Sagittal T2W image demonstrates thinning of cord with hydromyelia. Cord is also low lying and tethered; (C to E) Coronal T2W image, axial T1W, and T2W images show asymmetric split of cord (arrows) into two hemicords with bony spur (arrowhead) in between; and (F) Axial CT shows bony spur better (arrow). (CT: computed tomography; T1W: T1-weighted; T2W: T2-weighted)

causes of cord tethering. It may be noted that tethered cord syndrome is not a type of dysraphism, rather it is the clinical manifestation of a variety of dysraphic states.

Lumbosacral agenesis has also been classified into five different types depending on the nature and severity of agenesis. Type I is total sacral agenesis with some lumbar vertebra also missing. Type II is total sacral agenesis but the lumbar vertebrae are not involved while type III is subtotal sacral agenesis and at least S1 is present. Type IV is a hemisacrum whereas type V is coccygeal agenesis.[4]

Segmental Spinal Dysgenesis

Segmental spinal dysgenesis (SSD) is a rare form of dysraphic spinal state resulting from defective development of segment of notochord during preneurulation stage. This is characterized by segmental agenesis of the spine with dysgenesis of spinal cord at the level of bony abnormality. Severity of this anomaly varies from minimal segmental thinning of cord to complete loss of segment of spinal cord.[34]

CONCLUSION

Spinal dysraphism is a heterogeneous group of developmental abnormalities in which there is a defective closure of the neural tube. MRI is a single stop-shop imaging modality in majority of cases and also helps to classify them based on the commonly followed clinicoradiological classification proposed by Torotti et al. It is important for the radiologist and clinicians to be familiar with normal embryologic development of spine and MR findings of spinal dysraphism. Various other congenital anomalies are frequently associated and should be meticulously looked for when dysraphism is detected. **Box 5** summarizes the important points to be included in the MR imaging report in such cases.[25,27]

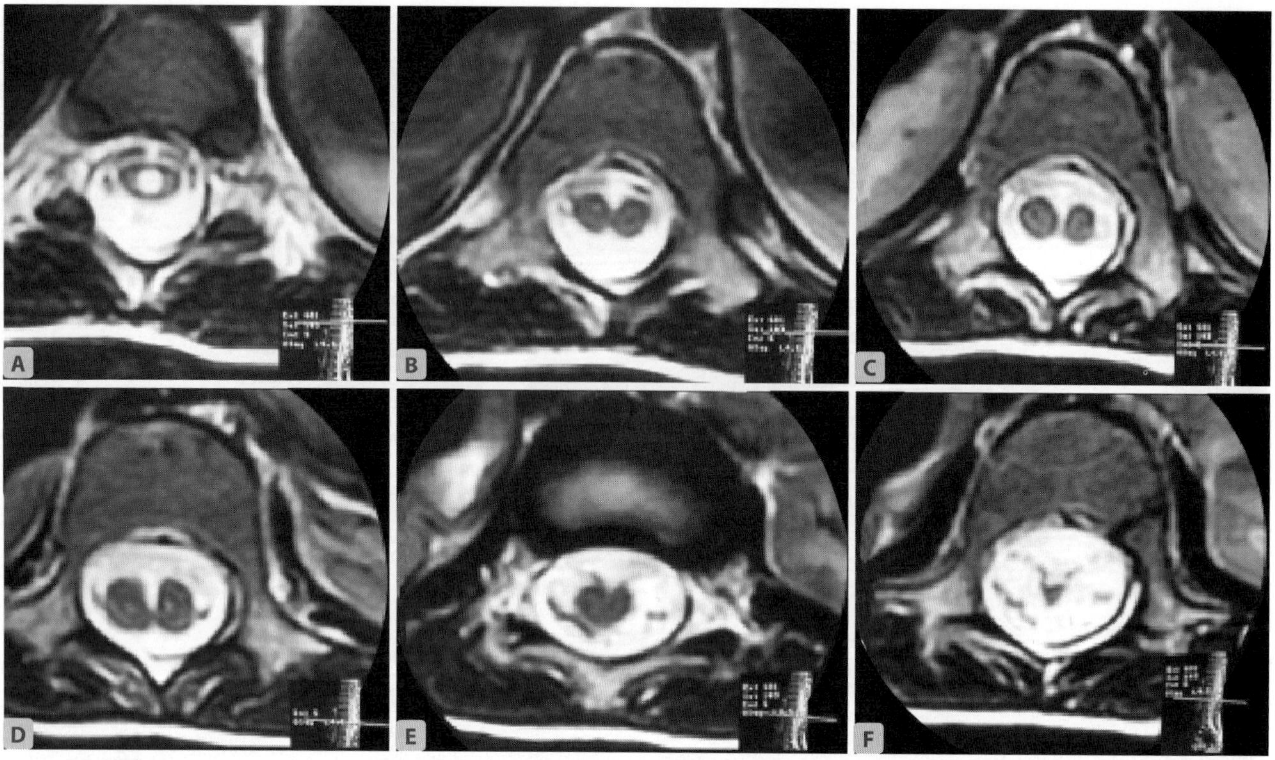

FIGS. 22A TO F: Type 2 split cord malformation (SCM) in a 10-year-old male. (A to F) Axial T2-weighted (T2W) images show two hemicords spur contained within a single dural sac. Syrinx is seen in the cord proximal to split and there is no bony/fibrous spur.

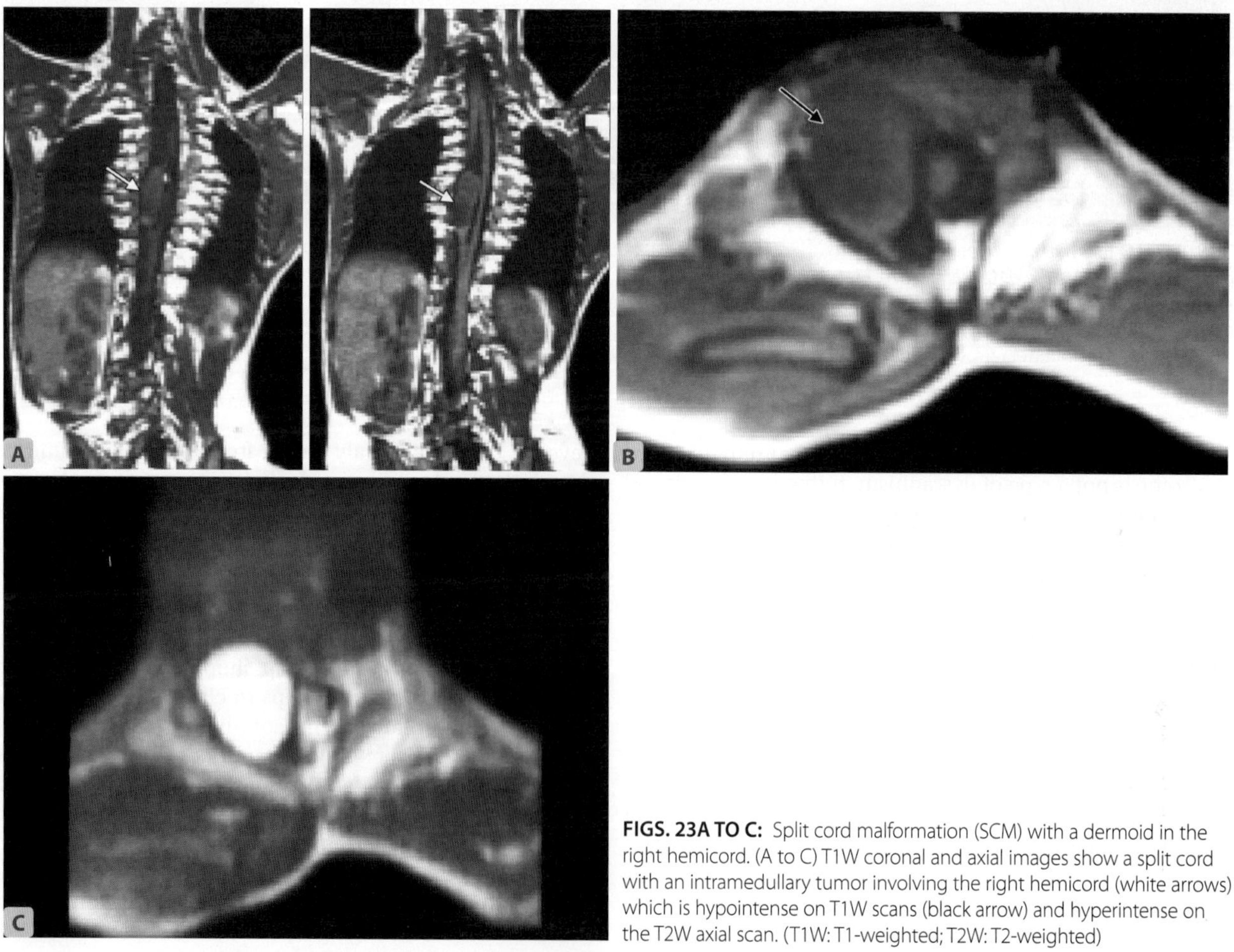

FIGS. 23A TO C: Split cord malformation (SCM) with a dermoid in the right hemicord. (A to C) T1W coronal and axial images show a split cord with an intramedullary tumor involving the right hemicord (white arrows) which is hypointense on T1W scans (black arrow) and hyperintense on the T2W axial scan. (T1W: T1-weighted; T2W: T2-weighted)

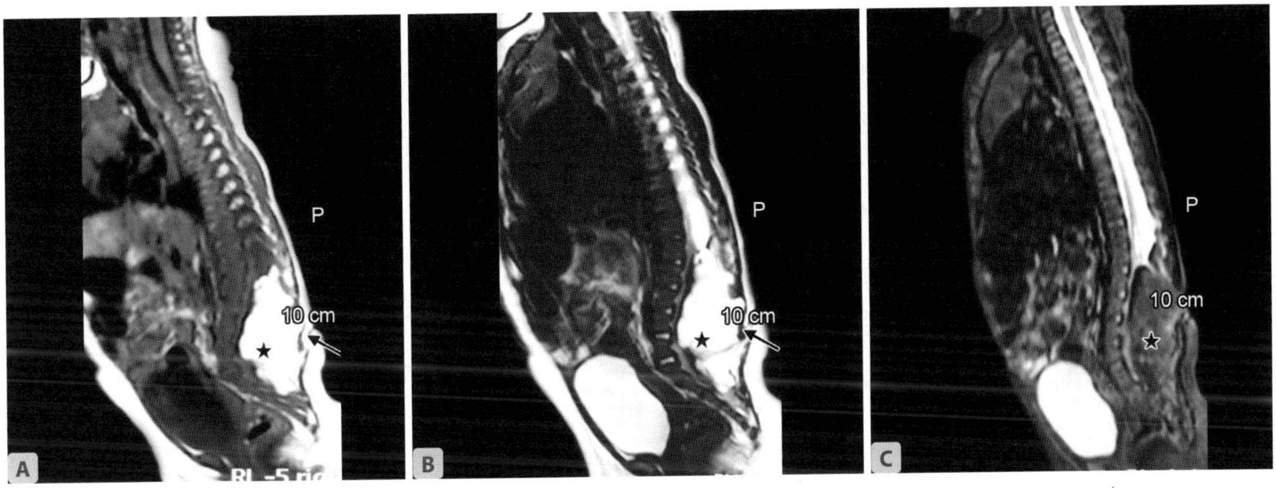

FIGS. 24A TO C: Dorsal dermal sinus (DDS) in a child with skin dimple and mass at back. (A to C) Sagittal T1W and T2W images show a hypointense linear tract (arrows) extending from skin till dura and terminates in a well-defined T1 and T2 hyperintense lesion (stars) showing homogeneous signal suppression on fat-suppressed image suggestive of intradural lipoma. (T1W: T1-weighted; T2W: T2-weighted)

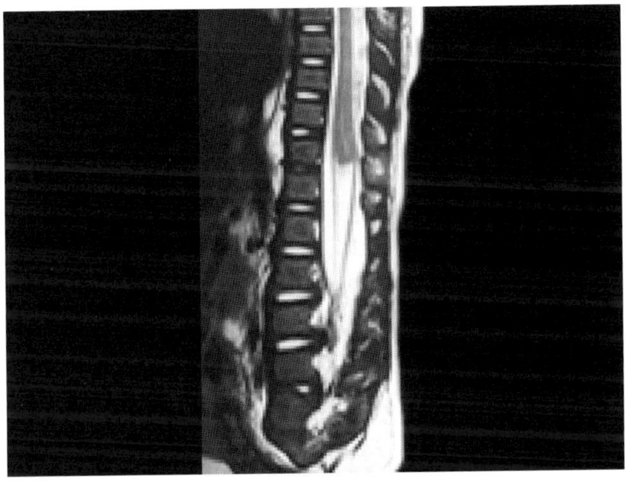

FIG. 25: Caudal agenesis type 1 in an 8-month-old male: Sagittal T2-weighted (T2W) image shows absence of the sacral segments below S1 with abrupt bulbous termination of cord at D12-L1 disk level with abnormal distal nerve roots.

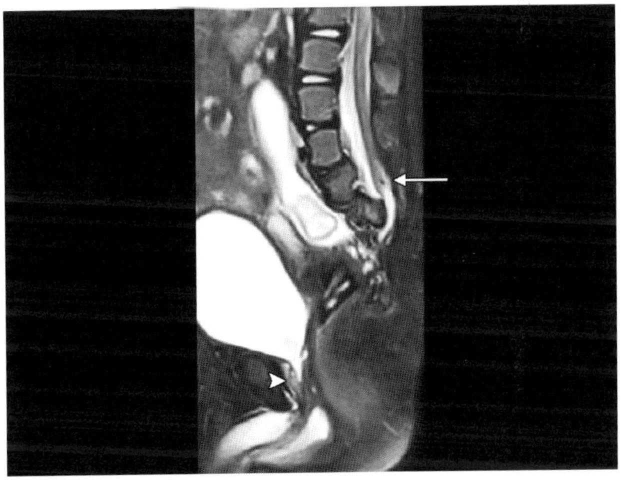

FIG. 26: Caudal agenesis type 2 in a 2-year-old male: Sagittal T2-weighted (T2W) image demonstrates abnormal low-lying cord reaching upto S1 (arrow) with agenesis of distal sacral segments. Bladder neck is patulous (arrowhead) suggestive of neurogenic bladder.

BOX 4: Common causes of tethered cord.

- Low-lying cord
- Postoperative fibrosis
- Intradural/filar terminale lipoma
- Tight filum terminale
- Lipomyelomeningocele and lipomyelocele
- Diastematomyelia
- Caudal agenesis

BOX 5: Reporting points to be included in postnatal magnetic resonance imaging (MRI) report.

- Types of dysraphism: Open/closed with/without subcutaneous mass and simple/complex in latter
- Exact type of dysraphism
- Status of overlying skin, subcutaneous fat, and posterior vertebral elements
- Tissue characterization of mass: Fluid only/lipoma/neural placode/dermoid/epidermoid
- Location of abnormality: Vertebral level and in relation to spinal canal (extraspinal component present or not)
- Location of lipoma–placode interface: Ventral subarachnoid space dilated or normal
- Status of spinal cord: Split cord, atrophy, and hydromyelia/syrinx
- Level of conus
- Cord tethering
- Filar thickness
- Vertebral anomalies and alignment
- Brain manifestations: Hydrocephalus, Chiari malformation, cortical dysplasia, and corpus callosum
- Genitourinary (kidneys, bladder) and anorectal anomalies
- Miscellaneous: Dural ectasia, meningitis

REFERENCES

1. Warder DE. Tethered cord syndrome and occult spinal dysraphism. Neurosurg Focus. 2001;10:e1.
2. Byrd SR, Darling CP, Mclone DG. Developmental disorders of the pediatric spine. Radiol Clin North Am. 1991;29:9-21.
3. Drolet B. Birthmarks to worry about. Cutaneous markers of dysraphism. Dermatol Clin. 1998;16:447-53.
4. Silverman FN. Spinal dysraphism. In: Silverman FN, Kuhn JP (Eds). Caffey's Pediatric X-ray Diagnosis, 9th edition. Philadelphia: Lippincott Williams and Wilkins; 1993. pp. 312-24.
5. Tortori-Donati P, Rossi A, Cama A. Spinal dysraphism: a review of neuroradiological features with embryological correlations and proposal for a new classification. Neuroradiology. 2000;42:471-91.
6. Tortori-Donati P, Rossi A, Biancheri R, Cama A. Magnetic resonance imaging of spinal dysraphism. Top Magn Reson Imaging. 2001;12:375-409.
7. Nievelstein NAJ, Hartwig NG, Vermeji-Keers C, Valk J. Embryonic development of the mammalian caudal neural tube. Teratology. 1993;48:21-31.
8. French BN. The embryology of spinal dysraphism. Clin Neurosurg. 1983;30:295-340.
9. Rossi A, Biancheri R, Cama A, Piatelli G, Ravegnani M, Tortori-Donati P. Imaging in spine and spinal cord malformations. Eur J Radiol. 2004;50:177-200.
10. Bulas D. Fetal evaluation of spine dysraphism. Pediatr Radiol. 2010;40:1029-37.
11. Von Koch CS, Glenn OA, Goldstein RB, Barkovich AJ. Fetal magnetic resonance imaging enhances detection of spinal cord anomalies in patients with sonographically detected bony anomalies of the spine. J Ultrasound Med. 2005;24:781-9.
12. Kumar J, Afsal M, Garg A. Imaging spectrum of spinal dysraphism on magnetic resonance: a pictorial review. World J Radiol. 2017;9:178-90.
13. Tortori-Donati P, Cama A, Fondelli MP, Rossi A. Le malformazioni di Chiari. In: Tortori-Donati P, Taccone A, Longo M (Eds). Malformazioni cranio-encefaliche. Turin: Minerva Medica; 1996. pp. 209-36.
14. McLone DG, Dias MS. Complications of myelomeningocele closure. Pediatr Neurosurg. 1991;17:267-73.
15. Scott RM, Wolpert SM, Bartoshesky LF, Zimbler S, Klauber GT. Dermoid tumors occurring at the site of previous myelomeningocele repair. J Neurosurg. 1986;65:779-83.
16. Cama A, Tortori-Donati P, Piatelli GL, Fondelli MP, Andreussi L. Chiari complex in children. Neuroradiological diagnosis, neurosurgical treatment and proposal of a new classification (312 cases). Eur J Pediatr Surg. 1995;5:35-8.
17. McLone DG, Knepper PA. The cause of Chiari II malformation: a unified theory. Pediatr Neurosci. 1989;15:1-12.
18. Fichter MA, Dornseifer U, Henke J, Schneider KT, Kovacs L, Biemer E, et al. Fetal spina bifida repair—current trends and prospects of intrauterine neurosurgery. Fetal Diagn Ther. 2008;23:271-86.
19. Hirose S, Farmer DL. Fetal surgery for myelomeningocele. Clin Perinatol. 2009;36:431-8.
20. Naidich TP, McLone DG, Fulling F. The Chiari II malformation. Part IV. The hindbrain deformity. Neuroradiology. 1983;25:179-97.
21. Pang D, Dias MS, Ahab-Barmada M. Split cord malformation, Part I: A unified theory of embryogenesis for double spinal cord malformations. Neurosurgery. 1992;31:451-80.
22. Pang D. Split cord malformation. Part II: Clinical syndrome. Neurosurgery. 1992;31:481-500.
23. Breningstall GN, Marker SM, Tubman DE. Hydrosyringomyelia and diastematomyelia detected by MRI in myelomeningocele. Pediatr Neurol. 1992;8:267-71.
24. Rufener SL, Ibrahim M, Raybaud CA, Parmar HA. Congenital spine and spinal cord malformations—pictorial review. AJR Am J Roentgenol. 2010;194:S26-37.
25. Kumar I, Sachan A, Aggarwal P, Verma A, Shukla RC. Structured MRI reporting in spinal dysraphism. Acta Radiol. 2020. [Online ahead of print].
26. Acharya UV, Pendharkar H, Varma DR, Pruthi N, Varadarajan S. Spinal dysraphism illustrated: Embroyology revisited. Indian J Radiol Imaging. 2017;27:417-26.
27. Reghunath A, Ghasi RG, Aggarwal A. Unveiling the tale of the tail: an illustration of spinal dysraphisms. Neurosurg Rev. 2019. [Online ahead of print].
28. Gadodia A, Sharma R, Jeyaseelan N, Aggarwala S, Gupta P. Prenatal diagnosis of mediastinal neurentric cyst with an intraspinal component. J Pediatr Surg. 2010;45:1377-9.
29. Sharma A, Sharma R, Goyal M, Vashisht S, Berry M. Diastematomyelia associated with intramedullary tumour in a hemicord: a report of two cases. Australas Radiol. 1997;41:185-7.
30. Barkovich AJ, Edwards MSB, Cogen PH. MR evaluation of spinal dermal sinus tracts in children. AJNR Am J Neuroradiol. 1991;12:123-9.
31. Schwartz ES, Rossi A. Congenital spine anomalies: the closed spinal dysraphisms. Pediatr Radiol. 2015;45:S413-9.
32. Nievelstein RAJ, Valk J, Smit LME, Vermeji-Keers C. MR of the caudal regression syndrome: embryologic implications. AJNR Am J Neuroradiol. 1994;15:1021-9.
33. Pang D. Sacral agenesis and caudal spinal cord malformations. Neurosurgery. 1993;32:755-79.
34. Tortori-Donati P, Fondelli MP, Rossi A, Raybaud CA, Cama A, Capra V. Segmental spinal dysgenesis. Neuroradiologic findings with clinical and embryologic correlation. AJNR Am J Neuroradiol. 1999;20:445-56.

CHAPTER

81

Imaging of Pediatric Joint Pathology

Anjali Prakash, Rajat Jain, Gaurav Shanker Pradhan, Jyoti Kumar

INTRODUCTION

Children are vulnerable to a diverse group of arthritis, some of which, though similar to the adult counterparts, have certain unique imaging features. The growing skeleton is different from the mature skeleton, a fact that is reflected in the appearance on imaging.

An immature skeleton has epiphyseal cartilage and growth plate (physis) both of which involute as the bones mature. The subchondral bone is lined by articular cartilage which remains present throughout life. The epiphysis is entirely cartilaginous in newborns, undergoing progressive ossification. Cartilage is not seen on radiographs and the use of ultrasound is also limited in its evaluation. Magnetic resonance imaging (MRI) is the investigation of choice for evaluation of the growing skeleton including cartilage. The cartilage displays intermediate signal intensity on T1-weighted image (T1WI) and is hypointense on fluid-sensitive sequences.

As the ossification starts, foci of high signal intensity are seen on fluid-sensitive sequences. As the child begins to walk, the weight-bearing portions of the epiphyseal cartilages present a decrease in their signal intensity on T2-weighted image (T2WI), more evident in the knees and the hips. During growth spurts, irregularity of the secondary ossification centers at the bone and/or cartilage junction is a normal finding. Progressive narrowing of physis is seen with bone maturation with centrifugal pattern and final formation of a physeal scar, which also fades over a period of time with only a linear area of low signal intensity persisting throughout the life.[1,2]

IMAGING MODALITIES

Radiographs

Radiographs remain the first line of investigation for patients with joint pathologies. Easily available and cost-effective, they are used for the initial, and in many cases, the final diagnosis, and also in follow-up of these patients. An important drawback of radiographs is its poor sensitivity to early changes with pre-erosive signs of inflammation such as synovitis and osteitis being undetectable. Inability to visualize the articular cartilage and the use of ionizing radiation are the other limitations.[3]

Ultrasound

Ultrasound is an attractive investigation for pediatric age group due to the absence of ionizing radiation, ease of availability, cost-effectiveness, and patient acceptability. Ultrasound of the joints allows assessment of effusion, synovitis, cartilage, soft tissues, and even bone erosions in many cases. Doppler adds to the diagnostic confidence by assessing blood flow to the joint, a marker of inflammation.

The real-time nature of ultrasound allows dynamic assessment of pathology such as developmental diseases of the hip. It is also used for guidance in joint aspirations and other therapeutic procedures.

CT

CT is an excellent imaging investigation for assessing osseous anatomy with a very high degree of sensitivity to detect cortical erosion, incomplete fractures, subtle periosteal reaction, and tiny foci of calcifications. Three-dimensional (3D) visualization of the anatomy in locations like the cervical spine is helpful. Despite having these advantages, the use of CT should be very judicious due to significant amount of ionizing radiation delivered in a single scan. There is limited soft-tissue resolution and changes in the bone marrow are not appreciated on CT.

MRI

MRI is the most useful imaging modality for detailed assessment of pediatric joint pathologies. It has excellent spatial and contrast resolution with the added advantage of not using radiation. MRI is very useful in evaluation of inflammatory arthropathies like juvenile idiopathic arthritis (JIA) and septic arthritis which are still in the pre-erosive stage, thereby allowing early treatment. Whole-body MRI is considered to be of use in pediatric rheumatology for evaluation of chronic recurrent multifocal osteomyelitis, arthritis, dermatomyositis, and connective tissue diseases.

Using an appropriate coil is essential in the MR imaging of a pediatric joint. Practical modification such as use of an adult wrist coil for elbow of a small child may be done. In the immature skeleton when the joint is undergoing progressive ossification with age, the cartilage appears relatively hyperintense and should not be misinterpreted as bone marrow edema on fluid-sensitive sequences. A cartilage-sensitive sequence is an essential component for joint imaging by MRI. The long acquisition time, need for sedation, poses an additional challenge in the pediatric age group.[4,5]

Nuclear Scan

Nuclear scans are extremely sensitive, but lack specificity in assessment of bone pathology. There is poor spatial resolution and the exposure to ionizing radiation is an additional problem. Increased uptake of the tracer is seen in the growing skeleton posing a challenge in interpretation.

JUVENILE IDIOPATHIC ARTHRITIS

Juvenile idiopathic arthritis is a broad term which covers several distinct categories and has replaced older nomenclature such as juvenile rheumatoid arthritis and juvenile chronic arthritis. An autoimmune systemic disease of the connective tissue that affects individuals at the developmental age, it is characterized by synovial inflammation and is the most common rheumatic complaint in children.[6]

The affected joint is painful, red, warm, swollen, and stiff with reduced motion. Some patients may present with systemic onset with intermittent spiking fever, migratory light pink rash over the trunk and extremities, and hepatosplenomegaly. Poor prognostic indicators are early hip and wrist involvement, a positive rheumatoid factor (RF) serology, severe, widespread involvement at initial presentation.

Etiopathogenesis

Juvenile idiopathic arthritis is an immune-mediated disease thought to be the result of a combination of genetic and environmental factors. Different associations between human leukocyte antigen (HLA) alleles and JIA categories have been reported. In combination with genetic factors, environmental triggers are also described in the pathogenesis of JIA. Infectious viral or bacterial agents are considered potential triggers. Ethnic differences are seen with Whites more affected than Asian or African individuals. Equal gender ratio is reported in ethnic groups such as Indian and black South Africans. The wrist is affected in 61% of patients with polyarticular JIA, being second only to the knee as the most frequently involved joint. Hips and wrist are the most vulnerable joints to radiographically visible destruction. Joint involvement begins with synovial inflammation, progressing to synovial hyperplasia and pannus formation. Pannus erodes the cartilage causing bone destruction and finally a stage of ankylosis.

Classification of Juvenile Idiopathic Arthritis

The International League of Associations for Rheumatology defines JIA as an arthritis with onset before the age of 16 years and lasting for at least 6 weeks. The diagnosis is established on the basis of the clinical presentation. It includes a heterogeneous group of arthritis which has been divided into several subtypes based on prevailing clinical signs in the first 6 months from the onset and laboratory findings **(Box 1)**.

BOX 1: International League of Associations for Rheumatology classification criteria for juvenile idiopathic arthritis (JIA).

- Systemic-onset JIA
- Pauciarticular or oligoarticular JIA (oligoarthritis), including persistent or extended arthritis
- Polyarticular rheumatoid factor-positive JIA
- Polyarticular rheumatoid factor-negative JIA
- Psoriatic JIA
- Enthesitis-related arthritis
- Other undifferentiated types of arthritis wherein:
  - The clinical picture of the disease does not meet the criteria for any of the aforementioned type
  - The clinical picture combines two or more JIA types

- *Systemic JIA*: The diagnosis is established based on signs of arthritis in at least one joint with concomitant or preceding fever lasting for at least 2 weeks as well as the presence of at least one of the following symptoms: Evanescent and erythematous rash, generalized lymphadenopathy, hepatosplenomegaly, or serositis.
- *Pauciarticular JIA*: It is the most common clinical subtype. It occurs typically in very young girls and is often associated with the presence of antinuclear antibodies. One to four joints affected within 6 months of onset of disease. The arthritis is asymmetrical and the knee joint is usually affected first followed by the ankle joint.
- *Polyarticular RF-positive JIA (seropositive JIA)*: Clinical signs and immune disorders presented by patients with this form of JIA resemble rheumatoid arthritis in adults. It is characterized by arthritis in ≥five joints during the first 6 months of the disease and positive immunoglobulin M (IgM) RF in the serum (two positive RF test results at least 3 months apart within 6 months of disease onset).
- *Polyarticular RF-negative JIA*: This form of JIA shows a bimodal peak with usual affection in older children. It is characterized by arthritis in small and large joints. The inflammatory process involves ≤five joints within the first 6 months from the onset with negative IgM RF.
- *Psoriatic juvenile idiopathic arthritis*: It is characterized by arthritis and psoriasis or arthritis and two or more of the following: Dactylitis, nail pitting or onycholysis, or psoriasis in a first-degree relative.
- *Enthesitis-related arthritis (ERA)*: It is the only form of JIA found to occur mainly in boys, usually older than 6 years of age. It presents with arthritis and/or enthesitis, with two or more of the following: Presence or history of SI joint tenderness or inflammatory low back pain; positive HLA-B27 antigen; male over 6 years of age at onset; acute (symptomatic) anterior uveitis; or a history of ankylosing spondylitis, ERA, sacroiliitis with inflammatory bowel disease (IBD), Reiter syndrome, or acute anterior uveitis in a first-degree relative.

- *Undifferentiated forms of JIA*: When the clinical presentation fits into no category or overlaps with at least two categories or overlaps with at least two of the other categories.

Imaging in Juvenile Idiopathic Arthritis

Although JIA remains a clinical diagnosis, imaging plays a critical role in excluding other causes of joint swelling, monitoring disease progression and treatment response, and evaluating potential complications. With the advent of newer biological therapeutic agents, the goal of JIA treatment is complete suppression of synovitis before the development of irreversible joint abnormalities. Although radiography remains the most commonly used imaging modality in the evaluation of JIA, early detection of inflammation is best achieved with use of contrast-enhanced (CE) magnetic resonance (MR) imaging and Doppler ultrasonography (USG), either of which can help in detecting inflammatory lesions before permanent joint destruction occurs and in monitoring disease progression and treatment response.[7-9]

Radiographs

Radiographic findings in early-stage JIA are often nonspecific and include soft-tissue swelling, joint effusion, and osteopenia **(Fig. 1)**. Osteopenia tends to be periarticular in the early stages of disease secondary to joint inflammation whereas in advanced-stage JIA, it can be diffuse due to decreased physical activity or steroid administration. For evaluation of the lower extremities, weight-bearing radiographs are recommended over supine images for detecting joint space loss, limb length discrepancy, or joint malalignment. Radiography is useful for predicting joint damage. Patient with erosions and joint space narrowing in the early phase of the disease will have a prolonged clinical activity and will be less likely to achieve clinical remission.

The radiographic features are detailed in the inset **(Box 2)**. Although JIA presents with many overlapping imaging features with adult rheumatoid arthritis, there are pathognomonic imaging findings which include:

- *Periosteal reaction*: Usually seen along the shafts of the proximal phalanges and metacarpals.
- *Joint ankylosis*: Articular ankylosis is reported to develop within 3–5 years of disease, if left untreated. Ankylosis may involve the wrist and interphalangeal joints. Fusion of apophyseal joints of the cervical spine is a characteristic finding.
- *Growth plate abnormalities*: As JIA occurs before skeletal maturation, alteration in growth plate is common. Enlarged epiphysis of distal femur leads to overgrowth of condyles and associated widening of intercondylar notch and squaring of patella **(Fig. 2)**.
- *Sacroiliitis*: It is seen in about 30% of children with ERA subtype of JIA.

Ultrasound

The primary anatomical structures in JIA evaluated with USG include:

- *Joint cavities, sheaths, and bursae for signs of synovitis*: Effusion, synovial thickening, hypervascularity, and increased synovial echogenicity as signs of chronic inflammation or fibrosis **(Fig. 5A)**.
- Intra- and extra-articular fat tissue for signs of inflammation such as increased echogenicity and increased blood flow.
- Hyaline cartilage, cartilaginous epiphyses, and subchondral bone for any damage (erosions, cysts, and scars after injuries).
- Ligaments, tendons, and entheses in evaluation of enthesopathies and tendinopathies (tenosynovitis, tendinitis secondary to tenosynovitis, tendon injuries, and enthesitis) **(Fig. 5B)**.

Ultrasonography enables the detection of subclinical synovitis (i.e., synovitis that is not manifested clinically)

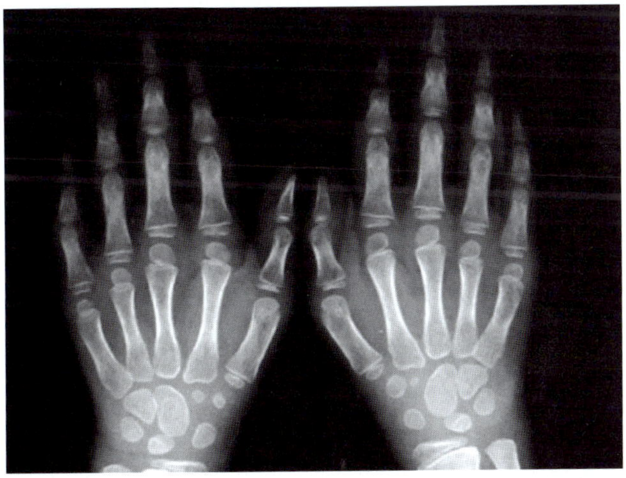

FIG. 1: Anteroposterior view of bilateral hands shows symmetric and bilateral periostitis along the proximal and middle phalanges in both hands, notably from the second to the fourth digits. Periarticular osteoporosis is also appreciated in this patient with juvenile idiopathic arthritis (JIA).

BOX 2: Radiographic findings in juvenile idiopathic arthritis (JIA).

Early findings:
- Joint effusion
- Soft-tissue swelling
- Osteoporosis—juxta-articular/diffuse
- Periostitis—periarticular region of phalanges, metacarpals, and metatarsals **(Fig. 3)**

Late findings:
- Joint space loss
- Joint malalignment—subluxations and dislocations
- Bony erosions—typically late manifestation if not seropositive/systemic onset **(Fig. 4)**
- Growth disturbances—epiphyseal overgrowth, premature physeal closure, short broad phalanges, metacarpals, metatarsal, TM hypoplasia, and leg length discrepancy
- Ankylosis—small joints of hands and feet, cervical spine
- Hypertrophic bursitis
- Synovial cysts—popliteal, bicipital, and subchondral
- Compression fractures—weight-bearing epiphysis

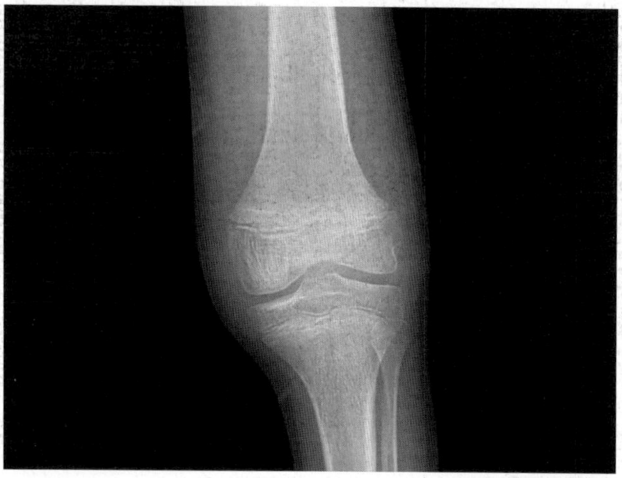

FIG. 2: Anteroposterior view of left knee shows condylar hypertrophy with widened intercondylar notch. Diffuse osteoporosis and growth recovery lines are also noted.

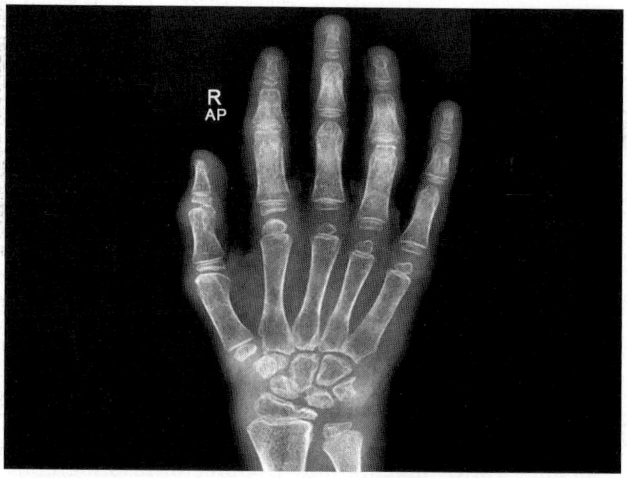

FIG. 3: Anteroposterior radiograph of the hand reveals juxta-articular osteopenia, erosions along the radial head epiphysis, and multiple erosions along the various carpal bones with soft-tissue swelling along the wrist, metacarpophalangeal, and proximal interphalangeal joints.

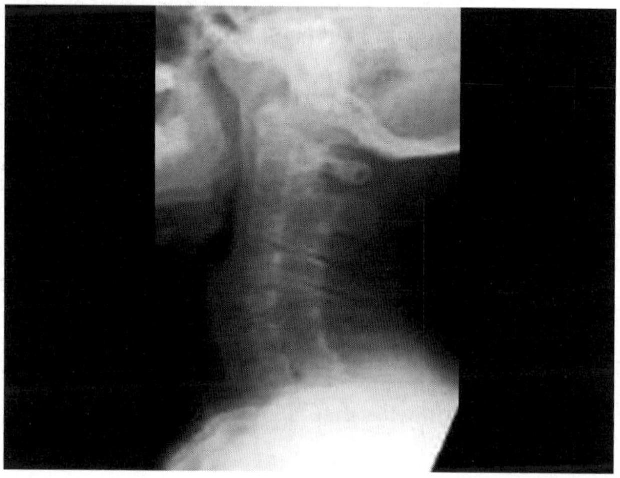

FIG. 4: Lateral cervical spine radiograph shows bony ankylosis at various levels due to long-standing juvenile idiopathic arthritis (JIA).

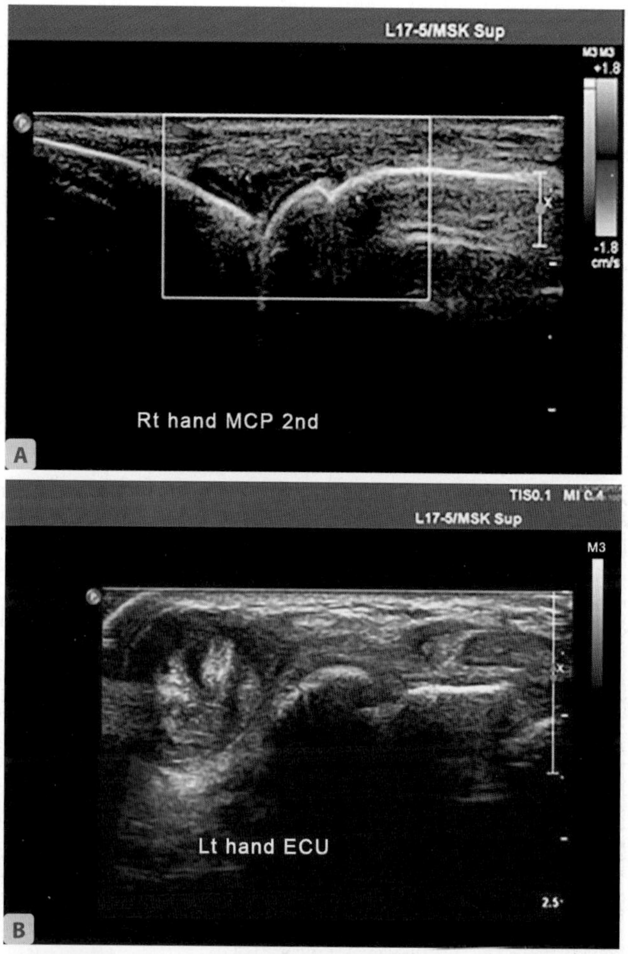

FIGS. 5A AND B: (A) Ultrasonography image at the level of right second metacarpophalangeal joint shows synovial thickening and hypervascularity as the sign of chronic inflammation; and (B) Ultrasonography image showing extensor carpi ulnaris tendon in a different patient with fluid along the tendon sheath—tenosynovitis.

in children with suspected JIA. The drawbacks are variability in the sensitivity of USG in identifying pre-erosive changes as seen in different studies, interobserver variability in detecting the disease manifestations, and inability to asses anatomically challenging joints such as temporomandibular joint (TMJ).

MR Imaging

Contrast-enhanced MR imaging is the most sensitive imaging technique for detecting synovitis. MR imaging can help detect synovitis before it is apparent at physical examination, a potentially important prognostic indicator **(Figs. 6A and B)**. The presence of bone marrow edema in the setting of JIA is considered a preerosive abnormality and an indication for initiating therapy to prevent permanent joint damage. Various MR imaging scoring systems have been proposed,

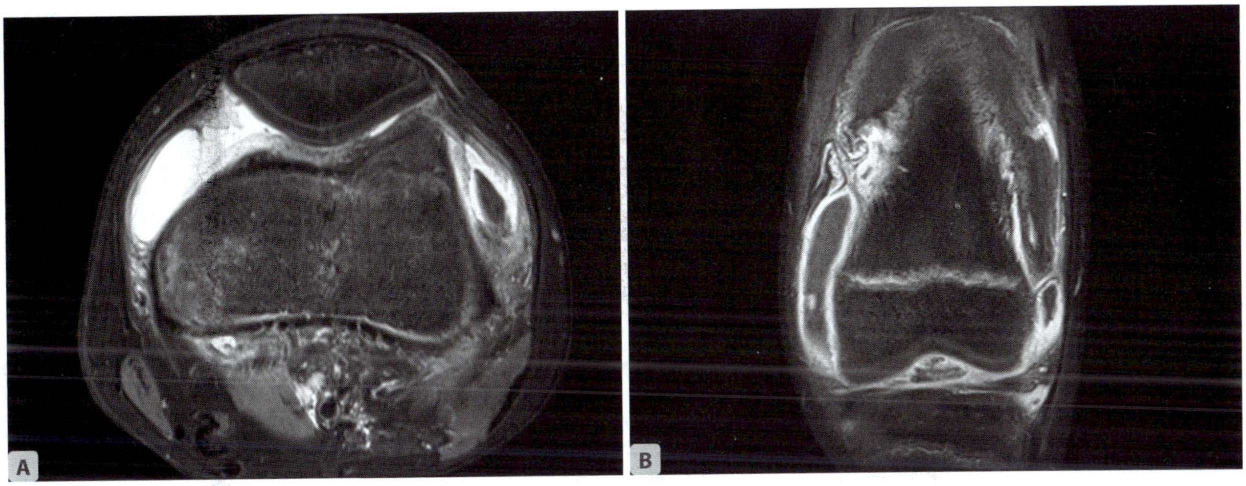

FIGS. 6A AND B: Axial PD-fat saturated (A) and postgadolinium coronal fat-saturated T1-weighted images (B) of a patient with long standing juvenile idiopathic arthritis reveals marked synovitis with joint effusion. Oedema along the lateral aspect of lateral femoral condyle represent pre-erosive changes.

some for individual joints such as wrist but further validation is required at a larger scale.[7]

Specific Joint Involvement in Juvenile Idiopathic Arthritis

A few joints such as TMJ and cervical spine are involved commonly in JIA.

Temporomandibular Joint

Temporomandibular joint involvement is more commonly seen in patients younger than 4 years. Active inflammation of TMJ is characterized by joint effusion, synovial enhancement, and bone marrow edema.

Contrast-enhanced MRI is the modality of choice to assess inflammatory changes of the TMJ. Presence of joint effusion, synovial enhancement, and bone marrow edema indicates active inflammation and should prompt escalation of systemic therapy or site-specific steroid injection under fluoroscopy or CT guidance.

Cervical Spine

Cervical spine involvement in JIA is usually silent and hence, MR imaging is found to be more useful than clinical examination in the detection of joint damage. Ankylosis of the apophyseal joints, usually involving C2–C3, is a characteristic finding. Odontoid process erosions due to atlantoaxial synovial proliferation can be seen in polyarticular JIA. Atlantodental interval widening due to inflammation at the atlantoaxial articulation with subsequent ligamentous insufficiency may be seen which can lead to atlantoaxial instability, which can be evaluated on flexion and extension radiographs.

Sacroiliac Joint

Sacroiliac joint inflammation is detected better by MR imaging than clinical examination which shows involvement after 5–10 years after the onset of symptoms. Synovial enhancement helps in the evaluation of disease activity and differentiation of active synovitis from burnt out disease.

Role of Imaging in Treatment

Ultrasound is used for guidance of intra-articular therapeutic injections and aspirations. Both US and MRI are used to follow-up patients who are in remission and clinically asymptomatic. Signs of inflammation in such patients are likely to show disease progression at follow-up.

IMAGING OF JUVENILE SPONDYLOARTHRITIS

Juvenile spondyloarthritis refers to a group of conditions characterized by SI joint involvement along with varying degree of enthesitis and arthritis, associated with HLA-B27 antigen with onset before the age of 16 years. The various diseases considered under this group are:[10,11]

- Juvenile ankylosing spondylitis (JAS)
- Juvenile psoriatic arthritis (JPA)
- Reactive arthritis
- Arthritis associated with IBD

Juvenile Ankylosing Spondylitis (Box 3)

Similar to adults, boys are more frequently affected with the usual age of onset being in early second decade. Involvement of axial skeletal is usually seen very late in the disease in contrast to the adult-onset ankylosing spondylitis, with arthritis and enthesitis being the more common articular manifestations in early disease.

Large joints of lower limb like hip and knee are more commonly affected with a more severe articular disease in comparison to adult counterpart. Common radiographic findings include progressive joint space narrowing and bone erosions. Involvement of the axial skeleton is not essential in making the diagnosis of JAS unlike the adult

BOX 3: Juvenile ankylosing spondylitis.

- More common in boys
- Involves large joints of lower limb
- Axial skeleton involvement seen in later course
- Spine involvement follows sacroiliac (SI) joint involvement
- Symmetric sacroiliitis

prototype and some patients never show involvement of SI joint. However, when seen, it is very similar to adult-onset disease. The changes are usually bilateral, although unilateral disease may be seen at presentation. As the disease advances, there is gradual narrowing of the joint spaces and ankylosis may be very rarely found in late-stage JAS. Vertebral involvement, if it occurs, almost always follows sacroiliitis in JAS. Thoracolumbar spine is most commonly affected in late-stage disease. Classic radiographic findings include sclerosis of vertebral corners, squaring of the vertebral bodies, syndesmophytosis, and ankylosis of the facet joints.

MRI is the preferred investigation for early diagnosis, which can detect the disease even in the pre-erosive phase by showing joint effusion, synovial thickening, and inflammation of bones and soft tissue. In advanced cases, cartilaginous and bone erosions can also be seen.

Juvenile Psoriatic Arthritis (Box 4)

Juvenile psoriatic arthritis is an uncommon disease, defined as persistent arthritis lasting for >6 weeks and with onset prior to age 16 years and either the presence of a psoriatic rash or, in the absence of rash, at least two of the following minor criteria:

- First-degree relative with psoriasis
- Nail pitting
- Onycholysis
- Dactylitis

Asymmetric oligoarticular arthritis, predominantly involving knee and peripheral joints of hand and feet, is the most common finding. The involvement of the hand is much more frequent than foot with a characteristic involvement of distal interphalangeal joint is typical. Association of peripheral erosions and periostitis may lead to the characteristic "mouse ear" appearance in short bones of hands and feet.

Early changes are difficult to appreciate on radiography. Osseous erosions, proliferative changes, periostitis, and enthesitis are common findings, seen late in the disease. Pencil-in-cup deformity, the hallmark of adult psoriatic arthritis, is rare in pediatric age group. Arthritis mutilans is also uncommon. When there is involvement of axial skeleton, sternoclavicular, manubriosternal, and sternocostal joints are affected in as much as one-fourth of the patients. Dactylitis, resulting in sausage finger if seen, is characteristic of JPA even when there are no dermatological manifestations. It is seen due to combination of soft-tissue inflammation, tenosynovitis, arthritis, and periostitis.

Contrast-enhanced MRI is the investigation of choice for assessing the extent of inflammatory changes in early disease as well as to monitor disease evolution.

BOX 4: Juvenile psoriatic arthropathy.

- Arthritis with psoriatic rash or specific dermatological manifestation
- Commonly involves peripheral joints of hand and feet
- Hand is more commonly involved than feet
- Mouse ear appearance
- Dactylitis (sausage finger) characteristic even in the absence of skin changes
- Asymmetric sacroiliitis

Arthritis Associated with Inflammatory Bowel Disease in Children

Approximately 10% of the pediatric patients with IBD have associated arthritic changes noted on imaging. These changes may precede the disease onset or may follow the enteropathy. Two distinct patterns of arthritis are noted:

1. Peripheral arthritis, without sex predilection
2. Axial spondyloarthritis with predominance of spondylitis and sacroiliitis, more common in males.

The arthritic activity usually parallels the severity of enteritis with asymmetric nondestructive oligoarticular arthritis being the most common pattern.

Among the peripheral joints, knees, ankles, and wrists are affected most often, followed by small joints of the hands and shoulders. The involvement of axial skeleton, though less common, is very similar to that found in JAS. Spondylitis and sacroiliitis can progress even if the enteritic changes are not severe.

Reactive Arthritis

Reactive arthritis usually follows an intestinal infection or a urogenital infection. Only a small group of patients show classic clinical triad of arthritis, urethritis, and conjunctivitis. Males are more commonly affected between the age group of 15–35 years with the involvement of younger age group being rare. The joints of lower limb are more frequently involved with usual monoarticular involvement. First interphalangeal joint involvement is typical. It is usually a self-limiting condition with no evidence of any viable microorganism in the aspirated fluid. Dactylitis, tenosynovitis, and synovial cyst may be seen however, erosive arthropathy is uncommon. In the pediatric age group, involvement of axial skeleton is much less common than adults. Sacroiliitis, if seen, is usually bilaterally symmetrical.

INFECTIOUS ARTHROPATHIES IN CHILDREN

Imaging of an infected joint has an ancillary role to joint aspiration which provides the definitive diagnosis. Accurate and prompt diagnosis is of utmost importance, so that structural damage can be prevented and permanent sequelae can be avoided.

Pyogenic/Septic Arthritis

Pyogenic arthritis refers to the bacterial infection of the joint. Clinically, there is fever, joint pain, and swelling of the affected joint. Boys are affected twice as frequently as girls. It is a medical emergency as it may lead to joint destruction and impairment, if not immediately and adequately treated.

Acute purulent infection of the joints is more common in infancy and early childhood because of greater blood flow to the joints during active growth. Hematogenous seeding is the most common cause and is related to an upper respiratory tract infection or pyoderma. Pyogenic arthritis usually presents as an acute monoarthritis, involving lower extremities in majority of the patients, mostly hips and knees. Infection may also spread from adjacent osteomyelitis in metaphysis (especially in hip, where the metaphysis is intra-articular) or from cellulitis, abscess, etc. During infancy, septic arthritis frequently complicates osteomyelitis because capillaries from the metaphysis traverse the physis into the epiphysis. Infants with immune dysfunction, indwelling catheters, and vascular lines are at increased risk.

Staphylococcus aureus is the most common cause of bacterial arthritis, with group B *Streptococcus* seen in neonates, *Haemophilus influenzae* in the 1–4 years age group. Children with chickenpox are at increased risk of developing septic arthritis and other musculoskeletal infections secondary to group A *Streptococcus*. Pneumococcal joint infection may be seen in children with splenic dysfunction. *Neisseria gonorrhoeae* leading to gonococcal arthritis may be found in neonates caused by birth canal infection.[12,13]

Pathology

The joint cartilage is avascular and the synovial fluid cushions, lubricates, and nourishes the joint cartilage. Bacteria may seed into the synovial space through the highly vascular synovial membrane. Initially, there is edema and hypertrophy of the synovial membrane with joint effusion, which distends the joint. Hyperemia and immobilization lead to demineralization and osteoporosis. The ensuing inflammatory reaction results in destruction of the cartilage matrix leading to reduction of the joint space. Inflammatory pannus destroys the articular cortex, which is eroded. Severe cases are characterized by massive destruction, separation of bone ends, subluxation, and dislocation. During recovery, bones recalcify and bony and fibrous ankylosis may occur.

Imaging

Radiography is the initial imaging modality and should be obtained in all patients even though this is quite insensitive and irreversible joint damage is usually present by the time that radiographic abnormalities become evident. Plain films may demonstrate joint space widening with adjacent soft-tissue swelling and disruption of normal tissue planes **(Fig. 7)**. It may show joint space loss and erosions with relative preservation of mineralization.

Radionuclide imaging is more sensitive than radiographs. A bone scan localizes the site of infection and is positive as early as 2 days after the onset of symptoms. In septic arthritis, there is increased articular activity in the blood flow and blood pool phases. Reduced uptake within the epiphysis may be as a result of ischemia.

Ultrasonography can clearly delineate the presence and nature of joint fluid by direct visualization and can be used to guide needle aspiration. It is particularly helpful for the detection of joint effusion in deep-seated joints such as the hip or shoulder where clinical examination is not effective **(Figs. 8A and B)**. USG can also demonstrate erosions and involvement of adjacent bursae and tendon sheaths. Power Doppler ultrasound has been used to differentiate septic arthritis from sterile synovitis.

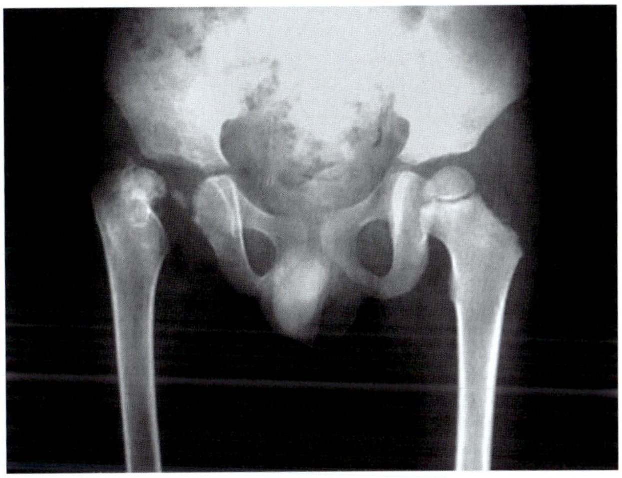

FIG. 7: X-ray pelvis erosions in right femoral head with dislocation and widening of joint space—septic arthritis.

CT has limited usefulness in the assessment of pyogenic arthritis in pediatric patients. It is usually performed as an adjunct to MRI for osseous assessment or to evaluate anatomically complex joints.

MRI is extremely sensitive for detection of even a very minimal effusion. Patients with both septic arthritis and transient synovitis may show joint effusion, intense enhancement, and hypertrophy of the synovial membrane. Patients with septic arthritis, however, also show signal abnormalities in adjacent bone marrow on fat-suppressed CEMRI, a finding not seen in patients with transient synovitis. The joint space becomes an abscess cavity **(Figs. 9A to C)**. Pyogenic abscess in a joint space can be differentiated from reactive fluid based on diffusion MR. A pyogenic abscess shows an increased signal intensity on diffusion-weighted imaging whereas a reactive effusion shows a low signal.

Differentiation of pyogenic from tubercular joint infection is important as treatment is different in both. Serology and joint fluid analysis form the basis of diagnosis. MR imaging may offer some clues to the diagnosis. A thin and smooth abscess rim favors tubercular arthritis whereas a thick and irregularly-enhancing rim is indicative of pyogenic arthritis.[12-15]

Tuberculous Arthritis

Tuberculosis (TB) of the skeletal system is widespread in our country and accounts for 15% of all (adults and children) patients of osteoarticular TB with hip involvement, being second to spine. It is typically a slowly progressive monoarthritis that affects weight-bearing joints such as the knees and hips.

Joint involvement, rather than isolated osteomyelitis, is more commonly seen in tubercular infection. This is due to transphyseal dissemination of an active tuberculous focus in

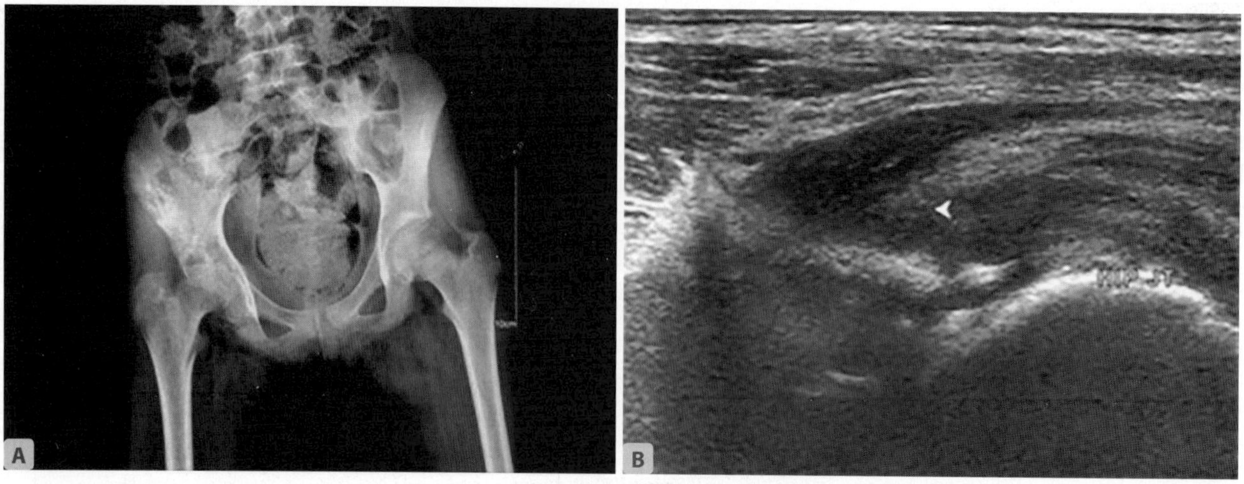

FIGS. 8A AND B: (A) X-ray—reduced right hip joint space with irregularity of articular outline; and (B) Ultrasound hip of the same patient shows disorganized joint with effusion that shows debris—a case of septic arthritis.

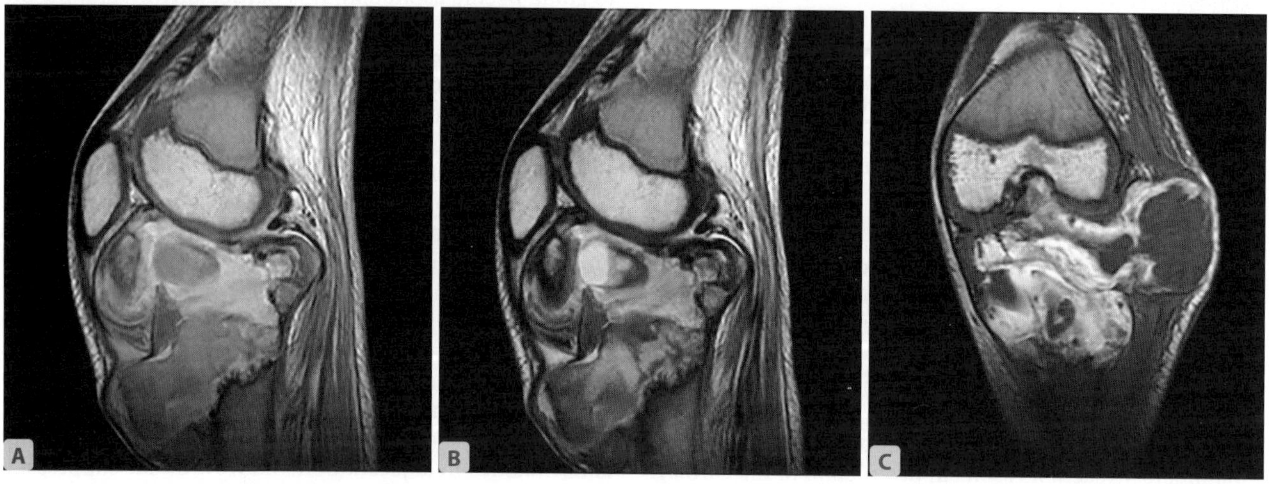

FIGS. 9A TO C: MRI knee sagittal images proton density (A) and T2-weighted (B) reveal destruction of proximal tibia with large erosions and loculated intraosseous collections, extending into joint; and (C) Postcontrast coronal scan reveals typical peripheral enhancement—septic arthritis.

the metaphysis of a long bone leading to both osteomyelitis and arthritis, characteristic of osteoarticular TB. There could be abscesses around the joint or adjacent to bone, which are known to rupture and lead to the formation of sinus tracts, characteristic of musculoskeletal TB **(Figs. 10A to D)**.

Radiography

Radiographic findings are nonspecific in early stage and may show joint space widening and soft-tissue swelling. The "Phemister triad" of periarticular osteoporosis, bone erosions, and preserved joint space is classic for tuberculous arthritis. Due to lack of proteolytic enzymes in tuberculous arthritis, joint space narrowing is a late finding. Periosteal reaction and cortical irregularity may be seen. Fibrous ankylosis may be seen due to progressive destruction of the subchondral bone and extensive osteochondral damage. When compared with pyogenic arthritis and osteomyelitis, tuberculous osteomyelitis lacks sclerosis and has much less periosteal reaction and sequestrum.

Ultrasonography

USG is very helpful in the assessment of tuberculous arthritis in children. Common findings include joint effusion, synovial thickening, hyperemia, and soft-tissue swelling. Soft-tissue abscesses can be identified with varied echogenicity depending on their content. Superficially located erosions may also be seen. It is also helpful in guiding invasive joint procedures.

Computed Tomography

CT scan is useful to demonstrate soft-tissue calcifications and bone sequestrum, the former being typical of chronic osteoarticular TB.

Magnetic Resonance Imaging

MRI can detect changes much earlier in the course of disease, revealing chondral loss, subchondral bone marrow edema, joint effusion, synovial thickening, and osseous erosions. CEMRI reveals intense enhancement of acutely inflamed

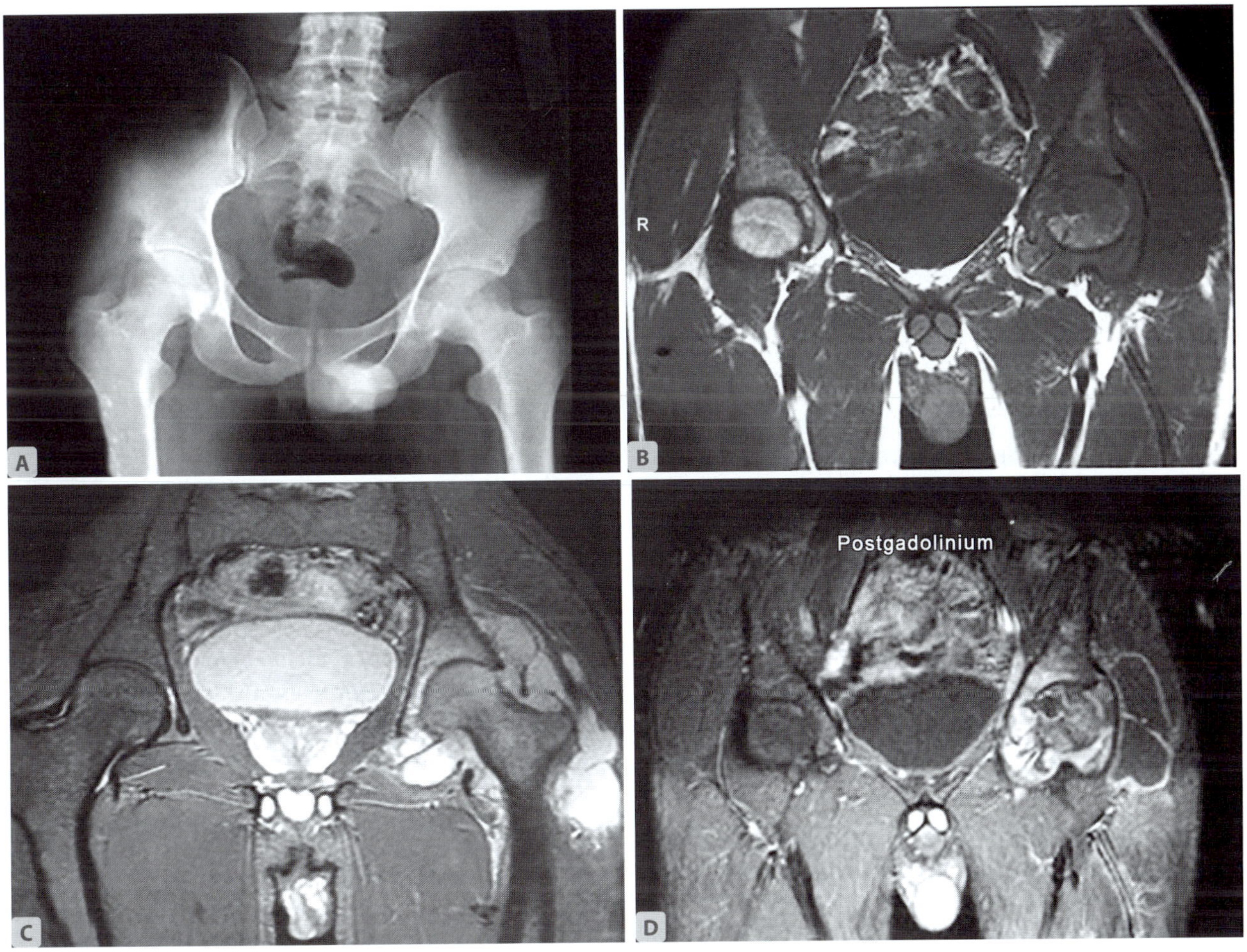

FIGS. 10A TO D: (A) X-ray pelvis—mild osteopenia on the left side with decrease in joint space; (B) MRI T1 coronal; (C) STIR coronal; and (D) T1 coronal postgadolinium. Marrow signal alteration with lytic lesion in left femoral head and acetabular margin, hypointense on T1, and hyperintense on T2, with cortical irregularity. Heterogeneous enhancement is noted. There is a large multilocular, peripherally enhancing collection in the adjacent muscles—TB hip (STIR: short tau inversion recovery; TB: tuberculosis)

synovium whereas chronically inflamed synovium exhibits minimal or no enhancement at all. Tuberculous tenosynovitis is commonly seen in the hand, with synovial thickening, fluid distension, and hyperintense material on T2WI within tendon sheaths. Intraosseous abscesses similar to pyogenic arthritis may be seen however, the presence of hypointense areas on T2WI usually indicates caseous transformation and is very suggestive of tuberculous osteomyelitis. "Rice bodies" can also be identified within the joints, bursae, and tendon sheaths.[16-18]

Transient Synovitis of Hip

Transient synovitis is a self-limited inflammatory condition specific to the hip. It affects boys more commonly than girls in all age ranges, but is more common between 3 and 6 years. Only 1% has bilateral disease. The etiology is unknown; some children have a preceding history of upper respiratory infection or trauma. Patients present with acute onset of pain, limp, and refusal to bear weight. None of the symptoms or laboratory investigation is pathognomonic. Erythrocyte sedimentation rate (ESR) may be raised and symptoms usually regress within 10 days with simple bed rest. Prolonged immobilization and traction are very rarely needed.

Transient synovitis is a diagnosis of exclusion with the most common differentials being traumatic synovitis, JIA, and Legg-Calvé-Perthes (LCP) disease. Treatment consists of rest and nonsteroidal anti-inflammatory drugs (NSAIDs). Long-term sequelae are rare.

Radiographs are usually normal, but may show joint effusion with mild widening of joint space. Sonography is sensitive to the presence of effusion **(Figs. 11A and B)**. Aspiration is required to rule out infection. On MRI, there is evidence of joint effusion, but there is no concomitant bony abnormality. Scintigraphy may demonstrate a transient decrease in isotope uptake for the 1st week followed by rebound hyperemia within a month. Biopsies performed on these joints reveal nonspecific synovial inflammation and hypertrophy with joint effusion and normal articular cartilage and joint capsule.[19,20]

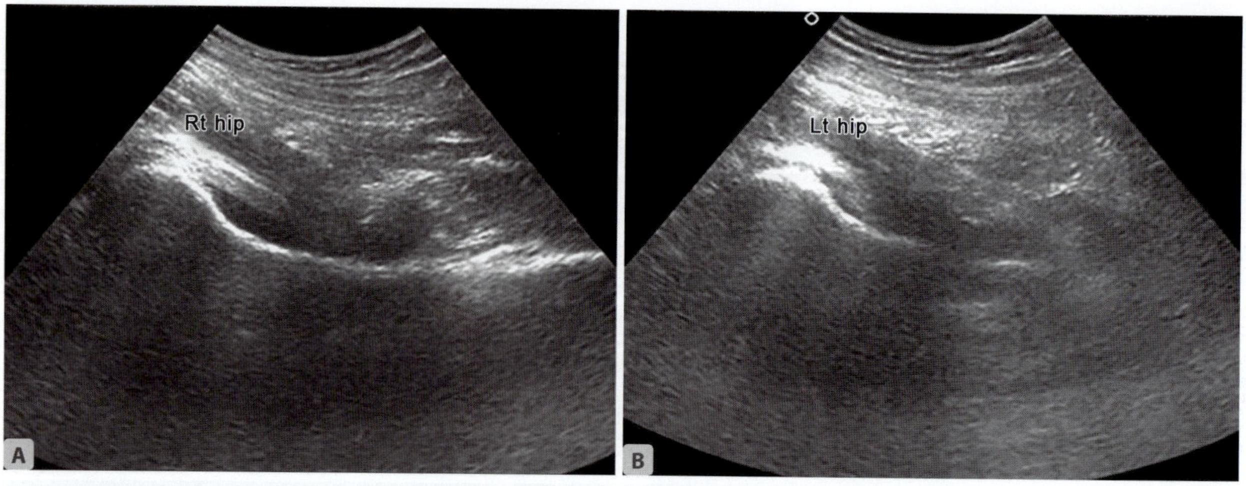

FIGS. 11A AND B: Ultrasonography (USG) anterior approach shows right hip effusion—transient synovitis of hip.

Hemophilic Arthropathy

Hemophilia is an inherited bleeding disorder characterized by functional deficiency of antihemophilic factor (AHF) VIII resulting in abnormality in blood coagulation. An X-linked recessive trait occurring in only males, who most often present in the first and second decades of life with joint changes, resulting from chronic repetitive bleeding into the bones and joints.

Pathologically, repeated episodes of intra-articular bleeding and inflammatory tissue response cause proliferation of synovium and erosion of cartilage and subchondral bone. The knee, ankle, and elbow are the most frequently involved joint and the affection is usually bilateral. To prevent hemophilic arthropathy (HA), prophylactic treatment of children with severe hemophilia should be started before joint damage sets in. The later the prophylaxis is started after the first incidence of hemarthrosis, the higher the risk of development of arthropathy.

Radiography

In the knee joint, radiographic features include periarticular osteoporosis, joint effusion (hemarthrosis) overgrowth of the femoral condyles with widening of the intercondylar notch, and patellar squaring. Frequently, articular cartilage erosions and subchondral cysts formation are seen. In advanced stages, uniform joint space narrowing and secondary degenerative arthritis set in. Similar findings are seen in other affected joints. Soft-tissue hematomas and rarely hemophiliac pseudotumor may be seen **(Figs. 12A to C)**.

The severity of symptomatic HA has been assessed with conventional radiography according to the Arnold-Hilgartner staging system **(Table 1)**.

MRI

The classical features on MR imaging include hemosiderin deposition best seen on gradient echo sequences and synovial hypertrophy on postgadolinium T1W sequences **(Figs. 13A to C)**. Hemorrhagic effusion, subchondral cyst formation, and bone edema are also noted.

Hemophilic arthropathy is nonseptic articular disorders that sometimes present a diagnostic challenge. The differentiation from JIA, the most common mimicker of HA, is based on absence of bony ankylosis/growth inhibition and frequent presence of pseudotumors in HA.[21,22]

Neuropathic Arthropathy

This is a destructive arthropathy due to repetitive, long-standing trauma. In children, it is related to myelomeningocele, syringomyelia, or congenital insensitivity to pain. The radiographic findings are related to hypertrophic synovitis and effusion, damage to the articular surface with debris formation, fracture, and dislocation. Growth plate widening and metaphyseal fragmentation may be seen as a result of growth plate injury.

DEVELOPMENTAL/MISCELLANEOUS ABNORMALITIES OF THE IMMATURE JOINT

In this section, following entities are covered:
- Developmental dysplasia of the hip (DDH)
- Developmental coxa vara
- Proximal femoral focal deficiency (PFFD)
- Legg-Calvé-Perthes disease
- Slipped capital femoral epiphysis (SCFE)
- Blount's disease
- Madelung deformity
- Pseudoarthritis

Developmental Dysplasia of the Hip

Normal hip growth occurs as a result of genetically determined balanced growth of the acetabular and triradiate cartilages and the presence of a properly located femoral head. Absence of a normal femoral head within the acetabulum during acetabular growth results in a flat shape of both the femoral head and acetabulum. The concave shape of the normal acetabulum is attributed to the presence of a spherical femoral head in close apposition to the acetabulum. Most acetabular

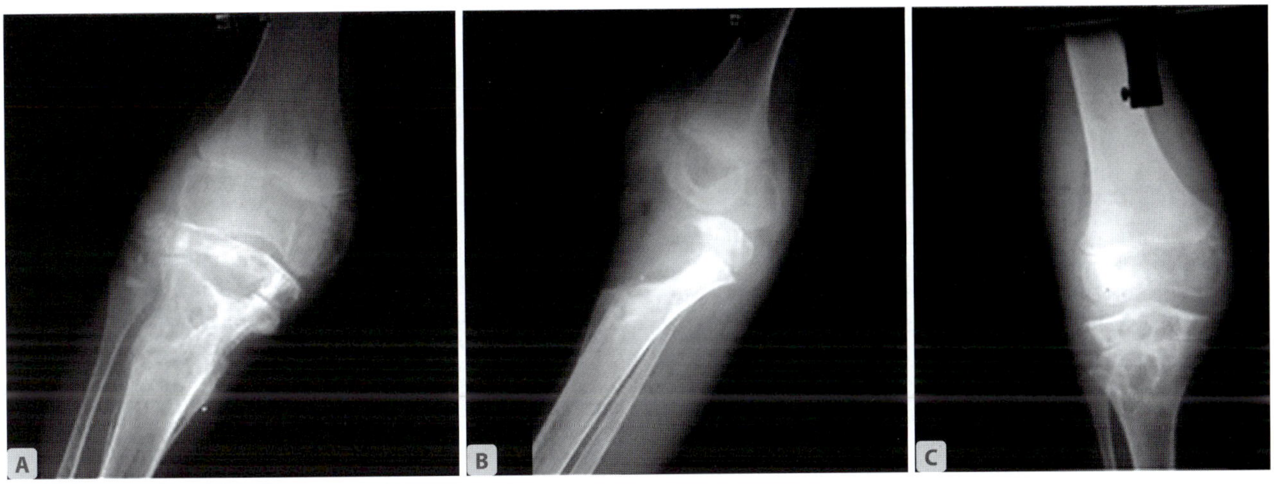

FIGS. 12A TO C: Radiograph of knee joint in a long-standing hemophilic arthritic patient reveals osteopenia, widened intercondylar notch, joint space narrowing, soft-tissue swelling, and pseudotumor formation.

TABLE 1: Arnold–Hilgartner staging system.

Stage	Findings
0	Normal joint
1	No skeletal abnormalities, soft-tissue swelling present Osteoporosis and overgrowth of epiphysis, no erosions, and no narrowing of cartilage space
2	Early subchondral bone cysts, squaring of patella, widening of intercondylar notch of distal femur or humerus, and preserved cartilage space
3	More advanced findings of stage 3, with narrowing of cartilage space
4	Fibrous joint contracture, loss of joint cartilage

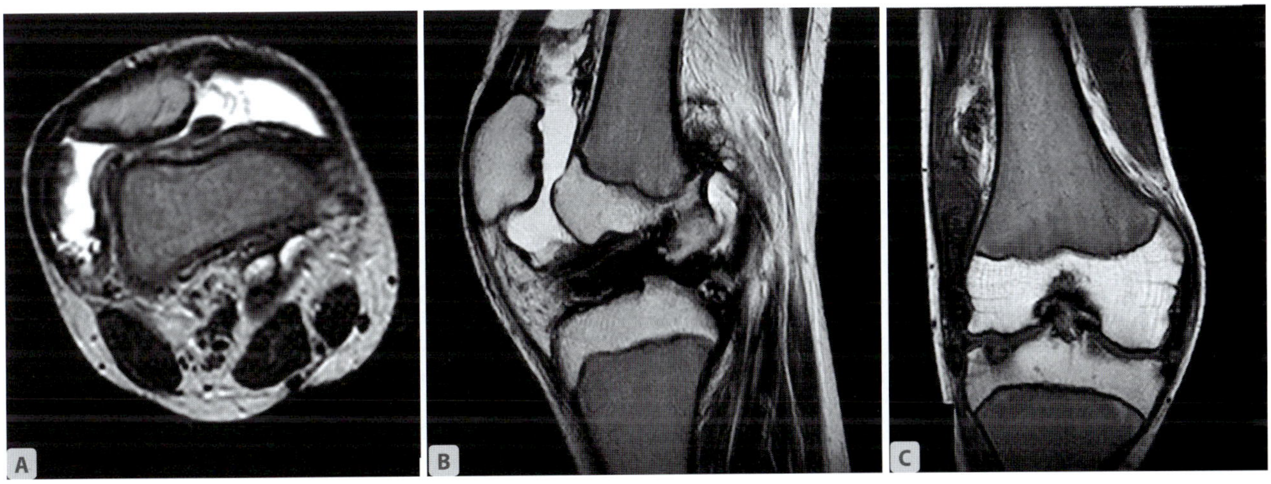

FIGS. 13A TO C: MRI knee in a known case of hemophilic arthritis reveals subarticular erosions with large joint effusion and thickened synovium with T2 hypointensity due to hemosiderin deposition.

development occurs by 8 years of age. The head, neck, and greater trochanter of the infant hip is cartilaginous with early ossification of the femoral head is seen between 3 and 6 months in girls and 6 and 9 months in boys.

Previously termed as "congenital dislocation of the hip", it is now referred to as DDH.[23] It is composed of two elements: (1) Instability; and (2) Abnormal morphology. Some authors observed that instability resulting in displacement of the femoral head prevents the acetabulum from developing properly while others found that a primary deficiency in development of acetabulum allows the hip to become displaced, creating instability.

The hip is at risk for dislocation at several critical periods in utero, including shortly after its formation, is complete at

12 weeks and at 18 weeks, when the hip muscles develop. The early in utero dislocations are often associated with other anomalies and are termed teratologic dislocations. These are fixed and secondary to paralysis from myelodysplasia, arthrogryposis, or other neuromuscular disorders.

Natural History and Pathology

The hip joint is entirely cartilaginous at birth. The normal concave cup-shaped acetabulum develops in response to the presence of a spherical femoral head. In DDH, there is a shallow saucer-shaped acetabulum that is not congruent with the femoral head and there is persistent femoral anteversion. Secondary changes can be observed in the surrounding soft tissue, with contractures, thickening of the ligamentum teres, increased pulvinar fat, and interposition of iliopsoas tendon and hip joint capsule. Soft-tissue adaptations can develop at the acetabular labrum with the formation of a neolimbus with superior migration of the femoral head; there is gradual eversion of the labrum with capsular tissue interposed between it and the outer wall of the acetabulum. In older infants with DDH, the labrum may be deformed, elongated, inverted, and may impede reduction. With abnormal pressure on the labrum, there is formation of fibrous tissue that merges with the hyaline cartilage of the acetabulum to form the neolimbus.[24]

The reported incidence of fixed dislocation is 1 in 1,000 whereas it is 0.4–0.6 in 1,000 for late dislocation, subluxation, and dysplasia. DDH is more common in girls (M:F = 1:6). The condition is usually unilateral (left:right::11:1), but both hips may be involved. Causes of DDH are multifactorial, with a combination of hormonal, familial, and mechanical factors. The hormonal factor may explain the 6:1 female–male incidence and 20% familial incidence. The mechanical factor involves in utero spatial constraint and compression of the fetus as can be seen in oligohydramnios and breech position. Other risk factors include talipes, arthrogryposis and spinal dysraphism, and generalized ligamentous laxity.

Early detection of DDH results in an excellent outcome, failing which the condition can cause significant long-term morbidity.

Clinical Examination

Developmental dysplasia of the hip may be suspected clinically in the newborn, when a physical examination reveals asymmetrical skin folds, shortened thigh, and irritability of the hip.

A "click" during the Ortolani reduction test performed by flexing the hip 90° with gentle abduction or an abnormal Barlow dislocation test performed by grasping the thigh in abduction with downward pressure on the hip indicates instability.

Radiological Diagnosis and Screening of Developmental Dysplasia of the Hip

The maximum potential for acetabular maturation is within the first 3 months of life; hence, DDH should be diagnosed and treated before this time. A certain amount of instability in the hips of newborns, representing capsular laxity, is normal in both boys and girls. This resolves spontaneously by 4 weeks. Delaying hip ultrasound till 6 weeks of age allows resolution of the same and hence ultrasound of clinically normal hips should be done at 4–6 weeks of age while a clinically unstable hip should be scanned at approximately 2 weeks.

The absolute indications for hip imaging include: (a) Family history of DDH; (b) Neonatal hip instability; (c) Limb shortening; and (d) Limitation of hip abduction in flexion.

The relative indications, if more than two are present, imaging should be done are: (a) Breech presentation; (b) First-born child; (c) Cesarean section; (d) Other congenital anomalies; and (e) Excessive fetal molding.

Imaging in Developmental Dysplasia of the Hip

Conventional Radiography

An anteroposterior (AP) projection is obtained with the infant placed, so that the pelvis is in neutral position and not rotated with hips slightly flexed. By 4–6 months, once the femoral head ossifies, radiographs become more reliable.

Before ossification, the site of nonossified epiphysis may be inferred as lying superior to the femoral epiphyseal plate. The superoinferior and lateral displacement of the femur can be determined by Perkin's line. The Shenton's line is disrupted in cases of dislocation **(Fig. 14)**. In dislocated hip, a line through the femoral shaft will point outside the acetabulum and will cross the spine at a higher level than normal as described in the Andrew and von Rosen method.

After ossification, from the age of 6 months onward, radiological diagnosis is usually easy. The femoral head is displaced upward and outward with delayed ossification of its epiphysis **(Fig. 15)**. The acetabulum is shallow with its roof sloping upward and outward with an increased acetabular angle. A false acetabulum can develop in a frankly dislocated hip and is a pathognomonic sign of dislocated hip.

Conventional radiography suffers from the following drawbacks—the cartilage is not directly visualized and its position has to be inferred from the bony landmarks, the standard radiographs are taken in a position in which subluxation is least likely to occur and the examination is static.

Ultrasonography

Sonography is now the primary imaging technique in the diagnosis and follow-up of DDH and has been shown to be more accurate than either clinical or radiographic assessment with sensitivity of 100% and specificity of 98%. Ultrasound examination has the following advantages—it visualizes the nonossified cartilage of the femoral epiphyses and the cartilaginous labrum and permits dynamic assessment of stability. It cannot be used over the age of 12 months due to acoustic shadowing from the developing ossification center of the epiphysis.[25,26]

The sonographic features to be noted in an infant hip include the following:

- Position of femoral head, its coverage, and change in position with stress
- Assessment of acetabular dysplasia
- Acetabular roof—horizontal or inclined
- Acetabular edge—sharp, rounded, or flattened

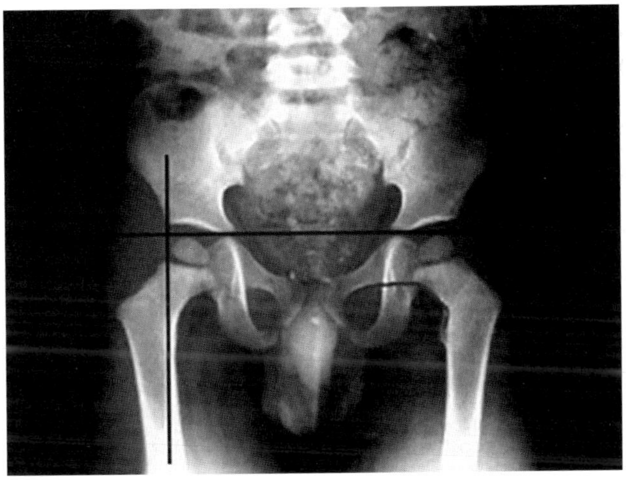

FIG. 14: X-ray pelvis showing acetabular angle and smooth unbroken Shenton's line. Hilgenreiner's line and Perkin's line are also depicted and femoral epiphysis lies in the medial inferior quadrant.

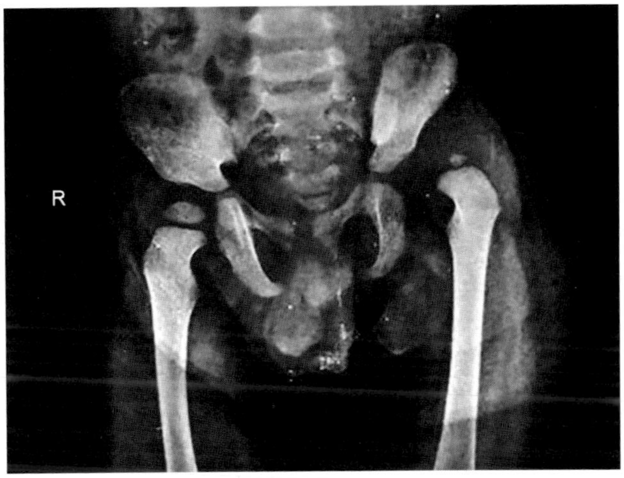

FIG. 15: Anteroposterior radiograph of pelvis reveals small dislocated femoral head with superolateral migration. Note interrupted Shenton's line and poorly developed acetabulum on left side.

- Acetabular fossa for presence of interposed soft tissues such as excessive fat or hypertrophied ligamentum teres
- Labrum—everted or inverted

The use of ultrasound in evaluation of DDH was first described by Graf in 1978. He assessed acetabular morphology and devised a classification system based on angles of inclination of the bony and cartilaginous roof **(Figs. 16A to C)**.

A static coronal image of the hip is obtained for interpretation. The baby is supported in a lateral decubitus position, knees slightly flexed. The hip is positioned in approximately 20° of flexion and slight internal rotation; this represents the neutral position for an infant. The transducer is positioned over the greater trochanter and held perpendicular to the skin and parallel to the table in order to obtain a coronal image of the acetabulum showing its maximum depth.

The cardinal landmarks are the inferior edge of the ilium, the lateral margin of the ilium projected as a horizontal line, and the acetabular labrum. The appearance of this standard plane has been likened to a "ball on spoon" appearance, with the femoral head representing the ball, the acetabulum representing the bowl of the spoon, and the ilium representing the handle of the spoon **(Fig. 17)**.

The proper coronal view contains three elements: (1) The echoes from the bony ilium should be in a straight line parallel to the transducer; (2) The transition between the os ilium and the triradiate cartilage should be seen definitively; and (3) The echogenic tip of the labrum should be in the same plane as the other two. Minor anterior or posterior adjustment may be required until the standard plane is obtained. False-positive diagnosis of dysplasia may be made when the transducer is not in midplane and is rotated anteriorly. Conversely, a dysplastic acetabulum may appear normal if the transducer is rotated posteriorly.

Graf demonstrated that in normal hips, the round, hypoechoic, and speckled femoral head lies centered in the acetabulum. His protocol had three lines drawn on the coronal view about the acetabulum from which the α and β angles could be measured. The first baseline A is drawn along the straight lateral margin of the ilium, where the perichondrium meets the ilium. A second inclination line B connects osseous convexity to labrum and the third roof line C connects the lower edge of acetabular roof medially to osseous convexity. One between acetabular roof line and baseline measures the α angle, which denotes inclination of the acetabular. A small α angle indicates a shallow bony acetabulum **(Figs. 18 and 19)**. The β angle is measured between the baseline and the line of inclination, giving an indication of coverage of femoral head by cartilaginous acetabular rim. A large β angle indicates lateral migration of femoral head. Classification of hip types on ultrasound studies is given in **Table 2**.[27]

Calculation of α and β angles is not possible if the femoral head is dislocated in anterior or posterior direction. Graf described types I and IIa/b as inherently stable and types IId, III, and IV as inherently unstable and found that it is only necessary to test for stability with type IIc **(Fig. 20)**.

Coronal images are also used to evaluate the position of the femoral head within the acetabulum. If the acetabular cup accommodates less than one-third of the femoral head, than acetabular dysplasia is definitely present and must be suspected, if only half to one-third is accommodated.

Harcke and Grissom advocated the use of dynamic sonography of the infant hip based on the premise that the position and stability of the femoral head are key factors in the diagnosis and management of DDH. If the femoral head is properly positioned and stability is achieved, then acetabular development will proceed.[28,29]

Pediatric radiologists are relying increasingly on the use of dynamic sonography as this allows real-time observation of maneuvers allowing a more accurate depiction of the femoral head in relation to the acetabulum as the hip position is changed. Hence, it allows not only depiction of DDH but is also able to assess whether a particular closed reduction is appropriate.

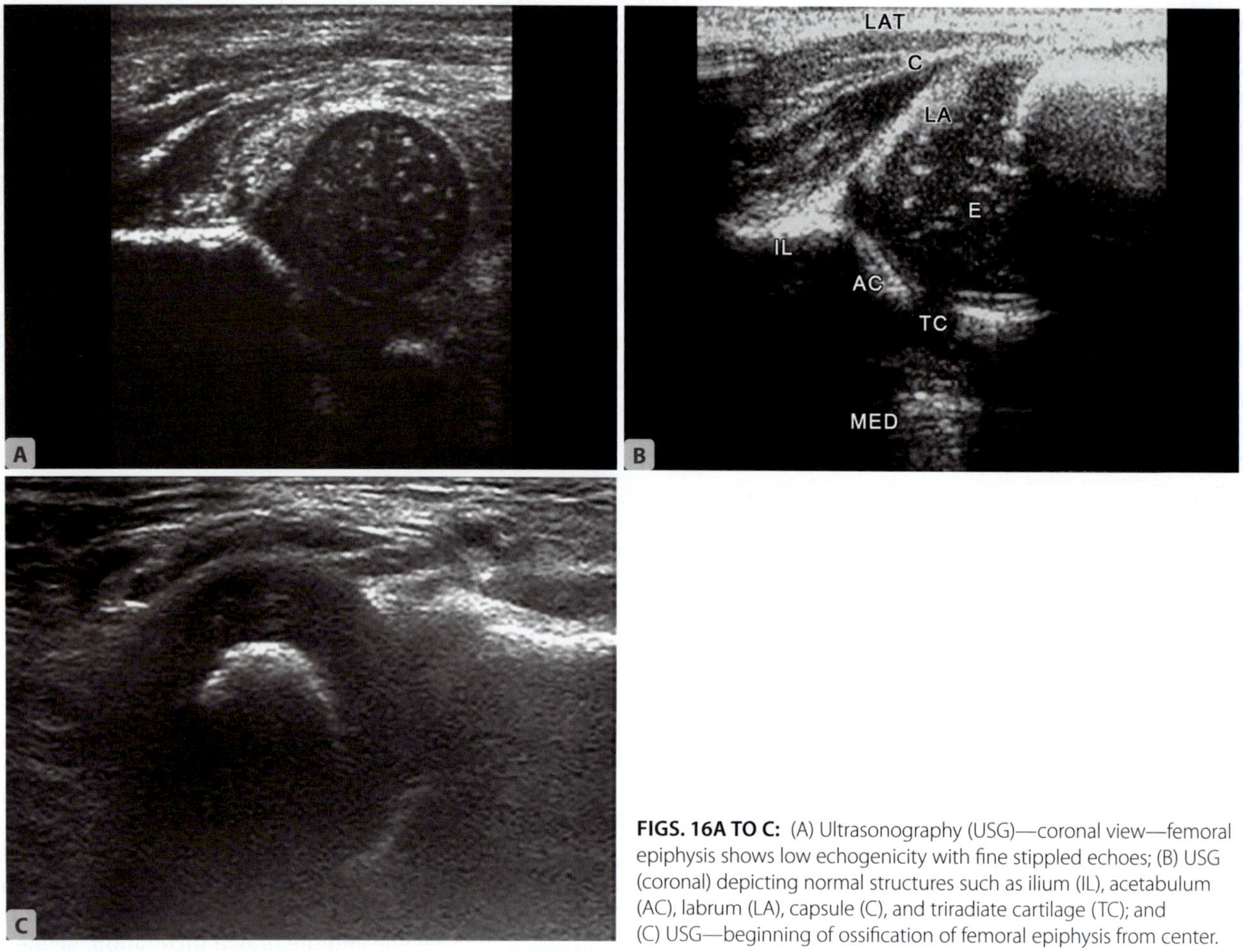

FIGS. 16A TO C: (A) Ultrasonography (USG)—coronal view—femoral epiphysis shows low echogenicity with fine stippled echoes; (B) USG (coronal) depicting normal structures such as ilium (IL), acetabulum (AC), labrum (LA), capsule (C), and triradiate cartilage (TC); and (C) USG—beginning of ossification of femoral epiphysis from center.

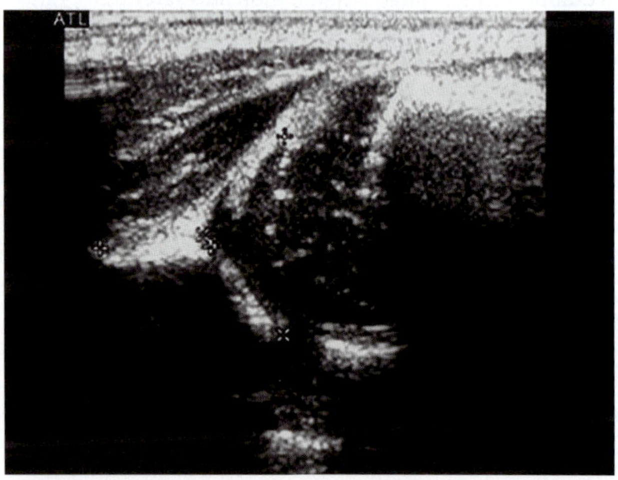

FIG. 17: Ultrasonography (USG): Coronal view "ball on spoon" appearance.

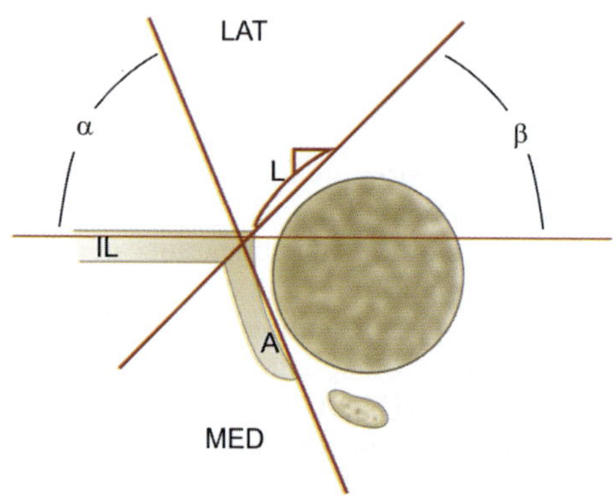

FIG. 18: Schematic diagram depicting straight bony iliac interface (IL), bony acetabulum (A) and echogenic labrum (L), and the α (alpha) and β (beta) angles are shown.

Sonography can also be used to monitor treatment of patients with DDH in a spica cast, brace, or Pavlik harness. The long axis anterior approach may be useful in a patient with a spica cast in which a window cannot be cut for lateral scanning. The window should be repositioned and the cast should be repaired to avoid posterior hip dislocation. The sonographic follow-up of patients being treated in a Pavlik harness is, however, easy as it permits movement within a safe zone while the degree of restriction prevents subluxation or dislocation. Improvement should be seen within 3 weeks of treatment. Duplex Doppler US has been used to assess vascularity of the femoral head in an infant undergoing abduction treatment.[30]

CT

CT is useful for the preoperative evaluation of DDH. CT is used for the detection of iliopsoas muscle deformity or intra-articular soft-tissue obstacles such as hypertrophied fibrofatty pulvinar which can make it difficult to achieve concentric reduction by the closed method and for the determination of femoral torsion and acetabular configuration. It can be performed even when the patient is in a cast and is most useful in postoperative assessment of reduction **(Figs. 21A and B)**.[31]

MRI

MRI is used in the evaluation of dysplasia of the hip when there is: (i) A complex dysplasia; (ii) There has been inadequate response to treatment; (iii) In late presentation; and (iv) In teratological dislocation. Axial and coronal MR images are most useful and small surface coils with high spatial resolution are necessary to evaluate DDH.

The value of MR imaging in preoperative planning is due to its ability to portray the cartilaginous part of the pelvis and also analyze the relationship of the femoral head to the acetabulum and labrum. The femoral head is variably laterally displaced in DDH with posterior and superior reduction. MR shows femoral head coverage in both coronal and axial planes without need for complex radiographic projections or magnification correction. MR imaging can show changes in the shape of the acetabulum, not demonstrated on CT, sonography, or radiography. In DDH, the acetabulum becomes elongated posteriorly or superiorly. The rim of the acetabulum becomes oval and the acetabular cartilage becomes thickened and may become displaced.

In the immediate postoperative period, MR imaging is useful in evaluation of proper reduction of the dislocated femoral head and its vascular health. Any obstruction to the reduction can be visualized, especially in cases where there is a history of failed closed reduction. These include a flipped labrum, prominent pulvinar and a redundant ligamentum teres, capsule or iliopsoas tendon, or transverse acetabular ligament, which may be interposed into the joint. Prominent pulvinar is visualized as fibrofatty material in the joint, which does not allow normal seating of the femoral head within the joint. There can be a small amount of pulvinar normally present with the head being slightly laterally displaced.

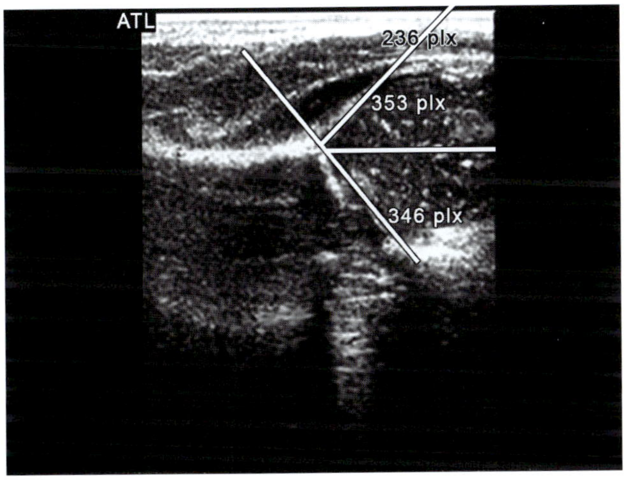

FIG. 19: Sonogram depicting baseline, inclination line, and acetabular roof lines—normal hip type I.

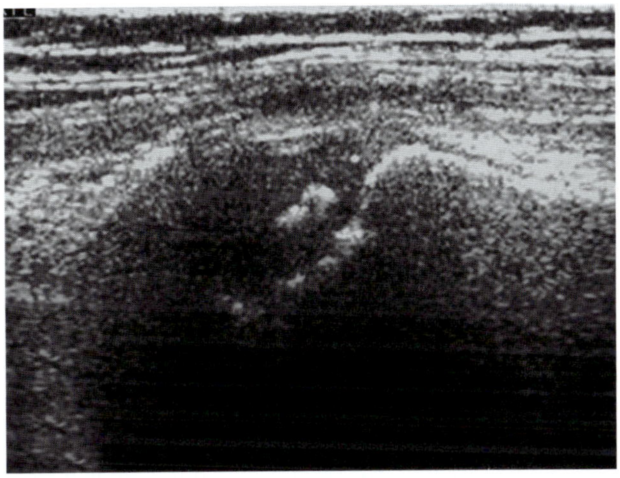

FIG. 20: USG: Gross superolateral hip dislocation with complete disruption in alignment with the acetabulum (type IV CDH). (CDH: congenital dislocation of the hip; USG: ultrasonography)

TABLE 2: Graf hip types.

Types	Description	α	β	Comments	Treatment
I	Normal hip	>60°	<55°	Stable	None
II	Concentric position:	–		–	–
	• Physiological immaturity (age <3 months)	50–60°	<77°	–	Observed till change to type 1
	• Delayed ossification (age >3 months)	50–60°	55–77°	–	Evaluation by orthopedic surgeon
	• Concentric position	43–49°	–	–	Evaluation by orthopedic surgeon
	• Subluxation	43–49°	>77°	Labrum everted	Required
		<43°	>70°	Bony roof deficient	Required
III	Low dislocation	–		Labrum everted	–
IV	High dislocation	Not measurable		Flat bony acetabulum	Required
		–		Interposed labrum	–

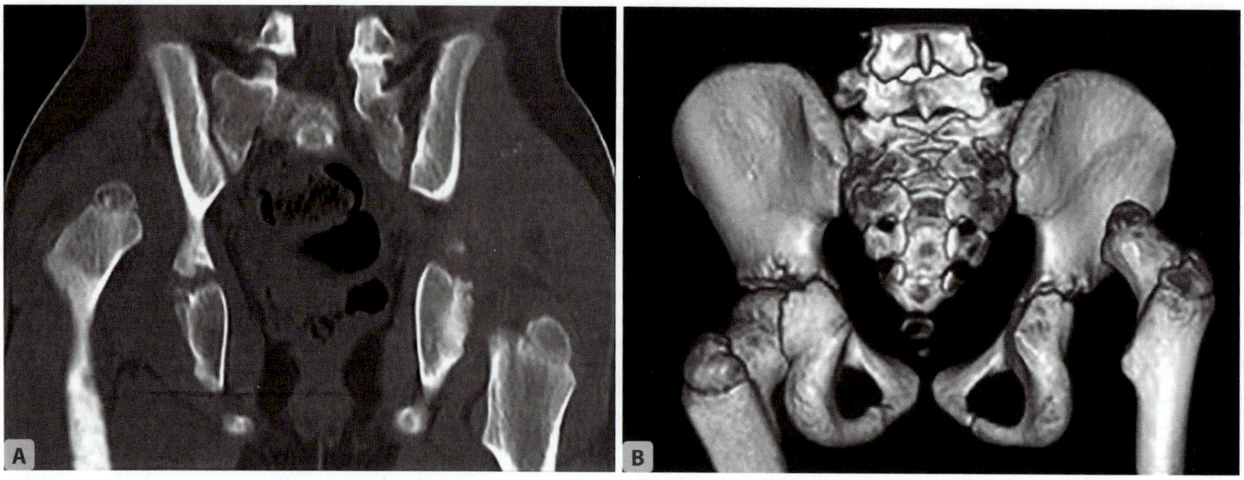

FIGS. 21A AND B: CTMPR (A) and VRT (B) show right femoral epiphysis dislocated superiorly and posteriorly. (CTMPR: computed tomography multiplanar reconstruction; VRT: volume rendering technique)

If the head is encompassed by the confines of the acetabulum and pointing at the triradiate cartilage, the pulvinar usually atrophies.

Recently, dynamic interventional MRI in an open configuration scanner has been used in the management of developmental dysplasia. The hip can be visualized during reduction and spica can be applied within the scanner itself.[32-35]

Differential Diagnosis of Developmental Dysplasia of the Hip

Radiographic features such as shallow acetabulum with high-angled roof lateral and cephalad displacement of the upper end of the femur and small ossification center for the head can be seen in congenital hypothyroidism. Following appropriate therapy, spontaneous resolution may occur.

Traumatic epiphyseal separation of the femoral neck in very young infants may simulate congenital dislocation. The possibility of trauma may be considered if there is history of an abnormal presentation/difficult labor. Acquired nontraumatic dislocation may develop in pyoarthrosis of hip. In such a case, there will be clinical signs of infection.

Proximal Femoral Focal Deficiency

Proximal femoral focal deficiency is a malformation in which complete growth and development of upper femur fails to occur. It encompasses a spectrum ranging from mild shortening of an otherwise normal femur to severe handicap of an absent femur, except for condyles accompanied by acetabular aplasia and muscular dysplasia.

Imaging

The radiographic findings consist of failure of development and delayed ossification of a lesser or greater part of the proximal femur. Hence, a short femur that is laterally situated and proximally displaced is demonstrated at birth. The distal femur is by definition always present **(Fig. 22)**. There is a misshapen femoral head and neck, upper end of disconnected distal femur is either bulbous or pointed. The femoral head is situated low in the acetabulum with a woolly outline **(Fig. 23)**. Secondary deformity of the acetabulum may result. In later cases, the greater trochanter will be found to curve like a beak and it may articulate with the ilium. Pelvis may show enlarged obturator foramen with a supra-acetabular bump or horizontal/dysplastic roof of the acetabulum.

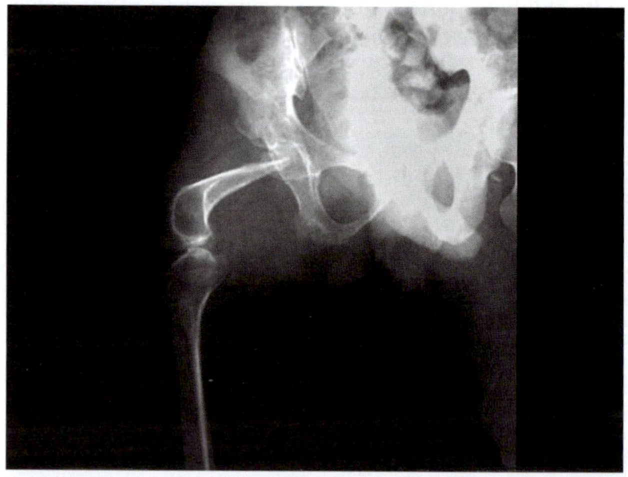

FIG. 22: X-ray pelvis: Focal femoral deficiency in the right side.

Hip sonography plays a role in the classification of PFFD and in confirming the location of the femoral head with respect to the acetabulum, especially when no proximal femur is seen on radiography. US may reveal a cartilaginous head and neck. USG may be useful in prenatal diagnosis and in infants to identify the femoral head. Mobility of the femoral head within the acetabulum may also be assessed.[36]

MR imaging can identify correctly the size and position of the femoral head present. Thin section coronal and axial imaging is of use in locating a small femur head. Continuity to the rest of the femur may also be assessed. Presurgical evaluation is important to guide the orthopedic surgeon in reconstruction. There may be a wide variation in the gap

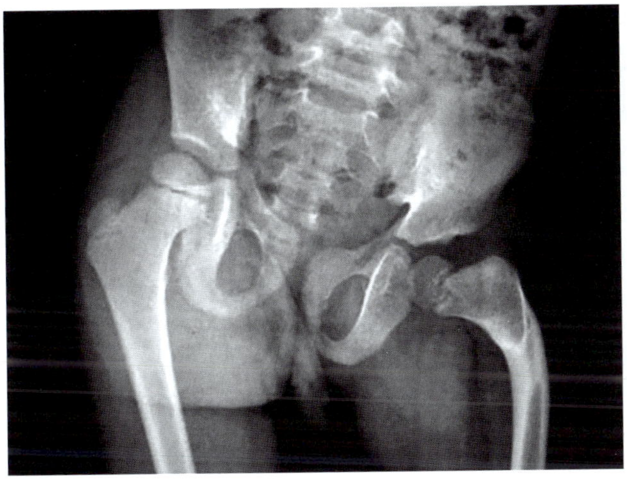

FIG. 23: Aitken class A proximal femoral focal deficiency (PFFD): Femoral head is present and connected to the shaft of femur.

between femoral head and subtrochanteric femur. The gap may be small with pseudoarthrosis or be filled with fibro-osseous tissue. It can also be devoid of any connective tissue. This and the resultant coxa vara deformity cannot be adequately seen on a radiograph as the gap is radiolucent.

The prognosis and treatment options depend on grading of the abnormalities. The most commonly used system is the Aitken classification which assigns types A to D to the abnormality depending on the presence or absence of the femoral head and the acetabulum and osseous integrity of the remainder of the femoral shaft.

The differential diagnoses of PFFD are:[37]

- Congenital short femur (no specific abnormalities of head, neck, and shaft)
- Congenital coxa vara—head, neck normal
- Developmental dysplasia of hip—Graf type 4
- Traumatic femoral capital epiphysiolysis in newborn which presents with pain plus edema of inguinal crease and upper thigh.

Legg–Calvé–Perthes Disease

Legg–Calvé–Perthes disease is a self-limiting osteonecrosis of the femoral head epiphysis which typically occurs between the ages of 3 and 12 years, more common in boys (M:F = 5:1). Both hips are involved in 15% of patients, with involvement being asymmetric. If there is asymmetric involvement, hypothyroidism or multiple epiphyseal dysplasias should be excluded. The first symptom is a limp sometimes painless, but usually associated with pain in groin, lateral hip, or knee.

The origin of LCP remains unknown. It is believed to represent multiple vascular occlusive episodes that involve the femoral head, causing changes of avascular necrosis (AVN) with a long ongoing process of vascular changes and repair. This differs from AVN seen in adults because in most cases, there is remodeling and healing with little residual deformity of the femoral head. If the age of the patient at the onset of disease is >9 years and the shape of femoral head at skeletal maturity is nonspherical, a worse outcome can be expected.[38]

BOX 5: Radiographic signs of Legg–Calvé–Perthes disease.

Early signs:
- *Joint effusion:* Widening of the medial joint space
- Asymmetrical femoral epiphyseal size (smaller on the affected side)
- Apparent increased density of the femoral head epiphysis
- Blurring of the physeal plate
- Radiolucency of the proximal metaphysis

Late signs:
- Fragmentation of femoral head
- Subchondral lucency—crescent sign
- Femoral head deformity with widening and flattening (coxa plana)
- *Proximal femoral neck deformity:* Coxa magna

Imaging

The goal of imaging in LCP disease is early diagnosis, assessment of the extent, and location of epiphyseal involvement and of the femoral head coverage. Imaging is also required to follow healing of the disease and measures sphericity of the femoral head at completion of healing.

Radiographs remain the mainstay of diagnosis, classification, and follow-up of the disease. Most children of LCP diseases present with an abnormal radiograph. The earliest radiographic abnormality includes asymmetry of the intergluteal fat planes, growth retardation, and reduced size of the capital femoral epiphysis. Subchondral fractures are noted and best seen in the frog-leg lateral view. Increased radiographic density of the femoral ossific nucleus occurs due to trabecular compression, dystrophic calcification in the debris, and creeping substitution. The classical triad comprises of condensation, collapse, and fragmentation. The amount of subchondral fissuring of the femoral head on the radiograph during the initial stages is thought to be predictive of later involvement of the femoral head. A poor prognosis is associated with subchondral fissuring >50% of the head **(Box 5)**.

Morphological changes related to epiphyseal necrosis may include articular surface flattening (coxa plana) and fragmentation. There may be lateral subluxation of the femoral head or loss of containment. This finding is due to cartilage thickening, joint effusion, and synovial thickening. Abnormality of the proximal femoral physis is also seen. This may be due to the primary ischemic insult or secondary to abnormal mechanical loads. Physeal abnormalities include increased undulation of the growth plate (W- or M-shaped, deepening of the growth plate, epiphyseal-metaphyseal osseous fusion, or physeal cystic changes which may lead to premature growth arrest of the femur) **(Figs. 24 and 25)**.

A radiographic staging for temporal evolution of the disease described by Waldenstrom is as follows:

- *Initial stage*—increased head socket distance, subchondral plate thinning, and dense epiphysis
- *Fragmentation stage*—subchondral fracture in homogeneous dense epiphysis, metaphyseal cysts
- *Reparative stage*—removal of sclerotic bone and replacement with normal bone, epiphysis more homogeneous

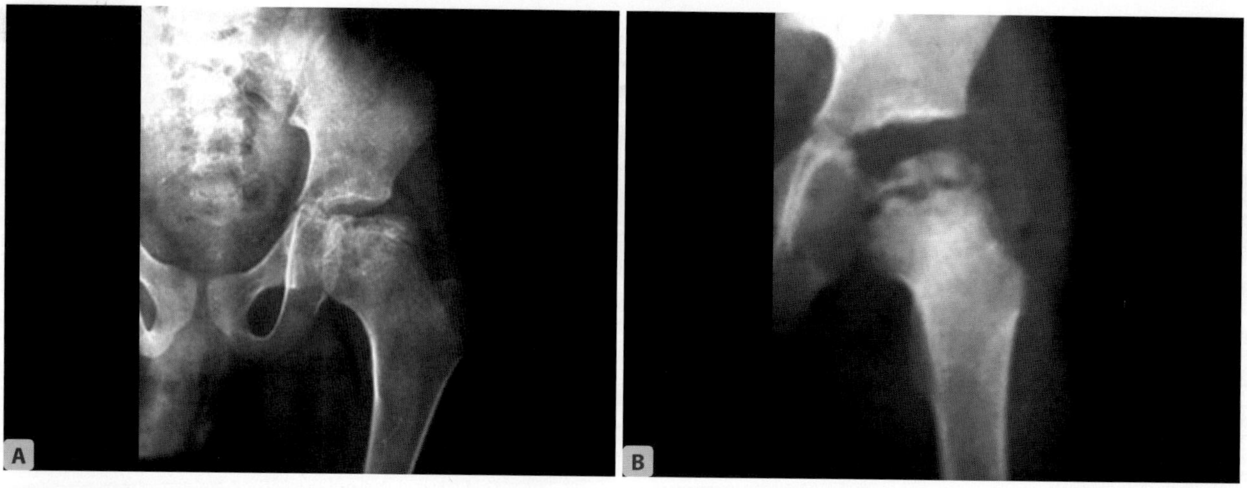

FIGS. 24A AND B: X-ray pelvis: Flattening and sclerosis with fissuring of femoral head and metaphyseal changes—Legg–Calvé–Perthes disease.

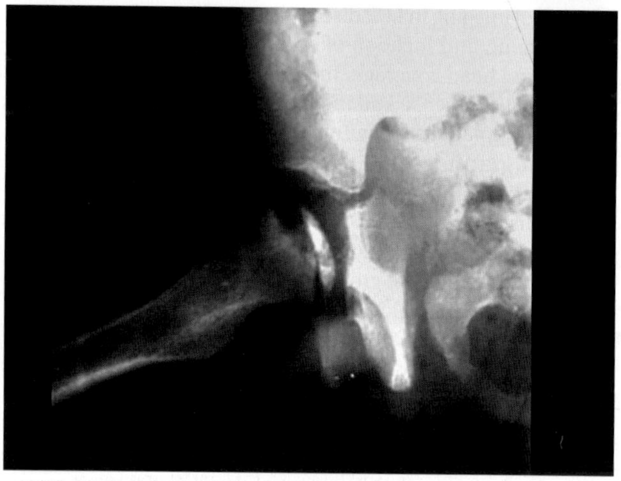

FIG. 25: X-ray left hip: Severe flattening of femoral head involving the entire epiphysis and sclerosis—Legg–Calvé–Perthes disease.

- *Growth stage*—approaches the final stage
- *Definitive stage*—final shape—congruent or incongruent hip joint

To classify the extent of ischemic process for purpose of prognostication based on plain X-rays, *Catterall* has described four groups: (1) Estimating the extent of involvement of the head by ischemia; (2) Deformity of the head by lateral displacement; (3) Collapse, and (4) Resorption of bone in the femoral head.

- *Group I*—only the anterior part of the epiphysis is involved. Collapse does not occur and healing begins from the periphery of the defect.
- *Group II*—more of the anterior epiphysis is involved which collapses and a dense sequestrum forms. The unaffected segment retains its height and reaches epiphyseal plate normally. Metaphyseal changes are minor and the involved segment heals by ossification from the periphery.
- *Group III*—only a small uninvolved part remains posteriorly. Subchondral fissuring is prominent. Speckled ossification occurs in cartilage around the nucleus. Metaphyseal changes are more and collapse and deformity are present.
- *Group IV*—the whole epiphysis is involved and flattened to a thin dense line. All quadrants are flattened and a mushroom deformity remains.

Herring system is based on the extent of involvement of the lateral pillar (LP) (LP is defined as the lateral most one-third of the femoral head).

- A—LP uninvolved.
- B <50% LP loss of height.
- B/C border group—narrow LP 75% original height, poorly ossified LP with at least 50% original height, or exactly 50% that is depressed relative to the central pillar.
- C—75% LP loss of height.

Sonography can be used as an adjuvant to other imaging modalities. The following parameters are assessed ultrasonographically: (i) Medial joint space; (ii) Epiphyseal changes and flattening, condensation, and fragmentation; and (iii) Metaphyseal changes such as fissures, widening, and sclerosis. The earliest ultrasound appearance is of hip joint effusion. Although this is a nonspecific finding, persistence of a hip joint effusion for >2 weeks should raise the possibility of LCP disease. Synovial thickening is often more marked than is seen in transient synovitis and thickening of the articular cartilage may be seen at an earlier stage. Ultrasound may demonstrate irregularity, flattening, and fragmentation of the capital femoral epiphysis, osteoid new bone, and recalcification in the healing phase. The articular cartilage thickens. Contrast-enhanced power Doppler has been used to demonstrate changes of the revascularization process in LCP, particularly within the physis.[39]

Scintigraphy is helpful in early stages of the disease. A focal area of decreased uptake is seen in the femoral head and the size of the scintigraphic defect is believed to correlate with the eventual amount of involvement of the femoral head.

CT and MRI

CT depicts changes of LCP disease. The area of femoral head necrosis is usually located in the superior anterior aspect with characteristic marginal sclerosis.

MR imaging is a sensitive and specific imaging technique for the evaluation of LCP disease. The condition can be diagnosed even in the setting of normal or equivocal radiographs. MRI helps in assessing the extent of cartilaginous involvement and the congruency of the joint.

The typical MR appearance in the avascular phase is the loss of the normally bright signal intensity of the femoral epiphysis on T1WIs **(Figs. 26A and B)**. Loss of signal may be subtle and needs to be compared to the contralateral hip **(Figs. 27A and B)**. T2W/short tau inversion recovery (STIR) imaging shows variable signal intensity including hyperintensity representing bone marrow edema. Curvilinear subchondral T2 hyperintensity and T1 hypointensity may be observed in the anterosuperior aspect of the femoral head. This finding, referred to as the *crescent or Caffey's sign*, suggests presence of a subchondral fracture. In LCP disease, there may be partial or complete nonenhancement of the proximal femoral epiphysis in the avascular phase. This is best depicted approximately 2 minutes after injection using subtraction techniques. Asymmetric involvement is noted with the anterior portion frequently and most prominently involved. There may also be flattening of the head. This is due to combination of necrotic trabecular bone collapse and resorption. Articular cartilage and labrum hypertrophy exist as they continue to derive nutrition from synovium. Periarticular T2/STIR hyperintensity and contrast enhancement may be seen due to associated synovitis.

In the revascularization and reparative phase of the disease, MRI reveals heterogeneous proximal femoral epiphyseal signal. Revascularized areas show T2/STIR hyperintensity and contrast enhancement which may persist on delayed imaging. Dynamic gadolinium-enhanced subtraction MR allows early detection of epiphyseal ischemia and accurate analysis of revascularization patterns which can aid therapeutic decision-making. Metaphyseal signal abnormality representing cartilaginous metaphyseal ingrowth indicates higher possibility of growth abnormalities. Subsequently, in the fragmentation stage, the involved area takes on speckled appearance, an indication of nonhomogeneous revascularization of necrotic zone. As revascularization and reossification progresses, the epiphysis regains a more uniform signal with healing, proximal femoral epiphyseal height is slowly restored, ossific fragments coalesce, and mature trabecular bone again constitutes the entire ossific nucleus. After approximately 6 years, the epiphysis shows normal MR signal.[40-44]

Prognostic evaluation of LCP disease by MRI has been proposed and takes into account the predictive value of four MRI indices—(1) extent of necrosis, (2) lateral extrusion, (3) physeal involvement, and (4) metaphyseal changes. As the extent of femoral head necrosis increases, overall prognosis worsens. Prognosis is also adversely affected by the involvement of the LP. Disturbance of the physis is the single most important predictor of growth disturbance. Extensive epiphyseal necrosis can sometimes be predicted by MRI in very early LCP disease. The two features predicting the same are: (1) Decreased signal intensity on both T1WIs and T2WIs covering over two-thirds of the epiphysis; and (2) Diffuse bone marrow edema of the femoral neck and metaphysis.

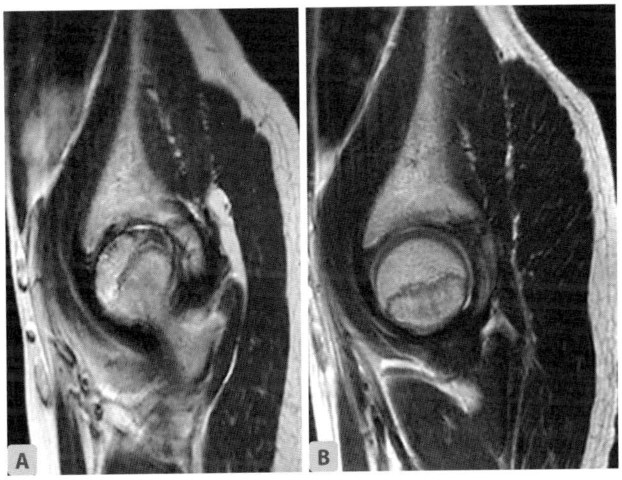

FIGS. 27A AND B: T1 sagittal of the affected (A) and normal (B) hip in a case of Legg–Calvé–Perthes disease seen as decrease in size of the femoral epiphysis on the affected side.

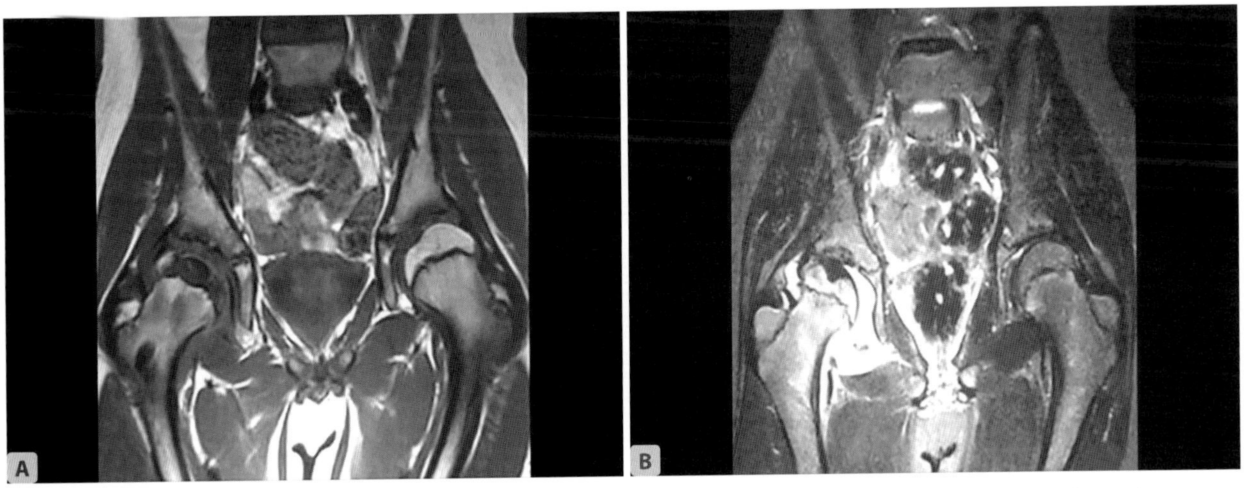

FIGS. 26A AND B: MRI-T1 coronal (A) and short tau inversion recovery (STIR) coronal (B) flattening of femoral head with loss of normal hyperintense signal of femoral epiphysis—Legg–Calvé–Perthes disease.

Factors that predict early degeneration of the hip joint include late age of disease onset and abnormal shape of the femoral head at the time of skeletal maturity.[45-51]

The main differential diagnoses of LCP are septic hip, juvenile chronic arthritis, and juvenile osteonecrosis (AVN due to a known cause—sickle cell anemia, thalassemia).

Slipped Capital Femoral Epiphysis (Box 6)

Slipped capital femoral epiphysis is an uncommon skeletal disorder of adolescence often overlooked because of its nonspecific presentation. It is a unique disorder because no other bone shows similar changes. It is usually seen during adolescent growth spurt in overweight children with the incidence of bilaterality being 25%. There is a morphological change in the relationship of the femoral head to the femoral neck centered at the physeal level probably caused by obesity. The femoral head becomes relatively retroverted at the physeal level placing the head and physis at a mechanical disadvantage when subjected to stress. It is a Salter–Harris type 1 fracture through the proximal femoral physis with displacement of the capital femoral epiphysis. In most cases, the displacement of the head is usually medial and posterior relative to the metaphysis.

The most common sign/symptom is limp, painful limitation of hip motion while walking/running. It coincides with adolescent growth and is related to endocrine disorders like hypothyroidism, pituitary dysfunction.

The slip is classified as stable or unstable with the criterion being the ability to bear weight with or without crutches. The incidence of complications is higher with unstable variety.

Imaging

Radiographs remain the prime method of diagnosing SCFE, though it may be difficult to diagnose on anterior projection alone. Medial displacement of the capital epiphysis is seen on the AP projection. A line drawn along the lateral border of the femoral neck (Klein line) in a normal individual intercepts the epiphyseal ossification center, so that a small portion of the head remains lateral to this line **(Figs. 28A and B)**. No part of femoral head ossification center is seen lateral to the line in SCFE. On the anterior projection, there may be mild widening, lucency, and irregularity of the physis. The femoral head may appear foreshortened and there may be apparent sclerosis in the regional femoral neck as the femoral head rotates posteriorly. In the frog-leg or true lateral position, the anterior and posterior corners of the epiphysis and metaphysis line up closely in a normal patient whereas they are displaced in SCFE **(Figs. 29A and B)**.

BOX 6: Slipped capital femoral epiphysis.

- Atraumatic Salter–Harris type 1 fracture through physeal plate
- Usually unilateral
- *Imaging features:*
    - Widened growth plate (prior to slip)
    - Posteromedial displacement of head during the slip
    - Decrease in neck shaft angle
    - Sclerosis and irregularity with a widened physis, if long-standing

Posterior displacement is seen on frog-leg lateral radiograph as medial displacement of epiphysis relative to metaphysis. Approximately 90° external rotation of femur on frog-leg lateral means what is actually a posterior displacement of epiphysis looks like medial displacement on radiograph. On the cross-table lateral radiograph with 25° flexion, it is seen as true posterior displacement of epiphysis. Metaphysis shows scalloping, irregularity, sclerosis, and posterior beaking. One needs to be careful when using opposite asymptomatic hip as control for radiographic evaluation of painful one as the opposite side may have unrecognized SCFE.[52-54]

Staging of radiographic findings is mild, moderate, and severe based on the displacement of ossification center by <1/3–1/3–2/3–>2/3 metaphyseal diameter.

Ultrasound may suggest malalignment of the capital femoral epiphysis relative to the metaphysis. The alignment of the epiphysis relative to the metaphysis should be assessed as part of hip ultrasound study. Joint effusion, which may accompany SCFE, is recognized by US.

CT demonstrates the slip and the reduced femoral anteversion; it may also demonstrate metaphyseal scalloping and beaking **(Figs. 30A to C)**.

MR imaging relies on identification of the morphological change at head/neck function and the abnormal signal intensity centered on the physis, indicating stress and edema. Physeal widening is a constant feature and can be seen on MR before being apparent on radiographs. 3D volume acquisition can be used to reconstruct sagittal oblique images along the axis of the femoral neck to identify any

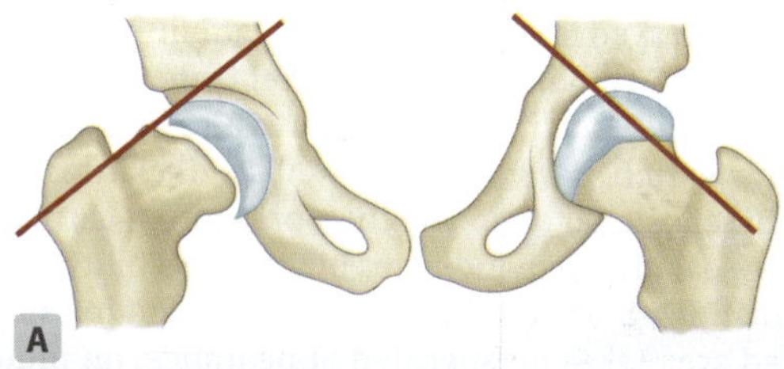

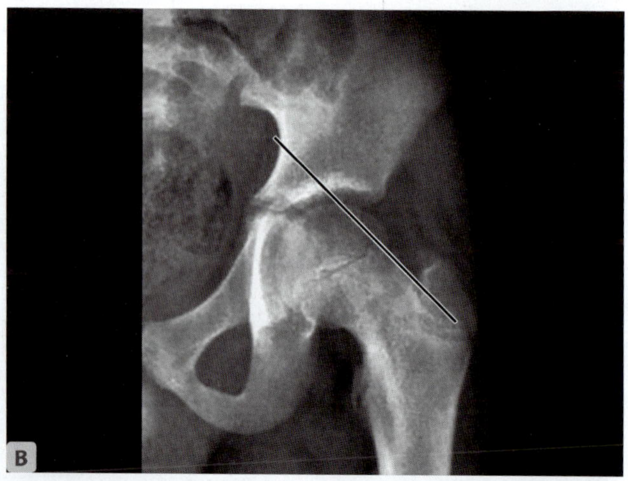

FIGS. 28A AND B: (A) Schematic representation of hip shows Klein's line that normally intersects lateral one-third of the femoral epiphysis on the left whereas in slipped epiphysis, no part of the epiphysis in lateral to it as seen on the right; and (B) X-ray pelvis depicting the normal position of the femoral head in relation to the Klein's line.

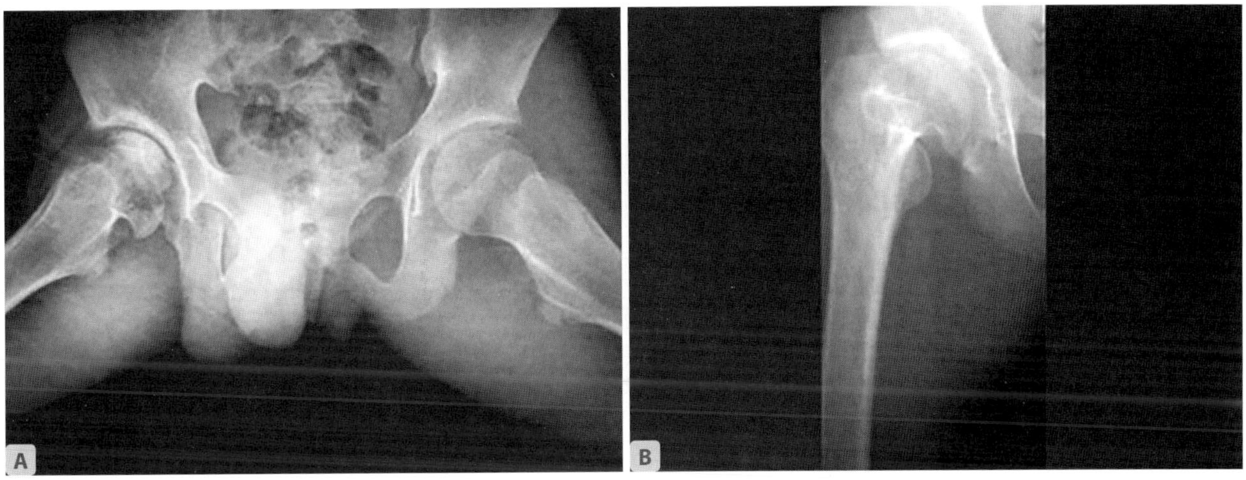

FIGS. 29A AND B: X-ray frog's leg view (A) and anteroposterior (AP) view (B)—shows medial and inferior displacement of the right capital epiphysis with widening of the physis.

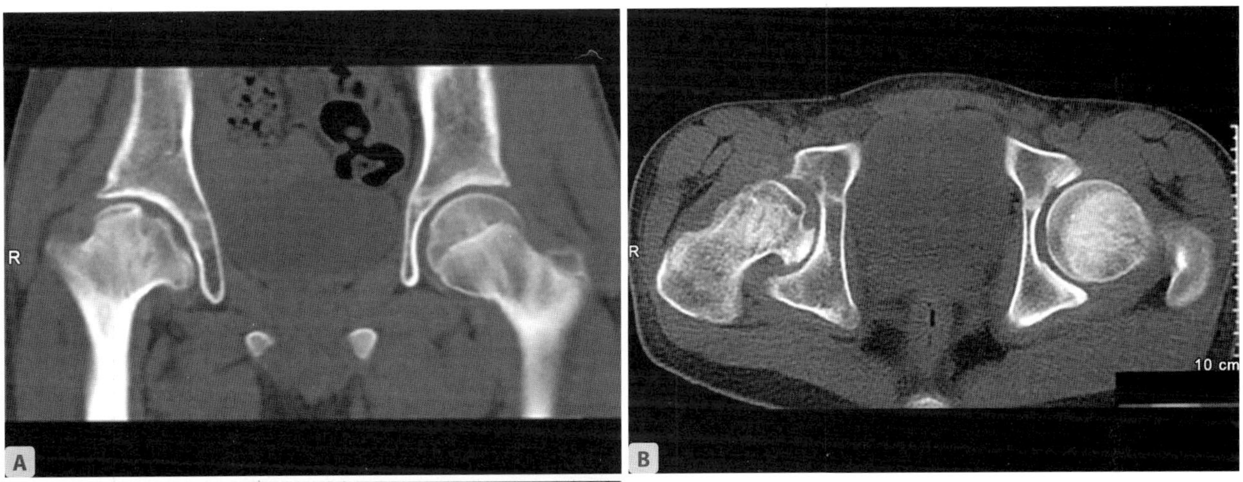

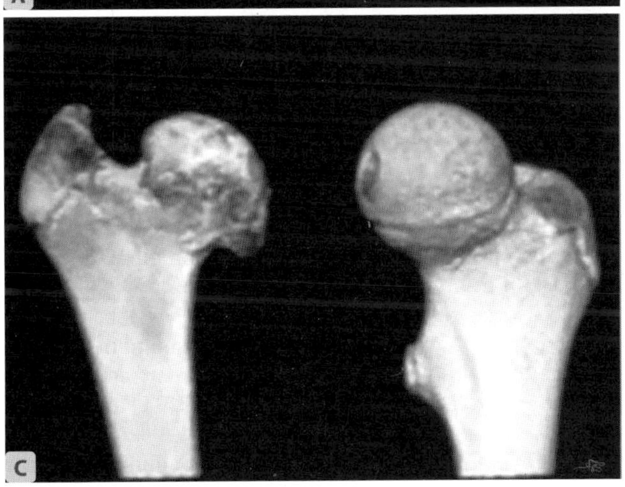

FIGS. 30A TO C: CT—coronal MPR (A), axial (B), and VRT (C) medial and posterior lip of the femoral epiphysis of the right hip with complication of avascular necrosis as seen by flattened head of femur. (MPR: multiplanar reconstruction; VRT: volume rendering technique)

retroversion. MR image can be oriented to a plane orthogonal to the plane of the physis to assess the width of the same. Physeal widening is seen on T1W MRI whereas synovitis and marrow edema are appreciated on T2WIs **(Figs. 31A and B)**. MRI can also demonstrate physeal widening in the center or posteromedial origin of the physis in a contralateral asymptomatic hip, providing for prophylactic treatment of the same. Hyperintensity on fluid-sensitive images at the physis is indicative of a chronic slip condition. Subtle abnormalities include edema on the metaphyseal side, usually at the extreme medial end of the physis.[53]

The complications of SCFE are AVN, occurring in 20–45% of cases and chondrolysis. Treatment consists of preventing further displacement and to cause closure of the physis.

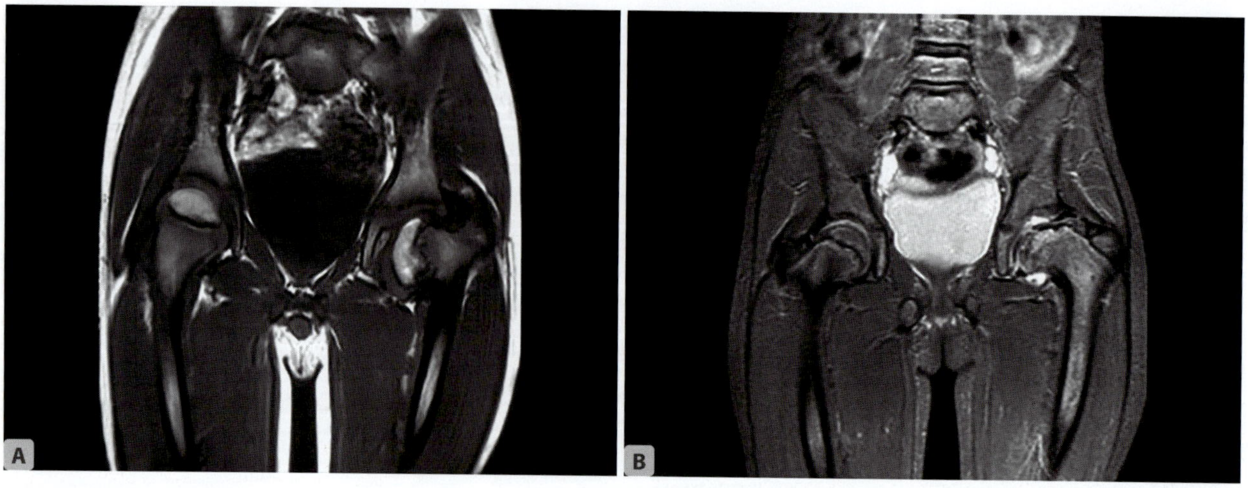

FIGS. 31A AND B: (A) MRI T1-weighted coronal; and (B) Short tau inversion recovery (STIR) coronal depicting widening and irregularity of the physis on the left side with physeal slip—slipped capital femoral epiphysis.

Chondrolysis is less common than AVN and is recognized by progressive thinning of the medial joint space on the radiographs. Premature closure of the physis of the greater trochanter is considered as predictive sign for chondrolysis.

The differential diagnosis includes:
- Legg-Calvé-Perthes disease—the patient is younger with irritable hip progressing to sclerosis and collapse of epiphysis.
- Osteoid osteoma
- Traumatic SCFE

Blount's Disease

Infantile tibia vara or Blount's disease is a developmental abnormality characterized by abnormal endochondral ossification of the medial portion of the proximal tibial physis. The characteristic radiographic findings include widening and irregularity of the medial tibial physis, varus deformity of the proximal tibia with medial and posterior downsloping of the articular surface, and prominent beaking of the medial metaphysis. The disease may be bilateral and symmetric. There may be functional movement restriction, joint instability, and premature osteoarthritis. MRI is helpful in detecting abnormalities of the epiphyseal cartilage and of the menisci as well as physical bars, thereby helping in surgical planning. The medial joint space appears wider than normal with thickened and hyperintense medial meniscus relative to the lateral meniscus.

Tarsal Coalition

Tarsal coalition is a congenital bridging of two or more tarsal bones. Three major types are found: (1) Fibrous (syndesmosis); (2) Cartilaginous (synchondrosis); and (3) Osseous (synostosis). More than one coalition can be found in the same extremity and bilateral disease occurs in up to half of the patients. Calcaneonavicular and talocalcaneal coalitions are the most common forms. Osseous coalition is generally readily apparent on cross-sectional imaging. Cartilaginous and fibrous coalitions may be more subtle on cross-sectional imaging, but generally are associated with some osseous deformity along the margin of the coalition. Most commonly, tarsal coalitions present in late childhood or adolescence. This is likely related to the fact that osseous coalitions usually ossify when patients are 8–16-year-old, leading to restricted motion and subsequent symptomatology.

Radiographs can show direct bony continuity in cases of osseous coalition whereas in cases of nonossified coalitions, the findings match with osteoarthritis seen as abnormally narrow and obliquely oriented joint spaces, whose surfaces are irregular and dysmorphic, often associated with subchondral sclerosis and cysts **(Box 7)**.

BOX 7: Radiographic signs in tarsal coalition.
- Dysplastic enlargement of the surfaces of the sustentaculum tali and of the adjacent talus
- Talar "beaks" may be seen in both talocalcaneal and in calcaneonavicular coalitions
- Absent middle facet sign
- C sign—curved line extending from the talar dome to the sustentaculum tali
- Anteater sign in calcaneonavicular coalition—elongation and hyperplasia of anterior process of calcaneum

Radiographs alone are insufficient for proper evaluation due to anatomic complexity of this region and CT and MRI are useful to both delineate the extent of the coalition and detect associated abnormalities. CT is the best for assessment of bone anatomy and providing information about the type, site, and extent of the coalition. Multiplanar reconstruction (MPR) and volume rendering technique (VRT) are especially useful for surgical planning.

MRI is helpful in showing all types of coalitions wherein an ossified coalition appears as a continuous bar that is isointense to the adjacent bones while a cartilaginous coalition shows an interposed band of signal intensity similar to that of the cartilage and a fibrous coalition displays low signal intensity in all sequences. Edematous changes of the juxta-articular bone marrow and of the soft tissues are frequently present. Both MRI and CT are helpful in demonstrating associated degenerative changes.[55]

Pseudoarthritis

Certain conditions like epiphyseal dysplasia mimic arthritis. Patients do not present with fever or any clinical sign of inflammation. Patients are normal at birth and slowly develop platyspondyly and intervertebral disk calcification. Marked deformities of the hip and knee joint are seen. Head of the femur remains cartilaginous till 5 years of age. The proximal femoral epiphysis is markedly flattened and irregular in shape, a progressive coxa varus deformity develops. On imaging, there is no evidence of joint effusion, synovial thickening, bone marrow enhancement, or soft-tissue edema.

CONCLUSION

The role of imaging in a suspected case of juvenile inflammatory arthritis is to detect signs of inflammation and to follow-up for disease activity and progression of disease. A case of suspected infection of the joint is a surgical emergency and guided arthrocentesis is important in cases with joint effusion.

REFERENCES

1. Jacobs P, Renton P. Congenital anomalies: Skeletal dysplasias; chromosomal disorders. In Sutton D(Ed): Textbook of Radiology and Imaging (4th edn). Churchill Livingstone. 1987;1:2-50.
2. Baheti AD, Iyer RS, Parisi MT, Ferguson MR, Weinberger E, Stanescu AL. "Children are not small adults": avoiding common pitfalls of normal developmental variants in pediatric imaging. Clin Imaging. 2016;40:1182-90.
3. Chauvin NA, Khwaja A. Imaging of inflammatory arthritis in children: status and perspectives on the use of ultrasound, radiographs, and magnetic resonance imaging. Rheum Dis Clin North Am. 2016;42:587-606.
4. Daldrup-Link HE, Steinbach L. MR imaging of pediatric arthritis. Radiol Clin N Am. 2009;47:939-55.
5. Collado P, Malattia C. Imaging in paediatric rheumatology: is it time for imaging? Best Pract Res Clin Rheumatol. 2016;30:720-35.
6. Christos Dimitriou, Grammatina Boitsios, Valérie Badot, Phu-Quoc Lê, Laurence Goffin. Imaging of Juvenile Idiopathic Arthritis. Radiol Clin N Am. 2017;55:1071-83.
7. Sheybani EF, Khanna G, White AJ, et al. Imaging of juvenile idiopathic arthritis: a multimodality approach. Radiographics. 2013;33(5):1253-73.
8. Azouz EM. Juvenile idiopathic arthritis: how can the radiologist help the clinician? Pediatr Radiol. 2008;38(Suppl 3):S403-8.
9. Ravelli A, Martini A. Juvenile idiopathic arthritis. Lancet. 2007;369(9563):767-78.
10. Aquino MR, Tse SM, Gupta S, Rachlis AC, Stimec J. Whole-body MRI of juvenile spondyloarthritis: protocols and pictorial review of characteristic patterns. Pediatr Radiol. 2015;45:754-62.
11. Herregods N, Dehoorne J, Joos R, Jaremko JL, Baraliakos X, Leus A, et al. Diagnostic value of MRI features of sacroiliitis in juvenile spondyloarthritis. Clin Radiol. 2015;70:1428-38.
12. Agarwal A, Aggarwal AN. Bone and joint infections in children: septic arthritis. Indian J Pediatr. 2016;83:825-33.
13. Jawin J, Hoffer F, Rand F, et al. Joint effusion in children with an irritable hip: Ultrasound diagnosis and aspiration. Radiology. 1993;1987:459.
14. Strouse PJ, Di Pietro MA, Adler RS. Hip Effusions: Evaluation with Power Doppler Sonography. Radiology. 1998;206:731-35.
15. Hopkins K, Li K, Bergmon G. Gadolinium DTPA enhanced magnetic resonance imaging of musculoskeletal infections processes. Skeletal Radiol. 1995;24:325.
16. Hong SH, Kim SM, Ahn JM, et al. Tuberculous versus pyogenic arthritis: MR imaging evaluation. Radiology. 2001;218:843-53.
17. Sawhney S, Jain R. Tuberculosis of the bones and joints. In Berry, Chowdhury, Suri (Eds): Diagnostic Radiology-Musculoskeletal and Breast imaging (1st edn). Jaypee Brothers 1998.
18. Chapman H, Murray RD, Stoken OJ. Tuberculosis of the bone and joints. Semin Roentgenol. 1979;19:266-82.
19. Lee SK, Suh KJ, Kim YW, et al. Septic arthritis, versus transient synovitis at MR imaging preliminary assessment with signal intensity alterations in bone marrow. Radiology. 1999;211:459.
20. Park JK, Kim BS, Choi G, et al. Distinction of reactive joint fluid from pyogenic abscess by diffusion-weighted imaging. J Magn Reson Imaging 2007;25(4):859-61.
21. Doria AS. State-of-the-art imaging techniques for the evaluation of haemophilic arthropathy: present and future. Haemophilia. 2010;16(Suppl 5):107-14.
22. Keshava SN, Gibikote S, Doria AS. Imaging evaluation of hemophilia: musculoskeletal approach. Semin Thromb Hemost. 2015;41:880-93.
23. Klisie PJ. Congenital dislocation of the hip: A misleading term. J Bone Joint Surg Br. 1981;63:38-42.
24. Kuhn JP, et al. Caffey's Pediatric Diagnostic Imaging. 10th edn 2277-9,2004: Mosby. The joints BabynPS, RansOm MD 2435-93.
25. Havije HT, Waller RS. Ultrasound screening for dysplasia of the hip (Letter). Pediatrics. 1995;95:799-800.
26. Zieger M. Ultrasound of the infant hip Part 2 validity of the method. Pediatric Radiol. 1986;16:488-92.
27. Graf R. Classification of hip joint dysplasia by means of sonography. Arch Orthop Trauma Surg. 1984;102:248.
28. Harcke HT, Lee MS, Born P, et al. Examination of the infant hip with real time ultrasonography. J Ultrasound Med. 1984;3:131.
29. Harcke HT, Grissom LE. Performing dynamic sonography of the infant hip. AJR Am J Roentgenol. 1990;155:837.
30. Rosendahl k, Toma P. Ultrasound in the diagnosis of developmental dysplasia of the new borns. The European approach. A review of methods, accuracy and clinical validity. Eur Radiol. 2007;17:1960-7.
31. Browing WH, Rosenkrantz H, Tarquinio T. Computed Tomography in congenital hip dislocation. J Bone Joint Surgery AM. 1982; 64:27-31.
32. Hubbard AM. Imaging of pediatric hip disorders. Rad Clin North Am. 2001; 39(4).
33. Dwek JR. The Hip: MR Imaging of Uniquely Pediatric Disorders. Radiol Clin North Am. 2009;47:997-1008.
34. Kawaguchi AT, Otsuka NY, Deigado ED, et al. Magnetic resonance arthrography in children with developmental hip dysplasia. Clin Orthop. 2000;374:235-46.
35. Tennant S, Kinmant C, Lamb G, et al. The use of dynamic interventional MRI in developmental dysplasia of the hip. J Bone Joint Surg B. 1999;81(3):392-97.
36. Grissom LE, Harcke HT. Sonography in congenital deficiency of the femur. J Paediatr Orthop. 1994;14:29-33.
37. Kayser R, et al. Proximalfocal femoral deficiency–rare entity in the sonographic differential diagnosis of developmental dysplasia of the hip. J Pedia tr. 2005;146(1):141.

38. Transient synovitis, septic hip, and Legg-Calvé-Perthes disease: an approach to the correct diagnosis. Pediatr Clin North Am. 2014;61:1109-18.
39. Doria AS, Guarniero R, Gunha FG, et al. Contrast enhanced power Doppler Sonography: Assessment of revascularization flow in Legg- Calve-Perthes' disease. Ultrasound Med Biol. 2002; 28(2):171-82.
40. Lahdes-Vasama T, Lamminen A, Merikanto J, et al. The Value of MRI in early Perthes' disease: An MRI study with a 2 year follow up. Pediatric Radiol. 1997;27(6):517-22.
41. De Sanctis N, Rega AN, Rondinella F. Prognostic evaluation of Legg-Calve-Perthes' disease by MRI-Pathomorphogenesis and new classification. J Pediatr Orthop. 2000;20(4):403-70.
42. Merlinic L, Combescure C, De Rosa V, et al. Diffusion–weighted imaging findings in perthes disease with dynamic gadolinium – enhanced subtracted (DGS) with MR correlation–a preliminary study. Pediatr Radiol. 2010;40(3):31.
43. Jaramillo D, Galen TA, Winalski CS, et al. Legg-Calve-Perthes' disease: MR imaging evaluation during manual positioning of the hip. Comparison with conventional arthrography. Radiology. 1999;212(2):519-25.
44. Dillman JR, Hernandez RJ. MRI of Legg-Calve-Perthes disease. AJR. 2009;193:1394-1407.
45. Mahnken AH, Staatz G, Ihme IV, et al. MR signal intensity characteristics in Legg-Calve-Perthes' disease value of fat suppressed (STIR) images and contrast enhanced T1 weighted images. Acta Radiol. 2002;43(3):329-35.
46. Lamer S, Dogeret S, Khairouni A, et al. Femoral head vascularization in Legg-Calve-Perthes' disease Comparison of dynamic gadolinium enhanced substraction MRI with bone scintigraphy. Pediatric Radiol. 2002;32(8):580-85.
47. Jaramillo D, Galen TA, Winalski CS, et al. Legg-Calve-Perthes' disease: MR imaging evaluation during manual positioning of the hip. Comparison with conventional arthrography. Radiology. 1999;212(2):519-25.
48. Dillman JR, Hernandez RJ. MRI of Legg-Calve-Perthes disease. AJR. 2009;193:1394-1407.
49. Mahnken AH, Staatz G, Ihme IV, et al. MR signal intensity characteristics in Legg-Calve-Perthes' disease value of fat suppressed (STIR) images and contrast enhanced T1 weighted images. Acta Radiol. 2002;43(3):329-35.
50. Lamer S, Dogeret S, Khairouni A, et al. Femoral head vascularization in Legg-Calve-Perthes' disease Comparison of dynamic gadolinium enhanced substraction MRI with bone scintigraphy. Pediatric Radiol. 2002;32(8):580-85.
51. Tiwari V, Gamanagatti S, Mittal R, Nag H, Khan SA. Correlation between MRI and hip arthroscopy in children with Legg-Calve-Perthes disease. Musculoskelet Surg. 2018;102:153-7.
52. Castriota-Scandfrberg A, Orsi E. Slipped capital femoral epiphysis ultrasonographic findings skeletal. Radiol. 1993;22(3):191-93.
53. Umans H, Liebling MS, Moy L, et al. Slipped capital femoral epiphysis: A physeal lesion diagnosed by MRI with radiographic and CT correlation. Skeletal Radiol. 1998;27(3):139-44.
54. Futami T, Suzuki S, Seto Y, et al. Sequential magnetic resonance imaging in slipped capital femoral epiphysis, assessment of prestep in the contralateral hip. J Paediatr Orthop B. 2001; 10(4):298-303.
55. Fayed LM, Johnson P, Fishman EK. Multidetector CT of musculoskeletal disease in pediatric patient; principles, techniques and clinical applications. Radiographics. 2005;25:603-61.

CHAPTER

82

Benign Bone and Soft-tissue Tumors and Conditions

Mahesh Prakash, Kushaljit Singh Sodhi, Anindita Sinha

INTRODUCTION

Benign bone tumor and tumor-like lesions are very common in children. More than half of all childhood bone neoplasms are benign.[1] It is important that radiologists recognize the typical imaging features of benign tumors, so that patient can avoid unnecessary diagnostic and surgical procedures.

The differential diagnosis of bone tumors can be narrowed, based on knowledge of age of the patient, gender, constitutional complaints, location of the lesion in body and bone, and general radiographic characteristics.[2] Plain film radiographs remain the primary tool for evaluating bone tumors. However, other imaging methods, particularly magnetic resonance imaging (MRI) and in some cases computed tomography (CT) and nuclear studies, provide support for initial diagnosis by demonstrating specific features.[1,2] Common benign bone lesions in children are osteochondroma, nonossifying fibroma, Langerhans cell histiocytosis, unicameral bone cyst, and aneurysmal bone cyst (ABC). Benign bone tumors and tumor-like lesions in children may be classified as follows:[1]

- *Cartilaginous tumors*:
  - Osteochondroma
  - Enchondroma
  - Chondroblastoma
  - Chondromyxoid fibroma
- *Osseous tumors*:
  - Osteoid osteoma
  - Osteoblastoma
- *Fibrous tumors*:
  - Nonossifying fibroma
  - Fibrous dysplasia
  - Osteofibrous dysplasia
- Langerhans cell histiocytosis
- Giant cell tumor (GCT)
- *Tumor-like lesions*:
  - Simple bone cyst
  - Aneurysmal bone cyst
  - Pseudotumor of hemophilia

CARTILAGINOUS TUMORS

Osteochondroma

Osteochondromas are common lesions of the growing skeleton, occurring in approximately 1% of the general population. It is the most common benign neoplasm and constitutes 20–50% of all benign tumors.[3] They arise from bony metaphysis with cartilage cap covering **(Fig. 1)**. These tumors are either pedunculated or sessile. The long axis of the osteochondroma pedicle or stalk is almost always directed away from the adjacent joint. The direct communication between the osteochondroma and the cortex and marrow cavity of the bone from which it arises is a distinctive feature that is particularly well-demonstrated on CT and MRI. T2-weighted (T2W) MR images are useful to demonstrate a cartilaginous cap **(Fig. 2)**. The cap can be quite thick in early childhood and like the normal physis, it becomes thinner with age. After epiphyseal

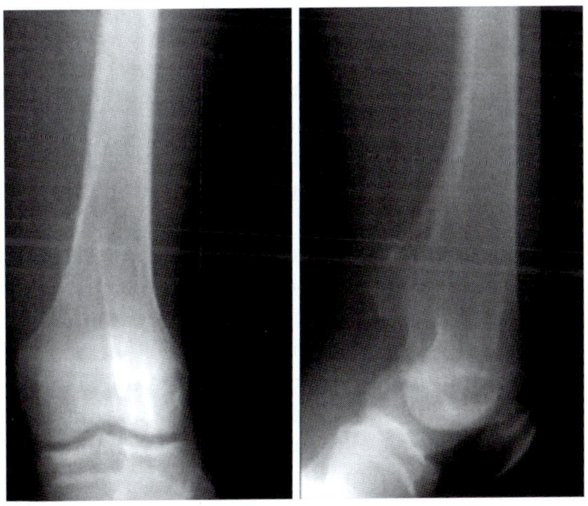

FIG. 1: Osteochondroma: Radiograph of lower end of femur [anteroposterior (AP) and lateral view] shows large well-defined bony outgrowth, with broad-based attachment to femur.

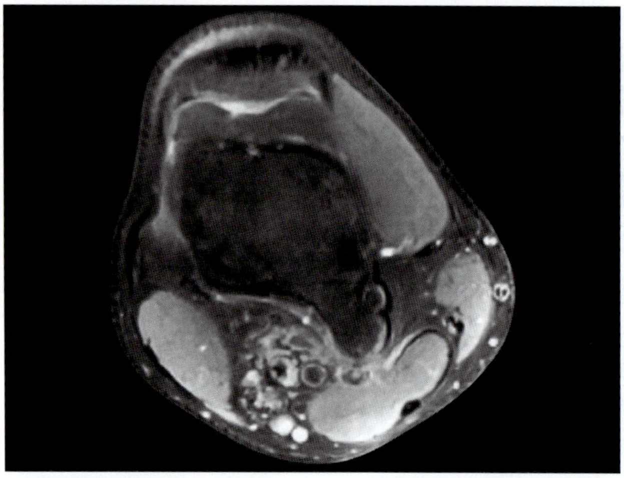

FIG. 2: Magnetic resonance imaging [T1-weighted (T1W) fat saturation]. Axial section of the same patient shows clear demonstration of continuity of marrow and cortex of host bone into osteochondroma with covering of cartilage cap.

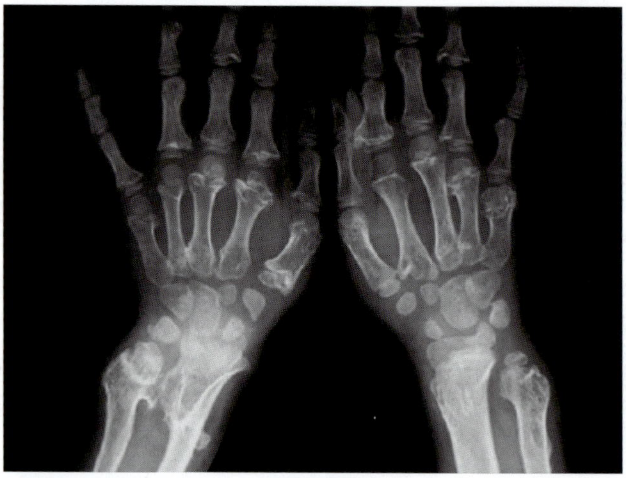

FIG. 3: Diaphyseal aclasis: Posteroanterior (PA) radiograph of bilateral hands shows multiple pedunculated osteochondromas, involving multiple bones of hands and forearm.

closure, growth of the osteochondroma ceases. Multiple osteochondromas occur as a manifestation of diaphyseal aclasis, an inherited disorder with autosomal dominance **(Fig. 3)**. Because most osteochondromas are asymptomatic, they are usually discovered incidentally. However, mechanical irritation of adjacent soft tissues or nerves, vascular injuries, fracture of the stalk, or malignant transformation can produce symptoms.

Malignant transformation into low-grade chondrosarcoma occurs in 1% of osteochondromas; however, the risk is 10–30% in cases of multiple osteochondromatosis.[3,4] Malignant trans-formation should be considered when the osteochondroma grows after epiphyseal closure. Malignancy occurs in the cartilaginous cap, which becomes thickened. The cap of an osteochondroma usually measures <1 cm in thickness whereas that of a chondrosarcoma often exceeds 2 cm.

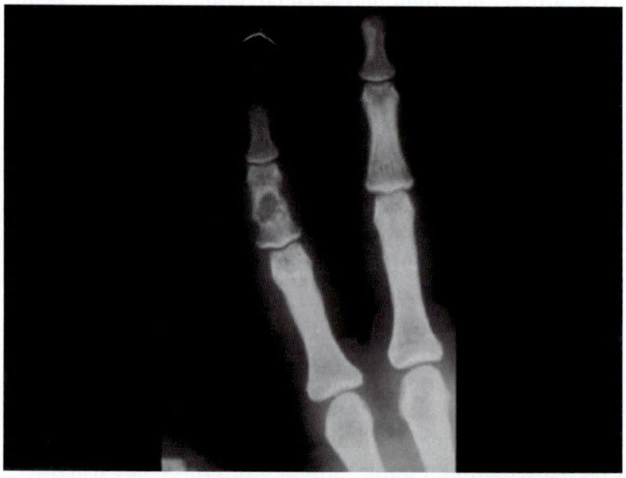

FIG. 4: Enchondroma: Radiograph shows a sharply demarcated expansile lytic lesion with pathological fracture in the middle phalanx of index finger.

Enchondroma

Enchondromas account for 12% of benign bone tumors.[3] These are most frequently located in the large and small tubular bones of the limbs, particularly those of the hand **(Fig. 4)**. Like other cartilaginous tumors, enchondromas exhibit a lobulated growth pattern that results in asymmetric expansion of the medullary cavity and endosteal scalloping. Tumor matrix may be radiolucent or show calcification. Characteristic cartilaginous ring and arc pattern of calcifications are seen on radiographs and CT images. On MR imaging, the tumor is isointense to muscle on T1-weighted (T1W) and exhibits a heterogeneous, predominantly high T2W signal.[5] Contrast-enhanced MRI may demonstrate a pattern of thin arcs and rings.

Ollier disease is a nonheritable disorder of cartilage proliferation in which enchondromas involve multiple bones, especially those of the hands and may result in severe skeletal deformity. Enchondromatosis accompanied by multiple hemangiomas is known as Maffucci syndrome. Calcified phleboliths may be demonstrated radiographically in the hemangiomatous soft-tissue masses. Lesions associated with both Ollier disease and Maffucci syndrome carry a significant risk of malignant degeneration (30–70%).[6]

Chondroblastoma

It is less common than enchondroma. Chondroblastoma is composed of primitive cartilage cells, usually occurs in the age group of 10–20 years. It is typically located in epiphysis and apophysis of bone, most often the proximal humerus, distal femur, or proximal tibia. On plain X-ray, chondroblastoma is an eccentric, lucent, and well-defined lesion with sclerotic borders. Periosteal reaction, far from the lesion, is another common feature suggesting an accompanying inflammatory process. Approximately, one-third of chondroblastoma has a calcified matrix which can be better seen on CT scan **(Fig. 5)**.

The tumor shows signal intensity similar to that of muscle on MR imaging; however, the rim of the tumor has

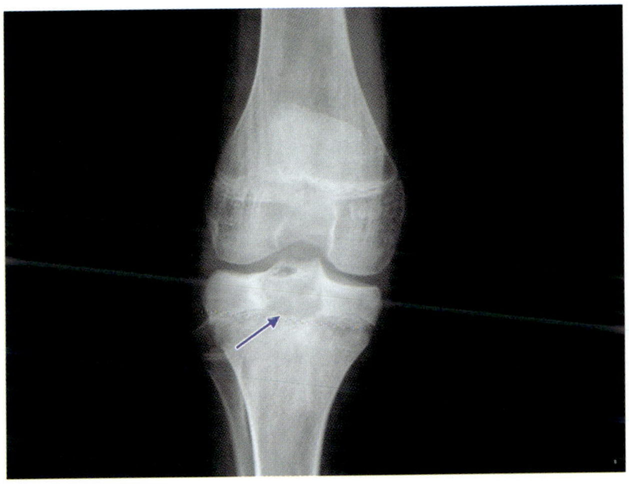

FIG. 5: Chondroblastoma: Plain radiograph of knee joint shows lytic lesion in epiphysis of upper tibia (blue arrow).

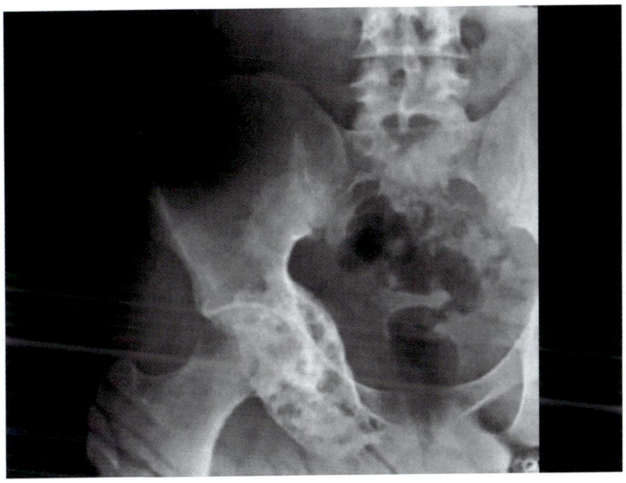

FIG. 6: Chondromyxoid fibroma: Radiograph of right hip shows large expansile lesion with sclerotic border involving right acetabulum.

lower signal intensity. On T2W images, the signal intensity of the tumor is low to intermediate. This tumor also shows extensive surrounding inflammation which may be confused with more aggressive lesion. Malignant transformation of chondroblastoma is extremely uncommon.[7]

Chondromyxoid Fibroma

Chondromyxoid fibroma is less common than chondroblastoma, affecting predominantly males in the age group of 15–35 years.[8] Histologically, it is composed of chondroid, myxoid, and fibrous tissue in varying amounts. The common locations of tumor are ilium and the bones of the knee and foot. These tumors are located characteristically in metadiaphyseal location unlike chondroblastoma and do not cross an open growth plate. On plain radiograph, it appears as a well-marginated central or eccentric lucent lesion, with sclerotic margins and cortical expansion **(Fig. 6)**. Half of the lesions may show parallel orientation to the long axis of the involved bone. Matrix calcification and periosteal new bone formation usually do not occur.

OSSEOUS TUMORS

Osteoid Osteoma

Osteoid osteoma is a fairly common tumor, accounting for approximately 10–12% of all benign tumors.[9] These tumors usually affect boys in the second decade of life. Clinically, most patients present with pain that is especially severe at night and relieved by aspirin or other nonsteroidal anti-inflammatory agents.

More than half of tumors are located in proximal femur and tibia. They occur less frequently in the upper extremities than in the lower extremities. Osteoid osteomas also frequently affect the tubular bones of the hands and feet. They are however, less common in the spine, where they affect the posterior arches of the vertebra. Histologically, the lesion consists of a nidus which is usually surrounded by dense sclerotic bone. The nidus contains interlacing trabeculae at various stages of ossification within a stroma of loose vascular connective tissue. Osteoid osteoma can be cortical (the most common type), cancellous or medullary, and subperiosteal. The latter two types produce less sclerotic bone than those in the cortex do, making radiologic diagnosis difficult.

Radiographically, the lesion appears as well-defined lytic lesion, surrounded by reactive sclerosis **(Figs. 7A and B)**. Solid or lamellated periosteal reaction is seen in 60% of patients. Nidus may be purely radiolucent or contain a dense center. Intra-articular osteoid osteomas may be either cancellous or periosteal and have little reactive bone or periosteal new bone formation.

Computed tomography is very useful in showing the nidus, which can vary in its degree of ossification. CT appears to display the nidus better than MRI. The tumor nidus typically shows hypo- to intermediate signal on T1W images and low to high signal on T2W images. The nidus shows enhancement with gadolinium.[10] Intra-articular osteoid osteomas produce joint effusions and synovial proliferation. Radionuclide bone scans have been used for many years to help diagnosis of osteoid osteomas. Bone scintigraphy, which is a highly sensitive method of detecting osteoid osteoma, typically shows increased flow to the lesion on immediate images and a focus of increased activity on skeletal equilibrium images with double density sign. Many times, osteomyelitis can mimic osteoid osteoma clinically as well as radiographically; however, presence of soft-tissue extension favors the diagnosis of osteomyelitis. The traditional treatment of choice has been surgical excision; however, it can also be successfully treated by radiofrequency ablation under image guidance.[11]

Osteoblastoma

Osteoblastoma constitutes 2–6% of all bone tumors and most commonly occurs in patients in the second and third decades of life.[12] This tumor is more common in males than in females. Histologically, the osteoblastoma is closely related to osteoid osteomas except that bony trabeculae are broader and longer with absence of surrounding sclerotic halo. Size is an important consideration in distinguishing between these

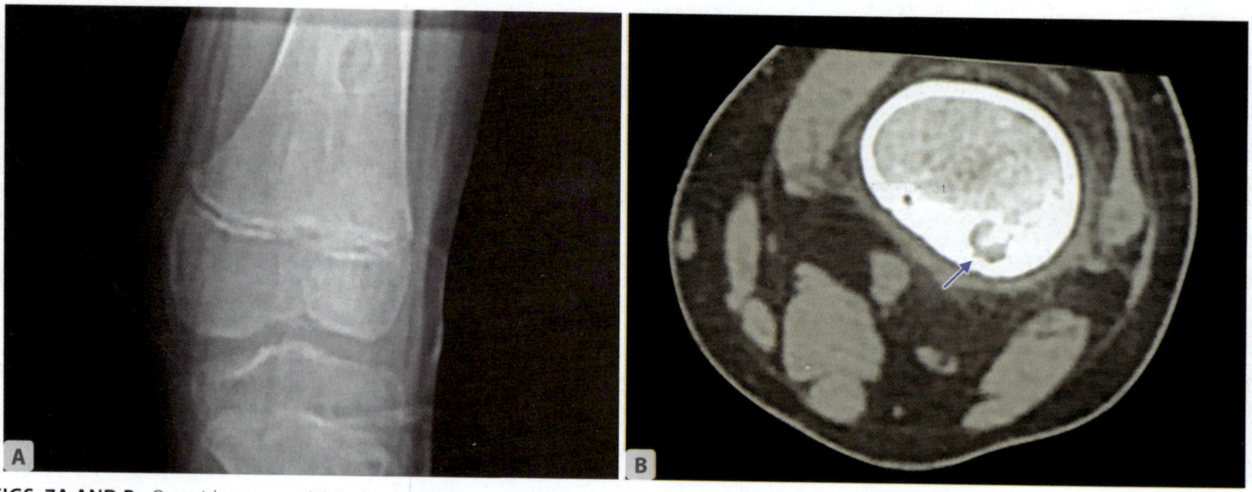

FIGS. 7A AND B: Osteoid osteoma. (A) Radiograph of knee joint shows lytic lesion with nidus in the lower end of femur; and (B) CT scan axial sections reveals well-defined lytic lesion with calcified nidus with adjacent sclerosis (blue arrow).

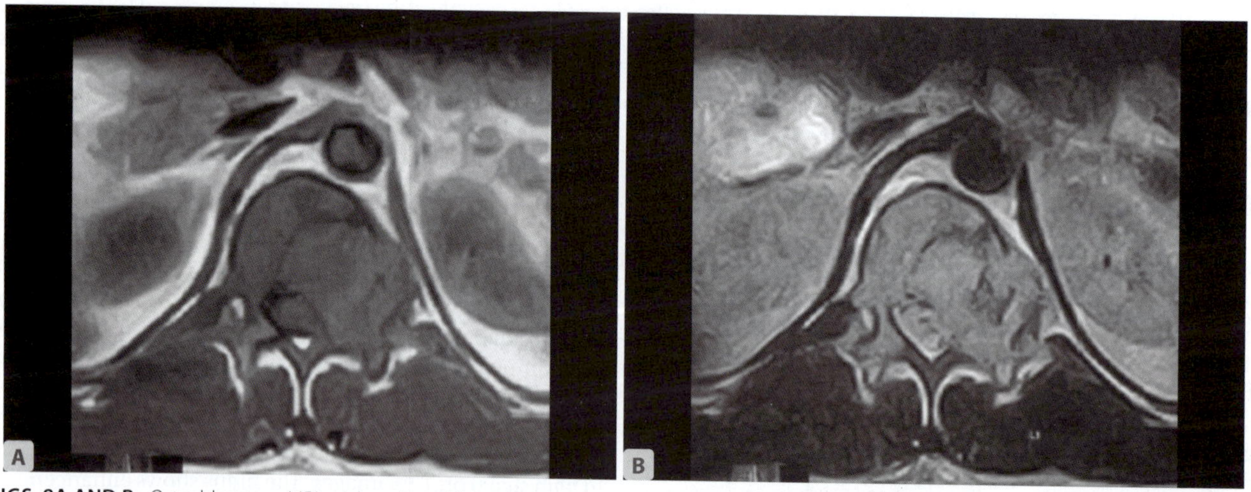

FIGS. 8A AND B: Osteoblastoma: MRI axial section, T1W and T2W images reveal heterogeneous signal lesion, predominantly involving posterior elements of vertebra with extension into spinal canal and left paravertebral location. (T1W: T1-weighted; T2W: T2-weighted)

two types of tumors. If the size of lesion is <1.5 cm in diameter, than it is likely to be osteoid osteomas whereas tumors >1.5 cm are usually osteoblastoma.

The most common location of osteoblastoma is spine where it classically affects posterior elements (33%)[12] **(Figs. 8A and B)**. The other common locations are proximal femur and talus. On plain X-ray, spinal osteoblastoma is osteolytic lesion with destruction of overlying cortex and may extend into the spinal canal. In the long bones, osteoblastoma appears radiologically as round or oval lucent tumors in the medulla. Periosteal reaction is common. Edema in the soft tissues or marrow appears hyperintense on T2W images, but the signal characteristics are not specific. Treatment is by surgical excision or curettage, but there is a moderate recurrence rate after these procedures.

FIBROUS TUMORS

Nonossifying Fibroma

Nonossifying fibroma is a benign fibroblastic mass that occurs in long bones of children and represents continuation of growth of fibrous cortical defect. It occurs eccentrically in the medullary cavity. The common location of lesion is in the bones around the knee joints. These lesions are usually asymptomatic and do not require specific treatment. On plain radiography, the lesion appears as well-marginated eccentric lytic lesion with scalloped margin **(Fig. 9)**. Its inner border is often sclerotic and may appear multilocular due to corrugations. Differential diagnosis includes unicameral bone cyst, ABC, fibrous dysplasia, and chondromyxoid fibroma. The signal intensity of nonossifying fibroma is equal

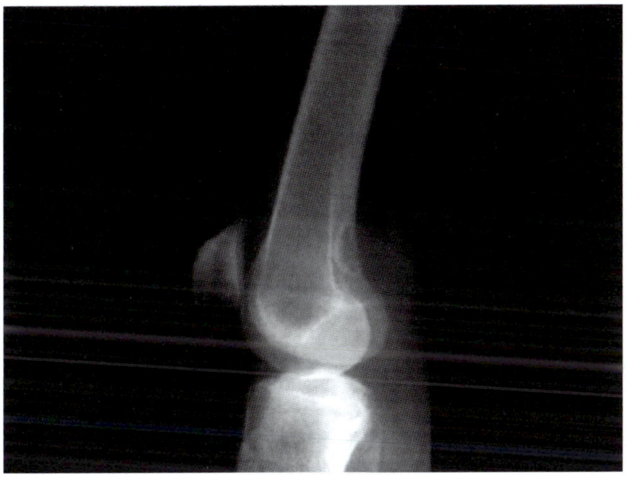

FIG. 9: Nonossifying fibroma: Radiograph of knee joint (lateral view) shows well-defined lytic lesion with sclerotic margin in characteristic location of lower end of femur.

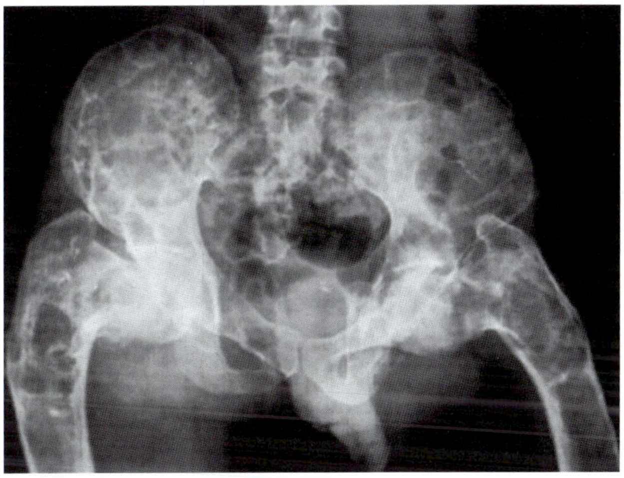

FIG. 10: Fibrous dysplasia: Radiograph of pelvis shows multiple lytic lesions involving all the visualized bones with characteristic Shepherd's crook deformity.

to or less than muscle on T1W MR images and hypointense to fat on T2W MR images. Postcontrast images usually show heterogeneous enhancement.

Fibrous Dysplasia

Fibrous dysplasia is disorder where bone is replaced by abnormal fibrous tissue. Fibrous dysplasia can be monostotic, polyostotic, monomelic, or polymelic. It is more common in young females. It is occasionally seen in the first decade of life. In a small percentage of cases (2–3%), fibrous dysplasia is associated with endocrine disorders, especially precocious puberty in girls (McCune-Albright syndrome).[13] Although it is not a true neoplasm, fibrous dysplasia involving a long bone may mimic a bone tumor or cyst. This type of fibrous dysplasia causes expansion of the medullary cavity of tubular bones, endosteal scalloping, and trabeculation. The margin is sclerotic. The lesion may appear as ground glass or radiolucent and this depends upon amount of fibrous tissue within the lesion. Bowing of the affected long bone may occur; when the affected bone is femur, the resulting deformity is called a "Shepherd's crook" **(Fig. 10)**. Thinning and destruction of the bony cortex may be seen on CT or MR images. Soft-tissue extension of the lesion is unusual. On T1W MR images, the signal intensity of fibrous dysplasia is similar to that of skeletal muscle. Although, the signal of pure fibrous tissue is hypointense on T2W images, the signal of fibrous dysplasia is variable.

Osteofibrous Dysplasia

It is a rare lesion that is usually confined to the tibia, but can also involve the fibula. Most cases occur during the first decade of life. On plain X-ray, the lesion appears as an eccentric, lucent, solitary, or multiloculated, lesion involving the anterior aspect of tibia. CT is very helpful in determining its intracortical location, an important feature in distinguishing osteofibrous dysplasia from fibrous dysplasia.[14]

HISTIOCYTOSIS X (LANGERHANS CELL HISTIOCYTOSIS)

Histiocytosis X is a syndrome that consists of group of clinical pathological entities: Eosinophilic granuloma, Hand-Schüller-Christian disease, and Letterer-Siwe disease. Eosinophilic granuloma is localized skeletal disease and is one of the commonly occurring bone tumors of boys in the first decade of life.[15] The skull is the most frequent location, followed by the femur, mandible, pelvis, ribs, and spine. The lesions are usually located in the medulla of the diaphysis and metaphysis and rarely involve the cortex and epiphysis. Multiple lesions occur in about 25% of cases.[15] Pain is most common presenting problem with local tenderness and palpable mass. Histologically, the tumors are composed of Langerhans cell histiocytosis containing their characteristic cleaved nuclei and electron microscopy reveals Birbeck granules in the cytoplasm adjacent to the cell membrane. Radiographic appearance is variable. The lesion in calvarium typically appears as well-defined lytic lesion with scalloped/beveled borders **(Fig. 11)**. Sometimes, a button sequestrum may be seen in the lesion. Most of the lesions in long bones appear as lytic lesion with well-defined borders; however, some of the lesions are permeative and associated with periosteal new bone formation **(Fig. 12)**. The later findings suggest aggressive behavior. MRI is a very sensitive, but nonspecific method of detecting eosinophilic granuloma. The lesion can be hypointense or hyperintense on T1W and hyperintense on T2W images, associated with extensive marrow and soft-tissue edema. Occasionally, there is cortical disruption with adjacent soft tissue seen on MRI **(Fig. 13)**. The natural history of isolated lesion is gradual healing.[16] Treatment depends upon the site, location, and multiplicity of lesion.

GIANT CELL TUMOR

Giant cell tumors are very rare in children under 15 years of age and commonly seen in girls.[17] Radiographically, these tumors

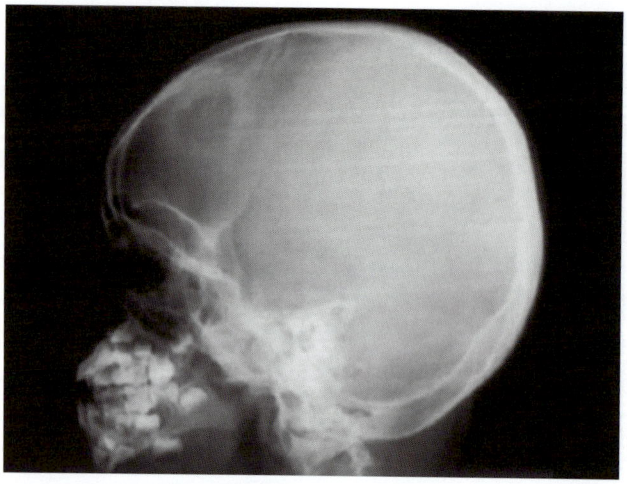

FIG. 11: Histiocytosis: Radiograph of skull (lateral view) shows well-defined lytic lesion with beveled margins in frontal lobe.

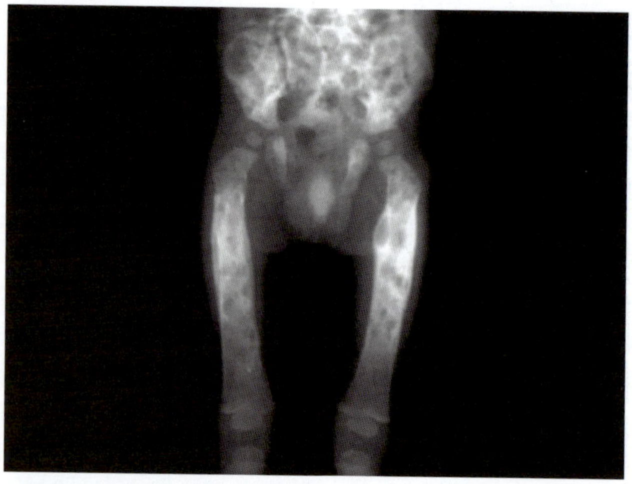

FIG. 12: Histiocytosis: Radiograph of the pelvis and upper femora shows multiple well-defined and ill-defined lesions with associated periosteal reaction in both femora.

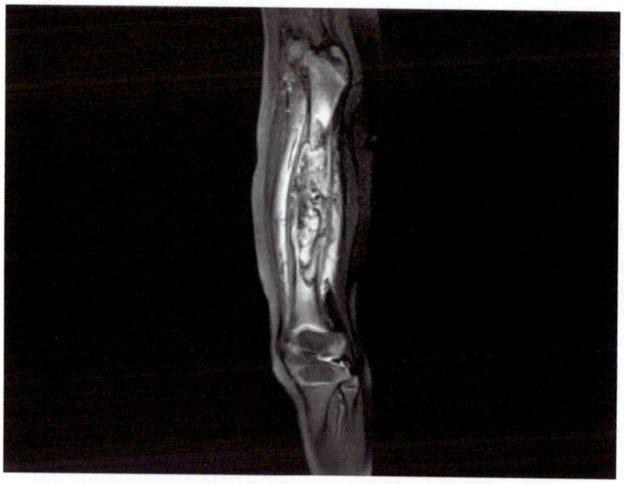

FIG. 13: Histiocytosis: MRI of femur shows large heterogeneous signal intensity lesion in diaphysis with cortical destruction, soft tissue, and periosteal reaction.

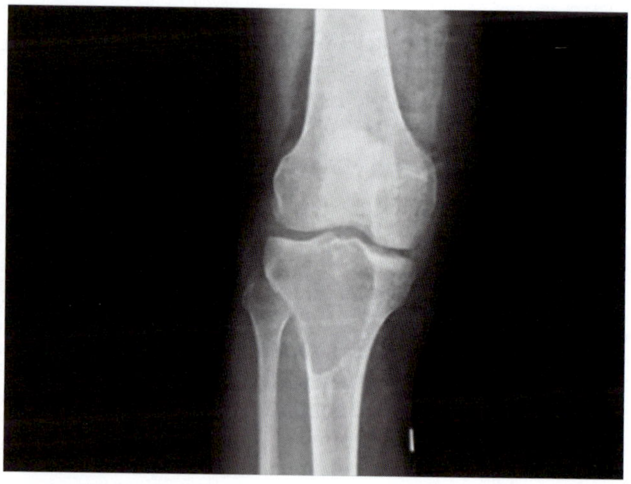

FIG. 14: Giant cell tumor: Radiograph of knee [anteroposterior (AP) and lateral view] shows large expansile eccentric lytic lesion in upper end of tibia, extending up to subchondral region.

are well-defined, eccentric lytic lesions usually located around the knee. The lesion usually shows nonsclerotic margin, cortical thinning without matrix calcification **(Fig. 14)**. GCT is located in the metaphysis and does not cross the open physis, but may extend to the subchondral bone if the physis is closed. On MRI, the lesion shows generalized hypointensity on T2W images. This T2 hypointensity may result from the tumor cellularity or from recurrent hemorrhage within the lesion. The solid portions of GCT enhance diffusely after gadolinium administration. Secondary, ABC formation can be seen in about 14% of GCT.[17]

TUMOR-LIKE LESIONS

Simple Bone Cyst

A bone cyst is a fluid-filled lesion with fibrous lining. It occurs in metaphysis of long bones and adjacent to physis in children and young adults. Common locations are proximal humerus and femur.[18] Calcaneum and ileum are less common sites. On plain radiograph, the lesion appears as moderately expansile, well-marginated with or without sclerosis **(Fig. 15)**. The cortex may be thinned out and may lead to pathological fracture. "Fallen fragment" sign may be seen, when there is piece of bone which migrates into the cavity and settles at the base. CT and MRI can confirm the cystic nature of the lesion. The fluid contents are usually of low intensity on T1W images and hyperintensity on T2W images. However, hemorrhage into the cyst can alter the signal characteristics of the lesion.[5,18]

Aneurysmal Bone Cyst

Aneurysmal bone cyst is solitary, expansile radiolucent lesion and generally located in metaphysis of long bones. Other sites are dorsolumbar spine, small bones of hand, feet, and pelvis. Pathologically, the lesion contains multiples cystic spaces containing various stages of blood. Radiologically, the lesion appears as expansile, lytic sharply circumscribed with

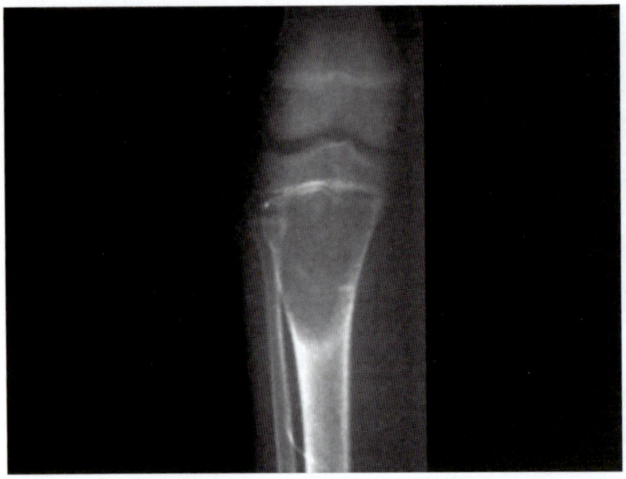

FIG. 15: Bone cyst: Radiograph of knee joint shows mildly expansile lytic lesion in metaphysis of tibia with thinning of cortex.

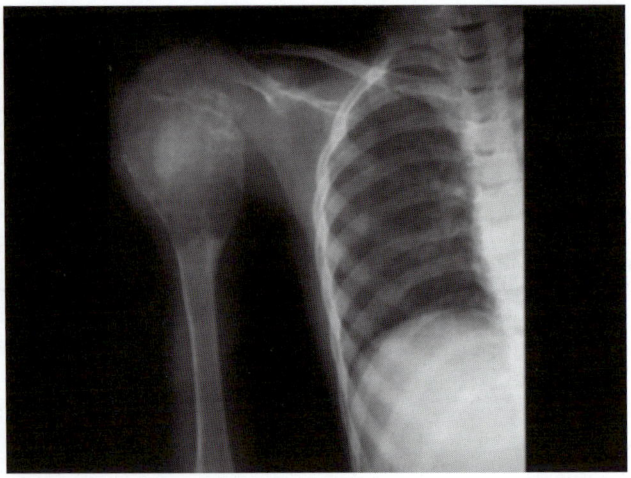

FIG. 16: Aneurysmal bone cyst: Radiograph of shoulder joint shows multiloculated expansile lytic lesion, involving upper end of humerus.

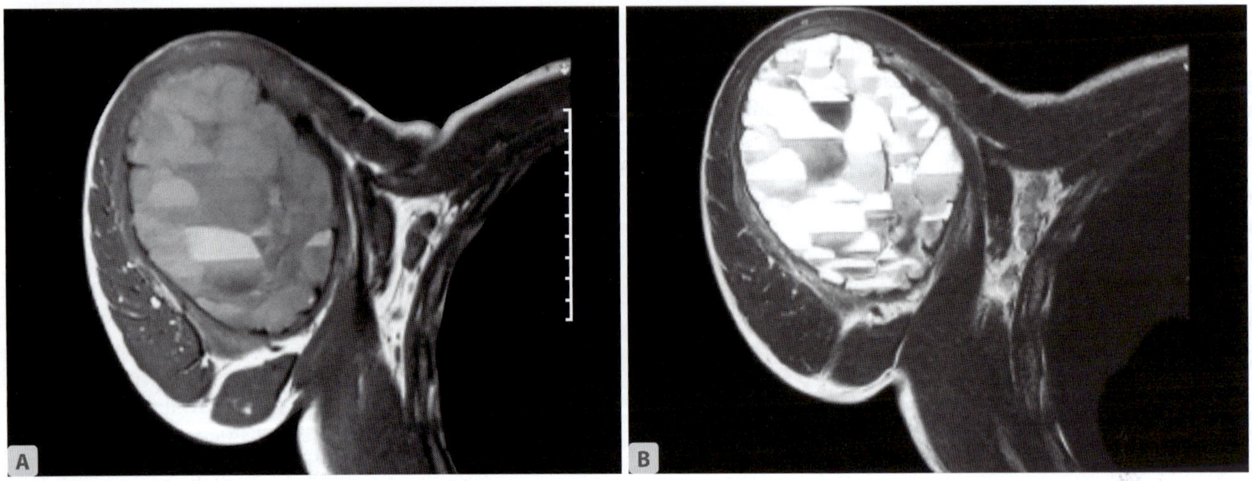

FIGS. 17A AND B: Aneurysmal bone cyst. (A and B) MRI of the same patient, axial T1W and T2W images show well-defined multiloculated expansile lesion with fluid-fluid/hemorrhage levels. (T1W: T1-weighted; T2W: T2-weighted)

thin cortex. The characteristic features are its ballooned out appearance and trabeculated appearance **(Fig. 16)**. CT may demonstrate fluid-fluid level and thin rim of bone overlying the lesion. MRI shows the various stages of blood products which appear as layers of different signal intensity on both T1W and T2W images[18] **(Figs. 17A and B)**. The differential diagnosis includes GCT, osteoblastoma, chondroblastoma, osteosarcoma, and simple bone cyst.

Pseudotumor of Hemophilia

Hemophilia is a bleeding disorder that occurs in males. Repetitive hemorrhage occurs close to muscle attachments without significant history of trauma. The common locations are iliopsoas and gastrocnemius muscles. Sometimes, there is intraosseous or subperiosteal hemorrhage, which can cause pressure erosion of bone. Plain X-ray shows pressure erosion/destruction of bone associated with large soft-tissue component **(Fig. 18A)**. Calcification within soft-tissue hematoma may be seen. MRI shows variable heterogeneous signal, in form of various stages of blood products **(Fig. 18B)**.

SOFT-TISSUE TUMORS

The diagnosis of soft-tissue tumors in pediatric age can be challenging due to broad spectrum of neoplasms, inflammatory conditions and pseudotumors, and developmental anomalies. Ultrasonography (USG) and MRI are very useful to characterize these tumors. However, for accurate diagnosis, we need to consider patient's age, clinical history, and physical examination. Ultrasound is excellent choice for the small and superficial soft-tissue lesions. Ultrasound provides some advantages like low cost, portability, lack of ionizing radiation, no need for sedation, and easy availability. Grayscale study should be performed by using highest frequency transducer available in the department. Color Doppler USG demonstrates the presence or absence of vessels within the lesion.

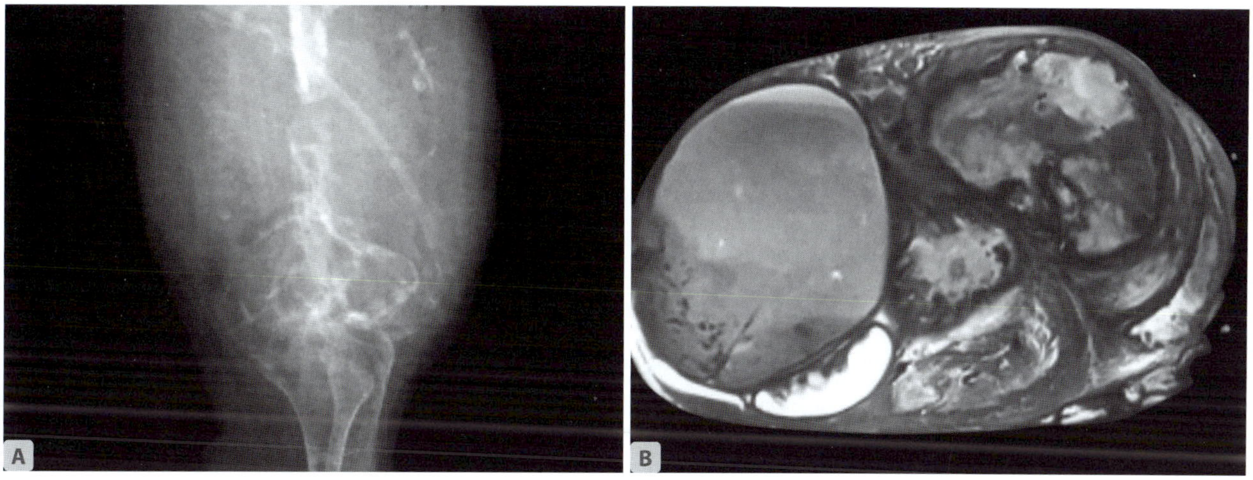

FIGS. 18A AND B: Pseudotumor of hemophilia. (A) Radiograph of lower end of femur shows lytic destruction of femur associated with large soft-tissue component and bony spicules; and (B) MRI of the same patient, fat saturation at T2-weighted (T2W) image shows large soft tissue with various stages of blood components.

Magnetic resonance imaging is the modality of choice for the evaluation of large and deep masses due to its multiplanar imaging capabilities, good tissue contrast resolution, and without radiation. MRI is useful for those cases in which ultrasound is not adequate/suboptimal. MRI should include the entire tumor, so as to demonstrate its margins. MR images of soft-tissue tumors have low specificity, are only occasionally helpful in differentiating between benign and malignant masses with certainty. Some imaging criteria on MRI have been postulated as indicators of malignancy. These include bigger size (>5–6 cm), low signal absence on T2W images, heterogeneous signal on T1W images, early contrast enhancement, initial rapid enhancement followed by a plateau or a washout phase, and adjacent bone invasion, neurovascular bundles, or both.[19]

Vascular Lesions

Vascular lesions are most common soft-tissue masses in children. Mulliken and Glowacki[20] divided them in two groups (hemangiomas and vascular malformations) based on physical examination, their clinical evolution, histology, and cellular kinetics. Hemangiomas are neoplastic lesions whereas vascular malformations are considered as errors of vascular morphogenesis. Categorization of a vascular lesion into one of these two groups is very useful for patient's management and prognosis.

Hemangioma

Hemangiomas are considered to be true neoplasms and they account for 7–10% of all benign soft-tissue tumors.[20] Hemangiomas may be localized or diffuse and are histologically benign. Capillary (usually cutaneous), cavernous, venous, and mixed types of hemangiomas have been described and classified according to the apparent origin of their vascular channels. Hemangiomas also contain variable amounts of nonvascular tissue and other elements, including fat, smooth muscle, fibrous tissue, myxoid stroma, and hemosiderin.

Ultrasonography, CT, MRI, and radiolabeled red cell scintigraphy can facilitate preoperative diagnosis. Radiographs are important for detecting associated osseous abnormality and the finding of calcified phleboliths on radiographs or CT images is an indication of a hemangioma **(Figs. 19A and B)**. On ultrasound, hemangioma appears as a well-defined mass of variable echogenicity.[21] Color Doppler may show high-flow pattern in proliferative phase; however, vascularity decreases in involuting phase. On T1W MRI images, hemangiomas are either isointense or when they contain sufficient fat, hyperintense to muscle. On T2W images, the lesions are well-defined and markedly hyperintense with serpiginous high signal zones that correlate with torturous vascular channels interlaced with lower intensity fibrous or fatty tissue. Phleboliths are hypointense on both T1W and T2W sequences.

Hemangiopericytoma is a rare soft-tissue tumor of low but unpredictable malignant potential that is believed to arise from vascular endothelial pericytes. These tumors are usually located in the thigh or the pelvic retroperitoneum, but can arise in any part of the body. Approximately, 10% of hemangiopericytomas occur during childhood and about one-third of these are congenital.[22] Congenital hemangiopericytoma can exhibit rapid initial growth, but spontaneous regression has also been reported. Microscopically, these tumors show endothelial proliferation with some similarity to hemangioma. Calcifications may be detected radiographically or by CT and the tumors are well-circumscribed. There may be partial destruction of adjacent bone. Hemangiopericytomas are very vascular lesions and show marked enhancement and frequently, central necrosis on contrast-enhanced CT images.

Like most soft-tissue sarcomas, hemangiopericytomas are isointense to muscle on T1W images and show high signal

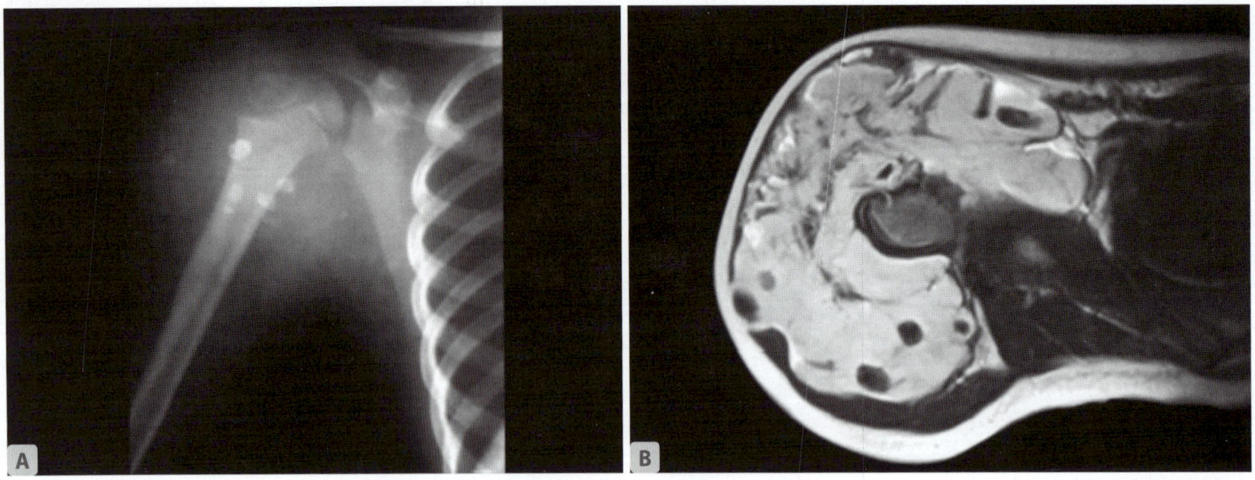

FIGS. 19A AND B: Hemangioma. (A) Radiograph of shoulder joint shows large soft tissue around the joint with phleboliths; and (B) MRI of same patient shows large lobulated soft tissue with multiple phleboliths.

on T2W and short tau inversion recovery (STIR) images and they enhance moderately with gadolinium.

Vascular Malformations

Vascular malformations are due to errors in vascular development which are always present at birth. They are classified as arteriovenous, venous, lymphatic, capillary, or mixed based on the main vascular channel within the lesion. Arteriovenous malformations (AVMs) are high-flow vascular malformations which show direct communication between the arterial and venous systems and no intervening capillary bed. These vascular lesions may be detected at child birth (40% of cases) and grow with the child.[23] They appear as multiple dilated tortuous channels on ultrasound diffusely involving subcutaneous tissues. This may not be well seen on grayscale USG, but are easily demonstrated with color Doppler. These AVMs have a high vascular density and spectral Doppler analysis demonstrates high velocity in the arteries **(Fig. 20)**, but usually a well-defined mass is not demonstarted.[21] These lesions appear as enlarged vascular channels associated with dilated feeding and draining vessels on MRI. The high-flow vessels seen as signal void on spin echo images or as high signal intensity on flow-enhanced gradient echo (GRE) images.

Venous malformations have characteristic feature of presence of anomalous ectatic venous channels which can be small and localized or extensive. Venous malformations usually show heterogeneous echogenicity, more commonly hypoechoic in comparison with the adjacent subcutaneous tissues on ultrasound. Phleboliths can be present in 16% of cases. Doppler ultrasound may detect slow flow within these lesions. Flow may not be detected which may reflect very slow flow or thrombosis. These lesions on MRI may appear as dilated tortuous veins or as lobulated masses, having multiple locules reflecting dilated venous spaces separated by thin septae. Venous malformations are iso- to hypointense to muscle on T1W images, hyperintense on T2W images. They show patchy contrast enhancement after the administration of intravenous gadolinium.[24]

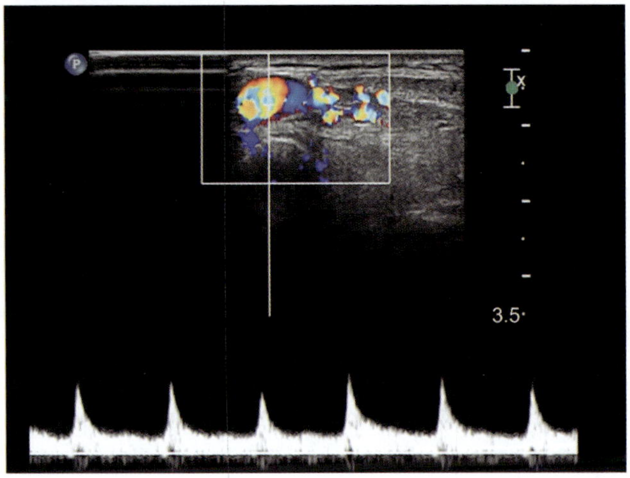

FIG. 20: High-flow vascular malformation in soft tissue having arterial flow spectral pattern.

Lymphangioma, most likely visible at birth, is more commonly seen in the head and neck region but also seen in the visceral organs, trunk, and extremities. Clinically, they are soft, smooth, and translucent masses. The macrocystic lymphatic malformations appear as well-defined, multicystic lesions on USG. CT scan will also show multicystic hypodense mass **(Fig. 21)**. These lymphatic malformations appear as well-defined cysts usually of low signal intensity on T1W images and high signal intensity on T2W images and often show fluid-fluid levels. Postcontrast images show only septal enhancement with no enhancement in cystic spaces. This is very helpful feature in the differentiation of these lesions from venous malformations.[24]

FIBROBLASTIC/MYOFIBROBLASTIC TUMORS

These tumors comprise a large number of mesenchymal tumors with both fibroblastic and myofibroblastic characteristics. Common lesions of this group are described here.

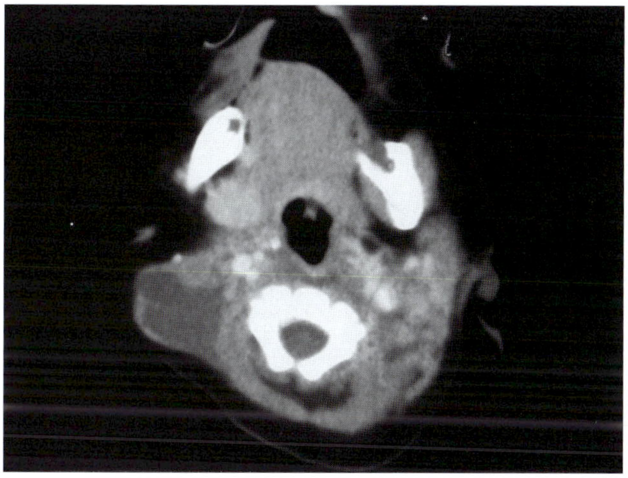

FIG. 21: Lymphangioma: CT scan, axial section in the neck region shows multiseptated cystic lesion.

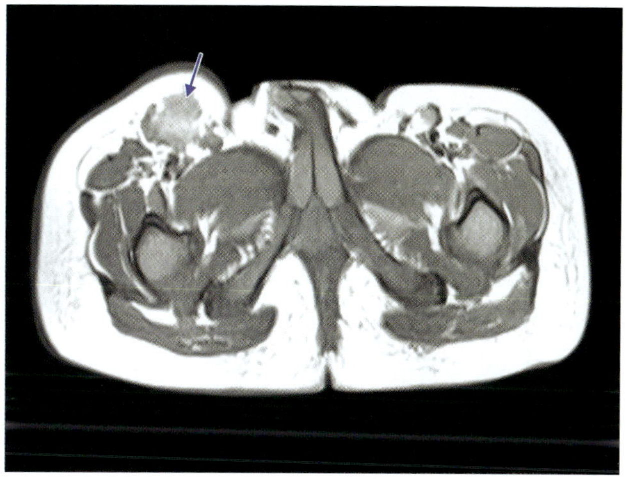

FIG. 22: Nodular fasciitis: MRI [T1-weighted (T1W)] axial image in the hip region shows heterogeneous signal soft-tissue lesion in subcutaneous plane in right upper thigh (blue arrow).

Nodular Fasciitis

This is an idiopathic, self-limited focal fibrous proliferation, most likely confined to the subcutaneous tissues. The common locations of nodular fasciitis include the upper extremities and trunk. Nodular fasciitis appears as a well-defined lesion with homogeneous/heterogeneous echotexture on USG. The MR imaging appearance of these lesions are variable. Commonly, they appears homogeneous isointense or slightly hyperintense to muscle on T1W images as a fascia-based lesions **(Fig. 22)**. They are hyperintense/heterogeneous on T2W images and show homogeneous contrast enhancement after gadolinium administration.[25]

Myositis Ossificans

Myositis ossificans is a reparative hypercellular lesion, composed of reactive hypercellular fibrous tissue and bone which is commonly localized and self-limiting. History of trauma is present in most of the cases. It often occurs more commonly in the thighs and arms which are often exposed to trauma. Plain X-ray may show heterogeneous calcification, adjacent to bony attachment **(Figs. 23A and B)**. CT is the modality of choice for diagnosis of myositis ossificans which picks up calcification very well. The appearance of myositis ossificans lesion changes with time. After 2 weeks of trauma, it appears as hypodense mass without calcification associated with edema of surrounding soft-tissues. Curvilinear peripheral calcification is usually seen after 4–6 weeks. Then after, progressive internal ossification/calcification occurs over the next several weeks and months.[26]

Myofibroma/Myofibromatosis

Solitary myofibroma is a benign fibrous tumor and commonly seen in children <2 years of age. It may present as a solitary or multiple nodules in the subcutaneous tissues or muscle or bone. The multicentric appearance is known as myofibromatosis. The myofibromatosis may have spontaneous regression; however, a high mortality is reported in multicentric cases with visceral involvement. The myofibromas have varied appearances on ultrasound but are often well-marginated with an anechoic center, reflecting central necrosis and having thick septa.[27] The myofibromas appear as of low signal intensity nodules on T1W images and a variable appearance on T2W MR images

Fibromatosis

Fibromatosis is a condition where benign proliferation of fibroblasts and myofibroblasts occurs with a marked production of collagen tissue. It shows infiltrative growth and a propensity for local tissue recurrence. These tumors are variably echogenic on ultrasound and their borders may be smooth or irregular. CT scan is useful to show extent of soft tissue and bony erosion **(Figs. 24A and B)**. On MR images, their appearance is also variable with a signal that is isointense or slightly hyperintense when compared with that of muscle on T1W images and either intermediate between muscles and fat or high signal on T2W images.[28]

Neurogenic Tumor

Most common neurogenic tumor arising from peripheral nerves in children is neurofibroma. Three types of neurofibroma have been described: (1) Localized, (2) Diffuse, and (3) Plexi-form types.[29] Localized neurofibroma is usually well-defined, encapsulated soft-tissue masses <5 cm in diameter. They are isointense to muscle on T1W and heterogeneous signal on T2W images and may show target pattern.[29] Plexiform neurofibroma is a diffuse mass involving multiple fascicles of nerve. These lesions can be deep, superficial, or combination of both, depending upon the location of tumor. Superficial types of lesions are more common, diffuse, and asymmetric in distribution and extend to skin surface **(Fig. 25)**.

Adipocytic Tumor

Common adipocytic tumors are lipoma, lipoblastoma, and lipomatosis of nerve in the pediatric age group. Liposarcoma is the most common type of soft-tissue sarcoma in adults, but rare in children.

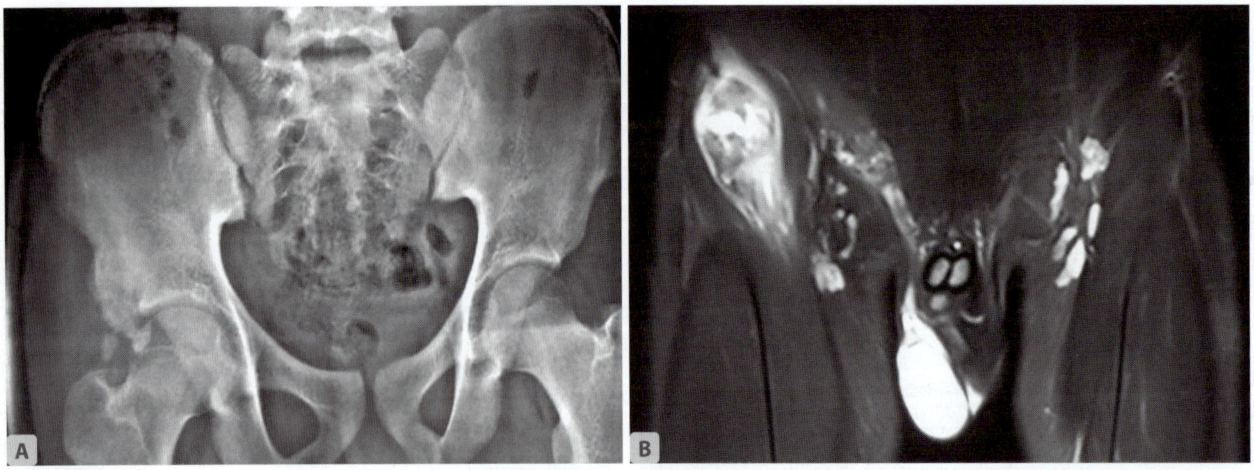

FIGS. 23A AND B: Myositis ossificans. (A) Radiograph of pelvis shows soft-tissue ossification adjacent to superior aspect of right acetabulum; and (B) MRI of same patient [fat saturated T2-weighted (T2W), coronal section] shows heterogeneous signal mass-like lesion with soft-tissue edema.

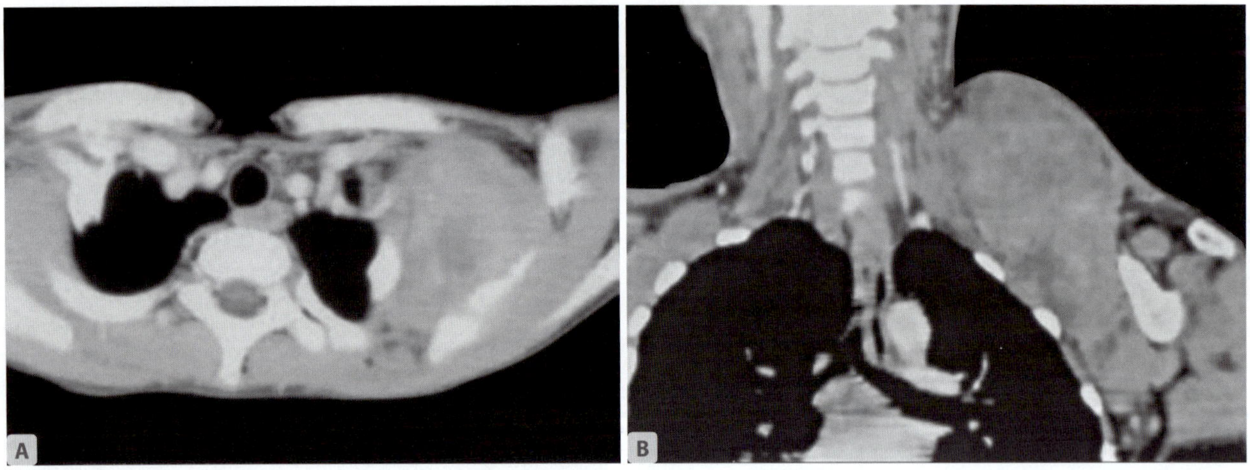

FIGS. 24A AND B: Fibromatosis: CT scan axial section (A) and coronal reformation (B) show large soft-tissue mass in the lower part of neck extending into axilla with erosion of adjacent scapula.

Lipoma

Common adipocytic tumors in children are lipomas. The common locations of lipomas are in the upper back, neck, proximal extremities, and abdomen. Lipomas are usually subcutaneous in children, although deep ones are not rare. These deep lipomas often require imaging. The lipomas have a variable appearance on ultrasound, with about two-thirds of cases demonstrating homogeneous echogenicity. About 60% show well-defined margins. The echogenicity of lipomas are so variable and hypoechoic, isoechoic, hyperechoic, and mixed echogenicity patterns of lipomas have been reported.[30] The lipomas have similar signal as subcutaneous fat on MRI and will show high signal intensity on T1W images and show fat suppression (low signal) on fat-suppressed images **(Fig. 26)**.

Lipoblastoma

Lipoblastoma is a tumor which contains mature adipocytes and lipoblasts in various stages of development. Lipoblastoma may represent up to 30% of adipocytic tumors in children.[31] It usually occurs in children <3 years of age and manifests as a painless, progressively growing soft-tissue mass. Lipoblastoma usually appears as a homogeneous, hyperechoic mass on ultrasound, although mixed echogenicity and fluid-filled spaces have also been reported in literature. The MR appearance reflects the amount of mature adipose tissue relative to lipoblasts and myxocollagenous stromal tissue. They can similar appearance like lipoma. The MR signal is heterogeneous when myxoid component is more and shows heterogeneous contrast enhancement. This imaging feature is indistinguishable from liposarcoma **(Fig. 27)**.[32]

Pseudotumors

These are nonneoplastic lesions and can present as soft-tissue mass. These include hematoma, fat necrosis, inflammatory lesions, and periarticular cysts.

Fat Necrosis

It is self-limiting entity and presents as small nontender subcutaneous nodule. The causes of fat necrosis include cold

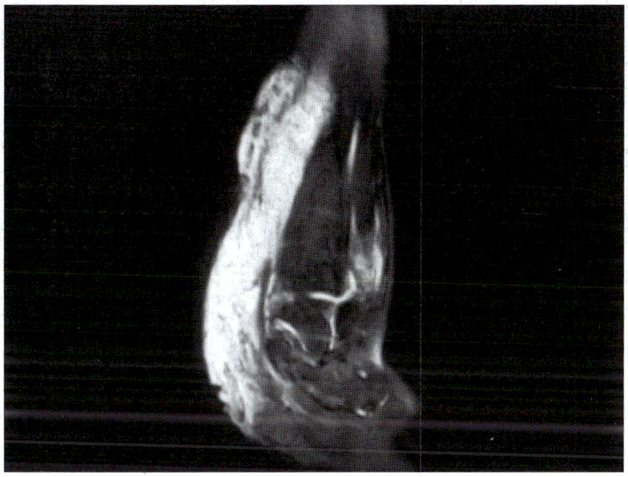

FIG. 25: Plexiform neurofibroma: MRI of leg shows large lobulated heterogeneous signal intensity lesion involving skin and deep soft tissue of leg.

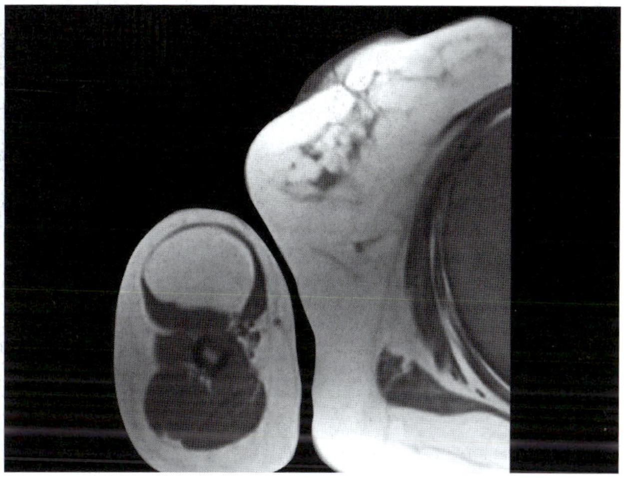

FIG. 26: Lipoma: MRI, axial section [T1-weighted image] shows well-defined lesion in anterior compartment of arm with similar signal intensity of subcutaneous fat.

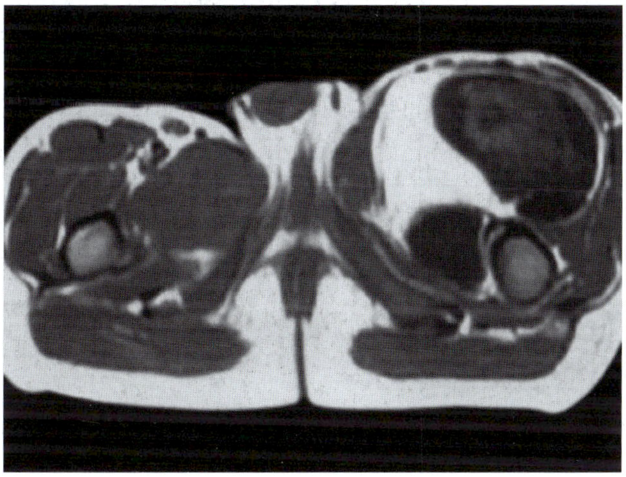

FIG. 27: Lipoblastoma: MRI, axial section [T1-weighted (T1W) images] of upper thigh, shows large soft-tissue mass in left upper thigh with signal intensity of fat as well as soft tissue.

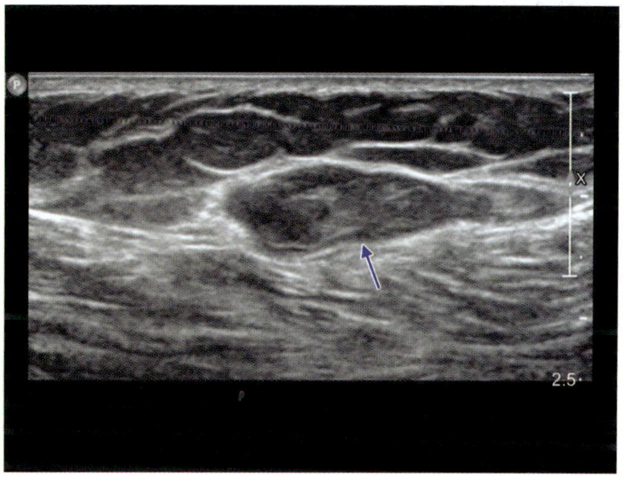

FIG. 28: Fat necrosis: Ultrasound image of thigh shows heterogeneous echotexture ill-defined area in subcutaneous fat (blue arrow).

exposure, trauma, injection, autoimmune disorders, and vasculitis. Common locations of fat necrosis are soft tissues overlying bone prominences in the back, shoulder, buttocks, thighs, and cheeks. Imaging findings on ultrasound is quite variable; however, predominantly it is a hyperechoic nodule with fuzzy margins **(Fig. 28)**. Fat necrosis appears as linear-shaped abnormal signal in subcutaneous tissue which is usually hypointense on T1W and hypo-/hyperintense on T2W images.[33]

Hematoma

Imaging of hematoma is usually not required; however, it may be needed when child is very symptomatic and in cases where clear history of trauma and bleeding disorders is not known. The imaging appearance of hematoma depends on the age of blood. Ultrasound is the initial investigation of choice. In acute stage, hematoma is hyperechoic; however, it becomes anechoic/heterogeneous in few days **(Fig. 29)**. MRI is useful and it can show hyperintensity on T1W images, hypointense on T2W images, and blooming on GRE sequences.[34]

Inflammatory Lesions

Cellulitis occasionally presents as soft-tissue mass. Ultrasound shows increased echogenicity of subcutaneous fat. On MRI, cellulitis appears as ill-defined T1 hypointense and T2 hyperintense area seen in subcutaneous tissue. Sometimes, aggressive infection leads to abscess formation in soft tissue. On ultrasound, abscess appears as hypoechoic fluid collection **(Fig. 30)**. MRI shows well-defined T1 hypointense and T2 hyperintense lesion with peripheral enhancement on postcontrast images **(Fig. 31)**.[35]

Periarticular Cysts

These include ganglion, synovial cyst, and meniscal cyst. Ganglion is cystic lesion which has fibrous capsule and

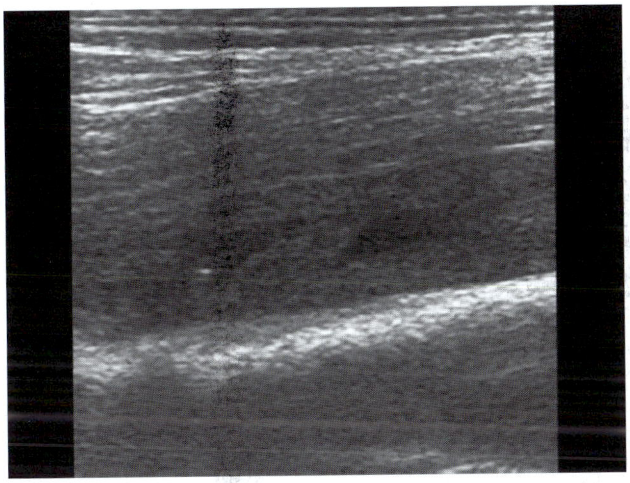

FIG. 29: Hematoma: Ultrasound image shows ill-defined heterogeneous echotexture lesion within the deep muscles of thigh, suggestive of hematoma.

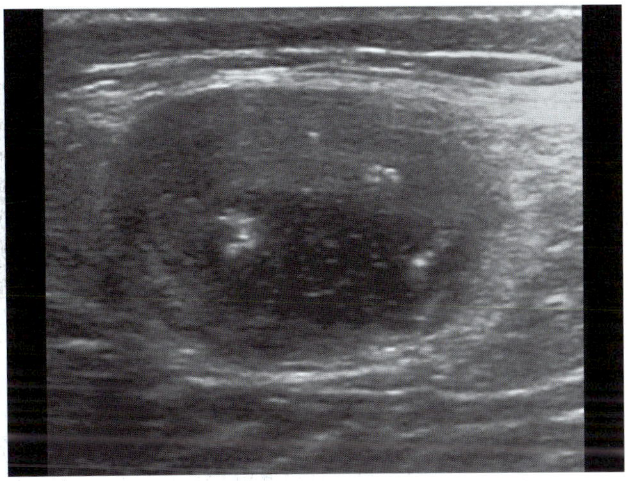

FIG. 30: Abscess: Ultrasound image shows well-defined collection in subcutaneous soft tissue with internal echoes suggestive of abscess.

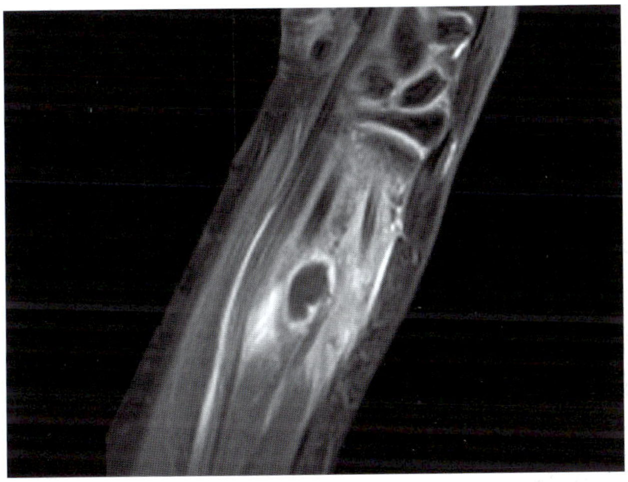

FIG. 31: Abscess: Contrast-enhanced MRI of forearm shows well-defined abscess with peripheral enhancement associated with surrounding inflammatory changes.

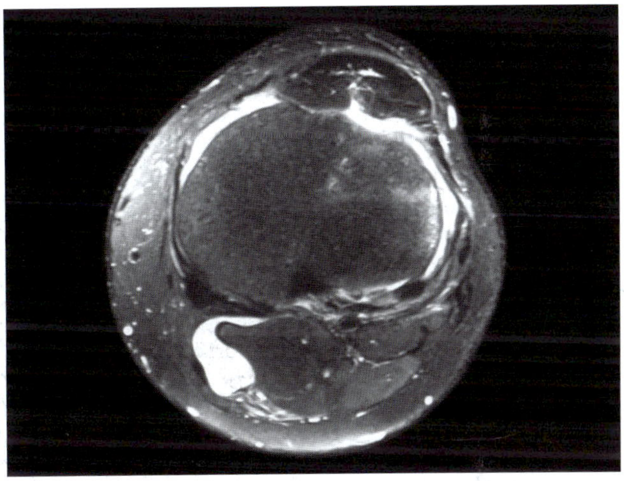

FIG. 32: Popliteal cyst: MRI, proton density fat saturated (PDFS) (axial section) of knee joint shows popliteal cyst in typical location.

composed of mucoid material. Imaging (USG and MRI) shows typical features of cyst; however, sometimes internal echoes and septae can be seen.[36] Synovial cyst is lined by synovial cells. Synovial cyst may communicate with joint space. Typical example of synovial cyst is popliteal cyst **(Fig. 32)**. Collection of fluid in the meniscus or parameniscal tissue is called meniscal cyst. It is associated with meniscus tear. MR imaging shows well-defined cyst/fluid collection in continuity with meniscus tear.[37]

Advance Magnetic Resonance Imaging

There has been advancement in MR imaging in last two to three decades with sequences like diffusion-weighted imaging (DWI), perfusion imaging (DWI), and spectroscopy. Most of them being used in diagnosis and management in malignant bone and soft-tissue tumors; however, some authors have tried these sequences in benign tumors also.

Diffusion-weighted Imaging

Diffusion-weighted imaging is a method of functional imaging.[38] DWI measures the Brownian motion of water at a microscopic level. Corresponding apparent diffusion coefficient (ADC) maps provide quantitative assessment of the diffusivity of the lesion. ADC is marker of cellularity and tumor density. High cellularity tumor has low ADC and low density tumor shows more ADC. Various authors have tried to differentiate benign and malignant bone tumors by using DWI and reported with good results with some overlap features.[39,40] Intraosseous infective focus can mimic other bony lesion in some cases. DWI can show diffusion restriction and low ADC value which can be very useful to differentiate these lesions **(Figs. 33A and B)**.

Perfusion-weighted Magnetic Resonance Imaging

Perfusion sequences provide insight of vascularity of tumor. The most common method of perfusion is dynamic contrast-

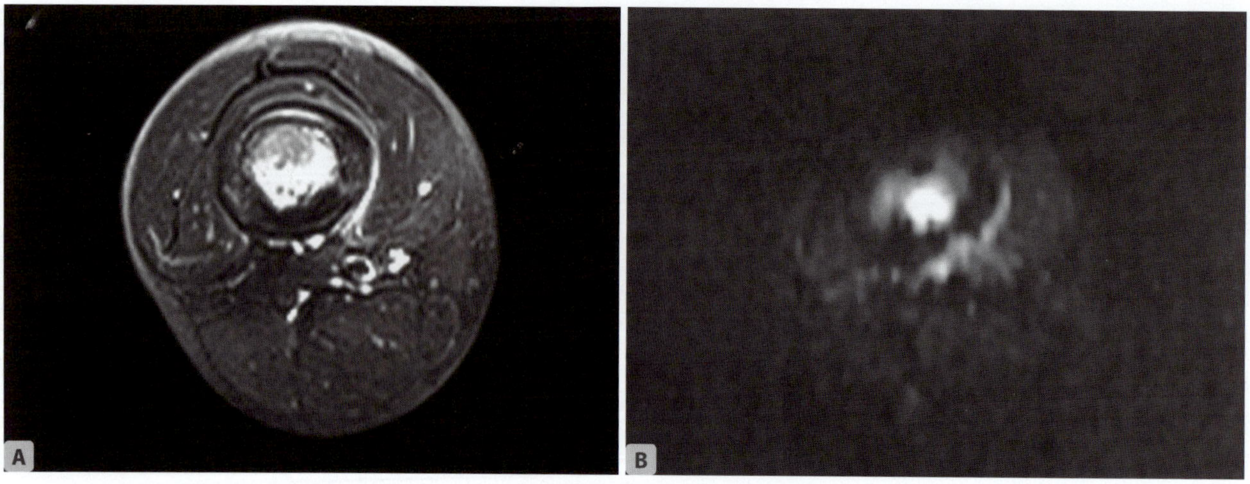

FIGS. 33A AND B: Diffusion-weighted imaging (DWI) in case of bony lesion. (A) Fat-saturated T2W axial shows T2 hyperintense intramedullary lesion in diaphysis of femur with periosteal reaction; and (B) DW image at same level shows diffusion restriction and lower ADC suggesting intramedullary infective lesion which was turned out as osteomyelitis later. (ADC: apparent diffusion coefficient; T2W: T2-weighted)

enhanced magnetic resonance (DCMR). This is done by using GRE sequence for particular volume of tumor after injecting intravenous contrast and creating time-intensity curve (TIC) and using semiquantitative measurements. Authors have used dynamic contrast-enhanced MRI (DCE-MRI) to differentiate malignant from benign bone lesions with good sensitivity and specificity.[41] Sometime osteoid osteoma can mimic chronic osteomyelitis on radiographs. Although CT is best to show nidus in osteoid osteoma; however, MRI can help by showing typical TIC curve by using DCE-MRI. Most osteoid osteoma shows arterial enhancement with rapid washout.[42]

Magnetic Resonance Spectroscopy

Proton MR spectroscopy is noninvasive method that forms molecular characterization of tumor. Some of the authors have shown choline peaks and different choline ratio for differentiating benign and malignant musculoskeletal tumors.[43,44] The method is technically challenging and may have overlapping features as choline may not be feature of tumor aggressiveness and malignancy.[45]

CONCLUSION

A wide spectrum of benign bone and soft-tissue tumor and conditions is seen in children. It is imperative for the radiologist to be aware of entire gamut of imaging findings, so as to avoid unwarranted biopsies and surgeries in these children. Plain radiograph continues to be first-line imaging modality of choice and is the cornerstone in diagnosis of pediatric benign bone tumors. MR imaging has emerged to become an integral part of diagnostic algorithm of these lesions, owing to its excellent soft-tissue resolution, multiplanar capabilities, and nonionizing nature.

REFERENCES

1. Fletcher BD. Benign and malignant bone tumor. In: Coley B (Ed). Caffey's Pediatric Diagnostic Imaging, 13th edition. Philadelphia: Mosby Elsevier; 2004.
2. Biermann JS. Musculoskeletal neoplasms in children. In: Sponseller PD, Shaughnessy JW, Rosemont IL (Eds). Orthopaedic Knowledge Update. United States: American Academy of Orthopaedic Surgeons; 2002. pp. 51-61.
3. Giudici MA, Moser RP, Kransdorf MJ. Cartilaginous bone tumor. Radiol Clin North Am. 1993;31:237-59.
4. Mirra JM, Picci P, Gold RH. Bone Tumors: Clinical, Radiologic and Pathologic Correlation. Philadelphia: Lea & Febiger; 1989.
5. Steven S, Srinivas K, Javicr B. MR imaging of tumors and tumor like lesions of upper extremity. Magn Reson Imaging Clin North Am. 2004;12:349-59.
6. Holtz P, Sundaram M. Enchondroma. Orthopedics. 1995;18:509-10.
7. Mermelstein LE, Friedlaender GE, Katz LD. Chondroblastoma. Orthopedics. 1997;20:67-71.
8. McGrory BJ, Inwards CY, Mcleod RA. Chondromyxoid fibroma. Orthopedics. 1995;18:307-10.
9. Bloem JL, Kroon HM. Osseous lesions. Radiol Clin North Am. 1993;31:261-65.
10. Assoun J, Riichardi G, Railhac JJ, Baunin C, Fajadet P, Giron J, et al. Osteoid osteoma: MR imaging versus CT. Radiology. 1994;191:217-36.
11. Bruners P, Penzkofer T, Günther RW, Mahnken A. Percutaneous radiofrequency ablation of osteoid osteomas: technique and results. Rofo. 2009;181:740-7.
12. Moulton JS, Bvaley SE, Biedel JS. Bone and soft tissue tumors. In: Edelman RR, Hesselink JR, Zlatkin MB (Eds). Clinical Magnetic Resonance Imaging, 2nd edition. Philadelphia: Saunders; 1996. pp. 2042-77.
13. Lucas E, Sundaram M, Boccini T. Polyostotic fibrous dysplasia. Orthopedics. 1995;18:311-3.

14. Zeanah WR, Hudson TM, Springfield DS. Computed tomography of ossifying fibroma of the tibia. J Comput Assist Tomogr. 1983;7:688-91.
15. Marin C, Warrier RP. Langerhan's cell histiocytosis. Orthop Clin North Am. 1996;27:615-23.
16. Copley L, Dormans JP. Benign pediatric bone tumors. Evaluation and treatment. Pediatr Clin North Am. 1996;43:949-66.
17. Murphey MD, Nomikos GC, Flemming DJ, Gannon FH, Temple HT, Kransdorf MJ. Imaging of giant cell tumor and giant cell reparative granuloma of bone: radiologic-pathologic correlation. Radiographics. 2001;21:1283-309.
18. Conway WF, Hayes CW. Miscellaneous lesions of bone. Radiol Clin North Am. 1993;31:339-58.
19. Brisse H, Orbach D, Klijanienko J, Fréneaux P, Neuenschwander S. Imaging and diagnostic strategy of soft tissue tumors in children. Eur Radiol. 2006;16:1147-64.
20. Mulliken JB, Glowacki J. Hemangiomas and vascular malformations in infants and children: a classification based on endothelial characteristics. Plast Reconstr Surg. 1982;69:412-22.
21. Paltiel HJ, Burrows PE, Kozakewich HPW, Zurakowski D, Mulliken JB. Soft-tissue vascular anomalies: utility of US for diagnosis. Radiology. 2000;214:747-54.
22. Auguste LJ, Razack MS, Sako K. Hemangiopericytoma. J Surg Oncol. 1982;20:260-4.
23. Frieden I, Enjolras O, Esterly N. Vascular birthmarks, other abnormalities of blood vessels and lymphatics. In: Schachner LA, Hansen RC (Eds). Pediatric Dermatology, 3rd edition. New York: Mosby; 2003. pp. 833-62.
24. Konez O, Burrows PE. Magnetic resonance of vascular anomalies. Magn Reson Imaging Clin North Am. 2002;10:363-88.
25. Leung LYJ, Shu SJ, Chan ACL, Chan MK, Chan CHS. Nodular fasciitis: MRI appearance and literature review. Skeletal Radiol. 2002;31:9-13.
26. Siegel MJ. Magnetic resonance imaging of musculoskeletal soft tissue masses. Radiol Clin North Am. 2001;39:701-20.
27. Koujok K, Ruiz RE, Hernandez RJ. Myofibromatosis: imaging characteristics. Pediatr Radiol. 2005;35:374-80.
28. Lee JC, Thomas JM, Phillips S, Fisher C, Moskovic E. Aggressive fibromatosis: MRI features with pathologic correlation. AJR Am J Roentgenol. 2006;186:247-54.
29. Stull MA, Moser RP, Kransdorf MJ, Bogumill GP, Nelson MC. Magnetic resonance appearance of peripheral nerve sheath tumors. Skeletal Radiol. 1991;20:9-14.
30. Fornage BD, Tassin GB. Sonographic appearances of superficial soft tissue lipomas. J Clin Ultrasound. 1991;19:215-20.
31. Miller GG, Yanchar NL, Magee JF, Blair GK. Lipoblastoma and liposarcoma in children: an analysis of 9 cases and a review of the literature. Can J Surg. 1998;41:455-8.
32. Murphey MD, Carroll JF, Flemming DJ, Pope TL, Gannon FH, Kransdorf MJ. From the archives of the AFIP: benign musculoskeletal lipomatous lesions. Radiographics. 2004;24: 1433-66.
33. Tsai TS, Evans HA, Donnelly LF, Bisset GS, Emery KH. Fat necrosis after trauma: a benign cause of palpable lumps in children. AJR Am J Roentgenol. 1997;169:1623-6.
34. Bush CH. The magnetic resonance imaging of musculoskeletal hemorrhage. Skeletal Radiol. 2000;29:1-9.
35. Faingold R, Oudjhane K, Armstrong DC, Albuquerque PAB. Magnetic resonance imaging of congenital, inflammatory, and infectious soft-tissue lesions in children. Top Magn Reson Imaging. 2002;13:241-61.
36. Seymour R, Lloyd DCF. Sonographic appearances of meniscal cysts. J Clin Ultrasound. 1998;26:15-20.
37. McCarthy CL, McNally EG. The MRI appearance of cystic lesions around the knee. Skeletal Radiol. 2004;33:187-209.
38. Einarsdóttir H, Karlsson M, Wejde J, Bauer HC. Diffusion-weighted MRI of soft tissue tumors. Eur Radiol. 2004;14:959-63.
39. Pekcevik Y, Kahya MO, Kaya A. Diffusion-weighted Magnetic Resonance Imaging in the Diagnosis of Bone Tumors: Preliminary Results. J Clin Imaging Sci. 2013;3:63.
40. Rao A, Sharma C, Parampalli R. Role of diffusion-weighted MRI in differentiating benign from malignant bone tumors. BJR Open. 2019;1:20180048.
41. Cao J, Xiao L, He B, Zhang G, Dong J, Wu Y, et al. Diagnostic value of combined diffusion-weighted imaging with dynamic contrast enhancement MRI in differentiating malignant from benign bone lesions. Clin Radiol. 2017;72:793.e1-9.
42. Chai JW, Hong SH, Choi JY, Koh YH, Lee JW, Choi JA, et al. Radiologic diagnosis of osteoid osteoma: from simple to challenging findings. Radiographics. 2010;30:737-49.
43. Fayad LM, Barker PB, Jacobs MA, Eng J, Weber KL, Kulesza P, et al. Characterization of musculoskeletal lesions on 3-T proton MR spectroscopy. AJR Am J Roentgenol. 2007;188:1513-20.
44. Fayad LM, Wang X, Salibi N, Barker PB, Jacobs MA, Machado AJ, et al. A feasibility study of quantitative molecular characterization of musculoskeletal lesions by proton MR spectroscopy at 3 T. AJR Am J Roentgenol. 2010;195:W69-75.
45. Ratnaparkhi CR, Tayade KA, Mitra KR. Magnetic Resonance Spectroscopy of Giant Cell Tumor of Bone. J Clin Diagn Res. 2018;12:TC07-10.

CHAPTER

83

Pediatric Malignant Bone and Soft-tissue Tumors

Ankur Goyal, Manisha Jana, Deep Narayan Srivastava

INTRODUCTION

Malignant bone tumors account for about 6% of all childhood malignancies,[1,2] though malignant soft-tissue tumors are rare in childhood. The most common malignant bone tumors include osteosarcoma and Ewing's sarcoma while rhabdomyosarcoma is the most common pediatric malignant soft-tissue tumor.[3,4] Most of the tumors affect the appendicular skeleton and result in significant morbidity and mortality. **Table 1** shows age distribution of common bone and soft-tissue tumors occurring in children. The most recent World Health Organization (WHO) classification of bone and soft-tissue tumors is the 4th edition (2013).[4] The various malignant bone and soft-tissue tumors are summarized in **Table 2**. Soft-tissue tumors are divided into various groups and each of these is subdivided into benign, intermediate (locally aggressive and rarely metastasizing type), and malignant types.

IMAGING MODALITIES

Plain Radiographs

Radiographs are the primary imaging modality in cases of bone tumors and often a specific diagnosis can be made on plain radiographs alone depending on location of the lesion (**Table 3**). The appearance of the lesion and the patient age remain important considerations for diagnosis. Most of the pediatric malignant bone tumors involve the metaphysis; however, Ewing's sarcoma and lymphoma have a propensity to involve diaphysis. The pattern of bone destruction is a pointer toward the aggressiveness of the lesion. Most malignant bone tumors present radiographically with a permeative lytic or moth-eaten pattern of bone destruction **(Figs. 1A and B)**.

TABLE 1: Age distribution of common pediatric bone and soft-tissue tumors.

Age	Bone tumor	Soft-tissue tumor
Less than 5 years	• Neuroblastoma metastases • Osteosarcoma • Ewing's sarcoma	• Rhabdomyosarcoma • Infantile fibrosarcoma • Kaposiform hemangioendothelioma • Granulocytic sarcoma
More than 5 years	• Osteosarcoma • Ewing's sarcoma • Lymphoma	• Rhabdomyosarcoma • Synovial sarcoma • Undifferentiated sarcomas

In cases of pediatric soft-tissue tumors, plain radiographs are often done as the first modality, though of limited importance. Clinical examination can often prove useful in evaluating small superficial lesions (e.g., lipoma), but for proper assessment of extent of most soft-tissue tumors, radiologic evaluation is imperative.

Sonography

Ultrasonography is useful for characterization of soft-tissue lesions, especially for superficial lesions.[5] Doppler can help in the assessment of vascularity of lesion and also for guided biopsies and in monitoring tumor response to chemotherapy. Ultrasound elastography may also be aid in differentiating between benign and malignant soft-tissue masses. Contrast-enhanced ultrasound provides real-time assessment of tumor vascularity without any radiation exposure or nephrotoxicity.

Computed Tomography

Among the cross-sectional imaging, role of computed tomography (CT) has considerably reduced after the introduction of magnetic resonance imaging (MRI). However, CT is superior to MRI in the detection and characterization of matrix mineralization, cortical changes, bone trabeculation, and periosteal reaction. Though soft-tissue resolution is poor, CT may demonstrate calcification, fat attenuation, and hyperdensity (suggesting hemorrhage) in soft-tissue masses. CT angiography may help in identifying arterial feeders as well as show vascular involvement **(Fig. 2A)**. Noncontrast CT of chest is also used in the detection of pulmonary metastases.

Magnetic Resonance Imaging

The role of MRI in pediatric bone tumors includes accurate assessment of the extent of the lesion, evaluation of skip

TABLE 2: Malignant bone and soft-tissue tumors as per the WHO classification 2013.

Bone tumors	Soft-tissue tumors
• *Osteogenic*: Osteosarcoma	• *Adipocytic*: Liposarcoma
• *Chondrogenic*: Chondrosarcoma	• *Fibroblastic/Myofibroblastic*: Fibrosarcoma
• Ewing's sarcoma	• *Skeletal muscle differentiation*: Rhabdomyosarcoma
• Undifferentiated high-grade pleomorphic sarcoma	• *Smooth muscle differentiation*: Leiomyosarcoma
• *Hematopoietic neoplasms*: Primary non-Hodgkin lymphoma, plasmacytoma, and myeloma	• *Chondro-osseous*: Mesenchymal chondrosarcoma, extraosseous osteosarcoma
• *Osteoclastic giant cell-rich tumors*: Malignancy in GCT	• *Pericytic*: Malignant glomus tumor
• *Notochordal tumors*: Chordoma	• Malignant peripheral nerve sheath tumors
• *Vascular tumors*: Angiosarcoma, epithelioid hemangioendothelioma	• *Vascular tumors*: Angiosarcoma, epithelioid hemangioendothelioma
• *Fibrogenic*: Fibrosarcoma	• *Tumors of uncertain differentiation*: Synovial sarcoma, alveolar soft part sarcoma, and extraskeletal Ewing's sarcoma
• *Rare*: Liposarcoma, leiomyosarcomas	• *Undifferentiated/Unclassified sarcomas*: Undifferentiated pleomorphic sarcoma

(GCT: giant cell tumor; WHO: World Health Organization)

TABLE 3: Common locations of primary malignant bone tumors.

Location	Tumors
Metaphysis	• Osteosarcoma • Metastases • Ewing's sarcoma • Lymphoma
Diaphysis	• Ewing's sarcoma • Lymphoma
Epiphysis	Aggressive giant cell tumor (rare)

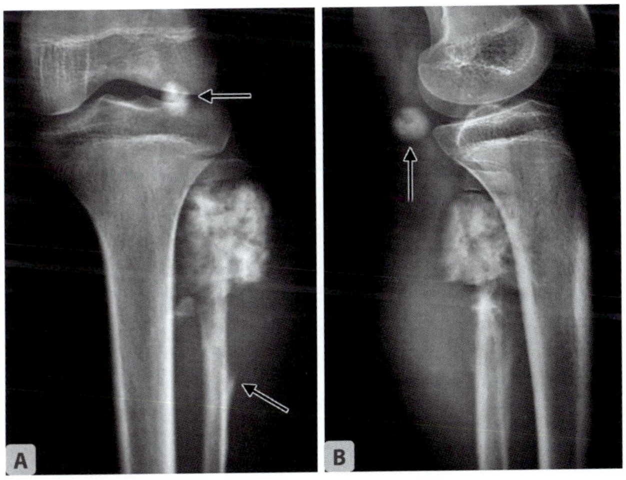

FIGS. 1A AND B: (A) Anteroposterior (AP) and (B) lateral radiographs of the left leg show permeative lytic destruction of proximal fibular metaphysis, cloud-like osteoid matrix, periosteal reaction, and Codman triangle (thin arrow), typical imaging features of a malignant bone tumor with large soft-tissue component. Metastatic popliteal lymph node (block arrow) also shows osteoid matrix. Histopathology: osteosarcoma.

lesions, and neurovascular and articular involvement **(Figs. 2B to F)**. T1-weighted (T1W) spin echo images remain the most important sequence to assess the intraosseous tumor extent **(Figs. 3A and 4A)**, owing to the contrast between normal hyperintense fatty marrow and hypointense tumor.[6] Inversion recovery sequence (short tau inversion recovery—STIR) sequence makes the tumor more conspicuous by suppressing normal marrow fat as the hyperintense tumor stands bright **(Figs. 3B and 4B)**. Postcontrast images (after gadolinium administration) can define the exact extent of the tumor, define viable tumor and the necrotic areas,[7] and help in tumor edema differentiation **(Fig. 2E)**.[8] Peritumoral edema can either be intraosseous or extraosseous and often show high signal on T2-weighted (T2W) or STIR images. In the bones, edema has poorly defined margin and often difficult to differentiate from the tumor mass. In the soft tissues, edema does not have mass effect and follows muscle and fascial planes.

Magnetic resonance imaging is the modality of choice for evaluation of soft-tissue lesions. In addition to accurately characterizing fat and blood, other paradigms like diffusion-weighted imaging, time-resolved MR angiography, and dynamic contrast-enhanced imaging provide additional diagnostically useful information—not to mention, better soft-tissue contrast and delineation of masses. Most of the malignant bone and soft-tissue tumors share common similar imaging features, e.g., they are hypointense on T1W and hyperintense on T2W images.[9-12] However, few lesions show characteristic signal intensities, e.g., fat-containing lesions are bright on T1W as well as T2W sequences and fibrous tumors may show hypointense signal on both T1 and T2W images. In bone tumors, the role of imaging is to identify that the likely diagnosis is malignant, suggest the likely histology, delineate local extent, and stage the malignant masses. The role of imaging in soft-tissue masses is to identify the benign masses and those with characteristic features, suggest differentials, stage the lesions, and to plan a way to sample the indeterminate ones.

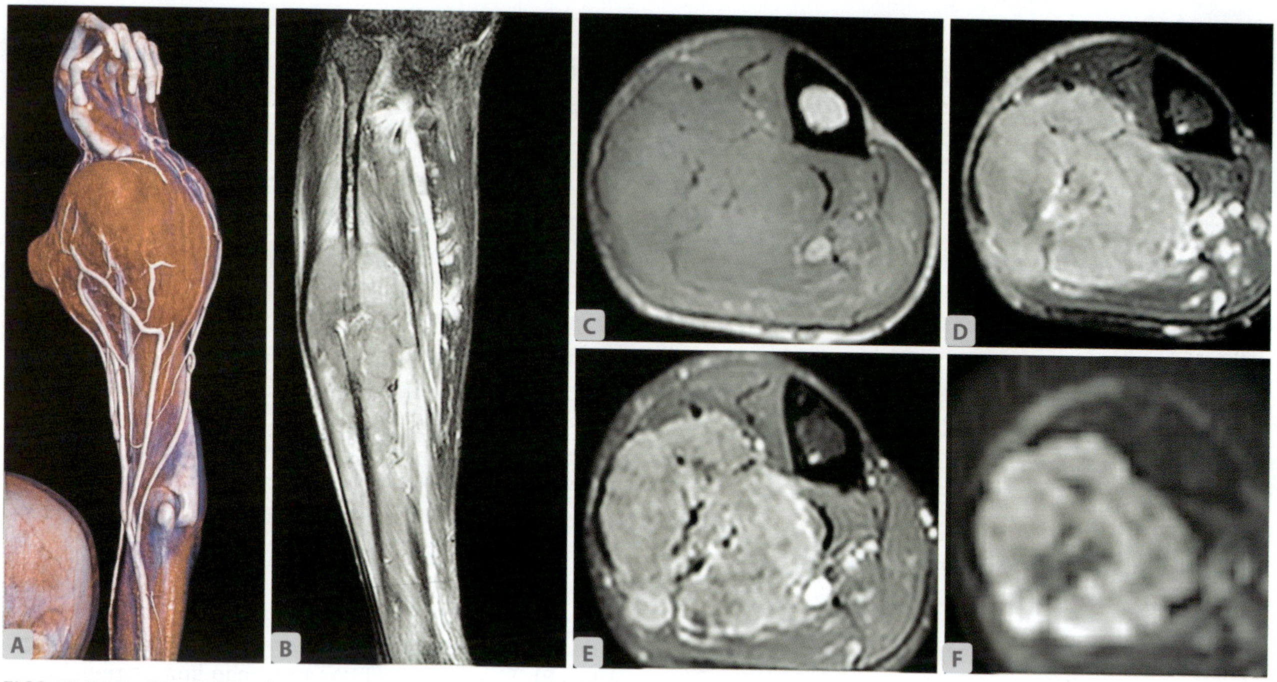

FIGS. 2A TO F: CT and MRI in bone tumors. (A) Volume-rendered image generated from CT angiography dataset in a case of osteosarcoma. Distal end of radius shows multiple feeders from radial and ulnar arteries; and (B to F) Different patient with Ewing's sarcoma of fibula. (B) STIR coronal; (C) Axial T1W; (D) T2W; (E) Postcontrast; and (F) High b-value diffusion-weighted images show homogeneous T2 hyperintense tumor with soft-tissue extension and marked diffusion restriction. (CT: computed tomography; MRI: magnetic resonance imaging; STIR: short tau inversion recovery; T1W: T1-weighted; T2W: T2-weighted)

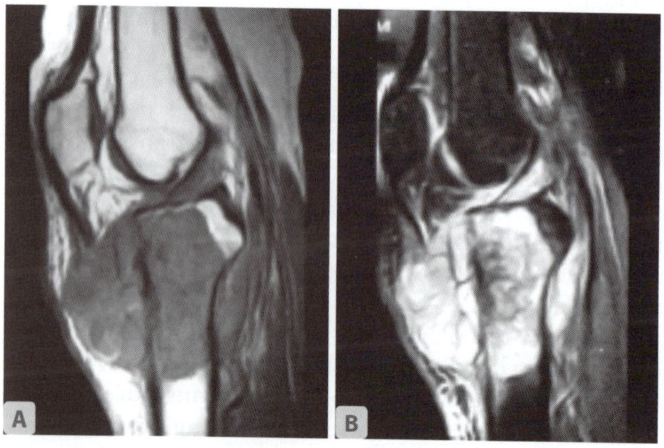

FIGS. 3A AND B: (A) Sagittal T1W and (B) T2W MR of a case of osteosarcoma. The tumor is hypointense in contrast to hyperintense fatty marrow on T1W and hyperintense on T2W fat-suppressed sequences. The tumor has an extra compartmental extension into the muscle plane. (MR: magnetic resonance; T1W: T1-weighted; T2W: T2-weighted)

Magnetic Resonance Imaging Techniques for Bone and Soft-tissue Tumors

The sequences should include T1W images in coronal or sagittal plane for accurate delineation of tumor extent **(Figs. 3A, 4A, and 4C)**, identify skip lesions, and articular involvement in bone tumors, if any. T2W fat-saturated or STIR images are useful for better demonstration of soft-tissue relationships with adjacent muscles, nerves, and vascular structures **(Figs. 3B, 4B, and 4D)**. Axial gradient-echo images **(Fig. 4E)** may be acquired to better depict the vessels in relation to the tumor.

In case of soft-tissue neoplasms, initial wide field of view images (STIR and T1W) are acquired in coronal plane. Then, axial T1W and T2W fat-suppressed (FS) images are acquired. T1W FS and T2W non-FS may also be needed in case of T1 hyperintense masses **(Figs. 5A to C)**. Diffusion-weighted imaging may aid in diagnosing malignant lesions. **Table 4** shows the suggested MRI protocol for evaluation of bone and soft-tissue tumors.

Role of Contrast-enhanced Magnetic Resonance Imaging

In primary bone tumors, contrast administration is usually not required because the role of MRI is for staging. However, in soft-tissue masses, contrast administration is often useful to assess lesion vascularity and identify solid-enhancing areas for sampling **(Figs. 5D to F)**. Dynamic contrast-enhanced MRI is useful in angiography and specifically helpful in detecting tumor recurrence,[13] which often shows early contrast enhancement and washout. MR angiography may also be done to look for vessel involvement in equivocal cases and also to identify feeders in case preoperative embolization needs to be done **(Figs. 5D to F)**. The time-intensity curves may correlate with malignant lesions or with assessing treatment response. In soft-tissue lesions, whenever contrast is administered, it may be useful to do dynamic acquisition because it gives additional useful information about the perfusion kinetics without adding significant time to the study.

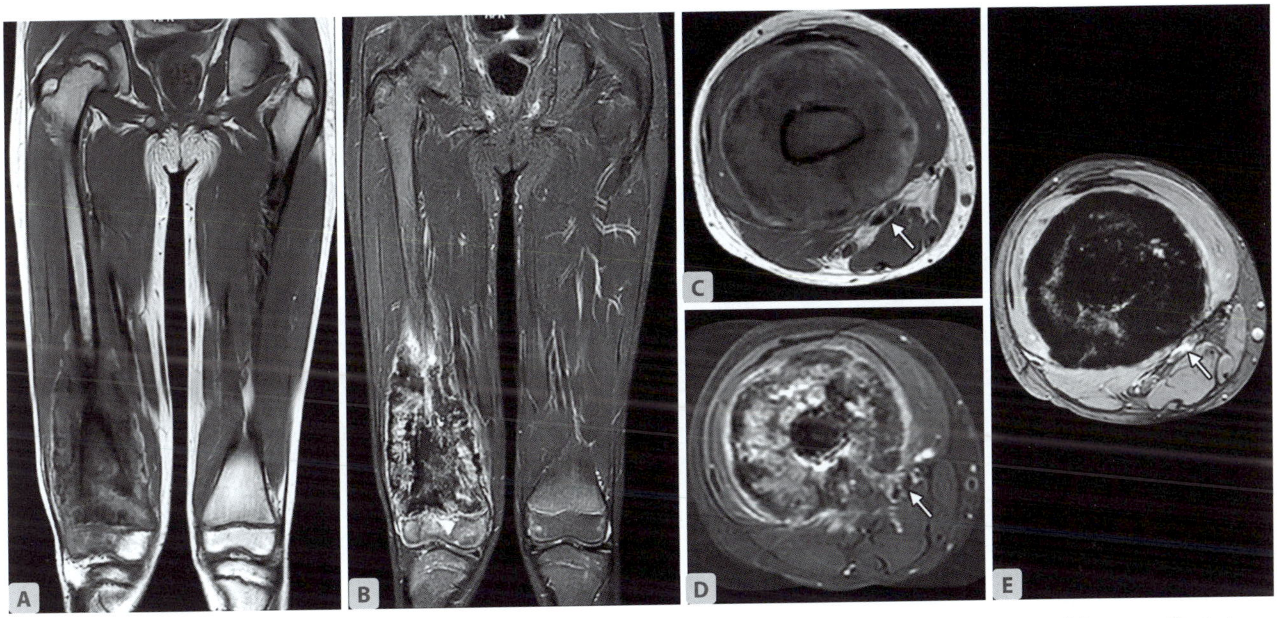

FIGS. 4A TO E: MRI in osteosarcoma right distal femur. (A and B) Coronal T1W and STIR images show craniocaudal extent of the tumor. The lesion does not involve the epiphysis and no skip lesions are seen; (C) Axial T1W; (D) T2W FS; and (E) Gradient-echo images show femoral vessels are normal (arrow) with preserved fat plane with the tumor. (FS: fat-suppressed; MRI: magnetic resonance imaging; STIR: short tau inversion recovery; T1W: T1-weighted; T2W: T2-weighted)

Other Magnetic Resonance Imaging Techniques

Diffusion-weighted Magnetic Resonance Imaging

Diffusion-weighted MRI may prove useful to rule out nontumorous conditions, suggest cellular areas to be targeted for biopsy and predict the tumor viability after treatment and hence, to reflect the response to treatment **(Fig. 2F)**.[13] After treatment, many times, the tumor bulk may not reduce significantly but the apparent diffusion coefficient (ADC) value increases[14] indicating response to treatment.

Dynamic Contrast-enhanced Magnetic Resonance Imaging

Dynamic contrast-enhanced MRI is a new addition in the imaging of malignant bone tumors, especially osteosarcoma. It measures the tumor viability by determining the contrast accumulation within the tumor. It is more useful for soft-tissue sarcomas. Dynamic contrast-enhanced MRI assessment of dynamic vector magnitude (based on contrast accumulation rate over time and maximal intensity of the tumor) and Kep (measure of the gadolinium exchange between the vascular and the interstitial space) tends to predict the outcome after the treatment.[15]

Magnetic Resonance Spectroscopy

In vivo proton MR spectroscopy is a promising modality in the evaluation of malignant bone and soft-tissue tumors. On MR spectroscopy, these tumors show choline peak (resonance at 3.2 ppm),[16] which is highly sensitive and specific.

STAGING OF MALIGNANT BONE AND SOFT-TISSUE TUMORS

The Enneking system of staging malignant bone and soft-tissue tumors[17] **(Table 5)** was based on three criteria: (1) extent of tumor [T1 suggests an intracompartmental tumor, T2 suggests an extracompartmental spread **(Figs. 3A and B)**], (2) presence or absence of metastases (M0 and M1, respectively), and (3) histologic grade of the tumor (low-grade G1, high-grade G2). Low-grade tumors (stage IA or IB, T1G1M0 or T2G1M0) are candidates for wide local excision or limb salvage surgeries. High-grade tumor (G2) without metastases is treated with radical surgeries like amputation.

In 1983, the American Joint Committee on Cancer (AJCC) developed another system of staging of bone and soft-tissue tumors depending on four criteria: (1) Extent of tumor (confined by bone cortex T1, with transcortical extension T2), (2) Nodal disease (N0 no nodal disease, N1 regional nodal spread), (3) Metastases (absence of metastases M0, presence of metastases M1), and (4) Histologic grade of tumor (G1—well-differentiated tumor, G2—moderately differentiated tumor, G3—poorly differentiated tumor, and G4—undifferentiated tumor). Bone and soft-tissue tumors are, thus, unique in the fact that these sarcomas are the only tumors where grade is taken into consideration for staging by the AJCC; in rest only, tumor, necrosis, and metastasis (TNM) staging exists.

The recent revision in this staging is the 8th edition, adopted in 2018 and there are multiple changes compared with prior editions.[18] Now, staging of bone sarcomas is different depending on location: spine, pelvis, and rest (trunk, appendicular skeleton, skull, and face). Similarly,

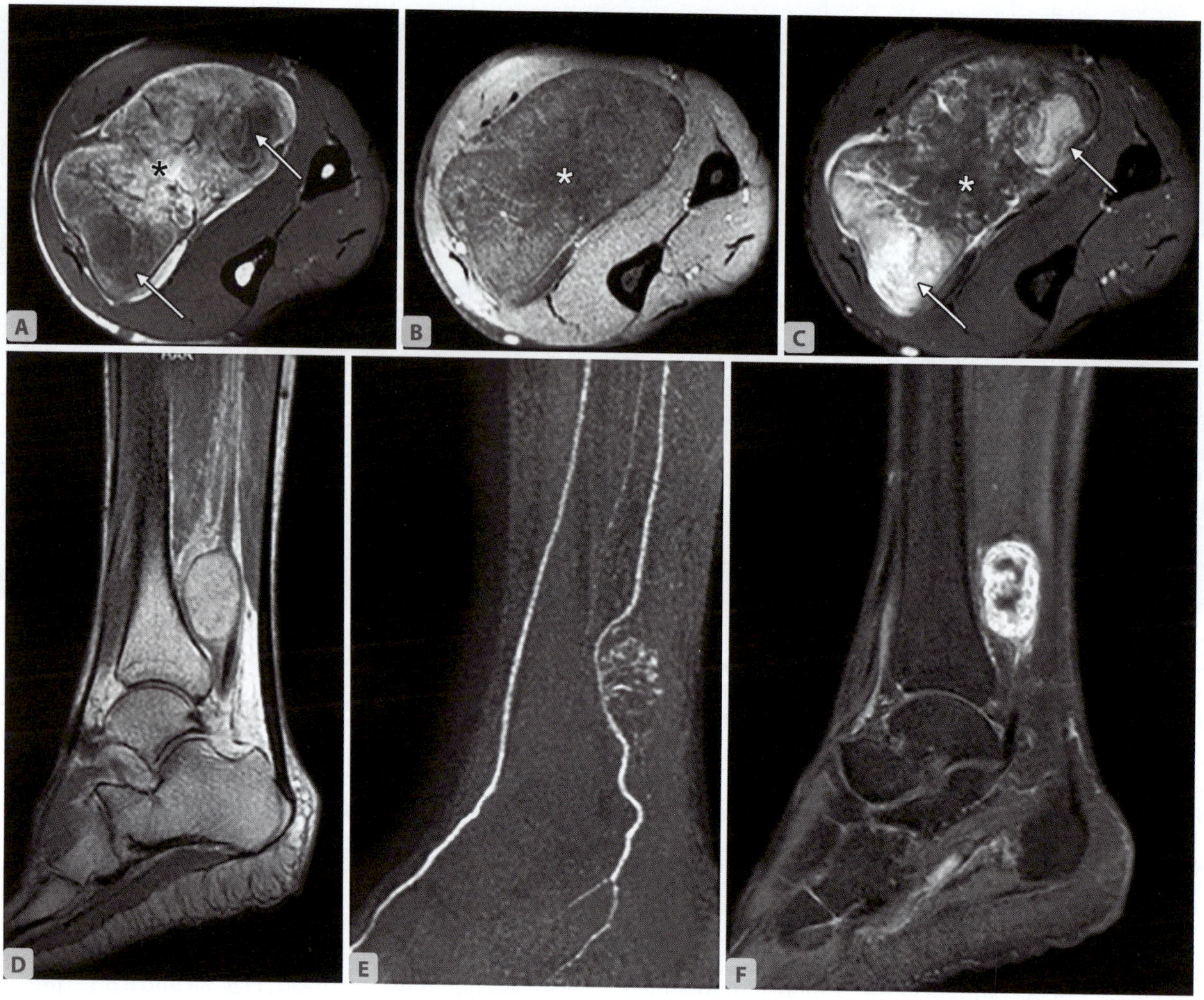

FIGS. 5A TO F: MRI in soft-tissue neoplasms. (A) Axial T1W; (B) T1W FS; and (C) T2W FS images of forearm show a large lesion in flexor compartment showing fat signal intensity areas (asterisks) and nonfatty soft-tissue areas (arrows) in a case of well-differentiated liposarcoma; and (D to F) Another patient with peripheral nerve sheath tumor arising from tibial nerve; (D) Sagittal T2W; (E) MR angiography; and (F) Postcontrast images show well-defined encapsulated oval lesion in continuity with the nerve with split fat sign and showing arterial feeders and intense heterogeneous enhancement. (FS: fat-suppressed; MRI: magnetic resonance imaging; T1W: T1-weighted; T2W: T2-weighted)

TABLE 4: Suggested MRI protocol for malignant bone tumors and soft-tissue tumors.

Suggested MRI protocol for malignant bone tumors	Suggested MRI protocol for soft-tissue tumors
• Large field of view (FOV) coronal T1W and STIR (include proximal and distal joint) • Axial T2W fat-suppressed (FS), T1W ± Gradient-echo (GRE) sequence (MEDIC) • Sagittal STIR/T1W *Optional*: • Diffusion-weighted imaging (DWI) • *Contrast-enhanced MRI*: To identify enhancing areas: usually in at least two planes • MR angiography for feeders/doubtful vascular involvement *Assessment of treatment response*: • Dynamic contrast-enhanced MRI • DWI	• Coronal T1W and STIR • Axial T2FS, T2, and T1 (±T1FS) • Sagittal STIR/T1W • Dynamic contrast-enhanced MRI/Time-resolved MR angiography • Postcontrast MRI in at least two planes (with option to subtract precontrast sequence from it) *Optional*: • DWI • Axial GRE sequence like MEDIC

(MEDIC: Multiple Echo Data Image Combination; MRI: magnetic resonance imaging; STIR: short tau inversion recovery; T1W: T1-weighted) for soft-tissue sarcomas, staging depends on location: trunk and extremity, head and neck, retroperitoneum, and viscera. Histological grading has been reduced to three grades instead of four grades: low grade (well-differentiated), intermediate and high grade (poorly differentiated), and latter two are clubbed together as high grade. Size of the lesion is a determining factor for T stage of both bone and soft-tissue sarcomas and depends on the location as well. Skip lesions in bone tumors (noncontiguous neoplastic lesions in the primary bone site) are considered T3 while metastases to other bones taken as M1b. Lymph node and extrapulmonary metastases (including bone metastases) have poorest prognosis in bone tumors, thus these are classified as stage IVb while lung metastases are classified as stage IVa. Depth of the lesion is no longer included in the staging of soft-tissue sarcomas. Primary bone lymphoma and myeloma are not included in the AJCC staging.

TABLE 5: Enneking staging for primary malignant bone and soft-tissue tumors.

Stages	Tumor	Metastases	Histologic grade
IA	T1 (intracompartmental tumor)	M0	G1
IB	T2 (extracompartmental tumor)	M0	G1
IIA	T1	M0	G2
IIB	T2	M0	G2
III	T1 or T2	M1	G1 or G2

MALIGNANT BONE TUMORS

Osteosarcoma

Osteosarcoma is the most common pediatric malignant bone tumor,[19] usually affecting children in the second decade. Patients with retinoblastoma, Li-Fraumeni syndrome, and prior radiation therapy are more prone to develop osteosarcoma. The usual clinical presentation is with a painful extremity mass. Serum alkaline phosphatase is increased in 50% of the patients.

Histologic subgroups in central osteosarcoma include conventional osteosarcoma (most common, subdivided into osteoblastic, chondroblastic, and fibroblastic), low-grade telangiectatic, and small cell type.[20] Conventional osteoblastic type is the most common. Low-grade type occurs in young adults and histologically mimics fibrous dysplasia. Surface osteosarcomas can be parosteal, periosteal, or high grade. Periosteal type occurs in second decade while parosteal type occurs late in third decade.

Plain radiographs are usually the first investigation performed. Osteosarcoma in pediatric age groups predominantly involves the metaphyses of long bones (femur and tibia most commonly involved). On radiographs, they present with a permeative lytic destruction with wide zone of transition, blastic lesion, or a mixed pattern **(Figs. 1 and 6)**. Often, there is an associated soft-tissue component, “sunburst” type of periosteal reaction, “Codman triangle” formation, and an osteoid tumor (cloud-like amorphous) matrix mineralization **(Figs. 1 and 6)**. Telangiectatic type presents as well-demarcated predominantly lytic lesion with aneurysmal expansion of the underlying bone and osteoid matrix is relatively less common.

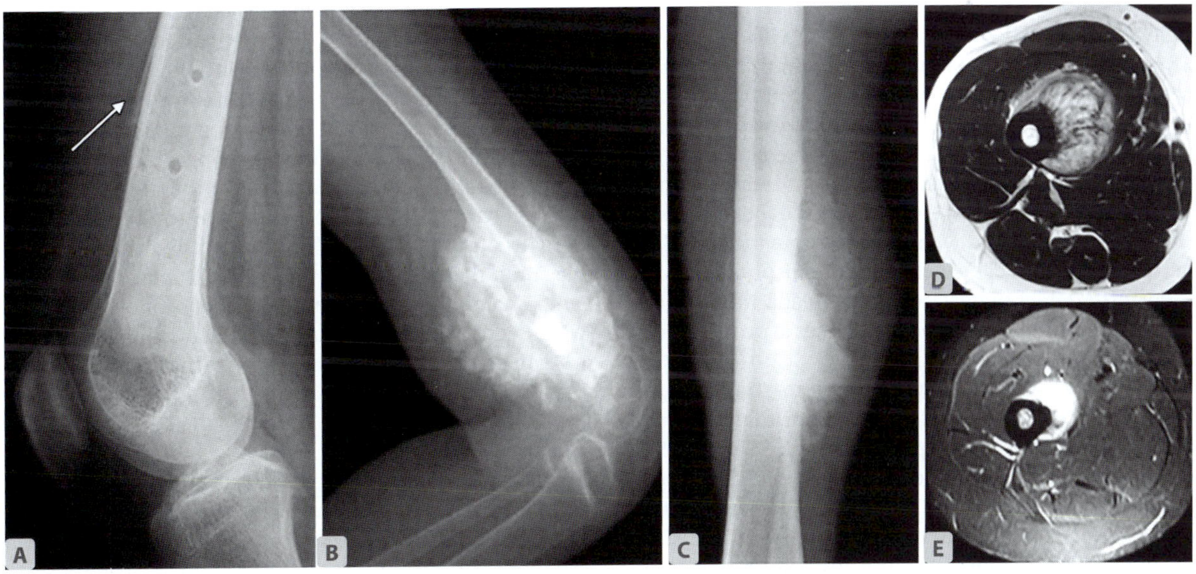

FIGS. 6A TO E: Variable appearances of osteosarcoma (OS). (A) Interrupted periosteal reaction (Codman triangle) (arrow); (B) Dense cloud-like osteoid matrix; and (C to E) Periosteal OS: Densely ossified extraosseous mass with broad base toward cortex; (D) Axial T2W and (E) T2W FS images show the cortical-based tumor along with marrow involvement. No cleft is seen with the cortex. (FS: fat-suppressed; T2W: T2-weighted)

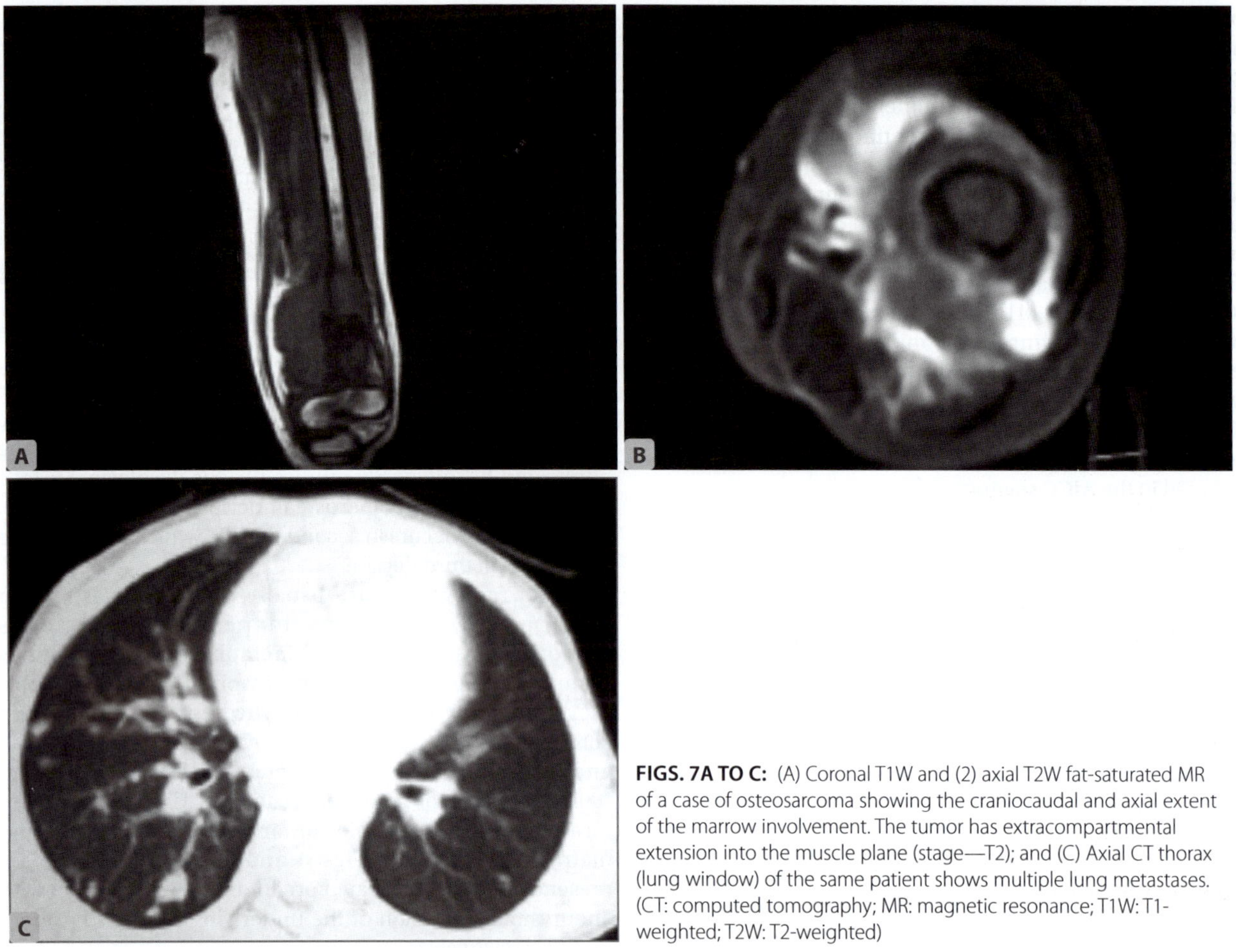

FIGS. 7A TO C: (A) Coronal T1W and (2) axial T2W fat-saturated MR of a case of osteosarcoma showing the craniocaudal and axial extent of the marrow involvement. The tumor has extracompartmental extension into the muscle plane (stage—T2); and (C) Axial CT thorax (lung window) of the same patient shows multiple lung metastases. (CT: computed tomography; MR: magnetic resonance; T1W: T1-weighted; T2W: T2-weighted)

Pathological fractures are more common in a telangiectatic variety which often presents with well-defined lytic involvement. Periosteal tumors present as broad-based diaphyseal masses causing extrinsic erosion of underlying thickened cortex and perpendicular periosteal reaction **(Figs. 6A to E)**. These wrap around the bone circumference. Parosteal tumors are separated from the underlying bone by a thin lucent line (cleft sign) and occur in the metaphysis.

The workup of a child with osteosarcoma includes CT of chest **(Figs. 7A to C)**, ^{99m}Tc methylene diphosphonate (MDP) bone scan (to detect metastases as it spreads via the bloodstream and about 20% may have metastases at presentation),[6] and MRI for the local tumor extent.

Magnetic resonance imaging tends to show accurate intramedullary extent of the tumor. Tumor mass is usually hypointense on T1W and hyperintense on T2W and STIR images. The osteoid matrix is dark on all sequences **(Figs. 4 and 7)**. The rare telangiectatic variety may present as purely lytic well-defined lesion without osteoid matrix and shows blood-fluid levels secondary to intratumoral hemorrhage[3] **(Fig. 8)**. Skip lesions within the same bone may be seen in 15% of cases.

Features to distinguish telangiectatic osteosarcoma from aneurysmal bone cyst include osteoid matrix, thick nodular septae, enhancing component, and progression on serial imaging. Osteosarcomas can occur in patients of retinoblastoma either due to genetic predisposition or as a result of radiotherapy **(Figs. 9A and B)**.

Survival and response to chemotherapy depends on the tumor burden which can be measured by tumor size. Histologic response to preoperative neoadjuvant chemotherapy (percent of necrosis) is the strongest predictor of survival.[21-23] Often, the tumor size remains unchanged after treatment and it is difficult to determine response based on the size criteria.[15] Newer MR imaging techniques which help in predicting tumor response include diffusion-weighted images and dynamic contrast-enhanced MRI. With treatment, the ADC of the tumor mass increases.[14]

Ewing's Sarcoma

Ewing's family of tumors includes classic Ewing's sarcoma, primitive neuroectodermal tumor (PNET), Askin tumor (PNET of the chest wall), extraosseous Ewing's tumor, and peripheral neuroepithelioma. All these tumors have a common neuroectodermal origin and frequently seen in children.

Classic Ewing's sarcoma is the second most common bone malignancy in children, predominantly seen in the second and third decade of life. Males and females have equal incidence. Usual clinical presentation is with local pain and swelling, often with constitutional symptoms. Laboratory investigations may show elevated erythrocyte sedimentation rate and leukocytosis; hence, the clinical picture often mimics osteomyelitis.

Metadiaphyses of the long bones and flat bones of pelvis are the most common site for Ewing's sarcoma. On plain radiographs, the tumor presents as a permeative lytic bone destruction with a wide zone of transition, cortical destruction **(Figs. 10A and B)**, onion-peel type of periosteal reaction, and often extensive noncalcified soft-tissue mass.[24] Saucerization of the outer cortex may occur due to erosions by tumor growth in the subperiosteal region. In cases of flat bone involvement, the soft-tissue component is larger than osseous destruction. CT scan, though not commonly indicated, can define the bony destruction **(Figs. 11 and 12)**. However, chest CT is done to detect pulmonary metastasis. Radionuclide study is useful in the detection of bone metastasis. The differential diagnoses include osteomyelitis and other malignant bone sarcomas. A characteristic feature of highly cellular aggressive round cell tumors (like Ewing's sarcoma and lymphoma) is presence of significant soft-tissue component with little cortical destruction. This occurs because neoplastic cells permeate through the small cortical vascular channels and haversian canals.

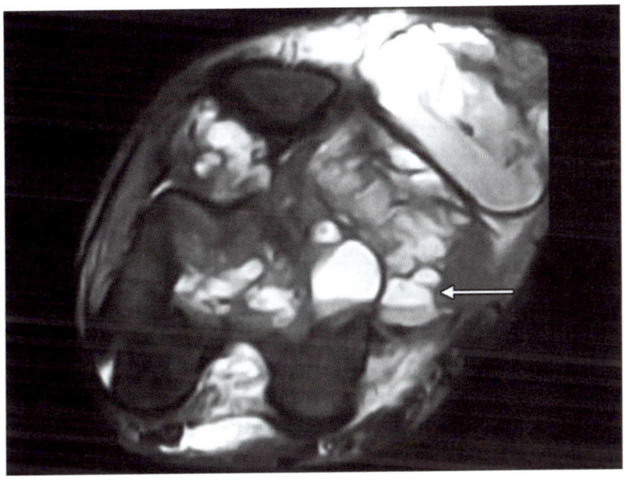

FIG. 8: Axial T2W fat-saturated MR image in a case of telangiectatic osteosarcoma showing multiple areas of blood-fluid levels (white arrow) suggesting intratumoral hemorrhage. (MR: magnetic resonance; T2W: T2-weighted)

On T1W-MRI, the mass is isointense to mildly hypointense; on T2W or STIR images, it is hyperintense **(Figs. 13A and B)** and shows variable contrast enhancement. The tumor is relatively homogeneous and cellular, thus appears only mildly hyperintense on T2W images and shows marked diffusion restriction. Skip lesions may be present in 14% cases.[24] The soft-tissue mass tends to decrease in size and undergoes necrosis with treatment. As with osteosarcoma, diffusion-weighted MRI and dynamic contrast-enhanced MRI can predict the response to neoadjuvant chemotherapy or radiotherapy.[23] Positron emission tomography (PET) is also used in monitoring response to therapy and metastatic disease.

Primitive neuroectodermal tumor of the chest wall (Askin tumor) **(Figs. 14 and 15)** usually presents with an intrathoracic extrapulmonary mass having single rib involvement and extrathoracic component. They are hypointense on T1W and hyperintense on T2W images, showing moderate contrast enhancement. Multiplanar imaging using MRI or CT is helpful in determining the extent of the soft-tissue mass.

Chondrosarcoma

Chondrosarcoma is rare in pediatric age group and should be differentiated from the chondroblastic variety of osteosarcoma. It predominantly involves the flat bones of pelvis and shoulder girdle followed by metaphyses of long bones, ribs, and spine. The tumors can either be primary or secondary. Secondary tumors may develop

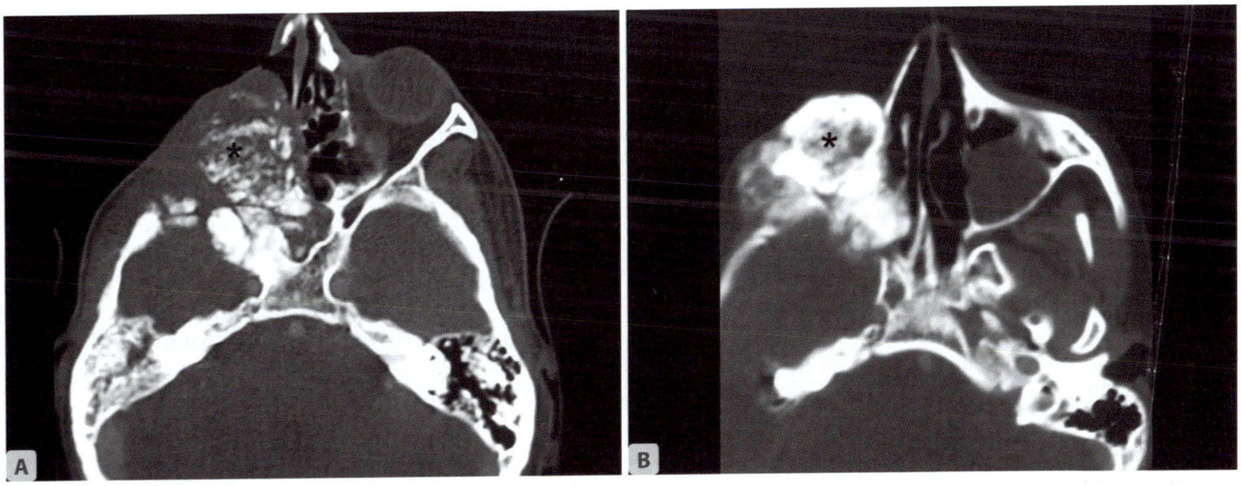

FIGS. 9A AND B: Osteosarcoma developing as a second primary tumor in a child with retinoblastoma. Computed tomography (CT) of the orbits bone window images: osteoblastic tumor arising from the lateral wall of right orbit. Note the dense cloud-like matrix (asterisk). Right globe is not visualized (enucleated).

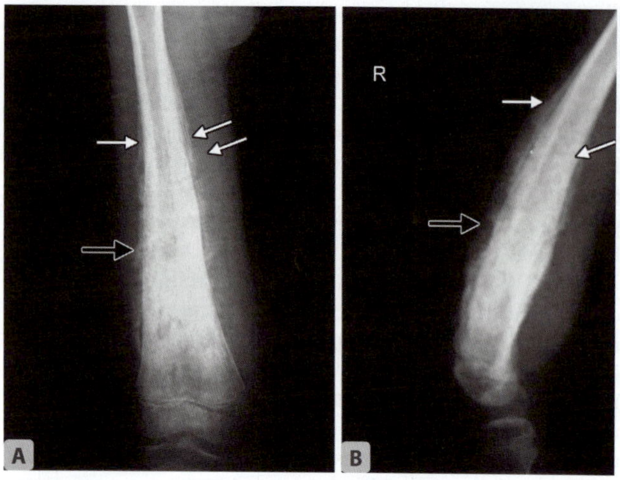

FIGS. 10A AND B: Ewing's sarcoma of femur in a 11-year-old boy. Ill-defined permeative involvement of lower femoral metadiaphyseal region with linear interrupted periosteal reaction (arrows) around and "sunburst" appearance (block arrows).

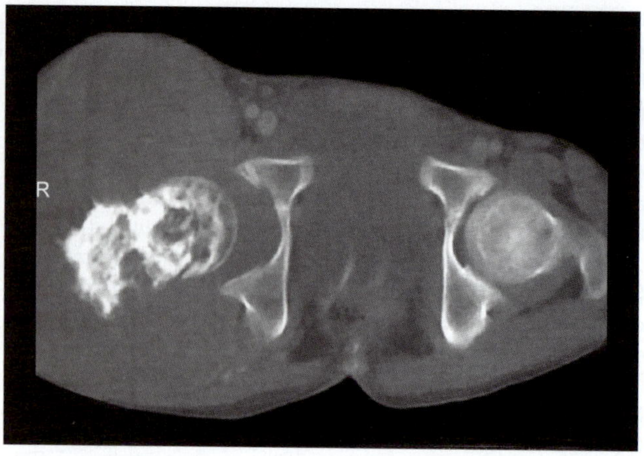

FIG. 11: PNET of the right femur; Axial CT scan bone window reconstruction reveals mixed lytic-sclerotic destruction of the right femoral head and neck with adjacent large soft tissue. (CT: computed tomography; PNET: primitive neuroectodermal tumor)

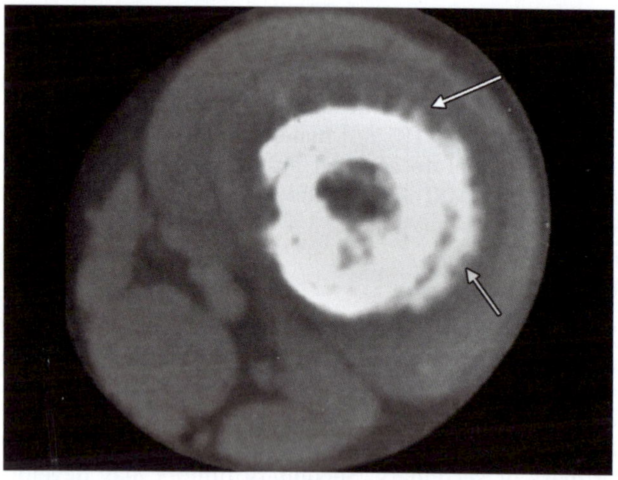

FIG. 12: Ewing's sarcoma; Axial computed tomography (CT) bone window reconstruction reveals permeative lytic destruction of the femoral diaphysis, with spiculated periosteal reaction (arrows) and associated soft tissue.

in osteochondromas, especially in genetic diseases like hereditary multiple exostosis where the risk of malignant transformation is approximately 2.7%.[25] On radiographs, they are usually expansile lytic lesions with variable matrix mineralization (chondroid rings and arcs or punctate type) **(Figs. 16A and B)**. On MR imaging, they show low signal intensity on T1W images. The signal on T2W images is variable, depending on the matrix mineralization. Cartilaginous matrix is characteristically bright on T2W images whereas areas of calcification and hemorrhage are hypointense.[26] The bright cartilaginous areas usually show peripheral/septal calcification.

The indicators of malignant transformation of osteochondromas and enchondromas include the following:

- Heterogeneity in mineralization/new lucency on radiographs
- Cortical destruction and/or soft-tissue mass
- Ill-defined margins
- Cartilaginous cap destruction or thickening (>2 cm in children)
- Any growth or increased pain after skeletal maturity
- Peritumoral edema
- Endosteal scalloping greater than two-thirds of the cortical width in long bones.

The conventional type of chondrosarcoma seldom occurs in children. Clear cell variant occurs in children and may mimic chondroblastoma because it tends to involve epiphyses of femur and humerus. Large areas of hemorrhage and cystic change can also occur. Mesenchymal, myxoid, and juxtacortical variants also involve younger age groups.

Lymphoma

Primary bone lymphoma comprises 5% of all children with lymphoma and most of them are high-grade B-cell non-Hodgkin lymphoma (NHL).[20] Usual locations include the spine and the long bones. On imaging, they commonly show permeative lytic destruction, sometimes with periosteal reaction and commonly associated with soft-tissue component. Frank cortical destruction is often not evident and the lesions are easily missed on radiographs.[27] Hodgkin's disease can cause sclerotic bony lesions and characteristic "ivory" vertebra. MRI reveals the marrow of the affected bone to be hypointense on T1W and mildly hyperintense on T2W images, enhancing after contrast **(Figs. 17A and B)**. For primary bone lymphoma, medullary cavity of a single bone should be involved without any lymphadenopathy or visceral involvement. CT chest and abdomen need to be done to exclude disseminated lymphoma.

Secondary bone lymphoma is more common than primary bone lymphoma, especially in children. The incidence can be as high as 25% in children. Secondary skeletal involvement in Hodgkin's disease is usually from contiguous lymph nodal spread and the lesions are more commonly sclerotic. In

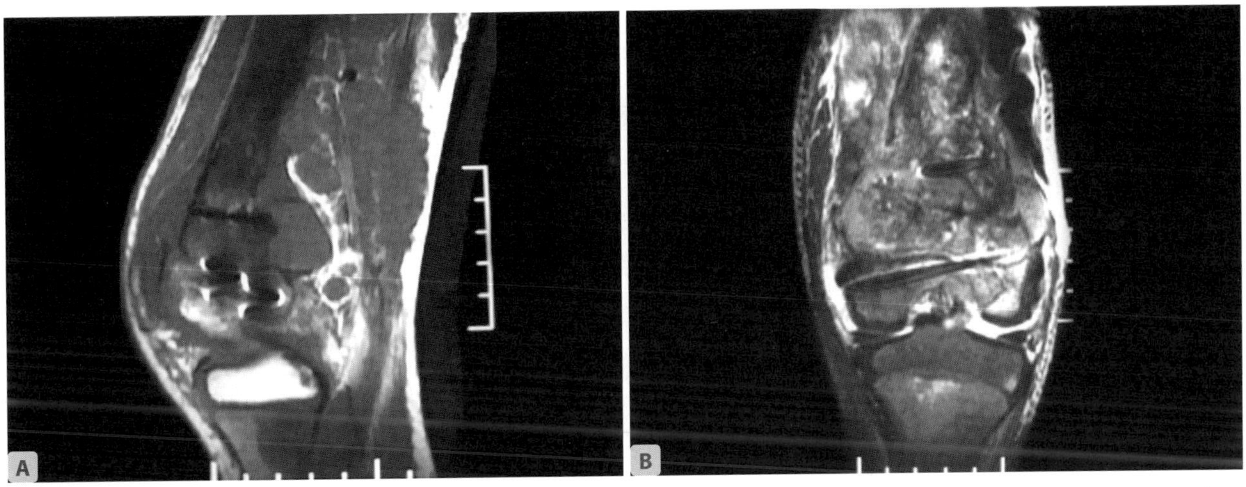

FIGS. 13A AND B: (A) Sagittal T1W and (B) coronal T2W MR of a case of Ewing's sarcoma. The tumor is hypointense on T1 and heterogeneously hyperintense on T2 with diffuse marrow infiltration and extraosseous spread. (MR: magnetic resonance; T1W: T1-weighted; T2W: T2-weighted)

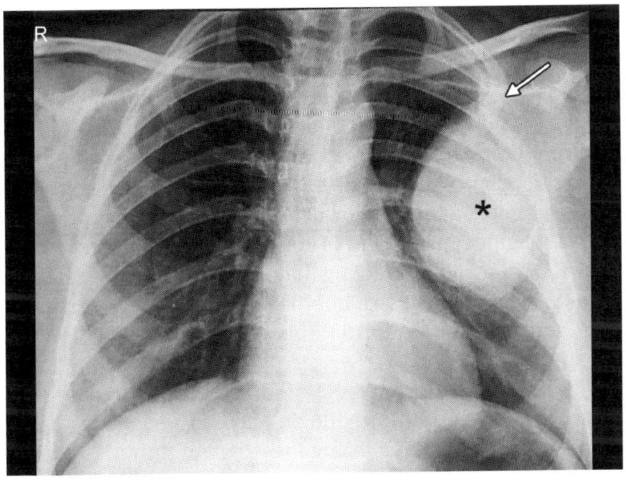

FIG. 14: Primitive neuroectodermal tumor (PNET) of the chest wall. Left-sided second rib shows expansile lytic destruction (arrow) with a large soft-tissue mass (asterisk).

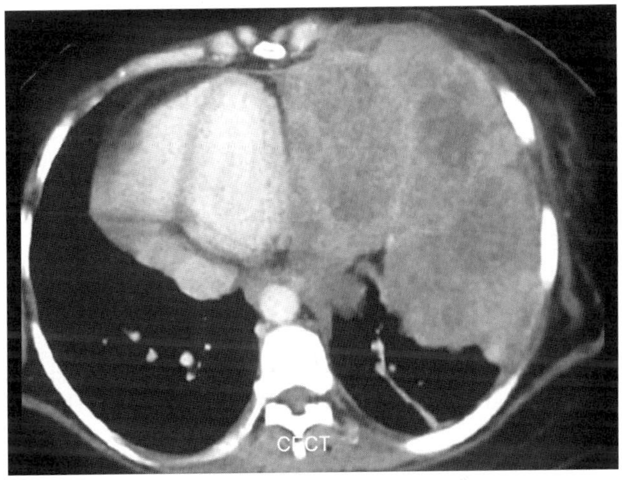

FIG. 15: PNET of the left thoracic wall (Askin tumor). Axial image of CECT thorax mediastinal window shows a large heterogeneous mass lesion in the left hemithorax with a small extrathoracic component. (CECT: contrast-enhanced computed tomography; PNET: primitive neuroectodermal tumor)

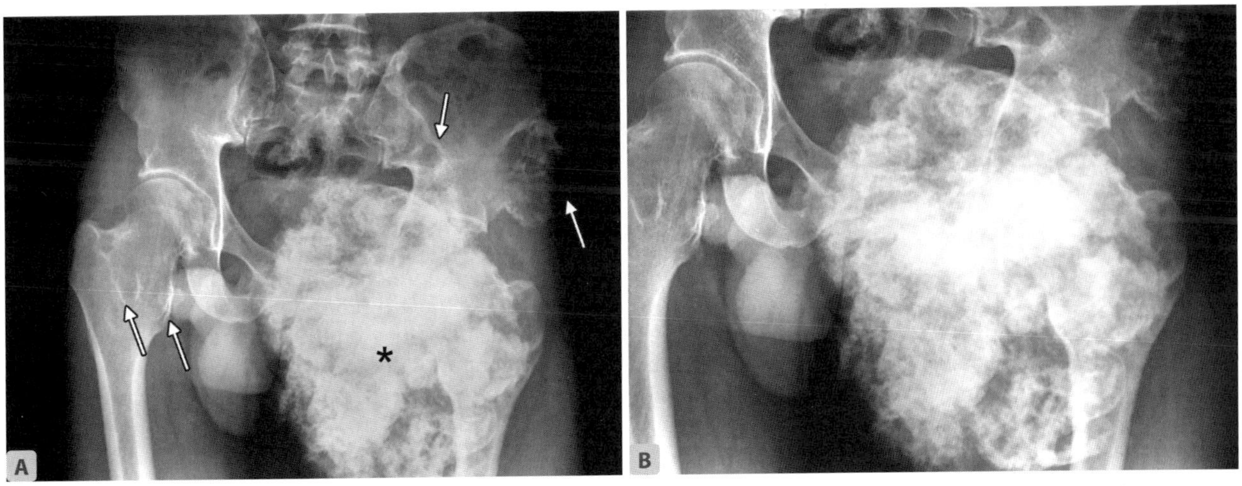

FIGS. 16A AND B: Chondrosarcoma in a child of hereditary multiple exostoses (HME). (A) Pelvic radiograph: multiple sessile osteochondromas (arrows) and a large mass overlying left pubic bone and proximal femur (asterisk); and (B) Magnified image: dense matrix mineralization having "ring" or "arc"-like appearance.

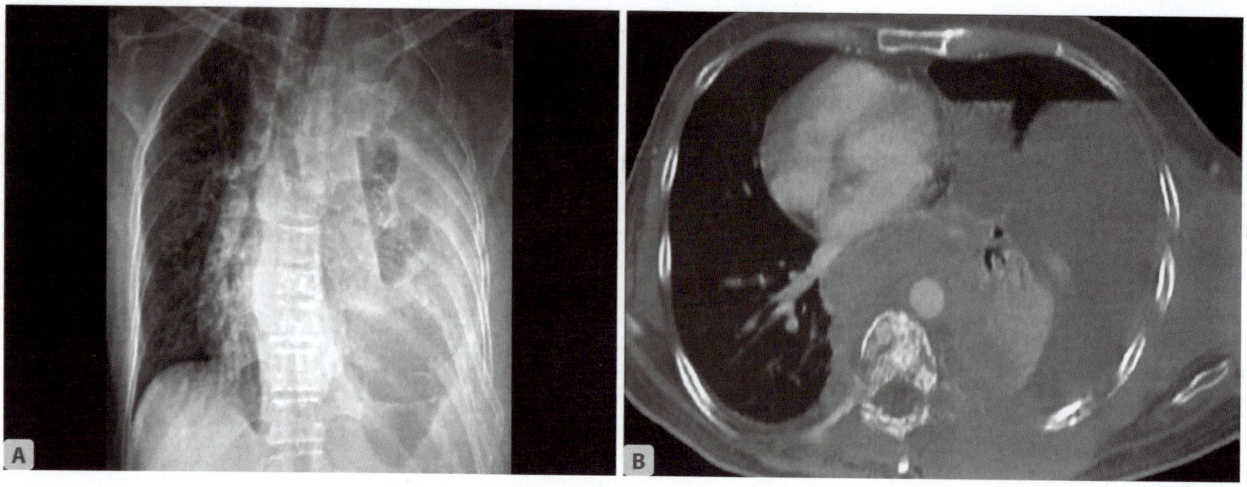

FIGS. 17A AND B: NHL of the left thoracic wall. (A) Chest radiograph reveals opaque left hemithorax with lytic sclerotic destruction of left 7th and 8th ribs as well as the 8th dorsal vertebral body; and (B) Axial CECT bone window of the same patient shows permeative lytic sclerotic bone destruction involving the vertebral body, posterior element, and the posterior ribs having a large soft-tissue component in the paraspinal locations and along posterolateral thoracic wall. (CECT: contrast-enhanced computed tomography; NHL: non-Hodgkin lymphoma)

secondary involvement by NHL, most commonly affected sites are pelvis, spine, and skull. The usual presentation is with permeative lytic destruction of bone with cortical destruction.

Metastases

Metastases to bone in pediatric age group commonly occur from primary tumors like neuroblastoma, Ewing's sarcoma, or osteosarcoma **(Figs. 18 and 19)**. Osseous metastases in osteosarcoma are usually blastic. Metastases from neuroblastoma show a "sunburst" type of periosteal reaction **(Figs. 18A to D)**. When occurring in the calvarium, they often give rise to sutural diastasis secondary to dural deposits **(Figs. 18A to D)**. These are enhancing lesions on MRI and show T2 hyperintensity **(Figs. 19A to C)**.

Other Rare Bone Sarcomas

Malignant fibrous histiocytoma has been renamed as undifferentiated high-grade pleomorphic sarcoma of bone and occurs very rarely in pediatric age group and usually affects the adolescents. Most common location includes metaphysis of a long bone. The radiographic findings range from geographic to permeative lytic destruction. Periosteal reaction is uncommon unlike other malignant tumors. MRI features are nonspecific. Fibrosarcoma may rarely affect the pediatric bones.

SOFT-TISSUE TUMORS

In the pediatric age group, most of the soft-tissue masses are benign; only 1–6% being malignant.[28] Rhabdomyosarcoma alone comprises more than half of the pediatric soft-tissue sarcomas.[3,4] In the infancy, fibrosarcoma is the most common and after that up to 14 years of age, rhabdomyosarcoma is the most common malignant soft-tissue sarcoma. This is followed by undifferentiated sarcomas and synovial sarcoma.[29] Clinicoradiological indicators which favor a benign etiology include younger age group, smaller size of the mass, well-circumscribed lesion, subcutaneous or fascial location, homogeneous signal on T2W imaging, no diffusion restriction, and no surrounding edema.[30] Sometimes, a malignant soft-tissue tumor may have well-defined margins with a pseudocapsule and homogeneous in signal intensity on MRI. Many times, imaging may be able to suggest a benign histological diagnosis like lipoma, epidermoid cyst, ganglion cyst, and vascular malformations and thus obviate the need of sampling.

The prime important role of imaging in malignant soft-tissue tumor is not to provide an accurate diagnosis, but to provide information regarding the extent of tumor, extension beyond fascial planes, adjacent bone, and neurovascular bundle involvement. Other important role of imaging includes response assessment after treatment. Differentiating a residual or recurrent tumor from posttreatment changes is the most challenging part in follow-up imaging. Both can present with high T2W signal intensity. Tumor recurrence is often associated with mass effect, diffusion restriction, and early contrast enhancement, whereas posttreatment changes lack these features.[31]

Rhabdomyosarcoma

Rhabdomyosarcoma **(Figs. 20 to 23)** accounts for 4–5% of all childhood cancers and 10–15% of solid tumors in the extremities.[32] It is a high-grade, small round cell neoplasm, with the more differentiated components resembling skeletal muscle cells. Imaging manifestation includes aggressive soft-tissue mass in a child without any fat component. The most common locations are the head and neck region (parameningeal and orbital), genitourinary tract (bladder and prostate), the retroperitoneum, and the extremities. The histologic subtypes include embryonal, alveolar, pleomorphic, and spindle cell/sclerosing types. Embryonal subtype is the most common with relatively better prognosis and commonly occurs in <5 years age group. However, this

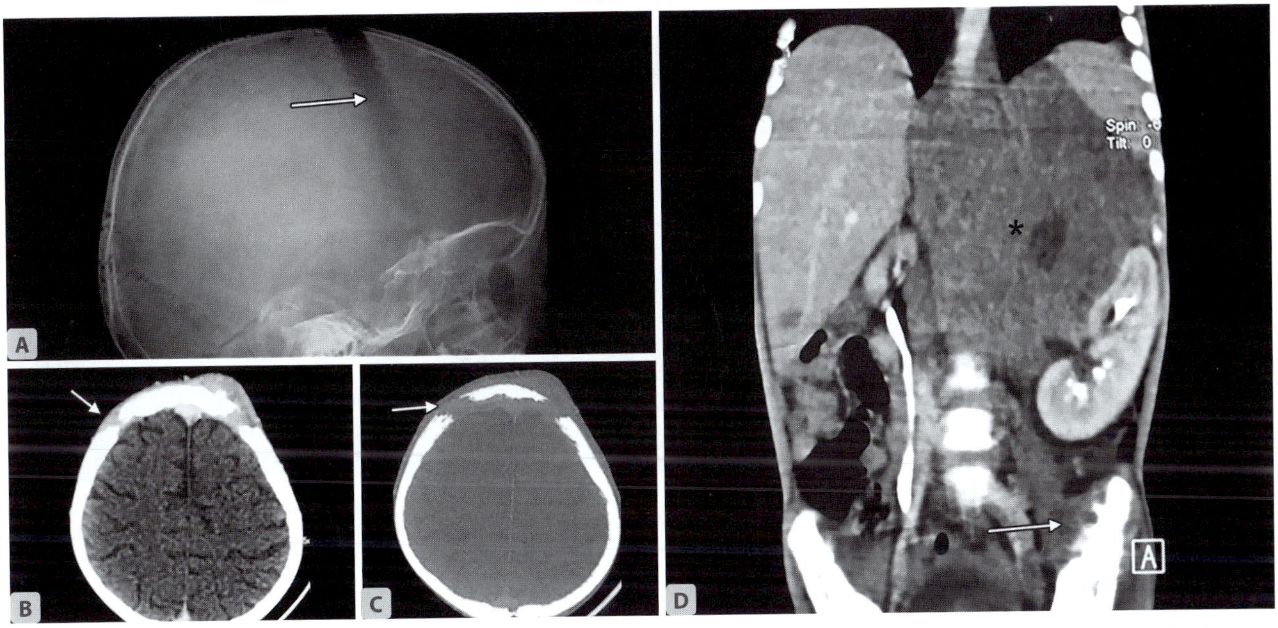

FIGS. 18A TO D: Skeletal metastases from left adrenal neuroblastoma. (A) Sutural diastasis on radiograph (arrow); (B and C) Enhancing dural metastases along sutures on CT (arrows); and (D) Left adrenal solid mass (asterisk) with adjacent organ invasion and bony metastasis to left iliac wing (arrow).

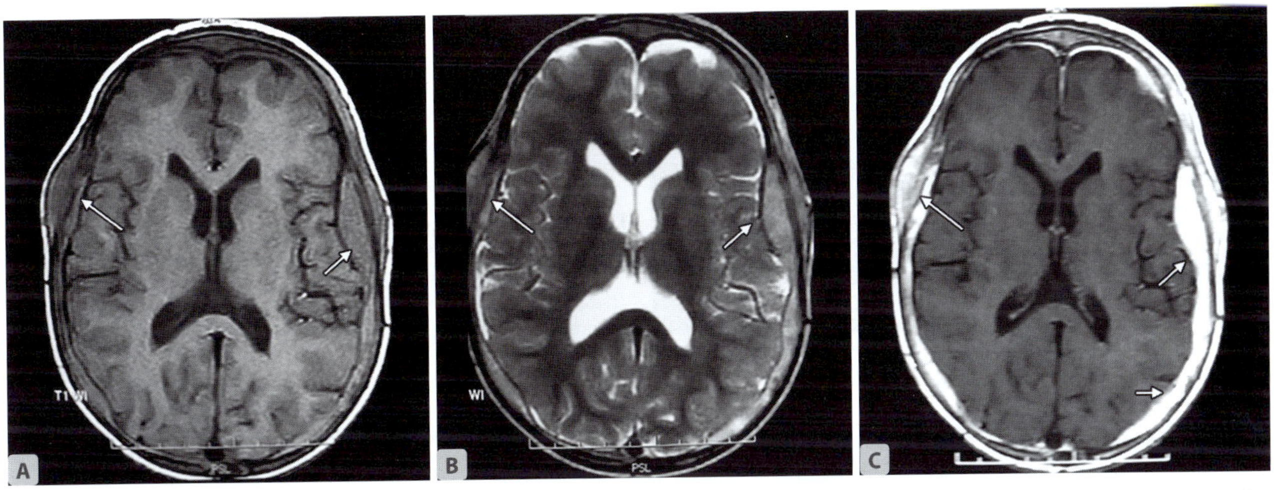

FIGS. 19A TO C: MRI appearance of skeletal metastases from adrenal neuroblastoma. (A) The dural deposits are hypointense on T1W images (arrows); (B) Intermediate on T2W images (arrows); and (C) Show homogeneous enhancement (arrows). (MRI: magnetic resonance imaging; T1W: T1-weighted)

type may cause bowing or destruction of the adjacent bones. Embryonal type is commonly homogeneous while alveolar and pleomorphic types show necrosis **(Figs. 20A and B)**. The alveolar subtype, which is relatively aggressive, is seen in the perineum and extremities of young adults. The prognosis of this tumor depends on the size, local invasion, nodal spread, and distant metastases. Tumor with a diameter <5 cm has better overall prognosis. Extremity tumors, which are usually of alveolar or pleomorphic subtype, have a poorer prognosis. Prognosis is better in case of proximal extremity tumors than distal tumors.[33] Complete resection is the treatment of choice and survival in unresectable tumors is poor.

On MR imaging, the tumor is isointense to muscle on T1W and hyperintense on T2W images and shows strong contrast enhancement.[30] Pleomorphic form may show ring-like enhancement. A specific type of embryonal rhabdomyosarcoma (RMS) is sarcoma botryoides (bunch of grapes-like submucosal lesions). It occurs in the walls of hollow viscera like bladder, vagina, nasopharynx, and bile duct.

Synovial Sarcoma

Synovial sarcoma **(Figs. 24 and 25)** is the most common nonrhabdomyosarcomatous soft-tissue sarcoma in the children. It is a high-grade tumor showing differentiation

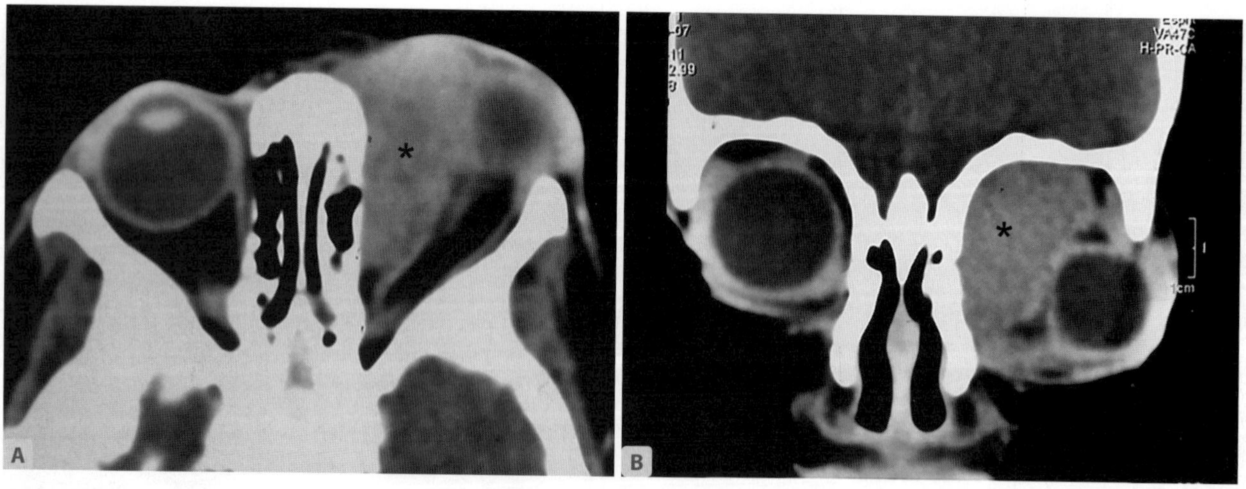

FIGS. 20A AND B: Embryonal RMS in a 4-year-old girl. (A) Axial and (B) Coronal CECT: Enhancing solid extraconal mass (asterisk) lesion causing abaxial proptosis. (CECT: contrast-enhanced computed tomography; RMS: rhabdomyosarcoma)

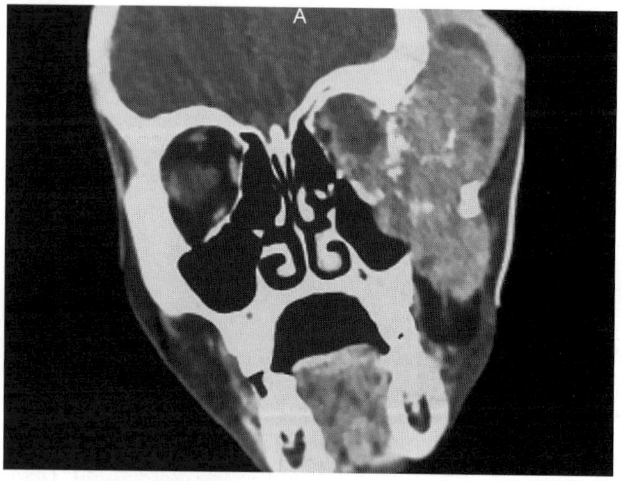

FIG. 21: Rhabdomyosarcoma in a child presenting with rapid onset proptosis and facial swelling. Contrast-enhanced computed tomography (CECT) orbit coronal reformatted image shows a large heterogeneously enhancing mass lesion causing destruction of the left zygoma and lateral maxillary and orbital wall.

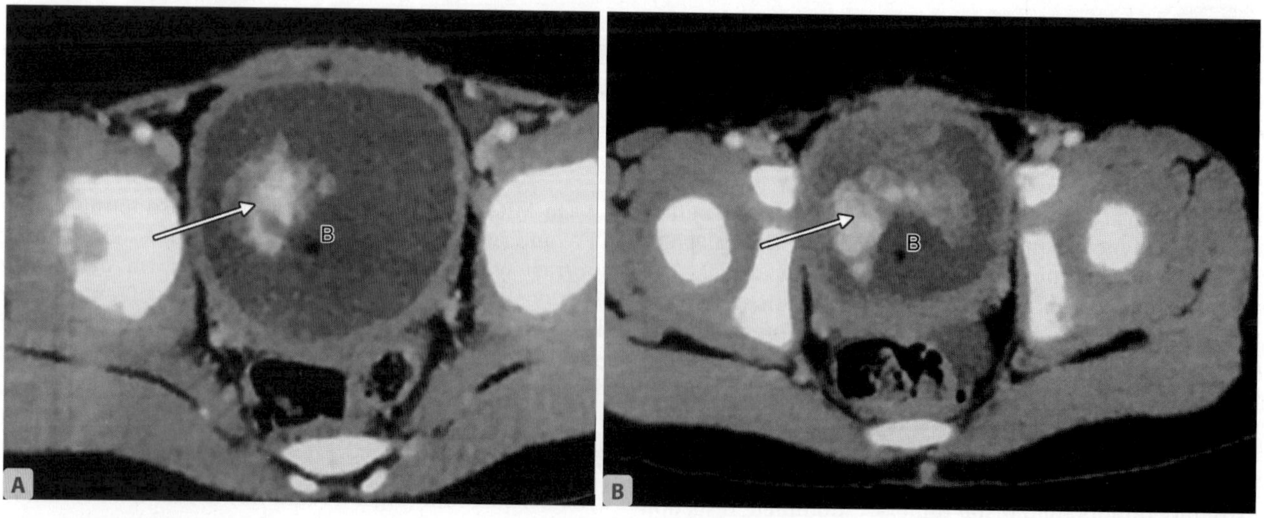

FIGS. 22A AND B: Bladder-prostate rhabdomyosarcoma (RMS) in a 4 year-old boy presenting with urinary retention. Enhancing frond-like intravesical mass (arrows) around the Foley bulb.

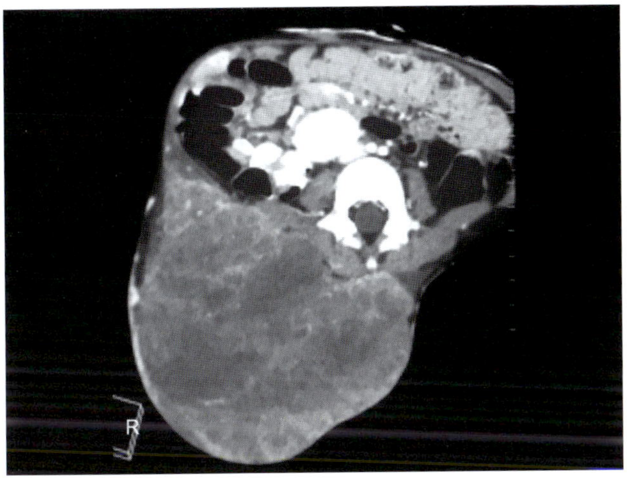

FIG. 23: Rhabdomyosarcoma in a child presenting with an enlarging back mass. Axial contrast-enhanced computed tomography (CECT) of abdomen shows infiltration of the mass into the paraspinal and posterior abdominal muscles on right side.

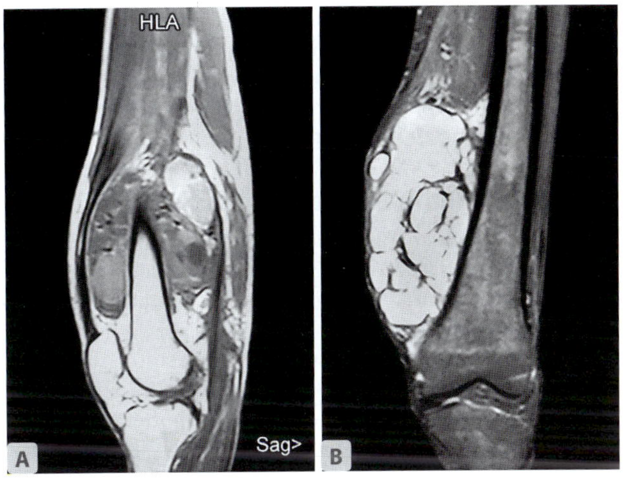

FIGS. 25A AND B: Synovial sarcoma. (A) Sagittal T1W and (B) coronal STIR images show presence of juxta-articular lobulated soft-tissue mass which is bright on T2W image and shows areas of hyperintensity on T1W image (suggesting hemorrhage). (STIR: short tau inversion recovery; T1W: T1-weighted; T2W: T2-weighted)

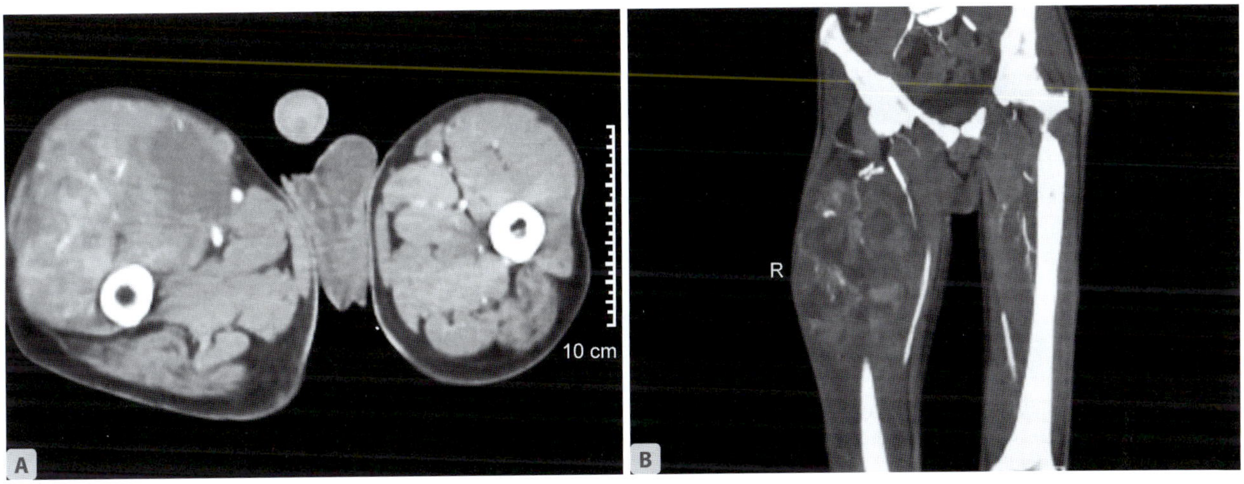

FIGS. 24A AND B: Synovial sarcoma in a 15-year-old child. (A) Contrast-enhanced computed tomography (CECT) thigh axial soft-tissue window and (B) coronal maximum intensity projection (MIP) images show a heterogeneous mass lesion in the extensor compartment, abutting and displacing the right superficial femoral artery.

of tumor cells into spindle cells resembling synoviocytes and not derived from synovial cells. As per the 2013 WHO classification, synovial sarcoma is included under the heading of tumors of uncertain differentiation. t(X;18) translocation is pathognomonic of synovial sarcoma. The usual location of this tumor is in periarticular regions (most common popliteal fossa), though it can occur in other places as well. These tumors commonly present as a painless extremity mass, most commonly around the knee joints. On imaging, they are well-defined, lobulated in outline, isointense to muscle on T1W, and heterogeneously hyperintense on T2W images, with areas of hemorrhage and fluid levels **(Figs. 25A and B)**.[34] Scattered calcification is seen in as high as one-third of the lesions.[35] Sometimes, the lesions are cystic, mimicking a ganglion cyst or Baker's cyst. The mixture of signal intensities on T2W images gives rise to "bowl of grapes" sign or triple sign.

Infantile/Congenital Fibrosarcoma

Infantile fibrosarcoma is the most common malignant soft-tissue tumor of infancy. The peak age group affected is <5 years, specifically in infants or neonates. These are usually large disfiguring masses, but biologic behavior is favorable than their adult counterparts. They rarely metastasize. They are isointense to muscles on T1W images and heterogeneously hyperintense on T2W images **(Figs. 26A and B)**.[36] Contrast enhancement is usually heterogeneous. In older children, the tumor behaves like those in adults, with a more aggressive course.[4] As per the recent WHO classification (4th edition, 2013), infantile fibrosarcoma is of intermediate malignant potential (rarely metastasizing) while adult and myxoid fibrosarcomas are malignant. Infantile fibrosarcoma mimics the more common vascular tumors and it may have skin discoloration as well; however, the enhancement is less marked without any enlarged feeding vessels or flow voids. There may be associated disseminated intravascular coagulopathy which may be clinically confused with Kasabach–Merritt phenomenon (latter occurs almost exclusively with kaposiform hemangioendothelioma). Adult fibrosarcomas occur in teenagers.

Other Malignant Soft-tissue Pediatric Tumors

Other soft-tissue malignant tumors in childhood include undifferentiated sarcomas, malignant vascular tumors, myxoid liposarcoma, granulocytic sarcoma, and tumors of uncertain differentiation.

Myxoid liposarcoma occurs in the deep soft tissues of the extremities of young adults. It has characteristic hyperintense signal on T2W images and also shows moderate–intense contrast enhancement. Fat signal is usually not evident on imaging.

Malignant vascular tumors include epithelioid hemangioendothelioma and angiosarcoma. However, these do not occur in children. Kaposiform hemangioendothelioma is borderline malignant vascular tumor of infancy with ill-defined margins, subcutaneous fat stranding, skin thickening, and osseous invasion. Other features are similar to hemangiomas (enhancing solid hypoechoic T2 hyperintense mass). Another helpful clinical feature is Kasabach-Merritt phenomenon (coagulopathy with thrombocytopenia) and this lesion constitutes 90% of the cases of this phenomenon.

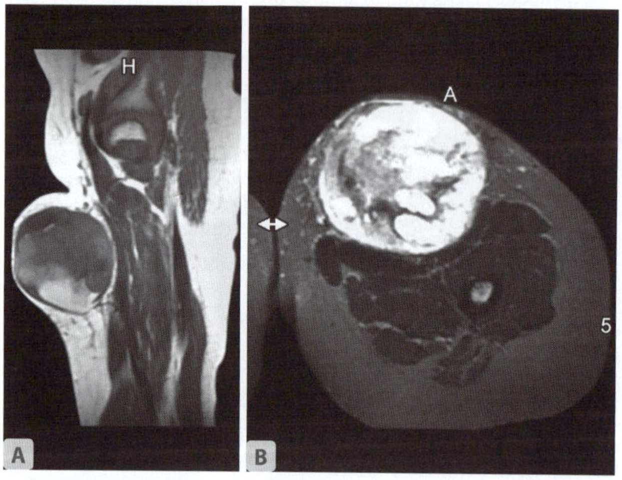

FIGS. 26A AND B: Infantile fibrosarcoma. (A) Sagittal T1W and (B) axial T2W FS images show a well-defined heterogeneous mass in subcutaneous region of thigh with areas of hemorrhage within. (FS: fat-suppressed; T1W: T1-weighted; T2W: T2-weighted)

Alveolar soft part sarcoma is a rare vascular mass occurring in young adults (girls more commonly) with high metastatic potential. The primary lesion is small pulsatile T2 hyperintense mass with flow voids within, usually in buttocks or thigh **(Figs. 27A and B)**. Punctate calcification foci can also occur. This lesion is included under the heading of tumors of uncertain differentiation as per the 2013 WHO classification. Other malignant tumors in this category which may rarely occur in children are epithelioid, clear cell sarcoma, and extraskeletal Ewing's sarcoma.

Tumors, previously known as malignant fibrous histiocytoma, are now categorized into *undifferentiated/unclassified sarcomas* and majority is included in undifferentiated pleomorphic sarcoma. These do not have any specific imaging features **(Figs. 28A and B)**.

Granulocytic sarcoma (also called chloroma) is seen in 5% cases of acute myeloid leukemia and contains primitive precursors of granulocytes. To begin with, they arise in bone marrow and traverse the haversian canals to extraosseous locations. The most common site is head and neck region **(Figs. 29 and 30)**. They are hyperdense on noncontrast-enhanced computed tomography (NCCT), isointense to muscle on T2W images, and show intense homogeneous enhancement.[37]

Malignant peripheral nerve sheath tumors may rarely occur in pediatric age group. These are hypodense on CT, hyperintense on T2W, and may show heterogeneity.

Extranodal soft-tissue lymphoma may be considered in the differential diagnosis of pediatric soft-tissue masses, if there is a history of congenital immunodeficiency or human immunodeficiency virus infection.

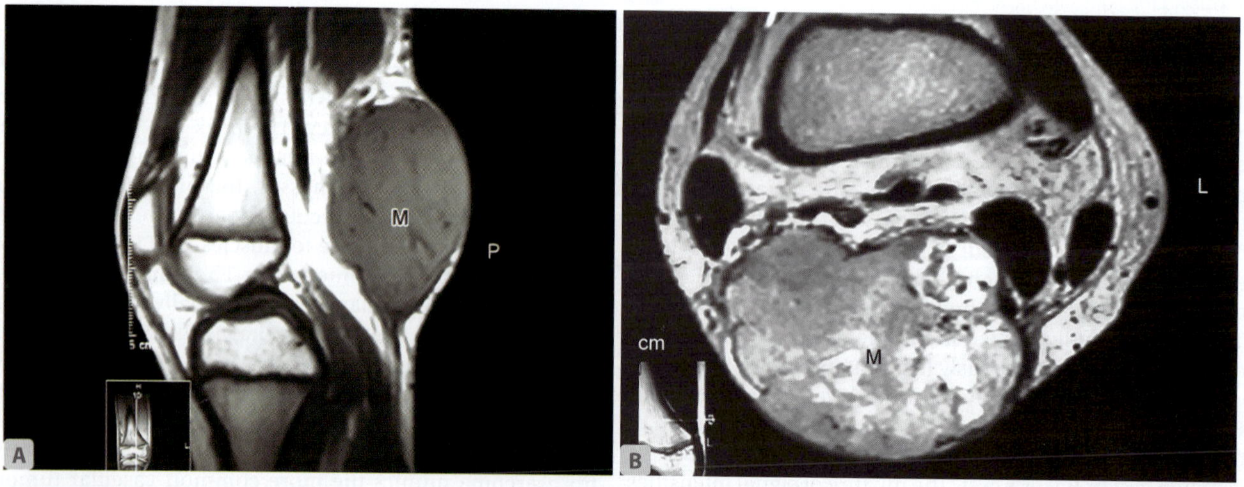

FIGS. 27A AND B: Alveolar soft part sarcoma in a 7-year-old boy; The mass (M) is hypointense on T1W and hyperintense on T2W MR images with few flow voids within. (MR: magnetic resonance; T1W: T1-weighted; T2W: T2-weighted)

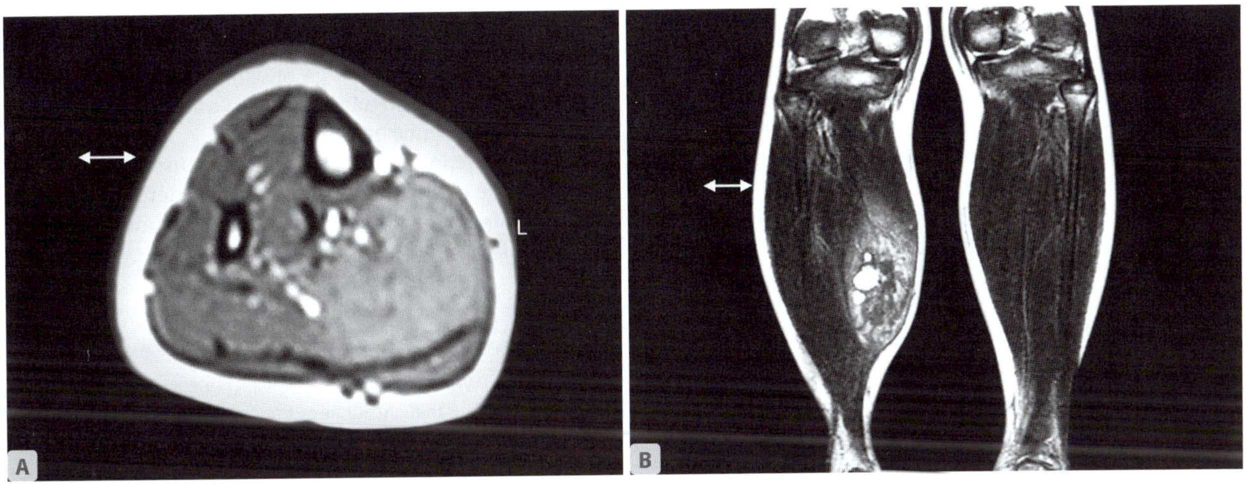

FIGS. 28A AND B: Undifferentiated pleomorphic sarcoma. (A) Axial T1W and (B) coronal STIR images show T1 isointense and T2 heterogeneously hyperintense intramuscular mass in the calf of a 6-year-old child. (STIR: short tau inversion recovery; T1W: T1-weighted)

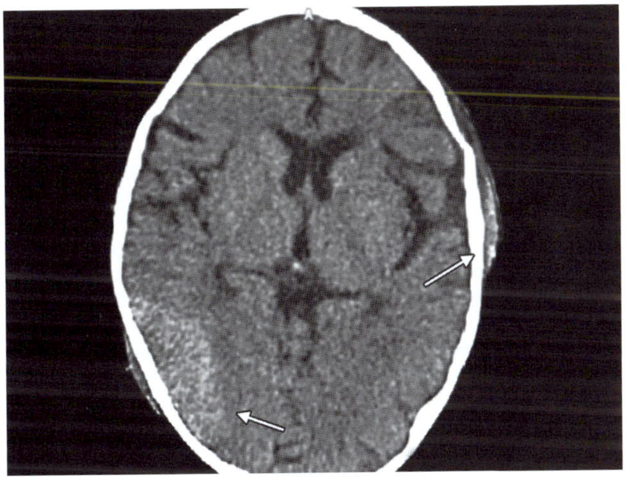

FIG. 29: Granulocytic sarcoma in a case of acute myeloid leukemia. Contrast-enhanced computed tomography (CECT) of head reveals multiple enhancing soft-tissue masses (arrows) involving the calvarium.

MIMICS OF SOFT-TISSUE SARCOMAS

Sometimes, benign neoplasms or even nonneoplastic conditions may simulate malignancy.[38] Hematomas can appear large and heterogeneous with hyperdense areas within which may be interpreted as enhancement. Large hematomas in patients with bleeding diathesis (hemophiliac pseudotumors) may appear aggressive and can occur within the bone or in soft tissues. Low-flow vascular malformations (venous and lymphatic malformations) and benign high-flow lesions (arteriovenous malformations and benign vascular tumors like infantile and congenital hemangiomas) can also mimic soft-tissue sarcomas. Lipoblastomas and fibrous hamartoma of infancy contain soft-tissue component and may be suspected to be malignant. Myositis ossificans can show rim enhancement with surrounding edema, masquerading like a malignant sarcoma. Other mimickers include fat necrosis, ganglion cyst, muscle hernias, giant cell tumor of tendon sheath, and benign nerve sheath tumors.

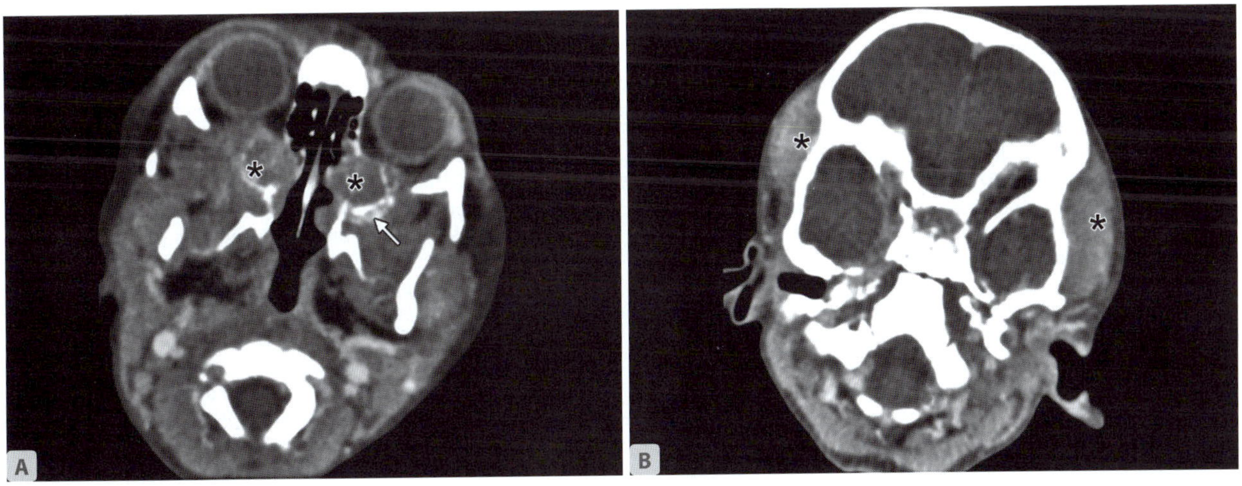

FIGS. 30A AND B: Granulocytic sarcoma in a 2-year-old boy with acute myeloid leukemia (AML). (A) Enhancing soft-tissue masses in bilateral maxillary sinuses (asterisk). Note the bone destruction (arrow); and (B) Enhancing soft-tissue deposits in bilateral temporal muscles (asterisk).

CONCLUSION

Though the pediatric malignant bone tumors account for about 6% of all childhood malignancies, malignant soft-tissue tumors are rare in childhood. The role of imaging is to diagnose an aggressive mass, assess the extent of the lesion, thus establishing the accurate stage and determining resectability. Plain radiographs are the most important tool in evaluating bone tumors. MRI offers better assessment of the bony and extraosseous extent and neurovascular involvement, the knowledge of which is crucial for surgery. CT scan of thorax and bone scans is required to determine the presence or absence of metastases.

Soft-tissue lesions in childhood are usually benign. The primary role of imaging is to assess the extent in a soft-tissue lesion, thus establishing the accurate stage and determining resectability.

REFERENCES

1. Wootton-Gorges SL. MR imaging of primary bone tumors and tumor-like conditions in children. Radiol Clin North Am. 2009;47:957-75.
2. Caudill JSC, Arndt CAS. Diagnosis and management of bone malignancy in adolescence. Adolesc Med. 2007;18:62-78.
3. Arndt CA, Crist WM. Common musculoskeletal tumors of childhood and adolescence. N Engl J Med. 1999;341:342-52.
4. Fletcher CDM, Bridge JA, Hogendoorn PCW, Mertens F. WHO Classification of Tumors of Soft Tissue and Bone, 4th edition. France: IARC Publications; 2013.
5. Stein-Wexler R. MR imaging of soft tissue masses in children. Radiol Clin North Am. 2009;47:977-95.
6. Hoffer FA. Primary skeletal neoplasms: Osteosarcoma and Ewing sarcoma. Top Magn Reson Imaging. 2002;13:231-400.
7. Meyer JS, Nadel HR, Marina N, Womer RB, Brown KL, Eary JF, et al. Imaging guidelines for children with Ewing sarcoma and osteosarcoma: a report from the Children's Oncology Group Bone Tumor Committee. Pediatr Blood Cancer. 2008;51:163-70.
8. Alyas F, James SL, Davies AM, Saifuddin A. The role of MR imaging in the diagnostic characterization of appendicular bone tumours and tumour-like conditions. Eur Radiol. 2007;17:2675-86.
9. Sun Y, Liu X, Pan S, Deng C, Li X, Guo Q. Analysis of imaging characteristics of primary malignant bone tumors in children. Oncol Lett. 2017;14:5801-10.
10. Kransdorf MJ, Murphy MD. Radiologic evaluation of soft-tissue masses: A current perspective. AJR Am J Roentgenol. 2000;175:575-87.
11. Rana KA, Meyer J, Ibrahim S, Ralls M, Kent PM. The role of imaging of malignant bone tumors in children and young adults. Curr Probl Cancer. 2013;37:181-91.
12. Jelinek J, Kransdorf MJ. MR imaging of soft-tissue masses: Mass like lesions that simulate neoplasma. Magn Reson Imaging Clin North Am. 1995;3:727-41.
13. Ahlawat S, Fayad LM. De Novo Assessment of Pediatric Musculoskeletal Soft Tissue Tumors: Beyond Anatomic Imaging. Pediatrics. 2015;136:e194-202.
14. Hayashida Y, Yakushiji T, Awai K, Katahira K, Nakayama Y, Shimomura O, et al. Monitoring therapeutic responses of primary bone tumors by diffusion-weighted image: Initial results. Eur Radiol. 2006;16:2637-43.
15. McCarville MB. New frontiers in pediatric oncologic imaging. Cancer Imaging. 2008;8:87-92.
16. Wang CK, Li CW, Hsieh TJ, Chien SH, Liu GC, Tsai KB. Characterization of bone and soft-tissue tumors with in vivo 1H MR spectroscopy: Initial results. Radiology. 2004;232:599-605.
17. Enneking WF, Spanier SS, Goodman MA. A system for surgical staging of musculoskeletal sarcoma. Clin Orthop. 1980;153:106-20.
18. Tanaka K, Ozaki T. New TNM Classification (AJCC Eighth Edition) of Bone and Soft Tissue Sarcomas: JCOG Bone and Soft Tissue Tumor Study Group. Jpn J Clin Oncol. 2019;49:103-7.
19. Longhi A, Errani C, De Paolis M, Mercuri M, Bacci G. Primary bone osteosarcoma in the pediatric age: state of the art. Cancer Treat Rev. 2006;32:423-36.
20. Vlychou M, Athanasou N. Radiological and pathological diagnosis of pediatric bone tumours and tumour-like lesions. Pathology. 2008;40:196-216.
21. Reddick WE, Wang S, Xiong X, Glass JO, Wu S, Kaste SC, et al. Dynamic magnetic resonance imaging of regional contrast access as an additional prognostic factor in pediatric osteosarcoma. Cancer. 2001;91:2230-7.
22. Bacci G, Ferrari S, Bertoni F, Picci P, Bacchini P, Longhi A, et al. Histologic response of high-grade nonmetastatic osteosarcoma of the extremity to chemotherapy. Clin Orthop Relat Res. 2001;386:186-96.
23. Provisor AJ, Ettinger LJ, Nachman JB, Krailo MD, Makley JT, Yunis EJ, et al. Treatment of nonmetastatic osteosarcoma of the extremity with preoperative and postoperative chemotherapy: a report from the Children's Cancer Group. J Clin Oncol. 1997;15:76-84.
24. Peersman B, Vanhoenakcker FM, Heyman S, van Herendael B, Stam M, Brys P, et al. Ewing's sarcoma: imaging features. JBR-BTR. 2007;90:368-76.
25. Czajka CM, DiCaprio MR. What is the Proportion of Patients With Multiple Hereditary Exostoses Who Undergo Malignant Degeneration? Clin Orthop Relat Res. 2015;473:2355-61.
26. Kaim AH, Hügli R, Bonél HM, Jundt G. Chondroblastoma and clear cell chondrosarcoma: radiological and MRI characteristics with histopathological correlation. Skeletal Radiol. 2002;31:88-95.
27. Krishnan A, Shirkhoda A, Tehrznzadeh J, Armin AR, Irwin R, Les K. Primary bone lymphoma: radiographic-MR imaging correlation. Radiographics. 2003;23:1371-87.
28. Bissett GS. MR imaging of soft-tissue masses in children. Magn Reson Imaging Clin North Am. 1996;4:696-719.
29. Loeb DM, Thornton K, Shokek O. Pediatric soft tissue sarcomas. Surg Clin North Am. 2008;88:615-27.
30. Moulton JS, Blebea JS, Dunco DM, Braley SE, Bisset GS, Emery KH. MR imaging of soft-tissue masses: diagnostic efficacy and value of distinguishing between benign and malignant lesions. AJR Am J Roentgenol. 1995;164:1191-9.
31. Siegel MJ. Magnetic resonance imaging of musculoskeletal soft tissue masses. Radiol Clin North Am. 2001;39:701-20.
32. Kim EE, Valenzuela RF, Kumar AJ, Raney RB, Eftekari F. Imaging and clinical spectrum of rhabdomyosarcoma in children. Clin Imaging. 2000;24:257-62.
33. Tabrizi P, Letts M. Childhood rhabdomyosarcoma of the trunk and extremities. Am J Orthp. 1999;28:440-6.
34. Jones BC, Sundaram M, Kransdorf MJ. Synovial sarcoma: MR imaging findings in 34 patients. AJR Am J Roentgenol. 1993;161:827-30.
35. Frassica FJ, Khanna JA, McCarthy EF. The role of MR imaging in soft tissue tumor evaluation: perspective of the orthopaedic oncologist and musculoskeletal pathologist. Magn Reson Imaging Clin North Am. 2000;8:915-27.
36. Eich GF, Hoeffel JC, Tschäppeler H, Gassner I, Willi UV. Fibrous tumors in children: imaging features of a heterogeneous group of disorders. Pediatr Radiol. 1998;28:500-9.
37. Stein-Wexler R, Wootton-Gorges SL, West DC. Orbital granulocytic sarcoma: An unusual presentation of acute myelocytic leukemia. Pediatr Radiol. 2003;33:136-9.
38. Navarro OM. Soft tissue masses in children. Radiol Clin North Am. 2011;49:1235-7.

CHAPTER

84

Congenital Brain Anomalies

Sameer Vyas, Vikas Bhatia, Ajay Kumar

INTRODUCTION

Congenital brain anomalies or malformation are frequently seen in pediatric neuroimaging practice. There has been description of >2,000 different congenital brain anomalies in the literature with reported incidence of about 1% of all live births. With advancement in imaging technique, especially magnetic resonance imaging (MRI), there has significant understanding and correlation among genetics, neuroimaging, and development of these anomalies. So, it is important for radiologist to be familiar with the imaging pattern of these anomalies to understand the genotype imaging phenotype correlation. MRI is modality of choice for detailed evaluation of these anomalies and computed tomography (CT) may be complementary in showing bony details and calcifications. In this chapter, various congenital brain anomalies have been discussed broadly under three groups: (1) Anomalies of dorsal prosencephalon development, (2) Anomalies of ventral prosencephalon development, and (3) Anomalies of the posterior fossa (midbrain-hindbrain development and craniocervical junction). Brief description of the various anomalies is provided with main emphasis on the characteristic neuroimaging finding of these anomalies.

ANOMALIES OF DORSAL PROSENCEPHALON DEVELOPMENT

These include anomalies of the cerebral commissures and malformations of cortical development.

Commissural Anomalies

Cerebral commissures are axonal bundles that arise from cortical neurons and connect the two cerebral hemispheres crossing the midline. These are the most common developmental brain anomalies affecting around 1.8 per 10,000 live births.[1] Commissural anomalies are identified in one-third of fetal brain malformations on MR imaging,[2] however the actual incidence may be high.

Variants of commissural malformation include:

- Complete agenesis of all commissures
- Complete agenesis of corpus callosum (CC) with agenesis of the hippocampal commissures
- Posterior agenesis with failure of the hippocampal commissure and posterior CC
- Failure of the anterior callosum to grow and the hippocampal commissure pushed posteriorly.

The anterior commissure and hippocampal commissure are typically affected when the CC develops abnormally.[3] Most commonly, the anterior commissure will be small and the hippocampal commissure absent in the setting of callosal agenesis.[3,4] A variety of syndromes are associated with corpus callosal agenesis as shown in **Table 1**.

Corpus Callosum Dysgenesis

In complete CC agenesis, all the five segments (rostrum, genu, body, isthmus, and splenium) are missing. There is absence of cingulate gyrus especially noted on sagittal scans, with the hemispheres demonstrating a radiating "spoke-wheel" gyral pattern **(Figs. 1A and B)** extending perpendicularly to the roof of the third ventricle.[4,5] On coronal sections, there is presence of a "high-riding" third ventricle. The lateral ventricles appear upturned with a pointed corner. Probst bundle is situated just inside the apex of each ventricle representing misdirected commissural fibers, which should have crossed the midline but instead course from front to back, indenting the medial walls of the lateral ventricles.[4]

The septi pellucidi are widely separated with parallel nonconverging lateral ventricles. The occipital horns are dilated and termed as colpocephaly. In case of CC hypogenesis, the spectrum of findings vary according to which

TABLE 1: A list of syndromes commonly associated with commissural anomalies.

Aicardi syndrome	Median cleft face syndrome
Apert syndrome	Nonketotic hyperglycinemia
Chiari II malformation	Pyruvate dehydrogenase deficiency
Dandy–Walker malformation	Oral-facial-digital syndromes
Fetal alcohol syndrome	Walker–Warburg syndrome

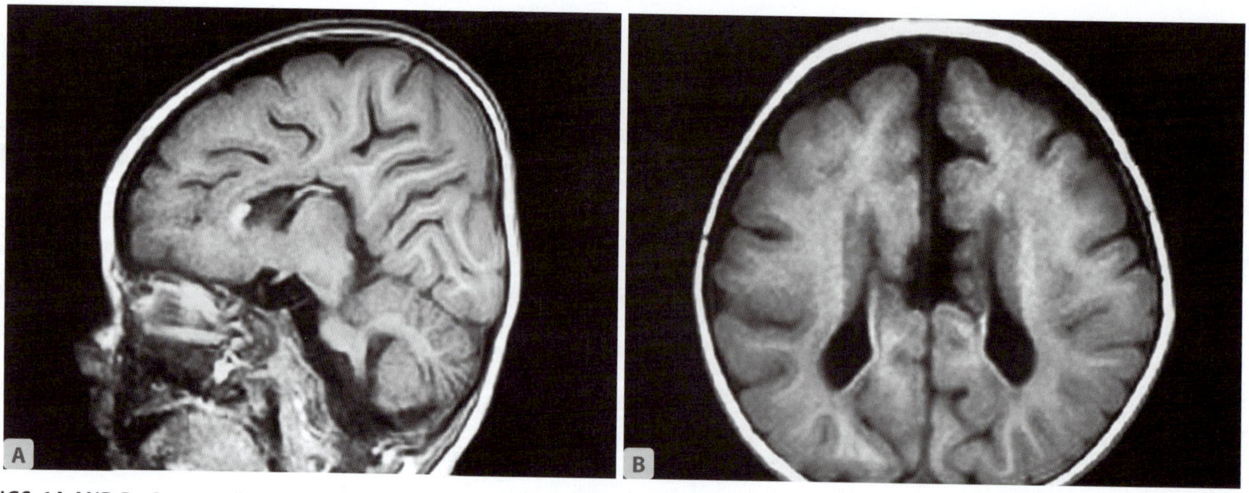

FIGS. 1A AND B: Corpus callosum (CC) agenesis: T1-weighted (T1W) sagittal and axial images depicting partial CC agenesis with radiating pattern of cerebral gyri and parallel alignment of lateral ventricles with colpocephaly.

segments are missing. The splenium is usually small or absent. Axial noncontrast-enhanced computed tomography (NECT) scans show parallel, nonconverging, and widely separated lateral ventricles **(Fig. 2)** with disproportionate enlargement of the occipital horns. On MRI, sagittal T1 and T2 scans best demonstrate complete CC absence or partial dysgenesis (complete CC agenesis).[4] A midline interhemispheric cyst **(Fig. 3)** may be present above the third ventricle. Such cysts can be ventricular outpouchings or separate structures that do not communicate with the ventricular system.[5] A classification system for interhemispheric cysts has been proposed as shown in **Table 2**.[5]

Associated azygous anterior cerebral artery (ACA) can be seen "wandering" upward in the interhemispheric fissure. Associated malformations of the eyes, hindbrain, and hypothalamic-pituitary axis are common.[4] Diffusion tensor imaging (DTI) is especially helpful in depicting CC agenesis with absent normal right-to-left encoded color of the CC and prominent front-to-back tracts of the Probst bundles. Summary of key imaging findings in CC agenesis is shown in **Table 3**.

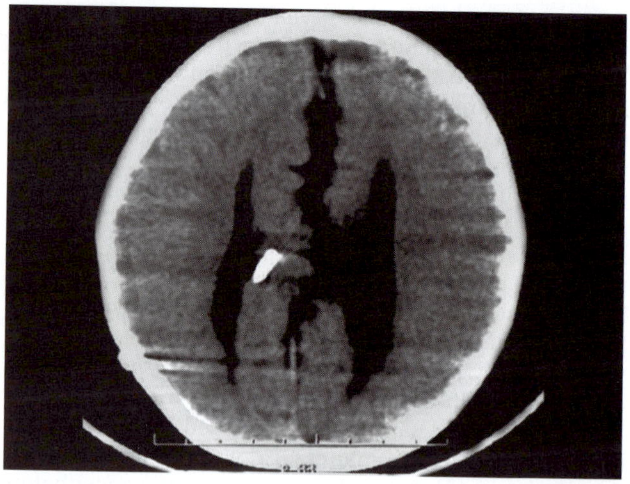

FIG. 2: Corpus callosum (CC) agenesis: Axial computed tomography (CT) sections show parallel configuration of the lateral ventricles. Absence of the CC leads to separation of the interhemispheric fissure. A shunt has been placed in the right lateral ventricle.

Corpus Callosum Hypogenesis

In partial agenesis, the rostrum and splenium are usually absent **(Fig. 4)**. The remaining CC can appear thick. The hippocampal commissure is typically absent, but the anterior commissure is generally preserved.[4] The major differential diagnosis of CC dysgenesis is destruction caused by trauma, surgery (callosotomy), or ischemia.

Malformations of Cortical Development

The three major stages of cortical development are: (1) Proliferation, (2) Neuronal migration, and (3) Postmigrational development.[5]

- *Malformations due to abnormal neuronal proliferation or apoptosis*:
  - *Decreased proliferation*: Microcephaly
  - *Cortical dysgenesis with abnormal proliferation (abnormal cell types) but without neoplasia*:

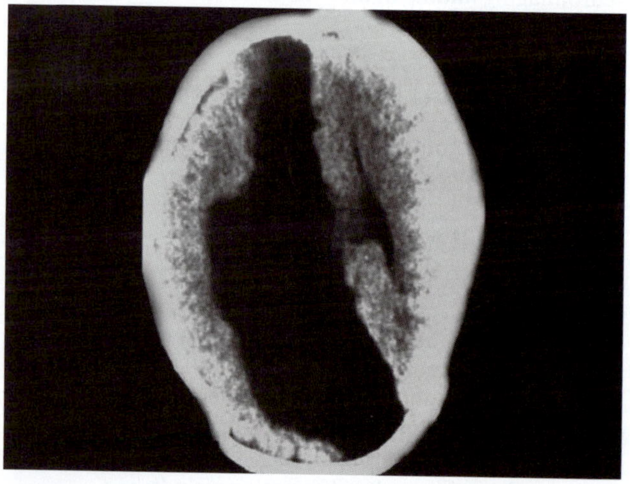

FIG. 3: Corpus callosum (CC) agenesis associated with an interhemispheric cyst which extends across the midline.

TABLE 2: Classification system for interhemispheric cysts.

Type 1	Communicate with ventricles	Associated anomalies
1a	• Isointense to cerebrospinal fluid (CSF) • Unilocular • Communicates with ventricles	Hydrocephalus
1b	• Isointense to CSF • Unilocular • Communicates with third ventricle	Thalamic fusion without subcortical heterotopia
1c	• Isointense to CSF • Unilocular • Communicates with lateral and third ventricle	Small ipsilateral cerebral hemisphere
Type 2	**No communication with ventricle**	
2a	• Isointense to CSF • Multilocular • No communication with ventricles	Hydrocephalus
2b	• Multiloculated • No communication with ventricles • Hyperdense on computed tomography • Hyperintense on T1MR	• Subependymal heterotopia • Polymicrogyria • Deficient falx cerebri
2c	• Isointense to CSF • Multilocular • No communication with ventricles	Subcortical heterotopia
2d	• Arachnoid cyst • Isointense to CSF • Unilocular • No communication with ventricles	None

TABLE 3: Key imaging findings in corpus callosum (CC) agenesis.

Findings	Imaging scan
High riding third ventricle	Coronal, sagittal
Interhemispheric cyst	Coronal, sagittal, and axial
Absent cingulate gyrus	Sagittal
Radiating gyri	Sagittal
Parallel nonconverging third ventricle	Axial
Probst bundle	Axial, coronal
Viking helmet	Coronal
Pointed upcoming lateral ventricles	Coronal
Rounded vertically oriented hippocampus	Coronal

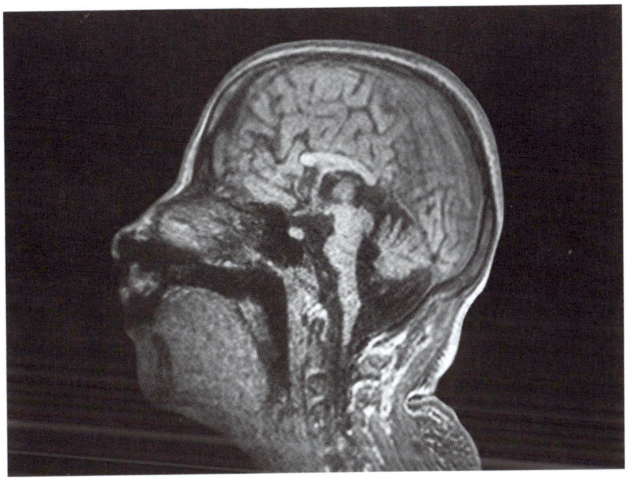

FIG. 4: Sagittal T1 3D MP-RAGE sequence shows absence of splenium of corpus callosum (CC). (3D: three-dimensional; MP-RAGE: magnetization-prepared rapid gradient echo)

        - *Normal brain size*: Cortical hamartomas of tuberous sclerosis and focal cortical dysplasia (FCD) types IIa, IIb
        - *Megalencephaly*: Hemimegalencephaly (HMEG) and dysplastic megalencephaly (DMEG) isolated or as part of overgrowth syndrome
    - *Cortical dysgenesis with abnormal cell proliferation*:
        - Cortical tubers
        - Focal cortical dysplasia (type IIb, Taylor type)
        - Hemimegalencephaly
- *Malformations secondary to abnormalities of neuronal migration*:
    - *Heterotopia*: Periventricular nodular heterotopia (PVNH)
    - *Lissencephaly (LIS) spectrum*:
        - Agyria
        - Pachygyria
        - Subcortical band heterotopia
    - Subcortical heterotopia and sublobar dysplasia
    - *Cobblestone malformations*:
        - Congenital muscular dystrophies (CMDs)
- *Abnormalities of postmigrational development*:
    - Polymicrogyria (PMG)
    - Schizencephaly
    - Focal cortical dysplasia (types I and III)
    - Postmigrational microcephaly

Malformations with Abnormal Cell Numbers/Types

Microcephalies

These can be primary microcephaly which is congenital and caused by a defect in brain development or secondary caused by an acquired disorder resulting from an insult such as ischemia, infection, maternal diabetes, and trauma that effect the early brain growth.[6] The incidence of primary microcephaly ranges from 1:10,000 to 30,000 and frequently present with mental retardation, developmental delay and seizures are the most common clinical symptoms.[5]

Types of microcephaly are summarized in **Table 4**.

The craniofacial ratio is decreased with slanted forehead and overriding sutures. The cortical surface can be variable with normal or moderately enlarged ventricles. The major challenge is in differentiating primary from secondary microcephaly with calcifications, cysts, gliosis, and encephalomalacia are more common in secondary microcephaly.[6]

Focal Cortical Dysplasia

Focal cortical dysplasia is a common cause of medically refractory epilepsy with accurate delineation that can result in good surgical resection. These are localized regions of nonneoplastic malformed gray matter (GM). The International League Against Epilepsy (ILAE) has established a three-tiered classification of FCD based on clinical, imaging, and neuropathologic findings (e.g., lamination disturbances or cytoarchitectural/cellular dysplasia) **(Table 5)**.[4,5]

The exact pathology and genetics are well-studied, however incompletely understood. Decreased expression of bone morphogenetic protein-4 (BMP-4) and increased expression of double cortin-like protein have been found in both FCDIIb. The mammalian target of rapamycin (mTOR) cascade abnormalities have been implicated as the cause of FCD.[7] The histopathologic hallmarks of FCD are disorganized cytoarchitecture and neurons with abnormal shape, size, and orientation. FCDs are the single most common cause of severe drug-resistant epilepsy in children and young adults. FCD type II is found in 15–20% of patients undergoing epilepsy surgery. FCD-associated seizures usually begin in the first decade, but can present in adolescence or even adulthood.[5,7] Standard MR images may miss the lesion. Hence, utilization of advanced techniques such as voxel-based morphometry, parametrical mapping, and texture analysis may increase detection of epileptogenic lesions. Functional imaging such as ictal single-photon emission computed tomography (SPECT), positron emission tomography (PET), and magnetoencephalography (MEG) can be useful in patients with normal MRI. Fusion and function images can be used for operative localization and surgery planning.[7] The major differential diagnosis of FCD (especially type IIb) includes neoplasm, tuberous sclerosis, and demyelinating disease.[7]

TABLE 4: Various types of microcephaly.

Types	Imaging findings
Microcephaly with simplified gyral pattern	• Simplified gyri with reduced number • Shallow sulci • Cortex is normal or thinned
Microlissencephaly	• Severe microcephaly • Simplified/smooth sulcal pattern • Extremely small brain • Cortex is thickened
Microcephaly with extensive polymicrogyria	• Small brain • Polymicrogyria

Hemimegalencephaly

It is a rare malformation characterized by enlargement and cytoarchitectural alteration of all or part of one cerebral hemisphere. It is considered as hemispheric FCD. Various syndromes are associated with HMEG in approximately one-third of cases such as Proteus, Klippel–Weber–Trenaunay, and epidermal nevus syndromes, neurofibromatosis (NF) type 1, and hypomelanosis of Ito.[8] The affected hemisphere is enlarged and dysplastic with abnormal gyral pattern, cortical dysgenesis, enlarged ipsilateral ventricle, and white matter hypertrophy. HMEG represents <5% of cortical dysplasias diagnosed on imaging. HMEG usually presents in 1st year of life with macrocephaly, developmental delay, and intractable seizures.[5]

TABLE 5: Various types of focal cortical dysplasia (FCD).

Types	Pathology	Imaging findings
FCD type I FCD type Ia FCD type Ib FCD type Ic	• Vertical (radial) persistence of developmental microcolumns • Loss of the horizontal hexalaminar structure • Both patterns of abnormal cortical layering	• Often subtle • Small focus difficult to detect • Mild hemispheric hypoplasia
FCD type II FCD type IIa FCD type IIb	• Altered cortical layering and dysmorphic neurons • Without balloon cells • With balloon cells	Localized area of increased cortical thickness **(Figs. 5A and B)** and a funnel-shaped area of blurred gray-white interface at the bottom of a sulcus, the "transmantle MR" sign. No DW restriction, no enhancement. Reduced NAA and increased myoinositol on MRS
FCD type III FCD type IIIa FCD type IIIb FCD type IIIc FCD type IIId	• Postmigrational disorder associated with principal pathologies such as ischemia, infection, trauma, etc. • Hippocampal sclerosis • Epilepsy-associated tumors • Vascular malformations • Other epileptogenic lesions	Imaging findings consistent with the associated pathology

(DW: diffusion-weighted; MRS: magnetic resonance spectroscopy; NAA: N-acetyl aspartate)

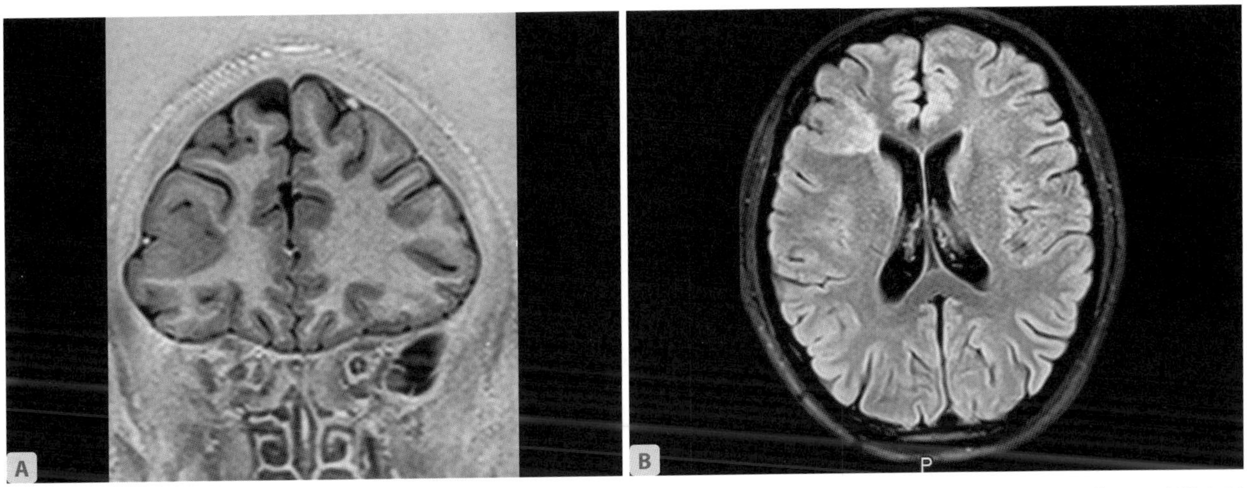

FIGS. 5A AND B: (A) 3D IR coronal images showing thickening of right middle frontal gyrus with blurred gray-white matter interface; and (B) Axial FLAIR images show presence of transmantle sign. (3D: three-dimensional; FLAIR: fluid-attenuated inversion recovery)

Imaging Features: It is characterized by an enlarged **(Fig. 6)** dysplastic hemisphere with thickened cortex and white matter abnormalities. The lateral ventricle usually appears enlarged. The posterior falx often appears displaced across the midline. Dystrophic calcifications may be seen commonly. Prominent superficial veins may be seen superficial to the dysplastic cortex. Myelination may be accelerated as seen on T1-weighted (T1W) scans. Associated heterotopias and PMG are usually associated.[4,5,8] The major differential diagnosis included FCD, tuberous sclerosis, and dysplastic tumors like gangliocytoma. Use of color fractional anisotropy (FA) maps can help in delineating the indistinct gray-white matter junction and hypermyelination which are characteristic finding in so characteristic of HMEG.

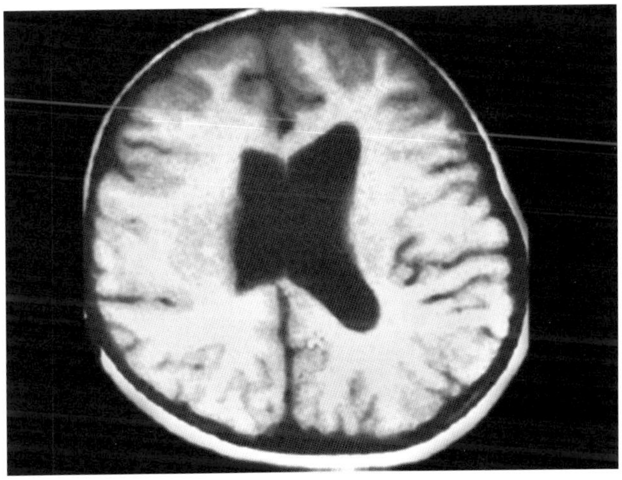

FIG. 6: Hemimegalencephaly (HMEG): T1-weighted image (T1WI) shows unilateral megalencephaly with a larger left hemisphere.

Abnormalities of Neuronal Migration

Heterotopias

These are characterized by arrest of normal neuronal migration along the radial glial cells. Different types based on location of heterotopic GM are PVNH and subcortical band heterotopia.[8]

Periventricular Nodular Heterotopia

Periventricular nodular heterotopia is the most common cortical malformation in adults characterized by more subependymal nodules of GM along the lateral walls of the ventricles. It can be unilateral or bilateral and focal or diffuse. Imaging characteristics are that they follow GM in signal intensity on all sequences with no enhancement on contrast administration **(Figs. 7A and B)**. They are usually round or ovoid and may give a "lumpy-bumpy" appearance to the ventricles. No calcification is seen. The major differential diagnosis is the subependymal nodules of tuberous sclerosis.[4] These are characterized by focal or mass-like rests of neurons in the deep cerebral white matter anywhere from the ependyma to the cortex. Imaging is characterized by focal, linear, or swirling masses anywhere from ependyma to the pia which is isointense to GM on all sequences with no calcification, edema, or enhancement. Associated portion of the affected hemisphere is hypoplastic with thin or dysplastic cortex. The major differential diagnosis is subcortical neoplasm such as gangliocytoma.[4,5] Occasionally, ribbon-like bands of GM (subcortical band heterotopia) form partway between the lateral ventricles and cortex giving a double cortex appearance **(Fig. 8)**.

Lissencephaly or Smooth Brain

In this condition, there is complete or partial absence of sulcation. Complete lack of gyri is termed as agyria and the presence of few, broad, and flat gyri is termed as pachygyria. Patient of LIS presents with dysmorphic facies, seizures, mental retardation, and microcephaly. Sonographic findings include a smooth surfaced cortex without sulcal or gyral formation. Sonography can only suggest the diagnosis of LIS, but the characteristic findings are more readily identifiable

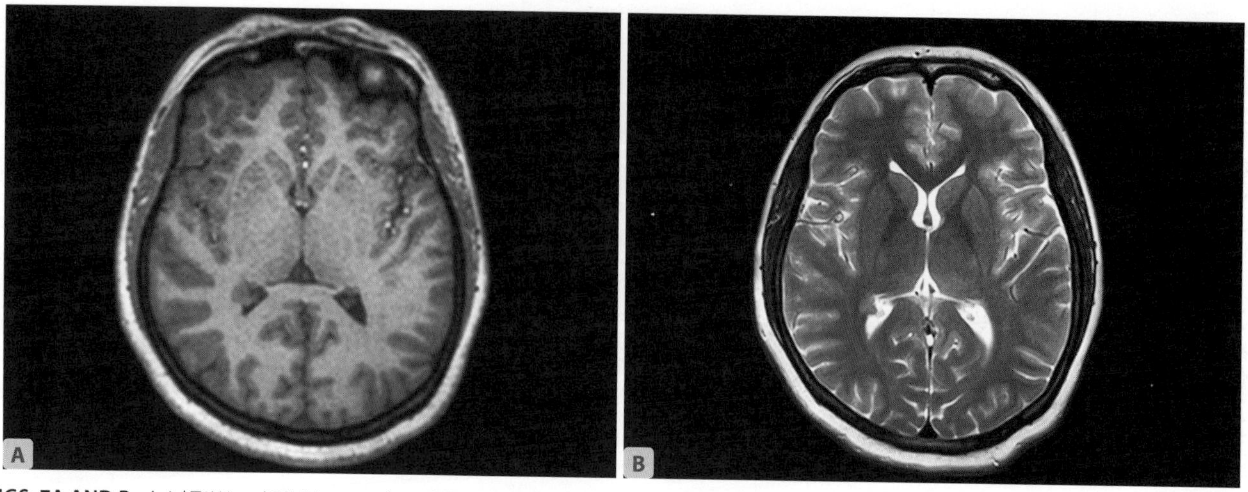

FIGS. 7A AND B: Axial T1W and T2W images show bilateral periventricular nodular heterotopia (PVNH) and subcortical heterotopias. (T1W: T1-weighted; T2W: T2-weighted)

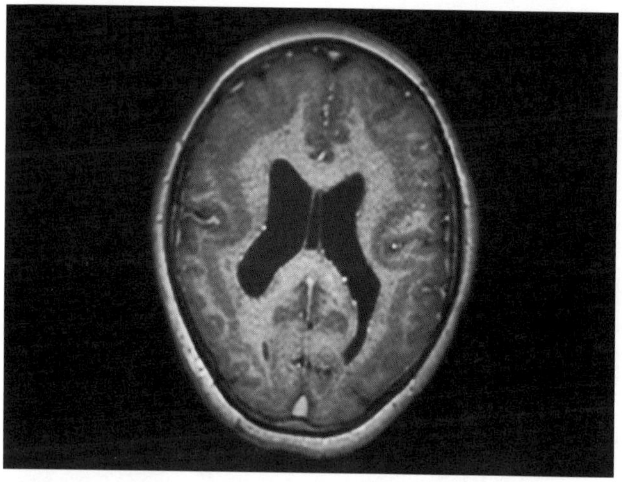

FIG. 8: Axial postcontrast T1-weighted (T1W) images showing band heterotopia.

on CT or MRI. Based on CT and MRI, various types of LIS have been described:[5]

- *Classic (type I) LIS (cLIS) (four-layer LIS/complete LIS)*: Brain surface lacks normal sulcation and gyration. Subcortical band heterotopia is also called "double cortex" syndrome and is the mildest form of classic LIS.
- *Cobblestone (type II) LIS (congenital muscular dystrophy)*: Uneven, nodular, and "pebbly" brain surface with ocular abnormalities.
- *Incomplete LIS*: True agyria with complete loss of all gyri is relatively uncommon. Most cases of cLIS show parieto-occipital agyria with some areas of broad, flat gyri ("pachygyria"), and shallow sulci along the inferior frontal and temporal lobes.
- *Variant LIS (vLIS)*: Thick cortex and reduced sulcation without a cell-sparse zone. Examples include X-linked LIS with callosal agenesis and ambiguous genitalia.
- Lissencephaly with cerebellar hypoplasia.

In classical LIS,[8] the MRI features are that of an abnormal contour and surface of the brain. The cerebral surface is smooth, devoid of sulci (agyric) or with few areas of pachygyria or with equal areas of pachygyria and agyria. The brain assumes a figure of eight appearance **(Fig. 9)** due to the bilateral shallow sylvian fissures. There is marked reduction in the white matter and the gray-white matter interface is smooth with loss of cortical white matter distribution.[9]

Differential diagnosis include extremely premature brain, microcephaly with simplified gyral pattern, cobblestone LISs type 2 LIS (LIS2) associated with CMDs, pachygyria, and cytomegalovirus (CMV)-associated LIS.[5]

Malformations Secondary to Abnormal Postmigrational Development

Polymicrogyria

It is secondary to abnormal postmigrational development and typically reflects infectious or ischemic insults. It is characterized by irregular cortex with numerous small convolutions and shallow or obliterated sulci.[8] Multiple factors such as infections (e.g., TORCH, Zika virus infection), intrauterine vascular insult, trauma, and metabolic disorders have been implicated. Bilateral perisylvian PMG **(Fig. 10)** is the most common location (61% of cases). These are followed by generalized, frontal **(Fig. 11)**, and parasagittal parieto-occipital sites. Associated heterotopia is seen in many cases. Multiplanar high-resolution thin section MR can demonstrate complete extent and detection of subtle lesions. Thickened cortex with nodular surfaces and irregular gray-white matter interfaces are the most characteristic finding.[5,9]

Schizencephaly

It is a form of migrational disorder characterized by abnormal columns of GM across the cerebral hemisphere.[5] The basic abnormality is a pial-ependymal seam (GM-lined cleft) which extends across full thickness of cerebral hemisphere from the ventricular system (ependyma) to the periphery (pial surface) of the brain. These clefts are usually perisylvian, but can occur anywhere in the brain. Two types have been described:

Type I or closed lip schizencephaly is characterized by a GM-lined pial-ependymal seam with both the lips opposed to each other. There is no intervening cerebrospinal fluid

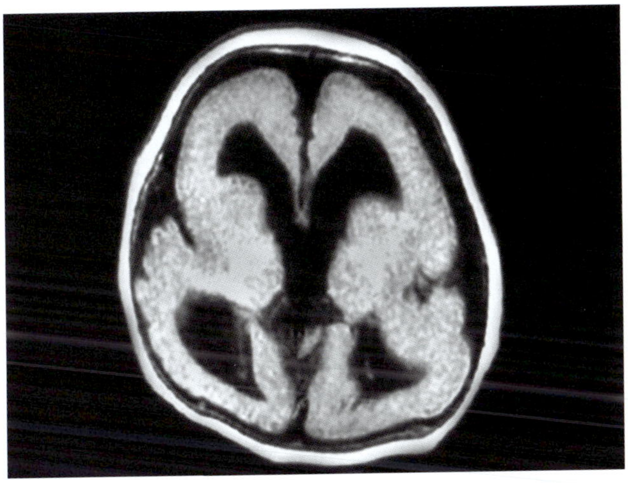

FIG. 9: Lissencephaly (LIS): Short repetition time (TR) axial MR section showing the shallow sylvian fissures giving a figure of eight configuration of the cerebral hemispheres.

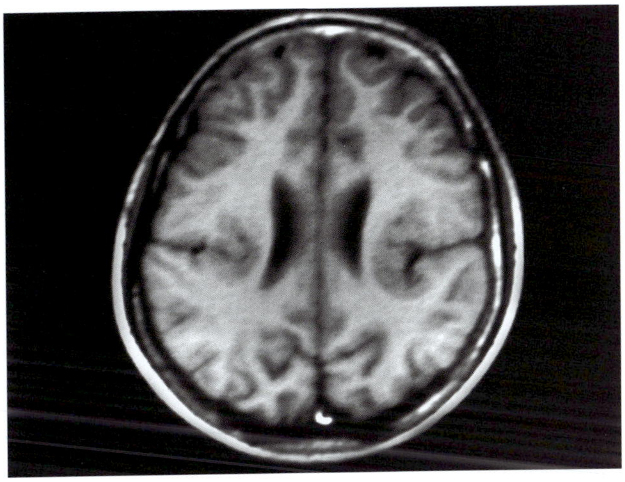

FIG. 10: Axial T1-weighted (T1W) MR image showing bilateral perisylvian polymicrogyria (PMG).

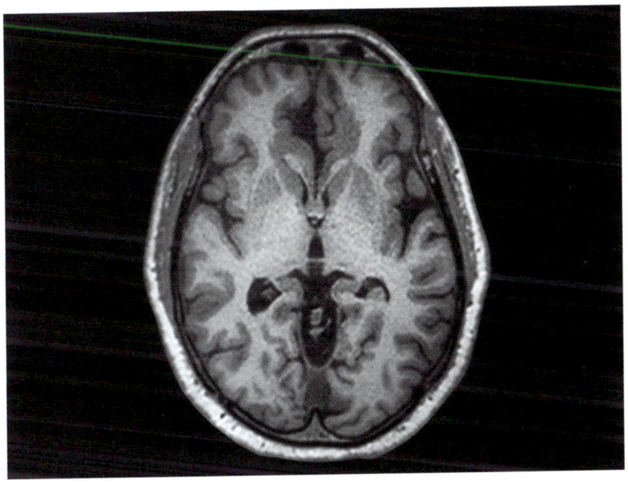

FIG. 11: Axial T1-weighted (T1W) MR image shows bifrontal polymicrogyria (PMG).

(CSF) cavity. The common site of involvement is the roof or lateral borders of lateral ventricle. MR or CT scan will show an outpouching or nipple at the ependymal surface of the cleft in closed lip schizencephaly. MRI demonstrates the full thickness of cleft and the pial-ependymal seam of GM **(Figs. 12A and B)**.

Type II or open lip schizencephaly in which the pial-ependymal seam is widened by a CSF cleft. CT and MRI show the CSF cleft extending from the ventricular system to the pial surface of brain. The CSF cavity is usually bilateral and symmetric. However, it may be asymmetric or even unilateral. Severe form of open lip schizencephaly presents with massive CSF cavities which communicate with the ventricular system and has an appearance which is a called "basket brain". This congenital malformation has a high association with absence of septum pellucidum, PMG, septo-optic dysplasia, and heterotopia[8] **(Figs. 12C and D)**.

ANOMALIES OF VENTRAL PROSENCEPHALON DEVELOPMENT

These include holoprosencephaly, arrhinia/arrhinencephaly, septo-optic dysplasia, isolated absence of the septum pellucidum, anomalies of the hypothalamic-pituitary axis, and anomalies of the eyes.

Holoprosencephaly

Holoprosencephaly is a congenital malformation characterized by incomplete cleavage and differentiation of the prosencephalon (forebrain) into cerebral hemispheres. Mutation of at least four different genetic loci has been identified to be associated with this condition and these are on chromosome 21, 2, 7, and 18.[5] Syndromic association of this condition is encountered in trisomy 13 (Patau syndrome) and trisomy 18 (Edwards syndrome). Embryogenesis of holoprosencephaly is postulated to be the lack of mesenchyme in the developing rostral neural tube, as a result of which the telencephalon does not separate from the diencephalon. The telencephalon does not develop in the two hemispheres and there is lack of cortical organization.[10]

There are three types of holoprosencephaly—(1) Alobar, (2) Semilobar, and (3) Lobar. Prenatal ultrasound (US) and postnatal CT or MRI can image the confluent ventricles and thalami adequately.

Alobar holoprosencephaly is the most severe form of holoprosencephaly. There is no differentiation of the frontal, occipital, or temporal lobes. The cerebral hemispheres are fused to form a small flat mass of tissue containing single crescent-shaped holoventricle. The flattened cerebrum occupies a small rostral segment of the calvarium. The calvarium is occupied with the large dorsal cyst which communicates with the holoventricle. Thalami may be fused with absence of interhemispheric fissure, falx cerebri, and septum pellucidum. The cerebellum and brainstem are relatively normal. This condition is associated with a severely

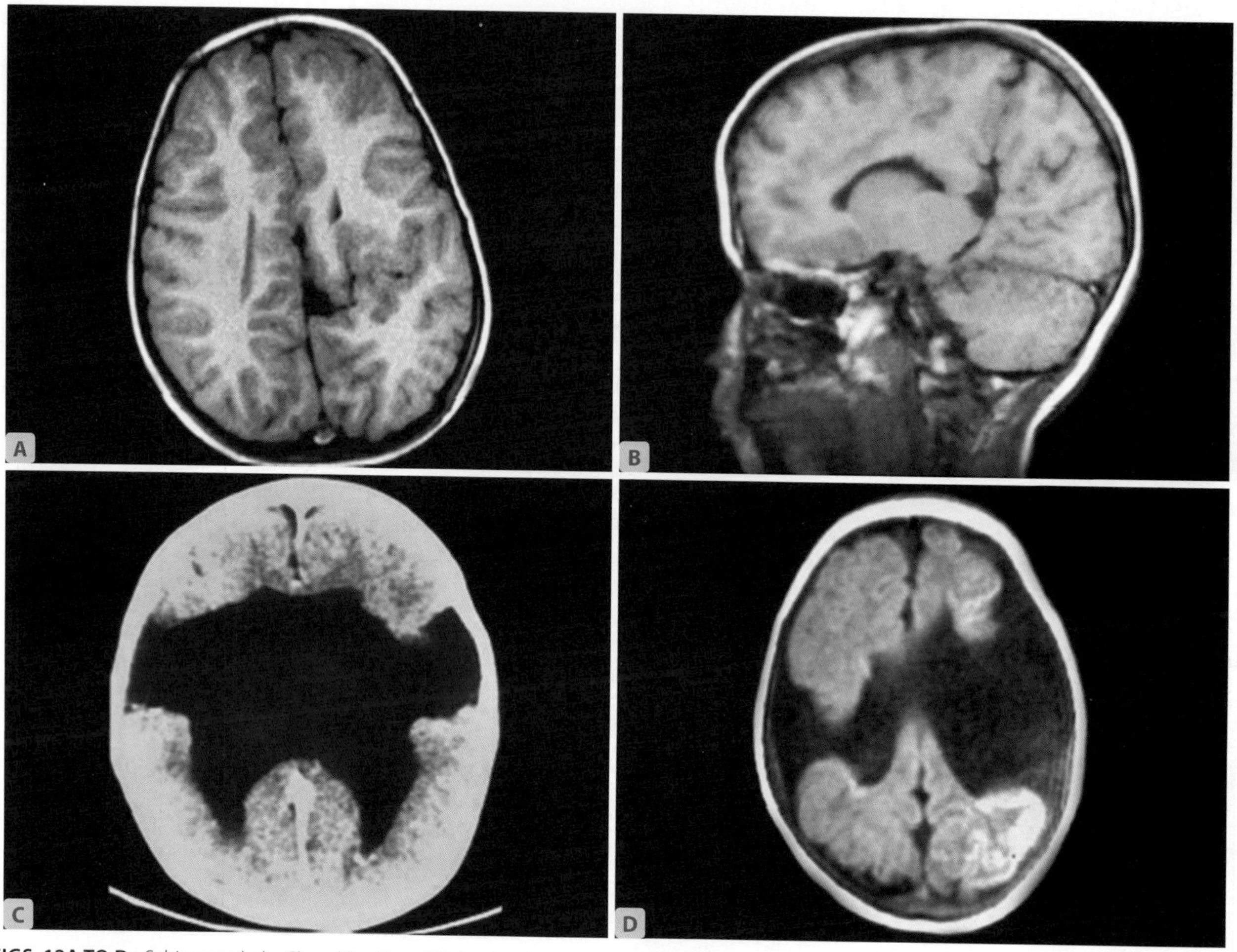

FIGS. 12A TO D: Schizencephaly: Closed lip. (A and B) Axial and sagittal T1W MR sections show deep extension of cerebral sulci reaching up till the ventricle with gray matter (GM) lining. Open lip: (C and D) Axial computed tomography (CT) and T1 MR sections show bilateral CSF clefts communicating with the lateral ventricles. (CSF: cerebrospinal fluid; T1W: T1-weighted)

dysmorphic facies, abnormal reflexes, and increased tone at birth.

Semilobar holoprosencephaly **(Fig. 13)** is a less severe form of holoprosencephaly. There is partial separation of the cerebral hemispheres with rudimentary temporal and occipital lobes. The frontal lobes are fused. There is a monoventricle with presence of the falx cerebri which is only partially seen posteriorly and suggestion of presence of an interhemispheric fissure. Septum pellucidum is absent and thalami are partially separated. The splenium of the CC is formed without the genu or body.

Lobar holoprosencephaly **(Figs. 14A and B)** is the least severe form. Brain appears normal, but the frontal horns remain fused with absence of septum pellucidum. Appearance of the frontal horns with angular corners is termed "box-like". Temporal and occipital horns are separated and are of normal size and shape. However, the bodies of the lateral ventricles may be closely apposed. Interhemispheric fissure is formed, but is shallow anteriorly. The thalami are separated.

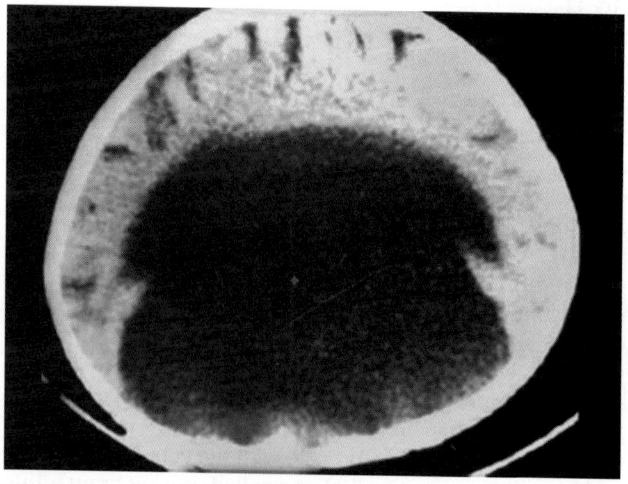

FIG. 13: Semilobar holoprosencephaly: Axial computed tomography (CT) section shows a monoventricle with a dorsal cyst and partially formed temporal lobes.

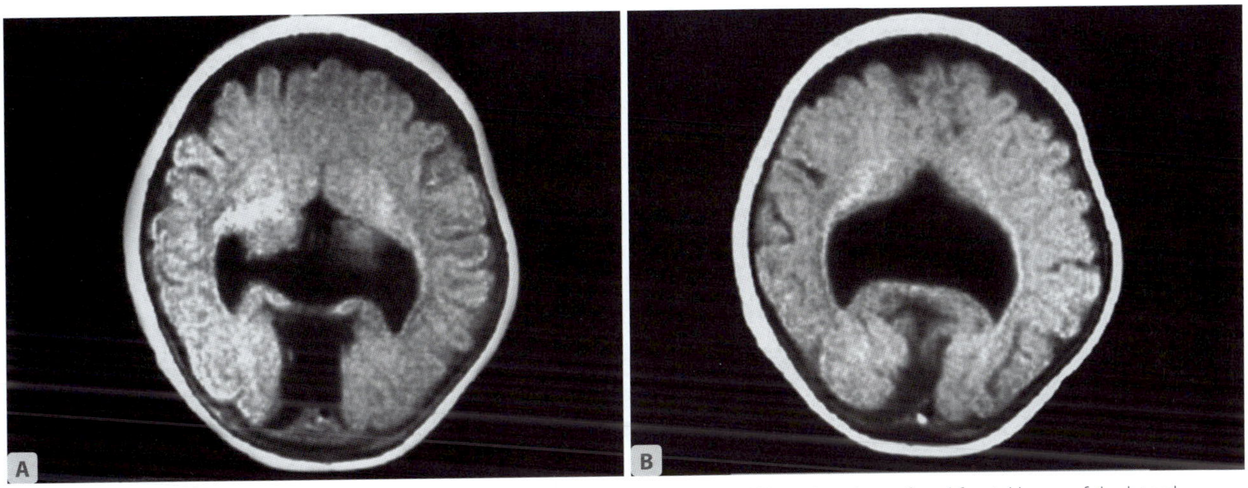

FIGS. 14A AND B: Lobar holoprosencephaly: Axial short repetition time (TR) sequence MR section shows fused frontal horns of the lateral ventricles. The cerebral hemispheres are well-formed, however, the anterior interhemispheric fissure is partially delineated.

Holoprosencephaly Variants

Middle Interhemispheric Variant of Holoprosencephaly (Syntelencephaly)

In this variant, only the mid sections are fused with normal separation of the anterior and posterior hemispheres by the falx and interhemispheric fissure. The basal ganglia and olfactory sulci appear normal.[4] The CC body is absent. The posterior frontal lobes are continuous across the midline on coronal images. On coronal imaging, a single common ventricle lacking a septum pellucidum is present. In most of the cases, the sylvian fissures course superiorly and meet in a coronal GM-lined fissure that is continuous across the midline.

Solitary Median Maxillary Central Incisor Syndrome

It is a rare malformation that consists of multiple (mainly midline) defects. Imaging findings range from isolated dental abnormalities with a single maxillary incisor and V-shaped palate to multiple complex abnormalities that involve the brain such as anomalies of the fornix, septi pellucidi and anterior CC, azygous anterior cerebral, and pituitary stalk hypoplasia.[4]

Septo-optic Dysplasia

Septo-optic dysplasia is believed to be a mild form of lobar holoprosencephaly and consists of absence of septum pellucidum with hypoplasia of the optic nerve and optic chiasma and hypoplasia of the hypothalamus. MRI shows these findings with clarity. In addition, abnormally squared or flattened frontal horns of the lateral ventricles and an enlarged anterior recess of the third ventricle may be seen. It may be associated with aqueductal stenosis, Chiari II malformation, schizencephaly, and CC agenesis. In addition, an association of hypothalamus-pituitary dysfunction is seen in two-thirds of the patients with this condition.[5,11]

Hydranencephaly

Hydranencephaly is an encephaloclastic porencephaly which results presumably secondary to in utero occlusion of either of the internal carotid arteries or infection such as CMV or due to a genetic cause. This results in infarction, necrosis, and destruction of the cerebral cortex. The cerebral hemispheres are replaced by a thin-walled membranous sac which is lined by glial tissue on the inside and leptomeninges on the outside. Diagnosis on US is easy as the falx cerebri, thalami, and cerebellar hemispheres are identified in the presence of the two large fluid-filled sacs.[12] Differential diagnosis includes severe hydrocephalus, in which a rind of remaining cortical mantle can be identified and alobar holoprosencephaly where absence of falx and presence of fused thalami clinches the diagnosis. CT or MRI may be done when US findings are equivocal **(Figs. 15A and B)**.

CONGENITAL ANOMALIES OF THE POSTERIOR FOSSA

Anomalies of Midbrain-hindbrain Development

With marked advancement in the neuroimaging techniques and genetic sequencing over the years, there has been better understanding of pathogenesis and classification of these posterior fossa brain anomalies.[13-15] These still remain challenging to the radiologist because of their complexity and less common incidence than supratentorial malformation. These anomalies may result from either inherited (genetic) or acquired (disruptive) factors.[16] Various classifications have been described in the literature based on neuroimaging, genetics, and developmental biologic criteria.[17-19] In this chapter, we will be discussing these malformation based on the neuroimaging features proposed by Doherty et al. as it is relatively simple and better for understanding as radiologist; though there may be limitation as neuroimaging-based approach is not exhaustive as genetic based.[19]

Based upon predominant involvement of the posterior fossa structure on neuroimaging, these can be broadly divided into four groups: (1) Predominantly cerebellar, (2) Cerebellar and brainstem, (3) Predominantly brainstem, and (4) Predominantly midbrain malformations **(Flowchart 1)**.

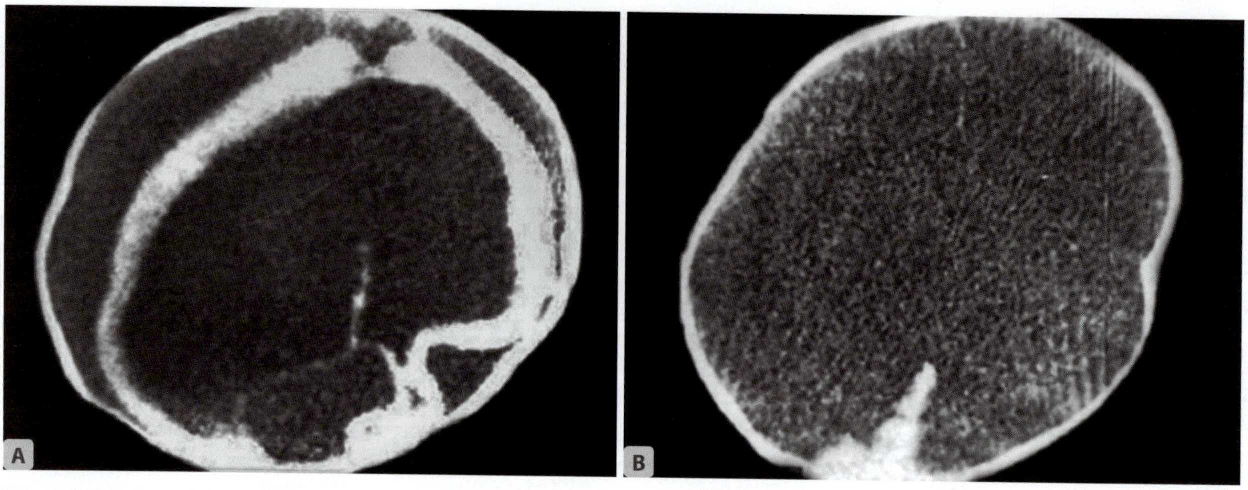

FIGS. 15A AND B: Hydranencephaly versus congenital hydrocephalus. (A) Axial computed tomography (CT) section shows presence of a preserved cortical mantle with interhemispheric fissure. Bilateral subdural collection favors the diagnosis of hydrocephalus; and (B) In hydranencephaly, the brain is replaced by a fluid-filled sac. No cortical mantle is identified.

FLOWCHART 1: Four different groups of congenital anomalies of the posterior fossa based on neuroimaging.

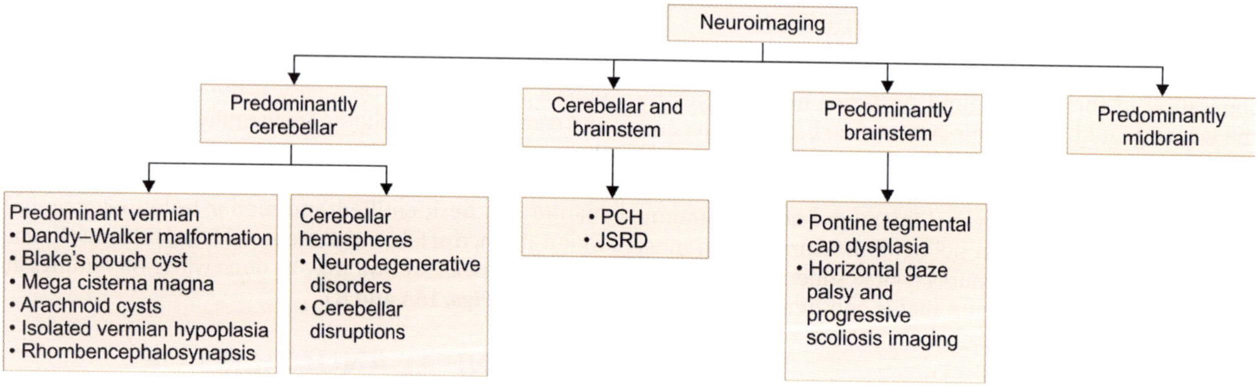

(JSRD: Joubert syndrome and related disorder; PCH: pontocerebellar hypoplasia)

Predominantly Cerebellar Anomalies

Cerebellar anomalies can be divided into those involving predominately the vermis or cerebellar hemispheres (bilateral or unilateral). These anomalies may be seen in the form of hypoplasia (decreased volume of cerebellum), dysplasia (morphological cerebellar abnormalities of foliation, fissuration, and of the cerebellar white matter architecture), or mixed of these. Predominant vermian involvement is common and seen in variety of disorders which may be grouped as cystic lesions of the posterior fossa [Dandy–Walker malformation (DWM), Blake pouch cyst, mega cisterna magna (MCM), and arachnoid cysts], isolated vermian hypoplasia, and rhombencephalosynapsis. Predominant cerebellar hemispheres involvement is uncommon and may be seen in neurodegenerative disorders like pontocerebellar hypoplasia (PCH) or developmental disorders like cerebellar disruptions.

Dandy–Walker Malformation

Dandy–Walker malformation is the most common posterior fossa malformation. Its occurrence is usually sporadic and less commonly as part of chromosomal anomalies or syndrome with a low recurrence rate (1–5%).[13] Patients with DWM usually present in the 1st year of life with features of increased intracranial pressure, most commonly with macrocephaly is the neonatal period. With antenatal sonography, cystic posterior fossa malformation is usually diagnosed in most of the patients. The prognosis of the DWM is variable and depends upon whether it is an isolated anomaly where it has usually good outcome or is associated with other brain anomalies (like callosal dysgenesis or malformation of cortical development) and systemic involvement (like cardiovascular, urogenital, or skeletal anomalies) where it has a poorer prognosis. The characteristic imaging feature **(Figs. 16A to C)** is combination of hypoplasia (or rarely agenesis) of the cerebellar vermis and cystic dilatation of fourth ventricle. The vermis is usually elevated and upwardly rotated and usually the inferior vermis is typically hypoplastic with variable involvement of the superior part. The morphology of the cerebellar hemispheres is usually normal and they may be displaced anterolaterally. Enlargement of the posterior fossa is usually seen due to cystic dilatation of the fourth ventricle with elevation of the tentorium, torcular, and transverse sinuses.

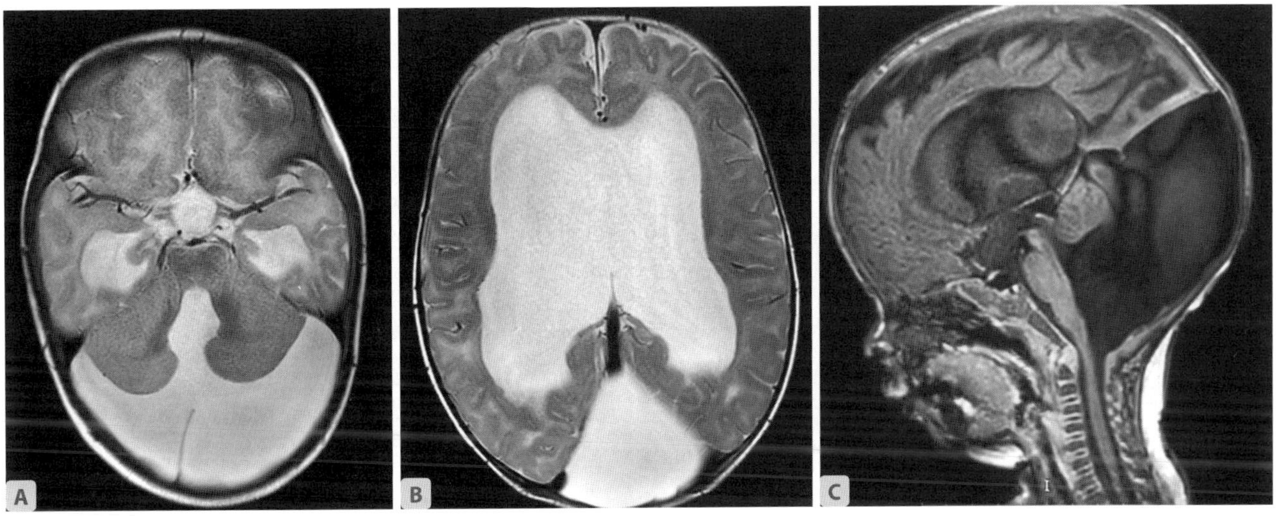

FIGS. 16A TO C: Axial T2-weighted (A and B) and sagittal T1-weighted (C) images showing Dandy–Walker Malformation. Posterior fossa is enlarged with a hypoplastic vermis in upward rotation (A and C). There is cystic dilatation of the fourth ventricle which is communicating with an enlarged posterior fossa and there is supratentorial hydrocephalus (B).

In DWM, hydrocephalus is seen in about 90% of patients and CSF flow studies provide better insight into the hydrodynamic changes due to DWM. Many different terminology has been used in the literature to classify the cystic posterior fossa malformations that do not meet the criteria for DWM like Dandy–Walker variant, Dandy–Walker complex, or Dandy–Walker spectrum. These nomenclatures are more subjective, lack specificity, and are confusing, so these should be avoided and morphologic description of the lesion should be used to describe these malformations. Neuroimaging plays a key role in identification and differentiation of various cystic posterior fossa malformations. Characteristic imaging findings of MCM is normal appearance of cerebellum and fourth ventricle, vermis and cerebellum are hypoplastic with enlarged posterior fossa and fourth ventricle in DWM, and in arachnoid cyst posterior fossa is normal along with vermis and fourth ventricle but occipital bone scalloping may be seen.

Blake's Pouch Cyst

Blake's pouch cyst (BPC) was described by Tortori-Donati et al. as a differential of cystic posterior fossa malformation. Embryologically, the roof of the fourth ventricle is divided by the choroid plexus into an anterior and a posterior membranous area. In normal development, communication of the Blake's pouch is established with the subarachnoid space through the foramen of Magendie by 8 weeks and with the foramen of Luschka by 4–5 months and when there is failure of the perforation of the foramen of Magendie, protrusion of the posterior membranous area of the fourth ventricular roof leads to cystic dilation of the fourth ventricle without cisternal communication which refers to persistent the BPC. It extends inferiorly and posteriorly from the vermis into the cisterna magna, with mild anticlockwise rotation of the cerebellar vermis and usually associated hydrocephalus but the cerebellum is usually normal. BPC cyst occurs sporadically with no reported recurrence. Most commonly BPC presents with hydrocephalus and macrocephaly in the neonatal period. The characteristic imaging feature is a posterior fossa cyst which is located posteriorly or inferiorly to the cerebellum. The choroid plexus inferior to the vermis is displaced anterosuperiorly by the cyst, which is helpful in differentiating from other posterior fossa cysts and better appreciated on sagittal contrast-enhanced MR images. In BPC, the posterior fossa is typically normal in size and no supratentorial anomalies are described, except hydrocephalus. Endoscopic third ventriculostomy is the treatment of choice in BPC associated with hydrocephalus.

Mega Cisterna Magna

Cisterna magna refers to the subarachnoid space in the posterior cranial fossa filled with CSF which is inferior to the cerebellum and posterior aspect of the medulla and is also known as posterior cerebellomedullary cistern. When the focal enlargement of cisterna magna is >10 mm with normal cerebellar vermis and fourth ventricle, then it refers to enlarged or MCM **(Figs. 17A and B)**. It is measured on midsagittal images from the posterior aspect of the cerebellar vermis to the inner aspect of the occipital bone. Usually, MCM is not associated with hydrocephalus and CSF flow studies have shown free communication with the fourth ventricle and the cervical subarachnoid space. Most authors agree that BPC and MCM result from a defect of the posterior membranous area whereas DWM results from a defect of the anterior membranous area. MCM results from delayed fenestration of the Blake's pouch whereas BPC occurs when there is no fenestration of the Blake's pouch. MCM is usually an incidental finding and represents a normal variant with no reported recurrence risk. Children with MCM have normal development and no follow-up imaging is required.

Posterior Fossa Arachnoid Cysts

Posterior fossa arachnoid cysts (PFACs) can occur either in the midline or lateral aspect of the posterior fossa and constitute about 10% of arachnoid cysts in children.

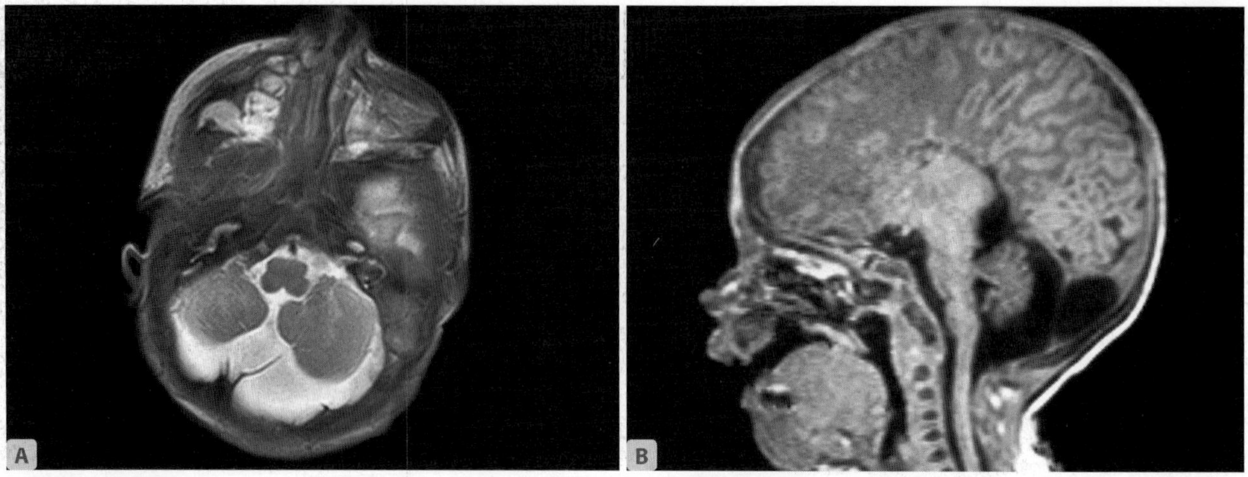

FIGS. 17A AND B: Axial T2-weighted (A) and sagittal T1-weighted (B) images showing marked enlargement of cisterna magna with normal cerebellar vermis and fourth ventricle. There is no hydrocephalus.

They are located inferior or posterior to the cerebellar vermis in a midline (retrocerebellar), superior to the vermis (supravermian), anterior or lateral to the cerebellar hemispheres, or anterior to the brainstem. Arachnoid cysts results from the duplications of the arachnoid membrane and there is no communication with the fourth ventricle and/ or cervical subarachnoid space. Children with PFAC may present with macrocephaly, signs of increased intracranial pressure, and developmental delay whereas in adults, these are usually asymptomatic and discovered incidentally. Rarely, these may be associated with hydrocephalus or remodeling (scalloping or thinning) of the overlying occipital bone. The characteristic imaging feature is well-circumscribed extra-axial cystic lesion which is isointense to CSF on all sequences. However, content of the cyst may vary, if there are proteinaceous content or hemorrhage in the cyst. The walls of the cyst are very thin and are not visualized at MRI.

Isolated Inferior Vermian Hypoplasia

Isolated inferior vermian hypoplasia refers to partial absence of the inferior portion of the cerebellar vermis. It is a pathologic condition and some authors refer it as Dandy-Walker variant which creates confusion and such terminology should be avoided. It may be an isolation condition with a favorable outcome and no recurrence risk or may be associated with other Mendelian syndromes with increased recurrence risk. The characteristic imaging feature is partial absence of the inferior vermis, which is better appreciated on midline images. The other structures of the posterior fossa are normal. For the prenatal diagnosis of isolated inferior vermian hypoplasia, fetal MRI is more sensitive and specific than sonography.

Rhombencephalosynapsis

It is a rare midline cerebellar congenital abnormality, characterized by absence of cerebellar vermis.[20] There is apparent fusion of the cerebellar hemispheres with continuity of the cerebellar hemispheres, dentate nuclei, and superior cerebellar peduncles. It is usually seen in isolation or rarely with other central nervous system (CNS) and extra-CNS malformations. It can be seen in patients in Gómez-López-Hernández syndrome (rhombencephalosynapsis with parietal/temporal alopecia and sometimes trigeminal anesthesia, towering skull shape, and dysmorphic features) and in patients with associated vertebral anomalies, anal atresia, cardiovascular anomalies, tracheoesophageal fistula, renal anomalies, and limb defects (VACTERL). The common clinical features are truncal and/or limb ataxia, abnormal eye movements, head stereotypies, and delayed motor development. Systemic involvement is rare, but patients may die in childhood or early adult life. The characteristic imaging feature **(Figs. 18A and B)** is agenesis or hypogenesis of the vermis with continuity of the cerebellar hemispheres, superior cerebellar peduncles, and dentate nuclei. Posterior coronal MR typically shows the horizontal folial pattern. Common associated CNS anomalies include hydrocephalus and forebrain abnormalities like absent olfactory bulbs, dysgenesis of the CC, and absent septum pellucidum.

Macrocerebellum

It is a rare entity and refers to an isolated and abnormal increase of the cerebellum size with no morphological or signal abnormalities. The clinical presentation of the entity is variable. On imaging, it is characterized by marked cerebellar enlargement with preserved architecture and shape. The cerebellar hemispheres are more commonly involved than the vermis.

Cerebellar Dysplasia

It is collective terminology which includes many cerebellar malformation and disruption having variable clinical and imaging features. They may be associated with cerebral malformations. Imaging features include disorganized foliation, abnormal fissuration (including defective, enlarged, or vertical fissures), and attenuated gray-white matter junction and white matter arborization. Cerebellar dysplasia may be focal which indicate disruptive lesion or global which indicate a malformation.

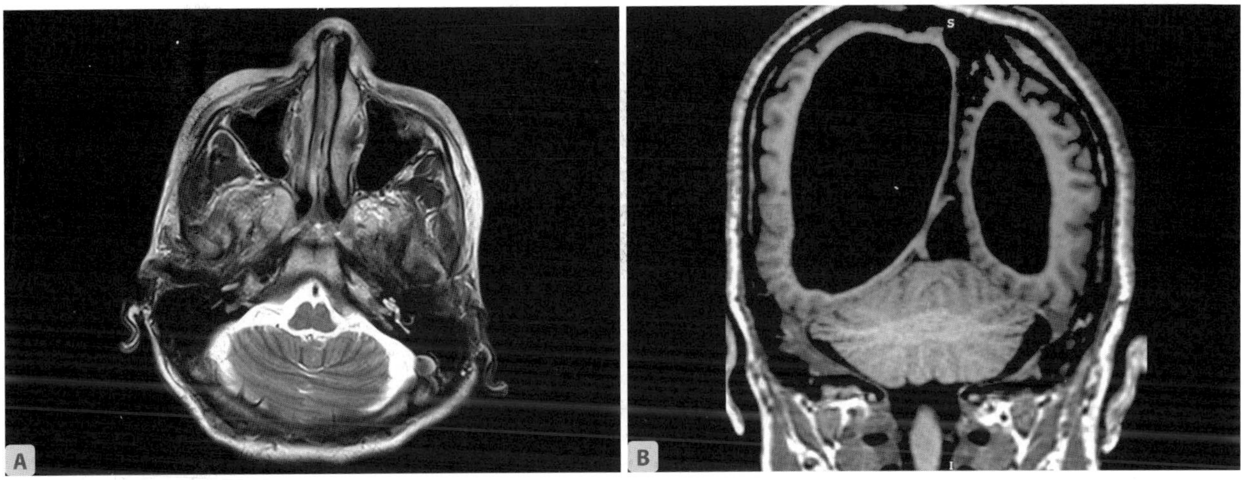

FIGS. 18A AND B: Axial T2 (A) and posterior coronal T1-weighted (B) MR image shows continuity of the cerebellar hemispheres without an intervening vermis, an abnormal transverse orientation of the cerebellar foliae with continuity of the cerebellar hemispheres.

Cerebellar Involvement in Migrational Disorders

Cerebellar and pontine abnormalities are described with migrational disorders, mutations in RELN and VLDLR, and mutations in tubulin genes. Clinical and imaging spectrum is variable.

Cerebellar and Brainstem Malformations

Important malformations under this spectrum include PCH type 1–10, Joubert syndrome, and CMDs due to defective dystroglycan O-glycosylation. Other included are glycosylation type 1a congenital disorder, CASK mutations, Joubert syndrome, cerebellar agenesis caused by a disruptive lesion or representing a malformation due to PTF1A mutations, vanishing cerebellum in Chiari 2 malformation (CM2), and cerebellar disruption secondary to prematurity.

Pontocerebellar Hypoplasia

It is a group of rare autosomal recessive neurodegenerative disorders caused by genetic mutations mainly with a prenatal onset. Peter G Barth first described them as a specific entity and is characterized by hypoplasia of the cerebellum and pons. Hitherto, 11 subtypes of PCH with different phenotypes and pathogeneses have been identified.[21] On imaging, they are characterized by severe hypoplasia or atrophy of cerebellum and pons. In addition, supratentorial structures are variably involved with motor and cognitive impairments. Coronal and sagittal MR images are very helpful in the evaluation of PCH. "Dragonfly" appearance is described for PCH that refers to flattened cerebellar hemispheres (the "wings") and a relatively preserved vermis (the "body") on coronal MR images.

Joubert Syndrome

Joubert syndrome is a rare inherited autosomal recessive disorder with recurrence may be seen in 25% in the affected family.[22] It shows heterogeneous clinical, genetic, and neuroimaging findings. Clinical features include hypotonia, ataxia, ocular motor apraxia, facial dysmorphism, neonatal breathing dysregulation, and intellectual disability of variable severity. Systemic involvement may be seen and six phenotypic subgroups have been described on the basis of involvement of kidneys (nephronophthisis), eyes (colobomas, retinal dystrophy), liver (congenital hepatic fibrosis), and bones (various forms of polydactyly). High morbidity and mortality are seen with renal and hepatic involvement. Correlation between phenotype-genotype is seen with identified associated 26 different genes so far, which encode for proteins of the nonmotile primary cilia, which play a key role in the development and functioning of various cells. In the brain, primary cilia are responsible for the neuronal cell proliferation and axonal migration in the cerebellum and brainstem. Characteristic neuroimaging finding for the Joubert syndrome was reported first by Maria et al. as "molar tooth sign" (MTS) **(Figs. 19A to D)** which refers to elongated, thickened, and horizontally oriented superior cerebellar peduncles, a deep interpeduncular fossa, and vermian hypoplasia. In addition, fourth ventricle is enlarged and distorted. Though MTS is radiological hallmark of the Joubert syndrome, it was found that MTS may be seen in other syndromes. So, all these syndromes were clubbed together and named as Joubert syndrome and related disorders (JSRDs) with mandatory diagnostic neuroimaging criteria of MTS and vermian hypoplasia. However, there is variable involvement of the supratentorial structures of the brain and the brainstem in about 30% of patients each. The brainstem may be involved in form of dysmorphic tectum and midbrain, thickening and elongation of the midbrain, and a small pons. The neuroimaging findings are of limited value in classifying patients with Joubert syndrome as no correlation has been found between neuroimaging findings and genotype. Absence of decussation of the superior cerebellar peduncles and corticospinal tract can be shown on DTI.

Congenital Muscular Dystrophies Owing to Defective Dystroglycan O-glycosylation

The "α-dystroglycanopathies" are a group of CMDs due to genetic mutations that have autosomal recessive pattern

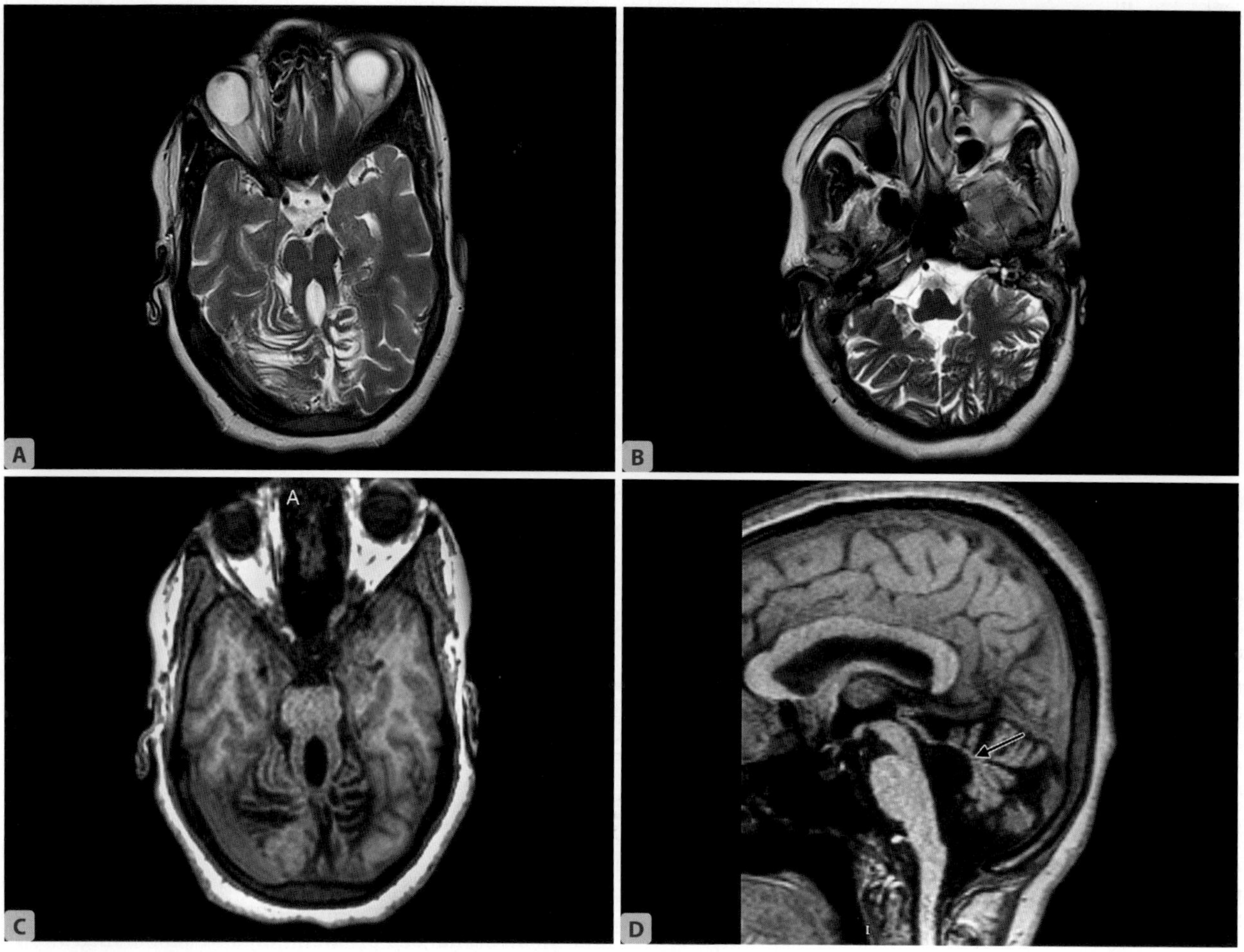

FIGS. 19A TO D: Axial T2- (A to C) and sagittal T1-weighted (D) images showing hypoplastic and dysgenetic vermis. Superior cerebellar peduncles is elongated, thickened, and horizontally oriented giving the characteristic molar tooth sign. In addition, there is with upward and posterior displacement of the fastigium (arrow).

inheritance. Various phenotype forms and clinical features have been described with involvement of the muscles, brain, and eyes. In brain, both supra- and infratentorial structures are involved variably. Supratentorial involvement is seen in the form of mild ventriculomegaly to severe hydrocephalus, white matter changes, PGM, and cerebral cortical abnormalities, including cobblestone LIS. Infratentorial involvement is seen in form of hypoplasia or dysplasia of cerebellum, cerebellar cysts, pontine hypoplasia, ventral pontine cleft, and pontomesencephalic kinking. In CMDs, these cerebellar cysts are a relatively specific finding for CMDs. Most likely, these cysts are formed from the portions of the subarachnoid space that were entrapped by the dysplastic cerebellar folia, especially at the interphase between normal and dysplastic cerebellar cortex.

Predominantly Brainstem Involvement

Abnormalities include pontine tegmental cap dysplasia (PTCD) and horizontal gaze palsy with progressive scoliosis (HGPPS).

Pontine Tegmental Cap Dysplasia

It is a rare disorder with characteristic clinical and pathognomonic neuroimaging features **(Figs. 20A and B)**. It is characterized by a flattened hypoplastic ventral pons and a cap-like dorsal pontine tegmental protrusion (the "cap").[23,24] The "cap" being representing an ectopic dorsal transverse pontine fiber projecting from the pontine tegmentum into the fourth ventricle. Additional features include partial absence of the middle cerebellar peduncles, vermian hypoplasia, a molar tooth-like aspect of the pontomesencephalic junction, and absent inferior olivary prominence. The PTCD is a sporadic malformation with unknown genotype and pathogenesis, but probably results from a defect in axonal guidance and/or migration. Its prognosis is variable. Clinical findings are characterized by the involvement of vestibulocochlear, facial, trigeminal, and glossopharyngeal nerves, resulting in hearing loss, facial paralysis, trigeminal anesthesia, and difficulty in swallowing. Systemic involvement may be seen in form of vertebral segmentation anomalies, rib malformations, and congenital heart defects. DTI shows absence of the transverse

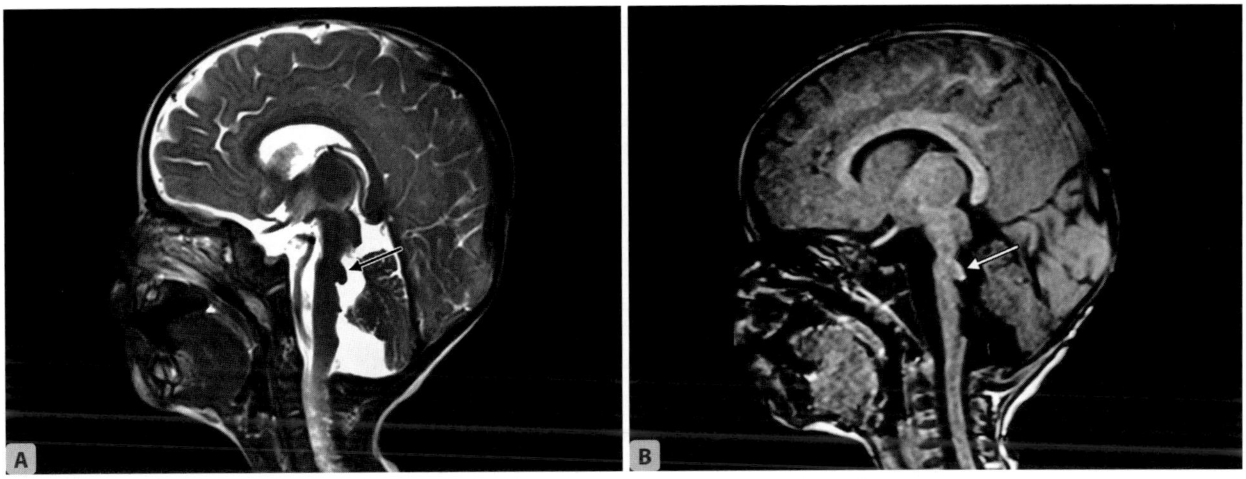

FIGS. 20A AND B: Sagittal T2 (A) and T1 (B) images showing a flattened ventral pons and a cap (arrows) covering the dorsal pons which is projecting into the fourth ventricle.

pontine fibers and the presence of a dorsal transverse axonal band at the level of the so-called cap in the dorsal pons. The dorsal ectopic axonal band most likely results from abnormal axonal guidance and/or neuronal migration.

Horizontal Gaze Palsy with Progressive Scoliosis

It is a rare autosomal recessive congenital disorder characterized by congenital absence of horizontal eye movements, preservation of vertical gaze and convergence, and progressive scoliosis developing in childhood and adolescence. It occurs due to mutation in *ROBO3* gene/chromosome 11q23-q25, which encodes a receptor required for axonal guidance.[25] MRI **(Figs. 21A to E)** shows brainstem hypoplasia with absence of facial colliculi, presence of a deep midline pontine cleft (split pons sign), and a butterfly shape of the medulla due to the missing prominence of the gracile and cuneate nuclei. DTI typically shows the absence of decussation of the corticospinal tracts, pontine sensory tracts, and superior cerebellar peduncles.

Predominantly Midbrain Malformations

There are relatively few disorders where predominant midbrain involvement has been described. Imaging shows abnormal configuration of the midbrain in form of transverse elongation or craniocaudal shortening of the brainstem. Variable clinical features are seen. Dysplasia of the diencephalic-mesencephalic junction with a butterfly-like contour of the midbrain on axial images has been reported by Zaki et al.

Anomalies of the Craniocervical Junction

Chiari malformations: Hans Chiari, in the late 19th century based on autopsy observations, divided group of hindbrain malformations which were associated with hydrocephalus into three types: Chiari 1–3. These were primarily associated with congenital caudal displacement of the cerebellum and/or brainstem. Depending on autopsy or imaging, these malformations are divided based on their morphology and severity of anatomic defects. Inferior displacement of the cerebellar tonsils is seen in Chiari 1 whereas herniation of the medulla and vermis with associated myelodysplasia is seen in Chiari 2. In Chiari 3, herniation of posterior fossa contents through a low occipitocervical bony defect. Chiari 4 terminology is no longer used as it was used for severe cerebellar hypoplasia or primary cerebellar agenesis and not a hindbrain herniation. In addition to these three described Chiari malformations, other terms are used to include the variants like Chiari 0 which refers to syrinx without frank tonsillar herniation, Chiari 1.5 which refers to caudal protrusion of brainstem in addition to the tonsils and Chiari 5 which refers to Chiari 2 plus occipital or high cervical myelomeningocele.

Type 1 Chiari malformation (CM1) or simply Chiari I refers to caudal cerebellar tonsillar ectopia. It is the least severe form of Chiari malformations and is often found incidentally. It is characterized by one or both pointed (peg-like, not rounded) cerebellar tonsils that project 5 mm or more below the foramen magnum, measured by a line drawn from the basion to the opisthion (McRae line). However, this precise distance criteria of CM1 is not agreed upon by investigator and they believe that additional abnormalities around the foramen magnum such as tonsillar deformity, effaced retrotonsillar CSF spaces, or altered CSF flow dynamics should also be present. Cervical spinal cord abnormalities, hydrosyringomyelia or simply syrinx, are common in CM1. The pathogenesis of CM1 is not well-known and is controversial. However, many factors like abnormal geometry of the bony posterior fossa, altered CSF dynamics, and genetics have been proposed. It is seen in all age groups with estimated prevalence of 0.6–1.0% in the general population. Clinical presentation varies with age and up to 50% of with CM1 patients diagnosed on imaging may be asymptomatic at the time of diagnosis. Common clinical presentations in children include oropharyngeal dysfunction (in children ≤2 years), occipital or posterior cervical headache or scoliosis (in 3–5 years), altered pain, temperature, and vibratory sensation in children with holocord syringohydromyelia.

Imaging features of CM1 include caudal tonsillar ectopia (≥5 mm below foramen magnum), pointed, peg-like tonsils with angled folia with crowding at foramen magnum, and

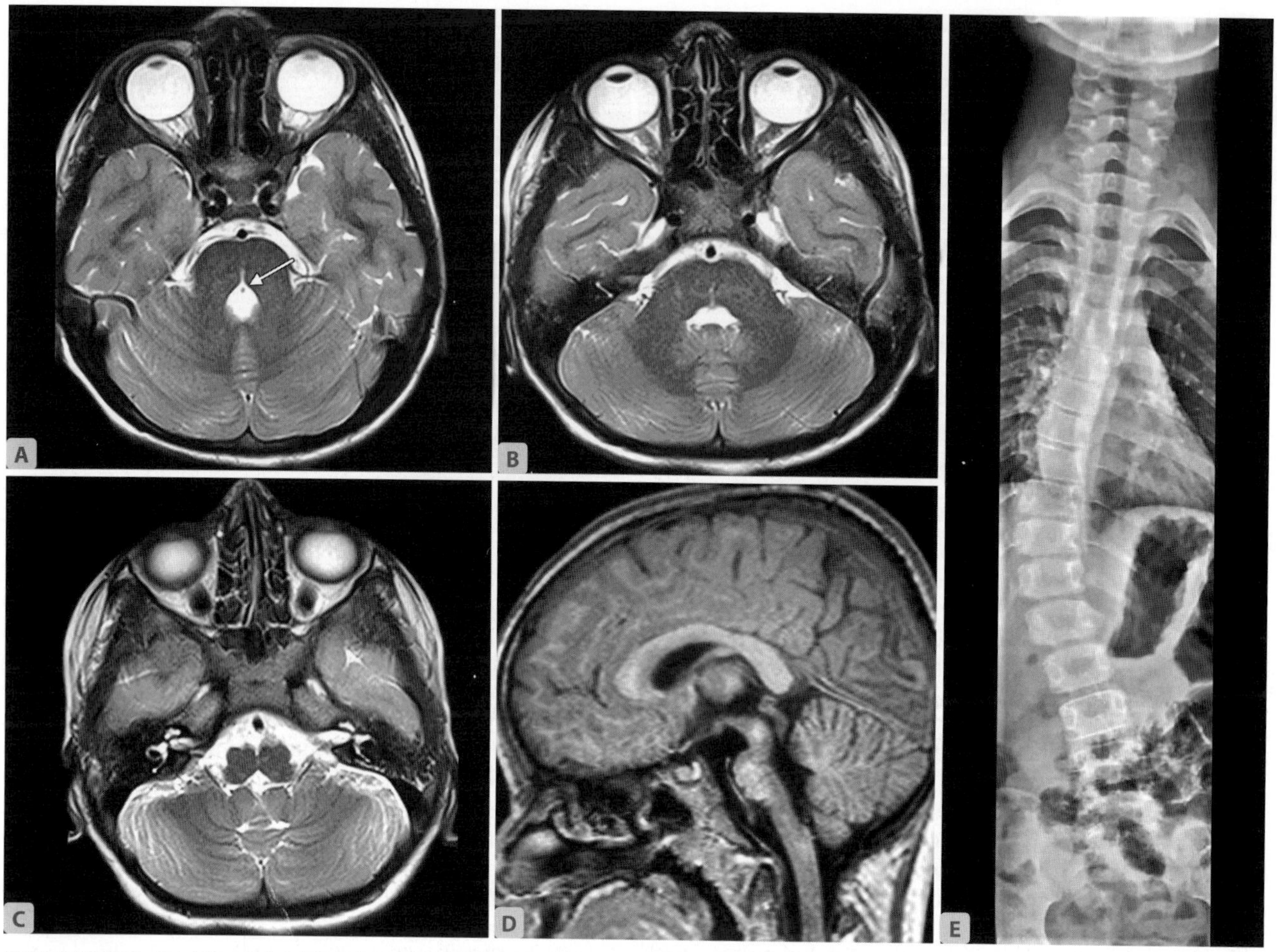

FIGS. 21A TO E: Axial T2-weighted (A to C), and mid sagittal T1-weighted images showing reduced volume of pons and medulla, midline deep clefting at dorsal aspect of pons (white arrow showing split pons sign, A), absent facial colliculi (B), butterfly configuration of medulla (C). X-ray AP view of whole spine (E) shows scoliotic deformity of thoracolumbar spine.

effaced CSF spaces **(Figs. 22A and B)**. In addition, syrinx is seen in symptomatic (40–80%) as well as asymptomatic (10–20%) patients with decreased or absent CSF flow at posterior foramen magnum.

Chiari 2 malformation or Chiari II refers to complex hindbrain malformation (cerebellar and brainstem herniation and a towering cerebellum) that is almost always associated with myelodysplasia (an open distal spinal dysraphism/myelomeningocele). The underlying cause of CM2 is an open neural tube defect (myelomeningocele) along with disorder of paraxial mesodermal abnormalities of the skull and spine. Leakage or redirected flow of CSF in utero leads to continued collapse of the fourth ventricle, which results in a hypoplastic posterior fossa and cerebellar/brainstem displacements. The other underlying causes are those factors which increase the risk of neural tube defects like maternal folate deficiency and methylenetetrahydrofolate reductase (MTHFR) mutations and teratogens such as anticonvulsants. In CM2, supratentorial abnormalities are commonly seen with hydrocephalus that is present in the most of the cases. Other anomalies include CC dysgenesis and GM anomalies such as PMG and heterotopias. At birth, presentation is usually myelomeningocele and hydrocephalus.

Imaging abnormalities in CM2 are seen in spine, brain, and skull **(Figs. 23A to C)**. In spine, myelomeningocele is almost always seen with half of the cases showing hydrosyringomyelia. In brain, small posterior fossa is seen with inferior displacement of medulla and vermis. Due to this, characteristic imaging findings include cervicomedullary kink and medullary spur, tectal beaking, towering and creeping cerebellum, and elongated fourth ventricle (soda straw appearance). Supratentorial findings include prominent massa intermedia, hydrocephalus or scalloped ventricles, if shunted, callosal dysgenesis, stenogyria, and GM heterotopias. Skull and dural abnormalities include lacunar skull, abnormal dura (tentorial incisura is widened and thinned with heart-shaped appearance, foramen magnum is gaping, and fenestrated falx with interdigitating gyri).

Chiari 3 malformation (CM3) or Chiari III is relatively rare with finding same as Chiari II but with a low occipital or upper cervical bony defect and meningoencephalocele

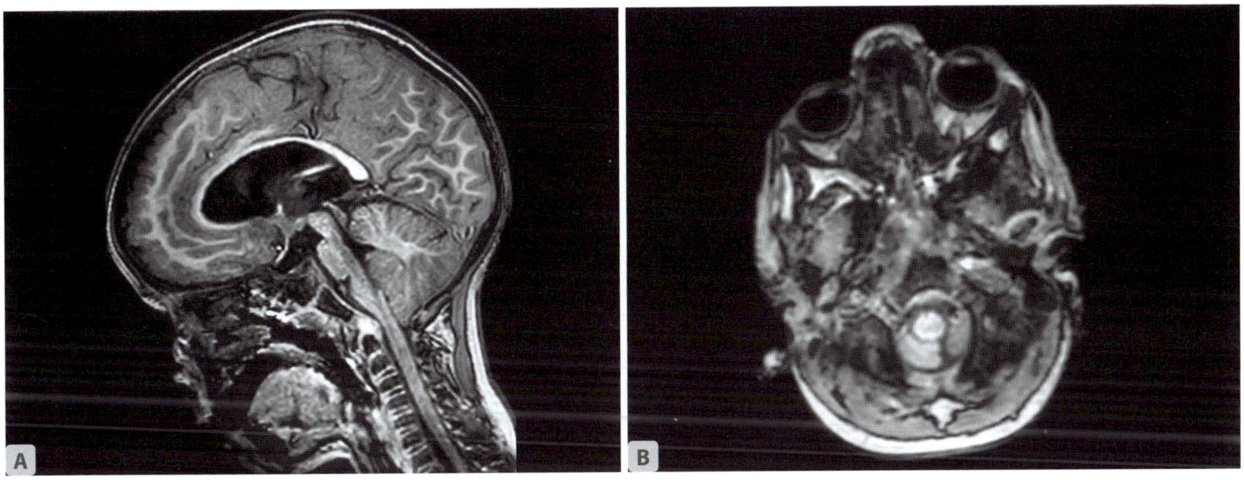

FIGS. 22A AND B: Sagittal (A) and axial (B) T1-weighted images in a young male man with classic Chiari 1 malformation shows a low-lying, pointed tonsil with crowding of the structures at foramen magnum with obliterated retrotonsillar cerebrospinal fluid (CSF) space.

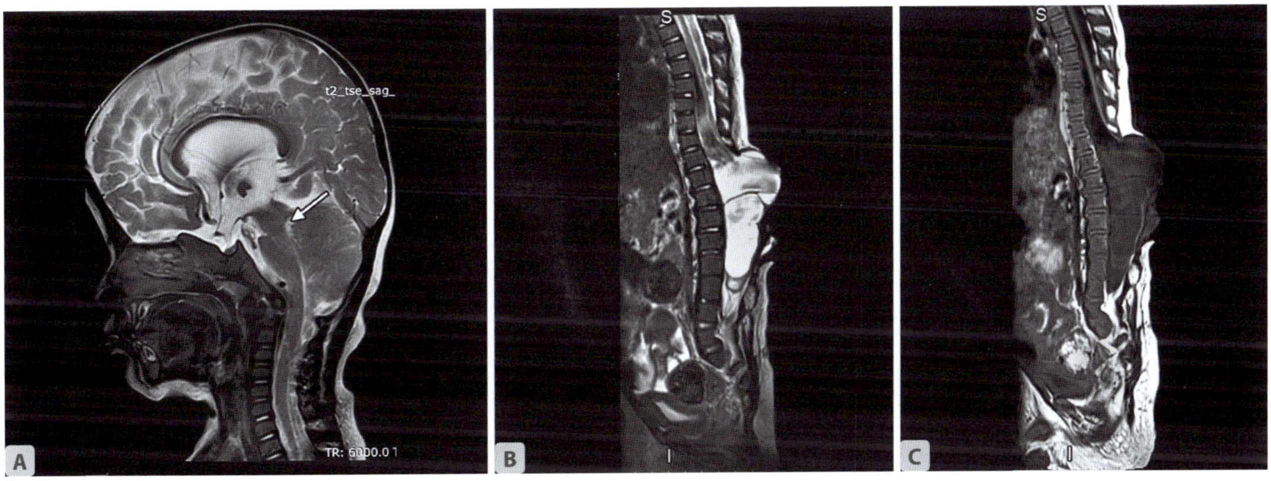

FIGS. 23A TO C: Sagittal T2-weighted MR images of the brain (A), and T2- (B) and T1-weighted (C) MR images of spine showing features of Chiari 2. Posterior fossa is small, fourth ventricle is elongated giving "soda straw" appearance, beaked tectum (arrow). Spinal cord is tethered with large myelomeningocele.

as compared to the lumbar/sacral myelomeningocele in Chiari II. In this malformation, posterior fossa is small and posterior fossa contents with meninges are variably displaced inferiorly. Imaging features in skull/dura and brain are almost similar to CM2 features. Variable contents of herniated cerebellum and/or brainstem are seen, which may be dysplastic.

CONCLUSION

MRI plays a pivotal role in identifying and characterising the various congenital anomalies of the brain. Systematic approach based on neuroimaging is helpful for diagnosing and better understanding the various disorders especially of the posterior fossa.

REFERENCES

1. Glass HC, Shaw GM, Ma C, Sherr EH. Agenesis of the corpus callosum in California 1983–2003: a population-based study. Am J Med Genet A. 2008;146A:2495-500.
2. Raybaud C, Levrier O, Brunel H. MR imaging of fetal brain malformations. Childs Nerv Syst. 2003;19:455-70.
3. Raybaud C, Girard N. The developmental disorders of the commissural plate of the telencephalon: MR imaging study and morphologic classification. Nerv Syst Child. 1999;24:348-57.
4. Barkovich AJ, Raybaud C. Syringomyelia. In: Barkovich AJ, Raybaud C (Eds). Pediatric Neuroimaging, 6th edition. Philadelphia: Lippincott Williams & Wilkins; 2018.
5. Osborn AG, Salzman KL, Jhaveri MD. Diagnostic Imaging: Brain, 3rd edition. Philadelphia: Elsevier; 2016.
6. Passemard S, Kaindl AM, Verloes A. Microcephaly. Handb Clin Neurol. 2013;111:129-41.

7. Engel J. Seizures and Epilepsy, 2nd edition. New York: Oxford University Press; 2013.
8. Abdel Razek AA, Kandell AY, Elsorogy LG, Elmongy A, Basett AA. Disorders of cortical formation: MR imaging features. AJNR Am J Neuroradiol. 2009;30:4-11.
9. Robertson R, Casuso PA, Truwit CL. Disorders of brain development. In: Atlas SW (Ed). Magnetic Resonance Imaging of the Brain. Philadelphia: Lippincott Williams & Wilkins; 2002. pp. 279-369.
10. Hahn JS, Barnes PD. Neuroimaging advances in holoprosencephaly: Refining the spectrum of the midline malformation. Am J Med Genet C Semin Med Genet. 2010;15:120-32.
11. Morishima A, Aranoff G. Syndrome of septo-optic pituitary dysplasia: The clinical spectrum. Brain Dev. 1986;8:233-35.
12. Byrd SE, Charles RF. Congenital brain malformations. In: Khun JP, Slovis TL, Haller JO (Eds). Caffey's Pediatric Diagnostic Imaging, 10th edition. St Louis: Mosby Year Book; 2004. pp. 506-29.
13. Bosemani T, Orman G, Boltshauser E, Tekes A, Huisman TA, Poretti A. Congenital abnormalities of the posterior fossa. Radiographics. 2015;35:200-20.
14. Barkovich AJ, Millen KJ, Dobyns WB. A developmental and genetic classification for midbrain-hindbrain malformations. Brain. 2009;132:3199-230.
15. Jissendi-Tchofo P, Severino M, Nguema-Edzang B, Toure C, Soto Ares G, Barkovich AJ. Update on neuroimaging phenotypes of mid-hind brain malformations. Neuroradiology. 2015;57:113-38.
16. Alkan O, Kizilkilic O, Yildirim T. Malformations of the midbrain and hindbrain: a retrospective study and review of the literature. Cerebellum. 2009;8:355-65.
17. Abdel Razek AA, Castillo M. Magnetic Resonance Imaging of Malformations of Midbrain-Hindbrain. J Comput Assist Tomogr. 2016;40:14-25.
18. Longo MG, Félix TM, Ashton-Prolla P, Vedolin LM. Brain imaging and genetic risk in the pediatric population, part 2: congenital malformations of the central nervous system. Neuroimaging Clin North Am. 2015;25:53-67.
19. Doherty D, Millen KJ, Barkovich AJ. Midbrain and hindbrain malformations: advances in clinical diagnosis, imaging, and genetics. Lancet Neurol. 2013;12:381-93.
20. Toelle SP, Yalcinkaya C, Kocer N, Deonna T, Overweg-Plandsoen WCG, Bast T, et al. Rhombencephalosynapsis: clinical findings and neuroimaging in 9 children. Neuropediatrics. 2002;33:209-14.
21. van Dijk T, Baas F, Barth PG, Poll-The BT. What's new in pontocerebellar hypoplasia? An update on genes and subtypes. Orphanet J Rare Dis. 2018;13(1):92.
22. Poretti A, Huisman TA, Scheer I, Boltshauser E. Joubert syndrome and related disorders: spectrum of neuroimaging findings in 75 patients. AJNR Am J Neuroradiol. 2011;32:1459-63.
23. Cadman CJ, Fraser L, McArthur C. Case 266: Pontine Tegmental Cap Dysplasia. Radiology. 2019;291:814-8.
24. Briguglio M, Pinelli L, Giordano L, Ferraris A, Germanò E, Micheletti S, et al. Pontine tegmental cap dysplasia: developmental and cognitive outcome in three adolescent patients. Orphanet J Rare Dis. 2011;6:36.
25. Bosley TM, Salih MA, Jen JC, Lin DD, Oystreck D, Abu-Amero KK, et al. Neurologic features of horizontal gaze palsy and progressive scoliosis with mutations in ROBO3. Neurology. 2005;64:1196-203.

CHAPTER

85

Hypoxic-ischemic Encephalopathy

Atin Kumar, Manisha Jana,
Devasenathipathy Kandasamy, Arun Kumar Gupta

INTRODUCTION

Neonatal encephalopathy following birth asphyxia or perinatal hypoxia is referred to as hypoxic-ischemic encephalopathy (HIE).[1] It is also often referred to as hypoxic-ischemic injury (HII). It represents the most common cause of neonatal encephalopathy. Exact incidence of HIE is not known but at most centers, incidence of perinatal hypoxic-ischemia is between 1.0 and 1.5%.[2]

The diagnosis of HIE is clinically suspected in a neonate in the setting of known perinatal stress. Presence of more than one of the following is a strong predictor of HIE in the right clinical setting—profound metabolic/mixed acidemia which results in a low cord pH (<7), a low Apgar score (<3) at 0 and 5 minutes after birth, abnormal early neurologic findings, and abnormal electroencephalography (EEG) soon after birth. The other etiologies of neonatal encephalopathy include various infections, metabolic disorders, congenital disorders, and trauma.[3] However, HIE needs to be differentiated from these disorders and diagnosed early as the current standard of therapy is controlled hypothermia which has to be instituted within a sensitive time window of <6 hours after the insult (presumed to be during birth). This is usually done before there is any time for imaging or diagnostic studies.[4,5]

Imaging plays a role to early detect the changes, assess the severity of the injury, and occasionally has a prognostic value. It, therefore, becomes mandatory for the pediatrician and the pediatric radiologist to understand the various imaging features with awareness of the limitations and advantages of each imaging modality.

Clinically, HIE has been graded into mild, moderate, and severe grades with prognosis directly related to the severity.[6] Approximately, 15–20% of neonates with hypoxic ischemia would die within the newborn period.[7]

NEUROIMAGING IN INFANTS WITH HYPOXIC-ISCHEMIC ENCEPHALOPATHY

Role of neuroimaging in the workup of infants with HIE is twofold:

1. Imaging of the pathologic lesions and their follow-up
2. Prediction of clinical outcome based on pathologic lesions observed on imaging.

Three important imaging techniques used for examination of the newborn brain are: (1) Sonography, (2) Computed tomography (CT), and (3) Magnetic resonance imaging (MRI). Although maturity of the neonatal brain and suspected pathology should dictate the choice of imaging, but expertise in conducting and interpreting the images on a particular diagnostic technique may decide the final selection of an investigation. Sonography, being widely available, possible even at cribside for sick babies, nonionizing, painless, not requiring sedation, or intravenous contrast, makes it an ideal screening modality in children. Depending upon the sonographic findings and the clinical status, further imaging protocol may be decided later.

It is a well-established fact that the pattern of cerebral injury in a newborn infant depends, to a great extent, on the maturity of the brain at the time of insult. It is generally agreed that the dividing line between the immature and the mature brain is around 36 weeks.[6-8]

Therefore, two broad groups, i.e., "below 36 weeks group—the premature neonate" and "at or above 36 weeks group—the term neonate" are discussed separately.

BELOW 36 WEEKS GROUP—THE PREMATURE NEONATE

Preterm neonates are much more prone to HIE than term neonates. It occurs because of increased chances of hypoxic insult due to very low birth weight (<1,500 g),[9,10] hyaline membrane disease, antepartum placental abruption, hypocapnia, twin pregnancy, septicemia, patent ductus arteriosus, and also due to poor autoregulatory capacity of the premature brain.[8,11-16]

Imaging features can be subdivided based on severity (and to some extent duration) of injury into two types: (1) Severe hypoxia versus mild-to-moderate, or (2) Partial asphyxia. It must be remembered that features of both severe and partial asphyxia may be seen together in any given patient.

Severe, Total Hypoxia

The most metabolically active regions within the brain in this period, i.e., the deep gray matter including thalami, basal ganglia, hippocampus, cerebellum, dorsal brainstem, and corticospinal tracts, are the areas of involvement. The thalami, anterior vermis, and the dorsal brainstem are the most frequently affected. The basal ganglia and perirolandic cortex myelinate at around 35–36 weeks of gestational age and therefore are less severely and less frequently involved than the thalami.[17] Acute profound hypoxia of short duration will spare the rest of the brain parenchyma. However, if this severe profound injury is prolonged, it leads to a catastrophic total brain injury involving the cerebral hemispheres besides the above metabolically active regions of the brain.

Cranial ultrasound (US) is the first modality performed in the preterm neonates for screening and diagnosis for HIE. It may be normal in the first 48 hours, but may show hyperechogenicity in the basal ganglia and thalami by the third day.[8] CT will similarly show hypodensity within the basal ganglia and thalami with their attenuation values close to that of white matter.

Magnetic resonance imaging is a sensitive modality to detect the changes of HIE. Diffusion-weighted images may show restriction of diffusion within the involved areas, most commonly the thalami, in the first 24 hours. The abnormalities on conventional MRI start appearing in the form of T1 and T2 hyperintensity in the thalami and basal ganglia from third day onward **(Figs. 1A to C)**. The restriction of diffusion reaches peak at around 3–5 days and then starts to "pseudonormalize" after a week. T2 shortening starts to occur after 1 week in the affected areas **(Figs. 2A and B)**. The T1 hyperintense signal may persist into the chronic stage **(Figs. 3A and B)**.

Mild-to-moderate Hypoxia

This is by far the most common pattern of insult to the premature neonatal brain. The two major pathological lesions observed in this setting are: (1) Hemorrhage, and (2) White

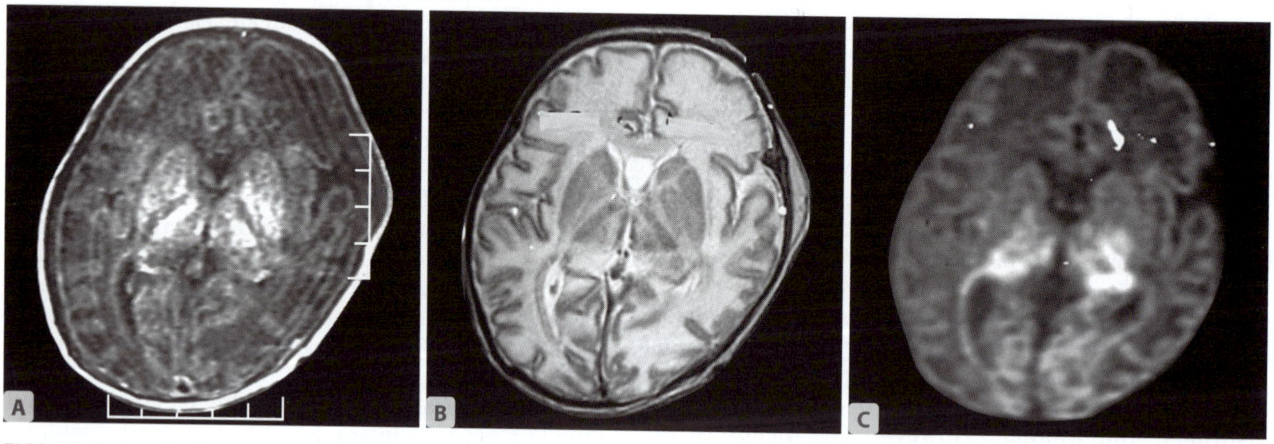

FIGS. 1A TO C: MRI of brain in a 6-day-old preterm neonate with perinatal asphyxia: (A and B) T1W and T2W images show hyperintense signal changes in bilateral thalami and posterior putamen; and (C) DWI shows restricted diffusion in involved areas. (DWI: diffusion-weighted imaging; MRI: magnetic resonance imaging; T1W: T1-weighted; T2W: T2-weighted)

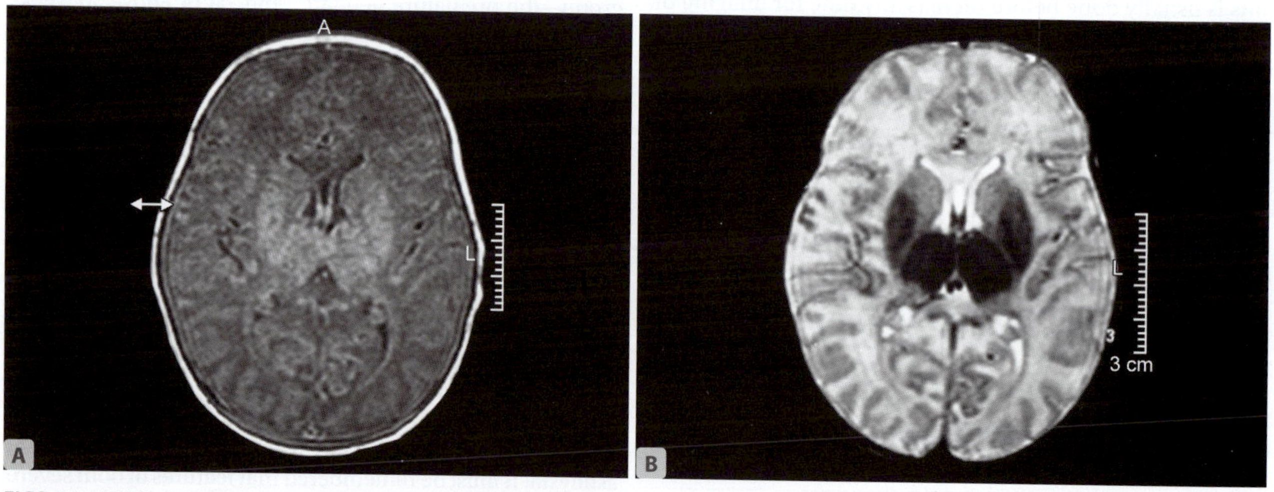

FIGS. 2A AND B: Axial MR images of a 9-day-old premature neonate. (A) T1 weighted image shows hyperintense signal changes in bilateral thalami and basal ganglia and (B) T2 weighted image shows hypointense signal in the same region.

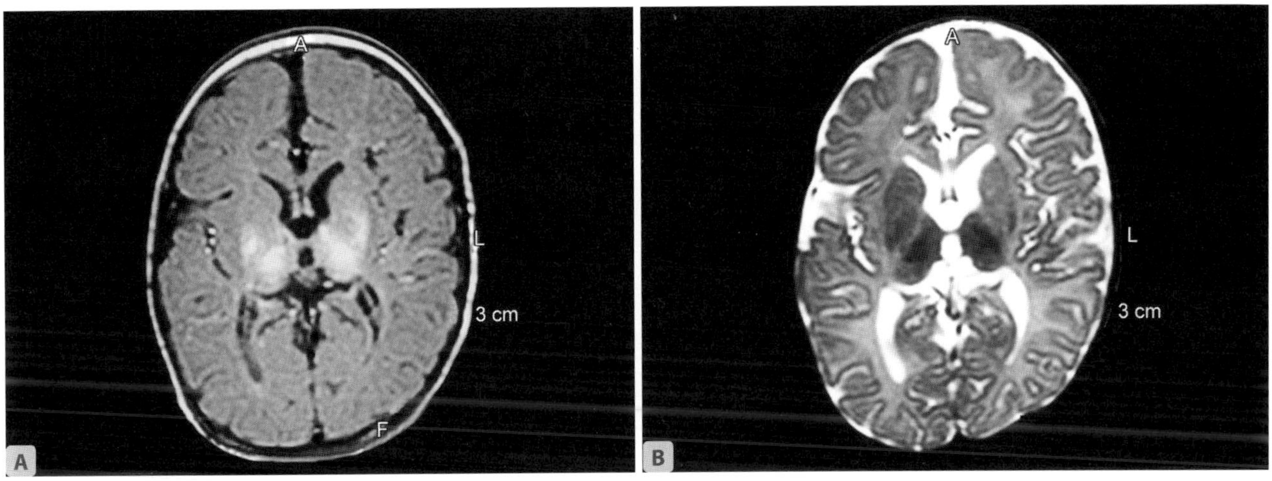

FIGS. 3A AND B: Axial MR images of a 2-month-old premature neonate: The (A) T1 weighted image shows hyperintense signal in the thalami and posterior putamen whereas the (B) T2 weighted image shows hypointense signal in these areas. The T1 hyperintensity may persist for months after the initial insult.

matter injury of prematurity or periventricular leukomalacia (PVL).[8]

Hemorrhage

Intracranial hemorrhage (ICH) in premature neonates is directly related to the degree of gestational immaturity. Germinal matrix (GM), the site of initial bleed, is a highly vascular area within the ventricular wall. GM is most prominent and active between 8 and 28 weeks of gestation.[8,18,19] Hemorrhage could be at germinal matrix hemorrhage (GMH), intraventricular hemorrhage (IVH), or parenchymal hemorrhage.[18-22]

Germinal Matrix Hemorrhage

Prematurity coupled with respiratory distress syndrome are the two main factors presumed to be responsible for hemorrhage in the immature brain. Following ischemic insult, when the ischemic tissue is reperfused, damaged cerebral autoregulation[23-25] associated with sudden rapid rise in cerebral blood flow or perfusion pressure as with handling, suction, and artificial ventilation leads to rupture of fragile weakened blood vessels in the germinal matrix bed.[8,18,19] The germinal matrix involutes by 34 weeks of gestation. The last portion of germinal matrix to involute is the ganglionic eminence located deep to the ependyma in the caudothalamic notch in the groove between the head of caudate nucleus and the thalamus. Hence, it is the most common site for GMH. It may also occur in the cerebellum from the germinal zones within the cerebellum and subependymal layer of roof of fourth ventricle.

Intraventricular Hemorrhage

IVH results either from rupture of a GMH into the ventricle or from choroid plexus bleeding. Depending upon the amount of bleeding and alteration in the cerebrospinal fluid (CSF) dynamics, ventricles may or may not show dilatation.

Parenchymal Hemorrhage (Periventricular Hemorrhagic Infarction)

It is typically unilateral, extensive, and always associated with IVH. Unlike hemorrhage occurring in an area of ischemia, periventricular hemorrhagic infarction (PVHI) occurs more anteriorly, roughly triangular in shape with apex of the triangle in the midline. GM and IVH cause compromise of terminal veins underlying GM leading onto congestion, thrombosis, and rupture of medullary veins draining the deep white matter. This leads to a hemorrhagic venous infarct in the periventricular parenchyma.[26] PVHI occurs about 24–48 hours after the onset of GMH and IVH. About 15% of patients with IVH develop PVHI.[22] On follow-up, such hemorrhage results in the development of a porencephalic cyst on imaging and hemiplegia on clinical examination.

Grading of Intracranial Hemorrhage

Papile et al.[20] proposed four grades of severity: (1) Grade (I) hemorrhage confined to GM in the subependymal region [subependymal hemorrhage (SEH) or GMH], (2) Grade (II) is associated with IVH but without ventricular dilatation, (3) Grade (III) IVH is associated with ventricular dilatation, and (4) Grade (IV) bleeding occurs into the brain parenchyma (PVHI). A number of other classifications followed, but none has been universally accepted so far due to their limitations.

Imaging of Intracranial Hemorrhage

Transfontanelle sonography is the most sensitive modality to detect SEH and IVH in the acute stage.[27,28] SEH is seen as a focal echogenic area at the head of caudate nucleus in the most anterior end of caudothalamic groove **(Fig. 4)**.[5,6,26] It is important to document the abnormality in two planes, since normal choroid plexus in the same area may be mistaken for SEH. Normal choroid plexus tapers as it extends anteriorly and disappears beyond foramen of Monro. On the other hand, in a GM bleed, there is prominent, bulbous enlargement of choroid

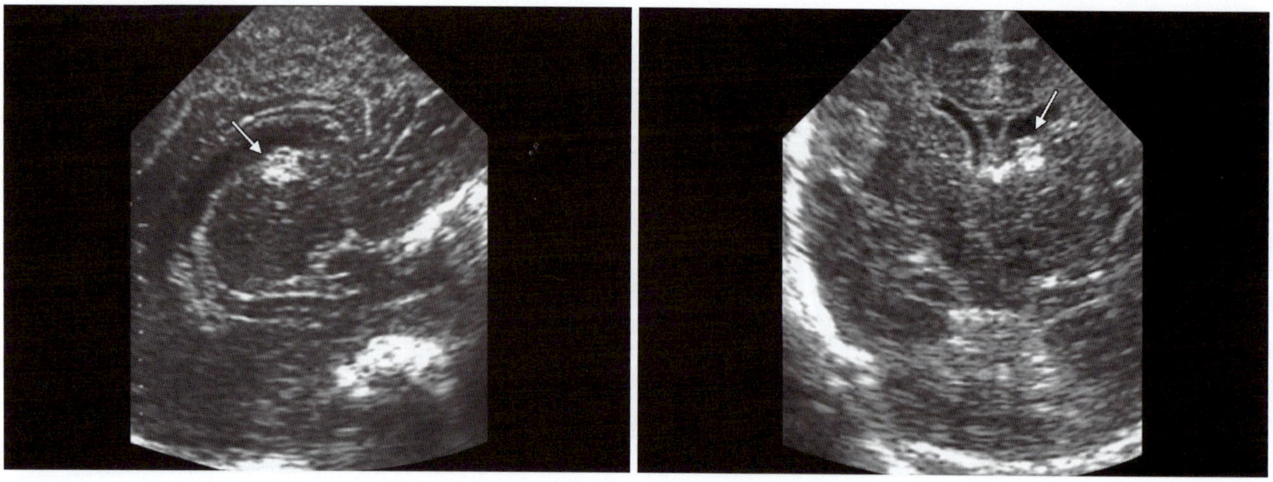

FIG. 4: Ultrasound: Grade II bleed subependymal hemorrhages (SEH) on left side (arrow). Note location of bleed at caudothalamic junction in sagittal view.

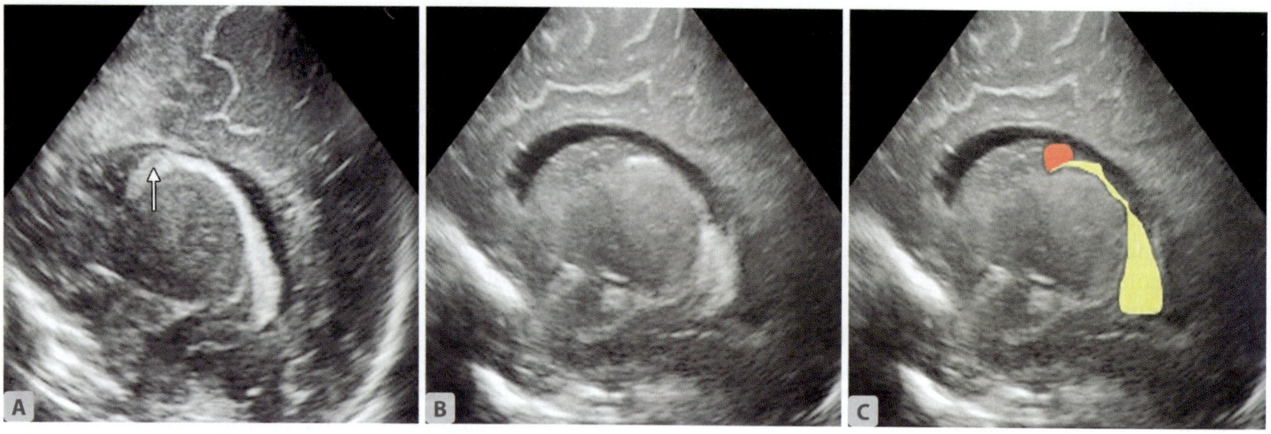

FIGS. 5A TO C: Grade I germinal matrix hemorrhage (GMH) versus normal choroid plexus on parasagittal images. (A) Grade I GMH seen as echogenicity extending to the caudothalamic groove (arrow). (B) Normal choroid plexus showing anterior tapering as it approaches the caudothalamic groove; and (C) Diagrammatic representation of normal choroid plexus (yellow) and GMH (red).

density which also extends beyond foramen of Monro **(Figs. 5A to C)**. On noncontrast computed tomography (NCCT) head, SEH is visible as a focal, high attenuating area. IVH is echogenic on sonography and the organized clot takes the shape of the ventricle which later shows dilatation **(Figs. 6A and B)**. With time, the clot becomes iso- and then hypoechoic. On NCCT, IVH is high attenuating initially becoming iso- and finally hypoattenuating. PVHI in the acute stage is brightly echogenic, unilateral, and clearly defined echogenicity on sonography.[8] with the apex of the triangle pointing toward the ventricle in the midline. Associated IVH is almost always present **(Figs. 7 and 8)**.

Subarachnoid hemorrhage (SAH) and hemorrhage in the posterior fossa and parieto-occipital area can be easily missed on the sonography. NCCT head is more sensitive in depicting these bleeds in the acute phase. On MRI, both T1-weighted image (T1WI) and even T2-weighted image (T2WI) may miss these bleeds in the acute stage.

On follow up, initially SEH becomes a subependymal cyst **(Figs. 9 and 10)** which may later disappear completely. IVH cast also resolves with time. Ventriculomegaly may be the only clue of an earlier episode of bleed. PVHI evolves into a porencephalic cyst which is usually in communication with the ventricle. With time, visibility of the hemorrhage, both on sonography and CT, decreases but on MRI visibility increases due to the formation of methemoglobin **(Figs. 11A and B)**. Also, MRI is more specific for assessing the time of hemorrhage.

Optimum time for sonographic detection of ICH secondary to HIE is between fourth and seventh day, by end of which 97% of hemorrhages will be visible.[27,28] In order to monitor for the development of hydrocephalus as a complication of IVH, sonography is recommended on the 14th day, and if negative, then at 3rd month.[27]

White Matter Injury of Prematurity/Periventricular Leukomalacia

The term PVL in literal terms means "white matter softening". A number of theories have been proposed for its pathogenesis.

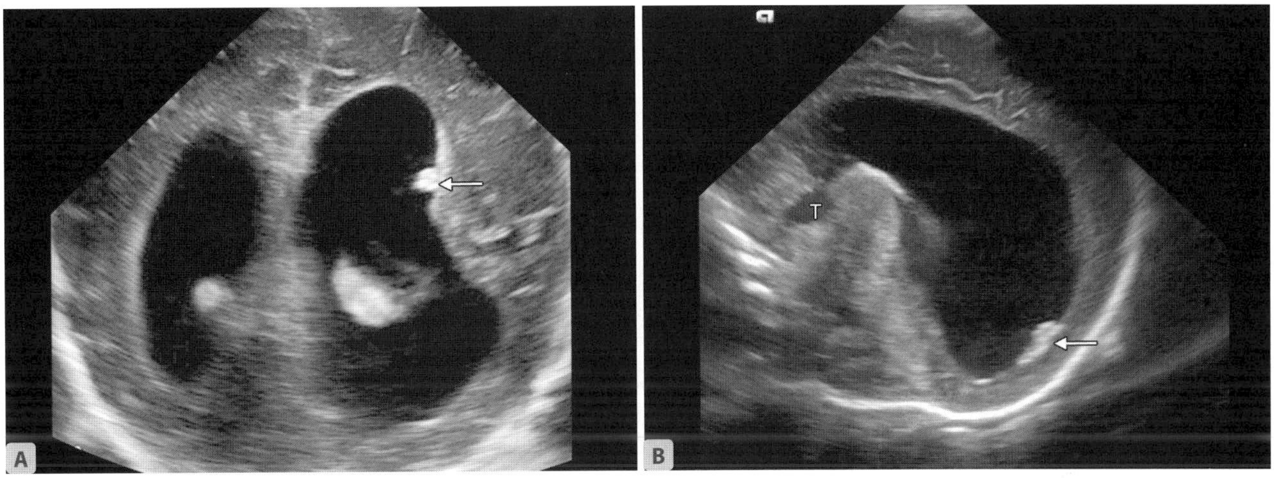

FIGS. 6A AND B: Intraventricular hemorrhage (IVH) with hydrocephalus. (A) Coronal and (B) midsagittal images reveal ventriculomegaly involving the lateral ventricles. Third ventricle (T) is normal. The clue toward the diagnosis of an IVH causing this ventriculomegaly is presence of echogenic adherent clot (arrows) along left lateral ventricle wall.

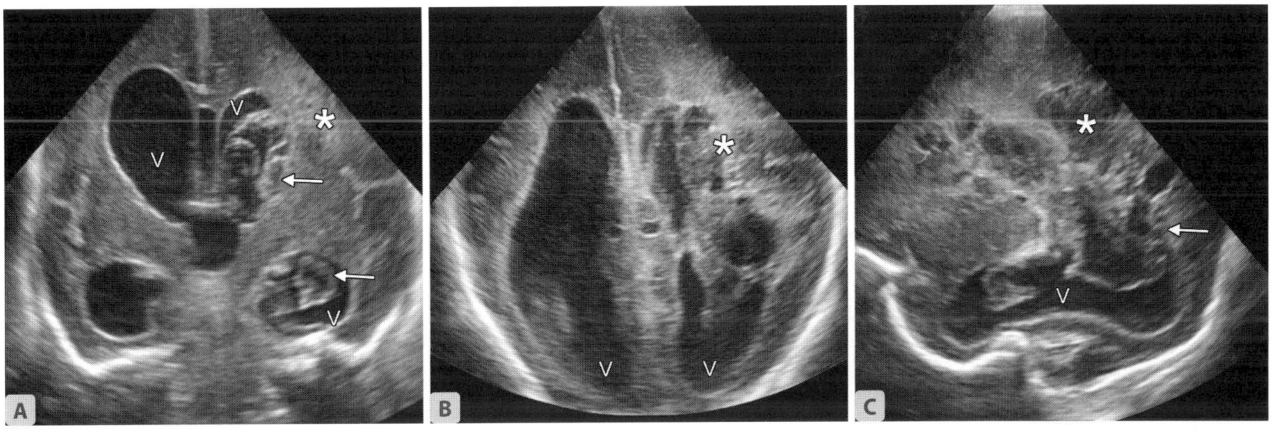

FIGS. 7A TO C: PVHI in a small for age, 35-week-old male neonate. (A) Anterior coronal image showing intraventricular clot (arrows) and echogenicity in left periventricular WM (asterisk). (B) Posterior coronal image showing the parenchymal component of PVHI (asterisk) and ventriculomegaly; and (C) Left parasagittal image showing extension of the parenchymal infarct (asterisk) into the ventricle (arrow). (PVHI: periventricular hemorrhagic infarction; V: lateral ventricles; WM: white matter)

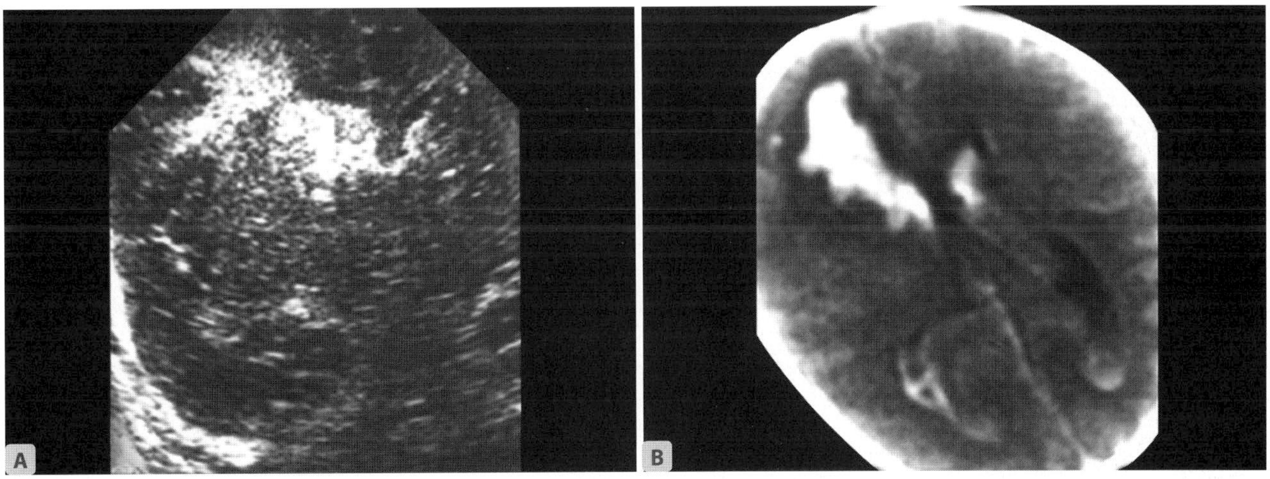

FIGS. 8A AND B: PVHI on right side. (A) US shows typical appearance of a triangular echogenicity extending from apex of frontal horn and associated IVH on right side; and (B) CT scan confirms the same finding. (CT: computed tomography; PVHI: periventricular hemorrhagic infarction; US: ultrasound)

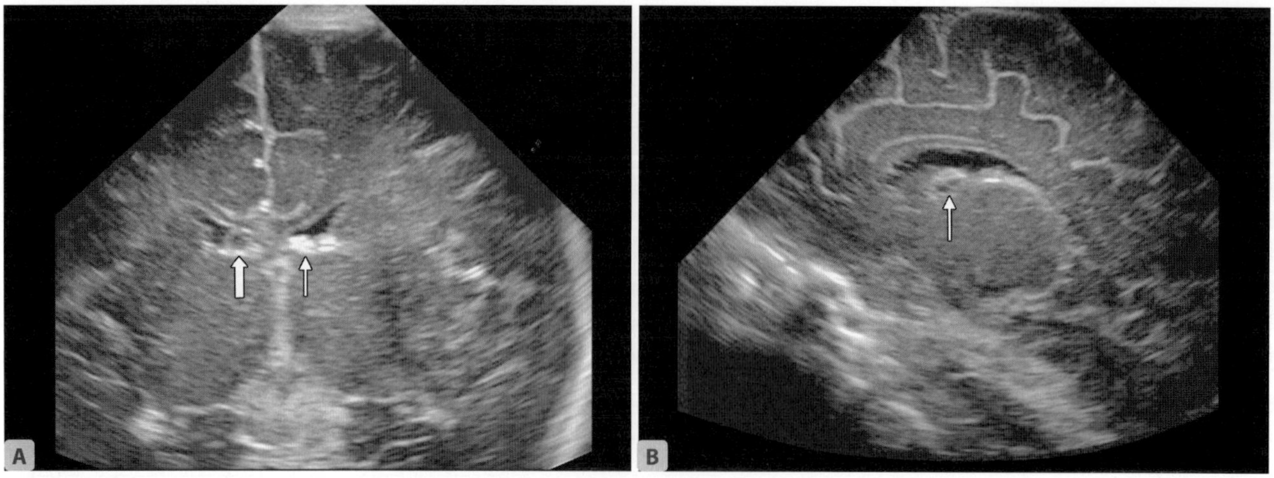

FIGS. 9A AND B: Grade I GMH of variable stage of evolution. (A) Coronal US image showing echogenicity along left caudothalamic groove (arrow) and a cyst on right groove (block arrow) suggestive of development of germinolytic cyst; and (B) Right parasagittal image showing the cyst in caudothalamic groove (arrow). (GMH: germinal matrix hemorrhage; US: ultrasound)

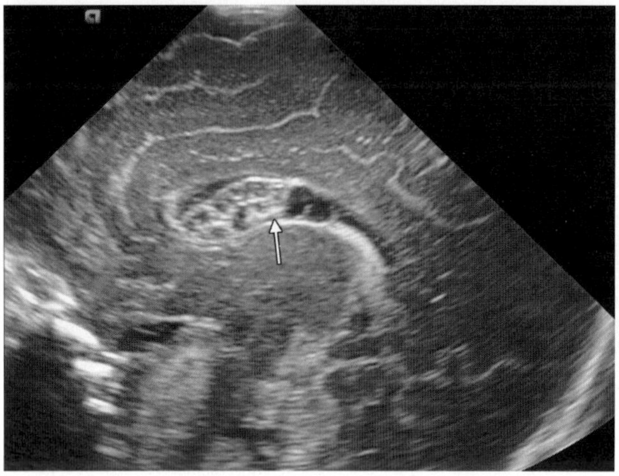

FIG. 10: Ultrasound sagittal image shows a complex cyst (arrow) developing in the resolving subependymal hemorrhage.

Unlike ICH, where prematurity is a clear risk factor for the development of PVL, a large number of ante- or perinatal events have been identified which may result in hypoperfusion to fetal cerebral tissue or injury to oligodendroglial cells and are thus important causative factors.[29-32] However, besides hypoxic-ischemic insult, other causes like infection, metabolic diseases, and hydrocephalus also can cause similar injury to the white matter. Also, the whole white matter may be involved, not just the periventricular white matter. Therefore, these insults are better termed as "white matter injury of prematurity" rather than PVL.

In a premature neonatal brain, the periventricular area is almost totally perfused by penetrating arteries that extend inward from the surface of the brain (ventriculopetal vessels). Junction of ventriculopetal and the ventriculofugal vessels (watershed area) exists in the periventricular region. In the event of any hypoxic-ischemic insult, therefore, this periventricular (watershed) area is at the highest risk.

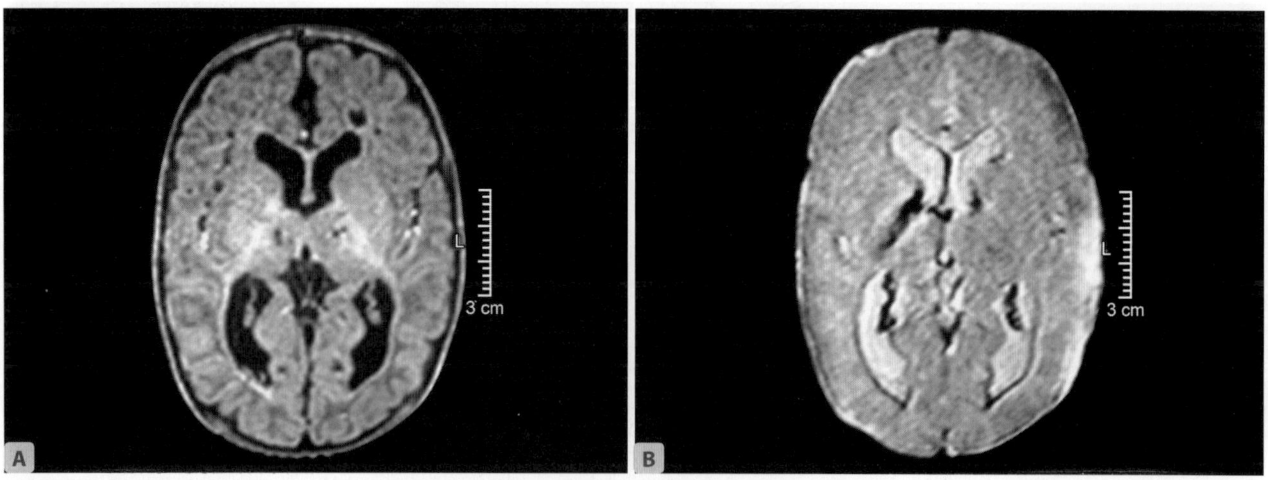

FIGS. 11A AND B: (A) Axial T1-weighted MR image in a premature neonate shows intraventricular hemorrhage (IVH) appearing hyperintense in the occipital horns (dependent part); and (B) The gradient T2-weighted image is more sensitive in detecting the bleed which is evident as hypointense signal lining the ventricular margins, choroid plexus, and right caudothalamic groove.

This combined with relative hypovascularity of the periventricularwhitematterthatplaysaroleinthedevelopment of PVL. Recently, it has been believed that presence of oligodendrocyte lineage cells pro-oligodendrocytes within this area makes them most susceptible to changes of hypoxia-ischemia. These cells mature into oligodendrocytes which are less prone to insult by around 32 weeks of age and hence, there is decreased frequency of PVL after this gestational age.[33,34] Also, toxins and excitatory amino acids, especially maternal chorioamnionitis,[35] may play a role in reducing local blood and energy supply and subsequent development of PVL.

Exact incidence of PVL is not clear and would vary depending upon the imaging modality used. Autopsy series report an incidence ranging from 25 to 75%. On sonography, incidence of PVL is reported to vary from 15 to 35%.[8,36-38]

Pathologically, the temporal sequence of events in the development of PVL are: coagulation necrosis in the first 24–48 hours followed by cavitation evolving over the next 2–4 weeks (when these cysts can be detected on US) and after several weeks, the cysts collapse and disappear completely with residual white matter atrophy and ventriculomegaly as the only evidence.[8,25] The ventricles have irregular lateral walls and cerebral cortex reaches up to the lateral ventricle wall. PVL may be purely ischemic or at times complicated by blood. Imaging features will, therefore, vary depending upon the time of imaging in relation to the ischemic insult and whether it is purely ischemic or complicated by hemorrhage.

Periventricular leukomalacia lesions could be focal or diffuse.[22] Classically, focal PVL lesions are distributed bilaterally, symmetrically, and primarily around the trigone areas, but may extend also to involve the frontal lobes adjacent to the foramen of Monro.[13,15,39,40] However, lesions may be visible only on one side on imaging and that should not exclude the diagnosis of PVL. Diffuse lesions involve the entire periventricular region.

Clinically, the characteristic neurological abnormality due to PVL is spastic diplegia[27,40] in about 5–15%. This is because the site of pathological lesions of PVL is located in the periventricular region from where also the corticospinal tracts descend. Tracts of lower limbs are located in the most medial region, i.e., closest to the PVL lesion and are thus first to be affected resulting in diplegia.[25,41] Visual impairment[42,43] and cognitive impairment[44] may occur without spastic diplegia.

Imaging of Early Periventricular Leukomalacia

Ultrasound Due to hemodynamically unstable state of most of these neonates, a cribside US in the intensive care unit (ICU)/nursery is usually the first investigation. Besides portability, the other advantages of US are: Nonionizing, no intravenous (IV) contrast, or sedation is required and can be repeated frequently without harmful effects. Addition of color Doppler and quantitative analysis[45] to two-dimensional (2D) imaging may improve information content. PVL should be suspected on US studies when increased echogenicity is present in the periventricular regions. On US, periventricular areas of increased echogenicity is visible within 24–48 hours of ischemic insult. However, there are two major potential pitfalls. Firstly, in normal newborns, also there is a periventricular increased echogenicity, so called "periventricular blush".[8] Secondly, brain edema also appears bright on US.[46,47] Therefore, presence of increased echogenicity in itself is not enough to diagnose PVL. Reliable sign of PVL is the presence of periventricular "flares". The brightness of echogenicity due to PVL "flare" is more than the normal periventricular echogenicity and approaches or becomes equal to that of adjacent choroid plexus. Also, the normal tissue architecture is lost.[8,48] However, this limits the capability of US[49-51] since a certain degree of subjective element creeps, especially in milder degrees of abnormality. "Periventricular flare" should be confirmed and documented in both the coronal and the parasagittal views.

If ischemic PVL is complicated by hemorrhage, then the abnormalities are readily detected by sonography. It is important to recognize that both, the edema as well as the hemorrhage, in the brain parenchyma will produce increased echogenicity on US. Differentiation is possible by observing the *degree of brightness* **(Figs. 12A and B)**. In these situations, CT and MRI help to differentiate between the two.

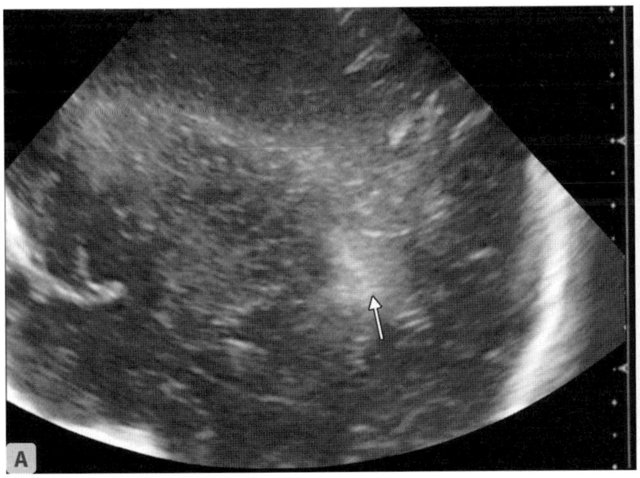

A

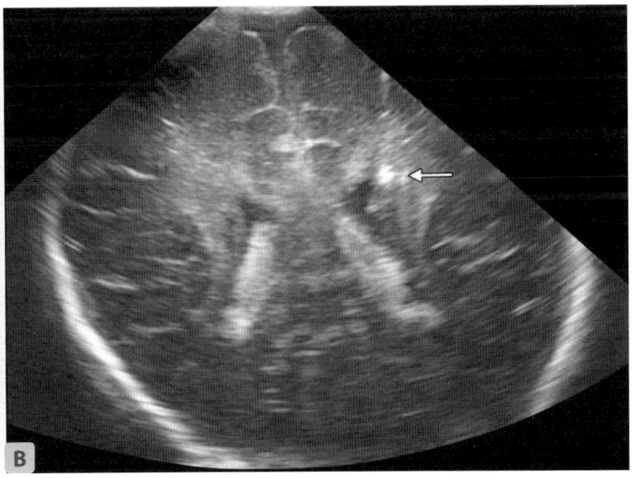

B

FIGS. 12A AND B: (A) Echogenic focal edema (arrow) in parieto-occipital white matter in a 35-week neonate; and (B) Focal parenchymal bleed (arrow), appearing "more bright" than edema in this 34-week neonate (different patient than A).

On follow-up, the flares may completely disappear, usually in about half of the patients, within 7–10 days. If, however, the flares persist beyond 1 week, then the term "persistent flares" are used and are considered as grade I PVL.[48] In about 10%, the flares may progress to the next pathological stage, i.e., cavitation, usually within 2–4 weeks **(Figs. 13A to D)**. Development of few, small cysts represents milder end of the spectrum of PVL, but multiple cysts is an indicator of a poor neurological prognosis with development of cerebral palsy.[27] Not only the size, but also the distribution of cysts is important for predicting the severity of clinical outcome.[52] Thus, cysts in the frontoparietal area have a better prognosis as compared to those in the posterior parieto-occipital region. Also, the cysts secondary to PVL need to be differentiated from other common causes of cysts seen in this age group like germinolytic cysts and connatal cysts **(Fig. 14)**.[53] US is superior to CT **(Figs. 15A and B)** for the detection of small cysts of PVL. However, MRI is a superior modality for detection of these cysts **(Figs. 16A and B)**.

Ultrasound also has been used to grade the PVL. The classification suggested by de Vries[48] is simple to use **(Table 1)**. The grading increases with extent and the severity of pathological lesions and is, therefore, directly related to the severity of neurological abnormality.

Computed Tomography Computed tomography has no added advantage over US and should be avoided because of the associated ionizing radiation exposure. The only exception where CT scores over US is differentiation of bleed from edema. However, since MRI can also differentiate the two and is generally more sensitive for other findings, it is the next preferred modality after US.

Magnetic Resonance Imaging The capability of MRI to detect subtle injuries, its superior contrast resolution, and its multiplanar potential makes it a far superior technique to US for detection of white matter abnormalities. With recent advances in MRI, ventilators, and anesthesia equipment hardware, the problems of feasibility of MRI in very sick and premature neonates have been largely overcome.[54]

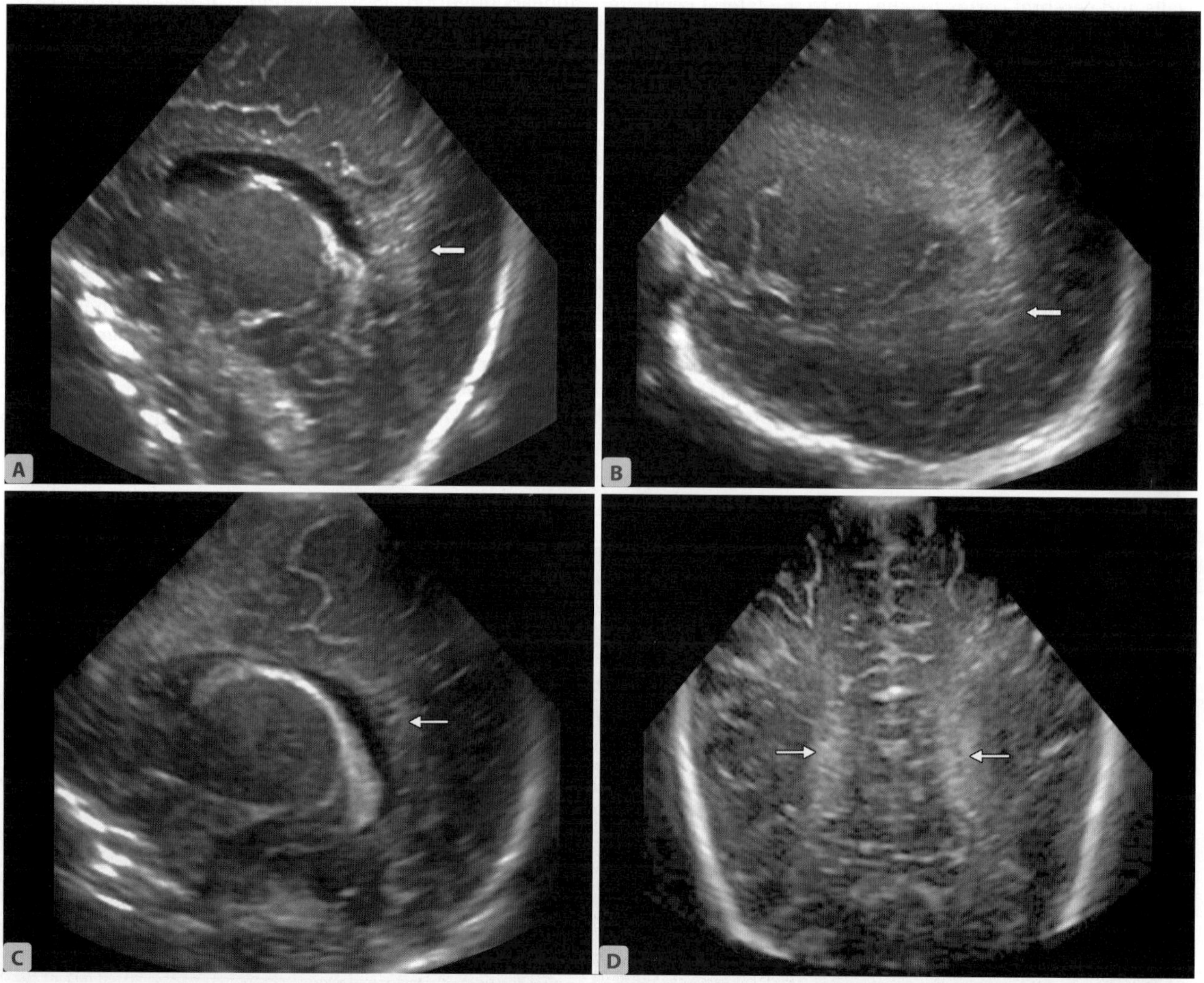

FIGS. 13A TO D: Periventricular leukomalacia (PVL) in various stages and grades. (A) Grade I: Persistent "flare" in periventricular white matter (WM) (arrow). (B) Grade II: Early changes of grade II PVL, note the development of cysts (arrow) within the echogenic area; and (C and D) Grade III: Multiple small cysts in parieto-occipital WM (arrows).

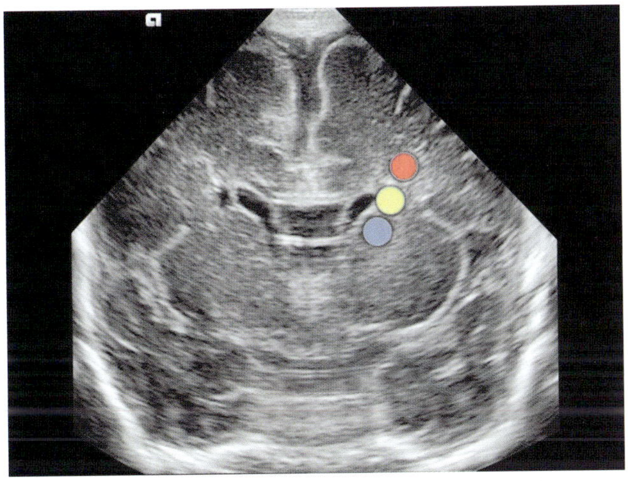

FIG. 14: Differentiating periventricular leukomalacia (PVL) cysts from other cysts in neonatal cranial ultrasonography. Red: Cystic PVL (above the level of the lateral margin of ventricle), Yellow: Connatal cyst/coarctation of lateral ventricle, a congenital variant anatomy, and Blue: Germinolytic cysts developing after EPH. In this patient: connatal cyst is seen on right side.

Early white matter injury appears as foci of T1 hyperintensity in the periventricular white matter by 3–4 days postinsult. These lesions are not evident on T2WIs at this time. Instead, T2WIs show diffuse hyperintense signal within the periventricular white matter. The T1 hyperintense foci subsequently become hypointense on T2WIs by 5–6 days. Hemorrhage also gives rise to T2 hypointense lesions but in this case, the hypointensity is more marked.

Advances in MRI have made it possible to diagnose early white matter injury. Diffusion-weighted imaging (DWI) in a number of studies has been found to be much more accurate than conventional MRI in the acute phase of PVL.[8,49,55,56] Recently, further advances have been made and studies using serial quantitative diffusion tensor MRI[57,58] have reported very high degree of accuracy in diagnosing early white matter injuries. In this technique, two parameters are assessed: (1) Apparent diffusion coefficient (ADC) mapping, and (2) Relative anisotropy of cerebral water. This method has been found so accurate that it is being nowadays used for white matter tractography.[59,60]

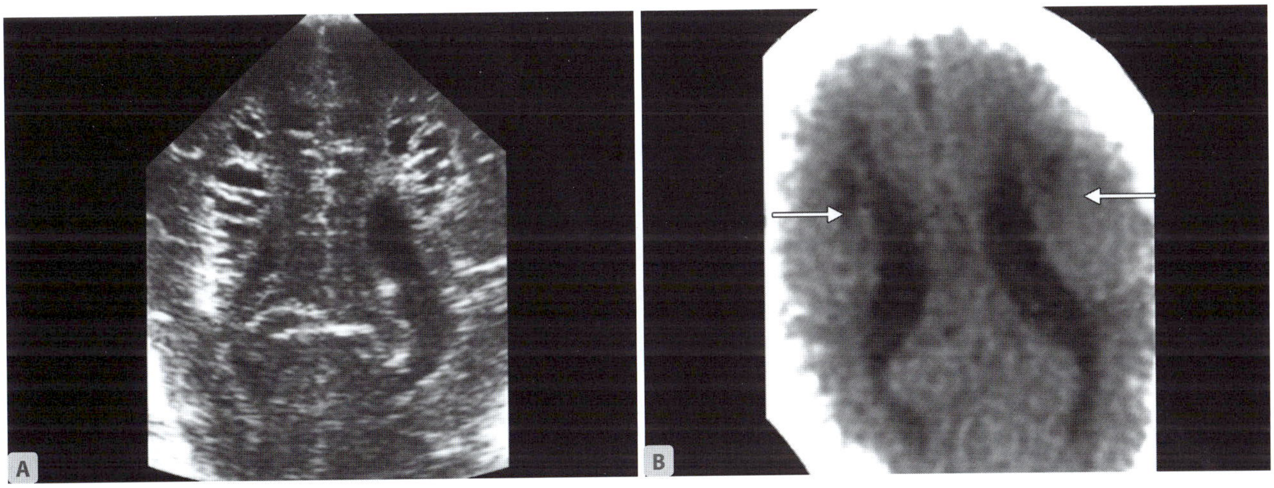

FIGS. 15A AND B: Extensive cystic periventricular leukomalacia (PVL). (A) Ultrasound (US) shows extensive cysts in bilateral periventricular white matter; and (B) CT scan of the same patient also shows the cystic PVL (arrows). Note that the cysts are better appreciated on US.

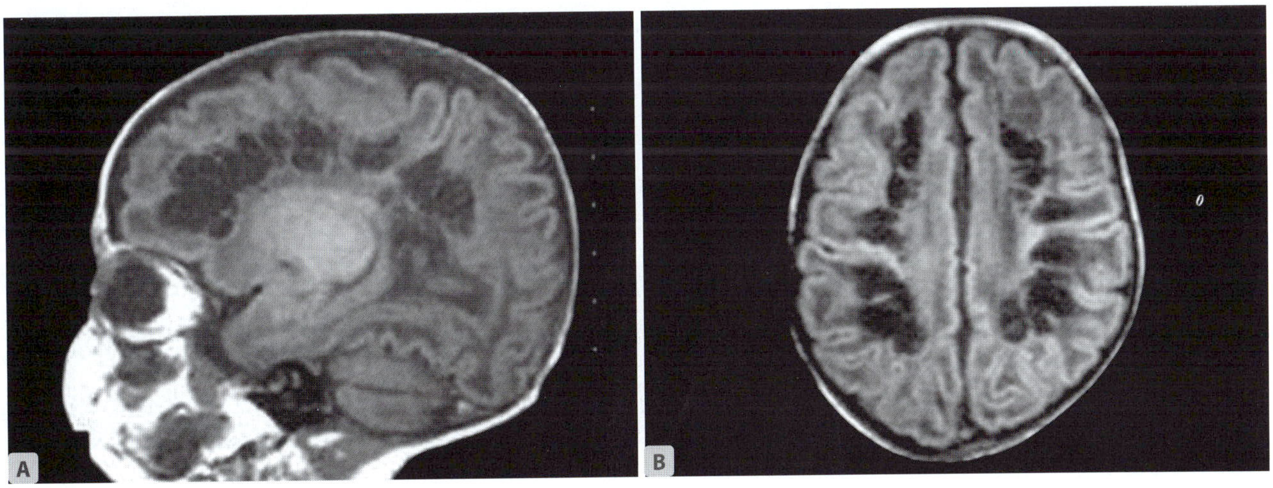

FIGS. 16A AND B: Extensive cystic PVL. (A) T1W sagittal and (B) FLAIR axial MR images show bilateral extensive cystic PVL. (FLAIR: fluid-attenuated inversion recovery; PVL: periventricular leukomalacia; T1W: T1-weighted)

Imaging of End-stage Periventricular Leukomalacia

After several weeks, usually 3 months onward, the cysts collapse and completely disappear. Diagnosis on US at this stage is very difficult, if not impossible. A characteristic triad of findings due to white matter collapse is seen both on CT and MRI[8,13,15,61] **(Figs. 17A and B)**. The triad consists of:

- Abnormally increased bilateral periventricular white matter signal intensity on a T2W sequence, most commonly in the trigone regions of lateral ventricles. This abnormal hypersignal intensity extends right up to the ventricular ependyma. This corresponds to gliosis and demyelination observed pathologically in late PVL. Important differential diagnosis of similar increased signal intensity includes normal, unmyelinated white matter (the terminal zones of myelination), myelinoclastic disorders, and postradiation or chemotherapeutic administration. However, by careful interpretation of the images in the proper clinical background, one can differentiate each of these conditions from one another and from PVL. The terminal zones of myelination is also seen as hyperintense on T2 and fluid-attenuated inversion recovery (FLAIR) images, but can be differentiated from PVL by the presence of a thin band of low signal between this hyperintensity and the ependymal margin of the ventricle. On coronal images, this terminal zone is triangular in shape with the apex of the triangle pointing superiorly.
- Marked loss of periventricular white matter in the regions of abnormal high signal intensity results in close approximation of the cortical sulci to the ventricles. Many a times, this may be the only clue of an end-stage PVL.
- Compensatory focal enlargement of the ventricle adjacent to the regions of abnormal high signal intensity with irregular outlines.

On MRI, two other findings may also be seen,[8] i.e., observation of delayed myelination and thin, atrophic corpus callosum particularly in the posterior body and splenium. However, it should always be remembered that all these above late stage signs on imaging may be caused by many different disorders such as ventriculitis (a common sequel of meningitis in infants), inborn errors of metabolism, hydrocephalus, and in utero events.[8] The diagnosis is best made in conjunction with a thorough past medical history.

In addition to PVL, two other distinct types of white matter abnormalities have been described in the premature neonates: (1) *Punctuate lesions,* and (2) *Diffuse excessive high signal intensity (DEHSI)*.[26,54] These are much better seen on MRI as compared to US. The *punctuate lesions,* though more common in premature neonates, may also be seen in term neonates. They are most frequently seen in the corona radiata, posterior periventricular white matter and the optic radiation, and rarely in deep gray matter. In some cases, they may represent the early and mild end of PVL spectrum. They are seen as T1 hyperintense and T2 hypointense lesions which occasionally show evidence of bleed on gradient sequences and restricted diffusion on DWI. These may regress with time. Their significance is still not fully understood and they may not always correlate with an adverse developmental outcome. In contrast, DEHSI refers to diffuse signal changes in deep white matter appearing hypointense on T1 and hyperintense on T2WIs. These signal changes are more profound than the normal appearances of unmyelinated white matter in the premature neonatal brain. It may be noted here that even in the normal developing brain, there are more distinct zones of high signal intensity on T2 and low signal intensity on TWIs.

TABLE 1: Grading of periventricular leukomalacia (PVL).

Grades of PVL	Description
Grade I	Periventricular echogenic areas, persistent for >7 days
Grade II	Periventricular echogenic areas, evolving into localized small frontoparietal cysts
Grade III	Periventricular echogenic areas, evolving into multiple cysts in the parieto-occipital white matter
Grade IV	Echogenic areas in the deep white matter, evolving into multiple subcortical cysts (multicystic encephalopathy)

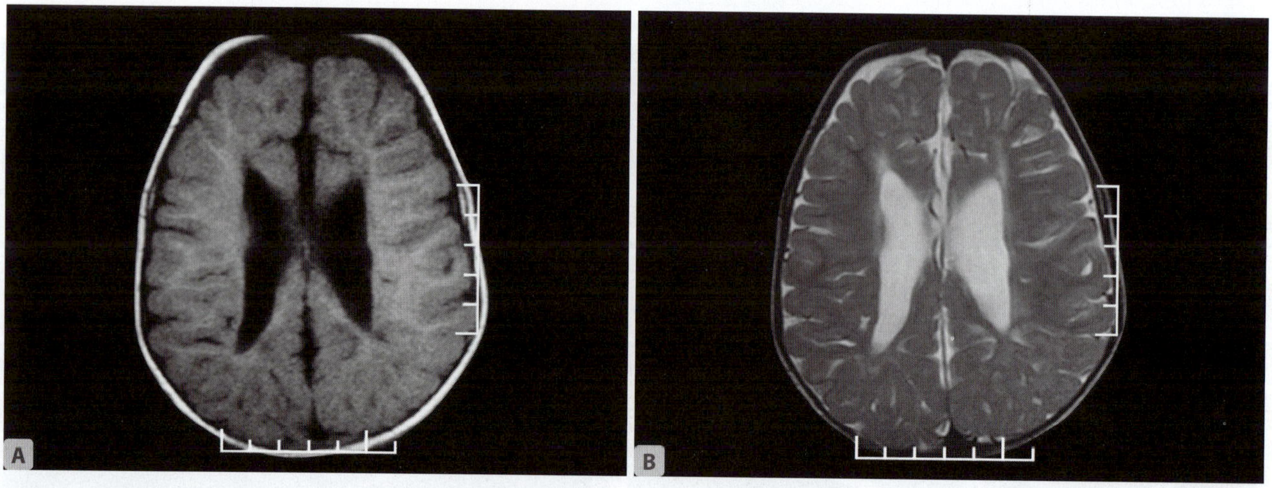

FIGS. 17A AND B: End-stage periventricular leukomalacia (PVL). (A) T1 and (B) T2-weighted axial MR images show loss of volume with signal changes in the deep periventricular white matter and ventricular dilatation with irregular margins.

These appear in the shape of caps anteriorly in the frontal white matter and arrowheads posteriorly in the peritrigonal white matter.[54] The DEHSI can be differentiated from these by being diffuse. Neonates with DEHSI have been shown to have impaired development in about 50% of the cases with rest leading onto develop normally.[26]

ABOVE 36 WEEKS GROUP—THE TERM NEONATE

Incidence of HIE in term neonates has decreased over the years and is reported to be about 1–2 per 1,000 live births.[8,62] Affected neonates may have significant neurologic abnormalities,[25] mental retardation,[25] or visual impairment.[63] HII in the term neonate usually occurs in association with antepartum risk factors either alone or in combination with intrapartum risk factors. Remaining few cases are associated with intrapartum factors alone or secondary to postnatal complications such as sepsis, shock, and respiratory distress.

With the maturity of the infant, three important anatomic changes occur:[8] (1) Involution and regression of the GM resulting in decreased incidence of ICH in term neonates in contrast to preterm neonates, (2) The site susceptible for HII changes. The watershed zone shifts from the earlier periventricular location in a preterm to a more peripheral location in the subcortical region, and (3) While earlier the response of the preterm brain to trauma was by liquefaction and resorption of the damaged brain, the mature brain responds to the same trauma by reactive astrogliosis.[8,64]

The pathological lesions and imaging characteristics due to HIE in infants beyond 34 weeks of gestation are again dependent on severity and duration of hypoxia and are divided into severe and mild-to-moderate groups.

Severe, Total Hypoxia

Severe hypoxia refers to sudden total loss of oxygenation as may be seen in abruption of placenta, prolapsed cord, or ruptured uterus. As seen in the preterm neonates, the deep gray matter including putamen, ventrolateral thalamus, hippocampus, dorsal brainstem, and lateral geniculate nuclei are the areas of involvement.[8] In contrast to preterm neonates, the basal ganglia involvement is more severe compared to thalami. The perirolandic cortex may also be affected. The remaining cortex is involved only with more prolonged profound insults leading to catastrophic total brain damage. In this type of injury, hypoxia is the predominant component of insult rather than hypotension.

Cranial US done within the first week has low sensitivity. It may show pattern of diffuse cerebral edema seen as diffuse increased echogenicity of brain with obliterated CSF spaces. US done after a week may show increased echogenicity of involved areas of basal ganglia, thalami, and brainstem **(Figs. 18A and B)**. Follow-up US shows diffuse cerebral atrophy.

Computed tomography is much less sensitive and specific than MRI. CT findings include decrease in the density of basal ganglia, cortex with subsequent loss of gray white matter differentiation **(Fig. 19)**. CT may also show evidence of diffuse cerebral edema evident as effacement of sylvian fissures and basal cisterns **(Fig. 20)**. It may be seen about 8 hours after insult and peak by 3–4 days.

Magnetic resonance imaging is the most sensitive modality for evaluation of HIE in the term neonate. Conventional T1 and T2WIs in combination with DWI depict the extent of damage. The conventional images may start showing findings from second day onward, but the abnormalities on these images are best visualized after a week.[8] DWI usually shows the abnormality within the first 24 hours when the conventional images are normal. However, the DWI done on the first day, though sensitive, underestimates the extent of injury which is seen to progress on these images to a peak on 3–5 days. The findings then subsequently "pseudonormalize" by the end of first week. DWI, however, can objectively categorize tissue injury based on values of ADC and subsequently predict outcome to a certain extent.[65,66] MR spectroscopy has been shown to be sensitive modality for detecting hypoxic damage in the early period within first 24 hours even when the DWI images are normal. Elevated choline, decreased N-acetylaspartate (NAA), increased lactate, and increased glutamine-glutamate

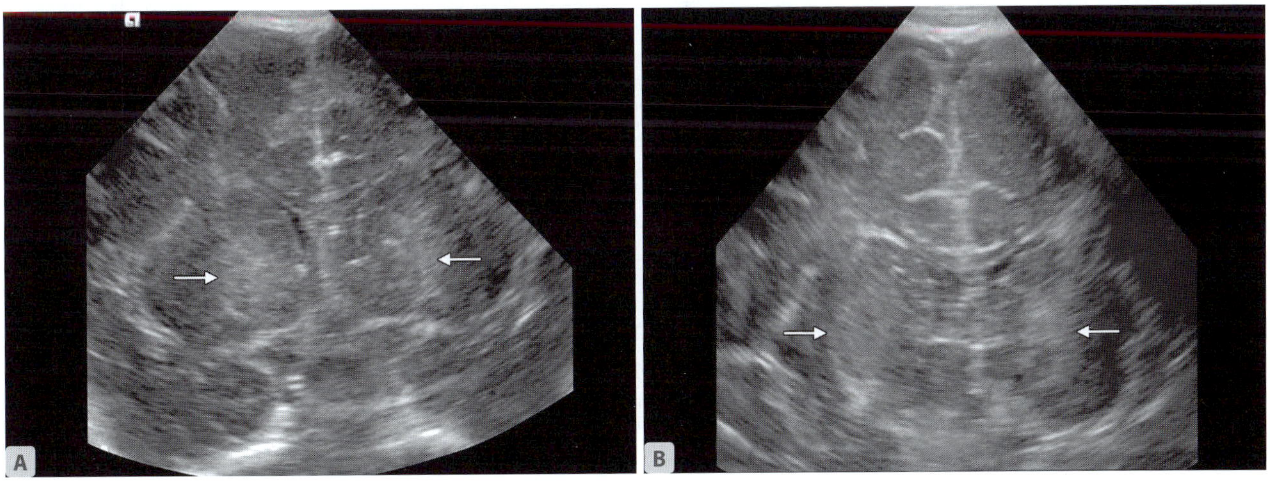

FIGS. 18A AND B: Echogenic basal ganglia in a two-term neonates (arrows). This is a poor prognostic marker.

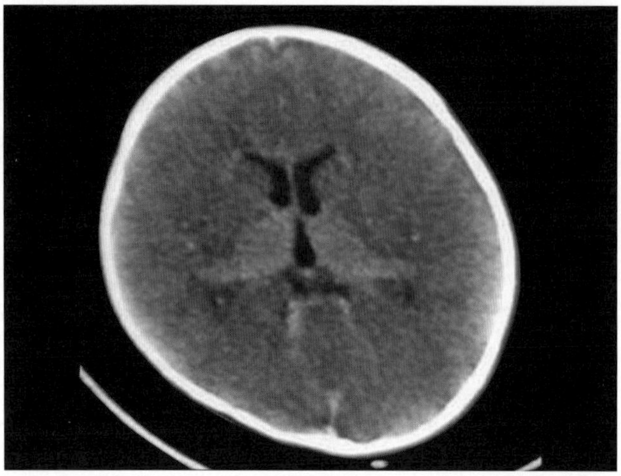

FIG. 19: Axial CT image in a term neonate with severe hypoxia shows diffuse hypodensity involving the cortical gray matter and basal ganglia with loss of gray-white matter differentiation.

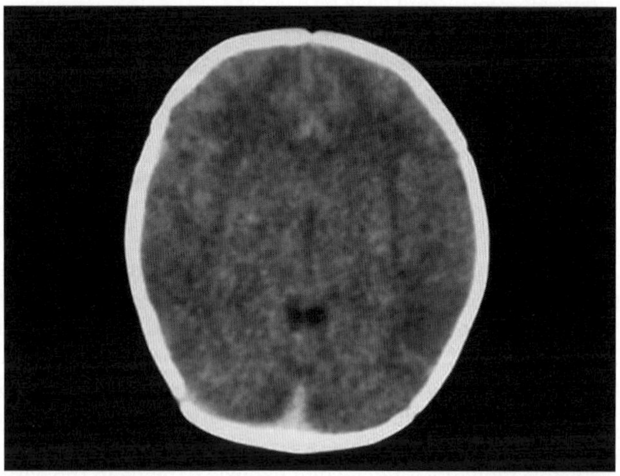

FIG. 20: Axial CT image in another term neonate with severe hypoxic injury shows diffuse cerebral edema with effacement of sulci, cisterns, and ventricles.

are seen. Lactate elevation seen as a lactate doublet (two sharp peaks) centered at 1.33 ppm is typically seen due to anaerobic glycolysis secondary to mitochondrial dysfunction. It can be detected as early as 4–8 hours after birth. But by the end of 24 hours, the lactate returns to normal—known as pseudonormalization. Subsequently, there occurs secondary energy failure which again leads to elevation of lactate after 24–48 hours which then peaks at around 5 days of life.[67] It should be noted that elevated lactate levels may be normally seen in preterm neonates making it a less useful investigation in these category compared to term neonates. Hence, it is important to interpret the magnetic resonance spectroscopy (MRS) taking into account the gestational age as well as day of acquisition after the insult. Increased lactate/NAA ratio observed on first day of life has been shown to be a very sensitive parameter for injury and may be considered as gold standard. It may be useful in identification of infants who may benefit from early therapeutic intervention.[67-71] Diffusion tensor imaging has also recently shown promise in detecting and timing these lesions by showing decreased fractional anisotropy (FA) values in the affected parts of brain which may be seen even after "pseudonormalization" on DWI.[65]

Magnetic resonance imaging findings include:

- T1 hyperintense basal ganglia—seen in the first 3 days of life. The posterior putamina are the most commonly involved. It should be remembered that mild T1 hyperintensity of the basal ganglia may be seen in normal infants also. Hence, it is important to see for associated findings of HIE.
- T1 hyperintense thalami—the signal change is subtle compared to that of the basal ganglia. When abnormal, the thalami show diffuse hyperintense signal on T1WIs **(Figs. 21A and B)**. This should be differentiated from the focal hyperintense signal seen within the posterolateral part of thalami in normal neonates corresponding to the myelination of ventrolateral thalamic nuclei just medial to the terminal portion of the posterior limb of internal capsule. Both the putamina and thalami appear hyperintense on T2WIs in the early period, but then

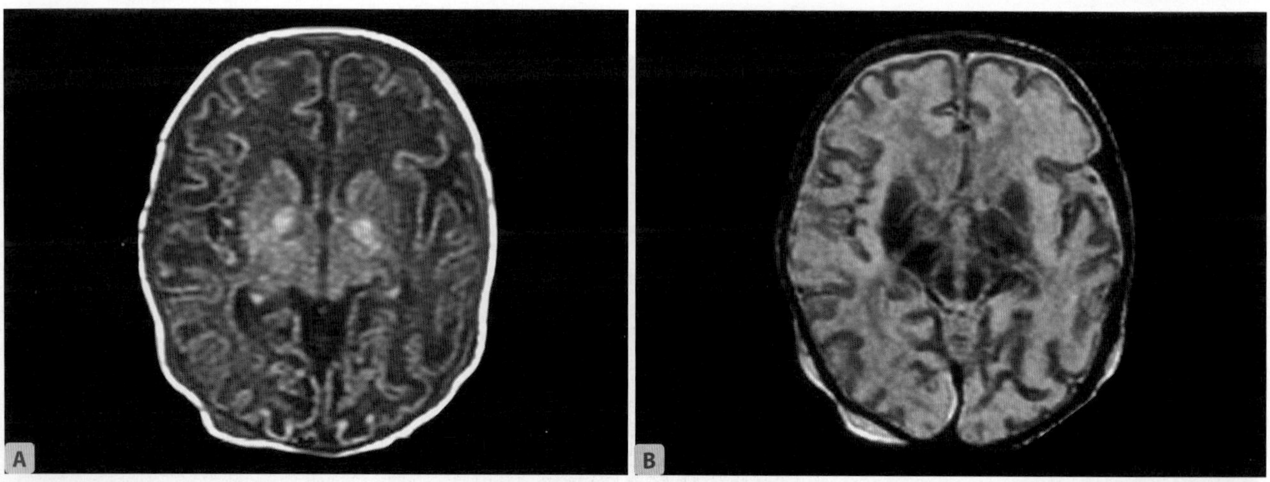

FIGS. 21A AND B: (A) Axial T1 and (B) T2-weighted MR images in a 6-day-old term neonate with severe hypoxic injury shows the thalami and basal ganglia appearing hyperintense on T1 and hypointense on T2. Also, note the loss of normal T1 hyperintense and T2 hypointense signal within the posterior limb of internal capsule.

progress to develop T2 hypointensity by the second week **(Figs. 21A and B)**. The T1 hyperintense signal within the basal ganglia, thalami, and also in the perirolandic cortex has been shown to persist for several months.

- "Absent posterior limb" sign—the posterior 50% of the posterior limb of internal capsule (PLIC) normally gets myelinated by 37 weeks of gestational age and is then seen as hyperintense on T1 and hypointense on T2WIs. Absence of these normal signal characteristics of the PLIC is a sensitive marker of hypoxia in a term infant (beyond 37 weeks of age). Although, it may be seen on the first day of life, it is usually best evident after 3–4 days. In doubtful cases, the signal characteristics of PLIC may be compared with the adjacent posterolateral putamen. In normal neonates, the PLIC appears more hyperintense than the posterolateral putamen on T1WIs. Reversal of this pattern is considered very sensitive for hypoxic damage. T2WIs showing loss of normal hypointensity in the PLIC that may be useful in case of doubt on T1 images, especially in the setting of abnormal hyperintense signal within the adjacent basal ganglia and thalami secondary to HII **(Figs. 22A and B)**.
- Abnormal DWI—restriction of diffusion may be seen in the basal ganglia, PLIC, and thalami in the affected neonates. As stated above, the abnormality may be seen within the first day, but usually peaks by about 4–5 days and starts to "pseudonormalize" by 7–10 days. Initial findings on DWI may underestimate the true extent of injury. Hence, a "normal" appearing DWI does not exclude insult.
- Profound global injury—involving both the cortical gray matter and subcortical white matter. It is seen much less commonly than the above four patterns and is seen when the profound insult is prolonged and persistent. In acute setting, it is visualized as hyperintense signal of the cerebral cortex on T1WIs. On DWI, it is seen as the "white cerebrum" contrast from normal appearing cerebellum. Since, it is usually symmetrical, it is easier to appreciate this restriction when comparing to normal cerebellum on coronal DWI images. It is usually fatal. Survivors show multicystic encephalomalacia on follow-up imaging **(Figs. 23A and B)**.
- Parasagittal gray and white matter injury—bilateral cortical and subcortical white matter necrosis in the parasagittal areas extending to involve the parieto-occipital areas of the brain.

Follow-up imaging in these neonates shows atrophy of the involved structures with T2 hyperintense signal, especially in the posterior putamina, ventrolateral thalami, and corticospinal tracts. Also appreciated is thinning of the corpus callosum in the region of the middle or posterior body, secondary to degeneration of the transcallosal fibers.

Prolonged, Partial Hypoxia

A mild-to-moderate acute hypoxia lasting <10 minutes usually does not lead to any significant effects over the brain parenchyma due to a fairly developed autoregulation mechanism, especially in the term neonates. A prolonged partial asphyxia refers to a more sustained (>15–25 min), but incomplete loss of oxygenation as seen in prolonged difficult labor with fetal bradycardia. It is also more common after hypotension, hypoglycemia, and infection. Hypotension plays a more major role in this type of insult rather than hypoxia. It results in shunting of blood to the vital brain structures including brainstem, basal ganglia, thalami, hippocampi, and cerebellum from the cerebral cortex and white matter which are not so metabolically active. Hence, these above vital brain structures are spared from injury whereas the watershed zones in cortical and subcortical areas get affected. Abnormalities are earliest seen on DWI (best evident as hypointensity on ADC maps) followed by findings on conventional T1 and T2WIs. T2WIs show cortical swelling and hyperintense signal within the gray and subcortical white matter with loss of gray-white matter differentiation. The parasagittal watershed zones are the most favored site of involvement, but the findings may be diffusely seen in the cerebral hemispheres **(Fig. 24)**. Follow-up imaging may show leukomalacia, especially in the subcortical areas. This pattern

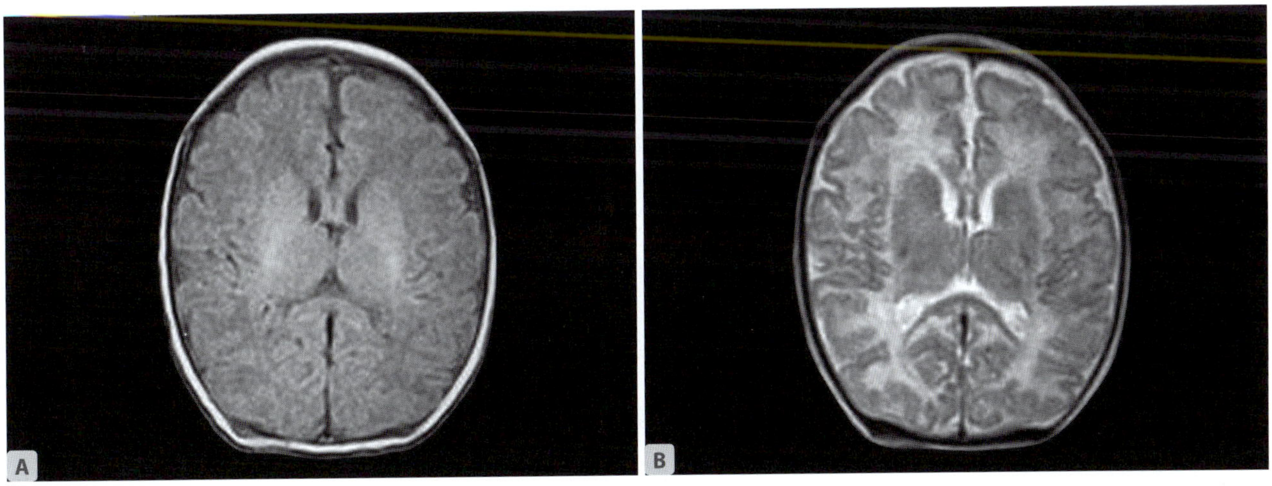

FIGS. 22A AND B: A 9-day-old term neonate with severe hypoxic injury shows lack of myelination of posterior limb of internal capsule on (A) T1-weighted and (B) T2-weighted axial MR images.

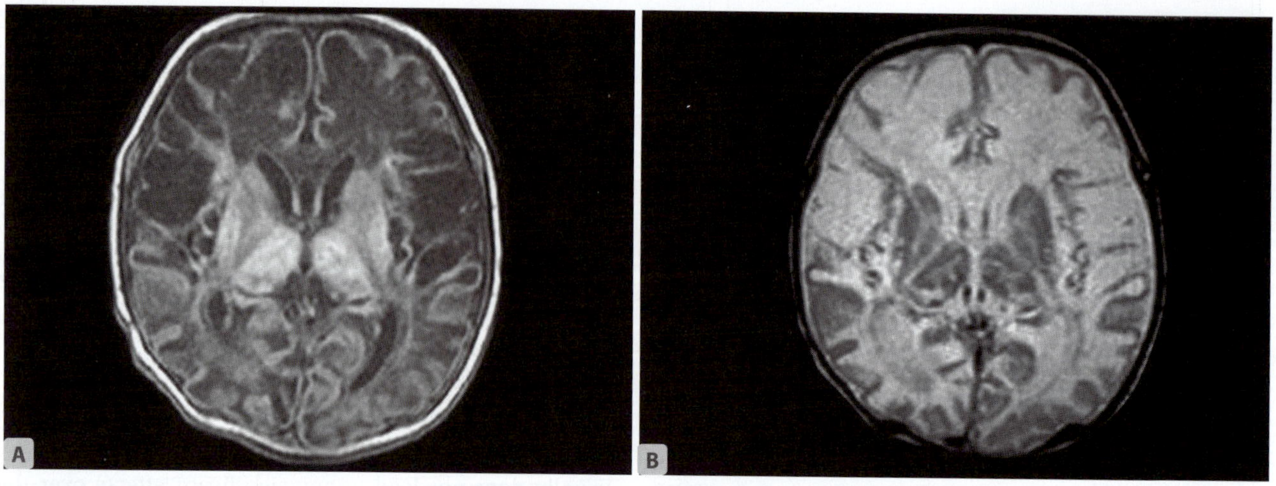

FIGS. 23A AND B: (A) T1 and (B) T2-weighted axial MR images of a 18-day-old term neonate with severe hypoxic injury shows diffuse multicystic encephalomalacia involving cortex and subcortical white matter. Also, note the persistent signal changes in the basal ganglia and thalami.

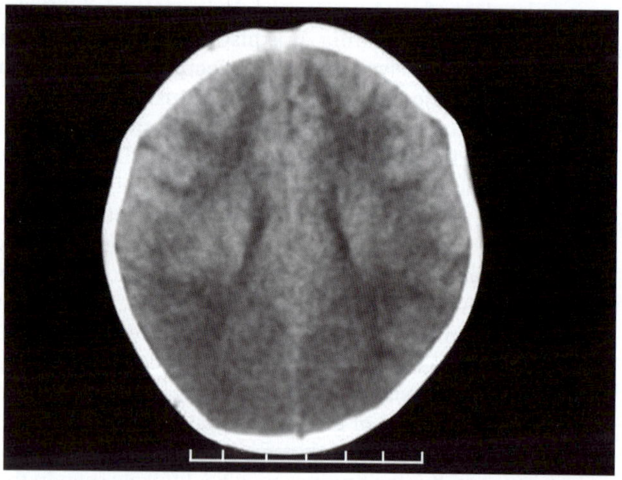

FIG. 24: Axial CT image of a 10-day-old term neonate with prolonged partial asphyxia shows hypodensity involving the watershed zones in the frontal and parieto-occipital regions.

is different from that of a premature neonate where there occurs PVL. Chronic sequelae may be in the form of ulegyria which is atrophy and thinning of the deep cortex at the depth of sulci leading to a characteristic "mushroom-shaped" gyri.

It is important to remember that any given patient may show imaging features suggestive of both severe and partial prolonged hypoxic insult.

HYPOXIC-ISCHEMIC INJURY IN POSTNATAL AGE GROUP

Rapid brain maturation is observed in the postnatal period and the brain becomes almost completed myelinated by 2 years of age. So, after 2 years of age, the hypoxic injury patterns are similar to those seen in adults. The usual causes for injury in this period are nonaccidental trauma, choking, drowning, and asphyxiation.

Severe, Total Hypoxia

Profound HII in children between 1 and 2 years of age affects the basal ganglia, hippocampi, lateral geniculate body, and cerebral cortex in the anterior frontal and parieto-occipital region. The perirolandic cortex and thalami are typically spared in contrast to their involvement seen in the perinatal period.[72] Infants below 1 year of age, however, may show an overlap between these categories and therefore may show involvement of thalami and perirolandic cortex along with involvement of basal ganglia, brainstem, and other cortical areas. Children above 2 years behave same as adults and basal ganglia, thalami, hippocampi, cerebellum, and cortical gray matter get affected **(Figs. 25A and B)**. Cortex may be diffusely involved or may be limited to perirolandic and parieto-occipital regions. Since cranial US is not feasible after the closure of anterior fontanel which occurs by about 4 months of age, CT and MRI are the mainstay of imaging in these children.

Computed tomography shows features of basal ganglia hypodensity with features of diffuse cerebral edema with relative sparing of perirolandic regions. Few affected children may also show "reversal sign" defined as white matter appearing hyperdense compared to the gray matter on CT. This results when diffuse edema in the brain leads to elevated intracranial pressure which causes partial venous obstruction and distension of deep medullary veins within the white matter. The "white cerebellum sign" may also be noted when the supratentorial brain parenchyma shows diffuse hypodensity and the brainstem and cerebellum are spared. This occurs due to redistribution of blood flow to the posterior circulation.

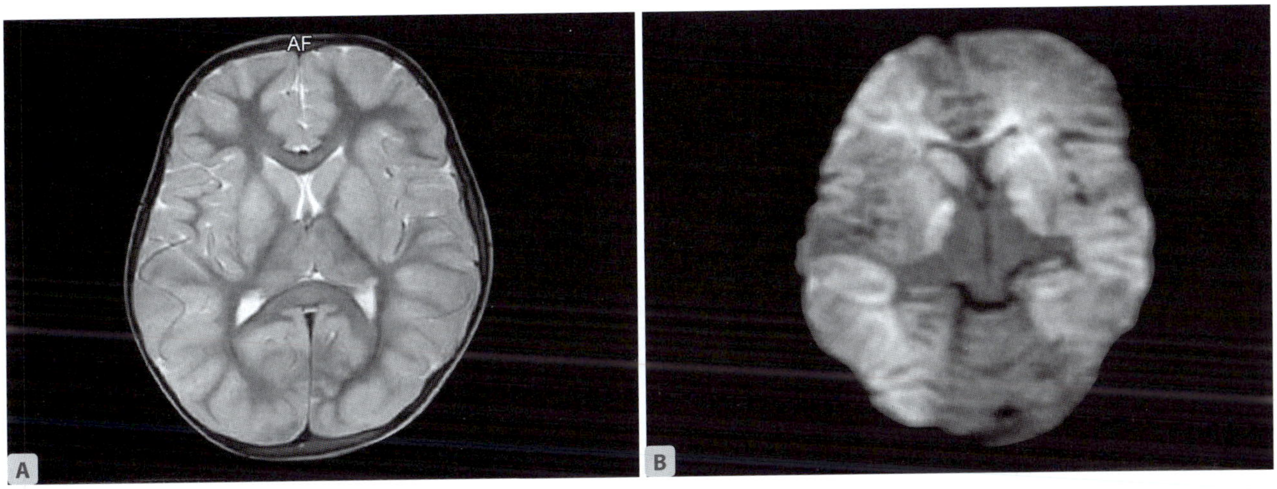

FIGS. 25A AND B: A 3-year-old girl with hypoxic injury. (A) Axial T2-weighted MR image shows hyperintense signal changes within the basal ganglia, thalami, and the cortical gray matter which show restricted diffusion on the diffusion-weighted imaging (DWI); and (B) Note the relative sparing of the cerebellum on the DWI.

Magnetic resonance imaging is more sensitive in showing abnormalities in the affected regions which are seen as hyperintense signal changes in the affected regions on T2WIs. DWI is most sensitive with abnormal signal detected within 24 hours.

Mild-to-moderate Hypoxia

The older infants and children below 2 years of age who suffer from mild-to-moderate hypoxia show involvement of cortex and subcortical white matter similar to the pattern seen in the neonates with partial prolonged hypoxia. The watershed zone infarcts are seen with relative sparing of the deep periventricular white matter. The CT and MRI features are similar to those described above. On follow-up imaging, T2-weighted MR images may show residual persisting hyperintensity within the involved regions, especially within the basal ganglia. T1WIs may show gyriform pattern of hyperintensity within the affected cortex representing cortical laminar necrosis.

IMAGING CHOICE FOR EVALUATION OF HYPOXIC-ISCHEMIC INJURY

Neonates with suspected HIE are usually hemodynamically unstable and very sick and therefore a cribside US in the ICU/nursery is usually the first investigation for screening. Besides portability, the other advantages of US are: Nonionizing, no IV contrast or sedation is required, and can be repeated frequently without harmful effects. Addition of color Doppler and quantitative analysis to 2D imaging may improve information content. However, limitations include low sensitivity and operator dependence. It has good positive predictive value, but a negative scan does not rule out injury and in a high-risk scenario, the neonate should be evaluated with MRI. CT, because of radiation exposure and low sensitivity in presence of unmyelinated white matter, is not preferred in the neonatal age group. MRI with conventional T1 and T2WIs along with DWI is the modality of choice for further evaluation. It is also more sensitive than US for early detection and mild changes, especially myelination abnormalities. If MRI is negative in the early period, MR spectroscopy may be performed or the MRI can be repeated after 3–4 days.[72]

In postnatal age group, especially after 4 months of age when anterior fontanel closes, cranial US is no longer feasible. In these children, NCCT can be performed as the first investigation. MRI may be required for negative scans with high suspicion or for better extent of the injury where CT is positive.

Technique and Timing of Magnetic Resonance Imaging

A typical MRI protocol for imaging of HIE should include T1, T2, DWI, and susceptibility-weighted imaging in axial plane, MR spectroscopy, and optional coronal plane DWI. Additional sequences may be obtained tailored to the findings in each case. The unmyelinated white matter in the neonate causes a poor differentiation between the cortex and white matter. This differentiation can be accentuated by increasing the repetition time (TR) in both T1 and T2 sequences. The TR in T1W sequence may be increased from the usual 400 to 800 ms whereas in T2W sequence, it may be increased from the usual 4,000 to 6,500 ms.[4,5]

On day 1, MR spectroscopy is the most useful technique. DWI may show changes, but these are typically subtle. On day 2, there occurs pseudonormalization of lactate, as discussed earlier, leading to decreased usefulness of MR spectroscopy. The DWI is the most sensitive sequence at this time including visual appearance, ADC values as well as FA values. The peak diffusion restriction is seen after 72 hours and it starts to decrease after 5 days leading to pseudonormalization by the end of 1 week. This period may be prolonged to 8–10 days, if therapeutic hypothermia was instituted in the neonate. The T1 and T2WIs start to show signal alterations on day 3 and show the best changes by the end of 1 week. After fifth day, T1 and T2 are the best sequences to see the extent of the injury.

Hence, imaging is best performed at 3–5 days when the imaging features are best visualized on all sequences. This will help to diagnose as well as assess the extent of damage. The imaging can be performed earlier within the first few hours in specific situations, if there is dilemma in the diagnosis and there is a need to start therapeutic hypothermia.

PREDICTION OF CLINICAL OUTCOME

After imaging, the second most important role of a pediatric radiologist in the workup of infants with HIE is to predict, if possible, the clinical outcome based on imaging findings at an early stage. This is a crucial, but difficult situation. A number of workers have used different imaging modalities and have reported various parameters to predict the clinical outcome.

Clinically, it has been observed that decreased rate of head growth during early months in a term neonate correlates closely with the neurological dysfunction and cerebral atrophy at a later stage.

Various studies based on imaging to predict the clinical outcome are as follows.

Ultrasound

Echogenic Thalamus

Normal thalamus and basal ganglia region have medium level echoes on US. In infants with HIE, characteristic increase in the echogenicity of these tissue has been reported,[73] usually in the second week after the episode of asphyxia. Visualization of this sign predicts poor prognosis and has been reported to be associated with mortality in 1% and long-term morbidity in 56%. A corollary to this is the recently described PLIC sign on US. Normally, PLIC is not separately seen on US. This sign is said to be positive when PLIC is separately visualized as a hypoechoic line between the abnormal hyperechogenic putamen and thalamus and implies a severe hypoxic injury.[74]

Cerebral Artery Doppler

Duplex scanning of the cerebral arteries has been studied, both in normal neonates as well as in those affected by perinatal asphyxia.[75,76] Resistive index (RI), the single most important Doppler parameter, has been used to measure the flow abnormality. Mean RI in normal healthy neonates is 75 and is inversely related to gestational age. With an RI of 60 as the critical level and all cases with values below 60 taken as abnormal, it has been observed that clinical outcome is poor even though 2D sonogram may appear normal. Thus, Doppler scanning of cerebral arteries may provide an easy and a reliable parameter on day 1 of life to predict the clinical outcome in a neonate with HIE.

Ultrasound Scoring System

Several authors have attempted in devising a scoring system on transcranial US.[77-80] In most cases, the scoring comprises of both gray matter and white matter findings. Most of the scores are found to correlate well with the neurodevelopmental outcome, especially when the US is performed between third and seventh day of life. These US scores have been shown as alternative to the gold standard MRI to correlate with the neurodevelopmental outcome.[74]

Computed Tomography

Reversal Sign

Presence of reversal sign, i.e., diffuse decreased attenuation of the cerebral cortex **(Figs. 24A and B)** with a relative preservation of density in the thalami, brainstem, and cerebellum, has been observed to be associated with poor prognosis[81] **(Fig. 21)**. Exact mechanism of this sign is not clear, although a number of theories have been put forward, e.g., mechanical factor, postischemic hypervascularity, distension of deep medullary veins, and high serum glucose level. The sonographic counterpart of reversal sign of CT is echogenic thalamus discussed earlier.

Diffuse Decreased Density

Diffuse low attenuation is a common finding, both in the preterm and term neonates,[8] affected by perinatal asphyxia. However, diffuse low attenuation in preterm (below 34 weeks of gestation) has no predictive value because there is very poor correlation with late neurologic sequelae. Reason for it is obvious, i.e., difficulty in differentiating pathological low attenuation from normal immature myelin tissue at this age. On the other hand, diffuse low attenuation in a term neonate is a very important prognostic predictor because it has a good correlation with poor clinical outcome.

Magnetic Resonance Imaging

Conventional Sequences

Delayed myelination is one of the hallmark of HIE which can be detected only on MRI. Studies have shown that delayed myelination in a term neonate in the first few days of life suggests significant perinatal asphyxia and hence poor prognosis. With the introduction of serial quantitative tensor MRI technique, assessment for white matter injury has become more reliable and at an early stage.[57-60] Delayed myelination on MRI may, therefore, be used as an early predictor of clinical outcome.

In mature term neonates, abnormal signal intensity within the PLIC has been found to be an excellent predictor of abnormal motor outcome. Asymmetrical involvement predicts hemiplegia and bilateral symmetrical involvement correlates with subsequent development of spastic diplegia or quadriplegia.[82] The severity of basal ganglia and thalamic lesions detected on MRI also has good correlate with severity and nature of cerebral palsy. The involvement of white matter exacerbates cognitive impairment and poor head growth.[83]

In premature neonates, finding of PVHI correlates well with development of hemiplegia in survivors whereas PVL correlates more with spastic diplegia. It has also been observed that most of the neonates with documented PVL on

US/CT along with DEHSI had neurologic abnormality.[84-86] Also, a general correlation between the neurological impairment and the severity of MR abnormalities was demonstrated. Abnormalities on MRI scan, therefore, can be used not only to predict the neurological deficit, but also its severity.

Magnetic Resonance Spectroscopy

Magnetic resonance spectroscopy has proved invaluable to detect early brain injury with good correlation between the degree of abnormality and the clinical outcome. Therefore, MRS may be used as a predictor of prognosis.

CONCLUSION

Hypoxic-ischemic encephalopathy is a relatively common clinical problem in the neonatal period. Pathological changes depend upon the gestational age. Imaging features, therefore, also differ in the preterm and term infants. Depending upon the gestational age and the abnormality suspected, a particular imaging modality is chosen.

Cranial ultrasound remains the first screening modality, especially in the premature neonate. However, MRI has a vast potential not only to detect subtle, early, and specific abnormalities, but also to predict clinical outcome based on imaging features in the first few days of life. MRS has also shown good promise in early detection of changes.

A close cooperation and teamwork are, therefore, required between the neonatologist and the pediatric radiologist to decide the imaging approach appropriate for the gestational age, suspected pathology, imaging facilities available, and the expertise, both in performing and interpreting the images, without duplicating the information and keeping the cost-benefit in view.

REFERENCES

1. Singh M. Hypoxic ischemic encephalopathy. In: Talukdar B (Ed). Essentials of Pediatric Neurology. New Delhi: New Age International (P) Ltd; 1997. pp. 95-107.
2. Legido A, Katoseos CD, Mishra OP, Delivoria-Papadopoulos M. Perinatal hypoxic ischemic encephalopathy: Current and future treatments. Int Pediatr. 2000;15:143-51.
3. Krishnan P, Shroff M. Neuroimaging in neonatal hypoxic ischemic encephalopathy. Indian J Pediatr. 2016;83:995-1002.
4. Varghese B, Xavier R, Manoj VC, Aneesh MK, Priya PS, Kumar A, et al. Magnetic resonance imaging spectrum of perinatal hypoxic-ischemic brain injury. Indian J Radiol Imaging. 2016;26: 316-27.
5. Ghei SK, Zan E, Nathan JE, Choudhri A, Tekes A, Huisman TAG, et al. MR imaging of hypoxic-ischemic injury in term neonates: pearls and pitfalls. Radiographics. 2014;34:1047-61.
6. Division of Neonatology. (2019). Teaching Files: Perinatal Asphyxia (Hypoxic Ischaemic Encephalopathy). California: Cedars-Sinai Medical Center; 2019.
7. Vannucci RC, Perlman JM. Interventions for perinatal hypoxic ischaemic encephalopathy. Pediatrics. 1997;100:1004-14.
8. Barkovich AJ. Brain and spine injuries. In: Barkovich AJ (Ed). Pediatric Neuroimaging, 4th edition. Philadelphia: Lippincott Williams & Wilkins; 2005. pp. 190-290.
9. Horwood LJ, Mogridge N, Darlow BA. Cognitive, educational, and behavioural outcomes at 7 to 8 years in a national very low birthweight cohort. Arch Dis Child Fetal Neonatal Ed. 1998;79:F12-20.
10. Emslie HC, Wardle SP, Sims DG, Chiswick M, D'Souza S. Increased survival and deteriorating developmental outcome in 23 to 25 week old gestation infants, 1990-4 compared with 1984-9. Arch Dis Child Fetal Neonatal Ed. 1998;78:F99-104.
11. Keeney SE, Adecock EW, McArdle CB. Prospective observations of 100 high risk neonates by high field (1.5 Tesla) magnetic resonance imaging of the central nervous system: I. Intraventricular and extracerebral lesions. Pediatrics. 1991;87:421-30.
12. Koeda T, Suganuma I, Kohno Y, Takamatsu T, Takeshita K. MR imaging of spastic diplegia: Comparative study between preterm and term infants. Neuroradiology. 1990;32:187-90.
13. Flodmark O, Roland EH, Hill A, Whitfield MF. Periventricular leukomalacia: radiologic diagnosis. Radiology. 1987;162:119-24.
14. Barkovich AJ, Westmark K, Partridge C, Sola A, Ferriero DM. Perinatal asphyxia: MR findings in the first 10 days. AJNR Am J Neuroradiol. 1995;16:427-38.
15. Flodmark O, Lupton B, Li D, Stimac GK, Roland EH, Hill A, et al. MR imaging of periventricular leukomalacia in childhood. Am J Roentgenol. 1989,152:583-90.
16. Huppi PS. MR in HIE. Clinical Perinatol. 2002;29:827-56.
17. Barkovich AJ, Sargent SK. Profound asphyxia in the premature infant: Imaging findings. Am J Neuroradiol. 1995;16:1837-46.
18. Hambleton G, Wigglesworth JS. Origin of intraventricular hemorrhage in preterm infant. Arch Dis Child. 1976;51:651-60.
19. Wigglesworth JS, Pape KE. An integrated model for hemorrhage and ischemic lesions in the newborn brain. Early Hum Dev. 1978;2:179-99.
20. Papile LA, Brustein J, Koffer H. Incidence and evolution of subependymal and intraventricular hemorrhage: A study of infants with birth weight less than 1500 gm. J Pediatr. 1978;92:529-34.
21. Gould SJ, Howard S, Hope PL, Reynolds EO. Periventricular intraparenchymal cerebral haemorrhage in preterm infants: the role of venous infarction. J Pathol. 1987;151:197-202.
22. Volpe JJ. Brain injury in the premature infant. Neuropathology, clinical aspects, and pathogenesis. MRDD Res Rev. 1997;3:3-12.
23. Del-Toro J, Louis PT, Goddard-Finegold J. Cerebrovascular regulation and neonatal brain injury. Pediatr Neurol. 1991;7:3-12.
24. Hill A. Current concepts of hypoxic-ischemic cerebral injury in the term newborn. Pediatr Neurol. 1991;7:317-25.
25. Volpe JJ. Hypoxic-ischemic encephalopathy: neuropathology and pathogenesis. In: Volpe JJ (Ed). Neurology of the Newborn, 3rd edition. Philadelphia: Saunders; 1995. pp. 279-313.
26. Rutherford MA, Supramaniam V, Ederies A, Chew A, Bassi L, Groppo M, et al. Magnetic resonance imaging of white matter diseases of prematurity. Neuroradiology. 2010;52:505-21.
27. Maria A, Gupta AK, Paul VK. Germinal matrix—intraventricular hemorrhage of the premature infants and PVL. In: Kalra V (Ed). Practical Paediatric Neurology. New Delhi: Arya Publications; 2002. pp. 36-8.
28. Gupta AK, Pradhan MK, Bhushan S, Paul VK, Berry M. Sonography in hypoxic-ischaemic encephalopathy. Indian J Radiol Imaging. 1998;8:45-56.
29. Zupan V, Gonzalez P, Lacaze-Masmonteil T, Boithias C, d'Allest AM, Dehan M, et al. Periventricular leukomalacia: Risk factors revisited. Dev Med Child Neurol. 1996;38:1061-7.
30. Verma U, Tejani N, Klein S, Reale MR, Beneck D, Figueroa R, et al. Obstetric antecedents of intraventricular hemorrhage and periventricular leukomalacia in the low-birth-weight neonate. Am J Obstet Gynecol. 1997;176:275-81.

31. Nelson K, Ellenberg J. Antecedents of cerebral palsy: Multivariate analysis of risk. N Engl J Med. 1986;315:81-6.
32. Maria A, Gupta AK. Periventricular leukomalacia: Brain injury in the premature infant. Childhood Disability Update. 2002;2:25-30.
33. Back SA, Luo NL, Borenstein NS, Levine JM, Volpe JJ, Kinney HC. Late oligodendrocyte progenitors coincide with the developmental window of vulnerability for human perinatal white matter injury. J Neurosci. 2001;21:1302-12.
34. Back SA, Han BH, Luo NL, Chricton CA, Xanthoudakis S, Tam J, et al. Selective vulnerability of late oligodendrocyte progenitors to hypoxia-ischemia. J Neurosci. 2002;22:455-63.
35. Perlman JM, Risser R, Broyles RS. Bilateral cystic periventricular leukomalacia in the premature infant: associated risk factors. Pediatrics. 1996;97:822-7.
36. Hesser U, Katz-Salamon M, Mortensson W, Flodmark O, Forssberg H. Diagnosis of intracranial lesions in very-low-birthweight infants by ultrasound: incidence and association with potential risk factors. Acta Paediatr Suppl. 1997;419:16-26.
37. Claris O, Besnier S, Lapillonne A, Picaud JC, Salle BL. Incidence of ischemic-hemorrhagic cerebral lesions in premature infants of gestational age < or = 28 weeks: a prospective ultrasound study. Biol Neonate. 1996;70:29-34.
38. Maria A, Gupta AK, Aggarwal R, Sreenivas V, Paul VK, Deorari AK. Incidence of periventricular leukomalacia among a cohort of very low birth weight neonates (<1500 g). Indian Pediatr. 2006;43:210-6.
39. McArdle CB, Richardson CJ, Hayden CK, Nicholas DA, Amparo EG. Abnormalities of the neonatal brain: MR imaging. Part II. Hypoxic-ischemic brain injury. Radiology. 1987;163:395-403.
40. Banker BQ, Larroche JC. Periventricular leukomalacia in infancy: a form of neonatal anoxic encephalopathy. Arch Neurol. 1962;7:386-410.
41. Weisglas-Kuperus N, Baerts W, Fetter W, Hempel MS, Mulder PG, Touwen BC, et al. Minor neurological dysfunction and quality of movement in relation to neonatal cerebral damage and subsequent development. Dev Med Child Neurol. 1994;36:727-35.
42. Pinto-Martin JA, Dobson V, Cnaan A, Zhao HM, Paneth NS. Vision outcome at age 2 years in a low birth weight population. Pediatr Neurol. 1996;14:281-7.
43. Uggetti C, Egitto ME, Fazzi E, Bianchi PE, Bergamaschi R, Zappoli F, et al. Cerebral visual impairment in periventricular leukomalacia: MR correlation. AJNR Am J Neuroradiol. 1996;17:979-85.
44. Roth SC, Baudin J, McCormick DC, Edwards AD, Townsend J, Stewart AL, et al. Relation between ultrasound appearance of the brain of very preterm infants and neurodevelopmental impairment at eight years. Dev Med Child Neurol. 1993;35:755-68.
45. Barr LL, McCullough PJ, Ball WS, Krasner BH, Garra BS, Deddens JA. Quantitative sonographic feature analysis of clinical infant hypoxia: A pilot study. AJNR Am J Neuroradiol. 1996;17:1025-31.
46. Vannucci RC, Christensen MA, Yager JY. Nature, time–course, and extent of cerebral edema in perinatal hypoxic-ischemic brain damage. Pediatr Neurol. 1993;9:29-34.
47. Grant EG, Schellinger D, Richardson JD, Coffey ML, Smirniotopoulous JG. Echogenic periventricular halo: normal sonographic finding or neonatal cerebral hemorrhage. AJR Am J Roentgenol. 1983;140:793-6.
48. de Vries LS, Eken P, Dubowitz LMS. The spectrum of leukomalacia using cranial ultrasound. Behav Brain Res. 1992;49:1-6.
49. Debillon T, N'Guyen S, Muet A, Quere MP, Moussaly F, Roze JC. Limitations of ultrasonography for diagnosing white matter damage in preterm infants. Arch Dis Child Fetal Neonatal Ed. 2003;88:F275-9.
50. Miller SP, Cozzio CC, Goldstein RB, Ferriero DM, Partridge JC, Vigneron DB, et al. Comparing the diagnosis of white matter injury in premature newborns with serial MR imaging and transfontanel ultrasonography findings. AJNR Am J Neuroradiol. 2003;24:1661-9.
51. Inder TE, Anderson NJ, Spencer C, Wells S, Volpe JJ. White matter injury in the premature infant: a comparison between serial cranial sonographic and MR findings at term. AJNR Am J Neuroradiol. 2003;24:805-9.
52. Graham M, Levene MI, Trounce JQ, Rutter N. Prediction of cerebral palsy in very low birthweight infants: prospective ultrasound study. Lancet. 1987;8559:593-6.
53. Salas J, Tekes A, Hwang M, Northington FJ, Huisman FJ. Head Ultrasound in Neonatal Hypoxic-Ischemic Injury and Its Mimickers for Clinicians: A Review of the Patterns of Injury and the Evolution of Findings Over Time. Neonatology. 2018;114:185-97.
54. Arthur R. Magnetic resonance imaging in preterm infants. Pediatr Radiol. 2006;36:593-607.
55. Bozzao A, Di Paolo A, Mazzoleni C, Fasoli F, Simonetti A, Fantozzi LM, et al. Diffusion-weighted MR imaging in the early diagnosis of periventricular leukomalacia. Eur Radiol. 2003;13:1571-6.
56. Roelants-van Rijn AM, Nikkels PG, Groenendaal F, van Der Grond J, Barth PG, Snoeck I, et al. Neonatal diffusion-weighted MRI imaging: relation with histopathology or follow-up MR examination. Neuropediatrics. 2001;32:286-94.
57. Arzoumanian Y, Mirmiran M, Barnes PD, Woolley K, Ariagno RL, Moseley ME, et al. Diffusion tensor brain imaging findings at term-equivalent age may predict neurologic abnormalities in low birth weight preterm infants. AJNR Am J Neuroradiol. 2003;24:1646-53.
58. Miller SP, Vigneron DB, Henry RG, Bohland MA, Ceppi-Cozzio C, Hoffman C, et al. Serial quantitative diffusion tensor MRI of the premature brain: development in newborns with and without injury. J Magn Reson Imaging. 2002;16:621-32.
59. Hoon AH, Lawrie WT, Melhem ER, Reinhardt EM, van Zijl PCM, Solaiyappan M, et al. Diffusion tensor imaging of periventricular leukomalacia shows affected sensory cortex white matter pathways. Neurology. 2002;59:752-6.
60. Melhelm ER, Mori S, Mukundan G, Kraut MA, Pomper MG, van Zijl PCM. Diffusion tensor MR imaging of the brain and white matter tractography. AJR Am J Roentgenol. 2002;178:3-16.
61. Baker LL, Stevenson DK, Enzmann DR. End-stage periventricular leukomalacia: MR evaluation. Radiology. 1988;168:809-15.
62. Hull J, Dodd KL. Falling incidence of hypoxic-ischemic encephalopathy in term infants. Br J Obstet Gynecol 1992;99:386-91.
63. Truwit CL, Barkovich AJ, Koch TK, Ferriero DM. Cerebral palsy: MR findings in 40 patients. AJNR Am J Neuroradiol. 1992;13:67-78.
64. Raybaud C. Destructive lesions of the brain. Neuroradiology. 1983;25:265-91.
65. Rutherford M, Srinivasan L, Dyet L, Ward P, Allsop J, Counsell S, et al. Magnetic resonance imaging in perinatal brain injury: clinical presentation, lesions, and outcome. Pediatr Radiol. 2006;36:582-92.
66. Hunt RW, Neil JJ, Coleman LT, Kean MJ, Inder TE. Apparent diffusion coefficient in the posterior limb of the internal capsule predicts outcome after perinatal asphyxia. Pediatrics. 2004;114:999-1003.
67. de Vries LS, Groenendaal F. Patterns of neonatal hypoxic-ischemic brain injury. Neuroradiology. 2010;52:555-66.
68. Hanrahan JD, Sargentoni J, Azzopardi D, Manji K, Cowan FM, Rutherford MA, et al. Cerebral metabolism within 18 hours of birth asphyxia: a proton magnetic resonance spectroscopy study. Pediatr Res. 1996;39:584-90.
69. Peden CJ, Cowan FM, Bryant DJ, Sargentoni J, Cox IJ, Menon DK, et al. Proton MR spectroscopy of the brain in infants. J Comput Assist Tomogr. 1990;14:886-94.
70. Holshouser BA, Ashwal S, Luh GY, Shu S, Kahlon S, Auld KL, et al. Proton MR spectroscopy after acute central nervous system injury: outcome prediction in neonates, infants, and children. Radiology. 1997;202:487-96.

71. Penrice J, Cady EB, Lorek A, Wylezinska M, Amess PN, Aldridge RF, et al. Proton magnetic resonance spectroscopy of the brain in normal preterm and term infants, and early changes after perinatal hypoxic-ischemia. Pediatr Res. 1996;40:6-14.
72. Huang BY, Castillo M. Hypoxic-ischemic brain injury: imaging findings from birth to adulthood. Radiographics. 2008;28: 417-39.
73. Connolly B, Kelehan P, O'Brien N, Gorman W, Murphy JF, King M, et al. The echogenic thalamus in hypoxic ischaemic encephalopathy. Pediatr Radiol. 1994;24:268-71.
74. Annink KV, de Vries LS, Groenendaal F, Vijlbrief DC, Weeke LC, Roehr CC, et al. The development and validation of a cerebral ultrasound scoring system for infants with hypoxic-ischaemic encephalopathy. Pediatr Res. 2020;87:59-66.
75. Seibert JJ, McCowan TC, Chadduck WM, Adametz JR, Glasier CM, Williamson SL, et al. Duplex pulsed Doppler US versus intracranial pressure in the neonate: clinical and experimental studies. Radiology. 1989;171:155-9.
76. Stark JE, Seibert JJ. Cerebral artery Doppler ultrasonography for prediction of outcome after perinatal asphyxia. J Ultrasound Med. 1994;13:595-600.
77. Tann CJ, Nakakeeto M, Hagmann C, Webb EL, Nyombi N, Namiiro F, et al. Early cranial ultrasound findings among infants with neonatal encephalopathy in Uganda: an observational study. Pediatr Res. 2016;80:190-6.
78. Leijser LM, Vein AA, Liauw L, Strauss T, Veen S, van Wezel-Meijler G. Prediction of short-term neurological outcome in full-term neonates with hypoxic-ischaemic encephalopathy based on combined use of electroencephalogram and neuro-imaging. Neuropediatrics. 2007;38:219-27.
79. Swarte R, Lequin M, Cherian P, Zecic A, van Goudoever J, Govaert P. Imaging patterns of brain injury in term-birth asphyxia. Acta Paediatr. 2009;98:586-92.
80. Trivedi SB, Vesoulis ZA, Rao R, Liao SM, Shimony JS, McKinstry RS, et al. A validated clinical MRI injury scoring system in neonatal hypoxic-ischemic encephalopathy. Pediatr Radiol. 2017;47:1491-9.
81. Han BK, Towbin RB, De Courten-Meyers G, McLaurin RL, Ball WS. Reversal sign on CT: effect of anoxic/ischemic cerebral injury in children. AJR Am J Roentgenol. 1990;154:361-8.
82. Rutherford MA, Pennock JM, Counsell SJ, Mercuri E, Cowan FM, Dubowitz LMS, et al. Abnormal magnetic resonance signal in the internal capsule predicts poor neurodevelopmental outcome in infants with hypoxic-ischemic encephalopathy. Pediatrics. 1998;102:323-8.
83. Rutherford M, Biarge MM, Allsop J, Counsell S, Cowan F. MRI of perinatal brain injury. Pediatr Radiol. 2010;40:819-33.
84. Cordes I, Roland EH, Lupton BA, Hill A. Early prediction of the development of microcephaly after hypoxic-ischemic encephalopathy in the full-term newborn. Pediatrics. 1994;93:703-7.
85. Han TR, Bang MS, Lim JY, Yoon BH, Kim IW. Risk factors for cerebral palsy in preterm. Am J Phys Med Rehabil. 2002;81:297-303.
86. van de Bor M, den Ouden L, Guit GL. Value of cranial ultrasound and magnetic resonance imaging in predicting neurodevelopmental outcome in preterm infants. Pediatrics. 1992;90:196-9.

CHAPTER

86

Craniospinal Sonography

Radhika Batra, Rashmi Dixit, Manisha Jana, Anjali Prakash, Devasenathipathy Kandasamy

PART A: CRANIAL SONOGRAPHY

INTRODUCTION

Cranial sonography is an essential diagnostic tool for assessing the neonatal and infant brain while the fontanels remain open therefore, it is best before the age of 12 months.[1] It is noninvasive, readily available, and reproducible. It is portable, can be done at bedside without sedation with little disturbance to the baby, and is relatively inexpensive. It is safe as it does not use ionizing radiation. Cranial sonography can be performed at an early stage and can be repeated, making it suitable for serial imaging for assessment of the evaluation of a lesion and the growth and maturation of the brain. Current ultrasound equipment allows rapid evaluation of infants in the intensive care nursery with excellent visualization of normal structures and a wide range of pathologies. However, cranial sonography has some limitations as image quality is dependent on the size of the acoustic window available and presence of scalp hair[2] **(Fig. 1)**.

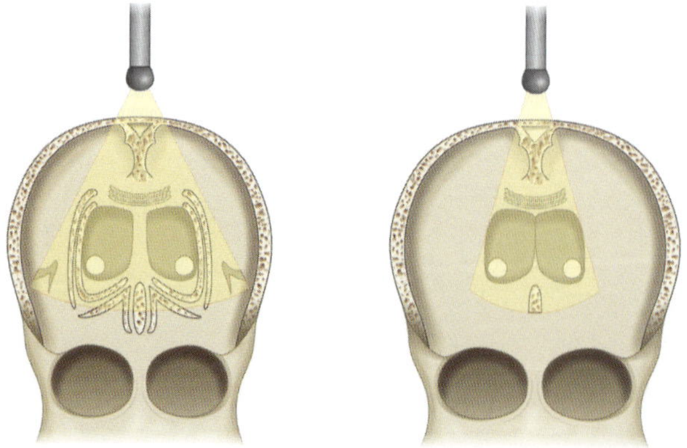

FIG. 1: Diagram showing the size of fontanel limiting the sonographic window.

INDICATIONS OF CRANIAL SONOGRAPHY[3]

- Screening for hemorrhage or parenchymal injury
- Follow-up of intraventricular hemorrhage (IVH) and posthemorrhagic ventricular dilatation
- Neonatal encephalopathy including hypoxic-ischemic encephalopathy (HIE)
- Congenital malformations of brain
- Follow-up of antenatally detected brain abnormalities
- Congenital or acquired brain infection including intrauterine infection
- Birth injuries such as fractured skull bones, subgaleal hemorrhage
- Assessment of preexisting neurological damage before neonatal extracorporeal membrane oxygenation (ECMO)
- Evaluation of babies following therapeutic hypothermia and ECMO
- Suspected metabolic disorders
- Monitoring in neonates on ventilatory support
- In cases of sudden deterioration in clinical condition, sudden drop in hemoglobin, necrotizing enterocolitis, and sepsis
- Signs and/or symptoms of central nervous system (CNS) disorders: Seizures, microcephaly, macrocephaly, hypotonia, and unexplained poor feeding at term.

EQUIPMENT

High frequency phased array transducers (5–7.5 MHz) with a small footprint are used for performing cranial ultrasounds. High-resolution images are obtained in preterm neonates by using a probe with a frequency of 7.5 MHz. If the size of the anterior fontanel (AF) is small, phased array transducers of small footprint and wide insonation angle (140°) are useful.[2] A transducer frequency of 7.5 MHz usually enables optimal visualization of the peri- and intraventricular areas of the brain. For evaluation of more superficial structures (cortex, subcortical white matter, subarachnoid spaces, and superior sagittal sinus) and/or in very tiny infants with small heads, it is advisable to perform an additional scan, using a higher frequency of up to 10 MHz. In larger and older infants, infants with thick curly hair or in order to obtain a better view of deeper structures (posterior fossa, basal ganglia in full-term infants), deeper penetration of the beam is required and scanning should be performed using a lower frequency probe (5 MHz).[4]

TECHNIQUE AND NORMAL ANATOMY

Cranial sonography is most successfully performed in a warm environment, when the baby is quiet or after feeding. Aseptic precautions like hand washing and transducer cleansing before and after the examination should be followed. It is essential to monitor the baby during the examination and body temperature should be maintained. After selecting the appropriate probe and preset for cranial sonography, the depth, gain, and time gain compensation settings are adjusted. Coupling gel is applied to the transducer and it is held firmly over the fontanel.[3]

Most cranial ultrasounds are performed through the AF which remains useful for scanning up to the age of 12–14 months.[1] Supplemental windows which can be used for cranial sonography include the posterior fontanel (PF), mastoid fontanel (MF), and temporal window (TW).

The AF is an excellent window to image the supratentorial part of the brain. The AF is located at the junction of coronal and sagittal sutures and remains open for the first 12–14 months of age. Pressure over the AF should be avoided, especially in an ill premature neonate. The transducer should be placed in the middle of the AF with the plane of the transducer passing from ear to ear; the marker on the transducer should point to the right side of the baby. The transducer is angled as far forward and backward as possible to scan coronal images in a sequential manner. After imaging in the coronal plane, the transducer is rotated through 90° to scan in the sagittal plane. The transducer should be parallel to the anteroposterior diameter of the cranial vault and the marker should point towards the baby's nose. Once the midline sagittal view has been obtained, the transducer should be angled laterally to the right and left to obtain parasagittal views. At least five standard images should be obtained in the sagittal and parasagittal planes. Imaging through a supplementary window should be performed if any abnormality is seen in the sagittal or coronal plane.[3]

Standard Views

Coronal Planes

There are six standard coronal planes **(Fig. 2)**. The images should be symmetric with the interhemispheric fissure in midline.

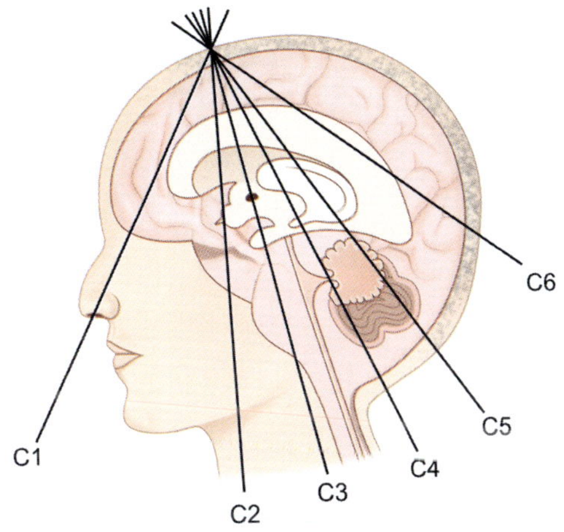

FIG. 2: Illustration demonstrates the six standard coronal planes obtained in neonatal cranial ultrasound through the anterior fontanel.

1. *Coronal plane C1* is at the level of the frontal lobes: The probe is angled as far forward as possible to see the frontal lobe.
2. *Coronal plane C2* is at the level of the frontal horns of lateral ventricles: The transducer is angled backward to assess frontal horns of lateral ventricles on either side of midline. The lateral ventricles are larger in preterm infants. The cavum septum pellucidum (CSP) is seen as a fluid-filled space between the frontal horns. The corpus callosum (CC) lies superior to the CSP giving rise to a tram line appearance. The caudate nucleus is present below the lateral ventricle.
3. *Coronal plane C3* is at the level of third ventricle, as the transducer is angled further backward, the third ventricle is seen between the lateral ventricles and CSP. The foramen of Monro may be seen on this view. The sylvian fissure is another important structure noted in this plane; it appears Y-shaped in term infants and is wide open in preterm infants.
4. *Coronal plane C4* is at the level posterior to foramen of Monro (level of cerebellum): This view is obtained as the transducer is angled further backward. The brainstem may be seen as a "Christmas tree" appearance on this view **(Fig. 3D)**. The cerebellum, quadrigeminal cistern, fourth ventricle, and cisterna magna are seen on this view.
5. *Coronal plane C5* is at the level of trigone of lateral ventricles: In this plane the trigones of lateral ventricles are seen, the choroid plexus fills the cavity of the lateral ventricles. The ventricular cavities should diverge laterally, if they are parallel CC dysplasia should be considered. The cavum vergae may be visible if present. "Peritrigonal blush" is seen in this plane (periventricular white matter is echodense, symmetric, and less echogenic than choroid plexus).
6. *Coronal plane C6* is at the level of occipital lobes, the parietal and occipital cortex is seen.[3]

Important intracranial structures seen on coronal sonograms are shown in **Figures 3A to F**.

Sagittal Planes

Five standard sagittal and parasagittal sections should be obtained through the AF **(Fig. 4)**.

Midline sagittal S1: This plane is obtained with the transducer in midline of AF. The CC, CSP, third and fourth

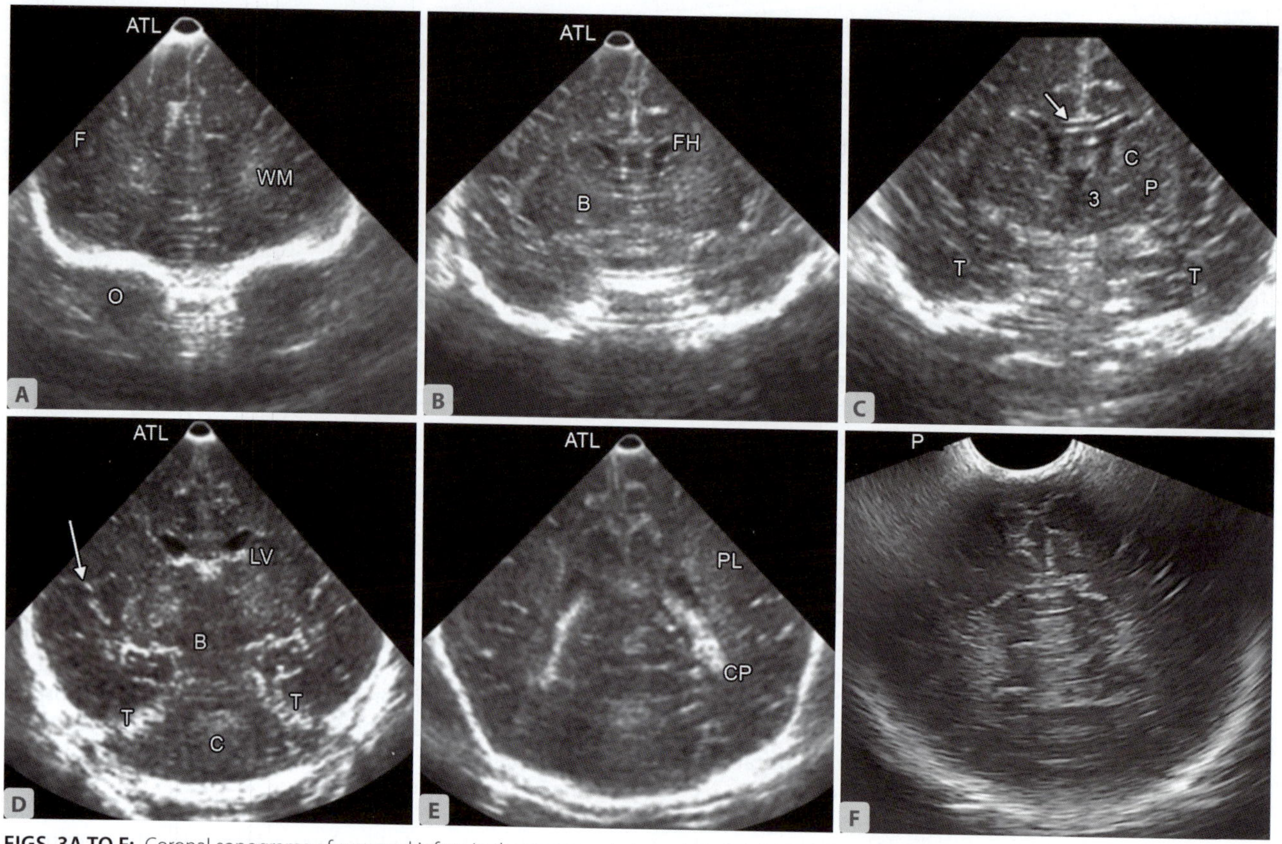

FIGS. 3A TO F: Coronal sonograms of a normal infant in the six coronal planes (C1–C6). (A) F: frontal lobes, WM: frontal white matter, and O: orbits; (B) FH: frontal horn of lateral ventricle, B: basal ganglia; (C) C: caudate nucleus, P: putamen, T: temporal lobe, 3: third ventricle, and white arrow points to the corpus callosum; (D) B: brainstem, T: tentorium, C: cerebellum, and white arrow points to the sylvian fissure; (E) PL: parietal lobe, CP: glomus of the choroid plexus. Note that the white matter of the centrum semiovale appears slightly more reflective than the gray matter; and (F) Level of occipital lobes.

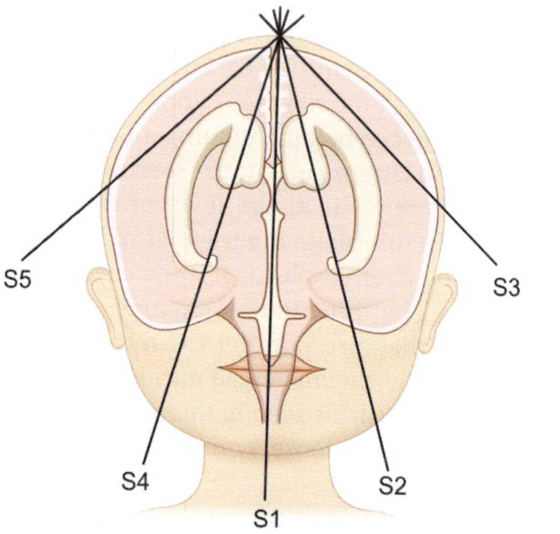

FIG. 4: Illustration demonstrates the five standard sagittal planes obtained in neonatal cranial ultrasound through the anterior fontanel.

ventricles, and vermis should be included in this view. CC is a hallmark of this view, seen as a longitudinal hypoechoic band bounded by callosal sulcus sweeping from front to back with the cingulate gyrus above and parallel to it.

Parasagittal through lateral ventricle S2 and S4: The probe is angled to the right and to the left to obtain parasagittal images. C-shaped lateral ventricle with choroid plexus within is the hallmark of this plane. Caudothalamic groove is a shallow inverted V-shaped depression between caudate nucleus and thalamus, the choroid plexus extends anteriorly into the caudothalamic groove and appears as a white dot. This should not be confused with hemorrhage.

Parasagittal through insula S3 and S5: These are the images superficial to the lateral ventricles. Sylvian fissure is the hallmark in this plane.[3]

Important intracranial structures seen on sagittal sonograms are shown in **Figures 5A to C**. **Table 1** enlists the various standard views which are useful to assess different pathologies while performing cranial ultrasound.

Supplemental Windows

Use of supplemental acoustic windows such as the PF, the TW, and the MF help in better visualization of brainstem and posterior fossa.

Posterior Fontanel

The PF is located at the junction of sagittal and lambdoid sutures and usually closes by about 3 months of age. The transducer is placed at the middle of the PF transversely to obtain the coronal view and it is rotated vertically to obtain

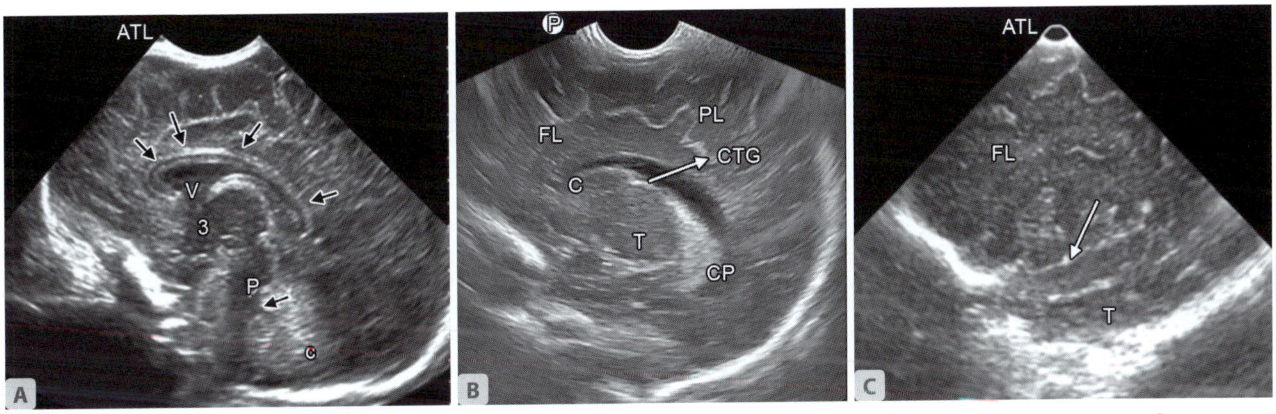

FIGS. 5A TO C: Sagittal (A) and parasagittal (B and C) scans of a normal infant. (A) V: cavum septum pellucidum and, 3: third ventricle, P: pons, arrows point to corpus callosum (B) C: caudate nucleus, T: thalamus, CTG: caudothalamic groove, CP: choroid plexus, FL: frontal lobe, and PL: parietal lobe; (C) FL: frontal lobe, T: temporal lobe, and white arrow points to the sylvian fissure.

TABLE 1: Standard views useful to assess different pathologies.

Standard view	Pathology to be assessed
Coronal plane C3	• Assess basal ganglia for edema, ischemia, and hemorrhage • Lenticulostriate vasculopathy
Coronal plane C5	• Choroid plexus cysts • Choroid plexus bleed • Corpus callosum dysplasia
Coronal plane C6	• Assess cerebral parenchyma for cystic periventricular leukomalacia and periventricular flare
Parasagittal planes S2 and S4	• Choroid plexus cysts • Choroid plexus hemorrhage • Assess basal ganglia • Lenticulostriate vasculopathy
Parasagittal planes S3 and S5	• Assess periventricular white matter • Periventricular flare • Cystic periventricular leukomalacia

the sagittal view. The occipital horns, occipital parenchyma, and cerebellum are well-visualized.[3]

Temporal Window

Temporal window is located approximately 1 cm above and anterior to the external auditory meatus. The probe is placed horizontally over it with the marker towards the nose and axial views can be obtained. The position should be adjusted to see the cerebellum and brainstem. Doppler flow measurement of circle of Willis can be done in this view.[3]

Mastoid Fontanel

Mastoid fontanel is located at the junction of posterior parietal, temporal, and occipital bones and it may not fuse until 2 years of age. The transducer is placed 1 cm posterior to the helix of the ear at a level approximately 1 cm above the tragus. Axial images are obtained with transducer parallel to orbitomeatal line. Coronal views are obtained with the transducer placed along the coronal suture. This helps in the visualization of the posterior fossa and midbrain.[3]

Supplemental windows are useful in:

- Large IVH to exclude posterior fossa hemorrhage
- Suspected congenital anomalies of posterior fossa
- Ventriculomegaly without obvious cause
- To enable Doppler flow measurements especially of middle cerebral artery (MCA).

CRANIAL DOPPLER SONOGRAPHY

The AF approach for Doppler US provides the most easily accessible view and reveals the best anatomic detail. A combination of coronal and sagittal scans allows identification of the major intracranial vessels including anterior cerebral artery (ACA) (A1 segment and distal segment), internal carotid artery, and basilar artery. The M1 segment of the MCA is not well-demonstrated as the direction of blood flow is nearly perpendicular to the Doppler beam. The internal cerebral veins and the vein of Galen are easily seen on the midsagittal view. The superior sagittal sinus and straight sinus can also be identified.[5]

The temporal approach through the thin squamous portion of the temporal bone provides detailed images of the midbrain and the vessels forming the circle of Willis. The proximal segments of the anterior and middle cerebral arteries and the M1 portion are well seen due to the more favorable Doppler angle. This approach can also be used in older children when the AF is closed.[5,6]

The brain is a low-resistance vascular bed and continuous forward flow should be seen throughout the arteries in systole and diastole. The resistive index (RI) of major intracranial arteries ranges from 0.6 to 0.8.[7] It is slightly higher (0.68–0.88) in infants <34 weeks of gestational age.[8] Besides pathological conditions, elevated RI may be seen with increased scanning pressure, high pass filter settings, and in the presence of a patent ductus arteriosus.

Doppler plays an important role in diagnosis and follow-up of brain damage secondary to ischemia, hemorrhage, infection, developmental disorder, and tumors. It is also used

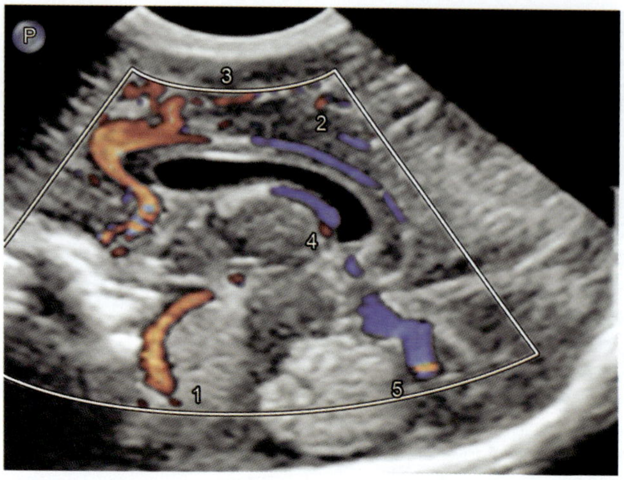

FIG. 6: Midline sagittal color Doppler scan showing (1) internal cerebral artery, (2) pericallosal artery, (3) callosomarginal artery, (4) internal cerebral vein, and (5) straight sinus.

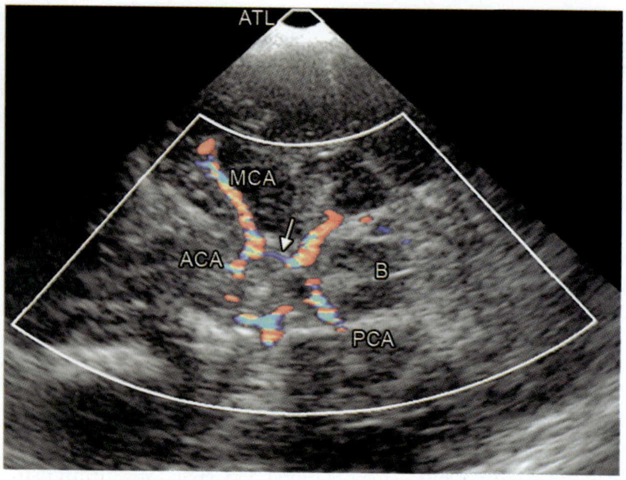

FIG. 7: Axial section through the squamous temporal bone showing the vessels of the circle of Willis. Arrow points to the posterior communicating artery. (ACA: anterior cerebral artery; MCA: middle cerebral artery; PCA: posterior cerebral artery)

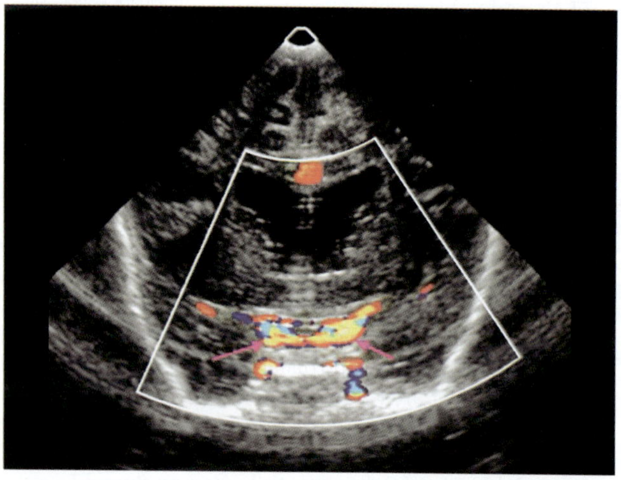

FIG. 8: Coronal CDFI scan showing ICA on both sides, arrow points to their bifurcation on both sides. (CDFI: color Doppler flow imaging; ICA: internal carotid artery)

for differentiation of a subarachnoid from subdural fluid collection and diagnosis of venous thrombosis.

The normal vascular anatomy as seen by color Doppler flow imaging (CDFI) is depicted in **Figures 6 to 8**.

NORMAL ANATOMIC VARIANTS

Cavum Septum Pellucidum and Cavum Vergae

During fetal life, there is a single continuous cystic structure in the midline of septum pellucidum. The part anterior to the foramen of Monro is called CSP and the part posterior to it is the cavum vergae. The structure closes from back to front, beginning at 6 months of gestation. At term, no cystic component is seen in the posterior part in 97% of infants, so that there is only a CSP at birth.[9] CSP is present in up to 50–61% of normal neonates. Usually, this disappears by 3–6 months of age; however, sometimes the CSP may persist into adulthood.

Cavum Veli Interpositi

This is a potential space between the choroid in the roof of the third ventricle (below) and the columns of the fornices (above). It appears as an anechoic, inverted, and pyramidal space posteroinferior to the splenium of CC, i.e., in the pineal region. It is not seen after 2 years of age.[10] Differential diagnosis includes arachnoid cyst, however, cavum veli interpositi lacks mass effect.

Frontal Horn Variants (Cysts)

Also known as coarctation of the frontal horns and connatal cysts, these represent cysts oriented exactly parallel to the frontal horns. They are usually bilateral and may show septations between them and the frontal horns.

Choroid Plexus Variants

Normal choroid plexus is seen in the roof of the third ventricle and extends into the lateral ventricles. The frontal and occipital horns have no choroid plexus and echogenic material seen in these sites suggests IVH. Considerable variations in the shape of choroid plexus are seen—lobular or bulbous variants frequently occur within the ventricular atria and lateral ventricles. Small choroid cysts are a common finding and are of no clinical significance.[11]

Hyperechoic White Matter Pseudolesion or Periventricular Halo

These are apparent periventricular echogenic areas that are visualized only in one plane of imaging. These artifacts are due to anisotropic effect. Therefore, a pathologic abnormality on cranial ultrasound should be noted in two planes.[12]

Minor asymmetry in frontal horns or bodies of lateral ventricles and mega cisterna magna are also normal anatomic variants.

INTRACRANIAL HEMORRHAGE

One of the most important roles of cranial ultrasound in infancy is the investigation of intracranial hemorrhage in the newborn. The patterns and etiology of hemorrhage are different in preterm and term neonates.

Hemorrhage in Preterm Neonate

The germinal matrix is the most common site of origin of intracranial hemorrhage in the preterm neonate. It occurs in 20–45% of preterm low birth weight neonates.[13,14] Preterm neonates with a gestational age of <32 weeks have immature autoregulation of their blood pressures. The neonatal brain is at risk due to lack of baroreceptors (that adults have) to keep pressures normal in the brain, despite hypotension or hypertension. Elevations in blood pressure cause dilatation of the neonatal intracranial vessels with the potential rupture of the fragile vessels at the germinal matrix. Hypotension leads to decreased flow into the brain and can result in hemorrhage from hypoxia and reperfusion injury.[15]

The germinal matrix consists of an area of neuronal and glial proliferation with many neuroblasts and a rich array of single cell-thick vessels. It appears at the 7th week of gestation in the subependymal layer of the ventricles. The cells of the germinal matrix migrate towards the periphery (cortex) during fetal brain development. Early in gestation, the germinal matrix lines the entire ventricular system and reaches its greatest size at 23 weeks of gestation **(Fig. 9)**. It starts to involute in the area of the third ventricle followed by involution at the temporal and occipital horns of the lateral ventricles by the end of second trimester. Only a small amount of germinal matrix remains by 28–32 weeks of gestation as a focal area at the caudothalamic groove. Involution of the germinal matrix is complete by 35–36 weeks.[16] The vessels are particularly vulnerable between 25 and 28 weeks of gestation and become less vulnerable as blood flow is shifted toward the cortex by 32–34 weeks. Veins of the germinal matrix are the likely source of hemorrhage.

Papile et al. classified germinal matrix hemorrhage (GMH) into four grades[17] **(Fig. 10)**:

1. *Grade I*: Subependymal hemorrhage (SEH)
2. *Grade II*: Intraventricular extension without hydrocephalus
3. *Grade III*: IVH with hydrocephalus
4. *Grade IV*: IVH with deep intraparenchymal hemorrhage with or without hydrocephalus.

Sonography is the most effective method for detecting this hemorrhage in the newborn period and for follow-up in subsequent weeks. Most hemorrhages (90%) occur in the first 7 days of life, only one-third occur in the first 24 hours. The recommended time for US screening in preterm neonates (<33 weeks) is around 7–10 days to detect GMH and evolving hemorrhage followed by a late scan at 1 month to detect cystic changes of periventricular leukomalacia (PVL) and hydrocephalus.[14]

The choroid plexus in a very premature infant may normally have a lumpy-bumpy appearance with prominent echogenicity; however, this should not be confused with an acute intraventricular clot. Echogenic choroid plexus can be differentiated from hemorrhage. Choroid plexus is not seen in the frontal horns anterior to the foramina of Monro or the occipital horns therefore, echogenic masses seen anterior to the foramina of Monro or in the occipital horns are clots. Doppler evaluation can also help as flow can be seen in the normal vascular choroid plexus and is absent within a hemorrhagic clot.

Grade I

These are small hemorrhages confined to the subependymal or germinal matrix area between the lateral ventricle and

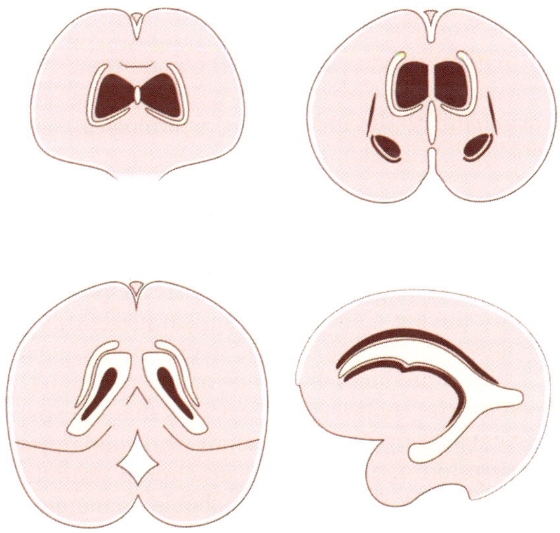

FIG. 9: Illustration shows the location and the extent of the germinal matrix (shaded in dark red).

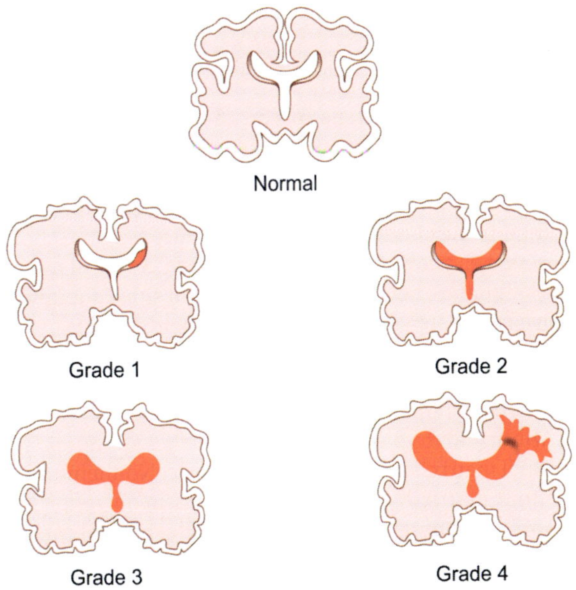

FIG. 10: Illustration demonstrating classification of intraventricular hemorrhage (IVH) by Papile.

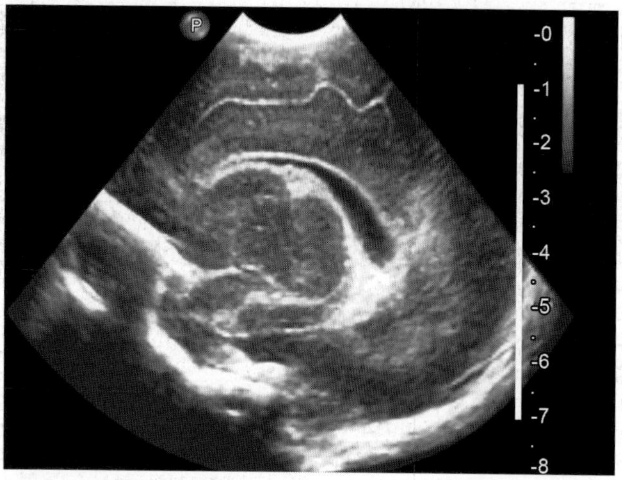

FIG. 11: Sagittal sonogram showing a small hyperechoic area in the caudothalamic groove with no evidence of hydrocephalus consistent with grade I periventricular hemorrhage.

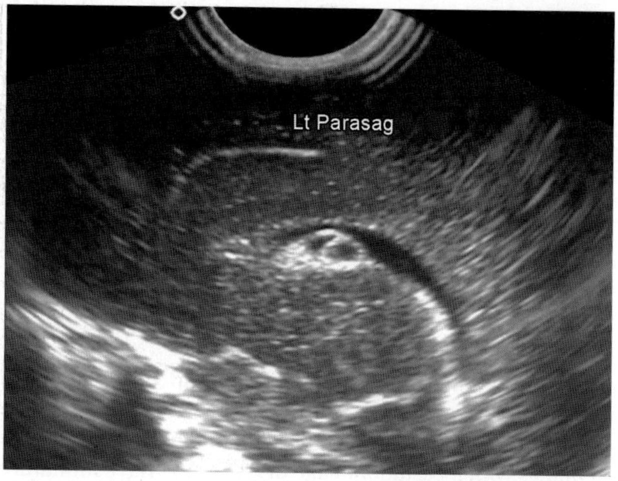

FIG. 12: Sagittal scan (of the same patient as in **Fig. 11**) after a week shows liquefaction of the hematoma with formation of subependymal cysts.

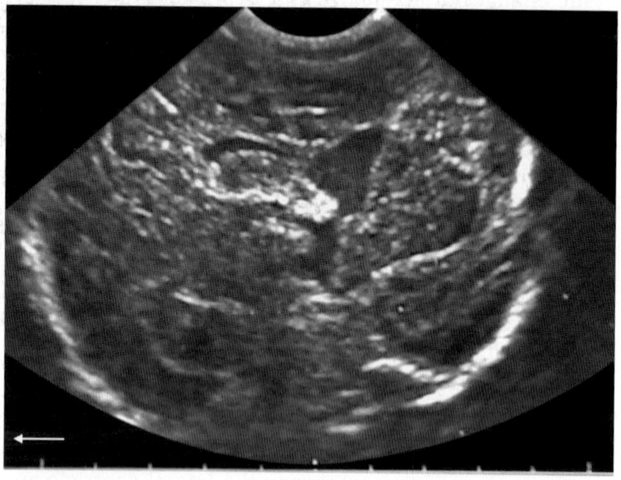

FIG. 13: Intraventricular clot in the left lateral ventricle extending to the third ventricle with mild prominence of the ventricular system, well seen on this coronal scan, suggesting grade II hemorrhage.

head of caudate nucleus or the caudothalamic groove[18] **(Fig. 11)**. They may be unilateral or bilateral. In the acute stage, this appears as a moderately or highly reflective area in the inferolateral wall of the frontal horn superficially resembling the choroid plexus but in a site where the choroid is absent, i.e., anterior to foramen of Monro. As the hematoma ages, it liquefies, becomes sonolucent, and subsequently may resolve completely or persist as a subependymal cyst or as a linear echo[5,6] **(Fig. 12)**. The neurological outcome of these children does not differ significantly from preterm infants with normal cranial ultrasound.

Abnormal hyperechogenicity of the subependymal germinal matrix is not always hemorrhagic. Nonhemorrhagic germinal matrix hyperechogenicity has been reported as an isolated finding or in association with cerebral infection [cytomegalovirus (CMV), rubella], extracerebral infection (especially rotavirus gastroenteritis), etc. The location is the same as with GMH, but the timing, appearance, and evolution are different. Nonhemorrhagic germinal matrix hyperechogenicity is seen primarily in near-term and term neonates, is teardrop shaped, and bilaterally symmetric whereas GMH occurs in premature infants predominantly in the first 2 weeks of life and tends to be round and asymmetric or unilateral. Also, nonhemorrhagic germinal matrix hyperechogenicity persists or evolves by germinolysis into subependymal pseudocysts with gliotic walls lacking hemosiderin whereas GMH liquefies and resolves by resorption, occasionally with hemosiderin-lined subependymal pseudocysts as residua.[19]

Grade II

This is an IVH with minimal or no significant ventriculomegaly at presentation. Before the blood has clotted, it is difficult to visualize in the ventricles, but subsequently it can be seen as hyperechoic material that fills a portion or whole of the ventricular system.[5,6] The clots may just produce an echogenic irregular outline/thickening of the choroid plexus **(Fig. 13)**. Small clots tend to settle in the dependent occipital horns in the supine infant and are difficult to detect through the AF approach. Use of PF or axial views may improve detection of IVH in normal-sized ventricles.[20] If blood extends into the cisterna magna, there is an increased risk of posthemorrhagic hydrocephalus.[14] The incidence of neurological deficits is marginally higher in this group.[21,22]

Grade III

Large IVHs result in significant ventricular dilatation at presentation. Large highly reflective areas fill the ventricular system producing a "cast-like" appearance. A chemical ventriculitis as a response to blood in the cerebrospinal fluid (CSF) typically produces thickening of the ependymal lining of the ventricle. Hydrocephalus occurs due to expansion of the ventricle by the blood along with impairment of CSF resorption at the level of arachnoid granulations **(Figs. 14A and B)**. Hydrocephalus should be monitored by serial ultrasound scans. In most cases, the hydrocephalus may resolve and approximately 34% of very low birth infants require shunting.[14,18] The clinical outcome with varying degrees of permanent neurological impairment is significantly worse in this group.

Grade IV

This consists of simultaneous intraventricular and intraparenchymal cerebral hemorrhage **(Fig. 15)**. It is usually located in the frontal or parietal lobes because it often extends from the germinal matrix. Grade IV IVH was once believed to be due to intraventricular blood, with or without ventricular dilation extending into the brain parenchyma. The definition has evolved since Volpe described the periventricular abnormality as a result of periventricular venous hemorrhagic infarction and stated that it was not from direct extension from the ventricular cavity. CDFI may be used to show initial displacement and gradual encasement and obstruction of the terminal veins by an enlarging GMH. This finding may be useful for early prediction of infants at risk for worsening intracranial hemorrhage.[23,24] The neurological sequelae in this group are usually severe and tend to be developmental delay and poor tone as opposed to spastic diplegia or quadriplegia in patient with ischemia in the same region.

Cerebellar hemorrhage can be seen in preterm infants, especially with birth weight <750 g. Hemorrhage is seen in germinal zones that exist within the external granule cell layer of the cerebellar hemispheres and in the subependymal layer of the fourth ventricle. Acute cerebellar hemorrhage appears (with clot development) homogeneously echogenic and with time, the clot becomes heterogeneous and eventually hypoechoic. Cerebellar hemorrhage can be detected with the MF views.

Subarachnoid hemorrhage may also occur in preterm newborns and is usually difficult to identify on ultrasound due to normal variation in the appearance of subarachnoid cisterns. It may be seen as widening of sylvian fissures with increased reflectivity.

Hemorrhage in Term Neonate

Hemorrhage in the term neonate may occur due to birth trauma and subdural hemorrhage (SDH) is the most commonly encountered lesion due to falcine or tentorial laceration while extradural hemorrhage is uncommon. Acute SDH appears as a highly reflective linear or elliptical collection that compresses the brain parenchyma. Transcranial scanning may be useful to demonstrate this lesion. Cerebellar hemorrhage is a reported complication of traumatic delivery in full-term neonates, in ECMO, or with coagulopathy. Posterior fossa hemorrhages are more difficult to demonstrate by the AF approach and the MF scanning is now routinely used. Subarachnoid hemorrhage may occur in neonates who have experienced asphyxia or trauma and may be the only

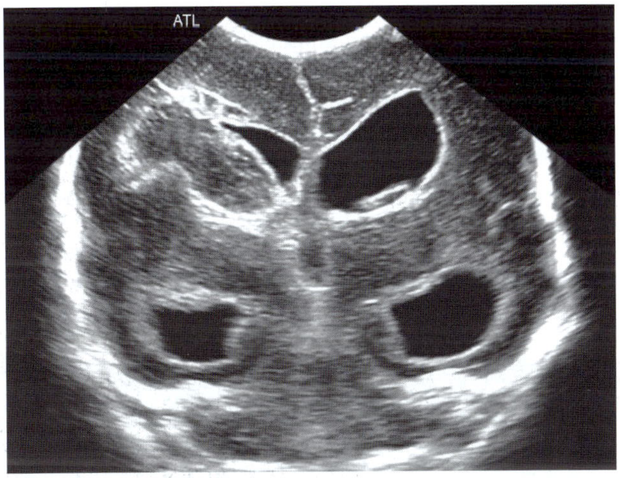

FIG. 15: Coronal sonogram showing marked dilatation of both lateral ventricles with intraventricular hemorrhage (IVH) and deep parenchymal hemorrhage (grade IV) on the left side and IVH (grade III) on the right side. The ependymal appears echogenic due to chemical ventriculitis.

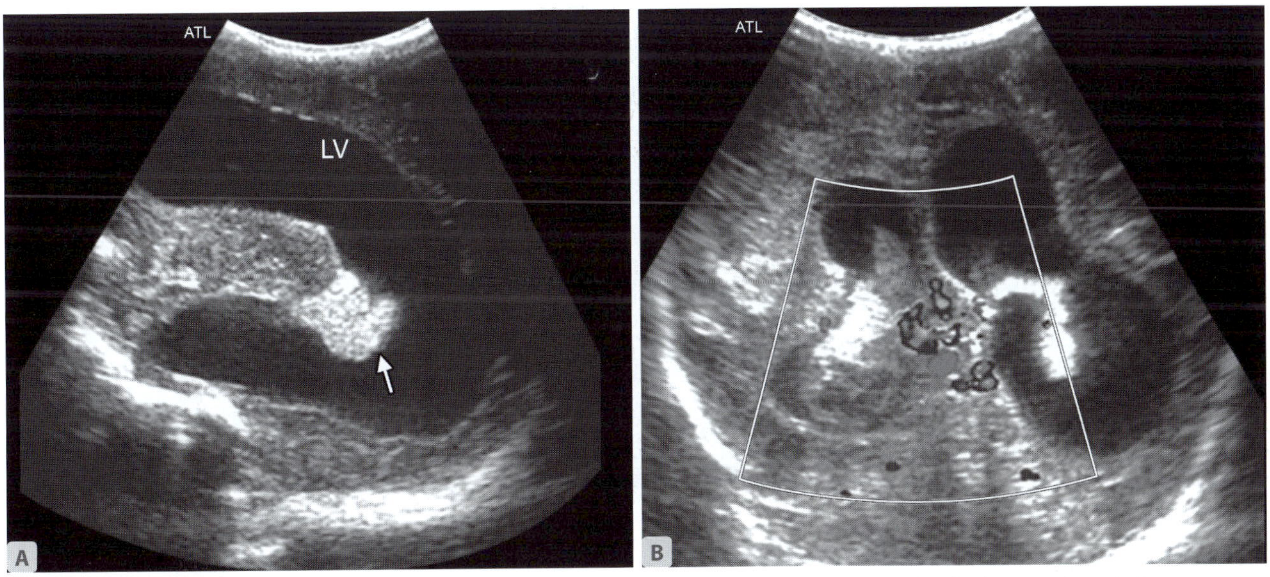

FIGS. 14A AND B: Sagittal and coronal sonograms showing grossly dilated lateral ventricles with enlarged and echogenic choroid plexus appearing avascular on color Doppler flow imaging (CDFI) consistent with hemorrhage.

hemorrhage in full-term neonates not at risk for GMH.[5,6] IVH has also been reported in term neonates probably arising from the choroid plexus or germinal matrix.[14,25,26]

HYPOXIC-ISCHEMIC INJURY

The pattern of brain injury may differ in preterm neonates and term neonates according to the severity and duration of hypoxia and degree of brain maturation however, some overlapping features may exist.

Hypoxic-ischemic Injury in Preterm Neonates

The hallmark of hypoxic-ischemic injury in preterm neonates is periventricular leukomalacia. It results from a relatively insidious cerebral parenchymal insult. The word "leukomalacia" is derived from "leukos" meaning white and "malacia" means softening. PVL is the leading cause of nonhemorrhagic neuropathological abnormality in the cerebral white matter of a premature neonate. PVL is more common in premature neonates than in term neonates and its incidence increases with decreasing gestational age. PVL most commonly occurs at 24–32 gestational weeks and in those with birth weight <1,500 g.[27]

The periventricular white matter (supplied by ventriculopetal penetrating arteries) is most vulnerable to hypoxic-ischemic injury in preterm neonates with immature brain. Mild-to-moderate hypoxic-ischemic injury results in PVL, which may be focal (seen adjacent to frontal horns and trigones) or diffuse. Progressive necrosis leads to loss of periventricular white matter, passive ventriculomegaly (irregular margins of the bodies and trigones of lateral ventricles), and thinning of CC. Cavitation and cyst formation are seen in end-stage PVL **(Figs. 16A to E)**. Periventricular cysts are usually ≤2–3 mm and larger cysts carry poorer prognosis.[28] Thalami, brainstem, and cerebellum in the immature brain have high metabolic activity and hence are more susceptible to injury in severe hypoxic-ischemic injury **(Figs. 17A to C)**.

Sonographic Grading of Periventricular Leukomalacia

Four grades of PVL were described by de Vries.[29,30]

1. *Grade 1 PVL* usually presents as an increase in echogenicity in the periventricular region, mainly around the trigone, lasting <7 days. These early sonographic findings are described as a periventricular flare. Interpretation may be difficult in the extremely premature neonate, in whom periventricular parenchyma is often echogenic.
2. *Grade 2 PVL* presents as persistent periventricular hyperechogenicity which lasts for >7 days.
3. *Grade 3 PVL* presents with relatively advanced parenchymal changes leading to microcyst formation. These changes

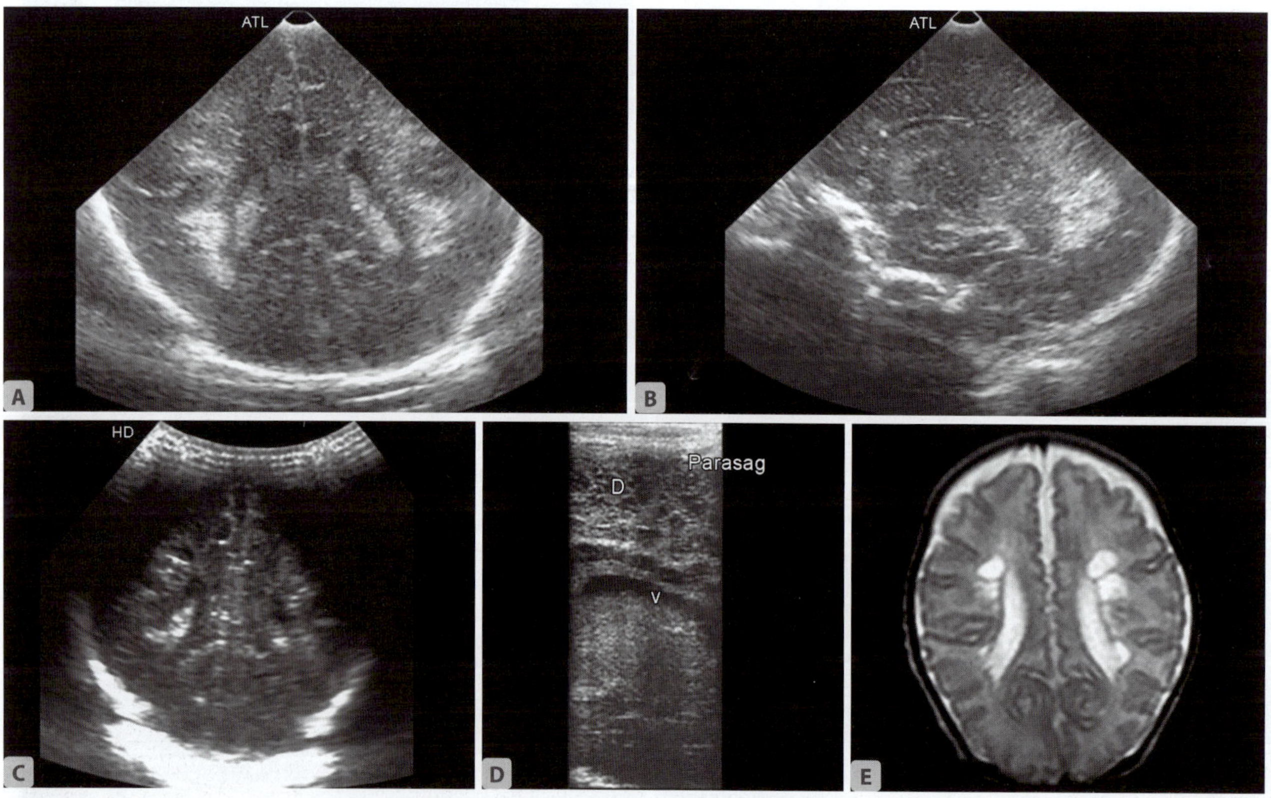

FIGS. 16A TO E: Serial cranial sonograms in a preterm neonate with birth asphyxia reveal periventricular areas of increased echogenicity most marked in the peritrigonal region on the initial coronal (A) and sagittal (B) scans; (C and D) Subsequent coronal and high-resolution sagittal scans reveal partial resolution of the abnormal echogenicity with development of multiple small periventricular cysts; and (E) Axial T2W MR image of the same child depicts the multiple periventricular cysts—consistent with cystic PVL. (PVL: periventricular leukomalacia; T2W:T2-weighted; MR: magnetic resonance)

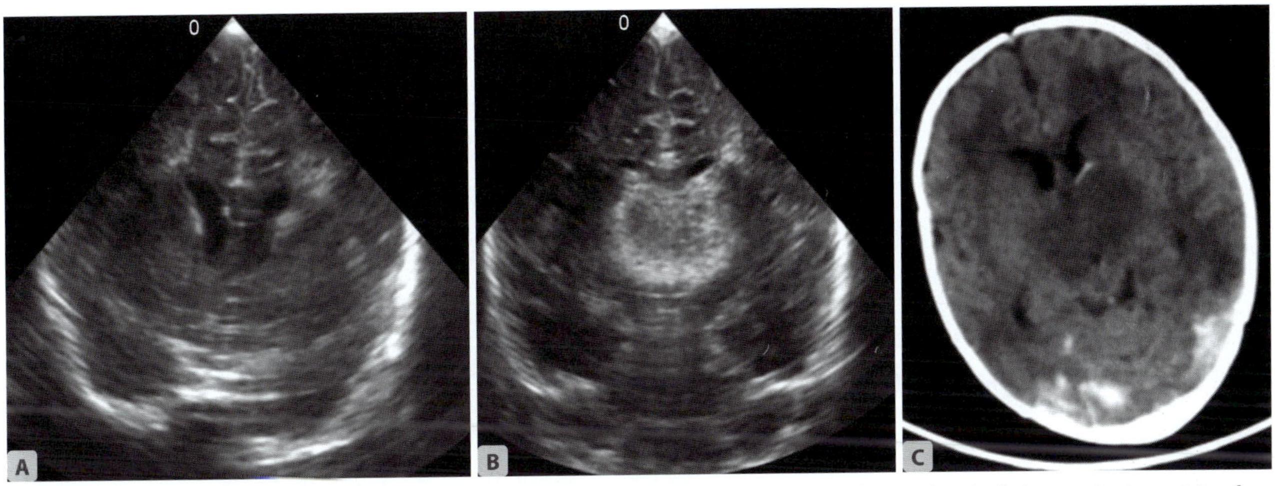

FIGS. 17A TO C: (A and B) Coronal sonograms showing abnormal bilateral periventricular echogenicity and markedly increased echogenicity of the thalami in a neonate with severe asphyxia; and (C) The axial CT section of the same shows both the thalami to be hypodense due to hypoxic injury. Note the presence of posterior fossa hemorrhages as well [not seen in ultrasound (US) scan through anterior fontanel].

are more evident in the parietal region and also extend to the frontal areas.

4. *Grade 4 PVL* presents with multiple coalescing cystic areas in the cerebral parenchyma. Grade 4 changes represent advanced cystic changes that reach up to the level of cortex.

Grades 3 and 4 changes are often associated with neurological sequelae such as diplegia and paraplegia in later life in up to 50% of patients.

Hypoxic-ischemic Injury in Term Neonates

Mild-to-moderate hypoxic-ischemic injury in term neonates causes parasagittal watershed zone infarcts between anterior/middle cerebral arteries and middle/posterior cerebral arteries. Involvement of the cortex and underlying subcortical white matter is seen. Severe hypoxic-ischemic injury results in injury to metabolically active tissues such as ventrolateral thalami, posterior putamina, hippocampi, brainstem, corticospinal tracts, and sensorimotor cortex **(Fig. 18)**. Basal ganglia injury is more common than parasagittal pattern and carries the worst prognosis. Severe global hypoxia may also lead to diffuse cerebral edema. Chronic HIE may reveal cortical atrophy and thinning (ulegyria) and multicystic encephalomalacia[28] **(Figs. 19A to C)**.

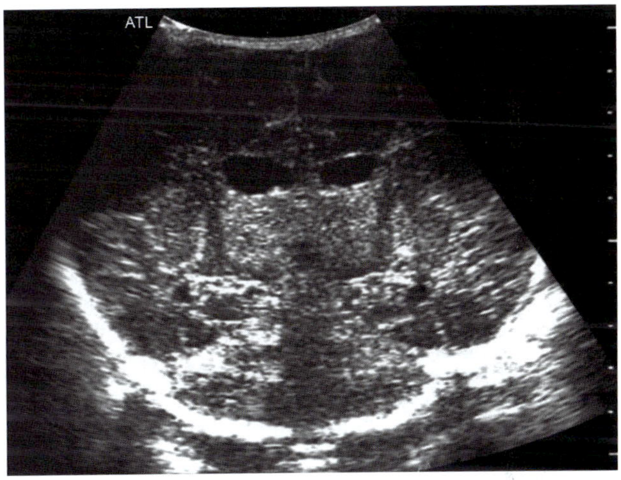

FIG. 18: Coronal sonogram showing increased echogenicity of bilateral thalami and basal ganglia in a term neonate with severe birth asphyxia.

Diffuse cerebral edema is a common result of hypoxic-ischemic events in full-term neonates. Initially, the brain edema causes slit-like ventricles with a diffusely echogenic brain. This echogenicity may cause silhouetting of the sulci, so that the sulci seem to disappear. The brain develops a diffusely reflective and featureless appearance due to a combination of edema and ischemic damage. Doppler evaluation of severely asphyxiated infants has demonstrated earlier and at times more focal abnormalities than on grayscale imaging alone. Doppler studies may be helpful, showing low resistance indices (<0.6) in the anterior and middle cerebral artery complexes with increased diastolic flow in the first 48 hours of asphyxia insult. This correlates with adverse neurological outcome. As cerebral edema worsens, cerebrovascular resistance increases resulting in dampening of diastolic blood flow velocities. The patterns of hypoxic-ischemic injury in premature and mature neonate are enlisted in **Table 2**.

HYDROCEPHALUS

Hydrocephalus is an excessive accumulation of CSF in the ventricular system, subarachnoid spaces overlying the brain, or a combination of both. It results when there is an imbalance between its production and absorption or an obstruction to the free flow of CSF.[31] Hydrocephalus may be considered to be communicating, i.e., extraventricular obstruction to CSF flow or noncommunicating, i.e., intraventricular obstruction to CSF flow, up to the level of the outlet foramina of the fourth ventricle. Common causes of extraventricular obstruction include hemorrhage and infection and causes of intraventricular obstruction include infection, hemorrhage, congenital anomalies [aqueductal stenosis, Dandy–Walker

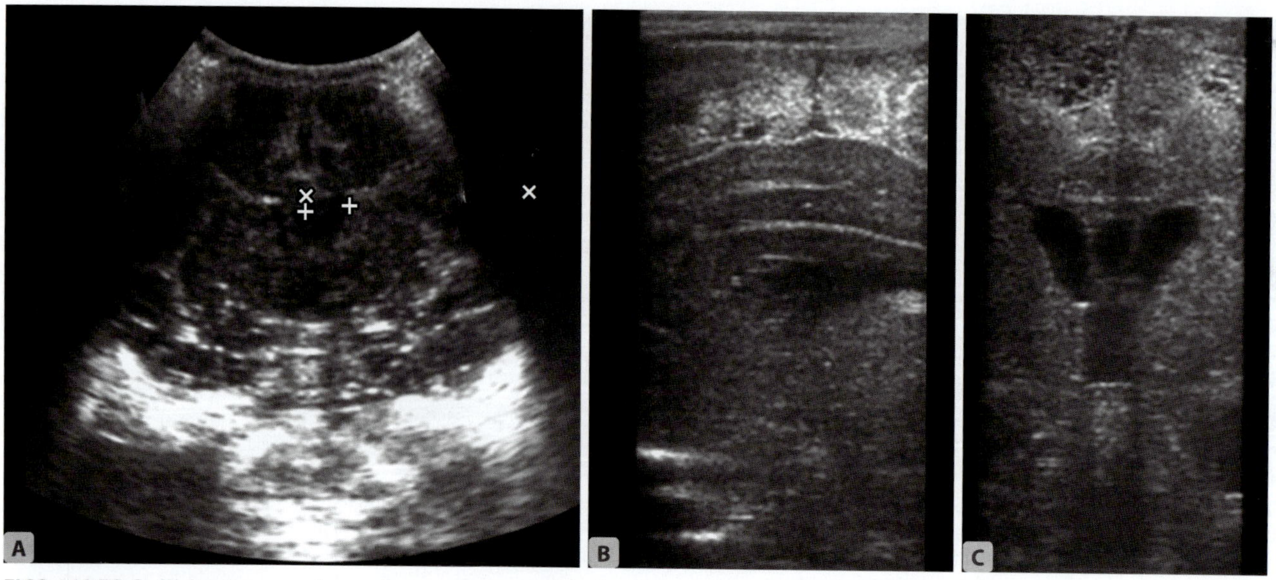

FIGS. 19A TO C: (A) Routine coronal scan of a term neonate with birth asphyxia appears unremarkable; (B) However, subsequent high-resolution sagittal scan shows marked increase in cortical and subcortical echogenicity; and (C) A coronal high-resolution scan at a later date demonstrates multiple subcortical cysts.

TABLE 2: Patterns of hypoxic-ischemic injury in premature and mature neonates.

Patterns of hypoxic-ischemic brain injury		
	Moderate	**Severe**
Premature neonate	Periventricular leukomalacia	Thalamic, basal ganglia, and brainstem
Term neonate	Parasagittal white matter in cerebral cortex	Thalamic, basal ganglia, brainstem, and perirolandic white matter

malformation (DWM)], and tumors. Rarely, excessive production of CSF may result in hydrocephalus as may be seen with choroid plexus papillomas.

Detection of Hydrocephalus and Ultrasound Measurement of Lateral Ventricles

Sonography is the preferred modality for the initial evaluation of an infant with suspected hydrocephalus. Often, hydrocephalus can be diagnosed in utero by 15 weeks of gestation. The size of the atrium and glomus remain constant in second and third trimesters. In utero, an upper limit of 10 mm for the ventricular atrium has been established.

On neonatal sonography, the ventricular system is well-defined with separation of the walls in preterm infants whereas in the full-term and older infant, the ventricles are less distended and ventricular walls are often apposed. The frequently used measurements include **(Figs. 20A and B)**:

- *Ventricular index (VI) (Levene index)*: This is the distance between the falx cerebri and the lateral wall of the lateral ventricles which is measured at the level of foramen of Monro in midcoronal plane. There is a reference range with each gestational age and it is considered normal if less than 97th centile, moderate if more than 97th centile, and severe if more than 97th centile + 4 mm.[3]
- *Anterior horn width (AHW)*: This is the diagonal width of frontal horns of the lateral ventricles which is measured in the same plane as the VI. It is more sensitive to mild ventricular dilatation. It is normal if <3 mm, mild ventriculomegaly is present if AHW is 3–5 mm, moderate ventriculomegaly if 6–10 mm, and severe ventriculomegaly if it is >10 mm.[3]
- *Thalamo-occipital distance*: This is the distance from the thalamus to the tip of the occipital horn and is measured in sagittal plane. This is important as mild lateral ventricular dilatation manifests first in the occipital horns.

Qualitative assessment of ventricular size is often used in practice. The most useful signs are progressive rounding and bulging of the superolateral angles of the frontal horns and dilatation of occipital horns.[32]

Frontal horn ratio, which is the ratio of the distance between the falx and the lateral wall of the frontal horn and the hemispheric width (measured in the third coronal plane), can also be used for detection of ventricular dilatation[32] **(Fig. 21)**.

Level of Obstruction

Sonography is also useful in determining the level of obstruction. Evaluation of the entire ventricular system should be done, so that the level at which there is a transition from a large to small ventricle can be identified. Dilatation of the lateral and third ventricles indicates an obstruction at the aqueductal level, most often secondary to IVH or infection or sometimes congenital, often an X-linked recessive trait. Regional flow imaging with color Doppler has been investigated as a method to exclude obstructive hydrocephalus. Free passage of CSF through the ventricles and out into the basal cisterns confirms the diagnosis of communicating hydrocephalus.

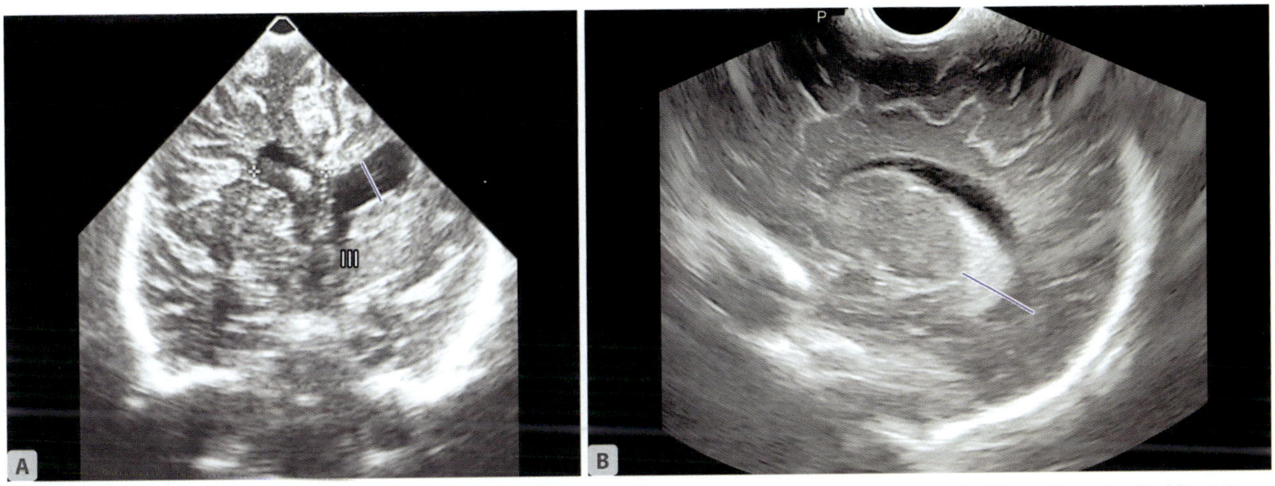

FIGS. 20A AND B: (A) Coronal scan depicting that the ventricular index is measured as the distance between the falx and lateral wall of frontal horn in a coronal plane (between the calipers in white), anterior horn width is measured as the distance between the medial wall and floor of lateral ventricle at the widest point (blue line); and (B) Sagittal scan depicts the measurement of thalamo-occipital distance (blue line).

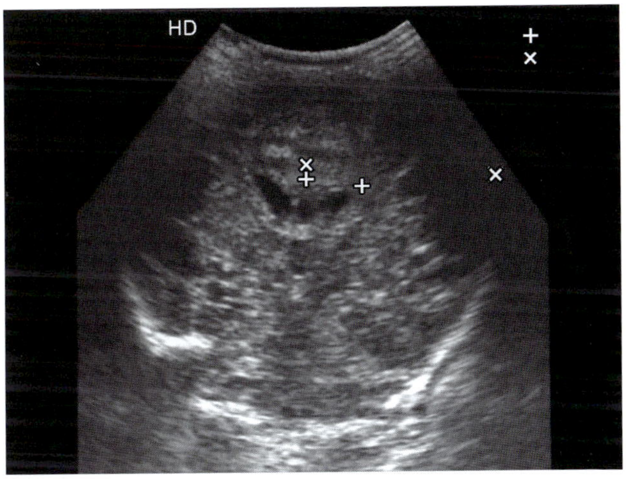

FIG. 21: Coronal section at the level of foramen of Monro depicting measurement of frontal horn ratio.

Doppler Imaging

Color Doppler flow imaging techniques may be helpful in evaluating CSF flow dynamics in infants with hydrocephalus. Microbubbles that are produced from CSF jets act as transient but efficient reflectors for ultrasound, enabling visualization of CSF flow. CSF flow produces a highly characteristic sinusoidal spectral Doppler waveform, indicative of cyclical to and fro motion of CSF within the ventricular system.[6] Examination of the ventricular system during cranial and abdominal compression may induce movement of CSF detectable with color flow or Doppler scanning.[33]

The effect of hydrocephalus on cerebral circulation can be evaluated and the RI correlated linearly with the intracranial pressure (ICP) in hydrocephalus, which is more important than the anatomic assessment of ventricular size alone. As the ICP rises, arterial flow tends to be more affected during diastole than during systole resulting in an increased pulsatility of flow. Increasing RI correlates well with elevation in ICP **(Figs. 22A and B)**. The RI decreases after ventriculoperitoneal shunting or tapping.[34,35] Doppler examination of the anterior or middle cerebral artery during fontanel compression may be useful in the early identification of infants with abnormal intracranial compliance prior to the development of increased ICP as shown by elevated baseline RI.[36] Increased pulsatility index (PI), decreased end-diastolic velocity, and slight decrease of systolic velocity have been noted, the parameters return to normal after drainage procedure. A strong correlation has been found between PI and size of cerebral ventricles. The ACA and MCA have the highest predisposition to early reaction to change of intracranial dynamics. The ACA lies close to the lateral and third ventricles and is, therefore, affected to a greater extent with ventricular dilatation.[37] In normal infants, CSF or blood flow can be readily displaced compensating for the small increase in volume caused by compression of AF resulting in no increase in ICP. In infants with hydrocephalus, however, this maneuver results in transient increased ICP and an acute increase in arterial pulsatility. **Table 3** enlists the reference values for RI and PI for cranial Doppler.[38]

Follow-up with Ultrasonography

Sonography is ideal for following ventricular size in infants who are on treatment for hydrocephalus, displaying the position of the shunt tube, and size of the ventricles. Following successful shunting, a fall in the arterial RI has also been demonstrated.

Benign Enlargement of Subarachnoid Space in Infancy

Another important type of hydrocephalus in infancy is the so-called benign communicating hydrocephalus which has also been described as benign external hydrocephalus of infancy or chronic subdural hygromas of infancy. It is characterized by an enlargement of the subarachnoid spaces >5 mm overlying the cerebral hemispheres, particularly over the frontal and temporal convexities. There is associated mild or moderate ventricular dilatation. The condition usually

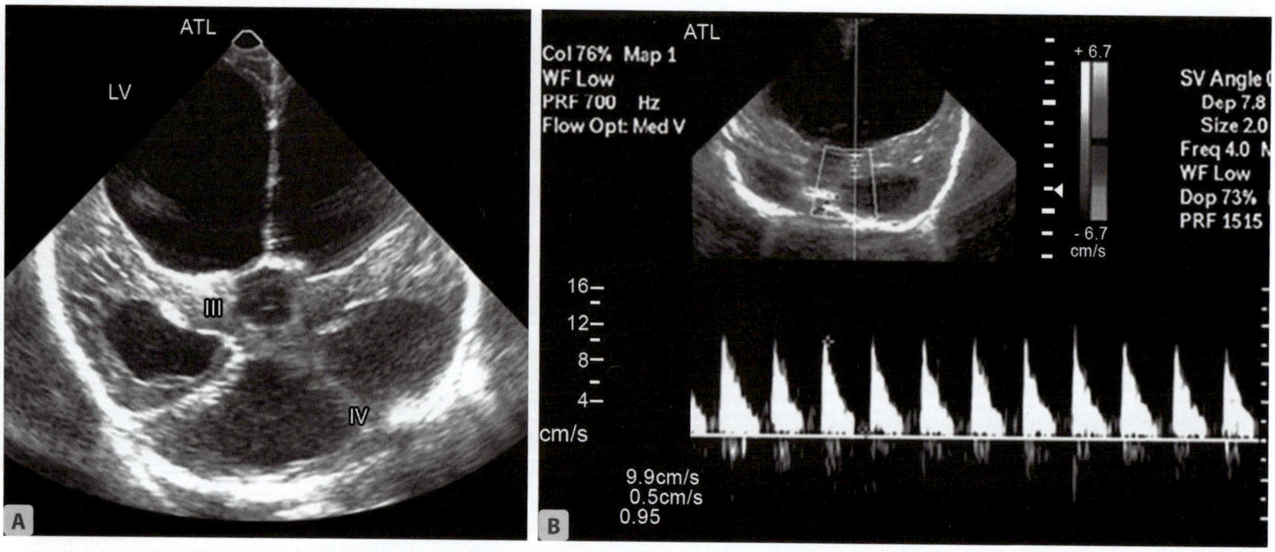

FIGS. 22A AND B: (A) Coronal sonogram showing generalized dilatation of the ventricular system; and (B) Color Doppler flow imaging of the same patient showing markedly elevated RI in the MCA suggestive of increased intracranial pressure. (MCA: middle cerebral artery; RI: resistive index)

TABLE 3: Reference values for resistive index (RI) and pulsatility index (PI) for cranial Doppler.

Parameters	Values

RI	• Normal: 0.6–0.85
	• Low <0.6 (low resistance, increased cerebral blood flow)
	• High >0.85 (high resistance, decreased cerebral blood flow)
	• In hydrocephalus indication for treatment:
	  ○ RI >0.7 without pressure by transducer
	  ○ RI >0.9 with pressure by transducer (inward pressure applied on anterior fontanel for 5 s and blood flow velocities are measured)

PI	Normal: 0.5–1.05

presents in the 1st year of life, the infant presenting with a large head. It is generally a self-limiting process that resolves without treatment by 2 years of age. The etiology is probably transient immaturity of the arachnoid granulations or villi.[39] In the past, excess fluid overlying the hemispheres has been misconstrued as being subdural hygromas of indeterminate etiology. However, both ultrasound and magnetic resonance imaging (MRI) can demonstrate that the excess fluid is actually in the subarachnoid space dipping into the sulci. This condition is also termed as benign enlargement of subarachnoid space (BESS) syndrome. Follow-up imaging is not required, but serial head circumference measurements should be obtained. The condition is not entirely benign, as it predisposes to extra-axial hemorrhage after minor head trauma and transient minor developmental delay occurs in a minority of cases during the period of most rapid head growth at 5–12 months of age.

The differential diagnosis of benign enlargement of the extra-axial fluid spaces includes cerebral atrophy (widened sulci, small or normal head circumference, proportionate ventricular enlargement), subdural collections (arachnoid neomembranes, echogenic fluid, displacement of bridging cortical veins within the subarachnoid space away from skull toward the brain), meningitis (thickened leptomeninges, echogenic fluid), and communicating hydrocephalus (larger ventricles).

Doppler imaging is useful in differentiating between BESS syndrome and subdural collections as superficial bridging cortical veins can be seen traversing the enlarged subarachnoid space differentiating it from a subdural collection.[40]

CONGENITAL BRAIN ANOMALIES

These may occur at any stage of brain development. Sonography may be the first modality used for an infant with a congenital brain malformation. Many anomalies can be diagnosed while in others it is useful in directing the patient to MR imaging which is the current standard of reference. The various congenital brain anomalies can be classified as:

- Disorders of organogenesis
- Disorders of diverticulation
- Disorders of sulcation and migration
- Disorders of histogenesis

Disorders of Organogenesis

Disorders of Neural Tube Closure

The first stage in brain development is neural tube closure in the 1st month of gestation, failure of which caudally causes myelomeningocele and cranially causes anencephaly or encephalocele. A myelomeningocele is very often associated with a Chiari II malformation. Aqueductal stenosis may also develop during neural tube closure in the first trimester. It often causes obstructive hydrocephalus and may lead to severe brain damage. Infants born with a myelomeningocele require a cranial examination to establish the baseline status of the ventricular system, which frequently enlarges following primary repair of the spinal lesion, due to change in CSF dynamics.

Chiari II Malformation

Sagittal sonograms demonstrate a small posterior fossa resulting in displacement of the cerebellar vermis, fourth ventricle, and medulla into the cervical canal with a medullary kink. The fourth ventricle is often poorly visualized as it is thin, elongated, compressed, and displaced into the upper spinal canal.

The degree of ventricular dilatation is variable at presentation but is usually progressive. The occipital horns and atria are disproportionately dilated compared to the frontal and temporal horns (colpocephaly). On coronal images, there is anterior and inferior pointing of the frontal horns referred to as "batwing configuration". The septum pellucidum may be partially or completely absent. The massa intermedia is enlarged and fills a dilated third ventricle. The interhemispheric fissure is often prominent in these patients. Sonography has been a reliable method for follow-up of shunting procedures and evaluation of hydrocephalus in the 1st year of life,[5] although abnormalities of the Chiari malformation are best appreciated on MRI.

Agenesis of the Corpus Callosum

Corpus callosum forms during the first 8–12 weeks of gestation. Depending on the timing of intrauterine insult, the development can be partially arrested or complete agenesis may occur and is frequently associated with major malformations. The bundles of Probst that failed to fuse persist as rounded masses on each side of the midline. The key sonographic findings are widely spaced lateral ventricles which are tiny anteriorly and enlarged posteriorly. The frontal horns are slit like, widely separated with concave medial margins, and superolateral peaks. The third ventricle is dilated and high placed and often associated with a dorsal cyst **(Fig. 23)**. On midline sagittal images, the sulci are arranged radially above the third ventricle.[5,6] It is difficult to diagnose partial agenesis on sonography.

Dandy-Walker Malformation

The imaging features include hypoplasia (or, rarely, agenesis) of the cerebellar vermis, which is elevated and upwardly rotated and dilatation of the cystic-appearing fourth ventricle, which may fill the entire posterior fossa. Both findings are present and are necessary for the diagnosis. The cystic structure within the posterior fossa is not the posterior fossa subarachnoid space or an arachnoid cyst; it represents the cyst-like dilatation of the fourth ventricle secondary to hypoplasia of the inferior cerebellar vermis. The cerebellar hemispheres are displaced anterolaterally. The posterior fossa is enlarged and elevation of the tentorium, torcular herophili, and transverse sinuses is seen. Additional malformations that may be associated with DWM include dysgenesis or agenesis of the CC, occipital encephalocele, polymicrogyria, and heterotopia (in 30–50% of individuals). Hydrocephalus is associated with DWM in about 90% of

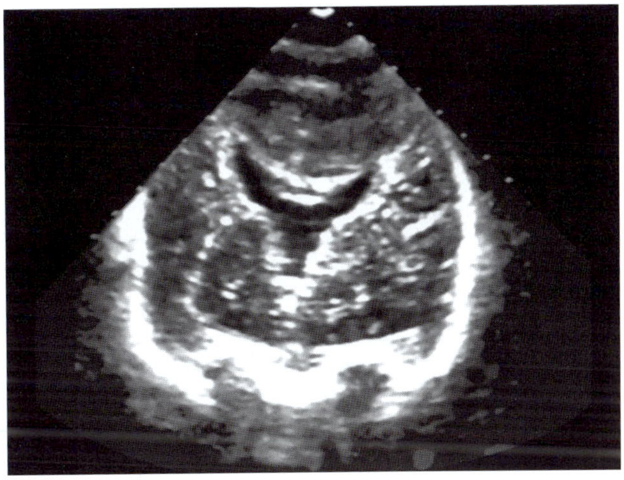

FIG. 23: Coronal sonogram showing frontal horns with concave medial borders and sharply angled lateral peaks. The third ventricle is also mildly dilated and slightly high placed, consistent with agenesis of corpus callosum.

patients **(Figs. 24A and B)**. Terms such as "Dandy-Walker variant", "Dandy-Walker complex", or "Dandy-Walker spectrum" have been used to classify malformations that do not meet the criteria for DWM however, these terms lack specificity and more detailed anatomic descriptors (e.g., inferior cerebellar vermis or global cerebellar hypoplasia) are preferred to be used.[41]

Disorders of Diverticulation

The second stage of brain development during the second month of gestation is diverticulation into two hemispheres, development of the pineal and pituitary glands as well as optic and olfactory tracts. Malformations include the spectrum from simple absence of the septum pellucidum to alobar holoprosencephaly. Since the face is formed at the same time, severe midline facial abnormalities are often present.[42]

Holoprosencephaly

A failure of midline cleavage of the prosencephalon causes failure of formation of separate cerebral hemispheres.

The most severe form of holoprosencephaly is alobar holoprosencephaly. On sonography, there is a single horseshoe or crescent-shaped monoventricle, which communicates with a large dorsal cyst. The thalami are fused and the third ventricle is absent, as are the CC and interhemispheric fissure. The cortex is thin with sparse convolutional markings and a smooth appearance to the brain surface. The cerebellum and brainstem are often spared. If Doppler is applied, absence of anterior cerebral arteries or occurrence of only a single vessel may be noted. There is absence of internal cerebral veins, the superior sagittal sinus, and straight sinus.[43]

Semilobar holoprosencephaly is the less severe variant. The single ventricle persists, but there may be separate occipital and temporal horns. Portions of the septum pellucidum and CC may be present posteriorly. The thalami are partially fused along the floor of the malformed third ventricle.

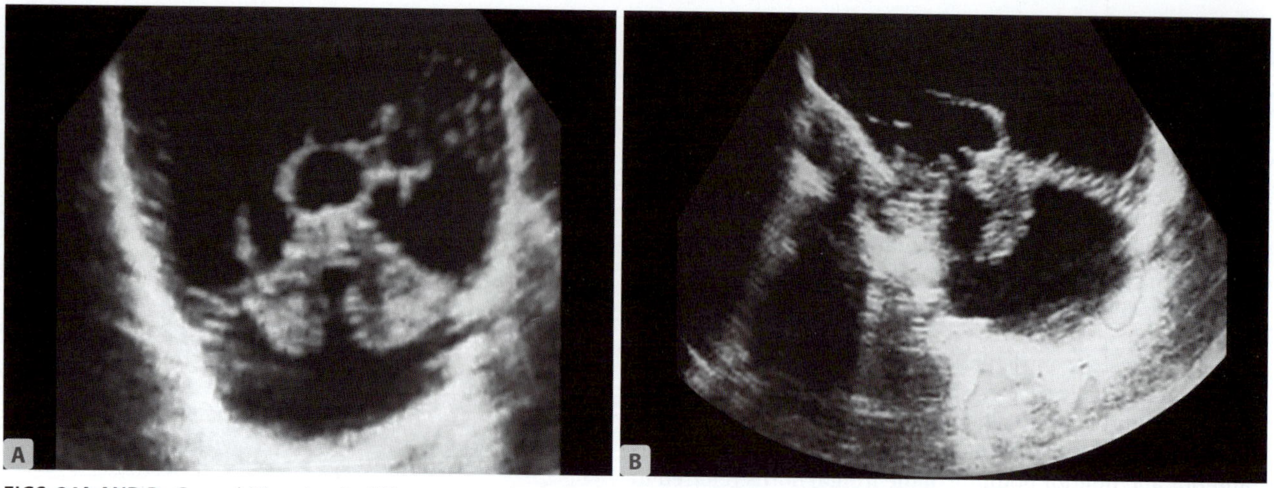

FIGS. 24A AND B: Coronal (A) and sagittal (B) sonograms showing a large posterior fossa cyst communicating with the fourth ventricle with hypoplastic vermis and cerebellar hemispheres which are displaced anterolaterally. Marked generalized hydrocephalus is present—findings consistent with Dandy–Walker malformation.

Lobar holoprosencephaly is the least severe form. There is nearly complete separation of the hemispheres with development of the falx and interhemispheric fissure, but the anteroinferior portion is incomplete and the frontal lobes are fused. The septum pellucidum is absent. The anterior horns of the lateral ventricles are fused and square-shaped, but occipital horns are separated. The third ventricle is usually present, separating the thalami and the splenium and body of CC are often present with absence of the genu and rostrum.

Pellucidal Agenesis and Dysgenesis

Absence of septum pellucidum is often associated with other malformations such as holoprosencephaly, septo-optic dysplasia, callosal agenesis, Chiari II malformation, etc. Secondary destruction is more common than primary agenesis and may occur following trauma, inflammation, or ventricular obstruction **(Fig. 25)**.[44]

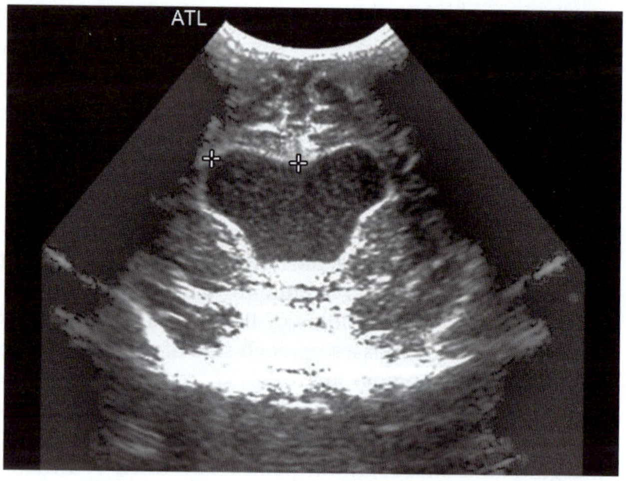

FIG. 25: Coronal sonogram showing hydrocephalus with low-level echoes within the ventricular system due to ventriculitis. Note the absence of septum pellucidum due to secondary destruction.

Disorders of Sulcation and Migration

These occur during the 3rd to 6th months of gestation and result when the neuronal cells fail to migrate to the cortex such that the cortex becomes too thick and/or too smooth or heterotopic nodules of gray matter are left in unusual places. Neuronal migration anomalies are best evaluated with MR imaging.

Schizencephaly

Schizencephaly is a developmental defect resulting in a brain cleft lined by gray matter, which is an asymmetric process resulting in a single or bilateral cleft extending from the surface of the brain to the ventricular system. The asymmetry suggests that in some patients, schizencephaly may represent an early insult during brain development. The lesions have been divided into two groups based on fused or separated lips of the clefts. Type I represents the closed lip schizencephaly and type II represents the open lip schizencephaly. The open-lipped type may be easily diagnosed by ultrasound where an echo-free cavity extends from the surface of the brain to fuse with the lateral wall of the lateral ventricle.[6] Type I schizencephaly may not be well seen with ultrasonography (USG).

Lissencephaly

In lissencephaly, the cerebral sulci and gyri fail to develop fully with a thick smooth four cell-layered cortex resembling an hourglass in the coronal plane. In type I lissencephaly, microcephaly, facial dysmorphism, and severe mental retardation are the rule. On ultrasound, the cerebral cortex resembles that of a 24-week fetus with no cerebral sulci, nearly absent operculization of the insula giving a figure of 8 appearance. Type II lissencephaly typically presents with macrocephaly, secondary to obstructive hydrocephalus. Ultrasound may help to identify the agyric cortex despite severe ventricular dilatation which may be difficult to identify on CT scanning.[6]

Disorders of Histogenesis

These may result in tumors, arteriovenous malformations, or cysts, but they are uncommon in infancy.

Tuberous Sclerosis

Central nervous system manifestations of tuberous sclerosis include hamartomas of the periphery of the brain parenchyma and benign subependymal tubers. Subependymal nodules are seen on sonography as small focal highly reflective nodules in the wall of the lateral ventricle. Echogenic lesions in the brain parenchyma represent peripheral hamartomas.[44]

Sturge–Weber Syndrome

Serpiginous echodensities due to leptomeningeal angiomatosis may be identified in the brain periphery associated with decreased cortical volume of the involved hemisphere, i.e., cortical hemiatrophy. Usually, the choroid plexus is enlarged due to the presence of angiomas within the structure.

Vascular Malformations

The most common intracranial vascular malformation presenting in the neonatal period is the vein of Galen malformation. Sonographic hallmark of the lesion is a midline echo-free or mixed echogenicity, pulsatile mass that blooms with color when Doppler modalities are applied. CDFI may be helpful in distinguishing the two most common types.[45] The choroidal type is characterized by multiple abnormal feeding vessels arising in the midbrain with venous drainage via the aneurysmally dilated vein of Galen and straight sinus. The infundibular type consists of an arteriovenous fistula with one or few arterial feeders draining directly into the vein of Galen.

Spectral Doppler imaging typically shows arterialization of venous flow and increased flow velocities with reduced pulsatility of arterial feeders. Whether embolization or surgery is planned, intraprocedural neurosonography is useful in evaluating completeness of therapy. After treatment, patients are generally monitored with Doppler sonography.[44]

DESTRUCTIVE BRAIN LESIONS

Porencephalic Cyst

A porencephalic cyst is an area of normally developed brain that has been damaged and heals with a lining of gliotic white matter. The resultant lesion usually communicates with the ventricles. On sonography, an anechoic cavity communicating with the ventricular system is seen. The term should ideally be restricted to true in utero causes of cystic brain damage[6] **(Fig. 26)**.

Focal or diffuse brain damage in neonates can result in areas of cystic encephalomalacia. These typically do not communicate with the ventricular system **(Fig. 27)**.[5,6]

Hydranencephaly

Occlusion of the supraclinoid internal carotid arteries between the 12th and 26th weeks of gestation results in destruction of the formed cerebral hemispheres. A fluid-filled membranous sac fills the calvarium but the falx is present, differentiating this condition from holoprosencephaly. Variable amounts of frontal and occipital lobes may be preserved. The thalami, basal ganglia, midbrain, and posterior fossa contents are essentially normal. On CDFI, flow in the internal carotid arteries is absent.[5,6] It can be difficult to differentiate hydranencephaly from severe hydrocephalus, but a thin rim of cortex should be visualized by sonography in hydrocephalus.[46-48] Macrocephaly is usual although the head may be normal or even small in size.

INTRACRANIAL INFECTION

Both prenatal and postnatal infections are a significant cause of morbidity and mortality in infants. Diagnosis is almost always suspected on clinical grounds, the role of imaging being to support the clinical diagnosis and reveal complications of infection.

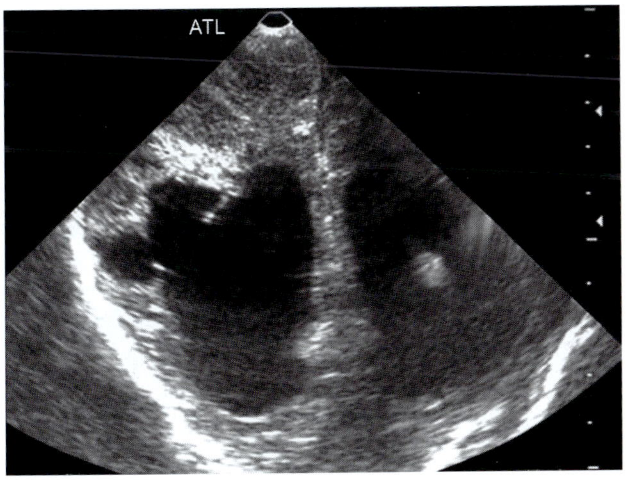

FIG. 26: Coronal sonogram showing dilated lateral ventricles with a porencephalic cyst communicating with the left lateral ventricle.

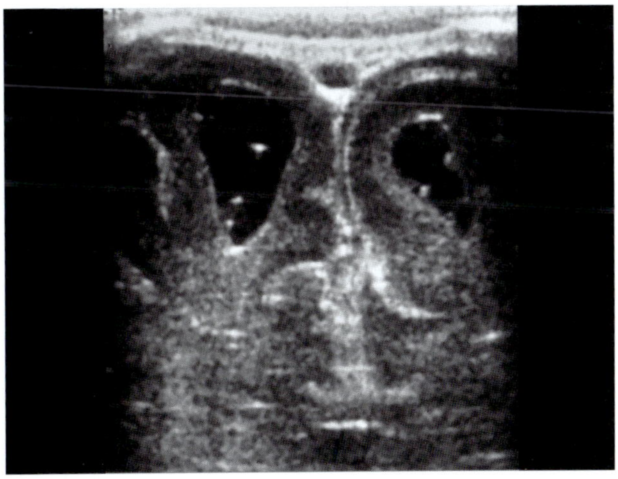

FIG. 27: Coronal sonogram showing well-defined anechoic areas representing cystic encephalomalacia in both frontal lobes.

Congenital Infections

The most frequent congenital infections are caused by the Toxoplasmosis, Other Agents, Rubella, Cytomegalovirus, and Herpes Simplex (TORCH) complex. The resultant pathology including parenchymal necrosis, vasculitis, and gliosis is similar in all these, though the severity and extent of disease may vary. CMV infection is the most common congenital infection. Calcifications occur in a characteristic periventricular location, when these are surrounded by a hypoechoic ring-like zone, the ultrasound finding is characteristic of CMV **(Fig. 28)**.[44] Calcifications may also occur in the basal ganglia, cortex, or subcortical region. Intracranial calcification is also seen in toxoplasmosis, which is the second most common congenital infection, with a predilection for basal ganglia, but more scattered calcification and periventricular calcification are also often seen. Herpes simplex type 2 is common in the neonate, resulting in diffuse encephalitis with loss of gray-white matter differentiation.

Acquired Infections

Pyogenic Meningitis

Group B streptococci and *Escherichia coli* are the most common bacterial organisms in the neonatal period and *Haemophilus influenzae* in infants (>3 months of age). Sonography may be normal in uncomplicated cases. It demonstrates increased reflectivity of the cerebral sulci, secondary to leptomeningeal inflammation and pus.[49,50] Cerebral vasculitis and thrombophlebitis may produce areas of cerebritis or infarction which are seen as echogenic areas in a segmental or gyral distribution.

Venous sinus thrombosis may also occur and can be detected using CDFI.[5] This may be associated with more complex patterns of brain injury, including venous ischemia and hemorrhage.

Extra-axial fluid collections are frequent findings in bacterial meningitis, especially *Haemophilus influenzae* infection. Subdural and subarachnoid collections may be echo-free or may have low-level echoes, the more reflective the collection, the more likely it is to represent empyema. CDFI may help to separate subdural and subarachnoid collections. Vessels on the surface of the brain are compressed onto the surface of the brain in subdural fluid collection whereas they traverse the fluid in subarachnoid collection, this is known as the "cortical vein sign".

Mild-to-moderate ventriculomegaly may occur as an early or late sonographic feature. In the acute stage, it probably represents a form of normal pressure hydrocephalus and is usually reversible. At a later date, it may occur due to obstruction to CSF flow at strategic points.

Involvement of the choroid plexus and spread to the ventricular system result in ventriculitis and hydrocephalus. The ventricular margins become more reflective, indicating generalized ependymitis. Particulate debris may be seen floating in the ventricles. Subsequently, septations and band adhesions appear resulting in complex multicompartmentalized hydrocephalus which is frequently resistant to effective shunting **(Fig. 29)**.

Abscess formation may occur in an area previously showing altered echogenicity due to cerebritis/infarction. This is seen as a well-marginated lesion with an echogenic rim and hypoechoic center. It may be associated with mass effect **(Fig. 30)**.

Tubercular Meningitis

Sonography in tubercular meningitis (TBM) may show echogenic sulci as in pyogenic meningitis, which is due to intense inflammatory exudates that accumulate in the depth of the sulci. TBM can also result in basal or occasionally parenchymal calcification and communicating hydrocephalus.[51,52] Aqueductal block and infarcts have been more frequently observed in TBM than pyogenic meningitis. Granulomas may also be seen as hypoechoic lesions with echogenic walls **(Fig. 31)**.[53]

NEOPLASMS AND CYSTS

Neoplasms

Neoplasms in the infant brain are rare and of all the tumors detected in the pediatric age group, only about 4% present

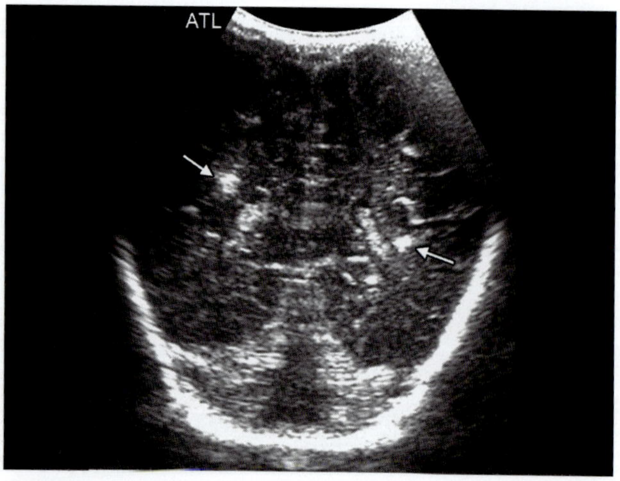

FIG. 28: Coronal sonogram showing bilateral periventricular echogenicities representing calcification in a case of cytomegalovirus (CMV) (white arrows).

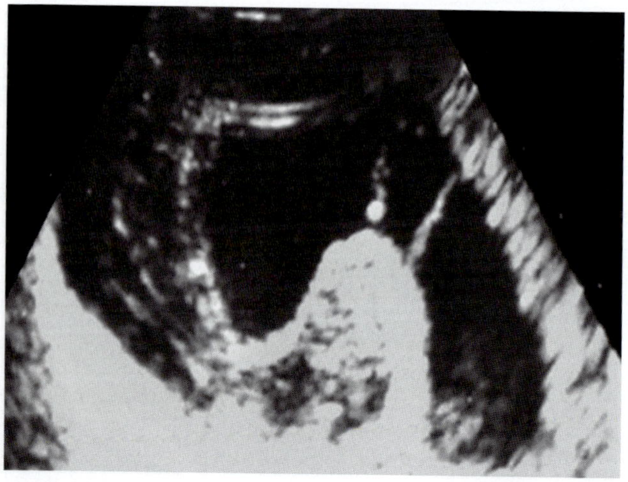

FIG. 29: Sagittal sonogram showing dilated lateral ventricle with multiple septations consistent with ventriculitis.

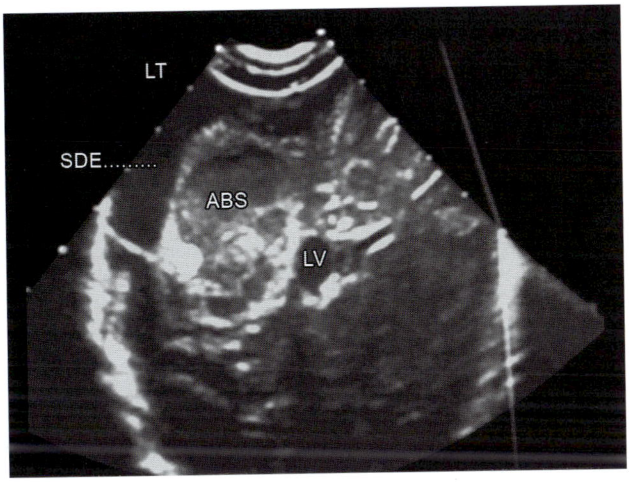

FIG. 30: Coronal sonogram showing a large round to oval lesion with hyperechoic walls and internal debris and mass effect suggestive of abscess in the left frontal lobe. A large subdural effusion is also present on the same side.

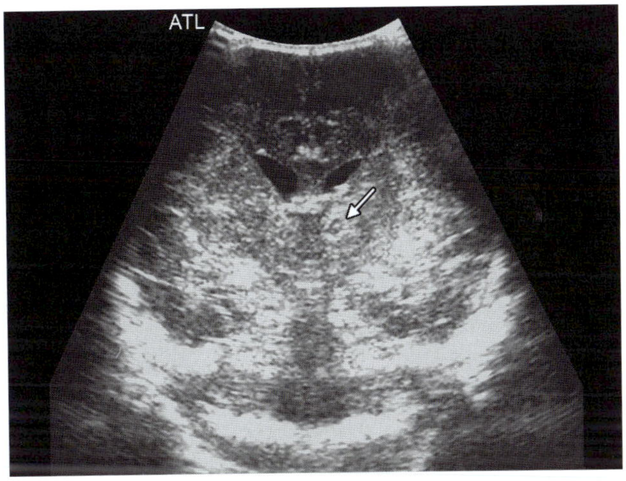

FIG. 31: Coronal sonogram in a patient with cerebrospinal fluid (CSF) findings suggestive of tubercular meningitis shows a small round hypoechoic granuloma with echogenic wall in the right thalamic region (white arrow).

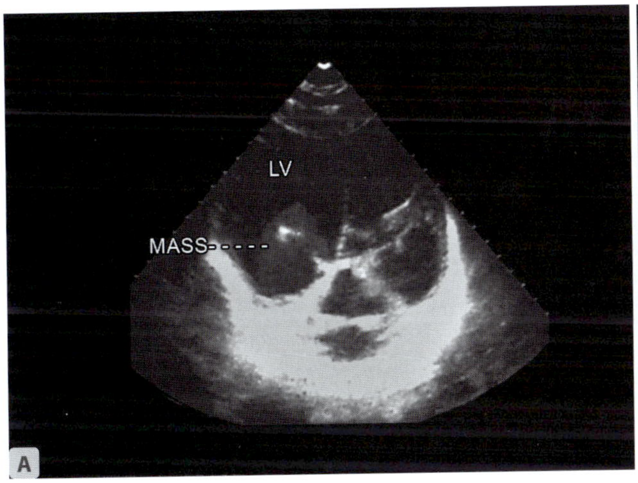

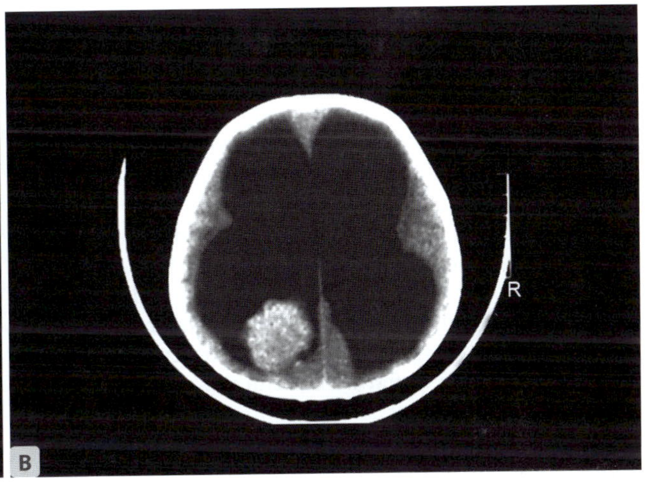

FIGS. 32A AND B: (A) Sonogram showing a mass in the left lateral ventricle with hydrocephalus; and (B) Contrast-enhanced computed tomography (CECT) of head of the same patient showing an intensely enhancing intraventricular mass consistent with choroid plexus papilloma.

during the 1st year of life. As neoplasms cause elevation of ICP, fontanels in affected infants may remain open for a longer time, enabling detection of the lesions with sonography. Tumors that present early are usually congenital. Congenital tumors can present with hemorrhage. Any hemorrhage noted in unusual circumstances or location should be investigated for an occult tumor, serial imaging is also helpful as hemorrhage resolves with time. Doppler can identify vascular components within a tumor. The majority of the brain tumors under 1 year of age are supratentorial and therefore accessible by ultrasound. The common neoplasms include teratomas, astrocytomas (usually from optic chiasm/nerves and hypothalamus), atypical teratoma/rhabdoid tumors, primitive neuroectodermal tumors, ependymomas, and choroid plexus papillomas **(Figs. 32A and B)**. The ultrasound appearance is variable and nonspecific but many are hyperechoic and further evaluation is required to characterize these lesions with computed tomography (CT) and MRI. The major use of ultrasound is in intraoperative localization of tumors.

Cysts

Besides porencephalic cysts, the other commonly encountered cysts include arachnoid cysts, choroid plexus cysts, subependymal cysts, and connatal cysts.

Arachnoid cysts are the most common true cysts of the brain, but they account for only 1% of all space-occupying lesions in children. They are located in the anterior middle cranial fossa, suprasellar region, posterior fossa, quadrigeminal region, cerebral convexities, and interhemispheric fissure in decreasing order of frequency. The cysts are seen as anechoic areas with discrete walls. Lesions abutting the ventricular system may cause obstructive hydrocephalus[54] **(Fig. 33)**.

Choroid plexus cysts are common and usually incidental findings. They range in size from <4 to 7 mm, are usually unilateral, and are located within the body of the choroid

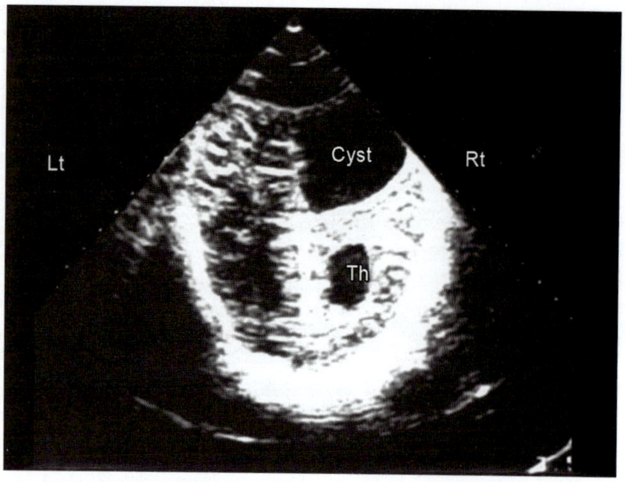

FIG. 33: Sonogram showing a large cyst in the right temporoparietal region with displacement of the cerebral hemisphere—arachnoid cyst.

plexus. These cystic lesions are of concern if encountered during pregnancy as they are associated with aneuploidy, particularly trisomy 18, especially if large (1 cm), bilateral, and associated with structural abnormalities, when the maternal age is ≥32 years or if the maternal serum screening results are abnormal. When detected postnatally, choroid plexus cysts are of no clinical significance in otherwise normal neonates. On high-resolution images, they appear spherical and may exhibit a double wall.

Subependymal cysts can be of two types, one is an acquired, posthemorrhagic cyst and the other is congenital and related to germinolysis. It may be difficult to differentiate between the two on sonography. The posthemorrhagic cystic lesions are most commonly seen in the caudothalamic notch and are found most frequently in preterm infants. They are usually tear-shaped and measure 2–11 mm in size. Congenital subependymal cysts may be due to hemorrhage, hypoxic-ischemic damage, or neurotropic infection. An association with congenital viral infections (mainly CMV and rubella), metabolic disorders (especially Zellweger syndrome), chromosomal abnormalities, and maternal cocaine consumption has been reported. However, subependymal cysts may be an isolated finding in otherwise healthy newborns.[54]

Connatal cysts are also referred to as coarctation of the lateral ventricles and frontal horn cysts. These are cystic areas seen adjacent to the superolateral margins of the frontal horns and body of the lateral ventricles. They are thought to represent a normal variant due to approximation of the walls of the frontal horns of the lateral ventricles proximal to their external angles. When the ventricular walls are close enough to touch each other, the most external portion of the ventricle acquires a rounded configuration, resulting in a cystic appearance.[54]

The differentiation of various types of cysts in the frontal horn area based on their location is discussed in **Table 4**. Diagrammatic representation of the distribution of cysts in periventricular region is shown in **Figure 34**.

TABLE 4: Differentiation of various types of cysts in frontal horn area according to their location.

Types of cyst	Location
Connatal cyst	At or just below the superolateral angles of frontal horn or body of lateral ventricles and anterior to foramen of Monro
Subependymal cyst	Below the external angles of frontal horn or body of lateral ventricles and posterior to foramen of Monro
Periventricular leukomalacia	Above the angles

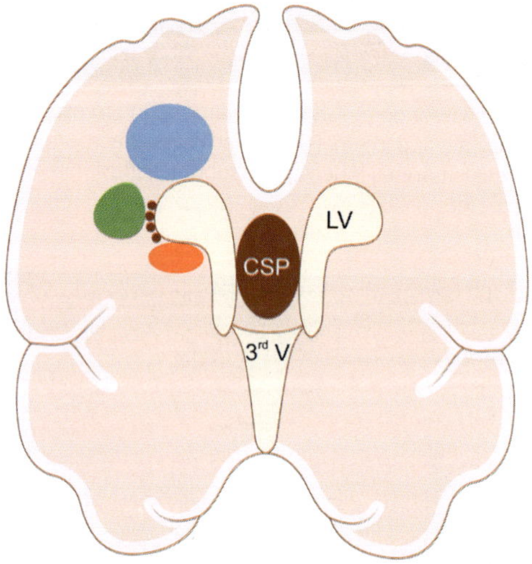

FIG. 34: Diagram in coronal plane through the lateral and third ventricles showing the location of different types of periventricular cysts. The red oval represents the posthemorrhagic subependymal cyst, green oval represents connatal cysts, blue oval shows location for cysts secondary to PVL, and the dotted line represents the external angle of lateral ventricle. (CSP: cavum septum pellucidum; PVL: periventricular leukomalacia)

EXTRACORPOREAL MEMBRANE OXYGENATION

Extracorporeal membrane oxygenation is commonly used to treat term infants with respiratory insufficiency. The infants are continuously heparinized during the procedure and are at risk for intracranial hemorrhage. Baseline sonograms are performed prior to ECMO and patients with severe anoxic-ischemic injury, large infarcts, or IVH more than grade 2 are not ECMO candidates. Ultrasounds are performed on a daily basis and any hemorrhage more than grade 1 is cause for discontinuing ECMO. Since hemorrhages occurring while the patients are anticoagulated are less echogenic than hemorrhages in babies with normal clotting factors, a high index of suspicion should be maintained to look for mass effect not seen on the previous day's neurosonogram.[44]

During venoarterial ECMO, the right common carotid artery and jugular vein are cannulated and ligated for vascular access and infants are placed on nonpulsatile partial cardiopulmonary bypass. Alterations in the intracranial hemodynamics are seen and as the amount of flow through the ECMO bypass circuit increases, arterial pulsatility decreases and may disappear, especially in association with severe cardiac dysfunction. During bypass, flow to the right MCA is via retrograde flow through A1 segment of right ACA and anterior communicating artery.

POST-TRAUMATIC INJURY

Subdural and epidural hematomas can be a difficult diagnosis on sonography and they present as unilateral or bilateral hypoechoic fluid collections. Imaging through the PF or foramen magnum may be needed for posterior fossa collection.[5,6]

Cephalohematomas are traumatic subperiosteal hematomas of the skull that usually result from birth injury. They are bound between the periosteum and cranium hence, they cannot cross sutures. On sonography, it is seen as a subperiosteal hemorrhage of moderate echogenicity and the underlying brain is usually normal.

The differentials for cephalohematomas are caput succedaneum and subgaleal hemorrhage. A caput succedaneum is a collection of blood under the skin and above the cranial aponeurosis, it occurs most commonly during birth and crosses suture lines. A subgaleal hemorrhage is situated under the cranial aponeurosis and above the periosteum and can cross suture lines.

MINERALIZING LENTICULOSTRIATE VASCULOPATHY

Diffuse hyperechogenicity seen in the region of the basal ganglia and thalamus in preterm neonates must be considered distinct from the linear pattern of hyperechogenicity encountered along vessels of the basal ganglia and thalami in mineralizing lenticulostriate vasculopathy. The pathologic correlate of this condition is hypercellular thickened vessel walls with intramural and perivascular deposits of basophilic material, iron, and calcium.

Mineralizing lenticulostriate vasculopathy is detected by USG in 0.4% of all neonates, 2–6% of ill neonates, 5% of preterm neonates, and 20% of very preterm neonates, but is typically occult on CT and MRI. It appears early in term infants and later in preterm infants, at a mean age of 1 month, as it tends to develop around the same postmenstrual age. On sonography, it appears as hyperechoic linear or branching tubular streaks in the basal ganglia and thalami **(Figs. 35A and B)**. It is bilateral in 40–80% of cases and is more common on the right than the left side when unilateral.

Mineralizing lenticulostriate vasculopathy was initially reported with neonatal TORCH infections [CMV, rubella, syphilis, human immunodeficiency virus (HIV)] and has subsequently been reported in association with numerous other disorders, including chromosomal abnormalities (trisomy 13, trisomy 21, unbalanced translocation of 11, mosaicism 46XX/47XXX, pericentric inversion of chromosome 2), asphyxia, fetal alcohol and drug exposure, neonatal IVH, neonatal lupus, neonatal hypoglycemia, antenatal glucocorticoid therapy, antenatal high-dose tocolytic magnesium sulfate ($MgSO_4$), encephalitis, hypothyroidism, twin-twin transfusion, diabetic fetopathy, cyanotic or low output cardiac disease (especially hypoplastic left heart syndrome), sialidosis, and rotavirus infection. It has also been reported in otherwise uncomplicated prematurity, but should not be regarded as merely an incidental finding and clinical correlation for associated conditions, such as infection, chromosomal disorder, or drug exposure should be done.[19]

Mineralizing lenticulostriate vasculopathy can resolve in 36–50% of cases.[19] Progression on USG can occur without clinical deterioration. Mineralizing lenticulostriate vasculopathy may be best regarded as a nonspecific marker of previous insult to the brain and the neurologic outcome is largely related to the associated conditions or comorbidities.

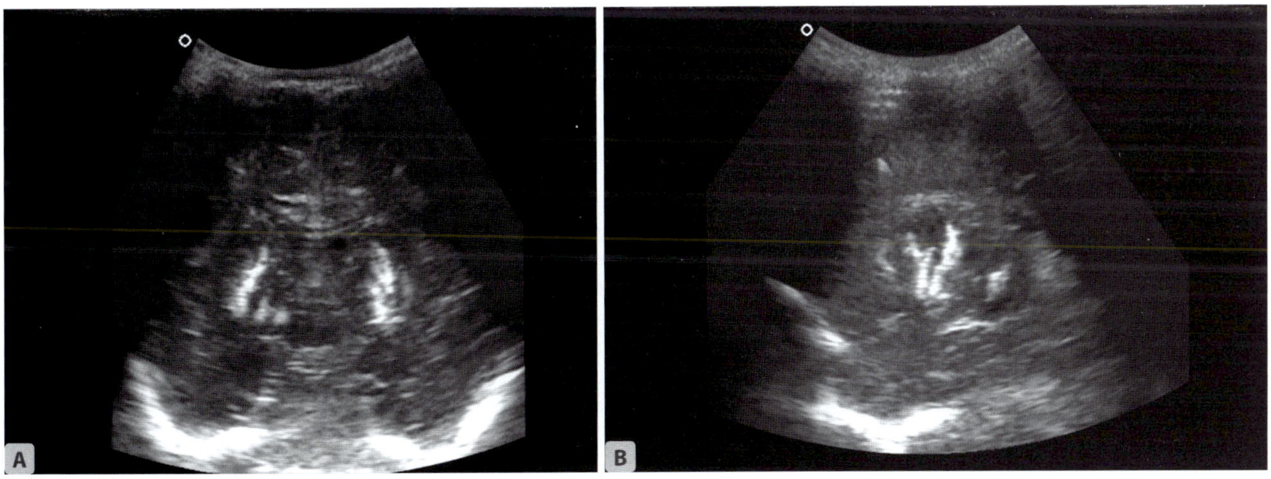

FIGS. 35A AND B: Coronal (A) and sagittal (B) sonograms showing branching linear echogenicities in the basal ganglia consistent with mineralizing vasculopathy.

LIMITATIONS OF CRANIAL SONOGRAPHY AND RECOMMENDATIONS FOR MRI

The limitations of cranial sonography include:

- Small acoustic windows can affect image quality and some structures and abnormalities remain difficult to visualize.
- Evaluation of superficial structures is difficult. Subtle aspects of cortical folding and extracerebral hemorrhage situated at the convexity of the cerebral hemispheres (i.e., subdural, epidural, and subarachnoid hemorrhages) may remain difficult to detect.
- Precise definition of posterior fossa abnormalities such as cerebellar hemorrhage and infarctions may not always be possible.
- Myelination is not visualized.
- Damage to the basal ganglia in term HIE and areas of focal infarction are usually detected, but they may not be defined well enough for precise prognostication.
- Diffuse white matter injury, as can occur in very preterm infants, may not be well-detected by cranial sonography.

Cross-sectional studies such as MRI of brain may be helpful in certain instances as it helps to depict brain maturation and can detect lesions in locations that are difficult to visualize with cranial sonography. It allows detection of diffuse and noncystic white matter lesions in preterm infants and diffusion-weighted imaging allows very early detection of hypoxic-ischemic brain injury.[4]

FUTURE PERSPECTIVES

Technological progress has led to an increase in the computational speed of US systems with introduction of new applications. "Ultrafast US" systems have been developed that can process 1,000s of frames per second and have revolutionized the temporal resolution and sensitivity. Quantitative mapping of cerebral vascular dynamics has been made possible by high-frequency imaging.[55]

Sensitive, specific, and safe bedside evaluation of brain perfusion is essential in the early diagnosis, treatment, and improved survival of neonates with hypoxic-ischemic injury. Contrast-enhanced ultrasound imaging is a technique in which intravenously injected gas-filled microbubbles generate enhanced ultrasound echoes from an acoustic impedance mismatch and can be used to assess hypoperfusion in the brain. Both qualitative and quantitative contrast-enhanced ultrasound evaluation methods can be used. Qualitative contrast-enhanced ultrasound evaluation of the brain involves subjective detection of focal or asymmetric perfusion abnormalities while quantitative contrast-enhanced ultrasound evaluation derives perfusion kinetic parameters from the contrast time intensity curve, which is a curve of contrast wash in as detected by an increase in the signal intensity over time.[56]

CONCLUSION

The valuable information obtained from cranial sonography reveals the importance of this safe, cost-effective, and accurate diagnostic modality to assess neurological findings in neonates and infants. It also helps to guide further management. Accurate technique and knowledge of normal anatomy and variations are essential for proper interpretation. Cranial sonography is an excellent tool for serial imaging in neonates and infants.

ACKNOWLEDGMENT

We would like to acknowledge the contribution of Dr Prince Das, Senior Resident in Department of Radiodiagnosis, Maulana Azad Medical College for making the diagrams for this chapter.

PART B: PEDIATRIC SPINAL SONOGRAPHY

INTRODUCTION

Neonatal and infantile spinal sonography (USG) is an extremely useful tool in the evaluation of suspected occult spinal dysraphism in neonates. Although MRI is the present reference standard for imaging in suspected spinal dysraphism in children, USG has its own edge, especially in neonates. While MRI provides an excellent soft-tissue characterization, it requires administration of general anesthesia. Prolonged examination time is also another drawback of MRI. USG, to the contrary, is a quick, easily available imaging modality which does not require the child to be anesthetized or sedated. With the advancements in US hardware and transducer technology, obtaining a very high-resolution image of smaller structures within the spinal canal has become possible.[57,58] Moreover, evaluation for cord tethering is much more conveniently done on USG, as most commonly adopted position for a spinal USG is prone position. This chapter will discuss the indications and technique of spinal USG and imaging findings in various pathologies.

INDICATIONS

Recommended indications for spinal USG are listed in **Box 1**.[59-70]

EQUIPMENT

Spinal USG should be performed using a high frequency linear transducer (5–12 MHz or higher). In neonates, owing to thin layer of subcutaneous tissue on the back, even a hockey-stick transducer (2–20 MHz) can be used for superior spatial resolution.[71] However, in presence of a large back mass, a convex (2–5 MHz) or a microconvex (2–7 MHz) transducer should be used. Microconvex transducer is preferable over a convex one due to its small footprint.

TECHNIQUE

Before starting spinal USG, the back of the infant should be carefully inspected. In presence of any skin defect over a back mass, spinal USG should be performed with caution so as not to introduce any infection in the CSF space. In such

BOX 1: Common indications for spinal ultrasonography (USG).[59-70]

- *Cutaneous stigmata associated with closed spinal dysraphism*:
  - Midline back swelling
  - Naevi/discoloration in midline in lower back
  - Tail-like appendage or skin tag
  - Hair tuft
  - Elevated discolored patch or hemangioma
  - Skin dimple
- Suspicion of tethered cord syndrome
- Suspected split cord malformation or syrinx
- Patients suspected of having caudal regression syndrome including patients having anorectal malformation or vertebral anomalies
- Detection of subdural hematoma
- Guidance for lumbar puncture[69]
- Postoperative assessment for cord[70]

situations, the transducer should be placed away from the skin defect[72] and cranial/caudal angulation should be utilized to get visualize the abnormality.

The infant should be peacefully lying on mother's lap or examination table, preferably in a prone position. When prone positioning is not feasible, lateral decubitus position can be adopted. Spinal USG should be performed in a systematic way, moving in one direction (cranial to caudal or vice versa). Scanning should be performed in both axial and sagittal plane. In the neonates and early infancy, unossified spinous process provides a good acoustic window. In presence of spina bifida, the gap in posterior spinal elements is more widened, providing even better acoustic window.

Gray-scale USG should be coupled with M-mode evaluation for the movement of the filum and the nerve roots. Real-time assessment of pulsatile movement of the filum and cauda equine nerve roots should always be done.

DETERMINATION OF VERTEBRAL LEVEL

Determination of vertebral level is of paramount importance in spinal USG. The lower level of spinal cord and thecal sac termination should be expressed in terms of vertebral level. There are several methods[73-75] for this:

- *Localization of lumbosacral junction*: This is the most commonly used and consistent method. On USG, lumbar vertebral bodies appear horizontal. In comparison, sacral vertebrae have a gentle upsweep and are seen as inverted L-shaped echogenic lines **(Figs. 36A and B)**. It is important to identify the transition and then count the vertebrae in a cranial direction.
- *Localization of the coccygeal vertebrae*: This is much less often performed. Coccygeal vertebrae tend to have a rounder shape compared to sacral vertebrae. However, this method is less consistent than the previous one.
- *Identifying the 12th thoracic vertebrae*: This is the last vertebra bearing ribs on the side. Counting of lumbar vertebrae can be done caudal to it.
- Identification of thecal sac termination (normally at S2 level)[75] and then counting cranially.

NORMAL ANATOMY

Spinal USG is most useful for the evaluation of the lumbosacral spine, compared to cervical or thoracic spine. Normal dural sac is seen as an echogenic line, lying underneath the unossified spinous process. Spinal cord is seen as a hypoechoic structure surrounded by anechoic CSF space **(Figs. 37 and 38)**. The spinal cord surface has an echogenic pial covering. Nerve roots are seen as echogenic structures, arranged in ventral and dorsal bundles. Conus medullaris is seen as an expansion of the lumbar spinal cord, having a tapered ending. Normal conus medullaris in a term neonate corresponds to the L2/L3 intervertebral disk level.[66,76-79] In preterm newborns, it may lie at a little lower level (midbody of L3). In such situations, a follow-up imaging should be done between term corrected age and 6 months.[66] Normal thecal sac terminates at S2 level.[75] Posterior elements of sacral vertebrae are mostly not ossified in a term neonate.

NORMAL VARIATIONS

While performing spinal USG, one should be aware of the normal variants which may mimic pathology. These are listed in **Table 5**.[5,80]

DISEASE ENTITIES

Spinal Dysraphism

Closed spinal dysraphism is the most common indication of spinal USG in a neonate/infant. Open spinal dysraphism usually does not need USG and is diagnosed clinically. Moreover, presence of a skin defect overlying the back mass may pose a risk of introduction of infection while performing USG **(Figs. 41A and B)**.

Closed spinal dysraphism can present either with a skin-covered back mass or without back mass. In the latter scenario, various cutaneous markers such as a sacral dimple, hairy tuft, and sinus tract may be present. USG is especially useful in both these situations. A sacral skin dimple, i.e., >2.5 cm from anus or associated with hair tuft is more likely to be associated with spinal dysraphism.[61]

Closed Spinal Dysraphism with Skin-covered Back Mass

This group includes lipomyelocele, lipomyelomeningocele, and terminal myelocystocele.

Lipomyelocele

There is a spina bifida along with a soft back mass comprising of fatty tissue and neural elements.[58,81-83] The junction of the neural tissue with fatty component (lipoma-placode interface) lies within the spinal canal and ventral CSF space is not enlarged **(Figs. 42A to E)**.

Lipomyelomeningocele

In this entity, the back mass consists of all three elements: (1) Neural tissue; (2) Fat; and (3) CSF.[58,81-83] The lipoma-placode

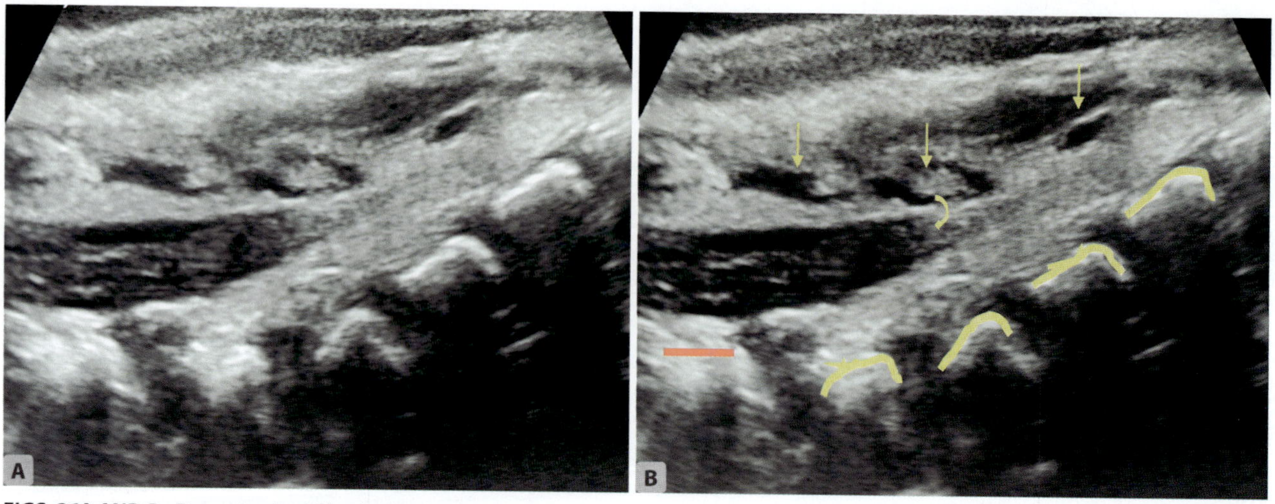

FIGS. 36A AND B: Determination of lumbosacral junction on sonography. Midsagittal image of lumbosacral region (A) and annotated image (B) showing horizontal orientation of L5 (red line) and gentle upward curve of sacral vertebrae (yellow lines). Posterior elements of sacral vertebrae (arrows) are not ossified. Also note that the thecal sac terminates at the level of S2 (normal) (curved arrow).

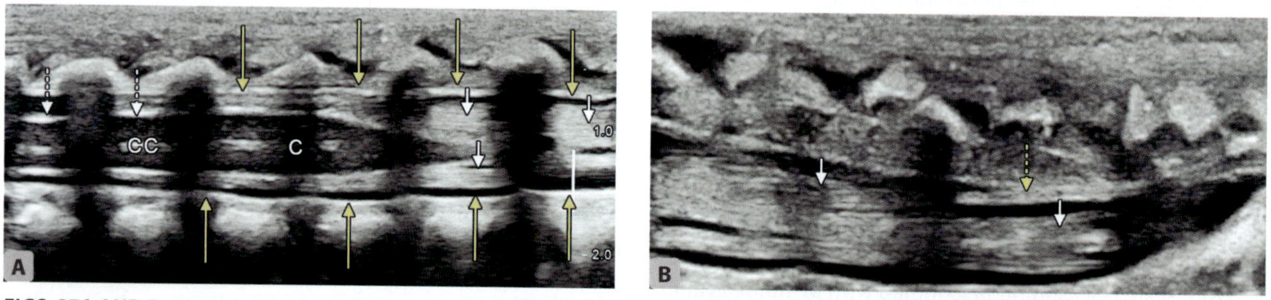

FIGS. 37A AND B: Normal sagittal spinal sonogram: (A) Image at the lumbar level shows conus medullaris (C) as an expansion of the lumbar cord, having a tapered ending. The cord appears hypoechoic, surrounded by a reflective pial covering (dotted arrow). The dural lining is shown with long arrows. Cauda equina nerve roots show uniform arrangement and echogenic appearance (small arrows). The central canal is seen as an echogenic line (CC); and (B) Image of a caudal level at lumbosacral junction shows the filum terminale (dotted arrow), cauda equina nerve roots (small arrows), and termination of thecal sac.

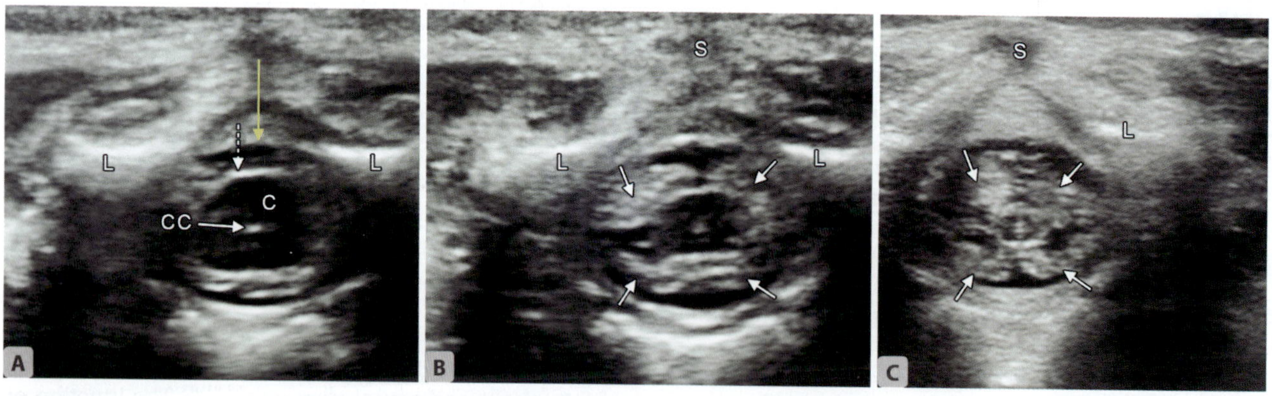

FIGS. 38A TO C: Normal axial sonogram of lumbar spine. (A) Image at the level of conus medullaris (A) shows conus (C) having an outer echogenic pial lining (dotted arrow). Outside the pial covering lies the clear CSF in subarachnoid space superficial to which lies the echogenic dural lining (long arrow); and (B and C) Images at more caudal level show uniform arrangement of dorsal and ventral nerve roots (small arrows). (CC: central canal; CSF: cerebrospinal fluid; L: lamina; S: spinous process)

TABLE 5: Normal variants in spinal ultrasonography **(Figs. 39 and 40)**.

Entity	Imaging features	Pathology which it mimics	Differentiating feature
Ventriculus terminalis[5,71,80]	Fusiform dilatation of the central canal in the terminal part of conus medullaris **(Fig. 39)**	Syrinx	• Location more caudal, in terminal conus • Regresses in few weeks after birth
Filar cyst[5,74,80]	Midline fusiform cystic lesion just below conus, within the filum terminale **(Fig. 40)**	• Syrinx • Arachnoid cyst	• Location within filum terminale
Cauda equina pseudomass[58,74]	Clumping of nerve roots on one side	Arachnoiditis with root clumping	• Visualized on lateral decubitus position of the infant • Disappears on prone positioning
Pseudosinus tract[74]	Hypoechoic linear tract from the tip of coccyx to a skin dimple, has no CSF within	Dorsal dermal sinus	• Location at the tip of coccyx (dorsal dermal sinus is usually more cranial) • No CSF within the tract

(CSF: cerebrospinal fluid)

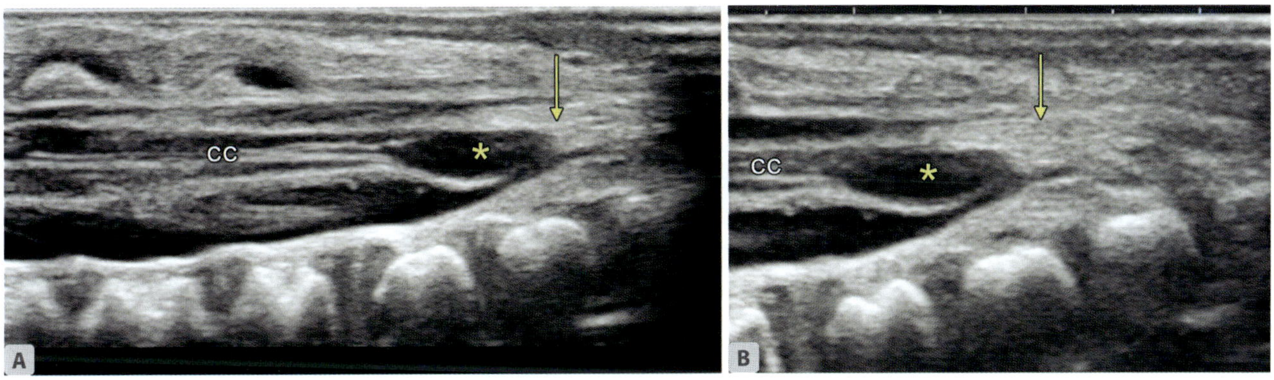

FIGS. 39A AND B: Ventriculus terminalis: The central canal (CC) is seen to continue with the fusiform cystic lesion (asterisk) at the terminal end of the cord. The cord is low-lying and tethered to an intraspinal lipoma (arrow).

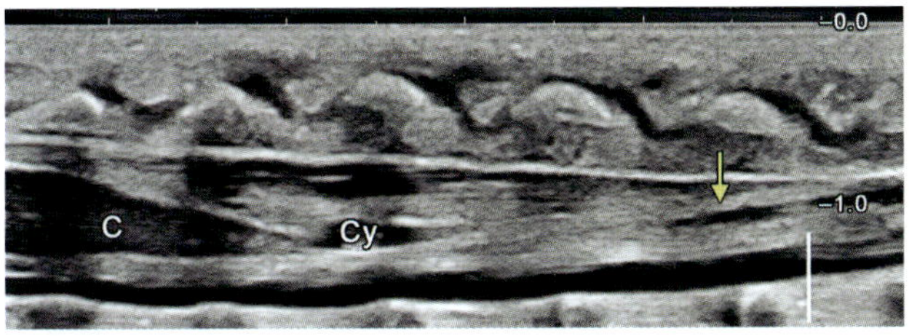

FIG. 40: Filar cyst: Note the typical location of the cyst (Cy): Midline, distal to the conus. It is located in the filum (arrow) and has a fusiform shape.

interface lies outside the spinal canal and the ventral CSF space is enlarged **(Figs. 43A to C)**.

Spinal Lipoma

They can be intradural or extradural. They can be associated with other closed dysraphism, vertebral anomalies, or tethered cord. On USG, they appear echogenic and on MRI, they follow fatty signal.[81,83]

Terminal Myelocystocele

In this entity, the neural element within the sac consists of distal cord/conus with a dilated central canal.

Closed Spinal Dysraphism without a Back Mass

Common entities of this group include fatty filum, filar lipoma, and split cord malformation.

Fatty Filum and Filar Lipoma

These result from abnormal retrogressive differentiation of the caudal cell mass and the distal part of neural tube. A minor aberration in this stage may result in persistence of fat in the filum **(Figs. 44A and B)**. The clinical significance of fat within the filum terminale depends on many other factors. Isolated fatty filum, especially if it is not thickened, is not considered to be clinically significant, as it can be seen in about 6% of normal autopsy specimens.[81] However, if fatty signal in the filum is associated with thickening (>2 mm), then it is significant[57,82,83] and can present with tethered cord syndrome. If the fatty tissue (appearing echogenic on USG) assumes the shape of a mass, it is called a filar lipoma. It can have a uniform echogenic or striated echogenic appearance **(Figs. 45A and B)**.

Dorsal Dermal Sinus

Ultrasonography can be useful in delineating the tract, its communication with the CSF space, and presence of CSF

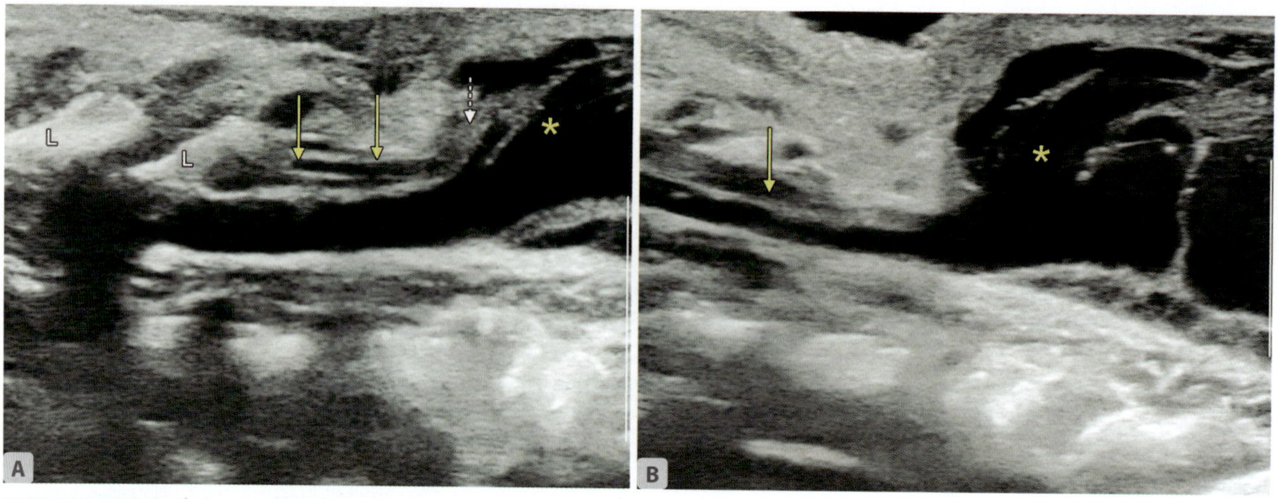

FIGS. 41A AND B: Performing spinal sonography in an open spinal dysraphism. If deemed essential, study can be performed by placing the transducer at a place away from the skin defect and visualizing the abnormality with a caudal transducer tilt (A and B). Note the defect in the posterior elements of spine, posteriorly placed spinal cord (arrows) within the spinal canal, and continuation of the neural placode (dotted arrow) and CSF (asterisk) within the back mass. (CSF: cerebrospinal fluid; L: lamina)

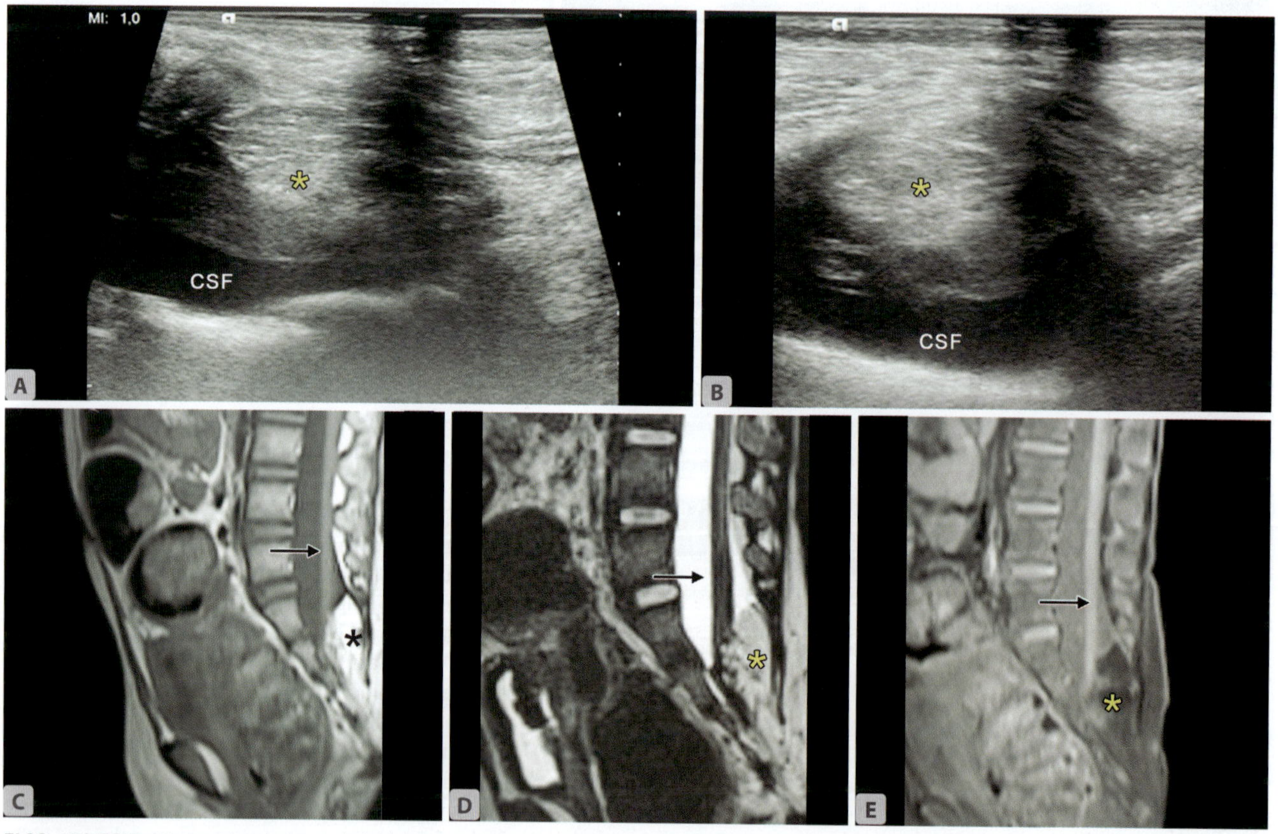

FIGS. 42A TO E: Lipomyelocele in a girl child presenting with soft back mass. (A and B) The ventral CSF space is enlarged and the intraspinal component of the lipomatous component appears echogenic (asterisk); (C) T1W; (D) T2W; and (E) T1W fat-suppressed images show a low-lying cord (arrow), tethered to the fatty intraspinal component (asterisk). (CSF: cerebrospinal fluid; T1W: T1-weighted image; T2W: T2-weighted image)

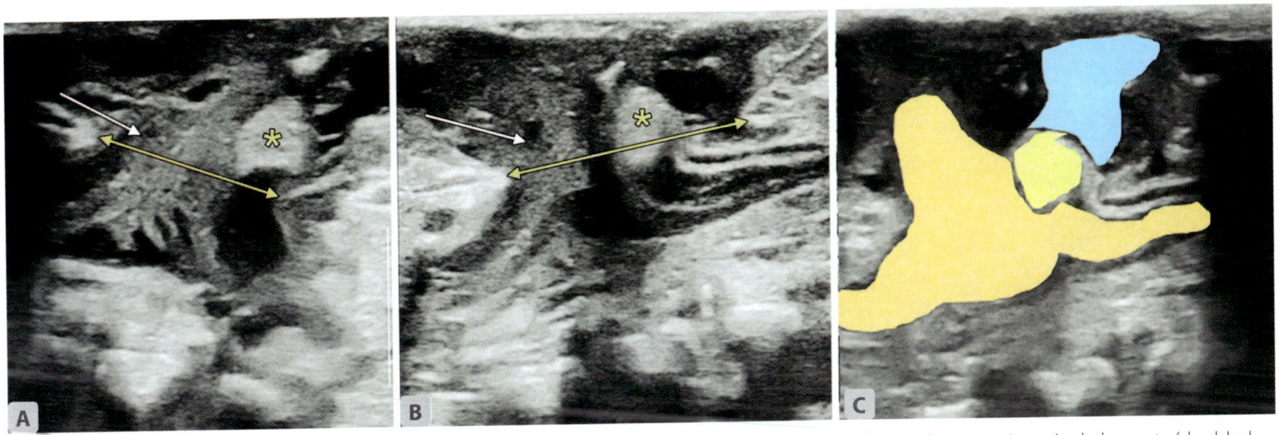

FIGS. 43A TO C: Lipomyelomeningocele: Axial (A) and sagittal (B) sonography images show the defect in the posterior spinal elements (doubled-edged arrow) and herniation of neural placode (arrow) in the back mass. Note the location of the fatty component (asterisk) at the caudal margin of the spinal defect; and (C) Diagrammatic representation of the sagittal image [neural tissue: Orange, fat: Yellow, and cerebrospinal fluid (CSF): Blue].

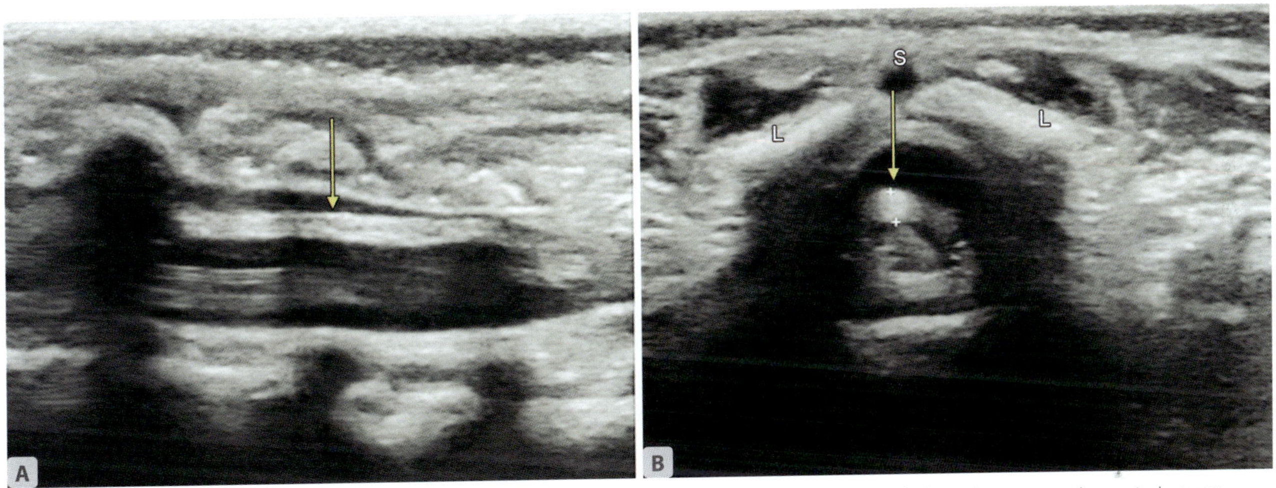

FIGS. 44A AND B: Fatty filum: Sagittal (A) and axial (B) sonography images reveal that the filum terminale (arrow) appears echogenic, but not thickened. If the thickness exceeds 2 mm, it is considered thickened and labelled filar lipoma. (L: lamina; S: spinous process)

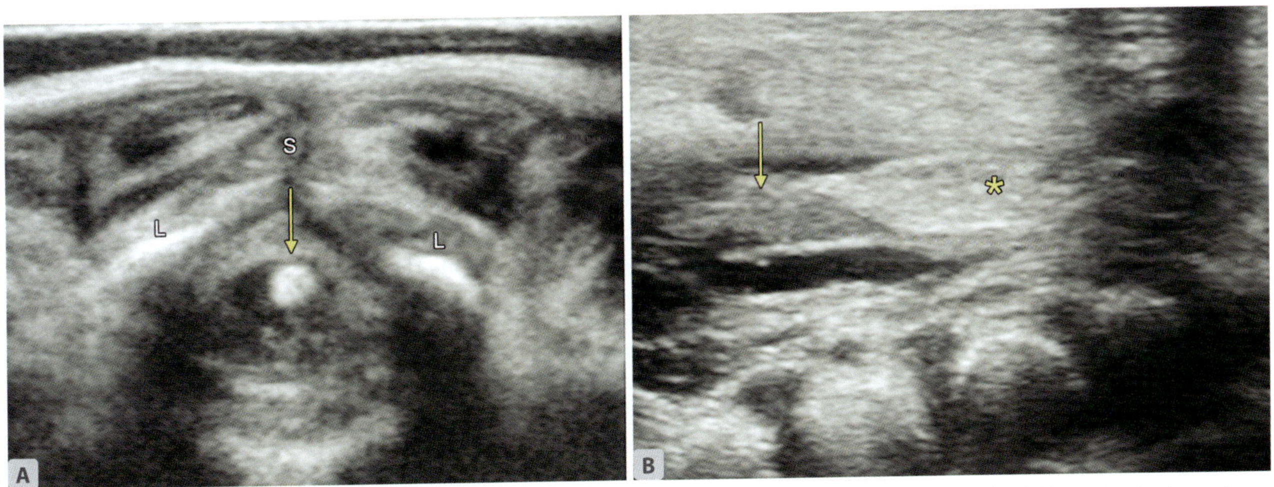

FIGS. 45A AND B: Variable appearances of filar lipoma. (A) Axial sonography image in a 10-day-old neonate reveals a thickened and echogenic filum (arrow); and (B) Sagittal image in another infant showing an echogenic mass (asterisk) in the location of filum terminale and spinal cord tethering (arrow). (L: lamina; S: spinous process)

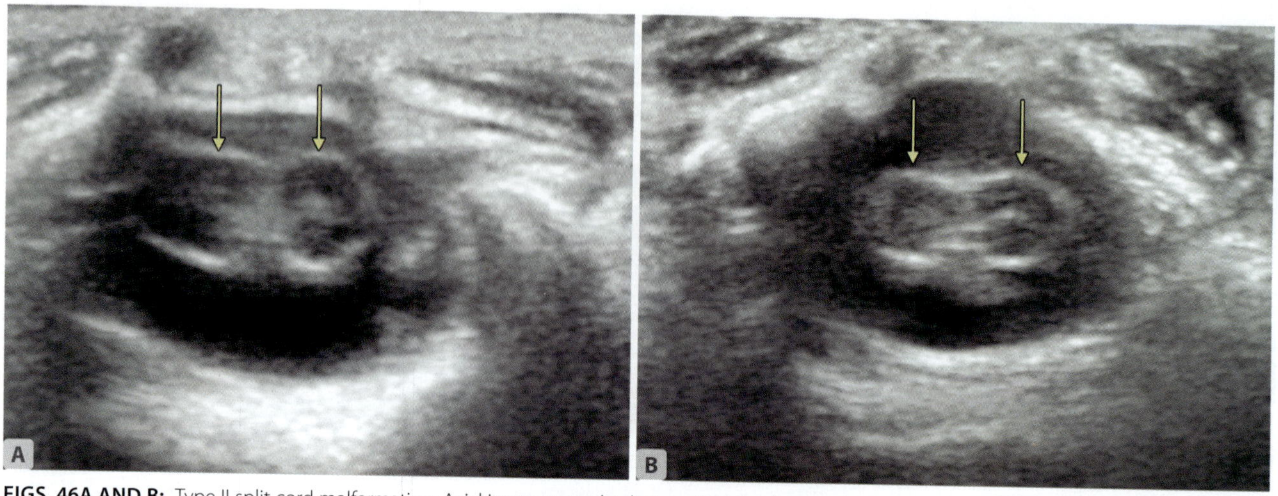

FIGS. 46A AND B: Type II split cord malformation: Axial images reveal splitting of the lumbar cord in two hemicords (arrows) in a single dural sac, each having its own central canal. No bony/fibrous septa is visible.

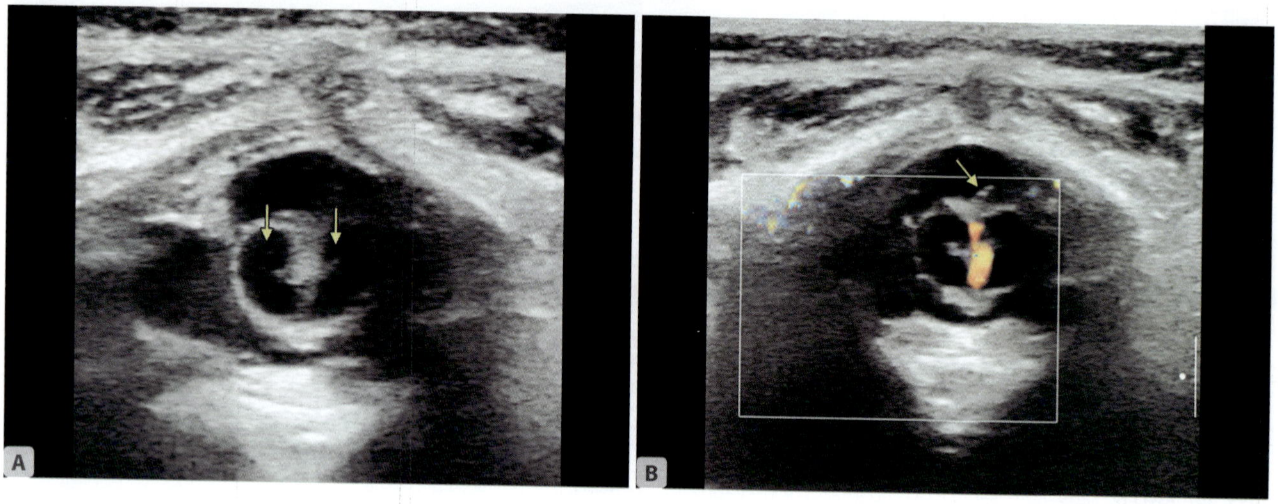

FIGS. 47A AND B: Type II split cord malformation. (A) Axial gray-scale sonography image reveals splitting of the lumbar cord in two hemicords (arrows); and (B) Doppler interrogation shows vascularity in the intervening septa (arrow).

within the tract.[58,83] Presence of fluid within the tract and a communication with CSF space differentiate it from a pseudosinus tract.

Complex Dysraphism

Split Cord Malformation

In this disease entity, the spinal cord is split into two hemicords **(Figs. 46 and 47)**, which may be separated by bony/fibrous septa and have two separate dural sheaths (type I) or have no bony/fibrous septa and lie within the same dural sac (type II). The hemicords usually unite again at a level caudal to the split. They can be associated with other anomalies (tethered cord, filar lipoma, myelomeningocele involving any hemicord, syrinx) as well **(Figs. 48A and B)**. Spinal USG is very accurate in delineating the split, presence/absence of septa, number of dural sacs, and other associated anomalies.[58] The role of USG here is 2-fold: Firstly, to accurately delineate the anatomy and associated anomalies and secondly, to rule out tethered cord in a postoperative scenario.

Caudal Regression Syndrome

Clinical and radiological manifestations of this syndrome can be very variable. The sacrum and lower lumbar vertebrae may show variable degree of dysgenesis.[58,71] On USG, the conus medullaris shows an abrupt transition, instead of normal tapered appearance **(Figs. 49A and B)**. The normal uniform arrangement of cauda equina nerve roots may be replaced by an abnormal arrangement of roots in two thick bundles.

Tethered Cord Syndrome

Tethered cord syndrome is a clinical diagnosis manifested by specific set of clinical symptoms.[58,84] They usually result from

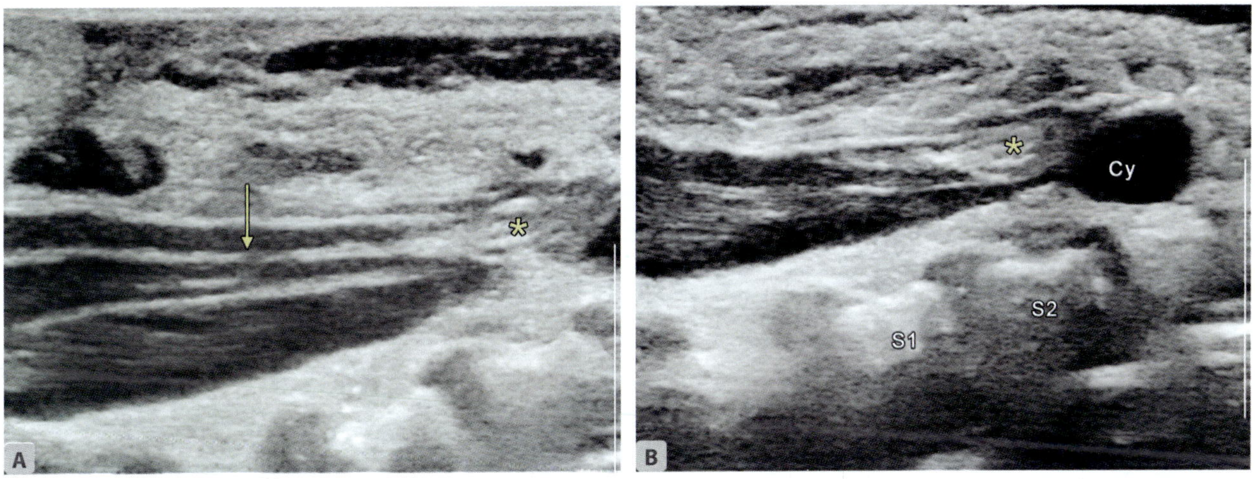

FIGS. 48A AND B: Associated anomalies in split cord malformation: Same patient as in **Figures 47A and B**. (A and B) Sagittal sonographic images at sacral level reveal a low-lying cord (arrow), tethered to a filar lipoma (asterisk). Note the lipoma has a striated appearance. Caudal to the lipoma, an arachnoid cyst (Cy) is also seen.

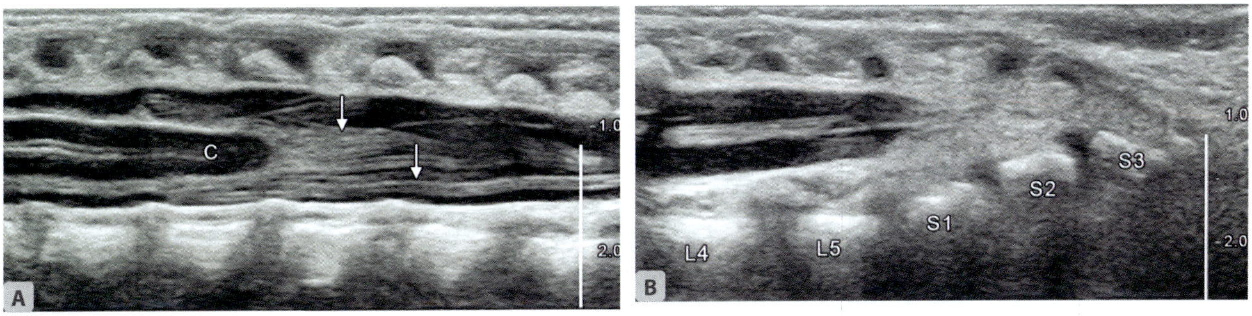

FIGS. 49A AND B: Caudal regression syndrome. (A) Sagittal sonographic images at lumbar reveal a rounded abrupt termination of conus medullaris (C). Cauda equina nerve roots are shown with arrows; and (B) Sagittal image at a more caudal level shows the sacrum to be dysmorphic. The S3 vertebra has an abnormal downward slope. S4 and S5 are absent. Note the normal lumbar vertebrae have a horizontal orientation.

an abnormally adherent distal spinal cord/filum terminale, which results in traction on the nerve roots. The clinical symptoms may not be evident in neonatal age or infancy, rather may present due to nerve traction as the child grows. Usual presentations include lower limb weakness, bladder and bowel dysfunction, abnormal gait, and reflexes. It can either be primary (congenital) or secondary (usually in postoperative scenario). The congenital causes of tethered cord may either be a tight filum terminale or tethering of cord to a mass (filar lipoma, dermoid, arachnoid cyst, myelocele, meningomyelocele).

Tight filum terminale is a congenital condition where the filum terminale is short, thick, and less elastic filum, which may otherwise look normal.[85] Tight filum terminale syndrome is the combination of a tight filum terminale and clinical presentation of tethered cord syndrome.[85]

On imaging,[58,83,85] tethered cord should be suspected **(Figs. 50A to C)** when there is:

- An abnormally dorsally or laterally located cord on USG performed in prone position.
- Less movement of conus/filum on real-time US.
- Thickened echogenic filum with reduced movement of conus/filum.

Associated mass lesion (filar lipoma, dermoid, arachnoid cyst) in the subdural/subarachnoid spaces can also cause tethering of cord **(Fig. 51)**.

Subdural Hematoma

Subdural hematoma in infant can be a result of birth injury/difficult delivery. Repeated attempts at lumbar puncture can also result in a hematoma.[69] Spinal USG can detect subdural hematoma as echogenic lesions outside the CSF space.[86] USG can be an important tool to ascertain whether there is thecal sac compression.

Infection

Although this is not a routine indication of spinal USG, inflammation of the meninges can be detected by the presence of debris in the subarachnoid space on spinal USG. It can also be associated with clumping of nerve roots secondary to arachnoiditis.[87]

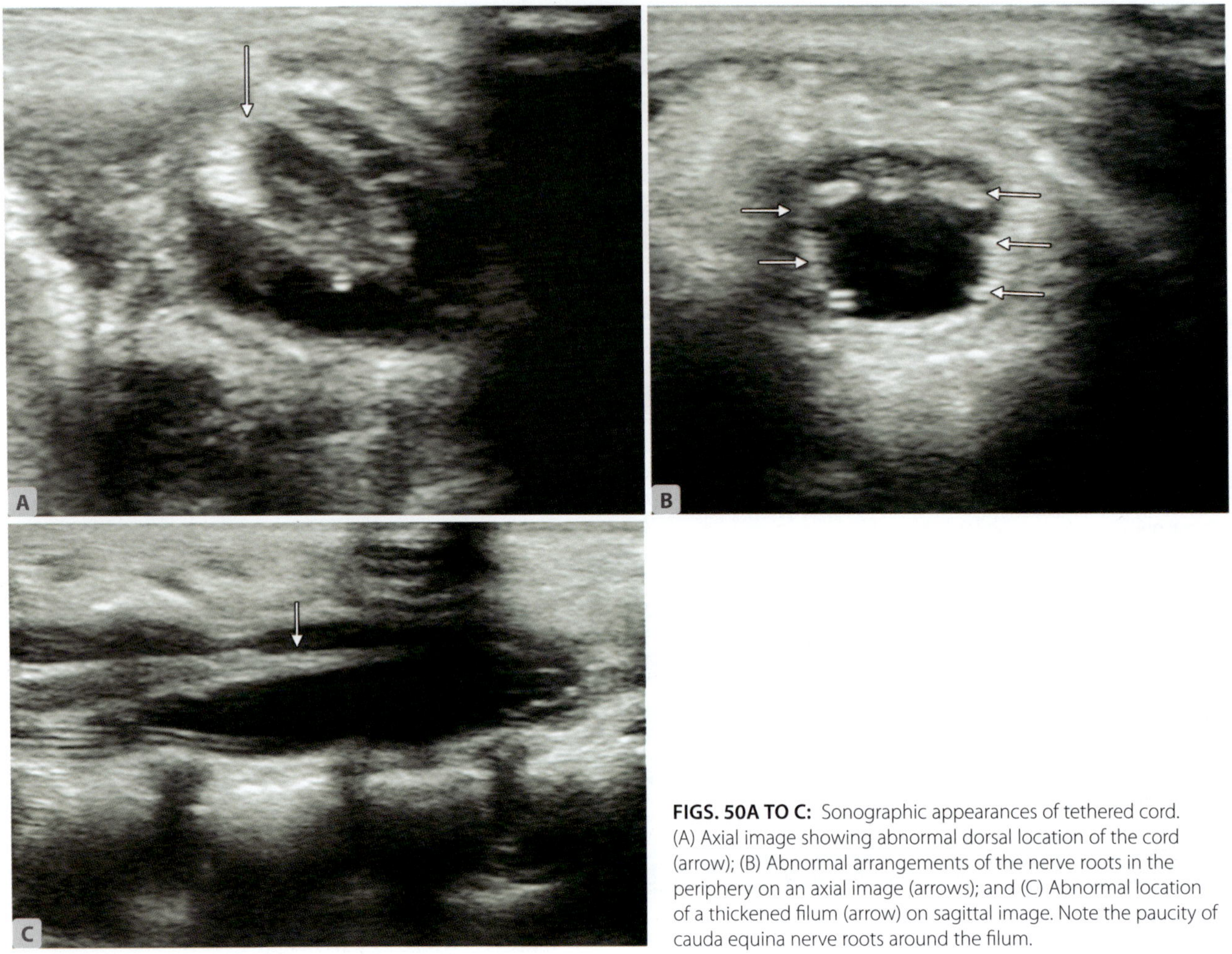

FIGS. 50A TO C: Sonographic appearances of tethered cord. (A) Axial image showing abnormal dorsal location of the cord (arrow); (B) Abnormal arrangements of the nerve roots in the periphery on an axial image (arrows); and (C) Abnormal location of a thickened filum (arrow) on sagittal image. Note the paucity of cauda equina nerve roots around the filum.

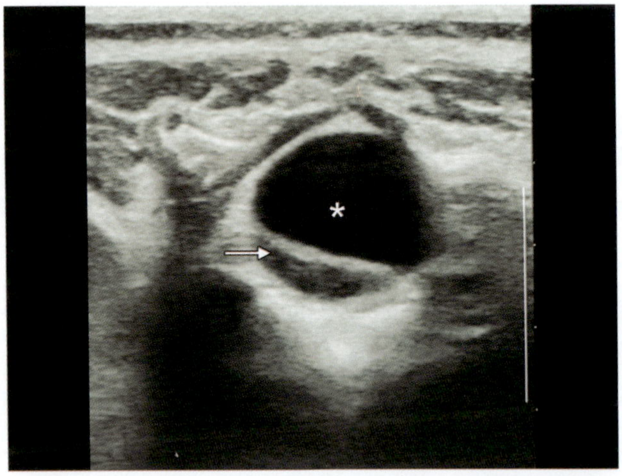

FIG. 51: Intradural arachnoid cyst: Axial image showing an anechoic lesion (asterisk) within the spinal canal causing compression of the spinal cord (arrow).

Other Indications

Real-time guidance for lumbar puncture is another indication of spinal USG. In infants younger than 6 months, when the spinous processes are not ossified, it may be difficult to decide the spinal level by palpation. In such cases, USG can guide puncture of the thecal sac and help avoid inadvertent injuries.[69]

CONCLUSION

Ultrasonography of neonatal and infantile spine is a useful investigation which can be used as a screening tool for closed spinal dysraphism, especially when there is lower back mass or skin stigmata. To the contrary, it is not recommended in open spinal dysraphism. With selection of proper transducer and following proper imaging technique, it can provide almost all clinically relevant information in closed spinal dysraphism.

REFERENCES

1. Gupta P, Sodhi KS, Saxena AK, Khandelwal N, Singhi P. Neonatal cranial sonography: a concise review for clinicians. J Pediatr Neurosci. 2016;11:7-13.
2. Bhat V, Bhat V. Neonatal neurosonography: a pictorial essay. Indian J Radiol Imaging. 2014;24:389-400.
3. James AC. Practical guide to neonatal cranial ultrasound (CrUS): basics. Paediatr Child Health. 2018;28:P424-30.
4. Meijler G. Neonatal Cranial Ultrasonography, 2nd edition. Berlin: Springer-Verlag; 2012.
5. Kaske TI, Rumack CM, Harlow CL. Neonatal and infant brain imaging. In: Rumack CM, Wilson SR, Charboneau JW, Levine D (Eds). Diagnostic Ultrasound: General Adult, 2nd edition. United States: Mosby; 1998. pp. 1443-501.
6. Jaspan T. The neonatal brain. In: Melre II, Cosgrove D, Dewbury K, Farrant P (Eds). Clinical Ultrasound: A Comprehensive Text, 2nd edition. London: Churchill Livingstone; 2001. pp. 1055-6.
7. Allison JW, Faddis LA, Kinder DL, Roberson PK, Glasier CM, Seibert JJ. Intracranial resistive index (RI) values in normal term infant during the first day of life. Pediatr Radiol. 2000;30:618-20.
8. Chadduck WM, Seibert JJ. Intracranial duplex Doppler: practical uses in pediatric neurology and neurosurgery. J Child Neurol. 1989;4:S77-86.
9. Farruggia S, Babcock DS. The cavum septi pellucidi: its appearance and incidence with cranial ultrasonography in infancy. Radiology. 1981;139:147-50.
10. Chen CY, Chen FH, Lee CC, Lee KW, Hsiao HS. Sonographic characteristics of the cavum velum interpositum. AJNR Am J Neuroradiol. 1998;19:1631-5.
11. Gupta JK, Cave M, Lilford RJ, Farrell TA, Irving HC, Mason G, et al. Clinical significance of fetal choroid plexus cysts. Lancet. 1995;346:724-9.
12. Grant EG, Schellinger D, Richardson JD, Coffey ML, Smirniotopoulous JG. Echogenic periventricular halo: normal sonographic finding or neonatal cerebral hemorrhage. AJR Am J Roentgenol. 1983;140: 793-6.
13. Hack M, Horbar JD, Malloy MH, Tyson JE, Wright E, Wright L. Very low birth weight outcomes of the National Institute of Child Health and Human Development Neonatal Network. Pediatrics. 1991;87:587-97.
14. Rumack CM, Drose JA. Neonatal and infant brain imaging. In: Rumack CM, Wilson SR, Charboneau JW, Johnson AM (Eds). Diagnostic Ultrasound, 3rd edition. United States: Mosby; 2005. pp. 1623-702.
15. Maller VV, Cohen HL. Neonatal Head Ultrasound: A Review and Update—Part 1: Techniques and Evaluation of the Premature Neonate. Ultrasound Q. 2019;35:202-11.
16. Volpe JJ. Intracranial hemorrhage: germinal matrix-intraventricular hemorrhage of the premature infant. In: Volpe JJ (Ed). Neurology of the Newborn, 5th edition. Philadelphia: Saunders; 2008. pp. 517-88.
17. Burstein J, Papile L, Burstein R. Subependymal germinal matrix and intraventricular hemorrhage in premature infants: diagnosis by CT. AJR Am J Roentgenol. 1977;128:971-6.
18. Kirks DR, Bowic JD. Cranial ultrasonography of neonatal periventricular/intraventricular hemorrhage: who, why, how, and when? Pediatr Radiol. 1986;16:114-9.
19. Guillerman RP. Infant Craniospinal Ultrasonography: Beyond Hemorrhage and Hydrocephalus. Semin Ultrasound CT MRI. 2010;31:71-85.
20. Babcock DS. Sonography of the brain in infants role in evaluating neurologic abnormalities. AJR Am J Roentgenol. 1995;165: 417-23.
21. Cooke RW. Early and late cranial ultrasonographic appearances and outcome in very low birth weight infants. Arch Dis Child. 1987;62:931-7.
22. Trounce JQ, Ratter N, Levene MI. Periventricular leucomalacia and intraventricular hemorrhage in preterm neonate. Arch Dis Child. 1986;61:1196-202.
23. Volpe JJ. Current concepts of brain injury in the premature infant. AJR Am J Roentgenol. 1989;153:243-51.
24. Taylor GA. Effect of germinal matrix hemorrhage on terminal vein position and patency. Pediatr Radiol. 1995;25:537-40.
25. Bergman I, Bauer RE, Barmada MA, Latchaw RE, Taylor HG, David R, et al. Intracerebral hemorrhage in the full-term neonatal infant. Pediatrics. 1985;75:486-96.
26. Chadha V, Mathur NB, Khaniju CM. Periventricular hemorrhage in term germinal matrix. Indian Pediatr. 1991;2:28.
27. Ahya KP, Suryawanshi P. Neonatal periventricular leukomalacia: current perspectives. Res Rep Neonatol. 2018;8:1-8.
28. Bano S, Chaudhary V, Garga UC. Neonatal Hypoxic-ischemic Encephalopathy: A Radiological Review. J Pediatr Neurosci. 2017;12:1-6.
29. Dammann O, Leviton A. Duration of transient hyperechoic images of white matter in very low birth weight infants: a proposed classification. Dev Med Child Neurol. 1997;39:2-5.
30. de Vries LS, Eken P, Dubowitz LM. The spectrum of leukomalacia using cranial ultrasound. Behav Brain Res. 1992;49:1-6.
31. Carey CM, Tullous MW, Walker ML. Hydrocephalus etiology, pathologic effects, diagnosis, and natural history. In: Cheek WR (Ed). Pediatric Neurosurgery, 3rd edition. Philadelphia: Saunders; 1994. pp. 189-201.
32. Brouwer MJ, de Vries LS, Pistorius L, Rademaker KJ, Groenendaal F, Benders MJ. Ultrasound measurements of the lateral ventricles in neonates: why, how, and when? A systematic review. Acta Paediatr. 2010;99:1298-306.
33. Winkler P. Color-coded echographic flow imaging and spectral analysis of cerebrospinal fluid (CSF) in infants. Part II. CSF-dynamics. Pediatr Radiol. 1992;22:31-42.
34. Seibert JJ, McCowan TC, Chadduck WM, Adametz JR, Glasier CM, Williamson SL, et al. Duplex pulsed Doppler US versus intracranial pressure in the neonate: clinical and experimental studies. Radiology. 1989;171:155-9.
35. Bada HS, Miller JE, Menke JA, Menten TG, Bashiru M, Binstadt D, et al. Intracranial pressure and cerebral arterial pulsatile flow measurements in neonatal intraventricular hemorrhage. J Pediatr. 1982;100:291-6.
36. Taylor GA, Phillips MD, Ichord RN, Carson BS, Gates JA, James CS. Intracranial compliance in infants evaluation with Dopper US. Radiology. 1994;191:787-91.
37. Branislav K. (2018). Cerebral Hemodynamics in Pediatric Hydrocephalus: Evaluation by Means of Transcranial Doppler Sonography. [online] Available from https://www.intechopen.com/books/highlights-on-hemodynamics/cerebral-hemodynamics-in-pediatric-hydrocephalus-evaluation-by-means-of-transcranial-doppler-sonography. [Last accessed September, 2020].
38. World Health Organization (WHO). (2019). Cranial ultrasonography. [online] Available from https://newbornwhocc.org/2019_pdf/Cranial_Ultrasonography-2019.pdf. [Last accessed September, 2020].
39. Wolpert EM, Barnes PD. Clinical principles in pediatric neuroradiology. In: Wolpert EM, Barnes PD (Eds). MRI in Pediatric Neuroradiology. Philadelphia: Mosby; 1992. pp. 41-80.
40. Soetaert AM, Lowe LH, Formen C. Pediatric cranial Doppler sonography in children: non-sickle cell applications. Curr Probl Diagn Radiol. 2009;38:218-27.
41. Bosemani T, Orman G, Boltshauser E, Tekes A, Huisman TA, Poretti A. Congenital abnormalities of the posterior fossa. Radiographics. 2015;35:200-20.
42. Kollias SS, Ball WAS. Congenital malformations of the brain. In: Bale JR (Ed). Pediatric Neuroradiology. Philadelphia: Lippincott-Raven; 1997. pp. 110-30.

43. Shuman WP, Rogers JV, Mack LA, Alvord EC, Christie DP. Real-time sonographic sector scanning of the neonatal cranium: technique and normal anatomy. AJR Am J Roentgenol. 1981;137:821-8.
44. Barr LL. Neonatal cranial ultrasound. Radiol Clin North Am. 1999;37:1127-46.
45. Tessler FN, Dion J, Viñuela F, Perrella RR, Duckwiller G, Hall T, et al. Cranial arteriovenous malformations in neonates: color Doppler imaging with angiographic correlation. AJR Am J Roentgenol. 1989;153:1027-30.
46. Pretorius DH, Russ PD, Rumack CM. Diagnosis of brain neuropathology in utero. In: Naidich WS, Quencer RM (Eds). Clinical Neurosonography. Berlin: Springer-Verlag; 1987.
47. Dublin AB, French BN. Diagnostic image evaluation of hydranencephaly and pictorally similar entities, with emphasis on computed tomography. Radiology. 1980;137:81-91.
48. Diebler C, Dulac D. Pediatric Neurology and Neuroradiology. Berlin: Springer-Verlag; 1987.
49. Han BK, Babcock DS, McAdams L. Bacterial meningitis in infants: sonographic findings. Radiology. 1985;154:645-50.
50. Chowdhary V, Gulati P, Sachdev A, Mittal SK. Pyogenic meningitis: sonographic evaluation. Indian Pediatr. 1991;28:749-55.
51. Das KM, Padmini P, Sachdeva S. Sonographic evaluation of intracranial abnormalities in neonates and infants. Indian J Radiol. 2013;1:193-8.
52. Ganeshan S, Dhawan SK, Mukherjee S. Ultrasound in infectious meningitis. Indian J Radiol. 1988;42:199-202.
53. Chowdhury V, Gulati P, Sachdev A. Sonography in pyogenic and tubercular meningitis: a comparative study. Indian J Radiol Imaging. 1991;1:7-10.
54. Epelman M, Daneman A, Blaser SI, Neira CO, Konen O, Jarrín J, et al. Differential diagnosis of intracranial cystic lesions at head US: correlation with CT and MR imaging. Radiographics. 2006;26: 173-96.
55. Dudink J, Steggerda SJ, Horsch S, eurUS.brain group. State-of-the-art neonatal cerebral ultrasound: technique and reporting. Pediatr Res. 2020;87:3-12.
56. Hwang M. Introduction to contrast-enhanced ultrasound of the brain in neonates and infants: current understanding and future potential. Pediatr Radiol. 2019;49:254-62.
57. Dick EA, Patel K, Owens CM, De Bruyn R. Spinal ultrasound in infants. Br J Radiol. 2002;75:384-92.
58. Nair N, Sreenivas M, Gupta AK, Kandasamy D, Jana M. Neonatal and infantile spinal sonography: a useful investigation often underutilized. Indian J Radiol Imaging. 2016;26:493-501.
59. Guggisberg D, Hadj-Rabia S, Viney C, Bodemer C, Brunelle F, Zerah M, et al. Skin markers of occult spinal dysraphism in children: a review of 54 cases. Arch Dermatol. 2004;140:1109-15.
60. Izci Y, Gonul M, Gonul E. The diagnostic value of skin lesions in split cord malformations. J Clin Neurosci. 2007;14:860-3.
61. Kriss VM, Desai NS. Occult spinal dysraphism in neonates: assessment of high-risk cutaneous stigmata on sonography. AJR Am J Roentgenol. 1998;171:1687-92.
62. Ozturk E, Sonmez G, Mutlu H, Sildiroglu HO, Velioglu M, Basekim CC, et al. Split-cord malformation and accompanying anomalies. J Neuroradiol. 2008;35:150-6.
63. Robinson AJ, Russell S, Rimmer S. The value of ultrasonic examination of the lumbar spine in infants with specific reference to cutaneous markers of occult spinal dysraphism. Clin Radiol. 2005;60:72-7.
64. Long FR, Hunter JV, Mahboubi S, Kalmus A, Templeton JM. Tethered cord and associated vertebral anomalies in children and infants with imperforate anus: evaluation with MR imaging and plain radiography. Radiology. 1996;200:377-82.
65. Medina LS, Crone K, Kuntz KM. Newborns with suspected occult spinal dysraphism: a cost-effectiveness analysis of diagnostic strategies. Pediatrics. 2001;108:E101.
66. Beek FJ, de Vries LS, Gerards LJ, Mali WP. Sonographic determination of the position of the conus medullaris in premature and term infants. Neuroradiology. 1996;38:S174-77.
67. Schumacher WE, Drolet BA, Maheshwari M, Horii KA, Nopper AJ, Newell BD, et al. Spinal dysraphism associated with the cutaneous lumbosacral infantile hemangioma: a neuroradiological review. Pediatr Radiol. 2012;42:315-20.
68. Drolet BA, Chamlin SL, Garzon MC, Adams D, Baselga E, Haggstrom AN, et al. Prospective study of spinal anomalies in children with infantile hemangiomas of the lumbosacral skin. J Pediatr. 2010;157:789-94.
69. Coley BD, Shiels WE, Hogan MJ. Diagnostic and interventional ultrasonography in neonatal and infant lumbar puncture. Pediatr Radiol. 2001;31:399-402.
70. Gerscovich EO, Maslen L, Cronan MS, Poirier V, Anderson MW, McDonald C, et al. Spinal sonography and magnetic resonance imaging in patients with repaired myelomeningocele: comparison of modalities. J Ultrasound Med. 1999;18:655-64.
71. Unsinn KM, Geley T, Freund MC, Gassner I. US of the spinal cord in newborns: spectrum of normal findings, variants, congenital anomalies, and acquired diseases. Radiographics. 2000;20:923-38.
72. American Institute of Ultrasound in Medicine (AIUM). (2016). AIUM Practice Parameter for the Performance of an Ultrasound Examination of the Neonatal and Infant Spine. [online] Available from https://www.aium.org/resources/guidelines/neonatalSpine.pdf. [Last accessed September, 2020].
73. Deeg KH, Lode HM, Gassner I. Spinal sonography in newborns and infants, part I: method, normal anatomy, and indications. Ultraschall Med. 2007;28:507-17.
74. Lowe LH, Johanek AJ, Moore CW. Sonography of the neonatal spine, part 1: normal anatomy, imaging pitfalls, and variations that may simulate disorders. AJR Am J Roentgenol. 2007;188:733-8.
75. Taveras JM, Ferrucci J, Dalinka M. Radiology: Diagnosis Imaging Intervention. Baltimore: Lippincott Williams & Wilkins; 2003.
76. DiPietro MA. The conus medullaris: normal US findings throughout childhood. Radiology. 1993;188:149-53.
77. Kesler H, Dias MS, Kalapos P. Termination of the normal conus medullaris in children: a whole-spine magnetic resonance imaging study. Neurosurg Focus. 2007;23:1-5.
78. Wilson DA, Prince JR. John Caffey Award: MR imaging determination of the location of the normal conus medullaris throughout childhood. AJR Am J Roentgenol. 1989;152:1029-32.
79. Zalel Y, Lehavi O, Aizenstein O, Achiron R. Development of the fetal spinal cord: time of ascendance of the normal conus medullaris as detected by sonography. J Ultrasound Med. 2006;25:1397-401.
80. Coleman LT, Zimmerman RA, Rorke LB. Ventriculus terminalis of the conus medullaris: MR findings in children. AJNR Am J Neuroradiol. 1995;16:1421-6.
81. Barkovich AJ. Normal development of the neonatal and infant brain, skull, and spine. In: Barkovich AJ. Pediatric Neuroimaging, 3rd edition. Philadelphia: Lippincott Williams & Wilkins; 2000. pp. 50-4.
82. Byrd SE, Darling CF, McLone DG. Developmental disorders of the pediatric spine. Radiol Clin North Am. 1991;29:711-52.
83. Lowe LH, Johanek AJ, Moore CW. Sonography of the neonatal spine: part 2, Spinal disorders. AJR Am J Roentgenol. 2007;188:739-44.
84. Hill CA, Gibson PJ. Ultrasound determination of the normal location of the conus medullaris in neonates. AJNR Am J Neuroradiol. 1995;16:469-72.
85. Selcuki M, Vatansever S, Inan S, Erdemli E, Bagdatoglu C, Polat A. Is a filum terminale with a normal appearance really normal? Childs Nerv Syst. 2003;19:3-10.
86. Leadman M, Seigel S, Hollenberg R, Caco C. Ultrasound diagnosis of neonatal spinal epidural hemorrhage. J Clin Ultrasound. 1988;16:440-2.
87. Nepal P, Sodhi KS, Saxena AK, Bhatia A, Singhi S, Khandelwal N. Role of spinal ultrasound in diagnosis of meningitis in infants younger than 6 months. Eur J Radiol. 2015;84:469-73.

CHAPTER

87

Infectious and Inflammatory Diseases of the Brain

Chirag Kamal Ahuja, Anuj Prabhakar, Paramjeet Singh

INTRODUCTION

Inflammatory disorders constitute a significant proportion of intracranial pathologies in children. Neuroinflammation may be a representation of response to a number of external and internal substrates namely infections, toxic metabolites, foreign elements, trauma, and as a result of autoimmunity. Microglial cells of the central nervous system (CNS) usually mediate this response. The blood–brain barrier distinctly blocks any infiltration of the CNS by immune cells, however its breach may initiate an immune response by extra CNS elements. Aimed at protecting the nervous system, the effect may, at times, initiate a widespread inflammation leading to local damage. The following chapter would highlight infections and other inflammatory disorders leading to changes in the brain along with their imaging manifestations.

NEUROINFECTIONS

Being a developing tropical nation, the major focus of medicine in pediatrics has been in the management of malnutrition and infections. Neuroinfections form a distinct category, which relies heavily on neuroimaging for diagnosis, prognosis, and follow-up of these patients. Role of imaging in CNS infections is to characterize the involvement of the various structures of the cranial cavity namely meninges, brain parenchyma, and cerebrospinal fluid (CSF) spaces to appropriately plan medical or surgical treatment. Imaging findings in unison with clinical and epidemiological considerations along with CSF analysis significantly facilitate diagnosis. The various imaging modalities available are computed tomography (CT) and magnetic resonance imaging (MRI). Other imaging modalities like fluorodeoxyglucose-positron emission tomography (FDG-PET) occasionally play a role.

Investigative Modalities

CT is often the first modality of investigation in CNS infection because patient often presents with nonspecific signs and symptoms such as fever or seizures. CT can depict the late parenchymal changes in supratentorial lesions and complications such as hydrocephalus very well. It also helps in ascertaining the origin as well as evolution of the infectious process. The adjoining bony structures are also better visualized namely the paranasal sinuses and middle ear cavity. CT serves well in segregating patients requiring urgent surgical management such as ventriculoperitoneal shunting, decompression for mass effect like in large abscesses, etc. The specific role of nonemergent CT comes in evaluation of calcifications such as in congenital Toxoplasmosis, Other Agents, Rubella, Cytomegalovirus, and Herpes Simplex (TORCH) infections and calcifications in parenchymal granulomas. However, as the CT findings in the early stage of infection are nonspecific and due to the limited resolution for peripheral and posterior fossa lesions, the evaluation of meningeal, cisternal, and infratentorial parenchymal lesions become difficult with contrast CT alone.

MRI plays a complementary role to the CT, but has now become the procedure of choice, wherever feasible and available, because of lack of bony artifacts and far superior soft-tissue resolution, which is clearly beneficial for visualizing the posterior fossa. MR clearly outscores CT for demonstrating small lesions, white matter, and meningeal pathologies. Advanced MR sequences often add tremendously to the imaging information. Diffusion-weighted imaging (DWI) is helpful in demonstrating complications of infections including abscess/empyema formation and changes of early ischemia and infarction. Other specialized sequences like proton MR spectroscopy and susceptibility-weighted imaging (SWI) help in providing an in vivo assessment of the biochemical changes within inflammatory lesions and the surrounding brain and the presence of hemorrhage/calcification/other susceptibility-inducing elements.[1] Yet there is considerable overlap between the various imaging findings, which may at times make specific diagnosis difficult. Laboratory data along with relevant CSF findings often help to reach a conclusive diagnosis.[2]

BACTERIAL INFECTIONS

Bacterial infection remains a major cause of morbidity and mortality in the pediatric population with long-term neurological sequelae. The most common form of acute bacterial CNS infection is meningitis (especially during the first 2 years of life) followed by intracranial abscesses and subdural and epidural empyemas. The various causative organisms are group B streptococci and *Escherichia coli* (first 2 weeks of life) and *Proteus mirabilis*, *Enterobacter cloacae*, *Klebsiella pneumonia*, and *Salmonella enteritidis* (infancy and childhood). **Table 1** highlights the age-wise etiology of meningitis in children.

Meningitis

The organisms resulting in meningitis reach and lodge in the meninges by one of these five routes:

1. Direct hematogenous spread
2. Passage through the choroid plexus
3. Rupture of superficial cortical abscesses
4. Penetrating trauma
5. Contiguous spread from the infected sinuses and middle ear

Except for rare occasions, the diagnosis of meningitis is made from clinical signs and symptoms and the results of lumbar puncture. Imaging in meningitis is not performed routinely other than to ensure the absence of hydrocephalus or abscess formation before a lumbar puncture is performed. Neuroimaging is indicated if the clinical diagnosis is unclear and if the meningitis is associated with persistent seizures or focal neurological deficit.[1] On cross-sectional imaging, thickened meninges showing continuous abnormal enhancement after contrast administration clinch the diagnosis of meningitis.[3] The enhancement can involve the dura-arachnoid complex (pachymeningitis) or pia and subarachnoid spaces (leptomeningitis). Contrast-enhanced MR is more sensitive imaging modality than contrast-enhanced CT in this regard **(Figs. 1A and B)**. Other imaging findings include inflammatory exudates in nonventricular CSF spaces especially along the convexity (clinical finding: tubercular meningitis where the exudates are more marked in the basal cisterns). They can be hypo-, iso-, or hyperdense on CT and may show variable enhancement. On MRI, purulent exudates of acute meningitis give appearance of "dirty" CSF, which may be better appreciated on fluid-attenuated inversion recovery (FLAIR) sequence. It may show diffusion restriction on DWI. Postcontrast T2 FLAIR and sometimes delayed contrast-enhanced T1-weighted image (T1WI) are better at depicting meningeal enhancement than routine postcontrast T1 scans. The major differential of bacterial meningitis is noninfectious meningitis including rheumatoid-related meningitis, IgG4-related disease, drug-related aseptic meningitis, and carcinomatous meningitis. Due to identical appearance on imaging, reliance on clinical and laboratory findings is often necessary.

Once the meningeal infection is established, neurological sequelae can be caused by a number of mechanisms. These include hydrocephalus, arteritis of penetrating cortical vessels leading to ischemic changes, brain abscess formation,

TABLE 1: Age-wise distribution of bacterial agents in meningitis.

First 2 weeks	3–6 weeks	7 weeks to 15 years	>15 years
Escherichia coli	*Streptococcus pneumoniae*	*Streptococcus pneumoniae*	*Streptococcus pneumoniae*
Enterococcus	*Haemophilus influenzae type b*	*Haemophilus influenzae type b*	*Neisseria meningitidis*
Group B *Streptococcus*	Group B *Streptococcus*	*Neisseria meningitidis*	*Streptococcus*
Listeria monocytogenes	*Neisseria meningitidis*	–	*Staphylococcus*
–	*Escherichia coli*	–	*Listeria monocytogenes*
–	*Listeria monocytogenes*	–	–

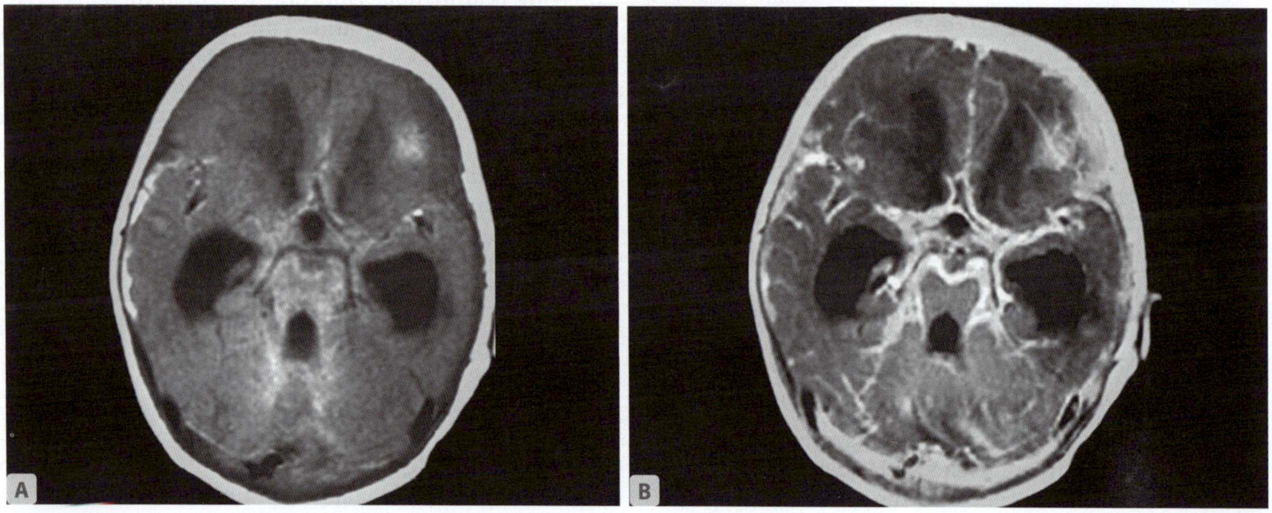

FIGS. 1A AND B: Meningitis: Noncontrast and contrast-enhanced short T1 MR sections showing intense leptomeningeal enhancement in case of meningitis.

subdural effusion, subdural empyema, ventriculitis, and venous thrombosis.

Hydrocephalus is demonstrated by all imaging modalities including ultrasound in the neonate. However, MR is most effective in localizing the level of obstruction, which is commonly of the extraventricular obstructive type.[4]

Subdural effusions are commonly encountered in meningitis, especially due to *Haemophilus influenzae (H. influenzae)*. Unlike empyemas, they are sterile reactive fluid collections over the frontal and temporal lobes. They are usually not surgically treated as they regress along with the meningitis. On CT scan, they appear isodense to CSF and may be slightly hyperintense to CSF on MR on T1- and T2-weighted sequences[5] **(Figs. 2A and B)**. They do not show diffusion restriction unlike subdural empyemas.

Subdural empyema **(Fig. 2C)** may occur as a complication of bacterial meningitis, especially associated with *Pneumococcus meningitis*. The reported incidence is 20% of all intracranial bacterial infections.[5] Apart from meningeal inflammation, the cause of empyema is spread of infection from the paranasal sinuses, middle ear, calvarial osteomyelitis, infection following shunt placement or craniotomy, or contamination of effusions. They are commonly located over the frontal lobes or close to the source of infection from the paranasal sinuses or middle ear.[6,7] On imaging studies, empyemas are seen as widening of extracerebral spaces which appear as hypo-/isodense crescentic or lentiform collection adjacent to the inner table **(Fig. 2C)**. On contrast administration (especially on CT), a thin curvilinear rim of enhancement is present demarcating the empyema. Mass effect may be evident with effacement of sulci, compression of ventricles, and midline shift. In infants, transfontanelle sonography using 7–10 MHz transducer will show empyemas as hyperechoic collections often with fibrinous strands and a thick hyperechoic inner membrane. Sterile effusion on the contrary appears anechoic.[7] On MR, there are no signal characteristics which can distinguish empyema from nonpurulent collections because they appear hyperintense to CSF on both T1- and T2-weighted images (T2WIs). However, as highlighted above, DWI can be a clincher. It is important to remember that any extra-axial collection associated with sinusitis, otitis, or orbital cellulitis is highly indicative of the presence of empyema. Empyemas are generally unilateral, however reactive effusion due to *H. influenzae* is usually bilateral.[7] Subdural empyema also needs to be differentiated from cystic hygroma (sterile, nonenhancing, nondiffusion-restricting subdural CSF collection secondary to an arachnoid tear) and chronic subdural hematoma (usually traumatic with susceptibility-weighted MRI aiding in differentiating due to "blooming" of the blood).

Ventriculitis **(Figs. 3A to C)** is the term for inflammation of the ependymal lining of one or more ventricles. The cause of ventriculitis is due to possible retrograde spread of infections from the basal cisterns or due to a rupture of a periventricular abscess or through the choroid plexus route. It may also be secondary to complications. In neonates, cranial sonography can demonstrate hyperechoic CSF or proteinaceous debris/septations **(Fig. 3A)**. On contrast-enhanced MR/CT, the ependymal lining of the ventricle shows smooth, thin, and linear mild-to-moderate enhancement which is pathognomonic of ventriculitis.[1,5] There may be ventricular encystment **(Fig. 3B)**. This should be differentiated from intraventricular spread of glioblastoma, primary CNS lymphoma or germinoma, or even metastases, which cause irregular nodular ependymal thickening and enhancement. There may be layering of dependent diffusion-restricting debris in the occipital horns **(Fig. 3C)**.

Venous thrombosis can affect deep veins, cortical veins, and dural venous sinuses as a complication of meningitis. Sinus thrombosis can be diagnosed on contrast-enhanced CT (CECT) as empty delta sign which is a triangle of decreased density in the posterior segment of the affected sinus.[5,8] On MR, acute thrombus is seen as hyperintensity on T1WI. Other than in the subacute phase, thrombi are sometimes

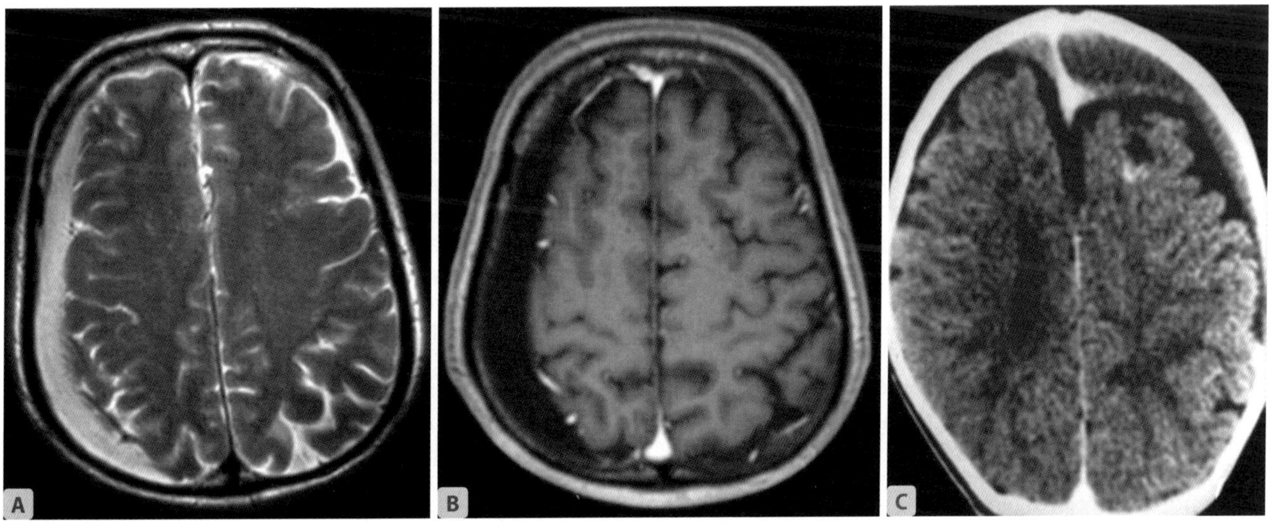

FIGS. 2A TO C: Sequelae of meningitis: Axial T2 (A) and postcontrast T1 (B) weighted MR images show right frontal subdural effusion in a patient of treated pyogenic meningitis isointense to cerebrospinal fluid (CSF) on both sequences; and (C) Subdural empyema appears as a extracerebral collection which is of higher density than ventricular CSF as observed on this contrast-enhanced CT scan.

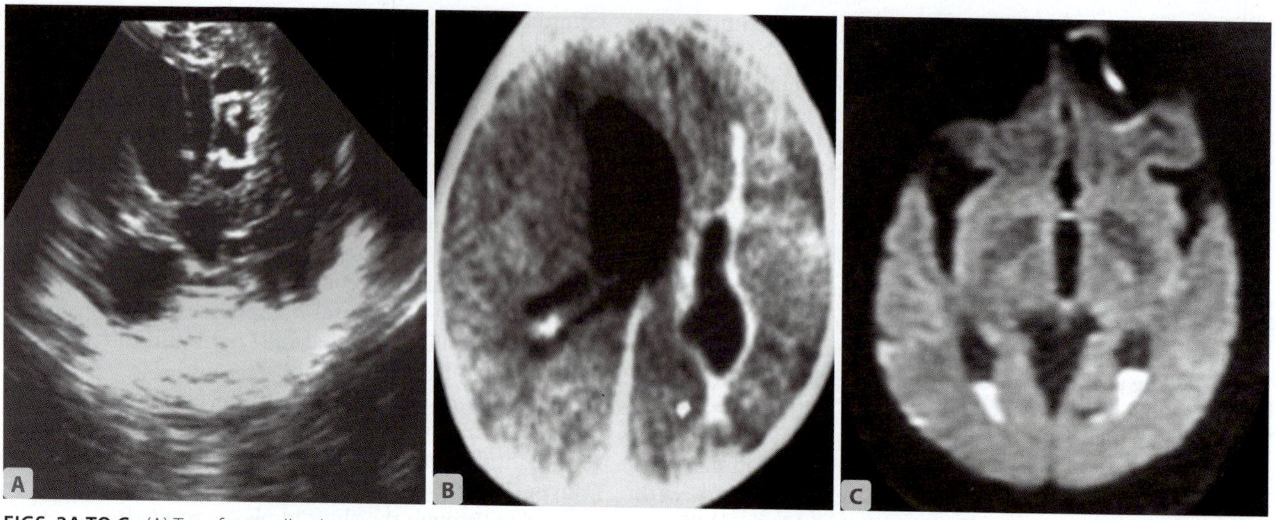

FIGS. 3A TO C: (A) Transfontanelle ultrasound showing increased echogenicity around the left lateral ventricle with internal septations suggesting ventriculitis; (B) Axial CT scan in another patient demonstrates ependymal enhancement as a hallmark of the same. Note contralateral ventricular dilatation due to obstruction of the foramen of Monro; (C) Axial diffusion-weighted MR image showing diffusion-restricting contents signifying pus in a patient of ventriculitis.

difficult to image.[1,5] However, a combination of appearance on FLAIR, DWI, SWI, and MR venography (MRV) usually increases the confidence of thrombus detection. MRV by phase-contrast technique is particularly useful in detecting venous thrombosis.[5] Venous infarcts resulting from cortical occlusions or venous sinus thrombosis result in signal changes in the subpial cortex and underlying white matter not conforming to an arterial distribution. There may be venous congestion and hemorrhage, restricted to the white matter or gray-white junction (clinical finding: cortical location of hemorrhage in the arterial infarct).

Arteritis occurs when the meningitis process spreads into perivascular space. The vessels exposed to the inflammatory exudates undergo thrombosis or spasm leading to arterial or venous infarctions. The arterial infarcts are seen as sharply demarcated areas corresponding to arterial territories on CT or MRI with diffusion restriction in the acute stage and gyriform enhancement in the subacute stage.[5]

Cerebritis and Brain Abscess

Cerebritis refers to inflammation of brain parenchyma as the initial manifestation of bacterial affliction of the brain. It is similar to encephalitis, a term conventionally used in viral involvement of the brain parenchyma. Cerebritis usually results from a direct spread of infection via the intracranial vessels through the otorhinologic route or meningitis or hematogenous route from a distant source (septic emboli). On imaging, it appears as an ill-defined heterogeneous area with nil to mild enhancement but appearing hyperintense on T2/FLAIR sequences. There may be patchy diffusion restriction. It eventually leads to formation of an abscess, if not appropriately contained by medical means. The common bacterial agents leading to abscess formation in immunocompetent patients are *Streptococcus*, *Staphylococcus*, and pneumococcal species. *Enterobacter* and *Klebsiella* are some other occasional organisms.[9]

Abscess implies encapsulated pus within the brain parenchyma due to coalescence of necrosis within the area of cerebritis. Most often brain abscess is solitary, but can be multiple in approximately 11–14% of cases and are usually secondary to cyanotic heart disease or middle ear infections. Infratentorial abscesses alone or in association with supratentorial abscesses are invariably otogenic in origin **(Figs. 4A and B)**. Overall, frontal and parietal lobes are the most common sites for abscess formation. Cross-sectional imaging helps in the diagnosis, localization, and in detecting complications of cerebral abscesses.

The evolution to abscess is a continuous process with eventual formation of a collagen capsule around the necrotic core. The transition from cerebritis stage to complete abscess formation has been characterized by four stages:

1. *Stage I (early cerebritis/focal suppurative encephalitis) (3–5 days)* consists of an inflammatory infiltrate of polymorphonuclear cells, lymphocytes, and plasma cells within the brain parenchyma with edema and petechial hemorrhages around this infiltrate.
2. *Stage II (late cerebritis/focal suppurative encephalitis with confluent central necrosis)* this is a stage (5–10 days) when focal necrosis of the brain becomes better defined. Encapsulation begins as vessels proliferate around the necrotic area with increasing deposition of reticulin, inflammatory cells, and minimal amount of collagen.
3. *Stage III (early capsule formation) (10–14 days)* is characterized by walling off the necrotic area by increasing deposition of collagen and reticulin. The capsule is better delineated than stage II. The surrounding edema tends to regress with partial resolution of the cerebritis.
4. *Stage IV (late capsule formation) (2–8 weeks)* is a stage when the encapsulation of the abscess by collagen deposition is complete. The abscess is well-defined and smaller than stage III. The wall is better delineated and thicker toward the cortex than medially toward the ventricles, possibly due to the increased vascularity of the

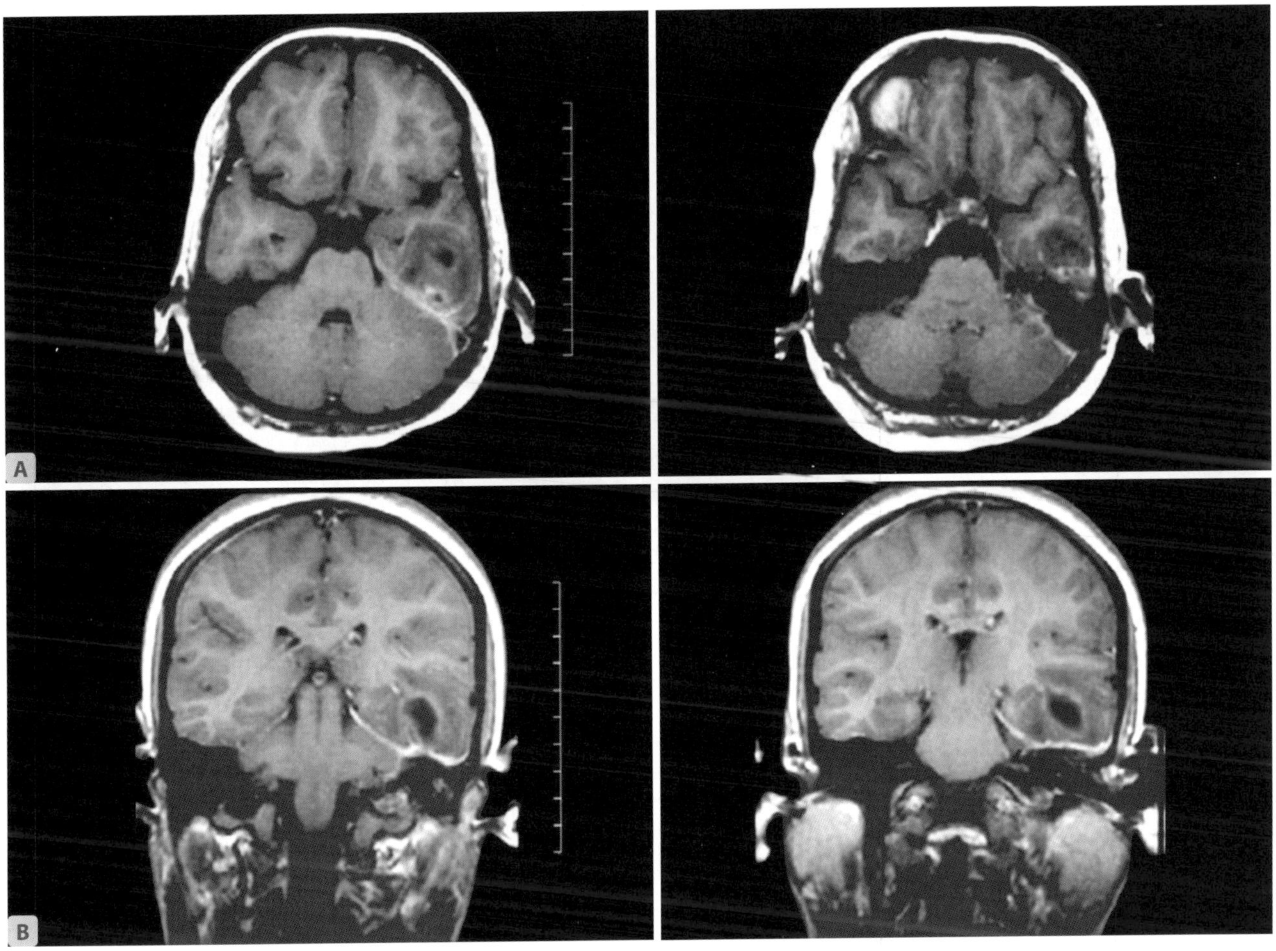

FIGS. 4A AND B: Otogenic brain abscess: Axial and coronal contrast-enhanced T1-weighted image (T1WI) showing enhancement within the middle ear cavity and there is enhancement of the leptomeninges over the petrous temporal bone. An ill-defined mixed intensity mass with peripheral rim-enhancing lesion is present in the overlying temporal lobe which is suggestive of an evolving brain abscess.

gray matter.[1,8] Daughter abscesses become apparent at this stage. Most patients present in the late cerebritis or stage of late capsule formation.[10,11]

The imaging features mirror the evolutionary stages of abscess formation **(Figs. 5A and B)**. On noncontrast CT (NCCT) scan, abscess appears hypodense with a barely discernible hyperdense wall. On contrast administration, the capsule or the wall of the abscess enhances usually measuring 5 mm or less in thickness. There is surrounding edema.[8]

On MR, all four stages can be recognized.[1,12] Stage I is heterogeneous on T1- and T2WI with patchy enhancement after contrast injection. In stage II, the abscess wall can be recognized as a hyperintense rim on T1WI. On T2WI, the rim is hypointense. Contents of the abscess are heterogeneous on both sequences. Abscess wall is shown to be thicker in stage II than stages III and IV. The abscess wall enhances moderately in this stage. Contents of the abscess may also show patchy enhancement with punctate areas of "blooming" on gradient recalled echo/susceptibility-weighted images and moderate-to-intense diffusion restriction on DWI. In stage III, the abscess wall will be hyperintense on both T1- and T2W sequences. Contents of the abscess are uniformly hypointense on T1WIs and hyperintense on T2WIs and abscess wall will enhance after contrast administration. The rim is thin, complete, and smooth with a "double rim" sign (outer hypointense and inner hyperintense relative to cavity contents) seen in 75% of cases on T2W and susceptibility-weighted MRI.[13] Stage IV abscesses show isointense walls on T1WI which are hypointense on T2WI. Contents of the abscess are iso-/hypointense on T1WI and hyperintense on T2WI; abscess walls enhance after contrast administration. Changes in the signal intensities in the wall of the abscess are believed to be reflecting the decreasing free water in the collagenous tissue.[12] The abscess cavity gradually collapses while the capsule thickens giving a "crenulated" appearance.

Role of proton MR spectroscopy lies in differentiation of abscesses from tumors.[14-17] Tumors show presence of choline peak with increased choline/creatinine and choline/N-acetylaspartate (NAA) ratios whereas abscesses show amino acids (0.9 ppm), lactate (1.3 ppm), acetate (1.9 ppm), and succinate (2.4 ppm) in the necrotic core. Attempts have been made to categorize MR spectral patterns with respect to underlying etiologic agents.[18] Presence of succinate and/or acetate signal resonances in addition to lipid/lactate and amino acids indicates infection by obligate anaerobes. Most obligate aerobes or facultative anaerobes show presence of lactate and amino acids, with or without lipids.[19]

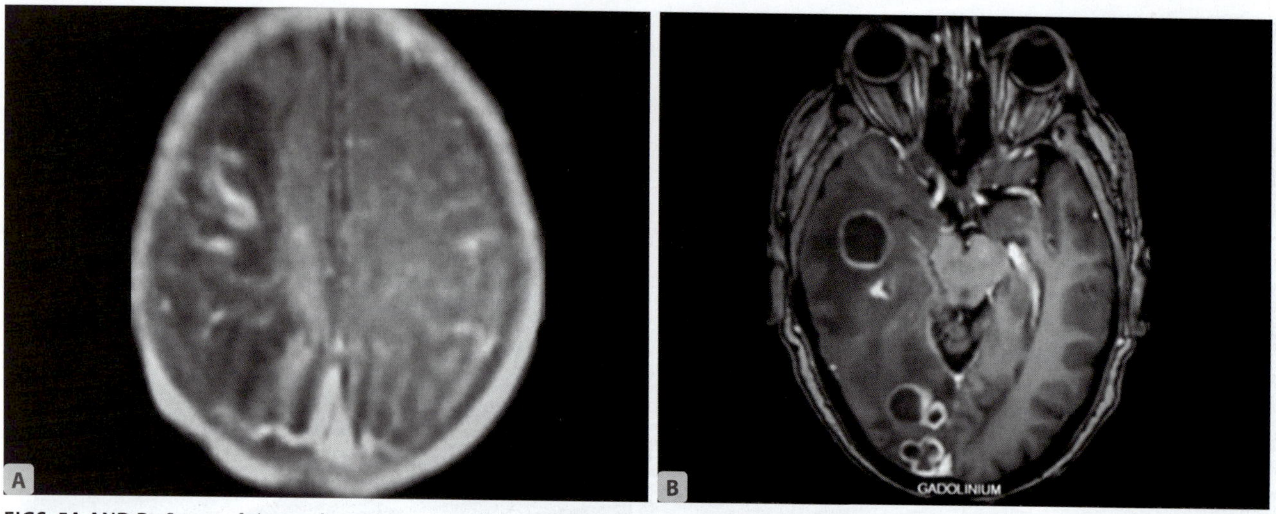

FIGS. 5A AND B: Stages of abscess formation: Axial gadolinium-enhanced MRI sections from different patients show (A) an area of cerebritis in the right frontal lobe and multiple abscesses with smooth capsule formation in right temporo-occipital lobe (B).

Complications of brain abscess include extension of the abscess into the ventricular system leading to ventriculitis and subarachnoid spaces leading to purulent leptomeningitis. Daughter abscesses may develop when due to poorly developed capsule, abscess ruptures into the adjacent parenchyma.

Cranial Tuberculosis

Central nervous system tuberculosis (TB) is of grave socioeconomic concern in developing countries.[20] CNS involvement occurs in 2–5% of all TB patients and in 10–19% of those with acquired immunodeficiency syndrome (AIDS)-related TB.[21,22] Coexistent pulmonary TB is often seen in 25–83% of cases of CNS TB. Adult TB is most often a postprimary infection whereas most cases in children are due to primary infection.[23]

The causative organisms belong to the *Mycobacterium* genus are rod-shaped, acid-fast bacilli of three subtypes of which *Mycobacterium tuberculosis* accounts for 98% of CNS TB. Atypical *Mycobacterium* constitutes the rest and *Mycobacterium leprae* virtually never involves CNS. CNS TB starts as a "rich" focus of tubercular bacilli in the subpial or subependymal surface of the brain. This focus ruptures into the subarachnoid space to cause meningitis and vasculitis. Intracranial TB manifests in three forms, viz., isolated meningeal involvement, isolated parenchymal form, and compound parenchymal/meningeal lesions.

Tuberculous Meningitis

Tuberculous meningitis (TBM) is the most common form of presentation of CNS TB in children in India constituting to about 75–80% of all cases. Two distinct pathogenetic mechanisms are believed to play a role in its causation. The more widely proposed method is thought to be rupture of a subependymal or subpial focus (Rich focus) into the CSF. The other involves direct penetration of meningeal vessel walls by hematogenous spread from a distant source (gastrointestinal or pulmonary).[23] Incidence of TBM is directly proportional to the prevalence of endemic TB. The diagnostic criteria of TBM on imaging are:[24]

- Enhancing basal exudates
- Progressive hydrocephalus
- Infarction in the striate cortex

Basal Exudates

In TBM, there is a thick, gelatinous exudate around the brainstem, extending into the basal cisterns and into the sylvian fissures **(Figs. 6A and B)**. NCCT scan or T1W MR images show these exudates as isodense (isointense) or hypodense (hypointense) areas in the basal cisterns.[1] Intense enhancement occurs after intravenous contrast administration **(*see* Figs. 1A and B)**. Exudates can be easily overlooked on T2W MR images because they will appear hyperintense similar to CSF and may not be clearly distinguishable from it.[23] The degree of involvement of meninges over the convexities and in the depth of sulci are better appreciated on MR than on CT. Meningeal enhancement can extend over the cerebral hemispheres with epicenter in the basal cisterns. There may also be an extension to involve the ventricular surface referred to as ependymitis. It has been seen that gadolinium-enhanced FLAIR is more sensitive in depicting meningeal enhancement than the standard T1W MRI. Rarely, there may be pachymeningeal involvement with focal thickening of the dura. Bhargava et al.[25] have graded the exudates as mild (+), moderate (++), and severe (+++). In mild grade, the cisterns are obliterated, but do not enhance; in moderate grade, increased attenuations are seen outlining the obliterated cisterns and in severe grade, there are copious and dense exudates with increased attenuation, filling, and enlarging the cisterns. In their study, this grading had a prognostic significance. Patients with severe degree of exudates had a longer duration of illness and carried a higher incidence of morbidity and mortality. Severe grade of exudates were seen to occur mostly in children. Carcinomatous meningitis is a close differential, which often

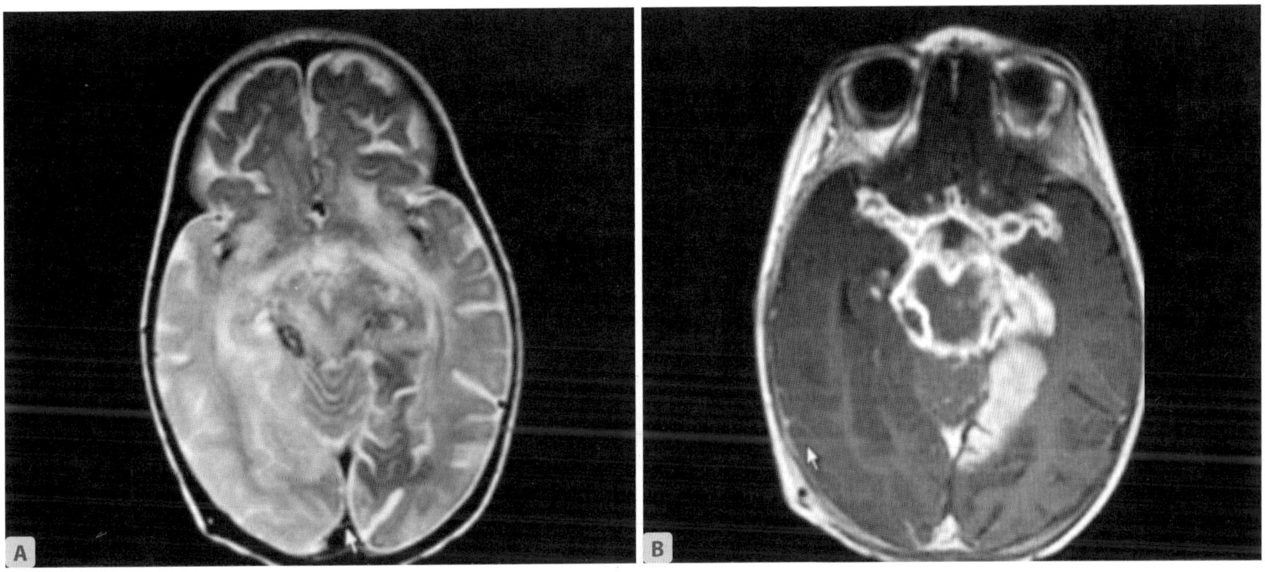

FIGS. 6A AND B: Tubercular meningitis: Axial T2 (A) and postcontrast T1 (B) weighted images demonstrating dense basal meningeal exudates and enhancement with left posterior cerebral artery (PCA) territory infarct secondary to meningovasculitis.

gives a "molten wax" appearance in a contextual clinical setting.

Cerebrospinal fluid analysis typically shows pleocytosis with low glucose and raised protein levels. Elevated adenosine deaminase (ADA) levels and polymerase chain reaction (PCR)/GeneXpert help in early detection when the other parameters are equivocal.

Cranial nerve involvement is seen in up to 30% cases of TBM. The commonly affected ones are optic nerve (opticochiasmatic arachnoiditis) and cranial nerves III, IV, and VII. MRI shows them to be enlarged with enhancement on postcontrast images.

Hydrocephalus

Communicating hydrocephalus is most commonly observed due to obstruction of flow of CSF by the exudates in the basal cisterns (e.g., suprasellar cisterns, ambient cisterns) and over the cerebral convexities and is therefore of the extraventricular obstructive type. Uncommonly, obstruction of the aqueduct by exudates or adjoining tuberculomas or ventricular entrapment by granulomatous ependymitis may result in intraventricular obstructive/noncommunicating hydrocephalus. Presence of hydrocephalus may precede the obliteration of basal cisterns by several weeks and is frequently associated with poor prognosis, especially in children. Presence of periventricular ooze suggests high-pressure hydrocephalus. The progress of hydrocephalus can be followed-up by sequential CT scans. The incidence of hydrocephalus increases with the duration of disease.[25-27]

Infarction

Inflammatory changes in arteries and veins result in meningovasculitis leading to formation of thrombi, which in turn cause multiple infarcts **(Figs. 6A and B)**. These vascular complications occur in 20–50% of cases.[28] These inflammatory changes may be caused by direct involvement by the bacilli or due to adjoining arachnoiditis or secondarily by reactive endarteritis leading to small vessel occlusions. The middle cerebral artery territory is the most common area where infarcts due to meningeal TB occur. Involvement of the perforating vessels arising from circle of Willis is common and it results in infarcts of the basal ganglia. The areas supplied by the medial striate and thalamoperforating arteries are specially affected in TBM and are termed as the medial TB zone as opposed to the area supplied by the lateral striate, anterior choroidal, and thalamogeniculate arteries which is termed the lateral ischemic stroke zone.[27-30] Infarcts appear as low density regions on CT and as areas of prolonged T1 and T2 relaxation time on MR. Apart from the regions described above, infarcts can also occur in the cerebral cortex due to involvement of cortical vessels but these are less common. Vessel wall MRI serves very well to document the involvement of the vessels with demonstration of nodular or granular lesions, related thickness and prominent enhancement in the wall, and lumen narrowing or occlusion.[31]

Detection of ischemic infarcts by MR is significantly higher as compared with CT.[32] MRI also helps in differentiating cerebritis from infarction. Infarction will appear bright with matching area of decreased signal on apparent diffusion coefficient (ADC) map on DWI. It is important to note that early cerebritis and infarction both appear as areas of increased signal intensity on conventional MR sequences however, cerebritis will, in time, evolve into an abscess and arterial infarction will confirm to distinct topographical lesion corresponding to arterial territories.[2] In addition, a large number of these infarcts are hemorrhagic in nature on MR finding which has not been well-documented on CT scans. MR angiography may be a useful modality in follow-up of patients with vasculitis secondary to TBM. The findings are similar to those seen on autopsy or conventional angiogram and consist of a triad of narrowing of the arteries at the base of the brain, narrowed or occluded small or medium-sized arteries associated with early draining veins, and wide sweep of pericallosal arteries secondary to hydrocephalus.[27-30]

Parenchymal Tuberculous Granulomas

Tuberculous granuloma (tuberculoma) is the most common form of parenchymal lesion.[24] Granulomas of TB occur at all ages. These may be solitary or more commonly multiple **(Figs. 7 and 8)**. Infratentorial lesions are more common in children.[33,34] Parenchymal tuberculomas appear as multiple conglomerate punctate or ring-enhancing lesions at the junction of gray and white matter.

On CT scan, tuberculomas appear as low- or high-density ring lesions which are rounded or lobulated and enhance after contrast administration. The walls of these ring lesions are irregular and of varying thickness. There is moderate to marked perilesional edema frequently seen with parenchymal tuberculomas.[35,36] One-third of patients may display a "target sign" which appears as central calcification or focal enhancement surrounded by a region of hypodensity and peripheral ring enhancement. This, however, is not pathognomonic.[37]

MR features of individual tuberculomas are dependent on whether the lesion is noncaseating, caseating with a solid center (solid caseation), or caseating with a liquid center (liquid caseation)[36] **(Table 2)**.

The noncaseating granuloma is hypointense on T1WI and hyperintense on T2WI. On contrast administration, the lesion usually shows homogeneous nodular enhancement **(Figs. 7A to D)**. The caseating granuloma with a solid center **(Figs. 8A and B)** appears hypointense to isointense on T1WIs and isointense to hypointense on T2WIs. The wall of the caseating TB granuloma often has a striking hypointense rim on T2WI, which enhances on administration of gadolinium. In vivo proton MR spectroscopy has shown presence of lipids in caseating granulomas, which characterizes this lesion.

Caseating granulomas with central liquefaction of caseous material appear hypointense on T1WI and hyperintense on T2WI with a peripheral hypointense rim on T2WI **(Figs. 8C and D)**. Enhancement of the rim occurs after gadolinium administration as in the granulomas with a solid center and is indistinguishable from pyogenic abscess on the imaging characteristics.

Differential diagnosis of parenchymal tuberculoma includes cysticercosis, pyogenic and fungal lesions, and foci of primary or metastatic neoplasia. Ring-enhancing lesions on CT in patients presenting with epilepsy present a diagnostic dilemma since granulomas of cysticercus and TB both have similar morphological appearances.

Rajshekhar et al.[38] have reported that it is possible to distinguish between solitary cysticercus granuloma and

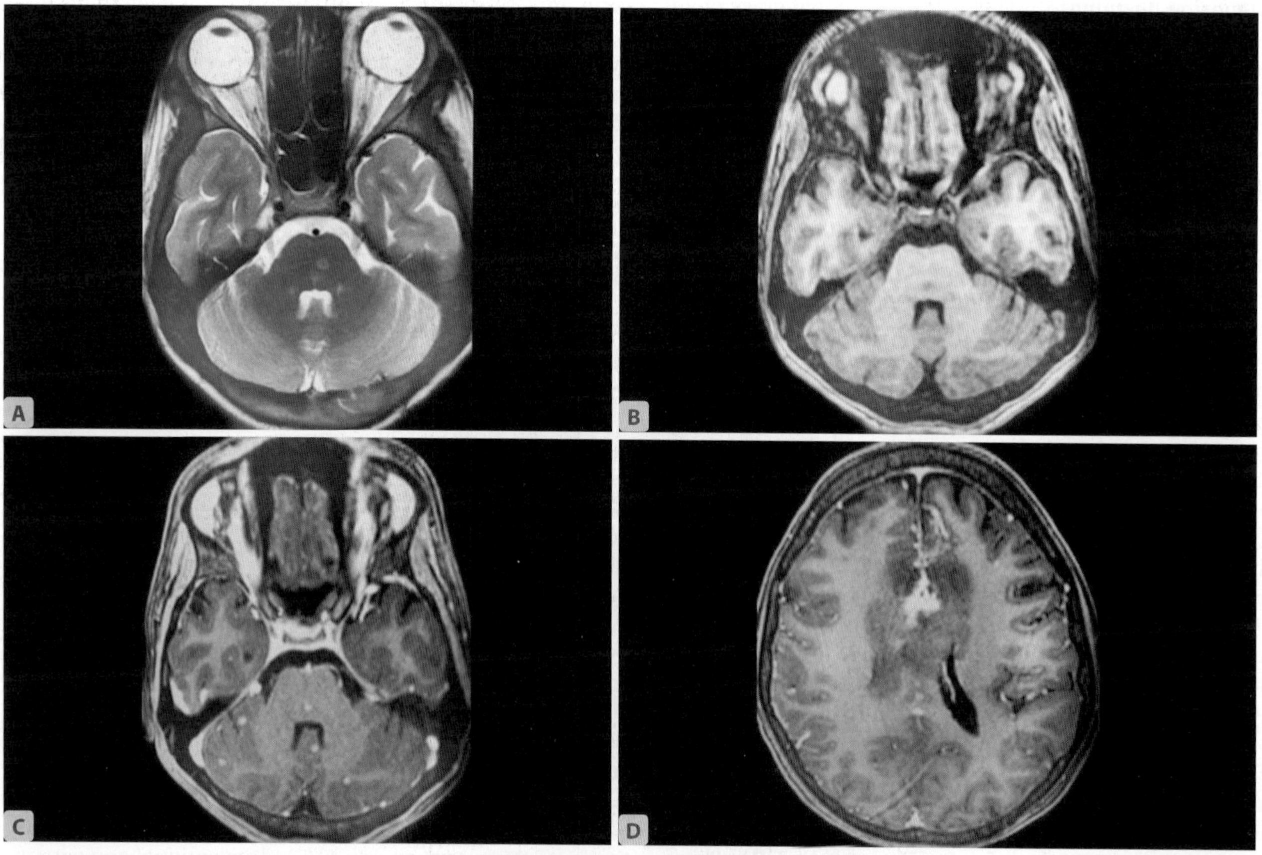

FIGS. 7A TO D: Noncaseating tuberculous granulomas: Axial T2W (A), non-contrast T1W (B) and post contrast T1W (C) MR images reveal multiple focal nodular enhancing lesions in the brainstem and cerebellar hemispheres suggesting granulomas. There is en-plaque meningeal based enhancing lesion along the anterior inter-hemispheric fissure (D) consistent with en-plaque tuberculoma in the same patient.

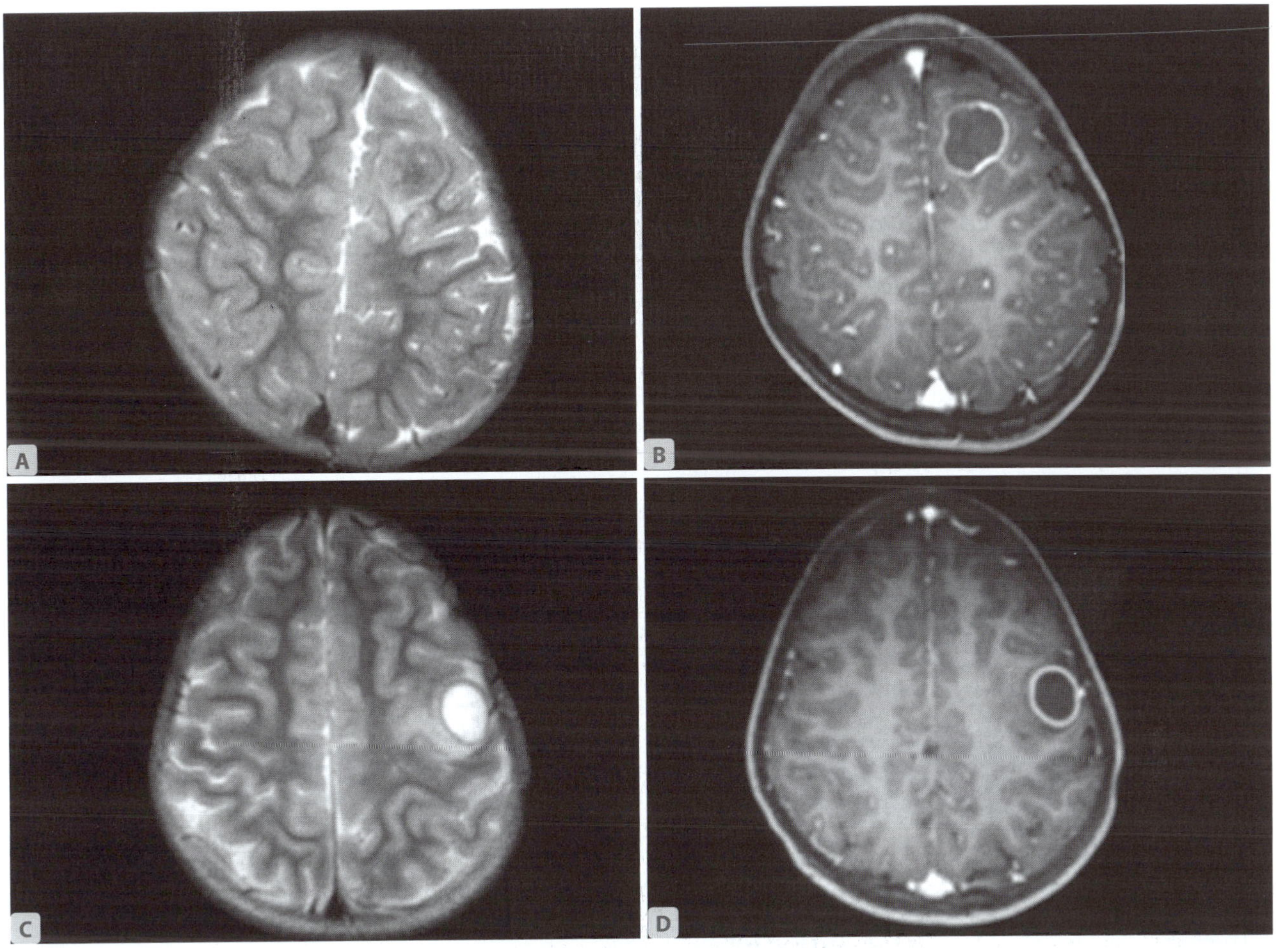

FIGS. 8A TO D: Tuberculous granuloma: Axial T2 (A and C) and postcontrast T1 (B and D) weighted MR images reveal T2-hypointense peripherally enhancing solid caseating tubercular granuloma (A and B) and T2-hyperintense rim-enhancing liquid caseating tubercular granuloma (C and D).

TABLE 2: MRI characteristics of intracranial tuberculoma.

Tuberculoma	T1WI	T2WI	Contrast-enhanced T1
Noncaseating	Hypointense	Hyperintense	Homogeneous nodular enhancement
Solid caseation	Hypo- to isointense core	Iso- to hypointense core with hypointense rim	Smooth ring enhancement
Liquid caseation	Hypointense	Hyperintense with hypointense rim	Smooth ring enhancement (resembling abscess)

(MRI: magnetic resonance imaging; T1WI: T1-weighted image; T2WI: T2-weighted image)

tuberculous granuloma in patients presenting with seizures on the basis of clinical signs and radiological (CT) findings. In patients with tuberculoma, there is evidence of raised intracranial tension with progressive neurological deficit. On CT scanning, the size of ring-enhancing lesion is usually >20 mm. Some of these may show irregular outlines, most of them cause midline shift. In contrast to this, neurocysticercus granuloma is <20 mm in size, rounded or oval in outline, and appears as disks or rings. There is no significant mass effect. These findings based on the size and shape of lesions in their study that had a specificity of 100% and 96%, respectively. They have also stressed the role of repeat CT scans after 8–12 weeks of anticonvulsant therapy to rule out enlarging lesions, which could be due to different etiologies. They advocated that all lesions >20 mm should be biopsied to reach definitive diagnosis. Lately, however, thin-section heavily T2W MR sequences have changed the imaging dimensions of a granuloma. The depiction of scolex has become the sine qua non of a cysticercus granuloma, which is characteristically absent in a tuberculoma. Coalescence which was considered a characteristic of a tuberculoma is now questioned as many cysticercus cysts give appearance of lesion conglomeration but are actually communicating with each other.

MR spectroscopy has also being playing a consistent role in distinguishing tuberculomas from pyogenic abscesses. Intracranial tuberculomas on proton MR spectroscopy primarily show peaks from lipids at 0.9 ppm and 1.3 ppm **(Figs. 9A to F)**.[39] The major difference between spectra of tuberculomas and pyogenic abscess is that although lipid and lactate peaks are found in both conditions, additional amino acid, acetate, and succinate peaks are more commonly seen in pyogenic abscesses as discussed above **(Figs. 10A to C)**.[40] Morales et al. have described a spectroscopy peak at 3.8 ppm as specific to tuberculoma helpful in differentiating it from malignant tumors.[41]

Compound Parenchymal and Meningeal Tuberculosis

Meningeal and meningocerebral forms of tuberculous pathology of the brain can coexist and in one series, they are the least common of all presentations.[35]

Rare presentation of intracranial TB includes tuberculous abscess and miliary TB. In general, true abscess formation is uncommon in CNS TB. Tuberculous abscess may be found more frequently in adults and immunocompromised patients.[33] Children are less commonly affected. Tuberculous abscess as opposed to tubercular granuloma is composed of pus teeming with tubercular bacilli which are few or absent in the latter. Tuberculous abscess is thin-walled **(Figs. 9A to F)**. Walls are smooth and regular in thickness and indistinguishable from pyogenic abscesses on CT and MR, although tuberculous abscesses are often multiloculated. Response to chemotherapy is variable, as TB abscesses may not resolve and may have to be treated surgically.[42-44]

Miliary tuberculomas in the brain may be a feature of generalized miliary TB and the primary focus may be

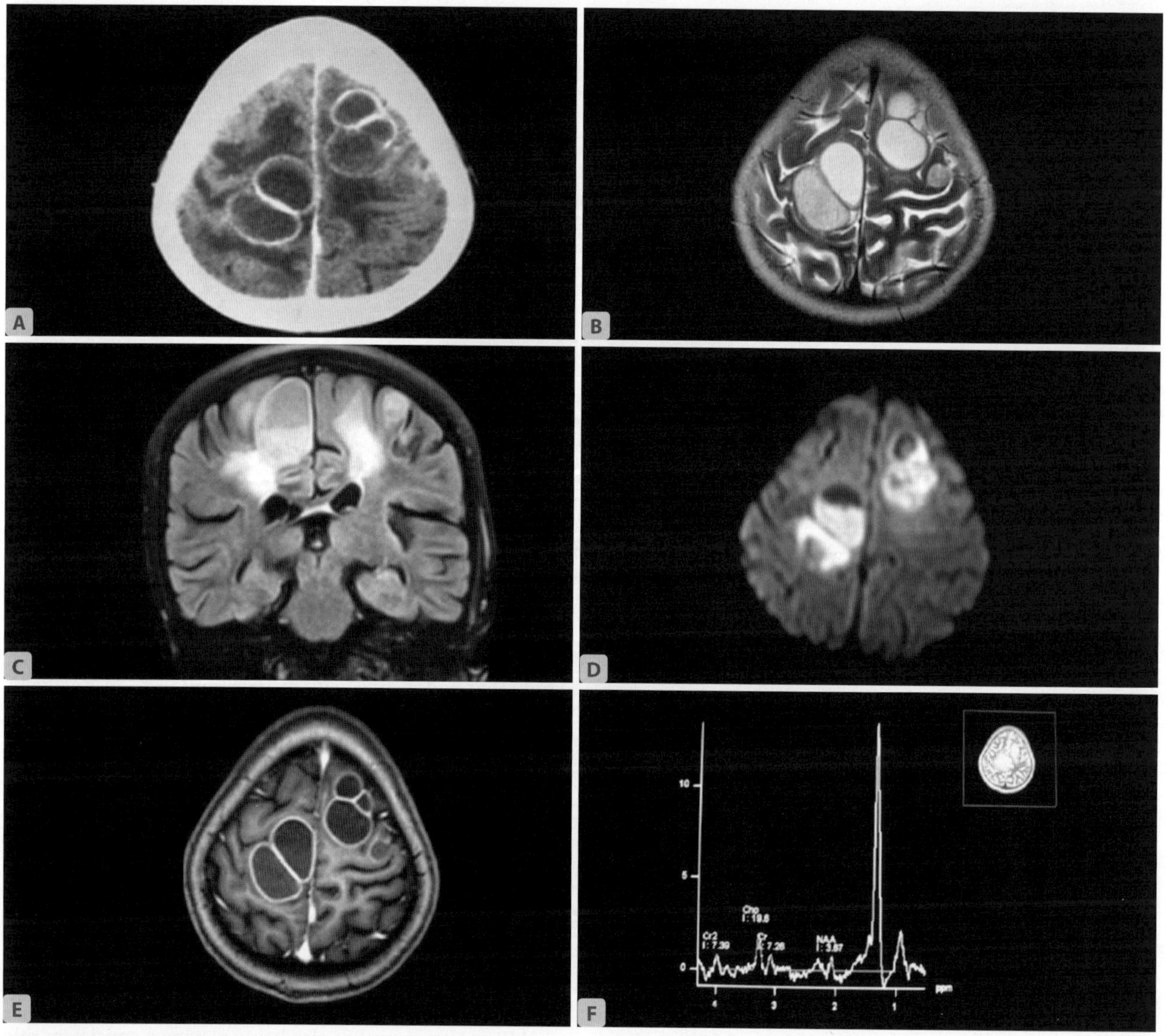

FIGS. 9A TO F: An 11-year-old child with multiple tubercular abscesses on antitubercular therapy. (A) CECT; (B) T2WI; (C) FLAIR; (D) DWI; and (E) CEMR images showing multiple conglomerate ring-enhancing lesions in bilateral high frontoparietal lobes. Few of these lesions are showing restriction on DWI suggestive of partially treated lesions. Single voxel MR spectroscopy done at TE = 30 showing lipid peak at 1.3 ppm (F). (CECT: contrast-enhanced computed tomography; CEMR: contrast-enhanced magnetic resonance; DWI: diffusion-weighted imaging; FLAIR: fluid-attenuated inversion recovery; T2WI: T2-weighted image; TE: echo time)

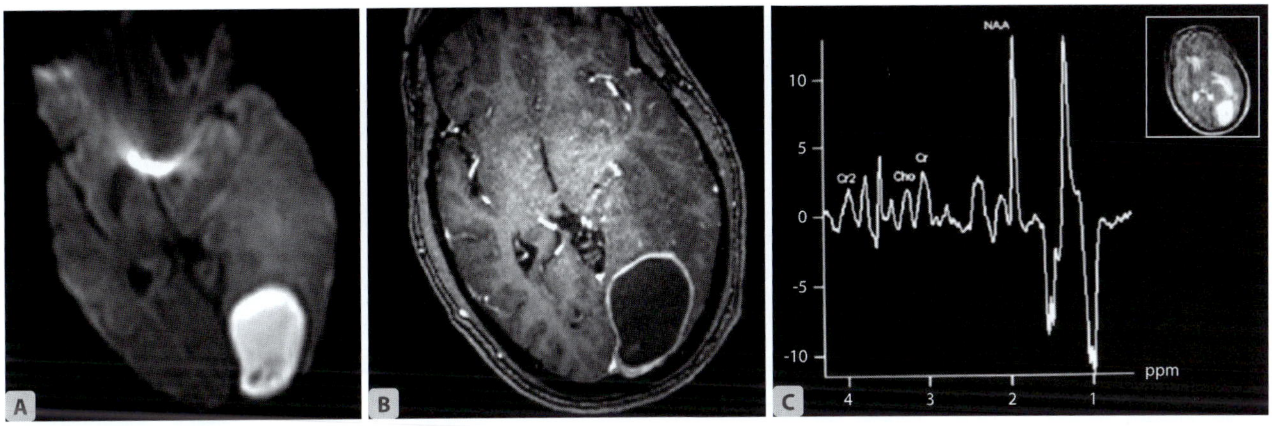

FIGS. 10A TO C: (A) The DW image shows restriction in the cavity of the lesion; (B) Pyogenic abscess in left occipital lobe; and (C) Single voxel MR spectroscopy of pyogenic abscess at TE 30 shows lipid lactate peak at 1.3 ppm and presence of acetate (1.9 ppm) and succinate (2.4 ppm) peaks. (DW: diffusion-weighted; TE: echo time)

found in the lung or elsewhere. They are distributed in the gray-white matter junction and in the distribution of the perforating vessels. They appear on CT as small round homogeneously enhancing lesions in the supra- and infratentorial compartments. On MR, they appear as high-intensity foci throughout the brain on T2WI. There is usually associated TBM. Their appearance may rarely precede the onset of meningitis. If treatment is successful, the lesions may disappear. Paradoxical response to treatment may occur with the lesions increasing in size and new lesions appearing during the course of therapy.[45,46]

Neurocysticercosis

Pediatric neurocysticercosis should be considered an endemic disease in the third world countries. It assumes significance in the wake of its presentation in the form of one of the most common cause of focal epilepsy. The disease is transmitted by encysted form of pork tapeworm, *Taenia solium*. To become clinically manifested, two hosts are needed to complete its life cycle. Humans are an intermediate host, acquiring the organism by accidental ingestion of tapeworm eggs from fecal contaminated substances. The eggs hatch in the small intestine, burrow into the mucosa, and penetrate the venules. Mature larvae, or cysticerci, develop after 60–70 days. Cysticercus can lodge anywhere in the human body, viz., brain, retina, skeletal muscle, heart, and subcutaneous tissues. However, the brain contributes to majority (60–90%) of these cases.

Clinical Features and Pathology

The expression of the disease is variable, although seizures have been reported in as high as 92% of patients. Headaches and focal neurological deficits are also common. The clinical symptomatology depends on the size, number, viability, location, and stage of the cysts. The abovementioned symptoms are secondary to the inflammatory reaction related to cyst degeneration. Pathologically, four patterns of intracranial involvement have been described: (1) Parenchymal, (2) Intraventricular, (3) Subarachnoid, and (4) Mixed type.[1,47]

The cysticercus larva in the CNS undergoes a regular life cycle from the vesicular form to involution. These parenchymal cysticerci are categorized according to Escobar's four pathological stages:[48,49]

1. *Vesicular stage*: The larva is viable with no or minimal inflammatory reaction in the surrounding tissue and hence the patient is usually asymptomatic. It is seen as a small marginal nodule projecting into a small cyst containing clear fluid. On imaging, a clearly marginated cyst with cyst fluid similar to the CSF signal intensity is seen on CT and MRI. A discrete, eccentrically placed scolex may be appreciated, better demonstrated on FLAIR, SWI, or heavily T2W sequences [constructive interference in steady state (CISS)/DRIVE/fast imaging employing steady-state acquisition (FIESTA)], and may show diffusion restriction. No contrast enhancement is seen in the cyst wall **(Figs. 11A and B)**.
2. *Colloidal vesicular stage*: As the larva begins to degenerate and the scolex shows signs of hyaline degeneration, the cyst shrinks in size, cyst fluid becomes turbid, and cyst wall becomes somewhat thick with presence of surrounding inflammatory reaction. At this stage, the child may become symptomatic with seizures or focal neurological deficits. The cyst is slightly hyperintense on T1WIs and markedly hyperintense on T2WIs **(Figs. 12A and B)**. There is associated contrast enhancement of cyst wall and perilesional edema. There may also be diffusion restriction, however the ADC values are not as low as seen in pyogenic abscesses.
3. *Granular nodular stage*: The cyst undergoes retraction and the scolex is transformed into a coarse mineralized granule and surrounding edema regresses gradually. The cyst may be seen as a nodular or a thick small ring-like enhancement. Occasionally, a target or bull eye appearance is seen with the calcified scolex in the center of the mass.
4. *Nodular calcified stage*: By this stage, the granulomatous lesion has contracted to a fraction of its initial size. On NCCT scans, a small, calcified nodule without mass effect or enhancement is typical. These are hypointense on T2W MRI and become apparent on gradient echo or SWI.

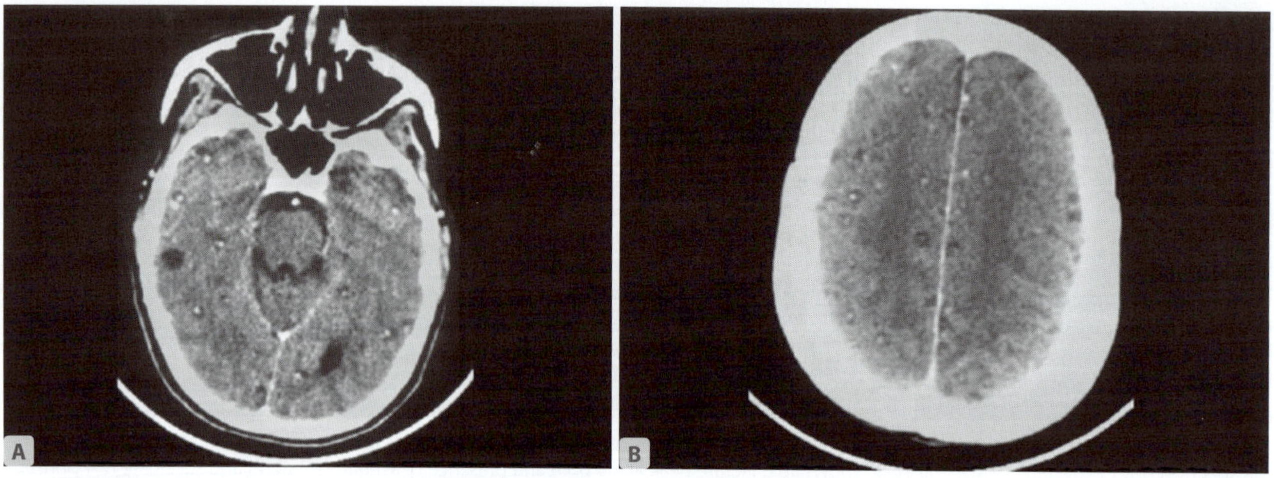

FIGS. 11A AND B: Diffuse intraparenchymal neurocysticercosis (NCC). (A and B) Contrast-enhanced computed tomography (CECT) axial sections showing multiple cystic attenuation lesions seen in bilateral cerebral hemispheres. These lesions are not associated either with perilesional edema or enhancement suggestive of vesicular stage of NCC. The scolices are seen as eccentric hyperdense foci within the cysts.

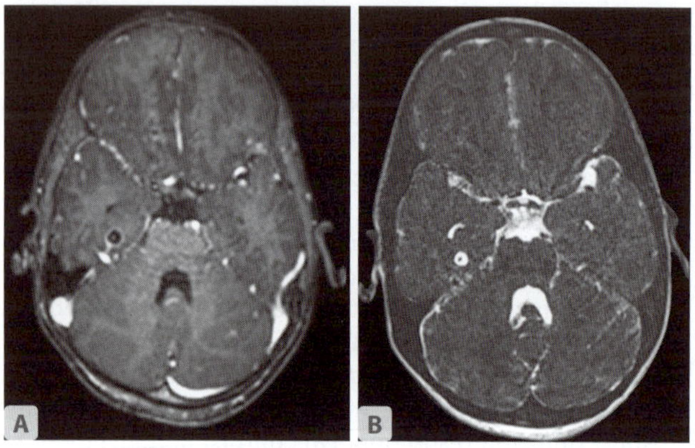

FIGS. 12A AND B: Neurocysticercosis—colloid vesicular stage: Axial contrast-enhanced T1 (A) and constructive interference in steady state (CISS) (B) images depicting the thin peripheral enhancement in the right temporal lobe lesion with exquisite demonstration of scolex on CISS.

It is to be noted that it is not necessary that the child would be deemed cured when the cyst reaches the calcified stage. Perilesional edema has been reported in a calcified lesion much later, which has led one to believe that the larval antigens are present in the granuloma, which when released, may trigger an inflammatory reaction.[48,49] Enhancing calcified lesions are also a risk factor for seizures.

Intraventricular Form

These are important to identify because affected patients can die from acute intraventricular obstruction. They are most commonly seen in fourth ventricle followed by lateral ventricle and third ventricle and can migrate from one ventricle from another ventricle and can be trapped in aqueduct of Sylvius to cause acute hydrocephalus. The MR imaging is superior to CT in imaging of these lesions. TIWIs 3 mm or less in thickness optimize detection of the scolex **(Figs. 13A and B)**. The use of steady-state sequences such as CISS can also be useful in finding intraventricular or cisternal cystic lesions. Sagittal and coronal plane images allow better appreciation of fourth ventricular lesions.[48]

Subarachnoid Form (Racemose Cysts)

These are multilobular, considered nonviable (therefore lacking scolex) cysts located in the subarachnoid space. They are most commonly seen in the cerebellopontine angle, the suprasellar region, the sylvian fissures, and the basilar cisterns. Although the lesions are sterile, these lesions can grow by proliferation of cyst wall. They may become multiloculated, resembling a cluster of grapes, hence referred to as the racemose variety. On CT scans, large cystic lesions are seen which may enhance after contrast administration. On MRI, multiple cysts of varying size, clustered together, are seen in the involved cisterns **(Figs. 14A to C)**. A combination of large cyst/cysts, multilobulation of a cyst, lack of mural nodule within the cyst, cisternal location, and leptomeningeal enhancement on MRI strongly suggest that the lesion is caused by racemose cysticercus, especially in endemic areas. A chronic leptomeningitis may accompany these cysts possibly due to leakage of cysticercus antigens into the CSF.[48] Some refer this to be leptomeningitic form of neurocysticercosis. There may be resultant arteritis leading to infarction of the basal perforating vessels. These racemose forms usually do not calcify.

Mixed Form

As the name indicates, mixed form is a combination of parenchymal and subarachnoid/intraventricular forms. The characteristics are similar to those individually described previously. In endemic regions, due to recurrent ingestions of ova, intracranial cysts are found in different stages of life cycle, i.e., anywhere from vesicular to calcified forms.

Hydatid Disease

Hydatid disease is caused by *Echinococcus granulosus* (*E. granulosus*) and less frequently by *Echinococcus multilocularis* (*E. multilocularis*) (referred to as alveolar

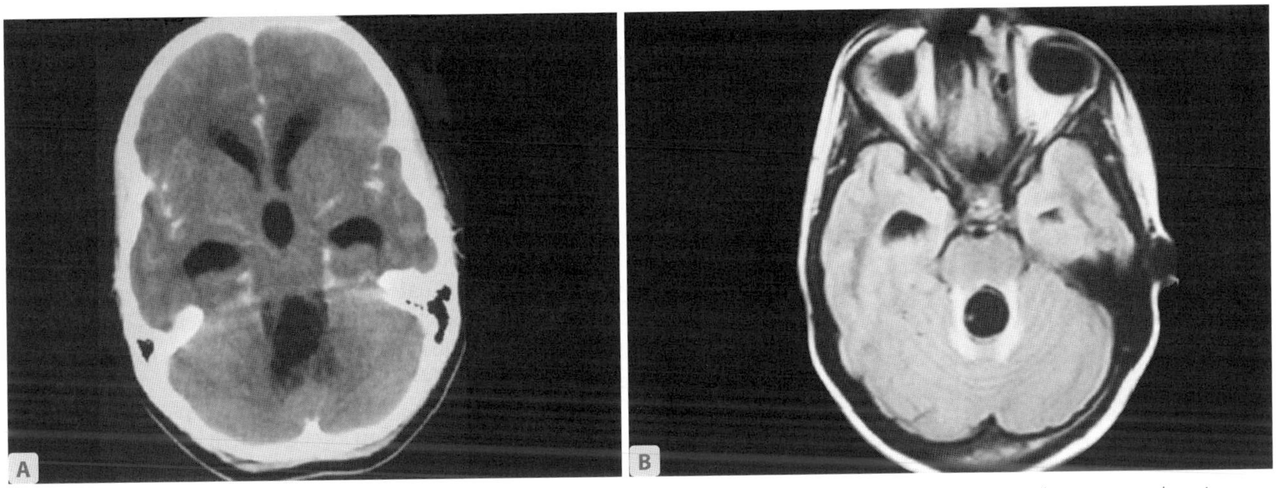

FIGS. 13A AND B: Intraventricular neurocysticercosis. (A) CECT image reveals presence of dilated supratentorial ventricular system and cystic lesion in fourth ventricle having enhancing eccentric nodular focus; and (B) FLAIR image delineates the scolex in the cystic lesion. (CECT: contrast-enhanced computed tomography; FLAIR: fluid-attenuated inversion recovery)

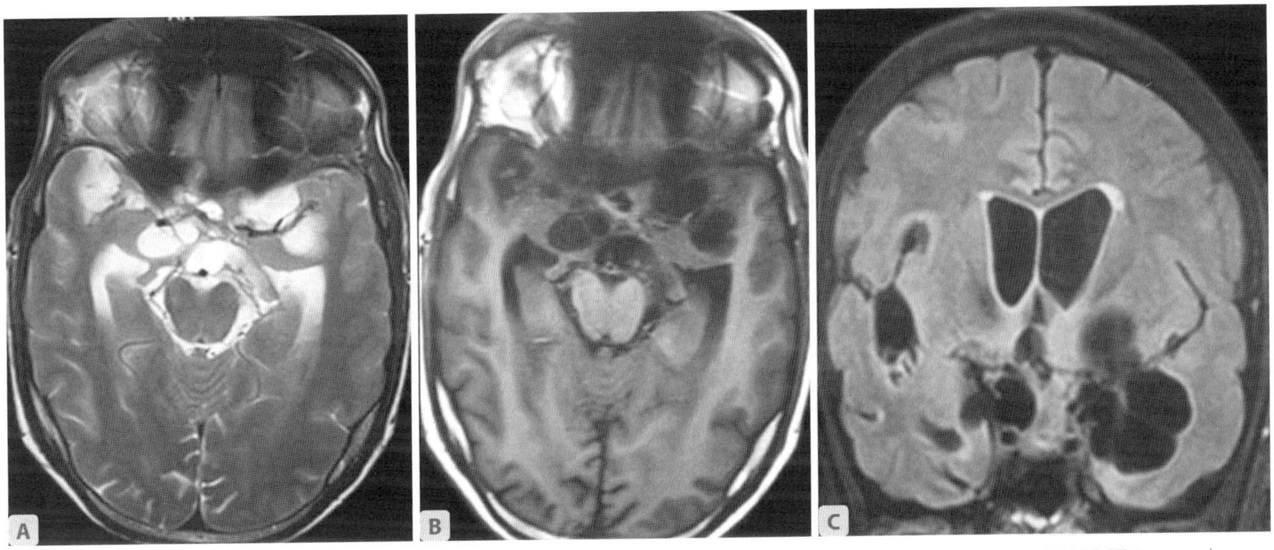

FIGS. 14A TO C: Racemose neurocysticercosis (NCC): Axial T2 (A), T1 (B), and coronal fluid-attenuated inversion recovery (FLAIR) (C) images show multiple cystic lesions in the basal cisterns with imperceptible walls leading to hydrocephalus.

echinococcosis). It is the second most common parasitic infection of the CNS. Human infection occurs by contact with definite host dog or by drinking or eating contaminated water or vegetables.

Ingested ova hatch in the gastrointestinal tract. Liberated embryos can then spread to virtually every organ or tissue via the portal and systemic circulation. They subsequently develop into cystic larva termed as hydatid cyst. CNS involvement occurs in 5% of cases as compared to liver (65–75%) and lung (15–20%). *E. granulosus* usually affect children unlike *E. multilocularis* which is seen in adults. The cysts are usually unilocular, solitary, and located in parietal lobes.[50,51] There can be associated "daughter cysts". The cyst wall has three layers: (1) Outer fibrous pericyst secondary to host reactions, (2) Middle laminated membranous ectocyst (mucopolysaccharide membrane), and (3) An endocyst (inner germinal layer).

CT shows presence of a thin-walled spherical CSF density cyst. Calcification of the wall is rare and enhancement is uncommon. The MR T2W sequence shows a typical thin low-signal intensity rim surrounding a high-signal intensity lesion. Sometimes detached membranes **(Figs. 15A and B)** or hydatid sand may be seen within the cyst. MR spectroscopy shows elevated lactate, succinate, and acetate peaks within the cyst. When the cyst ruptures, contrast enhancement and pericyst edema occur and secondary infection may ensue.

Other parasitic infections such as acquired toxoplasmosis, amebiasis, malaria, schistosomiasis, paragonimiasis, sparganosis, trichinosis, and trypanosomiasis are very rare and regionally localized. These present variably with necrotizing, hemorrhagic meningitis and angiitis (primary amebic meningitis—*Naegleria fowleri*) or parenchymal granulomatous inflammation (granulomatous amebic encephalitis—*Acanthamoeba* species). Congenital

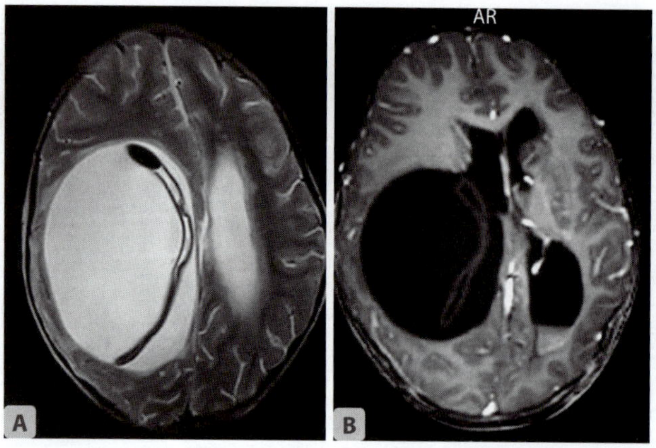

FIGS. 15A AND B: Hydatid cyst: Axial T2 (A) and postcontrast T1 (B) MR image showing a large right frontoparietal thin-walled cyst with T2-hypointense membranes floating within.

toxoplasmosis will be discussed under the section of congenital infections. For specifics of the rest of the parasitic infections, the readers are referred to specific texts elsewhere beyond this textbook.

VIRAL INFECTIONS

Viral infection of the CNS is usually diffuse or multifocal parenchymal inflammatory process known as encephalitis. Less commonly, it involves the meninges wherein it is referred to as meningoencephalitis. The parenchymal inflammation may be due to direct invasion by the virus or due to immune-mediated hypersensitivity process. Although a large number of viruses may affect the brain, all exhibit two common pathological processes—(1) neuronal degeneration and (2) inflammation. Imaging is required for early detection and accurate diagnosis because some patients may present with atypical clinical features and laboratory findings. MRI is widely accepted as a sensitive technique for the diagnosis of encephalitis and is very useful for detecting early changes.[52] The various viruses that infect the CNS are discussed below.

Herpes Simplex Encephalitis

Herpes simplex encephalitis (HSE) is the most common among sporadic encephalitis. Herpes simplex virus type 1 (HSV-1) causes 95% of all herpetic encephalitis. HSV type 2 is the cause of neonatal herpes encephalitis. Initial HSV-1 infection occurs in oro-/nasopharynx through contact via infected secretions. The virus gains entry into the lingual branches of the trigeminal nerve and lies dormant in the trigeminal ganglion. Later, it invades the brain along these cranial nerves. HSV-1 reactivation may occur spontaneously or be precipitated by various factors such as local trauma and immunosuppression. HSV-1 disease has a predilection for the limbic system and the lesions are localized to the temporal lobes, the insular cortex, subfrontal areas, and the cingulate gyrus. The pathological hallmark of HSV encephalitis is hemorrhagic necrotizing encephalitis, which results in severe edema and massive tissue necrosis. HSV-1 encephalitis has a characteristic sequential bilaterality, i.e., initial lesions are unilateral but are followed by less severe contralateral disease. Changes appear earlier on MR than on CT. The findings include gyral edema in the involved regions, which are better appreciated on T2WI and FLAIR sequences **(Figs. 16A to D)**. Contrast administration shows enhancement of the affected cortex and surrounding leptomeninges. As the disease progresses, T1 and T2 shortening develops secondary to hemorrhage and calcification also better appreciated on SWI as areas of blooming.[53,54] Diffusion-weighted sequences show patchy diffusion restriction, which sometimes is appreciable even when no other MR sequences demonstrate these changes. The gyral involvement is much more extensive and variable in HSV-1 infection of the infants.

Herpes simplex virus type 2 encephalitis, seen in neonates, is acquired from infection in maternal genital tract. The virus destroys the brain leaving the pial glial membrane, ependyma, and choroid plexus. Sonography of affected neonates shows diffuse hyperechogenicity of the brain without ventricular compression. As the disease progresses, the ventricles dilate and the encephalomalacic brain shows increasing hyperechogenicity. On MR, the lesions are nonspecific with shortened T1 and T2 relaxation times in all sequences, which persist for weeks or months. The changes are most marked in cortical gray matter.[53,54]

Japanese Encephalitis

Japanese encephalitis (JE) is a common viral infection in Southeast Asian countries. It causes seasonal epidemics with significant neurological manifestations. JE virus belongs to the arbovirus-flavivirus group. Clinical symptoms are in form of acute fulminant neurologic disease with fever, altered sensorium, and rapid development of focal neurologic signs. The virus induces formation of glial nodules and circumscribed necrolytic foci which predominantly involve the thalami, substantia nigra (SN), corpus striatum, cerebral cortex, brainstem, and cerebellum. The most consistently appreciated finding in JE is bilateral thalamic lesions with or without hemorrhages on MR imaging **(Figs. 17A and B)**. Although thalamic, SN, and basal ganglia lesions are characteristic of JE, temporal lobe involvement involving hippocampus sparing rest of temporal lobe may also be seen. This pattern of temporal lobe involvement with concurrent thalamic, SN, and basal ganglionic lesions allows its differentiation from HSE.[55,56]

The other viruses which infect the CNS are briefly discussed.

Varicella—CNS infection may result in meningoencephalitis, transverse myelitis (TM), and aseptic meningitis. Neuroimaging may often be negative. *Zoster* CNS infection may lead to encephalitis, myelitis, and neuritis. Five patterns of CNS involvement have been described: (1) Acute meningomyeloradiculitis, (2) Multifocal leukoencephalitis, (3) Ventriculitis, (4) Focal necrotizing myelitis, and (5) Necrotizing angiitis involving leptomeningeal arteries.[57] MRI shows clustered plaque-like lesions of demyelination, some showing enhancement. Increased T2 signal may be appreciated in the brainstem and supratentorial gray matter. Postvaricella encephalitis may take two forms:[58] (1) Bilateral, symmetric, and nonenhancing basal ganglia

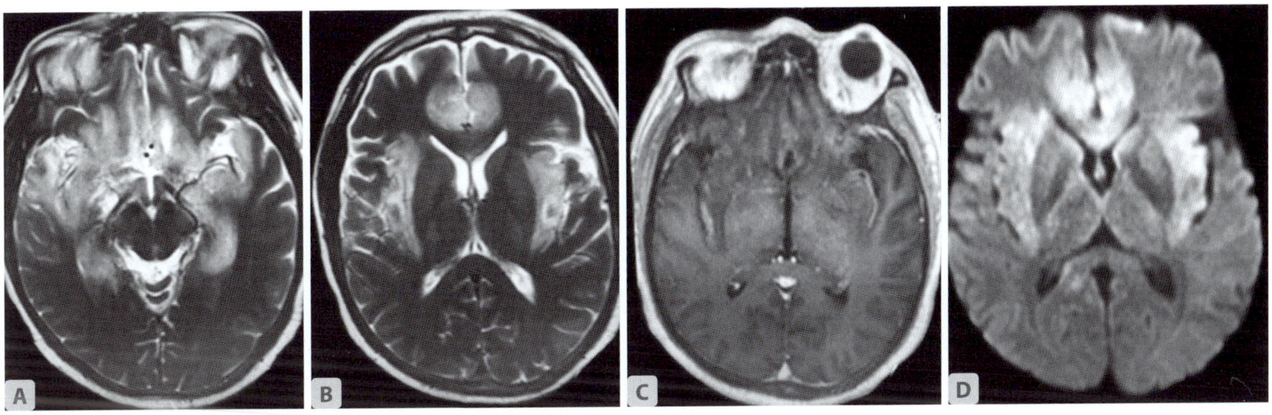

FIGS. 16A TO D: Herpes encephalitis: Axial T2W (A and B), postcontrast T1W (C), and diffusion-weighted (D) MR images showing hyperintensities involving bilateral medial temporal lobes, bilateral insular cortices, and cingulate gyri with mild patchy right insular enhancement and diffusion restriction. (T1W: T1-weighted; T2W: T2-weighted)

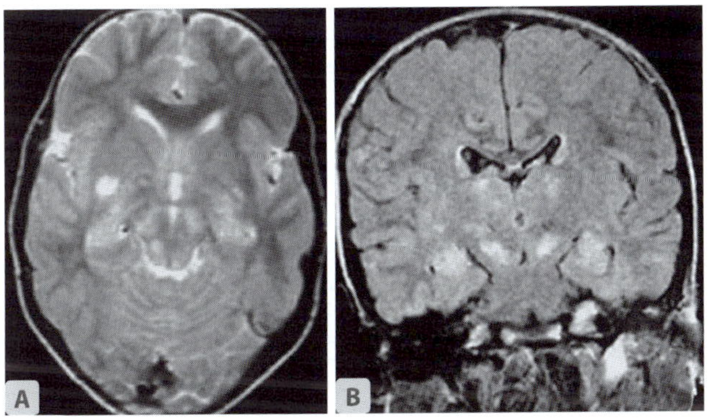

FIGS. 17A AND B: Japanese encephalitis: (A) T2W axial and (B) FLAIR coronal MR images showing hyperintensities involving bilateral thalami and substantia nigra. (FLAIR: fluid-attenuated inversion recovery; T2W: T2-weighted)

lesions (hypodense on CT and hyperintense on T2WI MRI); and (2) Diffuse, multiple gray and white matter lesions of similar imaging characteristics. Postvaricella arteriopathy is characterized by unilateral stenosing arteriopathy affecting the terminal internal carotid artery (ICA) and proximal anterior and middle cerebral arteries with occasional infarcts in corresponding territories.

Acute necrotizing encephalopathy is a severe life-threatening form of influenza-associated encephalitis caused by many viruses notably H3N2, H1N1, and coronavirus-2.[59,60] There is symmetric, often hemorrhagic necrosis involving thalami, midbrain tegmentum, and pons. SWI shows blooming, especially in thalami with some cases showing diffusion restriction.

Subacute sclerosing panencephalitis (SSPE) is a slow progressive infection by measles virus (*Morbillivirus* genus). The condition manifests after a latent period of 3–9 years after measles infection. Boys are affected more than girls. MRI is more sensitive in detection of the lesion and in assessing the extent of the disease. In the early stages, the lesion is usually located in the gray matter and subcortical white matter of the parietal and temporal lobes **(Figs. 18A to C)**. It is asymmetrical and bilateral. As the disease progresses, high-signal intensity in the centrum semiovale and periventricular white matter is observed. In the final stages of the disease, diffuse cortical atrophy develops with T2 prolongation in the brainstem. Basal ganglia involvement is seen in 20–35% of affected patients.[61] The disease causes eventual death of the patient.

Rasmussen (chronic focal) encephalitis is rare progressive encephalitis resulting in intractable seizures, progressive hemiparesis, and mental impairment. It is believed to result from a chronic viral infection or as an autoimmune phenomenon following HSV infection. Early imaging findings are unremarkable which, however, are seen as development of T2/FLAIR hyperintensities in the cortex or subcortical white matter of the affected hemisphere.[62] In due course, there ensues progressive cortical atrophy **(Figs. 19A and B)**.

Diffusion-weighted imaging plays a key role in demonstration of viral lesions. In the acute stage of encephalitis, there are areas of congestion, perivascular cuffing, and thrombus formation pathologically. These changes are responsible for the cytotoxic edema that leads to restricted diffusion and low ADC, changes that may not be picked up on conventional MR pulse sequences **(Figs. 20A to D)**. In the late acute and early subacute stages, the components of vasculitis and perivascular cuffing diminish, so the proportion of diffusion restriction decreases and ADC starts to increase. At this stage, due to vasogenic edema, the number and extent of the lesion will be more marked in T2 and FLAIR images.[63]

CONGENITAL INFECTIONS

Infections of the fetal nervous system differ from those of older children and adults in that the age of the fetus at the time of insult is more important than the nature of insult. In general, infections during the first trimester will result in congenital malformations seen in bilateral frontal and parieto-occipital lobe white matter whereas those that occur during the third trimester are manifested as destructive lesions.[1,64]

The transmission of infection is by two modes. Bacteria travel through the amniotic fluid whereas toxoplasmosis, syphilis, and viruses usually pass through the transplacental

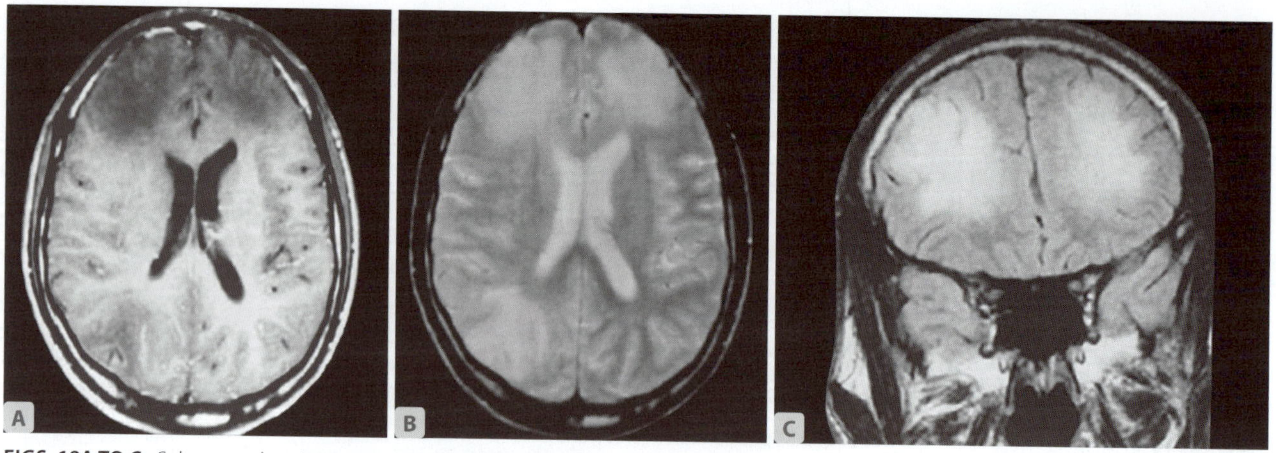

FIGS. 18A TO C: Subacute sclerosing panencephalitis. (A to C) T1-hypointense and T2 and fluid-attenuated inversion recovery (FLAIR) hyperintense lesions are seen in bilateral frontal and parieto-occipital lobe of white matter.

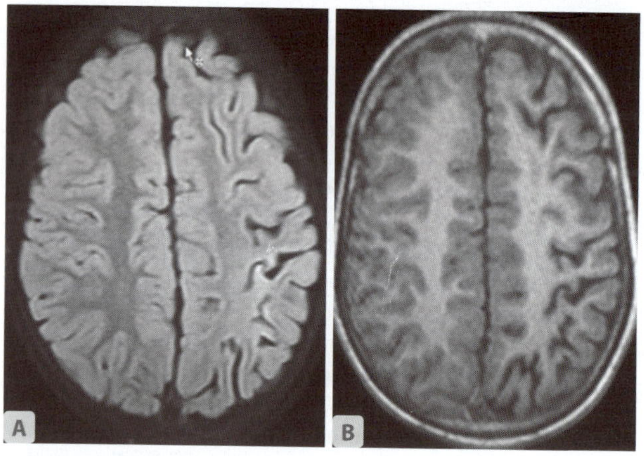

FIGS. 19A AND B: Rasmussen's encephalitis: Axial fluid-attenuated inversion recovery (FLAIR) (A) and T1-weighted (B) MR images reveal left cerebral cortical atrophy with mild signal changes in the underlying white matter.

circulatory route. These infections are referred to by the acronym TORCH. Others are congenital syphilis, Zika virus, and lymphocytic choriomeningitis virus.

Congenital Cytomegalovirus

Congenital cytomegalovirus (CMV) disease is the most common cause of CNS infection in neonates. It results from vertical transmission of the CMV from the mother to the fetus transplacentally. It can cause hematologic, neurologic, and developmental signs and symptoms.

Patients presumably infected during the first half of the second trimester have microcephaly, lissencephaly with a thin cortex, hypoplastic cerebellum, delayed myelination, marked ventriculomegaly, and significant periventricular calcification. Those infected in the middle of second trimester have more typical polymicrogyria and less ventricular dilatation. Patients infected near the end of gestation or in early postnatal period have normal gyral pattern and damaged periventricular or subcortical white matter with scattered periventricular calcification **(Figs. 21A to E)**. When the findings of dystrophic calcifications (in the germinal zone, cortical malformations, myelination delay, and cerebellar hypoplasia) are present in a child with developmental delay or seizures, a diagnosis of congenital CMV is considered.[1]

Congenital Toxoplasmosis

It is the second most common cause of congenital CNS infections. The infection may be generalized or localized to the CNS. The CNS findings are chorioretinitis, hydrocephalus, and seizure activity. The findings on cross-sectional imaging may be similar to those in CMV infection. Dystrophic calcifications located in basal ganglia, periventricular region, and cerebral cortex are seen. Microcephaly, large ventricles, and hydrocephalus can be seen. Absence of cortical and gyral malformations can be differentiating feature from CMV infection.

Neonatal Herpes Simplex Encephalitis

Herpes simplex virus type 2 encephalitis seen in neonates is acquired from infection in maternal genital tract. Sonography of affected neonates shows diffuse hyperechogenicity of the brain without ventricular compression. On MR, for the first 2 days, the lesions are patchy, widespread areas of prolonged T1 and T2 relaxation times in white matter, with restriction on DWI. Later, the changes are seen in cortical gray matter. As the disease progresses, cortex shows thinning, the ventricles dilate, and the encephalomalacia changes are seen in white matter and gyral or punctate calcifications are seen.

Rubella

Congenital rubella is transplacentally transmitted infection. Risk of fetal damage is highest during the first trimester and decreases subsequently. Infection results in microcephalic brain with cortical and basal ganglia calcifications. CT shows hypodensity throughout the white matter together with calcification in periventricular region, basal ganglia, and cortex. On MR, multifocal bright lesions will be seen on T2WI with delay in myelination. Predilection of the virus for vascular endothelium may cause thrombosis or hemorrhagic infarction.

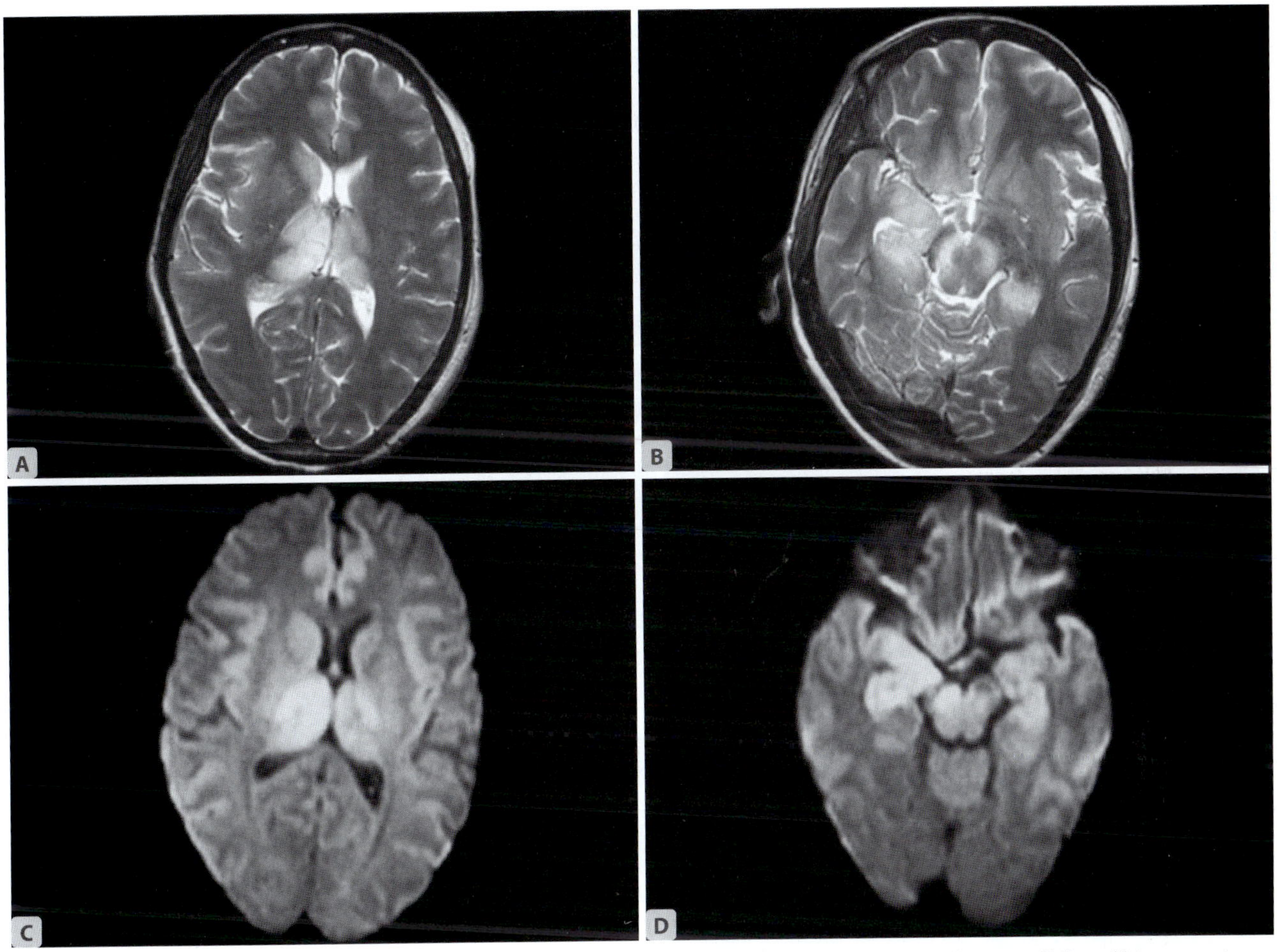

FIGS. 20A TO D: DWI on third day of illness in Japanese encephalitis. (A and B) The T2W images showing involvement of bilateral hippocampi, substantia nigra, and bilateral thalami; and (C and D) The diffusion-weighted images showing restriction in the involved areas. (DWI: diffusion-weighted imaging; T2W: T2-weighted)

Congenital Human Immunodeficiency Virus Infection

Human immunodeficiency virus (HIV) infection is a significant public health problem because of large number of HIV-infected women who are having children. Nearly 80% of all childhood HIV infections are maternally transmitted, although only one-third of HIV-positive mothers pass on the infection. CNS manifestations are primarily of two types: (1) Progressive encephalopathy; and (2) Static encephalopathy. Neuroimaging studies reveal meningoencephalitis, atrophy, and calcific vasculopathy. HIV encephalitis results in diffuse cerebral atrophy (90% of cases) and calcification of basal ganglia and subcortical white matter (33% of cases). Calcification is seen in those infected in utero and hence usually never seen below 1 year of age. HIV vasculopathy can result in infarcts.[65-67] Zika virus causes microcephaly, parenchymal calcifications (common at the gray-white matter junction), polymicrogyria, lissencephaly, and pachygyria.[68]

In contrast to adults, opportunistic infections and tumors are relatively rare (15% of cases), the most common neoplasm being lymphoma reported with 5% incidence and CMV and progressive multifocal leukoencephalitis (PML) are more common opportunistic infections. Proton MR spectroscopy has been used in pediatric patients. The NAA/creatinine ratio is normal in static disease and significantly lower in progressive encephalopathy patients.[69,70]

FUNGAL INFECTIONS

Fungal infections are uncommon in children. Fungal infection can be classified in two broad categories: (1) Those occurring in patients with lowered resistance as opportunistic infections, e.g., diabetes, leukemia, lymphoma, and in children on long-term cytotoxic, immunosuppressive, or antibiotic therapy; and (2) Those due to pathogenic fungi infecting healthy immunocompetent children. The former infections are generally due to *Aspergillus*, *Candida*, and *Mucormycosis* species and the latter are due to *Cryptococcus*, *Histoplasma*, *Coccidioides*, and *Blastomyces* species.[71,72]

The increased incidence of fungal infections of the CNS is being realized both in immunocompromised and immunocompetent individuals. Certain clinical syndromes are specific for certain fungal infections. The rhinocerebral form is the most common presenting syndrome with zygomycosis and skull base syndromes are often the presenting clinical syndromes in patients with sinocranial aspergillosis. Subacute and chronic meningitis in patients

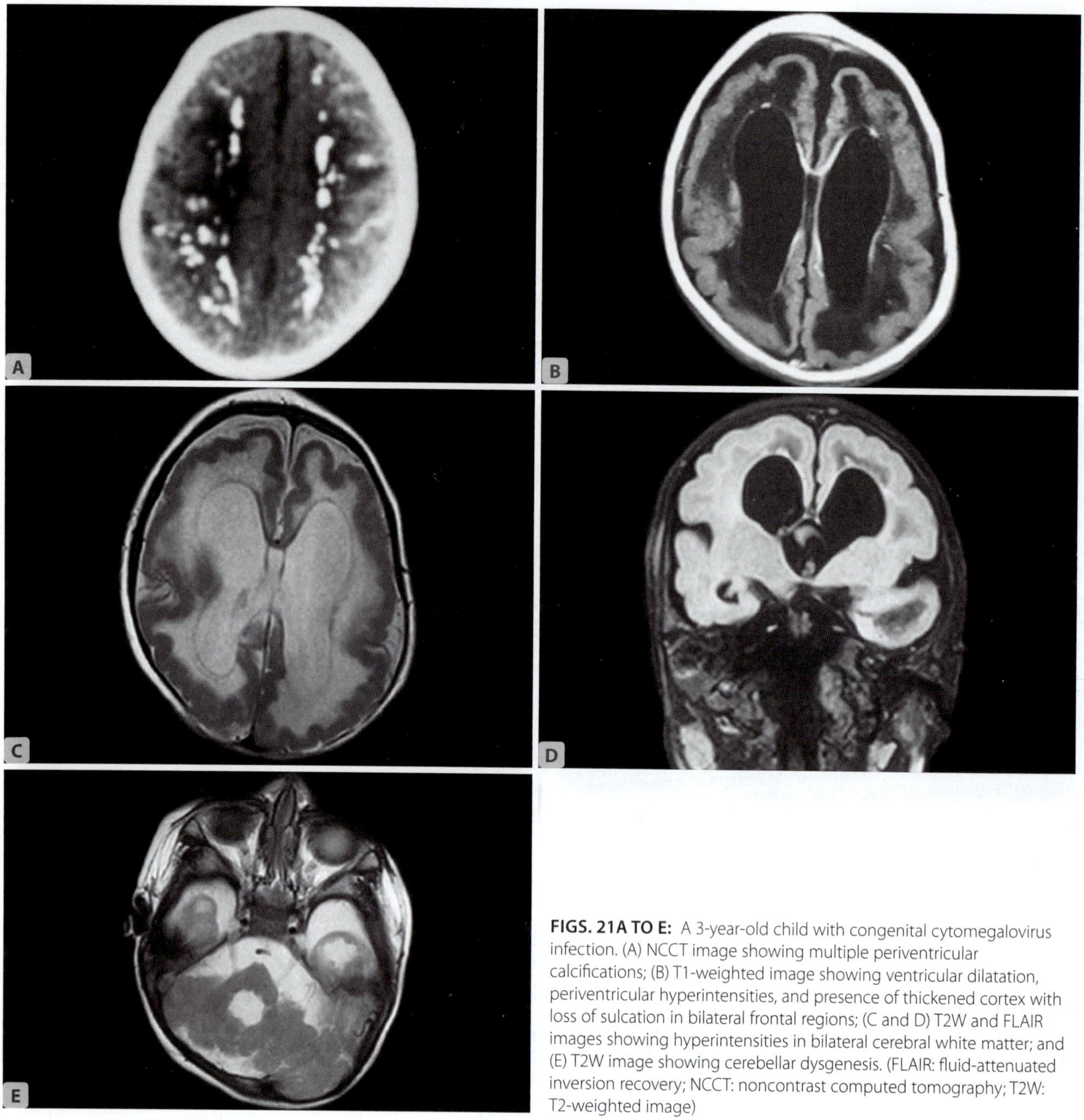

FIGS. 21A TO E: A 3-year-old child with congenital cytomegalovirus infection. (A) NCCT image showing multiple periventricular calcifications; (B) T1-weighted image showing ventricular dilatation, periventricular hyperintensities, and presence of thickened cortex with loss of sulcation in bilateral frontal regions; (C and D) T2W and FLAIR images showing hyperintensities in bilateral cerebral white matter; and (E) T2W image showing cerebellar dysgenesis. (FLAIR: fluid-attenuated inversion recovery; NCCT: noncontrast computed tomography; T2W: T2-weighted image)

with HIV infection is more likely to be due to cryptococcal infection.

Aspergillosis

Aspergillus is saprophytic opportunistic ubiquitous fungi found in soil and plants. *Aspergillus fumigatus* is the most common human pathogen.[73]

Central nervous system aspergillosis is a rare condition. The infection reaches the brain directly from the nasal sinuses or is hematogeneous from the lungs and gastrointestinal tract. Three pathological manifestations can occur with aspergillosis: (1) Infarction, (2) Abscess formation, and (3) Meningitis.[74]

The most distinct imaging characteristics at CT or MR imaging are multiple lesions with infarction or hemorrhage

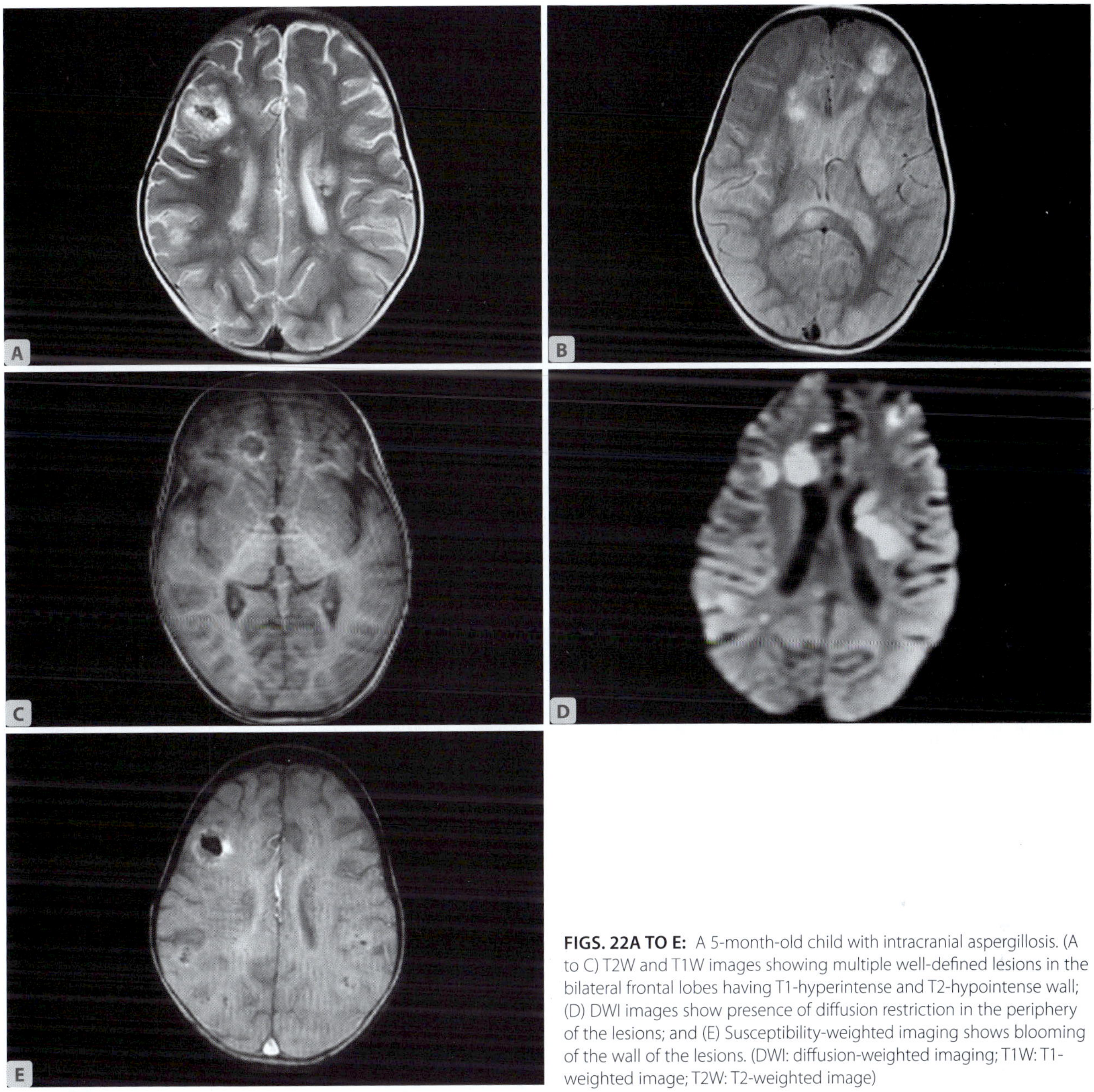

FIGS. 22A TO E: A 5-month-old child with intracranial aspergillosis. (A to C) T2W and T1W images showing multiple well-defined lesions in the bilateral frontal lobes having T1-hyperintense and T2-hypointense wall; (D) DWI images show presence of diffusion restriction in the periphery of the lesions; and (E) Susceptibility-weighted imaging shows blooming of the wall of the lesions. (DWI: diffusion-weighted imaging; T1W: T1-weighted image; T2W: T2-weighted image)

in a random distribution due to the angioinvasive nature of the fungus. *Aspergillus* abscesses are usually hypointense on T1WIs, but areas of high-signal intensity may be seen due to presence of iron, manganese, or methemoglobin. Hemorrhage occurs in approximately 25% of cases and contrast enhancement is usually minimal or absent. On T2WIs, peripheral low-signal areas may be seen which correspond to areas of hemorrhages **(Figs. 22A to E)**. On diffusion-weighted images, most lesions show peripheral areas of high-signal intensity suggestive of restriction of diffusion that are interspersed with dark foci which can be due to susceptibility artifact due to hemorrhagic or iron products.[74,75]

Mucormycosis

Mucormycosis is a life-threatening opportunistic fungal infection caused by one of the members of the Mucoraceae family. *Rhizopus oryzae* is the most common cause of infection.

The infection ensues when the hyphae invade the blood vessels disseminating hematogenously or may spread through the paranasal sinuses into the brain and orbits. Mucormycosis is more commonly seen in patients of diabetes, anemia, leukemia, uremia, and in those receiving steroids or chemotherapy. The rhinocerebral form is the most common

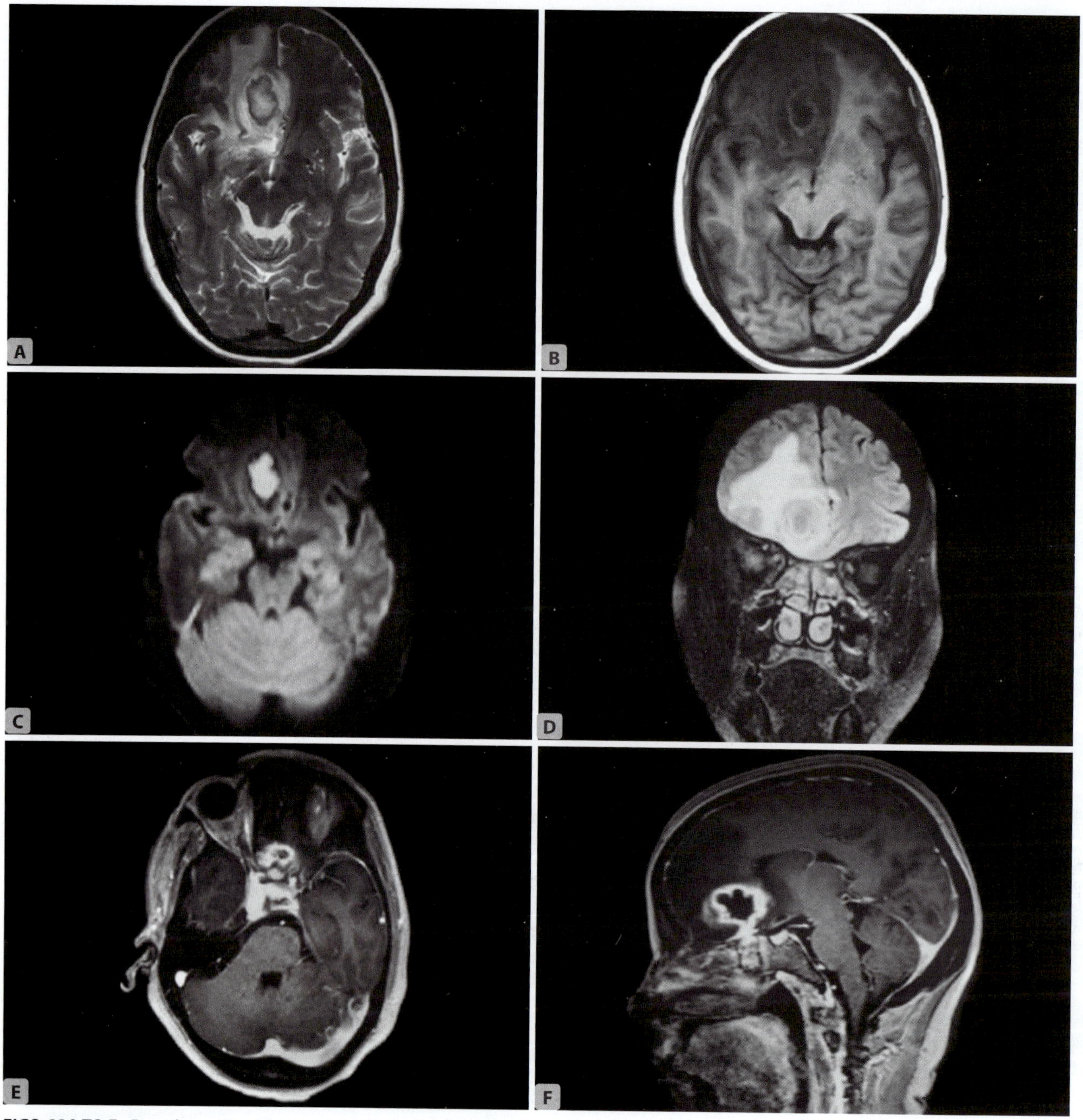

FIGS. 23A TO F: Fungal sinusitis with intracranial involvement. (A to C) Heterogeneous lesion with T2-hypointense rim and T1-isointense rim with central diffusion restriction; and (D to F) The fluid-attenuated inversion recovery (FLAIR) image shows hyperintense contents in the ethmoid sinuses with enhancement of the sinus contents, bilateral cavernous sinuses, and wall of the frontal abscess.

infection wherein the organism spreads directly through the cribriform plate via retrograde proliferation along vessels or through the superior orbital fissure or optic canal. Isolated CNS mucormycosis, a focal intracerebral infection, is rare and is most commonly seen in drug abusers.

Findings on CT and MR images include soft-tissue opacification of paranasal sinuses with absence of air-fluid levels **(Figs. 23A to F)**. There is usually associated bony erosion of the sinus walls. The sinus soft-tissue contents may have variable MR imaging characteristics, from hypointensity to hyperintensity on T2WI. There may be associated cavernous sinus thrombophlebitis and invasion of the cavernous ICA leading to arteritis and distal thromboembolism leading to infarcts related to vascular thrombosis, mycotic emboli, and fungal abscesses.[73,76]

INFLAMMATORY DISEASES

Inflammatory disorders of the pediatric brain include a wide range of diseases that are characterized by an insult secondary to autoimmunity. This group of diseases is now being recognized as an important cause of childhood morbidity.

Heterogeneous clinical and laboratory manifestations may delay the diagnosis. Hence, imaging plays an integral role in the management of these patients. Below, we will discuss some of the more common diseases.

Multiple Sclerosis

Multiple sclerosis (MS) is a chronic inflammatory disorder that involves the CNS. It results in inflammation and subsequently demyelination of both brain and the spinal cord. There are no large-scale studies evaluating the incidence of MS in the Indian pediatric population. However, data from the Western countries reveals that 3–5% of MS patients have onset below the age of 18 years. In <2% of patients, the disease onset is below 2 years of age.[77] The incidence of MS in pediatric patients may vary from 0.13 to 0.6 cases/100,000 children/year.[78]

There are various risk factors that may be associated with development of MS. There is a 2–5% risk of developing MS in first-degree relatives. This increases to 25–30% in monozygotic twins. Up to 200 susceptibility genes and 13 major histocompatibility complex (MHC) loci have been found to be associated with adult MS. One-third of the genetic variants found in adult MS are also associated with pediatric-onset MS. One of the main genetic risk factors for pediatric MS is HLA-DRB1*15:01 in the MHC class II. This particular genetic variant increases the risk of MS by three times. Environmental factors have also been implicated in the development of MS. Previous infection with Epstein–Barr virus has been associated with an increased risk of MS. Similarly, prior infection with HSV-1 may also be a contributory factor toward development of MS, depending upon the HLA-DRB1*15:01 status. Female sex, obesity, low levels of vitamin D, low iron intake, and exposure to smoking at home are also associated with an increased risk for MS.[79]

The clinical course of MS may be classified into three patterns namely—(1) Relapsing-remitting MS (RRMS), (2) Secondary progressive MS (SPMS), and (3) Primary progressive MS.[80] Younger patients have multifocal symptoms at presentation as compared to adolescents who have single focal symptoms like in adults.[81] The relapsing-remitting pattern is characterized by discrete episodes of neurological deficit with partial recovery between attacks. 98% of pediatric-onset MS cases fall into this category.[79] Pediatric patients are known to have more frequent and severe relapses of MS with shorter intervals between the first and second attacks when compared to adults.[82] However, the potential for complete recovery is higher initially.[79] Pediatric patients take longer to reach disability levels. However, they transition to secondary progressive MS at an earlier age as compared to adults.[80] There is progressive worsening in the secondary progressive MS pattern. Primary progressive MS patients show a slow, but progressive accumulation of disability without any discrete deficits or relapses. Such a progressive course is rare in children and should prompt further workup for an alternate diagnosis.[83]

The diagnosis of MS has been based on the McDonald criteria, which have undergone periodic revisions (2001, 2005, 2010, and 2017). The 2010 criteria have been evaluated in pediatric patients. These criteria have shown high sensitivity, specificity, and positive predictive value (PPV) (76%) in children older than 11 years. However, in younger children with a non-acute disseminated encephalomyelitis (ADEM)-like presentation, the PPV is reduced to 55%. This suggests that 2010 criteria must be used with caution in young patients. These criteria are also not applicable in patients who have an ADEM-like presentation.[84] The International Panel on diagnosis of MS revised the 2010 McDonald criteria in 2017. As compared to the 2010 criteria, the 2017 McDonald criteria demonstrated improvement in both accuracy and sensitivity.[85] However, the 2017 criteria have not been validated in children <12 years of age.

As per the International Pediatric MS Study Group (IPMSSG), MS may be defined by the presence of any of the following:[86]

- Two or more nonencephalopathic CNS clinical events separated by >30 days, involving more than one CNS area.
- Single clinical event and MRI features as per 2010 revised McDonald criteria for dissemination in space (DIS) and dissemination in time (DIT) (but criteria relative for DIT for a single attack and single MRI only apply to children ≥12 years and only apply to cases without an ADEM onset).
- Acute disseminated encephalomyelitis followed 3 months later by a nonencephalopathic clinical event with new lesions on brain MRI consistent with MS.

The criteria for clinically isolated syndrome (CIS) in pediatric population as per the IPMSSG are[86] (all are required):

- A monofocal or polyfocal, clinical CNS event with presumed inflammatory demyelinating cause.
- Absence of a prior clinical history of CNS demyelinating disease [e.g., absence of past optic neuritis (ON), TM, and hemispheric or brainstem-related syndromes].
- No encephalopathy (i.e., no alteration in consciousness or behavior) that cannot be explained by fever.
- The diagnosis of MS based on baseline MRI features is not met.

Clinically isolated syndrome in the pediatric population usually presents as ON, TM, or brainstem syndromes. The rate of conversion to MS is 13.8–32%. The risk is higher in children that have an abnormal associated brain MRI, bilateral ON, or recurrent ON.[87]

Imaging in Multiple Sclerosis

Protocols

MRI has become an important tool in the diagnosis and monitoring of MS. The protocols used for MS imaging must be standardized, not only for accurate diagnosis but also for follow-up. Evidence-based guidelines have been published by the Magnetic Resonance Imaging in MS (MAGNIMS) Study Group and the Consortium of MS Centers (CMSC).[88] Wherever possible, a 3T imaging system is recommended due to its superior capability for detection of both white and gray matter lesions. The spatial resolution should also be standardized for both diagnosis and monitoring with an in-plane resolution of ≤1 × 1 mm. The whole brain must be covered during acquisition. Orientation of the axial sequences should be along the subcallosal line. The slice thickness must be ≤3 mm with no interslice gap. The core sequences, for brain imaging, that must be performed include three-dimensional (3D)-T2, 3D sagittal T2W-FLAIR, two-dimensional (2D) axial diffusion-weighted images, and a 3D postgadolinium

FLASH (noninversion recovery) sequence. Other than these sequences, axial proton density, pre- and postcontrast axial T1 spin echo sequences, and SWI may also be performed.[89]

The cervical spine should also be covered along with brain imaging. Sagittal T2W and short tau inversion recovery (STIR) sequences should be performed (<1–3 mm slice thickness; no gap) followed by axial T2 and postcontrast axial T1 sections through the lesions (section thickness 5 mm; no gap). The rest of the spine may be imaged, if there are any clinical symptoms or signs.

Imaging of the orbit may be required to evaluate ON. Coronal STIR or fat-suppressed T2 followed by a coronal fat-suppressed T1 sequence (slice thickness ≤2 mm) should be acquired. The scan should extend up to the optic chasm.

Conventional MR Imaging

On T2W/FLAIR imaging, MS lesions appear as hyperintense round to ovoid lesions that surround medullary veins and radiate centripetally away from the wall of the lateral ventricle. This pattern of perivascular inflammation leads to a finger-like shape on axial images and is also known as "Dawson fingers" **(Figs. 24 and 25)**. The perivascular location of these lesions can be demonstrated using T2 and susceptibility imaging. Lesions that are larger in size have more hyperintense signal in the center and less hyperintensity peripherally. MS plaques are triangular in shape with a broad base toward the ventricles on sagittal images. The callososeptal interface is commonly involved. Alternating areas of hyperintensity along the ependyma may also be seen. This is known as the "ependymal dot-dash" sign. T2 turbo spin echo (TSE) sequence allows detection of both supratentorial and infratentorial white matter lesions and lesions within the spinal cord. However, it is insensitive toward cortical demyelination and gray matter abnormalities.[90] FLAIR images show a higher lesion load in the periventricular areas due to attenuation of the underlying CSF. Infratentorial lesions were evaluated in a cohort of patients suffering from CIS. It was seen that both cerebellar and brainstem lesions predict conversion to clinically definite MS. Brainstem lesions predicted progression of disability as well.[88] Spinal cord lesions are mostly seen in the upper cervical cord and also the lower thoracic cord. These lesions are usually wedge-shaped and are located in the lateral and posterior columns on the spinal cord **(Figs. 26A to D)**. Both gray and white matter are involved. Atrophy of the cervical spinal cord has also been seen and has been

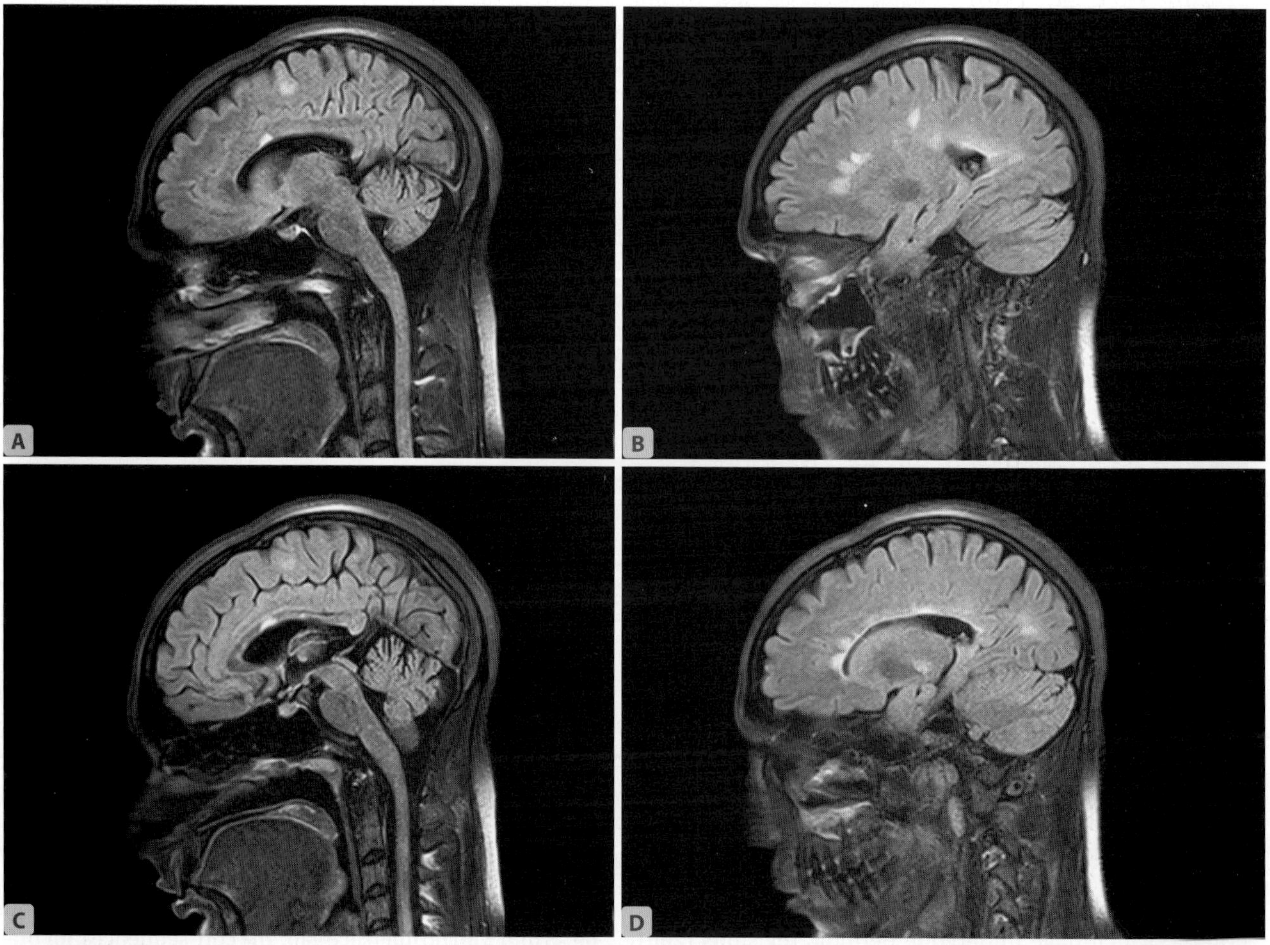

FIGS. 24A TO D: Multiple sclerosis: Sagittal fluid-attenuated inversion recovery (FLAIR) images (A to D) showing the characteristic distribution pattern of hyperintensities. The lesions are predominantly periventricular and triangular with a broad base toward the lateral ventricle (B and D). The corpus callosum and the callososeptal interface are also involved (C). Another lesion is seen as subcortical frontal white matter (A).

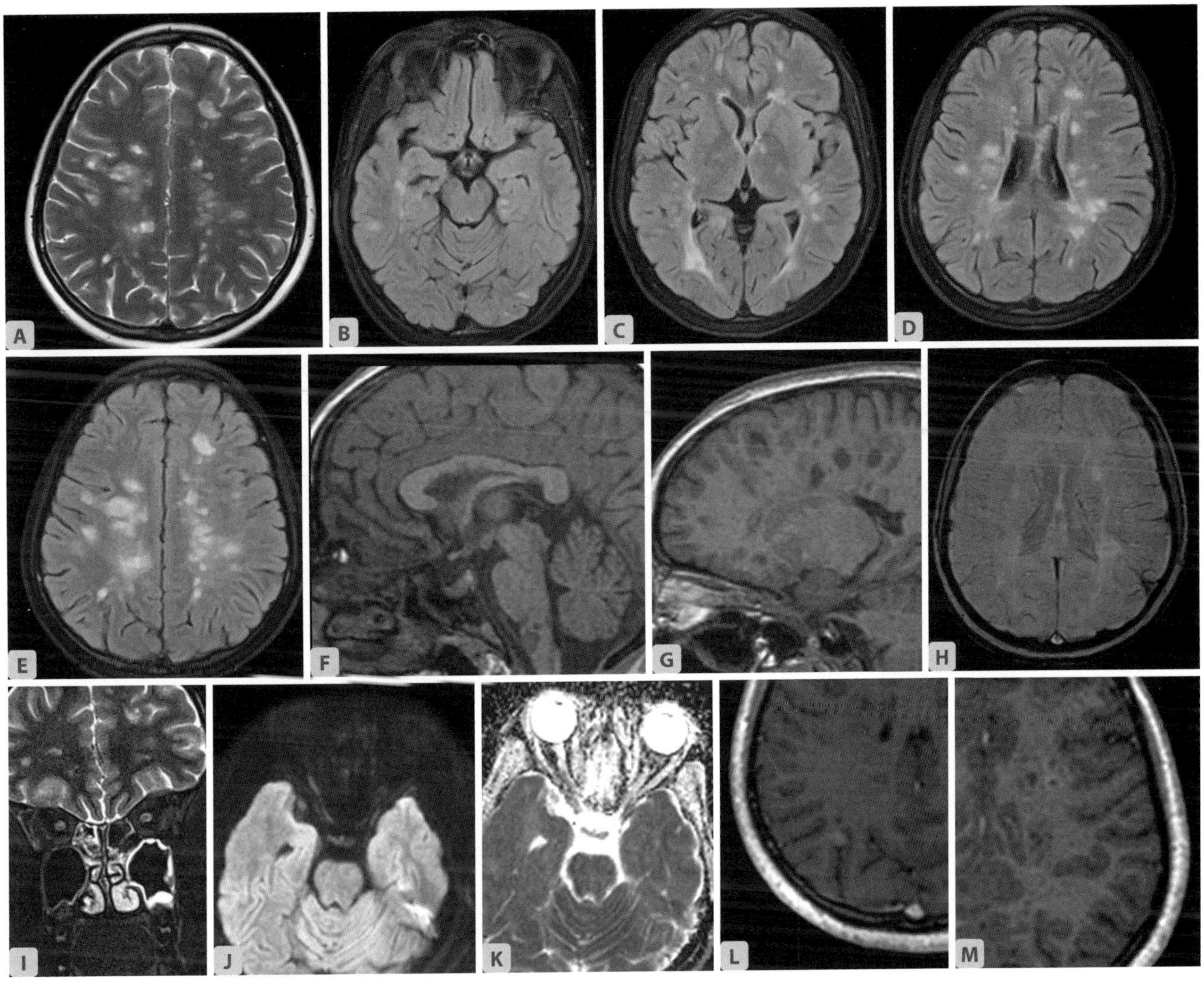

FIGS. 25A TO M: Relapsing-remitting multiple sclerosis (RRMS): Axial T2/FLAIR (A to E) images in a 16-year-old patient suffering from RRMS with relapse reveal multiple small ellipsoid and linear hyperintense lesions involving the periventricular, deep, subcortical white matter, corpus callosum, and the callososeptal interface. The lesions are isointense to hypointense on sagittal T1-weighted images (F to G). There is no evidence of hemorrhage on SWI (H). The right optic nerve shows hyperintense signal on T2 fat-saturated coronal image (I) with mild diffusion restriction (J and K). Subtle solid and ring enhancement is seen in a few of the subcortical (L) and deep white matter lesions (M), respectively. (FLAIR: fluid-attenuated inversion recovery; SWI: susceptibility-weighted imaging)

shown to be related to the clinical disability in these patients. Proton density-weighted images provide superior lesion to tissue contrast and are more useful for identification of periventricular lesions. This sequence is extremely useful in children <2 years of age due to incomplete myelination of the white matter.

Multiple sclerosis plaques are iso- to hypointense on TIW imaging. This hypointensity is representative of axonal destruction and is a predictor of subsequent disability. A subtle rim of mild hyperintensity may be seen around the hypointense "black holes" due to macrophage infiltration and lipid peroxidation. Volume loss with generalized atrophy and thinning of the corpus callosum are seen in advanced cases. Transient enhancement is seen at the time of active demyelination. Punctate nodular, linear, and rim patterns are seen. An incomplete rim of enhancement that is open toward the cortex may be seen in larger lesions. Leptomeningeal enhancement may be seen. Enhancement disappears within 6 months in >90% of the lesions. Acute plaques mostly show normal or increased diffusivity on DWI, however restriction of diffusion may be seen occasionally.

Imaging studies in pediatric MS cohorts have revealed that children have higher lesion burden on initial brain imaging when compared with adults, more so in the brainstem and cerebellum. Atypical imaging features are also found more commonly in children. The demyelinating lesions tend to be larger and more confluent with ill-defined borders and deep gray matter involvement. Tumefactive lesions (lesions >2 cm in size with surrounding edema) have also been described as initial brain imaging findings in young children with MS.[90]

Advanced Imaging Techniques

These include brain volumetry, magnetization transfer imaging, cortical imaging techniques, diffusion tensor imaging (DTI), MR spectroscopy, and SWI.

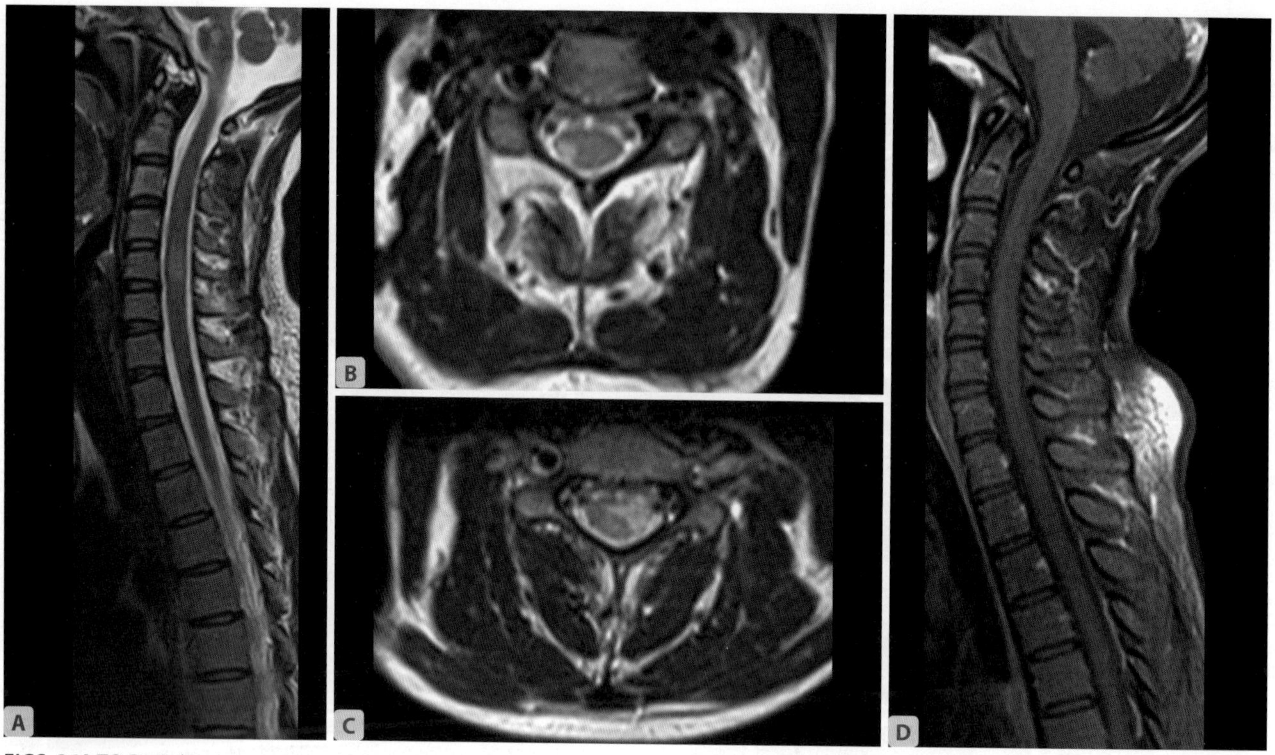

FIGS. 26A TO D: Relapsing-remitting multiple sclerosis (MS): Sagittal T2 (A), axial T2 (B and C), and sagittal postcontrast T1 (D) images reveal an area of short segment T2-hyperintensity at C4–C5 level. The lesion is posteriorly and laterally placed on axial images. There is no postcontrast enhancement.

Brain volumetry: This can be performed using high-resolution isotropic T1W sequences. Studies have shown that there is a significant reduction in global brain volume and thalamic volume in children and adolescents suffering from MS as compared to healthy controls. In addition, reduction in head size has also been seen, as pediatric MS patients do not have brain growth as per their age.

Magnetization transfer imaging: This technique is useful for quantifying the amount of microstructural damage within T2 lesions, the normal-appearing white matter, and the normal-appearing gray matter. There is a reduction in the total amount of myelin lipid and protein concentration in the brain due to inflammation in MS. Magnetization transfer ratio (MTR) imaging enables indirect detection of myelination. A fall in MTR implies that there is a reduction in the exchange of magnetization between bound protons and the surrounding free water. This suggests tissue destruction. Demyelinated MS white matter lesions show significant reduction in MTR as compared to the normal-appearing white matter. Reduction in MTR values has been observed in the normal-appearing white matter around the lateral ventricles in adults. Cognitive impairment has been seen to be associated with low whole-brain MTR. Reduced MTR in the normal-appearing brain tissue is a predictor of decline in memory performance also.[91] Yeh et al. have shown that adult patients in whom the onset of MS was in childhood had lower MTR values within the T2 lesions, normal-appearing white matter, and normal-appearing gray matter as compared to adult patients with adult-onset MS.[92] No difference has been found between MTR of normal-appearing white matter in pediatric MS patients when compared with healthy controls.[93]

Cortical imaging: Dedicated pulse sequences like double inversion recovery and phase-sensitive inversion recovery are more useful for evaluation of gray matter pathology as compared to conventional T2/PD, T2-FLAIR sequences. Cortical gray matter lesions may be seen in early stages of the disease and in radiological isolated syndrome also. The lesions may be juxtacortical involving both gray and white matter, subpial, and purely intracortical which do not involve the borders of the gray matter or gray matter lesions involving the full cortex but not the underlying white matter. Gray matter lesions are more difficult to detect on MRI as compared to white matter lesions as gray matter contains less myelin than white matter. It shows minimal glial reaction with no complement deposition or lymphocyte infiltration. The blood–brain barrier is also maintained.

Diffusion tensor imaging: This technique allows assessment of the microstructural integrity of white matter. The diffusion parameters that are evaluated include mean diffusivity (MD), axial diffusivity (AD), radial diffusivity (RD), and fractional anisotropy (FA). Reduced FA values indicate loss of white matter structural integrity. An increase in average MD and reduction in FA have been seen in normal-appearing white matter in children with MS. In another study, elevation of ADC with reduction of FA values has been seen in T2-hyperintense lesions involving the corpus callosum, posterior limb of internal capsule, and long association fibers.[90]

Reduction of FA in corpus callosum correlates with loss of cognitive performance and processing speed in pediatric MS patients.[93]

MR spectroscopy: This technique may help in differentiating RRMS from SPMS. The latter shows reduction in NAA in normal-appearing gray matter. An increase in choline and myoinositol levels with reduction in NAA and creatinine has been seen in children with MS. A citrulline peak at 3.15 ppm has been observed in 44% of children with MS in both involved and normal-appearing white matter.

Susceptibility-weighted imaging: In addition to the central vein sign that helps in diagnosing MS, reports have suggested that SWI may help to differentiate the initial lesion in pediatric MS from secondary ADEM. A higher percentage of FLAIR lesions also revealed abnormalities on SWI in patients who were finally diagnosed with MS as compared to cases of ADEM.[94]

Slowly evolving lesions may be seen in 57% cases of chronic MS. These lesions show a slow increase in size and are more commonly seen in patients who have had MS for a longer duration and in progressive MS. These lesions show hypointense rim on SWI. This rim may remain or it may gradually disappear. Such slowly evolving lesions are not seen in neuromyelitis optica (NMO) spectrum disorders (NMOSDs) or cerebrovascular diseases.[95]

Differential Diagnosis

There are various differential diagnoses for MS in children, especially at the time of the initial event. Certain red flags should prompt the radiologist to search for alternate diagnosis. Confluence and symmetry of white matter abnormalities may be indicative of a leukodystrophy. Foci of microbleeds/infarcts may suggest CNS vasculitis. Other differentials include NMOSDs, anti-myelin oligodendrocyte glycoprotein-immunoglobulin G (MOG-IgG) disease, and neuro-Behçet's disease.[96] The differences between MS, NMO, and anti-MOG disease are given in **Figure 27**.

Acute Disseminated Encephalomyelitis

Acute disseminated encephalomyelitis is an inflammatory event that is characterized by demyelination associated with encephalopathy and multifocal neurological findings. It occurs most commonly in childhood. The incidence ranges from 0.1 to 0.6/100,000 children/year. There is a slight male preponderance with male to female ratio ranging from 1.2:1 to 2.6:1. The average age at onset varies from 3.6 to 7 years. Like MS, the prevalence of ADEM increases with the increase in distance from the equator. Most of the patients suffering from ADEM have history of a prior viral illness (55–86%). Vaccination may also precede ADEM, although the risk is much lower (4–18% of ADEM cases). The excess risk is <1.16 case of ADEM per million vaccine doses.[97]

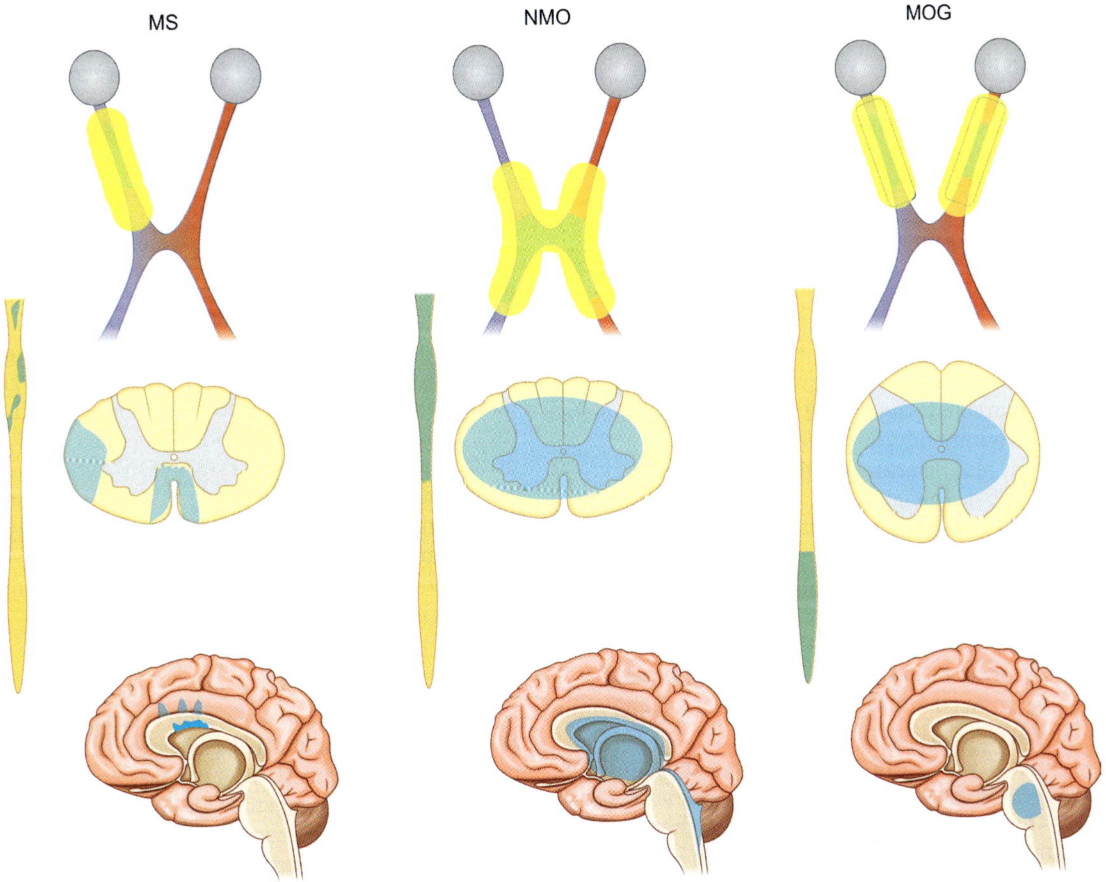

FIG. 27: Pictorial representation of areas of preferential involvement by MS, NMO, and anti-MOG antibody syndrome. (NMO: neuromyelitis optica; MOG: myelin oligodendrocyte glycoprotein; MS: multiple sclerosis)

Pathophysiology

Although the precise etiology of ADEM is not known, evidence of elevated CSF cytokines and chemokines has been found in patients of ADEM. It has been suggested that an inflammatory cascade is triggered due to molecular mimicry. The antigens that are thought to be targeted because of their similarity to the viral sequences include myelin basic protein (MBP), proteolipid protein (PLP), and MOG.[98] Mouse model data suggests that demyelination in ADEM may be caused primarily by T cells. T cells reactive to MBP and IgG antibodies against MBP, PLP, and MOG have been identified in ADEM patients. Anti-MOG antibodies have been identified in 33–66% of pediatric ADEM cases. These may activate complement and natural killer cells.

Clinical Features

Clinically, patients suffering from ADEM have features suggestive of encephalopathy with symptoms of TM, cerebellar involvement, seizures, or neurologic deficit. There is a latent period of approximately 12 days between the viral illness and onset of symptoms. This is followed by a prodromal phase that is characterized by fever, headache, and nausea. The prodromal phase lasts for 3–4 days after which neurological symptoms develop. Children with ADEM and anti-MOG antibodies have a higher likelihood of TM.[99] ADEM is a monophasic disorder. The active phase of inflammation lasts for approximately 3 months followed by both imaging and symptomatic improvement.

As per the IPMSSG, all of the following are required for the diagnosis of ADEM:

- An initial polyfocal, clinical neurological event which is presumably due to inflammatory demyelination.
- Encephalopathy that cannot be explained by fever.
- No emergence of new clinical and MRI findings after 3 or more months of disease onset.
- Abnormal brain MRI during the acute phase.

Imaging

The following findings are usually seen on a brain MRI **(Figs. 28A to F)**:

- Poorly demarcated, large (>1–2 cm), diffuse lesions that involve predominantly the white matter.
- Lesions may also be present in the deep gray matter (e.g., thalamus or basal ganglia).
- Rarely T1-hypointense lesions may also be seen in the white matter.
- Enhancement on postgadolinium imaging may be seen in 30% of the cases.
- Diffusion restriction may or may not be seen.
- There is sparing of normal-appearing brain tissue with no change in MTR and DTI parameters in normal brain parenchyma.

In fulminant cases with rapid clinical deterioration, multiple areas of necrosis and hemorrhage may be seen along with the demyelinating lesions (acute hemorrhagic leukoencephalitis). As compared to MS, there is absence of periventricular lesions and Dawson fingers. Thalamic and internal capsule involvement on MRI may help to differentiate ADEM from NMO.

Multiphasic Acute Disseminated Encephalomyelitis

It has been seen that 10% of children who have had an initial episode of ADEM may experience a relapse that may occur 2–8 years after initial illness. Multiphasic ADEM is defined as two episodes consistent with ADEM that are separated by a gap of 3 months and are not followed by any other event.[100] Any relapse after the second attack indicates a chronic disorder like MS or NMO. The IPMSSG has suggested that MS should be considered after an initial attack if the second event is nonencephalopathic, occurs 3 or more months after the initial event, and shows new MRI findings that are consistent with the revised radiologic criteria for dissemination in space.

Acute disseminated encephalomyelitis associated with ON has also been reported. The patient may suffer from a single attack on repeated attacks of ON. There is near-complete resolution of previous brain MRI findings with no new follow-up lesions. This phenotype is called ADEM-ON and has been found to be associated with anti-MOG antibodies.

If an initial episode of ADEM is followed by repeated episodes of ON, longitudinally extensive TM or area postrema syndrome, and the lesions on imaging are consistent with NMOSD, then a diagnosis of pediatric NMOSD must be considered. A positive anti-aquaporin-4 (AQP4) IgG titer greatly facilitates this diagnosis.[90]

Neuromyelitis Optica Spectrum Disorder

Neuromyelitis optica spectrum disorder is an autoimmune disease that is characterized by recurrent inflammation involving the optic nerves and spinal cord. Autoimmune antibodies (NMO-IgG) that target AQP4 receptors have been identified in a majority of adult patients suffering from NMO. Pediatric-onset NMO is rare. Only 3–5% of NMO cases have pediatric onset.

Pathophysiology

It is postulated that molecular mimicry occurs between human AQP4 and nonhuman sequences that resemble AQP4. The pathogenesis of NMO is thought to be mediated via the humoral immune system. AQP4, the target antigen for NMO-IgG, is concentrated in the spinal cord gray matter, periaqueductal and periventricular regions, and the astrocyte foot processes at the blood–brain barrier.[101] The area postrema is a preferential target. Astrocyte damage occurs due to binding of the antibody to astrocyte foot processes surrounding blood vessels. This leads to damage through complement and cell-mediated mechanisms, which cause demyelination, oligodendrocyte cell death, axonal injury, and microglial activation.[102]

Clinical Features

Optic neuritis, TM, and brainstem symptoms are commonly seen in NMO. In pediatric case series of NMO, ON was the presenting feature in 50–75% of cases and TM in 30–50% of cases, either alone or together. ON in NMOSD is bilateral, with involvement of optic chasm and has a relapsing course. The visual loss is more severe and the response to corticosteroids is also poor.

An ADEM-like picture with diffuse brain involvement has also been reported. NMO has also been described after

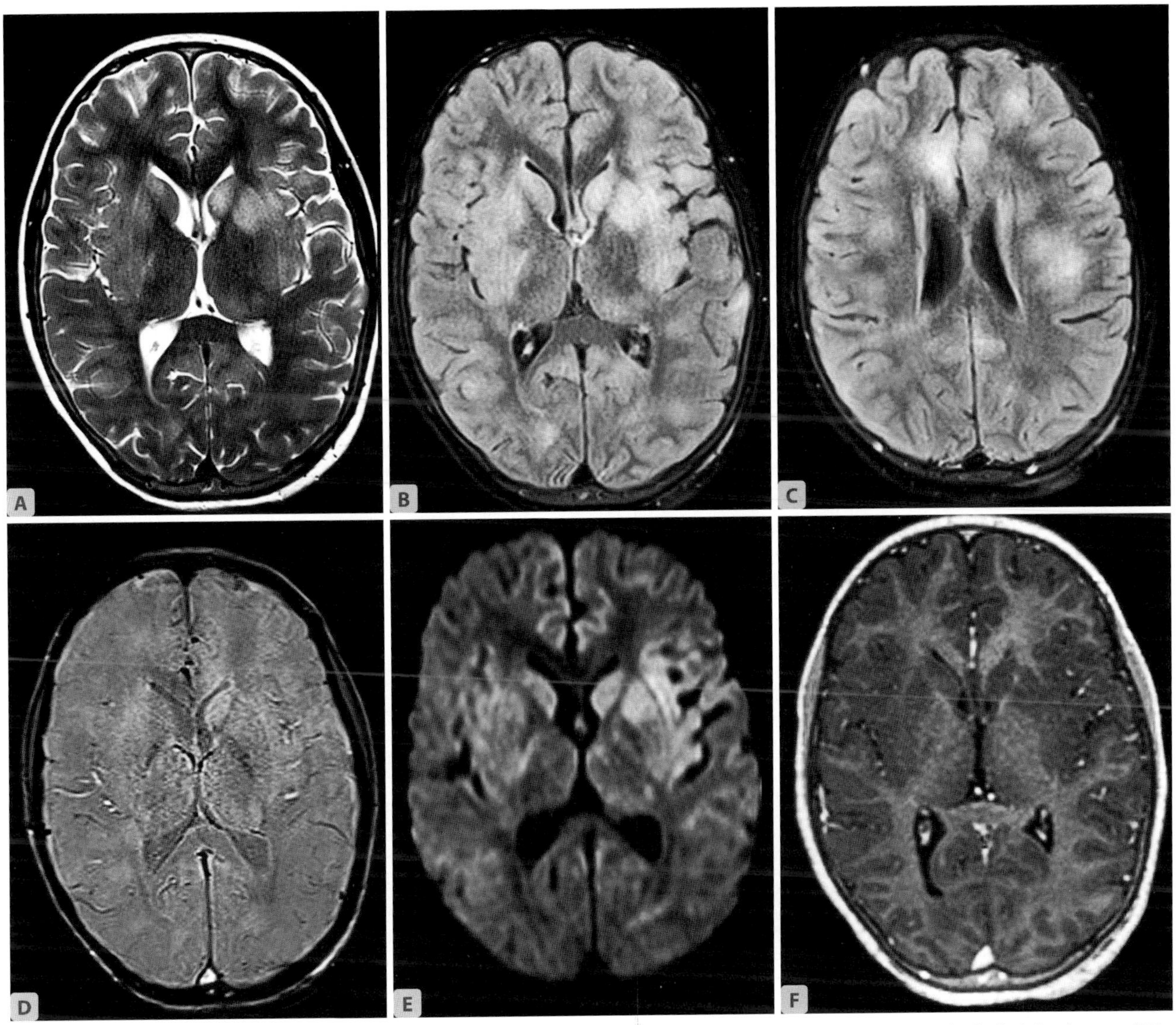

FIGS. 28A TO F: Acute disseminated encephalomyelitis (ADEM): Axial MRI of the brain in a 10-year-old child reveals multiple ill-defined areas of T2 (A)/FLAIR (B and C) hyperintensity involving bilateral basal ganglia, posterior limb of right internal capsule, left thalamus, and bilateral frontoparietal subcortical white matter. There is no hemorrhage or restriction on SWI (D) and DWI (E), respectively. Axial postcontrast T1 (F) does not reveal any enhancement. (DWI: diffusion-weighted imaging; FLAIR: fluid-attenuated inversion recovery; SWI: susceptibility-weighted imaging)

influenza, herpes infection and bone marrow transplant, and in association with another autoimmune disease. An area postrema syndrome with nausea, vomiting, and intractable hiccups may be seen. Brainstem involvement may lead to acute respiratory failure and death. Relapses occur in 90% of patients. Pediatric onset is associated with more frequent episodes of ON, more diffuse brain lesions, and lower mortality as compared to adult patients.

Revised IPMSSG consensus criteria for pediatric NMO require:

- Optic neuritis
- Transverse myelitis
- At least two of the following:
  i. MR imaging evidence of a contiguous spinal cord involvement extending over three or more segments
  ii. Aquaporin-4-IgG-seropositive status
  iii. Brain MR imaging not meeting diagnostic criteria for MS.

Imaging

As discussed above, the lesions are preferentially located at areas of high AQP4 expression like periventricular white matter along the third and fourth ventricles in the hypothalamus, diencephalon, and area postrema. Other involved regions include midbrain and cerebellum **(Figs. 29A to G)**. Postcontrast cloud-like pattern of enhancement can be seen in one-third of the cases with brain lesions. Acute brain lesions mostly resolve on posttreatment imaging. ON appears as thickening with high-signal intensity on T2W or STIR images in the optic nerves with postcontrast enhancement. There is preferential involvement of the posterior part of the optic nerve with extension of the signal change into the optic chiasm **(Figs. 29A to G)**. In chronic cases, thinning of the optic nerves is seen suggesting optic atrophy.

Acute TM occurs in mostly at the time of relapse. Spinal cord lesions are extensive, centrally located, and span a minimum of three segments. The lesions are hyperintense on T2 and may show patchy postcontrast enhancement. Cervical myelitis may also extend superiorly into the brainstem. T1-hypointense signal, suggesting cavitation and tissue necrosis, may also be seen.[103] Short segment TM may also be seen as the initial manifestation in up to 14.5% of cases.[104]

The differential diagnosis for NMO includes MS, ADEM, anti-MOG-related disorders, infections, and other autoimmune disorders such as systemic lupus erythematosus and Sjögren's syndrome.

Anti-myelin Oligodendrocyte Glycoprotein Syndromes

Myelin oligodendrocyte glycoprotein (MOG) is a glycoprotein that is found on the surface of the myelin in the brain and spinal cord. It is involved in the regulation of oligodendrocyte microtubule stability. MOG also plays a role in mediating complement cascade. Acquired demyelination syndrome with antibodies against MOG has been classified as a separate subgroup different from NMO and MS.[105]

The antibodies to MOG are produced peripherally. These reach the CNS after breakdown of the blood-brain barrier. Demyelination associated with anti-MOG antibodies may occur without any apparent predisposing illness. However, prior infection prodrome has been identified in almost 50% of patients. Anti-MOG antibody-related demyelination has been found to be associated with N-methyl-D-aspartate receptor (NMDAR) encephalitis, *Borrelia*, herpes simplex and Epstein-Barr virus infections, and rarely with relapsing MS. The age of onset of anti-MOG syndromes ranges from 6 to 70 years.

Clinical Manifestation

Optic neuritis is the most common presentation in adults, followed by myelitis and an ADEM-like presentation. ON in MOG-positive cases is severe, bilateral, and is associated with swelling of the optic nerve head. A relapsing course is common. 93% of patients have been seen to relapse when

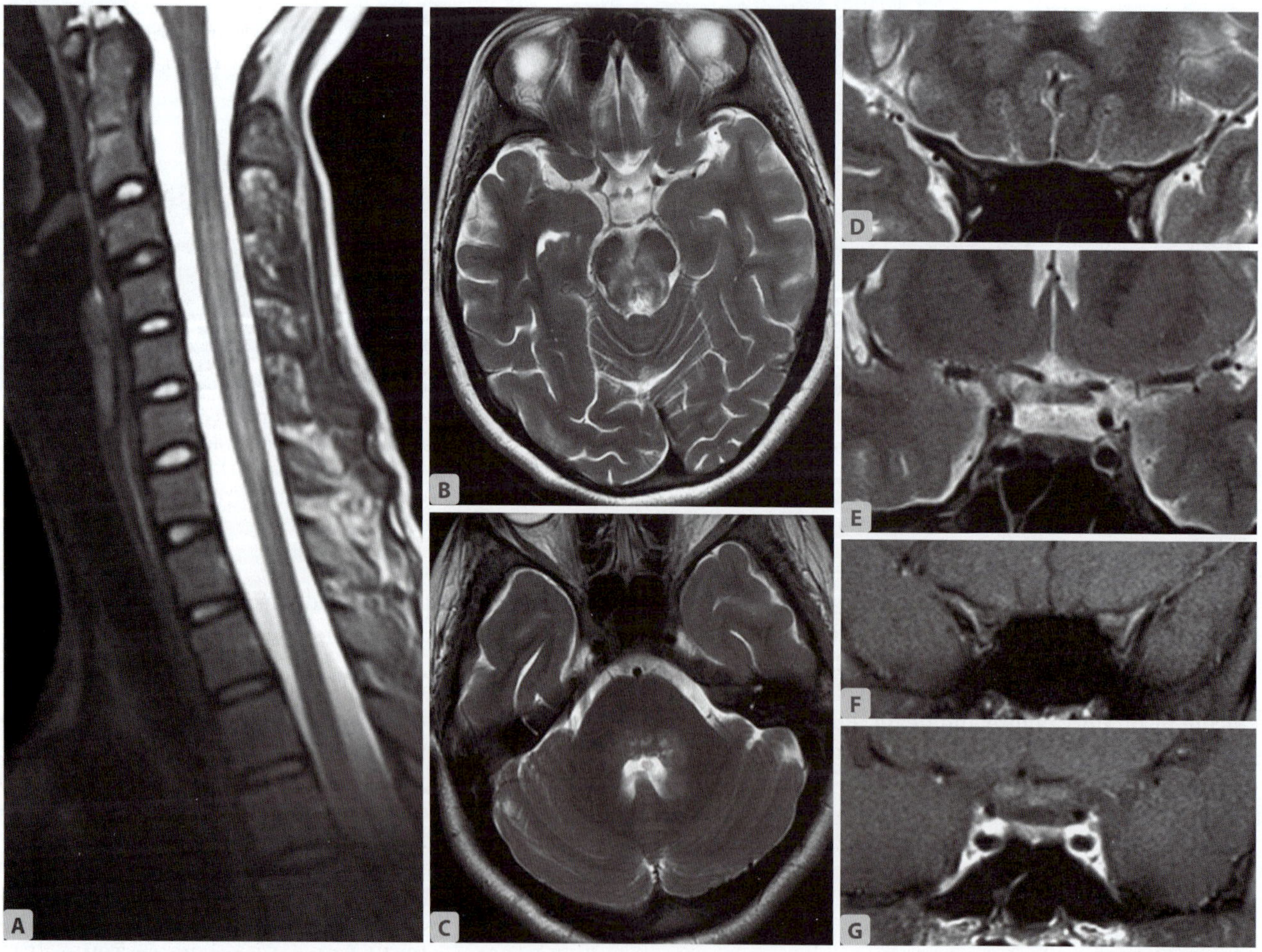

FIGS. 29A TO G: Neuromyelitis optica: Imaging in an aquaporin-4 antibody positive 15-year-old patient shows long segment cord hyperintensity on T2 sagittal section (A). Brain imaging revealed ill-defined T2-hyperintensities in the periventricular areas of the midbrain and pons (B and C). Coronal T2 (D and E) and postcontrast T1 images (F and G) show hyperintensity with enhancement involving the posterior intracanalicular segment of left optic nerve and the optic chiasm on the right side.

followed-up for duration of 8 years or more. In children, an ADEM-like presentation is more common.

Imaging

T2-hyperintense signal is seen in bilateral optic nerves. The retrobulbar and orbital segments are more commonly involved. The optic chiasm is very rarely involved. The optic nerve appears enlarged and tortuous. Optic disk edema may be seen. Restriction may also be seen on DWI **(Figs. 30A to H)**. Perioptic contrast enhancement, which may spread into the surrounding orbital tissue, may be seen in up to one-third of the cases. Optic atrophy may be seen on follow-up imaging with persistent T2-hyperintensity. Both long segment (two-thirds of the patients) and short segment (one-third of the cases) myelitis may be seen on spine MRI. Axial images show involvement of both gray and white matter with involvement of >50% of the surface area. Any part of the spinal cord may be involved, however conus medullaris involvement has been found to be very specific for anti-MOG antibody-related disorders. A sagittal linear hyperintensity with surrounding ill-defined hyperintense signal on T2 sagittal sections may also be seen. Patchy heterogeneous cloud-like enhancement with ill-defined margins is seen on postcontrast imaging. Well-defined foci of enhancement, meningeal enhancement, and linear ependymal enhancement may also be seen in some cases. On brain imaging, deep white matter and subcortical lesions are seen in the supratentorial white matter. Rarely, involvement of the brainstem, pons, cerebellar peduncles, and mesencephalon may also be seen. Cases showing an ADEM-like pattern with diffuse T2 hyperintensity involving the gray matter, subcortical white matter, deep gray matter, and white matter have also been reported. Multiple patchy areas of ill-defined cloud-like enhancement are seen on postcontrast imaging. Some of the active lesions may demonstrate diffusion restriction on DWI.[106] Focal discrete rounded white matter lesions are also seen in the corpus callosum. These are different from the Dawson fingers and the arch bridge pattern seen in MS and NMO, respectively.[107]

Autoimmune Encephalitis

Autoimmune encephalitis (AE) as a cause of pediatric encephalopathy is more common than previously seen. The disease may be activated by an infection, occult neoplasm, or vaccine. In cases of occult neoplasms, onconeural autoantibodies are formed that act against intracellular neuronal antigens. Encephalitic syndromes that do not have an association with an underlying tumor, but are due to autoantibodies to the surface or synaptic antigens in the brain, have also been described.[108] Currently, the most common autoantibodies known in children suffering from AE target the NMDAR, glutamic acid decarboxylase 65 (GAD65), and MOGs. Clinical presentation includes movement disorders, abnormal movements,

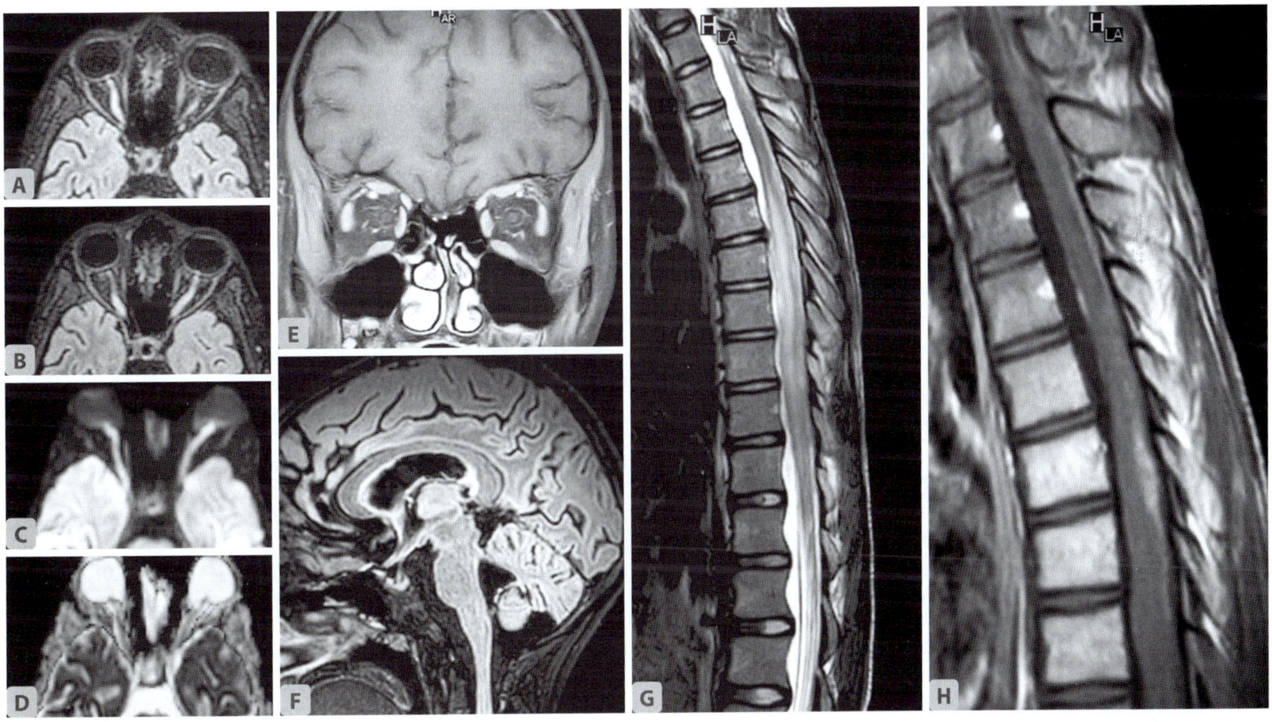

FIGS. 30A TO H: Anti-MOG antibody disease: A 16-year-old child presented with clinical features of optic neuritis and myelitis. Laboratory workup revealed positivity for anti-MOG antibodies. On imaging, the intraorbital and the retrobulbar segments of bilateral optic nerves revealed hyperintense signal on axial flair sections (A and B) with restriction on diffusion (C) and ADC (D) images. Perioptic nerve sheath enhancement was noted on coronal postcontrast T1 images (E). Small hyperintense focus was seen in the splenium of corpus callosum also (F). Sagittal T2 (G) and postcontrast sections (H) of the dorsal spine showed long segment involvement of the dorsal spinal cord with ill-defined peripheral enhancement. (ADC: apparent diffusion coefficient; MOG: myelin oligodendrocyte glycoprotein)

altered consciousness, seizures, cognitive decline, behavior changes, and psychiatric symptoms. Over 50% of patients may have a normal MRI at the time of presentation. In NMDAR encephalitis, T2-hyperintense signal may be seen in the cortex, basal ganglia, white matter, or the cerebellum. In GAD encephalitis, imaging may show lesions in the limbic system, cerebellum, and cortex. Cerebral atrophy may be seen in late stage of the disease. Imaging helps to rule out other differential diagnosis. The presence of known antibodies that are associated with AE in serum or CSF help in the diagnosis.[109]

CONCLUSION

Neuroinfections form an important category of pediatric CNS diseases, which are potentially treatable in the era of advanced antibiotics. MRI plays an important role in disease diagnosis and prognosis. Inflammatory disorders in children have a very wide spectrum. The diagnosis hinges upon a combination of clinical laboratory and imaging findings. Therefore, a comprehensive evaluation is essential in such patients. Correct diagnosis is essential, so that proper management can be instituted.

REFERENCES

1. Barkovich AJ. Infections of the nervous system. In: Benkovich AJ (Ed). Pediatric Neuroimaging, 4th edition. Lippincott: Williams and Wilkins; 2005. pp. 801-5.
2. Shih RY, Koeller KK. Bacterial, Fungal, and Parasitic Infections of the Central Nervous System: Radiologic-Pathologic Correlation and Historical Perspectives. Radiographics. 2015;35:1141-69.
3. Smirniotopoulos JG, Murphy FM, Rushing EJ, Rees JH, Schroeder JW. Patterns of Contrast Enhancement in the Brain and Meninges. Radiographics. 2007;27:525-51.
4. Friede RL. Developmental Neuropathology, 2nd edition. Berlin: Springer-Verlag; 1989.
5. Raybaud C, Girard N, Sevely A. Neuroradiologic pediatrique. In: Raybaud C, Girard N, Sevely A (Eds). Radiodiagnostic-Neuro-radiologic-Cppariel Locomotor. Paris: Elsevier Science; 1996. p. 26.
6. Moseley IF, Kendall BE. Radiology of intracranial empyemas, with special reference to computed tomography. Neuroradiology. 1984;26:333-45.
7. Courville CB. Subdural empyema secondary to purulent frontal sinusitis. Arch Otolaryngol. 1944;39:211-30.
8. Enzmann DR. Britt RH, Placone R. Staging of human brain abscess by computed tomography. Radiology. 1983;146:703-8.
9. Saini AG, Rathore V, Ahuja CK, Chhabra R, Vaidya PC, Singhi P. Multiple brain abscesses due to Enterobacter cloacae in an immune-competent child. J Infect Public Health. 2017;10:674-7.
10. Enzmann DR, Lyons BE, Carroll B, Placone RC, Rasor J, Britt RH, et al. Experimental brain abscess: enhanced sonography and pathologic correlation. AJNR Am J Neuroradiol. 1982;3:41-5.
11. Sze G, Zimmerman RD. The magnetic resonance imaging of infections and inflammatory diseases. Radiol Clin North Am. 1988;26:839-59.
12. Haimes AB, Zimmerman RD, Morgello S, Weingarten K, Becker RD, Jennis R, et al. MR imaging of brain abscesses. AJR Am J Roentgenol. 1989;152:1073-85.
13. Toh CH, Wei KC, Chang CN, Hsu PW, Wong HF, Ng SH, et al. Differentiation of pyogenic brain abscesses from necrotic glioblastomas with use of susceptibility-weighted imaging. AJNR Am J Neuroradiol. 2012;33:1534-8.
14. Kim SH, Chang KH, Song IC, Han MH, Kim HC, Kang HS, et al. Brain abscess and brain tumor: discrimination with in vivo H-1 MR spectroscopy. Radiology. 1997;204:239-45.
15. Martínez-Pérez I, Moreno A, Alonso J, Aguas J, Conesa G, Capdevila A, et al. Diagnosis of brain abscess by magnetic resonance spectroscopy. Report of two cases. J Neurosurg. 1997;86:708-13.
16. Venkatesh SK, Gupta RK, Pal L, Husain N, Husain M. Spectroscopic increase in choline signal is a nonspecific marker for differentiation of infective/inflammatory from neoplastic lesions of the brain. J Magn Reson Imaging. 2001;14:8-15.
17. Luthra G, Parihar A, Nath K, Jaiswal S, Prasad KN, Husain N, et al. Comparative evaluation of fungal, tubercular, and pyogenic brain abscesses with conventional and diffusion MR imaging and proton MR spectroscopy. AJNR Am J Neuroradiol. 2007;28: 1332-8.
18. Garg M, Gupta RK, Husain M, Chawla S, Chawla J, Kumar R, et al. Brain abscesses: etiologic categorization with in vivo proton MR spectroscopy. Radiology. 2004;230:519-27.
19. Pal D, Bhattacharya A, Husain M, Prasad KN, Pandey CM, Gupta RK. In vivo proton MR spectroscopy evaluation of pyogenic brain abscesses: a report of 194 cases. AJNR Am J Neuroradiol. 2010;31:360-6.
20. Muzumdar D, Vedantam R, Chandrashekhar D. Tuberculosis of the central nervous system in children. Childs Nerv Syst. 2018;34:1925-35.
21. Phypers M, Harris T, Power C. CNS tuberculosis: a longitudinal analysis of epidemiological and clinical features. Int J Tuberc Lung Dis. 2006;10:99-103.
22. Berenguer J, Moreno S, Laguna F, Vicente T, Adrados M, Ortega A, et al. Tuberculous meningitis in patients infected with the human immunodeficiency virus. N Engl J Med. 1992;326: 668-72.
23. Morgado C, Ruivo N. Imaging meningoencephalic tuberculosis. Eur J Radiol. 2005;55:188-92.
24. Wallace RC, Burton EM, Barrett FF, Leggiadro RJ, Gerald BE, Lasater OE. Intracranial tuberculosis in children: CT appearance and clinical outcome. Pediatr Radiol. 1991;21:241-6.
25. Bhargava S, Gupta AK, Tandon PN. Tuberculous meningitis—a CT study. Br J Radiol. 1982;55:189-96.
26. Fischbein N, Dillon W, Barkovich A. Tuberculosis. In: Fischbein N, Dillon W, Barkovich A (Eds). Teaching Atlas of Brain Imaging. New Delhi: Thieme Medical Publishers; 2000. pp. 165-8.
27. Bonafé A, Manelfe C, Gomez MC, Tager M, Massip P, Auvergnat JC, et al. Tuberculous meningitis. Contribution of computerized tomography to its diagnosis and prognosis. J Neuroradiol. 1985;12:302-16.
28. Leiguarda R, Berthier M, Starkstein S, Nogués M, Lylyk P. Ischemic infarction in 25 children with tuberculous meningitis. Stroke. 1988;19:200-4.
29. Hsieh FY, Chia LG, Shen WC. Locations of cerebral infarctions in tuberculous meningitis. Neuroradiology. 1992;34:197-9.
30. Reid H, Fallon RJ. Bacterial infections. In: Adams JH, Duchen L (Eds). Greenfields Neuropathology, 5th edition. New York: Oxford University Press; 1992. pp. 317-42.
31. Lu T, Zou Y, Jiang T, Yang Y, Wu A, Chen H, et al. Intracranial Artery Injury in HIV-negative Tuberculous Meningitis: A High-Resolution Vessel Wall Imaging Study. Clin Neuroradiol. 2020;30: 381-8.

32. Soni N, Kumar S, Shimle A, Ora M, Bathla G, Mishra P. Cerebrovascular complications in tuberculous meningitis—a magnetic resonance imaging study in 90 patients from a tertiary care hospital. Neuroradiol J. 2020;33:3-16.
33. Bhargava A, Tandon PN. Intracranial tuberculomas: a CT study. Br J Radiol. 1980;53:935-45.
34. Welchman JM. CT of intracranial tuberculomata. Clin Radiol. 1979;30:567-79.
35. Jinkins JR. CT of intracranial tuberculosis. Neuroradiology. 1991;33:126-35.
36. Jinkins JR. Gupta R, Chang KH. MR imaging of CNS tuberculosis. In: Goodman PC, Jinkins JR (Eds). Imaging of Tuberculosis and Craniospinal Tuberculosis. United States of America: Radiological Column of North America; 1995. pp. 771-89.
37. van Dyk A. CT of intracranial tuberculomas with specific reference to the "target sign". Neuroradiology. 1988;30:329-36.
38. Rajshekhar V, Haran RP, Prakash GS, Chandy MJ. Differentiating solitary small cysticercus granulomas and tuberculomas in patients with epilepsy. Clinical and computerized tomographic criteria. J Neurosurg. 1993;78:402-7.
39. Gupta RK, Vatsal DK, Husain N, Chawla S, Prasad KN, Roy R, et al. Differentiation of tuberculous from pyogenic brain abscesses with in vivo proton MR spectroscopy and magnetization transfer MR imaging. Am J Neuroradiol. 2001;22:1503-9.
40. Tyson G, Newman P, Strachan WL. Tuberculous brain abscess. Surg Neurol. 1978;10:323-5.
41. Morales H, Alfaro D, Martinot C, Fayed N, Gaskill-Shipley M. MR spectroscopy of intracranial tuberculomas: a singlet peak at 3.8 ppm as potential marker to differentiate them from malignant tumors. Neuroradiol J. 2015;28:294-302.
42. Whitener DR. Tuberculous brain abscess: report of a case and review of the literature. Arch Neurol. 1978;35:148-55.
43. Schaller MA, Wicke F, Foerch C, Weidauer S. Central Nervous System Tuberculosis: Etiology, Clinical Manifestations and Neuroradiological Features. Clin Neuroradiol. 2019;29:3-18.
44. Yang PJ, Reger KM, Seeger JF, Carmody RF, Iacono RP. Brain abscess: an atypical CT appearance of CNS tuberculosis. AJNR Am J Neuroradiol. 1987; 8:919-20.
45. Withman RR, Johnson RH, Roberts DL. Diagnosis of miliary tuberculosis by cerebral computed tomography. Arch Intern Med. 1979;139:479-80.
46. Gee GT, Bazan C, Jinkins JR. Miliary tuberculosis involving the brain: MR findings. AJR Am J Roentgenol. 1992;159:1075-6.
47. Carbajal JR, Palacios E, Azar-Kia B, Churchill R. Radiology of cysticercosis of the central nervous system including computed tomography. Radiology. 1977;125:127-31.
48. Suss RA, Maravilla KR, Thompson J. MR imaging of intracranial cysticercosis: Comparison with CT and anatomopathologic features. AJNR Am J Neuroradiol. 1986;7:235-42.
49. Suh DC, Chang KH, Han MH, Lee SR, Han MC, Kim CW. Unusual MR manifestations of neurocysticercosis. Neuroradiology. 1989;31:396-402.
50. Poeschl P, Janzen A, Schuierer G, Winkler J, Bogdahn U, Steinbrecher A. Calcified neurocysticercosis lesions trigger symptomatic inflammation during antiparasitic therapy. AJNR Am J Neuroradiol. 2006;27:653-5.
51. Gupta S, Desai K, Goel A. Intracranial hydatid cyst: a report of five cases and review of literature. Neurol India. 1999;47:214-7.
52. Koelfen W, Freund M, Gückel F, Rohr H, Schultze C. MRI of encephalitis in children: comparison of CT and MRI in the acute stage with long-term follow-up. Neuroradiology. 1996;38:73-9.
53. Demaerel P, Wilms G, Robberecht W, Johnnik K, Van Hecke P, Carton H, et al. MRI of herpes simplex encephalitis. Neuroradiology. 1992;34:490-3.
54. Tien R, Felsberg G, Osumi A. Herpes virus infections of the CNS: MR findings. AJR Am J Roentgenol. 1993;161:167-76.
55. Kumar S, Misra UK, Kalita J, Salwani V, Gupta RK, Gujral R. MRI in Japanese encephalitis. Neuroradiology. 1997;39:180-4.
56. Shoji H, Kida H, Hino H, Matsuura S, Kojima K, Abe T, et al. Magnetic resonance imaging findings in Japanese encephalitis. White matter lesions. J Neuroimaging. 1994;4:206-11.
57. Gray F, Bélec L, Lescs MC, Chrétien F, Ciardi A, Hassine D, et al. Varicella-zoster virus infection of the central nervous system in the acquired immune deficiency syndrome. Brain. 1994;117:987-99.
58. Darling CR, Larsen MB, Byrd SE, Radkowski MA, Palka PS, Allen ED. MR and CT imaging patterns in post-varicella encephalitis. Pediatr Radiol. 1995;25:241-4.
59. Chow CK, Ma CKL. Presentation and Outcome of Acute Necrotizing Encephalopathy of Childhood: A 10-Year Single-Center Retrospective Study From Hong Kong. J Child Neurol. 2020;35:674-80.
60. Dixon L, Varley J, Gontsarova A, Mallon D, Tona F, Muir D, et al. COVID-19-related acute necrotizing encephalopathy with brain stem involvement in a patient with aplastic anemia. Neurol Neuroimmunol Neuroinflamm. 2020;7:e789.
61. Brismar J, Gascon GG, Yon-Steyern KV. Subacute sclerosing panencephalitis. Neurology. 1996;47:1278-83.
62. Varadkar S, Bien CG, Kruse CA, Jensen FE, Bauer J, Pardo CA, et al. Rasmussen's encephalitis: clinical features, pathobiology, and treatment advances. Lancet Neurol. 2014;13:195-205.
63. Kiroğlu Y, Calli C, Yunten N, Kitis O, Kocaman A, Karabulut N, et al. Diffusion-weighted MR imaging of viral encephalitis. Neuroradiology. 2006;48:875-80.
64. Barkovich AJ, Girard N. Fetal brain infections. Childs Nerv Syst. 2003;19:501-7.
65. Kauffman WM, Sivit CJ, Fitz CR, Rakusan TA, Herzog K, Chandra RS. CT and MR evaluation of intracranial involvement in pediatric HIV infection: a clinical-imaging correlation. AJNR Am J Neuroradiol. 1992;13:949-57.
66. Spreer J, Enenkel-Stoodt S, Funk M, Fiedler A, de Simone A, Hacker H. [Neuroradiological findings in perinatally HIV-infected children]. Rofo. 1994;161:106-12.
67. States LJ, Zimmerman RA, Rutstein RM. Imaging of pediatric central nervous system HIV infection. Neuroimaging Clin N Am. 1997;7:321-39.
68. Radaelli G, Nunes ML, Soder RB, de Oliveira JM, Bruzzo FT, Neto FK, et al. Review of neuroimaging findings in congenital Zika virus syndrome and its relation to the time of infection. Neuroradiol J. 2020;33:152-7.
69. Lu D, Pavlakis SG, Frank Y, Bakshi S, Pahwa S, Gould RJ, et al. Proton MR spectroscopy of the basal ganglia in healthy children and children with AIDS. Radiology. 1996;199:423-8.
70. Pavlakis SG, Lu D, Frank Y, Bakshi S, Pahwa S, Barnett TA, et al. Magnetic resonance spectroscopy in childhood AIDS encephalopathy. Pediatr Neurol. 1995;12:277-82.
71. Singhi P, Saini AG. Fungal and Parasitic CNS Infections. Indian J Pediatr. 2019;86:83-90.
72. McCarthy MW, Kalasauskas D, Petraitis V, Petraitiene R, Walsh TJ. Fungal Infections of the Central Nervous System in Children. J Pediatr Infect Dis Soc. 2017;6:e123-33.
73. Jain KK, Mittal SK, Kumar S, Gupta RK. Imaging features of central nervous system fungal infection. Neurol India. 2007;55:241-50.
74. Tempkin AD, Sobonya RE, Seeger JF, Oh ES. Cerebral aspergillosis: radiologic and pathologic findings. Radiographics. 2006;26:1239-42.
75. Almutairi BM, Nguyen TB, Jansen GH, Asseri AH. Invasive aspergillosis of the brain: radiologic–pathologic correlation. Radiographics. 2009;29:375-9.

76. Smith AB, Rushing JR. Central nervous system infections associated with human immunodeficiency virus infection: radiologic–pathologic correlation. Radiographics. 2008;28: 2033-58.
77. Gordon-Lipkin E, Banwell B. An update on multiple sclerosis in children: diagnosis, therapies, and prospects for the future. Expert Rev Clin Immunol. 2017;13:975-89.
78. Waldman A, Ghezzi A, Bar-Or A, Mikaeloff Y, Tardieu M, Banwell B. Multiple sclerosis in children: an update on clinical diagnosis, therapeutic strategies, and research. Lancet Neurol. 2014;13: 936-48.
79. Langille MM, Rutatangwa A, Francisco C. Pediatric Multiple Sclerosis. Adv Pediatr. 2019;66:209-29.
80. Chou IJ, Wang HS, Whitehouse WP, Constantinescu CS. Paediatric Multiple Sclerosis: Update on Diagnostic Criteria, Imaging, Histopathology, and Treatment Choices. Curr Neurol Neurosci Rep. 2016;16:68.
81. Fisher KS, Cuascut FX, Rivera VM, Hutton GJ. Current Advances in Pediatric Onset Multiple Sclerosis. Biomedicines. 2020;8:71.
82. Benson LA, Healy BC, Gorman MP, Baruch NF, Gholipour T, Musallam A, et al. Elevated relapse rates in pediatric compared to adult MS persist for at least 6 years. Mult Scler Relat Disord. 2014;3:186-93.
83. Renoux C, Vukusic S, Mikaeloff Y, Edan G, Clanet M, Dubois B, et al. Natural history of multiple sclerosis with childhood onset. N Engl J Med. 2007;356:2603-13.
84. Sadaka Y, Verhey LH, Shroff MM, Branson HM, Arnold DL, Narayanan S, et al. 2010 McDonald criteria for diagnosing pediatric multiple sclerosis. Ann Neurol. 2012;72:211-23.
85. Hacohen Y, Brownlee W, Mankad K, Chong WK, Thompson A, Lim M, et al. Improved performance of the 2017 McDonald criteria for diagnosis of multiple sclerosis in children in a real-life cohort: Mult Scler. 2019. [Online ahead of print].
86. Krupp LB, Tardieu M, Amato MP, Banwell B, Chitnis T, Dale RC, et al. International Pediatric Multiple Sclerosis Study Group criteria for pediatric multiple sclerosis and immune-mediated central nervous system demyelinating disorders: revisions to the 2007 definitions. Mult Scler. 2013;19:1261-7.
87. Lee JY, Han J, Yang M, Oh SY. Population-based Incidence of Pediatric and Adult Optic Neuritis and the Risk of Multiple Sclerosis. Ophthalmology. 2020;127:417-25.
88. Dekker I, Wattjes MP. Brain and Spinal Cord MR Imaging Features in Multiple Sclerosis and Variants. Neuroimaging Clin N Am. 2017;27:205-27.
89. Traboulsee A, Simon JH, Stone L, Fisher E, Jones DE, Malhotra A, et al. Revised Recommendations of the Consortium of MS Centers Task Force for a Standardized MRI Protocol and Clinical Guidelines for the Diagnosis and Follow-Up of Multiple Sclerosis. AJNR Am J Neuroradiol. 2016;37:394-401.
90. Tenembaum SN. Pediatric Multiple Sclerosis. Neuroimaging Clin N Am. 2017;27:229-50.
91. Akbar N, Rudko DA, Parmar K. Magnetic Resonance Imaging of Multiple Sclerosis. 2017;1:14.
92. Yeh EA, Weinstock-Guttman B, Ramanathan M, Ramasamy DP, Willis L, Cox JL, et al. Magnetic resonance imaging characteristics of children and adults with paediatric-onset multiple sclerosis. Brain. 2009;132:3392-400.
93. Banwell B, Arnold DL, Tillema JM, Rocca MA, Filippi M, Weinstock-Guttman B, et al. MRI in the evaluation of pediatric multiple sclerosis. Neurology. 2016;87:S88-96.
94. Kelly JE, Mar S, D'Angelo G, Zhou G, Rajderkar D, Benzinger TLS. Susceptibility-weighted imaging helps to discriminate pediatric multiple sclerosis from acute disseminated encephalomyelitis. Pediatr Neurol. 2015;52:36-41.
95. Filippi M, Preziosa P, Banwell BL, Barkhof F, Ciccarelli O, De Stefano N, et al. Assessment of lesions on magnetic resonance imaging in multiple sclerosis: practical guidelines. Brain. 2019;142:1858-75.
96. Galardi MM, Gaudioso C, Ahmadi S, Evans E, Gilbert L, Mar S. Differential Diagnosis of Pediatric Multiple Sclerosis. Children. 2019;6:75.
97. Baxter R, Lewis E, Goddard K, Fireman B, Bakshi N, DeStefano F, et al. Acute Demyelinating Events Following Vaccines: A Case-Centered Analysis. Clin Infect Dis. 2016;63:1456-62.
98. Esposito S, Di Pietro GM, Madini B, Mastrolia MV, Rigante D. A spectrum of inflammation and demyelination in acute disseminated encephalomyelitis (ADEM) of children. Autoimmun Rev. 2015;14:923-9.
99. Cole J, Evans E, Mwangi M, Mar S. Acute Disseminated Encephalomyelitis in Children: An Updated Review Based on Current Diagnostic Criteria. Pediatr Neurol. 2019;100:26-34.
100. Pohl D, Alper G, Van Haren K, Kornberg AJ, Lucchinetti CF, Tenembaum S, et al. Acute disseminated encephalomyelitis: updates on an inflammatory CNS syndrome. Neurology. 2016;87: S38-45.
101. Lennon VA, Kryzer TJ, Pittock SJ, Verkman AS, Hinson SR. IgG marker of optic-spinal multiple sclerosis binds to the aquaporin-4 water channel. J Exp Med. 2005;202:473-7.
102. Tenembaum S, Chitnis T, Nakashima I, Collongues N, McKeon A, Levy M, et al. Neuromyelitis optica spectrum disorders in children and adolescents. Neurology. 2016;87:S59-66.
103. Lana-Peixoto MA, Talim N. Neuromyelitis Optica Spectrum Disorder and Anti-MOG Syndromes. Biomedicines. 2019;7:42.
104. Dutra BG, da Rocha AJ, Nunes RH, Maia ACM. Neuromyelitis Optica Spectrum Disorders: Spectrum of MR Imaging Findings and Their Differential Diagnosis. Radiographics. 2018;38:169-93.
105. Wynford-Thomas R, Jacob A, Tomassini V. Neurological update: MOG antibody disease. J Neurol. 2019;266:1280-6.
106. Denève M, Biotti D, Patsoura S, Ferrier M, Meluchova Z, Mahieu L, et al. MRI features of demyelinating disease associated with anti-MOG antibodies in adults. J Neuroradiol. 2019;46:312-8.
107. Salama S, Khan M, Levy M, Izbudak I. Radiological characteristics of myelin oligodendrocyte glycoprotein antibody disease. Mult Scler Relat Disord. 2019;29:15-22.
108. Barbagallo M, Vitaliti G, Pavone P, Romano C, Lubrano R, Falsaperla R. Pediatric Autoimmune Encephalitis. J Pediatr Neurosci. 2017;12:130-4.
109. Clinical approach to the diagnosis of autoimmune encephalitis in the pediatric patient. Neurol Neuroimmunol Neuroinflamm. 2020;7:e730.

CHAPTER

88

Pediatric Brain Tumors

Shailesh B Gaikwad, Ajay Garg

INTRODUCTION

In children, central nervous system (CNS) tumors are most common solid tumor and the leading cause of cancer-related mortality. 15–20% of all intracranial tumors occur in childhood. The peak age of occurrence of brain tumor in children is between ages of 4 and 8 years. Children below 2 years of age account for only 1–2% of all brain tumors.[1]

The molecular analysis has significantly advanced our understanding of the pathogenesis of childhood brain tumors. The World Health Organization (WHO) 2016 classification has incorporated molecular and genetic information to restructure the nosology brain tumors.

CLASSIFICATION OF CHILDHOOD TUMORS BASED ON TOPOGRAPHY[2]

The location of the tumor is a useful tool in the differential diagnosis and narrowing the list of possible tumors **(Table 1)**.

INFRATENTORIAL TUMORS

Medulloblastoma

Medulloblastoma (MB) is the most common infratentorial tumor in children, accounting for one-third of cases.[3] The great majority of MBs occurs in children between 5 and 15 years of age. The second peak occurs in adults, usually in the third and fourth decades of life. MBs typically occur in midline in the region of the vermis and inferior medullary velum (80% cases). In adults, MBs tend to occur in the cerebellar hemisphere. Approximately, 80% of patients with MB present with features of intracranial hypertension and the most common symptoms include headache, nausea, and vomiting. Cerebrospinal fluid (CSF) seeding occurs in approximately 40% of patients at the time of diagnosis.

Pathology

Medulloblastoma is most common embryonal tumor. Histologically, MBs are classified as classic, nodular or desmoplastic, MB with extensive nodularity, or as anaplastic/large cell variants. Over the past 5 years, considerable advances have been made in understanding MBs biology and genetics profiles.[4] The WHO 2016 update on classification of CNS tumors has incorporated histological and molecular schemes into the classification of MBs.[5,6]

Based on genomic characterization, MBs have four distinct molecular subgroups: (1) Wingless (WNT), (2) Sonic hedgehog (SHH), (3) Group 3, and (4) Group 4. Compared to tumor histology or clinical staging system, these molecular subgroups are more predictive of clinical behavior and outcome and are helpful in planning risk-adaptive treatment strategies.[4,6] Distribution of the different molecular subtypes between pediatric MB and adult MB are significantly different.[7] In pediatric MB, most common subgroup is group 3 (50–60%) followed by group 4 (10–30%), WNT (10–15%), and SHH (10-15%) while in adults MB, most common subgroup is SHH (50–60%) followed by group 4 (20–30%), WNT (10–15%), and group 3.[7]

Imaging

Medulloblastoma is a well-circumscribed vermian mass, centered near the midline. Typically, it fills the fourth ventricle and may extend midline inferiorly through the foramen of Magendie into the cisterna magna, rarely extend laterally through foramen of Luschka into cerebellopontine cistern. Characteristically, the tumor is hyperdense on nonenhanced CT scans due to hypercellularity and high nuclear-cytoplasmic ratio of the tumor cells **(Fig. 1A)**.[3] Up to one-fifth of cases may show foci of calcification. Enhancement on contrast administration is variable. Cystic and necrotic degeneration may occur, more so in adult MBs.

On MR imaging, MBs are typically hypo- to isointense on T1-weighted image (T1WI) and iso- to hypointense on T2-weighted image (T2WI) **(Fig. 1B)**. Cysts, hemorrhage, necrosis, and clump-like calcification may cause signal heterogeneity on T2WI **(Fig. 1C)**.[3] On diffusion-weighted MRI, characteristically MB shows a marked increase in the signal intensity **(Fig. 1D)** related to high cell density and the high nuclear-to-cytoplasm ratio of neoplastic cells.[8] However, the desmoplastic MB may have minimal or no diffusion restriction. Enhancement after contrast administration is

TABLE 1: Classification of brain tumor.

A. Infratentorial tumors				
	Cerebellum	**Brainstem**	**Fourth ventricle**	**Cerebellopontine angle**
	• Medulloblastoma	• Diffuse astrocytoma	• Ependymoma	• Ependymoma
	• Pilocytic astrocytoma	• Pilocytic astrocytoma	• Medulloblastoma	• Choroid plexus papilloma
	• Atypical teratoid rhabdoid tumor	• Diffuse midline glioma	• Pilocytic astrocytoma	• Astrocytoma
	• Hemangioblastoma	• Anaplastic astrocytoma	• Choroid plexus papilloma	
		• Glioblastoma (GBM)		
B. Supratentorial tumors				
	1. Cerebral hemispheres			
	Astrocytic tumors	**Oligodendroglial tumors**	**Ependymal tumors**	**Mixed neuronal-glial tumors**
	• Pilocytic astrocytoma	• Oligodendroglioma	• Ependymoma	• Ganglioglioma
	• Pleomorphic xanthoastrocytoma	• Anaplastic oligodendroglioma	• Embryonal	• Dysembryoplastic neuroepithelial tumors
	• Diffuse astrocytoma		• Atypical teratoid rhabdoid tumor	• Desmoplastic infantile tumors
	• Subependymal giant cell tumor (SGCT)		• Embryonal tumor with multi-layered rosettes C19MC-altered	
	• Anaplastic astrocytoma			
	• Glioblastoma			
	• Diffuse midline glioma			
	2. Intraventricular tumors			
	Lateral ventricle	**Third ventricle**		
	• Ependymoma	• Ependymoma		
	• Choroid plexus papilloma/ carcinoma (CPP/CPC)	• Astrocytoma		
	• Astrocytoma	• Choroid plexus papilloma		
	• Subependymal giant cell tumor	• Craniopharyngioma		
C. Pineal region tumors				
	Pineal parenchymal tumor	**Germ cell tumor**		
	• Pineoblastomas	• Pineal germinomas	• Diffuse midline glioma	
	• Pineocytomas	• Nongerminomatous GCTs		
	• Pineal parenchymal tumor of intermediate differentiation	• Teratoma		
	• Papillary tumor of the pineal gland	• Endodermal sinus tumor		
	• Pineal cysts	• Choriocarcinoma		
D. Sellar region				
	• Craniopharyngioma	• Pituitary adenoma	• Hypothalamic hamartoma	• Germinoma
	• Arachnoid cyst	• Epidermoid/dermoid	• Chiasmal/hypothalamic glioma	
E. Extraparenchymal tumors				
	• Meningioma	• Leukemia/lymphoma	• Arachnoid cyst	• Epidermoid/dermoid

variable as in CT scan **(Figs. 1E and F)**. At MR spectroscopy, MBs characteristically show taurine, detectable at short echo time (TE), and a high choline peak.[9]

At the time of diagnosis, up to one-third of MBs may show evidence of leptomeningeal dissemination which can be evaluated with contrast-enhanced MR imaging of the brain and the spine **(Fig. 1G)**.[3] In contrast to other malignancies, metastatic deposits in MB show less intense enhancement or may not enhance at all,[10] however they still show restricted diffusion.[11] Therefore, a diffusion-weighted sequence of brain and spine should be done in all cases of MBs to detect leptomeningeal dissemination.

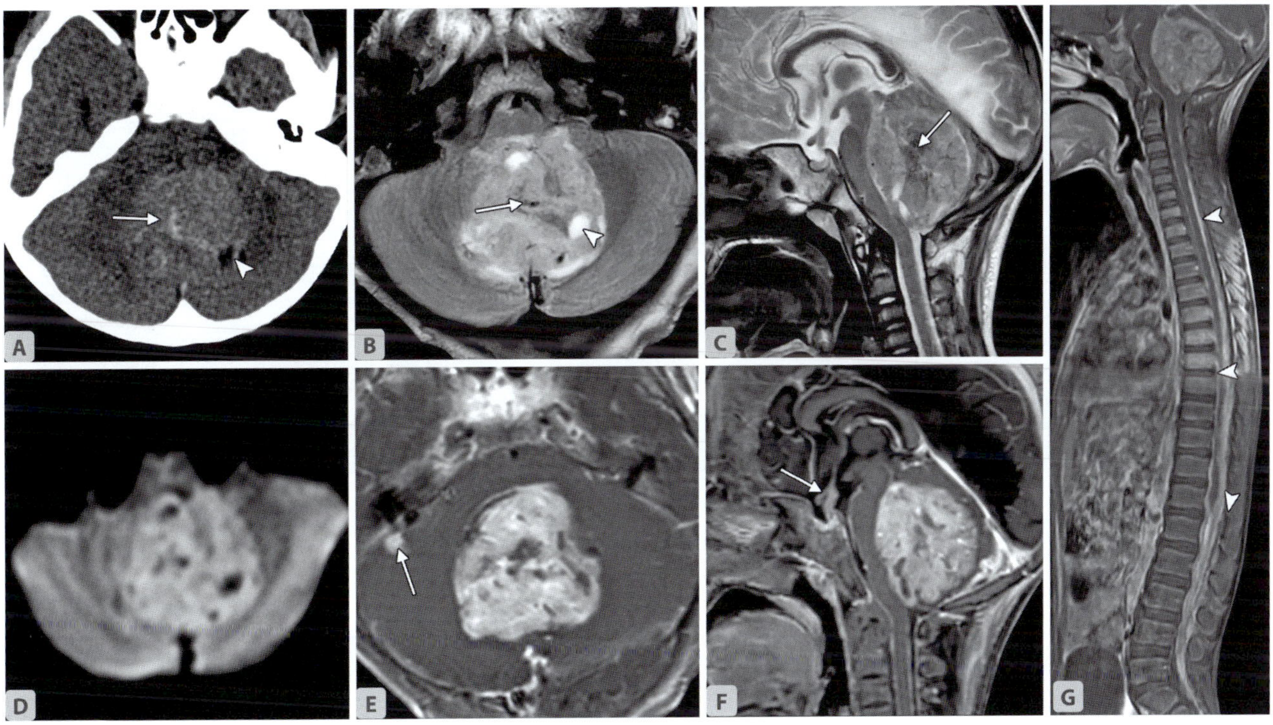

FIGS. 1A TO G: Type 3 medulloblastoma with leptomeningeal spread: Axial non-contrast CT scan (A) shows a hyperdense midline vermin mass with foci of hyperdense calcifications (small arrow in A) and a focal hypodense cyst (arrowhead in A). In axial (B) and sagittal (C) T2WI, the mass is hyperintense with hypointense (arrow in B and C) and hyperintense (arrowhead in B) areas corresponding to calcification and cyst, respectively as seen in CT. The mass is showing restricted diffusion in DWI (D). Postgadolinium axial (E) and sagittal (F) images of brain show intense enhancement of the mass along with leptomeningeal deposits in the right cerebellopontine angle cistern (arrow in E) and along pituitary stalk (arrow in F). Postgadolinium sagittal T1WI of the whole spine (G) shows diffuse leptomeningeal deposits (arrowhead in G) and enhancement of cauda equina nerve roots. (DWI: diffusion-weighted imaging; T1WI: T1-weighted image; T2WI: T2-weighted image)

Recently, there has been an attempt to predict molecular subtype of MBs based on imaging phenotype, a new emerging field of imaging known as radiogenomics. This is quite helpful when advanced molecular subtyping is not available. Wingless-type subgroup MBs are likely to be off-midline tumors that arise from the dorsal brainstem and cerebellum around the foramen of Luschka **(Figs. 2A to C)**.[12] These subtype of MBs may present either as isolated cerebellopontine angle mass, mass in region of foramen of Luschka, and midline fourth ventricle mass. These tumors are likely to contact dorsal brainstem. SHH subgroup of MBs typically occurs in adult and appears as off-midline intracerebellar tumors without any contact to brainstem **(Figs. 3A to C)**. Group 3 MBs are likely to present as midline intraventricular tumors, especially in children with small tumor size and prominent enhancement **(Figs. 1A to G)**. In addition, diffuse leptomeningeal spread at time of first presentation is also more likely to occur in group 3 MBs **(Figs. 1A to G)**. Group 4 MBs are likely to present as midline intraventricular tumors which show no or minimal enhancement **(Figs. 4A to C)**. MR spectroscopy may help differentiating various subgroups of MB. SHH MBs typically have high choline and lipid levels and low taurine and creatinine levels whereas group 3/4 MBs have been reported to have high taurine and low lipids and creatine levels.[13]

Molecular Subtypes

Based on genomic characterization, MBs have four distinct molecular subgroups. **Table 2** shows the demographic and imaging differences in various molecular subgroups of MBs.

Cerebellar Pilocytic Astrocytoma

Pilocytic astrocytomas (PAs) are well-circumscribed, slow growing, and the WHO grade I tumors of CNS arising from astrocytic precursor cells. They typically present between 5 and 15 years of age. They are generally located in the cerebellum (60%), hypothalamus-optic chiasmal region, brainstem, and less commonly from cerebral hemispheres. Classically, cerebellar PA manifests with waxing and waning headache. Truncal ataxia and dysdiadochokinesia are other cerebellar signs. They have an excellent prognosis with 90% of patients having 10-year survival rate after total resection.

Pathology

Pilocytic astrocytoma may be vermian or hemispheric in origin. Grossly, the cerebellar PA is usually sharply circumscribed with a very narrow zone of microscopic infiltration. Approximately, 50% of tumors are cystic with an enhancing mural nodule. Nearly 40% of tumors are mixed solid with cystic or necrotic components and the rest are purely

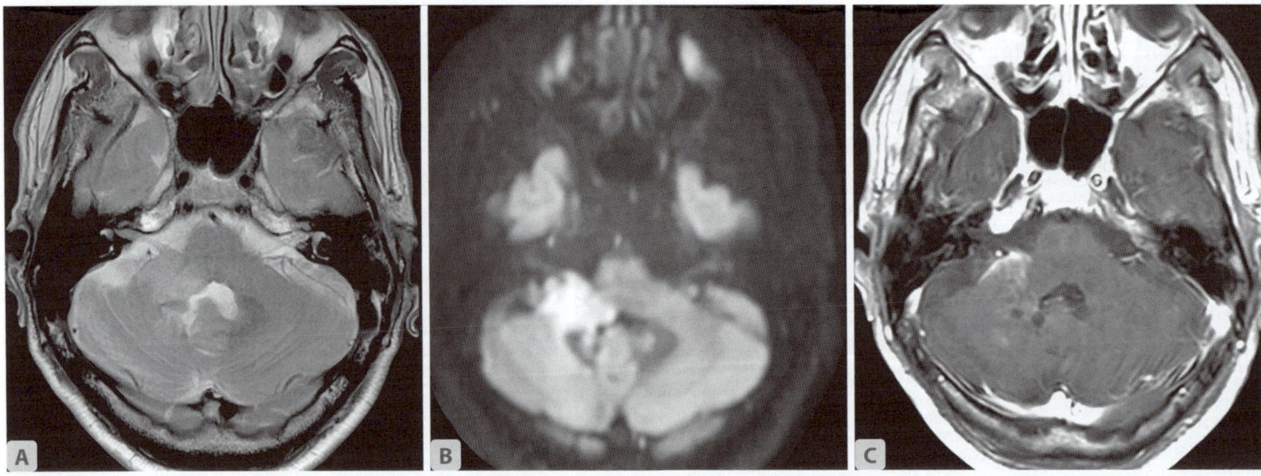

FIGS. 2A TO C: Wingless (WNT), medulloblastoma: Axial T2WI (A) shows characteristic location in CPA cistern/foramen of Luschka region with involvement of dorsal brainstem, restricted diffusion in DWI (B), and enhancement following contrast administration (C). (CPA: cerebellopontine angle; DWI: diffusion-weighted imaging; T2WI: T2-weighted image)

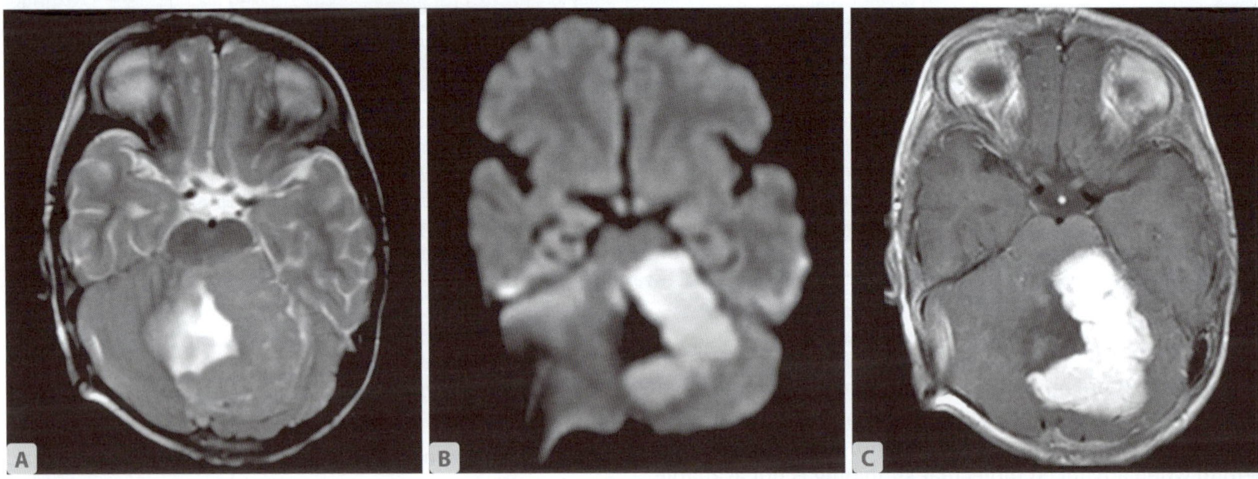

FIGS. 3A TO C: SHH medulloblastoma: Left hemispheric cerebellar tumor—isointense on T2WI (A), hyperintense on DWI images (B), and avidly enhancing in axial postgadolinium T1WI (C). (DWI: diffusion-weighted imaging; SHH: sonic hedgehog; T1WI: T1-weighted image; T2WI: T2-weighted image)

solid mass lesions. Unlike low-grade gliomas, the tumor capillaries lack an intact blood-brain barrier (BBB) and have open tight junction in the endothelial cells with fenestration, thereby have intense enhancement and production of the proteinaceous fluid that accumulates in the "cyst" of the tumor. Majority of pediatric infratentorial PAs have KIAA1549-BRAF fusion whereas majority of supratentorial PAs have BRAF V600E point mutation.[14]

Imaging

Classically, cerebellar PA appears as a cystic mass with an enhancing mural nodule or a mixed solid-cystic mass **(Figs. 5A to F)**. Solid portion is hypointense on T1WI (higher than CSF intensity) and hyperintense on T2WI and shows variable enhancement **(Figs. 5A to F)**. Cyst wall may or may not enhance. Typically, diffusion is facilitated in the solid-enhancing tumor component in comparison to MB and atypical teratoid rhabdoid tumor (ATRT). Peritumoral edema and intratumoral calcifications are usually absent. Hemorrhage can be present but rare.

On advanced imaging like MR spectroscopy and perfusion imaging, PAs mimic high-grade gliomas (HGGs). In magnetic resonance spectroscopy (MRS), choline is increased[15] and lipids/lactate is present. Similarly, relative cerebral blood volume (rCBV) is elevated in MR perfusion studies. Lack of edema and absence of hemorrhage in most of the cases are a helpful differentiating feature from HGG.

Ependymoma

Ependymomas (EPNs) account for 10% of childhood CNS neoplasms and 15% of infratentorial tumors. EPNs typically arise within or adjacent to the ependymal lining of the ventricular system and are thought to be derived from the radial glial cells in the subventricular zone. Approximately,

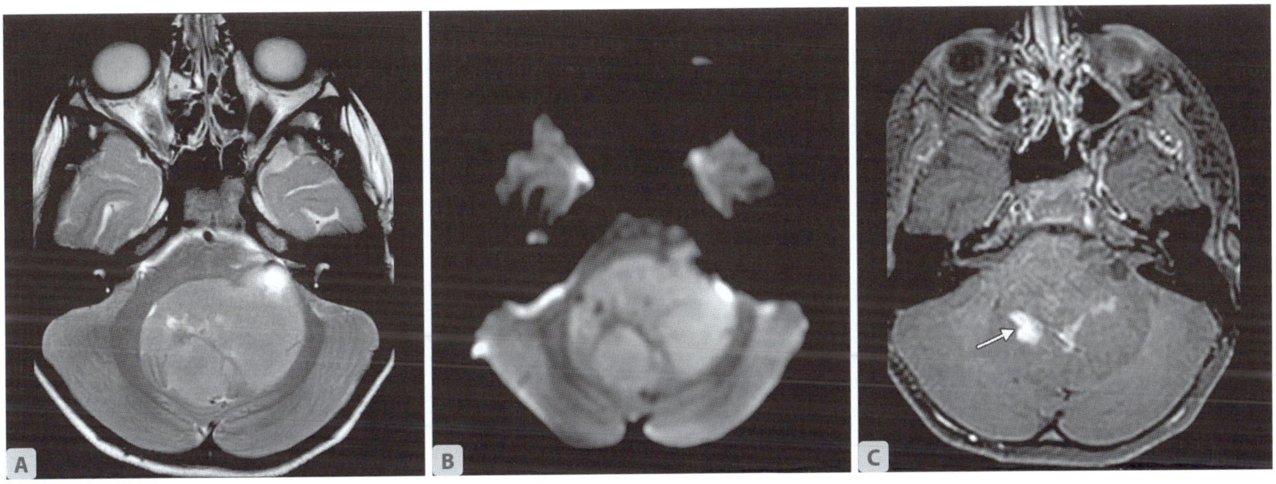

FIGS. 4A TO C: Group 4 medulloblastoma: Axial T2WI (A) shows a predominantly isointense midline mass with restricted diffusion in DWI (B) and focal central enhancement (arrow in C) in postgadolinium T1WI (C). (DWI: diffusion-weighted imaging; T1WI: T1-weighted image; T2WI: T2-weighted image)

TABLE 2: Main features of molecular subgroups of MBs

	WNT	SHH	Group 3	Group 4
Pediatric prevalence	Rarest, 10%	28–30% of all MBs	25–28%	Most common, 34–35%
Age	Children, peak between 10–12 years, uncommon <4 years	Dichotomous, <3 years and >16 years, rare in children	Infants and children but very rarely in adults	Rarely affect infants (0–3 years) and mainly affect children, with a peak age of 10 years
Location	Cerebellar peduncle/CPA cistern, centered on lateral recess of fourth ventricle	Cerebellar hemispheres or midline vermis, typically extraventricular	Mainly midline, immediate vicinity of the fourth ventricle	Mainly midline, immediate vicinity of the fourth ventricle
Prognosis	Best	Intermediate, strongly dependent on patient age, tumor histology and genotype, and metastatic status	Worst	Intermediate
Imaging features	T2-FLAIR hyperintense, hemorrhagic and cystic areas	T2-FLAIR isointense, hemispheric mass	• Midline tumors, ill-defined margins with prominent enhancement • Diffuse leptomeningeal spread at time of presentation, small tumor size (<35 mm with or without leptomeningeal spread)	Minimal or no enhancement
Histologic subtype	Classic (97%)	Essentially all desmoplastic/nodular, but also classic and LCA	Classic or LCA	Classic or LCA
Gender	M:F 1:1	Slight male predominance in infants	M:F 2:1	M:F 3:1
Cell of origin	Lower rhombic limb progenitors	GNPs from EGL and cochlear nuclei, SVZ stem cells	GNPs from EGL	Unknown
5-year survival	~95%	~60–80%	~40–50%	~75%
Adult tumor characteristics	~10–20% incidence, worst prognosis	~50–75% incidence, comparable outcome, exclusively intracerebellar growth, localization in the rostral cerebellum, and no brainstem contact	Extremely rare, worse prognosis	~20–30%, prognostic significance is unclear
Risk factors	–	SUFU-related basal cell nevus (Gorlin) syndrome (×20 times)	–	

(CPA: cerebellopontine angle; EGL: external germinal layer; FLAIR: fluid-attenuated inversion recovery; GNPs: granule neuron precursor; LCA: large cell anaplastic; MBs: medulloblastomas; SHH: sonic hedgehog; SVZ: subventricular zone)

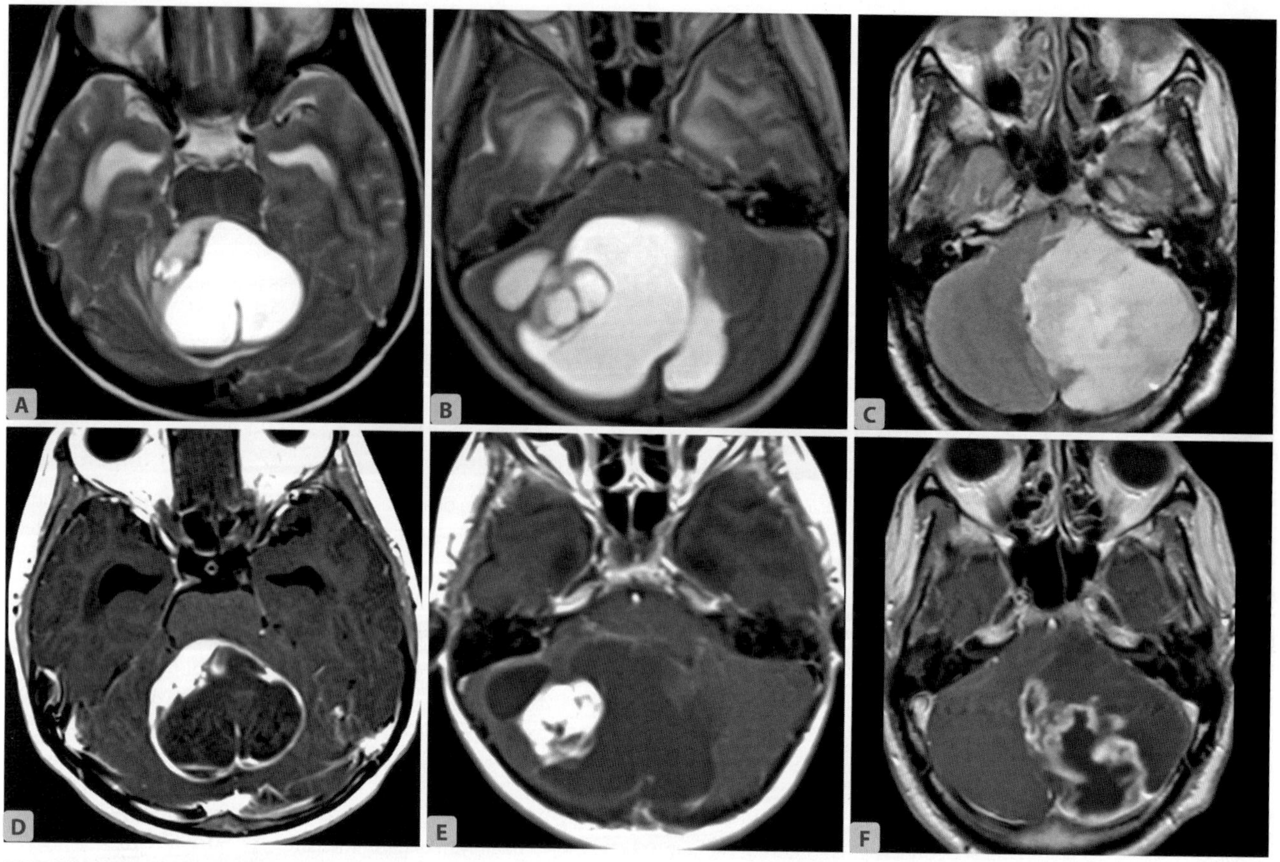

FIGS. 5A TO F: Pilocytic astrocytoma: Axial T2-weighted image (T2WI) (A) shows a cystic lesion with hyperintense mural nodule in the vermis. The cyst wall and mural nodule enhance following contrast administration (D). Axial T2WI (B) shows a cystic lesion with hyperintense mural nodule which enhances following contrast administration (E), no wall enhancement is seen. Axial T2WI (C) MR imaging reveals a well-defined hyperintense left cerebellar mass compressing the fourth ventricle and without any associated edema. On gadolinium administration, mass shows heterogeneous enhancement (F).

60% of the tumors present in infratentorial compartment, 30% in supratentorial compartment, and 10% in the spinal cord.[16] Infratentorial tumors are intraventricular, arising from ependymal lining of the fourth ventricle and foramina of Luschka while supratentorial tumors can be either intraventricular, typically in the lateral ventricles or parenchymal. Most patients present between ages of 1 and 5 years, with a second smaller peak occurring in the fourth decade. Nausea, vomiting, disequilibrium, and headaches are common presenting symptoms and ataxia and nystagmus are common presenting signs.

Pathology

Ependymomas arise from the cuboidal or columnar cells lining the ventricles and the central canal. In the infratentorial compartment, they arise from the floor of the fourth ventricle with a tendency to fill it or track along its lateral recesses into the cerebellopontine angle. The four histological types include: (1) EPN (grade II), (2) Anaplastic EPNs (grade III), (3) Subependymoma (grade I), and (4) Myxopapillary ependymoma (grade I). Anaplastic ependymomas have greater incidence of leptomeningeal spread at the time of diagnosis and have poorer prognosis.

Comprehensive genomic study has divided infratentorial EPNs in two prognostically different subgroups, PFA and PFB.[17] The group A tumors are found predominantly in younger children and have balanced genome. These tumors are laterally localized, displacing the brainstem laterally, and extending into the cerebellopontine cistern without infiltration of obex of the fourth ventricle. The group B EPN occurs in adults. These are midline tumor, typically located in the inferior half of the fourth ventricle, and may infiltrate the obex.

Imaging

At CT, EPNs are lobulated heterogeneous midline intraventricular masses with indistinct separation from the floor of the fourth ventricle and have calcification (up to 45%) **(Fig. 6)**.[18] Typically, EPN shows tumor extension through the fourth ventricular outflow foramina, a feature shared with MBs.[19] However, the extension through the foramina in MB is more bulbous and has more restricted diffusion compared to thin tongues of tissue and intermediate diffusion in EPNs. Rarely, EPNs may appear as isolated cerebellopontine angle mass, presumably arising from the ependymal cell rests.

At MRI, EPNs are heterogeneous with T1 hypointensity, T2 iso-/hyperintensity, and iso- to hyper fluid-attenuated inversion recovery (FLAIR) signal intensity **(Figs. 7A to E)** due to presence of calcification, hemorrhage, and cystic changes within the tumor **(Figs. 7A to E)**. Following contrast administration, they usually show intense mixed heterogeneous enhancement **(Figs. 7A to E)**; however, rarely, EPNs do not enhance.[20] The presence of calcifications within a lobulated heterogenous fourth ventricular mass is highly suggestive but not diagnostic of EPN. Diffuse leptomeningeal spread is seen in <10% of patients at diagnosis when ependymoblastomas [embryonal tumor with abundant neuropil and true rosettes (ETANTR)] are excluded **(Fig. 7E)**.[21] Though not always reliable, apparent diffusion coefficient (ADC) of EPNs is generally intermediate between that of PAs and MB.[22] On dynamic susceptibility contrast (DSC) perfusion MRI, EPN typically has markedly elevated perfusion (rCBV) and marked leakiness of contrast with poor return to baseline presumably due to presence of fenestrated blood vessels and an insufficient BBB.[23] Though characteristic, these findings are not pathognomonic and also may be seen in embryonal tumors.[15] Proton MR spectroscopy typically demonstrates elevated myoinositol (mI) levels in classic grade II EPNs.[24]

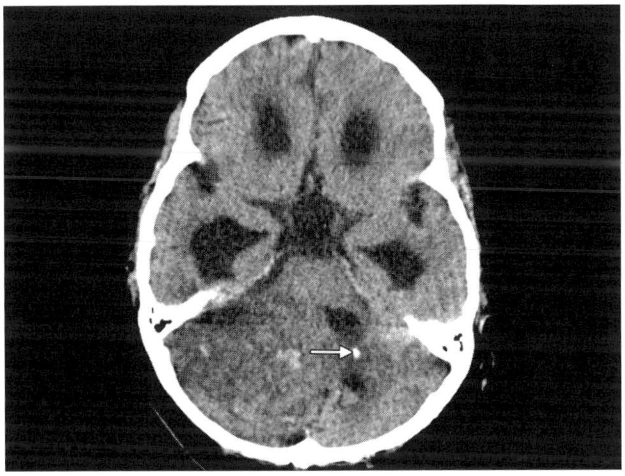

FIG. 6: Ependymoma. Noncontrast computed tomography (NCCT) shows a heterogeneous mass, which is predominantly hypodense with foci of calcification (arrows) in cerebellum.

Treatment for EPN to this date is maximal safe surgical resection followed by adjuvant radiotherapy.[25] The survival rates have seen limited improvement (~80%) in the last decade, with survivors suffering from the debilitating side effects of radiation-induced severe neurocognitive impairment and other radiation-induced complications.

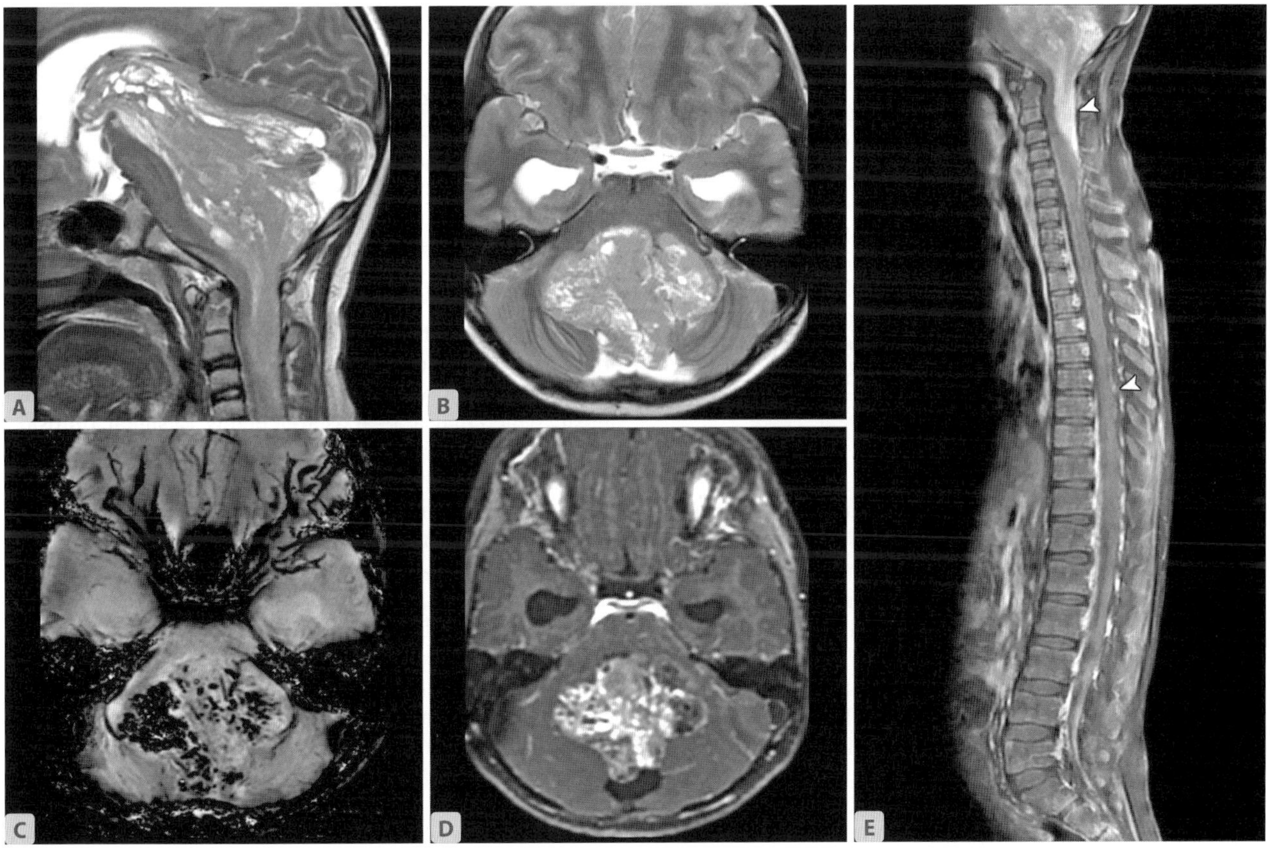

FIGS. 7A TO E: Ependymoma: Sagittal (A) and axial T2WI (B) shows an iso- to hyperintense mass filling fourth ventricle and extending superiorly into the third ventricle through aqueduct and inferiorly into cisterna magna and dorsal spinal subarachnoid space. SWI (C) shows multiple foci of susceptibility signal within the mass. Postgadolinium axial T1WI (D) shows avid enhancement of the mass. Postgadolinium sagittal T1WI of whole spine (E) shows focal leptomeningeal deposits (arrowheads in E). (SWI: susceptibility-weighted imaging; T1WI: T1-weighted image; T2WI: T2-weighted image)

Atypical Teratoid Rhabdoid Tumor

Atypical teratoid rhabdoid tumor is a highly malignant embryonal tumor primarily occurring in young children <3-year-old.[26] Approximately, two-thirds of ATRTs occur in the cerebellum, typically in the cerebellopontine angle, with invasion of surrounding structures. Approximately, one-fourth is supratentorial and 8% are multifocal.[27] Typically, infants present with lethargy, vomiting, and failure to thrive; older children may be symptomatic secondary to involvement of cranial nerves IV, VI, or VII such as head tilt, diplopia, or facial weakness. Approximately, one-third of the patients have subarachnoid dissemination (30%) at time of diagnosis. The prognosis is worse than that associated with MB, with a median survival of 12–24 months and 5-year overall survival of 30–40%.[28]

Pathology

Histologically, ATRTs are characterized by rhabdoid cells and are similar to that of other small round blue cell tumors; up to two-thirds also contain fields typical of primitive neuroectodermal tumors (PNETs).[29] Necrosis and a high rate of mitotic activity are common. In the WHO 2016 classification of CNS tumors, ATRT is genetically characterized by loss of either INI1 nuclear staining or loss of BRG1 staining.

Imaging

Tumors are typically large at presentation and associated with moderate-to-marked perilesional edema. Like MBs, these are highly cellular tumors, hyperdense on noncontrast-enhanced computed tomography (NCCT),[30] hypointense on T1WI, iso- to hypointense on T2WI, and show restricted diffusion **(Figs. 8A to D)**. Areas of necrosis, cyst formation, hemorrhage, and calcification may occur with various patterns of enhancement **(Figs. 9A to E)**.[29] Spinal imaging should to done to pick leptomeningeal spread. Neuroimaging cannot reliably differentiate ATRTs from MB. Unlike typical MB, ATRTs are more likely to be located offline, more heterogeneous, and rapidly growing. ATRT located in region of cerebellopontine angle may mimic WNT MB; however, the age of presentation is different.

Brainstem Gliomas

Brainstem gliomas constitute 10–20% of childhood CNS tumors, with a median age at diagnosis of 5–9 years without any sex predilection.[31] These are heterogeneous tumors, ranging from low-grade to high-grade lesions. Approximately, 80% of pediatric brainstem gliomas arise within the pons and around 20% arise in the medulla, midbrain, or cervicomedullary junction. Most pontine tumors are diffuse intrinsic pontine gliomas (DIPGs) and are generally high grade with local infiltrative pattern and are associated with poor prognosis. Approximately, 10–20% of nonpontine gliomas are high grade and are treated similarly to DIPGs. Multiple cranial nerve palsies, pyramidal tract signs, ataxia, and nystagmus are the usual presentation; shorter duration of symptoms (typically <3 months) in diffuse intrinsic pontine gliomas. Except in tectal gliomas, hydrocephalus is uncommon in brainstem gliomas. DIPGs have the worst prognosis.[32]

Pathology

Brainstem gliomas can be divided into the diffuse gliomas and focal gliomas (including dorsal exophytic, tectal, and cervicomedullary).[33] Diffuse brainstem gliomas are most often high-grade fibrillary gliomas with areas of anaplasia, necrosis, and hemorrhage and arise predominantly in the pons and less frequently in the medulla. On the contrary, focal brainstem gliomas are most often pilocytic or diffuse astrocytomas (DAs), or rarely, gangliogliomas (GGs) and typically arise in the midbrain and medulla as discrete, well-circumscribed tumors.

Advances in molecular genetics have revealed that nearly 80% of biopsied DIPGs harbor point mutations at position K27 in one of several histone-encoding genes. These neoplasms are defined as a new entity termed as "diffuse midline glioma H3 K27M mutant" in the revised 2016 update of the WHO classification of CNS tumors. Characteristically, they have diffuse growth pattern, located in midline (e.g., thalami, brainstem, spinal cord, third ventricle, hypothalamus, and pineal region),[6] and most often high-grade astrocytomas on histology.[34,35] Majority of these tumors have poor prognosis barring few exceptions. One must remember that "diffuse midline glioma H3 K27M mutant" is a pathological diagnosis and is not synonymous with the clinical and radiologic entity of DIPG, which does not require biopsy for diagnosis (and is often not biopsied) and behaves uniformly poorly, regardless of histologic grade or H3 K27M status.

Imaging

MR imaging is modality of choice for the evaluation of brainstem tumors. Typically, the DIPGs are centered in pontine tegmentum, ill-defined in outline, hypointense on T1WI, and hyperintense on T2WI **(Figs. 10A to D)** with occasional intratumoral heterogeneity. The tumor expands the pons and engulfs the basilar artery without any thrombosis. The signal changes may extend into the brachium pontis and cerebellum and/or adjacent brainstem and thalami. Contrast enhancement has been reported in approximately one-half of the cases and is often focal and nodular **(Figs. 10A to D)**. DIPG may contain focal areas of anaplasia and high cell density which may appear as area of low T2 signal, diffusion restriction, and focal or ring enhancement, area most suitable for biopsy. Approximately, 80% of DIPG harbor the histone H3 K27M mutation; however, imaging features like enhancement, infiltration, or peritumoral edema have failed to differentiate between DIPGs with or without the histone H3 K27M mutation.[36]

On MRI, focal brainstem gliomas most often appear as small (<2 cm), well-circumscribed masses that may be cystic, noninfiltrating, and without associated edema. They are typically isointense or hypointense on T1WI, hyperintense on T2WI, and enhance uniformly and avidly with intravenous contrast **(Figs. 11A to C)**. Diffusion tensor imaging (DTI) and white matter tractography are particularly useful in documenting axonal degeneration of the motor and sensory tracts in focal brainstem tumors. These imaging sequences may assist in surgical planning for biopsy or tumor debulking. Focal tumors of the midbrain can contain calcifications and enhance poorly with contrast. The other subtypes of focal

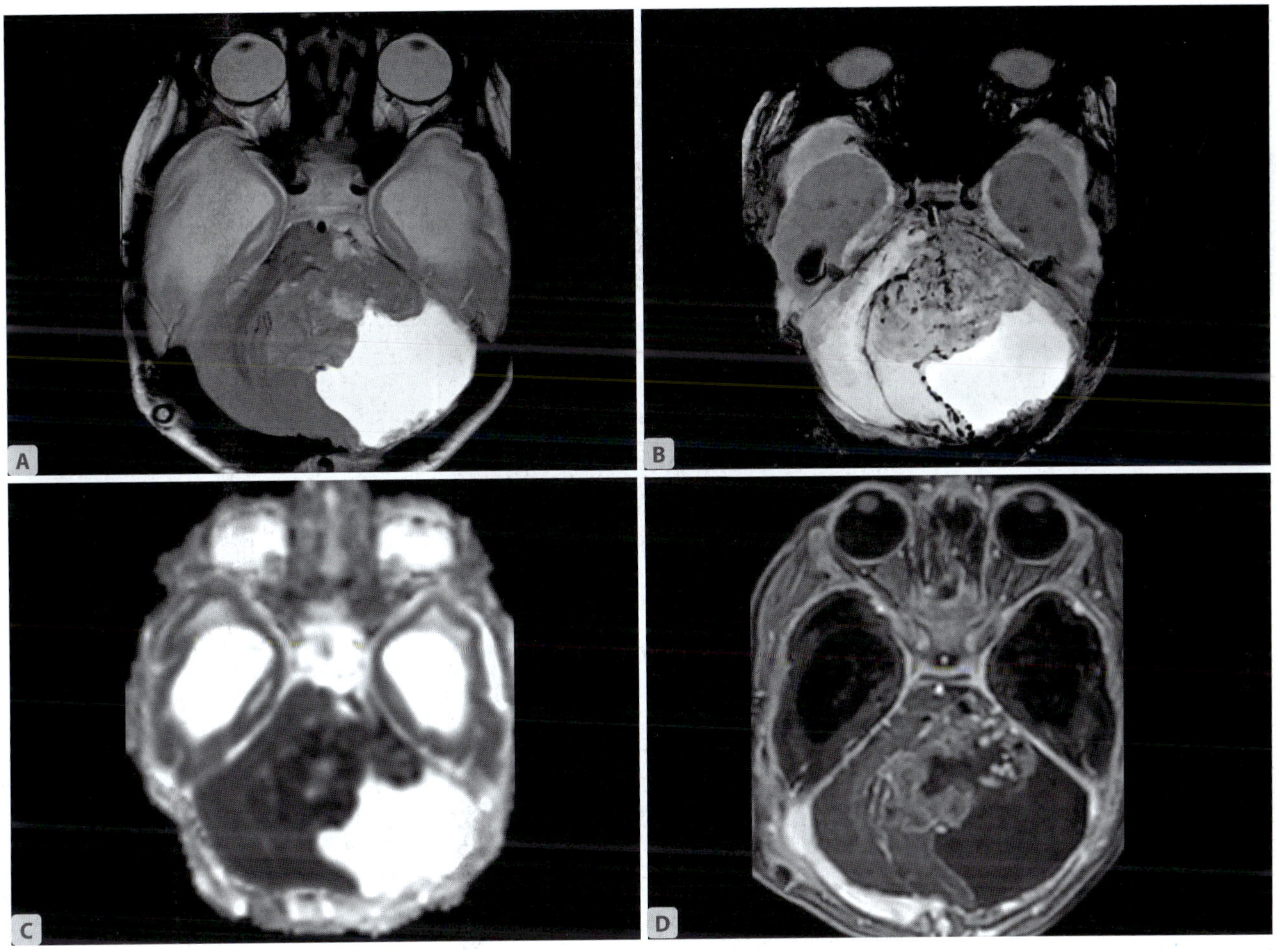

FIGS. 8A TO D: ATRT: A well-defined left cerebellar mass is seen without any plane between the tumor and the brainstem. The mass is isointense on axial T2WI (A), heterogeneous on SWI (B), and dark on ADC maps (C) suggesting restricted diffusion. Postgadolinium axial T1WI (D) shows heterogeneous contrast enhancement of the mass. (ADC: apparent diffusion coefficient; ATRT: atypical teratoid rhabdoid tumor; SWI: susceptibility-weighted imaging; T1WI: T1-weighted image; T2WI: T2-weighted image)

gliomas are tectal plate glioma **(Fig. 12A)** and cervicomedullary glioma **(Fig. 12B)**. Cervicomedullary gliomas typically include PAs and GGs. On imaging, cervicomedullary GGs are typically infiltrative and expansile solid masses with dorsal predominant "paintbrush" enhancement **(Fig. 12C)**.

Hemangioblastoma

Hemangioblastoma typically occurs in young and middle-aged adults and <20% occur in children. The tumors are usually located in the cerebellum (83–86%), brainstem (2–5%), and spinal cord (3–13%).[37] Hemangioblastomas occur both sporadically (75%) and as an important component of von Hippel–Lindau (VHL) disease (25%), along with retinal angiomas, endolymphatic sac tumors, renal cell carcinoma, pheochromocytomas, pancreatic cysts, and neuroendocrine tumors. Hemangioblastomas in VHL disease develop at an earlier age, often multifocal (20%), and have spinal cord tumor in approximately 50%.

Pathology

Classically, hemangioblastomas are well-circumscribed, cystic tumors with a mural nodule (60%) or completely solid (40%).

Imaging

On NCCT, hemangioblastoma usually appears as a well-circumscribed cyst with a mural nodule. The cyst is hypodense and nonenhancing whereas the mural nodule is iso- to hyperdense, abuts the pial surface, and shows strong homogeneous contrast enhancement. Solid hemangioblastomas are hyperdense on NCCT and homogeneously enhancing following contrast administration.

On MRI of hemangioblastoma, cyst is iso- to slightly hyperintense on T1WI and hyperintense on T2WI and nodule is hypointense on T1WI, hyperintense on T2WI **(Figs. 13A and B)**, and intensely enhancing after injection of gadolinium contrast material.[38] Vascular flow voids within and at the periphery of the tumor represent abnormal tumor vessels that are helpful in clinching the diagnosis. Peritumoral edema is usually slight or absent. Solid hemangioblastomas show multiple vascular flow voids and strong homogeneous enhancement **(Figs. 14A to D)**.

In perfusion MRI, hemangioblastomas have high rCBV ratios (around 11), which are significantly higher than those of metastases (around 5) and PAs.[39] Cerebral angiography is reserved for preoperative tumor embolization and shows dilated feeding arteries and a prolonged tumoral blush in the

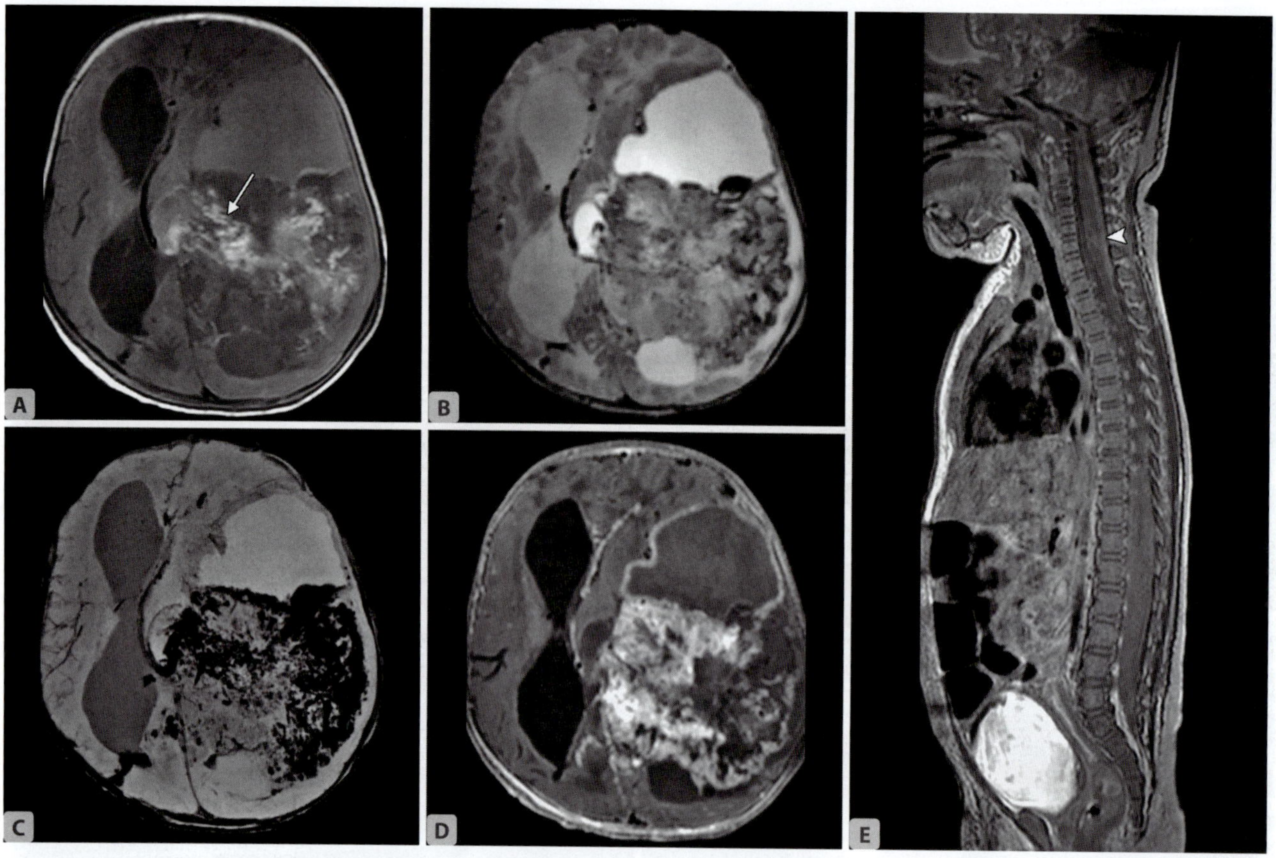

FIGS. 9A TO E: Supratentorial ATRT: Axial T1WI (A) and axial T2WI (B) show a heterogeneous solid cystic mass in left cerebral hemisphere with foci of T1 hyperintensity (arrow in A). The mass shows hypotense regions in SWI (C). Postgadolinium axial T1WI (D) shows heterogeneous contrast enhancement of the mass. Postgadolinium sagittal T1WI of whole spine (F) shows diffuse leptomeningeal deposits (arrowhead in E). (ATRT: atypical teratoid rhabdoid tumor; SWI: susceptibility-weighted imaging; T1WI: T1-weighted image; T2WI: T2-weighted image)

solid portion.[40] The other differential diagnosis of cyst with enhancing mural nodule in the infratentorial compartment is pilocytic astrocytoma which generally occurs at a younger age, not associated with intratumoral flow voids and show less increase in rCBV and permeability.

SUPRATENTORIAL TUMORS

Supratentorial tumors account for approximately 20% of brain tumors in children <14 years of age[41] and are more common than infratentorial region in children below 2 years and those older than 10 years.

Cerebral Hemisphere

Low-grade Tumors

Astrocytic Tumors

Pilocytic astrocytomas: In the supratentorial compartment, PAs most often arise from optic pathways—hypothalamus, optic nerve, optic chiasm, and less commonly in cerebral hemispheres. Nearly one-third of optic pathway gliomas (OPGs) are associated with neurofibromatosis type 1 (NF1) and such OPGs show a greater frequency of prechiasmatic involvement, presentation at a younger age, and better prognosis than those in patients without NF1.[42]

Imaging: Imaging features are like the infratentorial PA. MR reveals deeply located hemispheric mass, which is hypointense and hyperintense on T1WI and T2WI, respectively **(Figs. 15A to C)**.

Pleomorphic xanthoastrocytoma: Pleomorphic xanthoastrocytoma (PXA) is the WHO grade II neoplasm with median age of presentation of 20 years (range: early infancy to old age). Histologically, they are characterized by markedly pleomorphic cells with foamy xanthomatous cytoplasm, eosinophilic granular bodies, and prominent reticulin deposition. They are most often located in temporal lobe (39%) followed by frontal (18%) and parietal lobes (14%).[43] Typically, they have meningocerebral location, so commonly present with seizures.

Imaging: Most common morphology is a cystic tumor with enhancing mural nodule. The tumor is typically superficial in cortex with involvement of overlying meninges and scalloping of overlying inner table of skull. The imaging hallmark of PXA is a cyst with enhancing mural nodule with

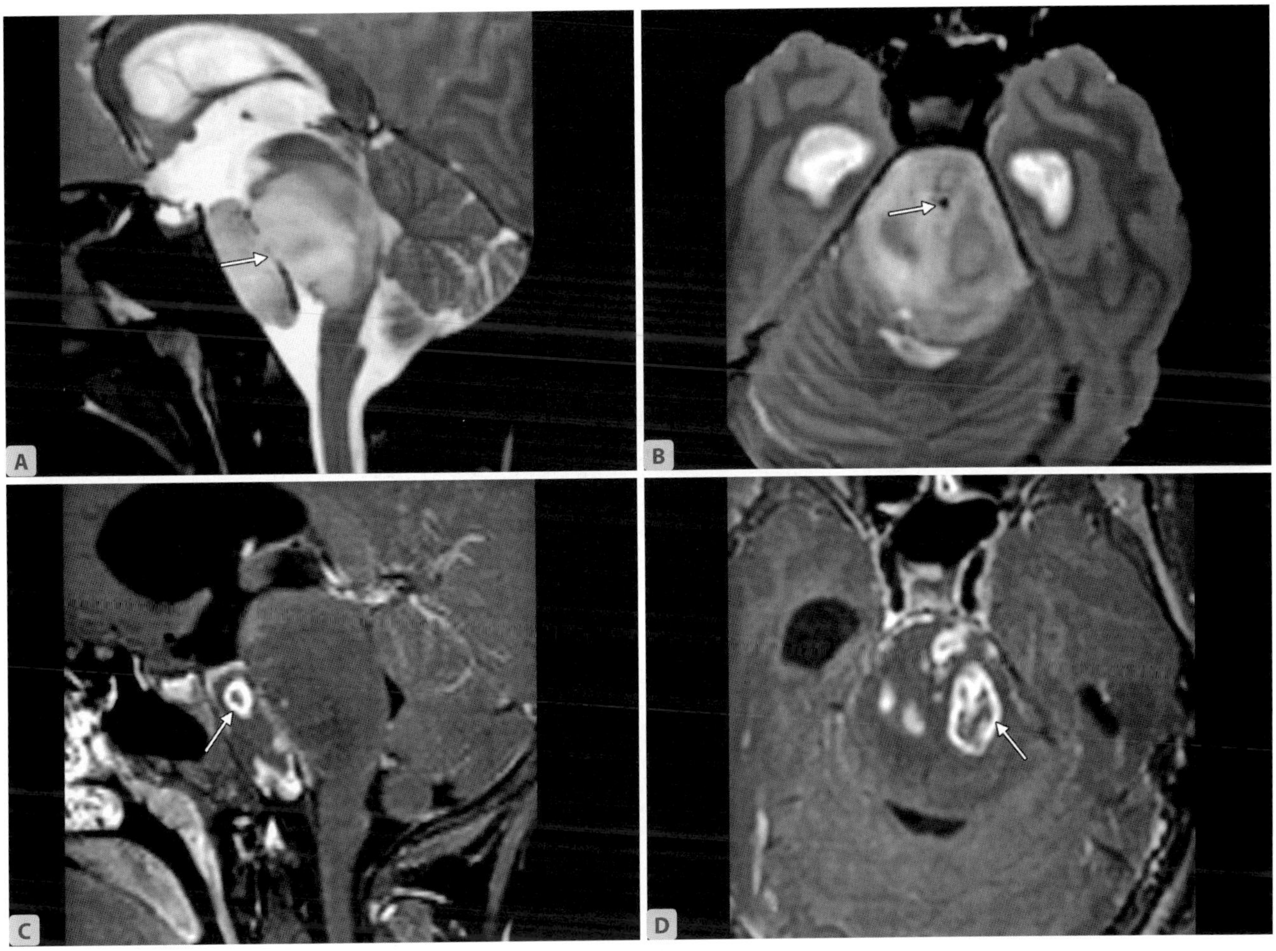

FIGS. 10A TO D: Diffuse pontine glioma: Sagittal (A) and axial T2-weighted image (T2WI) (B) shows diffuse pontine glioma causing expansion of pons, basilar artery encasement (arrows in A and B), and compression of the fourth ventricle with resultant hydrocephalus. The tumor contains final T2-hypointense areas (arrow in B) which show peripheral enhancement (C and D).

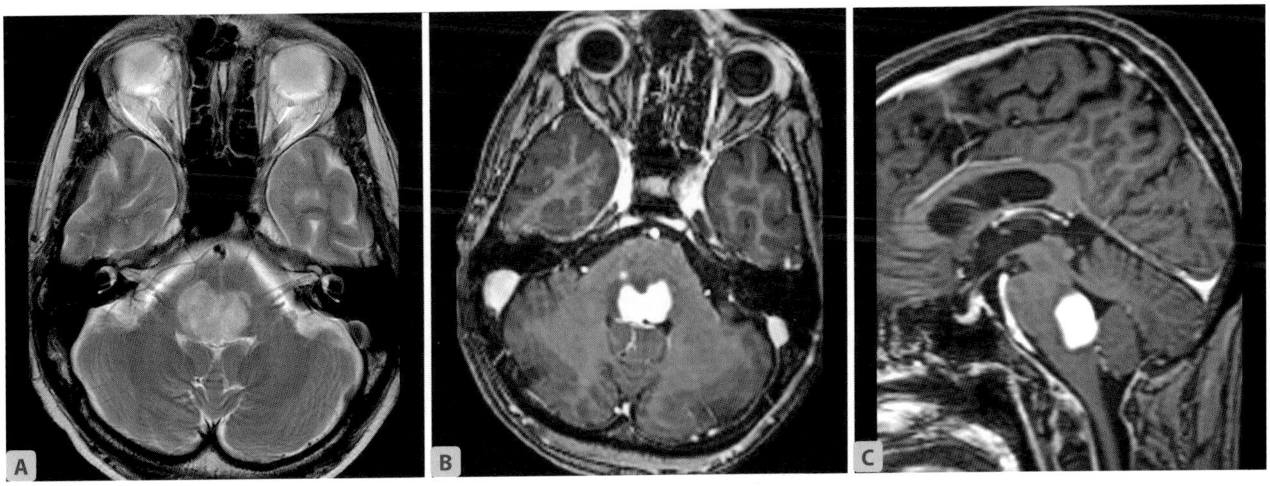

FIGS. 11A TO C: Dorsally exophytic brainstem glioma: Axial T2WI (A) shows a focal hyperintense mass originating from dorsal aspect of pons. The mass shows intense enhancement in axial (B) and sagittal (C) postgadolinium T1WI. (T1WI: T1-weighted image; T2WI: T2-weighted image)

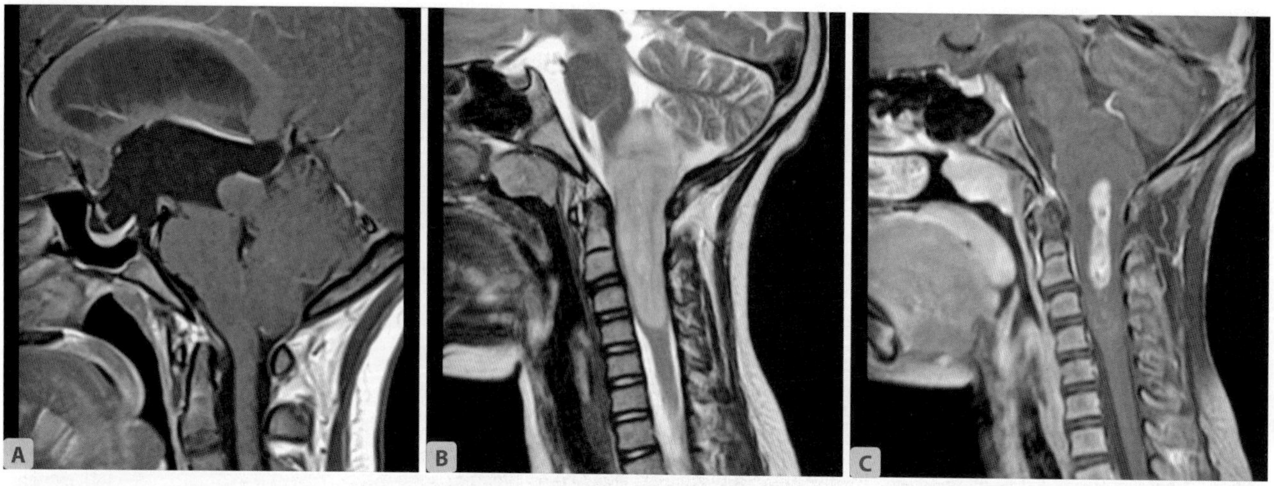

FIGS. 12A TO C: Tectal plate glioma. (A) and cervicomedullary glioma (B and C); Sagittal T1WI (A) shows nonenhancing tectal plate thickening causing aqueduct obstruction and resultant hydrocephalus suggestive of tectal plate glioma. Sagittal T2WI (A) and postgadolinium T1WI (B) well-circumscribed expansile T2-hyperintense mass involving cervicomedullary region with central enhancement in postgadolinium images suggestive of cervicomedullary glioma. (T1WI: T1-weighted image; T2WI: T2-weighted image)

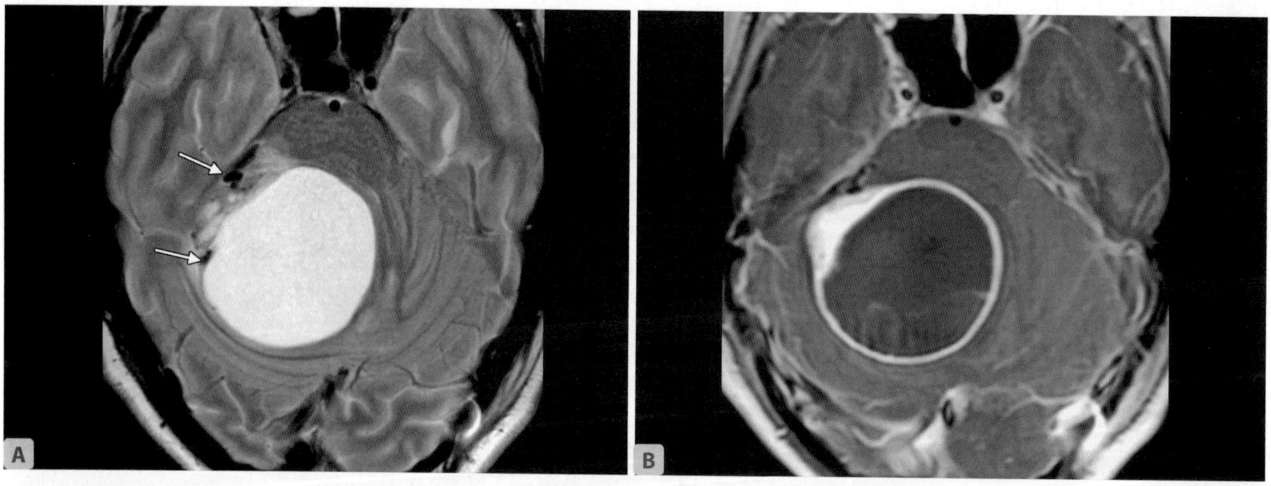

FIGS. 13A AND B: Typical hemangioblastoma: Axial T2WI (A) shows a cyst with a mural nodule without any perilesional edema in the right cerebellar hemisphere. Multiple vascular flow voids (arrows in A) are seen associated with mural nodule. Postgadolinium T1WI (B) shows intense enhancement of mural nodule along with cyst wall. (T1WI: T1-weighted image; T2WI: T2-weighted image)

associated adjacent meningeal enhancement and varying degree of perilesional edema.

Diffuse astrocytomas: DAs are the WHO grade II tumors and significantly less common than PA in children. They are most commonly located in frontal and parietal lobes.

Imaging: On MRI, the tumor is ill-defined, homogeneously hypointense on T1, and hyperintense on T2 without any diffusion restriction or enhancement **(Figs. 16A and B)**. On perfusion MRI, rCBV is low. Contrary to adult DAs, childhood DAs undergo malignant transformation in only 10% of cases.[44,45]

Subependymal giant cell tumor: Subependymal giant cell tumor (SGCT) is a benign WHO grade I mixed glioneuronal tumor with peak age of occurrence of 8–18 years. It occurs in 6–16% of patients with tuberous sclerosis and typically arising in the walls of the lateral ventricles near the foramen of Monro.[46] This tumor is also known as "ventricular tumor of tuberous sclerosis". These tumors may be responsive to treatment with the mammalian target of rapamycin (mTOR) inhibitors such as sirolimus and everolimus.

Imaging: CT shows hypo- to isodense mass in the region of foramen of Monro. Hydrocephalus and focal calcification are common. On MRI, SGCTs show mixed signal intensities on T1- and T2WI **(Figs. 17A and B)**.[46] Contrast enhancement is heterogeneous, but avid on both CT and MRI. Associated findings of tuberous sclerosis include presence of cortical tubers, subependymal nodules, and white matter lesions.

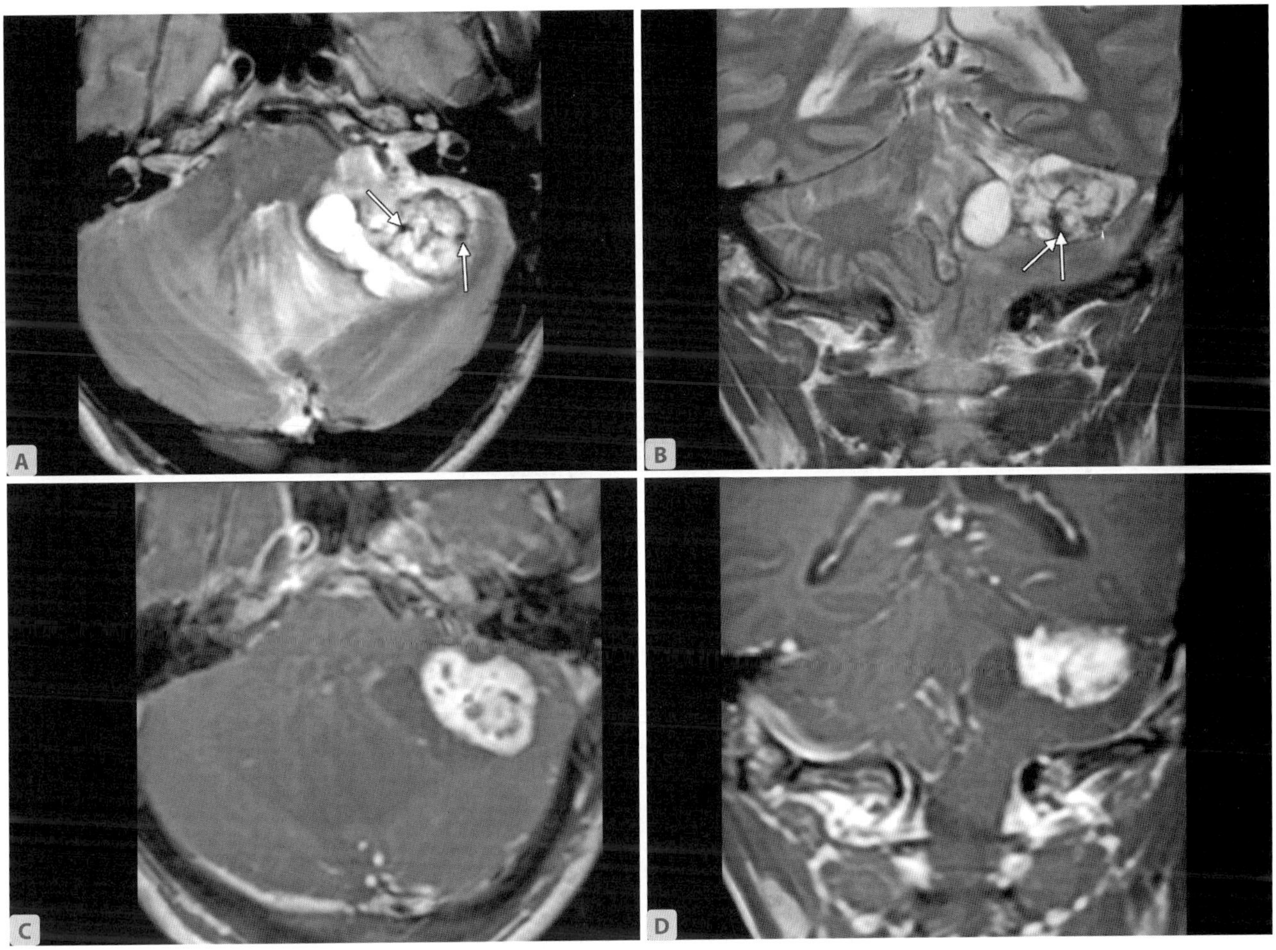

FIGS. 14A TO D: Atypical hemangioblastoma: Axial (A) and coronal (B) T2-weighted image (T2WI) shows a solid cystic mass with moderate perilesional edema in left cerebellar hemisphere. Multiple vascular flow voids (arrows in A and B) are seen associated with solid component. Postgadolinium axial (C) and coronal (D) show intense enhancement of solid component without any enhancement of cystic component.

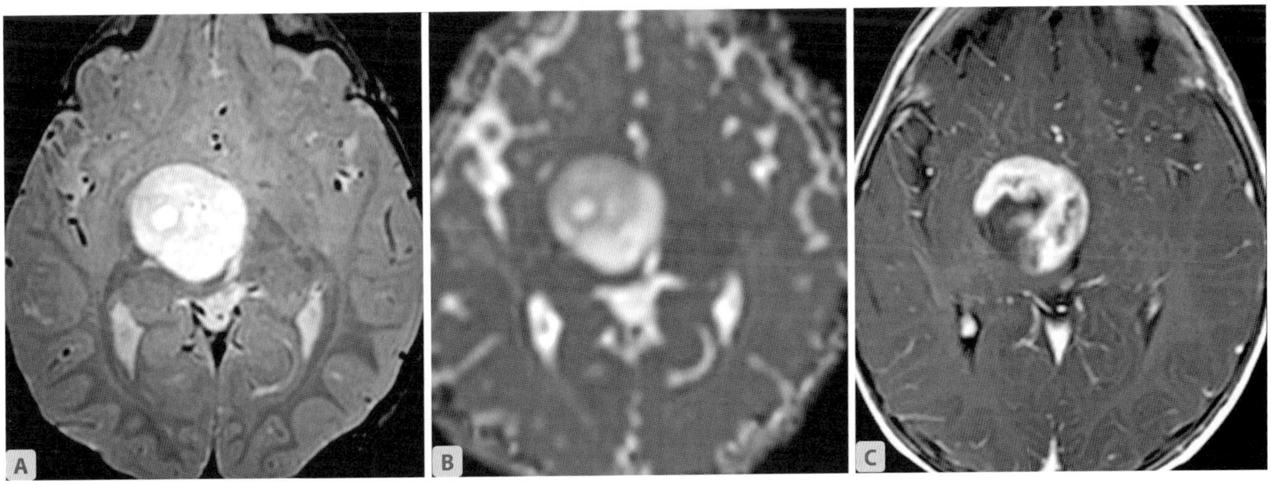

FIGS. 15A TO C: Thalamic pilocytic astrocytoma: Axial T2WI (A) shows a well-defined lesion in the right thalamus with any perilesional edema. The mass is hyperintense on ADC maps (B) suggesting facilitated diffusion. Postgadolinium axial T1WI shows intense enhancement. (ADC: apparent diffusion coefficient; T1WI: T1-weighted image; T2WI: T2-weighted image)

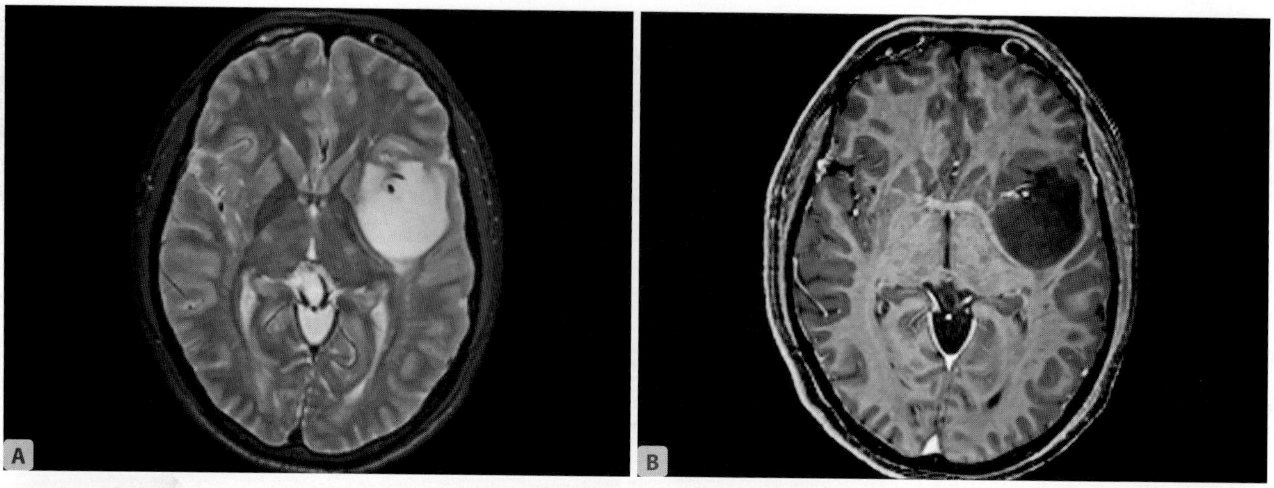

FIGS. 16A AND B: Diffuse astrocytoma: Axial T2WI (A) shows a well-circumscribed homogeneously hyperintense mass in left insular region without any enhancement in postgadolinium T1WI (B). (T1WI: T1-weighted image; T2WI: T2-weighted image)

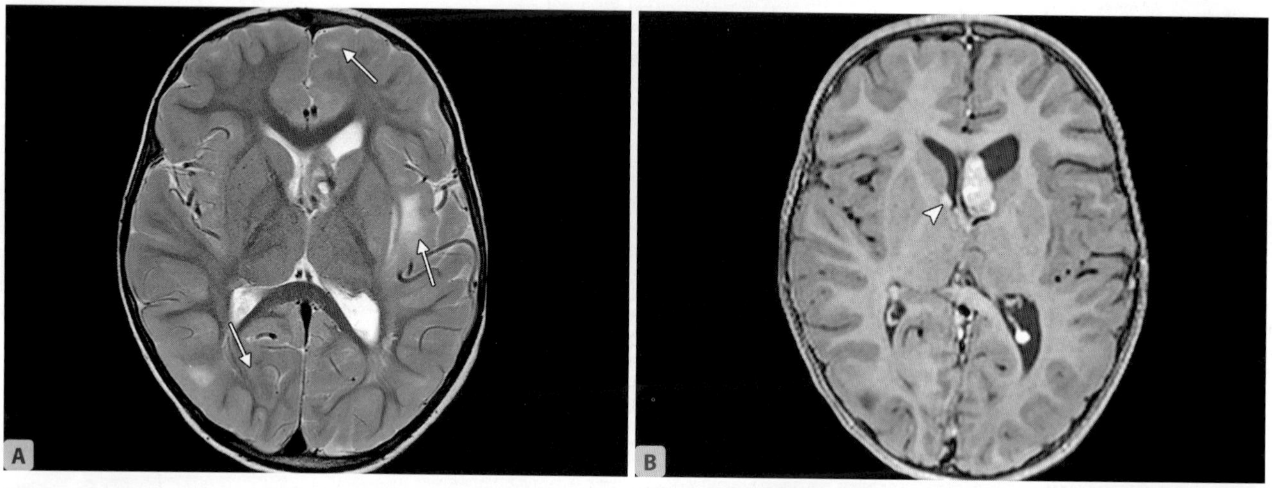

FIGS. 17A AND B: Subependymal giant cell tumor in patient with tuberous sclerosis: Axial T2WI (A) shows a heterogeneous mass near foramen of Monro with homogeneous enhancement in postgadolinium T1WI (B). The other stigmata of tuberous sclerosis are seen—multiple subcortical tubers (arrows in A) and enhancing subependymal nodule (arrowheads in B). (T1WI: T1-weighted image; T2WI: T2-weighted image)

Ependymal Tumors

Supratentorial ependymoma: Between 20 and 40% of childhood EPNs are supratentorial in location. The peak age of presentation is between the ages of 1 and 5 years and predominant in males. Seizures or focal neurologic deficits are common presentations of supratentorial EPNs.

Pathology: Histology is like infratentorial lesions. About 60% of the tumors are extraventricular, so subarachnoid seeding is uncommon. Supratentorial EPNs are more likely to have cystic component than infratentorial counterpart.

Imaging: The diagnosis of EPN should be considered in the presence of juxtaventricular hemispheric mass with focal calcification, cystic necrosis, and heterogeneous enhancement **(Figs. 18A and B)**. The tumor is heterogeneous in MRI due to presence of calcification, necrosis, and intratumoral hemorrhage.[47] High-grade astrocytoma and PNET are other diagnostic possibilities.

Oligodendrocytic Tumors

Oligodendroglioma: Oligodendroglioma (ODG) and anaplastic ODG are genetically defined, diffusely infiltrating gliomas that contain both an IDH1 or IDH2 mutation and 1p and 19q codeletion of chromosome arms. They are rare in children. They are typically slow growing hemispheric tumors with a propensity to involve the cortex. CT typically demonstrates a peripherally located hypodense tumor with calcifications (40–90%), cysts (20%), and calvarial erosions (17%). On MRI, ODGs usually have hypointense or mixed signal intensity on T1WI and hyperintense or mixed signal intensity on T2WI. Up to 50% of low-grade ODGs have some degree of contrast enhancement and contrast enhancement does not necessarily indicate high-grade (anaplastic)

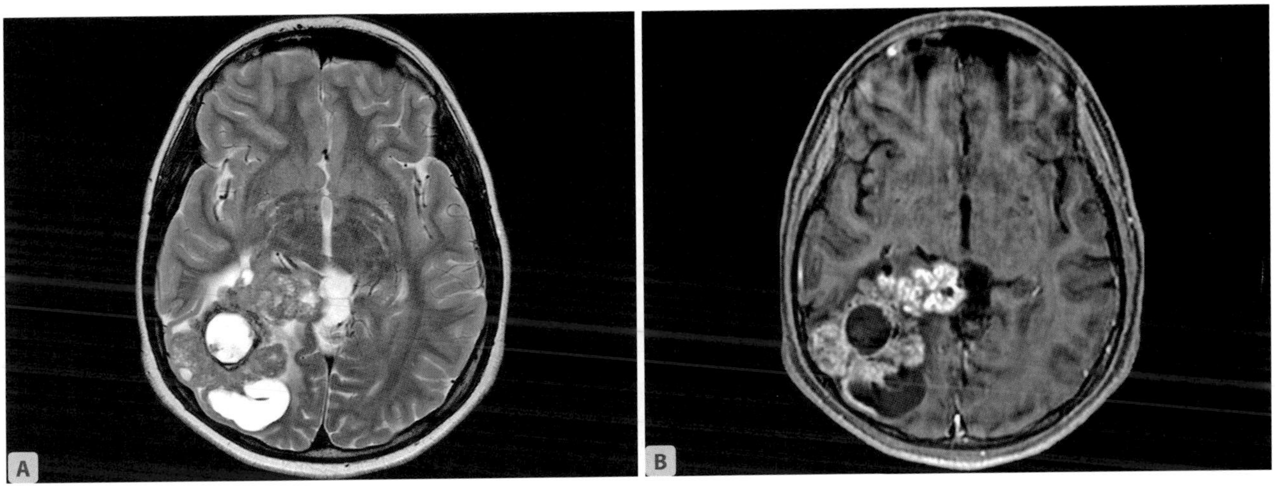

FIGS. 18A AND B: Supratentorial ependymoma: Axial T2WI (A) shows a heterogeneous cystic and solid mass with areas of calcification and perilesional edema in right occipital lobe with intense heterogeneous enhancement in postgadolinium T1WI (B). (T1WI: T1-weighted image; T2WI: T2-weighted image)

pathology. Compared with DAs, ODGs are more likely to have indistinct borders, cortical involvement, and inhomogeneous signal on T1WI and T2WI.[48]

Mixed Neuronal/Glioneuronal Tumors

Neuronal and mixed neuronal-glial tumors are characterized by a variable degree of neuronal and glial differentiation. Tumors in this category include dysembryoplastic neuroepithelial tumor (DNT or DNET), GGs and gangliocytomas, dysplastic gangliocytoma of the cerebellum (Lhermitte–Duclos disease), desmoplastic infantile astrocytoma (DIA)/GG, papillary glioneuronal tumor, rosette-forming glioneuronal tumor, diffuse leptomeningeal glioneuronal tumor (DLGNT), cerebellar liponeurocytomas, central and extraventricular neurocytomas, and paragangliomas.

They account for approximately 7% of all pediatric CNS tumors.

Gangliogliomas: GGs are mixed glioneuronal tumor that has a low-grade astrocytic component accompanied by collections of neoplastic ganglion cells. These tumors account for 1–4% of all childhood CNS tumors. GGs typically occur in children and young adults; the average age in most series is approximately 20 years. GGs are most often supratentorial and commonly located in the temporal lobes followed by the parietal lobe and the frontal lobe. GGs of temporal lobe typically present with drug refractory epilepsy and are the most common tumor associated with temporal lobe epilepsy.[49]

Imaging: Typically, GGs are mixed solid cystic mass with avidly enhancing solid component and calcification. On CT scan, the mass is hypodense (38%), mixed density (32%), and isodense (15%) or hyperdense (15%).[50] One-half of cases have cysts and approximately one-third have calcifications.[50] Remodeling of the skull may be present when the tumor is peripherally located. The enhancement is seen in 16–80% of GGs.[50]

The MR imaging appearance of GGs is nonspecific.[49,50] In general, the lesions are hypointense to isointense on T1 and hyperintense on T2 images **(Figs. 19A to C)**. Enhancement is highly variable, ranging from none to marked and may be solid or rim enhancement.

Dysembryoplastic neuroepithelial tumors: DNETs are benign mixed neuronal-glial neoplasm (WHO grade I) affecting children and adolescents and are clinically characterized by long-standing history of intractable focal epilepsy.[51] Key pathologic features of DNTs include the presence of entrapped cortical neurons, foci of dysplastic cortical organization, a multinodular architecture with components resembling astrocytoma or oligodendroglioma, and a columnar structure oriented perpendicular to the cortical surface.[52] The temporal lobe is the most common site (62%) followed by the frontal lobe (31%) and parieto-occipital lobe (9%).[51] They may also arise within the caudate nucleus, cerebellum, or pons. About 30% of tumors are associated with cortical dysplasia.

Imaging: On imaging, DNETs are well-circumscribed lesions that are based in and focally expand the cortex, sometimes extending into the white matter. At CT, the tumor is hypodense with calcific foci in 40% of cases.[53] Remodelling of the skull adjacent to the lesions may occur in long-standing lesions.[51] They are hypointense on T1WI and hyperintense on T2WI with no evidence of diffusion restriction **(Figs. 20A to C)**. Minimal or no edema and mass effect relative to the size of the lesion are seen.[54] About one-third of DNETs may show gadolinium enhancement, which is typically patchy and multifocal rather than diffuse. Gadolinium enhancement is variable, occurring in less than one-half of cases; enhancement is patchy and multifocal rather than diffuse.[51] A nonenhancing DNET may show contrast enhancement during follow-up without necessarily indicating malignant transformation. MRS may show increased mI.[55] Distinguishing features of DNET include a cortical tumor with thick nodular or gyral configuration with little or no edema and mass effect.

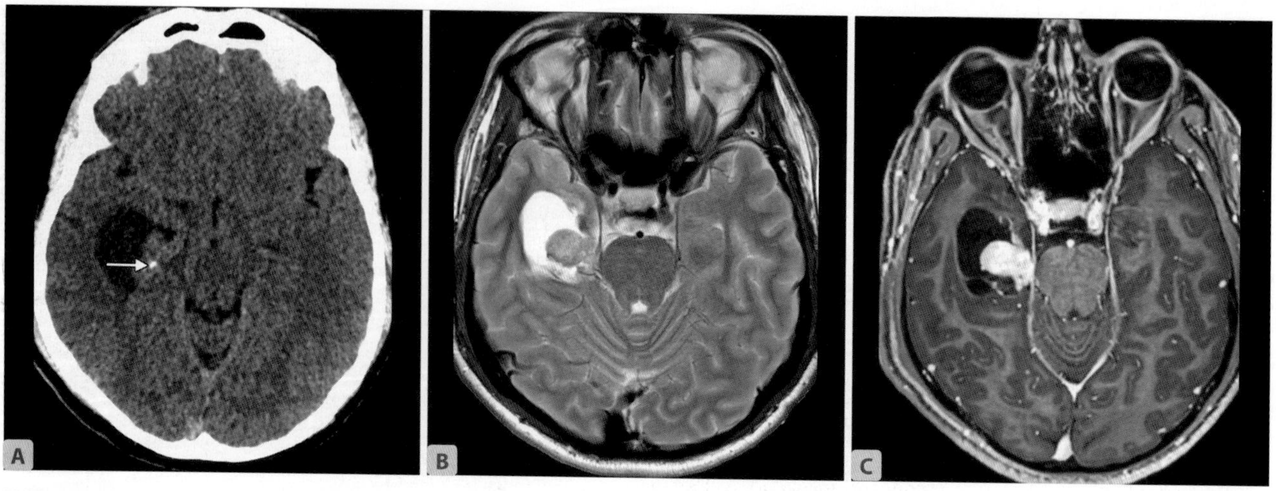

FIGS. 19A TO C: Ganglioglioma: NCCT head (A) shows a cyst with mural nodule containing focal calcification (arrow in A) in right medial temporal lobe. The nodule is hyperintense on axial T2WI (B) and enhances avidly in postgadolinium T1WI (C). (NCCT: noncontrast computed tomography; T1WI: T1-weighted image; T2WI: T2-weighted image)

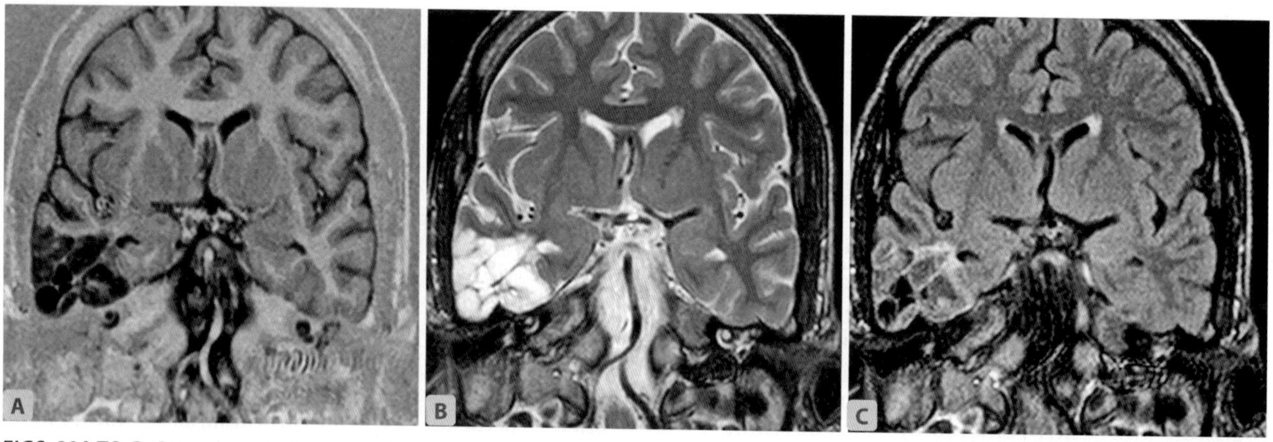

FIGS. 20A TO C: Dysembryoplastic neuroepithelial tumors: MRI shows a gyriform lesion in right middle and inferior temporal lesion without any mass effect or perilesional edema. The mass is hypointense on coronal T1WI (A), hyperintense on coronal T2WI (B), and shows partial signal suppression on coronal FLAIR images (C). (FLAIR: fluid-attenuated inversion recovery; T1WI: T1-weighted image; T2WI: T2-weighted image)

Desmoplastic infantile tumors: Desmoplastic infantile tumors (DITs) are benign, WHO grade I tumors, and include DIA and desmoplastic infantile ganglioglioma (DIG),[56] both having similar clinical presentations and imaging features. Pathologically, they are characterized by desmoplastic stroma along with neoplastic astrocytes only (DIA) or with neoplastic astrocytes and neuronal component (DIG).[57] Most tumors occur in children <18 months of age (peak: 3–6 months). Typically, tumors present as rapidly increasing head size with bulging fontanelle and rarely with seizures. Typically, the tumor is superficially located in frontal and parietal lobes. Growth into the subarachnoid space and adjacent meninges is uniformly present in these tumors.

Imaging: Typically, tumors are exceptionally large in size with predominant cystic component and cortical-based solid component which is nodular or plaque like. The cystic component is hypodense in CT scan, hypointense in T1WI, and hyperintense in T2WI in MRI **(Figs. 21A and B)**. The solid component has features of aggressive tumors—T2 hypointense and diffusion restriction, which are characteristic.[58] No necrosis is seen in solid component. No hemorrhage or calcification is seen. The solid component enhances avidly along with overlying meninges.[59] DITs are associated with no or minimal edema compared with the size of the mass.[49]

Differential diagnosis includes embryonal tumor with multilayered rosettes, EPN, and DA. Distinguishing features of DIT include a large cerebral mass with cystic component and enhancing solid component adjacent to meninges in an infant.

Angiocenteric glioma: Angiocentric glioma (AG) is a rare, slow-growing cerebral hemispheric tumors often associated

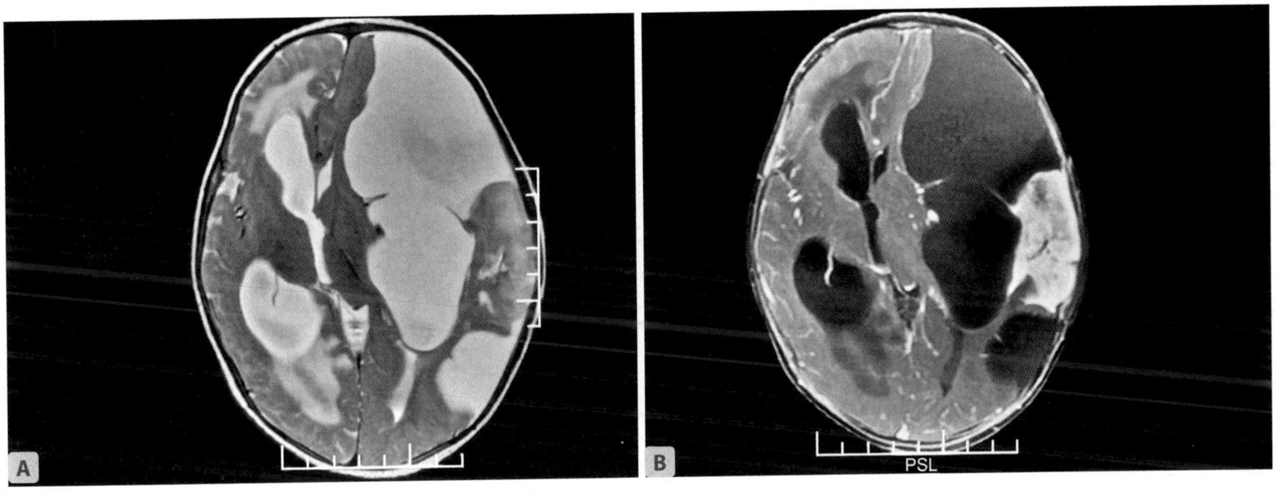

FIGS. 21A AND B: Desmoplastic infantile tumors: Axial T2WI (A) shows a large cystic mass with small solid component in left cerebral hemisphere causing midline shift. The solid component abuts and dial surface and enhances intensely in postgadolinium T1WI (B). (T1WI: T1-weighted image; T2WI. T2 weighted image)

with intractable epilepsy and occurs mainly in children and young adults.[56] The histological hallmark of AGs is perivascular pattern of growth. Most AGs are superficially located tumors that expand the cortex, hypointense on T1WI, hyperintense on T2WI, and do not enhance following gadolinium administration.[60] Their imaging hallmark is an intrinsic rim-like hyperintensity on T1WI and the stalk-like extension to the adjacent ventricle on T2WI which may not be seen in all cases.[61]

Diffuse leptomeningeal glioneuronal tumor: DLGNT is a newly designated tumor as of the 2016 revision of WHO CNS tumor classification. They have been previously known as primary leptomeningeal oligodendrogliomatosis or disseminated oligodendroglial-like leptomeningeal tumor of childhood. Median age is of 5 years (range: 5 months to 45 years). Patients usually present with signs and symptoms of raised intracranial tension due to hydrocephalus, cranial neuropathies, and leptomeningitis.

Imaging: MRI shows diffuse leptomeningeal thickening and enhancement, often most prominent along the spinal cord, posterior fossa, and brainstem. Intraparenchymal and intramedullary-enhancing nodules can also be seen. In addition, there may be countless small subpial cysts following CSF signal intensity (possible representing dilated perivascular spaces) **(Figs. 22A to D)**.[62] Also, there is often secondary hydrocephalus.

High-grade Tumors

Pediatric HGGs account for only 20% of all childhood brain tumors and approximately 44% of brain tumor-related deaths in children <14 years of age.[63] The pediatric HGGs are biologically distinct from adult HGGs with substantial differences in tumor location, contrast enhancement, and driver mutations. Approximately, 50% of pediatric HGGs harbor driver mutations involving histone (H) protein complex variants.

Astrocytic Tumors

High-grade astrocytic tumors include anaplastic astrocytomas (AAs) and glioblastoma (GBM).

Anaplastic astrocytoma: AAs are the WHO grade III neoplasms and account for about 2% of all CNS tumors in children.[64] Contrary to adult counterpart, majority of pediatric AAs are result of de novo mutations. They are most common in frontal and temporal lobe white matter. On imaging, tumor is ill-defined, hypointense on T1WI and hyperintense on T2WI with patchy enhancement. Compared to pilocytic or DAs, AAs have low ADC and high rCBV values.[65] On MRS, AAs show increased choline and decreased N-acetylaspartate (NAA), with decreased mI compared with the spectra of lower-grade gliomas.[65]

Glioblastoma: GBM is rare in children and accounts for about 3% of primary brain tumors.[66] Compared to adult GBM, survival is better in pediatric GBM.[67] Although GBM may arise anywhere in the neuroaxis, most are supratentorial and located in the frontal and temporal lobes. The key imaging feature of GBM is intense rim enhancement with central clearing indicative of necrosis, presence of hemorrhage in blood-sensitive sequences like susceptibility-weighted imaging (SWI), and marked peritumoral edema **(Figs. 23A to C)**. The solid component is hypercellular and shows diffusion restricted with low ADC values, increased perfusion and permeability parameters with high rCBV and Ktrans values, respectively, and usually enhances avidly with contrast.[65] On MRS, GBM typically has increased lactate and increased lipids due to anaerobic metabolism and presence of necrosis, respectively.[65]

Embryonal Tumors

Embryonal tumor with multilayered rosettes C19MC-altered: Embryonal tumor with multilayered rosettes (ETMRs) are highly malignant embryonal tumor with the median age of onset of approximately 2 years. The term, PNET, has been

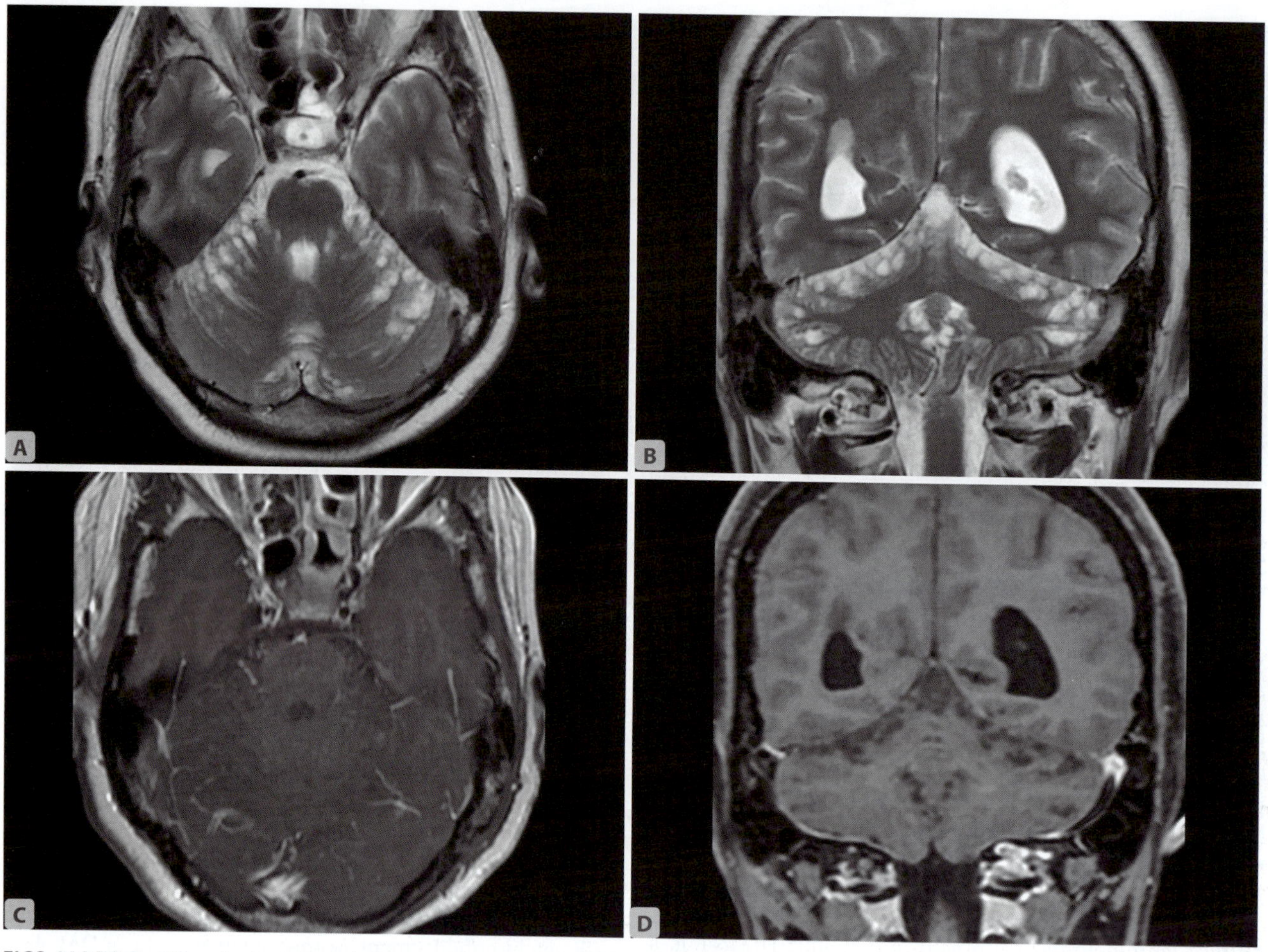

FIGS. 22A TO D: Diffuse leptomeningeal glioneuronal tumor: Axial (A) and coronal T2-weighted image (T2WI) (B) shows multiple subpial cysts in both cerebellar hemisphere which do not enhance following contrast administration (C and D).

removed in the new 2016 WHO classification of CNS tumors and now the tumor is genetically defined by presence of genetic alterations in the C19MC cluster of genes in tumors with variable histology.[6] Tumors previously labeled ETANTR, ependymoblastoma, and medulloepithelioma are all included in this group, provided they have evidence of C19MC amplification. In its absence, the tumor is called ETMR-NOS.

Embryonal tumor with multilayered rosettes most commonly arise in the supratentorial compartment, often in the frontal or parietotemporal lobes. Approximately, 30% of tumors arise in the cerebellum or brainstem. Patients may present with signs and symptoms of increased intracranial pressure or focal neurologic signs.

Imaging: Tumors are typically large (>5 cm) well-circumscribed masses with no or minimal peritumoral edema despite their large size.[68] Typically, they are heterogeneous masses on CT with associated calcifications in up to 70% of cases.[68] On MRI, they have mixed signal intensity on T1WI and T2WI due to presence of blood products, calcifications, and cystic changes **(Figs. 24A and B)**. FLAIR shows signal suppression in necrotic and cystic areas within the tumor. On diffusion-weighted imaging (DWI), the tumor shows restricted diffusion presumably due to high cellularity and nuclear-to-cytoplasmic ratio. The tumor shows heterogeneous contrast enhancement.[68] Perfusion MRI shows increased rCBV.[68] Subarachnoid dissemination can be seen in 40% of cases, necessitating the need to image the entire neuroaxis. Prognosis is dismal despite radiation therapy.

Sellar and Suprasellar Tumors

Tumors of the sellar region include pituitary tumors and craniopharyngiomas. Together, they account for approximately 15% of all pediatric CNS tumors.

Craniopharyngioma

Craniopharyngiomas are epithelial tumors that arise from remnants of Rathke's pouch. They constitute approximately 5–10% of brain neoplasms in children. They most commonly arise along the pituitary stalk in the suprasellar region (90%) and rarely completely intrasellar in location or within anterior third ventricle. The tumor has a bimodal age distribution, with one peak in children between 5 and 14 years old and a second peak in adults between 50 and 75 years of age. Most patients present with symptoms of headaches, visual

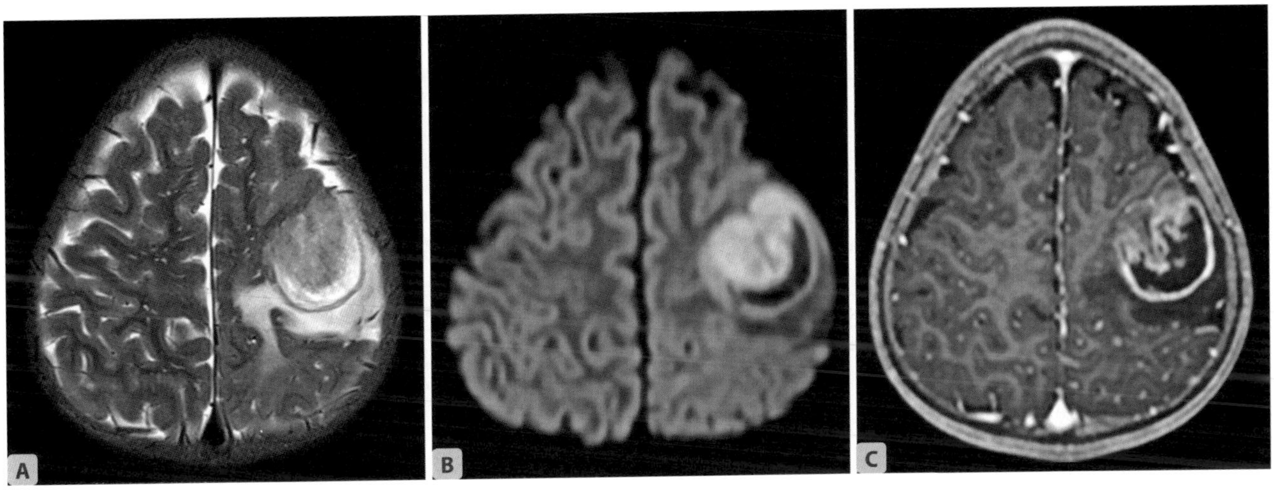

FIGS. 23A TO C: Glioblastoma: Axial T2WI (A) shows a solid cystic mass with perilesional edema in left posterior frontal region. The solid component shows restricted diffusion on DWI (B) and enhances intensely (C) in postgadolinium T1WI. (DWI: diffusion-weighted imaging; T1WI: T1-weighted image; T2WI: T2-weighted image)

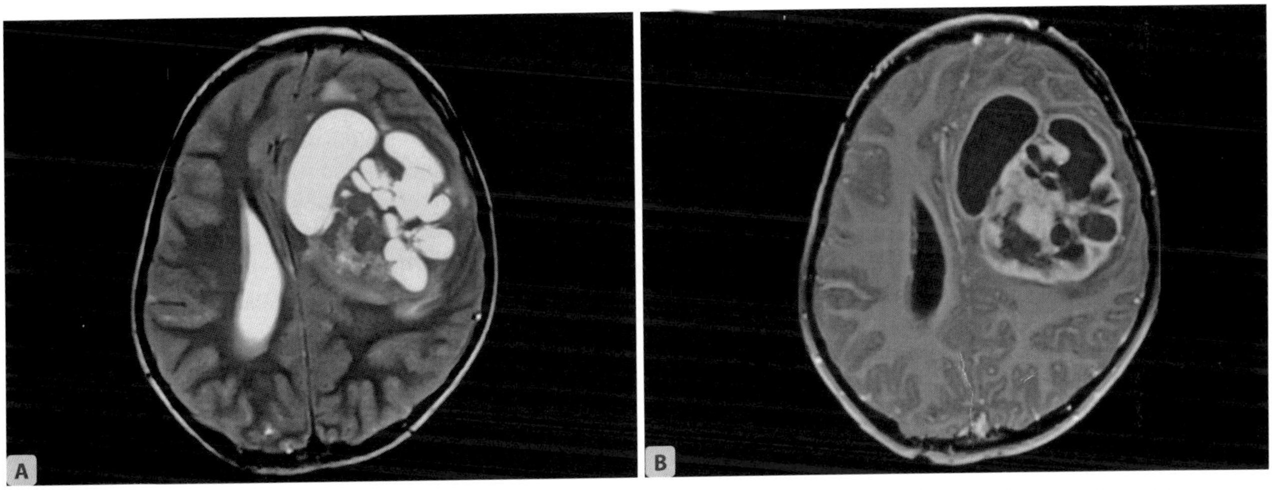

FIGS. 24A AND B: Primitive neuroectodermal tumor: Axial T2WI (A) shows a solid cystic mass without perilesional edema in left frontal lobe and causing midline shift. The mass shows heterogeneous enhancement in postgadolinium T1WI (B). (T1WI: T1-weighted image; T2WI: T2-weighted image)

disturbances, and endocrine dysfunction. Pathologically, two distinct subtypes are recognized: The adamantinous type, which tends to occur in children and the papillary variant, which tends to occur in adults.[69]

Imaging

On CT, craniopharyngiomas can be cystic, mixed cystic and solid, or solid tumors. The cyst has variable density depending on contents. Nodular or rim calcification is found in about 90% of cases.

MR imaging appearance of the tumor depends on the contents of the cyst. Cyst with high cholesterol content and/or subacute hemorrhage have high signal intensity on T1WI and T2WI **(Figs. 25A to C)** while cysts containing large amount of keratin are hypointense on T1WI. The solid component has mixed signal intensity on T1WI and T2WI reflecting presence of calcification and hemorrhage. Following contrast administration, the cyst wall may enhance and the solid component may show heterogeneous enhancement. Adamantinous type of craniopharyngioma is more likely to have lobulated shape, hyperintense cysts, vessel encasement, and recurrence whereas papillary type of craniopharyngioma is more likely to have round shape, hypointense cysts, and predominantly solid morphology.

Pituitary Adenomas

Pituitary adenomas represent <3% of all childhood intracranial neoplasms. In childhood, they are usually seen in adolescent males.[29] Adenomas measuring 10 mm or less are referred to as microadenomas and these tumors do not have suprasellar extension. Most microadenomas enhance less rapidly than surrounding normal pituitary tissue and therefore appear as hypointense areas on dynamic contrast-

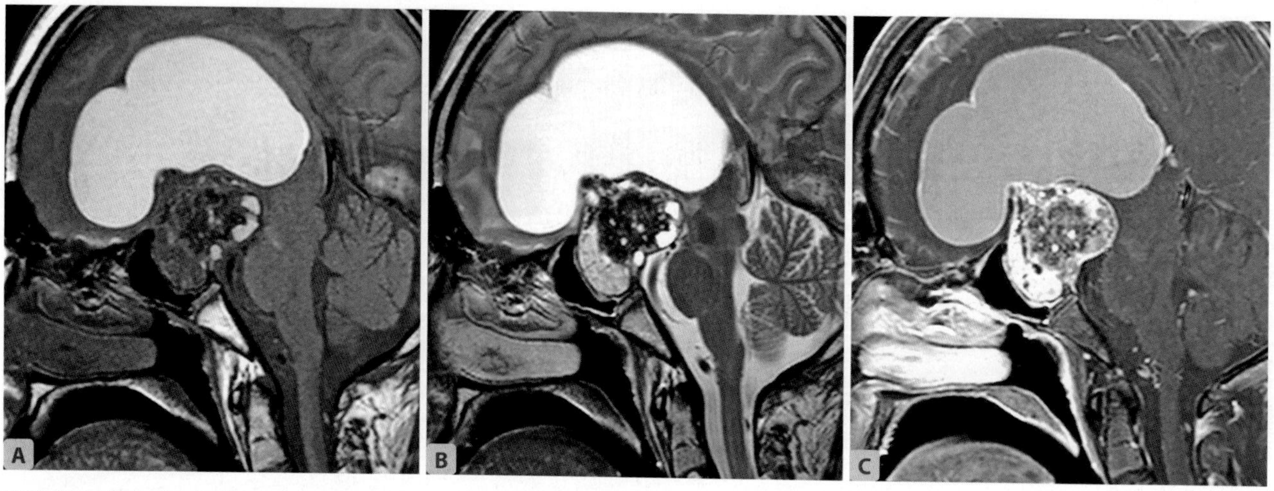

FIGS. 25A TO C: Craniopharyngioma: Sagittal T1WI (A) and T2WI (B) show a sellar-suprasellar solid cystic mass. The cystic component is hyperintense in both T1WI and T2WI. The solid component contains hypointense region in posterior half secondary to calcification. The solid portion enhances heterogeneously following gadolinium administration (C). (T1WI: T1-weighted image; T2WI: T2-weighted image)

enhanced MR studies. Macroadenomas are more common than microadenomas and enhance uniformly and intensely.

Chiasmatic/Hypothalamic Gliomas

Gliomas of the hypothalamus and posterior optic pathways represent 5% of pediatric brain neoplasms with 60% involving the optic chiasm and hypothalamus.[69] They represent 25–30% of pediatric neoplasm of suprasellar region.

Most chiasmatic/hypothalamic gliomas are PAs and rarely are GG. About 20–50% of these patients have clinical evidence or family history of NF1. The exact site of origin is almost impossible to determine since both hypothalamus and chiasm are involved regardless of origin. The mean age of presentation is 3 years. Patients usually present with impaired vision, headaches due to associated hydrocephalus, symptoms due to diencephalic syndrome, and endocrinopathies due to hypothalamic extension.

Imaging

MRI is crucial to differentiate this tumor from other suprasellar masses and to see the exact extent to the lesion and its relationship with adjacent vital structures. The tumor is usually solid with microcyst formation. Like PAs in other locations, tumor is typically iso- or hypointense on T1WI, hyperintense on T2WI, dark on diffusion trace images, and typically shows heterogeneous enhancement with a substantial cystic component **(Figs. 26A to D)**. The sella is usually normal. By contrast, PAs typically show heterogeneous enhancement with a substantial cystic component.

Pilomyxoid Astrocytoma

Pilomyxoid astrocytoma (PMA) is WHO grade II tumor, more aggressive myxoid variant of PA with mean age at diagnosis of 18 months. Majority of these tumors are in the hypothalamic/chiasmatic region and/or originate from the midline and tend to affect very young children. Most often, these are solid tumors and occasionally have a minimal cystic component.

On imaging, PMA is well-circumscribed solid tumor located in the region of chiasma/hypothalamus, isointense on T1WI, and enhances homogeneously. The necrosis is rare and peritumoral edema or parenchymal infiltration is absent.

Hypothalamic Hamartoma

Hypothalamic hamartomas are relatively rare tumor-like developmental malformations.[70] They are located in the region of the tuber cinereum, where they are attached to the floor of the third ventricle or suspended from the floor by a peduncle. There is a definite male predilection. They may be asymptomatic or present with symptoms of precocious puberty, gelastic (laughing or crying) and other types of seizures, developmental delay, and hyperactivity. Hypothalamic hamartomas associated with epilepsy are more likely to be sessile whereas those associated with precocious puberty may be pedunculated.[71] The size is variable ranging from few mm to giant (3–5 cm).

Imaging

Morphologically, these tumors can be sessile or pedunculated. On CT, hamartoma is a round or ovoid isodense mass that projects into the suprasellar or interpeduncular cistern. On MRI, mass is generally iso- to slightly hypointense on T1WI and isointense to slightly hyperintense on T2WI **(Figs. 27A and B)**.[71] It may contain patchy regions of slightly higher signal intensity on T2WI corresponding to fibrillary gliosis areas seen histologically. The mass does not enhance following gadolinium administration, a feature helpful in differentiating it from hypothalamic glioma.

Arachnoid Cyst

Arachnoid cysts are congenital lesions of the arachnoid membrane lined by arachnoid cells, specialized cells that

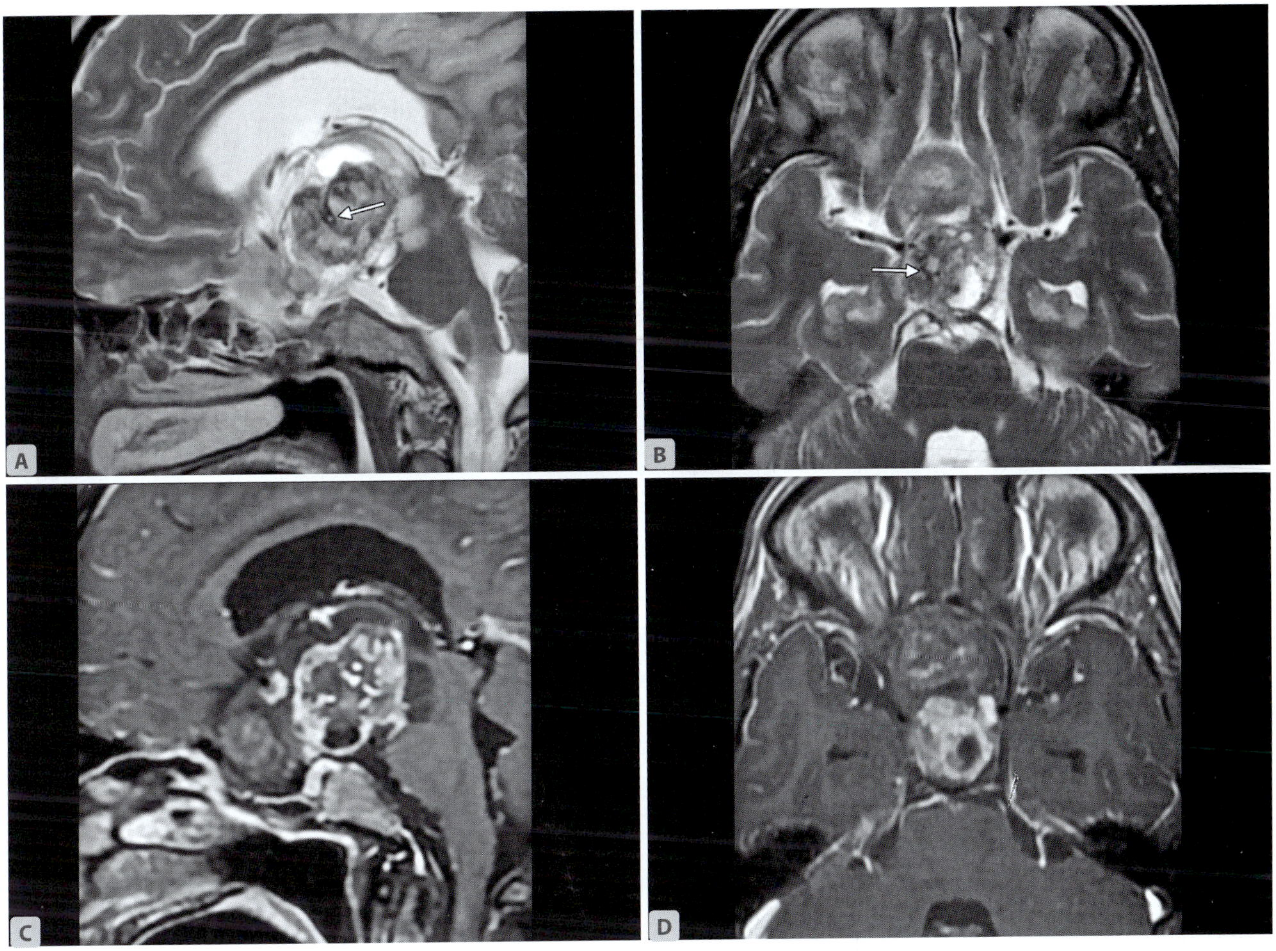

FIGS. 26A TO D: Chiasmal-hypothalamic glioma: Sagittal (A) and axial T2WI (B) shows a heterogeneous mass involving chiasma and hypothalamus with foci of T2 hypointensity in posterior portion (arrow in A and B). The posterior portion of mass shows heterogeneous enhancement in postgadolinium T1WI (C and D). (T1WI: T1-weighted image; T2WI: T2-weighted image)

contain enzymes for secretory activity. Therefore, true arachnoid cysts enlarge by accumulation of CSF secreted by these cells. Approximately, one-half of arachnoid cysts arise in the sylvian fissure; other common locations include cerebral convexity, suprasellar cistern, quadrigeminal cistern, cerebellopontine angle and posterior infratentorial midline cisterns, interhemispheric fissure, and anterior infratentorial midline cisterns. Only 5% of arachnoid cyst is symptomatic. Sylvian fissure cysts are commonly associated with seizures and headache.

Imaging

Arachnoid cysts on CT and MR are well-defined homogeneous unilocular masses that are like CSF density on all imaging modalities and pulse sequences **(Figs. 28A to C)**.[28] Large suprasellar cysts may cause hydrocephalus by obstructing the foramen of Monro. FLAIR is particularly useful in arachnoid cysts because the signal should be completely suppressed if the contents represent CSF.[28] Pulsation artifacts may occasionally be seen within the large cysts and are revealed as focal streaks of hypointensity on T2WI.[72] Subdural and intracystic hemorrhages may complicate middle cranial fossa cysts, either following trauma or spontaneously.

Pineal Region Masses

Pineal region tumors constitute about 3–8% of pediatric brain neoplasms[73] and include tumors arising from pineal parenchyma, ectopic germ cells, and arising from adjacent structures (posterior third ventricle, midbrain, and corpus callosum). All pineal region masses may present with Parinaud syndrome, obstructive hydrocephalus, precocious puberty, and diabetes insipidus. The imaging diagnosis of pineal region tumors can be challenging at times.

Intracranial Germ Cell Tumors

Intracranial germ cell tumors (GCTs) constitute approximately 3–4% of all pediatric CNS neoplasms. They are primarily seen in adolescents with median age of 12–14 years. They typically arise in midline locations and commonly affect the pineal and suprasellar regions. They can also arise in the basal ganglia, thalamus, cerebral hemisphere, and cerebellum.

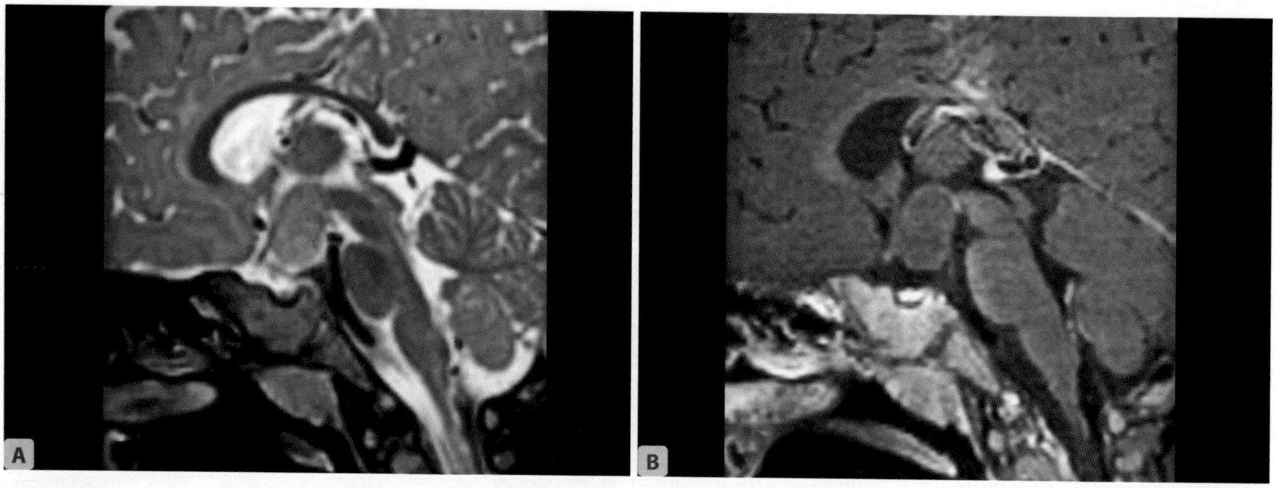

FIGS. 27A AND B: Hypothalamic hamartoma: Sagittal T2-weighted image (T2WI) (A) shows a mass in the suprasellar cistern abutting against floor of third ventricle. The mass is slightly hyperintense to gray matter on T2WI and does not show any enhancement after gadolinium administration (B).

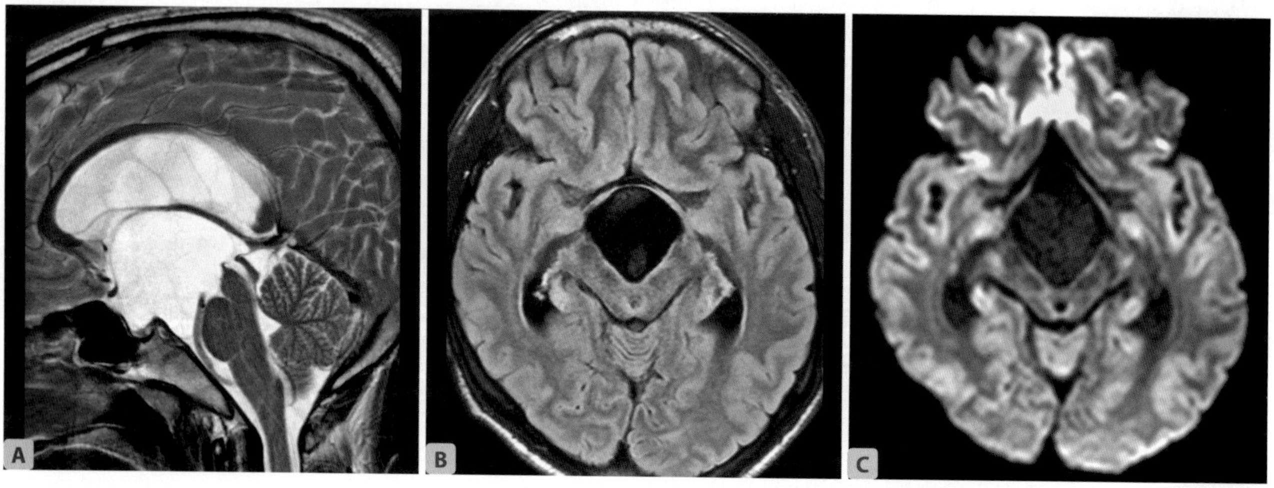

FIGS. 28A TO C: Suprasellar arachnoid cyst: Sagittal T2WI (A) shows a well-defined extra-axial cyst in suprasellar region. The cyst is isointense to the CSF, hypointense on FLAIR (B), and does not show diffusion restriction (C). (CSF: cerebrospinal fluid; FLAIR: fluid-attenuated inversion recovery; T2WI: T2-weighted image)

Intracranial GCTs are divided into germinomas and nongerminomatous GCTs (NGGCTs) which include embryonal carcinoma, endodermal sinus tumor (also known as yolk sac tumor), choriocarcinoma, teratoma (immature and mature teratoma, teratoma with malignant transformation), and mixed tumors with more than one element. Germinomas account for 60–65% of all pediatric intracranial GCTs. Approximately, 25% of NGGCTs are mixed and contain more than one histologic component. Intracranial GCTs can be further defined by tumor markers secreted into the CSF and serum as well as by the presence of histochemical markers on tumor cells.

Pineal Germinomas

Germinomas are the most common pineal tumors and constitute 60–65% of all GCTs in children. Synchronous pineal and suprasellar lesions have been reported in 6–12% of germinomas and are considered diagnostic. Primary pineal germinomas have slightly male predominance whereas suprasellar germinomas have female predominance. Germinomas are unencapsulated tumors with propensity to infiltrate adjacent structures and frequent subarachnoid seeding. Pure germinomas generally are associated with absent alpha-fetoprotein (AFP) and beta-human chorionic gonadotropin (HCG) levels in both CSF and serum.

Imaging

Pineal germinomas are well-circumscribed relatively homogeneous lesions that are not separable from the pineal body itself. Germinomas are typically hyperdense on NCCT, hypo- to isointense on T1WI and T2WI, and show restricted diffusion due to their high cellularity **(Figs. 29A to C)**. Typically, pineal germinomas engulf the pineal gland calcification. Intratumoral hemorrhage may be seen in these lesions. Among pineal regions tumors, germinomas are most likely to show bithalamic extension and thick peritumoral edema.[74] Germinomas and their metastases enhance markedly and homogeneously after intravenous (IV) contrast administration.

Pineal Teratomas

The second most common pineal GCTs are teratomas. They exclusively affect males and present in the first decade. They are most common congenital brain tumors, constitute >50% of cases. Pineal teratomas are extremely heterogeneous masses with irregular and lobulated margins. Histologically, teratomas are of three subtypes: (1) Mature teratoma, (2) Immature teratoma, and (3) Teratoma with malignant transformation.

Benign teratomas are typically well-defined, T1 and T2 mixed intensity masses with cystic areas, fatty tissue, and mineralization with minimal or absent perifocal edema **(Figs. 30A and B)**.[75,76] Both CT and MRI show heterogeneous or ring-like enhancement limited to the solid areas and along the walls of the cystic spaces. Immature teratomas are often larger than mature teratomas at presentation, infiltrate surrounding structures with perifocal edema, and more likely to have CSF dissemination.[75] Malignant teratomas have ill-defined margins, fewer cysts and calcification, and tend to involve adjacent tectum, the brainstem, and the splenium of corpus callosum.

Other Germ Cell Tumors

Choriocarcinoma, embryonal cell carcinoma, and endodermal sinus tumors are highly malignant tumors of pineal gland. Choriocarcinomas tend to bleed, a feature which differentiates it from other pineal tumors on imaging. Serologic and CSF analysis for tumor markers can aid in specificity of preoperative diagnosis. No definite imaging features are seen.

Pineal Parenchymal Tumors

Pineal parenchymal tumors (PPTs) constitute approximately 15–20% of all pineal region tumors and include pineocytomas (WHO grade I), pineal parenchymal tumor of intermediate differentiation (PPTID) (WHO grades II–III), pineoblastoma (WHO grade IV), and papillary tumor of the pineal region. Unlike germinomas, no sex predilection is seen in PPTs.

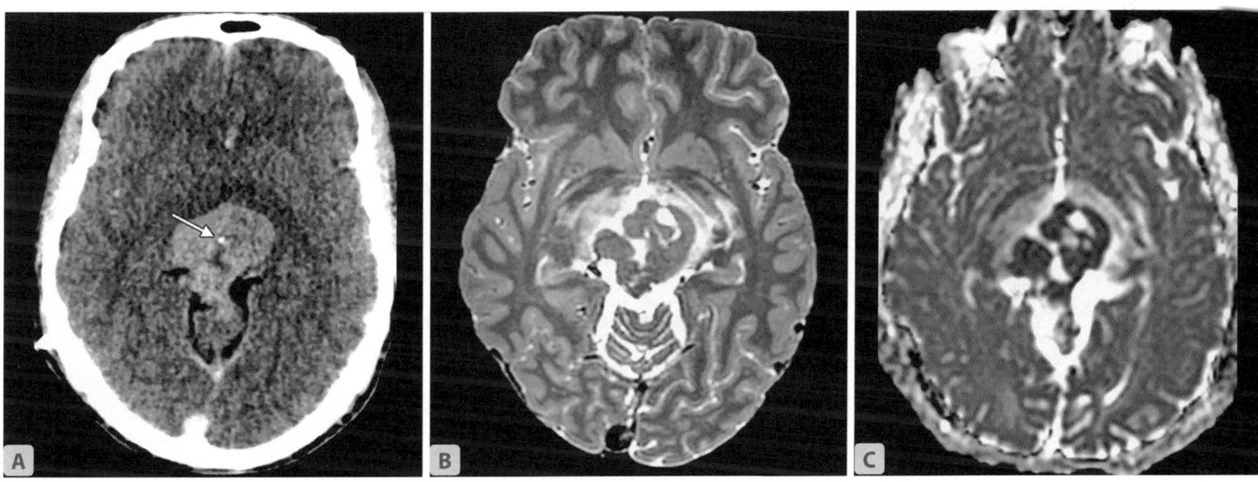

FIGS. 29A TO C: Pineal germinoma: Axial CT (A) shows a homogeneously enhancing pineal mass lesion engulfing pineal calcification (arrow in A). In MRI, the mass is isointense on T2-weighted image (T2WI) (B) and shows restricted diffusion (C).

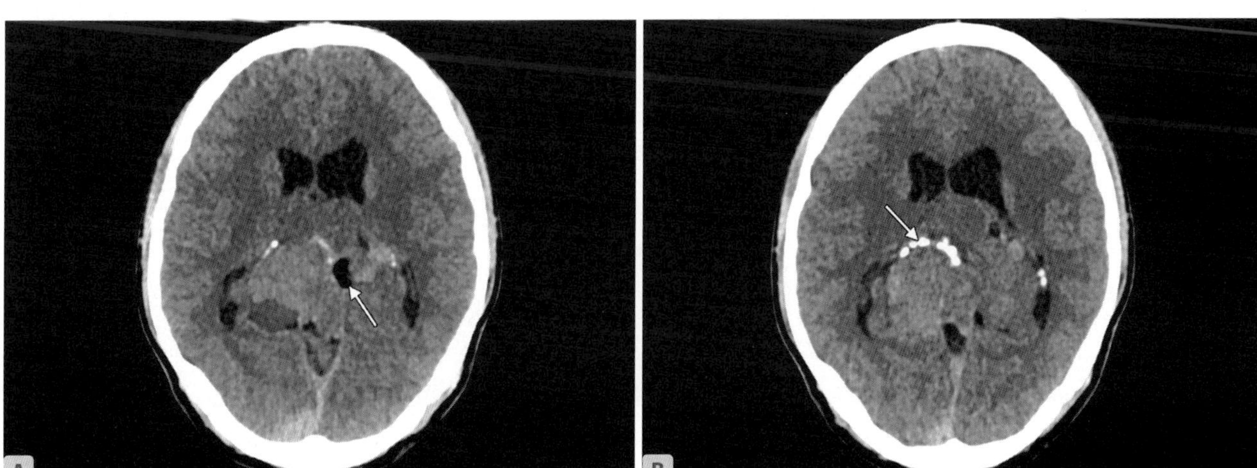

FIGS. 30A AND B: Pineal teratoma: Contrast-enhanced computed tomography (CECT) (A and B) shows a mixed signal intensity lesion in pineal region with foci of fat density (arrow in A) and calcifications (arrow in B).

Pineoblastomas

Pineoblastomas are highly malignant primitive embryonal tumor of pineal gland and account for 24–50% of PPTs. They tend to occur in young children with the mean age of presentation of 3 years. Typically, they are large (>4 cm), heterogeneous pineal mass with lobulated poorly defined margins, and almost all have obstructive hydrocephalus. Being hypercellular, solid portion is hyperdense on NCCT, iso- to hypointense to gray matter on both T1WI and T2WI, and shows restricted diffusion with low ADC values **(Figs. 31A to D)**. On CT, "exploded" peripheral calcification is seen in a large hyperdense mass. Enhancement is variable, ranging from none to intense enhancement. CSF dissemination on MRI is seen in 15–45% of cases.

Pineocytomas

Pineocytomas are slow-growing well-differentiated PPT of young adults. They are composed of small, uniform, and mature cells resembling pineocytes. The mean age of presentation is 35–40 years, but they may occur at any age including children and are almost exclusively found in females. Typically, they are well-defined mass that is <3–4 cm in size and may compress rather than invade the adjacent structures. On CT, they appear as well-circumscribed iso- to slightly hyperdense pineal mass that "explodes" pineal calcification peripherally. On MRI, the tumors are homogeneously hyperintense on T2WI and hypo- to isointense on T1WI **(Figs. 32A to D)**. Small tumors show homogeneous contrast enhancement whereas large tumors show heterogeneous contrast enhancement.

Pineal Parenchymal Tumor of Intermediate Differentiation

PPTID is a rare, intermediate-grade malignant tumor (WHO grade II or III) and was included first time as distinct entity in 2007 WHO classification of CNS tumors. They occur in middle-age and older patients as aggressive-looking pineal mass. These are moderately hypercellular tumors. Size varies from small (<1 cm) to large (~6 cm). CT scan shows "exploded" peripheral calcification, typical for PPTs. On MRI, large bulky tumor is heterogeneously hypointense on T1WI, heterogeneously hyperintense on T2WI, and hyperintense on DWI suggesting restricted diffusion and shows marked heterogeneous contrast enhancement.

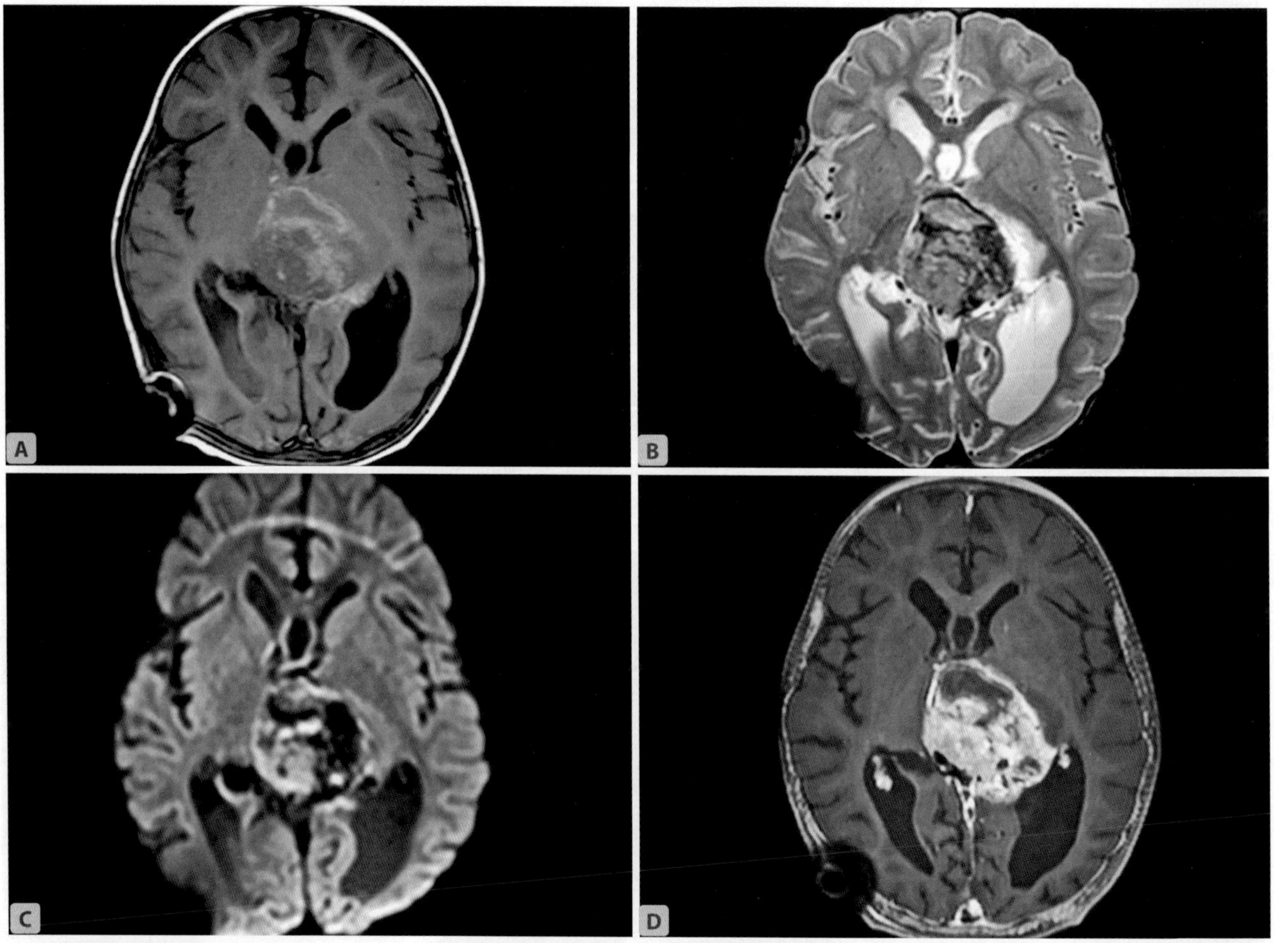

FIGS. 31A TO D: Pineoblastoma: Axial T1WI (A), T2WI (B), and DWI (C) show a large ill-defined pineal region mass. The lesions are iso- to hyperintense in T1WI (A), hypo- to isointense on T2WI, and show areas of diffusion restriction. Above features are suggestive of hypercellular mass with areas of hemorrhage. The mass enhances intensely with contrast administration (D). (DWI: diffusion-weighted imaging; T1WI: T1-weighted image; T2WI: T2-weighted image)

Papillary Tumor of the Pineal Gland

Papillary tumor of the pineal gland is rare tumors in pediatric population. On MRI, they are large, well-defined tumors with characteristic hyperintensity on T1WI **(Figs. 33A to D)**. They show heterogeneous contrast enhancement.

Pineal Cysts

Cystic lesions of the pineal gland are found in 21–41% of autopsy series and between 1.4 and 4.3% of cranial MR studies[77] and are usually incidental. Most are small (<1 cm) in size with minimal or no compression on tectum or aqueduct. The cyst may be multilocular and 25% have calcification in cyst wall. The cysts are iso- to slightly hyperintense to CSF on T1WI, T2WI, and FLAIR images.[77] Hemorrhage within the pineal cyst is rare and appears hyperintense on both T1WI and T2WI. The cyst wall is smooth, well-defined, <2 mm thickness, and enhances uniformly.[78] Over time, these cysts may enlarge in size and become symptomatic. Incidental typical pineal cysts on MRI may be followed clinically without further imaging.

Extraparenchymal Tumors

Choroid Plexus Papillomas and Carcinomas

Choroid plexus papillomas (CPPs) and choroid plexus carcinomas (CPCs) originate from choroid plexus epithelium. They constitute 5% of supratentorial pediatric tumors and <1% of all primary intracranial neoplasms. CPPs are most frequent in first year of life and present with hydrocephalus. CPCs make up 30–40% of choroid plexus tumors and occur mostly during first 5 years of life. Focal neurologic deficit resulting from adjacent brain invasion is the frequent presentation of CPCs. Male predominance is seen for both the tumors. Hydrocephalus frequently occurs with CPPs and may be secondary to obstruction of CSF pathways, adhesions resulting from hemorrhage, overproduction of CSF by tumor, or a combination thereof.

Pathology

The common site of origin for CPPs is the lateral ventricles; third and fourth ventricles are rarely involved in children.

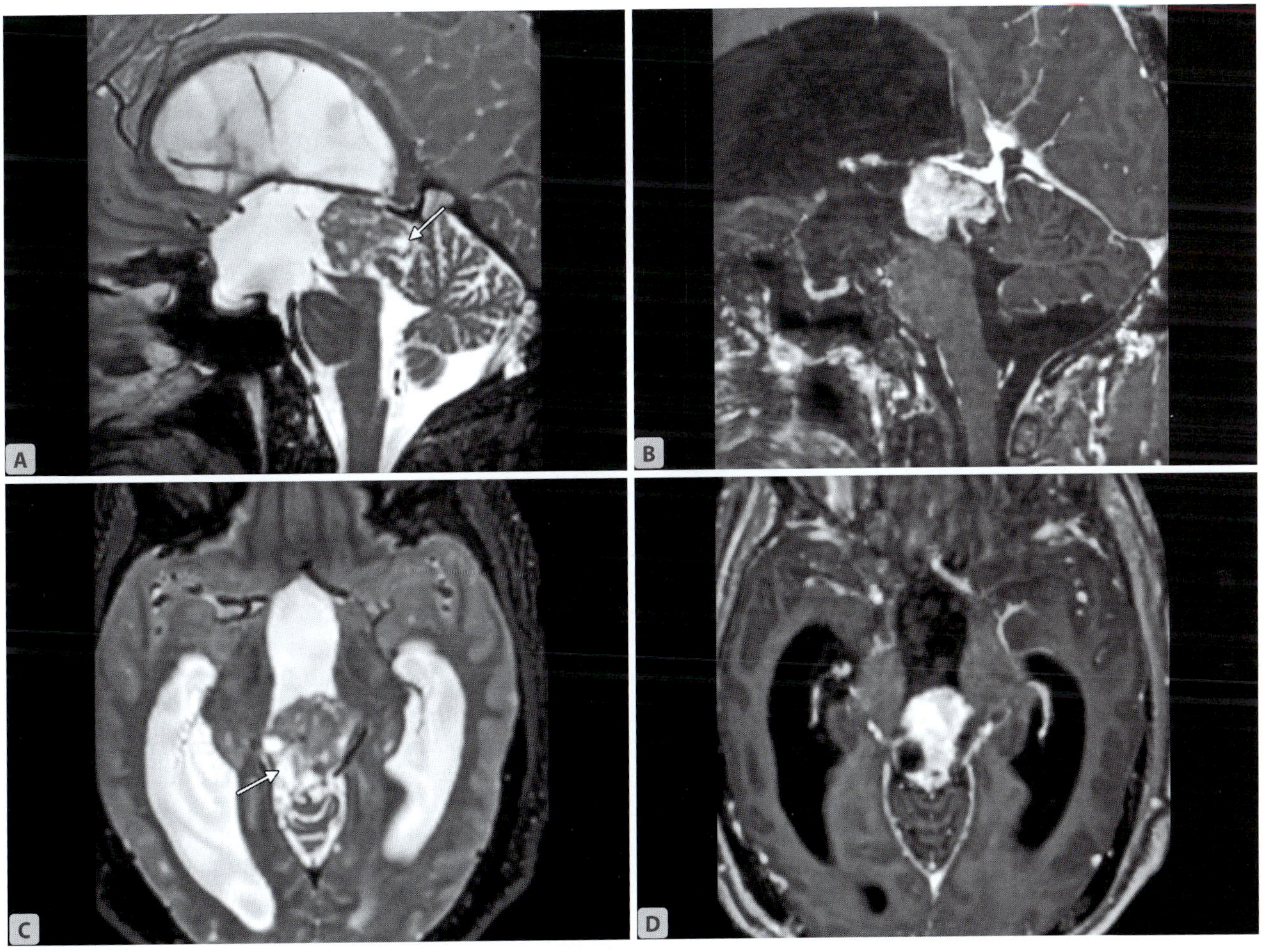

FIGS. 32A TO D: Pineocytoma: Sagittal (A) and axial (B) T2-weighted image (T2WI) shows a well-defined mass lesion in pineal region with cystic areas (arrow in A and C). The mass enhances intensely with contrast administration (B and D).

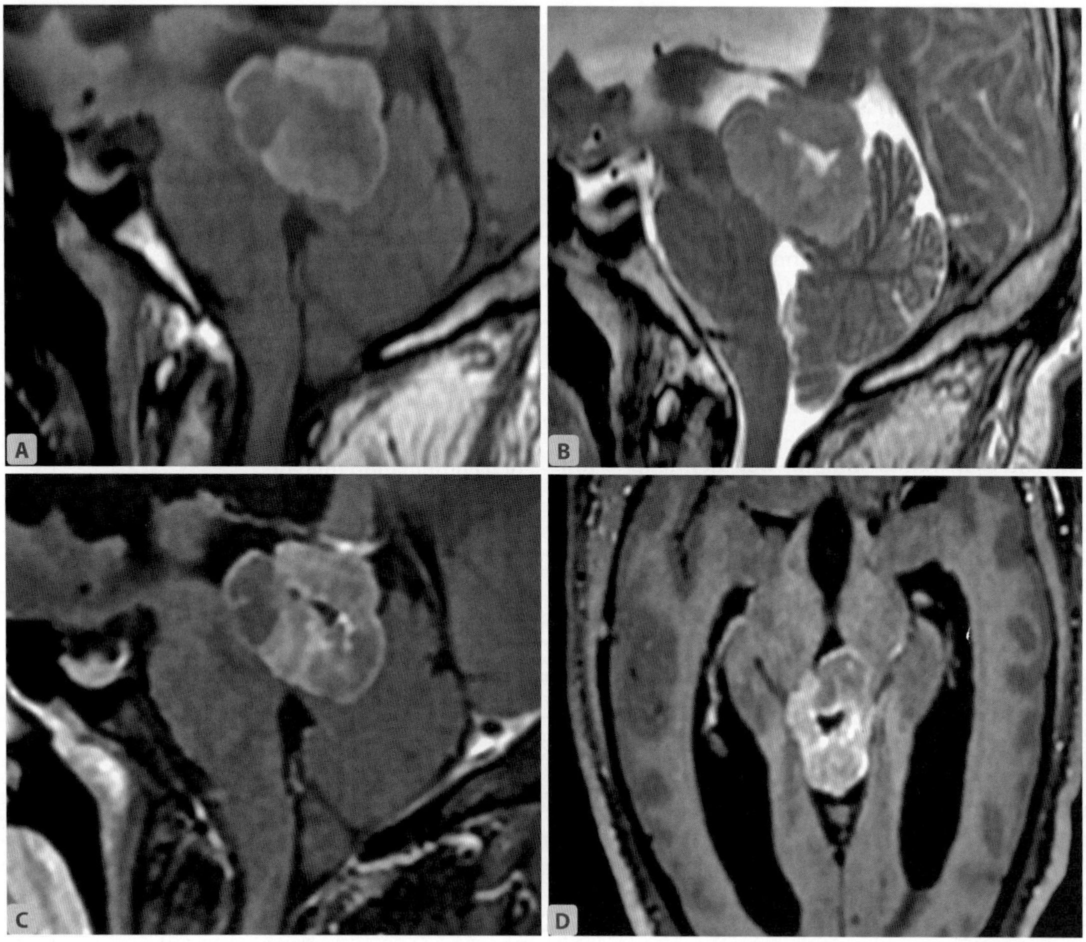

FIGS. 33A TO D: Papillary tumor of the pineal gland: Sagittal T1WI (A) and T2WI (B) show a well-defined mass lesion in pineal region. The mass is hyperintense on T1WI (A), isointense on T2WI (B), and mildly enhances heterogeneously with contrast administration (C and D). (T1WI: T1-weighted image; T2WI: T2-weighted image)

Fourth ventricle is the most common site of adult CPPs. CPPs are well-defined lobulated masses and cause enlargement of the involved ventricles. Foci of small hemorrhages and calcification may be found. Anaplastic papillomas frequently invade the brain and are difficult to differentiate from carcinomas. Metastasis through CSF pathways is common for both anaplastic papillomas and carcinomas.

Imaging

CPPs are typically isodense to hyperdense tumors with lobulated outline and foci of calcification on NCCT and intense enhancement on contrast administration. Anaplastic CPPs invade the ependyma and infiltrate into the adjacent white matter producing vasogenic edema. They are more irregular in outline and closely resemble CPCs. CPCs are much more aggressive than papillomas, irregular in contour, mixed density due to presence of cysts and hemorrhages on NCCT, and show variable enhancement. The invasive tumor invades the ventricular wall and involves underlying brain parenchyma.

At MRI, CPPs are homogeneous or heterogeneous cauliflower-like tumors. They are usually iso-/hypointense on both T1WI and T2WI and show avid enhancement following gadolinium administration **(Figs. 34A to C)**. Heavy clarified CPP may not show enhancement. Heterogeneous tumors contain areas of calcifications, intratumoral hemorrhage, and vascular flow voids.[79] Hydrocephalus is usually associated with CPP.[80]

Meningiomas and Related Tumors

Childhood meningiomas represent 1–4.2% of CNS tumors and 1.5–1.8% of all intracranial meningiomas. Childhood meningiomas have worse prognosis than adult counterparts due to surgical intervention limitation, association with neurofibromatosis, higher incidence of sarcomatous change, larger size, and limitation to use adjuvant radiotherapy and chemotherapy to treat the residual tumors in children.

Pathology

Pediatric meningeal tumors include meningioma, meningeal fibromas, meningeal sarcomas, and meningeal melanomas. Sylvian fissure meningiomas are common, lack a dural attachment, and originate from heterotopic meningeal

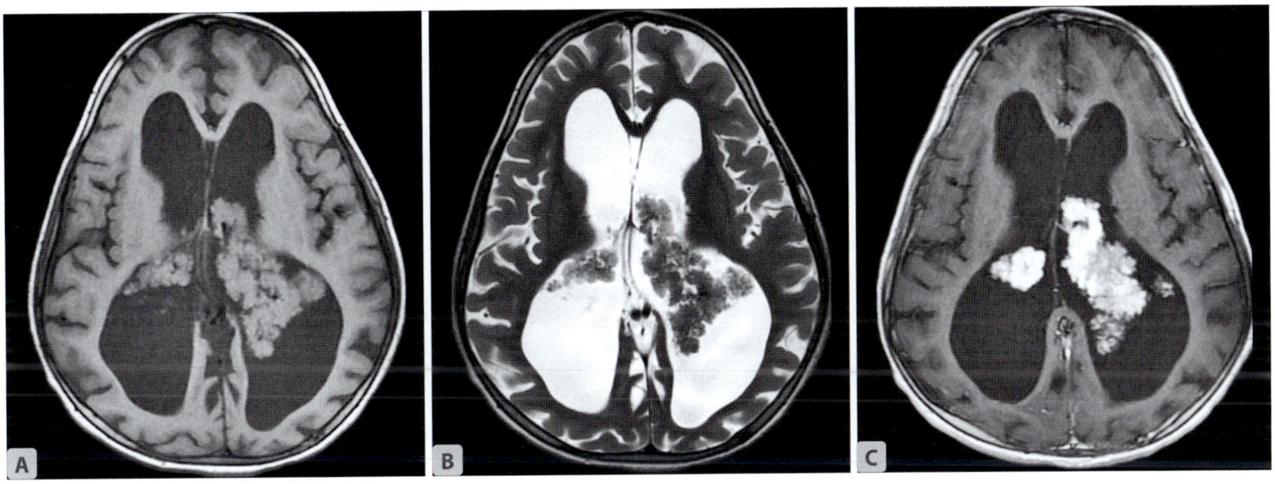

FIGS. 34A TO C: Choroid plexus papilloma: Axial T1WI (A) and T2WI (B) show a lobulated intraventricular mass in the atrial and body of both lateral ventricles (left > right). The mass is isointense to gray matter on T1WI (A), hypointense on T2WI (B), and shows intense enhancement following gadolinium administration (C). (T1WI: T1-weighted image; T2WI: T2-weighted image)

rests within the brain. Significant percentage of pediatric meningiomas is intraventricular.

Imaging

The tumors are iso- to hyperdense on NCCT and the solid portion shows diffuse enhancement on contrast injection. Heterogeneity is seen in about 50% of cases and is related to cystic changes and intratumoral calcification. A typical CT features should suggest a malignant tumor such as meningeal sarcoma or meningeal PNET. Intraventricular meningiomas originate from choroid plexus.[81]

On MR, meningiomas have well-circumscribed tumors isointense on T1WI and iso- to hyperintense on T2WI. Solid portions show uniform enhancement on infusion of paramagnetic substance **(Figs. 35A and B)**. Densely calcified areas may be very hypointense on pregadolinium T1WI whereas less densely calcified areas may be iso- to hyperintense on T2WI. At angiography, meningiomas usually have dual blood supply and meningeal branches from both internal carotid and external carotid arteries may feed the tumor.

Leukemia and Lymphoma

Meningeal and parenchymal metastatic disease from leukemia and lymphoma is extremely uncommon. Meningeal enhancement after contrast administration is found in 5% of leukemic patients with CNS symptoms. Granulocytic sarcoma is a solid tumor formed by deposits of blast cells outside bone marrow in systemic leukemia, usually the acute myeloid leukemia. On CT, they appear as iso- to hyperdense lesions that enhance homogeneously following contrast administration. In MRI, lesions are hypo- to isointense on T1WI, iso- to slightly hyperintense on T2WI, and hyperintense on DWI images suggesting diffusion restriction. The lesions enhance homogeneously and intensely following contrast on both CT and MR.

Epidermoid and Dermoid

Epidermoid and dermoid are congenital/developmental cystic lesions having lining of stratified squamous epithelium, with additional mesodermal elements such as hair, sebaceous, and sweat glands in dermoids.

Epidermoids are slightly more common than dermoids. They are most located in cerebellopontine angles cistern followed by parasellar region. On CT scan, epidermoids are hypodense with ill-defined borders and rarely enhancing. Rarely, epidermoid can be hyperdense on NCCT when they are termed as “white epidermoid”. Calcification is exceedingly rare. On MR, they are hypointense on T1WI and hyperintense on T2WI.[82] Occasionally, epidermoids are hyperintense on T1WI and then they need to be differentiated from the dermoid and lipoma. Chemical shift artifact is absent in epidermoids and a fat-saturation pulse sequence will suppress the high signal of dermoid and lipomas, but not of epidermoids. A lobulated mass with linear heterogeneities within the mass differentiates epidermoid from arachnoid cyst **(Figs. 36A to D)**. DWI will show arachnoid cyst having diffusion characteristic of fluid while epidermoids have diffusion characteristic of a solid lesion (similar to brain tissue).[83] Epidermoids are hyperintense on FLAIR while arachnoid cyst signal gets suppressed (isointense to CSF).

Dermoids are midline lesions and are most located in the parasellar, frontobasal region, or posterior fossa (vermis or fourth ventricle). Dermoids on CT are essentially fat density, extra-axial midline masses that do not enhance **(Figs. 37A and B)**. They may be associated with bone defect in nasofrontal or occipital region that points to the presence of a dermal sinus tract. CT is essential for detection of the calvarial defect while MR delineates the tumor better. Tumor is hyperintense on both T1WI and T2WI **(Fig. 38)**. Chemical shift artifact is present like lipomas. However, dermoids are less lobulated and displace rather than encase blood vessels

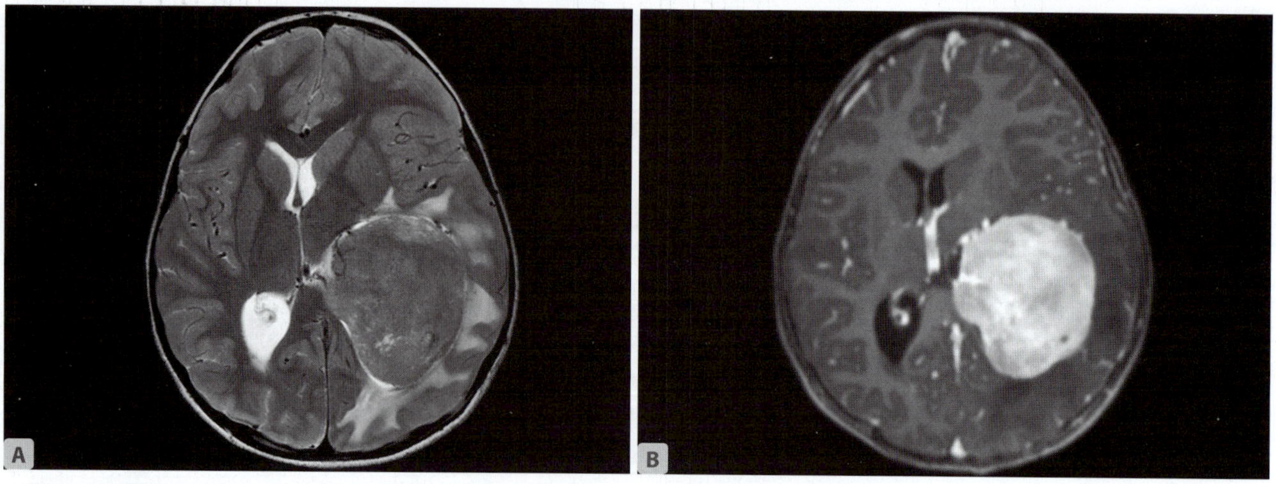

FIGS. 35A AND B: Intraventricular meningioma: Axial T2WI (A) shows well-circumscribed homogeneously isointense mass in atria of left lateral ventricle with intense homogeneous enhancement in postgadolinium T1WI (B). (T1WI: T1-weighted image; T2WI: T2-weighted image)

and neural structures in contrast to encasement of these structures by the lipomas.

Tumors of the Orbit and Neck Ocular Tumors

Retinoblastoma

Retinoblastoma is the most common intraorbital malignancy of childhood. Autosomal dominant inheritance is found in 10% of cases that are frequently bilateral. Up to 2–5% of patients with bilateral retinoblastoma will eventually develop pineoblastoma, the term trilateral retinoblastomas are then applied. Bilateral lesions are seen in 31% and 33% are multifocal.

Majority (80%) of retinoblastomas occur in children below 2 years of age. Soft-tissue sarcomas subsequently develop in 10–15% of affected patients. Leukocoria or "cat's eye reflex" is the usual clinical presentation in early childhood.

Imaging

CT shows a retinal mass with ill-defined margins and commonly associated with calcification (95%). Intracranial extension occurs through scleral lymphatics along the optic nerves. CT is the imaging modality of choice to detect calcification and identification of the tumor. MR is useful for detection of intracranial extension.

Differential diagnosis includes Coats' disease, which is a degenerative proliferative disease of retina. Retinal detachment and subretinal hemorrhage are a common complication of Coats' disease. Larval granulomatosis is caused by *Toxocara canis* infection and has CT appearance like Coats' disease. Both conditions lack calcification and therefore could be differentiated from majority of retinoblastomas containing calcification. Persistent hyperplastic primary vitreous is also associated with leukocoria, retinal detachment, and subretinal hemorrhage. Absence of calcification and hypoplastic affected globe are its major differentiating features from retinoblastoma.[84]

Vascular Tumors

Orbital hemangiomas and lymphangiomas are hamartomatous malformations. Capillary hemangiomas are the most common vascular masses, which typically present at birth and grow rapidly within first 6 months of life. They stop growing during the second year and subsequently involute over 5–6 years.

CT shows a diffuse, retrobulbar mass with ill-defined margins, and present extraconally, intraconally, or both. Contrast enhancement is diffuse. MR reveals a mass that is hyperintense to extraocular muscles and hypointense to fat on both T1WI and T2WI. Serpiginous flow void areas within the mass help to differentiate it from malignant masses such as rhabdomyosarcomas. Orbital enlargement is seen frequently.

Lymphangiomas present between the ages of 1 and 15 years. Recurrent hemorrhages within the mass cause recurrent episodic proptosis. On CT, lymphangiomas are heterogeneous, ill-defined masses with occasional phleboliths and heterogeneous enhancement. Recent hemorrhage appears hyperdense. On MR, lymphangioma appears as lobulated, multicystic mass, which is hypointense to muscle on T1WI and hyperintense to muscle on T2WI. Fluid-fluid levels, when present, are strongly suggestive of lymphangioma. Heterogeneous enhancement is seen on contrast administration. Cavernous hemangiomas are rare in children. They present as painless proptosis, which does not change with Valsalva maneuver, when compared with orbital varices. Cavernous hemangiomas are intraconal masses that spare the orbital apex and frequently have phleboliths within it. MR shows the mass as isointense on T1WI and hyperintense on T2WI compared to orbital muscles. Homogeneous contrast enhancement is noted on both CT and MR.[85]

Orbital Varices

Orbital varices are venous malformations located in the retrobulbar region. They present in older children or

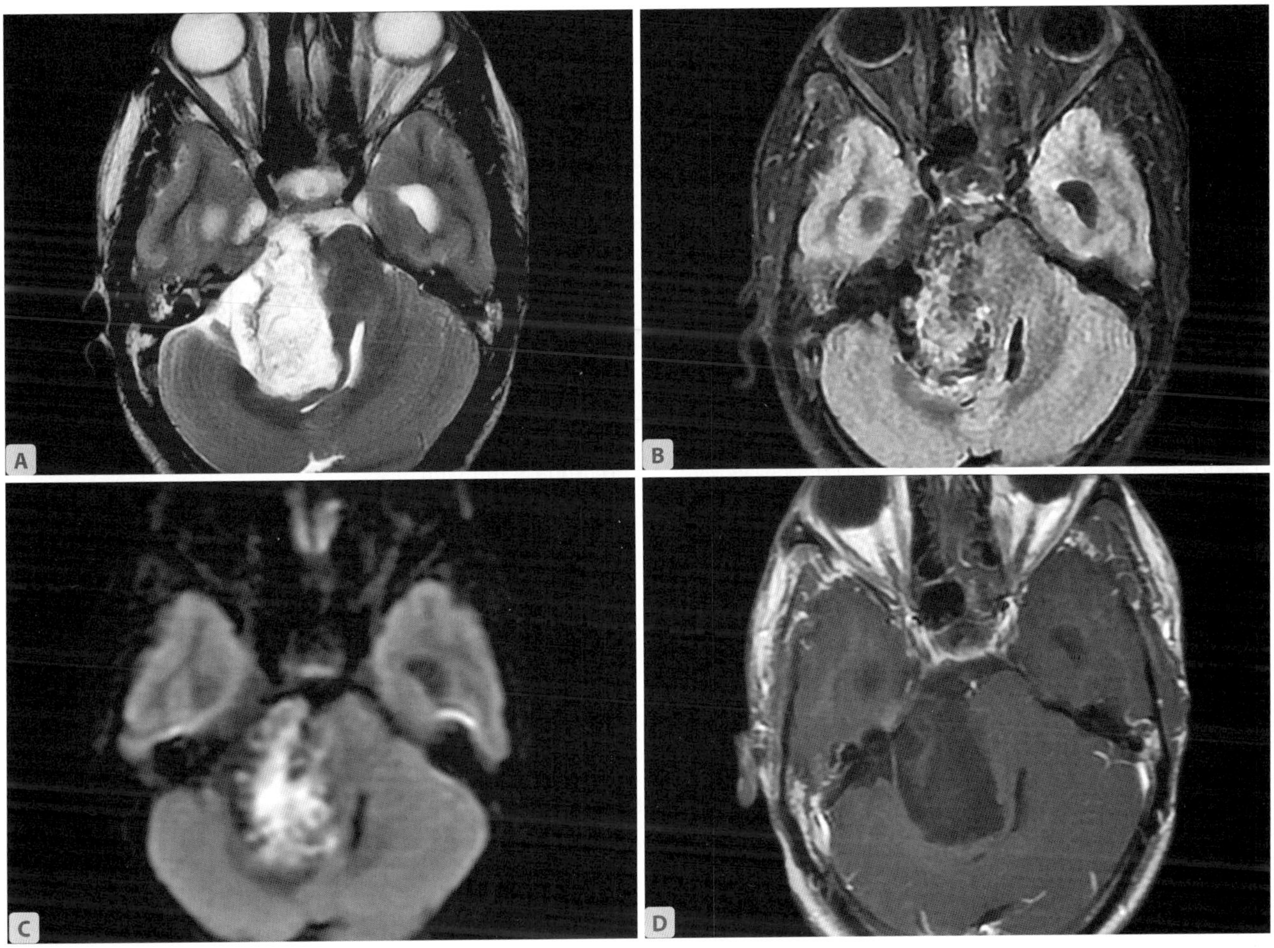

FIGS. 36A TO D: Epidermoid: Axial T2WI (A) shows a hyperintense mass in right cerebellopontine angle cistern. The mass shows internal heterogeneity, hyperintense in FLAIR images (B), and bright in DWI (C) suggesting diffusion restriction. No enhancement is seen following gadolinium administration (D). (DWI: diffusion-weighted imaging; FLAIR: fluid-attenuated inversion recovery; T2WI: T2-weighted image)

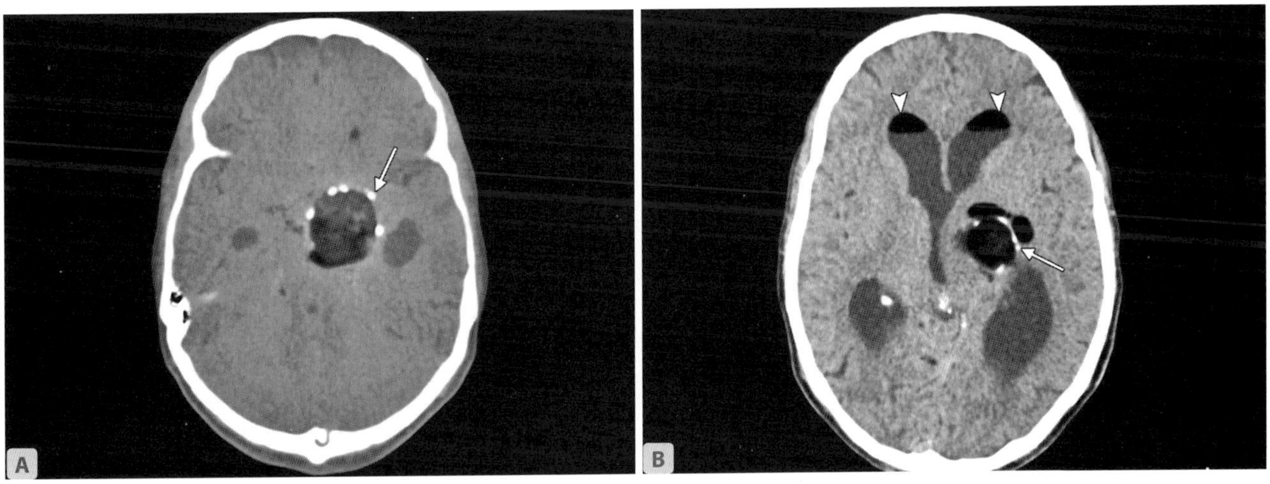

FIGS. 37A AND B: Ruptured parasellar dermoid: Noncontrast computed tomography (NCCT) scan shows a left parasellar mass of mixed signal density containing fat and peripheral calcification (arrow in A and B). Fat is also seen in nondependent position in both frontal horns (arrowheads in B).

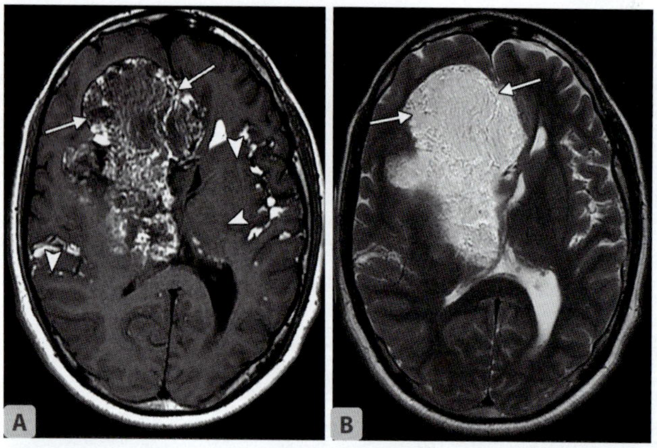

FIGS. 38A AND B: Ruptured dermoid: Axial T1-WI (A) and T2-WI (B) show hyperintense lesion in the right paramedian region (arrows in A and B). Multiple T1 hyperintense foci of fat signal intensity (arrowheads in A) are seen in bilateral sylvian cisterns.

adulthood. Classical presentation is intermittent proptosis, which increases on Valsalva maneuver on lying prone or on bending forward. CT and MR show a mass with curvilinear configuration, phleboliths, and dense enhancement after contrast administration. CT is a better modality since imaging can be performed during a Valsalva maneuver in short time.[85]

Neuroblastoma

Neuroblastoma is a common tumor of childhood, which involves the CNS either by direct extension, primarily in the spine or blood-borne metastases. Neuroblastoma metastases commonly involve the orbit and calvarium and rarely the brain. Unenhanced CT scan may show multiple intracranial hyperdense masses, some of which mimic intraparenchymal lesions. Bony spicules are seen radiating centripetally from the calvarium. Splitting the coronal and sagittal sutures is another characteristic finding in neuroblastoma. Coronal images are useful to verify a dural extradural location of these lesions. Primary neuroblastoma originates in the sympathetic chain of upper cervical or skull base portion. On MR, the tumor masses have intensity like soft tissues. Enhancement is marked and elevated periosteum also shows enhancement which helps to differentiate it from normal hematopoietic calvarium. Metastatic Ewing's sarcoma and leukemia cannot be differentiated from metastatic neuroblastoma to the skull base.[85]

Plexiform Neurofibroma

Plexiform neurofibroma is seen in the setting of NF1. They diffusely infiltrate the connective tissue and peripheral nerves of the orbit. Proptosis, visual loss, marked facial asymmetry, enlarged orbit, and dysplastic adjacent greater sphenoid wing are commonly found. The mass may extend through the superior orbital fissure into the cavernous sinus. The masses are isodense to extraocular muscles on CT. MR is preferred to CT, since cavernous sinus involvement and other manifestation of NF1 can be assessed well even without contrast.[85]

Rhabdomyosarcoma

Rhabdomyosarcoma is a common childhood malignancy, only next to intracranial brain tumors and retinoblastoma. Orbit and nasopharynx are commonly involved, followed by paranasal sinuses and middle ear, constituting 40% of all rhabdomyosarcomas. Primary intracranial rhabdomyosarcomas are rare, although cranial involvement is common from extension of extracranial tumors. Rhabdomyosarcomas are classified into three major groups depending on the site of origin—(1) Parameningeal, (2) Orbital, and (3) Other head and neck locations.

The parameningeal group consists of tumors originating in the middle nasopharynx, paranasal sinuses, and nasal cavity. Prognosis is extremely poor since tumor in this location commonly invades the skull or spread through the foramina at the skull base.

Orbital rhabdomyosarcoma spreads through orbital fissures in the cranium cavernous sinus and middle cranial fossa. The tumor is isodense on NCCT and enhances uniformly after IV contrast. Additionally, the involved foramina are expanded. MR findings consist of mass that is isointense on T1WI and hyperintense on T2WI as compared to muscle. Uniform enhancement is found following IV contrast. Fat-suppression technique with contrast is preferred for better delineation of the tumor from fat and muscle.[85]

Juvenile Angiofibroma

These tumors are benign but locally invasive lesions that arise in the sphenopalatine foramen, nasopharynx, or posterior nasal cavity. Adolescent boys are commonly affected. Local invasion is quite common.

Nasal obstruction and recurrent epistaxis are the frequent clinical presentation. Proptosis and cranial neuropathies are seen with intracranial extension of the tumor. CT shows a soft-tissue mass in the nasopharynx/pterygopalatine fossa, with well-circumscribed margins and homogeneous enhancement following IV contrast. It produces anterior bowing of posterior maxillary wall sinus. Sphenoid sinus extension is quite common.

MR shows a mass that is iso- to hypointense on T1WI and iso- to-hyperintense on T2WI as compared to muscles. Tumor vessels are seen as serpiginous flow void areas. Intense homogeneous enhancement of the tumor is a characteristic finding on IV contrast. Angiography reveals a very vascular tumor, mainly supplied by external carotid arteries. Endovascular embolization may be carried out to reduce intraoperative blood loss.[86]

CONCLUSION

Central nervous system is the second most common site of pediatric neoplasm. Infratentorial tumors account for 52% while 48% involve the supratentorial region. Aside from the initial recognition and characterization of these lesions, the mechanical effects and structural deformities resulting from intracranial neoplasms are also of great importance. Therefore, the neuroradiologists must be able to appreciate the consequences resulting from the combined effects of tumors and the associated edema, many of which are potentially life-threatening such as transtentorial herniation. For the optimal interpretation of MRI, it is essential for the neuroradiologists to be particularly familiar with neuropathology in addition to the requisite mastery of neuroanatomy, since imaging abnormalities reflect pathologic findings in these lesions.

REFERENCES

1. Miltenburg D, Louw DF, Sutherland GR. Epidemiology of childhood brain tumors. Can J Neurol Sci. 1996;23:118-22.
2. Karkavelas G, Tascos N. Epidemiology, histologic classification, and clinical course of brain tumors. In: Antonios D (Ed). Imaging of Brain Tumors with Histological Correlations, 2nd edition. Berlin: Springer-Verlag; 2002. pp. 1-10.
3. Koeller KK, Rushing EJ. From the archives of the AFIP: medulloblastoma: a comprehensive review with radiologic-pathologic correlation. Radiographics. 2003;23:1613-37.
4. Taylor MD, Northcott PA, Korshunov A, Remke M, Cho YJ, Clifford SC, et al. Molecular subgroups of medulloblastoma: the current consensus. Acta Neuropathol. 2012;123:465-72.
5. Wataya T, Hamasaki M, Taylor MD. [Molecular subgrouping and characterization analysis of medulloblastomas in a cohort of Japanese patients]. No Shinkei Geka. 2015;43:117-25.
6. Louis DN, Perry A, Reifenberger G, von Deimling A, Branger DF, Cavenee WK, et al. The 2016 World Health Organization Classification of Tumors of the Central Nervous System: a summary. Acta Neuropathol. 2016;131:803-20.
7. Kool M, Korshunov A, Remke M, Jones DT, Schlanstein M, Northcott PA, et al. Molecular subgroups of medulloblastoma: an international meta-analysis of transcriptome, genetic aberrations, and clinical data of WNT, SHH, Group 3, and Group 4 medulloblastomas. Acta Neuropathol. 2012;123:473-84.
8. Kotsenas AL, Roth TC, Manness WK, Faerber EN. Abnormal diffusion-weighted MRI in medulloblastoma: does it reflect small cell histology? Pediatr Radiol. 1999;29:524-6.
9. Moreno-Torres A, Martínez-Peréz I, Baquero M, Campistol J, Capdevila A, Arús C, et al. Taurine detection by proton magnetic resonance spectroscopy in medulloblastoma: contribution to noninvasive differential diagnosis with cerebellar astrocytoma. Neurosurgery. 2004;55:824-9.
10. Bühring U, Strayle-Batra M, Freudenstein D, Scheel-Walter HG, Küker W. MRI features of primary, secondary and metastatic medulloblastoma. Eur Radiol. 2002;12:1342-8.
11. Aboian MS, Kline CN, Li Y, Solomon DA, Felton E, Banerjee A, et al. Early detection of recurrent medulloblastoma: the critical role of diffusion-weighted imaging. Neurooncol Pract. 2018;5:234-40.
12. Patay Z, DeSain LA, Hwang SN, Coan A, Li Y, Ellison DW. MR Imaging Characteristics of Wingless-Type-Subgroup Pediatric Medulloblastoma. AJNR Am J Neuroradiol. 2015;36:2386-93.
13. Blüml S, Margol AS, Sposto R, Kennedy RJ, Robison NJ, Vali M, et al. Molecular subgroups of medulloblastoma identification using noninvasive magnetic resonance spectroscopy. Neuro Oncol. 2016;18:126-31.
14. Packer RJ, Pfister S, Bouffet E, Avery R, Bandopadhyayay P, Bornhorst M, et al. Pediatric low-grade gliomas: implications of the biologic era. Neuro Oncol. 2017;19:750-61.
15. Brandao LA, Poussaint TY. Posterior Fossa Tumors. Neuroimaging Clin North Am. 2017;27:1-37.
16. Pajtler KW, Witt H, Sill M, Jones DT, Hovestadt V, Kratochwil F, et al. Molecular Classification of Ependymal Tumors across All CNS Compartments, Histopathological Grades, and Age Groups. Cancer Cell. 2015;27:728-43.
17. Witt H, Mack SC, Ryzhova M, Bender S, Sill M, Isserlin R, et al. Delineation of two clinically and molecularly distinct subgroups of posterior fossa ependymoma. Cancer Cell. 2011;20:143-57.
18. Tortori-Donati P, Fondelli MP, Cama A, Garrè ML, Rossi A, Andreussi L. Ependymomas of the posterior cranial fossa: CT and MRI findings. Neuroradiology. 1995;37:238-43.
19. Blaser SI, Harwood-Nash DC. Neuroradiology of pediatric posterior fossa medulloblastoma. J Neurooncol. 1996;29:23-34.
20. Furie DM, Provenzale JM. Supratentorial ependymomas and subependymomas: CT and MR appearance. J Comput Assist Tomogr. 1995;19:518-26.
21. Vanuytsel L, Brada M. The role of prophylactic spinal irradiation in localized intracranial ependymoma. Int J Radiat Oncol Biol Phys. 1991;21:825-30.
22. Rumboldt Z, Camacho DL, Lake D, Welsh CT, Castillo M. Apparent diffusion coefficients for differentiation of cerebellar tumors in children. AJNR Am J Neuroradiol. 2006;27:1362-9.
23. Uematsu Y, Hirano A, Llena JF. [Electron microscopic observations of blood vessels in ependymoma]. No Shinkei Geka. 1988;16:1235-42.
24. Harris LM, Davies N, Macpherson L, Foster K, Lateef S, Natarajan K, et al. The use of short-echo-time 1H MRS for childhood cerebellar tumours prior to histopathological diagnosis. Pediatr Radiol. 2007;37:1101-9.
25. Merchant TE, Li C, Xiong X, Kun LE, Boop FA, Sanford RA. Conformal radiotherapy after surgery for paediatric ependymoma: a prospective study. Lancet Oncol. 2009;10:258-66.
26. Woehrer A, Slavc I, Waldhoer T, Heinzl H, Zielonke N, Czech T, et al. Incidence of atypical teratoid/rhabdoid tumors in children: a population-based study by the Austrian Brain Tumor Registry, 1996-2006. Cancer. 2010;116:5725-32.
27. Rorke LB, Packer R, Biegel J. Central nervous system atypical teratoid/rhabdoid tumors of infancy and childhood. J Neurooncol. 1995;24:21-8.
28. Fischer-Valuck BW, Chen I, Srivastava AJ, Floberg JM, Rao YJ, King AA, et al. Assessment of the treatment approach and survival outcomes in a modern cohort of patients with atypical teratoid rhabdoid tumors using the National Cancer Database. Cancer. 2017;123:682-7.
29. Agranovich AL, Ang LC, Griebel RW, Kobrinsky NL, Lowry N, Tchang SP. Malignant rhabdoid tumor of the central nervous system with subarachnoid dissemination. Surg Neurol. 1992;37:410-4.
30. Zuccoli G, Izzi G, Bacchini E, Tondelli MT, Ferrozzi F, Bellomi M. Central nervous system atypical teratoid/rhabdoid tumour of infancy. CT and mr findings. Clin Imaging. 1999;23:356-60.
31. Jallo GI, Biser-Rohrbaugh A, Freed D. Brainstem gliomas. Childs Nerv Syst. 2004;20:143-53.
32. Fischbein NJ, Prados MD, Wara W, Russo C, Edwards MS, Barkovich AJ. Radiologic classification of brain stem tumors: correlation of magnetic resonance imaging appearance with clinical outcome. Pediatr Neurosurg. 1996;24:9-23.
33. Fisher PG, Breiter SN, Carson BS, Wharam MD, Williams JA, Weingart JD, et al. A clinicopathologic reappraisal of brain stem tumor classification. Identification of pilocystic astrocytoma and fibrillary astrocytoma as distinct entities. Cancer. 2000;89:1569-76.

34. Buczkowicz P, Bartels U, Bouffet E, Becher O, Hawkins C. Histopathological spectrum of paediatric diffuse intrinsic pontine glioma: diagnostic and therapeutic implications. Acta Neuropathol. 2014;128:573-81.
35. Aihara K, Mukasa A, Gotoh K, Saito K, Nagae G, Tsuji S, et al. H3F3A K27M mutations in thalamic gliomas from young adult patients. Neuro Oncol. 2014;16:140-6.
36. Aboian MS, Solomon DA, Felton E, Mabary MC, Villanueva-Meyer JE, Mueller S, et al. Imaging Characteristics of Pediatric Diffuse Midline Gliomas with Histone H3 K27M Mutation. AJNR Am J Neuroradiol. 2017;38:795-800.
37. Ho VB, Smirniotopoulos JG, Murphy FM, Rushing EJ. Radiologic-pathologic correlation: hemangioblastoma. AJNR Am J Neuroradiol. 1992;13:1343-52.
38. Lee SR, Sanches J, Mark AS, Dillon WP, Norman D, Newton TH. Posterior fossa hemangioblastomas: MR imaging. Radiology. 1989;171:463-8.
39. Hakyemez B, Erdogan C, Bolca N, Yildrim N, Gokalp G, Parlak M. Evaluation of different cerebral mass lesions by perfusion-weighted MR imaging. J Magn Reson Imaging. 2006;24: 817-24.
40. Abo-Al Hassan A, Ismail M, Panda SM. Pre-operative endovascular embolization of a cerebellar haemangioblastoma. A case report. Med Princ Pract. 2006;15:459-62.
41. Jaimes C, Poussaint TY. Primary Neoplasms of the Pediatric Brain. Radiol Clin North Am. 2019;57:1163-75.
42. Seeburg DP, Dremmen MH, Huisman TA. Imaging of the Sella and Parasellar Region in the Pediatric Population. Neuroimaging Clin North Am. 2017;27:99-121.
43. Moore W, Mathis D, Gargan L, Bowers DC, Klesse LJ, Margraf L, et al. Pleomorphic xanthoastrocytoma of childhood: MR imaging and diffusion MR imaging features. AJNR Am J Neuroradiol. 2014;35:2192-6.
44. Nakamura M, Shimada K, Ishida E, Higuchi T, Nakase H, Sakaki T, et al. Molecular pathogenesis of pediatric astrocytic tumors. Neuro Oncol. 2007;9:113-23.
45. Pfister S, Hartmann C, Korshunov A. Histology and molecular pathology of pediatric brain tumors. J Child Neurol. 2009;24: 1375-86.
46. Jelinek J, Smirniotopoulos JG, Parisi JE, Kanzer M. Lateral ventricular neoplasms of the brain: differential diagnosis based on clinical, CT, and MR findings. AJNR Am J Neuroradiol. 1990;11:567-74.
47. Atlas SW, Lavi E, Fisher PG. Intraaxial Brain Tumors. In: Atlas SW (Ed). Magnetic Resonance Imaging of Brain and Spine, 3rd edition. Philadelphia: Lippincott; 2002. pp. 565-693.
48. Megyesi JF, Kachur E, Lee DH, Zlatescu MC, Betensky RA, Forsyth PA, et al. Imaging correlates of molecular signatures in oligodendrogliomas. Clin Cancer Res. 2004;10:4303-6.
49. Koeller KK, Henry JM. From the archives of the AFIP: superficial gliomas: radiologic-pathologic correlation. Armed Forces Institute of Pathology. Radiographics. 2001;21:1533-56.
50. Castillo M, Davis PC, Takei Y, Hoffman JC. Intracranial ganglioglioma: MR, CT, and clinical findings in 18 patients. AJR Am J Roentgenol. 1990;154:607-12.
51. Daumas-Duport C, Scheithauer BW, Chodkiewicz JP, Laws ER, Vedrenne C. Dysembryoplastic neuroepithelial tumor: a surgically curable tumor of young patients with intractable partial seizures. Report of thirty-nine cases. Neurosurgery. 1988;23: 545-56.
52. Daumas-Duport C. Dysembryoplastic neuroepithelial tumours. Brain Pathol. 1993;3:283-95.
53. Mano Y, Kumabe T, Shibahara I, Saito R, Sonoda Y, Watanabe M, et al. Dynamic changes in magnetic resonance imaging appearance of dysembryoplastic neuroepithelial tumor with or without malignant transformation. J Neurosurg Pediatr. 2013;11:518-25.
54. Zhang JG, Hu WZ, Zhao RJ, Kong LF. Dysembryoplastic neuroepithelial tumor: a clinical, neuroradiological, and pathological study of 15 cases. J Child Neurol. 2014;29:1441-7.
55. Fellah S, Callot V, Viout P, Confort-Gouny S, Scavarda D, Dory-Lautrec P, et al. Epileptogenic brain lesions in children: the added-value of combined diffusion imaging and proton MR spectroscopy to the presurgical differential diagnosis. Childs Nerv Syst. 2012;28:273-82.
56. Louis DN, Ohgaki H, Wiestler OD, Cavenee WK, Burger PC, Jouvet A, et al. The 2007 WHO classification of tumours of the central nervous system. Acta Neuropathol. 2007;114:97-109.
57. VandenBerg SR, May EE, Rubinstein LJ, Herman MM, Perentes E, Vinores SA, et al. Desmoplastic supratentorial neuroepithelial tumors of infancy with divergent differentiation potential ("desmoplastic infantile gangliogliomas"). Report on 11 cases of a distinctive embryonal tumor with favorable prognosis. J Neurosurg. 1987;66:58-71.
58. Bader A, Heran M, Dunham C, Steinbok P. Radiological features of infantile glioblastoma and desmoplastic infantile tumors: British Columbia's Children's Hospital experience. J Neurosurg Pediatr. 2015;16:119-25.
59. Fernandez C, Figarella-Branger D, Girard N, Bouvier-Labit C, Gouvernet J, Paredes AP, et al. Pilocytic astrocytomas in children: prognostic factors—a retrospective study of 80 cases. Neurosurgery. 2003;53:544-53.
60. Lellouch-Tubiana A, Boddaert N, Bourgeois M, Fohlen M, Jouvet A, Delalande O, et al. Angiocentric neuroepithelial tumor (ANET): a new epilepsy-related clinicopathological entity with distinctive MRI. Brain Pathol. 2005;15:281-6.
61. Ni HC, Chen SY, Chen L, Lu DH, Fu YJ, Piao YS. Angiocentric glioma: a report of nine new cases, including four with atypical histological features. Neuropathol Appl Neurobiol. 2015;41:333-46.
62. Gardiman MP, Fassan M, Orvieto E, D'Avella D, Denaro L, Calderone M, et al. Diffuse leptomeningeal glioneuronal tumors: a new entity? Brain Pathol. 2010;20:361-6.
63. Ostrom QT, de Blank PM, Kruchko C, Petersen CM, Liao P, Finlay JL, et al. Alex's Lemonade Stand Foundation Infant and Childhood Primary Brain and Central Nervous System Tumors Diagnosed in the United States in 2007-2011. Neuro Oncol. 2015;16:x1-36.
64. Kaatsch P, Rickert CH, Kühl J, Schüz J, Michaelis J. Population-based epidemiologic data on brain tumors in German children. Cancer. 2001;92:3155-64.
65. de Fatima Vasco Aragao M, Law M, de Almeida DB, Fatterpeaker G, Delman B, Bader AS, et al. Comparison of perfusion, diffusion, and MR spectroscopy between low-grade enhancing pilocytic astrocytomas and high-grade astrocytomas. AJNR Am J Neuroradiol. 2014;35:1495-502.
66. Perkins SM, Rubin JB, Leonard JR, Smyth MD, El Naqa I, Michalski JM, et al. Glioblastoma in children: a single-institution experience. Int J Radiat Oncol Biol Phys. 2011;80:1117-21.
67. Song KS, Phi JH, Cho BK, Wang KC, Lee JY, Kim DG, et al. Long-term outcomes in children with glioblastoma. J Neurosurg Pediatr. 2010;6:145-9.
68. Borja MJ, Plaza MJ, Altman N, Saigal G. Conventional and advanced MRI features of pediatric intracranial tumors: supratentorial tumors. AJR Am J Roentgenol. 2013;200:W483-503.
69. Sartoretti-Schefer S, Wichmann W, Aguzzi A, Valavanis A. MR differentiation of adamantinous and squamous-papillary craniopharyngiomas. AJNR Am J Neuroradiol. 1997;18:77-87.
70. Mittal S, Mittal M, Montes JL, Farmer JP, Andermann F. Hypothalamic hamartomas. Part 1. Clinical, neuroimaging, and neurophysiological characteristics. Neurosurg Focus. 2013;34:E6.
71. Freeman JL, Coleman LT, Wellard RM, Kean MJ, Rosenfeld JV, Jackson GD, et al. MR imaging and spectroscopic study of epileptogenic hypothalamic hamartomas: analysis of 72 cases. AJNR Am J Neuroradiol. 2004;25:450-62.

72. Atlas SW, Lavi E, Goldberg HI. Extra-axial brain tumors. In: Atlas SW (Ed). Magnetic Resonance Imaging of Brain and Spine, 3rd edition. Philadelphia: Lippincott; 2002. pp. 695-772.
73. Smirniotopoulos JG, Rushing EJ, Mena H. Pineal region masses: differential diagnosis. Radiographics. 1992;12:577-96.
74. Awa R, Campos F, Arita K, Sugiyama K, Tominaga A, Kurisu K, et al. Neuroimaging diagnosis of pineal region tumors-quest for pathognomonic finding of germinoma. Neuroradiology. 2014;56:525-34.
75. Tortori-Donati P, Rossi A. Pediatric Neuroradiology: Brain. Head, Neck, and Spine. United States: Springer Science and Business Media; 2005.
76. Parmar HA, Pruthi S, Ibrahim M, Gandhi D. Imaging of congenital brain tumors. Semin Ultrasound CT MR. 2011;32:578-89.
77. Mamourian AC, Yarnell T. Enhancement of pineal cysts on MR images. AJNR Am J Neuroradiol. 1991;12:773-4.
78. Barboriak DP, Lee L, Provenzale JM. Serial MR imaging of pineal cysts: implications for natural history and follow-up. AJR Am J Roentgenol. 2001;176:737-43.
79. Shin JH, Lee HK, Jeong AK, Park SH, Choi CG, Suh DC. Choroid plexus papilloma in the posterior cranial fossa: MR, CT, and angiographic findings. Clin Imaging. 2001;25:154-62.
80. Pencalet P, Sainte-Rose C, Lellouch-Tubiana A, Kalifa C, Brunelle F, Sgouros S, et al. Papillomas and carcinomas of the choroid plexus in children. J Neurosurg. 1998;88:521-8.
81. Hope JK, Armstrong DA, Babyn PS, Humphreys RR, Harwood-Nash DC, Chuang SH, et al. Primary meningeal tumors in children: correlation of clinical and CT findings with histologic type and prognosis. AJNR Am J Neuroradiol. 1992;13:1353-64.
82. Horowitz BL, Chari MV, James R, Bryan RN. MR of intracranial epidermoid tumors: correlation of in vivo imaging with in vitro 13C spectroscopy. AJNR Am J Neuroradiol. 1990;11:299-302
83. Bergui M, Zhong J, Bradac GB, Sales S. Diffusion-weighted images of intracranial cyst-like lesions. Neuroradiology. 2001;43: 824-9.
84. Price HI, Batnitzky S, Danziger A, Karlin CA, Goldberg L. The neuroradiology of retinoblastoma. Radiographics. 1982;2:7-23.
85. Bilaniuk LT, Zimmerman RA, Newton TH. Magnetic resonance imaging—orbital pathology. In: Newton TH, Bilaniuk LT (Eds). Radiology of the Eye and Orbit. United Kingdom: Clavadel; 1990. pp. 531-84.
86. Lloyd GA, Phelps PD. Juvenile angiofibroma: imaging by magnetic resonance, CT and conventional techniques. Clin Otolaryngol Allied Sci. 1986;11:247-59.

CHAPTER

89

Metabolic Disorders of the Brain

Sapna Singh, Jyoti Kumar, Rashmi Dixit

INTRODUCTION

Metabolic disorders are broadly divided into inborn errors of metabolism and acquired metabolic diseases. Acquired metabolic diseases usually occur in specific or suggestive clinical settings, such as kernicterus in neonatal hyperbilirubinemia, hypovitaminosis in malnutrition, or neonatal hypoglycemia in premature infants. Toxic encephalopathies are special, exogenous forms of acquired metabolic diseases.

Inborn errors of metabolism represent a vast complex group of pathologies. The cause is generally a mutation resulting in a biochemical alteration involving one or more metabolic pathways. The diagnosis of these disorders is often a challenge for all concerned with the care of the affected child. The presenting symptoms are usually nonspecific such as seizures, spasticity, ataxia, movement disorder, or delay in achieving the developmental milestones. Biochemical tests and genetic analyses are often negative. As a result, at least 60% of children with inborn errors of metabolism never receive a specific diagnosis despite extensive investigations.

MYELIN COMPOSITION

For an understanding of the various metabolic disorders, it is essential that a radiologist is familiar with the imaging appearance of the normal and abnormal myelination. Magnetic resonance imaging (MRI) is the most sensitive and specific neuroimaging tool for the detection and assessment of the various metabolic disorders.

Myelin is composed of a bilayer of lipids and proteins. The lipids constitute about 70% of the dry weight of the myelin membranes. While cholesterol, galactolipids, and phospholipids constitute the lipid layer, the myelin proteolipid protein (PLP) and myelin basic protein (MBP) are the major myelin proteins. Cholesterol (fat) has a short T1 while proteins cause a decrease in the T1 value of water. The resultant overall T1 shortening results in an increased signal on a T1-weighted (T1W) image. Thus, myelination will be seen as an area of increased signal or bright signal on a T1W image. Myelination also results in a loss of brain water as myelin lipids are hydrophobic. The loss in brain water results in a T2 shortening which will be seen as a decreased signal intensity or darker appearance on a T2-weighted (T2W) images. Hence, myelination is seen as an area of increased signal/bright signal on a T1W image and a decreased signal/dark signal on T2W image.

PROGRESSION OF MYELINATION

Myelination begins during the fifth fetal month and occurs in an orderly manner following the principles of phylogenetic development. It occurs first in the peripheral nerves followed by the spinal cord and lastly in the brain.[1] It is a dynamic process that occurs from caudal to rostral, dorsal to ventral, central to peripheral, and from proximal pathways to distal pathways (e.g., brainstem before supratentorial brain).[2]

The structures that are myelinated at birth are the medulla, dorsal midbrain, posterior limb of internal capsule, cerebellar peduncles, and ventrolateral thalamus **(Figs. 1A to D)**. The structures that get myelinated at 1 month are the pre- and postcentral gyri. By 3 months of age, the cerebellum and the motor tracts get myelinated. The pons matures by 3–6 months of age. The myelination proceeds in a caudal to rostral manner along the corticospinal tracts as well, that is from the pontomedullary location to the cerebral peduncles to the posterior limb of internal capsule and then the centrum semiovale. The subcortical white matter begins to show myelination by 3 months in the occipital white matter and then proceeds in a rostral manner to the frontal white matter. Similarly, the corpus callosum shows myelination in a caudal to rostral manner with the splenium getting myelinated by 4 months and the genu by 6 months **(Table 1)**.

On MR imaging, the brain changes appear at different times on T1W and T2W images possibly because of T1 shortening by the components of the developing myelin sheaths. The difference in the maturation rate makes T1W images more useful in the first 6–8 months and the T2W images thereafter. The T2W images depict changes that occur with water loss during myelination and are better seen after 6 months of age. The process of myelination is identified about 2 months earlier on a T1W image as compared to a T2W image. Inversion recovery sequences also give an excellent

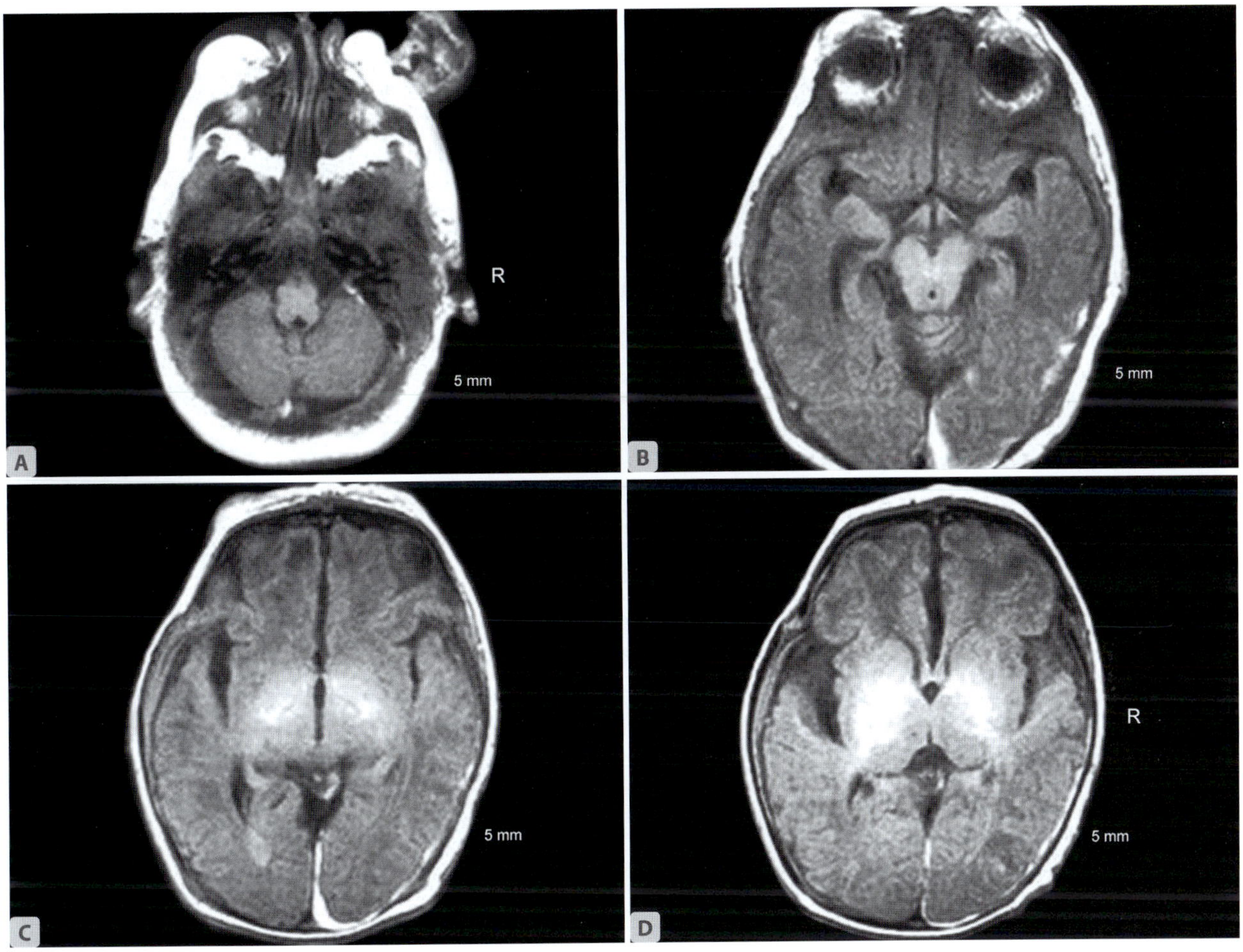

FIGS. 1A TO D: (A) Axial T1-weighted (T1W) MR images in a newborn depicting normal myelination as an area of increased signal intensity (bright) in medulla; (B) Dorsal midbrain; (C) Ventrolateral thalamus; and (D) In posterior limb of internal capsule.

TABLE 1: Normal milestones (Figs. 3A to D).

Structures	T1W	T2W
Cerebellar white matter	3 months	5 months
Splenium	4 months	6 months
Genu	6 months	8 months
Anterior limb of internal capsule	9 months	11 months
Frontal white matter	12 months	14 months
Adult pattern	9 months	18 months

(T1W: T1-weighted; T2W: T2-weighted)

depiction of the myelin deposition and are extremely helpful **(Figs. 2A to D)**.[3]

GRAY-WHITE MATTER DIFFERENTIATION

T2-weighted spin echo pulse sequences can distinguish gray and white matter in infants and demonstrate early progression of myelination. Although developmentally normal children show a spectrum of relative intensities of gray and white matter, their gray-white matter patterns fall into three distinct groups: (1) infantile, (2) isointense, and (3) early adult. At birth and first 6–8 months, the "infantile" pattern shows reversal of the normal adult pattern seen on T2W images, i.e., in neonates the white matter is hyperintense to gray matter. Children between the ages of 8–12 months demonstrate the transient "isointense" phase with poor differentiation of gray and white matter. The early "adult" pattern where gray matter has higher intensity than white matter is seen in all children over 12 months and may be seen as early as 10 months of age.[4]

A knowledge of the different terminologies used is imperative to understand the various disorders of myelination.

Delayed Myelination

This term is used when the myelination pattern observed is inappropriate for the age of the patient, i.e., it corresponds to a younger age. Since myelination is a very dynamic, active energy, and nutrient-dependent process, an interruption in the energy supply leads to a delay of myelination. A delayed myelination may, however, be reversible if the underlying causative factor is corrected.

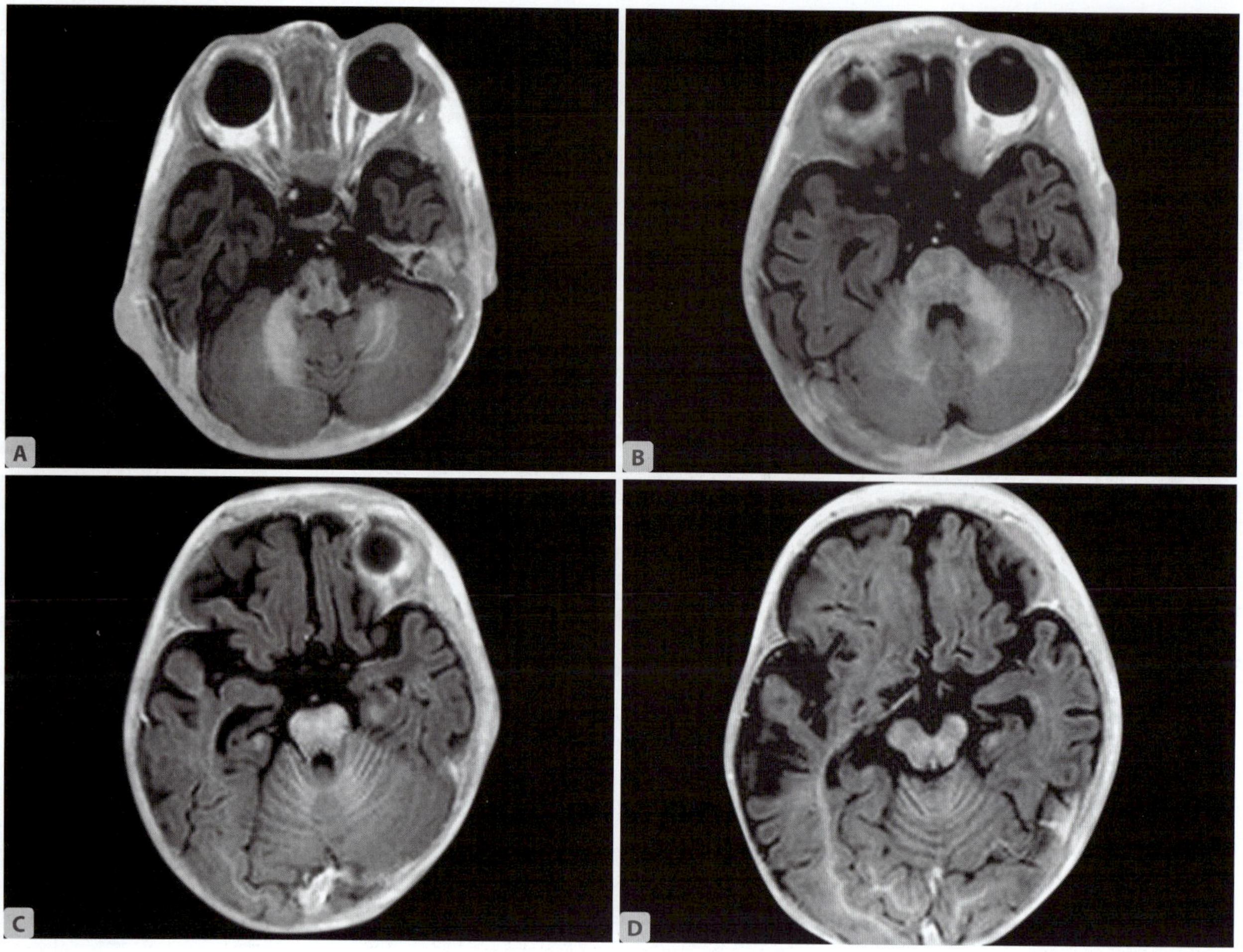

FIGS. 2A TO D: (A) Inversion recovery images in a 9-month-old infant showing normal myelin deposition in medulla and inferior cerebellar peduncles; (B) Pons and middle cerebellar peduncles; (C) Cerebellum; and (D) In midbrain.

Hypomyelination

The term is used when there occurs an actual arrest of myelination.[5] This is not reversible and indicates a permanent failure of myelination. A follow-up MRI would indicate no improvement, thereby differentiating it from delayed myelination. Pelizaeus–Merzbacher disease (PMD) is the classical example.

Demyelination

Demyelination refers to the loss of normal myelin. The normal preformed myelin breaks down secondary to toxins (exotoxins like chemotherapy), inflammation, ischemia, trauma, or due to functional changes in myelin. Multiple sclerosis is the classical example.

Dysmyelination

The term is used when there is a defect in the basic composition of myelin.[6] This defect can arise from an enzymatic deficiency that leads to abnormal accumulation of metabolites [very long-chain fatty acids in X-linked adrenoleukodystrophy (ALD), cerebroside sulfates in metachromatic leukodystrophy] or absence of a normal myelin component or due to defective myelin component, e.g., PLP in PMD.

CLASSIFICATION OF METABOLIC DISORDERS

Some methods of organizing the metabolic diseases from an imaging perspective are helpful to both the radiologist and the clinician as narrowing the differential diagnosis facilitates the clinical workup. Many classifications exist, all of them with the aim of facilitating the systematic approach of these diseases.

(A) Classification of Metabolic Disorders According to Brain Substance Involvement

The classification takes into account the dominance of substance involvement, i.e., gray matter, white matter, or both within the brain. This is usually best shown by MRI.[5,7]

Leukodystrophies

This group comprises the metabolic disorders that have a predominant involvement of the white matter.[8] The cause may be an inherited enzyme deficiency that causes abnormal formation, destruction, or turnover of myelin, e.g., lysosomal storage disorders, peroxisomal disorders, and mitochondrial disorders.

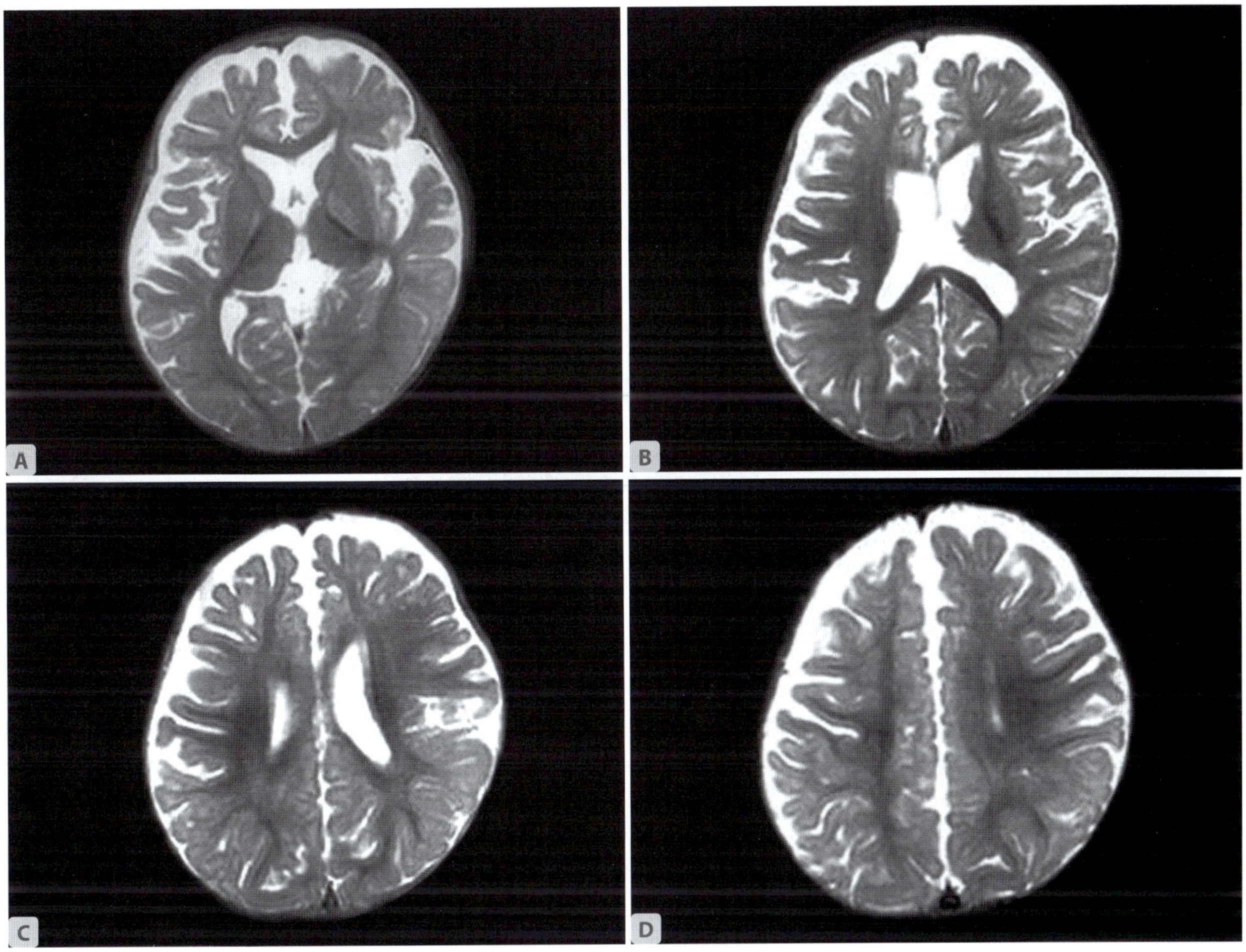

FIGS. 3A TO D: (A) Inversion recovery images in a 9-month-old infant showing normal myelin deposition in posterior and anterior limbs of internal capsule, genu of corpus callosum, and optic radiation; (B) Splenium of corpus; and (C and D) Peripheral white matter (occipital and parietal).

Poliodystrophies

This group comprises diseases that present with predominantly gray matter abnormalities. Some degree of white matter involvement, however, is often present. Classical disease categories are respiratory chain disorders (so-called "mitochondrial diseases") and organic acidopathies.

Pandystrophies

In this, there is involvement of both gray and white matter. The majority of the metabolic disorders fall into this category, since exclusive involvement of the gray or white matter structures is rare.

(B) Classification of Metabolic Disorders on the Basis of Organelle Disorder[9,10]

Lysosomal Storage Diseases with White Matter Involvement

- Metachromatic leukodystrophy (MLD)
- Krabbe disease
- Sphingolipidosis
- Fabry disease
- Gaucher disease
- Mucopolysaccharidosis (MPS)
- Niemann–Pick disease
- Fucosidosis
- Wolman disease and cholesteryl ester storage disease
- Ceroid lipofuscinosis

Peroxisomal Disorders

- X-linked ALD
- Zellweger syndrome
- Refsum disease
- Cerebrotendinous xanthomatosis
- Rhizomelic chondrodysplasia calcificans punctata
- Neonatal ALD
- Pseudoneonatal ALD
- Hyperpipecolic acidemia
- Abetalipoproteinemia

White Matter Disorders with Unknown Metabolic Defect

- Canavan disease
- Alexander disease

- Megalencephalic leukodystrophy with subcortical cysts
- Vanishing white matter disease/childhood ataxia with central nervous system (CNS) hypomyelination
- Pelizaeus-Merzbacher disease [metabolic bone disease (MBD)]
- Aicardi-Goutières syndrome
- Cockayne syndrome
- Congenital muscular dystrophy (Fukuyama type)

Mitochondrial Dysfunction with Leukoencephalopathy

- Mitochondrial encephalopathy, lactic acidosis, and stroke-like episodes (MELAS) syndrome
- Myoclonic epilepsy with ragged-red fibers (MERRF) syndrome
- Kearns-Sayre syndrome
- Leigh disease
- Leber's hereditary optic neuropathy (LHON)

In this chapter, the common metabolic disorders are described as per classification B. Following the classification, according to the cellular organelle dysfunction, the metabolic disorders can be described as mentioned below.

Lysosomal Storage Disorders

Metachromatic Leukodystrophy

Metachromatic leukodystrophy is an autosomal recessive disorder. It is the most common leukodystrophy and occurs due to the deficiency of the enzyme arylsulfatase A.[11] The enzyme is necessary for the breakdown of sulfatides, an important constituent of myelin sheath, which then accumulate in the myelin sheath, kidneys, gallbladder, and other viscera. A characteristic metachromatic reaction is obtained due to the accumulation of sulfatides within the glial cells and neurons. The name metachromatic is derived from the characteristic "metachromatic staining" seen in the nuclei of cells in MLD stained with Cresyl violet or toluidine blue. A brownish or reddish color rather than the normal blue color is seen due to the sulfatides.

Metachromatic leukodystrophy is diagnosed biochemically on the basis of an abnormally low level of arylsulfatase A in urine, peripheral blood leukocytes, or cultured fibroblasts. Diagnosis can also be made by sural nerve biopsy. Prenatal diagnosis can be achieved by assaying the activity of the enzyme in cultured amniotic fluid cells.

Clinical features: Three patterns of MLD are recognized—(1) The late infantile, (2) Juvenile, and (3) The adult forms depending on the age of the patient. The *late infantile form* is the most common seen in children between 12 and 18 months of age and is characterized by loss of milestones, motor weakness, and hypotonia followed by neurological deterioration.[12] There is deterioration in intellect, speech, and coordination. There is a rapid downhill course with quadriplegia, gait disturbances, blindness, and decerebrate posturing setting in. Death occurs within 6 months to 4 years after the onset of symptoms. The *juvenile form* begins later in life around 4 years of age and presents with poor school performance and emotional lability in addition to the other clinical features of the disease. The *adult form* is rare and is characterized by dementia followed by motor signs.

Pathologic findings: At autopsy, the surface of the brain appears atrophic, the white matter is shrunken and sclerotic, and the ventricles are dilated. Changes in the peripheral nerve myelin explain the polyneuropathy noted in MLD. The hallmark of the disease is metachromatic granules (20–30 mm in diameter) presumably derivatives of cerebroside sulfate.[12]

Imaging features (Box 1): The typical CT finding is a diffuse lucency of the white matter which is symmetrical and bilateral involving the centrum semiovale and the deep periventricular white matter **(Figs. 4A and B)**. There is a characteristic involvement of the corpus callosum as well. MRI shows symmetric confluent areas of high signal on T2W images in the periventricular and cerebellar white matter. An imaging hallmark of MLD is involvement of the deep periventricular white matter and sparing of the subcortical white matter **(Figs. 5A to C)**.[13,14] There is an occipital predominance of the signal abnormality in the late infantile form with a dorsofrontal progression of the disease. High signal intensity on T2W images along the posterior limbs of the internal capsule and the brainstem, i.e., along the corticospinal tracts, is another characteristic imaging finding. High signal intensity is also seen in the corpus callosum on T2W images **(Figs. 6A to D)**.[15] A tigroid pattern of myelination which consists of areas of normal white matter within the abnormal high signal intensity areas on T2W images is highly characteristic of this disorder.[16] Unlike the late infantile form, the juvenile and adult forms are characterized by a frontal preponderance of findings. Later in the course of the disease, cerebral atrophy with atrophic dilatation of the ventricles can be seen **(Figs. 7A to C)**. In the adult onset, the only imaging finding seen may be diffuse cerebral atrophy.[17]

Diffusion-weighted images (DWI) usually show signal abnormalities.[18,19] Moderate hypersignal is seen in the presumed progression zone of the demyelinating process. In the late stages, diffuse hyposignal is seen. The tigroid pattern is also sometimes conspicuous on the DWI.[20,21] Proton magnetic resonance spectroscopy (MRS) frequently demonstrates abnormality in the metabolic peaks before conventional MR imaging. The spectrum includes decrease in N-acetylaspartate (NAA), abnormal elevation of choline, myoinositol, and lactate peak **(Figs. 8A and B)**.[22] The elevation of myoinositol is highly suggestive of MLD.

BOX 1: Imaging findings in metachromatic leukodystrophy (MLD).

- High signal on T2-weighted MR images involving:
  - Deep periventricular white matter
  - Centrum semiovale
  - Corpus callosum
  - Cerebellar white matter
  - Corticospinal tracts
- Relative sparing of subcortical white matter
- Tigroid pattern of myelination

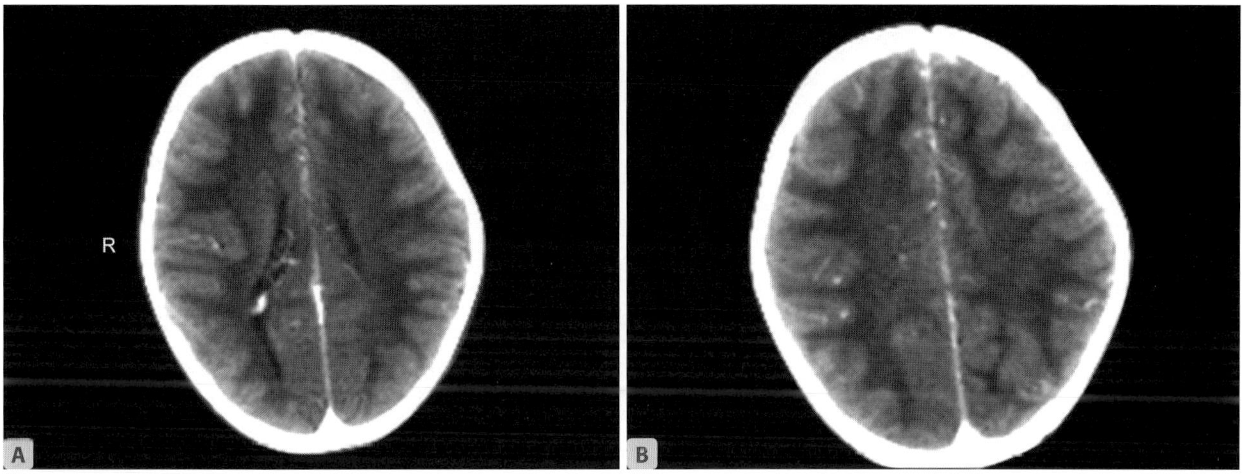

FIGS. 4A AND B: CT image in a 2-year-old child showing diffuse white matter hypodensity in periventricular location with relative sparing of the subcortical white matter—metachromatic leukodystrophy (MLD).

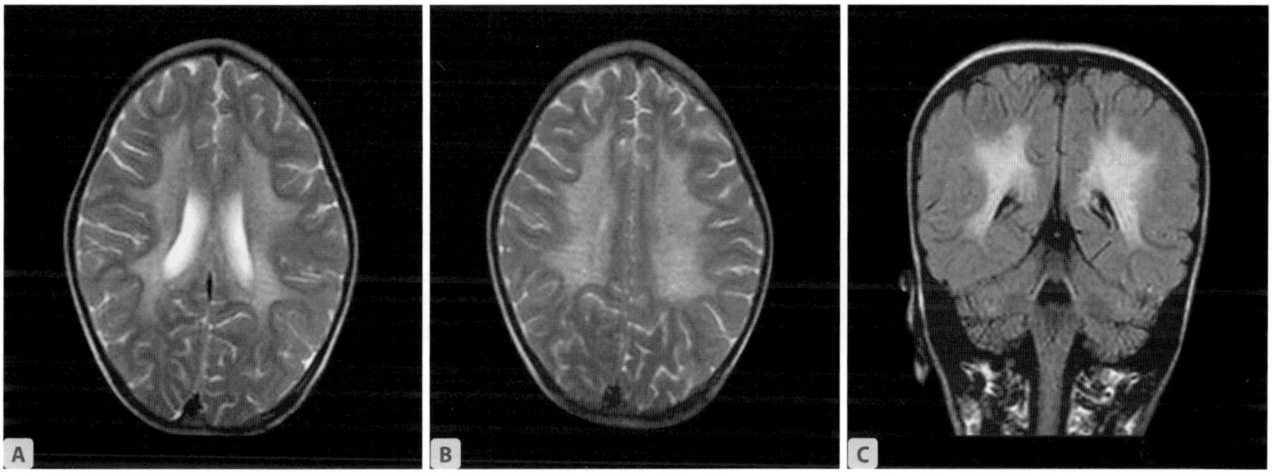

FIGS. 5A TO C: Axial T2W (A and B) and FLAIR coronal (C) MR images showing a symmetric pattern of high signal intensity in the deep periventricular white matter with relative sparing of the subcortical U-fibers. The tigroid pattern of white matter involvement is well seen (B)—metachromatic leukodystrophy (MLD). (FLAIR: fluid-attenuated inversion recovery; T2W: T2-weighted)

Krabbe Disease/Globoid Cell Leukodystrophy

Krabbe disease is an autosomal recessive disorder. It is caused by a deficiency of the lysosomal enzyme beta-galactocerebrosidase with resultant accumulation of cerebroside, a normal constituent of myelin. As soon as myelination commences and myelin turnover becomes necessary, cerebrosides accumulate in the lysosomes of macrophages within the white matter forming the globoid cells characteristic of the disease. The abnormal accumulation of beta-galactocerebrosidase and its derivative psychosine to toxic levels kills oligodendroglial cells. The diagnosis is made by demonstrating a deficiency of the enzyme in peripheral blood leukocytes.

Clinical features: There are two forms of the disease—(1) the early-onset form, and (2) the late-onset form.[23] The *early-onset form* begins before 2 years of age and has three phases. Irritability, fever, spasticity, and hypertonicity characterize first phase which is seen in the first 6 months of life followed by rapid deterioration in motor function, myoclonic jerks, hyperpyrexia, and opisthotonus. Decerebrate posturing and flaccid paralysis characterize the third phase with death occurring by 2 years of age. The *late-onset form* presents after 2 years of age and has a slower progression of the disease.

In the early-onset globoid cell leukodystrophy (GLD), cerebrospinal fluid (CSF) analysis always demonstrates an abnormally high protein level with a normal cell count. In the late-onset form, the protein level is not consistently high in CSF. Bone marrow transplantation has been shown to halt/reverse the neurologic manifestation of disease.[24]

Pathologic findings: The brain is small and weighs only 600–800 g. The white matter is rubbery to firm, but the cortex is relatively unaffected. The pathologic hallmark of Krabbe

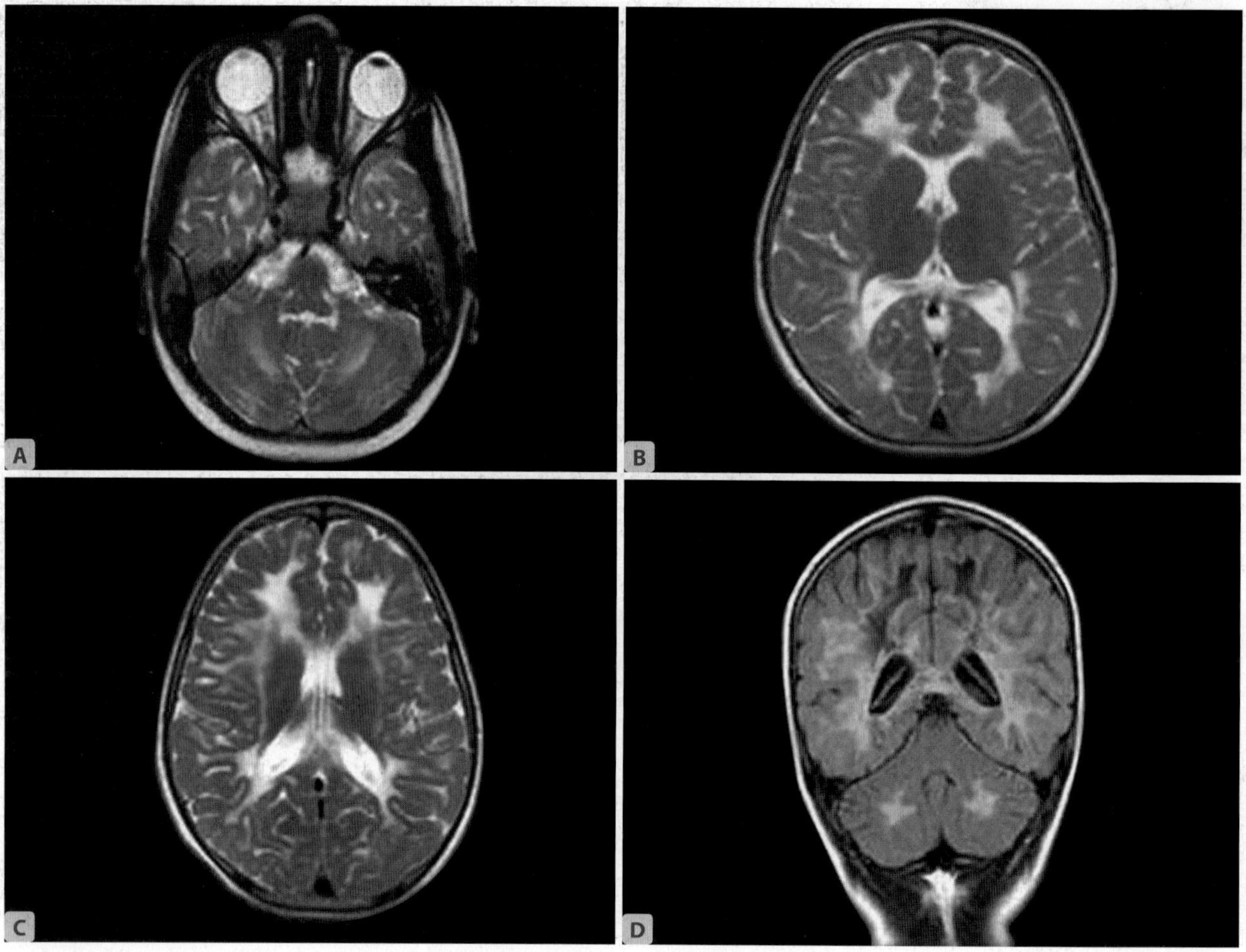

FIGS. 6A TO D: Axial T2W (A to C) and FLAIR coronal (D) MR images showing involvement of the deep periventricular white matter with relative sparing of the subcortical U-fibers. There is involvement of the posterior limbs of internal capsule (B), the cerebellar white matter (A and D), and the splenium of the corpus callosum (D)—metachromatic leukodystrophy (MLD). (FLAIR: fluid-attenuated inversion recovery; T2W: T2-weighted)

disease is a massive accumulation of large multinucleated cells containing periodic acid-Schiff (PAS)-positive material (globoid cells). There is complete myelin destruction with loss of oligodendroglia and marked astrogliosis.

Imaging features (Box 2): Hyperdense thalami, caudate nucleus, and corona radiata constitute the characteristic CT findings and the hyperdensity has been found to correspond to fine calcifications at autopsy. On MR, a high signal intensity on T2WI along the lengths of the corticospinal tracts constitutes the most characteristic imaging finding in both the early- and late-onset forms.[25] There is involvement of the parieto-occipital white matter and splenium of the corpus callosum **(Figs. 9A to E)**. The cerebellar white matter and the deep gray nuclei (dentate, basal ganglia, and thalami) may also be involved in the early-onset form, but not in the late-onset disease. Like MLD, Krabbe disease also involves the deep white matter with relative sparing of the subcortical white matter.[26]

The cranial nerves may be affected with evidence of thickened optic nerve seen on MR imaging and at autopsy. Optic nerve atrophy has also been described in late-onset form. Late-onset cases of GLD with primary involvement of the parietal periventricular white matter, splenium of corpus callosum, and corticospinal tracts may appear similar on imaging to ALD.[27,28] However, auditory pathway involvement is characteristic of ALD and is not seen in GLD.[29,30] MR imaging of the spine shows diffuse hypersignal within the spinal cord parenchyma. Nerve root enhancement may also be detected after intravenous contrast injection.

Diffusion-weighted images may show prominent hypersignal along the presumed progression zone of the demyelinating process like MLD **(Figs. 10A to D)**.[34,35] In the late stages, diffuse hyposignal is seen suggesting complete myelin loss. Diffusion tensor-derived anisotropy maps are useful as a quantitative evaluation of white matter abnormalities in these patients. Diffusion tensor imaging (DTI) scans are being studied as a potential tool for follow-up of patients before and after stem cell transplantation.[36-40] Perfusion MR techniques have also been used in the evaluation of white matter lesions in Krabbe disease. It shows a decreased intralesional cerebral blood volume.

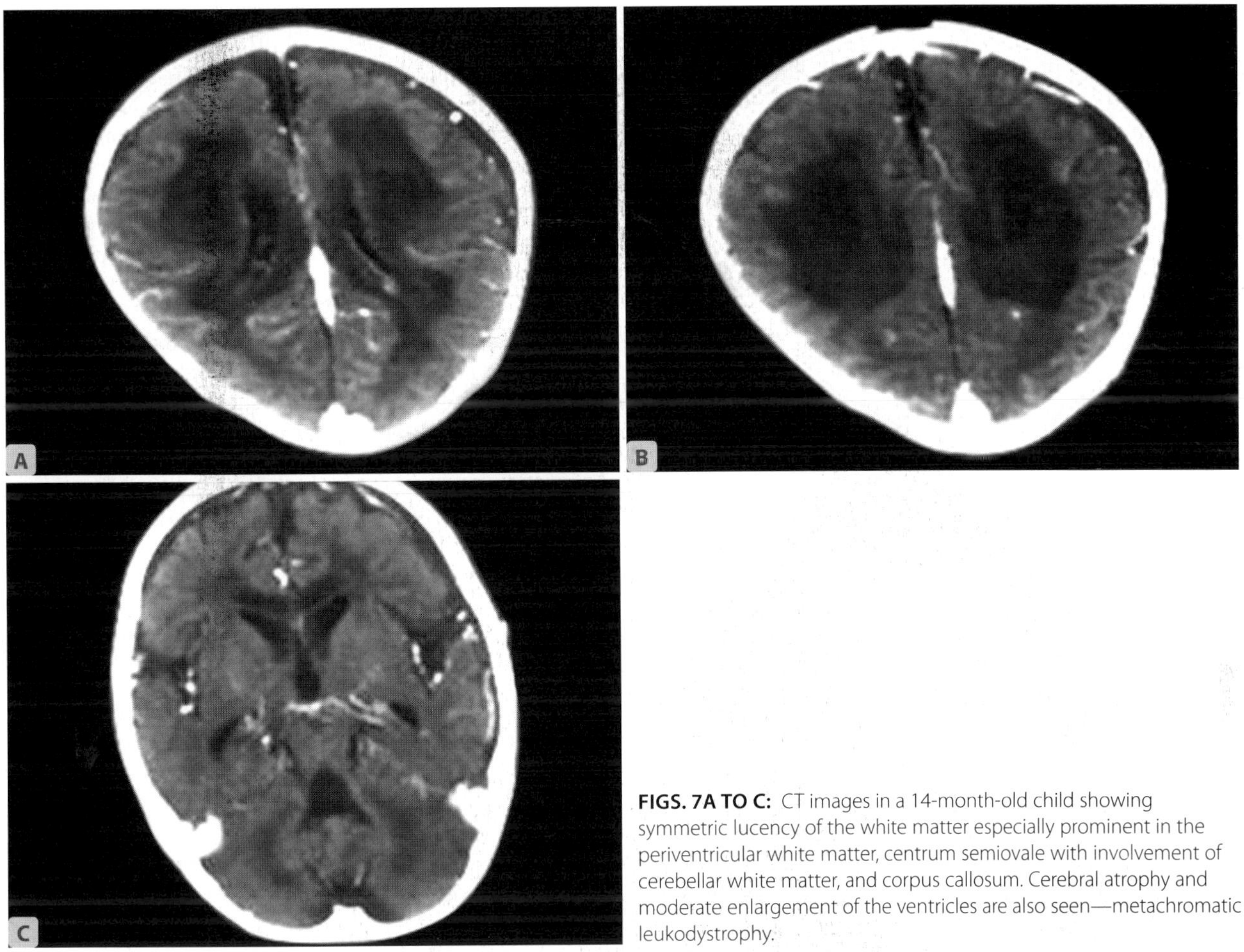

FIGS. 7A TO C: CT images in a 14-month-old child showing symmetric lucency of the white matter especially prominent in the periventricular white matter, centrum semiovale with involvement of cerebellar white matter, and corpus callosum. Cerebral atrophy and moderate enlargement of the ventricles are also seen—metachromatic leukodystrophy.

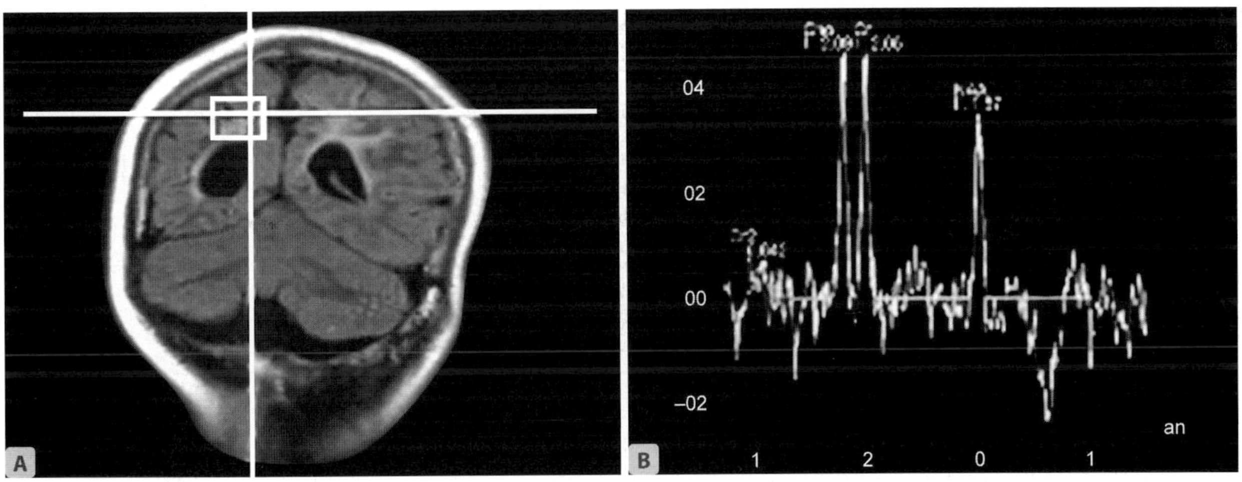

FIGS. 8A AND B: Coronal FLAIR images with voxel placement in the hyperintensity in frontal white matter shows abnormal elevation of choline peak—an early finding in MLD. (FLAIR: fluid-attenuated inversion recovery; MLD: metachromatic leukodystrophy)

Sphingolipidosis

The sphingolipidoses involve abnormal metabolism and accumulation of sphingolipids. Deficiency of hexosaminidase A alone results in GM2 gangliosidosis, the classic form of which is Tay-Sachs disease. Sandhoff disease is caused by a deficiency in both hexosaminidase A and B.[41] Clinical findings are identical to that of Tay-Sachs disease with additional findings of hepatosplenomegaly and bony deformities.

Clinical features: Onset of symptoms is between 3 and 6 months of age. The initial sign is an excessive startle reflex. A cherry red spot in the macula is almost always present at this stage and psychomotor regression then begins. Patients are macrocephalic and there is progressive psychomotor retardation, pyramidal and later extrapyramidal (choreoathetosis) signs, and generalized tonic-clonic seizures.

BOX 2: Imaging findings in Krabbe disease.[31-33]

- High signal on T2-weighted MR images:
  - Along corticospinal tracts
  - Cerebellar white matter
  - Deep gray nuclei (only in early-onset form)
  - Parieto-occipital white matter and splenium of the corpus callosum
  - Spinal cord parenchyma
- Optic nerve atrophy seen (late onset)

Imaging features: The imaging findings in Tay–Sachs and Sandhoff disease are quite similar. CT examination of the brain shows hyperdensities within the basal ganglia and/ or thalami due to calcifications. MR imaging is sensitive in demonstrating the widespread white matter changes within the cerebral hemispheres. All the white matter structures are involved except for the corpus callosum, the anterior commissure, and the posterior limbs of the internal capsules. The external and extreme capsules, the globi pallidi, and the putamina are all abnormal. The involved basal ganglia structures (putamina, caudate nucleus) are somewhat swollen particularly during the initial course of the disease. The thalami are spared and show low signal on T2W images. The cerebellar white matter often shows signal abnormalities on the T2W images and the hyperintensities are less prominent than supratentorially **(Figs. 11A to C)**. Typically, no abnormalities are seen within the brainstem and spinal cord. The overall lesion pattern in a macrocephalic infant can be highly suggestive of the disease.

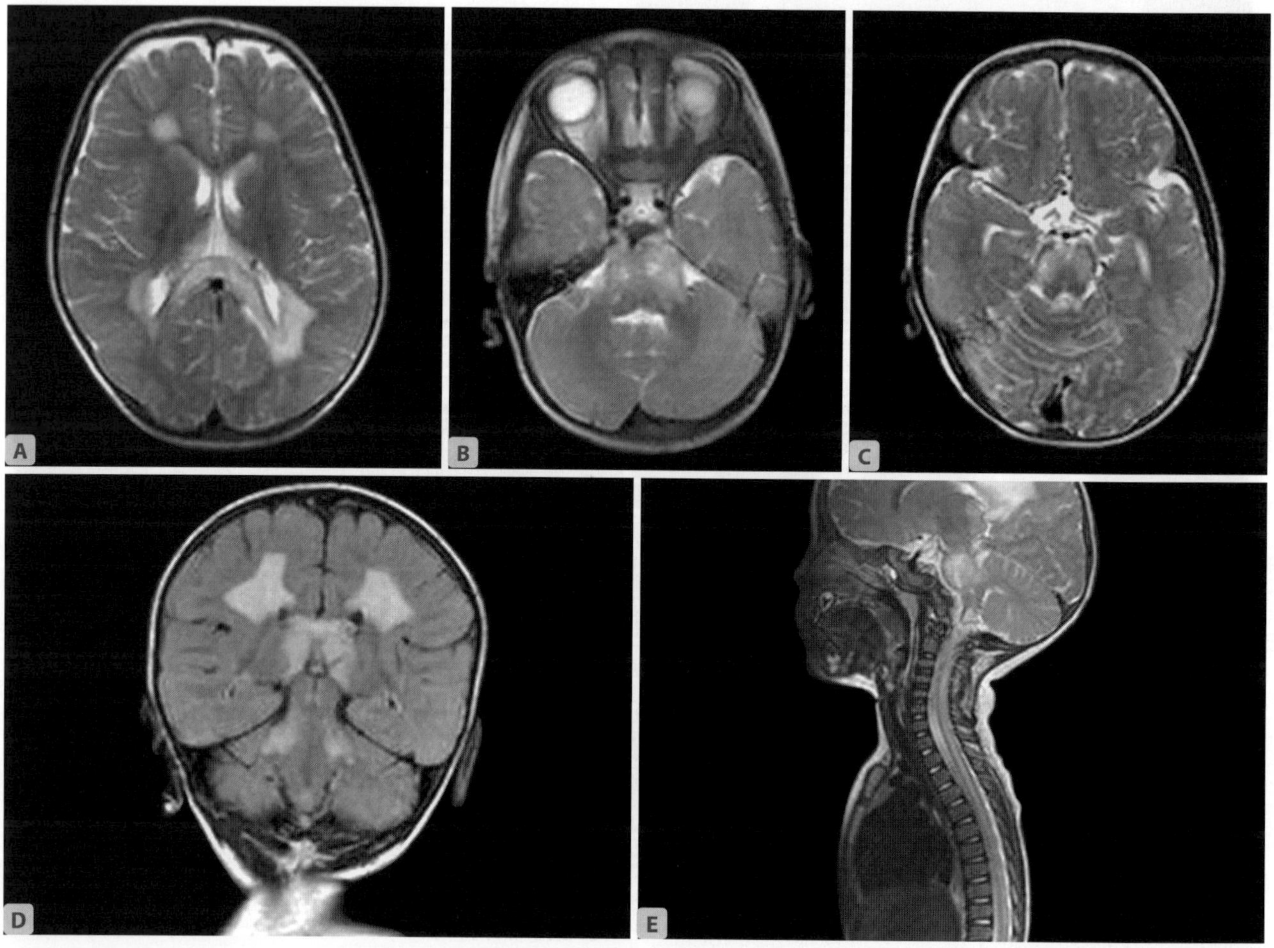

FIGS. 9A TO E: Axial T2W (A to C) and FLAIR coronal MR image (D) showing symmetric areas of white matter hyperintensity predominantly involving the parieto-occipital white matter with some involvement of the frontal white matter with relative sparing of the subcortical U-fibers (A and D). Involvement of the splenium (A) and the corticospinal tracts (B and C) is seen. Sagittal T2W MR image of the cervicodorsal spine (E) reveals high signal intensity within the spinal cord parenchyma—late-onset Krabbe disease. (FLAIR: fluid-attenuated inversion recovery; T2W: T2-weighted)

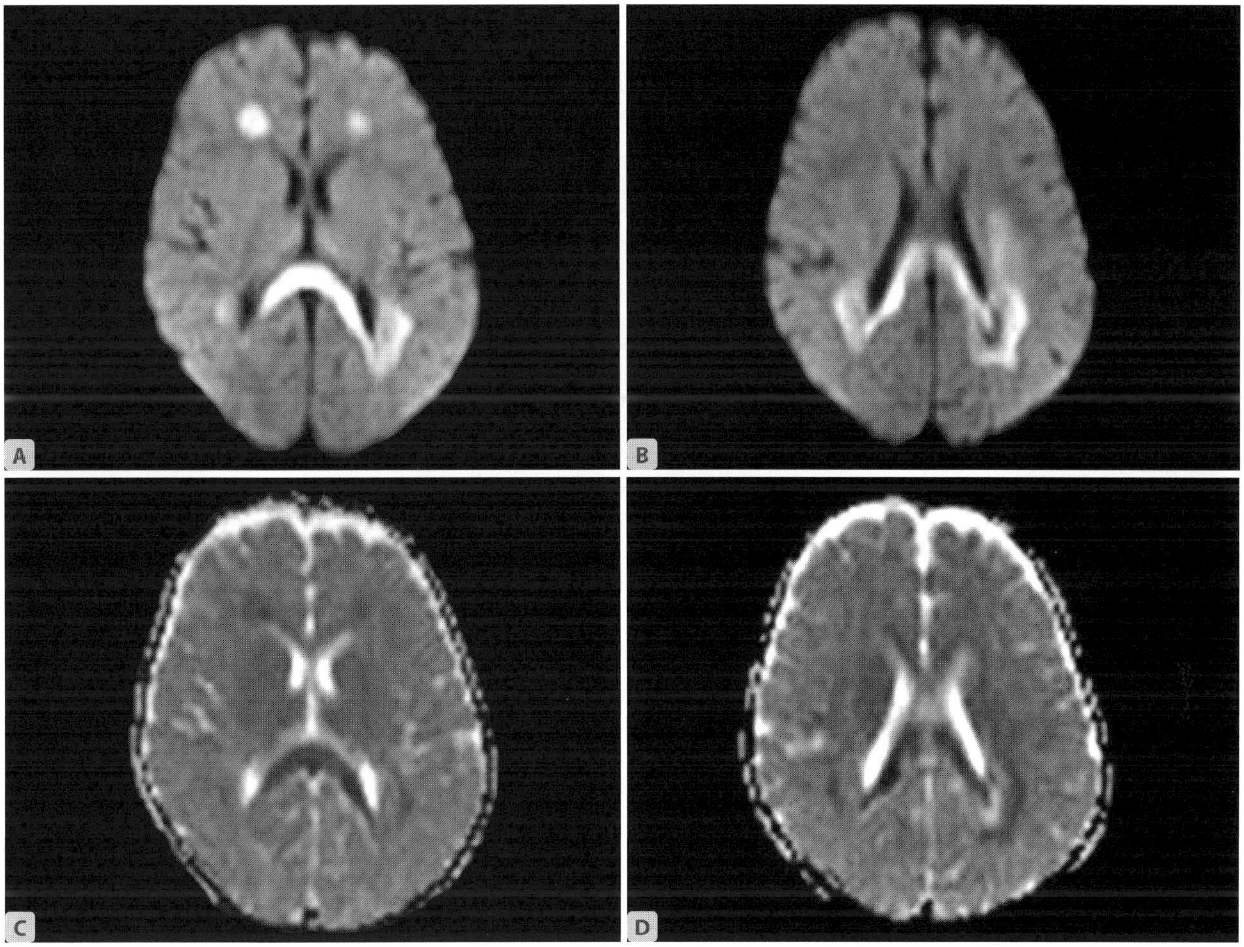

FIGS. 10A TO D: (A and B) Diffusion-weighted MR images in the same case showing a prominent hypersignal along the progression line of the demyelinating process reflecting the centrifugal gradient and the posteroanterior gradient of the disease process; and (C and D) Apparent diffusion coefficient (ADC) maps reveal a hyposignal suggestive of a restricted pattern of diffusion—Krabbe disease.

Diffusion-weighted images are usually quite unremarkable which suggest a slow demyelinating process. MR spectroscopy shows nonspecific alteration, the NAA peak is decreased, and the choline peak is increased. No lactate is identified.

Fabry Disease[42]

This is an X-linked recessive disorder due to deficiency of the lysosomal enzyme α-galactosidase A, which results in accumulation of glycosphingolipids in the vascular endothelium, smooth muscles, and neurons.

Clinical features: It typically presents late in childhood, but occasionally is not recognized until third or fourth decade of life. Early manifestations include a punctate telangiectatic skin and mucous membrane lesion followed by fever, weight loss, and pain in extremities and abdomen. Retinal, corneal, and conjunctival abnormalities are present early in the disease. Cardiac disease develops with age and is typically worsened by a systemic hypertension secondary to vascular disease. Patients may eventually present with transient ischemic attacks or strokes secondary to small vessel ischemia and focal infarcts.

Pathologic findings: Glycosphingolipids accumulate in the vascular endothelium particularly in the small vessels throughout the brain and spinal cord. Storage of lipids is seen within neurons of amygdala, hypothalamus, and the brainstem. Focal infarcts are frequently found in the basal ganglia and central white matter.

Imaging features: Early in the disease, small areas of high signal intensity are seen on long repetition time (TR) sequences, most commonly in the basal ganglia and periventricular white matter. The periventricular disease becomes more extensive and confluent with time and associated generalized loss of cerebral volume. Cerebral hemorrhage has also been reported.[42,43]

Gaucher Disease

Gaucher disease includes several autosomal recessive lipid storage diseases in which there is a deficiency of the lysosomal enzyme glucocerebrosidase.

Clinical features: Neurologic symptoms include seizures, developmental regression, spasticity, mental deficiency, incoordination, and tics.

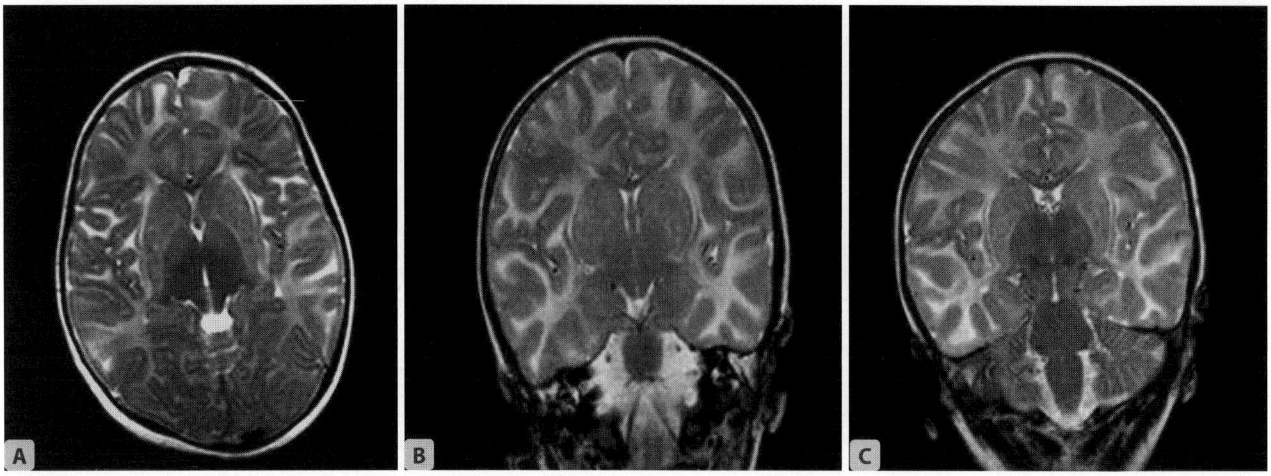

FIGS. 11A TO C: T2W axial (A) and FLAIR coronal (B and C) MR images showing extensive white matter changes in the supratentorial compartment with relative sparing of the infratentorial compartment. The basal ganglia (the putamina, caudate nucleus), the external, and the extreme capsules are all abnormal showing a high signal (A and B). The claustra are well-delineated due to the involvement of the external and extreme capsules (A). The thalami are spared and show low signal on the T2W images—Tay–Sachs disease.

Imaging features: CT and MR findings are similar to those of Fabry disease with atrophy, infarction, and occasional hemorrhage.

Mucopolysaccharidosis[44]

In MPS, impaired degradation of the various mucopolysaccharides (also known as glycosaminoglycans) causes variable combinations of coarse facies, short stature, bony defects, stiff joints, mental retardation, hepatosplenomegaly, and corneal clouding. All forms of MPS are autosomal recessive except MPS type II (Hunter syndrome) which is X-linked recessive. Imaging studies are usually performed when hydrocephalus or spinal cord compression is suspected. CT and MR reveal delayed myelination, atrophy, varying degrees of hydrocephalus, and white matter changes. In all types of MPS, the white matter abnormalities are manifested as sharply-defined foci in the corpus callosum and basal ganglia, isointense with CSF on all imaging sequences.[44] These represent enlarged perivascular spaces filled with mucopolysaccharide or CSF. With progression of the disease, the lesions become larger and more diffuse and resemble a leukodystrophy, reflecting the development of infarcts and demyelination. The atrophy and white matter changes become more progressive with time. Affected patients are commonly macrocephalic from a combination of hydrocephalus and mucopolysaccharide deposition within the brain, meninges, and skull.[45] A high incidence of intracranial arachnoid cysts has also been seen. The spine in MPS is usually imaged to determine the site and cause of cord compression which occurs frequently in MPS types IV and VI. The most common locations for cord compression are at the atlantoaxial joint. Atlantoaxial subluxation may occur in these patients as a result of laxity of transverse ligament in conjugation with hypoplasia of the odontoid.[46]

Magnetic resonance shows a shortened odontoid with a soft-tissue mass of variable size with intermediate signal on T1W and low signal on T2W images. The low signal on T2W images is a combination of unossified fibrocartilage and reactive changes. Another cause of cord compression at the C1–C2 level is dural thickening resulting from intradural deposition of collagen and mucopolysaccharides. This is seen as a thickening of the soft-tissue posterior to the dens with consequent cord compression. MR spectroscopy shows a decreased NAA/choline ratio and elevated glutamate, glutamine, and myoinositol.

Peroxisomal Disorders

Peroxisomes are responsible for the oxidation of very long chain and monosaturated fatty acids, the peroxisomal enzymes being involved in lysine metabolism, gluconeogenesis, and glutaric acid metabolism. The peroxisomal disorders can be broadly classified as—(i) defect in the formation and maintenance of white matter with X-linked ALD being the classical example, (ii) migrational disorders with Zellweger syndrome being the prototype, and (iii) development of neuronal degeneration such as cerebellar atrophy—the example being rhizomelic chondrodysplasia punctate.

X-linked Adrenoleukodystrophy

X-linked ALD is a peroxisomal disorder that affects the white matter of the CNS, adrenal cortex, and testes. This is the best known and most frequent of the peroxisomal disorders. It is a true leukodystrophy with no involvement of the gray matter structures.[47]

The genetic defect responsible for X-linked ALD is located in Xq28, the terminal segment of the long arm of the X chromosome.[48] X-linked ALD is caused by a deficiency of a single enzyme, acyl-CoA synthetase. The deficiency prevents the breakdown of very long-chain fatty acids which then accumulate in tissue and plasma. A rare form of ALD, neonatal ALD, is an autosomal recessive disorder characterized by multiple enzyme deficiencies. Adrenomyeloneuropathy probably represents a phenotypic adult variant of ALD and is characterized by adrenal insufficiency. Typically, the disease has slow progression, with survival into the eighth decade.[49]

Clinical features: The onset of symptoms is typically between 5 and 9 years. Since it is an X-linked disorder, it commonly affects male children. The presentation is with poor school performance, behavior problems, ataxia, visual and hearing problems, and decreasing mental functions. Seizures, spastic quadriparesis, and quadriplegia ensue with death occurring within the first few years of onset.[50]

Pathologic findings: The findings seen on histology correspond to the zones of activity seen on imaging studies.[51] The central zone of demyelination shows absent myelin sheath and oligodendroglia with glial stranding and scattered astrocytes. No active disease is seen in this zone. The next zone is of active inflammation and corresponds to the enhancing zone seen on postcontrast studies. This zone shows many macrophages filled with lipid. The outermost zone shows active myelin breakdown but no inflammation.

Imaging features (Box 3): The characteristic imaging findings include symmetric areas of T2W high signal involving the peritrigonal areas and the splenium of the corpus callosum.[52] The area of signal alteration spreads in a cephalad and outward direction to form a confluent mass involving almost the entire white matter **(Figs. 12A and B)**.[53] There is an involvement of the subcortical white matter very late in the disease with disease progression which is centrifugal and posteroanterior in nature **(Figs. 13A to C)**. The three zones of demyelination seen on histology are seen on imaging as well **(Figs. 14A and B)**.[54,55] The inner or central zone (zone of irreversible gliosis on histology) is seen as markedly hypointense on T1W MR and markedly hyperintense at T2W imaging. The intermediate zone (zone of active inflammation) is isointense on T1W images and shows rapid enhancement after contrast administration.[56] The outermost zone (zone of active demyelination but no inflammation) appears moderately hyperintense on long TR images with no evidence of contrast enhancement. Another characteristic imaging finding is the involvement of the pontomedullary corticospinal tract.[57] Rarely, there may be unilateral or predominant involvement of the frontal lobe white matter **(Figs. 15A to E)**.[58]

BOX 3: Imaging findings in adrenoleukodystrophy.

- High signal on T2-weighted (T2W) images involving:
  - Peritrigonal areas
  - Splenium of corpus callosum
  - Pontomedullary corticospinal tract
- Enhancement of active zone of inflammation—characteristic

Diffusion-weighted MR images also reveal the three distinct zones in the cerebral hemispheric white matter lesions. The burned out zone is hypointense, the intermediate inflammatory zone is moderately hyperintense, and the most peripheral demyelinating zone is very faintly hyperintense. MRS has a role in the prognostic assessment of ALD as it may become abnormal before the conventional MR findings.[59,60] On MRS, a decrease in NAA peak and an elevated choline peak are seen in cases of ALD **(Figs. 16A to D)**.[61]

Adrenomyeloneuropathy: Adrenomyeloneuropathy is not an independent disease entity; it is actually one of the clinical phenotypes of X-linked ALD. The age of onset is usually between 20 and 30 years but since both the clinical and the imaging findings are quite different from those in X-linked ALD, it is treated as a separate disease entity. Ataxia and paraparesis as well as peripheral neuropathy dominate the neurological presentation; mild cognitive disorder is often present as well.[62] Adrenal insufficiency is a frequent associated clinical finding.

On MR imaging, the lesions are predominantly found within the cerebellum and the brainstem. Both structures are atrophic. The brainstem signal abnormalities are significant, but the tegmental structures are relatively spared. The cerebellar white matter is diffusely abnormal. Involvement of the supratentorial white matter is limited mainly to the posterior limbs of the internal capsules and the splenium of the corpus callosum as well as the hemispheric white matter occasionally. Enhancement may also occur within the lesions after intravenous contrast injection. MR of the brain in adrenomyeloneuropathy may even be normal with

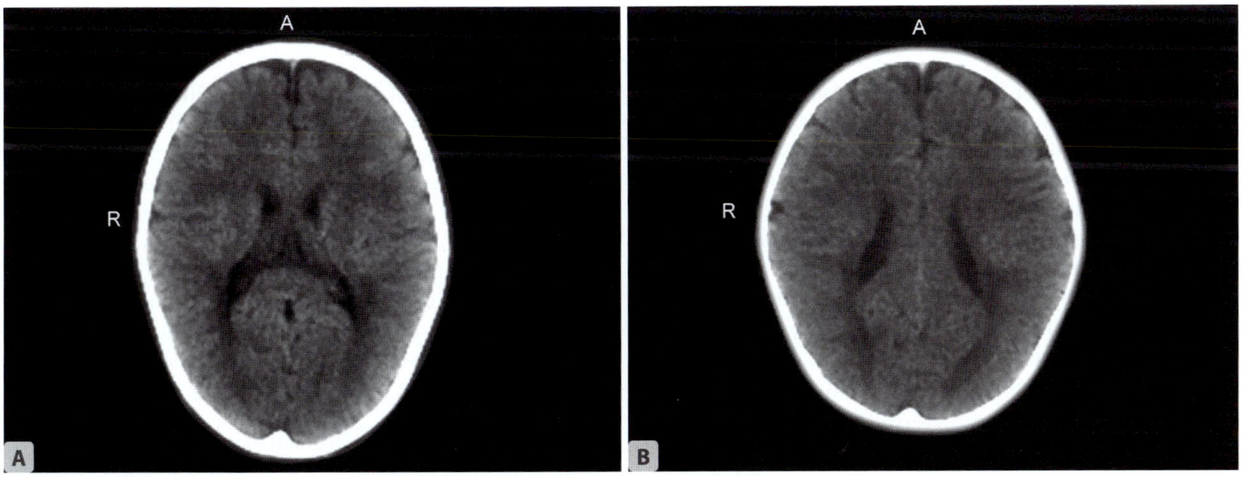

FIGS. 12A AND B: CT image in a child showing white matter hypodensity in the parieto-occipital and the peritrigonal areas—X-linked adrenoleukodystrophy.

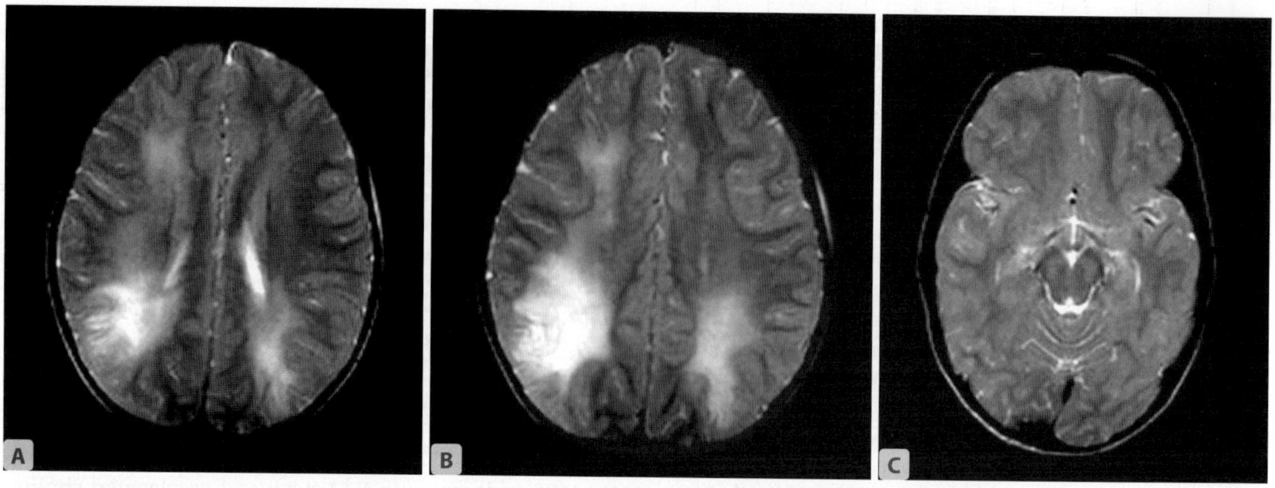

FIGS. 13A TO C: (A to C) Axial T2-weighted (T2W) MR images are showing extensive high signal abnormality in the peritrigonal regions in a bilateral symmetric pattern. Involvement of the corticospinal tracts is also seen (C)—X-linked adrenoleukodystrophy.

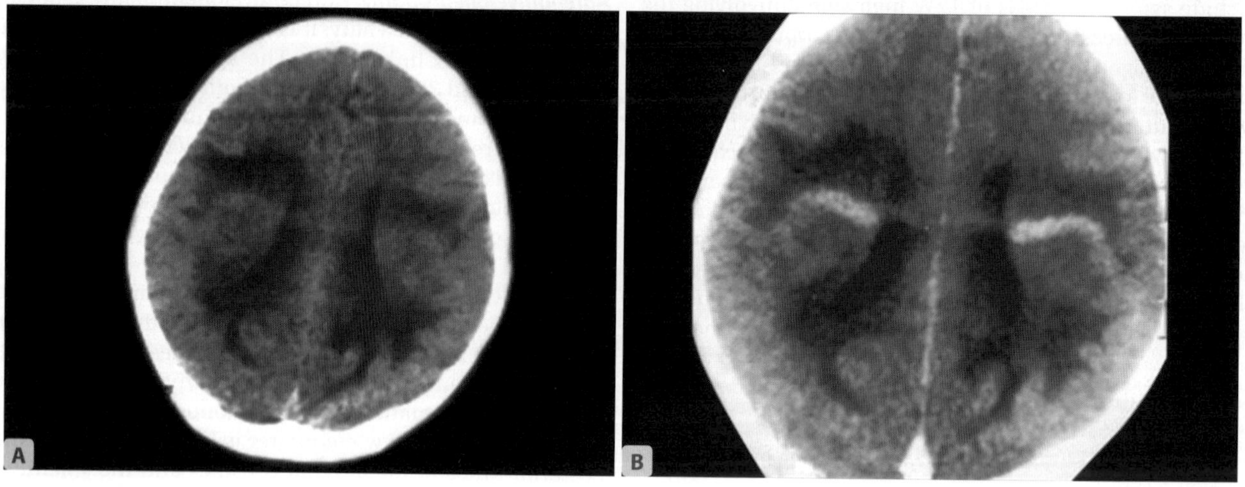

FIGS. 14A AND B: CT images showing symmetric areas of hypodensity in the peritrigonal regions extending across the splenium of the corpus callosum. These hypodensities are seen to extend outward and cephalad as a confluent lesion. Contrast enhancement is seen at the site of active inflammation—X-linked adrenoleukodystrophy.

neurologic involvement confined to the spinal cord and peripheral nerves.

Zellweger Syndrome

Zellweger syndrome or cerebrohepatorenal syndrome is an autosomal recessive disorder caused by multiple enzyme defects and characterized by liver dysfunction with jaundice, marked mental retardation, weakness, hypotonia, and craniofacial dysmorphism. It may lead to death in early childhood. The severity of the disease varies and is determined by the degree of peroxisomal activity.

Magnetic resonance imaging reveals diffuse demyelination with abnormal gyration that is most severe in the perisylvian and perirolandic regions.[63] The pattern of gyral abnormality is similar to that seen in polymicrogyria or pachygyria.

Magnetic resonance hallmarks of the disease are very markedly delayed myelination, brain atrophy, periventricular germinolytic cysts and bilateral symmetrical perisylvian cortical dysplasia (polymicrogyria), and gray matter heterotopias. The combination of these is pathognomonic of Zellweger syndrome.

Refsum Disease

This rare peroxisomal disorder is transmitted as an autosomal recessive condition and is caused by a deficiency of phytanic acid 2-hydroxylase which causes phytanic acid to accumulate in the myelin. The myelin, thus, affected has less viability. The infantile form is more severe. The affected children present with severe sensorineural deafness, retinitis pigmentosa, facial dysmorphism, hepatomegaly, growth retardation, and mental retardation. MRI may show diffuse white matter hyperintensity in the brain and in the cerebellum on T2W images. The involvement of the cerebellar white matter is more intense than in other conditions.[64]

Cerebrotendinous Xanthomatosis

In this condition, patients are deficient in a liver mitochondrial enzyme required for side chain oxidation of cholesterol to bile salts. The patients may show pyramidal and cerebellar

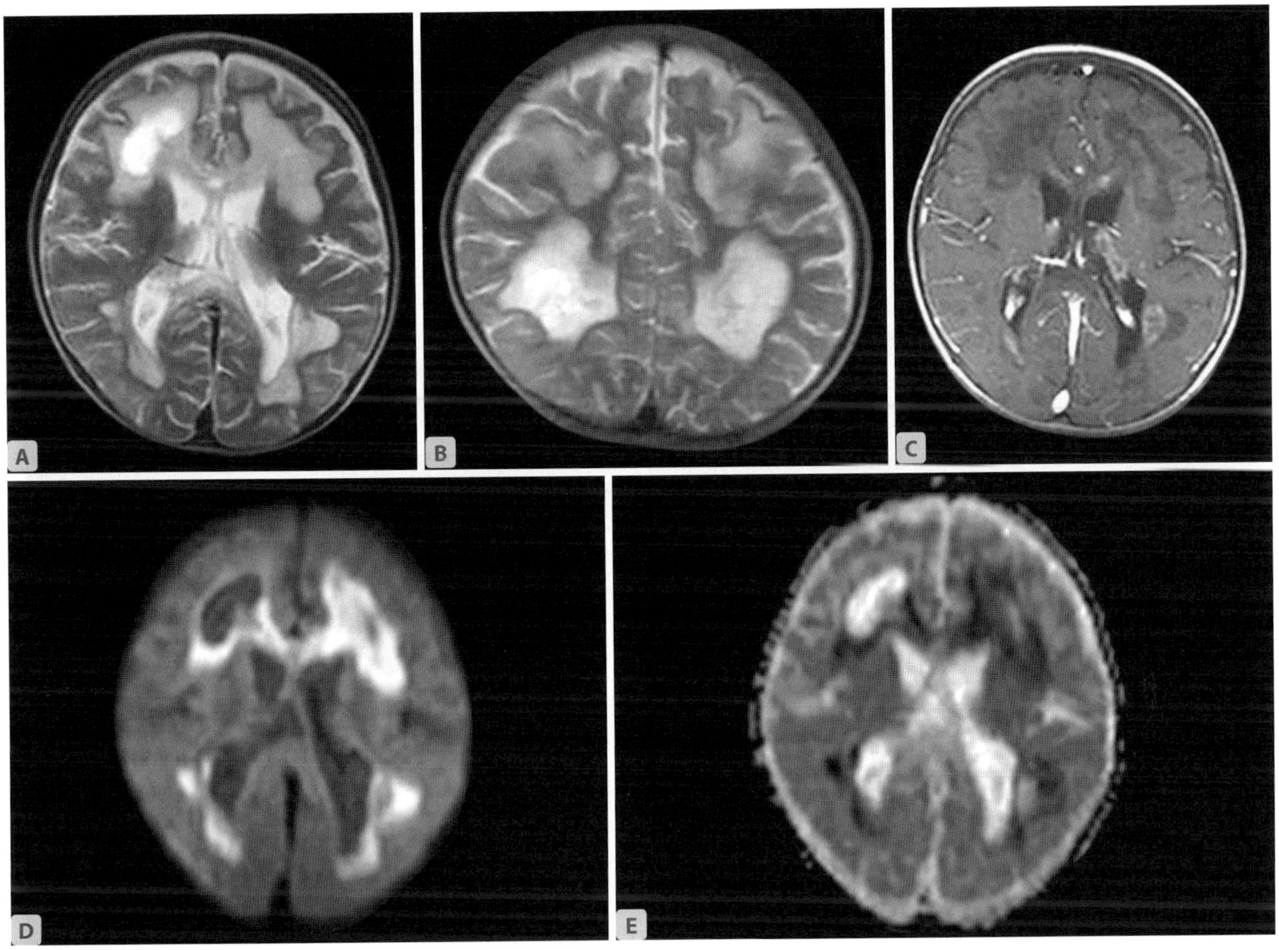

FIGS. 15A TO E: (A and B) Axial T2W MR images showing symmetrical parieto-occipital white matter lesions with sparing of subcortical U-fibers; (C) The intermediate zone of inflammation shows enhancement on the postcontrast images; and (D and E) Diffusion-weighted images show isotropically restricted water diffusion within the intermediate zone with faint hyposignal on the apparent diffusion coefficient image—X-linked adrenoleukodystrophy.

signs and may have mental retardation and usually present xanthomas in the Achilles tendon, the knees, and the elbows. CT may show decreased density in the cerebellum involving the region of dentate nuclei bilaterally. Hypointensity in the same areas is shown on MRI.[65]

Rhizomelic Chondrodysplasia Calcificans Punctata

This rare autosomal recessive disorder causes short limbs, dwarfism, abnormal facies, psychomotor retardation, congenital cataracts, and joint contraction. These patients usually die within the first year of life. The radiographs show finely stippled epiphysis. T2 MRI may show periventricular white matter and subcortical changes, particularly in the occipital region.[64]

Unclassified Leukodystrophies with Unknown Metabolic Defect

Canavan Disease

Also called spongy degeneration of the brain, Canavan disease is caused by the deficiency of the enzyme N-acetylaspartylase with resultant accumulation of N-acetylaspartic acid in the urine, plasma, and brain.[66] Canavan disease is an autosomal recessive disorder and the only disease in the body with a defect in NAA metabolism.[66,67]

Clinical features: Presentation is in early infancy as hypotonia followed by spasticity and cortical blindness. Macrocephaly or a large head size is another characteristic imaging finding. This may not be apparent in the first few months of life, but the head size enlarges above the 90th percentile by 6 months of age. Canavan disease has a progressive downhill course with a mean survival time of 3 years.

Pathologic findings: Grossly, the brain is heavy and soft with markedly increased water content. Canavan disease is characterized at pathologic analysis by extensive vacuolization that initially involves the subcortical white matter and then spreads to deep white matter. Normal myelin is absent and electron microscopy demonstrates increased water content within the glial tissue, described as having the texture of a wet sponge and dysmyelination.

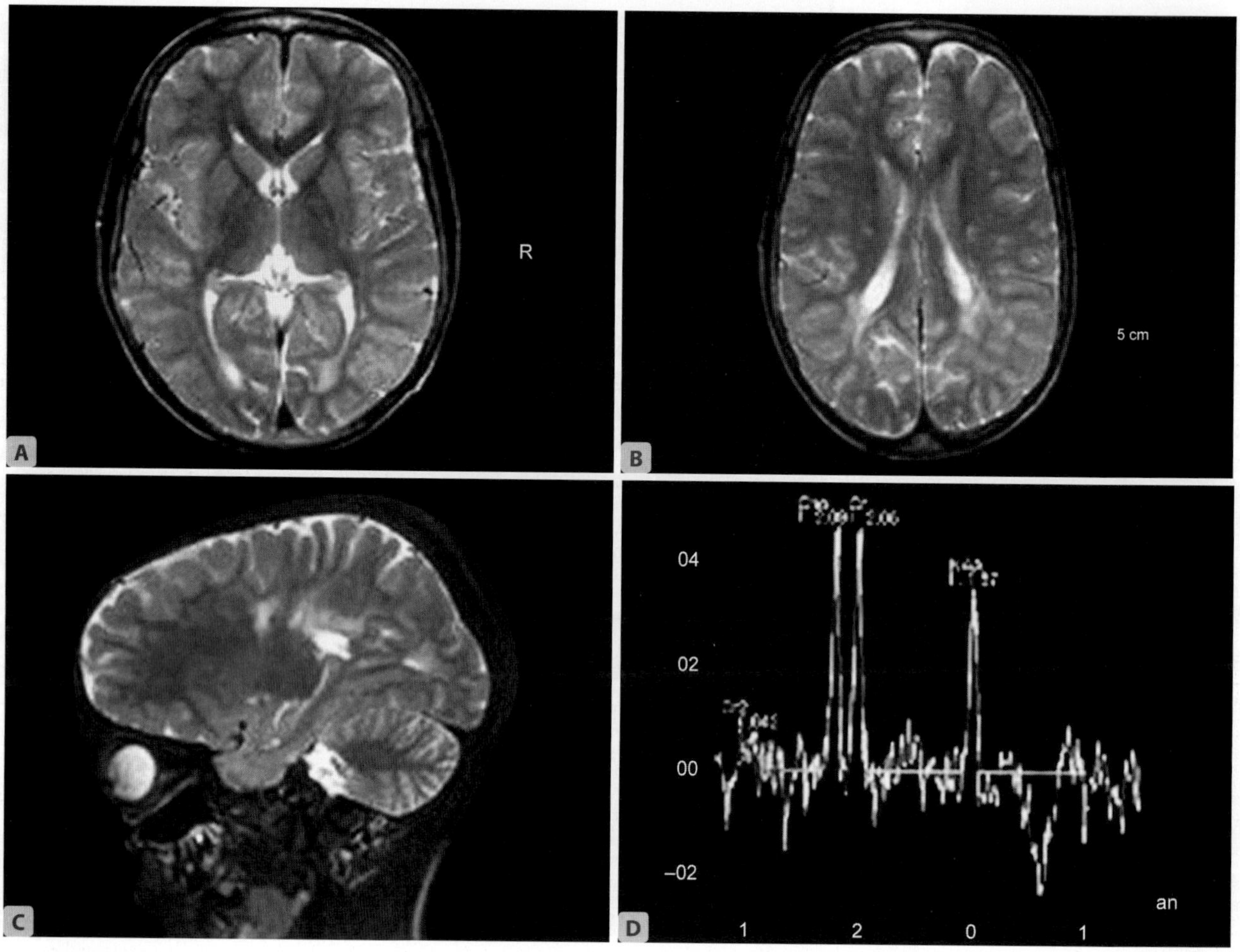

FIGS. 16A TO D: MR spectroscopy with voxel placement in the demyelinating zone in the peritrigonal region reveals a decreased N-acetylaspartate (NAA) and increased choline consistent with increased myelin breakdown—adrenoleukodystrophy.

Imaging features (Box 4): On CT and MR, there is a diffuse involvement of the cerebral and cerebellar white matter seen as an increased signal on T2W images **(Figs. 17A and B)**.[68] There is a predominant involvement of the subcortical U-fibers in Canavan disease unlike MLD and Krabbe disease where there is a relative sparing of the subcortical white matter. There is a centripetal progression of the disease with the central white matter becoming involved with disease progression.[69] There is a relative sparing of the corpus striatum (caudate nucleus and putamen), internal capsules, external capsules, and corpus callosum **(Figs. 18A to E)**. The thalamus and globus pallidus are, however, frequently involved. Atrophy is a late finding.[70,71]

There is evidence of restricted diffusion within the abnormal white matter structures [with increased signal on DWI and decreased signal on the apparent diffusion coefficient (ADC) maps], likely related to myelin edema or a "gelatinous-like" state of the extracellular space. On MR spectroscopy, there is a characteristic increase in NAA peak **(Fig. 19)**.[72]

BOX 4: Imaging findings in Canavan disease.

- High signal on T2W images involving:
  - Cerebral white matter which appears swollen
  - Subcortical U-fibers (in contrast to MLD and Krabbe disease)
  - Cerebellar white matter
  - Thalamus
  - Globus pallidus
- Relative sparing of corpus striatum, internal capsule, external capsule, and corpus callosum
- Increased NAA peak on MRS—pathognomonic

(MLD: metachromatic leukodystrophy; MRS: magnetic resonance spectroscopy; NAA: N-acetylaspartate; T2W: T2-weighted)

Alexander Disease

This leukodystrophy is a rare disorder with a sporadic occurrence and no known pattern of inheritance. It is also called fibrinoid leukodystrophy.[73]

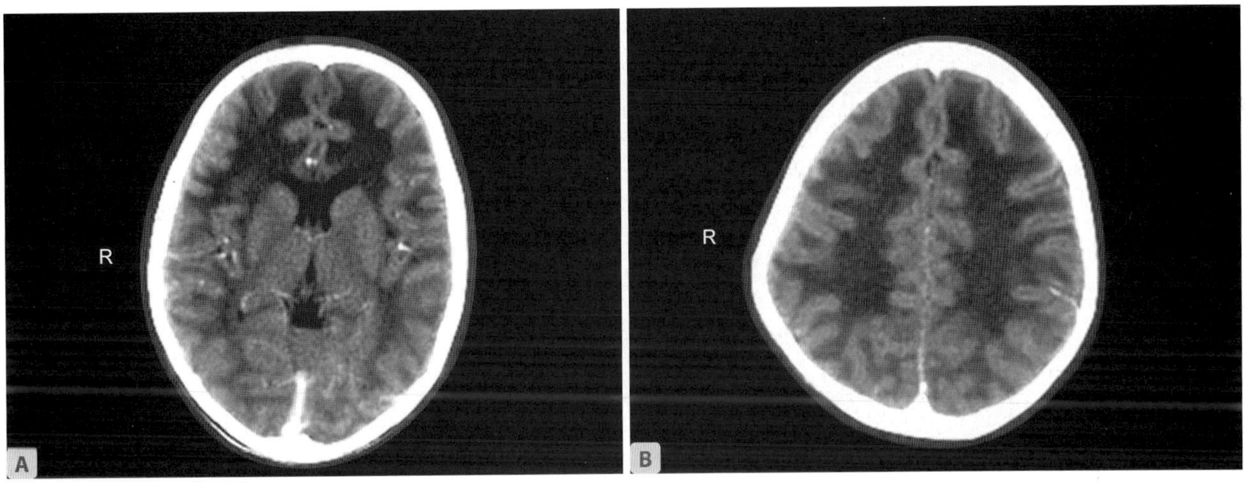

FIGS. 17A AND B: CT image in a child with macrocephaly showing diffuse white matter hypodensity with involvement of subcortical white matter—Canavan disease.

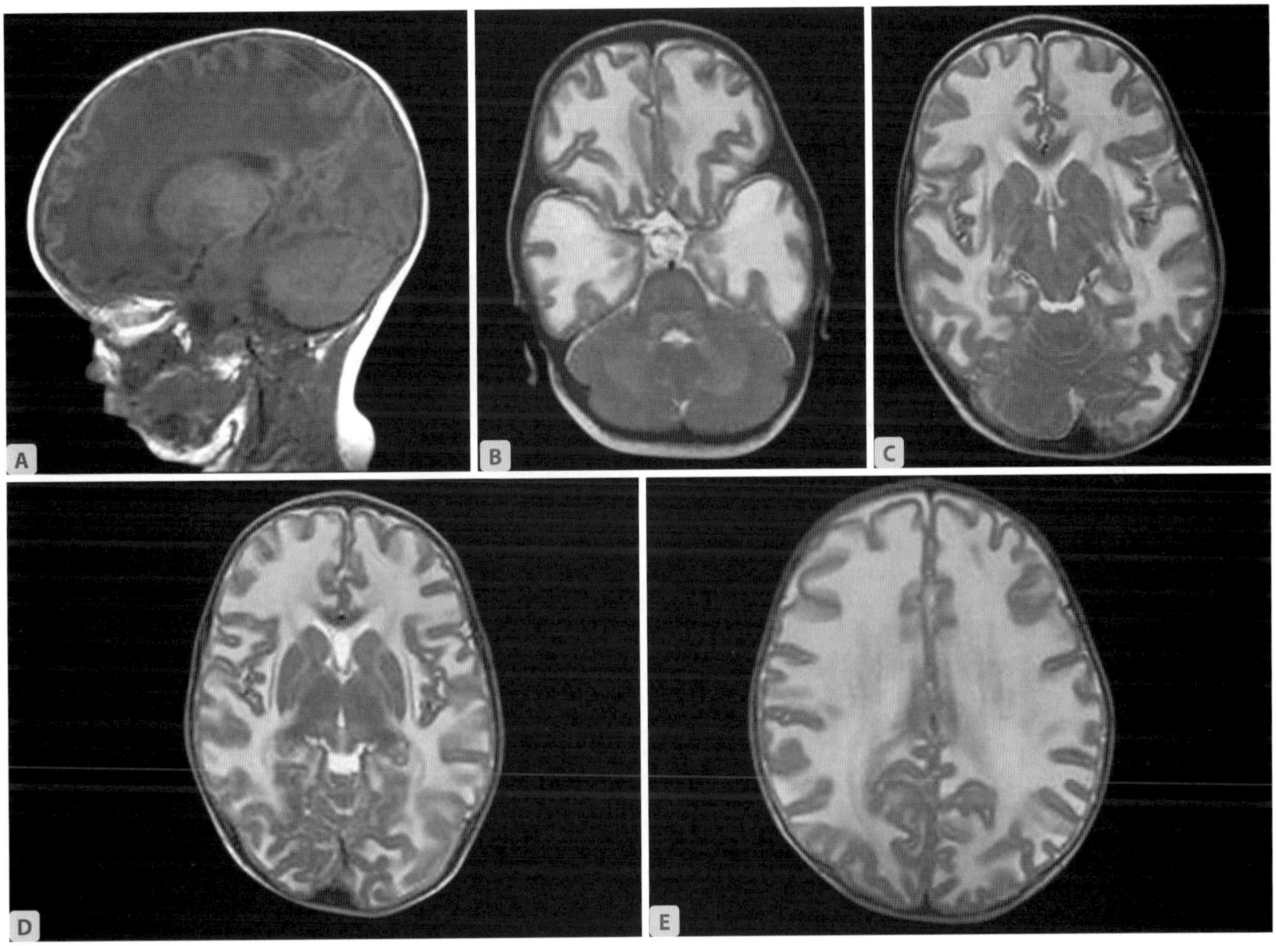

FIGS. 18A TO E: (A) Sagittal T1W MR image showing a widespread diffuse low signal throughout the cerebral white matter; (B and C) Axial T2W MR images reveal a high signal intensity in the white matter with extensive involvement of the subcortical U-fibers. There is involvement of the cerebellar white matter and the brainstem; (D) There is involvement of the globus pallidus with relative sparing of the corpus striatum; (E) The subcortical white matter appears swollen with broadened gyri—Canavan disease.

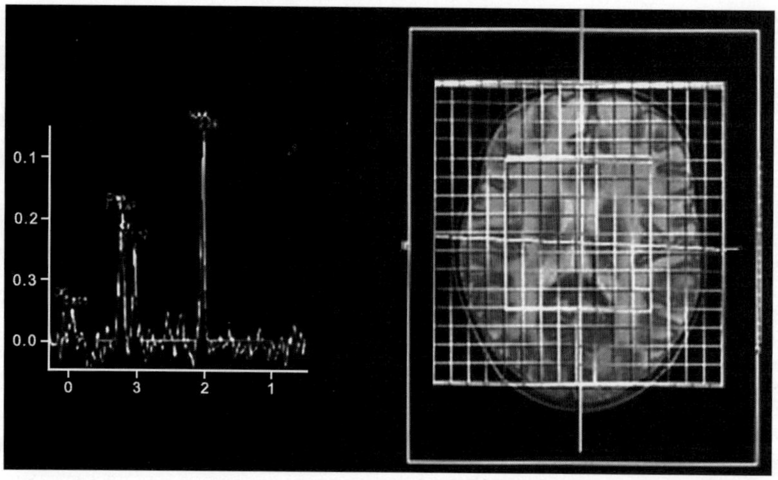

FIG. 19: MR showing a characteristic increase in N-acetylaspartate (NAA) peak—Canavan disease.

Pathologic findings: It is characterized at pathologic analysis by massive deposition of Rosenthal fibers seen as dense eosinophilic, rod-like cytoplasmic inclusions found in astrocytes in the subependymal, subpial, and perivascular regions.

Clinical features: Three clinical subgroups of the disease are recognized—(1) the infantile form, (2) the juvenile, and (3) the adult forms. Alexander disease is also a disorder where infants present with macrocrania or a large head size which occurs early in the disease. There is psychomotor retardation with seizures and death occurring within 2–3 years. A definite diagnosis requires a brain biopsy/autopsy. The *juvenile group* is characterized by onset of symptoms between 7 and 14 years of age with spasticity and bulbar palsy being common. The *adult form* is rare, occurs between second and seventh decades with the symptoms and clinical course mimicking multiple sclerosis.

Imaging features (Box 5): There is a predominant involvement of the frontal white matter which shows a high signal on the T2W images **(Fig. 20)**.[74] There is an early involvement of the subcortical white matter. A posterior progression into the parietal white matter is seen.[75] Internal and external capsules may also show signal alterations. Large cystic lesions are typically seen in the frontal and temporal lobes **(Figs. 21A to E)**. An enhancement of the tips of the frontal horns on the postcontrast images also constitutes a characteristic imaging finding.[74,75] Contrast enhancement may also be seen along the ependymal linings of the lateral ventricles, within the basal ganglia or even the dentate nuclei. Cystic dilation of the cavum septum pellucidum has been described. The occipital white matter and cerebellum are usually spared; however, involvement should not exclude the diagnosis. With disease progression, cavitation and atrophy of the white matter may be seen. Diffusion-weighted MR images may reveal a restricted pattern of diffusion **(Figs. 22A to E)**. When there is diffuse white matter signal abnormality and swelling in a patient with macrocephaly, the differential diagnosis is mainly between Canavan disease and Alexander disease.

BOX 5: Imaging findings in Alexander disease.

- High signal on T2-weighted (T2W) images in frontal white matter
- Early involvement of subcortical white matter
- Large cysts in frontal and temporal regions
- Enhancement of tips of frontal horns, ependymal lining of ventricles
- Cystic dilatation of cavum septum pellucidum

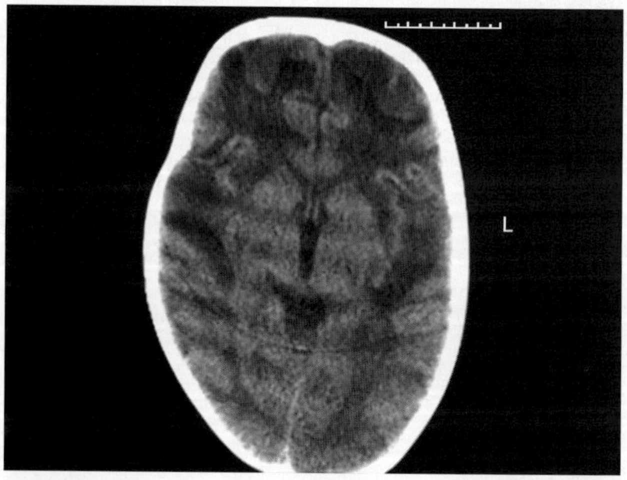

FIG. 20: CT scan showing bilateral symmetric low density areas within the frontal white matter and genu of the corpus callosum—Alexander disease.

Brain biopsy is usually necessary to establish the diagnosis. MR spectroscopy may show a lactate peak, decreased NAA, and elevated myoinositol.

Megaloencephalic Leukodystrophy with Subcortical Cysts

Clinical features: It was earlier called Van der Knaap disease. It is now called infantile-onset spongiform leukoencephalopathy with a discrepantly mild clinical course or megalencephalic leukodystrophy with subcortical

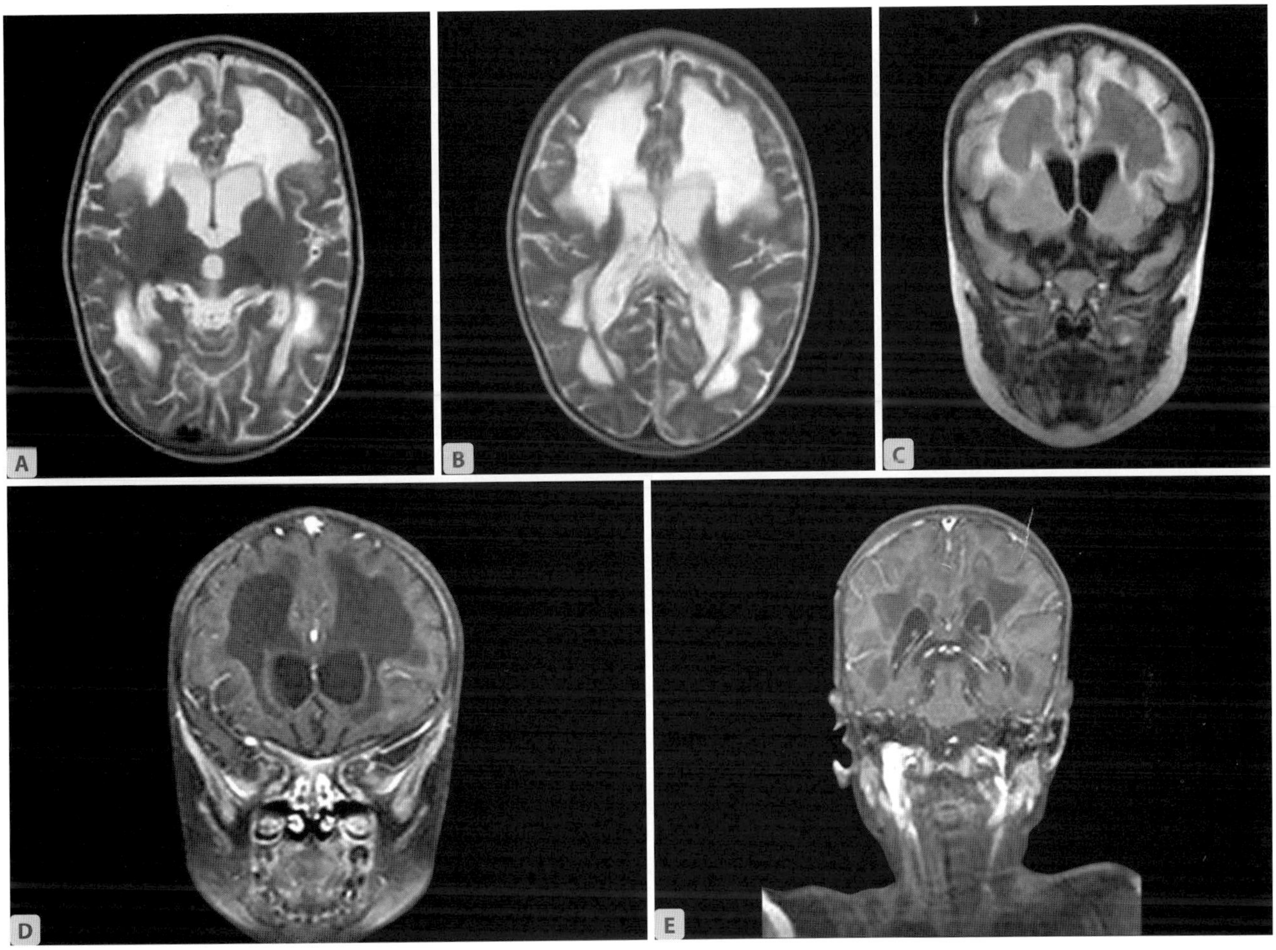

FIGS. 21A TO E: (A and B) Axial T2-weighted MR images revealing higher signal intensity in the frontal white matter than the parietal and occipital regions; (C) Fluid-attenuated inversion recovery (FLAIR) coronal image showing involvement of the subcortical U-fibers; and (D and E) Postcontrast MR images reveal enhancement of the ependymal lining of the frontal horns and also of the bodies of lateral ventricles—Alexander disease.

cysts. The disease has an autosomal recessive inheritance. The onset of the disease is usually during the first year of life, but usually it is diagnosed several years later. Patients present with macrocephaly.[76] The initial motor and mental development of the patients is either normal or slightly delayed. The disease is characterized by a slowly progressive course; in particular, ataxia, spasticity, gait disturbances, and in the later stage of the disease, mental deterioration and seizures develop. No peripheral neuropathy is detected. Laboratory tests fail to demonstrate any specific metabolic abnormality. Histologically, the findings are consistent with vacuolating myelinopathy.

Imaging features: The MR findings are pathognomonic. The brain is diffusely swollen during the early stage of the disease. In the later stages, sulcal and ventricular enlargement may be present. The white matter disease is always severe and it shows a clear centripetal progression pattern. The peripheral white matter structures of the cerebral hemispheres are the most severely involved, including widespread disappearance of the subcortical U-fibers and the presence of large subcortical cyst formation in the frontoparietal and the temporal regions **(Figs. 23A to C)**.[76] These subcortical cysts are best seen on the fluid-attenuated inversion recovery (FLAIR) images. These changes as well as the initial slight sparing of the periventricular and subcortical white matter in the occipital regions suggest an additional anteroposterior gradient **(Figs. 24A to E)**. The deep white matter structures, the corpus callosum, and the internal capsules are spared, but the external and extreme capsules are involved. The cerebellar white matter is involved, but much less markedly than the supratentorial white matter structures. Subtle signal changes may be present within the brainstem along the pyramidal tracts. The cortical and deep gray matter structures are normal. No abnormal signal enhancement is seen within the brain parenchyma after intravenous contrast injection.

Diffusion-weighted imaging shows prominent hyposignal within the subcortical cysts and somewhat decreased signal within the affected white matter. No definite hypersignal is seen within the nonaffected white matter structures or along the interface between the normal and abnormal areas.

The proton spectroscopic findings are nonspecific, the NAA peak is decreased, and the choline peak may be increased, but no abnormal metabolites are demonstrated.

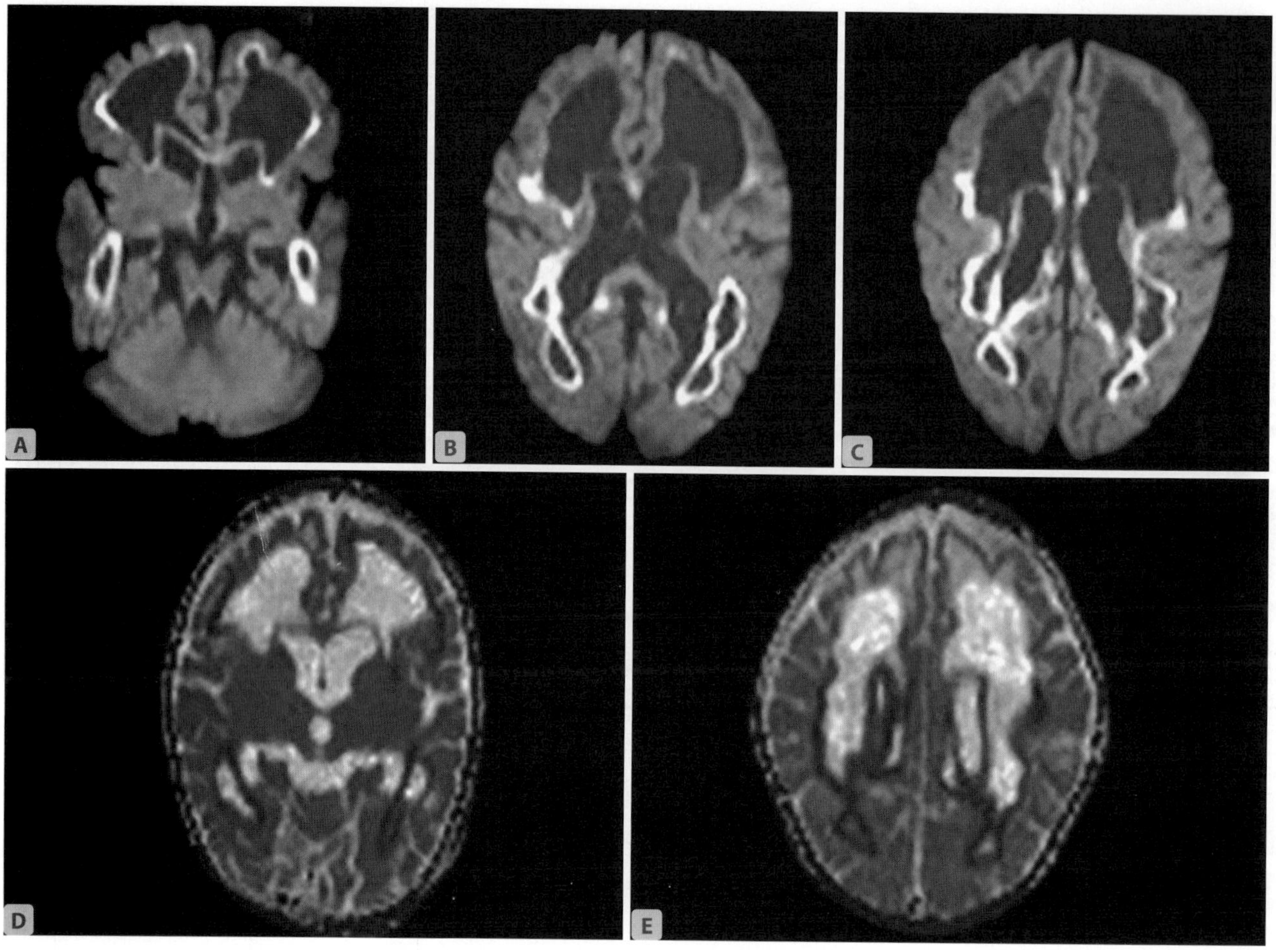

FIGS. 22A TO E: Diffusion-weighted MR (A to C) images revealing a restricted pattern of diffusion in the areas of signal abnormality with a hyposignal seen on the apparent diffusion coefficient (ADC) maps (D and E)—Alexander disease.

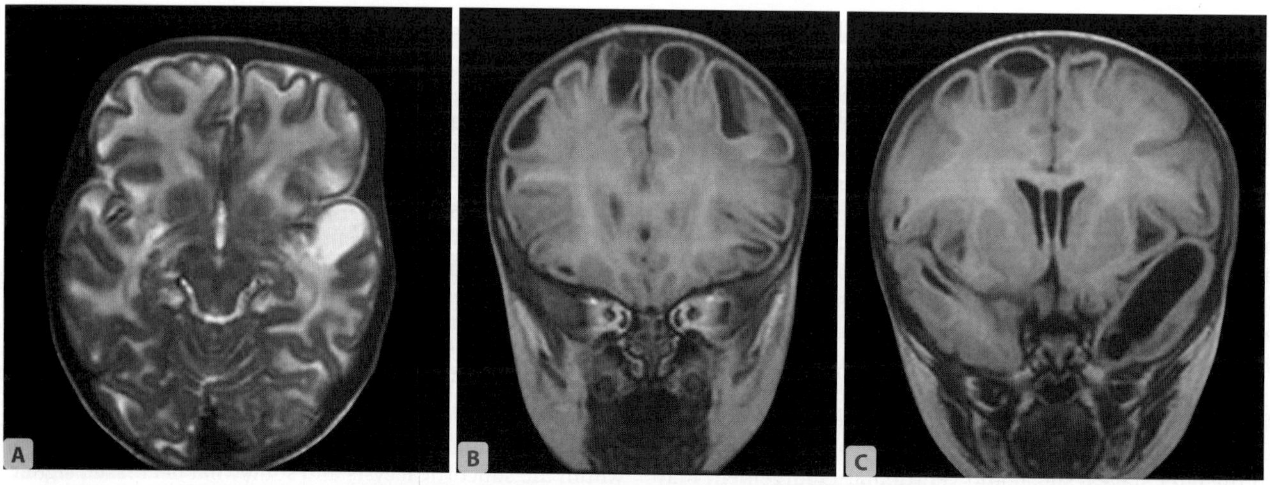

FIGS. 23A TO C: Axial T2W (A) and FLAIR coronal (B and C) MR images showing widespread involvement of the subcortical white matter. Subcortical cyst formation in the frontal and parietal regions is best seen on the FLAIR images (B and C)—Van der Knaap disorder. (FLAIR: fluid-attenuated inversion recovery; T2W: T2-weighted)

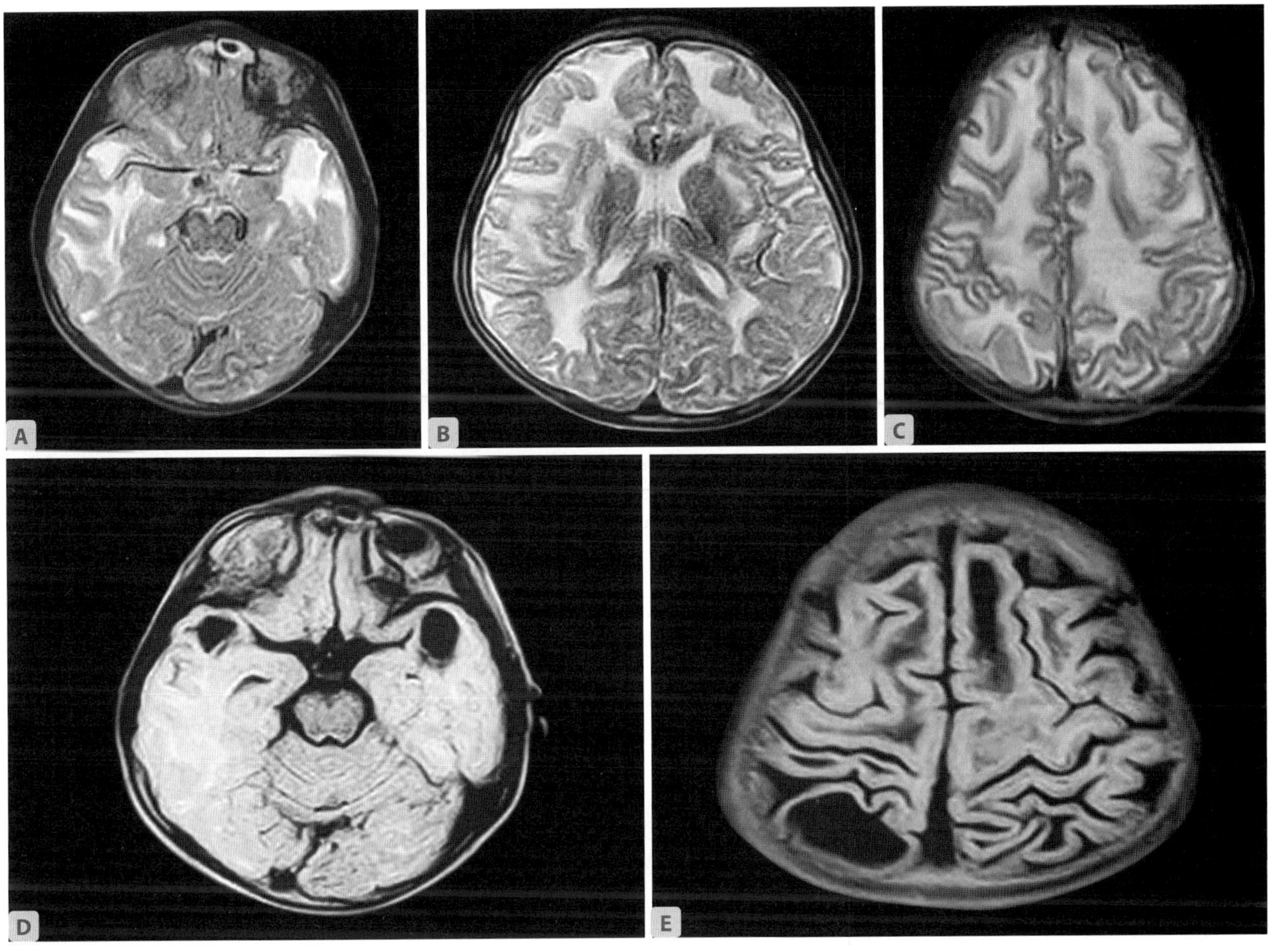

FIGS. 24A TO E: Axial T2W MR images (A to C) revealing extensive white matter changes with diffuse brain swelling with predominant involvement of the subcortical U-fibers (B and C). There is a relative sparing of the deep white matter structures, i.e., the corpus callosum and internal capsule (B). Signal changes are present in the brainstem along the pyramidal tracts (A) with relative sparing of the cerebellar white matter. Subcortical cyst formation is best seen on the FLAIR images (D and E)—Van der Knaap disease. (FLAIR: fluid-attenuated inversion recovery; T2W: T2-weighted)

Vanishing White Matter Disease/Childhood Ataxia with Central Nervous System Hypomyelination

Clinical features: This is a recently described, distinct clinical radiological entity. The disease is typically of childhood onset. Initially, the psychomotor development of the patients is normal. Affected patients present with ataxia, spasticity, and gait disturbance, but only mildly impaired mental capacities. The clinical manifestation of the disease seems to be preceded by minor head trauma or infection; the same factors are also responsible for episodes of deterioration. During the later stages of the disease, optic atrophy and mild epilepsy may develop. The disease is always progressive, but the disease course varies. The severe forms lead to death at a relatively young age (2–6 years), but patients with more moderate clinical phenotypes live up to adulthood.

Imaging features: The MR imaging findings are fairly characteristic. The brain appears to be slightly swollen, but some of the gyri are somewhat broadened. The lateral ventricles show mild-to-moderate dilatation. The white matter changes are very prominent; the signal properties of the affected myelin are practically identical to those of the CSF both on the T1W and T2W images.[77] The posterior limbs of the internal capsules are often involved whereas the anterior limbs are spared. The corpus callosum is also involved, with the exception of the outer rim. The cerebellum is usually slightly atrophic and the cerebellar white matter is mildly abnormal. In the brainstem, the posterior tegmental and the pyramidal tracts also show abnormal hypersignal. The gray matter structures including the basal ganglia are normal. MR spectroscopy of the affected gray matter shows decreased NAA, normal or slightly increased choline, and rather prominent lactate and glucose (at 3.43, 3.80 ppm) peaks. The affected white matter shows decreased NAA, choline, and creatinine peaks.[77]

Pelizaeus–Merzbacher Disease

This is best example of a hypomyelinating leukodystrophy caused by a lack of PLPs.[78] The PLP plays a role in the differentiation and survival of oligodendrocytes. PMD is an example of a sudanophilic leukodystrophy.

Clinical features: There are two forms of the disease—(1) the classic and (2) connatal forms. *Classic form* is less severe, begins in late infancy with X-linked inheritance. The *connatal form* which begins at birth is a more severe form of the disease with either an X-linked or an autosomal recessive inheritance. The connatal form is rarer as compared to the classic form. Nystagmus, abnormal eye movements, extrapyramidal hyperkinesias, psychomotor retardation, and spasticity constitute the classical presentation of the disease.

Pathologic findings: There is atrophy of the brain, most pronounced in the posterior fossa. Histologically, there is profound lack of myelin. There is astrocytosis and lack of oligodendroglia. The residual myelin preferentially remains around blood vessels giving rise to characteristic "tigroid" appearance. There is accumulation of sudanophilic droplets containing cholesterol and triglycerides in the white matter which is the histological hallmark of sudanophilic leukodystrophy.

Imaging Features: There is diffuse T2W high signal throughout the cerebral white matter involving the subcortical white matter **(Figs. 25A to C)**. There is a complete lack of normal myelination with no myelination seen even in the internal capsule—a structure that gets myelinated at birth.[79] A tigroid pattern of myelination may be seen which consists of small scattered foci of normal signal with the abnormal high signal white matter **(Fig. 26)**.[80]

Aicardi–Goutières Syndrome

This rare microcephalic disease is also called leukodystrophy with chronic CSF lymphocytosis and calcifications of the basal ganglia. The disease appears in the neonate or in early infancy. It is a relatively rapidly progressive, devastating disease, and characterized by delayed development and spasticity leading to death in a few months to years.

CT is an essential diagnostic modality in this disease since it almost always demonstrates calcifications within the basal ganglia and the periventricular white matter.[64] On MRI, the disease presents with an essentially supratentorial and very extensive white matter disease with possible cystic lesions in the temporal and parietal lobes. The internal capsules are somewhat less affected but are abnormal also. The brainstem and the cerebellar structures are spared.

Cockayne Syndrome

Cockayne syndrome is another sudanophilic leukodystrophy. The affected children may be normal until late in infancy and may live long enough to develop dwarfism. Transmitted as an

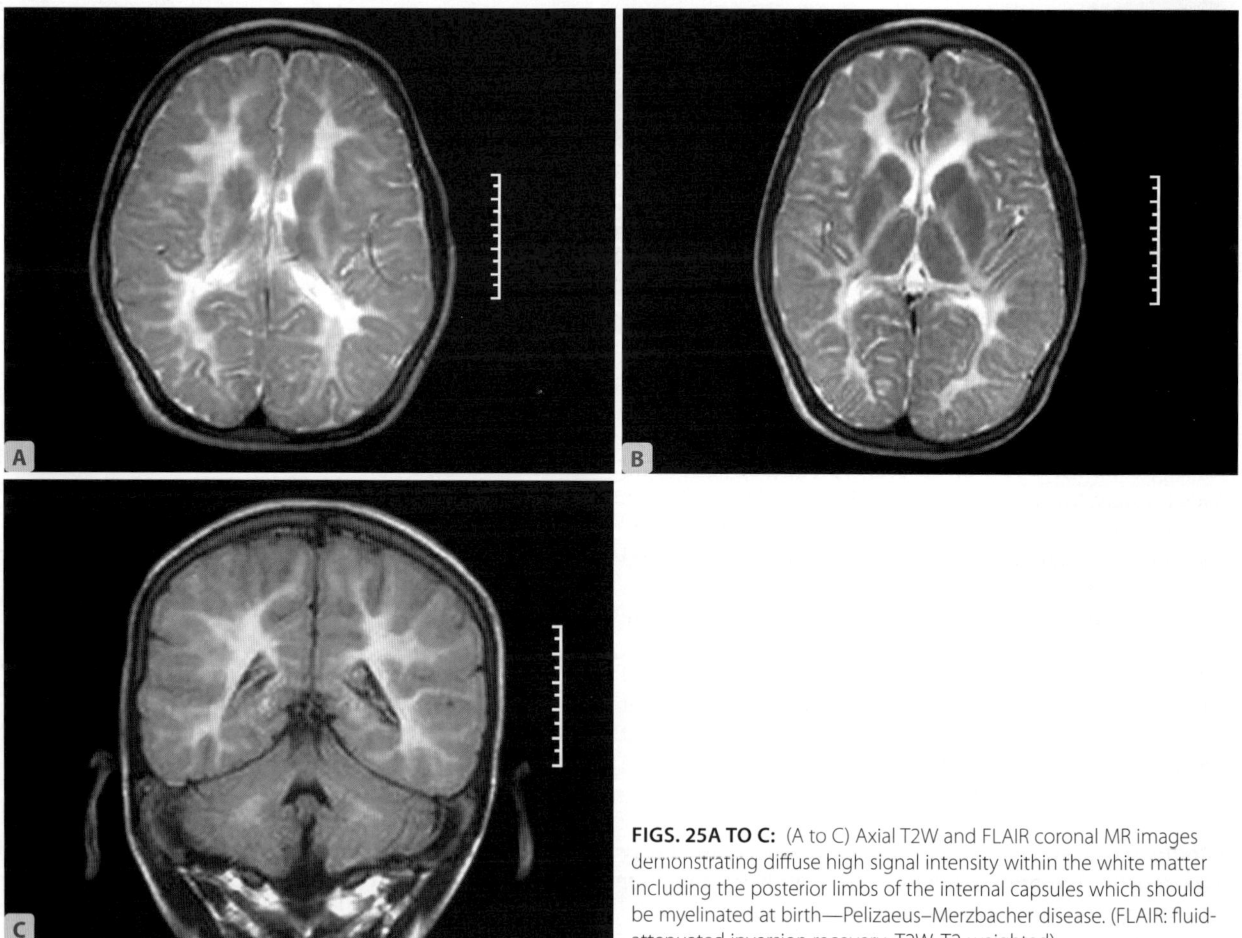

FIGS. 25A TO C: (A to C) Axial T2W and FLAIR coronal MR images demonstrating diffuse high signal intensity within the white matter including the posterior limbs of the internal capsules which should be myelinated at birth—Pelizaeus–Merzbacher disease. (FLAIR: fluid-attenuated inversion recovery; T2W: T2-weighted)

autosomal recessive trait, this syndrome consists of growth retardation, mental retardation, microcephaly, retinopathy, cutaneous photosensitivity, and ataxia. The pathologic changes are similar to other leukodystrophies. However, a significant difference is that small vessels become involved by mural and extramural colloid deposits which frequently contain iron and exhibit striking calcification. The deposits occur chiefly in the basal ganglia, the cerebral white matter, and the dentate nuclei of the cerebellum. There is extensive cortical calcification in both hemispheres.[64]

Proton MR spectroscopy may reveal no abnormal peak consistent with the absence of sclerosis and well-preserved axons. Diffuse or focal reduction in NAA consistent with axonal damage may be seen in more severe cases.[81,82]

The distinctive features of various leukodystrophies have been summarised in **Table 2**.

Mitochondrial Disorders/Defects of the Respiratory Chain

The term is used for a heterogeneous group of disorders caused due to a functional or structural defect of the mitochondria.

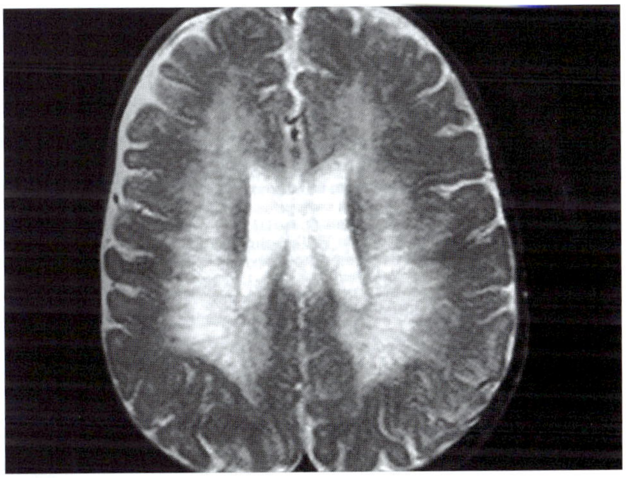

FIG. 26: Axial T2-weighted (T2W) MR image in an infant with slow psychomotor development with nystagmus and choreoathetoid movements revealing diffuse high signal intensity in the white matter with small scattered foci of more normal signal intensity within—tigroid pattern of myelination seen in Pelizaeus–Merzbacher disease.

The so-called respiratory chain is a complex multiunit system within the inner membrane of the mitochondria. Multisystem involvement is the rule in the diseases related to defect of the respiratory chain. It is an important clinical diagnostic clue. In respiratory chain deficiencies, practically any organ or tissue in any combination may be involved, the most frequently affected organs are, however, the CNS and the muscles (both skeletal and visceral).

Mitochondrial Encephalopathy, Lactic Acidosis, and Stroke-like Episodes Syndrome

Clinical features: Patients with MELAS syndrome usually appear healthy at birth with normal development, then exhibit delayed growth, episodic vomiting, seizures and recurrent strokes, and cortical blindness.[83] The age of onset is typically between 4 and 15 years, but early infantile and adult forms have also been reported. No ophthalmoplegia or heart block is seen. The stroke-like episodes are the result of a proliferation of dysfunctional mitochondria in the smooth muscle cells or small arteries giving rise to either permanent or reversible deficits. The disease course is progressive with periodic acute exacerbation. Systemic manifestations of the disease include cardiomyopathy and diabetes.

Pathologic findings: At electron microscopy, the affected tissue demonstrates an increased number of mitochondria which are enlarged and have lipid inclusions. Serum and CSF lactate levels are usually elevated. There is a proliferation of mitochondria in the endothelial cells and smooth muscles in pial arterioles and small arteries. The affected vessels are unable to dilate in response to an increased metabolic demand and this result in ischemia due to energy failure which is known as mitochondrial angiopathy.

Imaging features: The characteristic CT and MR findings of this syndrome are multiple infarct-like lesions.[84] The infarct-like lesions that result have a cortical or subcortical distribution in a bilateral symmetric or asymmetric manner. The lesions have a posterior predominance. Basal ganglia may also be involved and show chronic infarct, necrosis, and calcification. The infarct-like lesions of MELAS syndrome are different from a vascular infarct as these lesions are not restricted to any specific vascular territory and no occlusion is seen on angiography studies.[85] No restricted pattern is

TABLE 2: Distinctive features of various leukodystrophies.

Diseases	Age of onset	Head size	White matter changes [seen as high signal on T2-weighted image (T2WI)]	Gray matter changes	Subcortical involvement
Metachromatic leukodystrophy	1–2 years; 4–7 years (second peak)	Normal	Predominantly deep periventricular white matter	Often normal	Late
Adrenoleukodystrophy	5–10 years	Normal	Primary occipital and splenium of corpus callosum	Normal	Late
Canavan disease	1–2 years	Large	Diffuse involvement	Cystic changes in gray matter	Early
Alexander disease	<1 year	Large	Usually in frontal region	May show minimal changes	Early
Pelizaeus–Merzbacher disease	Late infancy	Normal/ Microcephalic	Tigroid pattern	Normal	Early

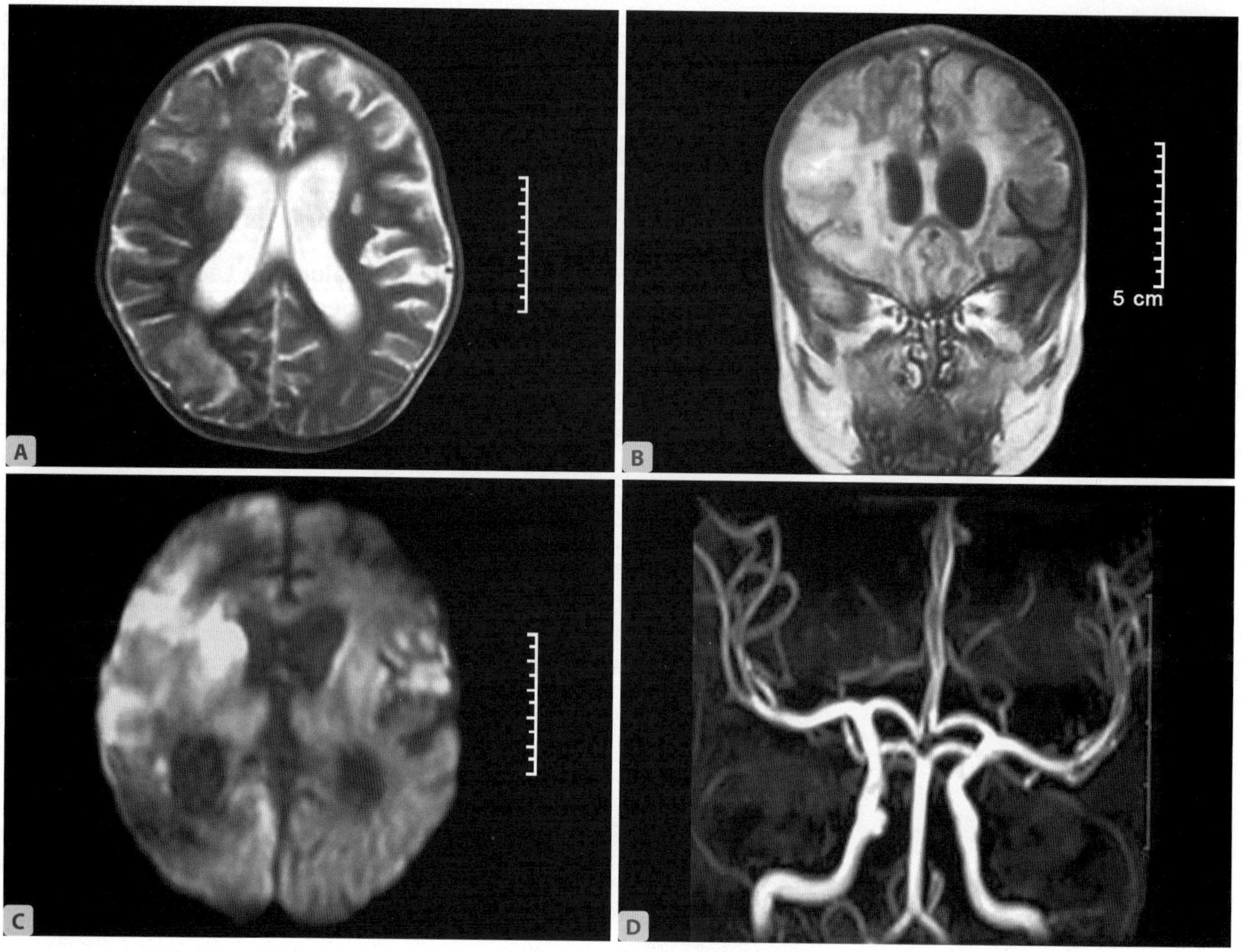

FIGS. 27A TO D: (A and B) Axial T2W and FLAIR coronal images showing asymmetrical infarct-like lesions involving the subcortical white matter and basal ganglia; (C) The lesions are not restricted to any specific vascular territory and show high signal on the ADC maps; and (D) MR angiography reveals no vascular occlusion—mitochondrial encephalopathy (MELAS). (ADC: apparent diffusion coefficient; FLAIR: fluid-attenuated inversion recovery; MELAS: mitochondrial encephalopathy, lactic acidosis, and stroke-like episodes; T2W: T2-weighted)

seen on the diffusion-weighted MR images in these lesions which substantiates the hypothesis that these lesions are due to an energy failure.[86] During the course of the disease, some of these lesions resolve with clinical improvement while new lesions appear in other regions.[87] This finding of multiple migrating infarct-like lesions not restricted to any specific vascular territory is unique to the MELAS syndrome **(Figs. 27A to D)**.[88,89]

Myoclonic Epilepsy with Ragged-red Fibers Syndrome

As the name suggests, patients usually present with myoclonus, weakness, ataxia, and generalized seizures. There are no strokes/infarct-like lesions as are seen in the MELAS syndrome. Conduction disorders of the heart and a short stature are some of the other features of the disorder.[90]

Pathologic findings: Muscle biopsy reveals ragged-red fibers in skeletal muscles. This finding implies degeneration of granular fibers and a proliferation of mitochondria.

Imaging features: A diffuse cerebral and cerebellar atrophy, signal abnormalities in white matter and deep gray matter constitute the imaging findings in MERRF syndrome. There may be calcification of the globus pallidus and dentate nucleus.

Kearns–Sayre Syndrome

An autosomal dominant mitochondrial disorder, Kearns–Sayre syndrome occurs more frequently in females.

Clinical features: The classic clinical triad of ophthalmoplegia, complete heart block, and retinal pigmentary degeneration is seen. Mental retardation and short stature may also be seen.[91]

Imaging findings: There is a predominant involvement of the subcortical white matter with relative sparing of the deep periventricular white matter.[91,92] High signal on T2W images can be seen in basal ganglia, the dorsal brainstem, and the cerebellar white matter **(Figs. 28A to C)**. Cerebral and cerebellar atrophy is another finding that may be seen on imaging.

Leigh Disease

Leigh disease is also known as subacute necrotizing encephalopathy. It is a progressive inherited neurodegenerative disease of infancy/early childhood.[93]

Clinical features: The clinical presentation includes hypotonia, psychomotor retardation, ataxia, and seizures. There may be dystonia, ophthalmoplegia, ptosis, and swallowing difficulties. Respiratory difficulties may also occur with acute respiratory failure being the cause of death in many cases.[94]

Pathologic features: Characteristic pathologic abnormalities include microcystic cavitation, vascular proliferation, neuronal loss and demyelination of the midbrain, basal ganglia and cerebellar dentate nuclei, and occasionally of the cerebral white matter.

Imaging features: The most characteristic imaging finding is a bilateral and symmetrical involvement of the putamen **(Figs. 29A to C)**.[95,96] Lesions may be seen in the globus pallidus and caudate nucleus as well but almost along with putaminal involvement. Additional sites of involvement include the periventricular white matter, substantia nigra, corpus callosum, periaqueductal region, brainstem, and gray matter in the spinal cord **(Figs. 30A to D)**.[97] Lesions in the lower brainstem that is the periaqueductal gray matter and the reticular formation in medulla account for the respiratory failure seen in this condition.[98] The dentate nuclei frequently show abnormalities. White matter lesions in the cerebral hemispheres are usually patchy and predominantly subcortical. The important differential diagnosis is organic acidopathies, but the presence of peculiar brainstem lesion in Leigh disease usually allows a confident differentiation.[99]

Proton MR spectroscopy with voxel placement in the basal ganglia typically demonstrates an abnormal lactate peak with a decrease in NAA/Creatine.[100] DWI may show a hypersignal during the acute metabolic attacks within lesion areas in the brainstem, the basal ganglia, and the dentate nuclei.[100]

Leber's Hereditary Optic Neuropathy

LHON presents with rapidly progressive visual loss due to degeneration of the optic nerves. The disease typically occurs in young adults. No skeletal muscle involvement has been described in this disease. MR imaging usually shows signal abnormalities within the distal intraorbital optic nerves. Putaminal lesions and scattered white matter lesions within the centrum cerebral hemispheric white matter may also be present.

In addition to the disorders of the cellular organelle, the various urea cycle defects and aminoacidopathies also constitute the spectrum of various metabolic disorders.

The distinguishing features of mitochondrial disorders have been summarized in **Table 3**.

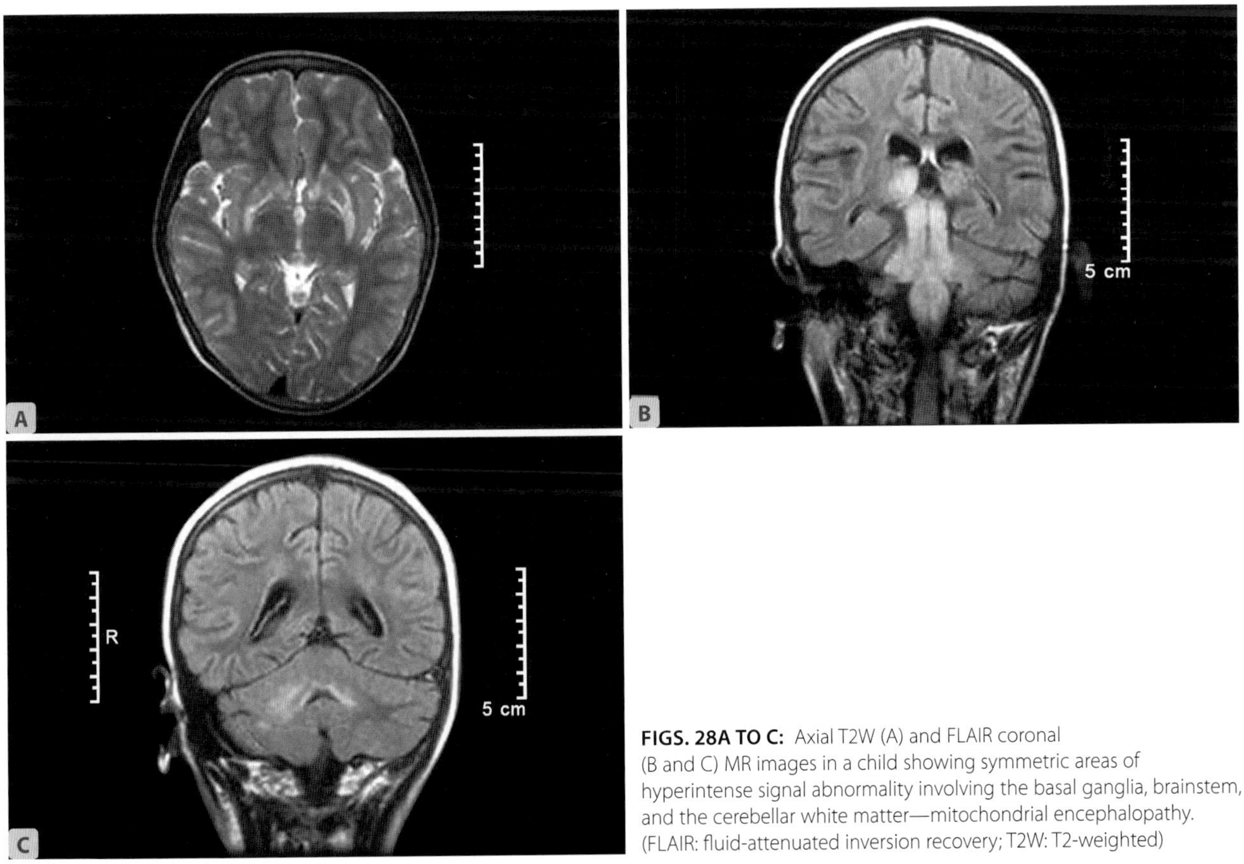

FIGS. 28A TO C: Axial T2W (A) and FLAIR coronal (B and C) MR images in a child showing symmetric areas of hyperintense signal abnormality involving the basal ganglia, brainstem, and the cerebellar white matter—mitochondrial encephalopathy. (FLAIR: fluid-attenuated inversion recovery; T2W: T2-weighted)

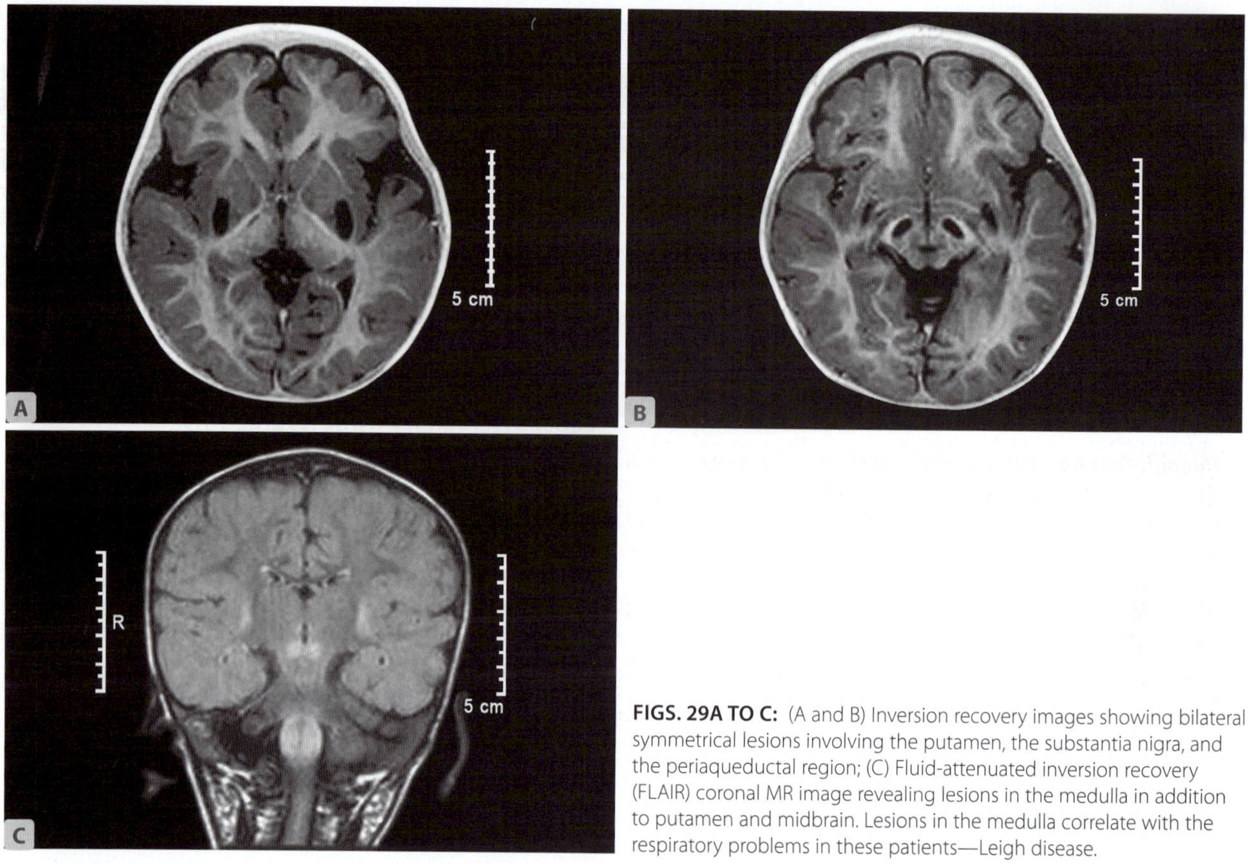

FIGS. 29A TO C: (A and B) Inversion recovery images showing bilateral symmetrical lesions involving the putamen, the substantia nigra, and the periaqueductal region; (C) Fluid-attenuated inversion recovery (FLAIR) coronal MR image revealing lesions in the medulla in addition to putamen and midbrain. Lesions in the medulla correlate with the respiratory problems in these patients—Leigh disease.

Disorders of Amino Acid Metabolism/ Aminoacidopathies

Urea Cycle Defects

The urea cycle is a complex metabolic process, the primary role of which is to convert the toxic ammonia into nontoxic urea. Urea cycle defects are characterized by autosomal recessive inheritance except ornithine carbamoyltransferase deficiency, which is X-linked. The urea cycle defects include carbamoyl phosphate deficiency, ornithine transcarbamylase deficiency, citrullinemia, and argininosuccinic aciduria. Hyperammonemia induces brain swelling and Alzheimer type II changes in astrocytes and chronic elevation leads to neuronal degeneration.

MR imaging findings in neonates with urea cycle defects are dominated by the prominent brain swelling and white matter signal changes related to vasogenic edema.[101] The myelinated white matter is less severely affected than the nonmyelinated areas **(Figs. 31A to H)**. Certain regions of cerebral cortex and deep gray matter show prolongation of T1 and T2 relaxation times on MR; in particular, the insular cortex (posterior more than anterior), perirolandic cortex, and basal ganglia (particularly the globi pallidi) show early T2 prolongation and swelling. The differentiation from hypoxic-ischemic injury can be made by the predominant globus pallidus and putaminal injury in urea cycle disorders in contrast to the predominant thalamic injury in hypoxic injury. MR spectroscopy reveals a characteristic elevated lactate (doublet centered at 1.33 ppm) and glutamate resonance at 2.2 and 2.6 ppm and at 3.75 ppm. The glutamate and glutamine resonances are best seen with short (20–30 ms) TEs.[102] As the case progresses, atrophy is often severe and may be multicystic.

Phenylketonuria

Classic phenylketonuria (PKU) is an autosomal recessive disorder caused by a deficiency in the enzyme phenylalanine hydroxylase which converts phenylalanine to tyrosine owing to which neurotoxic phenylketones accumulate. Two forms of PKU are known. The most frequent *classical phenylketonuria* is caused by deficiency of phenylalanine hydroxylase enzyme. The other more *malignant* and rare form is related to the deficiency of the tetrahydrobiopterin coenzyme which is also indispensable in the breakdown of phenylalanine into tyrosine.

The clinical and imaging manifestations of the two forms of PKU are different.

Classic Form of Phenylketonuria

Clinical Features: Infants are normal at birth but in the first year of life manifest with progressive cognitive delay, microcephaly, spasticity, recurrent eczematous rash, and a peculiar musty odor of the urine, skin, and hair. Seizures occur in about 25% of untreated patients.[103]

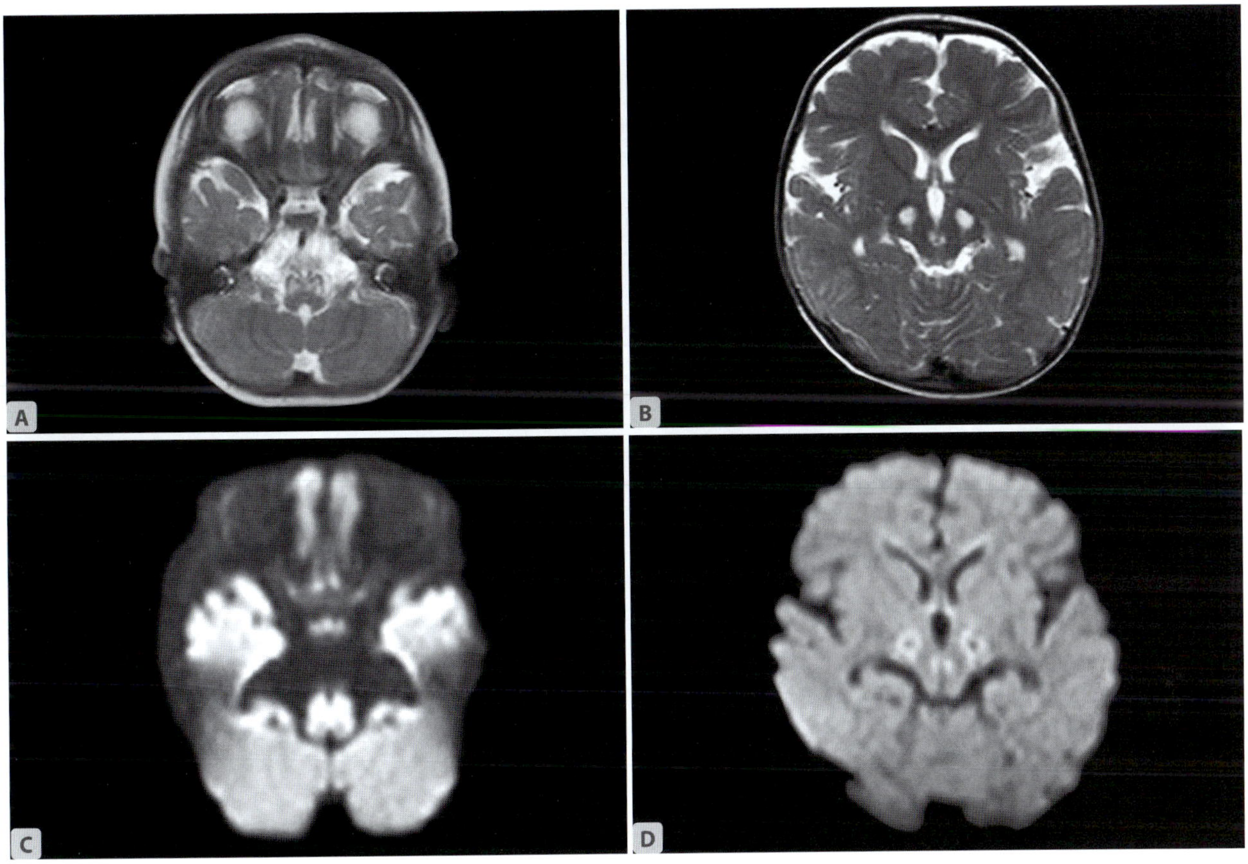

FIGS. 30A TO D: (A and B) Axial T2-weighted (T2W) images in a 20-month-old infant showing lesions in the medulla and symmetrical lesions in the substantia nigra and the periaqueductal region; and (C and D) These lesions reveal a restricted pattern of diffusion seen as hypersignal on the diffusion-weighted images during the acute metabolic crisis—Leigh disease.

Imaging findings: Imaging studies show primarily abnormal signal in the white matter that corresponds to the delayed and defective myelination. MR shows T2 prolongation that is predominantly found in the periventricular white matter in the initial stages. The subcortical white matter is involved later. Diffusion-weighted MR images obtained in the acute phase will show a reduced diffusion in the affected white matter due to spongiotic changes of myelin.[104] Proton MR spectroscopy shows the presence of a peak from elevated phenylalanine at 7.37 ppm. The size of the peak is useful for monitoring response to treatment.[105]

Malignant Form of Phenylketonuria

In the malignant form, microcephaly and delayed development are also typical but the disease, if not treated, often leads to death in early childhood. Neurologically, the patients present with prominent extrapyramidal signs (infantile parkinsonism, choreoathetosis, myoclonic, and grand mal seizures). Progressive pyramidal and bulbar signs develop in conjugation with severe cognitive deterioration.

In the biopterin-dependent form of PKU, CT examination shows calcifications at the level of the putamina and/or the globi pallidi as well as along the cortical-subcortical junction in the frontal regions somewhat similar to what may be seen in carbonic anhydrase II deficiency.

TABLE 3: Mitochondrial disorders: Distinguishing clinical features and MR findings.

Disorders	Clinical features	MR findings
MELAS	Episodic vomiting Cerebral blindness Hemiparesis Hemianopia	T2WI: High signal in subcortical WM, brainstem, basal ganglia, and cerebellum infarct-like lesions
MERRF	Myoclonus Ataxia Weakness	T2WI: High signal in deep GM and WM
KSS	Ophthalmoplegia Retinal degeneration Heart block CSF count >100 mg/dL	• T2WI: High signal in U-fibers, thalami, dorsal brainstem, and cerebellar WM • T1WI: High signal in basal ganglia
Leigh	Respiratory failure Visual/auditory problems Ataxia, weakness	T2WI: High signal in bilateral symmetric basal ganglia (particularly putamen), thalami, and dorsal brainstem

(CSF: cerebrospinal fluid; GM: gray matter; KSS: Kearns–Sayre syndrome; MELAS: mitochondrial encephalopathy, lactic acidosis, and stroke-like episodes; MERRF: myoclonic epilepsy with ragged-red fibers; T1WI: T1-weighted image; T2WI: T2-weighted image; WM: white matter)

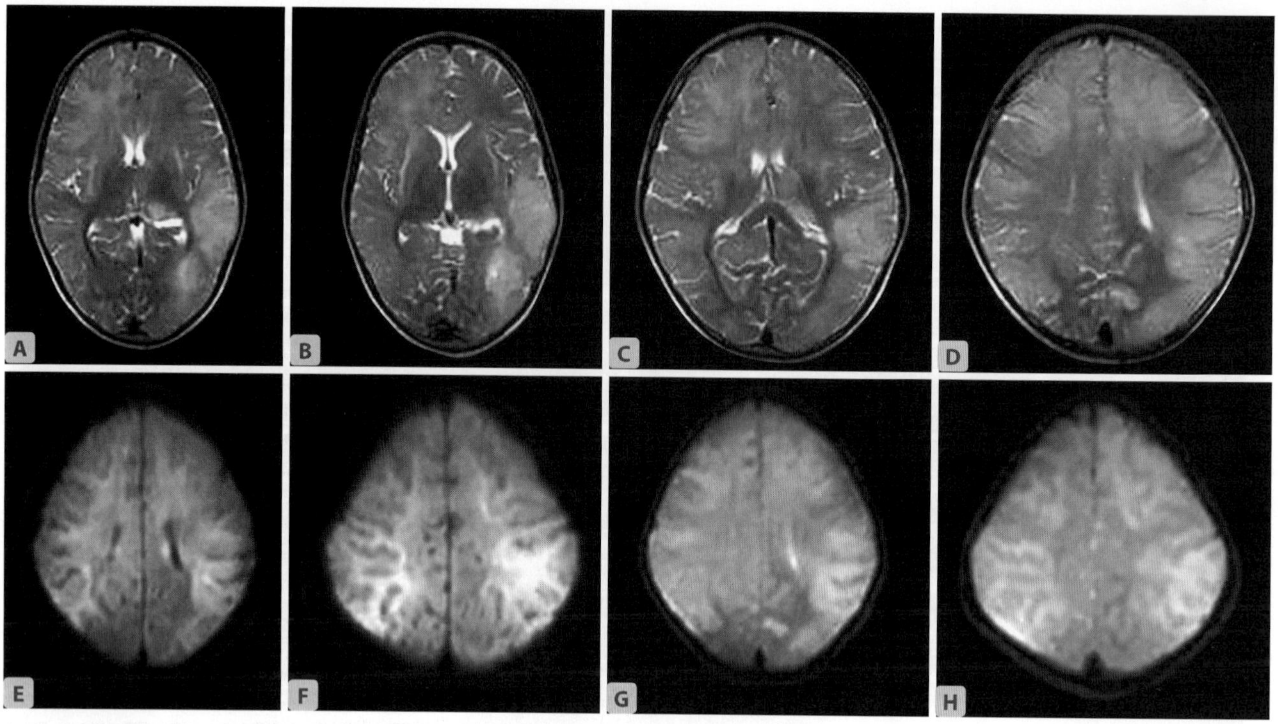

FIGS. 31A TO H: (A to D) Axial T2W MR images in a few months old infant showing a diffuse swelling of the brain. The unmyelinated white matter exhibits an abnormal increased signal intensity. There is a relative sparing of the myelinated optic radiation; and (E to H) Diffusion-weighted images and ADC maps do not reveal a restricted pattern consistent with vasogenic edema—urea cycle disorder. (ADC: apparent diffusion coefficient; T2W: T2-weighted)

The MR imaging study shows signal changes within the calcified areas: hyperintense on T1W and hypointense on T2W images. White matter lesions may be seen, sometimes they are diffuse and in other cases focal with cystic degeneration in the parieto-occipital regions.

Maple Syrup Urine Disease

Maple syrup urine disease (MSUD) is a genetically heterogeneous disorder caused by abnormal oxidative decarboxylation of the branched-chain amino acids such as leucine, isoleucine, and valine. Four clinical phenotypes are distinguished: (1) The classical, (2) The intermediate, (3) The intermittent, and (4) The thiamine responsive. The most severe form is the classical MSUD characterized by early postnatal onset and rapid progressive neurological deterioration leading to death, if untreated.

In the classic type, the infant is normal for about the first week. In the second week, the infant starts to eat poorly, fails to thrive, and develops hypotonia, lethargy, and vomiting.[106] Urine, sweat, and cerumen smell like maple syrup. The disease quickly progresses to coma, seizures, and death, if untreated. The severity of neurological sequelae is strongly correlated with the duration of the acute toxic phase in the neonatal period. Conventional MR imaging shows diffuse swelling of the brain.[106] This is mainly due to the vasogenic edema involving the nonmyelinated white matter structures. On the other hand, even more prominent signal changes are also present within the myelinated brain areas (posterior brainstem tracts, central cerebellar white matter, and posterior limbs of the internal capsules) representing myelin edema secondary to vacuolating myelinopathy.

The less severe forms of the disease with higher residual enzyme activity can present later in childhood with metabolic crisis resulting in lethargy, irritability, and vomiting that may progress to stupor or coma. An intermittent form may present later in life as attacks of transient ataxia, sometimes accompanied by cerebral edema. Tests during an attack show elevated leucine, isoleucine, and valine in blood as well as branched-chain amino acids in urine. Chronic management relies on dietary restriction of branched-chain amino acids.

Imaging findings: The neonatal form typically presents on the seventh day after birth. The imaging findings may be normal in the first ten days of life. Because classic MSUD presents in the neonatal period, it is one of the few metabolic diseases in which transfontanelle sonography may play a role in diagnosis. Cranial sonography may show a symmetric increase in the echogenicity of the periventricular white matter, basal ganglia, and thalami.[107] The CT and MR findings are quite characteristic revealing profound localized edema seen as increased signal on T2W images in the deep cerebellar white matter, dorsal brainstem, cerebral peduncles, inferior limb of the internal capsule, perirolandic white matter, and the globi pallidi **(Figs. 32A to E)**. The regions involved correspond to those that are myelinated or myelinating at the time of birth. Generalized edema of the cerebral hemispheres may be superimposed on the localized abnormalities particularly in the first weeks of life.[106]

Diffusion imaging is very useful in the acute stage as areas with MSUD edema (cerebellar white matter, dorsal brainstem, cerebral peduncles, corticospinal tracts, and globi pallidi) show reduced diffusion with ADC values falling to 20–30% of their normal values. Myelin edema presents with isotropically restricted water diffusion, hence there is high signal. The vasogenic edema is characterized by isotropically increased water diffusion which causes hyposignal on the diffusion-weighted images. The sharp contrast between the DWI signal properties of these edema types and the peculiar distribution of the pathological hypersignal (strictly limited to the myelinated white matter structures) results in a pathognomonic imaging pattern. After the acute phase of the disease has resolved, patients are left with a variable degree of brain damage dependent upon the time of initiation of the treatment. Proton MR spectroscopy in the acute phase of illness shows slight reduction of NAA and amino acid peak of leucine, isoleucine, and valine at 0.9 ppm on short echo time (TE).[108]

The intermittent and intermediate forms of MSUD have a more insidious clinical pattern. The first metabolic crisis may appear in late infancy or early childhood. The imaging findings are less characteristic. Typically, brain atrophy, delayed myelination and pathological signal changes within the upper brainstem structures, the thalami, the globi pallidi, and the centrum semiovale are observed. DWI also shows signal abnormalities in these areas, but they are often rather subtle. From the imaging point of view, the intermittent form of MSUD may, therefore, be somewhat similar to Canavan disease in the early stage but the clinical context and the laboratory findings allow easy differentiation.

In treated MSUD cases, the conventional MRI and the DWI findings rarely return to normal. Typically, variable but prominent residual abnormalities, including diffuse brain atrophy, delayed myelination, and structural lesions, are noted. The pattern of the structural lesions is very similar to those observed in the intermittent form of MSUD. Changes are also present in the hypothalamic structures, the dentate nuclei, and the cerebellar or the cerebral hemispheric white matter. Subtle residual DWI abnormalities may also be noted. In successfully treated cases, MR spectroscopy shows improvement but total normalization of the branched-chain amino acid peak complex is usually not achieved.

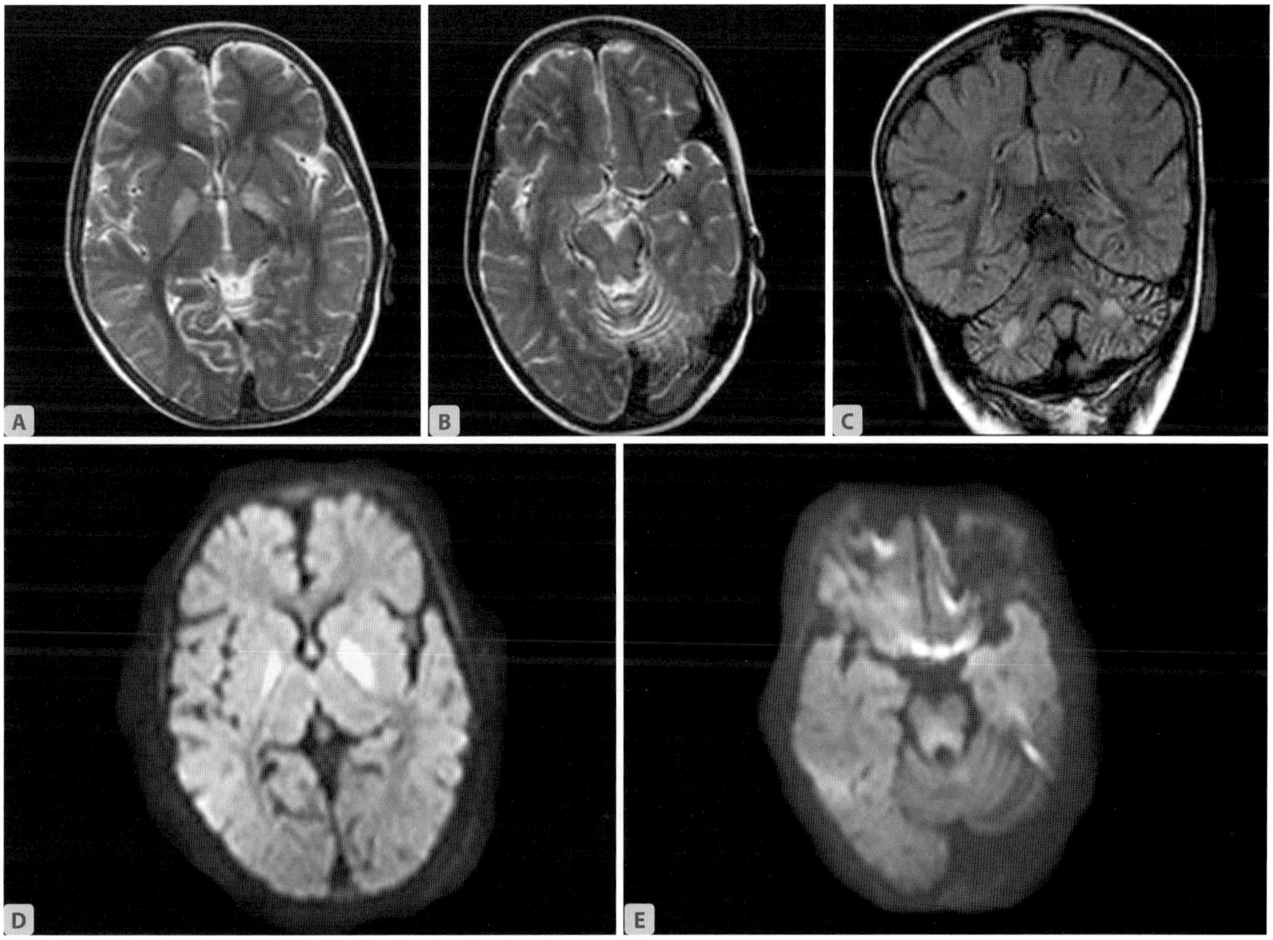

FIGS. 32A TO E: (A to C) Axial T2W and FLAIR coronal MR images revealing symmetric areas of signal abnormality in the globus pallidus, dorsal brainstem, and the deep cerebellar white matter; and (D and E) Diffusion-weighted MR images revealing restricted pattern of diffusion in the globi pallidi and dorsal brainstem—intermittent form of maple syrup urine disease. (FLAIR: fluid-attenuated inversion recovery; T2W: T2-weighted)

Classic Homocystinuria[109]

Classic homocystinuria is an autosomal recessive disorder caused by a defect in the enzyme cystathionine β-synthase resulting in elevations of homocysteine and methionine. This results in intimal irregularities that cause arteriosclerosis, arterial thromboembolism, and venous thrombosis in children and young adults. The excess homocysteine generates superoxide and hydrogen peroxide, changes coagulation factor levels (encouraging clot formation), prevents small arteries from dilating, and causes proliferation of smooth muscle cells in arterial walls.

Clinical Features

The findings include dislocation of lens, osteoporosis, thinning, and lengthening of long bones. Lens dislocation (ectopia lentis) is usually inferior which is the opposite of what is seen in Marfan syndrome. Untreated patients are at risk for seizures, psychiatric disorders, and thromboembolic events including stroke, myocardial infarction, and pulmonary emboli.

Imaging Features

Imaging studies reveal multiple cortical-subcortical and lacunar infarctions both within the cerebral and the cerebellar hemispheres. The disease may also present with a less specific, diffuse white matter involvement and the pattern is suggestive of "retrograde" demyelination.[109]

Nonketotic Hyperglycinemia

This is caused by a defect in glycine cleavage with resultant accumulation of glycine in the plasma, urine, and CSF. Two clinical phenotypes are known: (1) the more common neonatal type, which is characterized by practically absent glycine cleavage system activity and (2) the late-onset (infantile and juvenile) form, in which some residual glycine cleavage system activity is present. The neonatal form presents as lethargy and poor feeding after starting the protein feeds. The patients are hypotonic (glycine is an inhibitor neurotransmitter at the level of the lower motor neurons) and have frequent myoclonic seizures. This quickly progresses to persistent seizures, encephalopathy, and coma. Apnea is common and persistent hiccups have been described. The prognosis for the neonatal form is poor. The late-onset form has a milder and rather nonspecific clinical presentation.

Imaging Features

The imaging hallmarks of nonketotic hyperglycinemia are callosal abnormalities and delayed myelination.[110] The spectrum of morphological changes of the corpus callosum ranges from the rare true callosal dysgenesis to the more frequent callosal hypogenesis or hypoplasia, but some degree of abnormality is always present. The delay in myelination is increasingly evident with aging, if the infant and is probably associated with global hypomyelination. Cortical gyral abnormalities have also been described. Acute hydrocephalus may contribute to the severe clinical picture. In the chronic stage of the disease, progressive atrophy of the brain develops. Restricted diffusion is seen on the diffusion-weighted MR images.

MR spectroscopy is a useful adjunct to the MR workup of patients with suspected nonketotic hyperglycinemia, since the concentration of glycine is particularly elevated in the brain. Glycine resonates at the 3.55 ppm level. Proton MR spectroscopy reveals a glycine peak at 3.55 ppm. In order to separate the glycine peak from that of myoinositol which has a similar chemical shift, the spectrum should be obtained with a long TE. The myoinositol peak disappears on the long TE.

5,10-Methylenetetrahydrofolate Reductase Deficiency

5,10-methylenetetrahydrofolate reductase deficiency is the best known of the defects of folate metabolism. This form has an autosomal recessive inheritance. The onset of the disease is variable, it is more frequent in infants but later onset cases, including an adult form, are also known. Neurologically developmental delay is seen in conjugation with signs of spinal cord (combined degeneration of the cord) and peripheral nerve involvement.

MR imaging in 5,10-methylenetetrahydrofolate reductase deficiency may show rather prominent abnormalities in the brain. The cerebral white matter is diffusely normal, the lesions involve corpus callosum, the external and extreme capsules, the laminae medullares, and the anterior limbs of the internal capsules with sparing of the posterior limbs.[111] The cortico-spinal tracts within the centrum semiovale, the subcortical U-fibers in the occipital regions, and the optic radiations are also spared. The basal ganglia and the thalami are normal but the globi pallidi show increased signal intensity on the T2W images. Subtle signal changes may be present within the mesencephalon (hypersignal within the substantia nigra and the periaqueductal region) and the central tegmental tracts of the pons. The cerebellar white matter is not involved. DWI show hypersignal within the white matter lesions, due to vacuolating myelinopathy. The diffusion-weighted abnormalities (similar to the conventional MR imaging findings) may remain visible on follow-up studies even after a few years.

Organic Acidemias[112]

Many of the organic acidopathies fall into the group of devastating metabolic disease of the newborn, others have later and an often insidious onset. Typically, gray matter abnormalities dominate the imaging findings. White matter involvement may also be present which is usually less prominent. Occasionally, organic acidopathies present with a leukodystrophy-like presentation but gray matter lesions are always conspicuous.

Methylmalonic Acidemia

It is caused by a defect in methylmalonyl-CoA mutase. Acidosis and hyperammonemia can be severe and a single attack can cause permanent cognitive disability. Seizures, spasticity, behavior problems, and ataxia are common. Metabolic stroke with an acute decompensation can occur.

Imaging Findings during Metabolic Crisis

In methylmalonic aciduria, the most typical and often the sole abnormality is the symmetrical signal changes within the globi pallidi, which is associated with swelling. The caudate nuclei, the putamina, and the thalami are spared. The cortex is normal. During the acute metabolic crisis, DWI show hypersignal within the lesion areas. MR spectroscopy may show a small amount of lactate within the lesions. No disease-specific metabolites are demonstrated.

Imaging Findings after Metabolic Crisis

The globus pallidus lesions undergo necrotic changes; they are markedly atrophic and continue to show hypersignal on the T2W images **(Figs. 33A to C)**. Sometimes, mild cerebellar atrophy may be present and subtle signal changes within the dentate nuclei suggest some damage too. In early-onset cases, delayed myelination is frequently seen.

Differential diagnosis in bilateral globus pallidus disease without involvement of the other basal ganglia components includes methylmalonic aciduria, kernicterus, and carbon monoxide intoxication. In kernicterus, lesions of subthalamic nuclei are associated with globus pallidus lesions. Carbon monoxide intoxication is usually encountered in suggestive clinical settings.

Propionic Acidemia

It is also a disorder of organic acid metabolism. It is a relatively common organic acidopathy. The deficiency enzyme is propionyl-coenzyme A carboxylase. Clinical features include cognitive disability, cardiomyopathy, pancreatitis, osteoporosis, and movement disorders.

Imaging Findings

During metabolic crisis, diffuse brain swelling is seen. Signal abnormalities within the basal ganglia and the dentate nuclei are seen on the T2W images. Subtle signal changes may be present within the pulvinar of the thalami. The cerebral and cerebellar cortices are also affected. The involved gray matter structures are swollen at this stage. White matter structures also show signal changes, mainly subcortically, including the subinsular areas (external and extreme capsules). The corpus callosum, the internal capsule, and corticospinal tracts are spared. DWI usually show moderate signal increase within the involved gray matter structures and the subcortical white matter.

MR spectroscopy demonstrates lactate within the lesion areas consistent with impairment of energy metabolism resulting in anaerobic glycolysis. No disease-specific metabolites are identified.

Ethylmalonic Acidemia

Ethylmalonic aciduria typically presents with basal ganglia disease, but patchy white matter lesions may also be present

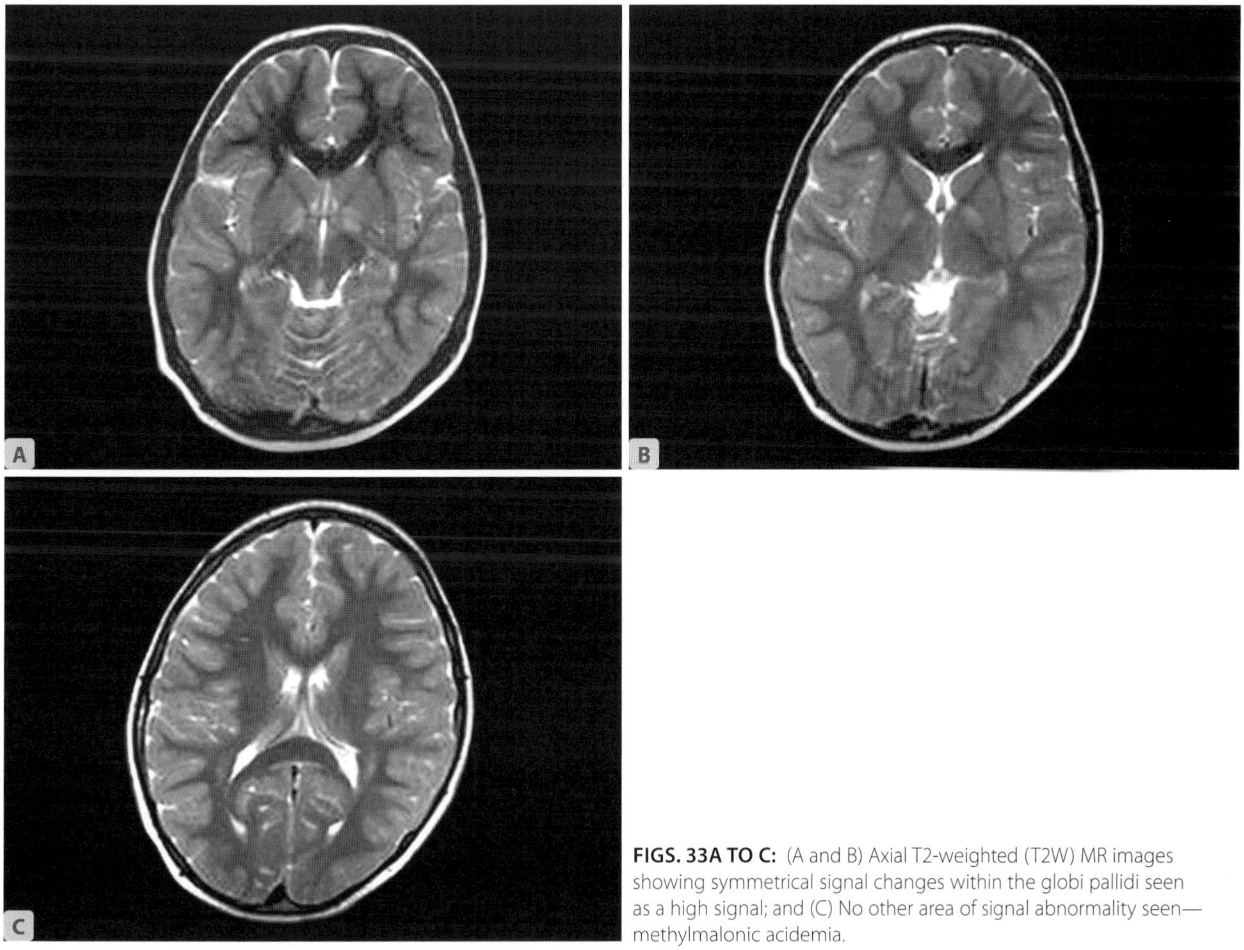

FIGS. 33A TO C: (A and B) Axial T2-weighted (T2W) MR images showing symmetrical signal changes within the globi pallidi seen as a high signal; and (C) No other area of signal abnormality seen—methylmalonic acidemia.

within the cerebral hemispheres. The signal changes within the heads of caudate nuclei and the putamina are patchy and inhomogeneous.[113] This may help to raise the possibility of the disease and differentiate it from other organic acidopathies. A distinct clinical feature of the disease is the widespread cutaneous petechiae and ecchymoses indicative of vasculopathy.

3-Methylglutaconic Aciduria

The disease has at least four clinical phenotype presentations. Type 2 has an X-linked inheritance, the other are autosomal recessive. The typical imaging presentation in types 1 and 4 of this metabolic disorder is, as in many other organic acidopathies, also the symmetrical bilateral basal ganglia disease.

Imaging Findings

During the acute stage of the disease, the basal ganglia are swollen and exhibit high signal on the DWI suggestive of cytotoxic edema. Sometimes, only the globi pallidi, the caudate nuclei, and the anterior parts of the putamina are involved; posteriorly they are spared. With the progression of the disease, the putaminal abnormalities become complete. In some cases, ill-defined, diffuse cerebral white matter signal changes are also present. During the metabolic crisis, the cerebellar cortex and the dentate nuclei may also show signal abnormalities. Cerebellar atrophy is a very characteristic imaging finding. The vermis is usually more affected than the cerebellar hemispheres. The association of cerebellar atrophy and basal ganglia disease is a suggestive imaging pattern of 3-methylglutaconic aciduria.

On MR spectroscopy, lactate is present within the lesion areas but no disease-specific metabolite is identified.

3-hydroxy-3-methylglutaryl-coenzyme A Lyase Deficiency

This is a relatively rare metabolic disorder of the L-leucine breakdown pathway. The disease may present with metabolic crisis with hypoglycemia or ketoacidosis. MR imaging usually reveals nonspecific abnormalities.

Since the disease usually starts in the early postnatal period or in early infancy, initially the gray matter abnormalities are easier to depict, since the white matter is not myelinated. Later, as the brain myelination progresses, the white matter changes, which correspond to demyelination become more apparent. The gray matter abnormalities involve the basal ganglia and the dentate nuclei. They are fairly subtle in most cases and do not seem to lead to necrosis if the disease is appropriately treated. The white matter abnormalities within the cerebral hemispheres are sometimes patchy, but usually confluent. The subcortical U-fibers are often spared. DWI shows faint hypersignal within the involved white matter structures.

MR spectroscopy invariably demonstrates disease-specific abnormalities with two abnormal peaks at the 1.3 and 2.4 ppm levels.

Glutaric Aciduria Type I

Glutaric aciduria type I is usually an insidiously developing metabolic disease. The disorder may be diagnosed during a metabolic crisis, which is typically triggered by a febrile illness.

In the clinically mild phenotypes, no parenchymal lesions may be seen. Patients with type 1 glutaric aciduria are usually macrocephalic. Another peculiar imaging finding is the bilateral enlargement of the sylvian fissures. They may correspond to arachnoid cysts or disturbed and incomplete opercularization. They are usually bilateral, but not necessarily symmetrical. Rarely, the abnormality is unilateral. These changes may be detected prenatally or in the early postnatal period by ultrasound. Macrocephaly and sylvian fissure abnormalities are present in both the clinically benign and malignant phenotypes.

Prominent brain atrophy may also develop. Chronic subdural hematomas are relatively frequently seen in glutaric aciduria type I without any evidence of significant head trauma in the clinical history.

The presence of bilateral sylvian fissure and temporal lobe CSF space enlargement and bilateral basal ganglia lesions in a macrocephalic child are almost pathognomonic of glutaric aciduria type I.[114] T2 prolongation is seen in the basal ganglia, most commonly the putamen, less commonly the caudate, and rarely the globus pallidus and periventricular white matter **(Figs. 34A to C)**.

MR spectroscopy may show lactate within the basal ganglia during the acute stage of the disease. Although the possible role of glutamine-glutamate complexes in the pathogenesis of basal ganglia disease has been raised (glutamine "excitotoxicity" or glutamine "suicide"), increased glutamine-glutamate levels have not been demonstrated within the basal ganglia by in vivo MR spectroscopy. The distinguishing features of various disorders of amino acid metabolism are summarised in **Table 4**.

DIFFERENTIATING FEATURES

There are various useful clinical and imaging findings that help to narrow the differential diagnosis. One of the important clinical findings is a large head size/macrocrania **(Box 6)** while an important imaging finding helpful in differentiation is those showing enhancement **(Box 7)**.

The integrated advanced MR imaging techniques such as DWI, DTI, and proton MR spectroscopy further enable to make an accurate diagnosis. **Box 8** shows leukodystrophies with restricted diffusion while **Box 9** enlists the peaks seen in various leukodystrophies.

Metabolic Disorders Primarily Affecting Gray Matter

Hallervorden–Spatz Disease

It is a rare metabolic disorder that is characterized by progressive gait impairment, gradually increasing rigidity of all limbs, choreoathetoid movements, dysarthria, and mental

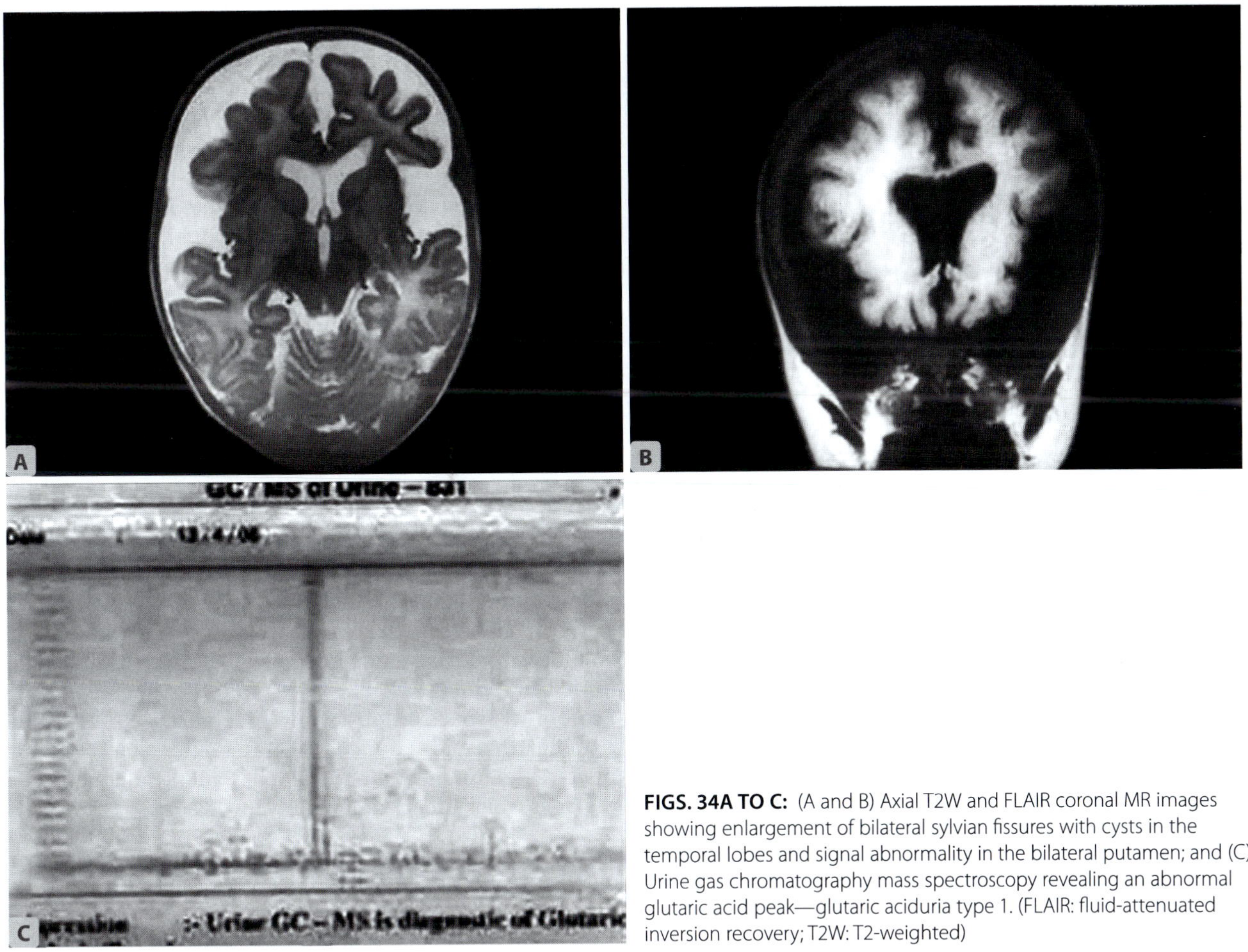

FIGS. 34A TO C: (A and B) Axial T2W and FLAIR coronal MR images showing enlargement of bilateral sylvian fissures with cysts in the temporal lobes and signal abnormality in the bilateral putamen; and (C) Urine gas chromatography mass spectroscopy revealing an abnormal glutaric acid peak—glutaric aciduria type 1. (FLAIR: fluid-attenuated inversion recovery; T2W: T2-weighted)

TABLE 4: Disorders of amino acid metabolism.

Diseases	Clinical findings	Imaging findings
Urea cycle defects	• Infancy: Lethargy, coma • Childhood: Episodic lethargy, confusion, ataxia, dysarthria, and coma	• Neonates: Brain swelling • Acute stages: Multifocal swollen areas of cortex and subcortical WM • Chronic stages: Diffuse atrophy, delay in myelination
Phenylketonuria	• Normal at birth • Developmental delay	Delay in myelination, increase signal on T2WI: Periatrial WM
Maple syrup urine disease	Neonate: Coma, seizures, and respiratory failure	Swelling and increase signal on T2WI: Brainstem, GP, and posterior limb of internal capsule
Nonketotic hyperglycinemia	Early infancy vomiting, seizures, and apnea	Decreased signal on T2WI: Periventricular WM, delay in myelination
Glutaric aciduria type I	• Infancy/childhood • Encephalopathy • Macrocephaly	Prominent extra-axial spaces, increase signal on T2WI: Bilateral caudate, putamen; delay in myelination

(GP: globus pallidus; T2WI: T2-weighted image; WM: white matter)

BOX 6: Leukodystrophies with a large head size/macrocrania.

- Canavan disease
- Alexander disease
- Megalencephalic leukodystrophy with subcortical cyst formation
- Glutaric aciduria type I
- Tay–Sachs disease

BOX 7: Leukodystrophies with enhancement.

- X-linked adrenoleukodystrophy
- Alexander disease
- Krabbe disease (cranial nerves, cauda equina)

BOX 8: Leukodystrophies showing restricted diffusion.

- Metachromatic leukodystrophy
- X-linked adrenoleukodystrophy
- Canavan disease
- Leigh disease
- Urea cycle disorders
- Maple syrup urine disorder
- Nonketotic hyperglycinemia

BOX 9: MR spectroscopy in leukodystrophies.

- *Lactate peak is seen in*:
  - Mitochondrial disorders
  - Krabbe disease
  - Alexander disease
  - Zellweger disease
  - X-linked adrenoleukodystrophy
  - Maple syrup urine disease
- *Increased N-acetylaspartate (NAA) peak*:
  - Canavan disease
- *Phenylalanine peak at 7.37 ppm*:
  - Phenylketonuria.
- *Branched-chain amino acids at 0.9 ppm*:
  - Maple syrup urine disease
- *Glycine peak at 3.56 ppm*:
  - Nonketotic hyperglycinemia
- *Glutamate/glutamine*: 2.55 ppm and 3.68–3.85 ppm
  - Urea cycle disorders

retardation. In the classic form, onset of symptoms occurs before the age of 10 years while the atypical form has an older age of onset.

The striking pathologic finding in affected patients is rust brown pigmentation of the globus pallidus and zona reticulata of substantia nigra. Iron is concentrated in these regions.

Imaging studies reflect the underlying pathology. CT scans show high or low density foci in the globi pallidi. MR imaging shows a pronounced hypointensity of both the globus pallidus and substantia nigra on T2W images resulting from iron deposition.

Imaging reveals a characteristic "eye of the tiger sign" with marked pallidal hypointensity peripherally and hyperintensity centrally. The hyperintense signal represents pallidal destruction and gliosis.

Neuronal Ceroid Lipofuscinosis

These are among the most common progressive encephalopathies of childhood. Eight types have been described and are grouped together because of similar pathologic and clinical presentation. The first symptom is loss of vision followed by progressive dementia, seizures, and progressive impairment of speech and motor function. Definitive diagnosis is made by chromosomal analysis or by electron microscopic analysis of lymphocytes from peripheral blood which shows characteristic curvilinear deposits.

Imaging Findings

There is variable cerebral and cerebellar atrophy associated with high signal rims around ventricles and low signal intensity in the thalami and globi pallidi on T2W images. The T2 changes appear to correlate with loss of myelin and gliosis of unknown origin. Thalamic atrophy develops later. MR spectroscopy shows a complete loss of NAA peak, marked reduction of creatine and choline, and elevation of myoinositol and lactate in gray and white matter.[115] Positron emission tomography (PET) and single-photon emission computed tomography (SPECT) are useful in establishing diagnosis of neuronal ceroid lipofuscinosis (NCL). Severe reduction of metabolism in the cortical and subcortical structures has been shown in 18F-fluorodeoxyglucose PET studies.

Rett Syndrome

Rett syndrome is a progressive neurodevelopmental disorder characterized by autistic-like behavior, gait, ataxia, irregular respiration, seizures, dementia, and microcephaly. On imaging, there is global reduction in gray and white matter volume with the largest reduction in the prefrontal, posterior frontal, anterior temporal cortices, and the caudate nucleus. Proton MR spectroscopy shows decreased NAA in older patients, more pronounced in gray matter than the white matter. The frontal and parietal lobes and insular cortex are the ones which are predominantly involved.

Disorders of Metal Metabolism

Wilson's Disease (Hepatolenticular Degeneration)

Wilson's disease results from an inborn error of copper metabolism and is transmitted in an autosomal recessive manner. It is characterized by a deficiency of ceruloplasmin, the serum transport protein for copper. As a result, copper is abnormally deposited in various tissues with resultant toxicity to these organs. Liver and brain are the most frequently involved with typical involvement of the lenticular nucleus.

Clinical Features

The peak age of presentation is between 8 and 16 years. Typical neurologic signs include tremor, rigidity, dystonia, gait difficulty, incoordination, and dysarthria. The Kayser-Fleischer ring, ring of green pigmentation in cornea, is virtually diagnostic of Wilson's disease.

Imaging Features

Typical sites of cerebral involvement are deep gray matter. Gray matter involvement is usually bilaterally symmetric in the putamen, caudate, thalamus, globus pallidus, dentate nucleus, pons and mesencephalon, and the claustra.[116] Involvement of the claustra is a very characteristic finding and an important differential diagnostic clue in Wilson's disease. The lesions are seen as hyperintensity on long TR images and reflect the pathologic changes of gliosis, edema, and/or necrosis. Mesencephalic involvement is characteristic, the so-called "face of the giant panda sign" **(Figs. 35A to C)**. This consists of high signal throughout the mesencephalon within the substantia nigra (mainly in the

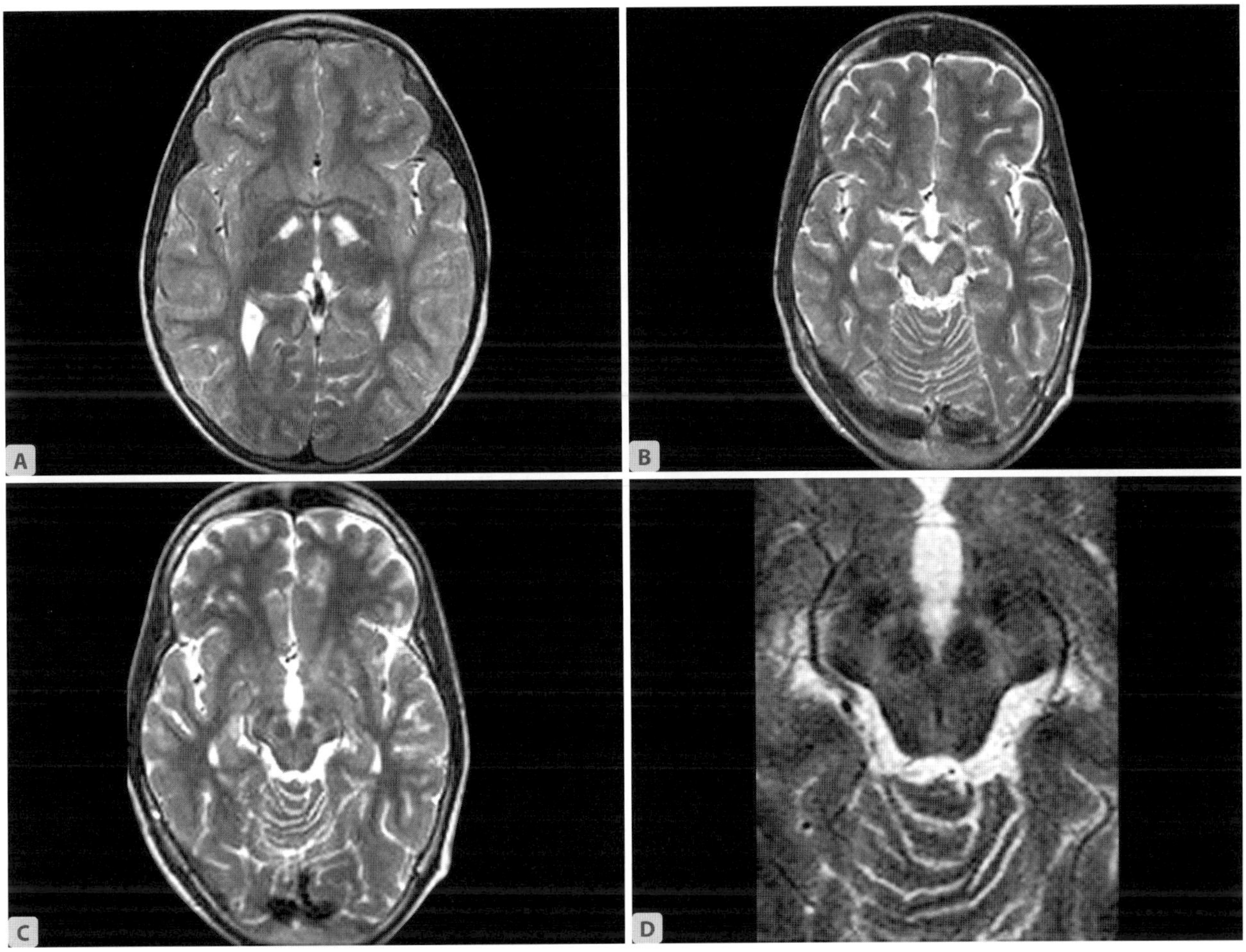

FIGS. 35A TO C: (A and B) Axial T2-weighted (T2W) MR images showing symmetrical signal changes in the putamen seen as a high signal; and (C) High signal is also seen within the substantia nigra and tegmentum with sparing of the red nucleus and tectum "face of giant panda sign"—Wilson's disease.

pars compacta) and the tegmentum of the mesencephalon in contrast with the normal or hypointense appearance of the red nuclei, the cerebral peduncles, and the tectum. Some of these lesions appear to improve or reverse during treatment. In contrast to gray matter lesions, white matter lesions, if present, are symmetric, located in the subcortical regions and are most common in the frontal lobes. The MR findings correlate well with neurologic findings. Lesion location is also useful. For example, dystonia correlates with putaminal lesions, dysarthria with both caudate and putaminal lesion, and distractibility of gaze fixation with frontal lobe involvement. MR spectroscopy shows a decrease in all the metabolites.[116]

Menkes Disease

Menkes disease is related to a defect at the level of the membrane copper transport mechanism.[117] One of the consequences of this is the impairment of the normal intestinal absorption of copper as a result of which a severe copper deficiency develops. On the other hand, transmembrane transport of copper is impaired therefore, copper cannot be delivered to copper-requiring enzymes and hence copper is trapped and accumulated in connective tissues. Serum copper and ceruloplasmin levels are low. The most important manifestations of the disease are, therefore, connective tissue abnormalities and progressive degeneration of the CNS, the latter due to global failure of copper-requiring enzymes, in particular cytochrome c oxidase.

The disease is of X-linked inheritance.[118] The onset of the disease is neonatal, but the patients are typically normal during the first 2 or 3 months of life. Then, there is loss of milestones, convulsions, hypotonia followed by spasticity, and eventually lethargy. Most affected children die during the first year of life. Menkes disease is often referred to as "kinky hair" disease because of the peculiar appearance of the hair.[119,120] Connective tissue abnormalities include bladder diverticulum, inguinal hernia, loose skin, hyperflexible joints, and vessel fragility.

At birth, the brain appears normal on MR imaging. During the course of the disease, rapidly developing atrophy and prominent delay of the myelination become obvious. Shrinking of the brain can be so marked that spontaneous subdural fluid collections (hygroma, subdural hematoma) frequently develop. On the T1W images, the basal ganglia exhibit hypersignal, similar to what is seen in chronic hepatic encephalopathies, including Wilson's disease. The cerebral vessels are usually tortuous and elongated; this can be seen on conventional images, but is better appreciated on MR angiography.

CONCLUSION

There are many different metabolic disorders, each of which has some distinctive features.[121-123] MR imaging is highly sensitive in determining the presence and assessing the severity of underlying abnormalities in patients with metabolic disorders.[124-128] Although the findings are often nonspecific, systematic analysis of the finer details of disease involvement may permit a narrower differential diagnosis, which the clinician can then further refine with knowledge of patient history, clinical testing, and metabolic analysis. MR imaging also has a role in monitoring the natural progression of various metabolic disorders and their response to therapy.

REFERENCES

1. Holland BA, Haas DK, Norman D, Brant-Zawadzki M, Newton TH. MRI of normal brain maturation. AJNR Am J Neuroradiol. 1986;7(2):201-8.
2. Hasegawa M, Houdou S, Mito T, Takashima S, Asanuma K, Ohno T. Development of myelination in the human fetal and infant cerebrum: a myelin basic protein immunohistochemical study. Brain Dev. 1992;14(1):1-6.
3. Barkovich AJ, Kjos BO, Jackson DE, Norman D. Normal maturation of the neonatal and infant brain: MR imaging at 1.5 T. Radiology. 1988;166(1):173-80.
4. Johnson MA, Pennock JM, Bydder GM, Steiner RE, Thomas DJ, Hayward R, et al. Clinical NMR imaging of the brain in children: normal and neurologic disease. AJNR Am J Neuroradiol. 1983;141(5):1005-18.
5. Dietrich RB. Maturation, myelination and dysmyelination. In: Stark DD, Bradley WG (Eds). Magnetic Resonance Imaging, 3rd edition. United States: Mosby; 1999.
6. Barkovich AJ, Jackson DE. MRI assessment of normal and abnormal brain myelinization. MRI Decisions. 1989;3(2):17-25.
7. Dietrich RB, Bradley WG. Normal and abnormal white matter maturation. Semin Ultrasound CT MR. 1988;9(3):192-200.
8. Dietrich RB, Bradley WG, Zaragoza EJ, Otto RJ, Taira RK, Wilson GH, et al. MR evaluation of early myelination patterns in normal and developmentally delayed infants. AJR Am J Roentgenol. 1988;150(4):889-96.
9. Becker LE. Lysosomes, peroxisomes, and mitochondria: function and disorder. AJNR Am J Neuroradiol. 1992;13(2):609-20.
10. Kendall BE. Disorders of lysosomes, peroxisomes, and mitochondria. AJNR Am J Neuroradiol. 1992;13(2):621-53.
11. Demaerel P, Faubert C, Wilms G, Casaer P, Piepgras U, Baert AL. MR findings in leukodystrophy. Neuroradiology. 1991;33(4): 368-71.
12. Kim TS, Kim IO, Kim WS, Choi YS, Lee JY, Kim OW, et al. MR of childhood metachromatic leukodystrophy. AJNR Am J Neuroradiol. 1997;18(4):733-8.
13. Suzuki K, Armao D, Stone JA, Mukherji SK. Demyelinating diseases, leukodystrophies, and other myelin disorders. Neuroimaging Clin N Am. 2001;11(1):15-35.
14. Kolodny EH. Sulfatide lipidosis: Metachromatic leukodystrophy. In: Scriver CR, Beaudet AL, Sly WS, Valle D (Eds). The Metabolic Basis of Inherited Diseases, 6th edition. New York: McGraw Hill; 1989.
15. Wolpert SM, Anderson ML, Kaye EM. Metabolic and degenerative disorders. In: Wolpert SM, Barnes PD (Eds). MRI in Pediatric Neuroradiology. United States: Mosby; 1992.
16. Nusbaum AO, Rapaleno O, Fung KM, Atlas SW. White matter diseases and inherited metabolic disorders. In: Atlas SW (Ed). Magnetic Resonance Imaging of the Brain and Spine, 94th edition. Lippincott: Williams and Wilkins; 2009.
17. Waltz G, Harik SI, Haufman B. Adult metachromatic leukodystrophy. Arch Neurol. 1987;44:225.
18. Faerber EN, Melvin J, Smergel EM. MRI appearances of metachromatic leukodystrophy. Pediatr Radiol. 1999;29(9):669-72.
19. Nowell MA, Grossman RI, Hackney DB, Zimmerman RA, Goldberg HI, Bilaniuk LT. MR imaging of white matter disease in children. AJR Am J Roentgenol. 1988;151(2):359-65.
20. Sener RN. Metachromatic leukodystrophy: Diffusion MR imaging findings. AJNR Am J Neuroradiol. 2002;23(8):1424-6.
21. Patay Z. Diffusion-weighted MR imaging in leukodystrophies. Eur Radiol. 2005;15(11):2284-303.
22. Kruse B, Hanefeld F, Christen HJ, Bruhn H, Michaelis T, Hänicke W, et al. Alterations of brain metabolites in metachromatic leukodystrophy as detected by localized proton magnetic resonance spectroscopy in vivo. J Neurol. 1993;241(2):68-74.
23. Suzuki Y, Suzuki K. Krabbe's globoid cell leukodystrophy: deficiency of galactocerebrosidase in serum, leukocytes, and fibroblast. Science. 1971;171(3966):73-5.
24. Zlotogora J, Chakraborty S, Knowlton RG, Wenger DA. Krabbe disease locus mapped to chromosome 14 by genetic linkage. Am J Hum Genet. 1990;47(1):37-44.
25. Loes DJ, Peters C, Kriwit W. Globoid cell leukodystrophy: distinguishing early-onset from late-onset disease using a brain MR imaging scoring method. AJNR Am J Neuroradiol. 1999;20(2):316-23.
26. Demaerel P, Wilms G, Vendue P. MR findings in globoid leukodystrophy. Neuroradiology. 1990;32:520.
27. Kolodny EH, Raghavan S, Krivit W. Late-onset Krabbe disease (globoid cell leukodystrophy): clinical and biochemical features of 15 cases. Dev Neurosci. 1991;13(4-5):232-9.
28. Lyon G, Hagberg B, Evard P, Allaire C, Pavone L, Vanier M. Symptomatology of late onset Krabbe's leukodystrophy: the European experience. Dev Neurosci. 1991;13(4-5):240-4.
29. Krivit W, Shapiro EG, Peters C, Wagner JE, Cornu G, Kurtzberg J, et al. Hematopoietic stem-cell transplantation in globoid-cell leukodystrophy. N Engl J Med. 1998;338(16): 1119-26.
30. Barone R, Brühl K, Stoeter P, Fiumara A, Pavone L, Beck M. Clinical and neuroradiological findings in classic infantile and late-onset globoid-cell leukodystrophy (Krabbe disease). Am J Med Genet. 1996;63(1):209-17.
31. Vanhanen SL, Raininko R, Santavuori P. Early differential diagnosis of infantile neuronal ceroid lipofuscinosis, Rett syndrome, and Krabbe disease by CT and MR. AJNR Am J Neuroradiol. 1994;15(8):1443-53.
32. Choi S, Enzmann DR. Infantile Krabbe disease: complementary CT and MR findings. AJNR Am J Neuroradiol. 1993;14(5):1164-6.
33. Jones BV, Barron TF, Towfighi J. Optic nerve enlargement in Krabbe disease. AJNR Am J Neuroradiol. 1999;20(7):1228-31.

34. Compston A. A new familial infantile form of diffuse brain-sclerosis. Brain. 2013;136(Pt 9):2649-51.
35. Baker RH, Trautmann JC, Younge BR, Nelson KD, Zimmerman D. Late juvenile-onset Krabbe's disease. Ophthalmology. 1990; 97(9):1176-80.
36. Loes DJ, Hite S, Moser H, Stillman AE, Shapiro E, Lockman L, et al. Adrenoleukodystrophy: a scoring method for brain MR observations. AJNR Am J Neuroradiol. 1994;15(9):1761-6.
37. Vasconcellos E, Smith M. MRI nerve root enhancement in Krabbe disease. Pediatr Neurol. 1998;19(2):151-2.
38. Kim MJ, Provenzale JM, Law M. Magnetic resonance and diffusion tensor imaging in pediatric white matter diseases. Top Magn Reson Imaging. 2006;17(4):265-74.
39. Provenzale JM, Escolar M, Kurtzberg J. Quantitative analysis of diffusion tensor imaging data in serial assessment of Krabbe disease. Ann N Y Acad Sci. 2005;1064(1):220-9.
40. McGraw P, Liang L, Escolar M, Mukundan S, Kurtzberg J, Provenzale JM. Krabbe disease treated with hematopoietic stem cell transplantation: serial assessment of anisotropy measurements—initial experience. Radiology. 2005;236(1): 221-30.
41. Okada S, O'Brien JS. Sandhoff's disease (GM2 gangliosidosis type 2): clinical, chemical, and enzyme studies in five patients. Pediatr Res. 1972;6(7):606-15.
42. Menzies DG, Campbell IW, Kean DM. Magnetic resonance imaging in Fabry's disease. J Neurol Neurosurg Psychiatry. 1988;51(9):1240-1.
43. Mirowitz SA, Sartor K, Prensky AJ, Gado M, Hodges FJ. Neurodegenerative diseases of childhood: MR and CT evaluation. J Comput Assist Tomogr. 1991;15(2):210-22.
44. Murata R, Nakajima S, Tanaka A, Miyagi N, Matsuoka O, Kogame S. MR imaging of the brain in patients with mucopolysaccharidosis. Am J Neuroradiol. 1989;10(6):1165-70.
45. Johnson MA, Desai S, Hugh-Jones K, Starer F. Magnetic resonance imaging of the brain in Hurler syndrome. AJNR Am J Neuroradiol. 1984;5(6):816-9.
46. Watts RW, Spellacy E, Kendall BE, du Boulay G, Gibbs DA. Computed tomography studies on patients with mucopolysaccharidoses. Neuroradiology. 1981;21(1):9-23.
47. Moser HW. Adrenoleukodystrophy: phenotype, genetics, pathogenesis and therapy. Brain. 1997;120(Pt 8):1485-508.
48. Bezman L, Moser HW. Incidence of X-linked adrenoleukodystrophy and the relative frequency of its phenotypes. Am J Med Genet. 1998;76(5):415-9.
49. Griffin JW, Goren E, Schaumburg H, Engel WK, Loriaux L. Adrenomyeloneuropathy: a probable variant of adrenoleukodystrophy I. Clinical and endocrinologic aspects. Neurology. 1977;27(12):1107-13.
50. Schaumburg HH, Powers JM, Raine CS, Richardson E. Adrenoleukodystrophy. A clinical and pathological study of 17 cases. Arch Neurol. 1975;32(9):577-91.
51. Powers JM, Liu Y, Moser AB, Moser HW. The inflammatory myelinopathy of adrenoleukodystrophy: cells, effector molecules, and pathogenetic implications. J Neuropathol Exp Neurol. 1992;51(6):630-43.
52. Jensen ME, Sawyer RW, Braun IF, Rizzo WB. MR imaging appearance of childhood adrenoleukodystrophy with auditory, visual, and motor pathway involvement. Radiographics. 1990;10(1):53-66.
53. Kumar AJ, Rosenbaum AE, Naidu S, Wener L, Citrin CM, Lindenberg R, et al. Adrenoleukodystrophy: correlating MR imaging with CT. Radiology. 1987;165(2):497-504.
54. Ono J, Kodaka R, Imai K, Itagaki Y, Tanaka J, Inui K, et al. Evaluation of myelination by means of the T2 value on magnetic resonance imaging. Brain Dev. 1993;15(6):433-8.
55. Melhem ER, Breiter SN, Ulug AM, Raymond GV, Moser HW. Improved tissue characterization in adrenoleukodystrophy using magnetization transfer imaging. AJR Am J Roentgenol. 1996;166(3):689-95.
56. Melhem ER, Loes DJ, Georgiades CS, Raymond GV, Moser HW. X-linked adrenoleukodystrophy: the role of contrast-enhanced MR imaging in predicting disease progression. AJNR Am J Neuroradiol. 2000;21(5):839-44.
57. Barkovich AJ, Ferriero DM, Bass N, Boyer R. Involvement of the pontomedullary corticospinal tracts: a useful finding in the diagnosis of X-linked adrenoleukodystrophy. AJNR Am J Neuroradiol. 1997;18(1):95-100.
58. Castellote A, Vera J, Vazquez E, Roig M, Belmonte JA, Rovira A. MR in adrenoleukodystrophy: atypical presentation as bilateral frontal demyelination. AJNR Am J Neuroradiol. 1995;16(4): 814-5.
59. Tzika AA, Ball WS, Vigneron DB, Dunn RS, Nelson SJ, Kirks DR. Childhood adrenoleukodystrophy: assessment with proton MR spectroscopy. Radiology. 1993;189(2):467-80.
60. Warren DJ, Connolly DJ, Wilkinson ID, Sharrard MJ, Griffiths PD. Magnetic resonance spectroscopy changes following haemopoietic stem cell transplantation in children with cerebral adrenoleukodystrophy. Dev Med Child Neurol. 2007;49(2): 135-9.
61. Wilken B, Dechent P, Brockmann K, Finsterbusch J, Baumann M, Ebell W, et al. Quantitative proton magnetic resonance spectroscopy of children with adrenoleukodystrophy before and after hematopoietic stem cell transplantation. Neuropediatrics. 2003;34(5):237-46.
62. Fatemi A, Smith SA, Dubey P, Zackowski KM, Bastian AJ, van Zijl PC, et al. Magnetization transfer MRI demonstrates spinal cord abnormalities in adrenomyeloneuropathy. Neurology. 2005;64(10):1739-45.
63. Barkovich AJ, Peck WW. MR of Zellweger syndrome. AJNR Am J Neuroradiol. 1997;18(6):1163-70.
64. Cheon JE, Kim IO, Hwang YS, Kim KJ, Wang KC, Cho BK, et al. Leukodystrophy in children: a pictorial review of MR imaging features. Radiographics. 2002;22(3):461-76.
65. Hokezu Y, Kuriyama M, Kubota R, Nakagawa M, Fujiyama J, Osame M. Cerebrotendinous xanthomatosis: cranial CT and MRI studies in eight patients. Neuroradiology. 1992;34(4): 308-12.
66. Matalon R, Michals K, Sebesta D, Deanching M, Gashkoff P, Casanova J. Aspartoacylase deficiency and N-acetylaspartic aciduria in patients with Canavan disease. Am J Med Genet. 1988;29(2):463-71.
67. Grodd W, Krägeloh-Mann I, Petersen D, Trefz FK, Harzer K. In vivo assessment of N-acetylaspartate in brain in spongy degeneration (Canavan's disease) by proton spectroscopy. Lancet. 1990;336(8712):437-8.
68. Patel PJ, Kolawole TM, Mahdi AH, Wright EA. Sonographic and computed tomographic findings in Canavan's disease. Br J Radiol. 1986;59(708):1226-8.
69. Brismar J, Brismar G, Gascon G, Ozand P. Canavan disease: CT and MR imaging of the brain. AJNR Am J Neuroradiol. 1990;11(4): 805-10.
70. McAdams HP, Geyer CA, Done SL, Deigh D, Mitchell M, Ghaed VN. CT and MR imaging of Canavan disease. AJNR Am J Neuroradiol. 1990;11(2):397-9.
71. Srikanth SG, Chandrashekar HS, Nagarajan K, Jayakumar PN. Restricted diffusion in Canavan disease. Childs Nerv Syst. 2007;23(4):465-8.
72. Lyon G, Fattal-Valevski A, Kolodny EH. Leukodystrophies: clinical and genetic aspects. Top Magn Reson Imaging. 2006;17(4): 219-42.

73. Borrett D, Becker LE. Alexander's disease: a disease of astrocytes. Brain. 1985;108(2):367-85.
74. Shah M, Ross JS. Infantile Alexander disease: MR appearance of a biopsy-proved case. AJNR Am J Neuroradiol. 1990;11(6):1105-6.
75. Trommer BL, Naidich TP, Canto MC, McLone DG, Larsen MB. Noninvasive CT diagnosis of infantile Alexander disease: pathologic correlation. J Comput Assist Tomogr. 1983;7(3): 509-16.
76. van der Knaap MS, Barth PG, Gabreëls FJ, Franzoni E, Begeer JH, Stroink H, et al. A new leukoencephalopathy with vanishing white matter. Neurology. 1997;48(4):845-54.
77. Sijens PE, Boon M, Meiners LC, Brouwer OF, Oudkerk M. 1H chemical shift imaging, MRI, and diffusion-weighted imaging in vanishing white matter disease. Eur Radiol. 2005;15(11):2377-9.
78. Seitelberger F. Neuropathology and genetics of Pelizaeus-Merzbacher disease. Brain Pathol. 1995;5(3):267-73.
79. Silverstein AM, Hirsh DK, Trobe JD, Gebarski S. MR imaging of the brain in five members of a family with Pelizaeus-Merzbacher disease. AJNR Am J Neuroradiol. 1990;11(3):495-9.
80. van der Knaap MS, Valk J. The reflection of histology in MR imaging of Pelizaeus-Merzbacher disease. AJNR Am J Neuroradiol. 1989;10(1):99-103.
81. Honkaniemi J, Kähärä V, Dastidar P, Latvala M, Hietaharju A, Salonen T, et al. Reversible posterior leukoencephalopathy after combination chemotherapy. Neuroradiology. 2000;42(12):895-9.
82. Kingsley PB, Shah TC, Woldenberg R. Identification of diffuse and focal brain lesions by clinical magnetic resonance spectroscopy. NMR Biomed. 2006;19(4):435-62.
83. Pavlakis SG, Phillips PC, DiMauro S, De Vivo DC, Rowland LP. Mitochondrial myopathy, encephalopathy, lactic acidosis, and strokelike episodes: a distinctive clinical syndrome. Ann Neurol. 1984;16(4):481-8.
84. Barkovich AJ, Good WV, Koch TK, Berg BO. Mitochondrial disorders: analysis of their clinical and imaging characteristics. AJNR Am J Neuroradiol. 1993;14(5):1119-37.
85. Allard JC, Tilak S, Carter AP. CT and MR of MELAS syndrome. AJNR Am J Neuroradiol. 1988;9(6):1234-8.
86. Kim IO, Kim JH, Kim WS, Hwang YS, Yeon KM, Han MC. Mitochondrial myopathy-encephalopathy-lactic acidosis-and stroke like episodes (MELAS) syndrome: CT and MR findings in seven children. AJR Am J Roentgenol. 1996;166(3):641-5.
87. Rosen L, Phillips S, Enzmann D. Magnetic resonance imaging in MELAS syndrome. Neuroradiology. 1990;32(2):168-71.
88. Ducreux D, Nasser G, Lacroix C, Adams D, Lasjaunias P. MR diffusion tensor imaging, fiber tracking, and single-voxel spectroscopy findings in an unusual MELAS case. AJNR Am J Neuroradiol. 2005;26(7):1840-4.
89. Wray SH, Provenzale JM, Johns DR, Thulborn KR. MR of the brain in mitochondrial myopathy. AJNR Am J Neuroradiol. 1995;16(5):1167-73.
90. Fukuhara N, Tokiguchi S, Shirakawa K, Tsubaki T. Myoclonus epilepsy associated with ragged-red fibres (mitochondrial abnormalities): disease entity or a syndrome? Light- and electron-microscopic studies of two cases and review of literature. J Neurol Sci. 1980;47(1):117-33.
91. Kearns TP, Sayre GP. Retinitis pigmentosa, external ophthalmoplegia, and complete heart block: unusual syndrome with histologic study in one of two cases. AMA Arch Ophthalmol. 1958;60(2):280-9.
92. Leutner C, Layer G, Zierz S, Solymosi L, Dewes W, Reiser M. Cerebral MR in ophthalmoplegia plus. AJNR Am J Neuroradiol. 1994;15(4):681-7.
93. Sandhu FS, Dillon WP. MR demonstration of leukoencephalopathy associated with mitochondrial encephalomyopathy: case report. AJNR Am J Neuroradiol. 1991;12(2):375-9.
94. DiMauro S, Servidei S, Zeviani M, DiRocco M, DeVivo DC, DiDonato S, et al. Cytochrome c oxidase deficiency in Leigh syndrome. Ann Neurol. 1987;22(4):498-506.
95. Chi JG, Yoo HW, Chang KH, Kim CW, Moon HR, Ko KW. Leigh's subacute necrotizing encephalomyelopathy: possible diagnosis by CT scan. Neuroradiology. 1981;22(3):141-4.
96. Berkovic SF, Karpati G, Carpenter S, Lang AE. Progressive dystonia with bilateral putaminal hypodensities. Arch Neurol. 1987;44(11):1184-7.
97. Koch TK, Yee MH, Hutchinson HT, Berg BO. Magnetic resonance imaging in subacute necrotizing encephalomyelopathy (Leigh's disease). Ann Neurol. 1986;19(6):605-7.
98. Medina L, Chi TL, DeVivo DC, Hilal SK. MR findings in patients with subacute necrotizing encephalomyelopathy (Leigh syndrome): correlation with biochemical defect. AJR Am J Roentgenol. 1990;154(6):1269-74.
99. Leigh D. Subacute necrotizing encephalomyelopathy in an infant. J Neurol Neurosurg Psychiatry. 1951;14(3):216-21.
100. Atalar MH, Egilmez H, Bulut S, Icagasioglu D. Magnetic resonance spectroscopy and diffusion-weighted imaging findings in a child with Leigh's disease. Pediatr Int. 2005;47(5):601-3.
101. Chen YF, Huang YC, Liu HM, Hwu WL. MRI in a case of adult-onset citrullinemia. Neuroradiology. 2001;43(10):845-7.
102. Connelly A, Cross JH, Gadian DG, Hunter JV, Kirkham FJ, Leonard JV. Magnetic resonance spectroscopy shows increased brain glutamine in ornithine carbamoyl transferase deficiency. Pediatr Res. 1993;33(1):77-81.
103. Pearsen KD, Gean-Marton AD, Levy HL, Davis KR. Phenylketonuria: MR imaging of the brain with clinical correlation. Radiology. 1990;177(2):437-40.
104. Phillips MD, McGraw P, Lowe MJ, Mathews VP, Hainline BE. Diffusion-weighted imaging of white matter abnormalities in patients with phenylketonuria. AJNR Am J Neuroradiol. 2001;22(8):1583-6.
105. Pietz J, Kreis R, Schmidt H, Meyding-Lamadé, Rupp A, Boesch C. Phenylketonuria: findings at MR imaging and localized in vivo H-1 MR spectroscopy of the brain in patients with early treatment. Radiology. 1996;201(2):413-20.
106. Brismar J, Aqeel A, Brismar G, Coates R, Gascon G, Ozand P. Maple syrup urine disease: findings on CT and MR scans of the brain in 10 infants. AJNR Am J Neuroradiol. 1990;11(6):1219-28.
107. Fariello G, Dionisi-Vici C, Orazi C, Malena S, Bartuli A, Schingo P, et al. Cranial ultrasonography in maple syrup urine disease. AJNR Am J Neuroradiol. 1996;17(2):311-5.
108. Jan W, Zimmerman RA, Wang ZJ, Berry GT, Kaplan PB, Kaye EM, et al. MR diffusion imaging and MR spectroscopy of maple syrup urine disease during acute metabolic decompensation. Neuroradiology. 2003;45(6):393-9.
109. Rossi A, Cerone R, Biancheri R, Gatti R, Schiaffino MC, Fonda C, et al. Early-onset combined methylmalonic aciduria and homocystinuria: neuroradiologic findings. AJNR Am J Neuroradiol. 2001;22(3):554-63.
110. Press GA, Barshop BA, Haas RH, Nyhan WL, Glass RF, Hesselink JR. Abnormalities of the brain in nonketotic hyperglycinemia: MR manifestations. AJNR Am J Neuroradiol. 1989;10(2):315-21.
111. Al Tawari AA, Ramadan DG, Neubauer D, Heberle LC, Awadi FA. An early onset form of methylenetetrahydrofolate reductase deficiency: a report of a family from Kuwait. Brain Dev. 2002;24(5):304-9.

112. Brismar J, Ozand PT. CT and MR of the brain in the diagnosis of organic acidemias. Experiences from 107 patients. Brain Dev. 1994;16 Suppl:104-24.
113. Ozand PT, Rashed M, Millington DS, Sakati N, Hazzaa S, Rahbeeni Z, et al. Ethylmalonic aciduria: an organic acidemia with CNS involvement and vasculopathy. Brain Dev. 1994;16(Suppl): 12-22.
114. Brismar J, Ozand PT. CT and MR of the brain in glutaric acidemia type I: a review of 59 published cases and a report of 5 new patients. AJNR Am J Neuroradiol. 1995;16(4):675-83.
115. Brockmann K, Pouwels PJ, Christen HJ, Frahm J, Hanefeld F. Localized proton magnetic resonance spectroscopy of cerebral metabolic disturbances in children with neuronal ceroid lipofuscinosis. Neuropediatrics. 1996;27(5):242-8.
116. Jayasundar R, Sahani AK, Gaikwad S, Singh S, Behari M. Proton MR spectroscopy of basal ganglia in Wilson's disease: case report and review of literature. Magn Reson Imaging. 2002;20(1):131-5.
117. Jacobs DS, Smith AS, Finelli DA, Lanzieri CF, Wiznitzer M. Menkes kinky hair disease: characteristic MR angiographic findings. AJNR Am J Neuroradiol. 1993;14(5):1160-3.
118. Patay Z, Blaser SI, Poretti A, Huisman TA. Neurometabolic diseases of childhood. Pediatr Radiol. 2015;45(3):473-84.
119. Mankad K, Talenti G, Tan AP, Gonçalves FG, Robles C, Kan EY, et al. Neurometabolic Disorders of the Newborn. Top Magn Reson Imaging. 2018;27(4):179-96.
120. Ibrahim M, Parmar HA, Hoefling N, Srinivasan A. Inborn errors of metabolism: combining clinical and radiologic clues to solve the mystery. AJR Am J Roentgenol. 2014;203(3):W315-27.
121. Reddy N, Calloni SF, Vernon HJ, Boltshauser E, Huisman TA, Soares BP. Neuroimaging findings of organic acidemias and aminoacidopathies. Radiographics. 2018;38(3):912-31.
122. Bray MD, Mullins ME. Metabolic white matter diseases and the utility of MR spectroscopy. Radiol Clin North Am. 2014;52(2):403-11.
123. Reichert R, Campos LG, Vairo F, de Souza CF, Pérez JA, Duarte JA, et al. Neuroimaging findings in patients with mucopolysaccharidosis: What you really need to know. Radiographics. 2016;36(5):1448-62.
124. de Oliveira AM, Paulino MV, Vieira AP, McKinney AM, da Rocha AJ, Santos GT, et al. Imaging patterns of toxic and metabolic brain disorders. Radiographics. 2019;39(6):1672-95.
125. Yang E, Prabhu SP. Imaging manifestations of the leukodystrophies, inherited disorders of white matter. Radiol Clin North Am. 2014;52(2):279-319.
126. Messing A, Brenner M, Feany MB, Nedergaard M, Goldman JE. Alexander disease. J Neurosci. 2012;32(15):5017-23.
127. Bhat M, Prasad C, Bindu PS, Aziz Z, Christopher R, Saini J. Unusual imaging findings in brain and spinal cord in two siblings with maple syrup urine disease. J Neuroimaging. 2013;23(4):540-2.
128. Sofou K, Steneryd K, Wiklund LM, Tulinius M, Darin N. MRI of the brain in childhood-onset mitochondrial disorders with central nervous system involvement. Mitochondrion. 2013;13(4):364-71.

CHAPTER

90

Pediatric Neck Lesions

Smita Manchanda, Ashu Seith Bhalla

INTRODUCTION

In the pediatric head and neck region, majority of the lesions are benign in nature, with congenital and inflammatory lesions accounting for a large number of these lesions. Even though many malignant tumors in children present as neck masses, they are responsible for only a small proportion. The common differentials of pediatric neck lesions are enlisted in **Box 1**. In this chapter, we will provide an overview of conditions that present as neck lesions in the pediatric age group along with a brief description of the entities specific to the neonatal period.

CONGENITAL

Branchial Cleft Anomalies

Introduction

The embryological precursors of the face, neck, and pharynx are the branchial arches. Anomalies of the branchial arches present as cysts, sinus, or fistulae in characteristic locations. These are the second most common congenital neck lesion, with the thyroglossal cyst being most common.

BOX 1: Etiology of neck masses in the pediatric age group.

- Congenital:
  - Branchial cleft anomalies, thyroid lesions (thyroglossal duct cyst, ectopic thyroid, congenital goiter), cervical thymus, dermoid and epidermoid cyst, and vascular lesions
- Inflammatory:
  - Lymphadenitis, deep neck infections
- Neoplasms:
  - Teratomas, lipoma, lipoblastoma, neurogenic tumors, neuroblastic tumors, rhabdomyosarcoma, inflammatory myofibroblastic tumor, juvenile nasopharyngeal angiofibroma, lymphoma, and epithelial malignancies
- Miscellaneous:
  - Desmoid infantile fibromatosis

Embryological Development of the Branchial Arches

Branchial arches are the embryological precursors of the ear and cartilage, bones, mucosal lining, blood vessels, and muscles of neck, face, and pharynx. Though six pairs of arches develop from the pharyngeal foregut in craniocaudal succession, the fifth arch is usually rudimentary/never forms and hence does not contribute to these anatomical structures. The embryological derivatives of arches I to IV and VI have been detailed in **Table 1**.[1]

Clinical Presentation

Branchial cleft cysts represent approximately one-fifth of cervical masses in children. Out of these, approximately 95% cases are second branchial arch anomalies and 1–4% cases are first branchial arch anomalies. The third and fourth arch anomalies are extremely rare. In approximately 2–3% of cases, these anomalies may be bilateral and then they are mostly familial.[2]

The clinical presentation can vary as follows (depending on the pattern of obliteration of any branchial tract):

- *Branchial cysts*:
  - Cyst forms when there is no communication with the inner mucosa or outer skin
  - Present in older children/young adults.
- *Branchial fistulas*:
  - A communication exists between two epithelialized surfaces, i.e., persistent pouch and cleft
  - Present in infants/young children.
- *Branchial sinus*:
  - Sinus is a blind-ending tract and may connect with either the skin (branchial cleft sinus) or with the pharynx (branchial pouch sinus).

Types

1. **Second branchial cleft anomalies**

   These commonly present as a fistula or cyst in the lower anterior or lateral region of the neck. Classically, swelling or opening is seen in the submandibular space or at the anterior border of the sternocleidomastoid muscle (SCM)

TABLE 1: Embryological derivatives of branchial arches.

Pharyngeal arch numbers	Supplying artery	Cranial nerve	Branchiomeric muscles	Skeletal derivatives	Adult derivatives
I	Maxillary artery	Trigeminal	Muscles of mastication	Malleus, incus, mandible, maxilla, zygomatic bone, palatine bone, squamous temporal bone, vomer, and Meckel's cartilage	Middle ear auditory tube
II	Hyoid artery, stapedial artery	Facial	Muscles of facial expression	Stapes, styloid process, lesser horn of the hyoid bone, and part of hyoid body	Supratonsillar fossa, tonsillar crypts
III	Carotid artery	Glossopharyngeal	Stylopharyngeus	Greater horn of hyoid, part of hyoid body	Thymus, inferior parathyroid glands
IV	Subclavian artery and aorta	Vagus and superior laryngeal nerve	Pharyngeal musculature, cricothyroid	Laryngeal cartilages	Superior parathyroid glands, postbranchial body
VI	Proximal pulmonary artery	Vagus and recurrent laryngeal nerve	Laryngeal musculature except cricothyroid	Laryngeal cartilages	-

Source: Adapted from Adams A, Mankad K, Offiah C, Childs L. Branchial cleft anomalies: a pictorial review of embryological development and spectrum of imaging findings. Insights Imaging. 2016;7:69-76.

within the lower part of the neck. However, these can occur anywhere along the course of the second branchial arch tract (from the skin overlying the supraclavicular fossa, between the external and internal carotid arteries, and entering the pharynx at the level of the tonsillar fossa).

- *Subtypes (by Bailey in 1929)*:[3]
  - *Type I*: Lies along the anterior surface of SCM, but deep to the platysma and is not in contact with the carotid sheath.
  - *Type II*: Most common subtype and lies anterior to SCM and posterior to submandibular gland. It is usually adjacent and lateral to the carotid sheath.
  - *Type III*: Extends medially between bifurcation of internal carotid artery (ICA) and external carotid artery (ECA) and is lateral to the pharyngeal wall.
  - *Type IV*: Lies deep to the carotid sheath within the mucosal space and it opens into the pharynx.
- *Imaging*:
  - *Ultrasonography (USG)*: Well-circumscribed, thin-walled, and anechoic cysts with evidence of compressibility, may contain internal echoes/internal debris[4] **(Fig. 1A)**.
  - *Computed tomography (CT)*: Cyst appears as a well-circumscribed, low-density, and thin-walled lesion. In cases of superadded infection, the cyst becomes thick-walled with localized inflammatory change and fat stranding. The location of the cyst is typically at the anteromedial border of the SCM (at junction of its upper and middle third), behind the submandibular gland, and lateral to the carotid space **(Fig. 1B)**.

    The external opening of a fistula is along the anterior border of the SCM (at the junction of its middle and lower third) and the internal opening lies in the region of the palatine tonsillar fossa **(Figs. 2A and B)**.
  - *Magnetic resonance imaging (MRI)*: Cyst is hyperintense on T2-weighted image (T2WI), variable signal intensity (SI) (low to high signal depending on the proteinaceous content of the cyst) on T1-weighted image (T1WI). Infected cysts will show thick enhancing wall with surrounding inflammatory changes. Fistulous tract can be well-demonstrated on MR fistulogram.
  - Bailey type III cysts classically have a tissue "beak" between the ICAs and ECAs.
  - *Management*: Management is surgical with complete excision and dissection of the cyst/sinus tract.

2. **First branchial cleft anomalies**

These are also present as cyst/fistula/sinus between the external auditory canal and submandibular area, but can occur anywhere along the course of the first branchial arch cleft. This course extends from a cutaneous opening in the submandibular triangle, ascending to the parotid gland region, and ending at the bony/cartilaginous junction of the external auditory canal. It can pass above/below the facial nerve.

Patient usually has a pit-like depression at the angle of mandible with purulent discharge with submandibular lymphadenitis (if infected). An inflammatory mass in the parotid region or drainage of mucus/pus from the external auditory canal in a young patient is also suggestive of first branchial arch anomaly.[5]

- Subtypes:[6]
  - *Type I anomalies*: Ectodermal in origin, seen as cystic masses adjacent to the external auditory canal.
  - *Type II anomalies*: Ectodermal and mesodermal in origin, clinically present as cyst/sinus/fistula in the region of angle of mandible.
- *Imaging*: Cystic lesion is seen in the parotid region with surrounding inflammation (if infected). The cyst

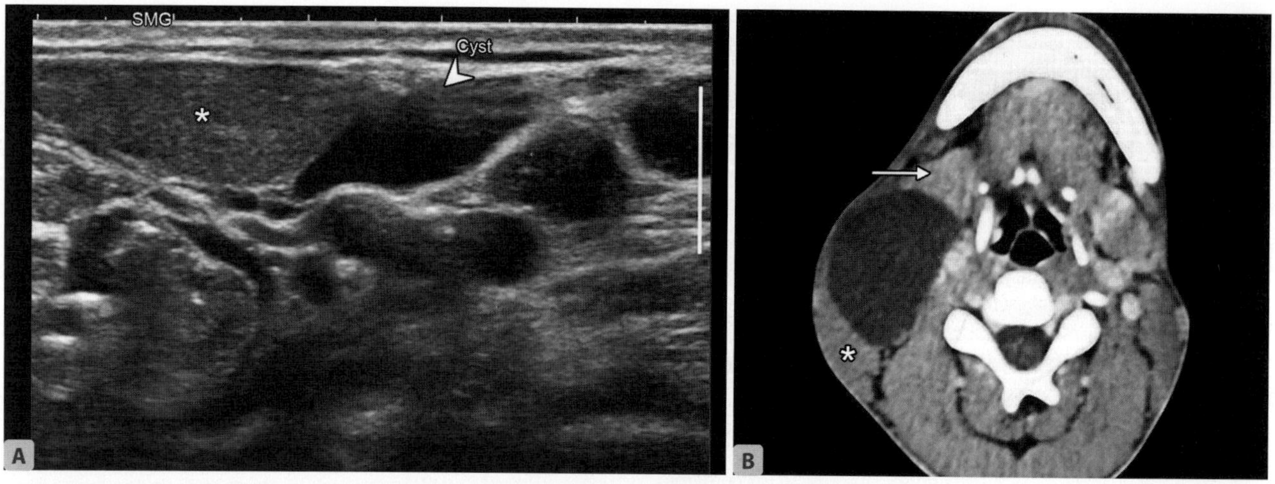

FIGS. 1A AND B: Second branchial cleft cyst type II. (A) Ultrasonography (USG) shows a lobulated cystic lesion (arrowhead) posterior to submandibular gland (asterisk); and (B) CECT shows a well-defined fluid attenuation lesion located posterior to the right submandibular gland (arrow) and anterior to the sternocleidomastoid muscle (SCM) (asterisk). (CECT: contrast-enhanced computed tomography)

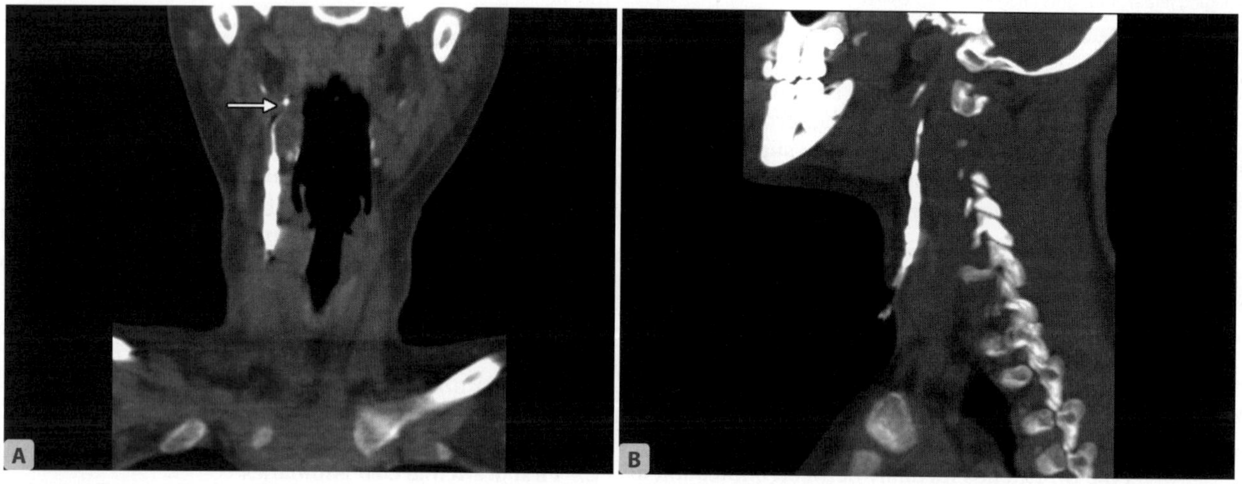

FIGS. 2A AND B: Second branchial fistula type IV. (A) Coronal MPR of CT sinogram. Linear contrast-filled tract in anterior neck extending from C6 vertebral level superomedially (arrow); and (B) Sagittal MIP image of CT sinogram. The tract is anterior to thyroid gland and extending along the right parapharyngeal space with internal opening in the oropharynx at the level of soft palate. (CT: computed tomography; MIP: maximum intensity projection; MPR: multiplanar reconstruction)

can lie superficial/within/deep to the parotid gland **(Figs. 3A and B)**. Delineation of the entire tract in case of a fistula or sinus by contrast sinogram or MRI is essential for preoperative mapping.

- *Management*: Management is surgical with complete resection of the sinus tract and utilizes a superficial parotidectomy approach with preservation of facial nerve. Excision of the cutaneous tract may require excision of part of skin and cartilage of the external auditory canal.

3. **Third and fourth branchial cleft anomalies**

In these sinus/fistulae, the external cutaneous opening in the supraclavicular area is similar to that of the second branchial cleft anomalies; however, internally the tract differs in the third and fourth branchial cleft anomalies. This tract enters the pharynx through the pyriform sinus, below the hyoid bone with third cleft anomalies above, and fourth pharyngeal cleft anomalies below the level of the superior laryngeal nerve. Fourth branchial cleft sinus/fistula tract presents as a sinus from the pyriform fossa apex along the tracheoesophageal groove to the superior aspect of left thyroid lobe. Recurrent abscess in the lower anterior neck/recurrent infective thyroiditis can be the clinical presentation in cases of repeated infection.

Third branchial cleft cysts are seen typically in the posterior cervical space, posterior to the SCM. Infected lesions present as posterior cervical space abscesses.

- *Imaging*: Attempt should be made to delineate the tract and barium studies in combination with CT/MR sinogram may be required.
- *Management*: Complete resection with open neck surgery is technically difficult because of the complex anatomical course. Endoscopic route with cauterization is preferred in some institutes.

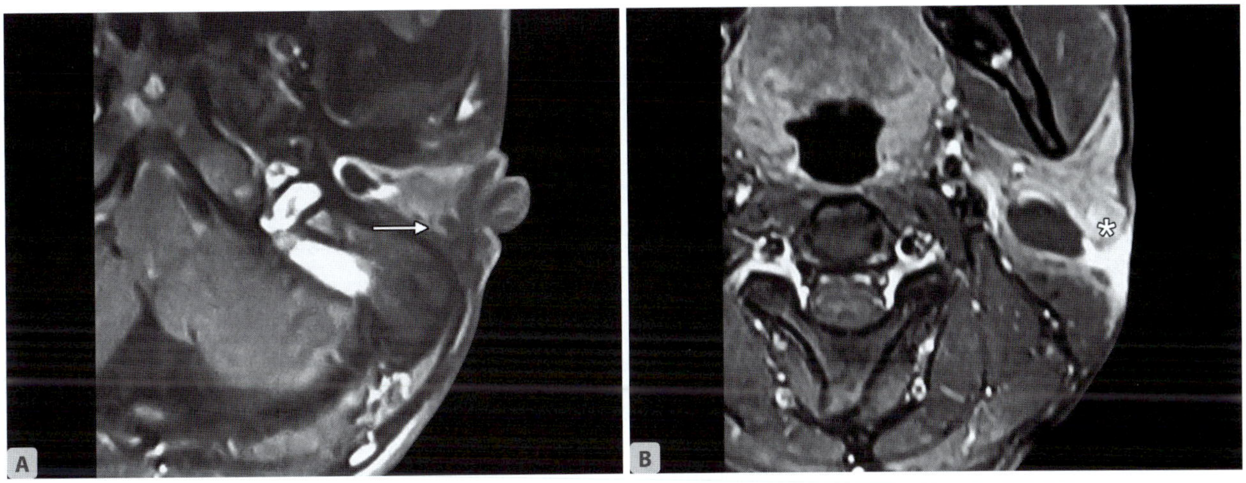

FIGS. 3A AND B: First branchial sinus. (A and B) Axial postcontrast T1-weighted images (T1WIs) of a child presenting with purulent ear discharge demonstrate a thick-walled sinus tract (white arrow) extending to the clinically apparent opening in the left external auditory canal. There is associated inflammation and abscess formation (asterisk) in the periparotid location.

TABLE 2: Common locations and differential diagnosis of branchial arch anomalies.

Types	Characteristic location	Key imaging differentials
First branchial cleft cyst	Cystic lesion in the parotid or periparotid region	• Parotitis/parotid abscess • Sialocoele • Lymphatic malformation • Lymphoepithelial cyst • Cystic pilomatrixoma
Second branchial cleft cyst	Cyst at anteromedial border of the sternocleidomastoid muscle behind submandibular gland and lateral to the carotid space	• Lymphadenopathy • Abscess • Lymphatic malformation
Third branchial cleft cyst	Cyst in the posterior cervical space	• Abscess • Lymphatic malformation • Infrahyoid thyroglossal duct cyst • Cervical thymic cyst • Cystic nodal metastases
Fourth branchial cleft cyst anomaly	• Sinus tract/fistula arising from the pyriform sinus, pierce the thyrohyoid membrane, and descend along the tracheoesophageal groove • Usually posterior to sternocleidomastoid and adjacent to thyroid gland	• Abscess • Cervical thymic cyst • Lymphatic malformation • Thyroglossal duct cyst • Thyroid colloid cyst • Recurrent thyroiditis

Source: Adapted from Adams A, Mankad K, Offiah C, Childs L. Branchial cleft anomalies: a pictorial review of embryological development and spectrum of imaging findings. Insights Imaging. 2016;7:69-76.

Differential Diagnosis

It is important to know the types of branchial arch malformations and their characteristic location as there are no pathognomonic clinical or imaging features. The evaluation of persistent cysts or fistulae in the head and neck region in typical locations should include appropriate history and examination with dedicated imaging evaluation. **Table 2** enlists the common locations and differential diagnosis of branchial arch anomalies.

Thyroid Anomalies

Thyroglossal Duct Cyst

These are the most common congenital midline cystic lesions in the neck. They can arise anywhere in the anterior neck along the course of the thyroglossal duct from the foramen cecum (at the base of tongue) to the pyramidal lobe of the thyroid gland. The majority are infrahyoid in location (65%) whereas about 20% are suprahyoid and 15% are seen at the level of the hyoid bone.[7] The usual clinical presentation is of a midline mass which moves with swallowing or protrusion of the tongue.

Imaging

The attachment to the hyoid bone and longitudinal extension into the tongue base is highly suggestive of thyroglossal duct cyst.

- *Ultrasonography*: Well-defined, anechoic, and unilocular cystic lesion. Internal debris may be seen in cases of infection/hemorrhage. Wall nodularity or solid component suggests malignancy.

  In comparison, the dermoid cysts are located in the submandibular or sublingual space and usually show a mixed internal echogenicity on USG.
- *Computed tomography and magnetic resonance imaging*: Fluid density/SI is noted within the lesion **(Figs. 4A and B)**. Complicated cysts show thick enhancing wall and septations. CT sinogram can be used to delineate the fistulous tract **(Figs. 5A and B)**.

Ectopic Thyroid

Ectopic thyroid tissue is identified along the path of descent of the thyroid and most commonly as lingual thyroid. The typical location for lingual thyroid is posterior to the foramen cecum at the base of the tongue.[8]

Imaging

Ultrasonography can document the echogenic appearance of the mass at base of tongue and also assess the orthotopic thyroid tissue. I-123 scintigraphy demonstrates uptake both in the ectopic location and normally located thyroid tissue (which at times may be minimal or absent). CT shows characteristic high attenuation of thyroid tissue **(Figs. 6A and B)**.

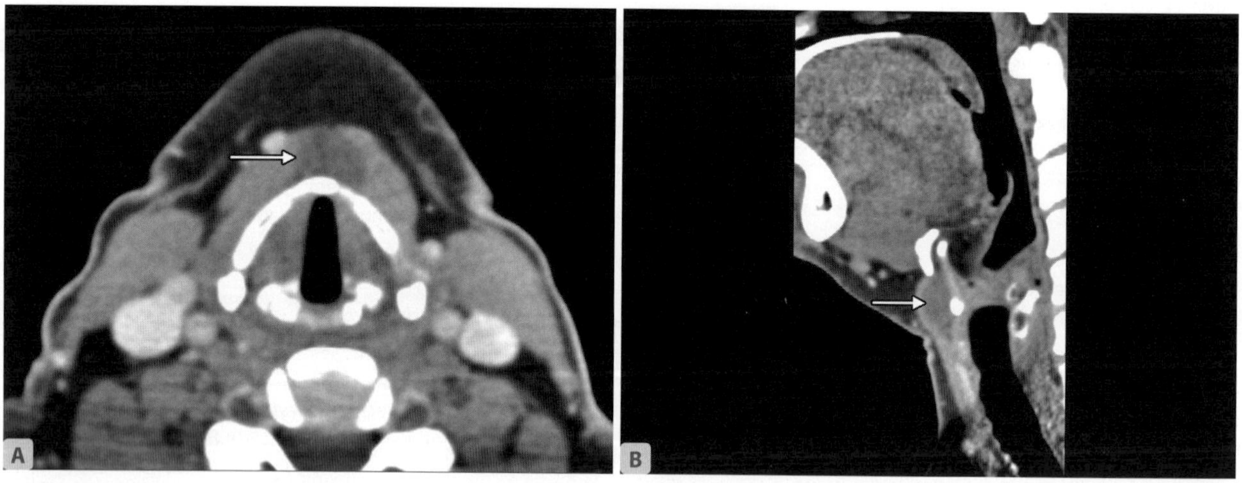

FIGS. 4A AND B: Thyroglossal duct cyst. (A and B) Axial and sagittal contrast-enhanced computed tomography (CECT) image demonstrating well-defined midline cystic lesion (arrows in A and B) in the infrahyoid location.

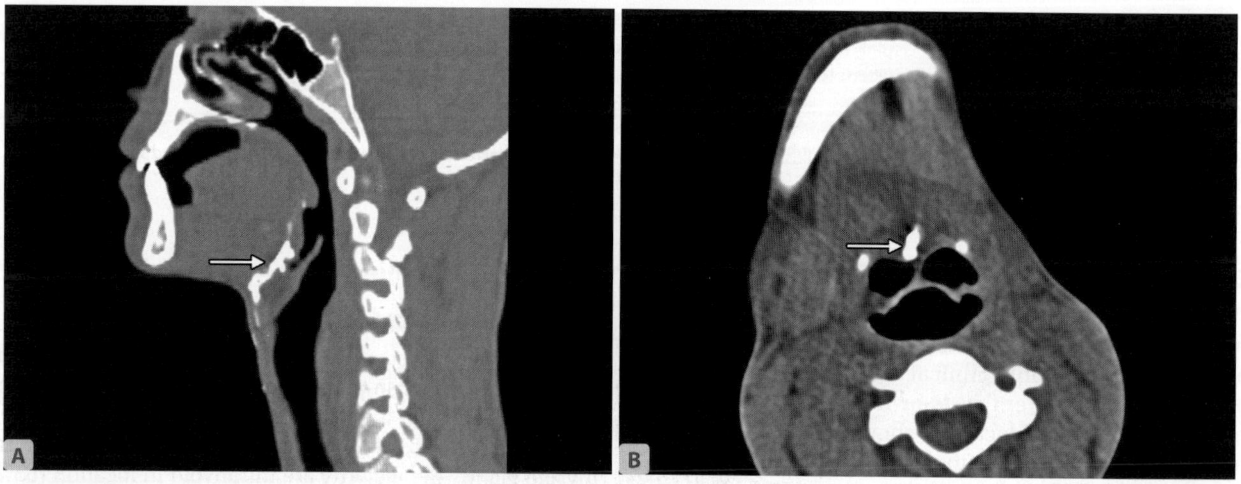

FIGS. 5A AND B: Thyroglossal duct fistula. (A) Sagittal MIP image of CT sinogram reveals a tract (arrow) extending from external opening in anterior neck midline at level of thyroid cartilage and ascending superiorly posterior to the hyoid bone; and (B) The tract is reaching up to the base of tongue (arrow) at level of foramen cecum. (CT: computed tomography; MIP: maximum intensity projection)

Congenital Goiter

Congenital goiter can present in the neonatal period as stridor and respiratory distress because of a diffusely enlarged thyroid gland compressing the trachea. On clinical examination, the neonate may have neck hyperextension and there may be history of a difficult vaginal delivery because of cervical dystocia. Impaired swallowing in the prenatal period can lead to polyhydramnios in utero.

The etiology can be hereditary (inborn errors in fetal hormone production) or due to nonhereditary causes [such as thyroid dysgenesis, maternal intake of antithyroid medicines, transplacental passage of maternal antibodies in Graves' disease, or rare mutations of thyrotropin (thyroid-stimulating hormone) receptors, i.e., McCune Albright syndrome].

Imaging

Antenatal USG evaluation: A diffusely and homogeneously enlarged thyroid gland with a circumference/diameter more than 95th percentile for period of gestation is suggestive of fetal goiter. On Doppler evaluation, peripheral vascularity is suggestive of an enlarged but inactive thyroid gland and central vascularity is likely representative of an overactive thyroid gland.[9]

Postnatal ultrasonography evaluation: Diffuse and homogeneous enlargement of the thyroid gland with narrowing of the adjacent airway.

Thymic Anomalies

Ectopic Cervical Thymus and Thymic Cyst

The pathway of thymic descent is from the angle of the mandible to the superior mediastinum and ectopic thymus can be seen at any point along this tract. Ectopic cervical thymus may present as a painless, midline, or lateral neck mass.[8]

Imaging (Figs. 7A and B)

Ultrasonography demonstrates characteristic "speckled appearance" of linear echogenic septa and scattered echogenic foci within normal thymus tissue. Continuity with normal thymus in the mediastinum establishes the diagnosis on cross-sectional imaging.[9] It is essential to identify this entity, as no intervention is required and it involutes like normal thymus. Cervical thymic cysts are rare cystic lesions within ectopic thymic tissue which have a characteristic cigar shape and demonstrate extension into the superior mediastinum.

Dermoid and Epidermoid Cysts

These have been described later in this chapter under the section on Teratomas.

Ranula

Ranula is a benign acquired cystic lesion that characteristically occurs in the floor of mouth. It is a mucus retention cyst which forms due to obstruction to the sublingual gland or minor salivary glands and is seen as a bluish mass in the floor of mouth.

Types

- *Simple ranula*: Within the sublingual space above the mylohyoid muscle
- *Plunging ranula*: Extends into the submandibular space around the posterior edge of the mylohyoid muscle.

Imaging

- *Ultrasonography*: Simple cystic lesion in the sublingual space. Infected ranula may have thick walls and internal debris **(Figs. 8A and B)**.
- *Computed tomography*: Fluid attenuating lesion in the characteristic location, walls of infected cysts may enhance. Surrounding fat stranding with inflammatory changes is seen in case of abscess formation.
- *Magnetic resonance imaging*: Typical fluid SI (T1 hypointense and T2 hyperintense), walls of infected cysts may enhance.

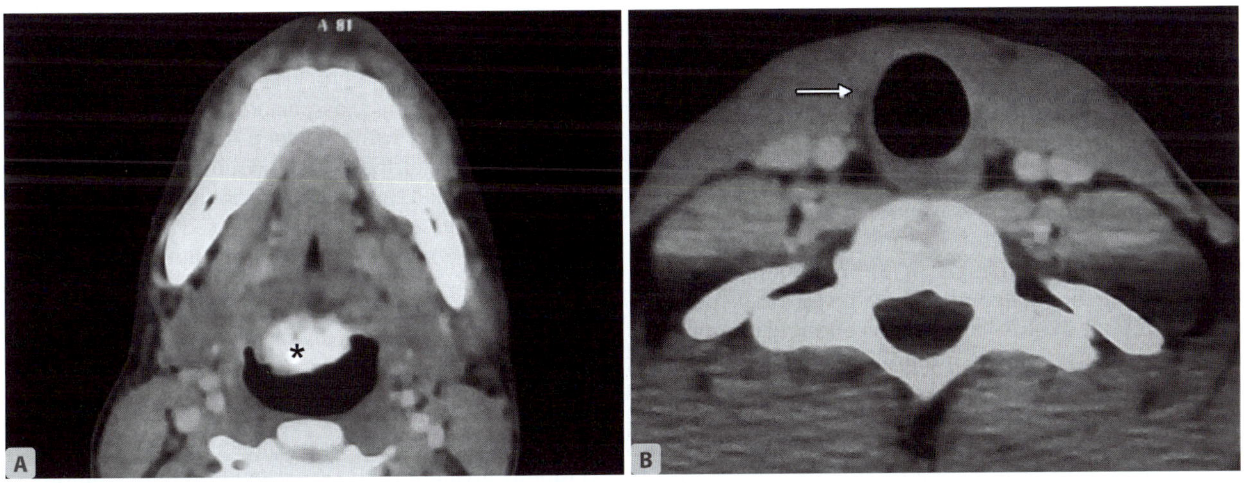

FIGS. 6A AND B: Lingual thyroid. (A) Axial contrast-enhanced computed tomography (CECT) scans demonstrate high-attenuation, well-defined mass (asterisk) in the midline base of tongue; and (B) Absence of normal thyroid tissue (arrow) in the lower neck.

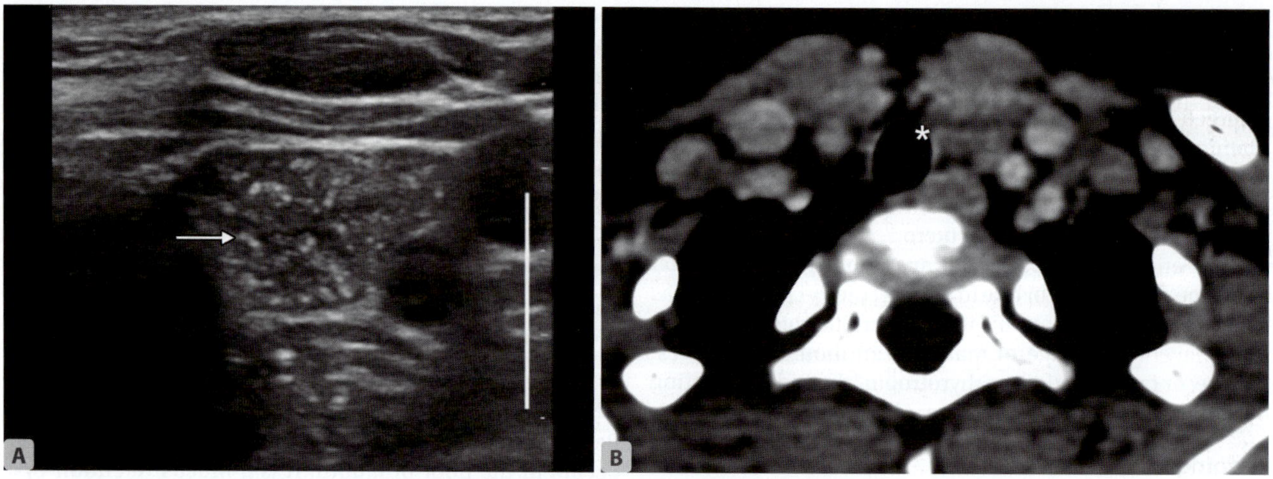

FIGS. 7A AND B: Cervical extension of thymus. (A) Ultrasonography (USG) of left supraclavicular swelling in a 7-year-old child reveals the typical "speckled appearance" of thymus (arrow); and (B) CECT revealed the swelling (asterisk) to be cervical extension of thymus. (CECT: contrast-enhanced computed tomography)

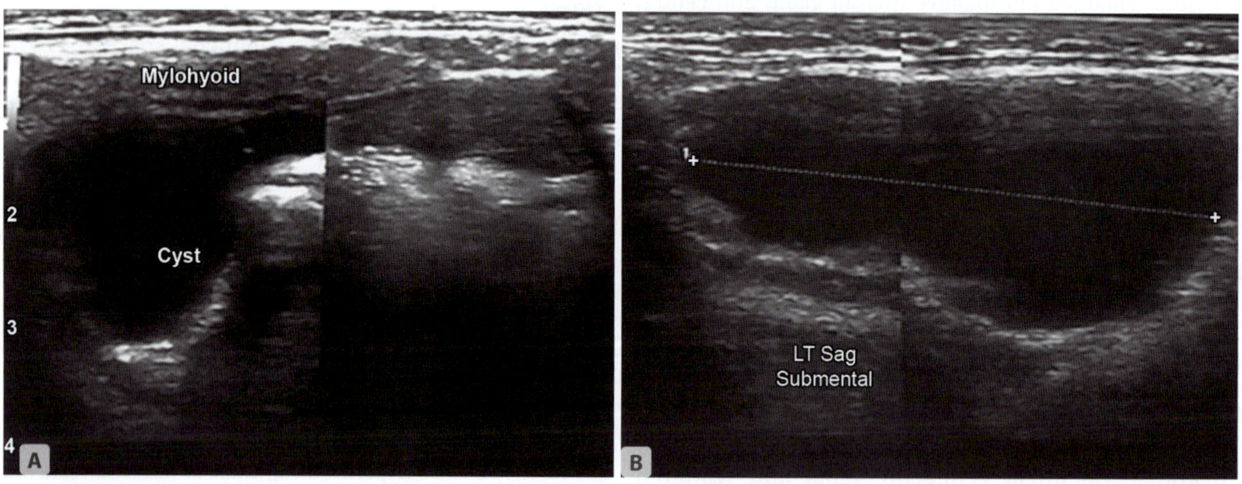

FIGS. 8A AND B: Ranula. (A and B) Ultrasonography (USG) images reveal a well-defined cystic lesion in the sublingual space deep to the mylohyoid.

Vascular Lesions

Vascular Malformations

This includes both low flow (capillary, venous, and lymphatic) malformations and high flow malformations (arteriovenous fistula and arteriovenous malformation).[10]

Low flow malformations are more common. These are multicystic transpatial lesions, most frequently seen in the posterior cervical triangle. With predominant venous component, hemorrhage and fluid levels may be seen because of prior hemorrhage or infection. Phleboliths are seen as hyperdense foci on CT and small signal voids on MRI and there is progressive contrast enhancement.[11]

Lymphatic malformations are multiseptated cystic and show no or only septal contrast enhancement **(Figs. 9A to C)**. These are more common in the first 2 years of life and can extend across facial boundaries. Large masses can extend into the axilla, mediastinum, orbit, and retropharyngeal space with airway compromise.

Infantile Hemangioma

Hemangiomas are benign vascular tumors. Superficial infantile hemangioma is associated with skin discoloration (strawberry mark) while in deep lesions overlying skin/mucosa may be normal. It is encountered during infancy or neonatal period, increases during the next few months, and then regresses. It is characterized by the following phases **(Table 3)**. Beta-blockers have shown to be effective in proliferating phase.[12] These tumors are often glucose transporter type 1 (GLUT1) positive.[13]

Congenital Hemangioma

Congenital hemangioma (CH) is almost fully grown at birth unlike IH which mostly grows postnatally. CH is of two forms: (1) rapidly involuting CH (RICH) and (2) noninvoluting CH (NICH). The main difference between IH, RICH, or NICH is the age of presentation/regression. CH like IH peaks soon after birth or in some instances have already begin to involute

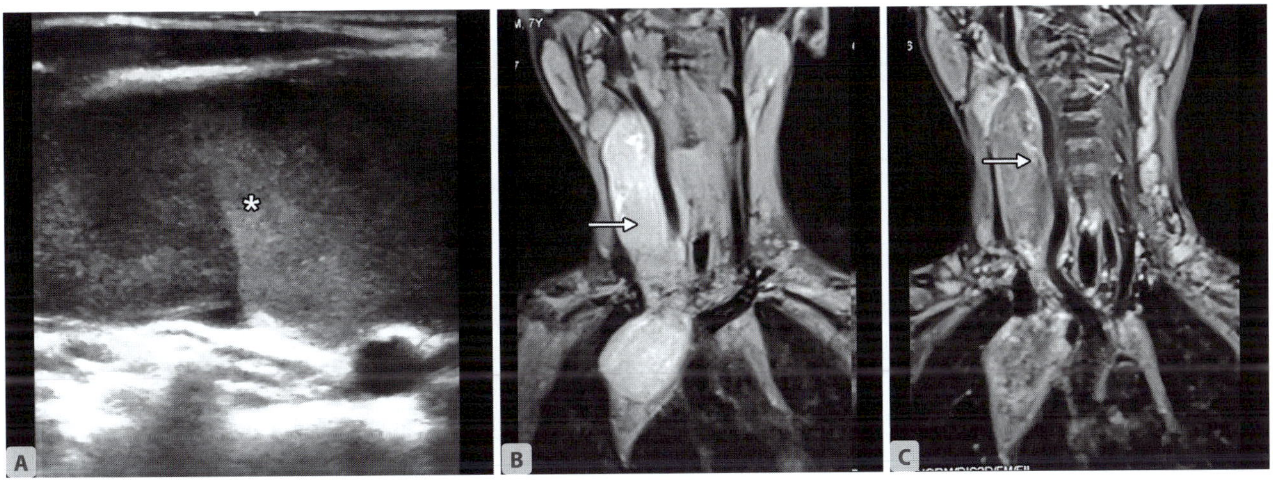

FIGS. 9A TO C: Lymphatic malformation. (A) Ultrasonography (USG) demonstrates a large multiloculated cystic lesion with echogenic debris, caused by internal hemorrhage (asterisk); (B) T2- weighted coronal MRI shows a large, multilocular, and trans-spatial cystic mass with mediastinal extension with hyperintense signal intensity (SI) (arrow); and (C) T1 fat-saturated postcontrast images reveal enhancement in the internal septa and wall (arrow) of the lesion. (MRI: magnetic resonance imaging)

TABLE 3: Imaging appearance of infantile hemangioma according to phases.

Phases	Period	Ultrasonography	Magnetic resonance imaging
Proliferative phase	• Neonatal/early infancy • Up to about 1.5 years of age	• Well-defined mass with variable echogenicity (low or high) **(Fig. 10)** • Lobulated • Doppler—arterial flow	• Well-defined • Lobulated • T1WI—hypo-/isointense • T2WI—hyperintense • Flow voids • Early, persistent enhancement
Involuting phase	• After 1 year • Continues for years • Slow regression	Decrease in size and vascularity	• Decrease in size • T2 hyperintensity and enhancement reduce • Fatty replacement

(T1WI: T1-weighted image; T2WI: T2-weighted image)

by that time. The rapidly involuting form completely regresses by about 1 year of age. NICH, on the other hand, appears early (vs. IH) and also does not regress.[14] CH tumors are usually GLUT1 negative.

While imaging features of CH and IH are broadly similar, CH displays some differences:

- More heterogeneity
- Ill-defined margins
- Aggressive features on angiography—aneurysms or arteriovenous shunts
- Calcification may be present.

Kaposiform Hemangioendothelioma

Kaposiform hemangioendothelioma (KHE) is so called due to its resemblance to Kaposi's sarcoma on pathology. It is a locally aggressive vascular neoplasm which occurs in infants or children. KHE has an association with Kasabach-Merritt syndrome (a consumption coagulopathy with thrombocytopenia). On imaging, the tumors are similar to hemangiomas but have ill-defined infiltrative margins and may show osseous invasion.[15] The tumor does not metastasize.

INFECTIOUS/INFLAMMATORY LESIONS

Lymphoid Hyperplasia

Enlargement of the Waldeyer's ring is frequently seen in children and a common cause of upper airway obstruction. Lateral radiographs of soft-tissue nasopharynx are obtained during nasal inspiration with closed mouth and neck extended for assessment of adenoid size and airway compromise. Adenoidal size is age dependent being maximum at 7–10 years of age and then declines.[8] This is measured by the adenoidal-nasopharyngeal (AN) ratio on a lateral radiograph of the nasopharynx (see Chapter 10).

Palatine tonsillar hypertrophy is seen as bilaterally symmetrical, smooth, and round masses in the oropharynx

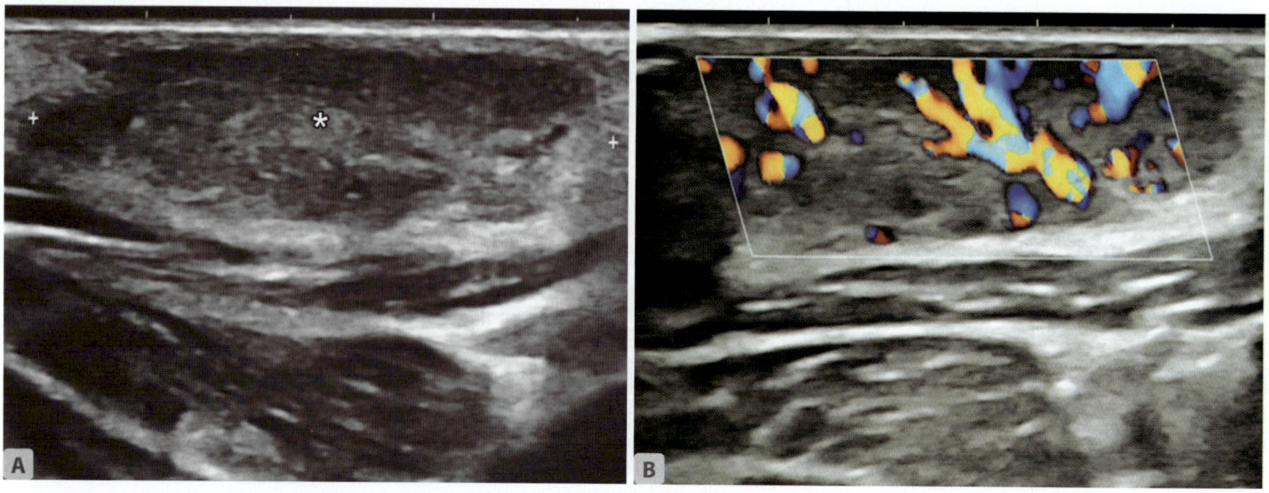

FIGS. 10A AND B: Hemangioma. (A) Ultrasonography (USG) shows well-defined mass (asterisk) with heterogeneous echotexture in the anterior neck subcutaneous plane; and (B) Color Doppler imaging shows intense color flow.

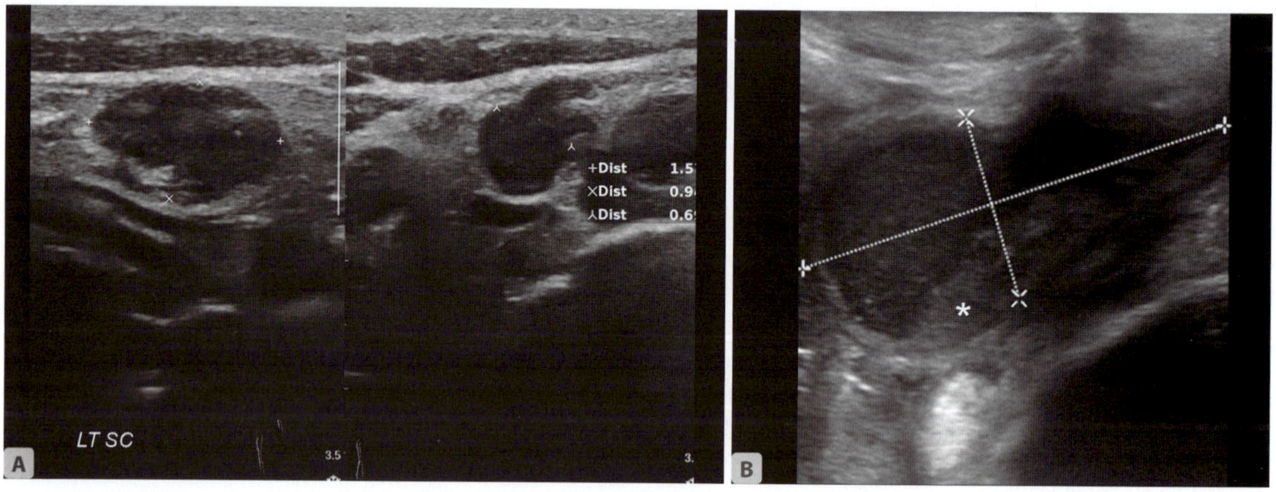

FIGS. 11A AND B: Lymphadenopathy and abscess formation. (A) Multiple, necrotic lymph nodes in left supraclavicular location in a case of nodal tuberculosis (TB); and (B) Neck abscess secondary to conglomeration of necrotic lymph nodes in another case of disseminated TB. Ultrasonography (USG) reveals a central hypoechoic fluid collection with internal debris, surrounded by a thick rim of solid tissue (asterisks).

with density similar to muscle on CT. These are isointense on T1WI and hyperintense on T2WI. Hypertrophic lingual tonsils are of similar morphology and seen in the base of tongue.

Lymph Node Enlargement

Lymph node enlargement is the most common cause of palpable neck mass in a child. Viral lymphadenitis is the most common etiology and presents as bilateral small cervical lymph nodes, typically levels I to III.[8] Causes include cytomegalovirus, infectious mononucleosis, rhinovirus, adenovirus, varicella zoster, herpes simplex virus (HSV), and enterovirus. Bacterial infection (*Staphylococcus aureus* and *Streptococcus*) in the oropharynx usually presents as acute, unilateral lymph node enlargement along the drainage pathway. Lymph nodes may suppurate and evolve into abscesses **(Figs. 11 and 12)**.

Deep Space Infections

The enlarged retropharyngeal nodes seen in nasopharyngeal and tonsillar infections can suppurate and present as retropharyngeal/parapharyngeal abscesses. The potential sources of infection are sinonasal tract, tonsil, throat, odontogenic disease, and middle ear.[10] Peritonsillar abscess (pus collection between fibrous capsule and pharyngeal constrictor muscle) occurs when bacterial tonsillitis transgresses the tonsillar capsule.[7] Retropharyngeal space infections can spread to the danger space and also inferiorly to the mediastinum.

Imaging

Lateral soft-tissue neck radiographs reveal thickened retropharyngeal soft tissue with smooth, anterior displacement of airway in cases of retropharyngeal abscess.

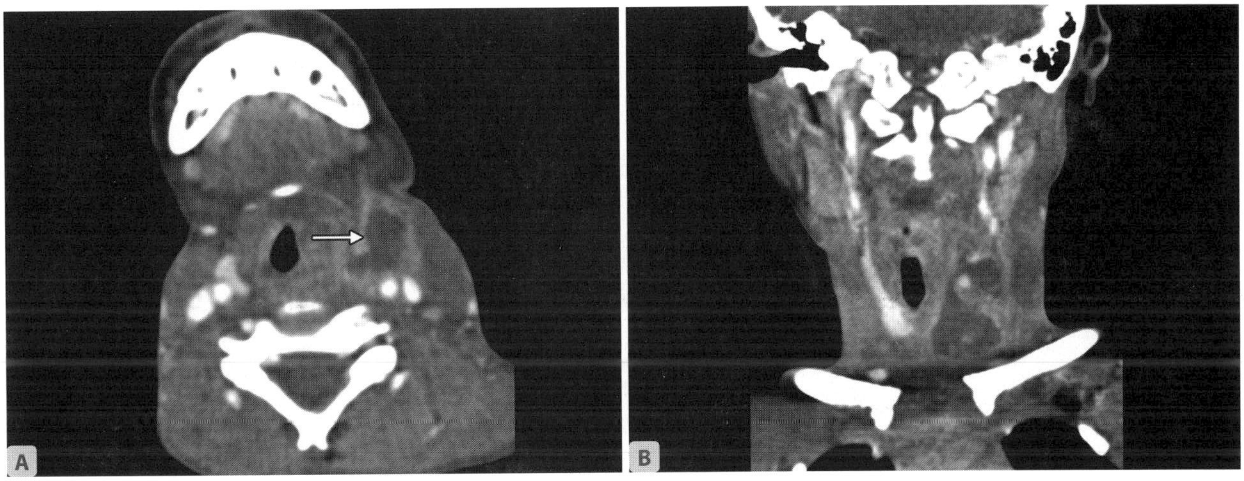

FIGS. 12A AND B: Superficial cervical abscess. (A and B) Contrast-enhanced computed tomography (CECT) axial and coronal shows a thick enhancing collection (arrow) in lower cervical subcutaneous plane and strap muscles anterior to thyroid lobe in left paramedian location with perilesional inflammatory changes.

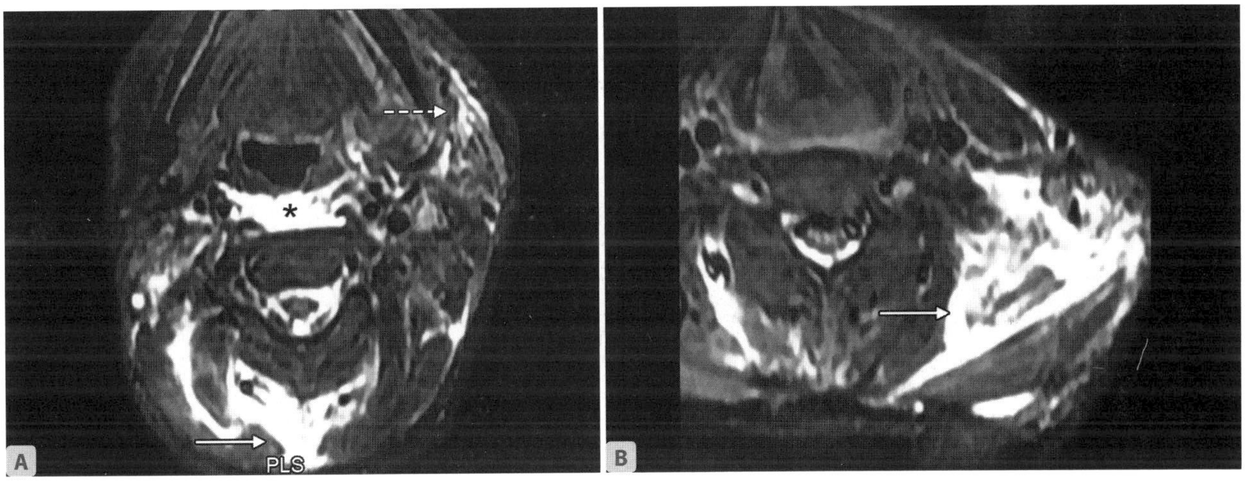

FIGS. 13A AND B: Deep space infection: Retropharyngeal abscess. (A and B) Axial T2FS MRI reveals a hyperintense collection (asterisk) in the retropharyngeal space with inflammatory changes in the masseter (dotted arrow in A), the posterior cervical space (arrow in B), and paraspinal muscles (arrow in A). (MRI: magnetic resonance imaging; T2FS: T2 fat-suppressed)

- *Ultrasonography*: Simple lymphadenopathy is seen as discrete, round-to-oval, and enlarged lymph nodes with preserved fatty hilum with increased blood flow. Suppurated lymph nodes have a necrotic hypoechoic center. Abscesses are hypoechoic to anechoic masses with an irregular, thick wall.
- *Contrast-enhanced computed tomography (CECT)*: This is the investigation of choice to assess deep space infections in the neck. Cellulitis is edema in the soft tissue and subcutaneous planes with obliterated fat planes.

  Abscess has characteristically central low attenuation and peripheral rim enhancement; however, this appearance usually overlaps with inflammatory changes and phlegmon.[8]
- *Magnetic resonance imaging*: Similar findings as CT, however the inflammatory changes are well-appreciated on the T2 fat-suppressed (T2FS) images **(Figs. 13A and B)**.

In the endemic regions, tuberculosis is an important cause of necrotic lymph nodes **(Figs. 11A and B)**, retropharyngeal collections, and cold abscess. Tuberculous lymphadenitis usually involves the posterior cervical, high internal jugular chain, and submandibular lymph nodes. In the early stages, there is homogeneous enhancement with or without a minimal amount of necrosis. It progresses to frank necrosis, which is the most common imaging manifestation of tuberculosis.[8] Necrosis is seen as low density on CECT and low SI on T1WI and high SI on T2WI. As the disease progresses, multiple nodes conglomerate and there is loss of adjacent soft-tissue planes. Cold abscess may form along with draining sinus tracts and fistulae. Healed tuberculous nodes show fibrocalcific changes.

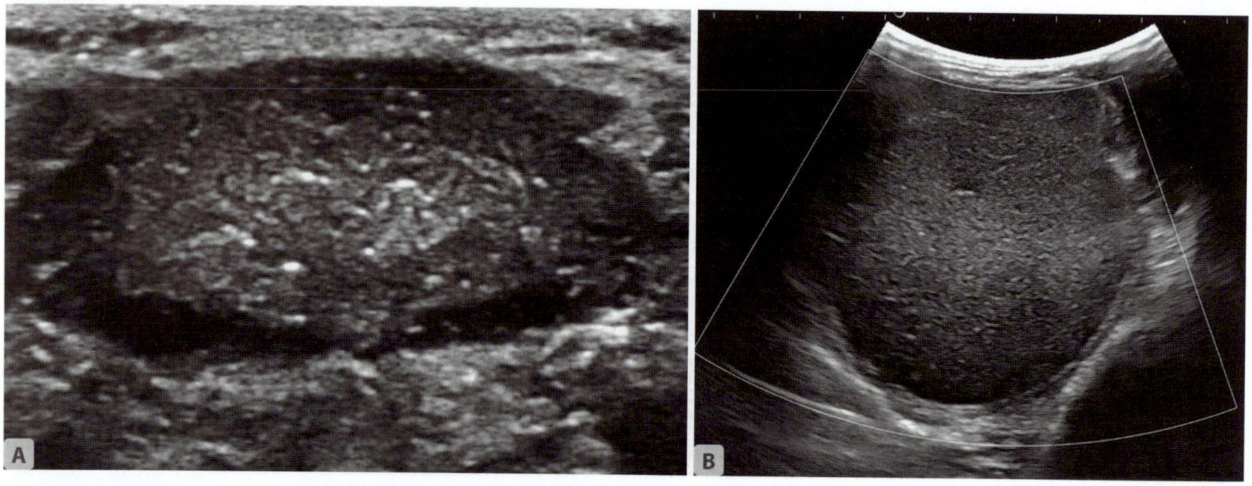

FIGS. 14A AND B: Dermoid and epidermoid cysts. (A) Dermoid cyst: Well-defined, midline cystic lesion in floor of mouth with coarse internal echoes; and (B) Epidermoid cyst: Large cystic lesion in the floor of mouth with internal debris.

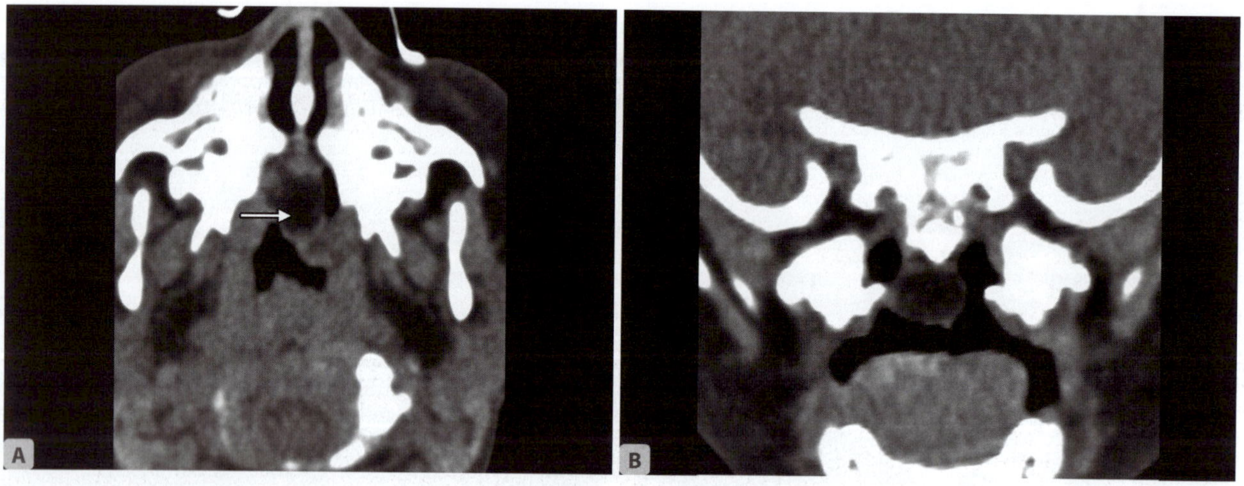

FIGS. 15A AND B: Midline dermoid cyst. (A and B) Axial and coronal noncontrast-enhanced computed tomography (NCCT) face show a well-defined midline fat attenuation cystic mass lesion (arrow) in the posterior part of hard palate. There was no evidence of intracranial extension of the mass.

NEOPLASMS

Teratomas

Teratomas are a form of germ cell tumors that comprise of components of all three germinal layers. Among these, epithelial components, along with its appendages (e.g., hair), give teratomas their characteristic imaging appearance. Teratomas are the most frequently encountered neck mass in the neonate/infant. They appear cystic, solid, or mixed on imaging, depending on its type.

Teratomas can be further classified as follows:

- Mature (cystic):
  - *Dermoid cyst*: Lining is squamous epithelium and skin adnexa in wall, cyst has internal echoes **(Fig. 14A)** or sac of marbles appearance
  - *Epidermoid cyst*: Lining is simple squamous epithelium, cyst has internal echoes **(Fig. 14B)**
  - *Teratoid cyst*: Lining is squamous epithelium and other tissues (muscle/bone/cartilage)
- Immature (solid)
- Malignant: Usually results from malignant transformation of dermoid cyst. This can be carcinoma/sarcoma/mixed.

The various sites of involvement of teratomas in the head and neck region and their imaging appearances are:

- *Dermoid cyst*:
  - All cystic teratomas are lined by squamous epithelium.
  - Dermoid cysts appear unilocular with nodules/solid component and calcification being less frequent.
  - These occur typically in a midline, suprahyoid location **(Figs. 15A and B)** with the floor of mouth being the most common site.[8]
  - Unlike solid teratomas, the cystic forms are often encountered in older children, adolescents, or even young adults. The presence of a unilocular cyst at a characteristic location that appears echogenic on USG, fat attenuation on CT, or hyperintense on T1WI is characteristic. The coalescence of fat into small nodules gives the "sac of marbles" appearance on ultrasound.

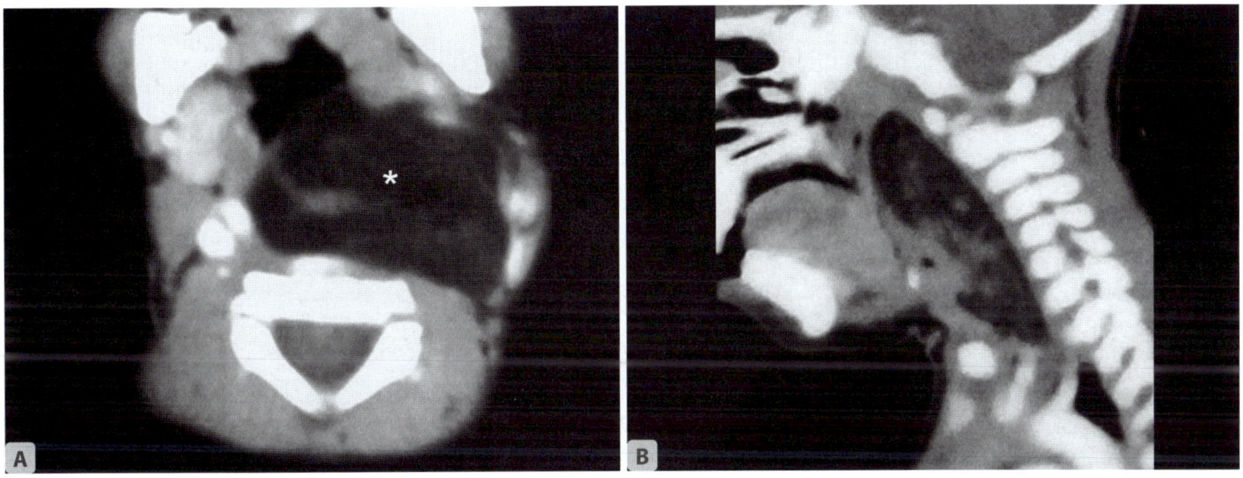

FIGS. 16A AND B: Left parapharyngeal space teratoma. (A and B) Axial and sagittal contrast-enhanced computed tomography (CECT) of neck shows a well-defined midline fat attenuation cystic mass lesion in the left parapharyngeal space (asterisk) with luminal compromise of the airway. There was no enhancing solid component.

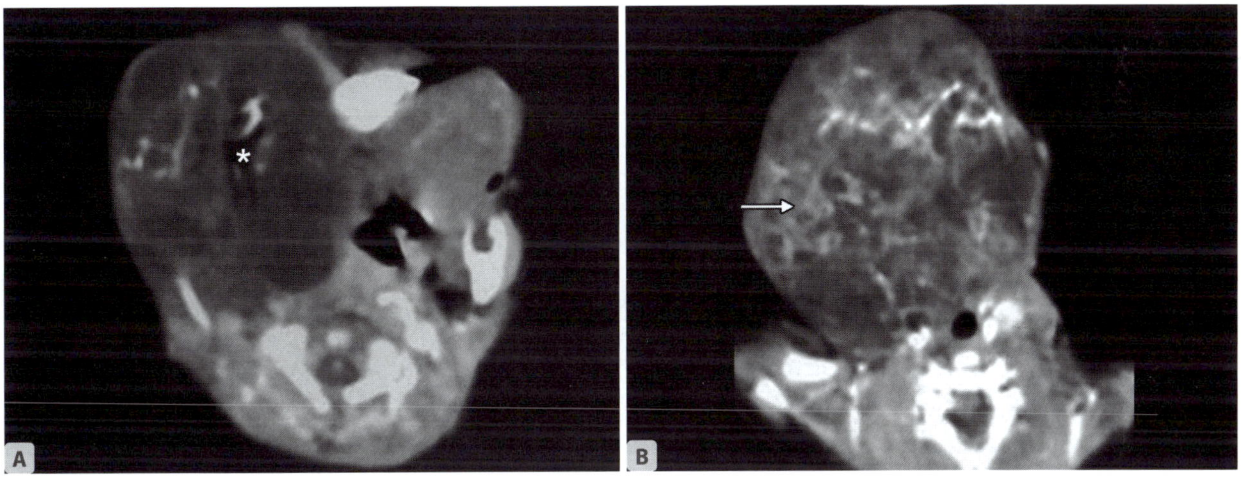

FIGS. 17A AND B: Immature teratoma. (A and B) Axial contrast-enhanced computed tomography (CECT) demonstrates a heterogeneous mass with areas of soft tissue, coarse calcification, and fat density (asterisk) with enhancing solid component (arrow).

- *Immature/mature teratomas seen in neonates/infants* ***(Figs. 16 and 17)***:
  - These occur in the anterior/lateral cervical space of the neck.
  - The tumors are often large in size and mixed cystic solid, with cysts being multilocular and showing variable density.
  - Calcifications may be seen within while presence of cartilage or bone is less frequent.
  - Large lesions result in airway/pharyngeal compression with babies encountering breathing or feeding difficulties.
  - Immature/mature teratomas may less frequently occur in orbit/paranasal sinuses.

Lipoma

Majority of adipocytic tumors are benign and lipoma is the most common, with liposarcoma being rare in children.[16] Numerous chromosomal aberrations have been reported in these tumors with HMGA2 protein truncation being one of these.[17] Most of these tumors do not cause pain unless they compress nerves. The classical lipoma on imaging displays an appearance of homogeneous fatty lesion similar to subcutaneous fat. Lipomas may have a capsule (encapsulated). Those without capsule can appear infiltrative with infiltrative intramuscular lipoma being one form. Characteristic fat attenuation on CT and fat SI on MRI is noted **(Figs. 18A and B)**.

Madelung Disease (Neck Lipomatosis)

Madelung-Launois-Bensaude syndrome or neck lipomatosis is a rare benign condition. There are multiple, symmetric, and nonencapsulated masses of fatty tissue which involve the neck and upper region of the trunk with proximal limb involvement.

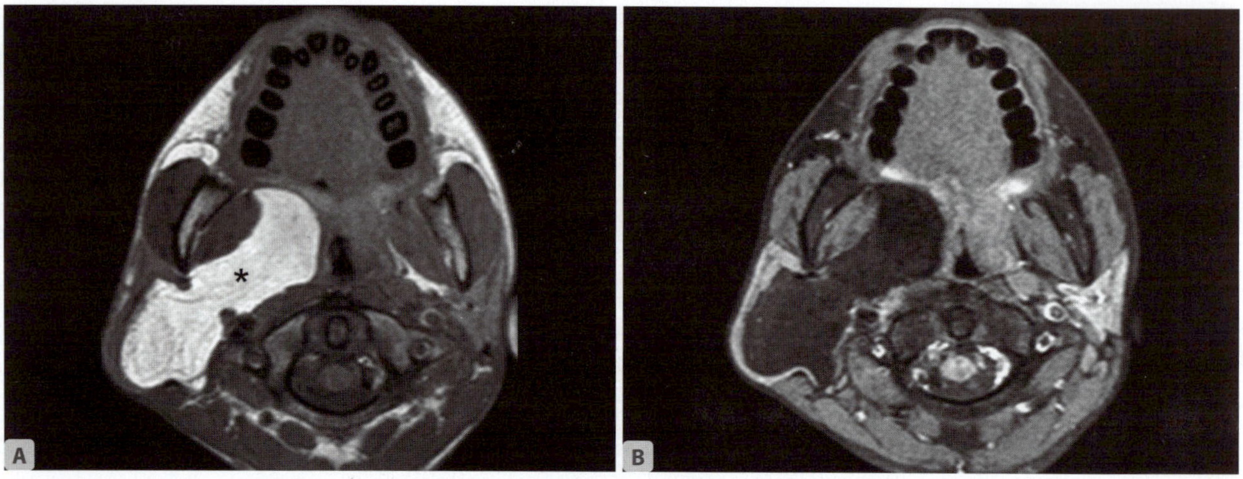

FIGS. 18A AND B: Lipoma. (A and B) Axial T1-weighted image (T1WI) and T1 fat-suppressed (T1FS) MR image show a well-defined lesion (asterisk) which is hyperintense on T1WI and uniformly suppressed on T1FS image in the right parotid and parapharyngeal space.

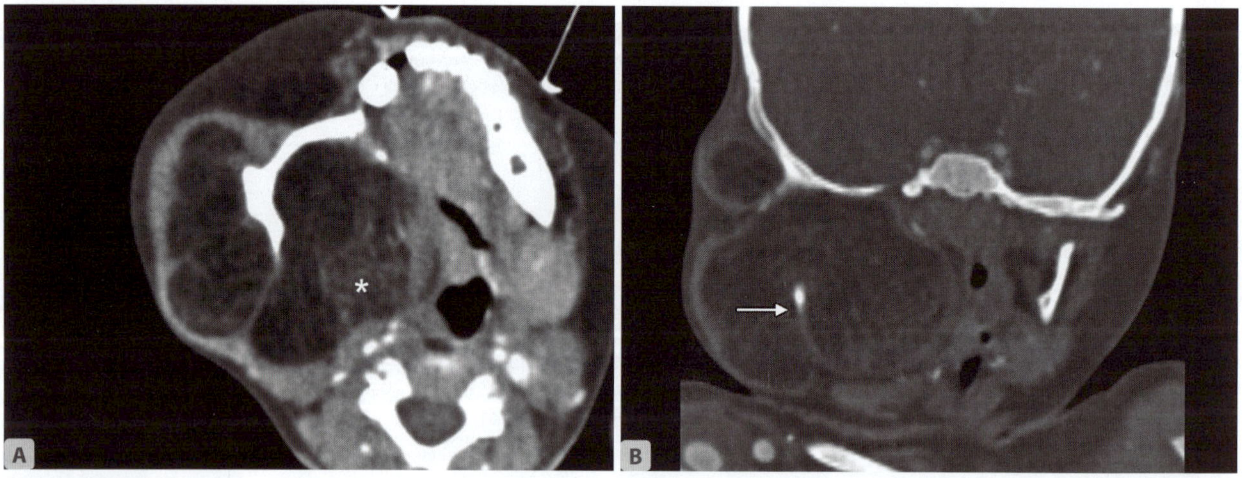

FIGS. 19A AND B: Lipoblastoma. (A) Axial contrast-enhanced computed tomography (CECT) image in an infant shows fat attenuation infiltrative lesion in right masticator and parapharyngeal space with septations within (asterisk); and (B) Coronal bone window shows thinning and scalloping of the lateral skull base and right hemimandible (arrow).

Lipoblastoma

Lipoblastoma is a rare tumor encountered typically in infants or early childhood (<3 years). It is mostly painless; however, nerve compression can result in pain or even Horner's syndrome (in cervicothoracic tumors) or thoracic cage compression in case of large tumors. Appendicular location is more common than trunk or head and neck.

Unlike lipoma, the tumor is composed of immature fatty tissue, which on MRI shows less hyperintensity (on T1WI) compared to mature fat. Also, there may be components of myxoid or fibrous tissues found within, further giving it a heterogeneous appearance **(Figs. 19A and B)**. The tumor is known to regress spontaneously or mature into a lipoma, as the child grows. Hence, this should be kept in mind when a decision regarding surgery or conservative approach is taken. On imaging and even histology, the lesion resembles a liposarcoma, however the typical age of presentation aids in the distinction. A diffuse, infiltrative form of the neoplasm is referred to as "lipoblastomastosis".[18]

Neurogenic Tumors

The most common neurogenic tumors are schwannomas and neurofibromas and they are usually found in the posterior triangle. The most common presentation is of a painless neck mass. Neurofibromas arise from the endoneurium whereas schwannomas develop eccentrically from the outer nerve sheath.[9] Majority of children with neurofibromas have neurofibromatosis type I.

Imaging

- *Ultrasonography*: Neurogenic tumors are well-circumscribed, homogeneous masses, and usually hypoechoic with posterior acoustic enhancement **(Fig. 20A)**. The internal vascularity is variable from mild-to-moderate. Neurofibromas characteristically demonstrate a target appearance (centrally hyperechoic and peripherally hypoechoic). Plexiform neurofibromas have diffuse peripheral nerve involvement rather than a focal lesion.[9]

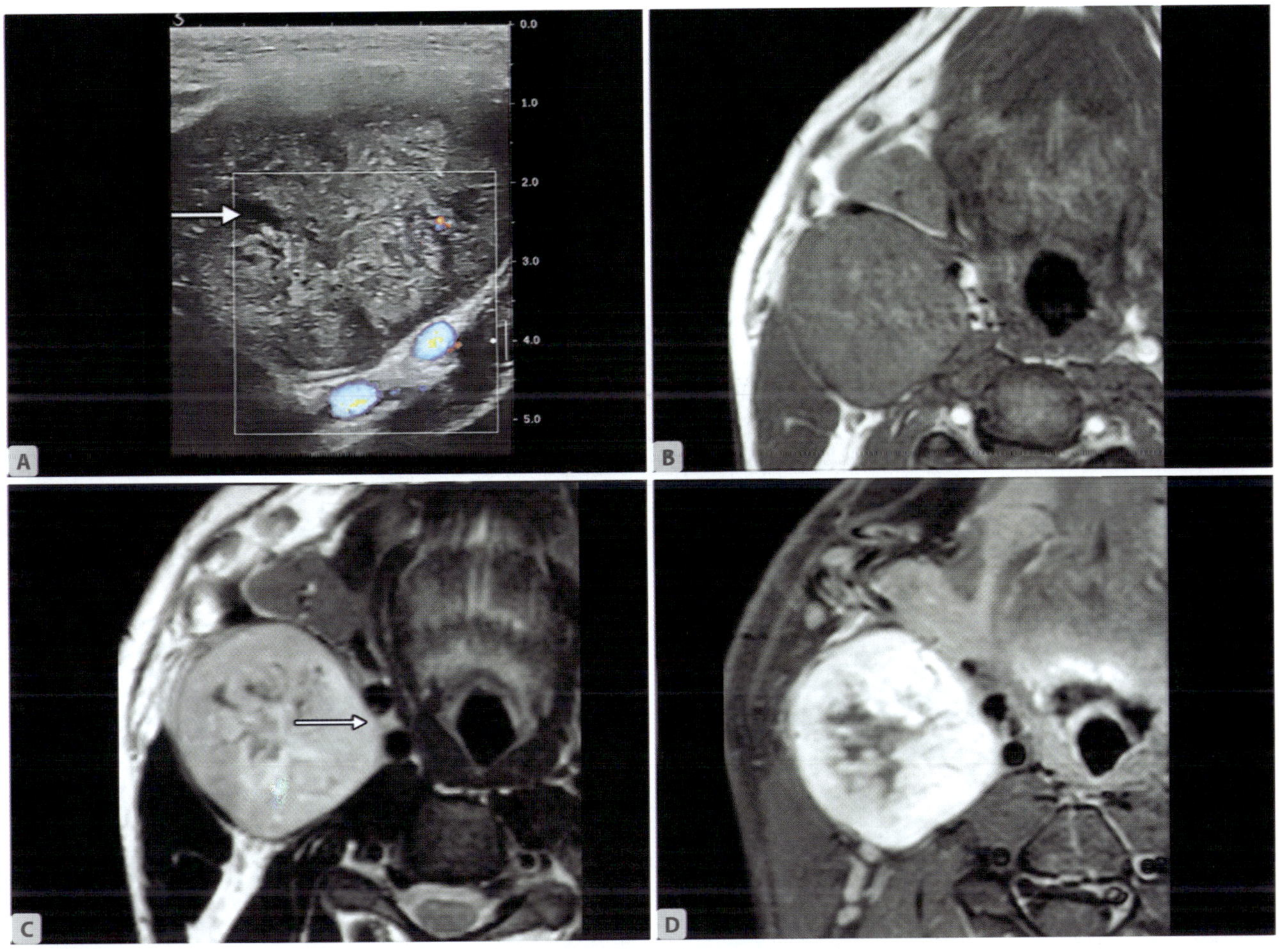

FIGS. 20A TO D: Schwannoma. (A) Ultrasonography (USG) shows a well-defined solid mass lesion in the right carotid space with areas of necrosis (arrow); and (B to D) Axial T1WI, axial T2WI, and postcontrast T1WI axial show an ovoid, right carotid space mass lesion displacing the vessels anteromedially (arrow). (T1WI: T1-weighted image; T2WI: T2-weighted image; USG: ultrasonography)

- *Computed tomography and magnetic resonance imaging*: These appear as well-defined, heterogeneous masses **(Figs. 20B to D)**. The larger lesions can involve skull base, orbits, and have intracranial extension. Neurofibromas show the "target" pattern of high peripheral SI and low central SI on T2WI **(Figs. 21A and B)**. Plexiform neurofibromas, on the other hand, are multilobulated masses along the course of a nerve (bag of worms appearance).[19]

Cervical Neuroblastoma

Neuroblastoma (NB) is a ganglion cell tumor and the third most common malignant tumor in pediatric age group, with cervical NB being responsible for <5% of all NB cases.[20] Metastases to neck and skull base from NB elsewhere are more common than primary cervical NB. There are three histologic variants of ganglion cell tumors: (1) NB is least differentiated, (2) Ganglioneuroblastoma is intermediate, and (3) Ganglioneuroma **(Figs. 22A to D)** is the most mature type with no metastatic potential.[10]

Clinical Presentation

Usually presents as a nontender lateral neck mass with symptoms related to external compression of adjacent structures. This includes swallowing difficulty (compression of esophagus), Horner's syndrome (cranial nerves), stridor (airway), and difference in right and left eye colors (heterochromia iridis).[9]

Imaging

- *Ultrasonography*: Appearance is of a solid complex or hypoechoic mass which may show calcification that usually arises posterior to the carotid sheath, with displacement/encasement of the internal jugular vein and carotid artery.[20]
- *Computed tomography*: The tumor appears as a heterogeneous mass with calcification, hemorrhage, or internal necrosis **(Figs. 23A and B)**.
- *Magnetic resonance imaging*: The appearance is of a heterogeneous lesion with mild T2 hyperintensity and

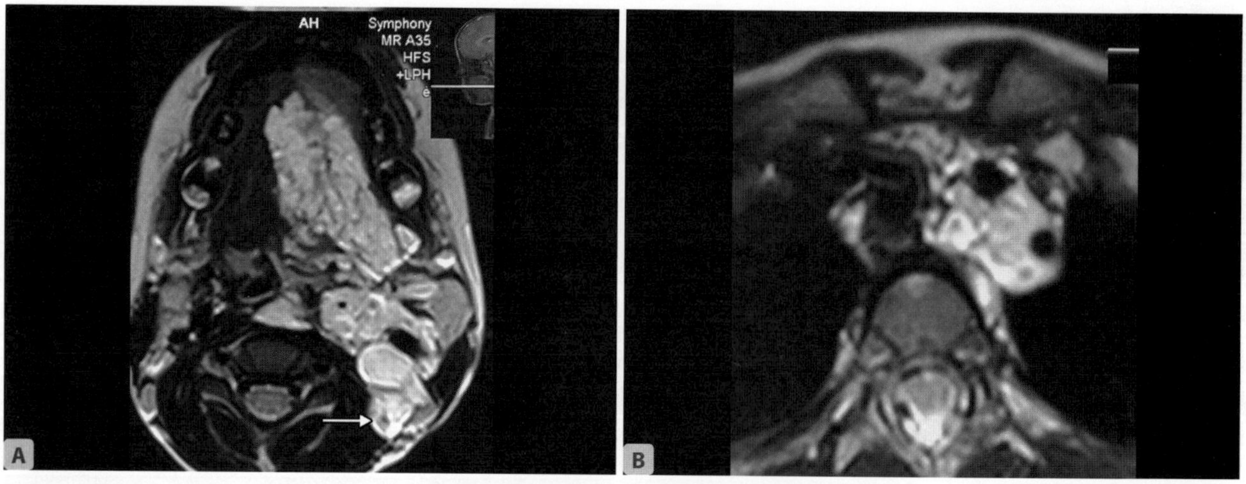

FIGS. 21A AND B: Plexiform neurofibroma. (A and B) Axial T2-weighted image (T2WI) reveals a large trans-spatial mass lesion with mediastinal extension. Lesion is T2 hyperintense with central T2 hypointensity suggestive of target sign (arrow in A).

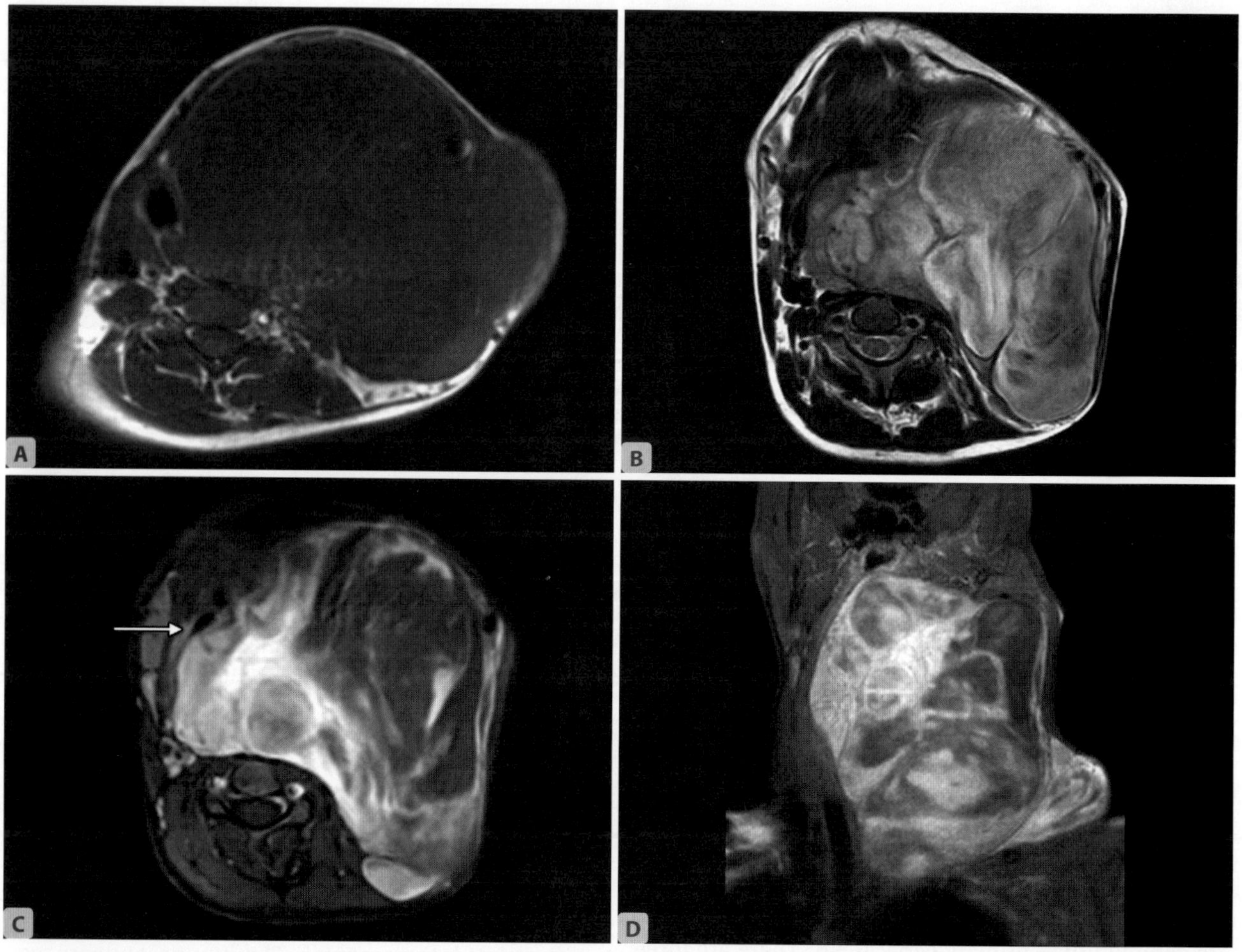

FIGS. 22A TO D: Ganglioneuroma. (A to D) Axial T1WI, axial T2WI, postcontrast T1WI axial, and coronal images reveal a large heterogenous trans-spatial mass lesion in the left cervical region from C1 level to sternoclavicular joint and causing significant airway compromise (arrow in C). Mass is T1 isointense, T2 hyperintense with heterogeneous enhancement. (T1WI: T1-weighted image; T2WI: T2-weighted image)

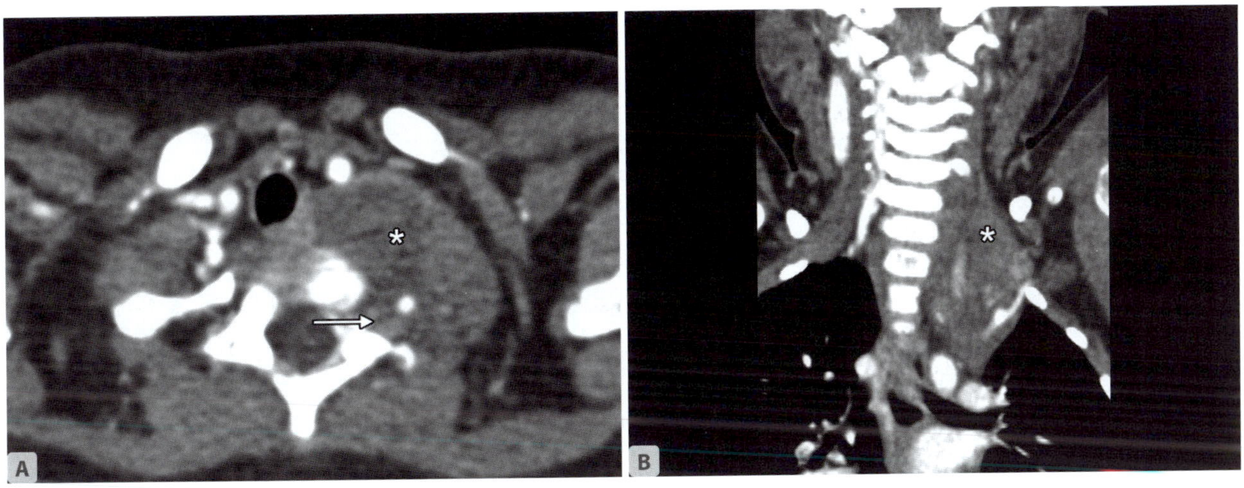

FIGS. 23A AND B: Cervicothoracic neuroblastoma (NB). (A and B) Axial and coronal contrast-enhanced computed tomography (CECT) demonstrates a heterogeneously enhancing lower cervical and upper mediastinal soft-tissue mass lesion (asterisks in A and B) with extension into the left foramen transversarium at D1 level (arrow in A).

marked contrast enhancement. Intraspinal extent, though not a common feature in cervical NB, should be carefully looked for.

Radionuclide imaging with m-iodobenzylguanidine (MIBG) is done in NB for assessing dissemination, though it is not required in the benign forms. The differential diagnosis for cervical NB includes vascular tumor, teratoma, lymphangioma, rhabdoid tumor, and sarcoma. Surgical excision is the treatment of choice after precise preoperative localization.

Rhabdomyosarcoma

Rhabdomyosarcoma (RMS) is frequent in the pediatric age group, particularly in children <10 years of age, among whom it constitutes about half of the soft-tissue sarcomas.[21] It is a high-grade, small round cell neoplasm, with the more differentiated components resembling skeletal muscle. On immunohistochemistry (IHC), tumors are positive for desmin and myogenin. The main differences between the major types are enlisted below:[22]

- *Embryonal RMS*:
  - More common (more than two-thirds)
  - Younger age group
  - Better prognosis
- *Alveolar RMS*:
  - Less than one-third cases
  - Older group
  - Worse prognosis

Head and neck region is the most common site (over one-third cases), followed by genitourinary or extremities. In the head and neck, masses may be orbital, parameningeal (involving skull base), or nonparameningeal. RMS is an aggressive neoplasm and is frequently metastatic with common sites being pulmonary, osseous, or lymph nodal. These can be associated with Li-Fraumeni syndrome or DICER1 syndrome among other predisposing factors.

The imaging appearance of RMS is nonspecific. It is the presence of a soft-tissue mass in described locations that is aggressive with no fatty component in a young patient that raises the suspicion **(Figs. 24A and B)**. Embryonal forms can cause bowing of adjoining bones while bone destruction is seen in up to one fifth of the patients. Calcification is uncommon. Necrosis is seen in alveolar and pleomorphic forms while the embryonal type is mostly homogeneous. MR signal is also nonspecific. The lesion may show flow voids. Contrast enhancement is moderate and the pleomorphic form may show "ring-like" enhancement.

Inflammatory Myofibroblastic Tumor

Inflammatory myofibroblastic tumor (IMT), earlier called inflammatory pseudotumor, is an intermediate-grade tumor (rarely metastasizing type). Up to one-fourth of the tumors recur postresection, but metastases are rare.[23] It is encountered most commonly in first to third decades of life with common sites being chest, head and neck, and abdomen. The tumor secretes interleukins which are inflammatory mediators and can hence be associated with systemic symptoms.

The tumor is composed of fibroblasts and myofibroblasts in combination with lymphocytes, plasma cells as well as eosinophils. It is this variable combination of fibrotic and cellular elements which will govern their imaging appearance, particularly the T2 signal. These tumors can be large and are characterized by moderate enhancement, which is characteristically persistent. Calcification is frequent.[24] Surgery is the treatment of choice, though recurrence is frequent. Chemotherapy is only employed in case of unresectable neoplasms.

Juvenile Nasopharyngeal Angiofibroma

Juvenile nasopharyngeal angiofibroma (JNA) is a benign but aggressive vascular tumor occurring in adolescent males. It usually presents with epistaxis and unilateral nasal obstruction. It arises from the sphenopalatine foramen and spreads to the pterygomaxillary fissure, pterygopalatine

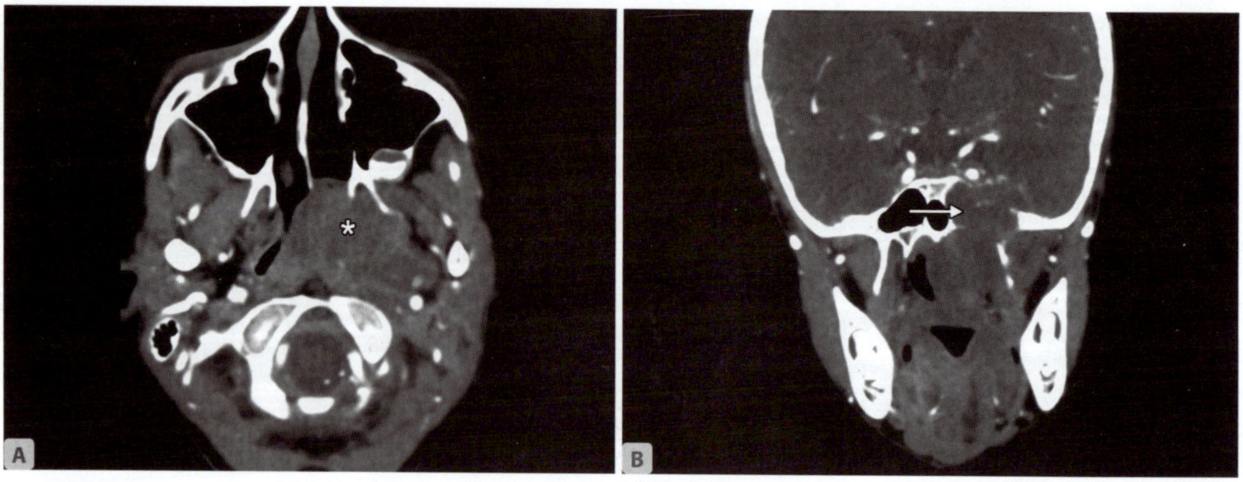

FIGS. 24A AND B: Rhabdomyosarcoma (RMS). (A and B) Contrast-enhanced computed tomography (CECT) axial and coronal images demonstrate a poorly defined, trans-spatial heterogeneously enhancing mass (asterisk) involving the nasopharyngeal mucosal, parapharyngeal, and masticator spaces with osseous invasion of the sphenoid bone (arrow) and intracranial extension.

fossa, infratemporal fossa, orbits, ethmoid and sphenoid sinuses, and cavernous sinus. Intracranial extension can occur through the superior orbital fissure or less frequently by direct invasion.[10]

Imaging

- *Contrast-enhanced computed tomography*: The appearance is of an intensely enhancing mass with extent as described above. CT delineates the osseous detail, including bony anatomy, erosion, and expansion **(Figs. 25A to C)**.
- *Magnetic resonance imaging*: Juvenile nasopharyngeal angiofibroma has low SI on T1WI, heterogeneous intermediate SI with flow voids on T2WI, and intense postcontrast enhancement with facilitated diffusion. The intracranial and intraorbital extension is also well-delineated on MRI.[11]

Lymphoma

It is the most common malignancy in children involving the extracranial head and neck region. Majority present as cervical nodal enlargement **(Figs. 26A and B)**. Non-Hodgkin's lymphoma may present with extranodal disease involving the Waldeyer's ring or the jaw.

Epithelial Malignancies

These are relatively less common in children, with nasopharyngeal carcinoma (NPC) and squamous cell carcinoma (SCC) in the setting of recurrent respiratory papillomatosis (RRP) being occasionally seen.

Nasopharyngeal Carcinoma

Benign enlargement of adenoids in children is a common entity and often NPC is not suspected till late in the course of the disease.[11] It is endemic in Southeast Asia, Southern China, and Mediterranean Basin. The childhood form of NPC is linked to Epstein–Barr virus (EBV) infection and has an undifferentiated histology. Characteristically, it presents as a painless upper neck mass (metastatic adenopathy) with or without nasal obstruction or bleeding.

On MRI, it is seen as a T2 hyperintense, mild-moderate homogenously enhancing mass in the posterolateral aspect of nasopharynx. Local extension into the pterygopalatine fossa, parapharyngeal space, and masticator space is commonly seen. Invasion of the central skull base with osseous erosion or widening of the petroclival fissure may be seen on CT.[25]

Cervical lymphadenopathy is seen in 80–90% of cases at presentation, with lateral retropharyngeal, high level II, and high level V nodes being commonly involved.[26] However, necrosis in these nodes is not seen as opposed to cervical nodes in adult NPC.

Squamous Cell Carcinoma in the Setting of Recurrent Respiratory Papillomatosis

Squamous cell carcinoma involving the larynx is very rare in the pediatric age group. Majority of the reported cases are transformed from the RRP with human papillomavirus (HPV) infection.[27] Papillomatosis is a condition associated with multiple papillomas. This condition typically affects children and young adults and is often limited to the larynx. It may involve the intrathoracic airways and also present with cavitating lung nodules and is referred to as RRP. Ill-defined soft-tissue thickening narrowing the upper airway with metastatic lymphadenopathy is usually seen **(Figs. 27A and B)**.

MISCELLANEOUS

Desmoid Infantile Fibromatosis

Desmoid infantile fibromatosis is a locally aggressive tumor encountered in children and young adults (it has a bimodal peak—one in first decade and then in third decade). It is common in extremities, truncal region, and less frequent in head and neck. If the lesion develops in a preexisting

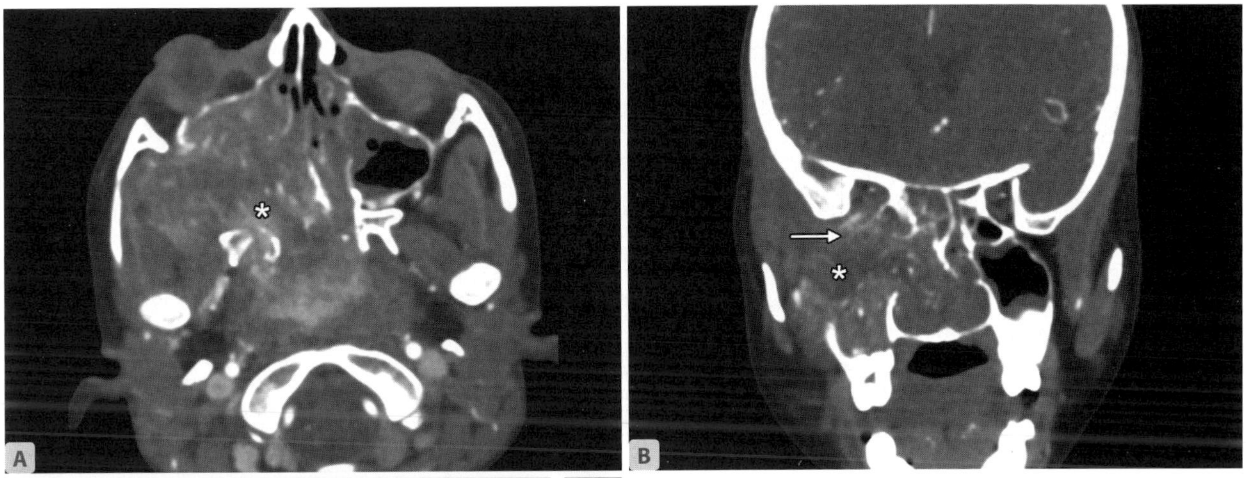

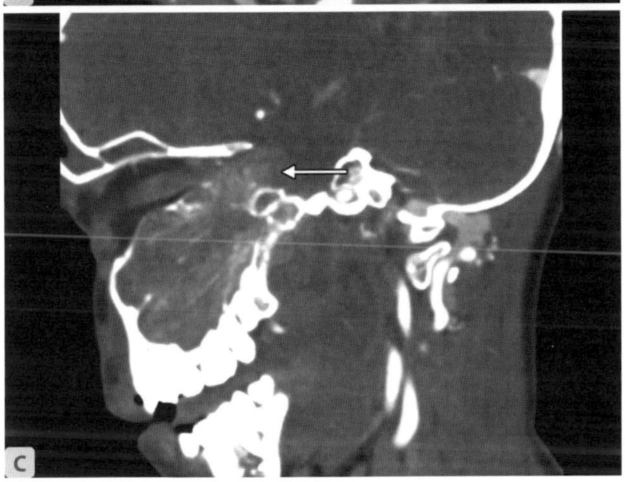

FIGS. 25A TO C: Juvenile nasopharyngeal angiofibroma (JNA). (A to C) Contrast-enhanced computed tomography (CECT) axial, coronal, and sagittal reveal an intensely enhancing heterogeneous mass lesion centered near right sphenopalatine foramen extending into right maxillary and ethmoid sinuses, posterior choana, and nasopharynx (asterisk in A). Laterally, the mass is extending into the pterygomaxillary fissure and masticator space (asterisk in B). There is widening of the inferior orbital fissure (arrow in B) and intracranial extension into the right temporal lobe (arrow in C).

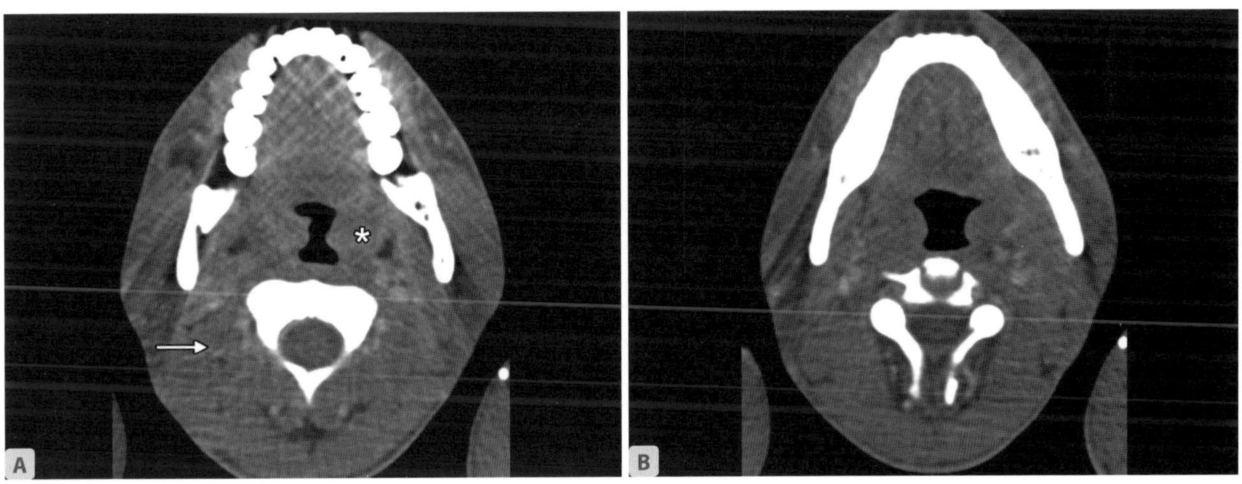

FIGS. 26A AND B: Burkitt's lymphoma. (A and B) Axial contrast-enhanced computed tomography (CECT) demonstrates internal jugular chain and posterior cervical (arrow) lymphadenopathy with tonsillar enlargement (asterisk in A).

fibroma, it has a more aggressive behavior. Association with familial adenomatous polyposis (FAP)/Gardner syndrome is described. Also, intra-abdominal lesions are more aggressive, compared to those in the head and neck or other sites.

Imaging

The masses can be well-delineated or infiltrative. The stroma of the tumors may predominantly have a stroma that is composed of collagen or one that is predominantly mucous.

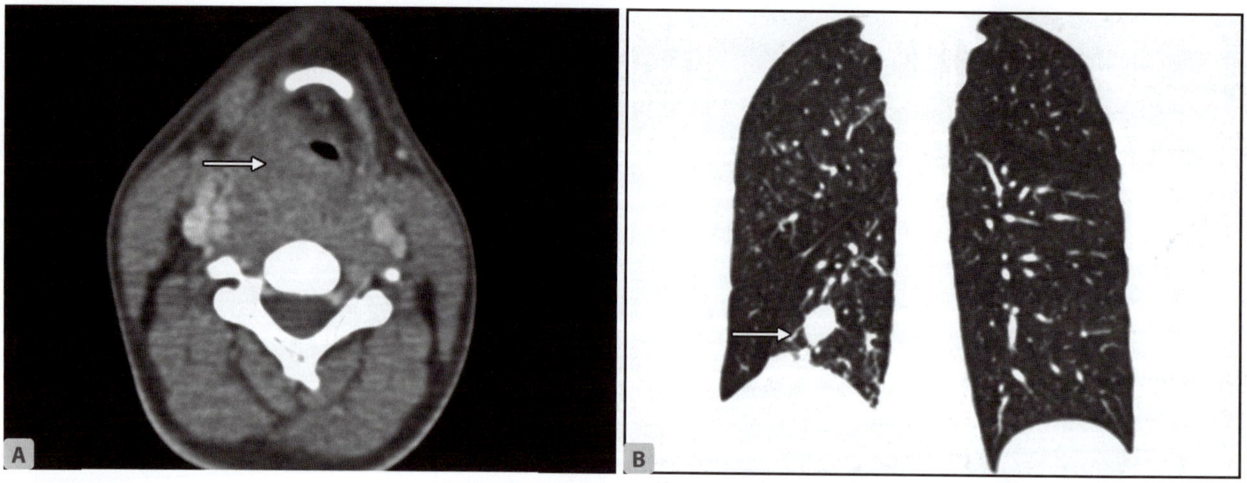

FIGS. 27A AND B: Squamous cell carcinoma (SCC) larynx in recurrent respiratory papillomatosis (RRP). (A) Axial contrast-enhanced computed tomography (CECT) of neck shows a large poorly enhancing supraglottic mass (arrow) in a young male with recurrent RRP; and (B) Coronal lung window CT chest reveals multiple large lung nodules in right lower lobe (arrow) with centrilobular nodules in right upper lobe due to aspiration.

Collagen-rich tumors are hypoechoic on USG and show posterior acoustic shadowing, have similar attenuation to muscles on CT, are T1 hypointense with variable T2 signal (collagen rich—hypointense, cellular—hyperintense) on MRI.

Mucous-rich tumors are also T1 hyperintense. Tumor may cause scalloping/pressure erosion of adjoining bone. Another sign described on imaging is the "fascial tail sign"—these results from extension of the neoplasm along the fascia.[28] Significant, heterogeneous contrast enhancement is seen on MR. Management is variable and includes surgical resection/chemotherapy.

NEONATAL NECK MASSES

The spectrum of lesions in the neonates is different from older children. These include vascular tumors, high-flow and low-flow vascular malformations, teratomas and other soft-tissue neoplasms, dermoid and epidermoid cysts, nasofrontal masses, and congenital goiter. The tumors include teratomas, primary cervical NB, and fibrous tumors (desmoid-type fibromatosis, fibromatosis colli, infantile fibrosarcoma, and fibrous hamartoma of infancy).[29]

Fibromatosis Colli

Also known as torticollis or wry neck, it presents as a distinct firm mass in the distal SCM in neonates after either vaginal or cesarean delivery. The right side and lower third of the muscles are more commonly involved. In approximately 10–20% of cases, congenital muscular torticollis may result due to the associated fibrosis.[7] USG reveals a hyperechoic or heteroechoic mass with a hypoechoic rim within the body of the SCM.[8] Spontaneous resolution is seen usually by 6–12 months of age. However, in some cases, it may lead to significant craniofacial asymmetry and scoliosis.

Melanotic Neuroectodermal Tumor of Infancy

Melanotic neuroectodermal tumor of infancy (MNTI) is a rare pigmented neoplasm of neural crest origin seen in infants. The majority of cases are seen in the maxilla and few in cranial vault. Though a benign tumor, it has aggressive nature and high recurrence rates.

Clinical Presentation

Painless, rapidly growing, and nonulcerative mass affecting the maxilla or other craniofacial structures. There may be feeding difficulties and aesthetic deformities.[30]

Imaging

- *Computed tomography*: Heterogeneously enhancing soft-tissue mass in the craniofacial skeleton with irregular lysis and adjacent hyperostosis/reactive sclerosis.
- *Magnetic resonance imaging* **(*Figs. 28A to C*)**: T1 hyperintensity is characteristic of melanin content. Subtracted images are required for assessment of contrast enhancement. T2 signal is heterogeneous and usually hypointense.[31]

Management is surgical resection; however, recurrence is seen in up to 15% of cases.[30]

CONCLUSION

In conclusion, familiarity with the spectrum of pediatric neck lesions and an algorithmic approach **(Flowchart 1)** allows an imaging-based diagnosis in a large proportion of patients.

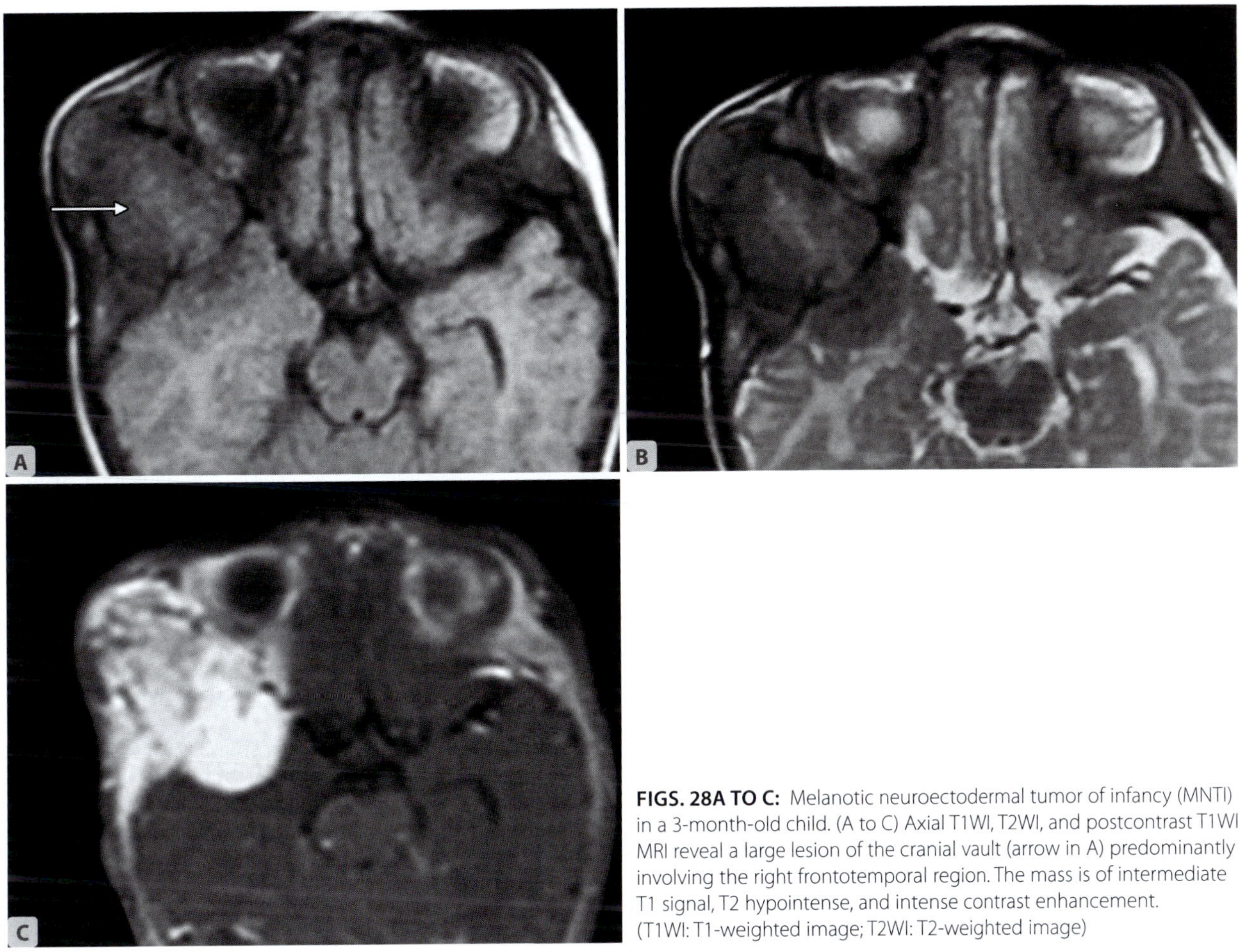

FIGS. 28A TO C: Melanotic neuroectodermal tumor of infancy (MNTI) in a 3-month-old child. (A to C) Axial T1WI, T2WI, and postcontrast T1WI MRI reveal a large lesion of the cranial vault (arrow in A) predominantly involving the right frontotemporal region. The mass is of intermediate T1 signal, T2 hypointense, and intense contrast enhancement. (T1WI: T1-weighted image; T2WI: T2-weighted image)

FLOWCHART 1: Algorithmic approach to pediatric neck masses.

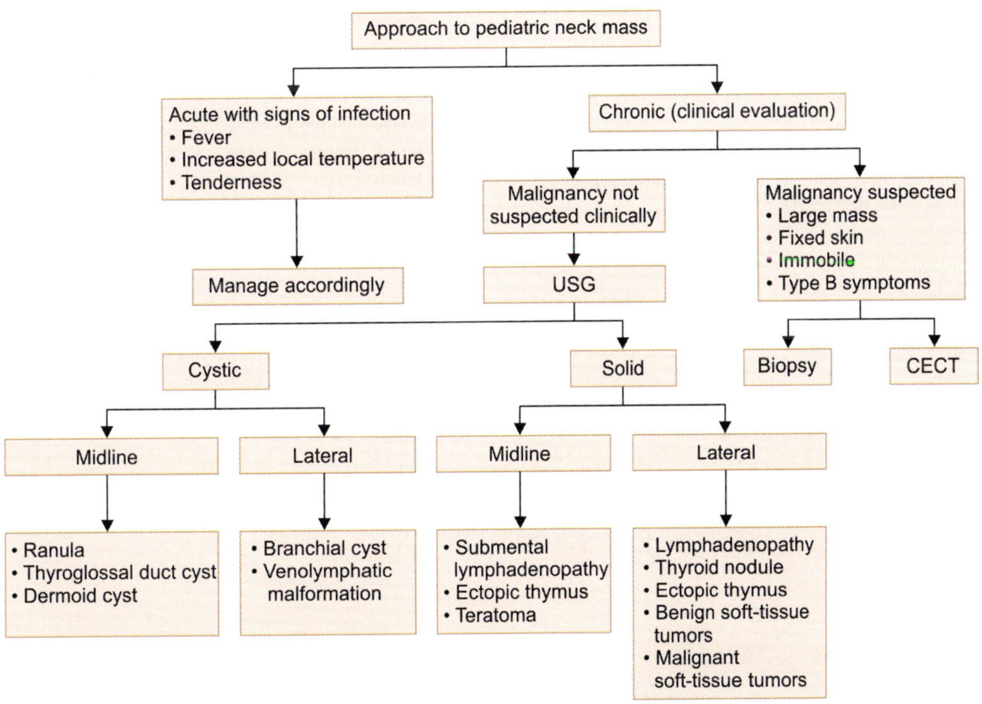

(CECT: contrast-enhanced computed tomography; USG: ultrasonography)

REFERENCES

1. Adams A, Mankad K, Offiah C, Childs L. Branchial cleft anomalies: a pictorial review of embryological development and spectrum of imaging findings. Insights Imaging. 2016;7:69-76.
2. Clevens R, Weimert T. Familial bilateral branchial cleft cysts. Ear Nose Throat J. 1995;74:419-21.
3. Bailey H. Branchial cysts and other essays on surgical subjects in the fascio-cervical region. London: H K Lewis & Company; 1929.
4. Ahuja A, King A, Metreweli C. Second branchial cleft cysts: variability of sonographic appearances in adult cases. AJNR Am J Neuroradiol. 2000;21:315-9.
5. Lowe LH, Stokes LS, Johnson JE, Heller RM, Royal SA, Wushensky C, et al. Swelling at the angle of the mandible: imaging of the pediatric parotid gland and periparotid region. Radiographics. 2001;21:1211-27.
6. Work W. Newer concepts of first branchial cleft defects. Laryngoscope. 1972;82:1581-93.
7. Malik A, Odita J, Rodriguez J, Hardjasudarma M. Pediatric Neck Masses: A Pictorial Review for Practicing Radiologists. Curr Probl Diagn Radiol. 2002;31:146-57.
8. Friedman ER, John SD. Imaging of Pediatric Neck Masses. Radiol Clin North Am. 2011;49:617-32.
9. Bansal AG, Oudsema R, Masseaux JA, Rosenberg HK. US of Pediatric Superficial Masses of the Head and Neck. Radiographics. 2018;38:1239-63.
10. Gujar S, Gandhi D, Mukherji SK. Topics in MRI: Pediatric Head and Neck Masses. Top Magn Reson Imaging. 2004;15:95-101.
11. Stern JS, Ginat DT, Nicholas JL, Ryan ME. Imaging of Pediatric Head and Neck Masses. Otolaryngol Clin North Am. 2015;48:225-46.
12. Léauté-Labrèze C, de la Roque DE, Hubiche T, Boralevi F, Thambo JB, Taïeb A. Propranolol for severe hemangiomas of infancy. N Engl J Med. 2008;358:2649-51.
13. Restrepo R, Palani R, Cervantes LF, Duarte AM, Amjad I, Altman NR. Hemangiomas revisited: the useful, the unusual and the new. Part 1: overview and clinical and imaging characteristics. Pediatr Radiol. 2011;41:895-904.
14. Restrepo R, Palani R, Cervantes LF, Duarte AM, Amjad I, Altman NR. Hemangiomas revisited: the useful, the unusual and the new. Part 2: endangering hemangiomas and treatment. Pediatr Radiol. 2011;41:905-15.
15. Gruman A, Liang MG, Mulliken JB, Fishman SJ, Burrows PE, Kozakewich HP, et al. Kaposiform hemangioendothelioma without Kasabach-Merritt phenomenon. J Am Acad Dermatol. 2005;52:616-22.
16. Bancroft LW, Kransdorf MJ, Peterson JJ, O'Connor MI. Benign fatty tumors: classification, clinical course, imaging appearance, and treatment. Skeletal Radiol. 2006;35:719-33.
17. Dreux N, Marty M, Chibon F, Vélasco V, Hostein I, Ranchère-Vince D, et al. Value and limitation of immunohistochemical expression of HMGA2 in mesenchymal tumors: about a series of 1052 cases. Mod Pathol. 2010;23:1657-66.
18. Gupta P, Potti TA, Wuertzer SD, Lenchik L, Pacholke DA. Spectrum of Fat-containing Soft-Tissue Masses at MR Imaging: The Common, the Uncommon, the Characteristic, and the Sometimes Confusing. Radiographics. 2016;36:753-66.
19. Lin J, Martel W. Cross-sectional imaging of peripheral nerve sheath tumors: characteristic signs on CT, MR imaging, and sonography. AJR Am J Roentgenol. 2001;176:75-82.
20. Abramson SJ, Berdon WE, Ruzal-Shapiro C, Stolar C, Garvin J. Cervical neuroblastoma in eleven infants—a tumor with favorable prognosis. Clinical and radiologic (US, CT, MRI) findings. Pediatr Radiol. 1993;23:253-7.
21. Jawad N, McHugh K. The clinical and radiologic features of paediatric rhabdomyosarcoma. Pediatr Radiol. 2019;49: 1516-23.
22. Leiner J, Le Loarer F. The current landscape of rhabdomyosarcomas: an update. Virchows Arch. 2020;476:97-108.
23. Coffin CM, Alaggio R. Fibroblastic and myofibroblastic tumors in children and adolescents. Pediatr Dev Pathol. 2012;15:127-80.
24. Patnana M, Sevrukov AB, Elsayes KM, Viswanathan C, Lubner M, Menias CO. Inflammatory pseudotumor: the great mimicker. AJR Am J Roentgenol. 2012;198:W217-27.
25. Yabuuchi H, Fukuya T, Murayama S, Sakai S, Okamura J, Fukuda T, et al. CT and MR features of nasopharyngeal carcinoma in children and young adults. Clin Radiol. 2002;57:205-10.
26. Stambuk HE, Patel SG, Mosier KM, Wolden SL, Holodny AI. Nasopharyngeal carcinoma: recognizing the radiographic features in children. AJNR Am J Neuroradiol. 2005;26:1575-9.
27. Zhang HK, Liu HG. Squamous cell carcinoma in the larynx in a 7-year-child. Pediatr Surg Int. 2011;27:1377-80.
28. Sargar KM, Sheybani EF, Shenoy A, Aranake-Chrisinger J, Khanna G. Pediatric Fibroblastic and Myofibroblastic Tumors: A Pictorial Review. Radiographics. 2016;36:1195-214.
29. Tranvinh E, Yeom KW, Iv M. Imaging neck masses in the neonate and young infant. Semin Ultrasound CT MR. 2015;36: 120-37.
30. Rachidi S, Sood AJ, Patel KG, Nguyen SA, Hamilton H, Neville BW, et al. Melanotic neuroectodermal tumor of infancy: a systematic review. J Oral Maxillofac Surg. 2015;73:1946-56.
31. Tan AP, Jacques TS, Mankad K, James G, Jeelani O, Slater O, et al. Melanotic neuroectodermal tumour of infancy: a case report and differential diagnosis. Neuroradiol J. 2018;31:434-9.

SECTION

4

Gastrointestinal and Hepatobiliary Imaging

CHAPTER

91

Imaging Techniques for Abdomen

Smriti Hari, Smita Manchanda

INTRODUCTION

The imaging techniques for evaluation of abdomen have evolved dramatically over the past few decades. Conventional radiographs and barium studies now have a limited role with the cross-sectional imaging modalities such as computed tomography (CT) and magnetic resonance imaging (MRI) being the mainstay of diagnosis. Ultrasound remains the first line investigation for suspected hepatobiliary and pancreatic pathologies. The recent advent of ultrasound contrast agents and elastography techniques has improved the diagnostic yield of ultrasound. The routine contrast-enhanced CT and MRI have been modified in the form of multiphase acquisition and enterography/colonography for an optimal delineation of hepatic/pancreatic and bowel pathologies respectively. There has been a significant advancement in the nuclear imaging studies with the advent of hybrid scanners like positron emission tomography (PET)-CT and PET-MRI that are capable of providing both anatomical and functional information.

CONVENTIONAL TECHNIQUES

Conventional radiographs of the abdomen are now limited to the emergency setting for the evaluation of suspected perforation and intestinal obstruction.

BARIUM STUDIES

Endoscopy is the investigation of choice for most esophageal pathologies with a complimentary role for barium studies. However, fluoroscopic barium studies **(Fig. 1)** are essential in the evaluation of motility disorders.

The stomach and duodenum are also best evaluated by endoscopy in cases of dyspepsia and abdominal pain. However, barium studies **(Fig. 2)** are required for assessing functional abnormalities like reflux and delayed emptying; submucosal masses and infiltrative processes. The barium/gastrografin oral contrast study is also the technique of choice for evaluation of early postoperative complications following gastric surgery.

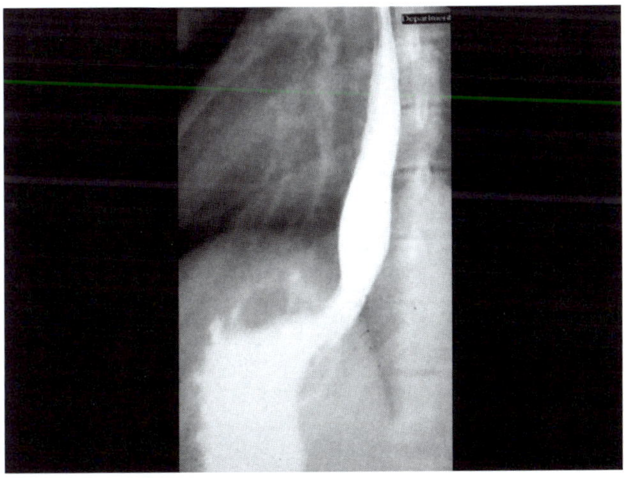

FIG. 1: The lower thoracic esophagus and gastroesophageal junction well seen in the distended state in a normal barium swallow.

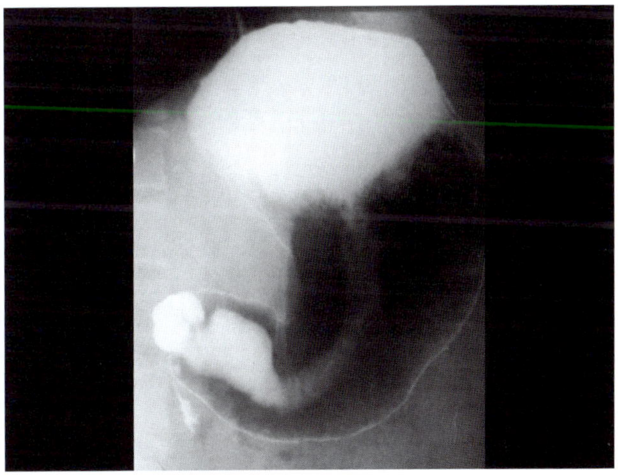

FIG. 2: Supine radiograph of double contrast barium swallow showing well-distended stomach and normal mucosal pattern.

For radiological evaluation of small bowel, both barium follow through **(Fig. 3)** and enteroclysis **(Fig. 4)**, are superior to CT/MRI examination in terms of demonstration of fine mucosal detail. The conventional enteroclysis has the advantages of shorter examination time, better distension of small bowel and better visualization of pathology but requires more radiologist time, greater technical skill, gives more radiation dose to patient and operator and is relatively uncomfortable for the patient. Small bowel follow through study is easy to perform, allows estimation of transit time and is more comfortable to the patient. However, complete and adequate distension of small bowel cannot be achieved in followthrough study.[1,2]

Colonoscopy is the investigation of choice for evaluation of colorectal diseases. However, barium enema **(Fig. 5)** is useful for delineating colonic caliber and configuration.[3] Also barium contrast enema is preferred in patients with question of large bowel obstruction, need for localization of colonic disease preoperatively or to assess the status of colon anastomosis.

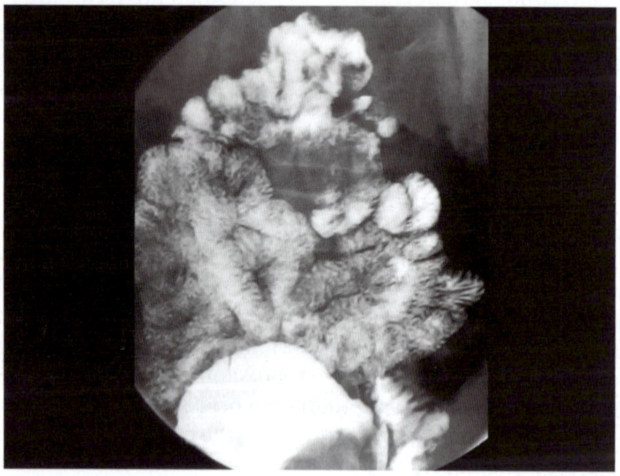

FIG. 3: Barium followthrough examination showing well-distended jejunal loops with normal villous pattern.

Prior to undertaking any barium procedure, appropriate medical history along with results of previous investigations (including imaging and endoscopic procedures) should be obtained. **Table 1** highlights the indications, contraindications, brief technique along with special modifications of the commonly performed barium procedures.[4-7]

ULTRASONOGRAPHY EVALUATION OF THE LIVER

Sonography is used as the initial imaging modality for suspected liver pathology.[8] It plays a vital role in the evaluation of focal liver lesions, screening for liver metastases in a patient with known malignancy, screening for hepatocellular carcinoma in the setting of hepatitis/cirrhosis, portal hypertension, surgical obstructive jaundice, hepatic veno-occlusive disease and preoperative work-up and postoperative follow-up of liver transplant patients. Sonography effectively differentiates a solid from a cystic lesion and provides significant information regarding the internal architecture of indeterminate lesions.

The addition of color Doppler flow imaging further helps in characterizing mass lesions and assessing patency of vessels.[9] Doppler is particularly helpful in liver transplants, Budd-Chiari syndrome and cirrhosis.

Technique

The liver is scanned in the supine or left decubitus position with a 3.5–5 MHz convex transducer in the transverse, sagittal and oblique planes, from a subcostal approach. The subcostal approach may not suffice in all patients and intercostal scanning may have to be done with a small footprint transducer.[9] This is especially true in shrunken cirrhotic livers. An attempt is made to delineate the venous landmarks so that all the liver segments can be identified and scanned sequentially.

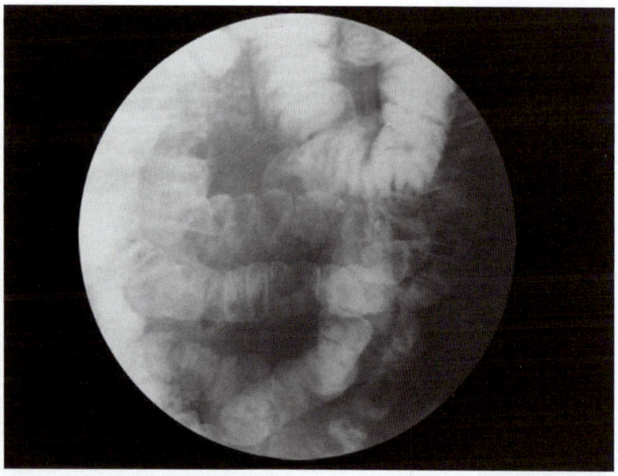

FIG. 4: Conventional small bowel enteroclysis showing normal distended jejunal and ileal loops in double contrast.

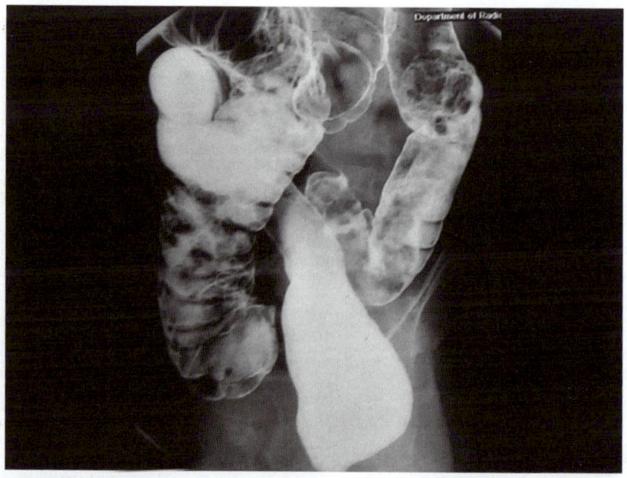

FIG. 5: Double contrast barium enema. Supine radiograph showing normal mucosal outline of the cecum, ascending colon, part of transverse colon and descending colon. The hepatic flexure and rectosigmoid colon are in a dependent position and hence seen in a barium-filled state.

TABLE 1: Commonly performed barium procedures.

Procedure	Indications	Contraindications	Patient preparation	Examination technique	Modifications
Barium swallow	• Dysphagia • Odynophagia • Reflux disease • Atypical chest pain	• Recent esophageal surgery • Recent gastric surgery • Recent trauma • Uncooperative patient	• Nil orally for a minimum of 2 hours prior to the procedure • No smoking	• Low density (60–95% weight per volume [weight/volume]) barium suspension is used • Esophagus anatomy and motility is evaluated under fluoroscopy • Spot images taken to document normal (barium-filled and mucosal relief views) and abnormal findings • Gastroesophageal junction is documented along with evaluation for reflux • *Double contrast:* Performed using a high-density (210–250% weight/volume) barium suspension along with an effervescent agent	*Water-soluble contrast agent*: In cases, where leak or perforation is suspected *Iso-osmolar or low-osmolar contrast or dilute barium*: In cases, where aspiration or esophageal-tracheal or bronchial fistula is suspected
Barium meal upper GI	• Suspected reflux • Epigastric pain/ discomfort • Dyspepsia • Upper GI bleeding • Anemia • Weight loss	• Recent esophageal surgery • Recent gastric surgery • Recent trauma • Uncooperative patient	• Nil orally after midnight, a day prior • No smoking	• Fluoroscopic evaluation of esophagus, stomach and duodenum • *Double contrast*: Performed using a high-density (210–250% weight/volume) barium suspension along with an effervescent agent • Spot images to document normal and abnormal findings • Barium-filled and mucosal relief views of esophagus, stomach and duodenum • Overhead images for full anatomical delineation of stomach	*Water-soluble contrast agent*: In cases, where leak or perforation is suspected
Barium follow-through	• Suspected small bowel obstruction • Unexplained GI bleeding • Malabsorption • Suspected enteric fistula • Abdominal pain • Diarrhea	• Uncooperative patient	• Nil orally after midnight prior to the procedure	• 600 mL of 50% weight/volume barium suspension • Oral administration over one hour • Fluoroscopic evaluation after 30 minutes and regular overhead radiographs in prone position • Spot compression views of any focal abnormality • Compression of accessible loops • Ileocecal junction demonstration • Peroral pneumocolon, if required for better delineation of distensibility of cecum and ileocecal junction	*Water-soluble contrast agent*: Preferred, if there is suspicion of bowel leak or obstruction

Continued

Continued

Procedure	Indications	Contraindications	Patient preparation	Examination technique	Modifications
Enteroclysis	• Recurrent small bowel obstructions • Unexplained weight loss or gastrointestinal (GI) bleeding • Anemia • Malabsorption	• Inability to pass catheter • Patient intolerance for catheter	• Nil orally after midnight before the procedure • Laxative may be given on the day prior to the examination • Enteroclysis catheter placed under fluoroscopic guidance and nasal anesthetic spray • Tip-positioned several centimeters beyond the duodenojejunal flexure	• Single-contrast examination • Medium-density barium suspension given via the tube to maintain adequate small bowel distension • Double-contrast examination • High-density barium suspension followed by 0.5% solution of hydroxypropyl methylcellulose, volume of room air • Administered under fluoroscopic guidance, double-contrast mucosal coating and optimal distention of small bowel • Infusion rate controlled to avoid excessive peristalsis • Avoid reflux of large amounts of this fluid into stomach • *Technique*: External compression, rotation and palpation • Separate overlapping bowel loops • Spot compression views • Overhead large-format • Images of completely distended small bowel	
Barium enema	• Abdominal pain • Diarrhea/ Constipation/Change in bowel habits • Gastrointestinal bleeding • Anemia • Abdominal masses • Weight loss • Fever or sepsis • History of previous colon polyp or neoplasm • Familial inheritance pattern diseases involving the colon	• Unexplained pneumoperitoneum • Toxic colon • Uncooperative patient • *Relative*: Rigid colonoscopy and biopsy	• Colon preparation to remove fecal matter and excess fluid • Dietary restriction • Hydration • Laxatives • Cleansing enemas	• Single-contrast enema • Low-density (15–25% weight/volume) barium suspension or water-soluble contrast • Spot compression views • Frontal views of entire filled colon • Lateral view of rectum • Angled-beam view of sigmoid colon • Postevacuation images • Double-contrast barium enema • Commercially available high-density (80% weight/volume or greater) barium suspension • Barium suspension and air introduced under fluoroscopic control • All segments of colon documented in double contrast • Overhead supine and prone radiographs of entire colon • Lateral view of rectum	*Water-soluble contrast*: • Immediate postoperative period • Suspected perforation • Bowel preparation not possible • Blind-ending colonic segments (e.g. Hartmann pouch) • May be therapeutic in cases of meconium ileus equivalent (cystic fibrosis)

(GI: Gastrointestinal).

Sonographic Anatomy

Liver parenchyma is imaged as fine homogeneous mid-level echoes interrupted only by fissures and vessels. The liver echogenicity is usually greater but may be equal to renal echogenicity. Hepatic veins **(Fig. 6)** are well-defined tubular structures without significant marginal echoes, whereas portal veins have echogenic walls due to fibrous and fatty tissue **(Fig. 7)**. Bile ducts run parallel to portal vein branches, but their location in relation to veins is variable, and the axiom that ducts are always anterior to portal vein branches is not correct. The state of art electronically focused ultrasound equipment demonstrates normal intrahepatic biliary radicles quite well and a bile duct must be at least 40% of the size of its neighboring portal vein branch for it to be considered dilated. Therefore, the mere visualization of parallel channels in the liver parenchyma does not indicate biliary dilatation.[9]

The gallbladder is located in the interlobar fissure and is well evaluated by ultrasound. The wall of the gallbladder should not be thicker than 3 mm in the fasting state. The common duct lies anterior to the portal vein at the porta hepatis and should be measured at the place where the hepatic artery crosses perpendicularly between them. This level has been used because of the consistent acoustic window provided by the surrounding liver, which ensures reproducibility of the measurement. The common duct should not be wider than 6 mm at this point.

On Doppler examination, the normal hepatic vein trace reflects the transmitted right heart pressure changes leading to flow reversal during the right atrial contraction **(Fig. 8)**. The portal vein trace is continuously antegrade with a mean peak velocity of 15–22 cm/s. The portal venous flow shows slight undulation related to the cardiac cycle and respiration **(Fig. 9)**.

Intraoperative Ultrasonography

Intraoperative and laparoscopic ultrasonography (US) are very useful techniques that have had major impact on patient management. A 5–7 MHz T-shaped linear array probe is used

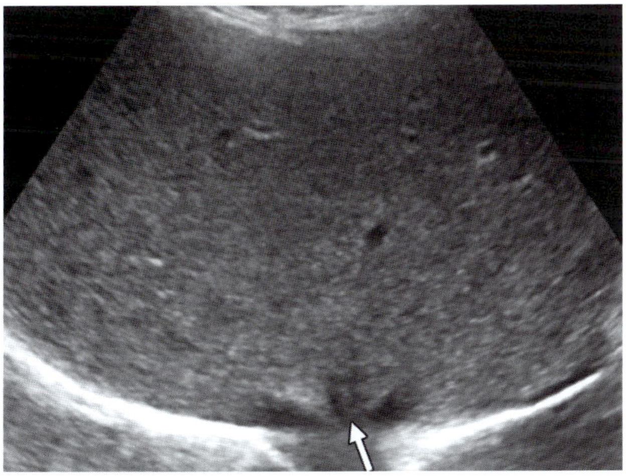

FIG. 6: Transverse US scan showing the three hepatic veins (arrow) joining the interior vena cava (IVC).

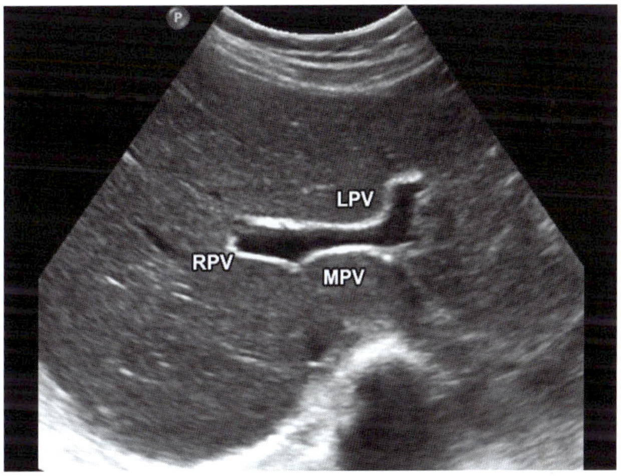

FIG. 7: Ultrasonography scan showing the bifurcation of main portal vein (MPV) into the right (RPV) and left portal veins (LPV).

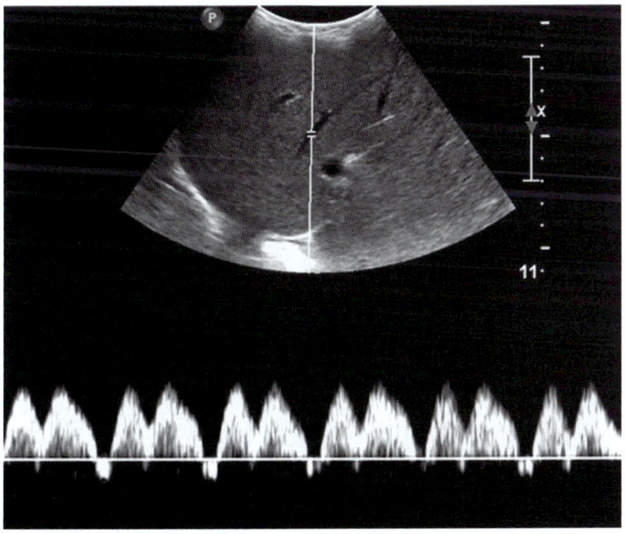

FIG. 8: Color Doppler flow imaging of hepatic vein showing normal triphasic flow pattern with a short phase of reversed flow.

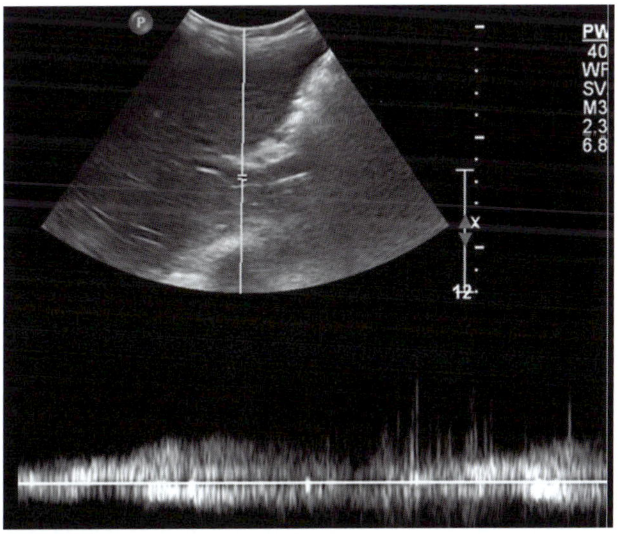

FIG. 9: Color Doppler flow imaging of portal vein showing continuous antegrade flow with minimal phasicity.

for intraoperative scanning. The probe can be sterilized using ethylene oxide gas sterilization. The probe is applied directly to the liver surface and no gel or acoustic coupling agent is necessary. The liver is scanned from the dome to the caudal edge and from left to right in a sequential manner. Color Doppler can be coupled with the grayscale scan and is very useful to identify vascular landmarks and assess their patency.

Intraoperative ultrasonography (IOUS) provides useful real time information to the surgeon and can alter the surgical approach. Current applications for IOUS include tumor staging, metastases evaluation, tumor ablation processes, evaluation of patency of vessels, intrahepatic biliary disease, and in liver transplantation.[9]

Endosonography

The development of endoscopic US (EUS) has rendered the gastrointestinal tract amenable to high resolution US examination and histopathologic sampling when required in the same session. Higher frequency probes (6–10 MHz) are used during EUS and the echoendoscopes have biopsy channels for performing fine-needle aspiration (FNA).[10] It is useful for assessing the depth of tumor invasion and sampling of smaller lesions and adjacent lymph nodes. It is being used to stage esophageal and stomach malignancies in many centers.

Similarly, transrectal ultrasonography can be used for staging of colorectal carcinomas. Anal endosonography is useful in patients with injury to the external anal sphincter and presenting with fecal incontinence.

Endoscopic US is also used for the characterization of cystic lesions of the pancreas by identifying the ultrasound morphology and performing FNA with cyst aspiration.[10]

USG Elastography

Elastography is a recent development, which gives a measure of tissue stiffness.[11,12] Depending on the deforming force applied and the method used to study the resultant deformation, it can be classified as:

- Static elastography
- Impulse elastography
  - Unidimensional transient elastography (Fibroscan)
  - Acoustic radiation force impulse (ARFI) imaging mode elastography
  - Shear wave elastography.

Acoustic radiation force impulse (ARFI) elastography gives a quantitative measure of the shear wave speed (in m/s) induced by acoustic radiation through an external vibrator. The measurement area is a 1 × 0.5 cm rectangle placed on the B-mode ultrasound image. These measurements are taken in the right lobe of liver through the intercostal space. Its main use is in the assessment of liver fibrosis and hepatic masses. However, this technique is not real time, does not give standard deviation and the size of the measurement area cannot be changed.[11]

Shear wave elastography measures the speed of shear waves that are produced in the tissue perpendicular to the direction of displacement when a focused ultrasound beam provides an acoustic 'push'. The acquisition is real time with simultaneous display of the B-mode image and the corresponding shear wave elastography image (two-dimensional box with elastography color map). The speed of shear waves is used to calculate the elasticity in kilopascals (kPa and real time measurements can be made by placing the Q box over the region of interest **(Fig. 10)**. The system generates the maximum, minimum and mean values along with the standard deviation. The size and position of the Q-box can be altered and in addition, retrospective measurements can be made with this system.

USG Contrast Agents

Contrast-enhanced ultrasound (CEUS) uses microbubble-based contrast agents to improve the echogenicity of blood. It has major clinical applications in echocardiography, hepatology and vessel evaluation. It can be easily peformed after baseline ultrasound in the same sitting and provides functional vascular information without the use of ionic radiation.

The microbubbles have an average diameter of 1–4 µm and they oscillate at ultrasound frequencies of 1–15 MHz. These nonlinear oscillations generate echoes which are detected by the imaging system. With the availability of phase modulation and amplitude modulation techniques, the sensitivity of ultrasound equipment for microbubble detection has consistenly improved in the last decade.[13]

Examples of commonly used contrast agents include SonoVue (sulfur hexafluoride microbubble) and Levovist (microcrystalline suspension of galactose and palmitic acid). The contrast agent is available in the lyophilized powder form, which is to be mixed with 5 mL of 0.9% normal saline and injected as a rapid IV bolus followed by 5–10 mL of saline flush. USG scanning is started immediately and

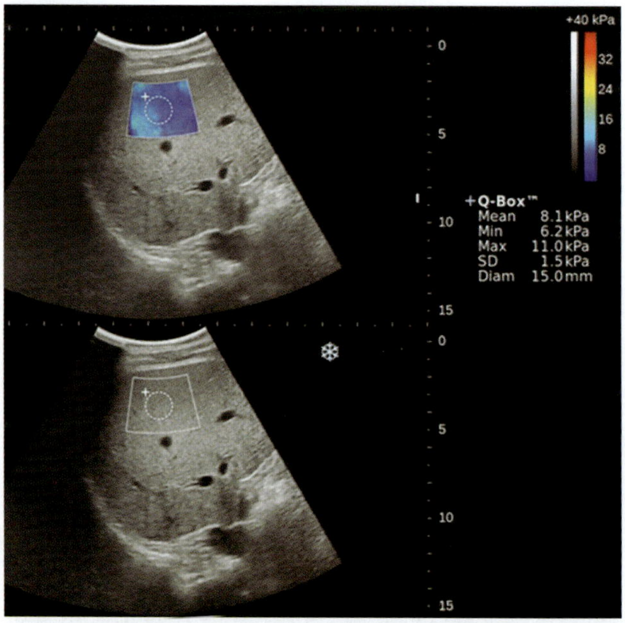

FIG. 10: Shear wave elastography of the liver seen as dual display. The color in the box corresponds to the velocity of the shear waves. The velocity is measured in kilopascals and is displayed in the vertical bar on the right.

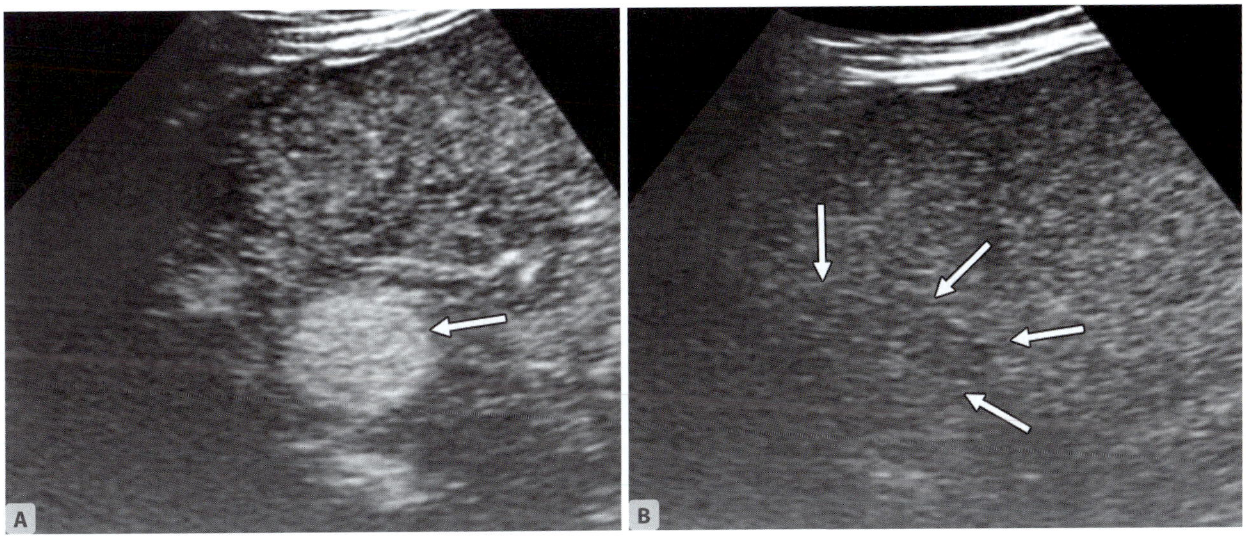

FIGS. 11A AND B: Small HCC in a 30-year-old man with chronic liver disease. (A) Arterial phase US image obtained 20 seconds after contrast material injection demonstrates diffuse homogeneous enhancement of the nodule (arrow); (B) Delayed phase US image obtained 192 seconds after injection shows washout (arrows).

takes approximately 4–5 minutes. For the evaluation of liver lesions, real time imaging is performed through the arterial, portal venous and parenchymal phases **(Figs. 11A and B)**. Contrast is seen to pass through the hepatic artery and its branches with liver echogenecity increasing from the arterial to the portal phase. Lesion echogenecity is compared to the parenchyma at the same depth and their enhancement pattern is compared with that of the blood pool.[13,14]

USG Image Fusion and Navigation

The higher end ultrasound machines provide integrated image fusion and instrument navigation capabilities. The image navigation system provides real time guidance for soft tissue biopsy and ablation procedures in ultrasound combining the cross-sectional data available. Image fusion techniques makes it possible to target those lesions which are not well visualized on USG but are seen on another modality like CT or MRI. The CT/MRI images of the patient are added onto the ultrasound fusion system. The two-dimensional cross-sectional images are then transformed into dynamic, fused imaging maps that combine CT or MR imaging with live ultrasound.

CT EXAMINATION OF THE ABDOMEN AND PELVIS

For complete CT evaluation of abdomen and pelvis, images are acquired in the axial plane from the dome of diaphragm to below the ischial tuberosities in suspended respiration. The slice thickness is 5 mm or less. CT examination is optimized for each patient according to the relevant history and clinical indication. This includes determining the need for non-contrast scan and planning of the study as a single phase or multiphase study.[15]

Enteric contrast agent is used for better delineation of bowel loops and can be administered orally, via nasogastric tube, per rectally or in varying combinations. Positive contrast agents include dilute barium (1–2%) and water-soluble iodinated contrast material (2–3%). These help to differentiate intraluminal from extraluminal pathology and detect suspected leaks. However, bowel wall enhancement characteristics are difficult to interpret when positive contrast agents have been used. Similarly, they also interfere with the 3D reformatted angiographic images and should not be used in cases of suspected GI bleed.[15,16]

Neutral contrast material is more useful when bowel wall characteristics need to be evaluated and in vascular studies. These include water and agents with water density like mannitol, lactulose and methylcellulose. However, the evaluation of abscesses and hypodense collections becomes more challenging with use of neutral contrast agents.

Negative contrast agents like air and carbon dioxide are used routinely in CT colonography for optimal colonic distension.

When single-phase acquisition is planned, intravenous nonionic iodinated contrast (100 mL of 350 mg I/mL) is administered and images are acquired after 50–70 seconds. When evaluating CT abdomen, care should be taken to use different widow width and window level settings for viewing the visceral organs, the intra-abdominal fat, bony anatomy and lung bases as well. Multiphase acquisition is planned according to the area of interest as described below.[15]

CT Evaluation of Hepatic Pathology

Multiphase CT scanning should be performed for the evaluation of liver pathology.

Multidetector CT Evaluation

Typically a *triple phase CT* is performed in case of suspected liver lesion.

Non-contrast scan has a limited role, and is of use predominantly in patients treated with TACE or other ablative therapies. It can help to assess post-contrast enhancement in patients with siderotic nodules of increased attenuation.

However, in order to keep the radiation dose low, most studies now do not recommend acquisition of the pre-contrast scan.[17,18]

Intravenous contrast is administered in a dose of 1.5–2 mL per kg body weight. The total iodine dose should be 525 mg iodine per kg or more; assuming iodine concentration of contrast to be 350 mg iodine per milliliter. Contrast should be administered at a flow rate of 3–4 mL/s using dual head mechanical injector and followed by saline flush. Most scanners now provide bolus-tracking software and passage of contrast through the descending aorta should be monitored to start the image acquisition.[19,20]

The images are acquired in the arterial, portal venous and delayed phases. The *early arterial phase* (about 10 seconds after the injection) is characterized by enhancement of the hepatic artery but not the portal vein. This phase is reserved for patients in whom CT angiography is required, such as potential transplant recipients, candidates for hepatic resection or cryoablation, or candidates for chemo-embolization.[21] CT angiography images can be created through three-dimensional reconstructions of the thin slice, isotropic images obtained in the early arterial phase. Water is preferred as the oral contrast agent for multiplanar CT angiography to allow optimal reconstructions from the 3D data sets. Maximum intensity projection, surface-shaded display, and volume-rendered techniques are used in the post-processing of CT angiography to depict vascular anatomy **(Figs. 12A and B)**.

The *late arterial phase,* which is acquired 20 seconds after contrast injection, is characterized by enhancement of hepatic artery, its branches and the portal vein.[22] This phase is critical for picking up hypervascular tumors. A combined CT angiogram/CT portogram can be obtained from the late arterial imaging phase and is used for delineation of the extrahepatic portal venous system in transplant cases and patients with pancreaticobiliary malignancy.[21] Venous compression, venous stenosis or thrombosis, and portal systemic venous collateral vessels can be displayed.

This is followed by the *portal venous* phase acquisition at 60–80 seconds after the start of injection of contrast. In this phase, there is peak parenchymal enhancement with optimal opacification of both the portal veins and the hepatic veins.[19,23]

The *delayed phase* is acquired to study the washout characteristics of liver lesions, capsular enhancement and to observe the delayed contrast enhancement of certain tumors like cholangiocarcinomas. This is acquired at 3–5 minutes post-contrast injection.[19]

The protocol has been summarized in **Table 2.**[19,23]

Dual Energy CT Evaluation

Triple-phase CT on a dual energy CT scanner is performed similarly as described above for the multidetector CT. The main advantage is generation of virtual unenhanced images

TABLE 2: Multidetector CT protocol (hepatic evaluation).

Intravenous Contrast:

Iodinated contrast medium: Iodine concentration 350 mg/mL
- Volume: 1.5–2 mL/kg
- Flow rate: 3–4 mL/s
- Bolus tracking software
- Mechanical injector with saline flush

Oral contrast: 600 mL tap water

Image acquisition:
- *Non-contrast phase*:
  - Before the injection of contrast material
  - In patients treated with ablative therapies
- *Late arterial phase*:
  - 20 seconds after start of injection
- *Portal venous phase*:
  - 60–80 seconds after start of injection
- *Delayed phase*:
  - >120 seconds after start of injection (3–5 min)

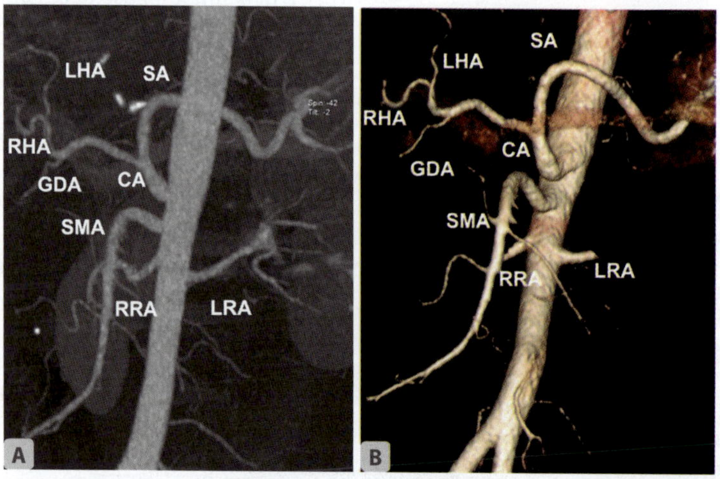

FIGS. 12A AND B: Coronal maximum intensity projection (MIP) (A) and volume rendered technique (VRT); (B) reconstructed from the axial MDCT images obtained during early arterial phase of contrast enhancement demonstrates abdominal aorta and its branches. (CA: celiac axis; SMA: superior mesenteric artery; SA: splenic artery; GDA: gastroduodenal artery; RHA: right hepatic artery; LHA: left hepatic artery; RRA: right renal artery; LRA: left renal artery).

without adding to the radiation dose **(Figs. 13A to D)**. These help to detect the presence of calcification and fat within lesions. Few studies have reported that it is feasible to quantity iron deposition in the liver, with dual energy CT.[24]

VOLUME ESTIMATION

Volume estimation of the liver **(Fig. 14)** helps in accurate planning of hepatic resection by delineating the exact 3D anatomy of the liver.[21] Estimation of liver volume using three-dimensional techniques, when combined with clinical and laboratory evaluation of liver function, can aid in predicting postoperative liver failure in patients undergoing resection, assists in embolization procedures, and planning of staged hepatic resection for bilobar disease.[25]

MULTIDETECTOR COMPUTED TOMOGRAPHY EVALUATION OF PANCREATIC PATHOLOGY

For the evaluation of the pancreas, multiphase acquisition **(Figs. 15A and B)** is recommended.[26]

The precontrast images are followed by the arterial phase at 17–25 seconds after the start of contrast injection. This phase is recommended wherever optimal delineation of the arterial supply is required.

The peak parenchymal enhancement of the pancreas is seen at 35–50 seconds after the start of contrast injection.

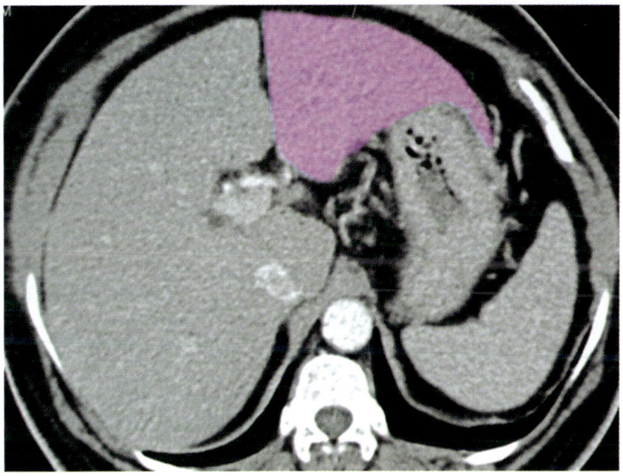

FIG. 14: CT volumetry in a patient planned for partial liver resection. Segments II and III are manually mapped out on contiguous axial slices and the volume is calculated using volumetric software.

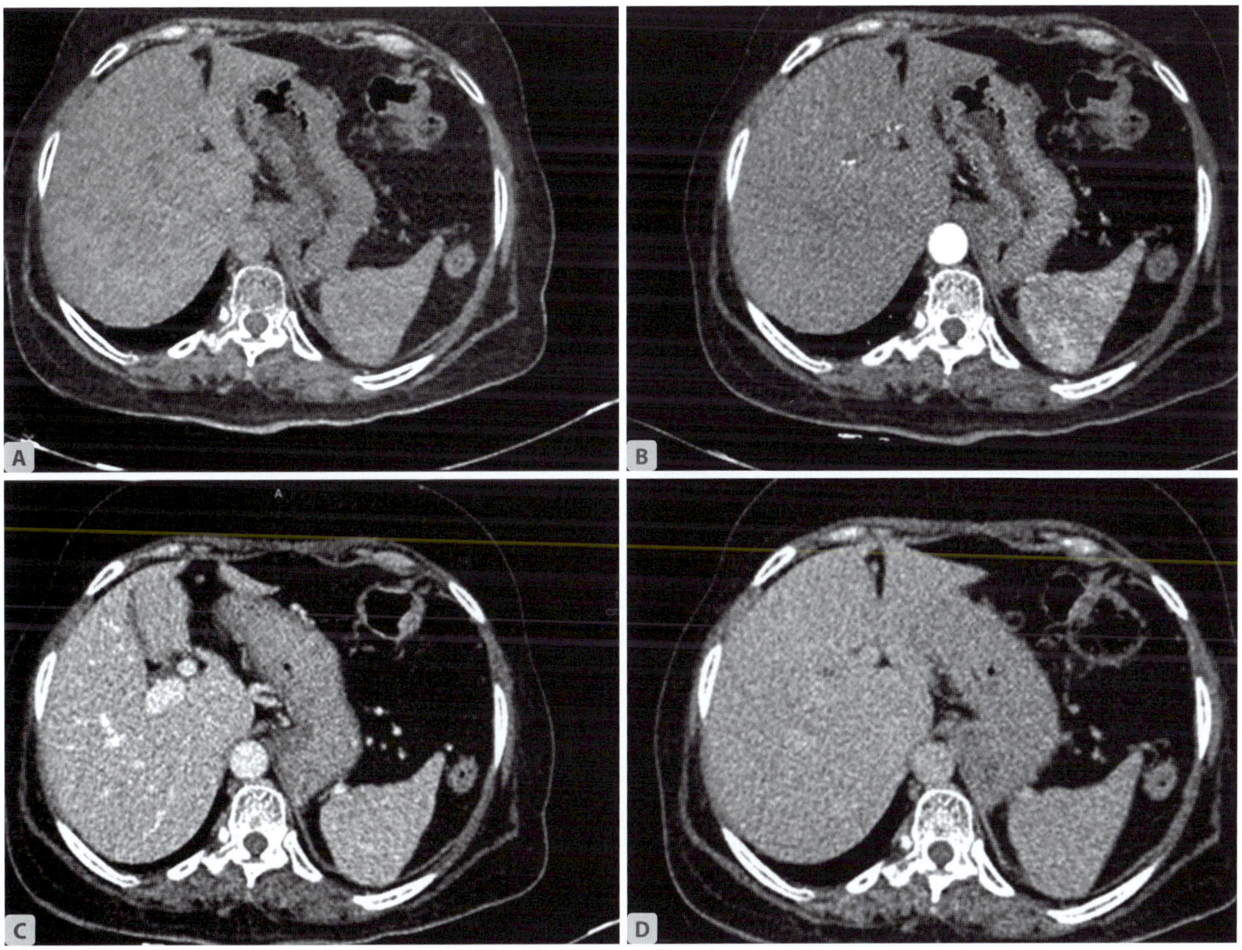

FIGS. 13A TO D: Multiphase CT acquisition for liver performed on a dual energy scanner. Virtual non-contrast (A); arterial (B); portal venous (C) and delayed (D) phase images reveal widening of the fissures in this known case of chronic liver disease. No focal lesion was detected.

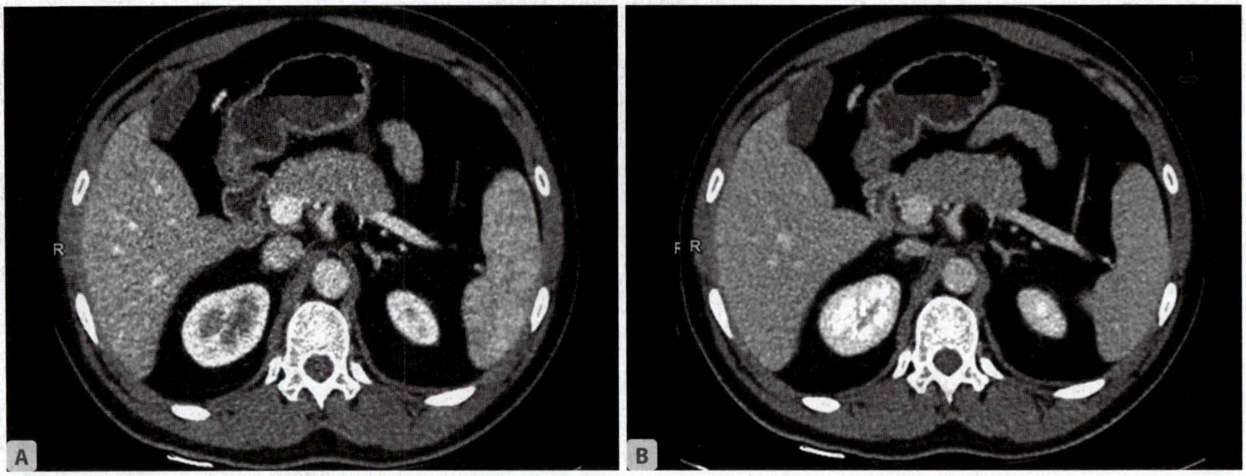

FIGS. 15A AND B: Multiphase CT acquisition for pancreas performed for suspicious lesion on USG. Pancreatic phase (A) is acquired at 35 seconds and portal venous phase (B) at 65 seconds after the injection of contrast medium. No focal lesion was detected.

TABLE 3: MDCT pancreatic protocol (image acquisition).

- *Arterial phase*:
  - 17–25 seconds after start of injection
  - For angiography images and arterial supply delineation
- *Pancreatic phase*:
  - 35–50 seconds after start of injection
  - Peak tumor-parenchymal attenuation difference
- *Portal venous phase*:
  - 55–70 seconds after start of injection
  - Venous involvement and metastases

TABLE 4: CT enterography protocol.

- Nil orally
- Intestine cleansing: Polyethylene glycol lavage
- *Oral contrast*:
  - 300 mL 20% w/v mannitol mixed with 1.5 L water
  - 500 mL mixture given orally every 15 minutes
  - Remaining solution: On table oral administration
- Scan performed at 50 minutes
- *Intravenous contrast injection*:
  - 100–120 mL @ 3–4 mL/sec
  - Single phase/Multiphase acquisition

This pancreatic phase is best for peak tumor-parenchymal attenuation difference. Curved multiplanar reformat (MPR) can be obtained along the pancreatic duct for showing relationship of the duct with the tumor **(Table 3)**.

The portal venous phase is acquired 55–70 seconds after the start of contrast injection and is ideal for depiction of venous involvement and liver metastases.[26,27] Minimum intensity projection (MinIP) images are used to delineate the anatomy of the pancreatic and biliary tree, which are seen as low-density structures.

BOWEL EVALUATION

CT Enteroclysis

Computed tomography (CT) enteroclysis involves the insertion of a nasojejunal tube under fluoroscopic guidance. The catheter tip is placed in the proximal jejunum and 1.5 L saline infused at 100 mL/min followed by on table infusion of 1.5 L saline with 100–120 mL intravenous contrast administration and single portal venous phase acquisition.[28] It has been replaced by CT enterography at most institutions.

CT Enterography

This is the preferred examination technique for the evaluation of small bowel pathology and is replacing traditional barium fluoroscopic studies, especially in cases of Crohn's disease.[29]

Neutral oral contrast agents are administered for optimal distension of small bowel. Bowel is prepared by prior fasting for 8 hours and intake of 50–100 mL of laxative diet solution (Polyethylene glycol lavage) one day prior to the study.[16] The neutral oral contrast agents used include water, mannitol, lactulose, methylcellulose, polyethylene glycol and 0.1% barium suspension. The CT attenuation of these agents is 0–30 HU and provides optimal contrast between bowel wall and lumen.[29]

The oral contrast should be consumed over 30–60 minutes. The protocol varies with institutions and a suggested protocol is given in **Table 4.**[16] Intravenous contrast is given (100–120 mL @ 3–4 mL/sec) and single-phase images are acquired between 50–70 seconds (either enteric or portal venous phase). However, in cases of obscure GI bleeding, both the arterial and portal venous phases must be acquired. Multiplanar reconstructions in the coronal plane **(Fig. 16)** better depict the anatomical relation of bowel loops and maximum intensity projection (MIP) images provide angiographic images for suspected GI bleed.[29]

CT Colonography

CT colonography **(Table 5)**[16] is a minimally invasive procedure for evaluation of the large bowel. It can be used as a screening, surveillance or diagnostic modality depending

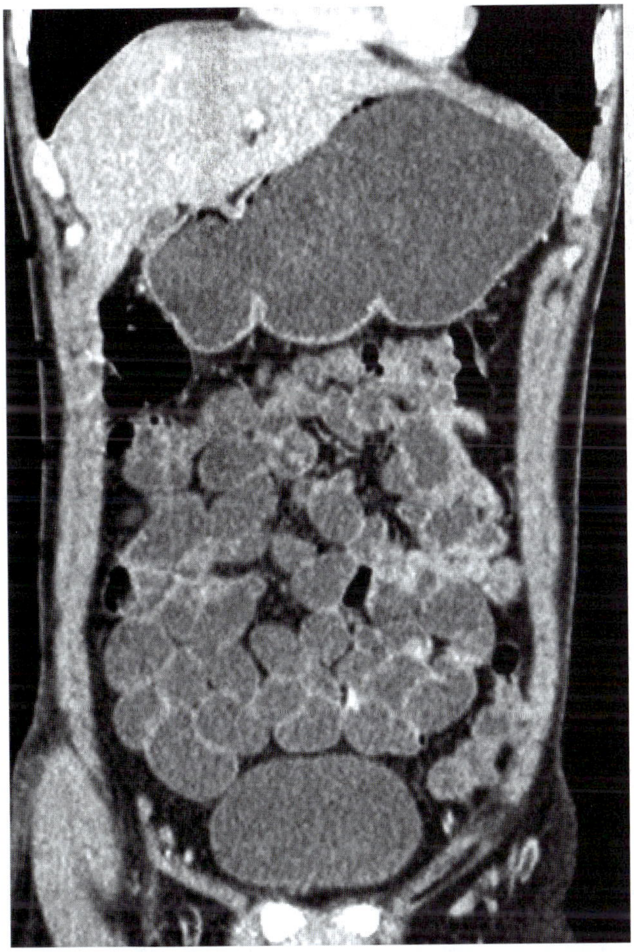

FIG. 16: CT enterography (coronal reformatted image) showing normal distension of the small bowel loops with no abnormal enhancement.

TABLE 5: CT colonography protocol.

- *Patient preparation*:
  - Low fiber diet
  - Adequate hydration
  - Intestinal cleansing: Polyethylene glycol lavage
- *Fecal tagging*: Oral administration of iodinated contrast or dilute barium
- Evacuation prior to the study
- *Colonic distension*: Carbon dioxide/Room air
- *Scanning*:
  - Precontrast images; prone position
  - 100–120 mL intravenous contrast administration
  - Portal venous phase acquisition; supine position

on the patient profile. Colonic preparation is essential and consists of low fiber diet (for 1–3 days), hydration and 50–100 mL of laxative diet solution (Polyethylene glycol lavage), one day prior to the study. Fecal tagging is usually performed with oral administration of water-soluble iodinated contrast or dilute barium. This is done to incorporate positive contrast into residual fecal material and increase its CT density. The increased density helps to distinguish fecal material from polyps or malignancy.[30]

The patient should be asked to evacuate prior to the study. Soft and flexible rectal catheter is inserted and the colon is insufflated with carbon dioxide (mechanical) or room air (manual). CT scout film should be taken to check the adequacy of colonic distension. Low dose pre-contrast scan is acquired in the prone position, followed by intravenous contrast administration. Images are then acquired at 50–70 sec in the portal venous phase in the supine position. Optimal colonic distension is indicated by pencil thin colonic wall with thin haustral folds. Axial and coronal reconstructed images can be analyzed using CAD software, wherever available.[16,30]

MAGNETIC RESONANCE IMAGING

Magnetic resonance (MR) imaging is an excellent imaging modality because of its high contrast resolution, multiplanar capability, sensitivity to blood flow and lack of ionizing radiation. Technical advances in MR hardware and software have allowed the introduction of faster pulse sequences without the motion artifacts that previously posed limitations to abdominal MR imaging. The use of parallel imaging techniques with multi-channel phased array coils has significantly reduced the scan time. MRI of the abdomen **(Table 6)** is now an important modality for imaging the abdomen encompassing a variety of sequences, which are continuously being improvised.[31]

Higher field strengths are preferred (1.5 T or 3 T) for abdomen evaluation. The advantage of 3T imaging systems is increased signal-to-noise ratio, better delineation of post-contrast enhancement and reduced time for chemical shift sequences (echo times of in and opposed phase sequences is less compared with 1.5 T). At the same time, in comparison to 1.5 T, 3 T scanners have increased specific absorption rate (SAR) and suffer from greater magnetic field inhomogeneity making images more prone to susceptibility and chemical shift artifacts.[32,33]

Phased array surface coil is used for abdomen evaluation. T1- and T2-weighted imaging is performed using breath-hold or respiratory triggered sequences. The acquisition is usually multiplanar with slice thickness of 5–8 mm and interslice gap not more than 3 mm. Either spin-echo (TSE or FSE) or gradient echo sequences can be used for T1-weighted imaging, with at least one in and out-of-phase gradient T1 sequence. T2-weighted images include either spin-echo sequences (TSE or FSE) or hybrid gradient and spin-echo (GRASE) sequences. Fat suppression is required during T2 weighted imaging, and can be achieved by chemical selective fat saturation, short tau inversion recovery (STIR), or spectral presaturation inversion recovery (SPIR). 3D sequences (both T1 and T2) are also available and provide higher SNR with better fat suppression. Intravenous contrast (gadolinium chelates) is used depending on the study protocol. Post-contrast administration, 2D or 3D T1-weighted sequences with fat suppression are acquired.[31]

Heavily T2-weighted magnetic resonance cholangio-pancreatography (MRCP) sequences are used for evaluation of the biliary and pancreatic ductal system. The sequences used are breath-hold rapid acquisition relaxation enhancement (RARE) or half-Fourier single-shot echo train

TABLE 6: MRI abdomen protocol.

• Fasting for 6 hours • Pelvic phased array surface coil • IV buscopan (1 mL~20 mg) • *Sequences*: - *T2WI*: Fat-suppressed; spin echo/hybrid sequence (axial, coronal) - Steady state fast field echo sequence: Axial - T1 in and opposed phase (axial) - DWI (b value 0, 400, 800) - T2 (multiecho) - *MRCP*: ▪ Breath-hold rapid acquisition relaxation enhancement (RARE) or half-Fourier single-shot echo train spin-echo sequence (thick slab acquisition) ▪ 3D respiratory-triggered T2- weighted FSE technique	• *Postcontrast (multiphase acquisition)*: - 2D or 3D T1-weighted sequences with fat suppression • *Pancreatic protocol*: - *Arterial phase*: 20 seconds after start of injection - *Portal Venous phase*: 45–65 seconds after start of injection - *Equilibrium phase*: 3–5 min after start of injection • *Hepatic Protocol:* - *Late arterial phase*: 20 seconds after start of injection - *Portal venous phase*: 60–80 seconds after start of injection - *Delayed phase*: >120 seconds after start of injection (3–5 min) - *Hepatobiliary phase*: Gadobenate dimeglumine (MultiHance): one hour postcontrast injection - *Gadoxetate (Eovist)*: 20 minutes postcontrast injection

spin-echo sequence as a thick slab acquisition **(Fig. 17)** in multiple projections or as multiple thin (less than 5 mm) slices in coronal or axial plane. 3D respiratory-triggered T2-weighted FSE techniques with maximum intensity projection (MIP) reconstruction **(Fig. 18)** can also be used.[31]

Diffusion-weighted imaging for abdomen uses single-shot echo-planar sequences, breath-held or respiratory triggered. At least two b-values are used (b = 0 to 50 s/mm^2 and b = 500 to 1,000 s/mm^2) and ADC maps are generated for proper interpretation. DWI has short acquisition time and is now a part of the routine protocol. In patients with contraindications to MR contrast this sequence is particularly advantageous.[16,31]

MRI of the Liver

MRI has evolved from a problem solving technique to first line investigative modality for liver lesions.

Pelvic-phased array surface coil is used with field of view including the entire liver. Acquisition is predominantly in the axial plane with additional coronal plane imaging to better depict the vascular anatomy and the hepatic dome.[34]

T1-weighted imaging is performed as in-phase and out-of-phase chemical shift gradient-recalled echo sequences prior to contrast administration. This is useful in evaluation of focal fat containing lesions and diffuse pathology like hepatic steatosis and iron overload.[35] In-phase (IP) and out-of-phase (OP) imaging is performed with a TE of 2.1 msec and 4.2 msec, respectively on 3T magnets. Both the images can be obtained in one TR by use of a double echo technique.[35]

T2-weighted images are acquired in the axial and coronal planes using a breath-hold or non-breath-hold technique. These include the accelerated fast spin-echo or single-shot accelerated fast spin-echo (half-Fourier single-shot turbo spin-echo (HASTE) or single shot fast spin-echo (SSFSE)) sequences. Respiratory compensation or respiratory triggering is employed whenever non-breath-hold sequences are used. An echo train length (ETL) of 16–20 provides optimal T2-weighted images in short scan time.[35] Echo-train spin echo sequences acquired as contiguous thin 2D sections or as a thick 3D volume slab, also form the basis for MR cholangiography.

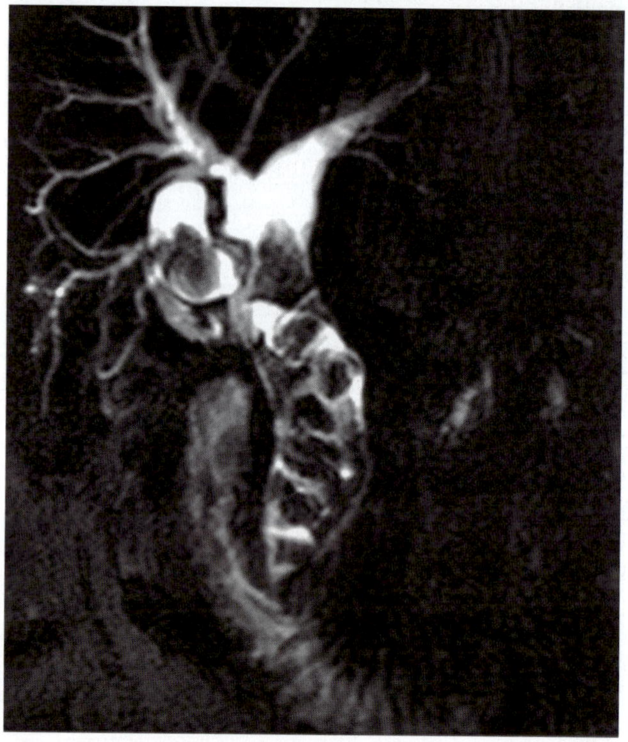

FIG. 17: Choledocholithiasis: Coronal thick slab projectional MRCP reveals multiple calculi in the common bile duct and right hepatic duct.

The TE of T2-weighted images is usually around 80-90 msec and longer TE (150–250 msec) T2W imaging can be used to differentiate between cysts and solid lesions.

The liver parenchyma appears homogeneous on both T1 and T2-weighted images. The liver shows moderate signal intensity on T1W images, similar to the pancreas but brighter than spleen and kidneys **(Figs. 19A and B)**. On T2W images **(Fig. 20)**, the liver appears dark and has signal intensity less than that of spleen.

Post-contrast administration, dynamic fat-suppressed MR imaging **(Figs. 21A to D)** is performed using a 2-D or 3-D technique. Contrast is administered at a dose of 0.1 mmol/kg at a rate of 2 mL/s and followed by saline flush.[36] Pre-contrast scan is followed by the acquisition of scans in the late arterial (20 seconds after administration of contrast), portal venous (60–80 seconds) and delayed (2–5 minutes) phases. The bolus timing technique (includes automated bolus detection system or fluoroscopic triggering) or acquisition of multiple repeated arterial-phase datasets is used for planning the arterial phase. Additional delayed images (more than 5 minutes) may be required in cases of hemangiomas, vascular malformations, or cholangiocarcinomas.[37,38] Subtracted images (subtraction of the pre-contrast scan from the postcontrast scan) should be generated in cases of T1 hyperintense lesions.

The use of hepatobiliary specific MR contrast agents is recommended for liver imaging. When gadobenate dimeglumine (Multihance) is used, one hour delayed scan is performed. However, with the use of gadoxetate (Eovist), hepatobiliary phase is obtained at 20 minutes post-contrast injection. This phase is used to document retention of contrast in lesions like focal nodular hyperplasia and to better delineate the biliary anatomy. However, it is important to obtain MRCP images (T2-weighted imaging of biliary tree) before biliary excretion of contrast, as the enhanced bile is not visualized on the MRCP images. For optimal time utilization, T2-weighted and diffusion-weighted images can be obtained after the injection of gadoxetate disodium.[34]

Diffusion-weighted images are obtained using echo-planar imaging (EPI) with breath held, free breathing, or respiratory-gated techniques. Imaging time can be reduced with the use of parallel imaging. DWI is performed with at least two b-values (b=20–50 s/mm^2 and b=400 to 1000 s/mm^2). The use of ADC maps and calculation of ADC values is recommended to identify T2 shine through effect, which can be a confounding factor in the interpretation of DW images. DWI is useful in characterization of focal liver lesions, liver fibrosis and screening of the entire abdomen for additional lesions. It is of particular use in patients with contraindications to MR contrast medium. However, it is important to view the DWI images in conjunction with the other sequences and amalgamate, its findings with the

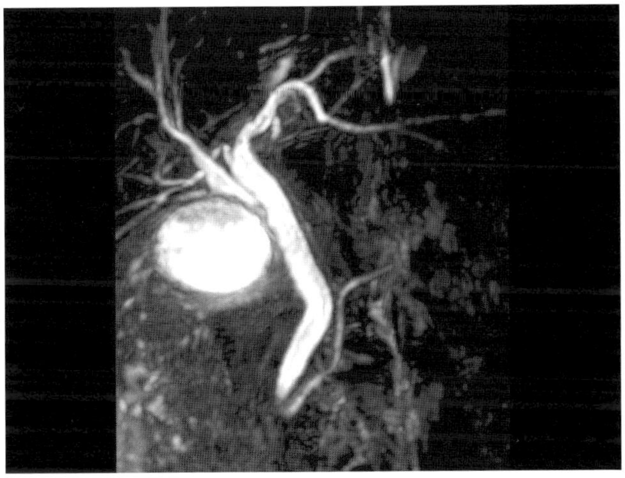

FIG. 18: MRCP (MIP) image showing normal intrahepatic biliary radicles, common bile duct and pancreatic duct in a case of carcinoma gallbladder.

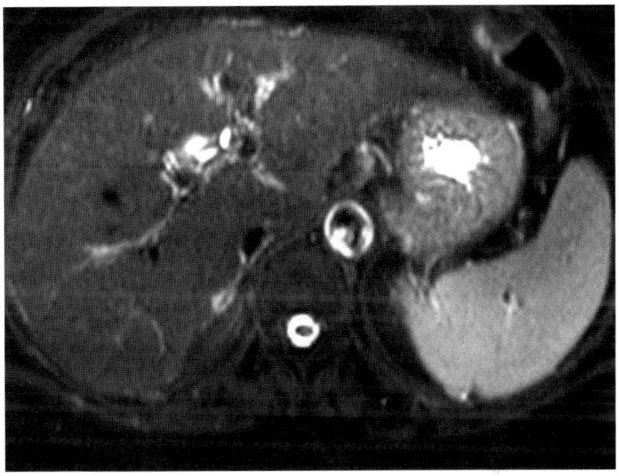

FIG. 20: Axial T2 WI fat-suppressed sequence reveals homogeneous signal intensity of the liver. Note the signal intensity of liver is less than that of spleen.

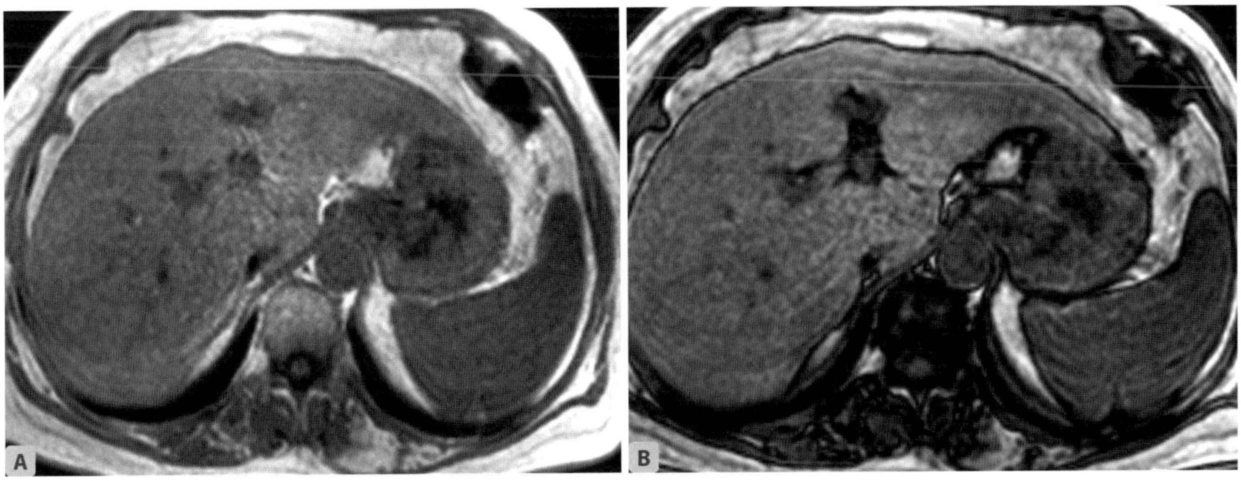

FIGS. 19A AND B: T1-weighted imaging for the liver. In-phase (A) and out-of-phase (B) chemical shift gradient-recalled echo sequences are performed prior to contrast administration. Liver shows homogeneous moderate signal intensity, greater than that of the spleen.

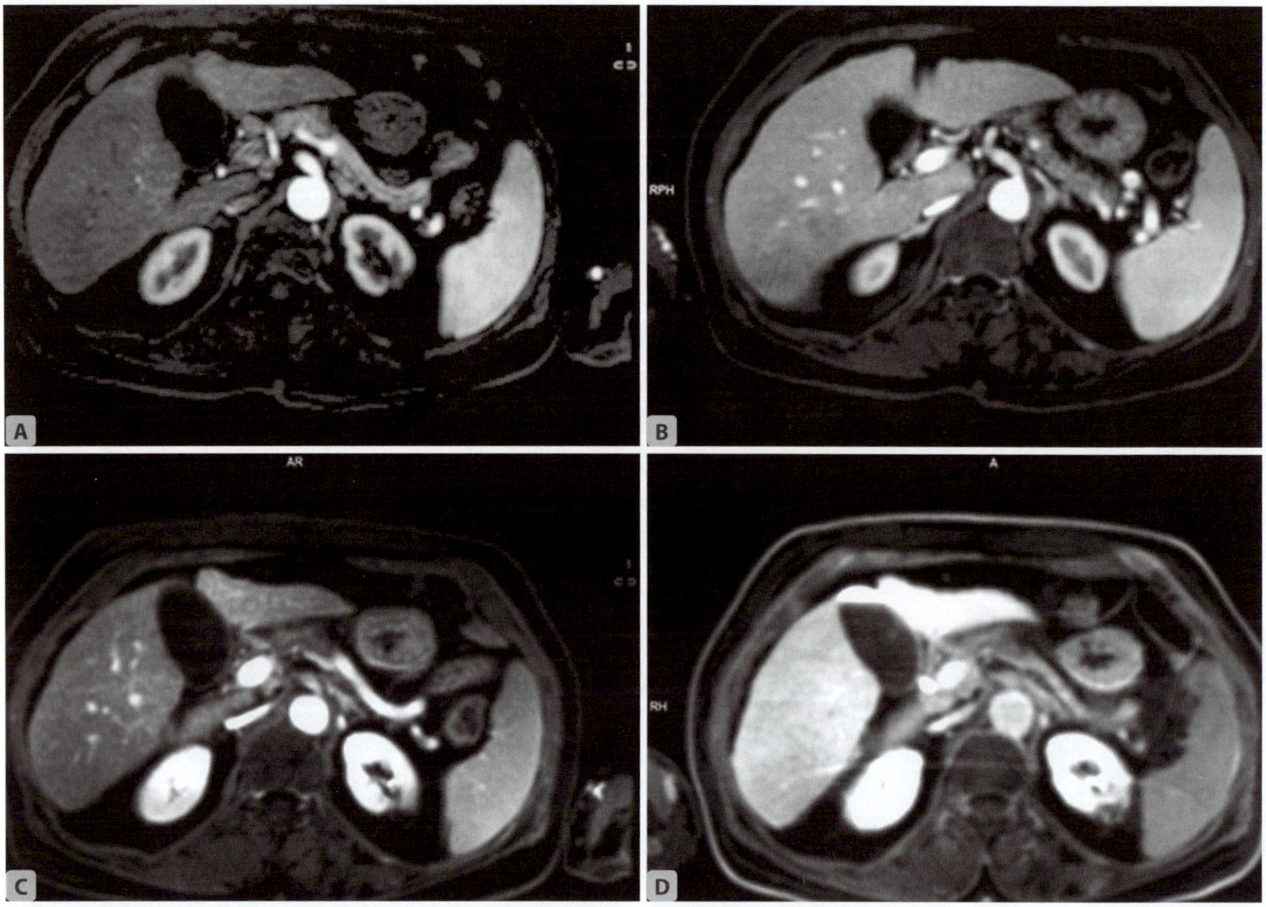

FIGS. 21A TO D: Multiphase MRI liver: Postcontrast (Gadobenate dimeglumine/Multihance) administration, T1-weighted fat-suppressed gradient echo images are obtained at 20 seconds (late arterial phase) (A); 65 seconds (portal venous phase) (B); 180 seconds (delayed phase) (C) and 1 hour (hepatobiliary phase) (D) in a patient of chronic liver disease. No focal lesion was detected.

morphology and enhancement characteristics for increased accuracy of diagnosis.[34]

MRI of Pancreatic Pathology

For the evaluation of pancreatic pathology, T1-weighted images are acquired as dual-echo GRE images in the axial plane and T2-weighted images as turbo spin-echo sequences in the axial and coronal plane. MRCP sequences using both 2D and 3D fast SE techniques are used to delineate the pancreaticobiliary anatomy. Intravenous gadolinium-based contrast medium is injected at a dose of 0.1 mmol/kg of body weight and dynamic scanning is performed. This includes the acquisition of arterial (20 sec after injection of contrast medium), portal venous (45–65 seconds) and equilibrium phase (3–5 min) images. Some authors recommend a coronal plane (parallel to the bifurcation of the portal vein) T1 GRE acquisition two minutes after the injection of contrast medium.[26,39]

MAGNETIC RESONANCE ENTEROGRAPHY

This is a noninvasive technique for the evaluation of small bowel pathology. Since there is no radiation exposure, it is the modality of choice for pediatric patients and monitoring of patients of inflammatory bowel disease.

Patient preparation includes fasting for 6 hours and intestinal cleansing as for CT enterography.

Biphasic contrast agents (hyperintense on T2-weighted and hypointense on T1-weighted sequences) are preferred as they provide maximal contrast with bowel wall on the post-contrast sequences. These include agents like water, mannitol, locust bean gum, low-dose barium, manganese compounds, and polyethylene glycol. The protocol varies with institutions and a suggested protocol is given in **Table 7**. Some centers advocate prone position as it decreases respiratory excursion and enables better separation of bowel loops.[16,40]

Images are acquired in both the axial and coronal planes **(Figs. 22A and B)**. T2W imaging can be performed as spin-echo sequence (TSE or FSE), gradient-echo (GRE) sequence, or a hybrid gradient and spin-echo (GRASE) sequence. Single shot technique is more useful as it is relatively insensitive to motion. Fat-suppressed sequences are preferred for the evaluation of active inflammation. T1 imaging can be performed as spin echo or gradient echo sequences with T1W 3D gradient-echo sequence having the advantage of short scan time allowing image acquisition within a single breath-hold.

"Cine imaging" of the bowel is real time, dynamic imaging of a predefined region of interest by employing a heavily T2W coronal slab or a single-shot steady-state free precession sequence. This is useful for the identification of fibrotic strictures.[40]

NUCLEAR IMAGING

Neuroendocrine tumors (NET) such as carcinoids and pancreatic NET express somatostatin receptors (SSTR) at the cell membrane.[41] Functional imaging uses the affinity of somatostatin receptor analogs for tissues, which express SSTR. There are six main subtypes of SSTR (1–5 including 2A and 2B) with SSTR-2 and SSTR-5 being the most commonly expressed in NET.

Octreotide scintigraphy (using octreotide labeled with indium 111) is the standard functional imaging modality for NET's. It is combined with single photon emission computed tomography for improved spatial resolution. It is also used to evaluate the response to treatment and for metastatic work-up of NET.[42] This technique has greater sensitivity for carcinoids and gastrinomas than insulinomas.[42]

Iodine 123 (^{123}I) MIBG scintigraphy: This technique uses Metaiodobenzyl guanidine, which is a norepinephrine analog and binds to the norepinephrine transporter in NET.

PET/CT: Newer analogs labeled with gallium-68 are now used in combination with PET-CT imaging. However, they have more affinity to the SSTR-2 receptors than to the SSTR-3 and SSTR-5 receptors. Compared with octreotide scintigraphy, PET/CT requires less time and has a higher spatial resolution. In addition, the production of 68Ga-DOTA peptides is relatively less costly as it does not require a cyclotron.

Three types of ^{68}Ga-DOTA-peptide analogs are available:

1. ^{68}Ga-DOTA-Phe^{1}-Tyr^{3}-Octreotide (TOC)
2. ^{68}Ga-DOTA-NaI^{3}-Octreotide (NOC)
3. ^{68}Ga-DOTA-Tyr^{3}-Octreotate (TATE)

Out of these, DOTA-NOC has good affinity for SSTR-3 in addition to SSTR-2 and SSTR-5 receptors and is preferred as a broad-spectrum agent.[43]

TABLE 7: MR enterography protocol.

- Fasting for 6 hours
- *Oral contrast*:
  - 300 mL of 20% mannitol mixed with 1.5 L of water
  - Administered in divided aliquots over 1 hour
- *Intravenous contrast*:
  - 0.1 mmol/kg of gadolinium-based agent
  - Single phase acquisition at 50 sec (enteric phase)
- IV buscopan (1 mL~20 mg): after acquisition of cine BTFE
- *Sequences*:
  - *Steady state fast field echo (Cine)*: Coronal
  - *Steady state fast field echo*: Axial
  - *T2W FS*: Axial, coronal
  - *T1W Non FS*: Axial
  - *DWI (b VALUE 0, 400, 800)*: Axial
  - Post-contrast T1W FS: Axial, coronal

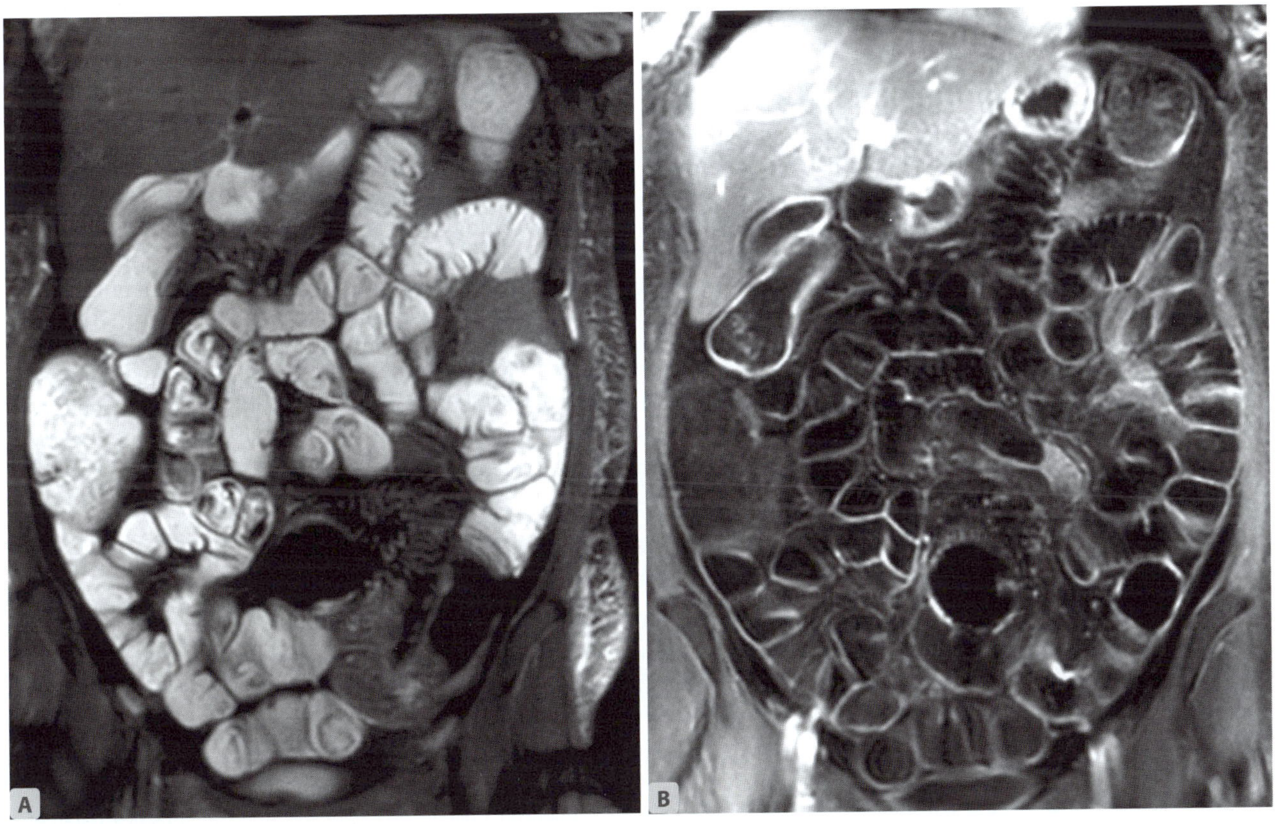

FIGS. 22A AND B: MR enterography: Coronal T2-weighted fat-suppressed fast spin echo (A) and post-gadolinium coronal T1 fat-suppressed gradient echo (B) acquisition shows good bowel distension and no abnormal enhancement.

^{68}Ga-DOTANOC PET enterography is useful for delineation of small bowel carcinoids.[16]

^{18}F FDG is also used as a glucose analog in FDG-PET (can be combined with CTE/CTC for evaluation of bowel neoplasms and inflammatory bowel disease) and ^{18}F DOPA is used as a catecholamine analog for DOPA PET in the evaluation of NET.[16,44]

ANGIOGRAPHY

Conventional hepatic/mesenteric angiography is now seldom used for diagnostic purpose as CT and MR imaging can generate high quality angiographic images in a non-invasive manner. The use of catheter angiography is now restricted to vascular interventions.

Technique

Coagulation profile and serum creatinine should be available prior to the procedure. The femoral artery is the preferred approach and Seldinger technique is used for the puncture. Angiography of the liver is performed by selective injections of the celiac axis and superior mesenteric artery (SMA) or one or more of their branches. A 5-French right angle or reverse curve catheter such as Cobra is commonly used. The volume of contrast used is about 20–30 cc injected at a rate of 5–6 cc per second. The portal venous system is visualized by injecting the splenic artery or SMA coupled with prolonged filming.

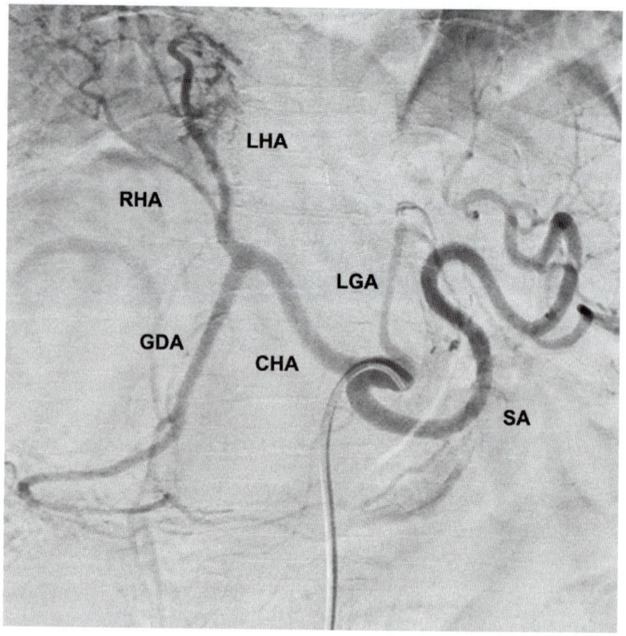

FIG. 23: Intra-arterial digital subtraction angiography (DSA) showing selective celiac axis injection, splenic artery (SA), left gastric artery (LGA), common hepatic artery (CHA), gastroduodenal artery (GDA), right hepatic artery (RHA) and left hepatic artery (LHA).

Anatomy

The celiac axis **(Fig. 23)** is the first major branch of the abdominal aorta and it gives rise to three major branches (the common hepatic, left gastric, and splenic arteries). The common hepatic artery gives rise to the gastroduodenal artery after which it becomes the proper hepatic artery. The proper hepatic artery divides into the right and left hepatic arteries, which further divide to supply the corresponding segments. The main branches of the gastroduodenal artery are the retroduodenal, superior pancreaticoduodenal and right gastroepiploic arteries. The splenic artery gives rise to short gastric branches and the left gastroepiploic artery. The superior mesenteric artery (SMA) arises approximately 1 cm caudad to the celiac trunk and supplies the small bowel through the inferior pancreaticoduodenal, jejunal, and ileal arteries. The right colon is supplied by the ileocolic, right colic and middle colic artery branches of the superior mesenteric artery forming an arcade (marginal artery of Drummond), which anastomoses with the branches of the inferior mesenteric artery (IMA). The branches of the IMA include left colic artery, sigmoidal artery, rectosigmoid artery and superior rectal artery.[45]

CONCLUSION

The imaging techniques for abdomen have evolved considerably in the past few years. Conventional radiographs and barium studies now have limited role in the evaluation of GI pathology. Recent advances in ultrasound like endosonography, elastography and contrast studies have significantly improved the diagnostic yield of a noninvasive and radiation free modality like ultrasound. Cross-sectional modalities such as CT and MRI remain the mainstay in the diagnosis and follow-up of most abdominal pathologies. A judicious use of the currently available imaging modalities is required for appropriate diagnosis and treatment of various abdominal diseases.

REFERENCES

1. Maglinte DDT, Sandrasegaran K, Chiorean M, Dewitt J, McHenry L, Lappas JC. Radiologic investigations complement and add diagnostic information to capsule endoscopy of small-bowel diseases. AJR. 2007;189:306-12.
2. Maglinte DDT. Capsule imaging and the role of radiology in the investigation of diseases of the small bowel. Radiology 2005; 236:763-7.
3. Halligan S, Robinson PJA. The large bowel: In: David Sutton (Ed). Textbook of Radiology and Imaging, 7th edn. Churchill Livingstone.
4. American College of Radiology. ACR practice parameter for the performance of esophagrams and upper gastrointestinal examinations in adults. *http://www.acr.org/~/media/5223A3FBC92E40378DF6E55FB8E6134B.pdf*. Accessed on September 07, 2016.
5. American College of Radiology. ACR practice parameter for the performance of a barium small bowel examination in adults. *http://www.acr.org/~/media/9408bdfc3c234e4287bd8610faafe3f1.pdf*. Accessed on September 07, 2016.
6. American College of Radiology. ACR–SAR practice parameter for the performance of an enteroclysis examination in adults.

http://www.acr.org/~/media/0CEECEA90E154EB99FC6562F1311E7E4.pdf. Accessed on September 07, 2016.

7. American College of Radiology. ACR practice parameter for the performance of fluoroscopic contrast enema examination in adults. *http://www.acr.org/~/media/ACR/Documents/PGTS/guidelines/Fluoroscopic_Contrast_Enema.pdf.* Accessed on September 07, 2016.
8. Kono Y, Mattrey RF. Ultrasound of the liver. The Radiologic Clinics of North America. 2005;43(5):815-26.
9. Gazelle GS, Saini S, Mueller PR, (Eds). Hepatobiliary and Pancreatic Radiology: Imaging and Intervention. New York, NY, USA: Thieme Medical Publishers, 1998.
10. Kusera JN, Kucera S, Perrin SD, Caracciolo JT, Schmulewitz N, Kedar RP. Cystic lesions of the pancreas: Radiologic endosonographic correlation. Radiographics. 2012; 32:E283-E301.
11. Frulio N, Trillaud H. Ultrasound elastography in liver. Diagn Interv Imaging. 2013;94:515-34.
12. Ferraioli G, Parekh P, Levitov AB, Filice C. Shear wave elastography for evaluation of liver fibrosis. J Ultrasound Med. 2014;33:197-203.
13. Unnikrishnan S, Klibanov AL. Microbubbles as ultrasound contrast agents for molecular imaging: Preparation and application. AJR. 2012;199:292-9.
14. Catalano O, Nunziata A, Lobianco R, Siani A. Real-time harmonic contrast material-specific us of focal liver lesions. Radiographics. 2005;25:333-49.
15. American College of Radiology. ACR–SPR practice parameter for the performance of computed tomography (CT) of the abdomen and computed tomography (CT) of the pelvis. *http://www.acr.org/~/media/ACR/Documents/PGTS/guidelines/CT_Abdomen_Pelvis.pdf.* Accessed on September 07, 2016.
16. Das CJ, Manchanda S, Panda A, Gupta AK, Sharma A. Recent advances in imaging of small and large bowel. PET Clin. 2016; 11:21-37.
17. Iannaccone R, Laghi A, Catalano C, et al. Hepatocellular carcinoma: role of unenhanced and delayed phase multi-detector row helical CT in patients with cirrhosis. Radiology 2005;234(2):460-7.
18. Doyle DJ, O'Malley ME, Jang HJ, Jhaveri K. Value of the unenhanced phase for detection of hepatocellular carcinomas 3 cm or less when performing multiphase computed tomography in patients with cirrhosis. J Comput Assist Tomogr. 2007;31(1):86-92.
19. Choi JY, Lee JM, Sirlin CB. CT and MR imaging diagnosis and staging of hepatocellular carcinoma: Part I. Development, growth, and spread: key pathologic and imaging aspects. Radiology. 2014;272:635-54.
20. McEvoy SH, McCarthy CJ, Lavelle LP, Moran DE, Cantwell CP, Skehan SJ. Hepatocellular carcinoma: Illustrated guide to systematic radiologic diagnosis and staging according to guidelines of the American association for the study of liver diseases. Radiographics. 2013;33:1653-68.
21. Oto A, Tam EP, Szklaruk J. Multidetector row CT of the liver. The Radiologic Clinics of North America. 2005;43(5):827-48.
22. Kim MJ, Choi JY, Lim JS, et al. Optimal scan window for detection of hypervascular hepatocellular carcinomas during MDCT examination. Am J Roentgenol. 2006;187(1):198-206.
23. Laghi A, Iannaccone R, Rossi P, Carbone I, Ferrari R, Mangiapane F. Hepatocellular carcinoma: Detection with triple-phase multi-detector row helical CT in patients with chronic hepatitis. Radiology. 2003;226:543-9.
24. Coursey CA, Nelson RC, Boll DT, Paulson EK, Ho LM, Neville AM. Dual-energy multidetector CT: How does it work, what can it tell us, and when can we use it in abdominopelvic imaging? Radiographics. 2010;30:1037-55.
25. Wigmore SJ, Redhead DN, Yan XJ, et al. Virtual hepatic resection using three-dimensional reconstruction of helical computed tomography angioportograms. Ann Surg. 2001;233:221-6.
26. Lee ES, Lee JM. Imaging diagnosis of pancreatic cancer: A state-of-the-art review. World J Gastroenterol. 2014;20:7864-77.
27. Chaudhary V, Bano S. Imaging of the pancreas: Recent advances. Indian J Endocrinol Metab. 2011;15:S25-32.
28. Manchanda SD, Prasad A, Sachdev N, De P, Abbas SZ, Baruah BP. Multidetector computed tomography (MDCT) evaluation of small bowel obstruction: pictorial review. Trop Gastroenterol. 2010;31:249-59.
29. American College of Radiology. ACR–SAR–SPR practice parameter for the performance of computed tomography (CT) enterography. *http://www.acr.org/~/media/99D260410DF44A3BA01F1AB716DE8F2F.pdf.* Accessed on September 07, 2016.
30. American College of Radiology. ACR–SAR–SCBT-MR practice parameter for the performance of computed tomography (CT) colonography in adults. *http://www.acr.org/~/media/A81531ACA92F45058A83B5281E8FE826.pdf.* Accessed on September 07, 2016.
31. American College of Radiology. ACR–SAR–SPR practice parameter for the performance of magnetic resonance imaging (MRI) of the abdomen (excluding the liver). *http://www.acr.org/~/media/8f5bc61adb114c5b9e46fe6914461d25.pdf.* Accessed on September 07, 2016.
32. Soher BJ, Dale BM, Merkle EM. A review of MR physics: 3T versus 1.5T. Magn Reson Imaging Clin N Am. 2007;15(3):277-90.
33. Leyendecker JR, Childs DD. Kidneys and MR urography. Magn Reson Imaging Clin N Am. 2007;15(3):373-82.
34. American College of Radiology. ACR–SAR–SPR practice parameter for the performance of magnetic resonance imaging (MRI) of the liver. *http://www.acr.org/~/media/6B520D299C0B4B018A90BE21A79D4F72.pdf.* Accessed on September 07, 2016.
35. Maniam S, Szklaruk J. Magnetic resonance imaging: Review of imaging techniques and overview of liver imaging. World J Radiol. 2010;2:309-22.
36. Arif-Tiwari H, Kalb B, Chundru S, Sharma P, Costello J, Guessner RW, Martin DR. MRI of hepatocellular carcinoma: an update of current practices. Diagn Interv Radiol. 2014;20:209-21.
37. Runge VM. A comparison of two MR hepatobiliary gadolinium chelates: Gd-BOPTA and Gd-EOB-DTPA. J Comput Assist Tomogr. 1998;22(4):643-50.
38. Soyer P, Bluemke DA, Reichle R, et al. Imaging of intrahepatic cholangiocarcinoma: 2. Hilar cholangiocarcinoma. Am J Roentgenol. 1995;165(6):1433-6.
39. Sandrasegaran K, Lin C, Akisik FM, Tann M. State-of-the-art pancreatic MRI. AJR. 2010;195:42-53.
40. American College of Radiology. ACR–SAR–SPR practice parameter for the performance of magnetic resonance (MR) enterography. *http://www.acr.org/~/media/99F8D0F593E64860AA3B1EC6CA1C758D.pdf.* Accessed on September 07, 2016.
41. Woodbridge LR, Murtagh BM, Yu DFQC, Planche KL. Midgut neuroendocrine tumors: Imaging assessment for surgical resection. Radiographics. 2014;34:413-26.
42. Virgolini I, Traub-Weidinger T, Decristoforo C. Nuclear medicine in the detection and management of pancreatic islet-cell tumours. Best Pract Res Clin Endocrinol Metab. 2005;19:213-27.
43. Sharma P, Singh H, Bal C, Kumar R. PET/CT imaging of neuroendocrine tumors with 68Gallium-labeled somatostatin analogues: An overview and single institutional experience from India. Indian J Nucl Med. 2014;29:2-12.
44. Sahani DV, Bonaffini PA, Castillo CFD, Blake MA. Gastroenteropancreatic neuroendocrine tumors: Role of imaging in diagnosis and management. Radiology. 2013;266:38-61.
45. Stallard DJ, Tu RK, Gould MJ, Pozniak MA, Pettersen JC. Minor vascular anatomy of the abdomen and pelvis: A CT atlas. RadloGraphlcs. 1994;14:493-513.

CHAPTER

92

Imaging a Patient with Dysphagia

Alpana Manchanda, Jyoti Kumar, Gaurav Shanker Pradhan

INTRODUCTION

Dysphagia is a common manifestation of many of the disorders affecting the esophagus. It is a nondescriptive term that literally means 'difficulty in swallowing'. It is defined as the subjective awareness of difficulty in swallowing or perception of obstruction of a solid or liquid bolus as it passes from the mouth to the stomach.[1] Dysphagia is considered to be clinically significant when such symptoms occur a minimum of several times a month. Dysphagia can result from functional or structural abnormalities of the oral cavity, pharynx, esophagus or gastric cardia. It may be further classified as oropharyngeal or esophageal (substernal), depending on the anatomic site of involvement. It is of utmost importance to differentiate between the two as their etiology, radiologic evaluation and management may vary greatly.[1]

EPIDEMIOLOGY

It effects nearly 22% of patients in the primary care setting; with two-thirds of the patients with dysphagia being more than sixty-five years of age.[2]

The diagnosis of dysphagia is important because of its associated morbidity and mortality. The elderly are at the highest risk of subsequent complications of dysphagia such as dehydration, weight loss, airway obstruction; the most dangerous being aspiration, which can be silent in up to 55% of patients.[2]

PHYSIOLOGY OF SWALLOWING

Swallowing is a complex activity which occurs in a coordinated manner to transport the ingested material from the mouth to the stomach. Normal swallowing is divided into oral, pharyngeal and esophageal stages and involves both voluntary and involuntary neuromuscular contractions starting from the mouth to the stomach.[2]

Oropharyngeal Stage

This stage is initiated by the contractions of the tongue and striated muscles of mastication which mix the food bolus with saliva and propel it from the oral cavity into the oropharynx. Once the food has left the oral cavity, swallowing is no longer under voluntary control. The bolus then activates the oropharyngeal sensory receptors which initiate the deglutition reflex which is a centrally-mediated wave of inhibition which precedes the peristaltic contraction. It not only propels the food through the pharynx and esophagus, but also prevents its aspiration (i.e. entry into the airway) and nasal regurgitation (retrograde flow into the nose). This is achieved in the following sequence of events—elevation of the soft palate which closes the nasopharynx, closure of the laryngeal vestibule which is critical for airway protection. This occurs as a result of upward and anterior movement of the larynx by the suprahyoid muscles. The epiglottis moves downwards to cover the airway. Finally the upper esophageal sphincter (UES) including the cricopharyngeus muscle relaxes due to which the bolus enters the cervical esophagus. The pharynx is cleared of the bolus by the sequential contraction of the pharyngeal constrictor muscles. The deglutition reflex lasts for approximately one second.[3]

Primary esophageal peristalsis is induced by a swallow at the pharyngesophageal junction. Caudad progression of a bolus is achieved by deglutitive inhibition.

Secondary peristalsis is induced by esophageal distension and initiates around the level of the aortic arch. It is a propulsive wave that occurs to clear the esophagus of any retained bolus.

Tertiary contractions are nonpropulsive and cause a variable degree of narrowing of the lumen. Between swallows, the esophagus is collapsed and the upper and lower esophageal sphincters are closed.

Esophageal Stage

The esophageal stage of swallowing begins once the bolus passes through the upper esophageal sphincter. In this phase, the peristaltic contractions of the smooth muscle of the thoracic esophagus propels the food towards the lower esophageal sphincter (LES) and stomach. The LES relaxes as soon as the swallow is initiated, which persists until the food bolus is propelled into the stomach.[3]

PATHOGENESIS OF DYSPHAGIA

The normal passage of the ingested bolus through the pharynx and esophagus depends on the size of the ingested bolus, size of the lumen, the force of peristalsis, deglutitive inhibition along with normal relaxation of the upper and lower esophageal sphincter during swallowing. When there is mechanical or structural cause to the dysphagia it is called *mechanical dysphagia*.

In contrast, *motor dysphagia* occurs due to weak peristaltic contractions or impaired deglutitive inhibition, causing nonperistaltic contractions and impaired relaxation of sphincters.[4]

Clinical Presentation

Dysphagia is a very nondescriptive term that can result from any problem from the proximal oral cavity to the proximal stomach.

A carefully taken history helps a physician to identify 80–85% of the causes of dysphagia. Specific questions such as the onset, duration, severity of dysphagia and any associated symptoms may help in narrowing the differential diagnosis to a specific diagnosis or to an anatomic or a pathophysiologic-related diagnosis.[5]

It is important to know if dysphagia is present during swallowing or at all times. Dysphagia which occurs during swallowing at all times without any organic cause is suggestive of globus hystericus. Dysphagia that occurs only for solids is likely due to a mechanical obstruction, while dysphagia for both solids and liquids is more likely to indicate a motility disorder.

Symptoms such as delayed or absence of swallow initiation, postswallow cough, nasopharyngeal regurgitation, repeated swallows to clear the bolus are indicative of oropharyngeal dysphagia.[6]

Abnormality of the oral phase of swallowing results in food dribbling from the mouth, difficulty in drinking or chewing, or difficulty in initiating a swallow. Soft palate insufficiency results in a nasal quality of voice or nasal regurgitation. Coughing or choking during swallowing indicates laryngeal penetration. Patients with pharyngeal dysphagia typically complain of a "lump in the throat" or of food "sticking in the throat" during swallowing. It may be caused by a functional abnormality such as cricopharyngeal dysmotility, amyotrophic lateral sclerosis or by a morphologic abnormality such as Zenker's diverticulum or pharyngeal tumor.[7]

A sensation of blockage at the level of the suprasternal notch or thoracic inlet raises the possibility of a cervical esophageal web, tumor or of extrinsic compression of the cervical or upper thoracic esophagus by an enlarged thyroid, mediastinal lymphadenopathy, or other mass lesion.[7] Substernal localization of dysphagia is usually due to a structural disorder such as reflux esophagitis, peptic stricture or Schatzki ring or motility disorder of the esophagus such as achalasia. A distal lesion (even carcinoma of the gastric fundus) may refer dysphagia proximally as far as the pharynx. The patient may complain of odynophagia (pain on swallowing) or chest pain. These symptoms may be due to esophageal spasm or other motor disorders, but may also be caused by infectious esophagitis, gastroesophageal reflux disease and ulcerated pharyngeal or esophageal tumors.

The duration and progression of symptoms also provide a clue to the etiology. Chronic and stable symptoms are suggestive of benign conditions such as peptic strictures, Schatzki's ring, while rapidly progressive symptoms associated with weight loss is suggestive of a malignant etiology. The timing of regurgitation in relation to swallowing or meals is also indicative of the underlying cause for example, regurgitation in between meals is suggestive of an underlying Zenker's diverticulum, while immediately after swallowing suggests esophageal retention of food.[6] (**Table 1**, lists the associated symptoms with possible etiologies of dysphagia).[4,5]

Dysphagia is also more common in patients with a history of gastresophageal reflux disease (GERD) than in those without GERD.[1]

Patients who develop dysphagia after a long history of reflux symptoms and those with poor control of symptoms

TABLE 1: Symptoms associated with possible etiologies of dysphagia.[4,5]

Symptoms	Possible diagnoses
Progressive dysphagia	Neuromuscular dysphagia
Sudden dysphagia	Obstructive dysphagia
Episodic dysphagia to solids	Lower esophageal ring
Difficulty in initiating swallow	Oropharyngeal dysphagia
Food sticks after swallow	Esophageal dysphagia
• Cough/choking-before, during or after swallow • In early phase of swallowing • In late phase of swallowing	• Indicative of aspiration • Neuromuscular dysphagia • Obstructive dysphagia
Weight loss: • In the elderly • With regurgitation	 • Carcinoma • Achalasia
Progressive symptoms: • Heartburn • Intermittent symptoms of dysphagia • Odynophagia	 • Peptic stricture, scleroderma • Rings and webs, diffuse esophageal spasm • *Esophagitis*: - Postradiation - Infectious - Pill induced
Chest pain with dysphagia	DES and related motor disorders
Worsening of pain by: • Solid food only • Solids and liquids	 • Obstructive dysphagia • Neuromuscular dysphagia
Regurgitation of old food	Zenker's diverticulum
Weakness and dysphagia	Stroke, muscular dystrophies, myasthenia gravis
Halitosis and dysphagia	Zenker's diverticulum
Dysphagia relieved with repeated swallows	Achalasia

may develop complications such as peptic stricture, Barrett's esophagus and even esophageal adenocarcinoma.[6] In young patients with history of atopy who present with dysphagia or obstruction to food bolus, eosinophilic esophagitis must be suspected and ruled out by endoscopic biopsy.

CAUSES OF DYSPHAGIA

These can be divided into two broad groups—mechanical and motor, involving oropharynx and esophagus **(Tables 2A to D)**.[4]

IMAGING TECHNIQUES IN THE EVALUATION OF DYSPHAGIA

As the anatomic structures and causes responsible for oropharyngeal and esophageal dysphagia are different, the approach to their evaluation also differ.[6]

Oropharyngeal dysphagia is evaluated by:
- Plain film
- Barium swallow
- Modified barium swallow/Videofluoroscopic Swallowing Study (VFSS)
- Nasopharyngeal-endoscopy
- Pharyngomanometry
- Cross-sectional studies (CT/MRI)

Esophageal dysphagia is evaluated by:
- Barium swallow
- Upper GI endoscopy

TABLES 2A TO D: Causes of dysphagia.

A: Mechanical oropharyngeal dysphagia	
• Zenker's diverticulum • Cricopharyngeal bar or stenosis • Cervical (mucosal) Web-Plummer-Vinson syndrome • Retropharyngeal abscess • Oropharyngeal tumor • Head and neck surgery • Stricture-caustic, postradiation	
B: Motor oropharyngeal dysphagia[6,8]	
1. Central nervous system	• Stroke • Parkinson's disease • Brainstem tumors • Alzheimer's disease • Drugs (Phenothiazines, benzodiazepines)
2. Degenerative diseases	• Amyotrophic lateral sclerosis • Huntington's chorea • Multiple sclerosis
3. Peripheral nervous system	• Spinal muscular atrophy • Guillain-Barré syndrome • Postpolio syndrome • Drugs (Botulinum toxin, cytotoxics)
4. Myogenic	• Myasthenia gravis • Dermatomyositis, polymyositis • Thyrotoxic myopathy • Drugs (amidarone, alcohol, cholesterol lowering drug)

Continued

Continued

C: Mechanical esophageal dysphagia	
1. *Intrinsic narrowing*	
i. Inflammatory/infective esophagitis	• Viral • Bacterial • Fungal • Caustic, chemical, thermal injury
ii. Webs and rings	• Congenital esophageal stenosis • Lower esophageal mucosal ring (Schatzki's ring)
iii. Benign strictures	• GERD and Barrett's esophagus • Peptic stricture • Caustic injury • Pill induced • Inflammatory (Candida, mucocutaneous lesions) • Postoperative or anastomotic • Postradiation
iv. Malignant stricture	
v. Foreign body	
2. *Extrinsic narrowing*	• Substernal thyroid • Posterior mediastinal mass • Vascular compression (aberrant right subclavian artery, right sided aorta, aortic aneurysm) • Enlarged vertebral osteophytes
D: Motor esophageal dysphagia[4]	
1. *Diseases of smooth muscles*	
i. Weak muscle contraction or LES tone	• Idiopathic • Scleroderma and related collagen vascular disease • Myotonic dystrophy • Metabolic neuromyopathy (amyloid/alcohol/diabetes) • Drugs (anticholinergics, smooth muscle relaxants)
ii. Enhanced muscle contraction	• Hypertensive peristalsis (nutcracker esophagus) • Hypercontracting lower esophageal sphincter (LES)
2. *Disorders of inhibitory innervation*	
i. Diffuse esophageal spasm (DES)	
ii. Achalasia	Primary, secondary (Chagas disease, carcinoma, lymphoma leading to pseudo-achalasia)
iii. Contractile (muscular/ lower esophageal ring)	

- Esophageal manometry
- Scintigraphy
- Cross-sectional studies (CT/MRI)
- Endoscopic ultrasound
- Intraesophageal pH measurement.

Even though there has been a decrease in the number of gastrointestinal fluoroscopic procedures, the number of contrast swallow studies have shown to increase.[9]

Barium studies and endoscopy are complementary investigations, but barium swallow is a useful first-line investigation for dysphagia. Its wide availability, non-invasiveness and it being a relatively inexpensive investigation are some of its advantages. It allows real-time continuous viewing of the bolus during transit from the oropharynx to the stomach and allows a good qualitative and functional assessment of the esophagus including the upper and lower esophageal sphincters.

A barium swallow may demonstrate an anatomical abnormality such as a stricture or mass lesion. It entails exposure to ionizing radiation and has poor sensitivity for subtle abnormalities, yet it is found to be more sensitive than esophagoscopy in detecting esophageal webs and rings.[6]

Examination Technique

Preparation: The pharynx, esophagus and stomach should be as free of fluid and secretions as possible to permit optimal mucosal coating during the barium study. The patient is instructed to fast overnight before the examination. The patient should avoid smoking or chewing gum as these activities may stimulate salivary and/or gastric secretions and impair mucosal coating.[7]

Plain Films

Although scout films are not obtained routinely, frontal and lateral plain films of the neck and chest may be helpful in cases of suspected foreign body, abscess, or fistula formation, and in the postoperative patient. The plain film may show fluid levels in the esophagus in a patient with achalasia. In major esophageal dilatation, the esophagus expands to the right, producing a mediastinal edge that runs from the neck to the diaphragm with a single indentation produced by the azygos vein.

Barium Studies

Examination of the pharynx and esophagus requires a dynamic evaluation of motility as well as double-contrast spot films to detect morphologic abnormalities. Cineradiography or videofluoroscopy should be used to study swallowing dynamics. The recordings may be reviewed later to analyse tongue movement, soft palate evaluation, epiglottic tilt, laryngeal closure, cricopharyngeal opening and pharyngeal peristalsis.

The routine barium examination of the esophagus should be a biphasic study combining upright double contrast and prone single contrast technique. In the double contrast phase, the aim is to achieve adequate gaseous distension of the lumen with a thin layer of high density barium coating the mucosa. Gaseous distension is improved by the patient swallowing effervescent agents. The patient is also instructed to swallow rapidly the high density barium. Rapid drinking causes air swallowing and thus, esophageal distension. In addition, it interrupts the esophageal peristalsis, thus resulting in esophageal hypotonia.

The effervescent agent may be omitted in patients with suspected esophageal infections or obstructing lesions (because it is painful and may cause artefacts).

Prone views of the upper esophagus best shows esophageal webs and indentations by aortic arch anomalies. Barium-filled views of the distal esophagus are important for the detection of hiatal hernias, strictures, webs or rings as these may not be visible in the erect double contrast phase. Next, the patient is turned to the right and gastroesophageal junction is monitored fluoroscopically to elicit spontaneous gastresophageal reflux. The cardia is best shown in double contrast with the patient in the recumbent right lateral position.

Provocative testing in an attempt to reproduce symptoms may be useful in a patient with solid food dysphagia who has a normal study with liquid barium. A barium impregnated solid bolus may hold up at a subtle stricture or induce spasm not seen with liquid bolus.

A tube esophagogram may be performed if there is marked aspiration or penetration.

Evaluation of a patient presenting with dysphagia includes detailed evaluation of the pharynx, esophagus, gastroesophageal junction and the cardia using double-contrast and single-contrast barium examinations.[7]

Evaluation of Pharynx

The patient is positioned erect in the right lateral position with the fluoroscopy table being vertical and asked to swallow approximately 10 mL of 250% w/v of barium sulfate (high density) suspension. A cine recording of the oral and pharyngeal phases of swallowing is done both in full-field lateral views as well as collimated views of the pharynx. In addition to this, two lateral spot films are obtained during phonation (patient is asked to say "eeeeeee...") and during suspended respiration respectively.[10]

The patient's position is then changed to a frontal position and the head tilted backwards till the mandible is superimposed over the occiput. In this position, cine recording of two additional swallows is done. Two frontal spot films are obtained during Valsalva maneuvere and during suspended respiration respectively **(Figs. 1A and B)**.

Evaluation of the Esophagus, Gastroesophageal Junction and Cardia

The patient is positioned erect in the left posterior oblique position with the fluoroscopy table being vertical and asked to swallow effervescent granules with approximately 10 mL of water. The patient is then asked to rapidly swallow a mouthful of 250% w/v of barium sulfate suspension. Spot films of the proximal and distal esophagus are obtained. In order to get proper double contrast views, the spot exposures should be timed with periods of optimal distension and coating **(Figs. 2A and B)**.

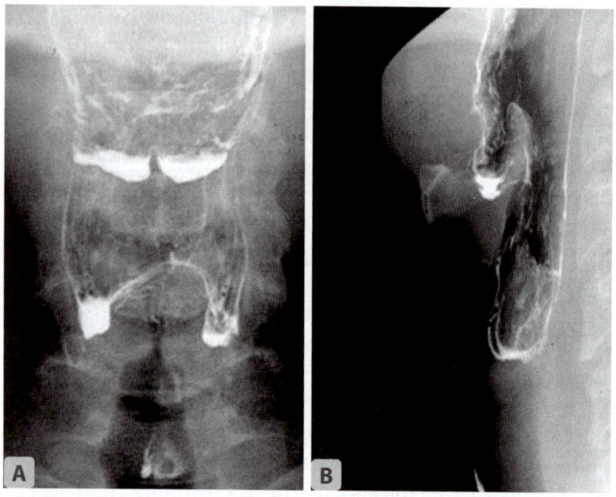

FIGS. 1A AND B: Spot views of the normal pharynx. (A) Frontal view shows normal smooth mucosal outline of the paired valleculae, pyriform sinuses and lateral walls of the hypopharynx; (B) Lateral view shows normal smooth mucosal outline of superimposed bilateral valleculae and pyriform sinuses.

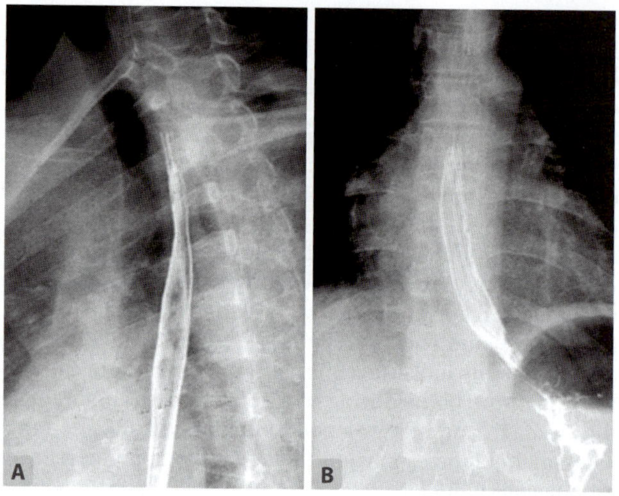

FIGS. 2A AND B: (A) Normal appearance of mid; and (B) Lower dorsal esophagus and gastroesophageal junction on Barium Swallow Study.

The fluoroscopy table is then made horizontal and the patient is asked to lie down in the right lateral position and spot films of the double contrast views of gastric cardia and fundus are obtained.

The patient is then turned prone in a right anterior oblique position and asked to swallow 100% w/v suspension of barium sulfate. Fluoroscopic examination of esophageal motility is done, along with spot exposures to obtain single contrast views of proximal and distal esophagus. In case of any abnormal esophageal motility detected, cine recording of additional swallows can also be done.

The patient is then asked to turn to his left side and then on to his back. The gastroesophageal junction is focused and monitored fluoroscopically as the patient is asked to slowly turn towards his right side in order to look for any spontaneous gastroesophageal reflux. If no spontaneous reflux is seen, then straight leg raising maneuver or Valsalva maneuver can be done to increase intra-abdominal pressure and gastroesophageal reflux is looked for.

Thus, there are several important principles in the evaluation of patients with dysphagia:[11]

- Radiographic evaluation of patients with dysphagia must include all structures involved in swallowing.
- If possible, the examination should be biphasic.
- Every patient should be examined in both the erect and recumbent positions.
- Each patient with dysphagia is different. Although there is a routine or basic examination, studies of patients with swallowing problems lend themselves to tailoring. Each examination is subtly altered on the basis of a short patient history taken by the radiologist. The routine examination is also modified by the clinical condition of the patient. The sicker the patient, less routine and more tailored the examination should be. The examination should be focused on answering a specific question such as "does the patient aspirate". The answer should not be just "yes" or "no" but "yes, for the following reasons". Aspiration may occur during swallowing due to a failure of laryngeal protection or after swallowing, for example, pharyngeal paresis may result in progressive retention of liquid in the pyriform sinuses and subsequent overflow aspiration, or gastroesophageal reflux may produce aspiration from esophagopharyngeal regurgitation of the refluxed material. Aspiration may also occur before swallowing if there is premature leakage from the mouth when the larynx is open and unprotected. The other important observation is whether the patient coughs during aspiration. With loss of sensory feedback, aspiration may be silent and not suspected clinically.

The Tailored Examination[7]

Recommended Approach

Patients with pharyngeal dysphagia or other symptoms localized to the pharynx, neck or suprasternal notch should undergo a careful radiologic examination of the pharynx with videofluoroscopic recordings and double contrast spot films. If the patient aspirates a substantial amount of barium, the examination should be terminated. If marked swallowing dysfunction occurs, particularly in stroke patients, a detailed study of the esophagus is unwarranted. However, patients with pharyngeal carcinoma have a significantly increased risk of synchronous esophageal carcinoma. Therefore, a double contrast examination of the esophagus should be performed in these cases. A normal pharyngeal study should always be followed by a careful examination of the esophagus and cardia to rule out more distal abnormalities causing referred dysphagia to the pharynx.

Conversely, patients with substernal dysphagia, odynophagia, reflux symptoms, or nonspecific chest pain should first undergo a detailed radiologic examination of the esophagus and cardia. Some esophageal disorders such as achalasia and gastroesophageal reflux disease may be associated with pharyngeal or cricopharyngeal dysfunction.

However, pharyngeal abnormalities virtually never cause referred dysphagia below the level of the thoracic inlet, so a limited pharyngeal study may be performed in patients with substernal symptoms.

Videofluoroscopic Swallowing Study

It is also known as modified barium swallow and is the standard of reference for evaluating the swallowing mechanism. Videofluoroscopic swallowing study (VFSS) is a dynamic fluoroscopic study performed with high frame rate image capture and is useful for evaluating the motility of oropharynx and hypopharynx. The study is often performed in conjunction with a swallowing therapist and provides information about swallowing function in response to therapeutic measures and necessary dietary requirements. The images can be reviewed later with referring physicians, speech language pathologist, patients and their family members to explain the management recommendations.[3] VFSS provides real time visualization of the oropharyngeal and esophageal structures, movement and coordination of swallowing. The study best detects aspiration during swallow. Even though VFSS is a gold standard for dysphagia, it can be normal in patients with early or slowly progressive disease. Hence, if patient discomfort persists inspite of normal VFSS, they should be followed up.

Nasopharyngoscopy

It is also known as fiberoptic endoscopic swallowing study. This technique allows direct visualization of lingual, pharyngeal and epiglottic movements during swallowing and also assesses the presence of any pharyngeal retention of fluids after swallowing.[6]

Pharyngeal/Esophageal Manometry

Manometry is the most sensitive and accurate technique to assess esophageal motility and diagnose esophageal motility disorders. The study entails positioning a pressure sensing catheter within the esophagus. Test swallows are given to the patient following which esophageal contractility is observed. The upper and lower esophageal sphincters appear as zones of high pressure that relax on swallowing while the intersphincteric esophagus shows peristaltic contractions.[12]

With advancements in technology, the conventional manometry has been replaced by high resolution manometry (HRM) with substantial improvement in its recording power and fidelity. Pressure measurement of 1 cm or less can be measured along the entire esophagus thereby providing detailed mapping of esophageal motor function including upper and lower esophageal sphincters.

The traditional line plot in manometry has further largely been replaced by the topographical or contour or color plot which aids in more rapid interpretation of results. The combination of HRM with topography, also called high-resolution esophageal pressure topography allows more precise measurement of esophageal pressures **(Fig. 3)**. It has been shown to have higher sensitivity (72%) for achalasia as compared to conventional manometry (56%).[6]

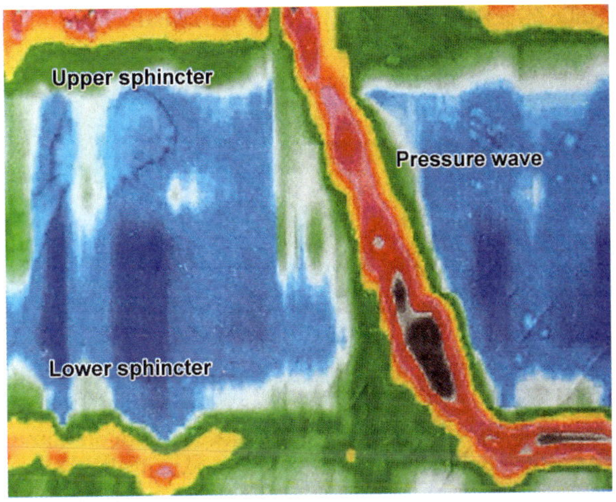

FIG. 3: Color plot depicting pressure waves of a normal swallow by esophageal manometry, also called high-resolution esophageal pressure topography.

Manometry is thus the "gold standard" test in diagnosing achalasia and esophageal spasm due to its high sensitivity in detecting pressure changes and its good correlation with bolus transit in these conditions.

Upper Gastrointestinal Endoscopy

Upper GI endoscopy not only provides direct visualization of the esophagus but also the oropharynx stomach and duodenum. It is the preferred investigation in patients with a history suggestive of mechanical obstruction and is useful in identifying intraluminal mass lesion, strictures, inflammatory disorders such as reflux disease, eosinophilic esophagitis and pill-induced ulceration.[6]

Endoscopes also have an instrumentation channel through which biopsy forceps, sclerotherapy catheters or balloon dilators can be passed and various therapeutic procedures can be performed simultaneously. Some of the advantages of endoscopy over contrast radiographic studies are:[12]

- Increased sensitivity for detection of mucosal lesions.
- Increased sensitivity in the detection of Barrett's metaplasia which is mainly identified by its abnormal color.
- Obtaining biopsy specimen of suspected abnormalities for histopathological evaluation.
- The ability to effectively dilate strictures, which may be peptic, anastamotic or radiation induced or esophageal web or Schatzki's ring is a therapeutic capability of this technique. Endoscopic-guided pneumatic dilatation and botulinum toxin injection at the LES are some of the therapeutic alternatives which can be performed in patients of achalasia who are not suitable for surgical myotomy.[6]

Though upper GI endoscopy has relatively low sensitivity and specificity in the evaluation of underlying motility disorder it can suggest underlying achalasia in the presence of a dilated esophagus with features of reduced contractions which occlude its lumen and a tight LES. In the setting of achalasia, endoscopy provides direct visualization of the gastresophageal junction and gastric cardia to detect any underlying carcinoma causing pseudoachalasia.

Esophageal Scintigraphy

Scintigraphy is a screening test used to detect an abnormality in the esophageal transit time. It involves the ingestion of a liquid or solid bolus labeled with a radionuclide such as ^{99m}Tc-DTPA. The radionuclide movement is recorded by a gamma camera which measures the esophageal bolus time and clearance. The investigation is not used much even though it has been reported to have a high sensitivity and specificity in detecting esophageal motor abnormalities.[6] Handling of radioactive material and radiation exposure, poor anatomical definition compared with barium swallow and a lack of well-defined diagnostic criteria are some of the reasons why scintigraphy is rarely used in the investigation of dysphagia.

Intraesophageal pH Monitoring

This investigation is done in the setting of suspected gastro-esophageal reflux disease (GERD). It can be performed in either of the two ways—a wireless pH—sensitive transmitter is anchored to the esophageal mucosa or a wire electrode is passed transnasally with the tip in the distal esophagus and an ambulatory 24–48 hours esophageal pH recording is done. The outcome is expressed as percentage and a pH value of less than 4 is indicative of recent acid reflux with values more than 5% indicative of GERD. Intraluminal impedance monitoring can be added to pH monitoring to detect reflux irrespective of whether it is acidic or not thereby increasing the sensitivity of the study.[12]

Endoscopic Ultrasound

Endoscopic ultrasound (EUS) combines an endoscope with an ultrasound transducer to create a transmural image of the tissue surrounding the endoscope tip. Its most important advantage in its greater resolution attributable to the proximity of the ultrasound transducer to the tissue being examined. There are two types of endoscopic probes-side viewing for imaging and at the tip for interventional purposes. The main esophageal application of endoscopic ultrasound are in the staging of esophageal cancer, in the evaluation of dysplasia in Barrett's esophagus and in the assessment of submucosal tumors.

Cross-sectional Imaging Studies

Imaging of the esophagus is challenging because the esophagus is a long tube, and poorly distensible, with a close relationship to many vital organs.[13]

Pharynx

Although the mucosal detail of the pharynx is studied best with barium contrast, the extraluminal anatomy is demonstrated in detail by CT, MRI and sonography. Axial techniques are therefore most useful as an adjunct to barium studies, particularly for tumor staging and the delineation of central and peripheral nervous system lesions producing pharyngeal dysfunction.

Esophagus

Although there is no absolute size of normal wall thickness, some authors define that the thickness should not exceed 3 mm in a well distended esophagus. Also, an eccentric thickening of the wall is suggestive of an underlying pathology.[6] Although, with increasing age, the esophageal caliber may increase, an anteroposterior (AP) diameter more than 10 mm and a transverse diameter greater than 24 mm are considered abnormal. Air may be seen in the esophagus in around 65% of normal population. However, an air-fluid level, fluid filled lumen or a lumen caliber more than 10 mm usually indicate obstruction or severe dysmotility.

Proper distension of the esophagus and stomach (by oral administration of effervescent granules and water) and optimally timed administration of intravenous contrast material are required to detect and characterize disease. Preoperative staging of esophageal carcinoma appears to be the main indication for MDCT. CT provides considerable information on the intramural and extramural extent of esophageal malignancy and is also an indispensable part of the planning for radiation therapy. CT and MRI have been used to stage esophageal carcinoma, because these techniques can reveal extraesophageal extension into adjacent mediastinal structures, including the trachea, bronchi, aorta, and pericardium, and can detect lymphadenopathy in the mediastinum. For assessing unresectability, CT and MR have comparable accuracy when using criteria such as tracheobronchial invasion and aortic invasion. However, CT appears more sensitive for detecting lymphadenopathy, particularly in the mediastinum.[14]

Though MR imaging is not routinely performed for esophageal pathology, the normal esophagus is well visualized in its entire length except the mid part which may be difficult to visualize as it is flattened behind the left atrium. On T1W images, the normal esophagus appears as a low signal intensity (SI) structure contrasted by high signal intensity of periesophageal fat. On T2W images, it appears as low signal intensity in contrast to high signal intensity of internal contents. Postcontrast MR images reveal moderate enhancement of the muscle layer of the esophagus. Use of phase array surface coils can provide high resolution MR images of individual layers of the esophageal wall. On high resolution T2W images the esophagus is seen as intermediate SI mucosa surrounded by high SI submucosa and low SI muscularis propria.[15]

FUNCTIONAL OROPHARYNGEAL ABNORMALITIES

Functional neuromuscular disorders (enlisted in **Table 2B**) can lead to the following pathophysiologic conditions with oropharyngeal dysphagia:

Laryngeal Penetration

During fluoroscopy, when the contrast material enters the laryngeal vestibule but does not pass below the level of the glottis through the true vocal cords, it is indicative of laryngeal vestibular penetration. In healthy people, spontaneous clearing of the contrast occurs from the laryngeal vestibule which is known as transient penetration or high penetration. It can arise from poor oral control of the bolus or from delayed initiation of the pharyngeal swallow.[3]

Aspiration

The term aspiration is used to describe the passage of foreign material including food and liquid through the true vocal cords into the trachea. Prevention of aspiration requires superior and anterior elevation of the larynx, closure of larynx and epiglottic tilt. These mechanisms can be evaluated at videofluoroscopy.[3] Aspiration can occur before, during or after swallow and is the most threatening symptom of oropharyngeal dysphagia.

Once aspiration has occurred, the immediate expected reflex is a cough due to excitation of recurrent laryngeal nerve receptors. In patients with dysphagia who present with aspiration, the cough response may be immediate, delayed or absent. The cough may also not be effective in throwing out material back into the hypopharynx. The severity of aspiration is determined subjectively by:

- The amount of material aspirated, i.e. minimal, moderate or severe.
- Quantification of the depth of aspiration.
- Response in terms of coughing.

The standard measure of severity of aspiration is the "8 point penetration aspiration scale" which includes both the depth of airway invasion (above or below the true vocal cords) and whether the material is ejected back into the hypopharynx or not. Silent aspiration is represented by a score of 8 in which material is aspirated below the true vocal cords without any overt clinical signs.

Postswallow Residue in the Pharynx

Following a swallow, the bolus may collect and remain in the valleculae and pyriform sinuses. This may be due to weak propulsion of bolus or inadequate opening of the upper esophageal sphincter. The residue in the pharynx may lead to secondary postswallow aspiration.

Cricopharyngeal Bar or Prominent Cricopharyngeus Muscle

The posterior indentation at approximately C5-C6 level by cricopharyngeus muscle normally effaces as a bolus passes through. Mild persistent indentation may be normal but more obvious prominence may be seen in patients with gastroesophageal reflux or functional or mechanical esophageal obstruction. It is postulated that acid reflux leads to edema, spasm and or hypertrophy of cricopharyngeus. On a contrast study on the lateral view it is seen as a smooth posterior bar-like or band-like protrusion into the lumen of the barium column at the junction of the hypopharynx and cervical (C5-C6 level) esophagus **(Fig. 4A)**. Cricopharyngeal bar may be seen in 5–10% of patients who are asymptomatic.

Extrinsic pharyngeal indentation caused by a cervical osteophyte may simulate cricopharyngeal prominence. Osteophytic impressions are fixed in position in relation to the spine, whereas cricopharyngeal indentations move with the pharynx and esophagus during swallowing.

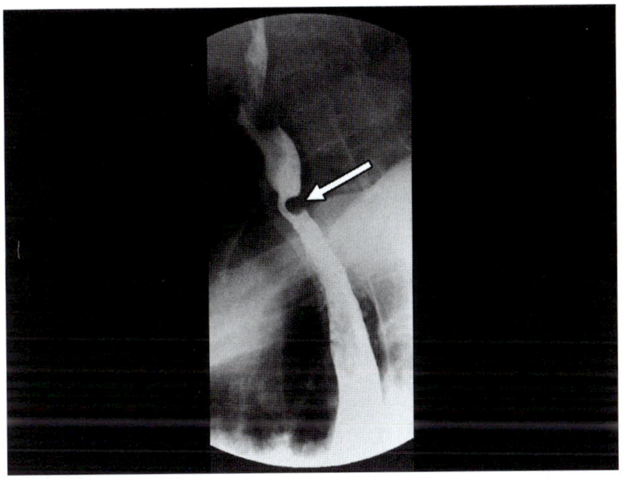

FIG. 4A: Prominence of the criocopharyngeus muscle seen as posterior indentation (arrow) on barium swallow study with mild proximal dilatation.

STRUCTURAL OROPHARYNGEAL ABNORMALITIES

Postcricoid Webs

Webs are thin mucosal folds that are located in the anterior wall of the lower hypopharynx and proximal few centimeters of the esophagus. They typically present with dysphagia to solids but deglutitive aspiration may occur due to their proximal location.[8] They have been reported to be twice as common in women than men and more easily appreciated on barium swallow than on endoscopy[8] wherein they are seen as eccentric but occasionally circumferential 1–2 mm wide shelflike filling defect **(Fig. 4B)**. Characteristic "jet effect" may be seen on contrast swallow when a large bolus passes through a web. They arise on the anterior wall and never on the posterior wall and are best seen on the lateral projection. As rapid peristalsis allows cervical webs to be visualized only for fraction of a second, cineradiography is required to demonstrate them. Differentiation must be made between webs and the submucosal venous plexus which is a normal structure on anterior wall and causes an impression that is effaced as the bolus distends the lumen.

Cervical webs have been linked to underlying conditions such as GERD, epidermolysis bullosa and possibly associated with iron deficiency anemia (Plummer-Vinson Syndrome).

Pharyngeal Diverticula and Pouches

Several types of diverticula may be seen on oropharyngeal and upper gastrointestinal barium studies such as pharyngeal diverticula and pouches, Zenker's diverticulum and Killian-Jamieson diverticulum. Zenker's diverticulum has been found to be the most common of them and frequently implicated in pharyngeal dysphagia. This develops secondary to fibrosis and loss of compliance of the cricopharyngeus muscle.[8] It occurs as a result of increase in intraluminal pressure associated with distal obstruction in the form of a stenotic cricopharyngeus muscle (upper esophageal

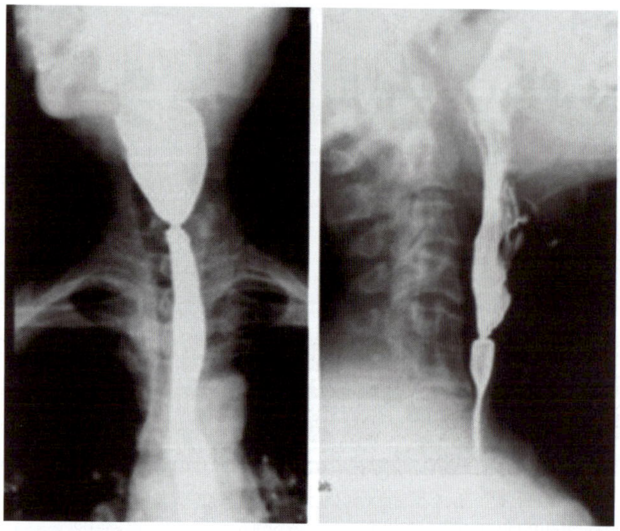

FIG. 4B: Barium swallow shows well-defined localized circumferential narrowing seen at the level of C5-C6 with minimal proximal dilatation—cricopharyngeal web.

sphincter). Zenker's diverticulum is a false diverticula which involves herniation of the mucosa and submucosa through the muscular layer of esophagus. It is a pouch that develops as an area of anatomic weakness in the posterior hypopharyngeal wall between the horizontal and oblique fibers of the cricopharyngeus muscle. It is seen on the lateral view as a bulge or true sac extending posteriorly from the posterior hypopharyngeal wall just above the cricopharyngeal impression. On the frontal view a Zenker's diverticulum is seen as a barium-filled sac below the arcuate lines of the pyriform sinuses. This area is known as the triangle of Killian or Killian dehiscence. The mouth of the Zenker's diverticulum is present immediately above the cricopharyngeal muscle. Imaging in three projections are required for confirmation and assessment of the severity of a Zenker's diverticulum, i.e. anteroposterior, lateral and oblique. In contrast, the Killian-Jamieson diverticula originates below the cricopharyngeus muscle.

Small Zenker's diverticulae are usually asymptomatic. Dysphagia occurs as the diverticulum fills preferentially with food and obstructs the lumen of the esophagus. There is regurgitation of pouch contents and often, aspiration as its overflows. Recurrent chest infection are hence common.

The treatment of choice for Zenker's diverticulum is cricopharyngeal myotomy, either alone or combination with pouch resection. In the elderly with significant comorbidity, cricopharyngeal dilatation can provide symptomatic relief and can be performed as an alternative treatment.

Oropharyngeal Tumors and their Surgery

Tumors of the head and neck such as those arising from the tongue, palate, pharynx, tonsil and glottis may present with dysphagia. The surgical resection of these cancers can cause complications such as anastomotic leak, vascular injury and cranial nerve damage which can result in dysphagia. The effect of head and neck cancer surgery on swallowing can vary markedly from person to person and depends on many factors such as the extent of surgical resection, whether flap reconstruction is required, the nature of component structures removed, i.e. cartilaginous, muscular or bony or whether surgery has resulted in damage to neural innervations.

In those undergoing surgery for oral cancer, the extent of tongue resection is the most important factor which determines the severity of dysphagia. This is because tongue base motion is very important in generating pharyngeal propulsive forces. Also, following laryngeal surgery the degree of preservation of tongue base motion is an important prediction of recovery of swallow function.[8]

The majority of malignant pharyngeal tumors are squamous cell carcinomas. Small tumors may be seen as a nodular mucosal surface en face or as an irregular contour. Radiographic findings in large, advanced tumors include intraluminal mass, mucosal irregularity and asymmetric distensibility. An intraluminal mass may be seen as an abnormal luminal contour, abnormally located extra-barium-coated lines, a focal area of increased radiodensity, or a filling defect in the barium pool. Mucosal irregularity is recognized by abnormal barium collections due to ulceration or by a nonuniform nodular surface pattern. Asymmetric distensibility may be due to an infiltrating tumor or extrinsic mass **(Figs. 5A and B)**. The value of double-contrast pharyngography in patients with a known carcinoma is to determine the size, extent and inferior limit of the pharyngeal tumor and the degree of functional impairment. Pharyngoesophagograms are also useful for detecting separate co-existing carcinomas of the pharynx and esophagus. Extraluminal extent of the tumor (e.g. invasion of the pre-epiglottic space or cartilage destruction) and lymphadenopathy are best assessed by CT and MR imaging. **(Figs. 6A to C)**.

Postradiation Stricture

Radiotherapy for malignancies of oral and pharyngeal region is known to cause severe nerve and muscle damage. Chemotherapy and radiotherapy both are known to produce esophageal strictures leading to dysphagia with a lower risk of development of strictures at doses less than 60 Gy.

Video fluoroscopy or contrast swallow study can depict the pharyngeal or esophageal strictures developing secondary to radiotherapy for a laryngeal malignancy. The stricture may vary from short, smooth to complete obliteration of the lumen.[3]

It is important to take a history of radiotherapy for an oral or neck surgery in the past as radiation-induced dysphagia is known to manifest clinically more than 10 years post-treatment.[8]

Retropharyngeal Abscess

Retropharyngeal abscess may occur secondary to tonsillar infection, suppurative lymphadenopathy, spread of tubercular infection from the prevertebral space to the retropharyngeal space or from perforating injury of the pharynx or esophagus. It is more often seen in small children who may present with fever, neck stiffness and dysphagia. On lateral plain radiograph of the neck, findings are an increase

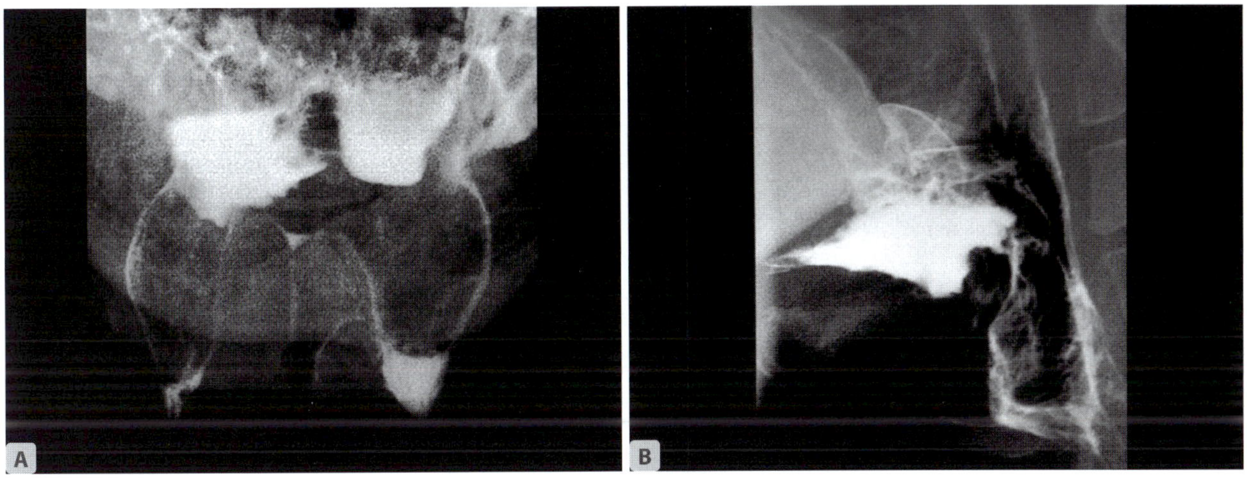

FIGS. 5A AND B: Contrast swallow. (A) Frontal; (B) Lateral spot views of the hypopharynx showing expansion and mucosal irregularity of the right vallecula by a malignant mass. The left vallecula and pyriform sinus appear normal—malignant right vallecular mass (SCC).

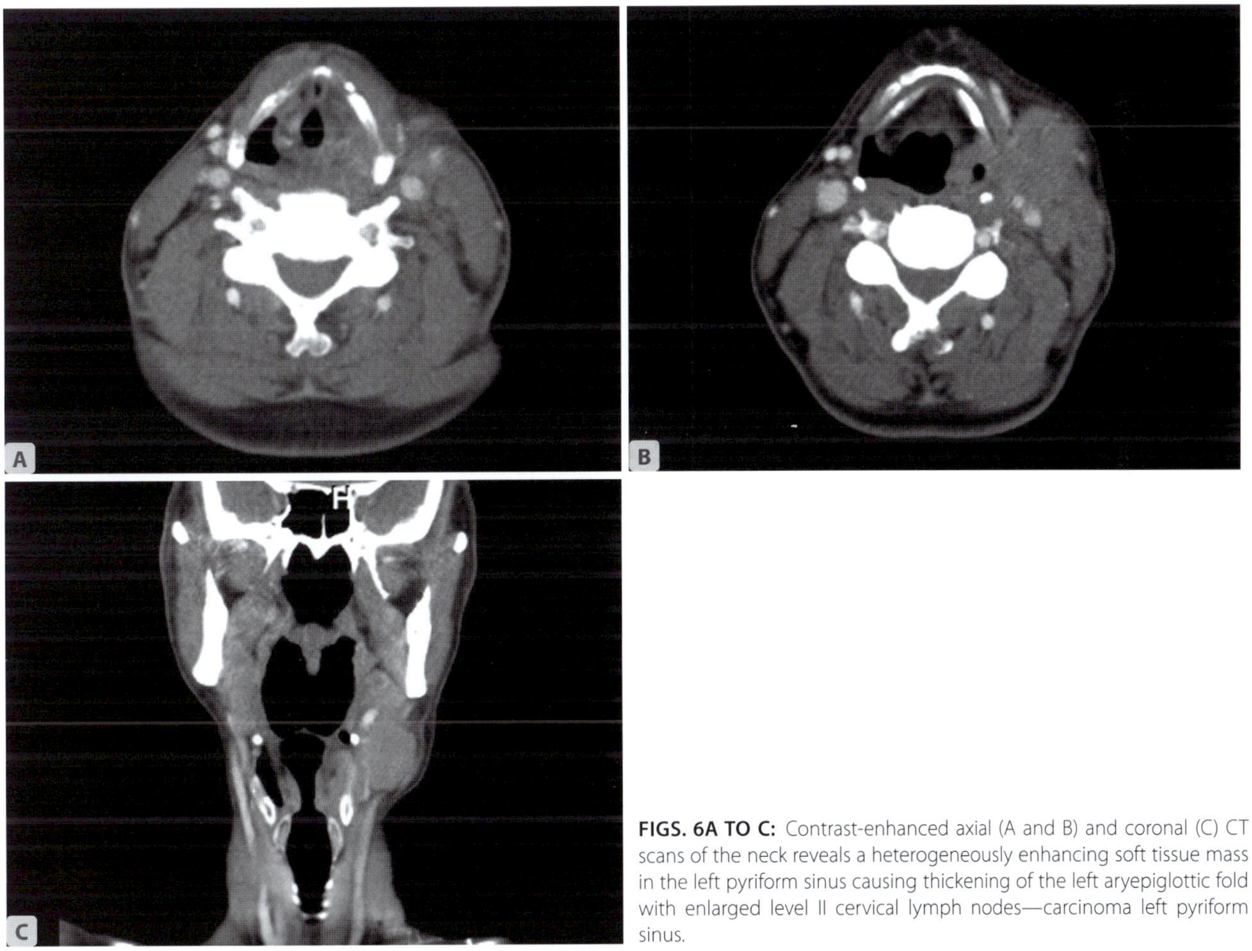

FIGS. 6A TO C: Contrast-enhanced axial (A and B) and coronal (C) CT scans of the neck reveals a heterogeneously enhancing soft tissue mass in the left pyriform sinus causing thickening of the left aryepiglottic fold with enlarged level II cervical lymph nodes—carcinoma left pyriform sinus.

in the retropharyngeal space, reversal of cervical lordosis and anterior displacement of the airway. The abscess may contain air and an air-fluid level may be seen. On CT, the abscess appears as an area of low attenuation with peripheral rim enhancement and on MR it is seen as high signal intensity on T2-weighted images **(Fig. 7)**.

Pharyngeal Foreign Bodies

A lateral radiograph of the neck taken at soft tissue exposure may show a radiopaque foreign body, but many impacted fish or chicken bones are poorly opaque. Evidence of perforation should be sought, including extraluminal gas and

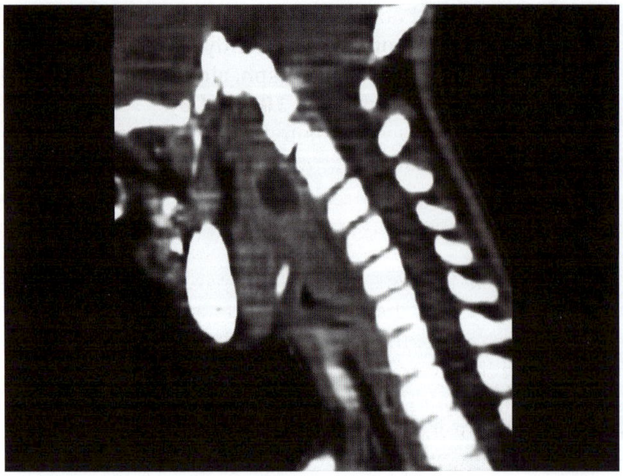

FIG. 7: Sagittal MPR image of CECT neck of a child with neck pain, fever and dysphagia shows a rim enhancing hypodense lesion in the retropharyngeal region causing compression of the oropharyngeal airway—retropharyngeal abscess.

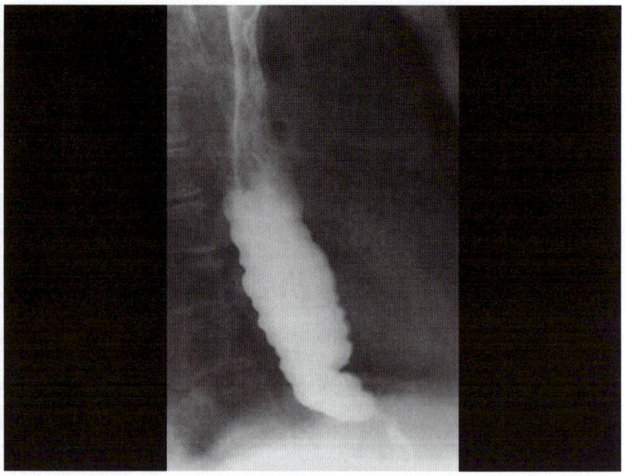

FIG. 8: Nonspecific esophageal motility disorder.

widening of the prevertebral soft tissues. A contrast swallow is performed with a small volume of low density barium, or water-soluble nonionic contrast if perforation is suspected. CT is an excellent investigation in localizing and identifying a foreign body, detecting complications such as perforation, collection or abscess formation and depicting involvement of adjacent structures.

ESOPHAGEAL MOTILITY DISORDERS

These disorders are those which are attributable to esophageal neuromuscular function and are commonly associated with dysphagia, chest pain or heart burn. The dysphagia is slowly progressive and occurs to both liquid and solid foods. The esophageal motility can be easily assessed at fluoroscopy with the patient in the prone right anterior oblique (RAO) position. Two to five individual swallows should be observed at fluoroscopy as the bolus passes. It is important to remember that in patients suspected of having an esophageal motility disorder, individual swallow should be evaluated, as a second or double swallow would interfere with primary peristalsis and limit evaluation of esophageal motility.

Specific motility disorders consist of diffuse esophageal spasm (DES), achalasia and scleroderma. However, the motility disorders may not fall into any of these categories and may occur in association with GERD.

PRIMARY MOTILITY DISORDER

Nonspecific Esophageal Motility Disorder

Motility abnormalities that do not meet the criteria of specific motility disorders fall into this broad category. Manometrically, abnormal peristalsis is seen in 20% of such cases. Peristalsis may be intermittently absent or of low amplitude. Lower esophageal sphincter dysfunction (incomplete relaxation) and frequent spontaneous or repetitive contractions are also detected. Radiologically a nonspecific disturbance of primary peristalsis and tertiary contractions are seen in 40–50% of cases **(Fig. 8)**.

Diffuse Esophageal Spasm

Clinical Presentation

Diffuse esophageal spasm is manifested by episodes of dysphagia and chest pain occurring due to abnormal esophageal contractions with normal lower esophageal sphincter (LES) relaxation on deglutition. Esophageal chest pain may closely mimic pain of angina. Features which suggest a pain of esophageal origin are it being unrelated to exertion, pain of prolonged duration which interrupts sleep, its relation to meals, relief with antacids and being accompanied by heartburn, dysphagia or regurgitation. All these presenting features also show overlap with cardiac pain. Both chest pain and dysphagia are also characteristic of peptic or infectious esophagitis. Hence, only after the more common entities mentioned above are excluded, that a diagnosis of diffuse esophageal spasm (DES) should be considered.[12]

Imaging Features

DES is characterized by the absence of primary peristalsis with simultaneous, spontaneous, repetitive, nonperistaltic uncoordinated esophageal contractions on manometry. The LES usually functions normally, although high resting pressures and incomplete relaxation may occur. It occurs in patients over 50 years of age and may be intermittent and noted mostly in the distal two-thirds of esophagus. Radiographically, there is loss of primary peristalsis in the distal esophagus. Nonperistaltic tertiary contractions are usually repetitive and simultaneous and may produce a corkscrew or rosary bead appearance **(Fig. 9)**. The findings are similar to those seen in nonspecific esophageal motility disorder. The clinical picture helps to distinguish the two conditions, because diffuse esophageal spasm is associated with chest pain. The esophagus is not usually dilated and the LES functions normally.

The radiological appearance of diffuse esophageal spasm is also known as pseudodiverticula or curling phenomena which can also be found with spastic achalasia.

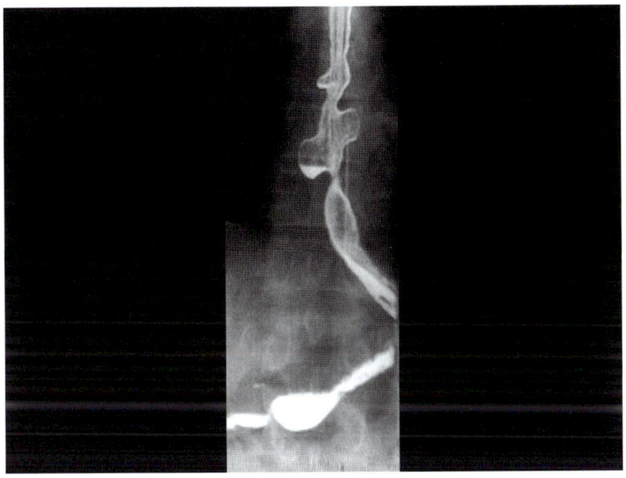

FIG. 9: 'Corkscrew' esophagus—nonpropulsive segmental contractions producing multiple areas of pronounced luminal narrowing with areas of sacculations.

Treatment

Various trials/treatment options for DES have been reported such as use of nitrates, calcium channel blockers, anxiolytics, with varying response. Surgery in the form of long myotomy or esophagectomy is generally not done.

Achalasia

Achalasia is an uncommon motility disorder of the esophagus characterized by a loss of primary esophageal peristalsis, incomplete relaxation of the lower esophageal sphincter in response to deglutition, increased resting LES pressure, and increased intraesophageal pressure.

All these lead to esophageal dilatation or megaesophagus. Of all the conditions associated with esophageal dilatation like achalasia, inflammatory narrowing, progressive systemic sclerosis (PSS) and carcinoma; achalasia causes the most severe generalized dilatation.[16]

Clinical Presentation

Achalasia can present at any age but is the most common in the 30–50 year age group. Dysphagia is usually worse with liquids than with solids, may initially be intermittent and eventually is persistent. It is diagnosed manometrically as esophageal aperistalsis and LES dysfunction, primary incomplete relaxation and elevated resting pressure. Esophageal dilatation is mild in the early stages, which may make radiographic diagnosis difficult.

Although the pathogenesis of achalasia is not known the most accepted theory is related to the paucity or absence of ganglion cells in the Auerbach's plexus in the distal esophageal wall.

Imaging Features

Plain chest radiographs are frequently sufficient for the diagnosis of achalasia. The esophagus is dilated with large amounts of retained food and fluid which may become markedly tortuous and present as a widened mediastinum mainly on the right side, adjacent to the cardiac shadow, often with an air-fluid level. Aspiration of the retained food from the dilated esophagus frequently leads to episodes of pneumonia. On an erect radiograph, air bubble of the gastric fundus is small or absent **(Figs. 10A and B)**.

Barium swallow with the patient erect demonstrates a variable degree of dilatation of the esophagus above a beak-like narrowing at the lower esophageal sphincter **(Figs. 11A and B)**. The sphincter opens intermittently under the force of the hydrostatic pressure of the barium column above it to allow bolus passage. A gradual, tapered, smooth, conical narrowing of the distal esophageal segment extending for 1–3 cm in length is known as bird's beak appearance and is the hallmark of achalasia. With the patient in erect position, sequential radiography can show small spurts of barium entering the stomach through the narrowed distal segment. The distal two-thirds of the esophagus, which contains smooth muscle is aperistaltic. Secondary stasis esophagitis is common. Esophageal carcinoma may develop which may be seen in 2–7% of patients with long standing achalasia. The carcinoma may develop in the mid esophagus secondary to stasis and irritation of esophagus. Whenever there is a worsening of symptoms in patients of achalasia, possibility of superimposed esophageal carcinoma is to be ruled out.[14]

It is essential that the patient with achalasia is examined in the recumbent position because in the erect position, gravity can simulate the effect of peristalsis and hide subtle abnormalities. Evaluation in the upright position is also necessary for the barium column to provide adequate hydrostatic pressure to force even small amounts of contrast into the stomach. In patients of achalasia, complete emptying of the esophagus does not occur even in the erect position. This is an important point to remember to differentiate from scleroderma radiologically, where emptying is usually normal in the erect position.[17]

Achalasia is diagnosed on barium swallow studies or esophageal manometry while the role of endoscopy is only in ruling out pseudoachalasia. Manometry is the most sensitive test in diagnosing achalasia as it identifies early disease before esophageal dilatation and food retention **(Fig. 12)**.[12] High resolution manometry identifies three subtypes of achalasia on the basis of pattern of pressurization in the aperistaltic esophagus: (1) Classic achalasia, (2) achalasia with compression and (3) spastic achalasia. All are characterized by impaired relaxation of the lower esophageal sphincter (LES) with absent peristalsis.

CT features of achalasia have been described by Rabuschka and colleagues[18] which consist of a moderate dilatation of the esophagus with a mean diameter of 4.5 cm at the carinal level, but having a normal wall thickness. They found that a normal wall thickness to be the most important feature that differentiates patients of achalasia from other esophageal diseases **(Figs. 13A to C)**. CT is routinely not indicated for the diagnosis of achalasia, but may be useful in confirming the diagnosis and detecting its complications. It may also suggest the presence of other diseases or superimposed benign or malignant processes.[16] The other causes of narrowing of the lower esophageal sphincter (LES) that may mimic achalasia are intrinsic or extrinsic neoplasm, peptic stricture and complications of scleroderma.

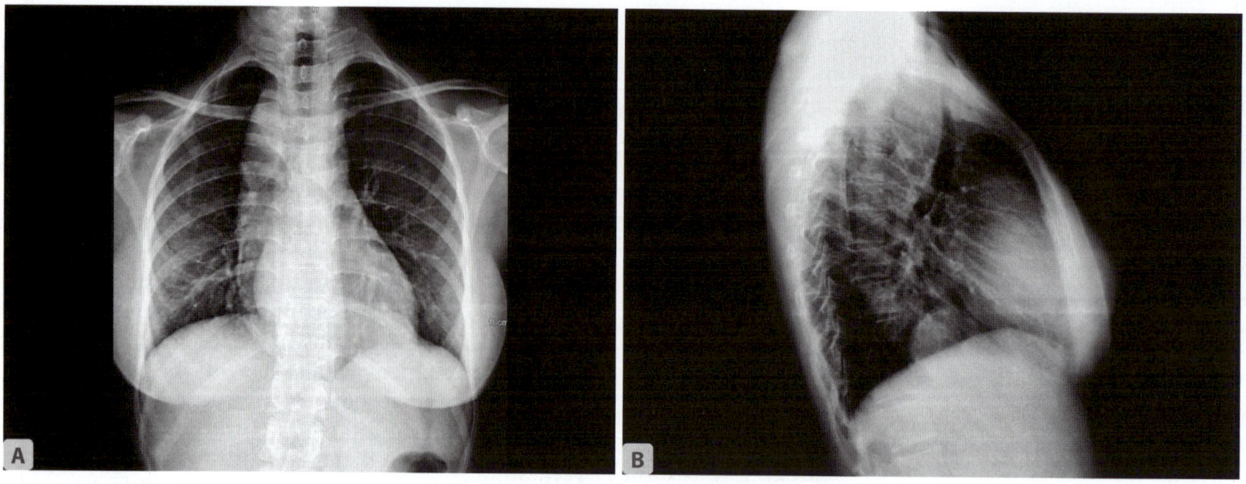

FIGS. 10A AND B: Chest (PA) erect (A) in a 21-year-old female with achalasia reveals a mediastinal shadow extending from the neck to the diaphragm on the right side due to markedly dilated esophagus. There is absence of air in the fundus of the stomach. Chest lateral (B) shows anterior displacement of the trachea by the dilated esophagus.

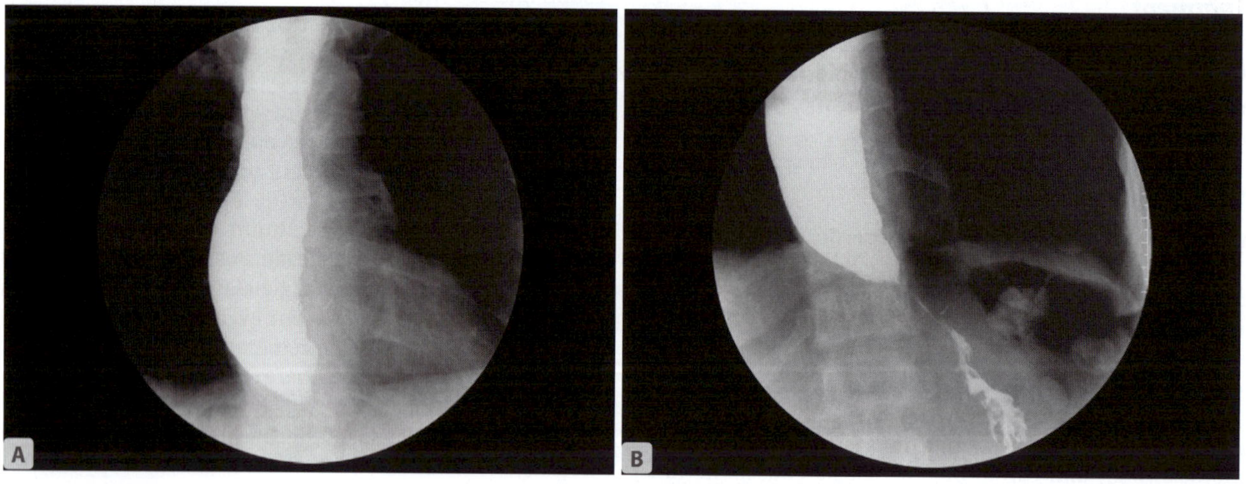

FIGS. 11A AND B: Barium swallow depicts. (A) A moderately dilated esophagus, (B) with a smooth conical narrowing of the distal esophagus: "Bird's beak" appearance-achalasia.

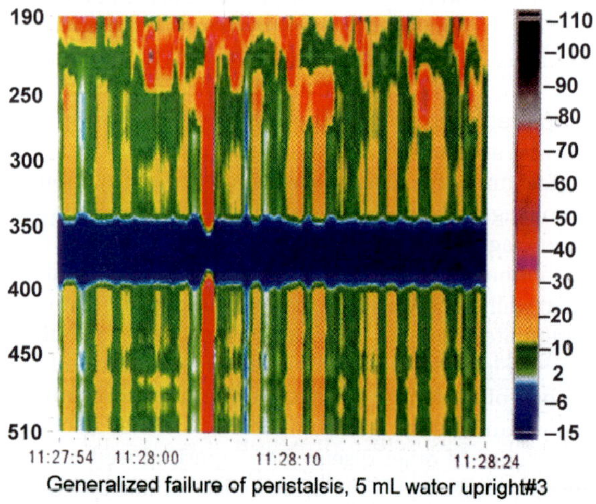

FIG. 12: Esophageal manometry in the patient with achalasia reveals absent esophageal peristalsis with incomplete relaxation of LES with high basal pressure.

Secondary achalasia refers to carcinoma of the gastric cardia or metastases involving the gastroesophageal junction resulting in a radiographic picture simulating achalasia. It is related to destruction of the intramural myenteric plexus. Secondary achalasia should be considered in older patients if symptoms are acute or if the tapered gastroesophageal junction shows mucosal nodularity or mass effect. Repeating the esophagogram after patient inhales amylnitrate may help to distinguish this entity from achalasia. This smooth muscle relaxant relaxes the lower esophageal sphincter in achalasia while in secondary achalasia the LES remains rigid and unchanged.

Treatment

Achalasia cannot be prevented or reversed. Therapy is directed at reducing lower esophageal sphincter pressure, so that gravity and esophageal pressurization promote esophageal emptying. Peristalsis is rarely known to return. LES pressure can be reduced by pharmacological therapy,

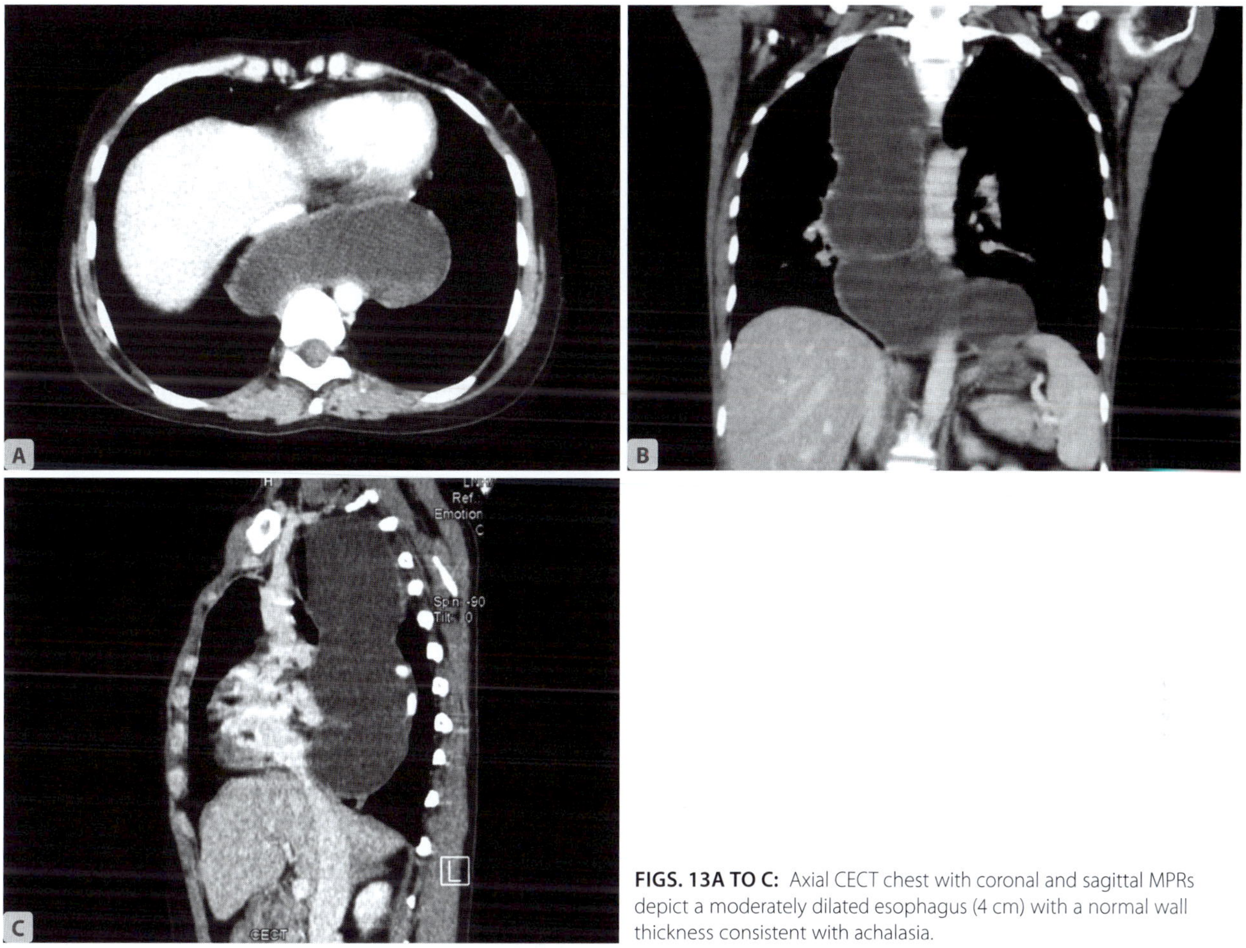

FIGS. 13A TO C: Axial CECT chest with coronal and sagittal MPRs depict a moderately dilated esophagus (4 cm) with a normal wall thickness consistent with achalasia.

forceful dilatation or surgical myotomy. Pharmacological therapy in the form of nitrates or calcium channel blockers are used as temporary therapies and are administered before eating. Botulinum toxin injected under endoscopic guidance into the LES inhibits acetylcholine release from the nerve endings and is known to improve dysphagia in about 66% of cases for at least six months.[12]

The most reliable therapies for achalasia are pneumatic dilatation and Heller's myotomy. Pneumatic dilatation is an endoscopic technique which uses a noncompliant, cylindrical balloon dilator positioned across the LES and inflated to a diameter of 3–4 cm. The reported accuracy of this technique ranges from 32–98%. Esophageal perforation is the major complication which can occur rarely. Heller's myotomy is the most effective surgical procedure for achalasia. It is performed laparoscopically, usually in conjunction with partial Nissen's fundoplication, with good to excellent results being reported in 62–100% of cases. The surgery involves incising the circular muscle fibers down to the mucosa and allowing the mucosa to protrude through.

In patients with advanced achalasia who fail to respond to the above surgical measures, esophageal resection with gastric pull up or interposition of a segment of transverse colon may be the only option other than a feeding gastrostomy.

SECONDARY MOTILITY DISORDER

Scleroderma

Scleroderma results from atrophy or degeneration of smooth muscle in the lower half to two-thirds of the esophagus with subsequent replacement of esophageal musculature by fibrosis. Neural elements and ganglion cells are normal. The upper third of the esophagus is composed of the striated muscles which is usually not effected by scleroderma. Hence, on a barium swallow a normal peristaltic wave may be seen in this region. In the distal two-thirds esophageal region as the disease progresses, mild uncoordinated tertiary contractions seen early in scleroderma may disappear. As the LES tone is severely decreased in scleroderma, drinking in the erect position allows the bolus to the propelled down the esophagus by the striated muscles i.e. pharyngeal constrictors and carried by gravity into the stomach. Due to the incompetent lower esophageal sphincter , there is reflux of acid secretions into the distal esophagus leading to peptic esophagitis and stricture formation, resulting in heartburn and severe dysphagia. Distal esophageal peristalsis is absent or diminished which contributes to the severity of reflux esophagitis **(Figs. 14A and B)**.

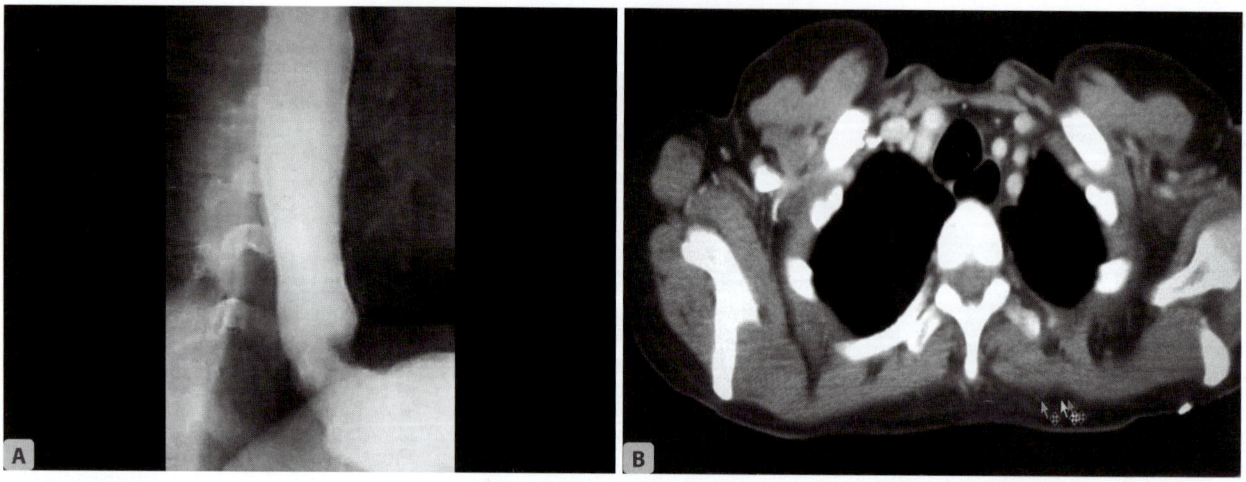

FIGS. 14A AND B: (A) Barium swallow spot film of lower dorsal esophagus showing dilated esophagus with patulous lower esophageal sphincter; (B) CT chest in the same patient shows dilated esophagus in a patient of scleroderma.

STRUCTURAL ESOPHAGEAL DYSPHAGIA

Esophagitis

Numerous etiologic factors may cause esophagitis. The most common cause is gastroesophageal reflux.

Gastroesophageal Reflux Disease and Barrett's Esophagus

Patients with gastroesophageal reflux disease usually complain of a variety of symptoms like heartburn, regurgitation, substernal pain and also dysphagia in some cases. On double-contrast esophagography, early changes of reflux esophagitis may be recognized as a fine mucosal nodularity or granular appearance of the mucosa in the distal third or half of the thoracic esophagus, occurring due to the presence of mucosal edema and inflammation during the early stages of reflux esophagitis. As the disease progresses, double-contrast esophagography may demonstrate shallow ulcers and erosions, thickened longitudinal folds, inflammatory polyps and scarring. Reflux esophagitis may be recognized also on mucosal relief views as lobulation or nodularity of slightly thickened longitudinal folds. Superficial ulceration occurs with increasing severity, seen as tiny, punctate, linear or irregular collection of barium associated with mounds of edema and fold thickening and distortion. The changes of reflux esophagitis involve a continuous area in the distal esophagus extending proximally from the gastroesophageal junction. Sparing of distal esophagus indicates another cause for the radiographic abnormalities.[19]

A stricture may develop with chronic gastroesophageal reflux disease, which is a smooth, tapered and concentric narrowing in the distal esophagus. Occasionally, the benign stricture is asymmetric due to scarring. Sacculations may form with severe scarring. Esophageal dysmotility and dilatation of the esophagus due to atony may also be seen in gastroesophageal reflux disease.

Barrett's esophagus represents acquired progressive columnar metaplasia of the squamous epithelium in the distal esophagus. It is a premalignant condition. It occurs in about 10% of patients with long-standing gastroesophageal reflux and reflux esophagitis. Most strictures of Barrett's esophagus appear as peptic-type distal esophageal stricture. However, a more specific but less common finding is a mid to upper esophageal stricture, often associated with a sliding hiatal hernia or gastroesophageal reflux. If Barrett's esophagus is suspected, patient should be kept under endoscopic surveillance with endoscopic biopsy performed as it carries a 100 fold increased risk of adenocarcinoma.[20]

Lower Esophageal Ring (Schatzki Ring)

A Schatzki ring is a thin, smooth, concentric, symmetric mucosal ring-like narrowing of the distal esophagus which marks the junction between the esophageal and gastric mucosa. The ring is constantly present and it does not change its position. However, Schatzki's ring is only seen on contrast swallow studies when the esophagus above and below it is dilated more than the width of the ring.It may be the result of gastresophageal reflux disease. These usually cause dysphagia when less than 13 mm in diameter but are usually asymptomatic when greater than 20 mm in diameter.[17]

The lower esophageal ring has been considered to be a transverse mucosal fold of non inflammatory origin. On barium studies it needs to be differentiated from a variant of ring-like peptic stricture with which it bears a resemblance. However, the ringlike peptic stricture is more asymmetric with tapered borders and generally longer than (greater than 4 mm) a Schatzki ring.[21]

Congenital Esophageal Stenosis

It is a rare condition which produces smooth fusiform narrowing of the esophageal lumen with varying degree of obstruction and proximal dilatation. Severe stenosis occurs in newborns and infants and usually requires surgery. However, a milder form of narrowing may go on till adulthood as patients adapt themselves to their eating habits to compensate for the stenosis. Its diagnosis can be made if a long concentric narrowing is seen in a patient with a long history of dysphagia often associated with recurrent food impaction with no other risk factors for developing esophageal stenosis.[17] On barium swallow the stenotic segment, usually in the mid-esophagus, may show mild narrowing with distinctive ring-like indentations ('ringed esophagus') in the region of the stricture. There are two schools of thought for this appearance. Some believe that the ring like indentations represent tracheobronchial remnants or cartilaginous rings in the wall of the esophagus. While others believe that it is an acquired condition which occurs secondary to gastroesophageal reflux disease.[21]

INFECTIOUS ESOPHAGITIS

Involvement of the esophagus by infective organisms such as *Candida* species, Herpes virus and cytomegalovirus (CMV) have become relatively common with the increase in use of immunosuppressive drugs for organ transplant as well as chronic inflammatory diseases, chemotherapy and acquired immunodeficiency syndrome (AIDS). In AIDS patients, infectious esophagitis is common when the CD4 count falls to <100. CMV esophagitis occurs only in immunocompromised patients, especially transplant patients.

Regardless of the cause of the infectious agents, odynophagia (painful deglutition) is a characteristic symptom of infectious esophagitis with dysphagia, chest pain and hemorrhage also being common. Odynophagia is uncommon with reflux esophagitis, hence its presence should always raise the suspicion of an alternative etiology.[12]

On CT scan, esophagitis appears as a long segment, uniform, circumferential esophageal wall thickening, often with a 'target sign'. The thickening is as a result of edema, infiltration by inflammatory cells and muscular spasm. The mediastinal fat plane is preserved in esophagitis while esophageal carcinoma usually shows asymmetrical wall thickening with extension into mediastinum. Berkovick and associates found 55% of patients with esophagitis showed an esophageal wall thickness of more than 5 mm with 17% of patients depicting a target sign.[22]

Candida Esophagitis

Candida albicans is the most common cause of infectious esophagitis. It usually occurs opportunistically in immunocompromised patients. *Candida* is normally present in the throat but can become pathogenic and produce esophagitis in the compromised host and is thought to result from downward spread of the fungus from the oropharynx to the esophagus. *Candida* esophagitis can also result from local esophageal stasis caused by severe esophageal motility disorders such as achalasia and scleroderma. Symptoms range from asymptomatic to severe dysphagia.

Imaging Features

Since it is a mucosal disease, it can be identified on double contrast barium examination. In the diagnosis of *Candida* esophagitis, double contrast esophagography shows a sensitivity of about 90%. The findings include discrete, linear, or irregular plaque like filling defects with intervening normal mucosa **(Fig. 15)**. These plaques are oriented longitudinally within the esophagus and may slough off resulting in ulcerations scattered on a background of plaques. In advanced disease, there may be coalescent plaques, which have been likened to a "cobblestone" or "snakeskin" appearance that correspond to the distinctive white plaques seen at endoscopy. Patients with AIDS may get a severe form of this disease, resulting in a grossly irregular or shaggy appearance secondary to extensive plaques and pseudomembranes that trap barium between them.

A newly described sign associated with esophageal candidiasis is the "foamy" esophagus seen on double contrast barium swallow study in the immunocompromised and in 25% of patients of esophageal stasis such as scleroderma, achalasia. It is characterized by the presence of multiple tiny, smooth, round lucencies (bubbles) of around 1–3 mm size that are intermingled with the barium suspension along the top of the barium column on upright views producing a layer of foam. The layer of foam may have a length ranging from 3 to 16 cm in the barium column. The pathophysiologic basis of the "foamy esophagus" is uncertain, but has been postulated to be produced directly by the fungal organisms that colonise the esophagus. These round lucencies in the foamy esophagus are bubbles, hence mobile and are usually distinguished radiographically from retained food or debris in the esophagus or diffuse nodularity of the esophageal mucosa. Undissolved effervescent granules used in a double contrast swallow may mimic the round lucencies seen in *Candida* esophagitis and hence should not be used in the initial swallows when candidial involvement is suspected.[22]

The CT findings of *Candida* esophagitis, though nonspecific and commonly seen in various kinds of esophagitis, are circumferential esophageal wall thickening of more than 5 mm, with relatively long segmental involvement. Enhanced scans may also depict the target sign (circumferential wall thickening and enhancing internal mucosa).[23]

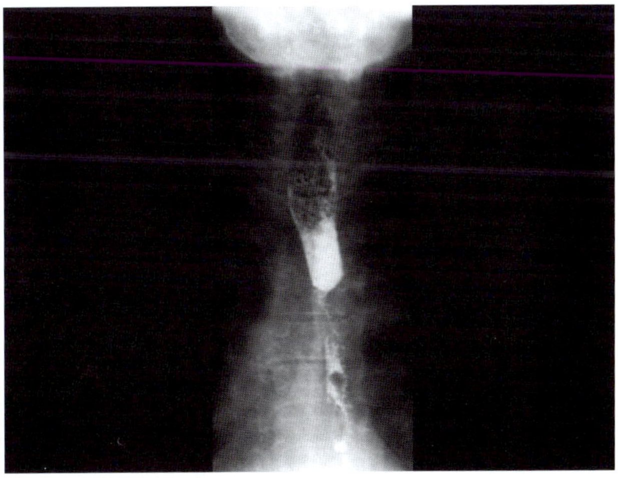

FIG. 15: *Candida esophagitis*: Esophagogram shows a shaggy contour with irregular plaque-like filling defects, seen above a stricture.

Viral Esophagitis

Herpes esophagitis manifests usually as multiple discrete superficial ulcers separated by normal mucosa. The ulcers may be punctate, linear or stellate and are surrounded by radiolucent halos due to edema. In the appropriate clinical setting, the presence of small, discrete ulcers without plaques should be highly suggestive of herpes esophagitis, because ulceration in candidiasis almost always occurs against a background of diffuse plaque formation. When cytomegalovirus and HIV infect the esophagus, large, shallow ulcers up to several centimeters in size are seen in the mid- and sometimes the distal esophagus. The ulcer is usually solitary, ovoid in shape and longitudinal in orientation with smooth margins and often surrounded by a thin radiolucent rim of edematous mucosa. Since the treatment of CMV and HIV esophagitis differs widely, endoscopy with biopsies and cultures is required to differentiate the two infections.[19]

Tuberculosis

Tuberculous involvement of the esophagus is rare. When present, it is usually secondary to current or previous tuberculous infection in other sites. The esophagus may become infected as a result of direct extension from adjacent mediastinal or hilar lymph nodes, vertebral bodies, aortic aneurysms, tuberculous pharyngitis or laryngitis, or by inoculation of swallowed sputum, hematogenous or lymphatic spread.[24]

Tuberculous lesions can occur in any segment of the esophagus. However, they are most common in the middle third, just proximal to the tracheal bifurcation, because of its proximity to the mediastinal lymph nodes around the bifurcation of the trachea.[25] The changes in the esophagus may result from pressure, adhesions or actual involvement of mucosal surface.[24] The most common feature is extrinsic compression of the esophagus, usually by a mass of lymph nodes **(Fig. 16)**. Although the esophageal mucosa is often intact in such cases, the adventitia is usually implicated and this may produce classical traction diverticulum. When the disease process involves the esophageal mucosa, a tumorous lesion or an ulcer may result. Sinus or fistula as a result of rupture of caseous lymph nodes may also occur. Tracheoesophageal or bronchoesophageal fistula and subsequent aspiration pneumonia or lung abscess may occur. A constricting lesion or kinking of the esophagus may be seen as a result of fibrosis.[25]

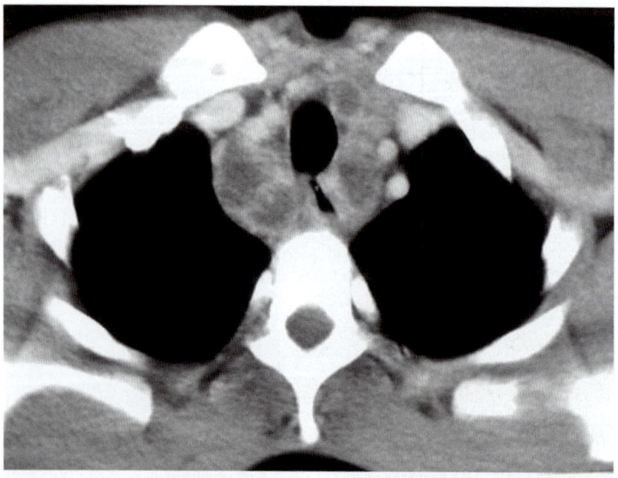

FIG. 16: CECT chest mediastinal window showing multiple variable sized rim enhancing necrotic mediastinal lymph nodes in bilateral paratracheal regions causing extrinsic compression of the esophagus—tuberculosis.

CT of the chest enables complete evaluation of the caseous mediastinal lymph nodes which surround and displace the esophagus and also depicts any fistulous tract extending from the esophagus to the nodal mass. The presence of amorphous gas in enlarged mediastinal lymph nodes in patients with tubercular lymphadenitis is suggestive of an esophageal nodal fistula.[12]

INFLAMMATORY ESOPHAGITIS

Corrosive/Caustic Esophagitis

Caustic ingestion can cause severe injury to the esophagus and stomach. The severity and extent of damage depends on the type, concentration, volume, physical form (solid or liquid) of the agent and duration of contact with the mucosa. Ingestion is usually accidental in children less than five years of age and intentional in adults. The most common cause is ingestion of a strong alkali (sodium or potassium hydroxide) present in drain cleaners, disc batteries, etc. The term 'lye' refers to substances which contain sodium or potassium hydroxide. Highly concentrated acids such as hydrochloric, sulfuric acid are contained in toilet cleaners, anti-rust compounds. Button batteries are highly concentrated alkaline solution which when lodged in the esophagus can cause burns within four hours and perforation within six hours.

The conventional school of thought is that acids preferentially damage the stomach as they are somewhat neutralized by the alkaline pH of the esophagus and alkalis injure the esophagus and spare the stomach. But extensive esophageal damage and perforation have been known to occur after acid ingestion.

Pathogenesis

Alkali ingestion results in a penetrating injury called liquifactive necrosis which spreads rapidly within seconds through the mucosa and wall of the esophagus resulting in esophageal perforation, mediastinitis and even death. This is most likely to occur with liquid preparations that coat larger mucosal surfaces. While solid lye preparation or alkaline batteries induce a more localized injury to the esophagus. The liquefactive necrosis usually lasts for 3–4 days with vascular thrombosis, mucosal inflammation, resulting in focal or extensive sloughing or ulceration. The esophageal wall becomes thinner in the next few weeks because of sloughing and development of granulation tissue and fibrosis. It takes 1–3 months for re-epithelialization be complete.

The likelihood of a stricture to develop depends on the depth of damage and the degree of collagen deposition.

Acid-induced injury produces a superficial coagulation necrosis that forms a protective layer over the mucosa. Being less viscous than alkaline solutions, they tend to pass quickly into the stomach. Patients of corrosive ingestion may complain of oropharyngeal, retrosternal or epigastric pain, odynophagia or dysphagia. Severe and persistent retrosternal or back pain may be indicative of esophageal perforation with mediastinitis.

Diagnosis and Staging

An upper GI endoscopy should be performed during the first 24 hours after caustic corrosive ingestion to assess the damage, establish the prognosis and guide further treatment. Endoscopy is contraindicated in a hemodynamically unstable patient, if there is severe respiratory distress or there is evidence of perforation.

An endoscopic grading system for corrosive esophageal injury has been developed for predicting clinical outcome, with grades 1 and 2A having an excellent prognosis while at the other end, grade 3B carrying a risk of early mortality in 65% cases. Patients with grades 2B and 3A are known to develop strictures in 70–100% cases.

Esophageal or gastric perforation can occur anytime during the first two weeks of ingestion. Water soluble contrast swallow should be performed to rule out the same. CT has been regarded more useful than endoscopy in assessing transmural damage and extent of necrosis and detecting perforation.

Sequelae of corrosive/caustic injury: Around one-third of patients of esophageal injury, mainly, those with grades 2B or 3 injuries, develop esophageal strictures. Dysphagia occurring due to stricture formation is generally seen two months after the corrosive injury. Barium swallow helps in evaluating the sequelae but is not able to differentiate if it is due to acid/alkali ingestion. Strictures secondary to corrosive injury are usually long, smooth and mostly involve the middle and distal esophagus **(Figs. 17A to C)**. But variable appearances of caustic/corrosive strictures have been described. They can be short, long or multiple with a smooth outline with nodular defects or scalloping due to focal areas of submucosal fibrosis. It is important to perform a contrast study up to the pylorus to rule out concomitant gastric injury which can occur from 20% to 62.5% cases in the form of antral ulceration, pyloric stenosis or frank gastric outlet obstruction.

Treatment

Esophageal strictures are treated by esophageal dilatations which should be performed 3–6 weeks after the initial injury because of the associated high incidence of perforation if attempted early. The goal is to dilate the esophageal lumen to 15 mm and to completely relieve dysphagia. Long and eccentric strictures may be managed by endoscopic dilatation under fluoroscopic guidance so as to minimize the risk of perforation.

There is an increased risk for the development of esophageal squamous cell carcinoma (SCC) in patients of caustic/corrosive ingestion. This risk is substantially higher in victims of chronic lye ingestion as compared to the general population.[21] The latent period is generally in decades. Hence, these patients should be followed up periodically to rule out the same, with endoscopic surveillance for cancer recommended for 15–20 years after ingestion.

Drug-induced or Pill Esophagitis

Drug-induced esophagitis is caused most commonly by ingesting antibiotics, such as tetracycline and doxycycline which cause only superficial ulceration. Other medications

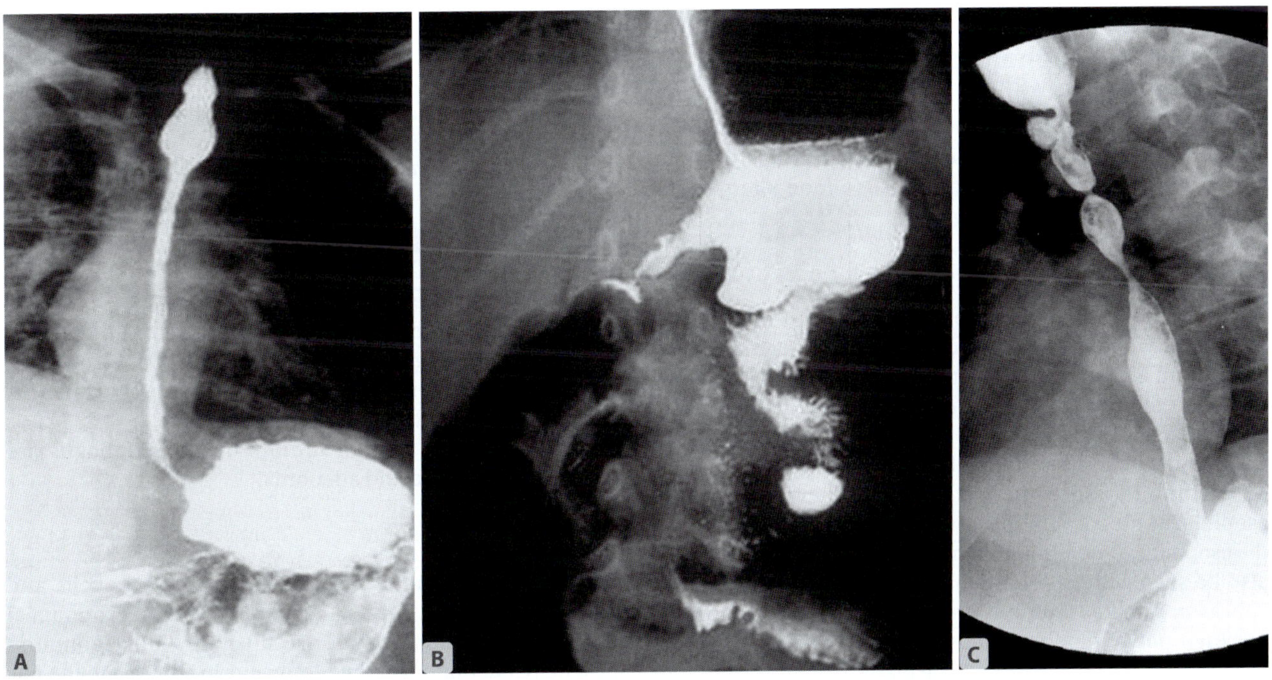

FIGS. 17A TO C: (A) Barium swallow showing a long stricture with nodular defects due to focal areas of submucosal fibrosis in a case of Caustic esophagitis; (B) The stomach shows narrowing of distal body and antrum with mucosal irregularity; Corrosive strictures in another patient showing (C) multiple, short, smooth strictures with proximal dilatation with diverticulum formation.

include potassium chloride, quinidine, ferrous sulfate and anti-inflammatory drugs. They generally get lodged in the esophagus at sites of extrinsic compression. These drugs may result in severe esophagitis and strictures may develop.

Clinical Presentation

When such drugs dissolve in the esophagus, they cause mucosal injury by creating an acid pH or by a direct irritant effect in the epithelium. Hold up of tablets in the esophagus is favored by swallowing pills while lying down, taking them without water, abnormal esophageal motility, and cardiomegaly. Symptoms are usually sudden in onset and consist of chest pain, odynophagia or dysphagia. The pain of drug/pill-induced esophagitis characteristically develops over a period of hours or will awaken the patient from sleep. A history of ingesting the pill obviates the need for any diagnostic testing. Endoscopy when performed, reveals localized ulceration or inflammation.

Drug-induced esophagitis usually involves the proximal or middle esophagus. A typical location is the aortic arch level, where tablets are delayed because of the aortic indentation on the esophagus and the low contractile force of peristalsis.

Imaging Features

The radiographic findings consist of luminal irregularity, frank ulceration and luminal narrowing. The ulcers are usually ovoid, occasionally linear and clustered circumferentially. A repeat study 7–10 days after withdrawal of the offending agent will show healing of ulcers. CT chest may sometimes show esophageal thickening consistent with transmural inflammation. The condition usually resolves within days to weeks, but symptoms may persist for months. In severe cases, stricture may develop, which may required dilatation.[19]

Eosinophilic Esophagitis

Eosinophilic esophagitis is an increasingly common inflammatory condition characterized pathologically by eosinophilic infiltration of the esophagus that is thought to occur as an inflammatory response to food allergens in susceptible individuals.

Clinical Presentation

The condition should be strongly considered in children and adults with long standing dysphagia and recurrent food impaction. Majority of the patients present with an atopic history of food allergy, asthmas eczema, allergic rhinitis or peripheral eosinophilia.

The diagnosis of eosinophilic esophagitis (EoE) is based on a combination of typical esophageal symptoms and esophageal mucosal biopsies demonstrating infiltration of the esophageal squamous epithelium with eosinophils. It can also be seen with gastroesophageal reflux disease (GERD). However, if the eosinophils are greater than 20 eosinophils per high power field on endoscopic biopsy, a diagnosis of eosinophilic esophagitis should be made.[26]

Imaging Features

Eosinophilic esophagitis may cause segmental or diffuse esophageal strictures that can be diagnosed with esophagoscopy. Strictures may occur most often in the upper to mid thoracic esophagus. It may be associated with distinctive ring-like indentation known as "ringed esophagus". An esophagus with a small caliber may instead be seen in this condition. The "small caliber esophagus" is a radiographic sign that has been described in 2010 by White, Levine et al at barium esophagography and is defined as an esophagus with a caliber of less than 20 mm. The involved segment of esophagus is long with variable length of narrowing having a mean length of 15.4 cm with smooth contours and tapered margins.[26]

Endoscopy needs to be performed for a definitive diagnosis.

Treatment

Treatment includes dietary modification, proton pump inhibitors, steroid therapy, dilatation of strictures. Esophageal dilatation must be cautiously performed in patients with strictures because of increased risk of esophageal mural disruption and perforation.[1,12]

Intramural Pseudodiverticulosis

It is an unusual condition in which inflammation leads to dilatation of the ducts of the deep mucous glands. Intramural pseudodiverticulosis may occur as a consequence of scarring and is associated with strictures in 90% of patients.

Imaging Features

Radiologically, they appear as tiny, flask-shaped outpouchings of contrast material, 1–4 mm in size arranged in clusters or longitudinal rows **(Fig. 18)**. Often the neck of the pseudodiverticula are not opacified and they appear to be separated from the esophageal lumen by 1 or 2 mm and appear to float outside the esophagus. The condition may be segmental or diffuse, and may be seen in association with a peptic stricture in the lower esophagus.

ESOPHAGEAL NEOPLASMS

Benign Esophageal Neoplasms

Benign tumors comprise 20% of esophageal tumors. The most common benign intramural neoplasm of the esophagus is leiomyoma. Others such as hemangioma, schwannoma, neurofibroma and glomus tumor are very rare.

Mucosal-based benign tumors of the esophagus are squamous papilloma and adenoma.

Leiomyoma

They are neoplasms of mature smooth muscle cells and account for more than 50% of all benign esophageal neoplasms.[14] Leiomyomas are also the most common mesenchymal tumors of the esophagus in contrast to the rest

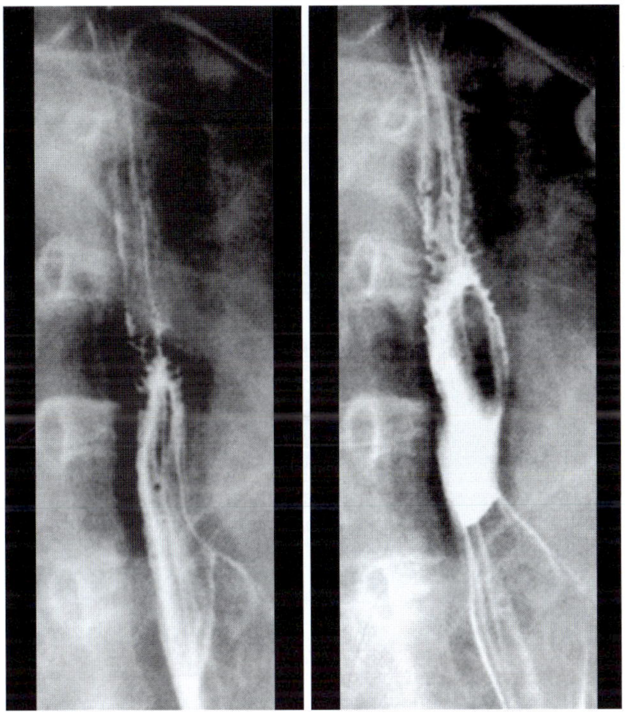

FIG. 18: Intramural pseudodiverticulosis: Tiny, flask-shaped outpouchings arranged in longitudinal rows produced by barium entering dilated esophageal glands, seen in the thoracic esophagus.

of the gastrointestinal tract, where gastrointestinal stromal tumors (GISTs) are more common.

Clinical Features

They occur mostly in adults, being twice more common in males than females. However, rarely they may also be seen in children. Most patients are asymptomatic, but dysphagia and pain may develop depending on the size of the lesion and how much the esophageal lumen is getting compromised. Those effected generally have symptoms of more than two years duration[27] and dysphagia to solids is the predominant symptom. On immunohistochemistry, esophageal leiomyomas can be distinguished from GISTs as leiomyomas are negative for CD117 and CD34.

Esophageal leiomyomas mostly involve the mid (60%) and lower (30%) third of the esophagus, where smooth muscle is present.[27] They may arise from the muscularis mucosa or muscularis propria layers of the esophageal wall. Majority of the leiomyomas (97%) are intramural with 10% of them showing circumferential growth pattern. These tumors are mostly solitary with a size of <3 cm. Multiple leiomyomas (leiomyomatosis) can be familial and often associated with Alport syndrome in children. Esophageal leiomyomatosis can occur on its own or be associated with leiomyomas of the tracheobronchial tree and genital tract in the pediatric age group.

Imaging Features

On double contrast barium studies, esophageal leiomyomas appears as smoothly marginated filling defect that forms an obtuse angle with the adjacent esophageal wall. This appearance is characteristic of a submucosal mass.[27] On cross-sectional imaging, it appears as a smoothly marginated exophytic intraluminal mass or as an eccentric esophageal wall thickening **(Figs. 19A and B)**. It shows soft tissue homogeneous attenuation which may occasionally contain calcification. Leiomyomas are iso to hypodense to muscle on non-contrast CT and slightly hyperintense on T2W MR imaging. They show homogeneous enhancement on contrast imaging without any necrosis.[14]

Endoscopic ultrasound (EUS) has a diagnostic accuracy of 89% in the diagnosis of esophageal leiomyomas as it is able to depict which layer of the esophageal wall is involved.[6] On EUS, leiomyoma is seen as homogeneous hypoechoic mass in the muscularis mucosa, submucosa or muscularis propria. On PET-CT, leiomyomas do not usually show avid uptake as these tumors have a low mitotic rate.[27]

Differential diagnosis of esophageal leiomyomas includes duplication cysts, gastrointestinal stromal tumors, lymphoma and hematogenous metastases. Duplication cysts usually manifest in childhood and appear as cysts on all imaging modalities. Calcification is a feature of leiomyomas, but may be seen in GISTs. Small GISTs may mimic leiomyomas as they too appear as homogeneous intramural masses. However, small leiomyomas are relatively more common. Large GISTs may be differentiated on the basis of necrosis or cyst formation in them. Esophageal lymphoma and metastatic disease generally occur in a setting of contiguous invasion or widespread disease.[27]

Treatment

Treatment for esophageal leiomyomas consists of removal in the form of endoscopic resection or surgical enucleation or conservative follow-up. These lesions have a benign course and usually do not recur after surgery.

Gastrointestinal Stromal Tumors

Esophageal gastrointestinal stromal tumors (GISTs) are uncommon mesenchymal tumors as compared to leiomyomas of the esophagus. Esophageal GIST, similar to other gastrointestinal stromal tumors in the gastrointestinal tract, are positive for C-KIT (a cell surface transmembrane tyrosine kinase also known as CD117) and CD34. These tumors have a malignant potential and have overlapping imaging features with esophageal leiomyomas. Hence, it is important for the radiologist to be familiar with the clinicopathologic and imaging features of these tumors for appropriate patient management.

Clinicopathological Features

Esophageal GISTs are more commonly encountered than previously thought. They occur more often in the lower dorsal esophagus, the site for abundant intrinsic distribution of the gastrointestinal stromal tumor progenitor cells, the interstitial cells of Cajal. The patients generally present late with symptoms of dysphagia because of their submucosal, exophytic location and are usually large at presentation. Patients may also have pain and cough due to the mass

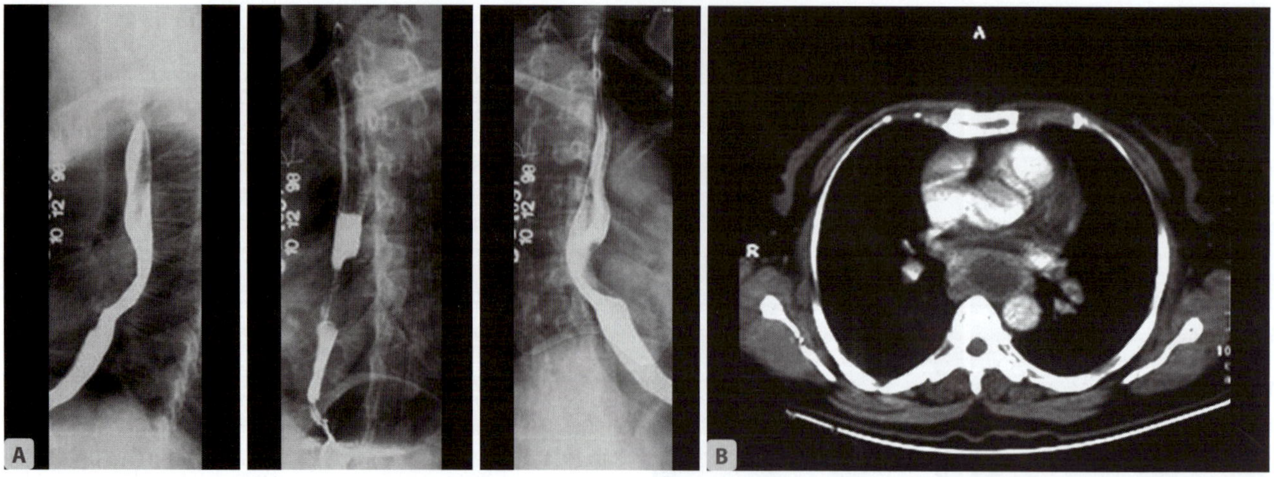

FIGS. 19A AND B: (A) Leiomyoma in the distal thoracic esophagus seen as a semilunar mass with intact mucosa, narrowing the barium column and widening the esophageal diameter; (B) CECT shows smooth hypodense mass seen indenting the esophageal lumen with intact fat planes around esophagus—leiomyoma.

TABLE 3: Differences between esophageal GISTs and leiomyomas.

	Esophageal GISTs	Esophageal leiomyomas
1. Tumor size	Larger (~5–6 cm)	Smaller (<3 cm)
2. Location	More frequently in distal esophagus	Mid (40%) and distal (50%) esophagus both locations
3. Barium swallow	Appears as smooth, submucosal nonobstructive filling defect	Appears as smooth, submucosal nonobstructive filling defect
4. CT scan	More heterogeneous attenuation	More homogeneous density
5. CECT	Moderately enhancing mass	Shows minimal to no enhancement
6. Ulceration	May be present. Seen on endoscopy or barium swallow study	No ulceration seen. Mucosa is normal
7. Calcification	Rare	Uncommon. Diffuse popcorn type
8. PET scan	FDG-avid tumor	Mild FDG uptake
9. Treatment	Surgical resection because of malignant potential/ adjuvant therapy or radiation	Resection/conservative follow-up if asymptomatic

effect exerted by the tumor on adjacent mediastinal structures.

Imaging Features

On barium studies GIST appears as a submucosal smoothly marginated mass. Ulceration may be seen in large GISTs on endoscopy or barium swallow study, while it is not a feature of esophageal leiomyomas.

On CT, esophageal GISTs appear as large, heterogeneous intramural soft tissue masses that are isoattenuating to muscles and show moderate postcontrast enhancement. Cystic areas are common in tumor larger than 4.5 cm while calcification is rare. Gastrointestinal stromal tumors show uniform FDG uptake on PET Scan.[28]

Treatment

Treatment consists of surgery alone or along with adjuvant imatinib (tyrosine kinase inhibitor) or radiation therapy. The table below **(Table 3)** lists the differentiating features between esophageal GIST and esophageal leiomyomas.[28]

Fibrovascular Polyp

Fibrovascular polyp is a rare, benign, tumor-like lesion of the esophagus composed of loose or dense fibrous tissue, adipose tissue and vascular structure. The polyp is covered by normal squamous epithelium. The components of fibrovascular polyp may vary from lesion to lesion and in different parts of the same lesion.

A fibrovascular polyp usually arises in the cervical esophagus near the level of the cricopharyngeus. It probably originates in the loose submuscular tissue of the cervical esophagus and gradually elongates over many years as it is dragged into the middle or distal third of the esophagus by esophageal peristalsis, until the intraluminal portion of the tumor becomes massive in size. Occasionally, it may even prolapse through the cardia into the gastric fundus.[29]

Clinical Features

Fibrovascular polyp generally occur in elderly with slowly progressive dysphagia over years. Other symptoms include vomiting, weight loss, respiratory difficulty likely due to compression of the adjacent trachea by the distended esophagus. Very rarely fibrovascular polyp with a long stalk may regurgitate into the pharynx or mouth, resulting in sudden death from laryngeal occlusion.[14]

Imaging Features

On plain chest frontal radiographs, fibrovascular polyps may be detected as a right sided superior mediastinal mass and on a lateral view may cause compression and anterior bowing of the trachea. It can be differentiated from achalasia due to lack of distension of the distal esophagus.

On barium swallow studies it typically appears as a smooth, expansile, sausage-shaped intraluminal mass that arises in the cervical esophagus and extends to the middle or distal third of the esophagus. It can show a lobulated appearance which if marked, can mimic a malignant neoplasm radiographically. The CT appearance can vary depending on the amount of fat and fibrovascular tissue in the lesion. If fat is the predominant tissue, the presence of an intraluminal esophageal mass with fat attenuation in it is considered a typical sign of a fibrovascular polyp. When oral contrast surrounds the mass on CT, it may help in determining the intraluminal location of the lesion.

MR further aids in characterizing the composition of a fibrovascular polyp. Fat within the mass, mucoid secretion and nonacute blood depict a high signal intensity on T1W images while soft tissue and muscle within the tumor appear as low signal intensity on T2W images.[14]

Treatment

Fibrovascular polyps do not usually undergo malignant degeneration. But still these lesions warrant a removal because of the progressive and debilitating nature of the symptoms. Also, because of the known risk of asphyxiation and sudden death due to the gigantic sizes it can grow to in the esophagus, it is imperative to surgically remove these tumors.

MALIGNANT ESOPHAGEAL NEOPLASMS

Majority (~80%) of the esophageal neoplasms are malignant. More than 90% of these are squamous cell carcinomas or adenocarcinomas which are epithelial neoplasms.

Esophageal Carcinoma: Squamous Cell Carcinoma and Adenocarcinoma

Both squamous cell carcinoma and adenocarcinoma are very aggressive malignant epithelial neoplasms which disseminate early because of lack of serosa in the esophagus. The non-epithelial malignant neoplasms are rare in comparison and include sarcomas, particularly leiomyosarcoma. Lymphoma, malignant melanoma and metastasis also involve the esophagus rarely.

Clinical Presentation

Histologically, the most common esophageal cancer is squamous cell carcinoma (SCC) in 90% cases. However, in recent years there has been a marked increase in the prevalence of esophageal *adenocarcinoma* due to increasing weight gain and obesity and it has been recently found to be the most predominant type of esophageal carcinoma with Barrett's esophagus seen in many of these patients.[1,14] Barrett's esophagus is the most important risk factor which is implicated in the development of esophageal adenocarcinoma. It is a premalignant condition where the normal stratified squamous epithelium of the esophagus is replaced by columnar epithelium secondary to chronic gastroesophageal reflux and reflux esophagitis. These patients may present with symptoms secondary to underlying gastroesophageal reflux disease (GERD). However, most patients have advanced malignancy at the time of presentation with symptoms of dysphagia, odynophagia, rapidly progressive weight loss being similar to that seen in patients with advanced squamous cell carcinoma. Esophageal adenocarcinoma is seen predominantly in males in the seventh decade. Most of them involve the distal third of the esophagus with consequent invasion of the stomach by direct extension across the gastroesophageal junction.

Major risk factors of *squamous cell carcinoma* are tobacco and alcohol intake with other predisposing factors being achalasia, lye strictures, Plummer-Vinson syndrome, coeliac disease and tylosis. Patients with achalasia have a much higher risk of developing esophageal cancer which is 9–28 times that of a person without achalasia. The secondary cancers developing in achalasia patients usually present late in the disease course and have a poor prognosis. They may appear as large, bulky mass within a markedly dilated esophagus. Squamous cell carcinoma is more common in males than females with peak age group of involvement being 60–74 years.[14,27] They are most commonly located in the middle third of esophagus, followed by the lower third and then the upper third. Patients present with progressive dysphagia and by the time dysphagia develops, the esophageal lumen is more than 50% compromised and two-thirds of the circumference of the esophageal wall is invaded by the tumor. Ulceration in the tumor can produce odynophagia and patients may have chest pain unrelated to swallowing if the tumor has invaded the mediastinum.[16]

Independent of staging, the prognosis of esophageal adenocarcinoma is better than SCC, with a 5-year survival rate after resection being 42% compared to 30% for SCC.[27]

Imaging Features

On barium contrast studies, esophageal adenocarcinoma may be indistinguishable from SCC on the basis of morphological findings. Advanced esophageal carcinoma present with a variety of morphologic abnormalities. They may appear as annular apple-core lesion with overhanging margins **(Fig. 20)**, irregular narrowed segment, smooth tapering stricture, bulky endophytic mass **(Fig. 21)**, large ulceration, varicoid infiltrate **(Fig. 22)**, or diffuse nodularity **(Fig. 23)**. Varicoid carcinomas are those in which submucosal spread of tumor produces thickened, tortuous, longitudinal defects

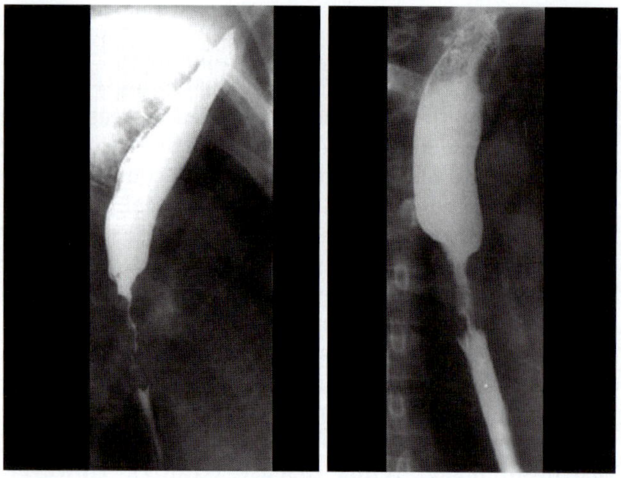

FIG. 20: Annular carcinoma in midportion of esophagus with circumferential infiltration and overhanging margins.

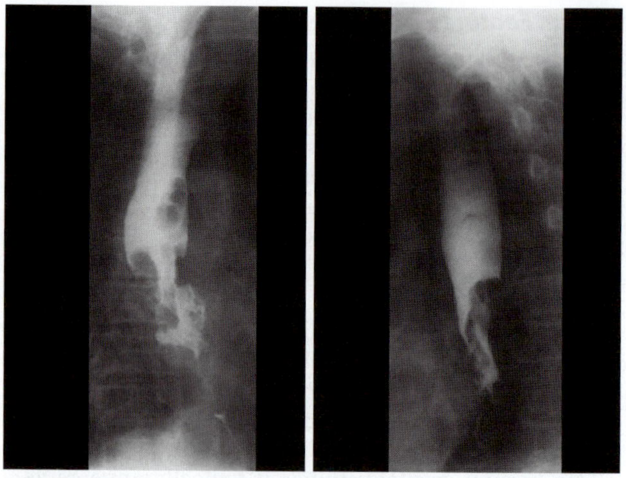

FIG. 21: Polypoidal filling defects with shouldering and irregular narrowing of lumen-carcinoma involving the mid and lower esophagus.

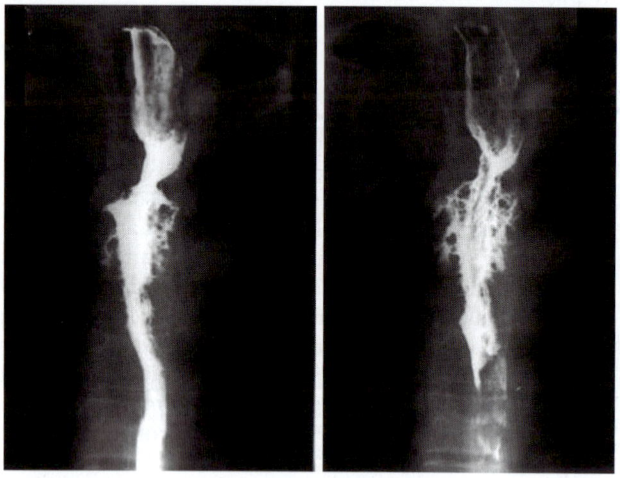

FIG. 22: Spot film of the esophagus at the level of aortic arch shows irregularity and nodularity of the mucosa with lymphatic infiltration-varicoid appearance in squamous cell carcinoma.

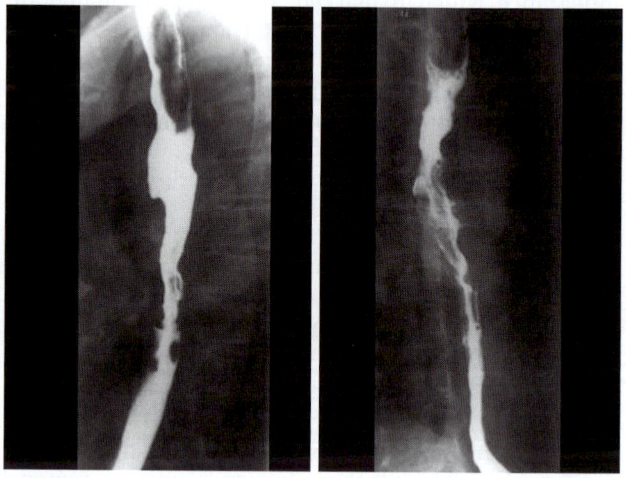

FIG. 23: Carcinoma involving mid esophagus with narrowing of lumen and diffuse nodular filling defects.

that mimic the appearance of varices. Varicoid tumors have a fixed configuration, whereas varices change in size and shape at fluoroscopy. In some cases, esophageal carcinoma spreads submucosally via the lymphatics and reappears at another site in the esophagus **(Figs. 24A and B)**. These satellite metastases may appear as polypoid, plaque-like, or ulcerated lesions separated from the primary tumor by normal mucosa.[19] Tumor also spreads subdiaphragmatically to the proximal stomach via submucosal lymphatics. Fistulization may occur spontaneously, or after radiotherapy.

On CT scans, esophageal carcinoma appears as a mass or wall thickening of soft tissue attenuation **(Figs. 25A to C)**. A recent study on dynamic CECT has shown that the optimal phase in depicting esophageal carcinoma in the late arterial phase as it best depicts the tumor enhancement and the attenuation difference between the tumor and the normal esophageal wall compared to early arterial and venous phases.[30]

On MR imaging the mass appears isointense to the residual esophageal wall on T1W images and intermediate or high signal intensity on T2W images. CT and MRI are both used for staging esophageal carcinoma and are both considered comparable for assessing resectibility in terms of mediastinal invasion, lymph node involvement and distant metastasis.[27] However, in routine clinical situations, CT is recommended.[14]

LEIOMYOSARCOMA

Leiomyosarcoma of the esophagus are rare, low grade malignant lesions accounting for less than 1% of all esophagal malignant neoplasms. They are characterised by slow growth and late metastasis, hence have a better prognosis than squamous cell carcinoma.

Leiomyosarcoma are seen in middle aged or older adults. Most of them are thought to arise de novo rather than from pre-existing leiomyomas.[30] They are usually located in the middle and distal thirds of the esophegas as the esophagus here is lined by smooth muscle. Leiomyosarcoma generally

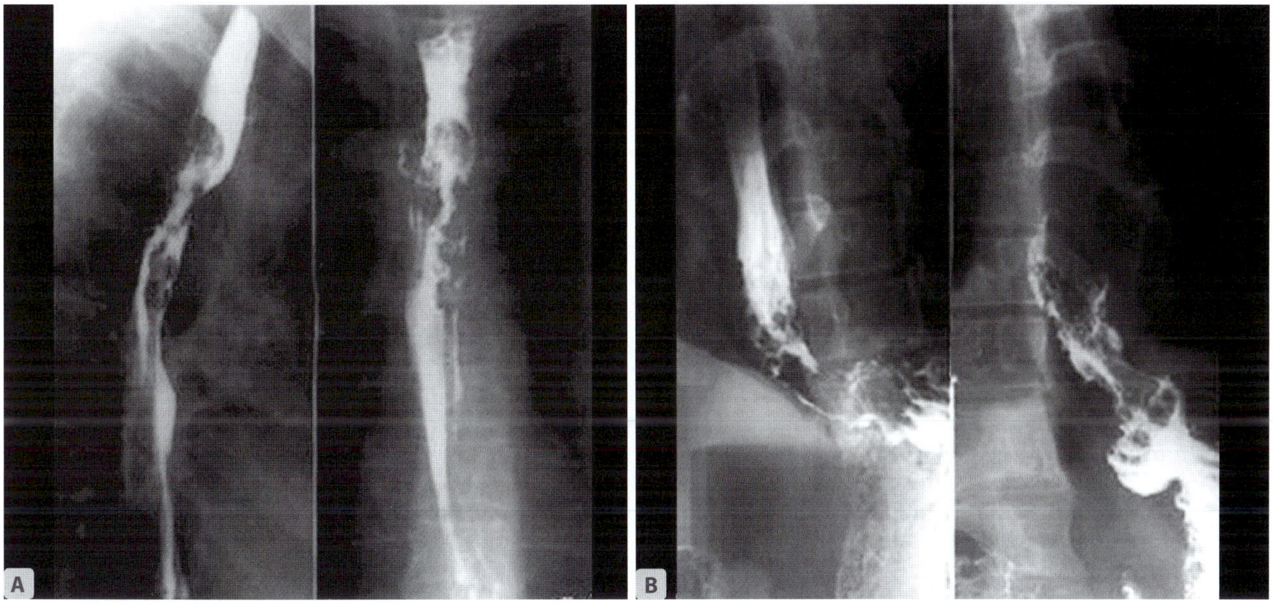

FIGS. 24A AND B: Carcinoma involving upper and mid esophagus in a circumferential manner. Another lesion is seen just above the esophagogastric junction—multicentric carcinoma.

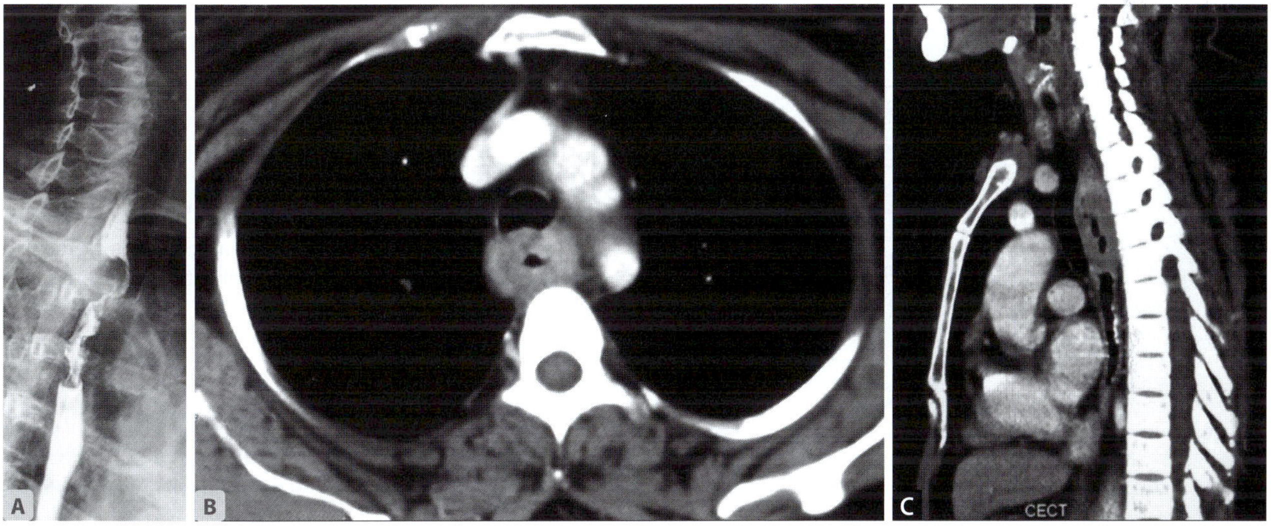

FIGS. 25A TO C: Barium swallow study (A) showing irregular area of luminal narrowing, ulceration with polypoid filling defect and shouldering involving upper dorsal esophagus; (B and C) axial and sagittal CECT reveals homogeneously enhancing circumferential mural thickening of the upper dorsal esophagus (D2-D5 level) with indentation of the trachea anteriorly. The periesophageal triangular fat pad is preserved: Carcinoma esophagus.

spread by direct extention into the mediastrinum or by hematogenous metastases.

Clinical Presentation

Patients present clinically with slowly progressive dysphagia and weight loss. But if tumor has a significant exophytic growth pattern without encroachment on the esophagus, dysphagia can be minimal or absent. GI bleeding can occur if the tumor ulcerates.

Imaging Features

Leiomyosarcoma may sometimes be detected on plain chest radiographs when they show a large exophytic component extending into the mediastinum. Two types of growth patterns have been described—polypoid or infiltrating. The typical appearance on barium studies is a submucosal mass that tends to be larger and more lobulated than benign leiomyoma and may sometimes contain areas of ulceration, cavitation or calcification **(Fig. 26)**.[31]

On CT, leiomyosarcomas of the esophagus are seen as thickening of the esophageal wall with a large soft tissue exophytic component showing central areas of low attenuation due to necrosis and extraluminal air due to ulceration. An infiltrating type of lesion may be indistinguishable from an infiltrative esophageal cancer.[14] On MR imaging the tumor may appear as a mass that is isointense to skeletal muscle on T1-weighted images and hyperintense on T2-weighted images.

Early treatment is essential as leiomyosarcomas have a better prognosis than squamous cell carcinoma.

LYMPHOMA

Esophageal lymphomas are very rare, accounting for less than 1% of all gastrointestinal lymphomas. Esophageal involvement usually occurs secondary to contiguous spread of lymphoma from the gastric fundus or direct invasion by adjacent lymphomatous lymph nodes. Primary lymphoma has been reported in patients of AIDS.[27]

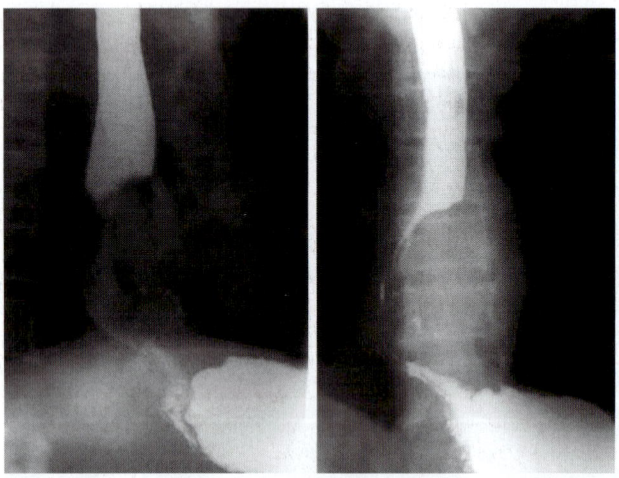

FIG. 26: Barium swallow shows a smooth extrinsic impression on the distal esophagus with a large exophytic component suggestive of an intramural mass—leiomyosarcoma.

Clinical Presentation

Patients may present with dysphagia but often these tumors may not produce symptoms and have known to be discovered at autopsy with widespread disease.[14]

Imaging Features

Lymphomas most often occur in the distal esophagus with variable appearance on imaging. On barium studies, they are commonly seen as irregular narrowing of the distal esophagus due to direct spread of the tumor from the proximal stomach. They may also appear as multiple submucosal nodules, polypoid or ulcerated lesions, enlarged folds or rarely as aneurysmal dilatation of the esophagus.[27]

On cross-sectional imaging, lymphomas can cause concentric or asymmetric thickening of the esophageal wall with or without mediastinal lymphadenopathy. A helpful point to remember is that an intact fat plane between the esophageal tumor and adjacent structures goes in favor of an esophageal lymphoma **(Figs. 27A to C)**.[27]

On EUS, the tumor most commonly appears as homogeneously hypoechoic transmural thickening. On PET scan it mostly demonstrates avid FDG uptake.

Treatment

Esophageal lymphomas are treated by a combination of chemotherapy and radiotherapy which have been found to be as effective as surgery.

SPINDLE CELL CARCINOMA

These tumors of the esophagus have both carcinomatous and sarcomatous components and are currently considered as a variant of squamous cell carcinoma.

Imaging Features

Majority of the spindle cell tumors are located in the middle and distal esophagus and are characterized by intraluminal growth rather than esophageal wall invasion.[27]

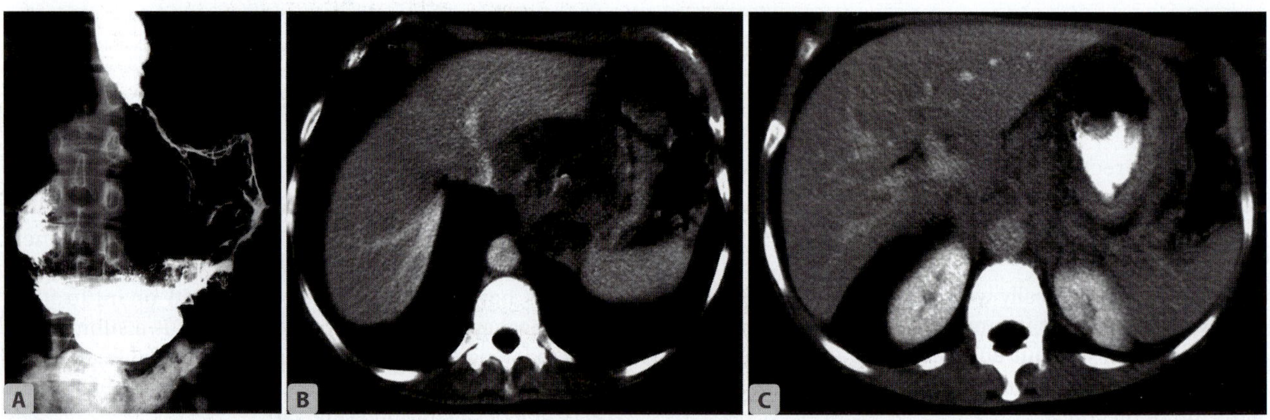

FIGS. 27A TO C: Barium swallow study (A) shows smoothly tapered narrowing of lower end esophagus with contiguous involvement of the proximal stomach. On CECT (B and C), there is bulky circumferential mass in the distal esophagus with diffuse infiltration into the stomach with preservation of fat planes: Primary esophageal lymphoma of lower end esophagus with contiguous involvement of proximal stomach.

On esophagography it seen as a large polypoid intraluminal mass which mainly expands the esophagus without causing obstruction. The CT appearance is of a large intraluminal mass without proximal dilatation or localized wall thickening. On MR imaging, these tumors show greater enhancement than the esophageal wall.

The differential diagnosis of spindle cell carcinoma includes leiomyosarcoma, fibrovascular polyp, primary malignant melanoma and squamous cell carcinoma. Fibrovascular polyp also appear as polypoid intraluminal masses. This can be differentiated from spindle cell carcinoma as they have a very smooth contour and arise from the cervical esophagus while spindle cell carcinoma are more lobulated and arise from mid dorsal esophagus.

PRIMARY MALIGNANT MELANOMA

These are very rare tumors of the esophagus which arise from malignant degeneration of the pre-existing melanocytes in the esophageal mucosa.

Imaging Features

On barium studies, primary malignant melanoma of the esophagus appear as polypoid intraluminal masses which expand the esophagus without causing significant obstruction. CT scan appearance is of a large intraluminal mass, surrounded by a rim of intraluminal air or contrast. They are not usually associated with lymphadenopathy.

SMALL CELL CARCINOMA

Small cell carcinoma is the most common histologic subtype of neuroendocrine carcinoma. It is a rare but aggressive malignant tumor of the esophagus which metastasizes early and resembles its counterpart in the lung.[27] The tumor usually expands the lumen of the esophagus.

Imaging Features

On contrast swallow it appears as a smoothly marginated, polypoid or fungating mass with ulceration. On CT, it shows irregular eccentric esophageal wall thickening and extensive lymph node metastasis to the mediastinum, supraclavicular region and abdomen. As spindle cell carcinoma is associated with extensive and distant metastasis, CT examination should include both the thorax and the abdomen.

STAGING OF ESOPHAGEAL CANCER

Staging of esophageal cancer is by the TNM classification which has been proposed by the American Joint Committee on Cancer (AJCC) has been revised in 2009 **(Table 4)**. It is the most widely accepted staging system for esophageal cancer and applies to all histologic types of carcinomas regardless of the pathologic type and longitudinal extent of tumor.

Accurate preoperative staging of esophageal cancer is difficult due to its proximity to other structures (aorta, trachea, left bronchus). The malignant nodes are also usually not enlarged and may arise some distance away from the tumor. Also, at time of diagnosis, unsuspected metastases may be present in 30% of cases. Hence, a number of different imaging modalities may be required for accurate staging such as endoscopy, CT, EUS and PET-CT. The multidisciplinary approach is crucial for planning appropriate treatment in patients of esophageal cancer.[32]

TABLE 4: Seventh edition (2009) of TNM staging system for esophageal cancer.

Category	TNM Staging
Tumor	Tis: High-grade dysplasia T1: Invasion of lamina propria, muscularis mucosae, or submucosa T2: Invasion of muscularis propria T3: Invasion of adventitia T4: Invasion of adjacent structures T4a: Resectable (pleura, pericardium, or diaphragm) T4b: Unresectable (aorta, vertebral body, or trachea)
Node	N0: Absent N1: 1–2 regional LNs N2: 3–6 regional LNs N3: ≥7 regional LNs
Metastasis	M0: Absent M1: Present

Initial diagnosis is usually with endoscopy as histological confirmation with biopsy is possible. A good quality double contrast swallow study can detect even early tumors. On a contrast swallow, if the appearance is of a symmetrical smooth narrowing, with gradual tapering to a normal caliber it is indicative of a benign stricture and malignancy can be ruled out safely. On the other hand, if a stricture shows ulceration, irregular mucosa, shouldering and shelf-like margins at fluoroscopy, it can be considered to be malignant at imaging.

Most of the patients undergo a CT scan at initial evaluation for staging. Even though CT is less sensitive than EUS and PET-CT, it is relatively specific for detecting locally advanced or metastatic disease. If these findings are picked up on CT, patient need not undergo further investigation for staging.

The introduction of the seventh edition of the TNM classification in 2009 has resulted in number of changes in the staging of esophageal cancer.[32] The changes which have been incorporated are:

- Tumors of the gastroesophageal junction (GEJ) have been reclassified as lower esophageal tumors if their epicenter is within 5 cm of the GEJ and they extend to involve the esophagus.
- T4 disease has been subdivided into resectable (T4a) and nonresectable (T4b) disease.
- Positive nodal disease has been subdivided into N1, N2 and N3 where N1 is 1–2 regional LN's, N2 is 3–6 regional LN's and N3 is ≥7 regional lymph nodes **(Fig. 28)**.

The spread of esophageal cancer to nodes occurs because of the longitudinal nature of lymphatic drainage. Hence, the revised manual defines regional lymph nodes which includes any paraesophageal lymph node from the cervical nodes to the coeliac nodes.

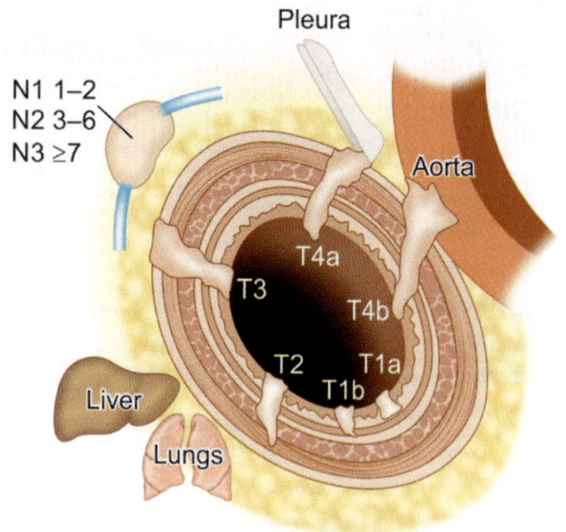

FIG. 28: Drawing illustrating the revised TNM staging system for esophageal cancer (seventh edition).

- Cervical or coeliac axis lymph node involvement are not classified as metastasis (i.e. M1a or M1b) any longer and have been reclassified in regional nodes.

Hence, the new N classification is similar to that used in staging of cancer stomach where N describes the number of cancer positive nodes.[33]

CT for Esophageal Cancer

Role of CT in local or T staging of esophageal malignancy is limited as it is not able to delineate the individual layers of the esophageal wall. Hence, CT is only used for distinguishing T1-T3 stage from T4 stage (i.e. invasion to other structures). Signs of T4 disease are:

- Tumor having an arc of contact of more than 90° with aorta;
- Loss of the triangular fat which is normally seen between the esophagus, aorta and vertebral column; and
- Nodular protrusion of the tumor into the airways.

CT and MR both detect macroscopic periesophageal fat invasion by the tumor with accuracy ranging from 88% to 100%. However, microscopic invasion of the same is not discernible on cross-sectional imaging. Periesophageal fat invasion on CT appears as strand like areas of soft tissue attenuation in the periesophageal fat plane **(Figs. 29A to D)**. On MR imaging, it appears as focal loss of bright signal of fat with periesophageal invasion having ill-defined, irregular margins. Though periesophageal fat infiltration adversely effects prognosis, it is not a contraindication to en-bloc resection of the tumor.[14]

While assessing mediastinal involvement on CT or MRI, accurate assessment of the tracheobronchial tree and aorta (T4 disease) is important as their invasion is a contraindication to surgical resection. The features of tracheobronchial invasion are displacement or indentation of the posterior wall of the trachea or the bronchus by the tumor mass as well as evidence of direct extension of the tumor into the lumen of the airway **(Figs. 30A to D)**. The reported overall accuracy of tracheobronchial tree invasion which has been described ranges from 88% to 97%. It is important to remember that an absent intervening fat plane can also be seen in normal persons and does not always suggest tumor invasion.

Picus et al. in 1983 defined the criteria for aortic invasion on CT which has an accuracy of more than 90%. Aortic invasion is diagnosed when the area of contact between the esophageal cancer and aorta is an arc of more than 90°. When area of contact is less than 45°; aortic invasion is considered to be absent while an area of contact of 45°–90° is considered indeterminate.[34]

The presence of pleural, pericardial diaphragmatic or gastric invasion are not considered contraindications to surgery as the involved area can be removed with the tumor at the time of surgery.

CT is relatively insensitive in nodal staging of esophageal cancer as majority of the malignant nodes are not enlarged (i.e. appear less than 1 cm in short-axis diameter). Also, benign inflammatory nodes may be larger than the cut-off criteria nodes may not be detectable if inseparable from the primary tumor and it may not be possible to accurately measure the number of lymph node metastasis if they are matted. The periesophageal, subcarinal, left gastric and coeliac regions are the common sites of nodal involvement by an esophageal cancer. The supraclavicular and retroperitoneal abdominal lymph nodes are the most frequently involved nonregional lymph nodes, i.e. metastatic nodes. The liver, lungs, bones and adrenal glands are the sites for distant metastasis.

Endoscopic Ultrasound for Esophageal Cancer

Endoscopic ultrasound (EUS) is the modality of choice for assessing the depth of penetration of the primary tumor through the esophageal wall. It is superior to CT/MRI and PET-CT for locoregional or T-staging of the tumor as the individual layer from which the tumor arises is well-visualized. In advanced tumor, if the stricture is too tight the EUS probe may not be negotiable. This indicates that the stage to be almost T3 or T4. Hence, a combination of CT and EUS should usually be performed for initial staging of patients with esophageal cancer.

For nodal disease, EUS has a higher sensitivity than PET or CT, but a lower specificity. *For evaluation of metastatic disease, EUS* does not have whole body coverage, hence it is to be used along with cross-sectional imaging for identifying the same.

PET-CT for Esophageal Cancer

PET-CT is the technique of choice for identifying metastases to nonregional lymph nodes and other tissues such as liver and skeletal muscle. It should be considered in all patients prior to radical treatment as it has the ability to correctly upstage up to 20% of patients. Even though most esophageal carcinomas appear FDG avid at PET-CT, the investigation has some limitations.[33]

- PET-CT has reduced spatial and contrast resolution which limits the entire anatomic extent of the primary mass to be evaluated.
- Not possible to assess the depth of local tumor invasion in most cases.

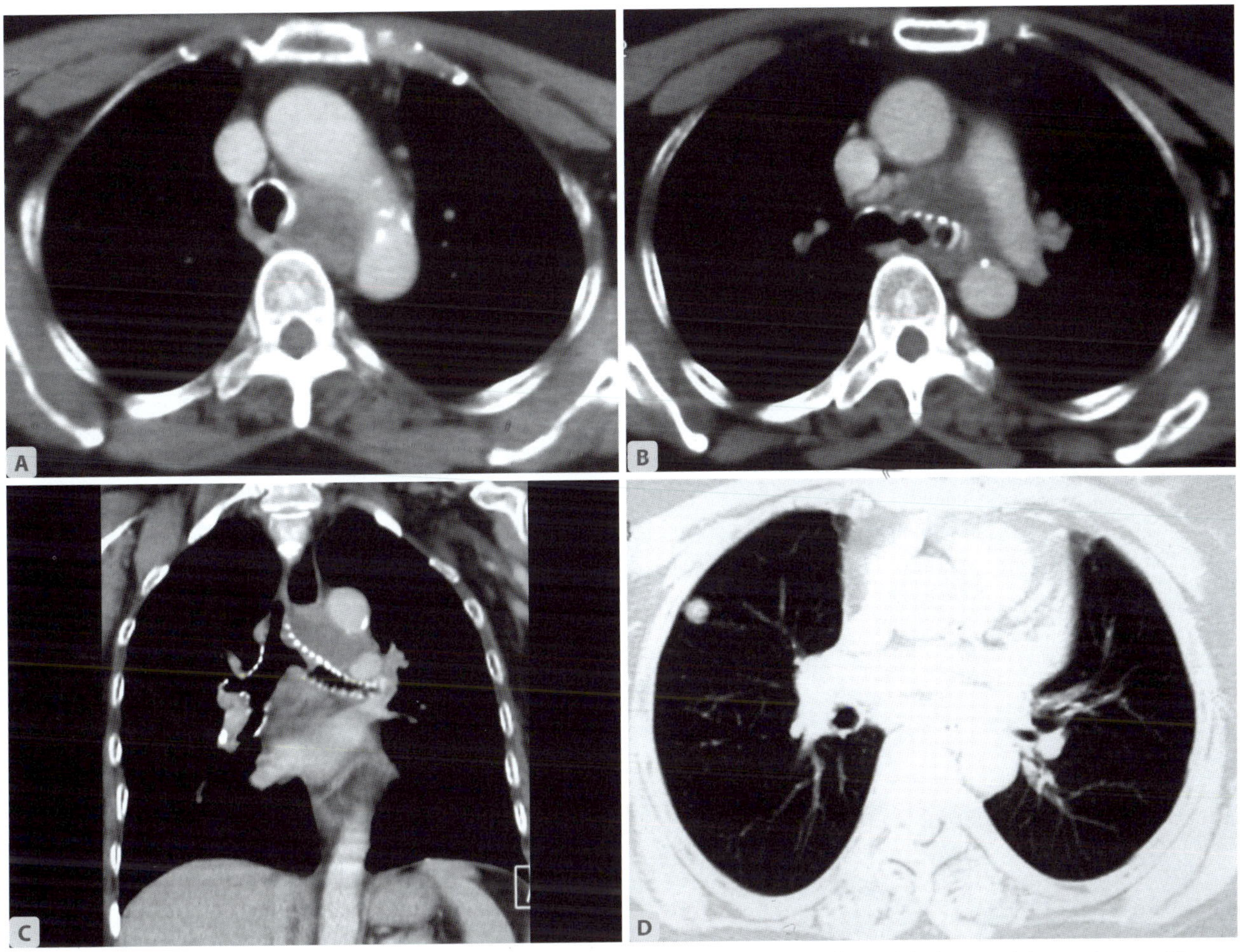

FIGS. 29A TO D: Contrast-enhanced CT chest in axial (A and B) and coronal planes reveals circumferential thickening of the esophagus with complete narrowing of its lumen with proximal dilatation at the level of carina (C). It is closely abutting the adjacent carinal wall, left pulmonary artery and descending aorta. (D) CT chest depicts a well-defined nodular opacity in the right upper lobe suggestive of a metastatic nodule. Carcinoma Esophagus—Stage IV.

- May not be possible to detect early stage carcinoma on PET-CT.
- It has limited role in assessing spread to locoregional lymph node.

However, for T or local staging, PET is not the investigation of choice. If a tumor is not detected on PET-CT, it is likely to be T2 or less in 70% of cases.[32]

In the Seventh edition of the TNM staging system, the biologic activity of the tumor, i.e. histologic grade, is a new cancer characteristic that has been introduced where it is categorized as G1 (well differentiated), G2 (moderately differentiated) and G3 (poorly differentiated). While the stage groupings in the Sixth edition were according to the anatomic T, N, and M classification only, the new stage groupings in the Seventh edition have been made according to the anatomic T, N, and M classification as well as nonanatomic cancer characteristics such as histopathologic cell type (SCC or adenocarcinoma), histologic grade (G1, G2 or G3) and cancer location (cervical, upper, mid or lower thoracic esophagus). These stage groupings have been introduced as they have been found to be consistent with data driven analysis and correspond to risk adjusted curves.[33] **Tables 5 and 6** give the stage groupings for esophageal adenocarcinoma and squamous cell carcinoma respectively.

Treatment

A primary tumor that is T1 or T2, i.e. confined to the esophageal wall is potentially curable by esophagectomy. However, most of the patients present with locally advanced disease and 20–30% have distant metastasis at the time of presentation. Those with periesophageal involvement (T3 stage) are treated with combined therapy in the form of neoadjuvant chemotherapy and radiotherapy followed by esophagectomy. T4 tumors are treated with definitive chemoradiotherapy, while patients with distant metastasis undergo palliative therapy.

EXTRINSIC NARROWING

Foreign Bodies

Foreign body ingestion is most commonly seen in children, those with psychiatric disorders, prisoners. In children, coins

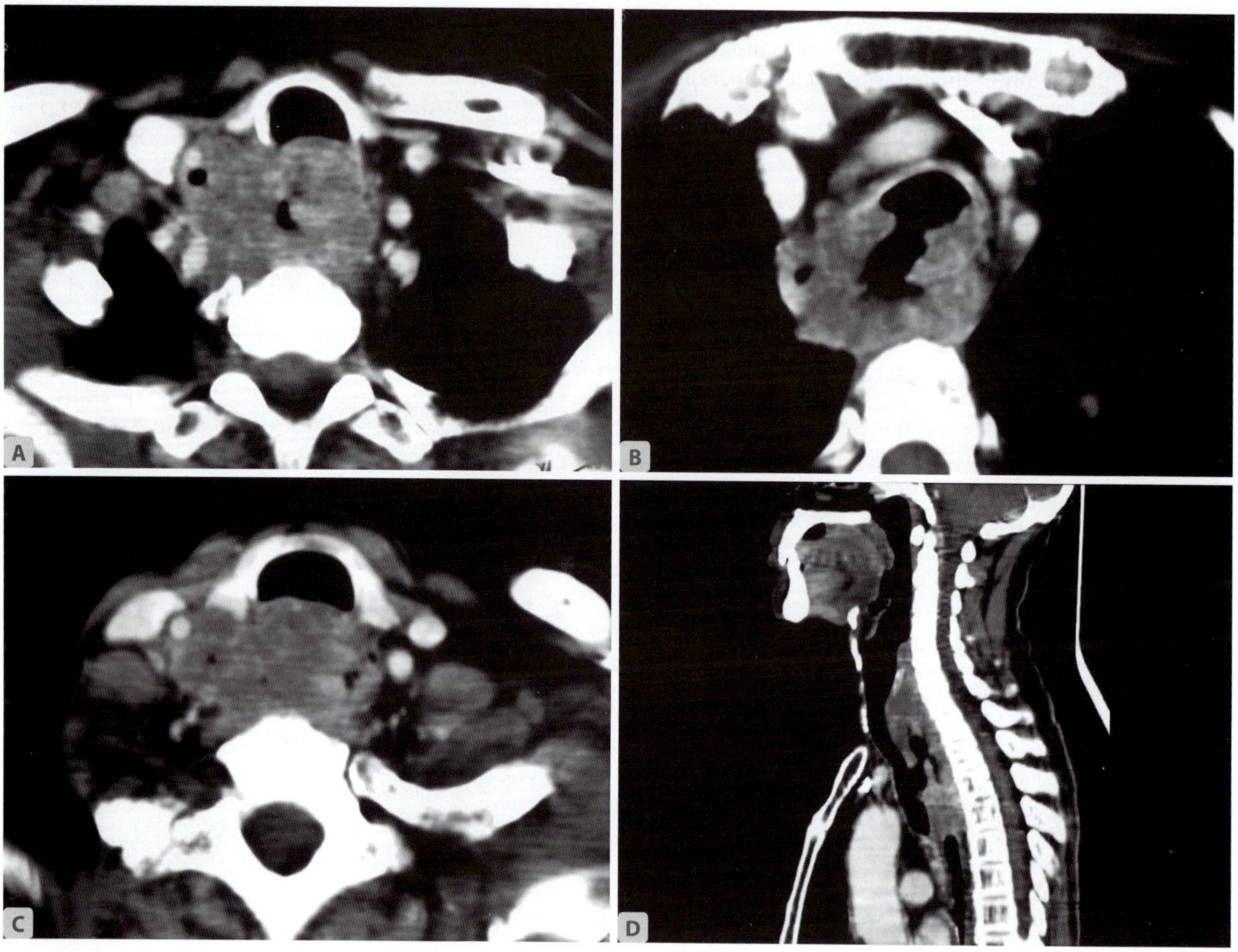

FIGS. 30A TO D: Axial (A to C) and sagittal (D) CECT reveals long segment asymmetric mass like mural thickening (~ 2.2 cm) of cervical, upper and mid thoracic esophagus (C6–D5 level) with infiltration and fistulous communication with posterior wall of trachea (B and D). There is partial encasement with loss of fat planes with right subclavian and proximal common carotid arteries (A and C): Squamous cell carcinoma (SCC) with tracheo-esophageal fistula.

TABLE 5: Stage groupings for adenocarcinoma.

	Stage				
	N0				
TM Category	**Grade 1-G2**	**G3**	**N1**	**N2**	**N3**
T1M0	IA	IB	IIB	IIIA	IIIC
T2M0	IB	IIA	IIB	IIIA	IIIC
T3M0	IIB	IIB	IIIA	IIIB	IIIC
T4M0			IIIC	IIIC	IIIC
T4a	IIIA	IIIA			
T4b	IIIC	IIIC			
Any T, M1	IV	IV	IV	IV	IV

(G: histologic grade).

are the most frequently ingested foreign bodies. Bones from fish and chicken are the second most common foreign body in both children and adults. Most frequently they get lodged in the hypopharynx or cervical esophagus and may be difficult to visualize endoscopically. Patients with history of foreign body

TABLE 6: Stage groupings for squamous cell carcinoma.

	Stage				
	N0				
TM Category	**G1**	**G2-G3**	**N1**	**N2**	**N3**
T1M0	IA	IB	IIB	IIIA	IIIC
T2M0			IIB	IIIA	IIIC
LE	IB	IA			
UME	IIA	IIB			
T3M0			IIIA	IIIB	IIIC
LE	IB	IIA			
UME	IIA	IIB			
T4M0			IIIC	IIIC	IIIC
T4a	IIIA	IIIA			
T4b	IIIC	IIIC			
Any T, M1	IV	IV	IV	IV	IV

(G: histologic grade; LE: lower esophagus; UME: upper and middle esophagus).

ingestion and impaction may present with symptoms such as dysphagia, odynophagia, foreign body sensation or food refusal. They are initially evaluated with plain radiographs of the neck, chest and abdomen. Barium studies are generally discouraged as they may hinder with attempts at endoscopic examination and retrieval later on. CT may be useful in select cases for definitive diagnosis or localization, prior to endoscopy or when perforation or another complication is suspected **(Figs. 31A to E)**.

Smooth foreign bodies, such as coins, buttons, dental crowns generally pass through the esophagus but may lodge in areas of normal anatomic narrowing at the thoracic inlet, aortic arch, or diaphragmatic hiatus. Sharp objects may arrest at any esophageal level. Metallic or dense foreign bodies are recognized on plain films of the neck or chest. Flat objects such as coins are oriented in the coronal plane of the esophagus in contrast to the sagittal plane orientation in the trachea. Obstructing foreign bodies may cause a gas-fluid level in the esophagus or tracheal displacement. Water-soluble contrast is indicated for the initial swallow to exclude perforation. Barium may be used for subsequent swallows. Cotton balls or marshmallows soaked in barium may be useful to demonstrate a small, hard-to detect foreign body. 80% of foreign bodies pass through the gastrointestinal tract spontaneously. If the diameter of the foreign body is too large to pass through the areas of esophageal narrowing, it lodges frequently at one of the three abovementioned areas of esophageal narrowing. Endoscopic removal of the obstructing foreign body may be required in such cases.

On plain frontal radiographs, coins can be differentiated from button batteries by their radiographic densities. While coins show homogeneous radiodensity, the ingested battery shows a central area of decreased density with a rim of increased density.[36]

A simple coin can be allowed to pass through the esophagus without worrying for any corrosive esophageal injury. However, button batteries need to be removed immediately by endoscopy, so as to prevent substantial damage to the esophagus. Due to its electrochemical properties, they can cause local cell death and mucosal necrosis. Complications secondary to ingestion of a button battery may range from local erosion to esophageal perforation to tracheoesophageal fistula. Fatal aortoesophageal fistulas have also been reported.

One must remember that proper history of the patient is very important as chronic impaction of a foreign body in the esophagus may produce features of erosion, fistula formation

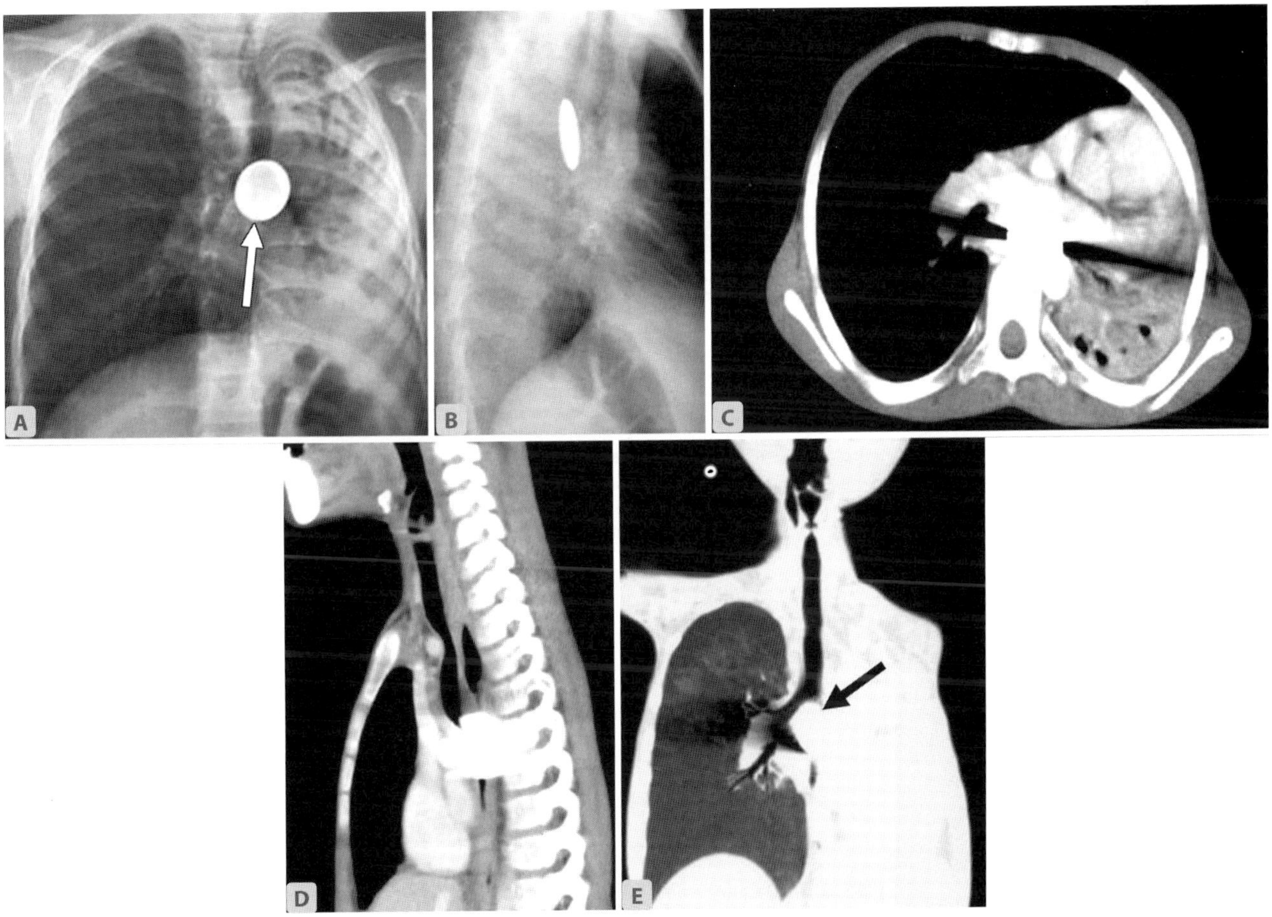

FIGS. 31A TO E: Impacted esophageal foreign body compressing airway: Frontal (A) and lateral (B) radiographs of chest reveal a well defined round radiopaque foreign body in the esophagus at the level of carina in the coronal plane on frontal X-ray (arrow in A) with associated volume loss of left lung. Contrast-enhanced axial (C) and sagittal MPR (D) images show a hyperdense foreign body giving streak artefacts impacted within the esophagus. (E) Coronal minimum intensity projection (MinIP) image shows near complete occlusion of left main bronchus (arrow) by the impacted esophageal foreign body with collapse of left lung.

and inflammatory reaction which may be similar to findings produced by a malignant process.[37]

Vascular Ring

Vascular ring is an aortic arch anomaly in which the trachea and esophagus are surrounded by vascular structures. The most common aortic arch anomaly is the left aortic arch with an aberrant right subclavian artery which occurs in 1 in 200 individuals.[38] The aberrant right subclavian artery arises from the diverticulum of Kommerell which is a persistence of the embryologic right aortic arch. In most cases, the aberrant right subclavian artery crosses posterior to the esophagus **(Figs. 32A to C)**. Patients are symptomatic at extremes of age with children usually presenting with tracheal obstruction or dysphagia. While in adults, aneurysms of aberrant subclavian artery or a prominent diverticulum of Kommerell can occur resulting in dysphagia, classically known as 'dysphagia Lusoria'.[36]

Enlarged Thyroid Gland

Mass effect due to enlarged thyroid gland is most often seen at the level of cervical esophagus. When the enlarged thyroid extends into the superior mediastinum it can result in a mass effect on the upper thoracic esophagus at esophagography. High resolution ultrasonography of the neck can confirm thyroid disease and CT neck apart from confirming helps in determining its extent **(Figs. 33A to C)**.

Enlarged Cervical Osteophytes

Cervical osteophytes are seen in around 20–30% of the elderly who may have neck stiffness and localized or radiating pain. However, large osteophytes have been known to cause dysphagia, odynophagia and globus symptoms. Dysphagia has also been found in patients of diffuse skeletal hyperostosis. The large osteophytes may impinge and mechanically compress the pharynx or upper esophagus causing obstruction **(Fig. 34)**. Another factor that can lead to dysphagia is the impaired tilting of the epiglottis over the laryngeal inlet by the mid cervical (C3-C4) osteophytes.

Retention of food and aspiration has been more often seen in patients with increased osteophytic size (>10 mm) that impinge on the pharynx than those without enlarged osteophytes.[39]

Cervical osteophyte-induced dysphagia is treated depending on the nature and severity of the disease. Sedation, anti-inflammatory drugs, muscle relaxants and appropriate

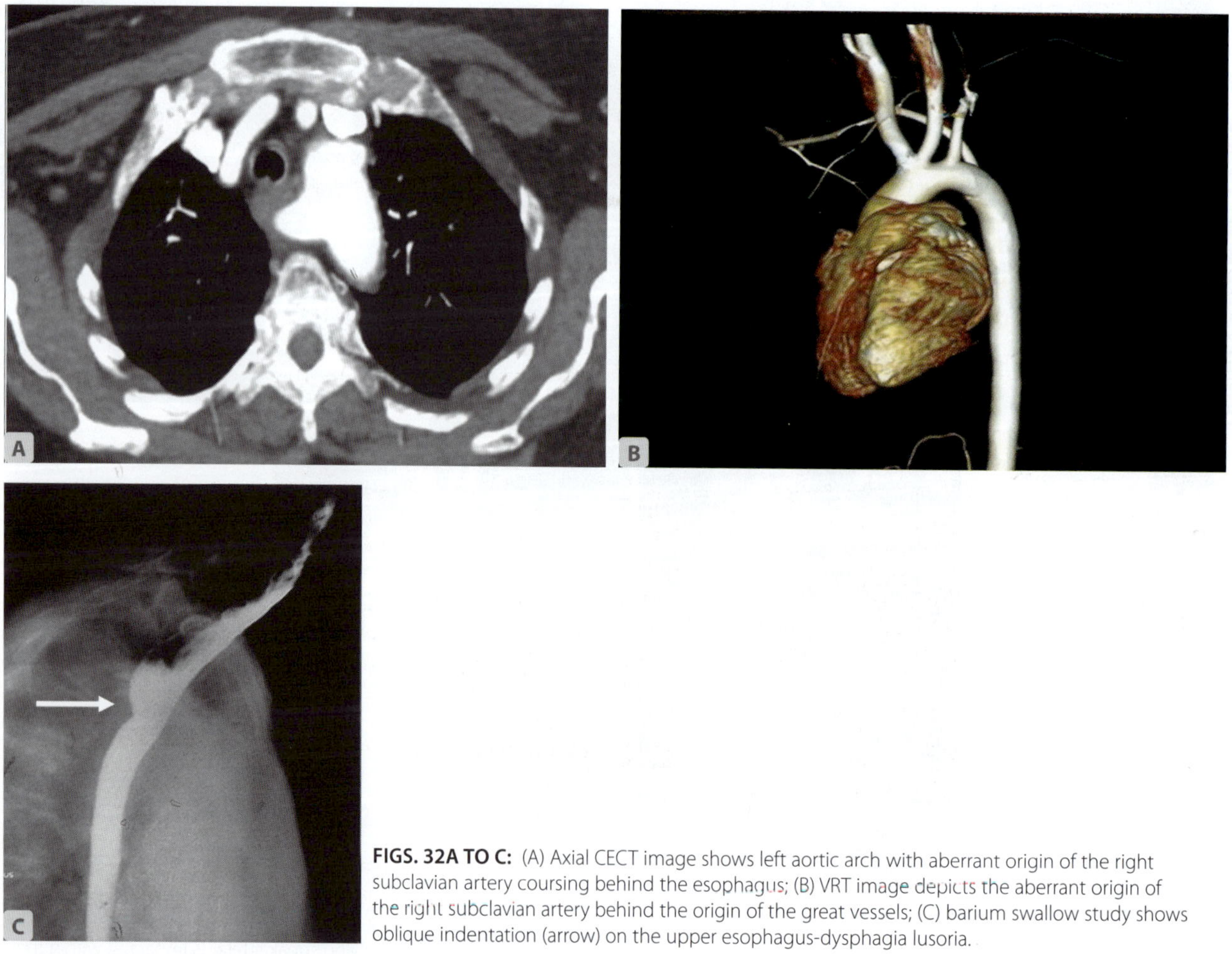

FIGS. 32A TO C: (A) Axial CECT image shows left aortic arch with aberrant origin of the right subclavian artery coursing behind the esophagus; (B) VRT image depicts the aberrant origin of the right subclavian artery behind the origin of the great vessels; (C) barium swallow study shows oblique indentation (arrow) on the upper esophagus-dysphagia lusoria.

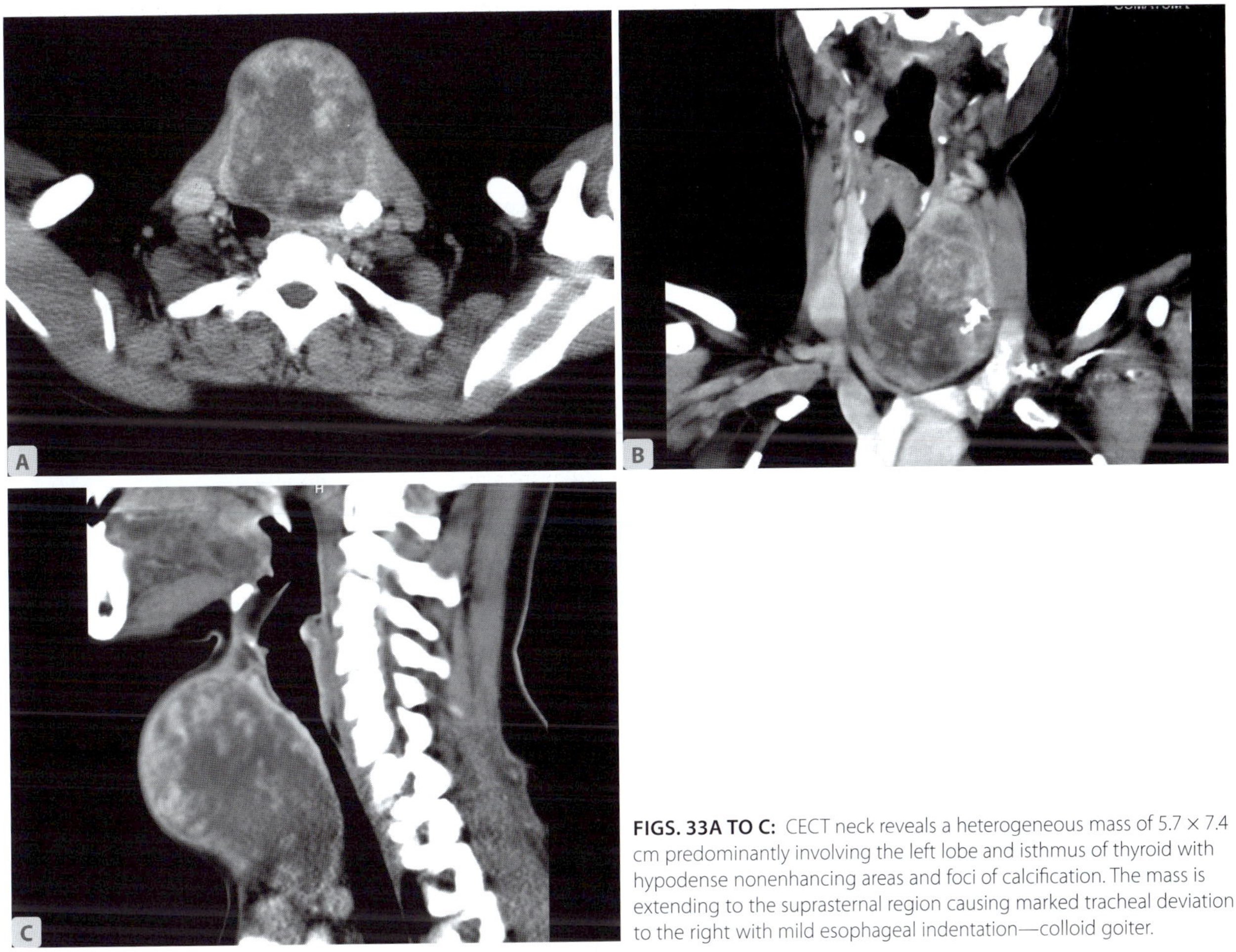

FIGS. 33A TO C: CECT neck reveals a heterogeneous mass of 5.7 × 7.4 cm predominantly involving the left lobe and isthmus of thyroid with hypodense nonenhancing areas and foci of calcification. The mass is extending to the suprasternal region causing marked tracheal deviation to the right with mild esophageal indentation—colloid goiter.

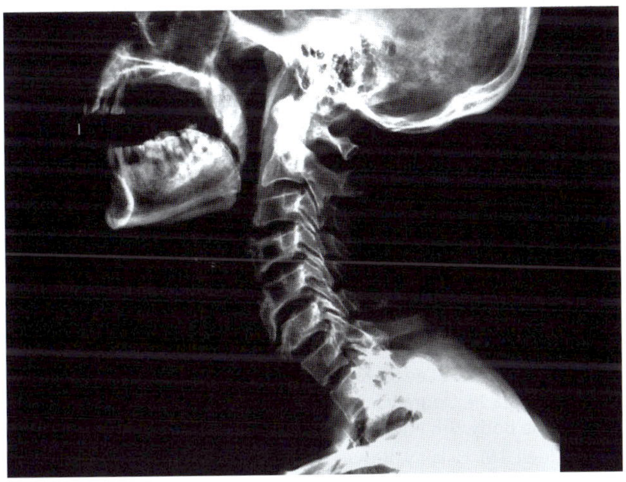

FIG. 34: X-ray lateral view cervical spine reveals enlarged osteophytes of C5, C6 vertebrae impinging on the esophagus.

soft diet are known to provide substantial relief. Surgical excision of large osteophytosis is reserved for patients with severe symptoms or those whose conservative treatment fails.

CONCLUSION

Dysphagia is a common problem and is generally due to an obstruction which may be either mechanical or functional. Patient demographics and symptomatology have an important role in determining the likely cause (i.e. oropharyngeal or esophageal) in around 85% of patients which helps in guiding subsequent investigation and management **(Flowchart 1)**. Knowledge of the radiological evaluation and imaging spectrum of the possible causes of dysphagia is essential for treatment planning.

FLOWCHART 1: Algorithmic approach to a patient with dysphagia.

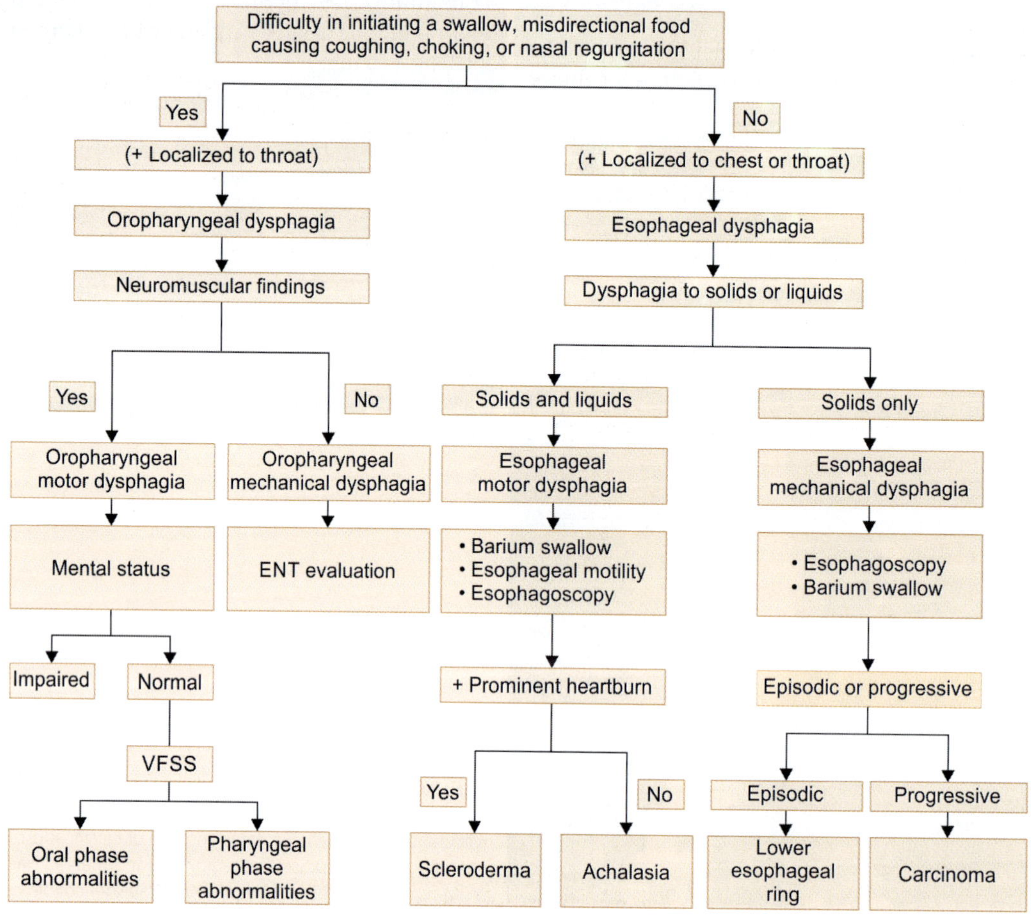

(VFSS: videofluoroscopic swallowing study; ENT: ear, nose and throat).

REFERENCES

1. Carucci LR, Turner MA. Dysphagia revisited: Common and Unusual causes. Radiographics. 2015;35:105-22.
2. Dodds WJ, Stewart ET, Logemann JA. Physiology and radiology of the normal oral and pharyngeal phases of swallowing. AJR. 1990;154:953-63.
3. Jaffer NM, Ng E, Au FW, Steele CM. Fluoroscopic evaluation of oropharyngeal dysphagia: anatomic, technical, and common etiologic factors. AJR. 2015;204:49-58.
4. Goyal RK. Alteration in gastrointestinal function. Dysphagia. In: Fanci AS, Kasper DL, Longo DL, et al (Eds). Harrison's Principles of Internal Medicine, 17th edition. McGraw Hill (Medical); 2008. pp. 237-42.
5. Spieker MR. Evaluating dysphagia. Am Fam Physician. 2000;61(12):3639-48.
6. Kuo P, Holloway RH, Nguyen NQ. Current and future techniques in the evaluation of dysphagia. Journal of Gastroenterology and Hepatology. 2012;27:873-81.
7. Levine MS, Rubesin SE. Radiologic Investigation of dysphagia. AJR. 1990;154:1157-63.
8. Cook IJ. Oropharyngeal dysphagia. Gastroenterol Clin N Am. 2009;38:411-31.
9. DiSantis DJ. Gastrointestinal fluoroscopy: what are we still doing? AJR; 2008.pp.1480-2.
10. Tao TY, Menias CO, Herman TE, McAlister WH, Balfe DM. Easier to swallow: Pictorial review of structural findings of the pharynx at barium pharyngography. Radiographics. 2013;33:E189-E208.
11. Jones B, Donner MW. Examination of the patient with Dysphagia. Radiology. 1988;167:319-26.
12. Kahrilas PJ, Hirano I. Disease of the esophagus. In: longo DL, Kasper DL, Jameson JL, et al (Eds). Harrison's Principles of Internal Medicine, 18th edition. McGraw Hill. 2012;292: 2427-37.
13. Ba-Salamah A, Zacheri J, Noebauer–Huhmann IM, et al. Dedicated multi-detector CT of the esophagus Spectrum of diseases. Abdom Imaging; 2007. p. 26.
14. Ha, HK, Park SH, Lee SS, Kim AY. Gastrointestinal tract– Esophagus In: Hagga JR, Dogra VS, Forsting M, et al (Eds). CT and MRI of the Whole Body, 5th edition. Mosby (Elsevier); 2009:30(2):1213-371.
15. Riddell AM, Hillier J, Brown G, et al. Potential of surface-coil MRI for staging of esophageal cancer. AJR. 2006;187:1280-7.
16. Jang KM, Lee KS, Lee SJ, et al. The spectrum of benign esophageal lesions: imaging findings. Korean J Radiol. 2002;3:199-210.
17. Eisenberg RL, Esophagus (Section-1). In: Eisenberg RL (Ed). Gastrointestinal Radiology. A Pattern Approach, 4th edition. Lippincolt Williams & Wilkins; 2003. pp. 3-150.
18. Rabushka LS, Fishman EK, Kuhlman JE. CT evaluation of achalasia. J Comput Assist Tomogr. 1991;15(3):434-9.

19. Pawa S, Prakash A. Imaging of the esophagus. In: Gupta AK, Chowdhury V, Khandelwal (Eds). AIIMS–MAMC–PGI's Comprehensive Textbook of Diagnostic Radiology. 1st edition. The Health Sciences Publisher (Jaypee); 2016;70(2):1139-57.
20. Leslie P, Carding PN, Wilson JA. Investigation and management of chronic dysphagia. BMJ. 2003;326:453-6.
21. Luedtke P, Levine MS, Rubesin SE, Weinstein DS, Larfer I. Radiologic diagnosis of benign esophageal strictures: a pattern approach. Radiographics. 2003;23(4):897-909.
22. Sam JW, Levine MS, Rubesin SE, Laufer I. The "foamy" esophagus: A radiographic sign of Candida esophagitis. AJR. 2000;174:999-1002.
23. Berkovich GY, Levine MS, Miller WT. CT findings in patients with esophagitis. Am J Roentgenol. 2000;175(5):1431-4.
24. Rosario MT, Raso CL, Comer GM. Esophageal tuberculosis. Dig Dis Sci. 1989;34:1281-4.
25. Nagi B, Lal A, Kochhar R, et al. Imaging of esophageal tuberculosis. Acta Radiologica. 2003;44:329-33.
26. White SB, Levine MS, Rubesin SE, Spencer GS, Katzka DA, Laufer I. The small-caliber esophagus: radiographic sign of idiopathic eosinophilic esophagitis. Radiology. 2010;256:127-34.
27. Lewis RB, Mehrotra AK, Rodriguez P, Levine MS. From the radiologic pathology archives: Esophageal neoplasms: radiologic-pathologic correlation. Radiographics. 2013;33:1083-108.
28. Winant AJ, Gollub MJ, Shia J, Antonescu C, Bains MS, Levine MS. Imaging and clinicopathologic features of esophageal gastrointestinal stromal tumors. AJR. 2014;203:306-14.
29. Levine MS, Buck JL, Pantongrag-Brown L, Buetow PC, Hallman JR, Sobin LH. Fibrovascular polyps of the esophagus: clinical, radiographic, and pathologic findings in 16 patients. AJR. 1996;166:781-7.
30. Umeoka S, Koyama T, Togashi K, Saga T, Watanabe G, Shimada Y, Imamura M. Esophageal Cancer: Evaluation with triple-phase dynamic CT-initial experience. Radiology. 2006;239(3): 777-83.
31. Levine MS. Esophageal cancer radiologic diagnosis. In: Gore RM (Ed.). The Radiologic Clinics of North America. 1997;35: 265-94.
32. Godfrey EM, Freeman AH. The esophagus. In: Adam A, Dixon AK, Gillard JH, Schaefer-Prokop CM (Eds.). Grainger and Allison's Diagnostic Radiology (A textbook of Medical Imaging), 6th edition. 2015;26(1):610-26.
33. Hong SJ, Kim TJ, Nam KB, et al. New TNM staging system for esophageal cancer: What chest radiologists need to know. Radiographics. 2014;34:1722-40.
34. Picus D, Balfe DM, Koehler RE, et al. Computed tomography in the staging of esophageal carcinoma. Radiology. 1983;146:433-8.
35. Bruzzi JF, Munden RF, Truong MT, et al. PET/CT of esophageal cancer: its role in clinical management. Radiographics. 2007;27:1635-52.
36. Hryhorczuk AL, Lee EY, Eisenberg RL. Esophageal abnormalities in pediatric patients. AJR. 2013;201:W519-32.
37. Young CA, Menias CO, Bhalla S, Prasad SR. CT features of esophageal emergencies. Radiographics. 2008;28(6):1541-53.
38. Gilkeson RC, Kolodny S. Thoracic Aorta in Hagga JR, Dogra VS, Forsting M, et al. (Eds). CT and MRI of the Whole Body, 5th edition. Mosby (Elsevier). 2009;1:1091-132.
39. Strasser G, Schima W, Schober E, et al. Cervical osteophytes impinging on the pharynx: importance of size and concurrent disorders for development of aspiration. AJR. 2000;174: 449-53.

CHAPTER

93

Tumors of Stomach and Duodenum

Gaurav Shanker Pradhan, Rashmi Dixit, Jyoti Kumar, Virendra Jain

INTRODUCTION

Stomach and duodenum can be involved by a wide variety of benign as well as malignant tumors. Benign tumors of the stomach and duodenum, though of more infrequent occurrence than malignant tumors, are sufficiently common to warrant attention.

Benign tumors of the stomach and duodenum are uncommon, with an incidence of 0.4% in autopsy series and 3–5% in upper endoscopic series, most of them performed for unrelated reasons. Over the recent years, the incidence of these lesions is rising due to a higher level of suspicion exhibited by clinicians, and the availability and wide application of diagnostic tools, such as gastrointestinal endoscopy. Most patients with benign stomach and duodenal tumors remain asymptomatic for long periods of time. Symptoms may be vague like abdominal pain or may manifest on account of large size of tumor, obstruction and bleeding. Patients with tumors at specific sites like at GE junction, ampulla of vater may present with dysphagia and jaundice respectively. Some benign polyps can have malignant potential while others may co-exist with a malignant lesion. So, proper evaluation, periodic surveillance and timely treatment hold the key to correct management.

Malignant tumors of the stomach and duodenum include adenocarcinoma, lymphoma, carcinoids and gastrointestinal stromal tumors. Most common among these are carcinoma of the stomach and lymphoma, other tumors are comparatively uncommon. Stomach and duodenum can also be secondarily involved by other malignancies, either by contiguous extension from tumors of the adjacent organs or by hematogenous dissemination. They often produce no specific symptoms when they are superficial and potentially surgically curable, although up to 50% of patients may have nonspecific gastrointestinal complaints such as dyspepsia. The lack of early pathognomic symptoms often delays the diagnosis. Consequently, 80–90% of patients present with locally advanced or metastatic tumors that have poor rates of resectability. High index of clinical suspicion especially in patients with risk factors for gastric malignancy, requires thorough evaluation and due surveillance, so as to pick up the disease at a very early stage.

Endoscopy is the modality of choice for evaluation of upper gastrointestinal tract, not just because mucosal detail is well appreciated but also because simultaneous biopsy of suspicious lesions can be performed. Amongst imaging modalities, barium meal upper gastrointestinal examination remains unsurpassed in the depiction of mucosal detail compared to other imaging modalities such as multislice computed tomography, virtual gastroscopy. This aided by fluoroscopic evaluation of peristaltic activity greatly improves diagnostic accuracy. On the other hand, cross-sectional modalities like CT and MRI are superior to barium examinations in depiction of wall of the viscera as well as extraluminal disease. FDG-PET scanning is useful in the staging and postoperative assessment of various malignancies.

GASTRIC POLYPS

Gastric polyps are classified histologically into three types:

- Epithelial polyps
- Hamartomatous polyps
- Mesenchymal polyps.

Epithelial Polyps

These are the most common type of gastric polyps and they are further divided in three types mainly—*fundic gland polyps (FGPs), hyperplastic polyps, and adenomatous polyps.* The incidence has increased in recent years due to increased number of endoscopic examinations. The prevalence and the type of the polyps also depend on the risk factors in the population under consideration. Hyperplastic and adenomatous polyps are encountered more often in an *H. pylori*-infected territory while fundic gland polyps are seen with increased proton pump inhibitor (PPI) usage.[1] They are usually asymptomatic, however, large polyps often become pedunculated and may erode surface epithelium, which may result in chronic blood loss and iron-deficiency anemia. Rarely they present with gastric outlet obstruction due to prolapsed large polyp into antropyloric region. The clinical importance of these polyps is because of the variable malignant potential and their co-occurrence with other risk factors for gastric malignancy. For these reasons polyps need to be biopsied or resected wherever possible, along with multiple biopsies from surrounding flat gastric mucosa.[2]

On barium images, these lesions are seen as ring shadow enface and small surface nodules forming acute angle on in profile view with the gastric wall. On CT they appear as single or multiple small uniform masses which shows enhancement on contrast enhanced images.

Fundic Gland Polyps

Fundic gland polyps (FGPs) are one of the most common polyps found in the stomach seen on upper GI endoscopy.[3] Sporadic FGPs are sessile polyps and are distributed exclusively in the body and fundus[4] of the stomach with the lesions varying from 1 mm to 8 mm in size, most commonly noted in middle-aged women.[5] Hypergastrinemia associated with a gastrinoma, Zollinger-Ellison syndrome, or long-term therapy with PPIs has been shown to be associated with fundic gland polyps. Few studies also conclude that sporadic FGPs are not associated with atrophic gastritis and have low prevalence of *Helicobacter pylori* infection.[6]

About 30–100% of patients with FAP have been reported to have gastric polyps.[4] Majority (95%) are FGPs while only remaining 5% are actually adenomatous polyps and arise from a mutation in the *APC* gene.[7]

Dysplasia is not common and usually of low grade. The risk factors for dysplasia include large polyp size, and presence of antral gastritis.[8] Polyps associated with PPI use have virtually no malignant potential.[1] As per current guidelines[4] polypectomy is not required for sporadic FGPs because of their low malignant potential. Biopsy is usually indicated at the initial endoscopy to rule out dysplasia or adenocarcinoma. FGPs >1 cm in size are resected assuming sampling error from forceps biopsy alone.[5]

Hyperplastic Polyps

These are the second most common gastric polyps after FGPs and typically occur in the sixth and seventh decades. These polyps are usually sessile or pedunculated, usually less than 2 cm.[4] The polyps are small and are usually multiple and are randomly distributed anywhere in the stomach, although antrum is the typical site.

These are the most common polyps and have a strong tendency to occur in the setting of inflammatory disorders such as chronic gastritis, *H. pylori* gastritis, pernicious anemia, gastric surgical site, bile reflux disease and chemical gastritis.[9,10] In most cases, in addition to polyp biopsy it is also advised to biopsy background flat mucosa to identify etiologic factors if any. 80% of the hyperplastic polyps have been seen to regress after treatment of *H. pylori* infection.[11] They appear as radiolucent filling defects if present on dependent posterior wall or as ring shadows with white rim of barium, if present on nondependent anterior wall. They are found most frequently in the antrum. They are usually smooth, dome-shaped, and measure between 0.5 cm and 1.5 cm in diameter, although they may be much larger. Large hyperplastic polyps often become pedunculated and may present with gastric outlet obstruction because the polyp may obstruct or prolapse through the pylorus.

Like FGPs, hyperplastic polyps also seem to have low neoplastic potential but they have a tendency to have synchronous cancers in the adjacent gastric mucosa especially if associated with chronic gastritis.[12]

Because of low risk of dysplasia and synchronous cancers there is confusion regarding the management of hyperplastic polyps. Recommendations of size criteria for polypectomy range from >2 cm as per few authors and >0.5 cm as per others.[13] Because of more risk of adenocarcinoma in the surrounding nonpolypoid flat tissue as compared to polyps per se, multiple biopsies from the flat uninvolved mucosa is recommended.[4]

Adenomatous Polyps

Adenomatous polyps are the precursor for gastric cancer and are divided into tubular, villous and tubulovillous distinctions histologically. These polyps are usually solitary and seen in the antrum, however can be seen anywhere in the stomach. They are commonly seen as sessile or flat lesions but the pedunculated form may be seen uncommonly. They are also seen in various polyposis syndromes like FAP, Gardner's syndrome,Turcot syndrome. These lesions are usually seen in relation to atrophic gastritis and in the background of intestinal metaplasia. *H. pylori* infection has not been seen associated with them. They vary in size from millimeters to centimeters[5] and larger size >2 cm and villous histology increases the risk of neoplasia (28–40%).[14]

They are premalignant with high-grade dysplastic changes and are currently redefined as noninvasive intraepithelial neoplasia (NiN).[15] It is hence recommended to remove the adenoma with further examination of entire gastric mucosa and biopsy if necessary.

Hamartomatous Polyps

These are mucosal polyps which can arise from any of the 3 embryonic layers and are composed of disorganized tissue in situ. These polyps are seen sporadically, though occasionally they occur as part of a syndrome such as Peutz-Jeghers syndrome, juvenile polyposis, etc. Although hamartomatous means non-neoplastic, they can coexist with adenomatous polyps.[16]

Peutz-Jeghers syndrome is an autosomal dominant hereditary disorder which characteristically has multiple hamartomatous polyps along the entire gastrointestinal system and mucocutaneous hyperpigmentation at the lips.[17] Gastric polyps are seen in 15–30% of the cases. Gastric syndromic polyps are however often indistinguishable from nonspecific gastric hyperplastic polyps and hence endoscopic, pathologic and clinical correlation is required for proper diagnosis.

Juvenile polyps and juvenile polyposis syndrome: These are mucosal tumors that consist of excess lamina propria and dilated cystic glands and hence are occasionally called inflammatory polyps or retention cysts due to these distended glands, inflammatory cells and edema.

These lesions are typically solitary pedunculated polyps and range from 3 mm to 20 mm in size. However, when multiple, a syndrome of juvenile polyposis should be considered.

The different subtypes are difficult to differentiate radiologically. These polyps if small are well circumscribed with smooth, nodular surface if seen en face and are seen to form acute angle with the gastric wall when viewed in profile on barium studies. Larger polyps have a lobulated surface and areas of erosion or ulceration mimicking malignant growth.[18]

Mesenchymal Polyps

These are polyps which arise from mesenchymal tissue and are usually beneath the surface epithelium and hence impart a nodular rather than polypoidal appearance. These include inflammatory fibroid polyps, gastrointestinal stromal tumors, leiomyomas and will be discussed in the later section of the chapter.

MALIGNANT GASTRIC NEOPLASMS

Malignant tumors of stomach and duodenum include adenocarcinomas, lymphoma, gastrointestinal stromal tumors and carcinoid with the most common malignancy being adenocarcinomas comprising 90–95% of all malignant gastric tumors.[1] Gastric malignancy is the second most common malignancy after lung cancer, in the world with incidence in males being twice as common as compared to females. Carcinoma of stomach is significantly more prevalent in Eastern Asia (Japan, Korea, China) and hence most of the early diagnostic techniques and management plans have been developed in Japan. The disease is picked up late especially in western world due to lack of mass screening programmes and vague symptoms like loss of appetite, loss of weight and epigastric pain or discomfort.

GASTRIC ADENOCARCINOMAS

Peak age of incidence for gastric cancers is between 50 and 70 years. It is equally distributed in the antrum, body and the fundus-cardiac region of the stomach with only 10% being diffusely infiltrative. The incidence of more aggressive carcinomas around the gastroesophageal junction has increased over the last two decades.[19] Though a marked reduction has been observed in the incidence of gastric carcinoma in North America and Western Europe in the last 50 years, 5-year survival rates are less than 20%, as most patients present late and are unsuitable for curative, radical surgery. There is an increased recognition of the association with *Helicobacter pylori* infection believed to increase the risk by 3-6 fold.[20] Other associated risk factors include inherited genetic component, pernicious anemia, adenomas, atrophic gastritis, patients having "A" blood group and those who have undergone gastrectomy. A number of dietary factors like salted, smoked and pickled food and food rich in nitrates also predispose a person for gastric cancer.[21]

Screening methods with variable success rates like-endoscopy, *H. pylori* antibody and serum pepsinogen testing are used at various places.[22]

Pathophysiology

Gastric carcinomas are classified according to cell types with adenocarcinoma being most common. Gastric adenocarcinomas are divided into 2 types. Type 1 adenocarcinomas are intestinal tumors and have well-formed glandular structures. This form of gastric carcinoma is more likely to involve the distal stomach and occur in patients with atrophic gastritis. It has a strong environmental association. Type 2 adenocarcinoma is a diffuse type, though cardia is commonly involved. Gastric wall infiltration is more pronounced in this type and patients have worse prognosis than type 1 tumors.

EARLY GASTRIC CANCER

The need for early gastric cancer (EGC) to be recognized as a separate entity originated in Japan, as there is high prevalence of gastric malignancy in the region and early detection and definitive treatment hold the key to successful outcome. These lesions are confined to the mucosa or submucosa irrespective of the nodal metastasis[23] (T1, any N) and are classified into 3 types as per Japanese system (elevated, superficial, shallow):[24]

1. *Type I:* Elevated lesions in gastric wall, protruding more than 5 mm into the lumen
2. *Type II:* Superficial lesions that are elevated (IIa, <5 mm), flat (IIb), or depressed (IIc)
3. *Type III:* Excavated, irregular ulcers with nodular, clubbed mucosal folds.

Limited literature is available for role of double-contrast barium upper GI examination in early gastric cancers.[25,26] With the widespread use of endoscopy, multiple endoscopic biopsies of suspicious lesions are considered the diagnostic procedure of choice for early gastric cancer. Recent advances of CT like multiplanar reformatting (MPR), surface shaded display, virtual gastroscopy, and dynamic contrast imaging have significantly improved the detection rate of type 1 EGC. On CT EGC lesions are commonly seen as focal enhancing thickening of the inner layer with visible low-attenuation outer layer and maintained perigastric fat planes. However, lesions without thickening or enhancement are likely to be missed.[1]

ADVANCED GASTRIC CANCER

Advanced gastric cancer (AGC) is the most commonly diagnosed form of gastric cancer seen in western world, defined as involvement of muscularis propria and beyond. The gross morphology of advanced lesions on imaging can be either polypoid, infiltrative or ulcerative with considerable overlap among them. The polypoidal lesions can have acute angle with gastric wall suggesting epithelial nature of the lesion.[1] Advanced gastric cancers are usually larger than 3 cm and most symptomatic patients present in this stage. Borrmann classified the advanced gastric cancers morphologically into 4 types.[27] Type 1 are polypoidal lesions, Type 2 are ulcerative, Type 3 are ulceroinfiltrative and Type 4 infiltrating linitis plastica type lesions.

Staging of Gastric Cancer

Tumor, node and metastasis (TNM) staging by the AJCC/UICC is the most commonly used staging system for gastric cancer. Two modifications have been made in their 7th edition *Tumor Staging Manual*. Firstly tumors arising at the gastroesophageal junction or gastric tumors which are crossing it but arising in the stomach <5 cm from GE junction are staged using the TNM system for esophageal cancer. Secondly, the stomach T categories **(Tables 1 and 2)**[28] have been harmonized with the T categories of the rest of gastrointestinal tract.[29]

The T stage, representing the extent of penetration through the gastric wall, is categorized in the **Table 1**.

N Staging

In the TNM staging system, the N category is defined on the basis of number of metastatic lymph nodes involved. As opposed to TNM staging the anatomical nodal stations are used in the Japanese system (JCGC 13th edn).[1]

The N stage, representing the number and site of draining lymph nodes involved, is categorized as follows:

- NX–Regional lymph nodes cannot be evaluated
- N0–No lymph nodes involved
- N1–Metastases in 1–2 regional lymph nodes
- N2–Metastases in 3–6 regional lymph nodes
- N3–Metastases in >7 regional lymph nodes
- N3a–7–15 regional lymph nodes
- N3b–16 or more regional lymph nodes.

TABLE 1: T-category (Gastric cancer).

- TX primary tumor cannot be assessed
- T0 no evidence of primary tumor
- *Tis carcinoma in situ*: Intraepithelial tumor without invasion of the lamina propria
- T1 tumor invades lamina propria, muscularis mucosae or submucosa
- T1a tumor invades lamina propria or muscularis mucosae
- T1b tumor invades submucosa
- T2 tumor invades muscularis propria
- T3 tumor penetrates subserosal connective tissue without invasion of visceral peritoneum or adjacent structures. T3 tumors also include those extending into the gastrocolic or gastrohepatic ligaments, or into the greater or lesser omentum, without perforation of the visceral peritoneum covering these structures
- T4 tumor invades serosa (visceral peritoneum) or adjacent structures
- T4a tumor invades serosa (visceral peritoneum)
- T4b tumor invades adjacent structures such as spleen, transverse colon, liver, diaphragm, pancreas, abdominal wall, adrenal gland, kidney, small intestine and retroperitoneum

Lymph node involvement and their localization are of paramount importance in deciding the surgical management. Lymph node metastases occur in approximately 80% of patients with gastric cancer. The frequency is related to the size and depth of the tumor with local perigastric nodes being involved first, followed by the regional (celiac, hepatic, left gastric, splenic) and distant (left supraclavicular and axillary) nodes. A wide range of values for accuracy have been reported on CT/MRI which vary with the threshold values of the size, margin, architecture and enhancement pattern. It is recommended to report all visible lymph nodes regardless of their size and to leave it to the histopathology for accurate N staging.[1] CT depicts 75% of nodes larger than 5 mm in diameter, but it does not depict tumor in normal-sized nodes. CT is not useful in distinguishing between enlarged nodes due to reactive changes and those due to tumor. The local nodes (N1) are located in the prepyloric region and in the gastrocolic and gastrohepatic ligaments. These nodes are removed by performing the standard gastrectomy procedure. The regional nodes (N2), located in the porta hepatis, hepatoduodenal ligament and peripancreatic region, are not routinely removed during gastrectomy procedure. So their detection is more important.

Recently it has been suggested that EUS and MDCT are comparable for both T and N staging and considered complementary techniques for loco regional staging.[30,31]

M Staging

The M stage, representing the presence of metastases, is categorized as follows:

- M0—No distant metastases
- M1—Distant metastases.

As the portal vein drains the stomach, the liver is the most common site for hematogenous metastases. Less common sites are the lungs, adrenal glands and kidneys. Bony and cerebral metastases are uncommon.

Intraperitoneal and omental metastases are common in advanced gastric cancer. They consist of nodules, localized fluid collections, irregular thickening and stranding of the mesentery and omentum. Ascites and small-bowel obstruction may also occur.

TABLE 2: TNM staging of gastric cancer.[28]

Stage of gastric cancer	TNM grades
0	Tis, No, Mo
1A	T1, N0, M0
1B	T1, N1, M0, T2, N0, M0
2A	T1, N2, M0, T2, N1, M0, T3, N0, M0
2B	T1, N3, M0, T2, N2, M0, T3, N1, M0, T4a, N0, M0
3A	T2, N3, M0, T3, N2, M0, T4a, N1, M0
3B	T3, N3, M0, T4a, N2, M0, T4b, N0 or N1, M0
3C	T4a, N3, M0, T4b, N2 or N3, M0
4	Any T, any N, M1

Imaging Features of Advanced Gastric Cancer

Upper GI endoscopy is the preferred technique for detection of gastric cancer which is also useful in obtaining histological confirmation of suspicious gastric lesions. Many cancers are picked up at asymptomatic level by this technique. However, due to limitation of evaluation of gastric wall and locoregional spread its role is limited.

Barium UGI Features

Malignant gastric ulcer is the most common presentation of gastric cancer on upper GI barium studies, hence it is important to differentiate benign from malignant ulcers **(Figs. 1A to C)**. Malignant ulcers are usually nonprojecting, with ulcer brim being wide and thick with central ulceration (Carman-Kirklin meniscus sign), distorted irregular radiating folds stopping well short of ulcer brim.[7] As opposed to malignant ulcers, a typical benign ulcer shows projecting ulcer **(Fig. 2A)** with an ulcer collar or mound with symmetrical radiating folds reaching up to brim of the ulcer **(Fig. 2B)**. There is also undermining of gastric mucosa noted in benign ulcers which is seen as a filling defect/lucent line rimming the ulcer crater on double contrast barium meal (DCBM) known as Hampton's line (Pathognomonic) **(Fig. 2C)**. Barium meal fluoroscopic procedures help in differentiating benign and malignant lesions and in evaluating response to treatment. However, the ease of direct visualization and choice of guided biopsy makes endoscopy a routine procedure of choice.[32]

Polypoid carcinomas are lobulated masses that protrude into the lumen. They may contain one or more areas of ulceration **(Fig. 3A)**. With ulcerated carcinomas, an irregular crater is located in a rind of malignant tissue. On profile view, these lesions are seen to be intraluminal as opposed to benign projecting ulcers, and on enface view, nodular distorted mucosal folds are seen converging to the edge of the ulcer **(Fig. 3B)**.

Infiltrative cancers on the other hand can have non-scirrhous or scirrhous (desmoplastic) histology. Non-scirrhous lesions have stomach wall thickening as well as rugal fold thickening in the form of nodularity or spiculation of the mucosa **(Fig. 4A)**. On the contrary aggressive scirrhous lesions exhibit wall thickening with loss of mucosal folds. If diffuse, scirrhous lesions are called linitis plastica. They cause narrowing of the stomach with a rigid structure (leather bottle stomach) and are better appreciated on fluoroscopic imaging than endoscopy **(Fig. 4B)**.[18]

In the lesions of the cardia, as distal esophagus is often involved, submucosal spread of tumors may result in pseudoachalasia or secondary achalasia with tapered, beaklike narrowing of the distal esophagus along with infiltration of the gastric cardia **(Figs. 5A to C)**.

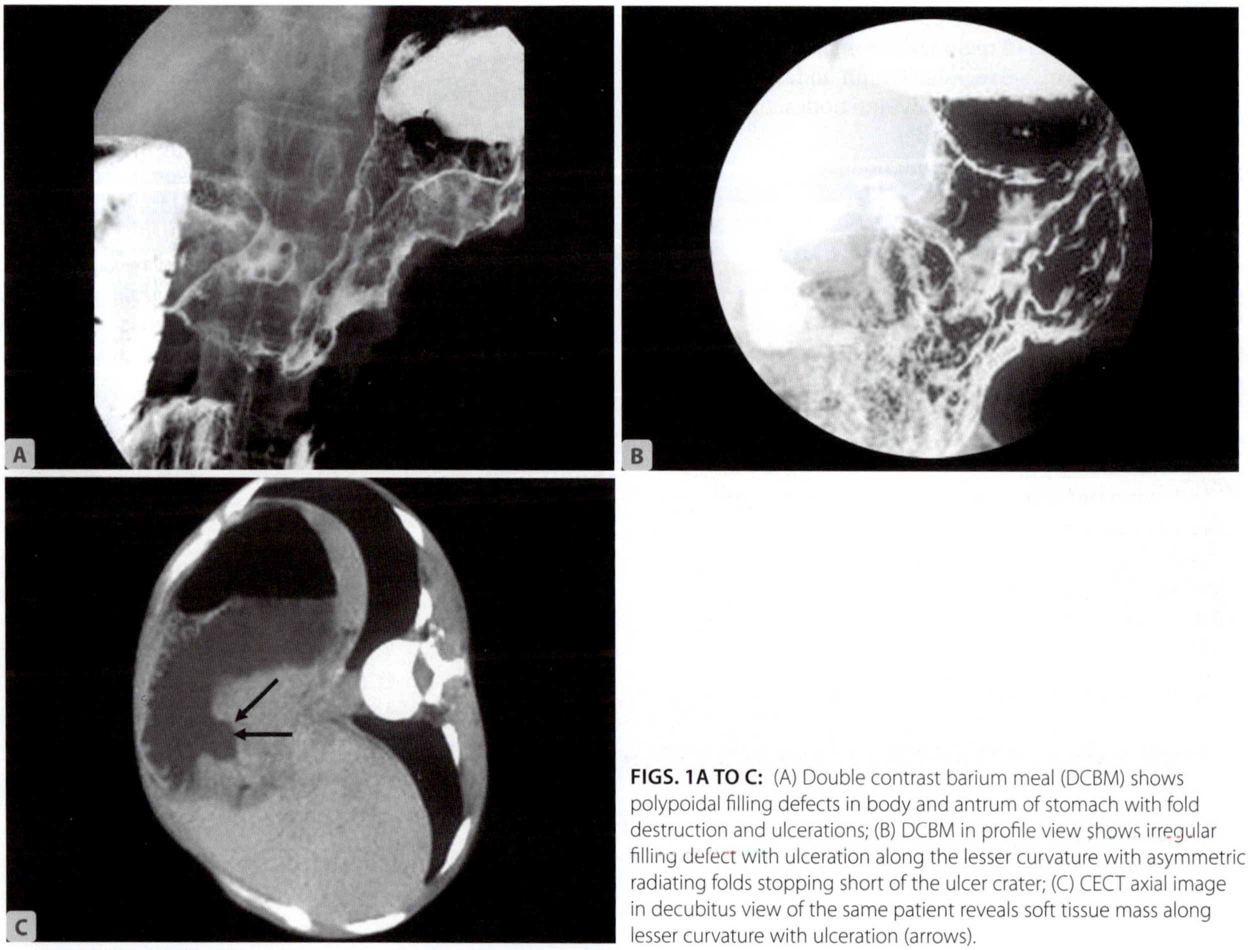

FIGS. 1A TO C: (A) Double contrast barium meal (DCBM) shows polypoidal filling defects in body and antrum of stomach with fold destruction and ulcerations; (B) DCBM in profile view shows irregular filling defect with ulceration along the lesser curvature with asymmetric radiating folds stopping short of the ulcer crater; (C) CECT axial image in decubitus view of the same patient reveals soft tissue mass along lesser curvature with ulceration (arrows).

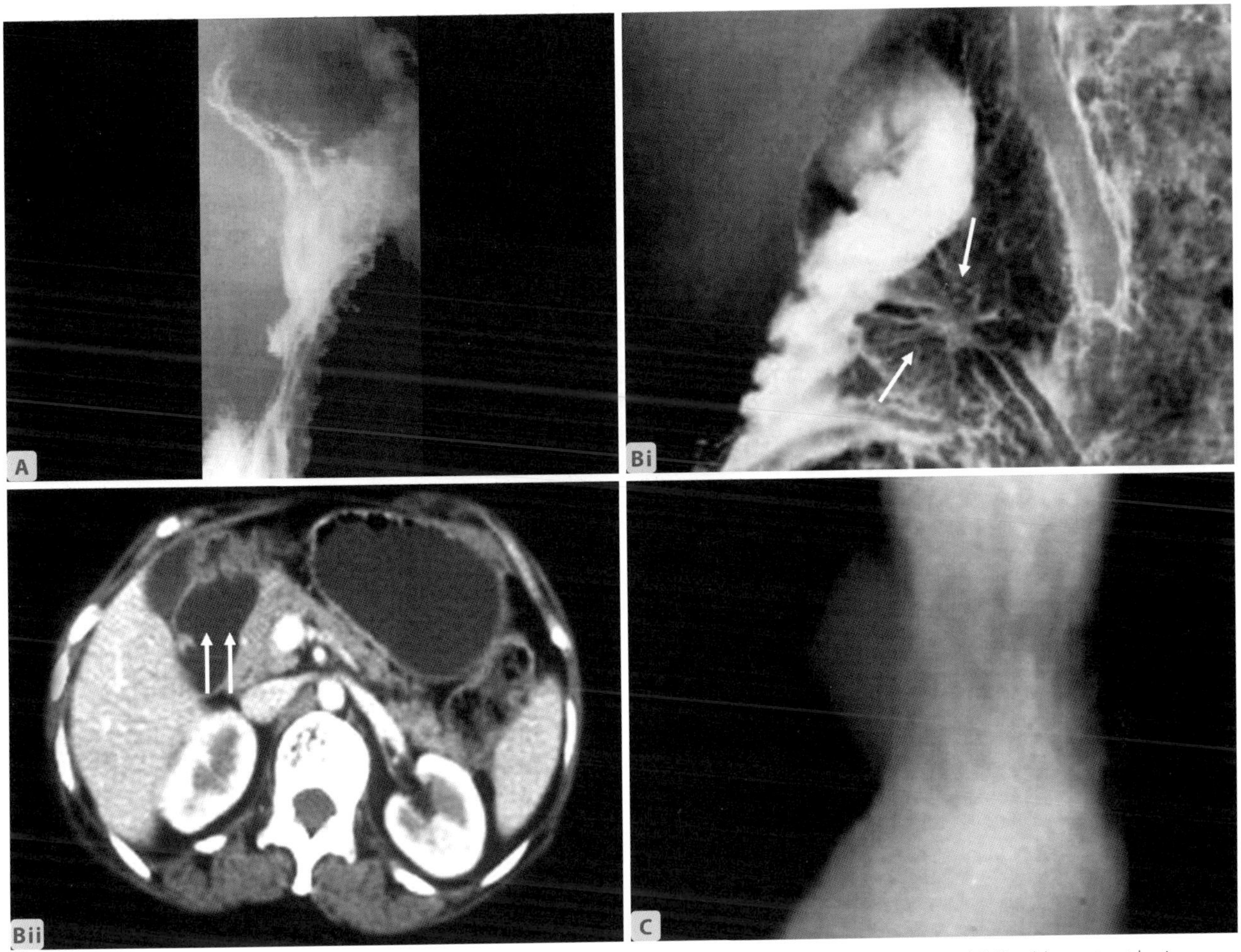

FIGS. 2A TO C: (A) Barium-filled crater seen projecting beyond the line of gastric contour on profile view; (Bi and ii) Double contrast barium meal study en face view showing a contrast-filled benign gastric ulcer along the anterior wall of stomach with the gastric folds seen reaching up to the ulcer margin. CECT of the same patient reveals mild gastric wall thickening in the antrum with ulceration; (C) Thin radiolucent line (Hampton's line) rimming the mouth of ulcer crater on profile view.

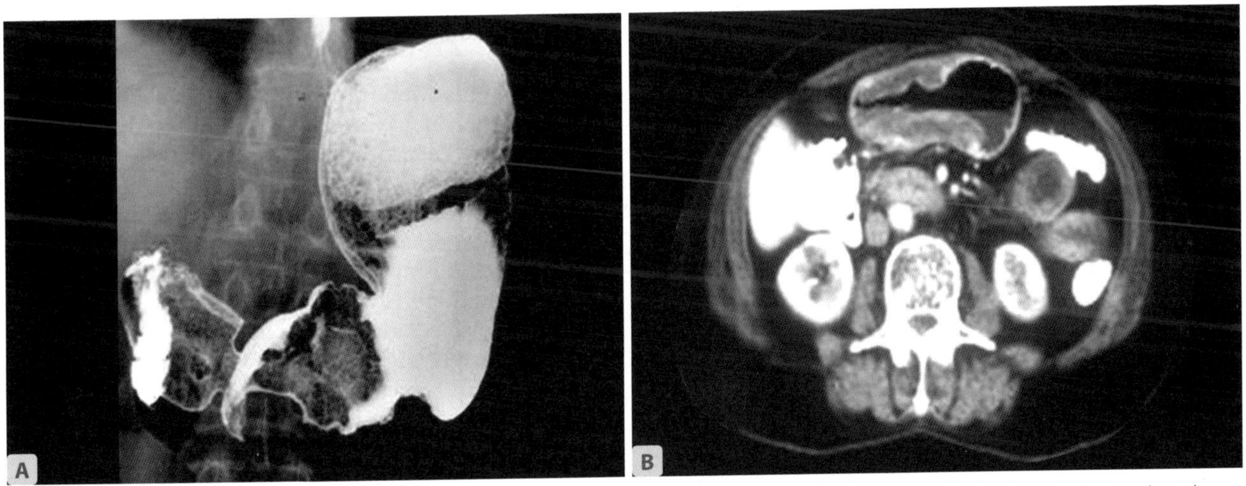

FIGS. 3A AND B: (A) Irregular polypoidal filling defect noted along greater and lesser curvature of the stomach distally on DCBM study with narrow string like pyloric canal and shouldering proximally. Visualized duodenum shows normal mucosal outline; (B) Heterogeneously enhancing polypoidal mural thickening noted in the gastric antrum on CECT. There is no perigastric extension noted.

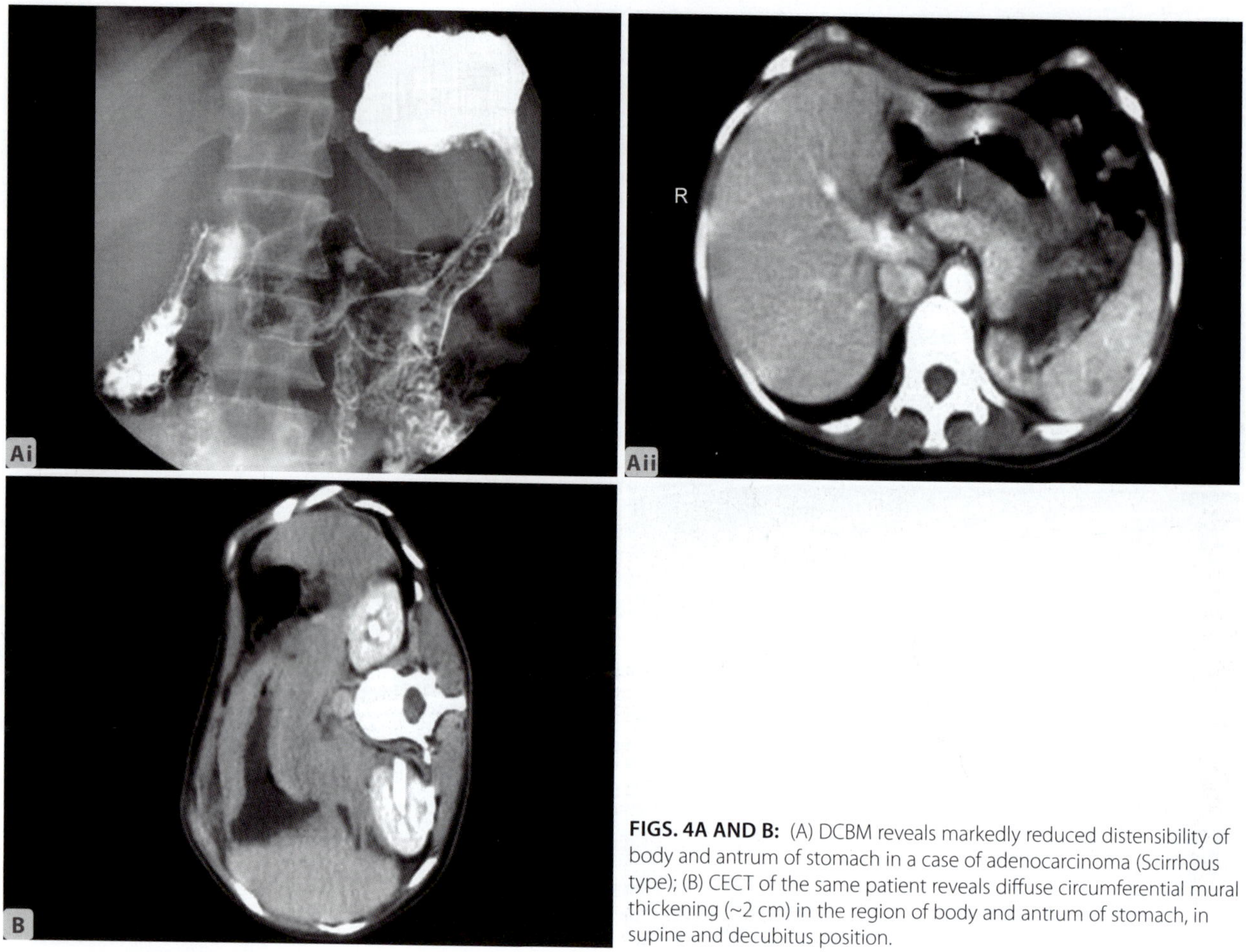

FIGS. 4A AND B: (A) DCBM reveals markedly reduced distensibility of body and antrum of stomach in a case of adenocarcinoma (Scirrhous type); (B) CECT of the same patient reveals diffuse circumferential mural thickening (~2 cm) in the region of body and antrum of stomach, in supine and decubitus position.

CT Features of Gastric Cancer

Computed tomography (CT) has become an indispensable tool for diagnostic evaluation of the stomach because of its superiority to barium studies over depiction of gastric wall as well as extra luminal disease. CT is used preoperatively, primarily to determine the stage and extragastric spread of a gastric carcinoma. MDCT with thin collimation (1.25 mm sections reformatted at 1 mm intervals) is performed using water as oral contrast agent. Water is preferred as an oral contrast agent over positive oral contrast medium, as enhancing gastric wall and subtle abnormalities can be well visualized and because it does not interfere with 3D imaging and CT angiography. Normal gastric wall is about 5–10 mm. In gastritis, the thickness is usually less than 10 mm while in carcinoma it is usually more than 10 mm. In lymphoma, gastric wall thickness is more than 20 mm. We also need to evaluate thickening on parameters like eccentric or circumferential lesion, focal or diffuse and whether the thickening shows enhancement. Stomach wall may however appear thickened if poorly distended and if obliquely oriented in the scan plane, like the GE junction and cardia which can be taken care of by adequate gastric distension (hydro-CT) or by changing patient position. Combination of unenhanced MDCT with air distension of stomach and dual phase contrast enhanced MDCT with water distension also improves the detection and T staging of the primary tumor. In addition, biphasic evaluation with early arterial phase is used to assess enhancement of the gastric wall while the portal venous phase is used to assess the liver parenchyma for metastases because they are mostly hypovascular **(Fig. 6)**.

CT scans may show focal wall thickening, ulcerations, polypoidal mass with or without ulceration or diffuse wall thickening. Mucinous carcinomas have low attenuation (high mucin content) and occasionally may contain calcification **(Figs. 7A and B)**. Transpyloric extension of antral lesion is seen in both carcinoma and lymphoma. Although more common in lymphoma, statistically carcinoma is more common overall hence it is not a reliable finding to differentiate the two. Usually there is focal wall thickening with mucosal irregularity or ulceration, which may show marked contrast enhancement (typically scirrhous carcinomas). Tumor invasion of the perigastric (T3) fat is seen as soft-tissue stranding and further extension involves adjacent structures (T4). AGC can also involve diaphragm, adrenal glands, peritoneal cavity and abdominal wall. Gastric carcinoma can metastasize to ovaries. These metastases are usually bilateral and are known as Krukenberg tumors **(Fig. 8)**.

Direct extension of the tumor into adjacent structures is relatively common. The pancreas is invaded via the lesser sac **(Figs. 9A and B)**, the transverse colon, via the gastrocolic

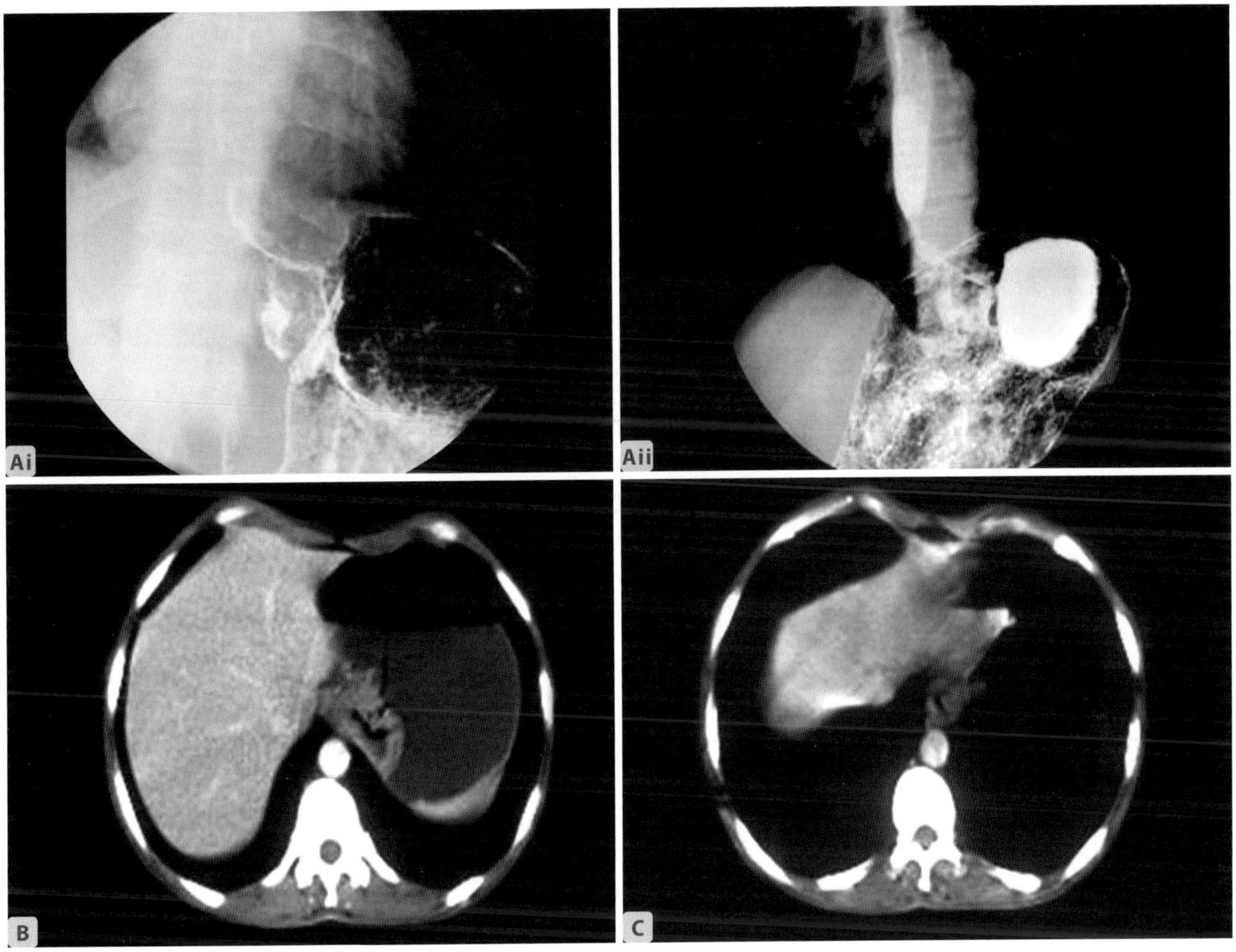

FIGS. 5A TO C: (A) Beak-like narrowing of GE junction with mass at gastric cardia with pooling of barium suggests ulceration on DCBM; (B and C) Axial CECT sections of the same patient reveal heterogeneously enhancing soft tissue mass at GE junction with ulceration in a patient of adenocarcinoma.

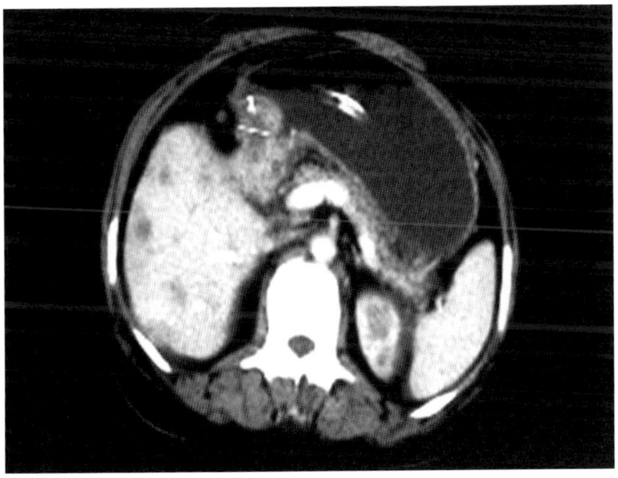

FIG. 6: CECT abdomen shows circumferential mural thickening of antropyloric region in a patient of adenocarcinoma with multiple non-enhancing hypodense lesions in the liver symptoms of metastasis.

ligament and the liver via the gastrohepatic ligament. Longitudinal spread to the distal esophagus occurs in as many as 60% of patients with carcinoma of the cardia. However, the duodenum is involved in only 5–20% of antral carcinomas[1] **(Fig. 9C)**. Left gastric nodes are consistently involved in most gastric cancers. The regional nodes (N2), located in the porta hepatis, hepatoduodenal ligament and peripancreatic region, are not removed by the routine gastrectomy procedure. So their detection is more important **(Figs. 10A and B)**.

Limitations of CT Scanning

Carcinoma in the region of the cardia is often missed on CT due to normal soft tissue thickening due to reflections of phrenicoesophageal ligaments and attachment of gastrohepatic ligament along lesser curvature. In double-contrast studies or on CT done after proper distension, normal anatomic landmarks are obliterated and replaced fallaciously by a plaque-like lesion. Moreover, loss of fat plane between the gastric wall and the left lobe of the liver may be seen.

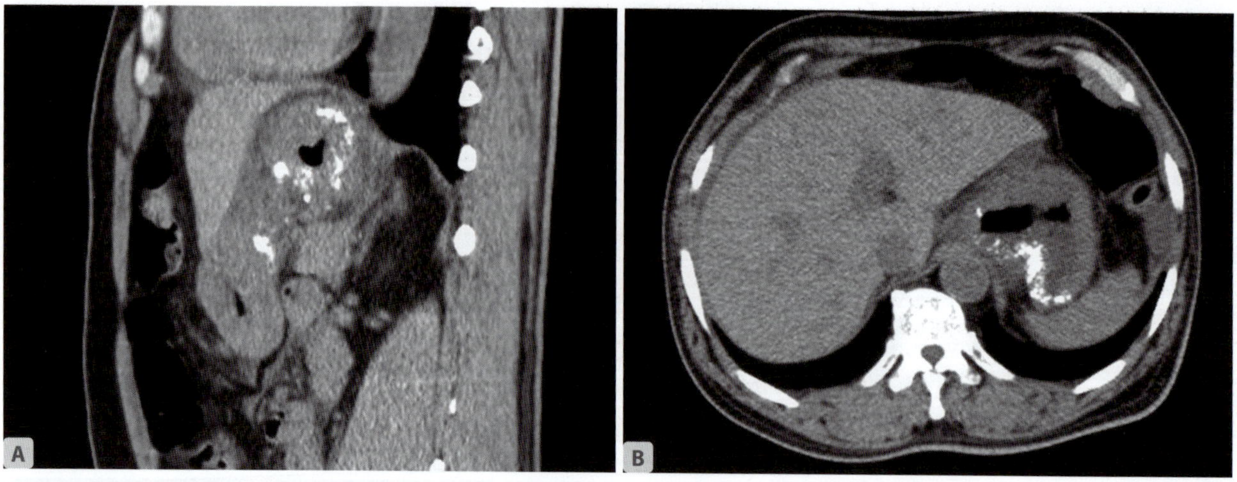

FIGS. 7A AND B: Noncontrast axial and sagittal scans of a patient with mucinous cystadenocarcinoma reveal diffuse thickening of the gastric wall with punctuate foci of calcification.

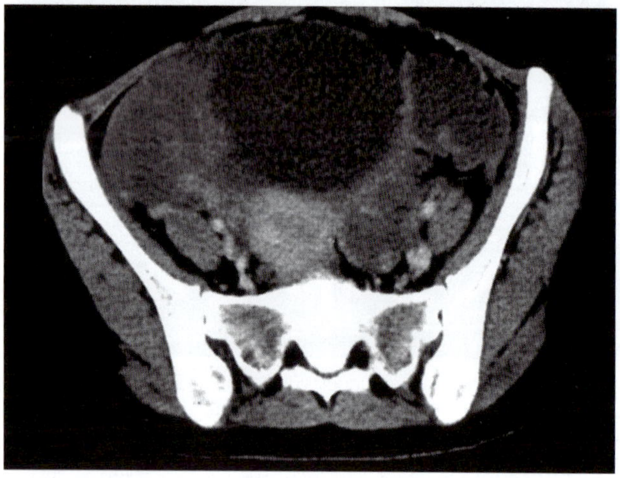

FIG. 8: In a postoperative case of carcinoma stomach, axial contrast-enhanced images reveals multicystic masses in bilateral adnexa suggests Krukenberg tumor in a postoperated case of recurrent gastric carcinoma.

On CT, T2 and T3 lesions may be difficult to distinguish. For AGC, the differentiation between serosal (T4A) versus the adjacent organ invasion (T4B) is more practical for surgeons for the planning of management. Focal change in the CT attenuation within the adjacent organs is required to make a diagnosis of adjacent organ invasion (T4b), not simply loss of intervening fat plane,[1] as loss of a fat plane between the tumor and pancreas may be due to an inflammatory reaction. In emaciated patients, loss of fat planes may simulate direct organ invasion and it is difficult to differentiate between T3 and T4 stage. CT may be inaccurate in assessing nodal involvement as small nodes may contain tumor, and large nodes may result from inflammatory causes. Further perigastric nodes may not be delineated, if the stomach is not well distended. CT may also fail to depict tiny omental and peritoneal deposits.

Inspite of inherent limitations, CT remains the staging modality of choice because it can help identify the primary tumor, assess for local spread, and detect nodal involvement and distant metastases.

Magnetic Resonance Imaging

Magnetic resonance imaging (MRI) provides better soft tissue resolution than CT and the fast-imaging technique is superior to CT in detecting serosal invasion. It is however, comparable to CT for T and N staging.[33] Since MRI is time consuming, costly and limited by motion artifacts it is not routinely used for diagnostic evaluation. Limited data is however, available for MRI of gastric lesions. The lesions show intermediate signal on T1W images compared to the surrounding normal mucosa and muscularis propria. Similar to CT, signal alteration on MR in adjacent organ implies involvement by tumor, rather than just loss of fat plane. Low signal intensity on T2W images and high signal intensity on opposed phase images are also noted.[34] MRI may be slightly better than CT for few T1 and T2 lesions but with similar results for T3-4 lesions, nodal and distant metastasis assessment. So now-a-days, MRI is predominantly used in patients where CT is contraindicated, like drug allergy and where there are concerns of radiation exposure.

Endoscopic Ultrasonography

The role of endoscopic ultrasonography (EUS) is to assess the depth of local invasion and the presence or absence of perigastric nodes. Unlike CT and MRI, EUS can depict stomach wall as 5 layered structure. This has improved the accuracy of local staging of gastric carcinomas on EUS as compared to CT and MRI. A gastric tumor is demonstrated as a hypoechoic mass with varying mural invasion. On endoscopic ultrasonography in T1 tumors, wall thickening is limited to the mucosa and submucosa. However, its depth may be overestimated because of the inflammatory response around the tumor, or underestimated because of microscopic spread.[35] Regarding N staging, involved nodes are rounder and more hypoechoic than normal nodes. EUS-guided FNAC can be done for lymph nodes although it is not a routine practice. Also EUS has limited role if there are long strictures, ulcerations and larger size lesions. It cannot evaluate distant

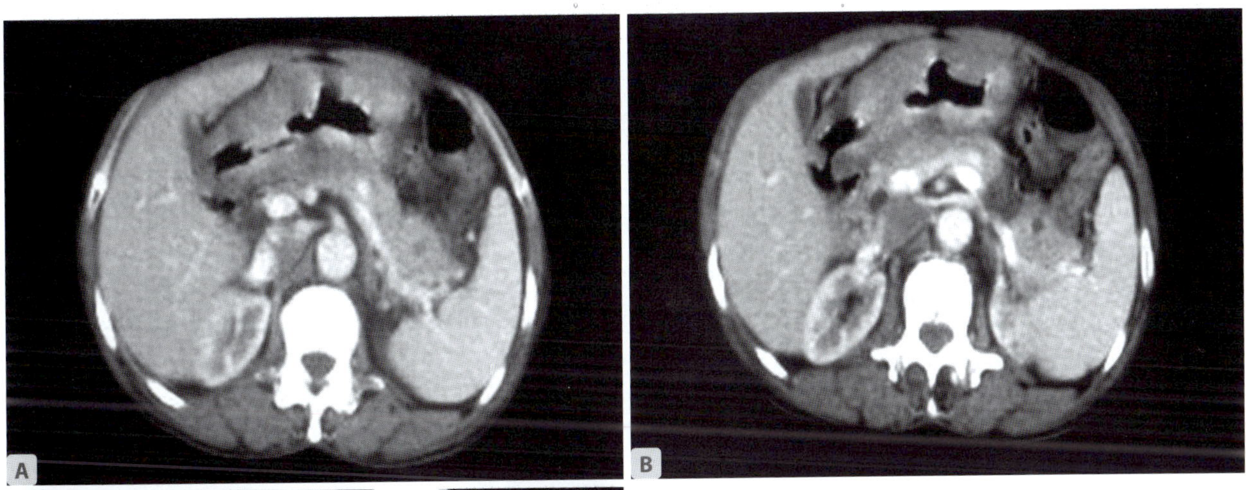

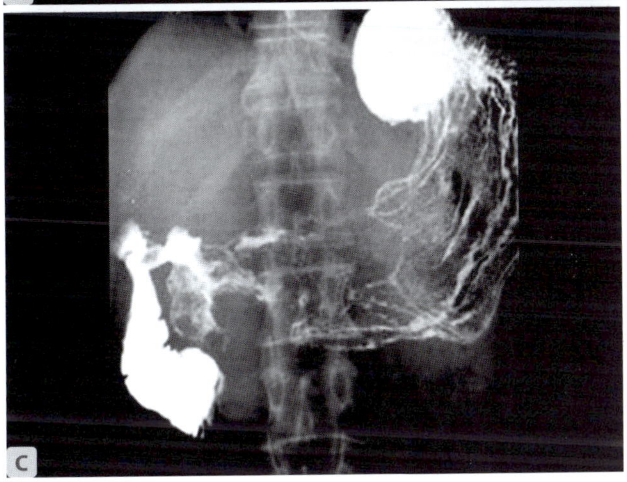

FIGS. 9A TO C: (A and B) CECT axial sections of a patient reveals irregular mural thickening of gastric body and antrum. Loss of fat planes with pancreas posteriorly suggests invasion; (C) Mass-like intraluminal filling defect with ulcerations in antropyloric region on DCBM with extension into first part of duodenum.

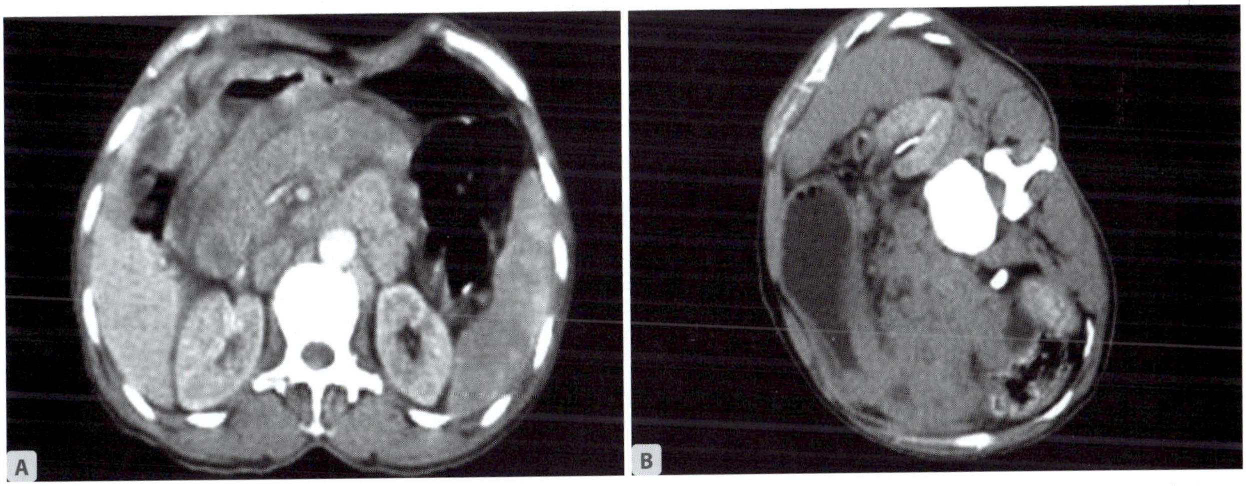

FIGS. 10A AND B: Supine and right lateral decubitus CECT scan showing mural thickening with heterogeneous enhancement in antropyloric region with multiple enhancing coeliac axis and aortocaval region lymph nodes (N1, N2).

metastasis and it is an invasive technique requiring lot of patient preparation and work-up.

Nuclear Imaging

FDG-PET depicts the primary tumor, but involved perigastric lymph nodes are not identified separately from the primary tumor because of poor spatial resolution. Mucinous, poorly differentiated adenocarcinomas and peritoneal metastasis can also be missed on FDG-PET on account of poor uptake. Superior spatial resolution of PET-CT makes it preferable over FDG-PET alone in detection of lymph nodes, metastasis and to evaluate therapeutic response. Diagnostic laparoscopy is highly sensitive for identifying peritoneal metastases and combined with laparoscopic ultrasound, peritoneal biopsy and ascitic cytology unnecessary surgeries can be avoided.[36]

Treatment and Prognosis

Gastric malignancy is an aggressive neoplasm with a 5-year survival rate of less than 20%, prognosis being correlated to the stage of the tumor at presentation. Surgical resection of the primary tumor and regional lymph nodes, if possible is the most definitive therapy. The important prognostic factors influencing survival in resectable gastric cancer are depth of invasion and the presence or absence of nodal metastases. Therefore, accurate staging of gastric cancer is essential because surgical resection is the treatment of choice for localized disease. Despite the accuracy of staging by CT a localized disease may be found unresectable and decision to proceed further is usually taken at laparotomy. Tumors within 5 cm of GE junction are treated with distal esophagectomy and partial gastrectomy combined with gastrojejunostomy. Localized tumors many a times are treated with neo-adjuvant chemotherapy to improve the chances of complete resection of tumor. Palliative surgery is sometimes indicated in advanced cancers to relieve obstruction at GE junction by placing stents.

CT also helps in detecting postoperative complications like afferent loop syndrome, anastomotic leaks and pancreatitis.

Differential Diagnosis

The differential diagnosis includes:

Gastric lymphoma in which the stomach remains pliable, despite large tumor bulk. Further, gastric lymphoma is associated with bulky lymphadenopathy extending below the renal hila, in contrast to adenocarcinoma.

GIST can also mimic the polypoidal form of adenocarcinoma, however GISTs are primarily exophytic and are usually not associated with lymphadenopathy.

Type III carcinoids are aggressive hypervascular masses with features of lymphatic and hematogenous invasion and can therefore mimic adenocarcinoma. So careful review is needed on CT scan to look for perigastric nodal or liver metastasis, which is uncommon in carcinoid tumors.

Metastasis present as multiple small submucosal masses which on having central ulceration give rise to "target or bull's eye" appearance. This can mimic malignant ulcer of adenocarcinoma.

In chronic gastritis, the gastric wall is thick and enhancing and can mimic adenocarcinoma, but the thickness is usually less than 10 mm. Further, there is no lymph node enlargement and the general clinical picture is of a relatively well preserved patient, as opposed to a cachectic patient suffering from malignant process.

Gastric Lymphoma

Gastric lymphoma constitutes 1–5% of the gastric malignancies. Lymphoma may involve GIT as primary malignancy or more commonly as a part of systemic illness and is considered the most common extranodal site for lymphoma. Gastric involvement is seen in about 50% cases and is the most common extranodal site of lymphoma overall.[35] Primary GIT lymphoma does not involve liver or spleen and is confined to stomach and the regional lymph nodes. Majority of lymphomas are non-Hodgkin lymphoma of B-cell type and there are only a few case reports of Hodgkin disease involving gastrointestinal system in literature.[37]

Primary gastrointestinal lymphomas usually affect one site. There are five diagnostic criteria, which have been described by Dawson[38] to make the diagnosis of a primary gastrointestinal lymphoma:

1. No palpable superficial lymph nodes.
2. No adenopathy on chest radiograph
3. Normal values of white cells in blood count.
4. Involvement of GI tract predominantly with involvement of drainage lymph nodes only if at all on laparotomy.
5. No lesions in the liver and spleen.

Patients frequently present with abdominal pain associated occasionally with malabsorption, abdominal mass and weight loss.

Modified TNM staging by European Gastrointestinal Lymphoma Study Group and Luguano staging[39] are two most commonly used staging protocols used for primary gastrointestinal lymphoma.

Most of lymphomas arise from mucosa associated lymphoid tissue (MALT) and have good prognosis as they remain localized for a long time. It is usually a low grade MALT lymphoma, however it can transform into intermediate or higher grade if not treated timely.[40] MALT lymphomas are now referred to as extranodal marginal zone B cell lymphoma (ENMZL), as they arise from the marginal zone of lymph node. Chronic *Heliobacter pylori* infection is associated with MALT lymphomas, and many low grade MALT lymphomas undergo regression with treatment of *H. pylori* infection. They may be low grade or high grade. Low grade lymphomas tend to spread superficially, accompanied occasionally by ulceration and manifest as small nodules with minimal mucosal thickening. Tumors <5 cm with <5 mitoses per high power field suggest low grade lymphoma. On the other hand, high grade lymphomas are usually large tumors, often >5 cms in size, polypoidal and associated with marked rugal fold thickening and have >5 mitoses per high power field. There is commonly necrosis within the tumor which may give rise to septated appearance and excavation may lead to communication with rest of the gastrointestinal tract or peritoneal cavity. Occurrence of hemorrhage may produce fluid-fluid level within the tumor. Direct invasion of adjacent organs or distant, omental and peritoneal metastasis may also occur.

T-cell lymphomas associated with enteropathy, Burkitt's lymphoma, etc are rare. Other risk factors for gastric lymphoma include inflammatory bowel disease, coeliac disease, HIV infection and immunosuppression after solid organ transplant.[41]

Diagnostic Imaging

Lymphoma can be focal or diffuse and involve any portion of the stomach. Though early lymphoma is confined to the mucosa and submucosa, gastric lymphomas are usually advanced at presentation and may mimic the appearances of gastric carcinoma.

Barium study and CT scan form the mainstay of diagnostic workup and radiographic findings of lymphoma parallel their gross morphological subtypes on both the techniques. The most common appearance is that of an infiltrating lesion with diffuse mural and fold thickening.

The CT reveals preservation of the perigastric fat planes even with a massive tumor. This favours the diagnosis of lymphoma over adenocarcinoma. Adenocarcinoma and lymphoma both are associated with lymphadenopathy, however bulky lymph nodes extending below the renal hila favor the diagnosis of lymphoma.[42] CT is also a better technique to diagnose complications like perforation, obstruction and fistulization. Moreover despite extensive infiltrative lesions stomach remains pliable and gastric outlet obstruction is uncommon in contrast to gastric adenocarcinoma.

The type of involvement can be infiltrative, ulcerative, polypoidal, nodular or a combination of above.

- *Infiltrative form*: Infiltration can be local or diffuse. It is associated with thick, nodular folds which are not effaced after hypotonic agent adminstration. Distensibility of stomach is maintained which helps in differentiation from linitis plastica due to adenocarcinoma. These patients are therefore less prone to develop gastric outlet obstruction[43] **(Figs. 11 and 12)**. Differential diagnosis includes Menetrier's disease, hypertrophic, lymphocytic and eosinophilic gastritis.
- *Ulcerative form*: Presence of ulcer accompanied by a polypoidal mass, absence of areae gastricae and associated rugal fold thickening are pointers of ulcerative form of lymphomatous involvement.
- *Polypoidal form*: There can be an intraluminal mass which may be lobulated or may present as submucosal mass. It may be associated with ulceration.
- *Nodular form*: These present as multiple submucosal masses. These often ulcerate giving "target or bull's eye" appearance.
- Extension to involve duodenum may be seen in about 40% cases **(Figs. 13A to C)**. Esophageal involvement is less common and seen in about 10% cases.[1]

The MRI is useful in evaluating bowel wall thickening along with organ and lymph node involvement. Lymphomatous masses are hypointense on T1 and hyperintense on T2 weighted images as they have high free water content. MR is helpful in evaluating treatment due to reduction in signal intensity on T2 as a result of reduced cellular and water content.

In the detection of low-grade and MALT lymphomas cross sectional imaging may be limited; which can be best overcome by staging EUS which accurately assesses the intramural infiltration, local node involvement, and response to therapy.[44]

Radionuclide imaging using FDG PET/PET-CT is helpful in evaluating lymph nodes as involved nodes show increased uptake, however its role is limited due to unpredictability and variability of degree of uptake in different subtypes.[45] FDG-PET is also found helpful in predicting the treatment response.

Metastatic Disease

Common tumors that metastasize to stomach include breast, malignant melanoma, lung, lymphoma and Kaposki sarcoma. These present as multiple small submucosal masses which on having central ulceration give rise to "target or bull's eye" appearance **(Figs. 14A and B)**. Differential diagnosis includes neurofibromas, pancreatic rest cells and leiomyomas.

Gastric and Duodenal Carcinoids

Gastrointestinal carcinoids are well differentiated endocrine neoplasms arising from specialized endocrine cells that populate the mucosa and submucosa of the gastrointestinal system. Hence theoretically they can be seen arising from any part of the gastrointestinal system and produce clinical symptoms depending on the type of the hormone they are secreting. Carcinoids arise most commonly from the distal ileum from enterochromaffin cells which produce serotonin. Usually they present as lymph nodal or liver metastasis.

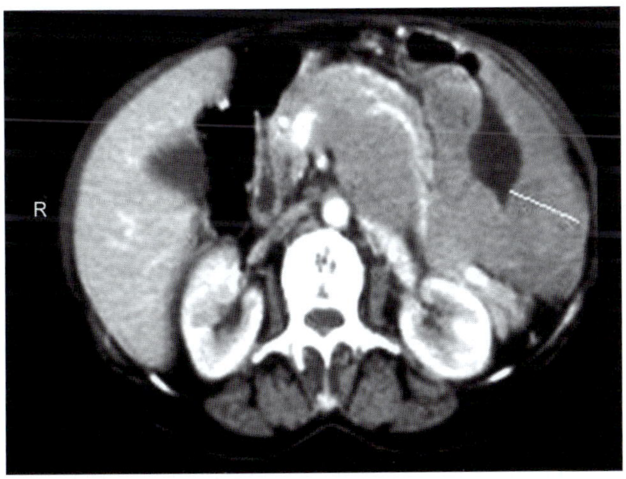

FIG. 11: Marked enhancing wall thickening (5 cm) noted in another patient of gastric lymphoma on CECT with multiple enlarged retroperitoneal nodes reaching up to renal hilum.

Courtesy: Dr Vinod G Maller, MAMC, New Delhi.

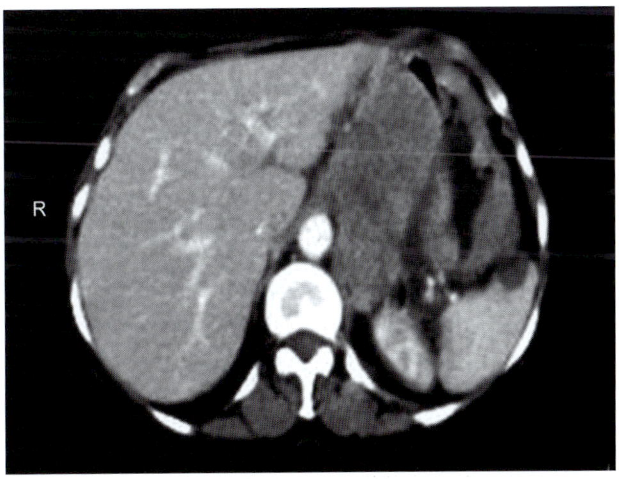

FIG. 12: Thick nodular folds in the region of gastric body along with enlarged lymph nodes noted in gastrohepatic ligament and paraaortic region. Note is also made of hypodense lesion in spleen.

Courtesy: Dr Vinod G Maller, MAMC, New Delhi.

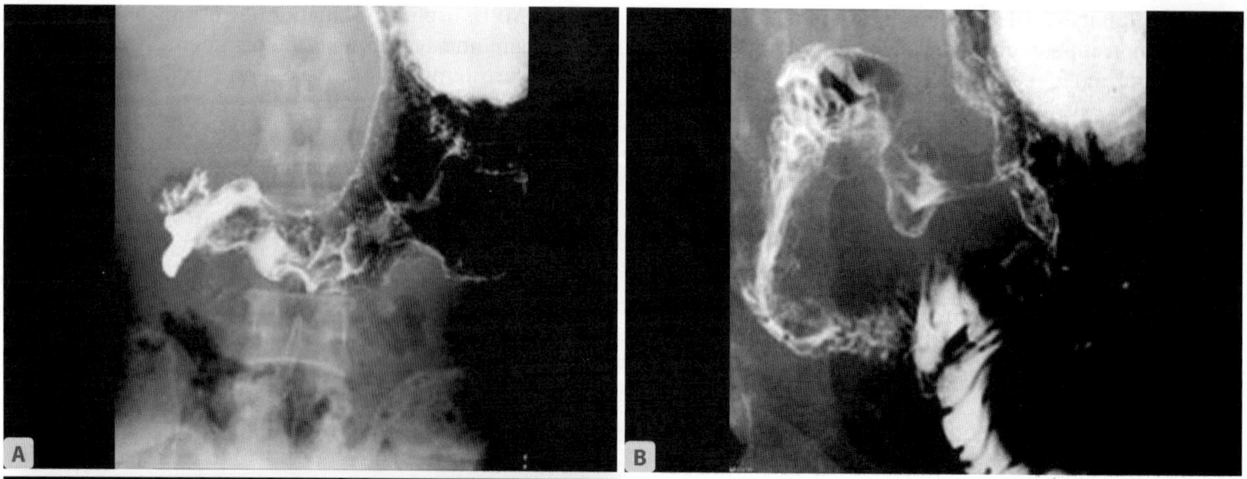
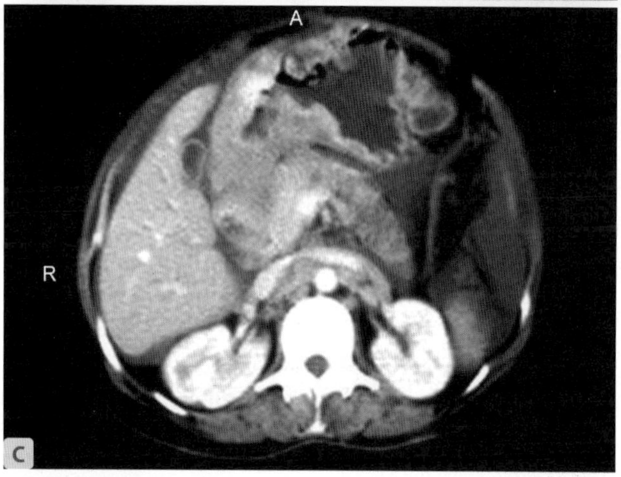

FIGS. 13A TO C: (A and B) Nodular filling defects noted on DCBM study in the distal body and antropyloric region with extension into duodenum in a patient of gastric lymphoma; (C) CECT of the same patient reveals enhancing mural thickening of distal body and antropyloric region. Enlarged aortocaval lymph nodes with ascites also seen.

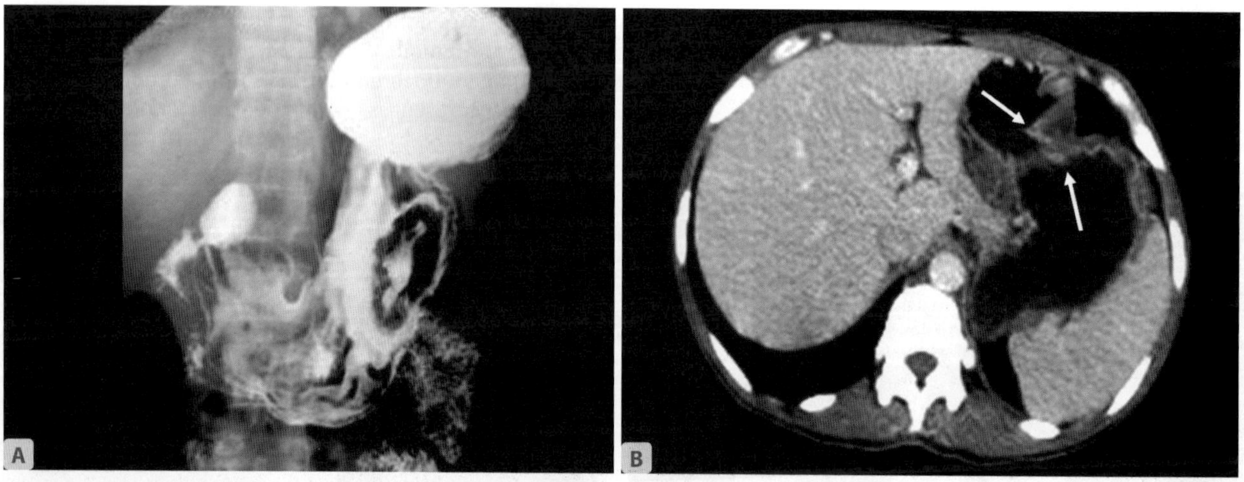

FIGS. 14A AND B: (A) Target/Bull's eye lesion—DCBM reveals a large filling defect in body of stomach with central pooling of barium; (B) CECT shows focal thickening of stomach wall in the region of body with central ulceration in a patient of submucosal metastasis from melanoma.

Carcinoids of the stomach, duodenum or colon are however a relatively rare entity. Majority of the gastric carcinoids arise from gastric body and fundus from oxyntic cells.[46]

Gastric carcinoids are primarily divided into three types depending on their clinical, imaging and pathological differences by Bordi et al.[47]

Type I: Most common (74%), female predominance at an older age, usually associated with autoimmune chronic atrophic gastritis and usually encountered during endoscopy performed usually for dyspepsia or anemia. Achlorhydria, pernicious anemia or gastric G-cell hyperplasia may be seen.

They are usually small (<1 cm) and seen as multiple smoothly marginated mucosal and submucosal masses in the body and fundus of stomach showing enhancement on CECT.

Type II: Usually associated with Zollinger-Ellison syndrome in patients of multiple endocrine neoplasia (MEN type-I). They usually present as recurrent nonhealing gastric or duodenal ulcers with marked mucosal fold and rugal thickening, abdominal pain, bleeding or diarrhea due to hypergastrinemia by gastrin producing neoplasms **(Fig. 15)**. They have a more marked propensity to metastasize than type I carcinoids.

They are also usually multiple but of variable size unlike type I carcinoids and can show ulceration. Smaller masses like in type-I can be missed on CECT **(Fig. 16)**.

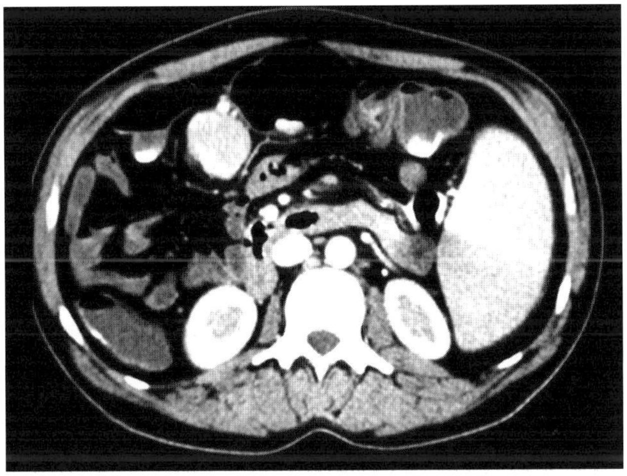

FIG. 15: A patient of gastrinoma showing heterogeneously enhancing mass lesion in relation to 2nd part of duodenum with intensely enhancing multiple nodular masses in the body and antrum region of stomach suggestive of multiple carcinoids.

Type III: Type III ECL-cell carcinoids represent 10–15% of the gastric carcinoids which usually does not have any associated hypergastrinemia or atrophic gastritis and usually present with signs and symptoms of aggressive mass like anorexia, weight loss, bleeding or pain abdomen.

It usually presents as large aggressive hypervascular solitary mass with exophytic component in the gastric fundus and body with features of lymphatic and hematogenous invasion on histopathology. So it needs a careful review on CT scan, to look for perigastric nodal or liver metastasis[46,47] **(Fig. 17)**.

The differentials for gastric carcinoids include other multifocal polypoidal masses like multiple hyperplastic polyps, adenomatous polyps in familial adenomatous polyposis syndrome, hamartomatous polyps in Peutz-Jeghers syndrome and juvenile polyposis for type I and II gastric carcinoids. Type III carcinoids can mimic adenocarcinoma, lymphoma, and gastrointestinal stromal tumors.

Majority of duodenal carcinoids are G cell type and they are also rare like gastric carcinoids. Patients with MEN 1 usually develop G cell carcinoids in 90% of the patients while D cell type usually associated with Neurofibromatosis type 1 (NF-1).

Gastrinomas usually present with abdominal pain, bleeding, recurrent nonhealing ulcers and diarrhea while somatostatin producing carcinoids are almost exclusively present around ampulla of Vater and hence present with obstructive symptoms like jaundice, pancreatitis or hemorrhage.

Duodenal carcinoids are usually small, homogeneous, 1-2 cm intramural or submucosal polypoid periampullary nodules which can show focal ulcerations. After adenocarcinoma, carcinoids are the second most common malignant tumors of the duodenum and may have similar syndromic associations as that of gastric carcinoid. Most of the tumors are small, however larger tumors (>1.5 cm in size) present with metastasis at the time of presentation.[48]

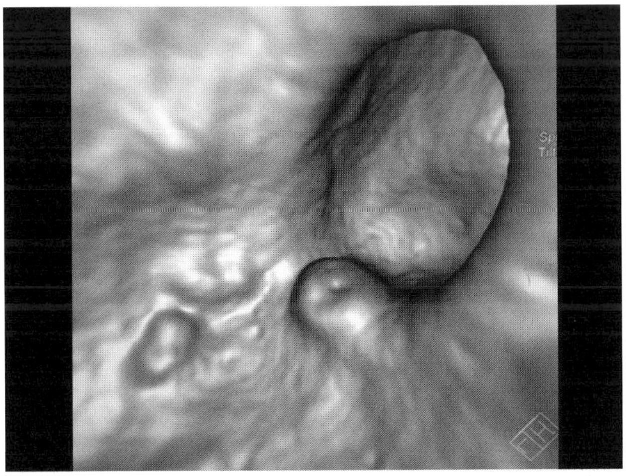

FIG. 16: Virtual gastroscopy of the same patient reveals multiple variable sized submucosal masses in the body and antrum of stomach with few of them showing central ulcerations.

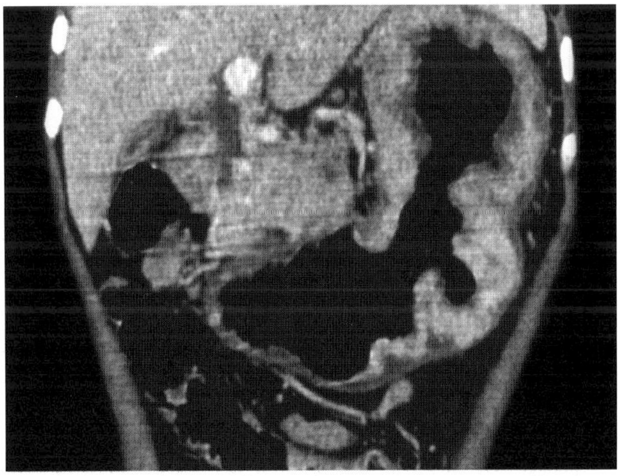

FIG. 17: Gastric carcinoid (Type-III)—CECT coronal reformat of another patient reveals diffuse mural thickening with irregular polypoidal lesions in the fundus and body of the stomach. There is a large heterogeneously enhancing mass lesion seen in the region of head of the pancreas.

Courtesy: Dr Prashant Nagpal, MAMC, New Delhi.

GASTROINTESTINAL STROMAL TUMOR

Etiopathogenesis

Gastrointestinal stromal tumor (GIST) is the most common mesenchymal neoplasm that can be found throughout the gastrointestinal tract with 60–70% of the tumors affecting the stomach.[49] Before the immunohistochemical tests were available, they used to be considered leiomyoma but the uniqueness of tumor being c-KIT (CD 117) positive helps to differentiate GIST from other neoplasms. 5% cases of GIST however do not show CD 117 immunoreactivity and rather harbor mutations for platelet derived growth factor receptor-alpha (PDGFR- alpha).[50]

They arise from pacemaker interstitial cells of Cajal normally present in myenetric plexus, which are responsible for peristalsis.[51] Because they arise from the deep muscularis propria, GISTs frequently have an exophytic or intramural pattern of growth. Endoluminal tumors although less common if present have features of intramural masses like smoothly circumscribed masses forming obtuse or right angles with the gastric wall.[52] Pressure necrosis can cause focal mucosal ulcerations in lesions larger than 2 cm which appears as "bull's eye" lesion on DCBM study.

Clinical Features

Clinical manifestations of the GIST depend on their size and location. Small lesions are discovered incidentally. Ulcerated lesions usually present with bleed in form of hematemesis, melena or iron deficiency anemia.[53] Larger masses usually present with abdominal pain and early satiety. However, because of predominantly exophytic nature of tumors, many of these patients remain asymptomatic until the tumors become quite large.[52]

Imaging Features

The typical CT appearance of small tumors are often of homogeneous density and that of large tumors is heterogeneously enhancing lobulated hypervascular exophytic mass with mucosal ulceration, central necrosis, hemorrhage, cavitation and areas of cystic degeneration[51] **(Figs. 18A to C)**. Ulcerations and fistulizations can be manifested as air and oral contrast within the lesion. 5–10% of the cases can show calcification. Size >5 cm, necrosis, mesenteric or contiguous organ infiltration and metastasis favors diagnosis of malignant GIST.[54,55] Rarely clumps of calcification can be seen. Nearly half of the patients present with metastasis in the advanced stages when the tumor has invaded the adjacent organs like colon, diaphragm and pancreas with deposits predominantly

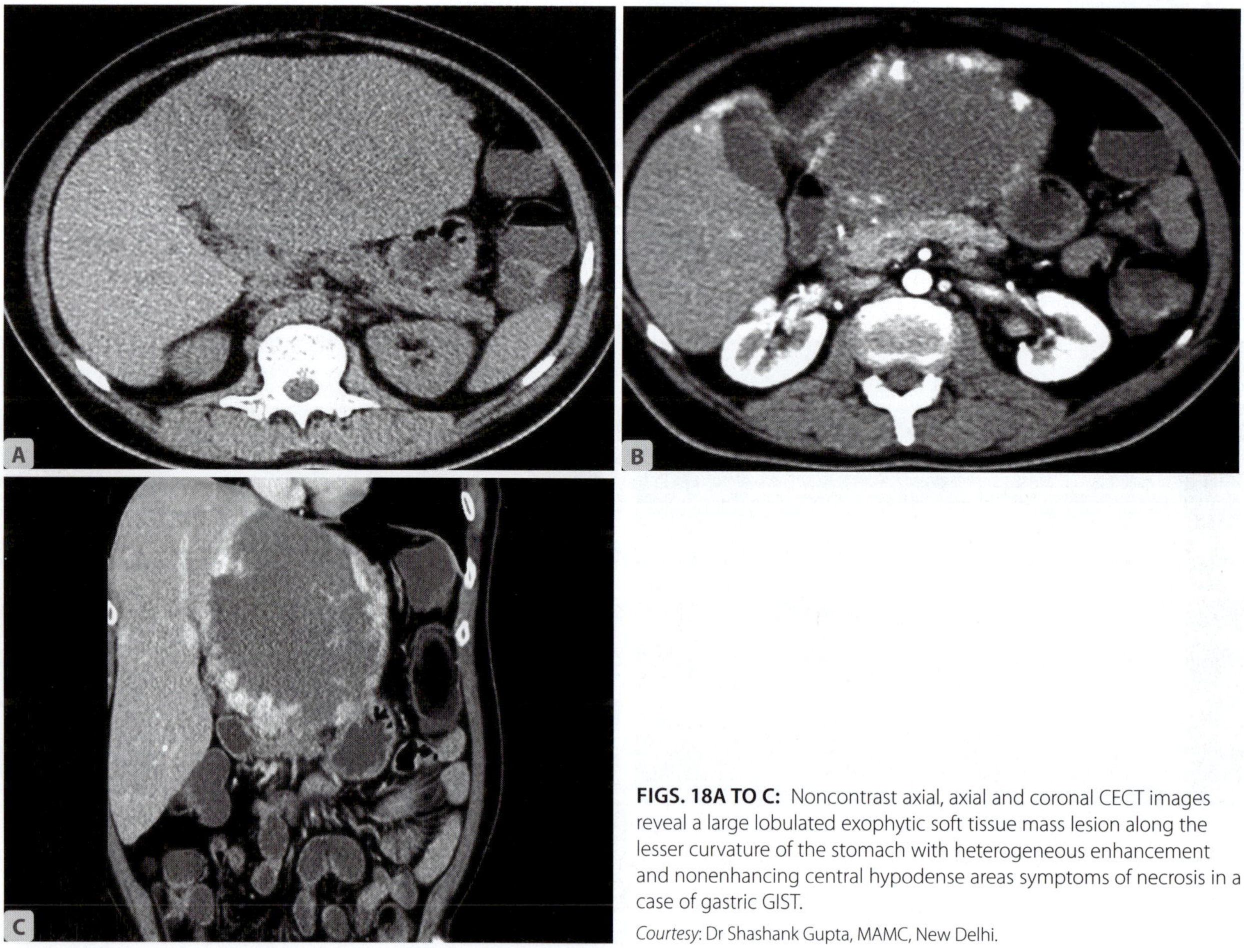

FIGS. 18A TO C: Noncontrast axial, axial and coronal CECT images reveal a large lobulated exophytic soft tissue mass lesion along the lesser curvature of the stomach with heterogeneous enhancement and nonenhancing central hypodense areas symptoms of necrosis in a case of gastric GIST.

Courtesy: Dr Shashank Gupta, MAMC, New Delhi.

seen in liver and peritoneum. Nodal metastasis is infrequent in GISTs.[56]

Differential diagnosis for GISTs can be neural tumors like schwannomas, true leiomyomas and small type 3 solitary carcinoid tumors. Immunoreactivity to c-KIT or DOG1 however can confirm the diagnosis.[57] Other tumors showing intramural growth like gastric adenocarcinoma or lymphoma can mimic a GIST. However, lymphadenopathy is rare for GISTs. Submucosal metastases to the stomach from melanoma or breast cancer can manifest as bull's-eye lesions, they can be single, however usually they are multiple.[52]

The GISTs smaller than 2 cm are generally considered benign with a very low risk of recurrence. However, no GIST can truly be labeled benign.[58] A definitive diagnosis is particularly important because advanced GIST can now be treated with a new tyrosine kinase inhibitor imatinib with a remarkable response and a prolonged survival.[59,60]

On CT, GISTs typically become homogeneous and hypoattenuating from heterogeneously hyperattenuating appearence, with disappearance of enhancing tumor nodules and tumor vessels in the early post-treatment period by Imatinib. There is development of myxoid degeneration and occasional areas of hemorrhage and necrosis can be seen within the healing tumor which can paradoxically increase the size of tumor. However with overall reduction in tumor enhancement this does not indicate tumor progression. The term *cystic change* is usually avoided while under treatment by Imatinib. Development of a nodule within the treated tumor is unique to GISTs and indicates recurrence regardless of changes in tumor size.[61]

Duodenal GIST

In institutional review of GIST, about 20% of GIST's occurred in duodenum as compared to rest of the gastrointestinal tract. They were larger than their gastric counterparts, with the majority occurring in 2nd part of duodenum. Association of duodenal GIST's with neurofibromatosis has also been noted.

Duodenal GIST often present with bleeding and, occasionally pain.[62] Similar to gastric lesions these lesions are seen as large heterogeneously enhancing, exophytic masses with central ulceration and filling of central cavity by oral contrast on CECT **(Figs. 19A to C)**.

In addition to medical treatment as described for gastric GIST's, surgical resection options include pancreaticoduodenectomy and segmental duodenectomy with preservation of pylorus.

Gastric Lipomas (Table 3)

Gastric lipomas are solitary submucosal lesions usually detected incidentally in asymptomatic patients. They are composed of mature fat cells surrounded by fibrous capsule.[63]

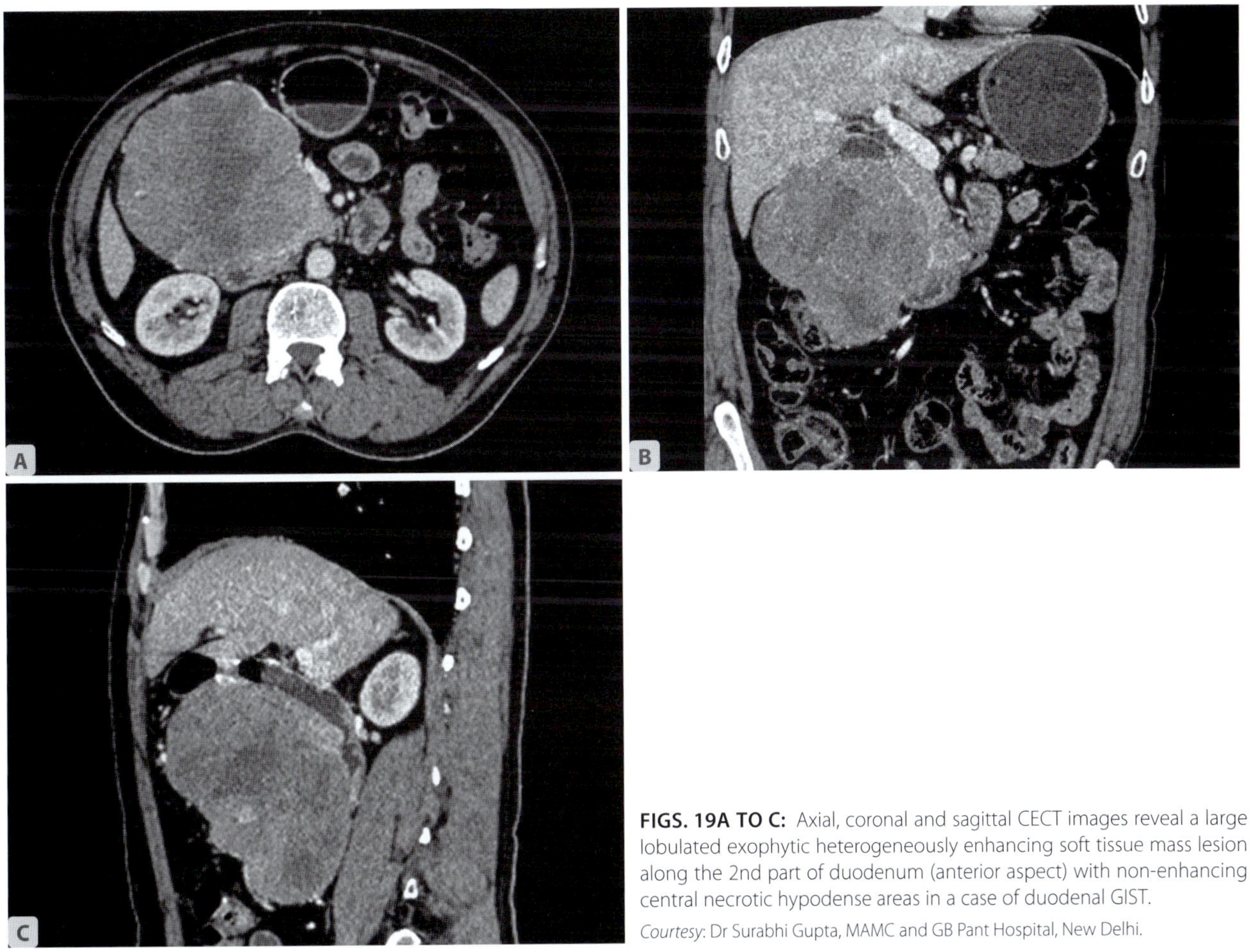

FIGS. 19A TO C: Axial, coronal and sagittal CECT images reveal a large lobulated exophytic heterogeneously enhancing soft tissue mass lesion along the 2nd part of duodenum (anterior aspect) with non-enhancing central necrotic hypodense areas in a case of duodenal GIST.

Courtesy: Dr Surabhi Gupta, MAMC and GB Pant Hospital, New Delhi.

TABLE 3: Other rare tumors and focal gastric lesions mimicking tumor.

Rare tumors	Other focal gastric lesions mimicking tumor
Gastric lipoma	Inflammatory pseudotumor/ myofibroblastic tumor
Leiomyoma/ leiomyosarcoma/ liposarcoma	Ectopic pancreatic rests/ myoepithelial hamartoma
Neurogenic tumors	Gastric duplication cyst
Glomus tumor	
Hemangioma	
Plasmacytoma	

Small tumors are asymptomatic although, larger tumors can present with abdominal pain and bleeding due to ulceration of overlying mucosa. Infrequently they can develop into pedunculated lesions which can intermittently prolapse through pylorus and cause obstruction.[61]

The most common location of gastric lipomas is gastric antrum. They appear as smooth submucosal masses on fluoroscopy, however can show central ulceration. They also can change size and shape with peristalsis being soft tissue lesions.[61] On CT they appear as solitary, submucosal, well demarcated lesion with homogeneous fat attenuation. Occasionally linear strands of soft tissue at the base or mild adjacent gastric wall thickening may be present.[47] On CT images, attenuation values of –70 to –120 HU are diagnostic of a lipoma.[63] Rarely, they can present with complications like ulceration, intussusceptions and hemorrhage.[64] So, they can present as masses of soft tissue attenuation rather than fatty attenuation.

Liposarcoma/Leiomyoma/Leiomyosarcoma

Liposarcoma originates in undifferentiated mesenchymal cells within the submucosal and muscularis of stomach wall. There is predominately exophytic growth and as a result, delay in diagnosis. Four forms of liposarcoma are differentiated, myxoid, round cell and pleomorphic variety. Necrosis, hemorrhage, fatty or cystic areas may occur within the mass depending on various types.

Leiomyomas and leiomyosarcomas are well circumscribed intramural tumors and predominate in the region of gastric cardia. The true leiomyomas are rare benign tumor of stomach and are negative for c-KIT and strongly and diffusely positive for desmin and smooth muscle actin.

Leiomyomas appear on CT as homogeneous, low attenuation masses with an endoluminal growth pattern.[65-67] They too can have central ulceration if >2 cm in size and hence includes GISTs and schwannomas as differentials. However, the malignant nature of leiomyosarcoma, is not easily distinguished by gross appearance and needs invasion and metastasis for the diagnosis **(Figs. 20A to C)**. Histological evaluation can only establish the final diagnosis in isolated cases. Sarcomas present mostly with bleeding due to hypervascular nature of tumor and central necrosis or massive mucosal erosion of the tumor and with partial obstruction if large. Endoscopically, the tumors appear as a smooth, submucosal mass over which the mucosal folds are stretched and effaced. Leiomyosarcomas can undergo hematogenous spread to the liver and lungs.[48]

Neurogenic Tumors of Stomach

These are benign submucosal neoplasms and comprise 4% of all benign gastric neoplasms and are nerve sheath tumors in origin (schwannoma).[68] They are believed to arise within the myenetric plexus in the muscularis propria. They are slow growing exophytic tumors which are mostly asymptomatic and because of this indolent growth these are usually discovered incidentally by cross sectional imaging or on endoscopy.[69] Carney's triad is associated with gastric neurogenic tumors along with pulmonary chondromas and extra adrenal paragangliomas.

Schwannomas arising mostly in the gastric body can have an exophytic or intramural growth, may be asymptomatic or present with pain, bleeding or obstruction if large.[70]

Neural tumors in the stomach usually appear on CT scans as submucosal masses (with or without ulceration) that are indistinguishable from other mesenchymal tumors. Gastric schwannomas are usually homogeneous, low attenuation masses. Hemorrhage, ulceration, calcification and cystic changes are rare unlike in schwannomas at other places which commonly shows cystic changes which help them in distinguishing from more heterogeneous GISTs. Contrast enhancement is variable. They usually show minimal to no significant enhancement on arterial phase but show delayed enhancement on equilibrium phase.[52]

Glomus Tumor

Neuromyoarterial receptors or glomus bodies are composed of modified smooth muscle cells and account for 2% of benign gastric tumors and arise nearly in all cases in muscularis propria.[71]

Their clinical presentation varies from asymptomatic nature of disease to various features like pain, hematemesis or melena.

They usually present in gastric antrum as hypervascular lesions.[66,71] These tumors are also soft tumors like lipomas on barium studies and can change in size and shape. However, strong arterial enhancement with persistence on delayed films differentiate from lipomas on CT.[1] The differentials for gastric glomus tumors include GIST, carcinoids, lipomas, metastasis, ectopic pancreas and sometimes due to specific peripheral nodular pattern of enhancement with delayed filling-in, hemangioma becomes a differential.[66,71]

Hemangioma

Another solitary vascular gastric tumor which comprises less than 2% of benign gastric lesions.[72] It is a debate whether these are true neoplasms or congenital malformations and are found to be associated with number of syndromes such as Klippel-Trénaunay syndrome, Maffucci syndrome, blue rubber-bleb nevus syndrome, or Osler-Rendu-Weber disease.

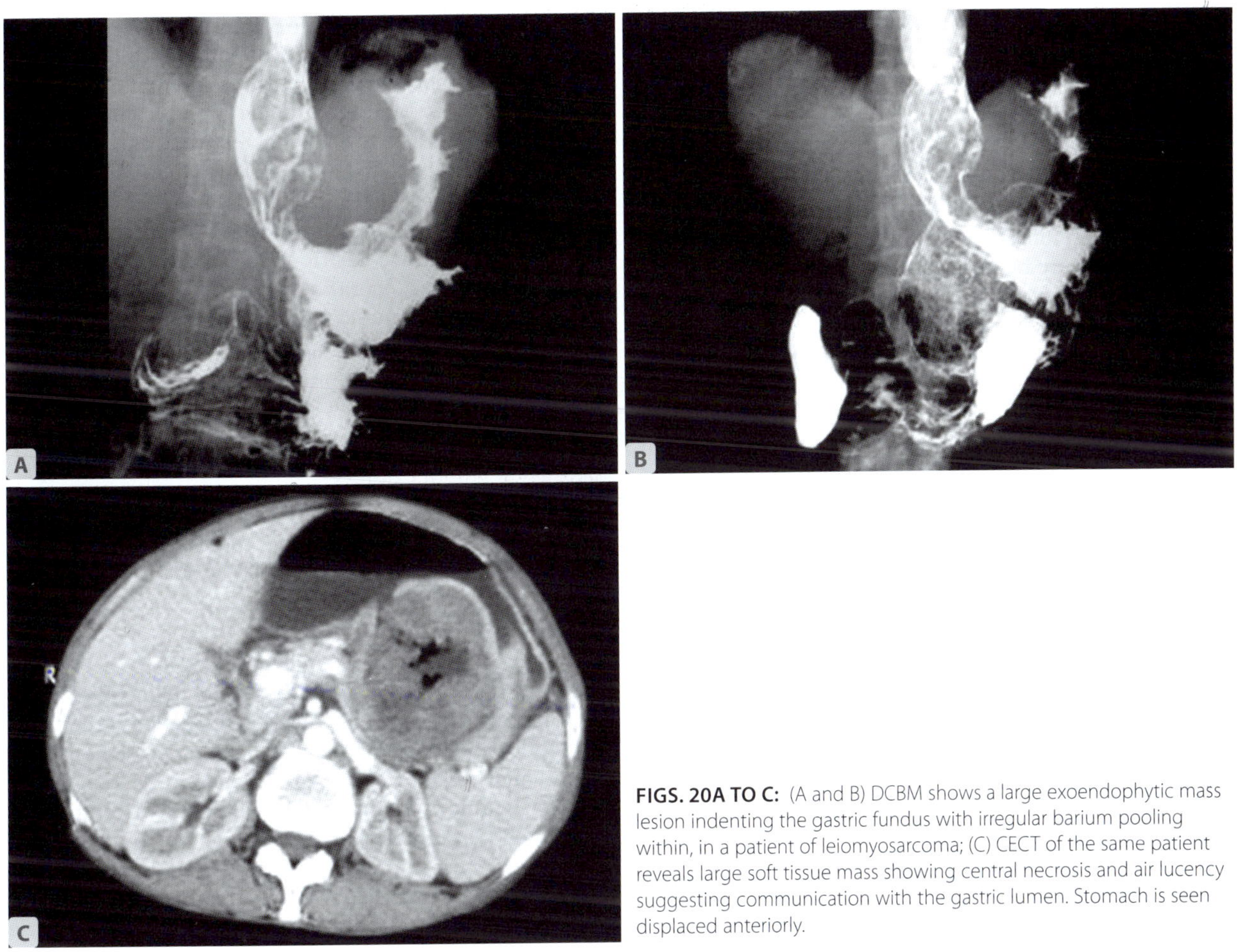

FIGS. 20A TO C: (A and B) DCBM shows a large exoendophytic mass lesion indenting the gastric fundus with irregular barium pooling within, in a patient of leiomyosarcoma; (C) CECT of the same patient reveals large soft tissue mass showing central necrosis and air lucency suggesting communication with the gastric lumen. Stomach is seen displaced anteriorly.

They are mostly seen in children and gradually involute with age. However, with the possibility of massive GI bleed they are usually resected.

They are seen as intramural masses on fluoroscopy and show avid enhancement on CT scan. Phleboliths, if seen in the lesion are considered pathognomonic.

Plasmacytoma

About 10% of extramedullary plasmacytomas occur in the gastrointestinal tract with primary gastric plasmacytoma accounting for five percent of them.

The diagnosis is established by absence of any visceral involvement elsewhere, apart from stomach. In addition there is no serum M protein and bone marrow infiltration. Four forms of primary gastric plasmacytoma include nodular, infiltrative, ulcerative and polypoidal variety. There is poor enhancement of the wall of stomach and diagnosis is established with immunohistological diagnosis of deep gastric tissue biopsy.

Other Focal Gastric Lesions Mimicking Tumor

A number of conditions can mimic the neoplastic processes in the stomach and hence their importance cannot be ignored given the implications for management.

Inflammatory Pseudotumor/Myofibroblastic Tumor

The term inflammatory myofibroblastic tumor or pseudotumor denotes a pseudosarcomatous inflammatory lesion that contains spindle cells, myofibroblasts, plasma cells, lymphocytes and histiocytes which can frequently be a benign lesion or have a more aggressive behavior with propensity of local recurrence and a low rate of metastasis. The pathogenesis of IMT remains unclear, although various allergic, immunologic, and infectious mechanisms have been postulated. The myofibroblastic tumor cells often show reactivity for anaplastic lymphoma kinase (ALK). ALK-negative IMFTs have been associated with older patient age at presentation and can manifest with distant metastases.[73] In most cases IMT features mimic malignancy on upper flexible endoscopy and radiological imaging. For that reason, most IMT cases require surgical exploration and complete resection to obtain an accurate microscopic diagnosis.

It is seen mostly in children or young adults. It occurs in the soft tissue of children and young adults and lungs are the most commonly affected site. It is rare in abdomen, but when present, it is seen along terminal ileum or greater curvature of stomach.[74]

On CT, IMFTs appear as enhancing, aggressive intramural masses,[75] which can invade through the gastric wall into the peritoneal cavity or nearby organs. They can also have ulcerations and calcifications at occasions.[76] GIST, solitary fibrous tumor and schwannomas hence make the differentials because of similar appearences on CT imaging.

Ectopic Pancreatic Rests/Myoepithelial Hamartoma

This is also known as heterotopic, accessory, or aberrant pancreas and is defined as pancreatic tissue lacking anatomic and vascular continuity with the main body of the gland.

These lesions are most commonly found incidentally in asymptomatic patients mainly along the greater curvature of prepyloric region of stomach and duodenum. Some patients present with abdominal pain, gastrointestinal bleeding, and obstruction due to complications like pancreatitis, pseudocyst, insulinoma, and pancreatic cancer.[77]

Ectopic pancreas may manifest as a submucosal mass in the stomach or duodenum and may easily be misinterpreted as another submucosal tumor such as gastrointestinal stromal tumor (GIST) or leiomyoma. They can appear as well defined submucosal masses on either single or double contrast barium studies and can even have central umbilication and rarely barium may even be seen to enter into rudimentary ductal system. However, the typical location (prepyloric antrum and duodenum), endoluminal growth pattern, ill-defined border, prominent enhancement of overlying mucosa, and a long diameter/short diameter ratio of greater than 1.4 are considered significant CT features for differentiating ectopic pancreas from other tumors.[78]

Magnetic resonance imaging (MRI) is diagnostic, as ectopic pancreas follows pancreatic signal and enhancement pattern on all sequences.[79] Usually these lesions are flat (LD/SD >1.4), however they can acquire ovoid form and protrude endoluminally after intra glandular cyst formation. Small cystic areas within the mass represent dilated anomalous ducts.[47]

Gastric Duplication Cyst

Duplication of the alimentary tract is a rare congenital anomaly with the gastric duplication cysts (GDCs) being rarest, representing only 4% of all alimentary tract duplications. The common age of presentation being the first decade with approximately 67% manifest within the first year of life.[80] Classically, barium studies show an intramural filling defect indenting the gastric contour. Typical NCCT appearance is a spheric to ovoid nonenhancing cystic lesion in close approximation to greater curvature. Occasionally marginal calcifications may be present. Contrast-enhanced CT scan typically demonstrates a thick-walled cystic lesion with enhancement of the inner lining. EUS can further add to the diagnosis by demonstrating an echogenic internal mucosal layer and a hypoechoic intermediate muscular layer making the diagnosis of GDC highly likely.

The essential criteria for diagnosis of a gastric duplication cyst includes—contiguity of the cyst wall with that of the stomach; smooth muscles in the cyst wall, which is continuous with the muscle of the stomach; and lining of the cyst wall by either gastric epithelium or any other type of gut mucosa.[81]

Majority of gastric duplications are cystic (80%) and do not communicate with lumen of the stomach. Few of them are tubular and may show some communication. It is defined as tubular when the lumen is contiguous with the stomach lumen and cystic when the lumen is not contiguous.

Because most of the duplication cysts occur along the greater curvature of the stomach, they can potentially compress the adjacent organs such as pancreas, kidney, spleen, and adrenal gland and hence lesions arising from these organs become the differential diagnosis of duplication cysts.

As with the native gastric mucosa, the cyst lining may undergo erosions, ulceration, bleeding and regenerative changes. In noncommunicating cysts pressure necrosis of the mucosa may be seen due to increased fluid production. These changes may lead to bleeding into the cyst or perforation into the peritoneal cavity. Duplication cysts have the potential for neoplastic transformation especially by production of oncofetal antigens which raises the problem of a precancerous condition in long standing cases.

DUODENAL FOCAL LESIONS

Introduction

Prevalence of small bowel malignancies are 50 times less common than colonic neoplasms, duodenal involvement is seen in approximately 20% of these neoplasms. Their peak incidence is between the sixth and eight decade of life with nearly equal frequency of symptomatic benign and malignant duodenal tumors and a near equal sex distribution. It is speculated that protective factors might play role in the low incidence of these tumors as compared to adenocarcinoma of the colon and stomach like secretory immunoglobulins, rapid transit with lack of bacteria, small intestinal hydroxylases that could neutralize potential carcinogens and alkalinity can prevent formation of potential carcinogen. Benign tumors abound in duodenal cap, there being almost equal preponderance of benign and malignant tumors in second part, while malignant tumors predominate in the remaining part of duodenum.[82]

Symptoms can vary from obstructive jaundice due to obstruction of the ampulla, partial duodenal obstruction, or from bleeding due to ulceration with resultant hematemesis or melaena. Patients may occasionally also present with pancreatitis, intussusception, and symptoms due to the effects of hormone production in case of neuroendocrine tumors.

Flexure defect pseudotumor is a normal finding that occurs due to bunching of mucosal folds at the apex of the duodenal bulb where there is sudden change in the direction of duodenum. Annular pancreas, a relative common congenital abnormality may be confused with annular carcinoma. A prominent notch like defect in the lateral wall of the second part of duodenum causing eccentric narrowing without any accompanying ulceration is quite suggestive of annular pancreas and intact mucosa on endoscopy and CT can also help differentiate it.[48]

Double contrast barium meal and in selected cases, hypotonic duodenography are helpful modalities in fluoroscopic diagnostic evaluation of duodenal pathologies.

Carcinoid, leiomyoma and leiomyosarcomas have already been discussed.

BENIGN DUODENAL TUMORS

Adenomas

Most common benign tumors in the duodenum are adenomas and are of three main types including adenomatous polyps, Brunner's gland adenomas, or villous adenomas. Villous adenomas are discussed under malignant tumors due to high rate of their malignant transformation. They can present with anemia due to chronic blood loss or intermittent jaundice/pancreatitis due to blockage of ampula of vater.

Adenomatous Polyps

These polyps of duodenum are sessile, nodular, or pedunculated and usually <1 cm in diameter. They are commonly associated with familial polyposis coli, Peutz and Jegher's syndrome Gardner's syndrome and have potential to transform into villous adenomas and adenocarcinomas. Surveillance is required and it is recommended to do periodic upper gastrointestinal endoscopies with numerous biopsies. The polyps which are considered suspicious like large lesions, ulcerated or bleeding lesions, lesions with white or firm areas, and lesions found to have tubulovillous components are better removed and radical treatment is performed only if an invasive carcinoma is detected.

Brunner's gland adenomas: These adenomas present as pedunculated polyps, circumscribed nodular hyperplasia or diffuse nodular hyperplasia and have very low malignant potential. Brunner's gland adenoma is usually single and presents as filling defect. Histologically they resemble Brunner's gland and produce mucus. Treatment includes endoscopic or local open resection.[48]

Lipomas

These are smooth submucosal masses which have a characteristic yellow appearance on endoscopy. Most remain fairly small, but some may become pedunculated, cause pain and bleeding due to mucosal erosion and obstruction especially intussusception in younger patients. They can change shape due to palpation, peristalsis and gravity.[82] Local excision is usually sufficient for symptomatic lesions **(Fig. 21)**.

Other Benign Tumors

Other benign duodenal masses include hemangiomas and lymphangiomas which are well circumscribed submucosal masses, and are composed of predominantly blood vessels or lymphatic vessels, respectively and can be multifocal. Emergency laparotomy may be required if bleeding from hemangiomas is massive. Other multifocal lesions are neurofibromas and schwannomas which are poorly circumscribed lesions with wavy, fibrillary elements, identical to lesions seen at other places. These lesions mostly present with bleeding and excision of all symptomatic lesions is advocated.

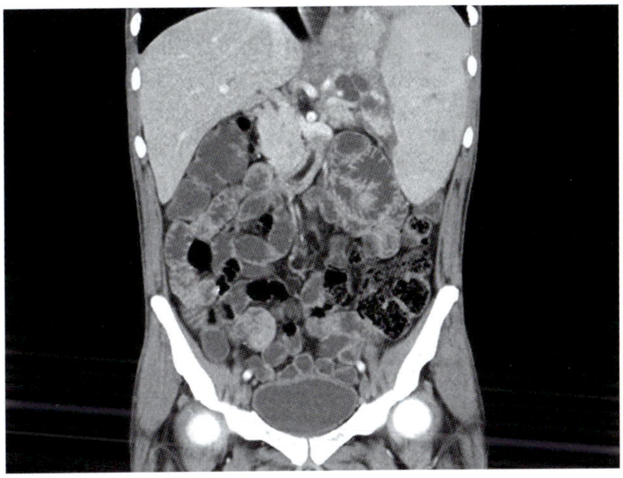

FIG. 21: Coronal CECT reveals a well-defined nonenhancing, submucosal hypodense lesion of fat attenuation seen along the 3rd part of duodenum extending along 4th part up to the DJ flexure suggestive of lipoma.

Malignant Duodenal Tumors

The common malignant lesions are adenocarcinoma, lymphoma, villous adenoma, GIST and carcinoid tumors. Associated malignancies are most often other adenocarcinomas of the intestinal tract, bladder carcinoma, and lymphomas. Squamous cell carcinoma of the duodenum is very rare and may arise in congenital anomalies such as duplications and diverticula. Most of the squamous cell carcinomas of the duodenum are metastatic tumors from other solid organs such as cervix or lung.[82] Close monitoring of all patients with duodenal tumors is therefore warranted.

Adenocarcinoma

Duodenum is most common site and accounts for 50% carcinomas of the small bowel overall however, primary adenocarcinomas of the duodenum is a rare entity and account for only 0.5% of all GI malignancies. *Perivaterian carcinoma* is a term that includes malignancies in and around ampulla, inclusive of malignancies of duodenum, ampulla, pancreas and distal common bile duct.

Adenocarcinomas can be ulcerating, infiltrating to polypoid and virtually all are mucin producing. The most common site is periampullary region, and approximately 20% of duodenal adenocarcinomas arise in villous adenomas. Rarely, they arise in a duodenal diverticulum or in patients with nontropical sprue.

Duodenoscopy is considered a more sensitive diagnostic procedure than barium studies or hypotonic duodenography as it detects small lesions that may otherwise be missed. An upper gastrointestinal series should however be performed to rule out synchronous small bowel lesions. Computed tomography is the preferred investigation to assess extraluminal spread, involvement of lymph nodes and distant metastasis. The lesion can be stenosing, polypoidal or ulceroinfiltrative and mostly present as nodular heterogeneously enhancing circumferential mural thickening **(Figs. 22A to C)**. If it involves ampulla, it causes dilatation of both main pancreatic duct and common bile duct giving "double duct sign".

The treatment of choice for adenocarcinoma of the duodenum is pancreatico-duodenectomy. Small tumors in the fourth portion of the duodenum only are however treated with distal duodenectomy and duodenojejunostomy.

Lymphoma

Although primary lymphoma of the duodenum is rare, the duodenum may be involved in systemic lymphoma, more so in AIDS patients.[82] Only 5% of all lymphomas are primary intestinal lymphoma and less than 10% of these are located in the duodenum. The only way to establish the diagnosis of primary lymphoma is to exclude the presence of the disease in other organs. Similar to gastric lymphoma most duodenal lymphomas are non-Hodgkin's lymphomas of B-cell origin. Only a few reports exist of Hodgkin's lymphomas or T-cell lymphomas. Involvement of the mesentery and the draining lymph nodes is common.

Lymphomas are difficult to distinguish from carcinoma preoperatively, though they tend to be larger than carcinomas. Often endoscopic biopsies are nondiagnostic as lymphomas arise in the submucosa. There may duodenal fold thickening, polypoidal masses and multiple nodules in patients of lymphoma. In advanced disease, however, perforation and multiple lesions are more common in lymphomas than in adenocarcinomas of the small bowel.

Lymphomas cause symptoms similar to those of duodenal and pancreatic carcinomas, and their appearance on computed tomography may be confused with pancreatic cancer. Histological cell type and grade help in deciding further management. Primary lymphoma of the duodenum is curable by surgery in only 40% of patients and unresectable cases of lymphoma requires radiotherapy and chemotherapy. Surgery in such cases is being used only to treat complications such has bleeding from high-grade lesions.

Villous Adenoma

Majority of the villous adenomas are located around ampulla and become symptomatic much earlier than other duodenal tumors due to obstructive jaundice. Approximately 40–50% of villous adenomas of the duodenum harbor adenocarcinomas, irrespective of the size of the tumor. Definite diagnosis of the villous adenomas is made by examination of entire tumor histologically after complete removal as 50% of the lesions are missed on endoscopic biopsy alone. Villous adenomas exhibit a characteristic 'cauliflower'or 'soap bubble' appearance on barium studies, caused by the trapping of barium in the crevices between the multiple frond-like projections of the tumor[1] **(Figs. 23A and B)**.

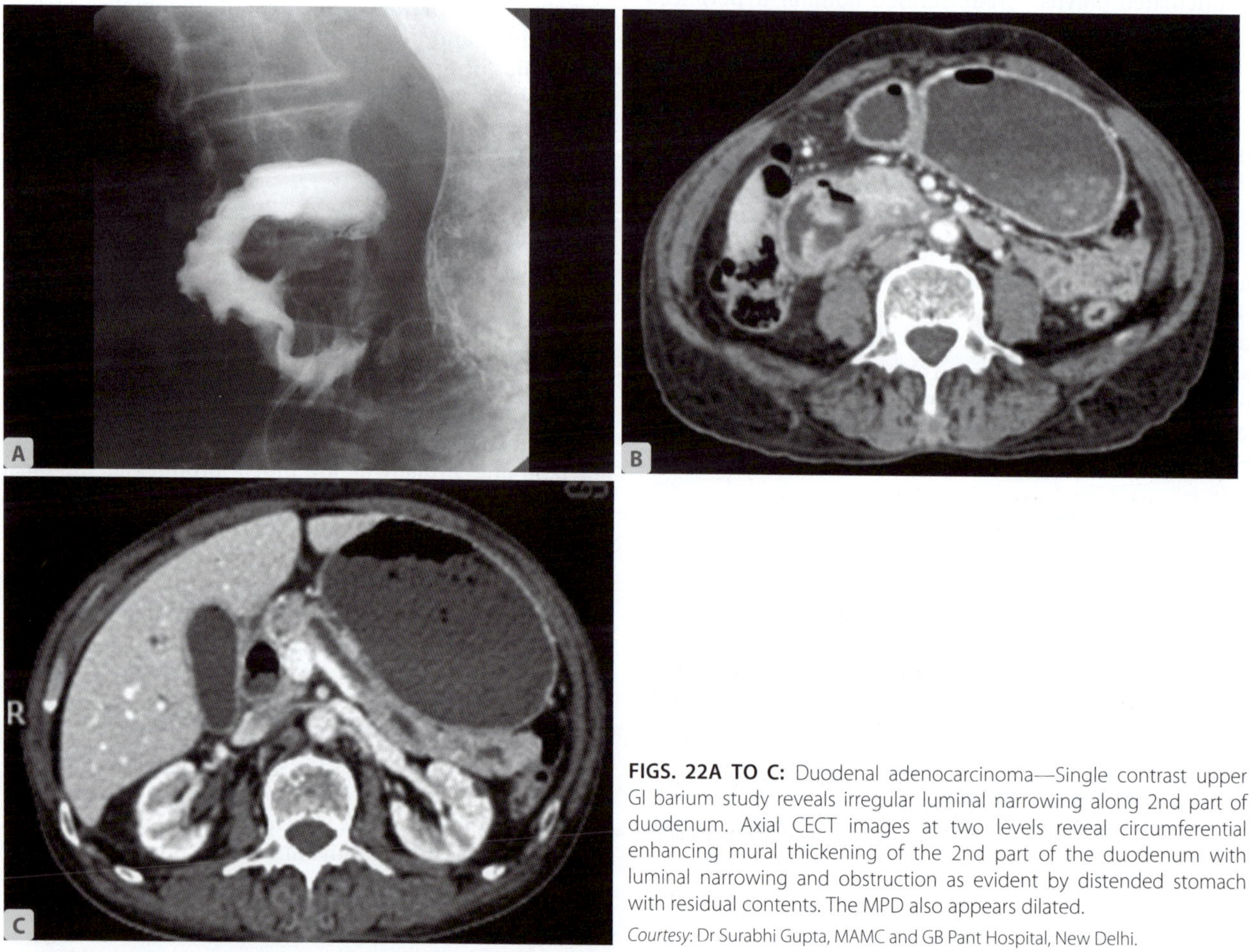

FIGS. 22A TO C: Duodenal adenocarcinoma—Single contrast upper GI barium study reveals irregular luminal narrowing along 2nd part of duodenum. Axial CECT images at two levels reveal circumferential enhancing mural thickening of the 2nd part of the duodenum with luminal narrowing and obstruction as evident by distended stomach with residual contents. The MPD also appears dilated.

Courtesy: Dr Surabhi Gupta, MAMC and GB Pant Hospital, New Delhi.

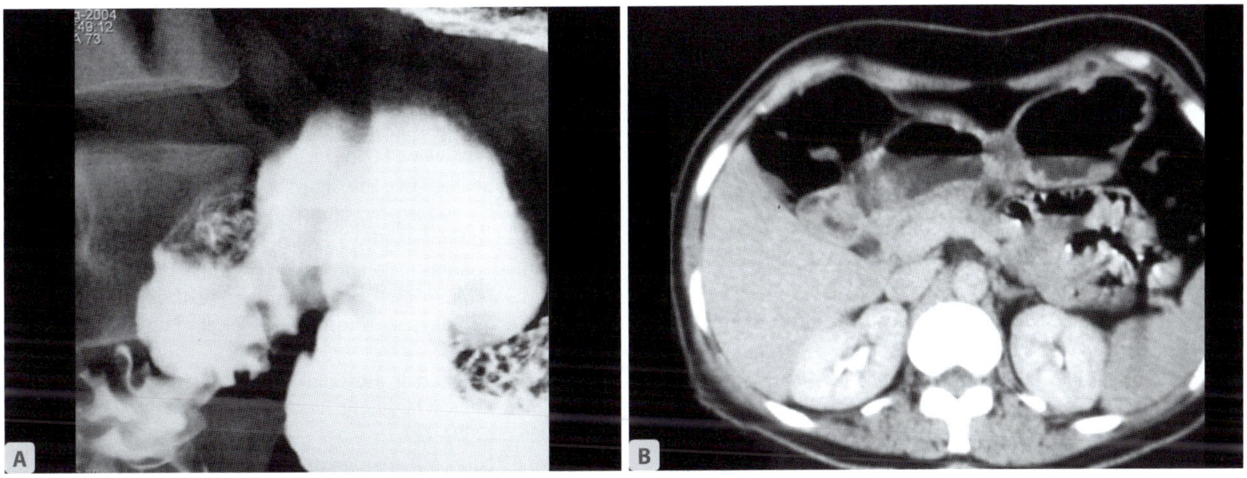

FIGS. 23A AND B: Villous adenoma: Polypoidal filling defect along lateral wall of duodenal bulb characteristic 'cauliflower' or 'soap-bubble' appearance on barium studies, caused by the trapping of barium in the crevices between the multiple frond-like projections of the tumor. CECT axial section reveals heterogeneously enhancing polypoidal mass lesion in first part of duodenum with nonenhancing fluid-filled hypodense linear areas symptoms of crevices between fronds with tracking of fluid in it.

Endoscopic resection is possible if the tumor is small and pedunculated. In all other cases duodenotomy is required. Since there is high incidence of co-existent malignancy, pancreaticoduodenectomy is the treatment of choice.

Secondary Involvement and Metastasis

Secondary involvement of duodenum by malignant process in adjacent viscera, like pancreas is fairly common and it is often not possible to distinguish a primary tumor of duodenum from a tumor of pancreas involving duodenum.[82]

Metastases to the duodenum can also occur and can present as filling defect with central ulceration and necrosis leading to classical "bull's eye" or "target" appearance. They are seen with metastasis from malignant melanoma **(Fig. 24)** and in patients with Kaposi's sarcoma.

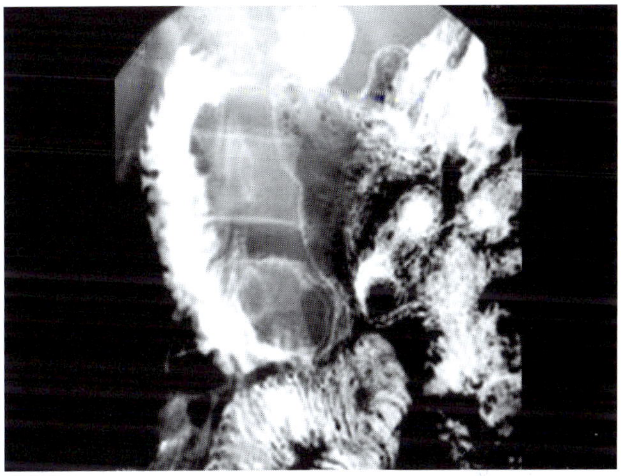

FIG. 24: Single contrast barium study showing large submucosal filling defect on enface view in the 3rd part of duodenum in a complaint of malignant melanoma symptoms of metastasis.

CONCLUSION

We should be aware of the advantages, pitfalls and limitations of the various imaging modalities in the diagnostic workup. Our aim should be to ensure early and accurate diagnosis of the tumors involving stomach and duodenum by judiciously using the various imaging modalities and techniques available and also ensure periodic surveillance for patients at risk.

REFERENCES

1. Grainger and Allison's Diagnostic Radiology—A Textbook of Medical Imaging, 5th edition, Churchill Livingstone; 2007.
2. Carmack SW, Genta RM, Graham DY, et al. Management of gastric polyps: a pathology based guide for gastroenterologists. Nat Rev Gastroenterol Hepatol. 2009;(6):331-41.
3. Stolte M, Sticht T, Eidt S, Ebert D, Finkenzeller G. Frequency, location, and age and sex distribution of various types of gastric polyp. Endoscopy. 1994;26(8):659-65.
4. Goddard AF, Badreldin R, Pritchard DM, Walker MM, Warren B. The management of gastric polyps. Gut. 2010;59(9):1270-6.
5. Chandrasekhara V, Ginsberg GG. Endoscopic management of gastrointestinal stromal tumors. Curr Gastroenterol Rep. 2011;13(6):532-9.
6. Shand AG, Taylor AC, Banerjee M, et al. Gastric fundic gland polyps in south-east Scotland: absence of adenomatous polyposis coli gene mutations and a strikingly low prevalence of *Helicobacter pylori* infection. J Gastroenterol Hepatol. 2002;17(11):1161-4.
7. el-Zimaity HM, Jackson FW, Graham DY. Fundic gland polyps developing during omeprazole therapy. Am J Gastroenterol. 1997;92(10):1858-60.

8. Bianchi LK, Burke CA, Bennett AE, Lopez R, Hasson H, Church JM. Fundic gland polyp dysplasia is common in familial adenomatous polyposis. Clin Gastroenterol Hepatol. 2008;6(2):180-5.
9. Abraham SC, Singh VK, Yardley JH, Wu TT. Hyperplastic polyps of the stomach: associations with histologic patterns of gastritis and gastric atrophy. Am J Surg Pathol. 2001;25(4):500-7.
10. Ohkusa T, Miwa H, Hojo M, et al. Endoscopic, histological and serologic findings of gastric hyperplastic polyps after eradication of *Helicobacter pylori*: comparison between responder and non-responder cases. Digestion. 2003;68(2-3):57-62.
11. Ljubicic N, Banic M, Kujundzic M, et al. The effect of eradicating *Helicobacter pylori* infection on the course of adenomatous and hyperplastic gastric polyps. Eur J Gastroenterol Hepatol. 1999;11(7):727-30.
12. Dirschmid K, Platz-Baudin C, Stolte M. Why is the hyperplastic polyp a marker for the precancerous condition of the gastric mucosa? Virchows Arch. 2006;448(1):80-4.
13. Ginsberg GG, Al-Kawas FH, Fleischer DE, Reilly HF, Benjamin SB. Gastric polyps: relationship of size and histology to cancer risk. Am J Gastroenterol. 1996;91(4):714-7.
14. Schmitz JM, Stolte M. Gastric polyps as precancerous lesions. Gastrointest Endosc Clin N Am. 1997;7(1):29-46.
15. Rugge M, Nitti D, Farinati F, et al. Non-invasive neoplasia of the stomach. Eur J Gastroenterol Hepatol. 2005;17:1191-6.
16. Calva D, Howe JR. Hamartomatous polyposis syndromes. Surg Clin North Am. 2008;88(4):779-817.
17. Beggs AD, Latchford AR, Vasen HF, et al. Peutz-Jeghers syndrome: a systematic review and recommendations for management. Gut. 2010;59(7):975-86.
18. Rubesin SE, Levine MS, Laufer I. Double-contrast upper gastrointestinal radiography: a pattern approach for disease of the stomach. Radiology. 2008;246:33-48.
19. Pisters PWT, Keslen DP, Tepper JE. Cancer of the stomach.In: Devita VT, Lawrence TS, Rosenberg SA (Eds), Cancer: principals and practice of oncology, 8th edition, Lippincott, Williams and Wilkins. 2008.pp.1043-79.
20. Parsonnet J, Friedman GD, Vandersteen DP, et al. *Heliobacter pylori* infection and the risk of gastric carcinoma. N Engl J Med. 1991;325:1127-31.
21. Ramon JM, Sera L, Cerdo C, et al. Dietary factors and gastric cancer risk: A case control study in Spain. Cancer. 1993;71:1731-5.
22. Hamashima C, Shibuya D, Yamazaki H, et al. The Japanese guidelines for gastric cancer screening. Jpn J Clin Oncol. 2008; 38:259.
23. Maruyama M, Baba Y. Diagnosis of the invasive depth of gastric cancer. Abdom Imaging. 1994;19:532-6.
24. Japanese Gastric Cancer Association. Japanese classification of gastric carcinoma—2nd English edition. Gastric Cancer. 1998. pp.10-24.
25. Low VH, Levine MS, Rubesin SE, et al. Diagnosis of gastric carcinoma: sensitivity of double-contrast barium studies. Am J Roentgenol. 1994;162:329-34.
26. Levine MS, Rubesin SE, Laufer I. Barium studies in modern radiology: do they have a role? Radiology. 2009;250:18-22.
27. Gore RM, Levine MS, Gahremani GG, et al. Gastric cancer: Radiologic diagnosis. Radiol Clin N Am. 1997;35:311-29.
28. Furukawa K, Miyahara R, Itoh A, et al. Diagnosis of the invasion depth of the gastric cancer using MDCT with virtual gastroscopy: comparison with staging with endoscopic ultrasound. Am J Roentgenol. 2011;197:867-75.
29. Washington K. Editorial: 7th edition of the AJCC Cancer Staging Manual: Stomach. Ann Surg Oncol. 2010;17:3077-9.
30. Kwee RM, Kwee TC. Imaging in local staging of gastric cancer: a systematic review. J Clin Oncol. 2007;25:2107-16.
31. Hwang SW, Lee DH, Lee SH, et al. Preoperative staging of gastric cancer by endoscopic ultrasonography and multidetector row computed tomography. J Gastroenterol Hepatol. 2010;25: 512-18.
32. Pradhan Gaurav S. Benign lesions of stomach and small intestine. AIIMS-MAMC-PGI's Comprehensive Textbook of Diagnostic Radiology, Jaypee Brothers Medical Publishers. 2016.pp. 1158-72.
33. Edelman Robert R, Hesselink John R, Zlatkin Michael B, Crees John S. Clinical Magnetic Resonance Imaging Vol-3, 3rd edition. 2006.pp.2684-721.
34. Kim Il Young. MR imaging of gastric carcinoma. In: Ismaili N (Ed). Management of Gastric Cancer. InTech. 2011. pp. 19-36.
35. Ghai S, Pattison J, Ghai S, O'Malley ME, Khalili K, Stephens. Primary Gastrointestinal Lymphoma: Spectrum of Imaging Findings with Pathologic Correlation. Radiographics. 2007; 27: 1371-88.
36. Lim JS, Kim MJ, Yun MJ, et al. Comparison of CT and 18F FDG-PET for detecting peritoneal metastases on the preoperative evaluation of gastric carcinoma. Korean J Radiol. 2006;7:249-56.
37. Isaacson PG. Gastrointestinal lymphomas of T and B-cell types. Mod Pathol. 1999;12:151-8.
38. Dawson IM, Cornes JS, Morson BC. Primary malignant tumors of the intestinal tract. Br J Surg. 1961;49:80-9.
39. Rohatiner A, d'Amore F, Coiffier B, et al. Report on a workshop convened to discuss the pathological and staging classifications of gastrointestinal tract lymphoma. Ann Oncol. 1994;5: 397-400.
40. Yoo CC, Levine MS, Furth EE, et al. Gastric mucosa-associated lymphoid tissue lymphoma: radiographic findings in six patients. Radiology. 1998;208:239-43.
41. Parsonnet J, Hansen S, Rodriguez L, et al. Recent developments in our understanding of gastric lymphoma. Am J Surg Pathol. 1996;20(Suppl I):S1-7.
42. Miller FH, Kochman ML, Talamonti MS, Ghahremani GG, Gore RM. Gastric cancer: radiologic staging. Radiol Clin North Am. 1997;35:331-49.
43. Ciftci AO, Tanyel FC, Kotiloglu E, Hicsonmez A. Gastric lymphoma causing gastric outlet obstruction. J Pediatr Surg. 1996;31: 1424-6.
44. Guglielmi G, Schiavon F, Cammarota T (Eds). Radiologia geriatrica, Springer; 2006.
45. Radan L, Fischer D, Bar-shalom R, et al. FDG avidity and PET/CT patterns in primary gastric lymphoma. Eur J Nucl Med Mol Imaging. 2008;35:1428-4330.
46. Levy AD, Sobin LH. Gastrointestinal Carcinoids: Imaging Features with Clinicopathologic Comparison. Radio Graphics. 2007;27:237-57.
47. Virmani V, Khandelwal A, Sethi V, Hill MF, Fasih N, Kielar A. Neoplastic stomach lesions and their mimickers: spectrum of imaging manifestations. Cancer Imaging. 2012;12:269-78.
48. Chappuis CW, Divincenti FC, Cohn I Jr. Villous tumors of the duodenum. Ann Surg. 1989;209:593-9.
49. Gong J, Kang W, Zhu J, Xu J. CT and MR imaging of gastrointestinal stromal tumor of stomach: a pictorial review. Quant Imaging Med Surg. 2012;2(4):274-9.

50. Heinrich MC, Corless CL, Duensing A, et al. PDGFRA activating mutations in gastrointestinal stromal tumors. Science. 2003;299(5607):708-10.
51. Lee NK, Kim S, Kim GH, et al. Hypervascular subepithelial gastrointestinal masses: CT-pathologic correlation. Radiographics. 2010;30:1915-34.
52. Kang HC, Menias CO, Gaballah AH, Shroff S, Taggart MW, Garg N, Elsayes KM. Beyond the GIST: Mesenchymal Tumors of the Stomach. Radiographics. 2013;33:1673-90.
53. Levy AD, Remotti HE, Thompson WM, Sobin LH, Miettinen M. Gastrointestinal stromal tumors: radiologic features with pathologic correlation. Radiographics. 2003;23(2):283-304.
54. Salamah AB, Prokop M, Uffmann M, Pokieser P, Teleky B, Lechner G. Dedicated Multidetector CT of the Stomach: Spectrum of Diseases. Radiographics. 2003;23:625-44.
55. Kim H-C, Lee JM, Kim KW, et al. Gastrointestinal stromal tumors of the stomach: CT findings and prediction of malignancy. AJR. 2004;183:893-8.
56. DeMatteo RP, Lewis JJ, Leung D, Mudan SS, Woodruff JM, Brennan MF. Two hundred gastrointestinal stromal tumors: recurrence patterns and prognostic factors for survival. Ann Surg. 2000;231(1):51-8.
57. Espinosa I, Lee CH, Kim MK, et al. A novel monoclonal antibody against DOG1 is a sensitive and specific marker for gastrointestinal stromal tumors. Am J Surg Pathol. 2008;32(2):210-8.
58. Demetri GD, Benjamin R, Blanke CD, et al. NCCN task force report: optimal management of patients with gastrointestinal stromal tumors (GIST)—expansion and update of NCCN clinical practice guidelines. J Natl Compr Cancer Netw. 2004;2:S1–26.
59. Joensuu H, Roberts PJ, Sarlomo-Rikala M, et al. Effect of the tyrosine kinase inhibitor STI571 in a patient with a metastatic gastrointestinal stromal tumor. N Engl J Med. 2001;344:1052-6.
60. Blanke C, Joensuu G, Demetri M, et al. Longterm follow up of advanced gastrointestinal stromal tumor (GIST) patients treated with imatinib mesylate (abstr). In: Proceedings of the 2004 Gastrointestinal Cancers Symposium: Current Status and Future Directions for Prevention and Management. Alexandria, Va: American Society of Clinical Oncology. 2004;43.
61. Hong X, Choi H, Loyer EM, Benjamin RS, Trent JC, Charnsangavej C. Gastrointestinal Stromal Tumor: Role of CT in Diagnosis and in Response Evaluation and Surveillance after Treatment with Imatinib. Radiographics. 2006;26:481-95.
62. Jayaraman MV, Mayo-Smith WW, Movson JS, Dupuy DE, Wallach MT. CT of the Duodenum: An Overlooked Segment Gets Its Due. Radiographics. 2001;21:S147-60.
63. Thompson WM, Kende AI, Levy AD. Imaging characteristics of gastric lipomas in 16 adult and pediatric patients. Am J Roentgenol. 2003;181(4):981-5.
64. Ferrozzi F, Tognini G, Bova D, et al. Lipomatous tumors of the stomach: CT findings and differential diagnosis. J Comput Assist Tomogr. 2000;24:854-8.
65. Miettinen M, Lasota J. Gastrointestinal stromal tumors: definition, clinical, histological, immunohistochemical, and molecular genetic features and differential diagnosis. Virchows Arch. 2001;438(1):1-12.
66. Hur BY, Kim SH, Choi JY, et al. Gastroduodenal glomus tumors: differentiation from other subepithelial lesions based on dynamic contrast-enhanced CT findings. Am J Roentgenol. 2011;197(6):1351-9.
67. Lee MJ, Lim JS, Kwon JE, et al. Gastric true leiomyoma: computed tomographic findings and pathological correlation. J Comput Assist Tomogr. 2007;31(2):204-8.
68. Park SO, Han JK, Kirn TK, et al. Unusual gastric tumors: radiologic pathologic correlation. Radiographics. 1999;19: 1435-46.
69. Raber MH, CMPZ des Plantes, Vink R, Vink R, Klaase JM. "Gastric schwannoma presenting as an incidentaloma on CT-scan and MRI," Gastroenterology Research. 2010;3(6): 276-80.
70. Hong HS, Ha HK, Won HJ, et al. Gastric schwannomas: radiological features with endoscopic and pathological correlation. Clin Radiol. 2008;63(5):536-42.
71. Miettinen M, Paal E, Lasota J, Sobin LH. Gastrointestinal glomus tumors: a clinicopathologic, immunohistochemical, and molecular genetic study of 32 cases. Am J Surg Pathol. 2002;26(3):301-11.
72. Levy AD, Abbott RM, Rohrmann CA Jr, Frazier AA, Kende A. Gastrointestinal hemangiomas: imaging findings with pathologic correlation in pediatric and adult patients. Am J Roentgenol. 2001;177(5):1073-81.
73. Coffin CM, Hornick JL, Fletcher CD. Inflammatory myofibroblastic tumor: comparison of clinicopathologic, histologic, and immunohistochemical features including ALK expression in atypical and aggressive cases. Am J Surg Pathol. 2007;31(4):509-20.
74. Bjelovic M, Micev M, Spica B, Babic T, Gunjic D, Djuric A, Pesko P. Primary inflammatory myofibroblastic tumor of the stomach in an adult woman: a case report and review of the literature. World Journal of Surgical Oncology. 2013;11:35.
75. Karnak I, Senocak ME, Ciftci AO, et al. Inflammatory myofibroblastic tumor in children: diagnosis and treatment. J Pediatr Surg. 2001;36(6):908-12.
76. Narla LD, Newman B, Spottswood SS, et al. Inflammatory pseudotumor. Radiographics. 2003;23:719-29.
77. Grendell JH, Ermak TH. Anatomy, histology, embryology, and developmental anomalies of the pancreas. In: Sleisenger and Fordtran's gastrointestinal and liver disease. Philadelphia, PA: Saunders. 1998.pp.761-71.
78. Kim JY, Lee JM, Kim KW, Park HS, Choi Y, Kim SH, Kim MA, Lee JY, Han JK, Choi BI. Ectopic Pancreas: CT Findings with Emphasis on Differentiation from Small Gastrointestinal Stromal Tumor and Leiomyoma. Radiology: 2009;252(1).
79. Okuhata Y, Maebayashi T, Furuhashi S, et al. Characteristics of ectopic pancreas in dynamic gadolinium-enhanced MRI. Abdom Imaging. 2008;35:85-7.
80. Singh JP, Rajdeo H, Bhuta K, Savino JA. Gastric Duplication Cyst: Two Case Reports and Review of the Literature. Hindawi Publishing Corporation Case Reports in Surgery. 2013, Article ID 605059, 4 pages.
81. Horne G, Ming-Lum C, Kirkpatrick AW, Parker RL. "High-grade neuroendocrine carcinoma arising in a gastric duplication cyst: a case report with literature review." International Journal of Surgical Pathology. 2007;(15)2:187-91.
82. Winfield RD1, Hochwald SN, Vogel SB, Hemming AW, Liu C, Cance WG, Grobmyer SR. Presentation and management of gastrointestinal stromal tumors of the duodenum. Am Surg. 2006;72(8):719-22; discussion 722-3.

CHAPTER

94

Small Bowel Tumors

Rashmi Dixit, Gaurav Shanker Pradhan, Anju Garg

INTRODUCTION

Tumors of the small bowel both benign and malignant are quite uncommon, this despite the fact the small bowel constitutes about 75% of the total length of the gastrointestinal tract and 90% of its mucosal surface. It also lies between two areas of high cancer risk, i.e. the colon and the stomach yet only about 3–5% of all GI tumors and less than 2% of all gastrointestinal malignancies arise in the small bowel.[1-3] However with advances in endoscopy and imaging an increasing number of small bowel tumors are being diagnosed.

About 40 different histologic types of tumors have been described in the small bowel. Although over 2/3 of lesions found at autopsy are benign, most symptomatic lesions and those detected at surgery tend to be malignant.[1] The major tumors are listed in **Table 1**.

TABLE 1: Small bowel tumors and polyps.

1. Epithelial Adenoma Carcinoma Neuroendocrine tumors/carcinoid Mixed carcinoid-adenocarcinoma Others
2. Nonepithelial/mesenchymal Lipoma Leiomyoma Hemangioma/lymphangioma Gastrointestinal stromal tumors (GIST) Leiomyosarcoma Kaposi's sarcoma Others
3. Lymphoid tissue Lymphomas
4. Neurogenic Neurofibroma Schwannoma
5. Secondary tumors/metastasis
6. Polyps

SMALL BOWEL CARCINOGENESIS–PATHOGENESIS

The exact reason for the low incidence of malignancy in the small intestine is not certain but several theories have been proposed including liquid contents of the small bowel causing less mucosal irritation, relatively rapid transit, lower bacterial load in small bowel and high levels of IgA due to increased lymphoid tissue.[1,4]

Certain syndromes or conditions are associated with increased incidence of specific histologic types of small intestine tumors, e.g. Peutz-Jeghers syndrome, familial adenomatous polyposis, Lynch syndrome and Gardner's syndrome predispose to adenoma and adenocarcinoma and von Recklinghausen's disease or neurofibromatosis to gastrointestinal stromal tumors. Gardner's syndrome also predisposes to multiple desmoid tumors.[1,4]

DIAGNOSTIC TECHNIQUES

The clinical presentation of most small bowel tumors is non-specific. The diagnosis is further challenged by lack of easy endoscopic access and relative rarity of disease leading to low index of suspicion. The various techniques available to evaluate the small intestine tumors are—conventional small bowel follow through examination, conventional enteroclysis, ultrasound, CT and MR (including CT and MR enterography and enteroclysis) and endoscopic techniques like capsule endoscopy, push enteroscopy.

Early diagnosis of small bowel tumors is challenging and currently there are no definite guidelines as to which technique should be used first, but it would be reasonable to use noninvasive imaging before more invasive and expensive endoscopic techniques are used.

Barium meal follow through may show some abnormal pattern in up to 83% cases of small bowel tumors however, direct evidence of presence of tumor is seen in only 30–44% cases. Enteroclysis has a sensitivity of 90–95% for the detection of small bowel tumors, but the technique is invasive and provides little information on mural and extramural extent of tumor.[5,6] With the advent of high end multiple detector computed tomography (MDCT) scanners and widespread use of CT enterography, conventional enteroclysis is rarely performed these days.

Ultrasound examination is generally not used for the primary diagnosis of small bowel tumors, however, because it is often the first investigation performed in nonspecific abdominal complaints it may detect a bowel mass especially when this is large. Malignant mass may be seen as asymmetric wall thickening, 'target lesion' or occasionally as a large exophytic mass where the organ of origin may not be clear like in gastrointestinal stromal tumors. Increased vascularity may be seen within the lesion on colour Doppler. Contrast enhanced ultrasound has also been used in bowel masses especially for follow-up of treated gastrointestinal stromal tumors. Associated findings such as nodal involvement and ascites can also be seen.[7]

Conventional CT has sensitivity of around 80% for small bowel tumors, however, CT/MR enterography have sensitivity of 85–95%.[4,8,9] CT enterography is generally the current standard practice given the excellent sensitivity to detect even small tumors due to superior tumor to background contrast enhancement owing to the use of neutral oral contrast. Due to its higher cost, lower spatial resolution as compared to CT and artifacts due to bowel motion MR enteroclysis/enterography is generally not used as a first line investigation unless radiation dose due to repeat examinations is a concern. However, MR of the gastrointestinal tract is gaining clinical acceptance. Cine sequences or MR fluoroscopy may also be performed during the exam allowing functional evaluation of small bowel as well. In some studies, MR enteroclysis was found to be more sensitive than CT enteroclysis in patients with Crohn's disease.[1,4]

Ultrasound and CT may also be used to guide percutaneous biopsy or needle aspiration .

^{18}F-FDG-PET/CT may be useful in patients with adenocarcinoma, lymphomas and sarcomas mainly for staging. PET-CT with octreotide analogs is useful in detection and staging of carcinoids.[4]

Hybrid PET-MRI is a promising new technique that has very limited availability as yet but appears to hold promise for evaluation of gastrointestinal malignancy. It combines the high contrast and spatial resolution of MR with the high sensitivity of PET and allows use of multiple sequences for combined functional and anatomical evaluation. This may allow for improved staging and restaging of disease status after treatment.[10]

Capsule endoscopy is a relatively new technique used by gastroenterologists, that can screen the entire small bowel. Capsule endoscopy may detect lesions not detected on standard push endoscopy and imaging. It has higher sensitivity to detect tumors and polyps than push enteroscopy which evaluates only the first 120 cm of the small bowel beyond the ligament of Treitz. However, some lesions may be missed due to poor bowel preparation, orientation of camera away from lesion and rapid or delayed small bowel transit. It is also not very accurate in exact localization and size estimation and is contraindicated in patients with bowel stricture, intestinal obstruction, swallowing and motility disorders.[4,5]

Balloon enteroscopy allows evaluation of the entire small bowel. Double balloon enteroscopy (DBE) has a sensitivity of about 86% in detecting small bowel tumors which is comparable with capsule endoscopy. The decision to use single or double balloon enteroscopy is the investigator's choice, as no definite advantage of single balloon enteroscopy has been demonstrated. Capsule endoscopy is less invasive and is generally preferred as the initial exam although the two can be complementary as abnormal areas can generally not be biopsied on capsule endoscopy. All endoscopic methods are limited in the evaluation submucosal and mural lesions.[4,5]

BENIGN TUMORS AND POLYPS

Adenoma

Adenomas represent the most common benign tumor of the small intestine. Histologically, these can be tubular, villous or tubulovillous. Although adenomas are benign they are considered premalignant. Large size and villous component are associated with an increased risk of malignant transformation. They may occur as a pedunculated polyp or sessile polypoid lesion, usually 2–3 cm in size.

On barium studies, when seen in profile, they are seen as smooth or lobulated lesions forming acute angles with the bowel wall. In pedunculated lesions the pedicle can also be visualized. Sometimes the surface may appear granular due to barium trapping in the interstices. They may act as a lead point for intussusception.[11,12]

Adenomas are difficult to appreciate on routine CT or MR but may be seen on CT/MR enteroclysis or enterography. On CT enteroclysis they are seen as well-defined soft tissue lesions with moderate enhancement on post-contrast images and a clear fat plane around the lesion **(Figs. 1A and B)**.[13,14] On MR enteroclysis adenomas are seen as homogeneously enhancing intraluminal masses on fat saturated postcontrast T1W images, while on T2W images they appear as low signal intensity intraluminal masses. Generally there is no proximal dilatation.[15,16]

Inflammatory fibroid polyps also known as Vanek's tumors are an important differential diagnosis which are predominantly located in the ileum and represent rare non-neoplastic pseudotumorous submucosal lesions of uncertain etiology. They can be sessile or pedunculated polypoid lesions. Histologically, IFPs consist of mass of loose fibrous connective tissue, with presence of inflammatory infiltrate consisting of large number eosinophils. On CT a well-defined, smooth, homogeneous, low attenuation, nonenhancing or hypoenhancing polypoid mass is seen **(Figs. 2A to C)**.[17]

Multiple adenomas can be found in the hereditary polyposis syndromes. A major risk factor is familial adenomatous polyposis (FAP) where 80% patients develop duodenal adenomas. Patients frequently develop jejunal and ileal polyps also.[4]

Treatment includes endoscopic resection for pedunculated tumors and surgical removal of large sessile tumors.[1,4]

Lipoma

Lipomas account for 15–20% of all small intestinal neoplasms. The small bowel is the most common site in the

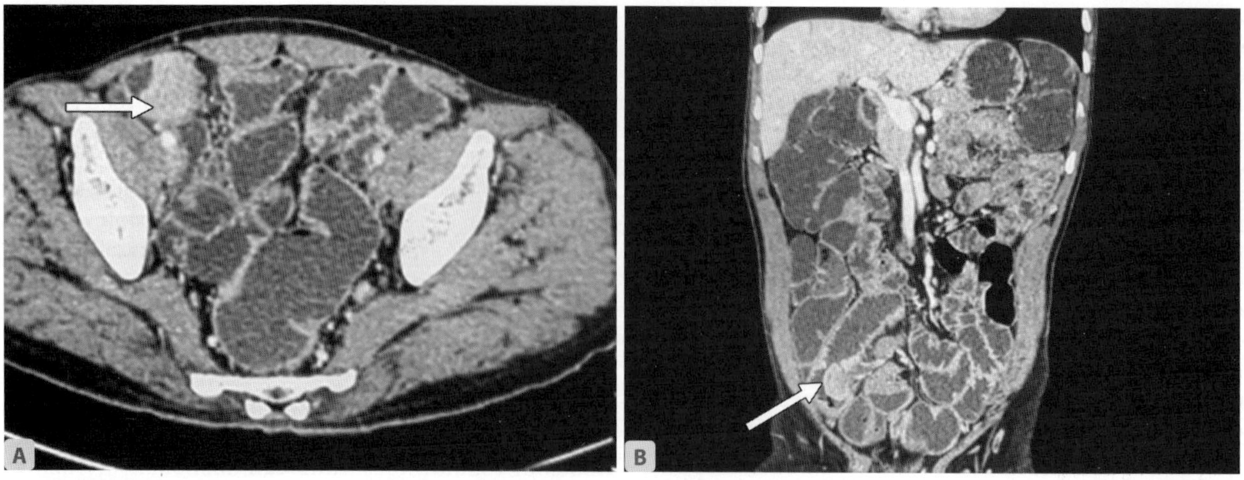

FIGS. 1A AND B: Small bowel adenoma: Axial (A) and coronal (B) CT enteroclysis images reveal a sessile polypoid moderately enhancing mass lesion in the ileum (arrows) with normal surrounding fat planes suggestive of an adenoma.

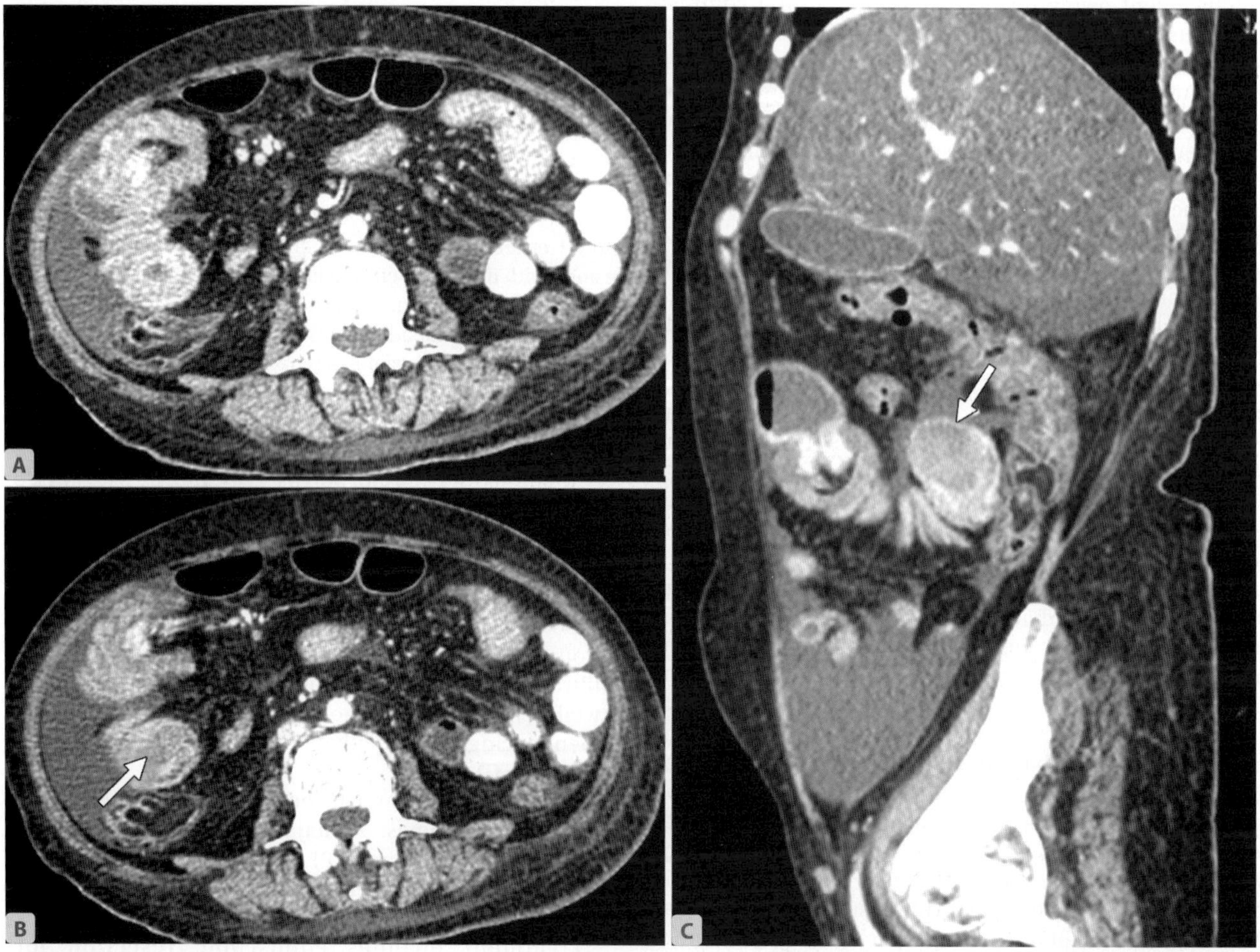

FIGS. 2A TO C: Inflammatory fibroid polyp: Axial (A and B) and sagittal (C) images show free fluid in the right paracolic region and telescoping of proximal ileum into a distal ileal loop along with a sleeve of mesenteric fat and vessels consistent with ileo-ileal intussusception. A well-defined poorly enhancing hypodense polyp is seen at the apex (arrows in B and C) which was proven to be an inflammatory fibroid polyp on histopathological examination.

gastrointestinal (GI) tract after the colon and within the small bowel ileum is the most common location. The vast majority of these are submucosal tumors that are composed of mature adipose tissue. About 5–10%, may be subserosal. Small lesions are mostly asymptomatic whereas larger lesions may produce intussusception, rarely surface ulceration may occur leading to gastrointestinal bleed.[13,16,18]

They can be sessile or pedunculated producing a sharply marginated ovoid or spherical polypoid defect on barium studies which may change shape with compression or on different views due to pliability. Sometimes the low density of fat may be apparent. Usually they are solitary but occasionally may be multiple. On CT lipomas are seen as a low density fat attenuation masses (between -60 to -120 HU) in the wall of the small intestine **(Figs. 3A to C)**. No contrast enhancement or nonfatty elements are seen, however, sometimes few linear strands of soft tissue attenuation may be seen at the base corresponding to prominent fibrovascular septae on histopathology. Such tumors may at times show surface ulceration and must not be mistaken for liposarcoma—the septae being presumably enlarged due to inflammation associated with the ulcer.[18] On MR enterography they are seen as well-circumscribed masses which are bright on T1W, match the signal on intra-abdominal fat on T2W images with signal suppression on fat saturated images and do not show contrast enhancement.[16]

Leiomyoma

True leiomyomas of the small intestine are extremely rare most lesions previously diagnosed as leiomyomas may actually represent gastrointestinal stromal tumors (GIST). They can be seen as round or crescentic predominantly submucosal masses showing homogeneous enhancement on CT or MR. They are virtually impossible to distinguish from small gastrointestinal stromal tumors on imaging. Occasionally intraluminal polyp or extraluminal masses may be seen.[1,13]

Hemangioma

Small bowel hemangiomas are rare most often situated in the jejunal submucosa and can be sessile, pedunculated or infilterative. Most lesions represent venous malformations rather than true tumors (hemangioma). Some cases can occur in association of syndromes like blue rubber bleb nevus and Klippel Trenaunay syndrome. In contrast to most other benign tumors most are symptomatic and commonly produce manifest or occult gastrointestinal bleed. Other symptoms include pain, obstruction due to intussusception and rarely perforation.[1,13]

On enteroclysis they may produce a nodular, pliable submucosal filling defect.[11] On contrast enhanced CT enterography they can be seen as intensely enhancing lesion

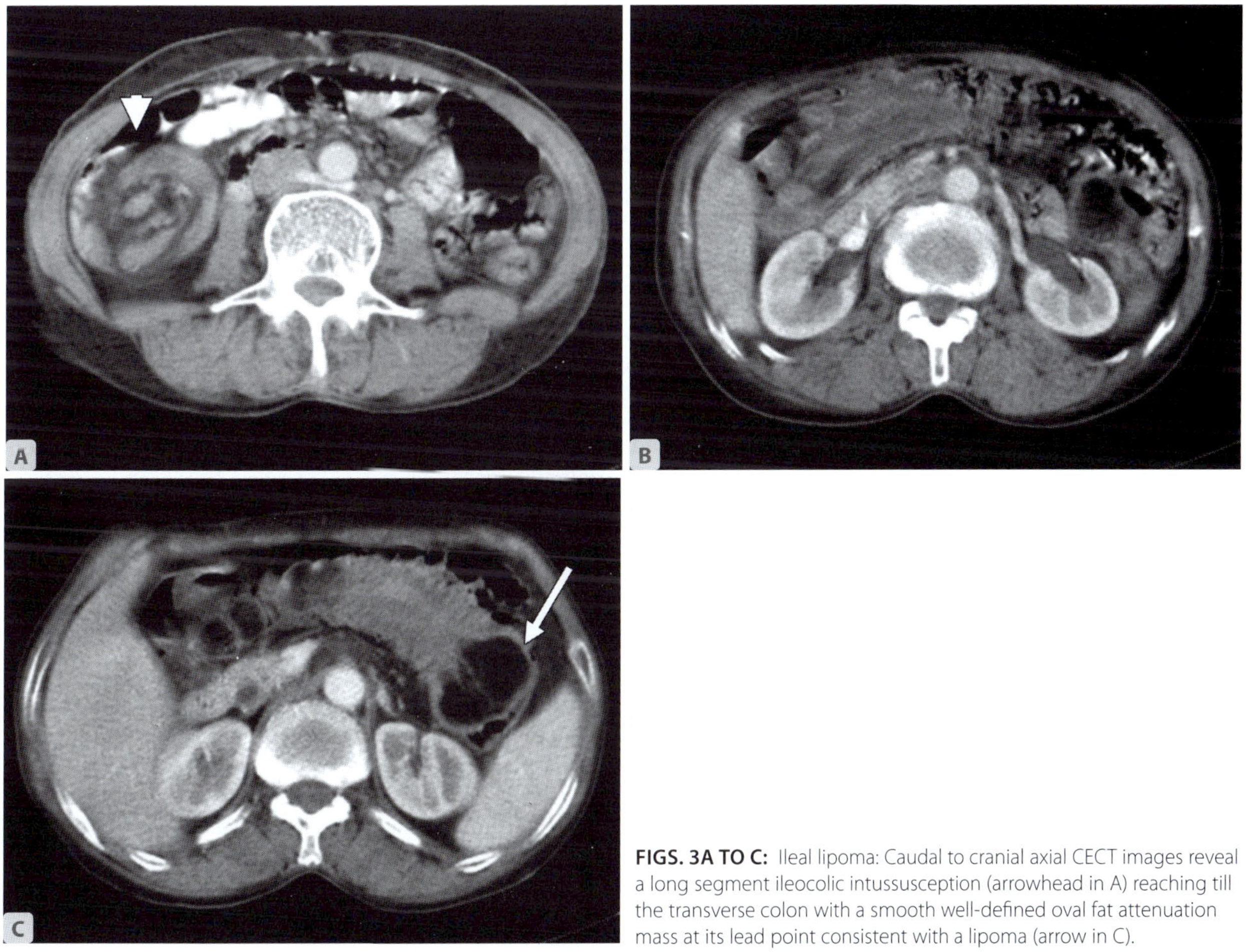

FIGS. 3A TO C: Ileal lipoma: Caudal to cranial axial CECT images reveal a long segment ileocolic intussusception (arrowhead in A) reaching till the transverse colon with a smooth well-defined oval fat attenuation mass at its lead point consistent with a lipoma (arrow in C).

with or without phleboliths. Progressive enhancement may be seen with multiphase CT.[19,20] On MR they are T1 hypointense, markedly hyperintense on T2W images with no loss of signal on fat saturated images. Nodular enhancement has been reported in the arterial phase and homogeneous enhancement in the delayed phase.[16]

Neurogenic Tumor

Neurogenic tumors are relatively rare arising from the intramural neural plexus. Most often these are nonplexiform neurofibromas occurring as well-defined subserosal masses on the antimesenteric border, difficult to detect on contrast examinations. They can be multiple especially in patients with neurofibromatosis. Occasionally they are submucosal when it is difficult to distinguish them from other submucoasl masses on imaging. Schwannomas usually occur as solitary masses. Plexiform neurofibromas can also involve the small bowel.[13]

POLYPOSIS SYNDROMES INVOLVING THE SMALL BOWEL

Although a number of polyposis syndromes can involve the small intestine the important ones are; Peutz-Jeghers syndrome; familial adenomatous polyposis generalized juvenile polyposis; and Cronkhite-Canada syndrome. These disorders are characterized by the presence of multiple polyps affecting all or parts of the gastrointestinal tract. They are distinguished by the way they can be inherited, location, associated extraintestinal symptoms and the microscopic appearance of the polyps.

Peutz-Jeghers Syndrome

Peutz-Jeghers syndrome (PJS) is a rare autosomal dominant syndrome but has incomplete penetrance.[1,11] It is associated with mutation of STK II tumor suppression gene resulting in hamartomas throughout the gastrointestinal tract. The characteristic feature of PJS polyp is the smooth muscle core arising from muscularis mucosae extending into the polyp. The polyps are most common in the small bowel and less so in the stomach and colon. They tend to be multiple and vary in size and shape. These can be sessile or pedunculated and produce intraluminal filling defects.[1,11,21]

The polyps, being firm are especially prone to intussusception and may cause bleeding as well **(Figs. 4A to D)**. Although the polyps of PJS, being hamartomatous, are benign, the syndrome is associated with a definitely increased risk of small bowel adenocarcinoma. It is not clear whether this arises from the polyp or from coexisting adenomas. PJS is associated with 10–18 fold increase in gastrointestinal cancers.[1,11]

In patients presenting with multiple polyps the presence of multiple cororectal polyps and duodenal polyps (adenomas) favors the diagnosis of familial adenomatous polyposis (FAP) while the presence of small number of large polyps in the distal duodenum and jejunum favors PJS.[1,11] Other associated findings which help to clinch the diagnosis of PJS include pigmented lesions on the buccal mucosa, lips and on the skin especially hands and feet.[1,21]

Management of these polyps may be done by enteroscopic clearance. Intestinal resection is limited to the necessary minimum when required. The primary aim of polyp removal is to present intussusception.[1]

Cowden's Disease[4,21]

Cowden's disease consists of gastric, small bowel and colonic hamartomas and facial trichilemmomas.

Familial Adenomatous Polyposis[1,4,21]

Familial adenomatous polyposis is an inherited, autosomal dominant syndrome characterized by the presence of multiple adenomatous polyps in the colon 80% of patients can also have adenomas involving the small intestine most common in the duodenum. Extra-intestinal manifestation of familial adenomatous polyposis (FAP) include osteomas of mandible, long bones and skull, thyroid malignancy, adrenal adenoma/carcinoma, CNS tumors (particularly medulloblastoma) and desmoid tumors.

Turcot's syndrome and Gardner's syndrome are also associated with multiple adenomatous small bowel polyps.

Cronkhite-Canada Syndrome[21]

It is characterized by several intestinal polyps of the inflammatory type, hyperpigmentation, dystrophy of nails, alopecia and diarrhea. The onset is usually after 40 years. The polyps are most commonly found in the small intestine and are generally not considered premalignant. The patient's main problem is usually malabsorption and protein loss.

Juvenile Polyposis[22]

Juvenile polyps are most often seen within first 10 years of life. The term juvenile however refers to the histology of the lesion and not the age of onset. Solitary lesions occur in the colon commonly presenting with bleeding per rectum. Juvenile polyposis is an autosomal dominant condition with multiple, i.e. more than 5 polyps throughout the colon (juvenile polyposis coli) but polyps can occur anywhere in the GI tract (generalized juvenile polyposis) usually presenting in adolescence or late childhood. The familial variety may be associated with an increased risk of GI cancer most often colonic.

MALIGNANT TUMORS

Adenocarcinoma

Adenocarcinoma of the small intestine is less common in Asia and developing countries than the western world where it accounts for 30–50% of small bowel malignancies. It occurs usually in the 6th–7th decade and is slightly commoner in males than females.[1,23]

The duodenum and proximal jejunum are the most sites for adenocarcinoma, the jejunum accounting for about 30% cases of adenocarcinoma small bowel (generally within 30 cm of ligament of Treitz) and the duodenum for 50%. Ileal involvement is seen only in 20% cases and is commoner in patients with Crohn's disease.[1,14,24]

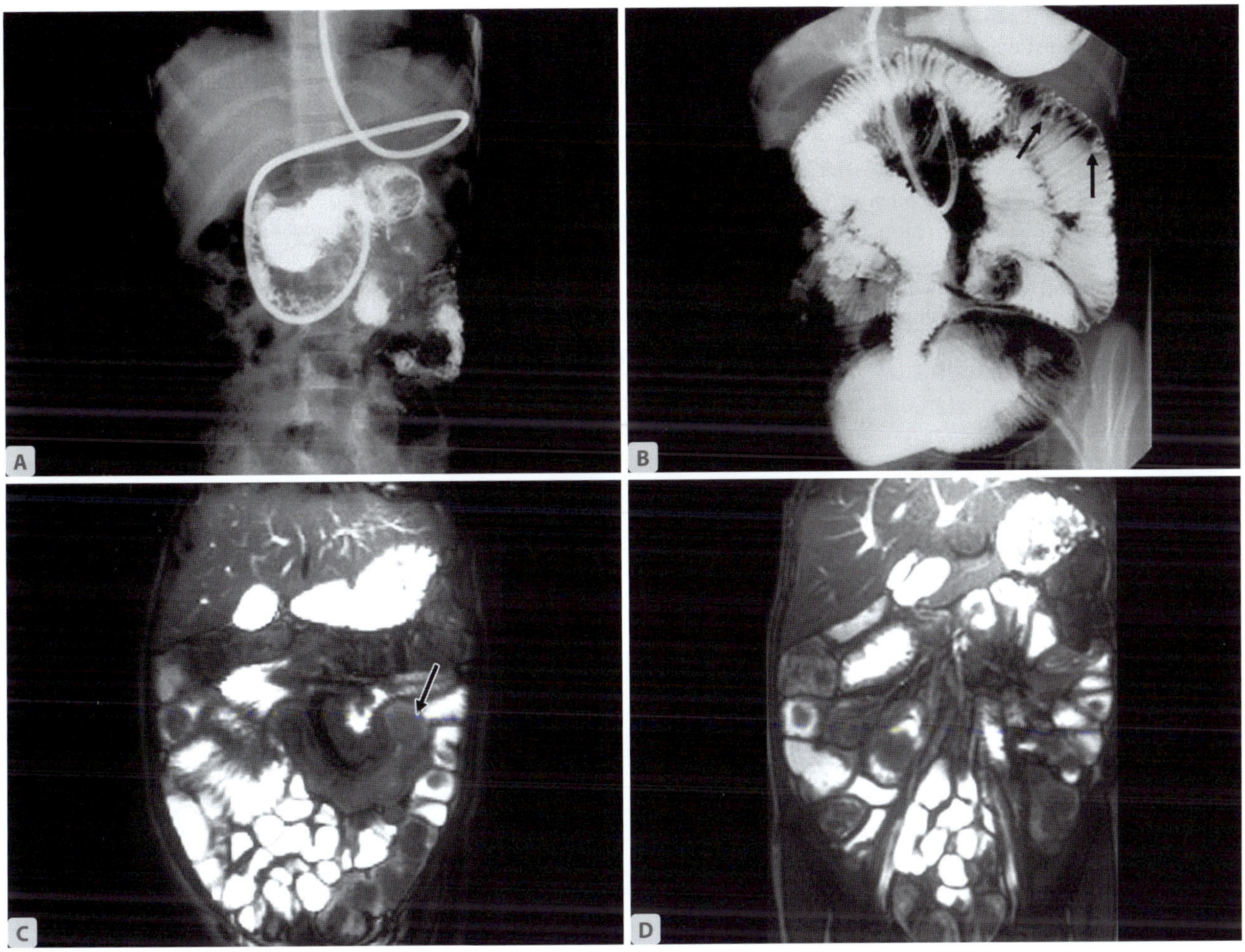

FIGS. 4A TO D: Peutz–Jegher's syndrome: Barium enteroclysis (A and B) in a patient with mucocutaneous pigmentation demonstrates multiple round to oval filling defects in the jejunum with jejuno-jejunal intussusception producing a coiled spring appearance in A. Coronal T2W (C and D) MR enteroclysis images of the same patient reveal multiple round to oval T2 iso to hypointense polyps in the jejunum. Jejuno-jejunal intussusception due to a polyp acting as a lead point is also well seen (arrow in C).

Etiopathogenesis

Risk factors and geographical distribution for adenocarcinoma of the small bowel are considered to be similar to colonic carcinoma. An increased risk of small bowel adenocarcinoma has been reported in colorectal cancer survivors. It is believed that an adenoma carcinoma sequence occurs in the small bowel as well. The presence of adenoma whether single or multiple is considered the most important risk factor for development of small bowel cancer. Syndromes such as familial adenomatous polyposis, Peutz-Jeghers syndrome, Lynch syndrome, Cowden's disease, Gardner's syndrome[1,24,25] and inflammatory disorders like Crohn's disease and celiac disease also predispose to development of adenocarcinoma. Some studies have shown an association with alcohol consumption, high animal fat intake, consumption of red meat and salt cured or smoked meat. Some urological procedures like ileal conduit of ileocystoplasty also increase the risk of adenocarcinoma.[1,24,25] No risk factor may be evident in most cases.

Clinical Presentation

Small bowel adenocarcinomas tend to become symptomatic later than the lesions located in the duodenum. The clinical features are nonspecific and include nausea, vomiting, pain abdomen, small bowel obstruction, weight loss and gastrointestinal bleed which may be occult. The nonspecific nature of clinical symptoms and uncommon nature of disease results in diagnostic delay.[1,26] Misinterpretation of radiological studies can also cause diagnostic delay.[1,26] As a result most lesions are already metastatic by the time they are diagnosed. Small intestinal mucosa, unlike the large bowel, contains lymphatics which extend till the luminal surface and invasion of mucosal tumors into these lymphatics may be responsible for early tendency to metastases.[1] A significant proportion of patients may present acutely with obstruction, massive gastrointestinal bleed or perforation.[1,24,26]

Imaging Features

On barium studies adenocarcinoma produces a short segment circumferential narrowing with mucosal irregularity and ulceration. The lesions tend to have overhanging margins—the so called "apple core" lesion **(Figs. 5A to D)**. These strictures have a fixed unchanging character on compression and with advanced lesions bowel obstruction is common.[11,26]

Differential diagnosis of small bowel strictures on barium include infective or inflammatory disorders like tuberculosis and Crohn's disease. These strictures do not have overhanging margins. In the case of Crohn's disease, associated adenocarcinomas of the terminal ileum, the tumor may resemble an inflammatory exacerbation of a fibrous stricture making the diagnosis difficult. It is unusual for lymphoma or gastrointestinal stromal tumors (GIST) to produce strictures, when they occur they tend to involve longer segment and are more pliable on fluoroscopy than adenocarcinoma. Occasionally small bowel metastases may produce lesions indistinguishable from adenocarcinoma.[11,26]

On CT/MR enteroclysis or enterography a small lesion may be seen as a polypoid mass which is indistinguishable from other benign tumors or polyps. Larger lesions may produce a discrete polypoidal mass or moderate wall thickening resulting in short segment annular narrowing with abrupt overhanging edges. Annular lesions are more common in the distal small bowel while polypoid lesions are more common in the duodenum. The high grade stenosis may result in proximal small bowel obstruction.[4,14,24] On T2W MR images, the mass may show a heterogeneous signal. Moderate post-contrast enhancement which is heterogeneous may be seen on CT or MR.[27] Marked diffusion restriction has been also reported on DW-MRI.[28] Occasionally, the lesions can be large and bulky mimicking lymphoma or gastrointestinal stromal tumors,[26-28] but bowel obstruction is unusual in lymphoma or gastrointestinal stromal tumors (GIST). The features favoring an adenocarcinoma include a short segment, solitary, stricturing lesion more common in the proximal small bowel

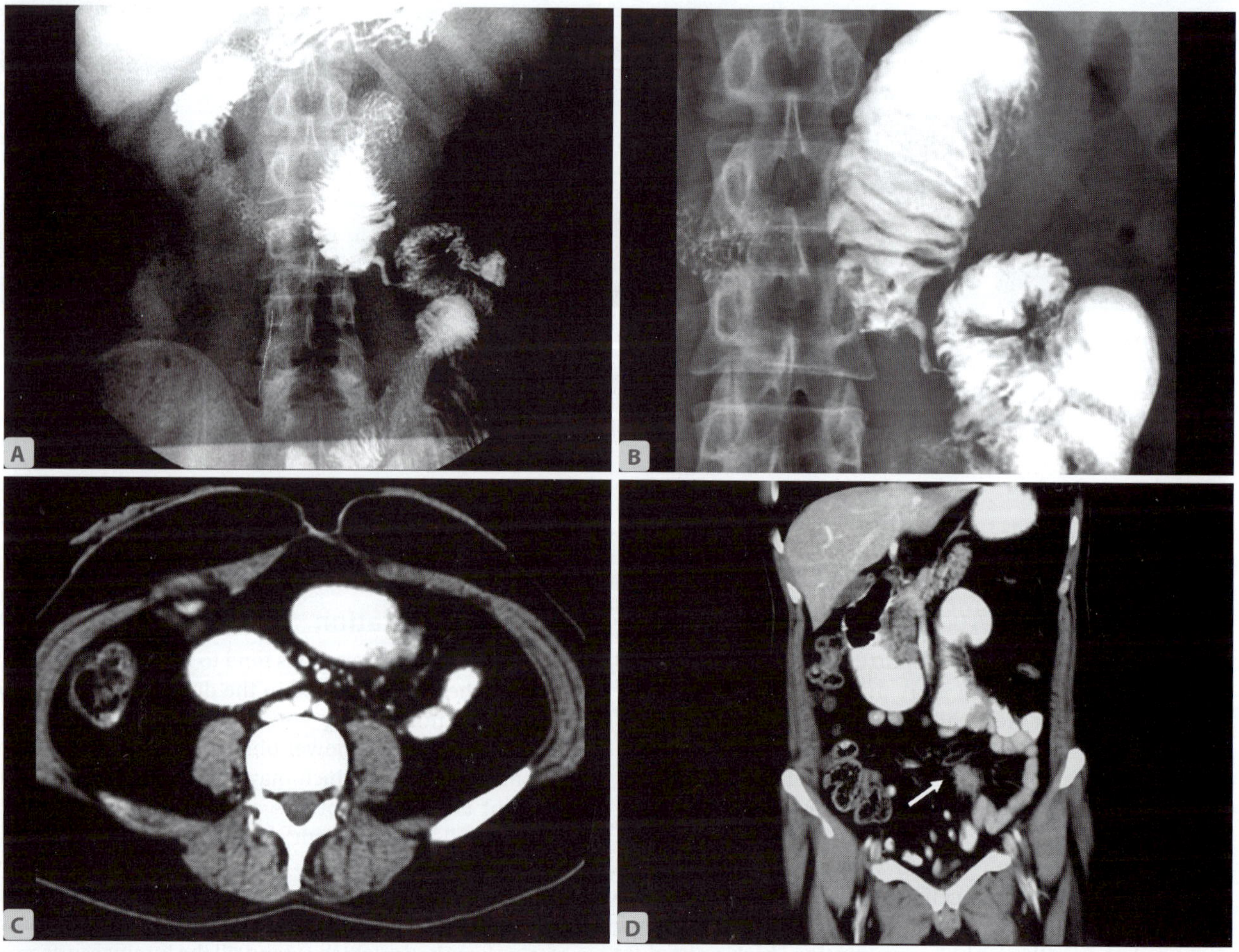

FIGS. 5A TO D: Adenocarcinoma jejunum: Barium meal follow through examination (A and B) showing a short segment tight stricture in the proximal jejunum with shouldering and mucosal irregularity—better appreciated on the magnified image (B). Axial and coronal CECT images (C and D) of the same patient depict homogeneously enhancing moderate wall thickening causing significant luminal narrowing with abrupt overhanging edges. Mesenteric lymphadenopathy is noted (arrow in D). Perivisceral fat appears normal.

with infiltration of perivisceral fat **(Figs. 6A to D)**.[16,26,27] The tumors are also FDG-avid and can be seen as increased activity on PET-CT.[29]

With advanced lesions invasion of mesentery and adjacent organs may occur. Retroperitoneal and mesenteric lymphadenopathy, hepatic and peritoneal metastases are the other findings that may be seen on cross sectional imaging.[26-28] DW-MR has been shown to be useful for detection of even small peritoneal metastases seen as nodular or linear areas of high signal on DW imaging which may be more easily seen with background suppression.[30,31] DW imaging has been reported to have high diagnostic accuracy especially when it is used in conjunction with oral and intravenous contrast enhanced MR.[30,32]

The key imaging findings are summarized in **Table 2**.

Staging and Prognosis

Once the diagnosis of small bowel adenocarcinoma is established a staging thoraco-abdominopelvic CT to search for metastasis is recommended. Upper gastrointestinal endoscopy and colonoscopy may also be done to look for predisposing genetic disease such as polyposis syndromes. Baseline plasma carcinoembryonic antigen (CEA) and carbohydrate antigen (CA) 19.9 should be done in advanced disease as the levels of these tumor markers have prognostic significance. Since most patients have advanced disease by the time diagnosis is made the prognosis is generally poor.

TABLE 2: Adenocarcinoma small bowel: Key imaging findings.
• *Site:* Duodenum, proximal jejunum
• *Barium:* Short segment stricture with shouldered margins
• *CT/MR*: Focal moderate wall thickening with overhanging margins
• Polypoid mass
• Heterogeneous moderate enhancement
• Associated findings
• Perilesional fat infiltration
• Lymphadenopathy
• Small bowel obstruction common

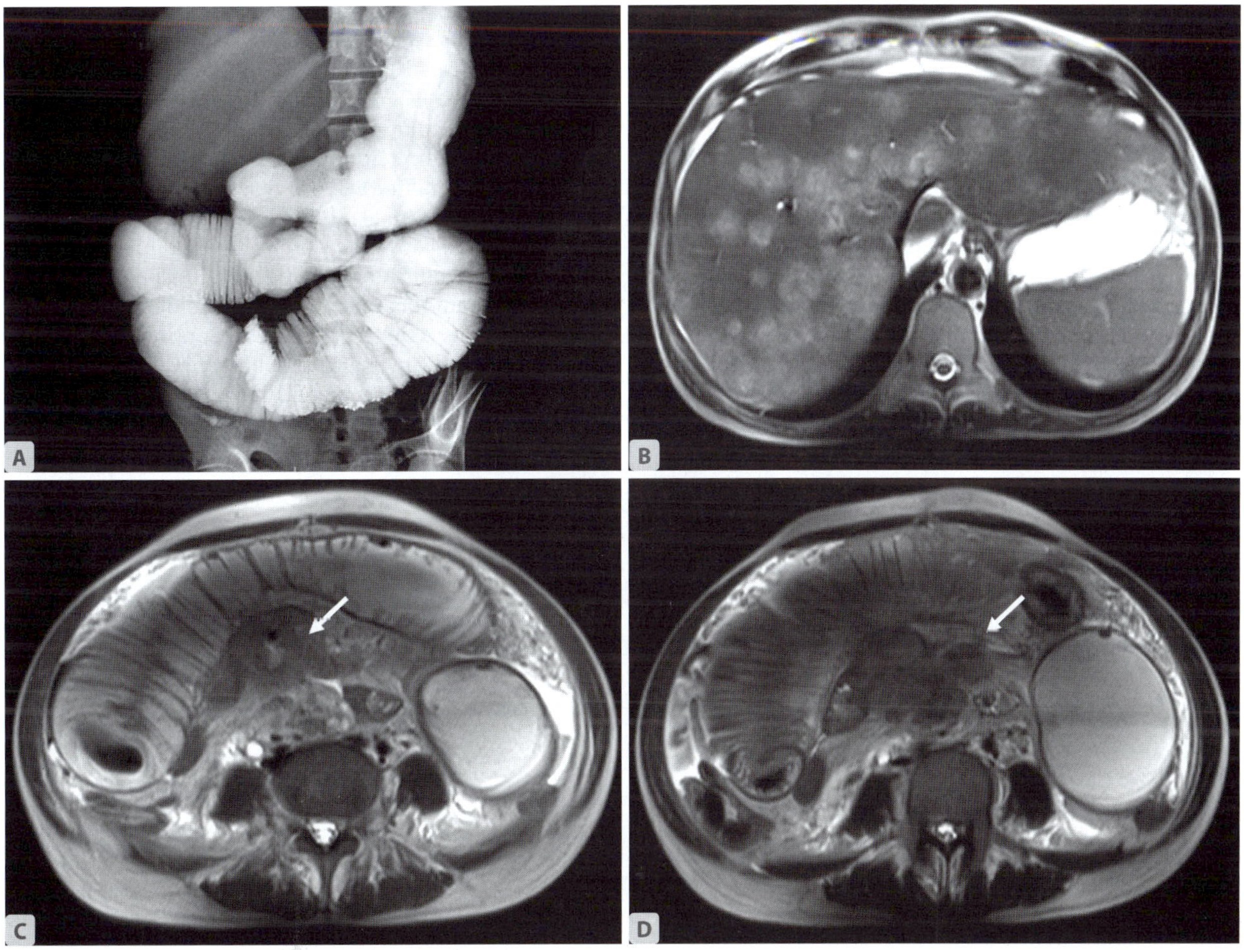

FIGS. 6A TO D: Adenocarcinoma jejunum with hepatic metastases: Barium meal follow through (A) reveals abrupt irregular narrowing of the jejunum producing complete obstruction and proximal dilatation. Cranial to caudal axial T2W MR images. (B to D) Images depict moderatecircumferential mural thickening of the jejunum in the same region with resultant marked luminal compromise (arrow in C) and adjacent lymphadenopathy (arrow in D). Multiple hepatic metastases and ascites are also noted.

Ileal or jejunal lesions have a slightly better prognosis than duodenal lesions.[1,24]

TNM staging system[33] is used to stage adenocarcinoma small intestine given in **Table 3**.

Treatment

Though surgical resection is the primary and the only potentially curative treatment option, very few cases are resectable at the time of diagnosis. Complete resection of the primary tumor with locoregional lymph node dissection is essential. The main prognostic factor for localized small bowel adenocarcinoma is lymph node invasion. Also, the number of positive lymph nodes have prognostic value in stage III disease, patients with more than 3 lymph nodes having a worse prognosis than those with only one or two positive lymph nodes.[24]

If following surgery the disease is found to be stage 0 or 1 no adjuvant treatment is recommended. For stage 2 disease with pT4 tumor or stage III disease adjuvant treatment is recommended. No standard adjuvant regimen has been defined to date due to lack of randomized controlled trials. Generally a chemotherapy regimen similar to that for colorectal cancer[34] is followed. Patients with advanced disease may be treated by chemotherapy or radiotherapy for palliation. Radiotherapy being mainly used for duodenal lesions. Stenting of the bowel strictures can also be done as a palliative measure.[24]

Carcinoid Tumors or Neuroendocrine Tumors

Carcinoid tumors were originally described by Langhans and Lubarsch[35,36] but Oberndorfer in 1907 was the first to use the term carcinoid or 'Karzinoide' meaning 'carcinoma like'.[37] This is because these tumors displayed less aggressive growth than seen with most other gastrointestinal carcinomas.[38] The current preferred nomenclature for these tumors is neuroendocrine tumors (NET) NETs are relatively rare neoplasms arising from Amine Precursor Uptake and Decarboxylation (APUD) cells of the diffuse endocrine system.[39] These cells have a number of antigens that are common with nerve elements (neuroendocrine markers) hence the term neuroendocrine is used for these cell types and tumors.[40,41] There are several types of diffuse endocrine cells in the gastrointestinal tract such as Gastrin or G cells, D cell (somatostatin producing cell), enterochromaffin or EC cell, etc. They represent largest number of neuroendocrine cells in the body, therefore, the gastrointestinal tract is the most common site of NETs accounting for 60–70% cases.[39]

Small bowel carcinoids are generally sporadic. Those associated with MEN—I are mostly foregut carcinoids while patients with NF1 typically have periampullary carcinoids.[42,43]

Etiopathogenesis

The incidence of carcinoids as reported in the western literature has increased over the last two decades. The distribution of tumors along the GI tract has also changed. The appendix is no longer considered most common site and the small bowel or the rectum are more commonly involved.[39]

Small bowel carcinoids account for 26–30% of all gastrointestinal carcinoids. Ileum is the most common site, the usual location being within 60 cm of ileocecal valve.[39,44] They occur most frequently between the fifth to seventh decades and some studies report a slightly higher incidence in males for small bowel carcinoids, others report equal incidence in males and females. Rarely NETs can arise in a Meckel's diverticulum.[41,45]

Majority of the jejunal and ileal carcinoids arise from the enterochromaffin (EC) cell type of endocrine cells in the crypts of Lieberkuhn also called Kulchitsky cell. Carcinoids are submucosal tumors which may produce intramural masses or protrude into the lumen forming polypoid nodules with occasional focal ulceration of the overlying mucosa. These nodules can cause intussusception. The primary intestinal tumors are usually small—generally not more than 3.5 cm but have already invaded the muscularis propria at the

TABLE 3: TNM staging of small bowel adenocarcinoma.

T stage		
Tis	Tumor limited to epithelium or carcinoma *in situ*	
T1	Tumor invades lamina propria submucosa or muscularis mucosa	
T2	Tumor extends into the muscularis propria	
T3	Tumor invades 2 cm or less into subserosa or into non-peritonealized perimuscular tissue (mysentery or retroperitoneum) surrounding the small bowel	
T4	Tumor invades into adjacent organs or extends through visceral peritoneum	
N stage		
N0	No lymph node involvement	
N1	Metastases in one to three regional lymph nodes	
N2	Metastases in four or more regional lymph nodes	
M stage		
M0	No distant metastases	
M1	Distant metastases present	
Stage 0	TisN0M0 (Carcinoma *in situ*)	Stage 3 N1 with any T M0
Stage 1	T1/T2N0 M0	Stage 4 Any T and N, M1
Stage 2	T3/T4 N0 nodes M0	

time of diagnosis in most cases. These infiltrative tumor cells extend through the muscularis propria forming tumor masses in the subserosa of the intestine extending into the adjacent mesentery. Local release of serotonin and other substances as well as the pattern of growth described above results in desmoplasia, which is most marked in the submucosa and adjacent mesentery. In addition mesenteric vessels close to the tumor as well as those far away may be thickened with focal occlusions or stenosis due to the vasoactive substances released or vascular invasion.[45]

Conventional argentaffin and argyrophil silver staining techniques can be used to identify the tumor cells as EC cells. More recently immunohistochemical markers for serotonin, substance P and other tachykinins have been used. These tumors are also strongly positive for general endocrine markers such as chromogranin A, neuron specific enolase and synaptophysin.[41,45]

Many pathologic classification systems have been proposed for carcinoid/NET. Based on their location and embryologic origin they were traditionally classified as foregut, midgut and hindgut[39,45] to emphasize clinicopathologic difference between these groups. However, this did not explain the heterogeneity in their biologic behavior following which a WHO classification was developed in 2000 and then modified in 2010. According to this system carcinoids are categorized under the generic term of neuroendocrine tumors (NET Gr I).[45] This is given in **Table 4**. This classification has clinical implications. Intermediate and high grade NETs are more likely to develop metastases so a shorter follow-up of 3 months is required for them than the usual follow-up at 6 months. Metastatic deposits from these tumors occur in lymph nodes, mesentery and liver and may become very large obscuring the primary tumor.[39,45]

Small bowel carcinoids are multiple in 30–40% of patients. A second primary malignancy (synchronous/metachronous) may present in gastrointestinal NET's. This is most frequent in the small intestinal NETs occurring in about 29% cases. Gastrointestinal adenocarcinomas are the most commonly associated malignancy others being prostate, breast, bronchus and bladder malignancies.[39]

Clinical Features

Most patients are asymptomatic because of the slow growing nature of these tumors. Symptoms may be related to the primary tumor, mesenteric involvement or metastatic disease. A long history of crampy abdominal pain, weight loss, fatigue or diarrhea and small bowel obstruction and very rarely obscure GI bleed may be seen.[45]

Carcinoid syndrome is seen in about 10% of all patients with gastrointestinal carcinoids and in around 17% of those with small bowel carcinoids. This occurs when vasoactive substance such as serotonin, kallikrein, bradykinin and prostaglandins produced by the tumor enter systemic circulation without metabolic degradation, which normally occurs in the liver. Patients with ileal carcinoids who have extensive hepatic metastases are most likely to develop carcinoid syndrome. The classic carcinoid syndrome consists of cutaneous flushing, diarrhea, abdominal pain, wheezing due to bronchospasm, palpitations and low blood pressure. This can be precipitated by alcohol, cheese, chocolate, exercise or emotional stress.[39,45] About 75% of patients with carcinoid syndrome develop carcinoid heart syndrome, i.e. right-sided valvular fibrosis and fibrosis of right cardiac chambers. Inactivation of the bioactive peptides in the lungs is thought to be responsible for left sided sparing.[39,45]

Laboratory tests that are useful in establishing the diagnosis of small bowel NETs/carcinoid include urinary 5 hydroxyindoleacetic acid (5-HIAA) a serotonin breakdown product which is elevated in 75% of midgut carcinoids and serum chromogranin A which is elevated in 80–90% of all gastrointestinal carcinoids (foregut, midgut and hindgut). The latter is also used to assess response to therapy.[39,45] In patients who have clinical features of carcinoid syndrome echocardiography is indicated to detect carcinoid heart disease which is an independent poor prognostic factor.[46]

TABLE 4: World Health Organization 2010 classification of neuroendocrine tumors (NETs).

NET type	Tumor classification
NET, grade I	Well-differentiated, low-grade, mitotic count <2 per HPF, Ki-67, index <3%
NET, grade II	Well-differentiated, intermediate-grade mitotic count 2–20 per HPF, Ki-67, index 3–20%
NET, grade III, small cell	Poorly differentiated, high-grade, mitotic count >20 per HPF, Ki-67 >20%, small cell features
NET, grade III, large cell	Poorly differentiated, high-grade, mitotic count >20 per HPF, Ki-67 >20% large cell features

Note: HPF, high power field; Ki-67 index refers to the % of cells which are +ve for Ki-67–a marker for cell proliferation.

Imaging

The imaging findings depend on primary tumor size, extent of mesenteric involvement and lymph node or hepatic metastases.

On barium studies/enteroclysis small carcinoids are generally not seen. When seen they produce mucosal elevations or rounded nodules with smooth overlying mucosa or surface ulceration producing a barium filled crater the so called 'bull's eye' or target appearance usually in the ileum. In the later stages, with bowel wall and mesenteric fibrosis,tethering and thickening of mucosal folds, rigidity, kinking, sharp angulations and narrowing of bowel loops is seen.[26]

While conventional abdominal CT has very low sensitivity for detection of small (<2 cm) lesions, multiphase helical CT with neural oral contrast, i.e. CT enterography or enteroclysis improve detection of smaller lesions because of improved tumor to background contrast.[47,48] The scan acquisition must be done earlier than usual, i.e. in the late arterial phase.[47,48] Some studies have reported that CT enteroclysis has a sensitivity of 100% for detection of small bowel carcinoids.Small ileal NETs may be seen as solitary or multiple hyperenhancing polyps, plaque like lesions or carpet lesions.[39,49]

Transmural extension of the tumor and associated mesenteric involvement and fibrosis are well seen on CT. About 50–75% cases of midgut carcinoids with median size of 3 cm have mesenteric masses more than 1.5 cm in size.[50,51] Transmural extension is seen on CT as concentric mural thickening with a focal soft tissue tumor mass adjacent to it. Deposits of carcinoid in the mesentery produce enlarged lymph nodes or masses which are commonly spiculated and produce mesenteric retraction. The soft tissue stranding or spiculation represents fibrosis rather than tumor infiltration and increases as the degree of fibrosis increases on histology. These masses may be much larger than the primary tumor and completely obscure it. Fine stippled or bulky and dense calcification may be seen in 40–70% of the mesenteric masses.[45,50] Histologically, this occurs in areas of mature fibrous scarring. The exact site of origin of mesenteric masses is not certain but they are usually thought to arise within the mesenteric fat or nodal tissue of small bowel mesentery.[52]

Mesenteric fibrosis angulates and kinks the involved intestine producing 'hair pin' bends—well appreciated on both axial images and multiplanar reconstructions **(Figs. 7A to E)**. It can also produce a 'spoke wheel' or 'sunburst' pattern of radiating mesenteric vessels.[45] 3D-CTA is a very useful technique to delineate full extent of the mesenteric mass and associated vascular involvement before surgical

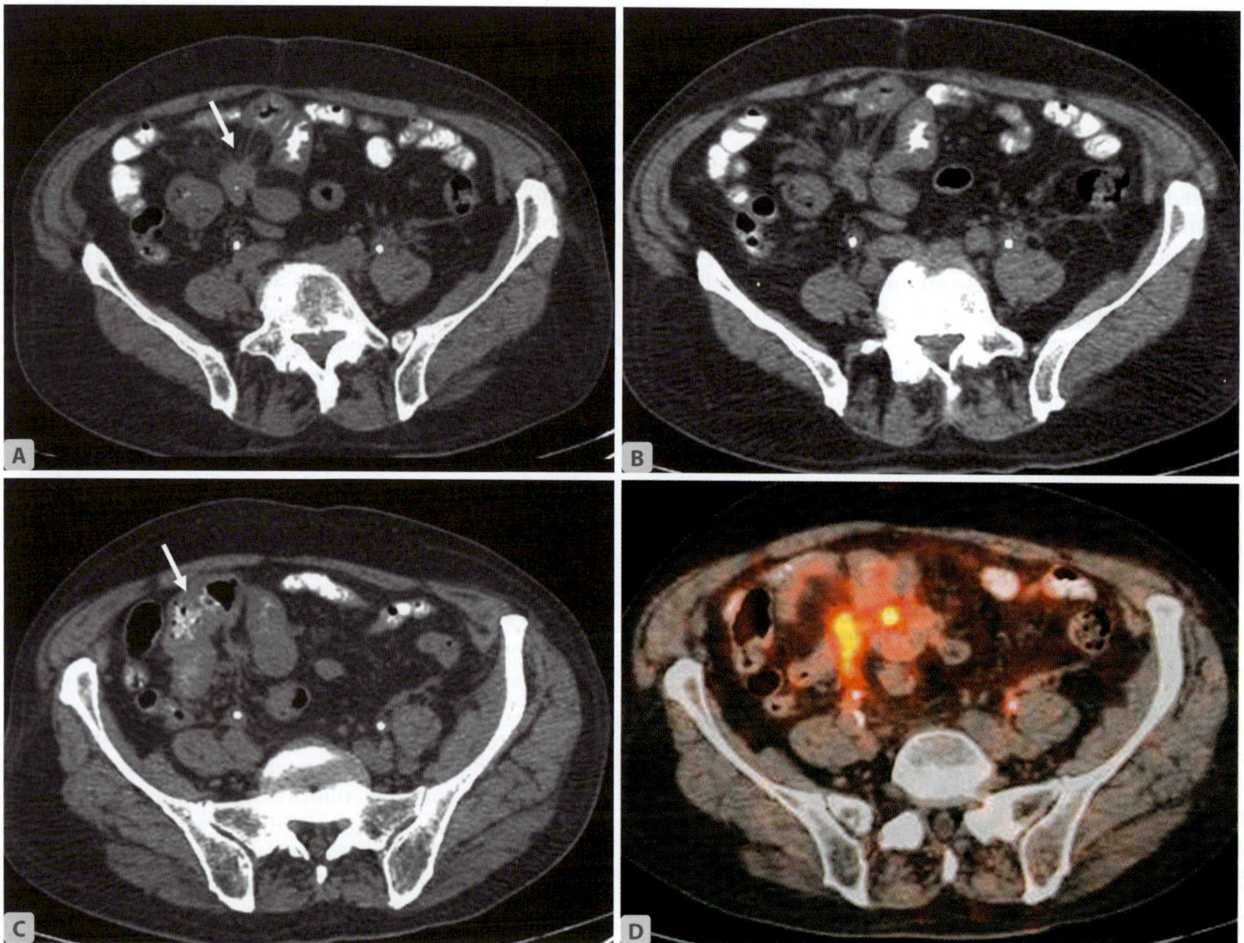

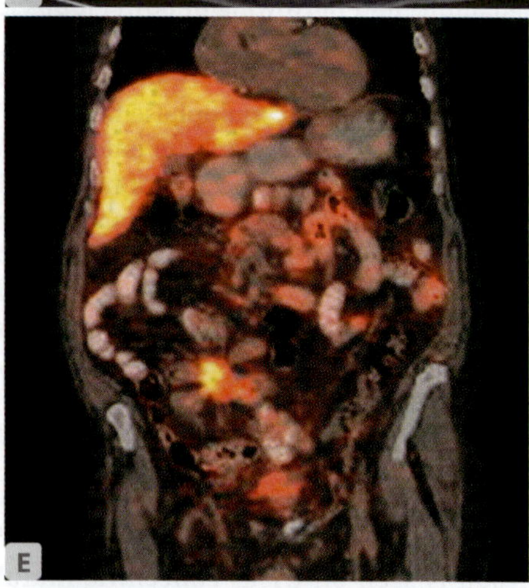

FIGS. 7A TO E: Small bowel carcinoid with mesenteric involvement and hepatic metastases: Axial (A to C) CT images with oral contrast depict a spiculated mesenteric mass with a speck of calcification, radiating soft tissue strands and mesenteric retraction (arrow in A). Adjoining small bowel loops are thickened and angulated (arrow in C). Bilateral ureteric stents are also noted. DOTANOC-PET–CT images (D and E) show intense uptake in the mesenteric mass and adjacent bowel and on the coronal image the spoke wheel arrangement of bowel loops around the mesenteric mass can be appreciated. Multiple metastatic lesions are also seen in the liver as areas of increased uptake.

planning. Occasionally signs of bowel ischemia may also be seen due to vascular involvement. Rarely, diffuse mesenteric or peritoneal disease can occur producing miliary peritoneal implants, large masses, mesenteric caking or ascites.[45,53]

On MR enterography or enteroclysis carcinoids may be seen as solitary or multiple nodular masses or nodular fold thickening appearing isointense to muscle on T1W images and iso to mildly hyperintense on T2W images with intense contrast enhancement. The mesenteric mass itself is isointense on both T1W and T2W images due to fibrosis, mesenteric extension resulting in stretching, fixing and angulation of small bowel loops. Calcification though not as well seen as on CT may be seen as signal voids.[16,54]

Nuclear medicine studies in gastrointestinal NETs help in staging the disease, detect additional sites of involvement before surgery and detect unknown primary in patients presenting with metastases. Somatostatin receptor scintigraphy (SRS) is performed using radiolabelled synthetic somatostatin analogue ^{111}I octreotide because NET's express somatostatin receptors especially subtypes II and V. Overall sensitivity of somatostatin receptor scintigraphy (SRS) in detecting tumor burden both primary and metastatic for gastroenteropancreatic (GEP) NETs is 80–90% however, the sensitivity in detecting occult primary in a patient presenting with metastatic disease is disappointingly low at 2–23%.[30] Some recent studies suggest that with the availability of DOTANOC–PET for comparison the sensitivity of SRS is substantially lower than that reported in earlier studies.[39,55]

PET-CT using tracers like ^{68}Ga labeled DOTATOC/DOTANOC which are octreotide derivatives and ^{11}C-5-hydroxytryptophan have higher sensitivity for tumor burden than SRS ranging from 93% to 97% while its sensitivity for localizing unknown primary is around 59% **(Figs. 7A to E)**.[45,56]

^{18}F-FDG PET/CT is not useful in diagnosing typical low grade NET's because of the low glycolytic rate but has a role in prognostication of poorly differentiated NET's (WHO grade 3 and 4). The tumors that are ^{18}F-FDG PET/CT avid have a poorer prognosis and more rapid disease progression than those with negative uptake.[57-59] These poorly differentiated tumors do not express somatostatin receptors. Thus, there is an inverse relationship in which DOTANOC PET/CT and FDG PET/CT findings are inversely related at either end of the NETs differentiation spectrum.[55]

Imaging of Metastatic Lesions

In the case of midgut carcinoids, metastases are more common as the tumor size increases with the reported incidences being over 70% with a tumor size exceeding 2 cm.[54] In the vast majority of cases the primary tumor is usually so small that it may not be apparent on imaging and secondary findings are more common. Hepatic metastases are the most frequent finding followed by tumor induced fibrosis causing kinking of small bowel mesentery.[54] Liver metastases are seen in about 40% of ileal lesions at initial presentation. On ultrasound, liver metastases may be hyperechoic. Contrast enhanced ultrasound may help in improving sensitivity of ultrasound from 68% to 99%. Since the metastases are generally hypervascular they are best seen on arterial phase imaging on CT or MR. Occasionally they can be necrotic and may calcify. MR has reportedly a higher sensitivity of 95.2% for detection of liver metastases than CT, USG or SRS.[54] In one study PET-CT using ^{68}Ga labeled DOTATOC/NOC was superior to all conventional imaging techniques like CT/MR for detection of osseous and nodal metastases but was not found to be significantly superior for detection of hepatic metastases.[45,54,55]

Retroperitoneal or mesenteric lymphadenopathy has been reported in 20–30% of midgut carcinoids.[54] In these patients with retroperitoneal lymphadenopathy, retroperitoneal fibrosis may occur resulting in ureteric obstruction at times.[54] Other less common sites of metastases include bones, lungs, peritoneal cavity and ovary.[39]

Differential Diagnosis

The differential diagnosis of small primary tumors includes gastrointestinal stromal tumor (GIST), adenoma or leiomyoma. Other lesions that need to be distinguished from carcinoid include lymphoma, adenocarcinoma, metastases, GIST and Kaposi's sarcoma. Presence of fibrosis and angulation of bowel loops is characteristic of carcinoid, however it may occur with mesenteric extension of adenocarcinoma or metastases. DOTANOC-PET-CT can be extremely useful when the diagnosis is not clear.

The mesenteric mass of carcinoid tumor may mimic sclerosing mesenteritis and it may be very difficult to distinguish these conditions preoperatively. The soft tissue mass in sclerosing mesenteritis may envelop the mesenteric vessels with collateral vessel formation however, the fat around the mesenteric vessels is preserved, the so called "fat ring sign" unlike in carcinoid.[16]

Table 5 summarizes the important imaging findings in carcinoid tumors.

Future Directions[16]

Cytogenetic studies may help to understand the malignant potential of carcinoids better. Some studies have shown that if the metastatic tumor is positive for transcription factor CDX-2 then the primary is likely to be in the midgut. In addition, if it is negative for other transcription factors including pancreatic and duodenum homebox factor (PDX-1) neuroendocrine secretory protein-55 (NESP-55) and thyroid transcription factor (TTF-1) the primary tumor is most likely located in the ileum. In such a patient it may be appropriate to plan a CT enterography while a pancreatic CT protocol may be more useful in pancreatic NETs.

TABLE 5: Carcinoid/NET key imaging findings.
• Site-distal ileum
• Intensely enhancing polypoid mass/bowel wall thickening
• Mesenteric mass with calcification and desmoplasia (spiculation)
• Mesenteric retraction
• Angulated or hair pin small bowel loops
• DOTANOC-PET avid

Treatment and Prognosis

Treatment depends on the extent of disease, symptomatology and receptor status. Localized small bowel NET's are treated surgically by removing the involved bowel and affected nodes. The entire bowel must be examined at surgery to rule out multiple lesions. Prophylactic cholecystectomy is recommended when treatment with somatostatin analogues is planned as these drugs cause impairment of gallbladder function with gallstones formation and cholecystitis. Even in patients with unresectable disease debulking may be carried out for symptomatic relief.

A multidisciplinary approach is required in patients with metastases. DOTANOC/DOTATOC-PET should be done if treatment with somatostatin analogues (octreotide/lanreotide/vapreotide) is planned to determine receptor status. Somatostatin analogue injections help to provide symptomatic relief in patients with carcinoid syndrome. They are also thought to inhibit the growth of tumors, hence have an important role in the treatment of carcinoid tumors with positive receptor status.

For limited liver metastases complete resection should ideally be done with curative intent. The various treatment options for extensive hepatic metastases include radiofrequency ablation (RFA), arterial embolization, chemotherapy, peptide receptor radionuclide therapy with ^{111}In, ^{90}Y or ^{177}Lu labeled octreotide analogues (DOTANOC-PET is useful in these patients to identify receptor status). Tyrosine kinase inhibitors and VEGF monoclonal antibodies are also being evaluated.[39]

Although carcinoids have a much less aggressive growth pattern than adenocarcinoma, the 5 years survival rate for small bowel carcinoids is about 54%. If complete surgical resection can be performed the survival rate improves greatly approaching 75%. The 5 years survival rate for patients with liver metastases in patients with few liver metastases (<5) is similar to those without metastasis and much better than in those with extensive hepatic metastases. In patients with distant metastases 5 years survival rate is below 20%.[47,54]

GASTROINTESTINAL STROMAL TUMORS

Gastrointestinal stromal tumors (GIST) are the most common nonepithelial or mesenchymal tumor of the gastrointestinal tract. The term was first used by Mazur and Clark.[60,61] Prior to 1983, these tumors were variably referred to as smooth muscle tumors; leiomyomas, leiomyosarcomas and leiomyoblastomas. However, they are distinct from true smooth muscle or neural tumors and are thought to arise from interstitial cells of Cajal. In 95% of patients, these tumors express KIT protein - CD117 a tyrosine kinase receptor which is the most important criterion for diagnosing GIST. Most GISTs are CD34 positive also. Immunoreactivity to KIT helps to differentiate gastrointestinal stromal tumors from true smooth muscle tumors.[60-62]

There is a small percentage of patients in whom the tumor does not show KIT mutation, instead mutations in the related tyrosine kinase platelet derived growth factor receptor alpha (PDGFR-α) are seen. A minority of gastrointestinal stromal tumors (GIST) have no KIT or PDG-FR and are known as 'wild type' GIST. The tumors seen in patients with neurofibromatosis are generally of the 'wild type' and have a low malignant potential.[63]

Clinical Features

The clinical presentation is extremely variable and depends on the size and location of tumors. Small gastrointestinal stromal tumors (GIST) may be discovered incidentally during radiological evaluation or surgery for another condition. Nausea, vomiting, abdominal pain, distension, palpable abdominal mass and feeling of satiety may occur with large masses.[64] Gastrointestinal bleeding from mucosal ulceration is a common manifestation of symptomatic gastrointestinal stromal tumors (GIST). This may be in the form of hematemesis melena or anemia due to occult bleed.[64]

Etiopathogenesis

The exact prevalence of gastrointestinal stromal tumors is difficult to ascertain however, it is estimated that there are about 5000–10,000 new cases every year.[62] Most patients are over 50 years at the time of diagnosis and there is no definite sex predilection. Ethnicity, race, occupation or geographic location have no association with gastrointestinal stromal tumors.

An increased incidence of GIST has been reported in patient with neurofibromatosis type 1 (NF1). Generally these patients have multiple small intestinal GISTs. Gastrointestinal stromal tumors are a probable feature of Carney's triad consisting of epithelioid leiomyosarcoma with paraganglioma and pulmonary chondroma. These do not necessarily occur at the same time. Other syndromes associated with GIST include Carney-Stratakis syndrome characterized by gastrointestinal stromal tumors (GIST) and paraganglioma and marked by germline mutations of succinate dehydrogenase (SDH) subunits A, B, C and D.[63,64]

Gastrointestinal stromal tumors (GIST) can arise all along the gastrointestinal tract, the stomach being the most frequent site followed by the small intestine. Any part of the small intestine can be involved. The esophagus is the only site in the gastrointestinal tract where leiomyomas are commoner than GIST accounting for 75% of mesenchymal esophageal tumors. Rarely, they can arise primarily in the omentum, mesentery and retroperitoneum.[64]

These tumors are well-circumscribed masses without a true capsule, size varying from few mm to over 30 cm. On gross pathology, cut surface is pink, tan or gray in color. Larger lesions can show focal areas of hemorrhage cystic degeneration and necrosis. GISTs arise from the outer muscular layer or muscularis propria of the gastrointestinal tract and tend to grow exophytically producing large masses arising from the intestinal wall and projecting into the abdominal cavity. Mucosal ulceration may be seen in a significant number of lesions as a component of the tumor extends to the mucosal surface.[64,65]

Histologically, these can be spindle cell, epithelioid or mixed cell types and on immunohistochemistry they express CD117 a transmembrane receptor for a growth factor called stem cell factor expressed on hematopoietic stem cells, myenteric plexus of adult gastrointestinal tract, etc. No gastrointestinal stromal tumor (GIST) can be unequivocally labeled benign although lesions less than 2 cm in size have a very low risk of recurrence and are mostly considered benign. Small bowel GISTs in general have a more aggressive course than gastric tumors hence the size threshold for estimating risk of metastases or recurrence may be smaller for small intestinal GISTs. Metastases tend to occur to the liver and peritoneum but do not involve the lymph nodes.[65,66]

Pediatric gastrointestinal stromal tumors (GIST) are extremely rare but constitute a distinct subset of GISTs which is associated with female predominance, lack of KIT/PDGFRA mutations, mainly gastric lesions which tend to be multicentric with lymph node metastases.[63]

IMAGING APPEARANCES

Although plain radiographs have no role in the diagnosis of gastrointestinal stromal tumors they may reveal a soft tissue haze due to the mass. Rarely irregular gas collections may be seen when the masses are cavitating with presence of air in the cavity.[65]

Ultrasound can detect large masses which appear heterogeneous due to areas of necrosis however, it may be difficult to identify the exact organ of origin (**Fig. 8**).[65]

On barium studies, due to a large extraluminal component these masses exhibit mass effect on the affected segment of intestine. A cavity or fistula communicating with the intestinal lumen hence filling with barium may be seen and rarely aneurysmal dilatation can be seen (**Figs. 9A to C**). Small lesions may produce submucosal masses indistinguishable from other benign submucosal

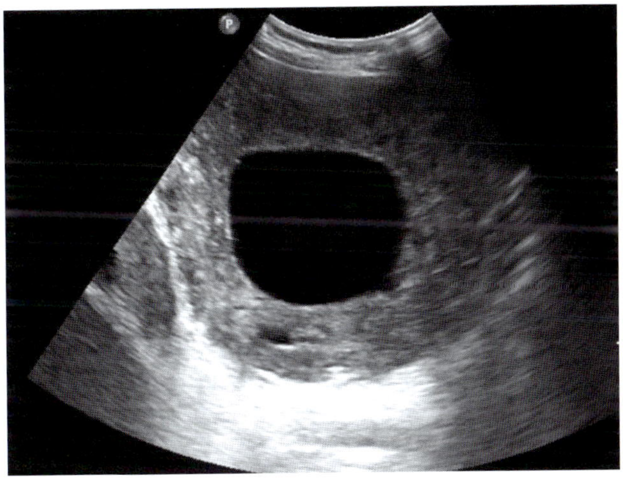

FIG. 8: Gastrointestinal stromal tumor: Grayscale ultrasound image reveals a large heterogeneous mass with a central area cavitation in a patient with GIST.

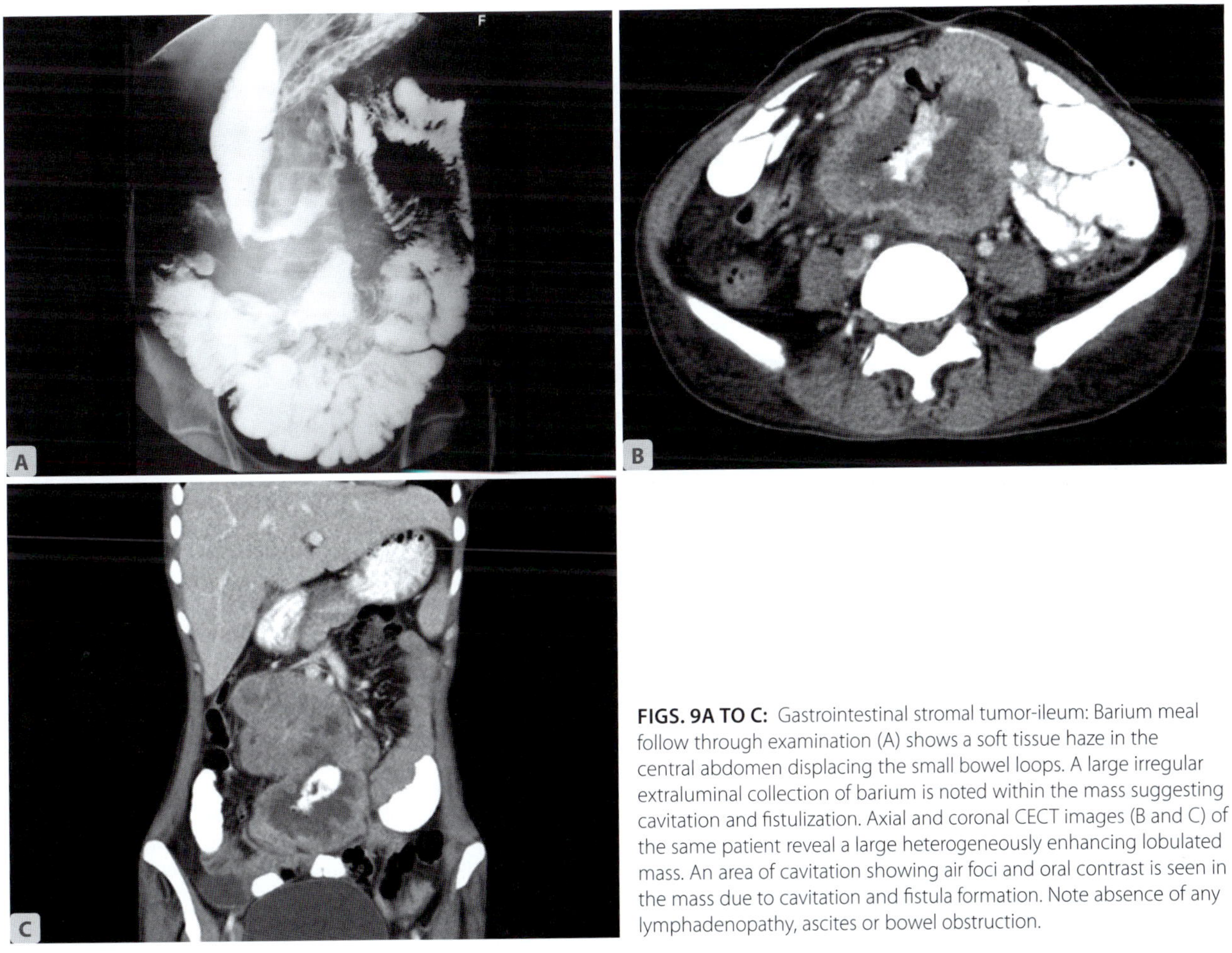

FIGS. 9A TO C: Gastrointestinal stromal tumor-ileum: Barium meal follow through examination (A) shows a soft tissue haze in the central abdomen displacing the small bowel loops. A large irregular extraluminal collection of barium is noted within the mass suggesting cavitation and fistulization. Axial and coronal CECT images (B and C) of the same patient reveal a large heterogeneously enhancing lobulated mass. An area of cavitation showing air foci and oral contrast is seen in the mass due to cavitation and fistula formation. Note absence of any lymphadenopathy, ascites or bowel obstruction.

lesions, sometimes mucosal irregularity due to ulceration can be seen.[64]

The CT is the mainstay for diagnosis and staging. The entire tumor including the mural, extramural and luminal component is well delineated on CT. In many cases the bulk of the tumor is extraserosal making its difficult to determine its origin from small bowel. The appearances are variable depending on the size and aggressiveness of the tumor, most lesions tend to be heterogeneous due to necrosis, hemorrhage or cystic degeneration and show inhomogeneous patchy enhancement following contrast administration **(Figs. 10A to C)**. Homogeneous attenuation is less commonly seen.[60,62,64,65] Calcification is rarely seen. Vascular supply is well-demonstrated on CTA using MIP or curved planar reconstructions. Usually the tumors displace adjacent organs but with advanced disease direct invasion of adjacent structures may be seen. Rarely the tumors may appear predominantly cystic and may be misdiagnosed as pseudocysts. Small GIST's usually produce homogeneous, submucosal or endoluminal polypoid masses.[60,62,64,65]

According to some reports nearly 50% of patients with gastrointestinal stromal tumors present with metastasis. Liver and peritoneal metastases are the most common occurring due to hematogeneous spread and peritoneal seeding respectively **(Figs. 11A and B)**. Less common sites of metastasis include lung, pleura and soft tissue. Lymph node metastases are distinctly uncommon.[60]

MR is indicated for evaluation of liver lesions indeterminate at CT, when CT is contraindicated and for surgical planning of rectal gastrointestinal stromal tumors. The MR appearances depend on the size, degree of necrosis and hemorrhage. The most common appearance is an exophytic bulky mass. Sometimes a protruding intraluminal mass or bidirectional growth pattern relative to the intestinal wall may be seen. The solid areas of the tumor are low signal on T1W images, high signal on T2W images and show enhancement after contrast administration. Areas of hemorrhage show variable signal intensity depending on the age of hemorrhage. Mesenteric masses in the case of gastrointestinal stromal tumors (GIST) tend to be smooth, without any spiculation.[16] DWI may reveal restricted diffusion with low ADC values **(Figs. 12A to F)**.[67]

^{18}F-FDG-PET/CT is also a highly sensitive technique for detection and staging of gastrointestinal stromal tumors but a small number of lesions are not FDG avid.[60]

The imaging findings are summarized in **Table 6**.

STAGING AND PROGNOSIS

Contrast-enhanced computed tomography (CECT) of the abdomen and pelvis is the imaging technique of choice for staging and follow-up. FDG-PET-CT/MRI is especially useful when early detection of tumor response to molecular targeted therapy is to be done. A TNM staging system for

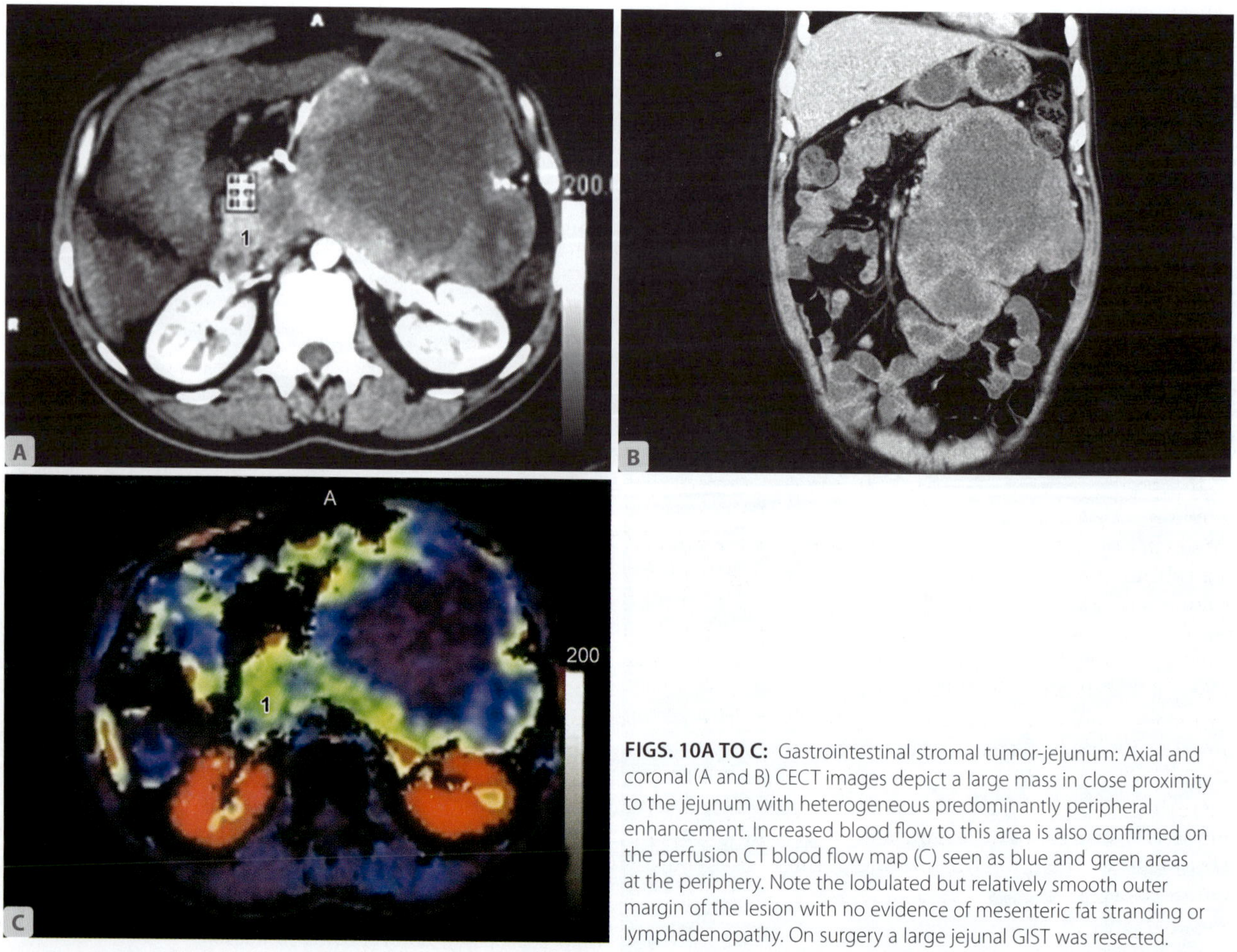

FIGS. 10A TO C: Gastrointestinal stromal tumor-jejunum: Axial and coronal (A and B) CECT images depict a large mass in close proximity to the jejunum with heterogeneous predominantly peripheral enhancement. Increased blood flow to this area is also confirmed on the perfusion CT blood flow map (C) seen as blue and green areas at the periphery. Note the lobulated but relatively smooth outer margin of the lesion with no evidence of mesenteric fat stranding or lymphadenopathy. On surgery a large jejunal GIST was resected.

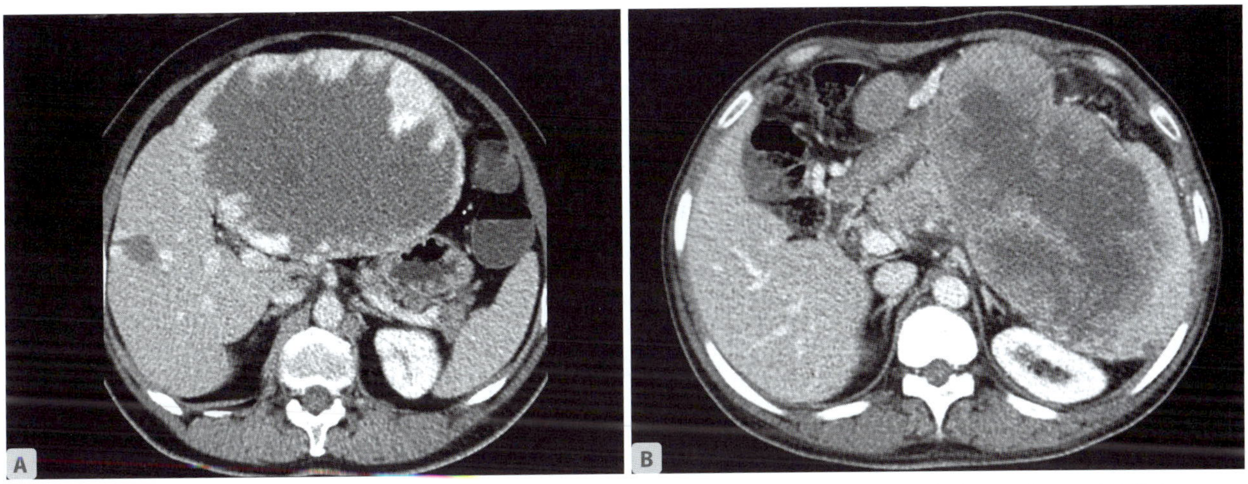

FIGS. 11A AND B: GIST with hepatic metastases: Metastasis to the left lobe liver in a patient with gastrointestinal stromal tumor (GIST) shows hypodense mass with multiple peripheral solid enhancing nodules on CECT. Also note the smaller lesion in the right lobe showing a similar appearance.

gastrointestinal stromal tumors (GIST) has been developed by AJCC in the 7th edition of the TNM staging system, however, it has several limitations and is generally not used.[63]

Several criteria have been proposed to prognosticate gastrointestinal stromal tumors. The term benign and malignant are not applied any longer since all gastrointestinal stromal tumors have some potential to behave in a malignant fashion.[63] Risk of recurrence is dependent on tumor size, mitotic index and site (i.e. location in gastrointestinal tract). Nongastric location is associated with poorer prognosis than gastric lesions. Some authors have stratified tumors into risk categories. Tumors less than 2 cm in size with a mitotic count < 5/50 HPF are categorized as very low-risk; and tumors >5 cm with a mitotic count of >5/50 HPF, tumors greater than 10 cm and any mitotic rate, while tumors of any size with a mitotic rate >10/50 HPF are classified as high-risk. Between these two lie low-risk and intermediate risk categories. Presence of rupture whether spontaneous or iatrogenic and male sex are independent adverse prognostic features.[63,68]

Treatment

Management of gastrointestinal stromal tumors requires a multidisciplinary approach. Tumors 2 cm or more in size should be surgically resected. The management of lesions that are <2 cm in size and discovered incidentally is controversial. The recommended standard treatment for localized tumors is complete surgical resection with clear margins with no lymph node dissection of clinically negative nodes. Although smaller tumors may be laparoscopically resected (if expertise is available) following the principles of oncologic surgery it is not recommended for large tumors due to higher risk of tumor rupture which has a very high-risk of recurrence. If the risk of relapse is substantial patient is put on adjuvant imatinib, a tyrosine kinase inhibitor (TKI) adjuvant treatment, close monitoring of treatment response is carried out during the treatment. Some authors recommend mutational analysis before adjuvant therapy since some subtypes may not be sensitive to TKI.[63]

Imatinib is also the standard treatment for inoperable and metastatic lesions. In case of confirmed nonresponse and disease progression or rarely intolerance to imatinib a second line TKI sunitinib may be used. Other drugs being tried include Regorafenib, sorafenib etc.[63]

RESPONSE EVALUATION AND SURVEILLANCE

Response evaluation to treatment is generally done on CT especially when ^{18}F-FDG-PET-CT/MR is not available and is generally done at 3 months. Traditional response evaluation criteria in solid tumors (RECIST) criteria based assessment of tumor response are insensitive in evaluating response to TKI as decrease in tumor size may take several months. Good response to imatinib is seen as lesions becoming homogeneous, hypoattenuating or hypodense, disappearance of enhancing nodules and tumor vessels. These changes represent a favorable effect even in the absence of anatomic decrease in size. Consistent similar signal changes on MR should also be considered as tumor response.[63] Choi et al. proposed CT response criteria which take into account both the tumor size and density.[69] A complete disappearance of lesion with no new lesions is considered complete response while a 10% decrease in diameter or 15% decrease in density with no new lesions is required for partial response.

A paradoxical increase in tumor size may occur during treatment this does not imply tumor progression in the absence of enhancing nodules. It may be caused by myxoid degeneration or hemorrhage. Hemorrhage may also produce an increase in tumor attenuation complicating the CT based assessment further. Sometimes intratumoral hemorrhage may be significant, producing possible decrease in hemoglobin levels in the first 4–8 weeks of imatinib therapy.[60] At times even the appearance of new lesions in the liver may be due to their becoming more apparent with decrease in density rather than true lesions.[60,63] Imatinib therapy may result in fluid retention which is the most common side effect. This may be seen as ascites, pleural effusion, pericardial

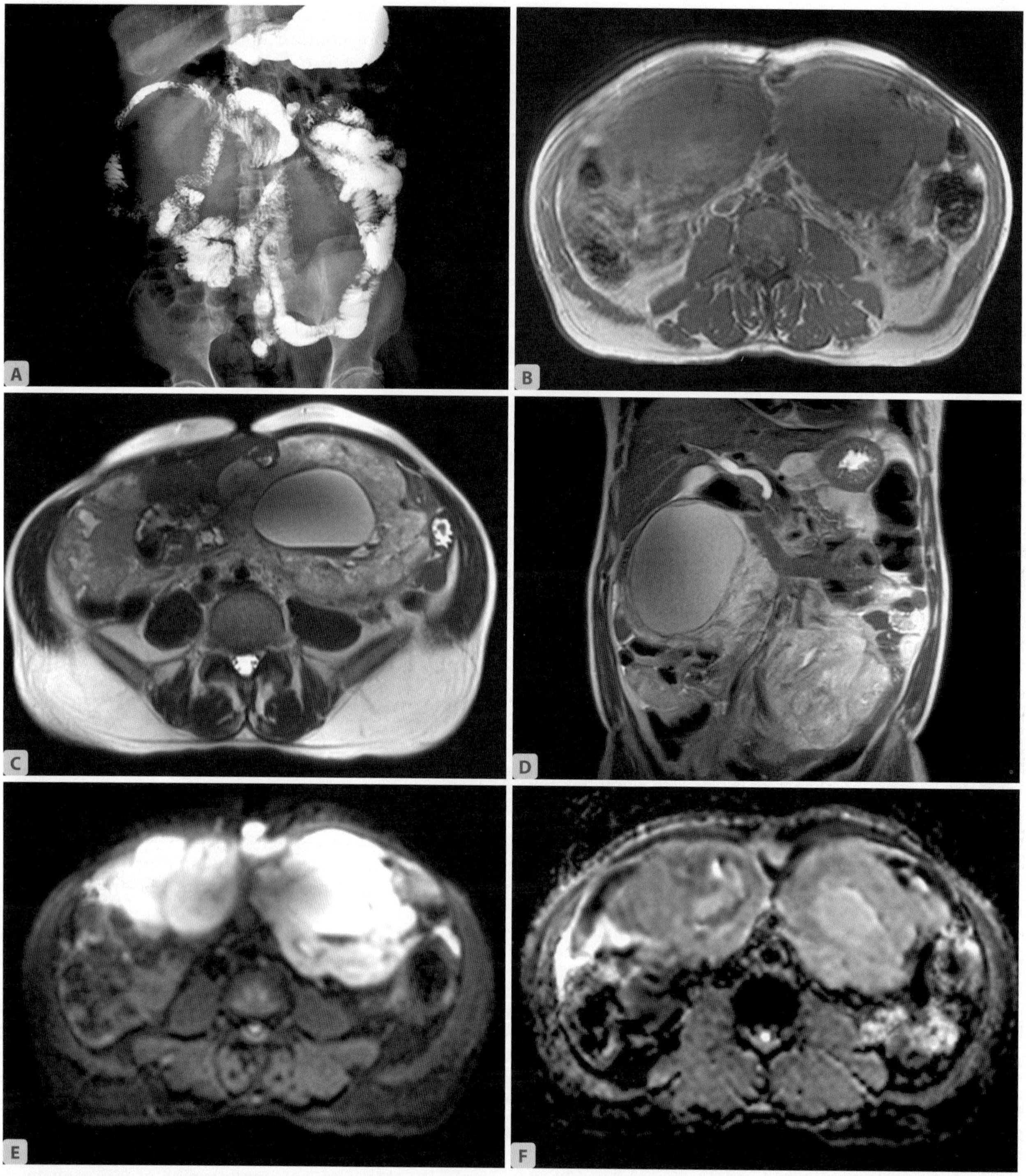

FIGS. 12A TO F: Gastrointestinal stromal tumor: Barium meal follow through examination (A) reveals evidence of extrinsic compression and displacement of small bowel loop around soft tissue masses. T1W (B); and T2W axial and coronal (C and D) MR images reveal T1W iso and T2W heterogeneously hyperintense masses in the mesentery in close proximity to the small bowel loops. A central area of cystic degeneration with fluid-fluid levels is seen in one of the lesions. (B) On DWI and ADC maps (E and F); there is evidence of restricted diffusion in the peripheral solid component appearing bright on DWI and dark on ADC maps. Note absence of lymphadenopathy or small bowel obstruction.

effusion or subcutaneous edema **(Figs. 13A and B)**. Hence, the presence of these on CT should not interpreted as new peritoneal disease.

Role of CT in early response evaluation is also being investigated, some studies reporting that decrease in attenuation of the tumor is seen within a month in most patients who respond to imatinib, in fact, it may be seen as early as 5 days after treatment. FDG-PET/MRI is extremely sensitive to detect early tumor response. A good response in the form of marked decrease in FDG uptake may be seen within 24 hours after a single dose. This may be very useful to identify early nonresponders. Even in patients showing a paradoxical increase in size on conventional CT due to hemorrhage or myxoid degeneration FDG-PET/CT can show no increase in metabolic activity resolving the dilemma.[60,63]

Other techniques that have been used include contrast enhanced ultrasound, perfusion CT and DW-MRI. On contrast enhanced ultrasound tumor response is seen as decreased tumor contrast uptake as early as day 5 or 7. Perfusion CT, has also been used to both prognosticate response to treatment and monitor treatment response with decrease in perfusion parameters such as blood flow and blood volume occurring with good response.[70,71] Using DW-MR some authors have reported that ADC values correlate closely with SUV parameters derived from PET-CT.

Surveillance is required for all cases as recurrence occurs in most patients even after complete resection, median time to recurrence being approximately 2 years. Generally recurrent disease first occurs in the liver or peritoneum. Criteria for progression include development of new lesions, increase in tumor size with new or enhancing nodules development of new lesions at previous site of disease and finally development enhancing nodules in hypoattenuating treated tumor even without increase in tumor size which is a typical pattern of progression seen in GIST **(Figs. 14A and B)**.[63]

TABLE 6: GIST key imaging findings.
• Site–stomach followed by small bowel
• Bulky exophytic heterogeneous mass
• Moderate heterogeneous enhancement
• Smooth lobulated outline
• Internal gas, cavitation and fistulization
• Lymphadenopathy distinctly uncommon
• Usually no obstruction

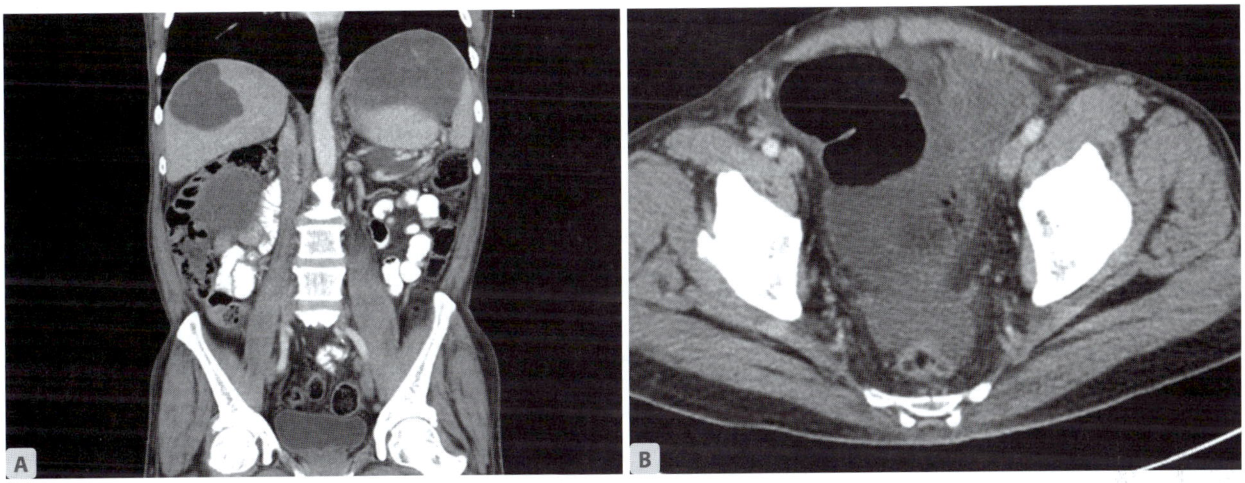

FIGS. 13A AND B: GIST on imatinib therapy: Coronal and axial CECT images of a patient with hepatic and peritoneal metastases from gastrointestinal stromal tumor (GIST) on imatinib reveal markedly hypodense lesions with no enhancing nodules consistent with a favorable response. Note the presence of free fluid in the pelvis due to fluid retention.

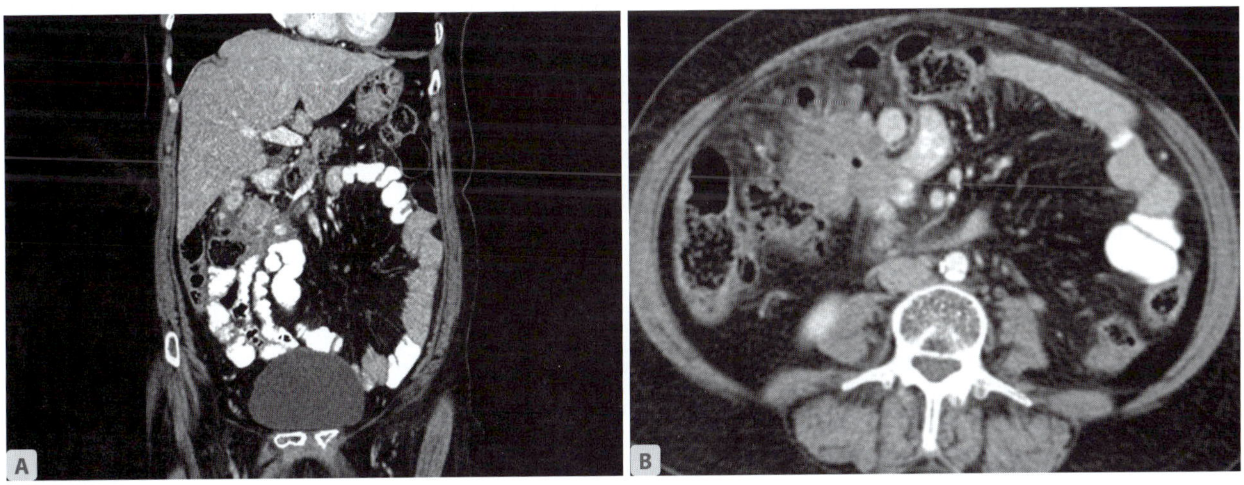

FIGS. 14A AND B: Recurrent jejunal gastrointestinal stromal tumor: Coronal and axial CECT images of an operated case of jejunal gastrointestinal stromal tumor showing a heterogeneously enhancing recurrent mass with irregular and spiculated margins at the site of previous disease involving the jejunum and adjacent transverse colon.

LYMPHOMA

Gastrointestinal tract is the most common site for extranodal non-Hodgkin's lymphoma (NHL) since the lymphoid tissue occurring in the mucosa, lamina propria and submucosa forms the largest collection of lymphocytes compared to any other immune organ in the body. Most GI tract lymphoid tissue is referred to as mucosa associated lymphoid tissue.[72-74]

Involvement of the gastrointestinal tract can be primary or secondary to generalized disease. Primary gastrointestinal non-Hodgkin's lymphoma constitutes 10–15% of all non Hodgkin's lymphomas and 30–40% of extranodal lymphomas. These generally involve only a single site. The criteria described by Dawson et al.[75] are used to define primary gastrointestinal disease. These are:

- Predominant involvement of gastrointestinal tract with lymph node involvement restricted to primary drainage area.
- No palpable lymph nodes.
- No liver or spleen involvement.
- Normal chest radiograph, i.e. no mediastinal lymphadenopathy.
- Normal peripheral white blood cell count.

Although this definition was developed before the availability of cross sectional imaging, it is still applicable.[72] Some authors however advocate a more liberal definition of primary gastrointestinal lymphoma as lymphomas that predominantly involve the gastrointestinal tract presenting with gastrointestinal symptoms notwithstanding the presence or absence of lymph node involvement.[76,77]

Secondary gastrointestinal tract involvement in generalized disease is much more frequent since lymphomas commonly arise in retroperitoneal and mesenteric lymph nodes. At autopsy gastrointestinal involvement has been reported in up to 50% cases although this may not be clinically evident.[75]

The primary form when diagnosed sufficiently early has a much better progress than systemic lymphoma with gastrointestinal involvement. However, in advanced cases it may be difficult to distinguish between primary and secondary involvement clinically, radiologically and even pathologically.[78]

ETIOPATHOGENESIS AND CLASSIFICATION

The incidence of non-Hodgkin's lymphoma is reportedly increasing due to increasing incidence of HIV infection and a variety of environmental factors.[78] Risk factors that have been identified in the pathogenesis of small bowel lymphoma include HIV infection, celiac disease, inflammatory bowel disease and immunosuppression after solid organ transplantation. The risk of lymphoma is 45–100 times in patients who have received allograft or marrow transplants. These tumors are commonly associated with Ebstein-Barr virus (EBV) infection and referred to as EBV related post-transplant lymphoproliferative disorder.[78] Gastrointestinal tract involvement is seen in one-fourth to one-third of patients with AIDS and involvement of stomach, small and large bowel has been reported with an almost equal frequency.[72,78]

Peak incidence is in the sixth decade of life with a slight male predilection of 3:2, a small peak is also noted around 10 years. Although uncommon in childhood, lymphomas constitute the most common gastrointestinal tumor in children.[78] Small bowel involvement represents about 1/3rd of the cases of gastrointestinal lymphoma and is the second most common site after the stomach. It is a common malignant tumor of the small bowel constituting about 20% of all malignant lesions. The distal ileum is the most common site likely due to the abundant lymphoid follicles in this region.[72,76,78]

The recent WHO classification of lymphomas has categorized lymphomas into two major types - B-cell lineage (including Hodgkin's lymphoma) and T-cell or NK (Natural Killer) cell lineage.[72] The various types under these two categories that may involve the small bowel are given in **Table 7**.

Most small bowel lymphomas like other gastrointestinal lymphomas are of the B-cell lineage. Although any histological subtype can occur diffuse large B-cell lymphoma (DLBCL) is the most common type of gastrointestinal lymphoma in adults. Extranodal marginal zone B-cell lymphoma (ENMZL), so named because it arises from the marginal zone of Peyer's patches, is found predominantly in the stomach but does occur in the small and large intestine also. ENMZL was previously referred to marginal zone lymphoma of mucosa associated

TABLE 7: Classification of small bowel/gastrointestinal lymphoma and clinical behavior.

B-cell	Clinical behavior prognosis	T-cell/NK cell	Clinical behavior prognosis
Diffuse large B-cell lymphoma (DLBCL)	Aggressive curable	Enteropathy associated T-cell lymphoma (EATL)	Poor prognosis due to abdominal complications
Extranodal marginal zone B-cell lymphoma (ENMZL)	Localized curable	Type I and II (EATL)	
Mantle cell lymphoma (MCL)	Moderately aggressive incurable		
Follicular lymphoma	Indolent to moderately aggressive incurable		
Burkitt lymphoma	Aggressive curable		
Hodgkin's lymphoma	Potentially curable		

lymphoid tissue (MALT lymphoma).[76] Immunoproliferative small intestinal disease (IPSID) also known as alpha chain disease is a subtype of extranodal marginal zone B-cell lymphoma found in the small bowel. It is thought to occur as a result of combination of genetic risk factors and chronic infection by *Campylobacter jejuni*. It affects young adults with almost equal sex incidence and is associated with poor socioeconomic status. Patients may show alpha heavy chain immunoglobulins in the serum. Infiltration of the bowel wall by plasma cells leads to protein losing enteropathy. It can transform to high grade Mediterranean lymphoma. This condition is common in the middle east, far east and Mediterranean region.[78] Mantle cell lymphoma (MCL) produces multiple lymphomatous polyposis first described by Cornes in 1961.[79] Burkitt's lymphoma is a highly aggressive B-cell lymphoma.[78]

T-cell lymphomas of the small bowel represent about 10–20% of primary intestinal lymphomas. Though a variety of T-cell lymphomas may involve the small bowel most of these are enteropathy associated T-cell lymphomas (EATL) occurring in refractory celiac disease.[72] A Swedish study has shown a 6.6 times higher risk of non-Hodgkin's lymphoma in patients with celiac disease, majority being primary gastrointestinal tract lymphomas of the T-cell type. These usually manifest over 60 years and are commoner in men. Besides non-Hodgkin's lymphoma, celiac disease is also a risk factor for small bowel adenocarcinoma, esophageal carcinoma and melanoma.[73]

WHO has classified enteropathy associated T-cell lymphoma or EATL as type I which is strongly associated with celiac disease and accounts for 80–90% of cases of EATL. Type II EATL is also referred to as monomorphic CD56+ve intestinal lymphoma which is not related to celiac disease although enteropathy like changes may be found on histology. Type I generally involves the jejunum and proximal ileum as the jejunum is the site where most villous damage and inflammation occur.[72,73,80]

Clinical Presentation

Clinical features of small bowel lymphoma are nonspecific. Patients may present with malaise, pain abdomen, weight loss, fever, lump abdomen, chronic diarrhea and occasionally gastrointestinal bleed and small bowel perforation.[72]

Imaging

Conventional small bowel follow through series or enteroclysis are rarely performed these days but are useful to show small polypoid lesions. On ultrasound, these tumors produce hypoechoic circumferential or asymmetric bowel wall thickening. Aneurysmal dilatation or intussusception may also be appreciated **(Figs. 15A and B)**.[78]

The CT is useful both for initial diagnosis, staging and in the follow-up after surgery or chemotherapy. CT enterography is more useful in lower grades of lymphoma where the wall thickening may be subtle. MR and MR enteroclysis provide similar information.[81]

Traditionally described radiological patterns[72,73,81] that are evident on barium studies and a well performed CT or CT/MR enterography are:

- Infiltrating form
- Polypoid form/multiple nodules
- Endoexoenteric form with excavation and fistulization
- Mesenteric invasive form.

Infiltrative Form

Circumferential infiltration of the bowel wall by lymphoma causes bowel wall thickening and subsequently distortion or effacement of folds. On barium studies submucosal infiltration by tumor causes loss or effacement of mucosal folds to produce a smooth featureless appearance. The bowel lumen is generally not narrowed, in fact it may be dilated, referred to as 'aneurysmal dilatation'. This implies a localized nonobstructive dilatation of bowel lumen with diameter more than 4 cm in areas of bowel wall thickening and is seen

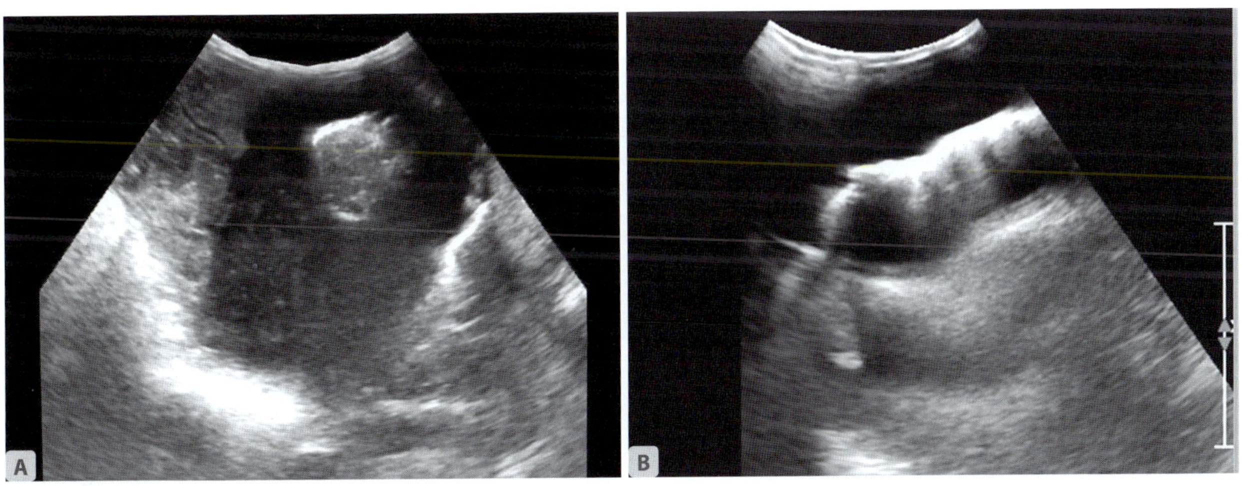

FIGS. 15A AND B: Lymphoma small bowel: Transverse and longitudinal ultrasound images reveal marked homogeneously hypoechoic bowel wall thickening with the dilated hyperechoic lumen in the center.

in about 31% of small bowel lymphoma. The underlying cause is the loss of bowel wall tone due to infiltration of submucosal myenteric plexus and muscularis propria by tumor **(Figs. 16A to C)**.[72,81]

On CT or MR there is marked homogeneous circumferential thickening of bowel wall with diameter greater than 2 cm, generally involving a long segment of bowel. The mural thickening results in separation of bowel loops which can also be appreciated on barium studies. The bowel wall attenuation is lower than or equal to muscle attenuation on CT **(Figs. 17A and B)**. On MR the wall tends to be iso on T1W and mildly hyperintense on T2W. These lesions tend to show

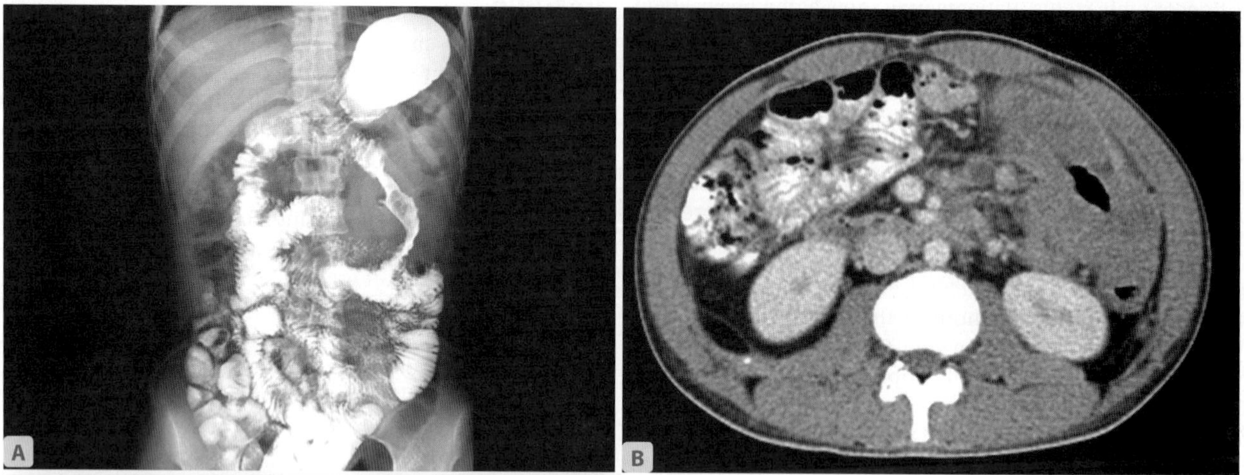

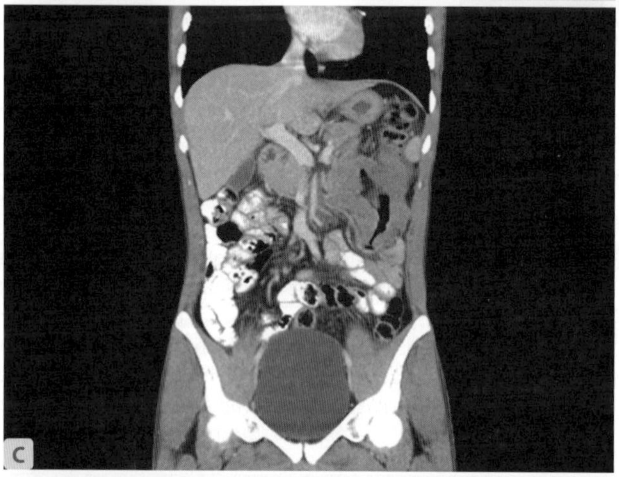

FIGS. 16A TO C: Lymphoma jejunum: Barium meal follow through examination (A) reveals an abnormal proximal jejunal loop showing a featureless appearance, fold thickening is noted along its proximal and distal aspect with separation of bowel loops due to the marked wall thickening which is appreciated on the axial and coronal CT images (C and D). The wall thickening is iso to hypodense to skeletal muscle with minimal enhancement typical of lymphoma. Note presence of mesenteric lymphadenopathy, absence of any obstructive features with aneurysmal dilatation of lumen. Radiological features consistent with an infiltrative variety of lymphoma.

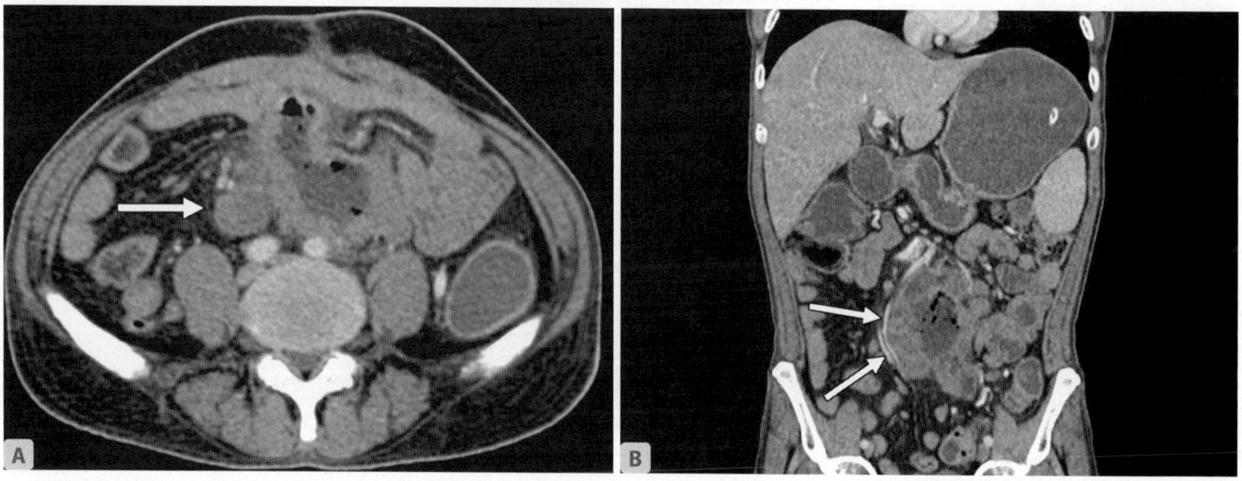

FIGS. 17A AND B: Lymphoma ileum: Axial and coronal CECT images reveal hypodense mildly enhancing wall thickening involving the ileum with aneurysmal dilatation of the lumen of the involved segment. Adjacent lymphadenopathy is also noted (arrow in A). The mesenteric vessels (arrows in B) are displaced by the mass but not encased or narrowed.

homogeneous enhancement which is generally less than that in other malignant tumors.[15,16] One study has reported lower ADC values in small bowel lymphoma compared with adenocarcinoma.[67,82]

This variety of lymphoma can generally be distinguished easily from carcinoma. The longer length of involvement, lack of luminal narrowing or the presence of aneurysmal dilatation, absence of obstructive features and a smooth mural contour with bulky mesenteric adenopathy favor the diagnosis of lymphoma. Obstruction is less common than with other tumors because non-Hodgkin's lymphoma does not evoke a desmoplastic reaction. Although aneurysmal dilatation is considered a characteristic feature of lymphoma it can be seen with gastrointestinal stromal tumors, metastatic disease and rarely adenocarcinoma.[72,73]

Polypoid Form

This form produces multiple or solitary polypoid filling defects ranging from few mm to 4 cm on small bowel barium examination. A polypoid lesion that is large enough may produce a homogeneous solid nodule protruding into the lumen on CT or MR without wall thickening or lymphadenopathy.[78] Generally the polypoid nature of nodules may not be apparent on CT and the only findings that may be seen are nonobstructive wall thickening and a mass lesion. The polypoid lesions may act as a lead point for intussusception.[73] This pattern is generally produced by mantle cell lymphoma but may also be produced by ENMZL and follicular lymphoma. The differential diagnosis of multiple/solitary polypoid lesions include intestinal polyposis syndromes, gastrointestinal stromal tumors, lipomas, adenomas or metastases. The inherited polyposis syndromes are much more commonly responsible for multiple gastrointestinal polyps than mantle cell lymphoma. A positive family history (though not always present), presentation during childhood or early adulthood and characteristic extraintestinal findings may help to establish the diagnosis of polyposis syndromes.[72]

Metastases are generally larger, more randomly distributed and may produce submucosal masses, 'bull's eye' or target lesions with central ulceration with pooling of contrast.[73]

Endoexoenteric Form

This form is associated with bowel wall thickening, a large lymphomatous mass showing exocentric growth and deep ulceration. There may be formation of sinus tracts to mesentery with resultant sterile abscesses or fistulization to other abdominal viscera.[73] Barium studies may show a large barium filled cavity along the mesenteric border of the affected bowel. CT reveals gross wall thickening, large cavitating mass with extraluminal contrast extending into the cavity which commonly shows fluid and debris.[73,83] Similar findings may be found with cavitating gastrointestinal stromal tumors and occasionally metastatic melanoma.[73]

Mesenteric Invasive Form

It is believed that this variety occurs due to direct extension of disease from affected mesenteric nodes. This produces bowel wall thickening with tethered and angulated folds contiguous with bulky mesenteric nodes. This is the variety most commonly associated with obstruction. On CT/MR a 'sandwich appearance' may be seen with mesenteric vessels forming the middle of the sandwich and surrounding conglomerate nodal/intestinal masses forming the outer layers **(Figs. 18A to C)**.[72,83]

Table 8 summarizes the most common imaging appearances of lymphoma.

Radiological Appearances of Some Specific Lymphoma Types

Hodgkin's lymphoma rarely involves the bowel with only isolated case reports being available. This may produce a stenotic mass as it produces fibrosis unlike NHL.[72]

T-cell lymphoma on barium studies, especially enteroclysis, may depict thickened nodular folds with ulceration and stricture formation usually in the jejunum but it can be multifocal. On CT/MR there may be only mild to moderate wall thickening which is better appreciated on CT/MR enteroclysis **(Figs. 19A and B)**. Associated lymphadenopathy and infiltration of mesenteric fat may also be seen. Perforation is much more common in this variety of lymphoma and is believed to be due to angiocentric growth of lymphoid cells with infiltration of vessel walls producing vascular occlusion and ischemic necrosis. It has been reported that perforation may be present in 16%–33% of patient with type I and type II EATL respectively.[73] Laparotomy may be required in as many as 50% patients for complications such as hemorrhage, perforation or obstruction.[72] This variety of lymphoma needs to be distnguished from other complications of celiac disease such as chronic jejunoileitis (CJI) and refractory celiac disease (RCD). CJI is a rare complication difficult to distinguish and considered by some to represent a low grade enteropathy-associated T-cell lymphoma. Findings of effacement of jejunal folds, small bowel wall thickening, intussusception, infiltration of mesenteric fat, lymphadenopathy and splenic atrophy have been reported on CT and MR in refractory celiac disease (RCD). FDG PET has an important role in distinguishing between RCD and EATL as 86–100% of EATL lymphomas show increased uptake. The 5 year survival for T-cell lymphomas at 25% is much worse than the 75% survival rate for B-cell lymphomas.[72,73]

Burkitt's Lymphoma

The endemic variety of Burkitt's lymphoma is associated with Ebstein-Barr virus (EBV) infection and commonly involves the head and neck region. Other variants include sporadic variety and that associated with HIV infection (the immunodeficiency associated variant). It is a very rapidly growing tumor, commonly occurring in children and usually affects the terminal ileum or ileo-cecal region in sporadic cases. Less commonly it may involve the stomach or colon peak age of occurrence is 11 years. The genetic defects identified include translocation and deregulation of *c-Myc* gene on chromosome 8. On histology a typical 'starry-sky appearance' is seen due to macrophage containing cellular debris lying scattered within dense sheets of lymphoid cells.[76,77]

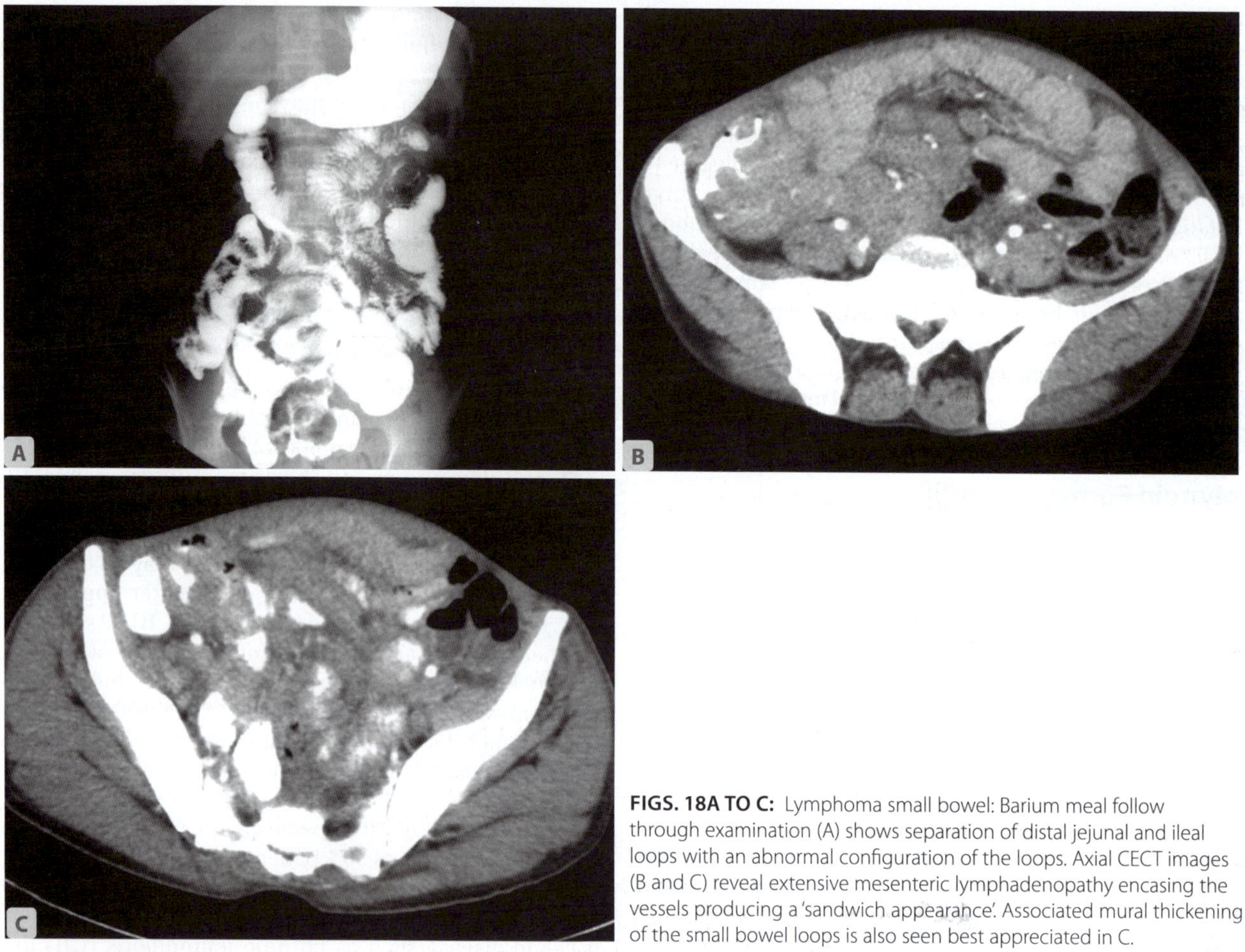

FIGS. 18A TO C: Lymphoma small bowel: Barium meal follow through examination (A) shows separation of distal jejunal and ileal loops with an abnormal configuration of the loops. Axial CECT images (B and C) reveal extensive mesenteric lymphadenopathy encasing the vessels producing a 'sandwich appearance'. Associated mural thickening of the small bowel loops is also seen best appreciated in C.

TABLE 8: Lymphoma key imaging findings.

• *Site*: Terminal ileum
• Long segment involvement
• *Barium*: Fold thickening/featureless appearance, aneurysmal dilatation
• *CT/MR*: Marked homogeneous hypodense/hypoattenuating wall thickening
• Minimal enhancement
• Smooth mural contour
• Associated findings
• Bulky adenopathy
• Bowel obstruction distinctly uncommon

Barium studies may show markedly thickened valvulae conniventes while grossly thickened bowel wall due to infiltration by tumor is seen on CT. There may be associated aneurysmal dilatation and intussusception with the thickened walls serving as the lead point. Diffuse lymphadenopathy, infiltration of the mesentery and peritoneum with peritoneal carcinomatosis may be seen. These tumors show high FDG uptake on initial scans due to their rapidly proliferating nature which reverts to normal following treatment **(Figs. 20A to F)**.

Endemic Burkitt's lymphoma is very chemosensitive and 5 years survival rates exceed 90% in children with localized disease. Sporadic and immunodeficiency associated Burkitt's are less sensitive to chemotherapy but 50–70% overall survival rate may be seen in adults after intensive chemotherapy.

Although radiological features of lymphoma are not specific to various pathogical types some radiologic pathologic correlation does exist[76] and is summarized in **Table 9**.

STAGING AND PROGNOSTICATION

Staging and response assessment systems in lymphoma have evolved over time owing to the introduction of radiation therapy, CT and FDG-PET/CT. ^{18}F-FDG-PET/CT along with a CECT has been recommended as a staging tool for all FDG avid lymphomas. For the non-FDG avid varieties a CECT is recommended. It is also an excellent tool to evaluate response after treatment before morphological changes become apparent.[84]

Lymphomas comprise an extremely heterogeneous group of tumors hence their metabolic activity and glucose uptake is variable with low grade NHLs showing lower glucose uptake than aggressive lesions. Low grade follicular lymphomas and indolent extranodal marginal zone B-cell lymphoma (ENMZL) may show very low FDG uptake making it difficult to

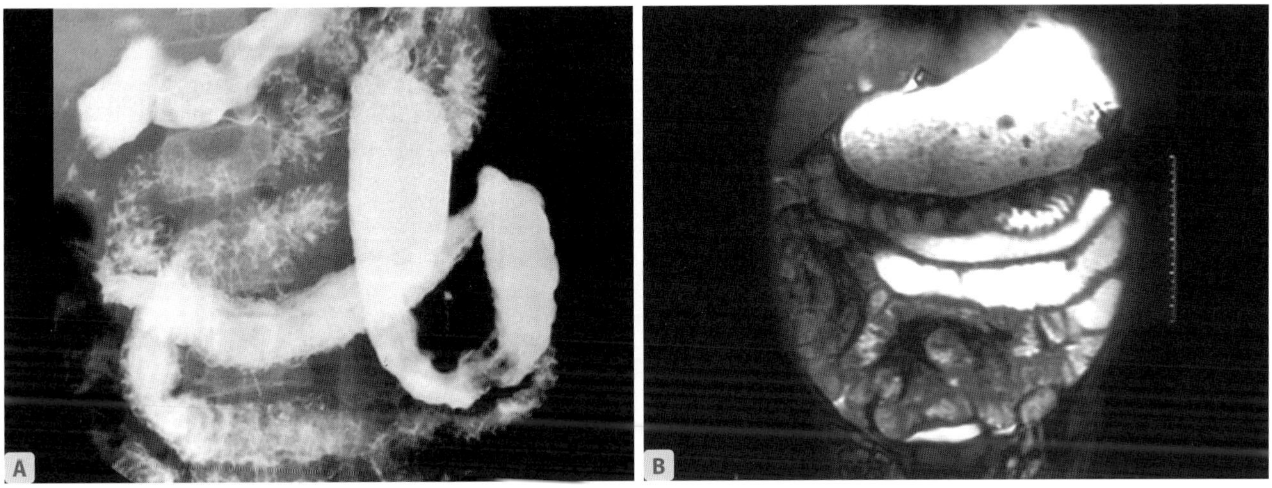

FIGS. 19A AND B: T-cell lymphoma jejunum: Barium enteroclysis (A) reveals nodular fold thickening in the jejunum with dilated featureless segment of jejunum in a patient with symptoms of malabsorption. Coronal T2W MR enteroclysis image (B) shows only mild wall thickening of the involved segments.

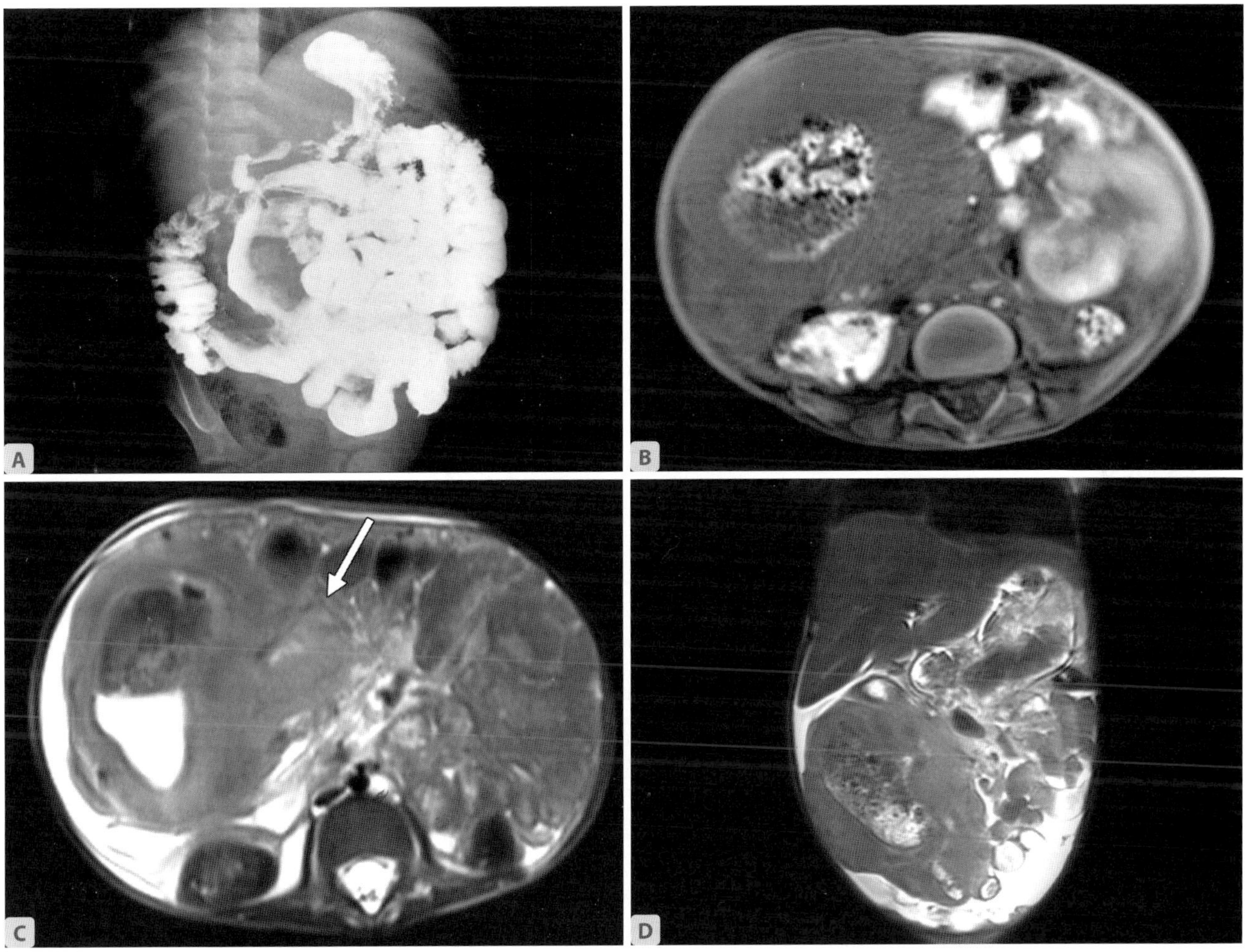

FIGS. 20A TO F: *Continued*

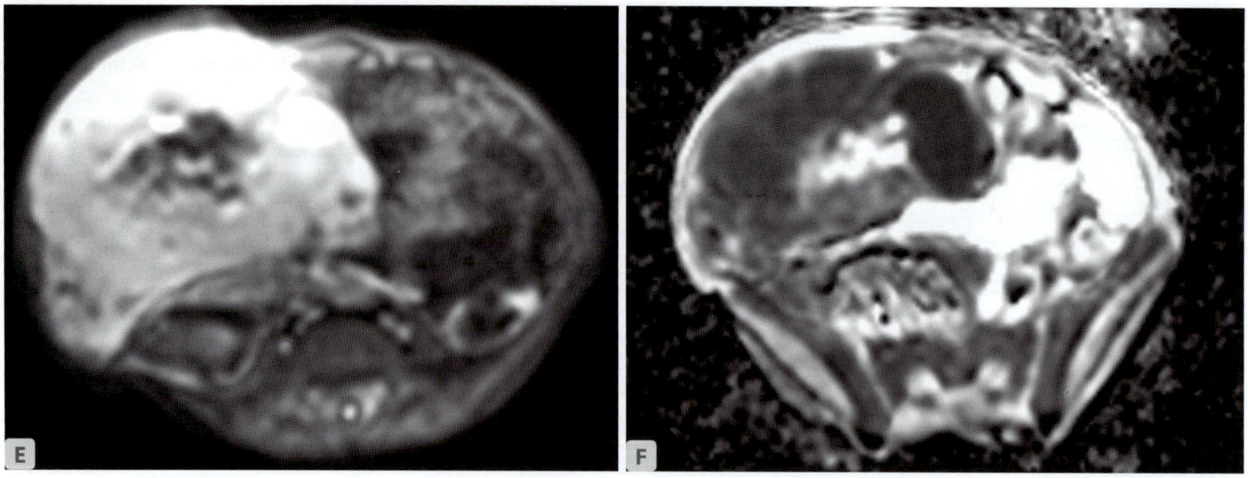

FIGS. 20A TO F: Burkitt's lymphoma: Barium meal follow through examination (A) of an 11-year-old boy presenting with a rapidly enlarging abdominal lump reveals long-segment effacement of mucosal folds resulting in a smooth featureless appearance of the distal ileum along with luminal dilatation. The presence of a significant extraluminal component is suggested by the surrounding soft tissue haze and displacement of bowel loops. T1W axial (B), T2W axial and coronal (C and D) depict marked wall thickening of the terminal ileum appearing hypointense on T1W images, mildly hyperintense on T2W images with evidence of diffusion restriction seen as bright signal on the DWI (E) and hypointense signal on ADC (F). Note the presence of ascites and adjacent lymphadenopathy (arrow in C).

TABLE 9: Correlation of radiologic findings with pathology in small bowel lymphoma.

Radiologic findings	Likely lymphoma type	Therapeutic options
1. Marked homogeneous nonobstructive bowel wall thickening, aneurysmal dilatation and bulky lymph nodes Site-distal ileum FDG-PET avid	DLBCL	Chemotherapy R-CHOP
2. *Barium*: Multiple small polyps *CT*: Polyps/nonobstructive bowel wall thickening and lymph nodes Site-distal ileum, colon and rectum Curvilinear areas of FDG-PET uptake	MCL Occasionally, ENMZL (more often in stomach/colon)	R-CHOP R-Hyper CVAD Consider stem cell transplant
3. Circumferential/asymmetric wall thickening polypoid mass FDG-PET avidity variable	MCL ENMZL	*H. pylori* +ve–antibiotics *H. pylori* –ve/resistant–chemotherapy
4. Nodular fold thickening Site-proximal jejunum, entire small bowel in young adult males from middle east	IPSID	Tetracycline based antibiotic Unresponsive to antibiotics CHOP
5. Tiny polyps/fold thickening in jejunum FDG PET—unreliable	Follicular lymphoma	Wait and watch Chemotherapy—fludarabine based
6. Bulky terminal ileal/ileo-caecal disease in a child, rapidly progressive Strongly FDG-PET avid.	Burkitt's lymphoma	Chemotherapy—Magrath regimen*, hyper-CVAD
7. Barium nodular fold thickening, ulceration *CT*: Long segment eccentric circumferential mild wall thickening perforation in up to 50%. Associated features of celiac disease. Site-proximal jejunum FDG-PET avid.	EATL	Anthracycline containing Combination chemotherapy—CHOP

*Magrath regimen, cyclophosphamide, doxorubicin, vincristine, methotrexate, ifosfamide, etoposide, cytarabine.

(CHOP: cyclophosphamide, doxorubicin, vincristine, prednisone; R: rituximab; Hyper-CVAD: cyclophosphamide, vincristine, doxorubicin, dexamethasone methotrexate, cytarabine; DLBCL: diffuse large B-cell lymphoma; ENMZL: extranodal marginal zone B-cell lymphoma; IPSID: immunoproliferative small intestinal disease; EATL: enteropathy associated T-cell lymphoma).

detect primary lesions. On the other hand diffuse large B-cell lymphoma (DLBCL), MCL, EATL, Burkitt's lymphoma and Hodgkin's disease are FDG avid. However, studies suggest that most low grade lymphomas can also be accurately staged with PET/CT.[84,85]

In some studies SUVmax (standard value uptake) varied greatly (between 3.2 and 43) among different lymphoma types. Aggressive lymphomas have a SUV max three times than that of indolent lymphoma on an average. A cut-off value of SUVmax at 10 reportedly had 71% sensitivity and 81% specificity in differentiating aggressive and indolent lymphomas.[84,85]

New tracers like ^{18}F fluorothymidine being evaluated for PET-CT may be useful to distinguish between high grade and low grade lymphoma and early response assessment.[81,83] Their uptake is dependent on cell proliferation rather than glucose metabolism. However, high physiological tracer uptake in the abdomen limits the usefulness of these tracers for imaging of abdominal and pelvic lymphomas.

Whole body of diffusion-weighted MRI (WB-DWMRI) has also been evaluated as a tool to stage and follow-up gastrointestinal lymphoma with reports suggesting comparable diagnostic value as FDG PET-CT.[82,86] In a study comparing DW-MRI and PET-CT, DW-MRI was found to be only slightly inferior to FDG PET/CT for staging FDG avid lymphomas but for lymphomas with variable FDG avidity such as MALT lymphoma, DWI was superior to both ^{18}FFDG-PET/CT and CECT (93.5% vs 64.5% sensitivity).[82,86] Thus WB-DW-MRI appears to be a promising tool for nodal and bone marrow of staging lymphomas. PET-MR Protocols are also being evaluated for lymphoma staging.[10]

A number of staging systems are available for GI lymphoma. The Mushoff modification of the Ann Arbor staging[87] is often used, however it suffers from the limitation that it does not address certain features specific to gastrointestinal lymphoma such as diffuse and incurable infiltration of the gastrointestinal tract.

An alternative staging system was first proposed by Blackledge and later modified by the international workshop in Lugano, Switzerland in 1994.[88] Lugano staging is a modification of the original Ann Arbor staging designed for the staging of primary GI lymphomas **(Table 10)**.

The Paris staging system[89] proposed by European Gastrointestinal Lymphoma Study (EGILS) Group in 2003 has become increasingly accepted. This is summarized in **Table 11**. The major advantage of this staging system is its ability to record the depth of tumor infiltration, specific lymphoma spread and extent of nodal involvement.

The prognosis of NHL is better than that adenocarcinoma as it remains confined to the bowel wall for a long time and because more effective chemotherapy is available. The adverse risk factors for GI lymphoma include advanced stage, involvement of para-aortic nodes, large tumor bulk, serosal penetration, and intestinal rather than gastric origin. Other poor prognostic factors include advanced age of patient and higher grade of lymphoma.[78,81]

Treatment

Treatment[83] usually consists of a combination of chemotherapy, surgery and radiotherapy and is summarized in **Table 8**.

TABLE 10: Lugano classification for GI lymphoma.

- *Stage I*: Tumor confined to gastrointestinal tract, single primary or multiple noncontiguous lesions
- *Stage II*: Tumor extends into the abdominal cavity from primary gastrointestinal site
- *Stage II1*: Local nodal involvement
- *Stage II2*: Distant nodal involvement
- *Stage IIE*: Penetration of serosa to involve adjacent organ or tissue
- *Stage III*: no stage III in this system
- *Stage IV*: Disseminated extranodal involvement or gastrointestinal tract lesion with supradiaphragmatic nodal involvement (CME lymphoma—12)
- Specify site of involvement, e.g. IIE pancreas. If both nodal and adjacent organ involvement—both subscript 1 or 2 and E is used, e.g. II2E (pancreas)

TABLE 11: Paris staging system for primary gastrointestinal lymphomas (TNMB).

Stage	Gastrointestinal lymphomas
TX	Lymphoma extent not specified
T0	No evidence of lymphoma
T1	Lymphoma confined to the mucosa/submucosa
T1m	Lymphoma confined to the mucosa
T1sm	Lymphoma confined to the submucosa
T2	Lymphoma infiltrates muscularis propria or subserosa
T3	Lymphoma penetrates serosa (visceral peritoneum) without invasion of adjacent structures
T4	Lymphoma invades adjacent structures or organs
NX	Involvement of lymph nodes not assessed
N0	No evidence of lymph nodes involvement
N1	Involvement of regional lymph nodes
N2	Involvement of intra-abdominal lymph nodes beyond the regional area
N3	Spread to extra-abdominal lymph nodes
MX	Dissemination of lymphoma not assessed
M0	No evidence of extranodal dissemination
M1	Non-continuous involvement of separate site in gastrointestinal tract (e.g. stomach and rectum)
M2	Non-continuous involvement of other tissues (e.g. peritoneum, pleura) or organs (e.g. tonsils, parotid gland, ocular, adnexa, lung, liver, spleen, kidney, breast, etc.)
BX	Involvement of bone marrow not assessed
B0	No evidence of bone marrow involvement
B1	Lymphomatous infiltration of bone marrow
TNM	*Clinical staging:* Status of tumor, node, metastasis, bone marrow
$_p$TNMB	*Histopathological staging*: Status of tumor, node metastasis, bone marrow
pN	The histopathological examination will ordinarily include six or more lymph nodes

B-cell Lymphoma

Anthracycline based chemotherapy is the mainstay in the treatment of intestinal DLBCL. Primary surgery may be required at times to establish the diagnosis, reduce tumor bulk, to manage complications from perforation, obstruction and for staging. Radiotherapy may be used when there is bulky residual disease or only partial resection has been possible.

Immunoproliferative small intestinal disease (IPSID) is initially treated with tetracycline and metronidazole. A wait and watch policy may be adopted for lower grades of lymphoma like follicular lymphoma.

T-cell Lymphoma

Owing to its rarity the treatment of primary T-cell lymphoma is not well-defined. A gluten free diet helps to reduce the risk of lymphoma in celiac disease. Primary surgery along with chemotherapy is generally recommended due to the risk of perforation, hemorrhage and obstruction. However, following surgery initiation of chemotherapy is usually delayed because of postoperative infection and the difficulty in healing due to malnutrition.

Kaposi's Sarcoma

Kaposi's sarcoma is a tumor commonly associated with AIDS. It is a low grade systemic vascular neoplasm involving skin in the form of pigmented cutaneous lesions, internal organs and lymph nodes. In AIDS associated Kaposi' sarcoma early involvement of intestine and lymph nodes is seen. Lesions of Kaposi's sarcoma tend to be multiple and are generally seen as elevated submucosal nodules in the jejunum and ileum. Small bowel folds may be diffusely thickened. The lesions generally show mild heterogeneous enhancement. Associated retroperitoneal and mesenteric lymphadenopathy is common. Differentiation from lymphoma may be very difficult although Kaposi's sarcoma is more focal and nodular.[15,16]

Leiomyosarcoma

True leiomyosarcomas of the small bowel arise from the smooth muscle of the small bowel wall or blood vessels and are very rare accounting for less than 15% of primary intestinal malignant tumors. Usually these are solitary being situated in the jejunum and ileum and most commonly in Meckel's diverticuclum. The growth pattern is mainly slow extraluminal growth resulting in late presentation. Usually tumors exceed 5 cm in size at presentation.[14,16]

On barium studies a predominantly extrinsic lesion with barium filled cavitation may be seen. On CT/MR they produce large heterogeneous masses with area of necrosis and cystic degeneration with rim enhancement. There can be associated cavitation or fistulization **(Figs. 21A to C)**. Liver and peritoneal metastasis may also be seen which tend

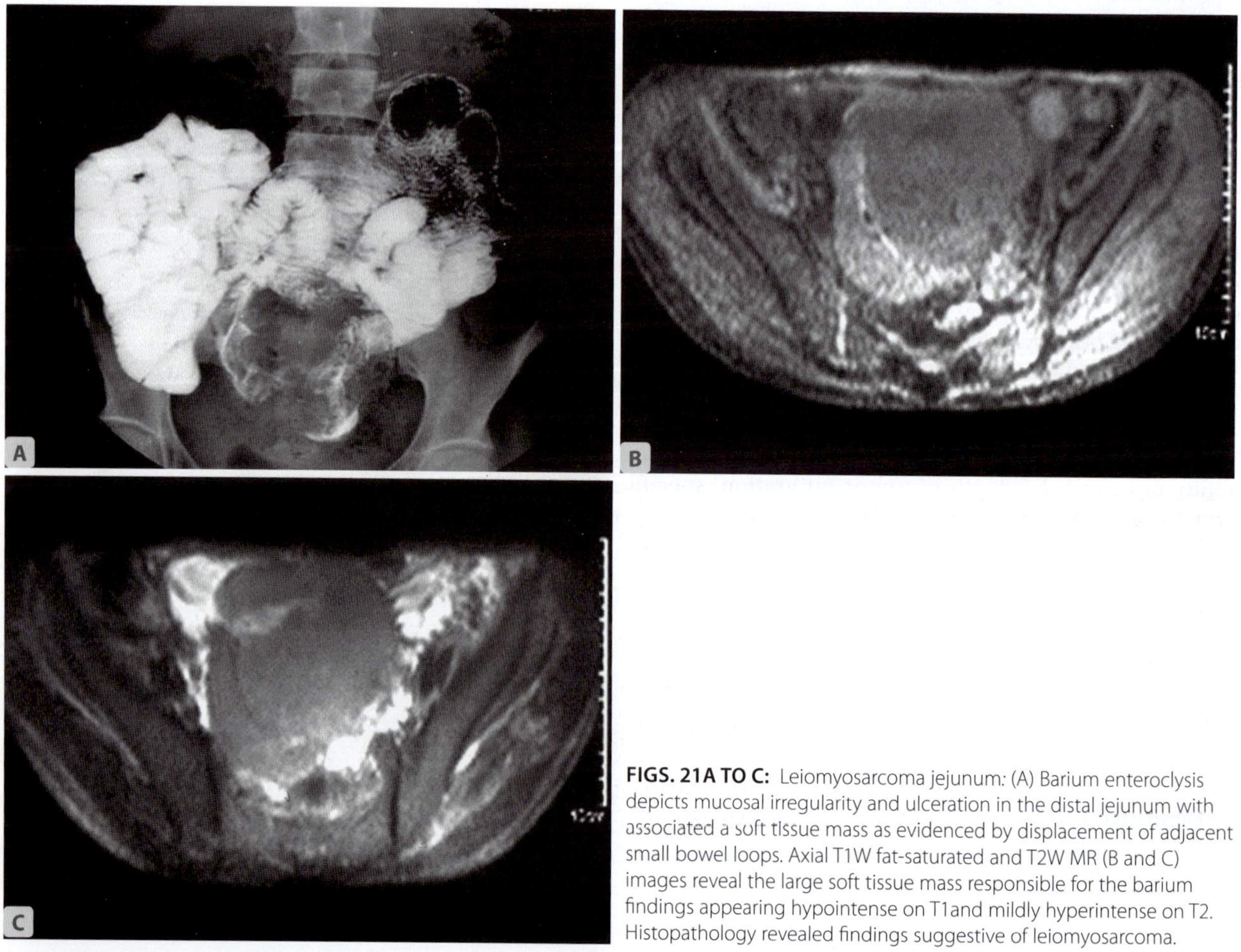

FIGS. 21A TO C: Leiomyosarcoma jejunum: (A) Barium enteroclysis depicts mucosal irregularity and ulceration in the distal jejunum with associated a soft tissue mass as evidenced by displacement of adjacent small bowel loops. Axial T1W fat-saturated and T2W MR (B and C) images reveal the large soft tissue mass responsible for the barium findings appearing hypointense on T1and mildly hyperintense on T2. Histopathology revealed findings suggestive of leiomyosarcoma.

to be large with peripheral rim enhancement due to central necrosis. On imaging these cannot be distinguished from GIST.[1,14,16]

Metastatic Neoplasms

Secondary metastatic involvement of the small bowel is commoner than primary and may account for nearly half of all small bowel tumors.[1] The major pathways for metastatic spread are hematogenous, direct extension, intraperitoneal seeding and lymphatic.[1] Tumors from the stomach, colon, ovary and uterus spread to the small bowel either by direct invasion or intraperitoneal spread while hematogenous metastases are seen in carcinoma breast, lung and melanoma.

The extraintestinal malignancy with the greatest propensity to metastasize to the bowel is melanoma. Small bowel is the most frequent site involved in the gastrointestinal tract owing to its rich blood supply. The vasa recti form a rich submucosal plexus on the antimesenteric border of the small bowel hence hematogenous metastatic deposits occur on the antimesentric border. Hematogeneous metastasis may produce solitary or multiple submucosal nodules on barium studies with or without central ulceration—'the bulls eye' appearance. On CT or MR these produce a short segment wall thickening or focal mass with contrast enhancement and at times may mimic primary neoplasm **(Figs. 22A to D)**.[1,14,16,28]

Intraperitoneal metastases most commonly arise from the colon or ovary. Transperitoneal seedling follows the circulatory pathway of peritoneal fluid. This fluid after flowing over the mesenteric recesses settles at the termination of small bowel mesentery in the ileo cecal region. Therefore transperitoneal metastases occur at the mesenteric border. They produce small contrast enhancing nodules along the serosal surface with disease progression they can encase the small bowel and cause obstruction. Gadolinium enhanced fat saturated MR has been shown to be more sensitive than CT to detect small tumor nodules **(Figs. 23A and B)**.[1,30,32]

Infiltration from advanced colonic, ovarian, pancreatic or biliary neoplasms can also involve the small bowel **(Figs. 24A to C)**.

CONCLUSION

Small bowel tumors are rare neoplasms, this combined with the nonspecific presentation and the relative difficulty in the evaluation of the small bowel makes early diagnosis of

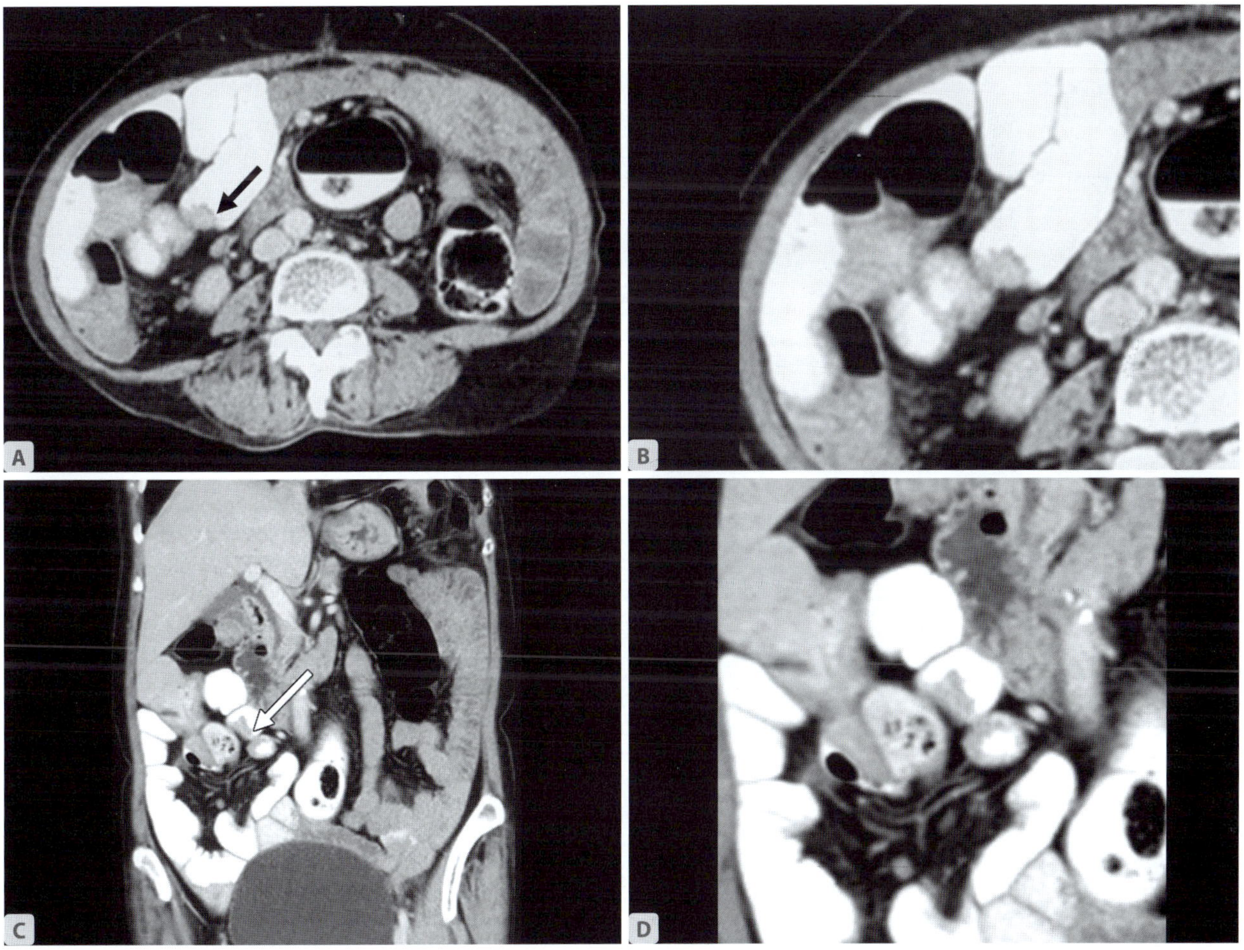

FIGS. 22A TO D: Metastases small bowel: Axial and coronal CECT images (A to D) in a patient of melanoma with hematogenous metastases reveals a focal polypoid intraluminal mass and wall thickening in the jejunum better seen on the magnified images (B and D) with mild dilatation of the loops.

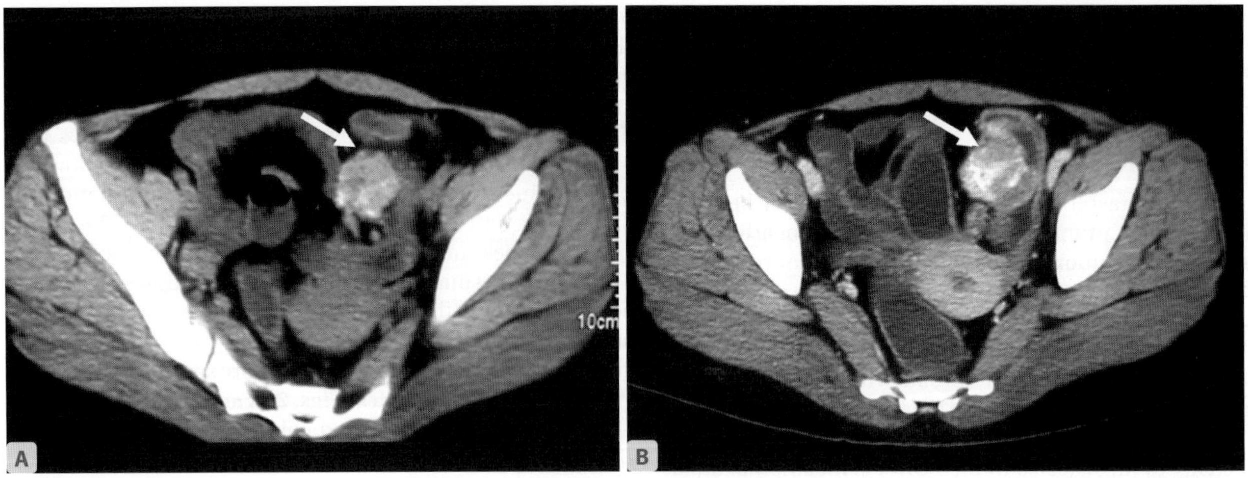

FIGS. 23A AND B: Metastases small bowel: Axial NCCT and CECT images show a serosal deposit on an ileal loop in the pelvis showing calcification and heterogeneous enhancement (arrows) in an operated case of adenocarcinoma ascending colon.

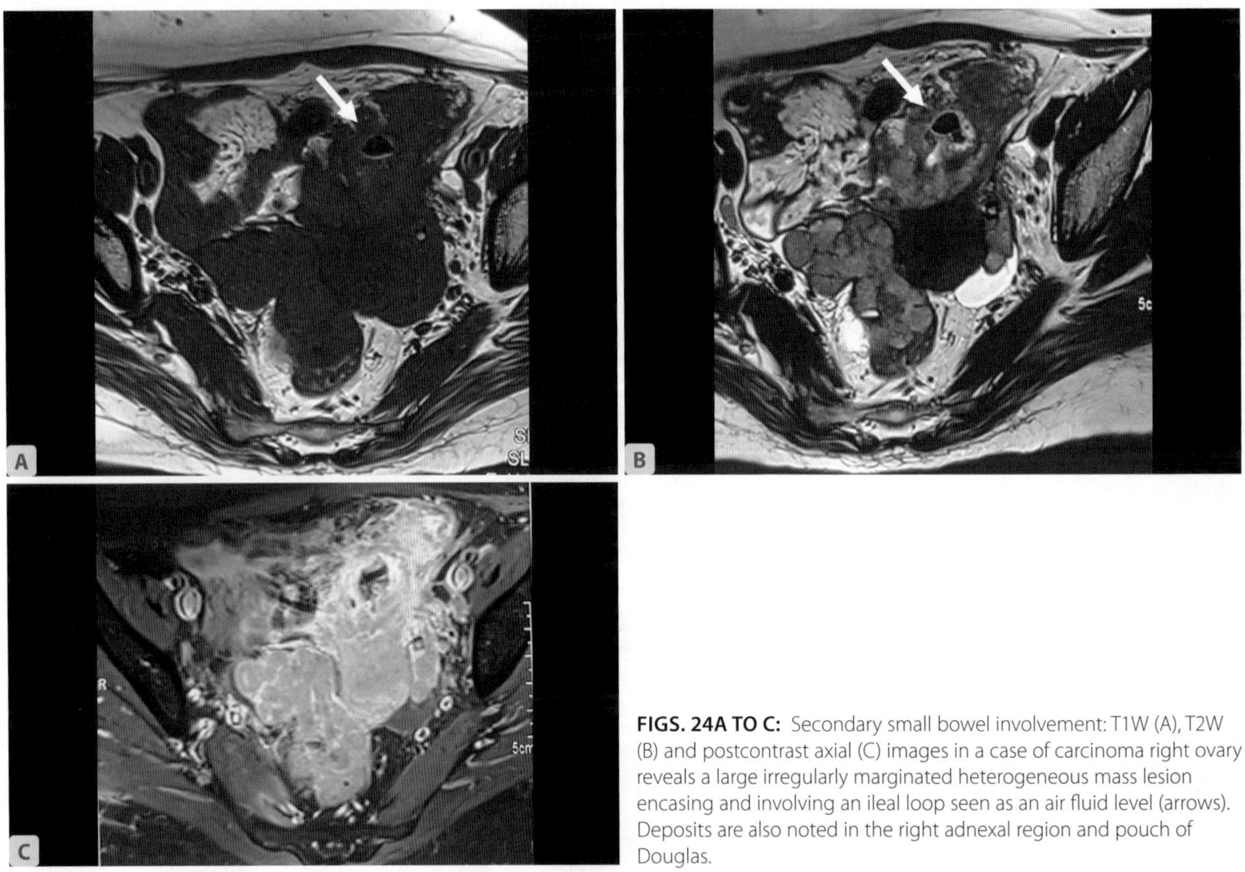

FIGS. 24A TO C: Secondary small bowel involvement: T1W (A), T2W (B) and postcontrast axial (C) images in a case of carcinoma right ovary reveals a large irregularly marginated heterogeneous mass lesion encasing and involving an ileal loop seen as an air fluid level (arrows). Deposits are also noted in the right adnexal region and pouch of Douglas.

these lesions difficult. Despite advances in endoscopy, the radiologist continues to play a key role in their diagnosis. The imaging features of various small bowel tumors may overlap with each other, however, recognition of certain characteristic features on imaging studies may help to narrow the differential. The radiologist therefore needs to be fully conversant with the imaging features of small bowel tumors and consider these as a differential diagnosis in the appropriate clinical and radiologic context to avoid delay in diagnosis.

REFERENCES

1. Xynopoulos D, Mihas AA, Paraskevas E, Dimitroulopoulos D, Heuman DM, Mihas AA. Small bowel tumors. Annals of Gastroenterology. 2002;15(1):18-35.
2. Martin RG. Malignant tumors of the small intestine. Surg Clin N Am. 1986;66:779-85.
3. Neugut AI, Jacobson JS, Suh S, Mukherjee R, Arber N. The epidemiology of cancer of the small bowel. Cancer Epidemiol Biomarkers Prev. 1999;7:243-51.
4. Pourmand K, Itzkowitz SH. Small bowel neoplasms and polyps current gastroenterology reports. 2016;18:23. doi 10.1007s11894.016.0497.xfghg
5. Hara AK, Leighton JA, Sharma VK, Height RI, Fleischer DE. Imaging of small bowel disease: comparison of capsule endoscopy, standard endoscopy, barium examination and CT. Radiographics. 2005;25:697-718.
6. Nolan DJ, Traill ZC. The current role of barium examination of the small intestine. Clin Radiol. 1997;52:809-20.
7. Wale A, Pilcher J. Current role of ultrasound in small bowel imaging: seminars in ultrasound CT and MRI. 2016;37(5): 482-97.
8. Pilleul F, Penigaud M, Milot L, et al. Possible small-bowel neoplasms: contrast-enhanced and water-enhanced multidetector CT enteroclysis. Radiology. 2006;241(3):796.
9. Pappalardo G, Gualdi G, Nunziale A, et al. Impact of magnetic resonance in the preoperative staging and the surgical planning for treating small bowel neoplasms. Surg Today. 2013;43(6):613.
10. Goh V, Prezzi D, Mallia A, Bashir U, Stirling JJ, John J, Charles-Edwards G, MacKewn J, Cook G. Positron Emission Tomography/ Magnentic Resonance Imaging of Gastrointestinal Cancers: Seminars in Ultrasound CT and MRI. 2016;37(4):352-7.
11. Levine MS, Rubesin SE, Laufer I. Pattern approach for diseases of mesenteric small bowel on barium studies. Radiology. 2008;249:2.
12. Rubesin SE. Simplified approach to differential diagnosis of small bowel abnormalities. Radiol Clin North Am. 2003;41: 343-64.
13. Lappas JC, Maglinte DD, Sandrasegaran K. Benign tumors of the small-bowel. Gore R, Levine M (Eds). Textbook of gastrointestinal radiology, 3rd edition. Philadelphia, PA: Saunders Elsevier; 2008. pp. 845-51.
14. Sailer J, Zacherl J, Schimaa W. MDCT of small bowel tumors. Cancer Imaging. 2007;7(1):224-33.
15. Masselli G, Polettini E, Casciani E, Bertini L, Vecchioli A, Gualdi G. Small-bowel neoplasm: prospective evaluation of MR enteroclysis. Radiology. 2009;251:743-50.
16. Masselli G, Colaiacomo MC, Marcelli G, et al. MRI of the small-bowel: how to differentiate primary neoplasms and mimickers. The British Journal of Radiology. 2012;85(1014):824-37.
17. CY Lee, MK Yuen. Inflammatory fibroid polyps causing intussusception in adult patients: Two case reports and review of literature focusing on radiological features. Hong Kong J Radiol. 2014;17:271-6.
18. Thompson WM. Imaging and Findings of Lipomas of the Gastrointestinal Tract American Journal of Roentgenology. 2005;184:1163-71.
19. Corsi A, Ingegnoli A, Abelli P, et al. Imaging of a small bowel cavernous hemangioma: report of a case with emphasis on the use of computed tomography and enteroclysis. Acta Biomed. 2007;78(2):139-43.
20. Huprich JE, Barlow JM, Hansel SL, et al. Multiphase CT enterography evaluation of small-bowel vascular lesions. American Journal of Roentgenology. 2013;201:65-72.
21. Buck JL, Harned RK. Polyposis syndromes. In: Gore RM, Levine MS (Eds). Textbook of gastrointestinal radiology, 2nd edition. Philadelphia, Pa: Saunders, 2000. pp. 1075-88.
22. Durno CA. Colonic polyps in children and adolescents. Can J Gastroenterol. 2007;21(4):233-9.
23. Brucher BL, Roder JD, Fink U, Stein HJ, Busch R, Siewert JR. Prognostic factors in resected primary small bowel tumors. Dig Surg. 1998;15:42-51.
24. Aparicio T, Zaanan A, Svrcek M, et al. Small bowel adenocarcinoma: epidemiology, risk factors, diagnosis and treatment. Dig Liver Dis. 2014;46:97-104.
25. Negri E, Bosetti C, La Vecchia C, Fioretti F, Conti E, Franceschi S. Risk factors for adenocarcinoma of the small intestine. Cancer. 1999;82:171-4.
26. Maglinte DD, Lappas JC, Sandrasegaran Malignant. Tumors of the small bowel. In: Gore R, Levine M (Eds). Textbook of gastrointestinal radiology, 3rd edition. Saunders Elsevier, Philadelphia, PA; 2008. pp. 853-69.
27. Masselli G, Gualdi G. Evaluation of small bowel tumors: MR enteroclysis. Abdm Imaging. 2010;35:23-30.
28. Faggian A, Fracella MR, D'Alesio G, Alabiso ME, Berritto D, Feragalli B, Miele V, Iasiello F, Grassi R. Small-Bowel Neoplasms: Role of MRI Enteroclysis: Gastroenterology Research and Practice Volume 2016, Article ID 9686815, 6 pages.
29. Cronin CG, Scott J, Kambadakone A, Catalano OA, Sahani D, Blake MA, McDermott S. Utility of positron emission tomography/ CT in the evaluation of small bowel pathology. Br J Radiol. 2012;85(1017):1211-21.
30. Sinha R, Rajiah P, Ramachandran I, Sanders S, Murphy PD. Diffusion-weighted MR imaging of the gastrointestinal tract: technique, indications, and imaging findings. Radiographics. 2013;33(3):655-76.
31. Kyriazi S, Collins DJ, Morgan VA, Giles SL, deSouza NM. Diffusion-weighted imaging of peritoneal disease for noninvasive staging of advanced ovarian cancer. Radiographics. 2010;30(5):1269-85.
32. Low RN, Sebrechts CP, Barone RM, Muller W. Diffusion-weighted MRI of peritoneal tumors: comparison with conventional MRI and surgical and histopathologic findings—a feasibility study. AJR. 2009;193(2):461-70.
33. Sobin LH, Gospodarowicz MK, Wittekind C. TNM classification of malignant tumors, 7th edition. Wiley Blackwell; 2009. pp. 153-9.
34. Cunningham D, Atkin W, Lenz HJ, et al. Colorectal cancer. Lancet. 2010;375(9719):1030-47.
35. Langhans T. Ubereinendrusenpolypimileum. Virchow Archiv Pathol Anatom Phys Klin Med. 1867;38:559-60.
36. Lubarsch O. Ueber den primaren krebs des ileum nebst bemerkungen uber das gleichzeitige vorkommen von krebs and tuberculose. Virchow Archiv Pathol Anatom Phys Klin Med. 1888;111:280-317.
37. Oberndorfer S. Karzinoide tumoren des dunndarms. Frankf Z Pathol. 1907;9:425-9.
38. Yao JC, Hassan M, Phan A, et al. One hundred years after "carcinoid": epidemiology of and prognostic factors for neuroendocrine tumors in 35,825 cases in the United States. J Clin Oncol. 2008;26:3063-72.
39. Ganeshan D, Bhosale P, Yang T, Kundra V. Imaging features of carcinoid tumor of gastrointestinal tract. Am J Roentgenol. 2013;201(4):773-86.
40. Rindi G, Bordi C. Highlights of the biology of endocrine tumors of the gut and pancreas. Endocr Relat Cancer. 2003;10:427-36.
41. Chang S, Choi D, Jin Lee S, Jae Lee W, Park M, Sang Won Kim, Da Keun Lee, Kee-Taek Jang. Neuroendocrine neoplasms of the gastrointestinal tract: classification, pathologic basis, and imaging features. Radiographics. 2007;27:1667-79.
42. Williams GT. Endocrine tumors of the gastrointestinal tract-selected topics. Histopathology. 2007;50(1):30-41.

43. Duh QY, Hybarger CP, Geist R, et al. Carcinoids associated with multiple endocrine neoplasia syndromes. Am J Surg. 1987;154(1):142-8.
44. Karatzas G, Kouraklis G, Karayiannakis A, et al. Ampullary carcinoid and jejunal stromal tumor associated with von Recklinghausen's disease presenting as gastrointestinal bleeding and jaundice. Eur J Surg Oncol. 2000;26(4):428-9.
45. Levy AD, Sobin LH. Gastrointestinal Carcinoids: Imaging Features with Clinicopathologic Comparison. Radiographics. 2007;27: 237-57.
46. Moller JE, Connolly HM, Rubin J, et al. Factors associated with progression of carcinoid heart disease. N Engl J Med. 2003;348:1005-15.
47. Kamaoui I, De-Luca V, Ficarelli S, Mennesson N, Lombard-Bohas C, Pilleul F. Value of CT enteroclysis in suspected small-bowel carcinoid tumors. AJR. 2010;194:629-33.
48. Horton KM, Kamel I, Hofmann L, Fishman EK. Carcinoid tumors of the small bowel: a multitechnique imaging approach. AJR. 2004;182:559-67.
49. Paulsen SR, Huprich JE, Fletcher JG, et al. CT enterography as a diagnostic tool in evaluating small bowel disorders: review of clinical experience with over 700 cases. Radiographics. 2006;26:641-57, discussion 657-62.
50. Woodard PK, Feldman JM, Paine SS, Baker ME. Midgut carcinoid tumors: CT findings and biochemical profiles. J Comput Assist Tomogr. 1995;19:400-5.
51. Bader TR, Semelka RC, Chiu VC, et al. MRI of carcinoid tumors: spectrum of appearances in the gastrointestinal tract and liver. J Magn Reson Imaging. 2001;14:261-9.
52. Pantongrag-Brown L, Buetow PC, Carr NJ, et al. Calcification and fibrosis in mesenteric carcinoid tumor: CT findings and pathologic correlation. Am J Roentgenol. 1995;164:387-91.
53. Maglinte DDT, Herlinger H. Small bowel neoplasms. In: Herlinger H, Maglinte DDT, Birnbaum BA (Eds). Clinical imaging of the small intestine, 2nd edition. New York, NY: Springer; 1999. pp. 377-438.
54. Reznek RH. CT/MRI of neuroendocrine tumors. Cancer Imaging. 2006;6(Spec No A):S163-77. doi:10.1102/ 1470-7330.2006.9037.
55. Hofman MS1, Lau WF, Hicks RJ. Somatostatin receptor imaging with 68Ga DOTATATE PET/CT: clinical utility, normal patterns, pearls, and pitfalls in interpretation Radiographics. 2015;35(2):500-16. doi: 10.1148/rg.352140164.
56. Pelage JP, Soyer P, Boudiaf M, et al. Carcinoid tumors of the abdomen: CT features. Abdom Imaging. 1999;24(3):240-5.
57. Adams S, Baum R, Rink T, Schumm-Drager PM, Usadel KH, Hor G. Limited value of fluorine-18 fluorodeoxyglucose positron emission tomography for the imaging of neuroendocrine tumors. Eur J Nucl Med. 1998;25:79-83.
58. Binderup T, Knigge U, Loft A, et al. Functional imaging of neuroendocrine tumors: a head-tohead comparison of somatostatin receptor scintigraphy, 123I-MIBG scintigraphy, and 18F-FDG PET. J Nucl Med. 2010;51:704-12.
59. Zalom ML, Waxman AD, Yu R, Lee J, Ih G, Wolin EM. Metabolic and receptor imaging in patients with neuroendocrine tumors: comparison of fludeoxyglucose-positron emission tomography and computed tomography with indium in 111 pentetreotide. Endocr Pract. 2009;15:521-7.
60. Hong X, Choi H, Loyer EM, Benjamin RS, Trent JC, Charnsangavej C. Gastrointestinal stromal tumor: Role of CT in diagnosis and in response evaluation and surveillance after treatment with Imatinib. Radiographics. 2006;26:481-95.
61. Mazur MT, Clark HB. Gastric stromal tumors: reappraisal of histogenesis. Am J Surg Pathol. 1983;7:507-19.
62. Sripathi S, Rajagopal KV, Srivastava RK, Ayachit A. CT features, mimics and atypical presentations of gastrointestinal stromal tumor (GIST). The Indian Journal of Radiology and Imaging 2011;21.3:176-81.
63. The ESMO/European Sarcoma Network Working Group Gastrointestinal Stromal Tumors: ESMO Clinical Practice Guidelines Ann Oncol. 2014;25 (Suppl 3):iii21-6.
64. Levy D, Remotti HE, Thompson WM, Sobin LH, Miettinen M. Gastrointestinal stromal tumors: radiologic features with pathologic correlation. Radiographics. 2003;23(2):283-304.
65. King DM. The radiology of gastrointestinal stromal tumors. Cancer imaging. 2005(5):150-6.
66. GJ, Badran M, Al-Muderis O, et al. Malignant gastrointestinal stromal tumor:distribution, imaging features and pattern of metastatic spread. Radiology. 2003;226:527-32.
67. Afifi AH, Ela AM, Albanna A. Feasibility of diffusion weighted MRI in evaluation of different small bowel pathology. Ejrnm. 2015;46:459-69.
68. Fletcher CD, Berman JJ, Corless C, et al. Diagnosis of gastrointestinal stromal tumors: a consensus approach. Int J Surg Pathol. 2002;10:81-9. [PubMed].
69. Choi H, Charnsangavej C, de Castro Faria S, et al. CT evaluation of the response of gastrointestinal stromal tumors after imatinib mesylate treatment: a quantitative analysis correlated with FDG PET findings. Am J Roentgenol. 2004;183:1619-28.
70. Schlemmer M, Sourbron SP, Schinwald N, Nikolaou K, Becker CR, Reiser MF, Berger F. Perfusion patterns of metastatic gastrointestinal stromal tumor lesions under specific molecular therapy. Eur J Radiol. 2011;77:312-8.
71. Lassau N, Lamuraglia M, Chami L, et al. Gastrointestinal stromal tumors treated with imatinib: monitoring response with contrast-enhanced sonography. Am J Roentgenol. 2006;187:1267-73.
72. Gollub MJ. Imaging of gastrointestinal lymphoma: Radiol Clin N Am. 2008;46:287-312.
73. Lewis RB, Mehrotra AK, Rodríguez P, Manning MA, Levine MS. From the radiologic pathology archives: gastrointestinal lymphoma: Radiologic and Pathologic Findings: Radiographics. 2014;34:1934-53.
74. Levine MS, Rubesin SE, Pantongrag-Brown L, Buck JL, Herlinger H. Non-Hodgkin's lymphoma of the gastrointestinal tract: radiographic findings. AJR. 1997;168(1):165-72.
75. Dawson I, Cornes J, Morson B. Primary malignant lymphoid tumors of the intestinal tract. Report of 37 cases with a study of factors influencing prognosis. Br J Surg. 1961;49:80-9.
76. Manning MA, Somwaru AS, Mehrotra AK, Levine MS. Gastrointestinal lymphoma: radiologic-pathologic correlation. Radiol Clin North Am. 2016:54(4):765-84.
77. Krol AD, le Cessie S, Snijder S, et al. Primary extranodal non-Hodgkin's lymphoma: the impact of alternative definitions tested in the comprehensive centre west population-based NHL registry. Ann Oncol. 2003;55(1):1-16.
78. Ghai S, Pattison J, Ghai S, O'Malley ME, Khalili K, Stephens S. Primary gastrointestinal lymphoma: spectrum of imaging findings with pathologic correlation. Radiographics. 2007;27:1371-88.
79. Cornes JS. Multiple lymphomatous polyposis of the gastrointestinal tract. Cancer. 1961;14:249-57.
80. Catassi C, Bearzi I, Holmes GKT. Association of celiac disease and intestinal lymphomas and other cancers. Gastroenterology. 2005;128:S79-86.
81. Lo Re G, Federica V, Midiri F, et al. Radiological features of gastrointestinal lymphoma. Gastroenterology Research and Practice. 2016;2016:2498143. doi:10.1155/2016/2498143.
82. Mayerhoefer ME, Karanikas G, Kletter K, Prosch H, Kiesewetter B, Skrabs C, et al. Evaluation of diffusion-weighted MRI for pretherapeutic assessment and staging of lymphoma: results of a prospective study in 140 Patients. Clin Cancer Res. 2014;20(11): 2984-93.

83. Ghimire P, Wu GY, Zhu L. Primary gastrointestinal lymphoma. World J Gastroenterol. 2011;17(6):697-707.
84. Allen-Auerbach M, de Vos S, Czernin J. The impact of fluorodeoxyglucose-positron emission tomography in primary staging and patient management in lymphoma patients. Radiol Clin N Am. 2008;46:199-211.
85. Schoder H, Noy A, Gonen M, et al. Intensity of 18 flurodeoxyglucose uptake in positron emission tomography distinguishes between indolent and aggressive non-Hodgkin's lymphoma. J Clin Oncol. 2005;23(21):4643-51.
86. Stecco A, Buemi F, Quagliozzi M, Lombardi M, Santagostino A, Saccheti GM, et al. Staging of primary abdominal lymphoma: comparison of whole-body MRI with diffusion-weighted imaging and 18F-FDG-PET/CT. Gastroenterology research and practice, vol. 2015, article ID 104794, 8 pages, 2015. doi:10.1155/2015/104794.
87. Musshoff K. [Clinical staging classification of non-Hodgkin's lymphomas] Strahlentherapie. 1977;153(4):218-21.
88. Rohatiner A, d'Amore F, Coiffier B, et al. Report on a workshop convened to discuss the pathological and staging classifications of gastrointestinal tract lymphomas. Ann Oncol. 1994; 5(5)397-400.
89. Ruskone-Fourmestraux A, Dragosics B, Morgner A, et al. Paris staging system for primary gastrointestinal lymphomas. Gut. 2003:52(6)912-3.

CHAPTER

95

Colorectal Tumors

Naveen Kalra, Mandeep Kang, Mahesh Prakash

INTRODUCTION

Colorectal tumors can be broadly classified as epithelial lesions, which include adenoma and adenocarcinoma; and nonepithelial or mesenchymal lesions, which include lipoma, leiomyoma, gastrointestinal stromal tumor (GIST), leiomyosarcoma and Kaposi's sarcoma. Other tumors are lymphoma, metastases and non-neoplastic benign polyps like hyperplastic and hamartomatous polyps. In this chapter, all these lesions will be discussed with particular focus on colorectal cancer.

EPIDEMIOLOGY

Colorectal cancer is the third most common cancer overall in both men and women. It is also the second leading cause of cancer deaths following lung cancer.[1] In men, it is the third most common cancer after lung and prostate cancer; and in women, it is the third most common cancer after lung and breast cancer.[2] The prevalence of colon cancer varies throughout the globe. While the incidence is high in North America, Europe and New Zealand, it is low in South America, Africa and Asia.[3] The reported incidence of colon cancer from eight population registries in India is 0.7–3.7/100,000 in men; and 0.4–3/100,000 in women with a higher incidence of rectal cancer (1.6–5.5/100,000 in men, 0–2.8/100,000 in women).[4] Colon cancer is more common in economically affluent populations, who have Western lifestyle practices like high intake of dietary fat, low intake of dietary fiber and sedentary lifestyle.[5] Minority (5.4%) of colorectal cancers occur in patients younger than 40 years.[5] The incidence of colorectal cancer rises after the age of 40 years with 90% of these cancers occur in persons more than 50 years old.[6] The median age at the time of diagnosis of colon and rectal cancer has been reported to be 71 years and 69 years respectively. Approximately, one half of the colon cancers occur in the rectum and sigmoid colon and these can be seen with the flexible sigmoidoscope.[7] There has been an increase in the right-sided lesions as opposed to the left-sided lesions. Distal lesions are more commonly found in men than in women.

RISK FACTORS

There are several risk factors, which are associated with the development of colorectal cancer. Primarily, these include dietary factors, hereditary factors, inflammatory bowel disease and other miscellaneous causes.

High-calorie, low-fiber diet rich in animal fats, including beef consumption is an important risk factor for the colon carcinogenesis. Excess intake of fat results in an increase in the level of fatty acids and free bile acids in the feces. This irritates the colonic mucosa and epithelial reparative proliferation ensues.[8] High fiber intake decreases exposure to the carcinogens by decreasing the fecal transit time. It also results in decreased bacterial-mediated conversion of primary to secondary bile acids by lowering the pH of the stool.[9]

There is an inverse relationship between the intake of calcium and of antioxidants such as vitamins A, C, E, selenium and colon cancer.[10] On the other hand, there is a direct relationship between alcohol consumption, smoking, hypergastrinemia in pernicious anemia patients, increased growth hormone level in patients with acromegaly and increased parathyroid hormone in patients with parathyroid adenomas, and the incidence of colorectal cancer.

Prior cholecystectomy has been reported to increase the risk of developing right-sided colon cancer in women by 1.5 times.[11] This is due to the deposition of potential carcinogens like bile salts and neutral sterols in the proximal colon while the distal colon is spared on account of their absorption proximally into the enterohepatic circulation. Prior ureterosigmoidostomy following cystectomy is also a potential risk factor for the development of adenocarcinoma at the site of anastomosis.

Occupational and environmental risk factors include exposure to asbestos, oils, printing materials, halogens, metal fumes, organic solvents, paint and dyes.

Radiation-induced colorectal cancers arise in rectum and sigmoid colon of patients with carcinoma of cervix, bladder and prostate. The latent period for such cancers is longer than 10 years with 3000 rad threshold value.[12] 1.5–9% of patients with colorectal cancer have been found to have a second synchronous cancer[13] and 5–8% subsequently develop a metachronous cancer.[14,15] The time interval between initial and metachronous cancer varies but the majority arises within 5 to 7 years of the index cancer.

Hereditary factors have been a subject of interest for colorectal cancer. Heredity has been shown to play a role in 5–6% of all colorectal cancers.[3] Familial adenomatous polyposis (FAP) is an autosomal dominant syndrome and is the result of germline mutation of the adenomatous polyposis coli gene. If a prophylactic colectomy is not performed in a patient with FAP, colorectal cancer always develops in these patients. Turcot's syndrome is a variant of FAP and in these patients, the extracolonic lesion is a brain tumor such as medulloblastoma.

In juvenile polyposis coli, there is a high incidence of colorectal neoplasia (dysplasia and adenocarcinoma) found in up to 20% patients at a relatively younger age (37 years).[10] Screening should be performed periodically in patients with Cronkhite-Canada syndrome, in which there are multiple juvenile polyps throughout the gastrointestinal tract except the esopahgus. These can undergo adenomatous and carcinomatous degeneration.

Hereditary nonpolyposis colorectal cancer or Lynch syndrome accounts for 4–6% of all colorectal cancers. In Lynch syndrome I, colorectal cancer is inherited as an autosomal dominant susceptibility with more metachronous and synchronous lesions. In Lynch syndrome II, there is an increased incidence of adenocarcinoma of endometrium, ovary and other organs in addition to colorectal cancer. The precursor lesion in Lynch-related colon cancer is a discrete proximal colonic adenoma. Right-sided colon cancer occurring at young age is the hallmark of Lynch syndrome. Colon cancers associated with Lynch syndrome have a better prognosis than other colorectal cancer varieties.[10]

Colon cancer in ulcerative colitis is uncommon, occurs in patients with pancolitis and constitutes about 1% of colorectal cancers. Patients with left-sided disease are at less risk. The risk begins to increase after 7–10 years of colitis. Actual risk of developing colorectal cancer is 0.5–2% after the initial 10 years of disease, 6.6% after 26 years, 11.4% after 32 years. Disease activity as such does not increase the risk of long-term colorectal cancer and lack of activity does not have a protective effect. The mean age of presentation in these patients is 40–45 years.[10]

The risk of developing adenocarcinoma of large and small bowel has been estimated to be 4 to 20 times more than that of general population in Crohn's disease. Most cancers develop in inflamed segments and in segments having strictures and fistulae. Excluded colon and rectum as well as bypassed small bowel segments are at particular risk. Multifocal carcinomas may be seen and are discovered late as they cannot be distinguished from benign strictures.[10]

PATHOGENESIS

Most colorectal cancers arise in adenomatous polyps.[16] Adenomas more than 1 cm in size have a higher risk of malignant transformation. The transition from benign adenoma to cancer usually takes 7–10 years. This adenoma-carcinoma sequence suggests that colon cancer is preventable if polypoid lesions larger than 1 cm are found and removed. This stresses the importance of screening programs for colon cancer.

In patients with inflammatory bowel disease, carcinoma evolves through a sequence of inflammation, dysplasia followed by carcinoma.

The malignant potential of an adenomatous polyp has four major determinants. These include size, presence of a stalk, villous architecture and degree of cellular atypia and dysplasia. Polyps less than 5 mm have little or no risk of malignant transformation, those between 1 and 2 cm carry a 5% risk and those which are more than 2 cm carry a 50% risk of harboring malignancy.[10] Sessile polyps are at higher risk for malignancy (>50%) than pedunculated polyps. In case a pedunculated polyp turns malignant, the invasion of the colonic wall by the cancer is rare if the length of the stalk is more than 2 cm. Adenomatous polyps are of three types—tubular, villous and tubulovillous. Malignant transformation is more likely with villous adenomas than with tubular adenomas.[17] This is because villous adenomas are usually sessile and penetration of the muscularis mucosa is more likely in a sessile polyp. Polyps with a greater degree of cellular atypia and dysplasia are more likely to become malignant.

CLINICAL FEATURES

Colorectal cancer is a slow-growing tumor. Therefore, symptoms may be absent or minimal at initial presentation. Symptomatic colorectal cancers usually present with evidence of bleeding. This may be in the form of occult blood in the stool, passage of frank blood per rectum or development of iron deficiency anemia. The symptoms depend upon the size and location of the tumor. Right-sided colon cancers usually grow to a large size before symptoms develop. This is because the right colon is more capacious and the contents are relatively fluid in consistency. Anemia and disordered bowel function are earlier findings in right-sided colon cancer. On the other hand, sigmoid cancers present, early as sigmoid colon is the narrowest portion of the large bowel and the cancer results in the obstruction to the passage of solid fecal matter early. These patients present with colicky, crampy abdominal pain that is relieved by a bowel movement. Left-sided colon cancers usually present with per-rectal bleeding or intestinal obstruction.

A feeling of incomplete bowel evacuation, persistent constipation or diarrhea and change in stool caliber should arouse suspicion of colorectal carcinoma in patients older than 40 years. Weight loss and anemia are seen in 50% of patients with colorectal carcinoma.

Patients with colorectal carcinoma usually have a normal physical examination. Sometimes, there may be a palpable mass or signs of intestinal obstruction. Palpable supraclavicular nodes may be seen with left-sided colon cancer and hepatomegaly may be present due to metastases. Among the laboratory investigations measurement of carcinoembryonic antigen (CEA) levels is a useful test. CEA is an antigen shed from the surface of tumor cells. Although not specific, CEA is a sensitive marker for colorectal cancer. The levels of serum CEA correlate with cancer stage and tumor size. Elevated preoperative CEA level predicts shorter disease-free survival.

PATHOLOGY

The gross morphology of the colorectal adenocarcinoma is related to its location. Large, polypoidal bulky masses overgrowing their vascular supply are seen in the cecum and ascending colon. They may also undergo necrosis. Tumors in the transverse and descending colon are ulcerated and infiltrative and have a large intramural component. Thus they are more invasive in nature. Tumors in the more distal colon and rectum are also infiltrative and have an annular constricting or 'napkin-ring' appearance. These tumors are the most biologically aggressive. In patients with inflammatory bowel disease, colon cancers are scirrhous, plaque-like or finely nodular.[18]

Malignancies of the large bowel are predominantly adenocarcinoma. Mucinous/colloid carcinomas are seen in the setting of inflammatory bowel disease and hereditary non-polyposis-related carcinoma in early age. They constitute 10 to 15% of the cancers with large lakes of mucin in which there is a scattered collection of tumor cells with signet ring cells. As the mucin is secreted within the interstitium of the gut wall, it dissects the wall, helps in the extension of the malignancy and worsens the prognosis. Calcification may occur in these tumors. Tumors that arise at the anorectal junction include squamous cell carcinoma, transitional cell carcinoma, cloacogenic carcinoma and melanocarcinoma.[10] They comprise less than 5% of malignant large bowel tumors. Primary lymphomas, carcinoid tumors and leiomyosarcomas comprise less than 0.1% of all large bowel tumors.[19] In addition, lymphoma, leiomyosarcoma and cancers of the breast, ovaries, prostate, lung and stomach can metastasize to the colon.

ROUTE OF SPREAD

There are five methods of tumor spread after the tumor has become invasive:

1. *Direct extension*: Direct invasion may occur along the tissue layers which provide the path of least resistance. As peritoneum represents a relative barrier, direct spread to neighboring intra-peritoneal organs is rare. After invading the visceral peritoneum, the tumor can spread to stomach, greater omentum, spleen, small bowel, another portion of the colon, uterus, bladder, fallopian tubes and ovaries. Retroperitoneal tumor may involve kidneys, pancreas, ureters and posterior truncal musculature. Rectal carcinoma after breaching fascia of Waldeyer may invade sacral plexus, sacrum and coccyx.[20] It may also invade internal iliac vessels and obturator musculature posterolaterally, and prostate, seminal vesicles, bladder, vagina and cervix anteriorly after compromising the fascia of Denonvillier's.
2. *Lymphatic spread*: Lymphatic spread occurs after the invasion of muscularis through submucosal lymphatics. Intramural spread of colorectal malignancy occurs to submucosal, muscular and subserosal lymphatics. The first sites of involvement are usually the epiploic and paracolic lymph nodes. The intermediate lymph nodes (along vascular branches) and principal lymph nodes (at origins of colonic blood vessels) generally show involvement later in the course of the disease. The prognosis worsens when multiple lymph nodes are involved.
3. *Hematogenous metastases*: There exists the potential for hematogenous metastasis if colorectal malignancy invades the rich capillary network of lamina propria. The most common route is through branches of portal vein. Thus liver is the most commonly involved organ. Distal rectum drains through tributaries of internal iliac vein, which finally drain into the inferior vena cava. Batson's vertebral venous plexus is another path of hematogenous spread. In 20–40% colorectal carcinoma patients, liver is the sole site of metastases. Metastases to the lung are seen in 20% of patients. In 4% of patients, the lungs are the sole site of metastases. Other sites are less common and include adrenal glands, bone, kidney, pancreas, spleen and central nervous system.
4. *Peritoneal seeding*: Intraperitoneal seeding may occur during operation because of breach in serosa. The anterior wall of rectosigmoid junction is the site of metastatic seedling. Eventually, both the parietal and visceral peritoneal surfaces will be involved leading to malignant ascities.
5. *Intraluminal implantation*: Intraluminal tumor spillage at surgery is a likely source of implantation metastases and anastomotic recurrence.[21] Anastomotic recurrences may also be due to incomplete tumor excision or a metachronous tumor.

STAGING

Staging of colorectal cancer has evolved over many years. In 1932, Dr Cuthbert E Dukes, a London-based pathologist, in a study of 215 patients with rectal cancers, found direct relationship between survival and depth of tumor penetration into the intestinal wall and lymph node metastasis.[22] The Astler and Coller modification of the Dukes classification is commonly employed to stage colonic neoplasm.

In this method, the staging is as follows:

A Tumor limited to the mucosa

B1 Tumor extending into, but not through, the muscularis propria

B2 Tumor penetrating the bowel wall, but without any lymph node involvement

C Tumor with regional lymph node involvement. This is divided into C1, in which the primary tumor is within the bowel wall and C2, in which the primary tumor has spread beyond the bowel wall.

Turnball introduced an additional staging category in 1967 as stage D further divided into stage D1, which included fixed cancers that had invaded adjacent organs and stage D2, in which distant metastases had occurred. Currently the American Joint Committee on Cancer (AJCC) and International Union against Cancer (UICC) have recommended staging by TNM classification.[23] Local tumor staging or T staging depends on the depth of tumor penetration into the bowel wall. The extent of mural invasion is important, as it has shown to influence prognosis independent of lymph node involvement.

Primary Tumor (T)

TX: Primary tumor cannot be assessed
T0: No evidence of primary tumor
Tis: Carcinoma in situ
T1: Tumor invades submucosa
T2: Tumor invades muscularis propria
T3: Tumor extending through the muscularis propria into subserosa or non-peritonealized pericolic or perirectal tissue
T4: Tumor directly invades other organs or structures (T4a) or perforates the visceral peritoneum (T4b).

Regional Lymph Node (N)

NX: Regional lymph nodes cannot be assessed
N0: No regional lymph node metastasis
N1: Metastasis in 1–3 pericolic or perirectal lymph nodes
N2: Metastasis in 4 or more pericolic or perirectal lymph nodes.

Distant Metastasis (M)

MX: Presence of distant metastasis cannot be assessed
M0: No distant metastasis
M1: Distant metastasis.

Stage Grouping

Stage 0	Tis	N0	M0
Stage I	T1	N0	M0
	T2	N0	M0
Stage II	T3	N0	M0
	T4	N0	M0
Stage IIIA	Any T	N1	M0
	Any T	N2	M0
Stage IV	Any T	Any N	M1

ROLE OF RADIOLOGY

Radiology plays an important role in screening for colorectal cancer. The purpose of doing imaging studies in patients with colorectal cancer is to provide the surgeon and the oncologist comprehensive and accurate assessment of the primary tumor, local and distant spread of the disease, synchronous lesions and to detect clinically occult complications. Radiology has a critical role after treatment of colorectal carcinoma in the detection of recurrent or residual disease, local and distant metastases and metachronous cancers.[24]

Screening for Colorectal Cancer

The American Cancer Society has recommended that one of the following five testing schedules should be adopted, beginning at 50 years of age:[25]

1. Yearly fecal occult blood test (FOBT) or fecal immunochemical test (FIT)
2. Flexible sigmoidoscopy every 5 years
3. Yearly FOBT or FIT, plus flexible sigmoidoscopy every 5 years
4. Double contrast barium enema every 5 years
5. Colonoscopy every 10 years.

Fecal occult blood test (FOBT) is the most widely available and least expensive screening test for colorectal cancer. Colorectal cancers bleed intermittently and the blood that is lost into the stool is broken down into hematin. Hematin reacts with guaiac and the commonly used hemoccult test is based on the guaiac reaction. False-positive reactions are caused by ingestion of meat, certain vegetables and aspirin. False-negative results occur as cancers only bleed intermittently. Moreover, it is thought that a polyp must be over 2 cm in size before it bleeds regularly. The sensitivity for detection of colon cancer is lower than 50% and nearly 90% of polyps are undetected by FOBT.[26]

Flexible sigmoidoscopy visually inspects the rectum and distal sigmoid colon. Therefore approximately only half of the colorectal cancers can be detected by flexible fibreoptic sigmoidoscopy alone. Though it is a safe and well-tolerated procedure and does not require sedation, it is relatively expensive and has the potential for transmission of disease by contaminated instruments.

Double-contrast barium enema (DCBE) is a widely available, inexpensive and simple test. However, in a study comparing DCBE to colonoscopy, it was found that the sensitivity of DCBE for polyps less than 0.5 cm was only 32%, for polyps 0.6 to 1 cm, was 53% and for polyps greater than 1 cm was 48%.[27]

Colonoscopy can directly visualize most colon cancers. The National Polyp Study and the Italian Mutlicenter Study showed reduction in the incidence of colorectal cancer among patients who had adenomas detected and subsequently removed on colonoscopy.[28,29] Colonoscopy is regarded as the gold standard for determining sensitivities of other examinations of the colon. However in a review of tandem or back-to-back colonoscopies, an average of 21% of adenomas were missed.[30] 26% of these adenomas were 1–5 mm and 2% of them were 10 mm or more in size. There are blind spots in the colon behind folds and around flexures. Colonoscopy also has the risk of perforation or hemorrhage in 1:500 examinations and a fatality rate of 1:5000 examinations. The completion rate of colonoscopy ranges from 55% to 95%.

Virtual colonoscopy is a novel noninvasive technique wherein a three-dimensional endoluminal image is generated after processing data acquired by multidetector helical CT using specialized computer software. In the American College of Radiology Imaging Network (ACRIN) study conducted at 15 study centers on 2600 asymptomatic participants, it was found that CT colonography has a 90% sensitivity and 86% specificity for detection of polyps measuring 10 mm or more in diameter.[31] Thus virtual colonoscopy performs well in detecting lesions larger than 1 cm which are actually clinically significant lesions. The entire colon is also evaluated by virtual colonoscopy. However, patients found to have significant lesions must undergo optical colonoscopy. The reported rate of complications with this technique is relatively small (0.08%).

Double-contrast barium enema and virtual colonoscopy will be discussed in detail in subsequent sections.

DIAGNOSTIC METHODS

Imaging modalities available are plain abdominal radiographs, barium enema, ultrasound including endoluminal and Doppler ultrasound, computed tomography/CT colonography, MRI/MR colonography and angiography.

Plain Radiographs

These are usually not very informative except for depicting complications of advanced colorectal malignancy like obstruction and perforation. Dilatation of colon and small bowel in cases of obstruction, thumb printing suggestive of ischemic colitis proximal to an obstructing lesion and free intra-peritoneal air in cases of perforation and pericolonic abscess formation may be detected on plain films. There may be a fistula with gallbladder or urinary bladder. Calcification of carcinomatous lesion or hepatic metastases may be evident. When advanced, bony invasion is easily diagnosed by identifying destruction of bone and presence of associated soft tissue mass. Lung metastases may also be seen on chest skiagram.

Barium Enema

The major advantage of barium enema is its ability to examine the entire colon. It is reasonably accurate, minimally invasive and requires no sedation. Complications related to the investigation are rare. DCBE has a 20% better sensitivity than single-contrast barium enema for detecting adenomatous polyps less than 1 cm in size.[32] However, this difference in the sensitivity of the two types of barium enema is not there when we consider the detection of colorectal carcinoma. The reported sensitivity of barium enema is in the range of 90–95% for the detection of significant (1 cm) size polyps and cancer.[33] The most important prerequisite for an accurate radiological examination is thorough bowel preparation with selection of an appropriate technique, strict quality control during the study and careful interpretation of the radiographs. The most effective regimen is combination of dietary manipulation, oral catheters and cleansing enema. About 10–40% of colonic carcinomas can be missed on initial barium enemas due to poor colon preparation.[34,35] Presence of fecal matter can mimic or mask polyps and cancers and account for the most common reason for false-positive findings on barium enema. The single contrast barium enema is simpler in concept than the double contrast study, but requires meticulous technique. The selection of the type of barium enema to be performed depends on the indication for the examination, sensitivity for detecting specific diseases and the age and physical condition of the patient.

The DCBE gives better information of mucosa with better detection of smaller lesions. It is the ideal technique in patients who are older than 40 years, who have a personal or family history of colonic polyps, cancer or inflammatory bowel disease, and a positive FOBT. Other indications are patients with previous ovarian, breast or cervical carcinoma and with prior pelvic irradiation.

Single-contrast barium enema is simpler and does not require rigorous maneuvers. Therefore, it is indicated in patients who are more than 70 years old, debilitated or uncooperative patients and in those patients where barium study is indicated for exclusion of obstruction or diverticulitis. Young patients with low likelihood of colon disease may also be candidates for single contrast study. Manual or mechanical compression of the colon during fluoroscopy and spot radiographs of the various segments are critical in detecting small polypoid lesions. Technique protocols should be followed, the adequacy of colon cleansing assessed, careful fluoroscopy performed, poor quality films repeated and additional films of questionable lesions should be obtained when needed.

Meticulous interpretation of the barium enema films is needed to avoid diagnostic errors due to presence of stool, air bubbles and diverticulae, or confusion of normal anatomic structures for an abnormality. False-negative errors are caused by perceptive lapses, technical problems, interpretive mistakes, or a combination of these factors. Perceptive errors can be reduced by close scrutiny, second review or retrospective review of the films especially for diagnosing colonic polyps and sigmoid colon malignancies. Accuracy of DCBE for evaluation of colorectal polyps is dependent on the location of the lesion and the size of the colonic polyps. As stated earlier, the sensitivity of DCBE is poor for polyps under 5 mm, improving for polyps 5–9 mm and is best for diagnosing polyps over 1 cm.

Complications of barium enema are uncommon. The rates of perforation for barium enema are documented at 1:25,00 to 1:12,500 and for mortality at 1:50,000.[36,37] Subsequent to a biopsy performed through a rigid scope, enema should be deferred for 2 weeks due to risk of perforation. Enema need not be postponed if biopsy is performed through a flexible sigmoidscope or colonoscope as the depth of biopsy does not extend beyond the muscularis mucosa. Recent endoscopic polypectomy precludes enema for 2–3 weeks. Barium and latex sensitivity, barium impaction, transient bacteremia, dehydration and inadvertent placement of the enema tip into vaginal vault are other complications which may also be encountered. Despite the risk of transient bacteremia, there is presently no recommendation to give prophylactic antibiotics.

Colorectal malignancies have a broad spectrum of morphological appearances on imaging. The mucosal surface can be seen en face, either in the barium pool or in air contrast. The normal mucosal surface is smooth. An abnormal mucosal surface may have a granular, finely nodular or ulcerated surface. Early carcinoma is usually seen as a sessile polypoid mass. The radiologic detection of early carcinoma is primarily an exercise in the detection of small polyps. There are two common types of colonic polyps, hyperplastic and adenomatous. Hyperplastic polyps have no malignant potential. Small polypoidal carcinomas may have a smooth outline and be radiographically indistinguishable from benign tumors **(Figs. 1 and 2)**. Barium enema cannot

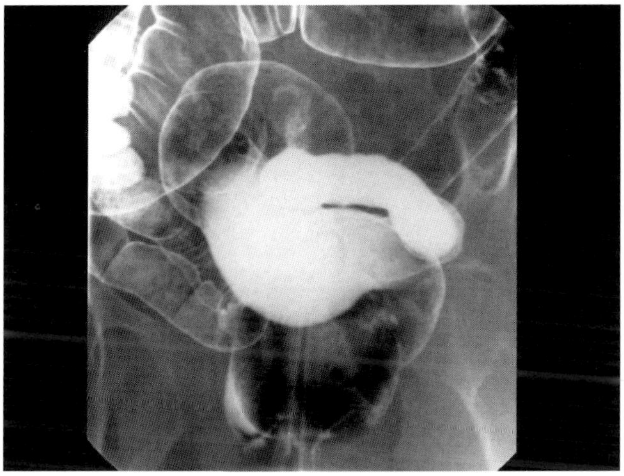

FIG. 1: Double-contrast barium enema DCBE shows a solitary, small, smooth polypoid lesion in the sigmoid colon which was malignant on histopathology.

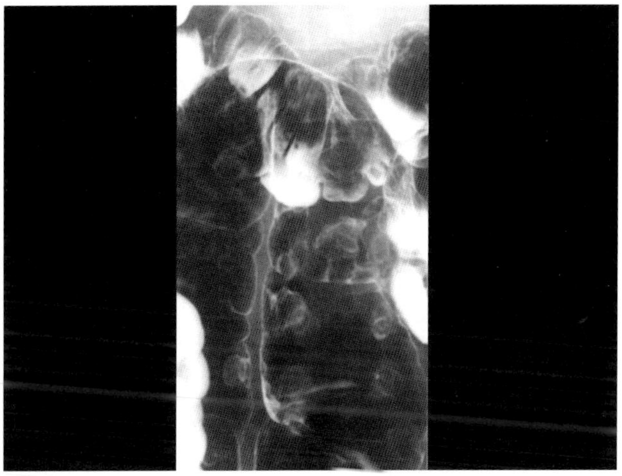

FIG. 2: DCBE in a patient with familial adenomatous polyposis showing multiple polyps in the colon.

determine accurately, whether polypoid lesions in the size range of 0.5–3 cm are benign or malignant. Whenever, possible polyps more than 1 cm in size are found, they must be removed by colonoscopic polypectomy followed by histological examination.

Pedunculated polyps are best demonstrated on erect or lateral decubitus views of the colon. Those arising from the nondependent wall of the colon give the appearance of 'Mexican hat' sign,[38] where the central ring represents the stalk and the outer ring represents the head of polyps. In these cases, a change in position of patients shows the stalk in profile and confirms the diagnosis.

Sessile polyps may vary in appearance from a small, smooth polypoidal lesion to a bulky, lobulated mass forming acute angles with the adjacent colonic wall. When viewed en face, they appear as filling defects in the thin barium pool if they arise from dependent wall and etched in white if present on the nondependent surface. However, they may be missed if too much of high-density barium is present in the lumen, obscuring the lesion. When viewed in oblique projections, sessile polyps manifest as 'Bowler hat' sign,[39] with the dome representing the head of polyps and brim representing base of the polyp. Although the 'Bowler hat' sign can be produced by a diverticulum, the direction of the dome helps to distinguish a polyp from a diverticulum. When the dome points away from the axis of the bowel, the lesion is a diverticulum; and when it points towards the lumen of the bowel, it is a polyp.

Certain criteria have been described to assess the risk of malignancy of polyps based on their imaging features which include sessile versus pedunculated appearance, size of the polyp, number of polyps, basal indentation and surface contour. 1 cm is the threshold size for increased cancer risk of a polyp. In case of pedunculated polyps a stalk length >2 cm is not associated with malignant invasion into the adjacent wall. Smooth basal indentation is related to geometric factors and can be present in both benign and malignant lesions. Presence of basal irregularity is most predictive of malignant lesion when it is broad and irregular in larger polyps. The smooth surface contour is unreliable in distinguishing benign from malignant polyps. Lesions that have an irregular, 'soap bubbly' surface generally have villous elements and are likely to have malignant degeneration in at least 50% of lesions.[40,41] The majority of colonic adenomas are tubular adenomas. They have varying degrees of villous change which increases as the polyp increases in size. At the other end of the spectrum are villous adenomas which have a frond-like surface. There may be a transition from tubular adenoma to tubulovillous adenoma to villous adenoma. The risk of malignancy is related to the proportion of villous change in an adenoma. As the barium gets caught in the frond-like protrusions which go hand in hand with the villous change, the surface of the polyp assumes a 'soap bubbly' or a 'lacy' pattern. The term 'carpet lesion' has also been used to describe a flat lobulated lesion that manifests due to an alteration in surface texture of the bowel. These are again tubular adenomas with varying degrees of villous change.

Once a polyp is detected, there is a 3.5% risk of synchronous cancer and a 20% chance of an additional polyp.[42] Therefore, the remainder of the colon should be examined meticulously.

Advanced colorectal cancers have various morphological types. These include polypoidal, annular, scirrhous and flat lesions. The polypoidal lesions protrude into the lumen and have an irregular outline **(Figs. 3A to D)**. They may cause bowel obstruction or intussusception. Annular cancers are short in length with abrupt transition between normal and tumor mucosa **(Figs. 4 and 5)**. The mucosa is destroyed and there may be heaped up edges or ulceration. A focal area of spasm may cause confusion on DCBE but the mucosal folds remain intact within the area of the spasm. The differential diagnosis of annular colonic narrowing includes adhesions, inflammation, diverticulitis, endometriosis, radiation changes, metastatic disease and primary adenocarcinoma. Semiannular or 'saddle' tumor involves only a portion of the wall and results in asymmetry of bowel lumen. En face, these tumors produce overlapping lines with an abnormal orientation on double-contrast studies. Scirrhous tumor causes marked mural thickening and smooth strictures with submucosal and

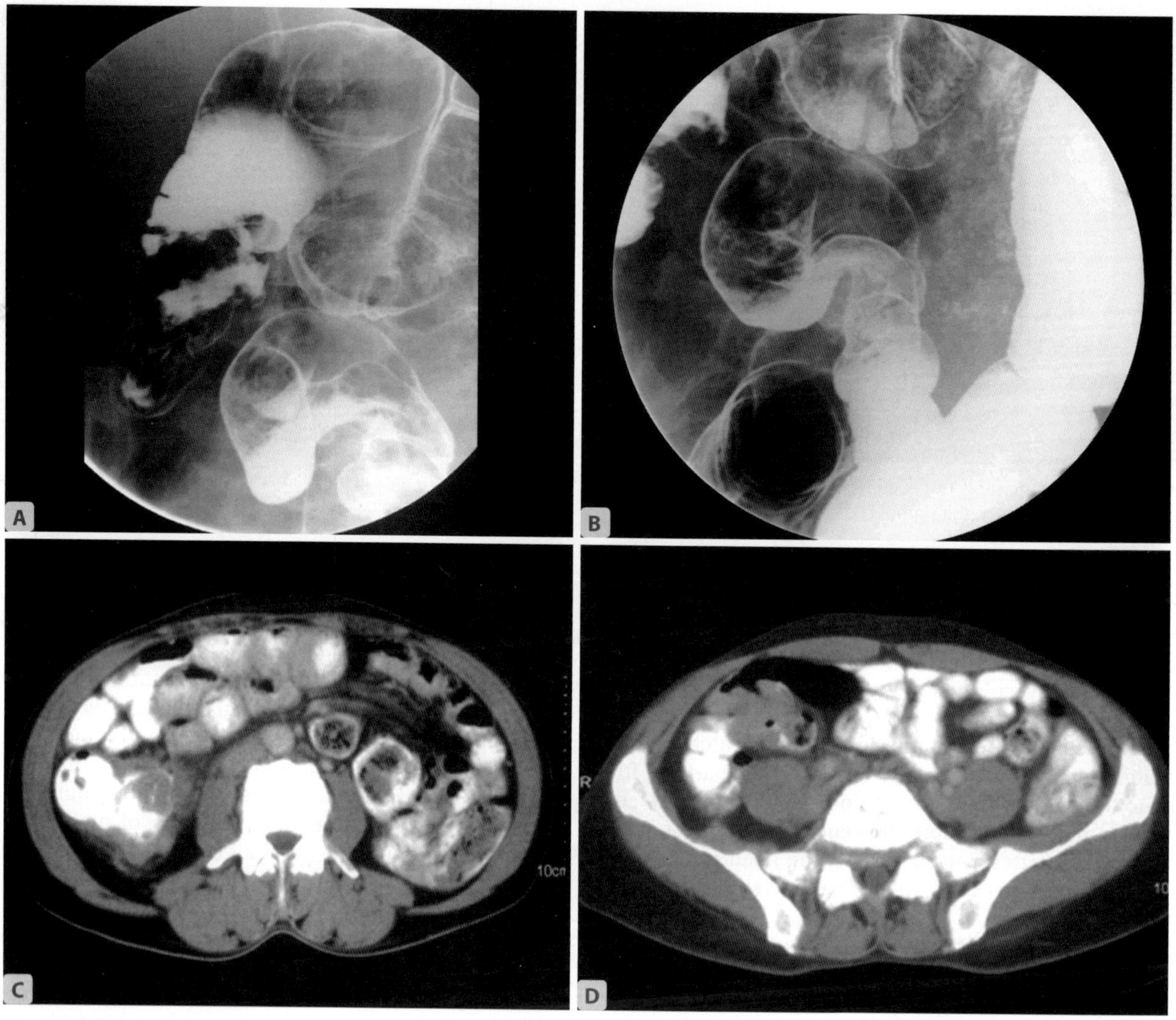

FIGS. 3A TO D: DCBE showing synchronous cancers in the ascending colon (A) and sigmoid colon (B). There is a short segment stricture in the ascending colon with a polypoidal component protruding into the colon. The sigmoid colon also shows a segment of narrowing. Axial CECT sections in the same patient showing circumferential mural thickening with a polypoidal component in the ascending colon (C). A similar lesion is also seen in the sigmoid colon with presence of ulcerations (D).

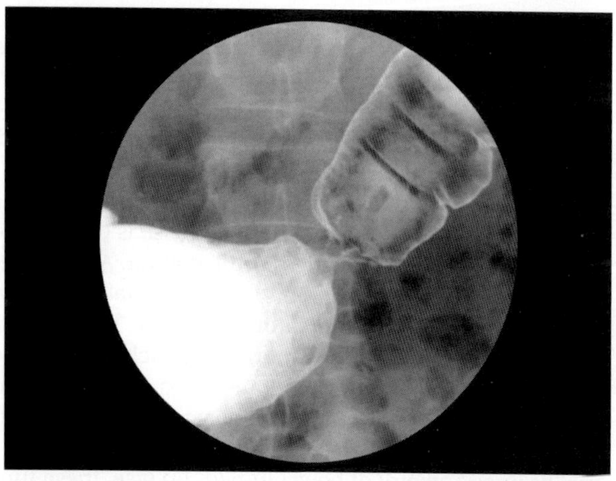

FIG. 4: DCBE showing a short annular stricture in the transverse colon with mucosal irregularity in a patient with colon cancer.

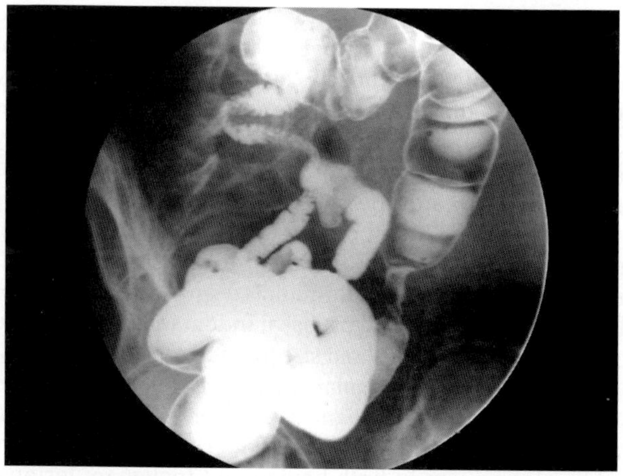

FIG. 5: Barium enema showing a stricture with mucosal irregularity in the descending colon in a patient with metachronous cancer. The patient had previous history of right hemicolectomy and ileotransverse anastomosis for carcinoma of ascending colon.

Courtesy: Professor B Nagi, Department of Gastroenterology, PGIMER, Chandigarh, India.

muscular invasion. Flat lesions are uncommon and usually occur in patients with long-standing ulcerative colitis. They can just result in abnormal lines on DCBE.

Problem Areas in Barium Studies

- *Distal rectum*: The catheter tip in the rectum can itself obscure plaque like or polypoidal lesions. Large internal hemorrhoids may mimic carcinoma, which appear on DCBE as thickened lobulated folds extending 3 cm or less from the anal verge or as cluster of small submucosal nodules in the rectum. However, low-lying rectal cancers that spread through the submucosa mimic hemorrhoids, but asymmetry of lesion and extent of rectal involvement suggests the diagnosis.
- *Ileocecal valve*: Tumors arising in this area have subtle findings which include widening, splaying, straightening or asymmetric lobulation of the valve. These may be missed on initial observation.
- The presence of diverticulosis may obscure lesions. In patients who have equivocal lesions in the sigmoid colon, a 'sigmoid flush' may be performed at the end by introducing a small amount of low-density barium into the rectum to demonstrate polypoidal lesions as filling defects in the thin barium pool.[43] Common errors in barium interpretation can be due to:
    - Failure to detect small filling defects in a pool of barium.
    - Insufficient distension or overdistension.
    - Incomplete cleansing prior to the study.
    - Poor adherence of barium resulting in poor mucosal coating.
    - Failure to detect a synchronous lesion in presence of one lesion. Satisfaction or distraction by finding one lesion may result in overlooking a synchronous lesion.
    - Lesions may be obscured by haustral folds or overlying bowel loops.
    - Perceptive errors, because of extraneous material such as feces, anatomic variation such as redundant bowel loops or presence of diverticulae.

As most colorectal carcinomas are slow-growing, it is assumed that if a carcinoma is found within 3 years of a previous normal barium enema study, the tumor was missed on the previous examination.[33,44,45]

Ultrasound

The appearance of bowel on ultrasound depends not only upon the structures of the individual segment but more importantly upon its content and degree of distension. The bowel may be collapsed, containing only a small amount of mucus (the mucus pattern), or may contain fluid or gas. The mucus pattern is the classical target appearance. Large bowel tends to produce a more complex pattern, because it contains small amount of fluid and gas even in the fasting state. Sometimes, the colonic contents are reflective with distal shadows due to suspended fecal material. In case of colorectal malignancy, bowel wall thickening may be visualized by ultrasound resulting in a target or 'pseudokidney' configuration **(Figs. 6A to C)**. Normal bowel wall thickness in the non-distended state is 5 mm, reducing to about 3 mm when bowel is distended. When the bowel wall is thickened, the mucus pattern changes to a thickened, sometimes irregular 'halo' of bowel wall, with highly reflective irregular center giving a 'pseudokidney' sign.[45] This sign is nonspecific but strongly suggests bowel pathology. The site of the involved bowel must be inferred from the position of the lesion in the abdomen. In inflammatory processes of bowel wall the multiple layers are retained with a large segment of involvement. However, in neoplastic process a short segment involvement with obliteration of bowel wall layers is seen. The exception is lymphoma in which the wall layers are preserved. The diagnostic accuracy of transabdominal ultrasound is improved by retrograde instillation of fluid into the colon. This procedure known as sono-colonography, enables an accurate evaluation of the colonic lumen, colonic wall and also of the surrounding connective tissue. According to a study done by Bernd[46] the sensitivity of the technique in the detection of colonic carcinomas was 94% and the specificity was 100%. Ultrasound (US) screening of abdomen helps to find out liver metastasis and retroperitoneal lymphadenopathy. Fine needle aspiration and core biopsy is also possible using US guidance. It is particularly valuable in patients where

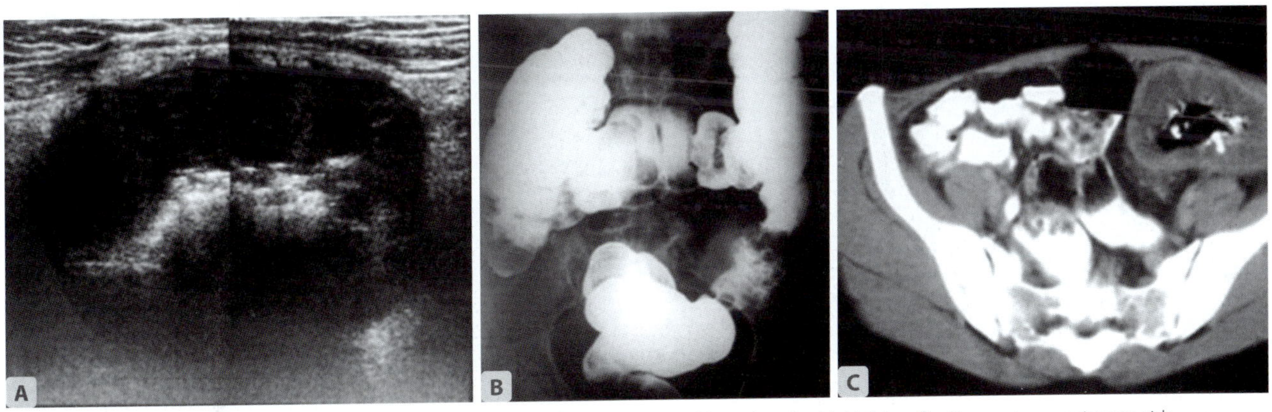

FIGS. 6A TO C: (A) Ultrasound of the lump in the left iliac fossa shows thickened bowel wall with highly reflective center consistent with 'pseudokidney sign; (B) Barium enema in the same patient shows a mass-like lesion with deep ulcerations in the region of descending colon; (C) Axial CECT section shows concentric mural thickening with ulcerations in the same segment.

confirmatory studies are either technically difficult or the findings are nonspecific.

Endorectal ultrasound (ERU): Evaluation of rectum with an endosonic probe was first done by Wilde and Reed in 1956.[45] The procedure is performed with an endorectally placed, rotating, high frequency transducer. If possible, the transducer should be passed proximal to the visualized tumor for complete assessment of mural involvement. The five layers of the rectal wall can be demonstrated as layers of alternating echogenicity with high-frequency transducers allowing an assessment of the depth of invasion of rectal tumors. The innermost ring is hyperechoic and represents the interface of the probe and the mucosa. The second ring is hypoechoic and is due to the muscularis mucosa. The third ring is hyperechoic and represents the submucosa. The fourth ring is again hypoechoic and is formed by the muscularis propria. The fifth ring is hyperechoic and is due to the perirectal fat or in areas of peritoneal reflection by the serosa and fat. Rectal carcinoma is seen as a hypoechoic mass with irregular borders interrupting the normal five-layer wall pattern. The accuracy of ERU in staging of colorectal carcinoma varies from 64% to 93%. Most of the errors are due to overestimates of the depth of invasion possibly as a result of co-existing inflammation. Tumor confined to the muscularis mucosa can be differentiated from tumor extending into the perirectal fat with invasion of adjacent structures and metastatic involvement of the perirectal lymph nodes **(Figs. 7A and B)**.

ERU may also help in differentiating benign villous adenomas from those with focal areas of invasive carcinoma. Glaser et al.[47] reported that benign villous adenoma appears hyperechoic and areas of invasive carcinoma appear hypoechoic. The presence of invasive carcinoma within a villous adenoma is determined by the involvement of the muscularis propria.[48] ERU can detect perirectal lymph nodes as small as 5 mm in size cannot be used to predict nodal involvement by malignancy. In fact, studies evaluating nodal metastasis based on the size of the lymph nodes have shown rather low accuracy rates. Nodal echo texture and morphology are the most often used criteria. Nodes which have sharply demarcated borders and an inhomogeneous hypoechoic pattern are more likely to be malignant unlike nodes with indistinct borders and a hyperechoic pattern. Limitation of ERU is in evaluating lymph nodes outside mesorectal fascia, lateral lymph nodes, distant metastasis, stenosing rectal carcinomas and tumors near the anal verge, which are difficult to visualize and may be missed. Other limitations of ERU include the inability to assess depth of penetration beyond the colonic wall as well as possible overestimation of tumor size in patients with extensive peritumoral inflammation or with preoperative radiation. Failure of the technique occurs in up to 15% of all rectal carcinomas.[45]

Transrectal US can distinguish three stages of disease based on TNM classification:

1. T1 tumor confined to mucosa and submucosa which does not interrupt the middle echogenic ring.
2. T2 tumor confined to rectal wall in which the outermost echogenic interface is intact.
3. T3 tumor which penetrates the perirectal fat and leads to disruption of outermost echogenic ring.

Doppler US may complement the US imaging by showing increased color flow, increased diastolic flow within tumor with low resistance waveform, as tumor vessels lack smooth muscle layer, thus offering little resistance **(Figs. 8A to E)**. A cut-off value of peak systolic velocity (PSV) greater than 25 cm/s is used to differentiate T3 and T4 tumors from T1 and T2 tumors and a PSV of more than 20 cm/s in lymph nodes is classified as malignant.

Computed Tomography

The primary aim of computerized tomography in imaging colorectal carcinoma is for preoperative staging, in assessing the postoperative complications and for the detection of tumor recurrence. It is estimated that up to 25% of patients with colorectal cancer have metastates at the time of

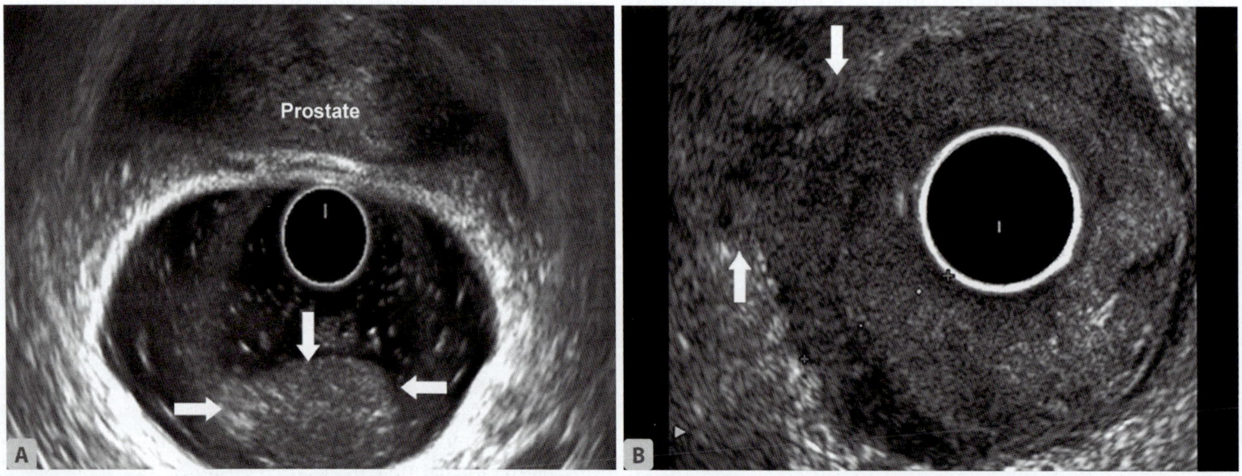

FIGS. 7A AND B: (A) EUS with radial echoendoscope shows polypoidal lesion (white arrows) with muscularis propria seen intact all around suggestive of T1 lesion; (B) EUS with radial echoendoscope shows involvement of all layers of rectum with infiltration of serosa and adjacent perirectal tissue (arrows) suggestive of T4 lesion.

Courtesy: Dr Surinder Rana, Department of Gastroenterology, PGIMER, Chandigarh, India.

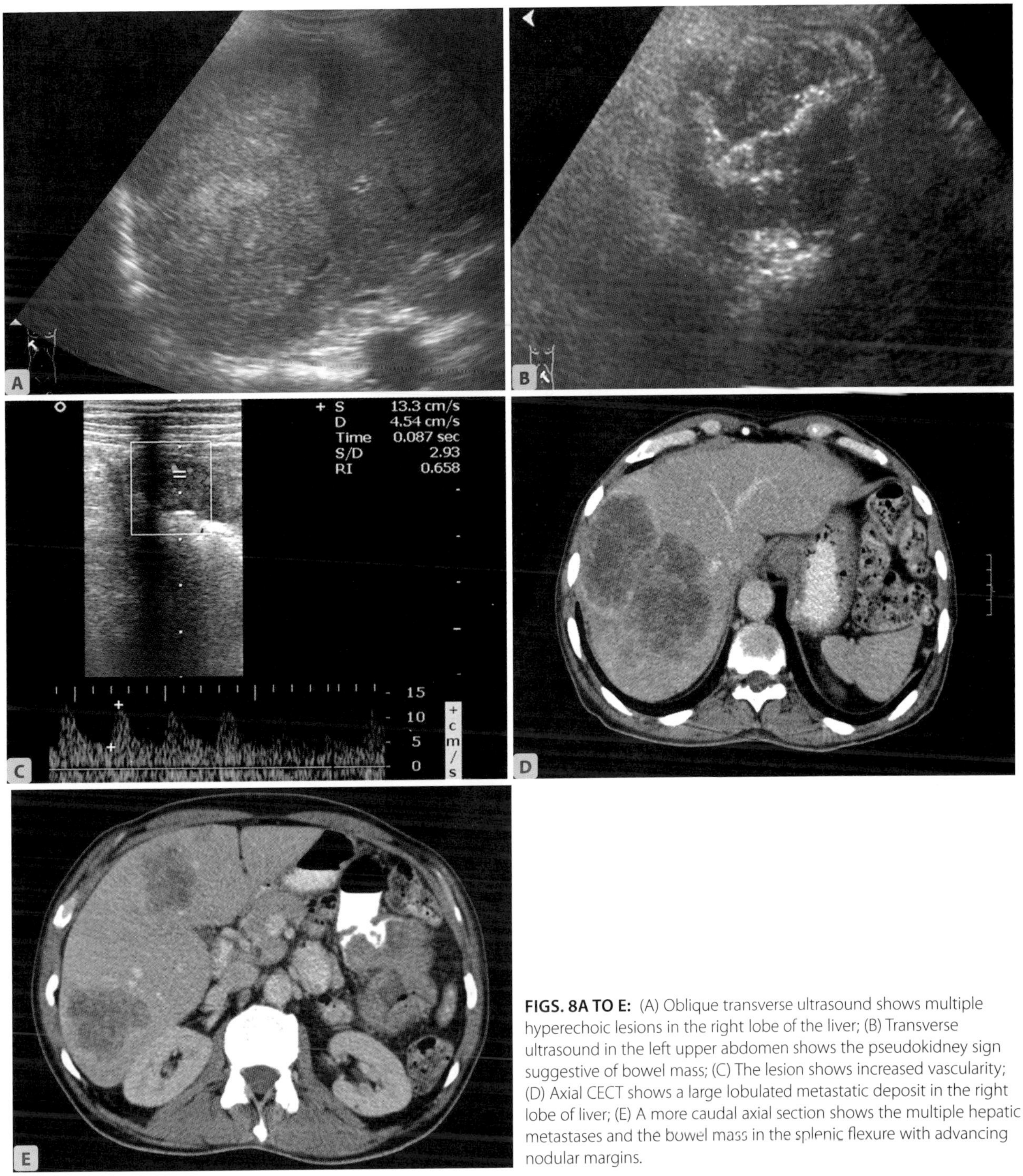

FIGS. 8A TO E: (A) Oblique transverse ultrasound shows multiple hyperechoic lesions in the right lobe of the liver; (B) Transverse ultrasound in the left upper abdomen shows the pseudokidney sign suggestive of bowel mass; (C) The lesion shows increased vascularity; (D) Axial CECT shows a large lobulated metastatic deposit in the right lobe of liver; (E) A more caudal axial section shows the multiple hepatic metastases and the bowel mass in the splenic flexure with advancing nodular margins.

diagnosis.[49] Therefore, staging technique should include both the primary colorectal neoplasm and sites of potential metastases.

Barium studies and colonoscopy/sigmoidoscopy provide excellent visualization of the mucosa. However, they cannot determine the depth of mural invasion by the tumor or the extent of metastatic involvement. Preoperative staging helps to assess tumor extent accurately to individualize therapy, assess risk of disease recurrence, and determine prognosis. CT and MRI have become the primary means for radiologic staging of colorectal carcinoma because of their ability to demonstrate the extent of wall invasion, extraluminal tumor spread, lymph node and distant metastasis. Complications of primary colonic malignancies such as obstruction, perforation and fistula formation can also be readily visualized with CT.

The accuracy of CT for colonic evaluation can be improved with several additional techniques including adequate cleansing of colon, administration of IV smooth muscle relaxants, distension of the colon with either air, carbon dioxide (CT colonography) or water and by having thin sections through the areas of tumor **(Fig. 9)**. A rectal enema may be given to delineate the descending colon and rectosigmoid region.

The normal wall thickening in a well-distended colonic segment is 3 mm, 3–6 mm is considered indeterminate, measurement greater than 6 mm is considered abnormal. Both the mucosal margin and outer colonic margin should be smooth and delineated by air/water-soluble contrast or pericolonic fat respectively. The rectum, rectosigmoid region, ascending and descending segments of the colon are relatively fixed structures and were, therefore, easily evaluated by conventional CT. Tumors in the flexures and transverse colon were less readily examined by conventional CT because bowel peristalsis and excursion of the diaphragm made these parts more difficult to evaluate. This has been overcome by the advent of fast helical CT scanners.

The primary bowel tumor is identified on CT as focal or circumferential wall thickening (>6 mm) with contour distortion or more frequently as a discrete mass. Occasionally, an intraluminal polypoid mass without wall thickening is seen. CT cannot depict the various layers of the bowel wall and cannot distinguish T1 from T2 stage. Sometimes, contrast-enhanced CT scan with rectal contrast can demonstrate a typical 'napkin ring' lesion of annular contricting malignancy and plaque-like lesion. Large masses may undergo central necrosis and appear as a soft tissue mass with central low attenuation. Mucinous primary adenocarcinoma may rarely contain calcification, however, this occurs more often in hepatic metastasis than in the primary tumor. Rectal and sigmoid cancers may appear as asymmetric nodular wall thickening that narrows the lumen. This appearance may mimic diverticulitis, especially if the tumor involvement of the wall has resulted in infiltration of the pericolic fat. However, presence of fluid in the root of the sigmoid mesentery and engorgement of adjacent sigmoid mesenteric vasculature favors the diagnosis of diverticulitis and presence of pericolic lymph nodes raises the suspicion of colon cancer. Pericolic lymph node adjacent to a segment of thickened colonic wall are seen much more frequently in cases of colon cancer than with diverticulitis. Thickening can occasionally appear symmetric and involve the entire circumference of the bowel wall. In such cases, it is difficult to differentiate malignant from benign causes of wall thickening, including inflammation and mural edema.

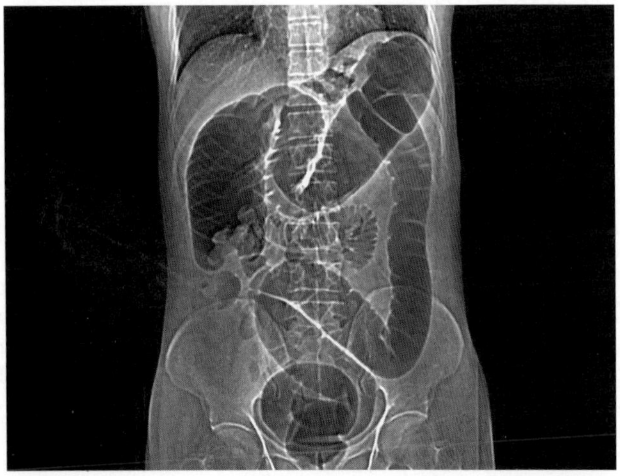

FIG. 9: Tomogram obtained before acquiring data for CT colonography shows the polypoidal mass lesion in the cecum. The rest of the colon is well distended with air.

The pericolonic and perirectal fat appear uniformly hypodense without soft tissue stranding on CT. Thickening of the perirectal fascia produces the 'halo sign' which can be seen with extension of tumor into perirectal fat. Invasion beyond the bowel wall should be suspected whenever a focal mass deforms the contour of the outer colonic wall with an advancing nodular margin with or without pericolonic soft tissue stranding **(Figs. 10 and 11)**. Extracolonic tumor spread is also suggested by the loss of fat planes between the large bowel and the surrounding muscles like levator ani, obturator internus, piriform, coccygeus and gluteus. Unfortunately, the loss of fat plane is a nonspecific sign in cross-sectional imaging and can also be seen with cachexia and lymphatic or vascular congestion, this interpretation must be made with caution.[50] However, invasion is definite when a tumor mass is seen to extend directly into the adjacent muscle with obliteration of fat planes with enlargement of the individual muscle. Occasionally an enhancing intramuscular mass is seen.

Spread to contiguous organs in the pelvis should also be interpreted with caution and diagnosed only if a major portion of the viscera is enveloped or if an obvious mass involves an adjacent organ **(Figs. 12A and B)**. Primary or recurrent colonic cancers can invade the small and large bowel, the seminal vesicles, sciatic nerve, prostate, bladder, uterus and ovaries and also cause hydronephrosis by obstructing the ureters. Fistula between tumor and adjoining viscera such as bladder can be demonstrated by either direct visualization of fistulous tract on CECT or demonstration of air within the bladder. Fistulation into uterovaginal areas, ischiorectal fossa and small bowel can occur. Colonic cancers can destroy the adjacent bone. Minor invasion of bone can present as cortical destruction. In advanced cases, soft tissue mass with destruction of bones of sacrum, coccyx and ilium can be seen.

Regional lymph nodes are the most common metastatic site of colorectal carcinoma. CT cannot distinguish benign from malignant lymphadenopathy. Metastatic foci may be found in normal-sized lymph nodes (<1 cm). Likewise reactive inflammatory lymph nodes are frequently larger than 1 cm resulting in false-positive assessment of nodal disease. Only lymphangiography or guided biopsy can give a definite diagnosis. Any nonenhancing mass in the perirectal fat should be considered to be malignant lymphadenopathy irrespective of the size as hyperplastic lymph nodes do not occur in this region.

Sites of distant metastasis generally include the liver, lung, adrenals, peritoneum, kidneys and bone marrow. The liver is the most common site of extranodal metastasis. On noncontrast CT scans, hepatic metastases are typically discrete, hypodense lesions of variable size, although foci of calcification can be seen within metastatic mucinous adenocarcinoma. Following a bolus IV injection of iodinated contrast, deposits often show early peripheral enhancement

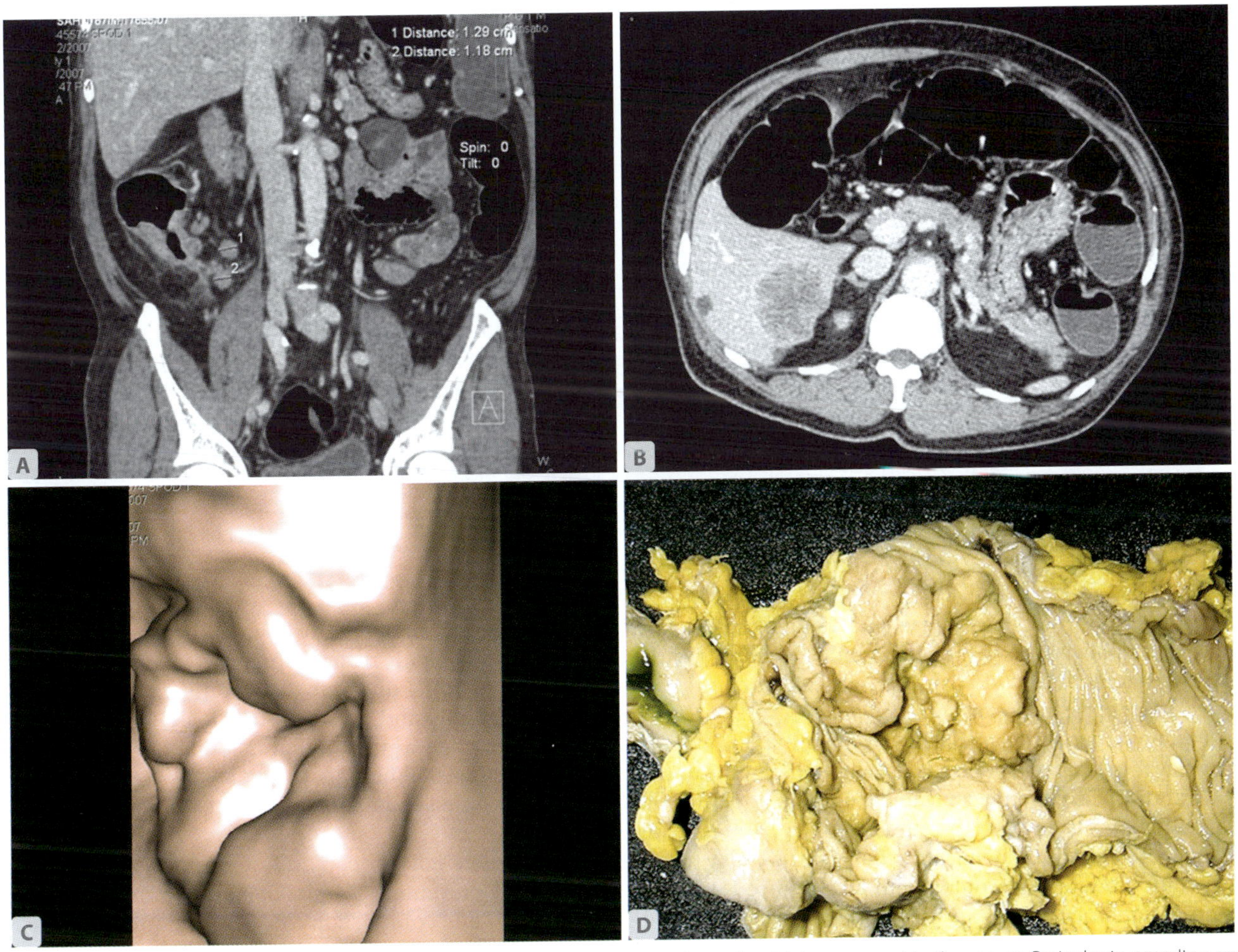

FIGS. 10A TO D: (A) Coronal MPR image shows concentric mural thickening with a polypoidal component in the cecum. Pericolonic stranding and multiple enlarged pericolonic lymph nodes are also seen; (B) Axial CECT section of the upper abdomen shows hypodense lesions in segment VI of liver suggestive of metastases; (C) CT colonoscopy endoluminal image shows the intraluminal irregular polypoidal growth; (D) Gross photograph of the ulceroproliferative growth involving the cecum which appears to be infiltrating up to the serosal fat.

Courtesy: Professor JD Wig, Department of General Surgery, PGIMER, Chandigarh, India.

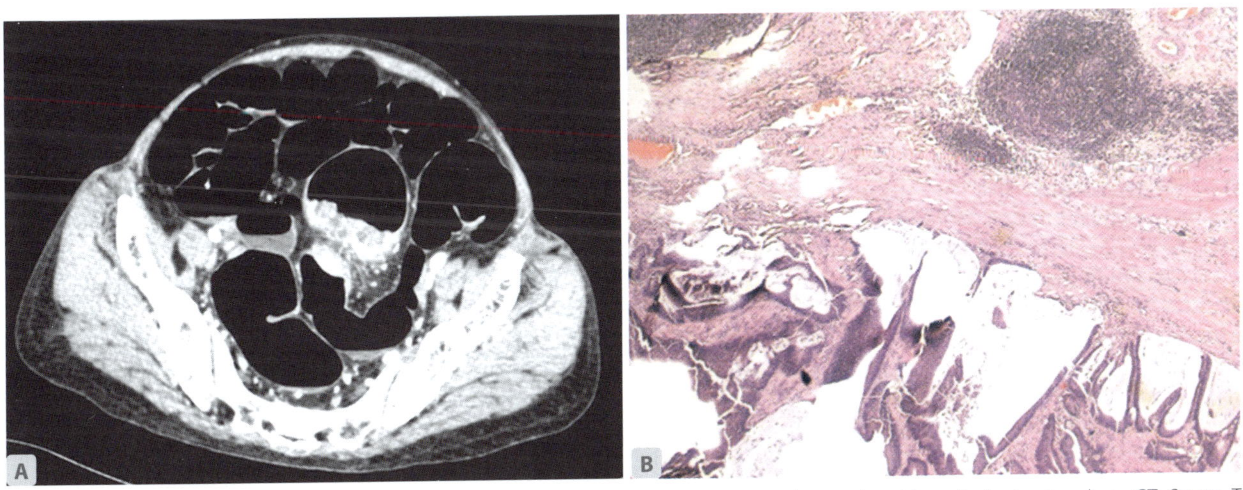

FIGS. 11A AND B: (A) CE-CTC image shows heterogeneously enhancing rectosigmoid growth with pericolonic stranding, CT Stage: T3; (B) Representative microphotograph of this T3 tumor showing infiltration through the muscularis propria into the subserosa consistent with stage T3. (H & E, × 250).

Courtesy: Professor K Vaiphei, Department of Histopathology, PGIMER, Chandigarh, India.

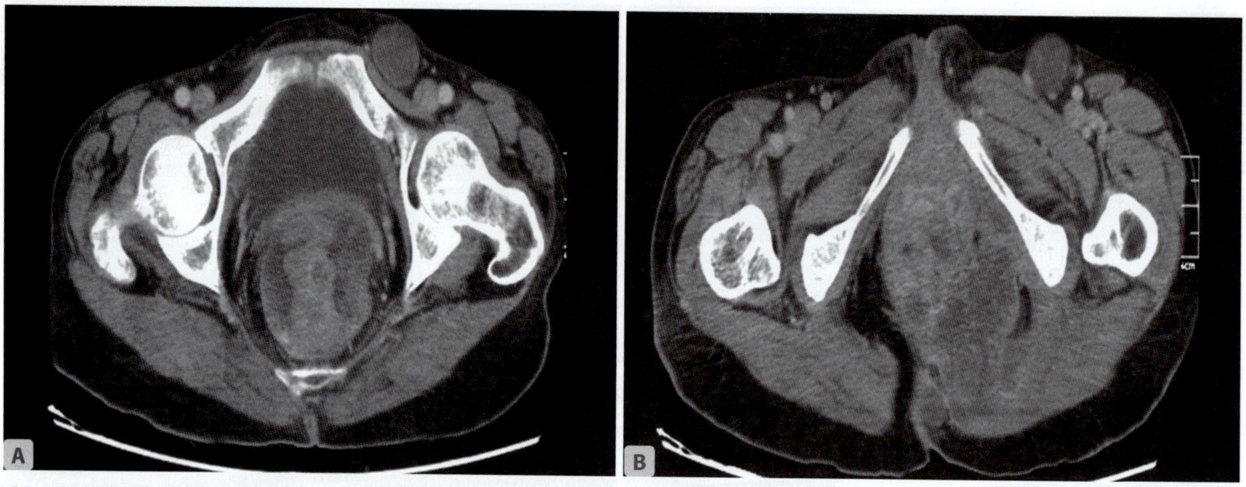

FIGS. 12A AND B: Axial CECT sections show a large heterogeneous mass in the rectum obliterating the lumen. The planes of the mass with the vagina, lateral pelvic wall and gluteal muscles on the left side are lost consistently with invasion. A large left inguinal lymph node is also seen.

or become uniformly hyperdense, go through an isodense phase and finally show washout of contrast. Scanning early in the dynamic phase to maximize liver-lesion contrast is critical to increase the lesion conspicuity.

Peritoneal carcinomatosis which is the result of spread of tumor over peritoneal surface, is usually well demonstrated by CT and appears as enhancing linear or nodular peritoneal thickening and is associated with ascites. In patients with disseminated disease, careful analysis of chest CT may reveal metastatic nodules. In women with an advanced stage of colon carcinoma, masses in the ovaries may be detected (Krukenberg's tumor).

CT scan is quite accurate in staging patients with advanced disease. Pitfalls occur in interpretation of scans in patients with less advanced tumors. Perforation/ulceration of colonic cancer can result in an inflammatory mass or abscess which obscures the underlying cancer. CT scan obtained after surgery or radiation therapy can demonstrate edema or hemorrhage of the pelvic structures simulating residual/recurrent disease.

CT staging is based on the combination of numerous findings like thickness of the colon wall, presence or absence of tumor spread to adjacent organs and presence or absence of metastases. Earlier studies have shown low accuracy (41–64%) for staging with conventional CT owing to low sensitivity of local tumor extent (53–77%) and of lymph node metastases (22–73%).[51] Recent studies have shown MDCT to be very useful in preoperative staging for colon cancer with accuracy of 4-slice CT being 83% for T-staging and 85% for N-staging.[52,53] In a study conducted at our Institute which was presented at the World Cancer Congress of UICC in 2008, the diagnostic accuracy for T-staging was 92.3% and for N-staging was 42.3%.[54] The lower specificity for lymph node metastases accounted for the lower accuracy of N-staging in this study **(Figs. 13A to D)**.

Computed Tomography Colonography

Computed tomography colonography (CTC) is an innovative technique that entails CT examination of the entire colon and computerized processing of the raw data acquired after colon cleansing and colonic distension. It was in 1994 that Vining and Gelfand from Bowman Gray University introduced CT colonography and exhibited the first CT colonography fly-through video at the annual meeting of the Society of Gastrointestinal Radiologists.[55]

The accepted indications for CT colonography are as follows:

- Incomplete colonoscopy due to an occlusive mass or stricture preventing examination of the proximal colon.
- Incomplete colonoscopy due to colonic tortuosity, adhesions, severe diverticular disease or patient intolerance of colonoscopy.
- Inability to perform colonoscopy due to requirement for anticoagulant therapy or risks of sedation.
- Patients who adamantly refuse to undergo colonoscopy but have a strong indication for diagnostic colonoscopy.

CT colonography is under analysis as a screening tool for colorectal cancer as it is relatively safe and has greater patient acceptance as compared with other available screening methods.

The contraindication for CT colonography are allergy to contrast, suspected colonic perforation, acute colonic infection (acute diverticulitis, severe infective colitis), acute lower GI bleeding, complete colonic obstruction, very recent colonic surgery (<1 week), medically unstable patients and refusal to undergo colonic preparation.

The technique involves colonic cleansing, colonic distension, image acquisition and post-processing of acquired data. For 'wet preparation' polyethylene glycol is used; while for 'dry preparation', phospho-soda is used. Adequate colonic distension is critical for increasing polyp conspicuity. This can be achieved by using room air or carbon dioxide. Colonic perforation is rarely seen (0.59–0.08%).[56] Advanced age and underlying colonic pathology are the risk factors for colonic perforation. Air can be administered easily, is available at no cost but is less well tolerated than carbon dioxide as it is not absorbed by the colonic mucosa. Carbon dioxide, on the other hand, is gradually absorbed by the colonic wall, resulting in diminished discomfort to the patient **(Fig. 14)**.

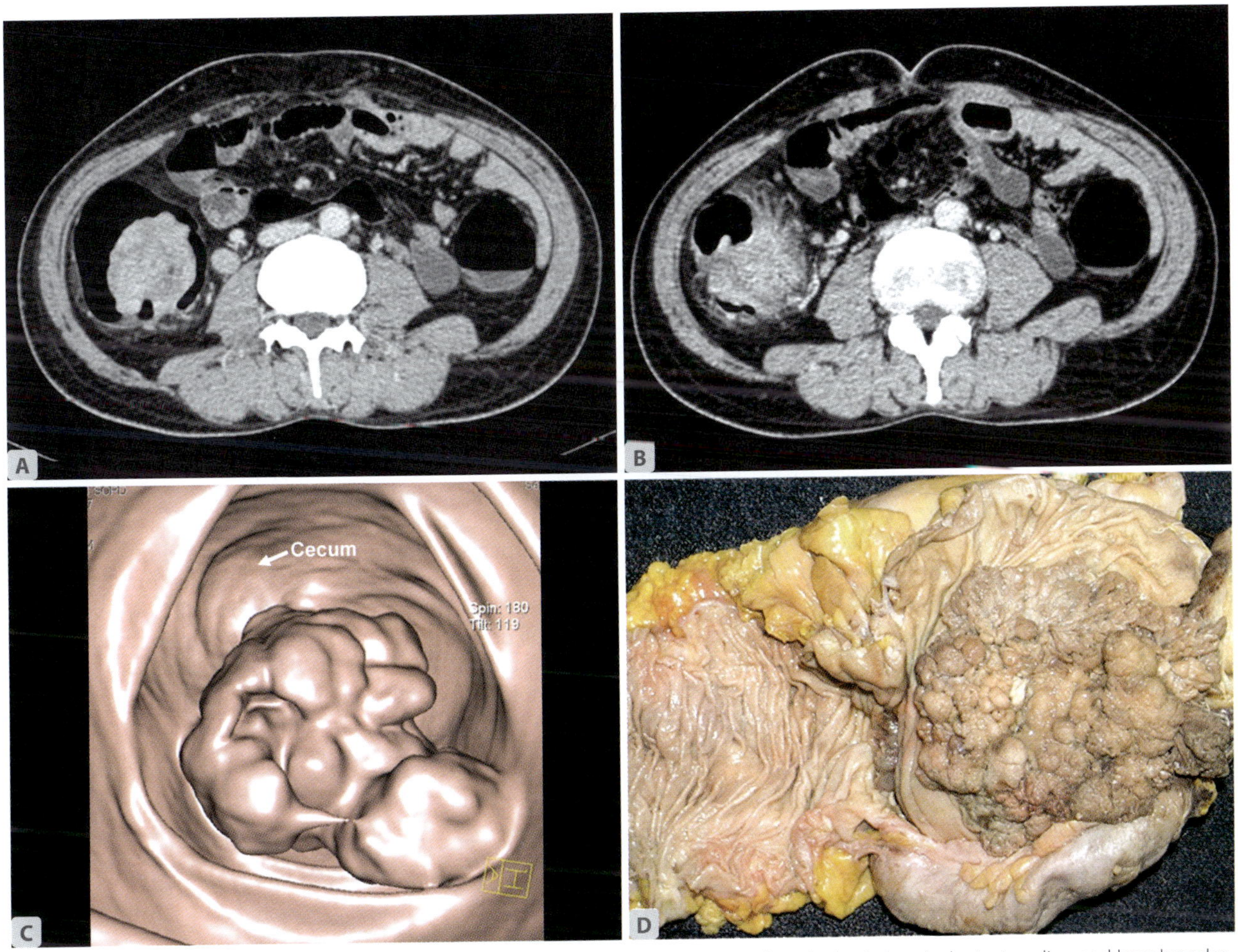

FIGS. 13A TO D: (A and B) Axial CE-CTC images show presence of polypoidal cecal growth with classical pericolonic stranding and lymph nodes—CT Stage: T3N2M0. Surgical Stage: T3N2M0. Histological stage: T3N0M0; (C) CT colonographic image of the same patient showing a polypoidal intraluminal cecal mass; (D) Gross photograph showing a proliferative tumor almost completely filling up the cecal lumen.

Courtesy: Professor JD Wig, Department of General Surgery, PGIMER, Chandigarh, India.

Image acquisition is done after colonic insufflation in supine and prone positions on a helical CT scanner using low-dose technique. The radiation dose is about half of the dose of a barium enema.[56] Intravenous contrast improves detection of medium-sized polyps (6–9 mm) especially in a suboptimally prepared colon.[57] After acquiring supine and prone scans, various software packages are used to display images in both 2D and 3D (endoluminal) views.

There are various mimickers of polyps which are potential pitfalls of CT colonography. These include adherent fecal matter, lipomas, inverted appendiceal stump, prominent ileocecal valve, inverted diverticulum and bulbous colonic folds. While some of these are due to technical errors on account of inadequate colon preparation or distension, others are due to perceptive errors.

In the first published study from India the sensitivity and specificity of CT colonography have been reported to be 65% and 77% respectively for lesions 1–5 mm; 97% and 83% respectively for lesions 6–9 mm; and 100% and 100%

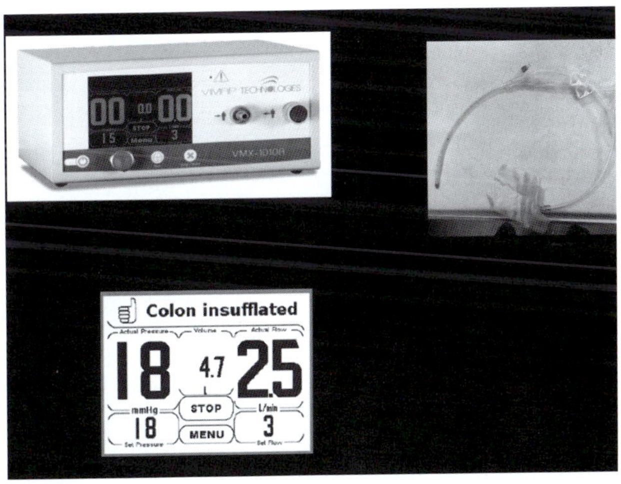

FIG. 14: CO_2 insufflation pump, insufflation tube catheter and the final message on the pump when the colon is completely insufflated.

respectively for lesions 10 mm or larger.[58] CT colonography scores over optical colonoscopy as it provides information about extracolonic findings. The incidence of significant extracolonic findings ranges from 6.8% to 21%.[56] A reporting system for CT colonography has been devised by the Working Group on Virtual Colonoscopy and has been termed 'C-RADS' or CT colonography reporting and data system.[59] The aim of this reporting system is to achieve standardization of reporting. The advances in CT colonography include fluid and fecal tagging to achieve 'prepless' studies by digital bowel cleansing using subtraction techniques. Computer-aided detection (CAD) software and novel 3D views that slice open and flatten the colonic wall are being developed.

Magnetic Resonance Imaging

Magnetic resonance imaging (MRI) can be used to detect and stage rectosigmoid tumors more accurately than tumors in the rest of the colon. This increased accuracy is due to the fixed position of the rectosigmoid colon in relation to the pelvis. Many refinements have been described including MRI using an endorectal coil, addition of IV gadolinium chelate and the use of oral and rectal contrast agents to achieve bowel distension. High-performance gradient, faster pulse sequences, and high-resolution MRI are now routinely available, producing additional improvement in MRI quality.

Presently, MRI using thin sections and phased-array coils can distinguish tumors localized to mucosa and submucosa (T1) and those that infiltrate the entire colonic wall (T2) with a reasonable accuracy (65–85%).[60] Detection of tumor improves if proper colon cleansing and adequate distension can be obtained with administration of air, water or supraparamagnetic contrast medium. Imaging in prone position helps to decrease motion artifacts with better depiction of rectal tumors.

The different layers comprising the bowel wall on gadolinium-enhanced T1-weighted fat-suppressed spin echo images are the high-signal intensity mucosa, low-signal intensity muscularis mucosa and lamina propria, high-signal intensity submucosa and low-signal intensity muscularis propria.

In T1W SE images, rectosigmoid tumors are seen as wall thickening with signal intensity similar to or higher than skeletal muscles (long T1). Perirectal fat has short T1 and hence appears bright on T1WI and rectal air has no signal, thus these tumors are very well delineated on T1W images and their extension beyond the colonic wall is well visualized. If polyps or tumor contain a large amount of mucin, signal intensity can be higher on T1WI.

Gadolinium enhancement makes lesions more conspicuous **(Figs. 15A to C)**. On gadolinium-enhanced spoiled gradient-echo (SGE) MR images with oral and rectal contrast,

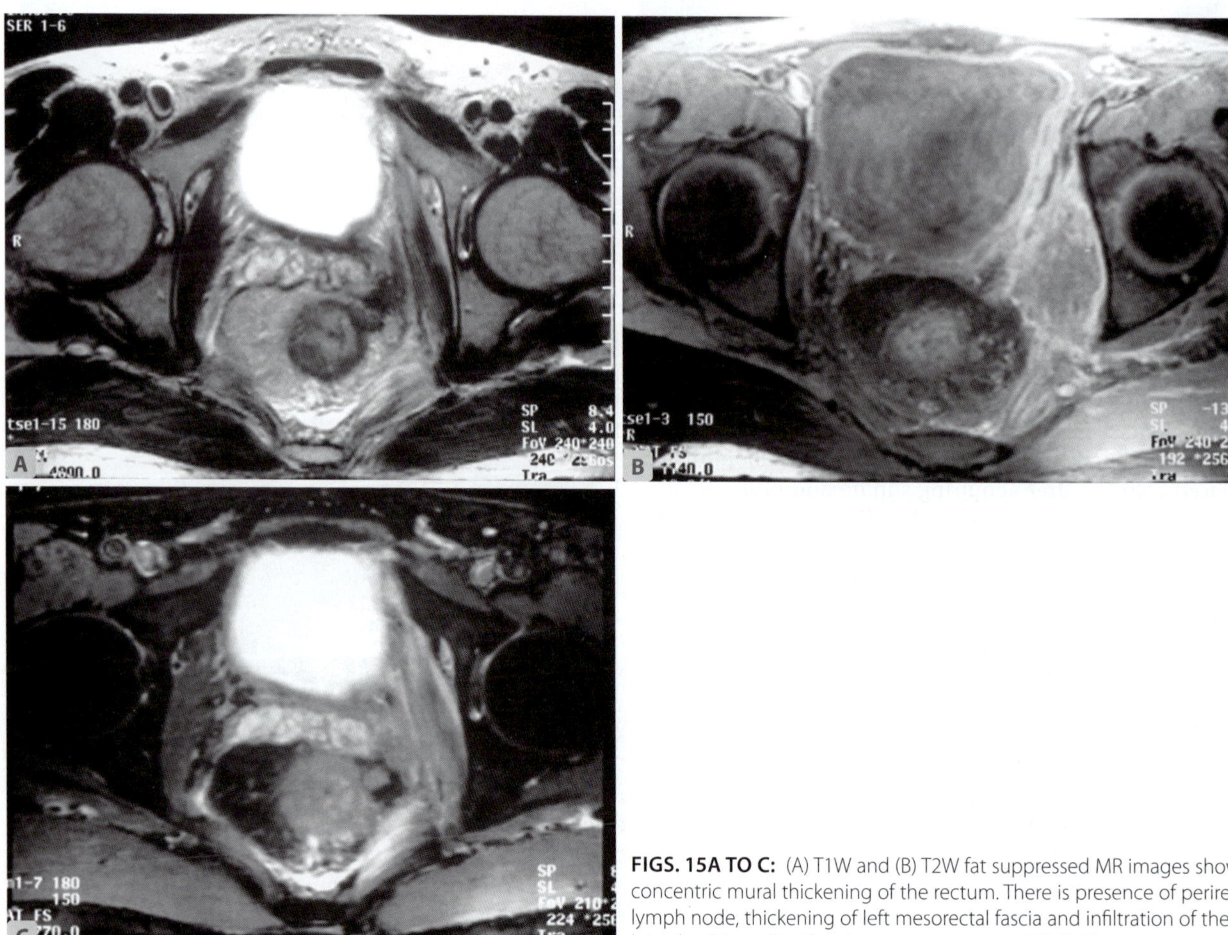

FIGS. 15A TO C: (A) T1W and (B) T2W fat suppressed MR images show concentric mural thickening of the rectum. There is presence of perirectal lymph node, thickening of left mesorectal fascia and infiltration of the lateral pelvic wall with enhancement seen on CEMR (C).

the lesion is depicted as an enhancing soft tissue mass or as mural thickening.

On T2W images, the lesion is hyperintense to the muscle, but as fat is also hyperintense, contrast between the tumor and perirectal fat is not adequate and hence T2W images are not as useful as T1W images for diagnosing extracolonic extension. T2W images provide good contrast between tumor tissue and surrounding pelvic wall muscles as tumor is hyperintense and muscle hypointense on T2WI.

Studies have shown that T2WI is superior to T1WI for evaluating the extent of tumor in relation to the rectal wall layers and the mesorectal fascia.[61,62] T2WI can demonstrate the mesorectal fascia better than T1WI. This has assumed importance since the introduction of total mesorectal excision (TME) for rectal cancer. In this, the entire mesorectal compartment is removed, which includes rectum, surrounding mesorectal fat with the perirectal lymph nodes and a thin fascia that envelopes the two former structures and is known as mesorectal fascia. The recurrence rate of cancer after TME is reported to be less than 10%.[63] MRI technique and image quality play a prominent role in T-staging and accuracy is dependent on obtaining high-resolution images (0.5 cm voxel size) perpendicular to the plane of the tumor.

For evaluation of cancers involving the anal sphincter, images in the coronal plane are particularly useful. Routine MR imaging cannot recognize tumor foci in normal-sized lymph nodes. A T1W SE sequence with fat suppression, readily demonstrates lymph nodes. Depicting tumor in normal-sized lymph nodes may require the use of additional contrast agent directed at imaging nodal metastasis. Invasion of adjacent organs is best seen on transverse or coronal MR images. Neither CT nor MRI can detect microinvasion.

Liver and adrenal metastases are as well demonstrated on MR as on helical CT. All extrahepatic anatomic sites must be evaluated carefully to assess for possible metastatic tumor. Peritoneal carcinomatosis is difficult to detect on MR images. Fat-suppressed, gadolinium-enhanced SGE MR images are most useful for extrahepatic imaging. Peritoneal deposits enhance slowly with gadolinium and are most conspicuous on delayed images obtained after 5 minutes delay. Surface implants on the liver may be detected by T2 WI without IV contrast material. The ability of MRI to depict subtle osseous metastases is an advantage compared with helical CT. MR imaging is superior to CT at distinguishing between fibrosis and recurrent cancer and could eliminate the need for biopsies.

More advanced MR technique includes the use of an endorectal surface coil which has the potential to allow differentiation of the bowel wall layers and thus permits more accurate 'T'-stage determination. Comparison of endorectal MR (ERMRI), ERUS and 3D-ERUS have shown an overall similar accuracy for depicting the transmural extent of the rectal cancer, 91%, 84% and 88% respectively.[64] In a comparison of ERUS, ERMRI and CT in rectal cancer, Kim et al.[65] have shown comparable accuracies of 81% for both ERUS and ERMRI for depth of tumor penetration which was superior to CT (65%).

Endorectal MRI does have some limitations. This technique cannot be performed in patients with severely stenotic infiltrating lesions. It is a rigid device with a small radial area of acceptable signal to noise imaging. It cannot adequately assess the mesorectal fascia and the circumferential resection margin (CRM).

Magnetic Resonance Colonography

Magnetic resonance (MR) colonography is based on the acquisition of MR datasets of the abdomen which optimizes visualization of the large bowel. Data is acquired during single breath-hold scans. The bowel is distended per rectally with water, barium, room air or CO_2. Spasmolytics are given intravenously before rectal filling. Patient preparation involves use of cathartics and enemas. 2D and/or 3D fast imaging with steady-state precession (FISP) is a useful sequence for MR colonography. 3D TIW images are also acquired before and after administration of gadolinium intravenously. A T1W 2D FLASH (fast low angle shot) sequence is also acquired in the axial plane for evaluation of adjacent abdominal organs. Axial, MPR and 'fly through' images are analyzed in both antegrade and retrograde directions. MR colonography has been reported to have 100% sensitivity for lesions larger than 10 mm and 89% for lesions 5–10 mm in size.[66] However, it has very limited accuracy for detecting lesions smaller than 5 mm.

The advantage of MR colonography over CT colonography is lack of ionizing radiation and superior soft tissue contrast. The disadvantages are lower spatial resolution, high susceptibility to motion artifacts, longer examination time and limited availability.

Arteriography

Arteriography has a limited value in colonic cancers. Its application is restricted to the investigation of patients with acute bleeding of apparent colonic origin with therapeutic embolization. The bleeding site may be demonstrated in patients with chronic low-grade blood loss. Arteriography with chemoembolization or radiofrequency ablation is also used for treating metastatic liver deposits in patients with colonic malignancies, who are not surgical candidates.

Immunoscintigraphy

Labeled anticarcinoembryonic antigen (CEA) monoclonal antibodies (MoAbs) have been used as *in-vivo* tumor localizing agents. Primary adenocarcinoma of colon and metastatic foci are seen as areas of increased radioactivity (hot spots). Depending on the size of tumor necrosis, liver metastases may appear as areas of intense, absent or intermediate uptake. The reported sensitivity of monoclonal antibody staging of colorectal cancer is 65–86% with specificity for detection of primary tumor, local recurrence and distant metastasis varying from 77% to 92%.[67]

Positron Emission Tomography

Fluorine 18-labeled deoxyglucose (^{18}FDG) is used, and there is a remarkably close correlation between tumor grade and glucose utilization. This method can be used for detection of distant, residual or recurrent disease **(Figs. 16 and 17)**. Malignant tissue demonstrates more rapid uptake with accumulation compared with normal tissue. Time activity curves of glucose utilization are generated for region of interest and pathologic areas are compared with surrounding normal tissue by generating a differential absorption ratio. Limitations of PET are decreased sensitivity in detecting colon lesion ≤10 mm in diameter and decreased tracer uptake by mucinous tumors. Nonspecific PET findings can result in negative impact on patient care in up to 9% patients.[68]

RECENT ADVANCES

These include PET/CT colonography and CT perfusion imaging for colorectal tumors. PET/CT colonography involves the combination of ^{18}F-FDG PET with CT colonography. It provides both anatomic and functional information. It has been used both for staging of colon cancer and for screening purposes.[69,70] The standard uptake value of malignant tumors has been reported to be between 4 and 20 with a mean of 9.[70]

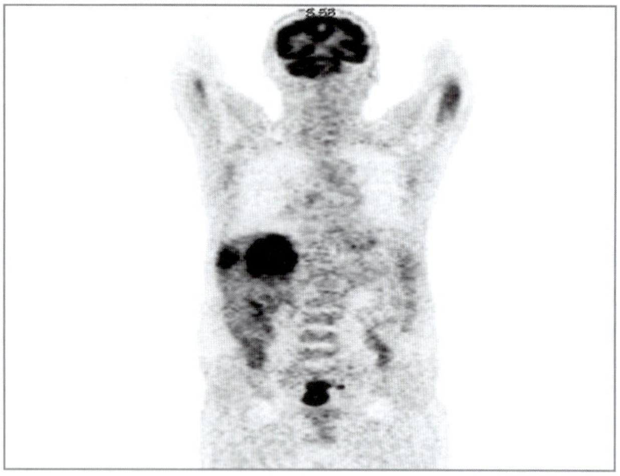

FIG. 16: Coronal PET image showing tracer avid rectal cancer with locoregional lymph node and liver metastases.

Courtesy: Professor BR Mittal, Department of Nuclear Medicine, PGIMER, Chandigarh, India.

Tumor perfusion of rectal cancer has been measured with first pass perfusion CT. Rectal cancers show higher blood flow (BF) and shorter mean transit time (MTT) compared with those of normal rectum. After chemotherapy and radiotherapy, responders show significant reduction in BF and increase in MTT.[71,72] Significant difference in baseline BF and MTT is seen between responders and nonresponders.

ACR RECOMMENDATIONS FOR COLORECTAL CANCER STAGING

The latest recommendations of the American College of Radiology (ACR) are based on the concept that for colon cancer, the role of imaging for locoregional staging (T and N stage) is of questionable utility. This is due to the fact that neoadjuvant therapy has not shown any survival advantage over surgery alone and the standard surgical approach is radical resection. On the other hand for rectal cancer, the surgical options are more varied and are dependent on the involvement or sparing of the sphincter, circumferential resection margin and peritoneal reflection. Neoadjuvant chemotherapy and radiation, in addition to surgical resection have been found to decrease local recurrence and improve survival. Hence there is a need for accurate preoperative staging of rectal cancer.

As per the ACR appropriateness criteria of 2016, MRI pelvis without and with IV contrast is most appropriate for locoregional staging of rectal cancer. CECT of the chest, abdomen and pelvis is most appropriate for the staging for distal metastases of colorectal cancer. The sensitivity and specificity of MRI for assessment of circumferential resection margin range from 94% to 100% and 85% to 88% respectively.[73,74] Locoregional staging is not routinely required for colon cancer. The most common sites of metastatic involvement are liver and lungs. Accurate depiction of number, size and distribution is the primary goal of colon cancer staging. Multiphase CECT or contrast-enhanced MRI with optimization of technique are best suited for diagnosing

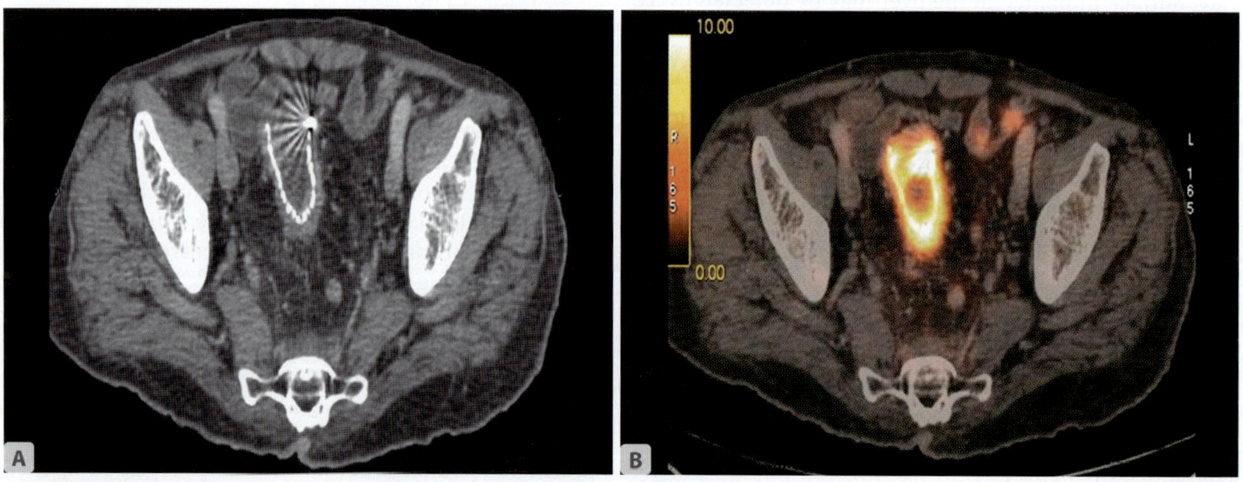

FIGS. 17A AND B: Axial CT (A) and PET-CT fusion image (B) in a patient postchemoradiation and postcolonic stent showing recurrent rectosigmoid thickening and locoregional lymph node. The bowel wall thickening showed more tracer uptake than the lymph node.

Courtesy: Professor BR Mittal, Department of Nuclear Medicine, PGIMER, Chandigarh, India.

liver metastases. MRI is more accurate in the setting of fatty liver and following neoadjuvant therapy. The use of chest CT, through controversial, is widely done along with CT or MRI of abdomen and pelvis. Only one quarter of pulmonary lesions found on CT are finally proven to be metastases. The routine use of PET-CT is not indicated for colorectal cancer.

OTHER EPITHELIAL TUMORS OF COLON

Squamous cell carcinomas are rare except in the rectum. Radiographic appearance is similar to adenocarcinoma and differentiation from other tumors is possible only by biopsy.

Cloacogenic carcinomas arise from transitional cloacogenic remnants of the anorectal junction. Radiographically the lesions are plaque-like and have a smooth or finely irregular surface. In profile, the borders form a tapered obtuse angle with the bowel wall. Ulceration is usually present. Since the lesions lie in the distal rectal areas, the catheter tip may completely obscure the lesion.

Carcinoid tumors present as submucosal lesions. The most common sites of colonic carcinoids are the rectum and cecum. They are seen as round, well-circumscribed masses **(Figs. 18A and B)**. Invasion of the bowel wall by tumor mass produces intense desmoplastic reaction and proliferation of fibrous tissue, resulting in contraction and kinking of the large bowel. Carcinoid tumors located in cecum and ascending colon are indistinguishable from adenocarcinoma on imaging.

NONEPITHELIAL TUMORS OF COLON

Mesodermal sarcomas of the large bowel are uncommon. They have a predilection for the rectal region. The lesions are usually rounded and lobulated but may be pedunculated. The tumors may grow extramurally and when the overlying mucosa ulcerates, necrosis and cystic cavitations can develop. Kaposi's sarcoma can involve any part of the gastrointestinal tract and presents as typical extramucosal mass or masses. On imaging, Kaposi's sarcoma is seen as a flat or plaque-like lesion, a small polypoid nodule or a polypoid submucosal lesion with or without umbilication.

Gastrointestinal stromal tumors (GISTs) arise from the interstitial cells of Cajal and express CD34. Only 1% of all GI tumors are of stromal origin and these are least commonly located in the colon. Small tumors are seen as sessile or pedunculated polyps. Large tumors may be seen as cavitating masses with a large extraluminal component or as submucosal masses with or without central ulceration **(Fig. 19)**. These lesions may mimic colonic lymphoma or carcinoma.

Colonic lipomas are uncommon benign tumors. Most lipomas are found in the right colon. About two thirds of these tumors are pedunculated. On barium enema, they are seen as smooth sessile or polypoidal lesions with a pedicle. Some of these lipomas may be lead points of intussusceptions. When this occurs, the lipomas may ulcerate and undergo fat necrosis resulting in CT attenuation more than fat. They are then confused with an intussuscepting carcinoma **(Figs. 20A to C)**.

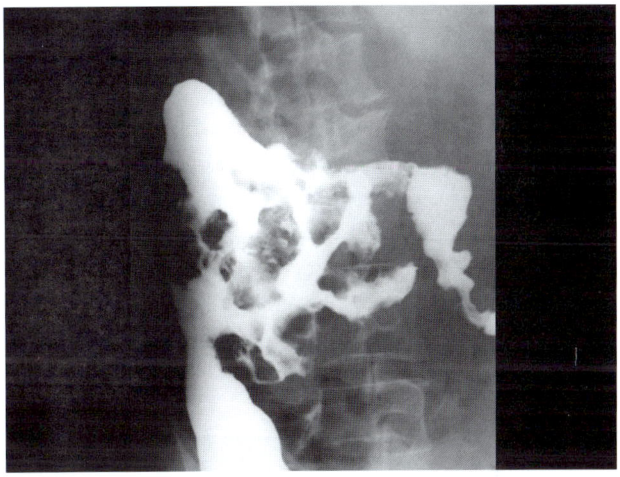

FIG. 19: Barium enema shows a large cavitatory mass lesion in the hepatic flexure with presence of deep ulcerations in a patient with leiomyosarcoma.

Courtesy: Professor B Nagi, Department of Gastroenterology, PGIMER, Chandigarh, India.

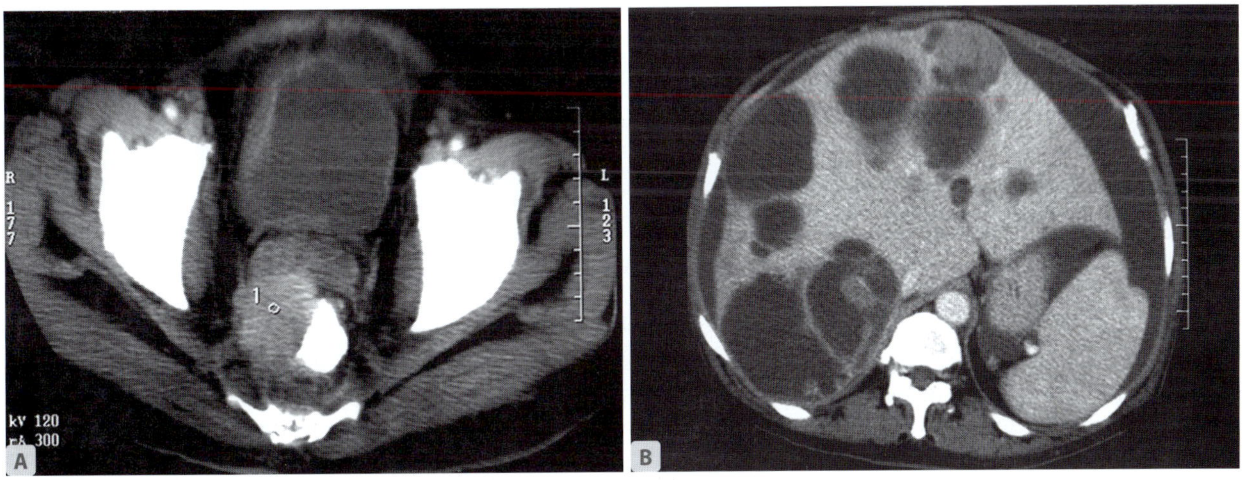

FIGS. 18A AND B: Axial CECT section shows a well-defined mass lesion along the right lateral wall of the rectum (A) with multiple cystic focal lesions in the liver (B) some of which are showing solid component in a patient with biopsy-proven carcinoid.

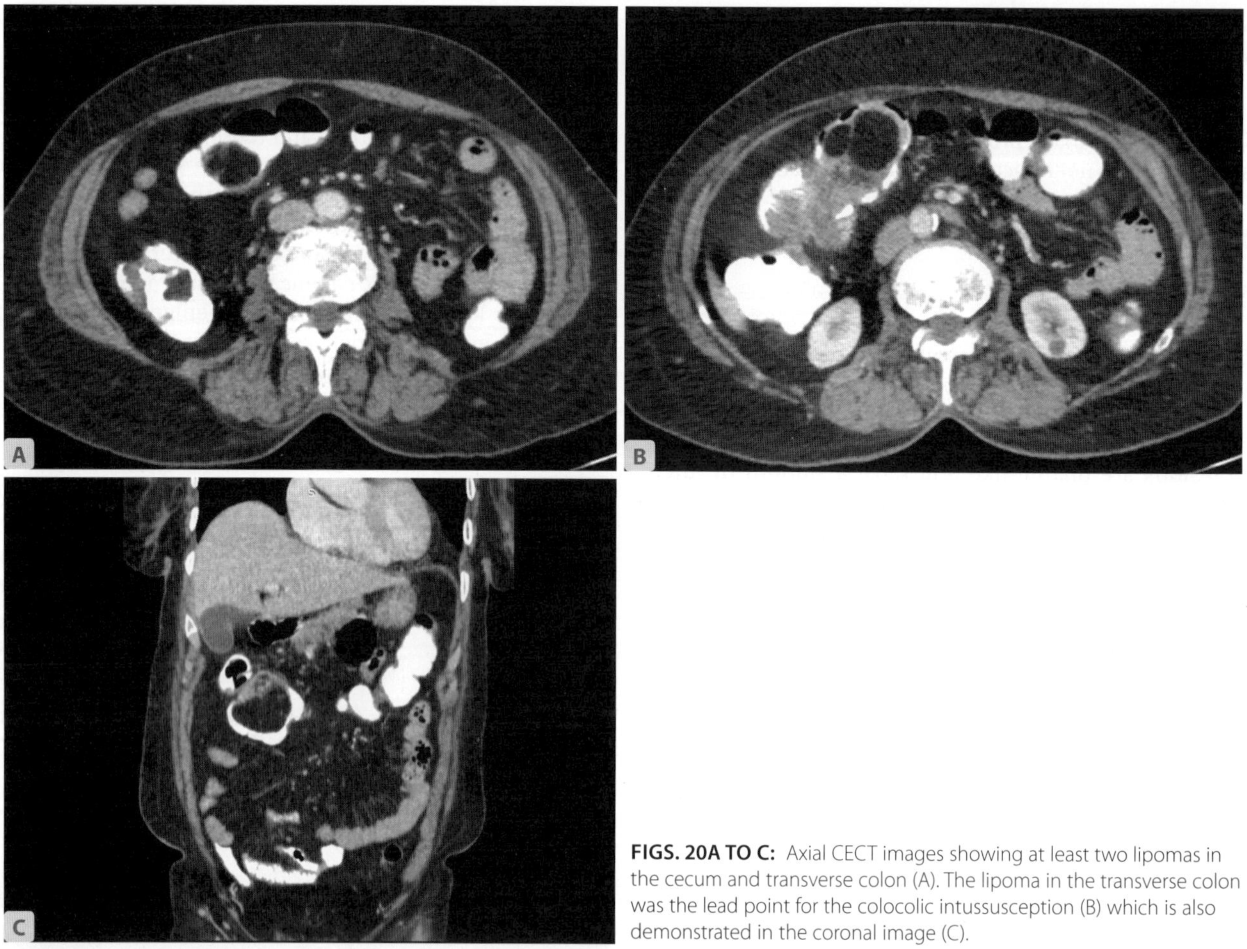

FIGS. 20A TO C: Axial CECT images showing at least two lipomas in the cecum and transverse colon (A). The lipoma in the transverse colon was the lead point for the colocolic intussusception (B) which is also demonstrated in the coronal image (C).

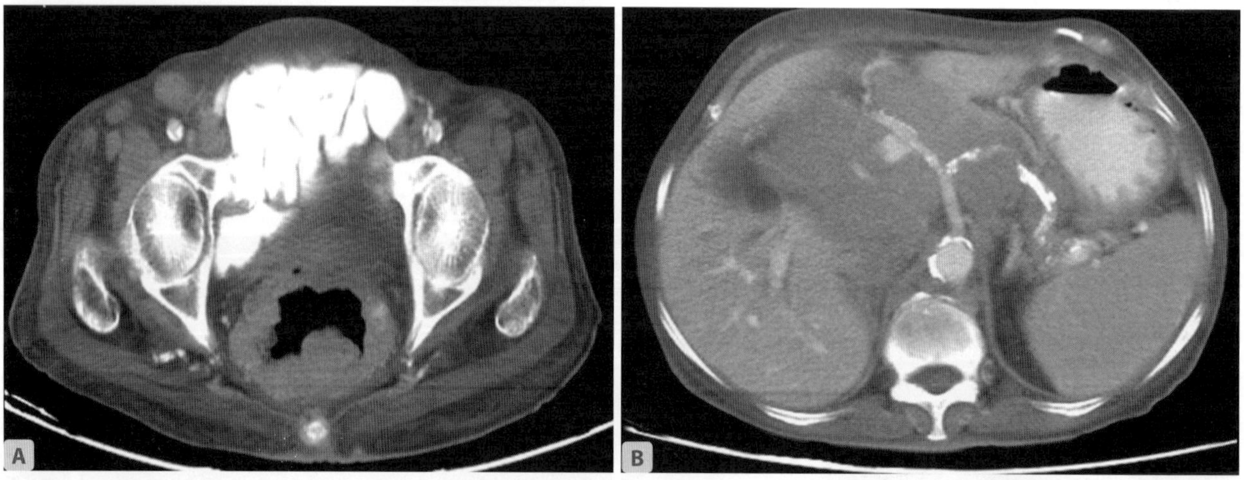

FIGS. 21A AND B: Axial CECT sections show concentric nodular mural thickening of the rectum (A) with conglomerate lymph nodal mass encasing the celiac trunk (B) in a patient with disseminated lymphoma.

Lymphoma of the colon is rare. The colon is the third most common primary site of lymphoma involving the gastrointestinal tract after stomach and the small bowel. As a primary lesion, lymphoma accounts for only 0.5% of all malignant tumors. Secondary involvement by lymphoma is usually multicentric **(Figs. 21A and B)**. The radiographic pattern may be localized or diffuse. In the localized form, the lesion is seen either as a polypoid mass that protrudes into the colonic lumen or as a constricting lesion that simulates an annular carcinoma. In the diffuse form, multiple small nodular lesions are seen. The defects are submucosal in origin with intact overlying mucosa. When lymphoma involves the mesentery, large masses may cause extensive compression on the colon.

SECONDARY TUMORS OF COLON

Tumors that commonly metastasize to colon include stomach, breast, pancreas and gynecologic pelvic malignancies. Infiltration of the colon by secondary tumors produces thickening of the colonic wall and mucosal folds. The classic radiographic appearances include indentations, spiculation, angulation, narrowing, displacement and fixation. Lymphogenous spread of tumors to the colon is characterized by the involvement of long segments, variable narrowing and loss of haustral markings. When metastases occur by the hematogenous route, as in melanoma, lesions present as smoothly marginated submucosal masses.

POSTOPERATIVE COLON AND RECURRENT CANCER

The radiologist should be aware of the various surgical techniques and postoperative anatomy for assessing the therapeutic response and for diagnosing tumor recurrence. In addition to the usual surgical resections like right hemicolectomy, extended right hemicolectomy, transverse colectomy, left hemicolectomy, sigmoid colectomy, the radiologist should be across more complex procedures such as Hartmann's procedure, anterior resection and abdominoperineal excision of rectum (APER).

Hartmann's procedure may be done for carcinoma of the sigmoid colon. It entails resection of the sigmoid and formation of the left-sided end colostomy. The rectum and distal sigmoid are closed off to form a rectal stump or Hartmann's pouch which is reattached to the colon within 3–6 months of the primary surgery. In anterior resection, the sigmoid and part of or the entire rectum, is resected. If the entire rectum is removed, that is, a low anterior resection is done, then a coloanal anastomosis is made. In case the entire rectum is not removed, a colorectal anastomosis is made. A temporary defunctioning stoma is usually made in cases of anterior resection. APER involves resection of the anus, rectum and part of the distal sigmoid colon through incisions made in the abdomen and perineum. This procedure is done for cancer of the distal third of rectum or anal canal and for salvage of the anal cancer that does not respond to chemoradiation.

T2-weighted MRI has been recommended for local restaging. Diffusion-weighted MRI adds to the response evaluation after chemoradiation **(Figs. 22A to E)**.[75,76] However, characterization of metastatic lymph nodes is challenging. Dynamic CEMR and perfusion CT assess the residual or recurrent tumor by showing contrast enhancement. The role of PET-CT is controversial. There are studies which show that irradiated rectal mucosa may show increased FDG uptake resulting in false-positive data.[77,78] Therefore, FDG PET is not recommended within the first four weeks after completion of chemoradiation.

POLYPOSIS SYNDROMES

Familial Adenomatous Polyposis Syndrome

It is the most common of the polyposis syndromes. Familial adenomatous polyposis syndrome (FAPS) is an autosomal-dominant disease and affects males and females equally. It is predominantly associated with development of adenomas in the colon which are small (80% are <5 mm in size) and sessile. Rectal sparing may be seen. Colonic carcinomas develop at around 40 years. The most common symptom is rectal bleeding and diarrhea. Treatment of choice is total colectomy with mucosal proectectomy and ileoanal anastomosis. Barium enema shows innumerable small sessile filling defects which carpet the entire colon. Extracolonic manifestations include fundal gastric polyps, premalignant gastric adenomas in the distal stomach and adenomas in the jejunum and ileum. Extraintestinal manifestations include sebaceous cysts, osteomas, fibrous tumors like desmoid, mesenteric fibromatosis and dental abnormalities (part of Gardner syndrome) and dental abnormalities. Congenital pigmented lesions of the retina are seen in >90% of patients with FAPS and may occur even before the colonic polyposis develops **(Fig. 23)**.[79] Several other tumors like medulloblastoma, meningioma, intracranial epidermoid cyst, papillary thyroid carcinoma and pancreatic carcinoma have been reported in patients with FAPS.

Peutz–Jeghers Syndrome

Peutz-Jeghers syndrome (PJS) is an autosomal dominant hereditary disease in which there are gastrointestinal hamartomas, mucocutaneous pigmentation and tumors outside the GI tract. Hamartomas is a non-neoplastic tumor composed of normal tissue elements. The hamartomatous polyps in PJS have a smooth muscle core from the muscularis mucosae, which is covered by the mucosa. The polyps may be the lead points of small bowel intussusceptions. The polyps are found in the jejunum, ileum, duodenum, colon and stomach in this order. They may be pedunculated or sessile. Pedunculated polyps are seen in the small bowel or colon while sessile polyps are seen in the stomach. The PJS polyps occur in clusters and not as carpet lesion.[80] Extraintestinal tumors include those of the pancreas, breast, ovary and uterus (adenoma malignum).

Cowden Disease (Multiple Hamartoma Syndrome)

Cowden disease is an autostomal dominant disease in which there are mucocutaneous lesions, thyroid gland abnormalities, breast cancer, GI tract hamartomatous polyps and abnormalities of the CNS. Facial trichilemmomas are pathognomic of Cowden disease. Hamartomatous polyps are seen as multiple, small, sessile lesions with segmental or diffuse distribution. They are seen in rectosigmoid colon, stomach, duodenum, small bowel and esophagus in this order. Hyperplastic and adenomatous polyps may also be present.

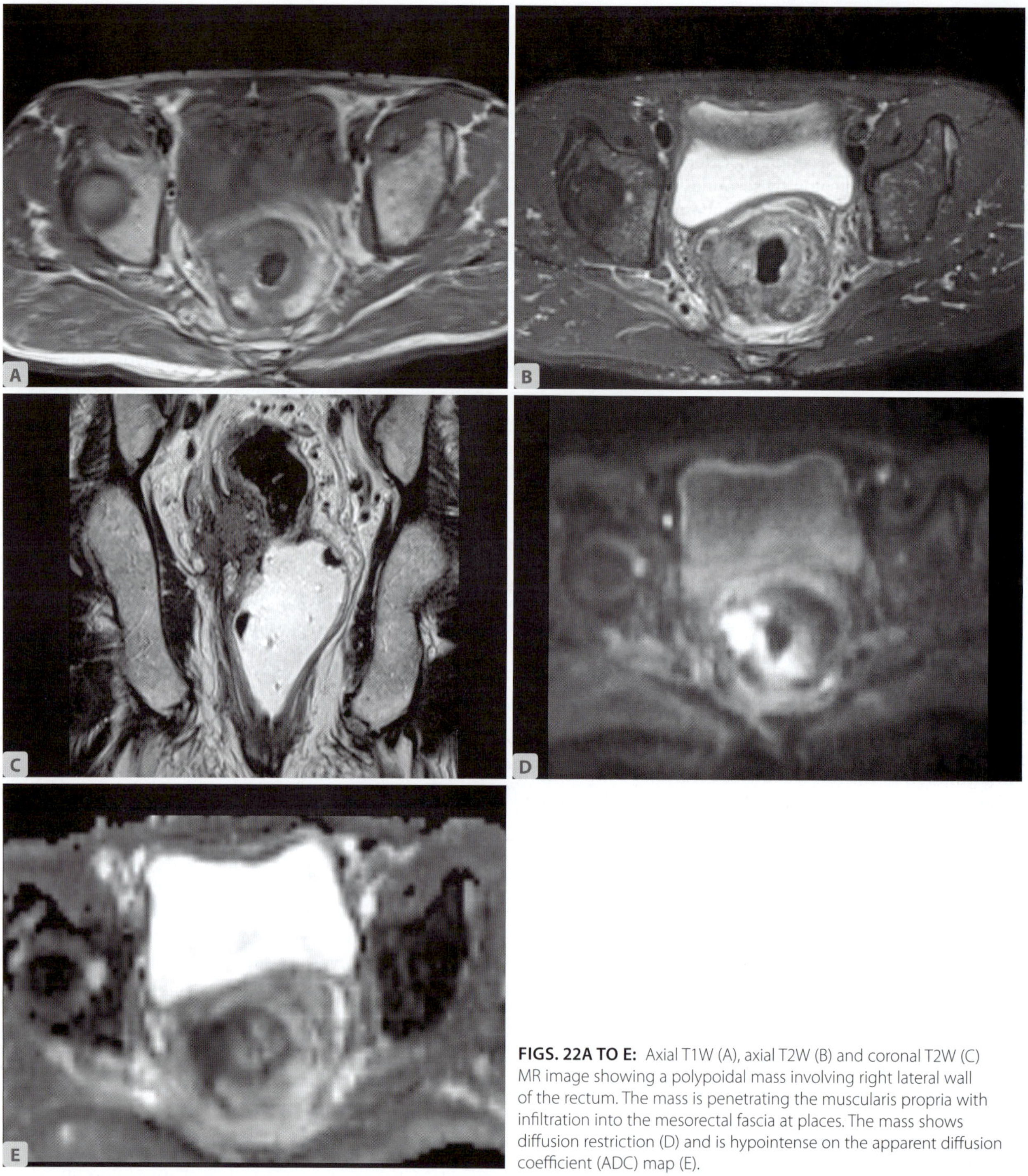

FIGS. 22A TO E: Axial T1W (A), axial T2W (B) and coronal T2W (C) MR image showing a polypoidal mass involving right lateral wall of the rectum. The mass is penetrating the muscularis propria with infiltration into the mesorectal fascia at places. The mass shows diffusion restriction (D) and is hypointense on the apparent diffusion coefficient (ADC) map (E).

Juvenile Polyposis

This is seen in the second decade of life. It is characterized by more than five juvenile polyps in the colon or rectum. The polyps can be seen throughout the GI tract as clusters. Juvenile polyps tend to be large lesions more than 1 cm in diameter. There can be sessile or pedunculated. Polyps are seen in the colon, stomach, small bowel and duodenum in this order.

Cronkhite–Canada Syndrome

Unlike the polyposis syndrome, Cronkhite-Canada syndrome (CCS) is not a familial disease. It is related to mental and physical stress. The lesions are predominantly inflammatory polyps.[81] Adenomatous, hyperplastic and hamartomatous polyps have also been reported. Polyps are seen as small, sessile or less commonly pedunculated lesions. They are seen in the stomach, small bowel and colon in this order. Ectodermal abnormalities of the hair, skin and nails occur after the onset of GI symptoms.

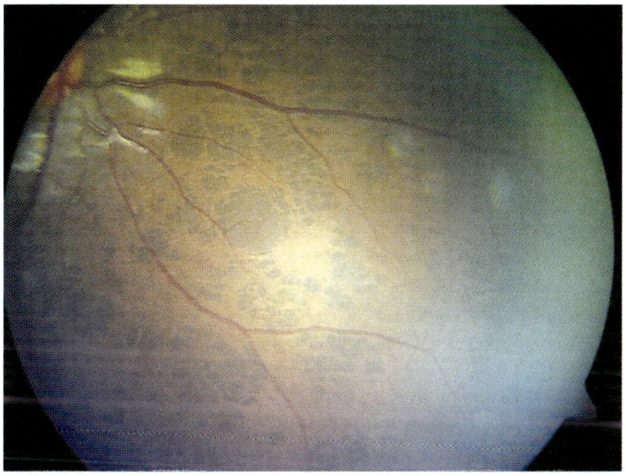

FIG. 23: Fundus picture showing sectoral hypertrophy of retinal pigment epithelium resembling animal footprints or pug marks.

Courtesy: Dr Subina Narang, Department of Ophthalmology, GMCH, Chandigarh, India.

CONCLUSION

Colorectal cancer is a unique malignancy as it represents a preventable disease. The adenoma-carcinoma sequence reiterates the need for screening for polyps which are precursors of colorectal cancer. Screening is of immense importance in countries which have high prevalence of colorectal cancer. Though this malignancy has a low prevalence in the Indian subcontinent, it is expected to increase as more people are adopting Western lifestyle and dietary habits.

Imaging plays a key role in the screening program as well as for detection and staging of colorectal cancer. For screening purpose, the radiological options include CT colonography. The high sensitivity of CT colonography for detecting clinically significant polyps >1 cm has been possible due to the spectacular advances in CT technology.

Endoscopic sonography, CT and MRI are the primary cross-sectional techniques used for staging of colorectal cancer. Of these modalities, MRI is preferred for the locoregional staging of rectal cancer and CECT is preferred for the staging of colorectal metastases.

REFERENCES

1. Jemal A, Siegel R, Ward E, et al. Cancer statistics, 2007. CA Cancer J Clin. 2007;57:43-66.
2. Seidman H, Mushinski MH, Gelb SK, et al. Probability of eventually developing and dying of cancers: United States, 1995. CA Cancer J Clin. 1985;35:36-56.
3. Theoni RF, Laufer I. Polyps and carcinoma of the colon. In: Gore RM, Levine MS (Eds): WB Saunders, Philadelphia. Textbook of Gastrointestinal Radiology; 2008.pp.1121-66.
4. Mohandas KM, Desai DC. Epidemiology of digestive tract cancers in India. Ind J Gastroenterol. 1999;18:118-21.
5. Potter JD, Slattery ML, Bostick RM, et al. Colon cancer: A review of the epidemiology. Epidemiol Rev. 1993;15:499-545.
6. Fleshner B, Slater G, Aufses AH. Age and sex distribution of patients with colorectal cancer. Dis Colon Rectum. 1989;32: 107-11.
7. Bond JH. Colonic tumors. Endoscopy. 1998;30:150-7.
8. Kritchevsky D. Colorectal cancer—the role of dietary fat and caloric restriction. Mutat Res. 1993;290:63-70.
9. Heilbrum LK, Nomura A, Hankin JH, et al. Diet and colorectal cancer with special reference to fiber intake. Int J Cancer. 1989;44:1-6.
10. Gore RM. Colorectal cancer: Clinical and pathologic features. Radiologic Clinics of North America. 1997;35:403-29.
11. McFaralane MJ, Welch KE. Gallstones, cholecystectomy and colorectal cancer. Am J Gastroenterol. 1992;87:1120-4.
12. Wilson RE, Donohue JH. Neoplasia of the colorectum. In: Phillips SF, Pemberton JH, Shorter RG (Eds). Raven Press, New York. The large intestine: Physiology, pathophysiology and disease; 1991. pp. 521-47.
13. Fenlon HM, McAneny DB, Nunes DP, et al. Occlusive colon carcinoma: Virtual colonoscopy in the preoperative evaluation of the proximal colon. Radiology. 1999;210:423-8.
14. Bulow S, Svendsen LB, Mellemgaard A. Metachronous colorectal carcinoma. Br J Surg. 1990;77:502-5.
15. Cali RL, Pitsch RM, Thorson AG, et al. Cumulative incidence of metachronous colorectal cancer. Dis Colon Rectum. 1993;36: 388-93.
16. Lane N, Fenglio CM. The adenoma-carcinoma sequence in the stomach and colon: I. Observation on the adenoma as precursor to ordinary large bowel carcinoma. Gastrointest Radiol. 1976;1:111-19.
17. Cooper HS, Deppisch LM, Gourley WK, et al. Endoscopically removed malignant colorectal polyps: Clinicopathologic correlations. Gastroenterology. 1995;108:1657-65.
18. Lev R, Lee M. Colorectal carcinoma: Pathology. In: Rustgi AK (Ed). Gastrointestinal cancers: Biology, diagnosis, and therapy. Lippincott-Raven: Philadelphia; 1995. pp. 379-98.
19. Dodd GD. Malignancies. In: Alimentary tract radiology. Margulis AR, Burhenne HJ (Eds), 4th edn. The CV Mosby Company; 1989. pp. 1051-92.
20. Gore RM, Meyers MA. Pathways of abdominal and pelvic disease spread. In: Gore RM, Levine MS, Laufer I (Eds). Textbook of Gastrointestinal Radiology. WB Saunders: Philadelphia; 1994. pp. 2352-66.
21. Turnbull RB. The no-touch isolation technique of resection. JAMA. 1975;231:1181-5.
22. Johnson RD, Geisinger KR. Colorectal adenocarcinoma: Staging and histopathology. Seminars in Roentgenology. 1996;31: 94-102.
23. Berlin JW, Gore RM, Yaghmai V, et al. Staging of colorectal cancer. Seminars in Roentgenology. 2000;35:370-84.
24. Silva AC, Hara AK, Leighton JA, et al. CT colonography with intravenous contrast material: varied appearance of colorectal carcinoma. Radiographics. 2005;25:1321-34.
25. Mandel JS. Screening for colorectal cancer. Gastroenterol Clin N Am. 2008;37:97-115.
26. Pamela M, McMahon G, Scott G. The case for colorectal screening. Seminars in Roentgenology. 2000;35:325-32.
27. Winawer SJ, Stewart ET, Zauber AG, et al. A comparison of colonoscopy and double-contrast barium enema for surveillance after polypectomy. National Polyp Work Group. N Engl J Med. 2000;342:1766-72.
28. Winawer SJ, Zauber AG, Ho MN, et al. Prevention of colorectal cancer by colonoscopic polypectomy. N Eng J Med. 1993;329:1977-81.

29. Citarda F, Tomaselli G, Capocaccia R, et al. Efficacy in standard clinical practice of colonoscopic polypectomy in reducing colorectal cancer incidence. Gut. 2001;48:812-15.
30. Van Rijn JC, Reitsma JB, Stoker J, et al. Polyp miss rate determined by tandem colonoscopy: a systemic review. Am J Gastroenterol. 2006;101:343-50.
31. Johnson CD, Chen MH, Toledano AY, et al. Accuracy of CT colonoscopy for detection of large adenomas and cancers. N Engl J Med. 2008;359:1207-17.
32. Gelfand DW. Colorectal cancer: Screening strategies. Radiology Clinics of North America. 1997;35:431-8.
33. Brady AP, Stevenson GW, Stevenson I. Colorectal cancer overlooked at barium enema examination and colonoscopy: A continuing perceptual problem. Radiology. 1994;192:373-8.
34. Ott DJ, Gelfand DW. How to improve the efficacy of the barium enema examination. AJR. 1993;160:491-5.
35. Ott DJ, Gelfand DW, Ramquist NA, et al. Causes of error in gastrointestinal radiology: II Barium enema examination. Gastrointest Radiol. 1980;5:99-105.
36. Gelfand DW, Ott DJ. Cost-effective screening for colorectal cancer. The radiologist's view. Primary Care and Cancer. 1992;12:11-3.
37. Stevenson GW. Normal anatomy and technique of examination of the colon: Barium, CT and MRI. In: Freeny PC, Stevenson GW (Eds): Margulis and Burhenne's Alimentary Tract Radiology. Mosby and Company, St Louis; 1994.p.692.
38. Laufer I, Kressel HY. Principles of double contrast diagnosis. In: Laufer I, Levine MS (Eds). Double-contrast gastrointestinal radiology. WB Saunders, Philadelphia; 1992.pp.9-54.
39. Youker JE, Welin S. Differentiation of true polypoid tumors of the colon from extraneous material: A new Roentgen sign. Radiology. 1985;84:610-5.
40. Boetow PC, Buck JL, Carr NJ, et al. Colorectal adeno carcinoma: Radiologic-pathologic correlation. Radiographics. 1995;15:127-46.
41. Delamarre J, Descombes P, Marti R, et al. Villous tumors of the colon and rectum: Double-contrast study of 47 cases. Gastrointest Radiol. 1980;5:69-73.
42. Bond JH. Polyp guideline: Diagnosis, treatment, and surveillance for patients with nonfamilal colorectal polyps. Ann Intern Med. 1993;119:836-43.
43. Lappas JC, Maglinte DDT, Kopecky KK, et al. Diverticular disease: Imaging with post-double contrast sigmoid flush. Radiology. 1988;168:35-7.
44. Kelvin FM, Gardiner R, Vas W, et al. Colorectal carcinoma missed on double contrast barium enema study: A problem in perception. Am J Roentgenol. 1981;137:307-13.
45. Dubbins PA. The small bowel and colon. In: Abdominal and general ultrasound. Cosgrove D, Meire H, Dewbury K (Eds). Churchill Livingstone. 1993;2:765-76.
46. Bernd L. Diagnosis of large bowel tumors by colonic sonography. The Lancet. 1990;20:144-6.
47. Glaser F, Schalg P, Harfarth C. Endorectal Ultrasonography for the assessment of invasion of rectal tumors and lymph node involvement. Br J Surg. 1990;77:883-7.
48. Hulsmans FH, Tio TL, Mathus-Vliegen EMH, et al. Colorectal villous adenoma: Transrectal US in screening for invasive malignancy. Radiology. 1992;185:193-6.
49. Scharling ES, Wolfman NT, Bechtold RE. Computed tomography evaluation of colorectal carcinoma. Seminars in Roentgenology. 1996;31:142-53.
50. Kalra N, Suri S, Gupta R, et al. MDCT in the staging of gallbladder carcinoma. Am J Roentgenol. 2006;186:758-66.
51. Regina GH, Beets T, Beets GL. Rectal cancer: Review with emphasis on MR imaging. Radiology. 2004;232:335-46.
52. Filippone A, Ambrosini R, Fuschi M, et al. Preoperative T and N staging of colorectal cancer. Accuracy of contrast-enhanced multidetector row CT colonography—Initial experience. Radiology. 2004;231:83-90.
53. Chung DJ, Huh KC, Choi WJ, et al. CT colonography using 16-MDCT in the evaluation of colorectal cancer. Am J Roentgenol. 2005;184:98-103.
54. Narayanan S, Kalra N, Bhatia A, et al. Staging of colorectal cancer using contrast-enhanced multidetector computed tomographic colonography. Singapore Med J. 2014;55:660-6.
55. Vining DJ, Gelfand DW. Non-invasive colonoscopy using helical CT scanning, 3D reconstruction and virtual reality. Presented in the syllabus of the 23rd annual meeting. Society of Gastrointestinal Radiologists. Maui (Hawaii); 1994.
56. Summerton S, Little E, Cappell MS. CT colonography: Current status and future promise. Gastroenterol Clin N Am. 2008;37: 161-89.
57. Bhatia A, Saxena AK, Kalra N, et al. Intravenous contrast enhanced computed tomography colonoscopy in children with suspected colonic polyps. Eur J Radiol. 2013;82:905-12.
58. Kalra N, Suri S, Bhasin DK, et al. Comparison of multidetector computed tomographic colonography and conventional colonoscopy for detection of colorectal polyps and cancer. Ind J Gastroenterol. 2006;25:229-32.
59. Zallis ME, Barish MA, Choi JR, et al. CT colonography reporting and data system: A consensus proposal. Radiology. 2005;236:3-9.
60. Brown G, Radcliffe AG, Newcombe RG, et al. Preoperative assessment of prognostic factors in rectal cancer using high-resolution magnetic resonance imaging. Br J Surg. 2003;90:355-64.
61. Beets-Tan RG, Beets GL, Vliegen RF, et al. Accuracy of magnetic resonance imaging in prediction of tumor-free resection margin in rectal cancer surgery. Lancet. 2001;357:497-504.
62. Brown G, Kirkham A, Williams GT, et al. High-resolution MRI of the anatomy important in total mesorectal excision of the rectum. Am J Roentgenol. 2004;182:431-9.
63. Heald RJ, Ryall RD. Recurrence and survival after total mesorectal excision for rectal cancer. Lancet. 1986;1:1479-82.
64. Hunerbein M, Pegios W, Rau B, et al. Prospective comparison of endorectal ultrasound, three-dimensional endorectal ultrasound and endorectal MRI in the preoperative evaluation of rectal tumors. Preliminary results. Surg Endosc. 2000;14:1005-09.
65. Kim NK, Kim MJ, Yan SH, et al. Comparative study of transrectal ultrasonography, pelvic computerized tomography and magnetic resonance imaging in preoperative staging of rectal cancer. Dis Colon Rectum. 1999;42:770-5.
66. Ajay W, Pelster G, Treichel U, et al. Dark lumen magnetic resonance colonography: Comparsion with conventional colonoscopy for the detection of colorectal pathology. Gut. 2003;52:1738-43.
67. Britton KE, Granowska M. The diagnostic role of radiolabelled antibodies. In: Murrary IPS, Ell PJ (Eds). Nuclear medicine in clinical diagnosis and treatment. Churchill Livingstone: Edinburgh; 1998. pp. 871-92.
68. Ramos E, Valls C, Martinez, et al. Preoperative staging of patients with liver metastases of colorectal carcinoma. Does PET/CT really add something to multidetector CT? Ann Surg Oncol. 2011;18:2654-61.
69. Kinner S, Antoch G, Bockisch A, et al. Whole-body PET/ CT colonography: a possible new concept for colorectal cancer staging. Abdom Imaging. 2007;32:606-12.
70. Gollub MJ, Akhurst T, Markowitz AJ, et al. Combined CT colonography and 18F-FDG PET of colon polyps: potential technique for selective detection of cancer and precancerous lesions. Am J Roentgenol. 2007;188:130-8.

71. Sahani DV, Kalva SP, Hamberg LM, et al. Assessing tumor perfusion and treatment response in rectal cancer with multi-section CT: initial observations. Radiology. 2005;234:785-92.
72. Bellomi M, Petralia G, Sonzogni A, et al. CT perfusion for the monitoring of neoadjuvant chemotherapy and radiation therapy in rectal carcinoma: initial experience. Radiology. 2007;244: 486-93.
73. Purkayastha S, Tekkis PP, Athanasiou T, et al. Diagnostic precision of magnetic resonance imaging for preoperative prediction of the circumferential margin involvement in patients with rectal cancer. Colorectal Dis. 2007;9:402-11.
74. Videhult P, Smedh K, Lundin P, Kraaz W. Magnetic resonance imaging for preoperative staging of rectal cancer in clinical practice: high accuracy in predicting circumferential margin with clinical benefit. Colorectal Dis. 2007;9:412-7.
75. Sun Ys, Zhang XP, Tang L, et al. Locally advanced rectal carcinoma treated with preoperative chemotherapy and radiation therapy: preliminary analysis of diffusion-weighted MR imaging for early detection of tumor histopathologic downstaging. Radiology. 2010;254:170-8.
76. Hein Pa, Kremser C, Judmaier W, et al. Diffusion-weighed magnetic resonance imaging for monitoring diffusion changes in rectal carcinoma during combined preoperative chemoradiation: preliminary results of a prospective study. Eur J Radiol. 2003;45: 214-22.
77. Konski A, Li T, Sigurdson E, et al. Use of molecular imaging to predict clinical outcome in patients with rectal cancer after preoperative chemotherapy and radiation. Int J Radiat Oncol Biol Phys. 2009;74:55-9.
78. Kalff V, Ware R, Heriot A, et al. Radiation changes do not interfere with postchemoradiation restaging of patients with rectal cancer by FDG PET/CT before curative surgical therapy. Int Radiol Oncol Biol Phys. 2009;74:60-6.
79. Iwamma T, Mishima Y, Okamoto N, et al. Association of congenital hypertrophy of the retinal pigment epithelium with familial adenomatous polyposis. Br J Surg. 1990;77:273-6.
80. Schumacher V, Vogel T, Leube B, et al. STK11 genotyping and cancer risk in Peutz Jeghers syndrome. J Med Genet. 2005;42:428-35.
81. Burke AP, Sobin LH. The pathology of Cronkhite-Canada syndrome polyps. Am J Surg Pathol. 1989;13:940-6.

CHAPTER

96

Ulceroconstrictive Diseases of the Gut

Devasenathipathy Kandasamy, Manisha Jana, Arun Kumar Gupta

INTRODUCTION

Imaging in ulceroconstrictive lesions of the gut has seen a paradigm change over the last few decades. While earlier conventional imaging studies relied predominantly on the luminal distension and opacification of the bowel lumen using positive oral contrast; newer modalities such as CT and MRI are capable of providing information on both intraluminal, as well as extrinsic abnormalities. CT enterography (CTE) and MR enterography (MRE) are unique imaging techniques having the combined advantages of both CT/MRI and enterography.

Plain Radiograph

The role of plain radiographs has diminished to a great extent because of the wider availability of cross-sectional modalities. They are useful only in a patient with acute or subacute intestinal obstruction, when they are often the first line modality. An erect abdominal radiograph can provide valuable information regarding the level and severity of bowel obstruction, and presence of pneumoperitoneum, although erect chest radiograph is the best method to detect the latter. Enteroliths can be seen sometimes proximal to the site of obstruction and presence of calcified lymph nodes can point towards the diagnosis of tuberculosis (TB). The drawback of this study is that it is often not helpful in detecting the etiology of obstruction. It plays no role in purely ulcerative disease entities.

Barium Studies

Barium meal follow through (BMFT) was the most widely used imaging technique for the evaluation small bowel until a few years ago. Constrictive lesions of the small bowel presenting as small bowel obstruction remain a challenge in diagnosis; as large part of the small bowel is not accessible by endoscopy. With the advent of better modalities such as multidetector computed tomography (MDCT) and MRI, the importance of BMFT has declined. BMFT, along with colonic evaluation by barium enema, can give valuable information regarding both small and large bowel obstructive lesions.[1] It is the best imaging technique to evaluate the mucosal details of small and large bowel. There are many classical signs described for TB and Crohn's disease (CD) on barium studies and they are good in demonstrating bowel narrowing, dilatation, mucosal ulcerations, kinking and clumping of bowel loops and fistulae **(Figs. 1 and 2)**. They are one of the few imaging techniques which are capable of studying the bowel motility which is an important parameter in bowel imaging. The evaluation of lesions in the ileum and cecum can be further enhanced by peroral pneumocolon (i.e. insufflation of air through the rectum).[2] Peroral pneumocolon can also provide valuable information regarding colonic pathologies.

Single contrast BMFT is usually performed with barium suspension having 66% w/v barium. With the technological advances in the field of fluoroscopic techniques, coupled with their wide availability and low radiation burden; most often the procedure is performed under fluoroscopic guidance nowadays. The major drawback in the evaluation of intestinal strictures by BMFT is the differentiation of a true stricture from a transient peristaltic contraction. In order to alleviate this drawback, enteroclysis (small bowel enema) came into practice; wherein the small bowel lumen is distended through a nasojejunal tube and using diluted barium. Enteroclysis yielded superior mucosal details compared to BMFT. Also, as the distension of bowel lumen was controlled and the luminal distension was visualized in real-time; this technique was superior to BMFT in the detection of subtle intestinal strictures. However, this technique entails ionizing radiation to the patient and the yield is also poor when compared with CTE or MRE. Hence, barium studies should be used only if CT or MR enterography is not available.

Single contrast barium enema and double contrast barium enema (DCBE) are two other important barium studies. While single contrast BE is adequate for delineating the strictures in the large bowel; DCBE is preferable in cases of suspected mucosal lesions such as in ulcerative colitis. However, colonoscopy is the primary modality of choice in the evaluation of patients with ulcerative colitis and imaging is not commonly performed for their evaluation.

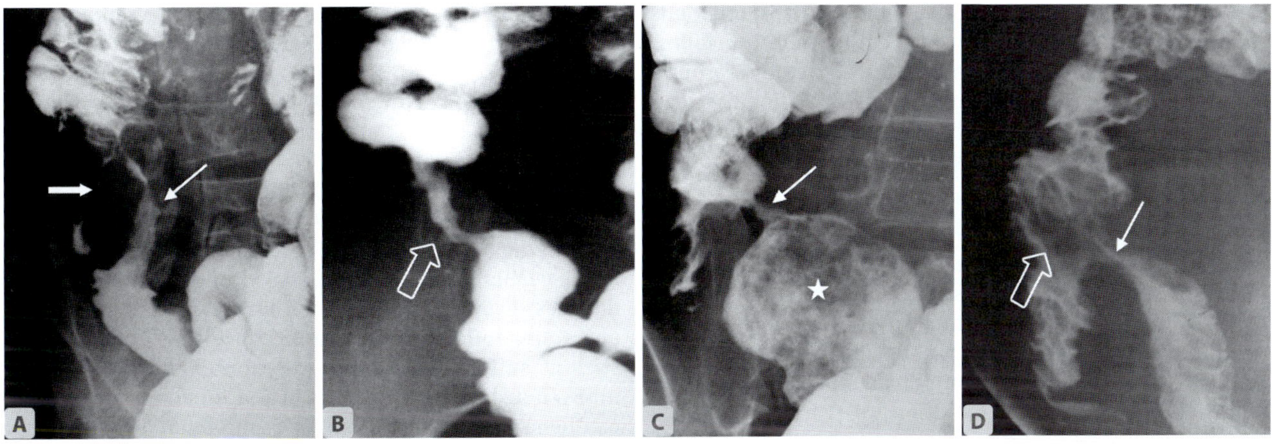

FIGS. 1A TO D: Ileocecal TB on barium studies: Barium meal follow through (BMFT) image (A) shows narrowing and mild mucosal irregularity (thin arrow) in the terminal ileum (string sign) with associated contracted cecum (thick arrow). BMFT image (B) of another patient shows narrowing of terminal ileum which is emptying directly into ascending colon (outlined arrow) with nonvisualization of cecum (Stierlin's sign). BMFT image (C) in a different patient shows fibrotic stricture in the terminal ileum (thin arrow) with proximal dilatation (star) and contracted cecum. BMFT image (D) of another patient shows mild gaping (thin arrow) and filling defect (outlined arrow) in the region of ileocecal valve (Fleischner's sign) due to edema of the valve.

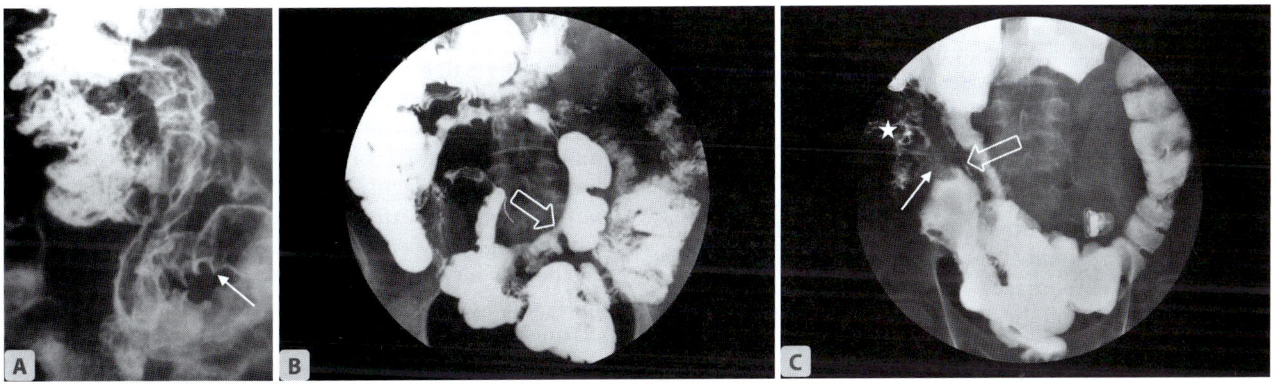

FIGS. 2A TO C: CD involving the small bowel: BMFT (A) showing mucosal irregularity in the terminal ileum and rose thorn ulcers (thin arrow). BMFT in another patient with CD (B) showing multiple strictures in distal ileum, shortening of mesenteric border and pseudosacculations in the antimesenteric border (outlined arrow). BMFT image (C) in a patient with CD showing narrowing of terminal ileum (thin arrow) with proximal dilatation, irregularity and narrowing of cecum (star). In one of the ileal loop there is a thin longitudinal extraluminal barium (outlined arrow) seen paralleling the bowel loop (double tracking) which is due to the presence of deep fissures in the bowel wall in CD.

CECT and CT Enteroclysis/CT Enterography

Contrast-enhanced CT (CECT) is the workhorse of imaging in suspected intestinal strictures. With the advent of newer generation fast MDCT scanners, CT can provide crucial information regarding mural/extraluminal findings in bowel pathology. CT enteroclysis combines the benefits of the two imaging modalities; good luminal distension similar to a conventional enteroclysis and visualization of extraluminal/transmural pathologies similar to CECT.[3] CT enterography (CTE) is a newer imaging technique wherein the luminal distension of small bowel is achieved without a nasojejunal tube; hence ameliorating patient discomfort arising from intubation. In this procedure either diluted mannitol/polyethylene glycol solution (PEG) is used as neutral oral contrast agent to distend the bowel loops. There are various protocols described for CTE in literature aimed at adequate bowel distension during scanning. The protocol given below is followed in our institute **(Table 1)**. CTE has been found to be a very sensitive tool in the diagnosis of inflammatory small bowel diseases; comparable to the capsule endoscopy.[4-6] Another important role of CTE is to rule out any strictures in the small bowel; prior to a capsule endoscopy; in order to avoid

TABLE 1: CT enterography protocol.

Preparation	6 hours fasting
Oral contrast	Water + Mannitol (300 mL of 20% mannitol in 1500 mL water)
Technique	450 mL at 60 min prior to scanning 450 mL at 40 min prior to scanning 225 mL at 20 min prior to scanning 225 mL at 10 min prior to scanning 250–300 mL on table just before scanning (plain water)

capsule impaction/retention.[6] Usage of ionizing radiation is an important drawback of CTE which limits its utility in follow up imaging. Radiation dose of a standard CTE study is around 15 mSv compared to 3-8 mSv for BMFT.[7,8] Radiation dose can be minimized by optimizing the scan parameters and using new techniques such as iterative reconstruction methods.

MRI/MR Enterography

Although CECT can provide a lot of diagnostic information in intestinal strictures; it comes with a high radiation burden; more so in patients of inflammatory bowel diseases who need repeated imaging.[9] MRI has the advantage of superior soft tissue contrast resolution; multiplanar imaging capability and lack of any ionizing radiation. MRI has the unique advantage of evaluating multiple paradigms such as T1 and T2 characteristics, diffusion restriction and pattern of contrast enhancement. In addition, new ultrafast sequences (True FISP - Cine MR) have made the real time evaluation of the small bowel possible; which is crucial for differentiating a stricture from a peristaltic contraction. MR enterography (MRE) has all the inherent advantages of CT enterography; with the additional benefit of being able to differentiate a fibrotic stricture from an active one. Diffusion weighted MRI (DWI) is also being increasingly used in cases of inflammatory bowel diseases.[10-13] The active lesions tend to show restriction of diffusion (hyperintense signal on high b value images). DWI can be an effective alternative to IV Gadolinium in the evaluation of lesion activity in inflammatory bowel diseases in patients in whom Gadolinium based contrast is contraindicated. Commonly used intraluminal contrast in MRE is diluted Mannitol, which can act as biphasic contrast agent. On the T2W images, it causes high signal intensity within the lumen and the bowel wall is seen as hypointense structure. On postcontrast T1W images, it serves as a 'negative' contrast agent and helps in better delineation of the wall enhancement against a dark lumen. The formulation of oral contrast and the timing of giving aliquots for MRE is the same as CTE protocol **(Table 1)**.

Ultrasonography and Contrast-enhanced Ultrasonography

Ultrasound (US) has limited role in the initial evaluation of intestinal obstruction; owing to gaseous abdominal distension which makes ultrasonographic visualization of bowel loops difficult. However, in cases of abdominal tuberculosis or inflammatory bowel diseases where the disease has been localized by other imaging modalities (such as CT or MRI); ultrasound is a useful tool for follow up evaluation. CT is associated with radiation burden, and MRI evaluation in children often needs sedation or general anesthesia. High-resolution US is an emerging technique to evaluate bowel disorders and it is very sensitive in detecting bowel wall abnormalities in the terminal ileum and ileocecal junction region. The spatial resolution of high resolution US is better than CTE or MRE and it can show wall thickening, dilated segment of bowel loop and bowel motility in real time. Increase in bowel and mesenteric vascularity can be detected on Doppler which is considered as a marker for disease activity in CD. Wide availability, repeatability and lack of radiation have made US an attractive technique in the evaluation of ulceroconstrictive bowel diseases. US is very sensitive to detect abnormalities in terminal ileum however for the evaluation of proximal small bowel loops the accuracy falls. Various studies across the globe have described a sonographic sensitivity and specificity for the diagnosis of CD ranging from 75 to 94% and 67 to 100%, respectively.[14,15]

Contrast enhanced ultrasonography (CEUS) is a recent advancement which has been evaluated and recommended in the evaluation of disease activity in inflammatory bowel diseases, distinguishing fibrous from inflammatory strictures, abscesses, and fistula.[16,17] It utilizes a special contrast agent such as sulfur hexafluoride microbubbles which is given intravenously to look for areas of abnormal enhancement. It can be used even in patients with renal impairment as the mode of excretion is via breath. Lack of expertise, limited availability of hardware and software for CEUS and contrast agent are the current limitations. The cine loops of CEUS can be processed using software and various quantifiable perfusion parameters can be obtained by placing region of interest (ROI) markers.

ABDOMINAL TUBERCULOSIS

Tuberculosis (TB) is one of the leading causes of death killing around 1.5 million people worldwide in 2014 and India constitutes 23% of all TB cases which is the highest in the world.[18] Abdominal TB constitutes about 17% of all inpatients admitted with the diagnosis of TB[19] Intestine is the sixth most common of all the extrapulmonary sites involved by TB.[20] TB is caused by *Mycobacterium tuberculosis* and abdominal TB generally includes involvement of gastrointestinal tract, lymph nodes, peritoneum and solid visceral organs of abdomen.

Gastrointestinal Tuberculosis

Gastrointestinal TB (GI TB) can present either with symptoms related to bowel like abdominal pain, vomiting, diarrhea and abdominal distension or systemic symptoms like fever, loss of appetite and weight.[21] The above symptoms of GI TB are not specific and can be seen in patients with CD. The role of imaging in differentiating GI TB and CD will be dealt later in this chapter. Apart from diagnosis, imaging is also useful in guiding FNAC or biopsy in patients where the diagnosis is uncertain on imaging alone. TB can involve any part of the gastrointestinal tract, but ileocecal region is most commonly involved (50–90%).[22,23] The other less commonly involved areas are ascending colon, jejunum, rest of the colon, rectum, duodenum, anal canal, esophagus and stomach in that order.[24,25]

Small Bowel Tuberculosis

Ileocecal region is by far the most common site for small bowel TB. There are various reasons hypothesized for this predilection which are as follows:

- Physiological stasis leading to longer contact
- Closer contact with tubercle bacilli
- Ileum is rich in lymphoid tissue
- Relatively neutral pH promoting bacterial growth.

Ileocecal TB has three morphological types—**ulcerative** (60%), **hypertrophic** (10%) and **ulcerohypertrophic** (30%). Ulcerative type is more common in immunocompromised individuals and hypertrophic type is more common in immunocompetent individuals. The ulcerohypertrophic form can closely mimic malignancy because of its morphology. The caseation necrosis occurring in the submucosal lymphoid tissue causes mucosal ulcerations whereas extensive inflammation and fibrosis in reaction to the bacilli leads to thickening in the hypertrophic type.

Before the advent of new cross-sectional techniques such as CTE and MRE, barium studies used to be the imaging modality of choice in suspected patients with ITB because of its unsurpassed ability to show the mucosal abnormalities. There are various signs on barium studies described in the different stages of ITB **(Fig. 1)**. Spasm, hypermotility, mucosal edema, edema of the ileocecal valve are the earliest signs of ileocecal TB. Fleischner or inverted umbrella sign which is due to the thickening of ileocecal valve with narrowing of terminal ileum is considered to be characteristic for ileocecal TB.[26] Stierlin's sign is due to rapid emptying of barium into cecum because of mucosal irritability **(Fig. 1)**. As the disease progresses there will be fibrosis and shortening of the involved bowel segment and napkin ring stenosis. This is called as string sign showing persistent narrowing of barium column in the area of stenosis **(Fig. 1)**. Cecum is pulled out of the right iliac fossa which is often referred to as pulled up cecum **(Figs. 3A to C)**. This also leads to contraction of cecum which can appear conical on imaging. Because of the cranial migration of cecum there is alteration in the angle between the terminal ileum and colon. The terminal ileum may appear hanging down and stretched from the contracted cecum which is called goose-neck deformity.

High resolution US can also show changes of GI TB in the form of abnormal wall thickening (>3 mm in distended state and >5 mm in collapsed state), inflammation in the surrounding mesentery and enlarged lymph nodes which may have calcification and necrosis. Bowel wall thickening is a nonspecific finding which can be seen in Crohn's disease, lymphoma, amoebiasis and carcinoma. However, TB commonly affects ileocecal junction and often the cecum is pulled up because of fibrosis. USG is optimal for the evaluation of ileocecal region wall thickening. However, USG is not sensitive to detect abnormalities in more proximal small bowel loops because of its inability to evaluate the entire length of bowel.

Contrast-enhanced CT is better than USG to detect and characterize small bowel TB which can show the bowel wall thickening, mesenteric changes and adenopathy **(Fig. 4)**. The necrosis in the nodes is better detected on

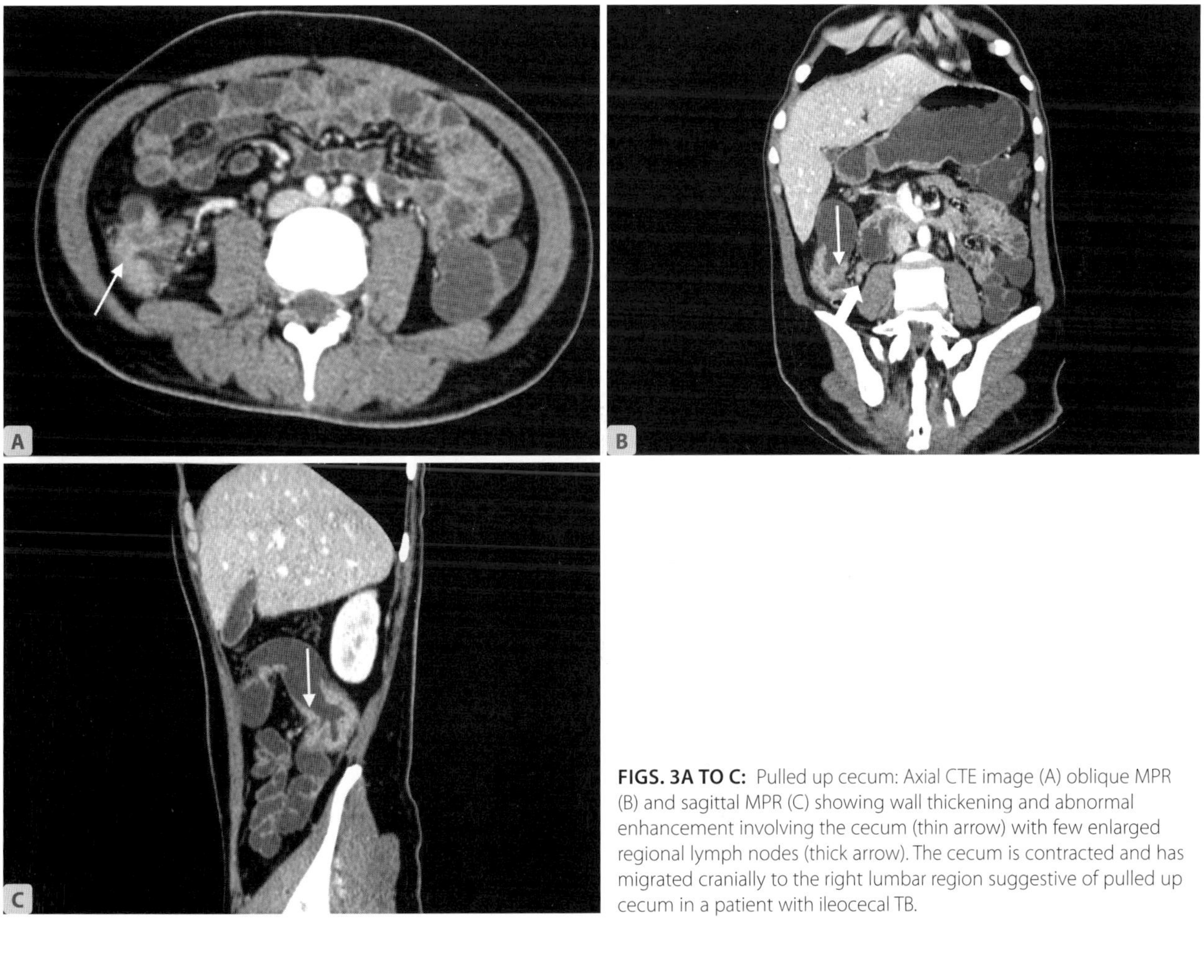

FIGS. 3A TO C: Pulled up cecum: Axial CTE image (A) oblique MPR (B) and sagittal MPR (C) showing wall thickening and abnormal enhancement involving the cecum (thin arrow) with few enlarged regional lymph nodes (thick arrow). The cecum is contracted and has migrated cranially to the right lumbar region suggestive of pulled up cecum in a patient with ileocecal TB.

CECT. Though it is not sensitive for detecting early mucosal changes, it can comprehensively evaluate most of the other features of abdominal TB such as peritoneal and solid organ involvement. CTE is a relatively new technique which is considered superior to conventional CECT in the evaluation of mucosal abnormalities and in the detection of subtle wall thickening and narrowing of lumen. In the early stage CTE may show nonspecific inflammatory changes in the form of stratified wall thickening in distal ileum, ileocecal junction and cecum which can later progress to more severe homogeneous wall thickening and narrowing leading to obstruction **(Figs. 5 and 6)**. It can also show clumping of bowel loops, adhesions, mesenteric changes and occasionally cocoon formation in which varying length of bowel loop is encapsulated by a thick fibrotic membrane **(Figs. 7A to C)**. Because of superior contrast resolution MRI or MRE can also be used to show the features of GI TB. Sometimes the inflammatory changes in the bowel wall and in the surrounding mesentery are better seen on MRI as compared to CT and the tubercular lesions are usually hypointense on T1W images and hyperintense on T2W images **(Figs. 8A to D)**. MRE may show wall thickening, lymphadenopathy, ascites, peritoneal thickening and other associated extraluminal findings. It also shows good correlation with barium meal follow through studies in detecting wall thickening and has the advantage of being a radiation free one-stop shop technique.[27] Most of these findings are common to both GI TB and CD which makes the diagnosis difficult. There are imaging features which

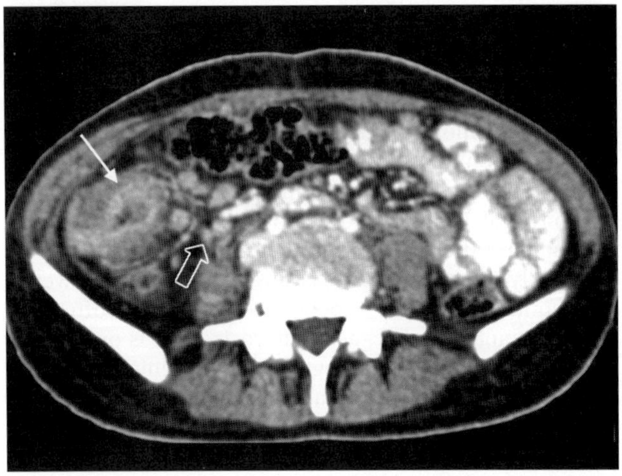

FIG. 4: Ileocecal TB: Axial CECT image showing circumferential wall thickening involving the cecum (thin arrow) with surrounding fat stranding and enlarged lymph nodes (outlined arrow). The above features are suggestive of TB.

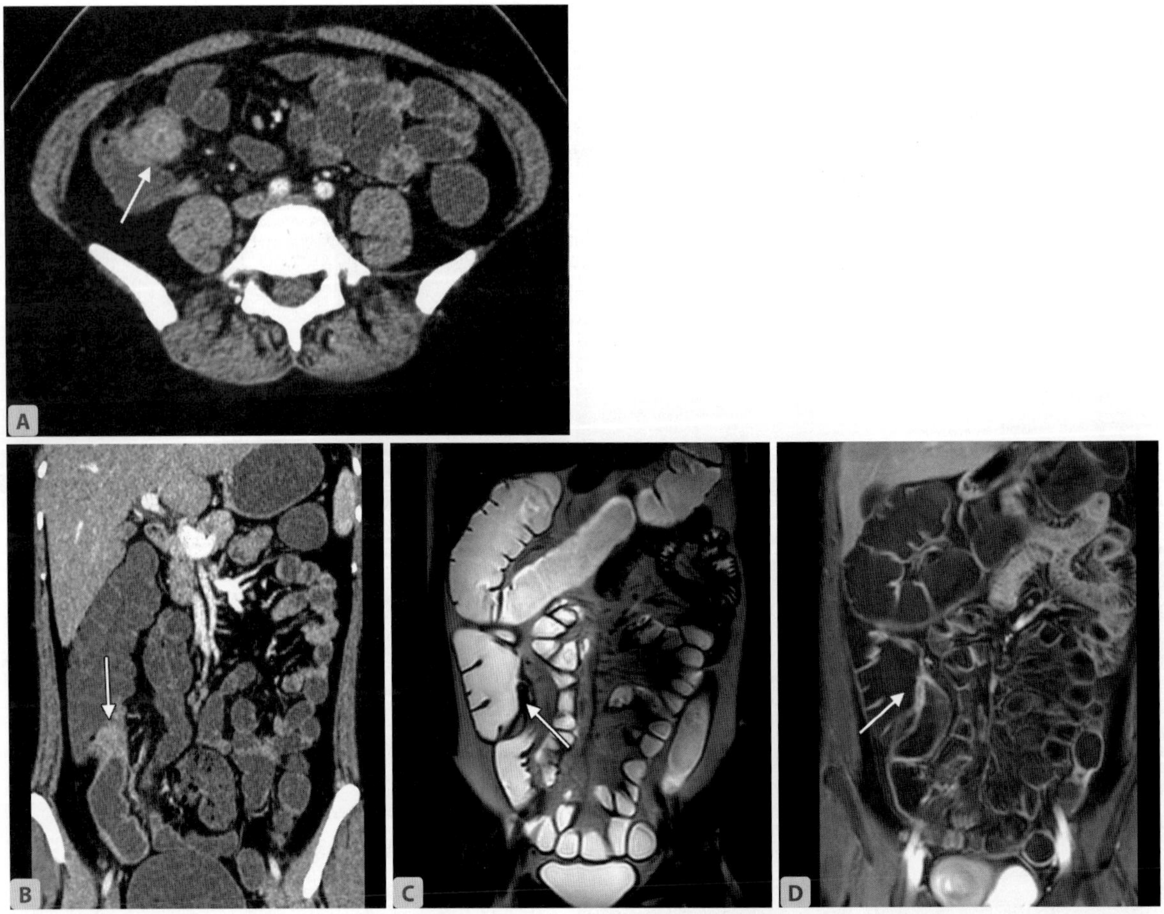

FIGS. 5A TO D: Fibrotic stricture in TB: CTE images (A and B) and MRE images (C and D) showing circumferential wall thickening involving the terminal ileum and ileocecal junction (thin arrow) causing mild proximal obstruction. The wall thickening is hypointense on T2-weighted image (C) and showing homogeneous enhancement on postcontrast image (D) suggestive of fibrosis.

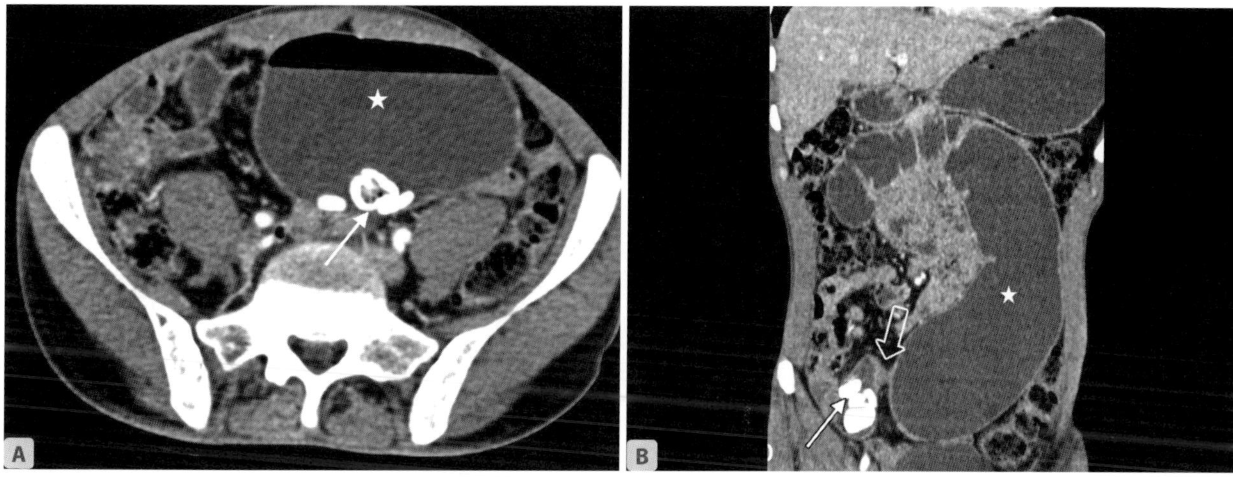

FIGS. 6A AND B: Small bowel obstruction with enteroliths: Axial CECT image (A) and coronal MPR (B) show a short segment ileal stricture (outlined arrow). There is marked proximal dilatation of small bowel with air-fluid level (star) suggestive of small bowel obstruction. Also noted is presence of multiple enteroliths (thin arrow).

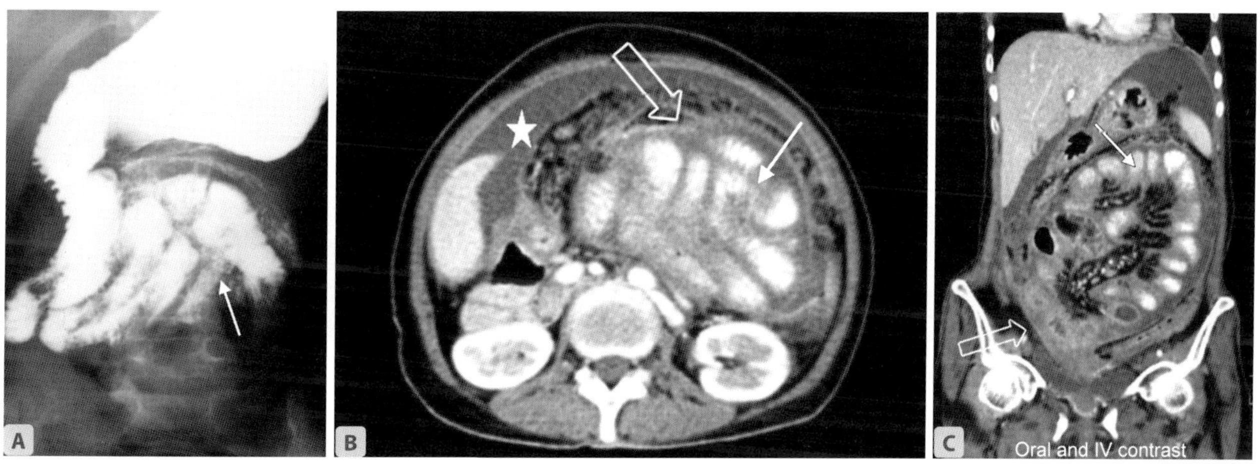

FIGS. 7A TO C: Sclerosing encapsulating peritonitis: Barium meal follow through (BMFT) (A) showing clumping and fixed position of the dilated small bowel loops (thin arrow) in the central abdomen. Axial CECT (B) and coronal MPR (C) image showing clumped dilated proximal jejunal loops which are encapsulated by a thick membrane (outlined arrow) all around suggestive of sclerosing encapsulating peritonitis (cocoon formation). There is associated loculated ascites (star) seen.

can help in this differentiation to a certain extent and are discussed later in this chapter.

Colonic and Anorectal TB

Colon is the second most common site of involvement in GI TB and isolated colonic involvement occurs in about 9% of patients.[28] Cecum is the commonest site followed by ascending colon. Colonic involvement usually presents with chronic pain in abdomen, rectal bleeding and alterations in bowel habit. On imaging colonic involvement presents as short or long segment thickening of the wall, ulcerations which are usually circumferential, and strictures with or without proximal dilatation. Occasionally, it can present with inflammatory polyps, bowel perforation or fistula formation. There may be other sites of involvement in the abdomen which can support the diagnosis. Barium enema can show the early mucosal abnormalities, ulcerations, spasm and stricture. Strictured area is seen as smooth narrowing producing an hour glass configuration as opposed to carcinoma colon which produces an apple core configuration. Colonic TB can closely resemble CD, ulcerative colitis, colonic carcinoma and amebic colitis.

Rarely, TB can involve the rectum and anal canal which can present as proctitis, strictures, fistula, ischiorectal fossa abscess, perianal fissures and warty growths. These findings are not specific for TB because they can occur in CD as well. Circumferential wall thickening because of tuberculous involvement can resemble carcinoma rectum. In doubtful cases, sampling should be done to confirm the diagnosis.

Duodenal Tuberculosis

It constitutes only about 2% of all GI TB and duodenum can be involved either by an extrinsic or intrinsic process.[29] Duodenum may be compressed or involved secondarily due to adjacent lymphadenopathy in which case barium studies can show widening of C-loop of duodenum and smooth

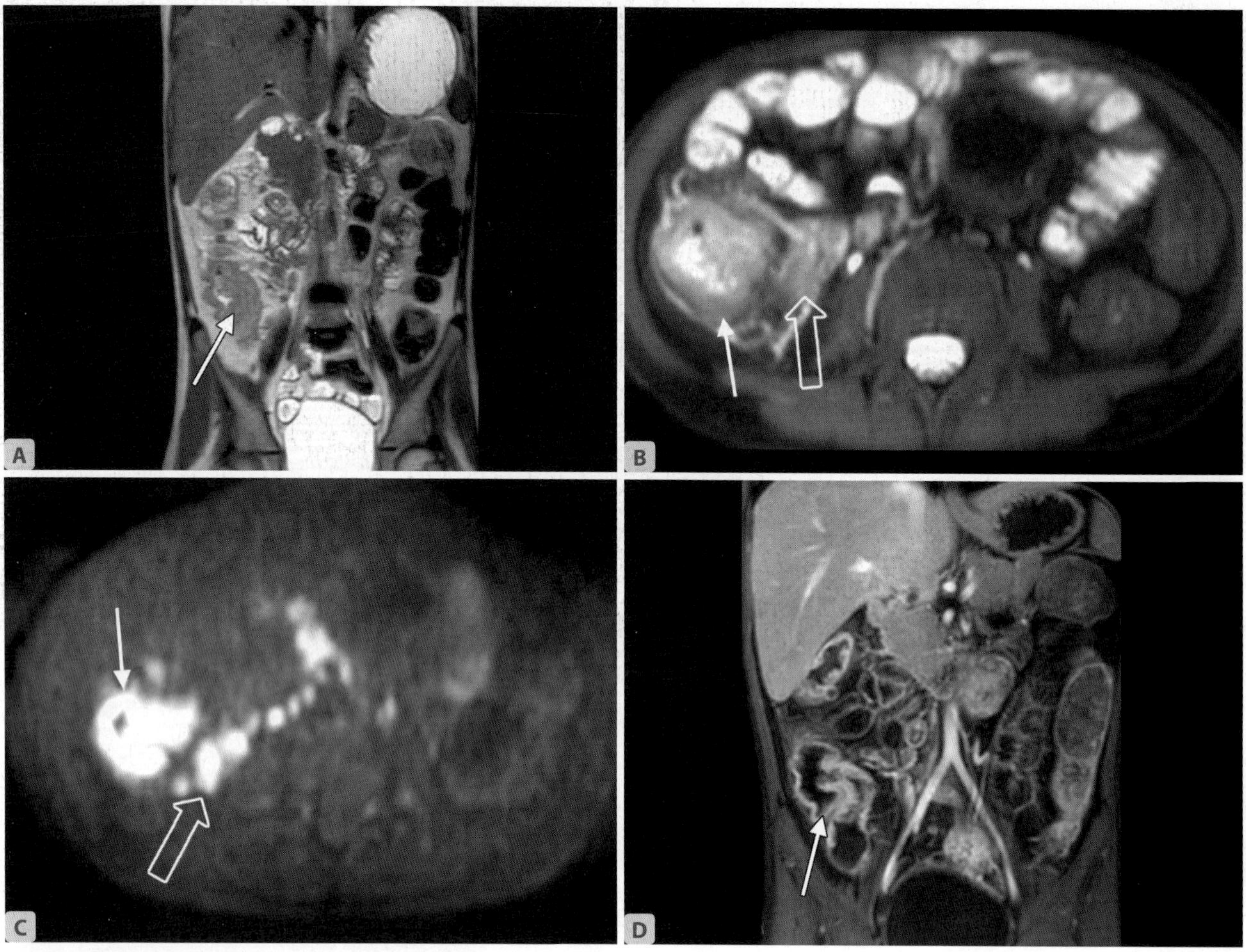

FIGS. 8A TO D: Ileocecal TB: MRE T2-weighted images (A and B) showing wall thickening which is hyperintense involving the ileocecal region (thin arrow) with enlarged regional lymph nodes (outlined arrow). The wall thickening shows diffusion restriction on diffusion weighted b-800 image (C) and hyperenhancement on post-gadolinium image (D) suggestive of active disease.

narrowing. Primary involvement can manifest either as ulcerative or hyperplastic form which can be seen on barium studies as ulcers, polyps, fistula formation and narrowing of lumen. CT may show thickening of the duodenal wall commonly involving the second and the third part, which may be associated with stricture and proximal dilatation **(Figs. 9A to C)**.[30] Duodenal TB can mimic CD, lymphoma and carcinoma and it is usually difficult to differentiate them. Biopsy is confirmatory for the diagnosis.

Gastric Tuberculosis

Stomach involvement by TB is exceedingly rare because of lack of lymphoid tissue in stomach, acidic environment and rapid emptying of gastric contents. Usually, spread of infection is via the hematogenous route or secondary to adjacent involved lymph nodes. Symptoms are very nonspecific like epigastric discomfort, vomiting and weight loss which can be seen in other diseases. Imaging features are usually nonspecific and depend on the nature of involvement. They are usually focal and commonly involve the antropyloric region of stomach. Ulcerative type can present with ulcer which can be seen on barium studies as a benign ulcer whereas the hypertrophic type can present with gross wall thickening which can mimic carcinoma or lymphoma. Stricture due to fibrosis can also be seen in the antropyloric region which can mimic CD. Occasionally, the entire stomach may be involved showing diffuse wall thickening and contracted stomach giving an appearance of linitis plastica. Diagnosis is usually confirmed on biopsy since the imaging features are not conclusive.

Esophageal Tuberculosis

Esophageal TB is a rare entity and it is usually secondary to adjacent mediastinal or pulmonary involvement. Tuberculous involvement of adjacent lymph node or vertebral body can spread to esophagus which is the commonest mode of spread.[29] Patients usually present with odynophagia, hematemesis and chest pain. Because of the close proximity with the lymph nodes, middle third of esophagus is the commonly involved site. Barium studies can show subtle findings such as ulcerations and mucosal irregularity. In advanced stages it may show stricture, traction diverticulum and sinus formation. Occasionally, there can be fistulous communication with the tracheobronchial tree. CT scan is more reliable in showing the extraluminal findings

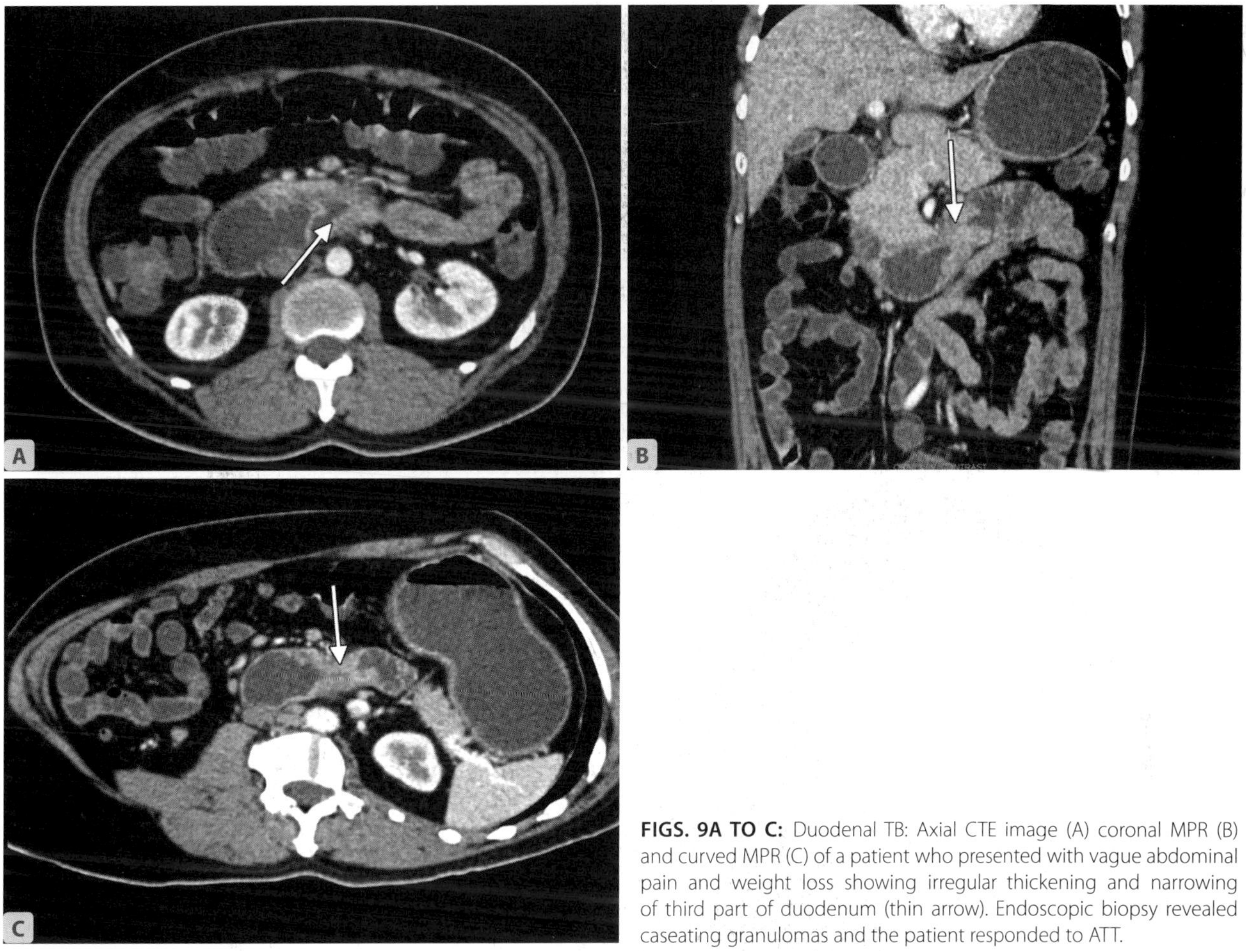

FIGS. 9A TO C: Duodenal TB: Axial CTE image (A) coronal MPR (B) and curved MPR (C) of a patient who presented with vague abdominal pain and weight loss showing irregular thickening and narrowing of third part of duodenum (thin arrow). Endoscopic biopsy revealed caseating granulomas and the patient responded to ATT.

and associated mediastinal and lung disease. It can closely mimic carcinoma esophagus because of which endoscopic sampling is necessary in almost all cases.

Extraintestinal Tuberculosis of Abdomen

Extraintestinal manifestation of TB can often be seen as associated findings in patients with GI TB. The salient features of extraintestinal TB will be covered briefly in this chapter.

Peritoneal Tuberculosis

Peritoneum is the most common location in the abdomen for involvement by TB, however, isolated involvement is relatively rare.[31] Most of the times it occurs in association with other sites of involvement. Involvement of peritoneum, mesentery and omentum are grouped under peritoneal TB. Spread of infection is either from rupture of involved lymph nodes or direct extension across the bowel wall. Peritoneal involvement manifests as thickening of the peritoneum (2–6 mm) with or without associated nodules. On USG the peritoneal thickening is seen as hypoechoic lesions and on CECT it is seen as smooth or nodular peritoneal thickening and enhancement. Contrast MRI may show the same features better mainly because of its superior contrast resolution and diffusion weighted MRI can also delineate this well. Ascites which can be either free or loculated is also a manifestation of peritoneal TB which can be seen in around 30–100% of patients.[32] USG is very sensitive in detecting ascites and also characterizing its nature. It is superior to CT in showing the septations and debris within the fluid. Usually high density ascites is seen in TB, but the density of ascites can range from water attenuation to high attenuation, depending on the amount of fibrin content and cellular debris.[33] Apart from characterizing ascites, imaging can also help in guiding aspiration of ascitic fluid for biochemical analysis. Tuberculous ascites usually shows low serum ascites albumin gradient (SAAG <1.1 g/dL) and elevated levels of adenosine deaminase (ADA) and lymphocytes. There are three types of peritoneal involvement based on the amount of ascites and associated features **(Figs. 10A to C)**:

1. Wet type—most common type, gross free or loculated ascites.
2. Fibrotic-fixed type—less common, with matted bowel loops, mesenteric masses and loculated ascites.
3. Dry-plastic type—rare, nodular dense fibrotic reaction of peritoneum.

Sclerosing encapsulating peritonitis (SEP) or cocoon is another manifestation of peritoneal TB in which a part or entire bowel loops or abdominal viscera is encapsulated by a fibrocollagenous membrane.[34] Barium studies may show

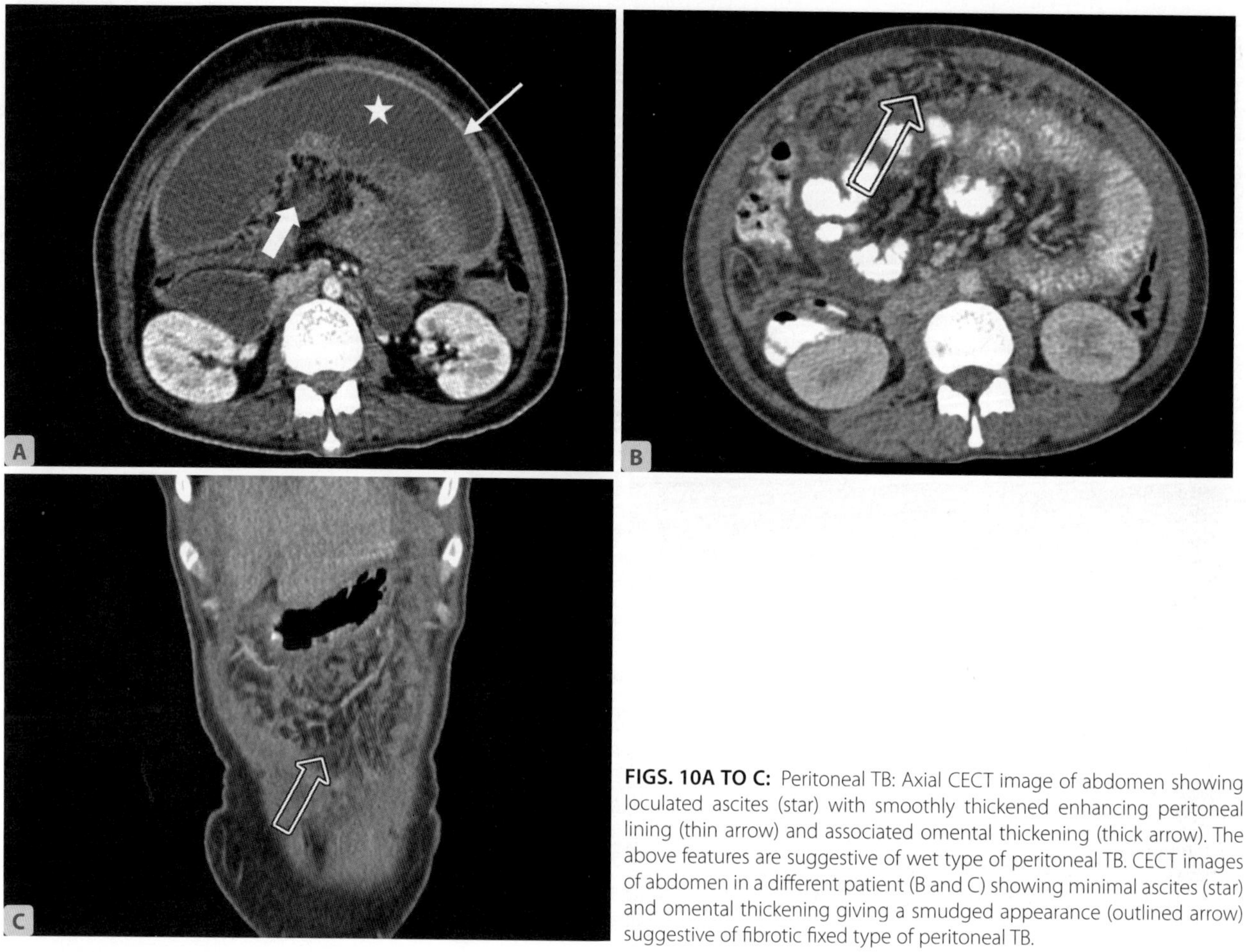

FIGS. 10A TO C: Peritoneal TB: Axial CECT image of abdomen showing loculated ascites (star) with smoothly thickened enhancing peritoneal lining (thin arrow) and associated omental thickening (thick arrow). The above features are suggestive of wet type of peritoneal TB. CECT images of abdomen in a different patient (B and C) showing minimal ascites (star) and omental thickening giving a smudged appearance (outlined arrow) suggestive of fibrotic fixed type of peritoneal TB.

clumping of bowel loops with or without obstructive features and CT scan show the membrane itself as a thick enhancing structure around the bowel loops **(Fig. 7)**. The other causes of SEP are chronic ambulatory peritoneal dialysis, ventriculoperitoneal shunts, sarcoidosis, gastrointestinal malignancies, etc.

Mesentery is frequently involved by TB and the appearance on imaging may be mild fat stranding, thickening, nodularity, diffuse infiltration or abscess formation.[31] Like mesentery, omental involvement may also show various imaging features. It may show a smudged, nodular thickening or caking of which smudged appearance is the most common type of involvement in TB **(Figs. 10A to C)**. Omental caking is a nonspecific finding and can be seen more commonly in peritoneal carcinomatosis.[31] CT scan is the preferred modality to evaluate the omental involvement and recently diffusion weighted MRI is also being evaluated in omental pathologies.[35]

Lymph Nodal TB

Mesenteric, omental, peripancreatic, periportal and upper retroperitoneal lymph nodes are commonly involved in TB **(Figs. 11 and 12)**. It is because these nodes are the regional draining sites for small bowel loops and proximal colon which are the common areas of involvement by TB.[33,36] The appearance of lymph node on imaging may vary depending on the stage of the disease. Enlarged lymph node with peripheral enhancement and central necrosis is the commonest type of appearance and is relatively specific for TB **(Figs. 11 and 12)**. However, central necrosis can be seen in malignancies, aggressive lymphoma and Whipple's disease.[36,37] Other less common appearances are homogeneous, heterogeneous or non-enhancement of the involved node. The nodes in TB tend to be matted and conglomerated because of periadenitis. Multiple normal-sized lymph nodes can also be a manifestation of TB, however not specific to TB. During the healing process the nodes can become smaller in size and become calcified. Enlargement of nodes, necrosis and calcification can be seen on both USG and CECT scan of which CT scan can provide a comprehensive evaluation of disease. Both can be used to guide sampling from the abnormal lymph nodes when imaging features are not conclusive. Enlarged nodes are seen as T1 hypointense and T2 hyperintense lesions on MRI. Necrosis and liquefaction in the center are seen as T2 hyperintensity within the node.

Visceral Solid Organ TB

Visceral organs such as liver, spleen and pancreas can be involved by TB and the usual route of spread is hematogenous.

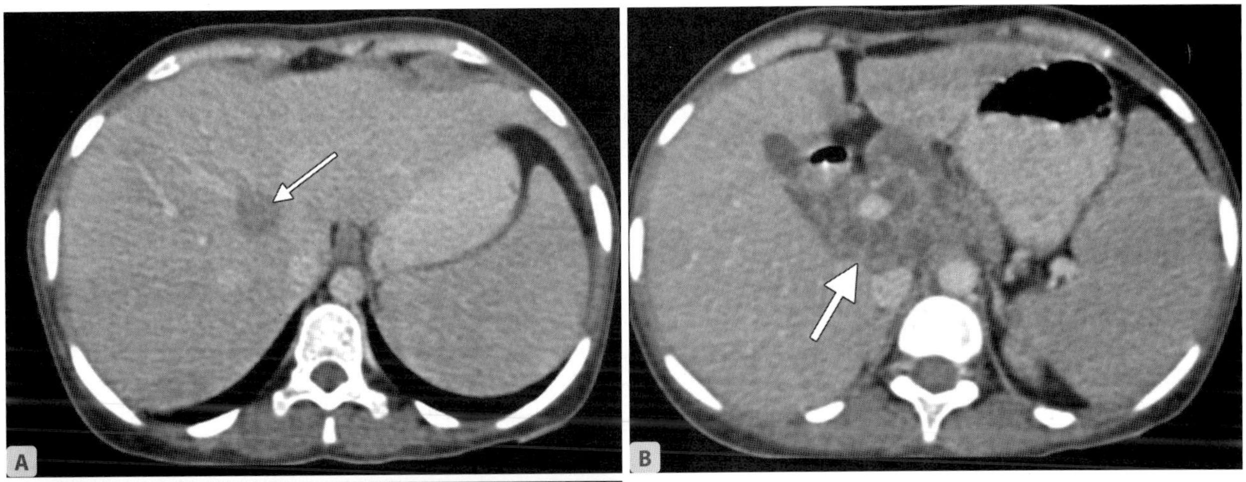

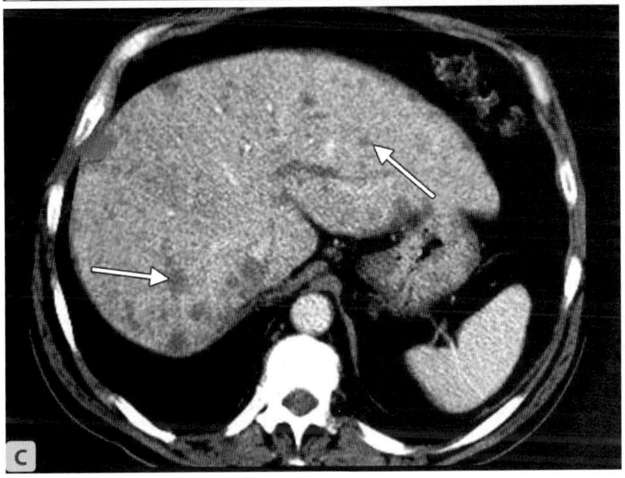

FIGS. 11A TO C: Liver and lymph nodal TB: Axial CECT images (A and B) showing a focal hypodense lesion in the liver (thin arrow) and multiple periportal and peripancreatic necrotic lymphadenopathy (thick arrow). These findings are consistent with macronodular type of liver lesions and lymph nodal involvement in TB. CECT image (C) of another patient showing varying sized focal lesions (thin arrow) involving both the lobes of liver (micro- and macronodular) in a patient diagnosed with TB.

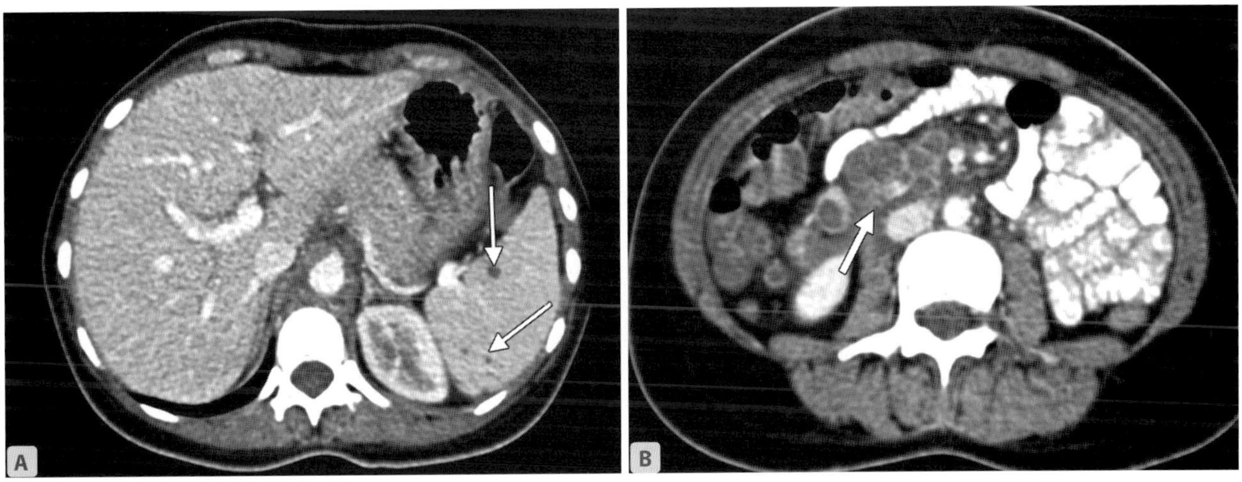

FIGS. 12A AND B: Splenic and lymph nodal TB: Axial CECT images of abdomen showing multiple hypodense lesions in the spleen (thin arrows) and multiple enlarged mesenteric lymph nodes which are showing peripheral enhancement and central necrosis (thick arrow). This patient responded to ATT confirming the diagnosis.

Hepatosplenic TB

Hepatosplenic TB usually occurs as a part of military TB and it is found in 80–100% of patients with miliary TB according to an autopsy series.[38] However, diagnosis on antemortem imaging is quite unusual. Hepatosplenic TB can manifest as micronodular or macronodular type **(Fig. 11)**. In micronodular type the lesions are tiny and often they are less than the resolving ability of routine imaging. Diffuse enlargement of liver and spleen may be the only manifestation of this type. Sometimes, with high resolution USG images these micronodular lesions can be visualized as hypoechoic lesions. In this regard, USG is superior to CT scan. Other differential diagnoses for this type are sarcoidosis, metastasis, fungal infection and lymphoma. In the macronodular type, lesions are usually 1-3 cm in size and they are seen as hypoechoic lesions on USG and hypoenhancing lesions on CECT **(Figs. 11 and 12)**. These nodular lesions are hypointense on T1W scans and hyperintense on T2W scans. DWI can also help in detecting these lesions as they show restriction of diffusion. To start with these lesions may be solid and as the disease progresses they become liquefied and the imaging appearance changes accordingly. They get calcified during the healing phase and in patients with compromised immunity the lesions can progress in size and can become an abscess.

Pancreatic TB

Pancreatic TB is very rare and only few cases are reported in literature. It is thought to be because of the pancreatic juice which provides protection against the tubercle bacilli.[39] The most common site of involvement is the head of pancreas. There are three types of patterns described which are diffuse, focal and multifocal. Lesions can be seen as heterogeneously hypoechoic on USG and heterogeneously hypodense mass lesion on CT scan. Calcification can also be seen in some lesions which can be used to differentiate from pancreatic carcinoma. There may be enlarged lymph nodes with necrosis seen in the vicinity of the pancreas. None of these features are diagnostic for TB and it is usually difficult to differentiate tuberculous lesion from carcinoma pancreas or other inflammatory mass lesions. Most often the diagnosis is apparent only after sampling or after surgical resection. However, recently there have been efforts to differentiate these lesions using CT pancreatic perfusion.[39] There is limited role of MRI in these patients and it can be used to differentiate it from cystic neoplasms of pancreas.

INFLAMMATORY BOWEL DISEASE

Inflammatory bowel disease comprises a group of bowel disorders characterized by idiopathic chronic inflammation of bowel. It includes mainly Crohn's disease and ulcerative colitis. Majority of the times based on the clinical and imaging features it is possible to classify these disorders into one of these two entities. However, in a small subset it is not possible to categorize them accurately and they are grouped as indeterminate colitis or inflammatory bowel disease unclassified. There is another entity called microscopic colitis which is distinctly different from Crohn's disease and ulcerative colitis and can present with chronic watery diarrhea.[40] Microscopic colitis which includes collagenous colitis and lymphocytic colitis usually has normal appearance on colonoscopy and imaging. Inflammation can only be seen on microscopy and hence the name microscopic colitis.

Crohn's Disease

Earlier Crohn's disease (CD) was considered to be a disease of the west and thought to be uncommon in India. Only few cases were reported in the past from India and this was due to the fact that the clinical and imaging features of CD closely resemble TB which is endemic here. Diagnosing CD with reasonable certainty was difficult under those circumstances. However, in the recent years with the improvement in sanitation standards coupled with better understanding of disease and advancements in the field of imaging have led to increase in the detection of CD.[41] The true incidence of CD in India is still not clear because of sparse data availability.

Crohn's disease is a transmural granulomatous inflammatory process of the bowel wall characterized by waxing and waning course and discontinuous involvement of the bowel, which can be complicated by fistulae and abscesses. It can affect any part of the GI tract, from the oral cavity to the anus, often involving multiple discontinuous segments. Small intestine involvement is seen in 70% of cases, most commonly at the terminal ileum and colonic involvement can be seen in up to 50% of which exclusive colonic involvement is seen in 15–20% of patients.[42] Patients present with pain abdomen, diarrhea, low grade fever and easy fatigability. Fecal calprotectin is a reliable marker of bowel inflammation but is nonspecific as far as the etiology of inflammation is concerned and can be elevated in GI TB also.

Imaging is an integral part of the evaluation for CD and it provides vital luminal and extraluminal information. Often imaging can differentiate active inflammatory CD from fibrostenotic CD which is in fact one of the main purposes of imaging in these patients apart from diagnosis and evaluating the extent of disease and its complications. The above differentiation is of paramount importance because the management for these two stages is very different. Active CD is managed by medical treatment whereas fibrostenotic CD may need surgical management.

Many attempts have been made to standardize the classification and scoring of severity of the disease. Montreal classification is one of these which is widely used in clinical practice and research to describe the disease phenotype in CD **(Table 2)**.[43] It describes the type, extent and behavior of disease and studies have proven the reliability of the classification.[44-46] Crohn's Disease Activity Index (CDAI) is another widely used tool for scoring the disease severity which

TABLE 2: Montreal classification of Crohn's disease.

Age at diagnosis (A)	
A1	16 years or younger
A2	17–40 years
A3	More than 40 years
Location (L)	
L1	Terminal ileum
L2	Colon
L3	Ileocolon
L4	Upper GI
Behavior (B)	
p-modifier for perianal disease, added as suffix to B	
B1	Nonstricturing, nonpenetrating
B2	Stricturing
B3	Penetrating

can be used to prognosticate CD and is useful in the follow-up of these patients.[47,48] Score of less than 150 is considered as remission of disease and score of more than 450 is considered as severe disease.

Imaging Features of Crohn's Disease

Imaging features of CD vary with the stage of disease process and the associated complications. Broadly, on imaging CD can be classified into four morphological subtypes:[49]

1. Active inflammatory subtype
2. Fibrostenotic subtype
3. Fistulising or perforating subtype
4. Reparative or regenerative subtype.

Double contrast barium enteroclysis was the imaging modality of choice before the emergence of cross sectional modalities like CTE and MRE. It is the best modality to show the aphthous ulcers seen in the active phase of disease as punctate collection of barium with surrounding radiolucent halo due to mucosal edema. When the disease progresses, the ulcers coalesce and form deep linear ulceration separating out the edematous mucosa **(Fig. 2)**. This is seen on barium studies as cobble-stoning. Later, the mesenteric border shortens due to fibrosis with formation of pseudosacculation along the antimesenteric border **(Fig. 2)**. Stenosis of the bowel loop with or without proximal dilatation and complications like bowel fistulization or contained perforation can also be seen on barium studies. In spite of the ability of double contrast barium to show the mucosal changes in great detail, the extraluminal changes of CD are not well evaluated for which the cross sectional modalities are better. In current practice barium studies are not routinely done for the diagnosis or follow up of CD. It may be done for few niche indications such as demonstration of aphthous ulcers, cobble-stoning of mucosa and fistula formation.[50] Ideal imaging modality for the evaluation of CD is CTE or MRE and the diagnostic performance of both the modalities are comparable for the detection of CD.[51-53] The choice between the two techniques depends largely on the local availability of equipment and expertise and few other clinical considerations. The radiation hazard involved in CTE and ability of MRE in differentiating active and fibrotic disease tilts the balance towards MRE in appropriate clinical scenario. When CD is suspected in a child or patient is being evaluated for response to treatment or follow-up imaging or there is suspicion of fistula, MRE is better than CTE. However, when CD is suspected in an elderly patient or clinical suspicion of CD is low or a diagnosis other than CD is suspected, CTE may be preferred over MRE because it is faster, reliable, relatively resistant to artifacts and gives consistent image quality.

Thickening of Bowel Wall

Bowel wall thickening is the most common finding in patients with CD **(Figs. 13 and 14)**. It is usually symmetrical and circumferential, most commonly involving the terminal ileum and the ileocecal junction. Often in CD, the degree of involvement of ileum is more than that of cecum.[54] Thickening of bowel wall is a nonspecific finding which can occur in both active inflammatory and fibrostenotic disease. In a distended bowel, wall thickness of more than 3 mm is abnormal. Single shot FSE or postcontrast sequence on MRE are the optimal sequences to look for wall thickening. This finding has high sensitivity and specificity in the range of 83–91% and 86–100%, respectively.[55] Wall thickening may reduce during the remission phase but, usually there will be some residual thickening compared to the normal segment. One pitfall of this finding is that bowel wall may apparently look thick when the bowel is collapsed. One should be careful not to label collapsed bowel loop as wall thickening.

Submucosal Edema

Submucosal edema leads to wall thickening and is usually seen as hypodense area on CTE and hyperintense area on T2 weighted sequence with or without fat suppression **(Figs. 13 to 15)**. Submucosal edema is a sign of active disease.

Bowel Wall Contrast Enhancement

Contrast enhancement of the involved segment can occur both in active inflammatory disease and in fibrostenotic phase. It is considered to be the earliest and the most

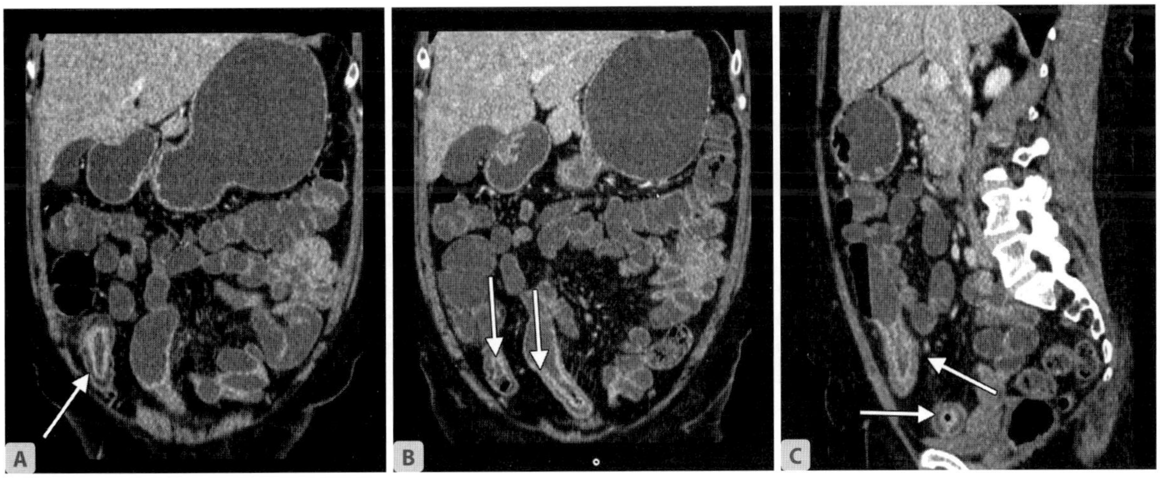

FIGS. 13A TO C: Stratified wall enhancement in active CD: Coronal CTE images (A and B) and sagittal MPR (C) showing thickening and stratified wall enhancement involving the ileal loops (thin arrow) which is a sign of active inflammatory stage of CD.

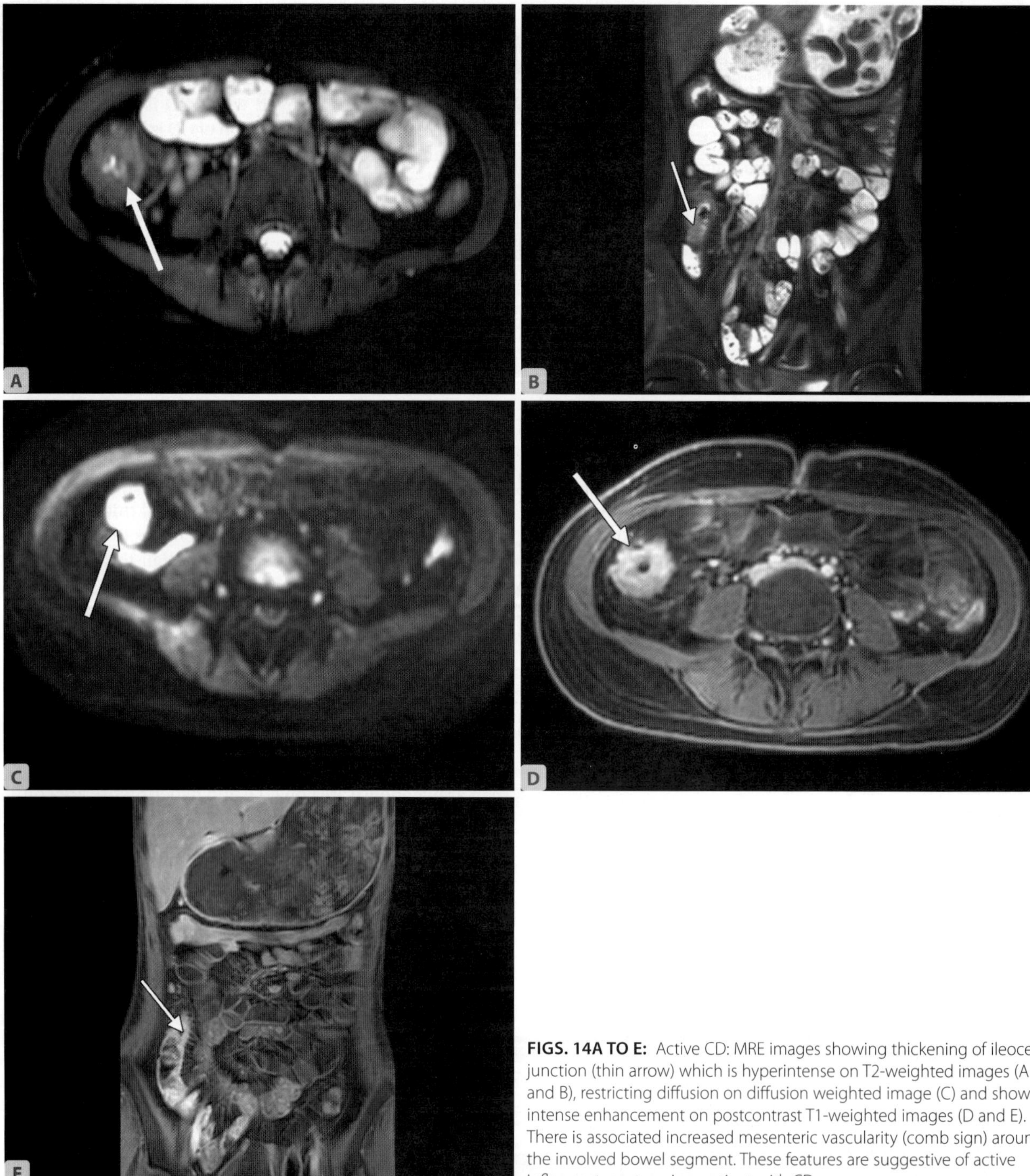

FIGS. 14A TO E: Active CD: MRE images showing thickening of ileocecal junction (thin arrow) which is hyperintense on T2-weighted images (A and B), restricting diffusion on diffusion weighted image (C) and showing intense enhancement on postcontrast T1-weighted images (D and E). There is associated increased mesenteric vascularity (comb sign) around the involved bowel segment. These features are suggestive of active inflammatory stage in a patient with CD.

sensitive sign for active CD.[56] It has been shown to correlate with the level of inflammation on histopathology. At the same time absence of abnormal enhancement almost excludes disease activity in CD.[57] Potential pitfalls in contrast enhancement are that the normal jejunal enhancement is more than ileal enhancement and collapsed bowel loops can show apparently increased enhancement. One should be aware of these pitfalls to avoid misinterpretation. There are three types of enhancement patterns described in CD-stratified, mucosal and homogeneous enhancement. Of the above types stratified bowel wall enhancement (target like) is specific for active inflammatory phase **(Figs. 13 and 15)**. Homogeneous enhancement is nonspecific and can be seen in both active and fibrotic phases **(Figs. 16 and 17)**. It is also known that often fibrosis and active inflammation can coexist and can present as varying features on imaging **(Figs. 18A to C)**. One promising alternative for contrast enhancement is diffusion weighted imaging in which the hyperintensity on trace images corresponds with active inflammation **(Fig. 14)**.[58] This technique is useful in patients

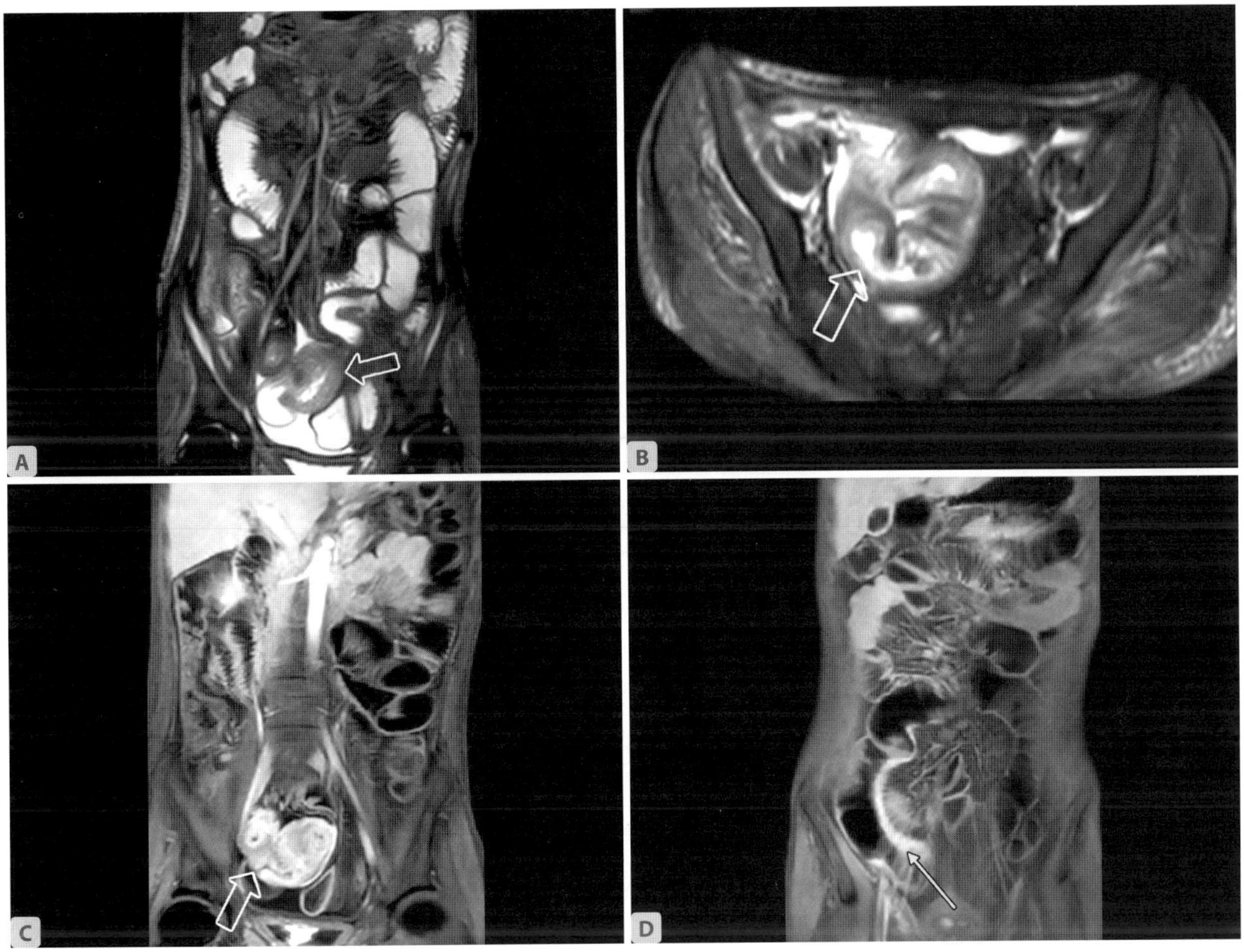

FIGS. 15A TO D: Active CD: Coronal MRE (A) and axial T2-weighted images (B) showing segmental wall thickening of a pelvic ileal loop (outlined arrow) which is showing T2 hyperintensity (A and B). Coronal postcontrast images (C and D) show stratified mural enhancement, asymmetrical wall thickening involving the mesenteric border of terminal ileum with intense enhancement (thin arrow). These findings are typical for active inflammatory stage of CD.

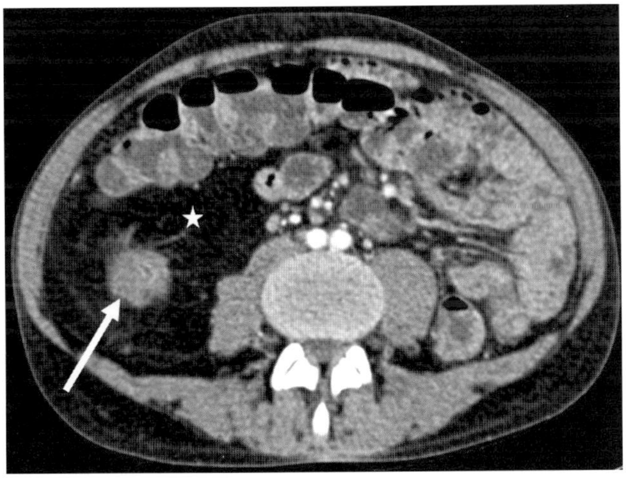

FIG. 16: Fat proliferation: Axial CTE image showing thickening of ascending colon (thin arrow) with surrounding fat proliferation (star). Minimal enhancement of the involved segment coupled with fat proliferation is suggestive of chronic fibrotic stage of CD.

where contrast cannot be administered for reasons like deranged renal parameters.

Submucosal Fat Infiltration

In patients with chronic inflammation there can be fat deposition in the submucosa which can appear markedly hypodense on CTE and loses signal on fat saturated sequences on MRE.[59,60] Although it is a nonspecific sign, the presence of submucosal fat infiltration in CD suggests chronicity.

Fibrosis

Recognising fibrosis on imaging is crucial for the management of CD because those patients are often considered for surgery as they are unlikely to benefit from medical therapy.[61] Fibrosis is a result of chronic inflammation which has a nonspecific appearance on CTE. MRE has an edge over CTE in this regard as fibrosis manifests as hypointensity on both T1 and T2-weighted images and shows progressive homogeneous enhancement in delayed phase **(Figs. 16 to 18)**.

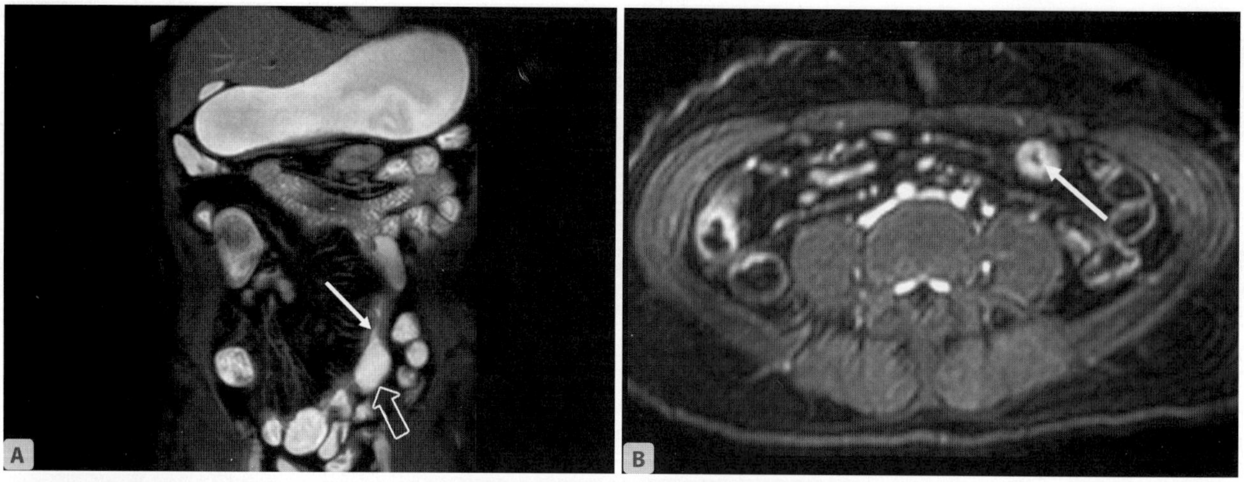

FIGS. 17A AND B: Pseudosacculations in fibrotic CD: Coronal T2-weighted image (A) of MRE study showing wall thickening and multiple segments of luminal narrowing involving the ileal loops (thin arrow). There are multiple pseudosacculations seen in the antimesenteric border (outlined arrow). Axial postcontrast T1 weighted image (B) shows homogeneous wall enhancement of the involved loop. The above imaging features are characteristic of fibrostenotic stage of CD.

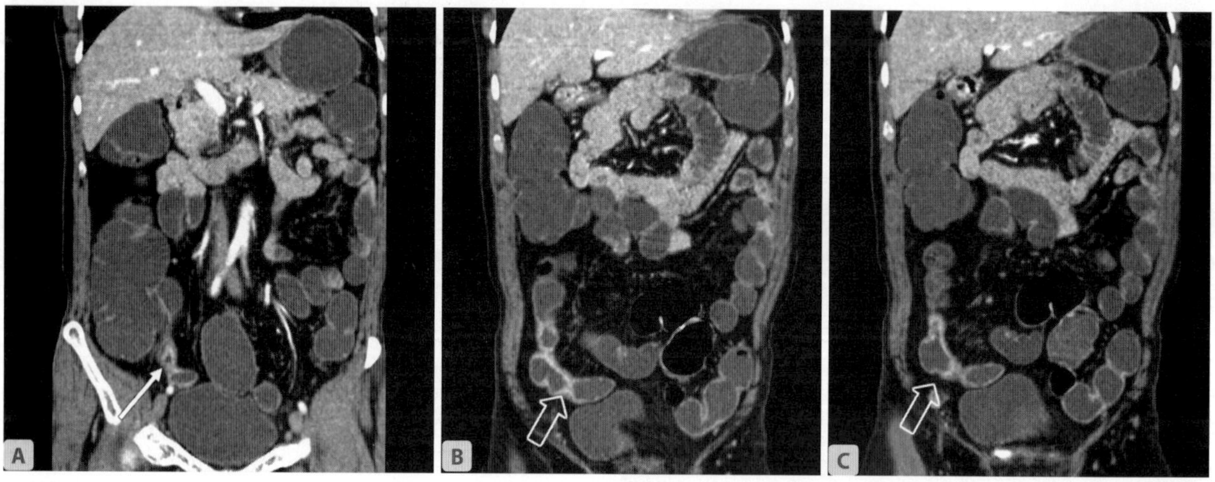

FIGS. 18A TO C: Coexisting active and chronic CD: Coronal CTE images (A to C) showing hyperenhancement with mural stratification (thin arrow) and pseudosacculation involving the antimesenteric border of distal ileum (outlined arrow). Mural stratification is a sign of active inflammatory stage whereas pseudosacculation is a sign of chronic CD.

Skip Lesions

This is defined as multifocal areas of involvement with normal healthy bowel in between. It is considered as an important sign to differentiate CD from other infective processes like TB but is not very specific.

Stenosis of Bowel Wall

Bowel wall narrowing in CD can be because of active inflammation leading to spasm or due to chronic fibro-stenosing disease. This differentiation can sometimes be difficult based on imaging because of overlapping features. Presence of stratified enhancement, wall edema and ulcerations favor active inflammation whereas prestenotic dilated bowel loop indicate a chronic process.

Comb Sign

Comb sign is a manifestation of prominent vasa recta due to increase in vascularity in the mesentery. It is regarded as one of the specific signs of active inflammation **(Figs. 14 and 19)**. This is best seen on TruFISP (BTFE) and postcontrast sequences.

Mesenteric Edema

It is due to inflammation and resultant edema in the mesentery secondary to bowel wall inflammation. It is also considered as a sign of active inflammation. It is seen as increased attenuation on CTE (mesenteric fat stranding) and increased intensity on fat saturated T2-weighted sequences. In severe cases minimal free fluid can also be seen.

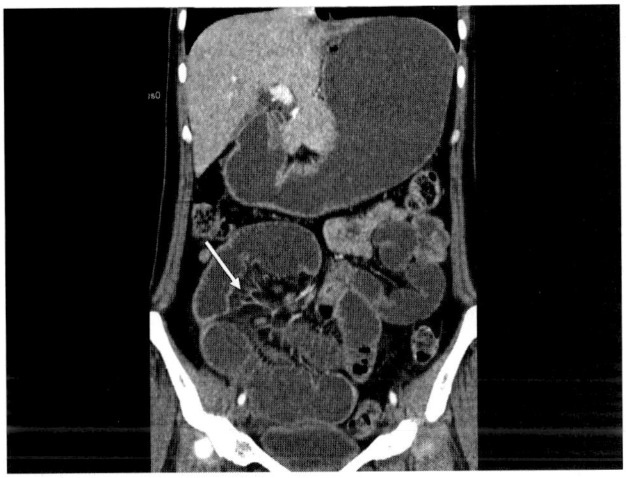

FIG. 19: Comb sign in active CD: Coronal CTE image showing a segment of dilated ileal loop with increased mesenteric vascularity (comb sign) (thin arrow) in a patient with CD. Presence of comb sign is a marker of active inflammatory stage of CD.

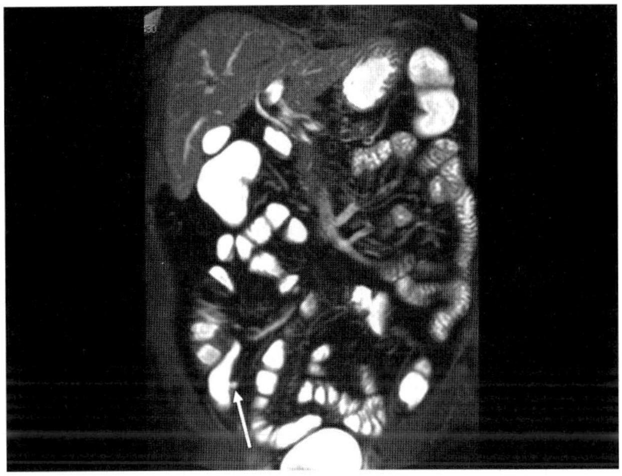

FIG. 20: Deep ulcer on CD: T2-weighted coronal image of MRE showing hyperintense outpouching (thin arrow) in the distal ileal loop suggestive of deep ulceration in a patient with CD.

Ulcerations

Ulcerations which are considered as a sign of active disease are sometimes seen on imaging especially on MRE when the loops are adequately distended **(Fig. 20)**. It may be seen as irregularity of the wall or thin linear hyperintensity extending into the wall. In a recent study, using high resolution MRE images, the sensitivity in detecting the mucosal features has been found to be in the range of 69–99% for superficial ulcers and 94–99% for deep ulcers.[62]

Abnormal Motility

Abnormal bowel motility is a known feature of active CD and sometimes it can be the early sign of disease. It can be classified into different patterns as follows:[63]

- Paralysis—when the involved segment does not show peristalsis
- Hypomotility—when the involved segment shows decreased motility
- Hypermotility—when the involved segment shows increased motility
- Intraluminal pendular movement—inefficient to and fro movement of bowel content.

The movement of the involved bowel loop is compared with the surrounding normal loops for any abnormality. If there is any abnormal movement of a segment, it has to be carefully studied in the other sequences on MRE to confirm the abnormality. Cine MR imaging which can be done as a part of MRE is the best way to evaluate bowel movement and it is found to increase the detection rate of lesions compared to standard MRE sequences.[63]

Abscesses, Sinuses and Fistulas

Abscesses, sinuses and fistulae developing in a patient with CD are considered as major complications and are also a sign of active disease. Abscesses are seen as hypodense lesion on CTE and hyperintense on T2-weighted sequences on MRE with the wall showing postcontrast enhancement. Sinuses and fistulae are seen as linear enhancing structures beyond the confines of bowel loop on CTE and MRE. In CD, there can be blind sinuses extending from the bowel wall, enteroenteric, enterocolonic, enterovesical, enterocutaneous or perianal fistula. A stellate configuration of bowel loops (star sign) which are adherent to each other is suggestive of enteroenteric fistula **(Fig. 21)**. The diagnosis of this entity has a bearing on management and may be an indication for initiating treatment with Infliximab. The sensitivity and specificity of CTE and MRE in detecting sinuses and fistulas is around 83% and 100% respectively.[60] However, MRE performs better in the diagnosis and evaluation of the extent of perianal

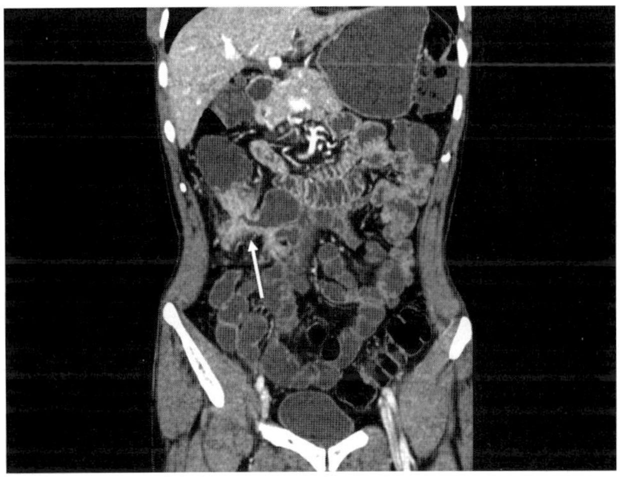

FIG. 21: Fistulizing stage of CD: Coronal CTE image showing abnormal thickening, distorted stellate configuration and communication between the small bowel loop and the ascending colon (thin arrow) suggestive of enterocolic fistula.

fistulae in relation to the internal and external sphincters **(Figs. 22A to D)**.[64,65]

Pseudodiverticulum Formation

This sign is a result of asymmetrical fibrosis and shortening of the mesenteric border leading to apparent sacculations along the antimesenteric border. It is usually seen in chronic CD and associated with other features of chronic disease **(Figs. 2, 17 and 18)**.

Fibrofatty Proliferation

It is seen in long standing CD as a result of chronic inflammation in bowel loops. It is seen as increased fat surrounding the involved bowel loops on all imaging modalities **(Fig. 16)**. This is a nonspecific finding and may be seen in any cause of chronic inflammation.

Reactive Lymphadenopathy

In India, enlarged regional lymph nodes with bowel wall thickening occur more commonly in TB. However, enlarged lymph nodes can occur in patients with CD also. However, lymph nodes in CD are usually less than 1cm in size. Mesenteric lymphadenopathy in CD is a nonspecific finding which can occur in both active and inactive disease. There is some evidence that the increased degree of nodal enhancement favors active disease in CD.[66]

Most of the features of CD described above are almost similar on CTE and MRE. Abnormalities such as submucosal edema, submucosal fat infiltration and fibrosis may appear as nonspecific hypoattenuation on CTE whereas they are more accurately characterized on MRE. The imaging features and their significance in differentiating active from fibrotic disease are listed in **Table 3**.

Imaging Features to Differentiate Intestinal TB from CD

Intestinal TB and CD have many features in common and their differentiation is difficult. This poses a greater problem in countries like India where TB is common and endemic. There is no single test which can reliably differentiate intestinal TB from CD. Hence a combination of clinical, endoscopic, imaging, histopathology and biochemical features should be used. Sometimes follow-up imaging and even a trial of anti-tubercular therapy may be required to differentiate between

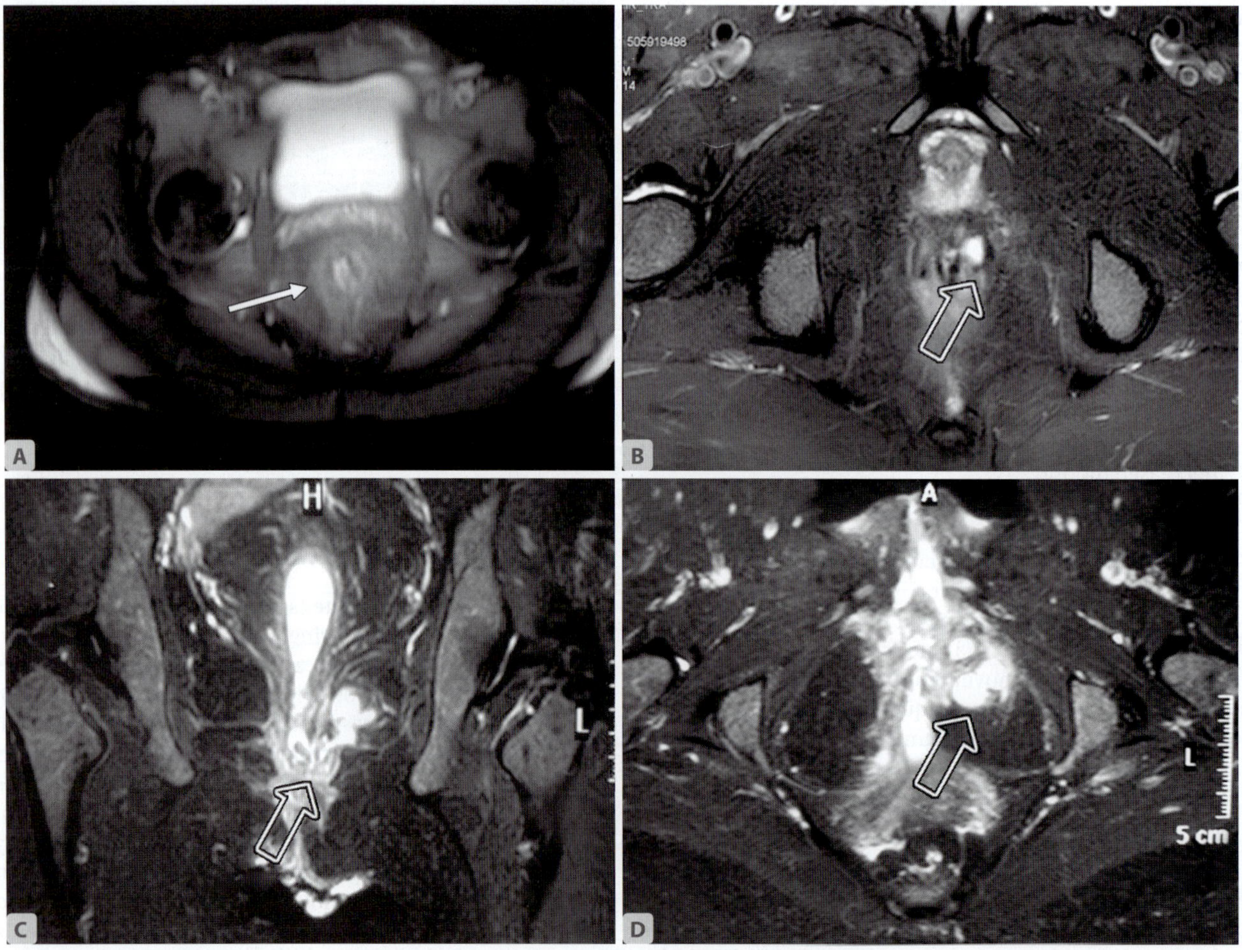

FIGS. 22A TO D: Perianal fistulas: T2-weighted MR images (A and B) of a patient with rectal involvement by CD (thin arrow) showing a small fistulous tract (outlined arrow) arising from the anal canal. T2-weighted images (C and D) of a different patient showing more complex fistulous tract and collections (outlined arrow) in left ischioanal fossa. Presence of fistula or sinus tract is a marker of active inflammatory stage in CD.

TABLE 3: Imaging features to differentiate active inflammatory from fibrostenotic disease in CD.

Active disease	Fibrotic stage	Nonspecific
• Submucosal edema • Early hyperenhancement • Stratified enhancement of wall • Comb sign • Mesenteric edema • Ulcerations • Abnormal motility • Abscesses, sinuses and fistulas	• Late progressive and homogeneous wall enhancement • Submucosal fatty infiltration • Fibrosis • Pseudodiverticulum • Fibrofatty proliferation	• Bowel wall thickening • Skip lesions • Bowel stenosis • Reactive lymphadenopathy

TABLE 4: Imaging features to differentiate GI TB and CD.

Imaging features	Intestinal TB	CD
Site of involvement	Cecum more than ileum	Ileum more than cecum
Length of involvement	Shorter segment	Longer segment
Multiple site involvement	Uncommon	Common
Skip lesions	Rare	Common
Type of wall enhancement	Homogeneous	Stratified
Mural stratification of wall	Rare	Common
Perianal fistula	Uncommon	Common
Mesenteric abscess	Very rare	Relatively common
Bowel fistulas	Rare	Relatively common
Strictures	Concentric	Eccentric with sacculations
Enteroliths	More common	Less common
Increased mesenteric vascularity	Uncommon	Common
Fibrofatty proliferation	Uncommon	Common
Mesenteric nodes	Large and necrotic	Small and homogeneous
Omental involvement	Often seen	Rare
Ascites	Frequent	Uncommon
Solid organ involvement	Relatively common	Very rare

Source: Modified and reproduced with permission from Sharma R, et al. Intestinal tuberculosis versus Crohn's disease: Clinical and radiological recommendations. Indian J Radiol Imaging. 2016;26(2):161-72.

them. Imaging is an important tool which is used routinely and the common imaging features used to differentiate both the entities are summarized in the **Table 4**.

Ulcerative Colitis

Ulcerative colitis (UC) is a characterized by superficial inflammation involving the colon. The colonic involvement in UC is symmetric and contiguous. Rectum is involved in almost all cases with varying length of proximal colonic involvement sometimes involving the entire colon (pancolitis).[67] Occasionally, terminal ileum can be affected and becomes edematous and dilated when the entire colon is involved and is called backwash ileitis. UC is well evaluated with colonoscopy and imaging is seldom used.

The earliest finding of UC on imaging is seen on double contrast barium enema (DCBE) as diffuse granular appearance of the mucosa because of inflammation and edema. This leads to thickening of wall and haustral folds. As the disease progresses to the submucosa, collar button ulcers develop. Collar button ulcers are not specific for UC because they can occur in other inflammatory diseases. In chronic disease, the colon shows narrowing and shortening and loses its haustral folds appearing featureless which is referred as lead pipe sign **(Figs. 23A and B)**.[68] When the mucosa gets denuded, residual mucosal mounds can develop into inflammatory pseudopolyps. Severe cases can be associated with backwash ileitis which may be seen as fixed and patulous ileocecal valve with dilated terminal ileum and granular appearance of mucosa. Because of chronic inflammation

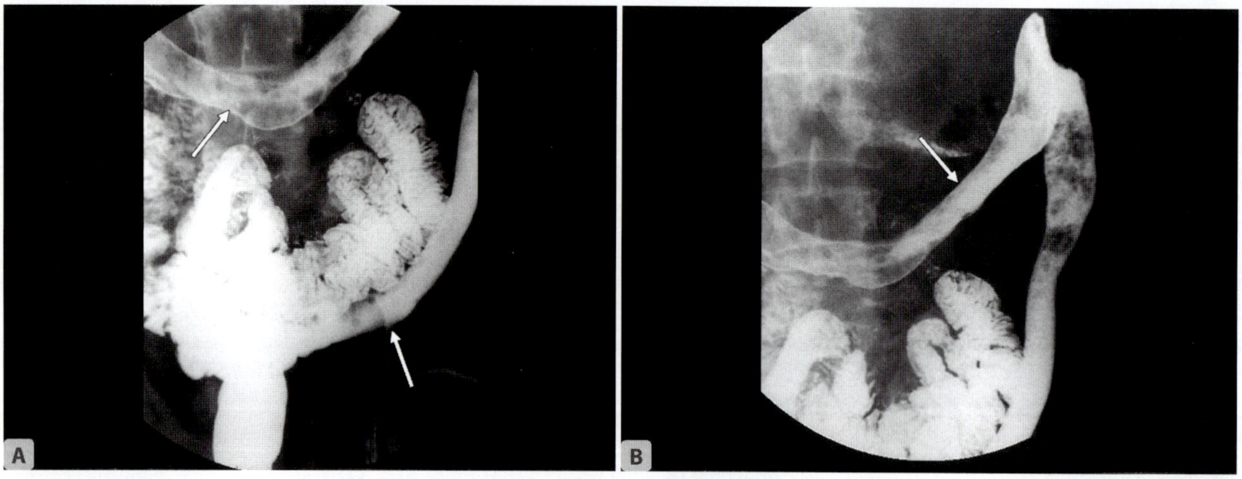

FIGS. 23A AND B: Lead pipe sign in chronic UC. Barium study images (A and B) of a patient with ulcerative colitis showing diffuse luminal narrowing and loss of haustrations (thin arrow) involving the entire colon without any skip areas. This featureless appearance of colon in chronic UC is known as lead pipe sign.

there may be increased presacral fat. One of the dreaded complication of UC is toxic megacolon which manifests as colonic dilatation more than 6 cm, thinning of wall and loss of haustrations. Plain radiography is usually diagnostic and barium studies are generally contraindicated because of the risk of perforation.

CT scan show the extraluminal changes of UC such as localized perforation, abscess, etc. CT is not sensitive in showing the early mucosal changes of UC. Inflamed bowel shows thickening and may show mural stratification. In chronic stage there may be narrowing of colon, alteration of haustral pattern and submucosal fat infiltration which can also be seen on CT. Narrowing of colon is usually because of benign strictures, however if there is asymmetry or eccentric thickening with focal loss of mural stratification, malignancy developing in UC should be suspected. The overall risk of developing malignancy in UC is 3.7% and in CD is around 2.9%.[69,70] Pericolonic fat proliferation is much better seen on CT scan rather than on conventional modalities.[67,68] Pericolonic fatty proliferation or creeping fat around the colon occurs more frequently in CD as compared to UC.[71,72] MRI is not routinely used for the evaluation of UC but it can show most of the features which are seen on CT scan. USG is an emerging technique for bowel evaluation which can show bowel wall thickening and mural stratification.

MISCELLANEOUS DISEASES

This category includes radiation enteritis, NSAID enteropathy, eosinophilic enteritis, etc. which will be discussed in brief.

Radiation Enteritis

Radiation enteritis occurs as a result of toxic effects of radiation (usually more than 3000cGy) to the bowel wall and to the vasculature. Radiation effects can be acute, subacute or chronic depending on the time of onset of manifestations after radiation therapy. Acute stage occurs within 2 months whereas subacute and chronic stages occur after 2 months and 12 months respectively. In the acute phase, imaging may

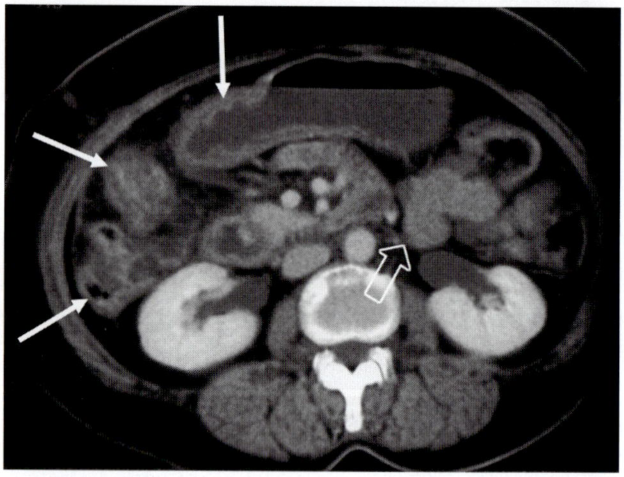

FIG. 24: Acute radiation enteritis. Axial CECT image of a patient who received radiotherapy for carcinoma gallbladder showing thickening of bowel loops with mural stratification and surrounding fat stranding (thin arrow) which are confined to the irradiated area. The bowel loops outside the irradiated area (outlined arrow) appear normal. These features are typical for acute radiation enteritis.

show spasm and edema of the involved bowel loops which can mimic other inflammatory conditions.[73] However, in radiation enteritis the involvement is limited to the irradiated area **(Fig. 24)**. In chronic stage there may be wall thickening, narrowing, ulceration and fat proliferation around the bowel. History of radiation and the area of involvement is the key to differentiate from other inflammatory diseases.

NSAIDs Enteropathy

Nonsteroidal anti-inflammatory drugs (NSAID) are one of the commonly prescribed drugs worldwide. They cause alterations in the protective mechanism of gut by affecting prostaglandin synthesis. It can affect the esophagus, stomach and small bowel and cause local complications. In esophagus and stomach it can cause multiple tiny mucosal erosions which may be seen on barium studies as focal collection of barium with surrounding halo due to edema around.[74,75] In the small bowel it can cause focal ulcers with associated wall edema in the acute phase. When the disease progress to chronic phase it can lead to ulcer and circumferential stricture which are typically thin and membrane like (mucosal diaphragm). They can cause bowel obstruction and lead to proximal bowel dilatation. Mucosal diaphragms are not specific to NSAID enteropathy because they can occur in other inflammatory diseases like CD.[74]

Eosinophilic Gastroenteritis

Eosinophilic gastroenteritis is a relatively uncommon entity which is characterized by patchy or diffuse infiltration of eosinophils in the bowel wall.[76] Majority of these patients have peripheral eosinophilia. Clinical features are nonspecific such as pain abdomen, vomiting or diarrhea. Gastric antrum is the most common site of involvement, however, it can also affect the duodenum and small bowel. It leads to mucosal fold thickening and submucosal infiltration which can be visualized on barium studies and CT scan. As the clinical and imaging features are nonspecific, the index of suspicion should be high to diagnose this condition and presence of peripheral eosinophilia is an important indicator.

CONCLUSION

In India where TB is endemic, it is often difficult to differentiate intestinal TB from CD only on the basis of clinical features. Imaging is an integral part of management of these patients and it can help in differentiating these two entities. A judicious combination of clinical, imaging, endoscopic and histological features should be used. Imaging also has an important role in the follow-up of these patients to look for complications and response to therapy. Hence, it is imperative for the radiologist to be aware of the imaging features so as to correctly diagnose these diseases and to avoid mismanagement.

REFERENCES

1. Maglinte DDT, Kelvin FM, O'Connor K, Lappas JC, Chernish SM. Current status of small bowel radiography. Abdom Imaging. 1996;21(3):247 57.
2. Nijhawan S, Kumpawat S, Mallikarjun P, Bansal RP, Singla D, Ashdhir P, et al. Barium meal follow through with pneumocolon: Screening test for chronic bowel pain. World J Gastroenterol WJG. 2008;14(43):6694.
3. Bender GN, Timmons JH, Williard WC, Carter J. Computed tomographic enteroclysis: one methodology. Invest Radiol. 1996;31(1):43-9.
4. Paulsen SR, Huprich JE, Fletcher JG, Booya F, Young BM, Fidler JL, et al. CT enterography as a diagnostic tool in evaluating small bowel disorders: review of clinical experience with over 700 cases. Radiographics. 2006;26(3):641-57.
5. Solem CA, Loftus EV, Fletcher JG, Baron TH, Gostout CJ, Petersen BT, et al. Small-bowel imaging in Crohn's disease: a prospective, blinded, 4-way comparison trial. Gastrointest Endosc. 2008;68(2):255-66.
6. Ha AS, Levine MS, Rubesin SE, Laufer I, Herlinger H. Radiographic Examination of the Small Bowel: Survey of Practice Patterns in the United States. Radiology. 2004;231(2):407-12.
7. Ilangovan R, Burling D, George A, Gupta A, Marshall M, Taylor SA. CT enterography: review of technique and practical tips. Br J Radiol. 2012;85(1015):876-86.
8. Mettler FA, Huda W, Yoshizumi TT, Mahesh M. Effective doses in radiology and diagnostic nuclear medicine: A catalog. Radiology. 2008;248(1):254-63.
9. Makanyanga JC, Taylor SA. Current and future role of MR enterography in the management of Crohn disease. Am J Roentgenol. 2013;201(1):56-64.
10. Kiryu S, Dodanuki K, Takao H, Watanabe M, Inoue Y, Takazoe M, et al. Free-breathing diffusion-weighted imaging for the assessment of inflammatory activity in Crohn's disease. J Magn Reson Imaging. 2009;29(4):880-86.
11. Oto A, Zhu F, Kulkarni K, Karczmar GS, Turner JR, Rubin D. Evaluation of diffusion-weighted MR imaging for detection of bowel inflammation in patients with Crohn's disease. Acad Radiol. 2009;16(5):597-603.
12. Oto A, Kayhan A, Williams JT, Fan X, Yun L, Arkani S, et al. Active Crohn's disease in the small bowel: evaluation by diffusion-weighted imaging and quantitative dynamic contrast-enhanced MR imaging. J Magn Reson Imaging. 2011;33(3):615-24.
13. Oussalah A, Laurent V, Bruot O, Bressenot A, Bigard MA, Régent D, et al. Diffusion-weighted magnetic resonance without bowel preparation for detecting colonic inflammation in inflammatory bowel disease. Gut. 2010;59(8):1056-65.
14. Chiorean L, Schreiber-Dietrich D, Braden B, Cui XW, Buchhorn R, Chang JM, et al. Ultrasonographic imaging of inflammatory bowel disease in pediatric patients. World J Gastroenterol. 2015;21(17):5231-41.
15. Levine A, Koletzko S, Turner D, Escher JC, Cucchiara S, De Ridder L, et al. ESPGHAN revised porto criteria for the diagnosis of inflammatory bowel disease in children and adolescents. J Pediatr Gastroenterol Nutr. 2014;58(6):795-806.
16. Dietrich CF, Cui XW, Schreiber-Dietrich DG, Ignee A. EFSUMB guidelines 2011: comments and illustrations. Ultraschall Med-Eur J Ultrasound. 2012;33(S 01):S11–21.
17. Dietrich CF. Comments and illustrations regarding the guidelines and good clinical practice recommendations for contrast-enhanced ultrasound (CEUS)–update 2008. Ultraschall Med-Eur J Ultrasound. 2008;29(S 04):188-202.
18. WHO | Global tuberculosis report 2015 [Internet]. WHO. [cited 2015 Nov 6]. Available from: *http://www.who.int/tb/publications/global_report/en/*.
19. Sircar S, Taneja VA, Kansra U. Epidemiology and clinical presentation of abdominal tuberculosis: a retrospective study. J Indian Med Assoc. 1996;94(9):342-4.
20. Marshall JB. Tuberculosis of the gastrointestinal tract and peritoneum. Am J Gastroenterol. 1993;88(7):989-99.
21. Sood R. Diagnosis of abdominal tuberculosis: role of imaging. J Indian Acad Clin Med. 2001;2(3):169-77.
22. Sharma MP, Bhatia V. Abdominal tuberculosis. Indian J Med Res. 2004;120(4):305-15.
23. Balthazar EJ, Gordon R, Hulnick D. Ileocecal tuberculosis: CT and radiologic evaluation. AJR. 1990;154(3):499-503.
24. Gulati MS, Sarma D, Paul SB. CT appearances in abdominal tuberculosis. A pictorial essay. Clin Imaging. 1999;23(1):51-9.
25. Ramesh J, Banait GS, Ormerod LP. Abdominal tuberculosis in a district general hospital: a retrospective review of 86 cases. QJM Mon J Assoc Physicians. 2008;101(3):189-95.

26. Carrera GF, Young S, Lewicki AM. Intestinal tuberculosis. Abdom Imaging. 1976;1(1):147-55.
27. Krishna S, Kalra N, Singh P, Kochhar R, Gupta R, Singh R, et al. Small-bowel tuberculosis: A comparative study of MR enterography and small-bowel follow-through. Am J Roentgenol. 2016;207(3):571-7.
28. Thoeni RF, Margulis AR. Gastrointestinal tuberculosis. In: Seminars in roentgenology [Internet]. Elsevier; 1979 [cited 2015 Sep 2]. p. 283-94. Available from: http://www.sciencedirect.com/science/article/pii/0037198X79900257.
29. Chong VH, Lim KS. Gastrointestinal tuberculosis. Singapore Med J. 2009;50(6):638-45; quiz 646.
30. Chavhan GE, Ramakantan R. Duodenal tuberculosis: radiological features on barium studies and their clinical correlation in 28 cases. J Postgrad Med. 2003;49(3):214-7.
31. da Rocha EL, Pedrassa BC, Bormann RL, Kierszenbaum ML, Torres LR, D'Ippolito G. Abdominal tuberculosis: a radiological review with emphasis on computed tomography and magnetic resonance imaging findings. Radiol Bras. 2015;48(3):181-91.
32. Akhan O, Pringot J. Imaging of abdominal tuberculosis. Eur Radiol. 2002;12(2):312-23.
33. Leder RA, Low VH. Tuberculosis of the abdomen. Radiol Clin North Am. 1995;33(4):691-705.
34. Jayant M, Kaushik R. Abdominal cocoon in a young man. World J Emerg Med. 2014;5(3):234-6.
35. Foti PV, Attinà G, Spadola S, Caltabiano R, Farina R, Palmucci S, et al. MR imaging of ovarian masses: classification and differential diagnosis. Insights Imaging. 2015;7(1):21-41.
36. Yang ZG, Min PQ, Sone S, He ZY, Liao ZY, Zhou XP, et al. Tuberculosis versus lymphomas in the abdominal lymph nodes: evaluation with contrast-enhanced CT. Am J Roentgenol. 1999;172(3):619-23.
37. Li DK, Rennie CS. Case Report Abdominal Computed Tomography in Whipple's Disease. J Comput Assist Tomogr. 1981;5(2):249-52.
38. Brauner M, Buffard MD, Jeantils V, Legrand I, Gotheil C. Sonography and computed tomography of macroscopic tuberculosis of the liver. J Clin Ultrasound. 1989;17(8): 563-8.
39. Yadav AK, Nadrajah J, Kandasamy D, Sharma R, Gamanagatti S, Garg PK. Volume perfusion computed tomography as an aid to diagnosis of pancreatic tuberculosis. Trop Gastroenterol. 2015;35(4):264-6.
40. Bohr J, Wickbom A, Hegedus A, Nyhlin N, Hultgren Hörnquist E, Tysk C. Diagnosis and management of microscopic colitis: current perspectives. Clin Exp Gastroenterol. 2014;7:273-84.
41. Makharia GK. Rising incidence and prevalence of Crohn's disease in Asia: Is it apparent or real? J Gastroenterol Hepatol. 2006;21(6):929-31.
42. Yacoub JH, Oto A. New magnetic resonance imaging modalities for Crohn disease. Magn Reson Imaging Clin N Am. 2014;22(1):35-50.
43. Silverberg MS, Satsangi J, Ahmad T, Arnott IDR, Bernstein CN, Brant SR, et al. Toward an integrated clinical, molecular and serological classification of inflammatory bowel disease: report of a Working Party of the 2005 Montreal World Congress of Gastroenterology. Can J Gastroenterol J Can Gastroenterol. 2005;19 Suppl A:5A–36A.
44. Spekhorst LM, Visschedijk MC, Alberts R, Festen EA, van der Wouden E-J, Dijkstra G, et al. Performance of the Montreal classification for inflammatory bowel diseases. World J Gastroenterol WJG. 2014;20(41):15374-81.
45. Dassopoulos T, Nguyen GC, Bitton A, Bromfield GP, Schumm LP, Wu Y, et al. Assessment of reliability and validity of IBD phenotyping within the National Institutes of Diabetes and Digestive and Kidney Diseases (NIDDK) IBD Genetics Consortium (IBDGC). Inflamm Bowel Dis. 2007;13(8):975-83.
46. Krishnaprasad K, Andrews JM, Lawrance IC, Florin T, Gearry RB, Leong RWL, et al. Interobserver agreement for Crohn's disease sub-phenotypes using the Montreal Classification: How good are we? A multicenter Australasian study. J Crohns Colitis. 2012;6(3):287-93.
47. Best WR, Becktel JM, Singleton JW, Kern F. Development of a Crohn's disease activity index. National Cooperative Crohn's Disease Study. Gastroenterology. 1976;70(3):439-44.
48. Peyrin-Biroulet L, Panés J, Sandborn WJ, Vermeire S, Danese S, Feagan BG, et al. Defining disease severity in inflammatory bowel diseases: Current and future directions. Clin Gastroenterol Hepatol. 2016;14(3):348-54.e17.
49. Maglinte DD, Gourtsoyiannis N, Rex D, Howard TJ, Kelvin FM. Classification of small bowel Crohn's subtypes based on multimodality imaging. Radiol Clin North Am. 2003;41(2):285-303.
50. Marshak RH. Granulomatous Disease of the Intestinal Tract (Crohn's Disease): Annual Oration in Honor of Benjamin H. Orndoff, MD, 1881-1971. Radiology. 1975;114(1):3-22.
51. Grand DJ, Beland MD, Machan JT, Mayo-Smith WW. Detection of Crohn's disease: comparison of CT and MR enterography without anti-peristaltic agents performed on the same day. Eur J Radiol. 2012;81(8):1735-41.
52. Lee SS, Kim AY, Yang SK, Chung JW, Kim SY, Park SH, et al. Crohn Disease of the Small Bowel: Comparison of CT Enterography, MR Enterography, and Small-Bowel Follow-Through as Diagnostic Techniques. Radiology. 2009;251(3):751-61.
53. Siddiki HA, Fidler JL, Fletcher JG, Burton SS, Huprich JE, Hough DM, et al. Prospective comparison of state-of-the-art MR enterography and CT enterography in small-bowel Crohn's disease. Am J Roentgenol. 2009;193(1):113-21.
54. Sharma R, Madhusudhan KS, Ahuja V. Intestinal tuberculosis versus crohn's disease: Clinical and radiological recommendations. Indian J Radiol Imaging. 2016;26(2):161-72.
55. Constantino CPL, Rodrigues RS, Neto JAO, Marchiori E, Araujo ALE, de Mello Perez R, et al. Computed Tomography and Magnetic Resonance Enterography Findings in Crohn's Disease: What Does the Clinician Need to Know From the Radiologist? Can Assoc Radiol J. 2014;65(1):42-51.
56. Fidler JL, Guimaraes L, Einstein DM. MR Imaging of the Small Bowel. Radiographics. 2009;29(6):1811-25.
57. Lawrance IC. Correlation of MRI-determined small bowel Crohn's disease categories with medical response and surgical pathology. World J Gastroenterol. 2009;15(27):3367.
58. Buisson A, Joubert A, Montoriol PF, Ines DD, Hordonneau C, Pereira B, et al. Diffusion-weighted magnetic resonance imaging for detecting and assessing ileal inflammation in Crohn's disease. Aliment Pharmacol Ther. 2013;37(5):537-45.
59. Elsayes KM, Al-Hawary MM, Jagdish J, Ganesh HS, Platt JF. CT Enterography: Principles, Trends, and Interpretation of Findings 1. Radiographics. 2010;30(7):1955-70.
60. Sinha R, Verma R, Verma S, Rajesh A. MR enterography of Crohn disease: part 2, imaging and pathologic findings. Am J Roentgenol. 2011;197(1):80-5.
61. Van Assche G, Dignass A, Panes J, Beaugerie L, Karagiannis J, Allez M, et al. The second European evidence-based Consensus on the diagnosis and management of Crohn's disease: Definitions and diagnosis. J Crohns Colitis. 2010;4(1):7-27.
62. Sinha R, Murphy P, Sanders S, Ramachandran I, Hawker P, Rawat S, et al. Diagnostic accuracy of high-resolution MR enterography in Crohn's disease: comparison with surgical and pathological specimen. Clin Radiol. 2013;68(9):917-27.
63. Froehlich JM, Waldherr C, Stoupis C, Erturk SM, Patak MA. MR motility imaging in Crohn's disease improves lesion detection compared with standard MR imaging. Eur Radiol. 2010;20(8):1945-51.

64. Haggett PJ, Moore NR, Shearman JD, Travis SP, Jewell DP, Mortensen NJ. Pelvic and perineal complications of Crohn's disease: assessment using magnetic resonance imaging. Gut. 1995;36(3):407-10.
65. Halligan S, Buchanan G. MR imaging of fistula-in-ano. Eur J Radiol. 2003;47(2):98-107.
66. Gourtsoyianni S, Papanikolaou N, Amanakis E, Bourikas L, Roussomoustakaki M, Grammatikakis J, et al. Crohn's disease lymphadenopathy: MR imaging findings. Eur J Radiol. 2009;69(3):425-8.
67. Roggeveen MJ, Tismenetsky M, Shapiro R. Best cases from the AFIP: Ulcerative colitis. Radiogr Rev Publ Radiol Soc N Am Inc. 2006;26(3):947-51.
68. Gore RM, Balthazar EJ, Ghahremani GG, Miller FH. CT features of ulcerative colitis and Crohn's disease. AJR. 1996;167(1):3-15.
69. Eaden JA, Abrams KR, Mayberry JF. The risk of colorectal cancer in ulcerative colitis: a meta-analysis. Gut. 2001;48(4):526-35.
70. Canavan C, Abrams KR, Mayberry J. Meta-analysis: colorectal and small bowel cancer risk in patients with Crohn's disease. Aliment Pharmacol Ther. 2006;23(8):1097-104.
71. Deepak P, Bruining DH. Radiographical evaluation of ulcerative colitis. Gastroenterol Rep. 2014;2(3):169-77.
72. Parente F, Greco S, Molteni M, Anderloni A, Bianchi Porro G. Imaging inflammatory bowel disease using bowel ultrasound. Eur J Gastroenterol Hepatol. 2005;17(3):283-91.
73. Addley HC, Vargas HA, Moyle PL, Crawford R, Sala E. Pelvic imaging following chemotherapy and radiation therapy for gynecologic malignancies. Radiogr Rev Publ Radiol Soc N Am Inc. 2010;30(7):1843-56.
74. McGettigan MJ, Menias CO, Gao ZJ, Mellnick VM, Hara AK. Imaging of Drug-induced Complications in the Gastrointestinal System. Radiogr Rev Publ Radiol Soc N Am Inc. 2016;36(1):71-87.
75. Frye JM, Hansel SL, Dolan SG, Fidler JL, Song LMWK, Barlow JM, et al. NSAID enteropathy: appearance at CT and MR enterography in the age of multimodality imaging and treatment. Abdom Imaging. 2015;40(5):1011-25.
76. Baig MA, Qadir A, Rasheed J. A review of eosinophilic gastroenteritis. J Natl Med Assoc. 2006;98(10):1616-9.

CHAPTER

97

Imaging of Ischemic Bowel Disease

Ajay Gulati, Naveen Kalra, Mandeep Kang

INTRODUCTION

Ischemic bowel disease occurs due to impaired arterial supply and/or venous drainage of splanchnic circulation, resulting in ischemic injury and altered bowel metabolism. Ischemic bowel disease present as complex spectrum of disorders with variable imaging manifestations depending upon time of onset, duration, severity of ischemic injury; the segment and length of bowel affected; vessels affected and status of collateral blood flow circuits. Ischemia may be acute or chronic; may be arterial or venous in origin. Ischemia may involve the small bowel, large bowel or both segments resulting in *mesenteric ischemia, colonic ischemia* and *ischemic enterocolitis* respectively. Variability in the above factors not only affects the clinical scenario, but also influences the management options, outcome and prognosis.

Bowel ischemia has numerous causes and variable presentations. Frequently patients complain of nonspecific symptoms. Classic triad of *abdominal pain, pyrexia and frank blood in stool* history is elicited only in less than one-third of the patients. Majority of the patients present with vague clinical symptoms including diarrhea, vomiting and abdominal discomfort.[1] Laboratory work up is often non-specific and time consuming. In the present modern era with advancements in imaging techniques, radiologists play a pivotal role in evaluation of bowel ischemia *by making an accurate diagnosis, and helping in treatment planning along with vital prognostic information*, as they are able to characterize and delineate the disease process.

ANATOMY OF SPLANCHNIC CIRCULATION

Relevant abdominal vascular anatomy knowledge is essential to understand and evaluate bowel ischemia; knowing the normal vascular pattern and its common anatomic variants is helpful in angiogram assessment and appropriate endovascular treatment planning. Splanchnic circulation consists of arterial supply and their collateral system; and venous drainage alternatively called as portal venous system.

Arterial Supply

Three major trunks arising anteriorly from abdominal aorta, namely *celiac axis, superior mesenteric artery, and inferior mesenteric artery* provide arterial supply to intra-abdominal viscera.

Celiac Axis

Celiac axis arises from aorta at T12 vertebral level, supply foregut derivatives such as liver, pancreas, spleen and bowel from stomach to 2nd part of duodenum by branching into *common hepatic artery, left gastric artery and splenic artery*. The common hepatic artery gives off gastroduodenal artery, right gastroepiploic artery and anterior superior pancreaticoduodenal artery branches. The splenic artery branches into left gastroepiploic artery and pancreatic artery **(Fig. 1)**.

Superior Mesenteric Artery

Superior mesenteric artery (SMA) arises from abdominal aorta at L1 vertebral level, supply midgut derivatives, from

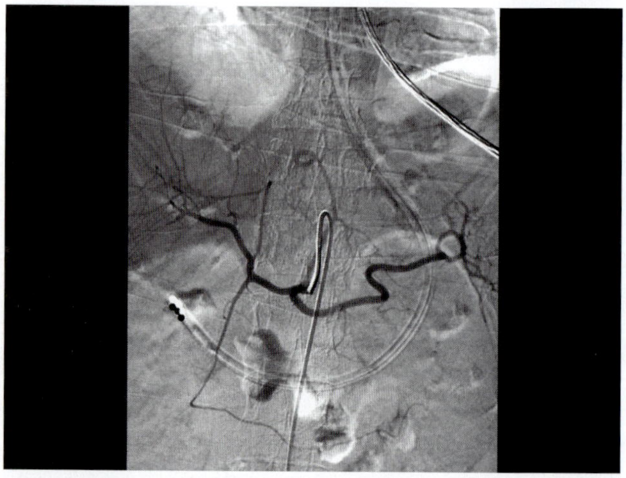

FIG. 1: Digital subtraction angiography (DSA) run of celiac axis trunk with its branches.

2nd part of duodenum till middle third of transeverse colon. Anterior and posterior inferior pancreaticoduodenal arteries, middle colic artery, right colic artery, ileocolic artery and numerous jejunal and ileal arteries arise from superior mesenteric artery. All these branches contribute to form multiple vascular arcades, from which straight vessels perforate bowel wall **(Fig. 2)**.

Inferior Mesenteric Artery

Inferior mesenteric artery (IMA) originates from anterior abdominal aorta at L3/L4 vertebral body level. Supply hindgut derivatives from distal third of transverse colon till proximal rectum, by left colic artery, sigmoidal arteries and superior rectal artery which are branched off from inferior mesenteric artery; distal rectum is supplied by hypogastric artery, which is a branch of internal iliac artery **(Fig. 3)**.

Collateral System

Abundant collateralization is seen between major mesenteric arterial trunks and the branches of mesenteric vascular arcades. These extensive collateral vessels are more conspicuous in the stomach, duodenum and rectum thereby accounting for inherent resistance to ischemia in these areas. The important collateral circuits:

- Pancreaticoduodenal arcade connecting celiac axis to superior mesenteric artery
- Marginal artery of Drummond
- Central anastomotic artery
- Arc of Riolan (aka the 'meandering mesenteric artery') are the potential conduits connecting superior mesenteric artery to inferior mesenteric artery **(Figs. 4A and B)**. Meandering artery connecting proximal middle colic artery of SMA with proximal left colic artery of IMA, may be visualized angiographically in presence of superior or inferior mesenteric artery occlusive pathology; hence it is essential to determine direction of blood flow within the meandering artery before dissecting any of the major mesenteric arteries.[1,2]

Portal Venous System

The small and large intestine is drained by superior and inferior mesenteric veins. Inferior mesenteric vein form

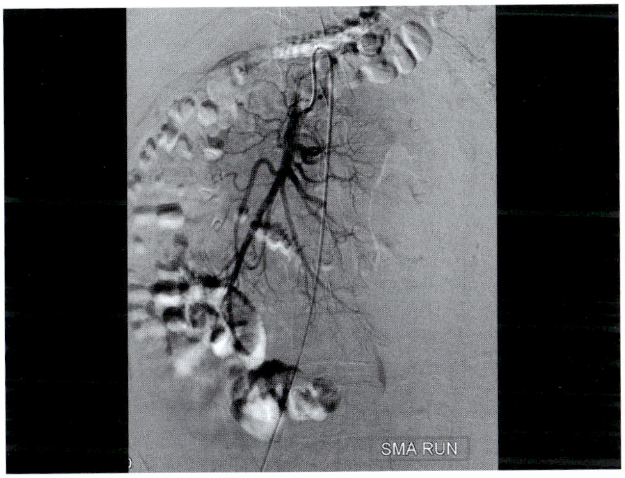

FIG. 2: DSA run showing superior mesenteric artery (SMA) and its branches.

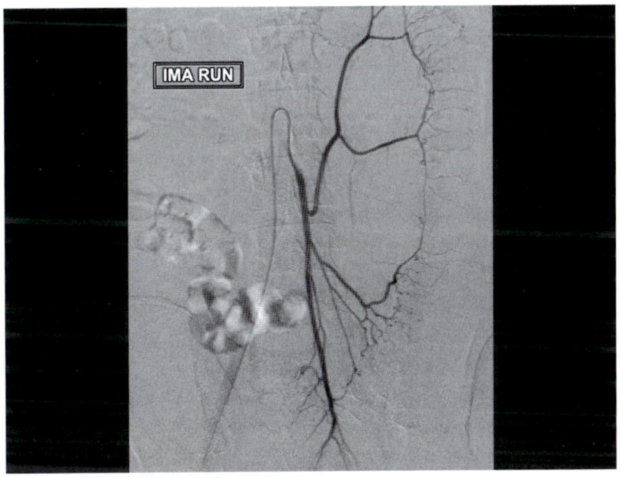

FIG. 3: DSA run showing inferior mesenteric artery (IMA) and its branches.

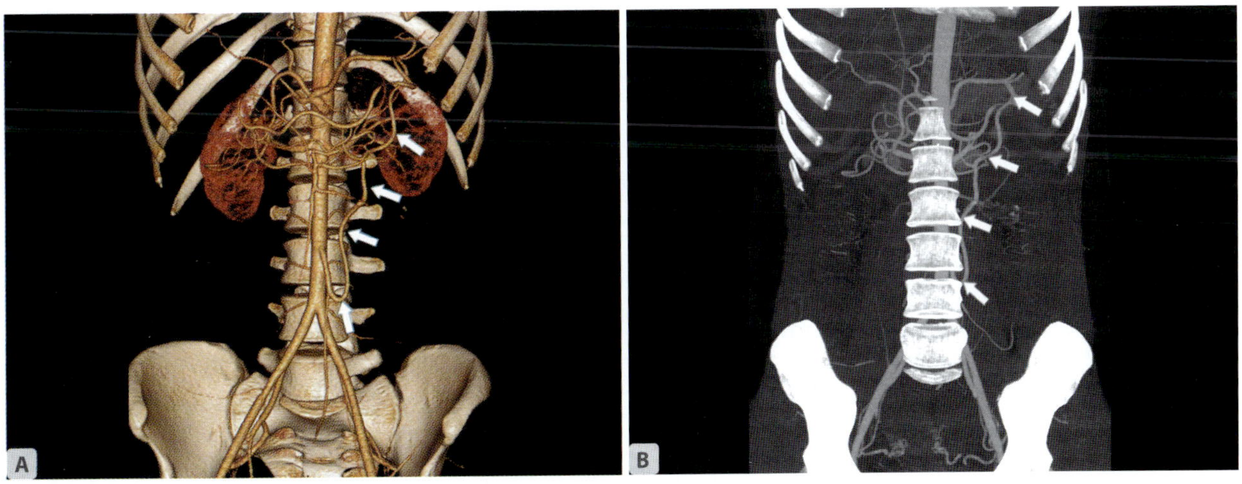

FIGS. 4A AND B: Coronal CT images (volume rendered and MIP) showing proximal superior mesenteric artery obstruction with arc of Riolan (arrows) reconstituting distal superior mesenteric artery (SMA) and its branches.

common channel with splenic vein and join superior mesenteric vein (SMV) to form portal vein.

ETIOLOGY

Ischemic bowel disease is classified based on the time of presentation, anatomic segment of bowel involved and etiopathogenesis of disease **(Table 1)**.

PATHOPHYSIOLOGY OF ISCHEMIC BOWEL DISEASE

Ischemic injury deprives nutrition and oxygen supply necessary for cellular metabolism and their intactness. Collateral vessels are recruited after major vessel occlusion due to arterial pressure drop distal to the occlusion and provide alternate pathway to maintain the viability of the bowel. However, after critical period of time, persistence of ischemia causes development of vasoconstriction in the obstructed bed, elevating the arterial pressure and hampering the collateral flow. Arterial obstruction cause vasospasm with subsequent loss of cellular integrity, whereas venous ischemia causes blood column stasis with edema and subsequently reduced arterial blood flow causing mucosal cellular detachment. The common outcome in both these conditions is intestinal necrosis and peritonitis in its natural course. Persistent hypoxia or reperfusion injury plays a central role in setting and propagation of ischemic injury through oxidant free radical damage. It is essential to understand, differentiate and define the nature of vascular obstructive pathology radiologically, as the prognosis significantly differs with a mortality rate of 89% in the arterial occlusion and 11% in the venous obstruction.[4]

Understanding the ischemic pathology is important as the radiological findings correlate with extent of disease process as shown in **Table 2.**[4] The acute bowel ischemia evolves over time and includes 3 stages based on the extent of bowel wall involved; further superinfection of the involved segment facilitates necrosis and perforation.[1] The first radiological change seen on CT is secondary to vasodilatation, which is manifested as diffuse wall hyperdensity on both arterial and venous phases. This implies that ischemia has yet not progressed to advanced stage and is possibly reversible, if treated expediently. If ischemia persists and is severe enough, leads to vasoconstriction thereby hampering the collateral flow, which manifests as reduced bowel wall enhancement. Persistence of ischemia leads to necrosis of the bowel wall causing proliferation and migration of microbial flora into the bowel wall resulting in pneumatoses intestinalis, air in mesenteric and portal veins and their branches. Subsequently advanced cases result in bowel perforation causing pneumoperitoneum, retropneumoperitoneum and ascites.[4]

Stage 1	Stage 2	Stage 3
• Reversible • Pathology limited to mucosa only	Pathology extends to submucosa and muscularis propria	• Transmural involvement • Highest mortality

TABLE 1: Bowel ischemia types and etiology.[3]

A. Mesenteric ischemia	
1. *Acute*:	
i. Occlusive (80%)	Thromboembolism
Occlusive arterial	Dissection/transection
Occlusive venous	Closed loop obstruction
(10–15%)	Thrombophilia and hypercoagulable states
	Hypotension and shock
ii. Nonocclusive (20–30%)	Drugs (ergots/cocaine)
	Atherosclerotic disease
2. Chronic	Arterial hyperplasia
	Vasculitides
B. Colonic ischemia	Nonocclusive causes such as hypotension and vasculitides Occlusive causes
C. Ischemic enterocolitis	Vasculitides Latrogenic/traumatic vascular injury

ACUTE MESENTERIC ISCHEMIA

Acute mesenteric ischemia is an abdominal emergency accounting for 5% of hospital admissions, which may be potentially life-threatening if not treated expediently. The reported mortality rate is high ranging ~60–80%, representing the extreme sensitivity of the small intestine to reduced blood supply.[5] Acute mesenteric ischemia results from occlusive and nonocclusive vascular pathology, and is further subclassified into arterial, venous or both categories depending upon the vascular structure involved. Understanding the pattern of bowel changes aids in accurate diagnosis and planning appropriate treatment.

TABLE 2: Radiopathological correlation of CT findings in ischemic bowel disease.

Pathologic events	CT imaging correlation
• Early vasodiltation • Vasoconstriction	• Wall hyperdensity (in both arterial and venous phase) • Absence/reduced bowel wall enhancement
Increased vascular permeability	• Bowel wall thickening • Bowel luminal dilatation
Mucosal cellular necrosis and microflora proliferation	• Pneumatoses intestinalis • Mesenteric/portal venous gas
Transmural bowel necrosis and bowel perforation	• Pneumoperitoneum • Retropneumoperitoneum • Ascites

Superior Mesenteric Artery Thromboembolism

The superior mesenteric artery is the most predisposed arterial trunk involved by the thromboembolic events due to anatomic factors including wide caliber and narrow take off angle at its origin. Most commonly embolus lodges in initial ~3 to 8 cm from its origin **(Figs. 5A to C)**. Embolic event related ischemic patient generally present acutely, whereas it is not uncommon for thrombotic patients to present subacutely due to antecedent partially occluding atherosclerotic plaques causing collateral development. This group of patients may present as mesenteric angina and chronic mesenteric ischemia, or may present acutely due to superimposed thrombus in background of atherosclerotic disease causing ambient radiological features. Thromboembolic events are usually seen with pre-existing cardiovascular comorbidities such as atrial fibrillation, myocardial infarction, complicated atherosclerotic plaques, mycotic aneurysm, vasculitis and arterial dissection.[6]

Venous Mesenteric Ischemia

Less commonly venous occlusion cause mesenteric ischemia accounting for ~10% of bowel ischemia. Venous occlusive ischemic disease is seen in relatively younger patents with mortality rate of ~10–40%.[5] Closed loop obstruction is the most common cause for venous bowel ischemia **(Figs. 6A and B)**. Venous thrombosis may also be seen in patients with hyper coagulable hematological disorders, vasculitides, and less frequently in pregnancy, OCP consumption and underlying inflammatory conditions like SLE.[1]

Nonocclusive Mesenteric Ischemia

Nonocclusive mesenteric ischemia is seen commonly with patients admitted in critical care units and is multifactorial in cause, constituting 20–30% of ischemic disease. Due to its uncertain etiology and compromised host status mortality rate is generally high ranging 30–90%. Systemic hypotension provoke autoregulation and homeostasis, preserving cardiac and brain blood supply along with associated splanchnic

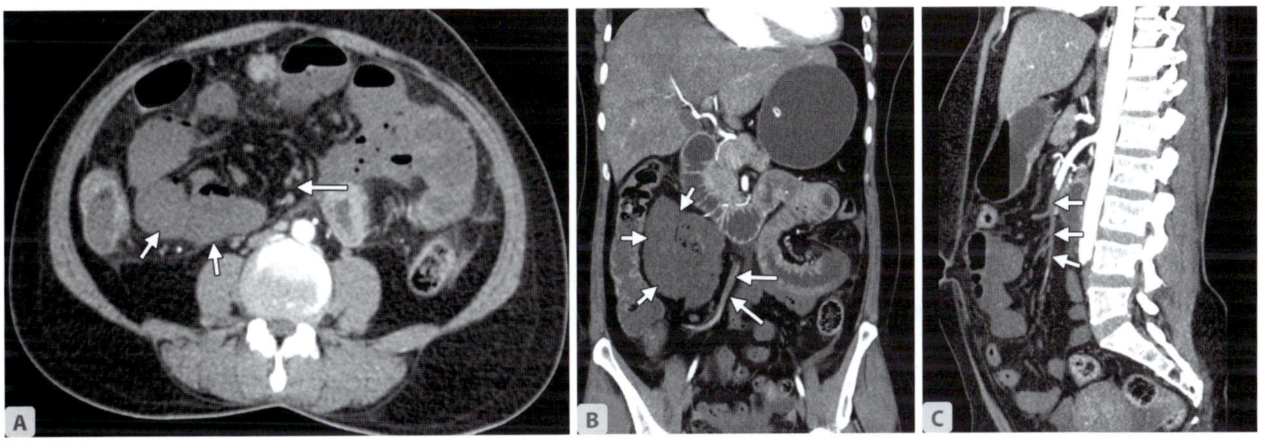

FIGS. 5A TO C: Axial, coronal, sagittal reconstructed CT images showing complete occlusion of the superior mesenteric artery (long arrows) with nonenhancing proximal small bowel loops in the right side of abdomen (short arrows).

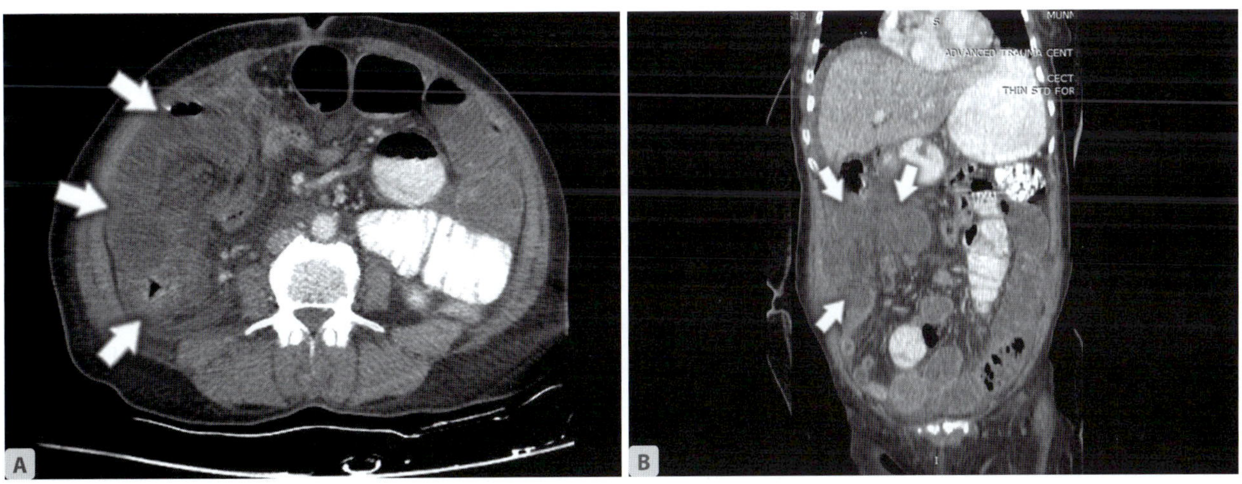

FIGS. 6A AND B: Venous ischemia secondary to closed loop (arrows) obstruction in the right upper quadrant with engorgement of vessels and fluid in the mesentery with thickened bowel wall.

vasoconstriction. Shock bowel injury generally seen with hypotensive and low cardiac output states. Any form of shock, renal failure with overly dialysis, drugs such as cocaine, amphetamines and ergotamines are attributed to causal role in nonischemic mesenteric ischemia.[1]

Imaging Modalities

Acute mesenteric ischemia patients generally present with vague clinical features and it is challenging to accurately diagnose this condition early, as it is utmost important to manage the condition timely, since the delay in the management will reflect in worse prognosis and higher mortality rates.

Plain radiographs may be the initial investigation preferred in patients presenting with acute abdomen. The findings are generally nonspecific and may demonstrate dilated bowel loops, thumb printing in early ischemic phase and may show pneumatoses, portal venous gas and pneumoperitoneum in advanced ischemic stage.[4] The sensitivity is significantly low and normal radiograph does not exclude ischemic bowel disease **(Fig. 7)**.[7]

Ultrasonography is the another common modality employed for evaluation of patients presenting with acute abdomen and its role is mainly to exclude other potential causes of acute abdomen. The diagnostic yield in patients with mesenteric ischemia is more often suboptimal due to gaseous distension of bowel loops causing technical difficulty in evaluation of mesenteric vasculature.[4]

In the present modern era with significant technological advancements, MDCT is the investigation of choice for evaluating patients with suspected ischemic bowel disease. It has nearly replaced conventional angiography for diagnostic purposes and aids in making the correct diagnosis, as well as excluding other alternative pathologies.[3] In patients with ischemia CT examination can help in understanding pathophysiology to accurately diagnose and to characterize arterial versus venous occlusive disease, grade the severity of the disease, help in planning accurate treatment and also provide vital prognostic information. Comprehensive assessment of the bowel wall, mesenteric vasculature and surrounding mesentery is essential for the overall estimation of the severity and extent of the disease.[8]

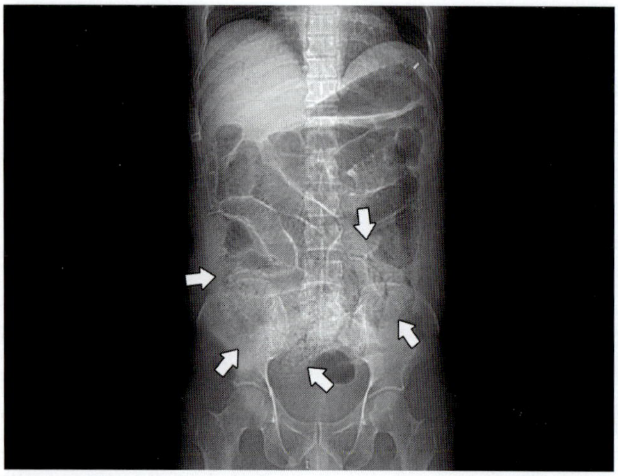

FIG. 7: Abdominal radiograph showing dilated bowel loops with pneumatosis intestinalis (arrows).

Technical Aspects

The study protocol consists of biphasic CT abdomen with an arterial phase (35–40 sec) performed for evaluating the arterial stenosis and occlusions, and venous phase (65–70 sec) for assessing the mesenteric venous system and various abdominal viscera for changes of ischemia. Nonenhanced CT has been shown to be of benefit in some studies in literature as it can better evaluate the submucosal hemorrhage, hyperdense clots and also provide baseline attenuation of the bowel.[1,4] However, this is controversial subject as it adds to the radiation burden and timeliness and therefore remains contentious issue.

Pearl

Biphasic protocol with both arterial and venous phases is the standard imaging protocol in all patients with suspected mesenteric ischemia and arterial phase should not to be excluded from the examination in order to achieve dose reduction.

The role of oral contrast is again controversial in literature and preference is individualistic. In patients presenting acutely CT is obtained only with IV contrast, to expedite the study, although these cases may be technically difficult to evaluate due to inadequate distension of the bowel loops. In patients presenting with more subacute features, neutral oral contrast is generally preferred by most radiologists as it is helps in better assessment of the bowel wall and also improves the assessment of vascular tree by various post processing techniques.[1] Present generation MDCT scanners allow volumetric data acquisition which can be further postprocessed by various dedicated computer softwares on work stations. MPR and 3D reconstructions help in better anatomical and vascular evaluation, and increase the confidence of the radiologist in making an accurate diagnosis.[4] Masking the bowel enhancement pattern and interference with 3D reconstruction is a major drawback of administration of positive oral contrast agents and is therefore not generally recommended.[1]

The administration with IV contrast material CT examination may reveal dilated and thickened bowel loops associated with ascites and mesenteric edema in initial stages of acute mesenteric ischemia, whereas pneumatoses, pneumoperitoneum and portal and mesenteric venous gas signify advanced ischemic stage **(Figs. 8A and B)**. CTA and its dedicated reconstruction techniques such as MIP (maximum intensity projection), tissue transition projections (TTP) and vessel probe (VP) are more specific and often demonstrate arterial occlusions as filling defect within the vessel lumen with/without associated collateral formation **(Figs. 9A and B)**[4]. Similarly venous thrombosis is identified as central filling defect with mural rim enhancement.[9]

CT features of nonocclusive mesenteric ischemia are overlapping with other inflammatory or infectious conditions involving the bowel, which makes it challenging to diagnose this condition. CT findings may be variable from focal

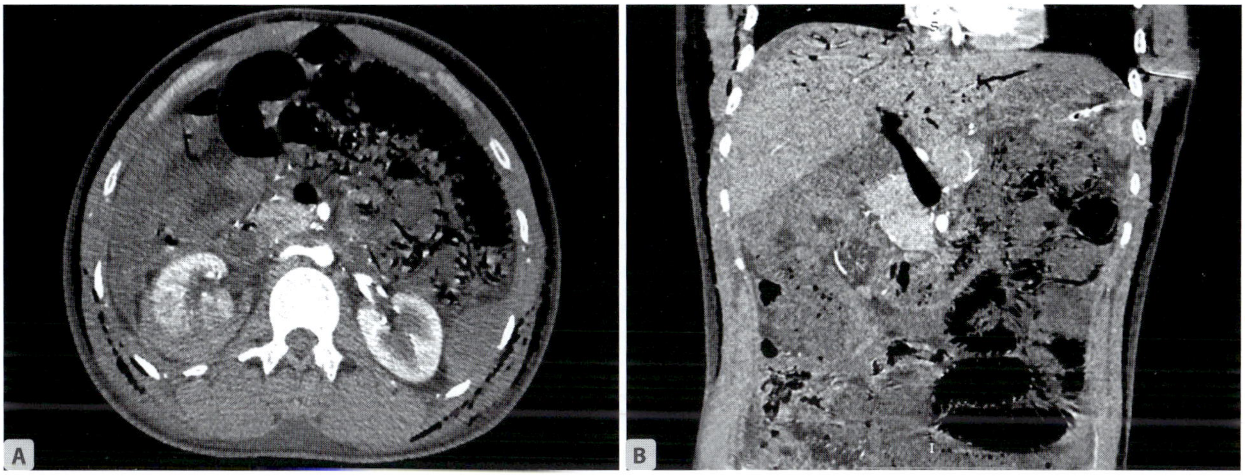

FIGS. 8A AND B: Patient of blunt trauma abdomen: Axial and coronal reconstructed CT images showing extensive pneumatosis, air in the mesenteric/portal venous branches and hemoperitoneum. Note is made of right renal contusion with perinephric hematoma.

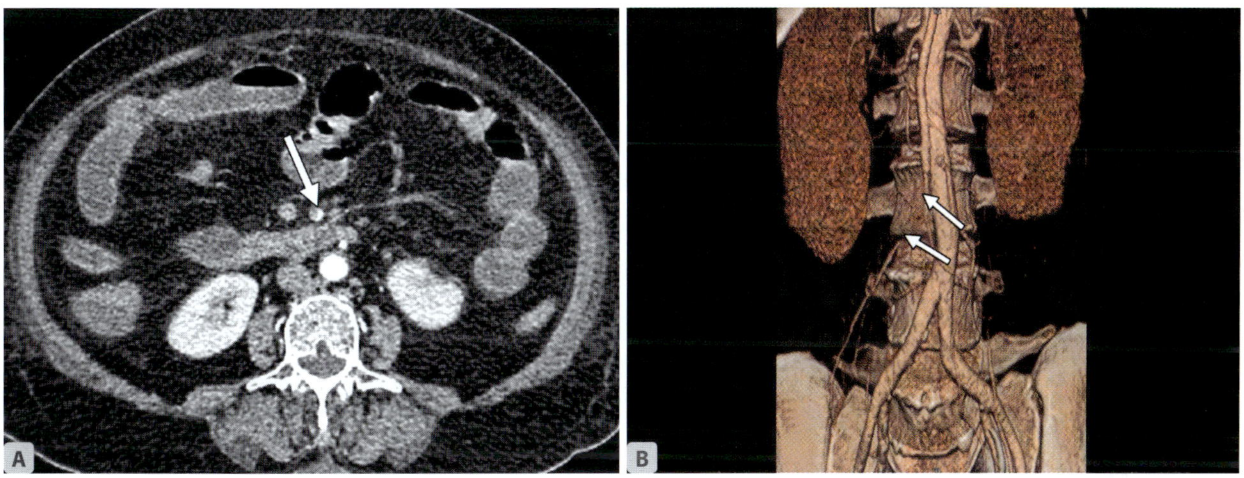

FIGS. 9A AND B: Axial, and volume rendered (VR) CT images showing occlusion of the branch of superior mesenteric artery (long arrows).

mucosal damage in watershed areas to the damage of entire bowel. Small bowel loops generally show mural thickening with hyperenhancement.[1] Usually there is normal appearing colon. Ancillary features like reduced caliber of inferior vena cava and abdominal aorta may be identified along with intraperitoneal fluid in hypoperfusion conditions.[13] Appropriate and confident diagnosis of nonocclusive mesenteric ischemia is possible by angiography, which may show narrowing of origins of SMA branches, irregularity and spasm of mesenteric arcades **(Figs. 11A to C)**.

Regardless of the etiology, CT imaging features represent obstructive state traits and are based on pathophysiologic state of the disease. Few pattern of traits may aid in differentiating occlusive and non occlusive causes **(Table 3)**. Arterial occlusion generally causes paper thin bowel wall and hypoattenuation; whereas venous occlusive disease result in markedly thickened oedematous bowel wall, early mesenteric fat stranding and marked luminal dilatation seen even in the early stages **(Figs. 12A and B)**. Similar changes are however seen in advanced cases of arterial ischemia progressed to transmural necrosis **(Table 4)**. Distinguishing CT imaging features of arterial and venous ischemia are enumerated in **Table 4**.[1,10]

Dual energy CT with iodine overlay technique may be useful in detecting subtle bowel wall enhancement to differentiate ischemia from infective/inflammatory bowel wall thickening.[11]

Conventional angiography (DSA) is the gold standard for the evaluation and treatment of arterial thromboembolism. Acute mesenteric thromboembolism is visualized as filling defect, occluding the arterial lumen with/without collateral channels. Assessment of the distal vascular occlusion and catheter directed intervention may be performed in suitably selected patients. Angiography is also suitable for cases in which diagnosis is uncertain on CT; however, angiography is mainly performed with an intent of therapeutic purposes for performing interventions like thrombolysis, aspiration of thrombus or vasodilatory medication administration in patients where diagnosis has already been made on CT.[12]

MR is another advanced modality which has been employed in patients with mesenteric ischemia, its role in cases of acute mesenteric ischemia is generally not advocated due to long imaging duration and critical status of the patients.[13] Patients with subacute/chronic features may be assessed by gadolinium enhanced MRA which can provide accurate assessment of the mesenteric vasculature

TABLE 3: Clinical and CT features of mesenteric ischemia.[1]

Features	Arterial occlusive ischemia	Venous occlusive ischemia	Nonocclusive mesenteric ischemia
Time of onset	Acute, chronic, acute on chronic	Acute or chronic	Acute or chronic
Predisposing conditions	Atrial fibrillation, recent myocardial infarction, atherosclerosis, aortic dissection, vasculitis, drugs like ergotamine and cocaine	Closed loop bowel obstruction and strangulation, hypercoagulable disorders, portal hypertension, pregnancy, malignancy, oral contraceptive pills (OCP)	Hypotension and shock, vasculitis, vasoconstricting drugs
Bowel wall status	May be thin in acute state or may be thickened with associated inflammation and edema	Edematous, markedly thickened bowel wall	Thickened bowel wall
Bowel wall enhancement	Depending on state of reperfusion, may nonenhance before reperfusion and may hyperenhance in reperfused state	Target sign with significant mucosal hyperenhancement **(Figs. 10A and B)**	Reduced enhancement
Mesenteric vasculature	Arterial stenosis/occlusion, aneurysm, dissection	Venous thrombosis	Nonspecific, with pruning of distal mesenteric vascular branches
Mesentery	Mesenteric fat stranding and free fluid in advanced stages	Significant mesenteric fat stranding and free fluid in early stages	Variable

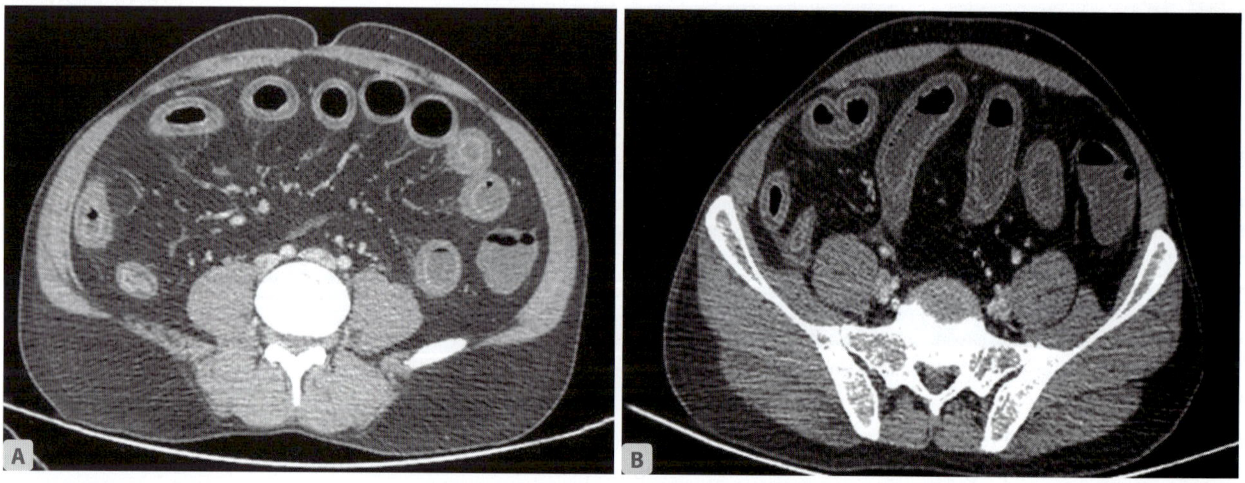

FIGS. 10A AND B: Axial CT images showing characteristic target sign with mucosal and serosal hyperenhancement in a patient of venous ischemia.

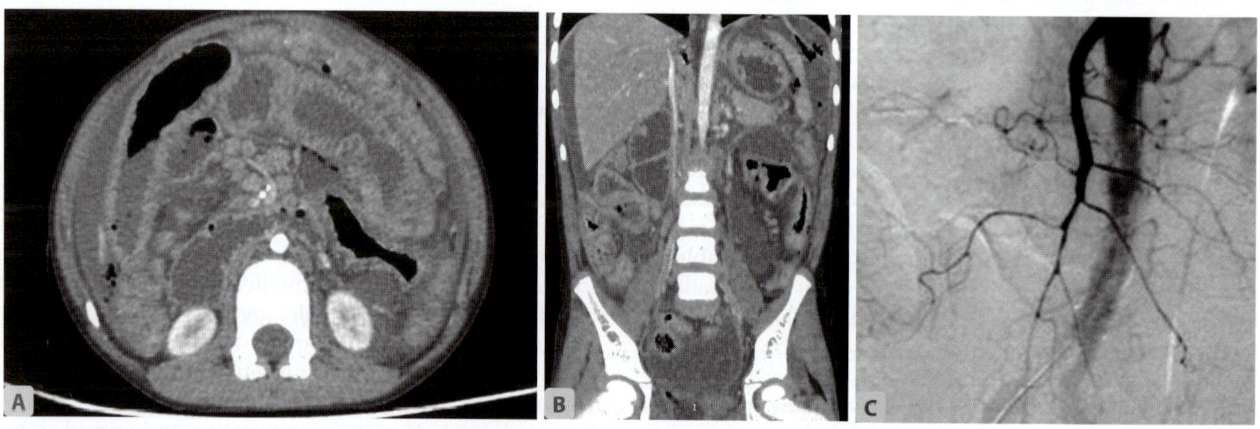

FIGS. 11A TO C: Patient of cardiogenic shock, CT Axial (A) and coronal (B) section showing reduced caliber of abdominal aorta with chinked IVC and showing diffuse concentric mural thickening involving bowel loops with ascites. DSA (C) SMA run showing reduced caliber and paucity of the distal branches with pruning.

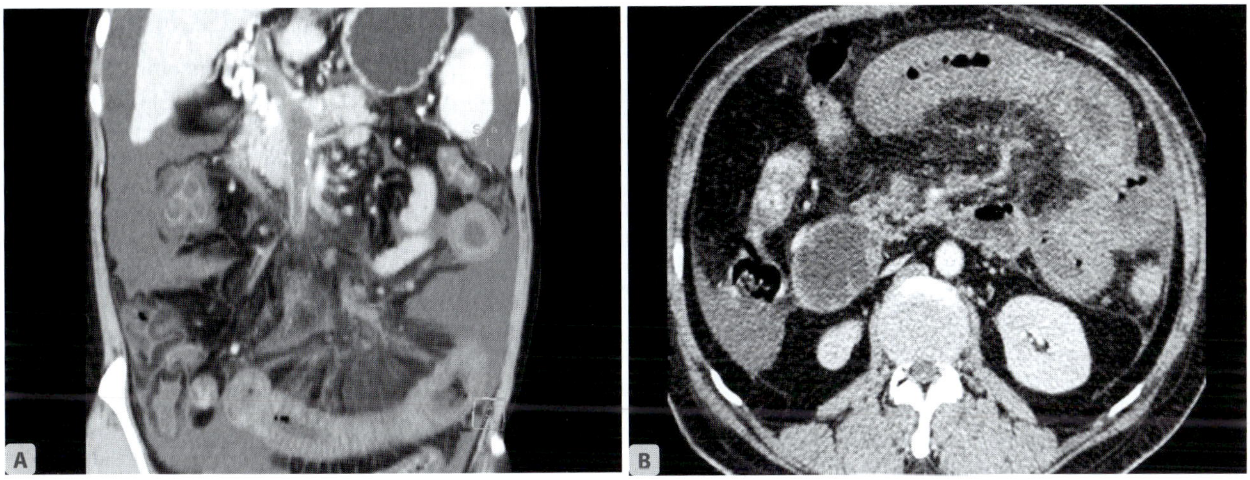

FIGS. 12A AND B: (A) Coronal CT image showing splenoportal thrombosis with thickened bowel loops and engorgement of mesenteric vessels suggestive of early venous ischemia; (B) Another patient of venous ischemia showing markedly thickened bowel wall with mesenteric changes.

TABLE 4: CT imaging features to differentiate arterial and venous occlusive ischemia.[10]

Arterial occlusion	Venous occlusion
Superior mesenteric artery (SMA) thrombosis	Superior mesenteric vein (SMV) thrombosis
No/subtle bowel wall enhancement	Hypo/Hyperdense bowel wall
Thinned out bowel wall	Significantly thickened bowel wall
Mucosal nonenhancement	Mucosal hyperenhancement
Bowel dilatation after transmural infarction	Dilated bowel lumen without infarction
Late mesenteric stranding, hemorrhage or edema	Marked early mesenteric fat stranding and hemorrhage

Note: Advanced cases of both arterial and venous ischemia show similar imaging manifestations such as air in mesenteric and portal venous system, pneumoperitoneum and retropneumoperitoneum.

TABLE 5: ACR appropriateness criteria for imaging acute ischemic bowel disease.[15]

Radiologic modality	Rating	Remarks
CTA abdomen with IV contrast	9	• Fast • Noninvasive • Evaluates other causes
Arteriography abdomen	8	Diagnosis and treatment in single procedure
X-ray abdomen	7	Initial tool to evaluate acute abdomen
MRA abdomen without and with IV contrast	7	• Time consuming • Limited benefits in distal thromboembolism and NOMI
US abdomen	6	• Better for venous occlusion • Assess other causes of abdominal pain
MRA abdomen without IV contrast	3	Lower sensitivity and specificity

Rating scale: 7, 8, 9 usually appropriate; 4, 5, 6 may be appropriate; 1, 2, 3 usually not appropriate.

comparable to CT evaluation. Experimental studies have shown that MR techniques may be able to differentiate between acutely ischemic and infarcted segments based on signal changes on T2 weighted images and postcontrast gadolinium images.[14]

American college of radiology (ACR) has formulated rating system for various radiological modalities aiding in systematic, appropriate and timely evaluation of suspected ischemia in various clinical conditions **(Table 5)**.

Treatment of Acute Mesenteric Ischemia

Immediately prompt treatment is instituted after established diagnosis of acute mesenteric ischemia and treatment aims at revascularization of the mesenteric vessels to prevent further bowel ischemia. Early medical supportive management include fluid resuscitation, naso gastric/orogastric tube decompression, and anticoagulation. Broad spectrum antibiotics must be administered and care must be taken to avoid vasoconstrictive drug administration especially in nonocclusive mesenteric ischemic patients. The emphasis of treatment has shifted from surgical approach to endovascular therapy in recent years.

In the presence of peritoneal signs, emergency laparotomy recommended, immediate surgical embolectomy or bypass with resection of nonviable bowel is essential and intraoperatively meticulous bowel assessment for its viability is necessary. A second look laparotomy may be required after emergency surgery owing to vasospasm of normal vascular tree, inadequate resection of ischemic segment, doubtful perfusion of bowel segments or the condition of the patient fails to stabilize.[16]

Catheter guided therapies are performed on patients without frank imaging and clinical features suggestive of gangrene/bowel necrosis; these may be in the form of aspiration embolectomy or catheter thrombolysis using rt-PA or urokinase. If atherosclerotic changes are noted in in the vessel wall, this procedure can be electively followed by a percutaneous transluminal angioplasty with or without stenting. PTA with stent placement is more effective in immediate and long-term vessel patency than PTA alone as stents offered additional structural support to the vessel wall leading to lesser repeat interventions.[17] Endovascular techniques have led to a decrease in surgery related complications including decreased amount of bowel resected leading to lower incidence of short bowel syndrome, lesser incidence of systemic complications and reduced mortality.[18]

Acute nonocclusive mesenteric ischemia can be treated in the same sitting in which diagnostic catheter angiography is done for confirmation of diagnosis. The typical treatment consists of administration of intra-arterial vasodilators like papaverine, nitroglycerin or glucagon. Intravenous high dose prostaglandin E1 is equally effective in management if transarterial catheterization is not feasible. However, these vasodilator drugs can lead to systemic hypotension which must be taken care during the procedure.[18]

The mainstay of treatment of venous mesenteric ischemia is systemic anticoagulation. Long-term maintenance therapy on anticoagulants has a higher chance of recanalization of occluded veins and lower incidence of recurrence. One of its complications can be bleeding in the gangrenous bowel, however this should not prevent or delay in administration of the systemic anticoagulant and bleeding has to be managed if it occurs. Transhepatic or transjugular cannulation of the SMV and thrombolysis with or without thrombectomy needs to be considered in acute or subacute venous occlusion depending on the severity of the condition to prevent bowel infarction. Adjunct transjugular intrahepatic portosystemic shunt (TIPS) can be created to improve the outflow of the venous system.[18]

CHRONIC MESENTERIC ISCHEMIA

Chronic mesenteric ischemia is an uncommon condition which generally affects elderly population often with widespread atherosclerosis. The diagnosis is often late in its course as atleast two of the three major mesenteric vascular trunks, should have significant luminal narrowing before developing symptoms **(Figs. 13A and B)**.[19] Central clue for making the diagnosis of chronic mesenteric ischemia is not only the presence of significant vascular stenosis, but also prominent and tortuous collateral conduits between the mesenteric trunks which maintain the bowel viability. Frequently patients with this condition will be elderly, fragile, females who experience postprandial abdominal pain, develop fear of food and often avoid meals resulting in chronic weight loss.[20,21] Widespread atherosclerosis of the abdominal vasculature is the most frequent cause of chronic mesenteric ischemia, other less common conditions like vasculitis, radiation vasculopathy and fibromuscular dysplasia also cause chronic mesenteric ischemia **(Figs. 14A and B)**.[19,22]

Imaging Modalities

Noninvasive imaging modalities such as US, CTA, MRI/MRA are employed for the evaluation.[12] Angiography has its role in further evaluation of equivocal diagnosis or if endovascular treatment is contemplated.[12] According to ACR appropriateness criteria for evaluation of chronic mesenteric ischemia, the preference of the imaging modalities is discussed in the **Table 6**.

CT and CT angiography is the primary diagnostic tool as it allows accurate diagnosis and excludes other alternative causes of the clinical condition. CTA allows confident depiction of vascular tree with occlusions/stenosis and collateral channel formation. Mesenteric vasculature is better demonstrated by 3D imaging techniques and other post-processing tools available in the modern work stations.

Duplex USG is another promising modality which has an important role in nonacute presentations. Sonography alongwith color and spectral Doppler correlation can detect hemodynamically significant stenosis in proximal CA and SMA **(Figs. 15A to D)**. Peak systolic velocity of >275 cm/s and >200 cm/s in SMA and celiac trunk respectively, are reliable indicators of 70% or more stenosis in the fasting state.[9,23] Comparison of pre- and postprandial peak systolic velocity may also suggest vascular occlusion.

MRA also been shown to have comparable accuracy to CTA for evaluation of stenosis in the mesenteric vessels. Noncontrast sequences (time of flight and phase contrast) can be employed in patients with renal function derangement in addition to the benefit of no radiation exposure. In chronic mesenteric ischemia, insufficient collateral channels may fail to meet the metabolic demands of bowel with decreased blood oxygenation in superior mesenteric vein or other mesenteric veins. This deranged physiology can also be assessed through MR perfusion techniques coupled with food challenge. Cine contrast phase imaging and MR oximetry can evaluate superior mesenteric vein flow and blood oxygenation respectively.[24] Decrease in superior mesenteric venous flow in phase contrast imaging and reduction in

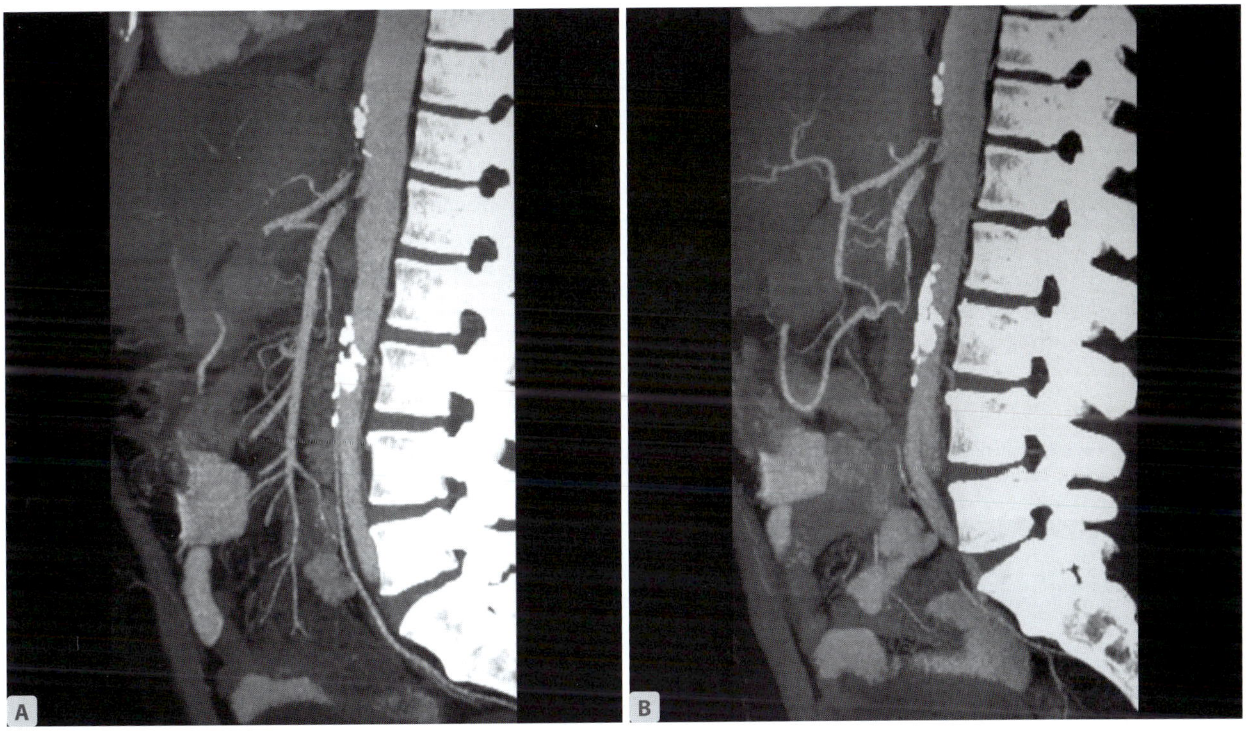

FIGS. 13A AND B: Patient of chronic mesenteric ischemia: Sagittal reconstructed CT images showing atherosclerotic changes with hemodynamically significant stenosis in the proximal celiac trunk and SMA.

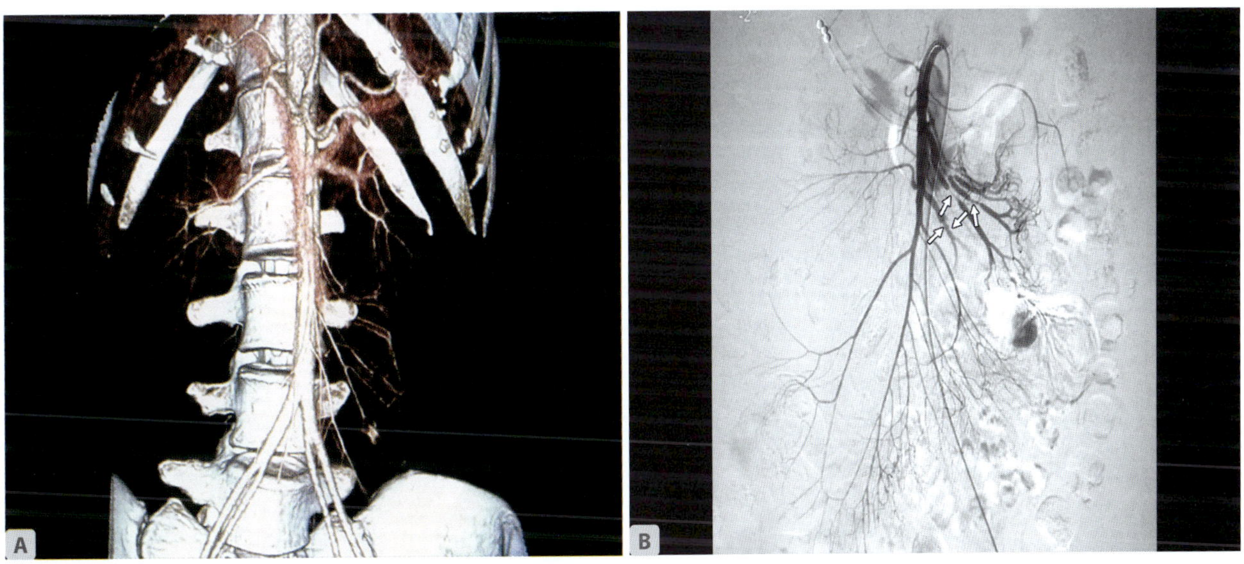

FIGS. 14A AND B: Patient of vasculitis with mesenteric angina: Volume rendered CT image showing subtle irregularity in the branches of SMA. DSA SMA run confirming the irregularities and multifocal narrowings in the branches of SMA.

superior mesenteric venous blood oxygenation level with resultant T2 value reduction after food challenge is noted with symptomatic chronic mesenteric ischemic patients.[24] However, lengthy acquisition time and inability to accurately evaluate the narrower caliber vessels such as IMA and other smaller branches are limitations in practice.

Treatment

Considering the individual patient anatomical factors and comorbities; life style changes surgery or endovascular treatment is advised, for relief of symptoms and to halt progression of chronic mesenteric ischemia into more acute events.[12,25,26] Angioplasty and stenting of the affected vascular

TABLE 6: ACR appropriateness criteria to evaluate chronic mesenteric ischemia.[15]

Radiologic modality	Rating	Remarks
CTA abdomen with IV contrast	9	• Fast • Noninvasive • Evaluate other etiology
Arteriography abdomen	7	Diagnosis and treatment in single procedure
US abdomen	7	• Better for venous occlusive cause • Evaluate other causes
MRA abdomen without and with IV contrast	7	• Time consuming • Limited role in distal thromboembolism and NOMI
X-ray abdomen	3	Normal study does not exclude ischemia
MRA abdomen without IV contrast	3	Lower sensitivity and specificity

Rating scale: 7, 8, 9 usually appropriate; 4, 5, 6 may be appropriate; 1, 2, 3 usually not appropriate.

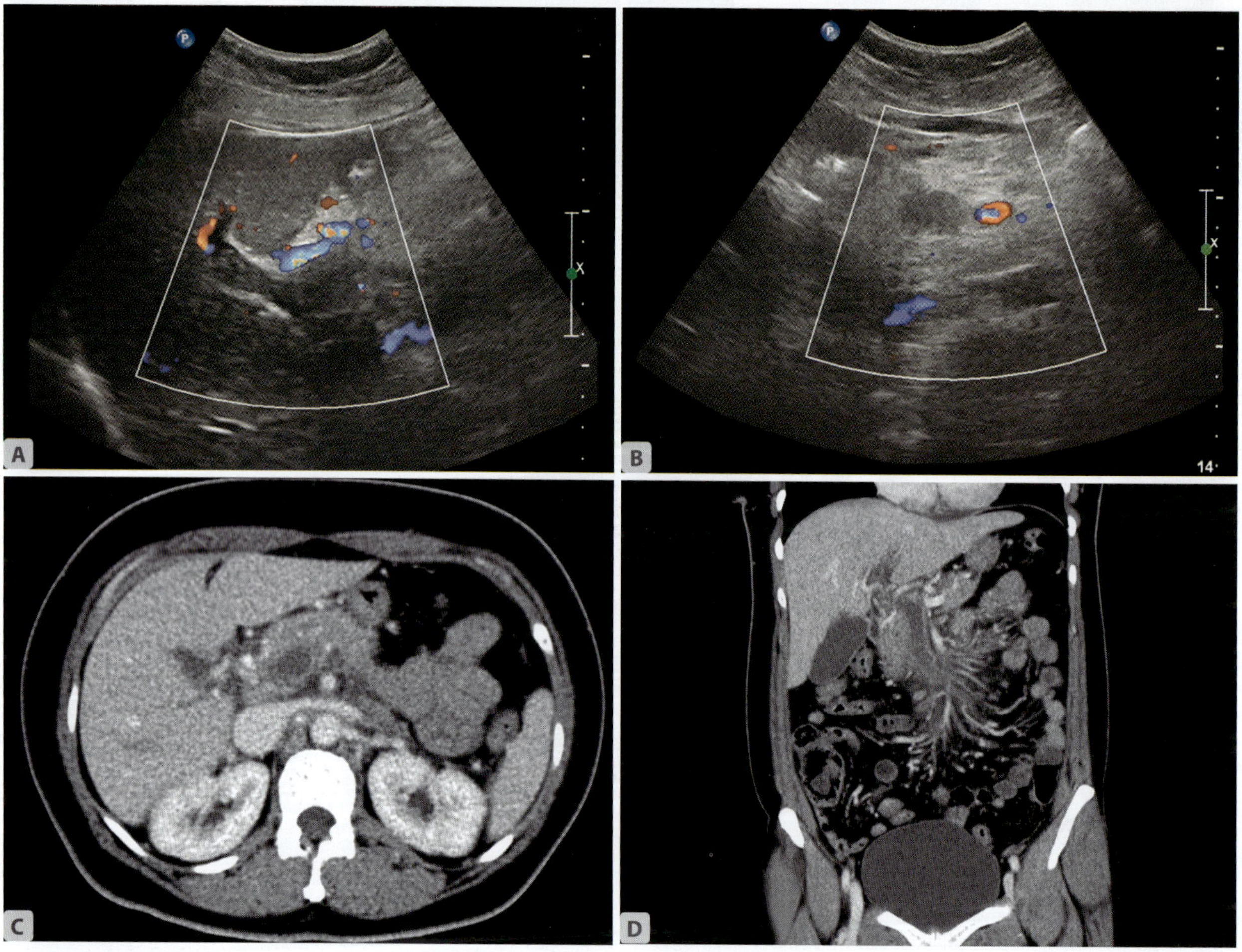

FIGS. 15A TO D: Doppler ultrasound images (A and B) showing dilated SMV and portal vein with no color filling suggestive of thrombosis; (C and D) Axial and coronal images confirming SMV and portal venous thrombosis.

segment are the endovascular procedures performed on affected vessels with high initial technical success rates of >90%. However, recurrent stenosis is not uncommon and reintervention is recommended **(Figs. 16A to F)**.[26-29] Endarterectomy, vascular bypass and arterial re implantation are the surgically available options for treating chronic mesenteric ischemia.[25] Revascularization of single vessel (usually SMA) is sufficient with long-term patency rate of 70-93%, despite multi vessel involvement.[25]

COLONIC ISCHEMIA

Colonic ischemia is the most common form of intestinal ischemia, usually seen in 7th decade of life, and second

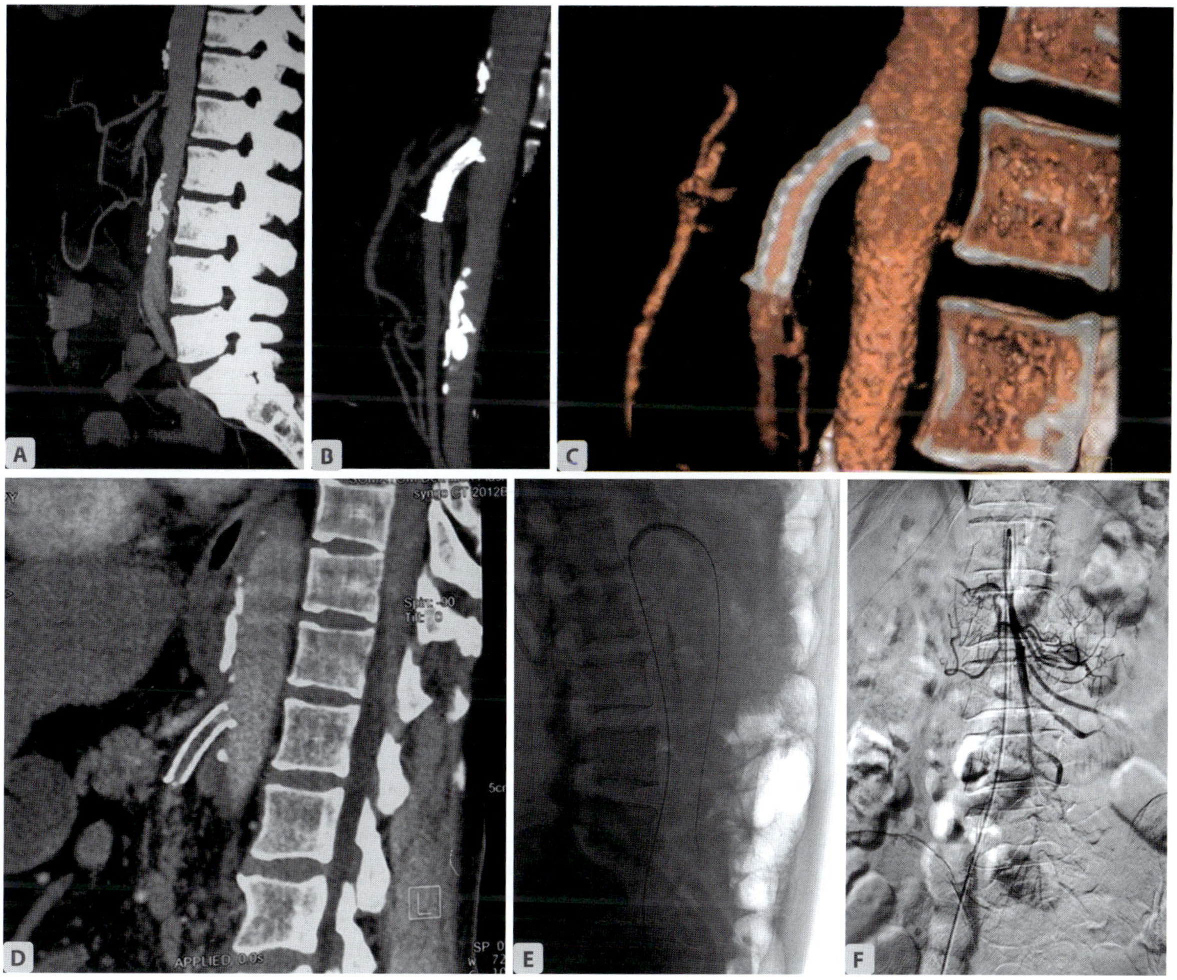

FIGS. 16A TO F: (A) Patient of chronic mesenteric ischemia with short segment stenosis involving proximal celiac trunk and SMA; (B and C) Metallic stenting performed in proximal SMA with good distal opacification; (D) Relapse of symptoms with CT repeated after 7 months showed in stent thrombosis with poor distal flow; (E and F) Reintervention with balloon dilatation performed across the stent with restored flow in the distal SMA and relief of symptoms.

Courtesy: Dr Vivek Gupta and Anupam Lal, Department of Radiodiagnosis, PGIMER, Chandigarh, India.

most frequent cause of lower gastrointestinal bleeding.[30] Underlying pathophysiologic changes are due to altered circulation, failing in meeting colonic metabolic demands. Most commonly vascular compromise results from non-occlusive etiology such as hypoperfusion states, vasculitis and other vasculopathy. Only 25% of patients are attributed to vascular occlusion.[31]

Vascular compromise can cause evolution of pathophysiologic changes in colon, may be seen sequentially as mucosal/submucosal damage, reversible colitis, ulcerative changes, stricture formation and gangrenous changes.[13,31] Patients usually present with mild lower abdominal pain and bloody diarrhea.[32] Water shed areas of colon such as Sudecks point and Griffith points in splenic flexure and sigmoid colon are more prone for ischemic changes.[33]

Diagnosis

Radiographic changes depends upon the underlying pathophysiology and severity of bowel necrosis. Plain abdominal radiographic features can vary from normal study to very severe damage resulting in pneumo/retropneumoperitoneum. Other features such as nonspecific ileus, thumb printing, transverse ridging and a haustration may be observed, occasionally pneumatosis or portal venous gas may be identified due to transmural bowel necrosis.[34,35]

Barium examination features vary with stage and degree of ischemic damage, serial changes in the barium study characteristics is the hallmark feature of colonic ischemia.[36-38] Features observed on barium studies may include thumb printing (most common), transverse ridging, spasm, ulceration, intramural barium and stricture formation.[34] Ultrasonography also demonstrates non specific bowel wall thickening and diminished color flow in involved bowel segment.[23]

CECT has become the gold standard investigation for diagnosing ischemic colitis which usually involves a specific segment of colon.[32] This is in contrary to the infective/inflammatory etiology which may be patchy or diffuse and is generally nonsegmental colonic involvement. Most common bowel segment affected is left colon;[32] CT features of ischemia include target/double halo sign, shaggy irregular contours, pneumatosis intestinalis, portal venous gas, peritoneal fluid, or pneumoperitoneum.[32] Limitations of CT evaluation is lack of specificity and difficult assessment of the bowel wall thickening secondary to inadequate bowel distension.[32] Also in colonic ischemia, initial imaging features cannot be utilised for definite prognostication.

Colonoscopic evaluation is the most sensitive diagnostic tool for colonic ischemia evaluation, and specific location and patchy segmental involvement may help in diagnosis. Favier classification is widely utilised by clinicians to make the diagnosis, to ascertain prognosis and to decide surgical intervention.[39,40]

Treatment

Correction of hypovolemia and treating primary cause is primary goal. Medical management consists of gastric rest, fluid and electrolyte management, administration of broad spectrum antibiotics and prophylaxis against venous thromboembolism. Resection of ischemic bowel with/without bowel anastomosis and/or cholecystectomy is the surgical management available for suitable patients.[32]

ACKNOWLEDGMENTS

Dr Muniraju M and Dr Akash Bansal, Department of Radiodiagnosis.

REFERENCES

1. Dhatt HS, Behr SC, Miracle A, Wang ZJ, Yeh BM, et al. Radiological evaluation of bowel ischemia. Radiol clin N Am. 2015;53:1241-54.
2. Gourley EJ, Gering SA. The meandering mesenteric artery: a historic review and surgical implications. Dis Colon Rectum. 2005;48(5):996-1000.
3. Upponi S, Harvey JJ, Uberoi R, Ganeshan A, et al. The role of radiology in the diagnosis and treatment of mesenteric ischemia. Postgrad med J. 2013;89:165-72.
4. Moschetta M, Telegrafo M, Rella L, Ianora AAS, Angelelli G, et al. Multidetector CT features of acute intestinal ischemia and their prognostic correlation. World J radiol. 2014;6(5):130-8.
5. Brandt LJ, Fuerstadt P. Intestestinal ischemia. Textbook of Sleisenger and Fordtran's Gastrointestinal and Liver Disease, 10th edition; volume 2:2076-2101.
6. Sandstorm CK, Ingraham CR, Monroe EJ, et al. Beyond decreased bowel enhancement: acute abnormalities of the mesenteric and portal vasculature. Abdominal Imaging. 2015;40(8):2977-92.
7. Oldenburg WA, Lau LL, Rodenberg TJ, et al. Acute mesenteric ischemia: a clinical review. Arch Intern Med. 2004;164:1054-62.
8. Furukawa A, Kanasaki S, Kono N, Wakamiya M, Tanaka T, Takahashi M, Murata K, et al. CT diagnosis of acute mesenteric ischemia from various causes. AJR. 2009;192:408-16.
9. Bradbury MS, Kavanagh PV, Bechtold RE, et al. Mesenteric venous thrombosis: diagnosis and noninvasive imaging. Radiographics. 2002;22(3):527-41.
10. Raman SP, Fishman EK, et al. Computed tomography angiography of the small bowel and mesentery. Radiol Clin N Am. 2016;54:87-100.
11. Fulwadhva UP, Wortman JR, Sodickson AD, et al. Use of dual energy CT and iodine maps in evaluation of bowel disease. Radigraphics. 2016;36:393-406.
12. Walker TG, Kalva SP, et al. Mesenteric ischemia. Semin Intervent Radiol. 2009;26:175-83.
13. Gore RM, Thakrar KH, Mehta UK, Berlin J, Yaghmai V, Newmark GM, et al. Clinical imaging, clinical gastro enterology and hepatology. 2008;6:849-58.
14. Wilkerson DK, Mezrich R, Drake C, Sebok D, Zatina MA. Magnetic resonance imaging of acute occlusive intestinal ischaemia. J Vasc Surg. 1990;11:567-71.
15. Oliva BI, Devarpanah AH, et al. ACR Appropriateness Criteria®—Imaging of Mesenteric Ischemia, 2012.
16. Klar E, Rahmanian PB, Bucker A, Hauenstein K, Jauch KW, Luther B. Acute mesenteric ischemia: a vascular emergency. Deutsches Arzteblatt International. 2012;109(14):249-56.
17. Landis MS, Rajan DK, Simons ME, Hayeems EB, Kachura JR, Sniderman KW. Percutaneous management of chronic mesenteric ischemia: outcomes after intervention. Journal of Vascular and Interventional Radiology. JVIR. 2005;16(10):1319-25.
18. Nicholas Fidelman AFA, Brooks D Cash, et al. ACR Appropriateness Criteria®—Radiologic Management of Mesenteric Ischemia, 2014.
19. Hohenwalter EJ, Heib RA, Patel PJ, et al. Chronic mesenteric ischemia: diagnosis and treatment. Semin Intervent Radiol. 2009;26:345-51.
20. Ujiki M, Kibbe MR. Mesenteric ischemia. Perspect Vasc Surg Endovasc Ther. 2005;17:309-18.
21. Kougias P, El Sayed HF, Zhou W, Lin PH. Management of chronic mesenteric ischemia. The role of endovascular therapy. J Endovasc Ther. 2007;14:395-405.
22. Sreenarasimhaiah J. Chronic mesenteric ischemia. Best Pract Res Clin Gastroenterol. 2005;19:283-95.
23. Reginelli A, Genovese EA, et al. Intestinal ischemia: US-CT findings correlations. Critical ultrasound journal. 2013;5:1-11.
24. Chow LC, Chan FP, Li KCP. A comprehensive approach to MR imaging of mesenteric ischemia. Abdom Imaging. 2002;27(5):507-16.
25. Schaefer PJ, Schaefer FKW, Mueller-Huelsbeck S, Jahnke T. Chronic mesenteric ischemia: stenting of mesenteric arteries. Abdom Imaging. 2007;32(3):304-9.
26. Atkins MD, Kwolek CJ, LaMuraglia GM, Brewster DC,Chung TK, Cambria RP. Surgical revascularization versus endovascular therapy for chronic mesenteric ischemia: acomparative experience. J Vasc Surg. 2007;45(6):1162-71.
27. Sharafuddin MJ, Olson CH, Sun S, Kresowik TF, Corson JD. Endovascular treatment of celiac and mesenteric arteries stenoses: applications and results. J Vasc Surg. 2003;38(4):692-8.
28. Matsumoto AH, Angle JF, Spinosa DJ, et al. Percutaneous transluminal angioplasty and stenting in the treatment of chronic mesenteric ischemia: results and longterm follow-up. J Am Coll Surg. 2002;194(Suppl 1):S22-31.
29. Sarac TP, Altinel O, Kashyap V, et al. Endovascular treatment of stenotic and occluded visceral arteries for chronic mesenteric ischemia. J Vasc Surg. 2008;47(3):485-91.
30. Paterno F, Longo WE. The etiology and pathogenesis of vascular disorders of the intestine. Radiol Clin North Am. 2008;46(5):877-85.
31. Balthazar EJ, Yen BC, Gordon RB. Ischemic colitis. Radiology. 1999;211:381-8.
32. Moszkowicz D, Mariani A, Trisallet C, et al. Ischemic colitis: the ABCs of diagnosis and surgical management. J Visc Surg. 2013;150(1):19-28.
33. Rogers AI, David S, et al. Intestinal blood flow and diseases of vascular impairment. In: Haubrich WS, Schaffner F, Berk JE (Eds). Gastroenterology, 5th edn, Philadelphia, Pa: Saunders. 1995. pp. 1212-34.

34. Parfitt JR, Driman DK. Pathological effects of drugs on the gastrointestinal tract: a review. Hum Pathol. 2007;38:527-36.
35. Wittenberg J, Athanasoulis CA, Williams LF, et al. Ischemic colitis: radiology and pathophysiology. AJR. 1975;123:287-300.
36. Gore RM, Calenoff L, Rogers LF. Roentgenographic manifestations of ischemic colitis. JAMA. 1979;241:1171-3.
37. Iida M, Matsui T, Fuchigami T, et al. Ischemic colitis: serial changes in double contrast barium enema examinations. Radiology. 1986;159:337-41.
38. Greenberg HM, Goldberg HI, Axel L. Colonic"urticaria" pattern due to early ischemia. Gastrointest Radiol. 1981;6:145-9.
39. Favier C, Bonneau HP, Tran Minh V, Devic J. Endoscopic diagnosis of regressive ischemic colitis. Endoscopic, histologic and arteriographic correlations. Nouv Presse Med. 1976;5:77-9.
40. Beppu K, Osada T, Nagahara A, et al. Relationship between endoscopic findings and clinical severity in ischemic colitis. Intern Med. 2011;50:2263-7.

CHAPTER

98

Gastrointestinal Hemorrhage: Imaging and Intervention

Deep Narayan Srivastava, Kumble S Madhusudhan, Shivanand Gamanagatti

INTRODUCTION

Gastrointestinal hemorrhage (GIH) is defined when bleeding occurs into any part of gastrointestinal tract (GIT), from esophagus to anal canal. It is a manifestation of various pathologies and is a serious symptom. It is associated with high morbidity and mortality, reaching up to 40% in severe cases.[1] The GIH may be acute or chronic/recurrent. Management of GIH involves multidisciplinary approach. The radiologist's role is in identifying the source and cause of bleeding and managing them with radiological interventions wherever needed.

CLASSIFICATION

The GIH may be upper (when the source of bleeding is proximal to ligament of Treitz) or lower, when the source is distal to it **(Box 1)**. Patients of upper gastrointestinal hemorrhage (UGIH) present with hematemesis (vomiting of blood) or melena (black tarry stools). For melena to occur (i.e. for stools to turn black) at least 60 mL of bleeding is needed and sufficient time should be available for blood to undergo degeneration by gastric and intestinal enzymes.[2] In lower gastrointestinal hemorrhage (LGIH), patients present with hematochezia, which is fresh blood in stools. However, this categorization is not absolute and may mislead the clinician.[3] Blood in gastrointestinal tract, due to cathartic properties, may rapidly reach the rectum and bleeding UGI source may present as hematochezia. Sometimes, due to slow colonic transit and bleeding rate, right colonic bleeding may present as melena. Occasionally, nasogastric tube may not show blood in cases of UGIH. Thus, evaluation of GIH should include both upper and lower GIT, till a source is identified.

Box 1: Classification of GIH.

Upper GIH	• Proximal to ligament of Treitz • From esophagus, stomach and duodenum
Lower GIH	• Distal to ligament of Treitz • From jejunum, ileum and colon (including rectum and anal canal)

Overt GIH is when bleeding can be visualized by the patient or by the clinician **(Box 2)**. Occult GIH is when bleeding is not macroscopic and there is positive stool occult blood test. Obscure GIH is a condition when patient has bleeding but UGIE and colonoscopy are negative. Obscure GIH may be occult or overt.[4]

Clinical Presentation

The patients of GIH present with hematemesis, melena or hematochezia.[5] Tachycardia and hypotension is seen when acute blood loss is greater than 500 mL.[3] Severe/massive GIH occurs when at least 15% of blood volume is lost and patients present with shock. Patients with chronic or recurrent GIH present with anemia. Patients may be asymptomatic for hemorrhage less than 100 mL/day.

Etiology

Various etiologies are identified which can cause GIH.[6] These have been listed in **Table 1**. One can see from the table, that most of the lesions do not need imaging for making a diagnosis. The source of bleeding may be arterial, venous

Box 2: Types of GIH.

Overt GIH	Hemorrhage is grossly visible
Occult GIH	Hemorrhage is microscopic (positive on stool occult blood test)
Obscure GIH	Hemorrhage is not detectable on UGIE or colonoscopy

TABLE 1: Etiology of GIH.

Upper GI bleed	Lower GI bleed
Peptic ulcer disease	Angiodysplasia
Varices	Diverticular disease
Gastritis/esophagitis/duodenitis	Neoplasms
Neoplasms	Colitis
Iatrogenic/postoperative	Iatrogenic/postoperative
Hepato-bilio-pancreatica	Hemorrhoids

or capillary. Thus appropriate investigation must be chosen depending on the suspicion.

Evaluation

Endoscopy is the initial diagnostic procedure performed in all cases of suspected GIH **(Box 3)**.[7] This includes upper gastrointestinal endoscopy (UGIE) for UGIH and colonoscopy for LGIH. The advantage of performing endoscopy in patients of GIH is in detection of the lesion responsible for bleeding and in managing them endoscopically wherever required. In addition, sampling of the lesion can be done wherever necessary. Various endoscopic treatment options include injection of epinephrine or alcohol, thermal ablations like electrocoagulation or laser therapy and mechanical placement of clips or bands. The sensitivity and specificity of UGIE in evaluation of UGIH are 92–98% and 30–100% respectively.[8] Colonoscopy has a variable accuracy of 45–90%.[9] There are few limitations of endoscopy. Performing an endoscopy in a sick patient is difficult and may take time. Blood in the GIT may obscure the bleeding source and therapy may be impossible. In colonoscopy, bowel preparation needed for proper visualization may not be possible in acute setting. Despite these drawbacks, it is still the first line of investigation as most of the lesions responsible of GIH may not be seen on imaging.

Wireless capsule endoscopy is useful in patients where the source is not identified on other endoscopic techniques. It is a noninvasive technique and is useful in patient with occult or chronic GIH, with a diagnostic yield of about 63%.[10] Since the study takes long time (patient preparation, capsule transit time and download of data), it is mainly used in chronic an intermittent GIH and not in acute GIH. Its major risk is retention of capsule proximal to an intestinal stricture which needs surgical treatment. Double balloon enteroscopy can help in visualizing up to distal small bowel with diagnostic yield of 40–80%.

IMAGING MODALITIES

Various imaging modalities are available in the workup of patients presenting with GIH. These have been described here. It is important for the radiologist to choose the right type of investigation depending on the clinical presentation and suspicion.

Indications

As described above, imaging is not needed in most patients presenting with GIH. The timing of imaging is also crucial in improving detection rates as bleeding is usually intermittent. Endoscopic diagnosis and management is sufficient. Also, in about 75% patients of UGIH and 80% patients of LGIH, the bleeding stops spontaneously and imaging may not detect any lesion. Thus about 20–25% patients of GIH require imaging.[3] Further, imaging may not identify a lesion in about 14% cases of UGIH and 20% of LGIH.[8] Thus, it is important to carefully define the indications for imaging in patients of GIH **(Box 4)**.

Radionuclide Studies

Radionuclide studies play role in the evaluation of patients with GIH with minimal risk and invasiveness to the patient.[11] The major indication is in cases where bleeding slow or intermittent as scanning can be done for longer periods. It is not useful in patients with massive continuous bleeding. It has variable accuracy and sometimes proximal or distal movement of the radionuclide between imaging sessions impair precise localization of the actual bleeding site.

The common radionuclides employed in patients with GIH are as follows:

^{99m}Tc Sulfur Colloid

It is cleared from the blood pool by the reticuloendothelial system. The half-life of the tracer in the blood pool is approximately 2.5–3 min. If active bleeding is occurring during this short time, the tracer extravasates into the bowel which can be identified on subsequent imaging. Although sulfur colloid scintigraphy can detect bleeding rates as low as 0.1 mL/min, this is possible only when there is active bleeding at the time of scan. In addition, isotope study can be repeated as often as required. The drawback is that bleeding into the hepatic or splenic flexures of the colon and UGIH will be obscured because of the overlap by normal accumulation of the tracer in liver and spleen.

^{99m}Tc-labeled Red Blood Cell

These labeled RBCs in circulation extravasate during bleeding and can be detected. They have longer half-life in circulation. The advantage is that images can be obtained up to 2 hours after the initial injection and hence is especially useful for evaluating intermittent GIH. The major limitation is that activity seen in the lower GIT, when it may have occurred from more proximal segments of small bowel and sources of bleeding may be missed if frequent views are not obtained. This has a sensitivity and specificity of 93% and 95% respectively for bleeding rates > 0.04 mL/min.[12]

^{99m}Tc-pertechnetate

It is used in cases where bleeding from Meckel's diverticulum is suspected. This tracer accumulates in ectopic gastric

Box 3: Routine investigations in GIH.

Clinical:
- Endoscopy/colonoscopy
- Enteroscopy/capsule endoscopy

Imaging:
- CT angiography/CT enterography
- Radionuclide scan
- Digital subtraction angiography

Box 4: Indications for imaging in GIH.

- Acute GIH when arterial source is identified on endoscopy
- Normal findings on endoscopy
- Hemobilia/hemosuccus pancreaticus on endoscopy
- Chronic/recurrent GIH
- Endoscopy not possible/difficult/failed
- Obscure or occult GIH

mucosa present in the diverticulum and helps in identifying the source of GIH.

Computed Tomography

Computed tomography (CT) scan is the corner stone in the evaluation of GIH.[13] It is easily available, has high spatial resolution and can detect bleeding as low as 0.3 mL/min. Faster scans are possible with multidetector CT. The timing of CT scan is important due to intermittent nature of GIH and should be done as soon as GIH is clinically diagnosed.[14] Signs of GIH on CT scan include direct sign like extravasation of contrast into bowel lumen (jet like or swirling; **Figs. 1A to C**) and indirect signs like pseudoaneurysm **(Figs. 2A to D)**, vascular malformation or tumors.

CT Protocol

This typically involves performing an arterial and a venous phases. Iodinated contrast material is injected at the rate of 4 mL/sec. Oral contrast is usually not necessary. Arterial phase [CT angiography—(CTA)] is done at about 25-30 seconds after injection of contrast. This should be a late arterial phase to help detect small lesions and source of bleeding. Automatic bolus triggering is used for this with region of interest in abdominal aorta and trigger attenuation of 150 HU. Time delay after triggering should be about 10-15 sec. This is followed by venous phase (60-70 sec). In cases of UGIH, arterial phase should include area from dome of diaphragm to iliac crest and venous phase, the entire abdomen, including pelvis. For LGIH, the entire abdomen from dome of diaphragm to symphysis pubis should be scanned in both phases. When a small bowel source is suspected, CT enterography should be performed with neutral oral contrast and both arterial and venous phases should be acquired. Plain scans may be done and it may show acute hematoma in the bowel lumen.

The sensitivity, specificity and accuracy of CT angiography in the detection and localization of GIH are 90.9%, 99% and 97.6% respectively.[15] In addition to routine baseline images, reviewing the coronal reconstruction, maximum intensity projections (MIP) and volume rendered images are useful in identifying the source of bleeding and the feeding artery if any **(Figs. 2A to D)**. Low kV acquisition (100 kV) may be done for improved contrast resolution. Wide window settings will help in reducing the beam hardening artifacts due to high iodine concentration. With the advent of CTA for diagnosis of source of GIH, the role of conventional angiography has been largely limited to endovascular interventions. The advantages of performing CTA prior to digital subtraction angiography (DSA) are many. These include:

- CTA helps to plan DSA by identifying the source artery and anatomical variations.
- This decreases number of DSA exposures
- CTA information allows faster catheterization of bleeding vessels
- It decreases the amount of contrast material used during angiography
- It reduces procedure time and radiation exposure

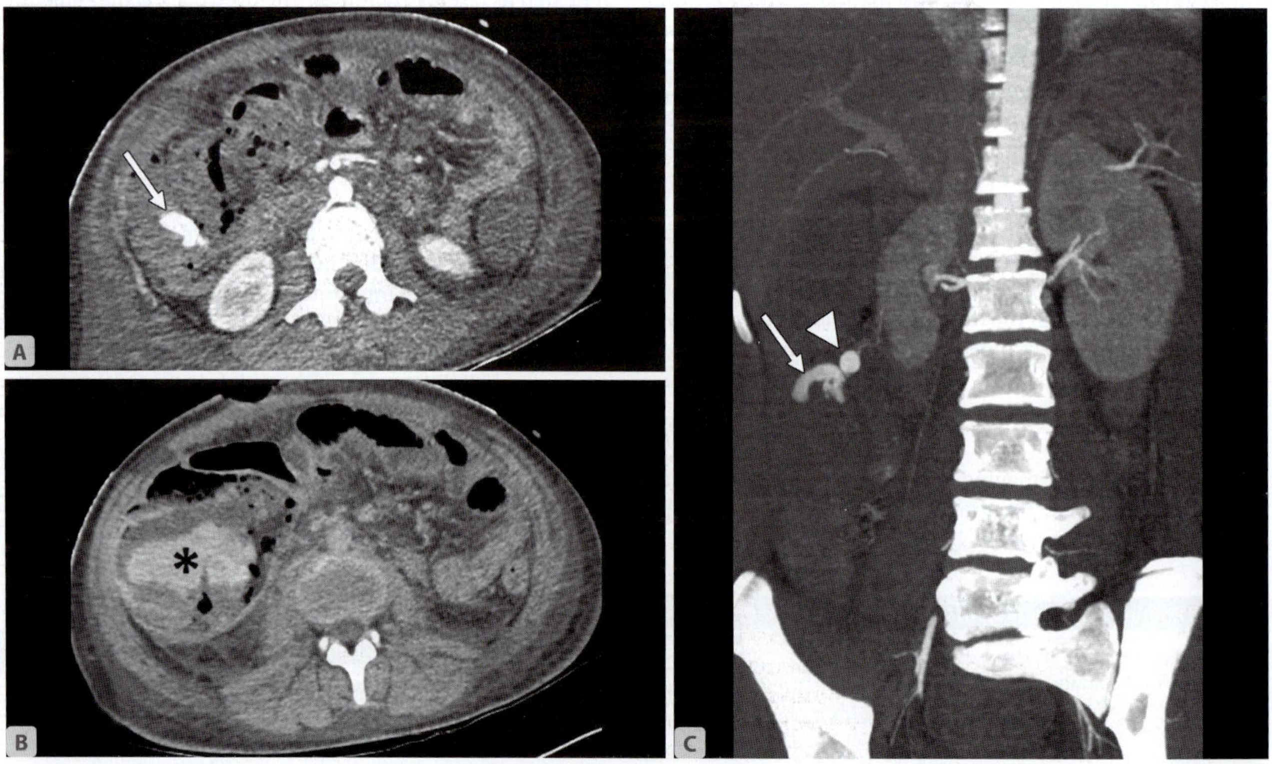

FIGS. 1A TO C: GIH presenting after ileal resection: Axial contrast-enhanced CT images in arterial phase (A) showing contrast extravasation into the ascending colon (arrow) from right colic artery with increase in extravasation in the venous phase (asterisk in B). Maximum intensity projection coronal image in arterial phase (C) also shows the pseudoaneurysm (arrowhead) with active extravasation of contrast (arrow).

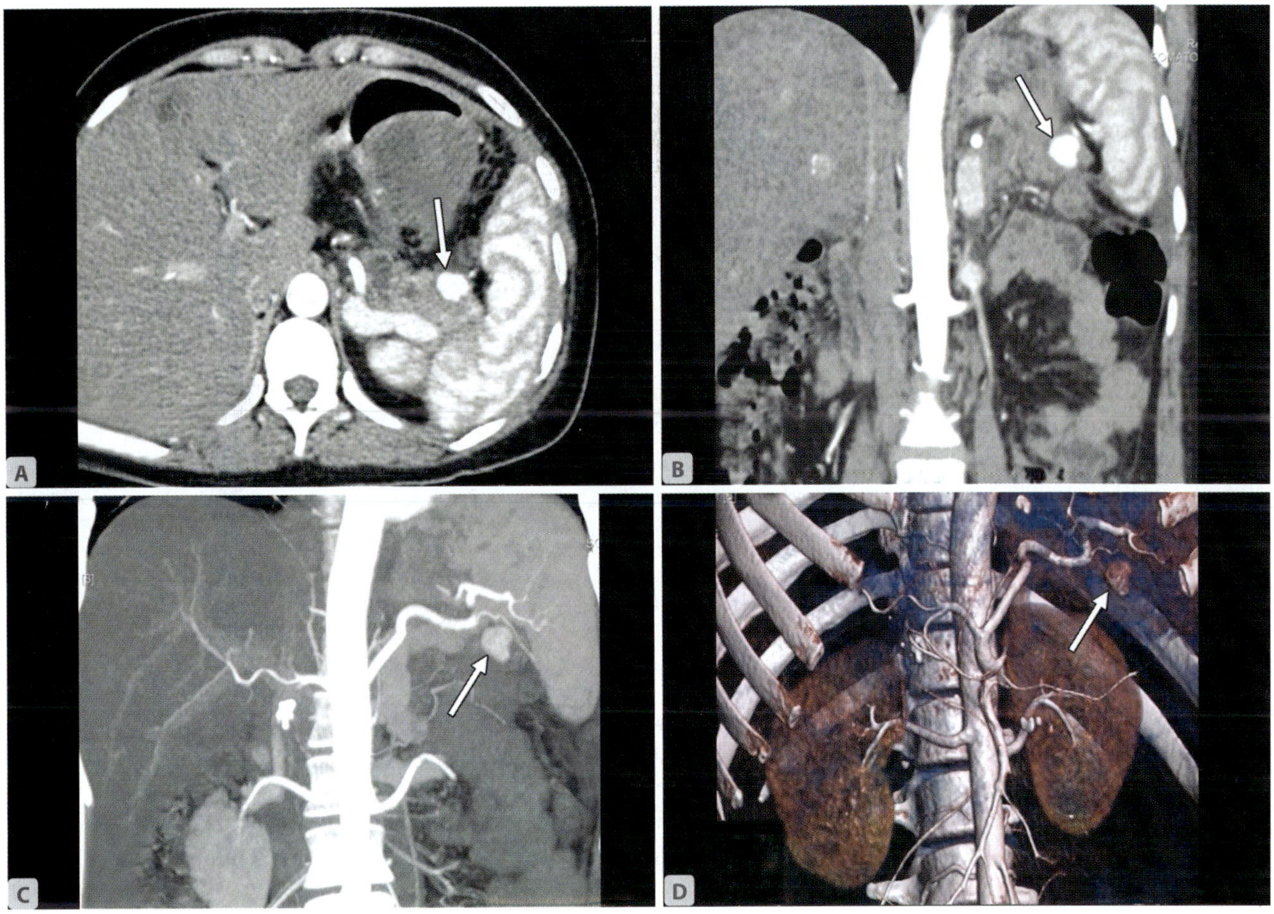

FIGS. 2A TO D: Chronic pancreatitis with GIH: Axial (A) and coronal (B) CT angiography images showing a pseudoaneurysm (arrow) arising from a branch of distal splenic artery. Coronal maximum intensity projection image (C) and 3D volume-rendered image (D) showing the pseudoaneurysm (arrow) and the source artery.

Dual energy CTA is a recent addition and helps in reducing radiation dose due to its capability of generating virtual non-contrast images. In a recent study by Sun et al, it was shown that dual energy CTA with virtual noncontrast images and iodine maps is an accurate screening method in patients with active GIH with lower radiation dose.[16]

Angiography

Angiography plays a significant role in the management of patients with acute GIH by localizing the actual site of active bleeding and transcatheter embolization of the bleeding artery.[17] The role of angiography in the diagnosis of cause of GIH has diminished because of wider availability of endoscopy and CT angiography. However, it remains a valuable tool in patients with recurrent or continued GIH in whom source has eluded all other investigations. Angiography is beneficial in patients who fail to respond to conservative or invasive endoscopic management. It is also valuable in patients who are unstable and are bleeding massively. Angiography in these situations can locate the bleeding vessel and provide access to transcatheter management either to obviate surgery or to stabilize the patient before surgery.[2]

Angiography is especially important in whom bleeding has continued after blind laparotomy.[18] In acute GIH, angiography detects the site if bleeding exceeds 0.5 mL/min (blood loss exceeds four units within 24 hours). If bleeding is intermittent and the patient is stable, other less invasive examinations can be used and emergency angiography is not required. Evaluation of recurrent hemorrhage may be time consuming and expensive if bleeding is intermittent. Provocative pharmacoangiography and carbon dioxide angiography may be useful in select situations.

Technical Details

The renal function should be normal because angiography requires large amount of contrast medium. If renal function is deranged, alternative contrast media like carbon dioxide can be used for angiography.

A flush aortogram may be done initially, but often it is avoided and direct selective and superselective arteriography is done. In flush aortogram, the tip of pigtail catheter tip is placed above the level of celiac axis and a total of about 40 mL of iodinated contrast agent is injected using a mechanical injector at the rate of 18–22 mL/sec. This is followed by selective and superselective studies using various visceral angiographic catheters. Flush aortograms are important, particularly in cases of suspected aortoenteric fistula. If a major splanchnic artery cannot be catheterized or identified, a lateral aortography is used to accurately demonstrate and catheterize major aortic branches.

In mesenteric studies, the flow rate for contrast injection should be approximately 10 mL/sec for the celiac, 8 mL/sec for the superior mesenteric artery and 3 mL/sec for the inferior mesenteric artery. The imaging must be rapid during the arterial phase (2–3 frames/sec) and reduced to (1 frame/2–5 second) for the capillary and venous phases. Imaging should be carried out up to at least 30 seconds, to identify slow extravasation, suspected venous occlusion and vascular malformations. The suspected bleeding artery should be catheterized first if there is prior CTA information. If not, then all major branches of celiac artery (gastroduodenal, hepatic and left gastric) and then superior mesenteric (middle colic, right colic, ileocolic, major jejunal/ileal branches) and inferior mesenteric arteries (left colic and superior rectal) are sequentially catheterized. Microcatheters (2.5–2.8F) should be used wherever possible for catheterizing smaller or tortuous arteries. The more selective the catheter is placed, the higher the probability that active bleeding will be recognized. The rate of blood loss must be at least 5–6 mL/min for it to be detected on the midstream flush aortogram. However, selective arteriography may reveal bleeding sources with rate of bleeding as low as 0.5 mL/min. DSA of mesenteric arteries may sometimes be suboptimal due to bowel gas and peristalsis. Such motion artifacts may be misinterpreted as contrast extravasation and hence antispasmodic drugs are sometimes used to reduce bowel peristalsis. The sensitivity of DSA is 63–90% and 40– 86% for UGIH and LGIH respectively and specificity is 100% and positive findings are seen in about 24–78% patients of GIH.[19]

In approximately 70% of patients with gastric mucosal hemorrhage, bleeding occurs from left gastric artery (LGA). Hence, it is essential that LGA be well opacified during selective angiography. The celiac axis angiogram would not suffice if the tip of the catheter is distal to the origin of the LGA, or if the LGA originates from the aorta. In bleeding duodenal ulcers, contrast extravasation is most commonly noted from the supraduodenal branch of gastroduodenal artery. In variceal bleeding, contrast extravasation is rarely demonstrated as contrast medium gets diluted by the time it reaches the bleeding veins. The purpose of angiography in variceal bleeding is very limited.

Angiographic Findings in GIH

- *Extravasation of contrast:* It is seen as a puddling or staining that persists beyond the capillary and venous phases.
- Delayed films may show opacified intestinal folds due to luminal extravasation of contrast medium.
- If the lumen of the gastrointestinal tract is filled with clotted blood, a 'pseudovein' appearance is often seen as the extravasated contrast flows through the clot to the most dependent part. However, unlike the venous phase, it persists for a much longer time.
- Other findings include pseudoaneurysm **(Fig. 3)**, arteriovenous fistula, abnormal blush, neovascularity or hyperemia.
- Because bleeding may be intermittent, and spasm may preclude opacification of the target vessel, repeat injection or repeat angiography may be required to show the bleeding vessel **(Figs. 4A to C)**.

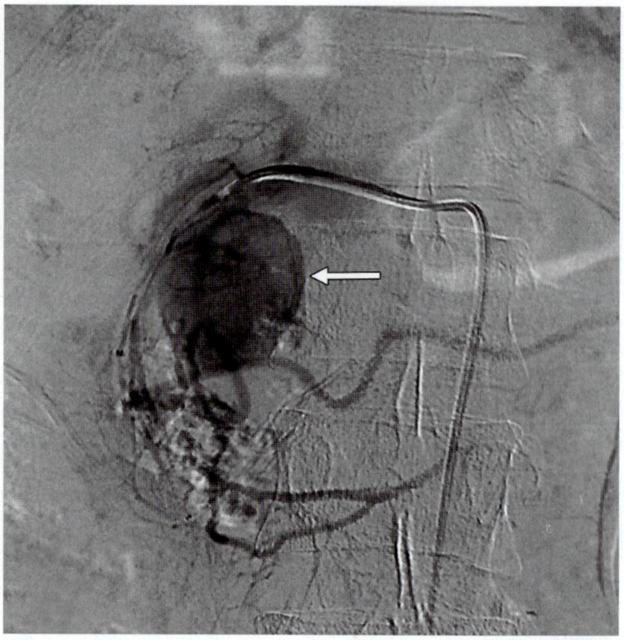

FIG. 3: DSA of gastroduodenal artery showing a large pseudoaneurysm (arrow) in a case of pancreatitis presenting with hematemesis.

Provocative angiography may be done in patients of GIH when no cause is found on routine imaging.[20] Here, heparin, tissue plasminogen activator (tPA) and vasodilator (tolazoline) are injected through the catheter into the artery. This is followed by DSA to demonstrate any bleeding source. This technique increases blood flow into the vessel, relieves vasospasm and lyses any small clot, and thus improves detection of bleeding lesion. Provocative angiography has been shown to identify a cause in up to 33% patients of GIH with normal routine DSA.[21]

Carbon dioxide angiography is useful in patients of renal failure and patients allergic to iodinated contrast agents. Carbon dioxide (CO_2) is an inert gas and easily dissolves in blood and is excreted by lungs.[22] It has low viscosity and has been suggested to be better in the evaluation of GIH.[23] It may be used in cases with high clinical suspicion and normal routine DSA.

Ultrasonography

Ultrasonography (USG) has limited role in the evaluation of patients with GIH. It specific situations like large superficial aneurysm/pseudoaneurysm and vascular abnormalities in solid organs (liver) color Doppler USG helps in detecting the lesion and may also guide if percutaneous intervention is needed. In addition, contrast enhanced USG assists in evaluating thickened segments of small bowel in patients with inflammatory bowel disease presenting with GIH.

Magnetic Resonance Imaging

Magnetic resonance angiography (MRA) has currently no role in the evaluation of acute GIH. Longer scan times, lower spatial resolution and need for breath hold limits its

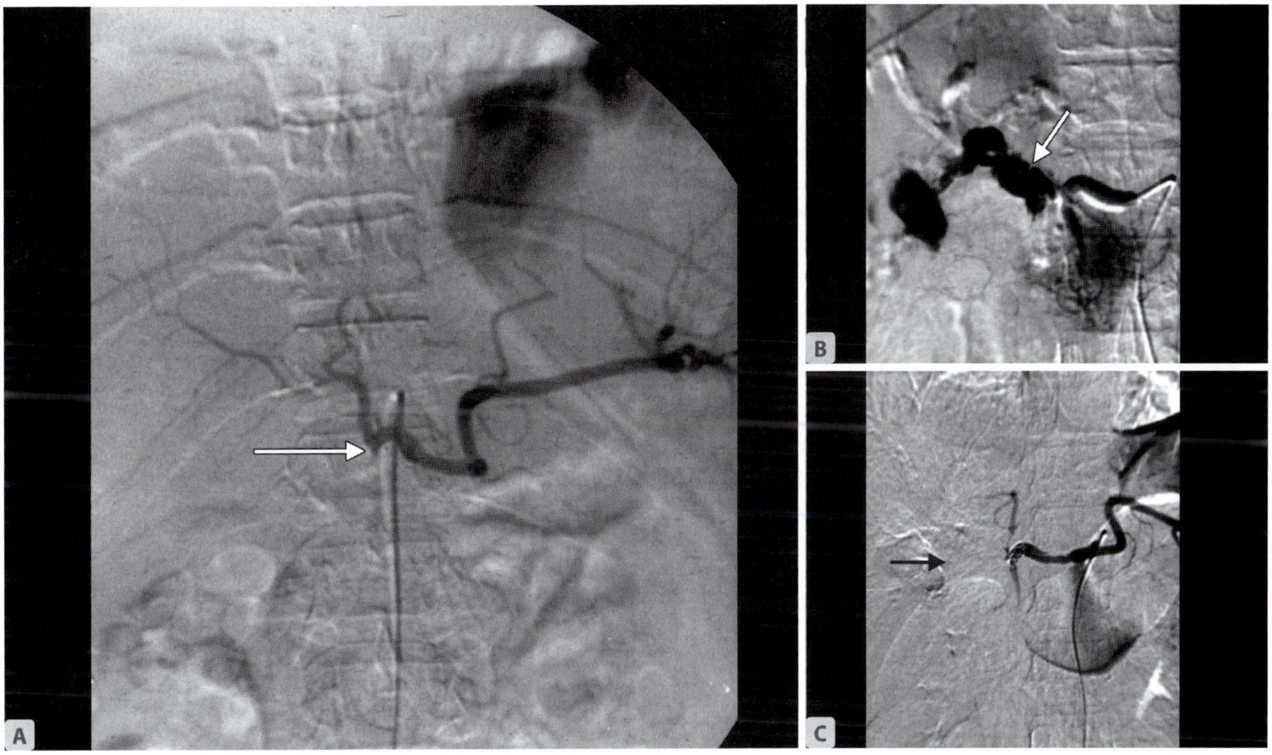

FIGS. 4A TO C: (A) Celiac artery angiogram in a case of GIH is showing spasm of gastroduodenal artery (arrow); (B) Hepatic artery angiogram showing extravasation of contrast in subhepatic area (arrow), and (C) Celiac artery angiogram after steel coil embolization not showing extravasation of contrast (arrow).

use in acute situations. However, in patients with chronic or recurrent GIH, MR enterography is useful in the evaluation of small bowel abnormalities such as inflammatory bowel disease, tumors, mesenteric ischemia and vasculitis.

RADIOLOGICAL INTERVENTIONS IN GASTROINTESTINAL HEMORRHAGE

After the bleeding site has been localized on imaging, minimally invasive angiographic procedures should be performed wherever possible to control the hemorrhage. This helps to avoid an emergency surgery in a patient with acute GIH. Endoscopic techniques like coagulation and mucosal injection of sclerosing agent controls bleeding in cases of ulcer and varices **(Box 5)**.

Radiological approaches used in the treatment of GIH include endovascular and percutaneous techniques.[24] Endovascular approach should be initially used in these patients as control is better and complications are fewer.

Box 5: Management of GIH.

Endoscopic
- Coagulation
- Sclerosant injection
- EUS-guided thrombin/glue injection

Radiological

Endovascular
- Embolization–coils, glue, plug, gelfoam
- Stents—stent graft, stent-assisted coiling
- Balloon remodeling

Percutaneous—thrombin or glue injection

Endovascular Approach

Endovascular embolization has been used for lesions of the stomach, colon and small bowel. It is especially useful in the treatment of bleeding pancreatic or hepatic artery pseudoaneurysms.[25] Here the target artery is catheterized superselectively and embolic agents are injected into the lesion or feeding artery to exclude the lesion from the circulation and thus control hemorrhage. The methods of endovascular treatment of pseudoaneurysm used include sandwich technique, proximal embolization, sac filling, stent assisted coiling, balloon remodeling and stent graft placement. The advantages are as follows:
- Control of bleeding is immediate
- Risk of visceral ischemia is minimal if embolization is superselective and collaterals are preserved.

Percutaneous Approach

This technique is used when endovascular approach fails or is not possible and in cases where the lesion is superficial and surrounded by solid parenchyma (e.g. intrahepatic pseudoaneurysm).[24] This is performed by direct puncture of the pseudoaneurysm by a thin needle (22G) under USG guidance followed by injection of embolic agent. The risks include rupture and non-target embolization.

Embolic Materials

Various embolic materials are available which are used in the management of GIH. These include permanent occluding agents like coils/microcoils, polyvinyl alcohol particles, n-butyl cyanoacrylate (nBCA or glue) and vascular plugs.[24,26] Temporary embolizing agents include gelatin sponge and autologous blood clot. Wherever a lesion is identified, permanent embolic agent should be used to avoid recurrence. Temporary agents may be used for per-operative and empirical (when bleeding source is not identified) embolization. The embolization in conjunction with vasopressin infusion is not recommended. The major risks of bowel embolization are ischemia and stricture formation, but these risks must be weighed against the high mortality rate of emergency surgery. Minimum amount of embolic material should be used to stop hemorrhage and should be injected as selectively as possible to avoid complications.

SPECIFIC SITUATIONS IN GASTROINTESTINAL HEMORRHAGES

Upper gastrointestinal hemorrhage (UGIH) can be differentiated from lower gastrointestinal hemorrhage (LGIH) by localizing the source of bleeding either proximal or distal to the ligament of Treitz. UGIH is 10 times more common than LGHI. Before imaging, a distinction must be made between UGIH and LGIH based on clinical findings.

Upper Gastrointestinal Hemorrhage

As described in **Table 1**, common causes (peptic ulcer disease, gastritis and varices) of UGIH account for up to 90% of all cases. Other less common causes include neoplasms of esophagus, stomach and duodenum, aortoenteric fistula, pancreatitis, hemobilia, arteriovenous malformations **(Figs. 5A to C)**, splanchnic arterial aneurysms and rarely mesenteric venous thrombosis and hepatobiliary and pancreatic tumors.[27,28] Acute UGIH due to penetration of a hepatic or left gastric artery aneurysm into the duodenal bulb **(Figs. 6A to D)** or stomach **(Figs. 7A to D)** is rare but has been reported.[29] Rarely primary blood dyscrasias, vasculitis, connective tissue disorders, hamartoma, jejunoileitis and uremia may also produce significant bleeding.[30]

Hemobilia

The causes are hepatic trauma, neoplasms, abscesses, hepatic artery aneurysm, laparoscopic and postoperative or interventional procedures of the liver **(Figs. 8 to 11)**. The presentation is characteristic, i.e. biliary colic, obstructive jaundice and UGIH. The diagnosis is made either on endoscopy by the appearance of blood from the ampulla of Vater or by diagnostic hepatic arteriography. The rupture of hepatic arterial branches and hepatic arterial aneurysms can be treated by angioembolization or surgical ligation of hepatic artery.[31]

Pancreatitis and Upper Gastrointestinal Hemorrhage

In pancreatitis a pseudocyst is frequently recognized on imaging, but a pseudoaneurysm is noted in less than 10% of cases. Intracystic hemorrhage has been reported in 6–10% of cases and this is due to extension of pancreatic inflammation to the nearby splenic artery. The pancreatic pseudocysts may present with the following five patterns of hemorrhage:[32]

1. Hemorrhage within the pseudocyst presenting with intermittent severe abdominal pain due to elevated intracystic pressure.
2. Gastrointestinal bleeding caused by fistula formation near the digestive tract.
3. Rupture into the peritoneum.
4. Hemorrhage caused by fistula formation with the bile duct.
5. Hemorrhage into the duodenum via the pancreatic duct (hemosuccus pancreaticus).

Celiac and superior mesenteric angiography should be done and selective arterial embolization may control the hemorrhage **(Figs. 12 and 13)**.

Lower Gastrointestinal Hemorrhage

Patients with lower gastrointestinal bleeding are usually older than those with gastric or duodenal lesions. Causes of

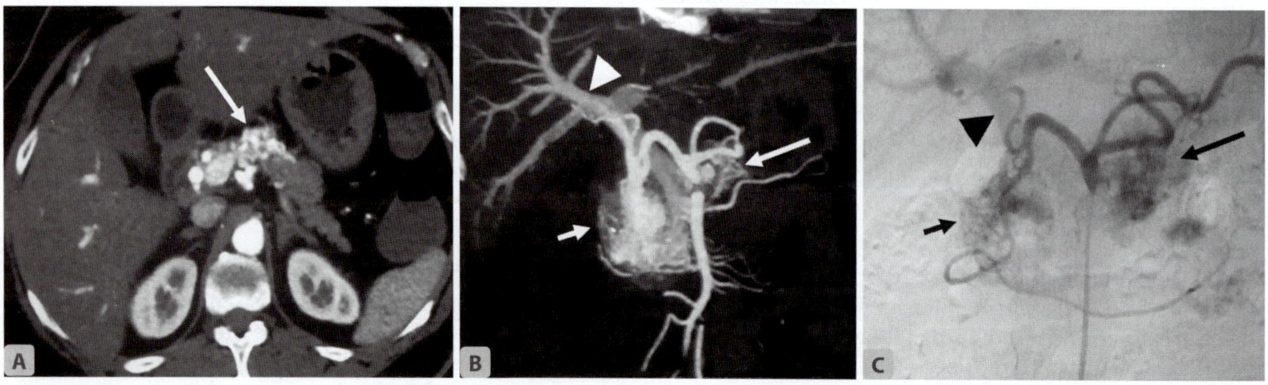

FIGS. 5A TO C: Pancreatic AVM. (A) Axial CT image in arterial phase showing cluster of vessels in the body of pancreas (arrow); (B) Coronal MIP image in arterial phase showing bunch of vessels at two locations, head (short arrow) and body (long arrow) region of pancreas with early filling of portal vein (arrowhead); (C) DSA of celiac artery showing the same two nidus, in head (short arrow) and body (long arrow) with arteriovenous shunting and opacification of portal vein (arrowhead). This was embolized preoperatively using PVA particles.

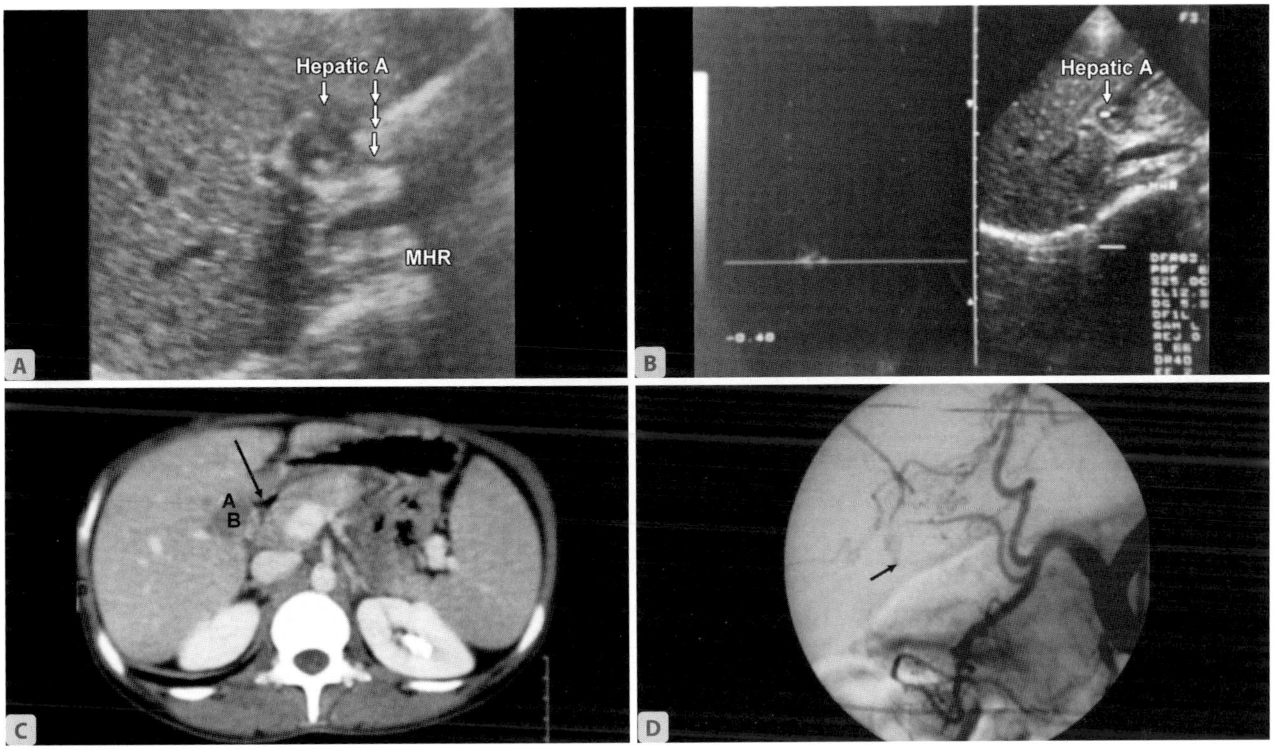

FIGS. 6A TO D: (A) Abdominal sonography showing a round, cystic mass at the porta; (B) Doppler sonography showing absence of signal in the echogenic area of the lesion; (C) Contrast-enhancing CT showing a low-attenuating area with an enhanced center lateral to second part at the duodenum (arrow). Selective celiac artery angiogram (D) is showing the aneurysm (arrow). At surgery, the partially thrombosed aneurysm was communicating to duodenal bulb.

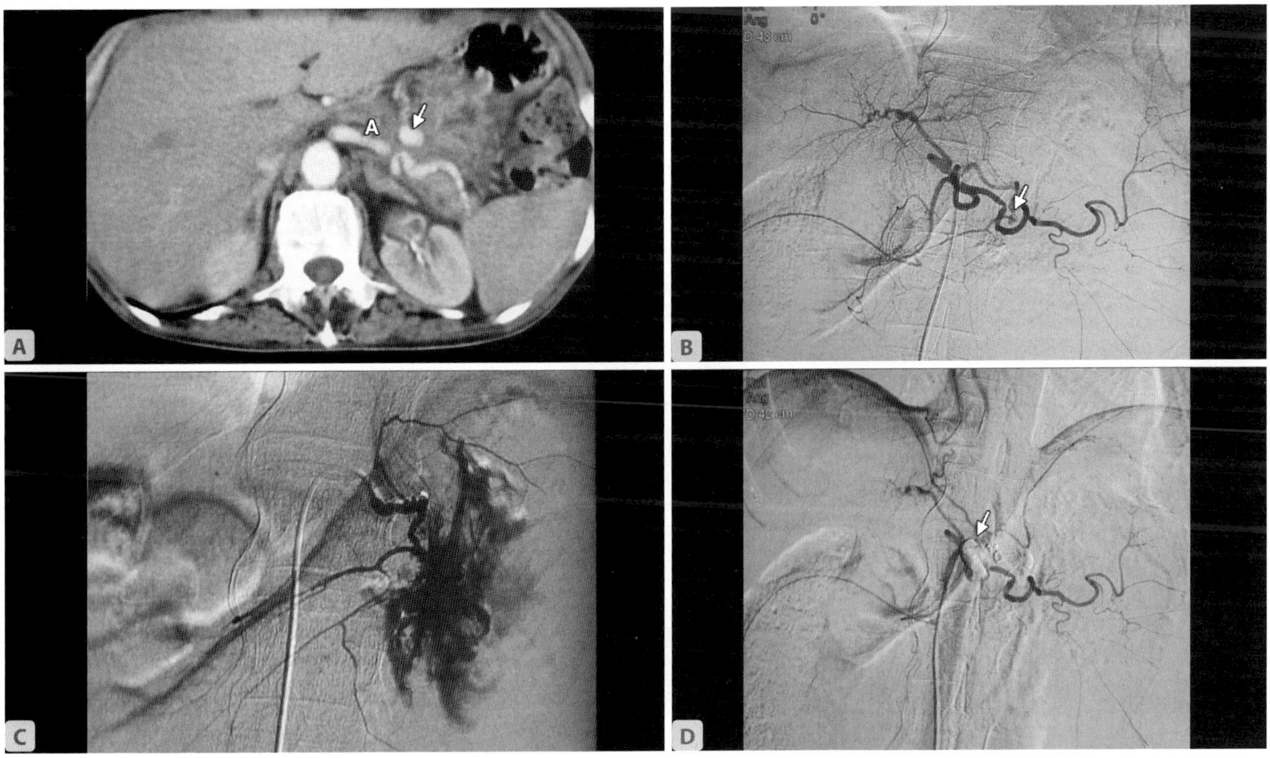

FIGS. 7A TO D: Contrast-enhanced arterial phase CT (A) and celiac artery angiogram (B) of a case of massive gastrointestinal hemorrhage is showing an enhancing aneurysm posterior to stomach (arrows). Selective left gastric artery angiogram (C) is showing leakage of contrast into stomach due to aneurysmogastric fistula. The left gastric artery was embolized (arrow) with steel coils (D) and partial gastrectomy was done later.

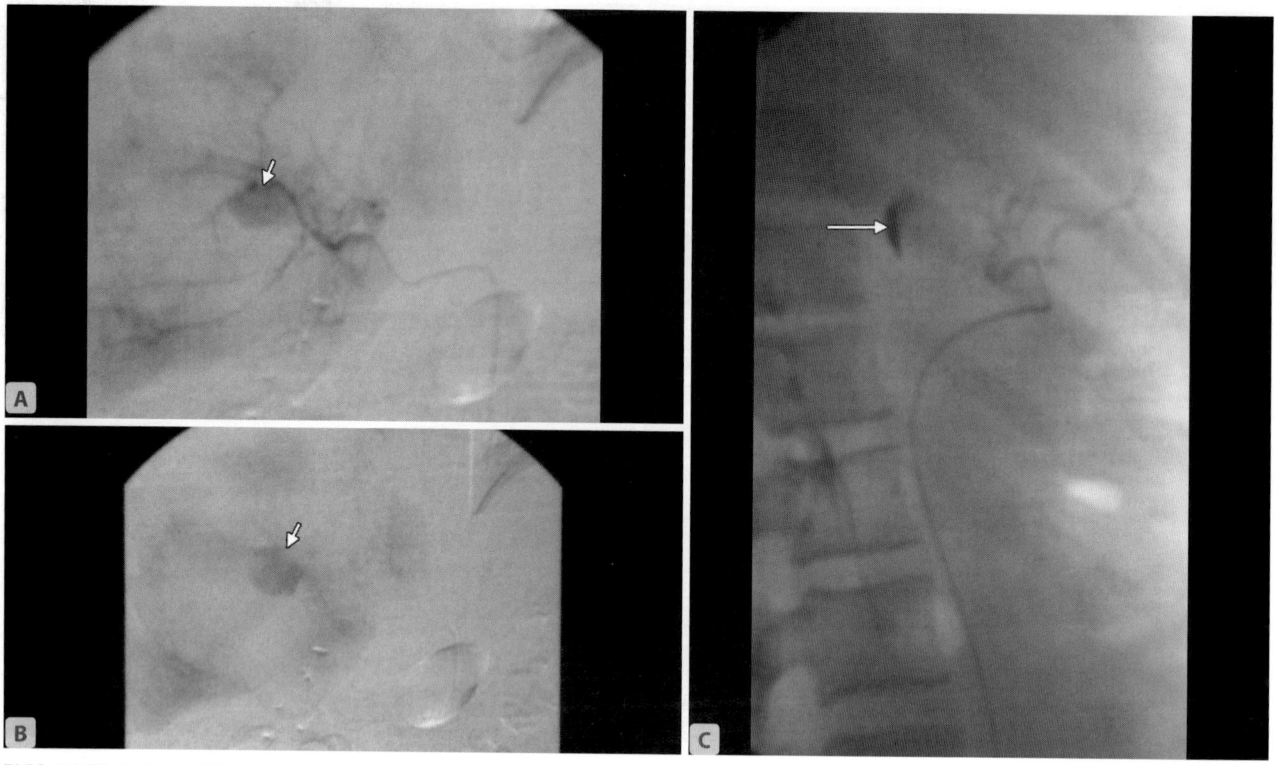

FIGS. 8A TO C: (A and B) Hepatic artery angiogram in a postoperative patient of road traffic accident showing extravasation of the contrast in the right lobe of liver (arrows); and (C) Lateral film showing pooling of contrast in a cavity (arrow).

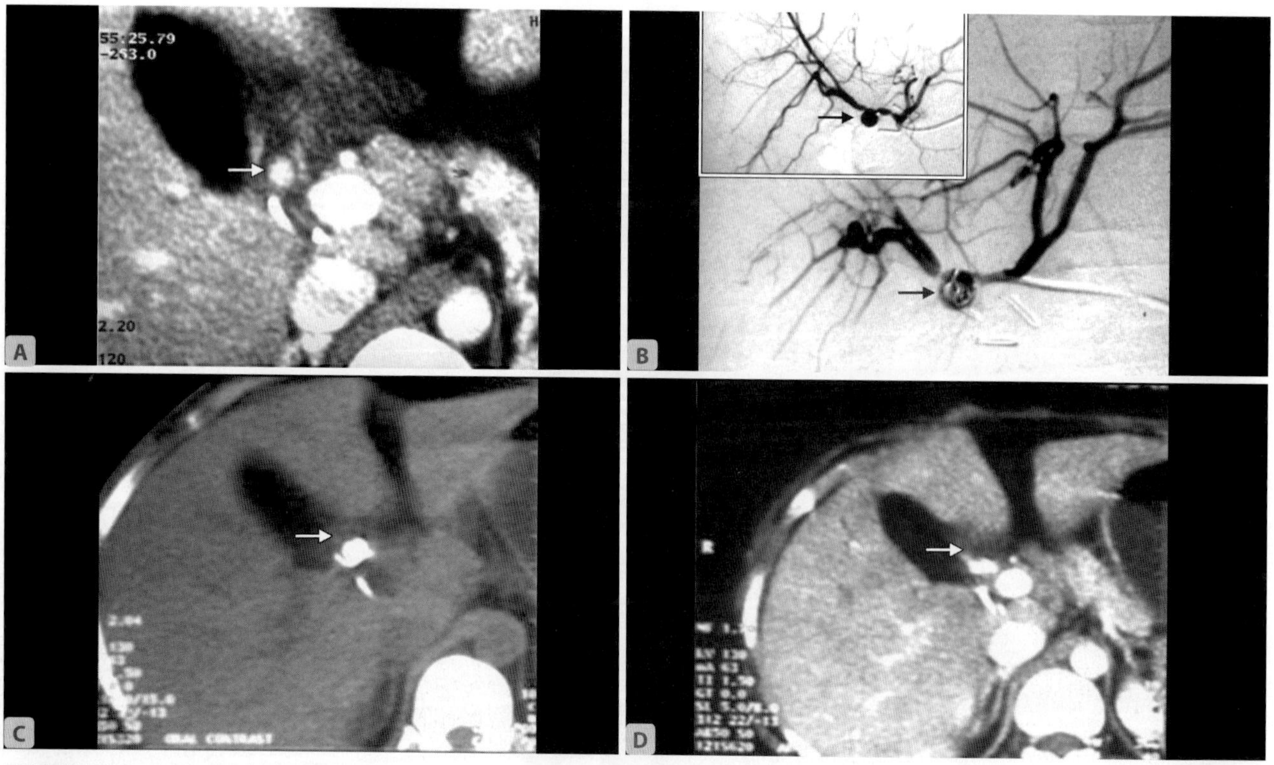

FIGS. 9A TO D: A 42-year-old woman with hemobilia following open cholecystectomy done two months ago shows right hepatic artery aneurysm (arrow) on CT (A) and hepatic angiography (B, inset). It was embolized using steel coils (B, arrow). Four months following embolization the noncontrast enhanced CT (C) shows aneurysm packed with coils (arrow). There is no enhancement of aneurysm on contrast-enhanced CT (D).

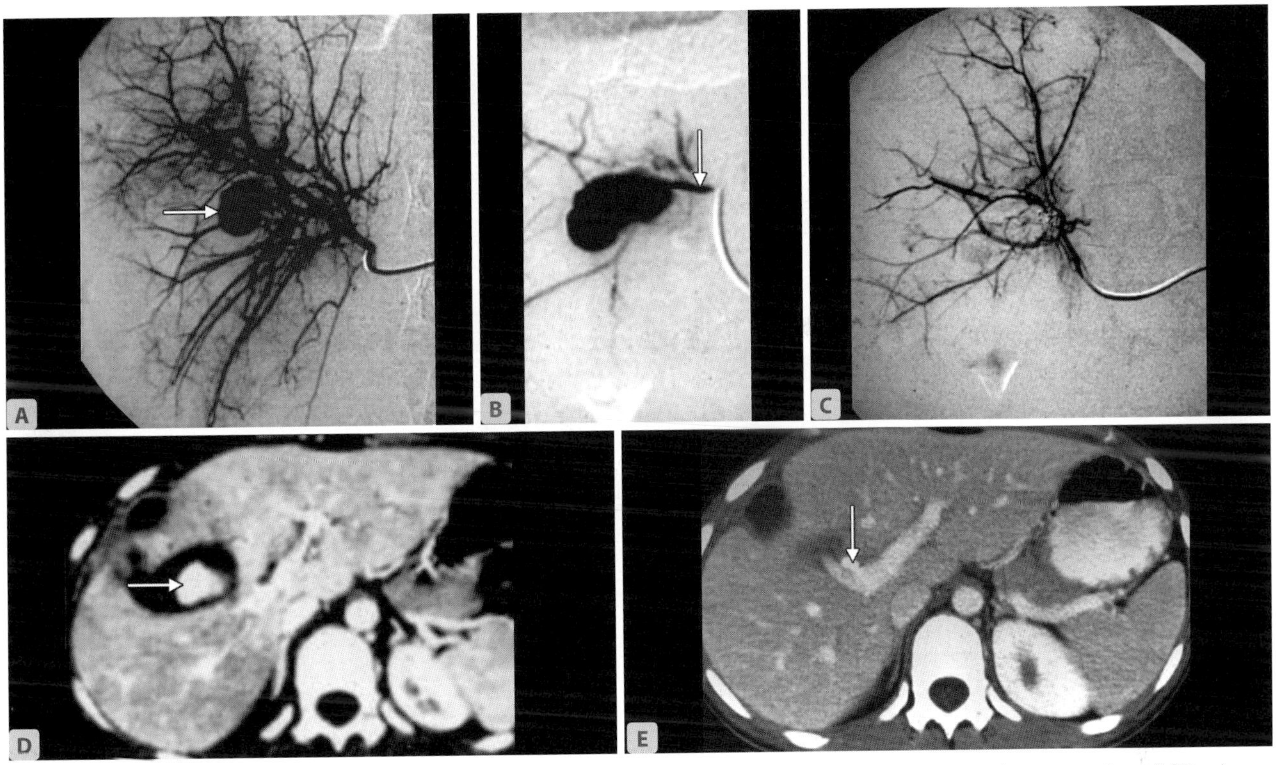

FIGS. 10A TO E: (A to C) Hepatic angiogram of a 28-years-old male a road traffic accident victim with a large pseudoaneurysm (arrow) filling by middle hepatic artery (arrowhead) was embolized with steel coil; (D and E) The aneurysm (arrow) and steel coil (arrowhead) are seen on pre- and postembolization three months CT.

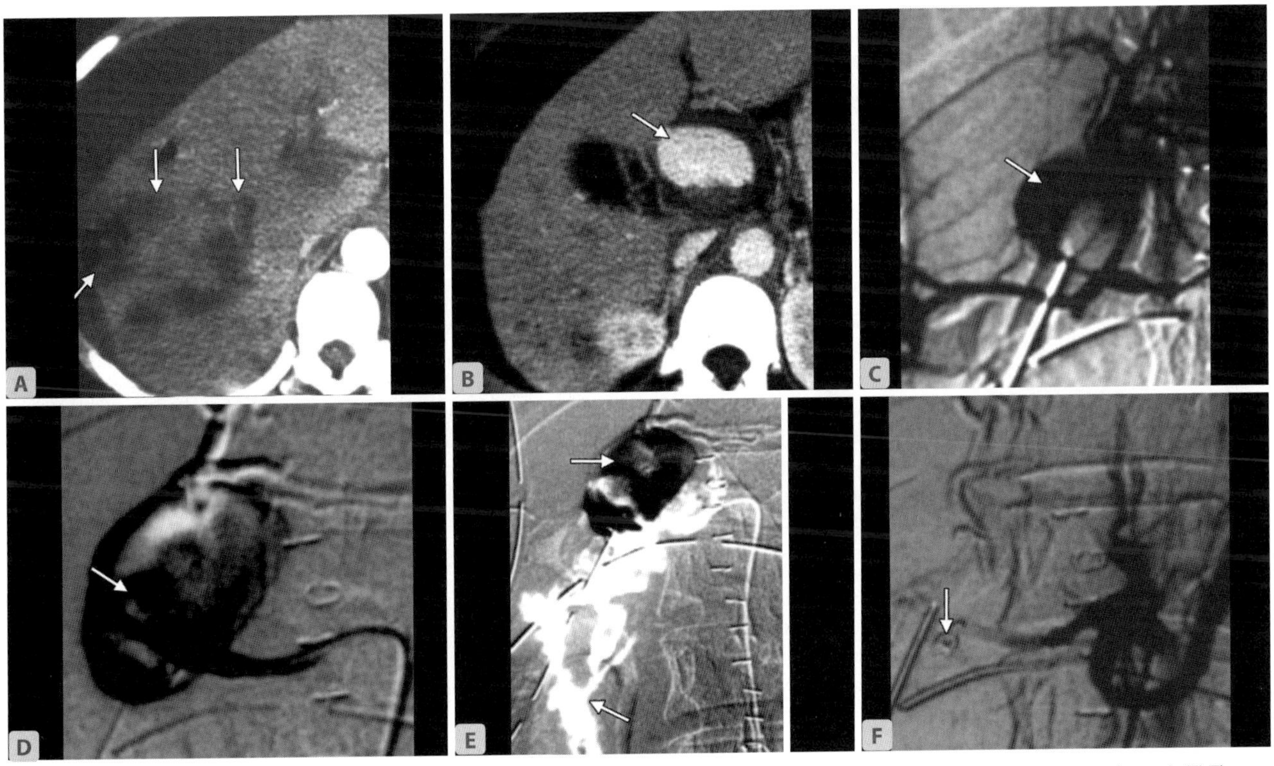

FIGS. 11A TO F: (A to D) A 35-year-old male with liver abscess (arrows) on treatment developed a large hepatic artery aneurysm (arrow); (E) There is simultaneous opacification of duodenum (arrows) due to communication of aneurysm to duodenum; (F) The hepatic artery was embolized using steel coils (arrow).

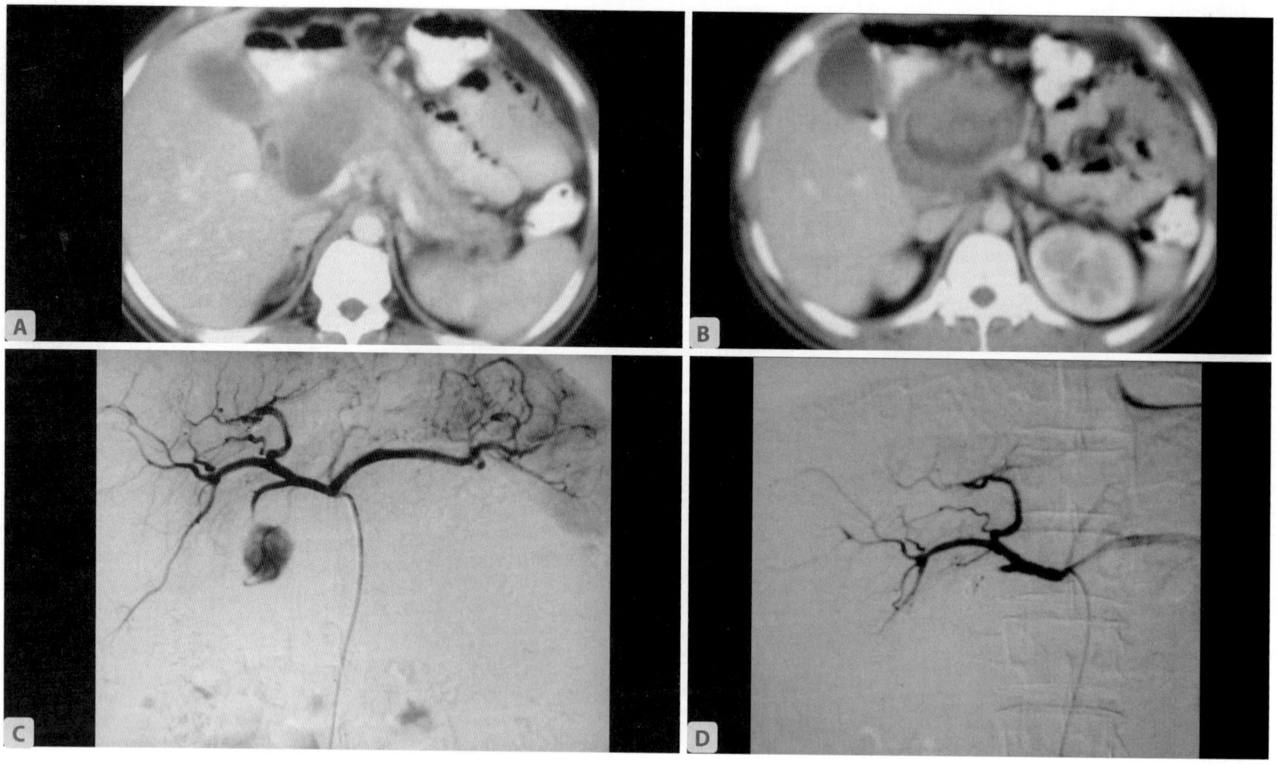

FIGS. 12A TO D: Contrast-enhanced CT (A and B) of a case of acute pancreatitis is showing a large pseudocyst with bleed and peripancreatic inflammation in head of pancreas. The pancreatic duct is dilated. Celiac artery angiogram (C) is showing an aneurysm of gastroduodenal artery. The artery was embolized with steel coils (D). Superior mesenteric angiogram was normal.

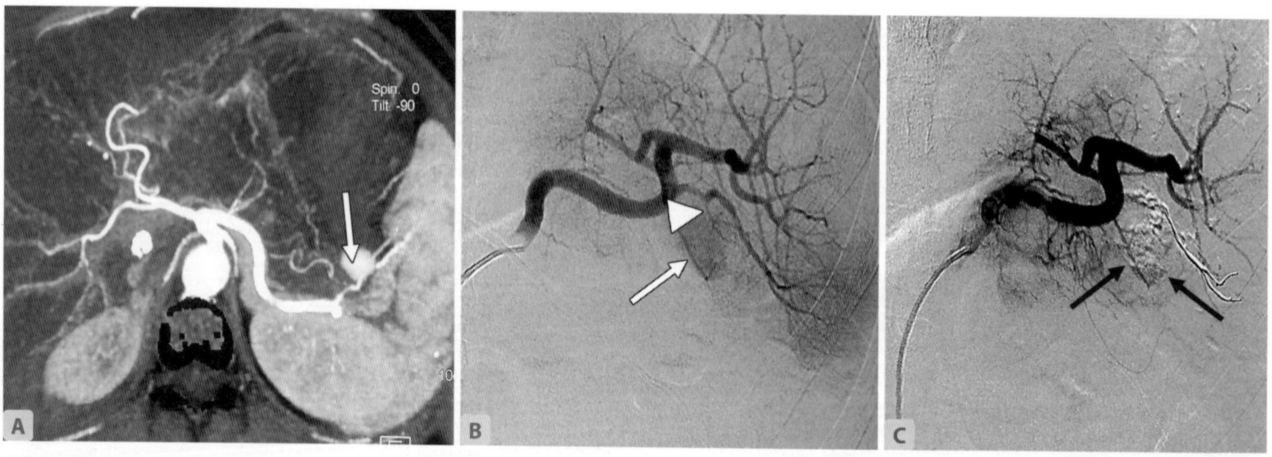

FIGS. 13A TO C: Splenic artery pseudoaneurysm: (A) MIP-CT image in arterial phase showing a contrast-filled outpouching (arrow) in the distal splenic artery; (B) DSA of splenic artery shows the pseudoaneurysm (arrow) arising from distal branch of splenic artery (arrow-head); (C) DSA after embolization with combination of coils and glue shows complete obliteration of the pseudoaneurysm (arrows).

LGIH in India are nonspecific ulcers (30%), enteric ulcers (15%), tuberculosis (6%), neoplasms (6%) and others (31%). In western literature the causes are diverticular (33%), colitis and ulcers (22%), neoplasms (20%), angiodysplasia and others (25%). Some of the causes of the LGIH are discussed below.

Colonic Diverticula

They are mostly seen in the left sided colon. Bleeding is typically abrupt in onset, massive and painless, and does not recur in 60% of patients. Active diverticular bleeding can be demonstrated either by direct endoscopic visualization or by filling of the bleeding diverticulum with contrast medium at the time of angiography.

Meckel's Diverticulum

It is a congenital anomaly of the distal ileum, present in about 2% of the population and is an important cause of acute hemorrhage in children and young adults. Although only about 15% of these diverticula contain gastric mucosa, half the lesions, which cause acute bleeding, contain gastric mucosa. The acid secretions from gastric mucosa result in peptic ulceration, most often in the ileal mucosa adjacent to the gastric mucosa and may lead to gastrointestinal bleeding.[33] ^{99m}Tc-pertechnetate radionuclide scans can detect these bleeding diverticula. Identifying normal Meckel's diverticulum is difficult on CT scan. It may show nodular enhancing mucosa in a tubular structure. Angiography can show the vessel supplying the area of abnormally increased contrast medium accumulation in the distal ileum. Vitelline artery is a separate branch of the superior mesenteric artery, which is specific to Meckel's diverticulum, but in 80% of diverticula this vessel is involuted and is replaced by a distal ileal branch **(Figs. 14A to E)**.[34]

Angiodysplasia

It is a mucosal telangiectasia, often multiple, usually involving the cecum or ascending colon. These lesions are often multiple and represent dilated pre-existing vascular structures (mucosal or submucosal venules). It is caused mainly by intermittent obstruction of venous outflow, but ischemia or toxic effects of bowel contents also have their role in its pathogenesis.

On angiography it is seen as a vascular tuft appearing in the arterial phase with an early opacification of a draining vein, and delayed emptying of a dilated and tortuous intramural vein. To diagnose bleeding from angiodysplasia, actual extravasation of contrast must be demonstrated. If extravasation is not detected, carcinoma or some other lesion should be considered, because about one-third of all elderly patients may have angiodysplasia without any history of bleeding. After angiographic diagnosis of the lesion, catheter may be left in place for arterial injection of methylene blue for intraoperative localization of the lesion. Treatment of incidentally found angioectasias is not indicated in patients with no history of LGIH.

Hemangioma and Arteriovenous Malformation

Gastrointestinal tract hemangioma and AVM are rare but can cause significant morbidity **(Figs. 5 and 15)**. The clinical presentation may be acute, recurrent or chronic. MR imaging is sometimes useful in the evaluation of extent of the colonic lesion.[35]

Tumors

These can bleed spontaneously, but such blood loss is more likely to be chronic and intermittent rather than massive. On angiography some tumors like leiomyomas and leiomyosarcomas, adenoma and Kaposi's sarcoma are hypervascular and typically have an intense capillary stain **(Figs. 16A and B)**.

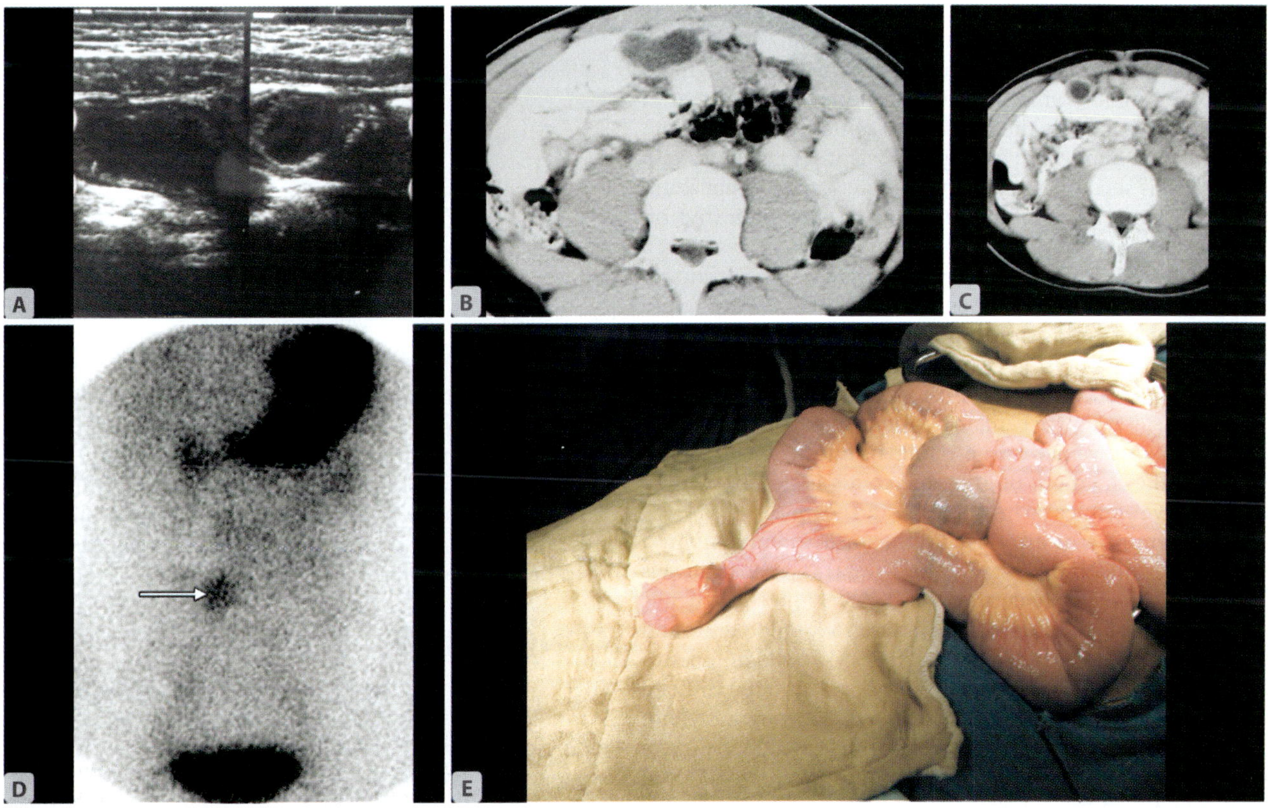

FIGS. 14A TO E: USG (A) showing a tubular, noncompressible, thick-walled blind ending structure in right paraumbilical region. On CECT (B and C) it was fluid filled with enhancing wall and showed active uptake of tracer (arrow) on 99mTc pertechnetate scan (D). The diagnosis of Meckel's diverticulum was confirmed at surgery (E).

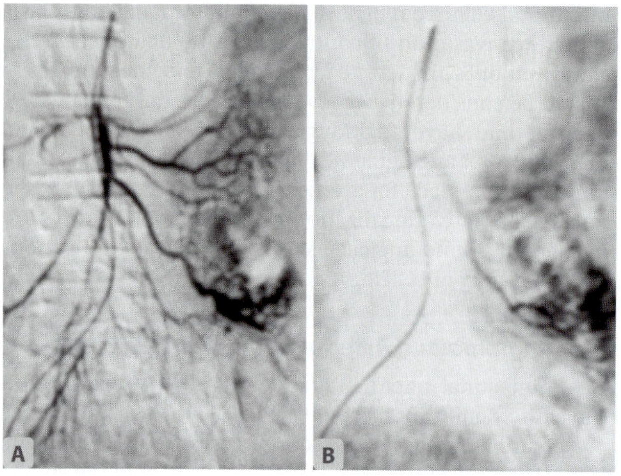

FIGS. 15A AND B: Superior mesenteric artery angiogram: (A) Early; (B) Delayed phase showing pooling of contrast in jejunal arteriovenous malformation.

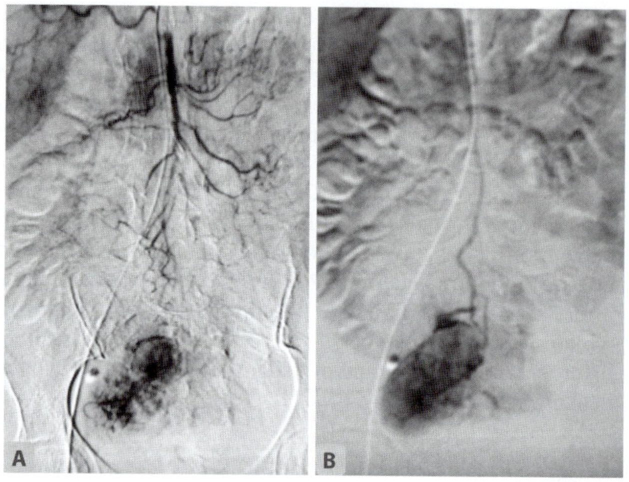

FIGS. 16A AND B: Superior mesenteric artery angiogram. (A) Early; (B) Delayed phase showing tumor vascularity in a case of ileal adenoma.

Inflammatory Bowel Diseases and Small Bowel or Colonic Ulcers

These produce nonspecific angiographic findings such as dilated arteries, mucosal outlining and sometimes pooling of contrast. Radiologic intervention is rarely needed.

Others

Mesenteric varices are rare and bleeding from these sites is unusual. The common location of these is in the rectosigmoid area. The most common cause of these varices is portal hypertension. Rarely these may be secondary to portal vein obstruction, congenital hepatic fibrosis (CHF), splenic vein thrombosis secondary to pancreatitis and splenorenal shunt block.[36] On angiography these can be demonstrated on delayed phase.

Ischemic colitis can be of occlusive or nonocclusive etiology. The occlusive causes are iatrogenic interruption of inferior mesenteric artery during aortic surgery, embolism, thrombosis, aneurysm of abdominal aorta, amyloidosis and vasculitis **(Figs. 17A and B)**.[37] Nonocclusive causes include low flow states due to cardiac dysfunction and hypovolemia. In the majority of patients, it is mild or transient. On barium enema, the hallmark of ischemic colitis is thumbprinting caused by submucosal hemorrhage and edema.

The rupture of arteriosclerotic aortic aneurysms into the small intestine (aortoenteric fistula) is almost always fatal. Rupture usually occurs after an arterial reconstructive surgery with fistula formation between synthetic graft and bowel lumen. A small bleed may precede a sudden massive hemorrhage from an aortoenteric fistula. It is often difficult to diagnose it angiographically and on CT angiography, but observation of a nipple-like projection or a pseudoaneurysm in the presence of a vascular graft is presumptive evidence of a fistula. Mycotic aneurysm of mesenteric vessels are rare and are usually managed by surgery **(Figs. 18A to C)**.

Acute portal hypertension may also result in severe variceal bleeding which may not be controlled by endoscopy.

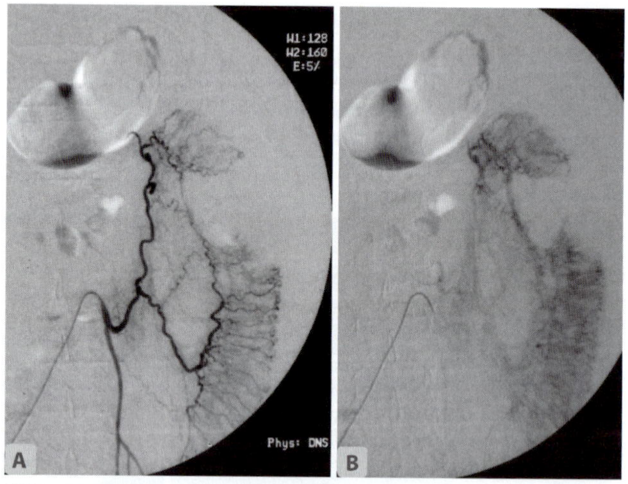

FIGS. 17A AND B: Inferior mesenteric artery angiogram: (A) Early; (B) Delayed phase showing avascular segment of descending colon.

Emergency transjugular intrahepatic portosystemic stent shunt (TIPSS) may be needed to save the patient. Bleeding fundal varices in patients with cirrhosis is difficult to manage by endoscopy and require an interventional procedure called balloon-occluded retrograde transvenous obliteration (BRTO) of varices. These procedures have been described elsewhere in the textbook.

CONCLUSION

GIH is a common clinical problem and needs a unified systemic approach by the physician, surgeon and radiologist with special expertise in vascular interventions. CT angiography should be the investigation of choice when endoscopy fails to diagnose the cause. DSA should be restricted to situations where interventions are required. In spite of many modern diagnostic techniques, quite often the cause of GIH remains undiagnosed.

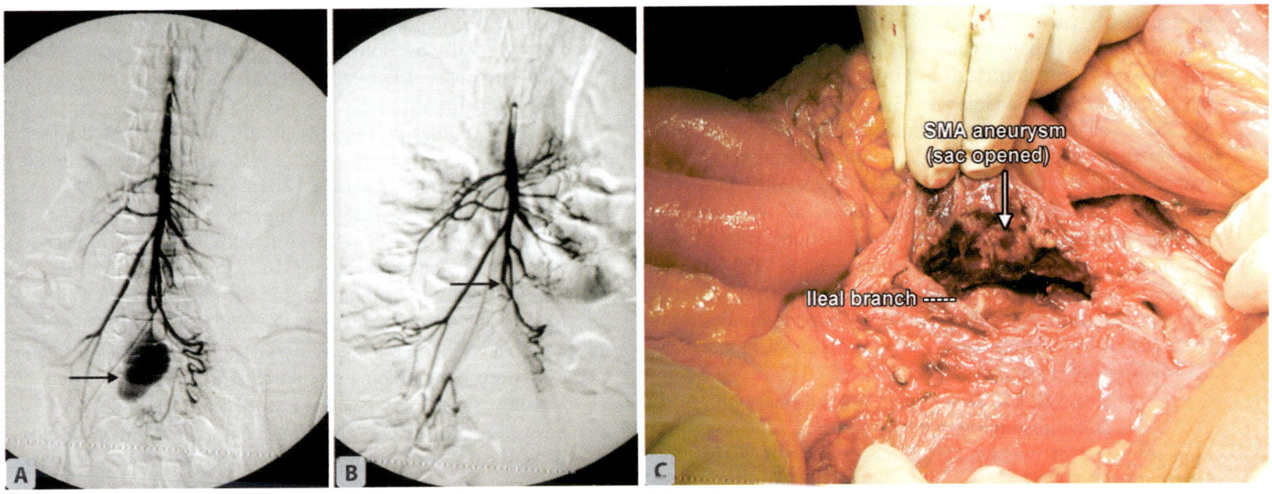

FIGS. 18A TO C: Superior mesenteric artery (SMA) angiogram (A) is showing a large aneurysm (arrow). The aneurysm was embolized (arrow) with steel coils (B) and later on surgically removed (C).

REFERENCES

1. Kennedy DW, Laing CJ, Tseng LH, Rosenblum DI, Tamarkin SW. Detection of active gastrointestinal hemorrhage with CT angiography: a 4(1/2)-year retrospective review. J Vasc Interv Radiol. 2010;21:848-55.
2. Huprich JE, Alexander JA, Mullan BP, Stanson AW. Gastrointestinal hemorrhage. In: Gore RM, Levine MS (eds.) Gastrointestinal Radiology, 4th edition. WB Saunders, Philadelphia; 2015.pp.2271-81.
3. Laing CJ, Tobias T, Rosenblum DI, Banker WL, Tseng L, Tamarkin SW. Acute gastrointestinal bleeding: Emerging role of multidetector CT angiography and review of current imaging techniques. Radiographics. 2007;27:1055-70.
4. Kim BSM, Li BT, Engel A, Samra JS, Clarke S, Norton ID, Li AE. Diagnosis of gastrointestinal bleeding: A practical guide for clinicians. World J Gastrointest Pathophysiol. 2014;5:467-78.
5. Whelan CT, Chen C, Kaboli P, Siddique J, Prochaska M, Meltzer DO. Upper versus lower gastrointestinal bleeding: a direct comparison of clinical presentation, outcomes, and resource utilization. J Hosp Med. 2010;5:141-7.
6. Lee EW, Laberge JM. Differential diagnosis of gastrointestinal bleeding. Tech Vasc Interv Radiol. 2005;7:112-22.
7. Manning-Dimmitt LL, Dimmitt SG, Wilson GR. Diagnosis of gastrointestinal bleeding in adults. Am Fam Physician. 2005; 71:1339-46.
8. Jaskolka JD, Binkhamis S, Prabhudesai V, Chawla TP. Acute gastrointestinal hemorrhage: radiologic diagnosis and management. Can Assoc Radiol J. 2013;64:90-100.
9. Strate LL. Lower GI bleeding: epidemiology and diagnosis. Gastroenterol Clin North Am. 2005;34:643-64.
10. Triester SL, Leighton JA, Leontiadis GI, Fleischer DE, Hara AK, Heigh RI, et al. A meta-analysis of the yield of capsule endoscopy compared to other diagnostic modalities in patients with obscure gastrointestinal bleeding. Am J Gastroenterol. 2005;100: 2407-18.
11. Mellinger JD, Bittner JG, Edwards MA, Bates W, Williams HT. Imaging of gastrointestinal bleeding. Surg Clin North Am. 2011;91:93-108.
12. Zuckier LS. Acute gastrointestinal bleeding. Semin Nucl Med. 2003;33(4):297-311.
13. Kim J, Kim YH, Lee KH, Lee YJ, Park JH. Diagnostic performance of CT angiography I patients visiting emergency department with overt gastrointestinal bleeding. Korean J Radiol. 2015;16:541-9.
14. Lee SM, Kim TO, Park HY, et al. Role of multi-detector row computed tomography for localisation of acute lower gastrointestinal bleeding. Korean J Gastroenterol. 2008;51:298-304.
15. Yoon W, Jeong YY, Shin SS, et al. Acute massive gastrointestinal bleeding: detection and localization with arterial phase multi-detector row helical CT. Radiology. 2006;239(1):160-7.
16. Sun H, Hou XY, Xue HD, Li XG, Jin ZY, Qian JM, et al. Dual-source dual-energy CT angiography with virtual non-enhanced images and iodine map for active gastrointestinal bleeding: image quality, radiation dose and diagnostic performance. Eur J Radiol. 2015;84(5):884-91.
17. Srivastava DN, Sharma S, Pal S, Thulkar S, Seith A, Bandhu S, et al. Transcatheter arterial embolisation in the management of hemobilia. Abdominal Imaging. 2006;31(4):439-48.
18. Jaeckle T, Stuber G, Hoffmann MH, Jeltsch M, Schmitz BL, Aschoff AJ. Detection and localization of acute upper and lower gastrointestinal (GI) bleeding with arterial phase multidetector row helical CT. Eur Radiol. 2008;18:1406-13.
19. Abbas SM, Bissett IP, Holden A, et al. Clinical variables associated with positive angiographic localisation of lower gastrointestinal bleeding. ANZ J Surg. 2005;75:953-7.
20. Kim CY, Suhocki PV, Miller MJ Jr, Khan M, Janus G, Smith TP. Provocative mesenteric angiography for lower gastrointestinal hemorrhage: results from a single-institution study. J Vasc Interv Radiol. 2010;21(4):477-83.
21. Ryan JM, Key SM, Dumbleton SA, Smith TP. Nonlocalized lower gastrointestinal bleeding: provocative bleeding studies with intra-arterial tPA, heparin, and tolazoline. J Vasc Interv Radiol. 2001;12(11):1273-7.
22. Madhusudhan KS, Sharma S, Srivastava DN, Thulkar S, Mehta SN, Prasad G, et al. Comparison of intra-arterial digital subtraction angiography using carbon dioxide by 'home made' delivery system and conventional iodinated contrast media in the evaluation of peripheral arterial occlusive disease of the lower limbs. J Med Imaging Radiat Oncol. 2009;53(1):40-9.
23. Cho KJ. Carbon dioxide angiography: Scientific principles and practice. Vasc Specialist Int. 2015;31(3):67-80.
24. Madhusudhan KS, Venkatesh HA, Gamanagatti S, Garg P, Srivastava DN. Interventional radiology in the management of visceral artery pseudoaneurysms: A Review of Techniques and Embolic Materials. Korean J Radiol. 2016;17(3):351-63.

25. Srivastava DN, Gandhi D, Julka PK, Tandon RK. Gastrointestinal hemorrhage in hepatocellular carcinoma: management with transhepatic arterioembolization. Abd Imaging. 2000; 25:380-4.
26. Madhusudhan KS, Gamanagatti S, Garg P, Shalimar, Dash NR, Pal S, et al. Endovascular embolization of visceral artery pseudoaneurysms using modified injection technique with N-butyl cyanoacrylate glue. J Vasc Interv Radiol. 2015;26(11):1718-25.
27. Srivastava DN, Sharma S, Yadav S, et al. Pedunculated hepatic hemangioma with arterioportal shunt treated with angioembolisation and surgery. Australas Radiol. 1998;42:151-3.
28. Falodia S, Garg PK, Bhatia V, Ramachandran V, Dash MR, Srivastava DN. EUS diagnosis of a left gastric artery pseudoaneurysm and aneurysmogastric fistula seen with a massive GI hemorrhage. Gastrointestinal Endoscopy. 2008; 68(2):389-91.
29. Gandhi D, Srivastava DN, Choudhary VP, Pande GK, Datta Gupta S. Haemangiolymphangiomatous hamartoma of jejunum: an unusual cause of massive gastrointestinal hemorrhage. Trop Gastroenterol. 2001;22(2):95-7.
30. Chandrasekhar W, Srivastava DN, Mathur M, Bhatnagar V. Angiographic and immunologic studies in acute necrotizing jejunoileitis. J Trop Pediatr. 2002;48(2):88-92.
31. Ibrahim AS, Allangawi MH, Al-Muzrakchi AM. Massive bleeding from an arteriovenous malformation in the gastric fundus following gastric biopsy treated by embolisation. Int J Clin Pract. 2003;57:354-5.
32. Rao RCK, Kumar A, Berry M. Pseudoaneurysm of anomalous right hepatic artery as a cause of hemosuccus pancreaticus. Gastrointest Radiology. 1987;12:313-4.
33. Choi SY, Hong SS, Park HJ, Lee HK, Shin HC, Choi GC. The many faces of Meckel's diverticulum and its complications. J Med Imaging Radiat Oncol. 2016.
34. Bree RL, Reuter SR. Angiographic demonstration of a bleeding Meckel's diverticulum. Radiology. 1973;108:287-8.
35. Kandpal H, Sharma R, Srivastava DN, Sahni P, Vashisht S. Diffuse cavernous hemangioma of colon: magnetic resonance imaging features. Report of two cases. Australas Radiol. 2007; 51:147-51.
36. Srivastava DN, Yadav S, et al. Emergency percutaneous occlusion of surgical portosystemic shunt using steel coils and balloon catheter. Am J Roentgenol. 1999;172:1453-4.
37. Srivastava DN, Gulati MS, Tandon RK. Colonic infarction in acute pancreatitis: an unusual cause of gastrointestinal hemorrhage. Am J Gastroenterol. 1998;93(7);1186-7.

CHAPTER

99

Imaging of Appendix

Anju Garg, Sapna Singh

INTRODUCTION

The vermiform appendix is present only in humans, certain anthropoid apes and the wombat. Morphologically, it is the undeveloped distal end of the large cecum found in many lower animals. It usually arises from the posteromedial wall of the cecum about 2.5–4 cm below the ileocecal valve **(Fig. 1)**.[1] Although the relationship of the base of the appendix to the cecum is essentially constant, the remainder of the appendix is free, which accounts for its variable location in the abdominal cavity. If the cecum occupies a relatively normal position, the retrocecal position of the appendix is the most frequent. More than 50% of the appendices are retrocecal or retrocolic in position as judged from both operative and postmortem reports. The next most frequent position is pelvic and rarer situations are preileal, postileal, splenic and pericolic **(Fig. 2)**. A recent imaging based study showed that only in 4% cases is the appendix located at the classic McBurney point[2] (junction of the lateral and middle third of the line between the anterior superior iliac spine and the umbilicus).

The appendix is invested with a mesentery called the "mesoappendix". The wall of the appendix is composed of the mucosa, submucosa, muscularis and serosa, similar to the rest of the intestine. There is a 'valve' at its orifice in the cecum which probably does not function in life. At postmortem examination total occlusion of the lumen of the appendix is seen in 3–4% cases, whereas almost total/partial obliteration is found in an additional 25%. In persons greater than 60 years of age, the lumen is obliterated in more than 50% cases and may represent a etrogressive normal change with age.[3]

NORMAL IMAGING APPEARANCE

On plain films a normal appendix cannot be visualized. A calcified appendicolith may sometimes be detected, incidentally, as a laminated density of variable size (0.5–6 cm) in the right lower quadrant **(Fig. 3)**. It may occur in unusual locations when the appendix is in an abnormal position.

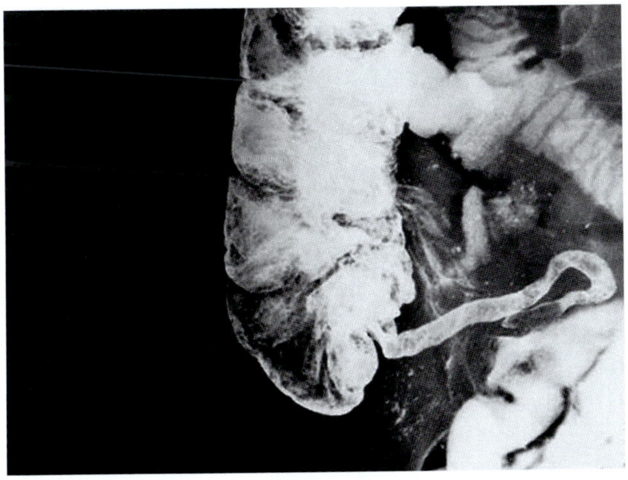

FIG. 1: Barium meal follow through study shows the origin of the appendix from the cecum below the ileocecal valve. A well-defined intraluminal filling defect is seen at its distal end due to a fecalith.

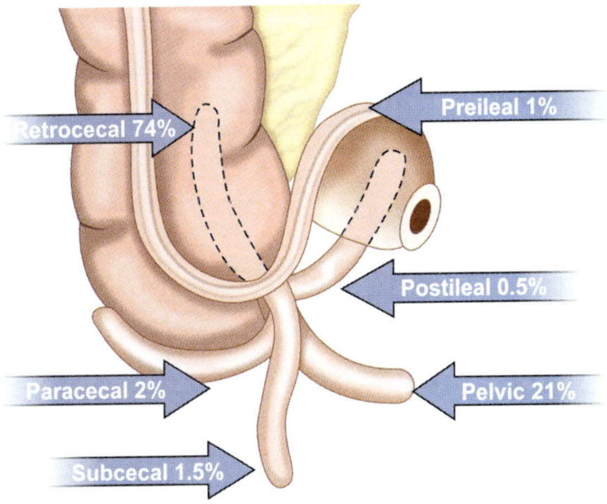

FIG. 2: The variable positions of the appendix.

The normal appendix fills with barium in 80–90% of barium studies and is seen as a thin, tubular structure with a convex, rounded tip. There may be filling defects seen within the barium filled appendix which can be due to noncalcified fecaliths, air bubbles, or mucus **(*see* Fig. 1)**. The presence of air bubbles within the lumen may be a normal finding specially in the subhepatic, vertically directed appendix.

Occasionally the appendix may not fill immediately at the time of a barium examination but may be seen to contain barium in delayed films. In approximately 10% of cases the normal appendix may not fill at all. In some cases barium may be persistently retained in the appendix for a period of weeks or months after the barium examination **(Figs. 4A and B)**. Retention of barium can rarely predispose to the development of acute appendicitis.[4,5]

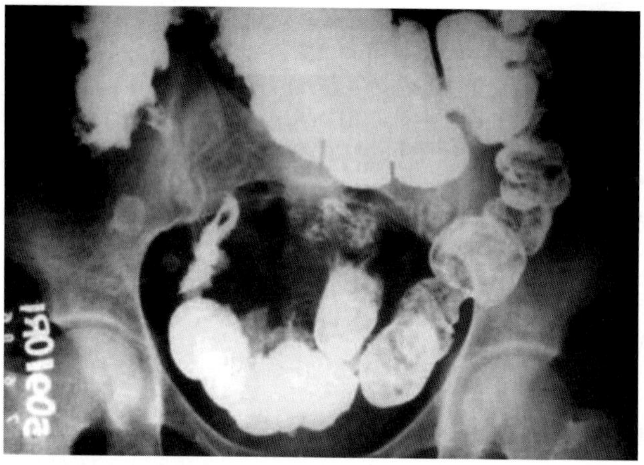

FIG. 3: Two appendicoliths can be seen in a noncontrast filled appendix on a barium study.

Sonography

In 1986, Puylaert[6] described a specific technique of graded compression applied with a high frequency transducer (> 5 MHz) for examination of the appendix. Using this technique the fat and bowel are displaced or compressed. This eliminates artefacts from bowel contents and reduces the distance from the transducer to the appendix, allowing the use of a high frequency probe with better image quality.

The normal appendix, when identified, is seen as a compressible, tubular, blind ended structure, of double layer wall thickness < 6 mm, with or without echogenic intraluminal material (gas or feces) with no evidence of peristalsis.[7] The typical lamellated appearance may be seen even in the normal appendix representing (from outer to inner) the echogenic outer serosa, the hypoechoic muscular layer, the echogenic submucosa, followed by the hypoechoic muscularis mucosae and the innermost echogenic mucosal lining[8] **(Figs. 5A and B)**.

During computed tomography (CT) of the abdomen visualization of a normal appendix depends in great measure on the amount of intraperitoneal fat, the adequate opacification of terminal ileal loops and cecum, the type and quality of CT examination, and the diligence of the examiner. The normal appendix can be identified in 67–100% of adults who undergo dedicated thin-section helical CT scan.[9-11] Although the normal appendix may be seen in most cases even on unenhanced scans, intravenous and oral contrast do increase the detection rate.

Depending on its orientation, the appendix appears as a small tubular or ring-like density in the right lower abdomen which is either collapsed or can be fluid or air filled and has a thin wall with a sharp outer contour **(Figs. 6A to C)**. It is enveloped by the homogeneous fat density of normal mesenteric structures and may be located in the pelvis or posterior to the right colon in the retrocecal position.

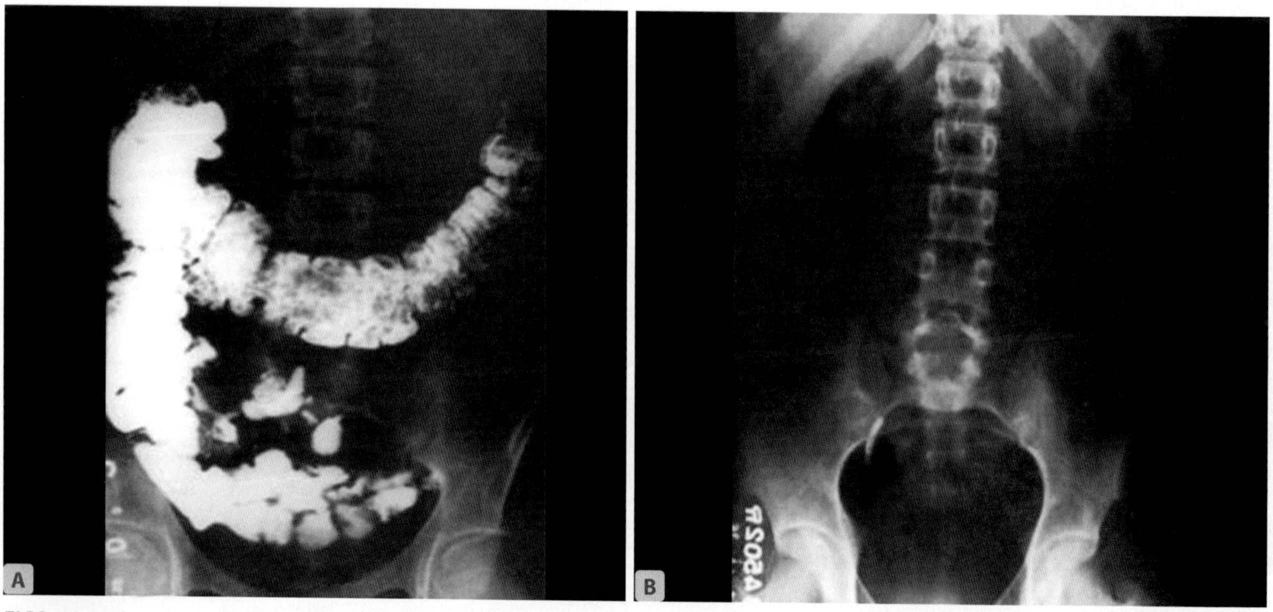

FIGS. 4A AND B: (A) Barium study showing a normally filling appendix; (B) Plain radiography done one month later shows retention of barium within the appendix.

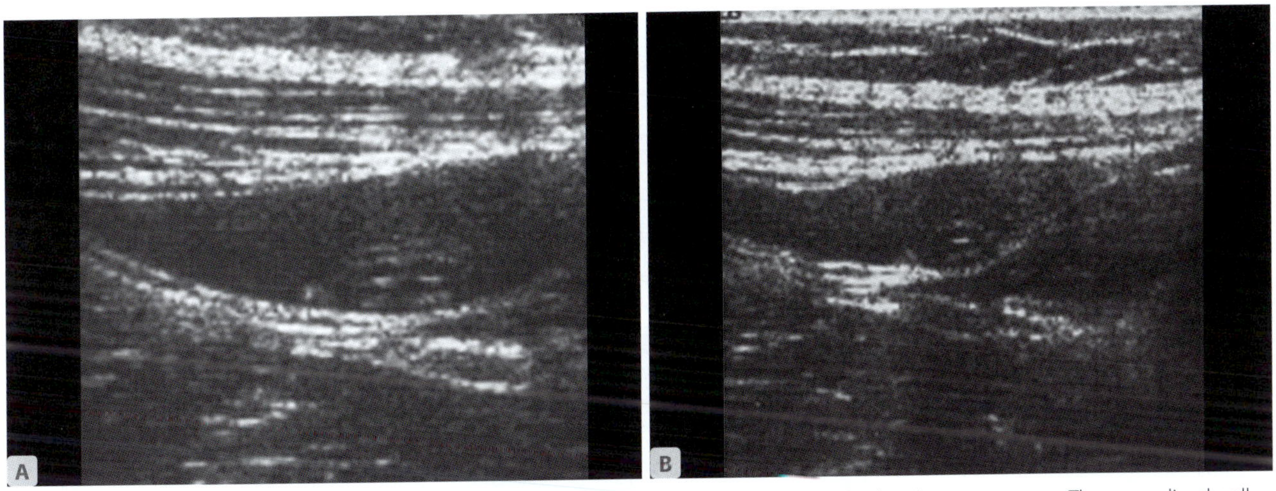

FIGS. 5A AND B: Sonographic visualization of the normal appendix in a case of ascites—longitudinal and transverse scans. The appendiceal wall shows the typical laminated appearance—the central hyperechoic interface of collapsed lumen, surrounded by the inner hypoechoic mucosa, echogenic muscularis propria bounded by the thin echogenic serosa. The total AP thickness of the appendix measured 3.8 mm.

The diameter of the appendix has been seen to range from 3 mm to 10 mm which overlap the values used to diagnose appendicitis.[12] Appendicoliths may be seen in asymptomatic individuals presenting as ring like or homogeneous calcific densities associated with a normal looking appendix. The presence of air, fecal matter, or calcifications in the appendix has no immediate clinical implications without the expected inflammatory changes indicative of appendicitis.

ACUTE APPENDICITIS

Acute appendicitis is the most common cause of acute abdominal pain requiring surgery. Early diagnosis is crucial to the success of therapy, which consists of surgical removal of the inflamed appendix before it perforates.

Pathophysiology

The pathogenesis of acute appendicitis is thought to relate to obstruction of its orifice.[13,14] Mechanical obstruction by fecalith or solid fecal material in the cecum is demonstrated in one-third of the cases. Occasionally tumors, parasites, foreign bodies, etc. may be incriminated. However, no obstruction is demonstrated in up to half of the patients with appendicitis.

Fecaliths, which result from the inspissation of fecal material and inorganic salts within the appendiceal lumen, are the most common cause of obstruction and are present in 11–52% of patients with acute appendicitis.[15,16] True appendiceal calculi (hard, noncrushable, calcified stones) are less common than appendiceal fecaliths (hard but crushable concretions) but have been shown to be associated more commonly with perforating appendicitis and periappendiceal abscess.[15]

A relation between viral infection and appendicitis has also been described. Viral infection can cause lymphoid hyperplasia or lymph node enlargement which in turn can obstruct the appendiceal lumen. Another theory is that viral infections can cause mucosal ulceration leading to bacterial invasion of appendiceal wall and subsequent appendicitis.[16,17]

As the secretions distend the obstructed appendix, the intraluminal pressure rises, eventually leading to ischemia, mucosal ulceration and invasion of the wall by intestinal bacteria. The inflammation commences as a catarrhal appendicitis with congestion of the mucous membrane and variable reaction in the submucosal, muscular and peritoneal layers. It progresses rapidly, specially in the presence of a fecalith and the infected, necrotic wall becomes gangrenous which may perforate within 24–48 hours.[18]

Rupture of the appendix with spillage of pus into the peritoneal cavity results in localized or generalized peritonitis. In most cases, the spill of pus is limited, being walled off by omentum, mesentery, bowel loops and adhesions. If this protective measure is successful an "appendicular mass" is formed which may be a phlegmon or, in cases of circumscribed pus collection, an appendiceal abscess. The abscess may be intraperitoneal or retroperitoneal. It is most often located in the proximity of the appendix, so that the inflammatory mass usually lies adjacent to the cecum and terminal ileum. Depending on the position of the appendix, this may be in the right iliac fossa or in the pelvis. When the appendix is abnormally located or is unusually long, the abscess can be anywhere in the abdomen. Abscesses have been described in the left lower quadrant, the right flank, the anterior abdominal wall, the lesser sac, and in the subhepatic and subdiaphragmatic spaces.

Clinical Picture

Acute appendicitis typically presents with diffuse abdominal pain, anorexia, nausea and vomiting with subsequent migration of pain to the right iliac quadrant. However, this typical presentation is seen in only 50-60% of patients. The cardinal signs of appendicitis are localized abdominal tenderness, muscle guarding, pain on percussion and rebound tenderness. Laboratory abnormalities include leukocytosis and an elevated C-reactive protein. The differential diagnosis of appendicitis includes a long list of common gastrointestinal and genitourinary disorders[19] **(Table 1)**.

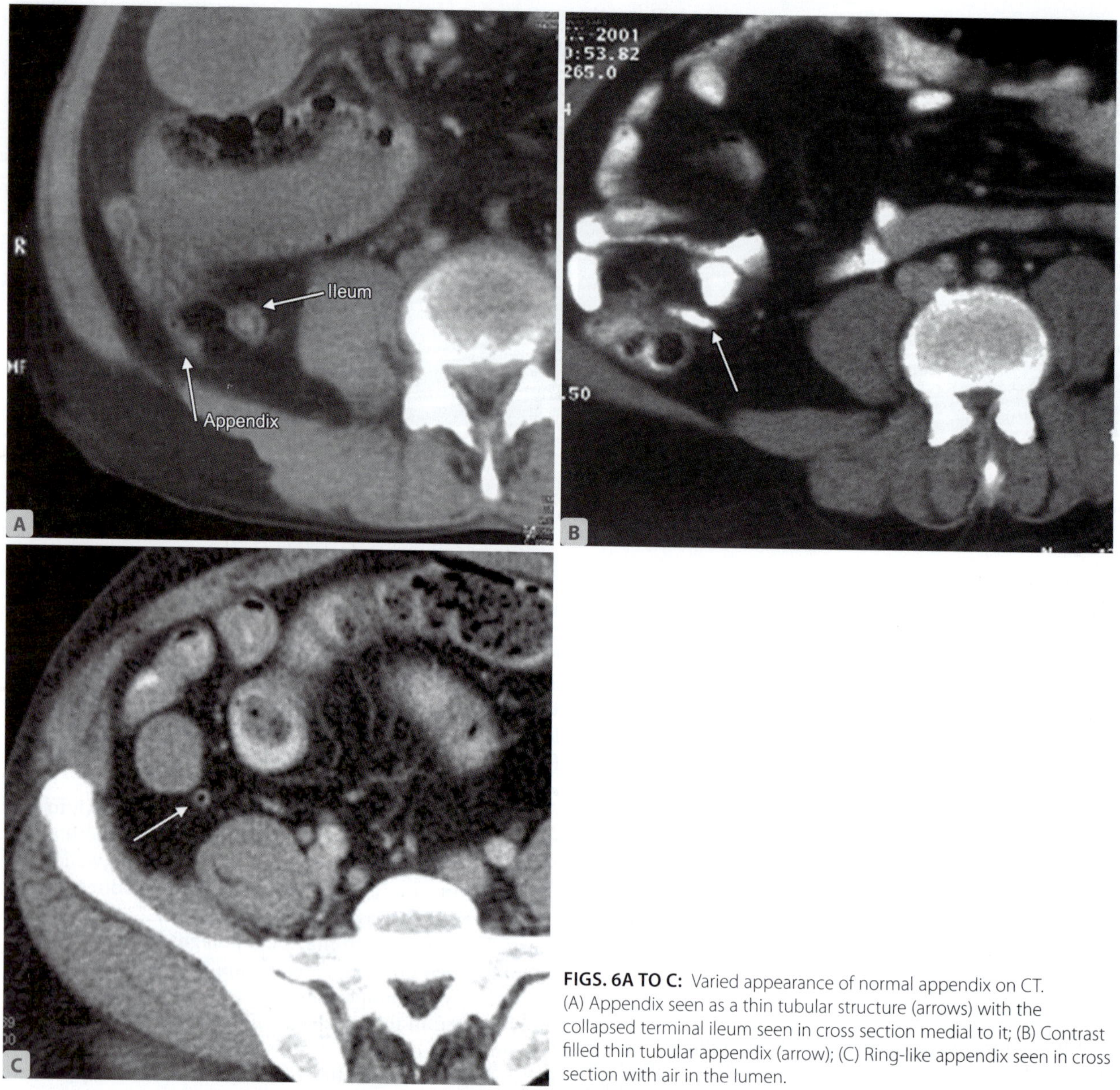

FIGS. 6A TO C: Varied appearance of normal appendix on CT. (A) Appendix seen as a thin tubular structure (arrows) with the collapsed terminal ileum seen in cross section medial to it; (B) Contrast filled thin tubular appendix (arrow); (C) Ring-like appendix seen in cross section with air in the lumen.

Imaging

Conventional Radiography

Plain abdominal radiographs are not indicated for clinically suspected appendicitis. Although they may be abnormal in approximately 50% of patients with acute appendicitis, they are not specific. The presence of calcified fecaliths (appendicoliths) is the single most important sign of appendicitis. Not only is their detection on the plain abdominal radiograph strong evidence of acute appendicitis, but their presence suggests perforation early in the course of the disease. Localized ileus, air-fluid level in cecum, cecal wall thickening and small bowel obstruction are other findings that can be seen on plain films.[20,21] Generalized paralytic ileus may occur in cases of perforated appendicitis but pneumoperitoneum is rare.

Ultrasonography

Ultrasonography is a widely available and inexpensive modality with the potential for highly accurate imaging in the patient suspected to have acute appendicitis.[22] In experienced hands US has reported sensitivities of 75–90%, specificities of 86–100%, accuracies of 87–96%, positive predictive values of 91–94% and negative predictive values of 89–97% for the diagnosis of acute appendicitis.[7,23-25]

Ultrasonography Technique

Puylaert's technique of using graded compression ultrasonography[6] is the most popular method of examination. It has a number of advantages. Firstly, it allows normal and gas filled loops of gut to be displaced from the field of view or compressed between the layers of musculature of the anterior and posterior abdominal wall. In contrast, abnormal loops of gut, or the obstructed appendix will be noncompressible and well seen on the grade dcompression image. This technique also allows for a successful examination of the patient who may have peritoneal irritation and sensitivity, as the compression is slow and gentle. Thirdly, the patient is able to provide input as to the point of maximal tenderness, which is often useful in focussing the examination in the correct area.[26] When a patient can self localize the site of maximal tenderness, there is a significant sonographic finding at this site in 94% of cases.[27]

Several additional maneuver have been shown to facilitate visualization of the appendix, e.g. applying pressure posteriorly to improve the degree of compression[28] or applying forceful upward sweeps with the transducer to displace the cecum and appendix upwards specially when the appendix is low lying or pelvic.[29] Turning the patient into the left lateral decubitus position is helpful in visualizing the retrocecal appendix.

Although high frequency linear probes are in wide use in patients suspected to have acute appendicitis, it has been reported that curvilinear probes work equally well and provide a slightly larger field of view and greater penetration. Transducers with a variable short focal zone and a frequency of 5–9 MHz have been recommended.[30] The use of harmonic imaging has also been shown to falicitate visualization of the appendix and the relevant surrounding structures.[31]

TABLE 1: Differential diagnosis of appendicitis.

- Acute mesenteric adenitis
- Acute gastroenteritis
- Crohn's disease
- Meckel's diverticulitis
- Diverticulitis
- Perforated peptic ulcer
- Intussusception
- Urinary tract infection
- Ureteral stone
- Ruptured Graafian follicle
- Epiploic appendagitis
- Endometriosis
- Ovarian torsion
- Ruptured ectopic pregnancy
- Pelvic inflammatory disease
- Ruptured hemorrhagic ovarian cyst
- Henoch-Schonlein purpura

Sonographic Findings

The inflamed appendix is seen as a blind ending, lamellated, a peristaltic tubular structure which is fixed, noncompressible and appears round on transverse sections. Traditionally appendicitis was diagnosed when its transverse diameter exceeded 6 mm. The threshold of 6 mm has a reported sensitivity of 98%,[32] however, sonographic studies of normal individuals show that up to 23% of normal patients have appendicular sizes > 6 mm.[33] Thus, the diameter of the appendix should be correlated with the associated findings, along with the clinical picture before a diagnosis of appendicitis is considered.

In early acute appendicitis-catarrhal stage-five layers can be identified **(Figs. 7A and B)**:

- A central, thin hyperechoic line representing the collapsed lumen and mucosal lining
- Hypoechoic layer (2–3 mm) representing the edematous lamina propria and muscularis mucosa
- Hyperechoic submucosa (2–3 mm)
- Hypoechoic muscular layer (2–3 mm)
- Outer most thin hyperechoic line representing the serosa.

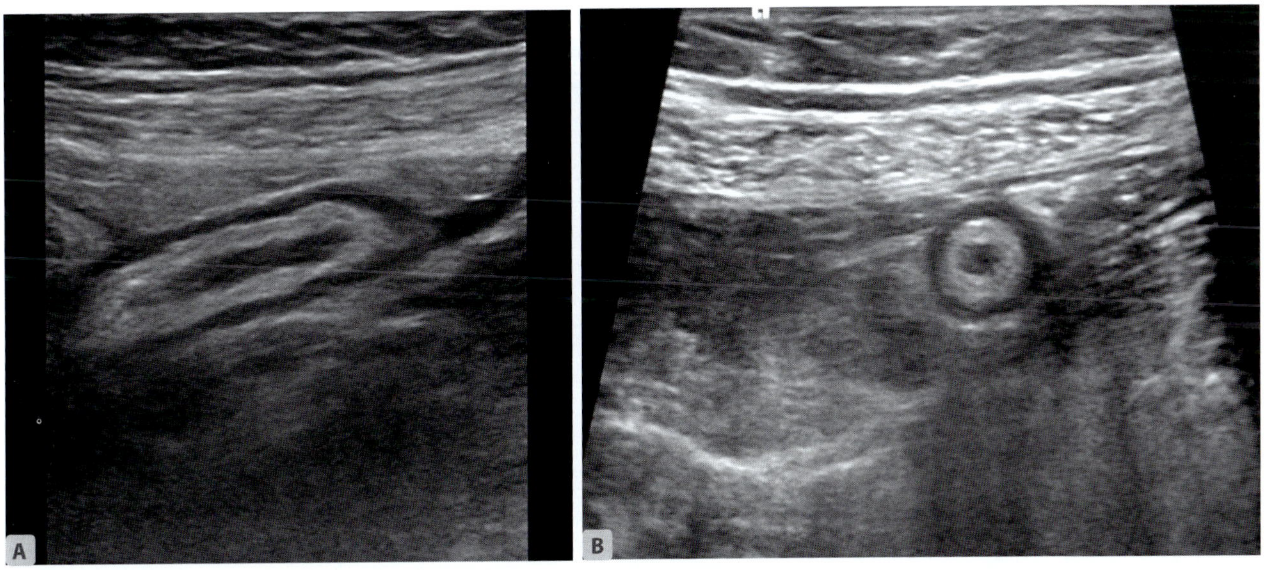

FIGS. 7A AND B: Acute appendicitis. (A) Oblique sonogram of right iliac fossa shows a blind-ending, tubular, layered, noncompressible inflamed appendix (maximal diameter 11 mm) which appears round on cross section; (B) Inflammatory changes can be seen as diffuse hyperechogenicity of the surrounding fat.

In the later suppurative stages, the lumen of the appendix gets distended with pus/fluid **(Fig. 8)** and there may be an increase in the thickness of the submucosa and muscular layer in the range of 3–6 mm.

Appendicoliths are seen as bright, echogenic foci with clean distal acoustic shadowing **(Figs. 9A and B)**. Their identification within the appendix or in the adjacent perienteric soft tissue after perforation is highly associated with a positive diagnosis. Failure to see an appendicolith is noncontributory. Inflammatory change in the adjacent fat appears bright and noncompressible and is a sonographic clue to the presence of appendicitis in doubtful cases. Enlarged mesenteric lymph nodes may be identified.

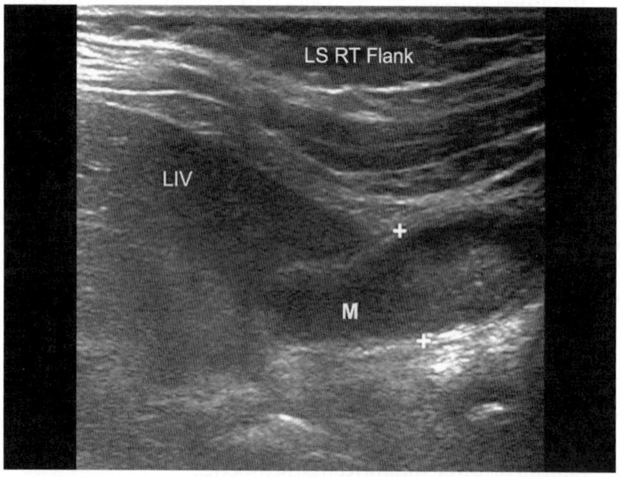

FIG. 8: Suppurative appendicitis in a subhepatic location. Longitudinal sonogram (LS) of right flank, in a 5-year-old boy, shows a markedly distended appendiceal lumen (++) with a fluid-debris level, just inferior to the liver (LIV).

An asymmetric thickening of the appendiceal wall suggests impending perforation **(Figs. 10A and B)**, whereas a focal/circumferential lack of visualization of the echogenic submucosa indicates perforation of the inflamed appendix. The lumen may or may not be distended.

An appendiceal mass is seen as a complex paracecal mass of mixed echogenicity and thickened paracecal fat. Phlegmonous change manifests as hypoechoic zones with poor margination within the inflamed fat **(Fig. 11)**. Liquefaction and abscess formation will manifest as an actual fluid component. Gas bubbles within a collection suggest either perforation or gas forming organisms. Sympathetic thickening of the adjacent terminal ileum and ascending colon can often be seen.[30]

Doppler Imaging

In cases of appendicitis, the presence of hyperemia in the appendiceal wall and adjacent mesoappendix **(Figs. 12A and B)** is a sensitive indicator of inflammation and can be well demonstrated on color Doppler.[34] The contribution of Doppler US is most evident in cases of equivocal grayscale US examination in which it is uncertain as to whether the imaged appendix is inflamed or normal.[35] When gangrenous changes supervene, color Doppler sonography may show decreased or no perfusion.

Pitfalls in Sonographic Diagnosis

Although ultrasound is highly specific for diagnosis of acute appendicitis, it requires considerable expertise. The most important cause for a false negative result is overlooking of the appendix. Peritonism may prevent graded compression in patients with perforation, or the dilated, air filled loops of a dynamic ileus can hide the appendix from view. Other causes are obesity, focal appendicitis of appendiceal tip, a gas filled appendix and a retrocecal position of the appendix.

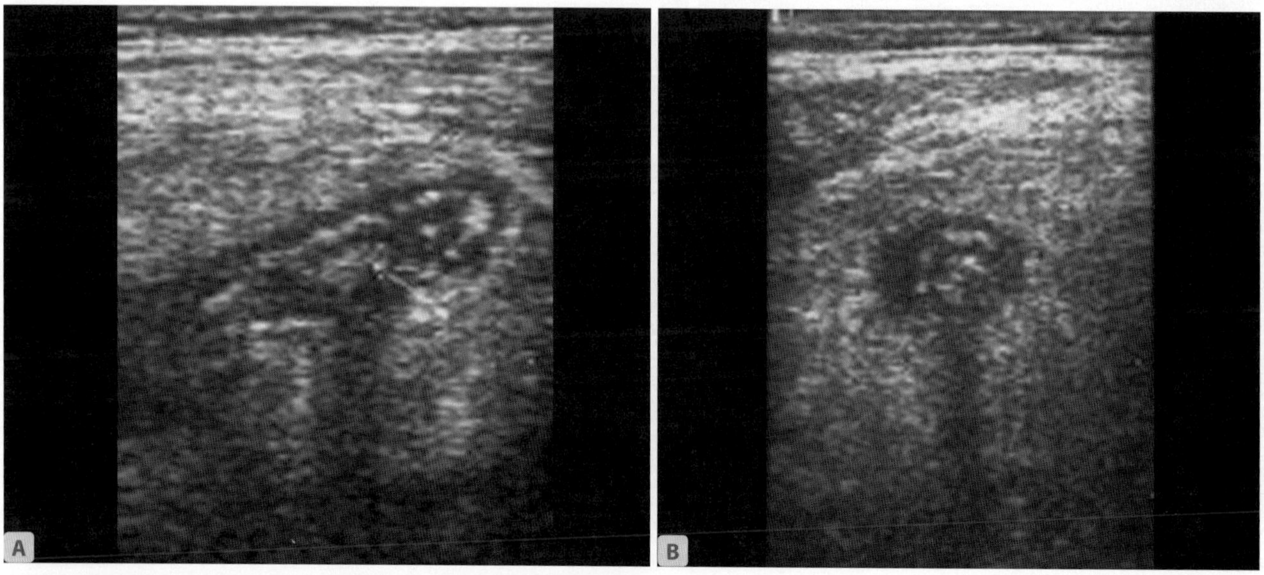

FIGS. 9A AND B: Acute appendicitis with appendicolith. (A) Longitudinal and (B) transverse sonographic images show an inflamed appendix with an appendicolith seen as an echogenic focus with distal shadowing within the lumen.

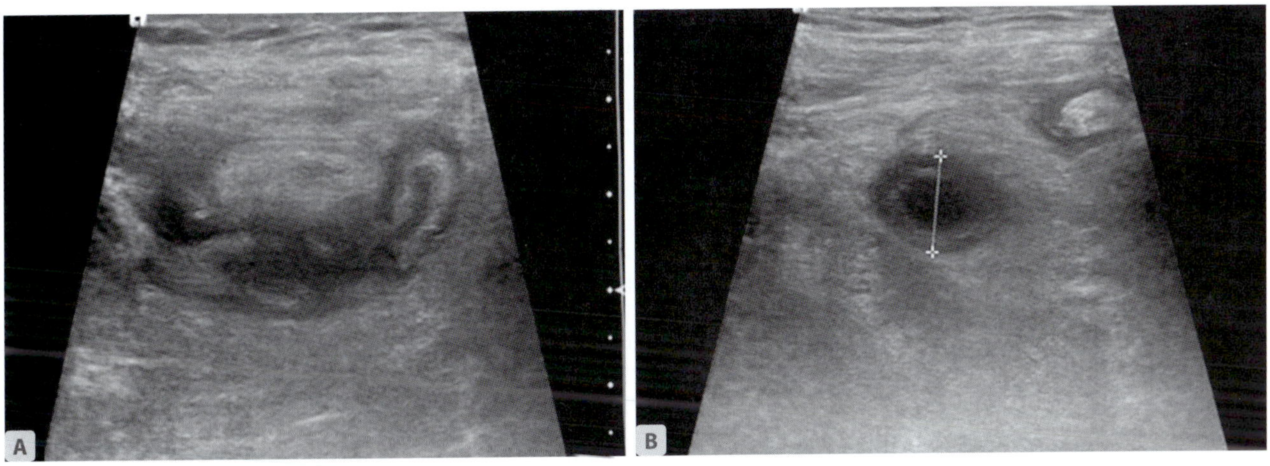

FIGS. 10A AND B: Acute suppurative appendicitis. (A) Longitudinal and (B) transverse sonographic images show a dilated appendix measuring 12 mm in diameter with a pus filled lumen and surrounding hyperechoic inflamed fat. The irregularly thickened echogenic submucosa suggests impending perforation.

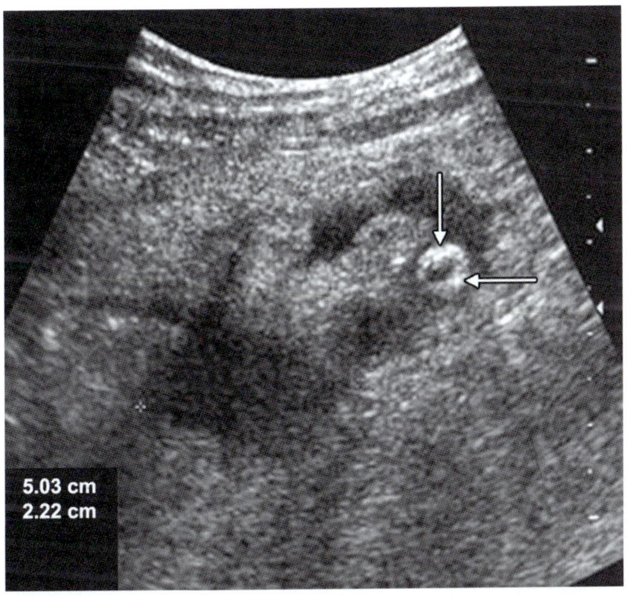

FIG. 11: Appendiceal mass: Sonography shows an ill-defined fluid collection and hyperechoic inflamed fat in the right iliac fossa with a small ring-shaped structure within it—the appendiceal remnant (arrows).

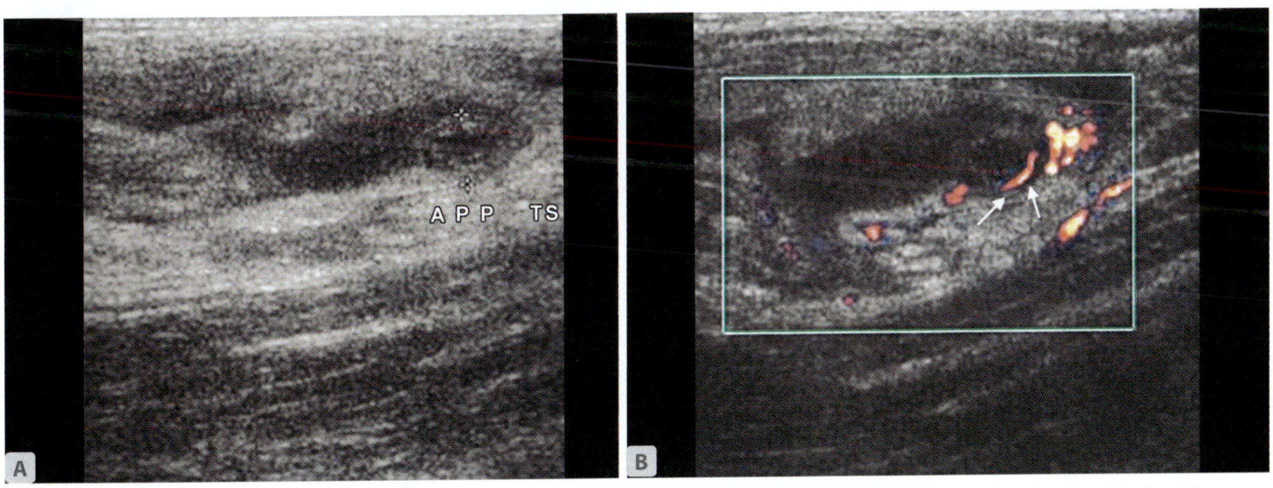

FIGS. 12A AND B: Color Doppler in acute appendicitis. Doppler demonstrates focally increased flow in the appendiceal wall and in the adjacent inflamed fat.

The appendix may be relatively thickened in cases of perforated peptic ulcer or sigmoid diverticulitis and a false positive diagnosis is possible. In some cases the terminal ileum or a dilated fallopian tube may be misinterpreted as the inflamed appendix. The appendicular diameter in children with cystic fibrosis may be more than 6 mm.

Computed Tomography

Computed tomography is a highly accurate and effective cross-sectional imaging technique for diagnosing and staging acute appendicitis. CT is readily available, operator independent and relatively easy to perform. It has reported sensitivities of 90–100%, specificities of 91–99%, accuracies of 94–98%, positive predictive values of 92–98% and negative predictive values of 95–100% for diagnosis of acute appendicitis.[30]

Computed Tomography Technique

Appendiceal CT protocols differ considerably with regard to the anatomic area to be included in the scan and to the use of intravenously, orally and rectally administered contrast material. The most popular and conservative approach is to perform helical CT scanning of the entire abdomen and pelvis with intravenous and oral contrast material. The main advantage of this technique is its ability to establish alternative or concurrent diagnoses. Scanning the entire abdomen also allows easy visualization of appendices in the nonstandard positions, including the right upper quadrant. The disadvantage of this technique is the time taken for the oral contrast to reach the cecum, which is essential for best results.

To overcome this drawback, simultaneous administration of rectal contrast has been recommended.[36] Not only does it shorten the delay of diagnosis, but the excellent visualization of the large bowel is helpful in identifying the appendix in difficult cases, in distinguishing bowel pathology from appendicitis and in distinguishing pelvic organs from bowel loops.

Rao et al. advocated a focussed appendiceal CT technique in which a limited helical CT study of the right lower quadrant is performed after the rapid administration of colonic contrast material.[10] This technique has proved to be as accurate as those techniques in which intravenous and oral contrast material are administered, while allowing scanning to be completed within 15 minutes in the majority of patients examined. It also reduces the radiation dose to approximately one-third that received in a full abdomen and pelvis examination. A limitation of this scanning method is that a minority of patients will require additional scanning of the proximal abdomen or of the distal pelvis to identify disease not included in the scanning field of view.

The fastest CT protocol has been promoted by Lane et al.[37,38] who have advocated use of nonenhanced helical CT of entire abdomen and pelvis. This examination may be performed in less than 10 minutes, does not expose the patient to the potential risks associated with iodinated contrast agents, requires no bowel preparation and represents the most cost effective imaging alternative to ultrasound. This procedure is most effective in patients with large body habitus, as diagnostic accuracy may be compromised in patients with little abdominal and intrapelvic fat.

CT Findings in Acute Appendicitis

A definitive CT diagnosis of acute appendicitis can be made if an abnormal appendix is identified or if a calcified appendicolith is seen in association with pericecal inflammation.[39,40] The inflamed appendix is seen as an enlarged, fluid filled, tubular structure associated with inflammatory stranding in the surrounding fat. Circumferential and symmetric wall thickening is nearly always present and is best demonstrated on images obtained with intravenous contrast enhancement **(Figs. 13A and B)**. The thickened wall usually enhances homogeneously, although mural stratification in the form of a target sign **(Fig. 14)** may be noted. Traditionally, the threshold diameter of 6 mm was

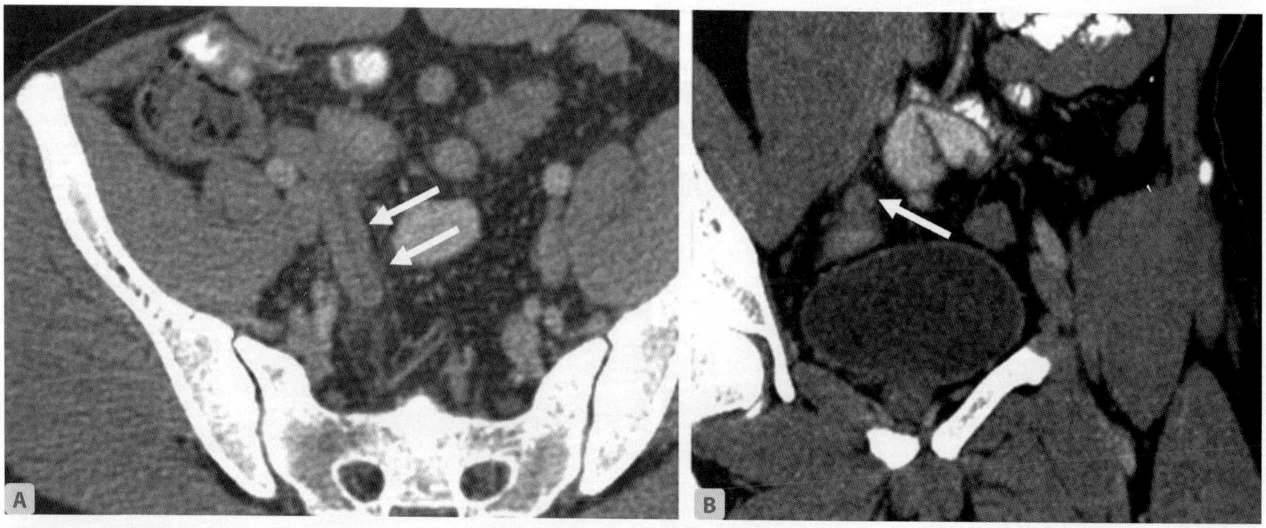

FIGS. 13A AND B: Appendicitis: A 27-year-old man with recurrent pain abdomen and negative US. CECT axial (A) shows the thickened, tubular, blind ending inflamed appendix (arrows) with subtle inflammatory stranding in the surrounding fat. The coronal oblique reformat (B) shows the inflamed appendix in cross section as a thickened ring (arrow). It measured 11 mm in diameter.

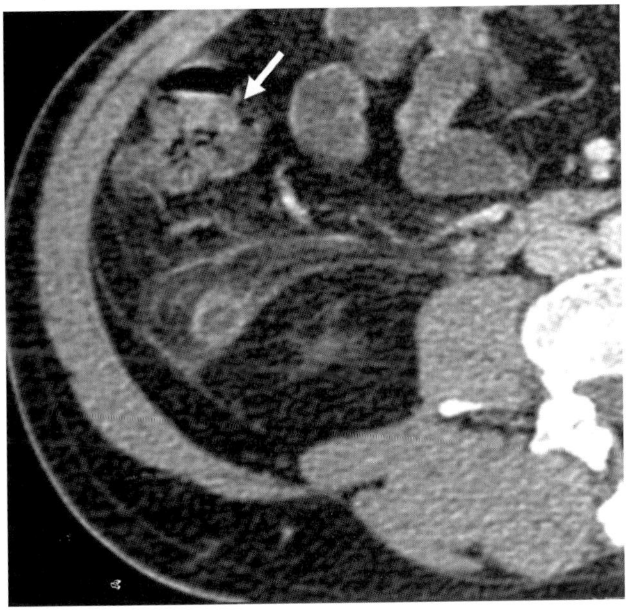

FIG. 14: Retrocecal appendicitis: CECT axial section shows the inflamed appendix as thickened, enhancing ringtarget sign—with marked surrounding inflammatory streaking. This was not seen on ultrasound as it was obscured by the cecum (arrow).

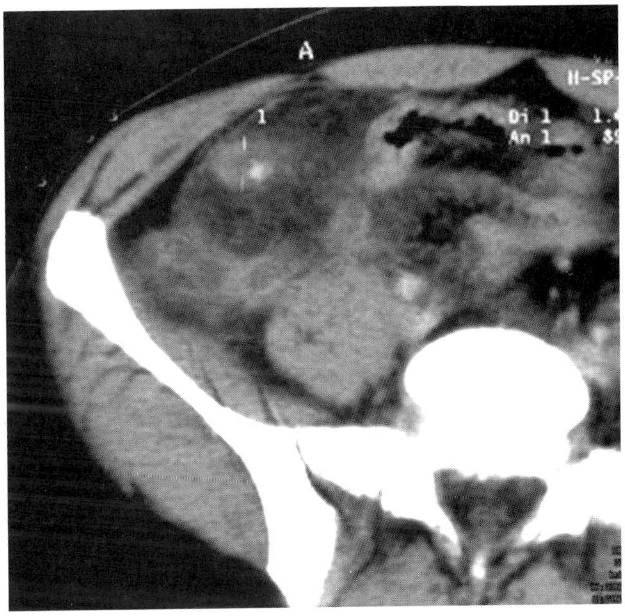

FIG. 15: Acute appendicitis: Axial CT section shows the appendix as a thick walled fluid filled structure (measuring 1.4 cm) with a small hyperdense focus within it—an appendicolith. Hazy, ill-defined, linear and streaky densities are seen in the adjacent mesentery due to severe peri-appendiceal inflammation.

used for diagnosis of appendicitis. However, it has been suggested that this may be too low, as studies in healthy adults have shown that the normal range of appendiceal size varies between 3 mm and 10 mm.[41] When the appendix diameter measures between 6 mm and 10 mm associated secondary changes such as fat stranding or cecal thickening should be present for a definitive diagnosis of appendicitis on CT. In the absence of secondary changes, a luminal diameter of 9 mm has been advocated as the threshold size for appendicitis.[42]

Linear fat stranding, local fascial thickening, and subtle clouding of the mesentery **(Fig. 15)** are characteristic findings of periappendiceal inflammation in nonperforated appendicitis; they may also be seen with microperforation. Other important findings include cecal apical thickening and the "arrowhead sign" **(Fig. 16)**. The latter finding occurs when cecal contrast material funnels symmetrically at the cecal apex to the point of appendiceal occlusion due to focal inflammatory thickening.[43] Another rare sign is the "cecal bar sign", which is seen when the inflamed cecal wall is interposed between cecal contents and a proximal obstructing appendicolith. Both, the arrowhead sign and the cecal bar sign can be seen only if positive contrast is present in the cecum.

Perforated appendicitis is usually accompanied by pericecal phlegmonor abscess formation **(Fig. 17)**. Associated findings include extraluminal air, marked ileocecal thickening, localized lymphadenopathy, peritonitis, and small-bowel obstruction. Contrast enhanced CT may be useful in cases of perforation by demonstrating the remains of a fragmented appendix. If the abnormal appendix is not seen, a specific diagnosis of appendicitis can be made by identifying an appendicolith with a periappendiceal abscess

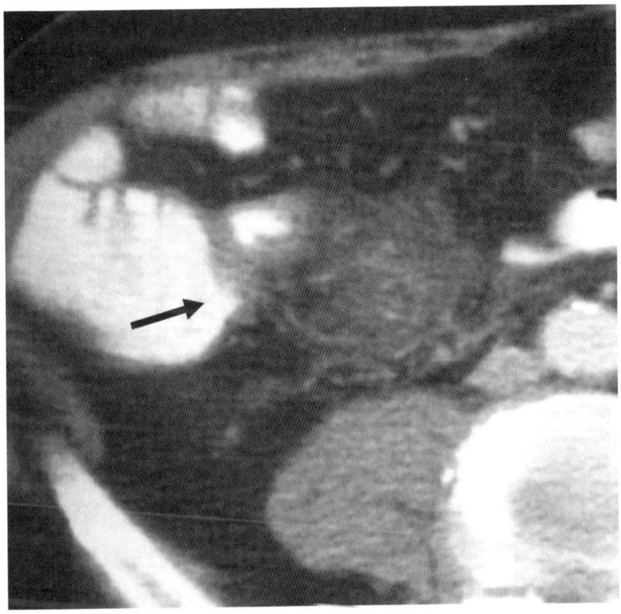

FIG. 16: Cecal arrowhead sign on CT: The focally thickened wall of the cecum seems to "funnel" the contrast material (arrow) towards the origin of the inflamed appendix.

or phlegmon. Appendicolith detection rates for helical CT are approximately twice those for conventional CT.[9,10,37]

Although a pericecal phlegmon or abscess is strongly suggestive of appendicitis, these are nonspecific findings that may be seen with other disease entities. If substantial inflammation is present within the right lower quadrant, it may be difficult to differentiate primary appendicitis with secondary inflammation of the cecum and terminal ileum from ileocolitis with secondary inflammation of the appendix.

The creation of multiplanar reformatted images increases the confidence in identifying both the normal and the inflamed appendix.[44] Some of the factors that cause difficulty in the diagnosis of appendicitis at axial CT can be overcome with MPR. Coronal MPR image can help clinicians and radiologists since it is analogus to a conventional abdominal radiograph. Oblique (coronal and sagittal) and curved MPRs along the axis of the appendix can show the entire length of the appendix often with an obstructing appendicolith between collapsed and inflamed segment **(Figs. 18A and B)**

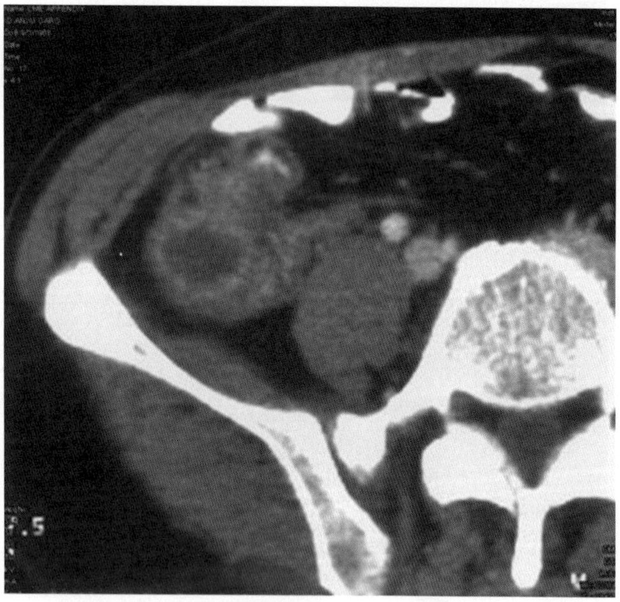

FIG. 17: CT of appendiceal abscess seen as a soft-tissue density mass with a central area of decreased attenuation in the right iliac fossa.

The CT findings of recurrent and chronic appendicitis are identical to those of acute appendicitis.[44] Distal appendicitis is diagnosed when CT reveals appendicitis that involves the distal, "upstream" aspect of the appendix, with a normal appearance of the proximal appendix and cecal apex. An obstructing pendicolith often is identified at the transition point between the normal and abnormal appendiceal segments. The proximal appendix in these cases may be collapsed or partially filled with contrast material or with air.

Pitfalls in CT Diagnosis

The paucity of intra-abdominal fat represents the most common reason for a false negative diagnosis. This can be overcome by good opacification of small bowel loops with oral contrast which allows their differentiation from a distended appendix. Abnormal enhancement of the appendiceal mucosa seen with intravenous contrast may also help in establishing the diagnosis of appendicitis in these cases. Other causes for false negative diagnosis may be the atypical presentations, e.g. tip appendicitis or stump appendicitis or atypical location of the appendix, e.g. in the inguinal or femoral canal.

Magnetic Resonance Imaging

Magnetic resonance imaging (MRI) is not routinely advocated in cases of suspected appendicitis. It can be useful in cases where sonography is nondiagnostic or equivocal and is an alternative modality for evaluation of pregnant and pediatric patients in whom exposure to radiation is a concern.

On MRI, the normal appendix is best seen on T2W images as a blind, tubular structure with a diameter of less than 7 mm, and a wall thickness less than 2 mm.[45] The inflamed appendix is also is best visualized on T2W sequences in the axial and coronal planes. T2W images are superior to T1W images because of better visualization of the bright signal intensity of inflammatory change associated with acute appendicitis.[46] The fat suppressed sequence in the axial plane shows the location of inflammation and free fluid collections better than other sequences although spatial resolution is less

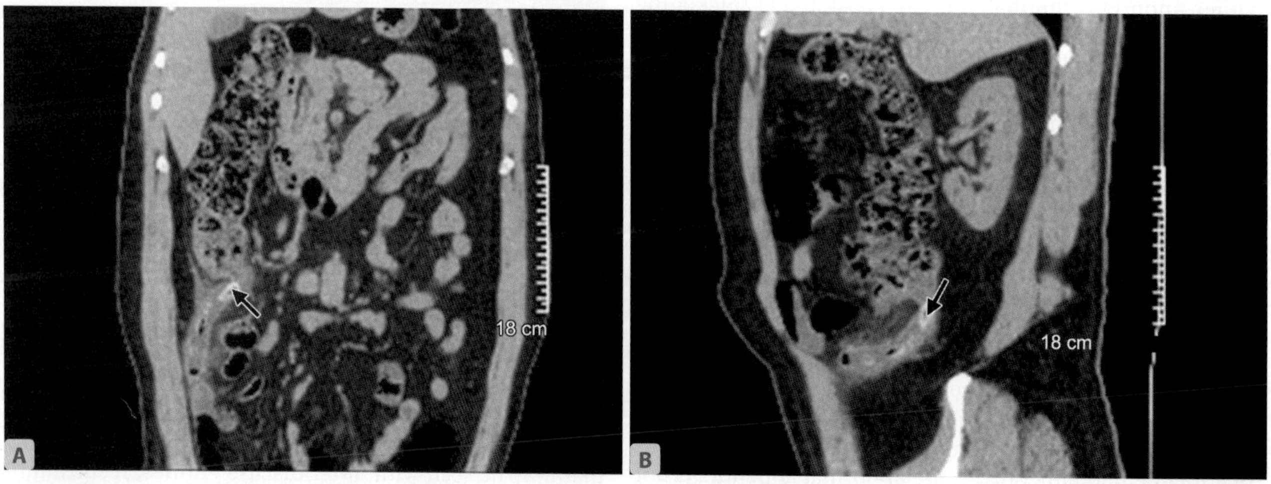

FIGS. 18A AND B: Coronal oblique and sagittal oblique reformats in another patient show the entire length of an enlarged, enhancing appendix arising from the cecum with an appendicolith (arrows) and few air lucencies within the lumen.

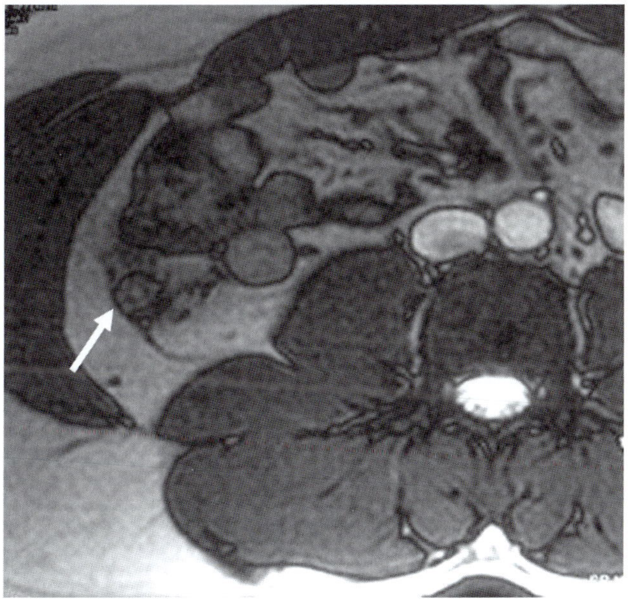

FIG. 19: MR-T2 weighted axial image showing a thickened, inflamed appendix in cross-section (arrow).

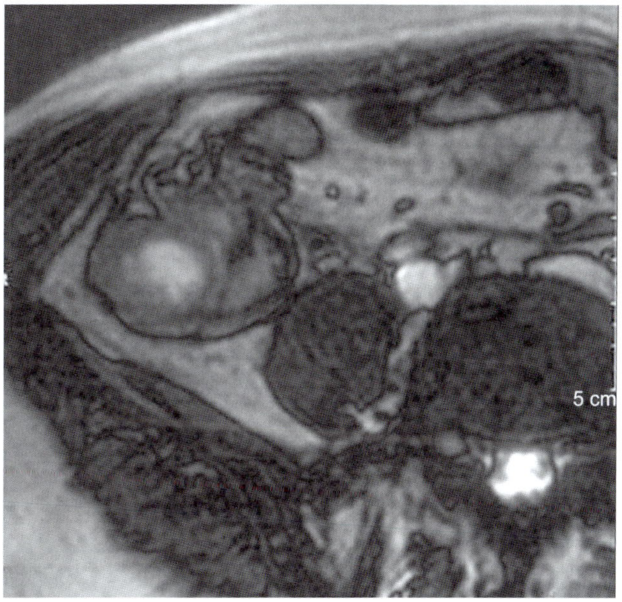

FIG. 20: MR-T2 weighted axial image in a case of appendiceal abscess shows a hyperintense fluid collection with a thick wall of lesser intensity.

as compared with T1W and T2W sequences. On fat saturated, gadolinium enhanced T1W images enhancement of the wall of the inflamed appendix is well seen.[47]

On T2W imaging, the thickened appendiceal wall is seen as a slightly hyperintense ring with a markedly hyperintense center representing intraluminal fluid **(Figs. 19 and 20)**. The cutoff threshold of the appendix is the same as for CT. Periappendiceal inflammation gives a marked hyperintense signal. Appendicoliths are difficult to demonstrate on MRI as they are seen as intraluminal structures without signal intensity on all sequences.

Diffusion weighted MR imaging and ADC quantification have also been found to be effective in detecting an inflamed appendix. The average ADC values in patients with non-perforated appendix have been found to be lower than normal control groups (1.01 × 10-3 mm^2/s vs 1.85 × 10-3 mm^2/s). ADC values were also found to be lower in cases of perforation as compared to nonperforated appendicitis (0.79 × 10-3 mm^2/s vs 1.11 × 10-3 mm^2/s). Thus, ADC values can be of help in the diagnosis of acute appendicitis and its complications.[48]

MR has the advantage of good visualization of the abnormal appendix and adjacent inflammatory process, the ability to identify appendicitis in atypical locations, operator independence and lacks exposure to iodinated contrast media. However, its drawbacks are long scan time, high cost, limited availability, inability to visualize an appendicolith, and limitations related to claustrophobia and metal artefacts.

WHICH MODALITY AND WHEN?

In almost 80% of the cases, acute appendicitis presents with typical findings and no imaging is required. In the rest of the patients, who are usually young, old or pregnant the clinical picture may be obscure and diagnosis is sometimes impossible until laparotomy. It is in this group of patients that imaging plays an important role and cross sectional imaging has a distinct advantage over clinical assessment.

A large number of studies have been performed to assess the comparative accuracy of US, CT and MRI in the diagnosis of acute appendicitis. Doria, et al performed a meta analysis of the studies published between 1986 and 2004.[48] CT had a pooled sensitivity and specificity of 94% and 95% respectively in children and 94% and 94% respectively in adults. Ultrasound had a pooled sensitivity and specificity of 88% and 94% respectively in children and 83% and 93% respectively in adults. Also, studies which compared US and CT directly confirmed that CT was more sensitive than ultrasound.

Gaitini D[49] reviewed studies which were performed between 2006 and 2011 comparing graded compression US and CT performance and using surgery or clinical follow-up as the standard reference. Her results are presented in **Table 2**. It was found that the sensitivity of US and CT ranged between 74–88% and 91–100% respectively, whereas the specificity ranged between 83–97% and 90–100% respectively, with higher US sensitivity in children than in adults. Pedrosa et al[50] compared the role of US and MRI in 148 pregnant patients suspected of appendicitis and found that US had a low sensitivity (36%) but excellent specificity (99%), whereas sensitivity and specificity of MRI was 100% and 93% respectively.

Although CT seems to have an advantage over ultrasound in detection of acute appendicitis, US is substantially less expensive than CT and does not use ionizing radiation. It is also more universally available in our country. However, it is operator dependent and a small but finite number of false negative results occur regardless of expertise **(Table 3)**. Nevertheless, it is still recommended as the initial imaging modality specially in children, followed by CT only if sonographic diagnosis is uncertain. This approach seems to

TABLE 2: US and CT performance for the diagnosis of acute appendicitis.

Publication	No. of patients	US sensitivity %	CT sensitivity %	US specificity %	CT specificity %
Van Randen A 2008[51]	671	79	91	83	90
Doria AS 2007[52]	4341 A	83	94	93	94
	9356 C	88	94	94	95
Poortman P 2009[53]	151 A	77	100	86	100
Gaitini D 2008[54]	420 A	74	100	97	99
Cuschieri J 2008[55]	3045 A	83	92		
Wan MJ 2009[56]	9356 C	88	97	94	94

(A: adults, C: children).

Source: Adapted from Gaitini D. Imaging acute appendicitis: state of Art. Journal of Clinical Imaging Science. 2011;3:1-9.

TABLE 3: Comparison of US, CT and MRI in imaging of acute appendicitis.

Feature	US	CT	MRI
Availability	High	Intermediate	Low
Oral contrast medium	No	Yes	No
Intravenous contrast medium	No	Yes (generally)	No
Sedation/general anesthesia	No	Yes (children)	Yes (children and claustrophobia)
Cost	Low	Intermediate	High
Speed	High	Low (contrast media ingestion)	Low
Operator dependence	High	Intermediate	Intermediate
Radiation exposure	No	Yes	No
Sensitivity	Intermediate	High	High
Specificity	High	High	High

Source: Adapted from Gaitini D. Imaging acute appendicitis: state of Art. Journal of Clinical Imaging Science. 2011;3:1-9.

have excellent accuracy with reported sensitivity of 94 to 99% and specificity of 94 to 95%.[57-61]

Computed tomography, being the best modality for showing the extent of inflammatory process, should be used in patients with a high likelihood of perforation. This includes elderly, immunosuppressed patients and those with prolonged clinical symptoms (>72 hours duration) or a high fever and marked leukocytosis. CT is also the preferred modality for obese patients, patients with right lower quadrant masses and in those with persistent pain but a negative ultrasound.

Ultrasound is also the initial imaging modality in pregnant women with suspected appendicitis. However, several factors may limit its usefulness; the appendix may be displaced and adequate graded compression may be difficult in the presence of the gravid uterus. In these cases MRI has emerged as a useful second line modality and has a reported high accuracy and low failure rate.[46,50]

TUBERCULOSIS OF THE APPENDIX

Primary involvement of the appendix by tuberculosis in which there is no detectable focus elsewhere is extremely rare. The appendix is more commonly involved secondary to ileocecal tuberculosis. Secondary involvement is also uncommon owing to the minimal contact of appendix with intestinal contents. Secondary involvement has been further classified as those secondary to:

- Local extension of ileocecal tuberculosis.
- Retrograde lymphatic spread from distant lesion in the cecum or ascending colon.
- Appendicular serositis/periappendicitis or peritoneal tuberculosis.

Majority of the patients present with symptoms of the associated intestinal lesion rather than acute appendicitis.

Radiological investigations do not establish the diagnosis which is always established by histopathology. Appendicectomy is advocated in all cases of appendicular tuberculosis as antitubercular drugs alone cannot control recurrent attacks of appendicitis. Antitubercular drugs are given with surgery to control local complications like sinus formation.[62]

MUCOCELE OF APPENDIX

Mucocele of the appendix is a descriptive term for an abnormal sterile, mucus accumulation distending the appendiceal lumen, regardless of the underlying cause. A precursor to the formation of a mucocele is obstruction of the appendiceal lumen which can occur due to fecalith, foreign body, carcinoid tumor, adhesions, endometriosis and mucinous cystadenoma or cystadenocarcinoma.[63]

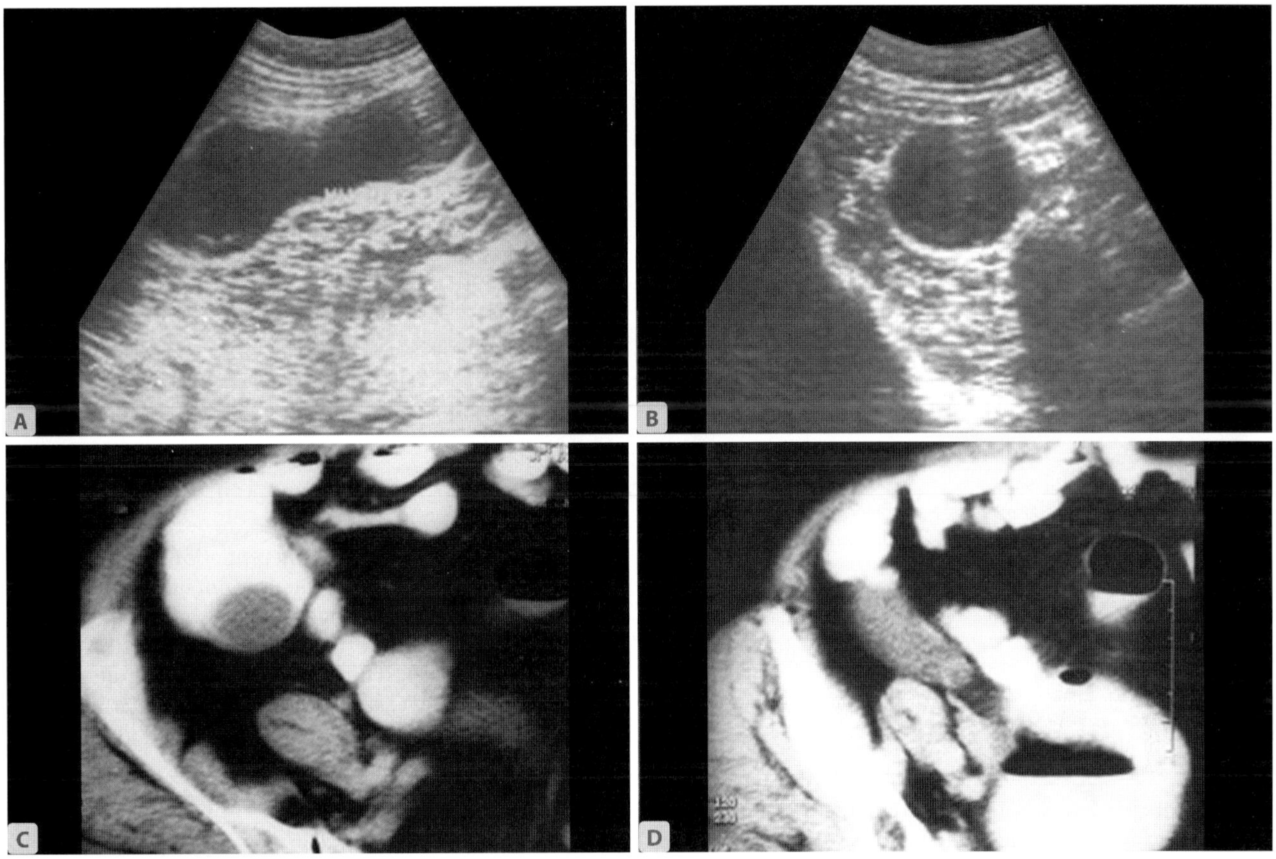

FIGS. 21A TO D: Mucocele of the appendix. (A and B) Axial and longitudinal views on sonography show a well-defined, thin walled, tubular, fluid-filled mass in the right iliac fossa; (C and D) Axial CECT scans show the mucocele invaginating into base of cecum.

Mucoceles associated with primary mucinous cystadenoma or mucinous cystadenocarcinoma, are also termed malignant mucoceles.

There is formation of a globular or reniform smooth walled, broad based mass invaginating the cecum, with frequent calcification in the wall or substance of the mass. It may be asymptomatic or patients may present with vague abdominal pain—acute or chronic, and rarely intermittent colicky pain caused by intussusception of the mucocele into the cecum.

Plain films may show a soft tissue mass, with or without rim calcification. Barium studies will show nonfilling of the appendix with a globular, smooth, broad based filling defect that invaginates into the cecum.[64] The cecum may be displaced laterally and/or cephalad depending on the size of the mucocele. Ultrasound demonstrates a cystic mass extrinsic to the solid viscera in the right lower quadrant, which may show internal echoes, layering or polypoid excrescences **(Figs. 21A and B)**. Peripheral rim calcification may be seen in some cases.[65,66] On computed tomography a round, sharply defined mass with or without calcification or septation is seen. Attenuation values range from near water density to soft tissue density (0–40 H) similar to the attenuation values seen in mucinous ascites and other proteinaceous fluids[67] **(Figs. 21C and D)**.

Myxoglobulosis is a rare variant of mucocele in which the appendix is filled with clusters of pearly white mucus balls intermixed with mucus.[68] These mucus balls may calcify to form spherules 1–10 mm in diameter which can be seen on plain films. Unlike appendiceal calculi, the calcified spherules in myxoglobulosis are usually annular and non- laminated, shift within the mucocele and can layer in the upright position.

The treatment of mucocele is at variance with acute appendicitis as many surgeons do not advocate laparoscopic appendicectomy in these cases. In fact, some believe that it is contraindicated because rupture of the mucocele with subsequent spillage of mucus into the peritoneal cavity can lead to pseudomyxoma peritonei which has a poor prognosis. If a neoplastic cause of mucocele is identified, right hemicolectomy rather than laparoscopic appendicectomy is advocated. Also the chances of failure of the laparoscopic procedure are higher with higher luminal diameters. It is thus important to differentiate between acute appendicitis with associated mucocele from acute appendicitis without mucocele. The CT findings that favor the diagnosis of a co-existing mucocele include a luminal diameter greater than 13 mm, cystic dilatation of the appendix and mural calcification. If these findings are visualized in a patient, the surgeon should be made aware of a co-existing mucocele since the surgical management is different.[69]

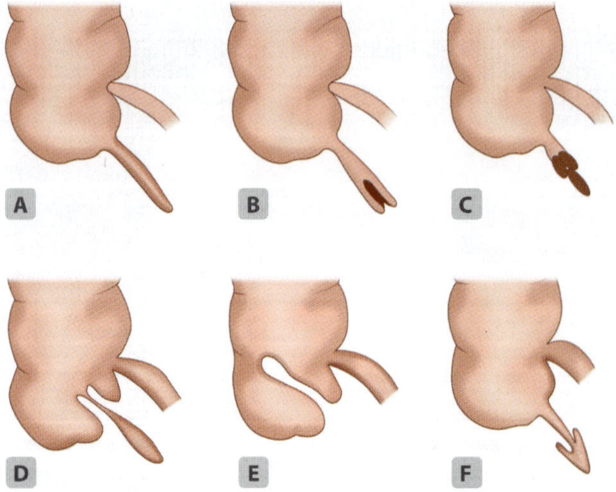

FIGS. 22A TO F: Types of simple primary appendiceal intussusception. (A) The normal appearance; (B, C and F) Variations of the appendicoappendiceal intussusceptions; (D) Incomplete appendiceal intussusception into the cecum (E) Complete appendiceal intussusception into the cecum. Only types D and E are visualized radiographically.

PRIMARY APPENDICEAL INTUSSUSCEPTION

This may present as an acute surgical emergency without time for preoperative diagnostic studies, or as a subacute recurring condition. Primary appendiceal intussusception (PAI) can also be asymptomatic and may be noted only during a barium enema examination **(Figs. 22A to F)**. It produces an oval, round, or finger like filling defect projecting from the medial wall of the cecum along with nonvisualization of the appendix.[70]

The radiographic pattern of PAI must be differentiated from mural and intramural cecal defects due to other causes like benign and malignant tumors of the cecum, inverted appendiceal stumps, appendiceal tumors or abscesses. Such a differentiation may be greatly aided if a specific attempt is made to fill and visualize the appendix by appropriate pressure over the cecum during the barium enema examination. Should the defect remain constant and homolateral to the ileocecal valve on two examinations, definite differentiation cannot be made between irreducible intussusception, appendiceal and cecal masses.

POSTOPERATIVE APPENDICEAL DEFECTS

Postoperative defects in the cecum following appendicectomy may be secondary to inversion of the appendiceal stump, ligation of the stump without inversion or complete resection of the appendix.[70]

The inverted appendiceal stump produces a filling defect in the tip of the cecum at the base of the appendix on barium enema examination which varies widely in size from several millimeters to 3 cm. The inverted stump is particularly prominent for several weeks after surgery owing to persistent edema and inflammation. The surface may be smooth, lobulated or irregular, so that differentiation from a mucosal lesion of the cecum is often difficult, if not impossible.

The importance of recognizing the defect lies in differentiating an inverted appendiceal stump from a significant lesion. The inverted stump rarely causes symptoms, although cases of ulceration and intussusception have been reported.

TABLE 4: Primary neoplasms of the appendix.[58]

- *Adenoma or adenocarcinoma (epithelial)*:
  - Mucinous
  - Nonmucinous (colonic type)
- *Carcinoid tumor*:
  - Classic
  - Tubular
  - Goblet cell
- Lymphoma
- *Other tumors (rare)*:
  - Ganglioneuroma
  - Pheochromocytoma
  - Mesenchymal tumors
  - Kaposi sarcoma

TUMORS OF THE APPENDIX

Primary appendiceal neoplasms are uncommon, being found in approximately 0.5–1% of appendicectomy specimens at pathological evaluation.[71] Approximately 30–50% of all appendiceal neoplasms will manifest clinically with signs and symptoms of acute appendicitis. Other clinical manifestations include an asymptomatic palpable mass, incidental imaging findings, intussusception, GI bleeding, ureteral obstruction or hematuria or increasing abdominal girth from pseudomyxoma peritonei.

Although rare, a variety of primary neoplasms can arise from the appendix **(Table 4)**. Collins reported an incidence of carcinoid 0.5%, adenocarcinoma 0.08% and benign tumors 4.3%.[3] Benign tumors are rarely picked up preoperatively because of their small size. The diagnosis is usually an incidental finding at surgery.

Carcinoids (a neuroendocrine tumor) are the most common and represent up to 60% of all appendiceal neoplasms. They are commonly seen in young adults. Over 70% of these tumors are found in the distal third of the appendix and are <1 cm in size.[72,73] Most carcinoids are discovered in appendices removed incidentally at surgery for another procedure or because of acute appendicitis. Appendiceal carcinoids arise from subepithelial neuroendocrine cells. Histologically, there are three types: classic type, tubular type and goblet-cell variety. Goblet-cell carcinoids are more aggressive and may represent a distinct subset of tumors with a malignant potential that is intermediate between carcinoids and adenocarcinomas.[74]

Computed tomography may not detect these tumors because of their small size. It may only show features of appendicitis. However, a larger tumor may be seen as a soft-tissue mass in the appendix with or without calcification.

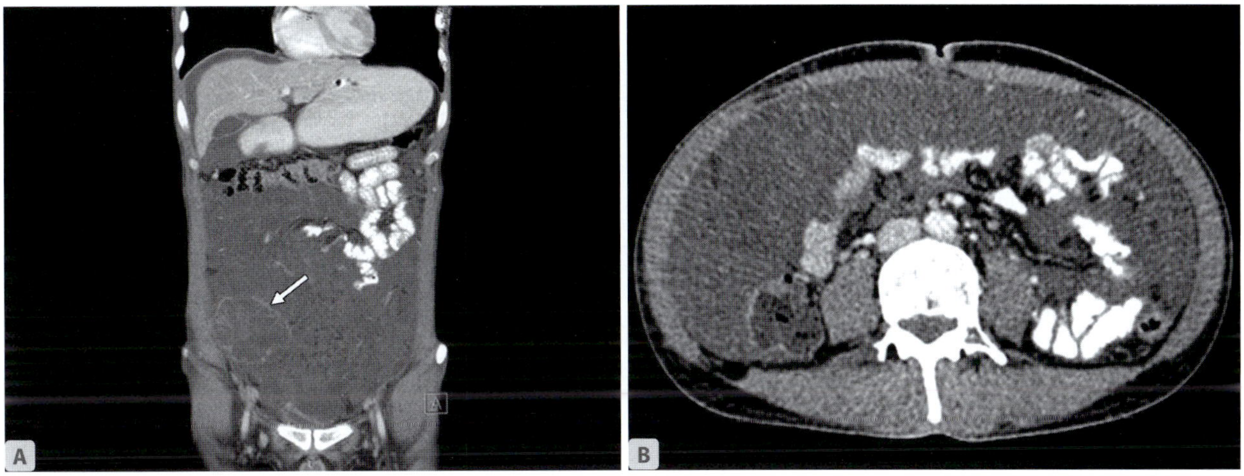

FIGS. 23A AND B: Pseudomyxoma peritonei from mucinous adenocarcinoma of the appendix manifesting as increasing abdominal girth in a 48-year-old man. Coronal (A) and axial (B) contrast-enhanced CT scans show a multiloculated mass in the right iliac fossa (arrow in A) with displacement and distortion of the bowel caused by diffuse intraperitoneal locules of pseudomyxoma peritonei which appear quite solid looking.

Mucinous cystadenomas and cystadenocarcinomas commonly present as mucoceles in case they cause luminal obstruction, or pseudomyxoma peritonei in case of rupture of mucocele or direct tumor extension into the peritoneal cavity.

On imaging it is rarely possible to see the tumor as it is generally very small. Features of mucocele (described above) or pseudomyxoma peritonei may be seen. Pseudomyxoma peritonei is a diffuse intraperitoneal accumulation of gelatinous ascites. Some investigators posit that nearly all true cases of pseudomyxoma peritonei are appendiceal in origin and that associated ovarian lesions usually represent metastatic disease, although this is controversial.[75,76] Ultrasound shows multiple solid appearing intraperitoneal masses displacing the bowel posteriorly, or a multiseptated ascites. Scalloping of the surface of the liver and spleen is a pathognomonic feature. Computed tomography shows characteristic low attenuation (<20 HU) masses throughout the peritoneal space displacing the bowel loops centrally and scalloping the surfaces of the liver and spleen **(Figs. 23A and B)**. MRI additionally enables differentiation between mucinous and fluid ascites on T2W images. Synchronous metastatic ovarian tumors may be seen in almost 40% of cases.

The *colonic (nonmucinous) adenocarcinomas* are much rare than the mucinous adenocarcinomas. These tend not to form mucoceles, rather they manifest clinically with appendicitis, related to malignant luminal obstruction.[72] At CT, a focal soft tissue mass that involves the appendix but does not show a mucocele formation is most characteristic.

Lymphoma of the appendix is mostly of the non-Hodgkin's variety. The appendix becomes massively enlarged but typically maintains its vermiform appearance. On US, diffuse hypoechoic mural thickening with a soft tissue attenuation on CT can be seen. Aneurysmal dilatation of the appendiceal lumen has also been described.[77]

Other neoplasms: Other rare neoplasms of the appendix can be the *neuroendocrine tumors* of the appendix including ganglioneuromas and paragangliomas. Diffuse ganglioneuromatosis has been described and is associated with neurofibromatosis type 1. Mesenchymal tumors of the appendix are rare and are generally benign. Leiomyomas, leiomyosarcomas and gastrointestinal stromal tumors may all arise from the appendiceal smooth muscle. Neurofibromas and schwannomas also rarely arise in the appendix. Kaposi sarcoma can occur in patients with acquired immunodeficiency syndrome (AIDS) and needs to be differentiated from AIDS-related lymphoma which may be difficult on imaging.[72]

REFERENCES

1. Buschard K, Kjaeldfaard A. Investigation and analysis of the position, fixation, length and embryology of the vermiform appendix. Acta Chir Scand. 1973;139:293-8.
2. Oto A, Ernst RD, Mileski WJ, et al. Localisation of appendix with MDCT and inference of findings on choice of appendecectomy incision. AJR. 2006;186:987-90.
3. Collins DC. 71,000 human appendix specimens. A final report summarising 40 years' study. Am J Proctocol. 1963;14:265.
4. Totty WG, Koehler RE, Cheung LY. Significance of retained barium in the appendix. AJR. 1980;135:753.
5. Vukmer GJ, Trummer MJ. Barium appendicitis. Arch Surg. 1965;91:630.
6. Puylaert JB. Acute appendicitis: US evaluation using graded compression. Radiology. 1986;158:355-60.
7. Abu-Yousef MM, Bleichaer JJ, Maher JW, et al. High resolution sonography of acute appendicitis. AJR. 1987;149:53-8.
8. Rioux M. Sonographic detection of normal and abnormal appendix. AJR. 1992;158:733-78.
9. Rao PM, Rhea JT, Novelline RA, et al. Helical CT technique for the diagnosis of appendicitis: prospective evaluation of a focussed appendix CT examination. Radiology. 1997;202:139-44.
10. Rao PM, Rhea JT, Novelline RA, et al. Helical CT combined with contrast material administered only through the colon for imaging of suspected appendicitis. AJR. 1997;169:1275-80.

11. Stillman CA, Katz DS, Lane MJ. The normal appendix: evaluation with unenhanced helical CT (abstr) AJR. 1999;172(Suppl):58.
12. Karabulut N, Boyaci N, Yagci B, et al. Computed tomography evaluation of the normal appendix: comparison of low-dose and standard dose unenhanced helical computed tomography. JCAT. 2007;31:732-40.
13. Wangensteen OH, Denins C. Experimental proof of the obstructive origin of appendicitis in man. Ann Surg. 1939;110:629-47.
14. Pieper R, Kager L, Tidefelt U. Obstruction of the appendix vermiformis causing acute appendicitis: an experimental study in the rabbit. Acta Chir Scand. 1982;148:63-72.
15. Nitecki S, Karmeli R, Sarr MG. Appendiceal calculi and faecoliths as indicators for appendicectomy. Surg Gyn Obstet. 1990;171:185-8.
16. Alder AC, Tomly TB, Wayne A. Association of viral infection and appendicitis. Arch Surg. 2010;145(1):63-71.
17. Shaw RE. Appendix calculi and acute appendicitis. Br J Surg. 1965;52:451-59.
18. Trimaur-Dahl J. Roentgen examinations in acute abdominal diseases. Springfield, IL, Charles C Thomas, 1960.
19. Thompson JP, Selvaraj D, Nicola R. Mimickers of acute appendicitis. J Am Osteopath Coll Radiol. 2014;3(4):10-21.
20. Soter CS. The contribution of the radiologist to the diagnosis of acute appendicitis. Semin Roentgen. 1973;8:375.
21. Graham AD, Johnson HF. The incidence of radio-graphic findings in acute appendicitis compared to 200 normal abdomens. Milit Med. 1966;131:272.
22. Jeffrey RB Jr, Laing FC, Townsend RR. Acute appendicitis: sonographic criteria based on 250 cases. Radiology. 1988;167: 327-29.
23. Jeffrey RB Jr, Laing FC, Lewis FR. Acute appendicitis: high-resolution real time US findings. Radiology. 1987;168:11-4.
24. Puylaert JBCM, Rutgers PH, Laosang RI, et al. A prospective study of ultrasonography in the diagnosis of appendicitis. N Engl J Med. 1987;317:666-9.
25. Sivit CJ, Newman KD, Boenning DA, et al. Appendicitis: usefulness of US in diagnosis in a paediatric population. Radiology. 1992;185:549-52.
26. Chesbrough RM, Burhard TK, Balsara EN, et al. Selflocalisation in US of appendicitis: an addition to graded compression. Radiology. 1993;187:349-51.
27. Chesbrough RM, Burkhard TK, Balsara ZN, et al. Selflocalization in US of appendicitis: an addition to graded compression. Radiology. 1993;187:349-51.
28. Lee JH, Jeong YK, Hwang JC, et al. Graded compression sonography with adjuvant use of a posterior manual compression technique in the sonographic diagnosis of acute appendicitis. Am J Roentgenol. 2002;78:863-8.
29. Lee JH, Jeong YK, Park KB, et al. Operator-dependent techniques for graded compression sonography to detect the appendix and diagnose acute appendicitis. Am J Roentgenol. 2005;184:91-7.
30. Birnbaum BA, Wilson SR. Appendicitis at the Millenium. Radiology. 2000;215:337-48.
31. Rompel O, Huelsse B, Bodenschatz K, et al. Harmonic US imaging of appendicitis in children. Pediatr Radiol. 2006;36(12):1257-64.
32. Kessler N, Cyteval C, Gallix B, et al. Appendicitis: evaluation of sensitivity, specificity, and predictive values of US, Doppler US, and laboratory findings. Radiology. 2004;230:472-8.
33. Rettenbacher T, Hollerweger A, Macheiner P, et al. Outer diameter of the vermiform appendix as a sign of acute appendicitis: evaluation at US. Radiology. 2001;218:757-62.
34. Quillin SP, Siegel MJ. Appendicitis: efficacy of colour Doppler sonography. Radiology. 1994;191:557-60.
35. Lim HK, Lee WJ, Kim TH, et al. Appendicitis: usefulness of colour Doppler US. Radiology. 1996;201:221-25.
36. O'Malley ME, Halpert E, Mueller PR, et al. Helical CT protocols for the abdomen and pelvis: a survey. Am J Roentgenol. 2000;175:109-13.
37. Lane MJ, Katz DS, Ross BA, et al. Unenhanced helical CT for suspected acute appendicitis. AJR. 1997;168:405-09.
38. Lane MJ, Liu DM, Huynh MD. Unenhanced helical CT for suspected acute appendicitis: experience in 300 consecutive patients (abstr) AJR. 1999;172(suppl):114.
39. Birnbaum BA, Balthazar EJ. CT of appendicitis and diverticulitis. Radiol Clin North Am. 1994;32:885-98.
40. Balthazar EJ, Megibow AJ, Siegel SE, et al. Appendicitis: prospective evaluation with high resolution CT. Radiology. 1991;180:21-4.
41. Tamburrini S, Brunetti A, Brown M, et al. CT appearance of normal appendix in adults. Eur Radiol. 2005;15:2096-103.
42. Daly CP, Cohan RH, Francis IR, et al. Incidence of acute appendicitis in patients with equivocal CT findings. Am J Roentgenol. 2005;184:1813-20.
43. Rao PM, Wittenberg J, McDowell RK, et al. Appendicitis: use of arrow head sign for diagnosis at CT. Radiology. 1977;202:363-6.
44. Kim HC, Dal MY, Jin W, et al. Added diagnostic value of multiplanar reformation of multidetector CT data in patients with suspected appendicitis. Radiographics. 2008;28(2): 393-406.
45. Singh A, Danrad R, Blake MA, et al. MR imaging of the acute abdomen and pelvis: acute appendicitis and beyond. Radiographics. 2007;27:1419-31.
46. Rao PM, Rhea JT, Novelline RA, et al. The computed tomography appearance of recurrent and chronic appendicitis. Am J Emerg Med. 1998;16:26-33.
47. Hoerman M, Paya K, Eibenberger K, et al. MR imaging in children with non-penetrated acute appendicitis: value of unenhanced MR imaging in sonography selected cases. AJR. 1998;171: 467-70.
48. Karul M, Berliner C, Keller S, et al. Imaging of appendicitis in adults. Fortsche Rontgenstr. 2014;186:551-8.
49. Giatini D. Imaging acute appendicitis: state of Art. Journal of Clinical Imaging Science. 2011;3:1-9.
50. Pedrosa I, Lafornara M, Pandharipande PV, Goldsmith JD, Rofsky NM. Pregnant patients suspected of having acute appendicitis: effect of MR imaging on negative laparotomy rate and appendiceal perforation rate. Radiology. 2009;250:749-57.
51. Van Randen A, Bipat S, Zwinderman AH, Ubbink DT, Stoker J, Boermeester MA. Acute appendicitis: meta-analysis of diagnostic performance of CT and graded compression US related to prevalence of disease. Radiology. 2008;249:97-106.
52. Doria AS, Moineddin R, Kellenberger CJ, Epelman M, Beyene J, Schuh S, et al. US or CT for diagnosis of appendicitis in children and adults? A meta-analysis. Radiology. 2006;241:83-94.
53. Poortman P, Oostvogel HJ, Bosma E, Lohle PN, Cuesta MA, de Lange-de Klerk ES, et al. Improving diagnosis of acute appendicitis: results of a diagnostic pathway with standard use of ultrasonography followed by selective use of CT. J Am Coll Surg. 2009;208:434-41.
54. Gaitini D, Beck-Razi N, Mor-Yosef D, Fischer D, Ben Itzhak O, Krausz MM, et al. Diagnosing acute appendicitis in adults: accuracy of color Doppler sonography and MDCT compared with surgery and clinical follow-up. Am J Roentenol. 2008;190:1300-6.
55. Cuschieri J, Florence M, Flum DR, Jurkovich GJ, Lin P, Steele SR, et al. The SCOAP Collaborative. Negative appendectomy and imaging accuracy in the Washington State surgical care and outcomes assessment program. Ann Surg. 2008;248:557-63.
56. Wan MJ, Krahn M, Ungar WJ, Caku E, Sung L, Medina LS, et al. Acute appendicitis in young children: cost-effectiveness of US versus CT in diagnosis-a Markov decision analytic model. Radiology. 2009;250:378-86.

57. Inceseu L, Coskun A, Seleuk MB, et al. Acute appendicitis: MR imaging and sonographic correlation. AJR. 1997;168:669-74.
58. Doria AS, Moineddin R, Kellenberger CJ, et al. US or CT for diagnosis of appendicitis in children and adults? A meta-analysis. Radiology. 2006;241:83-94.
59. Rybkin AV, Thoeni RF. Current concepts in imaging of appendicitis. Radiol Clin North Am. 2007;45:411-22.
60. Smink DS, Finkelstein JS, Garcia-Pena BM, et al. Diagnosis of acute appendicitis in children using a clinical practice guideline. J Pediatr Surg. 2004;35:392-5.
61. Hernandez JA, Swischuk LE, Angel CA, et al. Imaging of acute appendicitis. US as the primary imaging modality. Pediatr Radiol. 2005;35:392-5.
62. Singh MK, Arunabh, Kapoor VK. Tuberculosis of the appendix–a report of 17 cases and a suggested aetiopathological classification. Postgrad Med J. 1987; 63(774):855-7.
63. Higa E, Rosai J, Pizzimbono CA, et al. Mucosal hyperplasia, mucinous cystadenoma and mucinous cystadenocarcinoma of the appendix. A re-evaluation of appendiceal "mucocele". Cancer. 1973;6:1525-41.
64. Marohak RH, Gerson A. Mucocele of the appendix. Am J Digest Dis. 1960;5:49.
65. Dachman AH, Lichtenstein JE, Friedman AC. Mucocele of the appendix and pseudomyxoma peritonei. AJR. 1985;144:923-9.
66. Kim SH, Lim HK, Lee WJ, et al. Mucocele of the appendix: ultrasonographic and CT findings. Abdominal Imaging. 1998;23:292-6.
67. Madwed D, Mindelzun R, Jeffrey RB Jr. Mucocele of the appendix: imaging findings. AJR. 1992;159:69-72.
68. Lubin J, Berle S. Myxoglobulosis of the appendix. Arch Pathol. 1972;94:533.
69. Bennett GL, Tanpitukpongse TP, Macari M, et al. CT diagnosis of mucocele of the appendix in patients with acute appendicitis. Am J Roentgenol. 2009;192(3): W103–10.
70. Berk RN. Radiology of the appendix. In: Taveras JM, Ferucci JT (Eds). Radiology–Diagnosis—Intervention. Philadelphia: JB Lippincott Co. 1986;4(41).
71. Connor SJ, Hanna GB, Frizelle FA. Appendiceal tumors: retrospective clinicopathologic analysis of appendiceal tumors from 7,970 appendicectomies. Dis Colon Rectum. 1998;41: 75-80.
72. In't Hof KH, van der Wal HC, Kazemier G, Lange JF. Carcinoid tumour of the appendix: an analysis of 1,485 consecutive emergency appendectomies. J Gastrointest Surg. 2008;12: 1436-8.
73. Moertel CG, Weiland LH, Nagomey DM, et al. Carcinoid tumor of the appendix: treatment and prognosis. N Eng J Med. 1987;317:1699-1701.
74. Pickhardt PJ, Levy AD, Rohrmann CA, et al. Primary neoplasms of the appendix: radiologic spectrum of disease with pathologic correlation. Radiographics. 2003;23:645-62.
75. Carr NJ, Sobin LH. Unusual tumors of the appendix and pseudomyxoma peritoei. Semin Diagn Pathol. 1996;13:314-25.
76. Hinson FL, Ambrose NS. Pseudomyxoma peritonei. Br J Surg. 1998;85:1332-9.
77. Pickhardt PJ, Levy AD, Rohrmann CA, et al. Non-Hodgkin lymphoma of the appendix: clinical and CT findings with pathological correlation. AJR. 2002;78(5)1123-7.

CHAPTER

100

Diffuse Liver Diseases

Surabhi Vyas, Ashu Seith Bhalla, Arun Kumar Gupta

INTRODUCTION

Diffuse liver diseases encompass a wide spectrum of entities of diverse etiology. Diagnosis based on imaging alone is generally more difficult than in focal liver lesions, as their effect on normal liver architecture may be minimal. However, imaging can help in assessing the severity and extent of the diffuse liver diseases and to demonstrate sequela such as portal hypertension and neoplasia. The following conditions are included under the term diffuse liver diseases:

- Hepatic steatosis
- Hepatitis—viral, alcoholic, radiation induced
- Hemochromatosis and hemosiderosis
- Amyloidosis
- Wilson's disease
- Granulomatous diseases
- Cirrhosis.

HEPATIC STEATOSIS (FATTY LIVER)

Hepatic steatosis or fatty liver is a benign condition resulting from an excessive accumulation of triglycerides in the form of small or large vacuoles (micro/macrovesicular types) within the hepatocytes. Excess fat deposition in the liver may result from excess synthesis, decreased utilization, impaired release of hepatic lipoproteins and excess mobilization from fatty tissue.

The common causes are alcoholism, diabetes mellitus and obesity. One-third of asymptomatic alcoholic patients and up to 50% of patients with diabetes mellitus develop fatty liver.[1] Malnutrition, chronic illnesses, ileal bypass, drugs and toxins, total parenteral nutrition, inflammatory bowel disease, severe hepatitis, steroid intake, acquired immune deficiency syndrome and congestive heart failure can also result in fatty liver.

With increasing prevalence of obesity, hepatic steatosis has become a major source of liver dysfunction even though in most cases fatty liver is asymptomatic with normal liver function tests. Radiologist is frequently the first to suggest the diagnosis. Mild hepatomegaly with or without vague right upper abdominal pain can be present in symptomatic patients. In acute fatty liver associated with pregnancy or alcoholic binge, patients may present with jaundice, acute hepatic failure or even encephalopathy.

NAFLD-NASH Continuum

In contrast to the alcohol-induced fatty liver, the nonalcoholic fatty liver disease encompasses a spectrum of disorders ranging from nonalcoholic fatty liver (NAFL) in which the hepatic enzymes are either normal or minimally increased and histologically there is no evidence of hepatocyte damage. On the other end of the spectrum is nonalcoholic steatohepatitis (NASH) which is characterized by deranged liver enzymes with or without jaundice. Histologically there is evidence of scarring and fibrosis.[1] It is similar to alcoholic liver disease in clinical and biochemical features. The exact etiology of NASH is unknown, however it is seen more commonly in patients with certain medical conditions like diabetes, obesity, hyperlipidemias and insulin resistance, which together are often called metabolic syndrome.[2,3]

Ultrasonography

Ultrasonography (USG) reveals hepatomegaly, increased parenchymal echogenicity with impaired visualization of the normally echogenic walls of intrahepatic portal venous branches. There is increased attenuation and poor penetration of the sound beam resulting in poor visualization of the deeper portion of liver, the diaphragm, hepatic and portal veins **(Fig. 1)**. Echogenicity of the liver can be compared with that of adjacent kidney. The degree of echogenicity is roughly proportional to the degree of steatosis and tends to parallel biochemical and clinical dysfunction. Focal fat infiltration may produce single or multiple hyperechoic lesions, while areas of focal fat sparing appear hypoechoic in an otherwise hyperechoic liver. In the presence of fatty liver, hepatic hemangiomas may appear hypoechoic necessitating MR or CT for their differentiation **(Figs. 2A to C)**. Hepatic steatosis and fibrosis often coexist and produce similar US findings. On the basis of ultrasound findings, fatty liver may be graded qualitatively as:

Mild

Increased echogenicity with maintained differentiation of intrahepatic vessels, portal vein braches and diaphragm.

Moderate

Partially impaired demarcation of the portal vein and branches, diaphragm.

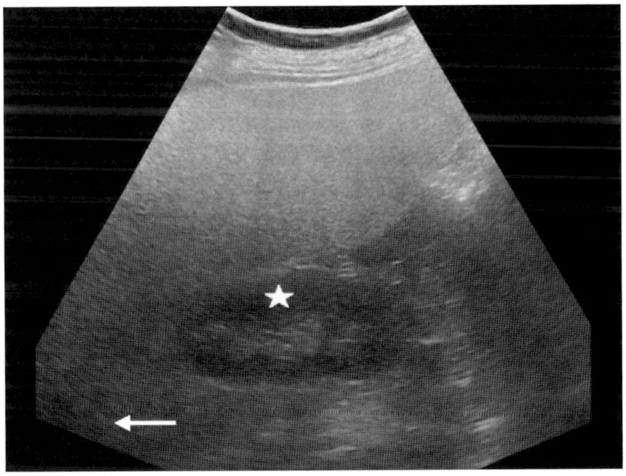

FIG. 1: Fatty liver: Increased echogenicity of the liver seen on ultrasound as compared to that of renal cortex (star). Note the poor depiction of diaphragm (arrow).

Severe

Markedly impaired demarcation of the portal vein branches and diaphragmatic contour.[4]

Quantitative assessment can be done by sonographic hepatorenal index (SHRI). In this method, a parasagittal image of the right lobe segment VI of liver and the right kidney is acquired. Region of interest (ROI) is placed on the liver parenchyma and renal cortex avoiding the vessels, renal pyramid and renal medulla. A numerical value based on the brightness/echogenicity in the selected pixel is assigned, and the ratio between the values of hepatic ROI to renal ROI is calculated to provide the SHRI.[5]

Ultrasound elastography is a noninvasive technique that assess the hardness of the target organ. The liver may show increased hardness in a variety of parenchymal disorders like parenchymal infiltrative disorders, cirrhosis, chronic inflammatory diseases and in congestive cardiac failure **(Figs. 3A and B)**. However, the liver stiffness may not increase in steatosis.

Computed Tomography

There exists an excellent correlation between the computed tomography (CT) attenuation of liver and the amount of fat deposition as determined on liver biopsy specimens.[6] Fatty liver is seen as reduced attenuation of the liver parenchyma **(Fig. 4)** Normal liver attenuation on unenhanced scans is

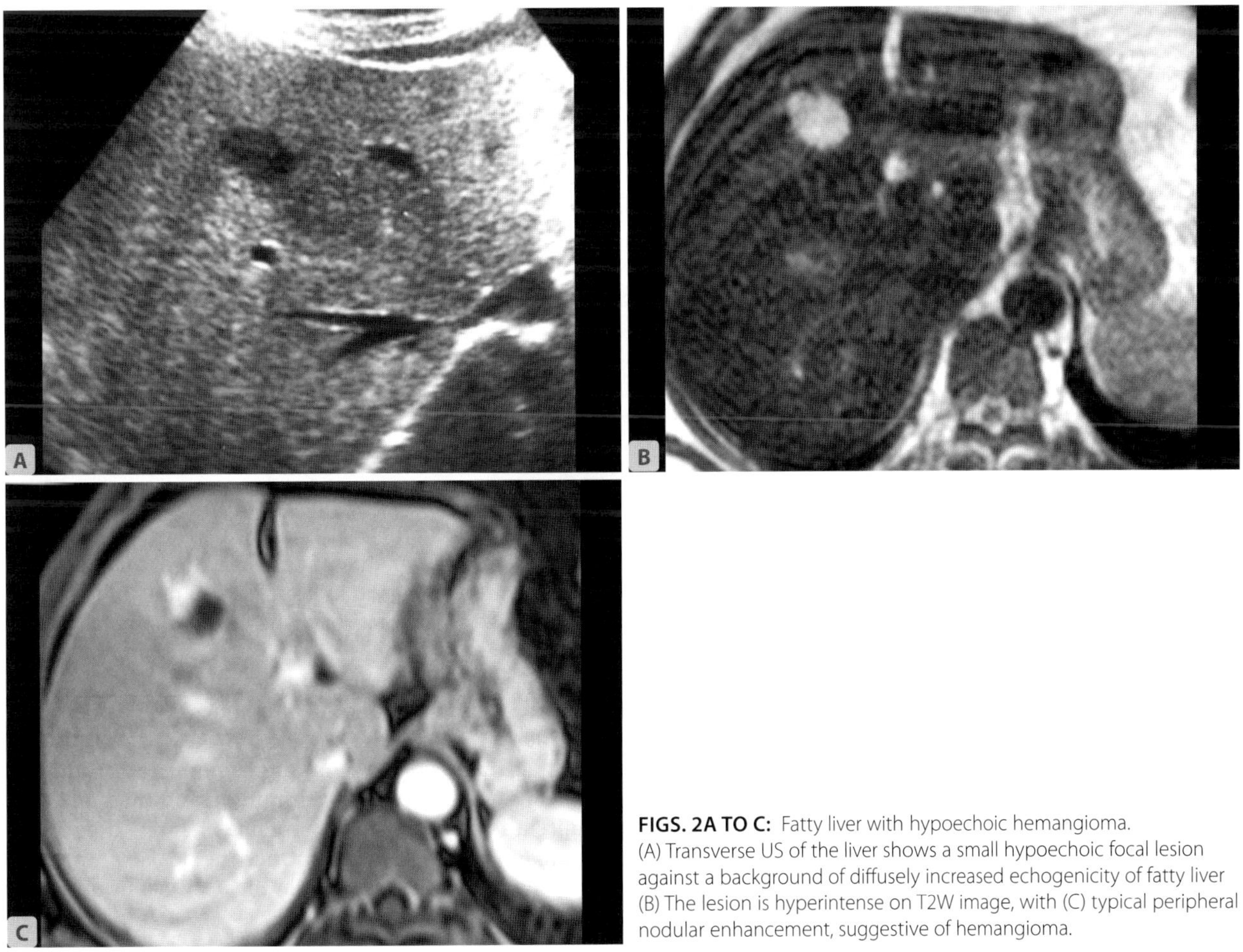

FIGS. 2A TO C: Fatty liver with hypoechoic hemangioma. (A) Transverse US of the liver shows a small hypoechoic focal lesion against a background of diffusely increased echogenicity of fatty liver (B) The lesion is hyperintense on T2W image, with (C) typical peripheral nodular enhancement, suggestive of hemangioma.

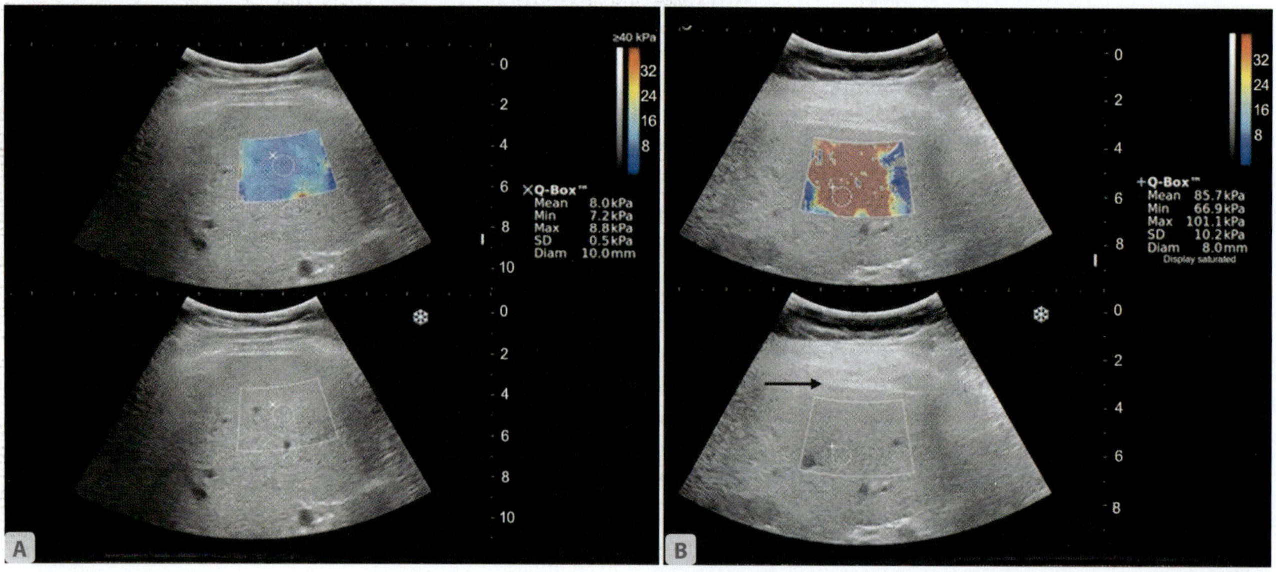

FIGS. 3A AND B: Shear wave elastography of liver showing a mean stiffness of 8 kPa, in case of mild fatty change (A), a higher value of 85.7 kPa in case of chronic liver disease (B). Also noted is irregularity of the hepatic surface in (B).

8–10 HU more than the spleen due to its glycogen content.[6] This relationship is reversed in fatty liver. A threshold CT attenuation value of 45 hounsfield units (HU) has been shown to be highly specific for moderate to severe steatosis.[7] The attenuation is often reduced below that of the normal portal vein and IVC so that these structures stand out prominently simulating contrast-enhanced image of the liver.[8] Unlike unenhanced scans, contrast enhanced CT is less reliable in the diagnosis of fatty liver.

Liver attenuation index (LAI) can also be calculated as mean liver attenuation–mean splenic attenuation to provide a numeric value. CT-LAI of more than 5 implies low probability of hepatic steatosis, whereas a value between minus 10 and 5 signifies moderate to severe fatty change. A value less than or equal to 0 correlates well with significant hepatic steatosis.[9] Another numeric value that can be used is hepatic-to-splenic attenuation ratio which if less than 0.8 or 1 is highly specific (specificity, 100%) for the diagnosis of moderate to severe (>30%) macrovesicular steatosis.[10]

Decreased attenuation in fatty liver can hamper the detection of hypodense liver lesions like abscesses or neoplasms. A confident CT diagnosis of focal fat infiltration can be made when it is lobar, segmental or wedge shaped. In such cases, the area of decreased attenuation typically extends to the liver capsule, without causing contour bulge and typically has a straight margin. However, MRI may be required for confident differentiation of nodular areas of fat deposition or fat sparing from focal mass lesions.

Dual energy CT (DECT) has a role in calculation of the hepatic fat (hepatic fat fraction-HFF), where various material decomposition algorithms allow creation of fat specific and virtual noncontrast images from the images acquired at tube potentials of 80 and 140 kVP. The liver attenuation is reduced at low energy level and increases at higher energy levels in hepatosteatosis. It has been reported that an increase in attenuation by more than 10 HU on higher kVP suggests fatty infiltration greater than 25% **(Figs. 5A to C)**.[11]

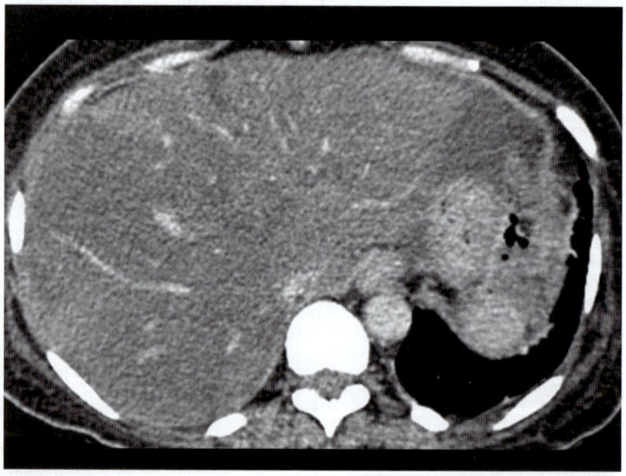

FIG. 4: Fatty liver: Axial CT image in a case of pancreatitis showing diffuse decrease in liver attenuation suggestive of fatty infiltration.

Magnetic Resonance Imaging

There are two magnetic resonance (MR) techniques used for hepatic fat estimation—MRI and MR spectroscopy (MRS). Both make use of the difference in the water and fat proton resonance frequencies to measure signal due to fat fraction (SFF i.e. signal fat fraction or proton density fat fraction (PDFF).

MRS is a direct method of estimating signal fat fraction, and since the resonance frequencies of both protons are different, so are their peaks on the spectral tracing. Usually a single voxel technique is employed. Multivoxel MR technique is limited by shimming and the inability to acquire a relatively longer sequence in single breath hold leading to breathing artifacts. Once the peaks of water and fat are identified, the areas under the peak can be quantified **(Fig. 6A)**.

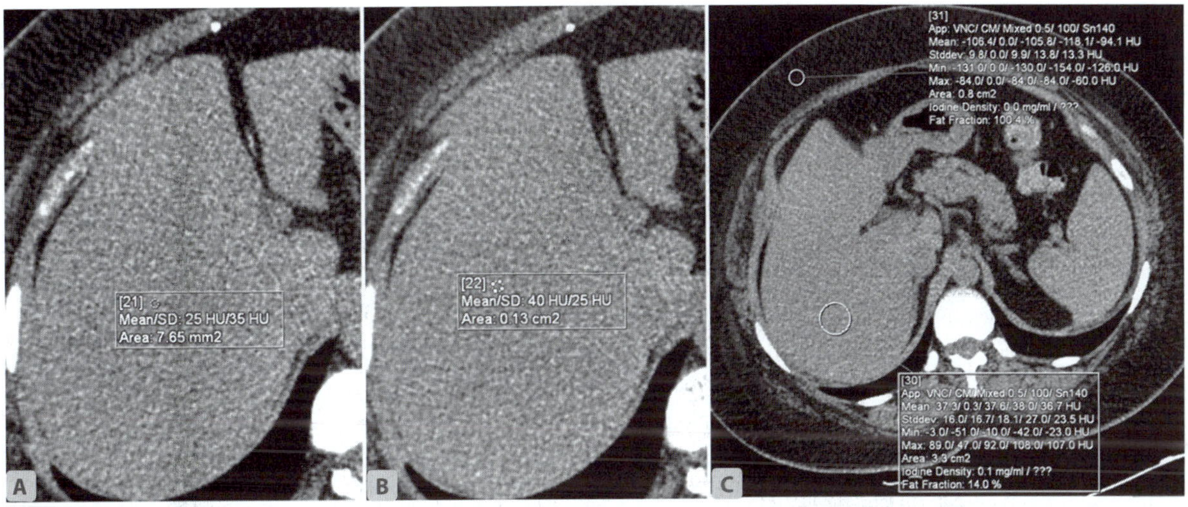

FIGS. 5A TO C: DECT hepatic steatosis at low keV (A) and higher keV (B) showing an increase in attenuation by more than 10 HU; (C) Liver fat fraction of 14% suggestive of steatosis. Note the fat fraction of subcutaneous fat is 100%.

Magnetic resonance imaging (MRI) based techniques for signal fat fraction estimation include chemical fat suppression, and chemical shift-based imaging. In the former, two sets of images are acquired, with and without fat suppression. However, the problem of inadequate fat suppression may preclude adequate signal suppression and thus the latter is preferred.

Chemical shift imaging is based on acquiring images at two echo times (TEs). Here fat suppression pulse is not employed. Loss of signal on the opposed phase image when compared with the in-phase image readily identifies excess fat containing areas in the liver **(Figs. 6B and C)**. With the in and opposed images, liver signal fat fraction (FF) may be calculated (proportion of the fat signal divided by the total (water + fat) signal, FF = fat signal/(fat signal + water signal). On a 1.5T scanner signals from fat and water are in phase every 4.6 ms, out of phase at 2.3 ms and at their multiples. At 3T, the signals are in phase at 2.3 ms and out of phase at 1.15 ms and their multiples thereafter. Chemical shift MR imaging is the investigation of choice in cases with focal nodular or multifocal fat deposition/sparing that may be confused with liver metastases on US or CT.

Although fatty infiltration may demonstrate increased signal intensity of liver on T1- and T2-weighted spin echo images this increase in signal may not be apparent even with massive fat deposition in liver.[12] Advanced MRI techniques based on 3D gradient echo imaging, are under evaluation for calculation of proton density fat fraction (PDFF), which allows quantitative evaluation of liver fat without the inherent limitations of the conventional chemical shift imaging which affect image quality such as choice of imaging parameters, field strength and coexisting biological factors like fibrosis, cirrhosis and iron overload.[13]

Contrast-enhanced MRI (CEMRI) using gadoxetic acid has been shown to have potential in differentiating simple steatosis from NASH, as the mean liver enhancement is found to be lower in NASH compared with simple steatosis likely due to increased hepatocyte volume reducing the sinusoidal space, and thereby the contrast uptake.[14] Similar observations have been seen by using USPIO, where poor hepatic uptake of USPIO has been seen in patients NASH than in simple steatosis.[15]

On cross-sectional imaging fat deposition is most often diffuse. Focal fat deposition and focal fat sparing are less common patterns that typically occur adjacent to the falciform ligament, fissure for ligamentum venosum, porta hepatis, gallbladder fossa and in the subcapsular portions of the liver. Their characteristic locations, geographic/wedge shape configuration with angulated margins, lack of mass effect, presence of normal blood vessels coursing through them and enhancement similar to normal liver help differentiate these from true lesions. When multifocal or nodular these may however, simulate true masses and may require chemical shift MRI for their confirmation **(Figs. 7A to E)**.

VIRAL HEPATITIS

Hepatitis is diffuse inflammation of the liver that can be divided into acute and chronic forms. The latter is in turn, subdivided into persistent and chronic active categories. Imaging is relatively nonspecific but can help to exclude biliary obstruction in acute hepatitis. In chronic hepatitis, imaging is useful in monitoring the progression of the disease, development of portal venous hypertension and complications such as hepatocellular carcinoma.

USG

In acute viral hepatitis, liver and spleen are frequently enlarged. Severe acute hepatitis may result in diffusely decreased parenchymal echogenicity against which the portal vein branches appear brighter than normal.[1] This pattern is seen in up to 60% of patients with acute viral hepatitis and is best appreciated in thin patients.[16] Gallbladder wall thickening or contraction or both, are other nonspecific findings seen in patients with hepatitis. Paradoxical response of gallbladder to fatty food may be seen as dilatation of gall bladder. Severe chronic hepatitis causes coarsening of parenchymal

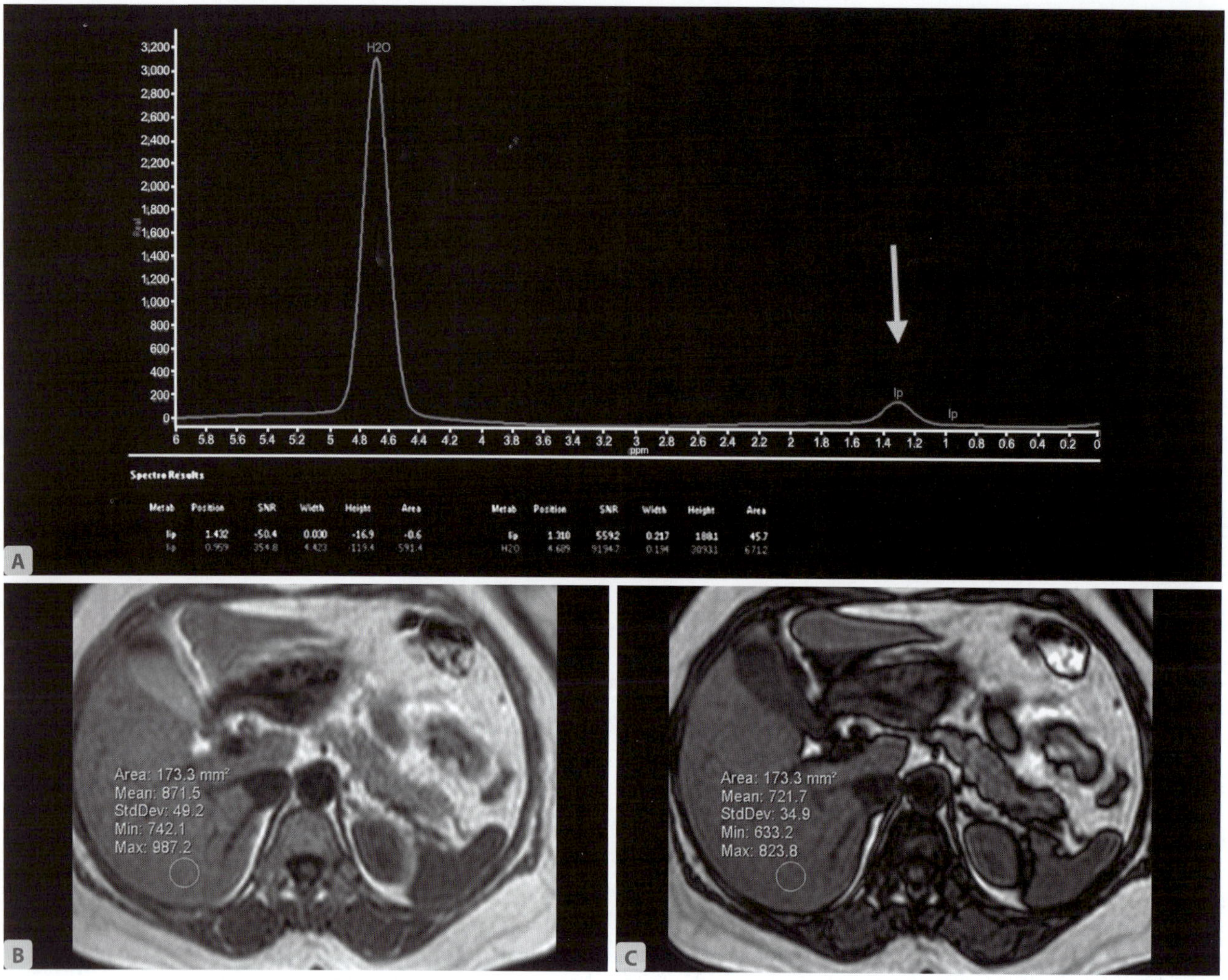

FIGS. 6A TO C: MRS spectrum in a case of fatty liver (A) showing a lipid peak at 1.3 ppm. Chemical shift MRI of fatty liver shows signal drop of liver parenchyma in the opposed-phase image (C) from in-phase image (B) due to steatosis.

echotexture and increased echogenicity resulting in poor visualization of portal venous branches. This finding, however, is nonspecific and is also seen in fatty infiltration and cirrhosis. Periportal lymphadenopathy may be seen in hepatitis.

CT

CT attenuation of liver is generally not altered in hepatitis unless fatty infiltration is present. Hepatomegaly, gallbladder wall thickening, and periportal hypodensity can be seen in acute hepatitis and periportal lymphadenopathy is commonly seen in chronic active hepatitis.

MRI

On MRI, the edematous liver in acute hepatitis may appear heterogeneous especially on T2-weighted images and early post contrast images. Periportal T2 hyperintense signal can also be seen. Likewise heterogeneous contrast enhancement and T2 hyperintensity signify severe ongoing inflammation in chronic hepatitis, while absence of patchy enhancement suggests low inflammatory reaction.[17] Progressive enhancement in the delayed phase suggests the presence of liver fibrosis in patients with chronic hepatitis.[18]

ALCOHOLIC HEPATITIS

Alcoholic liver disease manifests as three distinct but overlapping entities: fatty liver, alcoholic hepatitis and cirrhosis. Unlike acute viral hepatitis, liver echogenicity is increased in acute alcoholic hepatitis due to presence of concomitant fatty infiltration.

RADIATION HEPATITIS

In acute radiation hepatitis, CT shows a sharply defined, hypodense area in the liver corresponding to the radiation ports. This represents edema or fatty infiltration of the involved area. Clinically, onset is 2–6 weeks after therapy and is generally seen in patients receiving dose of more than 35 gray to the liver. The CT changes may be seen several weeks

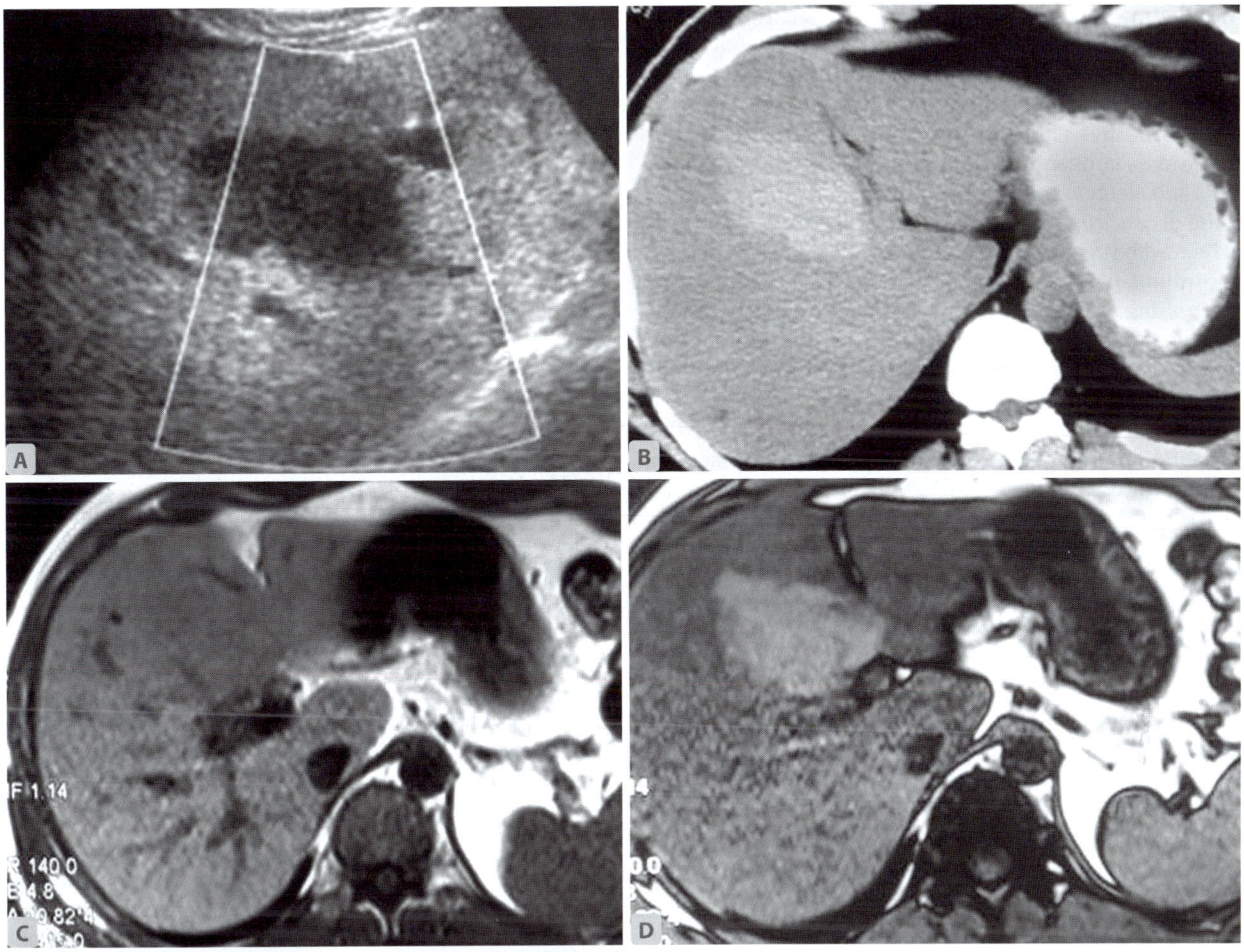

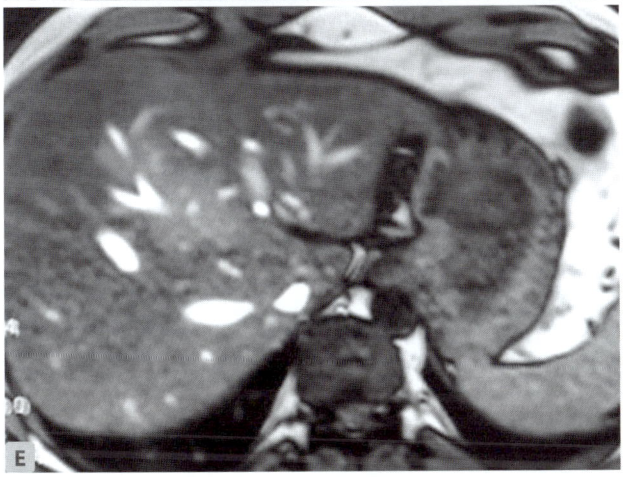

FIGS. 7A TO E: Fatty liver with focal fat sparing: US (A) reveals diffuse increase in liver echogenicity with a geographic hypoechoic area. NCCT (B) focal fat sparing seen as an area of increased attenuation against a background of diffusely hypodense liver. The focal area is located adjacent to the fissure for ligamentum teres. MR T1W in phase (C), opposed phase (D) images: The fatty liver parenchyma shows drop in signal intensity in the opposed phase image unlike the area of fat sparing which appears relatively hyperintense on the opposed phase image. True-FISP MR image (E) illustrates normal vessels coursing through the area of fat sparing.

after the initiation of the therapy and resolve by 3–5 months. Radiation hepatitis on MR imaging is seen as geographic areas of edema on T1- and T2-weighted images.[19]

HEMOCHROMATOSIS AND HEMOSIDEROSIS

Hepatic iron overload can be divided into parenchymal iron deposition (hemochromatosis) and reticuloendothelial iron deposition (hemosiderosis). In hemosiderosis, the excess iron (body iron stores 10–20 g) is derived from red blood cells typically due to repeated blood transfusions or hemolytic anemia. Because such iron is deposited primarily in the reticuloendothelial system (liver, spleen, lymph nodes, bone marrow) organ function is generally preserved.

Hemochromatosis on the other hand is a more severe form of iron accumulation (body iron stores up to 50–60 g) that adversely affects organ function. Hemochromatosis may be primary or secondary. Primary hemochromatosis is an autosomal recessive metabolic disorder of excessive iron absorption in duodenum/jejunum. The causes of secondary hemochromatosis include excess iron intake, anemia due to ineffective erythropoiesis requiring multiple blood transfusions, congenital transferrin deficiency, portocaval shunts and alcoholic cirrhosis.

The excess iron in hemochromatosis is stored as ferritin and hemosiderin in various organs including liver, pancreas, myocardium, joints, endocrine glands like pituitary and skin, in decreasing order of severity. Sometimes iron is deposited in spleen and kidneys. Brain and nervous tissues are spared. A fibrous tissue reaction is found wherever iron is deposited. Iron deposits are greatest in liver and pancreas where they can contain 50–100 times the normal amount of iron. The liver is the first organ to be damaged in hemochromatosis resulting in hepatomegaly in 95% symptomatic patients. Fibrosis is maximal in periportal areas resulting in micronodular pigment cirrhosis. Fatty change is unusual. Iron-induced interstitial fibrosis in the pancreas affects endocrine functions to a greater extent than exocrine functions. Skin hyperpigmentation and diabetes mellitus results in so called *bronze diabetes* in these patients. Splenomegaly is present in approximately 50% cases, arthropathy of small joints of the hand with or without evidence of chondrocalcinosis on radiographs occurs in 20–50% and cardiac involvement is the presenting complaint in 15% cases. Diminished sexual activity, loss of body hair and testicular atrophy can be seen due to decreased production of gonadotropins.

Primary hemochromatosis usually presents in fourth to sixth decade of life. It is ten times more frequent in males. Women are generally spared due to iron loss with menstruation and pregnancy. The disease responds favorably to treatment that includes venesection/removal of blood and iron chelators. However, once cirrhosis sets in, it is irreversible and is complicated by development of hepatocellular carcinoma in about one-third of patients despite adequate therapy.[20] Early diagnosis and treatment of hemochromatosis is therefore of vital importance.

USG

Ultrasonography (USG) only depicts nonspecific changes of cirrhosis in patients with hemochromatosis and therefore has no role in the diagnosis.

CT

Unenhanced CT shows an overall homogeneous increase in density of hepatic parenchyma. While normal liver attenuation is between 45 and 65 HU, in hemochromatosis this ranges from 70 to 135 HU. The intrahepatic vessels stand out against the background of hyperdense liver. A CT value of 70 HU or more on unenhanced scan is very sensitive and fairly specific indicator of severe iron overload **(Fig. 8)**,[12] although amiodarone treatment and glycogen storage disease can result in similar increased attenuation.

CT also demonstrates increased density in spleen, pancreas, adrenal and lymph nodes. The increased background liver attenuation in hemochromatosis may hamper detection of hepatocellular carcinoma in the postcontrast images but facilitates tumor detection in unenhanced scans.

Dual energy CT has a proven role in estimation of liver iron content (LIC). It is based on three material decomposition of iodine, water and iron, to provide virtual iron content (VIC) as well as providing a virtual nonenhanced image by commercially available postprocessing softwares.[21]

MRI

MR imaging is the most sensitive and specific imaging modality for demonstration of hepatic iron overload and also for follow-up of patients under treatment.[17] Gradient echo sequences are more sensitive than spin echo sequences. On MRI, hemochromatosis is characterized by dramatic loss of T1 and T2 signal of the liver (90%) and pancreas (20%) **(Fig. 9)**. A liver/paraspinal muscle (L/M) signal ratio below 0.6 on spin echo T2-weighted images is suggestive of severe iron overload. It correlates well with the amount of iron present in the liver.[12] Iron estimation can also be done by in

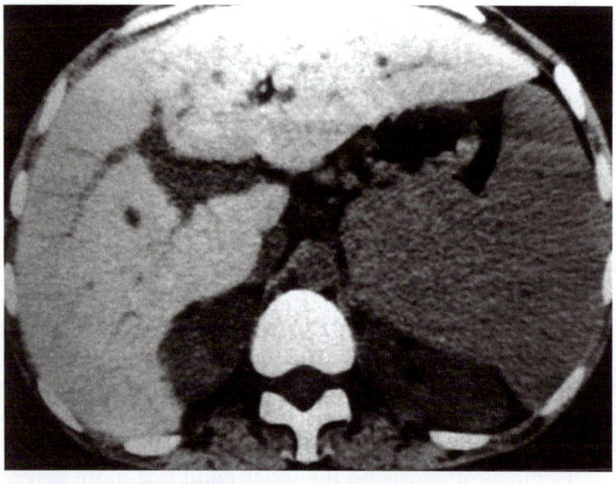

FIG. 8: Primary hemochromatosis: Unenhanced CT shows markedly increased attenuation of the liver parenchyma.

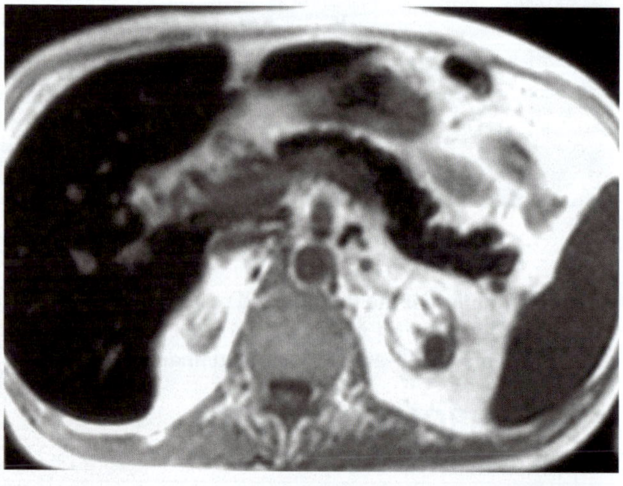

FIG. 9: Primary hemochromatosis: FSE T2W image reveals markedly hypointense signal of the liver and pancreas, while the spleen shows normal signal intensity.

and opposed phase imaging where contrary to what is seen in fatty infiltration, iron deposition results in loss of signal in the in phase image which conventionally is acquired at a longer TE than the opposed phase image **(Figs. 10A to C)**.

Another method of iron estimation is based on T2 relaxometry. This technique is based on spin-echo and gradient-echo sequences. MR images are acquired at progressively longer echo times (TE), and the rate of signal decay is mathematically estimated. This generates a cross-sectional map of T2 (in spin echo) or T2* (in gradient echo) relaxation rates. Once the T2 or T2* value is calculated, the liver iron concentration (LIC) in mg of elemental iron/g of liver tissue by dry weight can be estimated by validated calibration curves.[22] Liver iron content can also be calculated by signal intensity ratio (SIR) between the liver and the paraspinal muscles from a set of multiple GRE sequences with fixed TR, different TE and flip angles for 1.5 T scanners using an online calculator developed by University of Rennes.[23]

Iron overload coexisting with fat deposition may present a diagnostic challenge and requires careful evaluation in all sequences. In fat deposition, there is loss of signal on opposed phase images, whereas in iron deposition there is low signal on 'in phase' images. Moreover, in presence of focal fatty sparing or focal fatty change on a background of iron overload (pseudolesion) may require enhancement pattern characterization.

Decreased signal intensity in hemochromatosis is also demonstrated in pancreas and myocardium, and only occasionally in spleen. In transfusional siderosis, the signal intensity of both spleen and liver is diminished while the signal of pancreas remains unchanged as it is devoid of reticuloendothelial cells **(Figs. 11A and B)** his feature helps to differentiate transfusional siderosis from hemochromatosis.

AMYLOIDOSIS

Amyloidosis is a rare condition characterized by the deposition of an extracellular fibrillar protein in the organs. It may be primary or secondary. Primary amyloidosis is due to deposition of amyloid light chain protein (AL). It may occur without pre-existing disease or may be seen as a complication of multiple myeloma. Secondary amyloidosis is due to the deposition of amyloid A protein (AA) and is seen with chronic infections, rheumatoid arthritis, ulcerative colitis, Crohn's disease, malignant tumors and Hodgkin's lymphoma. Clinically, there is smooth, non-tender hepatomegaly. Hepatic function is usually preserved despite massive amyloid deposition.

Ultrasound is usually normal except for presence of hepatomegaly. Rarely US reveals a heterogeneous echotexture due to nonuniform deposition. Increased liver

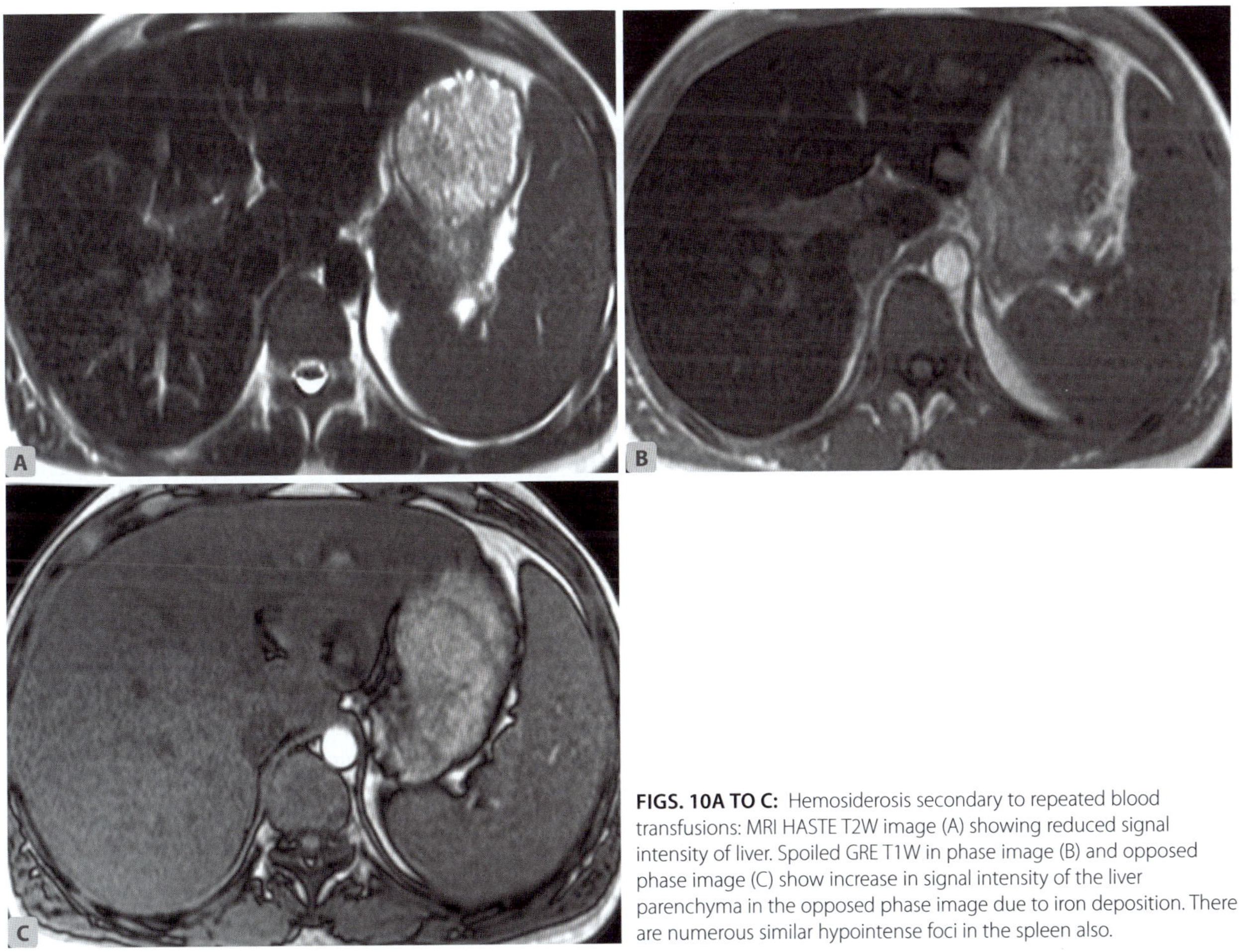

FIGS. 10A TO C: Hemosiderosis secondary to repeated blood transfusions: MRI HASTE T2W image (A) showing reduced signal intensity of liver. Spoiled GRE T1W in phase image (B) and opposed phase image (C) show increase in signal intensity of the liver parenchyma in the opposed phase image due to iron deposition. There are numerous similar hypointense foci in the spleen also.

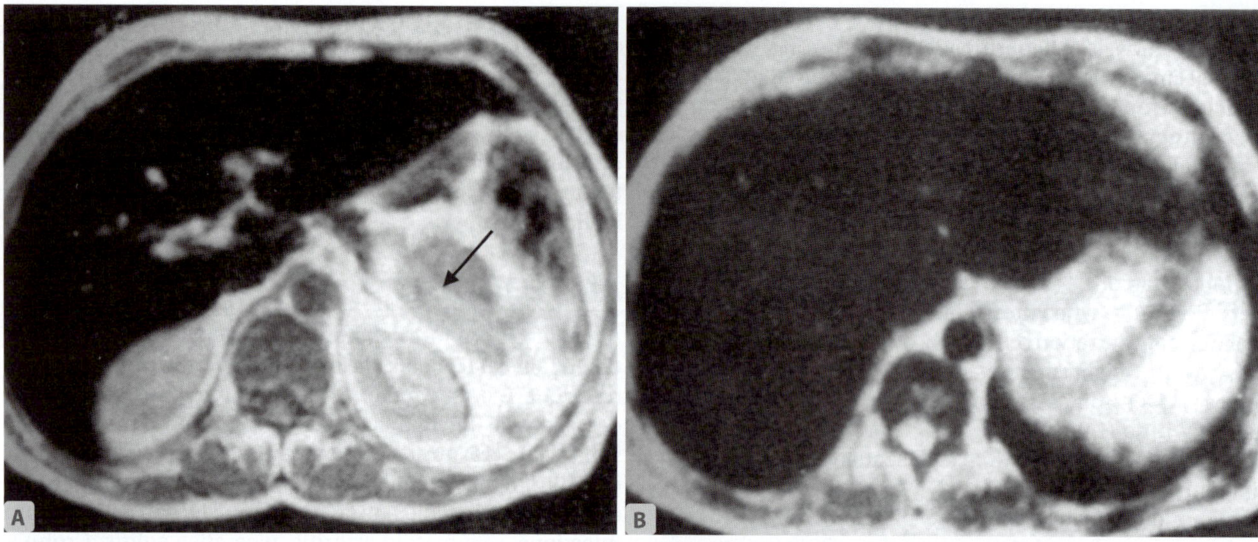

FIGS. 11A AND B: Hemosiderosis: Almost no signal intensity is seen on T1-weighted (A) and T2-weighted axial MR images (B). Normal signal intensity of the pancreas (↑) helps in differentiation from hemochromatosis. Spleen is not seen because of previous splenectomy in this patient.

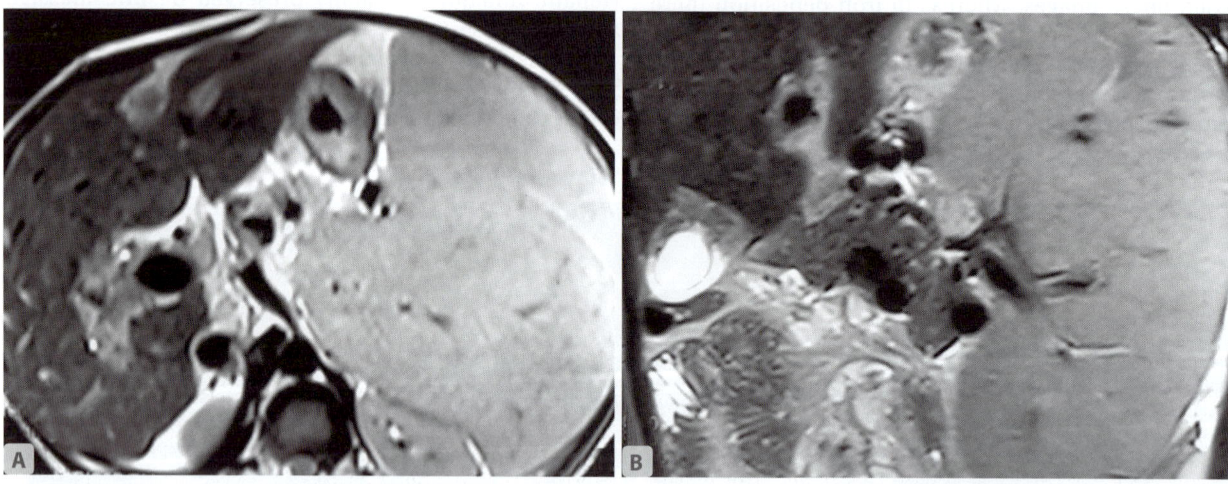

FIGS. 12A AND B: Wilson's disease: Axial (A) and coronal (B) TSE T2W image of a 15-year-old boy showing non-specific changes of liver cirrhosis with a shrunken liver and massive splenomegaly.

stiffness is seen on ultrasound elastography which may be due to the protein deposition.[24]

On unenhanced CT scans amyloid deposition results in hepatomegaly and generalized decreased attenuation. On contrast-enhanced scans, focal areas of decreased enhancement corresponding to nonuniform involvement may be seen. The involved areas may show contrast enhancement in the delayed phase. Concomitant decrease in splenic enhancement may help differentiate amyloid deposition from fatty liver in appropriate settings. MR imaging has little role in the assessment of hepatic amyloidosis as there is no significant change in the T2 signal of involved liver.[25] MRI elastography also reveals increased tissue stiffness.

WILSON'S DISEASE

Wilson's disease or hepatolenticular degeneration is a rare, inherited autosomal recessive disorder of copper metabolism characterized by impaired biliary excretion of copper. Initially the excess copper accumulates in the liver. Subsequently copper deposition occurs in the basal ganglia, renal tubules, cornea, bones, joints and parathyroid glands. The spectrum of liver injury in Wilson's disease is nonspecific and includes fatty infiltration, acute hepatitis, chronic active hepatitis, cirrhosis or massive liver necrosis. Development of HCC is extremely rare.

Most patients present in childhood or adolescence with liver disease before the onset of neurologic manifestations. They may have progressive jaundice, ascites or even fulminant hepatitis. Patients presenting after the age of 20 years can present with a clinical picture simulating chronic active hepatitis or with neurological symptoms like Parkinson like movement disorder and psychiatric disturbance. The Kayser-Fleischer ring is a characteristic corneal pigment that is invariably present. Early recognition is important as treatment with penicillamine and zinc can prevent toxic deposition of copper in the liver and brain. Imaging findings of cirrhosis, fatty liver are nonspecific **(Figs. 12A and B)**. Fatty infiltration and excess copper can cancel each other out in advanced Wilson's disease, so that a high CT density is usually not seen. Skeletal changes are seen in over 85% patients with Wilson's disease.[26] These include osteomalacia, chondrocalcinosis, premature osteoarthritis, anterior wedging of dorsal vertebrae, Schmorl's nodes, osteochondritis dissecans and a periosteal reaction at the trochanters.

On MRI, copper deposition has no ferromagnetic effect on the liver signal intensity as it exists intracellularly in bound form. The changes on MRI are similar to those of cirrhotic liver disease with contour abnormalities and regenerative nodules. A honeycomb pattern consisting of multiple low-intensity nodules surrounded by hyperintense septa on T2-weighted images may be seen. However, this finding is not specific to Wilson's disease.[27] Due to copper deposition T1 hyperintense and T2 hypointense nodules may be seen on MRI which may show resolution with chelation therapy.[28]

GRANULOMATOUS DISEASES

Granulomatous diseases denote the presence of a focal inflammatory process with the histological features of granuloma. The causes include various viral, bacterial, fungal and parasitic infections, sarcoidosis, granulomatosis with polyangitis (Wegener's), and toxic reaction to drugs and chemicals. Biochemical abnormalities in the form of elevated alkaline phosphatase (ALP) and gamma glutamyl transpeptidase (GGT) is frequently seen in various diffuse infiltrative diseases and alcoholic/viral chronic liver diseases.

Tuberculosis

Miliary tuberculosis is the most common form of hepatic tuberculosis. Usually it is not accompanied by radiological abnormalities because of its diffuse micronodular nature. Macronodular tuberculomas are uncommon and may be solitary or multiple. These are hypoechoic on ultrasound. CT scan shows hypodense masses with or without rim enhancement **(Fig. 13)**. Tubercular cholangitis and tubercular pyelophlebitis result from rupture of tubercular nodes/abscess and spread of caseous material into bile ducts and portal vein respectively. Both these conditions are rare. Multiple small intrahepatic calcifications with no associated masses seen on ultrasound and CT represent old healed granulomas.[12]

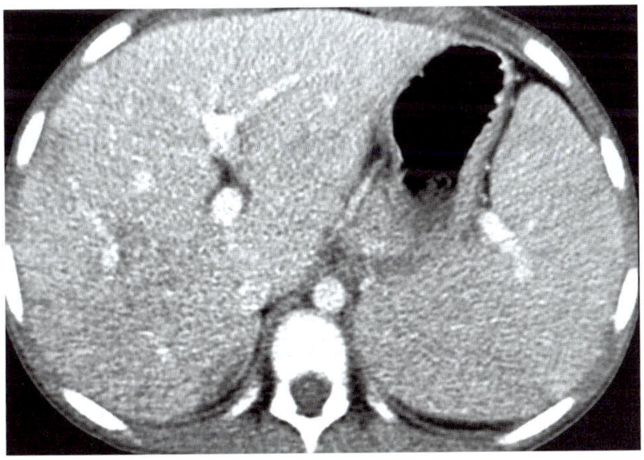

FIG. 13: Granulomatous disease: Contrast-enhanced CT of a young adult with disseminated tuberculosis reveals hepatosplenomegaly and ill-defined hypodense lesions in the right lobe of liver.

Sarcoidosis

Liver involvement occurs in 24–79% patients of sarcoidosis.[29] Clinically apparent liver disease is however rare. On imaging small (<2 mm) noncaseating granulomas are seen diffusely in the liver. Cross sectional imaging most frequently reveals hepatomegaly, often with associated splenomegaly. Less commonly granulomas are seen as nodular lesions 0.5–2 cm in size in the liver and spleen. These nodular lesions appear hypoechoic on US, hypodense on CT and hypointense on both T1- and T2-weighted MR images. Upper abdominal adenopathy is frequently associated in these patients. Occasionally, these nodes enlarge sufficiently to cause biliary obstruction at porta hepatis.

Schistosomiasis

It is a common parasitic infestation with high prevalence in endemic areas such as Africa, South America, Middle East, China and Japan. The adult worms release ova in portal and mesenteric veins, which embolize to the liver. The host reacts to the ova with a granulomatous inflammation, which is then replaced by fibrous tissue, leading to periportal fibrosis and portal hypertension. On ultrasound, periportal fibrosis is seen in the form of thick, echogenic bands replacing the normal portal venous walls, which radiate from porta hepatis to the periphery of the liver. These bands are seen as tubular, round or oval structures depending on the plane of the section. There may be evidence of portal hypertension. On unenhanced CT, the bands of periportal fibrosis are hypodense and they enhance markedly after contrast administration. They produce round, linear or branching patterns depending on the plane in which they are sectioned. The portal vein may not enhance, if it is thrombosed. Hepatic calcification, if seen, is fairly characteristic and has been termed as 'turtle back'.[30] It occurs within the capsule and hepatic parenchyma, perpendicular to the capsule looking like a septum. Sometimes the calcifications may be dense enough to be seen on the plain films.

Liver Fluke or Fasciola Hepatica

It is a trematode that infests cattle. Humans are accidental hosts. There is an acute phase of hepatic invasion that lasts for 1–3 months and a chronic phase of persistent adult flukes in the biliary tree. In hepatic fascioliasis, CT shows peripheral small, hypodense, serpentine or nodular lesions whose visibility is improved on dynamic or delayed enhanced CT. The tortuous peripheral channels correspond to the migratory tracts.[31]

There are many other causes of granulomatous infections, which include brucellosis, leptospirosis, syphilis, leishmaniasis, actinomycosis, aspergillosis and cryptococcosis. These are not associated with any specific radiological features.

CIRRHOSIS

Cirrhosis is a chronic disease of the liver, which is characterized by fibrosis, and nodular regeneration of the liver in response to hepatocellular necrosis. The etiology is diverse which includes viral hepatitis, alcoholism, prolonged cholestasis, hepatic venous outflow tract obstruction, malnutrition, cryptogenic cirrhosis, metabolic causes like hemochromatosis and Wilson's disease, various toxins and therapeutic agents. Cirrhosis is conventionally considered as an irreversibly scarred, end stage disease of the liver. Although the causes are many, the end result is same.[32] The response of the liver to the necrosis is limited, the most important being collapse of hepatic lobules, formation of diffuse fibrous septa and nodular re-growth of liver cells. The initiating hepatocyte injury leads to inflammation, structural collapse and fibrogenesis. The resulting fibrosis causes circulatory disturbances, portal hypertension and intrahepatic cholestasis. A vicious cycle is set-up whereby further hepatocyte injury occurs leading to progression of the disease. Morphologically cirrhosis is classified into micronodular and macronodular varieties. *Micronodular* disease is characterized by thick, regular septa, small regenerating nodules of uniform size, and involvement of every lobule. It may represent impaired capacity of re-growth as in alcoholism or malnutrition. *Macronodular* variety is characterized by septa and nodules of various sizes and presence of normal liver in between larger nodules.[32] There are many histological grading systems for categorizing hepatic fibrosis, *METAVIR* being the most common. It is a five point scoring system:

1. F0—no fibrosis
2. F1—portal fibrosis without septa
3. F2—few septa
4. F3—numerous septa without cirrhosis
5. F4—cirrhosis.[2]

A *regenerative nodule* is defined as a hepatocellular nodule containing one or more portal tracts located in a liver that is otherwise abnormal due to either cirrhosis or other severe disease. These nodules are present in all cirrhotic livers, and cirrhosis is classified on the basis of size of these on pathologic specimen as micronodular (less than equal to 3 mm), macronodular (more than 3 mm) or mixed. A *dysplastic nodule* is defined as a nodule of hepatocytes of at least 1 mm in diameter, with dysplasia of low or high grade but no histological criteria for malignancy. Dysplastic nodules are found in 15–25% of cirrhotic livers. Steatosis (fatty infiltration) can occur in either form, and either form may result in an enlarged or shrunken liver. *Focal confluent fibrosis* (or confluent hepatic fibrosis) refers to mass like fibrosis in advanced cirrhosis, associated with volume loss seen as retraction of overlying hepatic capsule or total shrinkage of segment or lobe.

Clinically, Child's classification is used to determine short-term prognosis. It takes into account jaundice, ascites, encephalopathy, serum albumin and nutrition status. In the Child-Pugh modification prothrombin time is used instead of nutritional status as a parameter. The total score classifies patients into grade A, B or C, with increasing severity of disease.[32] Complications of cirrhosis include portal hypertension, variceal bleeding, spontaneous bacterial peritonitis, coagulopathies, hepatic encephalopathy, hepatorenal syndrome and hepatocellular carcinoma (HCC). Risk of development of HCC in cirrhotic liver is approximately 3% per year. Although, cirrhosis of any etiology may lead to HCC, the risk is particularly high in cirrhosis which occurs secondary to viral hepatitis. Imaging studies play an important role in screening for HCC in cirrhotic patients.

USG

Liver is either enlarged or normal in size in the early stage of cirrhosis. A small shrunken liver is seen in advanced cases. Criteria for sonographic diagnosis include heterogeneously increased parenchymal echogenicity, decreased beam penetration through liver and poor depiction of diaphragm and intrahepatic portal venous walls. These features are common to both fatty infiltration and fibrosis and there is poor interobserver agreement on interpreting these finding. Echogenicity largely depends on gain settings; however, it can be compared with that of adjacent organs in cases of doubt. Normally, echogenicity of liver and renal cortex are almost equal or that of kidney is slightly lower than liver. In case the kidneys are diseased, comparison may be made with that of splenic echogenicity also as spleen has higher echogenicity than normal liver.

Morphological changes in cirrhosis include relative hypertrophy of the caudate lobe and segments 2, 3 of the left lobe and atrophy of the right hepatic lobe and segment 4 of left lobe. Sonographically, a right/left lobe ratio of sagittal diameters in midclavicular line and midline respectively of 1.3 or less can differentiate cirrhosis from normal liver with 93% accuracy, while a ratio of 1.4 or more excludes cirrhosis.[33] In advanced case of cirrhosis, accentuation of fissures, contour indentations, nodularity and regenerating nodules are seen. Regenerating nodules vary in size from 2 mm to 2 cm. These may be visible on US as hypoechoic nodules with echogenic border and are difficult to differentiate from small HCC on US. US scanning with a high frequency probe can depict a nodular liver contour even in early cirrhosis.[34] Atrophy of the liver, along with heterogeneous echotexture and poor beam penetration, however, limits the sonographic detection of small focal lesions in advanced cirrhotic liver. Sonography has a poor sensitivity in detection of HCC; it detects only 14% of lesions smaller than 2 cm and its sensitivity for detecting HCC during screening of cirrhotic patients is only 50%.[1,35]

Doppler evaluation is valuable as it provides hemodynamic information. Portal hypertension can be seen in the form of enlarged portal vein, diminution or reversal of portal venous flow and presence of portosystemic collaterals. Hepatic venous evaluation by Doppler is also helpful. Normal hepatic venous waveform is triphasic with a short phase of reversed flow. The fibrosis and decreased compliance of liver parenchyma leads to decreased amplitude of the phasic variations with loss of reversed flow. Alternatively, there may be a completely flat waveform. These features may be seen even in early stages of cirrhosis.[36] As the liver atrophies in end stage cirrhosis, hepatic veins may become attenuated and difficult to visualize. This can cause difficulties when the diagnosis of hepatic venous occlusion is being considered.[8]

The cirrhotic liver can be assessed noninvasively by three *ultrasound elastography* techniques, the transient elastography (fibroscan), acoustic radiation force impulse (ARFI) and shear wave elastography. The hepatic fibrosis correlates with the stiffness values generated on elastography such that value less than 6–7 kPa indicate no or mild fibrosis (F0-F1 METAVIR) and a value more than 12 kPa suggests cirrhosis (F3-F4 METAVIR) **(Fig. 3B)**.[3]

Contrast enhanced ultrasound using microbubble contrast agent has a role in characterizing focal liver lesions in cirrhotic liver and in screening of cirrhosis patients for hepatocellular carcinomas. It is a useful adjunct to CECT or CEMRI with the benefit of a real time contrast visualization without renal excretion of the contrast. Both dysplastic nodules and hepatocellular carcinomas show arterial phase hyperenhancement on CEUS, similar to CT and MRI.[37]

CT

Fatty liver is the most common CT feature of early cirrhosis. Morphological changes in advanced cirrhosis include an overall decrease in liver volume accompanied by atrophy of the right lobe and hypertrophy of left and caudate lobes. The dual arterial supply and shorter intrahepatic course of vessels supplying the caudate lobe along with the fact that caudate vein drains directly into the inferior vena cava permits better oxygenation and relative preservation of its function resulting in compensatory hypertrophy.[37] On the other hand it is postulated that alcohol and other toxins in the portal vein stream preferentially to the right hepatic lobe. Caudate lobe to right lobe size ratio has been proposed as an objective means of diagnosing cirrhosis. Three lines are drawn: Line 1 is parasagittal through the right lateral wall of main portal vein just caudal to its bifurcation, line 2 is parallel to line 1 through the medial margin of caudate lobe, and line 3 is perpendicular to these lines drawn midway between portal vein and IVC. The distances are measured on line 3. The distance between right abdominal wall and line 1 is right lobe size and distance between line 1 and line 2 is caudate lobe size **(Fig. 14)**. If the caudate lobe to right lobe ratio exceeds 0.65, cirrhosis is likely and it is definitive if it exceeds 0.73.[38] The hepatic fissure, gallbladder fossa and porta hepatis are widened due to parenchymal atrophy **(Fig. 15)**. These morphological changes are by and large similar irrespective of the underlying etiology of cirrhosis. However, patients with biliary cirrhosis and sclerosing cholangitis tend to have marked caudate lobe hypertrophy and often have atrophy of lateral segments of the left hepatic lobe in addition to atrophy of right lobe.

Cirrhotic liver often appears heterogeneous on both unenhanced and enhanced CT scans due to underlying fibrosis, iron accumulation, regeneration and altered portal venous flow.[8] Regenerating nodules and atrophy cause nodularity of liver contour. Ancillary CT features in cirrhosis include ascites, splenomegaly, enlargement of the hepatic artery, and evidence of porto-systemic collaterals, pericaval fat collection that may appear intraluminal on axial CT scans and increased attenuation of the mesenteric/retroperitoneal fat.

Regenerating nodules are usually less than 5 mm and are infrequently demonstrated on noncontrast CT, however may appear hyperdense if they contain iron (Siderotic nodules). These do not show arterial phase enhancement and remain isodense to minimally hypodense to the remaining parenchyma on portal venous phase.

Dysplastic nodules on the other hand measure 5–10 mm in size and show arterial phase enhancement due to progressive recruitment of hepatic arterial supply. The high grade dyplastic nodules may show portal venous washout similar to that of hepatocellular carcinomas.

Focal confluent fibrosis that is seen in 30% of patients with advanced cirrhosis can also simulate tumor appearing hypodense on unenhanced CT and isodense to slightly hypodense in contrast-enhanced CT. However, typical associated features including wedge-shaped lesion radiating from the porta hepatis, characteristic location in

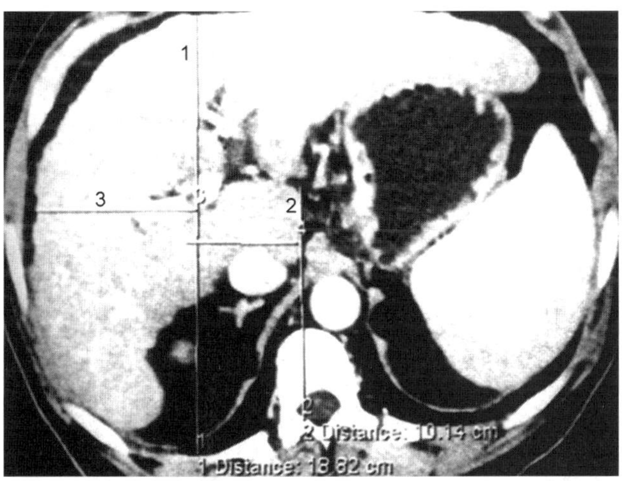

FIG. 14: CT scan shows method of measurements of right and caudate lobes. The diameters of right and caudate lobes are measured on line 3 as shown.

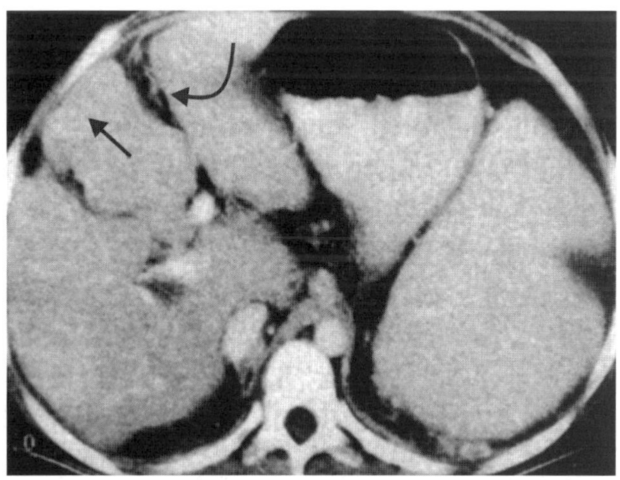

FIG. 15: Cirrhosis: Atrophy of the right lobe and hypertrophy of the caudate lobe with splenomegaly is seen on CT. Widened hepatic fissure (curved arrow), porta and nodularity of the contour of the liver (straight arrow) are also seen.

the anterior segments of right lobe and segment 4, delayed enhancement and focal retraction of the overlying liver capsule can help differentiate these from tumor. Similar to hepatitis, patients with cirrhosis can have enlarged upper abdominal lymph nodes and this finding is particularly common in patients with biliary cirrhosis and sclerosing cholangitis. Pseudocirrhosis results from distortion of the hepatic parenchyma due to treated multiple metastatic lesions, usually from breast carcinoma and can simulate changes of cirrhosis. Similar appearance may also result from pseudomyxoma peritonei or ovarian metastasis due to surface scalloping.

MRI

MR imaging can often detect cirrhosis at an earlier stage than US or CT.[1] In early cirrhosis, MRI demonstrates fine strands of fibrosis, which are seen as lace like hypointense fine network on heavily T2-weighted images. Out of phase spoiled gradient echo images are very sensitive in this regard. These fine fibrotic strands show progressive enhancement following intravenous gadolinium. Enlargement of hilar periportal space, which is a space anterior to right branch of portal vein, is considered as an early manifestation of cirrhosis. It is caused by atrophy of segment 4. Early detection of cirrhosis by MRI is of clinical importance as these patients may benefit from newer treatment options now available.[22] As cirrhosis progresses, MRI demonstrates all features which are seen on CT, including contour nodularity, relative right lobe atrophy and left/caudate lobe hypertrophy, splanchnic vessels enlargement, hepatic arterial enlargement, collaterals, splenomegaly and ascites. Expansion and widening of interlobar fissure is also seen.

Abnormal hepatic periportal intensity, which is seen as hyperintense rings or track marks surrounding the portal vein branches on T2-weighted images, can be seen in cirrhosis. It is a nonspecific finding and also seen in many biliary or hepatocellular diseases. Gamna Gandy bodies in spleen are seen as multiple, small, low intensity spots on gradient echo images. These represent hemosiderin deposits in collagen bundles and may be the result of small hemorrhages and can be seen in portal hypertension due to other causes like EHPVO.

MR imaging is the modality of choice for characterizing nodules in cirrhotic liver and can demonstrate regenerating nodules with greater sensitivity than any other modality. While only approximately 25% of regenerating nodules are seen on CT mainly due to their iron content, MR can demonstrate 50% regenerative nodules **(Figs. 16A and B)**.[1] Dysplastic nodules (previously called adenomatous hyperplastic nodules) represent premalignant intermediary phase in pathway of hepatocellular carcinogenesis **(Figs. 17A to D)**. The MRI appearance of regenerative and dysplastic nodules on various MRI sequences and enhancement phases is summarized in **Table 1**.

Focal confluent fibrosis has T1 and T2 signal similar to HCC, i.e. hypointense on T1 and hyperintense on T2-weighted images. It may show arterial phase enhancement, however persistent enhancement in delayed phase helps in differentiation from hepatocellular carcinoma. Moreover, as with CT, characteristic location and associated capsular retraction also helps in differentiation. MR imaging is useful in differentiating viral from alcoholic cirrhosis. Larger caudate lobe volume, presence of a notch in the outline of right posterior segment of liver and smaller size of regenerating nodules favors the diagnosis of alcoholic cirrhosis over virus induced cirrhosis.[39]

MR elastography (MRE) has a role in noninvasive evaluation, staging and follow-up of hepatic fibrosis. It is based on modified phase contrast sequence where a mechanical propagation wave is produced in soft tissues usually of frequency 60 MHz. The propagation of the wave in the tissue creates an elastogram using complex algorithms. In various studies MR elastography has shown good agreement with ultrasound elastography, liver biopsy and other biochemical markers of hepatic fibrosis.[40,41] The advantages of MR elastography over ultrasound elastography include ability to evaluate the entire liver and eliminating the sampling error of USE. Moreover, MRE is unaffected by obesity and presence of ascites, which are known confounders in US elastography.

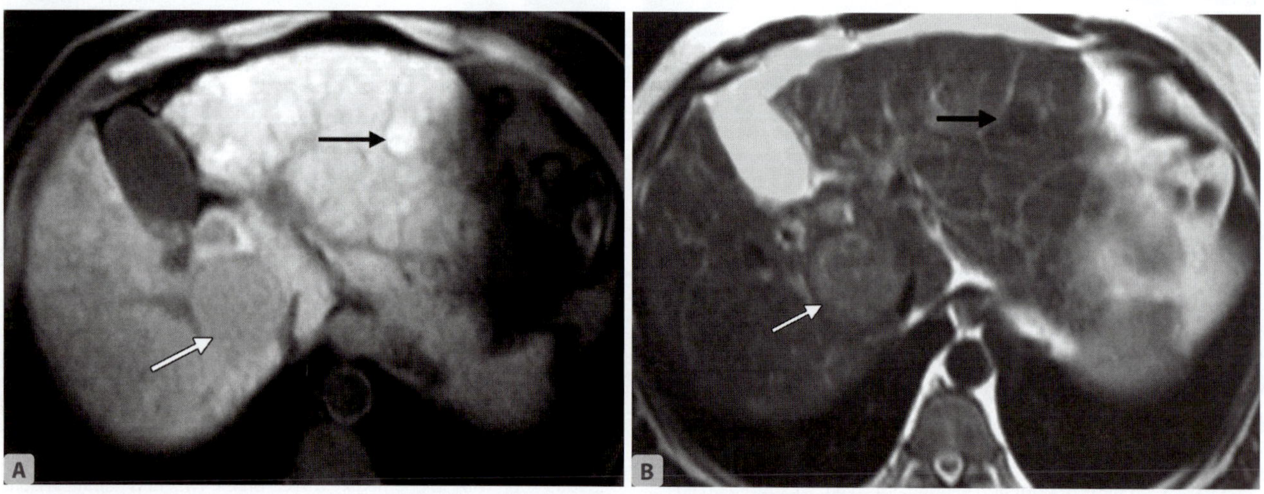

FIGS. 16A AND B: Cirrhosis with regenerative nodule and HCC: Axial T1W (A) and T2W (B) MR images shows a well-defined focal lesion in segment VIII of liver (white arrow) which is hypointense on T1 and hyperintense on T2W images suggestive of HCC. A regenerative nodule is also seen in segment II (black arrow) which appears hyperintense on T1 and hypointense on T2W images.

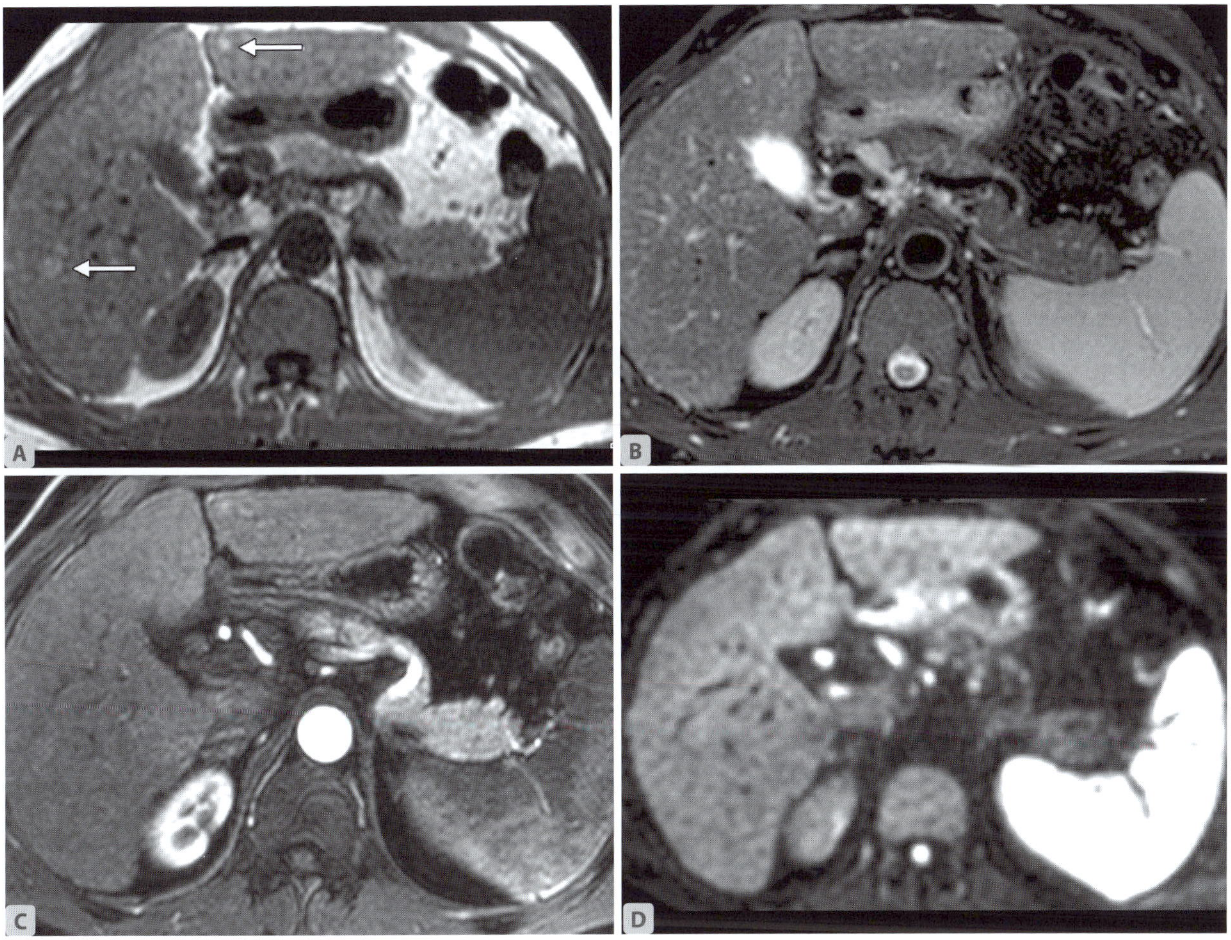

FIGS. 17A TO D: MRI findings of dysplastic nodules: In a patient of viral hepatitis related chronic liver disease showing irregular liver surface with multiple nodules (arrows) appearing hyperintense on T1W (A), isointense on T2W (B), with no arterial phase enhancement (C). Diffusion-weighted image (D) shows no areas of restricted diffusion.

TABLE 1: MRI features of nodules in liver cirrhosis.

	T1W	T2W	Arterial phase	Venous/Delayed phase
Regenerating nodule	Hyperintense	Iso- to hypointense	Isointense to liver	Isointense
Siderotic nodule	Hypointense	Hypointense	Isointense to hypointense	Iso- to hypointense
Low-grade dysplastic nodule	Iso- to hyperintense	Isohypointense	Isointense to liver	No washout
High grade dysplastic nodule	Iso- to hyperintense	Isohypointense	Hyperenhancing	No washout

MALIGNANT DIFFUSE LIVER DISEASES

Occasionally, a malignant process may diffusely involve the liver. Metastases, particularly from breast cancer, may give rise to diffusely increased heterogeneous echotexture on ultrasound. Hepatocellular carcinoma, lymphoma and leukemia can also be seen as diffusely altered echotexture of the liver. Diagnosis is difficult in such situations and may require biopsy in the appropriate clinical context.[6]

CONCLUSION

Diffuse liver diseases may result from a variety of causes, most important among which are alcoholic liver disease and viral hepatitis due to their wide prevalence, and complications like cirrhosis and hepatocellular carcinoma. Imaging plays an important role in diagnosis as well as management of diffuse liver diseases. Multiphase contrast enhanced CT remains the workhorse modality however MRI with its superior contrast resolution and higher sensitivity for lesion detection and characterization is the modality of choice in indeterminate lesions on CT. New modalities such as ultrasound elastography, contrast-enhanced ultrasound and MRI elastography have further enhanced the imaging evaluation of diffuse liver diseases.

REFERENCES

1. Gore RM. Diffuse Liver disease. In Gore RM, Levine MS (Eds): Textbook of Gastrointestinal Radiology, 3rd edn. Saunders Elsevier: Philadelphia; 2008.pp.1685-729.
2. The French METAVIR Cooperative Study Group Intraobserver and interobserver variations in liver biopsy interpretation in patients with chronic hepatitis C. Hepatology. 1994;20:15-20.
3. Ziol M, Handra-Luca A, Kettaneh A, et al. Noninvasive assessment of liver fibrosis by measurement of stiffness in patients with chronic hepatitis C. Hepatology. 2005;41:48-54.
4. Skoczylas K, Pawełas A. Ultrasound imaging of the liver and bile ducts–expectations of a clinician. Journal of Ultrasonography. 2015;15:292-30.
5. Borges VF, Diniz AL, Cotrim HP, Rocha HL, Andrade NB. Sonographic hepatorenal ratio: a noninvasive method to diagnose nonalcoholic steatosis. J Clin Ultrasound. 2013;41:18-25.
6. Park SH, Kim PN, Kim KW, et al. Macrovesicular hepatic steatosis in living liver donors: Use of CT for quantitative and qualitative assessment. Radiology. 2006;239:105-12.
7. Pickhardt PJ, Park SH, Hahn L, Lee SG, Bae KT, Yu ES. Specificity of unenhanced CT for non-invasive diagnosis of hepatic steatosis: implications for the investigation of the natural history of incidental steatosis. Eur Radiol. 2012;22:1075-82.
8. Lomas DJ. The liver. In: Grainger RG, Allison D, Adam A, Dixon AK (Eds): Diagnostic Radiology, 4th edn. Churchill Livingstone: London; 2001.pp.1237-76.
9. Lee SW, Park SH, Kim KW, et al. Unenhanced CT for assessment of macrovesicular hepatic steatosis in living liver donors: comparison of visual grading with liver attenuation index. Radiology. 2007;244:479-85.
10. Boyce C, Pickhardt P, Kim DH, et al. Hepatic steatosis (fatty liver disease) in asymptomatic adults identified by unenhanced low-dose CT. AJR. 2010;194(3):623-8.
11. Singh D, Das CJ, Baruah MP. Imaging of non alcoholic fatty liver disease: A road less travelled. Indian J Endocrinol Metab. 2013;17:990-5.
12. Venbrux AC, Freidman AC. Diffuse hepatocellular diseases. In: Friedman AC, Aachman AH (Eds). Radiology of the Liver, Biliary Tract and Pancreas. Mosby year book: St Louis; 1994.pp.49-167.
13. Reeder SB, Cruite I, Hamilton G, Sirlin CB. Quantitative assessment of liver fat with magnetic resonance imaging and spectroscopy. J Magn Reson Imaging. 2011;34(4):729-49.
14. Bastati N, Feier D, Wibmer A, et al. Noninvasive differentiation of simple steatosis and steatohepatitis by using gadoxetic acid–enhanced MR imaging in patients with nonalcoholic fatty liver disease: a proof-of-concept study. Radiology. 2014;271(3):739-47.
15. Smits LP, Coolen BF, Panno MD, et al. Noninvasive Differentiation between Hepatic Steatosis and Steatohepatitis with MR Imaging Enhanced with USPIOs in Patients with Nonalcoholic Fatty Liver Disease: A Proof-of-Concept Study. Radiology. 2016;278(3):782-91.
16. Tchelepi H, Ralls PW, Radin R, Grant E. Sonography of diffuse liver disease. J Ultrasound Med. 2002;21:1023-32.
17. Danet IM, Semelka RC, Braga L. MR imaging of diffuse liver disease. Radiol Clin North Am. 2003;41:67-87.
18. Martin DR, Semelka RC. Magnetic resonance imaging of the liver: review of techniques and approach to common diseases. Semin Ultrasound CT MR. 2005;26:116-3.
19. Semelka RC, Braga L. Armao D. Liver. In: Semelka RC (Ed). Abdominal Pelvic MRI. New York, Wiley-Liss; 2002.pp.33-318.
20. Kauffman JM, Grace ND. Hemochromatosis. In Weinstein WM, Hawkey CJ, Bosch J (Eds). Clinical Gastroenterology and Hepatology. Philadelphia, Elsevier-Mosby; 2005.pp.659-64.
21. Luo XF, Xie XQ, Cheng S, et al. Dual-Energy CT for patients suspected of having liver iron overload: can virtual iron content imaging accurately quantify liver iron content? Radiology. 2015;277(1):95-103.
22. Gandon Y, Olivie´ D, Guyader D, et al. Non-invasive assessment of hepatic iron stores by MRI. Lancet. 2004;363:357-62.
23. Online Gandon Y. Iron and liver. Available at: *www.radio.univ-rennes1.fr*
24. Lanzi A, Gianstefani A, Mirarchi MG, et al. Liver AL amyloidosis as a possible cause of high liver stiffness values. Eur J Gastroenterol Hepatol. 2010;22:895-7.
25. Srinivasan S, Tan YQ, Teh HS, Lee PJ, Khoo RN. Primary hepatic amyloidosis presenting as nodular masses on the background of diffuse infiltration and extreme liver stiffness on MR elastography. J Gastrointest Liver Dis. 2014;23:437-40.
26. Gitlin JD. Wilson's disease. In: Zakim D, Boyer TD (Eds). Hepatology: A Textbook of Liver Disease. Philadelphia, Saunders; 2003.pp.1273-88.
27. Vargas O, Faraoun SA, Dautry R, et al. MR imaging features of liver involvement by Wilson disease in adult patients. Radiol Med. 2016;121(7):546-56.
28. Hope TA, Ohliger MA, Qayyum A. MR imaging of diffuse liver disease: from technique to diagnosis. Radiol Clin North Am. 2014;52(4):709-24.
29. Karagiannidis A, Karavalaki M, Koulaouzidis A. Hepatic sarcoidosis. Ann Hepatol. 2006;5:251-6.
30. Fataar S, Bassiony H, Satyanatus P. CT of hepatic schistosomiasis. AJR. 1985;145:63-6.
31. Serrano MAP, Vega A, Oretega E, et al. CT of hepatic fascioliasis. J Comput Assist Tomogr. 1987;11:269-7.
32. Sherlock S, Dooley J. Hepatic cirrhosis. In: Sherlock S, Dooley J (Eds). Diseases of the Liver and Biliary System, 11th edn. Blackwell Science: Oxford; 2002.pp.365-8.
33. Goyal AK, Pokhrana DS, Sharma SK. Ultrasonic diagnosis of cirrhosis-reference to quantitative measurement of hepatic dimensions. Gastro Radio. 1990;15:32-3.
34. DeLeio A, Cestari C, Lomazz A, et al. Cirrhosis with sonographic study of the liver. Radiology. 1989;172:389-9.
35. Liu WC, Lim JH, Park CK, et al. Poor sensitivity of sonography in detection of hepatocellular carcinoma in advanced liver cirrhosis. Eur Radiol. 2003;13:1693-9.
36. Kemla A, Mural O, Umit C, et al. Hepatic vein Doppler waveform changes in early (child Pugh A) chronic parenchymal liver diseases. J Clin Ultrasound. 1997;25:15-1.
37. Giorgio A, Montesarchio L, Gatti P. Contrast-enhanced ultrasound: a simple and effective tool in defining a rapid diagnostic work-up for small nodules detected in cirrhotic patients during surveillance. J Gastrointestin Liver Dis. 2016;25(2): 205-11.
38. Giorgio A, Amoroso P, Lettieri G, et al. Value of caudate to right lobe ratio in diagnosis with US. Radiology. 1986;161:443-4.
39. Okazaki H, Ito K, Fujita T, Koike S, Takano K. Matsunaga N. Discrimination of alcoholic from virus-induced cirrhosis on MR imaging. AJR. 2000;175:1677-8.
40. Kim D, Kim WR, Talwalkar JA, et al. Advanced fibrosis in nonalcoholic fatty liver disease: noninvasive assessment with MR Elastography. Radiology. 2013;268:411-9.
41. Singh S, Venkatesh SK, Wang Z, et al. Diagnostic performance of magnetic resonance elastography in staging liver fibrosis: a systematic review and meta-analysis of individual participant data. Clin Gastroenterol Hepatol. 2015;13:440-51.

CHAPTER

101

Clinical Aspects of Liver Cirrhosis: A Perspective for the Radiologist

Shashi Bala Paul, Shivanand Gamanagatti, Arun Kumar Gupta, Subrat Kumar Acharya

INTRODUCTION

Cirrhosis is characterized by the formation of regenerative nodules leading to architectural distortion, advanced fibrosis, scarring in response to chronic liver injury and resulting in end stage liver disease.[1] Diagnosis of cirrhosis is histological and imaging has a limited role in determining the presence of cirrhosis. On the contrary, it plays a vital role in diagnosing advanced changes of cirrhosis and its sequelae, particularly, portal hypertension and hepatocellular carcinoma (HCC). Imaging modalities are also widely used for screening of this "at risk" population and for therapeutic procedures for complicated cirrhosis. It is therefore, imperative for the radiologists to be familiar with the clinical presentation, natural course and imaging features of cirrhosis.

EPIDEMIOLOGY

Precise prevalence of cirrhosis worldwide is difficult to ascertain and is unknown. It is estimated to be 0.15% in the United States and a similar burden has been reported from Europe.[1] In contrast, higher figures are observed in Asia and Africa due to the high prevalence of chronic viral infections of hepatitis B or C. Last three decades have seen the emergence of a new entity termed nonalcoholic fatty liver disease (NAFLD), the spectrum of which ranges from simple steatosis to nonalcoholic steatohepatitis (NASH). The later can progress from hepatic fibrosis to cirrhosis and hepatocellular carcinoma.[2]

Nonalcoholic steatohepatitis (NASH) affects about 5-7% of the general population and 30-40% of the patients with raised liver enzymes. It has become the most common cause of liver dysfunction in the developed and developing countries.[2] NAFLD/NASH has an association with metabolic syndrome comprising of truncal obesity, type 2 diabetes mellitus, dyslipidemia, hypertension and insulin resistance.

In India, the exact burden of cirrhosis is not known. Hepatitis B virus (HBV) infection has intermediate endemicity with nearly 4% of the population being chronic HBV carriers.[3] Frequency of hepatitis C virus (HCV) infections is just about 0.87% in the community[4] while the prevalence of NAFLD varies from 8% to 25%.[5] There has been an alarming increase in the prevalence of diabetes and obesity globally. In India too, obesity is rampant amongst the adolescents and about 90% of the obese have NAFLD. The prevalence of type 2 diabetes is around 10%, the highest in India.[6]

It is likely that cirrhosis prevalence could be an underestimate due to the fact that the compensated cirrhotics invariably lack overt symptomatology and remain undetected. Moreover, undiagnosed cirrhosis may be encountered in countries where problems of NASH and hepatitis C exist. It has been estimated that about 20% of the patients with hepatitis C and 10% of NASH patients could progress to cirrhosis. Up to 1% of the population could have cirrhosis diagnosed only on histology.[1]

CAUSES AND RISK FACTORS OF CIRRHOSIS

Multiple causes of cirrhosis are known **(Table 1)**.[7] These can invariably be identified by the patient's history combined with serological and histological investigations. In North America, approximately 75% of patients with cirrhosis are chronic alcoholics. Viral hepatitis and other identifiable causes are seen in about 15% of patients; the remaining 10% of cases are of idiopathic (cryptogenic) cirrhosis. In Asia and Africa, cirrhosis is associated predominantly with chronic viral hepatitis.[8]

In India, viral hepatitis is the dominant cause of chronic liver disease and 50% is due to HBV while 20% by HCV infection.[3,9] Identification of the etiology helps in predicting complications and aids therapeutic management. Regular (moderate) alcohol consumption, older age (>50 years) are important risk factors for developing cirrhosis in viral hepatitis, whereas, truncal obesity, older age, insulin resistance or type 2 diabetes, hypertension and hyperlipidemia are responsible for NASH.[1]

NATURAL HISTORY AND PROGNOSIS

The natural history of cirrhosis is related to its underlying etiology and the treatment. Cirrhotics tend to remain compensated for years before the features of decompensation

TABLE 1: Main causes of cirrhosis.[7]

Etiology	Examples
Infectious	• Hepatitis B, C, D • Schistosomiasis • Syphilis • HIV (sclerosing cholangitis)
Metabolic/ inherited	• Non alcoholic steatohepatitis (NASH) in association with the metabolic syndrome • Wilson's disease • Hemochromatosis • Alpha-1 antitrypsin deficiency • Glycogen storage disease • Cystic fibrosis • Tyrosinemia • Galactosemia • Fructose intolerance • Byler's disease • Mucopolysaccharidosis • Abetalipoproteinemia • Prophyria • Wolman's disease
Biliary disease	• Extrahepatic obstruction • Intrahepatic obstruction
Immunological	• Autoimmune hepatitis • Primary biliary cirrhosis • Primary sclerosing cholangitis
Vascular	• Veno-occlusive disease • Budd–Chiari syndrome • Cardiac failure • Hereditary hemorrhagic telangiectasia
Drugs and toxins	• Alcohol • Amiodarone • Dantrolene • Halothane • Isoniazid • Methotrexate • Methyldopa • Aflatoxin • Diclofenac • Hypervitaminosis A
Miscellaneous	• Indian childhood • Malnutrition • Sarcoidosis • Ischemia • Graft versus host disease

set in and once that happens, the mortality (without transplant) is as high as 85% in 5 years. The decompensation rates for hepatitis C and B are 4% and 10% yearly, respectively. Rapid decompensation generally develops in alcoholic cirrhosis if alcohol use is not discontinued. Mortality of cirrhotics with HCC is on the rise in most developed countries in contrast to the decreasing mortality trend of cirrhotics without HCC.[10]

PATHOLOGY

Histopathological changes of cirrhosis consists of inflammation, steatosis and progression to fibrosis which results in architectural distortion and development of a spectrum of nodules ranging from benign regenerating nodules to HCC.[11]

The nodular lesions are classified as regenerative, dysplastic or neoplastic according to the international nomenclature of hepatocellular nodules proposed in 1994.[12] Regenerative nodules represent a region of hepatic parenchyma that enlarges in response to necrosis and is surrounded by fibrous septa. The regenerative nodules are classified as micronodular (<3 mm), macronodular (>3 mm), or mixed forms. Macronodules rarely exceed 20 mm in size. When regenerative nodules contain iron, they are called siderotic nodules. Dysplastic nodules are classified as low or high grade on the basis of a spectrum of pathologic changes that include HCC. One such change is the appearance of a new vascular supply to the nodule, which becomes the dominant blood supply in large dysplastic nodules and small HCC.[13]

In the past, cirrhosis was labelled as an irreversible process of liver damage but recent studies have shown the reversal of cirrhosis by treating the underlying etiology at an early stage.[14]

TYPES OF CIRRHOSIS

Morphologically, cirrhosis is classified into micronodular, macronodular and mixed forms. Micronodular form is seen in cirrhosis due to chronic alcoholism, hepatitis C and biliary cirrhosis, and is characterized by the presence of regenerative nodules of relatively uniform and small size. Macronodular cirrhosis is a feature of chronic hepatitis B where the nodules are larger, coarser, and more variable in size. Mixed cirrhosis is a combination of both micronodular and macronodular forms in equal proportions.

CLINICAL PRESENTATION

Patients of cirrhosis present in either compensated or decompensated state. Compensated cirrhotics are often indolent and the disease may progress insidiously. Cirrhosis may be detected incidentally on routine clinical examination, biochemical screening, during abdominal surgery for some other ailment or on autopsy. About 30–40% of the cases of cirrhosis may be asymptomatic.[15] In the remaining, diagnosis is suspected when nonspecific symptoms like low-grade fever, general deterioration, anorexia, anemia, and weight loss appears.

Decompensated cirrhotics have clinical manifestations like jaundice, edema, coagulopathy, metabolic disturbances, gastroesophageal varices, ascites, spontaneous bacterial peritonitis, splenomegaly and hepatic encephalopathy **(Table 2)**.[16]

SEVERITY OF CIRRHOSIS

Grading of severity is on the basis of the Child Pugh Turcotte (CPT) classification[17] which takes into account the findings

TABLE 2: Clinical features of cirrhosis.[16]

	Description	Cause
Jaundice	Icterus	Compromised hepatocyte excretory function, occurs when serum bilirubin >20 mg/L
Spider angiomata	Central arteriole with tiney radiating vessels, mainly on trunk and face	Raised estradiol, decreased estradiol degradation in liver
Nodular liver	Irregular, hard surface on palpation	Fibrosis, irregular regeneration
Splenomegaly	Enlarge on palpation or in ultrasound	Portal hypertension, splenic congestion
Ascites	Proteinaceous fluid in abdominal cavity, clinically detected when >1.5 L	Portal hypertension
Caput medusae	Prominent veins radiating from umbilicus	Portal hypertension, reopening of umbilical vein that shunt blood from portal vein
Cruveilhier–Baumgarten syndrome	Epigastric vascular murmur	Shunts from portal vein to umbilical vein branches, can be present without Caput medusae
Palmar erythema	Erythema sparing central portion of the palm	Increased estradiol, decreased estradiol degradation in liver
White nails	Horizontal white bands or proximal white nail plate	Hypoalbuminemia
Hypertrophic osteoarthropathy/finger clubbing	Painful proliferative osteoarthropathy of long bones	Hypoxemia due to right-to-left shunting, portopulmonary hypertension
Dupuytren's contracture	Fibrosis and contraction of palmar fascia	Enhanced oxidative stress, increased inosine (alcohol exposure or diabetes)
Gynecomastia, loss of male hair pattern	Benign proliferation of glandular male breast tissue	Enhanced conversion of androstenedione to estrone and estradiol, reduced estradiol degradation in liver
Hypogonadism	Mainly in alcoholic cirrhosis and hemochromatosis	Direct toxic effect of alcohol or iron
Flapping tremor (asterixis)	Asynchronous flapping motions of dorsiflexed hands	Hepatic encephalopathy, disinhibition of motor neurons
Fetor hepaticus	Sweet, pungent smell	Volatile dimethylsulfide, especially in portosystemic shunting and liver failure
Anorexia, fatigue, weight loss, muscle wasting	Occurs in >50% of patients with cirrhosis	Catabolic metabolism by diseased liver, secondary to anorexia
Type-2 diabetes	Occurs in 15–30% of patients with cirrhosis	Disturbed glucose use or decreased insulin removal by the liver

of serum bilirubin, serum albumin, prothrombin time, presence of ascites and encephalopathy **(Table 3)**. Estimated child's score categorizes the severity of cirrhosis into CPT class A, B and C on the score of 6 and less, 7–9 and more than 10, respectively. CPT class also predicts the development of complications and response to treatment. The 1-year survival rates of CPT class A, B and C patients are 100%, 80% and 45% respectively.[18] The model for end stage liver disease (MELD)[19] has been developed which is based on parameters of serum creatinine, bilirubin and international normalized ratio (INR) and does not include features of portal hypertension. It provides better prediction of severity and short-term mortality.

TABLE 3: Child-Pugh classification for grading the child's score.[17]

Clinical and biochemical measurements	Points for increasing abnormality		
	1	2	3
Encephalopathy (grade)	None	I and II	III and IV
Ascites	–	Mild	Moderate
Bilirubin (mg/dL)	1–2	>2–3	>3
Albumin (g/dL)	>3.5	2.8–3.5	<2.8
Prothrombin time (seconds prolonged)	1–4	>4–6	>6
Total score	5–6 = Child's A	7–9 = Child's B	10 or more Child's C

DIAGNOSIS OF CIRRHOSIS

Liver biopsy is needed to confirm cirrhosis in patients with compensated liver function in whom the ultrasound (US) is usually normal. On the other hand, if clear signs of cirrhosis are present, like small, shrunken liver, ascites or coagulopathy, biopsy confirmation is not necessary.[1] Liver biopsy is the gold standard for diagnosing cirrhosis due to its ability to grade inflammation, steatosis and stage fibrosis. It also aids in establishing the etiology of cirrhosis in about 20% of the patients of unknown etiology. Degree of fibrosis is used as a quantitative

TABLE 4: METAVIR scoring.[20]

METAVIR fibrosis score		METAVIR activity score	
No fibrosis	F0	No activity	A0
Portal fibrosis without septa	F1	Mild activity	A1
Portal fibrosis with few septa	F2	Moderate activity	A2
Portal fibrosis with numerous septa without cirrhosis	F3	Severe activity	A3
Cirrhosis	F4		

measure and various staging methods are available. METAVIR scoring, a commonly used method, grades fibrosis from F0–F4 where the later denotes cirrhosis **(Table 4)**.[20]

Liver biopsy has a number of limitations as well. The procedure is invasive and associated with a significant level of morbidity and mortality. The biopsy sample represents 1/50,000 of the liver tissue and at times the sample may not be a representative of the overall disease as the disease has a nonhomogeneous pattern. The specimen smaller than 2 cm is almost always difficult to interpret. Additionally, there may be an inter or intraobserver variability. Thus, the sensitivity of liver biopsy is lower than 80% in detecting cirrhosis particularly in the macronodular type.[21]

The technique of obtaining liver biopsy varies from blind to image guided transabdominal approach, transjugular, and laparoscopic, open approach at surgery or autopsy. Use of ultrasound guidance aids in accurate targeting, reduce complication rate and improve the quality of samples.[22,23] The percutaneous route of liver biopsy is most commonly employed and in patients with increased risk of hemorrhage, a transjugular route is preferable.

Aspirin and other antiplatelet drugs are withheld one week before the scheduled procedure. Mild sedation is given prior and using local anesthesia, a 14/18 gauge needle is introduced under aseptic conditions into the last intercostal space as low and lateral, to avoid injury to the gallbladder and vascular structures. Biopsy is performed in sustained expiration to avoid penetrating the pleural space.

Contraindications to percutaneous liver biopsy are- an uncooperative patient, coagulopathy, massive ascites or generalized dilatation of the intrahepatic bile ducts which has an associated risk for choleperitoneum. Only 2–35% require hospitalization because of complications, of which pain and hypotension are the predominant causes. About 60% of the complications are encountered within 2 hours while 96% occur within 24 hours of the procedure. The mortality due to severe bleeding is extremely rare. In patients with moderate coagulopathy, the percutaneous liver biopsy can be performed with a prior transfusion of fresh plasma or platelets.

Short of biopsy, diagnosis of cirrhosis is formulated on the basis of clinical, biochemical, hematological, endoscopic and radiological findings. Clinical evaluation includes detailed history and physical examination. Presence of diabetes mellitus or hypertension is recorded. Investigations included complete blood count, liver function tests, blood sugar levels, lipid profile and serum alphafetoprotein. Viral markers for hepatitis B include HBsAg, total anti-HBc, HBeAg and HBVDNA while those for hepatitis C are anti-HCV and HCV RNA. Autoimmune markers are done, if the markers of hepatitis B and C are found negative. Radiological work-up comprises of an abdominal ultrasonography (US), multiphasic CT (MPCT) or MRI.

ENDOSCOPY

Endoscopy is routinely performed to look for the presence of esophageal varices. The size, extent and the appearance of varices is of immense relevance clinically. Grading of varices is done as the risk of bleeding increases with the size[24] and associated mucosal abnormalities.[25] The stomach and duodenum are also evaluated for features of gastropathy due to portal hypertension and associated ulcers are also looked for.

IMAGING IN CIRRHOSIS

Role of imaging in evaluation of cirrhosis is primarily for characterizing the morphologic manifestations of the disease, detection and quantitation of complications like ascites, portal hypertension, hepatic vein and portal vein thrombosis and detection of HCC. It is important to highlight that normal imaging findings do not exclude compensated cirrhosis. At the same time, in some patients with clinically unsuspected disease, the morphologic characteristics of the disease may be detected incidentally as part of screening strategies.

US is the most commonly used as it is widely available and inexpensive. Even though its role in determining the presence of cirrhosis is limited, it is often the first imaging modality. In the early stages of cirrhosis, liver appears normal in the majority of cases and often it is the advanced changes which are detected. These are, coarse, heterogeneous echo pattern of the liver, hypertrophied lateral segment of right lobe and caudate lobe, atrophy of medial segment of left lobe and the right lobe, liver surface nodularity, deep widened fissures, anteriorly placed gallbladder and shrunken size of the liver **(Figs. 1 and 2)**.

US is useful for detecting the complications of cirrhosis[26,27] It is the first imaging modality for suspected HCC, although its sensitivity and specificity is less than that of CT and MRI. Doppler US (DU) and Color Doppler are useful in the evaluation of vascular structures by virtue of their ability for prompt differentiation between vascular and nonvascular structures. DU is the technique for differentiating benign from malignant thrombus, evaluating portal or hepatic venous system and confirming suspected portal hypertension **(Figs. 3A to D)**.

Conventional CT and MRI are used to define the severity of cirrhosis. Findings in cirrhosis are variable. Early parenchymal changes in cirrhosis may be subtle and may not be detected. However, the early findings of enlarged hilar periportal space with increased fat in the porta hepatitis may be seen on MRI. Morphological changes of advanced cirrhosis as seen on ultrasound are better seen on CT and MRI **(Figs. 4A and B)**. The regenerative nodules occurring in cirrhosis are difficult to detect on CT. Multiphasic MRI is the reference modality for detection and characterization of the small liver

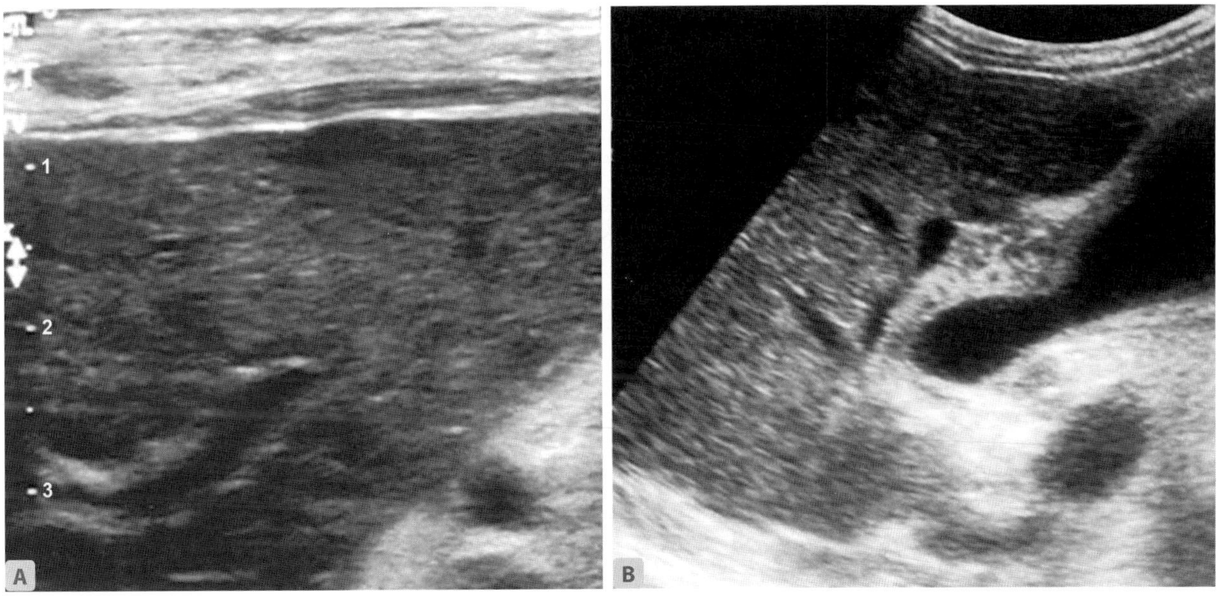

FIGS. 1A AND B: Changes of cirrhosis on US. (A) High frequency US depicting early changes of cirrhosis in the form of wavy and nodular outline of the surface of the liver; (B) In addition, the liver has coarsened echotexture. It is particularly useful to look for nodularity of the liver adjacent to the gallbladder.

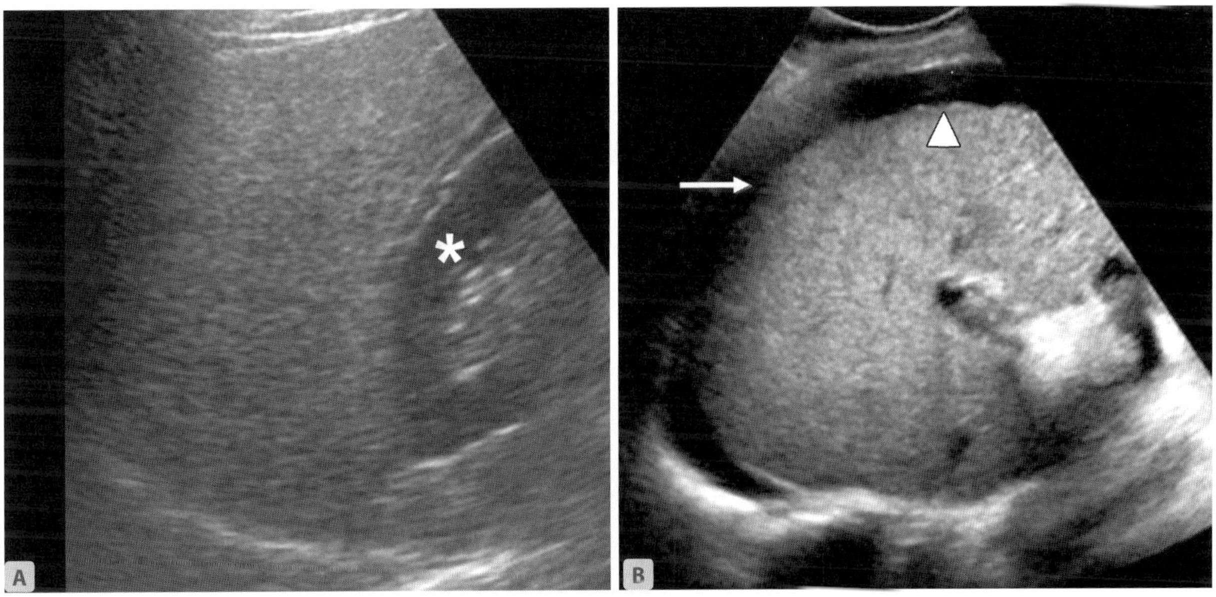

FIGS. 2A AND B: Late changes of cirrhosis on US. (A) Sagittal US image of the right lobe of liver showing increased echogenicity which is more than the right renal cortex (asterisk); (B) Small shrunken liver with surface nodularity (arrowhead) which is better appreciated due to the presence of ascites (arrow).

nodules in a cirrhotic liver, particularly early HCC **(Figs. 5A and B)** Moreover, specific MR sequences allow accurate detection of hepatic iron and fat content in hemochromatosis and liver steatosis as well.[28,29]

Since the emergence of the new concept of reversibility of changes of cirrhosis following treatment, the focus on accurate assessment of the grades of fibrosis in chronic liver disease has increased. The gold standard of biopsy being an invasive procedure, is unsuitable for repeated evaluation of therapeutic response. The last decade has seen the development of various noninvasive techniques for grading liver fibrosis. These are elastography techniques like transient elastography (Fibroscan), acoustic radiation force impulse (ARFI) quantification and 2D shear wave elastography (SWE) providing information regarding liver fibrosis by measuring the tissue stiffness.[30,31]

Transient elastography is one of the earliest and extensively used technique. It can reliably differentiate between significant fibrosis and mild fibrosis and also predict the occurrence of HCC on the basis of liver stiffness

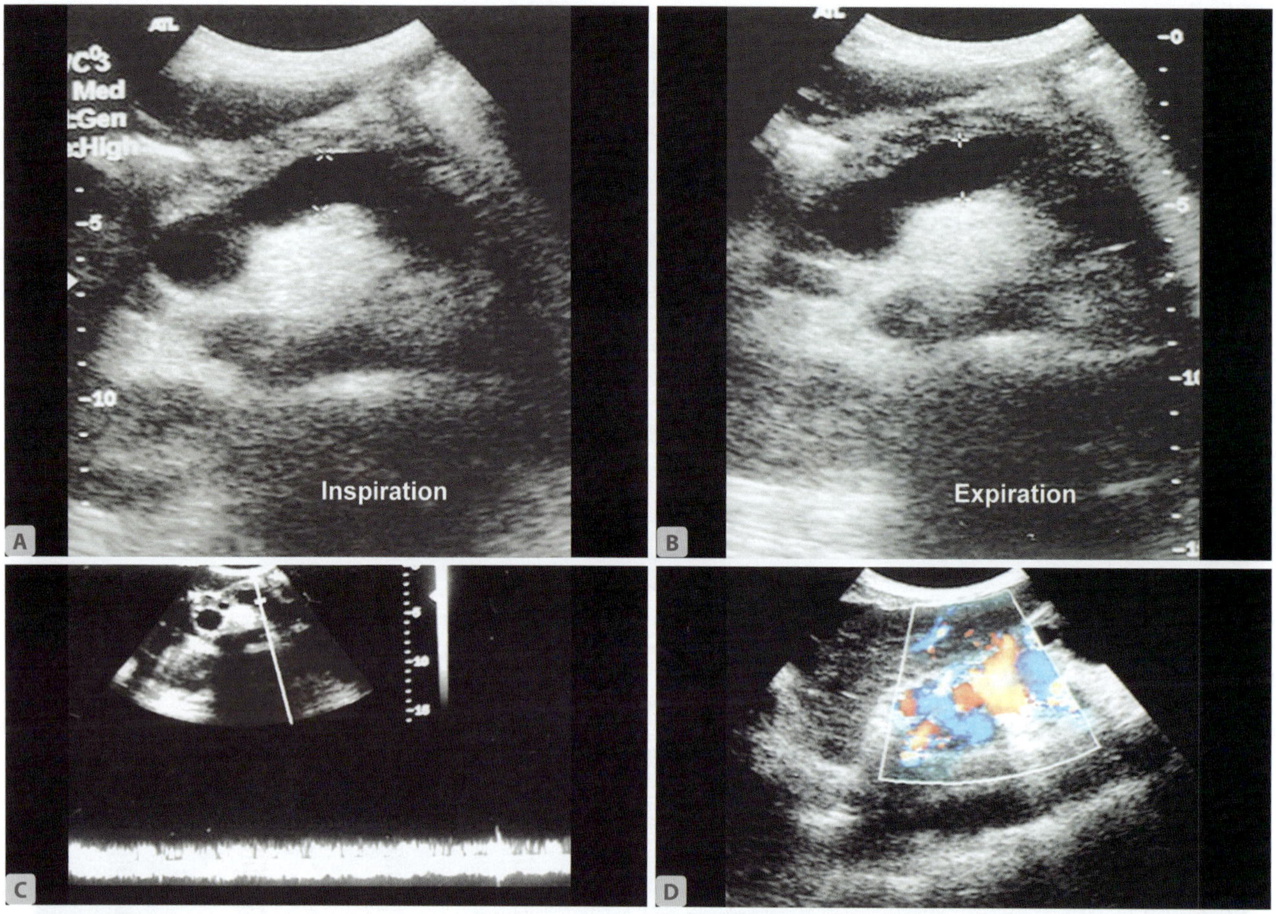

FIGS. 3A TO D: Cirrhosis with portal hypertension. (A and B) US of a known cirrhotic patient showing no appreciable change in size of the splenic vein during inspiration or expiration suggesting presence of portal hypertension; (C) Doppler of the same patient depicting dilated portal vein with continuous waveform without respiratory variation; (D) Color Doppler image of a different patient showing multiple gastric and perigastric collaterals with nodular left lobe of the liver.

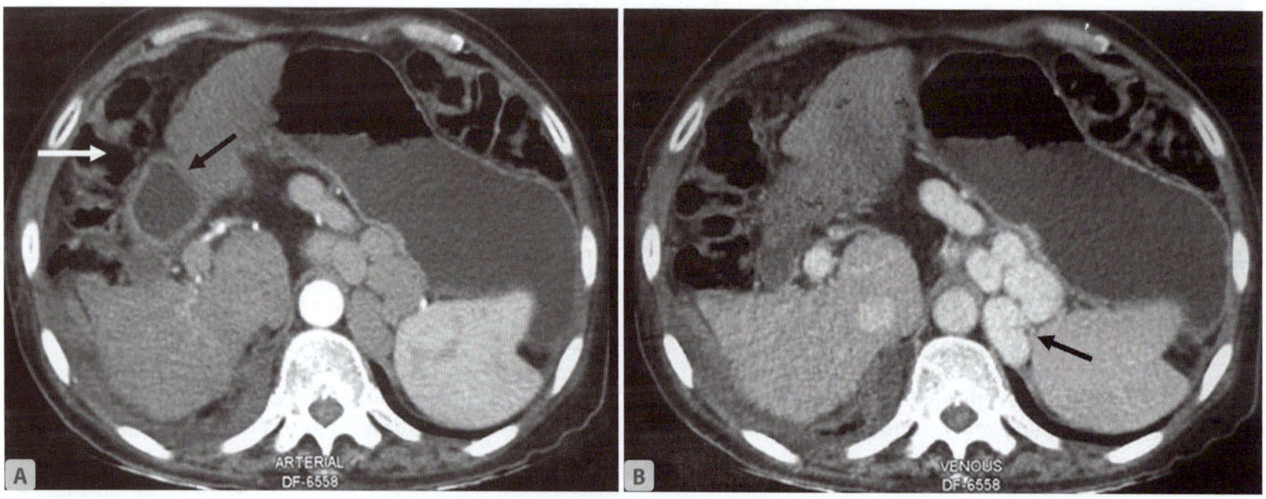

FIGS. 4A AND B: Cirrhosis with portal hypertension on multiphasic CT Liver. (A) Axial section arterial phase MPCT image showing a small, shrunken liver with deep widened fissures. There is atrophy of the right lobe and medial segment of left lobe with an enlarged caudate lobe. Colonic loop is interposed between the liver and the lateral abdominal wall (white arrow) and the gallbladder is placed anteriorly (black arrow); (B) Large, multiple perigastric and perisplenic collaterals are seen in the venous phase MPCT image (arrow).

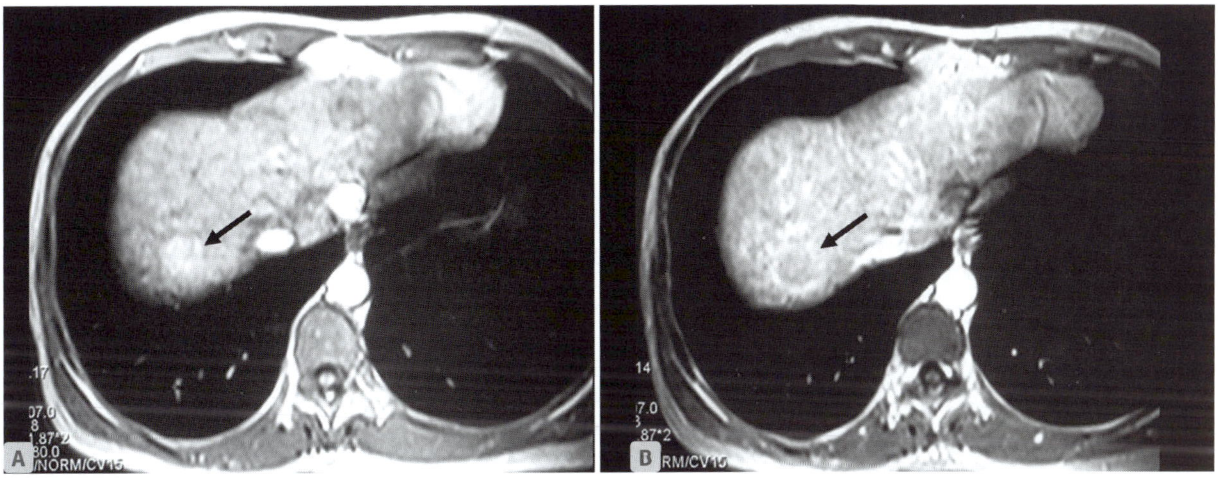

FIGS. 5A AND B: Characterizing nodules on multiphasic MRI liver: Axial arterial phase MRI image showing a cirrhotic liver with multiple variable sized nonenhancing (isointense) regenerating nodules and a solitary enhancing nodule (arrow, A) with washout in the delayed phase (arrow, B) suggestive of HCC.

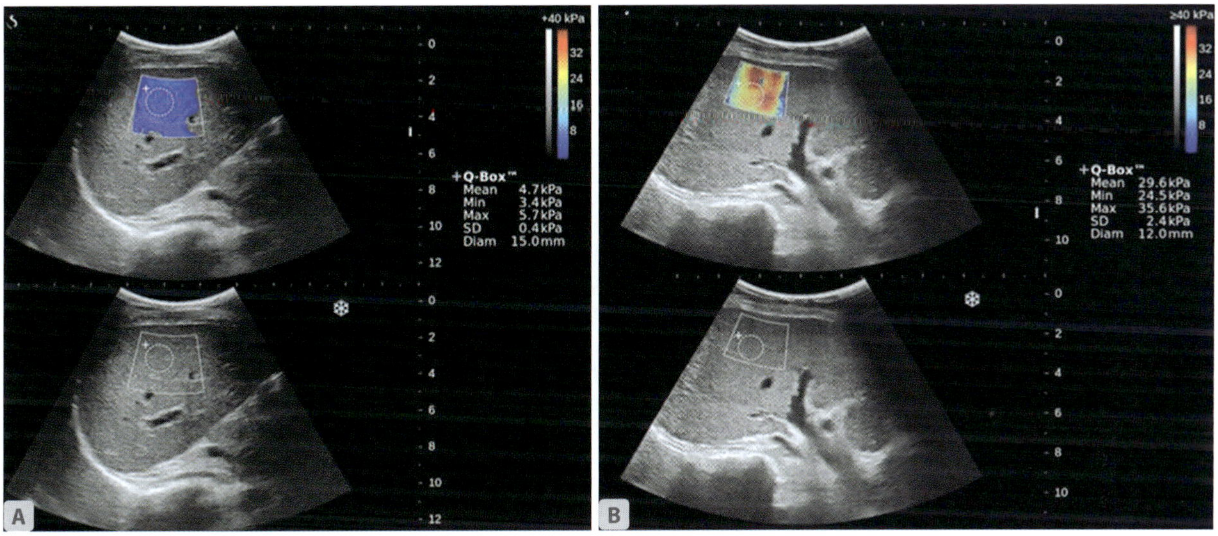

FIGS. 6A AND B: Estimation of liver fibrosis by SWE. (A) Simultaneous display of qualitative and quantitative SWE (a) and B mode US (b) of a chronic HBV patient—showing normal liver echogenecity (b) and depicting uniform deep blue color in the box with a mean stiffness value of 4.7 kPa. (a). The corresponding Metavir histological grade was F0 indicating absence of fibrosis; (B) Similar evaluation of another patient of chronic HCV showing an echogenic liver (b), and having colors of yellow, orange and red, with a mean elasticity of 29.6 kPa (a). The Metavir grade was F4, suggesting cirrhosis.

measurement.[32,33] With further refinements, ultrasound and MRI based elastography (MRE) techniques have been introduced with promising results. A meta-analysis on MRE has shown a sensitivity, specificity, AUROC of 92%, 96% and 0.98 respectively for differentiating advanced fibrosis and cirrhosis (more than F3) from less advanced fibrosis.[34] However, magnetic resonance elastography (MRE) has constraints of limited availability and high cost.

Ultrasound-based shear wave elastography (SWE) has gained immense popularity due to the easy availability and high diagnostic accuracy. It uses the combined information of the real time conventional ultrasound with both qualitative and quantitative liver stiffness assessment. Qualitative SWE refers to the display of various colors (vendor specific) corresponding to levels of tissue hardness in the small box placed at multiple sites in the liver. Similarly, the quantitative assessment is done by measuring the mean, maximum, minimum, standard deviation values of the shear wave speed in kilopascals or meters per second to provide the level of tissue stiffness interpreted as severity of fibrosis **(Figs. 6A and B)**. SWE estimates obtained from the right upper lobe show the best correlation with liver fibrosis severity on Metavir score on biopsy.[35] Recent meta-analysis containing 13 articles on SWE by Jiang T et al.[31] have reaffirmed the utility of SWE in estimating fibrosis. The pooled sensitivity and specificity for diagnosing advanced fibrosis (>F3) has been depicted as 0.89 ($p = 0.56$, 95% CI, 0.86–0.92, I2 = 0%), 0.86 ($p < 0.001$, 95% CI, 0.82–0.90, I2 = 75.73%) respectively.

COMPLICATIONS OF CIRRHOSIS

Recent advances have focused on prevention and treatment of complications of cirrhosis.

Major clinical challenges are the sequelae of portal hypertension which include ascites, hypersplenism, renal dysfunction (hepatorenal syndrome) and gastrointestinal hemorrhage. The latter occurs more frequently and is most dramatic. Prospective studies have shown that as large as 90% of patients of cirrhosis develop esophageal varices and a third of these bleed.[25]

More recently, there has been an increasing understanding of cirrhosis *per se* on the myocardial effects resulting in cirrhotic cardiomyopathy. Sepsis is known to occur in 30–40% of hospital admissions due to cirrhosis[36] and this leads to 30% excess mortality independent of the severity of the liver disease. Hematological, endocrine, pulmonary and cardiac complications are also encountered. Gallstones and peptic ulcer are more common in these patients. However, it is the development of HCC that is the most severe and fatal complication.

CIRRHOSIS AND HEPATOCELLULAR CARCINOMA

More than 80% of the HCCs arises in the cirrhotic liver. It is the fifth most common neoplasm in the world, and the third most common cause of cancer-related deaths.[37] Incidence of HCC ranges from 5 to 15 patients per 100,000 in Europe and United States, and between 27 and 36 patients per 100,000 in Asian countries in India, the estimated incidence is 1.6 % per year.[38] It affects 5% of the asymptomatic cirrhotics and 15–20% of patients with acute decompensation in both low and high incidence areas.[37] In a study on screening symptomatic patients of cirrhosis at the tertiary care hospital in India, 35.5% of cirrhotics were found to have coexistent HCC at their first presentation to the hospital.[39]

Since, by and large, it is only the patients of cirrhosis who develop HCC, it would be prudent to screen the patients of cirrhosis for the presence of HCC at diagnosis and keep them under surveillance for early detection of HCC so that they are amenable to curative therapy. The patient of cirrhosis is a potential candidate for screening as it fits with the generic criteria enunciated for cancer screening.[40] This criteria states that the disease must be common with substantial morbidity and mortality, a clear cut 'at risk' population be identifiable (e.g. cirrhosis), the screening tests must have a low morbidity, high sensitivity and specificity, there must be an established treatment therapy, and the screening program must be cost effective. Surveillance of cirrhosis patients can potentially lead to diagnosis of HCC at an early stage when the tumor might be amenable to resection, liver transplantation or percutaneous ablation. Hence, it is imperative to screen these patients and treat this fatal disease at early stages.

The population at risk for HCC is relatively easy to identify. If HCC is detected on screening, it should always be followed by therapy. Longitudinal studies on patients with cirrhosis of different etiologies have shown that male patients, older age and having sustained high serum alanine aminotransferase (ALT) levels are at an increased risk and have rapid development of HCC.[10,41]

Sherman and Colombo reviewed the guidelines pertaining to the screening strategies at length.[42] The American Association for the Study of Liver Diseases (AASLD) and the European Association for the Study of the Liver (EASL) suggested screening for all patients of cirrhosis irrespective of etiology. The ideal target population defined was all carriers of HBV, Asian men older than 40 years and females more than 50 years, African/North American Blacks older than 20 years and family history of HCC. It was also suggested by The Asian Pacific Association for the study of Liver (APASL) to extend the screening to patients with NAFLD and hepatitis C with bridging fibrosis, respectively.[43] The EASL-EORTC guidelines[44] later laid down a more stringent criteria for surveillance in 2012 recommending screening for Child-Pugh stage A and B, Child-Pugh stage C awaiting liver transplantation, noncirrhotic HBV carriers with active hepatitis or family history of HCC. The benefit of screening has been documented in an US-based mass screening study in Taiwan.[45] More than 90% of all incident HCC cases could be diagnosed and a 31% reduction in the age and sex adjusted mortality ratio in the screened population was documented in comparison to unscreened population at similar risk.

Screening Tests

US and Alpha Feto Protein (AFP) have been the screening tests used in most surveillance programs and in addition CT has been used in special situations. US and AFP are simple screening tests, easily available and safe. However, both have associated limitations as well.

AFP has been used as a marker of HCC for many years. However, only 60–70% of patients of HCC in USA and Europe and 80–90% of patients in Asia have elevated serum AFP.[46] AFP is reported to have a sensitivity of 39–65%, a specificity of 76–94% and a positive predictive value (PPV) of 9–50% in diagnosing HCC.[47-50]

As patients with clinically overt disease often have high levels of AFP, the conventional diagnostic level of AFP in HCC is >400 ng/mL.[51] AFP levels could also be elevated in the presence of chronic viral hepatitis with reactivation but without HCC. On the other hand, 'normal' serum levels of AFP (<20 ng/mL) is not an uncommon occurrence in association with small HCCs.[52] A correlation between the level of AFP and the size of HCC masses has also been observed, larger the mass, higher the serum AFP level.[39] A high cut-off value of AFP (>400 ng/mL) has no place if AFP is to be used as a screening test to detect early, small HCCs that invariably produce lower levels of AFP. Lower AFP cut-off levels of 20 ng/mL also show a low sensitivity of 41–65% and specificity of 80–94%.[47-50]

Role of AFP as a screening test has been studied at length and no utility of a single cut-off value in screening was found.[39] Accordingly, serum AFP estimation is no longer recommended due to its poor sensitivity and specificity.[1] However, AFP more than 400 ng/mL has been used for characterizing the liver mass as malignant and because of this fact, it was included in the diagnostic criteria for HCC by the European Association for the Study of the Liver (EASL).[53]

With the revision of the various guidelines for diagnosing HCC, importance of noninvasive modality of imaging has been increased while that of invasive biopsy has decreased. Reduced AFP cut-off level to more than 200 ng/mL was suggested subsequently by the AASLD guidelines in 2005[54] and later the AFP marker has been excluded as a surveillance or a diagnostic tool in the revised EASL guidelines of 2012[44] **(Flowchart 1)**.

Ultrasound is invariably the first screening test used for detection of HCC **(Figs. 7A to C)**. It is noninvasive, radiation free, less expensive and easily available. Imaging of a cirrhotic liver poses a real challenge to the radiologist. In advanced cirrhosis, liver is shrunken and therefore the sonographic window is usually limited. Additionally, the hepatic echotexture is heterogeneous due to the presence of fibrosis, fatty infiltration, parenchymal necrosis and myriads of micro- and macronodular cirrhotic regenerative nodules. Detection of HCC in such a background liver becomes a difficult task. Sensitivity of US for detecting HCC in patients of cirrhosis is low and ranges from 27% to 94% and specificity from 90% to 98%.[49,55,56]

Detection of HCC is directly proportional to its size, as the size increases, the sensitivity increases. For detection of less than 2 cm and more than 2 cm nodules, US sensitivity is 31.6% and 78.6% respectively while that of CT is 59% and 94.7% respectively. Hence, CT fares better than US in lesion detection and also has an additional advantage of better delineation of the extent of disease.[57]

Contrast-enhanced ultrasound (CEUS) is a recent addition to the imaging tools for evaluation of liver. By the use of ultrasound contrast agents (UCA), CEUS is able to overcome the limitation of lesion characterization by conventional US. Currently, second generation contrast agents are used and SonoVue (Bracco, Milan, Italy) is the only contrast agent available in India. It contains insoluble gases like sulfur hexafluoride (SF6) or perfluorocarbons and has a surface shell made of different substances like phospholipids, albumin or polymers providing better stabilization. Being blood pool agents, the UCA remains exclusively in the intravascular compartment providing detailed information of the intranodular hemodynamics on real time US and aiding in detection and characterization of the liver lesion. CEUS is now recommended by the World and the European Federation of Ultrasound as the first line imaging modality for liver lesions.[58] HCC exhibits typical enhancement patterns on CEUS quite similar to that seen on multiphasic CT/MRI. More than 90% of HCC are hyperenhancing in AP (arterialization) and 83–97% show washout (hypoenhancement) on DP **(Figs. 8A and B)**. CEUS has a sensitivity of 100%, specificity of 95.6%, PPV of 66.7%

FLOWCHART 1: Diagnostic algorithm and recall policy of European Association for the Study the Liver (EASL) 2012 guideline.[44]

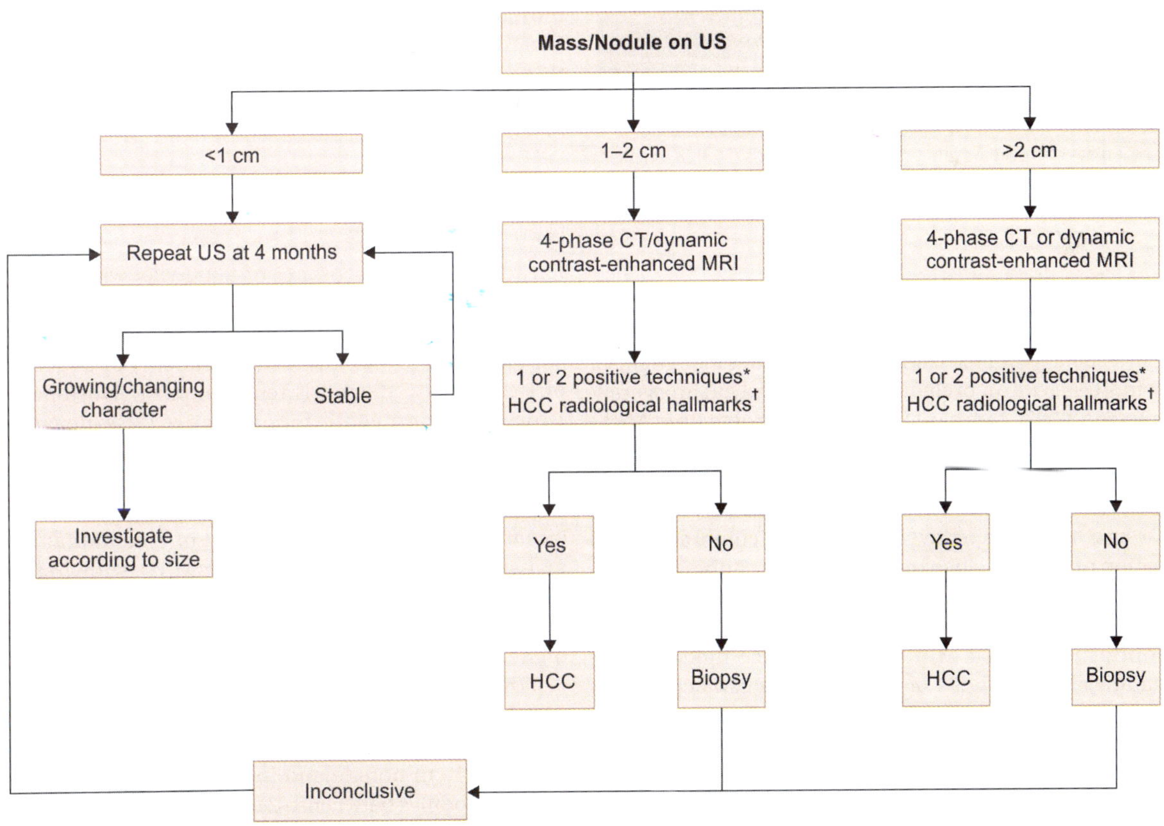

* One imaging technique only recommended in centers of excellence with high-end radiological equipment.

† Hepatocellular carcinoma (HCC) radiological hallmark: Arterial hypervascularity and venous/late phase washout.

Source: Adopted from European Association for the Study of the Liver.

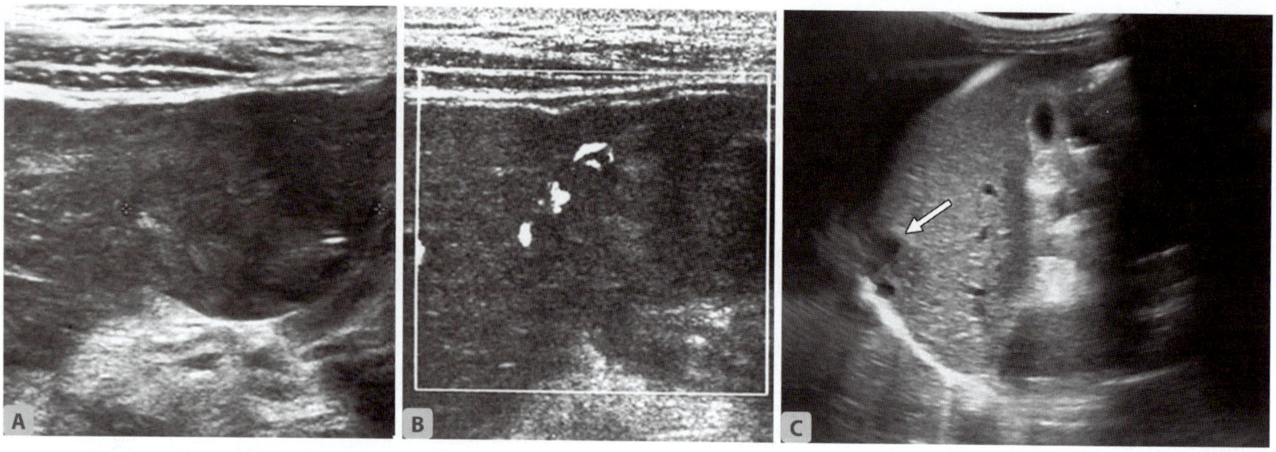

FIGS. 7A TO C: HCC detection on screening US. (A) High frequency screening US image of a patient with HCV cirrhosis, showing a 2.5 cm heterogeneously hypoechoic lesion in the left lobe of liver; (B) On power Doppler, a tortuous feeding artery is seen supplying the tumor; (C) US image of a decompensated HBV cirrhotic patient, showing a shrunken, echogenic liver with a small heteroechoic mass in the subdiaphragmatic location (arrow) suggestive of HCC in a cirrhotic liver.

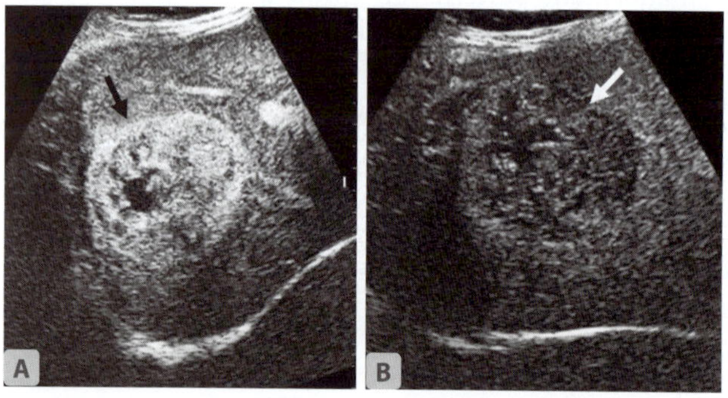

FIGS. 8A AND B: Typical pattern of HCC on CEUS. (A) Arterial phase CEUS image at 26 sec showing a large intensely enhancing mass in segment 7 mass of the liver with a small area of necrosis within (arrow); (B) The mass is showing hypoenhancement (washout) in the delayed phase at 284 sec (arrow).

and NPV of 100% in diagnosing HCC when compared to either histopathology or CT/MRI.[59] In a multicentric study[60] CEUS was 30.2% more sensitive in diagnosing malignancy, 16.1% more specific in excluding malignancy with an overall accuracy of 22.9% compared to CT and/or dynamic MRI. When comparing the three modalities with histology, CEUS has a higher sensitivity (95.5%) and specificity (75%) in comparison to CT (72.2% and 37.5% respectively) and MRI (81.8% and 42.9% respectively). Since the comprehensive evaluation of the entire hepatic parenchyma cannot be done in a short span of arterial phase of CEUS, this modality has not found place in the screening protocols for HCC.

Contrast-enhanced MRI is the reference modality for evaluation of the patients of cirrhosis as it can accurately characterize different stages of the cirrhotic nodules developing during hepatocarcinogenesis ranging from the benign regenerative nodules to dysplastic nodules and early HCC. MRI performs better than CT in the detection of nodules less than 2 cm.[61] However, MRI has a major disadvantage in terms of limited availability and high cost which is a limitation for its wide use in a developing country.

Surveillance Intervals

The optimal screening interval for HCC surveillance should depend on the information of the growth rate of HCC and the related premalignant lesions. According to studies on tumor growth, the reasonable interval is between 3 and 12 months.[62,63] Six months' surveillance interval allows most tumors to experience at least one doubling between surveillance intervals and allows ample opportunity to detect most tumors before they grow to more than 5 cm in diameter. Clearly, additional prospective studies are needed to validate this surveillance interval. Determination of this screening interval would have a direct implication on the stage of HCC detected and the cost effectiveness of the program.

Diagnosis of HCC and Protocol for HCC Surveillance

Earlier, the EASL protocol of 2000 was widely practiced world over.[53] It endorsed surveillance based on US and serum AFP every 6 months. In nodules smaller than 1cm, a 3 monthly follow-up was recommended. For larger nodules of 1–2 cm, HCC diagnosis required positive cytopathology. However, fine-needle biopsy has a false-negative rate of 30–40%.[64] It is important to note that a negative biopsy result, therefore, does not rule out malignancy. Further, a noninvasive diagnostic criteria was suggested for tumors larger than 2 cm which consisted of concomitant finding of two imaging techniques (CT, MRI) showing arterial hypervascularization, or by one positive imaging technique, showing hypervascularization associated with AFP level higher than 400 ug/L.[53]

The diagnostic criteria and recall policy for surveillance was later revised in 2012 by EASL[44] and the guidelines eliminated the role of AFP, recommended 4 monthly US for less than 1 cm nodule and introduced CT or MRI imaging even for nodules between 1–2 cm size. Thus greater emphasis has been attached to the imaging modalities subsequently and the role of biopsy has been reduced to situations where atypical imaging findings are encountered **(*see* Flowchart 1)**.

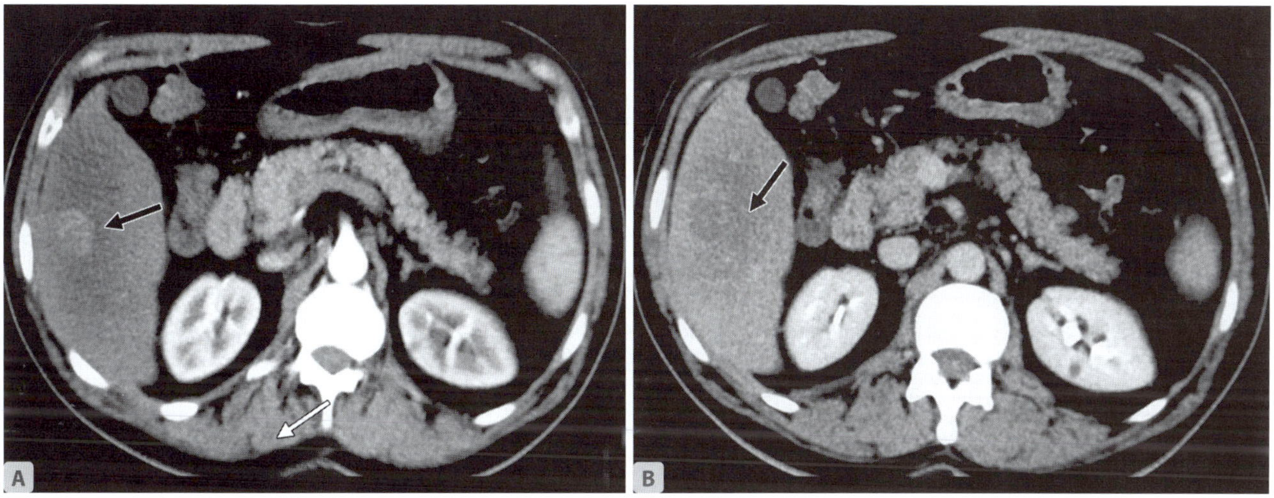

FIGS. 9A AND B: Typical pattern of HCC on multiphasic CT. (A) Arterial phase MPCT image depicting a small homogeneously enhancing mass in segment 6 of the liver (arrow,) with wash out in the delayed phase; (B) Liver has nodular margins suggesting presence of cirrhosis.

Typical imaging appearance of HCC is the presence of arterial phase enhancement followed by wash out in the venous or delayed phase of multiphasic CT/MRI. Larger tumors may also have small nonenhancing areas of necrosis in addition whereas the smaller tumors invariably are homogeneously enhancing in the arterial phase **(Figs. 9A and B)**.

Cost Effectiveness

The cost effectiveness of screening patients of cirrhosis depends on the incidence of HCC, efficacy of therapy and the age of the patient. In India, using the protocol of US and AFP six monthly and a yearly CT, the cost effectiveness of screening program from the patient perspective was ₹126,345 (US$ 2,808) for each HCC detected for local patients and ₹448,440 (US$ 9,965) for the outstation patients.[65] This cost per HCC case detected by the HCC surveillance program is exorbitant for low/middle income countries like India. Hence, measures for reducing cost need to be looked into.

TREATMENT OF CIRRHOSIS

Treatment is aimed at delaying the progression of disease and preventing the onset of complications. Delaying progression of compensated cirrhosis to decompensated status is important. A multifaceted approach is required for the management of these patients which includes treatment of the presenting signs and symptoms and the underlying cause of cirrhosis. Compensated cirrhotics need surveillance for developing HCC, screening for the presence of esophageal varices by upper GI endoscopy. Treatment of the etiology of cirrhosis is important. Specific therapy for hepatitis B or C infections, abstinence from alcohol to prevent progression to hepatic fibrogenesis and decompensation. Life style changes, weight loss, control of blood sugar levels in cases of diabetes are important in cases of NAFLD/NASH. Immunization for HAV, HBV, pneumococcal pneumonia and influenza are recommended. Protein calorie malnutrition needs redressal by encouraging small, frequent high protein meals. Some cases complain of fatigue, muscle cramps, sexual dysfunction which affect the performance status and quality of life. In them, a work up for anemia and thyroid function needs to be done.[66] Liver transplantation is recommended as an ultimate therapy for end stage liver disease. Survival rates following transplant at 1, 5 and 8 years are 83%, 70% and 61% respectively.[67]

TREATMENT OF COMPLICATIONS

Portal hypertension and its complications are managed with various radiological intervention procedures apart from surgery. Transjugular intrahepatic portosystemic shunt (TIPS) is indicated for control of active bleed refractory to sclerotherapy, intractable ascites, and an alternative to shunt surgery in high-risk patients and in cirrhosis due to hepatic venous outflow tract obstruction (HVOTO). Depending upon the site and extent of the venous block in HVOTO, various radiological procedure like angioplasty or stenting can be done to relieve obstruction.[68] Splenic artery embolization is considered these days for cases of hypersplenism since surgical splenectomy is associated with risk of morbidity.

HCC is the terminal, fatal complication of liver cirrhosis. Treatment of HCC is based on the Barcelona Clinic Liver Cancer (BCLC) staging classification **(Flowchart 2)** which links the stage of the disease with recommended treatment.[69]

Curative options of surgical resection and liver transplant are considered for BCLC stage 0 and stage A patients. A 5-year survival after resection can exceed 50% and in stage BCLC 0 (80–90%). The recurrence rate varies from 27% to 73%.

Liver transplant is considered in cases that fulfill the Milan criteria. Best results are seen within Milans criteria, where 4–5 years survival is seen in about 70–75%.[70] Locoregional therapies are the most widely used treatment option for HCC as most patients are not found suitable for surgery. Ablative procedures like radiofrequency ablation (RFA) or chemical ablation with ethanol (PEI) or acetic acid ablation (PAI) **(Figs. 10A to C)** have become the alternative

FLOWCHART 2: Barcelona Clinic Liver Cancer (BCLC) staging classification and treatment schedule.[69]

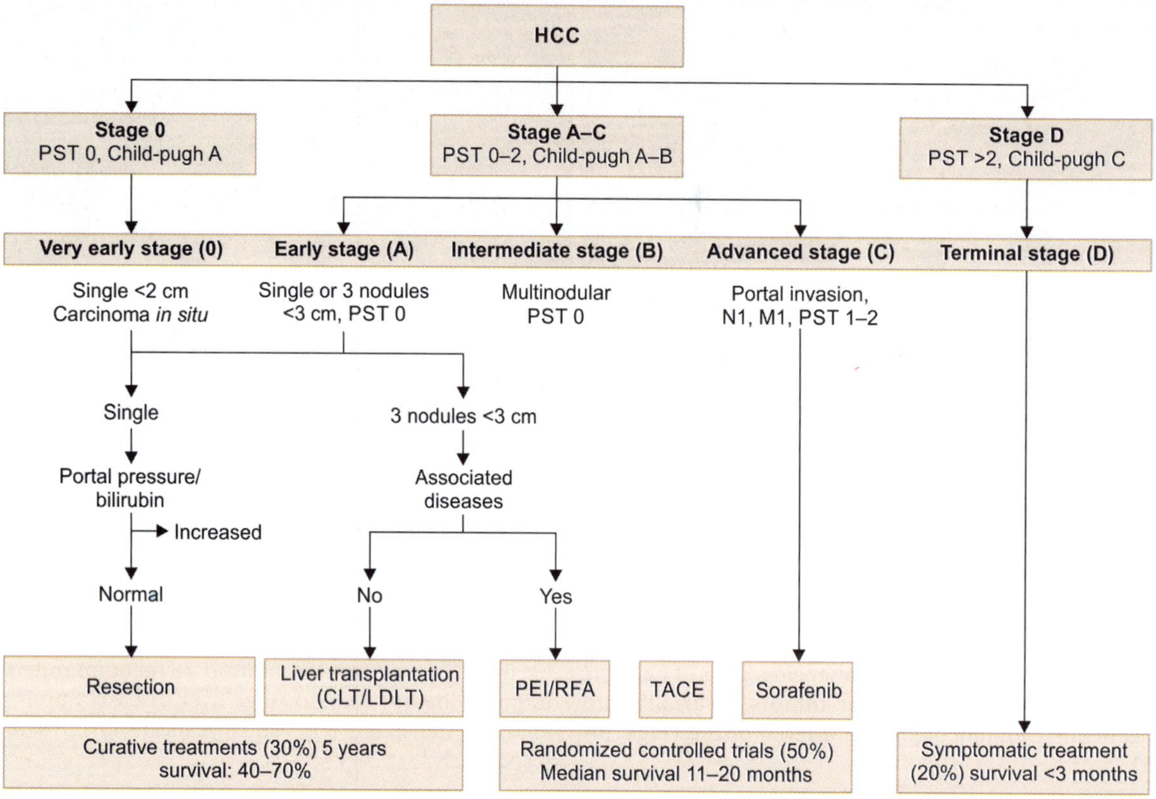

(PEI: percutaneous ethanol injection; CLT: cadaver liver transplant; LDLT: living donor liver transplant; M: metastases; N: Nodal stage; HCC: hepatocellular carcinoma; PST: Performance status; RFA: radiofrequency ablation; TACE: transarterial chemoembolization)

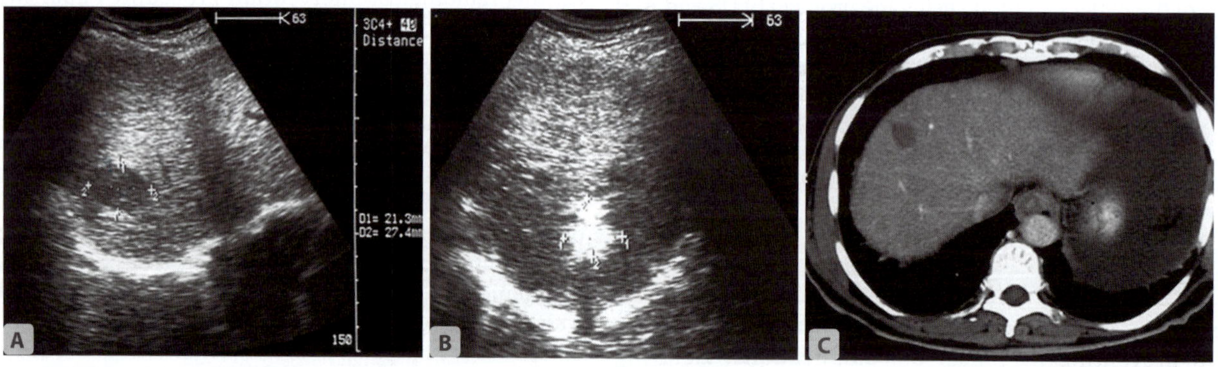

FIGS. 10A TO C: HCC treated with PAI. (A) US image of a patient of HBV cirrhosis showing a 2.5 cm hypoechoic lesion in the right lobe of the cirrhotic liver; (B) On subjecting to PAI, the lesion is completely hyperechoic on US immediately following PAI; (C) Follow-up CT at one year later shows that the ablative area has slightly reduced in size, is sharply demarcated with no residual or recurrent disease on the venous phase.

to surgery. Outcome of RFA is almost at par with surgery (5-year survival rates of 40–70%) in selected candidates.[71] Due to such good outcome, certain centers have made RFA as the first line of therapy for BCLC A stage HCC and the cumulative survival rates of 95.2%, 69.5% and 58% at 1, 3 and 5 years respectively have been documented.[72] For BCLC stage B, palliative option of chemoembolization (TACE) is offered. Two meta-analyses of the randomized controlled trials have confirmed the beneficial effects of prolonged survival post-TACE. Initial tumor burden is an important predictor of survival.[73,74]

Radioembolization using yttrium-90 microspheres or oral chemotherapy using targeted anticancer agents are recommended for BCLC C stage where portal vein is thrombosed. Limited availability and high cost is the biggest limitation. However, studies have shown that patients with Child-Pugh A disease, regardless of portal vein thrombosis, have derived maximum benefit, whereas those with

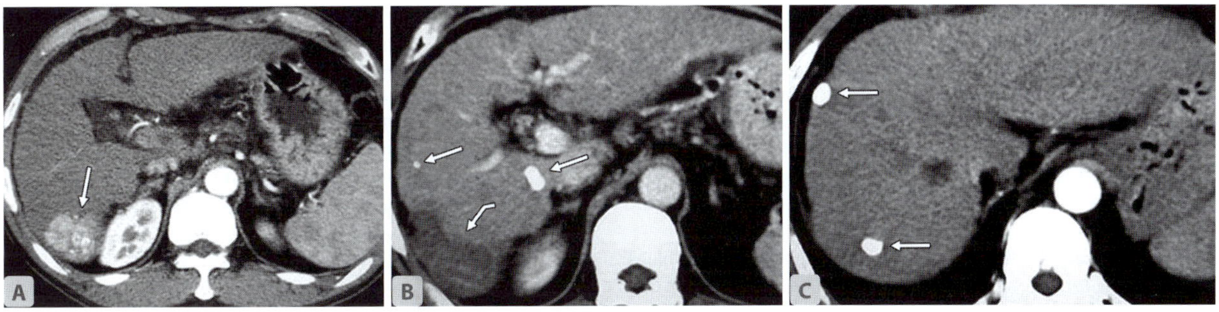

FIGS. 11A TO C: Combination treatment with RFA followed by TACE. (A) HBV cirrhosis patient found to have a small, solitary enhancing mass in segment 7 of liver on arterial phase CT, which was treated with RFA. At 18 months, multiple fresh lesions along with recurrence at the margin of the defect was noted and TACE was done; (B and C) Post TACE-CT images show all lesions covered with lipiodol (straight arrows and curved arrow respectively).

Child-Pugh B and portal vein thrombosis have had poor outcomes.[75] Rhenium too has been used in such patients with good results.[76] Sorafenib, an inhibitor of Raf kinase and tyrosine kinase activity of vascular endothelial growth factor, has been used to improve survival compared to patients undergoing supportive care.[77] The current trend is to resort to the multi-modality approach that is, combining regional and local therapies. This approach has been shown to produce better results than using single therapy alone.[78,79] Combinations tried are, TACE with RFA, TACE with PEI, TACE with PAI, or TACE with oral chemotherapy (Sorafenib) **(Figs. 11A to C)**. In advanced disease of BCLC D, the main stay of treatment is supportive therapy. However, oral chemotherapy too has been tried with little benefit.

CONCLUSION

Role of a radiologist is vital for patients of liver cirrhosis. Careful screening, early diagnosis, detection of life threatening complications and management by safe image-guided interventions has a significant impact on the outcome of the disease. Hence, understanding of the clinical profile, presentation, natural history and complications of this end stage liver disease is crucial for prolonging survival.

REFERENCES

1. Schuppan D, Afdhal NH. Liver cirrhosis. The Lancet. 2008;371: 838-51.
2. Review Team, LaBrecque DR, Abbas Z, et al. World Gastroenterology Organisation global guidelines: nonalcoholic fatty liver disease and nonalcoholic steatohepatitis. J Clin Gastroenterol. 2014;48:467-73.
3. Tandon BN, Acharya SK, Tandon A. Epidemiology of hepatitis B virus infection in India. Gut. 1996;38:S56-9.
4. Chowdhury A, Santra A, Chaudhuri S, et al. Hepatitis C virus infection in the general population: a community-based study in West Bengal, India. Hepatology. 2003;37:802-9.
5. Duseja A, Singh SP, Saraswat VA, et al. Non-alcoholic Fatty Liver Disease and Metabolic Syndrome - Position Paper of the Indian National Association for the Study of the Liver, Endocrine Society of India, Indian College of Cardiology and Indian Society of Gastroenterology. J Clin Exp Hepatol. 2015;5:51-68.
6. Williams CD, Stengel J, Asike MI, et al. Prevalence of nonalcoholic fatty liver disease and nonalcoholic steatohepatitis among a largely middle-aged population utilizing ultrasound and liver biopsy: a prospective study. Gastroenterology. 2011;140:124-31.
7. Guha IN, Iredale JP. Clinical aspects and diagnostic aspects of cirrhosis. Textbook of Hepatology: From Basic Science to Clinical Practice, 3rd edition. 2008;1:604-19.
8. Brown JJ, Naylor MJ, Yagan N. Imaging of hepatic cirrhosis. Radiology. 1997;202:1-16.
9. Panigrahi AK, Panda SK, Dixit RK, et al. Magnitude of hepatitis C virus infection in India: prevalence in healthy blood donors, acute and chronic liver diseases. J Med Virol. 1997;51:167-74.
10. Fattovich G, Stroffolini T, Zagni I, Donato F. Hepatocellular carcinoma in cirrhosis: Incidence and risk factors. Gastroenterology. 2004;127:S35-50.
11. Popper H. Pathological aspects of cirrhosis: A review. Am J Pathol. 1977;87:228-64.
12. International working party: Terminology of nodular hepatocellular lesions. Hepatology. 1995;22:983-93.
13. Kamel IR, Bluemke DA. Imaging evaluation of hepatocellular carcinoma. J Vasc Interven Radiol. 2002;13:S173-83.
14. Benyon RC, Iredale JP. Is liver fibrosis reversible? Gut. 2000;46:443-6.
15. Conn HO, Atterbury CE. Cirrhosis. Diseases of the liver. In: Schiff L, Schiff ER (Eds). Philadelphia; Lippincort. 1987. pp. 725-864.
16. Chung RT, Podolsky. Cirrhosis and its complications. In: Braunwald E, Hauser SL, Fauci AS, Longo DL, Kasper DL, Jameson JL (Eds). Harison's Principles of Internal Medicine. New York; 2001.pp.1754-61.
17. Pugh RN, Murray-Lyon IM, Dawson JL, et al. Transection of esophagus for bleeding esophageal varices. Br J Surg. 1973;60:646-9.
18. Infante-Rivard C, Esnaola S, Villeneuve JP. Clinical and statistical validity of conventional prognostic factors in predicting short-term survival among cirrhotics. Hepatology. 1987;7:660-4.
19. Wiesner R, Edwards E, Freeman R, et al. Model for end-stage liver disease (MELD) and allocation of donor livers. Gastroenterology. 2003;124:91-6.
20. Bedossa P, Poynard T. An algorithm for the grading of activity in chronic hepatitis C. The METAVIR Cooperative Study Group. Hepatology. 1996;24:289.

21. Gaiani S, Gramantieri L, Venturoli N, et al. What is the criterion for differentiating chronic hepatitis from compensated cirrhosis? A prospective study comparing ultrasonography and percutaneous liver biopsy. J Hepatology. 1997;27: 979-85.
22. Caturelli E, Giacobbe A, Facciorusso D, et al. Percutaneous biopsy in diffuse liver disease: Increasing diagnostic yield and decreasing complication rate by routine ultrasound assessment of puncture site. Am J Gastroenterol. 1996;91:1318-21.
23. Farrel RJ, Smidy PF, Pilkington RM, et al. Guided versus blind liver biopsy for chronic hepatitis C: Clinical benefits and costs. J Hepatol. 1999;30:580-87.
24. Lebrec D, et al. Portal hypertension, size of esophageal varices, and risk of gastrointestinal bleeding in alcoholic cirrhosis. Gastroenterology. 1980;79:1139-44.
25. North Italian Endoscopic Club for the Study and Treatment of Esophageal varices. Prediction of the first variceal haemorrhage in patients with cirrhosis of the liver and esophageal varices. A prospective multicenter study. New England Journal of Medicine. 1988;39:319:983-9.
26. Larcos G, Sorokopud H, Berry G, et al. Sonographic screening for hepatocellular carcinoma in patients with chronic hepatitis or cirrhosis: An evaluation. 1998;171:433-5.
27. Zweilbel WJ. Sonographic diagnosis of diffuse liver disease. Semin Ultrasound CT MRI. 1995;16:8-15.
28. Bonkovsky HL, Rubin RB, Cable EE, et al. Hepatic iron concentration: Noninvasive estimation by means of MR imaging techniques. Radiology. 1999;212:227-34.
29. Qayyum A, Goh JS, Kakar S, et al. Accuracy of liver fat quantification at MR imaging: comparison of out-of-phase gradient-echo and fat-saturated fast spin-echo techniques: initial experience. Radiology. 2005;237:507-11.
30. Ultrasound Shear Wave Elastography for Liver Disease. In: Piscaglia F, et al. A Critical Appraisal of the Many Actors on the Stage. Ultraschall in Med. 2016;37:1-5.
31. Jiang T, Tian G, Zhao Q, Kong D, Cheng C, Zhong L, Li L. Diagnostic accuracy of 2D-shear wave elastography for liver fibrosis severity: a meta-analysis. PLoS One. 2016; 11:e0157219.
32. Jung KS, Kim SU, Ahn SH, Park YN, Kim DY, Park JY, Chon CY, Choi EH, Han KH. Risk assessment of hepatitis B virus-related hepatocellular carcinoma development using liver stiffness measurement (FibroScan). Hepatology. 2011;53:885-94.
33. Wong GL, Chan HL, Wong CK, Leung C, Chan CY, Ho PP, Chung VC, Chan ZC, Tse YK, Chim AM, Lau TK, Wong VW. Liver stiffness-based optimization of hepatocellular carcinoma risk score in patients with chronic hepatitis B. J Hepatol. 2014;60:339-45.
34. Wang QB, Zhu H, Liu HL, Zhang B. Performance of magnetic resonance elastography and diffusion-weighted imaging for the staging of hepatic fibrosis: a meta-analysis. Hepatology. 2012;56:239-47.
35. Samir AE, Dhyani M, Vij A, et al. Shear-wave elastography for the estimation of liver fibrosis in chronic liver disease: determining accuracy and ideal site for measurement. Radiology. 2015;274(3):888-96.
36. Caly WR, Strauss E. A prospective study of bacterial infections in patients of cirrhosis. J Hepatol. 1993;18:353-8.
37. Llovet JM, Burroughs A, Bruix J. Hepatocelluar carcinoma. Lancet. 2003;362:1907-17.
38. Paul SB, Gulati MS, Sreenivas V, et al. Incidence of hepatocellular carcinoma among patients of cirrhosis of liver: an experience from a tertiary care centre in northern India. Indian J Gastroenterol. 2007;26,274-8.
39. Paul SB, Gulati MS, Sreenivas V, et al. Evaluating patients with cirrhosis for hepatocellular carcinoma: value of clinical symptomatology, Imaging and Alpha-fetoprotein. Oncology. 2007;72:117-23.
40. Prorok PC. Epidemiologic approach for cancer screening. Problems in design and analysis of trials. Am J Pediatr Hematol Oncol. 1992;14:117-28.
41. Benvegnu L, Fattovich G, Noventa F, et al. Concurrent hepatitis B and C virus infection and risk of hepatocellular carcinoma in cirrhosis. A prospective study. Cancer. 1994;74:2442-8.
42. Sherman M, Colombo M. Hepatocellular carcinoma screening and diagnosis. Semin Liver Dis. 2014;34:389-97.
43. Omata M, Lesmana LA, Tateishi R, Chen PJ, Lin SM, Yoshida H, et al. Asian Pacific Association for the Study of the Liver consensus recommendations on hepatocellular carcinoma. Hepatol Int. 2010;4:439-74.
44. European Association for Study of Liver; European Organisation for Research and Treatment of Cancer. EASL-EORTC clinical practice guidelines: management of hepatocellular carcinoma. Eur J Cancer. 2012;48:599-641.
45. Yeh YP, Hu TH, Cho PY, Chen HH, Yen AM, Chen SL, et al. Evaluation of abdominal ultrasonography mass screening for hepatocellular carcinoma in Taiwan. Hepatology. 2014;59: 1840-49.
46. Matsumoto Y, Suzuki T, Asadi T, et al. Clinical classification of hepatoma in Japan according to serial changes in serum alpha fetoprotein levels. Cancer. 1982;49:354-6.
47. Sherman M, Peltekian KM, Lee C. Screening for hepatocellular carcinoma in chronic carriers of hepatitis B virus: incidence and prevalence of hepatocellular carcinoma in a North American urban population. Hepatology. 1995;22:432-8.
48. Trevisani F, D'Intino PE, Morselli-Labate AM, et al. Serum alpha-fetoprotein for diagnosis of hepatocellular carcinoma in patients with chronic liver disease: influence of HBsAg and anti-HCV status. J Hepatol. 2001;34:570-5.
49. Gambarin-Gelwan M, Wolf DC, Shapiro R, Schwartz ME, Min AD. Sensitivity of commonly available screening tests in detecting hepatocellular carcinoma in cirrhotic patients undergoing liver transplantation. Am J Gastroenterol. 2000;95:1535-8.
50. Cedrone A, Covino M, Caturelli E, et al. Utility of alpha-fetoprotein (AFP) in the screening of patients with virus-related chronic liver disease: does different viral etiology influence AFP levels in hepatocellular carcinoma? A study in 350 western patients. Hepatogastroenterology. 2000;47:1654-8.
51. Daniele B, Bencivenga A, Megna AS, Tinessa V. Alpha fetoprotein and ultrasonography screening for hepatocelluar carcinoma. Gastroenterology. 2004;127:S108-12.
52. Johnson J. Tumor marker in the diagnosis and management of patients with hepatocullular carcinoma. Recent results in Cancer Research. 1986;100:68.
53. Bruix J, Sherman M, Llovet JM, et al. EASL panel of experts on HCC. Clinical management of hepatocellular carcinoma. Conclusion of the Barcelona 2000 EASL conference. European Association for the Study of Liver. J Hepatol. 2001;35:421-30.
54. Bruix J, Sherman M. Practice Guidelines Committee, American Associationfor the Study of Liver Diseases. Management of hepatocellular carcinoma. Hepatology. 2005;42:1208-36.
55. Bennett SL, Krinsky GA, Abitbol RJ, Kim SY, Theise ND, Teperman LW. Sonographic detection of hepatocellular carcinoma and dysplastic nodules in cirrhosis: correlation of pretransplantation sonography and liver explant pathology in 200 patients. Am J Roentgenol. 2002;179: 75-80.
56. Liu WC, Lim JH, Park CK, et al. Poor sensitivity of sonography is detection of hepatocellular carcinoma in advanced liver cirrhois: accuracy of pretransplantations sonography in 118 patients. Eur Radiol. 2003;13:1693-8.

57. Rao ARW, Chui AKK, Shi LW, et al. Sensitivity of radiological investigations in diagnosing hepatocellular carcinoma in cirrhotic liver. Transplantation Proceedings. 2003;35:348-9.
58. Claudon M, Dietrich CF, Choi BI, Cosgrove DO, Kudo M, Nolsøe CP, et al. Guidelines and good clinical practice recommendations for contrast enhanced ultrasound (CEUS) in the liver--update 2012: a WFUMB-EFSUMB initiative in cooperation with representatives of AFSUMB, AIUM, ASUM, FLAUS and ICUS. Ultraschall Med Stuttg Ger 1980. 2013;34:11-29.
59. Thakur S, Jhobta A, Dhiman DS, Sood RG, Chauhan A, Thakur CS. Role of contrast enhanced ultrasound in characterization of focal liver lesions. Egypt J Radiol Nucl Med. 2014;45:7-17.
60. Trillaud H, Bruel JM, Valette PJ, Vilgrain V, Schmutz G, Oyen R, et al. Characterization of focal liver lesions with Sono Vue (R) enhanced sonography: International multicenter-study in comparison to CT and MRI. World J Gastroenterol. 2009;15: 3748–56.
61. Burrel M, Llovet JM, Ayuso C, et al. MRI angiography is superior to helical CT for detection of HCC prior to liver transplantation: an explant correlation. Hepatology. 2003;38:1034-42.
62. Sheu J, Sung J, Chen D, et al. Growth rates of asymptomatic hepatocellular carcinoma and its clinical implications. Gastroenterology. 1985;89:259-66.
63. Barbara L, Benzi G, Gaiani S, et al. Natural history of small untreated hepatocellular carcinoma in cirrhosis: A multivariate analysis of prognostic factors of tumor growth rate and patient survival. Hepatology. 1992;16:132-6.
64. Durand F, Regimbeau JM, Belghiti J, et al. Assessment of the benefits and risk of percutaneous biopsy before surgical resection of hepatocellular carcinoma. J Hepatol. 2001;35:254-8.
65. Paul SB, Gulati MS, Sreenivas V, Madan K, Gupta AK, Mukhopadhyay S, Acharya SK. Economic evaluation of HCC surveillance program in India. Hepatol Int. 2008;2: 231-6.
66. Kamath PS, Shah VH. Overview of Cirrhosis, Sleisenger and Fordtran's Gastrointestinal and Liver Disease: Patho-physiology/Diagnosis/Management, 10th edn. PA: Elsevier Saunders. 2016;2:1254-60.
67. Roberts MS, Angus DC, Bryce CL, Valenta Z, Weissfeld L. Survival after liver transplantation in the United States: a disease-specific analysis of the UNOS database. Liver Transpl. 2004;204;10: 886-97.
68. Mukund A, Gamanagatti S, Acharya SK. Radiological interventions in HVOTO: Practical tips Tropical Gastroenterology. 2011;32:4-140.
69. Llovet JM, Di Bisceglie AM, Bruix J, Kramer BS, Lencioni R, Zhu AX, et al. Panel of Experts in HCC-Design Clinical Trials. Design and endpoints of clinical trials in hepatocellular carcinoma. J Natl Cancer Inst. 2008;100:698-711.
70. Mazzaferro V, Bhoori S, Sposito C, Bongini M, Langer M, et al. Milan criteria in liver transplantation for hepatocellular carcinoma: an evidence-based analysis of 15 years of experience liver transplantation. 2011;17:S44-S57.
71. Lencioni R, Cioni D, Crocetti L, et al. Early-stage hepatocellular carcinoma in patients with cirrhosis: long-term results of percutaneous image-guided radiofrequency ablation. Radiology. 2005;234:961-7.
72. Choi D, Lim HK, Rhim H, Kim YS, Lee WJ, Paik SW et al. Percutaneous Radiofrequency ablation for early stage hepatocellular carcinoma as a first line treatment: long term results and prognostic factors in a large single-institution series. Eur Radiol. 2007;17:684-92.
73. Camma C, Schepis F, Orlando A, et al. Transarterial chemoembolization for unresectable hepatocellular carcinoma: meta-analysis of randomized controlled trials. Radiology. 2002;224:47-54.
74. Paul SB, Gamanagatti S, Sreenivas V, et al. Trans-arterial chemoembolization (TACE) in patients with unresectable hepatocellular carcinoma: experience from a tertiary care centre in India. Indian J Radiol Imaging. 2011;21:113-20.
75. Salem R, Lewandowski RJ, Mulcahy MF, et al. Radioembolization for hepatocellular carcinoma using Yttrium-90 microspheres: a comprehensive report of long-term outcomes. Gastroenterology. 2010;138:52-64.
76. Kumar A, Srivastava DN, Chau TTM, et al. Inoperable hepatocellular carcinoma: transarterial 188 Re HDD-Labeled iodized oil for treatment—Prospective multi-center trial. Radiology. 2007;243:509-19.
77. Llovet JM, Ricci S, Mazzaferro V, et al. SHARP Investigators Study Group. Sorafenib in advanced hepatocellular carcinoma. N Engl J Med. 2008;359:378-90.
78. Yamakado K, Nakatsuka A, Ohmori S, et al. Radiofrequency ablation combined with chemoembolization in hepatocellular carcinoma treatment response based on tumor size and morphology. J Vasc Interv Radiol. 2002:13:1225-32.
79. Kurokohchi K, Watanabe S, Masaki T, et al. Combined use of percutaneous ethanol injection and radiofrequency ablation for the effective treatment of hepatocellular carcinoma. Int J Oncol. 2002;21:841-6.

CHAPTER

102

Benign Focal Lesions of Liver

Sapna Singh, Anjali Prakash

INTRODUCTION

A focal liver lesion is defined as a discrete abnormality arising within the liver. Owing to the advances in imaging, focal liver lesions are being increasingly detected. There has been an increase in the detection of focal lesions in the millimeter range. Characterization of these multitude of lesions detected becomes important as the diagnosis of the lesion as benign rather than malignant greatly alleviates patient's anxiety. State of the art multi detector computed tomography (CT) (MDCT) with its excellent spatial resolution and 3T magnetic resonance imaging (MRI) allows for a near isotropic imaging.[1,2] The lesions are usually categorized on the basis of their morphology, vascularity, enhancement patterns and specific functional characteristics.

Benign focal lesions of the liver can be classified as developmental, neoplastic, inflammatory and miscellaneous. The benign hepatic tumors can be broadly classified according to the cell of origin as:

Pathologic classification of benign liver tumors (Based on cell of origin)[3]

Hepatocyte
- Hepatocellular adenoma
- Hepatocellular hyperplasia
- Focal nodular hyperplasia
- Macroregenerative nodules
- Nodular regenerative hyperplasia

Bile duct epithelium (Cholangiocellular)
- Hepatic cysts
- Simple hepatic cysts
- Polycystic liver disease/congenital hepatic fibrosis
- Biliary cystadenoma
- Bile duct adenoma

Mesenchymal cells
- Mesenchymal hamartoma
- Hemangioma
- Infantile hemangioendothelioma
- Lymphangioma
- Lipoma/angiomyolipoma/myelolipoma
- Leiomyoma
- Fibroma

Heterotopic cells

Mesenchymal hamartoma and infantile hemangioendothelioma are benign liver tumors seen in the pediatric population. Abscess, hydatid disease and tuberculosis constitute the infective group while fatty infiltration, peliosis hepatis and inflammatory pseudotumor can be grouped as miscellaneous.

HEPATIC CYSTS

Hepatic cysts are benign developmental lesions showing no communication with the biliary tree. Seen in 5–14% of the general population, a definite female preponderance (female: male ratio of 5:2) is seen.[3]

Pathology

Hepatic cysts are also called bile duct cysts and are believed to originate from hamartomatous tissue.[4] Hepatic cyst is a solitary unilocular cyst with a lining composed of a single primary layer of cuboidal bile duct epithelium. Its wall is usually less than 1mm thick and is composed of fibrous tissue.

Clinical Features

These are usually asymptomatic and discovered incidentally at routine imaging. Large hepatic cysts can cause compression of adjacent intrahepatic ducts and may rarely be symptomatic.[4]

Imaging Features

On ultrasonography, a simple hepatic cyst is seen as a well-defined anechoic lesion with thin imperceptible walls. There is enhanced through transmission like cystic lesions elsewhere[5] **(Figs. 1 and 2)**. Thin septations may be present. Thick septations, calcifications, nodules and debris are not seen in a simple hepatic cyst but may be seen in a complicated cyst. Ultrasound is almost 100% accurate in the diagnosis of simple hepatic cysts.[5]

Computed Tomography

On CT, a simple hepatic cyst is seen as a well-defined, round to oval, intrahepatic lesion with water attenuation (10–15 HU).[6]

It has a homogeneous appearance with absence of any internal structures **(Fig. 3)**. The wall is thin and shows no evidence of contrast enhancement. Internal debris and contrast enhancement may however be seen in a cyst complicated by hemorrhage or infection.

Magnetic Resonance Imaging

On MRI, simple hepatic cysts are seen as well-defined homogeneous lesions with fluid signal intensity, hypointense on T1W and markedly hyperintense on T2W images[7] **(Figs. 4A and B)**. An increase in the signal intensity with increase in T2 weighting helps to differentiate these cysts from metastatic disease. A high signal on both T1 and T2- weighted images with a fluid level may be seen in the event of an intracystic hemorrhage. On diffusion weighted imaging (DWI), there is no restricted diffusion. These cysts show a decrease in signal intensity with increasing b values and are strongly hyperintense on apparent diffusion coefficient (ADC) sequence.

POLYCYSTIC LIVER DISEASE

When more than 10 cysts are present in the liver parenchyma, a polycystic disease should be considered. About 70% of patients with polycystic liver disease have autosomal dominant polycystic kidney disease while liver involvement occurs in 30–40% of patients with polycystic kidney disease.[8] Von Meyenberg's complexes and increased fibrous tissue are increasingly seen in the liver which surrounds the cysts in polycystic liver and autosomal dominant polycystic kidney disease.

CILIATED HEPATIC FOREGUT CYST

These cysts are congenital in origin and very rare. These are histologically similar to bronchogenic and esophageal duplication cysts.[9] They are usually solitary, seen more commonly in the medial segment of left lobe at the antero-superior margin or intersegmentally causing a bulge on the outer contour of the liver. A subcapsular location is

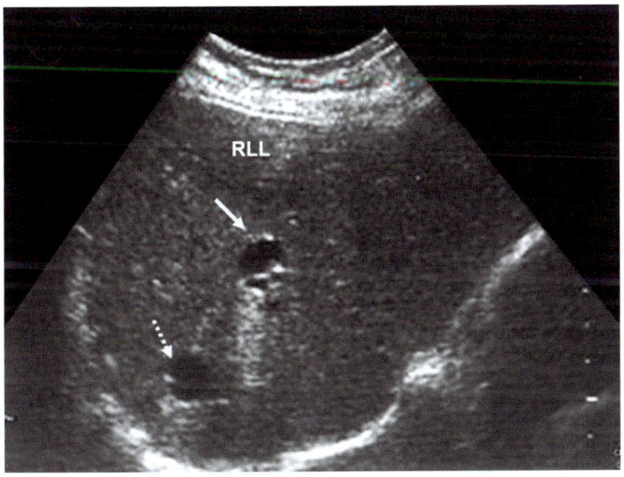

FIG. 1: Conventional US showing hypoechoic lesions in the right lobe of liver (RLL) with posterior acoustic enhancement and enhanced through transmission—simple liver cysts.

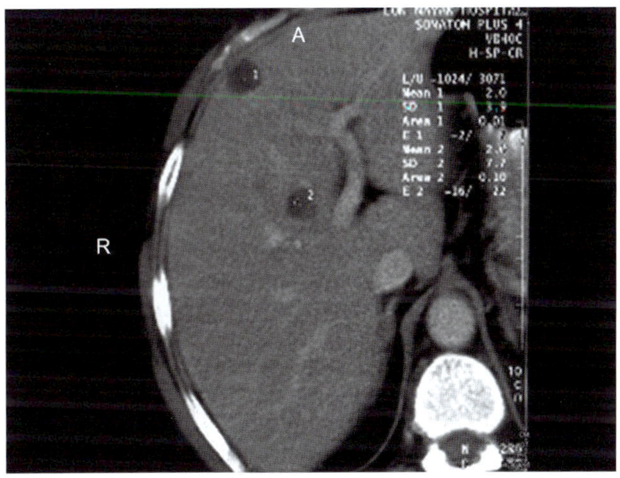

FIG. 3: Computed tomography (CT) image revealing small hypodense lesions in the liver having water attenuation—multiple simple liver cysts.

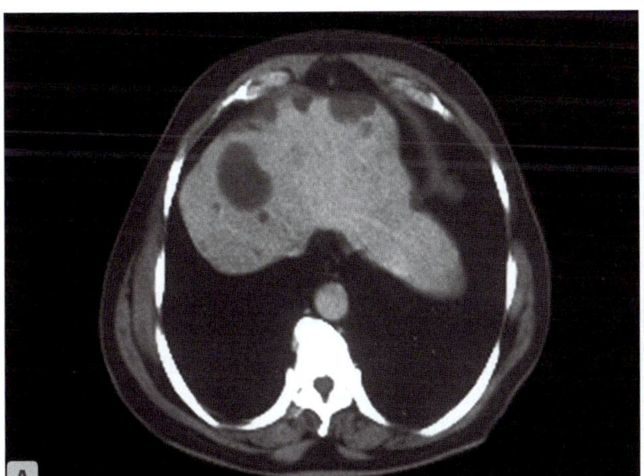

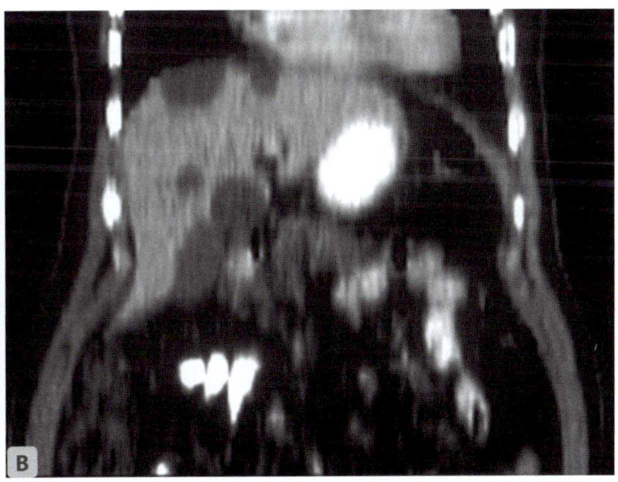

FIGS. 2A AND B: Computed tomography (CT) image revealing multiple hypodense cysts in the liver—simple liver cysts.

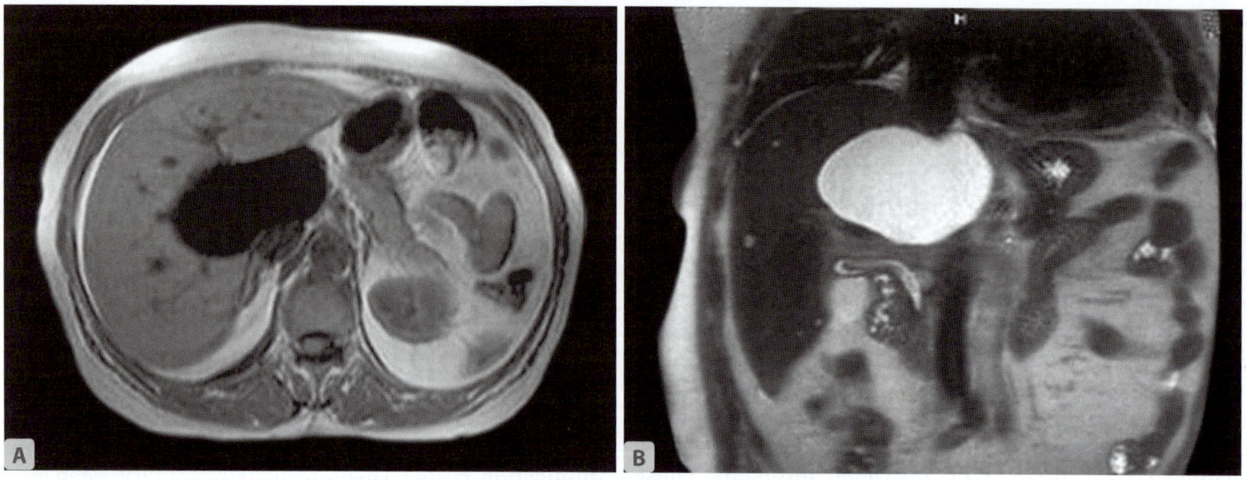

FIGS. 4A AND B: (A) T1W MR image showing a hepatic cyst as a homogeneous sharply marginated hypointense lesion; (B) T2W image reveals the cysts to be markedly hyperintense. Few smaller cysts are also seen in the periphery of the right lobe.

characteristic. Most of these cysts are asymptomatic and discovered incidentally. Rarely, obstructive jaundice and portal hypertension due to mass effect on the biliary system or portal vein may occur. They are usually unilocular and smaller than 3 cm. On T1-weighted imaging, these cysts have a variable signal intensity, depending on serous or mucinous content while on T2-weighted images, these are homogeneously hyperintense. No restricted diffusion or contrast enhancement is seen.[9] Very rarely, a malignant transformation may occur. An irregular wall thickness or solid component developing within the lesion should be viewed with suspicion. Owing to the risk of malignant transformation, though rare, a complete surgical excision is recommended.

PERIBILIARY CYST

The peribiliary cysts represent cystic dilatation of the glands in the bile duct walls. These are associated with cirrhosis, specifically with portal hypertension. On imaging, these cysts are seen as anechoic structures along the portal tracts and may be mistaken for a dilated bile duct. Presence of thin septa within the cysts helps to differentiate these cysts from dilated bile duct.[9] CT shows hypoattenuating structures and MR reveals the cystic nature of the lesions on T2W images.

BILIARY DUCT HAMARTOMAS

It is also called Von-Meyenberg's complexes. Bile duct hamartomas are cystic lesions typically less than 1.5 cm in diameter diffusely scattered throughout the liver parenchyma.[10]

Pathology

They do not communicate with the biliary tree and are believed to originate from the embryonic bile ducts that fail to involute. They are considered a part of the spectrum of fibropolycystic liver disease that also includes congenital hepatic fibrosis, autosomal dominant polycystic liver disease and Caroli's disease. Histologically, they consist of focally disordered collections of bile ducts surrounded by abundant fibrous stroma.

Clinical Features

Usually asymptomatic and discovered incidentally at imaging.

Imaging Features

The CT and MR demonstrate the cystic nature of the lesions hypointense on T1 and markedly hyperintense on T2W images. They are seen as multiple cyst like hepatic nodules diffusely scattered in both lobes of the liver and typically measuring 0.5–1.5 cm in diameter and usually showing no enhancement. Very rarely, thin rim enhancement corresponding to the compressed liver parenchyma is seen. At MR cholangiography, no communication with the biliary tree is seen. No enhancement is seen with the liver specific contrast agents as they lack communication with the biliary tree.

On DWI, biliary hamartomas show no evidence of restricted diffusion and behave as simple hepatic cysts, showing signal intensity loss with increasing 'b' values and appearing hyperintense on ADC sequences.

Differential Diagnosis

Bile duct hamartomas need to be differentiated from multiple simple cysts. Simple hepatic cysts have a regular outline while bile duct hamartomas exhibit irregular outline. Hamartomas are typically less than 1.5 cm in diameter and occur without any renal involvement.

BILIARY CYSTADENOMA

Biliary cystadenomas are rare tumors of biliary origin. They are multilocular cystic lesions with the majority (85%) being intrahepatic.[11] They occur predominantly in middle aged women, are usually large in size (1.5–35 cm), and well-defined, multiloculated solitary masses occurring predominantly in the right lobe. Multifocality is rarely seen.

Pathology

Biliary cystadenomas are thought to be premalignant lesions.[11] On pathology, lesions are subdivided on the presence or absence of ovarian stroma which is useful in prognostication. Histologically, they are similar to mucinous cystic neoplasm of the pancreas. Gross features include a multilocular appearance and a fibrous capsule while on microscopy a single layer of mucin secreting cells is seen to line the cyst wall.

Clinical Features

Owing to their slow growing nature, they present with non-specific symptoms such as abdominal pain. Jaundice may occur due to associated biliary obstruction. They may be completely asymptomatic and discovered incidentally.

Imaging Features

USG and CT

Biliary cystadenoma appears as a well-defined solitary multi-loculated cystic mass with thin septations. The septations may show fine calcifications and show enhancement on administration of intravenous contrast. The fluid within the tumor is usually mucinous in nature but may be proteinaceous, hemorrhagic, gelatinous or purulent due to infection.

Coarse calcifications, polypoid excrescences, nodular projections, thick septations are seen in biliary cystadeno-carcinomas rather than cystadenomas. Rarely, these tumors may communicate with the biliary tree and secrete mucinous material into the ducts.

MR Imaging

The lesions show fluid signal, hypointense on T1W and hyperintense on T2W images. A variable signal intensity is seen in the presence of hemorrhage and infection **(Figs. 5A and B)**. MR imaging can better demonstrate the relationship of the mass to the bile ducts or any intraductal tumoral extension.

Differential Diagnosis

A complex benign cyst, echinococcal cyst, cystic metastases, hematoma, undifferentiated sarcoma all constitute a differential diagnosis to these lesions. A percutaneous biopsy may be needed at times for a definite diagnosis. Resection of these lesions is usually complete and recurrence is rare.

HEMANGIOMA

Hemangioma is the most common benign neoplasm of the liver and is usually discovered incidentally. On routine cross sectional imaging studies, the reported incidence is 0.4% to 20%.[12] Hemangiomas range in size from a few millimeters to several centimeters; lesions larger than 10 cm are called giant hemangiomas. These are frequently located in a subcapsular location or in the vicinity of intrahepatic vessels though they may be located anywhere within the hepatic parenchyma. These are found more commonly in the right lobe and may rarely be pedunculated.

Pathology

On gross inspection, hemangiomas typically appear as soft reddish or bluish purple lesions. These are mesodermal in origin and are composed of blood filled cavernous vascular spaces lined by a single layer of endothelial cells supported by thin fibrous stroma. Depending on the size of the vascular spaces, hemangiomas are classified into two major types, the cavernous hemangioma and the capillary type, with cavernous type having large vascular spaces.[12] Thrombosis, fibrosis, calcification or ossification of the thrombus may occur due to slow blood flow within the spaces leading to involution. Involution is more common in lesions larger than 3 cm. Sclerosed hemangiomas represent the end stage of hemangioma involution and have obliterated and fibrosed vascular spaces. A hormonal influence has also been proposed in the etiopathogenesis as some hemangiomas enlarge during pregnancy while involution has been reported with corticosteroids.

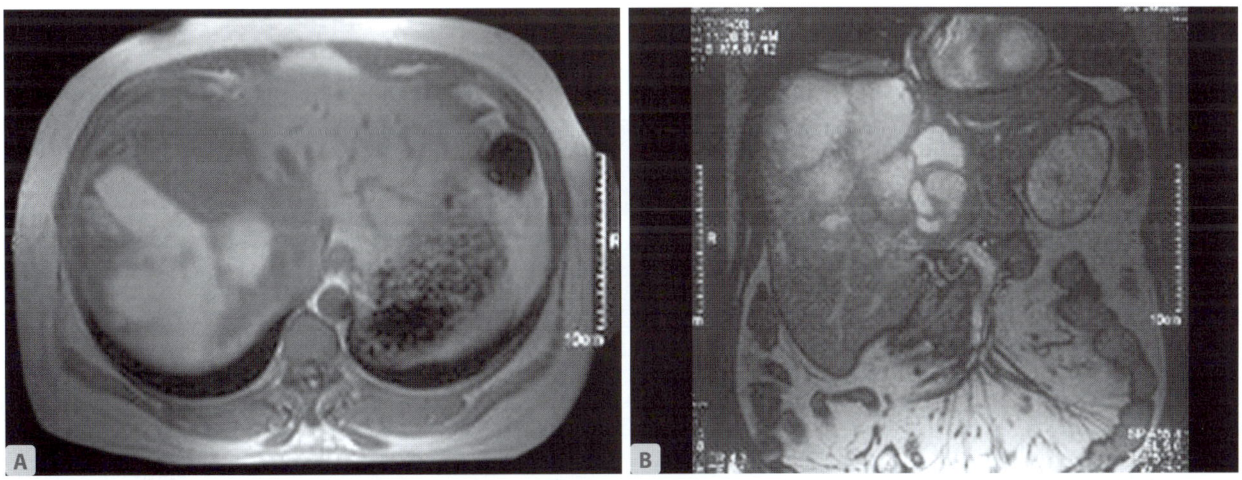

FIGS. 5A AND B: (A) T1W MR image depicting a multilocular cystic mass with variable signal due to the presence of fluid and hemorrhage/protein content; (B) T2W image showing the lesion to be high signal—biliary cystadenoma.

Clinical Features

Hemangiomas occur most commonly in the 4th and 5th decades of life and are more common in women.[13] Majority of the cases are asymptomatic and are discovered incidentally.[14] Rarely, patients may present with abdominal pain owing to the compression on adjacent organs caused by large hemangiomas. A very rare complication of hemangiomas is the Kasabach-Merritt syndrome in which patients present with fever, leukocytosis, thrombocytopenia and consumptive coagulopathy. Hemorrhage is seen very rarely and is the reason for a prophylactic resection.

Imaging Features

USG

A very distinctive imaging pattern is seen in lesions <2 cm in diameter. Sonography shows a well-circumscribed homogeneously hyperechoic lesion usually in a subcapsular location or in the vicinity of intrahepatic vessels **(Figs. 6 and 7)**. The echogenicity of hemangioma has been attributed to the interfaces between multiple vascular spaces. Larger lesions show a more heterogenous appearance owing to degeneration and fibrous replacement. On contrast US, a peripheral pooling or puddling of contrast expanding in a centripetal pattern followed by a complete fill in is seen.[15]

CT

On noncontrast scans, hemangiomas appear as low density lesions with well-defined lobulated margins. Following contrast administration, most hemangiomas show a characteristic peripheral nodular enhancement followed by a centripetal fill in and become isoattenuating with the liver parenchyma on delayed scans **(Figs. 8A to C)**. The initial peripheral nodular enhancement seen in hemangiomas in the arterial phase is isodense with the aorta, a finding which is 100% specific in differentiating hemangiomas from metastases. A peripheral centripetal fill in, coupled with delayed filling and persistence of enhancement constitute the diagnostic triad of hemangiomas by single level dynamic CT.[16,17] Though smaller lesions may show the characteristic imaging triad, larger lesions and giant hemangiomas exhibit nonenhancing areas corresponding

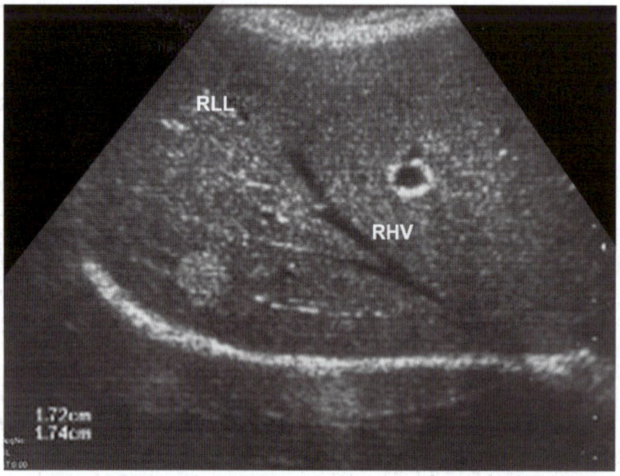

FIG. 6: US shows a well-circumscribed homogeneous hyperechoic lesion in the posterior segment of the right lobe of the liver—hemangioma.

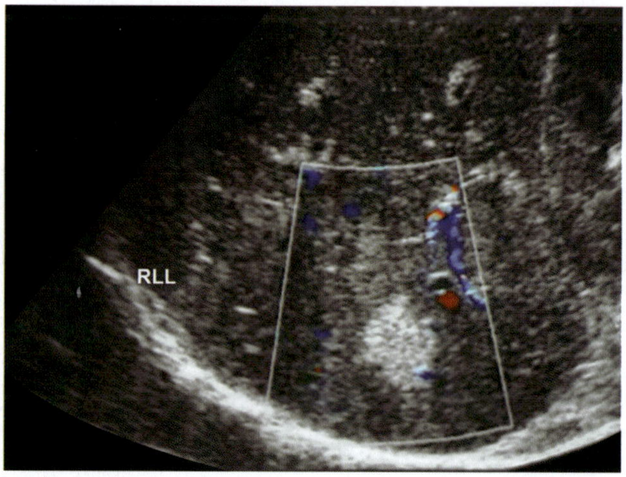

FIG. 7: Color flow imaging showing lack of internal vascularity in a hemangioma.

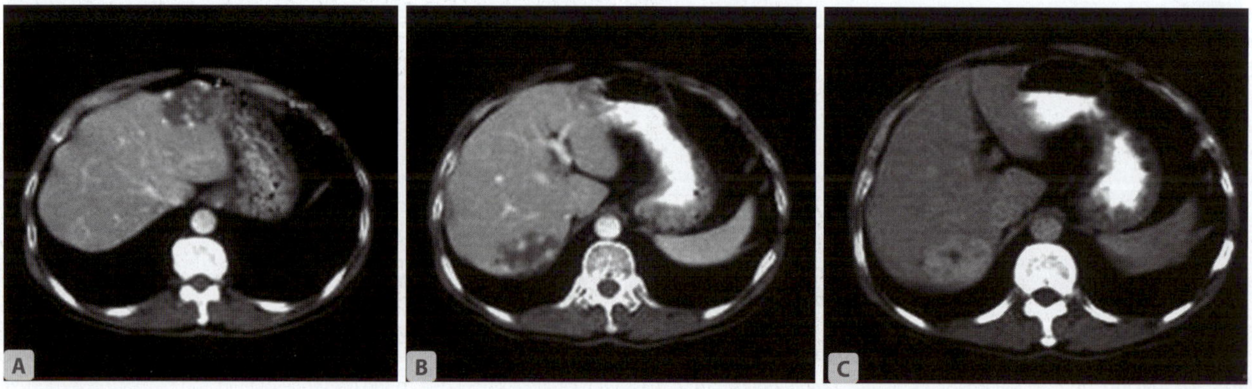

FIGS. 8A TO C: (A and B) Early phase CT (within 30 seconds) showing peripheral nodular enhancement in the hemangiomas; (C) Delayed phase enhancement 20 minutes later show complete fill in the hemangioma with a central fibrous scar seen in the larger one.

to scar tissue, cystic degeneration or myxoid changes. Similarly, sclerosed hemangiomas may not show the characteristic imaging pattern. Capsular retraction, volume loss, geographic margins and nodular areas of internal enhancement suggest the diagnosis of a sclerosed hemangioma.

MRI

On MRI, these are seen as well-defined lesions hypointense on T1 and markedly hyperintense on T2- weighted images. Hemangiomas show a characteristic increase in hyperintensity with increasing TE values which has been called the "light bulb appearance" **(Figs. 9A to D)**.

On administration of Gadolinium, three enhancement patterns have been described with reported specificities of 100% and diagnostic accuracy of 95%.[12]

Type 1

A uniform, fast and intense enhancement of the hemangioma in the arterial phase remaining hyperintense to the surrounding liver parenchyma on delayed post-contrast images constitutes a type 1 pattern.[18] A perilesional enhancement reflecting high flow in efferent perilesional veins is seen. This pattern is usually seen in small hemangiomas (<1.5 cm) also called "small flash filling" hemangiomas.

Type 2

Medium size hemangiomas (1.5–5 cm) usually show a type 2 pattern characterized by typical nodular peripheral enhancement in arterial phase followed by centripetal fill in seen on the portal venous phase (70s) and a complete homogeneous fill in on delayed image (3–5 minutes).

Type 3

Giant hemangiomas show a type 3 pattern in which there is a failure to completely fill in and no enhancement of the central scar even on very delayed images up to 15 minutes **(Figs. 10A to F)**.[19,20]

Hemangiomas need to be differentiated from hypervascular metastases which are T2 hyperintense and arterially enhanced. Metastases usually demonstrate a target pattern of enhancement rather than a discontinuous rim seen in hemangiomas. The arterial enhancing rim in metastasis shows a washout in the portal venous phase.

With hepatocyte specific agents (HSA), hemangiomas show a hypointense appearance during the hepatocyte phase owing to the lack of hepatocytes within the lesion.[21] Since hemangiomas lack Kupffer cells, one would expect no signal drop with superparamagnetic iron oxide (SPIO) agents (ferucarbotran, ferumoxide) on a T2W image but a delayed drop in signal intensity (10–40 minutes) is seen

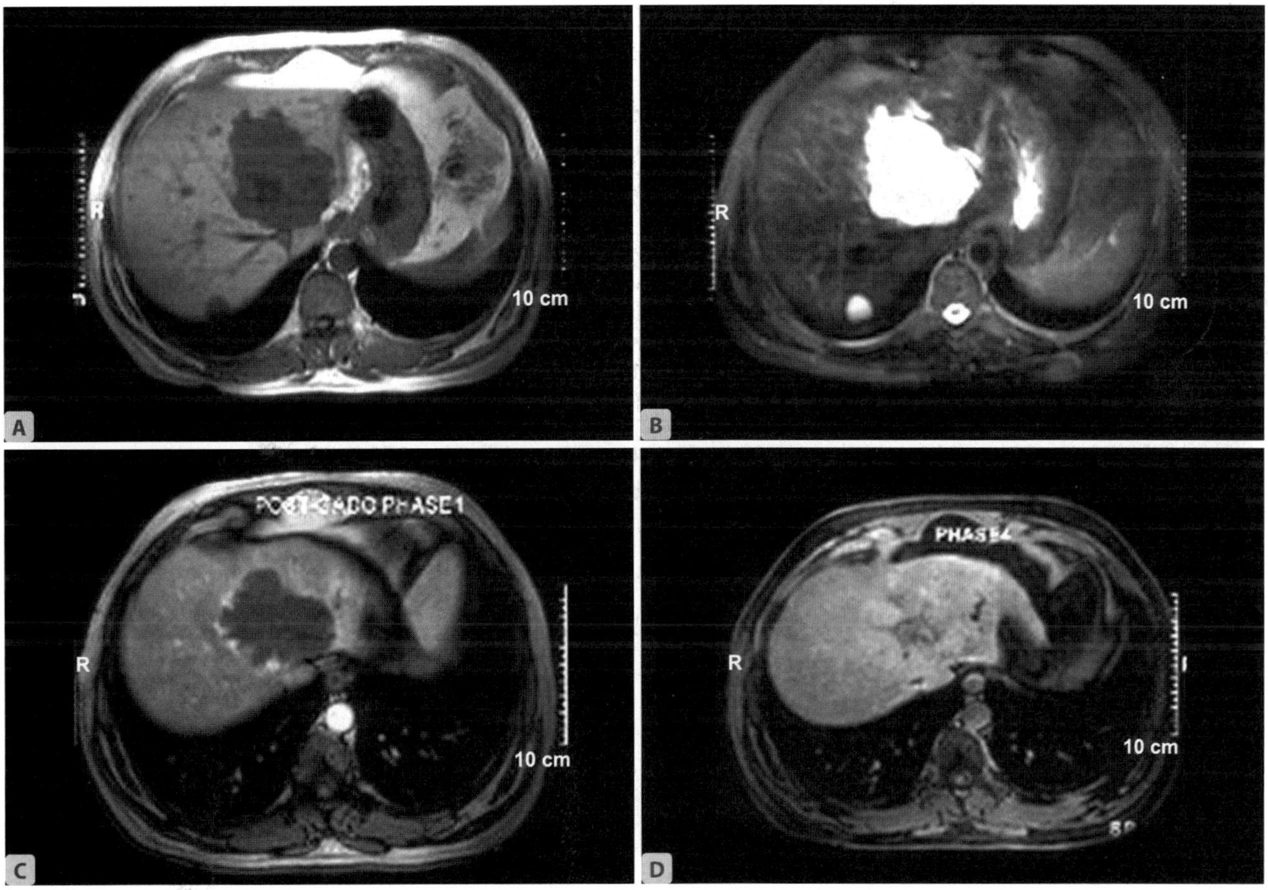

FIGS. 9A TO D: (A) T1 weighted MR image shows a well-demarcated lobulated hypointense lesion in the liver; (B) T2-weighted image reveals the lesion to be markedly hyperintense "light bulb appearance;" (C) Post-gadolinium image obtained within one minute of contrast administration shows peripheral enhancement within the lesion; (D) Delayed phase image shows centripetal fill in with a central scar-giant cavernous hemangioma.

owing to the blood pool phase of these agents. This blood pooling effect of SPIO is also seen in sclerosed or hyalinized type of hemangiomas. This finding helps to differentiate a hemangioma from metastases, as metastases do not show a drop in signal intensity as the blood pooling effect in metastases is negligible. On DWI, hemangiomas show a very high signal on ADC maps and a decrease in signal with increasing b values.[22] This pulse sequence along with contrast-enhanced MR can help in the differentiation between hemangiomas and cystic metastases.

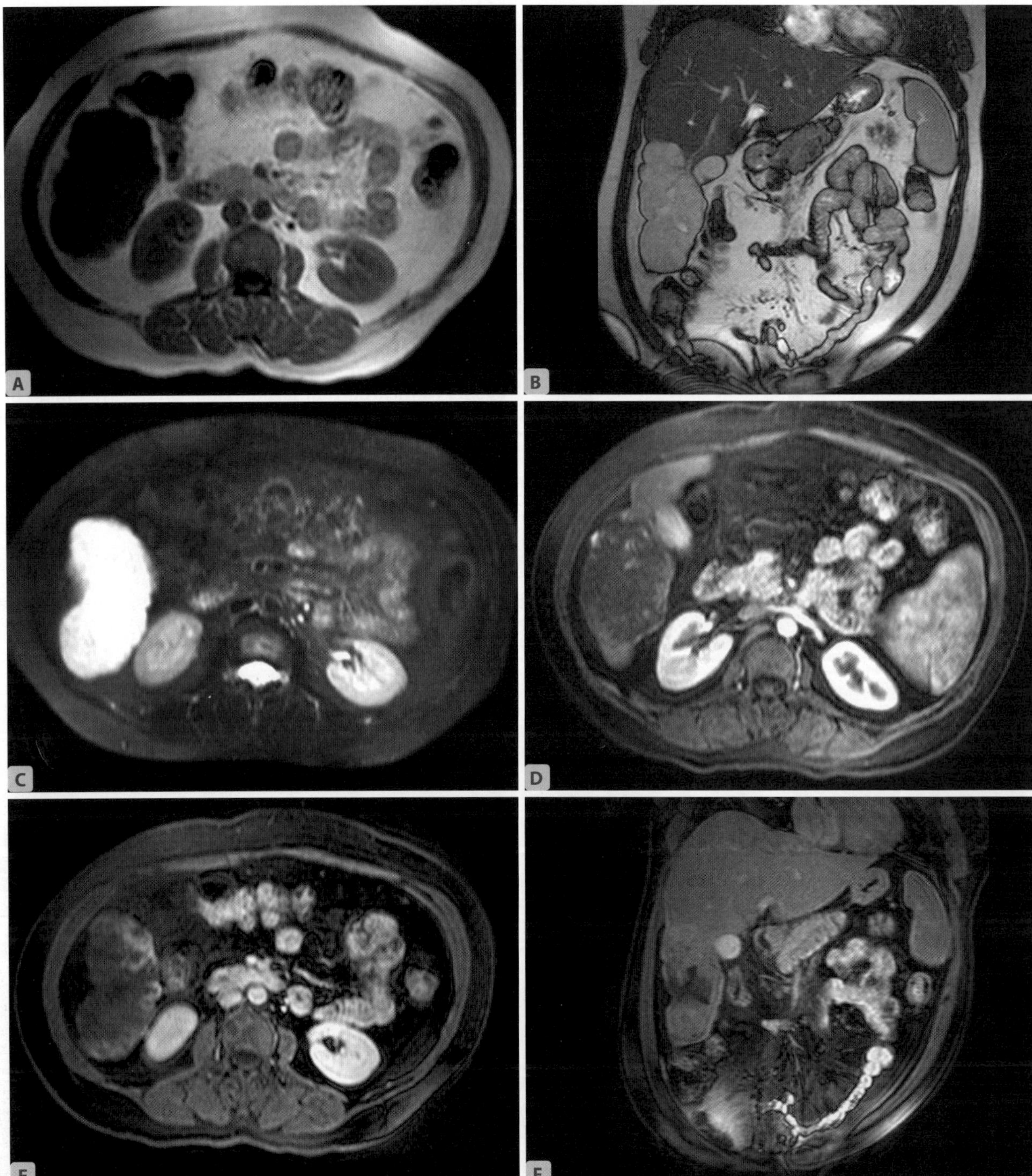

FIGS. 10A TO F: (A) T1W MR image showing an exophytic hepatic lesion hypointense on T1; (B) T2W image shows the lesion to be markedly hyperintense; (C) Marked hyperintensity seen with increasing TE value "light bulb appearance; (D and E) Postcontrast images showing the lesion with incomplete fill in; (F) No enhancement of the central scar seen even on delayed images—exophytic giant cavernous hemangioma.

FOCAL NODULAR HYPERPLASIA

It is the second most common benign liver tumor after hemangiomas, usually smaller than 5 cm with a mean diameter of 3 cm. When it involves an entire lobe, it is known as lobar focal nodular hyperplasia (FNH).[2]

Pathogenesis

A vascular etiology has been postulated as a congenital vascular malformation has been proposed to trigger hepatocyte hyperplasia. It has been suggested that hepatocyte hyperplasia occurs secondary to an increased arterial flow. This theory of pathogenesis is supported by the fact that FNH has been found in association with cavernous hemangiomas, vascular malformations elsewhere and with brain neoplasms.[12] As FNH is more common in women in 3rd–5th decade, a hormonal activity has also been proposed. Estrogens have been found to cause an increase in the size of the nodules (trophic effect). A regression in the size has been seen following the withdrawal of oral contraceptives suggesting a link between FNH and oral contraceptives (OCs).

Pathology

Focal nodular hyperplasia (FNH) is a well-circumscribed, nonencapsulated solitary lesion characterized by a stellate central scar. Histologically, it is composed of hepatocytes, bile duct elements, Kupffer cells and fibrous tissue. However, in FNH, the biliary elements are not connected with the normal biliary tree. FNH is classified into classic and nonclassic types. The classic form is the solid type containing the central scar. Malformed vessels and a nodular architecture are features of the classic type. Histologically, there are cellular areas of hepatic proliferation along with fibrosis. The nonclassic type is further subdivided as the (i) telangiectatic type (ii) FNH with cytologic atypia (iii) mixed hyperplastic and adenomatous FNH. A nodular architecture may be absent in the nonclassic form but it always shows bile duct proliferation. Of these, the telangiectatic variety is characterized by dilated blood filled spaces. In this type of FNH, the arteries are abnormal with a hypertrophic muscular layer and drain directly into the adjacent sinusoids. Necrosis and hemorrhage are common in this form. The other subtype contains areas of large cell dysplasia while the adenomatous form simulates an adenoma. Multiple lesions along with other lesions such as liver hemangiomas, meningiomas, astrocytomas, dysplastic systemic arteries and portal vein atresia constitutes the *multiple FNH syndrome.*[12]

Clinical Features

The FNH is more common in women in 3rd to 5th decade, though they occur at any age and in both males and females. Less than one third of the patients are symptomatic. Symptoms occur only when the lesions are very large in size and cause abdominal pain due to the expansion of Glisson's capsule or mass effect. Most of the lesions are asymptomatic and discovered incidentally on routine imaging.

Imaging Features

USG

FNH are usually seen as isoechoic homogeneous lesions usually identified only by the mass effect they exert **(Figs. 11A to C)**. Displacement of hepatic vessels may be the only identifiable abnormality. A hypoechoic halo seen around the lesion is due to the compressed liver parenchyma. Rarely they may be heterogeneous; a central scar may also be seen in larger lesions. When seen the central scar is usually hyperechoic. A stellate or spoke wheel pattern is seen corresponding to arteries running into radiating fibrous septa from the central scar on color Doppler. Spectral analysis reveals arterial waveform with a good diastolic flow and low resistive index. A continuous waveform from a draining vein may also be identified. On contrast-enhanced ultrosonography (CEUS), the lesion shows enhancement in the arterial phase and is isoechoic to the liver in the portal venous phase and beyond. On delayed imaging there is accumulation of contrast within the central scar.[23]

CT

FNH has been called a "stealth lesion" as it is not visualized on a noncontrast CT. It is a hypervascular lesion supplied by an enlarged anomalous hepatic artery and its drainage is always into the hepatic veins. The lesion shows intense enhancement in the arterial phase with a washout in the venous phase where it becomes isodense to the liver parenchyma. The central scar remains hypodense in the arterial or venous phases and shows accumulation of contrast only on the delayed images. The intratumoral vascularization of FNH is well demonstrated by 3D CT angiography which shows an arterial vessel leading directly into the lesion, lack of portal venous supply and presence of hepatic venous drainage.[24]

MRI

FNH shows a hypointense signal on T1W images and is hyperintense on T2W images. The central stellate radiating scar has a hyperintense signal on the T2W images owing to its vascular and myxoid tissue component. This is in contrast to the central scar seen in fibrolamellar hepatocellular carcinoma (HCC) which shows a low signal on both T1 and T2-weighted images owing to its fibrous nature.[25] A rapid enhancement in the arterial phase followed by a washout with the lesion becoming isointense in the venous phase is observed on administration of gadolinium. The central scar shows a delayed and persistent accumulation of contrast **(Figs. 12A to E)**.[26]

As a well-formed canalicular system is deficient in FNH, FNH shows a prolonged and excessive accumulation of Gd-BOPTA while adenomas show a hypointense appearance on delayed images owing to lack of bile ducts.[27,28] Other hepatocyte specific contrast agents like gadoxetate disodium can also be used. FNH contains Kupffer cells while adenomas do not. SPIO is a contrast agent that undergoes phagocytosis by the Kupffer cells. Hence in FNH there is a pronounced uptake of SPIO which shows a marked drop in signal intensity on T2W images while in adenomas a poor uptake of SPIO is seen due to lack of Kupffer cells.[29] SPIO also helps in differentiating between FNH and fibrolamellar HCC as the

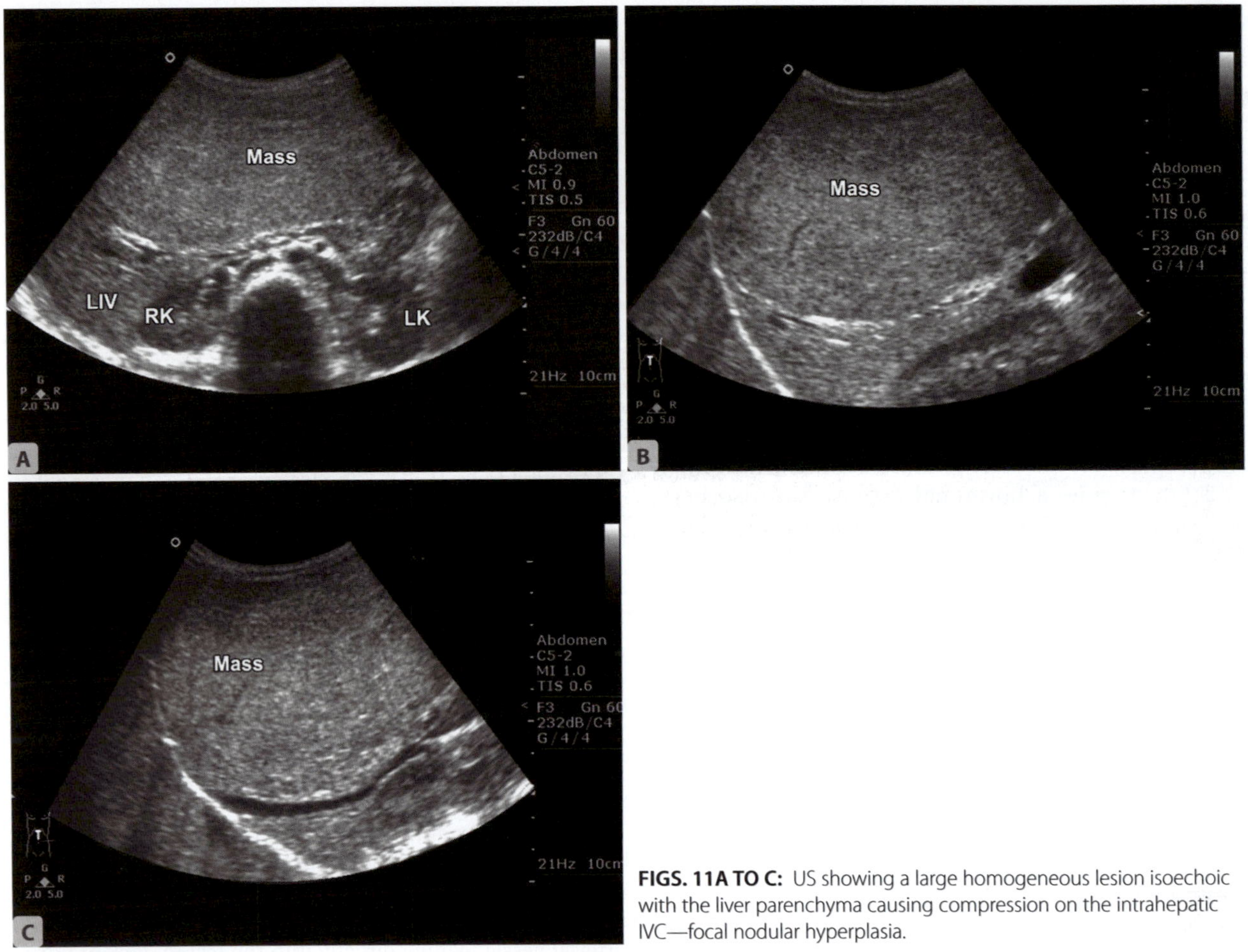

FIGS. 11A TO C: US showing a large homogeneous lesion isoechoic with the liver parenchyma causing compression on the intrahepatic IVC—focal nodular hyperplasia.

fibrolamellar carcinoma lacks Kupffer cells and shows no uptake of SPIO.

On DWI, FNH show a restricted diffusion with reported ADC values between 1 and 1.40 × $10^{-3}mm^2/s$ cm/s. However, these ADC values may also be seen in adenomas and malignant lesions.[22]

Differentiation between FNH and Hepatocellular Adenoma

FNH is usually managed conservatively while adenomas require resection due to their propensity for hemorrhage and hence the need for differentiation between FNH and adenomas.[2,3] A T1 isointensity, a homogeneous appearance, presence of central scar, a pronounced persistent hyperintensity with Gd-BOPTA, a marked uptake of SPIO are features suggestive of FNH while T1 hyperintensity, heterogeneity of the lesion, low uptake of SPIO and absence of enhancement with Gd-BOPTA are features of adenomas.

Differentiation between FNH and Fibrolamellar Carcinoma

A large size (>10 cm), tumor heterogeneity, a large scar (>2 cm), lymphadenopathy, invasion of adjacent vessels, calcification and metastases favors a diagnosis of fibrolamellar HCC.

	Focal nodular hyperplasia (FNH)	Hepatocellular adenoma (HA)	Fibrolamellar carcinoma
T1	Isointense	Hyperintense	Heterogeneously hypointense
Homogeneity	Homogeneous	Heterogeneous	Heterogeneous with central stellate calcification
Central scar	Present but < 2 cm, T2 hyperintense, rarely shows calcification	Absent	Large central scar > 2 cm, T2 hypointense, calcification common
Uptake of hepatocyte specific agents (HSA)	A pronounced persistent hyperintensity with HSA	Absence of enhancement	Absence of enhancement
SPIO	Pronounced uptake	Low uptake	No uptake
Invasion of adjacent organs	Absent	Absent	Present
Lymphade-nopathy	Absent	Absent	Present
Metastases	Absent	Absent	Present

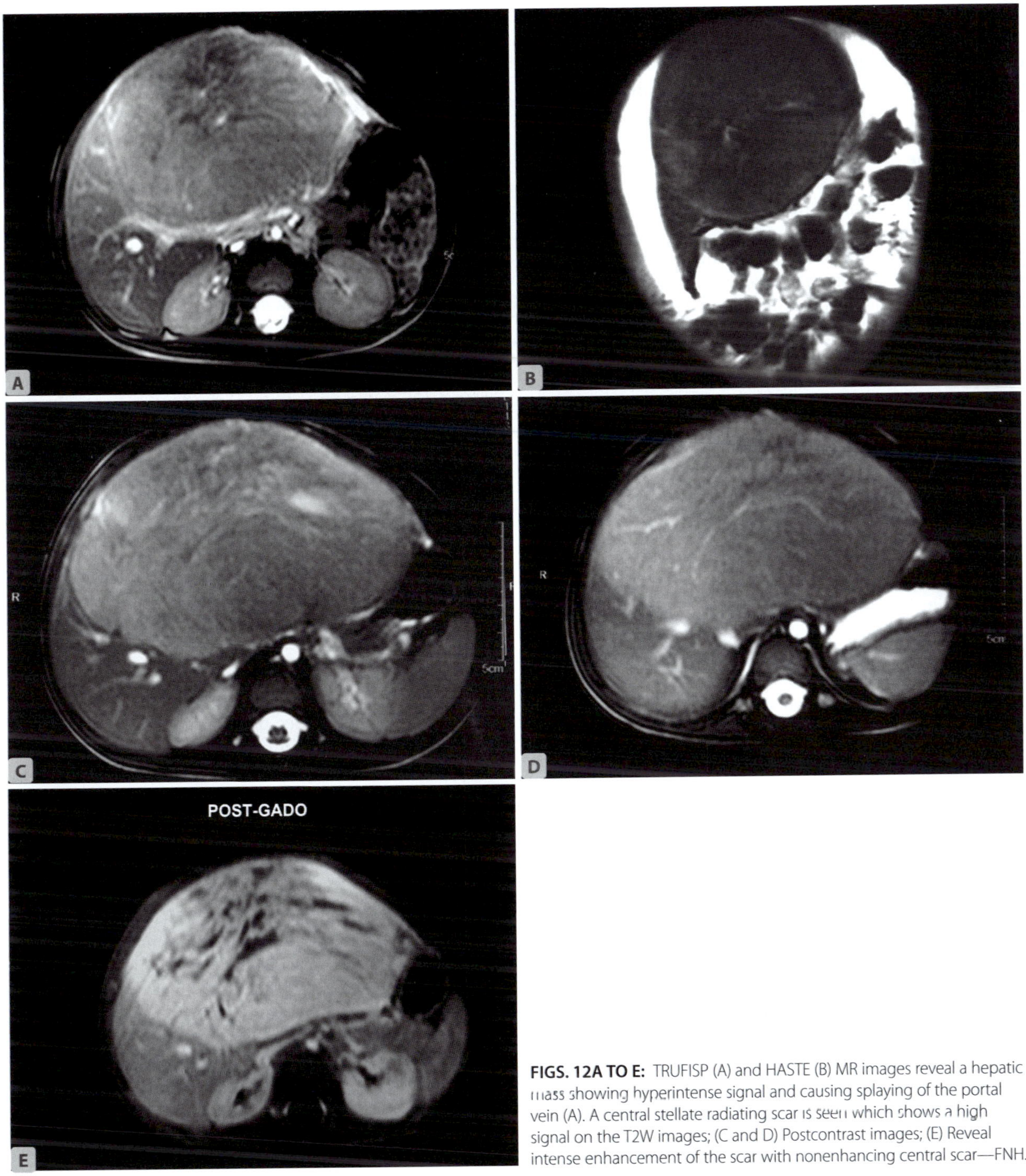

FIGS. 12A TO E: TRUFISP (A) and HASTE (B) MR images reveal a hepatic mass showing hyperintense signal and causing splaying of the portal vein (A). A central stellate radiating scar is seen which shows a high signal on the T2W images; (C and D) Postcontrast images; (E) Reveal intense enhancement of the scar with nonenhancing central scar—FNH.

HEPATOCELLULAR ADENOMA/ HEPATIC ADENOMA

Hepatocellular adenoma is an uncommon solid primary liver tumor. It is usually large in size (>10 cm) and is solitary. Hepatocellular adenomatosis is a rare condition in which multiple (>10) adenomas occur involving both lobes of liver.[30]

Pathogenesis

Although the exact pathogenesis is unknown, it is postulated that the development of adenomas, their number and size shows a definite relationship with the use of oral contraceptives in women and that of anabolic steroids in men. The dose and duration of intake also has a role with the annual incidence of adenoma reported to be 1 per million in women who have never been on oral contraceptives as compared to 30–40 per million in women on long term use.[31] Other associations include type I glycogen storage disease and Von-Gierke's disease where the possible mechanisms include glycogen/insulin imbalance and glycogen overload.[31]

Abnormalities of the hepatic vasculature like absence or occlusion of the portal vein or porto-hepatic venous shunts have also been proposed in the etiopathogenesis particularly in patients with adenomatosis where the adenomas are non-steroid dependent, more prone to hemorrhage and malignant degeneration and are progressive in size. A genetic alteration has also been suggested with mutation of the HNF-1α gene and a β-catenin mutation found in patients with adenomas.

Pathology

Histologically, adenomas consist of atypical hepatocytes with areas of bile stasis, necrosis or hemorrhage. The hepatocytes are typically arranged in cords. Adenoma cells are larger than normal hepatocytes owing to their glycogen and lipid content. Intracellular and intercellular lipid present in the tumor accounts for its yellow appearance on cut section and the presence of fat is useful in its diagnosis on imaging studies. Adenomas lack Kupffer cells and bile ductules.[31] *The notable absence of bile ducts is a key distinguishing feature between adenomas and FNH on histology*. The tumor lacks portal tracts and terminal hepatic veins which accounts for its propensity to hemorrhage. Owing to the lack of a portal venous supply, adenomas are perfused directly from peripheral arterial feeding vessels. The feeding arteries and the extensive sinusoids make adenomas a hypervascular lesion. The high arterial pressure coupled with a poor support from the connective tissue makes these tumors prone to hemorrhage which may spread into the liver or the peritoneal cavity due to the lack of a true tumor capsule.

Different subtypes of HCAs have been described, 50% of adenomas are classified into a *inflammatory subtype* characterized by inflammatory infiltrates, sinusoidal dilatation and thick walled arteries.[32] The inflammatory subtype was earlier called the telangiectatic variety. The second most common subtype (30–35%) is the HNF-1α inactivated type. HNF-1α subtypes are also called *steatotic adenomas* because of their diffuse lipid content.[12] The β-catenin mutated subtype accounts for 10–15% of cases, is usually seen in men and is associated with anabolic steroids. This subtype also carries the risk of malignant transformation.[32] The reported incidence of malignant transformation in adenomas is 7%.[12]

Clinical Features

Most are asymptomatic and discovered incidentally on routine imaging. Some may present with a right upper quadrant fullness, usually seen in larger lesions. The classical clinical presentation is however acute abdominal pain caused by spontaneous hemorrhage or rupture leading to hypotension and even death in some cases.

Imaging Features

USG

Adenomas are echogenic masses, the echogenicity being attributed to the fat and glycogen content. They may have a heterogeneous appearance due to areas of hemorrhage and fibrosis. One third of the lesions may show a pseudocapsule, seen as a hypoechoic peripheral rim on USG. Color Doppler US may reveal intratumoral arteries which is a helpful differentiating feature from FNH. On CEUS, perilesional arteries are seen as intense enhancement around the lesion, rapid intense enhancement followed by an isoechogenicity due to wash out is highly diagnostic of an adenoma.[33]

CT

On noncontrast scans, adenomas are seen as isodense or hypodense lesions **(Figs. 13A to D)** due to presence of fat and glycogen within.[34] They may be heterogeneous due to intratumoral hemorrhage. On contrast administration, an early and rapid enhancement is seen during the arterial phase with the lesion becoming isodense on the portal venous phase. The enhancement does not persist owing to an arteriovenous shunting. A pseudocapsule may be seen in the larger lesions as a hypodense rim on the noncontrast scans and a hyperdense rim on the equilibrium phase[35] **(Figs. 14A to F)**.

MRI

Adenomas are usually T1 isointense or hyperintense lesions due to the presence of fat or glycogen content. On administration of gadolinium, these lesions exhibit an intense enhancement in the arterial phase followed by an isointensity in the venous phase. The lack of uptake of hepatospecific MR contrast like Gd-BOPTA, MnDPDP and SPIO helps to differentiate an adenoma from FNH which shows a pronounced uptake.[36] It is important to differentiate an adenoma from a hepatocellular carcinoma since both may contain intralesional fat (up to 40% HCC) and both show arterial hyperenhancement. The clinical history including patient demographics, any risk factors for HCC as well as a cirrhotic liver background help in the differentiation.[37]

Since the HNF-1α inactivated subtype has the lowest risk of malignant transformation while the β-catenin mutated subtype has the highest risk, an attempt has been made by investigators to differentiate the subtypes on the basis of MR imaging.[12,32] Diffuse intralesional fat detected on chemical shift imaging (CSI) is characteristic of the HNF-1α inactivated subtype while marked T2 hyperintensity and strong arterial phase enhancement that persists on delayed images is highly suggestive of the inflammatory subtype. A characteristic "atoll sign" corresponding to a peripheral rim of hyperintensity and a central area of isointensity is seen in inflammatory hepatocellular adenomas (HCAs) resembling a coral atoll.[32] Scars and poorly defined T2 hyperintense areas suggest β-catenin mutated subtype.

Adenomas show a restricted pattern of diffusion though it may be seen in malignant lesions and FNH as well.[38] Management strategy for adenomas includes a lesion

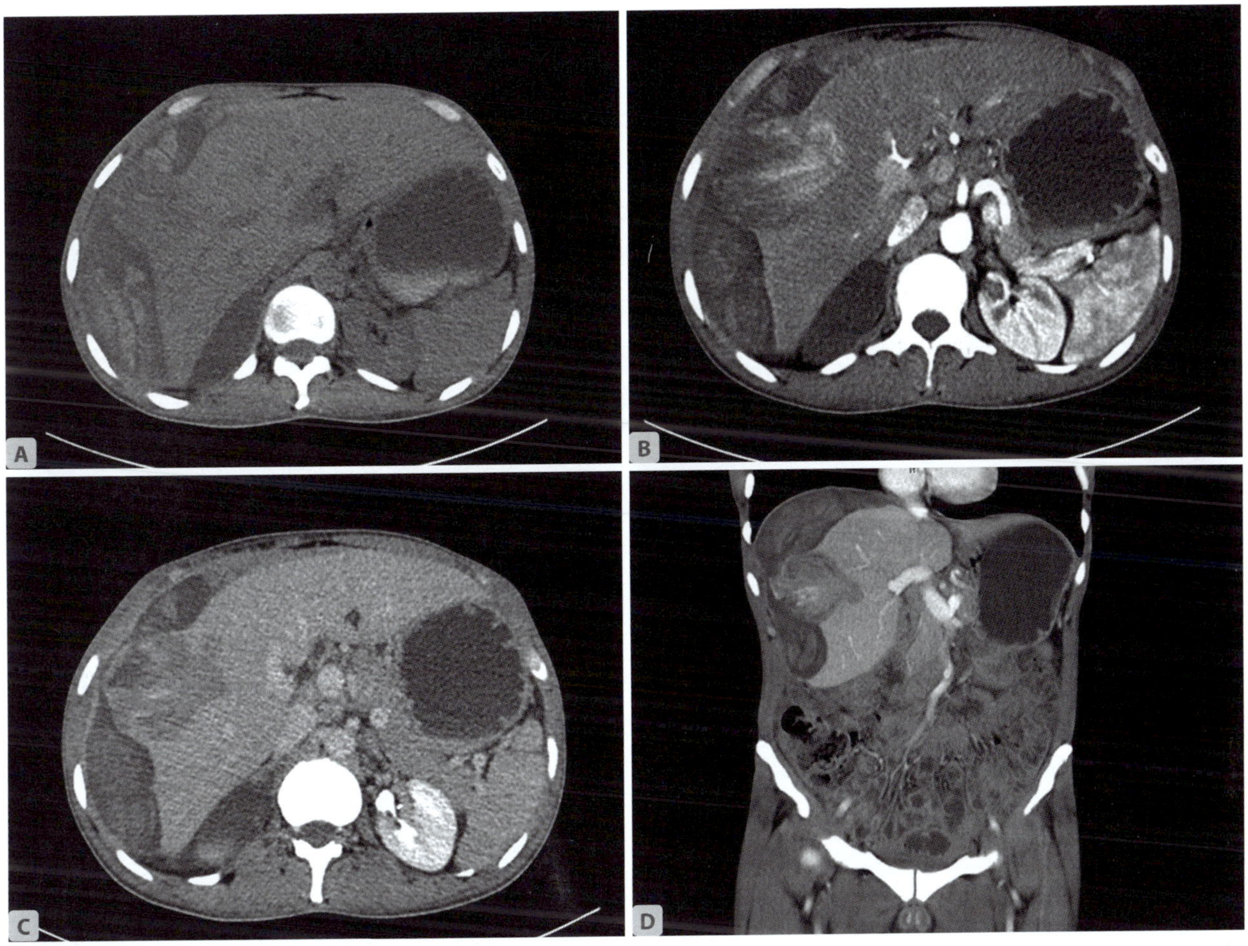

FIGS. 13A TO D: Noncontrast CT (A) shows a heterogeneous lesion in the liver with an exophytic component with evidence of subcapsular and subhepatic bleed. On contrast administration, an early and rapid enhancement in the arterial phase; (B) with the lesion becoming isodense in the portal venous phase; (C and D) is seen. Hepatocellular adenoma with hemorrhage.

characterization by MRI as (i) steatotic (ii) heterogeneous (iii) nonsteatotic. If the patient is on oral contraceptives or anabolic steroids, a discontinuation of these followed by repeat imaging at 3–6 months is recommended.[32] If the adenomas are seen to regress, a follow-up is indicated, while in the growing lesions further evaluation is warranted. Surgical resection is recommended for large lesions (>5 cm) and those found in association with glycogen storage disease owing to an increased risk of malignant transformation.

NODULAR REGENERATIVE HYPERPLASIA

Nodular regenerative hyperplasia (NRH) is a condition characterized by multiple nodules replacing the hepatic parenchyma without the formation of fibrous septa within the nodules. The absence of fibrosis differentiates this condition from the regenerating nodules of cirrhosis.

Pathogenesis

The causes of NRH are varied. Various myeloproliferative disorders, rheumatologic disorders, steroids and antineoplastic drugs have been implicated as the causative factors. Association with portal hypertension is also seen.[39]

Clinical Features

The mean age of occurrence is around 50 years with no gender predilection. Children may be affected by this disorder when associated with congenital absence of the portal vein.

Imaging Features

US

In most cases NRH is not seen on ultrasound, the lesions being isoechoic with the adjacent liver parenchyma.[40] At times, isoechoic or hypoechoic nodules are seen. Color Doppler demonstrates arterial supply within the nodules.

CT

The CT appearance of NRH may range from that of a normal liver to focal hypoattenuating nodules ranging from 0.1 to 3 cm. The nodules enhance homogeneously after administration of contrast.

MRI

The lesions are typically isointense to the liver parenchyma on T1-weighted image while on a T2-weighted image the nodules appear iso or hypointense. The nodules show enhancement in the arterial phase. On the portal venous

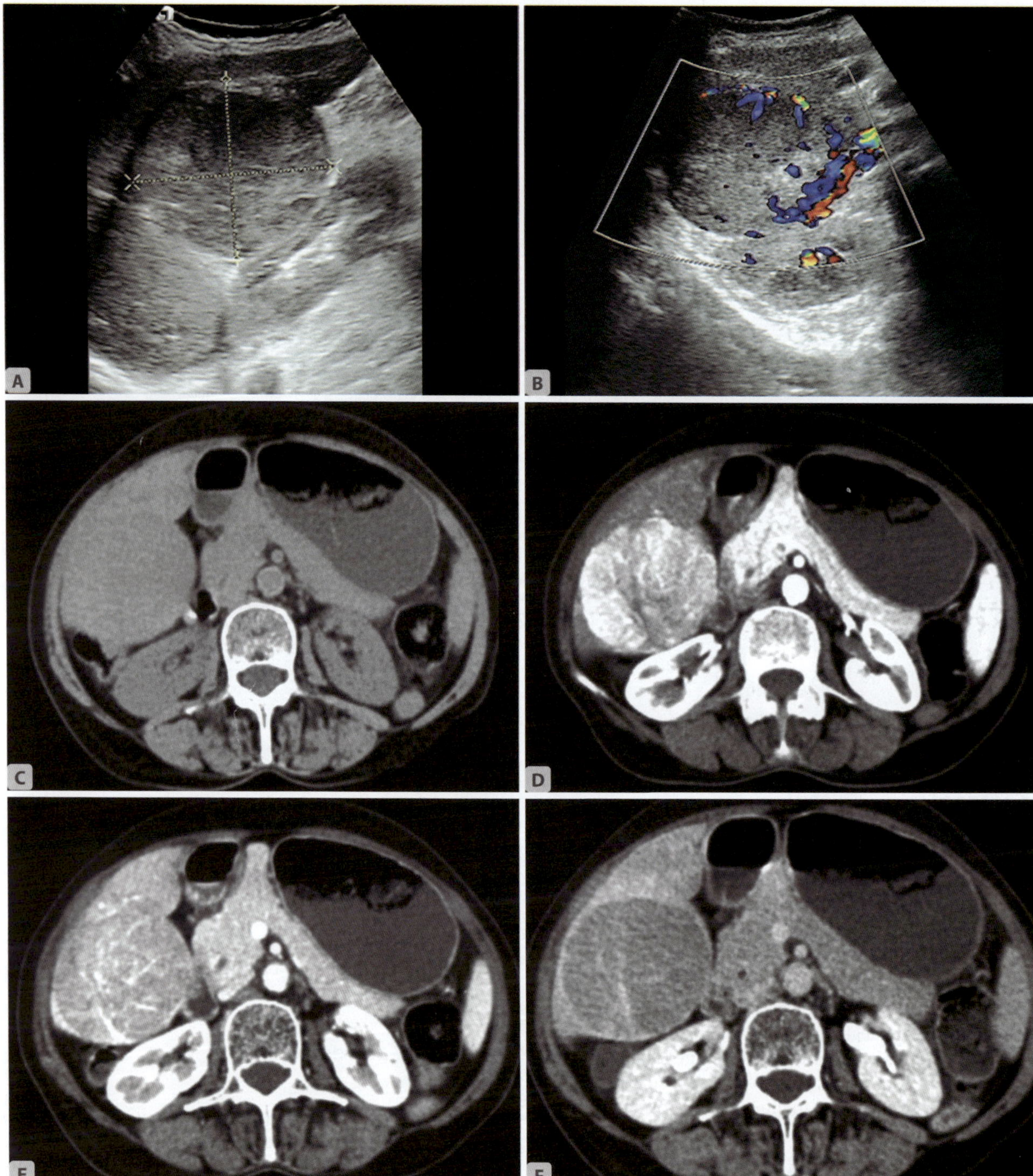

FIGS. 14A TO F: US showing a well-defined predominantly echogenic mass in the liver: with evidence of perilesional vascularity on color Doppler (A); NCCT scan (B); the mass to be isodense with the liver parenchyma, intensely enhancing in the arterial phase (C); becoming isodense in the portal venous phase (D); and hypodense in the equilibrium phase (E); Pseudocapsule can be seen in the delayed image as a hyperdense rim (F)—hepatocellular adenoma.

and equilibrium phases of contrast-enhanced dynamic MR imaging the lesions remain iso to slightly hyperintense.

On administration of Gd BOPTA, the lesions remain hyperintense owing to an abnormal biliary drainage. The presence of abundant Kupffer cells within the nodules accounts for a significant uptake of SPIO.

ADENOMATOUS HYPERPLASTIC NODULE

Adenomatous hyperplastic nodules (AHN) are benign but premalignant lesions usually seen in cirrhotic livers. They are also known as dysplastic nodules or macroregenerative nodules. They appear hyperintense on T1-weighted images and hypointense on T2W images. Dysplastic nodules that accumulate iron have a greater malignant potential owing to the tumor enhancing effects of iron.[41] Hepatocellular carcinoma (HCC) are hyperintense on T2W images, a finding that differentiates a dysplastic nodule from HCC. HCC are supplied by hepatic artery whereas dysplastic nodules have portal venous supply.[42]

The presence of "nodule within nodule appearance" consisting of a hyperintense nodule developing within a hypointense dysplastic nodule on T2W images is highly suspicious for the development of malignancy within the nodule.

PEDIATRIC LIVER TUMORS

Mesenchymal Hamartoma

Mesenchymal hamartoma is a benign cystic developmental lesion seen in the pediatric population. It is the second most common benign liver tumor occurring in the pediatric age group. Usually seen in children under the age of 2 years, it occurs twice as often in boys than girls.

Pathology

Mesenchymal hamartoma is a well-defined large encapsulated or pedunculated tumor.[43] It consists of gelatinous mesenchymal tissue with cyst formation and remnants of normal hepatic parenchyma and hence have a mixed solid cystic appearance in majority of the cases. They may have a predominantly cystic appearance if the cystic component predominates and solid appearance if the mesenchymal component predominates.

Clinical Features

Patients typically present with a gradually progressive enlarging abdominal distention. They may eventually develop vomiting, diarrhea or constipation as the mass enlarges. Respiratory distress may occur due to a mass effect on the diaphragm.

Imaging Features

USG

Usually seen as a well-circumscribed multilocular solid cystic lesion **(Figs. 15A and B)**. The cystic spaces are separated by echogenic septae.[44] The lesion may rarely have a solid appearance if the mesenchymal component predominates.

CT

It is seen as a multi-septated mass of water attenuation. The thin internal septations may show contrast enhancement. No calcification or hemorrhage is seen in these lesions **(Figs. 16A and B)**.

MRI

On MRI, the cystic component of the lesion is markedly hyperintense on T2W images while the mesenchymal (stromal) component is hypointense on both T1W images and T2W images **(Figs. 17A to C)**.[45,46]

INFANTILE HEPATIC HEMANGIOMA

Formerly, known as infantile hemangioendothelioma, infantile hepatic hemangioma is the most common benign hepatic tumor occurring in infants with females affected more commonly than males.[47]

Pathogenesis

Three subtypes of infantile hepatic hemangiomas have been described, the focal, multifocal and the diffuse types. While the focal subtype is thought to be the hepatic form of rapidly involuting congenital hemangioma (RICH), the multifocal subtype is thought to be the hepatic form of simple cutaneous hemangioma. The multifocal subtype is often associated with multiple cutaneous hemangiomas in the same patient. Histopathologic antibody staining of endothelial cells in RICH is negative for glucose transporter protein 1 (GLUT 1) while it is positive in the multifocal variety similar to the cutaneous infantile

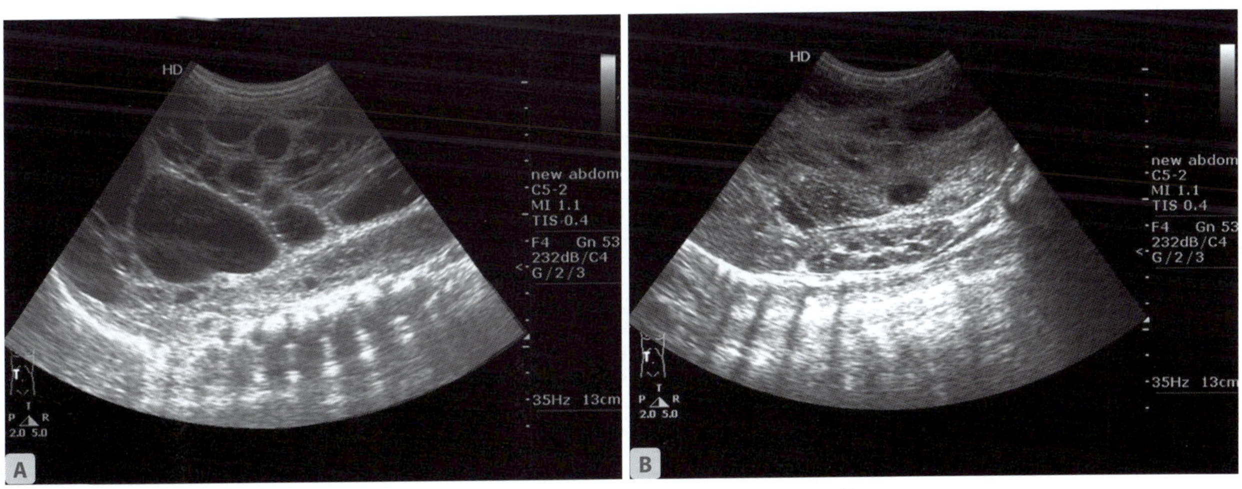

FIGS. 15A AND B: US shows a mixed solid cystic lesion within the liver in an infant—mesenchymal hamartoma.

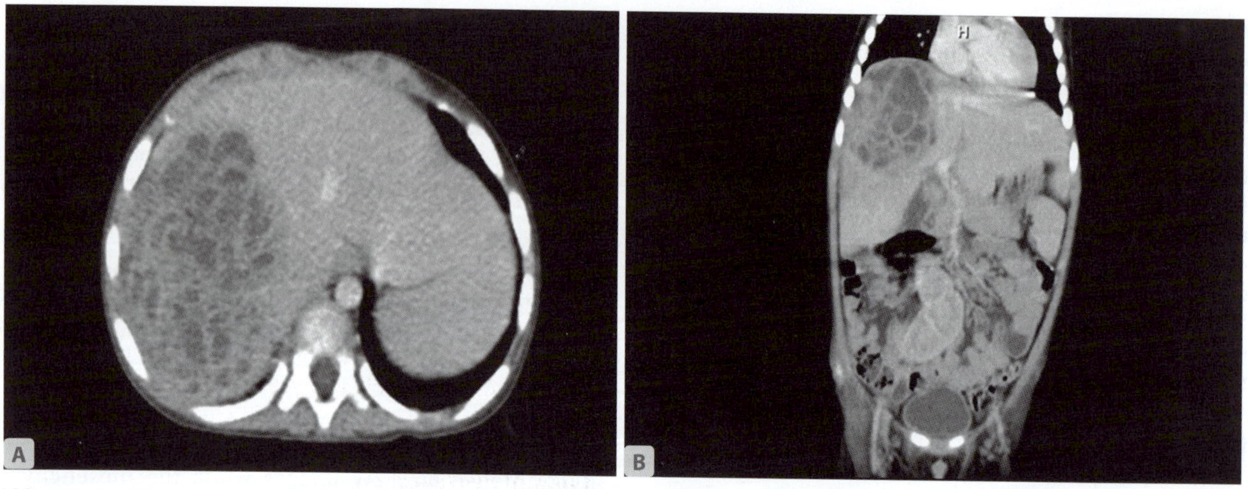

FIGS. 16A AND B: CT axial (A) and coronal (B) scans showing a multiseptated mass of water attenuation within the liver with the thin internal septations showing enhancement—mesenchymal hamartoma.

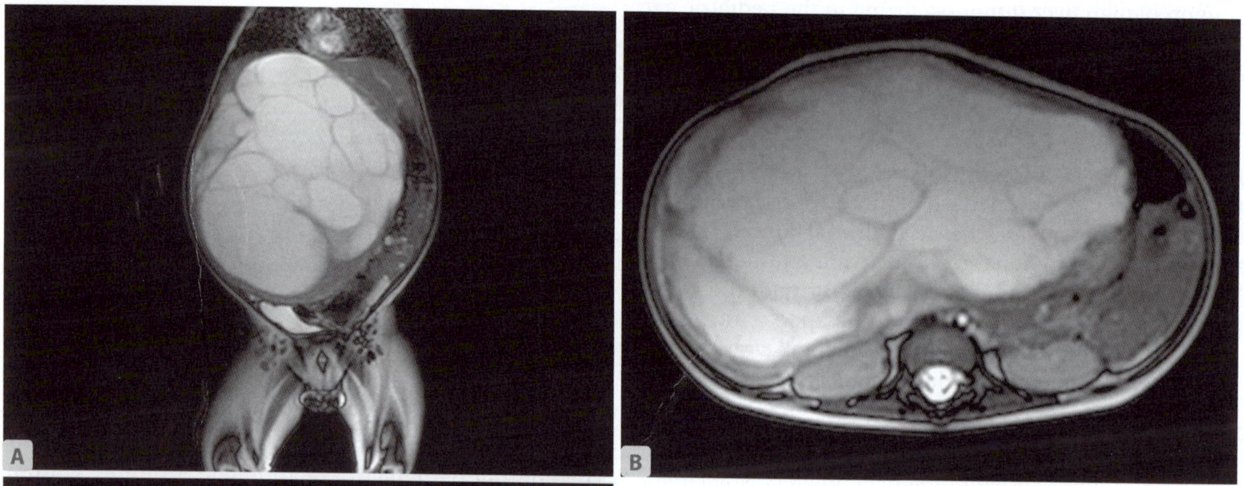

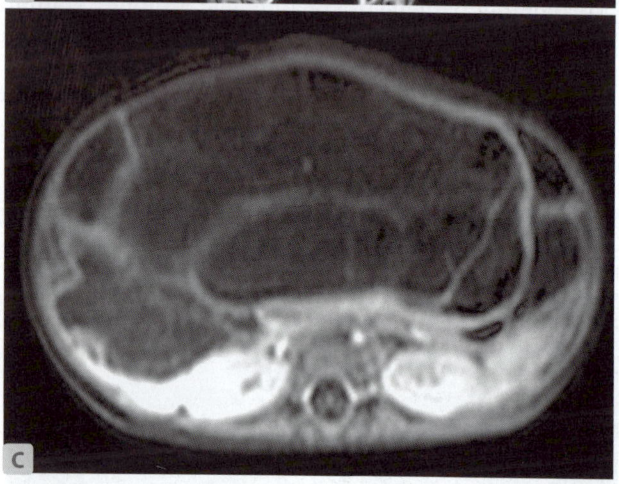

FIGS. 17A TO C: Coronal (A) and axial (B) T2W MR images showing a large multiloculated cystic lesion replacing the liver parenchyma. On contrast administration, the thin internal septations are seen to enhance (C)—mesenchymal hamartoma.

hemangioma. The diffuse subtype is characterized by almost complete replacement of the hepatic parenchyma by infantile hemangiomas. These patients present with a large palpable abdominal mass and high output failure due to arteriovenous shunting.

Pathology

On gross examination, the tumor is composed of multiple discrete round nodules measuring 2–15 cm in diameter. Microscopically, two histological types have been described—the type 1 has vascular spaces lined by endothelial cells and supported by reticular fibers. Type 2 has larger, irregular spaces lined by immature pleomorphic cells. The 2nd type has been reported to have some malignant potential.

Clinical Features

90% of these lesions occur during the first 6 months of life. Affected infants may present with a palpable abdominal mass and bruit. Arteriovenous shunting occurring within the lesion may cause congestive heart failure in these infants. Occasionally, spontaneous rupture may lead to a massive hemoperitoneum or rarely thrombocytopenia due to platelet sequestration (Kasabach-Merritt syndrome) may occur.

Imaging Features

Ultrasound

The lesions show variable echogenicity, it may be highly echogenic, hypoechoic or anechoic with echogenic septa. Like hemangiomas, the increased echogenicity is attributable to the multiple interfaces that exist between the vascular spaces. A narrowing of the abdominal aorta below the origin of the coeliac axis, a dilated coeliac axis and common hepatic artery and prominent draining hepatic veins forms a characteristic imaging finding of infantile hepatic hemangiomas seen on color Doppler. These vascular abnormalities do not occur in a malignant hepatic tumor.[48]

CT

Noncontrast scans show the liver to be enlarged with multiple hypodense lesions within. Calcification may be seen in 40% cases. Contrast enhancement reveals a peripheral and centripetal enhancement followed by a prolonged and persistent enhancement on delayed scans similar to that seen in hemangiomas **(Figs. 18A to C)**. CT angiography depicts the dilated coeliac axis artery and narrowing of the aorta below its origin.

MRI

The lesions are typically hypointense on T1W images and hyperintense on T2W images with the contrast enhancement pattern similar to hemangiomas.[49]

UNUSUAL BENIGN TUMORS OF THE LIVER

Lipomatous Tumors

These include lipomas, angiomyolipomas and myelolipomas depending on fat, myeloid and vascular tissue component.[50]

Pathology

On gross examination, lipomas are solitary, well circumscribed masses containing variable amount of adipose, smooth muscle tissue and thick-walled blood vessels. The presence of prominent hematopoietic tissue makes it a myelolipomas or angiomyolipoma.

Clinical Features

Angiomyolipomas are rare benign tumors of the liver. They usually do not cause any symptoms and are solitary. Rarely, patients may present with abdominal pain owing to bleeding within these tumors. Multiple liver angiomyolipomas which are progressive and symptomatic occur in association with Bourneville-Pringle syndrome.

Imaging Features

USG

This lipomatous tumors are highly echogenic on US owing to their fat content. Differentiation from hepatic hemangioma is difficult although a mixed hyper hypoechoic pattern may be seen at times.

CT

Fat attenuation values (–20 to –115 HU are) typically seen on the noncontrast scans with a variable enhancement seen on contrast administration depending on the vascular component within **(Fig. 19)**.[50]

MRI

These tumors are seen to have a high signal on both T1- and T2-weighted images owing to the fat content. On the fat suppressed sequences, signal suppression with a

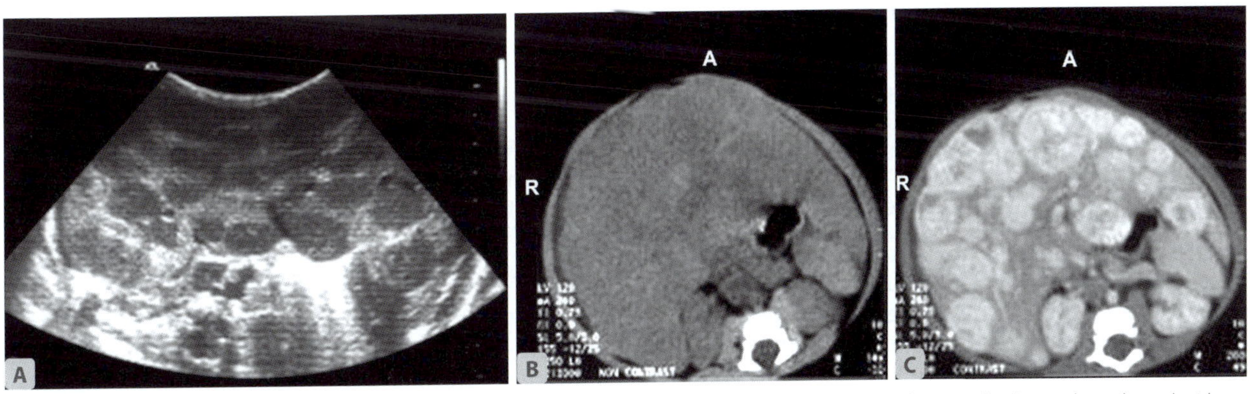

FIGS. 18A TO C: (A) US scan shows multiple hypoechoic lesions within the liver; (B) Noncontrast CT scan showing the liver to be enlarged with multiple hypodense lesions within; (C) Contrast-enhanced CT reveals peripheral and centripetal enhancement of the lesions—infantile hepatic hemangioma.

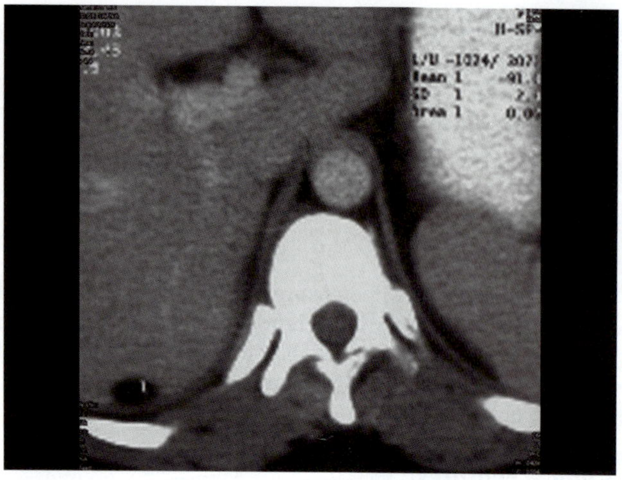

FIG. 19: CT image shows a small hypoattenuating lesion with fat attenuation value within the right lobe of liver—lipoma.

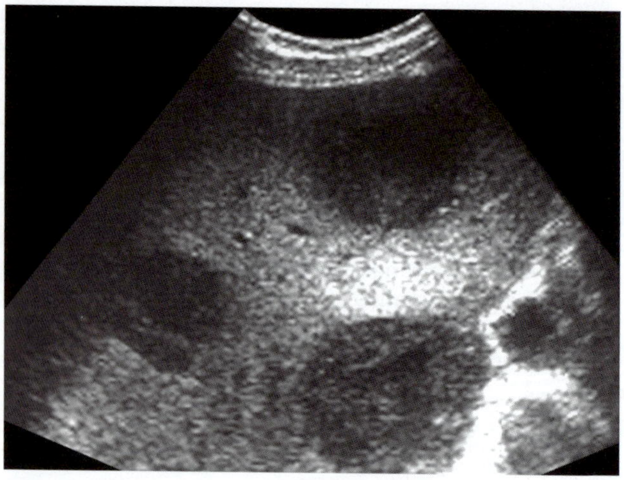

FIG. 20: US scan showing three lesions in the liver with well- defined walls and echoes within giving a solid appearance—pyogenic liver abscesses.

hypointense appearance is seen. A signal drop seen on the opposed phase images during chemical shift imaging (CSI) suggests the presence of both macroscopic and microscopic fat.

LEIOMYOMAS

Leiomyomas are extremely rare benign hepatic tumors. They arise from the smooth muscles as solitary, well-circumscribed masses. An association has been seen between HIV infection and leiomyomas as these have been reported in adults and children infected with the virus.

Imaging Features

USG

Leiomyomas appear as solid, hypoechoic masses with internal echoes.

CT

These appear as low attenuation masses on noncontrast scans with two distinct patterns of enhancement seen on contrast administration, a peripheral rim enhancement and a delayed homogeneous enhancement.

MRI

Leiomyomas are seen to have a hypointense signal on T1, a hyperintense signal on T2WI with an enhancement pattern similar to that seen on CT on contrast administration.

Paraganglioma

Paragangliomas are rare tumors of neural crest origin. Though usually seen along the sympathetic chain, these may very rarely be seen in the liver.[31] On imaging these are seen as well circumscribed lesions with intense contrast enhancement. Cystic areas and calcification may be seen.

INFECTIVE LESIONS

Bacterial (Pyogenic) Liver Abscess

A liver abscess may develop from several routes. The most common route is the biliary route owing to cholangitis secondary to obstructive biliopathy. Other routes include phlebitis of the portal or superior mesenteric vein secondary to appendicitis, diverticulitis, pancreatitis and other gastrointestinal infections. A direct extension from contiguous organs, arterial septicemia secondary to osteomyelitis, endocarditis, pneumonitis, a post-traumatic or an iatrogenic cause may also be the source of a liver abscess. A cryptogenic abscess may develop in patients with diabetes mellitus with no apparent source of infection. While abscesses of biliary origin are often multiple involving both lobes, abscess from the portal vein are often solitary and in 65% cases occur in the right lobe. *Staphylococcus* is the most common causative organism in children while *Escherichia coli* is the most common in adults.[51]

Clinical Features

The clinical symptoms include fever, pain in the right upper quadrant, nausea and vomiting and malaise. A tender hepatomegaly is seen with leukocytosis being the most common laboratory abnormality.

Imaging Features

Plain Film Findings

Elevation of the right hemidiaphragm, hepatomegaly, right pleural effusion and atelectasis may be seen in case of a large abscess.

USG

US can detect hepatic abscesses as small as 1.5 cm with a sensitivity of about 90%. They appear as well-defined lesions with thick, irregular walls **(Fig. 20)**. They are variable in echogenicity and are seen as anechoic in 50%, hyperechoic in 25% or hypoechoic in 25% cases.[52] Early lesions are hyperechoic and have well defined margins. Debris, septations, fluid-fluid level, air fluid level may also be seen. Echogenic foci with posterior reverberation artefacts are seen with gas producing organisms.

CT

On CT scans, abscesses are seen as low attenuation lesions with a characteristic peripheral rim enhancement **(Figs. 21A and B)**.[53] On administration of IV contrast, "double target sign" corresponding to perilesional edema and "cluster sign" representing coalescence of smaller lesions (<2 cm) to form a large abscess are characteristic features **(Figs. 22 and 23)**.[54] An air fluid level which is a specific sign of an abscess is seen in less than 20% of cases and may indicate an enteric communication.

MRI

These are seen as well-defined rounded lesions hypointense on T1W images, hyperintense on T2W images with intense peripheral rim enhancement on administration of contrast **(Figs. 24A and B)**. Peripheral edema seen as a high signal on T2W images is seen in only one third of the cases.[55] Diffusion weighted imaging of pyogenic abscesses shows a restricted pattern owing to the high cellularity and viscosity of pus.

AMOEBIC ABSCESS

Caused by the protozoan *Entamoeba histolytica*, amoebic liver abscess is the most common extraintestinal manifestation of amoebiasis. The organism may reach the liver from the colon, through the portal vein, via lymphatics or by direct extension.[56]

Pathology

The cavitary amoebic abscess occurs as the liver parenchyma is frankly destroyed. Initially, the lesion contains necrotic tissue including the viable organism. As the lesion becomes larger, central cavitation is apparent and the active organism lies in the necrotic tissue lining the cavity. Surrounding

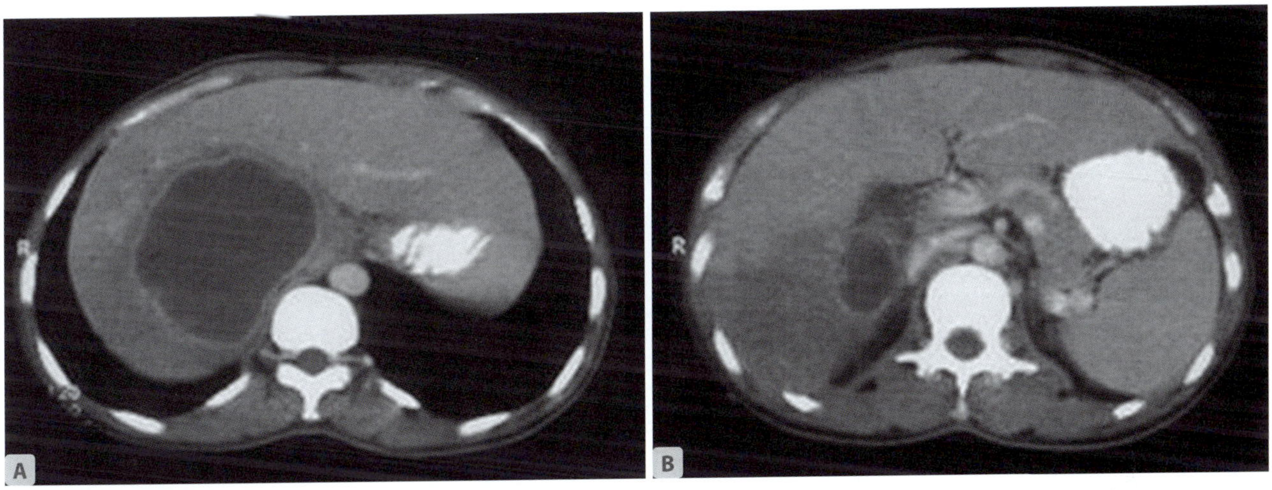

FIGS. 21A AND B: Contrast-enhanced CT showing irregular hypodense lesions in the liver with enhancing rim—pyogenic liver abscesses.

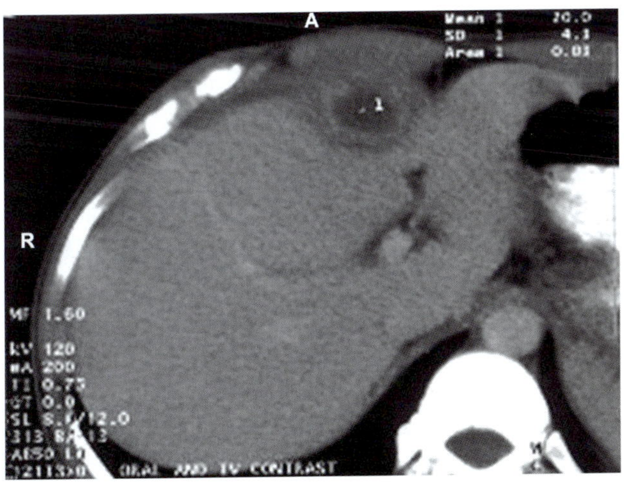

FIG. 22: Contrast-enhanced CT showing a hypodense lesion with perilesional edema giving a 'double target sign'—pyogenic liver abscess.

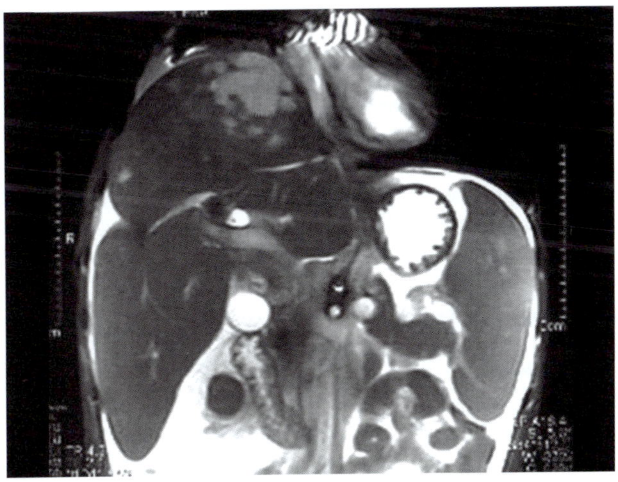

FIG. 23: MR image showing multiple small abscesses coalescing into a single cavity—"the cluster sign"—pyogenic liver abscesses.

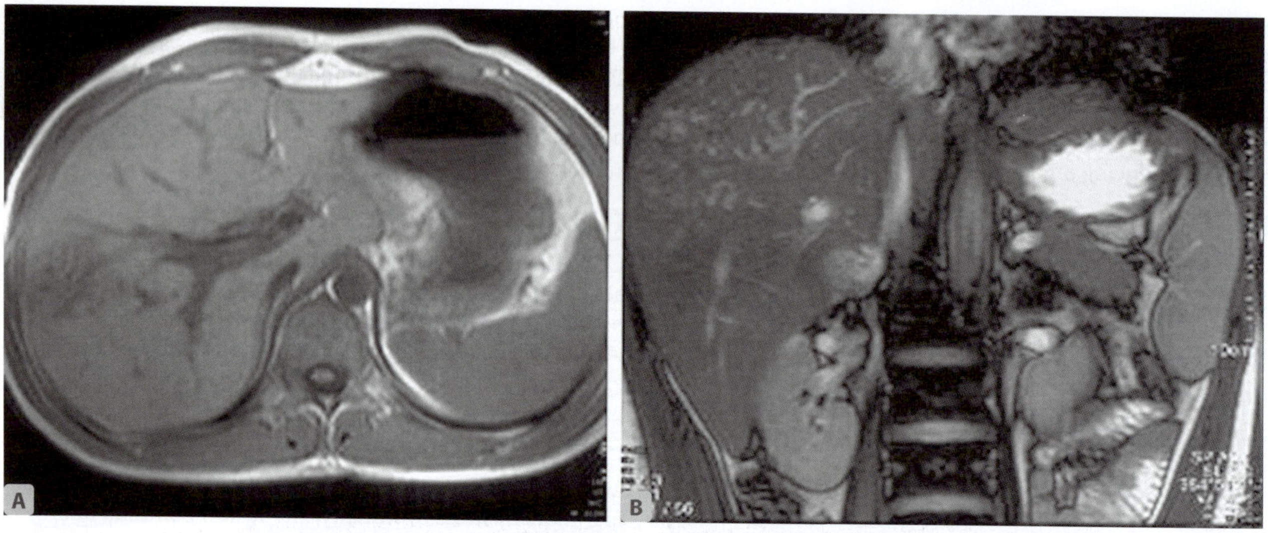

FIGS. 24A AND B: (A) T1 weighted MR image showing an ill-defined area hypointense in signal in the right lobe of liver; (B) T2-weighted image showing the area to have a high signal with multiple small lesions clustering together liver abscess.

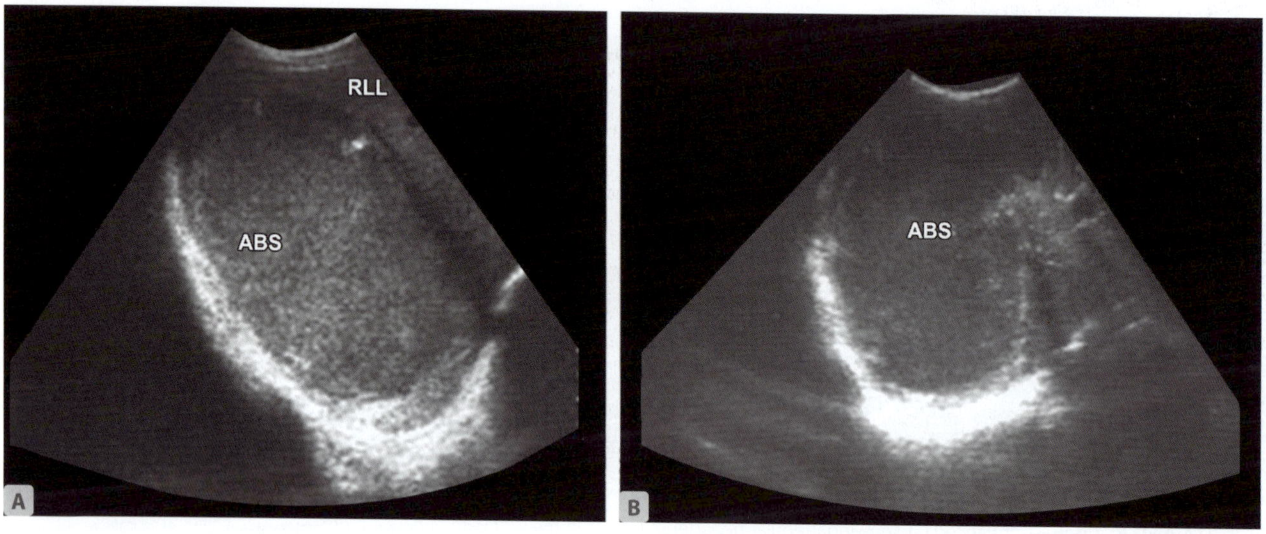

FIGS. 25A AND B: US showing a round hypoechoic lesion with low internal echoes within with absence of a well-defined abscess wall—amoebic liver abscess.

this layer is an inflammatory zone of hepatic parenchyma invaded by the organisms. Centrally, the cavity is often filled by a thick fluid that resembles "anchovy paste". Frequently solitary, the abscess is most commonly located in the right lobe being related to the venous drainage from the usually infected right colon, via the superior mesenteric vein to the portal vein preferentially flowing into the right lobe of liver.

Imaging Features

Ultrasound

Amoebic abscess is seen as a round to oval solitary lesion in the right lobe of liver, with fine low level echoes and usually in continuity with the diaphragm **(Figs. 25A and B)**. A round or oval shape and a hypoechoic appearance with fine echoes are sonographic findings that favor an amoebic over a pyogenic liver abscess.[57]

CT Scans

Amoebic abscess appears as a low attenuation lesion with evidence of rim enhancement on contrast administration. Lesions in the early stage of development have a solid appearance with older lesions being cystic in appearance.[58] A target appearance due to an outer rim of lower attenuation surrounding the enhancing rim may be seen.

Magnetic Resonance Imaging

The abscess cavity is seen to have a low signal on T1 and a high signal on T2W images. The central cavity is often

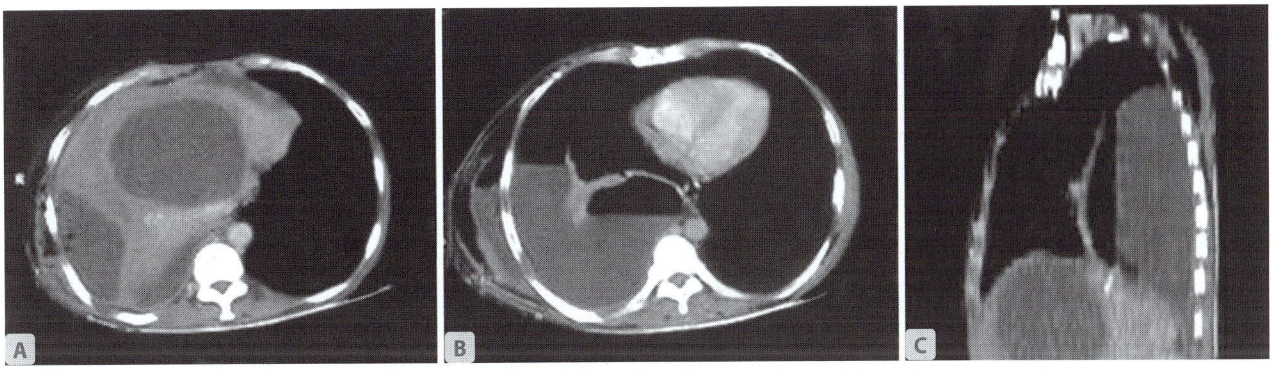

FIGS. 26A TO C: (A) Contrast-enhanced CT showing two abscesses in the liver with one of (A to C) lesions showing air loculi and indistinct margins; (B) A large hydropneumothorax is seen in the right pleural cavity; (C) Multiplanar reconstruction showing the communication between the abscess and the right hydropneumothorax—ruptured liver abscess.

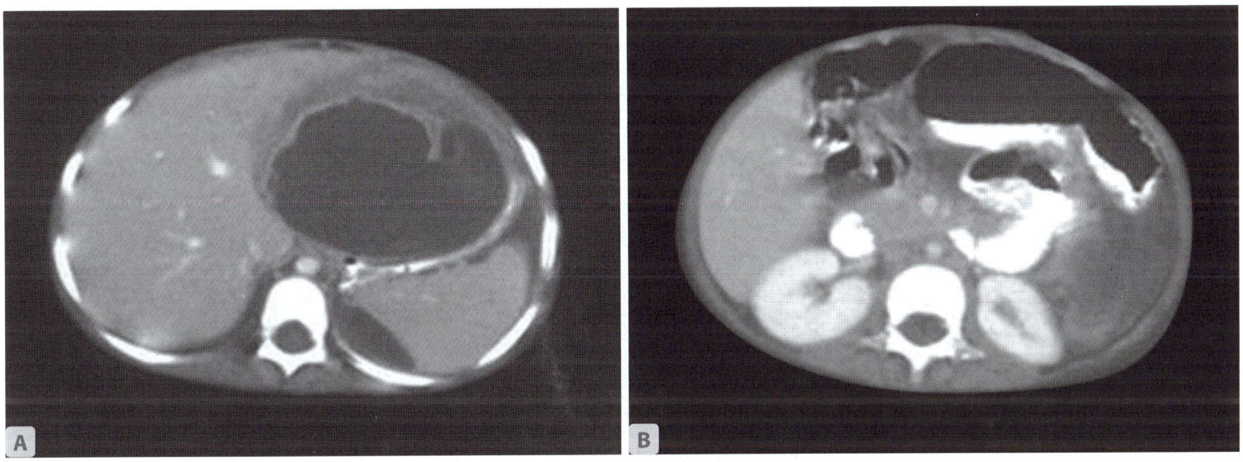

FIGS. 27A AND B: (A) Contrast-enhanced CT showing a large hypodense lesion with enhancing (A and B) rim in the left lobe of liver. Perilesional edema is noted. Fluid seen in the perihepatic and perisplenic region; (B) Fluid seen in the peritoneal cavity—intraperitoneal rupture of abscess.

surrounded by a rim of high signal intensity corresponding to hyperemic reactive zone. On contrast administration, this reactive zone shows evidence of enhancement.

Complications

The most common complication of a liver abscess is rupture through the diaphragm resulting in pleuropulmonary amoebiasis occurring in 20–35% of patients **(Figs. 26A to C)**. Complications include pleural effusions, empyema, consolidation, lung abscess and very rarely hepatobronchial fistula.[59] Rupture into the peritoneal cavity is another complication **(Figs. 27A and B)**. Rarely, abscesses located in the left lobe may rupture into the pericardial cavity which is a serious life-threatening complication leading to cardiac tamponade or shock **(Figs. 28A to D)**. A rare complication is rupture of abscess into the biliary tree.

FUNGAL HEPATIC ABSCESSES

Fungal hepatic abscesses are uncommon. Immunocompromised states like HIV, chemotherapy, lymphoma, etc. are considered to be the predisposing factors. Liver is involved secondary to hematogenous spread of mycotic infection in other organs, most commonly in the lungs. *Candida* is the most common causative organism.

Imaging Features

Sonographically, four major patterns of hepatic candidiasis are seen: (i) "wheel within a wheel", in which a peripheral zone surrounds an inner echogenic wheel (ii) "bull's eye", or target lesion in which a hypoechoic rim surrounds a hyperechoic center (iii) a "uniformly hypoechoic" appearance and (iv) "uniformly echogenic".

On CT scan, the most common pattern is multiple small, rounded hypoattenuating areas. Multiple punctate foci of increased attenuation due to calcification can be seen on NCCT.[60]

On MR, these lesions show increased signal intensity on T2-weighted images and STIR sequences.

HYDATID DISEASE

Hydatid disease is caused by the *Echinococcus granulosus*. Hydatid disease involves the liver in approximately 75% of cases with the right lobe more frequently involved.

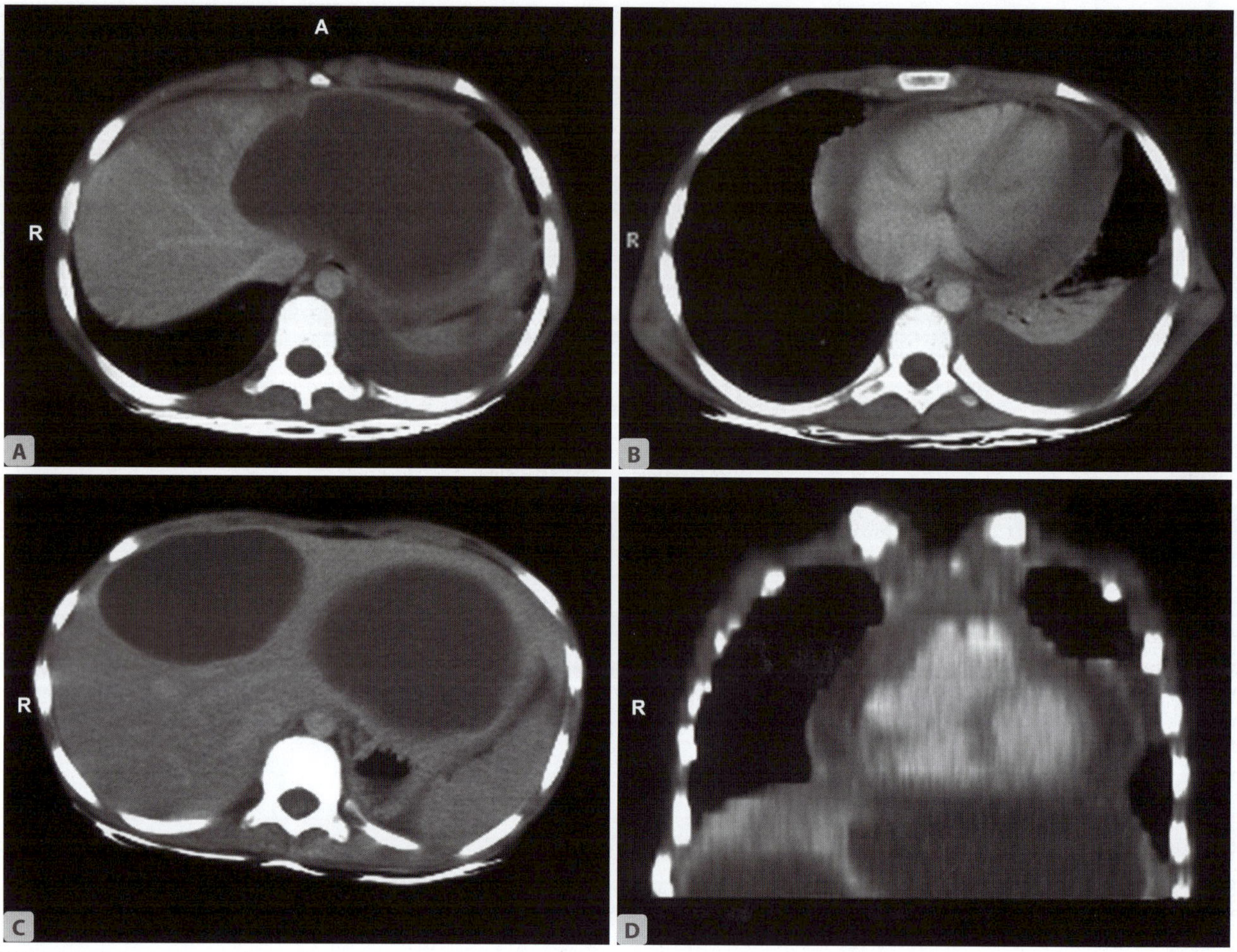

FIGS. 28A TO D: Contrast-enhanced CT sections reveal large abscesses in the liver with rupture of the left lobe abscess into the pericardium with pericardial and left pleural effusion—pericardial rupture of liver abscess.

Structure of Hydatid Cyst

The hydatid cyst is a trilaminated structure consisting of the pericyst, the ectocyst and the endocyst respectively. The pericyst is the outermost protective layer and comprises of modified host cells. The ectocyst allows passage of nutrients while the endocyst forms the true layer of the cyst, also known as the inner germinal layer. Daughter vesicles (brood capsules) that resemble a bunch of grapes arise from the inner germinal layer. Since the vesicles contain scolices, when they rupture the scolices pass to the cyst fluid forming a white sediment known as hydatid sand.[61]

Clinical Features

Classical symptoms of hydatid disease include abdominal pain and hepatomegaly. The majority may be asymptomatic and are discovered incidentally.

Imaging Features

Plain Film

Calcification is seen in 20–30% of hepatic hydatids, is usually seen in a curvilinear or a ring like pattern where the pericyst calcifies. Calcification of the pericyst, however, does not signify the death of the parasite which is usually represented by a dense complete calcification of the cyst.

Ultrasound

The sonographic patterns vary depending on the stage of evolution and maturity.

A well-defined anechoic cyst **(Fig. 29)** or a cyst with hydatid sand may be seen. The hydatid sand is seen as multiple echogenic foci within the cyst in a dependent position. Detachment of the endocyst from the pericyst may be either partial or complete. A partial detachment may produce a localized split in the cyst. Membranes are seen as serpentine, linear structures within the cyst giving rise to the "floating membranes" sign **(Fig. 30)**. An 'US water lily sign' is similar to the radiographic water lily sign seen in case of pulmonary hydatids.[62,63] A characteristic "honeycomb" pattern of cysts enclosed within cyst is seen in case of multiple daughter cysts from the germinal layer **(Fig. 31)**. The multiple septa seen represent the walls of the daughter cysts. A hydatid matrix of mixed echogenicity containing scolices, hydatid sand, membranes of broken daughter vesicles may be seen. Partial or complete

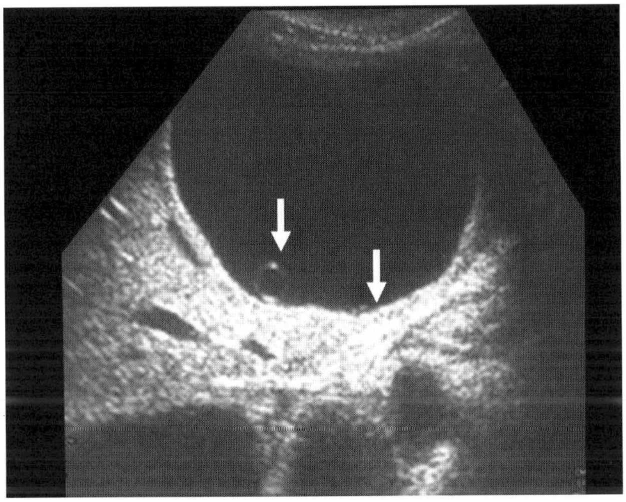

FIG. 29: US scan showing a well-defined anechoic cyst with a small cyst within—hydatid cyst.

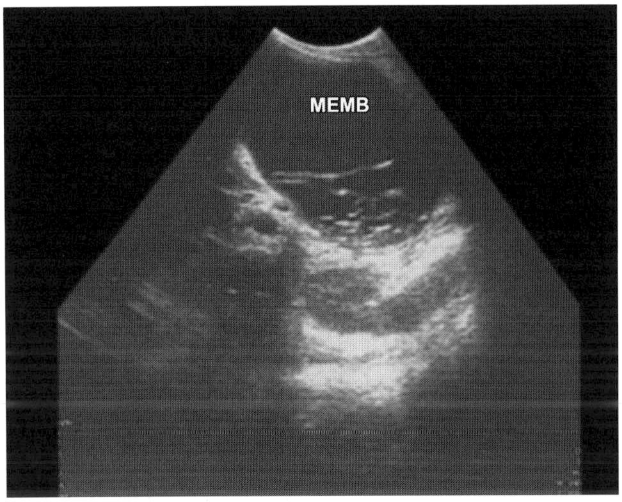

FIG. 30: US scan showing membranes as serpentine linear structures floating within a hydatid cyst.

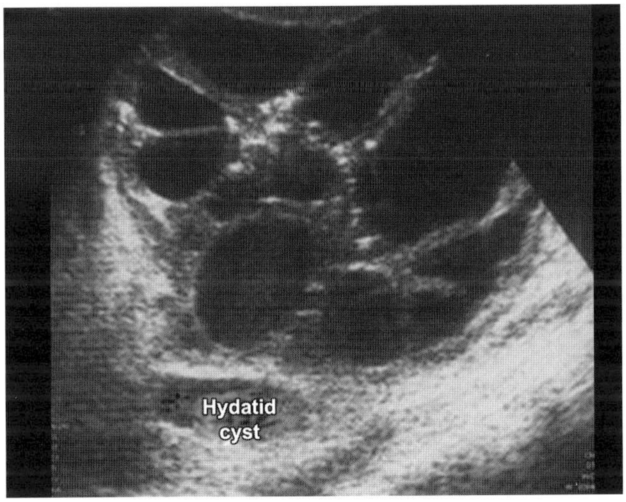

FIG. 31: US scan showing a characteristic appearance of cysts enclosed within a cyst giving rise to honeycomb pattern seen in a hydatid cyst.

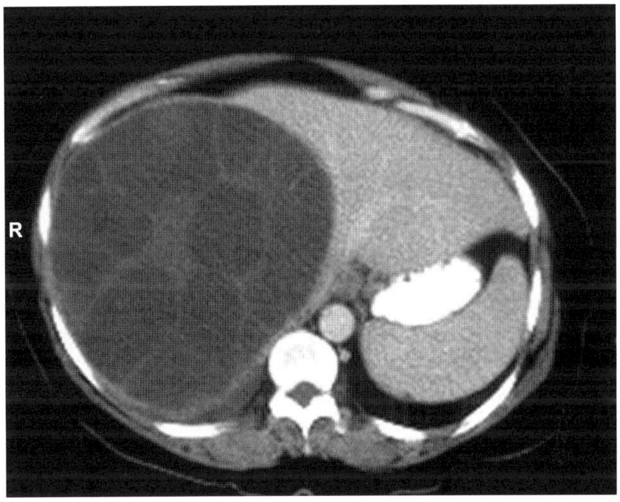

FIG. 32: CT scan showing the honeycomb pattern in a hydatid cyst with the multiple septae representing the walls of daughter cysts.

calcification of the cyst wall may occur and may be seen as hyperechoic contour with acoustic shadowing. Hydatid cysts may become diffusely hyperechoic once infected and lose their characteristic sonographic appearance.

USG has been used to monitor the response to medical treatment. A reduction in the size, membrane detachment, mural calcification and increased echogenicity all indicate a favourable response to the treatment.

CT

On CT scans hydatid cysts have a density of near water attenuation. Daughter cysts when present give the lesions a multilocular appearance or a honeycomb appearance with the multiple septa representing the walls of daughter cyst.[64] The fluid in the daughter cysts has a lower attenuation than that of the fluid in the mother cyst. On contrast administration, the cyst wall does not show enhancement. Only the internal septae enhance **(Fig. 32)**.

Detachment of the laminated membrane from the pericyst can be visualized as linear areas of increased attenuation or the membranes may be free floating within the cyst **(Fig. 33)**. Calcification in the cyst wall is also easily detected by CT scan **(Figs. 34A and B)**.

MRI

Hydatid cysts appear as hypointense on T1W images and hyperintense on T2W images. The hydatid fluid and sand have a high signal on T2W images.[65] A characteristic imaging finding on MRI is the presence of a low signal intensity rim on both T1- and T2W-images surrounding the cyst as the pericyst is rich in collagen. The internal architecture or the honeycomb pattern is also well seen on MRI **(Figs. 35A and B)**.[66] Floating membranes are seen as linear low signal intensity structures within the cyst. Degenerated cysts decrease in size and appear heterogeneous, solid or pseudotumor like.

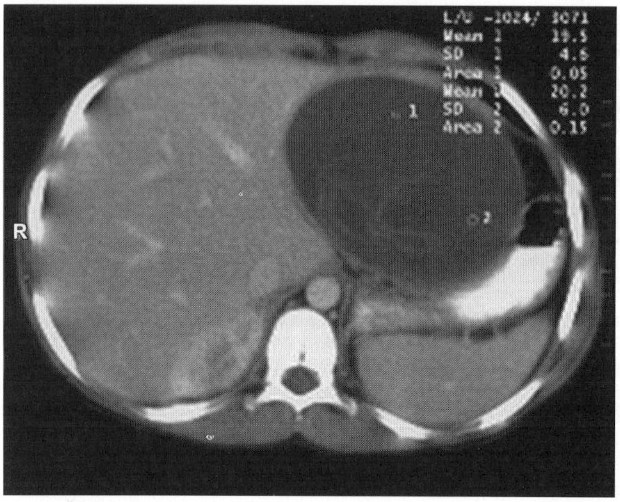

FIG. 33: Contrast-enhanced CT scan (CECT) showing detachment of the laminated membrane from the pericyst seen as linear areas of increased attenuation within the hydatid cyst.

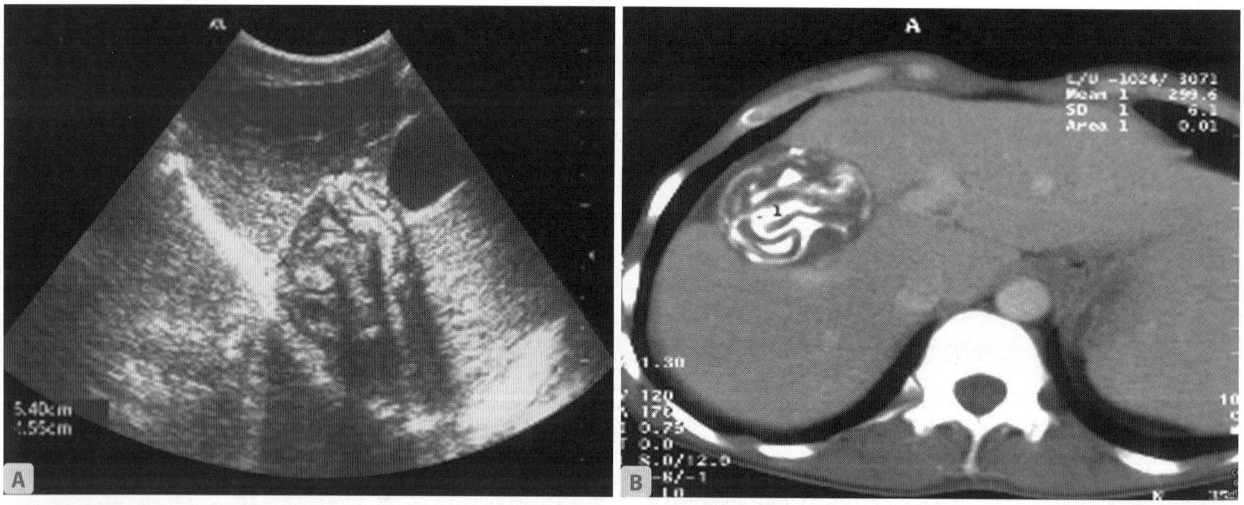

FIGS. 34A AND B: US (A) showing dense acoustic shadowing representing calcification in a hydatid cyst. CT (B) showing lamellar calcification in the membranes of the hydatid—calcified hydatid.

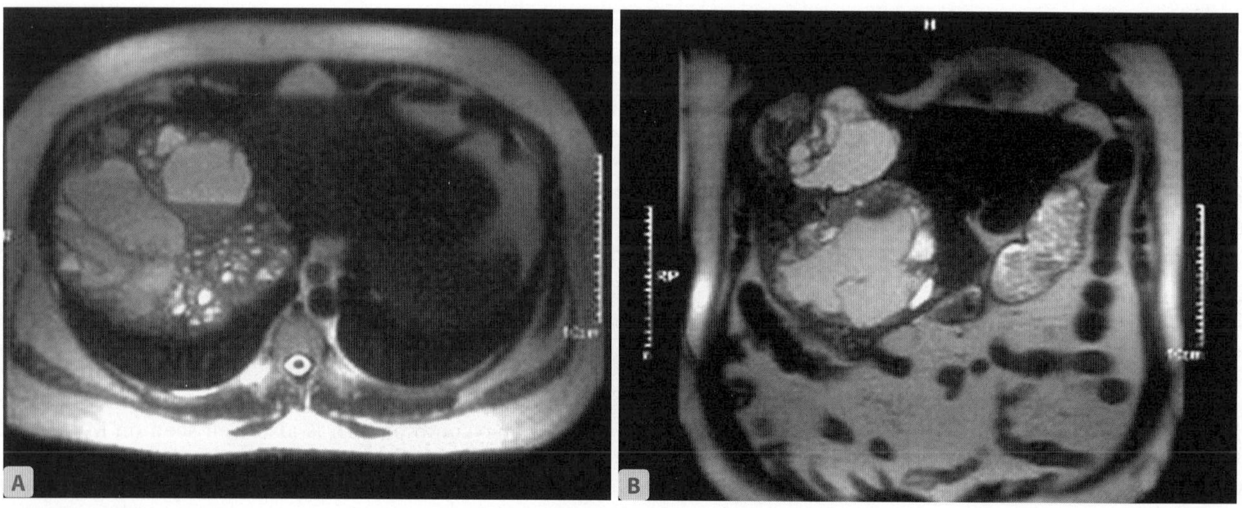

FIGS. 35A AND B: Axial (A) and coronal (B) MR images showing hepatic hydatids with multiple daughter cysts within appearing hyperintense on the T2-weighted images.

COMPLICATIONS OF HYDATID CYSTS

Intrahepatic Complications

These include cyst rupture and infection. In direct cyst rupture there is free spillage of the hydatid material into the peritoneal, pleural or visceral cavity. A direct cyst rupture can occur when both the pericyst and endocyst rupture in contrast to a contained rupture where only the endocyst ruptures and the pericyst remains intact. A passage of cyst contents into the biliary tree constitutes a communicating rupture.[67] On MR imaging rupture will be seen as interruption of the low signal intensity rim of the cyst wall and extension of the contents through the defect. Infection in the hydatid cyst can occur only when both the pericyst and endocyst rupture. Findings suggestive of an infection include a solid appearance, mixed pattern consisting of solid and fluid contents or air or air fluid levels within.

Peritoneal Seeding/Peritoneal Hydatidosis

Peritoneal seeding usually occurs secondary to hepatic hydatid disease through isolated cases of primary peritoneal echinococcosis can occur. The peritoneal cavity may be involved in 13% of the cases. Cysts are usually multiple, of varying sizes and may be located anywhere in the peritoneal cavity **(Figs. 36A to C)**.[68] An encapsulated multiloculated mass may be seen when the peritoneal hydatid disease grows and occupies the entire peritoneal cavity **(Figs. 37A to C)**.

Biliary Communication

The direct sign of rupture into the biliary tree is the visualization of the communication between the cyst wall and biliary radicles or the passage of hydatid cyst material into the biliary tree **(Figs. 38A to D)**. US can demonstrate echogenic linear filling structures without posterior acoustic shadow whereas CT can demonstrate high attenuation material in the biliary radicles or common bile duct. An air-fluid level or fat-fluid level are the indirect signs of a biliary communication.[69]

Other Complications

Hydatid cysts may grow exophytically to involve the bare area of the liver and the gastro hepatic ligament. Transdiaphragmatic thoracic involvement may be seen as pleural effusion, pulmonary lesion or chronic bronchial fistulas. Sagittal and coronal MR imaging is best to demonstrate the diaphragmatic defect and the migration of the hydatid cyst through it.[70] Perforation into the hollow

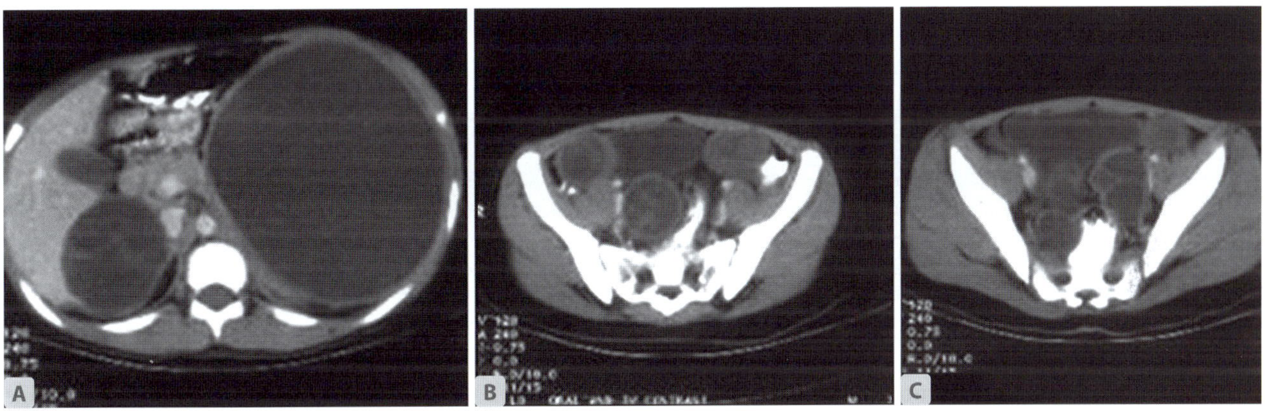

FIGS. 36A TO C: (A) CT scan showing hydatid cysts in the liver and spleen; (B and C) Multiple cysts of varying sizes seen in the peritoneal cavity—peritoneal seeding of hydatid cysts.

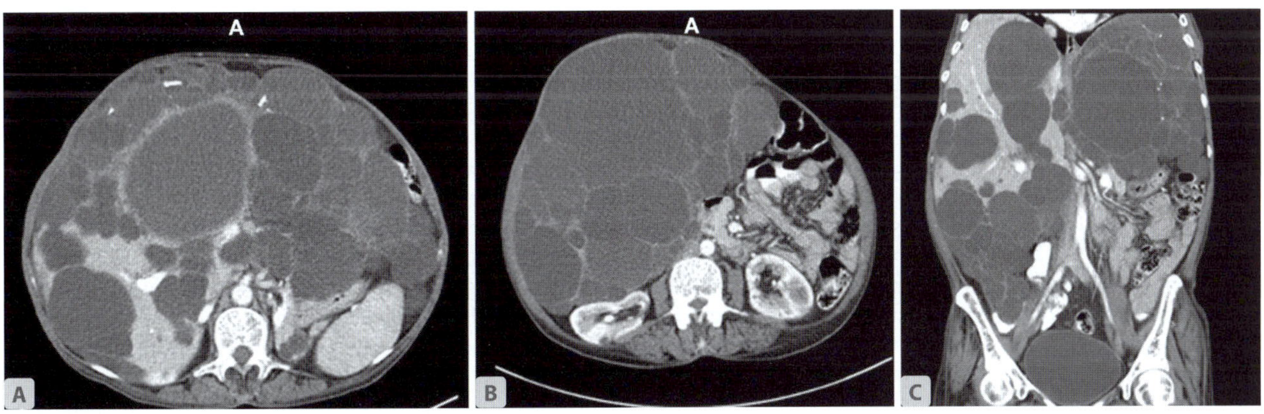

FIGS. 37A TO C: Contrast-enhanced CT scans revealing a multiloculated mass occupying the entire peritoneal cavity in addition to hydatid cysts within the liver—peritoneal hydatidosis.

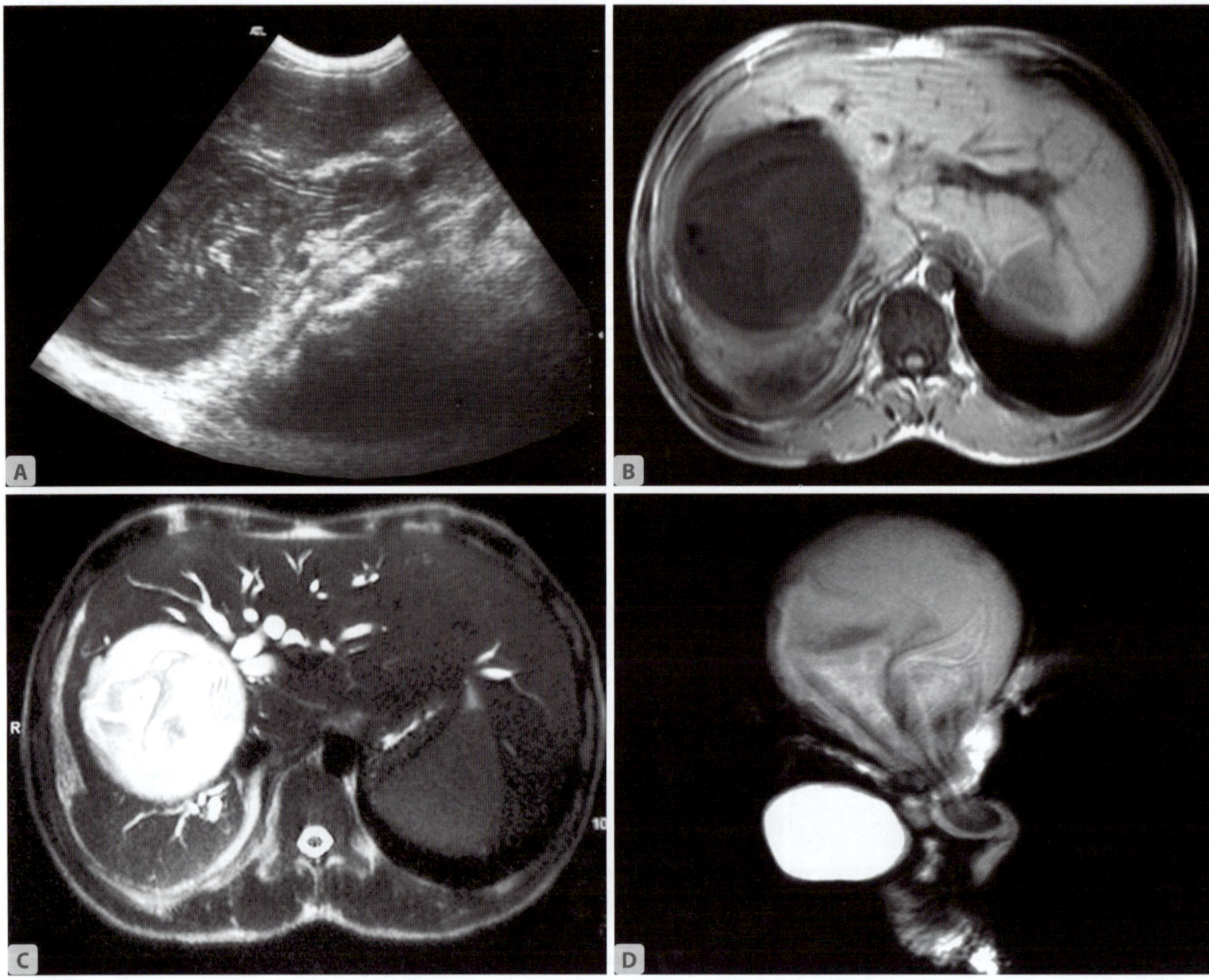

FIGS. 38A TO D: US (A) showing echogenic linear structures within the common bile duct. T1W (B) MR image showing the hydatid cyst as hypointense and T2W image (C) showing it as a hyperintense lesion with multiple linear low signal structures within s/o membranes. Passage of the cyst contents into the bile duct well depicted on the MRCP image—hydatid cyst with rupture into common bile duct.

viscera is an extremely rare complication seen in only 0.5% of cases. Patients may present with hydatidemesia or hydatidorrhea. Imaging may reveal an air-fluid level or orally administered contrast material inside the hollow viscus.[71] A portal cavernoma formation due to compression of the portal vein with secondary thrombosis is a rare complication. It is usually caused by hydatid cysts located in the caudate lobe.[72] Involvement of the abdominal wall may occur due to a direct communication between the cyst and the abdominal wall. An hour glass configuration may be seen due to the cysts passing through a small orifice.

HEPATIC ALVEOLAR ECHINOCOCCOSIS

The causative organism is *Echinococcus multilocularis*. It has a tendency to produce multilocular cysts anywhere in the organ or tissue with the liver being the most common site. Histologically, these cysts resemble alveoli rather than true cysts unlike hydatid cysts. These are usually 1–10 mm in diameter but may grow as large as 15–20 cm. They are usually solitary, multilocular or confluent.[73] The echinococcal cysts involve large regions of the hepatic parenchyma with an affinity for the porta hepatis with resultant portal hypertension and bile duct stenosis. Irregular margins, cystic and solid components and an in homogeneous enhancement pattern characterize the imaging appearances. Calcification begins in a scattered manner initially but eventually these become large calcified masses.

HEPATIC TUBERCULOSIS

Tuberculosis is a major cause of mortality and morbidity in the tropical countries and its incidence is increasing with the emergence of HIV and AIDS. Hepatic tuberculosis accounts for <1% of all tubercular infections,[74] being uncommon due to the low oxygen tension in the liver. The most common route of spread to the liver is hematogenous secondary to a tubercular focus elsewhere in the body resulting in a miliary pattern. Spread can also occur via the portal vein in cases of involvement of the gastrointestinal tract or via the lymphatic route in case of rupture of tuberculous lymph node along the portal tract.

Pathology

The histological hallmark of the disease is granuloma formation. Both caseating and noncaseating granulomas are seen. Presence of caseating epithelioid granuloma on histopathology is diagnostic of the disease.

Clinical Features

The disease may present at any age but is more common in young adults. Patients may present with high grade fever, weight loss, anorexia and upper abdominal pain. Rarely, patients may present with jaundice owing to biliary obstruction caused by periportal adenopathy.

Imaging Features

The disease can be classified into three forms: The parenchymal, serohepatic and tubercular cholangitis. The parenchymal form can be further subdivided as the micronodular and the macronodular pattern.[75]

Micronodular Form

This is the most common form of hepatic tuberculosis and usually occurs secondary to hematogenous dissemination.[76] A concomitant involvement of the lung may or may not be seen. The miliary hepatic lesions are randomly distributed throughout the hepatic parenchyma, are usually small in size and multiple. These may be at times, too small to be resolved by sonography and hepatomegaly may be the only imaging finding seen. A diffuse hypoechoic pattern of the liver parenchyma may be seen on sonography as the lesions are hypoechoic to the adjacent parenchyma.

On CT, the micronodular pattern is seen as microabscesses having a central hypodensity with peripheral rim enhancement on administration of contrast. This imaging appearance may mimic metastases, leukemic infiltration, lymphoma or fungal infections. Chronic lesions may calcify and the lesions may be seen as multiple echogenic foci with distal acoustic shadow on sonography or as multiple calcific foci on CT.

Macronodular Form

The macronodular form is less common than the micronodular variety.[77] Tubercular macronodules are also called pseudotumoral TB, tuberculomas or tubercular abscesses. These macronodules form as a result of conglomeration of miliary granulomas and may be seen as solitary or multiple complex hepatic masses. When solitary, the macronodular form may mimic a primary neoplastic lesion or other infective lesions. A "cluster sign" representing coalescence of multiple micronodular lesions into a macronodular lesion seen as a multiloculated cystic mass or a "target sign" representing a focus of calcification or enhancement in the center surrounded by low attenuation edema is highly suggestive but not pathognomonic of tubercular involvement.[78] At times, image guided biopsy is required for a definite histological diagnosis.[77]

Serohepatic Tuberculosis

This rare variety gives rise to a "frosted liver" owing to a predominant involvement of the subserosal plane of the liver. Imaging reveals multiple peripherally located conglomerated hypodense lesions with an overlying thickened enhancing capsule simulating sugar coating.[75] There may be associated bulky necrotic gastrohepatic and retroperitoneal adenopathy.

Tubercular Cholangitis

This can occur due to primary involvement of the biliary tree due to an extrinsic compression by periportal lymph nodes. Findings may vary from bile duct thickening, biliary dilatation and strictures with resultant obstructive biliopathy.[79]

HEPATIC SARCOIDOSIS

Liver involvement may be seen in 40–70% of patients with systemic sarcoidosis. The lesions are usually too small to be resolved by sonography and sarcoidosis may be seen as non-specific diffuse parenchymal heterogeneity, an increased parenchymal echogenicity or coarsening of the liver echotexture. CT and MRI will show the lesions as having a low attenuation with no enhancement seen on the post-contrast images.[74]

HEPATIC SCHISTOSOMIASIS

It is a serious parasitic infection of the humans usually having a chronic and insidious course. Hepatic involvement can occur due to *Schistosoma japonicum*, *Schistosoma mansoni* or *Schistosoma haematobium* infection. Patients may present with hematemesis due to portal hypertension or hematuria due to involvement of the urinary tract. Plain X-ray of the abdomen may show splenomegaly. Sonography may show periportal echogenicity due to fibrosis. Splenomegaly, collaterals and free fluid, i.e. features of portal hypertension can be seen. CT—A capsular or peripheral hepatic calcification is seen which is considered to be a hallmark of *Schistosoma japonicum* infection. Periportal areas of fibrosis may be seen as low density areas within the porta. Pseudoseptations within the liver, bands of calcification and liver notching are also characteristic imaging findings. MRI may show features of portal hypertension and low signal area within the porta due to fibrosis. Patients with schistosomiasis may develop hepatocellular carcinoma.

MISCELLANEOUS LESIONS

Fatty Infiltration

Fatty infiltration of the liver is a common occurrence resulting from increased deposition of triglyceride in hepatocytes. This arises from a variety of nutritional disturbances or toxic insults to the liver. These include obesity, nutritional deficiencies, diabetes mellitus, pregnancy, steroids, hepatotoxic drugs and alcoholism. The development of fatty infiltration is a dynamic process and changes may be seen in a few weeks of an insult and may regress within days. Most characteristically, the fatty involvement is uniform or geographic in distribution. However, occasionally it may be nodular or multifocal when it is indistinguishable from other focal hepatic lesions. Features suggesting the true nature of the process are sharp angular boundaries to the lesions and no evidence of displacement or effacement of venous structures. Chemical shift imaging on MRI will show focal fatty infiltration as an area of signal drop on the opposed phase images as compared to the in phase images.

Another well-recognized variant is focal sparing of small areas of normal liver in a more generalized fatty infiltration. The spared area appears as an echo-poor focal mass. A characteristic location for the spared area is the quadrate lobe anterior to the portal vein bifurcation or related to the gallbladder bed. The shape of the spared area or pseudomass is typically ovoid. Its location has led to the suggestion that the sparing relates to alteration of blood flow in this area.

Hematoma

The most common causes of hematoma are surgery and trauma. Hepatic lacerations, rib fractures and free fluid favor the diagnosis of a post-traumatic hematoma while iatrogenic hematoma usually occurs along a surgical plane. An intra or perihepatic hematoma can also occur due to bleeding in a hepatocellular adenoma. The CT appearance of a hematoma depends on the age of the blood products. While acute and subacute hematomas have a higher attenuation value due to aggregated fibrin components, a chronic hematoma has a fluid attenuation. On MRI subacute hematomas show a hyperintense signal on both T1- and T2-weighted images.[80] Gradient echo images are very sensitive for the detection of blood products.

Biloma

A rupture of the biliary system can produce bilomas. These can occur spontaneously, owing to trauma or following surgery. They can occur in an intrahepatic or perihepatic location. Pseudocapsule formation occurs due to the intense inflammatory reaction induced due to bile extravasation. On imaging bilomas appear as well defined cystic lesions within the porta. No septations or calcification are usually seen **(Figs. 39A to C)**. Clinical history, the location and imaging appearance helps in establishing the diagnosis.

Peliosis Hepatis

Peliosis hepatis is a benign vascular lesion characterized by sinusoidal dilatation and blood filled hepatic spaces. In 50% of cases, no cause can be found. In the remaining, the causative factors range from toxins (arsenic, PVC), drugs (steroids, oral contraceptives) to infections (*Bartonella*, tuberculous bacillus) and malignancies (HCC), renal and cardiac transplantation and diabetes.[80] A variable echogenicity with internal vascularity is seen on ultrasound. On noncontrast CT scans, a hypoattenuating area with an early brisk enhancement is noted on the postcontrast scans. Peliosis hepatis on MR is seen to be typically hypointense on T1 and hyperintense on T2W images.

Inflammatory Pseudotumor

Inflammatory pseudotumor (IPT) is a benign lesion consisting of inflammatory cells and fibrosis.[80] These may occur at all ages, they are more common in the young. Though the exact etiopathogenesis is unknown, it is postulated that they may occur secondary to an inciting hepatic infection. At US, inflammatory pseudotumors may appear as heterogeneous hyperechoic lesions with increased through transmission. These are seen as large hypoattenuating lesions on noncontrast CT. Contrast-enhanced CT reveals central hypodensity with thick peripheral hyperdensity **(Figs. 40A and B)**. The appearance may mimic a necrotic malignant mass. The hypodense center corresponds to inflammatory infiltrates while the hyperdense periphery corresponds to fibroblastic proliferation. The lesions are typically hypointense on T1W and hyperintense on T2W images.Contrast MRI reveals intense enhancement of the lesions with rapid washout and periportal involvement. It is difficult to differentiate this condition from a primary or metastatic neoplasm and biopsy may be required.[80]

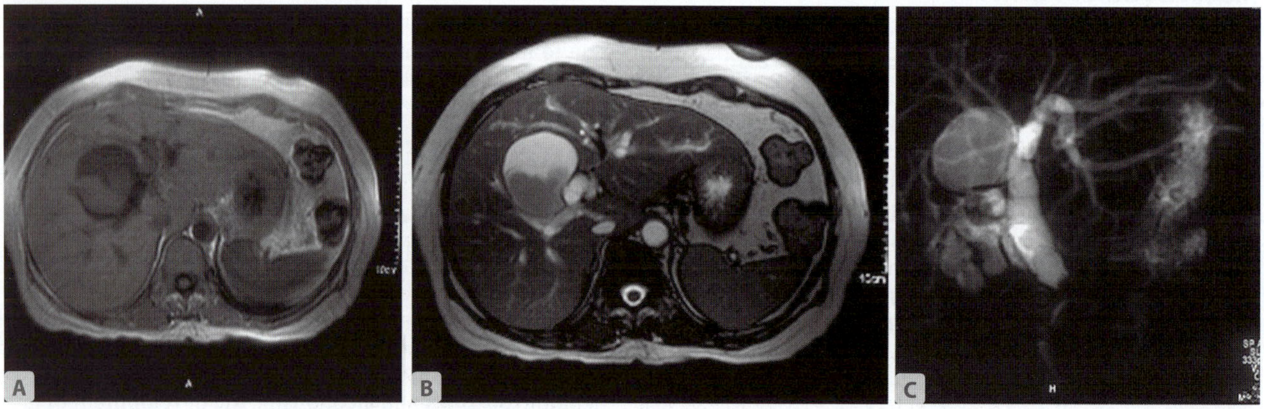

FIGS. 39A TO C: (A) MR image in a postcholecystectomy patient showing a well-defined hypointense lesion in the gallbladder fossa s/o biloma; (B) T2-weighted MR images shows a hyperintense signal in the cyst with a fluid-fluid level (due to inspissated bile/sludge); (C) MRCP image depicting the biloma.

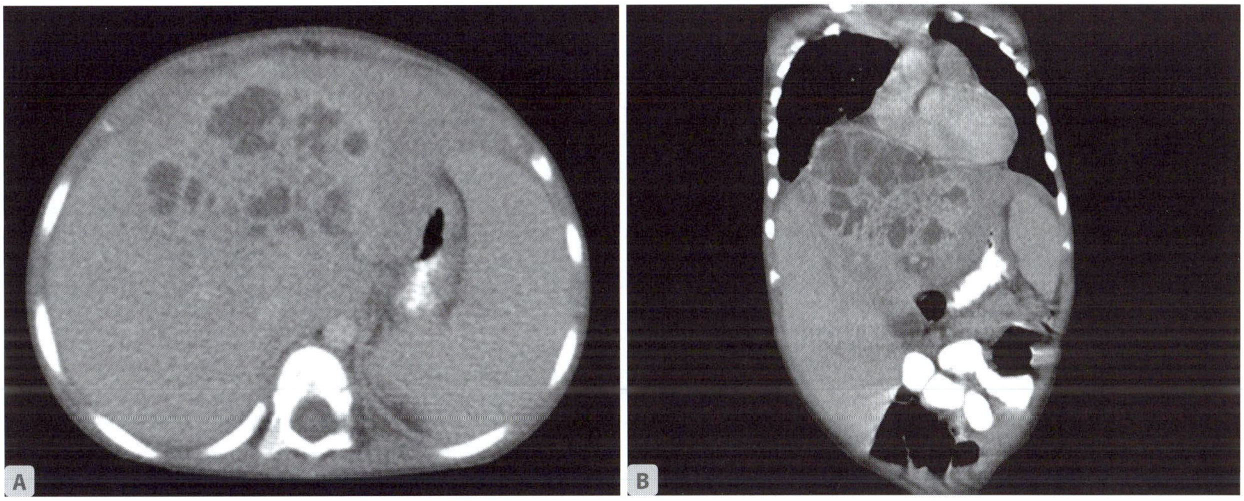

FIGS. 40A AND B: Contrast-enhanced CT reveals a mass with central hypodensity and thick peripheral hyperdensity in a child—inflammatory pseudotumor.

CONCLUSION

There are myriad benign hepatic lesions; however the majority often display fairly specific imaging characteristics which allow a confident diagnosis. Atypical manifestations and the less familiar rarer benign tumors may pose a diagnostic challenge. An accurate patient history and relevant clinical data are important. Advances in imaging techniques such as diffusion-weighted magnetic resonance (DWMR) imaging, chemical shift imaging and the use of hepatocyte specific MR contrast agents allow a better understanding of the lesion itself and allow for an improved lesion diagnosis.

REFERENCES

1. Ata Soy C, Akyar S. Multidetector CT contributions in liver imaging. Eur Radiol. 2004;52:2-17.
2. Winterer JT, Kotter E, Ghanem M. Detection and characterization of bengin focal liver lesions with multislice CT. Eur Radiol. 2006;16:2427-43.
3. Ros PR. Focal liver masses other than metastases. In categorical course on gastrointestinal radiology. Oak Brook III, RSNA Publications; 1999.
4. Van Sonnenberg E, Wroblicka JT, D'Agostino HB, et al. Symptomatic hepatic cysts: Percutaneous drainage and sclerosis. Radiology. 1994;190:387-92.
5. Dewbury KC. Benign focal liver lesions. In: Meire H, Cosgrove D, Dewbery K, et al (Eds). Abdominal and General Ultrasound (2nd edn) Churchill Livingstone; 2001.
6. Blumke DA, Fishman EK. Spiral CT of liver tumors. In: Fishman EK, Jeffrey RB (Eds). Spiral CT Principles, Techniques and Clinical Application (2nd edn) Lippincott Raven, 1998.
7. Mathieu D, Vilgrain V, Mahfouz A, et al. Benign liver tumors. Mag Reson Imaging Clin N Am. 1997;5:255-88.
8. Vachha B, Sun M, RM, Siewert B, et al. Cystic lesions of the liver. AJR. 2011;196:W 355-66.
9. Borhani AA, Wiant A, Heller MT. Cystic Hepatic Lesions: A review and an algorithmic approach. AJR. 2014;203:1192-1204.
10. Oto A, Tamm EP, Szklaruk J. Multidetector Row CT of the Liver Radiol Clin N Am. 2005;43:827-48.
11. Palacois E, Shannon M, Solomon C, et al. Biliary cystadenoma: Ultrasound, CT and MRI. Gastrointest Radiol. 1990;15:313-16.
12. Ba Ssalamah A, Baroud S, Bastati N, et al. MR Imaging of Benign Focal Liver Lesions. Mag Reson Imaging Clin N Am. 2010;18:403-19.
13. Matos AP, Velloni F, Ramalho, et al. Focal Liver lesions. Practical magnetic resonance imaging approach. World J Hepatol. 2015;16:1987-2008.
14. Birnbaum BA. Benign tumors of the liver: Hepatic haemangiomas. In: Margulis Burhennes (Eds) Alimentary Tract Radiology (5th edn), 1994.
15. Brannigan M, Burns PN, Wilson SR. Blood flow patterns in focal liver lesions at Microbubble enhanced US. Radiographics. 2004;24:921-35.
16. Powers C, Ros PR. Hepatic mass lesions. In: Haaga JR, Kanzieri CF, Gilkeson RC (Eds). CT and MR Imaging of the Whole Body (4th edn) Mosby, 2003.
17. Hanfusa K, Ohashi I, Himenso Y, et al. Hepatic haemangioma: Findings with two phase CT. Radiology. 1995;196:465.
18. Yu JS, Kim MJ, Kim KW, et al. Hepatic cavernous haemangioma: Sonographic pattern and speed of contrast enhancement on multiphase Dynamic MR Imaging AJR. 1998;71:1021-5.
19. Counbaras M, Weudum D, Cholley LM, et al. CT and MR Imaging features of pathologically proven Atypical Giant Haemangiomas of the liver. AJR. 2002;179:1457-63.
20. Danet IM, Semelka RC, Braga L, et al. Giant haemangioma of the liver: MR imaging characteristics in 24 patients. Magnetic Resonance Imaging. 2003;21:95-101.
21. Francisco FAF, Araújo ALE, Neto, et al. Hepatobiliary contrast agents: differential diagnosis of focal hepatic lesions, pitfalls and other indications. Radio Bras. 2014;47(5):301-9.
22. El-Badrawy A, Ashmallah GA, Tawfik Am, et al. Diffusion weight MR imaging of benign hepatic focal lesions. Open Journal of Radiology. 2014;4:136-43.

23. Kim TK, Jang HJ, Burns PN, Lavallee JM, Wilson SR. Focal Nodular hyperplasia and hepatic adenoma: differentiation with low mechanical index contrast enhanced sonography. Am J Roentgenol. 2008;190:58-66.
24. Brancatelli G, Federle MP, Katyal S, et al. Haemodynamic characterization of focal nodular Hyperplasia using three dimensional volume rendered multidetector CT angiography. AJR. 2002;179:81-5.
25. Macky MD, Frazer C, deBoer WB. Magnetic resonance features of focal nodular hyperplasia of the liver. Australasian Radiology. 1999;43:315-20.
26. Elsayes KM, Narra VR, Yin, et al. Focal hepatic lesions. Diagnostic value of enhancement pattern approach with contrast enhanced 3D gradient echo MR imaging. Radiographics. 2005;25:1299-1320.
27. Grazioli L, Morana G, Federle M, et al. Focal nodular hyperplasia: Morphologic and functional information from MR Imaging with Gadobenate Dimeglumine. Radiology. 2001;221: 731-9.
28. Ba Ssalamah A, Schima W, Schmook MT, et al. Atypical focal nodular hyperplasia of the liver: Imaging features of nonspecific and liver specific MR contrast agents. AJR. 2002;179:1447-56.
29. Beets Tan RGH, Van Engelshoven JMA, Greve JWM. Hepatic adenoma and focal nodular hyperplasia: MR findings with superparamagnetic iron oxide enhanced MRI. Clin Imaging. 1998;22:211-5.
30. Grazioli L, Federle MP, Ichikawa T, et al. Liver adenomatosis: Clinical, histopathologic, and imaging findings in 15 patients. Radiology. 2000;216:395-402.
31. Anderson SW, Kruskal JB, Kane RA, et al. Benign hepatic tumors and iatrogenic pseudotumors. Radiographics. 2009;29:211-99.
32. Cogley JR, Miller FH. MR Imaging of Benign Focal Liver Lesions. Radiol Clin N Am. *http//dx.doi.org*/10, 1016/ j. cl 2014.
33. Catalano O, Nunziata A, LobiancoR, Siani A. Real time harmonic contrast material specific US of focal liver lesions. Radiographics. 2005;25:333-49.
34. Horton KM, Blumke DA, Hruban RH, et al. CT and MR imaging of benign hepatic and biliary tumors. Radiographics. 1999; 19:431-51.
35. Tajima T, Honda H, Kuroiwa T, et al. Radiologic features of intrahepatic bile duct Adenoma: A look at the surface of the liver. J Comput Assist Tomography. 1999;23(5):690-5.
36. King LJ, Burkill GJC, Scurr ED, et al. Mn DPDP enhanced magnetic resonance imaging of focal liver lesions. Clinical Radiology. 2002;57:1047-57.
37. Bartolozzi C, Cioni D, Donati F, et al. Focal liver lesions: MR imaging—Pathologic correlation. Eur Radiol. 2001;11:1374-88.
38. Caraiani C, Chiorean L, Fenesan DI, et al. Diffusion weighted magnetic resonance imaging for the classification of Liver Lesions as Benign or Malignant. J Gastrointest. Liver Dis. 2015;24: 309-17.
39. Rha SE, Lee MG, Lee YS, et al. Nodular regenerative hyperplasia of the liver in Budd–Chiari Syndrome: CT and MR features. Abdom Imaging. 2000;25:255-8.
40. Quglia A, Tibballs J, Grasso A, et al. Focal nodular hyperplasia like areas in cirrhosis. Histopathology. 2003;42:14-21.
41. Krinsky GA, Lee VS, Nguyen MT, et al. Siderotic nodules at MR Imaging: Regenerative or Dysplastic J Comput Assist Tomography. 2000;24:773-6.
42. Bris FE, Bao Do AK, et al. Classification of hypervascular liver lesions based on hepatic artery and portal vein blood supply coefficients calculated from triphasic CT scans. Journal of Digital Imaging. 2015;28:213-33.
43. Ros PR, Goodman ZD, Ishak KG, et al. Mesenchymal hamartoma of the liver: Radiologic pathologic correlation. Radiology. 1986;158:619-24.
44. Ishak KG, Kabin L. Benign tumors of the liver. Med Clin North Am. 1975;59:995-1013.
45. Stanley P, Hall TR, Woolley MM, et al. Mesenchymal hamartomas of the liver in childhood: sonographic and CT findings. AJR. 1986;147:1035-9.
46. O'Neil J, Ros PR. Knowing hepatic pathology aids MRI of liver tumors. Diagn Imaging. 1989;11:58-65.
47. Ros PR, Rasmussew JF, Li KCP. Radiology of malignant and benign liver tumors. Curr Probl Diagn Radiol. 1989;18:95-155.
48. Srivastava DN, Mahajan A, Berry M, et al. Colour Doppler flow imaging of focal hepatic lesions. Australasian Radiology. 2000;44:285-9.
49. Keslar PJ, Buck JL, Selky DM. Infantile haemangioendothelioma of the liver revisited. Radiographics. 1993;13:657-70.
50. Prasad SR, Wang H, Rosas H, et al. Fat containing lesions of the liver: radiologic—pathologic correlation. Radiographics. 2005;25:321-31.
51. Brandborg LL, Goldman IS. Bacterial and miscellaneous infections of the liver. In: Zakim D, Boyer TD (Eds). Hepathology Philadelphia, WB Saunders, 1990.
52. Adeyiga AO, Lee EY, Eisenberg RL. Focal Hepatic Masses in Pediatric Patients. AJR. 2012;199:W422-40.
53. Halvovsen RA, Korobkin M, Foster WL, et al. The variable CT appearance of hepatic abscesses. AJR. 1984;141:941-6.
54. Jeffrey RB, Tolentino CS, Chang FC, et al. CT of small pyogenic hepatic abscesses: The cluster sign. AJR. 1988;151:487-9.
55. Balci NC, Semelhar RC, Noone TC, et al. Pyogenic hepatic abscesses: MRI findings on T1 and T2 weighted and serial Gadolinuim Enhanced Gradient Echo Images. J Magn Reson Imaging. 1999;9:285-90.
56. Gupta RK. Amoebic liver abscess. a report of 1000 cases. Int Surg. 1984;69:261-4.
57. Philips RL. Computed tomography and ultrasound in the diagnosis and treatment of liver abscesses. Australasian Radiology. 1994;38:165-69.
58. Radin DR, Ralls PW, Colletti PM, et al. CT of amoebic liver abscess. AJR. 1988;150:1297-1301.
59. Juimo AG, Gervez F, Angwafo FF. Extraintestinal amoebiasis. Radiology. 1992;182:181.
60. Shirkhoda A. CT findings in hepatosplenic and renal candidiasis. J Comput Assist Tomogr. 1987;11:795-8.
61. Beggs I. The radiology of hydatid disease. AJR. 1985;145:639-48.
62. Marti–Bonmati L, Menor Serrano F. Complications of hepatic hydatid cysts: Ultrasound, computed tomography and magnetic resonance diagnosis. Gastrointest Radiol. 1990;15: 119-25.
63. Von Sinner WN. New diagnostic sign in hydatid disease: Radiography, ultrasound, CT and MRI correlated to pathology. Eur J Radiol. 1990;12:150-9.
64. Pedroza I, Saiz A, Arrazola J, et al. Hydatid disease; Radiologic and pathologic features and complications. Radiographics. 2000;20:795-817.
65. Davolio SA, Canossi GC, Nicoli FA, et al. Hydatid disease: MR imaging study. Radiology. 1990;175:701-6.
66. Agildere AM, Aytekin C, Coskun M, et al. MRI of hydatid disease of the Liver: A variety of sequences J. Comput Assist Tomography. 1998;22(5):718-24.
67. De Diego J, Lecumberri FJ, Franquet T, et al. Computed tomography in hepatic echinococcosis. AJR. 1982;139:699-702.
68. Karavias DD, Vagianos CE, Kakkos SK, et al. Peritoneal echinococcosis. World J Surg. 1996;20:337-40.
69. Mendez JV, Arrazola J, Lopej J, et al. Fat–fluid level in hepatic hydatid cyst: A new sign of rupture into the biliary tree? AJR. 1996;167:91-4.

70. Gomez R, Moreno E, Loinaz C, et al. Diaphragmatic or transdiaphragmatic thoracic involvement in hepatic hydatid disease surgical trends and classification. World J Surg. 1995;19: 714-9.
71. Jain R, Sawhney S, Berry M. Hydatid disease: CT demonstration and follow-up of a cystogastric fistula. AJR. 1992;158:212.
72. Gil–Egea MJ, Alameda F, Girvent M, et al. Hydatid cyst in the hepatic hilum causing a cavernous transformation in the portal vein. Gastroenterol Hepatol. 1998;21:227-9.
73. Choji K, Fujita N, Chen M, et al. Alveolar hydatid disease of the liver: Computed tomography and transabdominal ultrasound with histopathological correlation. Clin Radiology. 1992;46: 97-103.
74. Chong V. Hepatobiliary tuberculosis: a review of presentations and outcomes. South Med J. 2008;101:356-61.
75. Yu RS, Zhang SZ, Wu JJ, et al. Imaging diagnosis of 12 patients with hepatic tuberculosis. World J Gastroenterol. 2004;10(11): 1639-42.
76. Tatco UR, Margarita AM, Santos M, et al. The many faces of Hepatic tuberculosis. WFPITB Corner. 2015;2:1-6.
77. Kakkar C, Polnaya AM, Koteshwara P, et al. Hepatic tuberculosis: a multimodality imaging review. Insights Imaging. 2015; 6:647-58.
78. Burrill J, William CJ, Bain G, et al. Tuberculosis: A Radiologic Review. Radiographics. 2007;27:1255-73.
79. Chong VH, Lim KS. Hepatobiliary tuberculosis. Singap Med J. 2010;51:744-51.
80. Alobaidi M, Shirkhoda A. Benign Focal Liver Lesions: Discrimination from malignant mimickers. Curr Probl Diagn Radiol. 2004;33:239-53.

CHAPTER

103

Malignant Focal Lesions of Liver

Raju Sharma, Kumble S Madhusudhan

INTRODUCTION

Imaging of the liver has undergone a paradigm shift during the last decade due to significant advances in technology and new contrast agents. This has led to greater understanding and better management of many diseases which affect the liver. The advent of ultrasound and MR elastography, dual energy CT and new MRI sequences and contrast agents (e.g. Gadoxetic acid) have increased the sensitivity for detection and accuracy for characterization of liver lesions.[1,2] Clinical information continues to be of paramount importance as it helps to tailor the imaging technique and narrows the differential diagnosis.

Malignant focal lesions of the liver are classified according to WHO as follows:[3]

- *Primary*:
  - *Hepatocellular tumors*:
    - Hepatocellular carcinoma (HCC)
    - Hepatocellular carcinoma, fibrolamellar
    - Hepatoblastoma, epithelial variants
    - Undifferentiated carcinoma
  - *Malignancies of mixed origin*:
    - Hepatoblastoma, mixed epithelial-mesenchymal
    - Combined hepatocellular-cholangiocarcinoma
  - *Bile duct lesions*:
    - Intrahepatic cholangiocarcinoma
    - Intraductal papillary neoplasm with invasive carcinoma
    - Mucinous cystic neoplasm
  - *Malignant mesenchymal tumors*:
    - Epithelioid hemangioendothelioma (EHE)
    - Angiosarcoma
- *Secondary*:
  - Metastatic deposits
  - Lymphoma.

Metastasis to the liver from an extrahepatic malignancy is by far the most common cause of a malignant hepatic neoplasm. Hepatic metastases are particularly common from primary malignancies of the gastrointestinal tract, breast and lung.

IMAGING TECHNIQUES AND ADVANCES

The imaging techniques used in the evaluation of focal liver lesions include ultrasonography (USG), computed tomography (CT), magnetic resonance imaging (MRI) and positron emission tomography (PET). Although ultrasonography is the initial imaging modality, most of the patients need further characterization by either multiphase contrast-enhanced CT or MRI. PET-CT is used in staging of the disease in case of liver metastases and lymphoma but not for the characterization of liver lesions. Recent advances in imaging techniques and contrast agents have further improved the accuracy of imaging in characterization of liver lesions.[4]

Elastography is a technique to assess the stiffness of tissues. Here either an external or an internal force is applied and the displacements of the tissue are subsequently measured. Various ultrasound elastography (USE) techniques are available including transient elastography (TE; fibroscan), acoustic radiation force impulse (ARFI) and 2D shear wave elastography (SWE).[5] TE and SWE give results directly in kilopascals whereas ARFI gives it in m/s (speed). Color coding is also done for different areas with different stiffness. USE may help in differentiation of benign from malignant focal liver lesions. Contrast-enhanced USG (CEUS) is a valuable technique for detection and characterization of focal liver lesions. Sulfur hexafluoride (Sonovue) is the widely used USG contrast agent. After contrast injection, dynamic imaging is done to assess the contrast flow characteristics within the lesion. Its limitations include operator dependence, difficulty in evaluating deeper lesions, lack of complete 3-dimensional information and difficulty in evaluating multiple lesions. It is also used to guide biopsies of liver lesions and in assessment of completeness of ablation of liver tumors immediately after the procedure. Other upcoming applications are quantitative perfusion imaging and molecular imaging. In the former, a time-intensity curve is generated and is useful in lesion characterization and assessment of treatment response of liver tumors. A recent addition is liver specific contrast agent—perflubutane (Sonazoid) which is taken up by Kupffer cells and normal liver shows uniform enhancement in Kupffer phase (15–120 min after injection). Focal liver lesions not containing Kupffer cells are seen as hypoechoic area in this phase. Thus, this helps in lesion detection and characterization.

Perfusion computed tomography (PCT) is a technique in which microvasculature of the tissue can be assessed after injection of intravenous contrast.[6] Improvement in the technology has resulted in larger coverage, reduced motion artifacts and radiation dose. This technique evaluates the vascularity of various tumors in liver and assists in making a diagnosis. It is also useful assessing response of tumors to chemotherapy and evaluating recurrence.

Dual energy computed tomography (DECT) is a recent addition to the existing imaging modalities.[7] In this technique, scan is done both at low energy (100 kVp) and high energy (140 kVp). The data obtained is then used in generation of iodine maps, virtual noncontrast images and material decomposition. Low kV images help in improving liver lesion detection by increasing the contrast to noise ratio. Iodine maps are useful in depiction of tumor vascularity in the liver based on iodine maps and iodine ratio and thus helps in differentiation of hepatic cystic/necrotic tumors from simple cysts and in assessing treatment response of tumors.[8]

MR elastography (MRE) is a technique similar to USE which uses shear waves to assess tissue stiffness.[4] Although, elastography is shown have role in differentiation of benign from malignant tumors, it is especially useful in differentiation of hepatic adenoma (softer) from focal nodular hyperplasia (stiffer) and hepatocellular carcinoma (softer) from cholangiocarcinoma (stiffer). They may also have a role in assessment of tumor response to chemotherapy. Liver specific MR contrast agents—Gadobenate dimeglumine and Gadoxetic acid are taken up by normal hepatocytes and excreted into the biliary tree in the hepatobiliary phase (60–90 min for gadobenate and 15–20 minutes for gadoxetic acid). Lesions not containing normal hepatocytes are seen as hypointense area. Thus, both these agents, in addition to initial dynamic contrast enhanced imaging, can be used in late phase imaging to improve lesion detection and characterization. Proton MR spectroscopy is also helpful in evaluation of focal liver lesions.[9] Studies have shown that malignant liver lesions show elevated choline compared to normal liver or benign lesions. Hepatocellular carcinomas after chemoembolization show reduction in choline on magnetic resonance spectroscopy and this may assist in evaluation of response. There is research still going on to improve the results by faster sequences, better hardware and faster processing.

PRIMARY MALIGNANT FOCAL LESIONS HEPATOCELLULAR CARCINOMA

Hepotocellular carcinoma (HCC) is the most common primary malignant neoplasm of the liver worldwide. The incidence varies, being more common in Africa and the far east. Etiology also varies among different population groups and the risk factors include hepatitis B and C infection, alcoholic cirrhosis, primary hemochromatosis, nonalcoholic fatty liver disease and exposure to carcinogens like aflatoxin. About 80% of cases of HCC arise in cirrhotic liver.[10] The 5-year cumulative HCC risk is 21% in hemochromatosis, 10% in hepatitis B virus infection, 8% in alcoholic cirrhosis and 5% in biliary cirrhosis.[11] Presence of multiple factors significantly increases the risk of HCC.[2] Any patient with chronic liver disease is at risk for the development of HCC with an annual incidence of 2–8%.[12,13] It is important to note that in patients with cirrhosis, in addition to HCC, there is an increased risk of development of intrahepatic cholangiocarcinoma.[14]

The HCCs which occur in cirrhotic liver are thought to arise in a stepwise fashion from a regenerating nodule which develops into a low grade dysplastic nodule, high grade dysplastic nodule which finally develops a focus of HCC to form early HCC and then progressed HCC.[15] The development of HCCs in liver without background cirrhosis is called *'de novo hepatocarcinogenesis'*.[16] Pathologically HCC may occur in three different forms: solitary, multifocal, or diffuse. In Asia, HCC usually presents as a well defined mass, either solitary or multifocal, associated with cirrhosis secondary to hepatitis B. In the west it usually presents as a diffusely infiltrating mass and has an association with alcoholic cirrhosis. Neovascularity is an important pathological characteristic of HCC. Capsule is seen in 65–82% of the lesions and encapsulated lesions have a better prognosis.[17]

Hepatocellular carcinoma frequently invades the portal vein (in about 40% cases) and less often the inferior vena cava and hepatic veins (15%).[2] Biliary invasion is uncommon. With various curative therapies now available (liver transplantation, hepatic resection, percutaneous ablative techniques, chemotherapy, immunotherapy), 5-year-survival rate is about 40–75%.[2]

The implementation of the screening programs has resulted in detection of HCC at an earlier stage **(Flowchart 1)**. Imaging is crucial for the diagnosis of HCC and biopsy is no longer performed.[18] The American Association for the Study of Liver Diseases (AASLD) recommends that if a mass >1 cm shows typical imaging features (arterial phase enhancement and washout in venous phase) on one modality [either Contrast-enhanced computed tomography (CECT) or Contrast-enhanced magnetic resonance (CEMR)] a diagnosis of HCC can be made. For lesions <1 cm, follow-up with USG should be done every 3 months to see if they progress or are stable.[18] Follow-up imaging is a must in all patients after treatment as recurrence rates are as high as 70% and most occur in the initial 3 years. This is done at 3-monthly intervals. Similar guidelines have also been suggested by National Comprehensive Cancer Network.[19]

Clinical Presentation

The clinical signs and symptoms are often obscured by the debilitating effects of cirrhosis. Upper abdominal pain, malaise, fever, weight loss, palpable mass and rapid deterioration of liver function in patients with long standing cirrhosis are possible indicators.

FLOWCHART 1: Diagnostic algorithm for suspected focal lesion in patients with chronic liver disease.

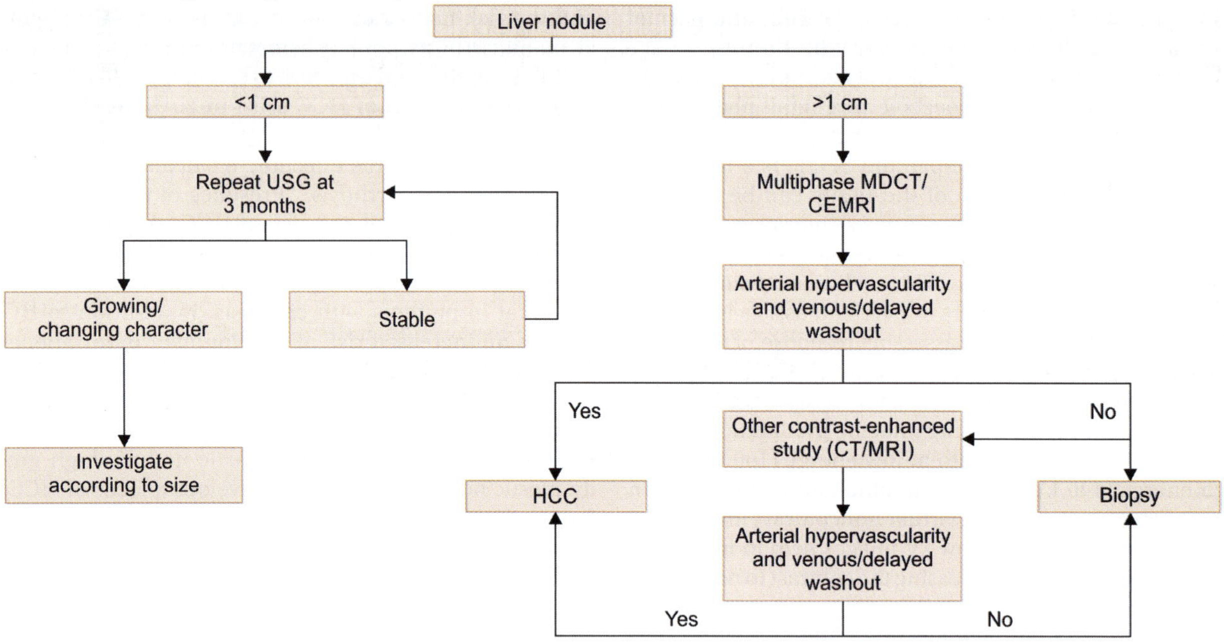

(MDCT: multidetector-row computed tomography; CEMRI: contrast-enhanced magnetic resonance imaging; USG: ultrasonography)

Source: Reproduced from AASLD Practice Guidelines 2010.

Alfa-fetoprotein (AFP) is a useful serum marker and is elevated in 50–70% cases. Serum levels more than 20 ng/mL are abnormal and levels above 1000 ng/mL are strongly suggestive of HCC.

Imaging in HCC

Imaging in HCC is a challenge as early diagnosis is critical for successful treatment. Lesions larger than 2 cm usually do not pose a diagnostic problem. However, nodules smaller than 2 cm often have nonspecific imaging features and create difficulties in diagnosis.[20] MRI scores over CT in detection of small HCCs in cirrhotic liver. The sensitivity of MRI and CT for detection of HCC is 81% and 68%, respectively. In addition differentiation of regenerative and dysplastic nodules from HCC, in cirrhosis, is vital for proper management.

Ultrasonography

Sonography being inexpensive and widely available is frequently used as the initial modality in the work-up of focal hepatic lesions. Recent advances in ultrasonography (USG) like liver specific ultrasound contrast agents and sonoelastography have increased its importance. The sensitivity of USG for detection of HCC ranges between 75% and 94% in various studies. However, sensitivity of USG for detection of HCC in the end stage cirrhotic liver is only about 50%, though the specificity has been reported to be as high as 98%. Most countries recommend a combination of USG and AFP every 6 months for HCC screening in high-risk patients.[18] Thus, any sonographically detected lesion in a cirrhotic liver should be evaluated according to the guidelines by American Association for Study of Liver Diseases.[18]

HCC has variable morphological presentations. Tumors can be solitary **(Fig. 1A)**, multifocal or diffusely infiltrating. The most common finding is a discrete lesion, either solitary or multiple. These lesions are usually hypoechoic, but are sometimes isoechoic and detected chiefly by virtue of a thin hypoechoic halo which corresponds to the tumor capsule. Encapsulated HCCs are more commonly seen in the Asian and Japanese population as compared to the west. Twenty-five percent of HCCs are echogenic.

The echo pattern has been shown to correlate with tumor morphology. Solid tumors without necrosis are hypoechoic whereas hyperechoic appearance is attributable to fatty metamorphosis, fibrosis, or sinusoidal dilatation **(Fig. 1B)**. The majority of small HCCs (<2 cm) are hypoechoic, whereas the larger HCCs are hyperechoic or of heterogeneous echo texture.

A less common pattern of HCC is diffuse parenchymal involvement with disorganization of the normal echo pattern. Multiple areas of decreased and increased echogenicity are present throughout the distorted liver without any distinct masses.

HCC has a propensity to invade the portal vein, hepatic vein or both, and this is depicted as echoes either partially or completely filling the lumen. Color Doppler flow imaging is a useful adjunct for detection of vascular invasion. The presence of arterial waveform within the thrombus indicates that it is neoplastic rather than bland thrombus. This distinction is vital because it has been shown that the presence of malignant portal vein thrombosis is the worst prognostic factor in predicting recurrence of HCC following surgical resection or liver transplantation. Color Doppler may also demonstrate intralesional vascularity in the form of a tangle of vessels within the tumor indicating hypervascularity

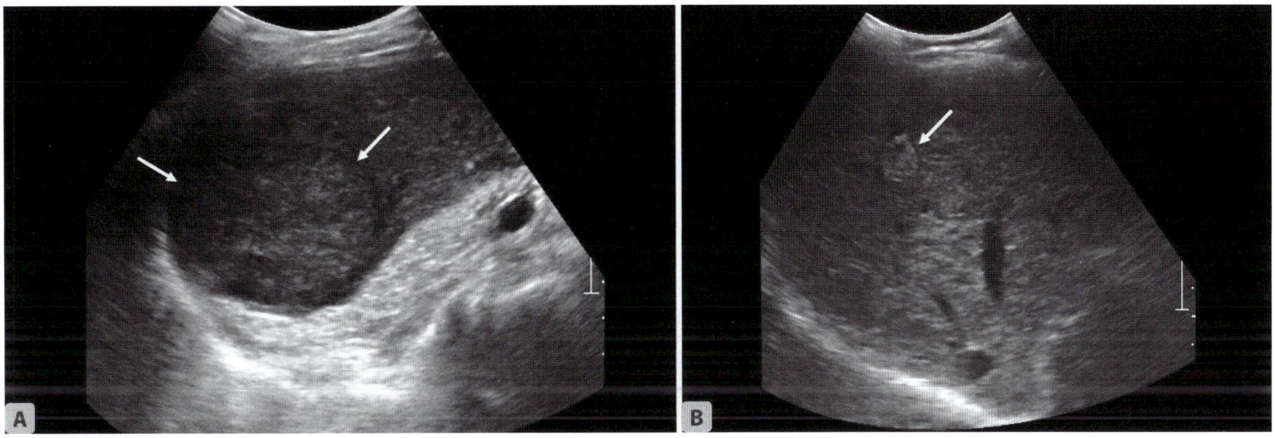

FIGS. 1A AND B: Sonographic appearance of hepatocellular carcinoma. (A) USG showing an isohyperechoic mass in the right lobe of liver (arrows) with normal background liver; (B) USG in a different patient with cirrhotic liver showing heterogeneous echotexture of parenchyma with an echogenic lesion (arrow) suggestive of HCC.

and arteriovenous shunting. A basket pattern of intralesional vessels, indicating internal vascularity and shunting, may be seen in up to 15% of cases.[21] However, there is a lot of overlap in Doppler patterns. Contrast-enhanced USG with sonovue (Bracco, Milano, Italy) shows early hyperperfusion of HCC with washout in portal venous phase.[22] Liver specific USG contrast agent (Sonazoid; GE healthcare, Norway) has been developed but it is currently not available in India. It is a perflubutane based microbubble and provides both dynamic and liver specific images.[23]

Computed Tomography

The advent of helical CT made it possible to perform multi-phasic examination of the liver in the arterial and portal venous phase with the same bolus of contrast. This has had a major impact on the detection and characterization of hypervascular lesions like HCC. Multidetector computed tomography (MDCT) has allowed faster scanning of liver, thus reducing respiration artifacts and has increased the spatial resolution substantially, leading to improvement in the characterization of smaller lesions. Also, with MDCT, good quality multiplanar reconstructions and CT angiographic images can be obtained. The latter enables proper planning of surgical resection or transplantation.

The liver receives 75–80% of its blood supply from the portal vein and 20–25% from the hepatic artery. On the other hand, most liver tumors receive the majority of their blood supply from the hepatic artery. HCCs have a rich arterial supply and are better visualized on the arterial phase. It has been reported that up to 11% of lesions may be seen only on the arterial phase as they become isodense on the portal venous phase. In addition, arterial phase imaging is useful in demonstrating arterialportal shunting (early enhancement of intrahepatic portal venous branches) and enhancement of portal venous thrombus confirming it to be tumor thrombus.[1,15]

The CT features are variable depending on the size, vascularity and growth pattern. The multiphasic CT scan includes a noncontrast phase, followed by arterial, venous and delayed phases. Late arterial phase should be done as HCC shows enhancement in this phase. On unenhanced CT, most HCCs present as solitary or multiple low attenuating lesions. Areas of fat density may be seen. In a fatty liver, HCC may be seen as a hyperdense lesion. On arterial phase images the hypervascular tumor shows intense enhancement throughout the tumor **(Figs. 2A to C)**. The lesions are frequently encapsulated and the capsule is seen as a hypodense rim. Larger tumors are often heterogeneous due to necrosis and hemorrhage **(Figs. 3A to C)**. Arterial phase may demonstrate the presence of arterioportal shunting **(Fig. 4)**. During the portal venous phase there is rapid washout and the lesion becomes isodense to hypodense to normal liver **(Figs. 2B and 3B)**. On delayed phase, images the capsule and fibrous septa may show prolonged enhancement **(Fig. 3C)**. Contrast washout has very high specificity (96%) for the diagnosis of HCC.[24] Dual energy CT generates iodine maps which helps in detecting subtle lesions **(Figs. 5A and B)**. Vascular invasion is common with HCC. Portal vein invasion is due to portal venous drainage of HCC. A tumor thrombus in portal vein is diagnosed if the main portal vein has a diameter of ≥ 23 mm (bland thrombus rarely causes portal vein dilatation) and the thrombus shows enhancement (typically called "threads and streaks") in arterial phase **(Figs. 6A and B)**. HCCs may also extend into the hepatic veins or IVC **(Figs. 7A to C)**. HCCs may occasionally rupture and may lead to hemoperitoneum. A ruptured HCC is hypodense on arterial phase images showing only peripheral rim enhancement with focal discontinuity ('enucleation sign').[2]

Imaging accuracy is often more limited in the cirrhotic liver due to architectural distortion, presence of regenerating nodules and hemodynamic alterations. Therefore, the detection of HCC in a cirrhotic liver may require several complementary imaging techniques. Since the imaging appearance of HCC can be variable it is said that any mass in a cirrhotic liver that does not fulfill criteria for a cyst or hemangioma should be considered an HCC until proved otherwise.

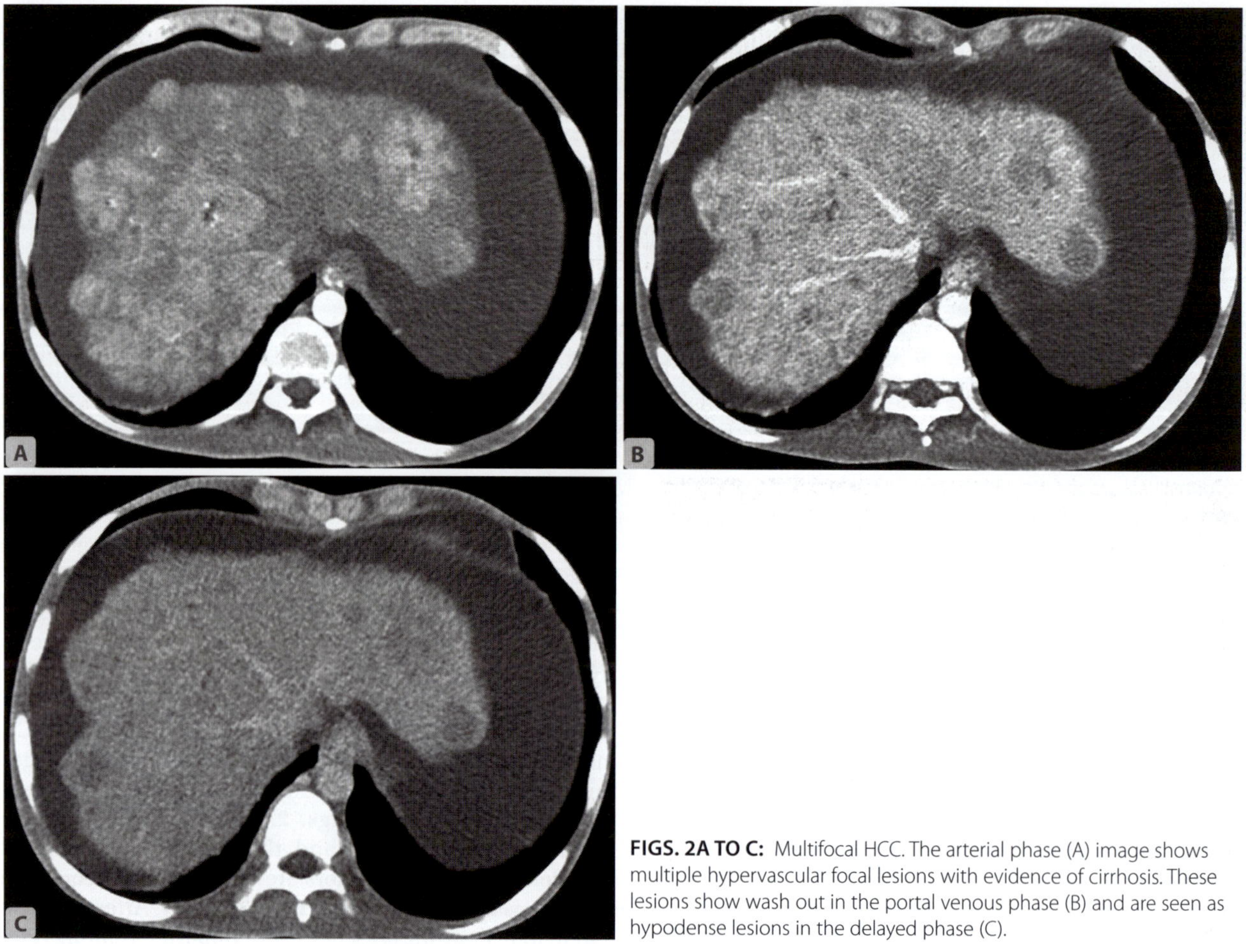

FIGS. 2A TO C: Multifocal HCC. The arterial phase (A) image shows multiple hypervascular focal lesions with evidence of cirrhosis. These lesions show wash out in the portal venous phase (B) and are seen as hypodense lesions in the delayed phase (C).

Magnetic Resonance Imaging

Magnetic resonance imaging (MRI) with its superior contrast resolution and multiple paradigms for lesion characterization is superior to CT for the evaluation of HCC in a cirrhotic liver. The MR appearance depends on the type of disease (solitary, multifocal or diffuse), the degree of fibrosis, amount of fat as well as on the presence of necrosis and hemorrhage.

Usually, HCC is hypointense on T1W images and mildly hyperintense on T2W images **(Figs. 8A to E and 9A to E)**. The presence of fat or hemorrhage may result in increased signal intensity on T1W images **(Fig. 8A)**. Encapsulated lesions have a hypointense rim on T1W images and a single or a double layered hypointense rim on T2W images. Fast gradient echo sequences allow the liver to be imaged in a breath hold and multi-phasic dynamic gadolinium-enhanced MR imaging has been shown to improve detection of HCC and is superior to dual phase CT. MRI frequently demonstrates HCCs, particularly tumors smaller than 1.5 cm, better than CT images. HCC is typically seen as a hypervascular mass with rapid washout. Tumors larger than 2 cm enhance in a heterogeneous fashion.[15]

The most sensitive sequence for detecting small HCC is the postgadolinium arterial phase on which small tumors enhance intensely. However, this feature is not specific as severely dysplastic nodules will also enhance. A more specific feature is washout of tumor below the signal of liver in venous or delayed phase with late enhancement of the capsule.[15] The arterial phase also allows distinction from metastatic disease because HCCs typically demonstrate enhancing stroma through the entire tumor whereas metastases have peripheral enhancement. However, metastases from hypervascular primaries (neuroendocrine tumors, renal cell carcinoma) may show similar enhancement and may pose diagnostic problem. The degree of vascularity in HCC may vary with the majority being hypervascular but some are hypovascular.

Diffuse infiltration with HCC may be subtle or simulate the appearance of chronic hepatitis or scarring. It may present as extensive hepatic parenchymal involvement with mottled punctate high intensity on T2W images and mottled enhancement on arterial phase images. Diffuse HCC is very frequently associated with portal vein thrombosis. MRI is useful in differentiation of tumor from bland portal vein thrombus. The hyperintense signal on T2W sequence is highly suggestive of tumor thrombus.[15] Other features favoring malignant thrombus include dilatation of the vein and contrast enhancement.

Liver specific MR contrast agents currently available include gadobenate dimeglumine and gadoxetic acid. Gadobenate dimeglumine (Gd-BOPTA) has the advantage of being both intravascular and hepatobiliary contrast agent.[15] Although it is mainly excreted by the kidneys, about 5% is

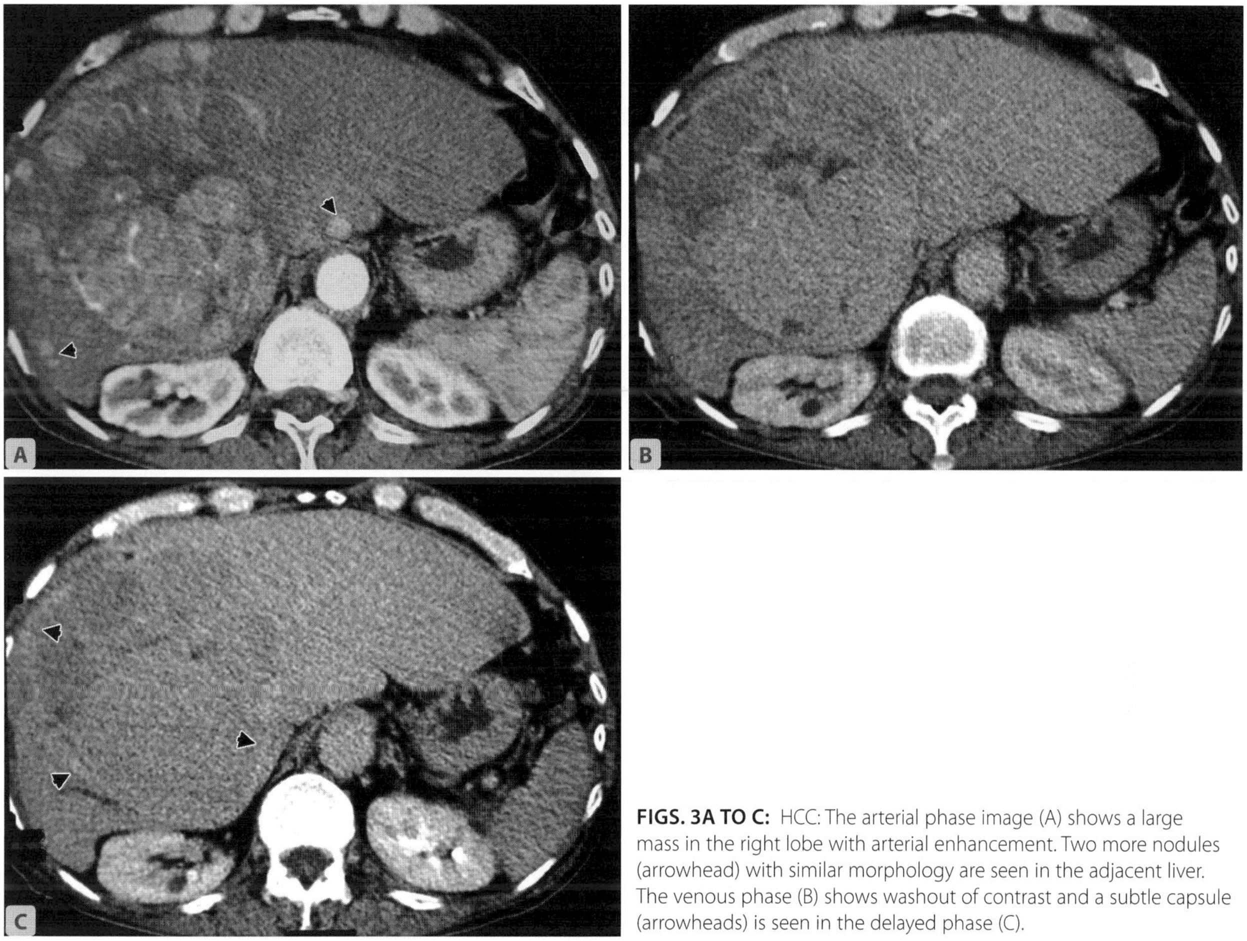

FIGS. 3A TO C: HCC: The arterial phase image (A) shows a large mass in the right lobe with arterial enhancement. Two more nodules (arrowhead) with similar morphology are seen in the adjacent liver. The venous phase (B) shows washout of contrast and a subtle capsule (arrowheads) is seen in the delayed phase (C).

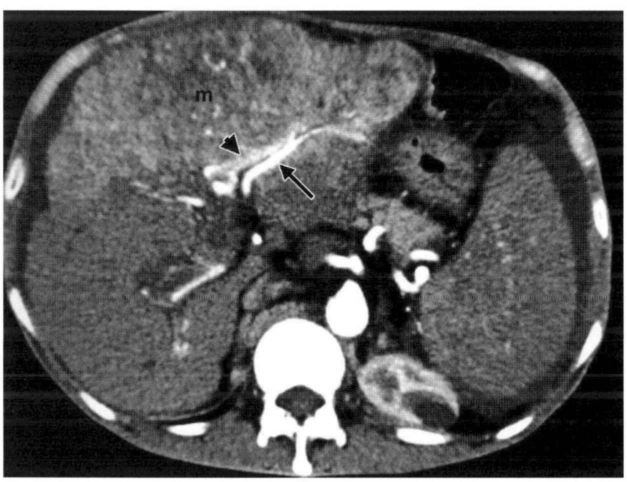

FIG. 4: Arterioportal shunt: The arterial phase CT image shows a large enhancing lesion (m) in the segments 3 and 4 of liver with contrast in the left hepatic artery (arrow) and left branch of portal vein (arrowhead) suggesting arterioportal shunting.

excreted in the biliary tree, which is prominently seen 60–120 minutes after intravenous injection. Gadobenate, is available in India and should be routinely used as a contrast agent for dynamic CEMR with an additional delayed scan taken at 1–2 hours after injection. Another liver specific contrast agent is Gadoxetic acid (Gd-EOB), which has about 50% hepatic excretion.[25] With this agent the hepatobiliary phase can be acquired at 15–20 min after contrast injection. Both these agents are taken up by functioning hepatocytes through organic anionic transport polypeptide (OATP) receptors and excreted into biliary canaliculi. Thus, lesion which do not contain hepatocytes are seen as hypointense areas compared to the enhancing normal liver parenchyma on hepatobiliary phase **(Figs. 10A to F)**. This hepatobiliary phase thus improves detection of the lesions. However, well-differentiated HCCs may also show uptake of the agent **(Fig. 9E)**.

Diffusion-weighted imaging (DWI) is increasingly being used in abdomen. The typical b-values used are 0, 400 and 800 s/mm^2. DWI has an important role in differentiation of benign from malignant liver lesions and improves the accuracy of contrast-enhanced MRI in detection of HCC with only a minimal time penalty.[26,27] HCCs show restriction of diffusion and this sequence may help in distinguishing it from other benign arterially enhancing lesions **(Figs. 9A to E)**.[28]

Various staging systems are available for HCC. The Barcelona Clinic Liver Cancer (BCLC) staging is the widely accepted one and it takes into consideration hepatic function (by Child-Pugh score), patient's performance status and tumor staging (tumor size and number and portal vein thrombosis) for disease classification.[29] In addition it also defines appropriate management for different disease stages. This is shown in **Flowchart 2**.

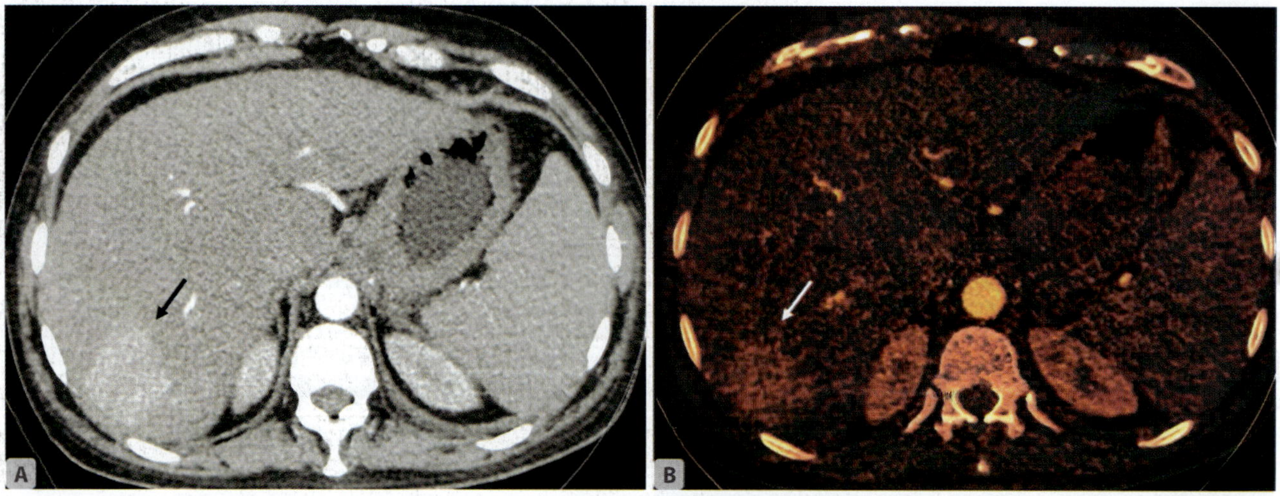

FIGS. 5A AND B: Dual energy CT appearance of HCC. (A) Axial CT scan in arterial phase showing enhancing lesion in segment 7 of liver (arrow); (B) Iodine map generated from dual energy CT data makes it easy to appreciate iodine uptake in the lesion (arrow).

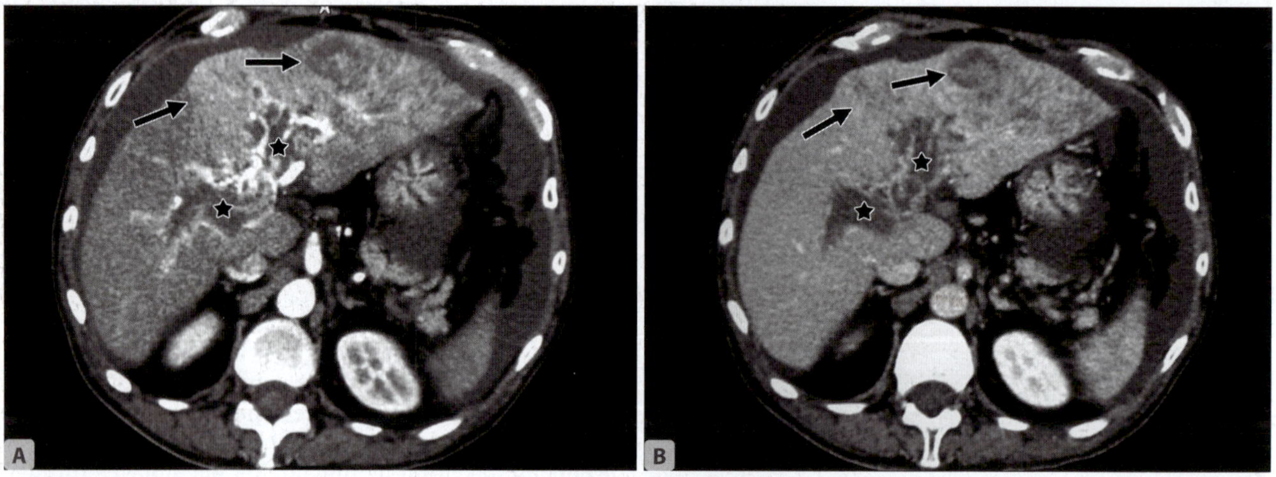

FIGS. 6A AND B: Portal vein thrombus: The arterial phase CT image (A) shows two enhancing lesions (arrows) in segments 3 and 4 of liver with arterioportal shunting. The portal vein in the venous phase image; (B) shows a large filling defect (stars) with 'thread and streak' pattern of enhancement suggestive of tumor thrombus.

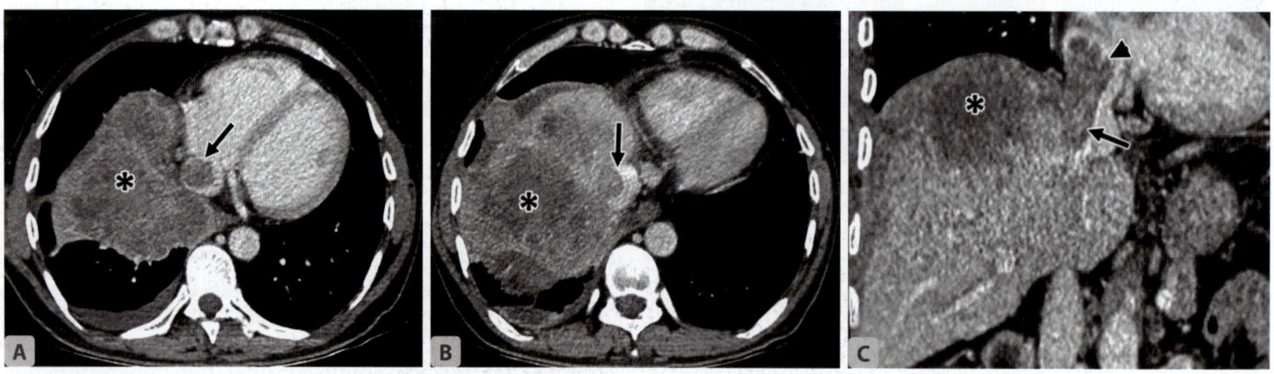

FIGS. 7A TO C: HCC with inferior vena cava extension. Axial (A and B) and coronal (C) contrast-enhanced CT scans in venous phase showing large mass in the liver (asterisk) with extension into the inferior vena cava (arrow) and right atrium (arrowhead in C).

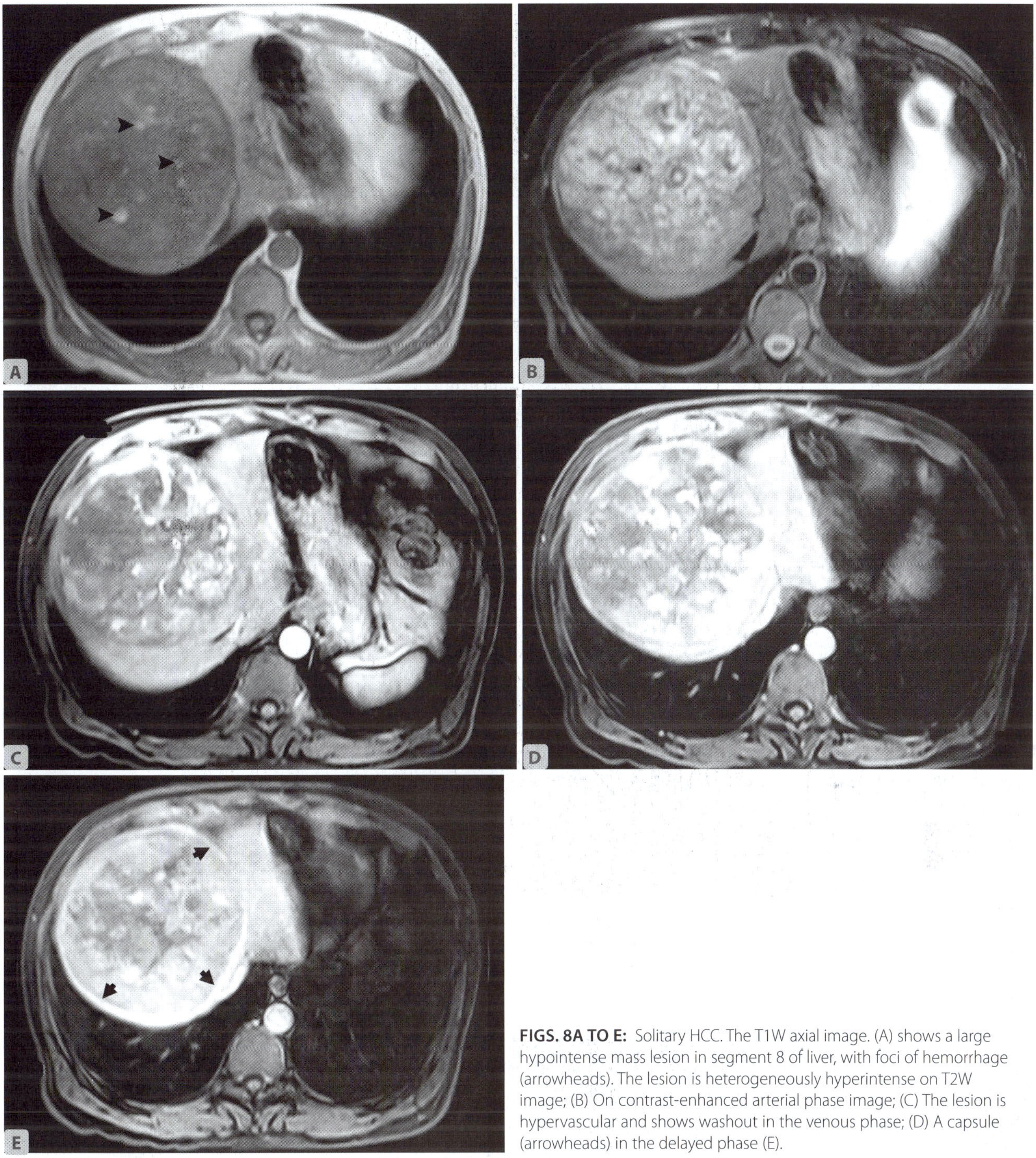

FIGS. 8A TO E: Solitary HCC. The T1W axial image. (A) shows a large hypointense mass lesion in segment 8 of liver, with foci of hemorrhage (arrowheads). The lesion is heterogeneously hyperintense on T2W image; (B) On contrast-enhanced arterial phase image; (C) The lesion is hypervascular and shows washout in the venous phase; (D) A capsule (arrowheads) in the delayed phase (E).

Differential Diagnosis of HCC

In a cirrhotic liver, regenerative nodules and dysplastic nodules are also common and these must be differentiated from HCC.[20,30] Regenerative nodules are usually isointense on both T1W and T2W images as they contain normal liver cells. They may be hyperintense on T1W images, which is due to the presence of protein, fat and copper **(Figs. 11A and B)**. Siderotic nodulesare hypointense on both T1W and T2W images, due to the presence of iron and fibrous content. They predominantly have portal venous blood supply and thus are isointense to normal liver on all three phases of CEMR. Dysplastic nodules, which are the precursors of HCC, are usually hyperintense on T1W and hypointense on T2W images. These too mostly (but not always) receive blood supply from portal veins and remain isointense on CEMR. A 'nodule within a nodule' appearance on T2W images (hyperintense focus in a hypointense nodule) is suggestive of HCC in a dysplastic nodule.[31] In doubtful cases, the features

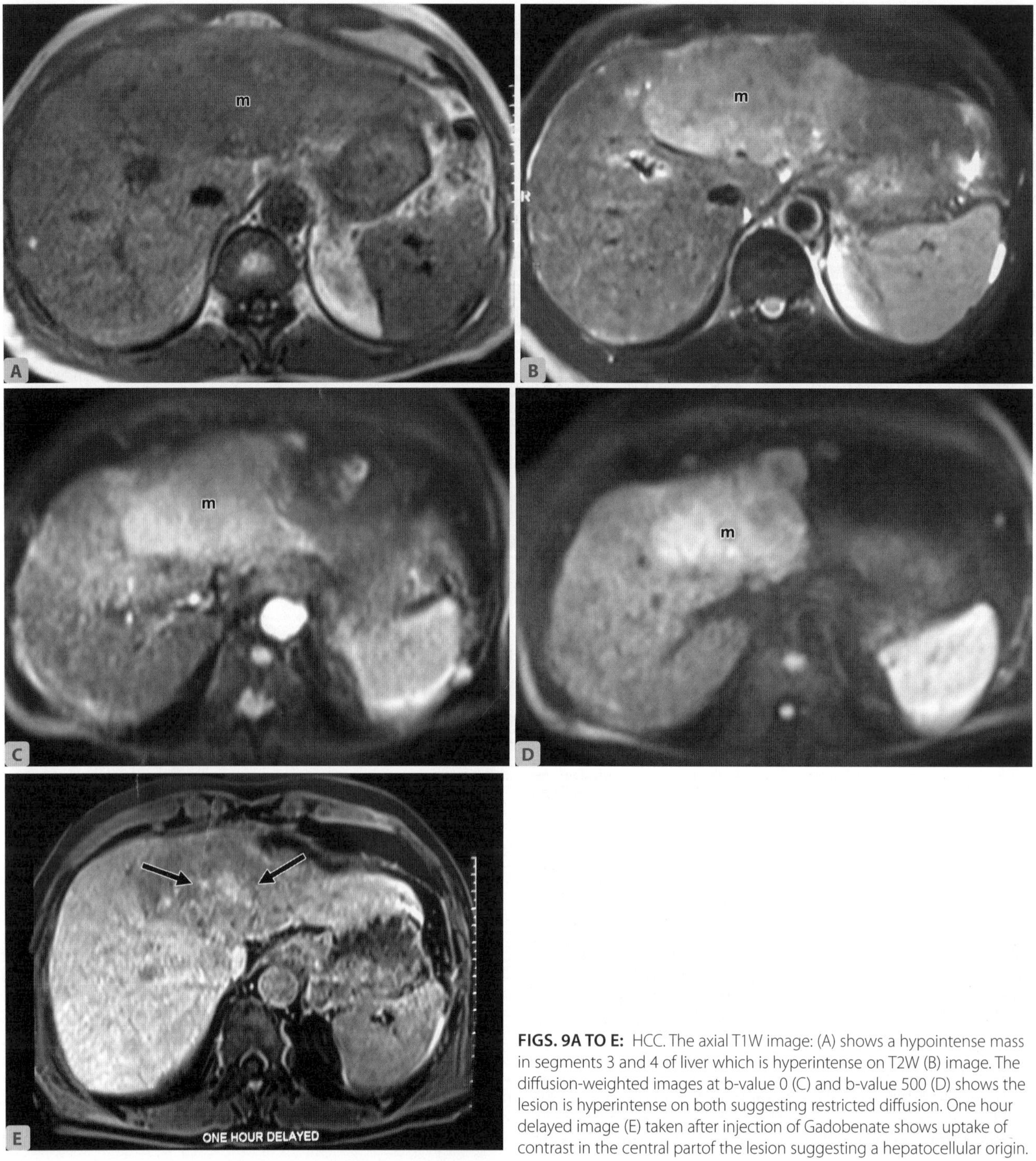

FIGS. 9A TO E: HCC. The axial T1W image: (A) shows a hypointense mass in segments 3 and 4 of liver which is hyperintense on T2W (B) image. The diffusion-weighted images at b-value 0 (C) and b-value 500 (D) shows the lesion is hyperintense on both suggesting restricted diffusion. One hour delayed image (E) taken after injection of Gadobenate shows uptake of contrast in the central partof the lesion suggesting a hepatocellular origin.

favoring HCC are size >2 cm, hyperintense T2W appearance, delayed washout, delayed enhancement of the capsule and rapid interval growth.

Other conditions which should to be differentiated from HCC include nodular regenerative hyperplasia (NRH), focal confluent fibrosis and nontumoros arterioportal shunt.[20] NRH is a non-neoplastic disease consisting of diffusely distributed regenerative nodules without associated fibrosis, occurring in noncirrhotic conditions like Budd-Chiari syndrome. These nodules are hyperintense on T1W images, hypo-to iso-intense on T2W images and often contain a central scar. They show arterial phase enhancement and differentiation from HCC is at times difficult. Focal confluent fibrosis may sometimes simulate tumors. It is often located in the anterior and medial segments of liver, and is wedge-shaped with base towards the liver capsule. It typically shows delayed enhancement, but occasionally arterial enhancement may be seen. The location of the lesion, shape and presence of atrophy with capsular retraction differentiate confluent fibrosis from HCC. Nontumoros arterioportal shunts are often seen in a

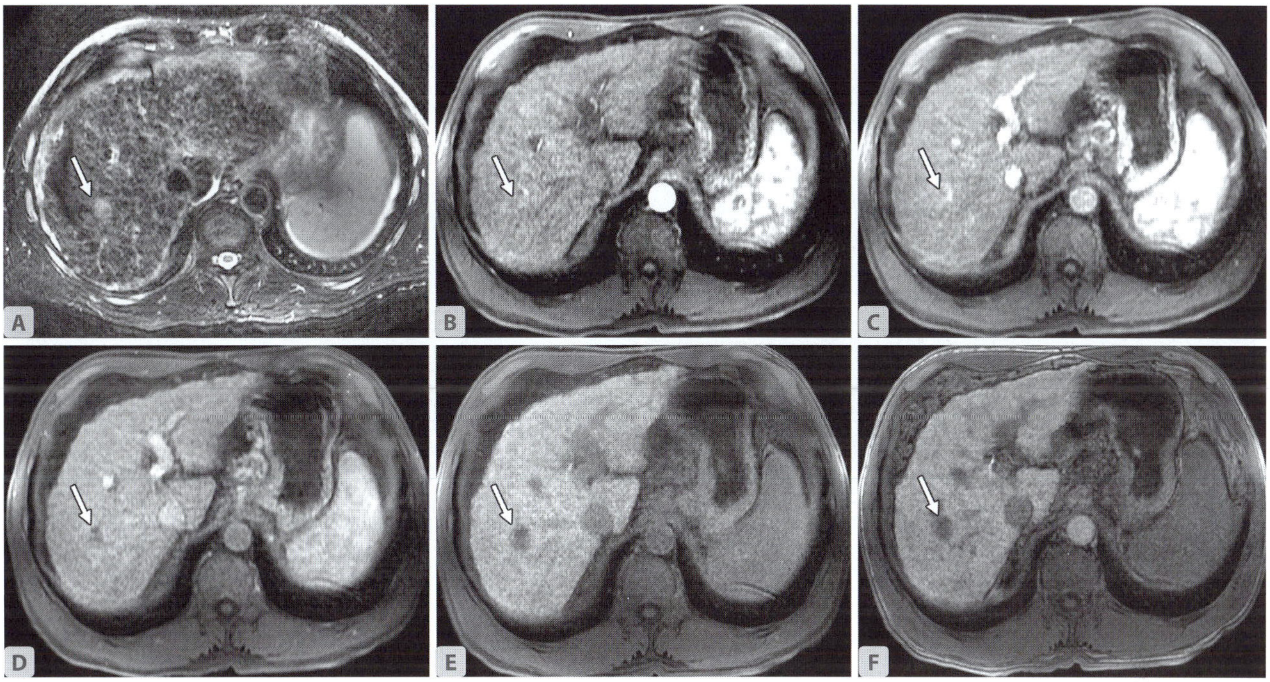

FIGS. 10A TO F: Gadoxetic acid-enhanced MRI. (A) T2W axial image showing a small hyperintense lesion in segment 7 of liver (arrow); (B) Arterial phase T1W image showing mild enhancement in the lesion (arrow); Venous (C) and Delayed (D) phase images showing contrast washout (arrow); Scans taken at 8 min (E) and 20 min (F) showing hypointense nature of the lesion (arrow) on hepatocyte phase suggesting no uptake of contrast by the lesion.
Courtesy: Dr Avinash Kambadakone, Dr Vinit Balyan, Massachusetts General Hospital, Boston.

FLOWCHART 2: Barcelona Clinic Liver Cancer (BCLC) staging system for hepatocellular carcinoma.

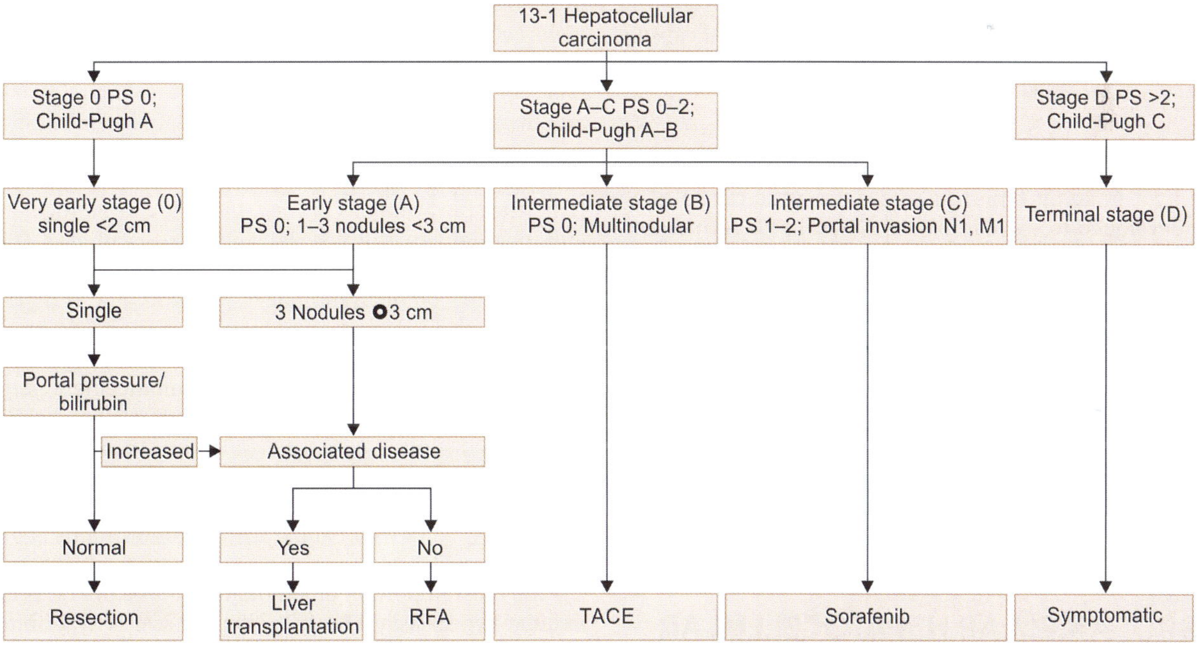

(M: metastasis; N: node stage; PS: performance status; RFA: radiofrequency ablation; TACE: transarterial chemoembolization)

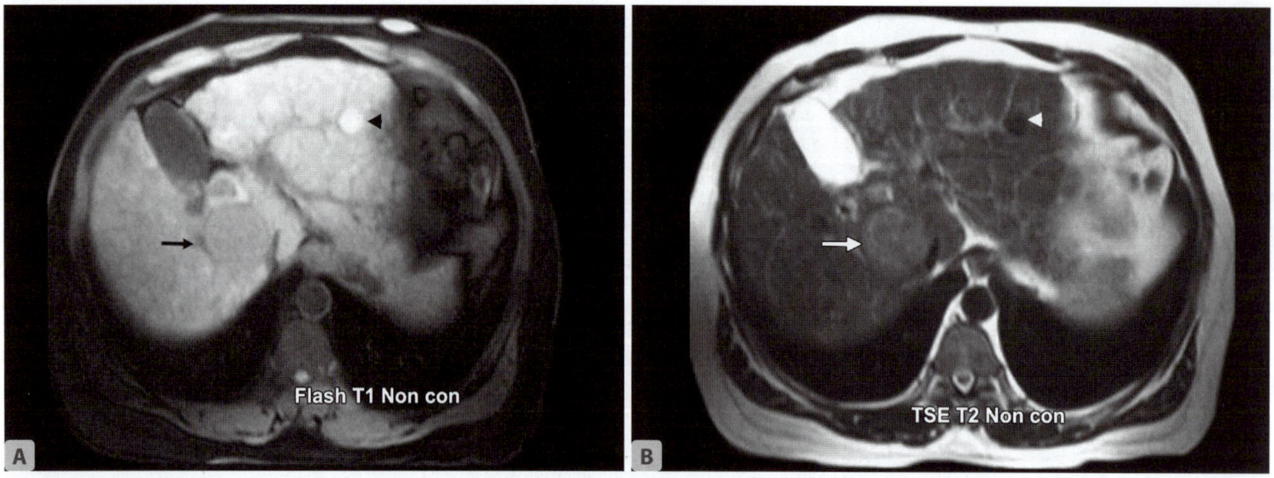

FIGS. 11A AND B: Regenerative nodule. Axial T1W image (A) shows a small hyperintense nodule (arrowhead) in left lobe which is hypointense on T2W image (B) suggestive of a regenerative nodule. In contrast to this, the segment 8 lesion (arrow) is hypointense on T1W image and mildly hyperintense on T2W image suggestive of HCC.

cirrhotic liver. They are subcapsular, wedge shaped and do not produce mass effect. They are isointense on T1W and T2W scans, and show intense enhancement on arterial phase images, but become isointense on portal venous and delayed phase.

Other differentials include intrahepatic cholangiocarcinoma, hypervascular metastases, flash filling hemangiomas and angiomyolipoma (especially epithelioid variety).

Imaging features favoring HCC in a cirrhotic liver include lesions >2 cm, enhancement in arterial phase, washout of contrast in venous or equilibrium phase, peripheral capsule in delayed phase, restriction of diffusion, hyperintense signal on T2W images and interval growth.[20]

Liver Imaging Reporting and Data System

The liver imaging reporting and data system (LI-RADS) was developed to standardize the CT and MRI techniques, terminology, diagnosis and reporting of HCC and other liver lesions in patients with chronic liver disease.[32] The focal lesions are categorized into LR1 to LR5, with LR1 being definitely benign and LR5 being definitely HCC. Major findings included in this system for diagnosis of HCC are size, arterial phase enhancement, washout, capsule and threshold growth. There are many ancillary features and tie breaker rules, the detailed discussion of which is beyond the scope of this chapter. The LIRADS version 2014 is the latest and is shown in **Flowchart 3**. The accuracy is above 80%. Further modification and simplification of classification is underway.

FIBROLAMELLAR HEPATOCELLULAR CARCINOMA

This is an unusual liver tumor found in young adults with a mean age of 25 years.[33,34] Patients do not have underlying cirrhosis nor are there any predisposing risk factors. It is frequently resectable and has a better prognosis than the usual HCC. The 5-year survival for fibrolamellar hepatocellular carcinoma (FLC) is 60% as compared to 30% for typical HCC. Serum AFP levels are typically normal. They usually present as a solitary large circumscribed mass that is partly or completely encapsulated. Satellite nodules are often seen. The major radiological clue to the diagnosis is the presence of central fibrous scar and central stellate calcification. Portal vein invasion, necrosis and hemorrhage are much less common than in typical HCC.[1,2]

On sonography, FLC is usually seen as a lobulated predominantly hyperechoic mass, although hypo and isoechoic forms have also been described **(Fig. 12A)**. Central hyperechoic nonshadowing areas with foci of shadowing correlate with the central scar and calcification within the scar. On unenhanced CT, FLC is a well-defined, lobulated and hypodense lesion. The central stellate calcification has been reported as a distinctive radiological feature and occurs in a high proportion (up to 68%) of these lesions **(Figs. 12A to D)**.[32] After intravenous contrast, FLC shows heterogeneous enhancement in the arterial and venous phases **(Figs. 12A to D)**. The scar does not show early enhancement but may enhance on delayed images.[2] On MRI, FLC is hypo- to isointense on T1W images and hyperintense on T2W images. The scar because of its fibrous nature, remains hypointense on T1- and T2-weighted images. The enhancement pattern on CEMR is similar to that seen on CT scans. On hepatobiliary phase, the lesion is hypointense to the surrounding liver parenchyma. The scar may be hyperintense. Although scar may be seen in other benign and malignant liver lesions, a large scar (>2 cm wide) along with fibrotic strands is more suggestive of FLC.[32]

The most important differential diagnosis of FLC is focal nodular hyperplasia (FNH). The central scar is hyperintense on T2W scans in FNH, but hypointense in FLC. Also, the scar of FLC shows calcification, but this is seen in <1.5% of cases of FNH. MRI with liver specific contrast agents is useful as FNH shows uptake of contrast in hepatobiliary phase unlike FLC.[1] The differentiation between the two is important as FNH is managed conservatively but FLC is treated surgically. Biopsy provides the diagnosis in difficult cases.[2] Other differentials

FLOWCHART 3: Liver imaging reporting and data system (LI-RADS) classification of liver lesions in patients of chronic liver disease.

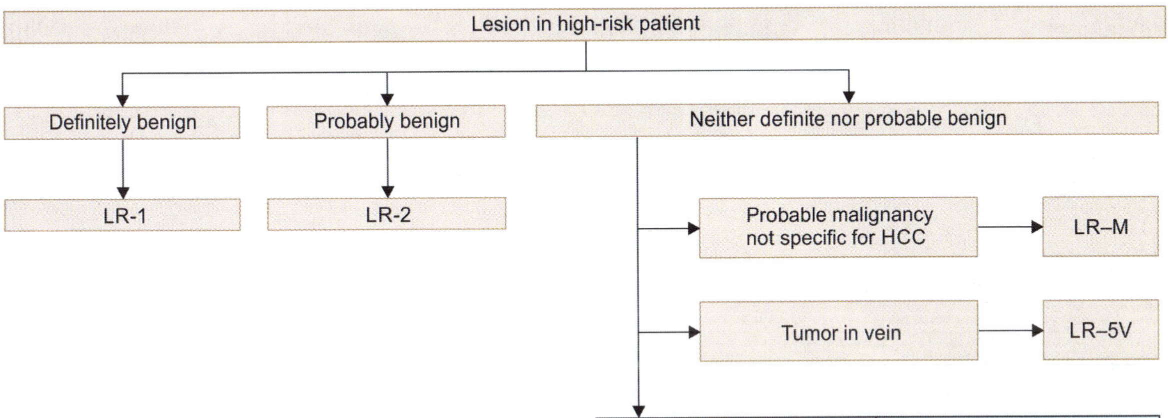

		Arterial phase hypo- or iso-enhancement		Arterial phase hyper-enhancement		
Diameter (mm)		<20	≥20	<10	10–19	<20
Washout	None	LR–3	LR–3	LR–3	LR–3	LR–4
Capsule	One	LR–3	LR–4	LR–4	LR–4/5	LR–5
Threshold growth	≥ Two	LR–4	LR–4	LR–4	LR–5	LR–5

include conventional HCC (differentiation is based on age, underlying liver disease, serum AFP levels) and intrahepatic cholangiocarcinoma (differentiation by enhancement characteristics, biliary dilatation).

Interventional Techniques

Many methods have been developed for the nonsurgical management of HCC employing angiographic and percutaneous techniques. These include hepatic arterial infusion chemotherapy and embolization and percutaneous techniques like ethanol ablation, and radiofrequency ablation. The details of these techniques are discussed in the chapter on Hepatic Intervention.

INTRAHEPATIC CHOLANGIOCARCINOMA

Intrahepatic cholangiocarcinoma is the second most common primary malignant hepatic tumor. It accounts for 10% of all cholangiocarcinomas and arises in small intrahepatic ducts. It has an increased incidence in patients with Caroli's disease, sclerosing cholangitis, intrahepatic calculi and inflammatory bowel disease. Cholangiocarcinoma typically produces extensive desmoplastic reaction.[2] Cirrhosis of liver may be a predisposing factor for intrahepatic cholangiocarcinoma (ICCA).

Patients present clinically with abdominal pain, anorexia and weight loss. Jaundice occurs only if major ducts are obstructed. A normal serum AFP may be helpful in suggesting ICCA rather than HCC.

Imaging

Sonographically, one or more hyperechoic, iso- or hypoechoic masses may be seen. Homogeneous hypoechoic pattern is the most common appearance **(Fig. 13)**. On Doppler USG the lesion is not very vascular. Dilated intrahepatic bile ducts distal to the mass are often seen.[1,2] On unenhanced CT, it is seen as a well-defined round to oval, hypodense mass. On multiphase contrast-enhanced CT, it typically shows thick irregular peripheral enhancement in the arterial or portal venous phase. A delayed central enhancement is often seen which may take 5–15 minutes and is thought to be due to the fibrous matrix of the tumor.[2] The mass may involve the portal vein branch with resultant atrophy of ipsilateral segment or lobe. The contralateral lobe may undergo hypertrophy. Hepatic capsular retraction, atrophy-hypertrophy complex and biliary dilatation adjacent to the mass are highly suggestive of ICCA (as these are rarely seen with HCC).[35] On MR imaging, the lesion appears hypointense on T1W and hyperintense on T2W images **(Figs. 14A to F)**. The central fibrous area may appear hypointense on T2W images. DWI shows restriction of diffusion. On CEMR, smaller lesions (2–4 cm) enhance homogeneously but those >4 cm show thick peripheral enhancement with centripetal progression **(Figs. 14A to F)**. On hepatobiliary phase (with gadoxetic acid or gadobenate dimeglumine) the lesion appears hypointense.[36] Occasionally, central fibrotic area may be hyperintense due to extracellular contrast retention. The primary angiographic finding in cholangiocarcinoma is serrated or serpiginous arterial infiltration. Large tumors may be mildly vascular but in small tumors arterial encasement is the only abnormality.

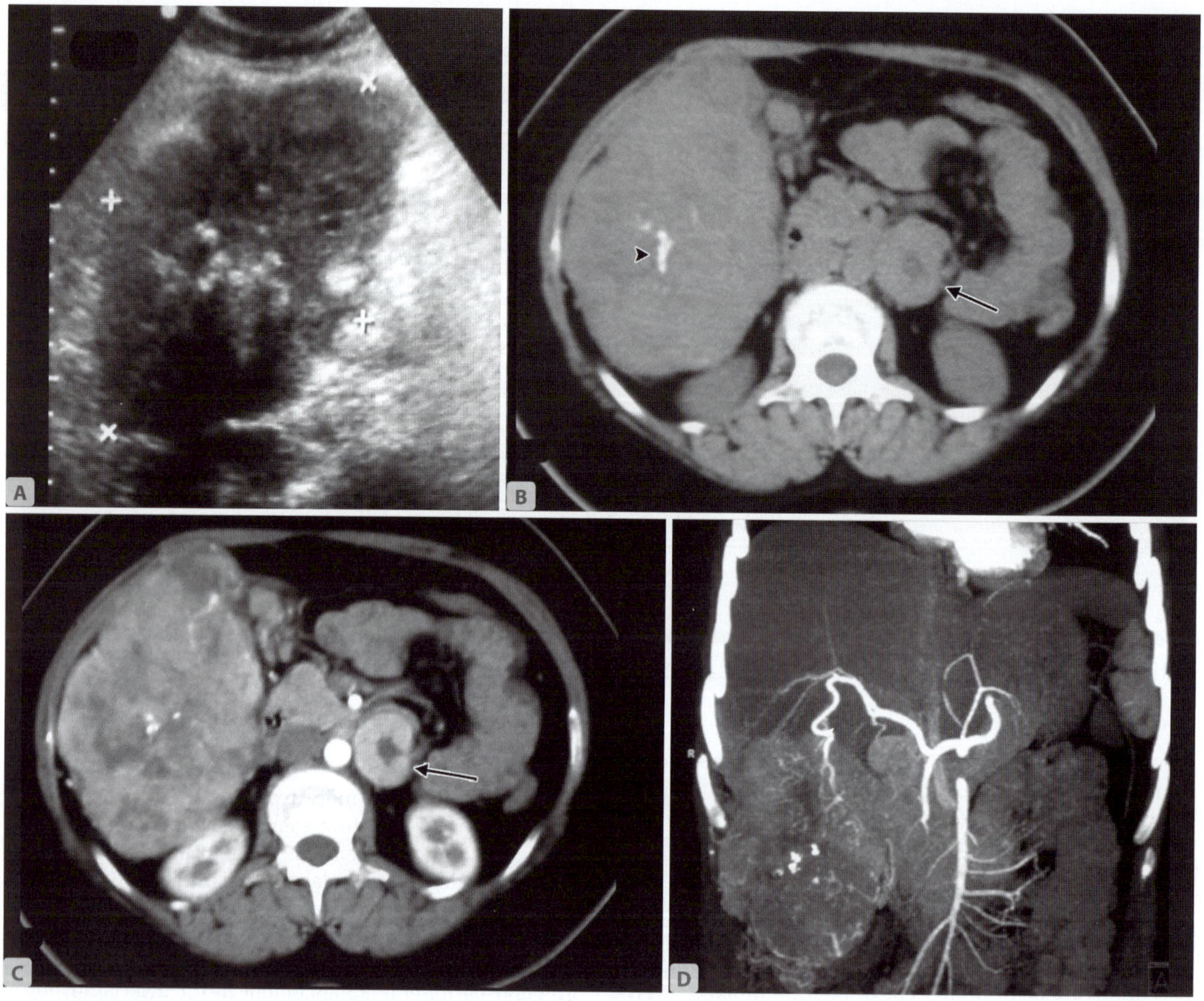

FIGS. 12A TO D: Fibrolamellar carcinoma: Ultrasonography (A) a hypoechoic mass in segment 6 of liver showing central calcification. Noncontrast CT scan; (B) hypodense mass in the liver with central calcification (arrowhead) and left para-aortic lymphadenopathy (arrow). Contrast-enhanced arterial phase CT image; (C) Heterogeneous enhancement with central scar showing calcification. The para-aortic node is showing intense enhancement (arrow). The CT maximum intensity projection image (D) shows a prominent feeder arising from the right hepatic artery (arrowhead).

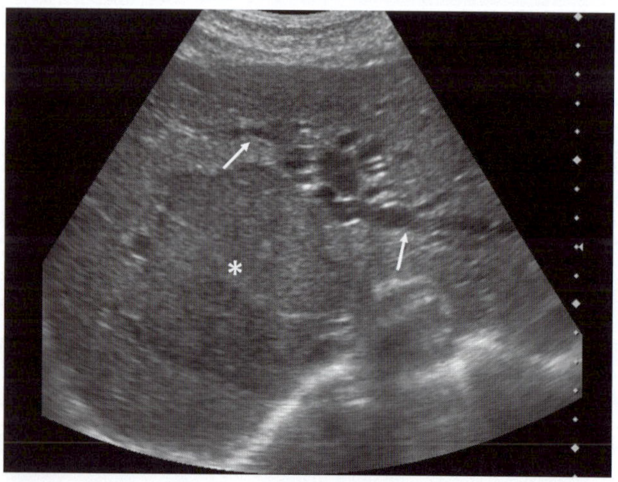

FIG. 13: USG of mass forming cholangiocarcinoma showing a large isohypoechoic mass in right lobe of liver (asterisk) with dilatation of biliary radicles (arrows).

The differential diagnosis include HCC, hemangioma and metastasis from gastrointestinal primary malignancy. The presence of capsular retraction, biliary dilatation, lobar or segmental atrophy, T2W hypointensity, peripheral thick band like enhancement in arterial phase and centripetal filling favour a diagnosis of ICCA. It is important to distinguish this tumor from HCC in a cirrhotic liver as patients with ICCA are taken off from the transplant list.

HEPATOCHOLANGIOCARCINOMA

Hepatocholangiocarcinoma (HCCA) is an uncommon biphenotypic malignancy.[33] It may be seen in patients of cirrhosis of liver and chronic viral hepatitis.[37] They have worse prognosis than HCC. The clinical presentation is nonspecific. Serum markers although not very helpful, diagnosis should be suspected if both AFP and CA19-9 are elevated. On imaging, morphological features of both HCC and ICCA are seen **(Figs. 15A to F)**.[38] The lesion may show peripheral

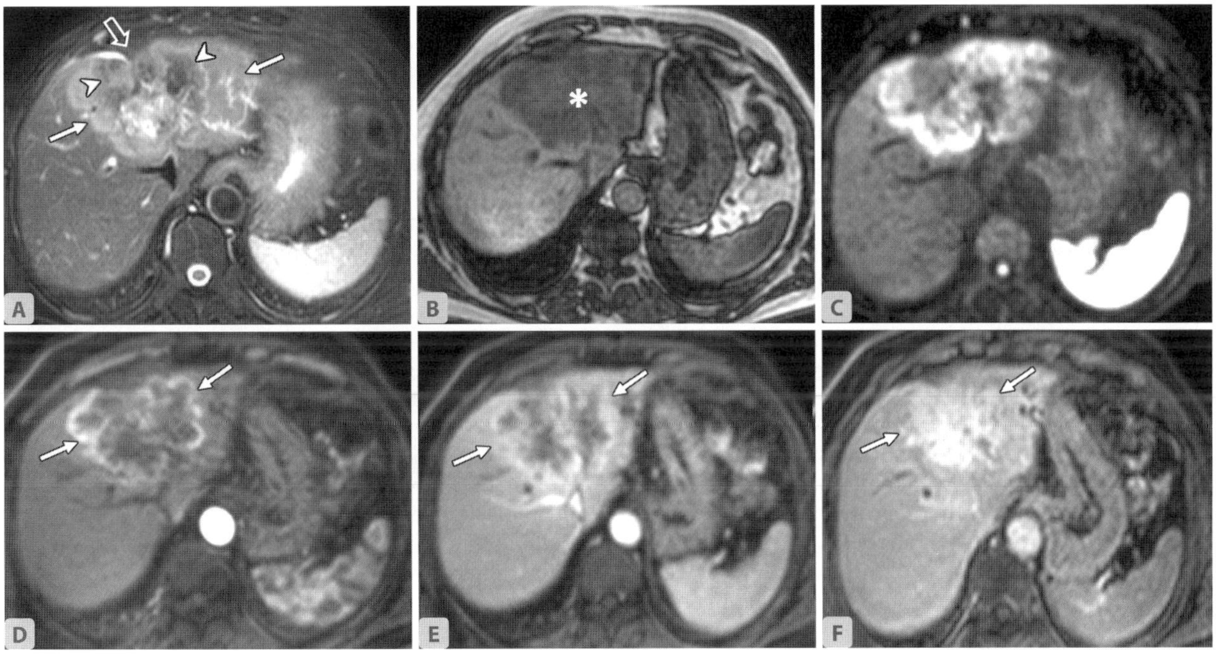

FIGS. 14A TO F: Mass forming cholangiocarcinoma. (A) Axial T2W fat-saturated image showing lobulated heterogeneous mass in left lobe of liver (arrows) with hypointense fibrotic areas (arrowheads) and retraction of capsule (block arrow); (B) Axial T1W image showing hypointense appearance of the lesion (asterisk); (C) Axial diffusion-weighted image (b-800) showing restriction of diffusion in the lesion; On contrast-enhanced images, the lesion shows thick smooth peripheral enhancement in arterial phase; (D) with gradual filling in of the lesion with contrast in venous; (E) Delayed; (F) Phases (arrows).

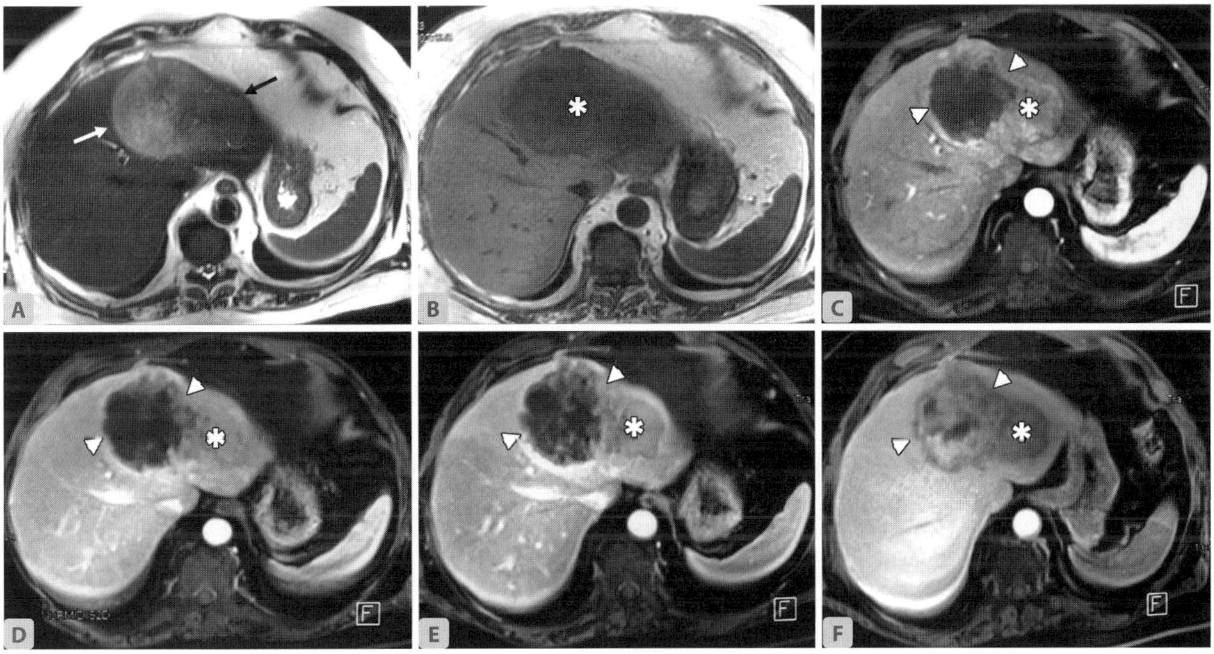

FIGS. 15A TO F: Hepatocholangiocarcinoma. (A) Axial T2W image showing a well-defined mass in the right lobe of liver with hyperintense (white arrow) and hypointense (black arrow) areas; (B) Axial T1W image showing homogeneous hypointense signal of the lesion; Dynamic contrast-enhanced T1W images showing the hepatocellular component (asterisk) with enhancement in arterial phase (C) and washout in venous (D) and delayed (E) phases with capsule formation (E). The cholangiocellular component (arrowheads) shows peripheral arterial enhancement (C) with gradual filling in of contrast in venous and delayed phases; (F) Axial T1W image in hepatobiliary phase shows hypointense hepatocellular component and retained contrast in cholangiocellular component due to fibrous matrix.

enhancement in the arterial phase with retention of contrast in the venous and delayed phases. Washout of contrast and capsular retraction may also be seen. Thus, more often, the enhancement characteristics follow more of ICCA than HCC. Biliary dilatation is uncommon. The lesion may show restriction of diffusion on DWI. However, whenever there is overlap of imaging features of HCC and ICCA in a liver lesion, HCCA should be suspected. Biopsy is needed for confirmation. It is important to differentiate HCCA from HCC as liver transplantation should be avoided in HCCA due to high recurrence.

BILIARY CYSTADENOCARCINOMA

Biliary cystadenocarcinoma is a rare tumor of bile duct origin and often develops due to malignant transformation of biliary cystadenoma.[39] They are more commonly seen in females in the age of 40–60 years. The clinical presentation is nonspecific and patients may present with abdominal pain or bloating, lump, vomiting or jaundice.[33] Anorexia and loss of weight may be present. Tumor markers such as cancer antigen (CA) 19-9 and carcinoembryonic antigen (CEA), may be elevated in some cases, but are not helpful in making a diagnosis.

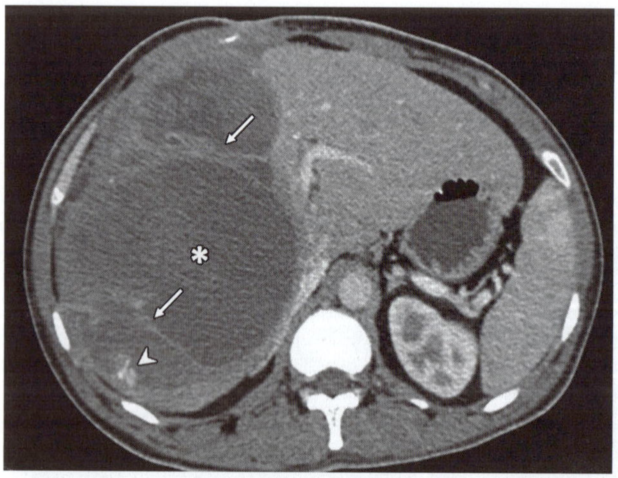

FIG. 16: Biliary cystadenocarcinoma. Contrast-enhanced CT scan showing a large cystic lesion in the right lobe of liver (asterisk) with thick enhancing septations (arrows) and enhancing mural nodule (arrowhead).

USG shows a variable-sized cystic lesion with multiple internal septations which appear thick and echogenic. Solid nodules may also be seen which may show internal vascularity. Contrast-enhanced CT or MRI shows the cystic lesion with enhancing thick septations **(Fig. 16)**. Enhancing solid nodules are seen which may show restriction of diffusion on DWI. Biliary communication or obstruction is usually not seen.

Differential diagnosis includes hydatid cyst and complicated liver cysts. Absence of enhancing septations and solid nodules may suggest that diagnosis but in most cases final diagnosis is possible only after surgical excision.

HEPATOBLASTOMA

Hepatoblastoma is the most common primary liver tumor of childhood.[34] It most commonly occurs in the first three years of life, whereas hepatocellular malignancies in children older than five years tend to be morphologically similar to those found in adults.

The most common presentation is a painless abdominal mass, however anorexia, weight loss, pain and jaundice can occur. Serum AFP levels are elevated in over 90% of patients.

Pathologically hepatoblastoma tends to be well defined, pseudoencapsulated, large, unifocal lesion. Less commonly multiple nodules or diffuse liver involvement may be seen. Calcification may be seen in up to one-third of patients.[2]

Imaging

The sonographic appearance of hepatoblastoma is of a large, inhomogeneous echogenic mass sometimes with calcification. Anechoic foci due to necrosis and a lobular pattern caused by septation may be seen.

CT most commonly demonstrates a well-defined hypodense mass with mild enhancement **(Figs. 17A and B)**. Involvement of portal vein and inferior vena cava (IVC) can be demonstrated. Three-dimensional reconstruction provides important information about vascular invasion. If this shows portal vein invasion and in very large lesions neoadjuvant chemotherapy is given to shrink the tumor away from portal

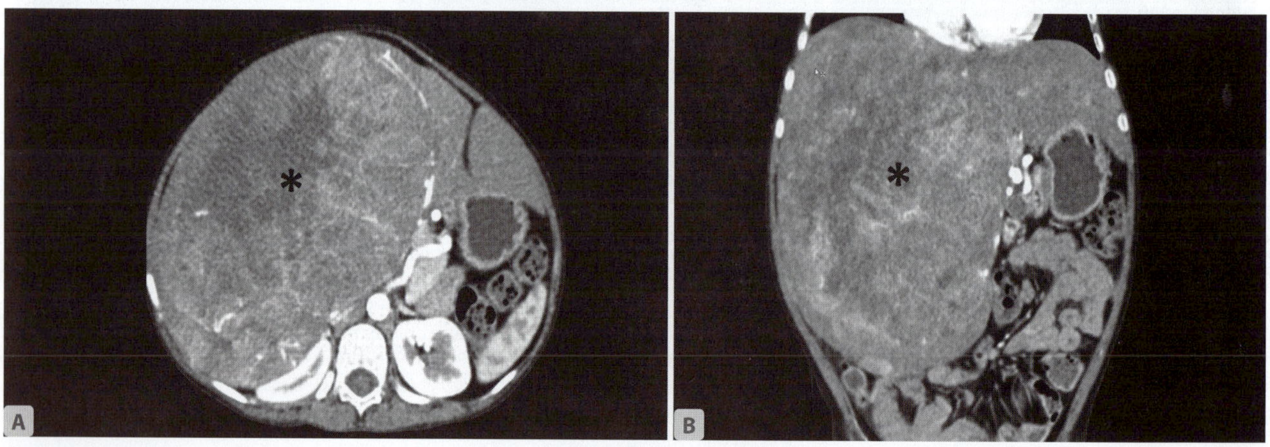

FIGS. 17A AND B: Hepatoblastoma. Axial (A) and Coronal (B) contrast-enhanced CT images showing a large mass replacing the right lobe of liver with central necrotic areas and peripheral enhancing areas in a 2-year-old child.

vein and then surgical excision is done.[40] Lung metastasis is common at presentation and CT scan of the chest is routinely performed before treatment. On MRI hepatoblastoma is seen as a lobulated mass that is hypointense on T1W and hyperintense on T2W scans. Internal septa are seen as bands of low signal intensity. On CEMR, immediate diffuse enhancement followed by washout is noted. DWI sequence is useful to pick up additional lesions.

EPITHELIOID HEMANGIOENDOTHELIOMA

Epithelioid hemangioendothelioma is a rare tumor of vascular origin which develops almost exclusively in adults, with slight female predominance. Pathologically multiple tumors are usually present that tend to grow and coalesce to form confluent masses. They are typically distributed in the periphery of the liver. They have better prognosis than angiosarcoma. Metastasis is seen in about 30% cases. Adjacent capsular retraction and calcification are frequently seen.[41,42]

Imaging

Sonographically, epithelioid hemangioendothelioma (EHE) usually presents as multiple peripheral hypoechoic masses. Hyperechoic and heterogeneous appearance has also been described. On unenhanced CT scan, multiple peripheral low attenuation lesions are noted. Calcification is infrequently present **(Figs. 18A to D)**. After intravenous contrast it shows peripheral enhancement surrounding the low attenuation fibrous core. Retraction of the overlying capsule is a common, though nonspecific, finding and should raise the possibility of this diagnosis. Large tumors are often associated with compensatory hypertrophy of the uninvolved lobes due to slow growth of these masses.[2] On MRI the lesion is hypointense on T1W images with a thin peripheral dark rim. T2W images show heterogeneously hyperintense lesion with or without low signal intensity peripheral rim **(Figs. 18A to D)**. Target appearance may be seen (hyperintense center with hypointense rim). Moderate peripheral and delayed central enhancement may be seen on CEMR. MRI is better than CT scan in characterization of EHE. Lollipop sign defined

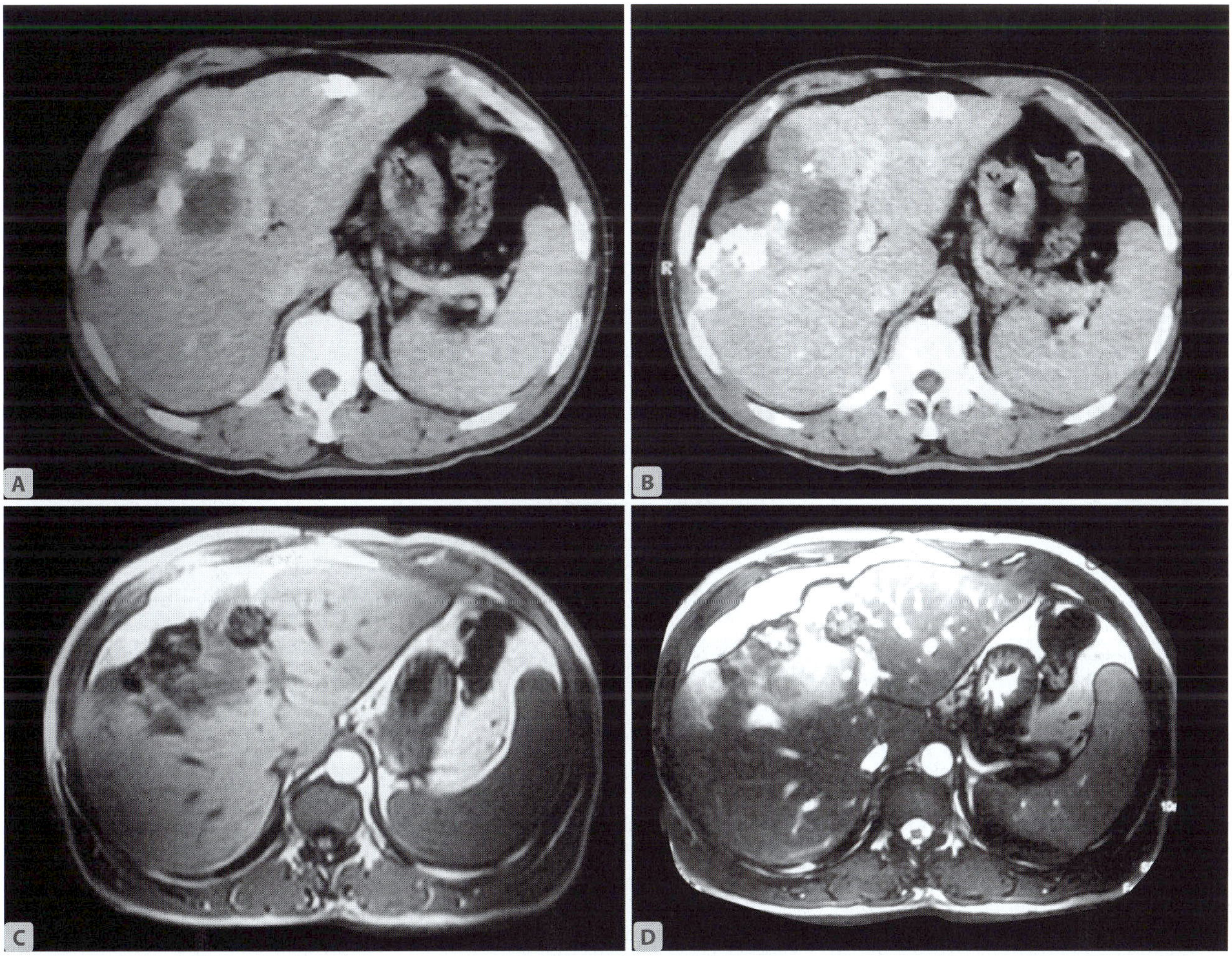

FIGS. 18A TO D: Epithelioid hemangioendothelioma. (A and B) CECT showing a hypodense mass in segments IVA and VIII with capsular retraction on the surface. Foci of calcification are seen in the lesion as well as another focus in the left lobe; (C) Axial gradient echo T1W scan shows that the mass is hypointense. The foci of calcification are markedly hypointense; (D) Axial T2W scan shows the mass is hyperintense with hypointense foci suggestive of calcification.

by a branch of a portal vein or hepatic vein leading to the periphery of an enhancing mass has been described in EHE. Target sign is seen on T2W, contrast-enhanced T1W and on DWI (peripheral restriction and central free diffusion).

Differential diagnosis includes mass forming intrahepatic cholangiocarcinoma, atypical hemangioma, confluent hepatic fibrosis and metastasis. Presence of confluent masses, target appearance on T2W, early peripheral enhancement and late central enhancement, and capsular retraction help in making a diagnosis. Biopsy is however needed in difficult cases.

ANGIOSARCOMA

Angiosarcoma is a rare tumor usually seen in adults in the fifth to seventh decade and is more common in males.[34] The risk factors include exposure to thorotrast, vinyl chloride, arsenic and steroids. Most of the angiosarcomas are multiple. Solitary lesions are unencapsulated and may contain blood-filled cystic areas. Clinical presentation is with weakness, loss of weight and appetite and abdominal pain. Thrombocytopenia may develop due to sequestration of platelets in large tumors.[2] Spontaneous rupture may be seen in up to 25% cases.

Sonography shows multiple or single hyperechoic masses. Anechoic areas due to necrosis and hyperechoic areas due to fresh hemorrhage may be seen **(Figs. 19A to F)**. On unenhanced CT angiosarcoma has a nonspecific low attenuation appearance. When the etiology is thorotrast exposure, background of high density reticular thorotrast laden parenchyma is seen. Marked peripheral enhancement is noted after administration of contrast. The enhancement may show a peripheral spread, usually with inhomogeneity on delayed scans. Differentiation from hemangioma may be difficult.[1,2] Presence of focal enhancing areas with attenuation less than aorta and peripheral ring-like enhancement (instead of globular) suggests angiosarcoma. Angiosarcoma is hypointense on T1W and heterogeneously hyperintense on T2W MRI **(Figs. 19A to F)**.[43] Fluid levels may be present representing internal hemorrhage. Dynamic CEMR shows an enhancement pattern similar to that of hemangioma. However, heterogeneous appearance on T2W images is unusual for hemangiomas.

On angiography, hepatic arteries supplying an angiosarcoma are of normal size and may show displacement but not encasement. A tumor stain appears at the periphery of the tumor and persists for a prolonged period.

SECONDARY MALIGNANCIES

METASTATIC DISEASE

The liver is second only to regional lymph nodes as a site for metastatic disease. It is far more common than primary liver cancer. The colon, stomach, pancreas, and breast are the common primary sites. Metastases are more common in the right lobe of the liver. Although the presence of liver metastases is a poor prognostic factor, the use of aggressive regimes in some subgroups can result in a better outcome. Over the past decade there has been increasing acceptance of liver resection as the best treatment for colorectal metastases. Successful outcome depends on knowledge of the size, number and location of the tumor burden and

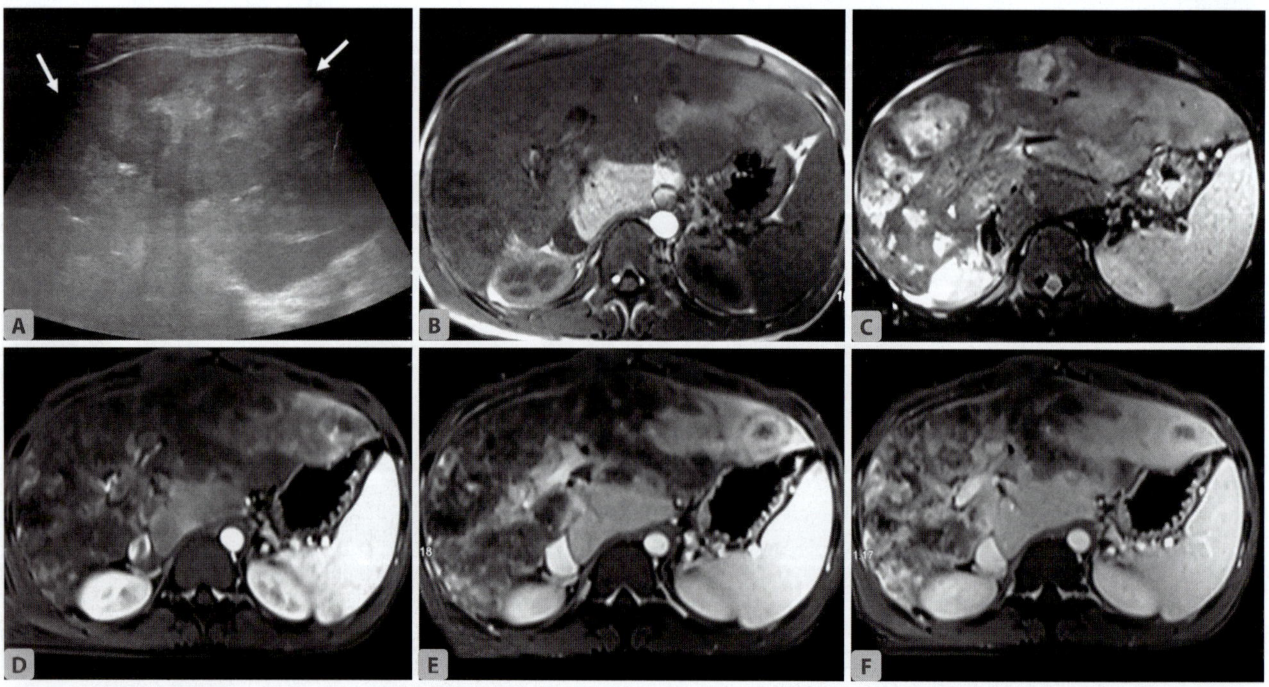

FIGS. 19A TO F: Angiosarcoma. (A) Ultrasonography showing multiple heteroechoic lesions in the liver (arrows); (B) Axial T1W image showing predominantly hypoechoic lesions replacing almost the entire liver; (C) Axial T2W fat-saturated image showing heterogeneous signal intensity of the lesions; Dynamic contrast-enhanced MRI in arterial (D), venous (E) and delayed (F) phases showing mild enhancement of the lesions in the arterial phase with gradual filling in of the lesions with contrast on venous and delayed phases.

accurate radiological assessment is essential to identify the subset of patients who would benefit from aggressive management.[1,2]

Many patients have hepatomegaly. Ascites, jaundice and varices may also be present. Liver function tests are normal in up to half of the patients and thus are unreliable for metastasis detection or follow-up. Thus, imaging is vital for diagnosis and follow-up of patients with liver secondaries.

Ultrasonography

This technique has variable sensitivity in detection of liver metastasis, ranging from 40–77%, and <20% for lesions under 1 cm.[44] Drawbacks include operator dependence, poor results in obese patients and in detecting small lesions near the dome and on the liver surface. Contrast-enhanced USG improves the accuracy of lesion detection.[1]

Hepatic metastases may be hypoechoic, hyperechoic, cystic or mixed echogenicity **(Figs. 20A to C)**. The most common pattern is hypoechoic with no distal shadowing or enhancement. This is produced by highly cellular and hypovascular lesions. Hyperechoic metastases are often seen with colonic and gastrointestinal malignancies and with vascular metastases from islet cell tumors, carcinoid, choriocarcinoma and renal cell carcinoma. They may be surrounded by a hypoechoic halo producing the bull's eye or target appearance **(Fig. 20)**. Presence of halo indicates an aggressive tumor and is commonly seen with bronchogenic carcinoma.[2] Calcification may be seen in mucinous metastases from colon and ovary. Cystic metastases are seen with adenocarcinoma of pancreas, ovary and colon.

On color Doppler imaging, metastases usually do not show intratumoral signal but a 'detour' pattern with a dilated portal vein meandering around the tumor nodules has been described. Intraoperative sonography is a very useful adjunct in patients who are candidates for surgical resection of metastases. It may show additional lesions in comparison with preoperative USG and CT scan.

Computed Tomography

The advent of multidetector CT has led to a lot of flexibility but has also added complexity to the imaging protocols for liver evaluation. Advantages include significant reduction in scan time, elimination of respiratory misregistration, improved Z axis resolution, better multiplanar and 3D reformats and it allows a more precise timing for evaluation of liver in different phases of contrast enhancement. It also helps in demonstration of a vein close to a lesion as this determines the response to radiofrequency ablation. Lesions in proximity to a vessel have higher chances of recurrence.

Since most metastases are hypovascular the usual protocol is to scan in the portal venous phase of enhancement **(Figs. 21A and B)**. Dual phase scanning may be useful for detection of metastases from hypervascular primaries such as renal cell carcinoma and islet cell tumors **(Figs. 22A and B)**. Although breast carcinoma metastases can be hypervascular, studies have not shown any added benefit of biphasic CT over portal phase CT for this indication.[2]

On unenhanced CT most metastases are hypodense to the liver parenchyma, whereas some are indistinguishable from normal liver. Small lesions are nodular and homogeneous, while larger lesions are more irregular, heterogeneous and with ill-defined margins. Calcification is common in mucinous GI tract carcinomas and in chemotherapeutically treated hypervascular lesions (e.g. carcinoid). After contrast administration, metastases from hypovascular tumors may have an enhancing rim that can be seen during arterial phase and occasionally during portal phase **(Figs. 23A and B)**. Lesions that do not have an enhancing rim show little if any enhancement during the arterial phase and become hypoattenuating during the portal phase.

Hypervascular metastases show moderate-to-intense enhancement during the arterial phase that may persist during the portal phase. However, most show a rapid washout and become iso- or hypodense to surrounding liver.

Magnetic Resonance Imaging

Liver metastases like most other liver lesions are hypointense to normal liver on T1W images and hyperintense on T2W images **(Figs. 24A to C)**. The use of fat suppression on T2W sequences, particularly fast spin echo T2W scans, is important as it improves the detection of subcapsular lesions. Morphological features have been shown to be useful in differentiating metastatic lesions from common benign

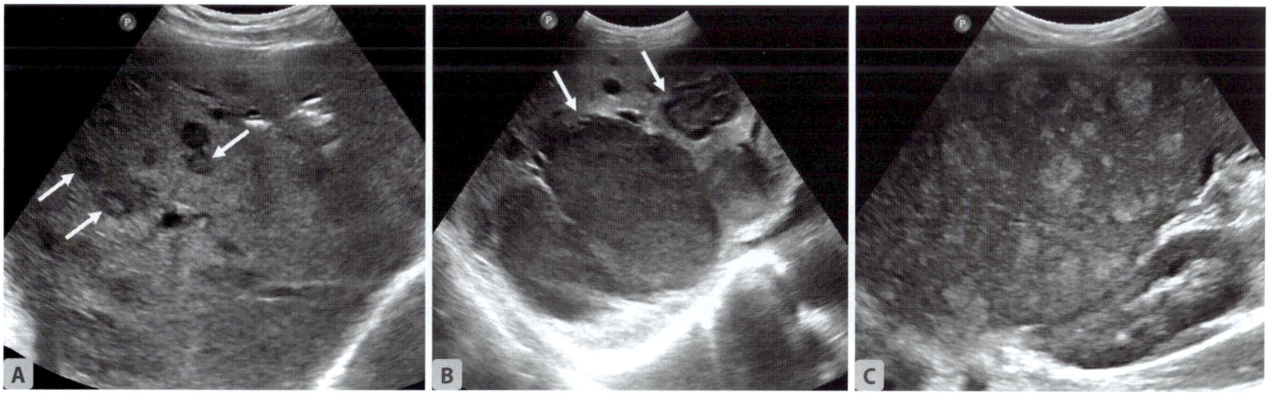

FIGS. 20A TO C: Metastases–Ultrasonography. (A) USG showing "target like" lesions (arrows) suggestive of metastases in a patient with lung carcinoma; (B) USG showing hypoechoic masses (arrows), which were metastases from carcinoma of colon; (C) USG of liver showing hyperechoic lesions suggestive of metastases in a patient with neuroendocrine tumor.

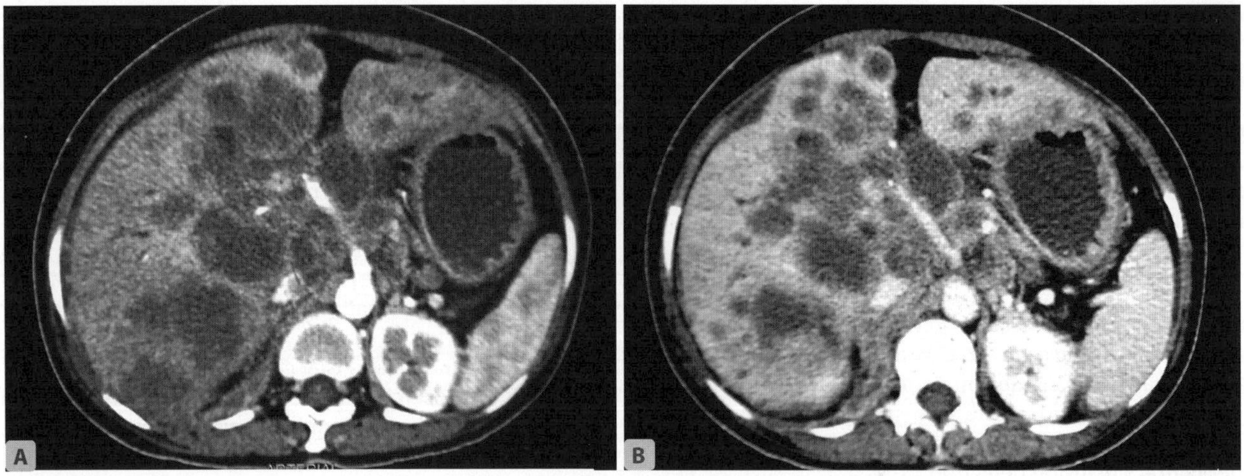

FIGS. 21A AND B: Hypovascular metastases: The contrast-enhanced arterial phase (A) and venous phase image (B) shows multiple hypodense lesions involving all segments of liver. The lesions do not show any enhancement in either of the phases.

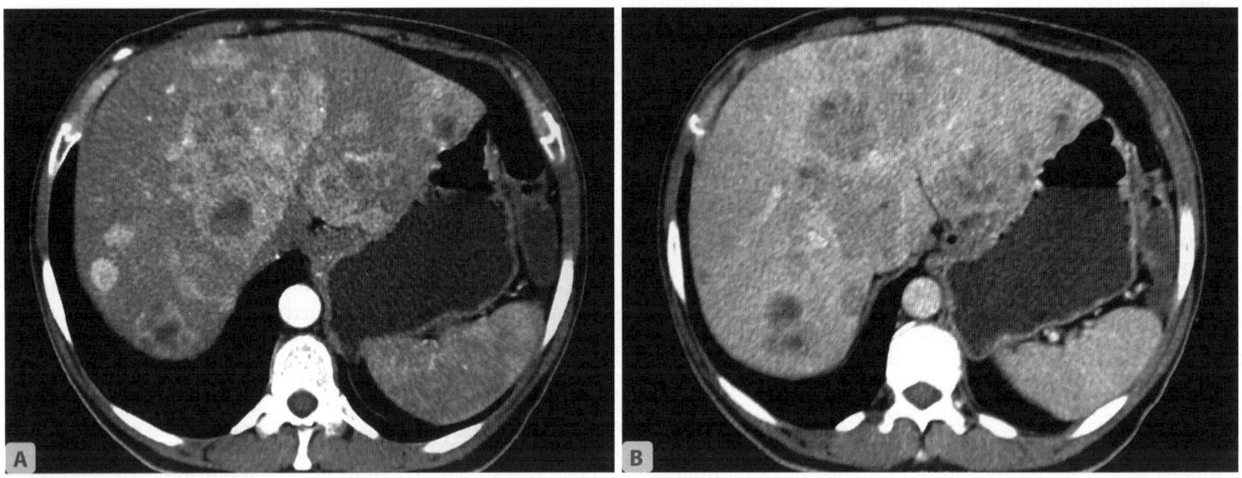

FIGS. 22A AND B: Hypervascular metastases: The contrast-enhanced arterial phase image (A) shows multiple intensely enhancing lesions in both lobes of a noncirrhotic liver with wash out seen in the venous phase (B).

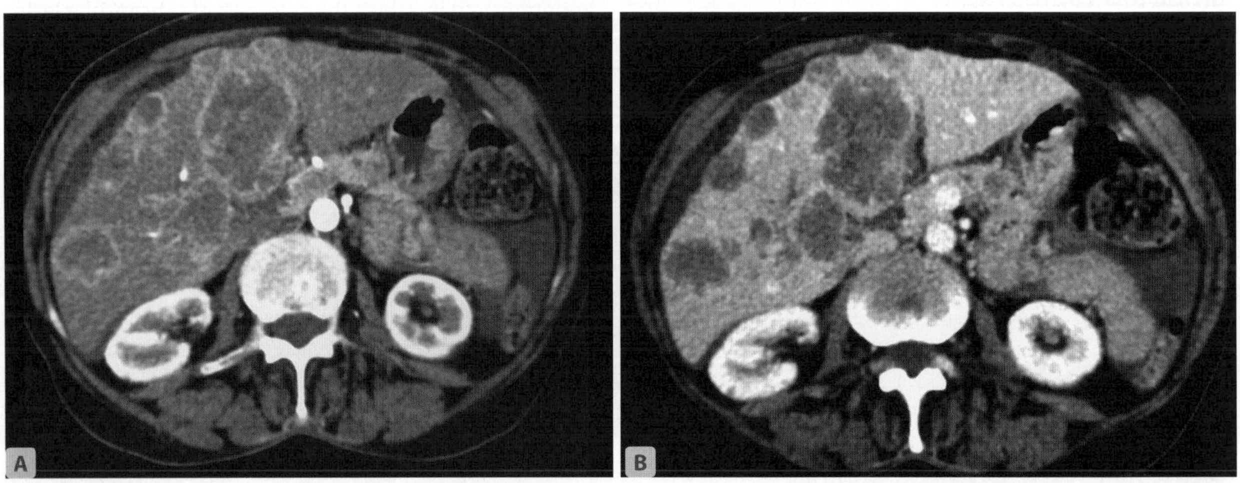

FIGS. 23A AND B: Rim-enhancing metastases. The contrast-enhanced arterial phase image (A) shows multiple rim-enhancing lesions with wash out seen in the venous phase image (B).

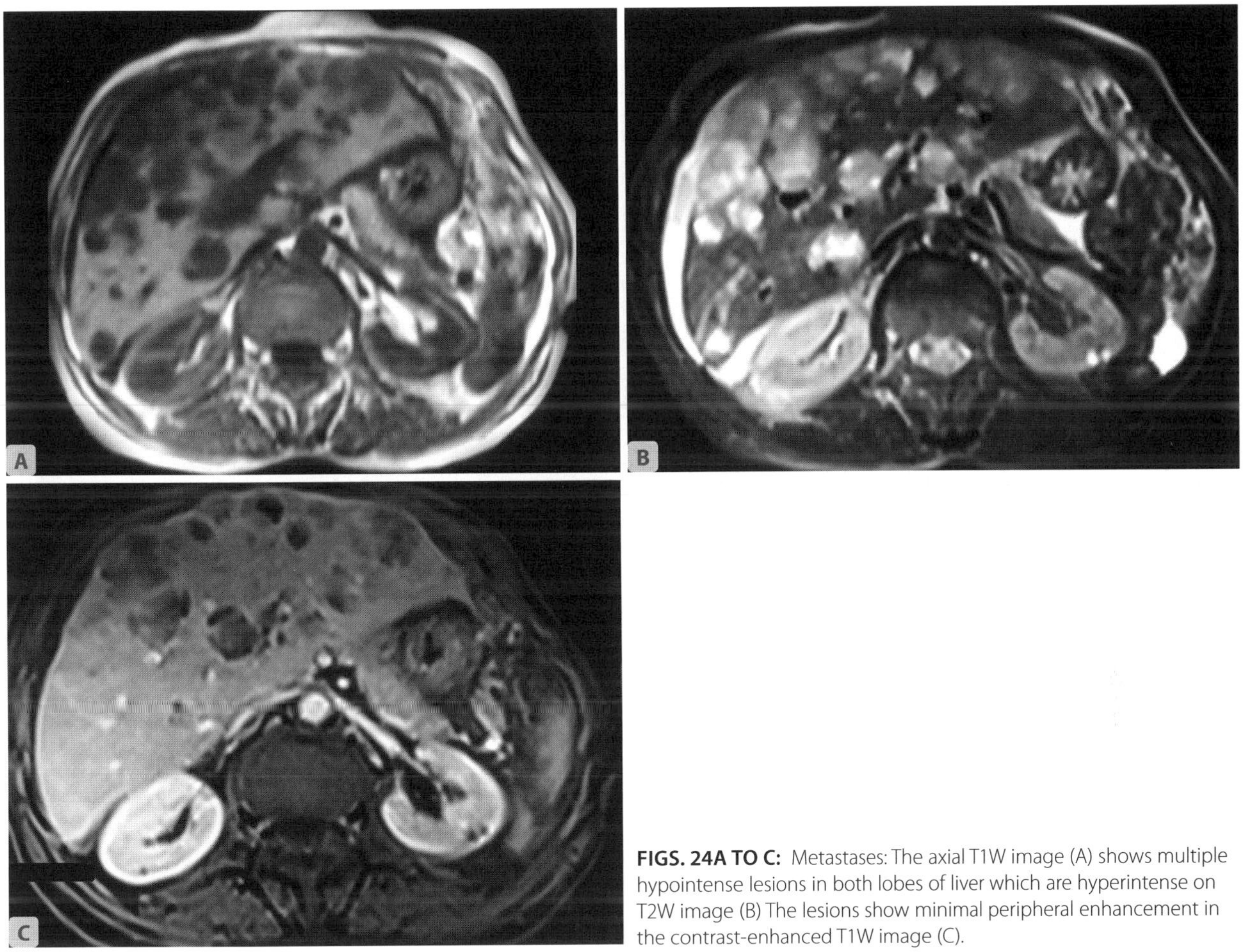

FIGS. 24A TO C: Metastases: The axial T1W image (A) shows multiple hypointense lesions in both lobes of liver which are hyperintense on T2W image (B) The lesions show minimal peripheral enhancement in the contrast-enhanced T1W image (C).

lesions such as hemangioma and cysts. Heterogeneous signal intensity and irregular or indistinct margins, smooth or irregular areas of high signal intensity surrounded by a ring of relatively lower signal intensity are said to be suggestive of metastatic disease. The acquisition of at least one sequence in the coronal plane is useful to evaluate the superior and inferior margins of the liver.

Six appearances of liver metastasis have been described on MRI.[2] Doughnut shape is usually seen with larger lesions, where the lesion is of low signal intensity on T1W images with central necrosis which has even lower signal. These lesions have target appearance on T2W image. Amorphous appearance is seen with heterogeneous masses with ill-defined margins. Peripheral halo is seen with some metastasis and represents either tumor infiltration or surrounding edema. Light bulb morphology, where the lesion is hyperintense on T2W images, is seen with cystic and hypervascular metastasis. Cauliflower appearance is typically seen with colorectal metastasis. Here the lesion has scalloped margins with enhancing periphery and internal septae.

Hypervascular metastases such as those from islet cell tumors, carcinoid and renal cell carcinoma are generally high in signal intensity on T2W images and show intense peripheral ring of enhancement immediately after gadolinium administration. This appearance may mimic hemangiomas. Dynamic serial gadolinium-enhanced MR is very helpful in differentiating these metastases from hemangiomas. Hemangiomas typically show early discrete nodular enhancement which shows a centripetal progression on delayed scans. Metastases often show a transient enhancement of the periphery with a peripheral washout on delayed scans. Enhancement of hypervascular metastases is better shown on MR than on CT images because of the higher sensitivity of MR to gadolinium chelates and the more compact bolus of contrast delivered to the hepatic parenchyma.[2] Hypovascular metastasis may show enhancing rim in arterial phase, with incomplete centripetal filling-in in delayed phase but remain hypointense in all the phases.

State-of-the-art MRI has a higher diagnostic accuracy and greater effect on patient management than CT scan. Diffusion weighted imaging is useful in detection of metastatic liver lesions.[27,45] Liver specific contrast agents such as gadobenate dimeglumine and gadoxetic acid improve lesion detection in hepatobiliary phase.[46] Despite the marked improvement in the accuracy of detection and characterization of metastatic disease, a significant number of lesions are found at surgery that goes undetected on preoperative imaging. These include subcentimeter and subcapsular lesions.

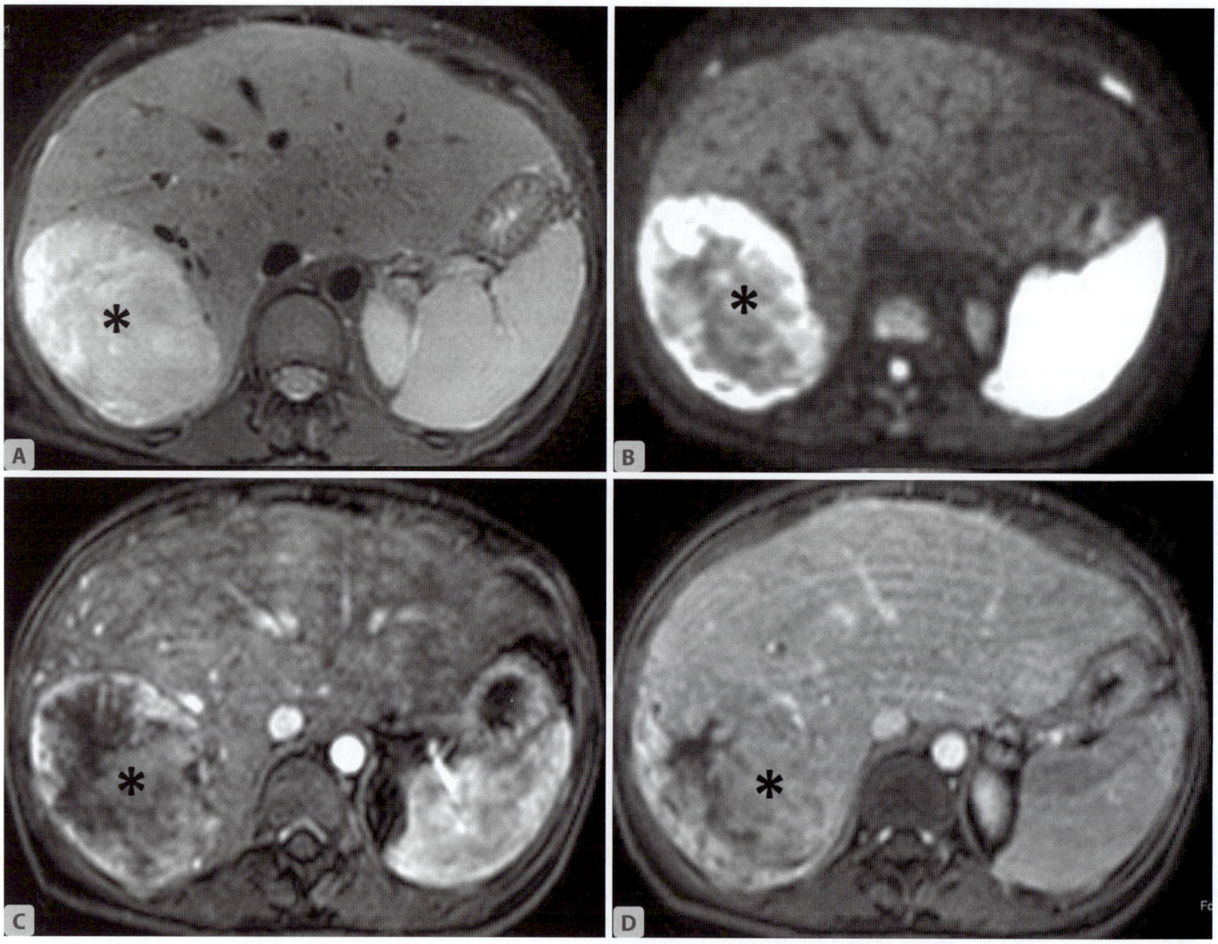

FIGS. 25A TO D: Primary hepatic lymphoma. (A) Axial T2W fat-saturated image showing well-defined hyperintense lesion in right lobe of liver (asterisk); (B) Diffusion-weighted image (b-800) showing restriction of diffusion within the lesion; Axial contrast-enhanced T1W image in arterial (C) and venous phases (D) showing heterogeneous contrast enhancement. Histopathology showed diffuse large B-cell lymphoma.

Differential Diagnosis

Multifocal HCC is an important differential for hypervascular liver metastases. Presence of background chronic liver disease, a capsule on delayed images and absence of a primary malignancy may suggest a diagnosis. However, differentiation may sometimes be difficult and sampling may become necessary. Multiple inflammatory granulomas (like tuberculosis and sarcoidosis) appear hypodense or hypointense on contrast-enhanced imaging studies, similar to metastasis. They usually do not show peripheral rim enhancement in the arterial phase. Clinical and laboratory details, presence of enlarged nodes and splenic lesions may help in making a diagnosis. Pseudotumoral nodular steatosis may mimic metastases; however, MRI is useful in making the diagnosis. There is characteristic signal drop within or in the margin of the lesions on the opposed phase T1W images.[47]

LYMPHOMA

Primary hepatic lymphoma is rare and most often of non-Hodgkin's (diffuse large B-cell type) type.[48] Primary hepatic lymphoma is much more common in organ transplant recipients treated with cyclosporine and patients with AIDS. The most common appearance is that of a solitary large mass, which is hypodense on unenhanced CT and does not enhance significantly after intravenous contrast. Tumors are moderately low in signal intensity on T1W scans and mild-to-moderately hyperintense on T2W scans, with marked diffusion restriction and show mild heterogeneous enhancement on immediate contrast enhanced MR images **(Figs. 25A to D)**.[1,2]

Secondary liver involvement in lymphoma is more common than primary lymphoma and occurs both in Hodgkin's disease and in non-Hodgkin's lymphoma. Diffuse infiltration is more common in Hodgkin's disease, whereas diffuse and nodular hepatic involvement is equally frequent in non-Hodgkin's lymphoma. Imaging findings are nonspecific and cannot be differentiated from other space occupying lesions.

PITFALLS IN THE DIAGNOSIS OF FOCAL LIVER LESIONS

Despite advances in imaging, there are several difficulties which can arise during the diagnosis of focal liver lesions.[46] Knowledge of these pitfalls is necessary for accurate diagnosis of liver lesions. Focal fatty infiltration or sparing may look like a focal lesion. But geographic nature of the lesion, presence of vessels within it and signal drop on opposed phase MRI assist in the diagnosis. Arterioportal shunts, which are sometimes seen in a cirrhotic liver, are seen as ill-defined areas of hyperenhancement in the arterial phase. There may be an adjacent enhancing small branch of portal vein. Isodense appearance on venous/delayed images, peripheral location and absence of discrete lesion on T2W images helps in its differentiation from HCC. Chronic superior vena caval obstruction results in opening up of collateral pathways and sometimes there are cavoportal collaterals which are seen as hyperenhancing area in the left lobe of liver in the arterial phase (hot spot sign). This may mimic hypervascular tumors of the liver. Focal confluent fibrosis is another entity which may mimic focal lesion in the liver. Presence of capsular retraction, location in segments 4, 7 or 8, wedge shape and enhancement in delayed phase suggest a diagnosis. Pseudotumor steatosis, as described above, is another entity which may cause difficulties in diagnosis.

CONCLUSION

Malignant focal lesions of the liver are common and imaging plays a vital role in detection and characterization. MRI is superior to CT for characterizing liver lesions. Many lesions have classical imaging appearances and in combination with clinical features, help in making the correct diagnosis often obviating the need for tissue diagnosis. Liver-specific contrast agents are useful and have potential role in diagnosis. Knowledge of pitfalls in imaging helps to reduce the chances of misdiagnosis. Biopsy may be required in difficult cases after discussion in multidisciplinary group meeting.

REFERENCES

1. Lamba R, Faranazapir G, Corwin MT, Khatri VP. Diagnostic imaging of hepatic lesions in adults. Surg Oncol Clin N Am. 2014;23:789-820.
2. Ros PR, Erturk SM. Malignant tumors of the liver. In: Gore RM, Levine MS (Eds): Textbook of Gastrointestinal Radiology, 4th edition. Philadelphia: Saunders; 2015.pp.1561-607.
3. Bosman F, Carneiro F, Hruban R, Theise N (Eds). Tumors of the liver and intrahepatic bile ducts. In: WHO classification of tumors of the digestive system, IARC, Lyon; 2010.
4. Van Beers BE, Daire JL, Garteiser P. New imaging techniques for liver diseases. J Hepatol. 2015;62:690-700.
5. Dewall RJ. Ultrasound elastography: principles, techniques, and clinical applications. Crit Rev Biomed Eng. 2013;41:1-19.
6. Kim SH, Kamaya A, Willmann JK. CT perfusion of the liver: principles and applications in oncology. Radiology. 2014; 272(2):322-44.
7. Agrawal MD, Pinho DF, Kulkarni NM, Hahn PF, Guimaraes AR, Sahani DV. Oncologic applications of dual-energy CT in the abdomen. Radiographics. 2014;34(3):589-612.
8. Gordic S, Puippe GD, Krauss B, Klotz E, Desbiolles L, Lesurtel M, Mullhaupt B, Pfammatter T, Alkadhi H. Correlation between dual-energy and perfusion CT in patients with hepatocellular carcinoma. Radiology. 2016;280:78-87.
9. GW ter Voert, L Heijmen, HWM van Laarhoven, A Heerschap. In vivo magnetic resonance spectroscopy of liver tumors and metastases. World J Gastroenterol. 2011;17(47):5133-49.
10. McGlynn KA, London WT. Epidemiology and natural history of hepatocellular carcinoma. Best Pract Res Clin Gastroenterol. 2005;19(1):3-23.
11. Fattovich G, Stroffolini T, Zagni I, Donato F. Hepatocellular carcinoma in cirrhosis: incidence and risk factors. Gastroenterology. 2004;127:S35-S50.
12. Llovet JM, Burroughs A, Bruix J. Hepatocellular carcinoma. Lancet. 2003;362:1907-17.
13. Kudo M. Real practice of hepatocellular carcinoma in Japan: conclusions of the Japan Society of Hepatology 2009 Kobe Congress. Oncology. 2010;78(Suppl 1):180-8.
14. Tyson GL, El-Serag HB. Risk factors for cholangiocarcinoma. Hepatology. 2011;54(1):173-84.
15. Choi JY, Lee JM, Sirlin CB. CT and MR imaging diagnosis and staging of hepatocellular carcinoma: Part I. Development, growth and spread: key pathologic and imaging aspects. Radiology. 2014;272(3):635-54.
16. Taguchi K, Asayama Y, Aishima S, et al. Morphologic approach to hepatocellular carcinoma development in man: de novo or the so-called 'dysplastic nodule-carcinoma' sequence? Oncol Rep. 2002;9(4):737-43.
17. Hanna RF, Aguirre DA, Kased N, Emery SC, Peterson MR, Sirlin CB. Cirrhosis-associated hepatocellular nodules: Correlation of histopathologic and MR imaging features. Radiographics. 2008;28:747-69.
18. Bruix J, Sherman M, American Association for the Study of Liver Diseases. Managementof hepatocellular carcinoma: an update. Hepatology. 2011;53(3):1020-2.
19. NCCN guidelines Version 2.2016. Hepatocellular carcinoma. NCCN.org.
20. Willatt JM, Hussain HK, Adusumilli S, Marrero JA. MR imaging of hepatocellular carcinoma in the cirrhotic liver: challenges and controversies. Radiology. 2008;247:311-30.
21. Brannigan M, Burns PN, Wilson SR. Blood flow patterns in focal liver lesions at microbubble-enhanced US. Radiographics. 2004;24:921-35.
22. Salvatore V, Gianstefani A, Negrini G, Allegretti G, Galassi M, Piscaglia F. Imaging diagnosis of hepatocellular carcinoma: recent advances of contrast-enhanced ultrasonography with sonovue. Liver Cancer. 2016;5: 55-66.
23. Takahashi M, Maruyama H, Shimada T, Kamezaki H, Sekimoto T, Kanai F, Yokosuka O. Characterization of hepatic lesions (≤ 30 mm) with liver-specific contrast agents: a comparison between ultrasound and magnetic resonance imaging. Eur J Radiol. 2013;82(1):75-84.
24. Marrero JA, Hussain HK, Nghiem HV, et al. Improving the prediction of hepatocellular carcinoma in cirrhotic patients with an arterially-enhancing liver mass. Liver Transpl. 2005;11(3): 281-9.
25. Filippone A, Blakeborough A, Breuer J, et al. Enhancement of liver parenchyma after injection of hepatocyte-specific MRI contrast media: a comparison of gadoxetic acid and gadobenate dimeglumine. J Magn Reson Imaging. 2010;31(2):356-64.
26. Xu PJ, Yan FH, Wang JH, Shan Y, Ji Y, Chen CZ. Contribution of diffusion-weighted magnetic resonance imaging in the characterization of hepatocellular carcinomas and dysplastic nodules in cirrhotic liver. J Comput Assist Tomogr. 2010;34(4): 506-12.

27. Calistri L, Castellani A, Matteuzzi B, Mazzoni E, Pradella S, Colagrande S. Focal liver lesions classification and characterization: what value do DWI and ADC have? J Comput Assit Tomogr. 2016 [Epub ahead of print].
28. Glockner JF. Hepatobiliary MRI: current concepts and controversies. J Magn Reson Imaging. 2007;25:681-95.
29. Arslanoglu A, Seyal AR, Sodagari F, Sahin A, Miller FH, Salem R, Yaghmai V. Current guidelines for the diagnosis and management of hepatocellular carcinoma: a comparative review. Am J Roentgenol. 2016;207:W1-11.
30. Park YS, Lee CH, Kim JE, Shin S, Park CM. Differentiation of hepatocellular carcinoma from its various mimickers in liver magnetic resonance imaging: what are the tips when using hepatocyte-specific agents? World J Gastroenterol. 2016;22:284-99.
31. Roskams T, Kojiro M. Pathology of early hepatocellular carcinoma: conventional and molecular diagnosis. Semin Liver Dis. 2010;30(1):17-25.
32. Shah A, Tang A, Santillan C, Sirlin C. Cirrhotic liver: What's that nodule? The LI-RADS approach. J Magn Reson Imaging. 2016;43(2):281-94.
33. Ganeshan D, Szklaruk J, Kundra V, Kaseb A, Rashid A, Elsayes KM. Imaging features of fibrolamellar hepatocellular carcinoma. AJR. 2014;202:544-52.
34. Sunnapwar A, Katre R, Policarpio-Nicolas M, Katabathina V, Erian M. Imaging of rare primary malignant hepatic tumors in adults with histopathological correlation. J Comput Assist Tomogr. 2016;40:452-62.
35. Choi BI, Lee JM, Han JK. Imaging of intrahepatic and hilar cholangiocarcinoma. Abdom Imaging. 2004;29:548-57.
36. Kang Y, Lee JM, Kim SH, et al. Intrahepatic mass-forming cholangiocarcinoma: enhancement patterns on gadoxetic acid-enhanced MR images. Radiology. 2012;264(3):751-60.
37. Bhagat V, Javle M, Yu J, Agrawal A, Gibbs JF, Kuvshinoff B, Nava E, Iyer R. Combined hepatocholangiocarcinoma: case-series and review of literature. Int J Gastrointest Cancer. 2006;37(1): 27-34.
38. Shetty AS, Fowler KJ, Brunt EM, et al. Combined hepatocellular-cholangiocarcinoma: what the radiologist needs to know about biphenotypic primary liver carcinoma. Abdom Imaging. 2014;39:310-22.
39. Lantinga MA, Gevers TJG, Drenth JPH. Evaluation of hepatic cystic lesions. World J Gastroenterol. 2013;19:3543-54.
40. Lu M, Greer ML. Hypervascular multifocal hepatoblastoma: dynamic gadolinium-enhanced MRI findings indistinguishable from infantile hemangioendothelioma. Pediatr Radiol. 2007;37:587-91.
41. Azzam RI, Alshak NS, Pham HP. AIRP best cases in radiologic-pathologic correlation: hepatic epithelioid hemangioendothelioma. Radiographics. 2012;32(3):789-94.
42. Lin J, Ji Y. CT and MRI diagnosis of hepatic epithelioid hemangioendothelioma. Hepatobiliary Pancreat Dis Int. 2010;9(2):154-8.
43. Bruegel M, Muenzel D, Waldt S, et al. Hepatic angiosarcoma: cross-sectional imaging findings in seven patients with emphasis on dynamic contrast-enhanced and diffusion-weighted MRI. Abdom Imaging. 2013;38(4):745-54.
44. Bartolotta TV, Taibbi A, Midiri M, et al. Focal liver lesions: contrast-enhanced ultrasound. Abdom Imaging. 2009; 34(2):193-209.
45. Kandpal H, Sharma R, Madhusudhan KS, Kapoor KS. Respiratory-triggered versus breath-hold diffusion-weighted MRI of liver lesions: comparison of image quality and apparent diffusion coefficient values. AJR. 2009;192(4):915-22.
46. Chen L, Zhang J, Zhang L, et al. Meta-analysis of gadoxetic acid disodium (Gd-EOB-DTPA)-enhanced magnetic resonance imaging for the detection of liver metastases. PLoS One. 2012;7(11):e48681.
47. Vilgrain V, Lagadec M, Ronot M. Pitfalls in Liver Imaging. Radiology. 2016;278(1):34-51.
48. Dhamija E, Madhusudhan KS, Shalimar, Das P, Srivastava DN, Gupta AK. Primary hepatic diffuse large B-cell lymphoma: unusual presentation and imaging features. Curr Probl Diagn Radiol. 2015;44(3):290-3.

CHAPTER

104

Interventional Radiology in Treatment of Liver Tumors

Deep Narayan Srivastava, Shivanand Gamanagatti, Shashi Bala Paul

INTRODUCTION

Liver is among the most common sites for primary and secondary tumors. Hepatocellular carcinoma (HCC) represents more than 90% of the primary liver tumors and is the second important cause of cancer related death. Its incidence and mortality is on the rise world over.[1] Metastatic liver tumors are even more common particularly in cases of colorectal carcinoma where about 20% of the cases have metastases at the outset and about half of them are likely to develop during its course.[2] Surgery remains the first line of therapy for these patients and the options of resection or liver transplant provide best outcomes of 5-year survival ranging from 60% to 80%.[3] However, the vast majority of these patients are unsuitable for surgery due to the advanced disease at diagnosis, poor liver reserve and performance status. Furthermore, limited infrastructure, organ shortage and long waiting period denies timely liver transplantation in many.

Over the last two decades, a large number of radiological interventions consisting of either ablative techniques or angiographic procedures have evolved, which are effective in prolonging survival **(Tables 1 and 2)**. Being widely available, safe and efficacious, these minimally invasive techniques have become widely popular and have emerged as the alternative therapeutic options to surgery for both primary and secondary liver malignancies. This chapter focuses on the armamentarium of the currently available image-guided interventional treatments used in the management of liver tumors.

TABLE 1: Radiological interventions for liver tumors.

1. Percutaneous ablative techniques
Chemical ablation: • Ethanol • Acetic acid *Thermal ablation:* • Radiofrequency ablation • Microwave ablation • Laser ablation • Cryoablation • High intensity focused ultrasound ablation *Nonthermal ablation:* • Irreversible electroporation (IRE) or nano knife
2. Intra-arterial procedures
• Transarterial embolization • Transarterial chemoembolization (TACE) • Transarterial chemotherapy (TAC) • Transarterial rhenium/Yttrium therapy (TART)
3. Portal vein embolization

TREATMENT OF MALIGNANT TUMORS

Hepatocellular Carcinoma

The treatment of HCC depends on the stage of the disease, severity of liver function and the performance status of the individual. The Barcelona Clinic Liver Cancer (BCLC) staging **(Flowchart 1)** is the most validated and widely used staging

TABLE 2: Survival rate of various interventional techniques, surgical resection and liver transplantation for treatment of HCC.

			Survival (%)				
Procedure	***No. of patients***	***1st year***	***2nd year***	***3rd year***	***5th year***	***7th year***	***10th year***
Surgical resection	25066	88.2	78.4	69.5	54.2	42.0	29.0
Transplant	183	74.2	69.3	63.4	56.7	NA	NA
Ablation	27150	92.8	81.4	68.6	45.6	29.8	15.7
TACE	19569	77.8	59.0	44.2	24.2	14.0	6.5

FLOWCHART 1: The Barcelona Clinic Liver Cancer Staging System.

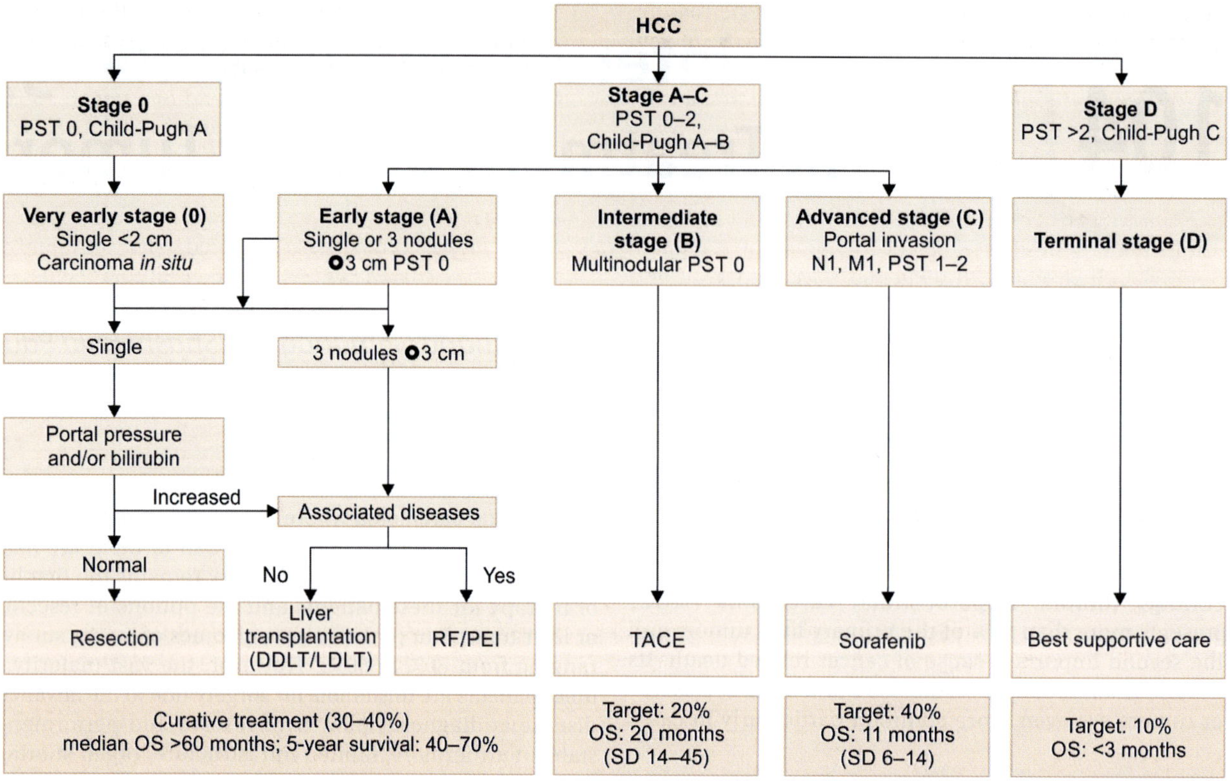

(HCC: hepatocellular carcinoma; LDLT: living donor liver transplantation; DDLT: deceased donor liver transplantation; TACE: transarterial chemoembolization; PEI: percutaneous ethanal injection; RF: radiofrequency; PST: performance status; SD: standard deviation)

for HCC. Besides staging the disease on the basis of these parameters, it also recommends the therapeutic options for all the different stages of HCC.[4] Amongst the interventional therapies, ablation and intra-arterial therapies are indicated for HCC of BCLC A and BCLC B/C stage respectively. Both these are termed locoregional therapies as they target exclusively the tumor tissue sparing the adjoining normal hepatic parenchyma.

Pretreatment Assessment for Locoregional Therapy

The evaluation includes laboratory studies, imaging and counseling of the patient. Laboratory studies include complete blood count, liver function tests, coagulation profile and AFP levels. Cross-sectional imaging by either multiphasic computed tomography (MPCT) or MRI is essential for staging of the disease. Treatment planning is done by careful appraisal of the imaging for the size, number and location of the tumors, presence of macrovascular (portal vein) invasion and extrahepatic disease. Holistic treatment needs to be done, which involves treating the tumor, the underlying tumor etiology (invariably is viral hepatitis) and the associated deranged liver function.

Percutaneous Ablative Therapy

Percutaneous ablation is the treatment recommended for unresectable early HCC. It aims at destroying the viable tumor tissue and creating a safety margin of 0.5–1 cm around. It is safe, easy to perform, well tolerated with very low major and minor complication rate. The best outcome of complete response following ablation varies and is related to the size of the tumor (90–100% in tumors of 2 cm, 50% in the tumors of 5 cm).[5] Hence, the real benefit of therapy lies in treating early, small tumors.

Selection Criteria for Ablation

Ideal HCC patients for ablation are those who are Child-Pugh class A/B cirrhosis, have performance status of 0–1, tumor size smaller than 5 cm (ideal < 3 cm), well-defined intrahepatic with hepatic parenchyma all around, solitary or multiple (not more than 3 in number) with absence of vascular invasion and extrahepatic disease.

Absolute contraindications to ablation are, presence of intravascular invasion, tumor located less than 1 cm from the main biliary duct, intrahepatic biliary dilatation, exophytic tumor or uncorrectable coagulopathy. Relative contraindications are the presence of extrahepatic metastases, bilioenteric anastomosis, superficial lesions, lesions close to gallbladder or any part of gastrointestinal tract, ascites, low platelet count (<50,000/mm^3, pacemaker/defibrillator, hepatic failure.[6]

- *Chemical ablation:* Chemical ablation involves the use of percutaneous ethanal injection (PEI) of either ethanol or percutaneous acetic acid injection (PAI) into the tumor. PEI is the earliest technique which has been extensively studied and its role in treating small HCCs has been well-established.[7] It is inexpensive and can be readily performed with imaging guidance without the use of any special equipment.

- *Mechanism of ethanol/acetic acid ablation:* Neoplastic and nonneoplastic tissue is made up of cellular, interstitial, and vascular compartments. Chemical agents with relatively low molecular weight, such as ethanol and acetic acid, when injected into the tumor, penetrates the cellular compartment remote from the point of injection, through the tumor interstitium. HCCs have extracellular volumes more than twice that of noncancerous liver. These factors result in a high interstitial fluid pressure and interstitial diffusion coefficient that favors easy diffusion of these low molecular weight agents.[8]

  As ethanol distributes through the tumor interstitium, its cytotoxic mechanisms are exerted through a combination of cytoplasmic dehydration, denaturation of cellular proteins, and small vessel thrombosis. These effects result in coagulative necrosis.

  The cytotoxic mechanisms of acetic acid are similar to those of ethanol, which include protein denaturation, dissolution of cellular basement membranes, and destruction of interstitial collagen.
- *Technique of chemical ablation:* Percutaneous chemical ablation is usually performed with real-time ultrasound (US) guidance and local anesthesia. A 20–22 gauge end-hole or conical tip multi-side-hole needle is used. Infusion is performed slowly in 0.1– 0.2 mL aliquots with continuous US monitoring. When the tumor becomes echogenic, the needle is withdrawn while injecting local anesthetic agent for local pain relief **(Figs. 1A to D)**.
- *Volume of alcohol and acetic acid injection:* Strength of the chemical agents used are 95% absolute alcohol (ethanol) or 50% acetic acid. The volume estimation is based on the volume of the tumor and a "surgical margin" of 1 cm beyond the periphery of the lesion. For PEI, the volume is calculated using formula: $V = 4/3\pi\,(r + 0.5)^3$, where V is the target volume of ethanol, r the radius of the lesion (in centimeters), and 0.5 for the correction for the additional "surgical margin". Multiple sessions are performed once or twice weekly and the number of treatment sessions varies according to the size of the lesion, the distribution of intralesional ethanol within the tumor and the condition of the patient.

  For PAI, the maximum total volume of acetic acid required to ablate the tumor is three times the maximum diameter of the tumor. This total dose is injected over multiple sessions (1–2 mL of acetic acid per tumor per session per week) under US guidance.
- *Advantage of PAI over PEI:* Both PAI and PEI are effective in treating small HCC less than 3 cm. PAI has high diffusion capacity and because of this smaller volume of acetic acid and fewer treatment sessions are required to achieve the same degree of cell kill as that with ethanol.[9] PAI has an advantage of infiltrating the tumor septae and capsule of tumors, whereas ethanol is unable to do so. Due to this limitation,

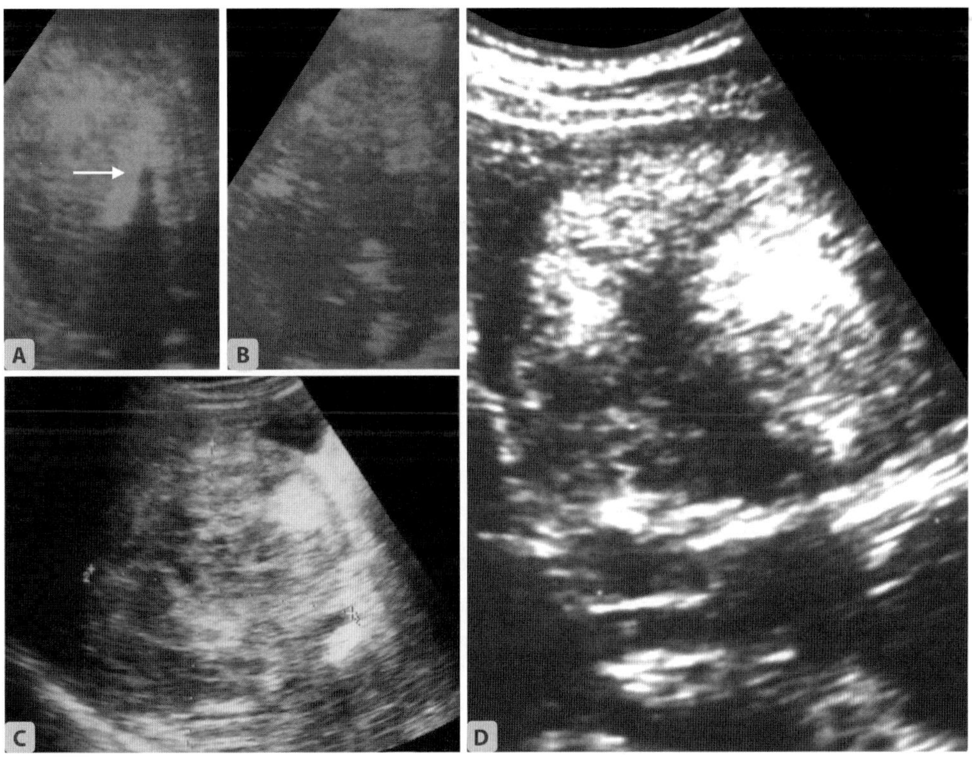

FIGS. 1A TO D: Percutaneous alcohol injection under ultrasound guidance in HCC: Alcohol is injected in the deepest portion (arrow) (A) followed by superficial portion (B) and (C) of the tumor with the help of a long needle (arrow). The perfused areas are seen as patches of hyperechogenicity (D).

PEI is unable to ablate the small satellite nodules and create a safety margin. The local recurrence rate of the tumor is therefore higher in PEI than PAI [37% and 8%, respectively ($P < 0.001$)].[10]

- *Complications:* PAI and PEI are safe procedures with low complication rate and no major complications. Minor complications in the form of transient pain, fever, transient renal failure (with acetic acid) may be encountered. Rarely, transient hemoglobinuria may occur immediately following PAI and this clears on its own. Major complications are rare which include hemorrhage, liver necrosis and abscess formation. Although PEI is performed with a small-caliber needle, substantial hemorrhage has been reported. Therefore, correction of underlying coagulopathy should be performed to a target international normalized ratio of 1.4 or less and a platelet count of 50,000/mm.[1,2]

- *Thermal ablation:* There are four types of thermal ablative techniques namely: Radiofrequency ablation, microwave ablation, cryoablation and laser ablation **(see Table 1)**. Among these, radiofrequency ablation (RFA) is the most widely used. The first experiments with thermal ablation of living tissue were described by d´Arsonval as early as 1868, while the use of thermal ablation for treatment of malignant hepatic lesions was first shown by McGahan et al. and Rossi et al. in 1990.[11,12] Since then, the technique has evolved as the most popular ablative technique world over.
  - *Principle of RFA:* The goal of RFA is to induce thermal injury to the tumor tissue by electromagnetic energy deposition. The patient is a part of a closed-loop circuit which includes an RF generator, an electrode needle, and a large dispersive electrode (ground pads). Radiofrequency energy is delivered as an alternating current at a frequency of 375-500 kHz within the tumor producing ionic agitation around the needle tip because of the relatively high electrical resistance of the tissue in comparison to the metal electrodes. This ionic agitation produces frictional heat around the electrode with resultant coagulative necrosis. The thermal damage is dependent on the tissue temperature achieved and the duration of heating. A temperature of 50-55°C for 4-6 minutes produces irreversible cellular damage.
  - *Types of RFA electrodes:* There are various types of electrodes which have either monopolar or bipolar technology. The difference between the two technologies is elaborated in **Table 3**. Bipolar and multipolar technology is the latest advance in the technique of radiofrequency ablation. This has eliminated the need of a grounding pad and is also more effective in ablating large areas.[13,14]

    The electrodes are broadly divided into the cooled tip or noncooled tip type depending upon the presence of the continuous cooling system. In the cooled tip type, there is continuous saline circulation through the electrode which produces cooling of the needle tip which prevents tissue charring. The heat is generated away from the electrode which results in coagulation necrosis of the tumor tissue.

TABLE 3: Monopolar versus bipolar RFA technology.

Monopolar system	*Bipolar system*
• Circuit is completed inside the patient (Patient is part of the complete circuit)	• Circuit is completed with the lesion
• Grounding pads are required	• No grounding pads
• Multiple lesions cannot be treated at same time	• Multiple lesions can be ablated at same time
• Arrhythmias may occur	

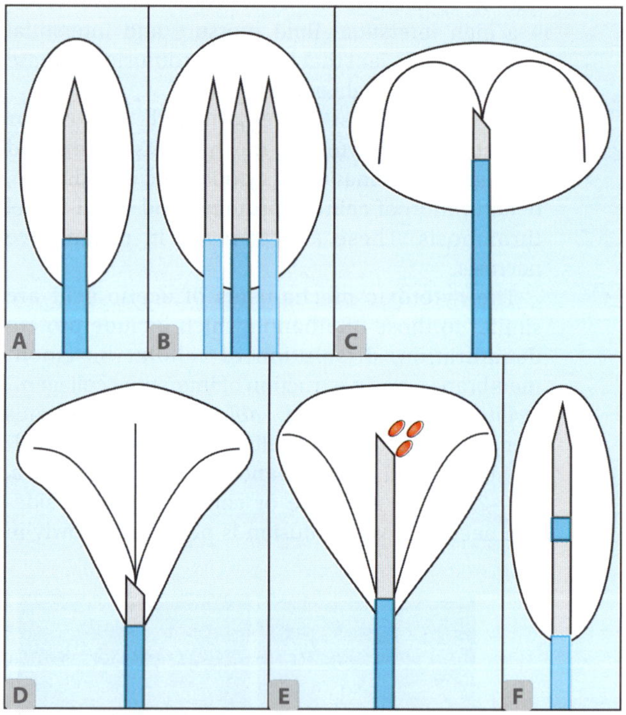

FIGS. 2A TO F: RFA electrode designs. (A) Monopolar single electrode; (B) Clustered electrode; (C) Tined electrode; (D) Multitined; (E) Saline perfused; (F) Bipolar single electrode.
Note: The area marked around each electrode represents the shape of ablating zone.

Based upon the array configuration, the electrodes may be single, clustered, multitined or saline perfused **(Figs. 2A to F)**.

  - *Patient selection:* RFA is ideally suited for smaller lesions less than 3 cm size. Although tumors up to 5 cm diameter can be ablated with RFA, but chances of complete ablation diminishes with increase in tumor diameter. The technique can also be used to treat multiple lesions and up to three lesions can be safely treated in single or multiple sittings. Lesions close to main branches of portal or hepatic veins are difficult to treat as continuous high blood flow in these vessels will have cooling effect because the thermal energy will be dissipated away, which is known as "heat sink effect". If the lesion is close to liver capsule or gallbladder, chances of peritonitis or cholecystitis respectively are high. For these reasons, lesions that do not have at least one centimeter of normal liver parenchyma separating it from the liver capsule, gallbladder, porta hepatis or major vessels are considered a relative contraindication for RFA. Such tumors close to critical structures require special procedures for ablation like saline instillation (5% dextrose water) or balloon occlusion of the larger vascular channel.[15]

Contraindications are similar to the other ablative procedures, like—extrahepatic metastatic disease, tumor volume more than 30% of the total liver volume, sepsis, severe debilitation and uncorrectable coagulopathies.

- *Technique of RFA:* RFA is usually performed with real-time ultrasound (US) guidance or computed tomography guidance, under intravenous sedation and standard cardiac, pressure, and oxygen monitoring.[7] To perform a typical ablation with monopolar RFA system, two grounding pads are placed on the patient's thighs to begin with. The radiofrequency probe is electrically insulated in its proximal part while the short distal part near the tip is uninsulated from where the electric current is passed into the tumor. The electrode is inserted into the lesion under either US or CT guidance. The RF generator is set for the wattage, timer, and temperature as per the device instructions (vendor specific). A pulsed RF energy is applied for 15–30 minutes, which causes a rise of the temperature at the target site from 80°C to 110°C. Once there is ionic agitation within the tissue, the microbubbles are seen forming around the electrode which make the lesion echogenic and obscures the tumor margins. After successful ablation, additional energy is applied during the withdrawal of the electrode under monitoring by real time ultrasound. This is done to prevent seeding of tumor cells in the probe track.
- *Post-RFA evaluation:* For immediate post RFA evaluation, contrast-enhanced sonography is useful for ascertaining the completeness of ablation. In situations of residual disease, reapplication of the radiofrequency electrode in the untreated area in the same sitting can be done to ensure complete response. Multiphasic CT of the liver within a few hours of the ablation is also helpful in gauging the completeness of ablation as well as evaluating any associated complications. However, the accuracy of immediate post RFA assessment scan is limited because of the presence of ablation-induced hyperemic rim around the ablated tumor tissue which mimics the appearance of residual viable tumor. The reactive hyperemia generally resolves in a months' time when more accurate assessment of tumor response can be made on imaging.
- *Complications:* RFA is a safe procedure with a mortality rate as low as 0.1–0.3% and the major complication rate of 2.2–3.1%. Minor complication rate ranges from 5% to 8.9%. Pain or fever is common and is usually self-limiting. Peritoneal hemorrhage, bile duct injury, hepatic abscess, intestinal perforation are some of the adverse outcomes rarely encountered.[16,17] Late complication of tumor seeding along the needle track is also known to occur but is highly uncommon (0.5–0.8%).
- *Limitations of RFA:* Complete tumor response is difficult to achieve in larger tumors more than 5 cm for which newer electrodes are coming into existence. Moreover combination of RFA with other available treatment modalities are being used for larger tumors with improved results.[18] Tumors adjacent to large blood vessels are difficult to treat due to the "heat-sink effect"—a perfusion-mediated tissue cooling reducing the extent of coagulation necrosis produced by thermal ablation.[19]

- *Microwave ablation:* Microwave ablation (MWA) uses electromagnetic waves generated from one or more thin microwave antennas that are applied directly to the tumor to create heat and friction that destroys the tumor.[20]

  The benefit of MWA over radiofrequency ablation (RFA) is the ability to do multiple ablations at the same time. MWA has the potential to destroy larger sized tumors faster and with less pain.
- *Cryoablation:* Cryoablation is another form of the ablative therapy in which the tumor is frozen and this results in cell death. The technique involves creation of an ice ball with subzero temperatures by circulating liquid nitrogen in a probe that is directly inserted into the tumor. As with other ablative therapies, CT, MR or ultrasound scanning provides precise guidance for the procedure. One of the major concerns of cryoablation is "Cryo shock", a fatal complication seen in large hepatic ablation occurring due to rapid release of cellular debris (inflammatory cytokine release) into the systemic circulation.[21] Cryoablation is more widely used in kidney, prostate, lung and bone than in liver tumors.
- *High-intensity focused ultrasound ablation:* High-intensity focused ultrasound (HIFU) is a noninvasive modality producing thermal ablation. The high frequency ultrasound beam is generated by ultrasound transducer which is arranged into a spherical form by an acoustic lens to create a focal point. The beam on reaching the focal point, delivers high temperature focused acoustic energy to the liver tumor producing tumor destruction at a temperature of 60°C.[22] General anesthesia is used and no needle placement within the tumor is required. HIFU is effective in tumors close to major vessels like inferior vena cava, portal or hepatic veins. Complete response can be achieved in 91% of tumors of <3 cm, and the 1 and 3 years survival rates are 87.7% and 62.4%, respectively.[22]
- *Laser ablation:* In this technique, the tumor is destroyed by the heat energy converted from light. Bare tip quartz fibers (300–600 μm) when inserted through multiple 21 gauge needles transmit laser light to the tumor. This light is absorbed and distributed within the tumor, converted to heat in the target tumor tissues and produce coagulation necrosis of the tumor. It is safe and highly effective in HCCs less than 4 cm and can also be used in patients with liver metastases.[23]
- *Nonthermal ablation—Irreversible electroporation:* Irreversible electroporation (IRE) is a new addition to the nonthermal ablative technique which is performed under CT guidance using short pulses of high voltage electrical energy through the electrodes for producing cellular damage in the tumor. Ninety pulses of 1000–3000 V/cm are delivered and a destabilizing electrical potential along

the cell membrane is generated leading to formation of permanent nanopores in the lipid bilayer. Cell death is incurred by irreversible disruption and increased cell permeability.[24] IRE is useful for treating hepatic tumors located close to the major vessels, bile ducts or hepatic veins.

Intra-arterial Procedures

Image-guided intra-arterial procedures are the most commonly used palliative treatment options for the patients of HCC as the vast majority have advanced disease at the outset which precludes the use of curative options. Being palliative in nature, the treatment invariably needs to be repeated in situations of disease progression or recurrences.

- *Transarterial chemoembolization (TACE):* TACE is used for treating patients of unresectable HCC of BCLC B stage,[4] unsuitable candidates for local ablative therapies of BCLC A stage and for downstaging the disease to make patients suitable for resection or transplant. Being palliative in nature, the primary goal of the therapy is to improve quality of life and prolong survival.

  The procedure of TACE is a combination of two steps—intra-artenal injection of chemotherapeutic drugs followed by embolization of the feeding supply to the tumor. In TACE, also called conventional TACE, the chemotherapeutic drug emulsion is prepared by mixing the chemotherapeutic drugs with lipiodol and the subsequent embolization is performed by either gelfoam pledgets or PVA particles **(Fig. 3)**.[25-27] This result in extensive necrosis of the hypervascular HCC as increased dose (up to hundred fold higher) of the chemotherapeutic agent is administered intra-arterially compared to systemic administration. The effect is further augmented by the additional embolization of the feeding arteries (branches from the hepatic arteries) causing ischemic necrosis of the tumor.

  - *Agents used:* Doxorubicin, epirubicin alone or in combination with cisplatin are the commonly used chemotherapeutic agents. Lipiodol, mixed with chemotherapeutic drugs to prepare emulsion, is used as a drug carrier. This drug emulsion is selectively retained within the tumor cells resulting in increased exposure of the neoplastic cells to the chemotherapeutic agents and also enhances the visibility of the emulsion on fluoroscopy.
  - *Patient selection:* Ideal candidates are patients of BCLC B stage. These patients are those who have a preserved liver function (Child-Pugh class A, B), multinodular tumors without vascular invasion or extrahepatic spread. Patients who have reduced liver function or hepatic failure (Child-Pugh C), have to be excluded for this treatment since the liver function may further deteriorate due to ischemic damage of the unaffected liver tissue leading to acute liver failure.
  - *Benefit of arterial embolization:* Arterial embolization induces selective ischemia which results in tumor necrosis and enhances the cytotoxicity of the anti-chemotherapeutic agents. Gelfoam embolization creates hypoxic environment in the tumor bed and tissue hypoxia inhibits the active efflux of the chemotherapeutic drug by making transmembrane P-glycoprotein, an ATP-dependent pump ineffective.
  - *Technique* **(Figs. 4A to F)**: Chemoembolization is performed in the angiography suite, under aseptic precautions with the patient under conscious sedation and through the percutaneous route. To begin with, diagnostic mesenteric and celiac arteriograms are performed using various preshaped polyurethane catheter (4 or 5F) with the digital subtraction technique to determine the vascular anatomy, feeding tumor supply and the portal blood flow. The placement of the catheter tip in the feeding artery, as close to the tumor as possible, is the most important technical factor undertaken for maximizing the treatment effect on the tumor and minimizing damage to nontumor hepatic tissue. Superior mesenteric arteriogram is done for detecting the presence of any hepatic arterial supply (accessory and aberrant) arising from the vessel as well as foe evaluating the patency of the portal vein. Depending upon the hepatic arterial branches arising from celiac artery, selective arteriography of the common, left and right hepatic arteries as per the case is done. The peripheral part of the large tumor, surface tumors, stenosis or occlusion of the hepatic artery or previously treated tumors may develop supply from the extrahepatic sources like parietal arteries, phrenic, internal mammary or intercostal arteries. Unusual origins of the various arterial supply to the tumor may be encountered, like the gastroduodenal artery arising close to the origin of the middle or left hepatic artery, the right gastric artery arising from right or proper hepatic artery or the left hepatic artery arising from the left gastric artery. Use of microcatheter and sometimes coil embolization of these vessels is performed to protect the stomach and duodenum from potential reflux of the chemotherapeutic and embolic agents. Microcatheter, coaxial system helps to reach the

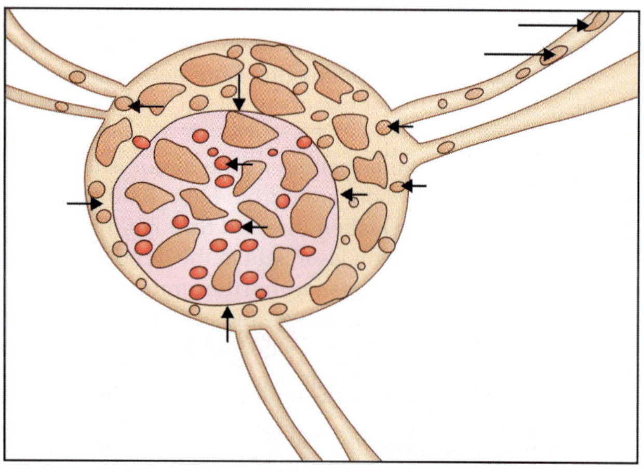

FIG. 3: Diagrammatic representation of transcatheter chemoembolization. Lipiodol is mixed with chemotherapeutic drug and is infused in hepatic artery followed by gelfoam embolization (long arrows) of the arterial branches. The dark area represents the tumor (small arrows).

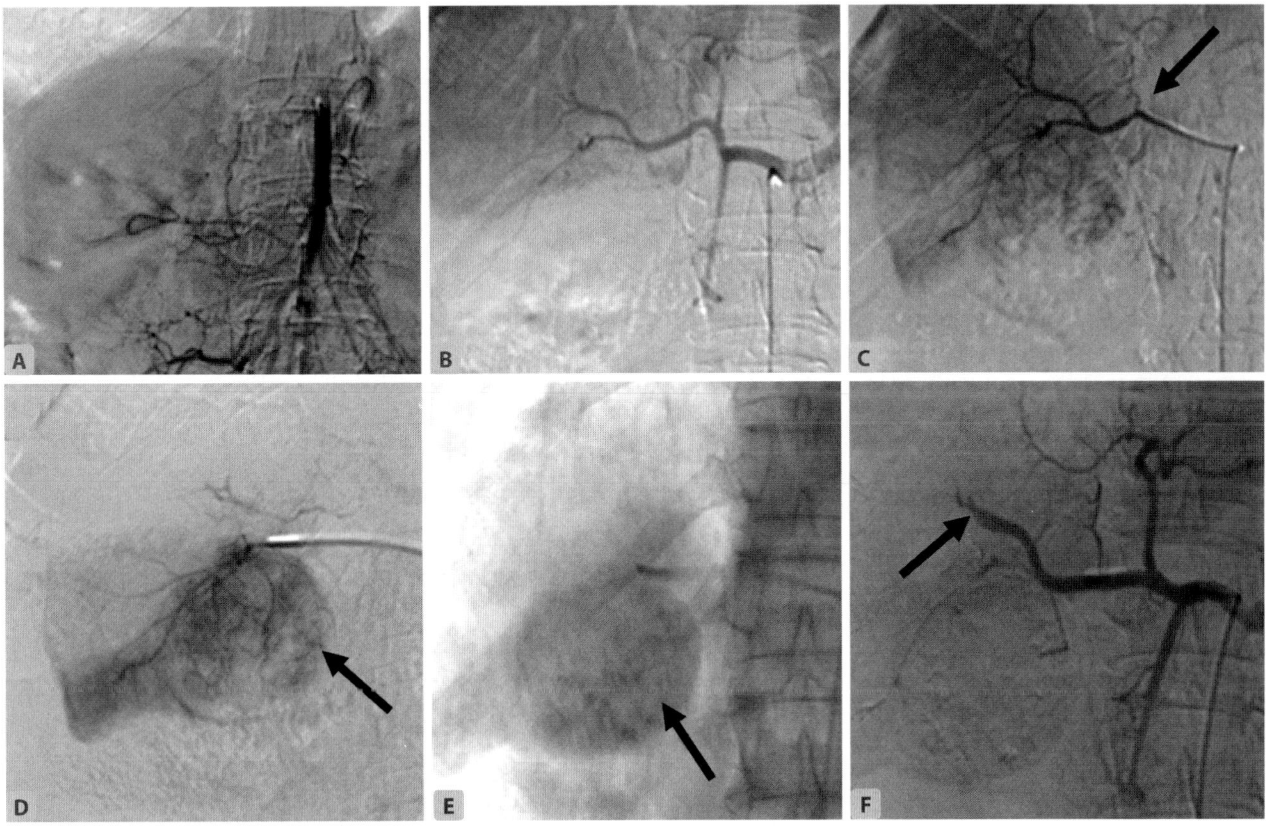

FIGS. 4A TO F: Various steps of angiographic technique of TACE: Initial SMA angiogram (A) performed to look for anomalous origin of hepatic artery, followed by celiac axis angiogram (B); Selective angiogram of the right hepatic artery (arrow) (C) showing abnormal tumor blush (arrow)(D), followed by injection chemotherapeutic emulsion into the tumor bed shows retention of lipiodol (arrow) (E) and stasis of blood flow (F) following gelfoam embolization (arrow).

tumor superselectively avoiding vessel spasm and dissection. After advancement of the microcatheter system to the appropriate segmental or subsegmental vessel supplying the tumor, the chemotherapeutic mixture is injected slowly at the rate of 1 mL/minute under continuous fluoroscopic observation avoiding reflux of chemotherapeutic agent into nontarget areas. There are no recommendations regarding the volume of emulsion to be injected with reference to the tumor size.

In case of multiple vascular feeders, the emulsion is injected into all the feeders superselectively in divided fractions. In case of significant arterioportal or arteriovenous shunting, a small amount of gelfoam is injected to block the shunt prior to the injection of chemotherapeutic emulsion. Subsequently, the feeding vessels are embolized by gelfoam pledgets to reduce the blood flow and also the wash out of chemotherapeutic agents into the systemic circulation.

If the tumor is very large in size, repeated sessions of TACE may be required to achieve complete response **(Figs. 5A and B)**. It is also important to search for any extrahepatic supply to the tumor in such cases.

- *Complications of TACE:* Postembolization syndrome is commonly encountered and is self-limiting. Major complications include hepatic insufficiency, liver abscess, ischemic complications (cholecystitis, bile duct necrosis, perforation of the alimentary tract), and renal dysfunction.

- *TACE using drug eluding beads (DEB-TACE):* The main target of TACE is to reduce systemic toxicity, increase the therapeutic efficacy and provide a sustained release of chemotherapy over time without damaging the healthy surrounding hepatic parenchyma. Recently, introduced novel technologies consisting of embolic microspheres have the ability to actively sequester doxorubicin hydrochloride from a solution and release it in a controlled and sustained fashion (DEB). They have been shown to substantially diminish the amount of chemotherapy that reaches the systemic circulation compared with lipiodol-based conventional TACE, thus significantly increasing the local concentration of the drug and achieving better tumor response rates.[28]
- *Transarterial radionuclide therapy (TART):* Hemodynamic principles and techniques of TART are similar to TACE. Internal radiotherapy by injection of isotopes like ^{131}Iodine+lipiodol, ^{188} Rhenium + lipiodol and ^{90} Yttrium (^{90}Y) into the hepatic artery has shown improvement in survival. ^{90}Y radioembolization can deliver extremely high levels of radiation (up to 150 Gy), with tolerable exposure to normal parenchyma. TART is a safe, effective and promising therapeutic option in patients with inoperable HCC **(Figs. 6A to E)**.

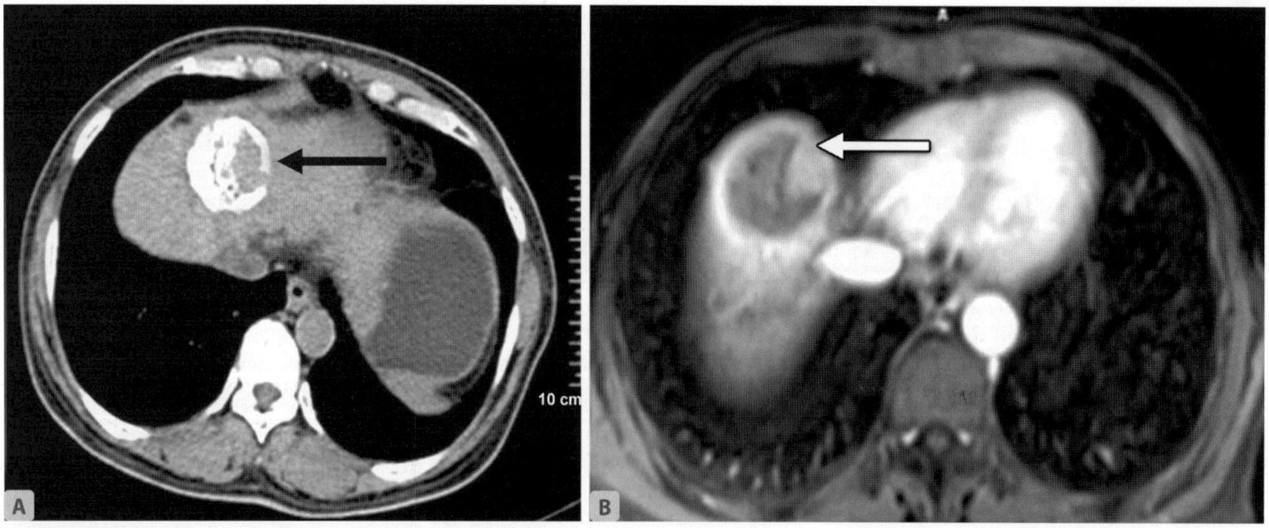

FIGS. 5A AND B: CT and MRI images of treated by TACE: Axial NCCT image (A) showing lipiodol defect on the medial aspect of the treated lesion (arrow). Postcontrast axial MR image (B) confirming the presence of enhancing component in the area of lipiodol defect (arrow) suggestive of partial response.

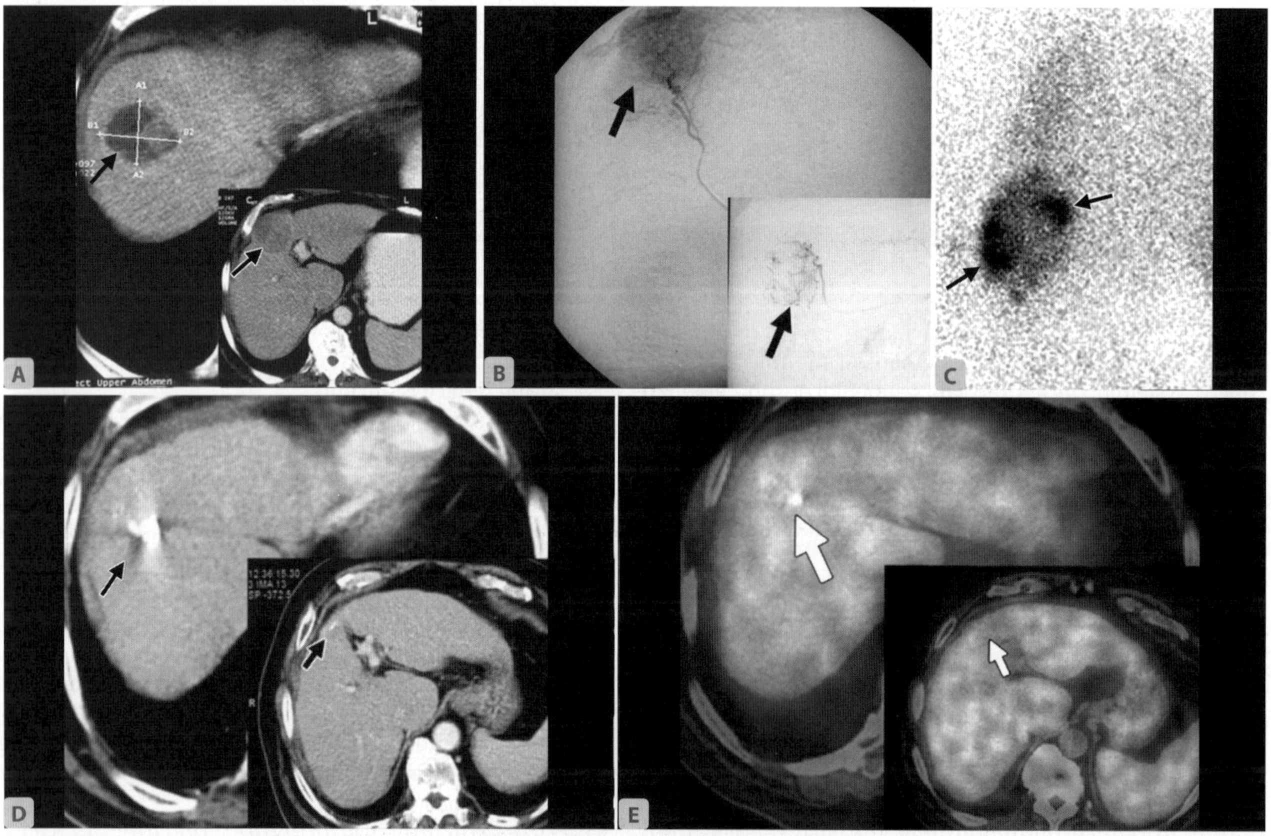

FIGS. 6A TO E: A 69-year-old man with two HCC lesions involving both lobes of the liver. Both lesions were completely ablated after two doses of 188Re HDD iodized oil at three-monthly intervals. At the time of this writing, the patient was alive and ambulatory with normal serum AFP levels and no evidence of mass at 3-year follow-up CT: (A) Pretherapy axial contrast-enhanced CT shows two lesions (arrows): One each in segments IV and VIII; (B) Angiogram shows increased vascularity in both lesions (arrows); (C) Post-treatment 188Re whole body scan shows radiotracer accumulation in the tumors (arrows), with faint visualization of lungs and no radiotracer uptake in the thyroid, gastrointestinal tract, or anywhere else; (D) Repeat CT obtained 3 months after the second dose shows complete disappearance of both lesions (arrows). Small radiopaque area in segment IV lesion (appearing to be enhancing HCC mass in larger arterial phase image) is actually a small amount of iodized oil, which was seen in all CT scanning phases (noncontrast, arterial, portal venous, and delayed); (E) Positron emission tomography/CT scan obtained 2 years after treatment also shows no evidence of residual or recurrent disease (arrows). Inset images show segment IV lesion.

The best candidate for TART is BCLC-Advanced stage C, i.e. HCC with portal vein tumor thrombosis (PVT).[29]

Combination Treatment

Currently, in cases with increased tumor burden or larger sized tumors, multimodality approach is being considered. The regional and local therapies are combined in the same patient to produce better results as compared to the use of single therapy.[30,31]

Ablative therapies of PEI or RFA are performed after the procedure of TACE in cases of small residual disease, TACE followed by oral chemotherapy is used for advanced HCC and in patients with postresection recurrence (s), RFA or TACE is undertaken frequently **(Figs. 7A to D)**.

Follow-up and Response Assessment after Locoregional Therapies for HCC

Clinical follow-up: Postprocedure, patients are followed up at 1–2 monthly intervals for the assessment of the liver function status and treatment side-effects if any. Liver and renal function tests, serum AFP (if elevated prior to treatment) and viral markers (depending upon the etiology of HCC) for monitoring of the hepatitis B or C activity status is undertaken. If a clinical suspicion of recurrence or disease progression arises on follow-up (features of decompensation or rise in AFP), imaging evaluation is asked for and the management done accordingly.

Imaging follow-up: Accurate assessment of tumor response is extremely important in oncology practice for prolonging survival. Imaging techniques of multiphasic CT and MR are generally recommended and lately, use of contrast-enhanced ultrasound (CEUS) has also been used with promising results.[32,33]

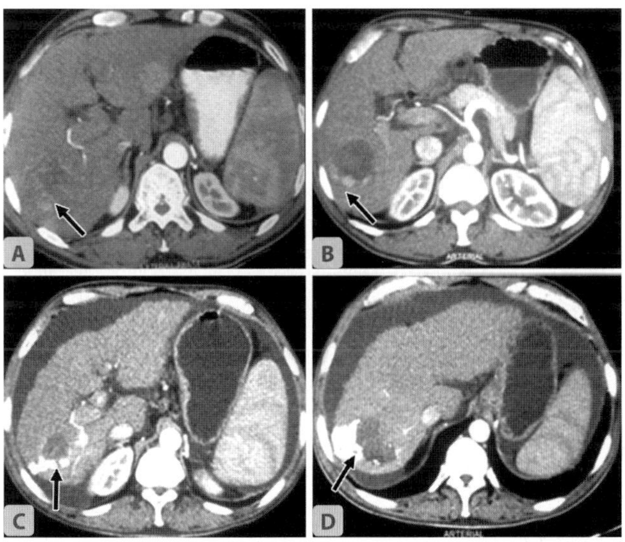

FIGS. 7A TO D: Combination treatment for HCC (RFA followed by TACE): Pre-RFA axial CT (arterial phase) image (A) showing arterial enhancing lesion (arrow) in segment VI treated by RFA. Post-RFA CT (arterial phase) image (B) showing peripheral nodular enhancing area (arrow) in segment VI lesion, which was subsequently treated by TACE. Post-TACE axial CT images (C and D) showing lipiodol deposition in the periphery of the lesion (arrows) corresponding to nodular enhancing area seen on image B. Findings are suggestive of complete response.

Due to the differences in the principles of imaging techniques, contrasts used, these modalities have some limitations, advantages and accuracies in the therapeutic assessment. Response evaluation entails detection of any viable tumor tissue which on contrast imaging techniques (CEUS, MPCT, MRI) is seen as an enhancing area at the tumor site, while the nonviable tissue lacks enhancement. One of the major limitations of MPCT is the difficulty in accurate assessment of the residual disease in post-lipiodol TACE patients. Lipiodol is radiodense and is seen as a hyperdensity in the tumor site on MPCT, the appearance that is similar to the hyperenhancing viable tumor tissue following contrast injection. This at times leads to masking of the small viable tissue on MPCT resulting in misinterpretation.

MRI has the highest accuracy in these patients as the assessment is not affected by the lipiodol presence.[34] Contrast sequences can be complimented with diffusion-weighted sequences (DWI) to improve the diagnostic accuracy. DWI helps to differentiate inflammatory enhancement (T2-shine through) from the viable tumor (diffusion restriction).[35] Evaluation by CEUS is also not hampered by the lipiodol presence and thus CEUS can diagnose even a small viable tissue with high accuracy.[36]

Multiphasic CT or MRI is done at 1, 3, 6 12 months post-procedure for detection of residual disease on the basis of mRECIST criteria.[37] Response assessment by this criterion is based on the percentage of necrosis, viable tumor tissue and not on the overall tumor size shrinkage. This is because the locoregional therapies produce tumor destruction and accurate interpretation of the viable and nonviable cells would give the true picture of efficacy of the therapy in the form of complete or partial response. According to the mRECIST criteria, tumor response is categorized as complete response (CR) is the disappearance of any intratumoral arterial enhancement in all target lesions, partial response (PR): >30% decrease in sum of diameters of all viable (enhancing) target lesions, progressive disease (PD) is >20% increase in the sum of diameters of all viable (enhancing) target lesions and any case that does not qualify for either PR or PD is stable disease (SD) **(Figs. 5 and 8)**.

If the imaging findings suggest PR or PD, then depending upon the disease stage at that point of time, the decision of further treatment is taken. When CR is achieved, the patient is kept under regular clinical and imaging follow-up. On MPCT/MRI, assessment of tumor morphology, resorption of ethiodized oil, overall liver size, development of new lesions or metastases is looked for.[38] Completely treated tumor invariably shrinks in size over period of time **(Figs. 9A to D)**.

Outcome of chemical ablation: PEI is highly effective in small HCCS of 3 cm size. Complete tumor response is encountered in about 80% of the cases and when the size increases to 5 cm, the complete response drops to 50%.[39] In Child's A with early HCC, a 5 years survival rate of 47–53% is seen following PEI.[40]

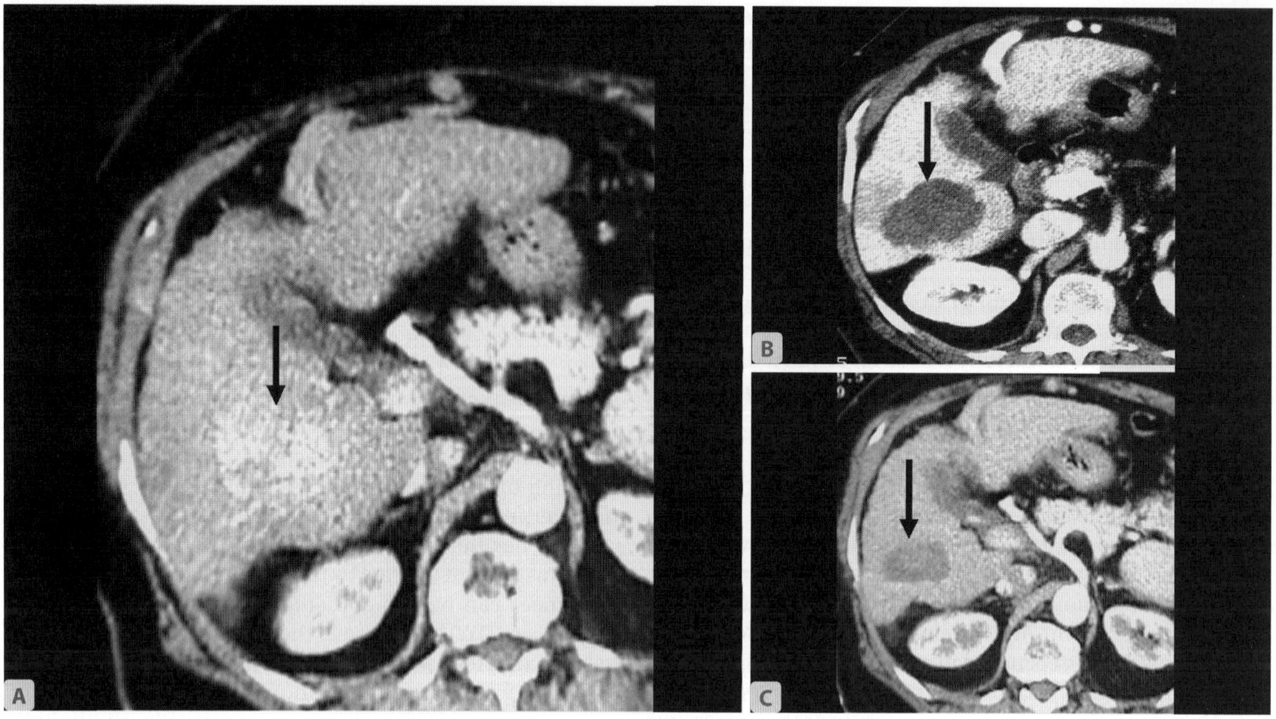

FIGS. 8A TO C: Preablation arterial phase CT liver showing vascular tumor (arrow, A) in segment VI, complete necrosis and reduction in size (arrow) at 1 year (B) and 2 years (C) after radiofrequency ablation. The patient died after two and half years due to hepatic failure secondary to advanced cirrhosis.

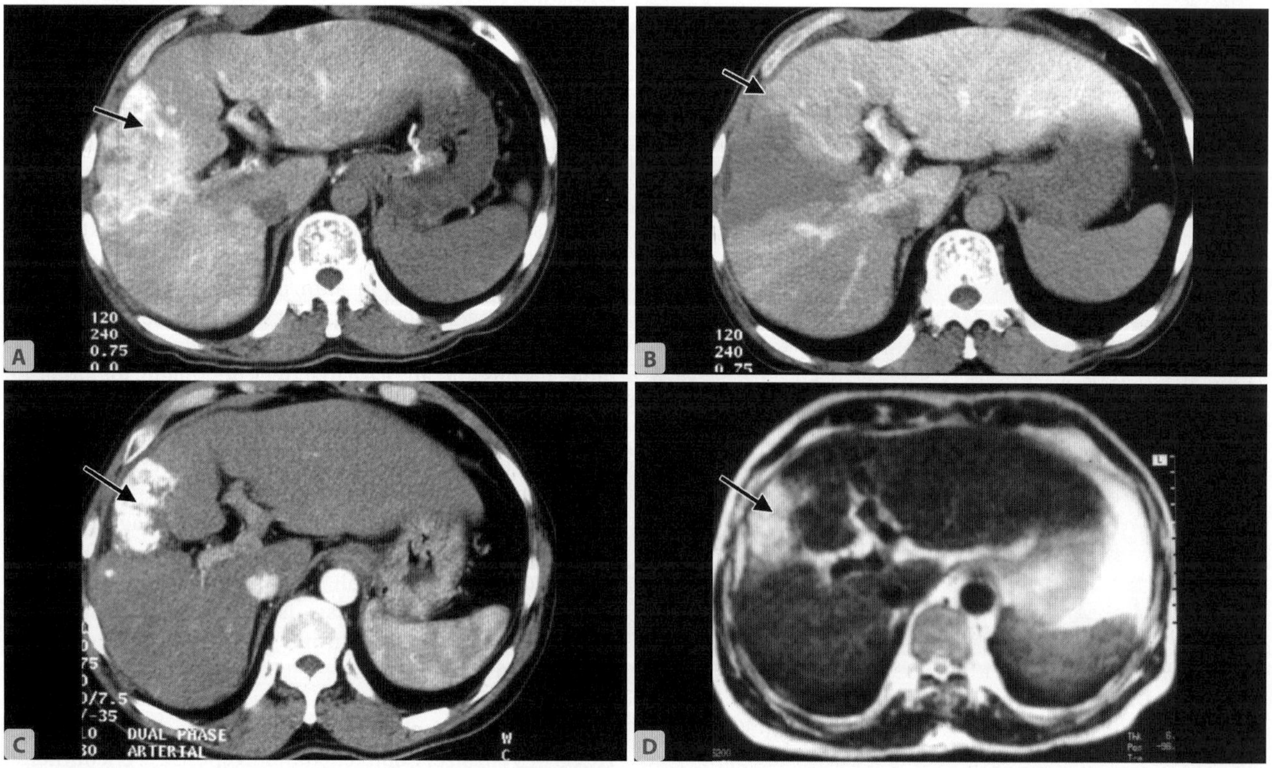

FIGS. 9A TO D: Pre- (A and B) and post-treatment CT (C) and MR (D) of liver showing vascular mass (arrows) in segments IV and V. The mass is reduced in size after TACE.

Limited studies on PAI are available. With PAI too, the response rates are better in small masses up to 3 cm. The local tumor recurrence rate is 51% at 1year and 74% at 3 years. The survival rate at 1 and 3 years is 84% and 51% respectively.[10] Combination of PEI or PAI with other treatments is being taken up for improving treatment outcomes of larger tumors.

Outcome of RFA: Like other techniques of ablation, the tumor response depends on the size, number and location of the tumor as well as the associated liver function. Several studies have reported the complete ablation rates of 80–90% in nodules <3 cm, 50–80% for 3-5 cm and as low as 25% in nodules >5 cm.[41] On comparing the outcome of RFA with surgical resection in multinodular HCC, a recent meta-analysis has shown a better survival benefit with resection than RFA, whereas in solitary small HCC of 2 cm, comparable results of RFA and resection have been observed.[42]

Outcome of transarterial chemoembolization: TACE is an effective procedure which produces significant tumor response and survival benefit despite tumor size in comparison to supportive care. A survival advantage of 82% and 63% for chemoembolization has been documented in comparison to 63% and 27% for supportive care at 1 and 2 years, respectively.[43,44] The largest Japanese cohort study has depicted a median survival of 34 months and a survival benefit at 1, 3, 5 and 7 years as 82%, 47%, 26% and 16%, respectively with negligible procedure-related mortality (0.5%).[45]

A study from India, TACE performed for relatively larger tumor size [up to16 cm (Mean size 6.6–3.92 cm], the cumulative survival rate at 1, 2 and 3 years was 66%, 47% and 36.4%, respectively.[46]

Outcome of DEB-TACE: As the DEB produce slow, sustained release of the chemotherapeutic drug, the liver toxicity as well as the systemic toxicity is less. Limited literature is available on long term follow-up. Improved local response and fewer treatment sessions are required with DEB-TACE in comparison to conventional TACE. Decreased frequency of postembolization syndrome with 100–300 mm versus 400–600 mm beads has also been documented. Less side effects leading to low hospitalization rates are seen.[47,48] In India, the biggest limitation of its use has been the high cost and limited availability.

Outcome of TART: As yet, there is limited evidence on the outcome of 90Y radioembolization in patients with unresectable hepatocellular carcinoma. The therapeutic efficacy essentially depends upon the radiation effects as opposed to the ischemia associated with chemoembolization or pure embolization. With 90Y, best outcomes occur in patients with preserved liver function (Child's A) regardless of PVT. Those with Child's B liver function and PVT, have poor outcomes.[29,49,50] The difference in survival between Child's A and B patients has been 17.2 months and 7.7 months; P= 0.002, respectively.[50] Rhenium used in one Indian multicentric trial depicted survival rates of 90.5% at 1 year and 30.5% at 3 years.[29]

Transcatheter arterial embolization (TAE): In this, tumor is embolized with intra-arterial temporary or permanent embolizing materials in single or multiple sessions. It has been proved to be a less effective palliative treatment especially for large and peripherally located HCC due to development of collateral circulation.

Transcatheter arterial embolization of the tumor may be done as an emergency procedure to reduce gastrointestinal hemorrhage in selected patients. Gastrointestinal hemorrhage from hepatocellular carcinoma (HCC) during the natural course of the tumor is unusual. The causes of massive intermittent gastrointestinal bleeding may be either due to varices or due to direct invasion of duodenum, transverse colon and stomach by the tumor. The variceal bleeding may be consequent to portal hypertension secondary to intra-tumoral arterioportal shunts **(Figs. 10A to D)**. These patients may respond well to TAE.[51] Some studies have shown that TAE is an effective method for palliative treatment in such patients.[51,52]

Portal Vein Embolization

Percutaneous portal vein embolization has become an important preoperative treatment in patients who undergo extensive liver resection due to hepatic malignancy. It is done when future liver remnant volume is less than 25% in case of normal back ground liver (less than 40% in case of cirrhotic patients). The aim is to occlude right portal vein either through ipsilateral or contralateral approach using various embolizing agents such as glue, PVA particles and coils. This results in compensatory hypertrophy of the future liver remnant and hence subsequent increase in the functional reserve of the liver and reduces postoperative hepatic failure. The procedure is done percutaneously using both ultrasound and angiography guidance. In normal livers, sufficient hypertrophy typically occurs within 2–4 weeks, whereas regeneration in patients with cirrhosis can take ≥4 weeks. This technique is mainly useful in noncirrhotic livers with malignant tumor confined to segments of one lobe **(Figs. 11A to D)**.[53]

Hepatic vein stenting: The association of Budd-Chiari syndrome and HCC is favored by two conditions. First, HCC can cause obstruction of the main hepatic veins or inferior vena cava due to endoluminal invasion by the tumor. This produces an acute or fulminant variant of Budd-Chiari syndrome, which has a poor prognosis. Second, HCC can develop in patients with chronic Budd-Chiari syndrome and accounts for 0.7% of all the cases of HCC. HCC is most common in patients with membranous obstruction of the vena cava. These patients can be managed effectively by combined interventional techniques; hepatic vein stenting or IVC dilatation to relieve the venous obstruction combined with transarterial chemoembolization for the hepatocellular carcinoma **(Figs. 12A to D)**.

TREATMENT OF METASTATIC DISEASES OF LIVER

Short of surgery, like HCC, interventional techniques of Ablation (commonly RFA) and intra-arterial chemotherapy is the standard treatment recommended for metastases to liver **(Figs. 13A to D)**.[54]

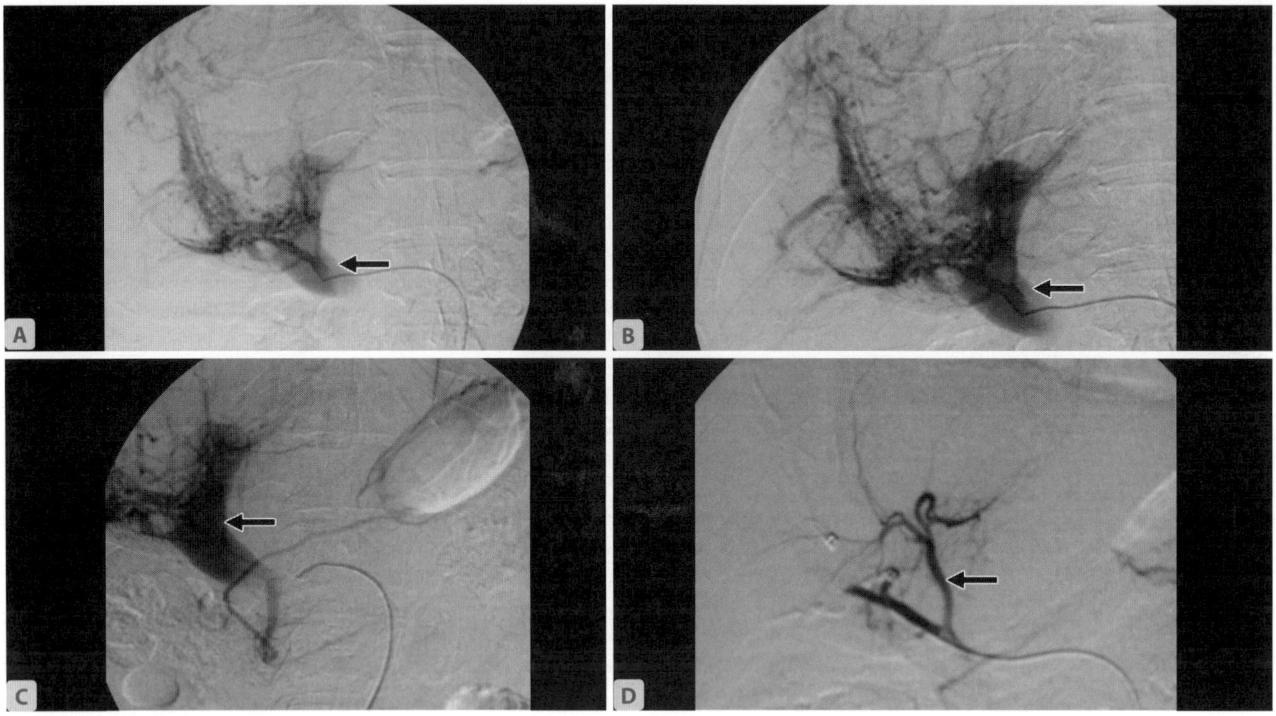

FIGS. 10A TO D: A 62-year-old male presented with massive upper gastrointestinal hemorrhage (GIH) due to variceal rupture secondary to intratumoral arterioportal shunts causing portal hypertension. The tumor (HCC) was embolized and GIH was stopped. Hepatic arteriograms (A to C) are showing tumor vascularity with simultaneous opacification of portal vein (arrows). The right hepatic artery branches were embolized with fiber steel coils. The postembolization angiogram is not showing opacification of portal vein; (D) The left hepatic artery was not embolized (arrow).

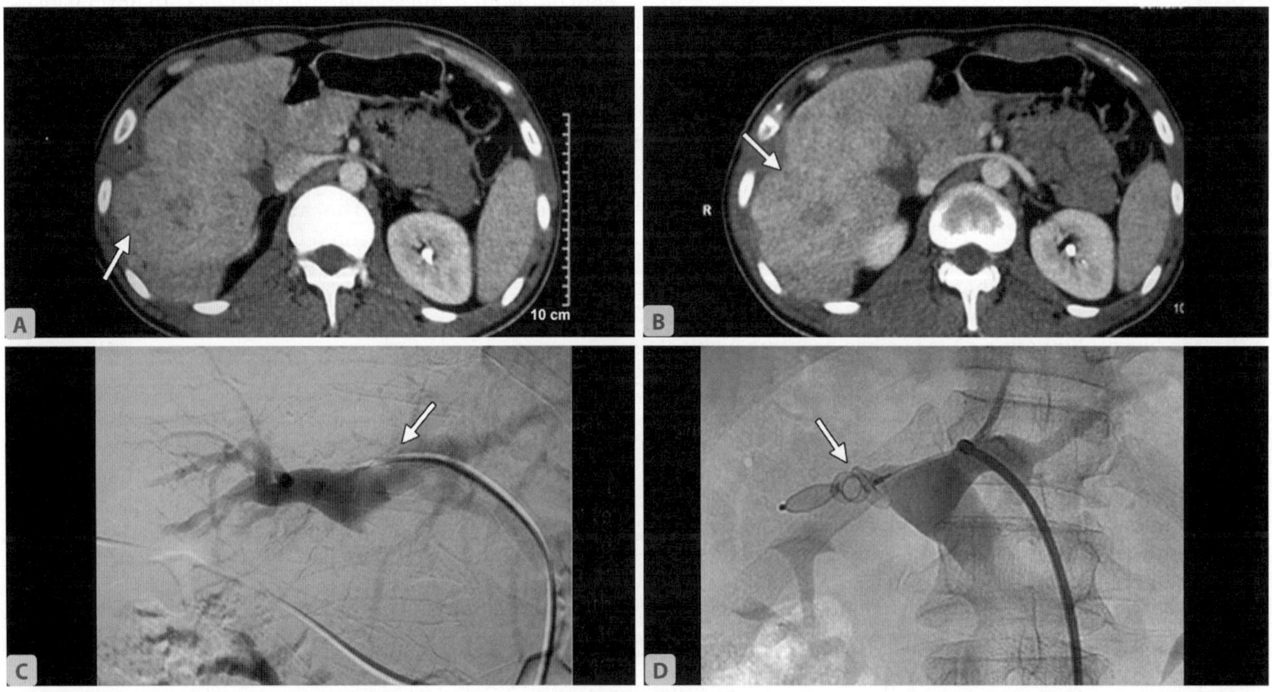

FIGS. 11A TO D: Right portal vein embolization for right lobe hepatocellular carcinoma planned for extended right hepatectomy: Axial CT images (A and B) showing large mass lesion in right lobe of liver (arrows), portal vein was accessed from left side (arrow) (C) and right portal vein was blocked using Amplatzer plug (arrow) (D).

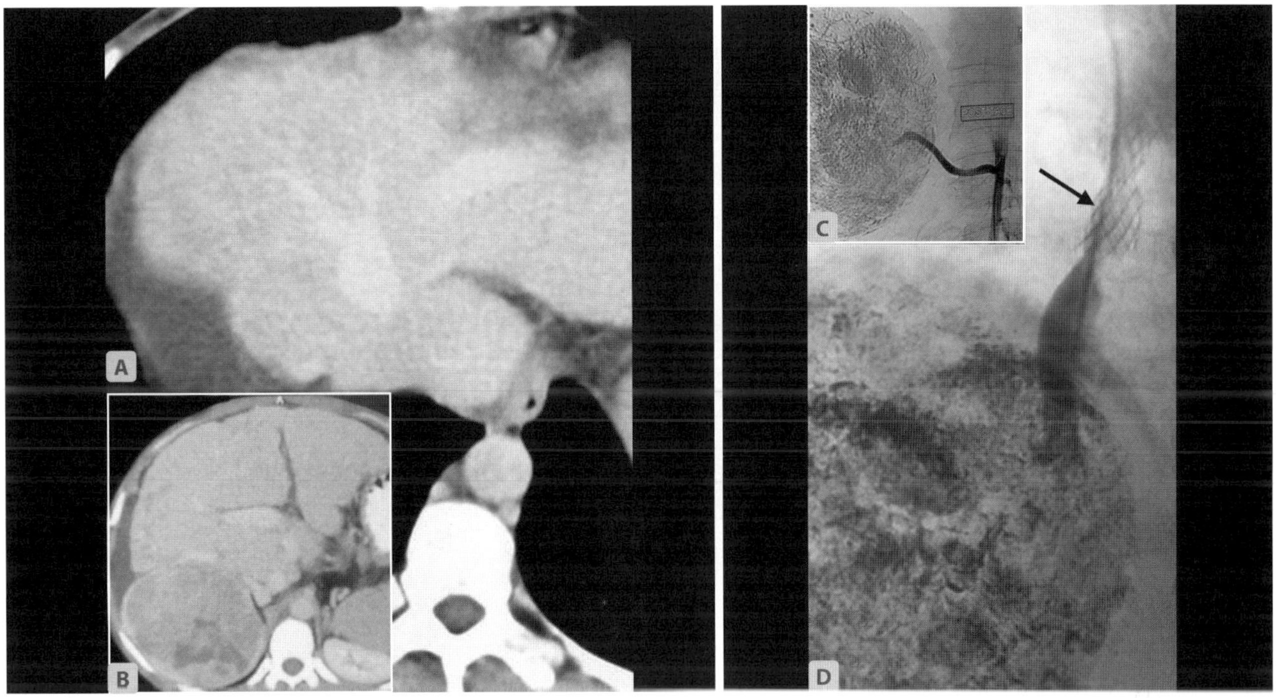

FIGS. 12A TO D: A 32-year-old male with HCC secondary to hepatic vein outflow tract obstruction (HVOTO) was treated with TACE and hepatic vein stenting. He developed lung metastases on one-year follow-up CT and is presently on systemic chemotherapy. Contrast-enhanced CT liver (A and B) showing right lobe HCC with HVOTO. The tumor was treated with chemoembolization (C) and HVOTO by right hepatic vein stenting (arrow) (D).

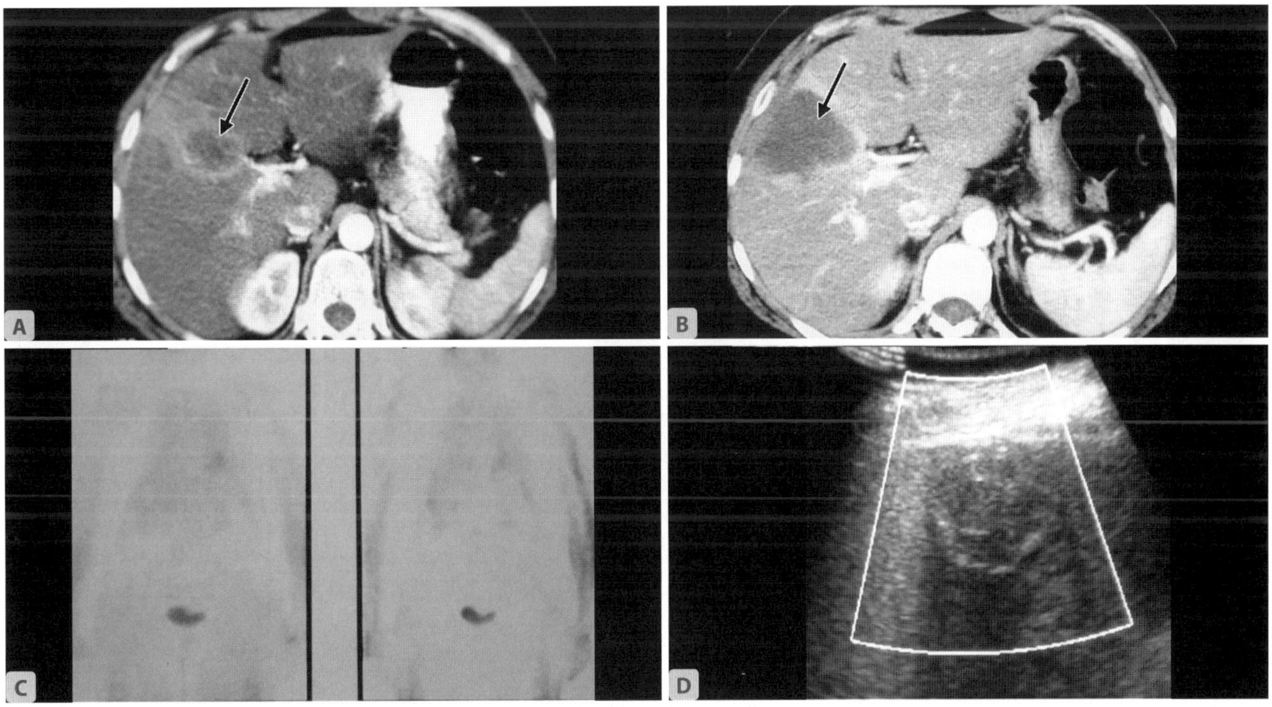

FIGS. 13A TO D: A 46-year-old female with single liver metastasis from carcinoma of breast (mastectomy done one year back) was treated with single session of RFA. Arterial phase CT (A) is showing single lesion (3.1 × 3 cm) in right lobe of liver (arrow). Post-PFA 3 months arterial phase CT (B) is showing complete ablation of tumor (arrow). Seven years follow-up PET (C) and color Doppler ultrasound (D) are normal.

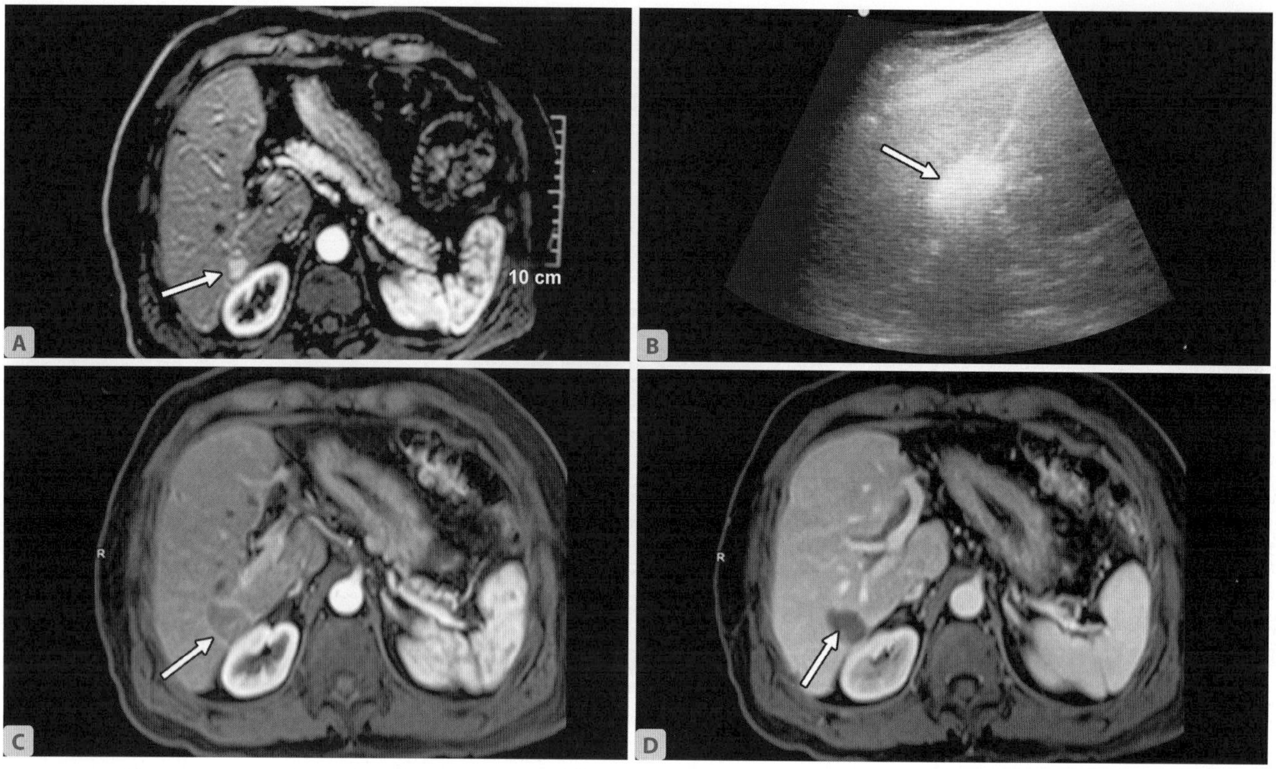

FIGS. 14A TO D: Radiofrequency ablation for hypervascular metastasis from neuroendocrine primary: Axial MR image (arterial phase) (A) showing small arterial enhancing lesion (arrow) in segment VI of liver which was ablated (arrow) under ultrasound guidance (B); Postablation axial MR images (C and D) showing complete necrosis of the lesion (arrows) suggesting complete response.

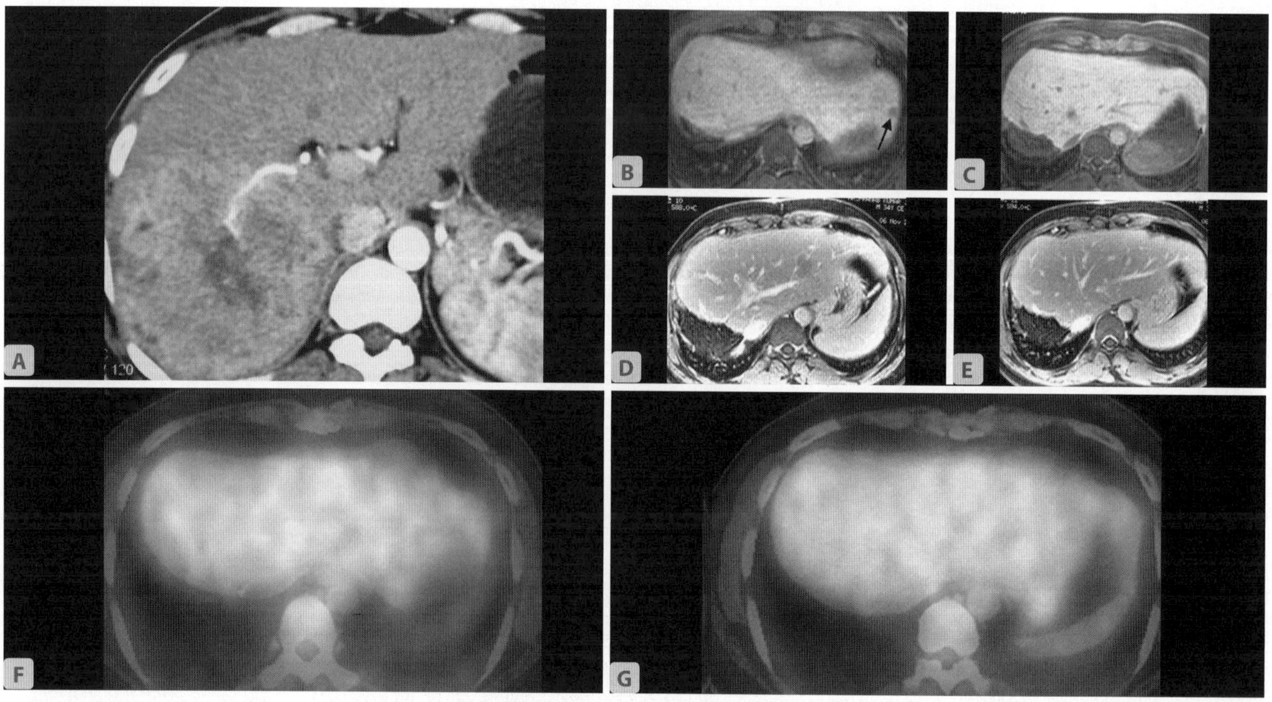

FIGS. 15A TO G: Arterial phase CT liver (A) is showing HCC in right lobe of liver. One year postright hepatectomy MR (B and C) is showing two metastatic deposits (arrow) in left lobe of liver. The lesions disappeared on follow-up MR (D and E) and PET/CT (F and G) after Re HDD[188] treatment.

Transarterial administration of anticancer drugs (Doxorubicin, cisplatin, 5-FU, mitomycin C, irinotecan), either alone or as hepatic arterial infusion (HAI), or combined with embolization of feeding artery [transarterial chemoembolization (TACE)] or bland vascular embolization (TAE) is used **(Figs. 14A to D)**. TART with Rhenium-188-HDD-lipiodol has also been used in the management of multiple intrahepatic recurrences after radiofrequency ablation and surgery of hepatocellular carcinoma **(Figs. 15A to G)**.[55-57]

TREATMENT OF BENIGN LIVER TUMORS

Hemangioma is the most common benign tumor of the liver. Cavernous hemangiomas are usually asymptomatic but may become symptomatic with rapid tumor enlargement. These patients may present with abdominal pain, fever, anemia, obstructive jaundice, hemobilia, spontaneous rupture with subsequent life-threatening hemorrhage, thrombocytopenia, hypofibrinogenemia and rarely portal hypertension either due to arterioportal fistula or pressure effect on portal vein.

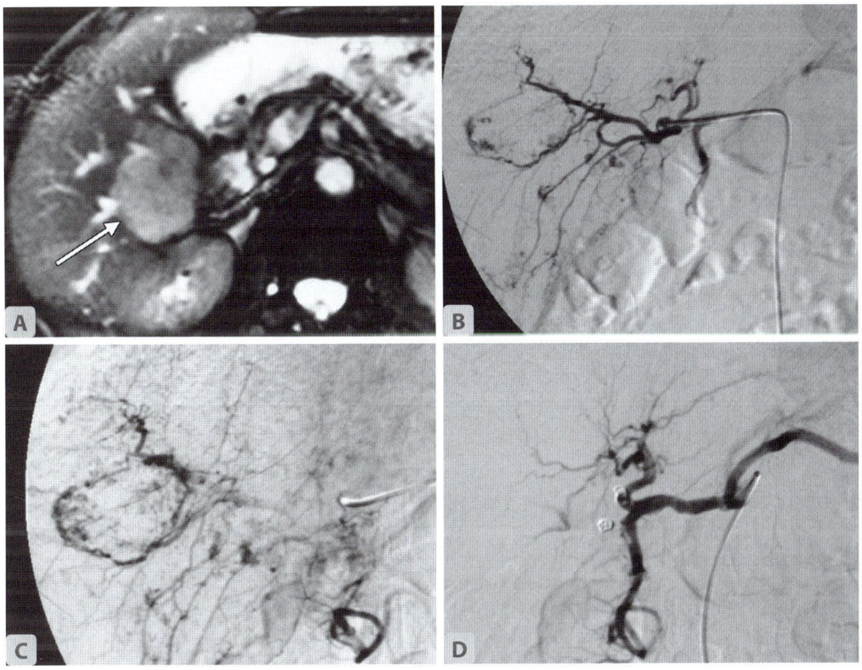

FIGS. 16A TO D: Large cavernous hemangioma of right lobe of liver extending up to porta hepatis causing recurrent pain and cholangitis was embolized. (A) MR image shows exophytic component of mass (arrow); (B and C) Hepatic artery angiograms show arterial supply from right hepatic artery; (D) Tumor was embolized with multiple steel coils and PVA particles. There was significant reduction in size of mass on follow-up imaging.

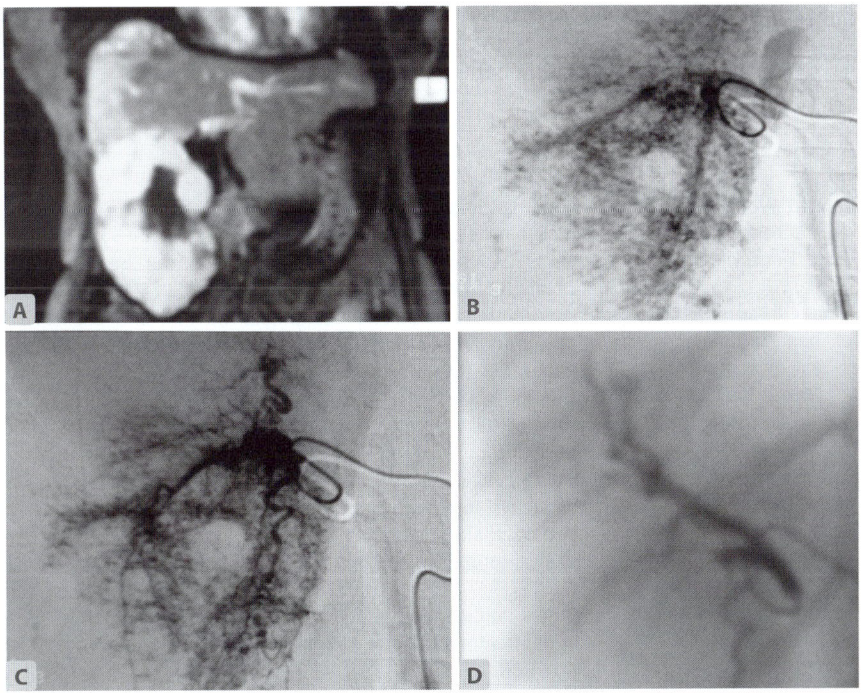

FIGS. 17A TO D: Large symptomatic pedunculated hepatic hemangioma was embolized preoperatively and surgically removed later. (A) Contrast MR image showing enhancing pedunculated mass in right lobe of liver with hypertrophied left lobe; (B and C) Right hepatic arteriogram showing large cavernous hemangioma with retrograde filling of portal vein; (D) Complete preoperative embolization of the tumor. The tumor was surgically removed with less blood loss.

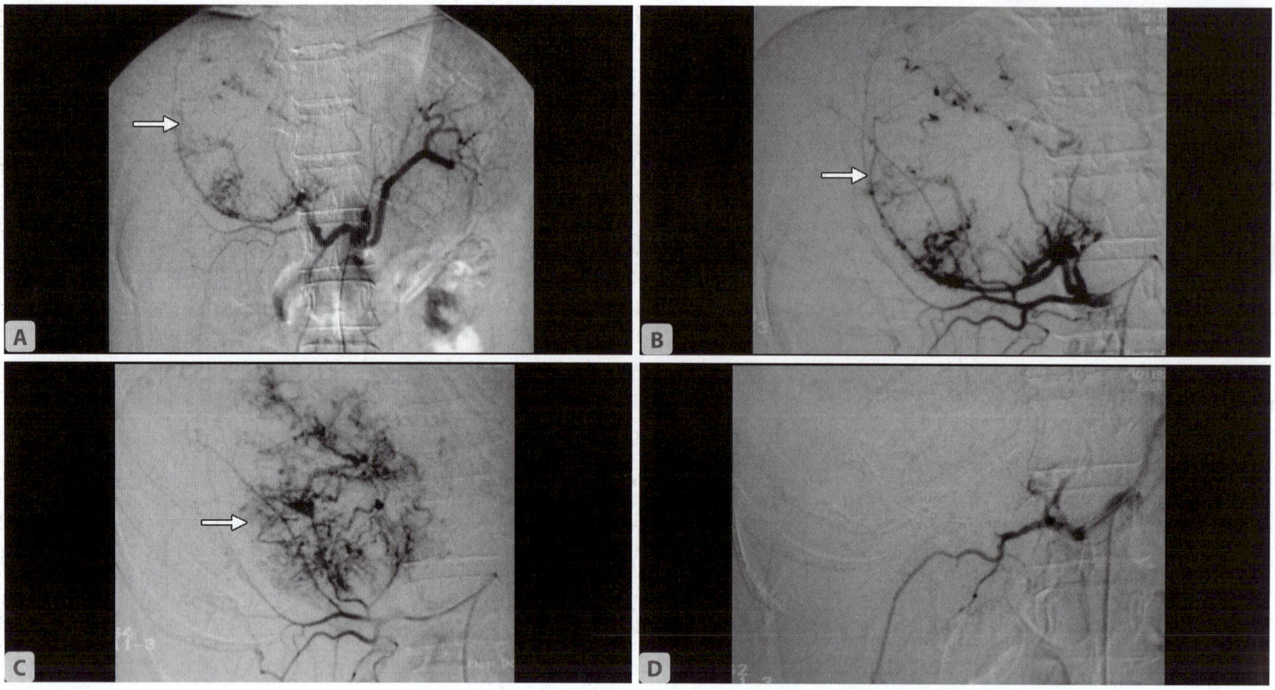

FIGS. 18A TO D: A 32-year-old female with hepatic adenoma left lobe of liver. Hepatic angiograms show (arrows) marked tumor vascularity (A to C). The tumor was embolized with gelfoam and the postembolization angiogram (D) is not showing tumor vascularity. Complete surgical removal of the tumor was done with less blood loss.

Hepatic artery embolization using both temporary and permanent occluding material may be indicated in the management of symptomatic hemangiomas, causing pressure symptoms or at high risk of bleeding **(Figs. 16 and 17)**. Various studies have shown that TAE of hepatic cavernous hemangioma is a useful procedure in the therapy of symptomatic hemangiomas.[58-60]

Preoperative embolization of focal nodular hyperplasia, hepatic adenoma or other vascular tumors may help in surgical removal of the tumor, by reducing intraoperative blood loss **(Figs. 18A to D)**.

CONCLUSION

Radiological interventions are established procedures and recommended therapeutic options for liver tumors. A variety of locoregional therapies are available which can be used in isolation or as a part of combination therapy. Treatment is based upon the clinical presentation, stage of the disease, liver function and the performance status of patient and varies from case-to-case. Decision and execution of treatment is a team work which aims at providing maximum patient benefit.

REFERENCES

1. International Agency for Research on Cancer: World Health Organization. GLOBOCAN 2012: Estimated cancer incidence, mortality, and prevalence worldwide in 2012. *http://globocan.iarc.fr* (Accessed January 20, 2015).
2. Lencioni R, Crocetti L, Cioni D, Della Pina C, Bartolozzi C. Percutaneous radiofrequency ablation of hepatic colorectal metastases: technique, indications, results, and new promises. Invest Radiol. 2004;39:689-97.
3. EASL-EORTC clinical practice guidelines: management of hepatocellular carcinoma. J Hepatol. 2012;56:908-43.
4. Llovet JM, Brú C, Bruix. Prognosis of hepatocellular carcinoma: the BCLC staging classification. Semin Liver Dis. 1999;19(3): 329-38.
5. Livraghi T, Bolondi L, Buscarini L, et al. No treatment, resection and ethanol injection in hepatocellular carcinoma: a retrospective analysis of survival in 391 patients with cirrhosis. Italian Cooperative HCC Study Group. J Hepatol. 1995;22: 522-6.
6. Foltz G. Image guided percutaneous ablation of hepatic malignancies. Semin Intervent Radiol. 2014;31:180-86.
7. Clark TW, Soulen MC. Chemical ablation of hepatocellular carcinoma. J Vasc Interv Radiol. 2002;13(9 Pt 2):S245-52.
8. Kapoor V, Thaete FL. Percutaneous ethanol and acetic acid ablation of hepatocellular carcinoma. Hepatocellular Cancer. Pages: 153-169. Publisher: Humana Press.
9. Ohnishi K, Nomura F, Ito S, Fujiwara K. Prognosis of small hepatocellular carcinoma (less than 3 cm) after percutaneous acetic acid injection: study of 91 cases. Hepatology. 1996;23: 994-1002.
10. Huo TI, Hiang YH, Wu JC, et al. Comparison of percutaneous and acid injection and percutaneous ethanol injection for hepatocellular carcinoma in cirrhotic patients. A prospective study. Scand J Gastroenterol. 2003;7:770-8.
11. Rossi S, Di Stasi M, Buscarini E, Cavanna L, Quaretti P, Squassante E, et al. Percutaneous radiofrequency interstitial thermal ablation in the treatment of small hepatocellular carcinoma. Cancer J Sci Am. 1995;1(1):73-81.

12. McGahan JP, Gu WZ, Brock JM, Tesluk H, Jones CD. Hepatic ablation using bipolar radiofrequency electrocautery. Acad Radiol. 1996;3:418-22.
13. Goldberg SN, Grassi CJ, Cardella JF, Charboneau JW, Dodd GD 3rd, Dupuy DE, et al. Society of Interventional Radiology Technology Assessment Committee and the International Working Group on Image-guided Tumor Ablation. Image-guided tumor ablation: standardization of terminology and reporting criteria. J Vasc Interv Radiol. 2009;20(Suppl 7):S377-90.
14. Seror O, N'kontchou G, Ibraheem M, Ajayon Y, et al. Large (> = 5.0—cm) HCCs: Multipolar RF ablation with three internally cooled bipolar electrodes initial experience in 26 patients. Radiology. 2008;248(1):288-96.
15. Yang W, Yan K, Wu GX, Wu W, Fu Y, Lee JC, et al. Radiofrequency ablation of hepatocellular carcinoma in difficult locations: Strategies and long-term outcomes. World J Gastroenterol. 2015;21(5):1554-66. doi: 10.3748/wjg.v21.i5.1554.
16. Livraghi T, Solbiati L, Meloni MF, et al. Treatment of focal liver tumors with percutaneous radiofrequency ablation: complications encountered in a multicenter study. Radiology. 2003;226:441-51.
17. Lahat E, Eshkenazy R, Zendel A, Zakai BB, Maor M, Dreznik Y, Ariche A. Complications after percutaneous ablation of liver tumors: a systematic review. Hepatobiliary Surg Nutr. 2014;3(5): 317-23.
18. Sheta E, El-Kalla F, El-Gharib M, Kobtan A, Elhendawy M, Abd-Elsalam S, Mansour L, Amer I. Comparison of single-session transarterial chemoembolization combined with microwave ablation or radiofrequency ablation in the treatment of hepatocellular carcinoma: a randomized-controlled study. Eur J Gastroenterol Hepatol; 2016.
19. Poch FG, Rieder C, Ballhausen H, Knappe V, Ritz JP, Gemeinhardt O, et al. The vascular cooling effect in hepatic multipolar radiofrequency ablation leads to incomplete ablation *ex vivo*. Int J Hyperthermia; 2016.pp.1-8.
20. Meloni MF, Chiang J, Laeseke PF, Dietrich CF, Sannino A, Solbiati M, et al. Microwave ablation in primary and secondary liver tumours: technical and clinical approaches. Int J Hyperthermia; 2016. pp. 1-10.
21. Kim GM, Won JY, Kim MD, Park SI, Lee DY, Shin W, et al. Cryoablation of hepatocellular carcinoma with high-risk for percutaneous ablation: safety and efficacy. Cardiovasc Intervent Radiol. 2016.
22. NG KK, Poon RT, Chang SC, et al. High-intensity focused ultrasound for hepatocellular carcinoma: a single center experience. Ann Surg. 2011;253:981-87.
23. Pacella CM, Bizzarri G, Francica G, Bianchini A, De Nuntis S, Pacella S, et al. Percutaneous laser ablation in the treatment of hepatocellular carcinoma with small tumors: analysis of factors affecting the achievement of tumor necrosis. J Vasc Interv Radiol. 2005;16(11):1447-57.
24. Davlos RV, Mir IL, Rubinsky B. Tissue ablation with irreversible electroporation. Annals Biomed Eng. 2005;33:223-31.
25. Tsochatzis EA, Germani G, Burroughs AK. Transarterial chemoembolization, transarterial chemotherapy, and intra-arterial chemotherapy for hepatocellular carcinoma treatment. Semin Oncol. 2010;37(2):89-93.
26. Davis CR. Interventional radiological treatment of hepatocellular carcinoma. Cancer Control. 2010;17(1):87-99.
27. Ramsey DE, Geschwind JH. New interventions for liver tumors. Semin Roentgenology. 2002;37:303-11.
28. Carter S, Martin Ii RC. Drug-eluting bead therapy in primary and metastatic disease of the liver. HPB (Oxford). 2009;11:541-50.
29. Kumar A, Srivastava DN, Chau TTM, et al. Inoperable hepatocellular carcinoma: transarterial 188Re HDD-Labeled iodized oil for treatment—prospective multicenter trial. Radiology. 2007;243:509-19.
30. Yamakado K, Nakatsuka A, Ohmori S, et al. Radiofrequency ablation combined with chemoembolization in hepatocellular carcinoma treatment response based on tumor size and morphology. J Vasc Interv Radiol. 2002;13:1225-32.
31. Yang M, Yuan JQ, Bai M, Han GH. Transarterial chemoembolization combined with sorafenib for unresectable hepatocellular carcinoma: a systematic review and meta-analysis. Mol Biol Rep. 2014;41:6575-82.
32. Lee JM, Yoon JH, Joo I, Woo HS. Recent advances in CT and MR imaging for evaluation of hepatocellular carcinoma. Liver Cancer. 2012;1:22-40.
33. Minami Y, Kudo M. Therapeutic response assessment of transcatheter arterial chemoembolization for hepatocellular carcinoma: ultrasonography, CT and MR imaging. Oncology. 2013;84(Suppl 1):58-63.
34. Guan Y-S, Sun L, Zhou X-P, Li X, Zheng XH. Hepatocellular carcinoma treated with interventional procedures: CT and MRI follow-up. World J Gastroenterol. 2004;10:3543-8.
35. Yuan Z, Li WT, Ye XD, Peng WJ, Xiao XS. Utility of diffusion-weighted imaging to assess hepatocellular carcinoma viability following transarterial chemoembolization. Oncol Lett. 2014;8:831 6.
36. Liu M, Lin MX, Lu MD, Xu ZF, Zheng KG, Wang W, et al. Comparison of contrast-enhanced ultrasound and contrast-enhanced computed tomography in evaluating the treatment response to transcatheter arterial chemoembolization of hepatocellular carcinoma using modified RECIST. Eur Radiol. 2015;25:2502-11.
37. Riccardo Lencioni R, Llovet JM. Modified RECIST (mRECIST) assessment for hepatocellular carcinoma. Semin Liver Dis. 2010;30:52-60.
38. Chung JC, Naik NK, Lewandowski RJ, Deng J, Mulcahy MF, Kulik LM, et al. Diffusion-weighted magnetic resonance imaging to predict response of hepatocellular carcinoma to chemoembolization. World J Gastroenterol. 2010;16(25): 3161-7.
39. Vilana R, Bruix J, Bru C, Ayuso C, Sole M, Rodes J. Tumor size determines the efficacy of percutaneous ethanol injection for the treatment of small hepatocellular carcinoma. Hepatology. 1992;16:353-7.
40. Lencioni R. Locoregional treatment of hepatocellular carcinoma. Hepatology. 2010;52:762-73.
41. Cucchetti A, Piscaglia F, Cescon M, Ercolani G, Pinna AD. Systematic review of surgical resection versus radiofrequency ablation for hepatocellular carcinoma. World J Gastroenterol. 2013;19:4106-18.
42. Duan C, Liu m, Zhang Z, Ma K, Bie P. Radiofrequency ablation versus hepatic resection for the treatment of early stage hepatocellular carcinoma meeting Milan criteria: a systematic review and meta-analysis. World J Surgl Oncol. 2013;11:190.
43. Llovet JM, Bruix J. Systematic review of randomized trials for unresectable hepatocellular carcinoma: chemoembolization improves survival. Hepatology. 2003;37:429-42.
44. Yamada R, Sato M, Kawabata M, Nakatsuka H, Nakamura K, Takashima S. Hepatic artery embolization in 120 patients with unresectable hepatoma. Radiology. 1983;148:397-401.
45. Takayasu K, Arii S, Ikai I, et al. Prospective cohort study of trans-arterial chemoembolization for unresectable hepatocellular carcinoma in 8510 patients. Gastroenterology. 2006;131:461-9.

46. Paul SB, Gamanagatti S, Sreenivas V, et al. Trans-arterial chemoembolization in patients with unresectable hepatocellular carcinoma: experience from a tertiary care centre in India. Indian J Radiol. Imaging. 2011;21:113-20.
47. Lammer J, Malagari K, Vogl T, et al. Prospective randomized study of doxorubicin-eluting-bead embolization in the treatment of hepatocellular carcinoma: results of the PRECISION V study. Cardiovasc Interv Radiol. 2010;33:41-52.
48. Prajapati HJ, Dhanasekaran R, El-Rayes BF, et al. Safety and efficacy of doxorubicin drug-eluting bead transarterial chemoembolization in patients with advanced hepatocellular carcinoma. J Vasc Interv Radiol. 2013;24:307-15.
49. Geschwind JF, Salem R, Carr BI, et al. Yttrium-90 microspheres for the treatment of hepatocellular carcinoma. Gastroenterology. 2004;127:S194-205.
50. Salem R, Lewandowski RJ, Mulcahy MF, et al. Radioembolization for hepatocellular carcinoma using Yttrium-90 microspheres: a comprehensive report of long-term outcomes. Gastroenterology. 2010;138:52-64.
51. Srivastava DN, Thulkar S, Sharma S, Pandey GK, Sahni P, Julka PK, Acharya SK. Therapeutic radiological interventional procedures in hepatocellular carcinoma. Indian J Gastroenterol. 2002;21:96-8.
52. Srivastava DN, Gandhi D, Julka PK, et al. Gastrointestinal hemorrhage in hepatocellular carcinoma management with transhepatic arterioembolization. Abdominal Imaging. 2000;25:1-6.
53. Madoff DC, Hicks ME, Vauthey JN, Charnsangavej C, Morello FA Jr, Ahrar K, et al. Transhepatic portal vein embolization: anatomy, indications, and technical considerations. Radiographics. 2002;22(5):1063-76.
54. Gunabushanam G, Sharma S, Thulkar S, Srivastava DN, et al. Radiofrequency ablation of liver metastases from breast cancer: results in 14 patients. J Vasc Interv Radiol. 2007;18(1):67-72.
55. Kumar A, Bal C, Srivastava DN, Thulkar SP, Sharma S, Acharya SK, et al. Management of multiple intrahepatic recurrences after radiofrequency ablation of hepatocellular carcinoma with rhenium-188-HDD lipiodol. Eur J Gastroenterol Hepatol. 2006;18(2):219-23.
56. Kumar A, Srivastava DN, Bal C. Management of postsurgical recurrence of hepatocellular carcinoma with Rhenium 188-HDD labeled iodized oil. J Vasc Interv Radiol. 2006;17(1): 157-61.
57. Srivastava DN, Madhusudan KS. Oncologic Imaging. Ind J of Medical and Paediatric Oncology. 2008;29(1):65-6.
58. Srivastava DN, Sharma S, Yadav S, et al. Pedunculated hepatic haemangioma with arteriportal shunt – treated with angioembolization and surgery. Australasian Radiology. 1998;2: 151-3.
59. Srivastava DN, Gandhi D, Seith A, Pande GK, Sahni P. Transcatheter arterial embolization in the treatment of symptomatic cavernous haemangioma of the liver: a prospective study. Abdominal Imaging. 2001;26:510-14.
60. Rammohan A, Sathyanesan J, Ramaswami S, Lakshmanan A, Senthil-Kumar P, Srinivasan UP, et al. Embolization of liver tumors: Past, present and future. World J Radiol. 2012;4(9):405-12.

CHAPTER

105 Imaging in Liver Transplant

Chandan J Das, Kumble S Madhusudhan, Deep Narayan Srivastava

INTRODUCTION

Liver transplantation is one of the boons in the history of medicine and has become the accepted treatment for patients with end stage liver disease with reported 1-year graft and patient survival rates of 80–95% and 5-year rates of 60–85%.[1] Unfortunately, there is inadequate availability of cadaveric liver grafts because of several limitations in organ donation, and hence transplantation of partial grafts from both living and deceased donors has become more popular in the last decade. There has been a paradigm shift in the various imaging techniques concomitant with the technical refinements in partial liver transplantation which allows precise as well as better understanding of donor and recipient anatomy prior to the transplantation.

Pretransplantation evaluation of the extent of liver disease, details of the vascular and biliary anatomy of potential recipients and donors are of paramount importance for successful liver transplantation. In this chapter, we will discuss the indications and contraindications of various types of liver transplantations, different surgical techniques and plethora of imaging modalities used for radiologic evaluation of donors as well as recipients. We also briefly discuss about imaging in various postoperative complications.

INDICATIONS AND CONTRAINDICATIONS FOR LIVER TRANSPLANTATION

The common indications for liver transplantation includes complications of cirrhosis, hepatocellular carcinoma, autoimmune hepatitis, chronic hepatitis B and C, cholestatic diseases like primary biliary cirrhosis and primary sclerosing cholangitis and metabolic diseases such as hemochromatosis and Wilson disease **(Table 1)**.[2]

There are few absolute and relative contraindications for transplantation. The absolute contraindications include uncontrolled ongoing sepsis, active abuse of alcohol or other substance, extrahepatic malignancy, severe cardiopulmonary disease, hepatopulmonary syndrome with severe pulmonary hypertension, lack of a psychosocial support system and some variants of cholangiocarcinoma. The relative contraindications include age > 65 years, human immunodeficiency virus (HIV) infection, hepatocellular carcinoma (HCC) (not fitting in established criteria), morbid obesity and psychologic instability.

TABLE 1: Common indications for liver transplantation.
• Cirrhosis with end stage liver disease and decompensation Hepatocellular carcinoma/hepatoblastoma
• Alcoholic liver disease
• *Hepatitis:* Autoimmune, chronic hepatitis B and C
• *Cholestatic diseases:* Primary biliary cirrhosis, primary sclerosing cholangitis
• *Metabolic diseases:* Hemochromatosis Wilson disease
• *Fulminant hepatic failure:* Viral/toxin/drug-induced

HOW TO SELECT PATIENTS?

Most of the patients have end-stage liver disease which is assessed by the model for end-stage liver disease (MELD) scoring system.[2,3] MELD is an objective way of assessing patients waiting for liver transplantation and is being used to prioritize the allocation of livers for transplantation. This scoring system, based on the patient's bilirubin, international normalized ratio (INR), and creatinine, was initially created to predict the 3-month mortality for patients with non HCC end-stage liver disease (ESLD) undergoing a Transjugular Intrahepatic Portosystemic Shunt (TIPS) procedure.[2,4] MELD scores range from 6 to 40, with 6 indicating the least sick patients and 40 indicating the sickest patients. It is generally thought that for liver transplantation wait-listing the patient should have at least 15 MELD points. Conversely it may be futile to contemplate transplantation for patients with MELD values closer to 40.

HEPATOCELLULAR CARCINOMA

Among patients with hepatocellular carcinoma (HCC), to be eligible for transplantation, the tumor must be grade 1 or grade 2, be solitary <5 cm, or may have up to 3 nodules with each < 3 cm, and there must be no extrahepatic metastases or evidence of macrovascular invasion. This is according to the Milan criteria which is accepted by most National deceased donor based transplant programs the world over.[5]

In the tumor, node, metastasis (TNM) staging system, T1 tumors may be any size as long as they do not extend into blood vessels. T2 tumors may be any size if they do extend into the blood vessels; they may also be classified as T2 if there are more than one and they are smaller than 5 cm. Tumors are characterized as T3 if larger than 5 cm. T4 tumors extend beyond the liver, except for the gallbladder. Transplant priority should be given to stage T2 disease because patients with T1 disease have high survival rates without transplantation, and those with T3 disease have a high rate of recurrence.[5]

Milan criteria is used for assessing transplant eligibility for small HCCs. According to Milan criteria, to be eligible for liver transplantation, patients with HCC should have a single tumor that is smaller than 5 cm or three or fewer tumors that are 3 cm or smaller. Similarly, the University of California San Francisco (UCSF) criteria is used for liver transplantation in patients with large tumors, i.e. they have a single tumor that is 6.5 cm or smaller or if three or fewer tumor nodules are present, with the largest being 4.5 cm or smaller. Recently, a cut off tumor volume of 115 cm^3 has been used for selecting candidates for transplantation showing enhanced accuracy of pretransplantation imaging.[6] Factors with high potential for recurrence after living donor liver transplantation (LDLT) include: a tumor larger than 6 cm, multiple nodules >3, disease that progresses after pretransplantation treatment, gross vascular invasion, and a tumor that is exposed to the liver surface.[7]

TYPES OF LIVER TRANSPLANTATION

Currently, there are 3 types of liver transplantation being performed: whole-liver cadaveric transplant, split-liver cadaveric transplant, and living donor liver transplant. Worldwide, the cadaveric or deceased donor liver transplantation (DDLT) is the most common type. It is also the most technically straightforward form of liver transplantation and has the advantages of full sized donor liver.

LIVING DONOR LIVER TRANSPLANTATION

Living donor liver transplant (LDLT) account for approximately 4.0% of the liver transplants performed in the last 10 years but accounts for more than 85% of the transplants being performed in our country. The advantages of LDLT include the elective nature of the procedure, good quality organ and lack of preservation injuries of the organ. The main disadvantage of this technique is the risk related to the healthy donor with a mortality risk of 0.15% to 0.20%, and postoperative complication rate of 20–40%. The residual donor liver must be more than 30% of the total donor hepatic volume to ensure adequate postoperative liver function, and the graft-to-recipient body weight ratio (GRWR) should be greater than 0.8 to minimize the risk of 'small-for-size' syndrome in the recipient.[8]

For an adult recipient, either a full-right or full-left hepatic graft (small adults < 50 kg) can be used. In the donor right hepatectomy, the liver is split on the right of the middle hepatic vein (MHV), close to Cantlie's line that connects the left border of the suprahepatic inferior vena cava (IVC) to the midpoint of the gallbladder fossa. Generally the MHV remains with the donor when the right side of the liver is harvested whereas it is harvested when left donor hepatectomy is performed.[9] Hence, variations in anatomy of the MHV are critical to the success of this operation and needs to be conveyed to the transplant surgeon beforehand. Left donor hepatectomy involves harvesting the MHV en-bloc to obtain an adequate sized-graft with good venous outflow as congestion of the paramedian segment (segment IV) in the recipient is avoided. As the right hepatic vein is dominant in most patients and caudate lobe usually remains in the donor, congestion of the remnant donor liver after removal of the MHV along with the left hemi liver usually is not clinically significant. The recipient left hepatic vein (LHV) and MHV can be enlarged and then anastomosed to the enlarged graft MHV-LHV confluence to provide unimpeded venous outflow to the graft after implantation. Left lateral segmentectomy (segments 2 and 3 with or without the caudate lobe) are suitable for children and smaller recipients (20–30 kg).[9,10]

Split-Liver Cadaveric Transplant is the least common type in which a single cadaveric liver is anatomically divided and transplanted into 2 recipients (usually one adult and 1 child).[10,11] The right lobe is given to an adult recipient whereas the left lateral segment is given to a child. Although this helps mitigate the shortage of deceased donor livers available, there are technical difficulties related to sharing of blood vessels/bile duct and a higher risk of complications in the adult recipient (bile leaks, cut surface bleeding, segment 4 necrosis). The most common cadaveric splitting technique involves a transection plane 1 cm to the right of the falciform ligament, resulting in a right extended graft (segments I and IV–VIII) used in adults, and a left lateral graft (segments II–III) for a pediatric recipient who are not larger than 30 kg. The common bile duct, main portal vein and inferior vena cava (IVC) are included in the right liver graft, and the main arterial trunk is part of the left liver graft. The biliary reconstruction of the left lateral graft usually entails a hepaticojejunostomy in the pediatric recipient.[10,11]

PREOPERATIVE IMAGING MODALITIES

Multidetector computed tomography (MDCT) and MRI are the workhorses of pretransplant imaging and has been used as complementary to each other in the evaluation of donor and recipient.

Multidetector Computed Tomography

Multidetector computed tomography (MDCT) is frequently used to evaluate the donor and recipient arterial as well as venous anatomy using intravenous contrast in the form of CT angiography (CTA). Donor liver fat content is also evaluated by unenhanced scan (by calculating the Hepatic attenuation index). Dual energy CT (DECT) scan has been increasingly used as virtual noncontrast image can be reconstructed from the set of enhanced images thus obviating the need of a true unenhanced scan reducing the dose of radiation. MDCT/CTA generates a huge amount of dataset which require dedicated postprocessing by vendor specific software for optimal evaluation of the anatomy—the hepatic arteries on three-dimensional or axial MIPs, the hepatic veins on axial MIPs, portal veins on coronal MIPs and volume renderings of the hepatic parenchyma. All these can be superimposed on one another for further delineation of the anatomy for the surgeons. MDCT should be judiciously used to reduce the radiation dose as donors are often young and healthy.

MR Imaging

MR imaging (MRI) coupled with magnetic resonance cholangiopancreatography (MRCP) is primarily performed to evaluate the biliary system. Hepatobiliary contrast agents such as Gd-BOPTA (Multihance, Bracco Diagnostics, NJ) can be used. The biliary tree is better seen on 3-dimensional heavily T2-weighted or 3-dimensional T1-weighted, postcontrast coronal oblique images. MRI can also be used to evaluate the hepatic parenchyma for characterizing incidental focal lesions and the degree of fatty infiltration.

Preoperative Imaging Evaluation

Recipient Evaluation

Imaging of the recipient liver should be performed as close to the time of transplantation as possible because tumors may grow rapidly, invade local structures, or metastasize, which may affect the stage of disease, management perspective, and surgical technique. Candidate eligibility is determined by the patient's MELD score to allow for candidate list prioritization based upon medical need. Imaging plays a pivotal role in the care of patients with HCC.[2] Imaging of the recipient consist of detailed evaluation and description of the arterial, portal venous and hepatic venous anatomy and the extent of tumor burden in HCC patients awaiting transplant.

For patients with liver lesions, the Organ Procurement and Transplantation Network (OPTN) or Liver Imaging Reporting and Data System (LI-RADS) criteria are used to characterize liver lesions as benign, suspicious for HCC, or definitely HCC.[12,13] The intrinsic signal intensity of the mass, enhancement and washout pattern, capsule appearance, and nodule architecture are frequently used to determine the likelihood that a nodule is HCC. Once the liver nodules are characterized, the Milan/UCSF criteria are used to determine transplant candidacy. Patients with HCC whose tumors are growing at a significant rate or who are expected to wait more than 6 months on the transplant list may be offered locoregional therapy, a practice known as "bridging to transplant". Occasionally. Some programs use down staging locoregional therapy for cases where the HCC lesions were beyond the standard listing criteria, provided there is no evidence of extrahepatic disease or macrovascular tumor invasion. In such patients there is a need for a 3-month waiting period post down-staging therapy (usually TACE/RFA) and re-imaging to see whether they fit the listing criteria before being considered for LT. This is accomplished by alcohol injection, thermal ablation (including radiofrequency and microwave ablation), transarterial radioembolization (TARE), and most commonly transarterial chemoembolization (TACE).[14] The choice of therapy is based on Barcelona Clinic Liver Cancer Staging (BCLC) Criteria, which take into account the number and size of HCC nodules, the patient's Child-Pugh score, and the patient's Eastern Cooperative Oncology Group (ECOG) performance status.[15] All the focal lesions should be described segment wise along with its relation with major vascular structures, the gallbladder, and central bile ducts because the outcome may be affected. If MDCT is indeterminate for a lesion characterization, contrast-enhanced MRI imaging should be performed to further characterize the lesion. It is also critical to perform CT chest and abdomen to exclude extrahepatic malignancy or spread.

Preoperative Imaging of the Living Donor Liver Transplantation Donor

Accurate preoperative depiction of donor anatomy is essential to determine the suitability of the donor so that hepatectomy may safely be performed without any risk to the donor and at the same time avoiding "small-for-size" syndrome in the recipient. This syndrome is characterised by poor bile production, delayed synthetic function, prolonged cholestasis, and intractable ascites and deranged coagulation which leads to septic complications and high mortality. To avoid small-for-size syndrome, the residual liver volume should exceed 30–35% of the total donor liver volume and the GRWR should be > 0.8 w.r.t the recipient.[16] Preoperative imaging of the living donor liver transplantation (LDLT) donor involves assessment of various features such as vascular and biliary anatomy for relevant variants, MHV anatomy, the hepatic parenchyma for degree of fatty infiltration, iron content, and focal hepatic lesions and last but not the least, calculation of liver volumes. Minor variations of anatomy can be tackled with advanced vascular surgical techniques.

In a study by Tsang et al. the various causes of donor unsuitability were recipient issues such as inadequate remnant volume (57.4%); steatosis (27.7%); a small-for-size graft (8.9%); and variations of biliary system (5%) hepatic artery (4%) and portal vein (1%) anatomy.[16]

Among the various imaging techniques, MDCT angiography is faster and more cost-effective than MR angiography and is used more often. Two-dimensional or three-dimensional reformations from MDCT in both arterial and portal venous phases provide the best methods of analysis. The MDCT protocol for liver donors vary with institutions. The protocol followed at our institution includes unenhanced CT followed by multiphase contrast-enhanced CT. In the unenhanced CT protocol, four 10 mm sections are obtained first followed by arterial and portal venous phase contrastenhanced CT. The details are given in **Table 2**.

Vascular Anatomy

Preoperative imaging of the hepatic artery, portal and hepatic veins involves identification of the vessels **(Figs. 1A to C)** and their variations and measuring the diameter at the site of the proposed anastomosis, since anastomosis of similar size decreases the risk of thrombosis or stenosis.

TABLE 2: MDCT protocol for LDLT donor evaluation.			
Phases	Iodinated contrast material	Delay	kVp
Unenhanced CT	—	—	120 kVp
Arterial phase	80–100 mL of with a concentration of 370 mg/mL @ 4–5 mL/s	30 s	100–120 kVp
Portal venous phase	80–100 mL of with a concentration of 370 mg/mL @ 4–5 mL/s	60–70 s	120 kVp

(MDCT: multidetector computed tomography; LDLT: living donor liver transplantation; CT: computed tomography)

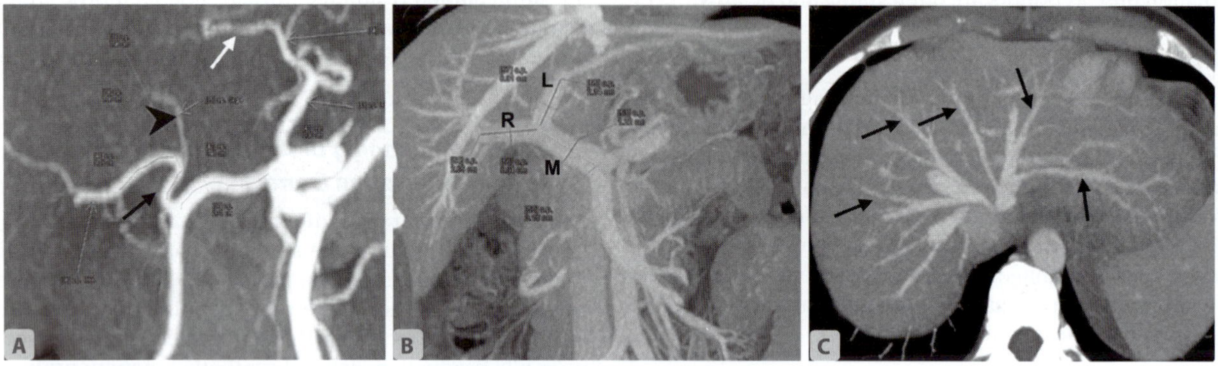

FIGS. 1A TO C: Preoperative work-up of liver donor. (A) CT scan in arterial phase showing right hepatic artery (black arrow) from celiac trunk and left hepatic artery (white arrow) from left gastric artery. Segment 4 branch (arrowhead) or middle hepatic artery is also seen. Caliber and length of the hepatic arteries should be measured. (B) Venous phase images showing densely opacified portal vein (M) with measurements of caliber and length of main as well as right (R) and left (L) branches. (C) Venous phase showing opacified hepatic veins and their tributaries (arrows) (segments 5 and 8 being important).

Hepatic Arteries

Normal hepatic arterial anatomy (Michel Type I) consisting of common hepatic artery arising from celiac axis and dividing into right and left hepatic artery is found in only 55% of the population.[17] Replaced right hepatic artery (RHA) from superior mesenteric artery (11%) and replaced left hepatic artery (LHA) from left gastric artery (10%) are other common variations.[17] The terms "aberrant" or "replaced" are used when the variant arteries substitute the normal artery whereas the variant artery that persists in addition to the normal one is termed "accessory." The most common arterial variant is an accessory right or left hepatic artery. As few of these variants are surgically relevant, hence variants should be mentioned in the report. A replaced or accessory RHA will affect right LDLT whereas a replaced or accessory LHA will affect full left or left lateral segment LDLT. Similarly, presence of middle hepatic artery (MHA) will affect both right as well as left LDLT. Diameter of RHA or LHA is also important as <2 mm diameter makes the future arterial anastomoses prone to thrombosis and microvascular techniques are often required.

Hepatic Veins

Hepatic venous variants are seen in 16–33% of the population and if not dealt with intraoperatively, these can lead to hepatic insufficiency in the donor or recipient if drainage to a liver segment is compromised.[18] Identification of the exact location and variation of the MHV is paramount for guiding surgical planning because the hepatectomy plane—which, in living donors, is to the right of the MHV along the gallbladder fossa—may be affected.[19] MDCT is frequently used to evaluate hepatic veins **(Fig. 2)**. The usual position of the MHV is between segments VIII and IV. The drainage of segment IVa and IVb should also be mentioned. It is important to determine if an accessory inferior right hepatic vein (RHV) as it is the most common venous variant. If there is accessory RHV(s) draining VI, VII and V, a separate anastomosis is needed to preserve drainage of these segments during a right LDLT. Similarly, the right lobe anterior sector segmental veins (V5 and V8) draining into MHV, need to be separately anastomosed to the recipient suprahepatic IVC to preserve drainage of these segments during right LDLT. This is especially needed when the right lobe graft is harvested without the MHV. When the right lobe graft is harvested with the MHV, in a MHV predominant system, care has to be taken to preserve the V4a tributary and terminal part of the MHV in the donor remnant liver.

The most common venous variant is an accessory right inferior hepatic vein (RHV) and if its caliber is 5 mm or more, then a separate anastomosis to the IVC is performed to prevent hepatic congestion. The distance in the coronal plane between the accessory inferior RHV and the right hepatic vein is crucial for the surgeon while planning the graft implantation.[20]

Portal Veins

Portal venous anatomic variants are less common, although a few surgically relevant variations exist. 3D CT images can help to find out the variation easily **(Fig. 3)**. Few critical

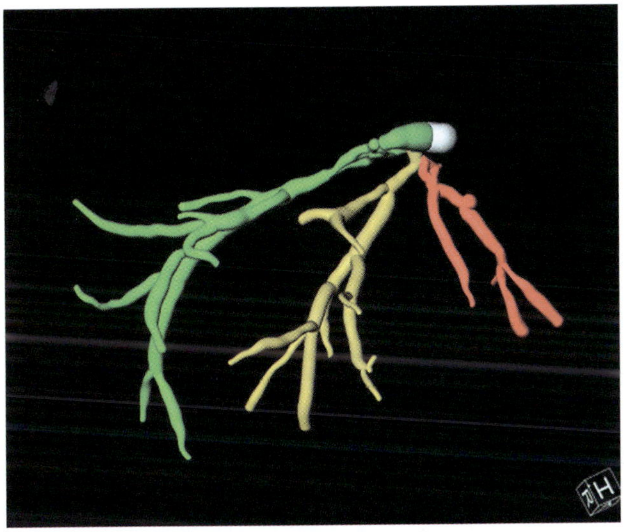

FIG. 2: Three-dimensional model of hepatic venous anatomy.

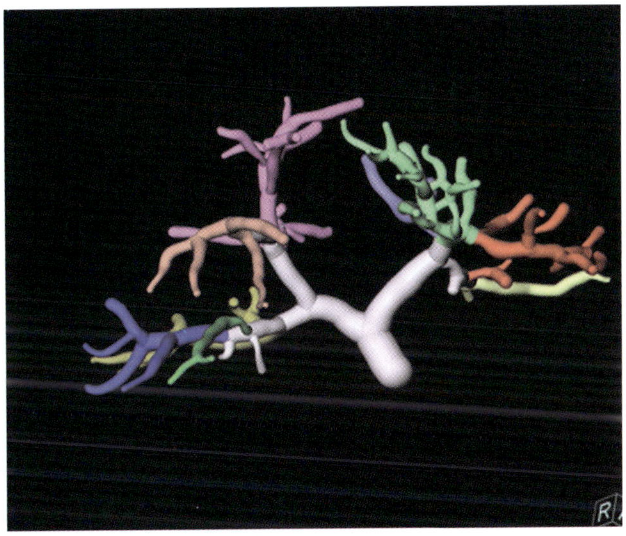

FIG. 3: Three-dimensional model of portal venous anatomy.

findings that can affect the transplant include left branch of portal vein (LPV) from right anterior branch of PV (RAPV) (affects Right LDLT, may be relative contraindication to donation) RAPV from LPV (affects left LDLT, may be relative contraindication to donation) and trifurcation into right posterior branch of PV (RPPV), RAPV, and LPV (affects both right and left LDLT; Right LDLT: must clamp and anastomose these separately; Left LDLT: RAPV from graft must be excluded).[21] There has been described association between portal venous and biliary system variants. Hence, if portal venous variants are identified, these should be examined closely to preclude associated biliary tree variations.[21]

Biliary Anatomy

A biliary anastomosis is usually between the donor common bile duct (CBD) and the recipient common hepatic duct (CHD) in a DDLT. Biliary variations are common seen in up to 33% of the population and if not identified preoperatively may result in biliary leaks and strictures leading to substantial morbidity or mortality in the donor and recipient in the postoperative period.[5] Biliary complications are the most common cause for morbidity after split and LDLT, occurring in up to 40% of patients.[21] Magnetic resonance cholangiopancreatography (MRCP) is useful for a detailed understanding of the biliary anatomy to prevent these types of complications.[22] Variations like right posterior hepatic duct (RPHD) or right anterior hepatic duct (RAHD) draining into left hepatic duct (LHD) are contraindication to left lobe donation whereas LHD draining into RAHD or RPHD are contraindication to right lobe donation. In order to prevent biliary complications and to be sure of the hilar ductal configuration during LDLT fluoroscopy-based intraoperative cholangiography (IOC) is essential before proceeding with the donor hepatectomy. IOC is repeated after graft removal to ensure there is no biliary leak and confirm that the calibre of the remnant ductal system is adequate.[22]

Liver Parenchyma

The final step of preoperative donor imaging is evaluation of the hepatic parenchyma to identify focal or diffuse liver disease (particularly steatosis), any incidental benign or malignant conditions that may preclude segmental donation and measurement of liver volumes **(Fig. 4)**.

Hepatic steatosis >30% precludes donation. NCCT findings consistent with this degree of steatosis include: hepatic density more than 10 HU lower than the spleen, hepatic density <40 HU and a hepatic-to-splenic density ratio of <0.8 **(Figs. 5A and B)**.[23] In MRI this degree of steatosis corresponds to 30% signal dropout on Dixon-type chemical shift imaging, with liver parenchymal signal drop-out normalized to the spleen. MR spectroscopy is considered to be better for estimating hepatic steatosis.

Finally, integrated software may be used to calculate the volume of the entire liver, the potential residual volume in the donor, and the potential volume in the recipient by performing virtual hepatectomy **(Figs. 6A to C)** from the MDCT data set. All the processed images of vascular tree, biliary system and liver parenchyma can be superimposed into a single presurgical liver model which can help as a guide map during surgery.

POSTOPERATIVE EVALUATION

Imaging of Post-transplant Complications

Multiple complications can be observed after liver transplantation. LDLT grafts recipient experience a higher rate of complications postoperatively as compared to recipients of whole-liver grafts. The role of imaging is to detect transplant related complication as well as to exclude other complications that can clinically mimic acute rejection. Postoperative evaluation starts USG plus Doppler daily for first week and twice weekly for next 2 weeks.

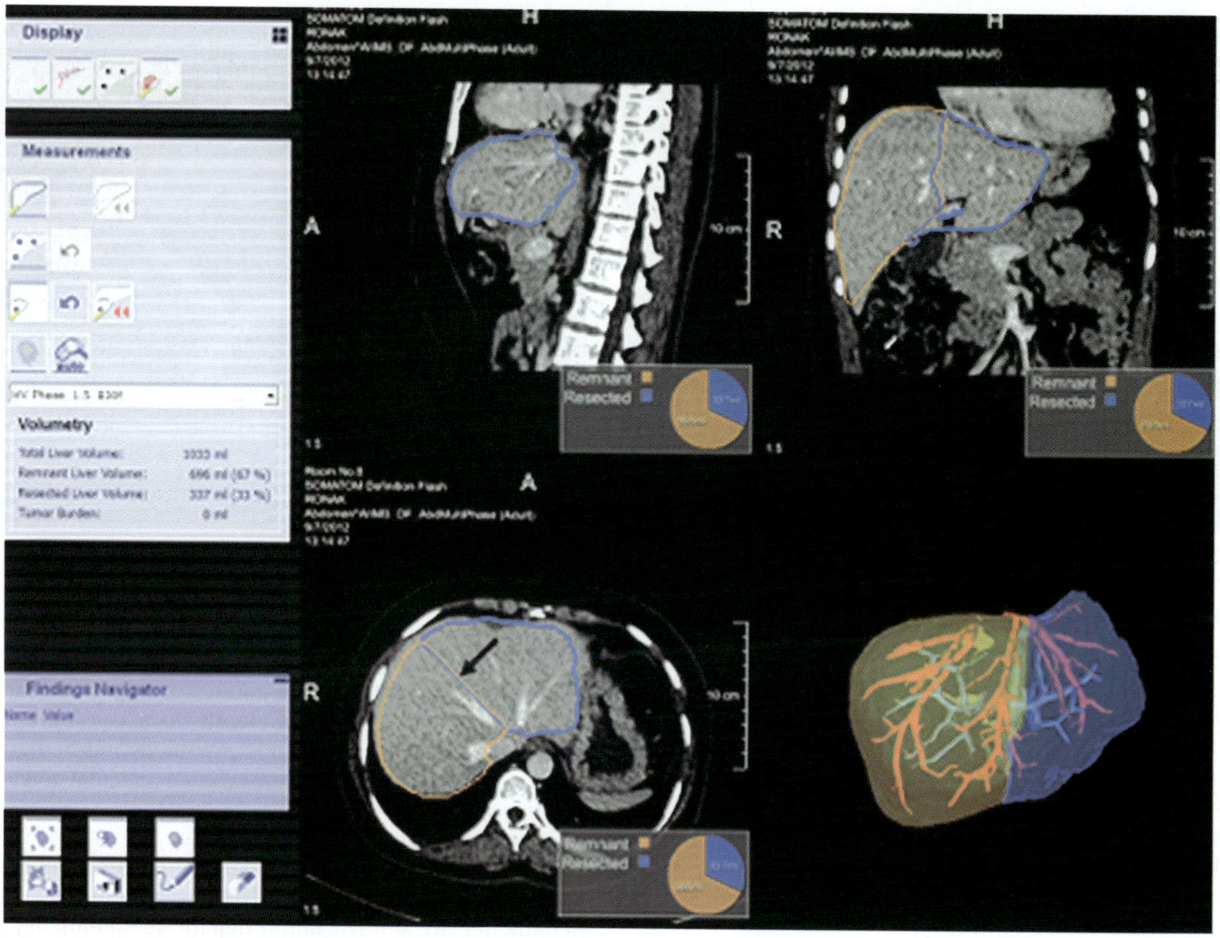

FIG. 4: Liver volumetry showing assessment of total liver volume using vendor specific software and generation of 3D model of liver. Note assessment of residual as well as donor liver volume separately by the software with line of division along the lateral margin of MHV (black arrow).

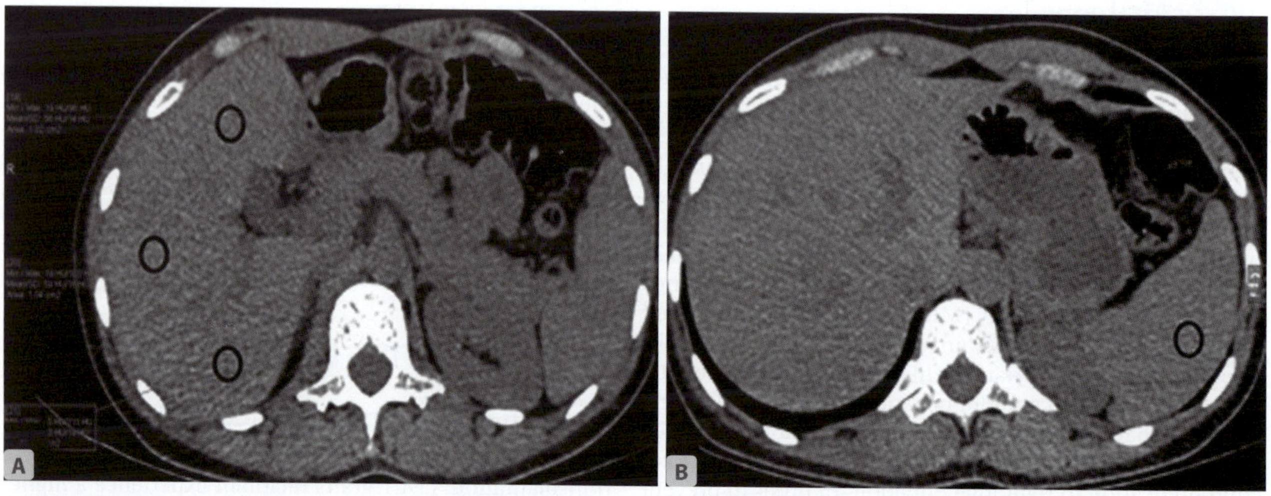

FIGS. 5A AND B: Liver attenuation index (LAI): Regions of interest (ROI) drawn on liver (25 ROI) and splenic (3 ROI) parenchyma avoiding vessels.

Assessment of hepatic vein **(Figs. 7A to C)**, hepatic artery **(Figs. 8A and B)**, IVC and portal vein are performed along with their various flow parameters. Any abnormality in USG/Doppler—further evaluation with CT/MRCP which are complementary to US and is reserved as a problem solving modality. An understanding of the strengths and weaknesses of each imaging modality will aid in early diagnosis and treatment. Knowledge of the location of various anastomosis is important because stenosis usually occurs in the anastomotic site.

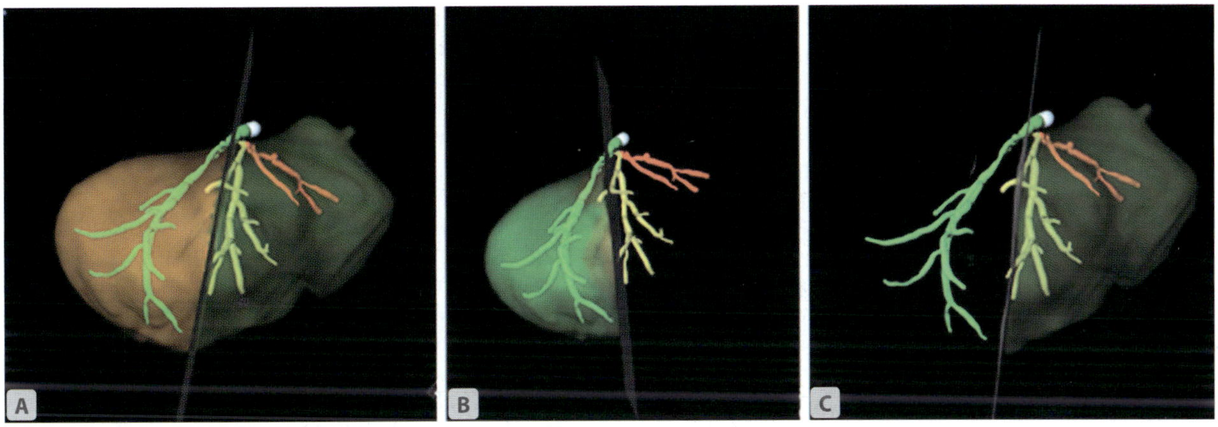

FIGS. 6A TO C: Virtual hepatectomy: Three-dimensional reconstructed CT images of the entire donor liver (A) showing the plane of hepatectomy which passes to the right of the middle hepatic vein, through segment VIII. The potential residual donor liver (B) and the donor segment (C) is also shown.

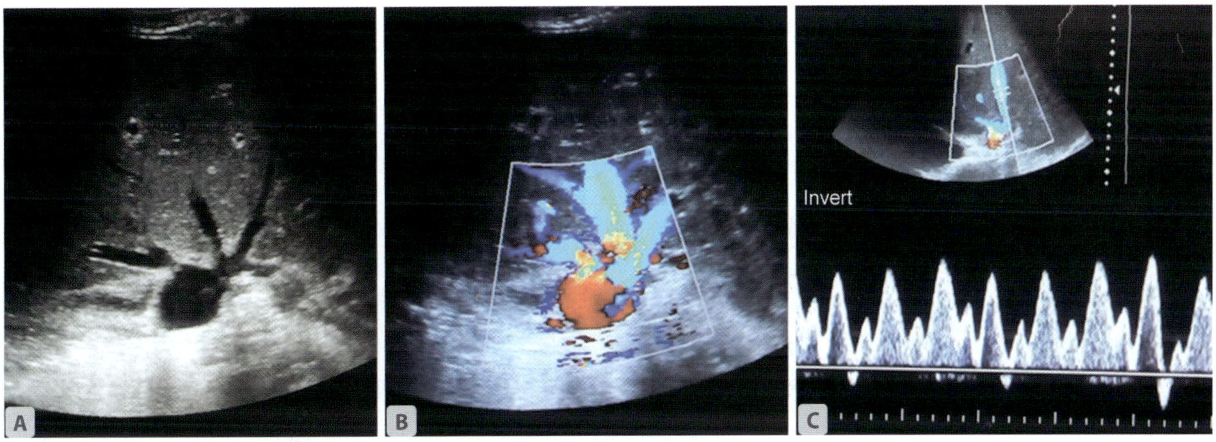

FIGS. 7A TO C: Postoperative ultrasonography: Hepatic veins. Grayscale (A), color flow (B) and Doppler trace (C) images show normal and patent hepatic veins and inferior vena cava.

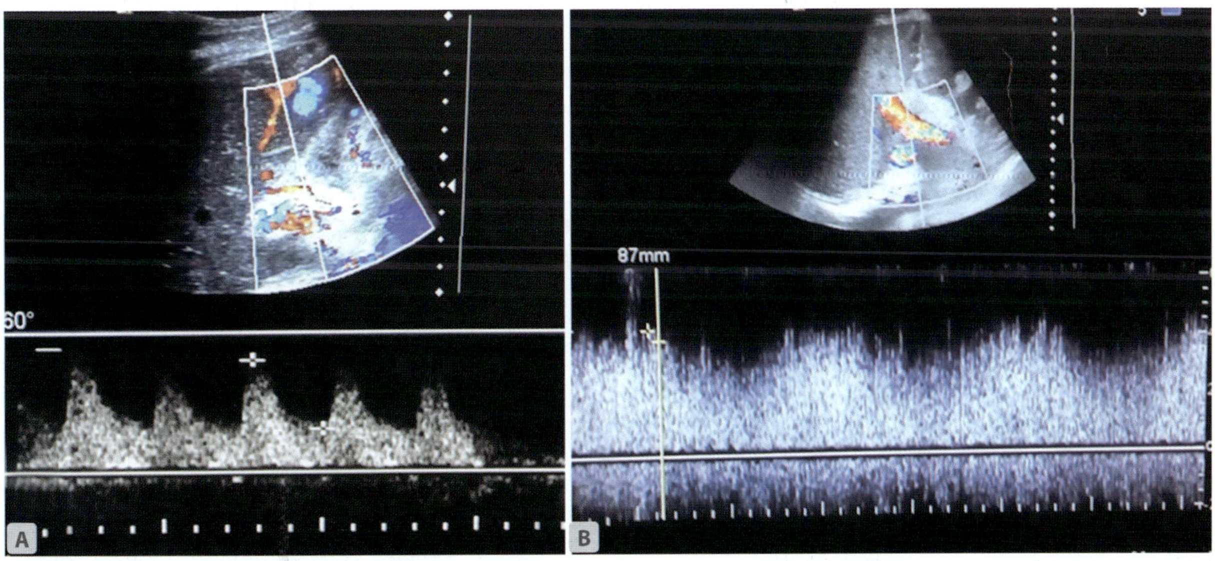

FIGS. 8A AND B: Postoperative ultrasonography. (A) Color Doppler image shows normal hepatic artery with low resistance flow. (B) Color Doppler image shows normal portal vein with undulating spectral waveform.

Hepatic Artery

Hepatic artery complications include thrombosis **(Figs. 9 and 10)**, stenosis, and pseudoaneurysm.[24] Hepatic artery thrombosis (HAT) and stenosis can lead to biliary ischemia leading to a nonanastomotic biliary stricture or a biloma. In orthotopic liver transplantation, the donor celiac axis is anastomosed to the recipient hepatic artery at either the bifurcation into left and right hepatic arteries or the origin of the gastroduodenal artery. In order to pre-empt and pick up HAT in the early post-transplant period (1st week post-transplant) serial Doppler sonographic evaluations are mandatory. In the event of any ambiguity, arterial patency has to be confirmed by CT angiography when required. The radiologist has a crucial role to play in the diagnosis as treatment usually consists of emergent thrombectomy or retransplantation.[25]

Portal Venous

Portal vein complications include thrombosis and stricture **(Figs. 11A and B)** at anastomotic site.[26] In orthotopic liver transplantation, portal vein anastomosis is most often end to end between the donor and recipient portal veins. Complications may occur due to faulty surgical technique, discrepancy between the calibres of the donor and recipient portal veins, hypercoagulable state, and history of previous thrombosis.

HV and IVC

Complications include IVC stenosis and thrombosis and hepatic vein stenosis.[27] Anastomosis of the donor and recipient IVCs can be end to end, with resection of the recipient retrohepatic IVC and anastomosis of the donor IVC superiorly and inferiorly to the recipient IVC. With living donor liver transplantation, the donor hepatic vein is anastomosed to the recipient IVC.[27] Strictures/kinking can occur in these levels of anastomosis and can affect the graft venous outflow.

Biliary Tree

The most common types of biliary complications are bile duct stricture and bile leak causing biloma.[28] Other complications include bile duct obstruction, stone formation, biliary

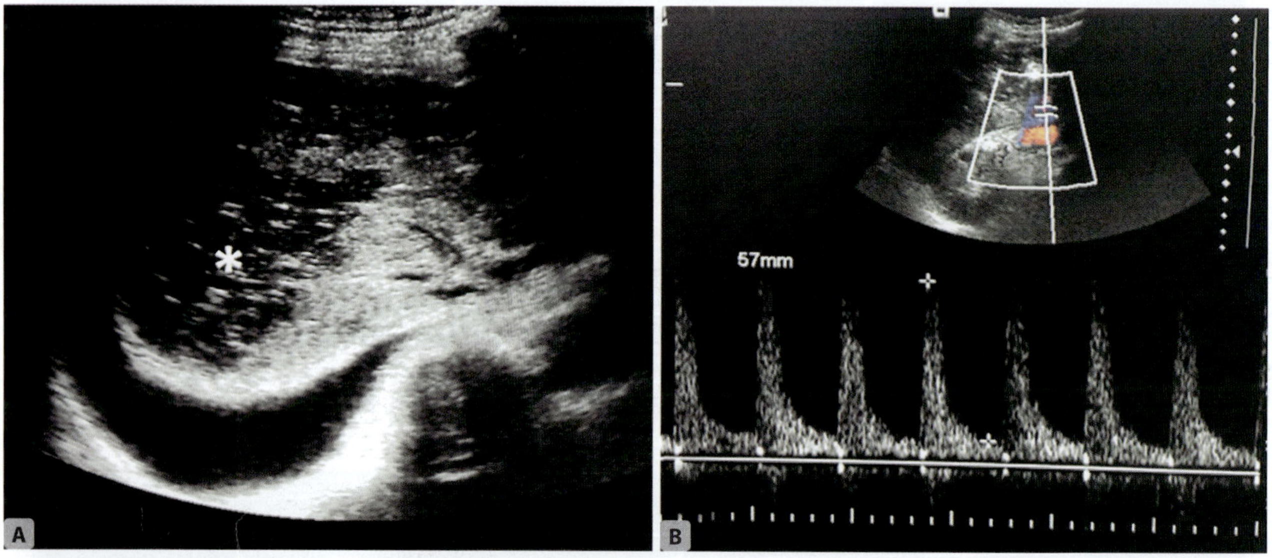

FIGS. 9A AND B: Hepatic artery thrombosis: Postoperative day 2 of a patient after cadaveric liver transplantation. (A) Grayscale ultrasonography shows a wedge-shaped hypoechoic area (asterisk) suggestive of infarct. (B) Color Doppler image at porta shows high resistance flow in hepatic artery proximal to the thrombosis.

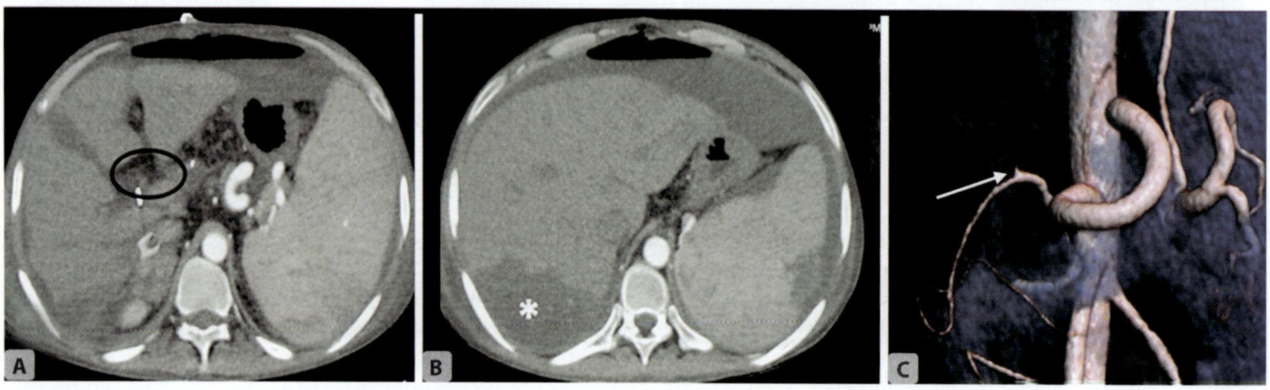

FIGS. 10A TO C: Hepatic artery thrombosis: CT angiography images show nonvisualization of hepatic artery at porta (ellipse in A) with hypodense area in right posterior segments suggesting infarct (asterisk in B). Volume-rendered image (C) shows abrupt cut-off of the hepatic artery with a small stump (arrow).

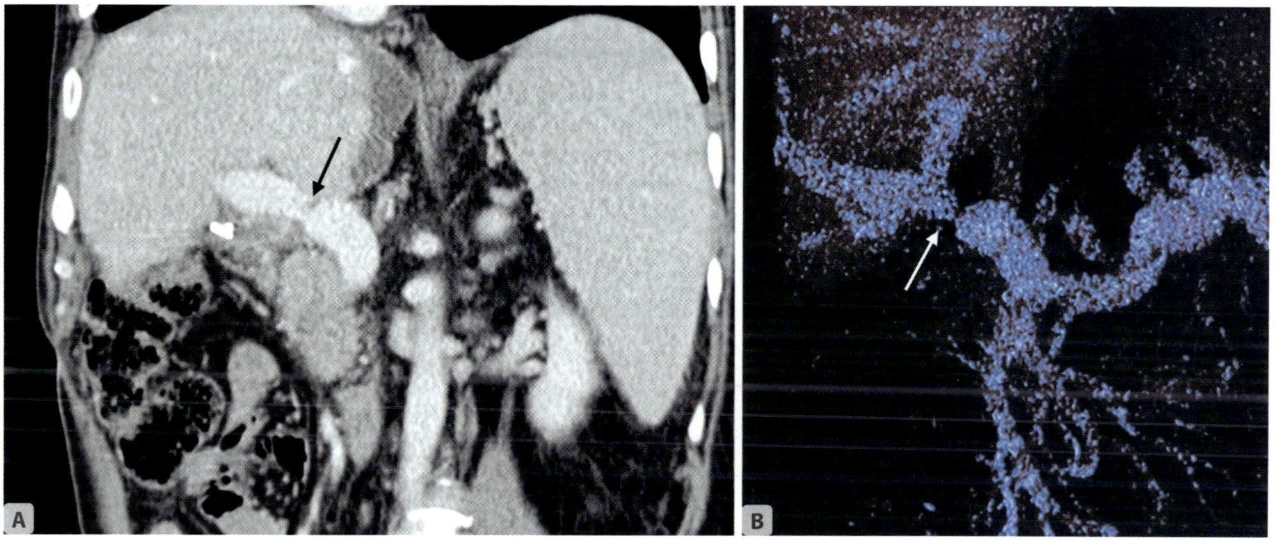

FIGS. 11A AND B: PV narrowing: Coronal (A) and volume rendered (B) contrast-enhanced CT images show short segment portal vein stenosis (arrow) with dilated splenic vein and splenomegaly, suggesting portal hypertension.

necrosis, and cholangitis. Biliary complications are more common with right-lobe liver donor transplantation. Scintigraphy is commonly used for the detection of bile leak whereas MRCP is very useful for bile duct obstruction. US has a lower sensitivity for detecting biliary complications.[29] Knowledge of the anastomotic site is important because stenosis may occur at this site **(Fig. 12)**. Non anastomotic strictures can occur in patients who have faced delayed graft hepatic artery stenosis or thrombosis and in whom immediate attempts at revascularization have failed. Biliary problems related to ischemic cholangiopathy are also more commonly observed in marginal deceased donor grafts especially from donations following cardiac death. The most common form of deceased donation in our country is donation after brain death (DBD).

Other complications include hematoma, abscess, infection, recurrent hepatitis, splenic infarct, recurrent malignancy, and post-transplantation lymphoproliferative disorder. Imaging also has an important role to play in their management.[30]

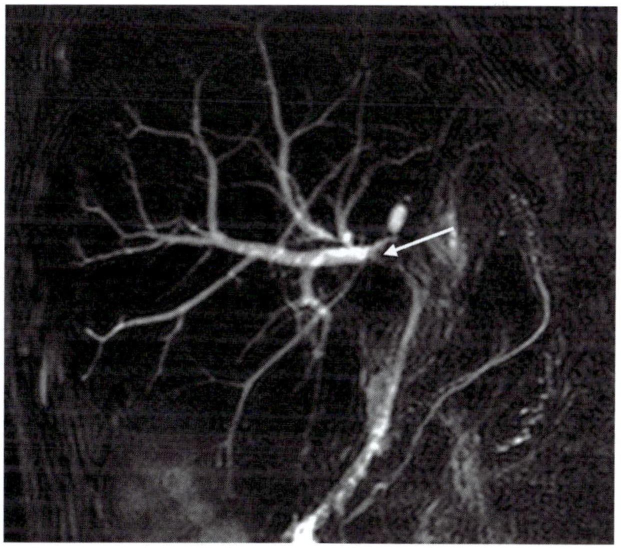

FIG. 12: Biliary stricture: MRCP in patient after right lobe liver donor liver transplantation showing short segment narrowing of bile duct (arrow) at the site of anastomosis with mild intrahepatic biliary radicle dilatation.

CONCLUSION

Preoperative imaging in potential liver transplant donor and recipient with CT and MRI is important for candidate selection and for preoperative evaluation of the liver parenchyma, vascular and biliary anatomy in the setting of LDLT. Multiphase liver CT is the modality of choice for pre-transplantation assessment of living donors and recipients whereas MRCP is commonly used for evaluation of biliary tree. Understanding the indications for transplantations and the common surgical techniques are important for a thorough assessment and can help the radiologist to craft a succinct and meaningful report **(Table 3)** which needs to be conveyed to the transplant surgeon. This report with the sets of reconstructed images and 3D model helps the surgeon perform liver transplant in a safe manner thus avoiding post-transplant complications. Imaging is also useful for the detection of various post-operative complications and long-term follow-up for transplant viability.[31]

ACKNOWLEDGMENTS

Authors sincerely acknowledge Dr Peush Sahni, Dr Sujoy Pal and Dr Nihar Ranjan Dash from Department of Gastrointestinal Surgery, All India Institute of Medical Sciences (AIIMS), New Delhi, India.

TABLE 3: Checklist for living donor MDCT reporting.
Liver size (craniocaudal) • Any evidence of acute or chronic liver disease • Any focal lesions: Yes/No (If yes, describe the number, size, segment and nature of the lesions) • Any biliary obstruction or IHBD
Liver fat estimation (on unenhanced or VNC images): • Mean liver attenuation (in HU) • Mean splenic attenuation (in HU) • Liver attenuation Index (in HU) • Do the intrahepatic vessels appear hypoattenuated compared to the liver parenchyma: Yes/ No
Liver volume analysis: • Total liver volume (in cc) • Graft volume (in cc) • Donor remnant liver volume (in cc) • Donor remnant liver volume (in percentage of total liver volume)
Hepatic arterial anatomy: • *Right hepatic artery (RHA)*: – Vessel of origin – Diameter at origin (in mm) – Length before first sectional division (in cm) – *Any vascular thrombus*: Yes/No (If yes, mention the degree of occlusion) • *Left hepatic artery (LHA)*: – Vessel of origin – Diameter at origin (in mm) – Length before first sectional division (in cm) – *Any vascular thrombus*: Yes/No (If yes, mention the degree of occlusion) • *Segment IV artery origin*: RHA/LHA/others (mention) • *Any variant vascular anatomy*: Yes/No (If yes, specify according to Michael classification) • *Accessory RHA/ LHA/ segmental artery (if any)*: – Vessel of origin – Diameter at origin (in mm) – Length before first division (in cm)
Portal venous anatomy: • *Main portal vein (MPV)*: – Length before first division (in cm) – *Any evidence of portal hypertension*: Yes/ No – *Any thrombus*: Yes/No. If yes, mention the extent (length and degree of luminal compromise), duration (acute versus chronic), nature (bland vs. malignant) and presence of collaterals • *Right portal vein (RPV)*: – Length before first sectional division (in cm) – Diameter at origin (in mm) – *Any thrombus*: Yes/No • *Left portal vein (LPV)*: – Length before first sectional division (in cm) – Diameter at origin (in mm) – *Any thrombus*: Yes/No • *Any variant vascular anatomy*: Yes/No. If yes, specify according to Nakamura classification. If type C, mention the distance between the ostium of the right anterior and posterior sectional portal veins (in cm) • Accessory RPV/LPV (if any)
Hepatic venous anatomy: • Diameters at IVC ostium in mm – Right hepatic vein (RHV) – Common middle hepatic vein (MHV) and left hepatic vein (LHV) stump (mention otherwise if separate) • *Any major (> 4 mm) segment V/ VIII tributaries into MHV*: Yes/ No. If yes, mention the number • *Any major segment VI/VII drainage into segment V/VII veins or MHV*: Yes/ No. If yes, describe • *Any accessory inferior RHV*: Yes/ No. If yes, specify the number of veins and the vertical distance between these veins and the RHV in cm • *Any thrombosis of IVC*: Yes/ No. If yes, mention the site, extent and nature
Other abdominal organs: Normal/ abnormal. If abnormal, specify
Ascites or lymphadenopathy: Yes/ No
Visualized lung bases and bone: Normal/abnormal. If abnormal, specify

REFERENCES

1. Ioannou GN. Development and validation of a model predicting graft survival after liver transplantation. Liver Transpl. 2006;12(11):1594-606.
2. United Network for Organ Sharing. National Data Report. *http://www.unos.org/*. Accessed September 23, 2016.
3. Koffron A, Stein JA. Liver transplantation: indications, pretransplant evaluation, surgery, and post-transplant complications. Med Clin North Am. 2008;92(4):861-88, ix.
4. Kamath PS, Wiesner RH, Malinchoc M, et al. A model to predict survival in patients with end-stage liver disease. Hepatology. 2001;33(2):464-70.
5. Singh AK, Cronin CG, Verma HA, Boland GW, Saini S, Mueller PR, Sahani DV. Imaging of preoperative liver transplantation in adults: what radiologists should know. Radiographics. 2011;31(4):1017-30.
6. Toso C, Trotter J, Wei A, et al. Total tumor volume predicts risk of recurrence following liver transplantation in patients with hepatocellular carcinoma. Liver Transpl. 2008;14(8):1107-15.
7. Woo HY, Jang JW, Choi JY, et al. Living donor liver transplantation in hepatocellular carcinoma beyond the Milan criteria. Liver Int. 2008;28(8):1120-8.
8. Marelli L, Grasso A, Pleguezuelo M, et al. Tumour size and differentiation in predicting recurrence of hepatocellular carcinoma after liver transplantation: external validation of a new prognostic score. Ann Surg Oncol. 2008;15(12):3503-11.
9. Woo HY, Jang JW, Choi JY, et al. Living donor liver transplantation in hepatocellular carcinoma beyond the Milan criteria. Liver Int. 2008;28(8):1120-8.
10. Tanaka K, Yamada T. Living donor liver transplantation in Japan and Kyoto University: what can we learn? J Hepatol. 2005;42(1):25-8.
11. Foster R, Zimmerman M, Trotter JF. Expanding donor options: marginal, living, and split donors. Clin Liver Dis. 2007;11(2):417-29.
12. Broering DC, Wilms C, Lenk C, et al. Technical refinements and results in full-right full-left splitting of the deceased donor liver. Ann Surg. 2005;242(6):802-12; discussion 812-3.
13. Rosenkrantz AB, Campbell N, Wehrli N, et al. New OPTN/UNOS classification system for nodules in cirrhotic livers detected with MR Imaging: Effect on hepatocellular carcinoma detection and transplant allocation. Radiology. 2015;274(2):426-33.
14. Liver imaging reporting and data system. Available at: *http://www.acr.org/quality-safety/resources/LIRADS*. Accessed May 24, 2016.
15. Prasad MA, Kulik LM. The role of bridge therapy prior to orthotopic liver transplantation. J Natl Compr Canc Netw. 2014;12:1183-91.
16. Forner A, Gilabert M, Gruix J, et al. Treatment of intermediate-stage hepatocellular carcinoma. Nat Rev Clin Oncol. 2014;11:525-35.
17. Tsang LL, Chen CL, Huang TL, et al. Preoperative imaging evaluation of potential living liver donors: reasons for exclusion from donation in adult living donor liver transplantation. Transplant Proc. 2008;40(8):2460-2.
18. Michels NA. Blood supply and anatomy of upper abdominal organs. Philadelphia, PA: Lippincott, 1955.
19. Fan ST, Lo CM, Liu CL. Technical refinement in adultto-adult living donor liver transplantation using right lobe graft. Ann Surg. 2000;231:126-31.
20. Sahani D, Mehta A, Blake M, Prasad S, Harris G, Saini S. Preoperative hepatic vascular evaluation with CT and MR angiography: implications for surgery. RadioGraphics. 2004;24(5):1367-80.
21. Erbay N, Raptopoulos V, Pomfret EA, Kamel IR, Kruskal JB. Living donor liver transplantation in adults: vascular variants important in surgical planning for donors and recipients. AJR. 2003;181(1):109-14.
22. Sahani D, D'souza R, Kadavigere R, et al. Evaluation of living liver transplant donors: method for precise anatomic definition by using a dedicated contrast enhanced MR imaging protocol. Radiographics. 2004;24:957-67.
23. Itamoto T, Emoto K, Mitsuta H, et al. Safety of donor right hepatectomy for adult-to-adult living donor liver transplantation. Transpl Int. 2006;19(3):177-83.
24. Piekarski J, Goldberg HI, Royal SA, et al. Difference between liver and spleen CT numbers in the normal adult: its usefulness in predicting the presence of diffuse liver disease. Radiology. 1980;137:727-9.
25. Orons PD, Sheng R, Zajko AB. Hepatic artery stenosis in liver transplant recipients: prevalence and cholangiographic appearance of associated biliary complications. AJR. 1995; 165(5):1145–9.
26. Singh AK, Nachiappan AC, Verma HA, Uppot RN, Blake MA, Saini S, Boland GW. Postoperative imaging in liver transplantation: what radiologists should know. Radiographics. 2010;30(2):339-51.
27. Nghiem HV. Imaging of hepatic transplantation. Radiol Clin North Am. 1998;36(2):429-43.
28. Uzochukwu LN, Bluth EI, Smetherman DH, et al. Early postoperative hepatic sonography as a predictor of vascular and biliary complications in adult orthotopic liver transplant patients. AJR. 2005;185(6):1558-70.
29. Fulcher AS, Turner MA. Orthotopic liver transplantation: evaluation with MR cholangiography. Radiology. 1999;211(3):715-22.
30. Zemel G, Zajko AB, Skolnick ML, Bron KM, Campbell WL. The role of sonography and transhepatic cholangiography in the diagnosis of biliary complications after liver transplantation. AJR. 1988;151(5):943-6.
31. Dupuy DE, Costello P. Cross-sectional imaging of liver transplantation. Semin Ultrasound CT MR. 1992;13(5):399-409.

CHAPTER

106

Imaging and Interventions in Hepatic Venous Outflow Tract Obstruction

Naveen Kalra, Ujjwal Gorsi, Niranjan Khandelwal

INTRODUCTION

Hepatic venous outflow tract obstruction, Budd-Chiari syndrome (BCS), is a rare disorder of hepatic venous outflow obstruction which may involve the hepatic veins, inferior vena cava (IVC) or both and is characterized by structural and functional abnormalities of the liver. It affects 1 in 100,000 population worldwide. The disease is more common in Northern India, South Africa and Japan as compared to the Western countries. The term 'Budd Chiari' was coined after George Budd, who reported three cases of hepatic vein thrombosis in 1845 and Hans Chiari, who described obliterating endophlebitis of the hepatic veins in 1899.[1]

BCS is classified into three types based on the level of venous occlusion.[2] In type I, involvement is at the level of IVC alone, in type II, it is at the level of hepatic veins and type III is the mixed type with involvement of both IVC and hepatic veins.

CLINICAL PRESENTATION

The clinical course of BCS is determined by the degree of hepatic venous outflow obstruction and the rapidity with which it develops. Usually the clinical presentation of the syndrome is nonspecific. Large and sudden blockage of veins results in acute BCS, which is characterized by severe abdominal pain, ascities, jaundice, tender hepatomegaly and rapidly developing hepatic failure over a period of few days to few weeks. Subacute BCS is the most common clinical type, has an insidious onset and may take as long as 3 months to become asymptomatic. The development is slow and during the period decompressive collaterals develop. Thus subacute BCS does not present with esophageal bleed. On the other hand, when there is still more insidious gradual venous outflow obstruction it leads to chronic BCS which is characterized by the development of postsinusoidal portal hypertension, prominent abdominal veins, upper GI bleed, pedal edema, ascities and large nodular liver developing over a period of several months. Acute BCS is mostly reported from western countries, whereas cases of chronic BCS are reported mainly from Japan, China, South Africa and India. Differentiation of acute and chronic forms of the disease is important for determining the prognosis and planning the treatment. In patients with acute form, the prognosis is poor with high mortality if not treated, whereas chronic form is less ominous and 50% patients are alive after five years.[3]

ETIOPATHOGENESIS

The BCS is classified as primary when the obstruction to hepatic venous outflow is due to a primary venous thrombosis, stenosis or web. It is classified as secondary when the obstruction is caused by extensive compression by tumor, cyst or abscess.[4] These lesions obstruct venous outflow by invasion of the lumen or by extrinsic compression. Most of the patients of BCS have an underlying inherited or acquired hypercoagulable state. Myeloproliferative disease is the most common thrombotic disorder detected. The other conditions associated with BCS are JAK2 V617F mutation, Factor V Leiden mutation, oral contraceptive pills, pregnancy, antiphospholipid antibodies, paroxysmal nocturnal hemoglobinuria, protein C and S deficiency. JAK2 V617F mutation may be detected in 30–50% of patients with BCS.

The etiology of BCS also has geographical variation.[5] In Asian countries, the most common causes are web or membranous obstruction of the IVC (MOVC), pregnancy and infections, while in the West, primary myeloproliferative disorders, hypercoagulable states, steroidal contraceptives and tumors are responsible in majority of cases. While earlier studies from India found isolated IVC obstruction to be the most common disease type, recent studies found the combination of IVC and hepatic vein obstruction to be the most common type.[6] Rarely, BCS may occur due to malignant thrombosis of the IVC or main hepatic veins secondary to hepatic, renal and adrenal neoplasms.[7] Hepatocellular carcinoma can produce an acute fulminant variant of BCS by causing obstruction of the main hepatic veins or inferior vena cava due to endoluminal invasion by the tumor. However, in 30–50% of patients etiology remains unidentified.[5]

Initially when the hepatic veins occlude, the sinusoidal and portal pressures increase and there is hepatic congestion **(Fig. 1A)**. This increase in sinusoidal pressure leads to hypoxic injury to hepatocytes which results in noninflammatory centrilobular cell necrosis especially in perivenular zones. In case the hepatocyte damage is massive, the patient presents with fulminant BCS. In case the damage is insidious, the liver slowly develops fibrosis and later cirrhosis **(Fig. 1B)**. The patient will then present with portal hypertension and ascites.

Liver biopsy differentiates BCS from veno-occlusive disease (VOD) which is due to nonthrombotic obstruction of hepatic vessels by subendothelial swelling on account of injury of sinusoidal wall **(Fig. 1C)**. The cause of VOD is toxic agents and it is also associated with bone marrow transplantation. Cyclophosphamide is the most common causative agent. VOD is also known as sinusoidal obstruction syndrome.

DIAGNOSTIC TECHNIQUES

The recent advances in imaging techniques have enabled delineation of the exact vascular abnormalities and their treatment resulting in better and improved survival rates in patients of BCS. The available therapeutic options include medical treatment; radiological interventional methods like balloon angioplasty, stent placement, transjugular intrahepatic portosystemic shunt (TIPS) and surgical treatment which includes portosystemic shunts and liver transplantation. Imaging thus plays a crucial role in diagnosis and management. Till recently, IVC venography, hepatic venography and liver biopsy alone or in combination were the definitive investigations available for anatomic and hemodynamic evaluation in patients of BCS, but these procedures are invasive and have risk of complications particularly in patients with coagulation abnormalities. Lately, several noninvasive imaging modalities like ultrasound, CT and MRI are being increasingly used in the diagnosis of BCS as they can depict the hepatic vascular anatomy accurately without catheterization and thereby guide management decisions. The current chapter will discuss the role of these newer investigations in evaluating the hepatic veins, IVC and liver parenchyma in diagnosis of BCS and various interventional techniques used for treating this condition.

EVALUATION OF HEPATIC VEINS IN BUDD-CHIARI SYNDROME

Real-time sonography is currently considered the investigation of choice for initial evaluation of BCS. The technique demonstrates the morphological hepatic changes as well as thrombosis or occlusion of hepatic veins or IVC. Simultaneously adjacent organs can also be assessed.

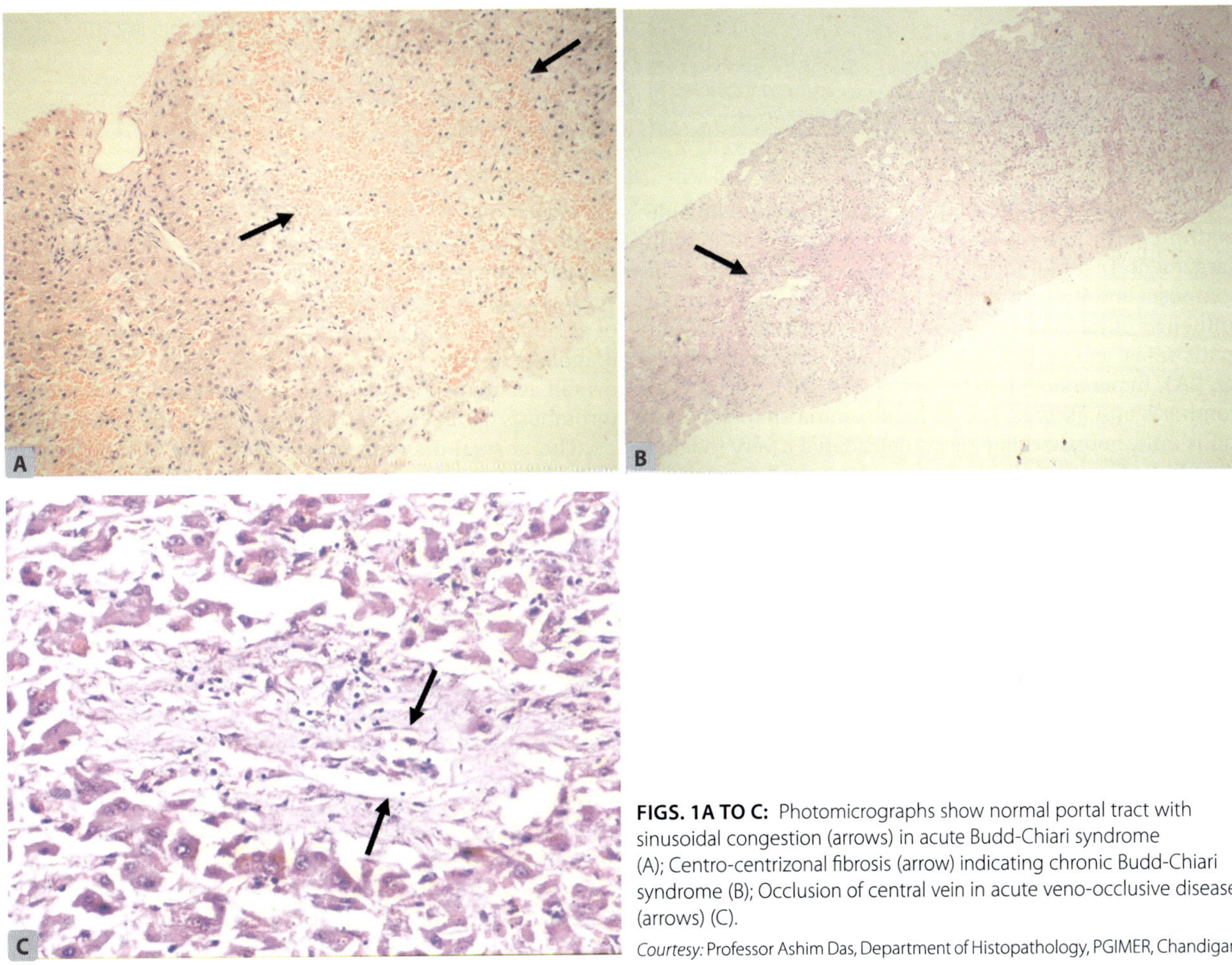

FIGS. 1A TO C: Photomicrographs show normal portal tract with sinusoidal congestion (arrows) in acute Budd-Chiari syndrome (A); Centro-centrizonal fibrosis (arrow) indicating chronic Budd-Chiari syndrome (B); Occlusion of central vein in acute veno-occlusive disease (arrows) (C).

Courtesy: Professor Ashim Das, Department of Histopathology, PGIMER, Chandigarh.

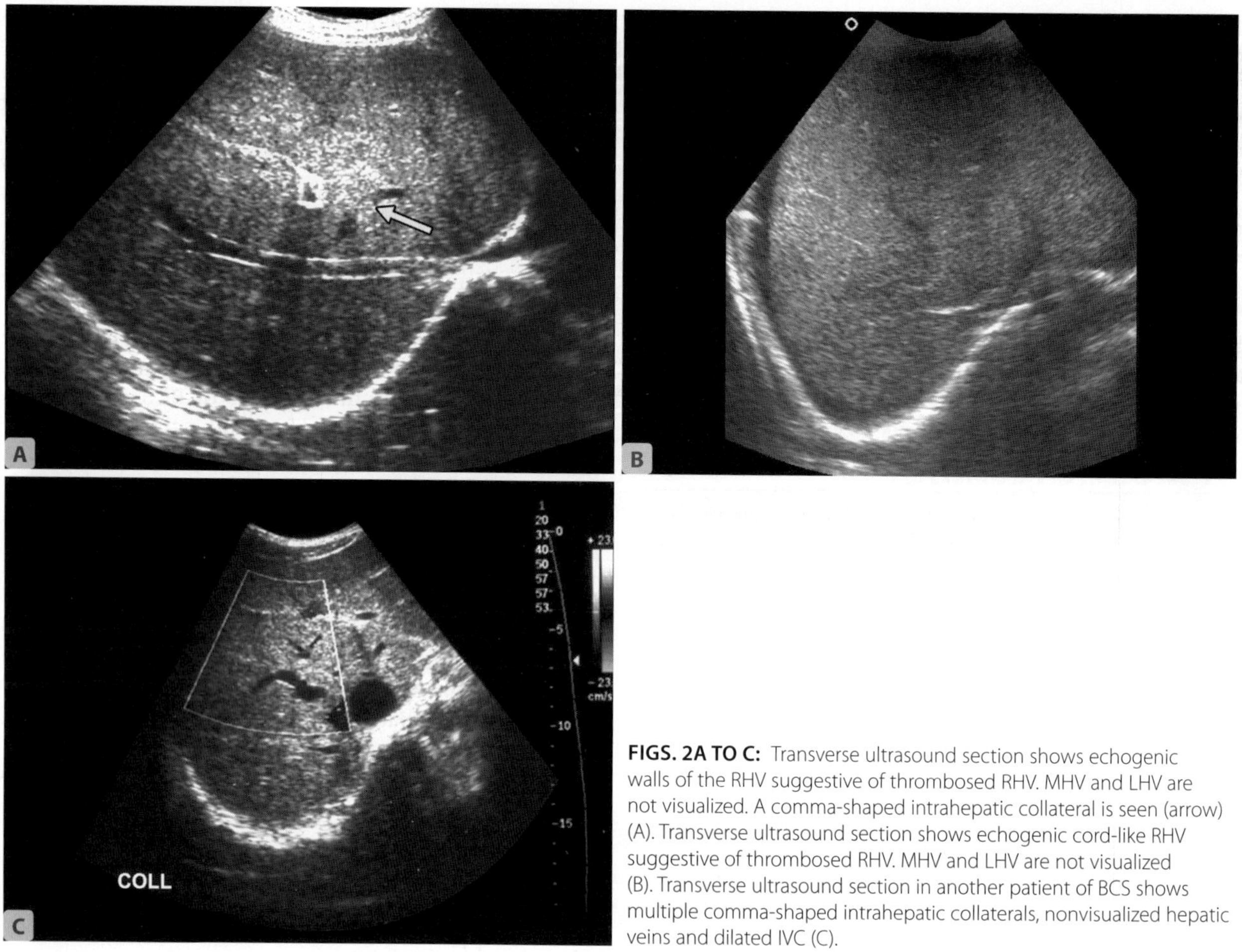

FIGS. 2A TO C: Transverse ultrasound section shows echogenic walls of the RHV suggestive of thrombosed RHV. MHV and LHV are not visualized. A comma-shaped intrahepatic collateral is seen (arrow) (A). Transverse ultrasound section shows echogenic cord-like RHV suggestive of thrombosed RHV. MHV and LHV are not visualized (B). Transverse ultrasound section in another patient of BCS shows multiple comma-shaped intrahepatic collaterals, nonvisualized hepatic veins and dilated IVC (C).

The various findings depicted by routine ultrasound include hepatomegaly, heterogeneous liver and caudate lobe enlargement. In addition, findings that suggest hepatic vein thrombosis on ultrasound (US) include nonvisualization of confluence of hepatic veins with IVC, distorted or absent hepatic veins, stenosed hepatic veins with thick wall echoes **(Fig. 2A)**, hyperechoic hepatic veins **(Fig. 2B)**, portal vein thrombosis and ascities. Presence of comma shaped veno-venous intra-hepatic collaterals is considered a very reliable sign of BCS **(Fig. 2C)**.[8-13] Subcapsular venous collaterals may also be seen. In case only the hepatic vein occlusion is the cause of BCS, at least two of the hepatic veins must be blocked for clinically evident disease.[14]

Liver is generally enlarged but may be normal in size or shrunken in advanced cases of chronic BCS. Right lobe may show atrophy with hypertrophy of the left lobe. Echotexture of liver is homogenously hypoechoic in acute BCS and non-homogeneous in chronic BCS. The surface of the liver may reveal fine nodularity due to cirrhotic changes. Caudate lobe enlargement is a common feature and a useful pointer towards the diagnosis, seen in 82–91% of the cases but is a nonspecific sign as it can be seen in cirrhosis due to other causes.[15]

Caudate lobe enlargement is explained by the fact that it has separate veins which are not affected by the thrombotic process and drain directly into the IVC just distal to the ostia of the main hepatic veins. This segment of the liver thus receives uninterrupted supply of hepatotropic agents like insulin. Caudate lobe drainage serves as an outflow for intrahepatic venous collaterals. It has been reported that visualization of a caudate vein >3 mm in diameter strongly suggests the diagnosis of BCS in an appropriate clinical setting.[16] The overall accuracy of ultrasound for detecting hepatic venous thrombosis has been found to be 70–87% in the literature.[11,17]

The normal diameter of the right and middle hepatic veins is less than 10 mm while that of the left hepatic vein is less than 9 mm.[18] Though US has been extremely useful for evaluation of hepatic veins, it does not provide any information about blood flow in hepatic veins or IVC or portal vein. The technique has limitations in cases of swollen and nodular, or shrunken and scarred liver in which veins may be obscured within the hepatic parenchyma. Detection of intraluminal webs, thrombosis or membranes is also limited. Poor delineation of extrahepatic collaterals and possibility of an inadequate study due to bowel gas are other limiting factors.

Color flow duplex Doppler US combined with real-time imaging has increased the sensitivity and specificity of diagnosis of BCS as it allows better visualization of hepatic veins by automatically adding flow information. Doppler waveform of hepatic veins in healthy individuals is a triphasic waveform (two negative waves and one positive) **(Fig. 3A)**.[19]

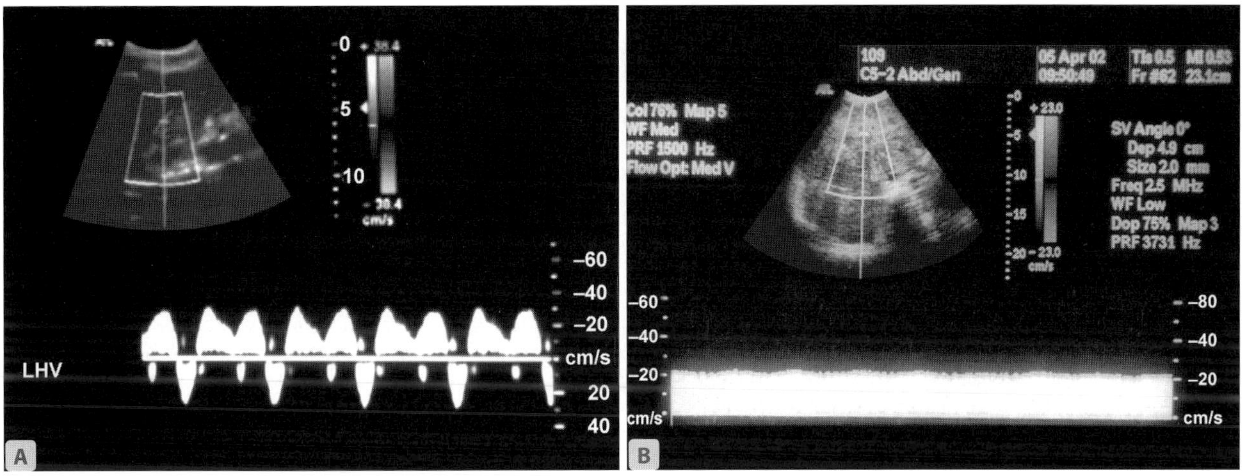

FIGS. 3A AND B: Normal pulsed Doppler tracing in the left hepatic vein (LHV) shows the triphasic waveform. The antegrade flow occurs during the ventricular systole and atrial diastole while retrograde flow occurs during the atrial systole (A); Doppler US with color box placed in the region of RHV and MHV in a patient of BCS shows no flow in RHV. MHV shows uniphasic flow (B).

Loss of the normal triphasic waveform is seen in BCS as well as in cirrhosis. Presence of flat waveform (uniphasic flow) without flutter or absent or reversed flow in hepatic veins are the most reliable signs of hepatic vein thrombosis **(Fig. 3B)**. Veins that may be nonvisualized on real-time ultrasound due to compression by hepatic nodules may reveal flow on color flow ultrasound and thus prove to be normal.[12] 3D ultrasound can also be used to show the entire morphology of the IVC and the hepatic veins.[18]

Magnetic resonance (MR) has also been used for evaluation of hepatic veins.[20] T2 weighted gradient echo sequence or multiphase contrast-enhanced images are needed for the evaluation of vessels and collaterals. MR has particular advantage of being able to show hepatic veins in three dimensions but its ability to determine the degree of flow is limited in the routine MR sequences. In our experience color flow Doppler US is superior to MR for evaluation of hepatic veins as the ostial narrowing can be better detected by US. The angiographic techniques used for delineation of the hepatic veins include IVC graphy with retrograde hepatic vein cannulation, percutaneous hepatography (injection of contrast in the hepatic parenchyma under fluoroscopy with serial filming to visualize the hepatic veins entering into IVC) **(Fig. 4)** and direct hepatic venography under US guidance. These techniques are the most definitive but are reserved for patients being considered for angioplasty or stent placement where exact delineation of the length of stenosed segment is mandatory for deciding the management. In BCS there is a collateral circulation between the tributaries of the hepatic veins which forms a 'spider web'. In the initial stage these collaterals are fine giving rise to a 'fine spider web'. With long standing BCS, these collaterals form a 'coarse spider web'.[21] Arteriography if performed in a patient with BCS would show larger diameter of the hepatic artery as compared to the splenic artery since the blood supply to the liver by the hepatic artery is increased.[22]

Scintigraphy and CT have also been used for the diagnosis of BCS. Scintigraphy may reveal increased uptake by caudate lobe and left lobe, patchy uptake of radionuclide in the rest of the liver giving the appearance of hot spots. On CT, presence of enlarged caudate lobe with low attenuation areas elsewhere in the liver, atrophy of right lobe, nonvisualization of hepatic veins and irregular surface of the liver may be seen. On CECT presence of patchy hepatogram, areas of linear, irregular or wedge-shaped hypoattenuation particularly in the peripheral portions of liver due to fibrosis and parenchymal destruction indicate hepatic venous thrombosis. Dynamic CT may demonstrate thrombus within the hepatic veins and comma shaped intrahepatic collaterals **(Fig. 5A)**. Presence of areas of hypoattenuation surrounded by areas of increased enhancement can simulate presence of intra-hepatic mass lesion. Although there is limited literature about the role of MDCT in BCS, the availability of volume imaging and 3D reconstructions **(Fig. 5B)** will provide a useful adjunct to axial images in the near future.[22]

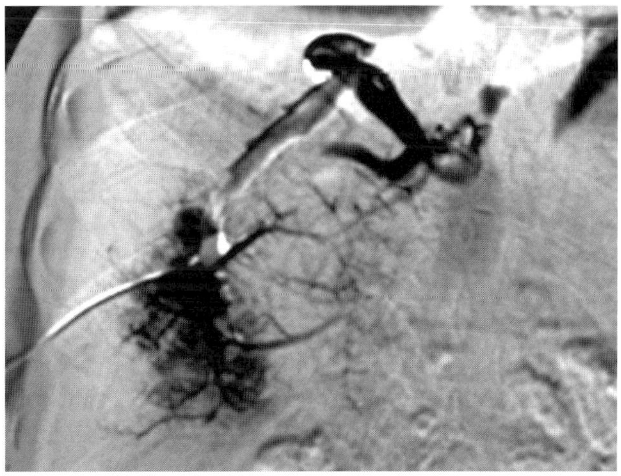

FIG. 4: Percutaneous hepatography shows nonopacification of the hepatic veins. There is filling up of multiple intrahepatic collaterals some of which have 'spider web' configuration.

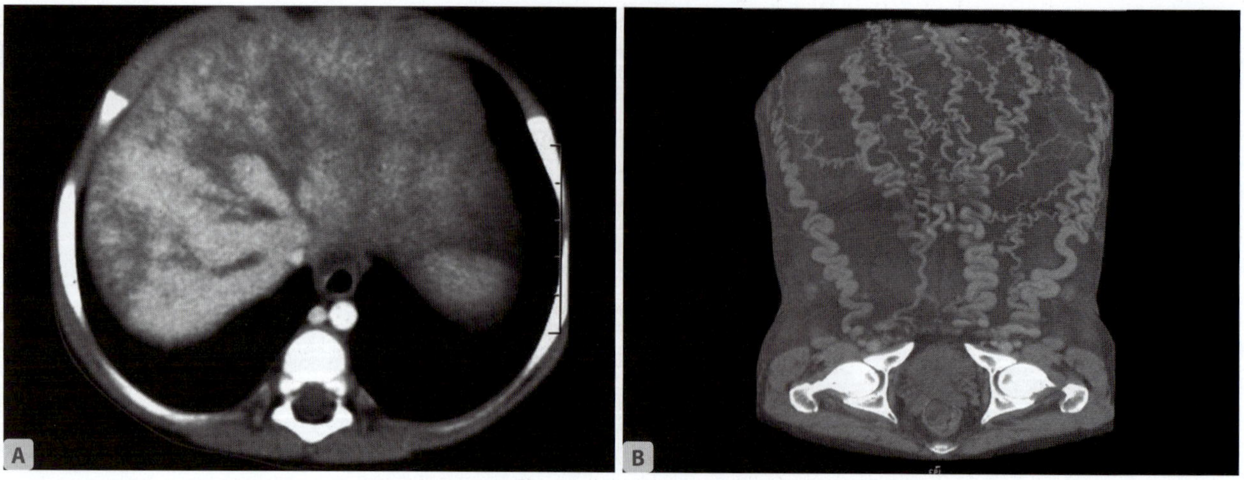

FIGS. 5A AND B: CECT in a patient of BCS shows patchy hepatogram: The right hepatic vein and middle hepatic vein are thrombosed while the left hepatic vein is not visualized (A); MDCT reconstructed image shows multiple parietal wall collaterals in a patient with type III BCS (B).

EVALUATION OF INFERIOR VENA CAVA IN BUDD-CHIARI SYNDROME

Evaluation of IVC is an important and essential component of the imaging evaluation of a patient suspected to have BCS for two reasons. Firstly, IVC obstruction alone or in combination with hepatic vein obstruction may itself lead to BCS. Secondly, patency of IVC must be established before deciding upon the surgical procedure to be undertaken such as portocaval/ mesocaval shunt when IVC is patent and mesoatrial shunt when IVC is obstructed.

Incidence of IVC obstruction in BCS varies from 33% to 56%.[23,24] IVC can be obstructed in its intrahepatic portion, suprahepatic portion or both. The causes of IVC obstruction are membranes, tumor thrombus and caudate lobe hypertrophy.[11,23,24] Suprahepatic obstruction is generally due to short segment stenosis or IVC webs. Intrahepatic IVC obstruction is most commonly due to compression from the enlarged caudate lobe. Chronic thrombosis of the IVC can evolve into calcification.[22]

Webs are visualized as dome shaped thin linear filling defects on contrast venography and MR angiography. On real-time imaging they appear as hyperreflective linear foci best seen in deep inspiration **(Figs. 6A to D)**. Whether these webs represent congenital lesions or they are the result of thrombotic process is an issue which remains disputed.[25] It seems quite plausible to assume that both IVC web and segmental stenosis actually represent the spectrum of same pathological process, i.e. thrombosis.

On real-time ultrasound, short segment stenosis is seen as an area of narrowing and the caliber of IVC is dilated proximal to the obstruction with loss of phasic variation with respiration **(Figs. 7A and B)**. Long segment narrowing of the IVC due to caudate lobe enlargement is well depicted. When the IVC obstruction is due to tumor thrombi, extension of the tumor into the IVC is well demonstrated. However, ultrasound is unable to determine the length of stenosis, webs can be missed and the hemodynamic significance of IVC narrowing cannot be assessed. Possibility of poor study due to bowel gas is also a limiting factor.

Color Doppler US combined with real-time imaging is superior to grayscale imaging as it provides better assessment of IVC impairment by adding flow information. The normal flow pattern of IVC is a triphasic waveform. The flow abnormality can be seen in the form of either absent (IVC occlusion), reversed or uniphasic flow (stenosis).[12,26] Turbulent flow may be seen at the site of short segment stenosis.[26,27]

The IVC venography has been considered the gold standard for evaluation of inferior vena cava. However, in patients of BCS, it has certain limitations particularly for evaluation of hepatic veins. Diagnosis of hepatic vein occlusion is inferred when there is failure to cannulate the hepatic veins selectively at the time of catheterization. Thus, over diagnosis of hepatic vein thrombosis may result even when failure of cannulation is due to technical failure. The other limitations of IVC graphy include nonvisualization of IVC distal to obstruction due to diversion of contrast into the collaterals. Thus, in case of suprahepatic obstruction due to web/membrane visualization of IVC above and below the lesion may require double catheter study. Lastly the intrahepatic collaterals which form important parameters for diagnosis of chronic BCS are not detected with IVC graphy.

Recently MR venography has shown a great potential by overcoming many of the limitations of IVC venography. MR venography accurately depicts the site and cause of IVC obstruction with clear delineation of IVC both above and below the obstruction **(Fig. 8)**.[17,20] MR is excellent for detection of both intra- and extrahepatic collaterals, portal vein obstruction and detection of tumor thrombi within the IVC. Incidence of portal vein thrombosis in BCS is 5–20%.[26,27]

Five Types of Collateral Pathways Develop in Budd-Chiari Syndrome[28]

1. Left renal-hemiazygous pathways
2. Vertebrolumbar azygous pathways
3. Intrahepatic collaterals
4. Superficial abdominal wall collaterals
5. Inferior phrenic-pericardiophrenic collaterals.

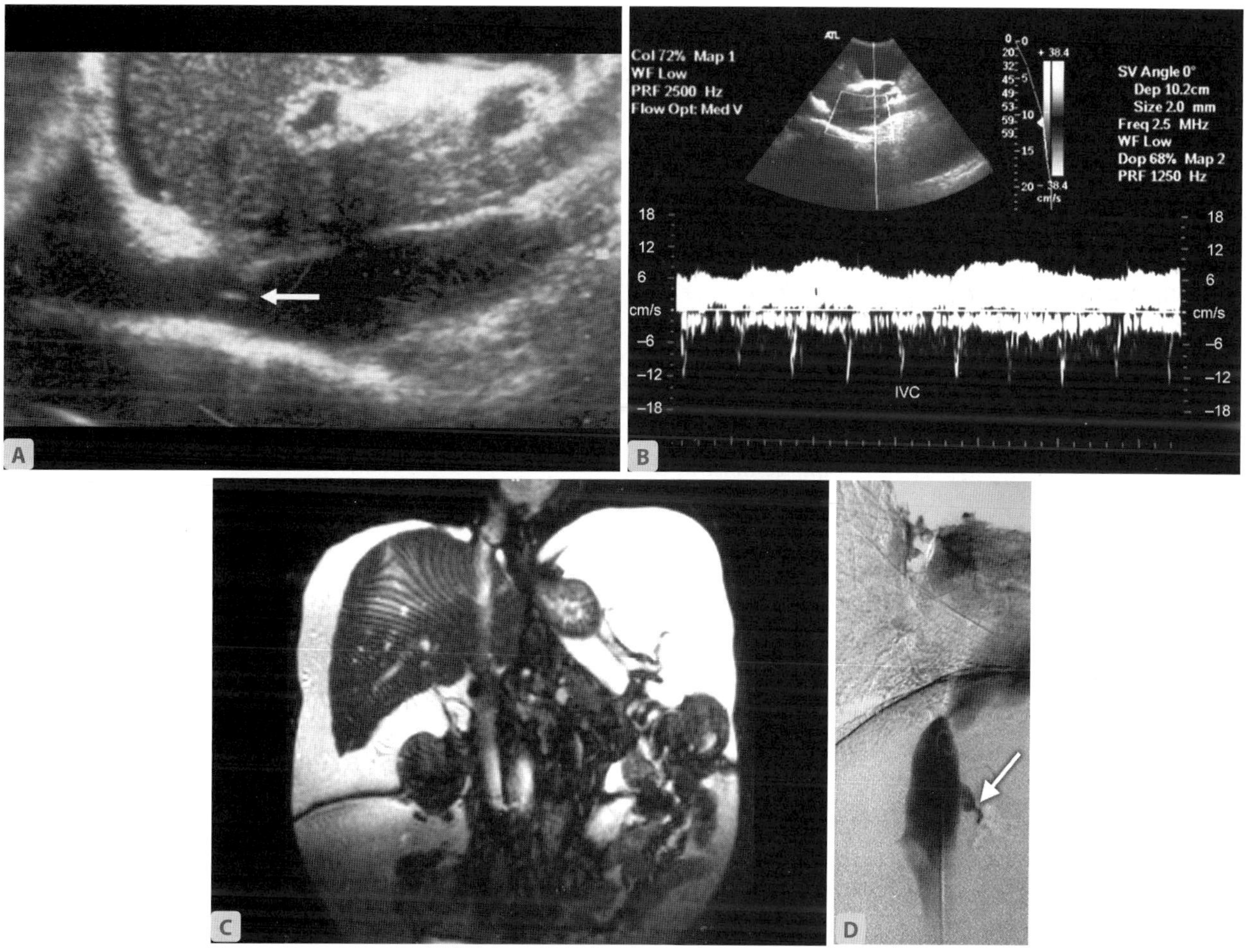

FIGS. 6A TO D: A 60-year-old male presenting with abdominal distention. Sagittal US showing echogenic linear area in IVC proximal to cavoatrial junction suggestive of a web in IVC (arrow) (A). There is uniphasic flow with fluttering seen in the IVC (B). Coronal FLASH flow sensitive MR image shows a hypointense linear signal in the IVC proximal to cavoatrial junction suggestive of a web in the suprahepatic portion (C). IVC graphy lateral view shows dome-shaped obstruction of suprahepatic IVC with a jet of blood flowing into right atrium confirming the presence of web. There is filling up of an intrahepatic collateral (arrow) (D).

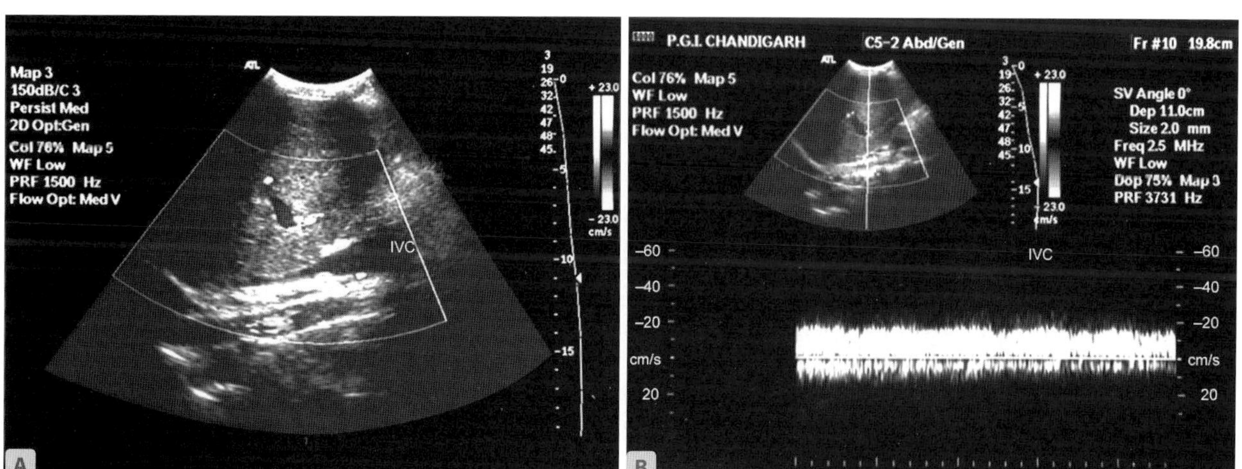

FIGS. 7A AND B: Dopplers show a smooth long segment narrowing in the intrahepatic portion of IVC with loss of the normal phasic variation and a uniphasic flow pattern.

Intrahepatic collaterals have been noted in 80–93% cases of BCS[12,27,29] and are seen as comma shaped bridging veno-venous collaterals which reveal flat waveform on color Doppler ultrasound.

ASSESSMENT OF LIVER PARENCHYMA IN BUDD-CHIARI SYNDROME

As a result of hepatic venous or IVC obstruction there is ischemic damage to the liver cells resulting in severe congestion, centrilobular necrosis followed by fibrosis and cirrhosis. In acute BCS, congestion predominates whereas patients of chronic BCS are more likely to develop cirrhosis and regenerative nodules.[24] Since the obstruction of the hepatic veins is usually asynchronous, liver biopsy may show areas of congestion and hyperplastic enlargement in the recently affected areas and fibrosis with atrophy in the older affected segments. As the distribution of the disease in the liver is inhomogeneous liver biopsy may even be normal.[30]

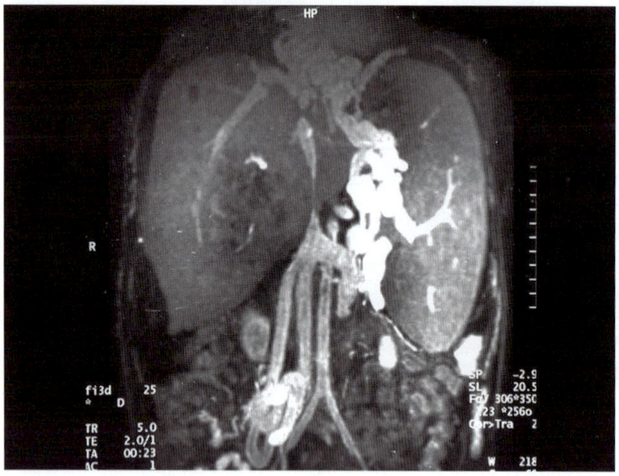

FIG. 8: Coronal contrast-enhanced MR venography shows long segment narrowing of IVC in intrahepatic portion with filling defect proximal to cavoatrial junction. There are multiple collaterals in the retroperitoneum and at the splenic hilum.

Development of regenerative nodules in BCS is known to occur in response to focal loss of portal perfusion and hyper arterialization in areas with preserved hepatic venous outflow.[22] Incidence of nodules greater than 5 mm have been seen on histology in 40–80% of patients.[27,31] Although the question of possible malignant transformation of the large regenerative nodule remains unsettled, it is generally believed that HCC is extremely rare in patients presenting with BCS due to hepatic venous obstruction alone. However, it may be co-existent in patients of BCS due to IVC obstruction particularly MOVC.[24] The obstruction may make the hepatocytes more susceptible to the action of environment carcinogens. HCC in BCS accounts for 0.7% of all cases of hepatocelluar carcinoma.[32] Differentiation of HCC from regenerative nodules is important. US and conventional CT are both poor modalities for detection of these nodules. On the other hand MRI and biphasic CT have been reported to be more reliable.[7,33,34]

Benign regenerative nodules which are hyperintense on T1WI and iso- to hypointense on T2WI are likely to be benign **(Figs. 9A and B)** compared to HCC nodules which are hypointense on T1WI and hyperintense on T2WI **(Figs. 10A and B)**. Multiple (>10) and small (<4 cm) lesions are suggestive of benignity.[7] On biphasic CT large regenerative nodules are markedly and homogeneously hyperattenuating on arterial phase images and remain slightly hyperattenuating on portal venous phase images.[22,34] On histopathology these nodules have normal or hyperplastic hepatocytes, arteries extending radially from the center of the nodule and a central scar in the larger nodules.[31,35] The imaging characteristics of this scar may be similar to those of the scar found in focal nodular hyperplasia on dynamic imaging.[31]

Liver biopsy has been used in the past to differentiate acute from subacute and chronic BCS. A liver biopsy is required only if radiological imaging is inconclusive.[36] Differentiation is important for deciding the plan of treatment. Acute BCS

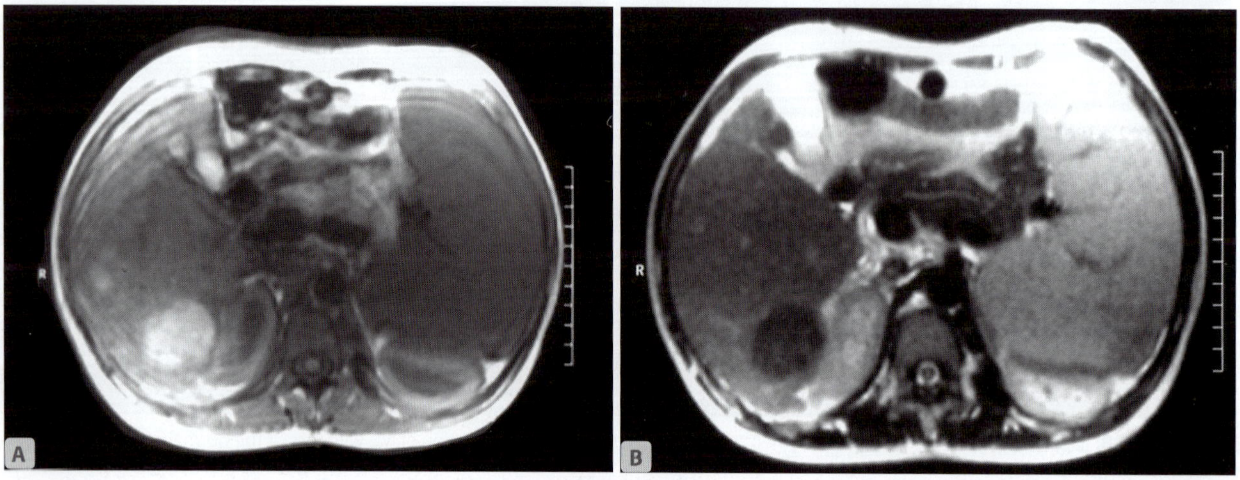

FIGS. 9A AND B: (A) Axial T1W FLASH image shows single large hyperintense nodule and multiple small hyperintense nodules of varying sizes in the liver. The hyperintensity of the nodules on T1WI is suggestive of their benign nature; (B) Axial T2W HASTE image at the same level depicts the hypointense signal of the large nodule. Smaller lesions are not seen, probably due to being isointense to the liver parenchyma.

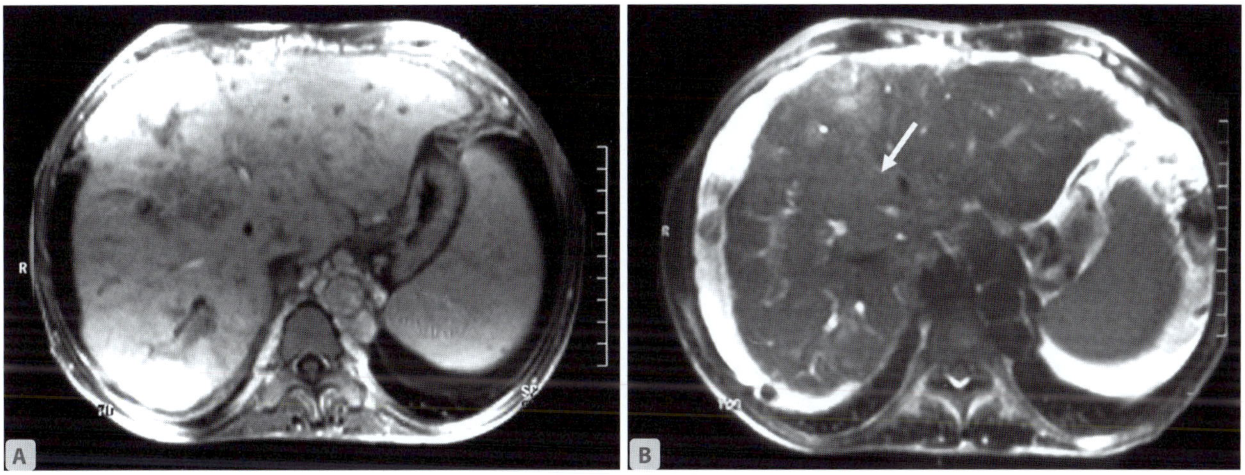

FIGS. 10A AND B: Axial T1W FLASH MR image at the level of hepatic veins shows irregular outline of liver with multiple ill-defined hypointense focal lesions in the liver. Ascites is seen (A); Axial T2W HASTE image at the same level shows that the lesions are isointense to hyperintense in signal (arrow). FNAC proved these lesions to be HCC (B).

may be treated by infusion of thrombolytic substances at the site of block followed by stenting whereas, chronic BCS requires the creation of a shunt between the hepatic veins and portal vein by transjugular intrahepatic portosystemic shunt procedure. MRI and dynamic CT have shown potential to determine the chronicity of the hepatic changes.[17,37,38]

A study by Noone et al.[17] has described the role of MRI in differentiation of acute, subacute and chronic BCS. In their experience in acute BCS there is decreased signal intensity on T1WI and heterogeneously increased signal intensity on T2WI peripherally with decreased enhancement of peripheral liver after gadolinium administration **(Figs. 11A to C)**. These changes were attributed to acutely increased tissue pressures and edema in the peripheral portions of the liver because of hepatic venous obstruction thus causing diminished inflow of blood. As the duration of disease increases there is reversal of flow in the portal vein and development of small collaterals permitting egress of blood. Thus in subacute BCS the signal characteristics on T1 and T2-weighted images are similar to those observed in patients with acute disease, however, periphery shows marked heterogeneous enhancement unlike to that seen in acute BCS. In chronic BCS there is no parenchymal edema and this stage is characterized by changes of fibrosis. Thus, there is no differential signal intensity and enhancement between peripheral and central liver. Using that criteria, in a study conducted at our institute 13 out of 20 cases of chronic BCS were correctly diagnosed with MRI **(Figs. 12A and B)**.[39]

Abnormal patterns of parenchymal enhancement have also been reported on triphasic helical CT in different stages of BCS in a study by Camera et al.[38] They found abnormal enhancement of the caudate lobe in the arterial phase, the 'fan shaped pattern', in all cases of acute BCS. Later a 'flip-flop' pattern develops in which the central liver becomes hypodense compared to the peripheral liver. On the other hand 'patchy pattern' of enhancement was seen in patients of subacute and chronic BCS.

In conclusion, ultrasound with color flow Doppler imaging is the modality of choice for initial diagnosis of BCS. When combined with MR and MRA, need for diagnostic IVC venography can be obviated which can be reserved for patients where surgical or radiological intervention is being contemplated. The role of dynamic helical CT in BCS also appears promising.

MANAGEMENT OF BUDD-CHIARI SYNDROME

The treatment modality for BCS is determined by the status of hepatocyte necrosis and the stage of the disease. Nonsurgical management of BCS such as radiological intervention alone or in combination with medical management is indicated in patients, where biopsy shows no evidence of hepatocyte necrosis.

The medical management includes treatment for ascites by diuretics or paracentesis and control of gastrointestinal bleeding with balloon tamponade or sclerotherapy. Systemic thrombolytic therapy has been shown to have varying outcome. Treatment with heparin alone has been followed by recanalization of thrombosed hepatic veins and of thrombosed portal vein when associated with thrombosed hepatic veins. Patients with fulminant disease who are not responding to systemic thrombolysis may benefit from local direct pharmacological and mechanical thrombolysis.[40]

Treatment of BCS by radiological intervention was first described in 1974 by Eguchi et al. who reported the successful balloon membranotomy for obstruction of the inferior vena cava.[41] The aim of the radiological interventions is the restoration of hepatic blood outflow by means of repermeation of the obstructed hepatic veins or IVC or by portosystemic shunting. The methods include balloon angioplasty, stent insertion and TIPS (transjugular intrahepatic portosystemic

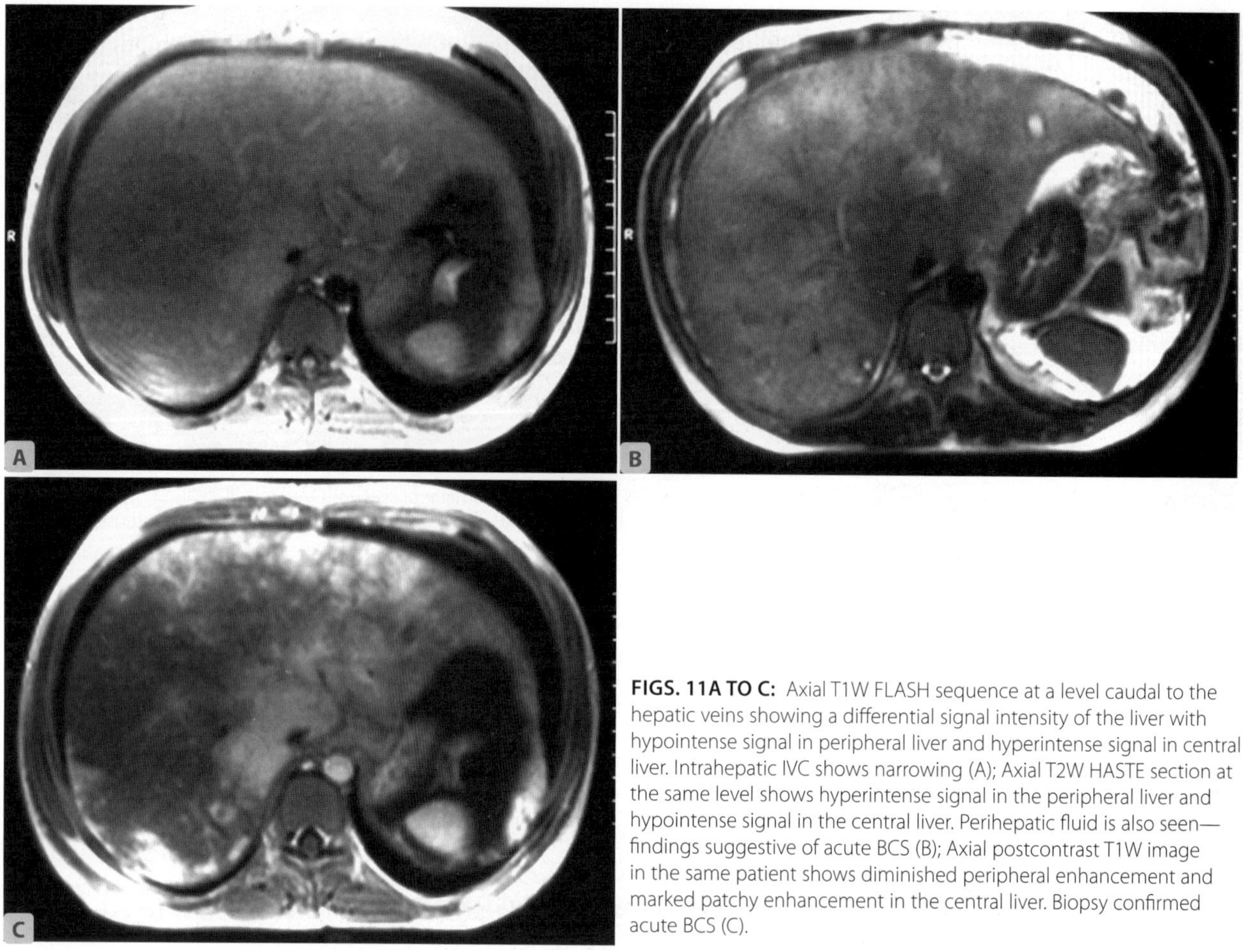

FIGS. 11A TO C: Axial T1W FLASH sequence at a level caudal to the hepatic veins showing a differential signal intensity of the liver with hypointense signal in peripheral liver and hyperintense signal in central liver. Intrahepatic IVC shows narrowing (A); Axial T2W HASTE section at the same level shows hyperintense signal in the peripheral liver and hypointense signal in the central liver. Perihepatic fluid is also seen—findings suggestive of acute BCS (B); Axial postcontrast T1W image in the same patient shows diminished peripheral enhancement and marked patchy enhancement in the central liver. Biopsy confirmed acute BCS (C).

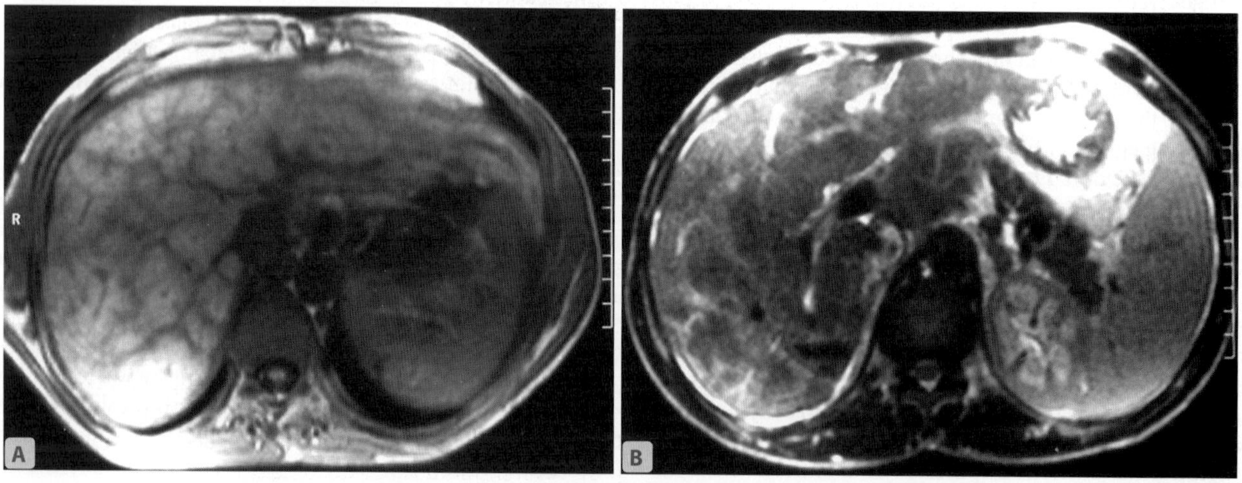

FIGS. 12A AND B: Axial T1W FLASH and T2W HASTE MR images show uniformly heterogeneous signal intensity of the liver. There is no differential SI of the peripheral or central liver seen. Hepatic veins are not visualized—a case of chronic BCS due to hepatic vein thrombosis and IVC stenosis.

shunt). IVC interventions should preferably be done using the femoral route as negotiation across narrowed segments is easier when this route is used. The abnormal segment or web is crossed using a guide wire and then serial dilatation is done with a balloon catheter **(Figs. 13A to D)**. Stenting is rarely required due to the large lumen of the IVC. Balloon angioplasty is also used for short length stenosis of the hepatic veins. This results in immediate relief of the obstruction. However, the recurrence following this procedure is common. Griffith, et al.[42] in their study of 18 patients found that restenosis occurred in all patients treated with angioplasty when followed for longer than 10 months. The use of wall stents has

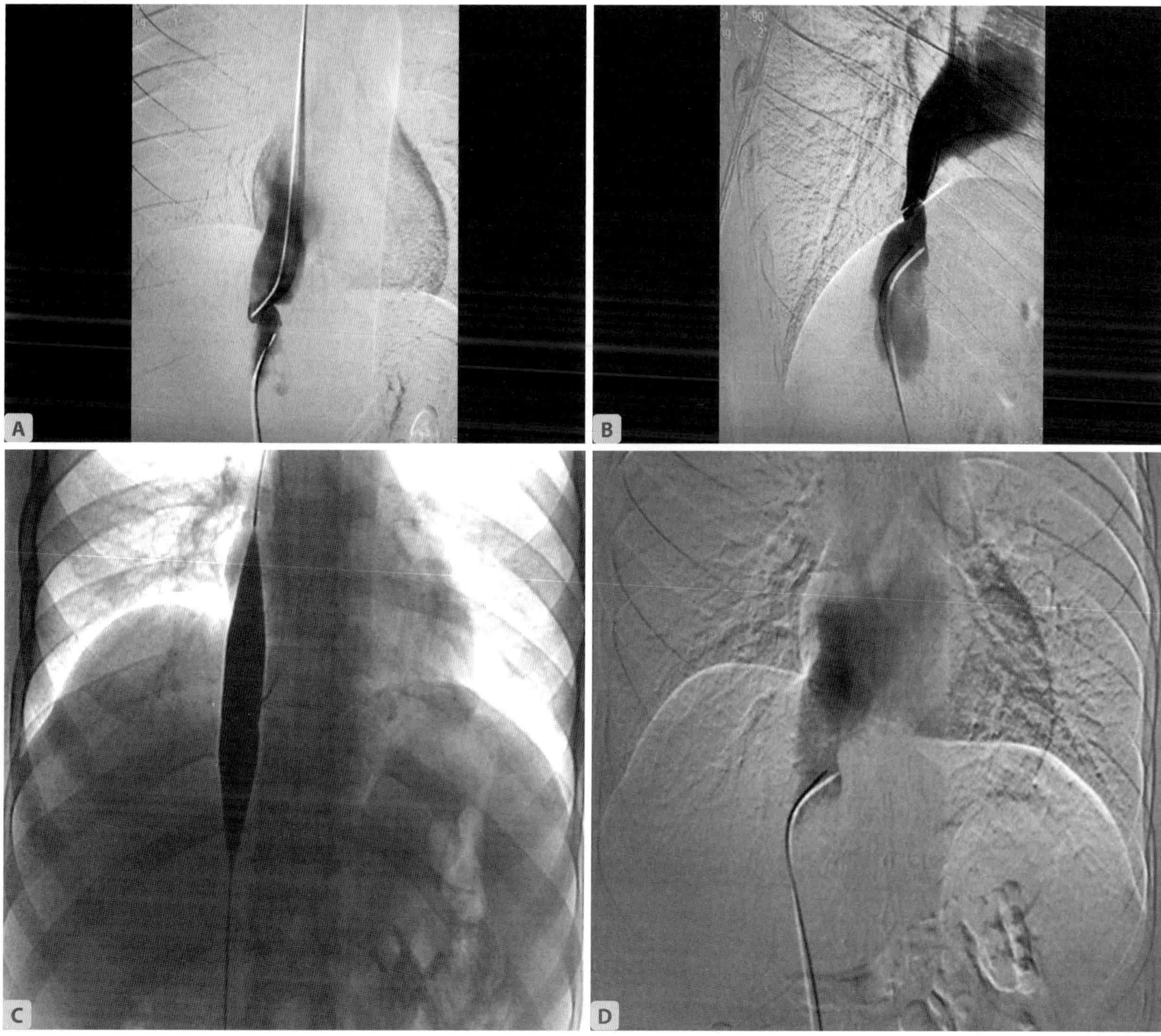

FIGS. 13A TO D: IVC venography in AP (A) and lateral (B) views with contrast injection from both the jugular and femoral access catheters showing a short segment stenosis of the IVC; The stenosis was crossed with a guidewire from the femoral access. Subsequently a balloon catheter was used for dilatation of the narrowing (C); Contrast injection through the femoral catheter shows no residual stenosis (D).

resulted in better long-term patency rates of the order of 80–90% over a one year follow-up period **(Figs. 14A to F)**.[27,43,44] Baijjal, et al.[45] performed percutaneous angioplasty followed by primary stent placement in their study of 9 patients with IVC obstruction. There was residual stenosis of about 9–40% after the procedure. Revascularization was successful in all patients and the IVC remained patent during the follow-up period (3–31 months).

Surgical management of BCS is indicated in patients with features of congestion, hepatocyte necrosis and fibrosis on liver biopsy. Decompressive surgical shunts like portocaval and mesocaval shunts relieve the sinusoidal congestion and thus halt the ongoing hepatocyte necrosis. The rationale for the side to side portocaval shunts is to transform the portal vein into an outflow tract for the hepatic circulation. A portocaval or mesocaval shunt is successful if the portal vein minus infrahepatic IVC pressure is >10 mm Hg. If this pressure gradient is <10 mm Hg, these infrahepatic surgical shunts should not be done.[21] These shunts are associated with a 25% mortality rate and shunt thrombosis which may occur in 10–25% of patients. Stenosis of the shunt is a late complication and is amenable for percutaneous balloon dilatation with or without stenting **(Figs. 15A to C)**. In patients who have intrahepatic IVC abnormality these classical infrahepatic portocaval shunts do not work unless a stent is inserted in the IVC to correct the pressure gradient. Such patients require a suprahepatic shunt, i.e. mesoatrial shunt between the SMV and the right atrium. The criteria for the mesoatrial shunt are reduction of IVC diameter more than 75% or a caval atrial gradient exceeding 20 mm Hg.[46] These shunts are, however, associated with poorer results and a higher incidence of shunt thrombosis.

Successful treatment of BCS with TIPS was described in 1993 by Peltzer et al. and Ochs et al.[47,48] This involves the

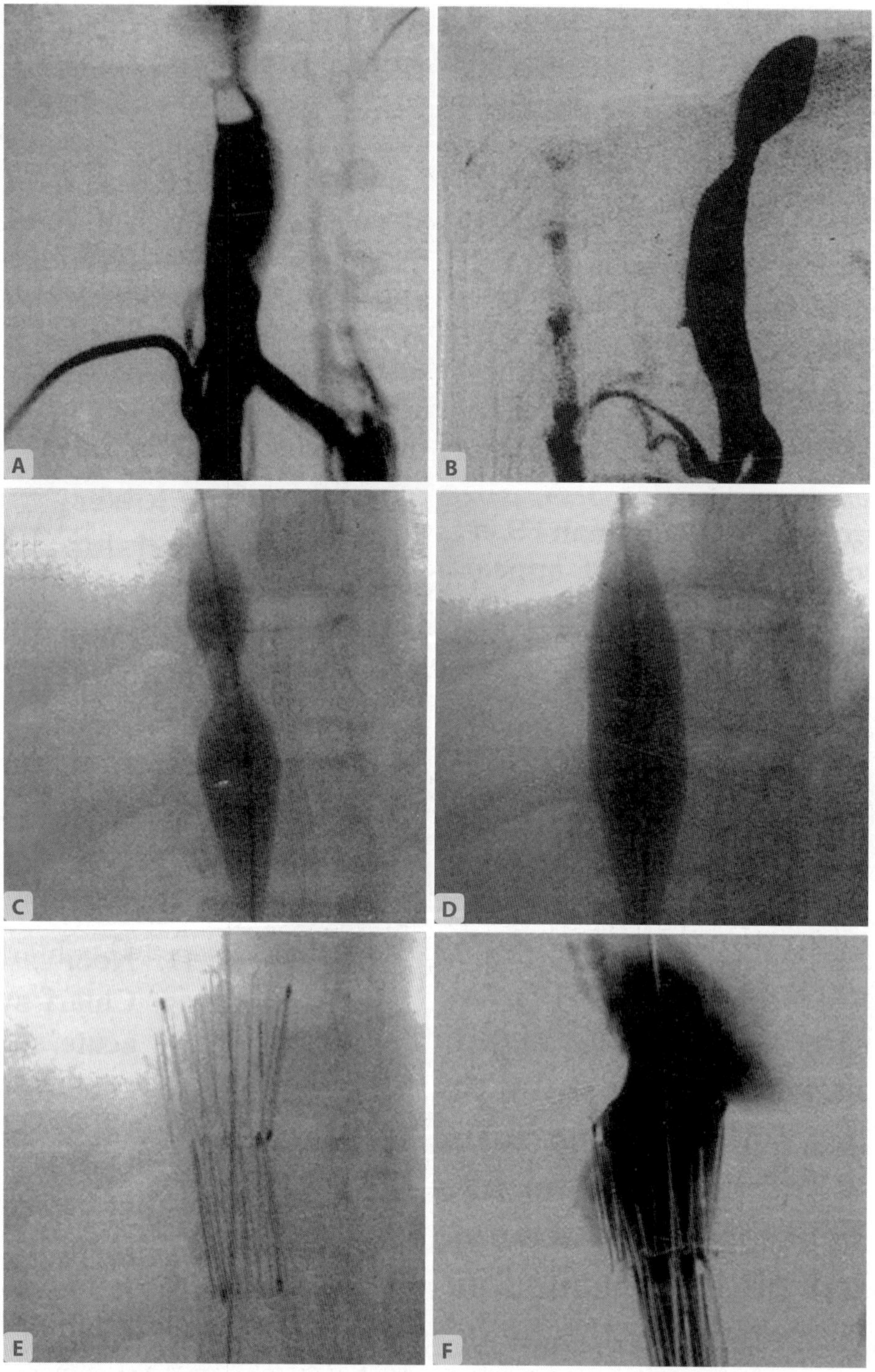

FIGS. 14A TO F: Percutaneous stent placement in a patient with short segment stenosis of intrahepatic IVC. IVC graphy images in AP (A) and lateral (B) views show the short segment narrowing of the intrahepatic IVC and filling up of multiple paravertebral collaterals. The stenosed segment was predilated with a balloon (C and D). This was followed by stent placement across the stenosis (E and F). Check angiogram shows free flow of contrast across the IVC into the right atrium.

placement of an intrahepatic shunt connecting a hepatic vein stump through the liver to a branch of the portal vein **(Figs. 16A to D)**. The shunt can also be created between the suprahepatic IVC and the portal vein when no hepatic vein stump is available. The transcaval approach is also technically more feasible in BCS. This is because the liver is enlarged and the intrahepatic IVC is surrounded by liver parenchyma providing stability for the transcaval direct intrahepatic portosystemic shunt (DIPS). These shunts may be created using a transjugular approach but a combined percutaneous and transhepatic approach may also be required **(Figs. 17A to E)**. In BCS the liver parenchyma is

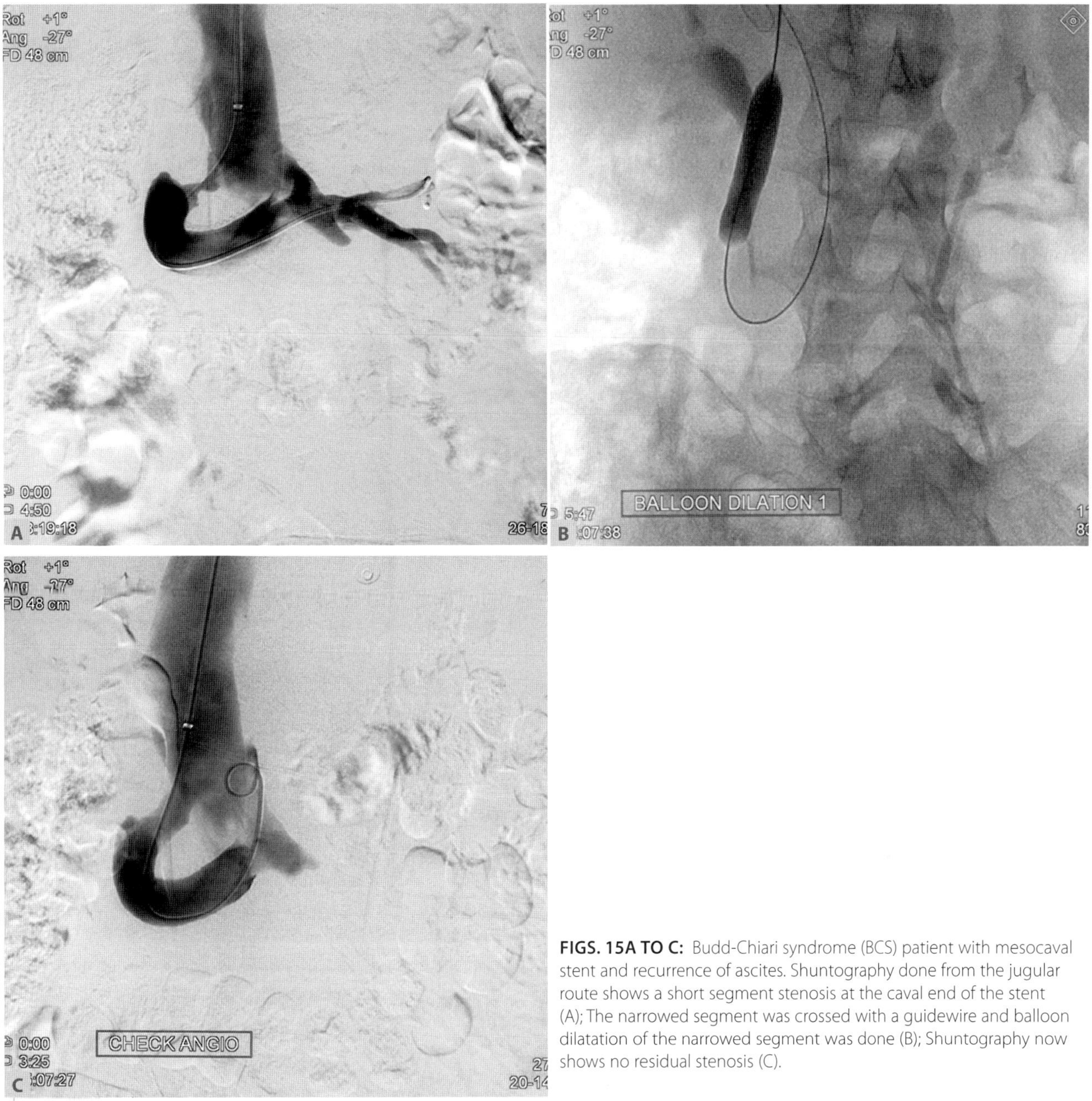

FIGS. 15A TO C: Budd-Chiari syndrome (BCS) patient with mesocaval stent and recurrence of ascites. Shuntography done from the jugular route shows a short segment stenosis at the caval end of the stent (A); The narrowed segment was crossed with a guidewire and balloon dilatation of the narrowed segment was done (B); Shuntography now shows no residual stenosis (C).

also relatively soft unlike that in other causes of cirrhosis.[49] The primary patency rate of these shunts has also increased with the use of polytetrafluoroethylene (PTFE) covered stents. The advantages of TIPS are its minimal invasiveness and the lower mortality rate as compared with surgical shunting. In addition, intrahepatic caval stenosis can also be bypassed by using TIPS which is not possible with the surgical shunts. This essentially functions as a portoatrial shunt. The most frequent complication of TIPS is hepatic encephalopathy which can occur in up to 30% of patients but can be treated medically. Other complications include stenosis or occlusion requiring revision in about 70% of cases by 6 months, intraperitoneal bleed, liver failure and subcapsular hematomas. The 6- and 12-month patency rates were 100% and 85.7% respectively for stent graft compared with 16.7% and 0% for bare stents.[49] Surgical options are now usually reserved for patients with failed radiological interventions. Some studies have suggested that an early use of TIPS in selected cases may have a survival advantage.[50,51] However, a study from India found that angioplasty and not TIPS, is of utility to the majority of BCS patients. The authors also reported that Child class and response to interventional treatment are important predictors of survival in BCS patients.[52]

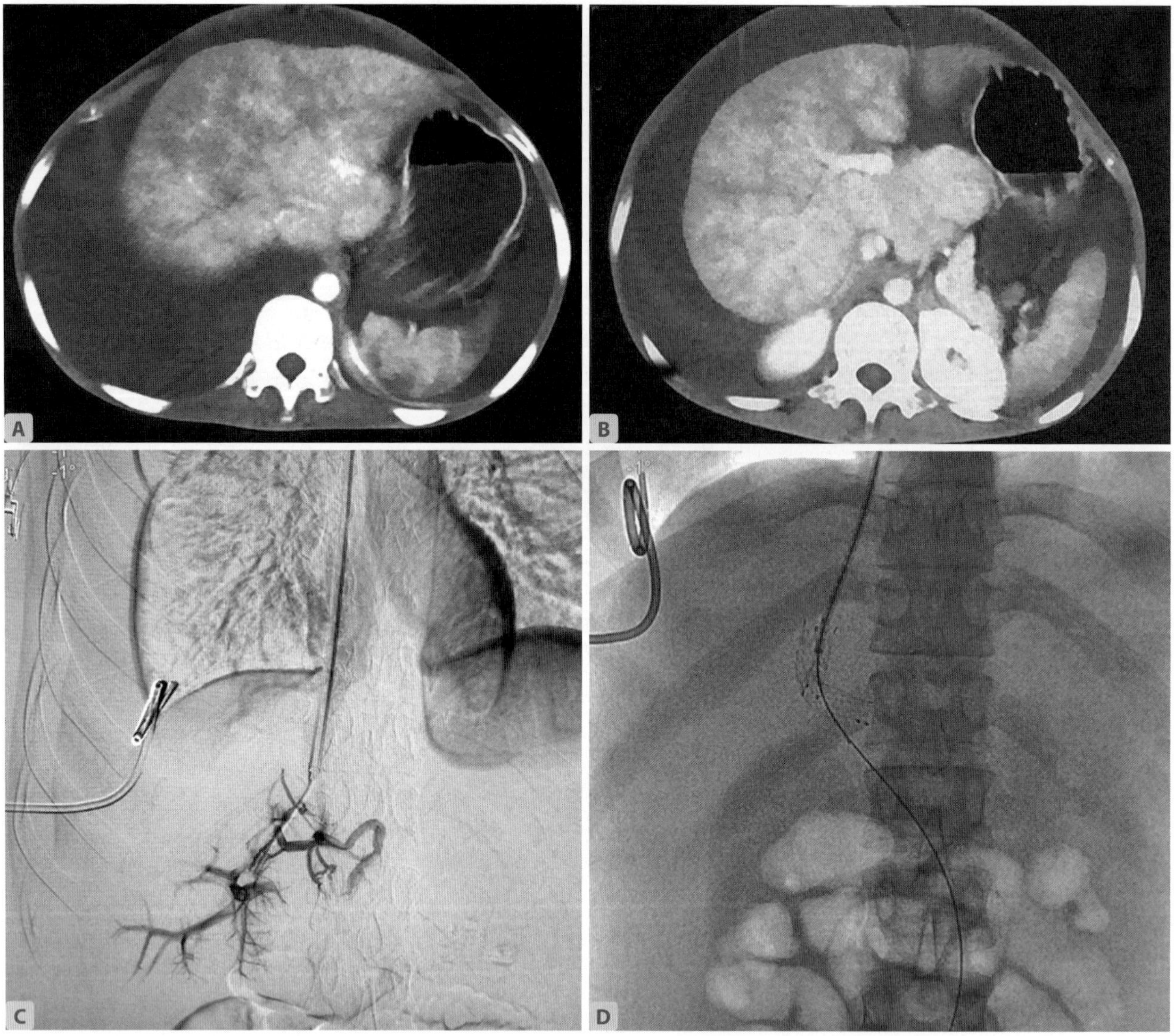

FIGS. 16A TO D: Contrast-enhanced CT scan showing mosaic attenuation of liver parenchyma with attenuated hepatic veins and normal caliber portal vein (A and B); there is gross ascites and right pleural effusion. Using the transjugular approach the hepatic vein stump was cannulated with a sheath. A puncture needle was advanced through the sheath and the liver parenchyma into the right branch of portal vein (C); Subsequently a calibrated pigtail catheter was advanced in the track. This was followed by balloon dilatation of the track. The stent was then placed in the track over an exchange guidewire (D).

It is imperative after any radiological intervention in BCS to continue long-term anticoagulant therapy in order to maintain the INR (international normalized ratio) around 2.5.[40,53] It is also important to have a regular three monthly follow-up in the first year using color Doppler. Subsequently the patients may be kept on a six monthly follow-up regimen.

The first liver transplant for BCS was performed in 1974. Liver transplantation is indicated for patients with fulminant hepatic failure, those who deteriorate after shunt procedure and in cirrhotics with end stage disease. In fact orthotopic liver transplantation is considered the only curative treatment for BCS.[43] Significant fibrosis and cirrhosis on liver biopsy with poor hepatocellular reserve can only be managed by transplantation. It is a useful option in patients with a hereditary thrombophilia state such as protein C, protein S, and antithrombin III deficiency which can be corrected with liver replacement. Ten-year survival rates up to 75% have been reported after liver transplantation.[27,54]

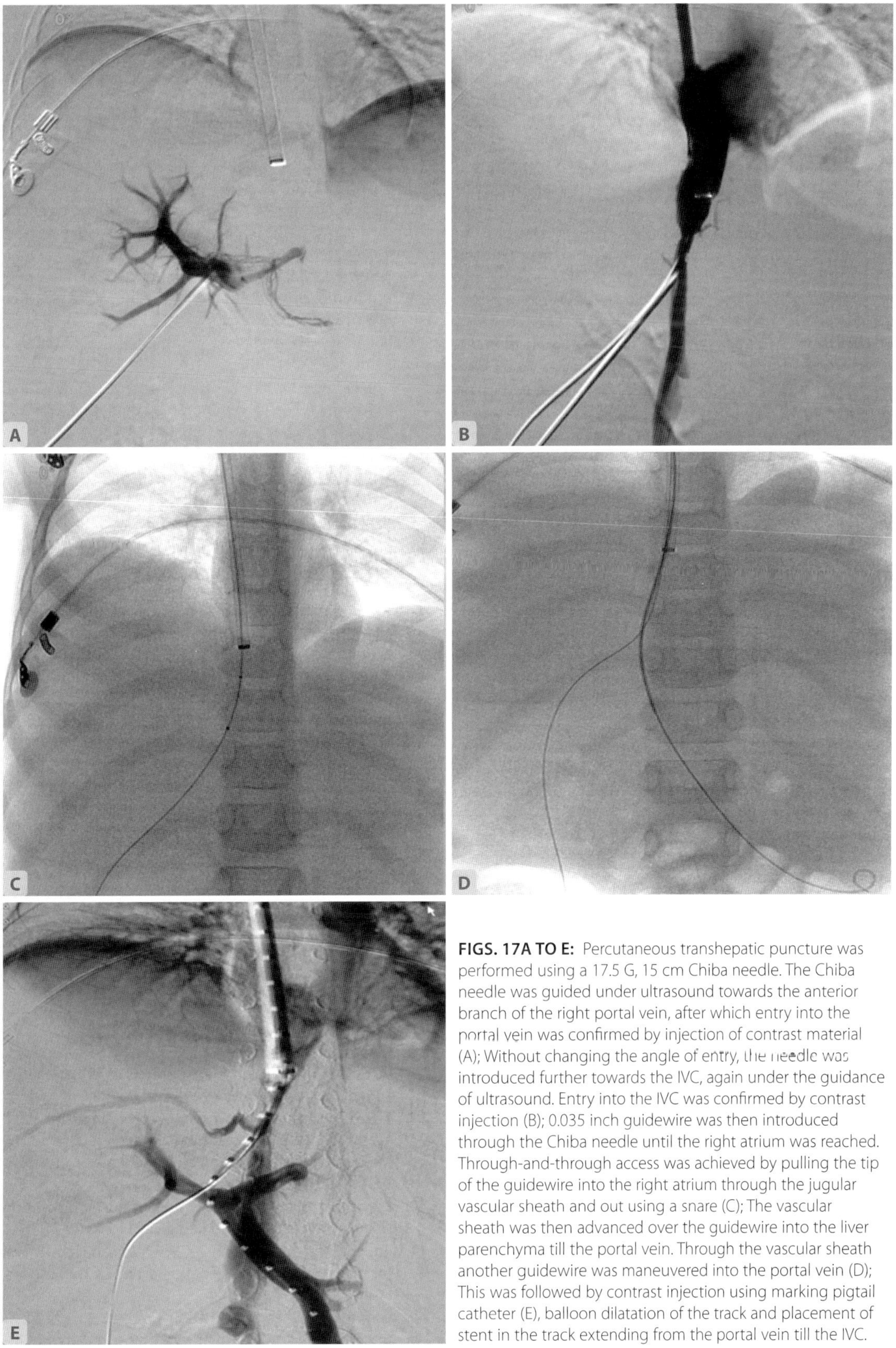

FIGS. 17A TO E: Percutaneous transhepatic puncture was performed using a 17.5 G, 15 cm Chiba needle. The Chiba needle was guided under ultrasound towards the anterior branch of the right portal vein, after which entry into the portal vein was confirmed by injection of contrast material (A); Without changing the angle of entry, the needle was introduced further towards the IVC, again under the guidance of ultrasound. Entry into the IVC was confirmed by contrast injection (B); 0.035 inch guidewire was then introduced through the Chiba needle until the right atrium was reached. Through-and-through access was achieved by pulling the tip of the guidewire into the right atrium through the jugular vascular sheath and out using a snare (C); The vascular sheath was then advanced over the guidewire into the liver parenchyma till the portal vein. Through the vascular sheath another guidewire was maneuvered into the portal vein (D); This was followed by contrast injection using marking pigtail catheter (E), balloon dilatation of the track and placement of stent in the track extending from the portal vein till the IVC.

REFERENCES

1. Ferral H, Behrens G, Lopera J. Budd-Chiari syndrome. AJR. 2012;199;737-45.
2. Patil P, Deshmukh H, Popat B, et al. Spectrum of imaging in Budd-Chiari syndrome. J Med Imaging Radiat Oncol. 2012;56:75-83.
3. Mulholland JP, Fong SM, Kafaghi FA, et al. Budd-Chiari syndrome: Diagnosis with ultrasound and nuclear medicine calcium colloid liver scan following nondiagnostic contrast CT scan. Australas Radiol. 1997;41:53-6.
4. Sharma V, Aggarwal A, Singla R, et al. Giant Hemangioma causing Budd-Chiari syndrome. Journal of Clinical and Experimental Hepatology. 2014;4:380-1.
5. Mahmoud A, Elias E. Advances in hepatology—new approaches to the Budd-Chiari syndrome. J Gastroenterol Hepatol. 1996;11:1121-3.
6. Eapen CE, Mammen T, Moses V, et al. Changing profile of Budd-Chiari syndrome in India. Indian J Gastroenterol. 2007;26:77-81.
7. Vilgrain V, Lewin M, Vons C, et al. Hepatic nodules in Budd-Chiari syndrome: imaging features. Radiology. 1999;210:443-50.
8. Arora A, Sharma MP. Recent trends in the diagnosis and treatment of Budd-Chiari syndrome. J Assoc Physicians India. 1992;40:533-6.
9. Floyd JL. The radiographic gamut of Budd-Chiari syndrome. Am J Gastroenterol. 1981;76:381-7.
10. Menu Y, Alision D, Lorphelin JM, et al. Budd-Chiari syndrome: US evaluation. Radiology. 1985;157:761-4.
11. Powell-Jackson PR, Karani J, Ede RJ, et al. Ultrasound scanning and 99mTc sulphur colloid scintigraphy in diagnosis of Budd-Chiari syndrome. Gut. 1986;27:1502-6.
12. Chawla Y, Kumar S, Dhiman RK, et al. Various imaging diagnostics in Budd-Chiari syndrome, liver cirrhosis and carcinoma-Duplex Doppler sonography in patients with Budd-Chiari syndrome. J Gastroenterol Hepatol. 1999;14:904-7.
13. Makuuchi M, Hasegewa H, Yamazaki S, et al. Primary Budd-Chiari syndrome: ultrasonic demonstration. Radiology. 1984;152:775-9.
14. Musa Aydini, Yusuf Bayraktar. Budd-Chiari syndrome: etiology, pathogenesis and diagnosis. World J Gastroenterol. 2007;13(19):2693-6.
15. Lupescu IG, Dobromir C, Popa GA, et al. Spiral computed tomography and magnetic resonance angiography evaluation in Budd-Chiari syndrome. J Gastrointestin Liver Dis. 2008;17:223-6.
16. Bargallo X, Gilabert R, Nicolau C, et al. Sonography of the caudate vein: value in diagnosing Budd-Chiari syndrome. Am J Roentgenol. 2003;181:1641-5.
17. Noone TC, Semelka RC, Siegelman ES, et al. Budd-Chiari syndrome: spectrum of appearances of acute, subacute and chronic disease with magnetic resonance imaging. J Magn Reson Imaging. 2000;11:44-50.
18. XU K, Ren K, Chen Y, et al. Application and evaluation of non-invasive examination for Budd-Chiari syndrome. Chinese Medical Journal. 2007;120:91-4.
19. Ohta M, Hashizume M, Tomikawa M, et al. Analysis of hepatic vein waveform by Doppler ultrasonography in 100 patients with portal hypertension. Am J Gastroenterol. 1995;89:170-5.
20. Kane R, Eustace S. Diagnosis of Budd-Chiari syndrome: comparison between sonography and MR angiography. Radiology. 1995;195:117-21.
21. Kamath PS. Budd-Chiari syndrome: Radiologic findings. Liver Transplantation. 2006;12:S21-2.
22. Brancatelli G, Vilgrain V, Federle MP, et al. Budd-Chiari syndrome: spectrum of imaging findings. Am J Roentgenol. 2007;188: W168-76.
23. Datta DV, Saha S, Singh SA, et al. Chronic Budd-Chiari syndrome due to obstruction of the intrahepatic portion of the inferior vena cava. Gut. 1972;13:372-8.
24. Dilawari JB, Bambery P, Chawla Y, et al. Hepatic outflow obstruction (Budd-Chiari syndrome)—Experience with 177 patients and a review of the literature. Medicine (Baltimore). 1984;73:21-36.
25. Kage M, Arakawa M, Kojiro M, et al. Histopathology of membranous obstruction of the inferior vena cava in the Budd-Chiari syndrome. Gastroenterology. 1992;102:2081-90.
26. Bolondi L, Gaiani S, Li Bassi S, et al. Diagnosis of Budd-Chiari syndrome by pulsed Doppler ultrasound. Gastroenterology. 1991;100:1324-31.
27. Valla DC. Hepatic vein thrombosis (Budd-Chiari syndrome). Semin Liver Dis. 2002;22:5-14.
28. Cho OK, Koo JH, Kim YS, et al. Collateral pathways in Budd-Chiari syndrome. CT and venographic correlation. Am J Roentgenol. 1996;167:1163-7.
29. Clain D, Freston J, Kreel L, et al. Clinical diagnosis of Budd-Chiari syndrome. A report of six cases. Am J Med. 1967;43:544-54.
30. Janssen HL, Garcia-Pagan JC, Elias E, et al. Budd-Chiari syndrome: review by an expert panel. J Hepatol. 2003;38:364-71.
31. Maetani Y, Itoh K, Egawa H, et al. Benign hepatic nodules in Budd-Chiari syndrome. Radiologic-pathologic correlation with emphasis on the central scar. Am J Roentgenol. 2002;178:869-75.
32. Tanju S, Erden A, Ceyhan K, et al. Contrast-enhanced MR angiography of benign regenerative nodules following TIPS shunt procedure in Budd-Chiari syndrome. Turk J Gastroenterol. 2004;15:173-7.
33. Brancatelli G, Federle MP, Grazioli L, et al. Benign regenerative nodules in Budd-Chiari syndrome and other vascular disorders of the liver: radiologic-pathologic and clinical correlation. Radiographics. 2002;22:847-62.
34. Brancatelli G, Federle MP, Grazioli L, et al. Large regenerative nodules in Budd-Chiari syndrome and other vascular disorders of the liver: CT and MR imaging findings with clinicopatholgic correlation. Am J Roentgenol. 2002;178:77-883.
35. Cazals-Hatem D, Vilgrain V, Genin P, et al. Arterial and portal circulation and parenchymal changes in Budd- Chiari syndrome: a study in 17 explanted livers. Hepatology. 2003;37:510-9.
36. Valla DC. Prognosis in Budd-Chiari syndrome after reestablishing hepatic venous drainage. Gut. 2006;55:761-3.
37. Artia T, Matsunaga N, Kobayashi H. Budd-Chiari syndrome: Peripheral abnormal intensity of the liver on magnetic resonance imaging. Clin Radiol. 2000;55:640-2.
38. Camera L, Mainenti PP, Di Giacomo A, et al. Triphasic helical CT in Budd-Chiari syndrome: patterns of enhancement in acute, subacute and chronic disease. Clin Radiol. 2006;61:331-7.
39. Kalra N, Virmani V, Singh P, et al. Imaging of Budd-Chiari syndrome (electronic exhibit presented at the 109th Annual Meeting of the American Roentgen Ray Society, 2009 at Boston, USA).
40. Mukund A, Gamangatti S. Imaging and interventions in Budd-Chiari syndrome. World J Radiol. 2011;28:169-77.
41. Eguchi S, Takeuchi Y, Asano K. Successful balloon membranotomy for obstruction of the hepatic portion of the inferior vena cava. Surgery. 1974;76:837-40.
42. Griffith JF, Mahmoud AEA, Cooper S, et al. Radiological intervention in Budd-Chiari syndrome: techniques and outcome in 18 patients. Clin Radiol. 1996;51:775-84.

43. Lopez RR, Benner KG, Hall L, et al. Expandable venous stents for the treatment of the Budd-Chiari syndrome. Gastroenterology. 1991;100:1435-41.
44. Pisani-Ceretti A, Intra M, Prestipino F, et al. Surgical and radiologic treatment of primary Budd-Chiari syndrome. World J Surg. 1998;22:48-53.
45. Baijjal SS, Roy S, Phadke RV, et al. Management of idiopathic Budd-Chiari syndrome with primary stent placement: early results. J Vasc Interv Radiol. 1996;7:545-53.
46. Orloff MJ, Orloff MS, Daily PO. Long-term results of treatment of Budd-Chiari syndrome with portal decompression. Arch Surg. 1992;127:1182-7.
47. Peltzer MY, Ring EJ, LaBerge JM. Treatment of Budd-Chiari syndrome with a transjugular intrahepatic portosystemic shunt. J Vasc Interv Radiol. 1993;4:263-7.
48. Ochs A, Sellinger M, Haag K, et al. Transjugular intrahepatic portosystemic stent shunt (TIPS) in the treatment of Budd-Chiari syndrome. J Hepatol. 1993;18:217-25.
49. Gandini R, Konda D, Simonetti G. Transjugular intrahepatic portosystemic shunt patency and clinical outcome in patients with Budd-Chiari syndrome: covered versus uncovered stents. Radiology. 2006;241:298-305.
50. Liu L, Qi XS, Zhao Y, et al. Budd-chiari syndrome: current perspectives and controversies. Eur Rev Med Pharmacol Sci. 2016;20:3273-81.
51. Mancuso A. Budd-Chiari syndrome management: timing of treatment is an open issue. Hepatology. 2014;59:1213.
52. Shalimar, Kumar A, Kedia S, et al. Hepatic venous outflow tract obstruction: treatment outcomes and development of a new prognostic score. Aliment Pharmacol Ther. 2016;43:1154-67.
53. Faraoun SA, Boudjella Mel A, Debzi N. et al. Budd-Chiari syndrome: an update on imaging. Clin Imaging. 2016;40: 637-46.
54. Mentha G, Giostra E, Majno PE, et al. Liver transplantation for Budd-Chiari syndrome: a European study on 248 patients from 51 centres. J Hepatol. 2006;44:520-28.

CHAPTER

107

Imaging Approach to Obstructive Biliopathy

Anjali Prakash, Rashmi Dixit

Imaging a patient with jaundice is done primarily to rule out obstruction of the bile ducts. This can be due to a block at any level, the hilar/perihilar level or at the low/mid duct level. The causes can be malignant, mainly due to pancreatic carcinoma, cholangiocarcinoma, metastasis, and gallbladder carcinoma. Among the benign cause of obstruction choledocolithiasis is the most common.

In a majority of patients, clinical findings such as age, pain, systemic symptoms such as itching, and biochemistry determines the type of jaundice. Breakdown of hemoglobin leads to formation of bilirubin which is conjugated in liver to form a water soluble compound, which is excreted in urine as urobilinogen. Presence of urobilinogen points to jaundice having a posthepatic cause or mechanical obstruction.

Imaging in a patient with obstructive biliopathy is required to answer the following questions, apart from documenting the presence of obstruction:

- Where is the obstruction? What is the anatomical level of obstruction?
- What is the cause of obstruction?
- If the cause is malignant, is it resectable? If unresectable, to decide the suitable route for palliative stenting.

IMAGING MODALITIES

Ultrasound

This is the initial modality to be used in a patient who presents with jaundice. It is cheap, noninvasive, easily available, does not use radiation, and dynamic evaluation is possible.

Dilated intrahepatic ducts are the imaging hallmark in a patient of obstructive jaundice. The bile ducts are seen as tubular structures adjacent to the portal vessels. The right and left ducts are routinely visualized at sonography **(Fig. 1)**. The intrahepatic ducts measure 2–3 mm centrally, the detection of the more peripheral intrahepatic ducts is seen with obstructive biliopathy **(Figs. 2A and B)**. The normal caliber of the common hepatic duct is considered up to 6 mm, in patients without history of biliary disease. There is an increase in diameter with increasing age and after cholecystectomy reaching up to 10 mm, however a ductal diameter of 7 mm or above is suspicious for obstruction and warrants a search for the cause.[1,2] In patients with history of cholecystectomy, a duct diameter of <4 mm has a high negative predictive value for choledocolithiasis.

In a majority of patients with obstructive biliopathy, bile duct dilatation will be seen on imaging. However, in a small percentage, there may be an obstruction without biliary duct dilatation. This may be seen in patients of choledocolithiasis, postoperative stricturing and sclerosing cholangitis. There is a time lag of 4–5 days after obstruction for the intrahepatic ducts to dilate after extrahepatic obstruction.[3] A dilated duct can be seen after passage of calculus. Not all dilated ducts imply obstruction, as in cases of choledochal cyst there is dilatation of duct but no obstruction.

The ultrasound technique should include (apart from a routine scan), a subcostal view in suspended inspiration; proximal common bile duct and porta hepatis are best seen on a subcostal view whereas distal common bile duct is best evaluated by using the epigastric window. An impacted calculus can be detected by slight rotation of the transducer. Ultrasound has certain limitations. Excessive bowel gas and

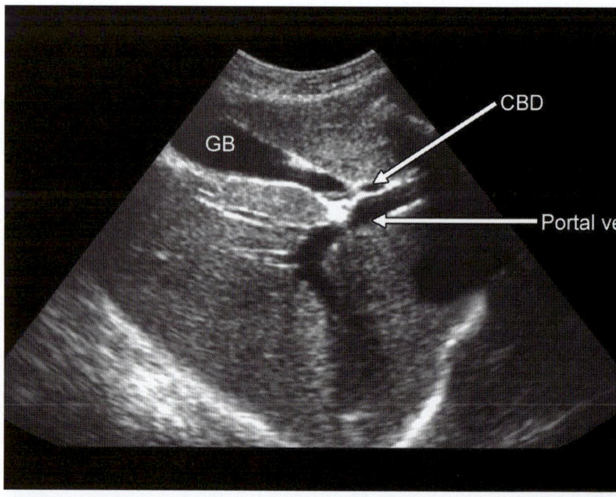

FIG. 1: Ultrasound of right hypochondrium-subcostal view-normal common bile duct (CBD) anterior to the portal vein. (GB: gallbladder).

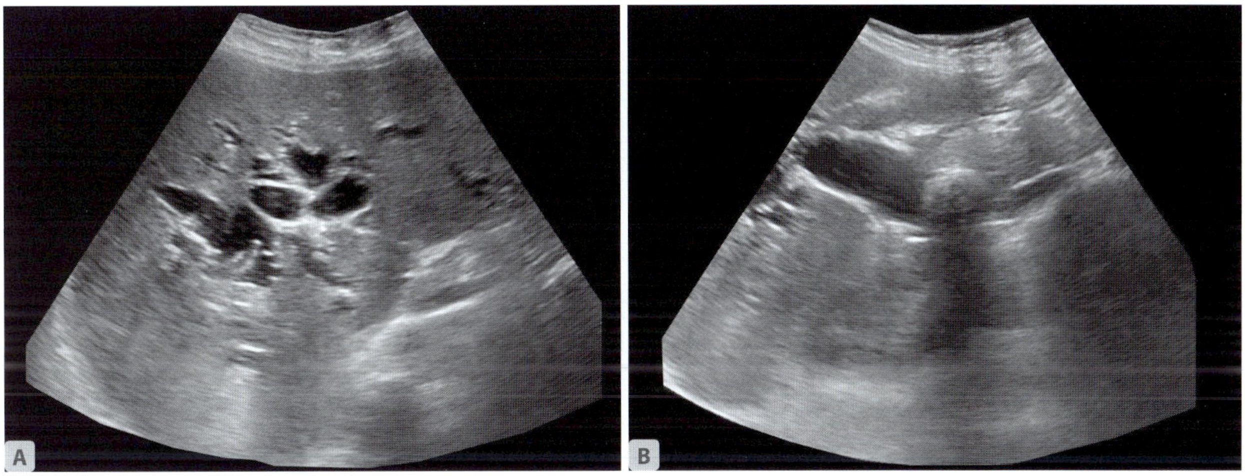

FIGS. 2A AND B: Ultrasound—dilated intrahepatic biliary radicals (A) in a case of choledocholithiasis (B), a large calculus is seen in common bile duct with distal shadowing.

body habitus may hamper visualization of the biliary system. The technique may be optimized[4] by:

- *Changing the patient position*: This will alter relative position of the bowel gas.
- *Compression of epigastrium*: This may displace bowel loops.
- Changing the sonographic window and the use of water in stomach and duodenum to provide an acoustic window may be used.
- Harmonic imaging increases the contrast between duct and the liver parenchyma with enhanced visualization of the lumen, wall and contents of the duct.

The reported sensitivity of ultrasound in defining the level of obstruction and cause ranges from 27% to 95% and from 23% to 88% respectively.[4,5] This wide variation underlines the fact that ultrasound is an operator-dependent modality.

Computed Tomography

Computed tomography (CT) is the imaging modality of choice in imaging a patient of obstructive jaundice, when a pancreaticobiliary malignancy is suspected.

The CT for a patient of obstructive jaundice should be a multiphasic study tailored to the clinical scenario and the ultrasound. It includes a late arterial phase, pancreatic phase at 45 seconds (whenever a pancreatic pathology is suspected), portal venous phase, and a delayed phase.

The CT helps to differentiate malignant from benign stricture. The zone of transition from a dilated to nondilated or non visualized duct provides the clue for the cause. Abrupt termination of the bile duct is a sign of malignancy whereas a gradually tapering duct indicates a benign process. Focal eccentric wall thickening of bile duct prior to obstruction is a sign of cholangiocarcinoma. There can be an associated mass lesion **(Figs. 3 to 6)**. Hyperenhancement of bile duct wall may be seen in both benign and malignant obstruction.[6]

In malignant obstruction, imaging has to determine resectability. In malignant hilar block, the proximal extent, i.e. extension into left/right hepatic ducts according to Bismuth classification, patency of portal veins, presence of secondaries needs to be evaluated. In malignant low obstruction due to periampullary or pancreatic carcinoma, the factors to be evaluated are the tumor size, vascular involvement, lymph node and hepatic metastasis. A meta-analysis has shown that CT has a higher accuracy than ultrasound and magnetic resonance imaging (MRI) in the diagnosis and in the determination of resectability of pancreatic cancer. CT does not have similar accuracy in assessing resectability of cholangiocarcinomas, it is limited in its ability in detecting small peritoneal deposits, secondaries in normal sized nodes and the intraductal extent of tumor.[7]

The CT may detect biliary calculi, if they are partially calcified or have bilirubinate in a sufficient quantity to render them hyperattenuating **(Fig. 7)**. CT is insensitive to cholesterol calculi. Biliary stones are usually seen as soft tissue density or a ring like density surrounded by lower density bile. In cases of suspected biliary calculus, noncontrast CT is to be done as contrast may obscure the calculus. Thin sections with a collimation <2.5 mm and tube kvp at 140 kv may help in demonstrating biliary calculi. CT is not the preferred modality for detection of biliary calculi.

Computed tomography has a reported sensitivity of 96–100% in detection of obstruction and level of obstruction is identified in nearly all cases whereas cause is identified in 70%.[8] The drawback of CT is the use of radiation and the need for IV contrast.

COMPUTED TOMOGRAPHY INTRAVENOUS CHOLANGIOGRAPHY

This investigation was used to study the biliary ductal system. There is very limited availability of the contrast (available in a few countries only, not available in India) and as the contrast has certain amount of toxicity, the examination has limited indications, in some cases of live hepatic donation for transplantation, to evaluate biliary anatomy. Certain variants of biliary anatomy are contraindications in hepatic transplant.

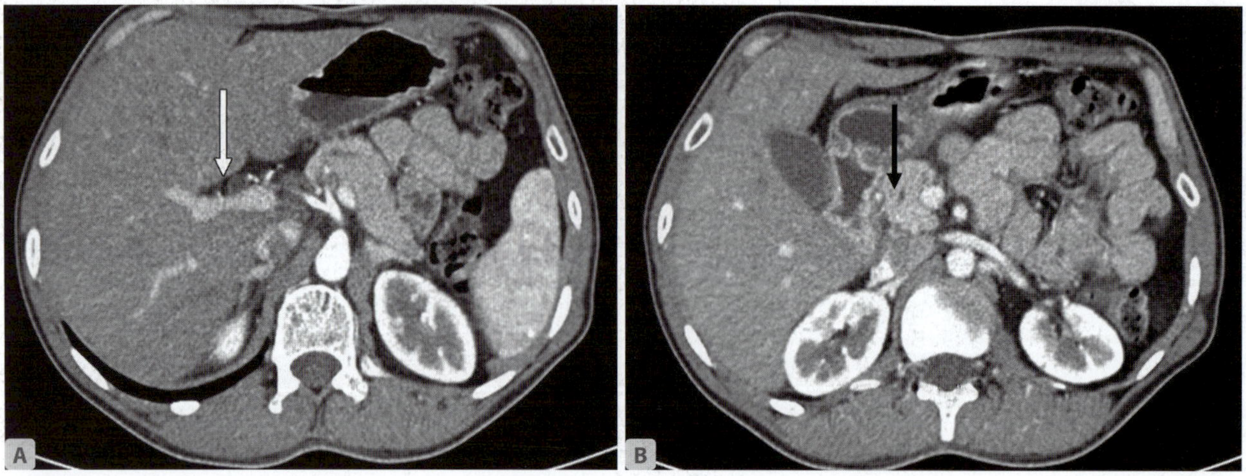

FIGS. 3A AND B: CT upper abdomen—normal caliber of CBD at porta hepatis (A), in the intrapancreatic part (B).

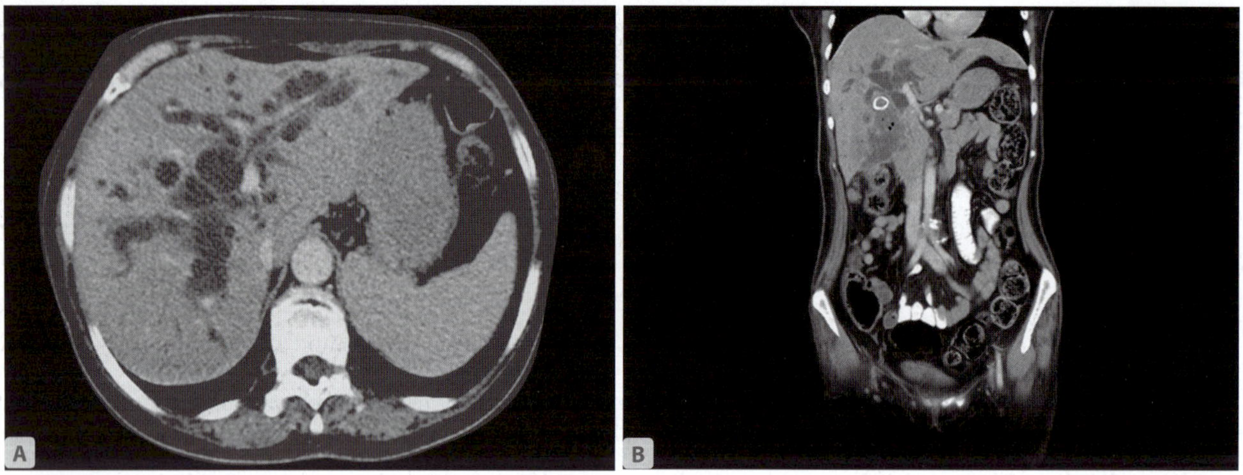

FIGS. 4A AND B: CT upper abdomen—axial (A) and coronal reformat (B). Intrahepatic biliary ductal dilation with a mass in the gallbladder fossa with cholelithiasis—a case of gallbladder malignancy.

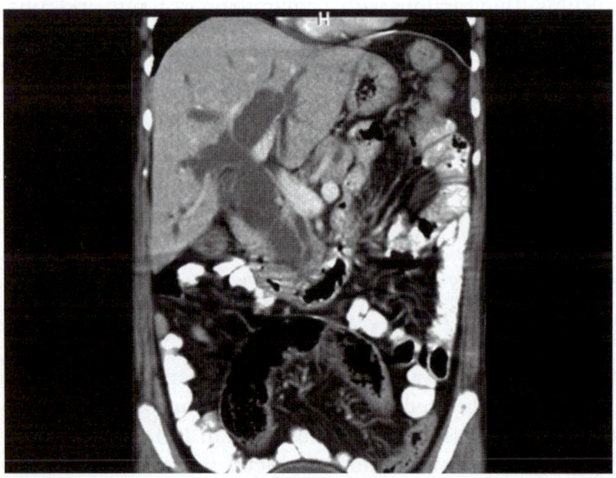

FIG. 5: CT coronal MPR—double duct sign—dilatation of both common bile duct and pancreatic duct in a case of carcinoma head of pancreas.

Intravenous contrast that is preferentially excreted by liver is given by slow infusion followed by CT after 30 minutes. Opacification of bile ducts is noted. The contrast used is Meglumine iotroxate (Biliscopin™) which has a better safety profile, than other IV biliary agents. The technique requires normal liver function and fails in patients with elevated bilirubin levels. CT intravenous cholangiography (CT-IVC) is a functional study as there is excretion and passage of contrast into the bile ducts.[9,10]

Magnetic Resonance Cholangiopancreatography

Magnetic resonance imaging (MRI) and magnetic resonance cholangiopancreatography (MRCP) have emerged as a primary imaging modality for evaluating the biliary ducts and the pancreatic duct. The examination can be done in jaundiced patients unlike CT-IVC. Contrast material is not routinely required and there is no sedation required.

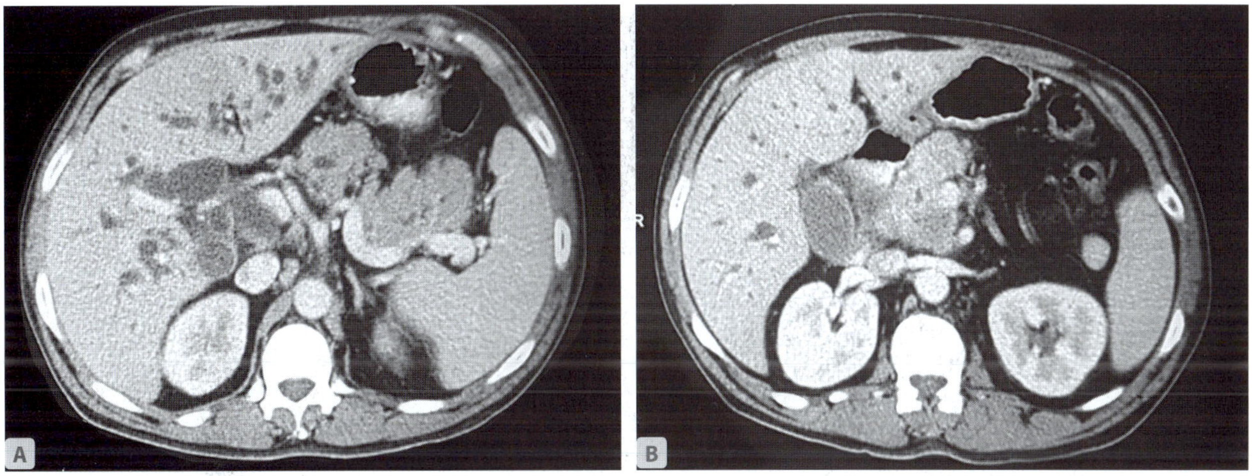

FIGS. 6A AND B: CECT abdomen-dilatation of intrahepatic duct (A), Common bile duct due to a hypoenhancing mass in head of pancreas (B).

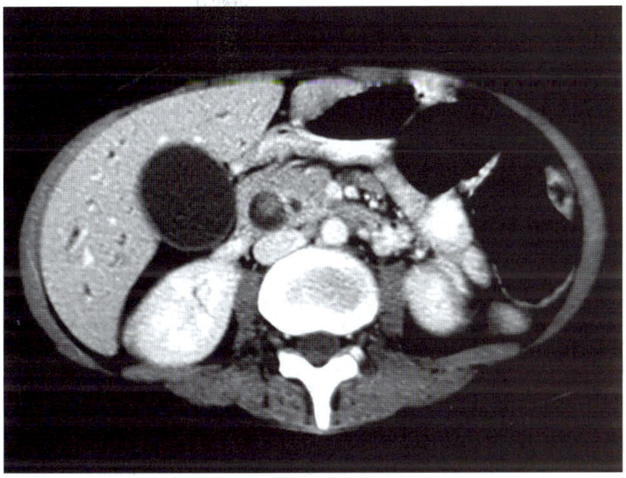

FIG. 7: CECT abdomen-calculus noted in common bile duct with upstream dilatation.

It is the preferred modality in pregnant patients with suspected hepatobiliary disease as there is no radiation exposure.

The two most commonly used sequences are T2-weighted turbo spin echo sequence and 2D single shot fast spin echo (SSFSE). 3D respiratory triggered fast spin echo provides greater details with 3–4 minutes acquisition. Luminal abnormalities are better evaluated with thin slab images. Biliary calculi appear as signal void areas, irrespective of their chemical composition **(Figs. 8 and 9)**. The sensitivity of MRCP in detection of calculi is dependent on the size of the calculus. Sensitivity for small stones, i.e. <3 mm is less than 50%, this increases to 67–100% with calculi >10 mm in size.[11,12] A bile duct filled with calculi may also look like a stricture. Interpreting 3D maximum intensity projection (MIP) images alone without interpreting 2D acquisition may lead to overlooking of small calculi due to superimposition effects on MIP images. Artefacts due to MR technique or in postprocessing may mimic pathology. Surgical clips or pneumobilia may look like a signal void. Indention by an adjacent artery; usually the right hepatic artery may mimic a stricture. All signal voids should be seen in at least two orthogonal planes for a confident diagnosis of calculus.

Sensitivity of MRI in differentiating benign and malignant stricture varies between studies (30–98%).[13,14] Malignant strictures are long due to infiltrative pattern of growth, irregular with asymmetric dilatation of the biliary radicals and there may be presence of a mass **(Fig. 10)**. Benign strictures are short in length, show gradual smooth tapering with a regular border.

The sensitivity decreases in patients with history of cholangitis or biliary intervention as inflammatory soft tissue may mimic a mass. MRI and MRCP has a higher sensitivity than CT in determining nature of hilar stricture. Lesions at the ampulla may however, be missed.

The MRCP has an advantage over endoscopic retrograde cholangiopancreatography (ERCP) that it demonstrates biliary ducts above the level of stricture, which ERCP cannot. This can help guide a planned management with ERCP. MRCP is useful in patients with biliary enteric reconstructions. However, no functional information is provided and it has an inferior resolution to ERCP. The biggest drawback is that no therapeutic intervention is possible.

The MRCP has a reported accuracy of 96–100% for level and 90% for cause of obstruction.[13,14]

CONTRAST-ENHANCED MAGNETIC RESONANCE CHOLANGIOGRAPHY

T1W imaging is done after intravenous (IV) administration of contrast gadolinium ethoxybenzyl diethylenetriamine penta-acetic acid-Gd-EOB-DTPA/Gadobenate disodium. Imaging is done in the hepatobiliary phase. Thin sections are obtained to generate MIP images. The study fails in cases of raised serum bilirubin as there is poor excretion of contrast. This is used in cases of biliary leaks and choledochal cysts.

ENDOSCOPIC ULTRASOUND

This is performed by combined endoscopy and ultrasound. Endoscopes are introduced via transgastric or transduodenal

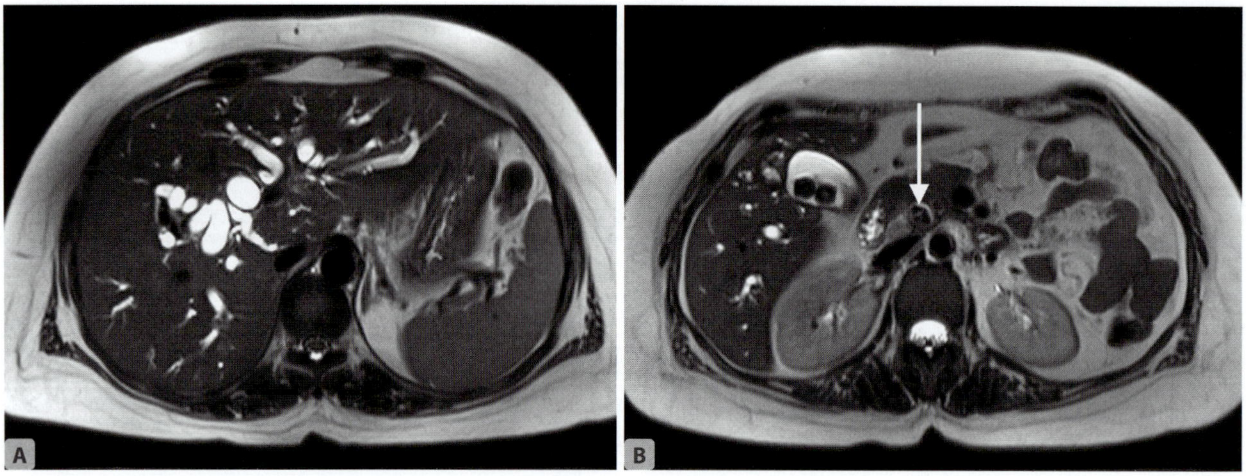

FIGS. 8A AND B: MRI-TRUE FISP sequence—dilated intrahepatic biliary radicals (A) in a case of cholelithiasis with choledocholithiasis. A large calculus is seen in common bile duct as a signal void (arrow marked in B).

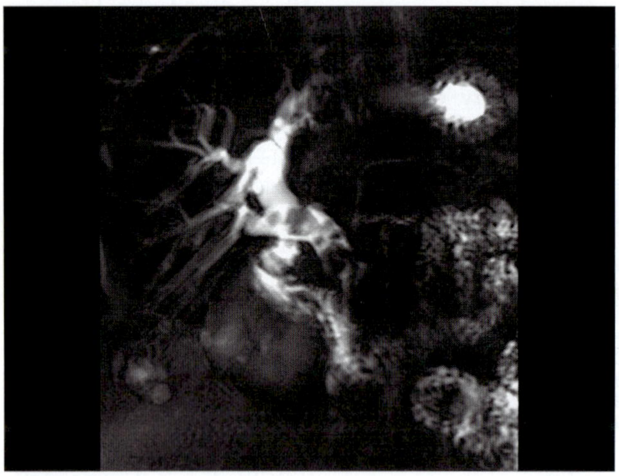

FIG. 9: MRCP-HASTE thick slab coronal—multiple calculi seen as signal voids in the common bile duct with dilatation of CBD and the intrahepatic bile ducts.

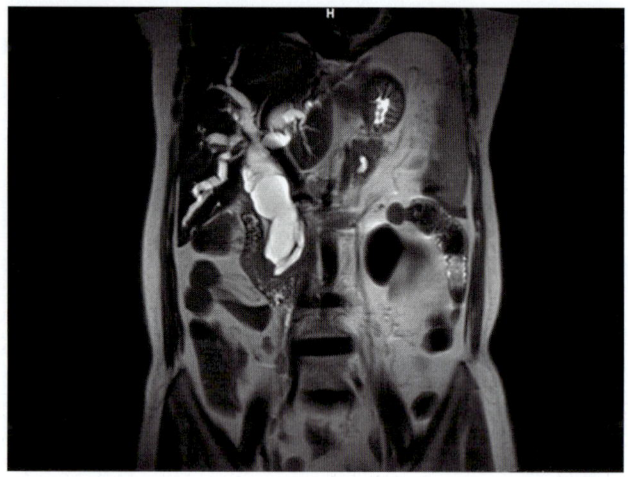

FIG. 10: MRI-T2W coronal image-dilatation of both common bile ducts, pancreatic duct in a case of pancreatic carcinoma.

route and using a water balloon system for acoustic coupling. The frequency range is between 7.5 MHz and 12 MHz, with a depth of penetration of 8–10 cm.

Endoscopic ultrasound (EUS) does not use radiation, unlike ERCP, is less invasive, can diagnose most causes of obstructive jaundice, and provide tissue sampling. However, EUS is not easily available, there is operator dependence. Presence of surgical clips, stents and aerobilia may hamper visualization. The most important drawback is that therapeutic option is not possible at the same time unlike in ERCP.

Endoscopic ultrasound is useful in detecting small biliary calculi, especially within non dilated ducts. It is equal to MRCP/ERCP in detection of calculi.

The EUS is used in the detection of pancreaticobiliary malignancies and in obtaining biopsy. It has a higher sensitivity than all other imaging modalities in the diagnosis of pancreatic tumors. This is especially useful in small (<3 cm) pancreatic tumors, those that will benefit from surgical resection. EUS has a reported sensitivity of 92% in T stage and 82% for N staging in pancreatic malignancy.[15] EUS is more accurate than CT and angiography in detecting invasion of portal vein, splenic vein and of the confluence. It has a similar sensitivity as dual phase CT in detection of pancreatic malignancy; however it is better in lesions less than 15 mm in size. These are the lesions most amenable to surgical resection.

The EUS has a sensitivity of 97% and a specificity of 88% in determining the cause of extrahepatic obstruction.[14,15]

FUNCTIONAL IMAGING

Scintigraphy-99mTc hydroxyiminodiacetic acid (HIDA) is the radiotracer used as it is excreted in bile. It is not a sensitive modality in assessing the level or cause of obstruction. The tracer may not be excreted in patients with high bilirubin level. This is not routinely used as MRCP/CT have higher resolution and provide comprehensive evaluation.

DIRECT CHOLANGIOGRAPHY

This includes endoscopic retrograde cholangiopancreatography and percutaneous transhepatic cholangiogram. Both investigations are invasive. There is a reported sensitivity of 100% in the detection of obstruction; these remain the gold standard for the evaluation and of biliary leaks and for subtle luminal changes. However, no extraluminal information can be obtained with either.

The ERCP is done after cannulation of the ampulla after a duodenoscope is introduced. Contrast is introduced in both biliary and pancreatic ducts. ERCP has a sensitivity of 90–96% and specificity of 98% in the detection of calculi.[14,16] There is reduced sensitivity in detection of small stones in a dilated bile duct. Air bubbles may be misinterpreted as calculi. Treatment in the form of sphincterotomy, balloon and basket removal of stones can be done via the same route.

The ERCP has a definite role in diagnosis and management of pancreaticobiliary tumors. Long strictures, with irregular margins, asymmetric dilatation and presence of mass point towards a malignant stricture.

Endoscopic tissue sampling like brush cytology, fine needle aspiration and forceps biopsy are available, with nearly 100% specificity though with moderate sensitivity (20–60%). Palliation of malignant obstruction can be done using a plastic or metal stent.

The ERCP carries significant morbidity (10%-pancreatitis) and a 0.4% mortality. The other drawbacks include cost of equipment, availability of trained personnel, need for conscious sedation. It is not possible to visualize ducts proximal to the obstruction. ERCP is now used for treatment and not for primary diagnosis.

Percutaneous Transhepatic Cholangiography

This has been almost completely replaced by MRCP/ERCP and is now used in transhepatic biliary intervention as a route for biliary decompression. The liver is punctured with a 22 gauge Chiba needle to enter an intrahepatic biliary duct after checking the coagulation profile. Contrast is then injected to opacify the biliary system and visualize the site of obstruction. The success of this procedure is dependent on the ducts being dilated, being almost 100% when the ducts are dilated and 75% in a nondilated system.[17,18]

The reported complication rate is <5%, and these are biliary leaks, bile peritonitis, hemobilia, sepsis, etc. PTC is reserved for patients with failed ERCP or to provide palliation in unresectable hilar tumors.

PET-CT

The index SUV (standardized uptake value) max, that measures glucose uptake shows a significant difference of value between benign and malignant causes of obstructive jaundice. Pancreatic cancer has a high uptake of the tracer, however tumors like infiltrating cholangiocarcinoma show low uptake. Combining PET with conventional imaging like CT, MRI increases the sensitivity and accuracy when compared with conventional imaging alone.[19]

INTRADUCTAL ULTRASOUND

This is done using a flexible, thin (2 mm) probe which is introduced via the endoscope into the pancreatic and biliary duct. The ducts are filled with fluid to provide acoustic coupling. The frequencies range from 12 MHz to 30 MHz providing high resolution but limited penetration. It is superior to EUS in evaluation of proximal biliary ducts. Intraductal ultrasound (IDUS) increases ability of ERCP in distinguishing benign from malignant cause of obstruction. A sessile tumor, size of tumor >10 mm and interrupted wall structure on IDUS favour malignancy. Heterogeneous and irregular bile duct thickening and invasion of vessels is seen in malignant obstruction. Lack of availability, operator expertise, low penetration remain a drawback.

IMAGING ALGORITHM IN OBSTRUCTIVE JAUNDICE

The American College of Radiology (ACR) has categorized patients with jaundice into three categories:[14]

1. High likelihood of mechanical obstruction. This has been further subdivided into benign and malignant obstruction
2. Low likelihood of obstruction
3. Intermediate likelihood.

The ACR has further suggested the most appropriate imaging modality in each scenario and ranked them on a scale of 0–10 with the most appropriate being.[10]

Imaging in a case of obstructive jaundice starts with transabdominal ultrasound. Once biliary dilatation is seen then the anatomical level of obstruction is to be determined. The differential diagnosis would be based on this and will guide further investigations **(Flowcharts 1 to 3)**.

In patients where choledocolithiasis is detected on ultrasound, ERCP is the next modality which is used for stone extraction. MRCP may be used to provide a roadmap to the endoscopist.If obstruction is found on ultrasound with history of biliary colic, and no cause is found, the second test should be MRI + MRCP.

Endoscopic ultrasound is to be done in patients in whom MRCP is normal, and especially in cases of nondilated ducts. If there is no clinical suspicion of calculus or colic then ultrasound should be followed by a biphasic

FLOWCHART 1: Imaging pathway in a case of jaundice with suspected biliary colic.

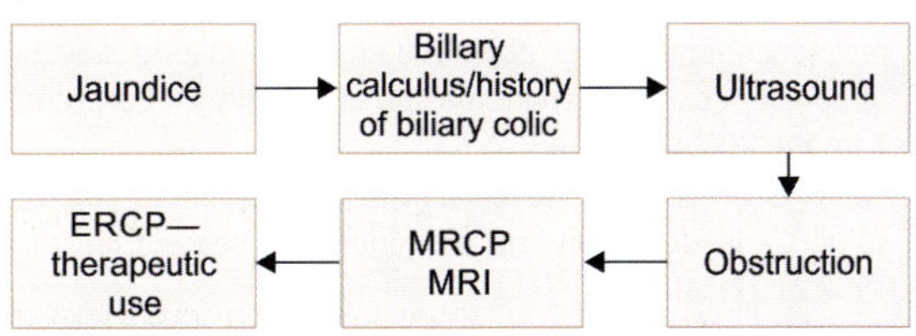

(MRCP: magnetic resonance cholangiopancreatography; MRI: magnetic resonance imaging)

FLOWCHART 2: Imaging pathway in a case of jaundice with suspected malignancy.

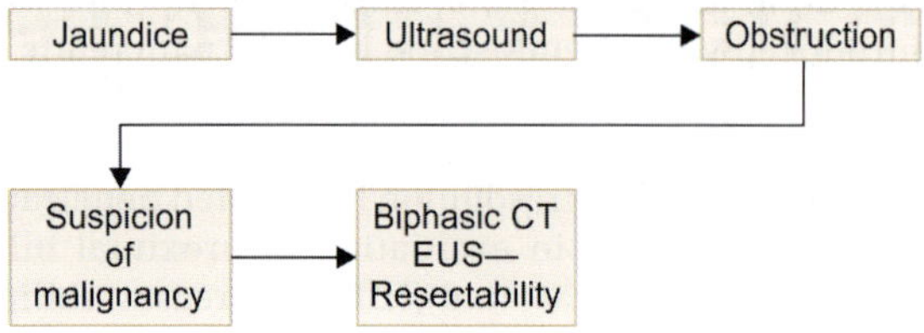

(CT: computed tomography; EUS: endoscopic ultrasound)

FLOWCHART 3: Imaging pathway in a case of jaundice with no features of obstruction on ultrasound.

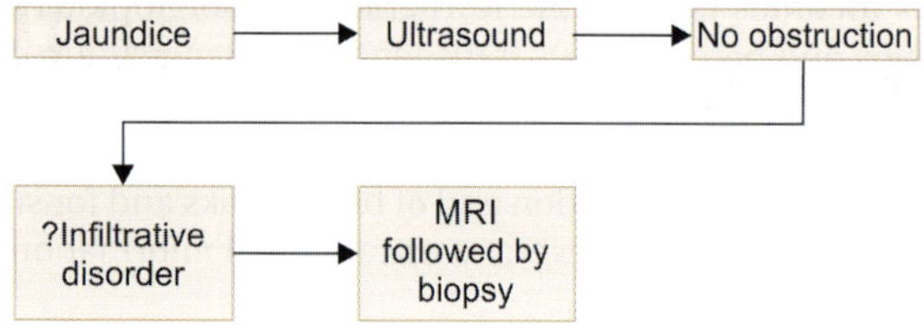

(MRI: magnetic resonance imaging)

CT for assessing the point of obstruction, resectability and staging in cases of malignancy. EUS is also used to assess resectability by evaluating vascular involvement in cases of pancreatic head tumors and in periampullary malignancy. Image (by ultrasound and CT)-guided biopsy or fine needle aspiration can be done. In the cases where surgical resection is planned, a preoperative biopsy is not considered appropriate. In cases where palliation is being considered, biopsy is to be deferred till after decompression to prevent bile leaks. Direct cholangiography is reserved as a therapeutic option.

If no mechanical obstruction is found, an infiltrative disorder needs to be looked for on MRI, followed by biopsy.

CONCLUSION

Obstructive biliopathy is a common clinical problem. Four questions have to be addressed while imaging these patients (inset). The choice of the modality used depends on the clinical scenario, the modalities available, the local expertise, the institutional and referring physician's preference and patient criteria.

Obstructive biliopathy—imaging questions?

- Is there obstruction?
- What is the level of the block?
- What is the cause of obstruction?
- If the cause is malignant, is it resectable?

REFERENCES

1. Bowie JD. What is the upper limit of normal for the common bile duct on ultrasound: how much do you want it to be? Am J Gastroenterol. 2000;95(4):897-900.
2. Horrow MM, Horrow JC, Niakosari A, et al. Is age associated with size of adult extrahepatic duct: Sonographic study.Radiology. 2001;221(2):411-4.
3. Rudralingam V, Sukumar SA. Imaging of the jaundiced adult. Imaging. 2013;22:51415473.
4. Turner MA, Fulcher AS. Gallbladder and biliary tract; normal anatomy and examination techniques. In: Gore RM, Levine MS (Eds). Textbook of gastrointestinal radiology, 2nd edition. Philadelpia. PA: WB Saunders; 2000.pp.1250-76.
5. Mittelstaedt CA. Ultrasound of the bile ducts. Semin Roentgenol. 1997;32:161-71.
6. Choi SH, Han JL, Lee JM, Lee KH, et al. Differentiating malignant from benign common bile duct stricture with multiphasic helical CT. Radiology. 2005;236:173-83.
7. Bipat S, Phoa SS, Van Delden OM, Bossuyat PM, et al. Ultrasonography, computed tomography and magnetic resonance imaging for diagnosis and determining resectability of pancreatic adenocarcinoma: a meta-analysis. J Comput Assist Tomogr. 2005;29:438-45.
8. Wyatt SH, Fishman EK. Biliary tract obstruction: the role of spiral CT in detection and definition of disease. Clin Imaging. 1997;21:27-34.
9. Ahmetoglu A, Kosucu P, Kul S, et al. MDCT cholangiography with volume rendering for the assessment of patients with biliary obstruction. AJR. 2004;183:1327-32.
10. Hyodo T, Kumano S, Kushihata F, Okada M, et al. CT and MR cholangiography: advantages and pitfalls in perioperative evaluation of biliary tree. Br J Radiol. 2012;85(1015):887-96.
11. Ishizaki Y, Wakayama T, Okada Y, Kobayashi T. Magnetic resonance cholangiography for evaluation of obstructive jaundice. Am J Gastroenterol. 1993;12:2072-7.
12. Kim JH, Kim MJ, Park SI, Chung JJ, Song SY, et al. Using kinematic MR cholangiopancreatography to evaluate biliary dilatation. AJR. 2008;190(2):396-405.
13. Romagnuolo J, Bardou M, Rahme, et al. Magnetic resonance cholangiopancreatography: a meta-analysis of test performance in suspected biliary disease. Ann Intern Med. 2003;139(7):547-57.
14. Lalani T, Couto CA, Rosen MP, Baker ME, Blake MA, et al. ACR Appropriateness Criteria® jaundice. [online publication]. Reston (VA), American College of Radiology (ACR); 2012.p.9.
15. Gress F, Hawes R, Savides T, et al. The role of EUS in the preoperative staging of pancreatic cancer: a large single center experience. Gastrointest Endosc. 1999;50:786-91.
16. Jailwala J, Fogel EL, Sherman S, Gottlieb K, et al. Triple tissue sampling at ERCP in malignant biliary obstruction. Gastrointest Endosc. 2000;51:383-90.
17. Ferrucci JT, Mueller PR, Harbin WP. Percutaneous transhepatic biliary drainage: technique, results and applications. Radiology. 1980;135:1-13.
18. Cotton PB, Speer AG. Risks and benefits of percutaneous transhepatic biliary drainage. Gastroenterology. 1987;93:667-8.
19. Wang S, Wu H, Wang Q, Zhou W, et al. 18F-FDG PET/CT in differentiating malignant from benign origins of obstructive jaundice. Hepatobiliary Pancreat Dis Int. 2015;14:516-22.

CHAPTER

108

Inflammatory Pathologies of the Biliary Tract

Anmol Bhatia, Ajay Gulati, Uma Debi

INFLAMMATORY CONDITIONS OF THE GALLBLADDER

Acute and chronic inflammatory conditions involving gallbladder are amongst the common causes of acute abdomen. Imaging helps in an early diagnosis and detection of complications in patients with gallbladder inflammatory disorders, thereby reducing morbidity and mortality. This part of the present chapter deals with chronic gallbladder inflammatory conditions. The acute inflammatory conditions have been covered in the chapter on nontraumatic acute abdomen.

Chronic Cholecystitis

Chronic cholecystitis is one of the most common inflammatory conditions of gallbladder and is seen to occur in the background of cholelithiasis in almost all of the patients. Patients usually present with history suggesting recurring episodes of acute cholecystitis and/or biliary colic, while few patients may be totally asymptomatic previously.[1] There is associated gallbladder dysmotility as evidenced by poor gallbladder ejection fraction on ultrasound.

The most commonly seen findings on cross-sectional imaging include cholelithiasis and thickened gallbladder wall. The gallbladder is usually contracted, and pericholecystic inflammation is mostly absent **(Fig. 1)**.[2]

Complications related to chronic cholecystitis include:

- Acute cholecystitis **(Figs. 2A and B)**.
- Gallbladder malignancy.
- *Cholecystoenteric fistula:* T his results in the passage of gallbladder calculi into the bowel loops resulting in bowel obstruction, which is termed as gallstone ileus. The passed out stones in the small bowel usually get stuck up in the terminal ileal loops near the ileocecal junction; they may however, be found in any location throughout the small bowel as well as in large bowel loops also.[3] Identification of Rigler's triad (which consists of gallstone in an abnormal/ectopic location, pneumobilia, and features of intestinal obstruction) on plain radiographs at times may be helpful in making the diagnosis. Rigler's triad, however, is seen in a small number of patients only.[3]

Xanthogranulomatous Cholecystitis

It is an inflammatory syndrome characterized by thickened gallbladder wall with intramural nodules,[4,5] which are formed by the occlusion and later on rupture of the Rokitansky–Aschoff sinuses. This leads to extravasation of bile into the wall inciting an inflammatory response, characterized histologically by the presence of fibroblasts, histiocytes, and multinucleated giant cells. Xanthogranulomatous cholecystitis is known to occur commonly in elderly population, but can occur across a wide range of age group.[6]

The most common findings on ultrasound (US) and computed tomography (CT) in xanthogranulomatous cholecystitis include gallbladder calculi and focal or diffuse gallbladder wall thickening. Inflammatory fat stranding may also be seen in pericholecystic region. Intramural hypoechoic areas on US and hypoattenuating nodules/bands on CT are highly specific for diagnosing xanthogranulomatous cholecystitis **(Figs. 3A to D)**.[5] Xanthogranulomatous cholecystitis many-a-times is a close mimicker of gallbladder

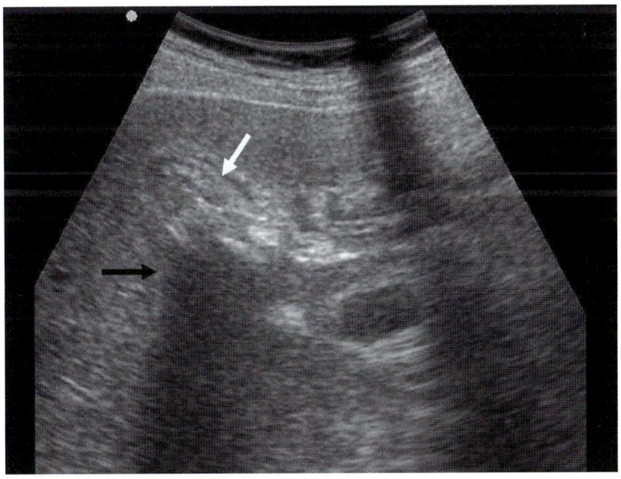

FIG. 1: Chronic cholecystitis. Ultrasound image showing contracted gallbladder with diffusely thickened wall (white arrow) and distal acoustic shadowing (black arrow) caused by multiple small calculi in its lumen.

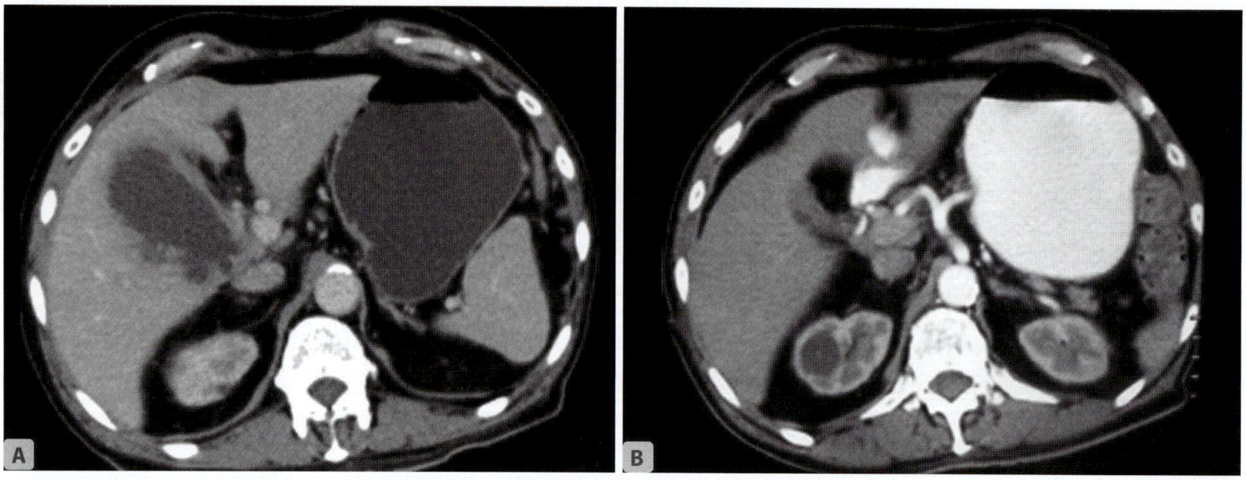

FIGS. 2A AND B: Acute on chronic cholecystitis. (A) Axial CECT image shows distended gallbladder with mural thickening and irregularity at places suggesting acute cholecystitis. Fat stranding is also seen in the adjacent fat; (B) Follow-up CT after 7 months shows shrunken gallbladder.

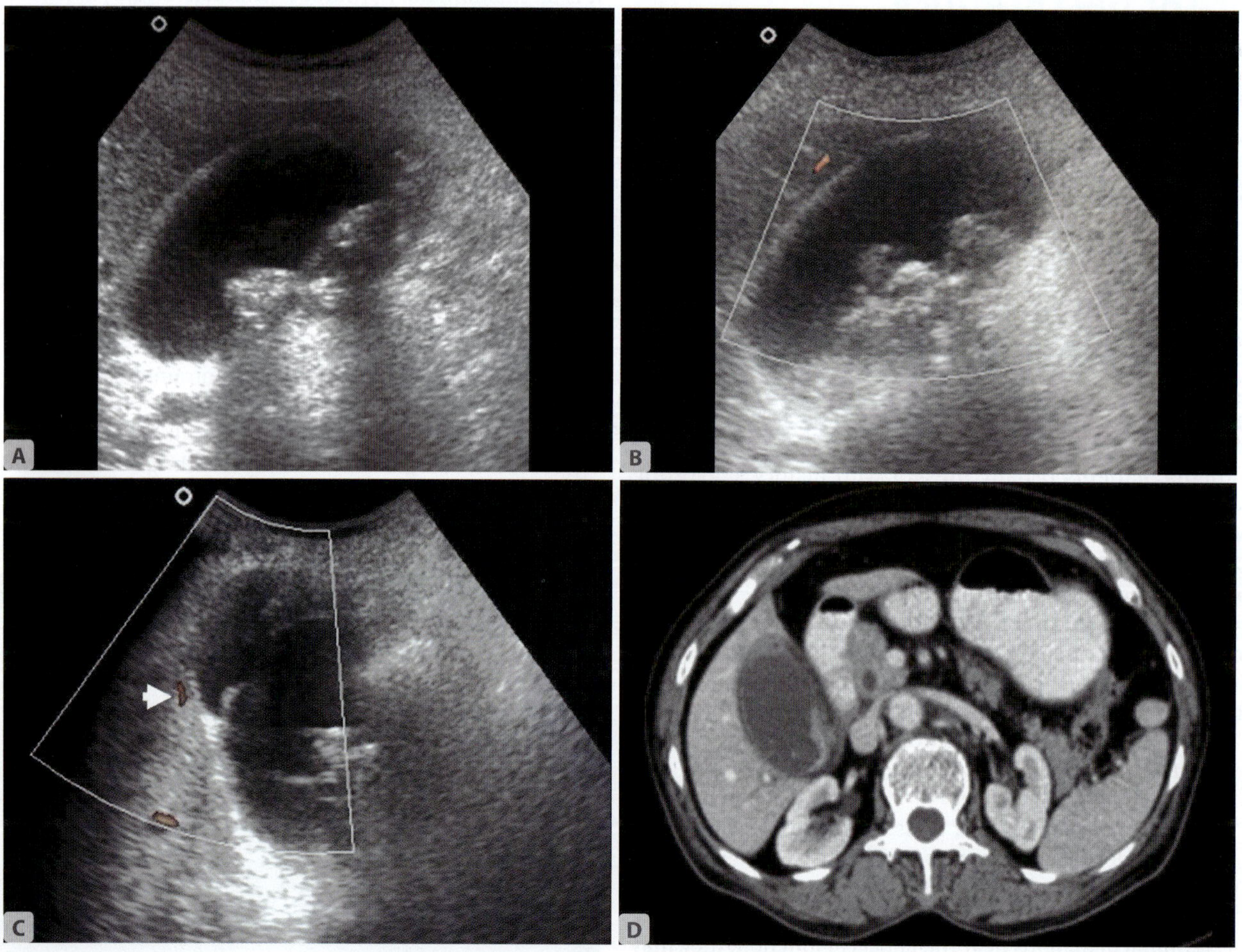

FIGS. 3A TO D: Xanthogranulomatous cholecystitis. (A) Grayscale ultrasound image showing cholelithiasis with thickened gallbladder wall. (B) Color Doppler (B) and power Doppler (C) images showing vascularity adjacent to the thickened wall (arrowhead in C). (D) Axial CECT image showing hyperattenuating inner wall and hypoattenuating outer wall. FNAC was suggestive of benign etiology with possible xanthogranulomatous foci.

carcinoma on US and CT,[4] while xanthogranulomatous cholecystitis is also associated with an increase in the risk of gallbladder malignancy.[4,6]

Complications encountered in xanthogranulomatous cholecystitis are gallbladder perforation, biliary fistula, liver abscess, stricture within the biliary ducts, and ascending cholangitis.[6] Open cholecystectomy is the preferred option in xanthogranulomatous cholecystitis due to adhesions and associated fibrosis, which make the laparoscopic surgery often unsuccessful.

INFLAMMATORY CONDITIONS OF THE BILIARY TREE

Imaging of biliary tract inflammation has undergone many changes in the last two decades. Due to availability of better diagnostic modalities and treatment options, some entities which were common before have become rare. Advances in cross-sectional imaging have led to an increase in the number of investigations for establishing the diagnosis. There has been evolution of new notions for the occurrence of the inflammatory pathologies affecting the biliary tree resulting in new entities that the radiologists need to know. This part of the present chapter aims to discuss these varying aspects of the biliary tract inflammation.

FIRST ASPECT: ENTITIES WHICH WERE COMMON IN THE PAST AND NOW RARELY SEEN

AIDS-related Cholangiopathy

The biliary tree is affected by human immunodeficiency virus (HIV) in patients having CD4 count of <100/mm^3, and the patients usually have pain in the right hypochondrium along with abnormal liver function tests, which are nonspecific. The alkaline phosphatase (ALP) level is elevated more than twenty times the normal value, while the bilirubin levels may be normal or show mild elevation. Abnormal liver function tests can occur due to a variety of causes which include drug-related reactions and hepatitis. Fever with chills may be indicative of systemic infection, whereas jaundice occurs only when there is severe hepatic dysfunction or significant common bile duct (CBD) obstruction. Imaging, therefore, has an important role to play to assess HIV patients suspected to have hepatobiliary involvement.[7,8]

Acquired immunodeficiency syndrome (AIDS) cholangiopathy is one of the causes of secondary sclerosing cholangitis due to opportunistic infections involving the biliary system, or damage to autonomic nerves or ischemia, but can also occur due to direct invasion of lining of the biliary tract by HIV.[7,8] In majority of the patients, no definite pathogen is isolated/identified; while a gamut of organisms have been implicated, which include *Mycobacterium avium* complex (MAC), herpes simplex virus, *Cryptosporidium parvum*, and cytomegalovirus. It needs to be differentiated from parenchymal liver processes such as MAC infection, for which imaging and biopsy need to be done to establish the diagnosis.[7-9]

Imaging features **(Figs. 4A to E)** *include*:

- Acalculous cholecystitis.
- Dilatation of intrahepatic and extrahepatic biliary ducts, predominantly involving left side ductal system.
- Irregular thickening and pruning of the CBD with areas of saccular dilatations.
- Papillary stenosis.

Diagnosis is confirmed by duodenal or ampulla biopsy, with the typical findings of biliary inflammation and the detection of involved organisms. The various treatment options available are sphincterotomy, stricture dilatation, and biliary stenting. Antimicrobial therapy is based on the specific pathogen involved.[7]

DISEASES KNOWN IN THE PAST WITH INCREASED DETECTABILITY IN THE PRESENT ERA

Primary Sclerosing Cholangitis

Primary sclerosing cholangitis (PSC) is an idiopathic, chronic, fibrosing inflammatory disorder affecting the biliary radicles leading to obstruction of bile ducts, cholestasis, progressing to biliary cirrhosis. It has a strong association with ulcerative colitis, which is seen in 70% of patients.[10] It is thought to be an autoimmune process due to its association with other autoimmune disorders including mediastinal fibrosis, Sjögren syndrome, and retroperitoneal fibrosis.[11,12]

Diagnostic criteria include:

- *Typical cholangiographic abnormalities:* Multifocal, intrahepatic strictures involving the biliary ducts alternating with normal-sized ducts producing a beaded appearance **(Figs. 5A and B)**.
- *Clinical, biochemical, and liver histology findings:* About 75% patients present with progressive fatigue, pruritus, or jaundice.[13] Elevated serum bilirubin and ALP is seen in most of the patients, with ALP rise at least three times the normal range.[13,14] Liver biopsy shows inflammatory fibrosis (nonspecific) involving the portal tracts with a scarcity of bile ducts. Therefore, the histology is considered for confirmation only in case there is a suspicion of PSC.
- *Excluding the secondary causes of sclerosing cholangitis:* This includes a gamut of disorders including chronic bacterial cholangitis following strictures or stones in the biliary system, parasitic infections, AIDS cholangiopathy, ischemia because of drugs like floxuridine or hepatic arterial thrombosis, intrahepatic cholangiocarcinoma, liver metastases, hepatobiliary surgery, as well as congenital disorders of the biliary system.

ERCP, which has been the gold standard for diagnosis of PSC, is associated with risk of cholangitis following bile stasis and biliary injury because of presence of sacculations with increased stiffness of the biliary system **(Figs. 6A and B)**. MRCP has been shown equivalent to ERCP for detecting and localizing the levels of obstruction in the biliary system, and can be helpful in establishing the diagnosis as well as help in planning for an intervention.[15]

The role of MRI/MRCP in PSC imaging is to address the following three aspects:

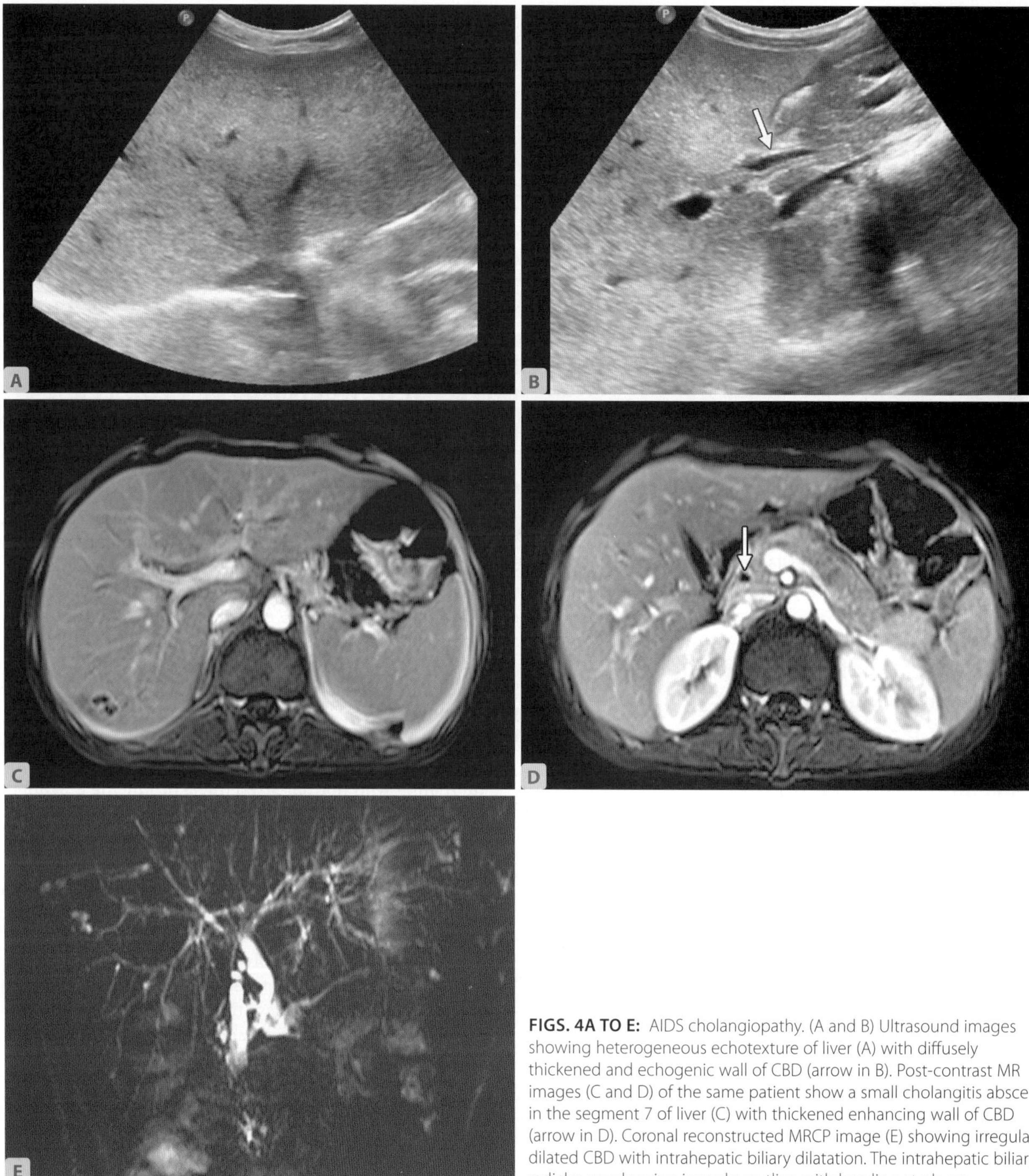

FIGS. 4A TO E: AIDS cholangiopathy. (A and B) Ultrasound images showing heterogeneous echotexture of liver (A) with diffusely thickened and echogenic wall of CBD (arrow in B). Post-contrast MR images (C and D) of the same patient show a small cholangitis abscess in the segment 7 of liver (C) with thickened enhancing wall of CBD (arrow in D). Coronal reconstructed MRCP image (E) showing irregularly dilated CBD with intrahepatic biliary dilatation. The intrahepatic biliary radicles are showing irregular outline with beading at places.

1. *Evaluation of intrahepatic and extrahepatic components of biliary system:* The pressure created by the injected contrast during ERCP maximally distends the biliary ducts, thereby making minimal changes and narrowing due to strictures, particularly in the peripheral system to be evaluated, while for involvement of the ducts alone MRCP is likely to miss the minimal changes of PSC. But, if more central strictures are present which are obstructing the flow of contrast during ERCP, MRCP shows upstream ductal involvement.
2. *Morphologic findings in the liver parenchyma supporting PSC diagnosis:* Liver in later stages of PSC shows markedly prominent lobulations of caudate lobe, left lobe atrophy, regenerative nodules (predominantly central in location), and enlarged lymph nodes may be seen in perihepatic location.[12-14] Postcontrast late arterial phase imaging shows peripheral hyperenhancing areas which occur due to a transient hepatic attenuation difference. This indicates increase in the arterial flow compensating for the decreased flow from portal venous

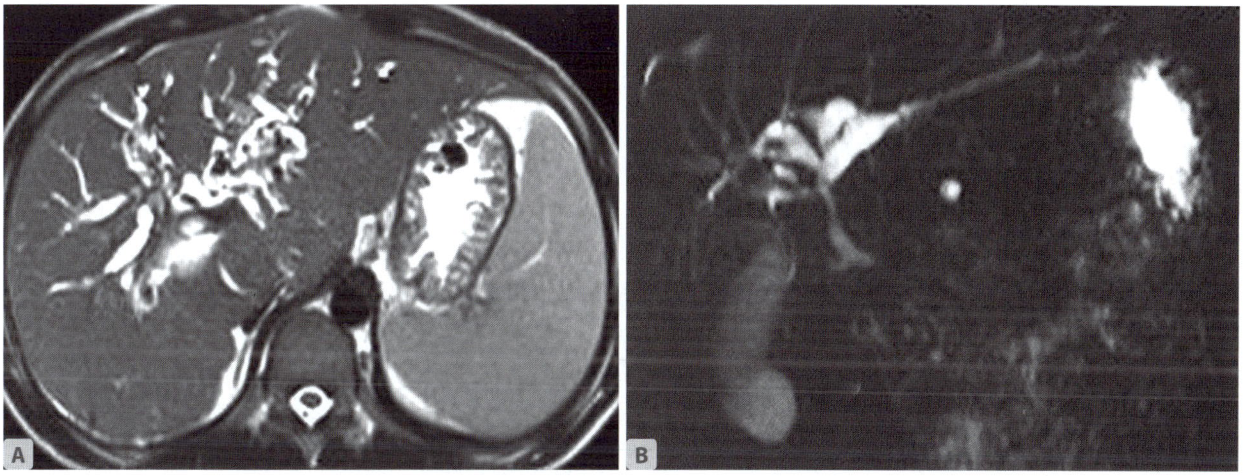

FIGS. 5A AND B: Primary sclerosing cholangitis. Axial T2-HASTE image (A) showing bilobar intrahepatic biliary dilatation. Coronal reconstructed MRCP image (B) showing multifocal strictures involving the biliary radicles with areas of dilatation.

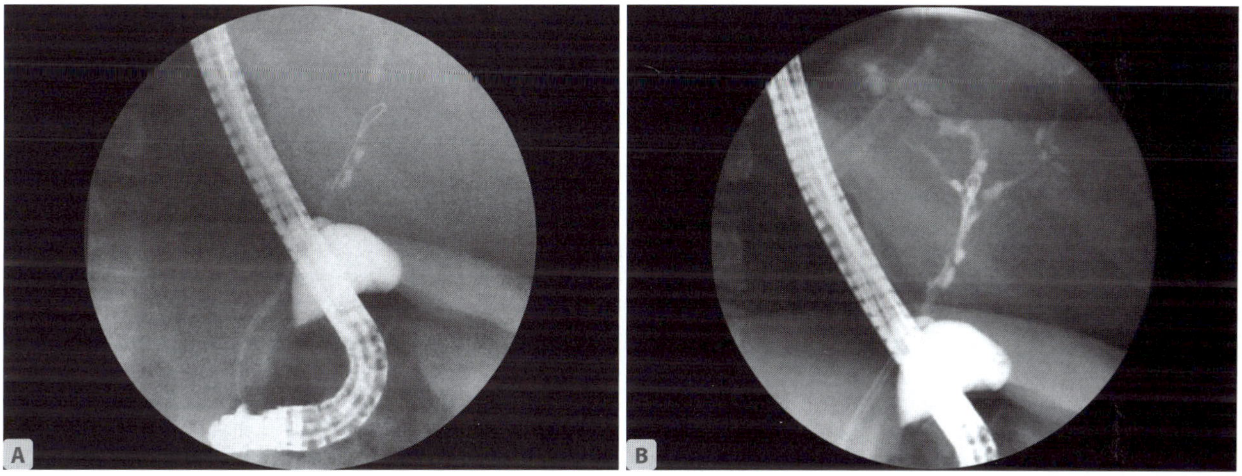

FIGS. 6A AND B: Primary sclerosing cholangitis. ERCP images (A and B) with guidewire showing multifocal segmental narrowing and dilated segments of the biliary ducts and CBD along with sacculations in CBD.

system in areas where there is obstruction of the biliary channels.[8,12,14] Hyperintensity can be seen on T2WI along the portal tracts, occurring due to combination of fibrosis, inflammatory infiltrate and lymphatics.[15] This may again show enhancement on postcontrast delayed phase scans.

3. *To diagnose cholangiocarcinoma:* MRI is also useful to detect cholangiocarcinoma, which is known to occur in 10-15% of PSC.[8] This tumor shows peripheral enhancement on arterial phase images with diffuse enhancement on delayed scans.

Secondary Processes Simulating PSC

These include ascending cholangitis occurring due to strictures, congenital anomalies of the bile duct, calculi, AIDS-related cholangiopathy, oriental cholangiohepatitis, and ischemia following iatrogenic insult or intra-arterial chemotherapy.

Nonsclerosing pathologies can also mimic PSC at ERCP, which include polycystic liver disease, metastases, cirrhosis, multifocal hepatocellular carcinoma (HCC) and cholangiocarcinoma. Cross-sectional imaging is therefore warranted to differentiate these nonsclerosing pathologies from PSC.

Ascending Cholangitis

It is caused by bacterial infection, usually by gram-negative enteric bacteria in an obstructed biliary system. The most common causes of obstruction include strictures, calculi, and papillary stenosis. Ascending cholangitis is a clinical diagnosis, and hence the role of imaging is find out the underlying cause of the obstruction. Also, findings of biliary enhancement on imaging help to corroborate with the clinical symptoms **(Fig. 7)**. Patients usually present with the Charcot triad of pain, fever and jaundice. Increased ductal pressure results in the injury of the walls of the ducts which leads to reflux infected bile into the portal triads, thereby forming liver abscess.[15]

Oriental Cholangiohepatitis

It is a parasitic infection of the biliary system in which the patients present with recurrent episodes of pain, fever, and jaundice. Endemic areas, like Southeast Asia, are most commonly affected where parasites like *Ascaris lumbricoides* and *Clonorchis sinensis* inhabit the biliary ducts and later on lead to ductal injury and formation of strictures.[15] It is considered synonymous with recurrent pyogenic cholangitis.

Imaging findings[15] include:

- Multifocal strictures with dilated intrahepatic bile radicles.
- Calculi within the intrahepatic biliary radicles **(Figs. 8A and B)**.
- Disproportionately dilated extrahepatic biliary system, which is not related to strictures or calculi.
- Branching pattern in a right-angled fashion, with reduced degree of arborization.
- Bile lakes or cholangiectasis.
- Primary pigmented stones (in 80% patients), liver abscess, and cholangiocarcinoma (in 2.5%–5.0% patients) are the complications which may be seen.

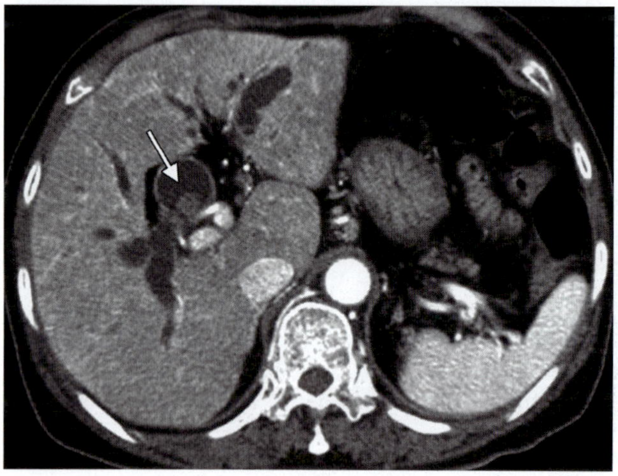

FIG. 7: Ascending cholangitis. Axial CECT image showing bilobar IHBRD with enhancing walls of the dilated radicles suggestive of cholangitis. In addition, there is presence of a calculus (arrow) in CHD.

Chemotherapy-induced Cholangitis

This usually is seen following intra-arterial infusion of chemotherapeutic drugs like floxuridine, in cases of liver metastases form colorectal cancer as a palliative treatment. This occurs due to a large amount of drug extraction during the first pass through the liver, leading to an inflammatory reaction as well as fibrosis around the portal triads mimicking PSC at imaging. Bile duct strictures are known to occur within 2 months of the initiation of the treatment and seen in up to 15% of patients. Strictures are seen at the division of the common hepatic duct (CHD), and distal common bile duct (CBD) is spared.[16]

NEW CONCEPTS

The era of autoimmune disease lead to evolution of the new insights in the inflammatory conditions of the biliary tract. Primary biliary cirrhosis (PBC) has been a well-known entity, but diseases which have been included in this list are autoimmune hepatitis, overlap syndromes, IgG4-related disease and eosinophilic cholangitis.

Primary Biliary Cirrhosis

Primary biliary cirrhosis (PBC) occurs due to inflammation of the medium and small sized biliary radicles/ducts, having components of acute as well chronic inflammation resulting in features of cholestasis clinically. It typically affects women (>90% of cases) between 30 and 65 years of age. Elevated antimitochondrial antibodies (more specific) and antinuclear antibodies (less specific) are characteristic findings in serology. It usually occurs in association with other autoimmune disorders, like inflammatory bowel disease,

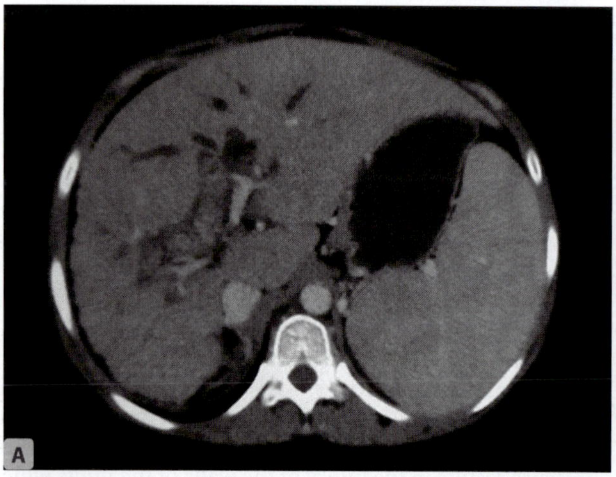

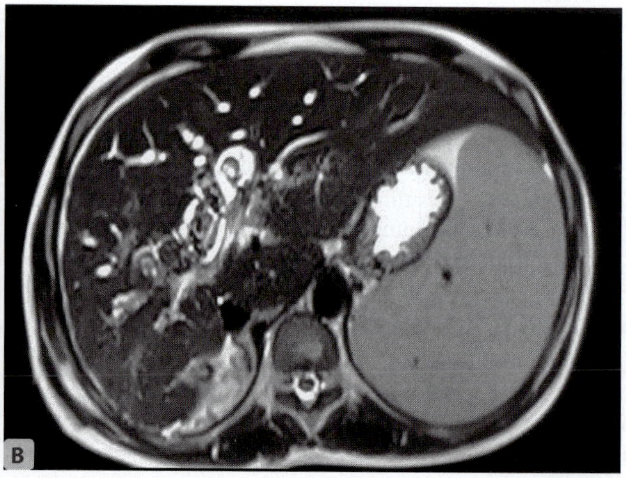

FIGS. 8A AND B: Oriental cholangiohepatitis. An 18-year-old female came with history of recurrent attack of abdominal pain, fever and jaundice. Axial CECT image (A) showing multiple large calculi within the dilated biliary ducts, which are seen signal voids within the ducts on axial T2WI (B).

Sjögren's syndrome, calcinosis, raynaud phenomenon, esophageal dysmotility, sclerodactyly and telangiectasia (CREST) syndrome, etc.

Imaging is not needed in most of the cases of PBC. The biliary tract abnormalities are reflection of the secondary changes of developing cirrhosis. However, when there is a diagnostic dilemma, imaging may be helpful in providing valuable information. On MRI, a fairly specific periportal halo sign is best seen on postcontrast T1W-FS portal venous phase or delayed scans.[17] It is seen with less conspicuity on T2WI as a low signal halo surrounding a high-signal-intensity center.[17] Hepatocellular carcinoma may be seen as a complication in around 5% of patients.

Autoimmune Hepatitis and Overlap Syndromes

Overlap syndrome is defined as a combination of PBC and autoimmune hepatitis, or PSC and autoimmune hepatitis. Autoimmune hepatitis leads to a more inflammatory reaction than seen in cases of PBC or PSC, where there is more cholestasis. Chronic inflammation in cases of autoimmune hepatitis begins in the periportal region and breaches the periportal plate thereby extending into the adjacent parenchyma. Autoimmune hepatitis affects younger women (15–40 years old) population, 3–4 times than men.[18,19]

A diagnosis is established when the work-up for the different causes of hepatitis is negative and abnormal findings are seen on serology with raised ANA, anti-SMA, or antibody to LKM 1.[18] Liver biopsy is required as an adjunct to establish the diagnosis and assessing the degree of inflammation.

MRI shows areas showing increased enhancement in liver parenchyma in early stages of the disease; and later on the varying degrees of fibrosis, generalized volume loss, and locoregional lymphadenopathy.[19] Up to 18% of patients with autoimmune biliary disorder have two diseases simultaneously.[20] The greater degree of inflammation in cases of autoimmune hepatitis warrants the use of immunosuppressive treatment in the patients with overlap syndrome.[20]

IgG4-related Biliary Involvement

IgG4-related disorder includes cholangitis; inflammatory pseudotumor; and IgG4 hepatopathy, which includes portal inflammation and/or interface hepatitis, lobular hepatitis, obstruction of large bile ducts, portal sclerosis, and canalicular cholestasis.[21,22] It is seen in up to 88% of cases of autoimmune pancreatitis, and the bile ducts are seen to be commonly involved after the involvement of pancreas in IgG4-related disorder. Involvement of the

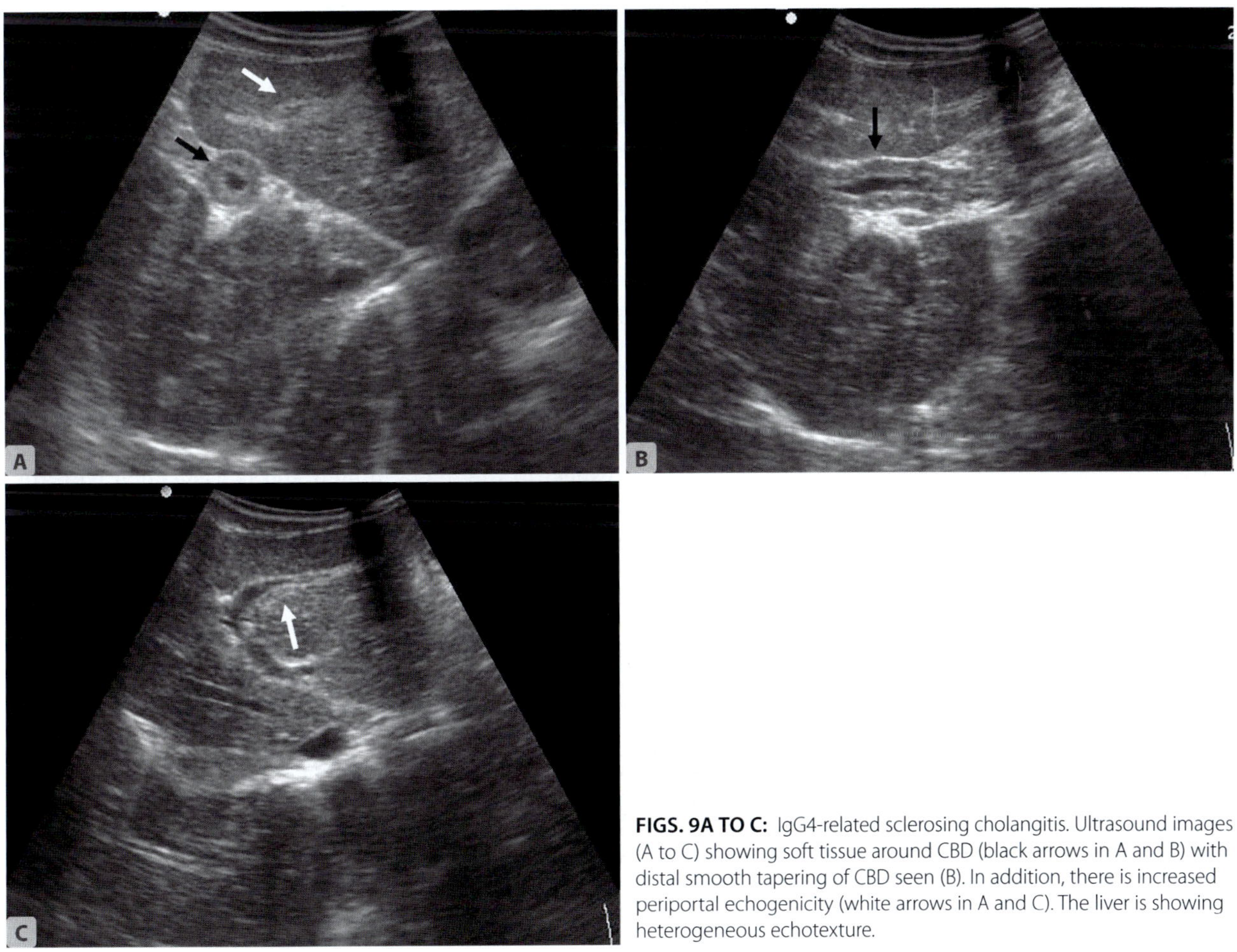

FIGS. 9A TO C: IgG4-related sclerosing cholangitis. Ultrasound images (A to C) showing soft tissue around CBD (black arrows in A and B) with distal smooth tapering of CBD seen (B). In addition, there is increased periportal echogenicity (white arrows in A and C). The liver is showing heterogeneous echotexture.

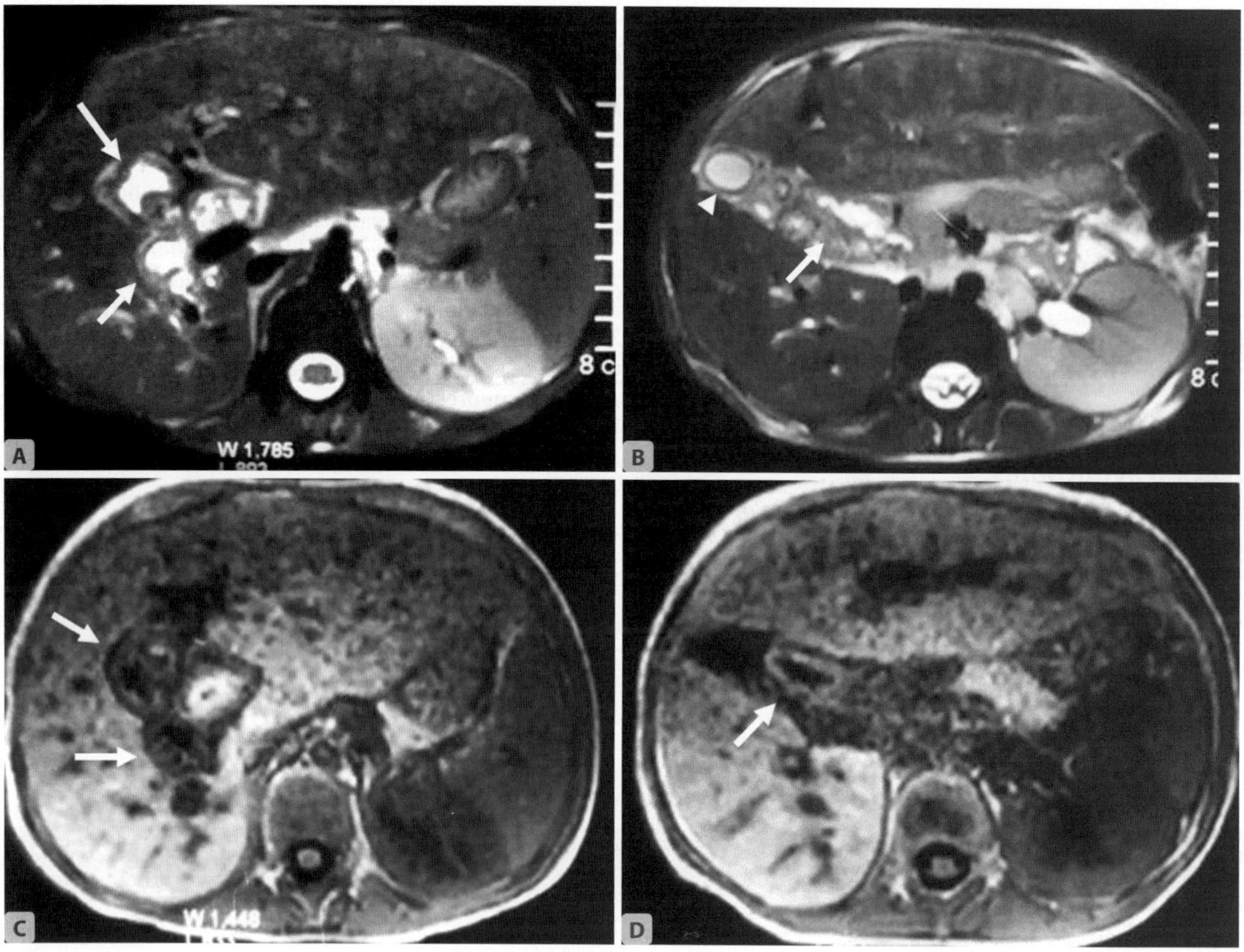

FIGS. 10A TO D: IgG4-related sclerosing cholangitis. MR images of the patient in Figure 9 showing diffusely heterogeneous signal intensity of the liver with increased periportal signal on T2WI (A and B). Soft tissue is seen around the biliary radicles (arrows in A and C) as well as around CBD (arrows in B and D) which is relatively hyperintense on T2WI (A and B) and isointense on T1WI (C and D). In addition, the wall of gallbladder is also thickened (arrowhead in B) suggesting acalculous cholecystitis.

biliary tree alone without the involvement of other organs is known to occur.

On cross-sectional imaging, the involved segments of the biliary tree show thickened walls with enhancement on contrast-enhanced scans, luminal narrowing, and stenosis. MRCP or ERCP shows the location and the degree of involvement and are useful in assessing the response to the treatment. Involvement of region of the porta with a soft tissue mass may simulate cholangiocarcinoma.[23]

Distinguishing between IgG4-related disease and overlap with primary sclerosing cholangitis may be challenging for the radiologist as the imaging findings in IgG4-related disease are not diagnostic. Clinically, primary sclerosing cholangitis occurs in the third to fourth decades and patients are typically less symptomatic than in IgG4-related sclerosing cholangitis, in which they have a more acute presentation of a smaller duration. Multifocal, short, band like strictures are seen in PSC, while the strictures of IgG4-related disease are typically long and show a continuity with segments of prestenotic dilatation. Isolated strictures involving the distal CBD only are also seen.[24]

The soft tissue around the common bile duct is another important diagnostic finding **(Figs. 9A to C)**. The soft tissue in primary sclerosing cholangitis is present to a lesser extent than in IgG4-related cholangitis. The inflammatory reaction of IgG4-related disease is centrifugal with respect to the ductal lumen and is associated with tiny fibroinflammatory nodules, while that in PSC is centripetal and is associated with degeneration and destruction of lining of the biliary tree.[25]

IgG4-related inflammatory hepatic pseudotumors have been classified as either fibrohistiocytic or lymphoplasmacytic by Zen et al.[26] depending on the histopathology. Lymphoplasmacytic type is more strongly associated with IgG4-related disease.[26]

On CT, homogeneous delayed enhancement has been considered an important imaging finding of IgG4-related disease.[27] On MRI, the lesions are hyperintense on T2WI, and isointense to hypointense on T1WI with variable contrast enhancement patterns **(Figs. 10A to D)**.[28] The differential diagnosis on imaging can be hepatocellular carcinoma, lymphoma and cholangiocarcinoma.

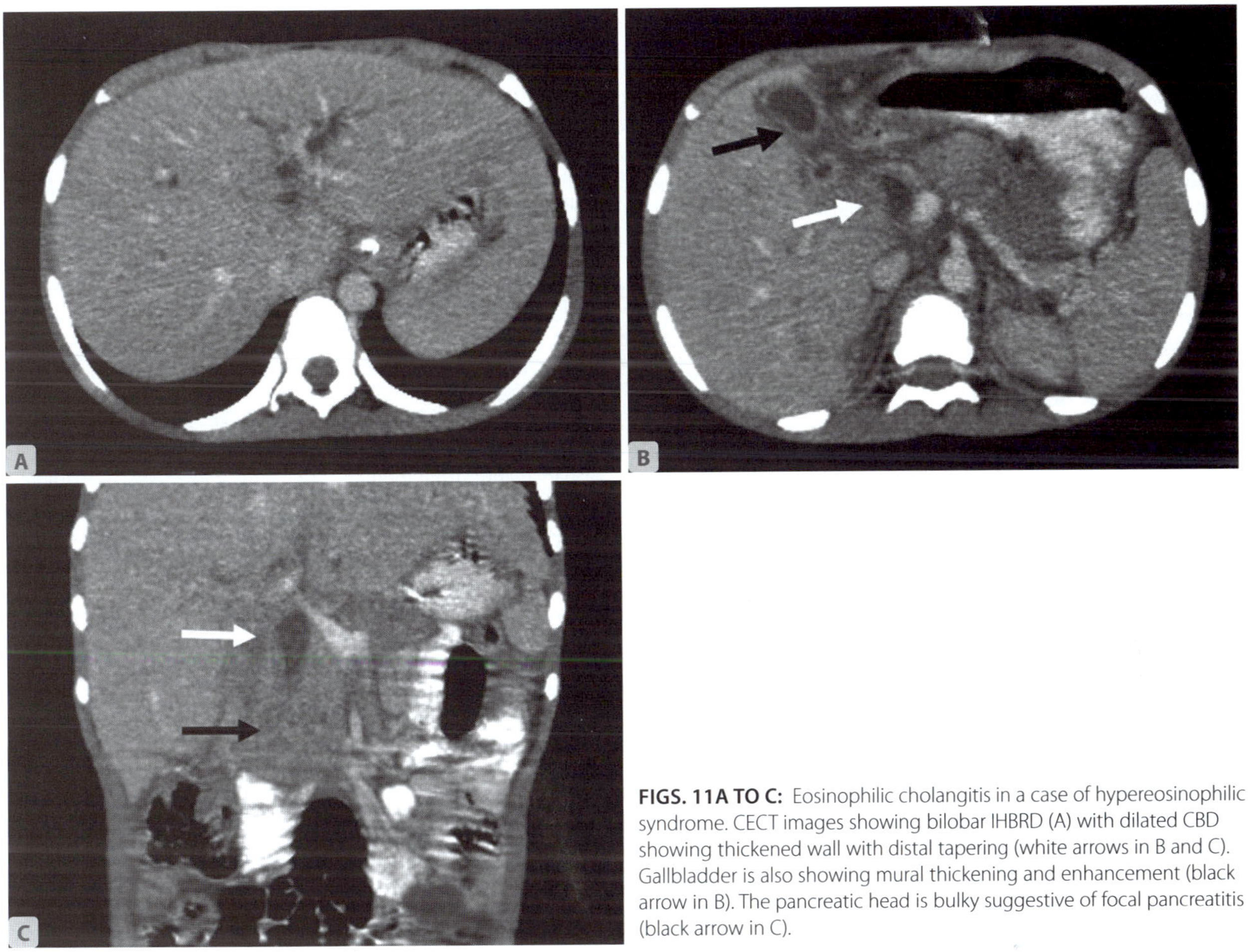

FIGS. 11A TO C: Eosinophilic cholangitis in a case of hypereosinophilic syndrome. CECT images showing bilobar IHBRD (A) with dilated CBD showing thickened wall with distal tapering (white arrows in B and C). Gallbladder is also showing mural thickening and enhancement (black arrow in B). The pancreatic head is bulky suggestive of focal pancreatitis (black arrow in C).

Involvement of the gallbladder, manifests as diffuse acalculous cholecystitis **(Fig. 10B)**, which can be seen in up to 25% of patients with IgG4-related sclerosing pancreatitis having concurrent IgG4-related sclerosing cholangitis. Though the imaging appearance of acalculous cholecystitis is nonspecific, there is extramural involvement predominantly with associated subserosal inflammatory nodular changes in IgG4-related disease.

Eosinophilic Cholangitis

It is usually seen in cases of eosinophilic gastroenteritis with radiologic and histologic features suggesting cholecystitis, chronic hepatitis, or cholangitis **(Figs. 11A to C)**. The patients rapidly respond well with corticosteroids.[15]

CONCLUSION

The gamut of biliary inflammatory disorders has changed and multiple etiologic factors for the inflammation of biliary tract have been proposed. Radiologists should be aware of these changing concepts regarding various pathophysiologic mechanisms and also understand the different approaches to imaging, as well as imaging findings of the various conditions involving the biliary tract.

REFERENCES

1. Raptopoulos V, Compton CC, Doherty P, et al. Chronic acalculous gallbladder disease: multi-imaging evaluation with clinical–pathologic correlation. AJR. 1986;147:721-4.
2. Yun EJ, Cho SG, Park S, et al. Chronic gallbladder carcinoma and chronic cholecystitis: differentiation with two-phase spiral CT. Abdom Imaging. 2004;29:102-8.
3. Bruljevac M, Busic Z, Cabrijan Z. Sonographic diagnosis of gallstone ileus. J Ultrasound Med. 2004;23:1395-8.
4. Chun KA, Ha HK, Yu ES, et al. Xanthogranulomatous cholecystitis: CT features with emphasis on differentiation from gallbladder carcinoma. Radiology. 1997;203:93-7.
5. Parra JA, Acinas O, Bueno J, Güezmes A, Fernández MA, Fariñas MC. Xanthogranulomatous cholecystitis: clinical, sonographic, and CT findings in 26 patients. AJR. 2000;174:979-83.
6. Roberts KM, Parsons MA. Xanthogranulomatous cholecystitis: clinicopathological study of 13 cases. J Clin Pathol. 1987;40:412-7.

7. Keaveny AP, Karasik MS. Hepatobiliary and pancreatic infections in AIDS: part II. AIDS Patient Care STDS. 1998;12:451-6.
8. Mahajani RV, Uzer MF. Cholangiopathy in HIV-infected patients. Clin Liver Dis. 1999;3:669-84.
9. Barthet M, Chauveau E, Bonnet E, et al. Pancreatic ductal changes in HIV-infected patients. Gastrointest Endosc. 1997;45:59-63.
10. Wiesner RH, LaRusso NF. Clinicopathologic features of the syndrome of primary sclerosing cholangitis. Gastroenterology. 1980;79:200-6.
11. Chapman RW, Jewell DP. Primary sclerosing cholangitis: an immunologically mediated disease? West J Med. 1985;143:193-5.
12. Crippin JS. Primary sclerosing cholangitis: etiology and immunology. Eur J Gastroenterol Hepatol. 1992;4:261-5.
13. Ueno Y, LaRusso NF. Primary sclerosing cholangitis. J Gastroenterol. 1994;29:531-43.
14. Lindor KD, Wiesner RH, MacCarty RL, Ludwig J, LaRusso NF. Advances in primary sclerosing cholangitis. Am J Med. 1990;89:73-80.
15. Vitellas KM, Keogan MT, Freed KS, et al. Radiologic manifestations of sclerosing cholangitis with emphasis on MR cholangiopancreatography. RadioGraphics. 2000;20:959-75.
16. Shea WJ Jr, Debas BE, Goldberg HI, Hohn DC, Ferrell LD, Kerlan RK. Sclerosing cholangitis associated with hepatic arterial FUDR chemotherapy: radiographic-histologic correlation. AJR. 1986;146:717-21.
17. Wenzel JS, Donohoe A, Ford KL III, et al. Primary biliary cirrhosis: MR imaging findings and description of MR imaging periportal halo sign. AJR. 2001;176:885-9.
18. Czaja AJ, Freese DK. Diagnosis and treatment of autoimmune hepatitis. Hepatology. 2002;36:479-96.
19. Bilaj F, Hyslop WB, Rivero H, et al. MR imaging findings in autoimmune hepatitis: correlation with clinical staging. Radiology. 2005;236:896-902.
20. Schramm C, Lohse AW. Overlap syndromes of cholestatic liver diseases and autoimmune hepatitis. Clin Rev Allergy Immunol. 2005;28:105-14.
21. Zen Y, Harada K, Sasaki M, et al. IgG4-related sclerosing cholangitis with and without hepatic inflammatory pseudotumor, and sclerosing pancreatitis-associated sclerosing cholangitis: do they belong to a spectrum of sclerosing pancreatitis? Am J Surg Pathol. 2004;28:1193-203.
22. Umemura T, Zen Y, Hamano H, et al. IgG4 associated autoimmune hepatitis: a differential diagnosis for classical autoimmune hepatitis. Gut. 2007;56:1471-2.
23. Vlachou PA, Khalili K, Jang HJ, Fischer S, Hirschfield GM, Kim TK. IgG4-related sclerosing disease: autoimmune pancreatitis and extrapancreatic manifestations. RadioGraphics. 2011;31:1379-402.
24. Nakazawa T, Ohara H, Sano H, et al. Cholangiography can discriminate sclerosing cholangitis with autoimmune pancreatitis from primary sclerosing cholangitis. Gastrointest Endosc. 2004;60:937-44.
25. Cheuk W, Chan JKC. IgG4-related sclerosing disease: a critical appraisal of an evolving clinicopathologic entity. Adv Anat Pathol. 2010;17:303-32.
26. Zen Y, Fujii T, Sato Y, Masuda S, Nakanuma Y. Pathological classification of hepatic inflammatory pseudotumor with respect to IgG4-related disease. Mod Pathol. 2007;20:884-94.
27. Naitoh I, Nakazawa T, Ohara H, et al. IgG4-related hepatic inflammatory pseudotumor with sclerosing cholangitis: a case report and review of the literature. Cases J. 2009;2:7029.
28. Anderson SW, Kruskal JB, Kane RA. Benign hepatic tumors and iatrogenic pseudotumors. RadioGraphics. 2009;29:211-29.

CHAPTER

109

Malignant Pathologies of Biliary Tree

Ujjwal Gorsi, Ajay Gulati, Mandeep Garg

INTRODUCTION

Biliary tract malignancies are the second most common hepatobiliary malignancy after hepatocellular carcinoma. These tumors can arise from any part of the biliary tract from smallest intra hepatic ductule to ampulla of Vater.[1] Most of the tumors that arise in biliary tree are adenocarcinomas as they occur as a consequence of malignant transformation of simple columnar epithelium which lines whole of the biliary tree and gallbladder.[2] Gallbladder cancer is the cancer arising from the gallbladder and the cystic duct. Cholangiocarcinoma can either be intrahepatic or extra hepatic. Cancer arising from the ampulla of Vater is included under the category of periampullary carcinomas which also include cancers arising from the terminal most common bile duct, head of pancreas and the duodenal bulb as they have similar clinical and radiological features and also the similar management.[3]

Patients with malignancies of biliary tree present clinically with symptoms of jaundice and right upper quadrant pain which are similar to many other benign conditions affecting the biliary tract. It is of paramount importance for the radiologist to be aware of imaging features of biliary tract malignancies so as to diagnose these tumors with certainty. In most of the instances, there is no single imaging test that will answer all clinical questions so multimodality imaging becomes necessary. The techniques routinely used to evaluate biliary tree pathologies include ultrasonography (USG), multidetector computed tomography (MDCT), magnetic resonance imaging (MRI) with magnetic resonance cholangiopancreatography (MRCP), endoscopic retrograde cholangiopancreatography (ERCP) and endoscopic ultrasound (EUS).

GALLBLADDER CARCINOMA

Gallbladder carcinoma is the cancer arising from gallbladder and cystic duct.[1] It is a notoriously lethal malignant tumor that is often discovered late.

Epidemiology

Gallbladder cancer is the seventh most common malignancy of the gastrointestinal tract and the most common malignant neoplasm of the biliary tree.[4] Some geographic areas have a high incidence of gallbladder cancer, including South America and India. The incidence of gallbladder cancer increases with age with more than 90% of patients being older than 50 years; the peak incidence is 70–75 years.[5]

In India, prevalence of gallbladder cancer is high in northern and northeastern states of Uttar Pradesh, Bihar, Orissa, West Bengal and Assam.[6] It is two times higher in women than men. In northern India cities, it is the most common digestive cancer in women.[7]

Risk Factors

Most common risk factor which is associated with gallbladder cancer is cholelithiasis with chronic inflammation and there are studies showing increase in risk of developing cancer as the size of stones increases.[8,9] Porcelain gallbladder is also a risk factor for developing gallbladder malignancy, however risk is not up to 22% which was reported in earlier studies[8] but between 7% and 15% as shown by newer studies.[10-12] Primary sclerosing cholangitis, congenital anomalous pancreaticobiliary duct junction and gallbladder polyps (solitary and symptomatic polyp >1 cm) are also associated with increased risk of developing gallbladder carcinoma. Other associations that are frequently implied include typhoid carrier state, chronic bacterial infections affecting gallbladder, and exposure to certain carcinogens.[8]

Pathological Features, Staging and Prognosis

Most carcinomas of the gallbladder are adenocarcinoma (85–90%) and can be papillary, tubular, mucinous, or signet cell type.[13] In gallbladder, most common location for the tumor to originate is fundus (60%) followed by body (30%) and neck (10%).[14] The gallbladder has unique anatomic features as its wall does not contain sub mucosa and at its hepatic attachment and along liver surface, there is no serosa. In addition, connective tissue of gallbladder is continuous with the interlobular connective tissue of the liver.[14] These anatomical features promote early local invasion into liver.

Gallbladder carcinoma is staged surgically by the depth of invasion, extension of disease into adjacent structures, involvement of lymph nodes, and presence of metastases

TABLE 1: TNM staging classification for gallbladder cancer (AJCC, 7th Edition).

TX	Primary tumor cannot be assessed		
T0	No evidence of primary tumor		
Tis	Carcinoma *in situ*		
Tla	Tumor invades lamina propria		
Tlb	Tumor invades muscular layer		
T2	Tumor invades perimuscular connective tissue		
T3	Tumor perforates serosa or directly invades the liver and/or one other adjacent organ		
T4	Tumor invades main portal vein or hepatic artery or invades multiple extra hepatic organs		
NX	Regional nodes cannot be assessed		
N0	No regional nodal metastasis		
N1	Metastasis to nodes along the cystic duct, common bile duct, hepatic artery and/or portal vein		
N2	Metastasis to periaortic, pericaval, superior mesenteric artery, and/or celiac artery lymph nodes		
M0	No distant metastasis		
MI	Distant metastasis		
Stage 0	Tis	N0	M0
Stage I	T1	N0	M0
Stage II	T2	N0	M0
Stage IIIA	T3	N0	M0
Stage IIIB	T1-3	N1	M0
Stage IVA	T4	N0-1	M0
Stage IVB	Any T	N2	M0
	Any T	Any N	M1

by the American Joint Committee on Cancer TNM staging system **(Table 1)**.[15]

Strongest prognostic factor gallbladder cancer is tumor stage. In a study, about 2500 patients with gallbladder malignancy from hospital cancer registries were analyzed and survival was related to tumor stage. 5 year survival for Stage 0 patients was 60%, for Stage I patients 39%, 15% for Stage II patients, 5% for Stage III patients and only 1% for Stage IV patients.[16]

IMAGING MODALITIES

The USG is often the initial imaging modality for suspected gallbladder cancer and many times it is on USG that a diagnosis of clinically unsuspected gallbladder malignancy will be suggested. The diagnostic accuracy of USG in gallbladder cancer is more than 80%, but it main limitation is its inability to stage the tumor.[17] Endoscopic USG can illustrate the depth of tumor invasion better and thus can overcome this limitation. In addition it helps in characterizing polypoid lesions involving gallbladder.[18] Dynamic contrast enhanced MDCT or MRI with MRCP are most useful imaging modalities for better depiction of the tumor morphology as well as staging. MRI may differentiate adenomyomatosis or xanthogranulomatous cholecystitis from gallbladder cancer, which may not be possible with other modalities. MRCP provides more detailed information than ultrasound or CT about biliary involvement of the tumor. In addition, adding diffusion-weighted imaging to the standard MRI protocol may improve sensitivity for distinguishing gallbladder cancers from other benign gallbladder diseases, which present with wall thickening.[19]

Radiological Findings

Radiologic Evaluation of the Primary Tumor

On imaging, gallbladder carcinoma can present as three patterns echoing the similar histologic patterns: a mass replacing or obscuring the gallbladder (most common), Intra luminal polypoid mass and mural thickening or irregularity of the wall of the gallbladder.[20]

Carcinoma Manifesting as a Gallbladder Fossa Mass

Most common presentation of gallbladder carcinoma is a large mass obscuring or replacing the gallbladder. This pattern is seen in 40–65%.[20] A large mass in gallbladder fossa that fills the lumen of gallbladder or replaces it and is seen invading the adjacent liver parenchyma is likely to be a gallbladder carcinoma.[21]

On USG, heterogeneous hypoechoic mass is seen in gallbladder fossa. Hyper echoic foci may be seen with in this mass, which are commonly due to calculi but may also represent porcelain gallbladder or tumor calcifications.[22]

On noncontrast CT gallbladder carcinoma is hypodense.[23] On MRI, on T1-weighted sequences gallbladder carcinomas hypo- to isointense and hyperintense on T2-weighted sequences.[20] On CT or MRI, after contrast administration, in early arterial phase, periphery of the mass may show enhancement which can be intense and irregular. During portal venous and delayed phases, contrast enhancement may be retained in fibrous stromal components of gallbladder carcinoma **(Figs. 1A to C)**. This feature helps in differentiating this tumor from large hepatocellular carcinomas (HCC) which may occur near the gallbladder fossa as HCC shows contrast material washout.[24] Other differential diagnoses include intra hepatic cholangiocarcinoma and metastasis to gallbladder fossa.[25]

Carcinoma Manifesting as a Polypoid Mass

Gallbladder carcinoma can present as intra luminal polypoid mass in 25% of cases and is more likely to be confined to the gallbladder at the time of diagnosis. These lesions are usually homogeneous and can be hyperechoic, isoechoic or hypoechoic on sonography and do not cast an acoustic shadow aiding in differentiation from gallstones. Necrosis or calcification is uncommon and the tumor shows homogeneous enhancement **(Figs. 2A to D)**. Small polypoid malignancies can be indistinguishable from cholesterol polyp, adherent noncalcified stone, adenoma, tumefactive sludge or blood clot. Polyps should be removed surgically if the size exceeds one cm, associated calculi are present, age of the patient is more than 50 years and the patient is

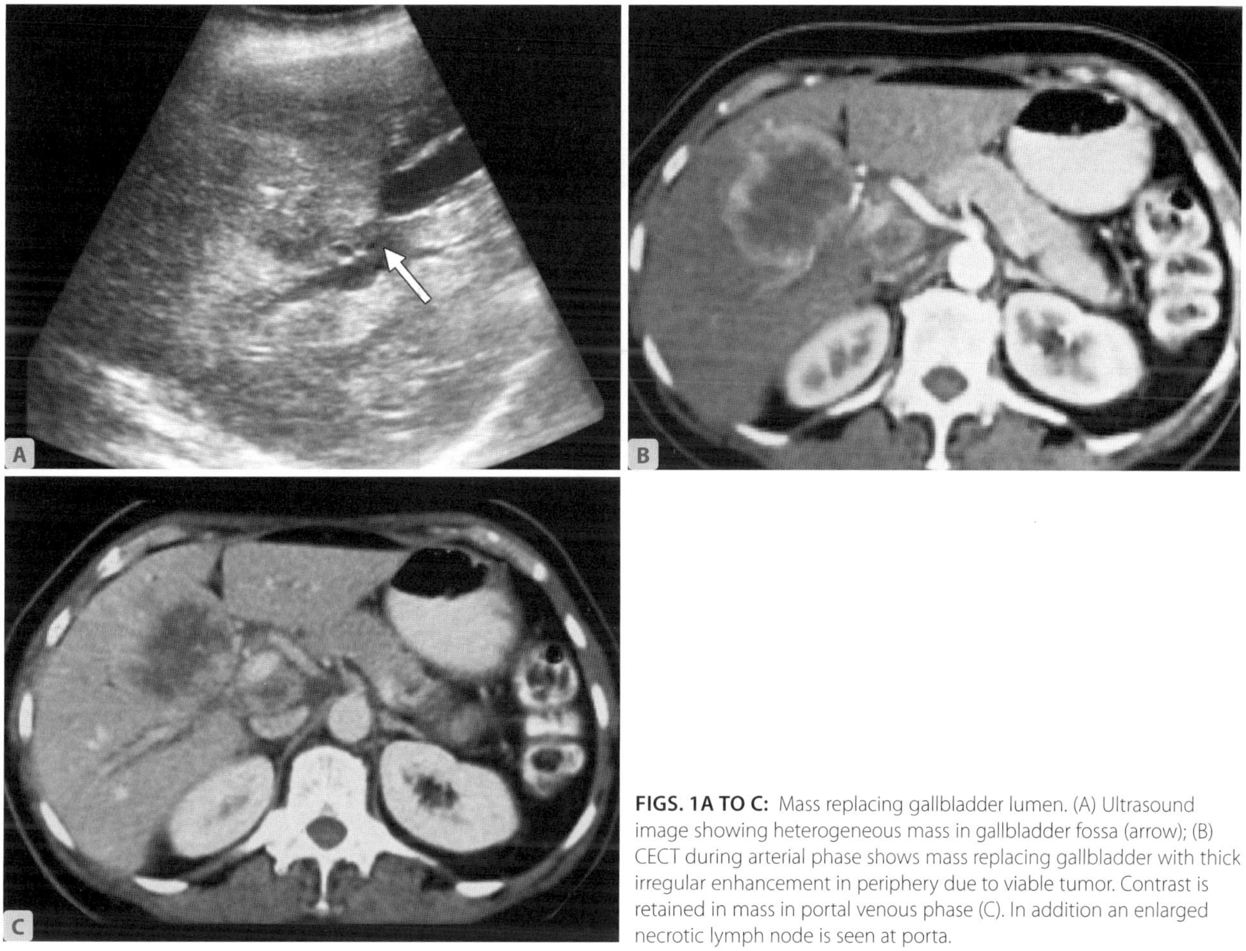

FIGS. 1A TO C: Mass replacing gallbladder lumen. (A) Ultrasound image showing heterogeneous mass in gallbladder fossa (arrow); (B) CECT during arterial phase shows mass replacing gallbladder with thick irregular enhancement in periphery due to viable tumor. Contrast is retained in mass in portal venous phase (C). In addition an enlarged necrotic lymph node is seen at porta.

symptomatic. Sludge is usually mobile when patient's position is changed, is more echogenic than tumor and does not show vascularity unlike tumor.[26]

Carcinoma Manifesting as Mural Thickening

The least common and most difficult to diagnose presentation of gallbladder malignancy is mural thickening which may be focal or diffuse.[27] The thickness of gallbladder wall up to 3 mm or less is considered normal and early lesions confined to the mucosa or slightly raised lesions are generally not picked up on ultrasound.[28] Gallstones can obscure subtle wall thickening associated with early malignancy. In general, benign entities, which include acute and chronic cholecystitis, adenomyomatosis, hepatitis, low protein states, inadequate distension and other causes, will cause diffuse mural thickening.[27] CT is inferior to ultrasound in depicting mucosal irregularity, mural thickening, and cholelithiasis however CT scores over ultrasound in evaluating the thickening of those portions of the gallbladder wall which are obscured by gallstones or mural calcification on USG.[28]

On contrast-enhanced MDCT, thick (>2.5 mm) and strong enhancement of the inner wall and irregular contour of the affected wall are considered significant predictors for malignancy while evaluating gallbladder wall thickening **(Figs. 3A to D)**.[29-31] When CT shows focal or irregular mural thickening of the gallbladder, careful inspection of the images should be done to look for bile duct dilation, local invasion, lymphadenopathy or metastasis[30] as presence of these help in predicting malignancy. Multiplanar reformatted images of MDCT scans are valuable for demonstrating extent of gallbladder cancers as well as relationship with adjacent organs.[27]

On MRI mural thickening will be hyperintense on T2-weighted sequences. Studies have demonstrated that diffusion-weighted MRI can improve the diagnostic capability for gallbladder wall thickening or polypoid lesions by demonstrating high signal on high b value diffusion-weighted imaging and a lower apparent diffusion coefficient value of gallbladder cancers than that of benign gallbladder diseases.[19]

Pathways of Tumor Spread

Pathway of gallbladder cancer spread include: Direct invasion of the liver, hepatoduodenal ligament, duodenum, or colon; lymphatic spread to regional and retroperitoneal lymph nodes; intraductal tumor extension; hematogenous spread to the liver and peritoneal spread **(Fig. 4)**. Distant metastases are unusual.

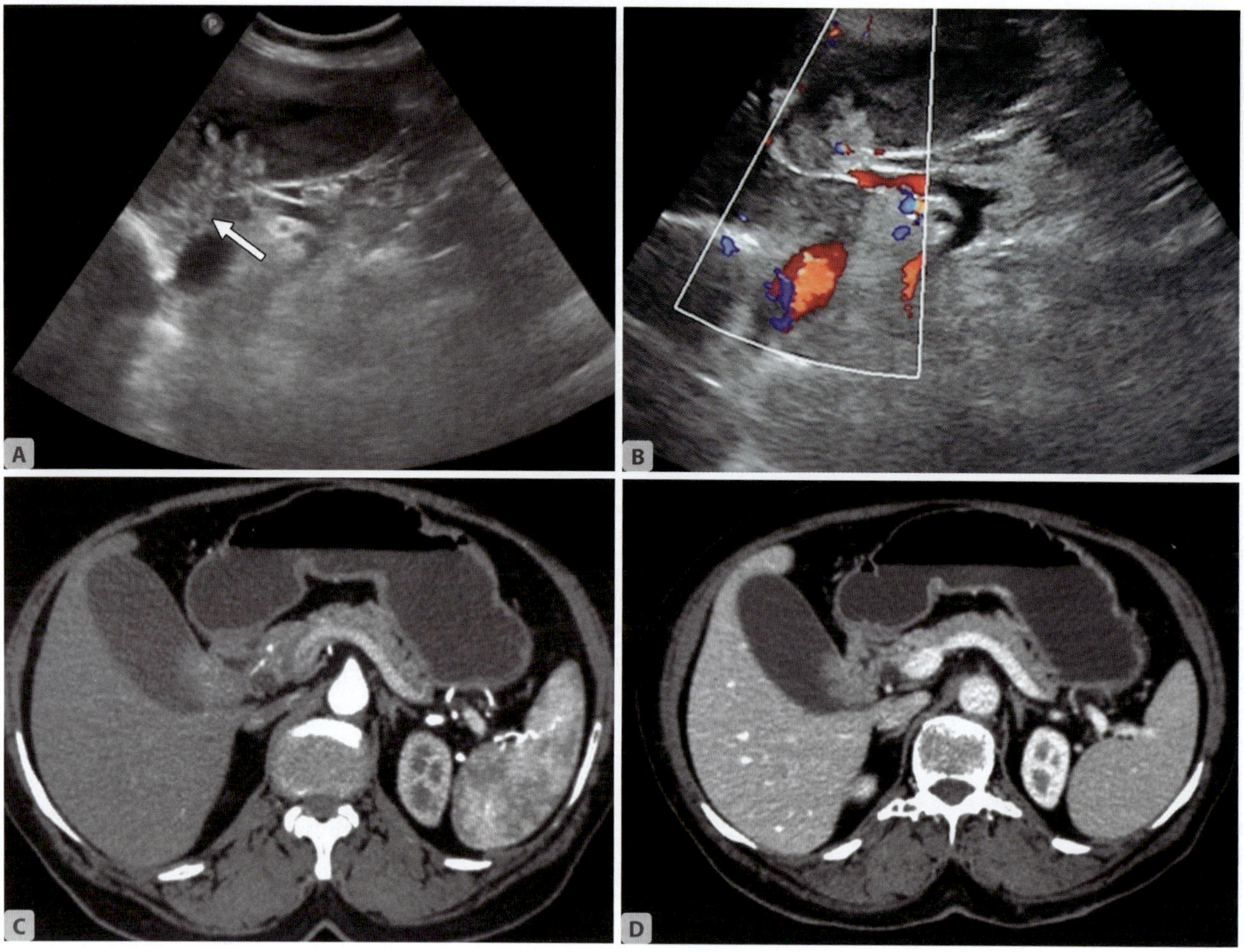

FIGS. 2A TO D: Intraluminal polyp. (A) Grayscale ultrasound image showing echogenic polypoid lesion in region of gallbladder neck (arrow) with no posterior acoustic shadow; (B) Color Doppler shows vascularity with in the lesion. CECT during arterial phase (C) and venous phase (D) shows homogeneously enhancing polypoid lesion with no arterial hypervascularity and no extension outside the gallbladder.

Gallbladder carcinoma spreads most commonly by direct invasion of the liver.[32] Invasion of the gastro hepatic ligament may lead to biliary obstruction at the porta hepatis. Compression of common bile duct (CBD) by lymphadenopathy, intra ductal tumor growth and choledocholithiasis are other causes of biliary obstruction in a patient of gallbladder malignancy.

There is a rich lymphatic drainage of gallbladder which facilitates rapid spread to lymph nodes most commonly at the porta hepatis, peri pancreatic and para aortic region. In determining the T stage of gallbladder carcinoma, MDCT has a accuracy of up to 84%.[29] MDCT has accuracy of 85% in predicting respectability.[33] Sensitivity and specificity of multi phasic MRI with MRCP in detecting hepatic invasion, lymph node metastasis and bile duct invasion is 87.5% and 86%, 60% and 90%, and 80% and 100%, respectively.[34]

OTHER MALIGNANT GALLBLADDER NEOPLASMS

Metastasis to the gallbladder are rare but may occur. Among the most common primary malignant neoplasms which may present as gallbladder metastasis are melanoma, breast carcinoma, hepatocellular carcinoma, and lymphoma.[24] Most of the times it is not possible to differentiate between metastatic neoplasms and primary gallbladder carcinoma except that gallstones will be seen less frequently in patients with metastases.

Cholangiocarcinoma

Cholangiocarcinoma is a malignant tumor arising from the epithelium of bile duct which is usually diagnosed late and is associated with poor outcome.

Epidemiology

Cholangiocarcinoma is the second most common primary hepatobiliary malignancy after hepatocellular carcinoma. This malignancy has poor prognosis. 5-year survival rate is less than 5%.[35] Its incidence shows distinct geographic variation, with the highest prevalence in far east and Southeast Asia,[36] where liver fluke infection and choledocholithiasis are common. Men are affected more often then women with a male-to-female ratio of 1.3: 1. Most of the tumors are diagnosed between 50 and 70 years.[37]

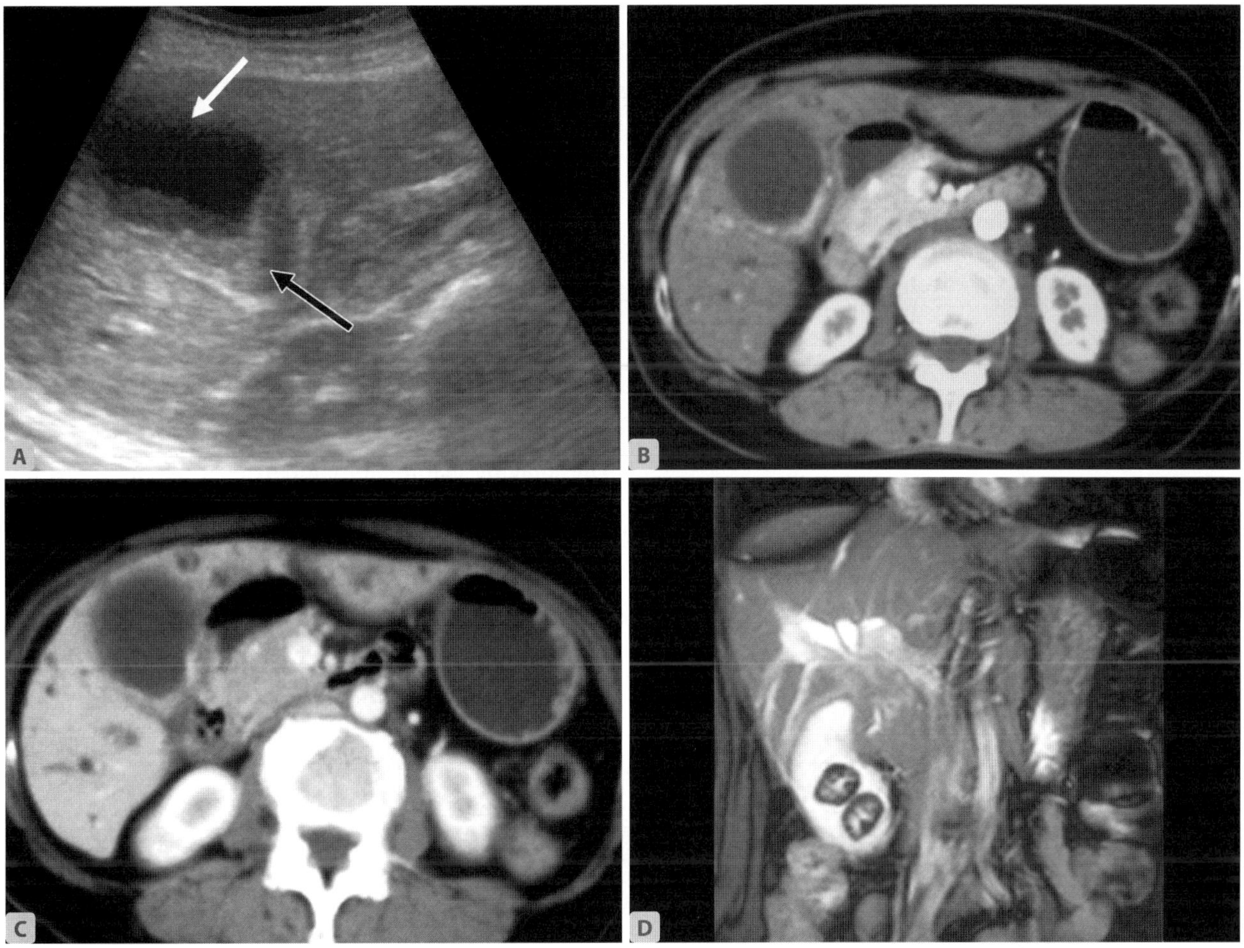

FIGS. 3A TO D: Asymmetric mural thickening. (A) Grayscale ultrasound image showing distended gallbladder (white arrow) and asymmetric irregular mural thickening involving gallbladder neck; CECT during arterial phase (B) and portal venous phase (C) shows layered pattern of enhancement of gallbladder wall thickening with hyperattenuating inner wall; (D) T2 axial TrueFisp coronal image depicting mural thickening in gallbladder neck and calculi in gallbladder.

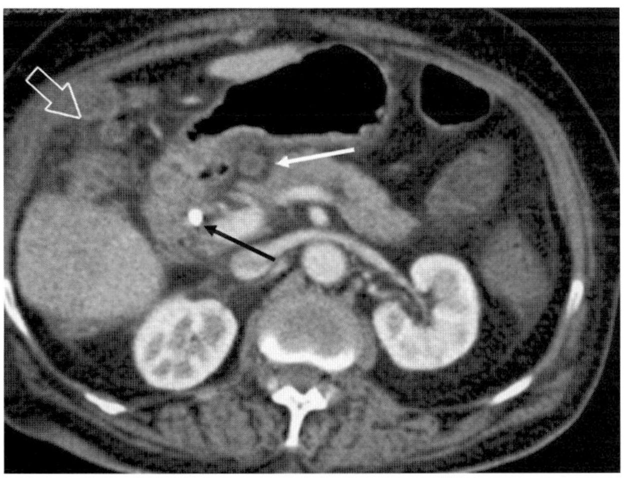

FIG. 4: CECT image showing multiple peritoneal deposits (block arrow) from a gallbladder carcinoma (not shown). Also seen is a metastatic necrotic peripancreatic lymph node (arrow). CBD stent is seen *in situ* (arrow).

Risk Factors

Risk factors for developing cholangiocarcinoma include primary sclerosing cholangitis (PSC), choledochal cyst, congenital hepatic fibrosis, hepatolithiasis, familial polyposis, liver flukes, chronic typhoid carriers and a history of exposure to thorotrast.[38] Patients who have cystic bile duct disorders (Caroli's disease and choledochal cyst) have a life time incidence of cholangiocarcinoma which may range from 6% to 30%.[39] A higher prevalence of positive anti-hepatitis C antibody is associated with this tumor. Cirrhotic patients have ten-fold higher risk of developing cholangiocarcinoma than the general population.[36,40]

Pathology and Classification

More than 95% of cholangiocarcinomas are adenocarcinoma originating from bile duct epithelium and are well or moderately differentiated adenocarcinomas. These tumors tend to have early perineural invasion and are often associated with desmoplastic reaction.[41]

Cholangiocarcinoma are classified based on their anatomical location as intrahepatic or extrahepatic cholangiocarcinoma with the later being more common. Intrahepatic cholangiocarcinoma is also called peripheral cholangiocarcinoma. A tumor that arises peripheral to the secondary bifurcation of the left or right hepatic duct is considered an intra hepatic cholangiocarcinoma. Extra hepatic cholangiocarcinomas are classified into hilar and distal tumors. Hilar cholangiocarcinomas occur at or near the primary biliary confluence where as distal cholangiocarinoma arise from extra hepatic bile duct above the ampulla of Vater.[27] Perihilar disease is most common and represents about 50%, of cholangiocarcinoma cases. Distal disease account for 40%, and intrahepatic disease less than 10% of cholangiocarcinoma cases.[42] From a treatment point of view, these types are considered as distinct entities. Intrahepatic tumors are treated with hepatectomy, hilar malignancies are managed with resection of the bile duct, preferably with hepatectomy where as extrahepatic tumors are treated similar to periampullary malignant neoplasms with pancreato duodenectomy.[27]

On the basis of morphology, cholangiocarcinoma are classified into three types:

1. Mass-forming type which often shows necrosis and fibrosis in the center and accompanying satellite nodules.
2. Periductal infiltrative type, which present as tumor growth along the bile duct longitudinally often resulting in concentric mural thickening and upstream biliary tree dilatation and may be associated with dense fibroblastic reaction.
3. Intra ductal growing papillary cholangiocarcinoma which present as intra luminal papillary tumors which may involve intrahepatic or extrahepatic bile ducts. This tumor leads to obstruction and dilation of the bile ducts due to abundant much in production. The primary tumor is usually small but may result in multiple tumors involving adjacent segments of bile ducts as it can spread superficially along the mucosal surface.[43,44]

Radiological Findings

The imaging features of cholangiocarcinoma depend on tumor location and type.

Intrahepatic Cholangiocarcinoma

Mass-forming intrahepatic cholangiocarcinoma most commonly presnt on imaging as well-defined mass with irregular borders.[45,46] It lacks the fibrous capsule found in hepatocellular carcinoma (HCC). Peripheral intrahepatic cholangiocarcinoma are usually large at presentation

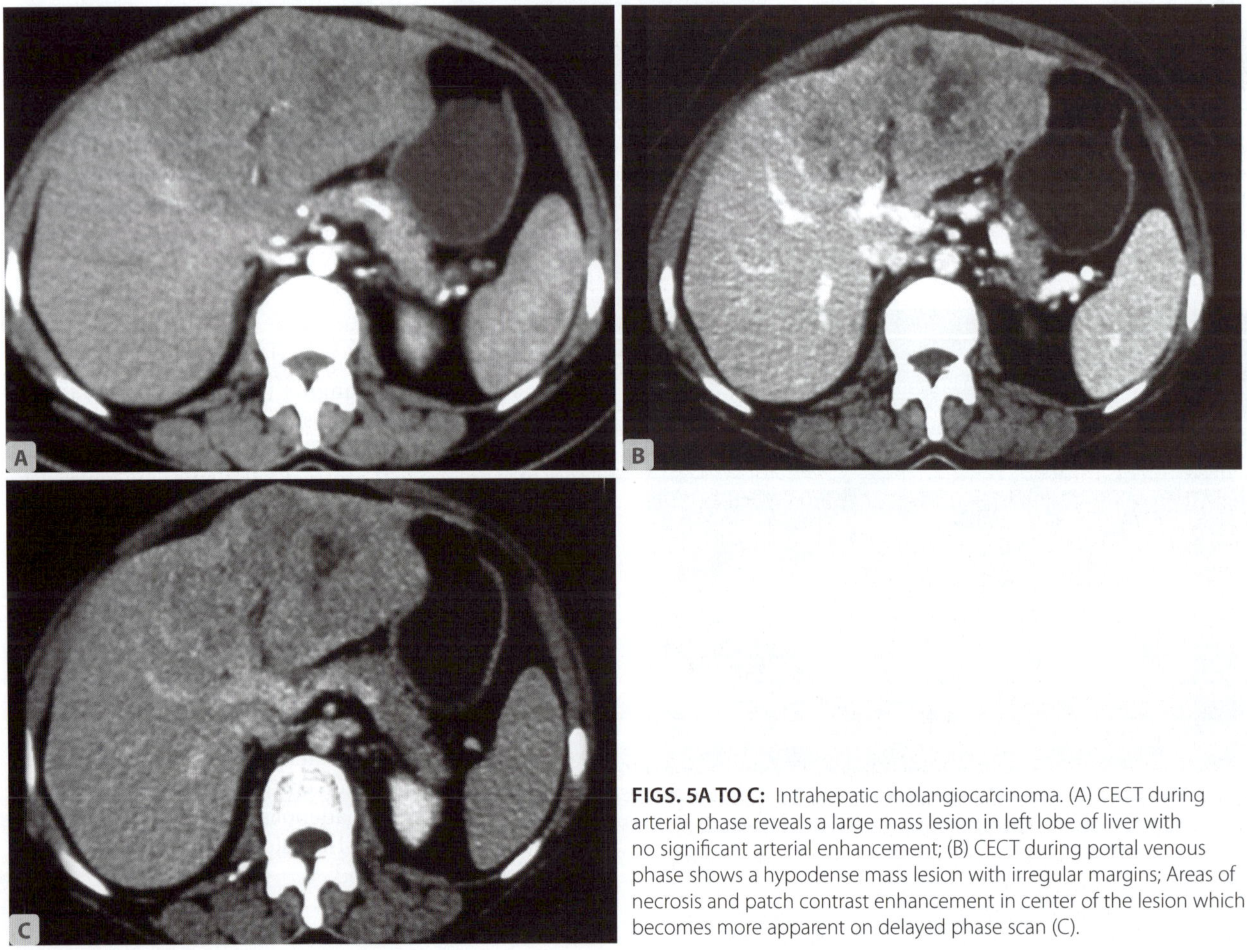

FIGS. 5A TO C: Intrahepatic cholangiocarcinoma. (A) CECT during arterial phase reveals a large mass lesion in left lobe of liver with no significant arterial enhancement; (B) CECT during portal venous phase shows a hypodense mass lesion with irregular margins; Areas of necrosis and patch contrast enhancement in center of the lesion which becomes more apparent on delayed phase scan (C).

because symptoms occur late. Ultrasonography reveals a hypoechoic, isoechoic or hyper echoic mass, which may be homogeneous or heterogeneous. Unenhanced CT reveals a hypodense solitary mass that may have satellite lesions. Focal intrahepatic biliary ductal dilatation, segmental atrophy and capsular retraction may be seen. On MRI, intrahepatic cholangiocarcinoma is hypointense on T1-weighted images and hyper intense on T2-weighted images.[47] On enhanced CT/MRI, the tumor may shows thin rim or thick band of peripheral and patchy enhancement in early phase corresponding to active tumor growth. The central area of the tumor, due to its fibrous composition, does not enhance during early phase but may show enhancement during the delayed phase, a feature which may help to differentiate it from HCC **(Figs. 5A to C)**.[48] The delayed enhancement may be bright enough to simulate hemangioma.

Peripheral cholangiocarcinoma can also be of periductal infiltrating type or intra ductal polypoidal type and these may cause segmental bile duct dilatation and lobar atrophy **(Figs. 6A to C)**. Polypoidal (papillary) variant can occasionally produce abundant mucin similar to IPMT of the pancreas. This can result in gross dilatation of the bile duct. Demonstration of direct continuity of tumor with bile ducts helps differentiate this entity from biliary cystadenocarcinoma. Hypovascular metastases can have an enhancement pattern similar to that of peripheral cholangiocarcinomas. Absence of a known primary malignant neoplasm, relatively large tumor size, and bile duct dilation suggest a diagnosis of cholangiocarcinoma rather than metastases.[45]

Hilar Cholangiocarcinoma (Klatskin's tumor)

Hilar cholangiocarcinoma are usually periductal infiltrating type and most often arise at the primary confluence or in the proximal common hepatic duct. Sonographic findings include intrahepatic bile ductal dilatation with or without isolation of right and left sided ducts and lobar atrophy. Definite mass is rarely seen on US and demonstration of dilated intrahepatic ducts without any evidence of extrahepatic dilatation alone should raise the suspicion of hilar cholangiocarcinoma. Sometimes tumor may be seen on sonography as bile duct wall thickening and less commonly may be seen as a polypoidal lesion. The tumors are moderately echogenic, reflecting the fibrous nature of the tumor. MDCT with its multi planer abilities is superior to USG in identification of these small tumors.[49] Although the tumor appears hypodense to liver in both unenhanced and enhanced CT scans, the focally thickened bile duct wall due to infiltrating tumor may appear hyper dense to the liver in the arterial and portal venous phase. In keeping with their fibrous rich stroma, delayed enhancement can be seen 8–15 minutes after contrast injection.[50] Cholangiocarcinoma are isointense/hypointense

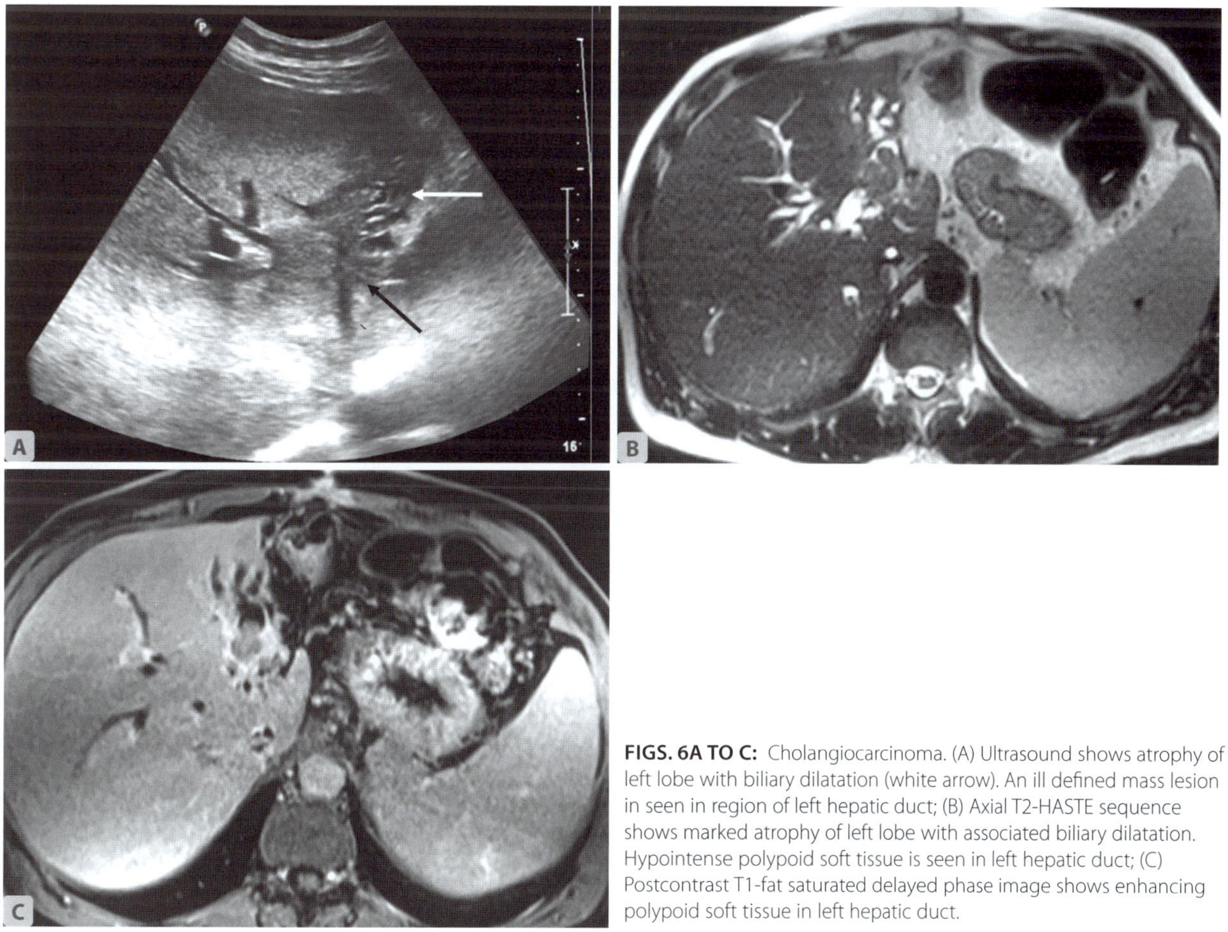

FIGS. 6A TO C: Cholangiocarcinoma. (A) Ultrasound shows atrophy of left lobe with biliary dilatation (white arrow). An ill defined mass lesion in seen in region of left hepatic duct; (B) Axial T2-HASTE sequence shows marked atrophy of left lobe with associated biliary dilatation. Hypointense polypoid soft tissue is seen in left hepatic duct; (C) Postcontrast T1-fat saturated delayed phase image shows enhancing polypoid soft tissue in left hepatic duct.

on T1-weighted images while T2 signal varies from markedly hyperintense to only mildly increased signal in fibrous tumors. Lobar hepatic atrophy is seen in one fourth of patients with cholangiocarcinoma and this finding coupled with biliary dilatation is strongly suggestive of cholangiocarcinoma. Atrophy results from long standing biliary obstruction or portal venous involvement and results in crowding of dilated bile ducts and volume loss most often affecting the left lobe of liver.[48] Contiguous invasion of the liver parenchyma and hepatoduodenal ligament is frequent in Klatskin tumors. Lymph nodal metastases can be seen in peri portal and peri pancreatic regions. Retroperitoneal adenopathy, proximal intestinal obstruction and peritoneal dissemination occur in advanced stages. Diagnostic percutaneous transhepatic cholangiography (PTC) and ERCP are now less commonly employed for cholangiocarcinoma. The involved ducts appear stenosed with smooth shouldering or irregular tapering. MDCT and cholangiography provide complimentary information as superficial (mucosal) involvement is better assessed on direct cholangiography while submucosal/extra mucosal involvement and areas not opacified on cholangiography are better seen on CT. Contrast enhanced MRI with MRCP can provide most comprehensive tumor staging.[51] EUS with EUS-guided FNA is increasingly being used for characterizing biliary strictures and assessing extent of periductal involvement and lymph nodal metastasis.[52] Hilar cholangiocarcinomas are commonly periductal infiltrating type though intra ductal papillary tumor may also be seen. The intra ductal tumors are hyperdense on noncontrast CT (NCCT) images and are hypodense on postcontrast images as they lack fibrotic stroma. These tumors when multiple can be confused with calculi. Contrast enhancement in these tumors help in differentiating these tumors from stones.[53,54]

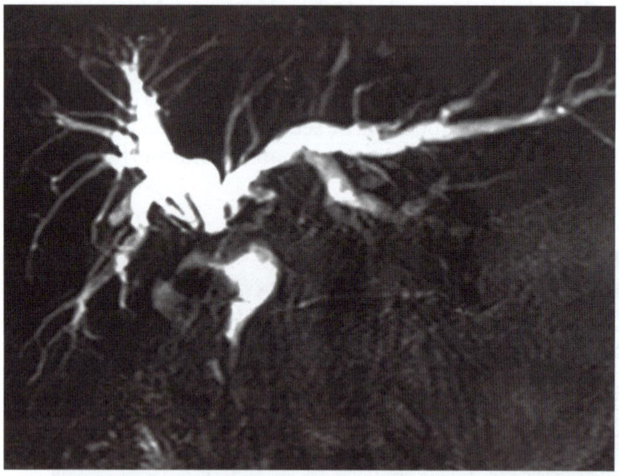

FIG. 7: Perihilar cholangiocarcinoma type 1: Coronal reconstructed MRCP image showing abrupt cut off of common hepatic duct with proximal biliary dilatation.

Nonresectability of hilar cholangiocarcinoma is suggested by:[55,56]

- Severe bilateral involvement of the secondary confluence
- Involvement of the main portal vein
- Involvement of both branches of the portal vein
- Bilateral involvement of the hepatic artery and portal vein
- Vascular involvement on one side of the liver and extensive bile duct involvement on the other side.

Perihilar cholangiocarcinoma are graded according to modified Bismuth-Corlette classification. The original Bismuth-Corlette system[57] classified perihilar cholangiocarcinoma into three types: type I, tumor distal to the confluence of the left and right hepatic ducts; **(Fig. 7)** type II, tumors involving the main biliary confluence and the main left or right ducts but not extending into the secondary level of ductal confluences; **(Figs. 8A and B)** type III, extension into the confluence of either the left or right hepatic ducts. The modified Bismuth-Corlette system[58] divided type III hilar cholangiocarcinoma into types IIIa and IIIb and added a type IV. Type IIIa is tumor extension beyond the confluence of the right hepatic duct into secondary biliary radicles, type IIIb involves similar extension into the left hepatic ductal system **(Fig. 9)**. Type IV signifies tumor extension to bilateral secondary biliary radicles **(Figs. 10A to C)**.

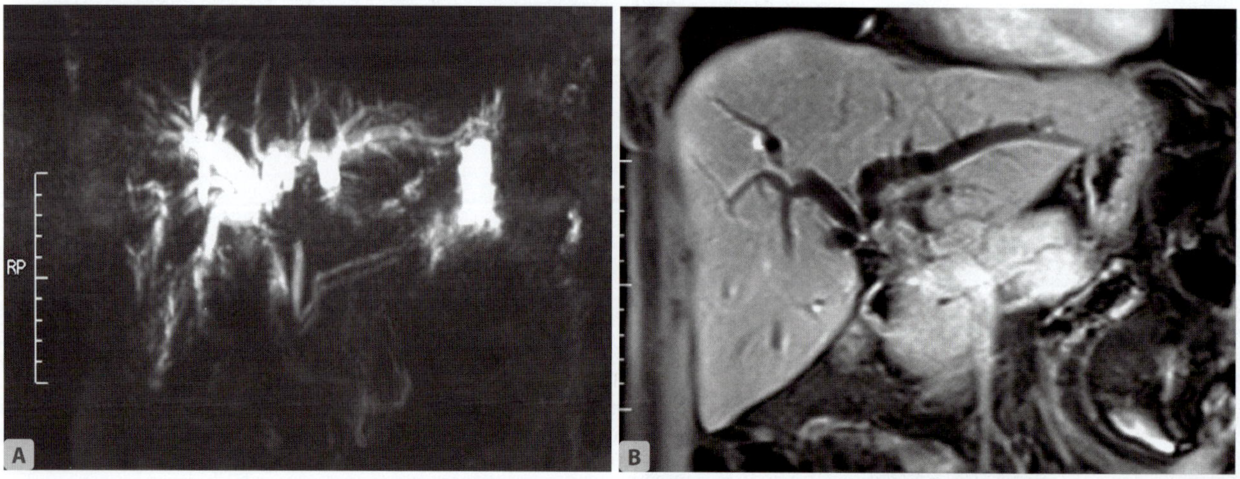

FIGS. 8A AND B: Perihilar cholangiocarcinoma type 2. (A) Coronal reconstructed MRCP image showing stricture involving the common hepatic duct and primary biliary confluence; (B) Postcontrast T1-fat saturated image showing ill defined poorly enhancing soft tissue at primary biliary confluence.

Distal Cholangiocarcinoma

Distal cholangiocarcinoma is the tumor arising from common bile duct between the origin of cystic duct and the ampulla of Vater. Tumors arising from ampulla are not included in distal cholangiocarcinomas.[44] These are usually small and have better prognosis than perihilar cholangiocarcinomas. Imaging features include biliary dilatation proximal to an abrupt obstruction. Mass itself is rarely demonstrated on imaging hence differentiation from benign strictures may not be possible. Cholangiocarcinoma should be suspected when abrupt obstruction of common bile duct is seen without visualization of a mass or calculus and the pancreas is normal in the absence of history of previous surgery. Carcinoma of the pancreas is more likely if the mass is seen near head of the pancreas.[59] Even with all imaging modalities, differentiating between benign and malignant biliary strictures is sometimes difficult. Longer and thicker involvement by the stricture, irregularity of lumen, asymmetric narrowing, hyper enhancement in portal venous phase, periductal soft tissue mass, and enlarged lymph node are associated with malignant stricture.[60] ERCP and EUS are important for complete evaluation of these tumors. EUS-FNA is very useful to predict unresectability.[61]

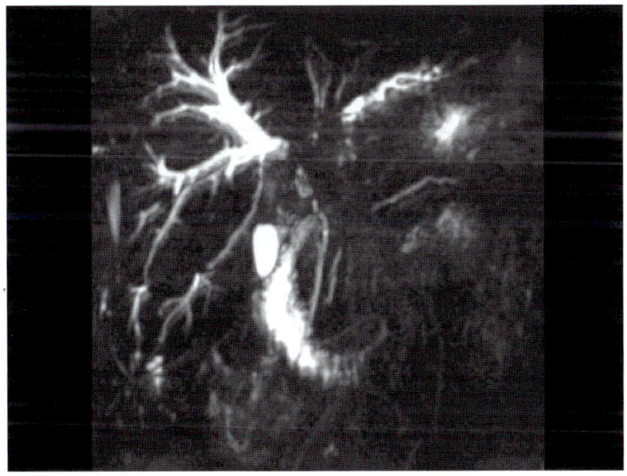

FIG. 9: Perihilar cholangiocarcinoma type 3b: Coronal reconstructed MRCP image showing stricture involving main biliary confluence and extending into left secondary confluence.

Periampullary Carcinoma

Periampullary carcinomas are those tumors arising from or within 1 cm of the papilla of Vater and include ampullary, pancreatic, bile duct, and duodenal malignancies.[3] It is often impossible by imaging or even by histologic examination to know the origin of tumor with certainty. Patients with familial adenomatous polyposis have higher incidence of these

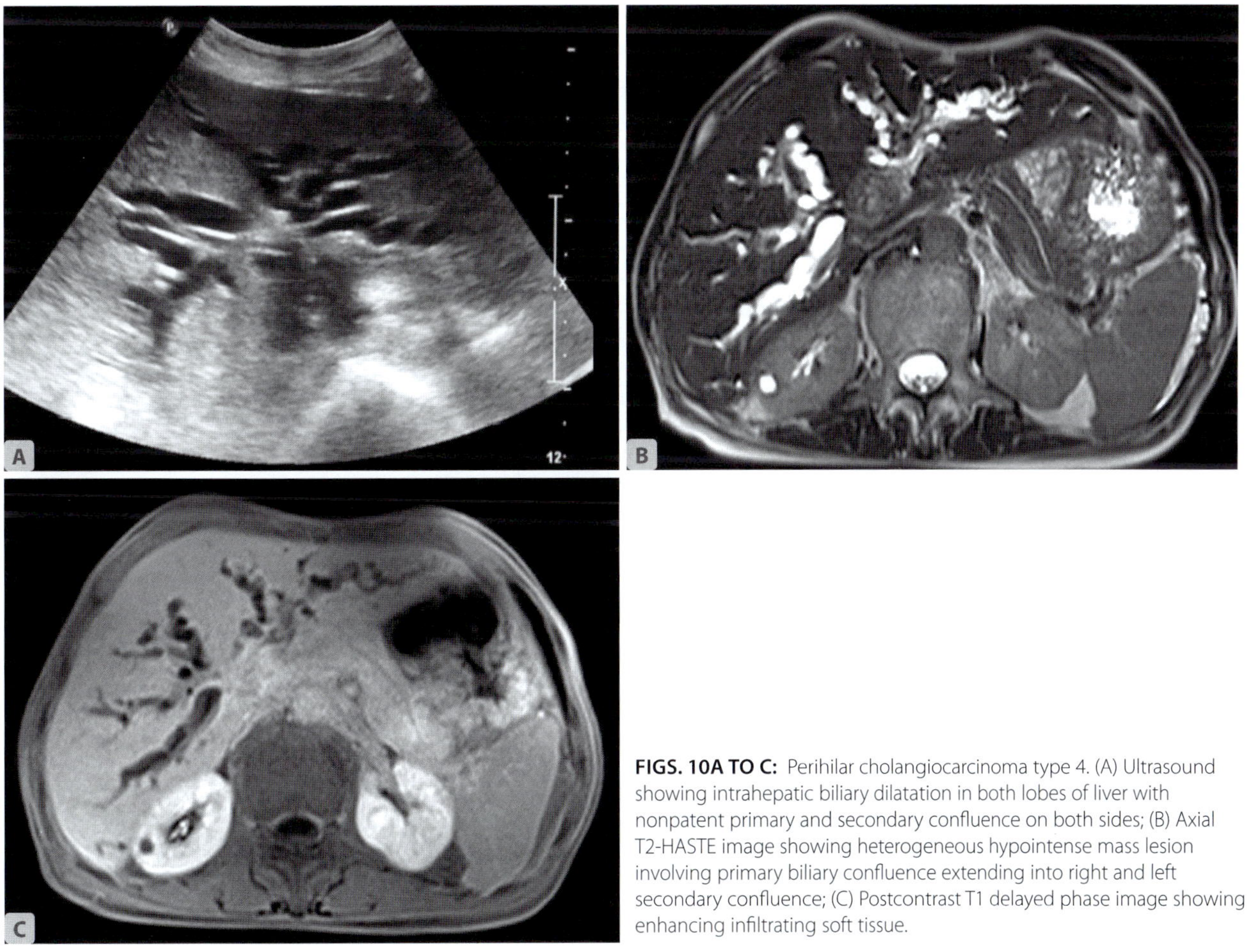

FIGS. 10A TO C: Perihilar cholangiocarcinoma type 4. (A) Ultrasound showing intrahepatic biliary dilatation in both lobes of liver with nonpatent primary and secondary confluence on both sides; (B) Axial T2-HASTE image showing heterogeneous hypointense mass lesion involving primary biliary confluence extending into right and left secondary confluence; (C) Postcontrast T1 delayed phase image showing enhancing infiltrating soft tissue.

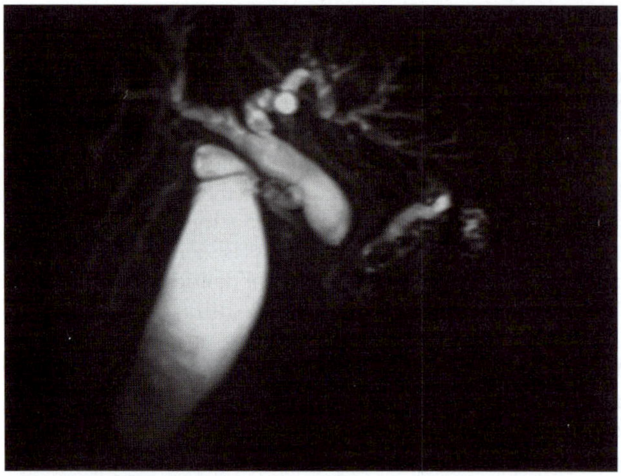

FIG. 11: Periampullary carcinoma: Coronal reconstructed MRCP image showing biliary dilatation with dilatation of both CBD and MPD (Double duct sign).

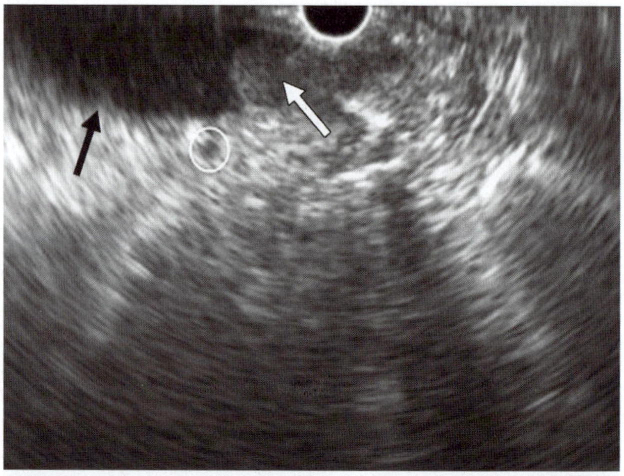

FIG. 12: Periampullary carcinoma: Endoscopic ultrasound image using linear EUS probe shows dilated CBD (black arrow) and polypoid hypoechoic mass in terminal CBD (white arrow). MPD (encircled) is not dilated. Findings are consistent with terminal bile duct cholangiocarcinoma.

Courtesy: Dr SS Rana, Department of Gastroenterology, PGIMER, Chandigarh, India.

tumors and are often preceded by duodenal or ampullary adenomas.[62] These tumors are usually of lower grade than proximal biliary malignancies. Periampullary tumors may not be seen on imaging, in which case a dilated common bile duct and dilated main pancreatic duct with abrupt termination in the head of pancreas is usually seen **(Fig. 11)**. Dilation of common bile duct is observed in 75% of cases, and pancreatic ductal dilation is seen in 67%.[62,63] On imaging if periampullary tumors are visualized they tend to be small and are likely to have a polypoidal growth pattern **(Fig. 12)**. Nodal and hepatic metastasis are rare at the time of diagnosis.

On T1-weighted images, periampullary tumors are usually hypo intense. On immediate postgadolinium T1-weighted images, these lesions will show low signal intensity due to their hypo vascular character compared with background pancreatic tissue.[63] On two minute delayed images, a thin rim of peripheral enhancement may be seen. ERCP though invasive will permit biopsy and stent placement. Sensitivity of EUS in detecting small periampullary tumor matches that of ERCP and is better than CT **(Fig. 13)**.[64] EUS shows the depth of invasion into the duodenum and local extension of the tumor. It may be the most accurate modality for assessing local staging of ampullary tumors.[65]

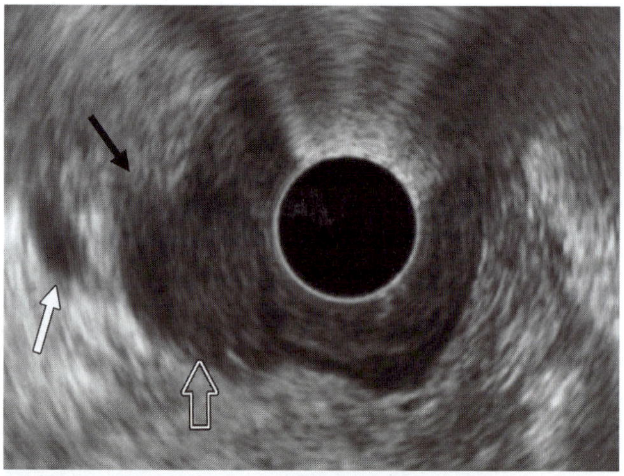

FIG. 13: Periampullary carcinoma: Endoscopic ultrasound (EUS) image using radial EUS probe shows dilated CBD (black arrow), dilated MPD (white arrow) and hypoechoic mass in ampulla (block arrow). Findings are consistent with ampullary carcinoma.

Courtesy: Dr SS Rana, Department of Gastroenterology, PGIMER, Chandigarh, India.

Malignant Cystic Bile Duct Neoplasms: Cystadenocarcinoma

Biliary cystadenoma and cyst adenocarcinoma are rare cystic neoplasms lined by mucin secreting columnar epithelium. They are usually seen in middle-aged women. Most cystadenomas and cyst adenocarcinomas are intrahepatic masses that are hypoechoic on ultrasound and are hypodense on CT. These cystic lesions can be unilocular or multilocular.[66] Mural nodules, papillary growths and septations are seen both in cystadenoma and cyst adenocarcinoma though cyst adenocarcinomas show papillary excrescences and solid portions more often.[66] The differential diagnosis of these tumors includes hepatic cysts, hydatid cysts, liver abscesses, cystic metastases, hematoma, cystic sarcomas, and choledochal cysts.[66]

OTHER MALIGNANT NEOPLASMS OF THE BILE DUCTS

In adults, metastasis, lymphomas, leiomyosarcomas, and carcinoid tumors can rarely occur in the bile ducts. Embryonal rhabdomyosarcoma is the second most common cause of jaundice in the pediatric population after choledochal cyst. Sonography and CT will show intra hepatic duct dilation and a soft tissue mass in the region of the common bile duct or porta hepatis. On MRCP, grape like filling defects are seen in dilated CBD which may show enhancement.[67]

CONCLUSION

Malignancies of the biliary tract are often discovered late. USG is the initial imaging modality whenever a biliary tree malignancy is suspected. MDCT with multi planer reformations, MRI with MRCP, ERCP and EUS all have a role to play in early detection, characterization, staging and preoperative planning of these highly lethal tumors. It is important for the radiologist to be aware of imaging features of malignant pathologies of biliary tree so as to play critical role in their management.

REFERENCES

1. Cleary SP, Dawson LA, Knox JJ, et al. Cancer of the gallbladder and extra-hepatic bile ducts. Curr Probl Surg. 2007;44:396-482.
2. Craig JR, Peters RL, Edmondson HA. Tumors of the liver and intra hepatic bile ducts. In: Atlas of Tumor Pathology. 2nd series. Fascicle 26. Washington, DC: Armed Forces Institute of Pathology; 1989.
3. Heinrich S, Clavien PA. Ampullary cancer. Curr Opin Gastroenterol. 2010;26(3):280-5.
4. Jemal A, Siegel R, Xu J, et al. Cancer statistics, 2010. CA Cancer J Clin. 2011;60:133-4.
5. Kiran RP, Pokala N, Dudrick SJ. Incidence pattern and survival for gallbladder cancer over three decades—an analysis of 10301 patients. Ann Surg Oncol. 2007;14:827-32.
6. Nanda Kumar A, Gupta PC, Gangadharn P, et al. Geographic pathology revisited: development of an atlas of cancer in India. Int J Cancer. 2005;116:740-54.
7. Dhir V, Mohandas KM. Epidemiology of digestive tract cancers in India IV. Gallbladder and pancreas. Indian J Gastroenterol. 1999;18:24-8.
8. Sheth S, Bedford A, Chopra S. Primary gallbladder cancer: recognition of risk factors and the role of prophylactic cholecystectomy. Am J Gastroenterol. 2000;95:1402-10.
9. Tazuma S, Kajiyama G. Carcinogenesis of malignant lesions of the gallbladder. The impact of chronic inflammation and gallstones. Langen becks Arch Surg. 2001;386:224-9.
10. Khan ZS, Livingston EH, Huerta S. Reassessing the need for prophylactic surgery in patients with porcelain gallbladder: case series and systematic review of the literature. Arch Surg. 2011;146(10):1143-7.
11. Schnelldorfer T. Porcelain gallbladder: a benign process or concern for malignancy? J Gastrointest Surg. 2013;17:1161-8.
12. Stephen AE, Berger DL. Carcinoma in the porcelain gallbladder: a relationship revisited. Surgery. 2001;129(6):699-703.
13. Henson DE, Albores Saavedra J, Corle D. Carcinoma of the gallbladder. Histologic types, stage of disease, grade and survival rates. Cancer. 1992;70:1493-7.
14. Albores Saavedra J, Henson DE. Tumors of the gallbladder and extra-hepatic bile ducts. Atlas of Tumor Pathology, Fascicle 22, 2nd Series. Washington, DC: Armed Forces Institute of Pathology, 1986.
15. Edge SB, Byrd DR, Compton CC, et al. AJCC Cancer Staging Manual, 7th ed. Chicago, Springer; 2010.pp.211-7.
16. Donohue JH, Stewart AK, Menck HR. The national cancer data base report on carcinoma of the gallbladder, 1989–1995. Cancer. 1998;83:2618-28.
17. Bach AM, Loring LA, Hann LE, et al. Gallbladder cancer: Can ultra sonography evaluate extent of disease? J Ultrasound Med. 1998;17:303-9.
18. Soyer P, Gouhiri M, Boudiaf M, et al. Carcinoma of the gallbladder: imaging features with surgical correlation. AJR. 1997;169:781-4.
19. Ogawa T, Horaguchi J, Fujita N, et al. High b-value diffusion-weighted magnetic resonance imaging for gallbladder lesions: Differentiation between benignity and malignancy. J Gastroenterol. 2012;47:1352-60.
20. Levy AD, Murakata LA, Rohrmann CA. Gallbladder carcinoma: radiologic–pathologic correlation. RadioGraphics. 2001;21:295-314.
21. Rodríguez-Fernádez A, Gómez-Río M, Medina-Benitez A, et al. Application of modern imaging methods in diagnosis of gallbladder cancer. J Surg Oncol. 2006;93:650-64.
22. Tsuchiya Y. Early carcinoma of the gallbladder: macroscopic features and sonography findings. Radiology. 1991;179:171-5.
23. Franquet T, Montes M, Ruiz de Azua Y, et al. Primary gallbladder carcinoma: imaging findings in 50 patients with pathologic correlation. Gastrointest Radiol. 1991;16:143-8.
24. Yoshimitsu K, Honda H, Kaneko K, et al. Dynamic MRI of the gallbladder lesions: differentiation of benign from malignant. J Magn Reson Imaging. 1997;7:696-701.
25. Furlan A, Ferris JV, Hosseinzadeh K, et al. Gallbladder carcinoma update: multimodality imaging evaluation, staging, and treatment options. AJR. 2008;191:1440-7.
26. Wilbur AC, Sagireddy PB, Aizenstein RL. Carcinoma of the gallbladder: color Doppler ultrasound and CT findings. Abdom Imaging. 1997;22:187-9.
27. Choi BI, Lee JM. Neoplasms of the Gallbladder and Biliary Tract. In: Richard M Gore, Marc S Levine (Eds): Textbook of Gastrointestinal Radiology. 4th edn. Saunders Elsevier; 2015.pp.1402-26.
28. Onoyama H, Yamamoto M, Takada M, et al. Diagnostic imaging of early gallbladder cancers: retrospective study of 53 cases. World J Surg. 1999;23:708-12.
29. Kim SJ, Lee JM, Lee JY, et al. Accuracy of preoperative T-staging of gallbladder carcinoma using MDCT. AJR. 2008;190:74-8.
30. Kim SJ, Lee JM, Lee JY, et al. Analysis of enhancement pattern of flat from cholecystitis. AJR. 2008;191:765-71.
31. Sandhu MS, Yoganand K, Kalra N, et al. Radiological evaluation of the enhancement patterns of thickened gallbladder wall to differentiate benign from malignancy. PGIMER study.
32. Kondo S, Nimura Y, Kamiya J, et al. Mode of tumor spread and surgical strategy in gallbladder carcinoma. Langenbecks Arch Surg. 2002;387:222-8.
33. Kalra N, Suri S, Gupta R, et al. MDCT in the staging of gallbladder carcinoma. AJR. 2006;186:758-62.
34. Kaza RK, Gulati M, Wig JD, et al. Evaluation of gallbladder carcinoma with dynamic magnetic resonance imaging and magnetic resonance cholangiopancreatography. Australas Radiol. 2006;50:212-7.

35. Mosconi S, Beretta GD, Labianca R, et al. Cholangiocarcinoma. Crit Rev Oncol Hematol. 2009;69:259-70.
36. Shaib Y, El-Serag HB. The epidemiology of cholangiocarcinoma. Semin Liver Dis. 2004;24(2):115-25.
37. Henson DE, Albores-Saavedra J, Corle D. Carcinoma of the extra hepatic bile ducts: histologic types, stage of disease, grade, and survival rates. Cancer. 1992;70:1498-501.
38. Sainani NI, Catalano OA, Holalkere NS, et al. Cholangiocarcinoma: current and novel imaging techniques. Radiographics. 2008;28:1263-87.
39. Tyson GL, El-Serag HB. Risk factors for cholangiocarcinoma. Hepatology. 2011;54:173-84.
40. Sorenson HT, Friis S, Olsen JH, et al. Risk of liver and other types of cancer in patients with cirrhosis: a nationwide cohort study in Denmark. Hepatology. 1998;28:921-5.
41. Khan ZR, Neugut AI, Ahsan H, et al. Risk factors for biliary tract cancers. Am J Gastroenterol. 1999;94:149-52.
42. DeOliveira ML, Cunningham SC, Cameron JL, et al. Cholangiocarcinoma: thirty-one-year experience with 564 patients at single institution. Ann Surg. 2007;245: 755-62.
43. Nakanuma Y, Sato Y, Harada K, et al. Pathological classification of intra hepatic cholangiocarcinoma based on a new concept. World J Hepatol. 2010;2:419-27.
44. Razumilava N, Gores GJ. Classification, diagnosis, and management of cholangiocarcinoma. Clin Gastroenterol Hepatol. 2013;11:13-21.
45. Heller SL, Lee VS. MR imaging of the gallbladder and biliary system. Magn Reson Imaging Clin N Am. 2005;13:295-311.
46. Choi BI, Lee JM, Han JK. Imaging of intra hepatic and hilar cholangiocarcinoma. Abdom Imaging. 2004;29:548-57.
47. Choi BI, Han KJ, Kim TK. Benign and malignant tumours of the biliary tract. In: Gazelle GC, Saini S, Meuller PR (Eds). Hepatobiliary and pancreatic radiology. New York, 1st edn, Thieme; 1998. pp.630-76.
48. Loyer FM, Chin H, DuBrow RA, et al. Hepato cellular carcinoma and intra hepatic peripheral cholangio carcinoma. Enhancement patterns with quadruple phasehelical CT. Radiology. 1999;212:866-71.
49. Choi BI, Lee JH, Han MC. Hilar cholangiocarcinoma. Comparative study with sonography and CT. Radiology. 1989;172:689-92.
50. Motohara T, Semelka RC, Bidar TR. MR cholangio pancreatography. RCNA. 2003;41:89-96.
51. Yeh TS, Jan YY, Tseng JH, et al. Malignant perihilar biliary obstruction: MRCP findings. Am J Gastroenterol. 2000;95:432-40.
52. Nguyen K, Sing JT Jr. Review of endoscopic techniques in the diagnosis and management of cholangiocarcinoma. World J Gastroenterol. 2008;14:2995-9.
53. Lee JW, Han JK, Kim TK, et al. CT features of intra ductal intra hepatic cholangiocarcinoma. AJR. 2000;175:721-5.
54. Kim JE, Lee JM, Kim SH, et al. Differentiation of intra ductal growing type cholangiocarcinomas at biliary MR imaging with MR cholangiography. Radiology. 2010;257:364-72.
55. Ahrendt SA, Pitt HA. Biliary tract. In: Townsend CM, Beauchamp RD, Evers BM, Mattox KL (Eds): SabistonTexbook of Surgery (17th edn) Philadelphia: Saunders Elsevier, 2004.pp.1112-43.
56. Manfredi R, Masselli G, Maresca G, et al. MR imaging and MRCP of hilar cholangiocarcinoma. Abdom Imaging. 2003;28:319-25.
57. Bismuth H, Corlette MB. Intra hepatic cholangioenteric anastomosis in carcinoma of the hilus of the liver. Surg Gynecol Obstet. 1975;140:170-8.
58. Bismuth H, Nakache R, Diamond T. Management strategies in resection for hilar cholangiocarcinoma. Ann Surg. 1992;215:31-8.
59. Choi SH, Han JK, Lee JM, et al. Differentiating malignant from benign common bile duct stricture with multi phasic helical CT. Radiology. 2005;236:178-83.
60. Park MS, Kim TK, Kim KW, et al. Differentiation of extra hepatic bile duct cholangiocarcinoma from benign stricture: Findings at MRCP versus ERCP. Radiology. 2004;233:234-40.
61. Mohamadnejad M, DeWitt JM, Sherman S, et al. Role of EUS for preoperative evaluation of cholangiocarcinoma: a large single-center experience. Gastrointest Endosc. 2011;73:71-8.
62. Dittrick GW, Mallat DB, Lamont JP. Management of ampullary lesions. Curr Treat Options Gastroenterol. 2006;9:371-6.
63. Kim JH, Kim MJ, Chung JJ, et al. Differential diagnosis of peri ampullary carcinomas at MR imaging. Radiographics. 2002;22:1335-52.
64. Skordilis P, Mouzas IA, Dimoulios PD, Alexandrakis G, Moschandrea J, Kouroumalis E. Is endosonography an effective method for detection and local staging of the ampullary carcinoma? A prospective study. BMC Surg. 2002;2:1.
65. Kubo H, Chijiiwa Y, Akahoshi K, Hamada S, Matsui N, Nawata H. Pre-operative staging of ampullary tumours by endoscopic ultrasound. Br J Radiol. 1999;72:443-7.
66. Choi BI, Lim JH, Han MC, et al. Biliary cyst adenoma and cyst adenocarcinoma: CT and sonographic findings. Radiology. 1989;171:57-61.
67. Tireli GA, Sander S, Dervisoglu S, Demirali O, Unal M. Embryonal rhabdomyosarcoma of the common bile duct mimicking choledochal cyst. J Hepatobiliary Pancreat Surg. 2005;12:263-5.

CHAPTER

110

Biliary Interventions

Mandeep Kang, Naveen Kalra, Anupam Lal

INTRODUCTION

The past few decades have witnessed a revolution in minimally invasive surgeries and techniques with image guided interventions having emerged at the forefront of these developments. Percutaneous biliary interventions had their origin way back in 1921 when direct puncture of the gallbladder was first performed to opacify the biliary tree. This was followed by reports describing percutaneous direct puncture of the biliary tree. The technique of percutaneous biliary drainage for the relief of obstructive jaundice was introduced in the 1970s[1-3] followed by percutaneous cholecystostomy in the 1980s.[4-6] The development of biliary stents has further enlarged the scope of percutaneous applications in the management of biliary diseases.[7-11]

In the present day, percutaneous biliary interventions include percutaneous transhepatic cholangiography (PTC) and biliary drainage (PTBD) for the diagnosis and management of biliary obstruction and percutaneous cholecystostomy. This route can also be used for percutaneous transhepatic cholangioscopy or biliary ultrasonography; biopsy of the biliary duct, cholangioplasty for benign biliary strictures and as an access for the removal of bile duct calculi, the application of intraluminal brachytherapy or radiofrequency ablation.

PERCUTANEOUS TRANSHEPATIC CHOLANGIOGRAPHY

Percutaneous transhepatic cholangiography (PTC) is a diagnostic procedure which involves placement of a fine needle into a peripheral biliary radicle under image guidance followed by contrast injection to opacify the biliary tree. The procedure is used for:[8,12]

- To define the level of obstruction in patients with obstructive biliopathy.
- To evaluate for presence of suspected choledocholithiasis.
- To determine the etiology of cholangitis.
- To evaluate suspected bile duct inflammatory disorders.
- To demonstrate the site of bile duct leak.
- As the preliminary step for draining the biliary tree (most common indication).

Although PTC has been shown to be an effective technique which reliably demonstrates the level of obstruction, it is more invasive and painful than endoscopic retrograde cholangiopancreatography (ERCP). It also involves the risk of significant complications such as hemoperitoneum and bile peritonitis. Hence, PTC is nowadays reserved for patients in whom an ECRP is not possible due to anatomy altering surgeries or following unsuccessful cannulation of the common bile duct.

Preprocedure Evaluation and Preparation

The initial workup of a patient with obstructive biliopathy includes a clinical evaluation with history taking, physical examination and pertinent laboratory tests. Cross sectional imaging such as ultrasonography, CT and MRI should be performed to provide information about the level of obstruction of the biliary tree and to determine the cause. Coagulation parameters including prothrombin time, prothrombin time index (>75%) and the international normalized ratio (≤1.5) as well as platelet count (>50–75,000) should be checked prior to the procedure and corrected with fresh frozen plasma or platelets if deranged.

Antibiotics are routinely administered in all patients as bacteremia and sepsis can develop during the procedure. Broad spectrum antibiotics covering both gram-positive and gram-negative organisms should be started prior to the procedure. A venous access should be secured and an informed consent obtained after explaining the procedure completely to the patient and attendants.

Conscious sedation should be used for adequate pain control. Over dosage of the sedative should be avoided as the patient needs to follow the instructions of the operator such as breath holding. General anesthesia may however be required in selected cases.[12-14]

Technique

With the patient lying supine on the fluoroscopy table, the upper abdomen is cleaned and draped. The skin puncture site is anesthetized with a local anesthetic (2% lidocaine) up to the liver capsule. If the peripheral biliary radicles are dilated they can be punctured under ultrasonographic guidance. If not dilated, the procedure is performed under fluoroscopic guidance. Most PTCs are performed from the right mid-axillary approach through an intercostal space which is caudal to the costophrenic sulcus. This can be identified on fluoroscopy on deep inspiration. A 15 cm fine (22G) Chiba needle is advanced into the liver aiming for the right lateral aspect of the 12th thoracic vertebral body. After the stylet is removed, the needle is slowly withdrawn while injecting a small amount of contrast. When contrast is seen to opacify the biliary tree, needle withdrawal is stopped and cholangiography performed to delineate the biliary anatomy. If the first puncture is unsuccessful a second or third puncture can be made by changing the needle angulation once the needle tip is near the liver capsule.

The success rates for PTC are reported to be more than 90% in a dilated system and 67–80% in a nondilated system. Major complications are seen in 3.5–10% of procedures and include sepsis, cholangitis, bile leak, hemorrhage or pneumothorax.[12-15]

PERCUTANEOUS TRANSHEPATIC BILIARY DRAINAGE

Percutaneous transhepatic biliary drainage (PTBD) is a therapeutic procedure that consists of sterile puncture of a peripheral biliary radicle under image guidance followed by placement of a catheter or stent for internal or external drainage of bile. Percutaneous therapy of bile duct lesions is often a staged procedure, requiring multiple sessions to achieve the therapeutic goals.[8]

Indications for Biliary Drainage

The presence of cholestasis, whether due to benign or malignant etiology, predisposes to biliary infection. Secondly, protracted hyperbilirubinemia causes impairment of the renal function. The surgical morbidity and mortality rates are also high (40–60% and 15–25% respectively) in the setting of hyperbilirubinemia, therefore decompression should be done as early as possible in patients with obstructive biliopathy. Malignancy causing biliary obstruction is often unresectable at the time of diagnosis and palliative therapy is the only management option possible. A normalized liver function is also required for the administration of chemotherapy. Biliary drainage thus will not only normalize liver function, restore the physiological drainage of bile into the duodenum, prevent the development of cholangitis and sepsis but also improve the nutritional status and quality of life of the patient.[7,9,10]

Common causes of benign biliary obstruction include choledocholithiasis, sclerosing cholangitis, and inflammatory conditions such as pancreatitis, iatrogenic causes (post-laparoscopic cholecystectomy, liver transplantation or anastomotic strictures) and infections such as HIV infection, oriental and parasitic cholangitis.[15] The common causes of malignant biliary obstruction include gallbladder carcinoma, cholangiocarcinoma, carcinoma of the pancreas and metastatic disease.[10,16]

The indications include:

- To decompress the obstructed biliary tree
- To dilate benign biliary strictures
- To remove bile duct stones
- To divert bile from and stent bile duct defects
- To stent malignant strictures.

There are no absolute contraindications for the procedure. Deranged coagulation parameters are a relative contraindication and should be corrected prior to the procedure with platelets or fresh frozen plasma. The presence of gross ascites with presence of perihepatic fluid is also a relative contraindication which requires to be drained before performing a PTBD.[14,16]

PATIENT PREPARATION

The patient preparation and preprocedure work-up are as for PTC. The endoscopic route is preferred for drainage, particularly in lesions involving the mid or distal common bile duct (CBD) as it is associated with a decreased complication rate. However, with lesions involving the hilum, the percutaneous approach is associated with a higher success rate and is therefore preferred. In cases of failed ERCP or where ERCP is not possible due to anatomy altering surgeries, PTBD is the only approach available.[10,11,16,17]

Preprocedure Imaging

Cross-sectional imaging with contrast enhanced computed tomography (CECT) and magnetic resonance imaging (MRI) with magnetic resonance cholangiopancreatography (MRCP) should be performed prior to the procedure. These will help identify the level and cause of obstruction and aid in planning the approach to percutaneous management.[7,10] When there is obstruction beyond the hilum of the liver, only one access is required. The left system is accessed from an anterior, subxiphoid approach while the right is accessed from the midaxillary approach using as caudad an intercostal space as possible, well below the costophrenic sulcus. Whether to use a left or right approach is largely a matter of individual or institutional preference, when both sided biliary radicles are adequately dilated. When the drainage is required for a longer period of time, most patients are more comfortable with a subxiphoid catheter rather than a right intercostal catheter. Other advantages of a left approach include a less painful procedure which is technically easier to perform (limited respiratory excursion of the left lobe of liver in comparison to the right and a shorter route to be traversed through the hepatic parenchyma), decreased pleural complication rate and less likelihood of catheter dislodgement, again due to less respiratory excursion of the left lobe as well as the fact that the patient finds it easier to look after a percutaneous catheter which is in front of his/her eyes rather than on one side of the body. The disadvantage of the left approach is the increased radiation dose to the operator's hands.

In cases of hilar obstruction with isolation of the biliary radicles, careful assessment has to be done of the CECT/MR as well as by preprocedure ultrasonography to assess the degree of biliary dilatation. One also has to look for obstruction of the secondary confluence, both right and the left as well as for multilevel isolation which may be present in the setting of metastatic disease. One also has to assess the approach to the segmental duct to be punctured for any mass or cyst in the path of the needle. At least 25–30% of the liver parenchyma should be drained with a single catheter as placement of multiple catheters increases the morbidity and mortality in a patient.[7,10]

If the procedure is done for palliative purposes for the relief of jaundice, drainage of one lobe is enough. However, in the presence of cholangitis, if drainage of one side does not relieve the symptoms, the other side will also need to be drained. In case of parenchymal atrophy of one lobe or segment, it is not useful to drain that lobe/segment as the procedure is unlikely to improve the hepatic function. In case of segmental isolated obstructions, if the patient is not in cholangitis, one should not drain that segment as once a drainage catheter is placed, it becomes virtually impossible to withdraw the access due to bacterial contamination and the patient will be left with an unneeded, potentially problematic catheter.[7,10,18]

Technique

The procedure is performed under conscious sedation with the patient placed supine on the fluoroscopy table. The first step of the procedure is performing a PTC. If the peripheral biliary radicles are sufficiently dilated, sonographic guidance may be used to puncture the selected segmental duct. After cleaning and draping the chosen puncture site, the skin is anesthetized by infiltrating with 2% lidocaine and a small skin incision given using a surgical blade. The underlying soft tissues should be dissected free as this will ease the subsequent drainage catheter insertion.[14] In a dilated system, a 18G puncture needle with a diamond tip is used to enter the selected biliary radicle as peripherally as possible.

Allowing a small amount of bile to drain after the puncture before injecting contrast is beneficial as it prevents over-distension of the biliary system which can result in bacteremia and sepsis. A little contrast is injected to opacify the biliary tree and to confirm that the needle tip is completely within the biliary system. If contrast is seen pooling at the puncture site, it signifies that the tip is within the parenchyma. If contrast is seen entering a tubular system with rapid dissipation, it denotes placement of the needle tip within a vascular structure. In both these situations, the needle has to be carefully repositioned. Once there is backflow of bile and contrast injection opacifies the biliary tree, a 0.032 or 0.035 inch hydrophilic guidewire is passed through the needle and manipulated into the biliary tree towards the liver hilum **(Figs. 1A to C)**.[10,14]

After safely anchoring the guidewire, the needle is withdrawn and a 4F or 5F sheath or cannula introduced. The slippy hydrophilic guidewire can then be exchanged for a stiffer (Teflon coated) guidewire over which a 7F or 8F drainage catheter can be placed after dilatation of the tract with fascial dilators **(Figs. 2A and B)**. If the tip of the catheter

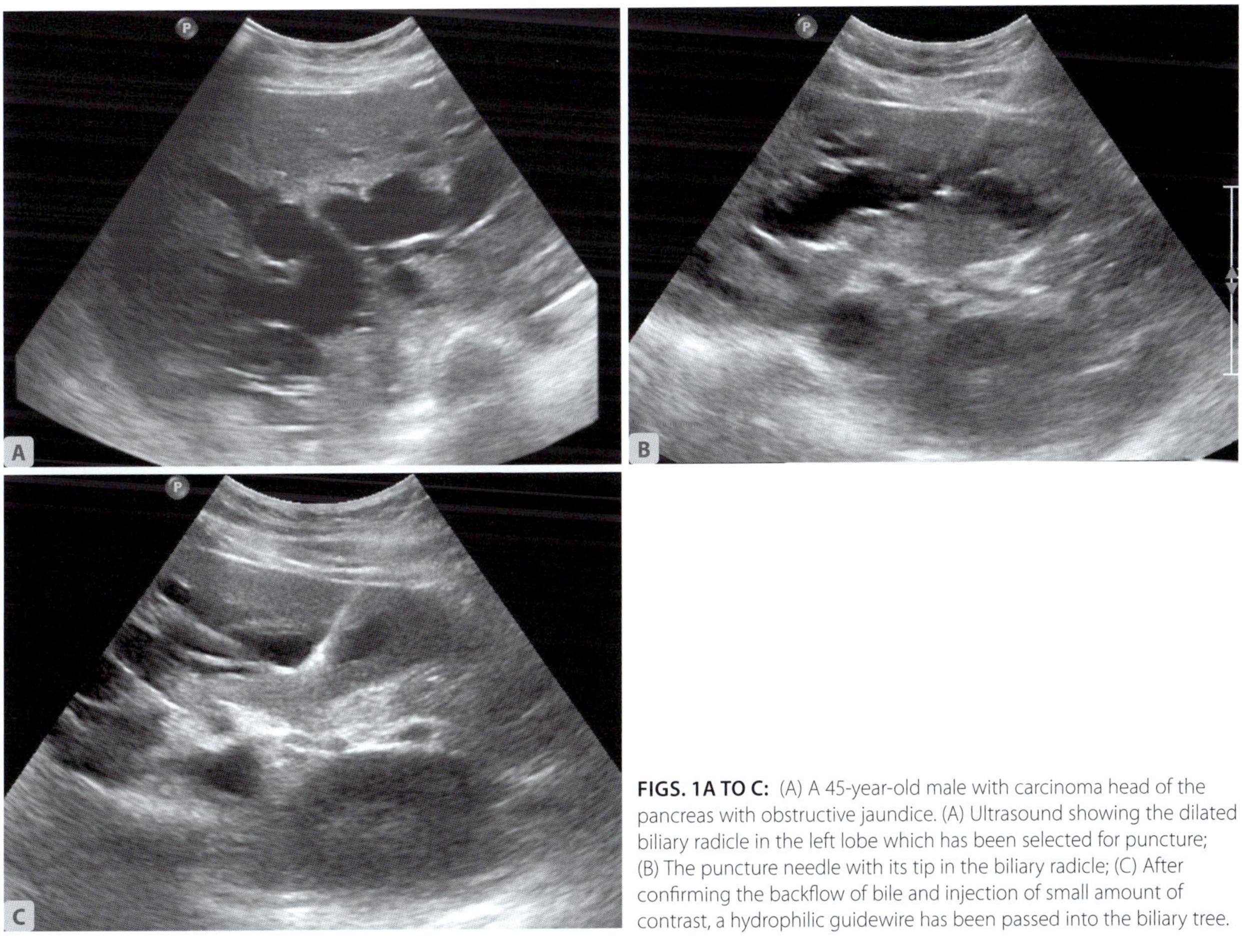

FIGS. 1A TO C: (A) A 45-year-old male with carcinoma head of the pancreas with obstructive jaundice. (A) Ultrasound showing the dilated biliary radicle in the left lobe which has been selected for puncture; (B) The puncture needle with its tip in the biliary radicle; (C) After confirming the backflow of bile and injection of small amount of contrast, a hydrophilic guidewire has been passed into the biliary tree.

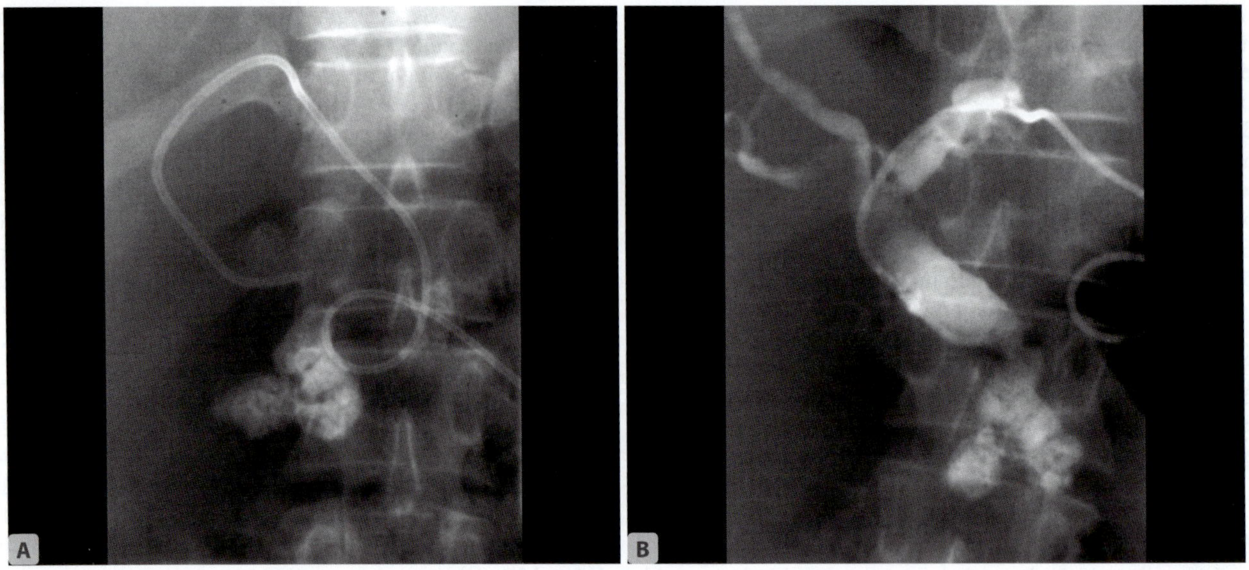

FIGS. 2A AND B: External biliary drainage: A 52-year-old male with chronic calcific pancreatitis with obstructive jaundice. (A) An 8F PTBD catheter has been placed via the left duct approach into the CBD for external drainage; (B) Cholangiogram shows a complete block of the distal CBD.

is in the CBD, a catheter of the pigtail type is placed. If the tip of the catheter is in an intrahepatic duct an angled catheter is selected. A self-locking catheter is usually used to prevent accidental slippage. The catheter should also be secured to the skin surface by using a suture or commercially available skin anchoring devices. The catheter is then attached to a drainage bag and left for gravity drainage.

Fluoroscopic Guidance

Fluoroscopic guidance can be used in patients with or without biliary dilatation for performing PTBD. There are two methods by which the procedure can be done. In the one step method, a 21G chiba needle is used for the puncture as for PTC. A 0.018" guidewire is then passed through the needle and manipulated into the biliary tree. The needle is then removed and a 4F percutaneous access set manipulated over the guidewire. The sheath of the access set allows passage of a 0.035" stiff guidewire and the rest of the procedure is as described under US guidance.[7]

In the two step method, a 22G chiba needle is used for puncture of the biliary radicle. After opacification of the biliary tree a second 18G puncture needle is used for re-puncture of a suitable biliary radicle.[14] This allows passage of a 0.035 guidewire and the rest of the procedure is as described earlier.

Minimal contrast injection and minimal possible manipulation should be done on the initial day of procedure to place an indwelling catheter to avoid over distension of the biliary tree and cholangiovenous reflux.

Two points should be kept in mind while doing the procedure. The site of puncture of the biliary radicle should be as far as possible from the obstructing lesion so as to allow safe anchorage of the external drainage catheter. Also, a longer passage makes subsequent internal drainage easier to perform. Secondly, the puncture should not be done in deep inspiration as the liver will move caudad, thereby causing a difference in the level between the site of punctures of the skin surface and the liver. Therefore, the puncture should be performed in shallow inspiratory breath-hold.

Internal and External Drainage

Internal drainage should ideally be attempted 48–72 hours after the initial PTBD. This allows decompression of the biliary system and therefore, straightening of the course of the wire. Secondly, this time allows the inflammatory changes to subside, particularly the edema around the obstructing lesion.[3,10,19] Injection of contrast through the drainage catheter at this stage will demonstrate the true picture of the type of obstruction whether beak shaped, tapered or flat-shaped. The drainage catheter is replaced with a 4F or 5F angiographic or biliary manipulation catheter with a curved or angled tip over a stiff guidewire. The stiff guidewire is then changed for a soft, angled or J-tip hydrophilic guidewire. If the site of obstruction is beak shaped or tapered, the tip of the catheter is wedged into the beak and the soft hydrophilic guidewire is gently pushed through the obstruction. On the other hand, if the site of obstruction is flat or irregular it may be better to keep the catheter a little proximal to the obstruction and gently probe the area with the hydrophilic guidewire, while simultaneously rotating the tip of the angled catheter into different directions.[10,20]

Once the guidewire successfully crosses the stenosis, it is manipulated into the duodenum along with the catheter. The slippy guidewire is then exchanged for a stiff guidewire over which a 8.3F ring biliary catheter or 10F pigtail catheter is placed with the loop in the duodenum **(Fig. 3)**. Contrast injection to check that side holes are present both proximal and distal to the obstruction and no side-holes are within the hepatic parenchyma completes the procedure **(Figs. 4A and B)**. The catheter should initially be left to external biliary drainage while ensuring adequate hydration of the patient. It can be capped to allow internal drainage once the bile is clear from blood or debris and the patient is afebrile. Once the "capping test" is successful with no fever, pain or vomiting, the patient can be discharged to home with the instruction to open the cap and attach an external drainage bag in the event of any of the above complications, and to report back to the hospital as soon as possible.

Postprocedure Management

Patients who have undergone biliary drainage procedures require in-patient admission for at least 24 hours following the procedure. The patient needs to be closely monitored as the procedures can cause bacteremia and sepsis. Vital signs should be checked every 15 minutes for one hour, every 30 minutes for 2 hours, hourly thereafter for 4 hours, and then 6 hourly for 4 hours. Biliary output can range from 400 to 800 mL every 24 hours, so adequate hydration needs to be taken care of. Adequate analgesics need to be administered for controlling the post procedural pain. Appropriate antibiotics also need to be continued for at least 48 hours after the procedure.[14]

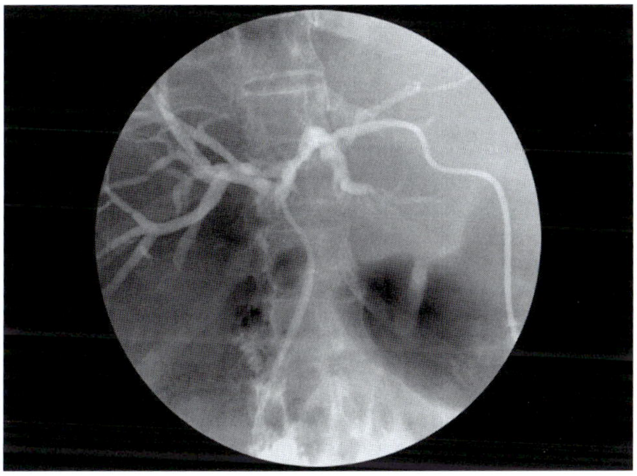

FIG. 3: External-internal biliary drainage: A 55-year-old female with carcinoma gallbladder with obstructive jaundice. Cholangiogram shows complete block of the common hepatic duct just distal to the confluence. An external-internal drainage has been instituted with the distal catheter tip placed in the second part of duodenum.

Follow-up of Biliary Catheters

Patients who have undergone percutaneous biliary drainage procedures require close monitoring and regular follow-up to be able to detect catheter migration or obstruction at an early stage. Bile output, color and body temperature should be recorded every day and a watch kept on the serum bilirubin and amylase levels. The normal daily output of bile is 400–800 mL and it is clear and yellow in color. Any decrease in the output, change in color or increased turbidity are signs of cholangitis. Regular sonographic examination to look for any dilated intra-hepatic radicles which denote undrained ducts or development of catheter obstruction should be performed. Some authors advocate daily, gentle, forward flushing of the catheter with 5–10 mL of normal saline or sterile water to prevent collection of debris which causes catheter blockage. Pericatheter leakage is usually due to occlusion of the catheter or dislodgement and requires flurosocopic evaluation and correction of the problem. Catheter blockage will also cause the serum bilirubin values to rise. Catheters should ideally be exchanged every 2–3 months to prevent blockage or breakage.[14]

Biliary Stenting

Biliary endoprostheses may be either plastic or metallic and various kinds of both types are available. An external drainage tube can be uncomfortable or of psychological disadvantage to the patient particularly in cases of malignant obstruction. An internal stent also prevents the complications of pericatheter biliary leakage or slippage.

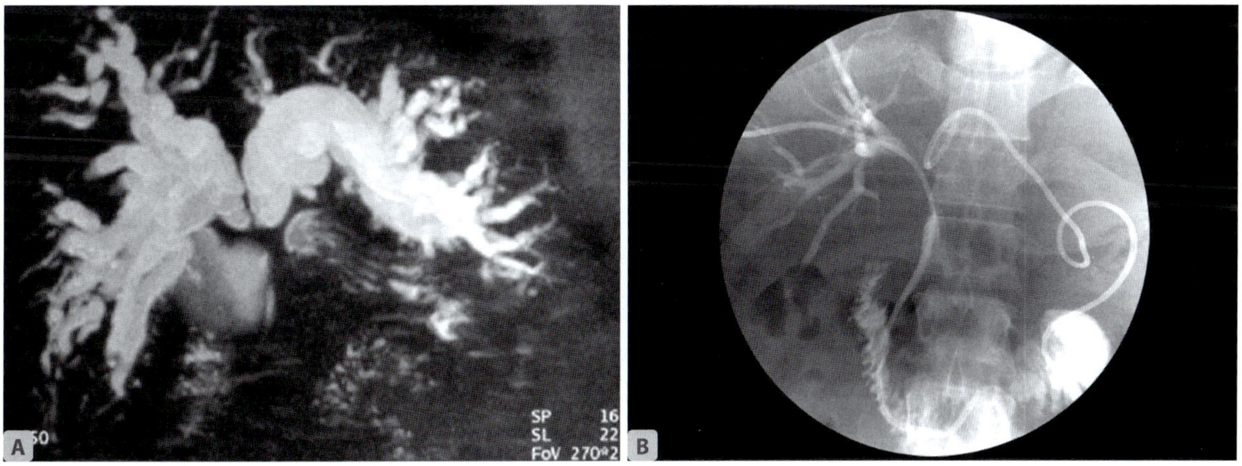

FIGS. 4A AND B: A 45-year-old male with carcinoma gallbladder with obstructive jaundice. (A) MRCP MIP image shows a hilar block with isolation of the biliary radicles; (B) An external-internal catheter has been placed in the right ductal system with its tip in the third part of duodenum. Check cholangiogram after the procedure confirms that side-holes are present both above and below the strictured segment. An external drainage catheter is seen in the left ductal system with its tip lying just proximal to the confluence.

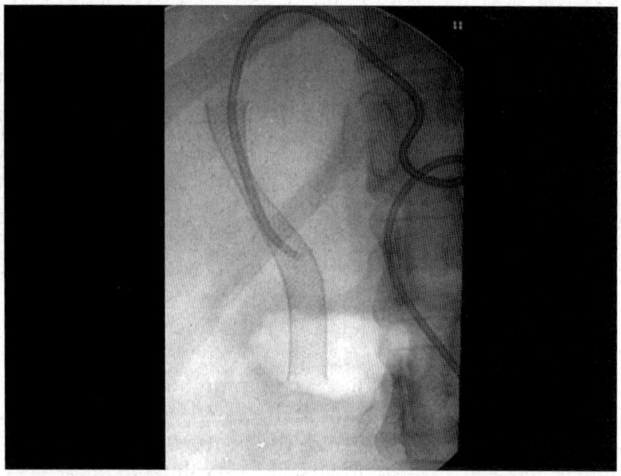

FIG. 5: (A) 63-year-old male with carcinoma head of the pancreas causing obstructive jaundice. A single, self-expanding metallic stent has been placed in the CBD.

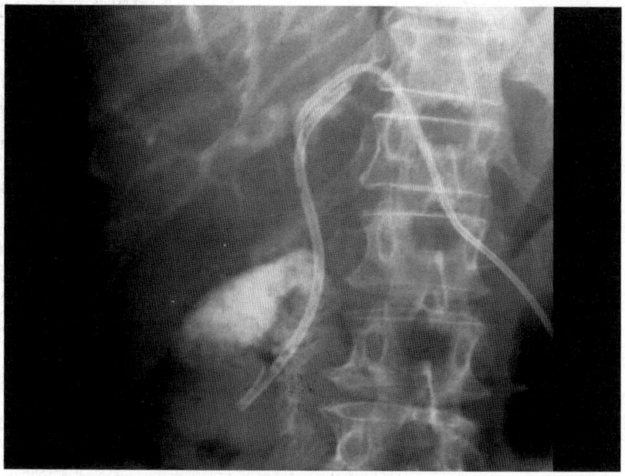

FIG. 6: A 58-year-old male with carcinoma head of the pancreas. A single plastic biliary stent has been placed across the stricture. An external drainage catheter has been left in place as a safety measure in the immediate postprocedure period.

The disadvantage of stents is the need for performing a new procedure (PTBD or ERCP) in case of stent obstruction.

Metallic stents are used almost exclusively for the palliative management of unresectable biliary malignant obstruction. The major advantage of metallic stents is that they can be inserted in a contracted state through a small calibre tract and can achieve a large lumen (up to 10 mm) following expansion **(Fig. 5)**. They are available as self-expanding metallic stents (SEMS) or balloon-mounted stents. These stents are less prone to migration and show a better patency rate than plastic stents.[7,21,22] The disadvantages include the high cost and difficulty in removal. Plastic stents are cheap but have many disadvantages including early occlusion, frequent migration and a traumatic insertion procedure due to the large tract size required **(Fig. 6)**. Because of the large calibre, endoscopic insertion is done more frequently than the percutaneous route.[23,24]

Most physicians prefer to allow internal drainage for a few days prior to stent placement. However, if the passage through the stricture has been relatively atraumatic without significant hemorrhage or debris, stenting can be done in the same sitting as the internal external drainage.[25]

A super-stiff guidewire is passed through the internal-external drainage catheter and securely looped in the duodenum. The catheter is removed and an appropriate introducer sheath placed. If a self-expanding metallic stent is being used, some workers prefer to balloon dilate the stricture prior to stent deployment.[14] It is advisable to over-stent the stricture with the proximal and distal ends of the stent at least 1–1.5 cm beyond the strictures limits.[21] Once the stent is at the appropriate site, as evidenced by the position of the radio-opaque markers at the ends of the stent, it is deployed. Since SEMS have a thermal memory, they will gradually expand to their maximum width within 24 hours after deployment once they achieve body temperature. A safety 8F biliary drainage catheter is then placed with its tip within the stent and the guidewire removed **(Figs. 7A to E)**. The external drain is capped after 24 hours and if the patient tolerates the "capping", a check cholangiogram is performed to confirm adequate drainage through the stent, following which the external catheter is removed.[9,14]

A single stent normally suffices for short segment strictures in the CBD. For longer strictures, one may need to place two telescoped stents (one stent overlapping with the other). In cases of hilar obstruction, bilateral stents may be required which can be placed in either a 'T' or 'Y' configuration. When placing in a 'Y' configuration, it is advisable to place the lower ends of the stents at the same level in the common bile duct **(Figs. 8A and B)**.[7,26] This parallel arrangement may prevent complete expansion of the stents at the level of the liver hilum, so other workers advocate using a "stent within stent" deployment technique. In this technique, the second stent is placed through the mesh of the first stent.[27] This technique is also said to prevent displacement of the stents. The advantage of 'T' stenting is that only a single percutaneous access is required thereby decreasing the complication rate **(Figs. 9A and B)**. However, at times the stricture cannot be crossed to the contralateral side, thereby necessitating the second puncture.[28] No significant difference has been reported between using the 'T' or the 'Y' configurations in terms of rates of technical success, complications or stent patency.[28] Multiple stents may be required in cases of involvement of the secondary confluences (Bismuth type III or IV strictures).[7]

The reported patency rate for palliative metallic stents in malignant obstructions is about 50% at 6 months.[17] Stent blockage occurs because of tumor in growth through the mesh of the stent or tumor over growth at the ends of the stent, biliary sludge and debris.[10,17] In an effort to limit tumor ingrowth, covered stents coated with polyurethane, silicone or expanded polytetrafluoroethylene (ePTFE) were developed. These stents are not integrated within the biliary wall and therefore, are prone for migration. Secondly, the openings of the side branches or cystic duct may be blocked

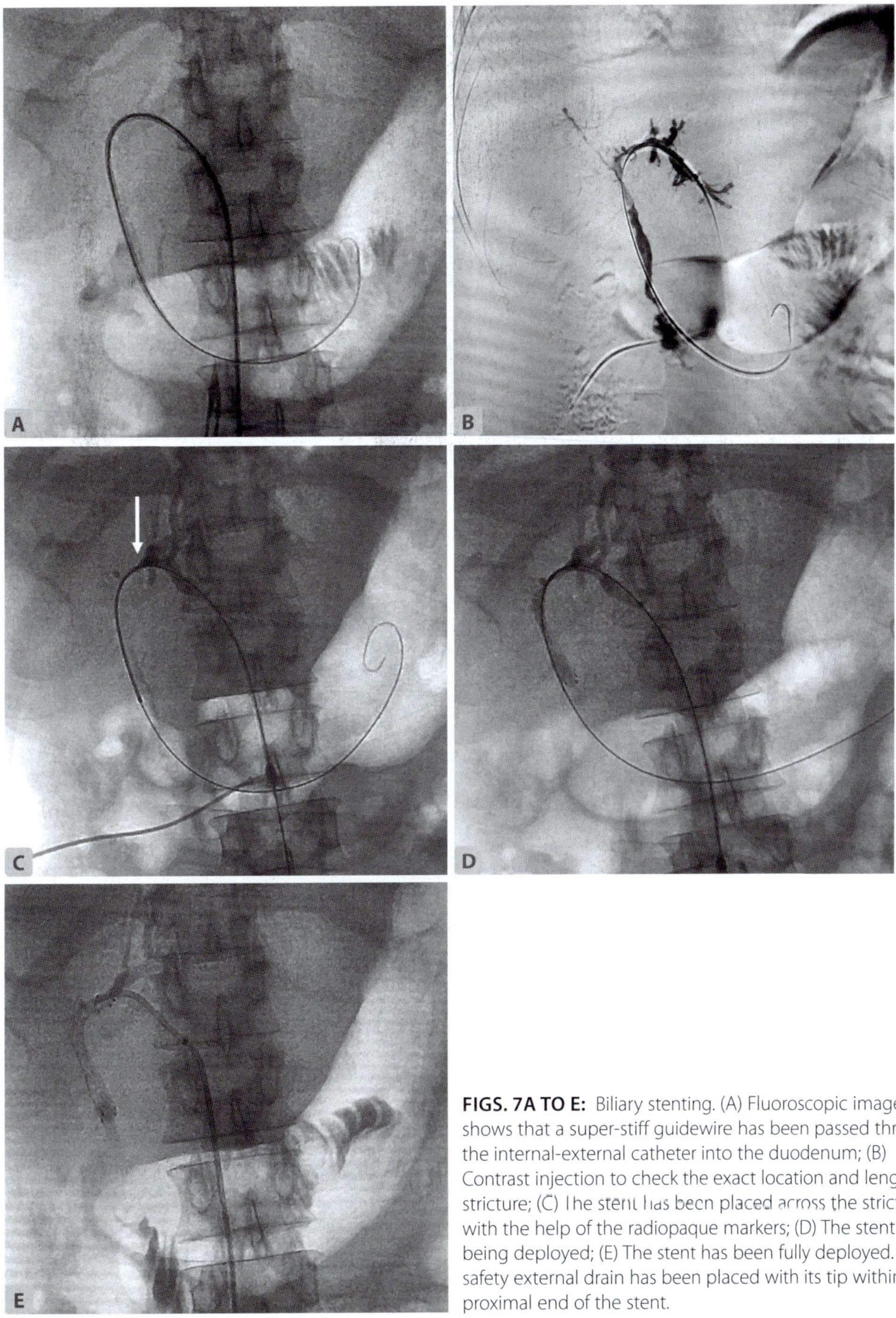

FIGS. 7A TO E: Biliary stenting. (A) Fluoroscopic image shows that a super-stiff guidewire has been passed through the internal-external catheter into the duodenum; (B) Contrast injection to check the exact location and length of stricture; (C) The stent has been placed across the stricture with the help of the radiopaque markers; (D) The stent is being deployed; (E) The stent has been fully deployed. A safety external drain has been placed with its tip within the proximal end of the stent.

by the stent, resulting in a higher complication rate of cholangitis, cholecystitis or pancreatitis.[29] Stent obstruction requires a repeat procedure with either placement of an internal—external drain or a fresh stent through the lumen of the obstructed stent.

Results and Complications of Biliary Drainage

Successful biliary drainage is defined as placement of a drainage tube or stent to provide continuous drainage of bile. The reported rates are 95% in dilated ducts and 70% in non-dilated ducts for placement of external drainage catheters. Of these, about 90% of cases successfully undergo internal-external drain placement.[8]

The complication rate for PTBD can be substantial and depends upon the pre-procedure patient status and diagnosis. The rate is higher in cases with malignant obstruction, cholangitis or coagulopathy. Major complications include hemorrhage, shock due to injection of contrast medium or sudden biliary decompression,

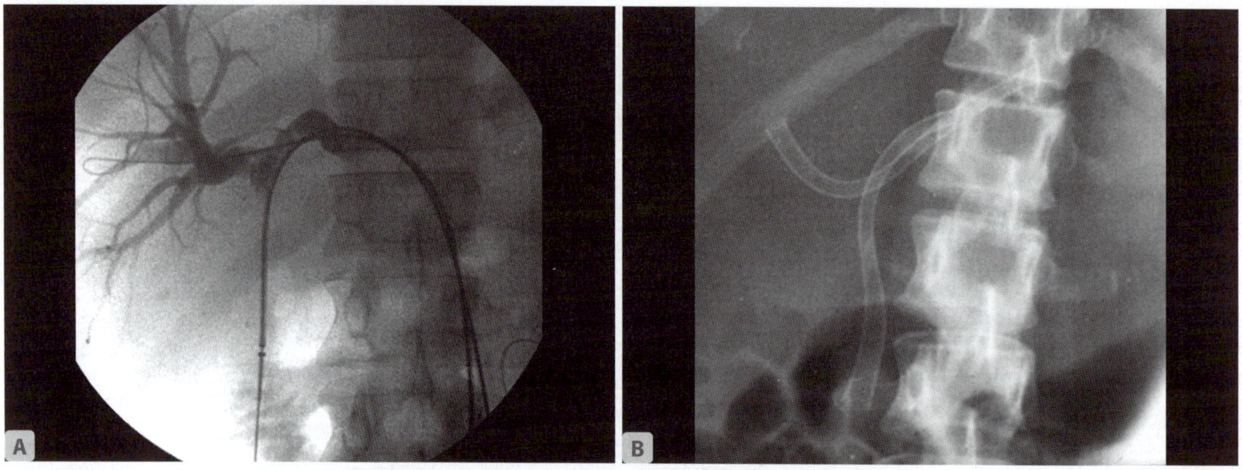

FIGS. 8A AND B: T-stenting in a 38-year-old female with hilar block due to carcinoma gallbladder. (A) An internal-external drain is present on the left side along with a left-to right drain. A stiff guidewire has been anchored in the right ductal system and a stent placed across the hilar stricture into the duodenum; (B) Two metallic stents have been placed across the hilar stricture in a "T" configuration.

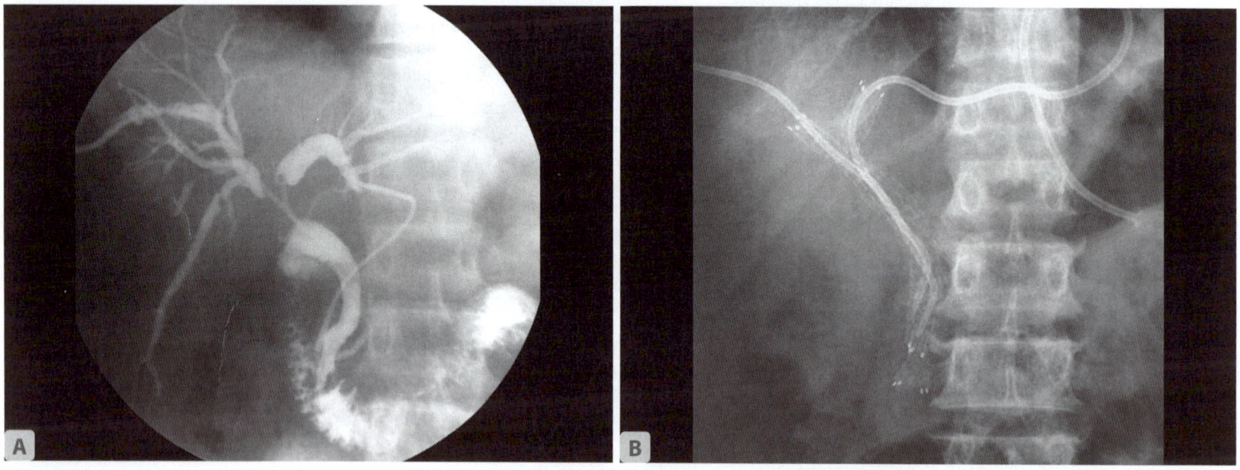

FIGS. 9A AND B: Y-stenting in a 58-year-old male with hilar obstruction due to cholangiocarcinoma. (A) Cholangiogram shows an internal-external drainage catheter placed via left and right ductal systems; (B) Two metallic stents have been placed parallel to each other in a "Y" configuration.

sepsis and bile peritonitis due to slippage of catheter. The hemorrhage may be due to venous or arterial injury. Hemobilia following the procedure is common and usually resolves within 48–72 hours but may require clamping of the catheter or change to a larger bore catheter.[25] If hemobilia persists, a CT angiogram should be done. If the scan shows a pseudoaneurysm or active extravasation of contrast, it can be managed with embolization. Pancreatitis can occur after internal-external drainage and may be due to edema of the common bile duct or obstruction of the main pancreatic duct by the catheter. Pneumothorax or pleural effusion can result from inadvertent transpleural puncture. Cholangitis can develop if there is blockage of the catheter or if some intrahepatic ducts remain undrained. The reported rate of major complications is 2.5–10% while the reported mortality is 0–3%.[7]

INTRALUMINAL PROCEDURES THROUGH PERCUTANEOUS TRANSHEPATIC BILIARY DRAINAGE

Various procedures can be performed using the access available through the percutaneous biliary drainage route. Diagnostic procedures include endobiliary tissue sampling for histopathological analysis. This can be done by using a cytological brush or endoluminal forceps through an 8F sheath after internal external drainage.[30]

Palliative therapies can be performed through the PTBD access route in an effort to improve the quality of life, life expectancy and stent patency. These include brachytherapy, radiofrequency ablation and photodynamic therapy. High dose rate intraluminal brachytherapy (ILBT)

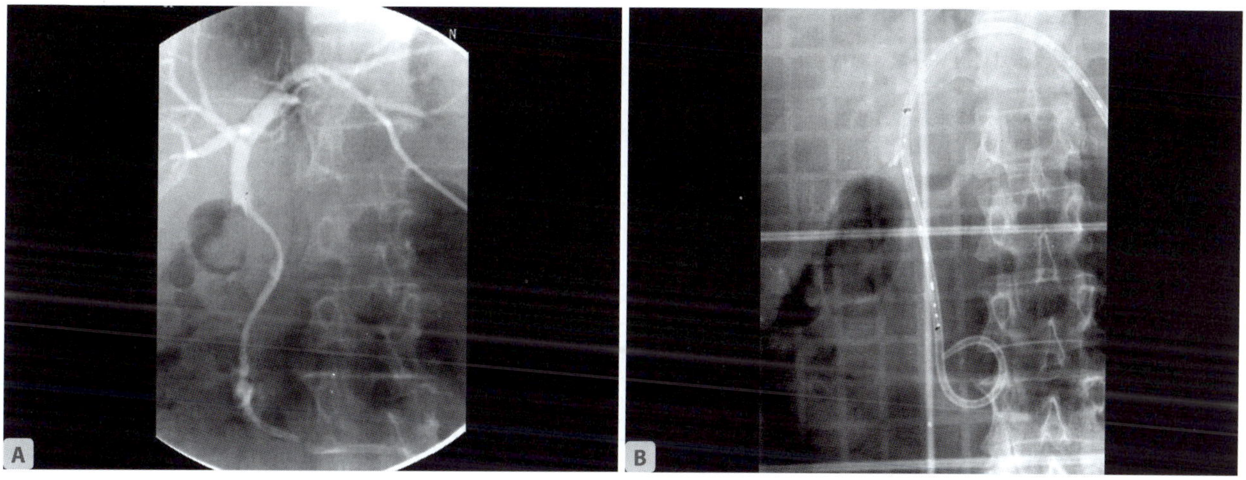

FIGS. 10A AND B: Intraluminal brachytherapy in a 41-year-old female with carcinoma gallbladder. (A) Cholangiogram after internal-external drainage demonstrates a 4 cm stricture in the mid CBD; (B) A 10 F pigtail catheter has been placed with its in the duodenum. Simulator film shows placement of the brachytherapy catheter within the pigtail catheter with its distal end 1 cm beyond the distal end of the stricture.

using Iridium-192 can be delivered selectively to the tumor whilst avoiding the side effect of external radiotherapy. This treatment can be offered in patients who have a single tumor with an overall stricture length of less than 6 cm and the absence of distant disease. The drainage catheter is replaced by the brachytherapy catheter over a stiff guidewire and positioned with its tip 1 cm beyond the distal end of the stricture. The unit is programmed to treat the stricture length and 1 cm beyond and proximal to the stricture **(Figs. 10A and B)**. Studies have shown a significant improvement in the quality of life when ILBT is combined with PTBD with improved stent patency.[31,32]

Similarly, a radiofrequency probe can be introduced through a sheath and the active part placed across the stricture **(Fig. 11)**. RF energy is applied in the range of 8–15 watts for 2 minutes at each level. The procedure has been shown to be safe, whether it results in improved stent patency requires further larger studies to be done.[33] Photodynamic therapy using laser has also been described.[34]

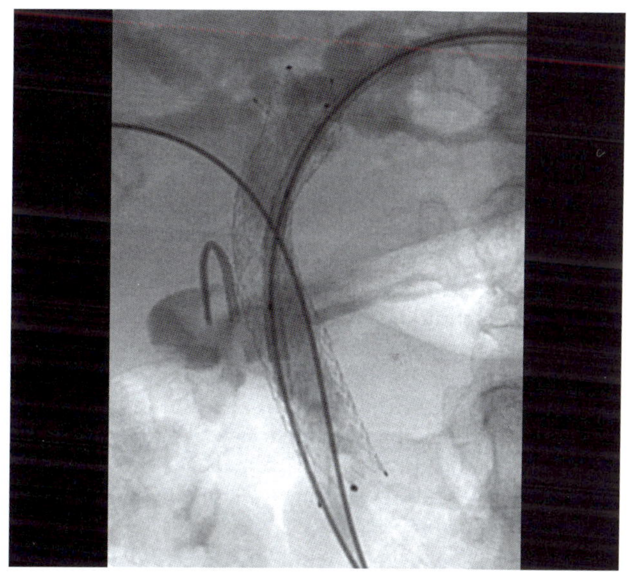

FIG. 11: Intraluminal radiofrequency ablation in a malignant hilar stricture. The radiofrequency probe has been placed through a sheath across the stricture.

Courtesy: Dr Shyamkumar N Keshava, Christian Medical College, Vellore, Tamil Nadu, India.

Percutaneous Transhepatic Cholangioplasty

Most benign biliary strictures are treated surgically with creation of biliary enteric anastomoses. A considerable number suffer recurrence of the stricture after surgical treatment and these are even more difficult to treat surgically. Balloon dilatation of these strictures is a therapeutic option. The technique consists of replacing the internal-external drainage catheter with a balloon catheter. The stricture is inflated with a 8–10 mm balloon for at least 10 minutes and a large diameter catheter is placed across the stricture to induce nonstenosed fibrosis **(Figs. 12A and B)**. It is recommended that three to six balloon inflations be performed at intervals of three weeks with upsizing of the drainage catheter at each sitting. Once cholangiograms show free flow of contrast across the stricture, the catheter is retracted proximal to the stricture and capped. The patient is monitored for a few days to ensure that the bile is flowing internally. The external catheter is removed if the patient remains asymptomatic. Success rates of 70–93% have been reported in literature.[35,36]

PERCUTANEOUS CHOLECYSTOSTOMY

Percutaneous cholecystostomy may be used as a temporizing measure in patients of acute cholecystitis who are critically ill and therefore cannot undergo surgery.[4-6,37] After the patient's condition is stabilized, cholecystectomy as the definitive treatment will still be required. However, in acalculous cholecystitis, percutaneous drainage may be the

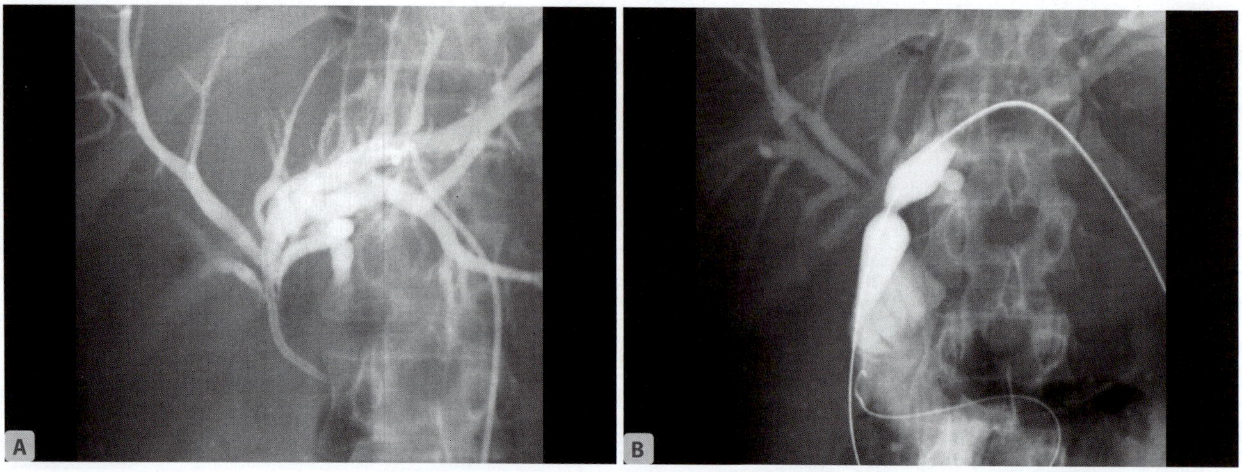

FIGS. 12A AND B: Balloon dilatation of a benign biliary stricture in a case of postoperative choledochojejunostomy stricture. (A) 8F drainage catheter has been placed across the stricture with its tip in the jejunal loop from the left duct approach; (B) Balloon catheter has been placed over the stricture and inflated. Note the "waist" formation in the balloon due to the tight stricture.

only treatment required. Cholecystostomy can also provide a means of accessing the biliary tree in patients with obstructive jaundice in whom the bile ducts are not dilated and the level of obstruction is distal to the insertion of the cystic duct.

Technique

The gallbladder is punctured under US guidance. There are two approach routes available for puncturing the gallbladder. The transhepatic route is usually preferred as the transperitoneal approach carried a greater risk of biliary leak with bile peritonitis. Using the transhepatic route, the gallbladder is punctured where it is fixed to the liver, generally at the junction between the cephalic and middle third of the body. In the transperitoneal approach, the gallbladder is punctured at the point where it lies closest to the anterior abdominal wall. The trocar technique is generally used for direct puncture while the seldinger technique is preferred for the transhepatic route.

An 18G needle is used to puncture the gallbladder and sample collected for gram staining and culture. A small amount of contrast is then injected to opacify the gallbladder for the subsequent steps for which flurosocopic guidance is used. A J-shaped soft tip guidewire is then inserted through the needle and coiled within the lumen. After dilating the tract, a 7F or 8F catheter having an anchor mechanism or of the pigtail type is placed within the gallbladder lumen and sutured to the skin. The catheter is left to drain by gravity **(Figs. 13A to C)**.

If surgery is not considered as in acalculous cholecystitis, the catheter can be removed once the patient's signs and symptoms resolve and a sufficient time has elapsed for the tract to mature. This is said to be at least two weeks when the transhepatic route is used and three weeks when the transperitoneal approach is used. Removal of the catheter before tract maturation may result in leakage of bile and peritonitis.[38,39]

Complications

The complications which can occur following percutaneous cholecystostomy include bile peritonitis, hemobilia and gallbladder perforation. Vasovagal reaction due to tube placement can be managed with atropine. Hemorrhage can at times be fatal. Minimal manipulation should be done at the time of initial drainage to avoid complications.[40] Reported mortality rates range from 3% to 36% depending on the co-morbid conditions.[14]

CONCLUSION

In conclusion, percutaneous biliary procedures are a well-established method of management of patients with obstructive jaundice. PTBD and stenting offer a safe and effective method for the palliative treatment of malignant biliary obstruction. Newer intraluminal palliative techniques hold the promise of improvement in the patient's quality of life and improved stent patency rates. Percutaneous cholangioplasty is a safe and effective therapeutic procedure for benign biliary strictures. Percutaneous cholecystostomy is a life-saving management option in critically ill patients.

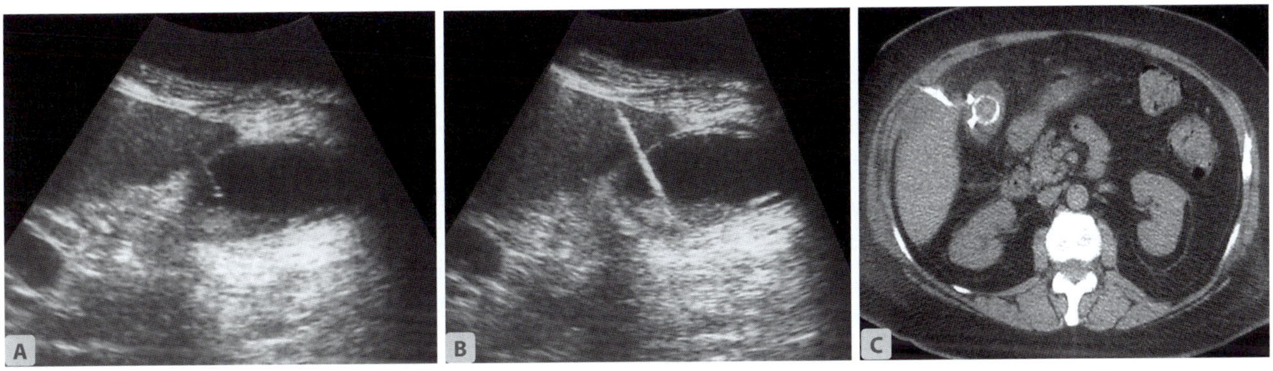

FIGS. 13A TO C: Percutaneous cholecystostomy in a case of empyema of the gallbladder. (A) Sonogram demonstrates the tip of the puncture needle in the lumen of the gallbladder placed via the transhepatic approach; (B) A stiff guidewire has placed and coiled in the lumen; (C) Follow-up CT axial image demonstrates the loop of the pigtail catheter in the lumen of the gallbladder.

REFERENCES

1. Molnar W, Stockum AC. Relief of obstructive jaundice through percutaneous transhepatic catheter—a new therapeutic method. AJR. 1974;122:356-67.
2. Ferrucci JT Jr, Mueller PR, Harbin WP. Percutaneous transhepatic biliary drainage: technique, results and applications. Radiology. 1980;135:1-13.
3. Mueller PR, Van Sonnenberg E, Ferrucci JT Jr. Percutaneous biliary drainage: Technical and catheter related problems in 200 procedures. AJR. 1982;138:17-23.
4. Hamy A, Visset J, Likholatnikov D, et al. Percutaneous cholecystostomy for acute cholecystitis in critically ill patients. Surgery. 1997;121:398-404.
5. Lee KT, Wong SR, Cheng JS, et al. Ultrasound guided percutaneous cholecystostomy as an initial treatment for acute cholecystitis in elderly patients. Dig Surg. 1998;15:328-32.
6. Davis CA, Landercasper J, Gundrsen LH, et al. Effective use of percutaneous cholecystostomy in high risk surgical patients: techniques, tube management, and results. Arch Surg. 1999;134:727-31.
7. van Delden OM, Laméris JS. Percutaneous drainage and stenting for palliation of malignant bile duct obstruction. Eur Radiol. 2008;18:448-56.
8. Saad WEA, Wallace MJ, Wojak JC, Kundu S, Cardella JF. Quality improvement guidelines for percutaneous transhepatic cholangiography, biliary drainage, and percutaneous cholecystostomy. J Vasc Interv Radiol. 2010;21:789-95.
9. Tapping CR, Byass OR, Cast JEI. Percutaneous transhepatic biliary drainage (PTBD) with or without stenting—complications, re-stent rate and a new risk stratification score. Eur Radiol. 2011;21:1948-55.
10. Madhusudan KS, Gamanagatti S, Srivastava DN, Gupta AK. Radiological interventions in malignant biliary obstruction. World J Radiol. 2016;8(5):518-29.
11. Pu LZCT, Singh R, Loong CK, de Moura EGH. Malignant biliary obstruction: Evidence for best practice. Gastroenterol Res Pract. 2016;Epub 2016 Feb11.
12. Harbin WP, Mueller PR, Ferrucci JT Jr. Transhepatic cholangiography: complications and use patterns of the fine-needle technique: a multi-institutional survey. Radiology. 1980;135(1):15-22.
13. Mueller PR, Harbin WP, Ferrucci JT Jr, et al. Fine-needle transhepatic cholangiography: reflections after 450 cases. AJR. 1981;136:85-90.
14. Rosenblatt M, Aruny JE, Kandarpa K. Transhepatic cholangiography, biliary decompression, endobiliary stenting and cholecystectomy. In: Handbook of Interventional Radiologic procedures, 3rd edn. Lippincott, Williams and Wilkins, Philadelphia, Kandarpa K, Aruny JE (Eds). PA. 2002;19106 USA.
15. Fidelman N. Benign biliary strictures: Diagnostic evaluation and approaches to percutaneous treatment. Tech Vasc Interv Radiol. 2015;18(4):210-7.
16. Baijal SS, Dhiman RK, Gupta S, et al. Percutaneous transhepatic biliary drainage in the management of obstructive jaundice. Trop Gastroenterol. 1997;18:167-71.
17. Tsetis D, Krokidis M, Negru D, Prassopoulos P. Malignant biliary obstruction: the current role of interventional radiology. Ann Gastroenterol. 2016;29:33-6.
18. Inal M, Akgül E, Aksungur E, Seydaoğlu G. Percutaneous placement of biliary metallic stents in patients with malignant hilar obstruction: unilobar versus bilobar drainage. J Vasc Interv Radiol. 2003;14(11):1409-16.
19. Madhusudan KS, Gamanagatti S, Gupta AK. Imaging and interventional in hilar cholangiocarcinoma: a review. World J Radiol. 2015;7:28-44.
20. Kücükay F, Okten RS, Yurdakal M, et al. Percutaneous management of malignant biliary disease: factors influencing the ability to overcome the stricture. Diagn Interv Radiol. 2011;17:169-73.
21. Lammer H, Hausegger KA, Fluckiger F, et al. Common bile duct obstruction due to malignancy: treatment with plastic versus metal stents. Radiology. 1996;201:167-72.
22. Moss AC, Morris E, MacMathuna P. Palliative biliary stents for obstructing pancreatic carcinoma. Cochrane Database Syst Rev. 2006;CD004200.
23. Moss AC, Morris E, Leyden J, MacMathuna P. Do the benefits of metal stents justify the costs? A systematic review and meta-analyses of trials comparing endoscopic stents for malignant biliary obstruction. Eur J Gastroenterol Heaptol. 2007;19:1119-24.
24. Mukai T, Yasuda I, Nakashima M, et al. Metallic stents are more efficacious than plastic stents in unresectable malignant hilar biliary strictures: a randomized controlled trial. J Hepatobiliary Pancreat Sci. 2013;20:204-22.
25. Inal M, Akgül E, Aksungur E, Demiryürek H, Yağmur O. Percutaneous self-expandable uncovered metallic stents in malignant biliary obstruction. Complications, follow-up and re-interventions in 154 patients. Acta Radiol. 2003;44:139-46.

26. Lee M, Dawson SC, Mueller PR, Saini S, Lu DS, Goldberg MA, Gazelle GS. Failed metallic biliary stents: causes and management of delayed complications. Clin Radiol. 1994;49:857-62.
27. Gwon D, Ko G, Kim JH, et al. Percutaneous bilateral metallic stent placement using a stent-in-stent deployment technique in patients with malignant hilar biliary obstruction. AJR. 2013;200:909-14.
28. Kim CW, Park AW, Won JW, Kim S, Lee JW, Lee SH. T-configured dual stent placement in malignant biliary hilar obstructions with a newly designed stent. J Vasc Interv Radiol. 2004;15:713-7.
29. Gwon D, Ko G, Yoon H, et al. Safety and efficacy of percutaneous Y-configured covered stent placement for malignant hilar biliary obstruction: a prospective pilot study. J Vasc Interv Radiol. 2012;23:528-34.
30. Xing GS, Geng JC, Han XW, Dai JH, Wu CY. Endobiliary brush cytology during percutaneous transhepatic cholangiodrainage in patients with obstructive jaundice. Hepatobiliary Pancreat Dis Int. 2005;4:98-103.
31. Aggarwal R, Patel FD, Kapoor R, Kang M, Kumar P, Sharma S. Evaluation of high-dose rate intraluminal brachytherapy by percutaneous transhepatic biliary drainage in the palliative management of malignant biliary obstruction—a pilot study. Brachytherapy. 2013;12:162-70.
32. Chen Y, Wang XC, Yan ZP, et al. HDR-192 Ir intraluminal brachytherapy in treatment of malignant obstructive jaundice. World J Gastroenterol. 2004;10:3506-10.
33. Mizandari M, Pai M, Xi F, et al. Percutaneous intraductal radiofrequency ablation is a safe treatment for malignant biliary obstruction: feasibility and early results. Cardiovasc Interv Radiol. 2013;36:814-9.
34. Lee TY, Cheon YK, Shim CS. Current status of photodynamic therapy for bile duct cancer. Clin Endosc. 2013;46:38-44.
35. Fidelman N. Benign biliary strictures: Diagnostic evaluation and approaches to percutaneous treatment. Tech Vasc Interv Radiol. 2015;18(4):210-7.
36. Gwon DI, Ko GY, Ko HK, Yoon HK, Sung KB. Percutaneous transhepatic treatment using retrievable covered stents in patients with benign biliary strictures: mid-term outcomes in 68 patients. Dig Dis Sci. 2013;58(11):3270-9.
37. Boggi U, DiCandio G, Campatelli A, et al. Percutaneous cholecystostomy for acute cholecystitis in critically ill patients. Hepatogastroenterology. 1999;46(25):121-5.
38. Kiviniemi H, Makela JT, Antio R, et al. Percutaneous cholecystostomy in acute cholecystitis in high risk patients: an analysis of 69 patients. Int Surg. 1998;83(4):299-302.
39. Hatjidakis AA, Karampekios S, Prassopoulos P, et al. Maturation of the tract after percutaneous cholecystostomy with regard to the access route. Cardiovasc Interv Radiol. 1998;21:36-40.
40. Pang KW, Tan Ch, Loh S, et al. Outcomes of percutaneous cholecystostomy for acute cholecystitis. World J Surg. 2016;02 (Epub ahead of print).

CHAPTER

111

Acute Pancreatitis: Imaging and Interventions

Kumble S Madhusudhan, Raju Sharma

INTRODUCTION

Acute pancreatitis (AP) is defined as acute inflammation of pancreas. The inflammation may extend beyond the pancreas to the surrounding fat and other organs as well and infrequently results in a systemic inflammatory response syndrome and organ failure. Mild type of pancreatitis is seen in about 80% patients and the severe variety in 20%.[1] Severe acute pancreatitis has high mortality reaching up to 30%.[2] The incidence of acute pancreatitis is rising due to increase in the incidence of obesity, gallstone disease and alcoholism.[3] Hence, early recognition and diagnosis of this condition is critical for judicious management. Recently, there has been a change in the terminology related to this disease and awareness of the features of revised classification and the role of radiologist in diagnosis and management is important.

PATHOPHYSIOLOGY

Pancreas secretes many enzymes; autodigestion of pancreatic parenchyma by these enzymes results in acute pancreatitis.[4] In normal pancreas, this is prevented by various natural defence mechanisms in pancreas. Whenever, there is pancreatic injury (e.g. alcohol) or increase in ductal pressure (e.g. gallstone), there is increase in secretion of activated proteolytic enzymes (trypsin, amylase, lipase) and increased permeability which result in increased concentration of these enzymes within the parenchyma **(Fig. 1)**. This leads to autodigestion of the pancreatic parenchyma and peripancreatic regions. A vicious cycle is initiated with more destruction of pancreatic cells and more release of enzymes.[4] This incites inflammation and increases cytokine production which is responsible for systemic manifestations. Lipase results in fat necrosis and saponification of peripancreatic fat.

ETIOLOGY

The two common causes of acute pancreatitis are alcohol intake and gallstone disease. These two together constitute 70–80% of cases of acute pancreatitis.[5] Other uncommon causes include abdominal trauma, drugs (azathioprine, tetracycline, thiazides), iatrogenic (post-endoscopic interventions), hypercalcemia, hyperlipidemia, tumors (periampullary carcinoma) and infections (mumps, coxsackie B virus). No cause is identified in about 10–15% cases (idiopathic).[5]

REVISED ATLANTA CLASSIFICATION

The original Atlanta classification was presented in the year 1992 to classify the types of pancreatitis, its severity and complications and was mainly based on clinical criteria.[6] Since then, there has been improvement in understanding of the disease, imaging techniques and treatment options. Also, the classification was inadequate, ambiguous and did not include radiological criteria. Thus there was a need for revising the classification which was done in 2012 **(Flowchart 1)**.[7] For the radiologists, the important aspect is the different morphological types of pancreatitis and CT criteria for various named fluid collections.[8] This revised classification is specific for acute pancreatitis and does not apply to chronic pancreatitis, acute on chronic pancreatitis and groove pancreatitis, which have different pathophysiology and outcome.

The following are the salient features of the revised Atlanta classification **(Flowchart 1)**.

Diagnosis

The diagnosis of AP is made when any two of the following three features are fulfilled:

1. Characteristic pain of acute pancreatitis (epigastric pain, radiating to the back)
2. Elevated serum amylase or lipase levels more than at least three times the normal levels
3. Typical imaging features of acute pancreatitis.

Thus acute pancreatitis is often a clinical diagnosis (when first two features are fulfilled) and imaging is needed only when clinical features are atypical.

Types of Acute Pancreatitis

Acute interstitial edematous pancreatitis (AIEP): In this type, there is inflammation in and around the pancreas, with or

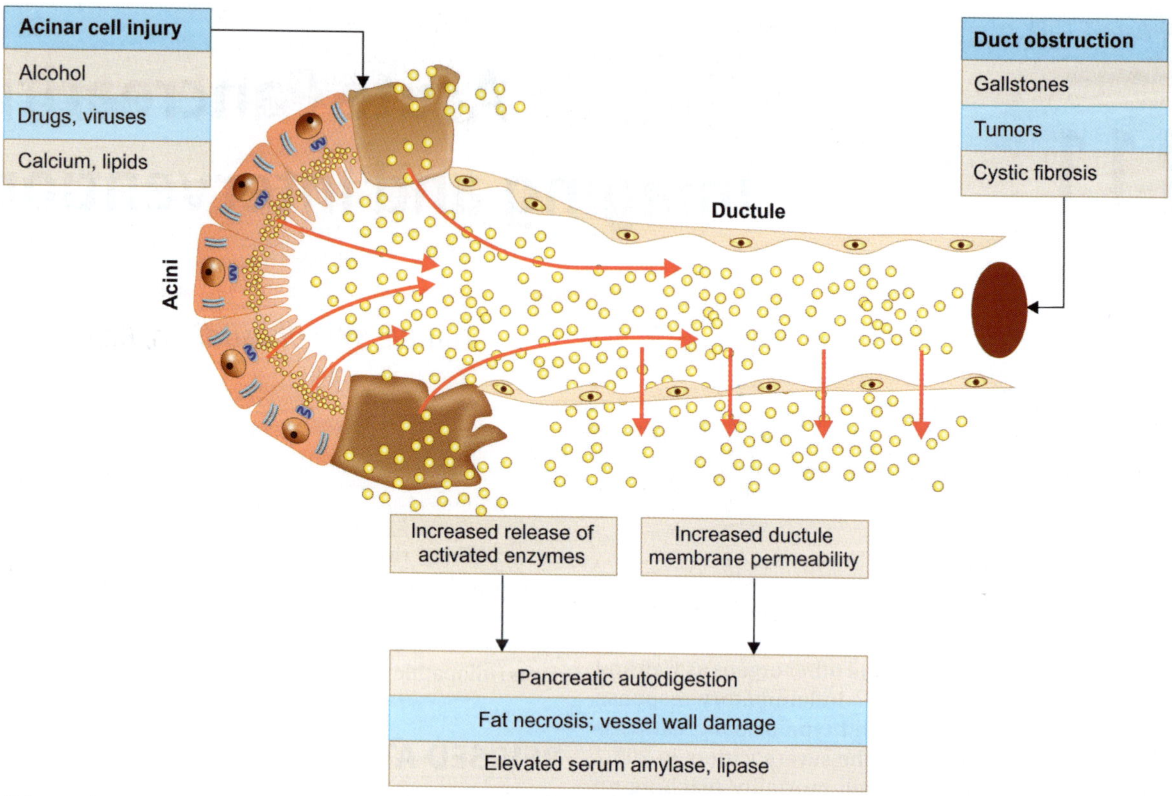

FIG. 1: Schematic diagram showing the pathophysiology of acute pancreatitis.

FLOWCHART 1: The nomenclature used in revised Atlanta classification.

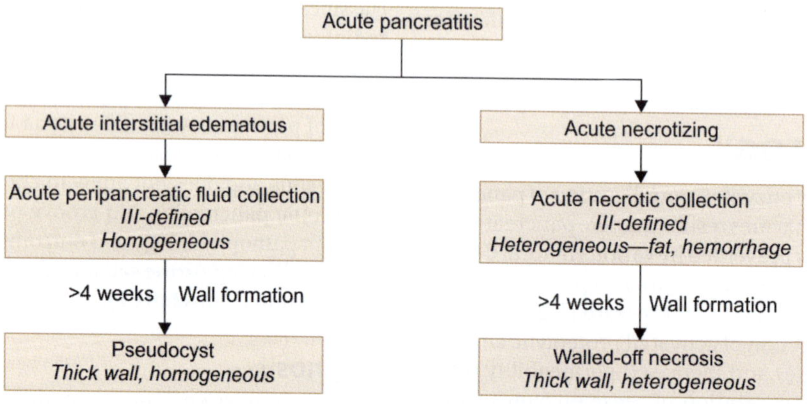

without fluid collections. However, no pancreatic or peripancreatic necrosis is seen. This has good prognosis and has a mortality under 3%.[9]

Acute necrotizing pancreatitis (ANP): This, as the name suggests, is associated with pancreatic and/or peripancreatic necrosis. This has variable prognosis, ranging from complete recovery to mortality, which is seen in up to 30% cases.

Phases of Acute Pancreatitis

Acute pancreatitis is divided into two phases due to biphasic clinical course. *Early phase* occurs in first week and is associated with systemic inflammatory response syndrome (SIRS) or multiorgan failure which may cause mortality.[2] In *late phase* (after first week), there are other complications such as infection or sepsis which are common causes of mortality. Imaging plays an important role in the late phase of the disease.

Nomenclature

The terminology has now been defined to allow uniformity among the radiologists and referring clinicians **(Figs. 2A to D)**.[5]

Acute Peripancreatic Fluid Collection (APFC)

This is seen in AIEP and is defined as simple fluid collection in peripancreatic location with ill-defined walls and

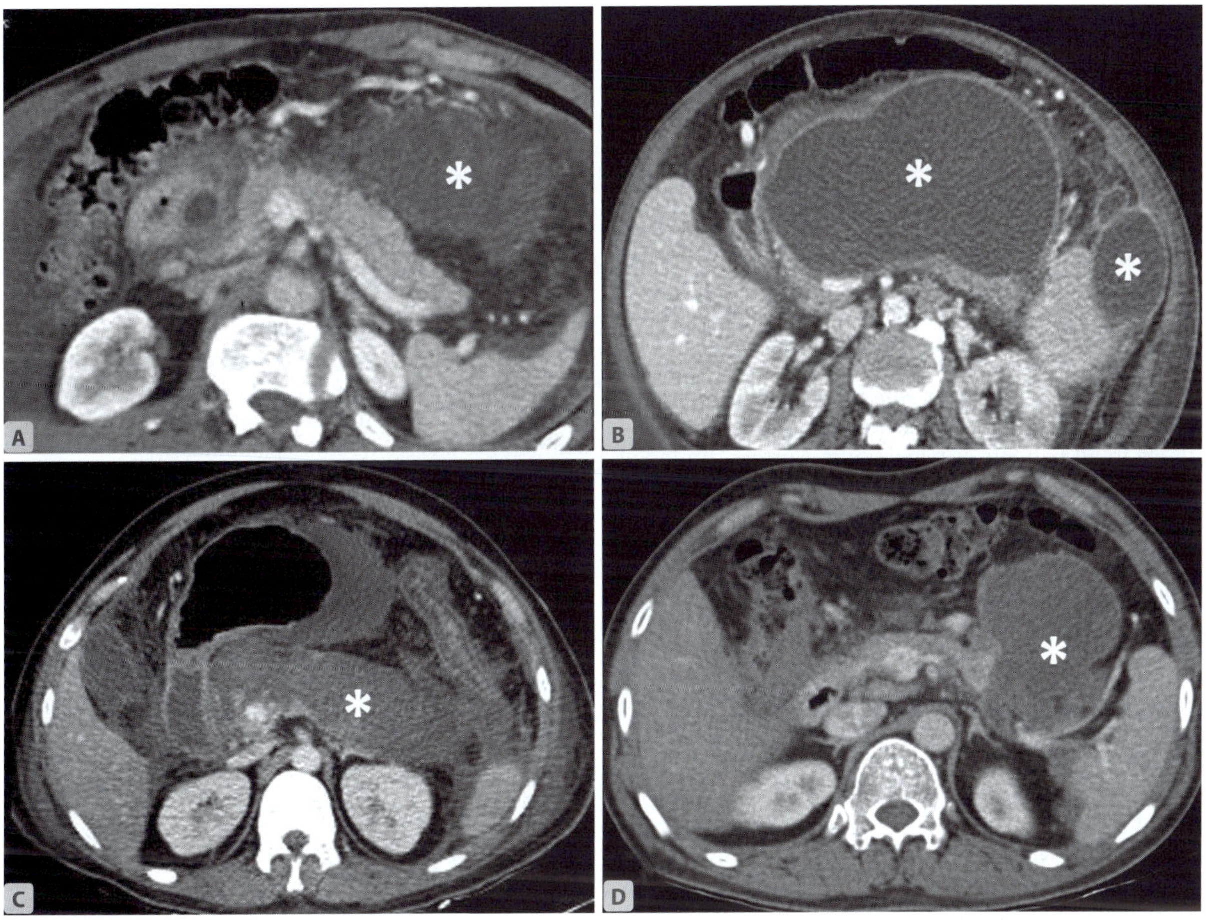

FIGS. 2A TO D: Nomenclature of collections (asterisks) according to revised Atlanta classification on contrast-enhanced CT scan: (A) Acute peripancreatic fluid collection; (B) Pseudocyst; (C) Acute necrotic collection; and (D) Walled-off necrosis.

homogeneous low density appearance and limited by fascial planes or peritoneal reflections. This is seen less than 4 weeks from the onset of the disease.

Acute Necrotic Collection (ANC)

This is seen in ANP and is a heterogeneous ill-defined collection of fluid within or around the pancreas. This is seen less than 4 weeks from the onset of the disease.

Pseudocyst

This is seen after 4 weeks of illness in the setting of acute edematous pancreatitis and is seen as a well-defined homogeneous low density fluid collection with well-defined wall.

Walled-off Necrosis (WON)

This is ANC after 4 weeks duration and is seen as a heterogeneous thick-walled collection.

It is important to understand that these terms have relevance in disease management. After 4 weeks, there is walling off of the collection with liquefaction in case of WON which determines successful intervention. Also, by convention, acute peripancreatic fluid collection (APFC) and pseudocyst are not seen in acute necrotizing pancreatitis (ANP) and acute necrotic collection (ANC) and WON are not seen in acute interstitial edematous pancreatitis (AIEP). The terms like pancreatic pseudocyst, phlegmon, pancreatic abscess and hemorrhagic pancreatitis are not used anymore.

TABLE 1: Classification of severity of acute pancreatitis.

Severity of acute pancreatitis	
Mild	No organ failure/local complications
Moderately severe	Local complications and/or organ failure <48 hours
Severe	Organ failure >48 hours

Classification of Severity

Based on severity (clinical and on imaging), acute pancreatitis can be divided into mild, moderately severe and severe **(Table 1)**. *Mild pancreatitis* is not associated with organ failure or any local or systemic complications. *Moderately severe pancreatitis* is defined when there is transient organ failure (lasting <48 hours) or local/systemic complications in the form of symptomatic collections or systemic inflammatory response syndrome (SIRS) requiring prolonged hospital stay or interventions. *Severe pancreatitis* is characterized by persistent organ failure (for >48 hours) with or without local or systemic complications. This has prognostic importance as almost all patients of mild pancreatitis recover in a week whereas patients with severe pancreatitis have high morbidity and mortality.[10] However, the correlation is not absolute. About 5% of patients with mild pancreatitis may have significant complications with mortality of 1–2% and about 30% of severe pancreatitis may have a benign course.[9]

IMAGING TECHNIQUES

Imaging plays an important role in the management of patients of acute pancreatitis. However, it is not done routinely in all patients of pancreatitis. Further, timing of imaging is also important.

Indications (Table 2)

As discussed above, the diagnosis of acute pancreatitis can often be made clinically. Imaging is needed when the abdominal pain is not typical or when serum amylase level elevation is borderline. Here, imaging will help in confirming or excluding a diagnosis of acute pancreatitis.[11]

In AIEP, imaging after diagnosis is not necessary as most patients have an unremarkable self-limiting course. Only when complications are clinically suspected, imaging is needed during the course of the disease. In ANP, imaging is often needed, usually in the first week, to define the extent of necrosis. Subsequently, imaging is done when complications are suspected, patient is not improving, there is organ failure, drop in hemoglobin, gastrointestinal bleed or features of sepsis. Imaging thus plays a role in severity assessment, evaluation of complications and guiding management.[8]

Plain Radiography

Plain radiography has a very limited role in the diagnosis of acute pancreatitis. It may show sentinel dilated jejunal/duodenal loop in the left hypochondrium due to ileus. Other signs include colon cut-off (dilated large bowel till splenic flexure), gasless abdomen, obliteration of left psoas shadow and elevated hemidiaphragm.[12] Calcifications may be seen in a patient with chronic calcific pancreatitis. More important role of abdominal radiograph is in excluding other causes of acute abdomen such as bowel perforation and acute small bowel obstruction.

TABLE 2: Indications for imaging.

Indications for imaging in acute pancreatitis
Doubtful/inconclusive clinical diagnosis
Interstitial edematous pancreatitis:
• Organ failure
• Local complications
Necrotizing pancreatitis:
• Initial baseline scan (after 5–7 days)
• Persistent organ failure or SIRS
• Fever/elevated leukocyte count
• Patient deterioration
• Requirement of interventions
• Gastrointestinal bleed/Hb drop

(SIRS: systemic inflammatory response syndrome)

Ultrasonography

Ultrasonography (USG) is often the initial investigation of choice in patients with acute abdomen. Normal pancreas shows intermediate echogenicity uniformly; it may appear hyperechoic due to fatty infiltration, which typically happens with age. The normal thickness of pancreatic parenchyma is about 20–25 mm in head and tail regions and 15–20 mm in the body region.[13] The normal pancreatic duct is less than 3 mm in size and shows smooth outline.

Frequently, due to extensive inflammation (especially in ANP) and ileus, pancreas is not visualized and diagnosing acute pancreatitis is difficult.[14] Although USG has lower sensitivity and specificity for diagnosis of acute pancreatitis, its major advantage is that it is radiation free and may be repeated whenever needed. It mainly helps in detection of gallstones, bile duct calculi, biliary obstruction and assessing the extent of liquefaction of collections which help in planning drainage procedures.[15] USG is also useful in guiding diagnostic and therapeutic interventions. Additional advantages include that it can be used in children and in bedside assessment of acute pancreatitis.[15]

Computed Tomography

Computed tomography (CT) scan occupies the centre stage of imaging in acute pancreatitis and has high accuracy (80–90%).[14] It is performed as a contrast-enhanced CT (CECT) scan after injecting intravenous-iodinated contrast agent and acquiring scans in the portal venous phase (60–70 seconds) after the beginning of contrast injection. An arterial phase (25–30 seconds) is acquired, whenever there is suspicion of gastrointestinal or extraluminal hemorrhage, pancreatic mass or mesenteric ischemia.[5] Pancreatic phase (40–50 seconds) has been suggested by some instead of portal venous phase as the pancreas enhances most during this phase.[16] In patients with renal failure or those with allergy to iodinated contrast agents, non-contrast CT or MRI may be done. Oral contrast is usually not necessary, when the patient presents with acute abdomen. However, during follow-up, positive oral contrast helps in evaluation of bowel loops and differentiate a distended fluid-filled bowel from fluid collection. Plain scans are usually not necessary, although it may help in detecting calcification and hemorrhage. The scan is done from the level of diaphragm to symphysis pubis initially. Subsequent follow-up scans may be limited to upper abdomen (diaphragm to iliac crest). Coronal and sagittal reformats are useful in defining the extent of inflammation and collections. Normal pancreas appears as homogeneously enhancing tissue with smooth outline. There may be lobulations uncommonly. As age progresses, fatty infiltration may be seen in the parenchyma.

The CT scan should be typically performed after atleast 72 hours of onset of pain as parenchymal necrosis is well-defined by this time. A CT scan done in very early stage of the disease may miss necrosis and will not accurately assess the severity.CECT is also the modality of choice when pancreatitis occurs in patients over 40 years of age to exclude a possible tumor causing secondary pancreatitis.

Magnetic Resonance Imaging

The role of MRI in acute pancreatitis is limited. The long scan times needed and difficulty in breath-holding in these sick patients often results in poor image quality. Faster sequences may still provide answers in select situations. Further, the high cost, need for MR compatible monitors in critically ill patients and limited availability has resulted in limited usage.[15] Specific indications include patients with renal failure or allergy to iodinated contrast agents, children and pregnant patients. It is also used in the evaluation of biliary tree for presence of any obstructing calculus, to assess for liquefaction of a necrotic collection prior to planning drainage and in evaluation of communication of pancreatic duct with collection. Diffusion weighed imaging (DWI) may help in differentiation of infected from sterile necrotic collection. Non-contrast MRI with DWI is better than non-contrast CT scan and should be preferred wherever possible.

The typical sequences include T1W gradient echo (in-phase and opposed phase), T2W spin echo-fat saturated, thick slab T2W rapid recovery and DWI sequences **(Table 3)**. Oral contrast is not necessary. Intravenous gadolinium is necessary when evaluating necrotizing pancreatitis, to assess the extent of necrosis.

IMAGING APPEARANCE

Acute Interstitial Edematous Pancreatitis

On USG, the pancreas appears hypoechoic and bulky **(Fig. 3)**. There may be a hypoechoic rim of inflammation or fluid around the pancreas. Fluid collections may be seen in the peripancreatic regions. Abnormal pancreas is seen in 33-90% of patients of acute pancreatitis.[17]

Contrast-enhanced computed tomography shows diffuse or focal (20%—head or tail) enlargement of the pancreas with mild heterogeneous contrast enhancement **(Figs 4A and B)**.[5] Non-enhancing areas are not seen in the parenchyma. The lobulated outline of pancreatic parenchyma may be lost. There is soft tissue stranding and hypodensity in the peripancreatic fat with thickening of anterior pararenal and lateroconal fascia. There may be associated fluid collections (APFC), seen as ill-defined homogeneous low density areas, ascites and pleural effusion, often left sided. The pancreatic duct is usually normal, unless acute inflammation occurs in the background of chronic calcific pancreatitis. As the disease progresses, most of the patients (80%) improve without any complications. About 10-20% progress to form pseudocysts after about 4 weeks of illness, which also resolve in most patients.[18] In some patients, pseudocyst may result in symptoms when intervention becomes necessary. Secondary infection is very rare.

MRI also shows diffusely bulky and edematous pancreas appearing hypointense on T1-weighted and hyperintense on T2-weighted images **(Figs. 5A and B)**.[19] Fluid collections may be seen in the peripancreatic region. Otherwise, inflammation is seen as ill-defined feathery hyperintense areas on T2-weighted images in peripancreatic regions. Thickening of anterior pararenal and lateroconal fascia is seen with hyperintense signal on T2W. Associated findings include gallstones, calculi in common bile duct with biliary dilatation and dilated pancreatic duct in cases of acute inflammation occurring in the background of chronic pancreatitis. DWI may show restriction of diffusion of the entire pancreas.

Acute Necrotizing Pancreatitis

Ultrasonography is less sensitive in the evaluation of ANP. Depending on the extent of necrosis, pancreas may be variably visualized. There may be fluid collections, appearing hyperechoic or isoechoic, in the lesser sac, perinephric and paracolic regions **(Fig. 6)**. In later stages, hypoechoic fluid collection may be seen in these areas.

In ANP, CECT is critical in defining the extent of parenchymal necrosis as it determines prognosis. The scans should ideally be done between 5 and 7 days after the onset of

TABLE 3: MRI sequences used in the evaluation of acute pancreatitis.

MRI sequences	
Axial T1W	Anatomy; pancreatic edema
Axial T2W FSE–FS	Pancreatic/peripancreatic edema; liquefaction of collections
Coronal T2W–FS	Pancreatic/peripancreatic edema; liquefaction of collections CBD
Axial SSFP	Vascular assessment
DWI	Infected necrosis; debris in collection
MRCP	Biliary tree and pancreatic duct evaluation
Contrast enhanced T1W–FS	Evaluation of pancreatic necrosis

(FSE: fast spin echo; FS: fat-suppressed; CBD: common bile duct; SSFP: steady-state free precession; DWI: diffusion-weighted imaging; MRCP: magnetic resonance cholangiopancreatography)

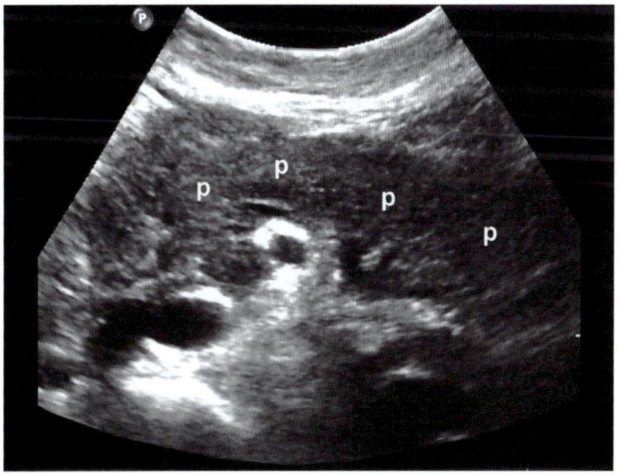

FIG. 3: Ultrasonography of a patient with acute interstitial edematous pancreatitis showing diffusely bulky and hypoechoic pancreas (p).

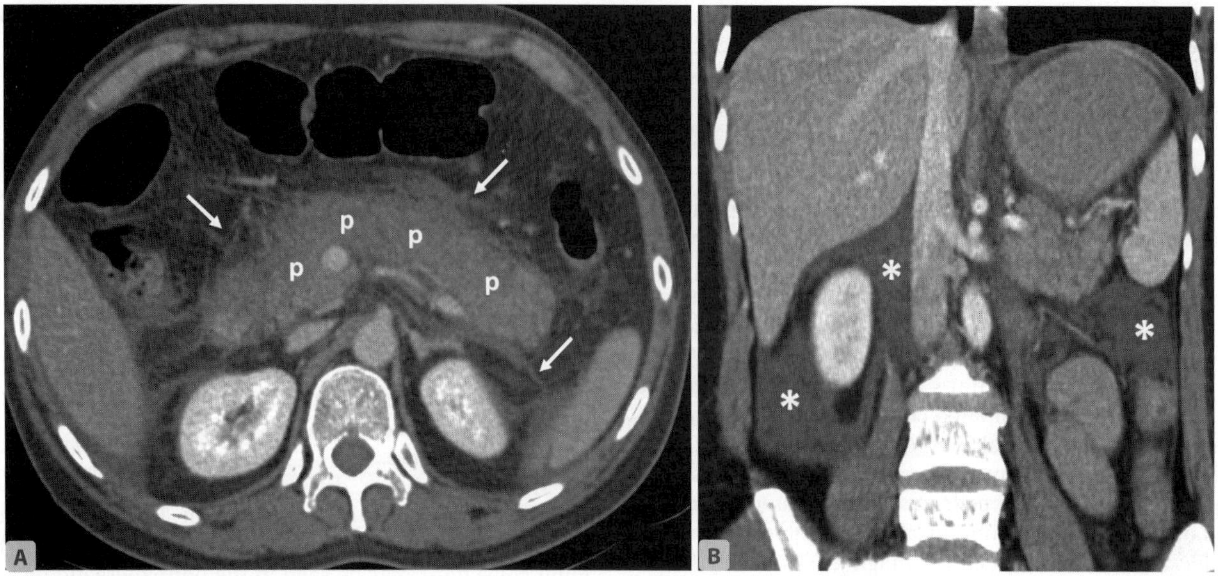

FIGS. 4A AND B: Contrast-enhanced CT scan of a patient with acute interstitial edematous pancreatitis: Axial (A) and coronal (B) images show diffusely bulky pancreas (p) with peripancreatic fat stranding (arrows). Acute peripancreatic fluid collections are seen in the coronal image (asterisks).

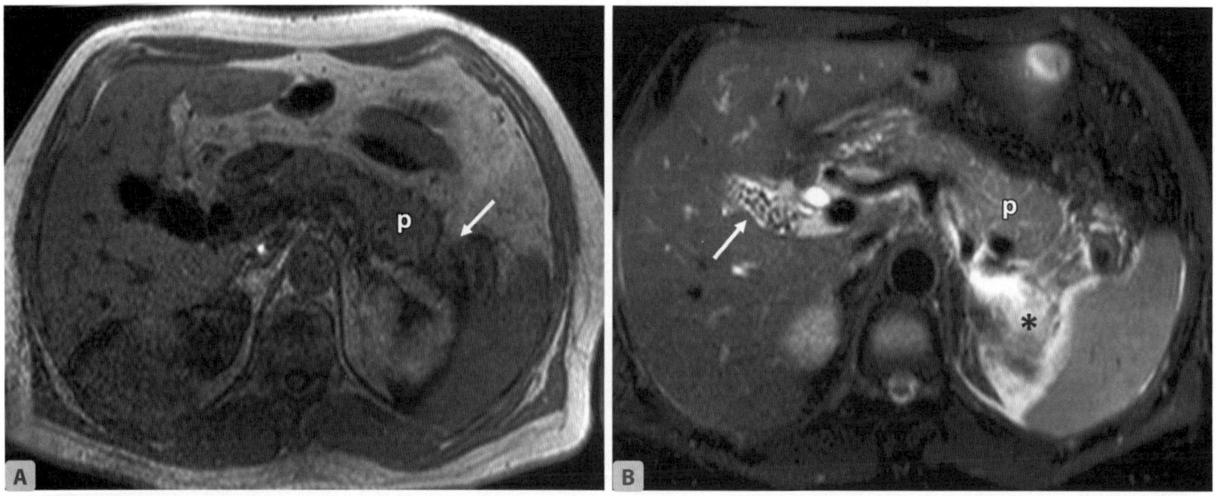

FIGS. 5A AND B: MRI in a patient with acute interstitial edematous pancreatitis: Axial T1-weighted (A) and T2-weighted fat saturated (B) images showing bulky body and tail of pancreas (p) with peripancreatic inflammation (hypointense on T1W—black arrow; hyperintense on T2W—asterisk). Note gallstones in B (white arrow).

the disease.[19] In addition to the features of AIEP, non-enhancing areas suggesting necrosis are seen in the parenchyma **(Figs. 7A and B)**. On MRI, the necrotic tissue is frequently hypointense on both T1- and T2-weighted images prior to liquefaction **(Figs. 8A and B)**. Similar to CT, parenchymal necrosis shows no contrast enhancement. The collections seen in the peripancreatic regions are heterogeneous and often contain areas of fat. They are ill-defined initially (ANC) and gradually get walled-off and liquefy over 4 weeks (WON). Since it is a necrotic collection, it acts as a nidus for secondary infection to develop. Presence of infection is suggested when air-foci are seen in the collection on CECT scan.

The necrosis can be of three types according to the revised Atlanta classification. They include pancreatic necrosis only, peripancreatic necrosis only and combined pancreatic–peripancreatic necrosis.[5,19]

Pancreatic necrosis alone is the least common type, seen in less than 5% of cases. Here, the necrosis is confined to the pancreatic parenchyma and appears as a hypoenhancing/non-enhancing area **(*see* Fig. 2C)**. The extent of necrosis has prognostic significance and is a part of CT severity index (vide infra). The necrosis usually liquefies as it evolves and may show a defined wall, when it is called walled of pancreatic necrosis. This, depending on the size may resolve

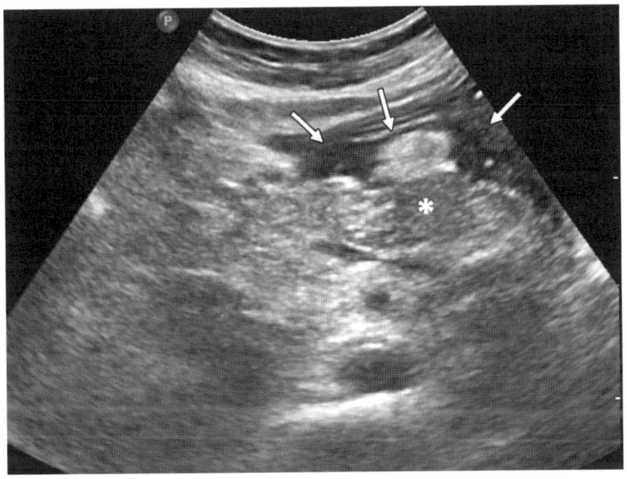

FIG. 6: Ultrasonography of a patient with acute necrotizing pancreatitis showing diffusely bulky and heteroechoic pancreas with hypoechoic area in the body (asterisk) and peripancreatic collection with debris (arrows).

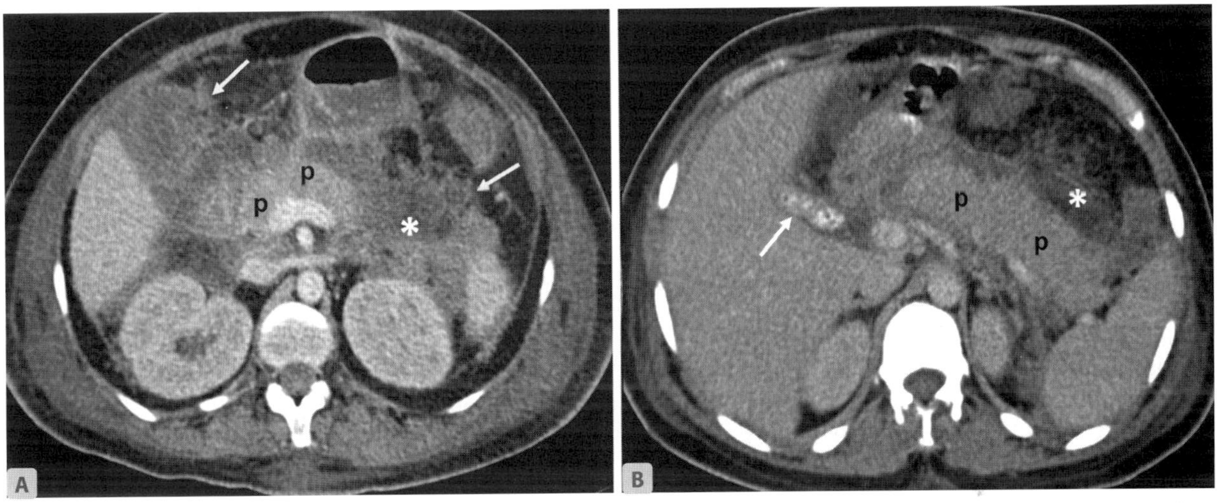

FIGS. 7A AND B: Contrast-enhanced CT scan of a patient with acute necrotizing pancreatitis: (A) Axial image showing pancreatic (asterisk) and peripancreatic (arrows) necrosis with areas of fat density. Normal enhancing pancreas (p) is seen; (B) Axial image showing normal enhancing pancreas (p) with isolated peripancreatic necrosis (asterisk). Note calcified calculi in the gallbladder (arrow in B).

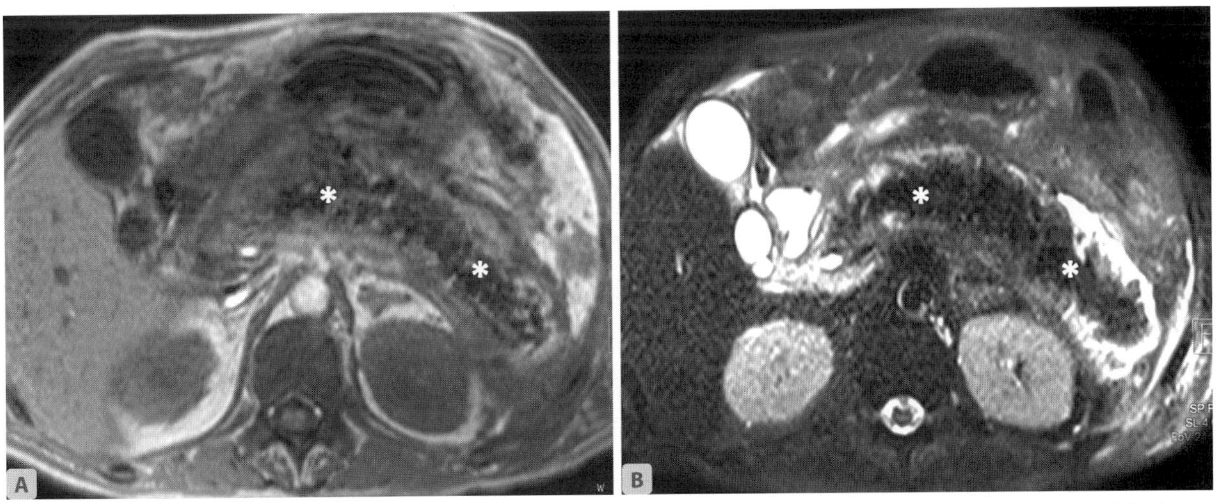

FIGS. 8A AND B: MRI in acute necrotizing pancreatitis: Axial T1-weighted (A) and T2-weighted fat saturated (B) images showing diffusely bulky pancreas with hypointense necrotic area (asterisks) and peripancreatic fat stranding.

spontaneously, may persist or may undergo complications (infection, hemorrhage, mass effect) at which point intervention becomes necessary.

Peripancreatic necrosis is the second most common type of finding, where necrosis is limited to peripancreatic regions. This is typically seen as heterogeneous areas of low density (usually 20–40 HU) on CECT, with areas of fat, hemorrhage or soft tissue density within **(Fig. 7B)**.[8] The usual locations include lesser sac, perinephric and paracolic regions. Initially they are called acute necrotic collection which gradually liquefies and in about four weeks becomes walled-off necrosis. However, liquefaction may be difficult to identify on CT and USG or MRI may be needed. A recent study suggested that volume of extrapancreatic necrosis has prognostic significance and a volume greater 100 mL is associated with higher incidence of organ failure and infection and poor prognosis.[20]

Combined pancreatic and peripancreatic necrosis is the most common type of necrosis seen in about 80% of patients. The imaging features are a combination of both the types described earlier **(Fig. 7A)**.

SEVERITY ASSESSMENT SCORES

Various clinical scores are used in the assessment of severity of acute pancreatitis as they help in determining prognosis. The clinical scores have modest accuracy and include Marshall scoring, Ranson's scoring and bedside index for severity in acute pancreatitis (BISAP).

There are various radiological scoring systems available to predict the severity of acute pancreatitis.[21] The scores used by the radiologist are Balthazar grade and CT severity index (CTSI) **(Fig. 9)**.[22] Balthazar graded acute pancreatitis from A to E **(Table 4)**. CT severity index includes the extent of parenchymal necrosis, giving 2 points for <30% necrosis, 4 points for 30–50% necrosis and 6 points for >50% necrosis in addition to Balthazar grade. A CTSI score of 7–10 suggests poor prognosis, 4–6 intermediate and 1–3 indicates good prognosis. This scoring has high correlation with clinical outcome with a sensitivity of 71% and specificity of 93%.[23] A modified CTSI was suggested by Mortele et al,[24] which is defined in **Table 5**. Studies, however, have suggested no significant difference between CTSI and modified CTSI in terms of prognostication of the disease.[23] Another scoring system by de Waele et al,[25] which relies mainly on extrapancreatic findings such as ascites, pleural effusion, retroperitoneal inflammation and mesenteric inflammation [Extra Pancreatic Inflammation on CT (EPIC) score], has limited clinical utility. Recent comparative studies have shown that CT scoring systems are similar to clinical scoring systems in accurately predicting severity of acute pancreatitis.[10,26] However, a study quantifying the extrapancreatic necrosis in patients with ANP showed significant correlation of its volume with clinical outcome.[20]

COMPLICATIONS

Acute pancreatitis is associated with wide range of complications which can broadly be classified into vascular and non-vascular complications **(Table 6)**.[18]

Nonvascular Complications

Symptomatic collections are the most common complication of acute pancreatitis. These collections may be acute peripancreatic collections, pseudocysts or walled-off necrosis.[18] Symptoms develop when these collections get infected or when they compress adjacent structures

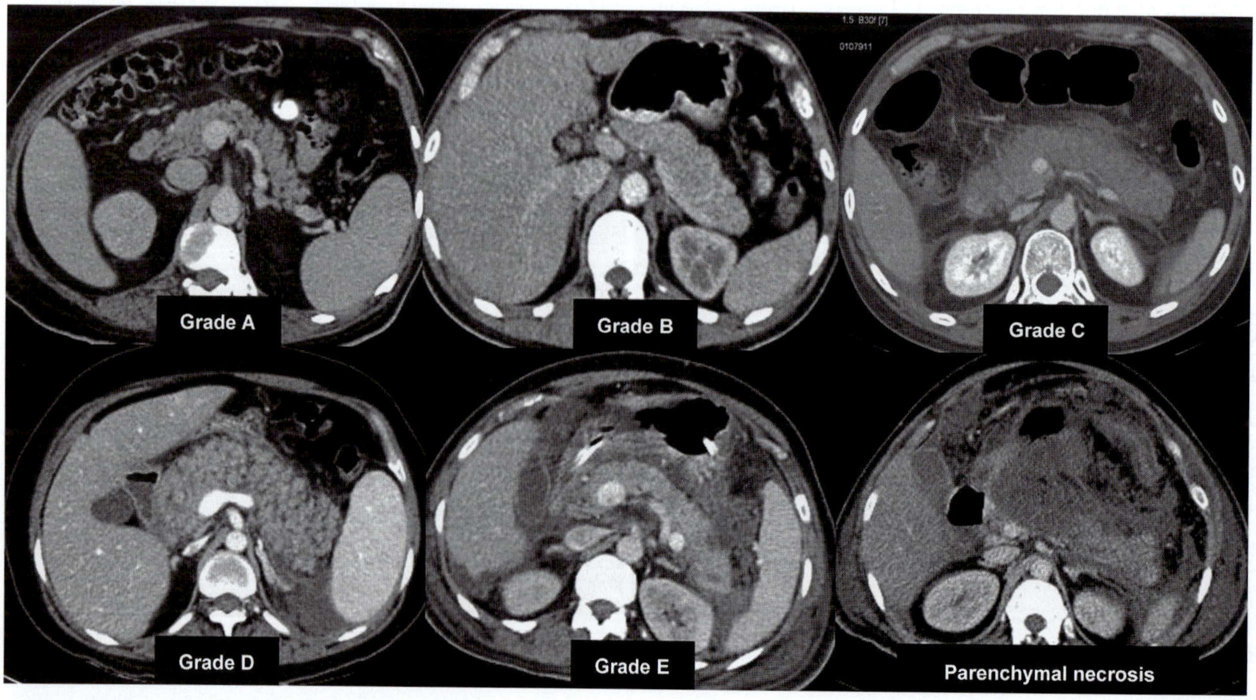

FIG. 9: Balthazar grade and CT severity index.

(Figs. 10A to C). Infection commonly occurs in necrotic collection, and is seen as a fluid density area with air foci within. However, air in infected necrosis is seen in about 20–40% cases.[27] Further, air foci may occur due to prior intervention or fistulous communication with the bowel. In the absence of air foci, diagnosis of secondary infection is done based on clinical suspicion or needle aspiration. Collections may be seen at variable locations with common locations being peripancreatic region, perisplenic, perigastric, perihepatic, paracolic and perinephric areas. Rarely, they may be seen in the mediastinum, within the spleen or liver and in the psoas muscle. Ascites is also commonly seen. The revised Atlanta classification defines five types of collections, acute peripancreatic fluid collection, acute necrotic collection, pseudocyst, walled-off necrosis and post-necrosectomy pseudocyst **(*see* Fig. 2A to D)**. Other terms such as pancreatic abscess, phlegmon and collection are not used. Pancreatic abscess is same as infected necrosis, but the latter terminology is better and has implications in drainage.

Acute peripancreatic fluid collection (APFC) is seen in AIEP, in the first 4 weeks of illness. It is seen on CECT as ill-defined homogeneous low density areas, often with feathery margins. On MRI, it is seen as an ill-defined homogeneous, non-encapsulated hyperintense area on T2-weighted images and hypointense area on T1-weighted images. This is an exudative fluid collection and contains only fluid and inflammatory cells without necrosis. It may or may not have

TABLE 4: CT severity index.

CT grade	*CT finding*	*Score*
A	Normal pancreas	0
B	Pancreatic enlargement	1
C	Pancreatic and peripancreatic inflammation	2
D	Single peripancreatic fluid collection	3
E	2 or more fluid collections ± gas	4
% Necrosis		***Score***
0		0
<30%		2
30–50%		4
>50%		6

TABLE 5: Modified CT severity index.

Imaging feature	*Score*
Pancreatic inflammation	
Normal pancreas	0
Intrinsic pancreatic abnormalities with or without inflammatory changes in peripancreatic fat	2
Pancreatic or peripancreatic fluid collection or peripancreatic fat necrosis	4
Pancreatic necrosis	
None	0
≤30%	2
>30%	4
Extrapancreatic complications	
One or more of pleural effusion, ascites, vascular complications, parenchymal complications, or gastrointestinal tract involvement	2

TABLE 6: Complications of acute pancreatitis.

Vascular	*Nonvascular*
Arterial: • Pseudoaneurysms • Rupture (Contrast extravasation)	*Collections*: • Infected necrosis • Walled off necrosis/ pseudocyst
Venous: • Acute thrombosis (SV, SMV, PV) • Collateralization—varices	Bowel necrosis/perforation Pancreatic ascites Pancreatic fistula

(PV: portal vein; SMV: superior mesenteric vein; SV: splenic vein)

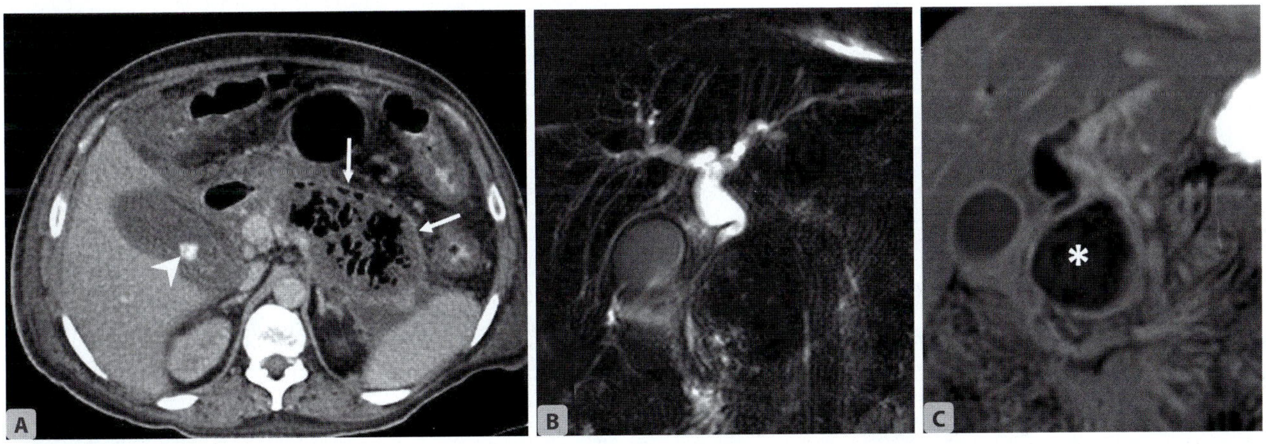

FIGS. 10A TO C: Complications—collections. (A) Axial contrast-enhanced CT image showing necrotic collection in the pancreatic bed—lesser sac region with multiple air foci suggesting secondary infection (arrows). Gallstone is also seen (arrowhead). (B and C) MRCP (B) and coronal contrast-enhanced T1W (C) images showing walled-off necrosis in the head of pancreas (asterisk) causing compression of distal common bile duct with proximal dilatation.

communication with side branches of pancreatic duct. It resolves spontaneously in most patients and intervention is not necessary. It must be differentiated from ascites which is seen in perihepatic, perisplenic and pelvic regions.

Pseudocyst is the collection which is seen in AIEP, after four weeks. This develops from an APFC, when it forms a wall around it. Thus, no necrosis is seen within it. On CECT, it is seen as a well-defined homogeneous low density collection with relatively thick walls. On MRI, it is seen as homogeneously hyperintense on T2W images. No restriction of diffusion is seen. Imaging may or may not show communication of the pseudocyst with pancreatic duct. The collection contains pancreatic juice and high amylase, which helps in making a diagnosis in difficult situations. Most of the pseudocysts resolve and infection is rare. Intervention is needed only if they are symptomatic.

Acute necrotic collection (ANC) is seen in ANP, in the initial four weeks of the disease. This may be seen in the pancreas or peripancreatic region. This develops as a result of leak of pancreatic enzymes which results in fat necrosis and saponification. Unlike APFC, it is seen as an ill-defined heterogeneous density area, often with foci of fat and/or hemorrhage within on CECT. But, early in the stage of the disease, prior to fat necrosis, it may appear homogeneous, and is difficult to differentiate from APFC. MRI is useful as the collections are seen as variable signal intensity (hyperintense and hypointense areas) on T2W images. DWI often shows diffusion restriction. As time progresses, ANCs may resolve spontaneously (20%), get infected (20%) or develop into walled-off necrosis (60%). Resolution of ANC is size dependent, majority of those less than 2 cm resolve spontaneously and most of those larger than 5 cm persist.[28]

Walled-off necrosis (WON) develops from ANC in ANP after 4 weeks. As the name suggests, there is a thick non-epithelial wall formed around the necrotic collection. The collection, depending on the extent of liquefaction, may be homogeneous or heterogeneous. Although, on CECT, it appears as homogeneous or heterogeneous collection with thick walls, the extent of liquefaction is difficult to assess. MRI or USG is helpful for this. USG shows the liquefied portion as anechoic area with internal echoes **(Figs. 11A to D)**. On MRI, the liquefied component appears as hyperintense on T2W and the necrotic component as iso-hyperintense on T1W and hypointense on T2W images **(Figs. 12A and B)**. Intervention is frequently needed for this collection. When a WON is fully liquefied, it may mimic pseudocyst on imaging. This differentiation is important as it has management implications. Pseudocyst is seen only in extrapancreatic location, associated with AIEP, and may be associated with dilated pancreatic duct due to compression, unlike WON where duct is necrosed and is decompressed due to drainage into the collection. Sometimes the term *disconnected duct syndrome* is used where a collection is formed due to necrosis of the pancreatic duct in the neck or body region **(Fig. 13)**. This seen in up to 30% of patients of ANP and is usually treated by either drainage or pancreatic resection.

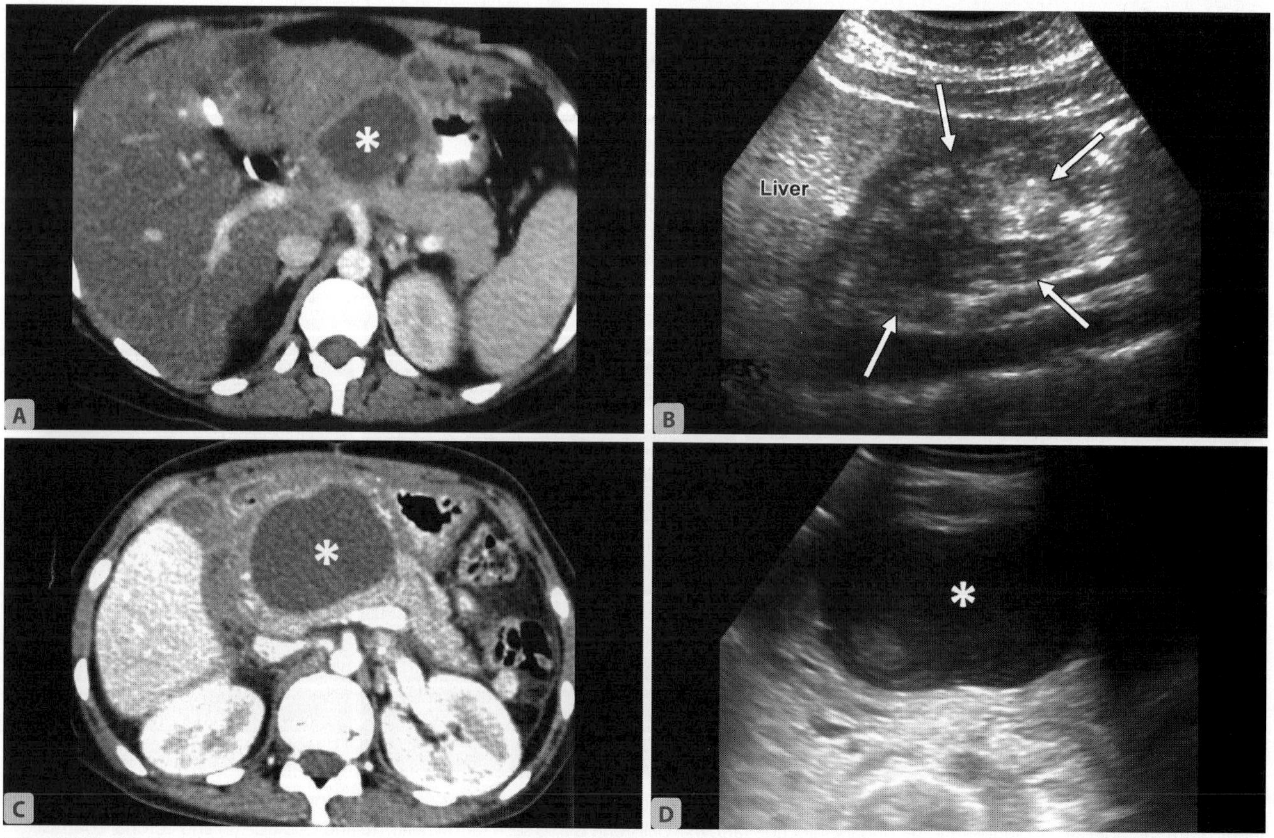

FIGS. 11A TO D: Assessment of liquefaction by ultrasonography: (A and C) Contrast-enhanced CT scans show similar looking walled of necrosis (asterisks). However, ultrasonography shows one is solid looking and not liquefied (arrows in B) and the other is fully liquefied (asterisk in D).

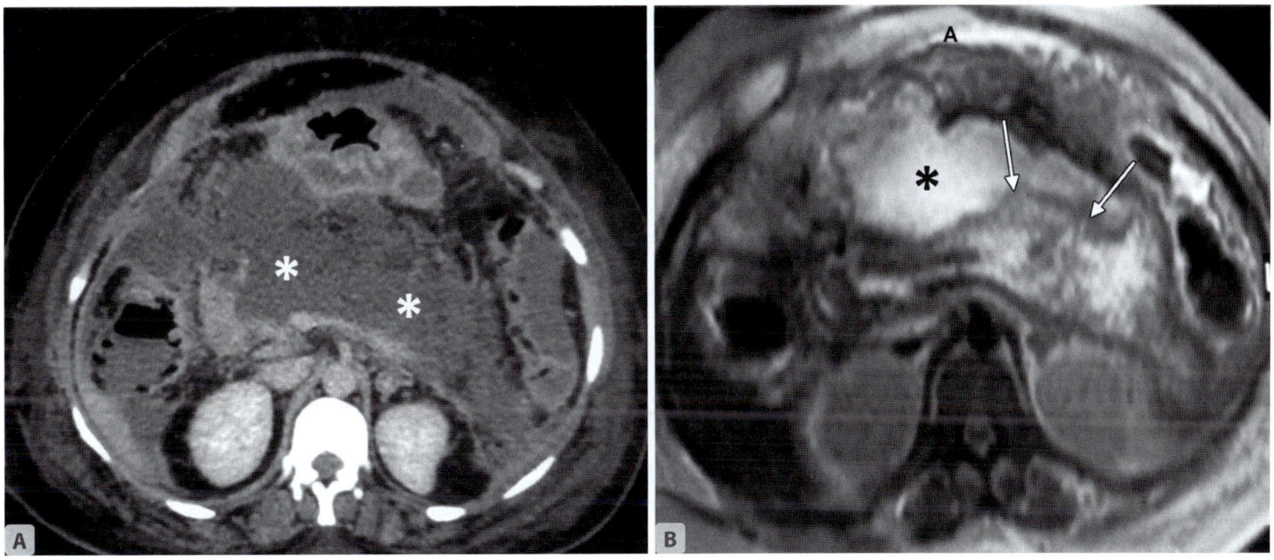

FIGS. 12A AND B: Assessment of liquefaction by MRI: (A) Contrast-enhanced CT scan shows large relatively homogeneous necrotic collection without definitive information on liquefaction (asterisks). (B) However, T2W-MR image shows both liquefied (asterisk) and non-liquefied (arrows) areas.

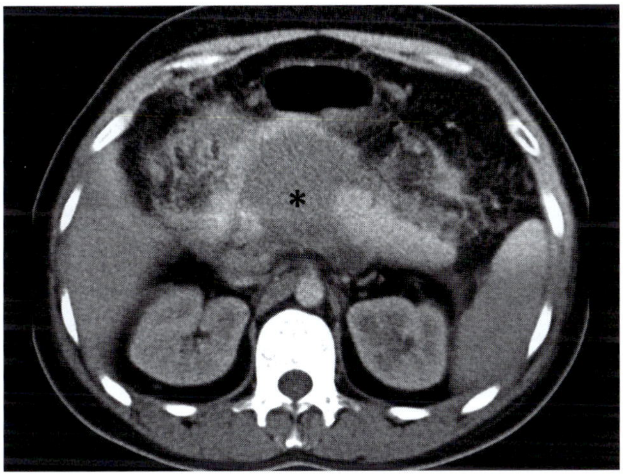

FIG. 13: Axial contrast-enhanced CT scan in a patient with ANP showing full thickness necrosis of pancreatic neck and body with walled-off collection (asterisk), suggesting disconnected duct syndrome.

Post-necrosectomy pseudocyst develops as a long-term complication after surgical necrosectomy of the pancreatic/peripancreatic necrosis. This may be seen either in the pancreas or in extrapancreatic location. This occurs as a result of disconnected duct syndrome due to necrosis in the head and body of pancreas. After necrosectomy, there is oozing of pancreatic juice from tail to form a collection at the site of necrosectomy, resulting in pseudocyst. On imaging, it is similar to the pseudocyst described above. Intervention is needed if symptomatic.

Infected necrotic collection is diagnosed on CECT scan when there are air foci in the collection **(Fig. 10A)**. In the absence of air foci, DWI or aspiration may help in making a diagnosis.

Bowel ischemia and necrosis are a rare but serious complications of acute pancreatitis.[29] They are seen typically in patients of ANP due to extension of inflammation along the mesentery to involve the vessels in the mesentery and walls of the bowel. Transverse colon and splenic flexure are the most common sites.[30] The involved bowel segment shows circumferential wall thickening with maintained stratification on CECT scan **(Figs. 14A and B)**. As the inflammation progresses, bowel necrosis and perforation may occur which is seen as pneumoperitoneum and extraluminal leak of oral contrast on CECT scan. Other complications include bowel obstruction and ileus.

Pancreatic fistula is a complication which develops as a result of necrosis of pancreatic ductal walls. This results in leak of pancreatic secretions causing persistence of collections. Such collections have high amylase levels on sampling. Management involves endoscopic stenting or surgery.

Other abdominal complications include cholecystitis, pancreatic duct strictures and splenic infarcts. Extra-abdominal complications are also seen, most common being pleural effusion. This is mostly reactive but may be gross causing respiratory symptoms. Lungs may show non-cardiogenic pulmonary edema in severe cases. Rarely, there may be fat embolism and patient may present with neurological symptoms.

Vascular Complications

Vascular complications may involve arterial or venous structures. Involvement of arteries may result in arteritis and erosion of the arterial wall by pancreatic enzymes which may lead to formation of pseudoaneurysms, rupture and thrombosis. Arterial hemorrhage and pseudoaneurysms are seen in up to 5% of patients with acute pancreatitis and are usually solitary.[31] It most commonly involves the splenic artery (60–65%; **Fig. 15A**), followed by the gastroduodenal artery (20–25%; **Figs. 15B and C**).[32] Other arteries involved include left gastric, hepatic, inferior pancreaticoduodenal and gastroepiploic arteries. Since these pseudoaneurysms are prone to rupture, which has very high mortality, immediate management is necessary. CT angiography (from dome of

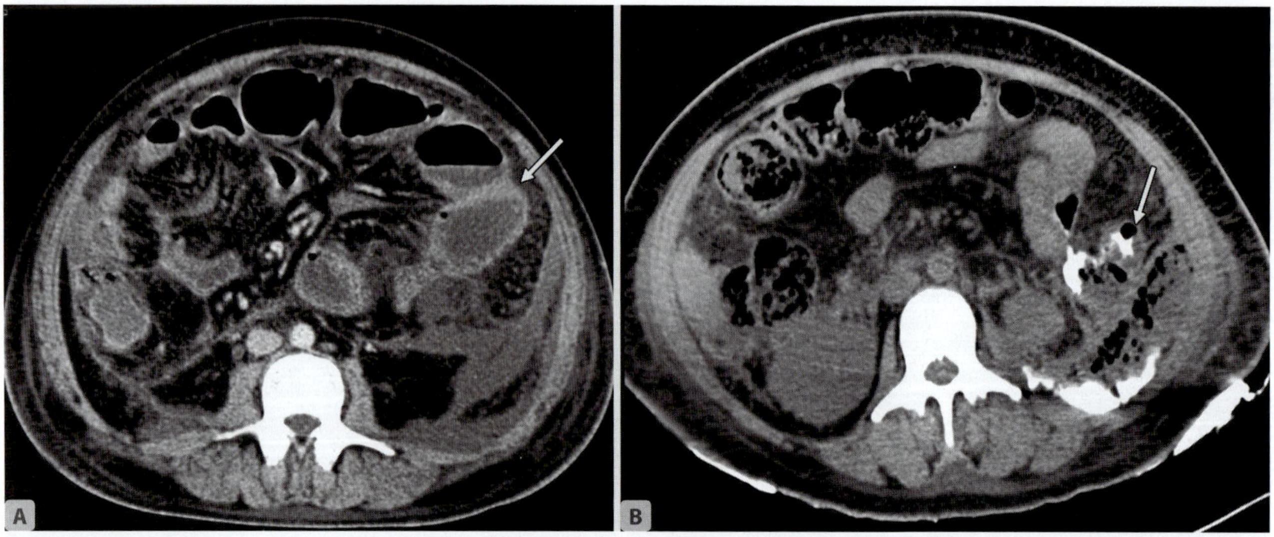

FIGS. 14A AND B: Bowel necrosis: (A) Axial contrast-enhanced CT scan shows circumferential thickening of descending colon (arrow). After drainage of paracolic collection percutaneously, there was feculent discharge in the drain; (B) Tubogram performed by injection of contrast into the drainage catheter shows contrast in the descending colon (arrow) suggesting perforation and fistula.

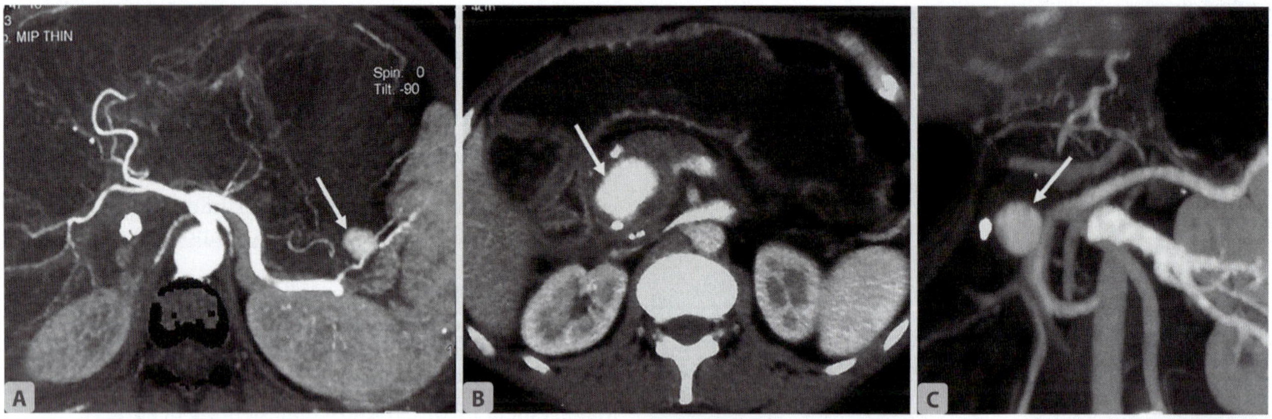

FIGS. 15A TO C: Pseudoaneurysm: (A) Maximum intensity projection (MIP) of CT scan in arterial phase shows a pseudoaneurysm arising from distal splenic artery (arrow); (B and C) Axial and coronal MIP contrast-enhanced CT images show a pseudoaneurysm in the region of head of pancreas, arising from gastroduodenal artery (arrow).

diaphragm to iliac crest) should be done in all cases where there is gastrointestinal bleed, hypotension or drop in hemoglobin. On imaging, plain CT scan may be done to show hemorrhage (high density area) in the collection **(Figs. 16A and B)** or in the adjoining bowel loops. The angiography images show a variable-sized smooth or irregular contrast filled out pouching from an artery or its branch. Sometimes the feeding artery may not be clearly seen due to spasm. Pseudoaneurysms with a very narrow neck may not opacify in the arterial phase, and may fill in the venous phase. Hence, both arterial and venous phases are needed in the evaluation of hemorrhage in patients of acute pancreatitis.[32]

Venous complications most commonly include thrombosis of splenic vein, portal vein and superior mesenteric vein which may result in formation of perigastric and splenic hilar collateral venous channels and portal hypertension. Splanchnic vein thrombosis is seen in about 2% patients of acute pancreatitis and about half of the patients with ANP.[33,34] Splenic vein thrombosis is the most common, accounting for over 80% of the cases. Diagnosis is mostly made on CECT. In the initial stage, thrombosis is seen as filling defect within the enhancing splenic vein **(Figs. 17A and B)**. Subsequently, as the thrombosis evolves, there is complete obstruction of the vein with opening up of short gastric and omental collaterals. Splenomegaly and splenic infarcts may also be seen. There may be thrombosis of the main portal vein and superior mesenteric vein which may be replaced by collaterals.

MANAGEMENT

Management of patients of acute pancreatitis involves multiple disciplines with a team approach. The gastroenterologists, gastrointestinal surgeons and radiologists all play an important role. In patients with AIEP and ANP, initial management is mostly conservative with the role of radiologist being in imaging, whenever necessary. The management involves nutritional support (oral for AIEP and enteral for

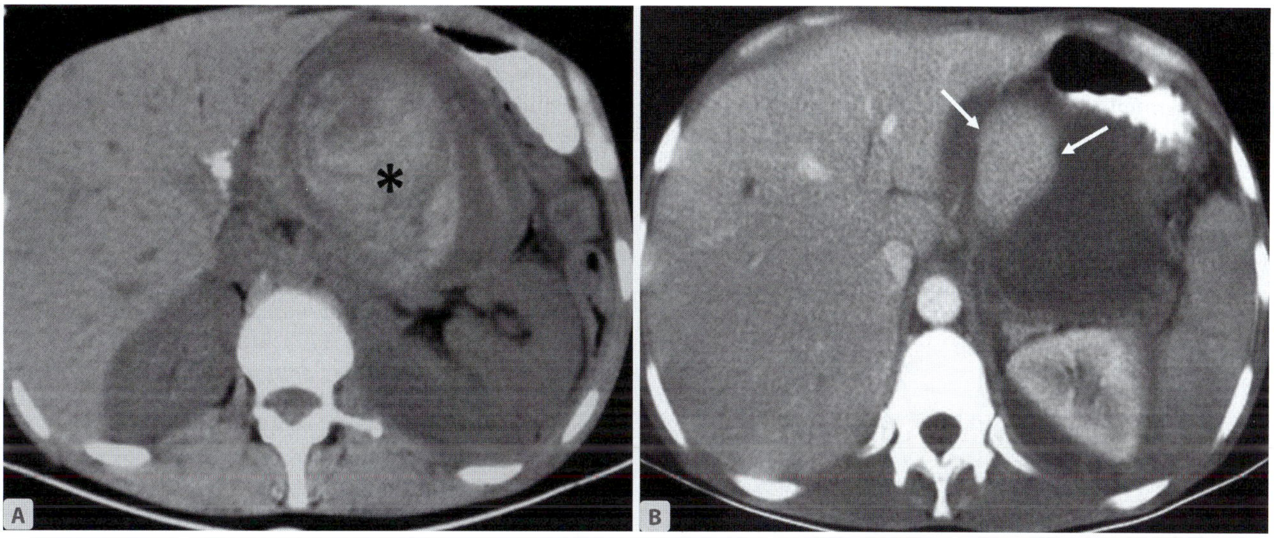

FIGS. 16A AND B: Pseudoaneurysm. (A) Noncontrast CT scan showing hyperdensity (asterisk) within a peripancreatic collection suggesting acute hemorrhage; (B) Late arterial phase CT scan showing an oval pseudoaneurysm (arrows) arising from splenic artery.

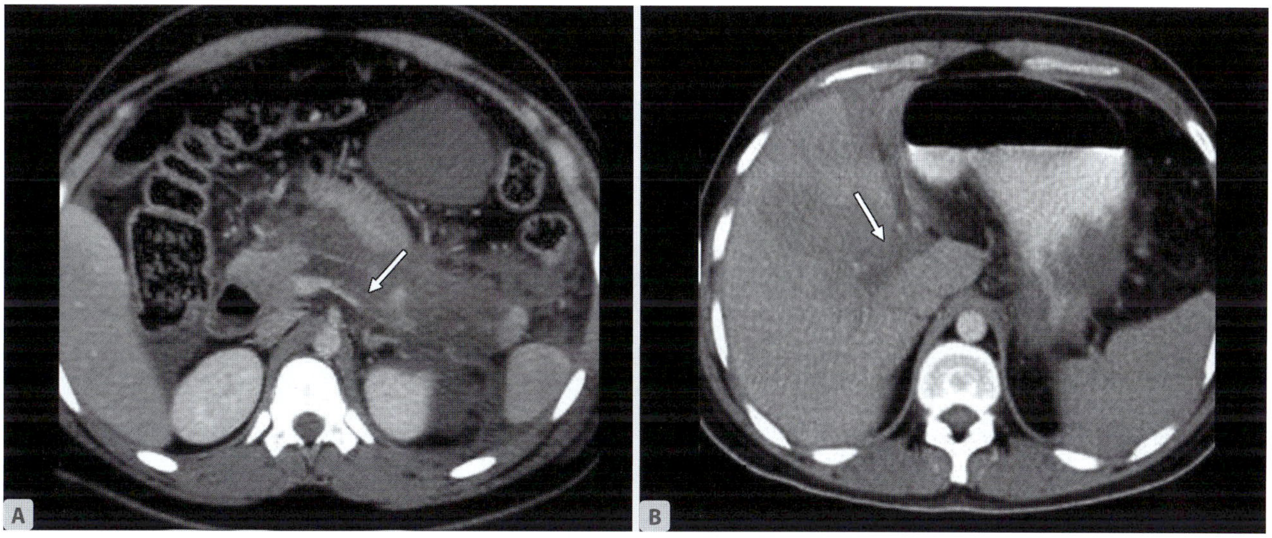

FIGS. 17A AND B: Venous thrombosis. (A) Contrast-enhanced CT scan showing a case of necrotizing pancreatitis with thrombosis of splenic vein seen as hypodense filling defect with in its lumen (arrow); (B) Contrast-enhanced CT scan in a case of acute pancreatitis showing non-enhancement of portal vein (arrow) suggesting thrombosis.

ANP), fluid resuscitation, pain control and mobilization.[35] ERCP may be done when there is biliary obstruction, calculi or cholangitis. There is no role for prophylactic antibiotics. In resolving phase, if there is a persistent pseudocyst (in AIEP) causing symptoms, it is usually managed by endoscopic or surgical cystogastrostomy. Percutaneous drainage may be needed occasionally. Radiological interventions play an important role in managing patients of ANP presenting with complicated collections and hemorrhage.

Radiological Interventions

Radiological interventions are broadly classified into vascular and nonvascular procedures.

Non-vascular procedures form the major bulk of radiological interventions in patients with acute pancreatitis. This predominantly involves drainage of collections. It is important to understand that any collection seen in acute pancreatitis does not need drainage. Specific indications for drainage include infection, mass effect, symptoms, non-improvement or deterioration of symptoms and large collections (>5 cm) which are persistent (>6 weeks).[36] A sterile collection should not be drained unless it is causing symptoms like pain, abdominal distension, vomiting or jaundice **(Fig. 10B)**. Secondary infection is mostly seen with necrotic collection, in up to 33% cases and is typically seen between 2nd and 4th week of onset of illness.[37] This occurs mostly due to translocation of microbia from the bowel into the collection.[38] Diagnosis of infected collection is based on clinical (fever, persistent/new organ failure) and lab parameters (leukocytosis) and by imaging (air within the collection on CECT; **Fig. 10A**). Although diagnostic aspiration of fluid may help in detection of infection, it is not routinely practiced due to high false negative rate (20-25%).[39] Mass effect due to collections may result in gastric outlet obstruction (due to duodenal compression), biliary dilatation (due to compression of bile duct), hydronephrosis (compression of ureters) and portal hypertension with multiple venous collaterals (compression of splenoportal axis).[16] It is important that a retroperitoneal route is used

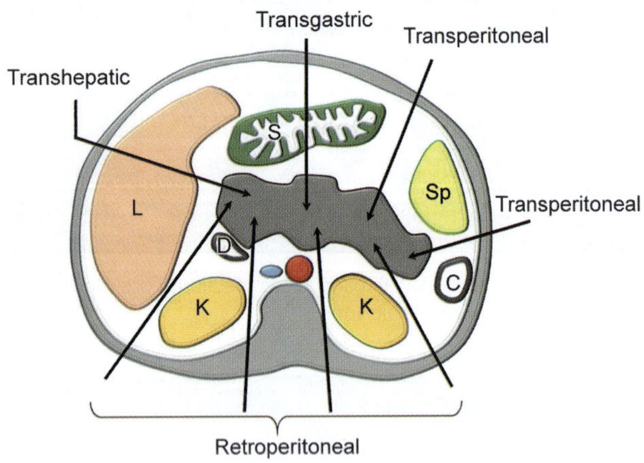

FIG. 18: Schematic diagram showing various approaches used to drain pancreatic collection. (C: colon; D: duodenum; K: kidneys; L: liver; S: stomach; Sp: spleen).

for drainage of collections and traversing the bowel should be avoided as it is unsafe and may give false positive results due to contamination. DWI and FDG-PET (with labeled autologous leukocytes) may be useful in differentiation of sterile and infected necrosis. Infected necrosis is associated with high morbidity and mortality (25-70%).[40]

An infected necrotic collection should always be drained.[36] However, the timing of drainage is important for its success. Usually, collections begin to liquefy after 3-4 weeks of the onset of illness. Hence, drainage should be planned after this time. This may be confirmed by either USG or MRI whenever possible as CECT is a poor investigation for assessment of liquefaction. There are various approaches used for drainage of collections in acute pancreatitis **(Fig. 18)**. Most common and the preferred approach is through the retroperitoneum, typically through the anterior pararenal space. This approach is associated with less complications, allows better drainage by gravity and the same tract can be used when endoscopic or minimally invasive surgical necrosectomy is done. Other approaches used include transgastric, paraspinal, transperitoneal and transhepatic. Mediastinal collections should be drained through paraspinal extrapleural approach. Saline injection may be necessary for avoiding lung or pleural puncture. The technique of drainage used is either the Seldinger technique or trocar technique. The imaging guidance used is either USG or CT scan **(Figs. 19A to D)**. When the collection is deep seated, in the lesser sac—anterior pararenal space and retroperitoneal

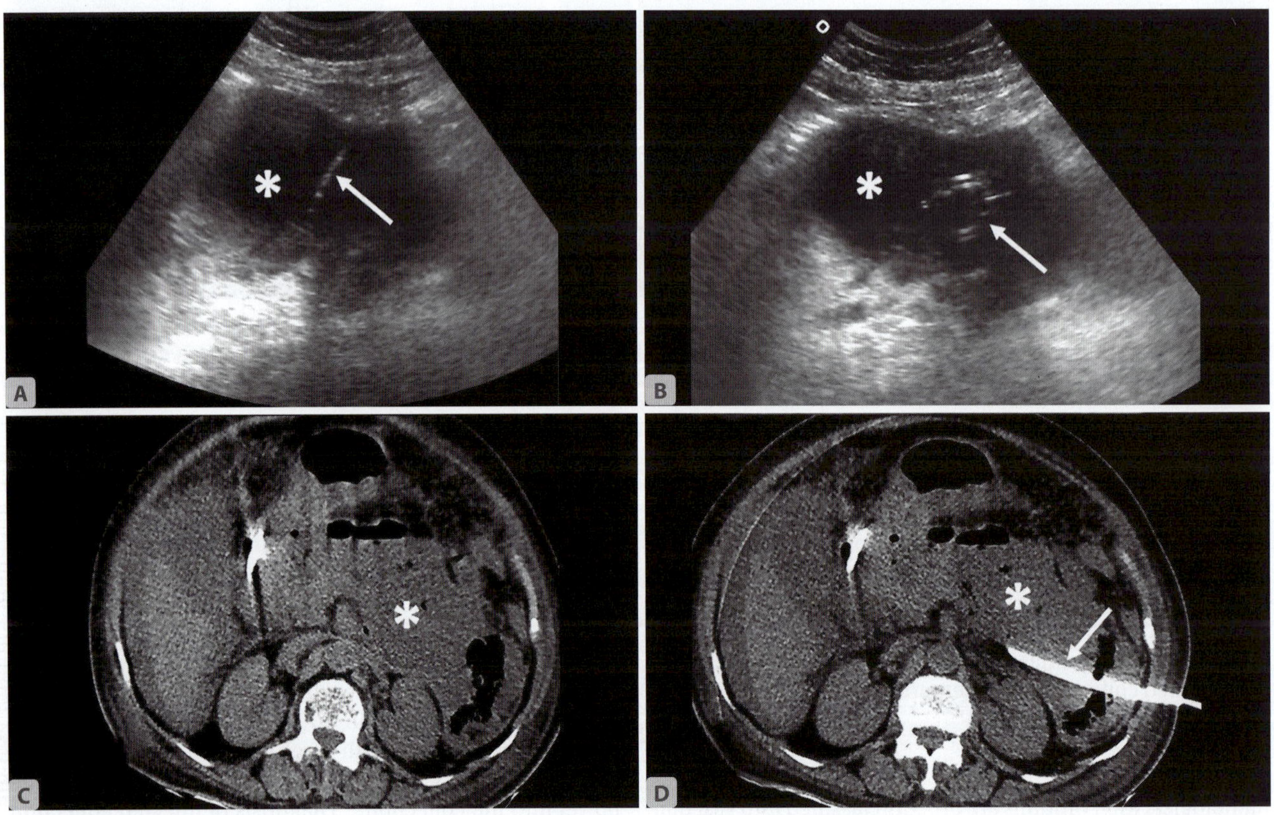

FIGS. 19A TO D: (A and B) Ultrasound-guided drainage of lesser sac collection (asterisk). Trocar with pigtail catheter is seen in A (arrow) with pigtail catheter in position in B (arrow); (C and D) CT-guided drainage of collection (asterisk). A lesser sac collection is seen with air pockets in C and catheter inserted in D (arrow).

approach is needed or when there is extensive air in the collection, CT guidance is preferred. In cases where the collection is visible on USG and liquefied, in sick patients when bedside procedure is needed and in superficial collections, USG guidance should be used.

The size of drainage catheter initially used is 10/12F. Subsequently, this needs serial upgradation through 16F, up to 20 or 24 F **(Figs. 20A to D)**. Once the initial catheter is inserted, exchanges are done over a stiff guidewire. Usually, Malecot catheter is preferred over pigtail catheter as the former has wide holes to allow drainage of thick necrotic debris. Once the catheter is inserted, regular flushing atleast twice a day with 10–20 mL saline is needed to allow free drainage. In some patients, simple drainage alone is sufficient in clearing all the collections. In rest of the patients, collections persist and further interventions in the form of percutaneous endoscopic necrosectomy, surgical necrosectomy or video-assisted retroperitoneal debridement are needed (*step-up approach*).

Other interventions performed in patients of acute pancreatitis include drainage of ascites, drainage of pleural effusion and percutaneous cholecystostomy (for biliary decompression).

Vascular interventions mostly involve embolization of pseudoaneurysms.[41] This can be done by three different approaches. Firstly, through the endovascular route, which is most commonly used. Second is the percutaneous approach, done for pseudoaneurysms within solid organs and superficial locations. Last is the endoscopic ultrasonography (EUS) guided route used when the previous two approaches fail or are not possible. Endovascular embolization has over 90% technical and clinical success rates in treatment of pseudoaneurysms of acute pancreatitis. But ongoing inflammation may be a problem and may result in recurrence. Coils are the most commonly used embolizing agents. Other agents used include glue n-butyl cyanoacrylate (nBCA) and thrombin. The latter is used often with percutaneous or EUS approaches.

The *endovascular* embolization is usually done through transfemoral route. It is important that a CT angiogram is done in all these cases as it will help to identify the source artery responsible for bleeding and also identify anatomical variations. This will reduce the time of the procedure and radiation exposure. When the source artery is known, the artery is catheterized using a 5F catheter (RC1; Cook). After initial angiogram acquired with catheter tip placed in proximal larger arteries (celiac, hepatic, splenic or superior mesenteric origin), distal catheterization of smaller arteries is done with microcatheter to avoid injury to the arteries. Once the neck is identified, embolization procedure should be done. It is important to note that gastroduodenal, splenic, left gastric and hepatic arteries have collateral circulation and hence 'sandwich' technique of embolization should be used **(Figs. 21 and 22)**. Here, embolization of segment of artery

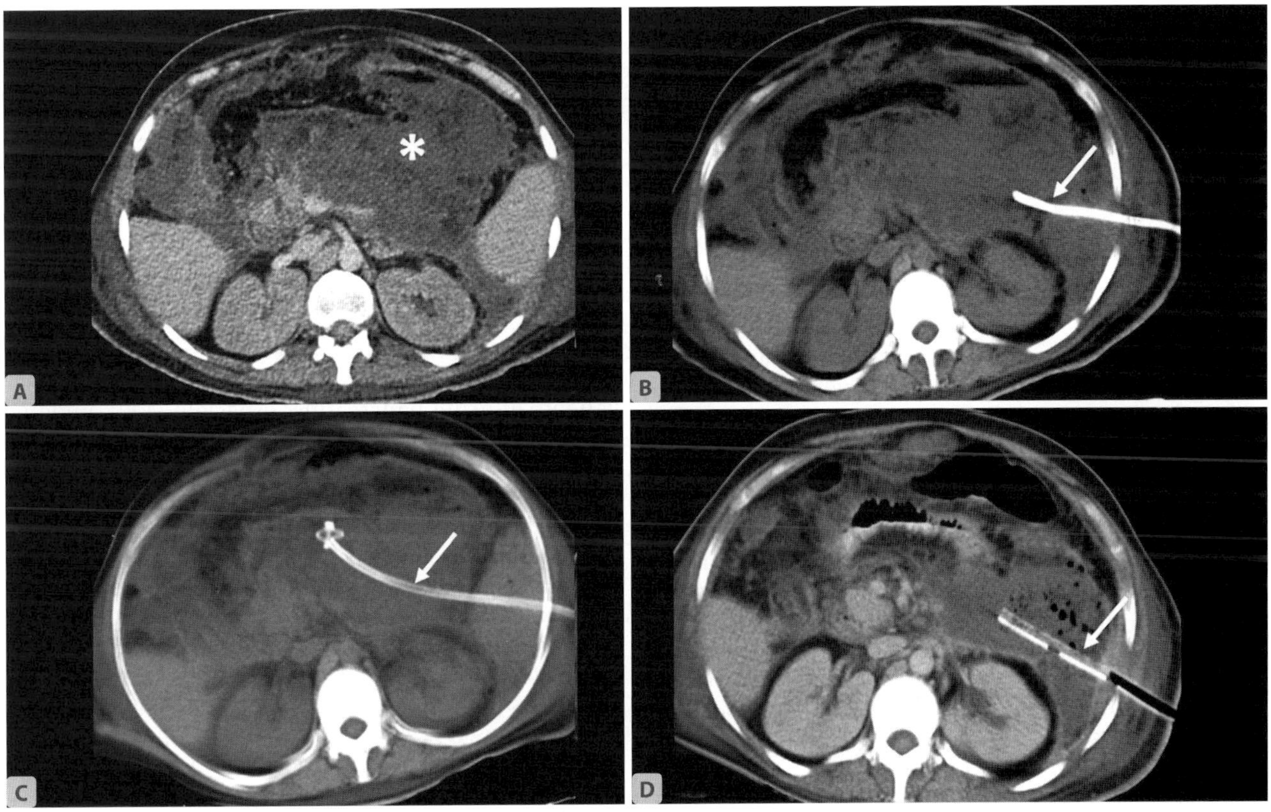

FIGS. 20A TO D: Serial upgradation of catheters under CT guidance. (A) Contrast-enhanced CT image showing necrotic collection in lesser sac (asterisk); (B) Collection with 12F pigtail catheter in situ (arrow); (C) Catheter upgraded to 16F Malecot catheter (arrow); (D) 20F drainage catheter within the collection (arrow).

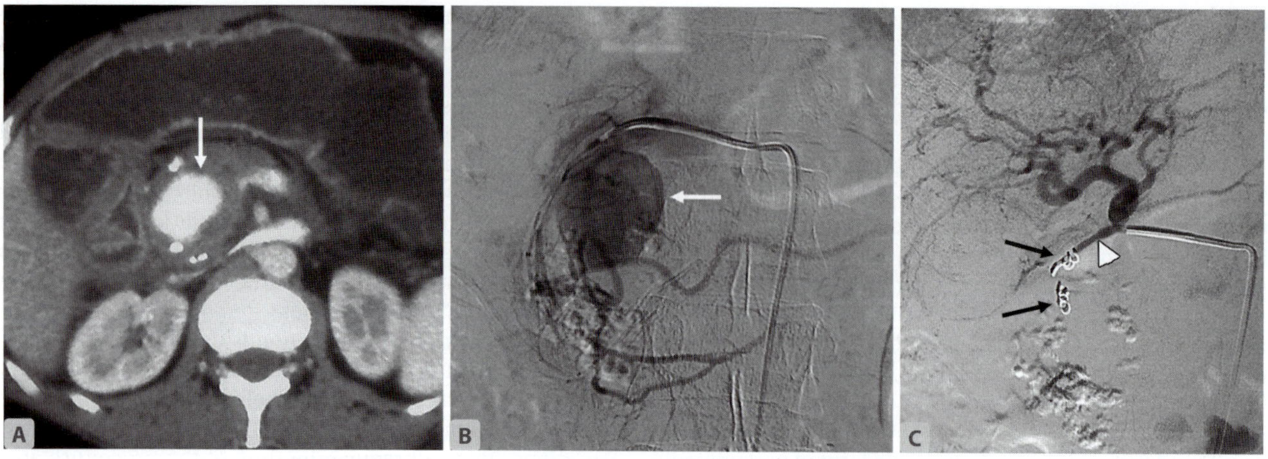

FIGS. 21A TO C: Embolization. (A) Contrast-enhanced CT scan shows a pseudoaneurysm arising from gastroduodenal artery (GDA, arrow); (B) Digital subtraction angiography (DSA) of gastroduodenal artery shows the pseudoaneurysm (arrow); (C) DSA after proximal and distal coiling (arrows) of GDA (arrowhead) shows complete embolization of the pseudoaneurysm.

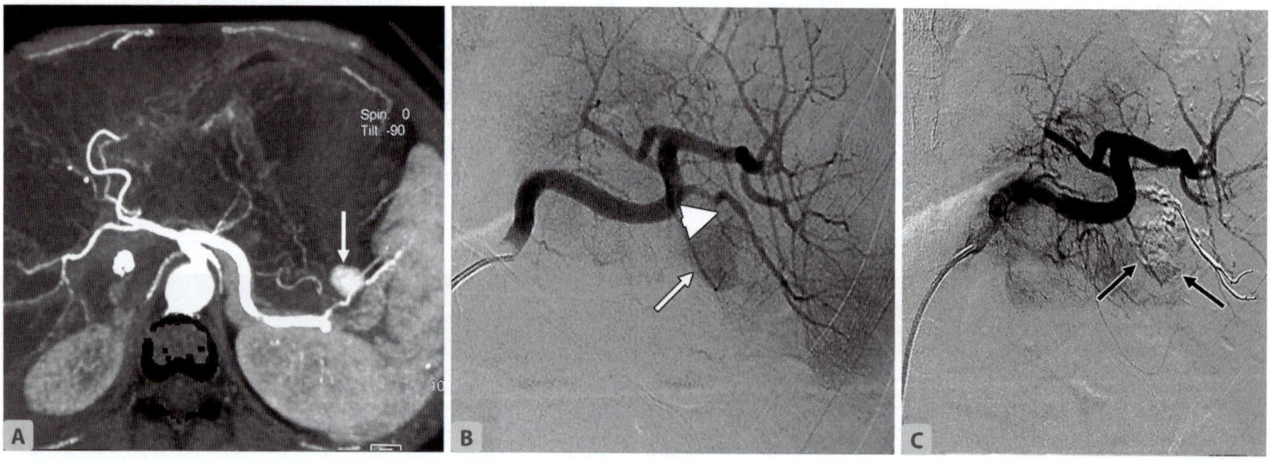

FIGS. 22A TO C: Splenic artery pseudoaneurysm: (A) MIP-CT image in arterial phase showing a contrast-filled outpouching (arrow) in the distal splenic artery; (B) DSA of splenic artery shows the pseudoaneurysm (arrow) arising from distal branch of splenic artery (arrowhead). (C) DSA after embolization with combination of coils and glue shows complete obliteration of the pseudoaneurysm (arrows).

distal to the neck of pseudoaneurysm and proximal to it is done so that there is no refilling from collaterals. This will isolate the pseudoaneurysm from the systemic circulation and thrombosis ensues. Microcoils (platinum coils) with fibers are used for embolization through either 'anchor' technique (anchoring the tip of microcoil into a smaller branch) or 'scaffolding' technique (using a stiffer coil initially like steel coils). They cause thrombosis by causing mechanical obstruction and due to the presence of thrombogenic fibers. n-BCA may also be used in specific situations like when optimal catheterization of the artery is not possible, when there are multiple feeders to the pseudoaneurysm or when there is coagulation derangement.[42] In *percutaneous* approach, the pseudoaneurysm is directly punctured using a 21G/22G needle under USG guidance.[41] Once the backflow of blood is confirmed, the embolic agent (thrombin or n-BCA) is injected under USG guidance. Thrombosis of the pseudoaneurysm occurs immediately and can be confirmed with color Doppler.

RADIATION EXPOSURE

Patients of acute pancreatitis, especially ANP, undergo multiple CT scans during the course of their admission which significantly increases radiation exposure. In a study by Ball et al. it was shown that the median number of CT examinations in patients of ANP was five and mean effective dose was 63 mSv.[43] Patients who underwent DSA were further exposed to more radiation. They also suggested that management decisions infrequently followed the CT scan. Thus it is important to avoid unnecessary CT scans in patients of acute pancreatitis. Alternate modalities like USG or MRI which are free of radiation should be used, wherever possible. Even during follow-up CT scan, low kV (100 kV) helps in reducing radiation dose. CT-guided procedures may be performed under low kV with scan area limited to the region of interest. Awareness of this problem and methods to reduce it is critical to prevent significant radiation exposure.

ADVANCES IN IMAGING

Ultrasound elastography may be a simple radiation-free tool to diagnosis acute pancreatitis. In patients with acute pancreatitis, there is increase in pancreatic stiffness. Measurement of pancreatic stiffness on sonoelastography may be a helpful bedside technique to diagnose acute pancreatitis in difficult cases. A recent study has shown that acoustic radiation force impulse (ARFI) is an accurate non-invasive tool in diagnosing acute pancreatitis and is comparable to CECT scan.[44]

Contrast-enhanced USG (CEUS) is being used in assessment of areas of necrosis in patients with ANP with accuracies equal to contrast enhanced CT scan.[45] The sensitivity and specificity of CEUS for diagnosing acute pancreatitis are 90% and 99% respectively. Thus it is a cost-effective method and can be used in patients where iodinated contrast agents cannot be used. The limitations are same as those for B-mode USG.

CT perfusion is a new imaging technique which has application in evaluation of acute pancreatitis. Perfusion CT (PCT) involves continuous acquisition of sections through the pancreas over a period of 2–3 minutes after intravenous contrast injection. The acquired images are then processed to generate various perfusion parameters. In acute pancreatitis, the role of perfusion CT is in the predicted severe variety. PCT done early in the course of the disease (within 48 hours) shows areas of hypoperfusion which on follow-up show necrosis.[46] Thus, perfusion CT is helpful in predicting the areas of necrosis prior to their development and may open new therapeutic options to prevent this ominous development.

Dual energy CT scan (DECT) has been shown to be useful in evaluation of pancreatic diseases. In patients with acute necrotizing pancreatitis, DECT in portal venous phase may help in assessment of areas of hypoperfusion and necrosis in the pancreatic parenchyma with improved contrast to noise ratio.[47] DECT thus may have potential in better identifying and defining necrotic areas.

All these advanced techniques are in the early stages of research and more evidence is needed to use them in routine practice.

SUMMARY

Acute pancreatitis is a disease with high morbidity. Early detection is important for judicious management. Knowledge of the revised Atlanta classification helps understanding the disease and defining various stages and terms uniformly. Imaging should be done only when indicated and whenever possible, modalities without radiation should be used. Diagnosis of various complications often requires high index of suspicion. Radiologist plays a critical role in both diagnosing these complications and in managing them, wherever necessary.

REFERENCES

1. Wu BU, Banks PA. Clinical management of patients with acute pancreatitis. Gastroenterology. 2013;144(6):1272-81.
2. Banks PA, Bollen TL, Dervenis C, et al. Classification of acute pancreatitis-2012: revision of the Atlanta classification and definitions by international consensus. Gut. 2013;62:102-11.
3. Lankisch PG, Apte M, Banks PA. Acute pancreatitis. Lancet. 2015;386(9988):85-96.
4. Elfar M, Gaber LW, Sabek O, Fischer CP, Gaber O. The inflammatory cascade in acute pancreatitis: relevance to clinical disease. Surg Clin N Am. 2007;87:1325-40.
5. Bollen TL. Acute pancreatitis: international classification and nomenclature. Clin Radiol. 2016;71:121-33.
6. Bradley III EL. A clinically based classification system for acute pancreatitis. Summary of the International Symposium on Acute Pancreatitis, Atlanta, GA, September 11 through 13, 1992. Arch Surg. 1993;128:586-90.
7. Banks PA, Bollen TL, Dervenis C, et al. Classification of acute pancreatitis 2012: revision of the Atlanta classification and definitions by international consensus. Gut. 2013;62(1):102-11.
8. Thoeni RF. The revised Atlanta classification of acute pancreatitis: its importance for the radiologist and its effect on treatment. Radiology. 2012;262(3):751-64.
9. Singh VK, Bollen TL, Wu BU, et al. An assessment of the severity of interstitial pancreatitis. Clin Gastroenterol Hepatol. 2011;9(12):1098-103.
10. Bollen TL, Singh VK, Maurer R, et al. A comparative evaluation of radiologic and clinical scoring systems in the early prediction of severity in acute pancreatitis. Am J Gastroenterol. 2012;107:612-9.
11. Bharwani N, Patel S, Prabhudesai S, et al. Acute pancreatitis: the role of imaging in diagnosis and management. Clin Radiol. 2011;66(2):164-75.
12. Merkle EM, Gorich J. Imaging of acute pancreatitis. Eur Radiol. 2002;12(8):1979-92.
13. Sirli R, Sporea I. Ultrasound examination of the normal pancreas. Med Ultrasound. 2010;12(1):62-5.
14. Turkvatan A, Erden A, Turkoglu MA, Secil M, Yener O. Imaging of acute pancreatitis and its complications. Part 1: Acute pancreatitis. Diagn Interv Imaging. 2015;96(2):151-60.
15. Bollen TL, van Santvoort HC, Besselink MG, et al. Update on acute pancreatitis: ultrasound, computed tomography, and magnetic resonance imaging features. Semin Ultrasound CT MR. 2007;28(5):371-83.
16. O'Connor OJ, McWilliams S, Maher MM. Imaging of acute pancreatitis. AJR. 2011;197(2):W221-5.
17. Balthazar EJ. Acute pancreatitis: assessment of severity with clinical and CT evaluation. Radiology. 2002;223:603-13.
18. Turkvatan A, Erden A, Turkoglu MA, Secil M, Yuce G. Imaging of acute pancreatitis and its complications. Part 2: Complications of Acute Pancreatitis. Diagn Interv Imaging. 2015;96(2):161-9.
19. Theoni RF. Imaging of acute pancreatitis. Radiol Clin N Am. 2015;53:1189-208.
20. Meyrignac O, Lagarde S, Bournet B, et al. Acute pancreatitis: extrapancreatic necrosis volume as early predictor of severity. Radiology. 2015; 276:119-28.
21. Delrue LJ, De Waele JJ, Duyck PO. Acute pancreatitis: radiologic scores in predicting severity and outcome. Abdom Imaging. 2010;35:349-61.
22. Balthazar EJ, Robinson DL, Megibow AJ, et al. Acute pancreatitis: value of CT in establishing prognosis. Radiology. 1990;174:331-6.
23. Bollen TL, Singh VK, Maurer R, et al. Comparative evaluation of the modified CT severity index and CT severity index in assessing severity of acute pancreatitis. AJR. 2011;197:386-92.

24. Mortele KJ, Wiesner W, Intriere L, et al. A modified CT severity index for evaluating acute pancreatitis: improved correlation with patient outcome. AJR. 2004;183:1261-5.
25. De Waele JJ, Delrue L, Hoste EA, et al. Extrapancreatic inflammation on abdominal computed tomography as an early predictor of disease severity in acute pancreatitis: evaluation of a new scoring system. Pancreas. 2007;34:185-90.
26. Sharma V, Rana SS, Ravi SK, et al. A study of radiological scoring system evaluating extrapancreatic inflammation with conventional radiological and clinical scores in predicting outcomes in acute pancreatitis. Ann Gastroenterol. 2015;28:397-402.
27. van Baal MC, Bollen TL, Bakker OJ, et al. The role of routine fine-needle aspiration in the diagnosis of infected necrotising pancreatitis. Surgery. 2014;155(3):442-8.
28. Kloppel G. Acute pancreatitis. Semin Diagn Pathol. 2004;21(4):221-6.
29. Gardner A, Gardner G, Feller E. Severe colonic complications of pancreatic disease. J Clin Gastroenterol. 2003;37:258-62.
30. Van Minnen LP, Besselink MG, Bosscha K, et al. Colonic involvement in acute pancreatitis: a retrospective study of 16 patients. Dig Surg. 2004;21:33-8. discussion 39-40.
31. Mortele KJ, Mergo PJ, Taylor HM, Wiesner W, Cantisani V, Ernst MD, Kalantari BN, Ros PR. Peripancreatic vascular abnormalities complicating acute pancreatitis: contrast-enhanced helical CT findings. Eur J Radiol. 2004;52(1):67-72.
32. Kirby JM, Vora P, Midia M, Rawlinson J. Vascular complications of pancreatitis: imaging and intervention. Cardiovasc Intervent Radiol. 2008;31:957-70.
33. Easler J, Muddana V, Furlan A, et al. Portosplenomesenteric venous thrombosis in patients with acute pancreatitis is associated with pancreatic necrosis and usually has a benign course. Clin Gastroenterol Hepatol. 2014;12(5):854-62.
34. Harris S, Nadkarni NA, Naina HV, et al. Splanchnic vein thrombosis in acute pancreatitis: a single-center experience. Pancreas. 2013;42(8):1251-4.
35. Working Group IAP/APA Acute Pancreatitis Guidelines. IAP/APA evidence-based guidelines for the management of acute pancreatitis. Pancreatology. 2013;13:1-15.
36. Bharwani N, Patel S, Prabhudesai S, Fotheringham T, Power N. Acute pancreatitis: the role of imaging diagnosis and management. Clin Radiol. 2011;66:164-75.
37. van Santvoort HC, Bakker OJ, Bollen TL, et al. A conservative and minimally invasive approach to necrotising pancreatitis improves outcome. Gastroenterology. 2011;141(4):1254-63.
38. Fritz S, Hackert T, Hartwig W, et al. Bacterial translocation and infected pancreatic necrosis in acute necrotising pancreatitis derives from small bowel rather than from colon. Am J Surg. 2010;200(1):111-7.
39. Rodriguez JR, Razo AO, Targarona J, Thayer SP, Rattner DW, Warshaw AL, et al. Debridement and closed packing for sterile or infected necrotizing pancreatitis: insights into indications and outcomes in 167 patients. Ann Surg. 2008;247:294-9.
40. Shyu JY, Sainani NI, Sahni VA, et al. Necrotizing pancreatitis: diagnosis, imaging, and intervention. Radiographics. 2014;34:1218-39.
41. Madhusudhan KS, Venkatesh HA, Gamanagatti S, Garg P, Srivastava DN. Interventional Radiology in the Management of Visceral Artery Pseudoaneurysms: A Review of Techniques and Embolic Materials. Korean J Radiol. 2016;17(3):351-63.
42. Madhusudhan KS, Gamanagatti S, Garg P, Shalimar, Dash NR, Pal S, Peush S, Gupta AK. Endovascular Embolization of Visceral Artery Pseudoaneurysms Using Modified Injection Technique with N-Butyl Cyanoacrylate Glue. J Vasc Interv Radiol. 2015;26(11):1718-25.
43. Ball CG, Correa-Gallego C, Howard TJ, Zyromski NJ, House MG, Pitt HA, Nakeeb A, Schmidt CM, Akisik F, Lillemoe KD. Radiation dose from computed tomography in patients with necrotizing pancreatitis: how much is too much? J Gastrointest Surg. 2010;14(10):1529-35.
44. Göya C, Hamidi C, Hattapoğlu S, Çetinçakmak MG, Teke M, Degirmenci MS, Kaya M, Bilici A. Use of acoustic radiation force impulse elastography to diagnose acute pancreatitis at hospital admission: comparison with sonography and computed tomography. J Ultrasound Med. 2014;33(8):1453-60.
45. Ardelean M, Şirli R, Sporea I, Bota S, Martie A, Popescu A, Danila M, Timar B, Buzas R, Lighezan. Contrast-enhanced ultrasound in the pathology of the pancreas: a monocentric experience. Med Ultrason. 2014;16(4):325-31.
46. Yadav AK, Sharma R, Kandasamy D, Bhalla AS, Gamanagatti S, Srivastava DN, Upadhyay AD, Garg PK. Perfusion CT: can it predict the development of pancreatic necrosis in early stage of severe acute pancreatitis? Abdom Imaging. 2015;40(3):488-99.
47. Yuan Y, Huang ZX, Li ZL, Song B, Deng LP. The value of dual-source dual-energy CT with iodine overlay in the diagnosis of acute necrotizing pancreatitis. Sichuan Da Xue Xue Bao Yi Xue Ban. 2012;43(4):597-600.

CHAPTER

112

Chronic Pancreatitis and its Variants

Anupam Lal, Manphool Singhal, Mandeep Kang

INTRODUCTION

Pancreatitis, the acute form is the most common benign condition affecting the pancreas, and in most cases, it resolves without significant structural or functional impairment. In contrast, chronic pancreatitis (CP) is a progressive fibro-inflammatory disease. This results in irreversible structural changes in the pancreas with progressive loss of the lobular morphology, deformation of the large ducts and changes in the arrangement and composition of the islets. These changes ultimately manifest as ductal obstruction, destruction of acini and the islets of Langerhans, causing loss of exocrine and endocrine functions. Patients may present with abdominal pain, nausea, vomiting, weight loss, diarrhea, and diabetes. The classic clinical triad of CP is exocrine and endocrine pancreatic dysfunction with recurrent episodes of abdominal pain.

ETIOPATHOGENESIS

The risk-factors associated with CP are multi-factorial, including environmental factors (alcohol, tobacco and nutrition), hereditary (mutations), ductal obstruction and autoimmune causes. In adults, the most common etiology attributed to CP is alcohol consumption (70–80% cases).[1] Development of CP is linked/associated with the dose and duration of alcohol consumption; however, recent epidemiological studies and animal experiments suggest that alcohol alone is not sufficient to induce CP and other environmental and genetic factors also play important role. Overall, less than 10% of heavy alcohol consumers develop alcohol-induced CP, nevertheless consumption of lesser quantities may also lead to pancreatic injury and may have an impact on the progression of the disease.[2,3]

Malnutrition remains the most common cause of CP in general population worldwide.[1] Among the hereditary causes, cystic fibrois and mutation of trypsinogen gene are well recognized. Pancreatic or periampullary neoplasms, sphincter of oddi dysfunction, ampullary stricture and congenital lesions like abnormal pancreaticobiliary junction and pancreatic divisum are also important causes of CP. Other causes of CP include hypercalcemia, hyperparathyroidism and hyperlipidemia. Whatever be the cause, the end result is pancreatic fibrosis, which usually takes several years to develop.

In children, the cause of CP is not ascertained in most cases hence labelled as idiopathic (up to 30% of cases). It is thought that hereditary and tropical pancreatitis is responsible for the majority of cases of chronic childhood pancreatitis.[4]

CLASSIFICATION OF CHRONIC PANCREATITIS

Large Duct Pancreatitis versus Small Duct Pancreatitis

There are two pathological subtypes of chronic pancreatitis: *Large duct* and *small duct pancreatitis*, which represent two ends of the same spectrum but have different pathological and radiological features and thus their management also varies.

Large duct pancreatitis is characterized by dilatation and dysfunction of the large ducts (MPD >7 mm) and diffuse pancreatic calcifications. These manifestations are easily recognizable on the imaging. Men are usually more commonly affected as compared to females. Clinical presentation is steatorrhea and abdominal pain. Treatment with replacement of pancreatic enzymes is not effective and the patients usually require surgical or endoscopic drainage to alleviate symptoms.

On the other hand, *small duct pancreatitis* (MPD <3 mm) occurs more in women and is usually not associated with pancreatic calcification. Imaging is essentially normal; therefore, a high index of suspicion is needed for diagnosis. Abdominal pain is the predominant symptom and steatorrhea is rare. Patients may respond to replacement of pancreatic enzymes. Traditionally, radical pancreatic resectional procedures have been carried out for small duct CP.

The longitudinal V-shaped excision of the ventral pancreas has also shown promising results for diffuse small duct CP.[5]

CP may also be classified according to major predisposing risk factors as either (1) toxic-metabolic, (2) idiopathic, (3) genetic, (4) autoimmune, (5) recurrent and severe acute pancreatitis, or (6) obstructive (TIGAR-O system).[6]

Radiologically, three major forms of CP are recognized:

1. *Calcifying chronic pancreatitis:* It is characterized by acinar destruction and perilobular fibrosis with acute and chronic inflammatory cells, leading to pancreatic parenchymal calcification and intraductal calculi. Etiopathogenesis to begin with is precipitation of proteinaceous material in the pancreatic ducts, which form protein plugs that subsequently calcify. Subsequent to the site of obstruction (by protein plugs or fibrosis) the pancreatic duct and smaller pancreatic ductules dilate. The main pancreatic duct shows a chain-of-lakes appearance due to alternating stenoses and dilatation. In approximately half of patients with chronic calcific pancreatitis, the pancreatic parenchyma may contain cuboidal epithelium lined cysts containing pancreatic enzymes of varying sizes (several millimeters to 5 cm). Clinically, this form presents as recurrent episodes of abdominal pain. Alcohol and tobacco are implicated for this form of CP. Other forms of calcifying CP can be hereditary, tropical, idiopathic, and senile.
2. *Obstructive chronic pancreatitis:* This form of CP is due to persistent obstruction of the pancreatic duct (tumor or ductal stricture) leading to atrophy of the distal pancreas. The prominent histologic changes are periductal fibrosis and subsequent ductal dilatation. These changes can either be focal or diffuse depending upon the site of pancreatic ductal obstruction. Focal changes in this form are much more common than other forms of CP. Diffuse changes occur when pancreatic duct or ampulla is obstructed. Intraductal calculi are rare. The pancreatic duct is dilated, and the pancreas is normal in size, atrophic, or focally and/or globally enlarged. Abdominal pain is usually absent, though occasionally the patients present with acute pancreatitis.
3. Autoimmune pancreatitis (AIP) is part of a chronic systemic sclerosing disease characterized by lymphoplasmacytic inflammatory process involving the pancreas and other organs. AIP unlike other forms of CP shows focal, segmental or diffuse narrowing of MPD and non-visualization of side branches on ERCP. The narrowing can also be seen in the lower end of common bile duct (CBD) causing biliary dilatation. On imaging, it may appear as diffuse (duct destructive) or as pseudotumoral lesions.

DIAGNOSIS

Evaluation of CP usually needs a battery of tests. Biochemical investigations are used to assess the endocrine and exocrine function of the pancreas. Fecal elastase 1 (FE 1) is one of the commonly used indirect methods but has low sensitivity.[7] Tubed secretin test is a direct method which involves prolonged intubation and serial collection of pancreatic juice after hormonal stimulation. It is considered as a reference standard for the evaluation of exocrine function of pancreas.[8]

Radiological investigations are primarily used for evaluation of structural changes and complications of CP.

Imaging Modalities

Usually a combination of imaging is required with different imaging modalities having their own advantages and limitations and the role of imaging is to help confirm the diagnosis, assess disease severity, detect complications, and provide a "road map" for interventional procedures.

Abdominal Radiographs

Abdominal radiographs are not routinely done for the evaluation of CP. Often pancreatic calcifications are incidentally detected on radiographs done to rule out other causes for abdominal pain and thus the diagnosis suspected. CP is manifested on abdominal radiographs as multifocal calcifications typically seen across the spine along the course of pancreas **(Fig. 1)**. Since calcifications are usually seen in the advanced cases and only in certain types of CP, radiographs are not a sensitive investigation. Typical pancreatic calcifications, however if seen on radiographs are pathognomonic of CP.

Endoscopic Retrograde Cholangio-pancreatography

Endoscopic retrograde cholangio-pancreatography (ERCP) is considered as the gold standard for the diagnosis of CP because of its superior spatial resolution and its ability to depict the ductal system in distended state. Side branch abnormalities in early CP may be detected. ERCP is an invasive procedure and has inherent procedure-related complications; hence this modality is mostly used with intent of therapeutic interventions. On ERCP, diameter of normal main pancreatic duct (MPD) varies with the region of pancreas—up to 4 mm in head, 3 mm in body and 2 mm in tail region. Side branches join the MPD at right angles in alternating fashion. Early CP is seen on ERCP in the form of irregularity and dilatation of side branches **(Fig. 2)**. These changes are more severe along with dilatation, loss of normal tapering and irregularity of MPD as the disease progresses **(Fig. 3)**. In advanced stages, alternate dilatation and stenosis of MPD can give the appearance of chain of lakes **(Figs. 4 and 5)**.

The Cambridge classification of CP based on ERCP is used to group patients into equivocal, mild, moderate or marked type. The status of MPD, side branches, presence of calculi and ductal strictures are taken into account in Cambridge classification.[9]

Cambridge Classification

Score 1 (Cambridge Class 0)

- Severity: normal
- Good quality ERCP/US or CT visualizing whole gland without abnormal signs.

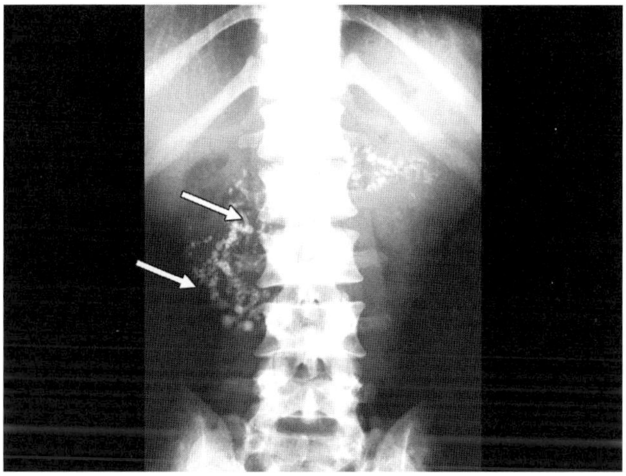

FIG. 1: Chronic calcifying pancreatitis: Plain radiograph abdomen showing calcifications along the course of pancreas. Note a pancreatic stent in situ (arrows).

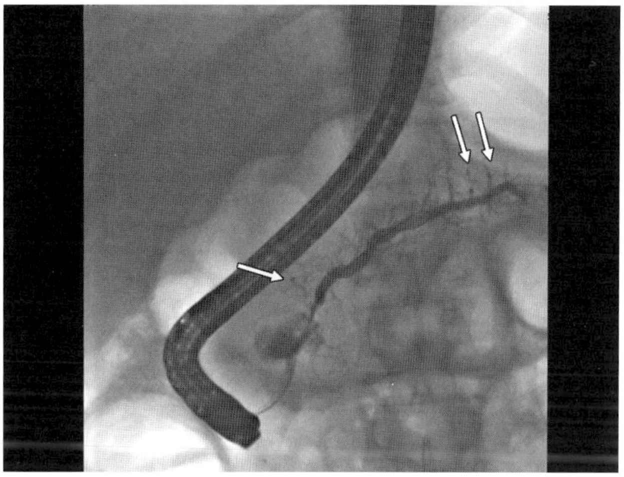

FIG. 2: Endoscopic retrograde cholangio-pancreatography (ERCP): Early changes of chronic pancreatitis showing mild irregularity of side branches (arrows). Main pancreatic duct (MPD) is not dilated.

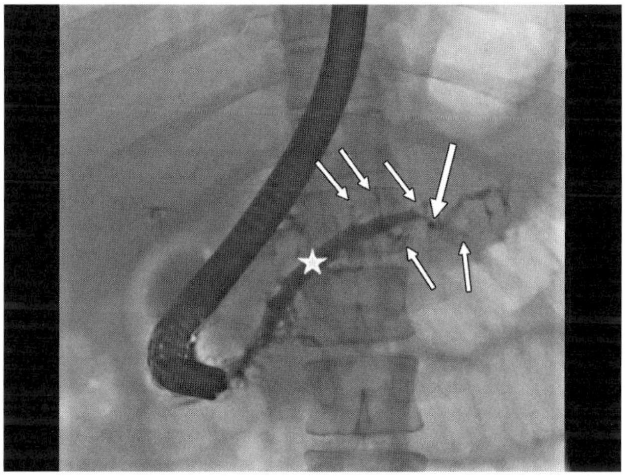

FIG. 3: ERCP: MPD is dilated (star). Note narrowing of MPD in tail region (long arrow) and multiple abnormal side branches (arrows).

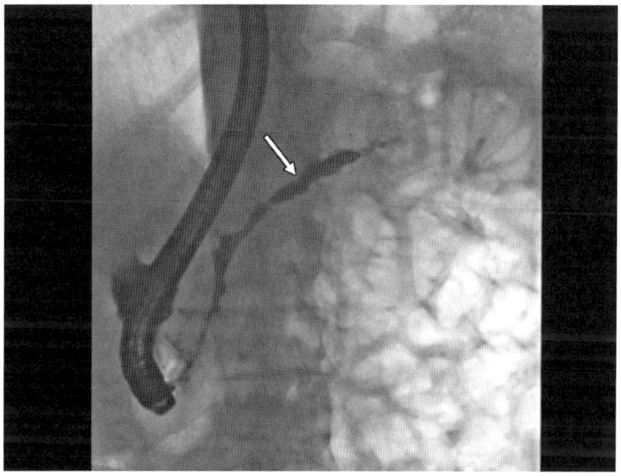

FIG. 4: ERCP: MPD (arrow) showing multiple strictures and irregular dilatation with truncated and abnormal side branches.

Score 2 (Cambridge Class 0)

- Severity: equivocal
- ERCP: <3 abnormal branches
- *US/CT*: abnormal sign—main pancreatic duct 2 to 4 mm diameter, gland 1 to 2 × normal.

Score 3 (Cambridge Class I)

- Severity: mild
- *ERCP*: 3 or more abnormal branches
- *US/CT*: 2+ abnormal signs: cavities <10 mm, duct irregularity, focal acute necrosis, parenchymal heterogeneity, increased echogenicity of duct wall, contour irregularity of head/body.

Score 4 (Cambridge Class II)

- Severity: moderate
- ERCP: >3 side branches plus abnormal main duct
- US/CT: as score 3.

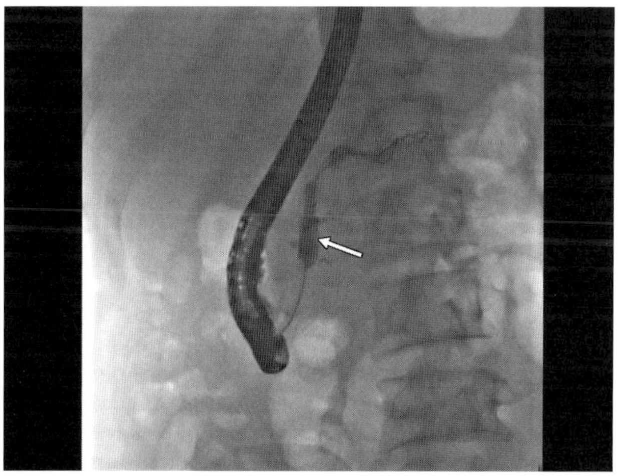

FIG. 5: ERCP: Multiple strictures of MPD (chain of lakes appearance). Note abnormally dilated side branches in head region and non-opacification of side branches in body and tail region.

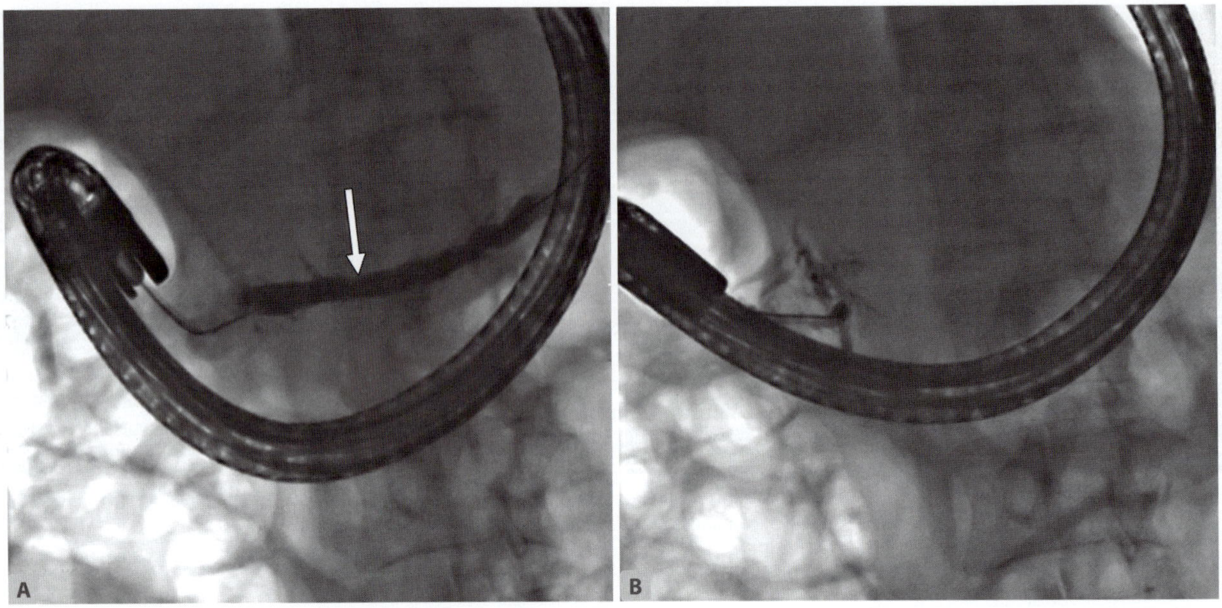

FIGS 6A AND B: Pancreatic divisum, ERCP Images (A and B). Cannulation of minor papilla (A) shows opacification of entire dorsal duct which is mildly dilated (arrow) with truncation of some side branches. Cannulation of major papilla shows only part of ventral duct draining part of head and uncinate process of pancreas. Also note the long route taken by the endoscope required for cannulation of minor papilla.

Score 5 (Cambridge Class III)

- Severity: severe
- ERCP: all of above, plus 1 or more of: large cavity >10 mm, intraductal filling defects, duct obstruction (stricture), duct dilation or irregularity
- US/CT: all of above, plus 1 or more of: large cavity >10 mm, intraductal filling defects, duct obstruction (stricture), duct dilation or irregularity, calculi/pancreatic calcification, contiguous organ invasion.

ERCP is also helpful in diagnosing other obstructive causes of CP such as ampullary lesions, intraductal neoplasms and congenital anomalies such as pancreatic divisum **(Figs. 6A and B)** or annular pancreas.

Ultrasonography

Trans-abdominal sonography: It is usually the first and initial imaging modality as most patients present with abdominal pain or discomfort. Sonographic evaluation is often challenging due to obscuration of pancreas by bowel gases. Maneuvers such as distending the stomach with water, changing position of patient and visualizing the tail of pancreas through splenic window are helpful. It is also important that the patient should be fasting adequately to reduce bowel gases.

USG appearance of pancreas varies with the stage of CP. In early stage, pancreas appears heterogeneous due to focal areas of intervening hypoechogenicity which are areas of focal inflammatory changes **(Fig. 7)**. At this stage only with a very high index of suspicion, the diagnosis can be suggested. In moderate-to-severe stages the changes become more marked and appreciable in most cases. In advanced disease, the changes of CP are easily appreciated in the form of irregular dilated main pancreatic duct (MPD) with pancreatic and intraductal calculi and associated atrophy of pancreas **(Fig. 8)**. USG is useful for detection of complications like pseudocysts, venous thrombosis or arterial pseudoaneurysms.

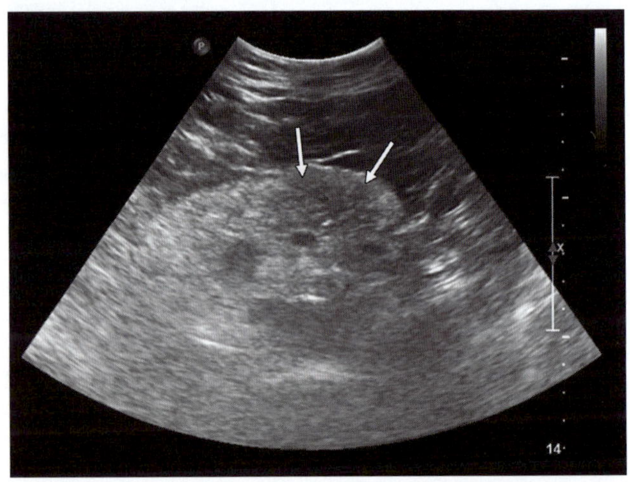

FIG. 7: Early chronic pancreatitis: Transabdominal USG image showing subtle ill-defined hypoechoic areas in pancreatic body (arrows).

Endoscopic Ultrasound (EUS)

Pancreas by the virtue of its location proximal to lumens of stomach and duodenum allows EUS to obtain high-resolution imaging without interference by bowel gas, which usually is the limiting factor for comprehensive evaluation by trans-abdominal USG. EUS allows recognition of early changes and several other features of CP which cannot be appreciated with other imaging modalities **(Fig. 9)**. These include hyperechoic margins of the pancreatic duct, subtle lobularity of the parenchyma, small cystic changes in the parenchyma, and side branch duct ectasia.[10] Currently, EUS is

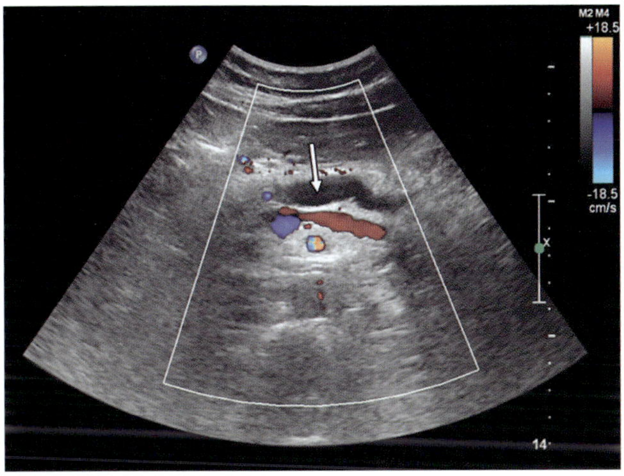

FIG. 8: Advanced changes of chronic pancreatitis: USG with color Doppler shows dilated MPD (arrow) with atrophy of pancreas. (MPD: main pancreatic duct).

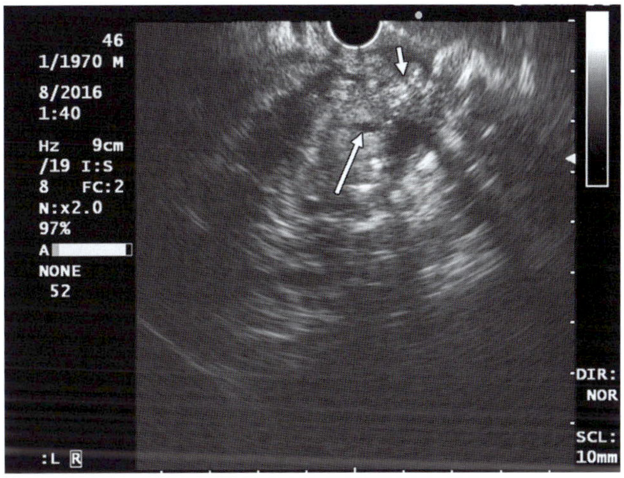

FIG. 9: Chronic pancreatitis: EUS image showing calcifications (arrow) in pancreatic head and mildly dilated MPD (long arrow).

considered to be the best imaging modality which can detect early chronic pancreatitis.[11]

Ultrasound elastography has also been used to evaluate the extent of fibrosis (stiffness) of pancreas and can be used along with trans-abdominal and endoscopic ultrasound. Retroperitoneal location of pancreas and close proximity to aorta (effect of aortic pulsations) are major hindrance for evaluation of pancreas with elastography. With advancing technology and improvement in equipment design, elastography may become a very useful imaging modality for early detection of chronic pancreatitis such as parenchymal edema recognized as change of tissue stiffness.[12] Also, elastography may contribute to early detection of pancreatic cancer in patients with CP.

Computed Tomography

Computed tomography (CT) is the imaging modality of choice for the evaluation of CP. The pancreatic calcifications are best seen on CT **(Fig. 10)**. It also plays a pivotal role in follow-up after medical or/and surgical treatment. The complete evaluation of CP on CT is optimally done using a multiphase protocol which includes unenhanced scan, arterial phase and a parenchymal phase scan. Pancreatic calcifications/calculi are detected on unenhanced scan and detection of arterial complications and arterial mapping are done using the arterial phase. Pancreatic parenchymal and ductal evaluation, pseudocysts and focal lesions are best evaluated using the parenchymal phase scans.

Normal pancreas on CT appears as a homogeneous structure with smooth lobulated borders. Inflammation in pancreas leads to focal or diffuse hypodensity and surrounding fat stranding. The characteristic features of CP are atrophy of pancreas, ductal dilatation and multiple parenchymal and intraductal calcifications.[13] In the early stage of CP, the MPD and side branches changes are not noticeable on CT and the contrast enhancement is also relatively homogeneous. With disease progression multifocal fibrotic changes lead to heterogeneity of enhancement as the normal parenchyma

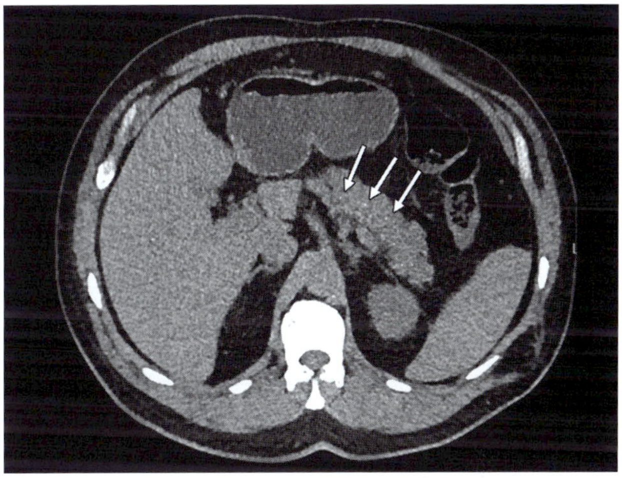

FIG. 10: Alcohol-induced chronic pancreatitis: CT axial image showing subtle pancreatic calcifications (arrows) in pancreatic body and tail region.

enhances earlier in the venous phase, whereas the fibrotic areas show delayed enhancement.

The pancreatic head is the most common location of parenchymal calcifications. The calcification can vary in size and morphology and the degree of calcification is directly proportional to the duration of the disease. Calcifications are seen early in alcoholic CP and certain hereditary pancreatitis as compared to obstructive CP.[13] Alcohol-related CP shows calcification in 20–40% of patients and it is usually seen after 5–10 years.[3] The MPD shows segments of stenosis alternating with dilatation containing multiple calculi of varying sizes and irregular morphology **(Figs. 11 and 12)**. In patients with cystic fibrosis having CFTR mutations, the calcifications appear late and they are smaller when compared to other genetic mutation. The stones in genetic mutation-related CP other than cystic fibrosis are usually round or oval in shape measuring more than 2–3 cm. On CT, they have a

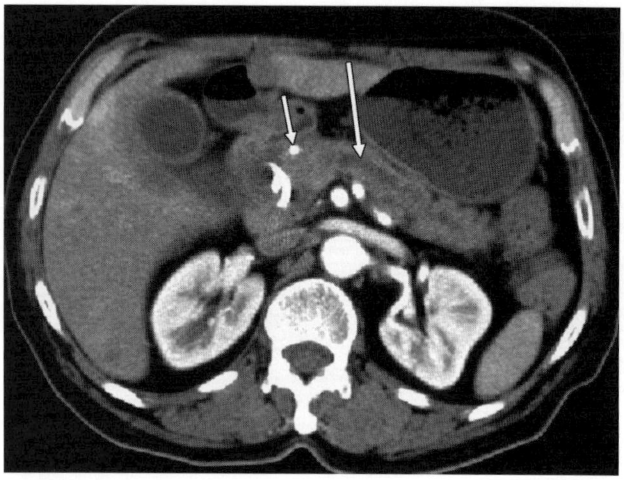

FIG. 11: Chronic pancreatits, CT axial image showing calcification (arrow) and dilated MPD (long arrow). An inflammatory mass is seen in head region obstructing the MPD. Note biliary stents in situ.

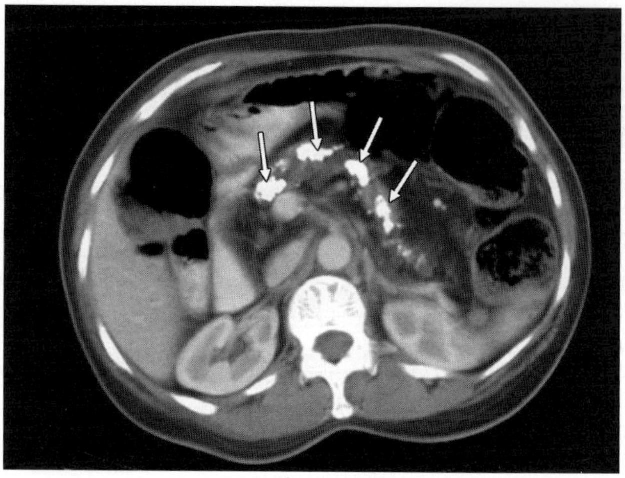

FIG. 12: Chronic pancreatitis—CT axial image: Large pancreatic ductal calculi (arrows) with atrophy and fatty replacement of pancreas.

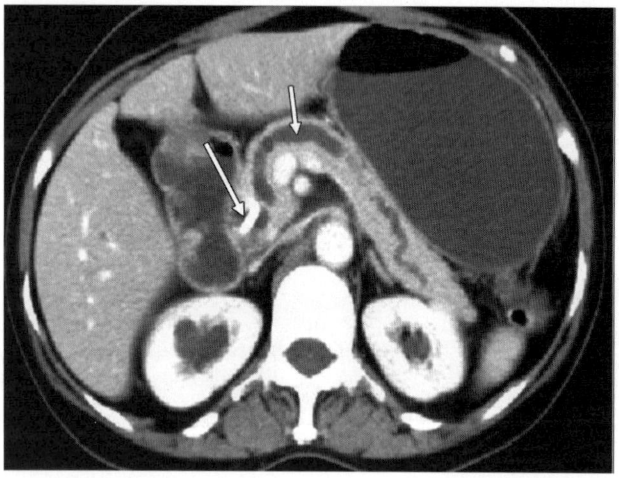

FIG. 13: CT image showing ill-defined hypoenhancing lesion at ampulla (periampullary CA) obstructing the MPD (arrow). Note biliary stents in situ (long arrow).

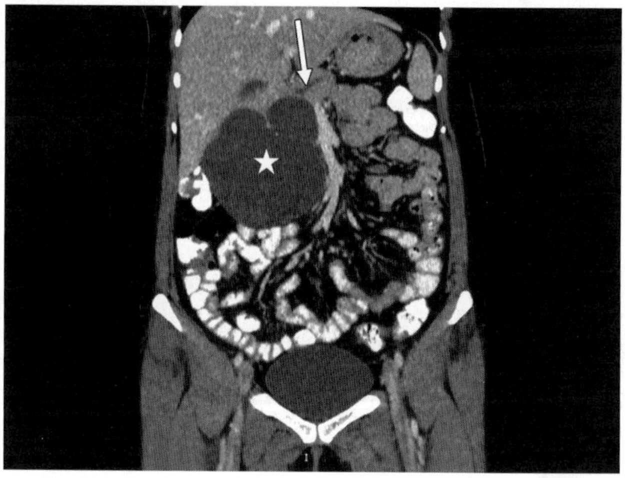

FIG. 14: CT coronal reformatted image: Large mucinous cystadenoma (star) causing pancreatic ductal obstruction (arrow).

typical appearance with hypodense center and hyperdense periphery which is due to the lack of calcium in the center. It is often referred to as Bull's eye stone.[14] These stones are usually arranged linearly within the dilated MPD. The above features of multiple large round to oval bull's eye stones should point towards the diagnosis of CP secondary to genetic mutations. Tropical pancreatitis which is predominantly a disease of developing countries also presents with parenchymal atrophy, ductal dilatation and large calculi which can reach up to 5 cm in size and can extend into side branches.[15] This finding is in contrast to alcoholic CP in which calcifications are small and speckled. CT in this scenario has an edge over MRI in giving a specific diagnosis.

In patients with obstructive CP the MPD is dilated, however, parenchymal or intraductal calcifications are usually not seen. Another important role of CT is to evaluate the cause for obstructive CP. Focal lesions such as pancreatic adenocarcinoma, periampullary carcinoma, and rarely non-functioning neuroendocrine tumors can lead to MPD obstruction and cause repeated attacks of pancreatitis eventually presenting as CP **(Fig. 13)**. Cystic tumors of pancreas such as serous, mucinous and intraductal tumors can also cause obstructive form of CP **(Fig. 14)**. CT is very helpful in characterising these solid tumors and to some extent cystic tumors.

Pancreatic divisum is one of the common congenital causes for CP for which the modality of choice is MRI. However, in advanced stages CT can recognize the changes due to pancreatic divisum. The inflammatory, fibrotic changes and the ductal changes are limited to the dorsal part of pancreas whereas the ventral pancreas appears normal.

CT has the ability to evaluate the complications related to CP. The prevalence of pancreatic pseudocysts in chronic pancreatitis is 20% to 40%.[16] Pancreatic pseudocysts most commonly arise in patients with alcoholic chronic pancreatitis (70–78%).[17] Pseudocysts are cystic lesions with a wall and usually they are well defined. They can be seen in peripancreatic region, intraperitoneal, retroperitoneal or

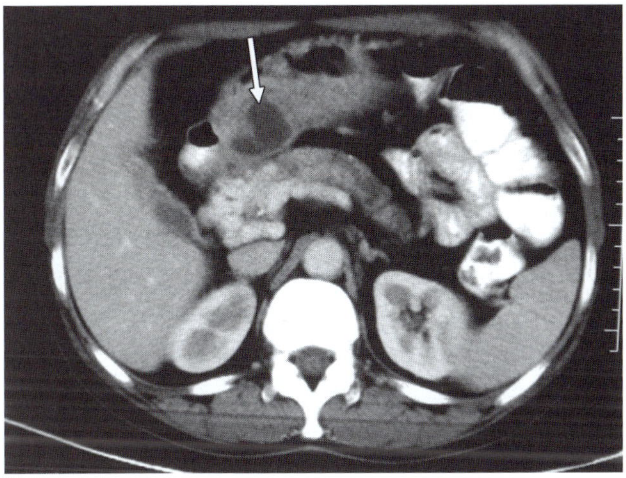

FIG. 15: CT image showing a duodenal intramural pseudocyst (arrow). Changes of chronic pancreatitis are evident.

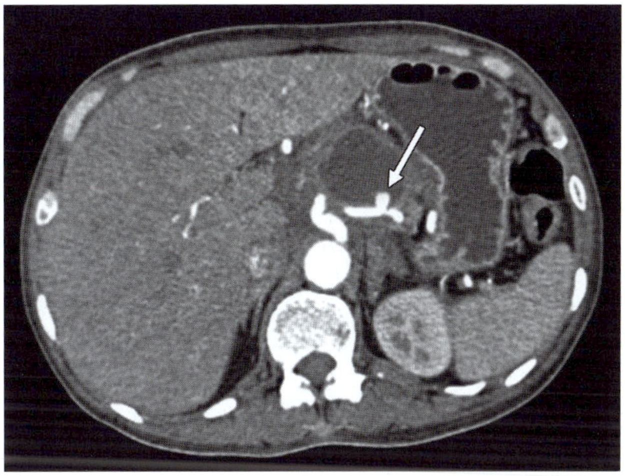

FIG. 16: Chronic pancreatitis: CT axial image showing splenic artery pseudoaneurysm (arrow) projecting into pseudocyst.

even in remote locations like chest. In CP, pseudocysts are generally formed during the evolution of peripancreatic fluid collections after an episode of pancreatitis **(Fig. 15)**. Pseudocysts are closely mimicked by retention cysts which occur in pancreas as a result of obstruction to MPD or side branch by calculi or as a result of fibrosis. The resulting cystic lesions are seen on CT as non-enhancing well-defined lesions and they are not necessarily associated with an acute episode of pancreatitis. Pseudocysts along with peripancreatic inflammation can involve the venous structures in the vicinity leading to phlebitis and thrombosis. These complications can be seen in splenic, superior mesenteric and portal vein and are seen as filling defects or occlusion on contrast-enhanced CT. The resulting portal hypertension which is usually limited to left side (segmental portal hypertension) can lead to the development of multiple collaterals. When the inflammation involves the arteries in the vicinity, it can cause formation of pseudoaneurysms **(Fig. 16)**. In CP, gastroduodenal, pancreaticoduodenal and splenic arteries are the most common to be involved. They can rupture and bleed into peritoneal cavity, bowel or biliary system and present an acute emergency. Sometimes they are detected on routine imaging in which case they have to be treated at the earliest to prevent catastrophic complications. Pseudoaneurysms are best seen on arterial phase CT scan when the concentration of contrast in arteries is at its peak. They can be missed on routine portal venous scan which makes the arterial phase acquisition important in this scenario.

Sometimes in CP, pancreatic fistula can develop with the peritoneal cavity or even pleural cavity. It can occur secondary to rupture of pseudocyst. On CT, they are seen as ascites or pleural effusion, however, the actual fistula site may not be demonstrated on CT scans. Biliary complications due to CP can manifest as fistula or inflammatory strictures which are better evaluated with MRCP.

Evidence from several case-control, cohort, and record linkage studies confirms that patients with CP are at increased risk of pancreatic cancer, although only about 5% of patients with common forms of pancreatitis will develop pancreatic cancer. Patients with early onset of pancreatitis, as in HP, have a high risk of developing pancreatic cancer.[18] Pancreatic carcinoma in patients with CP can mimic inflammatory mass forming chronic pancreatitis, focal AIP and groove pancreatitis. Reliable distinction between these lesions on imaging is quite challenging and is not always possible. Advances in CT techniques in the form of perfusion CT have added another dimension to the diagnostic capability of CT scanners. Perfusion CT is novel technique in which scans of a particular area are acquired in quick succession. The data collected is postprocessed and the contrast dynamics of the given area is depicted as color coded maps. Perfusion parameters such as blood flow and blood volume can be quantified. There are promising reports in which researchers have used perfusion CT to differentiate pancreatic carcinoma from mass forming chronic pancreatitis.

Lack of information on the exocrine function of pancreas, limited contrast resolution and exposure to radiation are the most important limitations of CT. Also CT does not have specific imaging characteristics in most cases on the basis of which an etiologic factor can be identified.

Magnetic Resonance Imaging

MRCP has replaced ERCP for the diagnostic imaging of biliary and pancreatic ducts. In MRCP, heavily T2 weighted sequences are used to image fluid-filled structures. MR has the additional advantage of having excellent contrast resolution without using ionizing radiation.

Normal pancreas is the most T1 hyperintense structure in abdomen due to the presence of proteinaceous secretion within the gland **(Fig. 17)**. T1 fat saturated sequence is a very sensitive sequence for the identification of any focal lesion within the pancreas as many of the focal lesions appear hypointense and they are easily recognized. Similarly any inflammation in pancreas leads to drop in signal on T1 weighted sequences.

In early stages of CP, because of the inflammation and onset of fibrosis there is drop in T1 signal. The gland may be

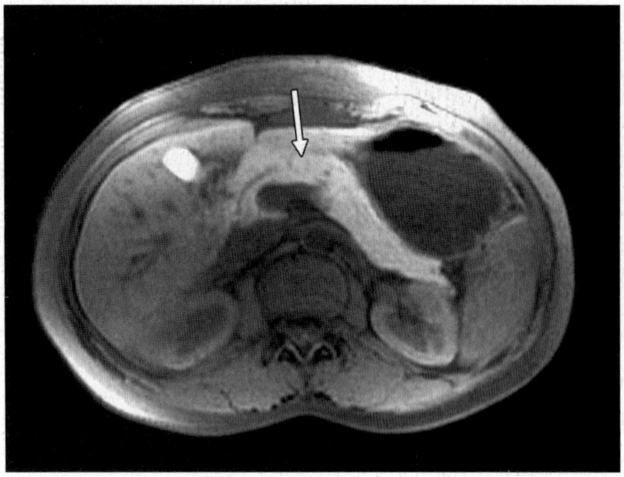

FIG. 17: T1 fat saturated MR image showing homogeneous hyper intense signals of pancreas (arrow).

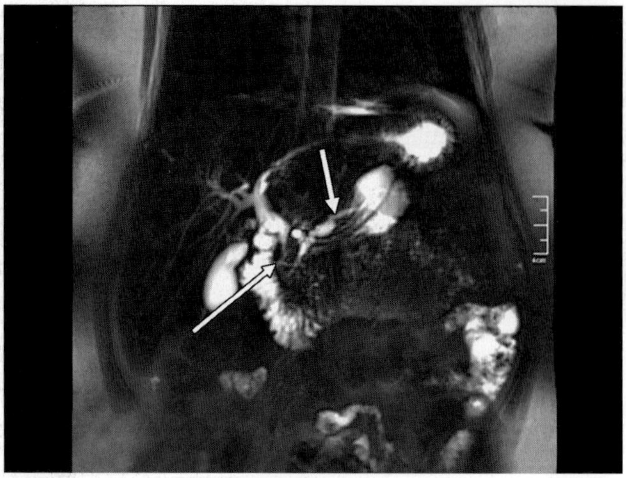

FIG. 18: Chronic pancreatitis: MRCP image showing multiple strictures (arrow) with irregular dilatation of MPD (arrow). Note stricture at lower end of CBD (long arrow).

heterogeneous because of focal areas of inflammation and fibrosis. There is heterogeneous and delayed enhancement in the post-contrast images because of fibrosis and this delayed enhancement compared to the normal pancreas is considered as an early marker of CP.

The ductal changes are better visualized on MRCP as compared to CT scan; however, subtle side branch changes can be missed. The ductal findings of early disease can range from normal looking MPD to mild irregularity of MPD and side branches **(Fig. 18)**. With progression of disease, there is progressive glandular atrophy and poor enhancement in portal venous phase and increased enhancement in delayed phase. Severe ductal changes in the form of irregular dilatation of both MPD and side branches along with interposed strictures give the appearance of chain of lakes on MRCP. MR is also good in depicting the associated complications such as pseudocysts and fistula. Intraductal calcifications are seen as filling defects in the hyperintense background of fluid. The sensitivity of MR for small calcification is limited when compared to CT scan.

MR is excellent modality to detect ductal abnormalities such as pancreatic divisum **(Fig. 19)**, and any solid or cystic focal lesion causing obstructive type of CP. It can also differentiate CP from other mimics like intraductal papillary mucinous neoplasms (IPMN) and other variants such as groove pancreatitis and AIP.

It is challenging to differentiate mass-forming chronic pancreatitis from pancreatic adenocarcinoma even on MRI. 'Duct penetrating sign' on MRCP, which means that a normal or smoothly stenotic MPD is seen to penetrate the mass, has been reported to be associated with inflammatory mass rather than carcinoma.[19] It has a reported sensitivity of 85% and specificity of 96%. Recently, diffusion weighted imaging (DWI) has been used to accurately differentiate mass-forming pancreatitis from carcinoma.[20] The role of 5-fluorodeoxyglucose-positron emission tomography (FDG-PET) in this scenario still remains controversial.

One of the major limitations of MRCP in the evaluation of CP is the lack of functional information and inability to image

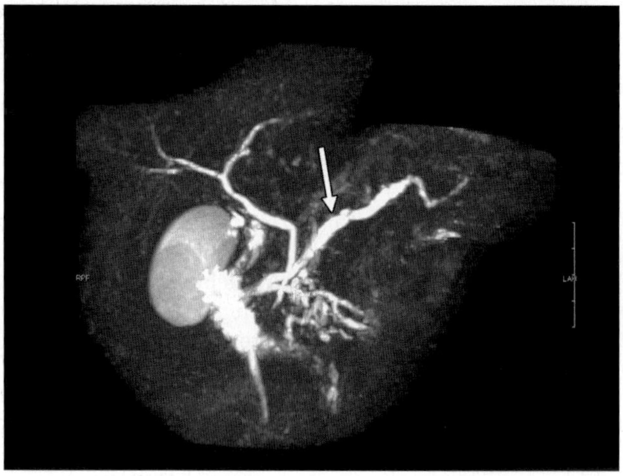

FIG. 19: Pancreatic divisum: MRCP image showing the main pancreatic duct (arrow) crossing horizontally the CBD and opening into minor papilla.

the ductal system in distended state. This drawback can be overcome by using secretin and acquiring serial MR images which is known as secretin enhanced MRCP or secretin stimulated MRCP (S-MRCP).[21] Secretin causes transient increase in the tone of sphincter of Oddi and increased secretion of bicarbonate-rich fluid. Patient should be fasting for 4–6 hours and a negative oral contrast is administered 30 minutes before the study to suppress the signals from pre-existing fluid in the duodenum. Baseline images are taken and secretin is injected as a slow intravenous injection to prevent the side effects. After injection, T2-weighted images are acquired every 30 seconds for a period of 15 minutes. This leads to the dilatation of MPD and the maximum dilatation occurs at 2–5 minutes after which the sphincteric tone decreases and MPD diameter comes to baseline after 10 minutes. The pancreatic secretions can be seen in the duodenum and can be graded in quantitative or semi-quantitative manner and reflect the exocrine function of the pancreas. The MPD should show an increase of at least 1 mm compared to baseline in patients with normal sphincter, absence of which would imply impaired ductal compliance. In normal pancreas the side branches are not visualized after secretin, whereas in patient with early CP because of subtle fibrosis, the side branches can show dilatation which are not otherwise seen on conventional MRCP. This is an important advantage of S-MRCP as it distends the MPD so that even the subtle abnormalities are better shown akin to ERCP. For the same reason, it is superior to conventional MRCP in delineating ductal anomalies such as pancreas divisum.

The exocrine function can be graded as follows: fluid confined to duodenal bulb is grade 1, confined to first and second part of duodenum is grade 2 and fluid reaching into the third part is grade 3. Grade 3 is considered normal and grades 1 and 2 are considered as impaired exocrine function. This quantification is found to consistently correlate with fecal elastase 1 values. Thus s-MRCP has the capability to provide both the structural and functional information which is crucial for the management of these patients.

Diffusion weighted imaging (DWI) is also used for the evaluation of CP using the apparent diffusion coefficient (ADC) values.[20] ADC of pancreas in patients with CP was found to be less than in normal patients. It is because of the decreased exocrine reserve of pancreas leading to decreased water diffusion and fibrosis which can by itself restrict diffusion. ADC values can potentially be used as an indicator of fibrosis and its extent in patients with CP which can be used to predict the outcome in patients who undergo surgery. Furthermore, DWI may be combined with S-MRCP to study the increase in ADC with the administration of secretin which increases secretion and hence promotes water diffusion.[21,22] In normal patients, the ADC is expected to increase in the early part of the s-MRCP study. This can be a potential method of quantification of exocrine function of pancreas in future.

MISCELLANEOUS TYPES OF CHRONIC PANCREATITIS

Autoimmune Pancreatitis

Autoimmune pancreatitis (AIP) is a pancreatic involvement in IgG4-related diseases which have been recently recognized as a distinct identity in the year 1995 by Yoshida et al.[23] It accounts for about 10% of all cases of chronic pancreatitis. On histology, lymphoplasmacytic infiltration is seen around the veins and ducts sparing the arterioles. Awareness of imaging features is of paramount significance for radiologists as correct diagnosis obviates unnecessary delay in treatment and surgeries. Accurate diagnosis is thus desirable as the disease responds dramatically to immune-suppressive therapy (mostly steroids). Diagnosis is usually established by typical imaging findings supplemented with raised serum immunoglobulin G4 (IgG4) levels and histopathology.

Men are affected twice as frequently as women with varying age of presentation (14 to 77 years), however, most patients at presentation are about 50 years of age.[24] AIP characteristically almost never presents with typical acute episodes of pancreatitis. Patients may present with jaundice, abdominal pain and weight loss, and diabetes mellitus.[24]

Various extra-pancreatic manifestations associated with AIP are biliary system (68–88%), where it presents with smooth strictures of biliary system (seen in up to 90% of patients), bowel (about 17%) (most commonly, ulcerative colitis), salivary glands (sialadenitis-12 to 16%), kidneys (4–35%) and retroperitoneal fibrosis (3–8%).[25] Strictures of more proximal bile ducts are also known and may resemble primary sclerosing cholangitis and therefore distinction of both is important as strictures due to AIP demonstrates dramatic response to steroid therapy while those of sclerosing cholangitis show a poor response to steroid treatment. Pulmonary involvement may be seen in the form of parenchymal nodules and infiltrates or mediastinal lymphadenopathy. Autoimmune prostatitis may be seen as an infrequent extra-pancreatic manifestation. Renal parenchymal involvement in the form of small peripheral cortical nodules, round lesions, well-defined wedge-shaped lesions, or diffuse patchy involvement may be seen and are important supporting clue for diagnosing autoimmune pancreatitis.[25]

Based on the current understanding, AIP has two distinct subtypes: *Type 1* is known as lymphoplasmacytic sclerosing pancreatitis (LPSP), which is characterized by elevated serum IgG4 levels, abundant infiltration with IgG4 positive cells and extrapancreatic involvement. *Type 2* is known as idiopathic duct centric pancreatitis (IDCP). LPSP is more common in Eastern countries whilst IDCP is more common in the Western world. Typical feature of IDCP is the presence of granulocyte epithelial lesions (GEL). Unlike type 1, IDCP usually does not have elevated serum levels of IgG4 and infiltration by IgG4-positive cells. In addition, extrapancreatic involvement is not seen in IDCP except that it can be associated with inflammatory bowel disease. Recurrence is common in AICP but rare in IDCP.

The Japan Pancreatic Society criteria based on imaging features: Serology or histopathology is one of the most commonly used criteria for the diagnosis of AIP. Various serological tests suggested are: Serum gamma globulin, IgG4, antilactoferrin antibody (ALA), anti-carbonic anhydrase II antibody (ACA II), anti-smooth muscle antibody (ASMA), and antinuclear antibody (ANA).[26]

In 2011, an International Consensus Diagnostic Criteria (ICDC) was developed based on the various existing and commonly used criteria. ICDC is considered to be the most sensitive and specific criteria for diagnosing AIP. ICDC is based on the imaging features of pancreatic parenchyma, ducts, serology, involvement of other organs, histology and response to steroid therapy.

CT scan is the diagnostic modality of choice and on imaging three distinct patterns (diffuse, focal and multifocal) have been described.[27] *Diffuse pattern* which is the most common type is seen as featureless or sausage-like pancreas because of the loss of lobular architecture **(Figs. 20 to 22)**. The involved pancreas is homogeneous and the MPD is either non-dilated or diffusely narrowed which is a characteristic finding in AIP. Calcification is rare unlike other types of chronic pancreatitis. There can be a hypoattenuating rim with associated fat stranding and foreshortening of pancreatic tail.

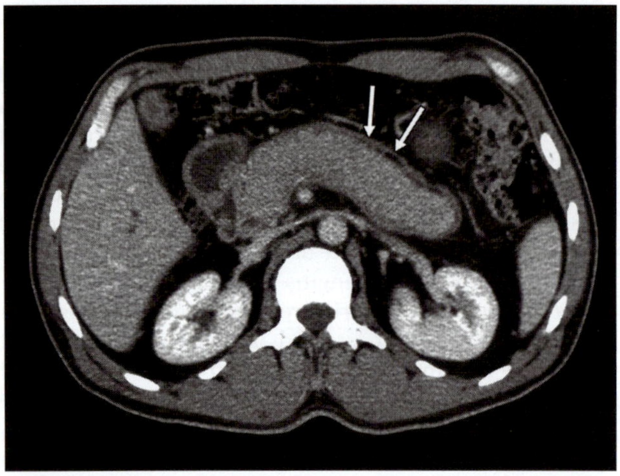

FIG. 20: Autoimmune pancreatitis: Axial CT image showing diffusely enlarged pancreas with loss of lobulations and peripheral hypoenhancing rim (arrows).

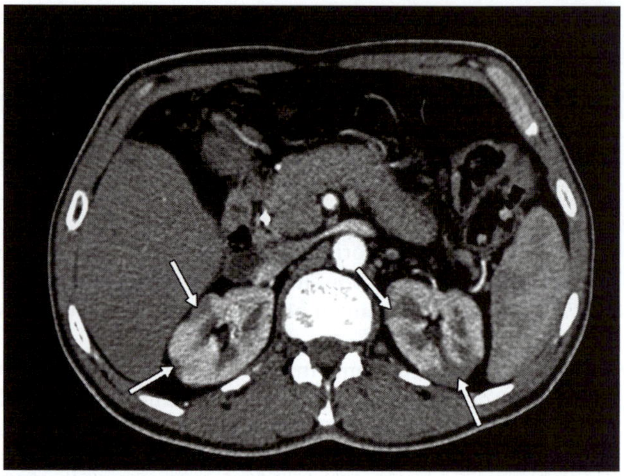

FIG. 21: Autoimmune pancreatitis: Axial CT image showing multple hypoenhancing wedge-shaped lesions in both kidneys (arrows).

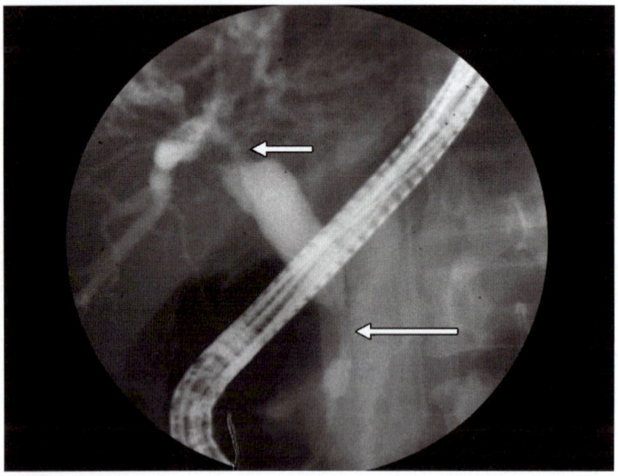

FIG. 22: Autoimmune pancreatitis: Endoscopic retrograde cholangiopancreatography (ERCP) image showing a hilar (arrow) and lower common bile duct (CBD) (long arrow) stricture.

The rim shows a characteristic delayed enhancement. On ERCP, characteristic finding is focal, segmental or diffuse narrowing and irregularity of MPD. MRI can show a mildly enlarged pancreas with loss of signal intensity on T1-weighted images and mild hyperintensity on T2-weighted images. After contrast administration the involved part of the pancreas shows delayed enhancement. The rim around the pancreas is hypointense on both T1- and T2-weighted images and shows delayed enhancement. MRCP can show features similar to ERCP and it can also show associated strictures in biliary tree.

The *focal* type of AIP can present as a focal mass lesion on all imaging modalities mimicking carcinoma pancreas. Even the clinical presentation may simulate and confuse with pancreatic cancer as some of these patients may have elevated carcinoembryonic antigen and cancer antigen 19-9 levels. Focal type can also present with upstream dilatation of MPD, however, the dilatation is less severe when compared to carcinoma pancreas. Delayed enhancement in AIP is another feature which differentiates it from carcinoma pancreas.

Positron emission tomography with 2-[fluorine 18] fluoro-2-deoxy-d-glucose can be useful, if imaging is equivocal and there is need to differentiate autoimmune pancreatitis from pancreatic cancer. On PET, AIP demonstrates heterogeneous pattern with multofocal areas of uptake in the pancreas. Extra-pancreatic uptake in lachrymal or salivary gland, biliary system, retroperitoneal space, or prostate gland provide important clue to diagnosis.[28]

Groove Pancreatitis

Groove pancreatitis is a rare type of CP which is localized to the pancreaticoduodenal groove. Exact etilogy is not known but factors such as duodenal ulcer, gastric resection, duodenal wall cysts, pancreatic heterotopia, pancreatic ductal obstructions have been implicated. Groove pancreatitis, cystic dystrophy of duodenum and paraduodenal wall cysts have many features in common and hence they are collectively categorized as paraduodenal pancreatitis.

Two forms of groove pancreatitis have been recognized: *"segmental"* and *"pure" form.* Typically the former involves the head of pancreas with formation of scar tissue within the groove, while in latter only groove is affected sparing the pancreatic head.[29] Patients usually present with duodenal and biliary obstruction. Biliary strictures are seen in majority (50% of cases).[29]

On imaging a soft tissue density is seen within the pancreaticoduodenal groove that usually shows delayed enhancement (fibrosis) and small cystic lesions along the medial wall of the duodenum **(Fig. 23)**. MR imaging is superior for characterization of these findings and post-gadolinium scans may show delayed enhancement of the mass.[30]

Groove pancreatitis may mimic pancreatic malignancy. Displacement of gastroduodenal artery towards pancreatic head, with associated cystic changes of duodenal wall which occurs in groove pancreatitis and abrupt cut-off of

MPD which occurs in carcinoma pancreas can be helpful in differentiation.

Chronic Pancreatitis in Cystic Fibrosis

There is chloride channel CFTR gene mutation in cystic fibrosis (autosomal recessive inherited disease). This leads to dysfunction of chloride channels which fail to add enough fluid in pancreatic glandular secretions causing inspissations of secretions, obstruction to the flow within pancreatic ducts and triggers the disease process.

In pediatric population, cystic fibrosis is the most common cause of exocrine pancreatic insufficiency with occurrence of one in 2500 children.[31,32] Clinical presentation are failure to thrive, fat intolerance, abdominal pain, bloating, and flatulence.[32] Glucose intolerance is quite common (seen in up to 50% of cases); however, transformation to frank diabetes mellitus is noted in 13% only.[32] Presentation in form of acute pancreatitis is rare.[33] Histopathologic evaluation demonstrates inflammation in the pancreas with widespread loss of acinar cells, fatty replacement of the pancreatic parenchyma and interstitial fibrosis. The severity of exocrine dysfunction usually correlates with degree of pancreatic fatty infiltration.

Pancreatic calcifications indistinguishable from those in other forms of chronic pancreatitis may be seen. USG may show atrophic pancreas with increased echogenicity secondary to fatty replacement. On CT, fat replacement with or without pancreatic atrophy is the most common and a characteristic finding **(Figs 24 and 25)**.[34] Other findings include calcification, cysts and ductal strictures, beading, and dilatations. Acute pancreatitis are rarely seen. Pancreatic cystosis is a rare manifestation of cystic fibrosis, where the entire pancreas is replaced by multiple cysts of varying sizes. On MR imaging and MR cholangiopancreatography, findings are the same and thus preferred in children due to lack of radiation exposure.

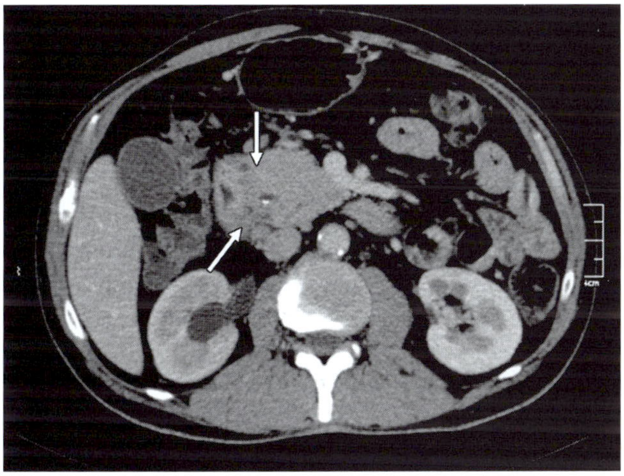

FIG. 23: Groove pancreatitis: CT axial image showing hypoenhancing sheet-like soft tissue in pancreaticoduodenal groove (arrows). Note presence of tiny cysts within this soft tissue and mildly bulky head of pancreas.

Hereditary Pancreatitis

Hereditary pancreatitis is an autosomal dominant disease that occurs due to mutation of the cationic trypsinogen gene (PRSS1) that leads to increased auto-activation of trypsinogen.[35,36]

Children between the ages of 5–10 years are commonly affecte where it presents with epigastric pain.[37] Hereditary pancreatitis is an uncommon cause of recurrent and chronic pancreatitis (less than 1%) and should be suspected in any patient who has suffered at least two unexplained attacks of acute pancreatitis.[35,38]

In its chronic form are: significant pancreatic atrophy, pancreatic calcifications, and calculi are seen.

Hereditary pancreatitis is associated with more than 50 fold increased risk of development of pancreatic cancer which otherwise is low in other form of CP (15–25-fold increased risk).[39]

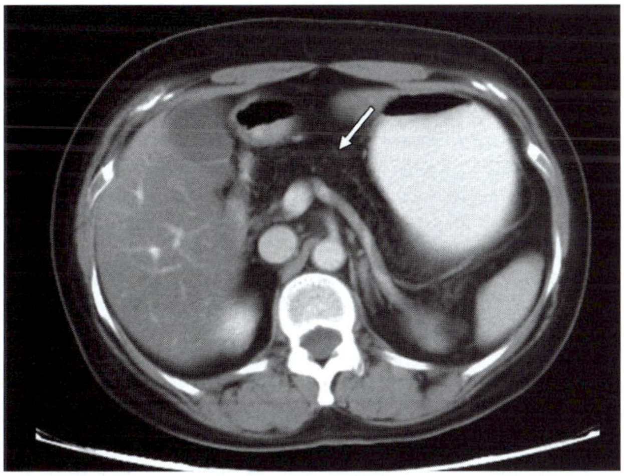

FIG. 24: Chronic pancreatitis in cystic fibrosis: CT image showing diffuse lipomatous transformation of pancreas (arrow).

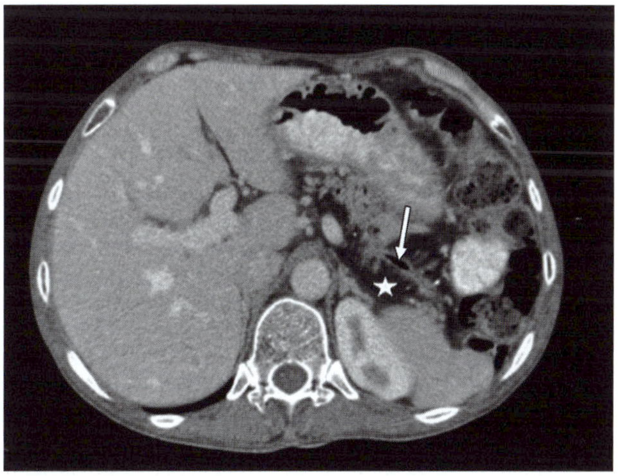

FIG. 25: Chronic pancreatitis in cystic fibrosis: CT image showing focal dilatations of MPD (arrow) and fatty transformation of pancreas (star). Note changes of CP in side branches.

Tropical Chronic Pancreatitis

Tropical chronic pancreatitis (TCP) has a typical geographic distribution and usually restricted to countries having tropical climate. Protein energy malnutrition, pancreatic ductal anomalies, food toxicities (chronic cyanide toxicity from cassava), and genetic predisposition (SPINK 1 N34S mutation and CFTR mutation) are implicated in its etiology.[40] TCP affects young population (mean age–12.5 years) with a slightly male predilection (male-to-female ratio, 1.6–5:1).[41] It is characterized by large intraductal calculi and development of insulin-requiring diabetes mellitus within 10 years of onset in about two-thirds of patients (fibrocalculous pancreatic diabetes).[42] Ketosis is rare in these individuals but there is higher incidence of pancreatic malignancy, which most frequently occurs in the pancreatic body and tail.[43] There is no association with alcohol consumption, biliary tract disease, and biochemical or structural predisposing factors for pancreatitis.

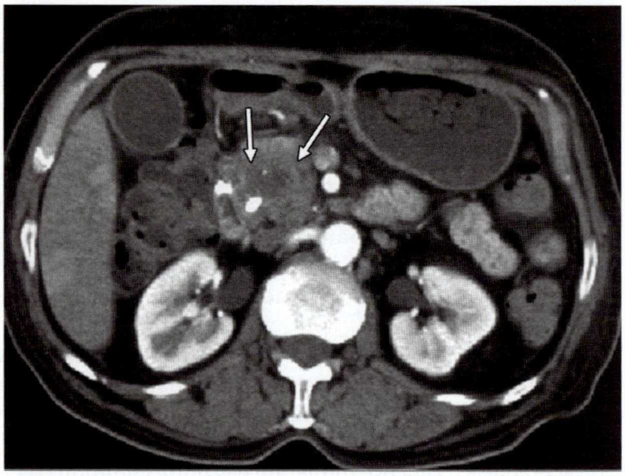

FIG. 26: Malignant change in CP: Pancreatic head show multifocal calcifications consistent with chronic pancreatitis. There is marked atrophy of pancreatic body and tail and contour deformity of head. An ill-defined hypodense lesion (arrows) is seen in pancreatic head which was confirmed to be adenocarcinoma on FNAC.

Chronic Pancreatitis and Pancreatic Adenocarcinoma

Association of pancreatic cancer and chronic pancreatitis is seen only in 1–2% of cases.[44] On imaging, it may be difficult to differentiate a focal mass of CP from pancreatic carcinoma **(Fig. 26)**. One should suspect pancreatic malignancy when an abnormal contour bulge or change in the morphology in the form of mass effect and alteration or disappearance of pre-existing calcification is detected in the setting of CP. Duct penetrating sign in this setting is useful in distinguishing an inflammatory mass from malignancy. Findings that favor diagnosis of carcinoma pancreas are: grossly dilated MPD, locoregional or distant lymphadenopathy, metastases, and vascular encasement or invasion.

Pancreatic perfusion CT can generate perfusion parameters which help in this distinction. The blood flow and blood volume are reduced in both inflammatory mass and carcinoma, the values usually are much lower in carcinoma than in inflammatory mass. Diffusion weighted imaging is also emerging as a helpful tool, in which carcinoma is shown to have a more marked diffusion restriction. FDG-PET CT has also been used for the same purpose with varying degree of success.

ACKNOWLEDGMENT

Professor SK Sinha, Department of Gastroenterology, Postgraduate Institute of Medical Education and Research (PGIMER), Chandigarh, India for ERCP images.

REFERENCES

1. Owyang C. Chronic pancreatitis. In: Yamada T (Ed). Textbook of Gastroenterology. Philadelphia, Pa: Lippincott Williams & Wilkins; 2003.p.2062.
2. Lankisch MR, Imoto M, Layer P, DiMagno EP. The effect of small amounts of alcohol on the clinical course of chronic pancreatitis. Mayo Clin Proc. 2001;76:242-51.
3. Dufour MC, Adamson MD. The epidemiology of alcohol-induced pancreatitis. Pancreas. 2003;27:286-90.
4. Vaughn DD, Jabra AA, Fishman EK. Pancreatic disease in children and young adults: evaluation with CT. RadioGraphics. 1998;18(5):1171-87.
5. Yekebas EF, Bogoevski D, Honarpisheh H, et al. Long-term Follow-up in Small Duct Chronic Pancreatitis: A Plea for Extended Drainage by "V-Shaped Excision" of the Anterior Aspect of the Pancreas. Annals of Surgery. 2006;244(6):940-8.
6. Etemad B, Whitcomb DC. Chronic pancreatitis: diagnosis, classification, and new genetic developments. Gastroenterology. 2001;120(3):682-707.
7. Brydon WG, Kingstone K, Ghosh S. Limitations of faecal elastase-1 and chymotrypsin as tests of exocrine pancreatic disease in adults. Ann Clin Biochem. 2004;41(1):78-81.
8. Bian Y, Wang L, Chen C, et al. Quantification of pancreatic exocrine function of chronic pancreatitis with secretin-enhanced MRCP. World Journal of Gastroenterology: WJG. 2013;19(41):7177-82.
9. Sarner M, Cotton PB. Classification of pancreatitis. Gut. 1984;25(7):756-9.
10. Seicean A. Endoscopic ultrasound in chronic pancreatitis: Where are we now? World Journal of Gastroenterology: WJG. 2010;16(34):4253-63. doi:10.3748/wjg.v16.i34.4253.
11. Ito T, Ishiguro H, Ohara H, et al. Evidence-based clinical practice guidelines for chronic pancreatitis 2015. J Gastroenterol. 2016; 51(2):85-92.
12. Kawada N, Tanaka S. Elastography for the pancreas: Current status and future perspective. World Journal of Gastroenterology. 2016;22(14):3712-24.
13. Luetmer PH, Stephens DH, Ward EM. Chronic pancreatitis: reassessment with current CT. Radiology. 1989;171(2):353-7.
14. Graziani R, Frulloni L, Cicero C, Manfredi R, Ambrosetti MC, Mautone S, Pozzi Mucelli R. Bull's eye pattern of pancreatic-duct stones on multidetector computed tomography and gene-mutation-associated pancreatitis (GMAP). Radiol Med. 2012;117(8):1275-86.

15. Barman K, Premalatha G, Mohan V. Tropical chronic pancreatitis. Postgraduate Medical Journal. 2003;79(937):606-15.
16. Arthet M, Bugallo M, Moreira LS, Bastid C, Sastre B, Sahel J. Management of cysts and pseudocysts complicating chronic pancreatitis. A retrospective study of 143 patients. Gastroenterol Clin Biol. 1993;17:270-6.
17. Ammann RW, Akovbiantz A, Largiader F, Schueler G. Course and outcome of chronic pancreatitis. Longitudinal study of a mixed medical-surgical series of 245 patients. Gastroenterology. 1984;86:820-8.
18. Raimondi S, Lowenfels AB, Morselli-Labate AM, Maisonneuve P, Pezzilli R. Pancreatic cancer in chronic pancreatitis; aetiology, incidence, and early detection. Best Pract Res Clin Gastroenterol. 2010;24(3):349-58.
19. Ichikawa T, Sou H, Araki T, Arbab AS, Yoshikawa T, Ishigame K, Haradome H, Hachiya J. Duct-penetrating sign at MRCP: usefulness for differentiating inflammatory pancreatic mass from pancreatic carcinomas. Radiology. 2001;221(1):107-16.
20. Sandrasegaran K, Nutakki K, Tahir B, Dhanabal A, Tann M, Cote GA. Use of diffusion-weighted MRI to differentiate chronic pancreatitis from pancreatic cancer. AJR. 2013;201(5):1002-8.
21. Manfredi R, Pozzi Mucelli R. Secretin-enhanced MR Imaging of the Pancreas. Radiology. 2016;279(1):29-43.
22. Wathle GK, Tjora E, Ersland L, Dimcevski G, Salvesen ØO, Molven A, Njølstad PR, Haldorsen IS. Assessment of exocrine pancreatic function by secretin-stimulated magnetic resonance cholangiopancreaticography and diffusion-weighted imaging in healthy controls. J Magn Reson Imaging. 2014;39(2):448-54.
23. Yoshida K, Toki F, Takeuchi T, Watanabe S, Shiratori K, Hayashi N. Chronic pancreatitis caused by an autoimmune abnormality: proposal of the concept of autoimmune pancreatitis. Dig Dis Sci. 1995;40(7):1561-8.
24. Kim KP, Kim MH, Song MH, Lee SS, Seo DW, Lee SK. Autoimmune chronic pancreatitis. Am J Gastroenterol. 2004;99(8):1605-16.
25. Takahashi N, Kawashima A, Fletcher JG, Chari ST. Renal involvement in patients with autoimmune pancreatitis: CT and MR imaging findings. Radiology. 2007;242(3):791-801.
26. Khalili K, Doyle DJ, Chawla TP, Hanbidge AE. Renal cortical lesions in patients with autoimmune pancreatitis: a clue to differentiation from pancreatic malignancy. Eur J Radiol. 2008;67(2):329-35.
27. Kawamoto S, Siegelman SS, Hruban RH, Fishman EK. Lymphoplasmacytic sclerosing pancreatitis (autoimmune pancreatitis): evaluation with multidetector CT. RadioGraphics. 2008;28(1):157-70.
28. Ozaki Y, Oguchi K, Hamano H, et al. Differentiation of autoimmune pancreatitis from suspected pancreatic cancer by fluorine-18 fluorodeoxyglucose positron emission tomography. J Gastroenterol. 2008;43(2):144-51.
29. Stolte M, Weiss W, Volkholz H, Rösch W. A special form of segmental pancreatitis: "groove pancreatitis." Hepatogastroenterology. 1982;29(5):198-208.
30. Irie H, Honda H, Kuroiwa T, et al. MRI of groove pancreatitis. J Comput Assist Tomogr. 1998;22(4):651-5.
31. Witt H. Chronic pancreatitis and cystic fibrosis. Gut. 2003;52 (suppl 2):ii31–41.
32. Gore MD, Fernbach SK. Pancreatic insufficiency and cystic fibrosis. In: Gore RM, Levine MS, Laufer I (Eds). Textbook of gastrointestinal radiology. Vol 2. Philadelphia, Pa: Saunders; 1994.pp.2187-92.
33. De Boeck K, Weren M, Proesmans M, Kerem E. Pancreatitis among patients with cystic fibrosis: correlation with pancreatic status and genotype. Pediatrics. 2005;115(4):e463–9.
34. Soyer P, Spelle L, Pelage JP, et al. Cystic fibrosis in adolescents and adults: fatty replacement of the pancreas—CT evaluation and functional correlation. Radiology. 1999;210(3):611-5.
35. Efthimiou E, Crnogorac-Jurcevic T, Lemoine NR, Brentnall TA. Inherited predisposition to pancreatic cancer. Gut. 2001;48(2):143-7.
36. Steinberg WM, Barkin J, Bradley EL 3rd, DiMagno E, Layer P. Workup of a patient with familial pancreatic cancer. Pancreas. 1999;18(3):219-24.
37. Efthimiou E, Crnogorac-Jurcevic T, Lemoine NR Brentnall TA. Inherited predisposition to pancreatic cancer. Gut. 2001;48(2).143-7.
38. Ellis I, Lerch MM, Whitcomb DC. Consensus Committees of the European Registry of Hereditary Pancreatic Diseases, Midwest Multi-center Pancreatic Study Group, International Association of Pancreatology. Genetic testing for hereditary pancreatitis: guidelines for indications, counseling, consent and privacy issues. Pancreatology. 2001;1(5):405-15.
39. Ghaneh P, Costello E, Neoptolemos JP. Biology and management of pancreatic cancer. Gut. 2007;56(8):1134-52.
40. Bhatia E, Choudhuri G, Sikora SS, et al. Tropical calcific pancreatitis: strong association with SPINK 1 trypsin inhibitor mutations. Gastroenterology. 2002;123(4):1020-25.
41. Balakrishnan V, Sauniere JF, Hariharan M, Sarles H. Diet, pancreatic function, and chronic pancreatitis in south India and France. Pancreas. 1988;3(1):30-5.
42. Petersen JM. Tropical pancreatitis. J Clin Gastroenterol. 2002;35(1):61-6.
43. Chari ST, Mohan V, Pitchumoni CS, Viswanathan M, Madanagopalan N, Lowenfels AB. Risk of pancreatic cancer in tropical calcifying pancreatitis: an epidemiologic study. Pancreas. 1994;9(1):62-6.
44. Levine E. Carcinoma of the pancreas presenting as acute pancreatitis: CT diagnosis. Gastrointest Radiol. 1981;6(1):29-33.

CHAPTER

113

Pancreatic Cancer Imaging

Ankur Goyal, Raju Sharma

INTRODUCTION

Pancreatic cancer is an aggressive malignancy with dismal prognosis. Strategically located deep in the retroperitoneum, it can potentially involve many crucial arteries, veins and nerves catering to liver, spleen, stomach and bowel.[1] Ductal adenocarcinoma is the most common nonendocrine pancreatic malignancy. After colorectal malignancies, pancreatic carcinoma is the second most common malignancy of the gastrointestinal tract. Pancreatic adenocarcinoma is the fourth most common cause of cancer-related deaths in the US. There have been lot of advances in the imaging and surgical management of pancreatic malignancies. Nevertheless, patient survival is dismal owing to early lymphatic and perineural spread.[2] Pancreatic carcinoma has a propensity to spread via celiac and mesenteric neural plexus and this results in preclinical dissemination.

The clinical presentation is vague, thus contributing to delay in diagnosis. The patients usually present with abdominal pain, anorexia, weight loss, nausea and jaundice. Age of presentation is middle age or elderly. Jaundice is a common presenting symptom in tumors of pancreatic head region whereas lesions of the body and tail present with abdominal pain and weight loss. Pancreatic carcinoma should also be suspected in diabetic patients with unusual manifestations such as late age of onset, abdominal symptoms and continuing weight loss.[3] It is important to differentiate ampullary cancers from the ductal adenocarcinomas, since the former have a much better prognosis and longer survival.[4] The serum levels of CA 19-9 are often elevated. Activating mutations in k-ras oncogene are present in more than 90% cases.[5]

The risk factors for pancreatic cancer include cigarette smoking, alcohol, high body mass index, chronic pancreatitis and occupational exposure to chemicals. Recently, there has been substantial increment in knowledge of the molecular biology of the disease. R0 surgical resection (negative margins) is the only treatment modality which can prolong survival in these patients; though even with surgery, mean patient survival is 2 years and thus long-term survival is lacking. Whipple surgery is a major intervention and is associated with postoperative morbidity. Thus, imaging is very important to diagnose malignancy and also to assess resectability. Accurate preoperative staging is essential for optimal management.

IMAGING MODALITIES

Multidetector computed tomography (MDCT) is the investigation of choice for diagnosis and staging of pancreatic cancer.[6] Thin sections, multiplanar reformation and high spatial resolution enable accurate delineation of tumor extent on MDCT. Transabdominal sonography may also detect larger lesions and depict local invasion, however the accuracy is much less. Magnetic resonance imaging (MRI), endoscopic ultrasound (EUS) and positron emission tomography–CT (PET-CT) are also useful in the diagnostic assessment of pancreatic malignancy.

Sonography

Ultrasound (US) abdomen is the most commonly used initial imaging modality for evaluation of abdominal pain and jaundice. It not only diagnoses obstructive jaundice but also localizes the level of obstruction and helps in suggesting the cause. Common benign diseases such as cholelithiasis and choledocholithiasis may be easily diagnosed. Though small pancreatic lesions may be easily missed on US, larger lesions can usually be seen and secondary evidence such as pancreatic ductal dilatation may also be evident. US can also provide real-time guidance for percutaneous sampling; although endoscopic route is preferred. Disadvantages are operator dependence and proper evaluation of pancreas may not be feasible because of obesity or bowel gas.

Multidetector Computed Tomography

Helical CT on a scanner with multiple rows of detector (16 or more) is the workhorse for workup of patients with suspected pancreatic cancer. A dedicated protocol is essential to accurately detect and stage pancreatic cancers **(Flowchart 1)**. The examination starts with neutral oral contrast given over 15–30 minutes for gastroduodenal distension. This enables proper visualization of the pancreas and ampullary region. Intravenous nonionic iodinated

FLOWCHART 1: MDCT protocol for pancreatic cancer imaging

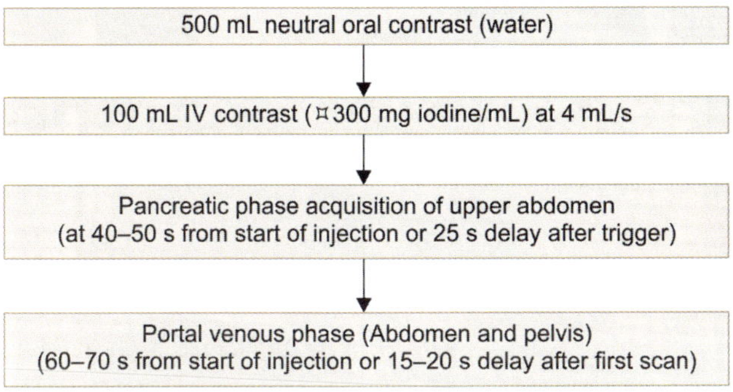

contrast is injected via rapid bolus at 4 mL/s using a pressure injector and a biphasic breath-hold acquisition is done.

The first acquisition is done in the late arterial/pancreatic phase, usually 40–50 seconds from the start of contrast injection. If contrast triggering is used, then typically a delay of 20–25 seconds is optimal, after the threshold attenuation is reached in the region of interest (ROI) (descending thoracic aorta in this case). The rapid contrast injection produces intense enhancement of the normal pancreas in this phase and thus the hypovascular ductal carcinomas are demonstrated well. The pancreatic phase scan should include the liver and pancreas (upper abdomen). Hypervascular lesions (like neuroendocrine tumors), hypervascular liver metastases, as well as flow-related phenomena (arterial hyperenhancement in case of pancreatic cancer liver metastases) are well seen in the late arterial phase. Subtle surrounding perivascular infiltration is also well seen.[7]

The second acquisition is portal venous phase at 60–70 s from the start of contrast injection and covers the entire abdomen and pelvis. The portal venous system is well opacified and the splanchnic viscera show homogeneous parenchymal contrast enhancement (CE). Former enables assessment of vascular involvement while the latter enables detection of hypoenhancing liver metastases. The scan coverage in this phase may include chest as well for complete staging.

Careful analysis of thin sections and three dimensional (3D) reconstructions on a workstation is key to accurate imaging assessment. Coronal and curved multiplanar reformations help to evaluate the status of common bile duct and pancreatic duct in relation to the tumor **(Figs. 1A to D)**. Postprocessing of volumetric dataset serves to highlight local invasion along blood vessels.

Magnetic Resonance Imaging

The MRI has similar accuracy to MDCT in staging of pancreatic cancers with the advantage of absence of radiation exposure.[8] The excellent contrast resolution more than makes up for the lower spatial resolution than MDCT. High resolution fast imaging of pancreas has become feasible owing to multichannel coils, parallel imaging, higher magnetic field strength (3T) and other advancements in MRI technology.

Fat-supressed (FS) T1-weighted (T1W) images demonstrate the normally hyperintense pancreatic parenchyma very well. Pancreatic cancers are hypointense on T1W, intermediate signal on T2W and show diffusion restriction on diffusion-weighted MR imaging (DW MRI). The latter manifests as retained high signal on the high b-value image and dark signal on the apparent diffusion coefficient (ADC) map. ADC map also enables quantification and pancreatic carcinoma is associated with lower ADC values compared with remaining parenchyma.[9] Heavily T2W sequences like HASTE employed in MR cholangiopancreatography (MRCP) enable exquisite demonstration of pancreatic and biliary ducts enabling detection of subtle areas of narrowing. Similar to CT, multiphasic scanning after contrast administration enables detection of pancreatic cancer in the late arterial phase and accurate staging in the portal venous phase. Ideally, MRI for evaluation of pancreatic cancer should include post-contrast multiphasic acquisition. However, noncontrast MR sequences can provide sufficient information in majority of the cases; and thus MRI is the modality of choice in patients with renal insufficiency where contrast administration is undesirable.

Magnetic resonance imaging is also a problem solving modality in case of small lesions and subtle liver metastases. The latter are best detected on diffusion-weighted MRI (DWI) **(Figs. 2A and B)**. DW MRI is useful in detection of small lesions as well as post-therapy response assessment. Absence of exposure to ionizing radiation is another advantage of MRI. Disadvantages include high cost, limited availability and long examination time.

Endoscopic Techniques

Side-viewing endoscopy is often employed for evaluation of periampullary malignancies, especially when small mass is not visible on CT or MRI but there is ductal dilatation.

Endoscopic ultrasound (EUS) may aid in detection of small lesions, may depict subtle vascular involvement and nodal spread, as well as guide sampling **(Figs. 3A and B)**. The advantage of this route of sampling is that the needle track falls within the field of surgical resection. The role of EUS is complimentary to CT for staging.[3] However, it is invasive and not widely available.

Endoscopic retrograde cholangiopancreatography (ERCP) with brush cytology is indicated when no mass is seen on imaging and stenting is to be done for palliation. Nowadays, ERCP is done only with the purpose of biliary decompression.

Positron Emission Tomography–Computed Tomography

Functional positron emission tomography (PET) imaging may be used as per institutional preference, in high-risk patients to detect metastases; but it is not a substitute for diagnostic CT/MRI.[3] It may be more helpful in follow-up assessment where post-therapy alterations may pose problems. It may prove useful in identifying unexpected sites of recurrence. However, the exact role of this modality in evaluation of pancreatic carcinoma is still evolving.

Recent Advances

Ultrasound elastography is a new technique which may be employed for detection of pancreatic cancers. Owing to

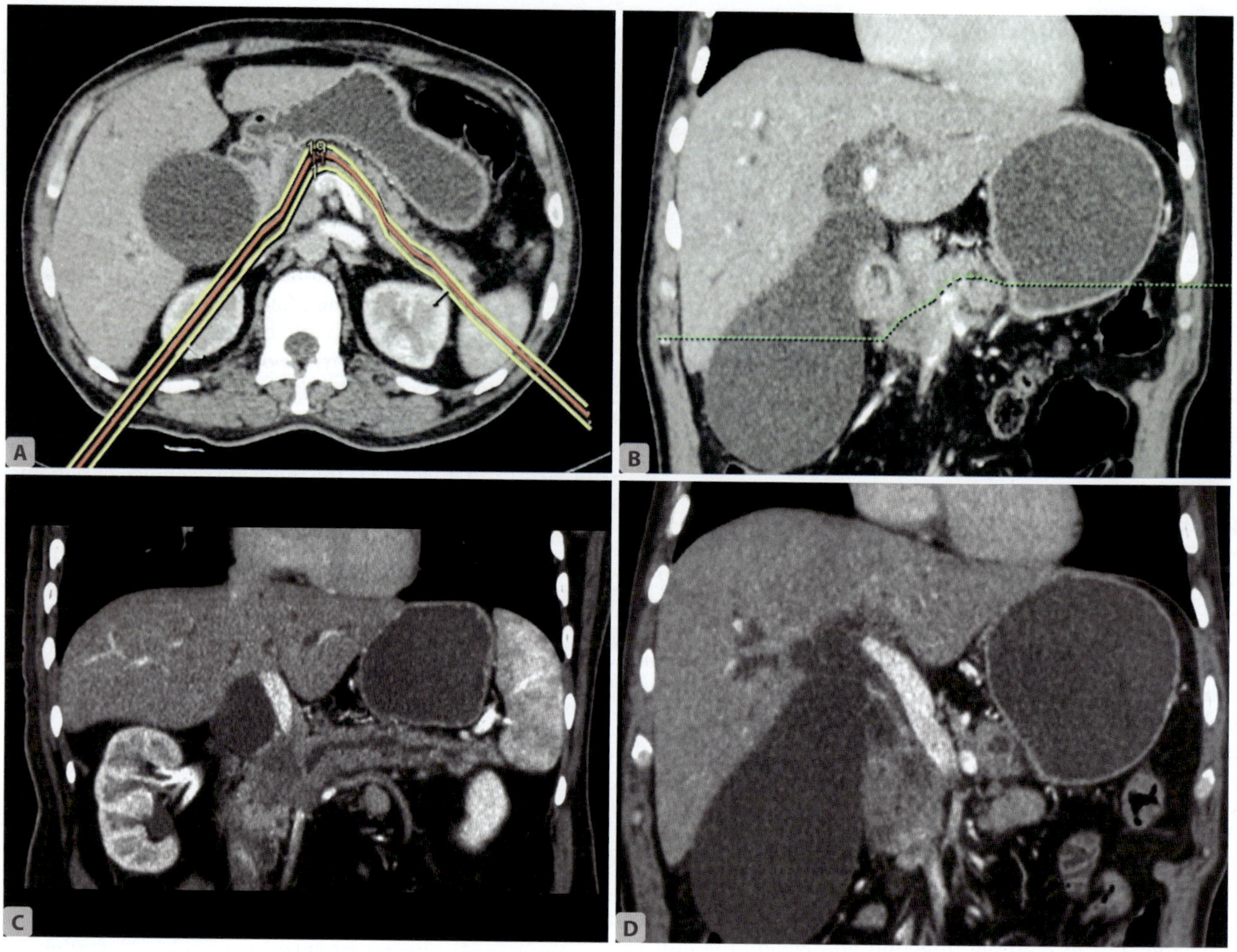

FIGS. 1A TO D: Utility of curved multiplanar reformations (MPR): Axial (A) and coronal (B) CT images demonstrate the planning of curved MPR along the pancreas. Resultant image (C) depicts the hypodense mass in the head with abrupt cut-off and upstream dilatation of pancreatic duct. Curved MPR better delineates the mass in relation to pancreatic duct in a single image compared to orthogonal coronal image (D).

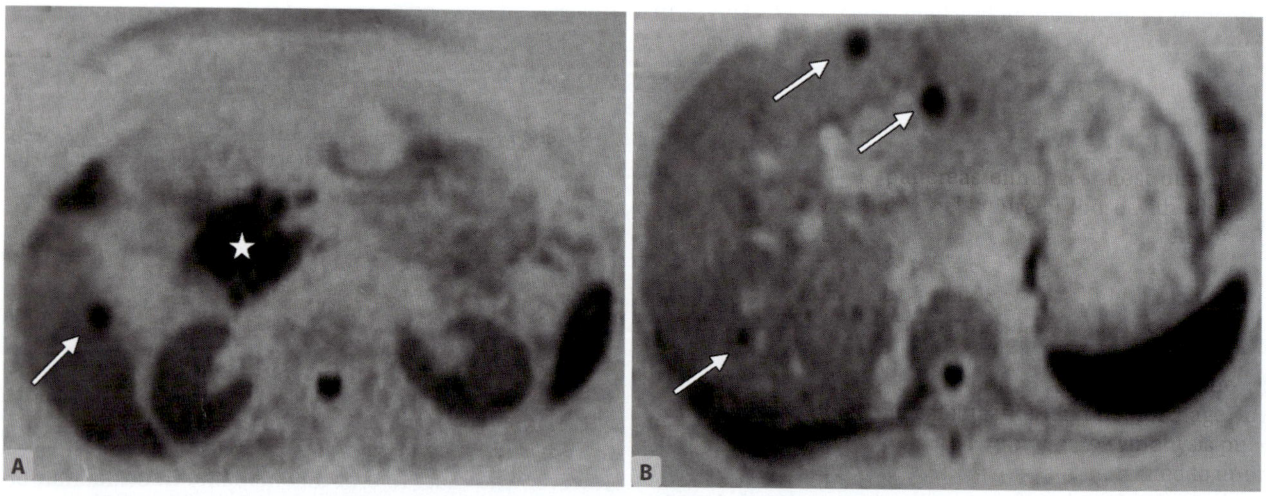

FIGS. 2A AND B: Utility of diffusion-weighted MRI in detecting small liver metastases. Contrast-inverted high b value (1000 s/mm^2) axial DW images (A and B) depict marked restriction of diffusion in the pancreatic head mass (asterisk) and multiple small liver metastases (arrows).

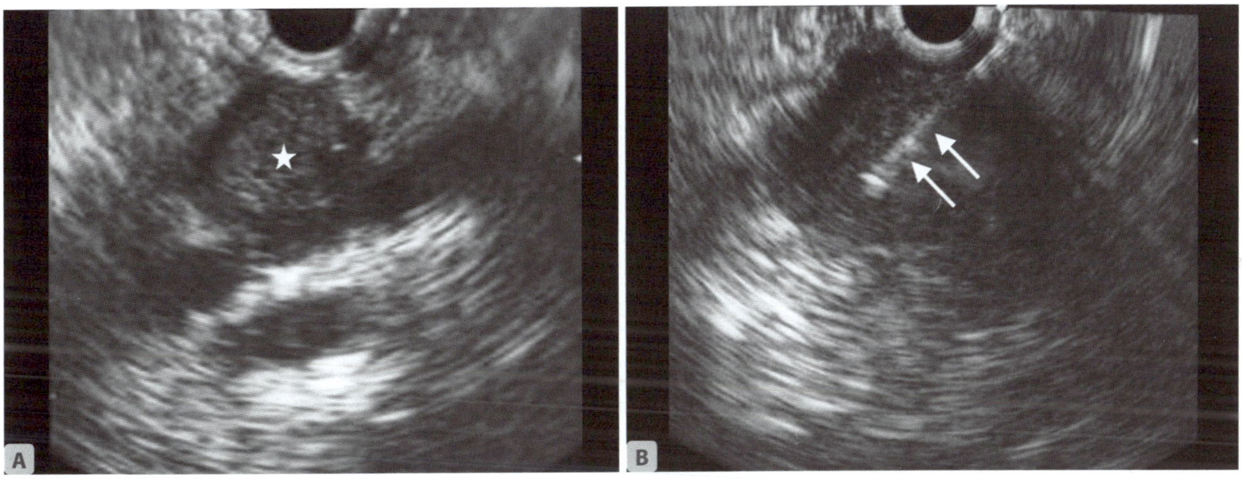

FIGS. 3A AND B: Endoscopic ultrasound (EUS) in evaluation of pancreatic carcinoma: EUS image (A) clearly shows the pancreatic head mass (asterisk) and (B) depicts sampling using EUS guidance (arrows denote the needle).

deep location and small size of pancreas, elastography has been considered difficult and less reliable. However, it is a promising modality for distinction between benign and malignant lesions and for screening in high-risk patients.[10] It can be performed through transabdominal or endoscopic routes. Contrary to shear wave elastography (SWE), strain elastography requires application of external pressure. Manual compression is however not effective for pancreas and strain generated by aortic pulsations is used instead. Thus it requires the probe, pancreas and aorta to be in the same line.[10] Also, pancreatic body can be well evaluated but not head and tail regions. SWE can be performed for the entire pancreas but not currently available via endoscopic route.[10] Pancreatic adenocarcinoma appears as hard heterogeneous lesion while chronic pancreatitis is soft and heterogeneous.[10,11] Neuroendocrine tumors are seen as hard homogeneous lesions.

Contrast-enhanced USG (CEUSG) employs microbubble contrast media which are excreted via lungs and thus can be used in patients with renal dysfunction. This is especially useful along with EUS to confirm areas of abnormality. Ductal adenocarcinoma commonly appears as hypoenhancing lesion relative to the surrounding pancreas.[12] Mass-forming chronic pancreatitis is isoenhancing or hyperenhancing while neuroendocrine tumors are hyperenhancing.[12]

Perfusion CT involves scanning the region of interest (pancreas) multiple times over a short span after rapid bolus contrast injection. In addition to color coded maps, many quantitative parameters such as blood flow, blood volume, mean transit time, time to peak, etc. are generated which are more representative of the contrast kinetics and vascularity of the lesion. This technique has a potential role in detection of small isodense pancreatic lesions **(Figs. 4A to D)**[13] and in assessment of post-therapy response. The basis of the latter use is that chemotherapeutic agents target tumor neo-angiogenesis and thus reduction in vascularity indicates response to therapy. Perfusion CT parameters, (especially blood flow) may also help to differentiate adenocarcinoma from mass forming chronic pancreatitis (MFCP).[14] The main drawback is increased radiation exposure.

Dual-energy CT scanners enable generation of virtual noncontrast images from a single acquisition. Also, lower keV dataset can be generated which offers superior contrast resolution while higher keV images have better signal-to-noise ratio (SNR) **(Figs. 5A to D)**.[15]

The *DW MRI* is now part of routine abdominal MR protocols in most of the institutions worldwide. The simple way of quantifying the diffusion restriction is based on the monoexponential model which generates a single ADC value based on combination of both diffusion and perfusion effects. Recently, biexponential-based estimation of the intravoxel incoherent motion (IVIM) parameters has been employed, with generation of separate diffusion and perfusion metrics. Perfusion fraction (f) has been shown to be markedly reduced in pancreatic ductal adenocarcinomas[16-18] and postulated to be superior than diffusion in differentiating from mass-forming chronic pancreatitis.[16,17] Another method which has been proposed is the non-Gaussian kurtosis model, which takes into account tissue heterogeneity (kurtosis effects).[9] Corrected diffusion coefficient (D_k) has been found to have highest accuracy for differentiation of adenocarcinoma and remaining pancreatic parenchyma.[9]

IMAGING FINDINGS (TABLE 1)

Pancreatic cancers are solid scirrhous tumor with reduced perfusion compared to normal parenchyma. They are infiltrative and incite surrounding inflammation and desmoplastic reaction. These lesions tend to obstruct and constrict the ductal structures, causing jaundice and pancreatitis. Pancreatic head is the most common location (60–70% cases) and thus biliary obstruction is frequent in pancreatic adenocarcinomas. Head is the part of pancreas to the right of SMV while body is to the left. Also, head lesions are detected at a relatively earlier stage because of biliary obstruction, whereas body and tail lesions may grow large before producing significant symptoms. Thus, lesions in the body and tail region are large at presentation and have areas of necrosis/hemorrhage within. Pancreatic carcinoma

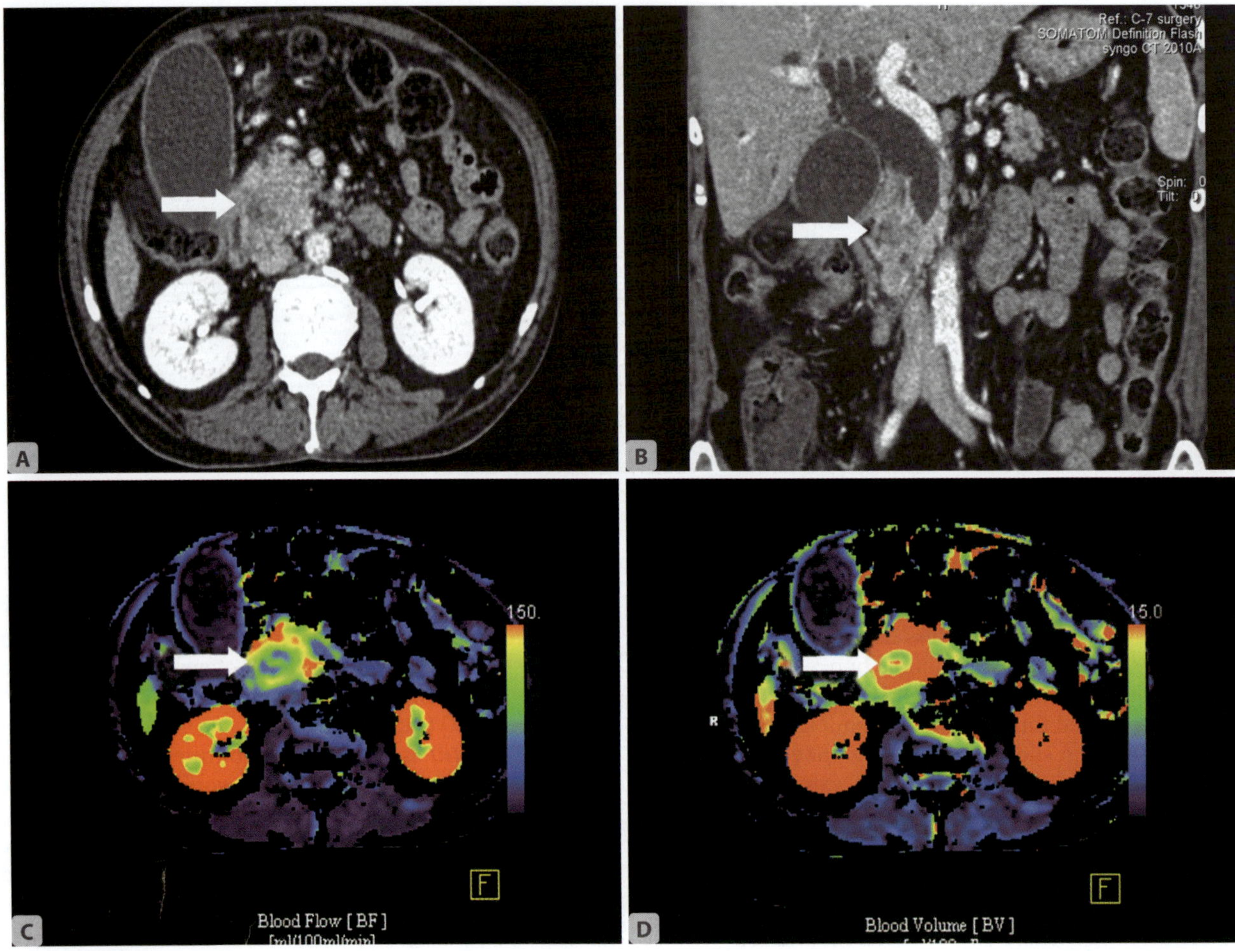

FIGS. 4A TO D: Role of perfusion CT in isodense masses: Axial (A) and coronal (B) contrast-enhanced CT images show an ill-defined mass in pancreatic head, which is mildly hypodense to the surrounding parenchyma (arrows) with dilated common bile duct. Axial blood flow (C) and blood volume (D) color maps (derived from perfusion CT) enable a much clearer depiction of hypovascular mass, distinct from adjacent parenchyma (arrows).

commonly metastasizes to the liver, peritoneum, lungs and bones.

Pancreatic cancers are usually solid hypoechoic on ultrasound and upstream ductal dilatation (diameter of pancreatic duct >2 mm) may be seen **(Figs. 6A to D)**. Margins are ill-defined and irregular. On color Doppler examination, no significant internal vascularity is seen. Larger lesions may have necrosis within and show infiltration of surrounding structures. Lesions in the pancreatic head often result in biliary dilatation **(Figs. 6A to D)**.

On the late arterial phase CT or MRI, the masses are hypodense in more than 90% cases **(Figs. 7A to D)**.[19] In addition to the attenuation difference, larger masses also produce a contour bulge of the pancreas **(Figs. 7A to D)**, and the fat planes with adjacent structures may be lost. 5–10% of the pancreatic carcinomas are isodense to the surrounding parenchyma **(Figs. 7A to D)** and thus difficult to detect based on attenuation values.[20] The problem is further compounded because these isodense cancers are frequently small (<2 cm) and may not deform the pancreatic contour.

MRI is useful in such cases with lesion being hypointense on T1W FS images, against background hyperintense parenchyma. MRI may visualize up to 79% of isodense pancreatic lesions **(Figs. 8A to D)**.[19] T2W images depict the mass as having intermediate signal intensity and are not much helpful in demonstrating the mass; but heavily T2W images depict ductal dilatation and obstruction quite well. Calcification is unusual in pancreatic adenocarcinoma. Pancreatic adenocarcinomas show heterogeneous diffusion restriction on DW MRI and their ADC values are lower than surrounding parenchyma **(Figs. 9A to E)**. Addition of DWI to conventional sequences increases the sensitivity of detection of pancreatic cancer.[21]

The secondary findings include dilatation of the pancreatic duct with or without biliary dilatation **(Fig. 10)**. Biliary dilatation occurs in case of lesions located in the pancreatic head as well as may occur due to metastatic lymph node enlargement compressing the suprapancreatic portion of common bile duct. The pancreatic duct may be abruptly cut off with upstream dilatation and may be the only clue to diagnosing small isodense and non-contour deforming

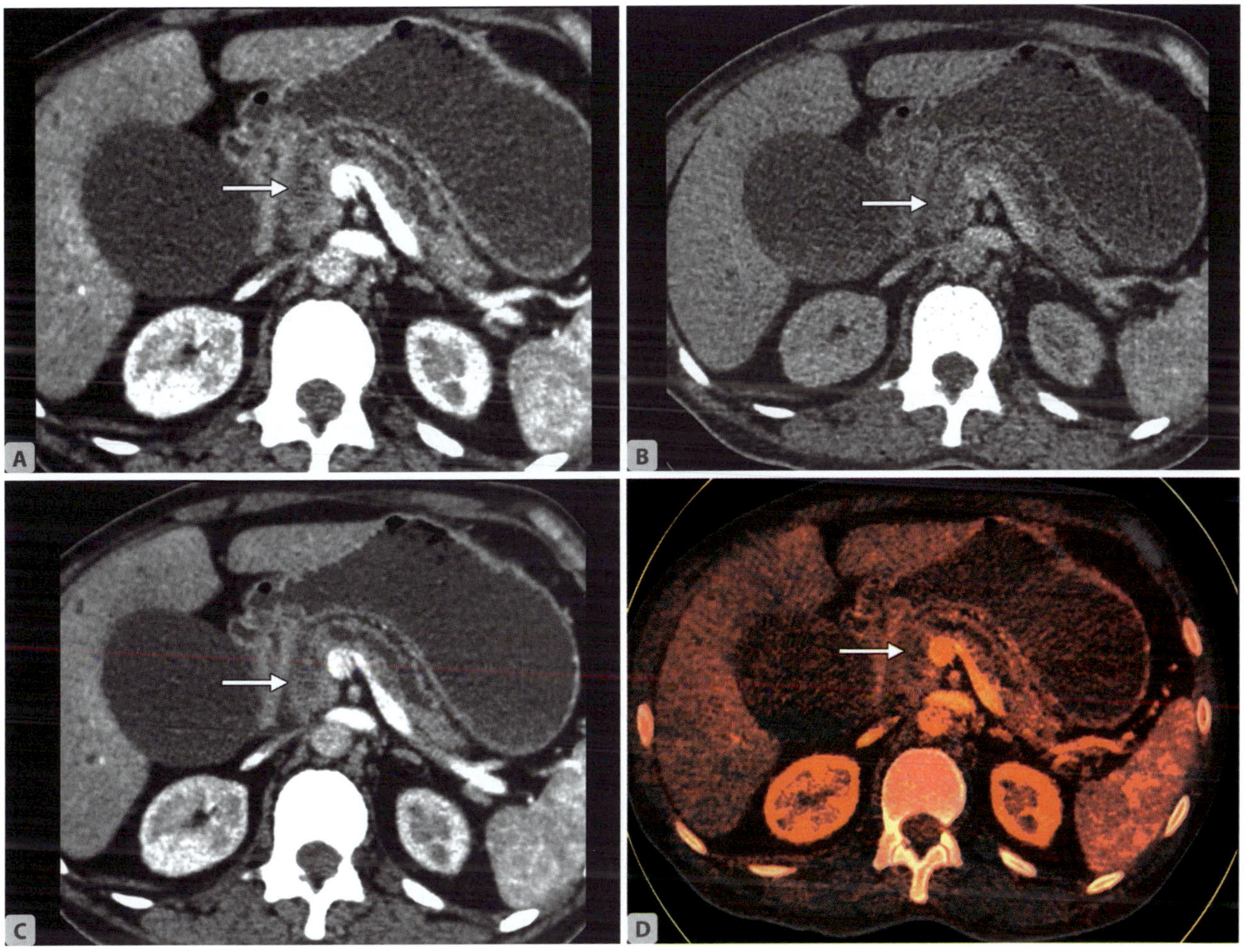

FIGS. 5A TO D: Dual-energy CT (DECT) in pancreatic mass evaluation: Axial monochromatic CECT images generated from dual-energy dataset: 70 keV image (A) gives better demonstration of mass (arrow) compared to 100 keV image (B), however is noisy. Optimal contrast image (C) derived by mixing of the datasets yields high contrast as well as low noise. Iodine map (D) depicts the hypodense mass distinct from the enhancing parenchyma as well as cut-off of pancreatic duct.

TABLE 1: Imaging features of pancreatic carcinoma.
• *Sonography*: - Solid - Hypoechoic - Irregular ill-defined margins - Usually no demonstrable internal vascularity
• *CT*: - Mildly enhancing lesion which appears hypodense relative to brightly enhancing normal pancreatic parenchyma - Contour bulge
• *MRI*: - T1 hypointense mass against background hyperintense *pancreas*: Diffusion restriction - Mass enhances less than surrounding parenchyma in pancreatic phase
• *Secondary signs*: - Upstream pancreatic ductal dilatation with/without atrophy - Contour bulge (in larger lesions) - Local infiltration - Biliary dilatation in head lesions

lesions **(Figs. 10A to D)**.[22] *Double duct sign* is seen in cancers located in the pancreatic head and represents dilatation of both pancreatic and biliary ducts due to obstruction of both PD and adjacent intrapancreatic part of common bile duct **(Fig. 11)**. Long standing lesions may cause distal parenchymal atrophy as well.

Rarely, pancreatic cancer may present as single or multiple episodes of acute pancreatitis, secondary to ductal obstruction.[23] In these cases, inflammatory changes predominate and may mask the underlying lesion. Disproportionate enlargement of the head, significant dilatation of the pancreatic duct with abrupt change in caliber, focal pancreatitis distal to obstruction and recurrent pancreatitis in the absence of risk factors may raise the suspicion of an underlying malignancy **(Figs. 12A and B)**. Many times, the lesion may be diagnosed only on follow-up scans when the inflammatory changes have subsided.[23]

Both pancreatic phase and venous phase images are important for accurate assessment of staging. A characteristic feature of liver metastases from pancreatic adenocarcinomas is flow-related phenomenon, seen on the late arterial phase images **(Figs. 13A to D)**. This can either be in the form of

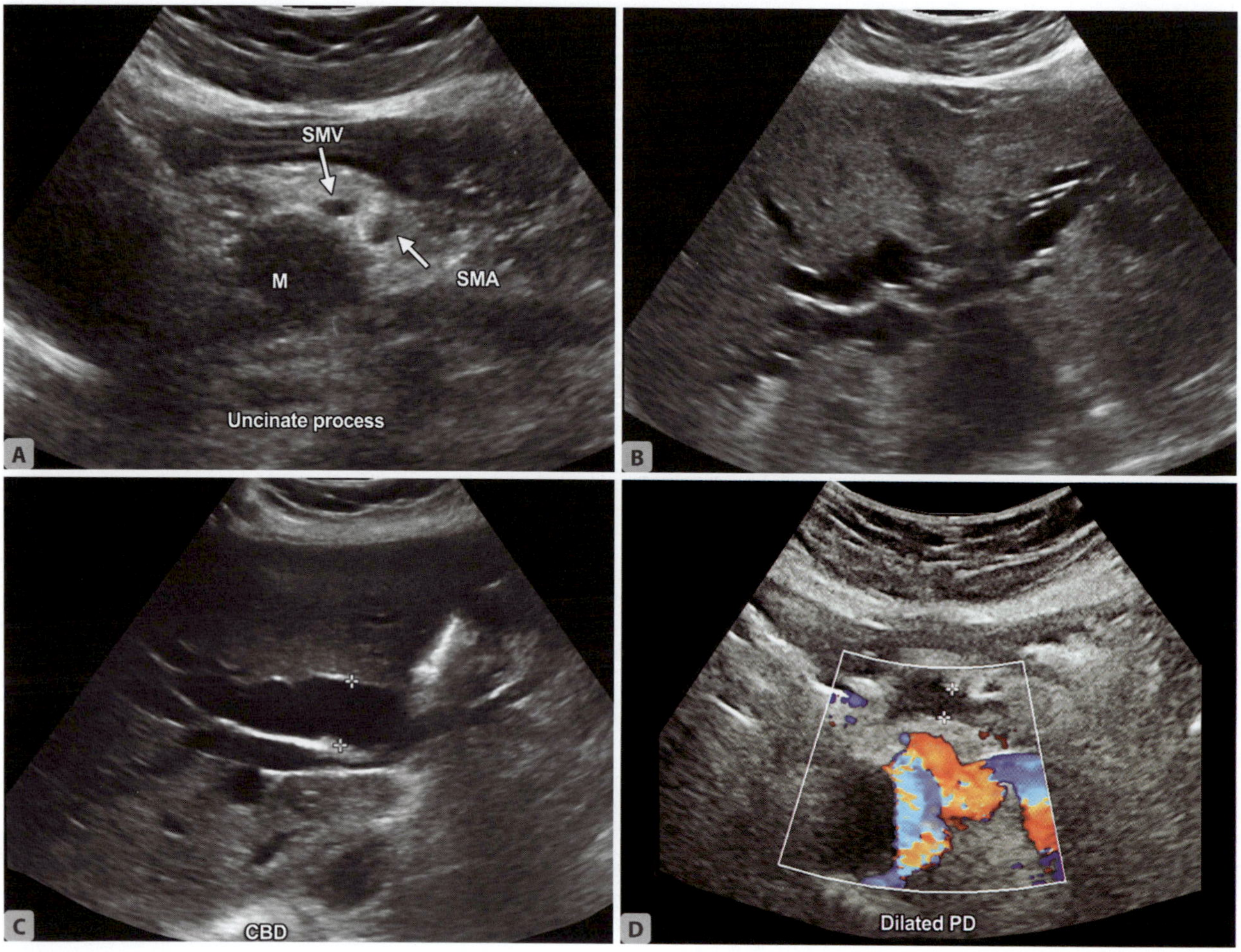

FIGS. 6A TO D: Sonography in pancreatic cancer: Gray-scale ultrasound image (A) shows solid hypoechoic mass lesion in the head and uncinate process of pancreas (M) with irregular margins. Superior mesenteric vessels (SMA and SMV) are seen separately; USG image (B) shows bilobar intrahepatic biliary radical dilatation and (C) depicts dilated common bile duct (cursors); Color Doppler image (D) shows dilated pancreatic duct (PD) (cursors).

thin peripheral contrast enhancement around hypodense metastases or perfusion abnormalities like transient hepatic attenuation difference. Liver metastases are best detected on T2W and diffusion-weighted MR sequences. Peritoneal dissemination is suggested by the presence of ascites, omental thickening and peritoneal nodularity. Peritoneal nodules are better visualized on DW MRI and PET-CT **(Figs. 14A to C)**.

PANCREATIC CANCER VARIANTS

Other than ductal adenocarcinoma, there are few rare variants which constitute around 10% of the pancreatic tumors.[24]

Acinar cell carcinoma is also a malignant epithelial tumor with slightly better prognosis and has a propensity to metastasize to lymph nodes and liver. Jaundice is usually not seen. These tumors are solid, can reach large size, and do not cause ductal dilatation even in advanced stage. Similar to adenocarcinomas, these are hypoenhancing; but in contrast, they show well-defined margins.

Mucinous colloid carcinoma also has better prognosis than adenocarcinoma. It shows T2 hyperintensity owing to mucin within. Adenosquamous carcinoma has both glandular and squamous components and is a histological diagnosis with worse prognosis. Anaplastic carcinomas are large tumors, common in the tail of pancreas. They may show marked contrast enhancement and have central areas of necrosis, and thus may mimic neuroendocrine tumors. These are aggressive lesions which usually present with lymphadenopathy and metastases.

DIFFERENTIAL DIAGNOSES

Focal pancreatitis (including autoimmune type) is an important diagnostic consideration especially because secondary changes of upstream ductal dilatation or atrophy may be seen.[25] *Mass-forming chronic pancreatitis (MFCP)* is chronic inflammation usually involving the pancreatic head. History of repeated episodes of acute abdomen and presence of calcifications indicates underlying chronic calcific pancreatitis. Pancreatic duct in the latter shows long smooth narrowing or irregular beaded appearance. The "Duct penetrating sign" refers to nonobstructed attenuated duct, which traverses the mass instead of getting cut-off and is used to differentiate an inflammatory pancreatic mass from

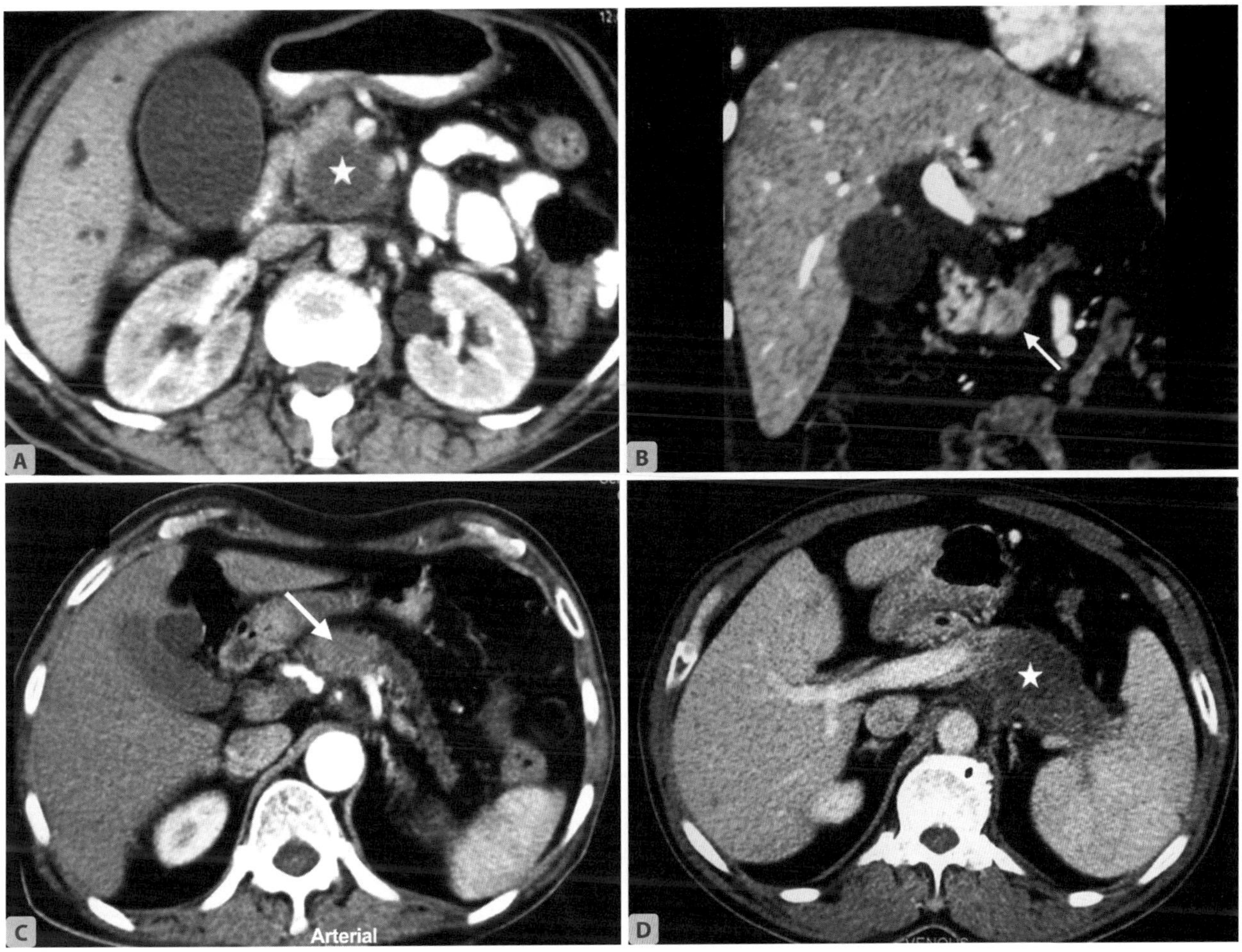

FIGS. 7A TO D: CT images of different patients showing pancreatic carcinoma with variable morphology in different locations. Axial CECT image (A) shows a hypodense mass lesion in the uncinate process of pancreas (star), abutting the superior mesenteric artery. Coronal CECT image (B) shows isodense mass lesion in the pancreatic head (arrow) with atrophy of distal pancreatic parenchyma and pancreatic ductal prominence. Axial CECT image (C) demonstrates isodense mass in the neck of pancreas (arrow) without contour bulge, but with pancreatic ductal dilatation. Axial CECT image (D) shows large hypodense mass lesion in the distal body and tail of pancreas with areas of necrosis within (star).

malignancy **(Figs. 15A to D)**.[26] Also, chronically inflamed pancreas demonstrates greater enhancement than tumor in the pancreatic phase imaging. Ratio of the diameter of dilated pancreatic duct to the maximum width of the abnormal part of gland greater than 0.5 favors carcinoma. DW MRI and perfusion CT can also help to differentiate focal chronic pancreatitis from malignancy.[14,27] EUS may be helpful in these cases and guided sampling may be done.

Autoimmune pancreatitis is characterized by elevated serum IgG4 levels and is treated with steroids and does not require surgery. The focal form can mimic malignancy on imaging. Absence of pancreatic duct dilatation, diffuse involvement, halo-like peripancreatic smooth hypodensity and extrapancreatic manifestations of IgG4-related sclerosing disease may help in differentiating from carcinoma.[27] The pancreatic and biliary ducts may show irregular wall thickening and enhancement.[28] Homogeneous enhancement (similar to surrounding parenchyma) and duct penetrating sign may help in differentiating mass-forming autoimmune pancreatitis from carcinoma.[29] It may be noted that diffusion restriction with low ADC values can be seen in autoimmune pancreatitis also due to dense lymphoplasmacytic infiltration and thus ADC values overlap with that of pancreatic malignancy.[29]

Paraduodenal/groove pancreatitis is a type of chronic focal inflammation localized to the space between the pancreatic head and the second part of duodenum. It is seen more often in middle aged men with history of alcohol abuse. Imaging appearance is in the form of ill-defined sheet-like thickening and bulky pancreatic head with delayed enhancement. There is a pure form which affects only the pancreatoduodenal groove and a segmental form which affects the groove and may extend medially to involve the pancreatic head. Cystic changes may be seen especially in the medial duodenal wall along with duodenal wall thickening **(Figs. 16A to C)**.[30] Thus, it comes in the differential diagnosis of periampullary and pancreatic head malignancies. Pancreatic ductal dilatation is usually not seen.

Despite all imaging advancements and even with sampling, focal pancreatitis may be difficult to differentiate

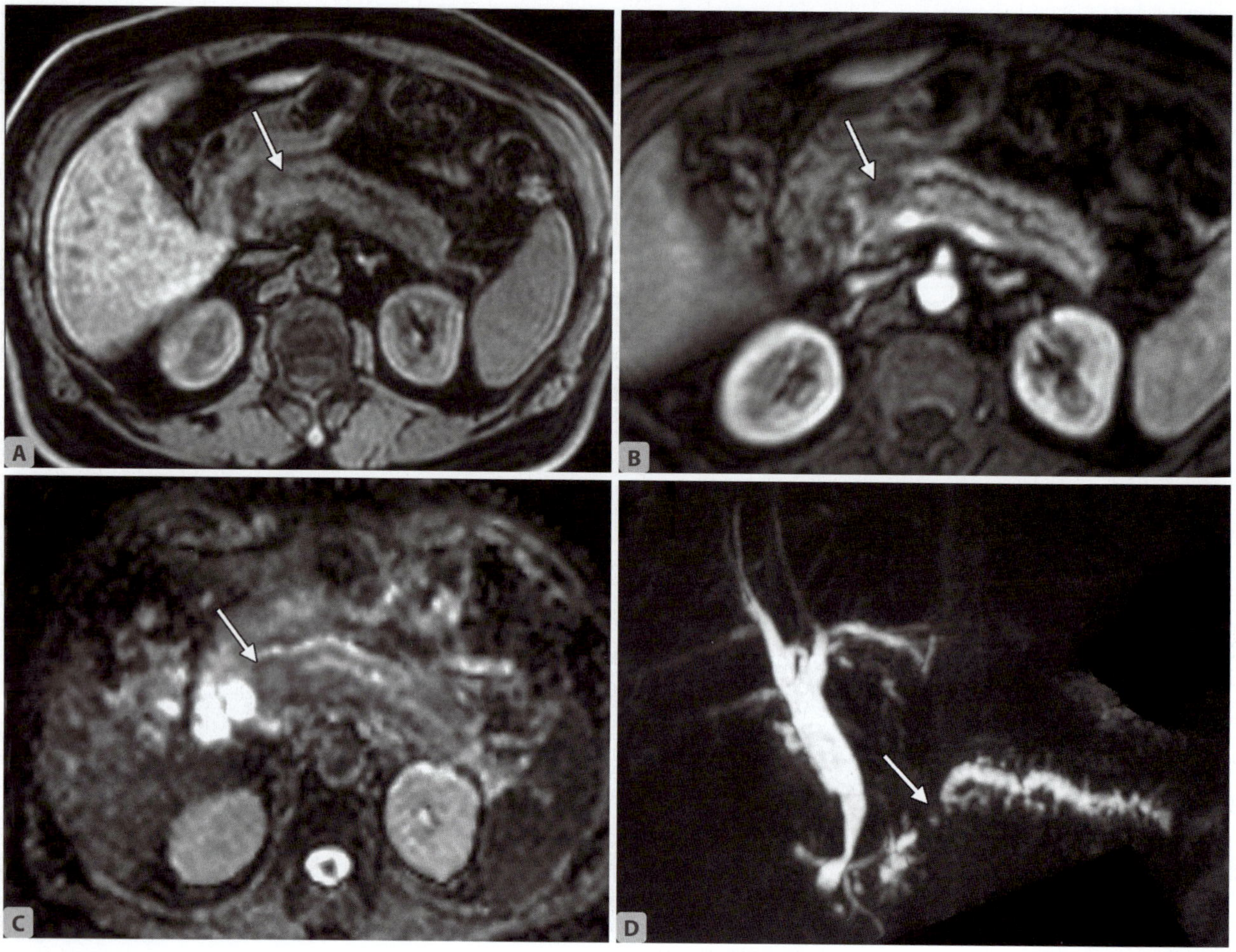

FIGS. 8A TO D: Utility of MRI in small lesions. Axial T1-weighted (T1W) fat-supressed (FS) image (A) shows an ill-defined small isointense mass in the pancreatic head-neck region (arrow) which is hypoenhancing compared to rest of parenchyma on postcontrast pancreatic phase imaging (B), with pancreatic ductal dilatation. Axial apparent diffusion coefficient (ADC) map (C) shows the lesion is dark (arrow), suggesting restricted diffusion. Projectional MRCP image (D) depicts abrupt cut-off of the main pancreatic duct (arrow). There is diffuse irregular dilatation of main pancreatic duct and side branches due to background chronic pancreatitis.

from carcinoma and they may occasionally coexist. Relatively spared pancreatic parenchyma in the background of atrophic gland in chronic pancreatitis may also mimic pancreatic malignancy.

Neuroendocrine tumors are usually small in size and show hypervascularity on the pancreatic phase imaging. Ductal dilatation is uncommon, as opposed to pancreatic carcinomas. Nonfunctional neuroendocrine tumors are large and heterogeneous with areas of necrosis and calcification within **(Figs. 16A to C)**. They may appear similar to ductal adenocarcinomas in the body and tail region because the latter also have large heterogeneous appearance. *Cystic pancreatic tumors* also come in the list of differentials in this scenario.

Metastases to pancreas are not common and most of these patients have metastatic lesions elsewhere in the body also. Primary malignancies which can metastasize to the pancreas include lung, breast and renal carcinomas and melanomas. Metastases can be solitary, multiple or diffuse infiltrating. Usually, they are multiple and well-defined but may mimic pancreatic carcinoma when occur singly. Enhancement characteristics are similar to the primary lesion (hypervascular in renal carcinomas and melanomas).

Lymphomatous involvement of the pancreas occurs frequently by direct infiltration from adjacent enlarged lymph nodes and is more common in non-Hodgkin's lymphoma. Other manifestations include single/multiple homogeneous focal masses showing little contrast enhancement. Ductal dilatation is infrequent, as is necrosis and calcification. Pancreatic head is commonly involved and diffuse involvement of the entire pancreas may also occur.

Occasionally *gastrointestinal tumors* from the stomach and duodenum may also mimic the imaging appearance of pancreatic cancer. *Tuberculosis* is another confounder, especially in developing countries.

STAGING OF PANCREATIC CANCER

After diagnosis, the next step is to assess the resectability of the lesion and also patient's suitability for pancreaticoduo-

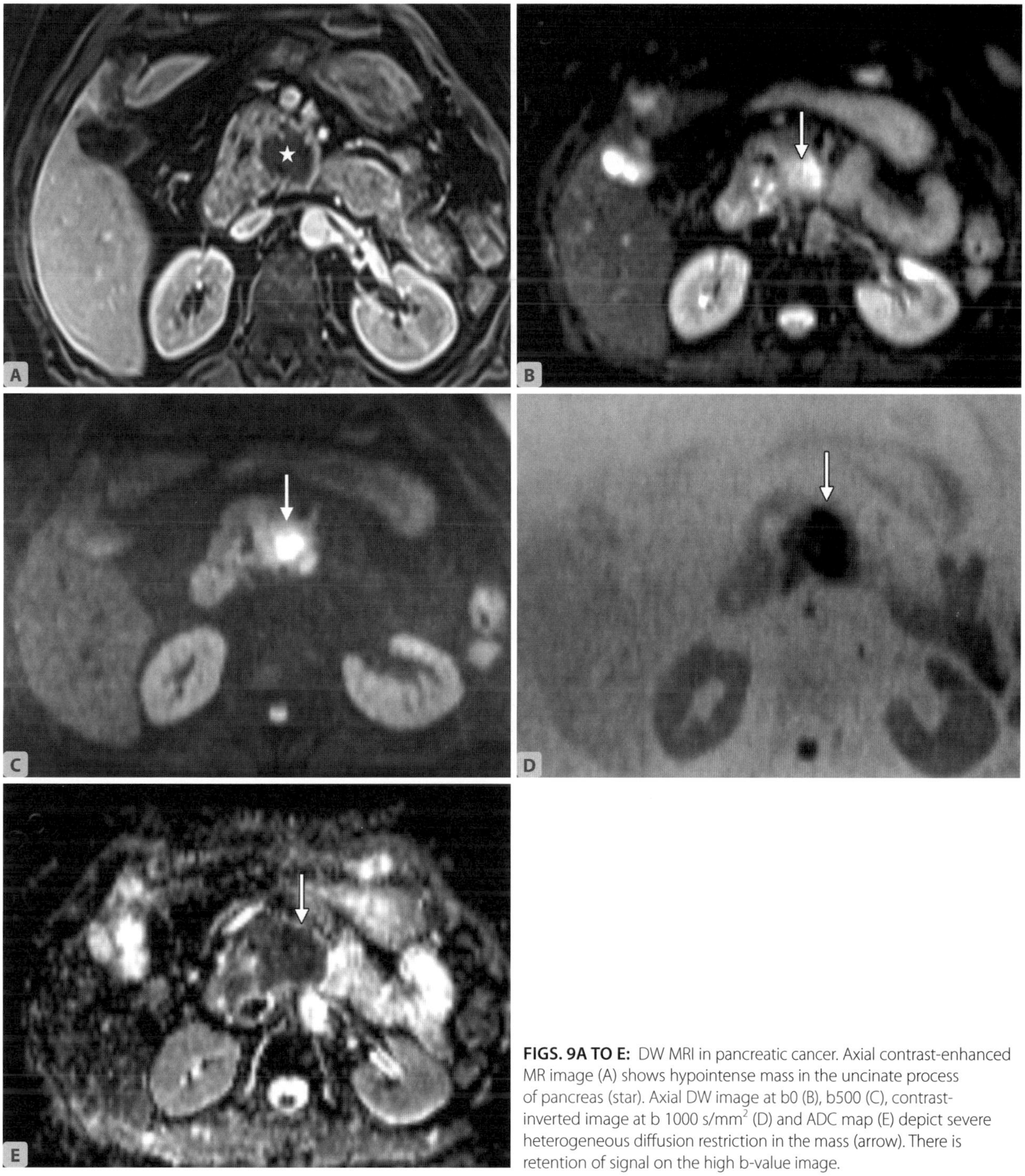

FIGS. 9A TO E: DW MRI in pancreatic cancer. Axial contrast-enhanced MR image (A) shows hypointense mass in the uncinate process of pancreas (star). Axial DW image at b0 (B), b500 (C), contrast-inverted image at b 1000 s/mm^2 (D) and ADC map (E) depict severe heterogeneous diffusion restriction in the mass (arrow). There is retention of signal on the high b-value image.

denectomy. Surgery is beneficial only if R0 resection (negative margins on pathology) is possible. Thus, it is important to avoid unnecessary laparotomy in rest of the patients since there is little survival benefit. The criteria to determine resectability rely more on specificity than sensitivity to avoid denying the benefit of surgery to potentially resectable patients. CT and MRI are equally accurate in the staging of pancreatic cancers.

The spread of pancreatic cancer depends on its location. Anteriorly located head lesions spread towards gastroduodenal and common hepatic arteries while posterior lesions cause early involvement of SMV-PV and replaced/accessory right hepatic arteries (arising from SMA). SMV is more commonly involved in head lesions, compared to SMA. This is because SMV is nearer to the head and also because arteries have thick muscular walls compared to thin walls of veins. Tumors located in the uncinate process have a propensity to grow along jejunal branches of SMA and SMV and thus perineural spread is common. Tumors located in

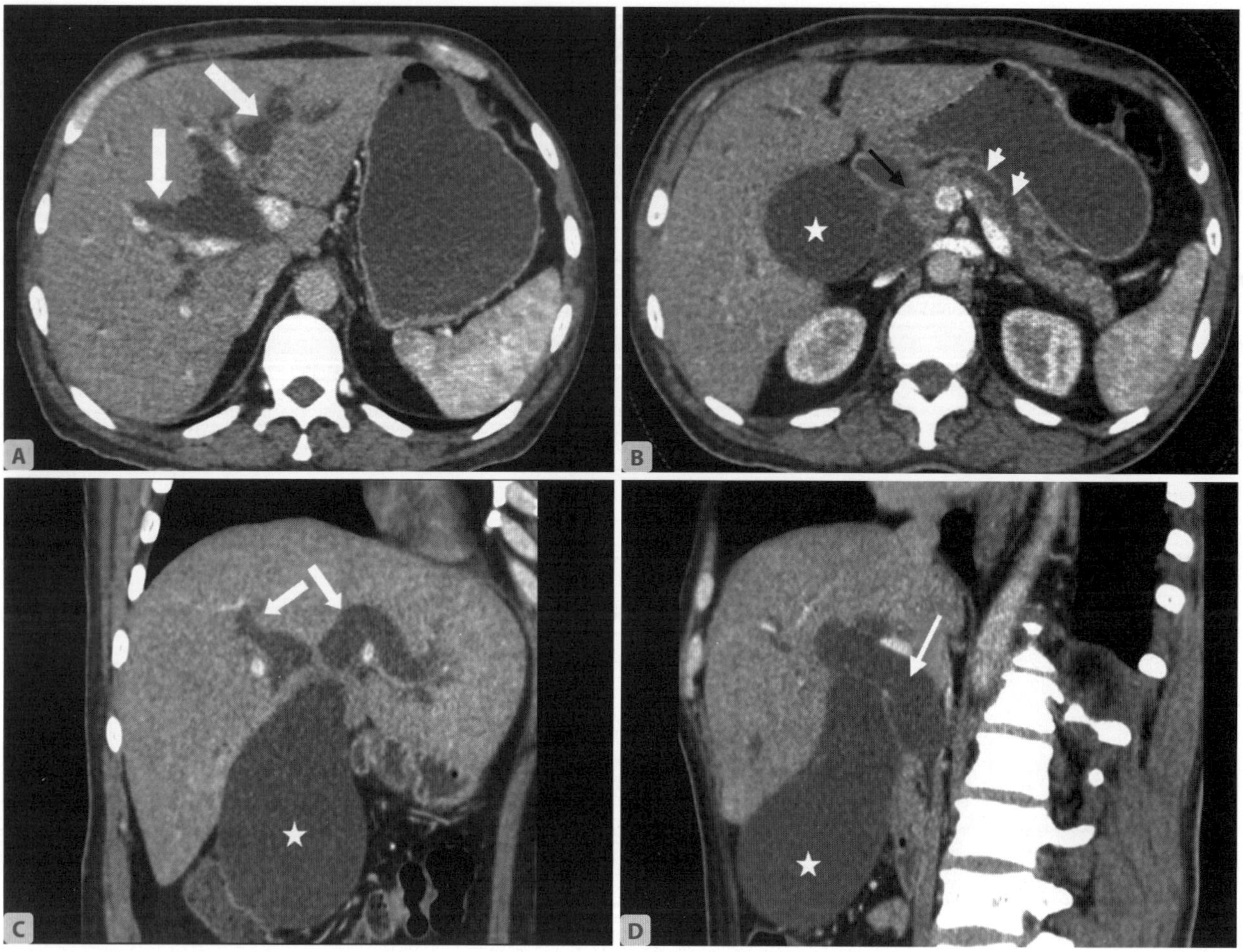

FIGS. 10A TO D: Secondary findings in pancreatic cancer: Axial (A and B), oblique coronal (C) and oblique sagittal (D) CT images in the pancreatic phase show dilatation of intrahepatic biliary radicals (solid arrows), common bile duct (white arrows), gallbladder (star) and pancreatic duct (arrowheads). These secondary signs help in the detection of small isodense mass in the pancreatic head (black arrow).

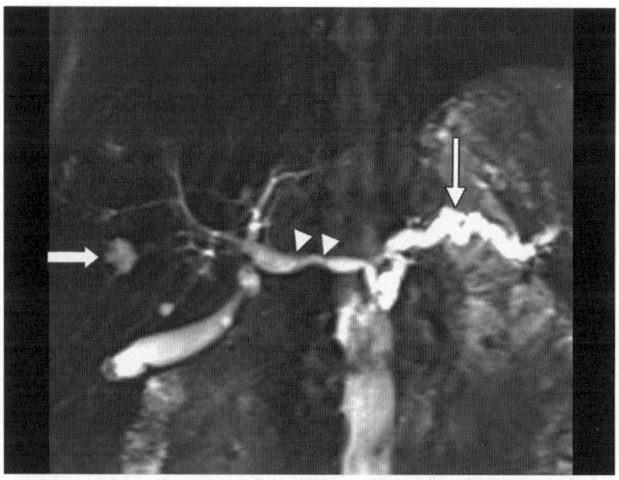

FIG. 11: Projectional MRCP image shows dilatation of both pancreatic (arrow) and biliary ducts (arrowheads) along with mild dilatation of intrahepatic biliary radicals. Few cholangiolar abscesses are also seen in the right lobe (solid arrow) due to obstructive cholangitis.

the body and tail region have a tendency to infiltrate splenic vessels and hilum of the spleen. In advanced cases, stomach, gallbladder and duodenum may also get involved.

There are three categories as per National Comprehensive Cancer Network (NCCN) criteria: resectable, borderline resectable and unresectable **(Table 2)**.[3,31] Location of the tumor and vascular involvement are the important determining factors for categorization. It is important to note that arterial encasement (contact >180 degrees or half the arterial circumference in cross-section) is an important criterion of unresectability of the pancreatic mass.[32] Infiltration of the surrounding structures (stomach, transverse colon, spleen, etc.) does not make the tumor unresectable, though surgery becomes more extensive.[31]

The lesion is *resectable* **(Figs. 17A and B)** if there is neither extrapancreatic infiltration nor distant metastases. Thus there is a clear fat plane separating the tumor from main arteries (celiac axis, common hepatic artery CHA and superior mesenteric artery SMA). The contact with the surrounding veins (superior mesenteric

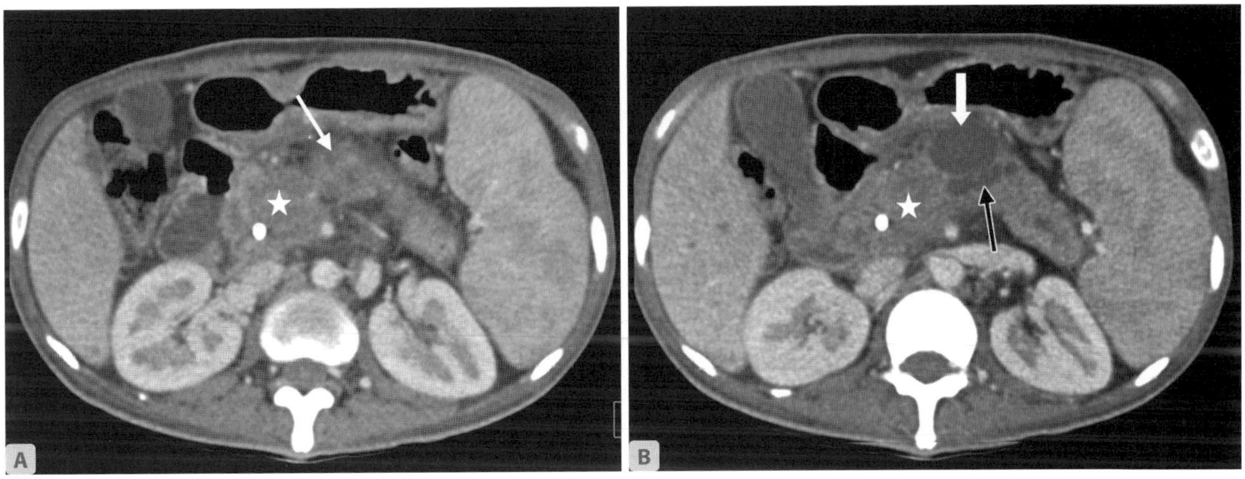

FIGS. 12A AND B: Pancreatic cancer causing acute pancreatitis with biliary stent *in situ*. Axial CECT images depict bulky heterogeneous mass in the pancreatic head region (star) with heterogeneity in the proximal body (white arrow). Former was ductal adenocarcinoma while latter was focal pancreatitis secondary to obstruction. Note is made of peripancreatic fat stranding in (A), peripancreatic fluid collection (solid arrow) and pancreatic ductal dilatation (black arrow) in (B).

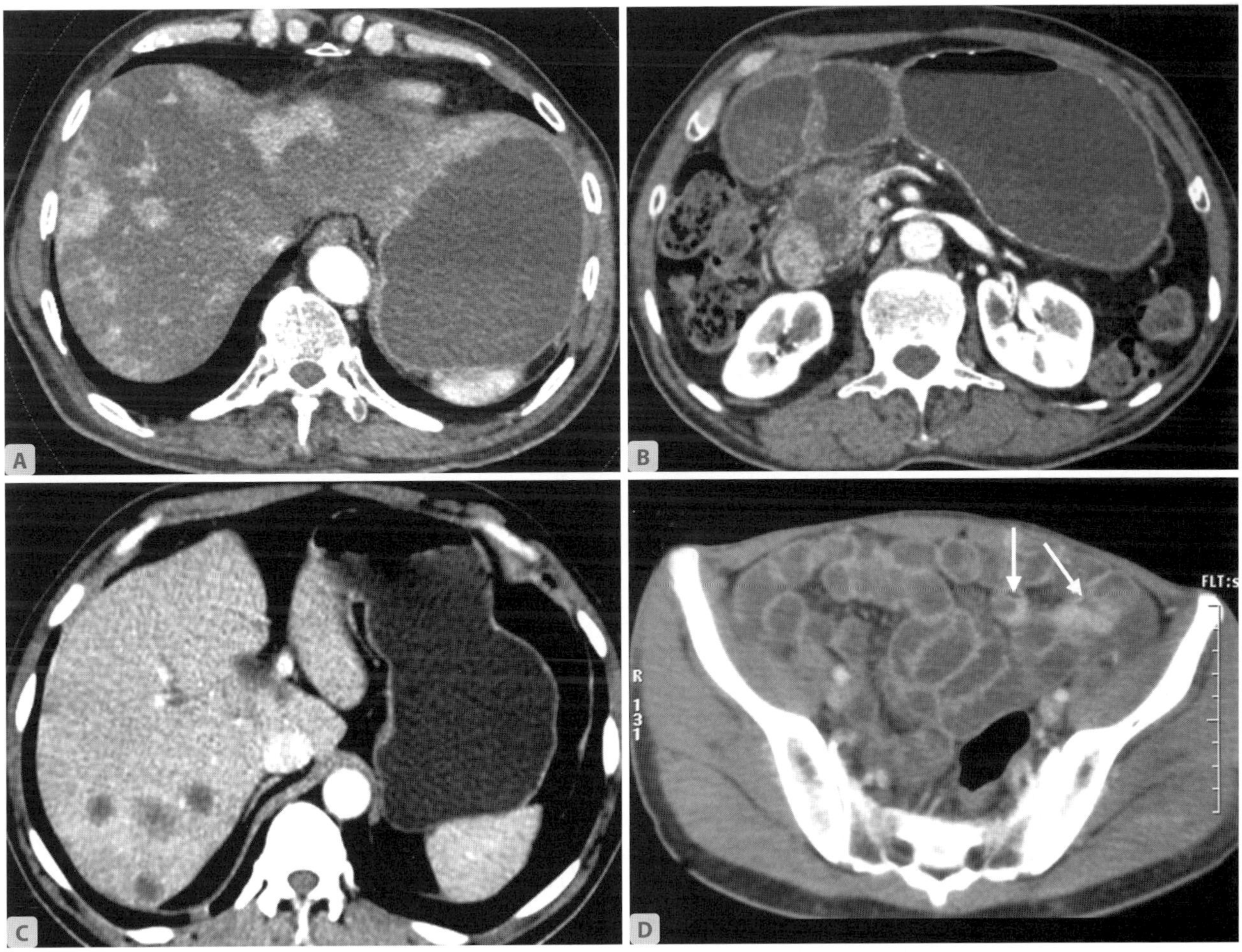

FIGS. 13A TO D: Liver and peritoneal metastases in pancreatic carcinoma. Late arterial phase axial CT image (A) shows multiple liver lesions with surrounding hyperenhancement and transient hepatic attenuation difference. Axial CT image at lower level (B) depicts a large heterogeneous pancreatic head mass. Axial CT image in a different patient (C) shows multiple hypodense liver metastases in the venous phase. Same patient as (C) also showed multiple areas of eccentric bowel wall thickening (arrows in D), suggesting serosal metastases.

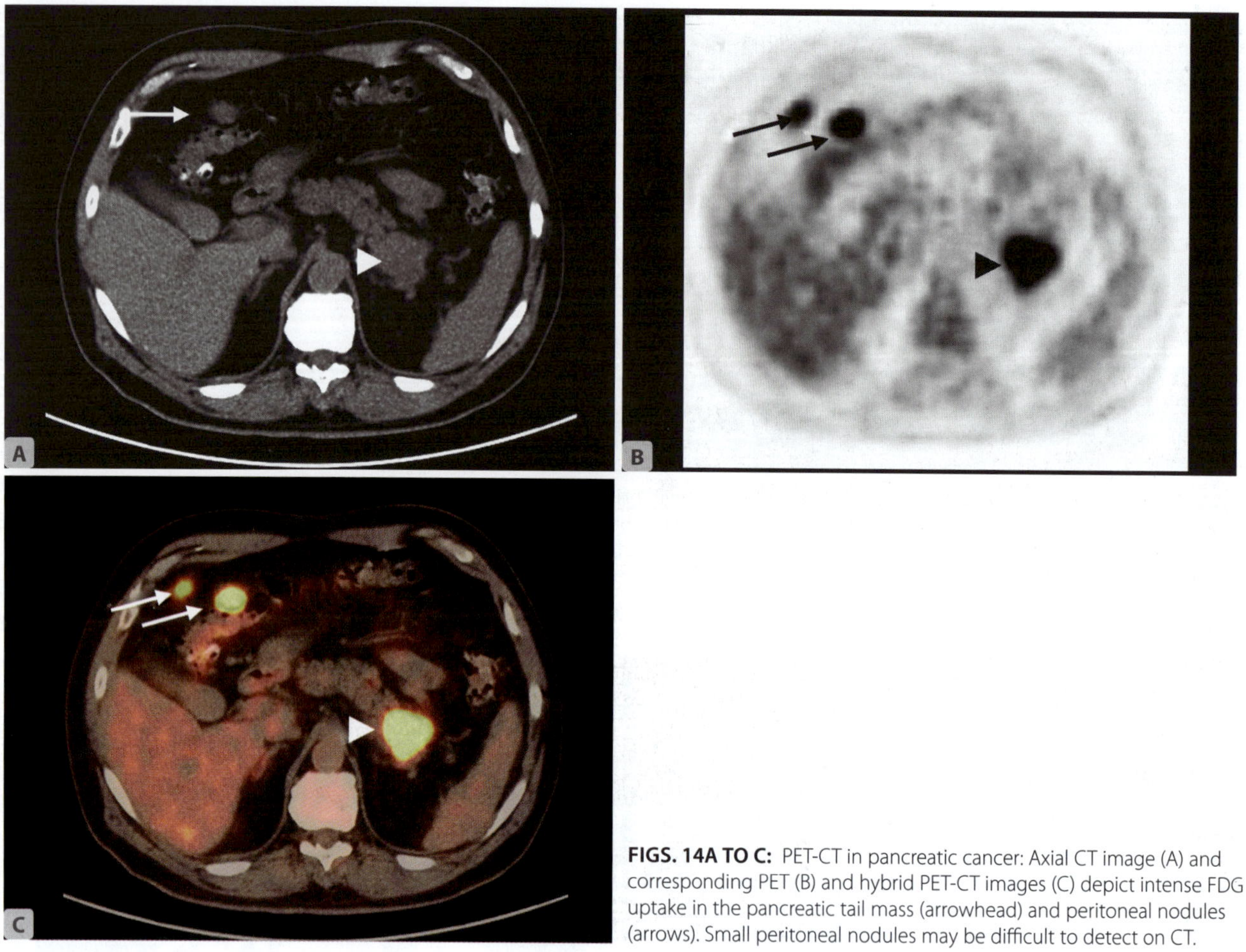

FIGS. 14A TO C: PET-CT in pancreatic cancer: Axial CT image (A) and corresponding PET (B) and hybrid PET-CT images (C) depict intense FDG uptake in the pancreatic tail mass (arrowhead) and peritoneal nodules (arrows). Small peritoneal nodules may be difficult to detect on CT.

vein SMV and portal vein PV) is also absent or there is just abutment (≤180 degrees contact without contour irregularity). No venous encasement or tumor thrombus is seen.

Unresectable tumors **(Figs. 18A to F)** either have distant metastases (including nonregional lymphadenopathy) or local invasion. Liver and peritoneal cavity are the common sites of metastases. Arterial invasion is in the form of encasement (contact >180 degrees circumference) of SMA, celiac axis or contact with first jejunal branch of SMA. Unresectable venous involvement includes unreconstructible SMV-PV due to infiltration/occlusion or contact with the most proximal draining jejunal branch into SMV.

Borderline resectability **(Figs. 19A to C)** in terms of venous involvement includes encasement or abutment of short-segment SMV-PV (usually up to 2 cm) with contour irregularity or venous thrombosis but amenable to surgical reconstruction. The prerequisite for reconstruction is that the two venous ends should have single lumen and thus branches cannot be attached to a single lumen.[1] Arterial involvement criteria are tabulated in **Table 2**.

Identifying variant vascular anatomy is also important and should be conveyed to the surgeon. Tumor contact with variant vessels (replaced right hepatic artery from SMA, low origin of CHA from celiac axis with abnormal course inferior to portal vein, high insertion of jejunal branches on SMV near PV confluence) can make resection/reconstruction difficult.[33]

Few authors have tried to correlate the appearance of venous contact of the tumor to the likelihood of successful R0 resection.[34–36] Latter is successful in those having smooth mass effect or unilateral focal mass effect with narrowing of SMV-PV. Patients with bilateral narrowing and circumferential encasement have high probability of positive surgical margins. Encasement of SMV leads to 'tear-drop' shape of the vein and suggests unresectability **(Figs. 20A to D)**.[37] Dilated peripancreatic vessels has been suggested to indicate surrounding local invasion.[38]

Metastatic lymph nodes can be identified by size criteria (>1 cm in short axis), morphology (round shape) and/or presence of central hypodensity (necrosis). Unequivocal lymph node enlargement beyond the extent of Whipple resection (i.e. except celiac axis) makes the mass unresectable. For lesions in the pancreatic head and neck, nodes along celiac axis, peripancreatic and periportal regions can be removed during surgery.[39] For body and tail cancers, nodes along CHA, celiac trunk, splenic vessels and splenic hilum come in the operative field. If nodal involvement is confirmed at surgery, then adjuvant chemotherapy is indicated.

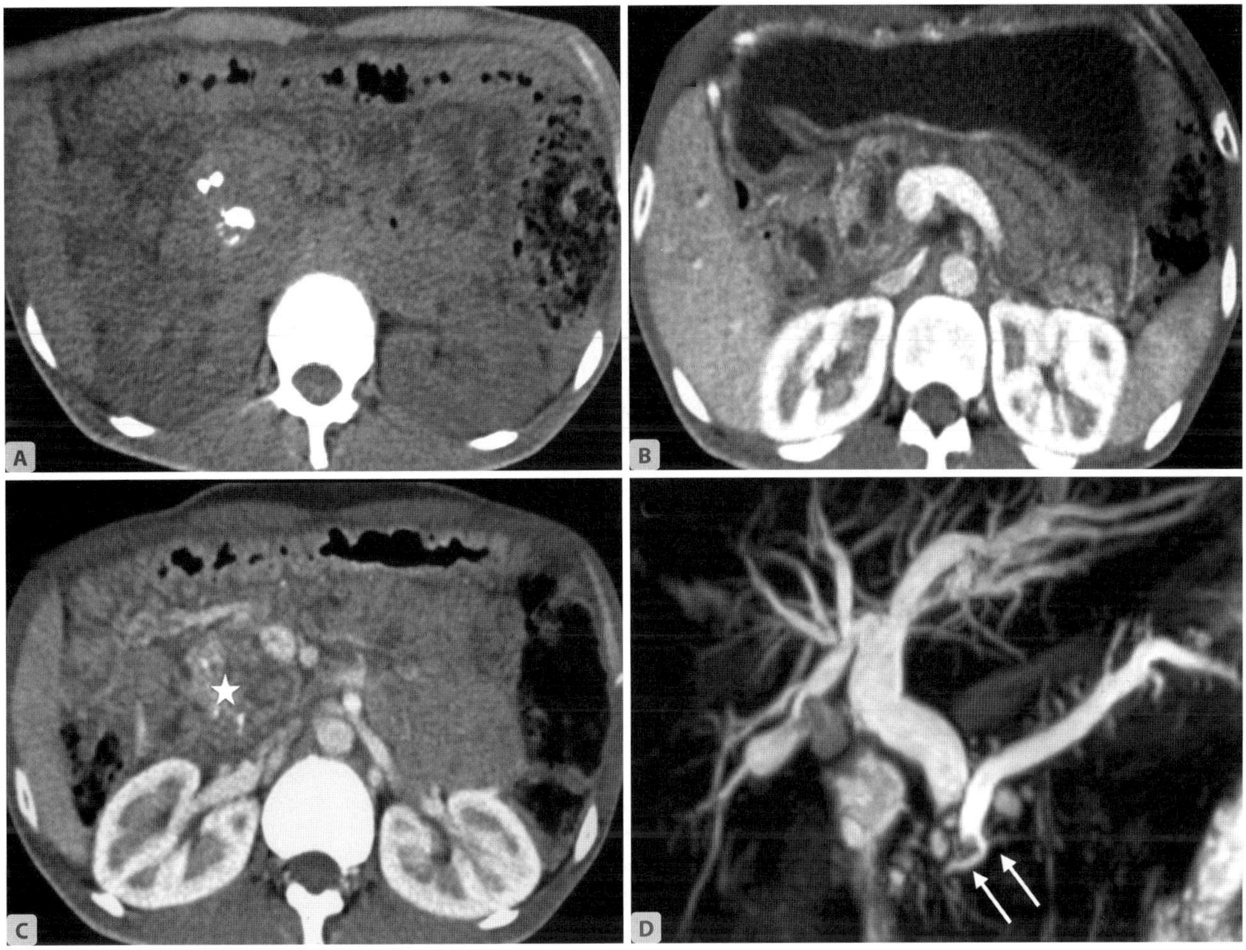

FIGS. 15A TO D: Mass-forming chronic pancreatitis: Axial noncontrast CT image (A) depicts multiple foci of calcification in the region of pancreatic head. Axial CECT images (B and C) show bulky heterogeneously enhancing head (star) with dilated pancreatic and common bile ducts. However, there is no abrupt cut-off of the ducts and the narrowed pancreatic duct can be seen to course through the head region (arrows in D), suggesting duct penetrating sign. EUS sampling confirmed focal chronic pancreatitis.

The overall accuracy of MDCT in predicting resectability of pancreatic cancer is 88–93%.[40] The problem areas include microscopic peritoneal implants and metastases to normal-sized lymph nodes.[41] Former are even more difficult to detect in the absence of ascites. Some centers routinely perform laparoscopy just prior to surgery to detect these peritoneal metastases. In cases of mismatch between surgery and imaging, metastases were found to be the most common cause of unresectability, rather than local invasion.[1] CT is very accurate in diagnosing unresectable disease (89–100% positive predictive value); however, accuracy is lower for predicting resectability (45–79%).[42]

Perineural invasion is a hallmark of ductal adenocarcinomas, although it may be seen in ampullary cancers and cholangiocarcinoma as well.[43] Perineural invasion may be suggested on CT when there is direct soft tissue infiltration along a known perineural pathway and has poor prognosis. The most common route of spread is along the plexus pancreaticus capitalis for cancers of the pancreatic head and uncinate process.[44] Plexus pancreaticus capitalis 1 (posterior hepatic plexus) extends from the right celiac ganglion, courses behind the portal vein up to upper medial border of uncinate process.[44] This is involved in pancreatic head lesions. Plexus pancreaticus capitalis 2 extends from SMA plexus, courses along posteroinferior pancreaticoduodenal artery and jejunal trunk of SMV, reaching up to the uncinate process. This plexus is usually involved in cancers of the uncinate process. Anteriorly located tumors of the head region may infiltrate along gastroduodenal artery plexus (anterior pathway), extend to plexus of CHA and hepatoduodenal ligament, and reach the right celiac ganglion and SMA plexus.[24] Literature regarding radiologic-pathologic correlates of perineural invasion is lacking but this has the potential to become an important criterion of unresectability.

Tumor node metastasis (TNM) staging system is not widely used since management depends on the resectability criteria as delineated above. However, it is used to assess the clinical prognosis and generate survival data.[31] The latest TNM staging system is shown in **Table 3** (American Joint Committee on Cancer AJCC, 7th edition).

The EUS may also be helpful in suggesting vascular invasion. The features suggesting vascular invasion include loss of normally hyperechoic vessel wall, vessel irregularity/occlusion and direct visualization of intravascular thrombus.[45]

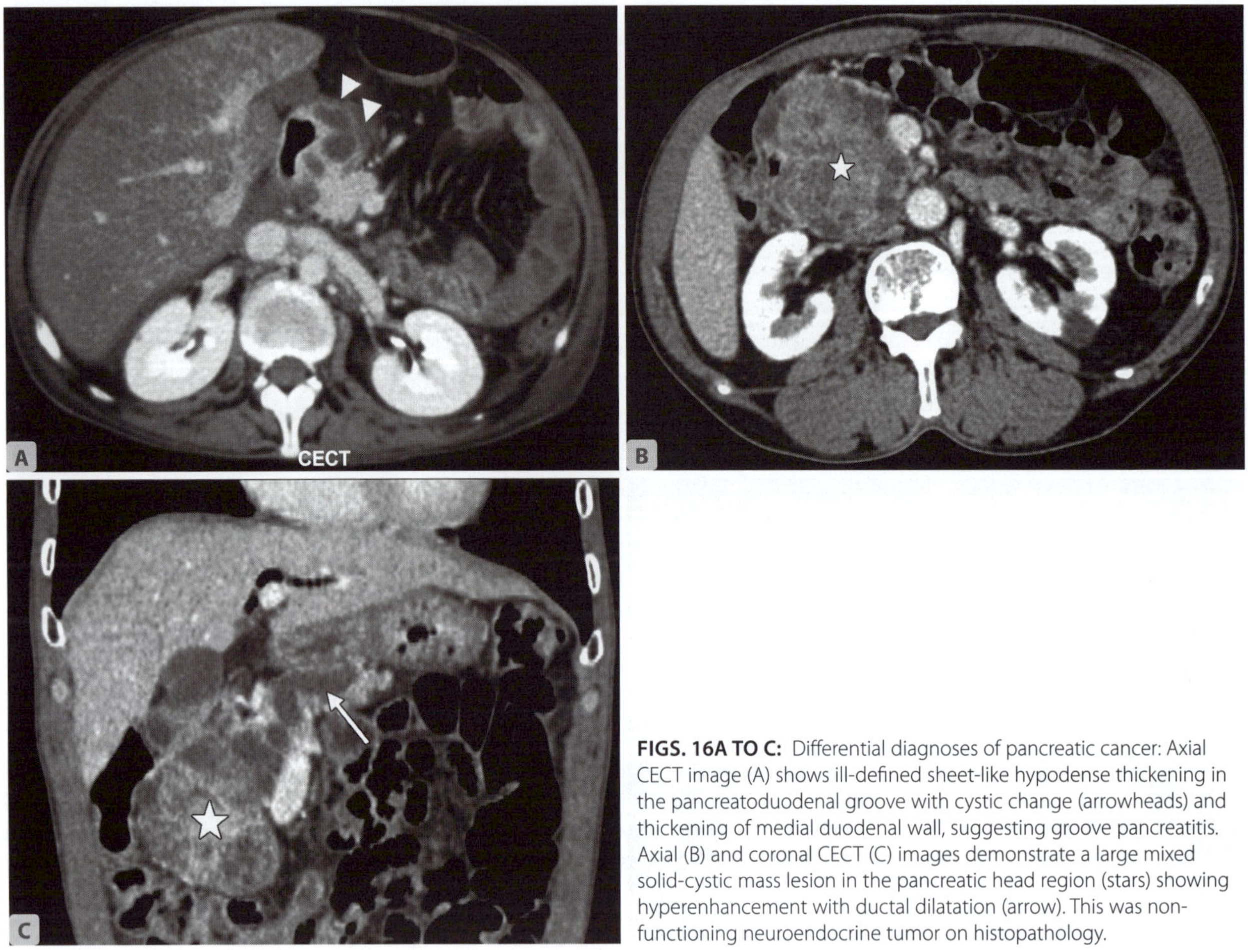

FIGS. 16A TO C: Differential diagnoses of pancreatic cancer: Axial CECT image (A) shows ill-defined sheet-like hypodense thickening in the pancreatoduodenal groove with cystic change (arrowheads) and thickening of medial duodenal wall, suggesting groove pancreatitis. Axial (B) and coronal CECT (C) images demonstrate a large mixed solid-cystic mass lesion in the pancreatic head region (stars) showing hyperenhancement with ductal dilatation (arrow). This was non-functioning neuroendocrine tumor on histopathology.

TABLE 2: Imaging criteria of resectability of pancreatic carcinoma.

	Arterial	***Venous***
Resectable	No arterial contact with tumor	No contact or only abutment of SMV-PV without irregularity and distortion
Borderline resectability	• Tumor contact with CHA without extension to celiac axis proximally or hepatic artery bifurcation distally (so as to allow for surgical reconstruction) • SMA abutment • Variant arterial anatomy with tumor contact • Celiac axis abutment in pancreatic body/ tail lesions* • Celiac axis encasement without involvement of aorta and with intact uninvolved GDA*	• Encasement or abutment of SMV-PV with contour irregularity or venous thrombosis but suitable vessel available proximal and distal for surgical reconstruction • Tumor contact with IVC
Unresectable	• Encasement of SMA, celiac axis • Celiac axis abutment in pancreatic head lesions • Extensive encasement of CHA (surgical reconstruction not possible) • Contact with first jejunal branch of SMA • Any contact with aorta	• Unreconstructible SMV-PV due to infiltration/occlusion • Contact with the most proximal draining jejunal branch (into SMV)

* Some institutions may consider these criteria to indicate unresectable disease.
Distant metastases, including nonregional lymphadenopathy also make the disease unresectable.

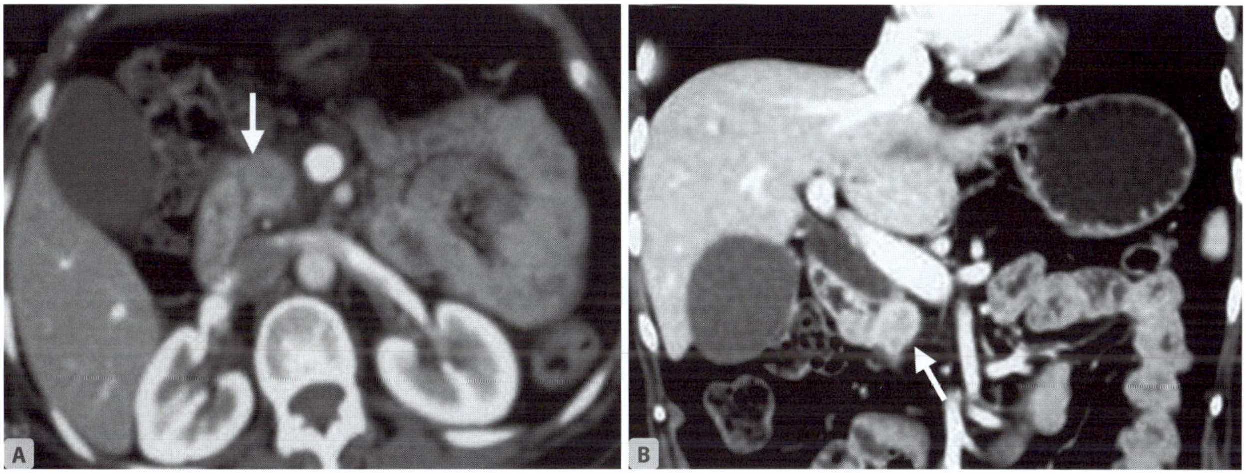

FIGS. 17A AND B: Resectable pancreatic cancer: Axial (A) and coronal (B) CECT images shows small pancreatic head mass (arrows) with clearly maintained fat planes with superior mesenteric vessels.

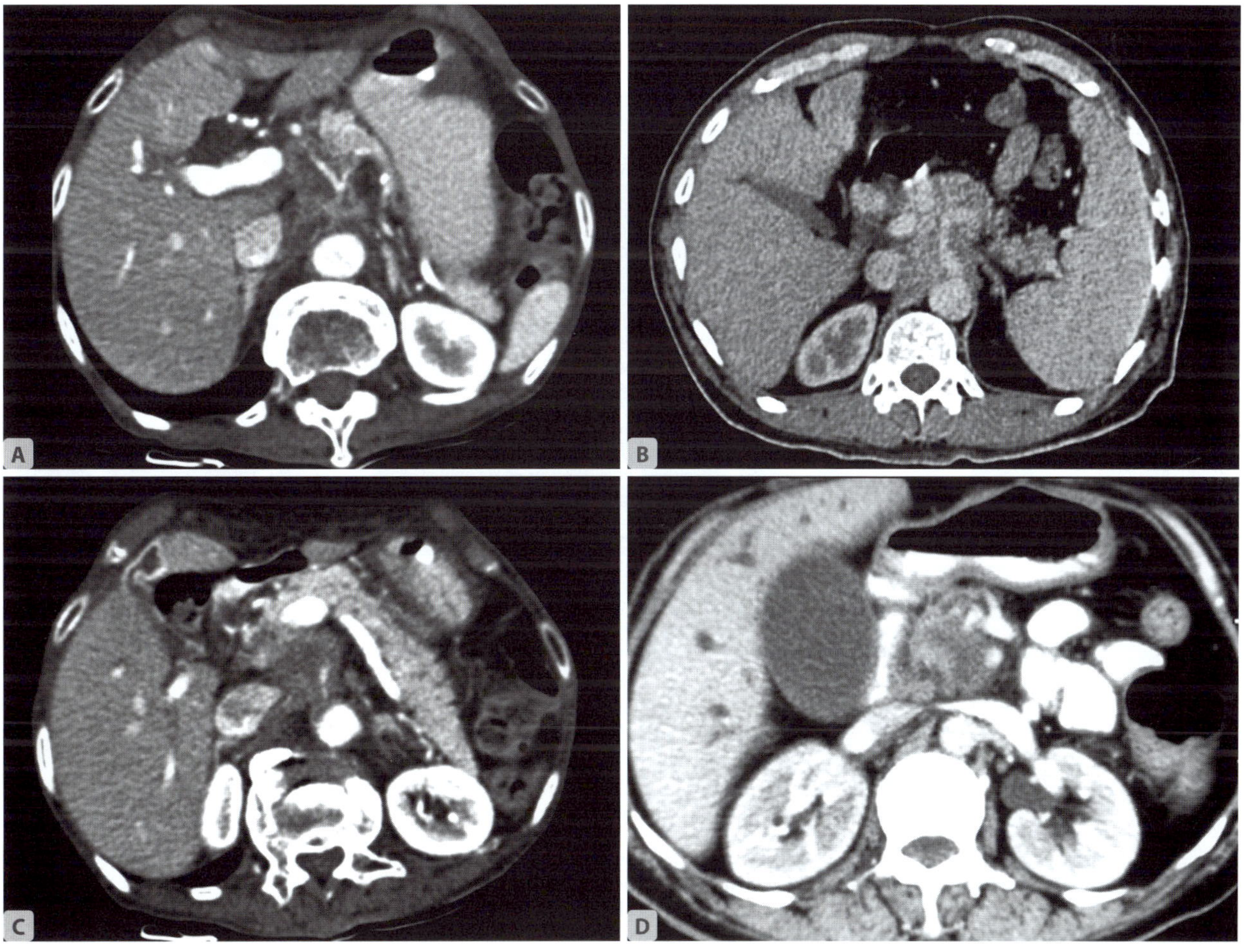

FIGS. 18A TO F: *Continued*

SAMPLING

The EUS-guided FNA of biopsy is preferred over CT/USG-guided percutaneous sampling because of better yield, safety and lower risk of peritoneal seeding. When clinicoradiologic findings are typical, then biopsy proof is not mandatory and an equivocal biopsy should not delay surgery in patients suspected to have pancreatic cancer. Nevertheless, tissue diagnosis is necessary before neoadjuvant therapy and in

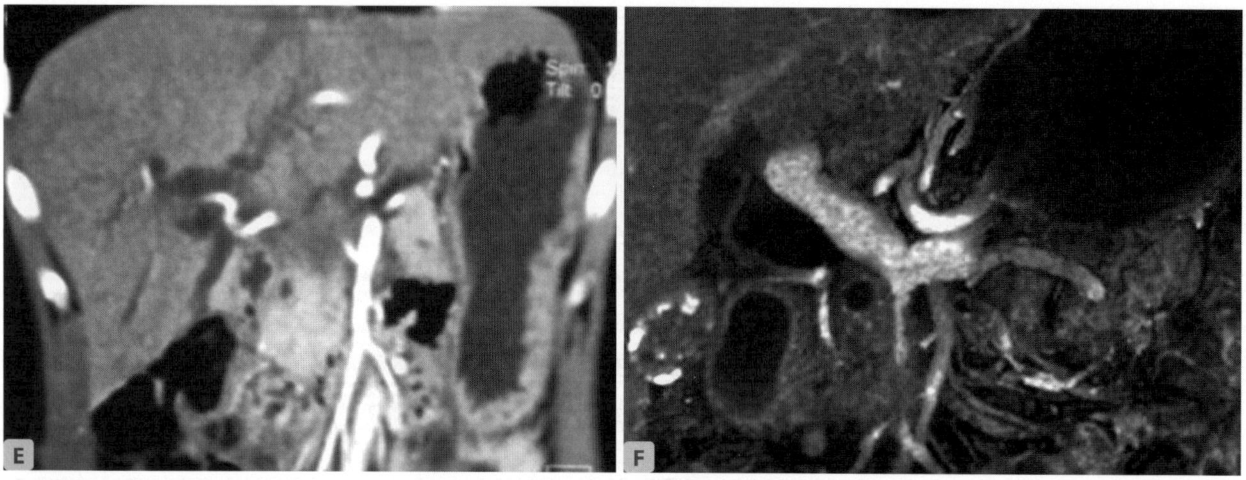

FIGS. 18A TO F: Unresectable pancreatic cancer: Axial CECT images depict encasement of celiac artery and common hepatic artery (A), encasement of celiac trunk and contact with aorta (B), encasement and irregular narrowing of SMA (C) and encasement of both SMA and SMV (D). Coronal CECT image, maximal intensity projection (MIP) in late arterial phase (E) depicts tumor encasement of replaced right hepatic artery (arising from SMA). Coronal MIP image generated from postcontrast MR images (F) shows encasement with irregularity of SMV with extension up to the jejunal branch, precluding surgical reconstruction.

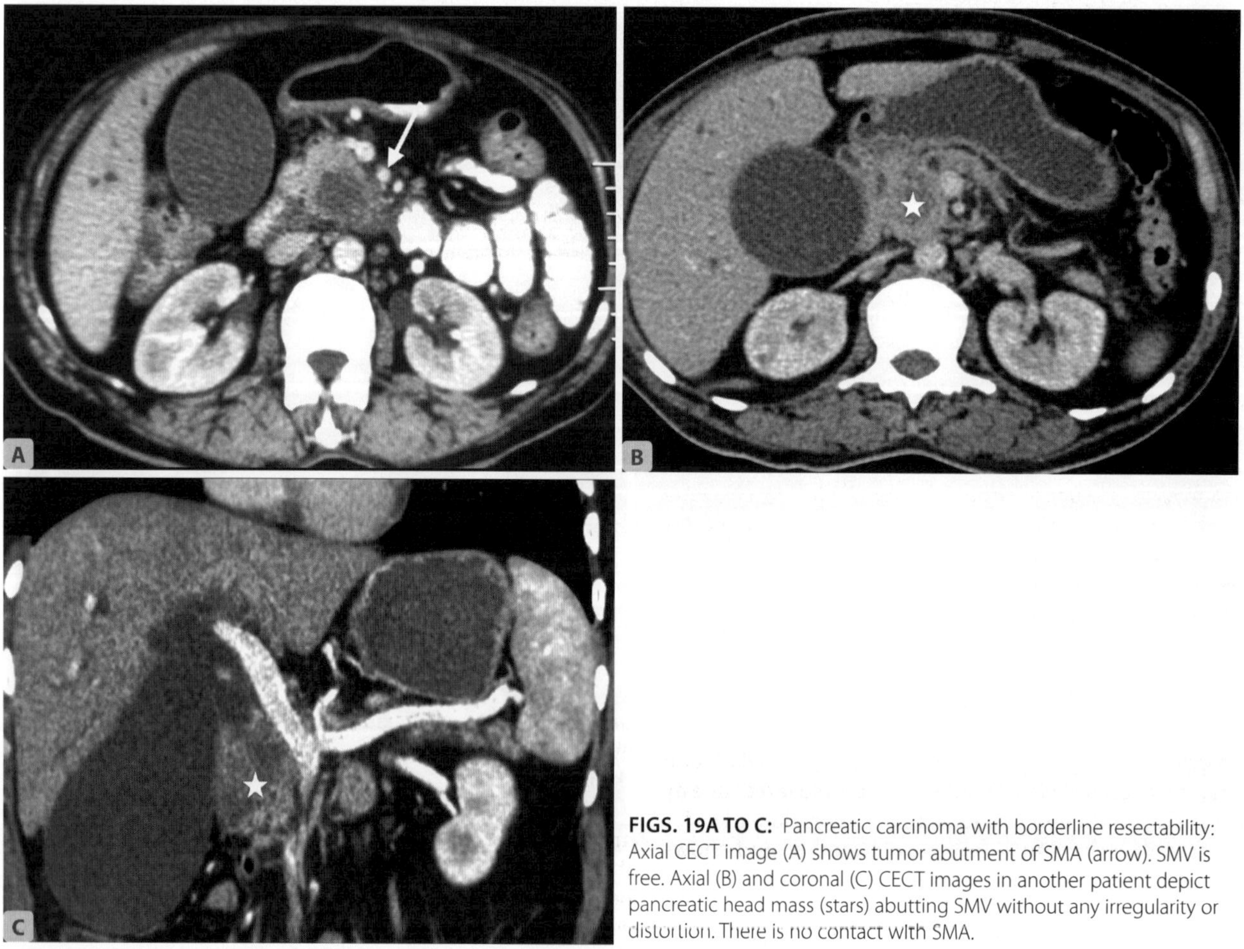

FIGS. 19A TO C: Pancreatic carcinoma with borderline resectability: Axial CECT image (A) shows tumor abutment of SMA (arrow). SMV is free. Axial (B) and coronal (C) CECT images in another patient depict pancreatic head mass (stars) abutting SMV without any irregularity or distortion. There is no contact with SMA.

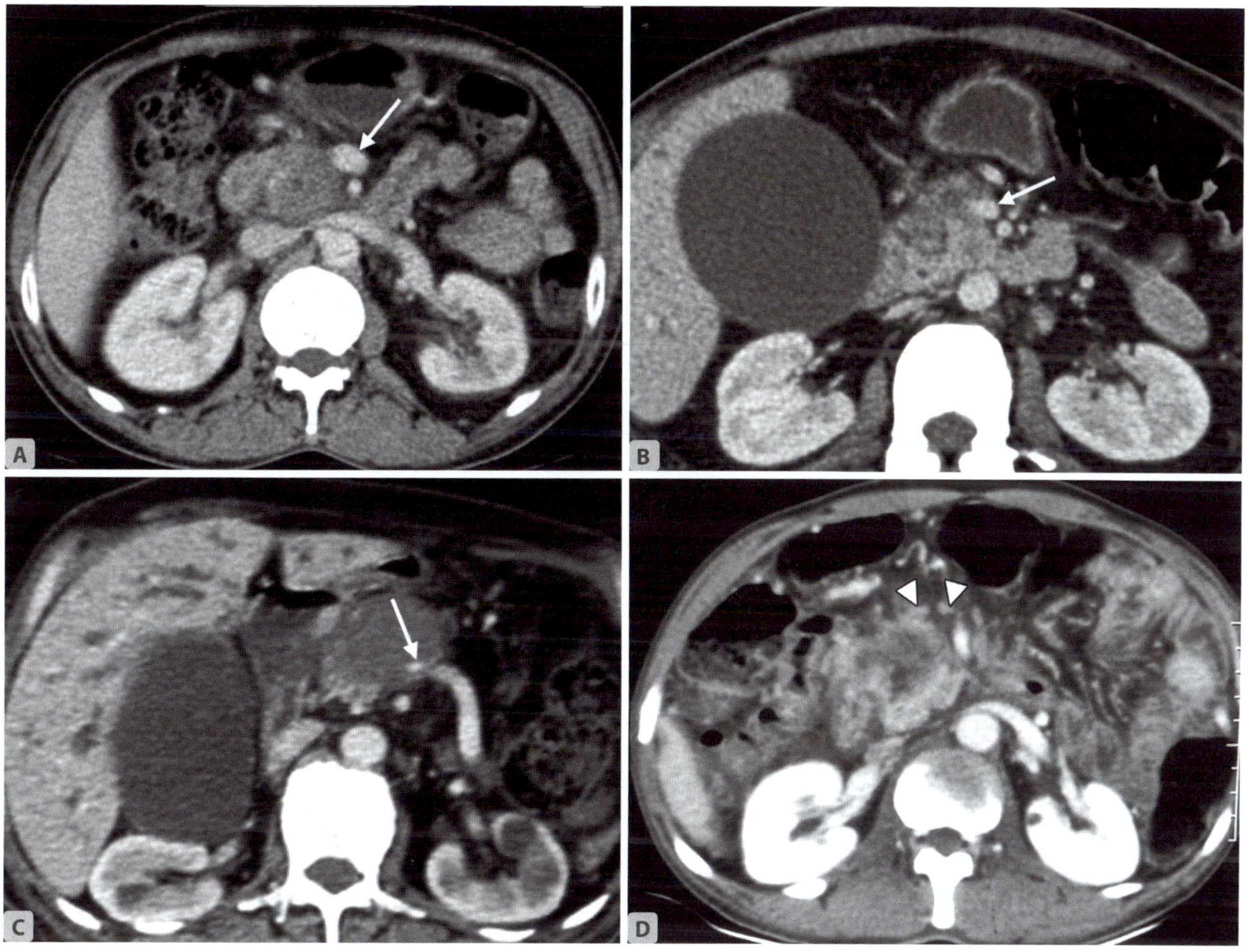

FIGS. 20A TO D: Spectrum of SMV involvement in pancreatic carcinoma: Axial CECT images show abutment of SMV (arrow) (A), encasement of SMV (arrow) with deformed contour (B), irregular narrowing of SMV (arrow) due to complete encasement (C) and nonvisualization of SMV (D) due to complete thrombosis and presence of collaterals (arrowheads).

patients with unresectable disease. Sampling of equivocal lymph nodes can also be done under EUS guidance.

Staging laparoscopy may be beneficial in patients deemed resectable by CT but otherwise at increased risk for dissemination. The additional lesions (usually peritoneal metastases) detected on preoperative laparoscopy may alter the management in 4–15% patients.[46]

BIOMARKERS

The most validated and studied biomarker is CA 19-9, but is nonspecific, being elevated in multiple hepatobiliary and pancreatic malignancies. It may also be elevated in any biliary obstruction and infections. It is a poor biomarker for screening but has value as prognostic marker and shows correlation with staging and survival.

k-ras gene mutations are common in patients with pancreatic carcinoma and are associated with poor prognosis.[47] Detection of k-ras mutations in the peripheral blood may indicate tumor burden and serve as prognostic biomarker.[47]

FOLLOW-UP IMAGING

Clinical follow-up is recommended every 3–6 months for the first 2 years after surgery and annually thereafter. CA 19-9 and CT can be done annually for detection of recurrence.

For locally advanced or metastatic disease on treatment (chemotherapy and/radiotherapy), serial CT follow-up is advised. Routine portal venous phase acquisition is sufficient, unless surgery is contemplated; for which dedicated pancreatic protocol is required.[3] Conventionally, size of the target lesions has been the main criterion of response evaluation.[24] Whether the lesion has become resectable comes next.

Early detection of nonresponders (to chemotherapy and/radiotherapy) is the key research area, considering the cost and toxicity associated with these therapies. This becomes even more relevant because change in size takes considerable time. Functional imaging modalities like PET-CT, perfusion CT/MRI and diffusion MRI may have a role in early response assessment. Treatment induces necrosis, and thus is expected to reduce the metabolic activity [indicated

TABLE 3: TNM Staging (AJCC 4th edition) of pancreatic carcinoma.

T-stage TX: Primary tumor cannot be assessed T0: No evidence of primary tumor Tis: Carcinoma *in situ* T1: Tumor limited to the pancreas, 2 cm or less in the greatest dimension T2: Tumor limited to the pancreas, >2 cm in the greatest dimension T3: Tumor extends beyond the pancreas but without involvement of celiac axis or SMA T4: Tumor involves the celiac axis or SMA
N-stage NX: Regional lymph nodes cannot be assessed N0: No regional lymph node metastasis N1: Regional lymph node metastasis
M-stage MX: Distant metastasis cannot be assessed M0: No distant metastasis M1: Distant metastasis
Stage 0: Tis N0 M0 Stage IA: T1 N0 M0 Stage IB: T2 N0 M0 Stage IIA: T3 N0 M0 Stage IIB: T1-3 N1 M0 Stage III: T4 Any N M0 Stage IV: Any T Any N M1

by standardized uptake values (SUV)] on PET scan, reduce the perfusion parameters and increase the apparent diffusion coefficient (ADC) values on DW MRI. However, differentiating post-treatment changes from viable tumor is difficult. This becomes even more challenging because treatment induces inflammatory changes which may mimic tumor infiltration on conventional imaging and also show increased metabolic uptake. DW MRI and perfusion imaging may have a role in this scenario. Comparison with previous imaging is also of paramount importance in these cases.

Assessment of resectability postneoadjuvant therapy is difficult because post treatment inflammation and fibrosis may mimic local vascular infiltration. Thus, the imaging accuracy decreases in detecting resectable disease.[39] This poses a practical problem in patients who receive neoadjuvant therapy after being diagnosed to have borderline resectable disease on initial CT. It has been found that radiological downstaging to resectable disease is rare (0.8%), though a significant proportion (66%) of such patients are actually found to have resectable disease at surgery.[48] Thus International Study Group of Pancreatic Surgery (ISGPS) recommends that in all patients with neoadjuvant therapy, exploratory laparotomy with attempted resection should be done, provided there is no progression on follow-up imaging.[49]

TABLE 4: Structured reporting format for suspected pancreatic malignancy.

Pancreatic lesion present: Y/N	• Location—head/neck/body/tail • Size • Enhancement relative to pancreas (in pancreatic phase)—hypo/iso/hyper • Misc—necrosis/calcification/none • Contour bulge—yes/no • Confined to pancreas with clear fat planes—yes/no • PD dilatation—yes with atrophy/yes without atrophy/no • Biliary dilatation—yes/no • GB status • Diagnosis—adenocarcinoma/others (specify differentials)
Status of arteries	• Arterial contact—yes/no • Celiac axis—no contact/abutment/ encasement • CHA—no contact/abutment/ encasement Surgically reconstructible—yes/no • SMA—no contact/abutment/ encasement Surgically reconstructible—yes/no • Contact with first jejunal branch of SMA—yes/no • GDA—involved/free • Aorta—involved/free • Variant arterial anatomy with tumor contact—yes/no • Significant atherosclerosis at origin of celiac axis/SMA—yes/no
Status of veins	• Venous contact—yes/no • Least distance to SMV • SMV—no contact/abutment/ encasement Surgically reconstructible—yes/no • Contact with the most proximal draining jejunal branch (into SMV)—yes/no • PV—no contact/abutment/encasement Surgically reconstructible—yes/no • Length of venous involvement • Contact with IVC—yes/no
• Adjacent structure infiltration • Adenopathy—yes/no (site) • Metastases—yes/no (liver/peritoneal/others—specify) • Ascites—yes/no	
ADV- EUS +/– sampling/MRI	

STRUCTURED REPORTING

Following a structured format for reporting pancreatic multiphasic CT examinations enables better evaluation of pancreatic cancer and optimal surgical planning.[50] Surgeons find it easier to understand the objective terms used in structured reporting format and are more likely to have all the information needed for surgical planning from these structured reports.[50] A sample structured reporting template for reporting suspected pancreatic malignancies is given in **Table 4**. The main problem with narrative reporting is that some of the key descriptors may be missing and the standardized lexicon may not be used, thus contributing to ambiguity in management.

FLOWCHART 2: Imaging and management protocol in a patient suspected to have pancreatic malignancy.

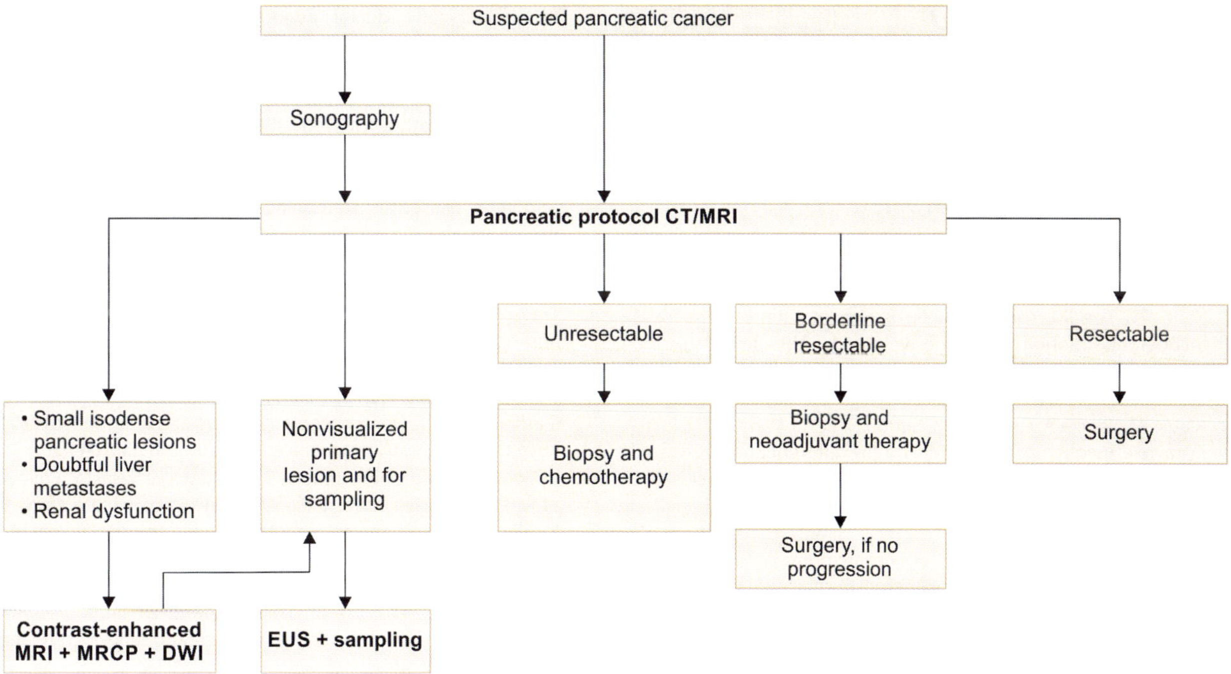

CONCLUSION

Early detection, accurate characterization and staging is essential for optimal management of pancreatic cancer, and imaging plays a crucial role. Sonography is frequently performed as the first investigation for evaluation of these patients. Both MDCT and MRI perform equally well in the detection and staging of pancreatic malignancies with CT being the most validated modality owing to faster acquisition and high spatial resolution. MRI is equally accurate and may have an edge in case of smaller lesions, demonstrating relationship with ducts and in cases where intravenous contrast cannot be given. DW MRI is very sensitive in detection of liver metastases. EUS provides limited but detailed information and plays a role in image-guided sampling. **Flowchart 2** shows imaging and management algorithm in a patient suspected to have pancreatic malignancy. Structured reporting improves evaluation and provides accurate assessment of the status of vessels, and better communication with the surgeon.

NCCN panel recommends that all diagnostic and surgical management decisions must involve multidisciplinary consultations in high volume centers. Imaging also plays a role in post-therapy response assessment and this is the field of active research, especially on newer and functional imaging modalities.

REFERENCES

1. Tamm EP, Balachandran A, Bhosale PR, Katz MH, Fleming JB, Lee JH, et al. Imaging of pancreatic adenocarcinoma: update on staging/resectability. Radiol Clin North Am. 2012;50(3): 407-28.
2. Jeffrey RB. Pancreatic cancer: radiologic imaging. Gastroenterol Clin North Am. 2012;41(1):159-77.
3. NCCN Clinical Practice Guidelines in Oncology. Pancreatic Adenocarcinoma. Version 1.2016. nccn.org.
4. Allema JH, Reinders ME, van Gulik TM, van Leeuwen DJ, Verbeek PC, de Wit LT, et al. Results of pancreaticoduodenectomy for ampullary carcinoma and analysis of prognostic factors for survival. Surgery. 1995;117(3):247-53.
5. Almoguera C, Shibata D, Forrester K, Martin J, Arnheim N, Perucho M. Most human carcinomas of the exocrine pancreas contain mutant c-K-ras genes. Cell. 1988;53(4):549-54.
6. Kinney T. Evidence-based imaging of pancreatic malignancies. Surg Clin North Am. 2010;90(2):235-49.
7. Kaneko OF, Lee DM, Wong J, Kadell BM, Reber HA, Lu DSK, et al. Performance of multidetector computed tomographic angiography in determining surgical resectability of pancreatic head adenocarcinoma. J Comput Assist Tomogr. 2010;34(5):732-8.
8. Schima W, Ba-Ssalamah A, Goetzinger P, Scharitzer M, Koelblinger C. State-of-the-art magnetic resonance imaging of pancreatic cancer. Top Magn Reson Imaging TMRI. 2007;18(6):421-9.
9. Kartalis N, Manikis GC, Loizou L, Albiin N, Zöllner FG, Del Chiaro M, et al. Diffusion-weighted MR imaging of pancreatic cancer: A comparison of mono-exponential, bi-exponential and non-Gaussian kurtosis models. Eur J Radiol Open. 2016;3:79-85.
10. Kawada N, Tanaka S. Elastography for the pancreas: Current status and future perspective. World J Gastroenterol. 2016;22(14): 3712-24.
11. Iglesias-Garcia J, Larino-Noia J, Abdulkader I, Forteza J, Dominguez-Munoz JE. EUS elastography for the characterization of solid pancreatic masses. Gastrointest Endosc. 2009;70(6):1101-8.

12. Gonçalves B, Soares JB, Bastos P. Endoscopic Ultrasound in the diagnosis and staging of pancreatic cancer. GE Port J Gastroenterol. 2015;22(4):161-71.
13. Klauss M, Stiller W, Fritz F, Kieser M, Werner J, Kauczor HU, et al. Computed tomography perfusion analysis of pancreatic carcinoma. J Comput Assist Tomogr. 2012;36(2):237-42.
14. Yadav AK, Sharma R, Kandasamy D, Pradhan RK, Garg PK, Bhalla AS, et al. Perfusion CT—can it resolve the pancreatic carcinoma versus mass forming chronic pancreatitis conundrum? Pancreatol Off J Int Assoc Pancreatol IAP Al. 2016.
15. Klauss M, Stiller W, Pahn G, Fritz F, Kieser M, Werner J, et al. Dual-energy perfusion-CT of pancreatic adenocarcinoma. Eur J Radiol. 2013;82(2):208-14.
16. Kang KM, Lee JM, Yoon JH, Kiefer B, Han JK, Choi BI. Intravoxel incoherent motion diffusion-weighted MR Imaging for characterization of focal pancreatic lesions. Radiology. 2013;270(2):444-53.
17. Klauss M, Lemke A, Grünberg K, Simon D, Re TJ, Wente MN, et al. Intravoxel incoherent motion MRI for the differentiation between mass forming chronic pancreatitis and pancreatic carcinoma. Invest Radiol. 2011;46(1):57-63.
18. Re TJ, Lemke A, Klauss M, Laun FB, Simon D, Grünberg K, et al. Enhancing pancreatic adenocarcinoma delineation in diffusion derived intravoxel incoherent motion f-maps through automatic vessel and duct segmentation. Magn Reson Med. 2011;66(5):1327-32.
19. Kim JH, Park SH, Yu ES, Kim M-H, Kim J, Byun JH, et al. Visually isoattenuating pancreatic adenocarcinoma at dynamic-enhanced CT: frequency, clinical and pathologic characteristics, and diagnosis at imaging examinations. Radiology. 2010;257(1): 87-96.
20. Prokesch RW, Chow LC, Beaulieu CF, Bammer R, Jeffrey RB. Isoattenuating pancreatic adenocarcinoma at multi-detector row CT: secondary signs. Radiology. 2002;224(3):764-8.
21. Park MJ, Kim YK, Choi S, Rhim H, Lee WJ, Choi D. Preoperative detection of small pancreatic carcinoma: value of adding diffusion-weighted imaging to conventional MR imaging for improving confidence level. Radiology. 2014;273(2): 433-43.
22. Goodman M, Willmann JK, Jeffrey RB. Incidentally discovered solid pancreatic masses: imaging and clinical observations. Abdom Imaging. 2012;37(1):91-7.
23. Shanbhogue AKP, Fasih N, Surabhi VR, Doherty GP, Shanbhogue DKP, Sethi SK. A clinical and radiologic review of uncommon types and causes of pancreatitis. RadioGraphics. 2009;29(4): 1003-26.
24. Sharma R, Kandasamy D. Imaging of pancreatic cancer. In: Garg PK (Eds). ECAB clinical update—pancreatic tumors. 2013th edn. Elsevier Health Sciences.
25. Lee H, Lee JK, Kang SS, Choi D, Jang KT, Kim JH, et al. Is there any clinical or radiologic feature as a preoperative marker for differentiating mass-forming pancreatitis from early-stage pancreatic adenocarcinoma? Hepatogastroenterology. 2007;54(79):2134-40.
26. Ichikawa T, Sou H, Araki T, Arbab AS, Yoshikawa T, Ishigame K, et al. Duct-penetrating sign at MRCP: usefulness for differentiating inflammatory pancreatic mass from pancreatic carcinomas. Radiology. 2001;221(1):107-16.
27. Coakley FV, Hanley-Knutson K, Mongan J, Barajas R, Bucknor M, Qayyum A. Pancreatic imaging mimics: Part 1, imaging mimics of pancreatic adenocarcinoma. AJR. 2012;199(2):301-8.
28. Sahani DV, Sainani NI, Deshpande V, Shaikh MS, Frinkelberg DL, Fernandez-del Castillo C. Autoimmune pancreatitis: disease evolution, staging, response assessment, and CT features that predict response to corticosteroid therapy. Radiology. 2009;250(1):118-29.
29. Choi SY, Kim SH, Kang TW, Song KD, Park HJ, Choi YH. Differentiating mass-forming autoimmune pancreatitis from pancreatic ductal adenocarcinoma on the basis of contrast-enhanced MRI and DWI findings. Am J Roentgenol. 2016;206(2):291-300.
30. Blasbalg R, Baroni RH, Costa DN, Machado MCC. MRI features of groove pancreatitis. AJR. 2007;189(1):73-80.
31. Al-Hawary MM, Francis IR, Chari ST, Fishman EK, Hough DM, Lu DS, et al. Pancreatic ductal adenocarcinoma radiology reporting template: consensus statement of the Society of Abdominal Radiology and the American Pancreatic Association. Radiology. 2014;270(1):248-60.
32. Callery MP, Chang KJ, Fishman EK, Talamonti MS, William Traverso L, Linehan DC. Pretreatment assessment of resectable and borderline resectable pancreatic cancer: expert consensus statement. Ann Surg Oncol. 2009;16(7):1727-33.
33. Lall CG, Howard TJ, Skandarajah A, DeWitt JM, Aisen AM, Sandrasegaran K. New concepts in staging and treatment of locally advanced pancreatic head cancer. AJR. 2007;189(5):1044-50.
34. Ishikawa O, Ohigashi H, Imaoka S, Furukawa H, Sasaki Y, Fujita M, et al. Preoperative indications for extended pancreatectomy for locally advanced pancreas cancer involving the portal vein. Ann Surg. 1992;215(3):231-6.
35. Raptopoulos V, Steer ML, Sheiman RG, Vrachliotis TG, Gougoutas CA, Movson JS. The use of helical CT and CT angiography to predict vascular involvement from pancreatic cancer: correlation with findings at surgery. AJR. 1997;168(4):971-7.
36. Chun YS, Milestone BN, Watson JC, Cohen SJ, Burtness B, Engstrom PF, et al. Defining venous involvement in borderline resectable pancreatic cancer. Ann Surg Oncol. 2010;17(11):2832-8.
37. Hough TJ, Raptopoulos V, Siewert B, Matthews JB. Teardrop superior mesenteric vein: CT sign for unresectable carcinoma of the pancreas. AJR. 1999;173(6):1509-12.
38. McNulty NJ, Francis IR, Platt JF, Cohan RH, Korobkin M, Gebremariam A. Multidetector row helical CT of the pancreas: effect of contrast-enhanced multiphasic imaging on enhancement of the pancreas, peripancreatic vasculature, and pancreatic adenocarcinoma. Radiology. 2001;220(1):97-102.
39. Pietryga JA, Morgan DE. Imaging preoperatively for pancreatic adenocarcinoma. J Gastrointest Oncol. 2015;6(4):343-57.
40. Li H, Zeng MS, Zhou KR, Jin DY, Lou WH. Pancreatic adenocarcinoma: the different CT criteria for peripancreatic major arterial and venous invasion. J Comput Assist Tomogr. 2005;29(2):170-5.
41. Sai M, Mori H, Kiyonaga M, Kosen K, Yamada Y, Matsumoto S. Peripancreatic lymphatic invasion by pancreatic carcinoma: evaluation with multidetector row CT. Abdom Imaging. 2010;35(2):154-62.
42. Brennan DDD, Zamboni GA, Raptopoulos VD, Kruskal JB. Comprehensive preoperative assessment of pancreatic adenocarcinoma with 64-section volumetric CT. Radiogr Rev Publ Radiol Soc N Am Inc. 2007;27(6):1653-66.
43. Makino I, Kitagawa H, Ohta T, Nakagawara H, Tajima H, Ohnishi I, et al. Nerve plexus invasion in pancreatic cancer: spread patterns on histopathologic and embryological analyses. Pancreas. 2008;37(4):358-65.
44. Deshmukh SD, Willmann JK, Jeffrey RB. Pathways of extrapancreatic perineural invasion by pancreatic adenocarcinoma: evaluation with 3D volume-rendered MDCT imaging. Am J Roentgenol. 2010;194(3):668-74.
45. Yusoff IF, Mendelson RM, Edmunds SEJ, Ramsay D, Cullingford GL, Fletcher DR, et al. Preoperative assessment of pancreatic malignancy using endoscopic ultrasound. Abdom Imaging. 2003;28(4):556-62.
46. Pisters PW, Lee JE, Vauthey JN, Charnsangavej C, Evans DB. Laparoscopy in the staging of pancreatic cancer. Br J Surg. 2001;88(3):325-37.

47. Tao L, Zhang L, Xiu D, Yuan C, Ma Z, Jiang B. Prognostic significance of K-ras mutations in pancreatic cancer: a meta-analysis. World J Surg Oncol. 2016;14:146.
48. Katz MHG, Fleming JB, Bhosale P, Varadhachary G, Lee JE, Wolff R, et al. Response of borderline resectable pancreatic cancer to neoadjuvant therapy is not reflected by radiographic indicators. Cancer. 2012;118(23):5749-56.
49. Bockhorn M, Uzunoglu FG, Adham M, Imrie C, Milicevic M, Sandberg AA, et al. Borderline resectable pancreatic cancer: a consensus statement by the International Study Group of Pancreatic Surgery (ISGPS). Surgery. 2014;155(6):977-88.
50. Brook OR, Brook A, Vollmer CM, Kent TS, Sanchez N, Pedrosa I. Structured reporting of multiphasic CT for pancreatic cancer: potential effect on staging and surgical planning. Radiology. 2015;274(2):464-72.

CHAPTER

114

Cystic Pancreatic Tumors and Neuroendocrine Tumors of Pancreas

Jyoti Kumar, Alpana Manchanda, Sapna Singh

CYSTIC PANCREATIC TUMORS

Cystic pancreatic tumors are a diverse group of lesions with different clinical presentation, histology, biologic behavior and prognostic implications. Imaging plays a key role in stratifying the risk in these patients, and hence, deciding upon the treatment options and appropriate follow-up strategy. Most of these tumors are picked up incidentally and increasing use of cross-sectional imaging techniques and their improved resolution have led to a 20-fold increase in the incidental detection of these lesions.[1] This has led to an increase in surgery for these tumors. In many instances, these resected lesions turn out to be benign and the surgery is actually unjustified.[2] Few of these tumors, especially when large, have characteristic imaging features that can aid in differentiation of these cystic masses. However, smaller lesions can have indeterminate findings on imaging and management protocols may still be confusing.[3]

Imaging Modalities

Both multidetector computed tomography (MDCT) and magnetic resonance imaging (MRI) are widely used in characterizing the cystic lesions of pancreas. MDCT is usually the primary modality of investigation with high spatial and temporal resolution. Its wide availability and ease of interpretation are the other advantages. CT also shows calcification within lesions to a greater advantage than MRI. In various studies, the accuracy of MDCT (56–85%) has been found to be comparable to MRI in characterizing cystic pancreatic lesions.[4-6]

Magnetic resonance imaging (MRI), on the other hand, has superior soft tissue and contrast resolution. Hence, it is an excellent technique to assess internal morphological features of cystic tumors, especially small cystic tumors measuring <3 cm.[7] Three-dimensional magnetic resonance cholangiopancreaticography (MRCP) is an effective tool in detecting communication of the lesion with the pancreatic duct. Sainini et al. showed a higher accuracy of MR in revealing ductal communication as compared to CT (100% versus 75% sensitivity).[7] As MR does not involve radiation, it is the preferable modality for follow-up of young patients with cystic pancreatic tumors.[8]

Endoscopic ultrasound (EUS) is an excellent technique to depict internal morphology of cystic lesions, showing internal septations and nodularity to a greater advantage, and hence assessing the aggressiveness of the pathology. It also enables sampling of fluid and solid contents of the lesion.[9] However, this is an invasive technique and highly operator dependent. It allows limited evaluation of the pancreatic tail region. It is used predominantly when CT and MR findings are indeterminate and in asymptomatic cysts as symptomatic cysts would anyways warrant a resection.

Clinical Presentation

Most of these cystic tumors are picked up incidentally during work-up for other nonrelated conditions.[9] Symptomatic cystic tumors mostly present with abdominal lump and pain. Jaundice and pancreatitis may result from biliary/pancreatic ductal communication. If it is an advanced cystic malignancy, patients may present with symptoms of pain, weight loss or jaundice.[3,9]

Classification

Cystic tumors of pancreas may be classified into relatively common cystic tumors and rare cystic tumors **(Table 1)**. The common cystic tumors may be serous cystadenoma, mucinous neoplasms (mucinous cystic neoplasm and intraductal papillary mucinous neoplasm) or solid pseudopapillary neoplasm. The rare cystic tumors include lymphangioma, teratoma, paraganglioma or solid tumors which have undergone cystic degeneration such as adenocarcinoma, neuroendocrine tumors and metastases.[10]

Morphological Classification

On the basis of imaging appearances, pancreatic cystic lesions can be classified into four major categories—unilocular appearance, microcystic lesion, macrocystic lesion and cysts with solid component **(Figs. 1A to D) (Table 2)**.[10]

Unilocular cysts include cysts with no internal septation, calcification or nodularity. Although inflammatory pseudocysts are the prototype example, cystic tumors that may uncommonly have a unilocular appearance are intraductal papillary mucinous neoplasms (IPMNs)

TABLE 1: Classification of cystic pancreatic tumors.

Common Cystic Tumors
- Serous cystadenoma
- *Mucinous neoplasms*:
  - Mucinous cystic neoplasm
  - Intraductal papillary mucinous neoplasm
- Solid pseudopapillary neoplasm

Rare Cystic Tumors
- Lymphangioma
- Teratoma
- Paraganglioma
- Cystic degeneration of solid tumors such as adenocarcinoma, neuroendocrine tumors and metastases

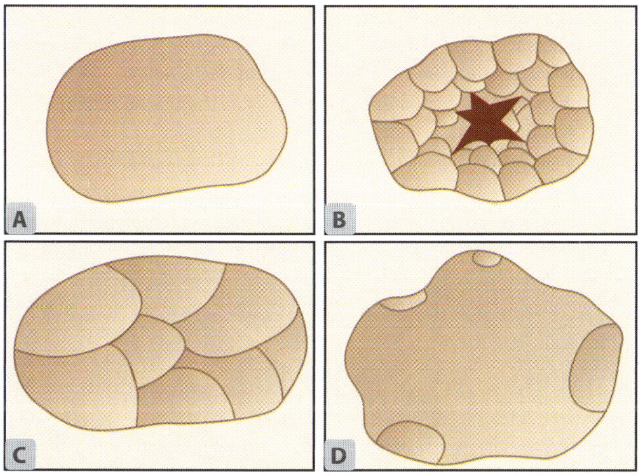

FIGS. 1A TO D: Morphological classification of cystic lesions: (A) Unilocular cyst with no internal septations; (B) Microcystic appearance with formation of multiple small cysts (>6 in number, <2 cm in size); (C) Macrocystic lesion with larger and fewer cysts; (D) Cyst with solid mural nodule.

and serous cystadenoma. Since pseudocysts are the most common cystic lesions of pancreas, correlation with history of acute or chronic pancreatitis is of paramount importance. Microcystic lesions are cysts with internal septations resulting in formation of mutiple tiny cysts which are usually more than 6 in number and <2 cm in size. The main example of a microcystic lesion is serous cystadenoma. Macrocystic lesions are multilocular cysts with fewer loculi (<6 cm) which are larger in size (>2 cm). The characteristic example of a macrocystic lesion is mucinous cystic neoplasm (MCN) and side branch IPMN. Cystic lesions with a solid component may be unilocular or multilocular. Mucinous cystic neoplasms or intraductal papillary mucinous neoplasm may have this appearance.[10]

Serous Cystadenoma (Table 3)

Serous cystadenoma accounts for 1–2% of exocrine pancreatic tumors. About 80% of these lesions occur in older women, with an average age of 65 years.[11–13] There is a slight preponderance of these tumors in the head region but they can be seen to

TABLE 2: Morphological classification of cystic pancreatic tumors.

- Unilocular
- Microcystic
- Macrocystic
- Cystic lesions with solid component

TABLE 3: Key points of serous cystadenoma.

- Mostly in older women; average age 65 years
- Increased incidence in von Hippel–Lindau disease
- Typically microcystic in appearance with lobulated outline
- Central scar seen in 30% cases and when seen is pathognomonic
- Only hypervascular cystic tumor of pancreas
- Benign tumor with no malignant potential

occur throughout the pancreas. These lesions are mostly asymptomatic, and hence can become large at presentation. The larger lesions may result in mass effect and nonspecific abdominal discomfort. Since these are benign lesions with no malignant potential, surgery is not indicated unless the large size (>4 cm) of the lesion mandates surgery because of its mass effect and resultant symptoms or rapid growth (approximately 2 cm/year).[14–16] In cases of von Hippel-Lindau disease, there may be an increased incidence of serous cystadenomas.[14]

These are typically microcystic lesions showing a honeycomb appearance on gross inspection. These are well-circumscribed lesions with lobulated outline and are not encapsulated. These fine external lobulations result from the larger cysts in the periphery of the lesion in this microcystic tumor. These lesions may have a central scar with or without stellate calcification. Although seen in only 30% of serous cystadenomas, it is considered pathognomonic when present.[9]

On ultrasound, these lesions are seen as lobulated lesions with hypoechoic cysts and hyperechoic fibrous component. Calcification may be seen within the fibrous scar when present. However, the lesion may appear solid due to multiple interfaces of the septations within the lesion.[3]

On CT, the lobulated microcystic appearance can be appreciated. Central stellate scar with calcification may be seen **(Fig. 2)**. The lesion may have a solid appearance because of the tiny size of these cyst separated by multiple septations. On contrast administration, the septae and scar enhance avidly with persistent enhancement on delayed images. Absence of ductal obstruction or invasion of surrounding structures confirms the benign nature of these lesions as these tumors displace surrounding structures rather than invade them.

MRI can aid in delineating the microcystic appearance of these tumors to a greater advantage when these are seen as high signal intensity structures on T2-weighted images **(Figs. 3A to C)**. The fibrous component is seen as hypointense on T1- and T2-weighted images. On contrast administration, the scar and septae show intense enhancement on the arterial phase with persistent enhancement on the delayed images, which helps to differentiate these tumors from hypervascular neuroendocrine tumors of pancreas which show washout on delayed images.[3]

Uncommonly, serous cystadenomas may have a macrocystic or oligocystic appearance (in less than 10% of cases) **(Fig. 4)**.[10] In these cases, mucinous cystic neoplasm is a close differential. In a study by Cohen-Scali et al. presence of a combination of any 3 of the following imaging features could help distinguish between the two entities with a specificity of 100%—location in head region, lobulated outline, wall thickness <2 mm and absence of wall enhancement. These findings favor the diagnosis of serous cystadenoma.[17]

Mucinous Cystic Neoplasm (Table 4)

Mucinous cystadenoma accounts for approximately 2.5% of exocrine pancreatic tumors.[18] Mucinous cystic neoplasms are most frequently encountered in middle-aged women with an average age of 50 years, slightly lesser than that of serous cystadenomas. These are known to occur almost exclusively in women with a frequency of approximately 99.7%.[3,19]

Patients may be symptomatic due to mass effect caused by the neoplasm although they are asymptomatic in 75% cases.[20] These neoplasms have a malignant potential and hence are considered surgical lesions. On histology, these could range from benign mucinous cystadenoma, borderline mucinous cystic tumor, mucinous neoplasm with carcinoma *in situ* to a frankly malignant mucinous cystadenocarcinoma. The stromal elements of these tumors are similar to ovarian stroma unlike IPMNs which have ductal origin stroma. Sampling of the lesion may not be an accurate method of differentiating between benign and malignant lesions as

TABLE 4: Key points of mucinous cystic neoplasm.

- Almost exclusively in women
- Average age 50 years, slightly lesser than serous cystadenoma
- Typically macrocystic in appearance with smooth outline
- Curvilinear calcification is considered specific for the diagnosis
- Thick wall, mural or septal calcification and internal enhancing soft tissue component are predictive of malignancy
- Unlike IPMNs which are also macrocystic, there is no ductal communication

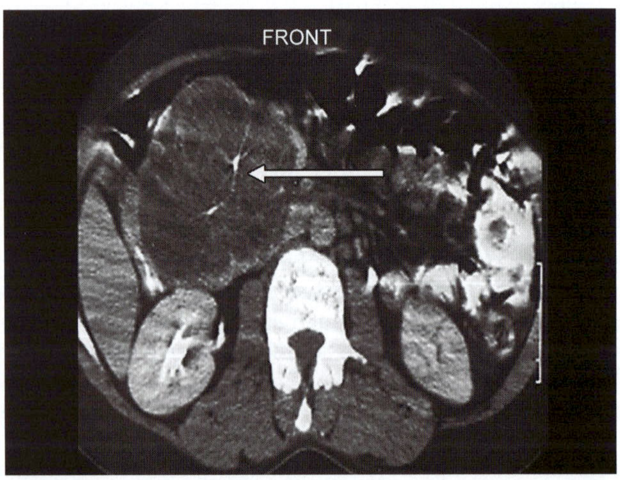

FIG. 2: Serous cystadenoma in a 62-year-old woman: Axial CECT image reveals a microcystic lesion with lobulated outline in the pancreatic head region. Central scar with stellate calcfication (arrow) is seen in this case which is pathognomonic for the lesion.

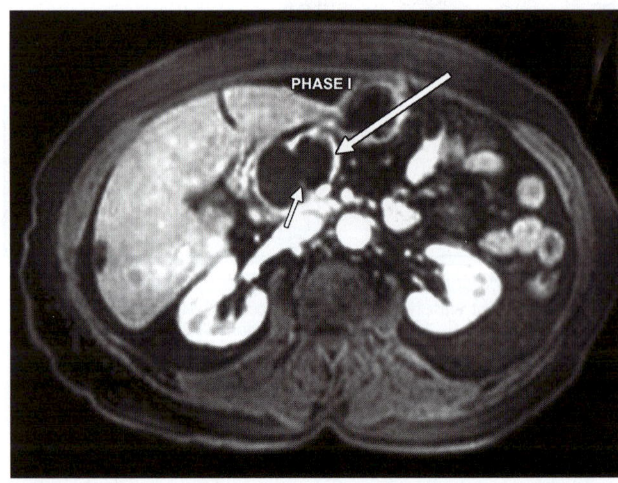

FIG. 4: Macrocystic serous cystadenoma in a 55-year-old man: A lobulated macrocystic lesion is seen in the head region of pancreas (long arrow) on this axial T1-weighted postgadolinium MR image. Thin septal enhancement (short thin arrow) is seen.

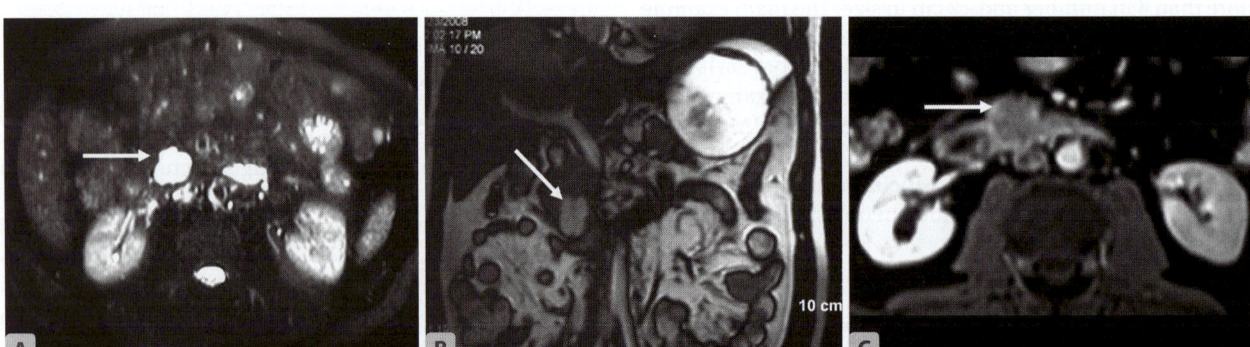

FIGS 3A TO C: Serous cystadenoma in a 60-year-old male: A microcystic lesion with lobulated outline is seen on axial HASTE (A) and coronal True FISP images (B) with internal septations within. Postcontrast arterial phase image (C) reveals subtle enhancement of the septae. (HASTE, Half-fourier acquisition single-shot turbo spin-echo; True FISP, True fast imaging with steady state precession).

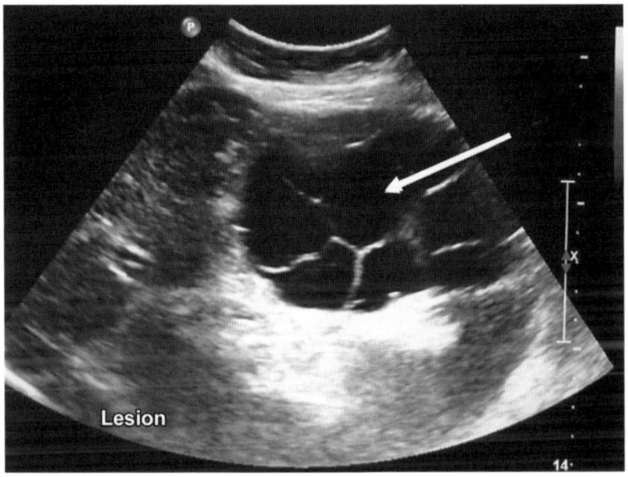

FIG. 5: Mucinous cystic neoplasm in a 52-year-old woman: US images shows a well-marginated macrocystic mass arising from the pancreatic tail.

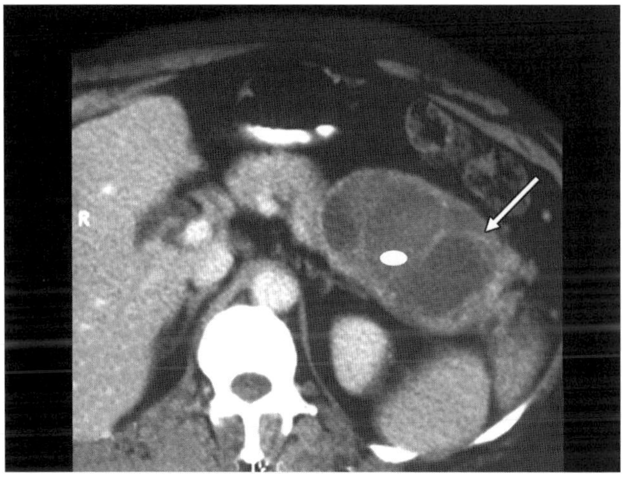

FIG. 6: Mucinous cystic neoplasm in a 51-year-old woman: Axial CECT image depicts a well-circumscribed macrocystic lesion in pancreatic tail (arrow) with variable attenuation of the internal contents of the cyst (dot) which could be due to proteinaceous contents.

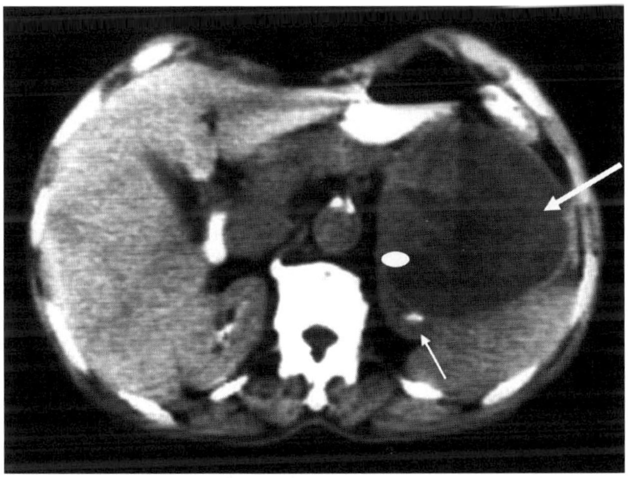

FIG. 7: Mucinous cystic neoplasm in a 48-year-old woman: CECT image showing a unilocular thin-walled cystic mass in the pancreatic tail (arrow) with small peripheral calcification in the inferior part of the cyst (short thin arrow).

different parts of the lesion may have different configuration of epithelium.[21]

These neoplasms are most commonly macrocystic in appearance. On ultrasound, a well-circumscribed multicystic mass is often seen which may have septations, mural nodules or calcification **(Fig. 5)**. Rarely, debris or hemorrhage may be seen within these cysts.[3]

On CT, these are well-defined encapsulated lesions with smooth outline **(Fig. 6)**. Calcification may be seen along the septae or wall of the lesion **(Fig. 7)**. This may be seen in approximately 15% of cases. Curvilinear calcification along the wall of the lesion is considered specific for this diagnosis.[22] On contrast administration, the wall is seen to enhance along with septae and mural nodules. In a study by Procacci et al.[23] the following imaging features were predictive of malignancy—thick wall, mural or septal calcification and internal enhancing soft tissue component.

MR can better delineate the internal morphology of the lesion. On T2-weighted imaging, the lesion is usually seen as hyperintense fluid-filled multiloculated lesion with hypointense wall. The signal intensity of the cyst, however, may be variable due to proteinaceous contents of the cyst. The wall and septations enhance on contrast administration, more so on the delayed images due to fibrous nature of the wall **(Figs. 8A and B)**. If the lesion results in pancreatic ductal obstruction, concomitant pancreatitis may result which may be seen as glandular atrophy, ductal dilatation and decreased signal on T1-weighted images with delayed enhancement.[3,24]

Side branch IPMNs are a close-imaging differential diagnosis. Patient demographics and absence of ductal communication in MCNs can help in differentiating the two entities. Although they do not communicate with ductal system, they can result in ductal obstruction, especially when aggressive. MCNs are most commonly encountered in body and tail region of pancreas wheras the uncinate process is the typical location of side branch IPMN.[9,21]

Intraductal Papillary Mucinous Neoplasm (Table 5)

Intraductal papillary mucinous neoplasms (IPMNs) are also mucinous tumors arising from ductal epithelium and may be main duct, side branch or mixed type. Around 70% of these lesions are encountered in men with a mean age of 65 years.[25,26]

These lesions have a variable degree of aggressiveness with risk of malignancy being higher in main duct and mixed type IPMNs than side branch IPMNs.[27,28] The pathological spectrum ranges from benign adenomas to invasive carcinomas.

Main duct IPMN does not fall into the category of a cystic pancreatic neoplasm and mainly presents as ductal dilatation. It is the side branch IPMN which generally presents as a pleomorphic cystic lesion communicating with the pancreatic duct. The cystic lesion is actually the mucin distended side branch which is affected by the pathology. Communication with pancreatic duct is the most important

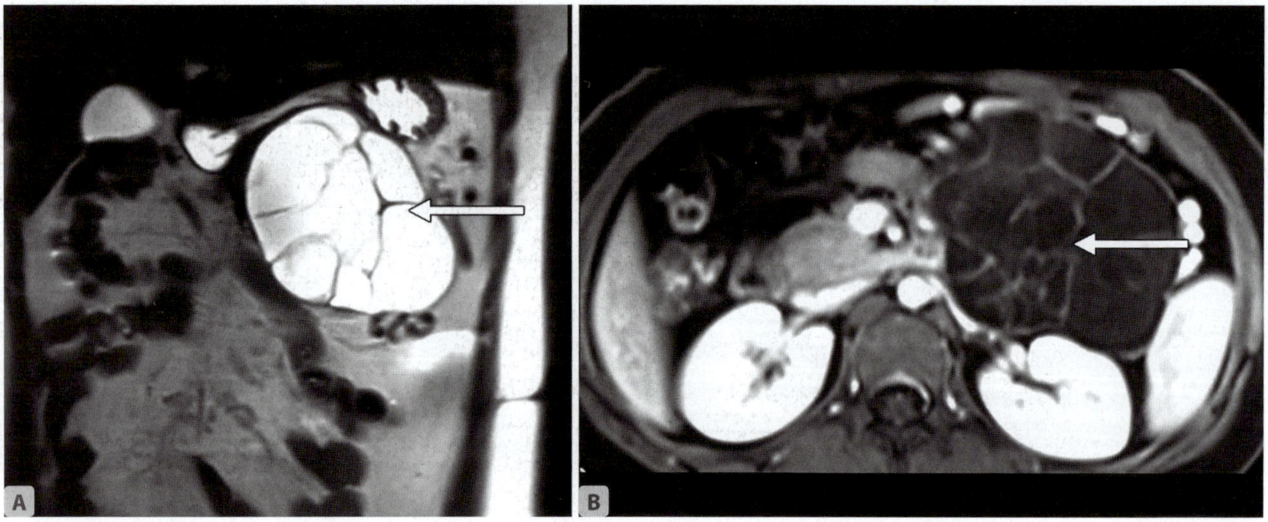

FIGS. 8A AND B: Macrocystic neoplasm in a 52-year-old woman: Coronal HASTE (A) and axial postgadolinium (B) images reveal a well-circumscribed macrocystic neoplasm in the tail region of pancreas with enhancing septae.

TABLE 5: Key points of intraductal papillary mucinous neoplasm.

- Around 70% are seen in men with an average age of 65 years
- Can be main duct, side branch or combined type
- Side branch IPMNs present as cystic pancreatic lesions
- Uncinate process is the classical site of side branch IPMN
- Communication with pancreatic duct is pathognomonic of this cystic tumor
- Copious mucin extruding from bulging papilla on endoscopy is highly suggestive
- Side branch lesion of size >3 cm, main duct component, enhancing soft tissue, enhancing MPD wall and dilatation of CBD are pointers towards aggressive nature

(MPD: main pancreatic duct; CBD: common bile duct)

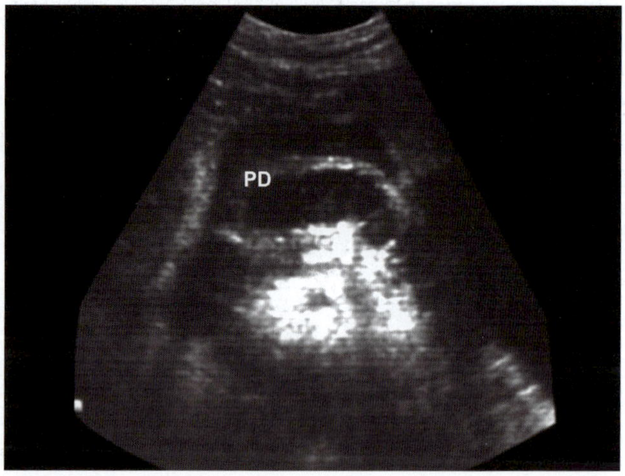

FIG. 9: Main duct IPMN in a 55-year-old male: US image depicts a markedly dilated main pancreatic duct with few-filling defects within.

imaging feature which is in contrast to other cystic neoplasm of pancreas. Serous cystadenoma, mucinous cystic neoplasm or solid pseudopapillary neoplasm generally do not show any communication with the pancreatic duct.[21]

On ultrasound, main duct IPMN is seen as dilatation of pancreatic main duct **(Fig. 9)** whereas a well-defined cystic mass may be seen in the case of a side branch IPMN. Communication of the cystic lesion with pancreatic duct cannot be appreciated on ultrasound in most cases. Other ancillary features such as mural nodularity, mucin globules or septations may be seen on ultrasound depending on the aggressive nature of the lesion. As ultrasound features are most often nonspecific, further imaging is required to evaluate these lesions.[3,21]

On CT, a side branch IPMN appears as a pleomorphic cystic lesion most often in the uncinate process, which is the classical site **(Figs. 10A and B)**. Communication with pancreatic duct is best seen on curved multiplanar reformatted images. Main duct IPMN is seen as diffuse or segmental dilatation of the pancreatic duct **(Fig. 11)**. Septations, and filling defects may be seen within the dilated duct **(Figs. 12A to C)**. The filling defects may either be mucin globules or soft tissue component associated with a more aggressive lesion; these may be differentiated using contrast-enhanced imaging, where soft tissue enhances and mucin globules do not enhance.[3,21]

MRI with MRCP remains the modality of choice to depict communication of the lesion with the pancreatic duct. The side branch lesion is seen as hyperintense on T2-weighted images and hypointense on T1-weighted images. In main duct IPMN, the duct is dilated with no obvious obstructive lesion or narrowing. The duct may be dilated diffusely or only involving a segment. Papillary bulging may be evident due to copious mucin production by the tumor.[12] Copious mucin extruding from a bulging papilla seen on correlative endoscopic examination is considered highly suggestive of the diagnosis.[29] Combined duct IPMNs are seen as dilatation of both main pancreatic duct and its side branches.

Various features on imaging can be the pointers towards the aggressive nature of the pathology. These include main duct dilatation >10 mm, diffuse or multifocal involvement of main pancreatic duct, cystic lesion of size more than 3

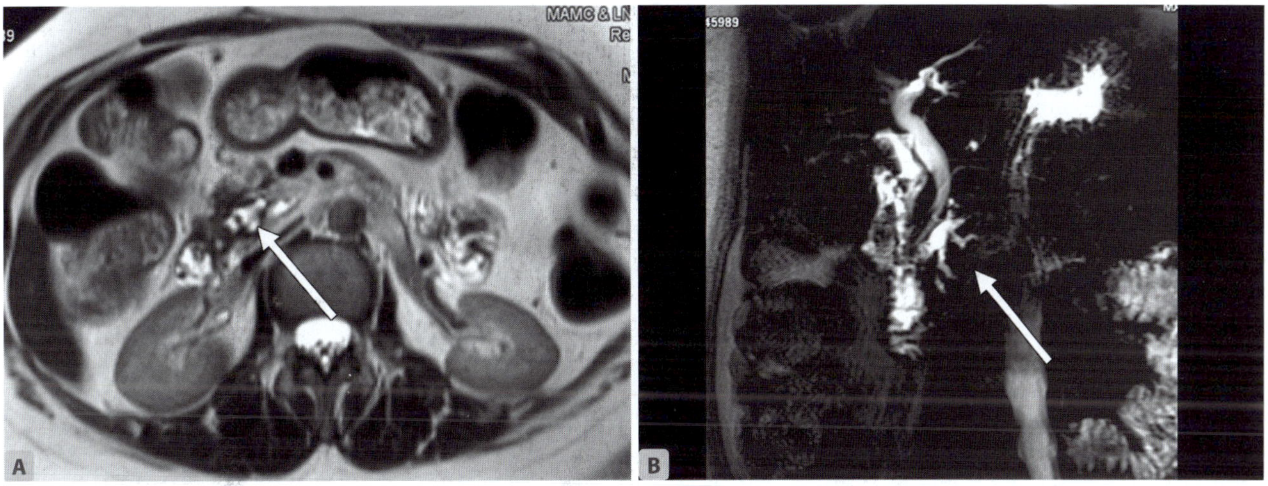

FIGS. 10A AND B: Side branch IPMN in 56-year-old woman: Axial HASTE image (A) reveals multiple cystic lesions in the region of head and uncinate process (arrow). On rare thick slab coronal image (B), multiple dilated side branches (arrow) are seen in pancreatic head region communicating with the pancreatic duct.

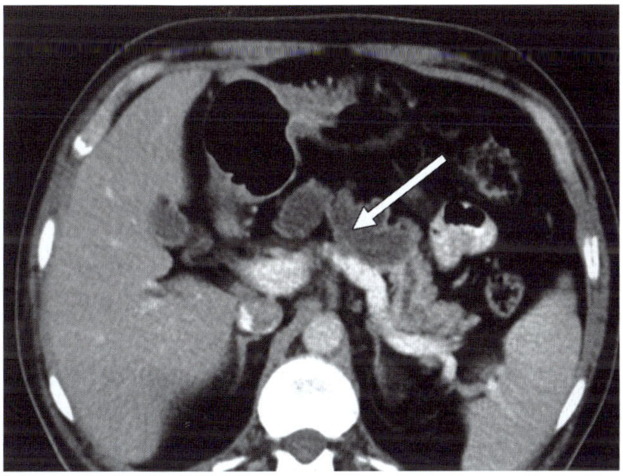

FIG. 11: Main duct IPMN in a 55-year-old male: There is segmental dilatation of the main pancreatic duct (arrow) in the pancreatic body region in this case of segmental main duct IPMN.

cm in case of a side branch lesion, increasing size of these cystic lesions, presence of enhancing soft tissue component or enhancing MPD wall, and dilatation of common bile duct.[3]

Main duct IPMN can be confused with chronic pancreatitis, which can also have duct dilatation and parenchymal atrophy. Presence of irregular beaded appearance of duct with stricture formation and presence of ductal calculi favor the diagnosis of chronic pancreatitis. Bulging papilla and enhancing nodules within the lesion are pointers to the diagnosis of IPMN.

Solid Pseudopapillary Neoplasm (SPN) (Table 6)

This is a rare pancreatic tumor with approximately 1000 cases reported in literature.[30] This is seen to occur mostly in young women with a mean age of 25 years.[31] It is seen most often in the tail region of pancreas.[32]

This tumor is mostly asymptomatic and usually detected when large in size. The average size at detection is 9.3 cm.[33] Larger masses may present with symptoms due to mass effect. These are tumors with low malignant potential and vascular invasion and metastastic disease can be seen in aggressive cases. Treatment is generally surgery and survival rates are as high as 96% even with solid pseudopapillary carcinoma.[3]

On imaging, SPN is a well-demarcated encapsulated lesion. Ultrasound features are nonspecific with a large complex attenuation mass with or without through transmission **(Fig. 13)**.

On CT, these are seen as well-defined encapsulated masses which have a combination of solid and cystic components **(Fig. 14)**. Areas of hemorrhage are commonly seen. The capsule and solid component enhance on contrast administration.[31]

Areas of hemorrhage can be better seen on MR imaging, appearing hypointense on T2-weighted images and hyperintense on T1-weighted images.[31] Hemorrhagic and cystic degeneration is mostly seen in the central part of the lesion while solid component is seen at the periphery. The capsule can be seen as hypointense on T1- and T2-weighted images, which is a key feature on imaging. On contrast administration, solid portions are seen to progressively enhance.[3] Cantisani et al. reviewed 19 cases of SPN and found early and intense enhancement of the capsule which blends with the rest of the solid component during later phases,[34] in most cases of SPN.

UNCOMMON CYSTIC PANCREATIC TUMORS

Cystic Endocrine Tumors

Endocrine tumors are discussed in detail in the latter half of the chapter.

These are usually solid tumors which may undergo cystic or necrotic degeneration. Most of these cystic lesions

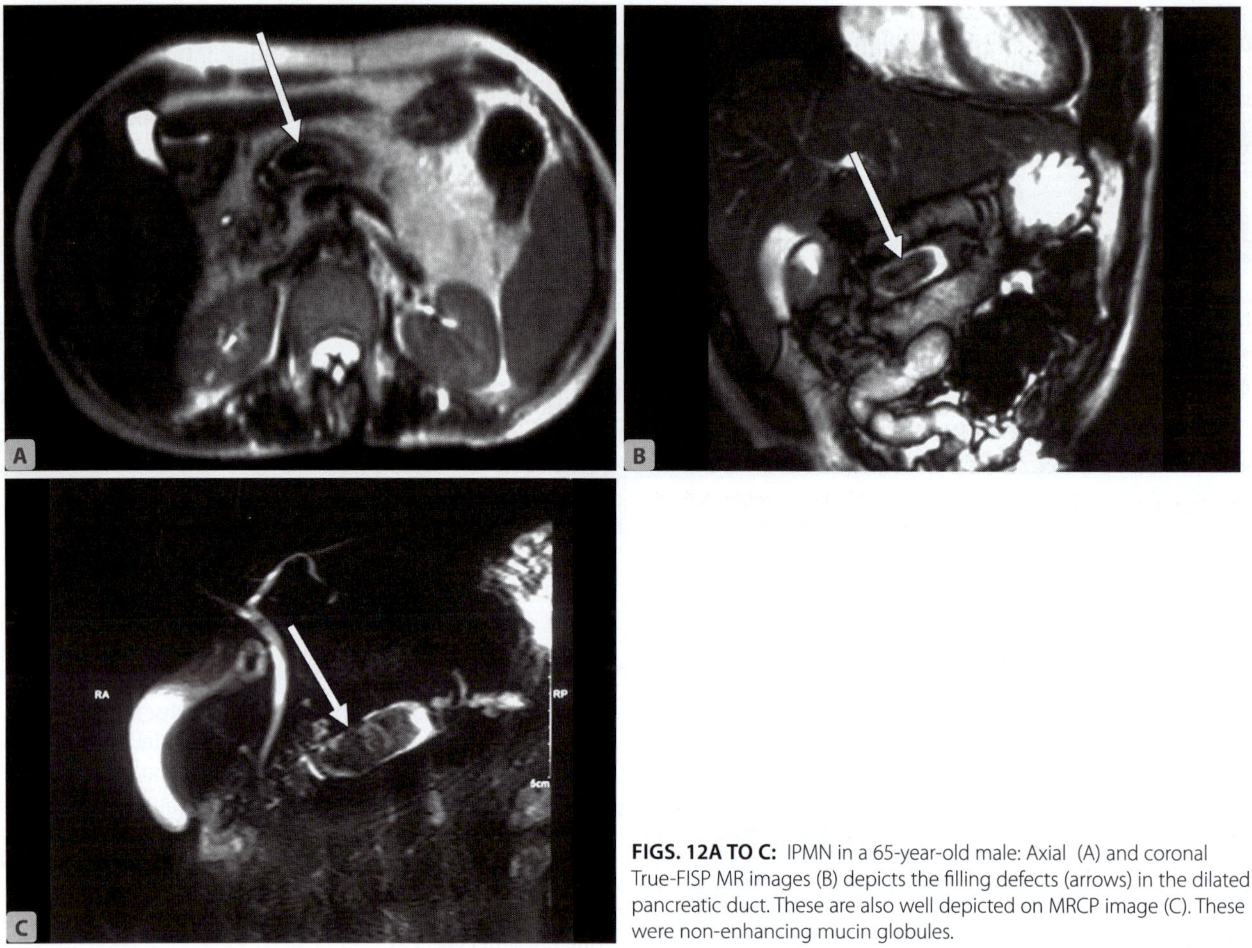

FIGS. 12A TO C: IPMN in a 65-year-old male: Axial (A) and coronal True-FISP MR images (B) depicts the filling defects (arrows) in the dilated pancreatic duct. These are also well depicted on MRCP image (C). These were non-enhancing mucin globules.

TABLE 6: Key points of solid pseudopapillary neoplasm.

- Mostly seen in young women with a mean age of 25 years
- Encapsulated lesion
- Combination of solid and cystic components
- Areas of hemorrhage commonly seen
- Tumors with low malignant potential and vascular invasion and metastastic disease can be seen in aggressive cases
- Survival rates are as high as 96% even with solid pseudopapillary carcinoma after complete surgical resection

are the nonsyndromic variety and if syndromic, they are the noninsulin producing tumors. These are generally larger at presentation than the solid variants. One fourth of these cases may be associated with multiple endocrine neoplasia type 1 (MEN I) and the rest are usually sporadic.[35]

These are mostly seen in the body and tail region of pancreas. Solid component of these masses can show hypervascular enhancement on imaging in the arterial phase although this may not be seen in all cases.

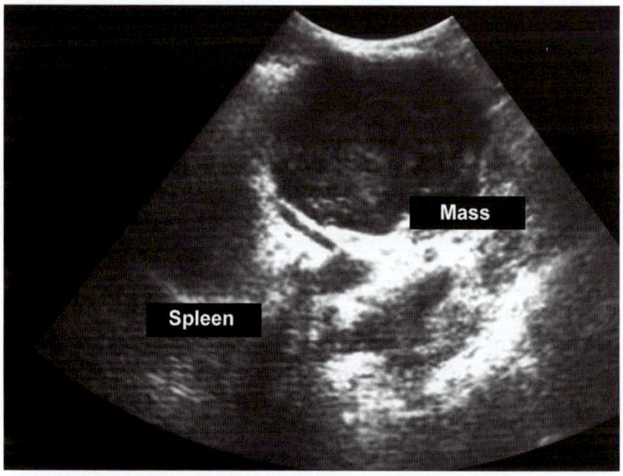

FIG. 13: Solid papillary epithelial neoplasm in a 32-year-old woman: Transverse sonogram image showing a mixed solid cystic mass in the pancreatic tail.

Cystic Metastases

Cystic metastases to pancreas most often arise from renal cell carcinoma and lung carcinoma. These are usually seen in late stages of disease when hematogenous metastases are also found at multiple other sites. An exception here is metastases from renal carcinoma where isolated pancreatic metastases have been encountered.[36]

Cystic Teratoma

Cystic teratoma is a very rare tumor with only few cases reported in literature. They can have varied imaging

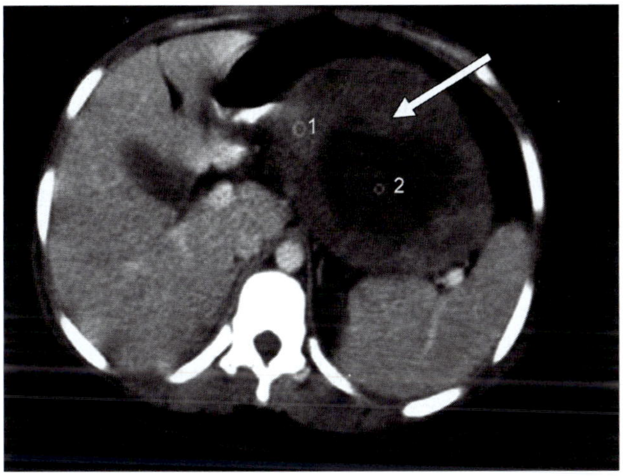

FIG. 14: Solid pseudopapillary neoplasm in a 32-year-old woman: Axial CECT image depicts a large well-circumscribed heterogeneous mass (arrow) with internal necrotic component in the region of pancreatic tail.

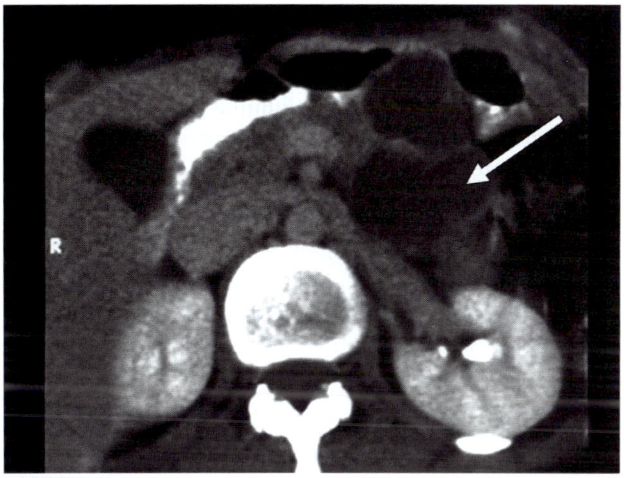

FIG. 15: Lymphangioma in a 30-year-old woman: CECT image shows a well-circumscribed multicystic mass (arrow) with thin septations within abutting the pancreatic tail.

appearances as they can be composed of up to 3 germinal layers. Teratomas are generally well-defined lesions with a variable internal appearance. These could range from predominantly cystic to mixed cystic solid to pure soft tissue masses. They may have fatty elements and areas of calcification. Various studies have shown that although these masses may abut vascular or biliary structures, they generally do not result in invasion or obstruction of these structures.[37,38]

Lymphangiomas

Although lymphangiomas are benign tumors, they may be locally invasive. Less than 1% of lymphangiomas may be seen in abdomen as most of them are encountered in neck and axilla.[39]

These are mostly seen in women with no age predilection. These are usually seen as multiloculated cystic lesions which may abut the pancreas or may be attached to pancreas by a pedicle **(Fig. 15)**. Hemorrhage or infection can occur within the cysts leading to complex attenuation or signal intensity.[3]

Endoscopic Ultrasound (EUS)/EUS-guided Fluid Characteristics of Cystic Lesions

In the evaluation of pancreatic cystic lesions, when the diagnosis is indeterminate on cross-sectional imaging, endoscopic ultrasound can be done to further characterize the internal morphology of these lesions. The diagnostic accuracy of endoscopic ultrasound has been found to be variable in various studies. The largest prospective study by by Brugge et al.[40] reported an accuracy of 50% in detecting septations and mural soft tissue on endoscopic ultrasound.

The additional benefit of EUS is guided fine needle aspiration of cyst fluid that may be done along with the diagnostic procedure. Although it increases the risk of certain complications such as pancreatitis and hemorrhage, it generally carries a favorable benefit to risk ratio.[41]

On fluid analysis, thick viscous fluid with high mucin content is seen in mucinous neoplasms (MCNs and IPMNs) while the fluid is thin and clear in serous cystadenoma.

The amylase levels may be raised in IPMNs (>2000 u/mL) as they involve the pancreatic ductal system and are typically low in serous cystadenomas (<250 U/L) and mucinous cystic neoplasms. Level of carcinoembryonic antigen (CEA) is raised in mucinous neoplasms (generally more than 192 mg/mL) and low in SCA (generally less than 5 ng/mL); hence CEA is used as tumor marker to differentiate between mucinous and non-mucinous cystic tumors. Other tumor markers such as CA 125 and CA 72-4 are raised in malignant transformation of mucinous neoplasms. Presence of glycogen is a specific marker for SCA.[3,8]

Management Guidelines

The treatment approach is usually selective, weighing the benefit-risk ratio in each patient. Various factors such as patient's age, tumor location and associated comorbidities need to be considered before a decision is made regarding patient management strategy. Surgery is generally indicated when there is a confident diagnosis of mucinous cystic neoplasm, IPMN with main duct component, side branch IPMN with features suspicious for malignancy, solid pseudopapillary neoplasm and serous cystadenoma when its size is larger than 4 cm or when it is symptomatic.[31] For asymptomatic SCA, annual imaging surveillance is generally considered optimal. Cystic lesions without septations/nodules can be followed up at 6 months and 1 year and then annually for 3 years. Cystic lesions with complex features can be followed up at more closer intervals.[3] On follow-up imaging, increasing cyst size, development of complex features within these cysts or new onset symptoms in this period are worrisome features that may point towards malignant transformation and resection may be considered in good surgical candidates.[31]

PANCREATIC NEUROENDOCRINE TUMORS (TABLE 7)

Pancreatic neuroendocrine tumors (pNETs) are rare tumors and account for only 1-2% of pancreatic neoplasms.[42] Since they are known not to arise from islet cells but from ductal cells that undergo endocrine differentiation, the term islet cell tumors is no longer preferred.[43] These are mostly seen between 40 and 60 years of age.[44]

These tumors may or may not be associated with symptoms due to hormone production, and hence, may be termed functioning and nonfunctioning respectively. The common functioning tumors may be insulinoma, gastrinoma, glucagonoma, VIPoma and somatastainoma.[44] While functioning tumors present with various hormonal symptoms, nonfunctioning tumors present with clinical features of mass effect or due to systemic metastases. Hence, functioning tumors are small at presentation, whereas non-functioning tumors are larger at presentation. It is these larger tumors that have a greater propensity to undergo necrotic/cystic change. Extensive cystic change with a thin peripheral rim can be encountered in 5-10% of cases.[44,45] They may be sporadic or associated with various syndromes such as multiple endocrine neoplasia I, von-Hippel Lindau syndrome, neurofibromatosis and tuberous sclerosis.[46]

As per the WHO 2010 classification system, these have been graded into well-differentiated grade 1 and grade 2 tumors and poorly differentiated grade 3 tumors. This grading has been done based on their mitotic count and cell proliferation (measured as Ki-67 labeling index).[47]

On US examination, these may be seen as well-defined hypoechoic masses. The larger tumors may be more heterogeneous with necrotic/cystic change. Presence of peripancreatic nodes and liver metastases are pointers towards malignancy. Hypervascular pattern may be noted on contrast-enhanced US.[44]

At CT, pNETs are well-circumscribed hypervascular tumors which enhance brightly on late arterial phase images **(Figs. 16A to C)**. However, they may not always be hypervascular, especially the nonfunctioning tumors.[45] Larger tumors can undergo necrotic/cystic degeneration. Cystic appearing neuroendocrine tumors can be differentiated from other cystic lesions of pancreas on the basis of the hypervascular nature of the peripheral rim. This hypervascular rim may be seen in 90% of cystic pNETs in a study by Ligneau et al.[48] In various studies, it has been shown that arterial phase images have a higher sensitivity for detecting pNETs (83–89%) than venous phase images (11–76%).[49,50] However, some tumors may only be seen on venous phase images.[44] Calcification may also be seen in pNETs and is more frequent in nonfunctioning tumors.[45] Lymph node and liver metastases may be seen in malignant pNETs and these are also hypervascular in nature, and hence, more appreciable on arterial phase images.[44]

On MRI, pNETs appear hypointense to the pancreatic parenchyma on T1-weighted images and hyperintense on T2 WI. Tumors with more fibrous content may have intermediate or hypointense signal on T2-WI. pNETs are generally seen as hypervascular masses with homogeneous, heterogeneous or rim enhancement. Heterogeneous/rim enhancement is seen in necrotic tumors. Liver metastases are hypointense on T1 and hyperintense on T2 WI. Liver and lymph node metastases may also show prominent enhancement. With liver specific contrast agents, these metastases are seen as hypointense lesions on hepatocyte phase imaging.[44,51]

If these cross-sectional modalities are unable to depict these tumors, then endoscopic US and nuclear imaging studies may be performed. Sensitivity with endoscopic US may be as high as 94% although, it has poorer performance in the tail region of pancreas.[52]

Nuclear medicine studies can depict the primary tumor, evaluate metastases and also receptor status for planning therapy. Nuclear imaging scans are based on the expression of somatostatin receptors in these tumors, and Octreotide is the most commonly used somatostatin analog. Scintigraphy techniques using octreotide include planar imaging as well as single photon emission computed tomography (SPECT). Octreotide scans have highest sensitivity for gastrinomas and lowest sensitivity for insulinomas depending upon the expression of somatostatin receptors.[45] PET scan has better spatial resolution than scintigraphy. Octreotide is conjugated with the chelator tetra-azacyclododecanetetra-acetic acid (DOTA) and is used for imaging as well as therapy of pNETs. Ga^{68} DOTA-TOC (DOTA-tyrosine-3-octreotide) and Ga^{68} DOTANOC (DOTA-1-NaI-octreotide) (DOTA-NOC) are the most frequently used analogs for depiction of the primary tumor as well as metastases.[44]

TABLE 7: Key points of pancreatic neuroendocrine tumors (pNETs).

- Rare tumors, mostly seen between 40–60 years of age
- May be functioning or non-functioning
- Hypervascular tumors which enhance brightly on arterial phase imaging
- Calcification may be seen and is more frequent in nonfunctioning tumors
- Peripancreatic nodes and liver metastases are pointers towards malignancy
- Metastases are also hypervascular in nature

Specific Features of Various pNETs (Table 8)

Insulinomas are the most common functioning tumors and account for more than 40% of functioning endocrine tumors of pancreas. These are usually smaller than other functioning as well as nonfunctioning tumors of pancreas due to the dramatic clinical symptomatology associated with these tumors. Most of these tumors (90%) are less than 2 cm in size and 40% are even smaller than 1 cm.[53] Since they are discovered early, they also usually carry the best prognosis. The characteristic Whipple's triad of their presentation

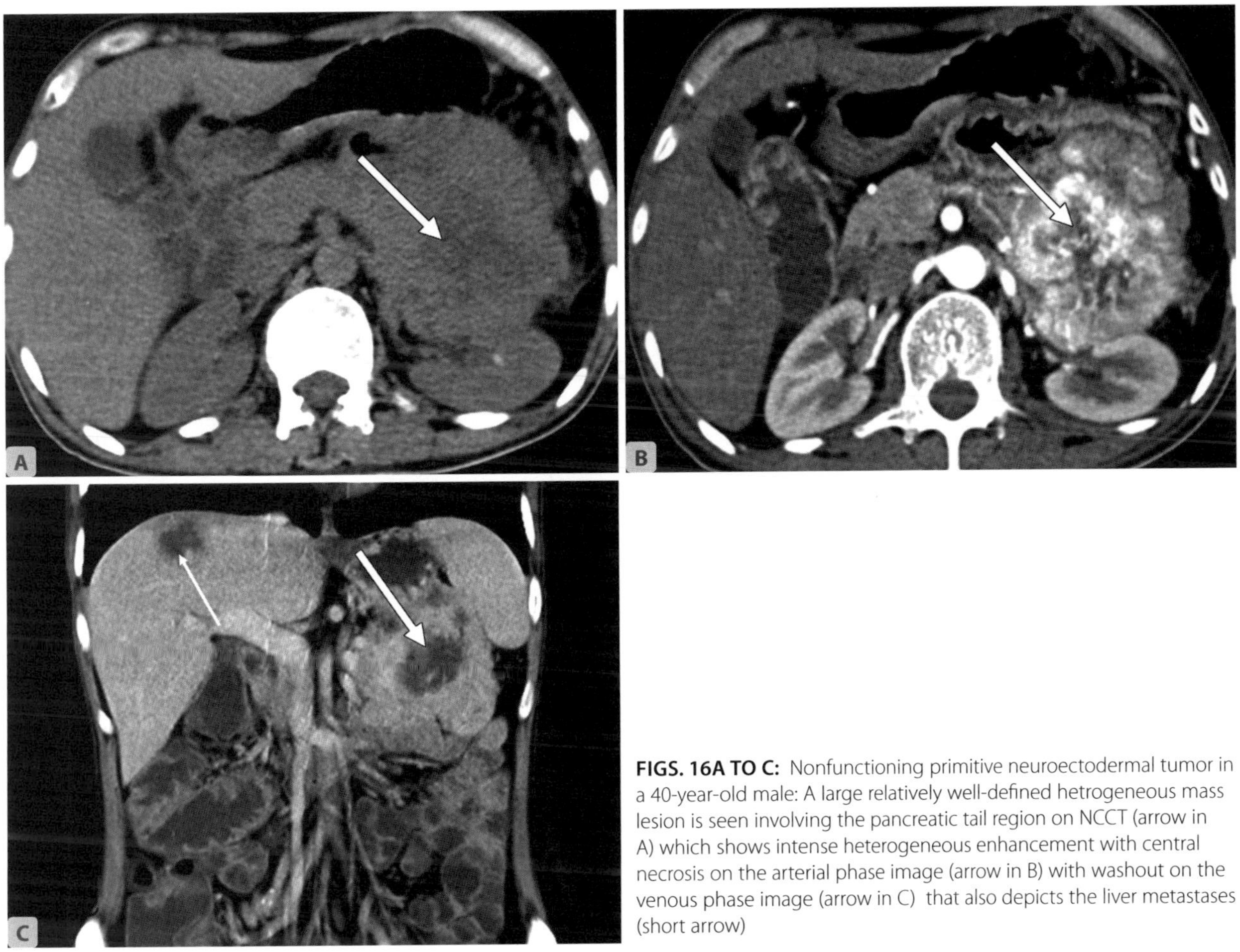

FIGS. 16A TO C: Nonfunctioning primitive neuroectodermal tumor in a 40-year-old male: A large relatively well-defined hetrogeneous mass lesion is seen involving the pancreatic tail region on NCCT (arrow in A) which shows intense heterogeneous enhancement with central necrosis on the arterial phase image (arrow in B) with washout on the venous phase image (arrow in C) that also depicts the liver metastases (short arrow)

includes the following symptoms: low blood glucose level, symptoms of hypoglycemia and relief of symptoms on administering glucose.[54] These are evenly distributed through the head, body and tail region of pancreas. Multiple lesions may be seen with MEN1 syndrome.[44]

Gastrinomas are the second most common functioning pNETs after insulinomas. These are mostly encountered in pancreatic head region and have an average size of 3–4 cm. These are most often seen in the gastrinoma triangle region, which is bounded by the following three points—junction of cystic and common bile duct, junction of 2nd and 3rd parts of duodenum and junction of neck and body of pancreas **(Fig. 17)**. Their somatostatin receptor concentration is also high and hence these are more readily depicted on nuclear imaging techniques than insulinomas. Gastrin levels in these patients are usually markedly elevated to more than 1000 pg/mL resulting in increased gastric acid production and peptic ulcer disease. Zollinger–Ellison syndrome refers to a triad of a gastrinoma, increased secretion of gastric acid and peptic ulcers in unusual locations (e.g. postbulbar duodenum, jejunum). Up to 60% of these tumors may be malignant.[44,55]

Glucagonomas are the third most common pNETs. These are usually large at presentation with an average size of 5–6 cm. These are most often seen in pancreatic body and tail region. Most of these tumors are malignant. Clinically, they present with 4D syndrome which includes dermatitis, diabetes, deep vein thrombosis, and depression.[44,53]

VIPomas are rare tumors that can be pancreatic or extrapancreatic in origin. Extrapancreatic tumors may arise from sympathetic ganglia of the retroperitoneum or mediastinum and even from stomach, small bowel, colon and liver. Symptoms result from excessive production of Vasoactive Intestinal peptide (VIP), a hormone that is not normally secreted by the pancreas. VIP prevents intestinal reabsorption and promotes intestinal secretion of water and electrolytes and these patients then present with watery diarrhea, hypokalemia and achlorhydria (WDHA syndrome). Most of these tumors are seen in tail region and are malignant tumors with an average size of approximately 5 cm.[44,56]

Somatostatinomas are rare tumors which can present with diabetes mellitus, steatorrhea, diarrhea, weight loss. Other hormones that may very rarely be produced by these

TABLE 8: Classification of pNETs.

- *Non-functioning pNETs*:
  - Generally larger in size as they present late with features of mass effect or systemic metastases
  - Evenly distributed throughout pancreas
- *Functioning pNETs*:
  - *Insulinomas*:
    - Most common functioning tumors
    - Characteristic Whipple's triad with low blood glucose, symptoms of hypoglycemia and relief of symptoms on administering glucose
    - Evenly distributed through head, body and tail region
    - Multiple lesions in MEN 1 syndrome
  - *Gastrinomas*:
    - Second most common
    - Most often seen in gastrinoma triangle
    - Zollinger Ellison syndrome constitutes a triad of gastrinoma, increased gastric acid production and peptic ulcers in unusual locations
  - *Glucagonomas*:
    - Third most common pNET
    - Mostly in pancreatic body and tail region
    - Present with 4D syndrome—dermatitis, deep vein thrombosis, diabetes and depression
  - *VIPomas*:
    - Rare tumors; pancreatic or extrapancreatic in origin
    - Mostly seen in tail region
    - WDHA syndrome—watery diarrhea, hypokalemia amd achlorhydria
  - *Somatostatinoma*:
    - Rare tumors
    - Can present with diabetes mellitus, diarrhea, steatorrhea, weight loss

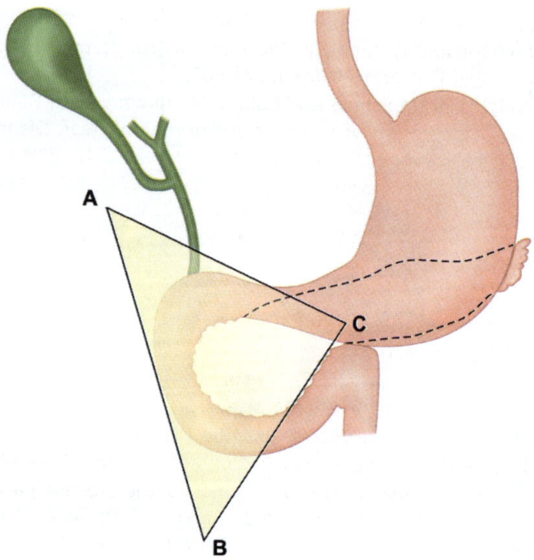

FIG. 17: Gastrinoma triangle region: This region is bounded by the following three points—junction of cystic and common bile duct (A); junction of 2nd and 3rd parts of duodenum (B); and junction of neck and body of pancreas (C).

functioning pNETs are adrenocorticotropic hormone, serotonin, growth hormone, and calcitonin.[44]

Nonfunctioning tumors may secrete pancreatic polypeptide, and have no associated hormonal symptoms. These are more common than functioning endocrine tumors of pancreas. They are seen evenly distributed throughout the pancreas. These are generally larger than functioning tumors as they present late with features of mass effect. These have greater propensity for necrotic and cystic degeneration. Calcification may also be seen in these tumors.[44,57]

Poorly differentiated endocrine cancers are extremely rare tumors and carry a prognosis much worse than well-differentiated tumors. The tumors usually are fatal within 1 year of detection. They are mostly seen in elderly men. On imaging, they are ill-defined masses with local invasion and distant metastases at presentation. They are mostly seen in the pancreatic head region. On nuclear imaging, octreotide scan has lower sensitivity for these cancers as they have poor expression of somatostatin receptors whereas FDG-PET scan can yield better results.[44]

CONCLUSION

Cystic tumors of pancreas can have overlapping imaging features. Patient demographics and few salient morphological features can help to narrow differential diagnosis on imaging. Endoscopic US and cyst aspiration may prove useful in indeterminate lesions.

Pancreatic neuroendocrine tumors can have a varied presentation but similar imaging features. They are generally indolent in behavior except for poorly differentiated endocrine cancers. Somatostatin analog nuclear imaging techniques can help us narrow our differential diagnosis, and also enable receptor-guided therapy as these confirm the presence of soamtostatin receptors on these tumors.

REFERENCES

1. Khalid A, Brugge W. ACG Practice Guidelines for the Diagnosis and Management of Neoplastic Pancreatic Cyst. Am J Gastroenterol. 2007;102:2339-49.
2. Allen PJ, Jaques DP, D'Angelica M, et al. Cystic lesions of the pancreas: selection criteria for operative and nonoperative management in 209 patients. J Gastrointest Surg. 2003;7(8): 970-7.
3. Dewhurst CE, Mortele KJ. Cystic lesions of the pancreas: Imaging and Management. RCNA. 2012;50:467-86.
4. Laffan TA, Horton KM, Klein AP, et al. Prevalence of unsuspected pancreatic cysts on MDCT. American Journal of Roentgenology. 2008;191(3):802-7.
5. Procacci C, Biasiutti C, Carbognin G, et al. Characterization of cystic tumors of the pancreas: CT accuracy. Journal of Computer Assisted Tomography. 1999;23(6):906-12.
6. Martin RCG, Klimstra DS, Brennan MF, Conlon KC. Solid-pseudopapillary tumor of the pancreas: a surgical enigma. Annals of Surgical Oncology. 2002;9(1):35-40.

7. Chang MK, Kyung SK, Jin SC, Kim H, Woo JL, Byong RK. Solid pseudopapillary tumor of the pancreas suggesting malignant potential. Pancreas. 2006;32(3):276-80.
8. Jani N, Hani BM, Schulik RD, Hruban RH, Cunningham C. Diagnosis and management of cystic lesions of the pancreas. Diagnostic and therapeutic endoscopy. 2011; *doi: 10.1155/2011/478913.*
9. Sahani DV, Kambadakone A, Macari M, Takahashi N, Chari S, Fernandez-del Castillo C. Diagnosis and management of cystic pancreatic lesions. AJR. 2013;200:343-54.
10. Sahani DV, Kadavigere R, Saokar A, Fernandez-del Castillo C, Brugge WR, Hahn PF. Cystic pancreatic lesions: A simple imaging-based classification system for guiding management. Radiographics. 2005;25:1471-84.
11. Fernandez-del Castillo C, Warshaw AL. Cystic tumors of the pancreas. Surg Clin North Am. 1995;75:1001-16.
12. Kalb B, Sarmiento JM, Kooby DA, Adsay NV, Martin DR. MR imaging of cystic lesions of pancreas. Radiographics. 2009;29:1749-65.
13. Solicia E, Capella C, Kloppel G. Tumors of the exocrine pancreas. (3rd series, fasc. 20) In: Rosai J, Sorbin L (Eds). Atlas of tumor pathology. Armed Forces Institute of Pathology, Washington, DC; 1997.pp.31-144.
14. Kanno A, Satoh K, Hamada S, et al. Serous cystic neoplasms of the whole pancreas in a patient with von Hippel-Lindau disease. Intern Med. 2011;50:1293-8.
15. Buck JL, Hayes WS. From the Archives of the AFIP. Microcystic adenoma of the pancreas. Radiographics. 1990;10:313-22.
16. Colonna J, Plaza JA, Frankel WL, et al. Serous cystadenoma of the pancreas: clinical and pathological features in 33 patients. Pancreatology. 2008;8:135-41.
17. Cohen-Scali F, Vilgrain V, Brancatelli G, et al. Discrimination of unilocular macrocystic serous cystadenoma from pancreatic pseudocyst and mucinous cystadenoma with CT: initial observations. Radiology. 2003;228:727-33.
18. Scott J, Martin I, Redhead D, et al. Mucinous cystic neoplasms of the pancreas: imaging features and diagnostic difficulties. Clin Radiol. 2000;55:187-92.
19. Crippa S, Roberta S, Warshaw A, et al. Mucinous cystic neoplasms of the pancreas is not an aggressive entity: lessons from 163 resected patients. Ann Surg. 2008;247:571-9.
20. Sarr MG, Murr M, Smyrk TC, et al. Primary cystic neoplasms of the pancreas: neoplastic disorders of emerging importance: current state-of-the-art and unanswered questions. J Gastrointest Surg. 2003;7(3):417-28.
21. Sidden CR, Mortele KJ. Cystic tumors of the pancreas: Ultrasound, computed tomography, and magnetic resonance imaging features. Semin US CT and MRI; 2007.pp.339-56.
22. Loftus EV, Olivares-Pakzad BA, Batts KP, et al. Intraductal papillary-mucinous tumors of the pancreas: clinicopathologic features, outcome and nomenclature. Gastroenterology. 1996; 110:1909-18.
23. Procacci C, Carbognin G, Accordini S, et al. CT features of malignant mucinous cystic tumors of the pancreas. Eur Radiol. 2001;11:1626-30.
24. Zhong N, Zhnag L, Takahashi N, et al. Histological and imaging features of mural nodules in mucinous pancreatic cysts. Clin Gastroenterol Hepatol. 2011;10:192-8.
25. Ohashi K, Murakami Y, Maruyama M. Four cases of mucin producing cancer of the pancreas on specific findings of the ampulla of Vater. Prog Dig Endosc. 1982;20:348.
26. Kawamoto S, Horton KM, Lawler LP, et al. Intraductal papillary mucinous neoplasm of the pancreas: can benign lesions be differentiated from malignant lesions with multidetector CT? Radiographics. 2005;25:1451-68.
27. Tanaka M. Intraductal papillary mucinous neoplasm of the pancreas: diagnosis and treatment. Pancreas. 2004;28(3): 282-8.
28. Taouli B, Vilgrain V, Vullierme M, et al. Intraductal papillary mucinous tumors of the pancreas: helical CT with histopathologic correlation. Radiology. 2000;217:757-64.
29. Barral M, Soyer P, Dohan A, Laurent V, Hoeffel C, Fishman EK, Boudiaf M. Magnetic resonance imaging of cystic pancreatic lesions in adults: an update in current diagnostic features and management. Abdominal imaging. 2014;39:48-65.
30. Casadei R, Santini D, Calculli L, et al. Pancreatic solid-cystic papillary tumor: clinical features, imaging findings and operative management. JOP. 2006;7:137-44.
31. Choi JY, Kim MJ, Kim JH, et al. Solid pseudopapillary tumor of the pancreas: typical and atypical manifestations. AJR. 2006;187: 178-86.
32. Morgan DE. Cystic lesions of the pancreas. Semin Roentgenol. 2009;44(4):255-65.
33. Balthazar EJ, Subramanyam BR, Lefleur RS, et al. Solid and papillary epithelial neoplasm of the pancreas: Radiographic, CT, sonographic, and angiographic features. Radiology. 1984;150: 39-40.
34. Cantisani V, Mortele KJ, Levy A, et al. MR imaging features of solid pseudopapillary tumor of the pancreas in adult and pediatric patients. AJR. 2003;181:395-401.
35. Horton KM, Hruban RH, Yeo C, et al. Multi-detector row CT of pancreatic islet cell tumors. Radiographics. 2006;26:453-64.
36. Eidt S, Jergas M, Schmidt R, et al. Metastasis to the pancreas: an indication for pancreatic resection. Langenbecks Arch Surg. 2007;392:539-42.
37. Koomalsingh KJ, Fazylov R, Chorost MI, et al. Cystic teratoma of the pancreas: presentation, evaluation and management. JOP. 2006;7:643-6.
38. Seki M, Ninomiya E, Aruga A, et al. Image-diagnostic features of mature cystic teratomas of the pancreas: report on two cases difficult to diagnose preoperatively. J Hepatobiliary Pancreat Surg. 2005;12:336-40.
39. Koenig TR, Loyer EM, Whitman GJ, et al. Cystic lymphangioma of the pancreas. AJR. 2001;177:1090.
40. Brugge WR, Lewandrowski K, Lee-Lewandrowski E, et al. Diagnosis of pancreatic cystic neoplasms: a report of the cooperative pancreatic cyst study. Gastroenterology. 2004; 126(5):1330-6.
41. Frossard JL, Amouyal P, Amouyal G, et al. Performance of endosonography-guided fine needle aspiration and biopsy in the diagnosis of pancreatic cystic lesions. American Journal of Gastroenterology. 2003;98(7):1516-24.
42. Eriksson B, Oberg K. Neuroendocrine tumours of the pancreas. Br J Surg. 2000;87:129-31.
43. Oberg K. Genetics and molecular pathology of neuroendocrine gastrointestinal and pancreatic tumors (gastroenteropancreatic neuroendocrine tumors). Curr Opin Endocrinol Diabetes Obes. 2009;16:72-8.
44. Lewis RB, Lattin GE, Paal E. Pancreatic endocrine tumors: radiologic-clinicopathologic correlation. Radiographics. 2010;30.
45. Kartalis N, Pozzi Mucelli RM, Sundin A. Recent developments in imaging of pancreatic neuroendocrine tumors. Ann Gastroenterol. 2015;28(2):193-202.
46. Metz DC, Jensen RT. Gastrointestinal neuroendocrine tumors: pancreatic endocrine tumors. Gastroenterology. 2008;135:1469-92.
47. Rindi G, Arnold R, Bosman FT, et al. Bosman FT, Carneiro F, Hruban RH, Theise ND. WHO classification of tumors of the digestive system, 4th edn. Lyon: IARC Press; Nomenclature and classification of neuroendocrine neoplasms of the digestive system; 2010.pp.13-4.

48. Ligneau B, Lombard-Bohas C, Partensky C, et al. Cystic endocrine tumors of the pancreas: clinical, radiologic, and histopathologic features in 13 cases. Am J Surg Pathol. 2001;25(6): 752-60.
49. Fidler JL, Fletcher JG, Reading CC, et al. Preoperative detection of pancreatic insulinomas on multiphasic helical CT. AJR. 2003;181(3):775-80.
50. Gouya H, Vignaux O, Augui J, et al. CT, endoscopic sonography, and a combined protocol for preoperative evaluation of pancreatic insulinomas. AJR. 2003;181(4):987-92.
51. Thoeni RF, Mueller-Lisse UG, Chan R, Do NK, Shyn PB. Detection of small, functional islet cell tumors in the pancreas: selection of MR imaging sequences for optimal sensitivity. Radiology. 2000;214(2):483-90.
52. Zimmer T, Scherübl H, Faiss S, Stölzel U, Riecken EO, Wiedenmann B. Endoscopic ultrasonography of neuroendocrine tumours. Digestion. 2000;62(suppl 1):45–50.
53. Mansour JC, Chen H. Pancreatic endocrine tumors. J Surg Res. 2004;120(1):139-61.
54. Whipple AO, Frantz VK. Adenoma of islet cells with hyperinsulinism: a review. Ann Surg. 1935;101(6):1299-1335.
55. Zollinger RM, Ellison EH. Primary peptic ulcerations of the jejunum associated with islet cell tumors of the pancreas. Ann Surg. 1955;142(4):709-23; discussion, 724-8.
56. Ghaferi AA, Chojnacki KA, Long WD, Cameron JL, Yeo CJ. Pancreatic VIPomas: subject review and one institutional experience. J Gastrointest Surg. 2008;12(2):382-93.
57. Hruban RH, Pitman MB, Klimstra DS. Tumors of the pancreas. In: Silverberg SG, Sobin LH (Eds). AFIP atlas of tumor pathology, 4th edn. Washington, DC: American Registry of Pathology, 2007.

CHAPTER

115

Nontraumatic Acute Abdomen

Mandeep Kang, Anmol Bhatia, Anindita Sinha

INTRODUCTION

Acute abdomen is defined as a clinical syndrome characterized by acute abdominal pain of sudden onset.[1] Patients with an acute abdomen comprise the largest group presenting to the surgical emergency department.[2] Identification of patients who require surgery is crucial for timely management and reducing the associated morbidity and mortality. Acute abdomen may be due to variety of diseases which may involve the gastrointestinal system, biliary tree, solid viscera or genitourinary system. Acute appendicitis is the most common cause of an acute abdomen, particularly in young adults. In a review of 10,682 patients presenting with an acute abdomen, acute appendicitis accounted for 28% of cases, followed by acute cholecystitis (9.7%), small bowel obstruction (4.1%), gynecologic disorders (4%), acute pancreatitis (2.9%), renal colic (2.9%), peptic ulcer disease (2.5%), cancer (1.5%), diverticular disease (1.5%) and a variety of less common conditions (9%).[3] In about one-third of cases, the cause of the abdominal pain remains indeterminate or nonspecific. On account of the considerable overlap of symptoms and signs in an acute abdomen, the clinical accuracy for the specific diagnosis is low, ranging from 50% to 65%.[4] This limitation emphasizes the importance of imaging in the diagnostic work-up of the acute abdomen.

The various imaging modalities available for investigating the acute abdomen include plain films, contrast studies, ultrasound (US), computed tomography (CT), and magnetic resonance imaging (MRI). The choice of the initial modality to be used should be guided by the disease suspected on clinical grounds, for example, plain radiographs continue to be the initial imaging modality in cases of intestinal obstruction and perforation.[2] Contrast examinations have a limited role. An upper GI series with water soluble contrast may be performed in cases of suspected perforation or a contrast enema may be required to confirm a colonic obstruction.

Ultrasound is the ideal screening modality for suspected hepatobiliary disease or for suspected pelvic pathology such as ectopic gestation or acute pelvic inflammatory disease (PID). It is also indicated for the initial evaluation of a patient with right lower quadrant pain especially in young women.[5] In cases of suspected intestinal obstruction, it may at times be difficult to differentiate between mechanical obstruction and paralytic ileus on plain radiographs. US is of special value in such a situation as it demonstrates increased peristalsis in cases of mechanical obstruction, whereas presence of dilated, atonic loops suggest the diagnosis of paralytic ileus. US is also helpful in localizing intra-abdominal abscesses, particularly in the solid viscera.

The introduction of multidetector computed tomography (MDCT) has impacted imaging of all organs of the body, especially the abdomen.[6] Because of the greater speed of Zee-Axis coverage and thinner sections with 3D reconstruction now available, MDCT has become the imaging modality of choice for evaluation of the acute abdomen. It provides a comprehensive view of all the intra-abdominal solid and hollow viscera, as well as the peritoneum, mesentery, lymph nodes and retroperitoneum. Data can be acquired in different phases making MDCT an ideal modality for evaluation of suspected mesenteric ischemia or vascular disorders such as abdominal aortic aneurysms. Low dose unenhanced CT has replaced excretory urography as the screening method of choice for the evaluation of renal colic in most centers.[6] Recent improvements in resolution and development of faster breath-hold sequences have drastically increased the utility of MRI in evaluation of the gut.[7] However, MRI is still not routinely used for evaluation of an acute abdomen except in situations where iodinated contrast cannot be administered or in pregnant patients.

COMPUTED TOMOGRAPHY TECHNIQUE

The technique used for acquisition of the image data set is of paramount importance for accurate diagnosis and should be tailored according to the most likely clinical diagnosis. Oral contrast is routinely administered to all patients in the form of 800–1000 mL of 2% iodinated contrast or dilute barium solution over a period of 45 minutes prior to the study. Negative oral contrast (plain water) is preferred in suspected mesenteric ischemia to adequately distend the bowel lumen. Oral contrast is withheld in patients with renal, ureteric or biliary calculi or patients in whom CT angiography is contemplated such as aortic dissection, aneurysm rupture, etc. Per rectal contrast is given in patients with suspected pelvic or large bowel pathology. Intravenous contrast, preferably nonionic iodinated contrast, helps in better depiction of inflammatory as well as neoplastic pathology, enables differentiation of lymph nodes from vessels and detection of vascular complications. 100–120 mL of contrast is injected at a rate of 2.8–3.5 mL/second and images routinely obtained in the portal venous phase at a delay of 70 seconds. Arterial phase imaging or dual energy scanning can be added, depending on the most likely clinical diagnosis. Scanning should be performed from the domes of the diaphragm to the pubic symphysis using a slice thickness of 5–10 mm which can be retrospectively reconstructed to thinner sections for various 3D reconstructions.

Plain Radiographs in Evaluation of the Acute Abdomen

Plain radiographs still remain an important initial investigation in the evaluation of a patient with acute abdomen. Interpretation of these radiographs represents a formidable challenge to the radiologist, as the findings may be nonspecific, confusing or even misleading at times.[2] Abdominal plain films are of greatest value in cases of hollow viscus perforation and intestinal obstruction.

Perforation

In the past, a minimum three film radiographic series was recommended for evaluation of an acute abdomen. This included a supine film of the abdomen and erect radiographs of the abdomen and chest **(Figs. 1A to C)**. More recently, it has been demonstrated that the erect film of the abdomen can be eliminated from the initial series without significant loss of the diagnostic information.[8] The upright chest film is ideal for demonstrating free air as the X-ray beam strikes the hemidiaphragms tangentially at their highest point and at an optimal exposure. Classical studies have shown that as little as 1 mL of free air can be detected below the right hemidiaphragm provided the patient has been in an erect position for at least 10–15 minutes prior to obtaining the radiograph.[9,10] The chest radiograph may also reveal chest diseases such as pneumonia, pulmonary or myocardial infarction which may mimic an acute abdomen. If the patient cannot sit or stand up a left lateral decubitus film will demonstrate air between the opacity of the liver and the abdominal wall. If the patient is too ill to roll over, a cross-table lateral view of the abdomen is obtained **(Fig. 2)**.

Various signs of pneumoperitoneum can be seen even on supine films if carefully searched for. The signs include "Rigler's or "double wall" sign describing visualization of both the mucosal and serosal aspect of the bowel wall due to presence of intra- and extraluminal air **(Fig. 3)**. The falciform ligament may be outlined by air in the epigastrium just to the right of the midline. The "football" sign is due to presence of large quantity of air which fills the peritoneal cavity. The lateral umbilical ligaments may be visualized in the lower abdomen known as the "inverted V" sign. Free air in morrison's pouch may be seen as an oval radiolucency in the subhepatic region. The right upper quadrant may appear radiolucent due to air collecting between the anterior surface of liver and the abdominal wall. The under surface of the central part of the diaphragm may be visualized—the "cupola" sign.[11] Retroperitoneal perforation of a duodenal ulcer results in air outlining the renal or psoas shadows **(Fig. 4)**. Large bowel may also perforate into the retroperitoneal space resulting in mottled extraluminal air lucencies. Plain films are inferior to CT for the detection of free intraperitoneal air. Supine abdominal films may detect free air in only about 60% of the cases, whereas CT can reliably detect even small amounts of free air which is usually seen just beneath the anterior abdominal wall or in the peritoneal recesses. Viewing the scan at wide window settings (lung window) increases the sensitivity of CT for the detection of free air.[9]

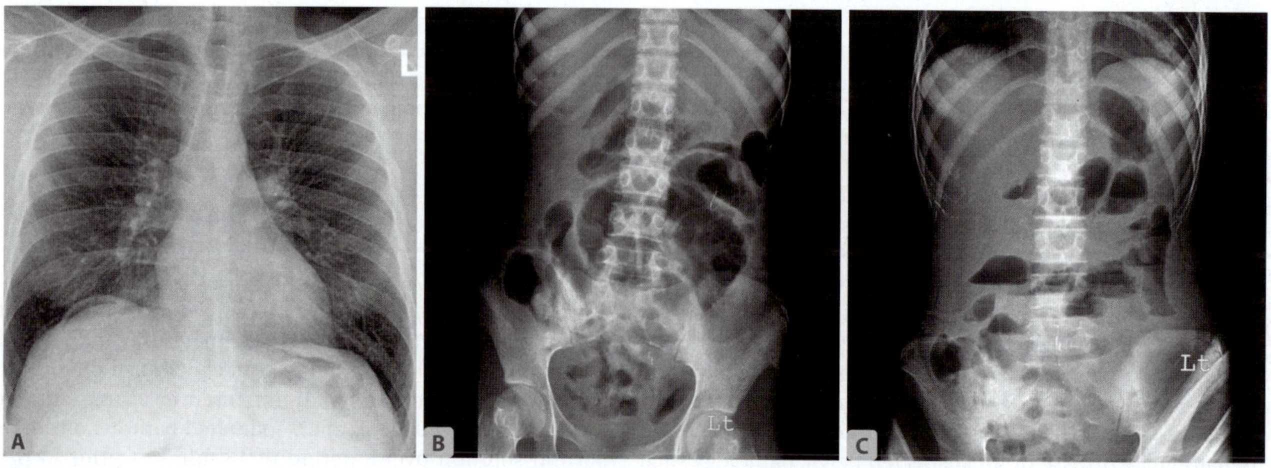

FIGS. 1A TO C: Abdominal series (Three views of the abdomen): (A) Chest X-ray reveals absence of free air under the domes of diaphragm; (B) Supine film shows dilated jejunal and ileal loops with no air in the large bowel; (C) Erect film demonstrates multiple air-fluid levels in a case of distal small bowel obstruction.

Intestinal Obstruction

The diagnosis of intestinal obstruction may be correctly suggested on the basis of plain films alone in nearly 80% of the cases. Additional imaging with US and CT is required in equivocal cases and also to determine the level and cause of obstruction.

In mechanical obstruction, plain films reveal dilated, gas-filled bowel loops with air-fluid levels proximal to the obstruction with collapsed loops with absence of air distal to the obstruction **(Figs. 1A to C)**. Dilatation of both small and large bowel loops from stomach to rectum indicates a diagnosis of paralytic ileus. It may not always be possible to differentiate between mechanical obstruction and paralytic ileus. A lateral view to look for air in the rectum may aid in the differentiation, however CT or contrast studies may be required in equivocal cases.[2,9]

Distinction between small and large bowel loops on plain films is based on the central position of the small bowel, presence of valvulae conniventes in the jejunum and tubular featureless appearance of the ileum. The dilated loops measure between 3 cm and 5 cm. The valvulae conniventis form thin, 1–2 mm complete rings at intervals of 1 mm. In contrast, the large bowel loops are located peripherally, usually measure more than 5 cm in diameter and display haustral markings that are incomplete, 2–3 mm wide and occurring at intervals of 1 cm.[12] The erect film in a normal person usually displays 2–3 fluid levels in the small bowel which does not exceed 3 cm in caliber. Dilated fluid-filled loops of small bowel may be identified as oval or round soft tissue densities.[2] At times the bowel loops proximal to the site of obstruction may get completely filled with fluid resulting in a gasless abdomen. When a tiny amount of gas accompanies a large amount of intraluminal fluid, small gas bubbles get trapped between the valvulae conniventis resulting in the "string-of-beads" sign[2] **(Fig. 5)**. This appearance is virtually diagnostic of mechanical obstruction as it is never seen with paralytic ileus.

Strangulating obstruction is a mechanical obstruction caused when two limbs of a loop are incarcerated within a hernia so as to cause vascular compromise by compression of the mesenteric vessels. Presence of thumb-printing due to submucosal edema or hemorrhage should suggest ischemia in the loops. If left untreated, the ischemia may progress causing breach of the mucosa, intramural air, air in the mesenteric and portal veins and frank perforation which are all ominous signs.

Intramural air in the form of parallel streaks of gas along the bowel wall or as rings may also be seen in infants with necrotizing enterocolitis. This appearance should not be confused with the bubbly appearance of pneumatosis coli which is a benign condition affecting the colon in adults.

The causes of intestinal obstruction vary with the age of the patient. In neonates and infants, the usual causes of obstruction are congenital conditions such as hypertrophic pyloric stenosis, duodenal stenosis or atresia, ileal atresia, etc. Duodenal atresia shows the typical "double-bubble" sign. In young children, intussusception or Ladd's bands are common causes of obstruction. Intussusception may be seen as a mass-like soft tissue shadow with a crescent of gas surrounding the leading edge. A barium examination will reveal the coil-spring appearance of the intussuscipiens with the "claw" sign **(Fig. 6)**.

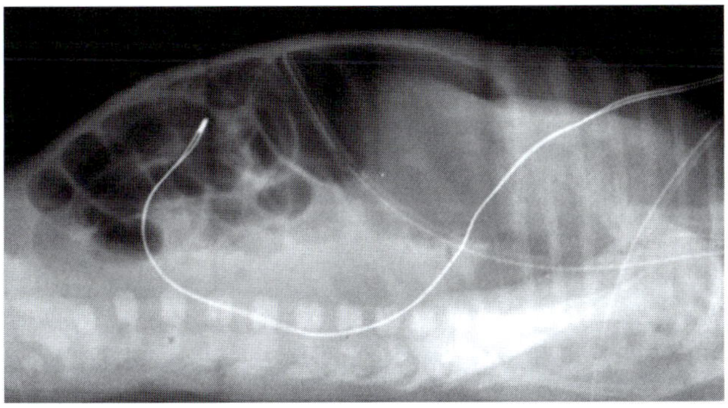

FIG. 2: Cross-table lateral view of a premature neonate reveals free intraperitoneal air in a case of necrotizing enterocolitis.

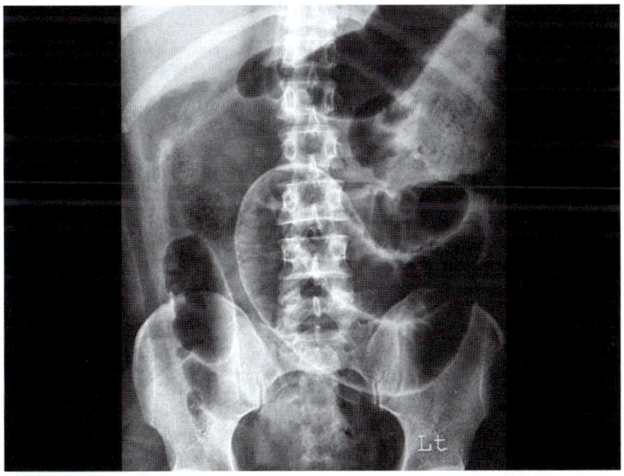

FIG. 3: X-ray of abdomen, supine film. Both the inner and outer walls of the small bowel loop are visualized due to the presence of free intra-peritoneal air. Air is also seen in the subhepatic region (Morrison's pouch).

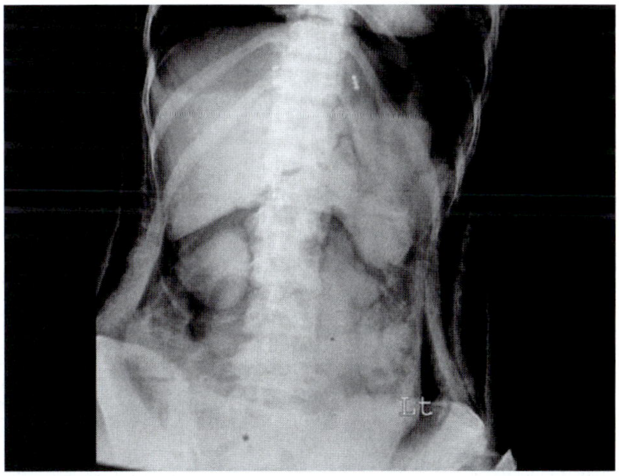

FIG. 4: Plain radiograph abdomen, erect film shows large amount of free air in the upper abdomen. In addition, air is also seen outlining the right kidney signifying retroperitoneal perforation of a duodenal ulcer.

In adults, adhesions and hernias account for more than 80% of small bowel obstructions. Other causes include an intraluminal obturation by neoplasm, gallstone or bezoar or a volvulus due to twisting of the gut around its mesentery. Sigmoid volvulus is generally seen in the older age group. The distended ahaustral sigmoid loop assumes an inverted "U" shape with its apex under either dome. The opposed inner walls of the loops appear as a single line giving the "coffee bean" appearance **(Fig. 7)**. Cecal volvulus generally occurs in younger individuals. The cecum twists and inverts so that its pole and appendix lie in the left upper quadrant.

In mechanical large bowel obstruction, the small bowel loops also dilate if the ileocecal valve is incompetent. However, if the ileocecal valve is competent, it can result in gross gaseous distension of the cecum with the attendant dangers of ischemia and perforation.

MISCELLANEOUS CONDITIONS

Apart from perforation and intestinal obstruction, plain films may sometimes reveal important findings which may clinch the diagnosis or indirectly suggest the possible diagnosis such as:

- Presence of intramural and intraluminal gas in patients of gangrenous cholecystitis.
- Presence of air in the biliary tree with small gut obstruction due to gallstone ileus caused by erosion of the gallstone into the duodenum.
- Presence of localized duodenal ileus (sentinel loop), dilated transverse colon with "colon cut-off" in case of acute pancreatitis.
- Presence of extraluminal mottled gas in patients with abdominal abscess.
- Presence of soft tissue mass with obliteration of properitoneal fat line in the right lower quadrant and scoliosis with convexity to the left in patients of acute appendicular abscess.
- Presence of gas in the perinephric region in cases of emphysematous pyelonephritis.
- Presence of intestinal pneumatosis or portomesenteric air in mesenteric ischemia.

ROLE OF CROSS-SECTIONAL IMAGING IN SPECIFIC DISEASE ENTITIES

Acute Appendicitis

In the majority of patients, the clinical picture is typical and patients undergo laparotomy without any imaging. Imaging is needed only in equivocal cases or when the clinical diagnosis is in doubt. In about one-third of patients, presentation of acute appendicitis is atypical. Conversely, other conditions may also mimic appendicitis resulting in a false negative laparotomy rate of 20% which rises to 35–45% in young women of reproductive age in whom distinction from acute PID and other gynecological conditions such

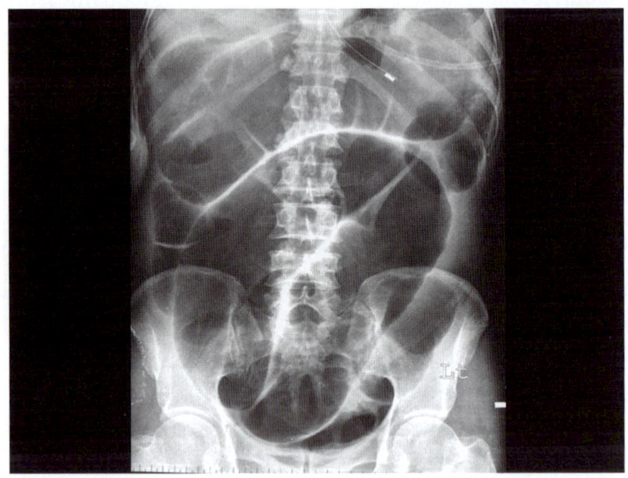

FIG. 7: X-ray of abdomen, supine view shows a hugely dilated a haustral loop arising from the pelvis with the "coffee-bean" sign in a case of sigmoid volvulus.

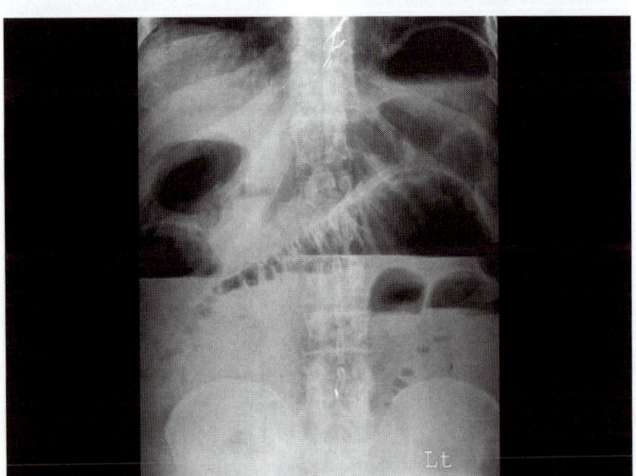

FIG. 5: X-ray of abdomen, erect view shows multiple air-fluid levels in the proximal jejunal loops with "string of beads" sign.

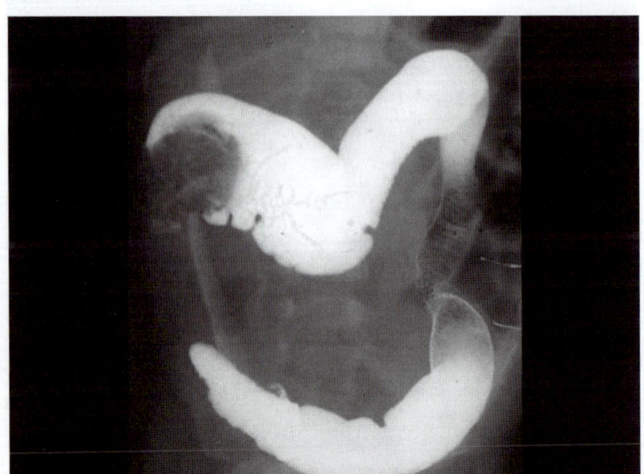

FIG. 6: Barium enema in a case of large bowel obstruction shows a crescentic intraluminal filling defect in the hepatic flexure with a soft tissue mass due to ileocolic intussusception.

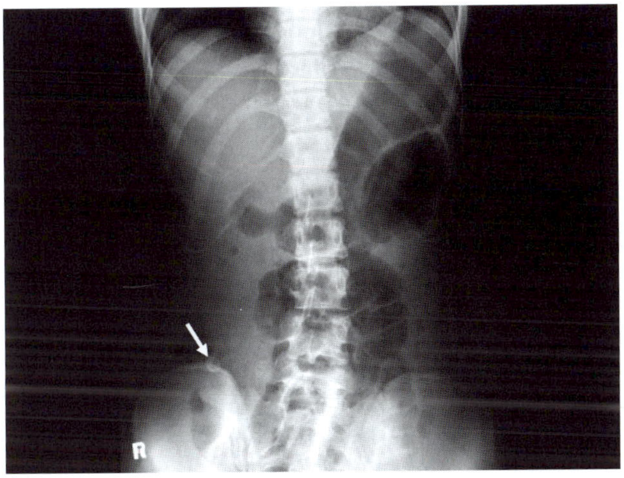

FIG. 8: X-ray of abdomen showing a paucity of gas in the right side with an appendicolith (arrow).

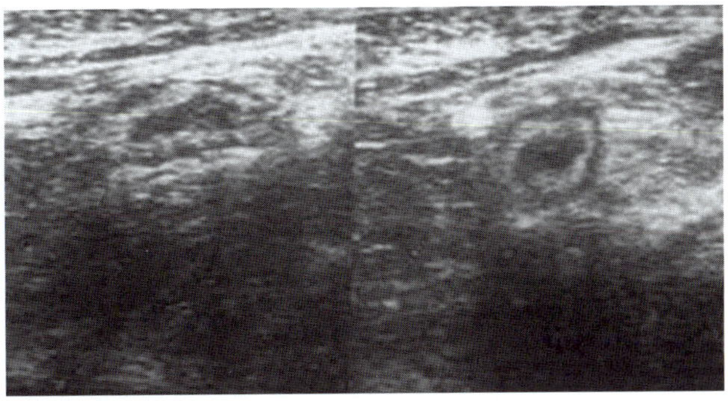

FIG. 9: Longitudinal and transverse sonograms showing the classical target lesion in the right iliac fossa due to inflamed, incompressible appendix with thickened walls.

as torsion of ovarian cyst is difficult on clinical grounds alone.[13] On plain radiography, although the presence of an appendicolith strongly suggests appendicitis, it is visualized on properly exposed radiographs in only 14% of all patients with appendicoliths **(Fig. 8)**.[8] At barium enema, lack of appendiceal visualization and presence of a cecal mass impression are nonspecific findings and not definitely diagnostic of appendicitis. Filling of the appendix up to its bulbous tip virtually excludes appendicitis, however, the appendix may not fill completely in up to one-third of normal individuals.[14] US is the screening modality of choice for initial evaluation in suspected appendicitis, followed by CT in selected cases. Graded compression sonography using high frequency linear transducers is a highly accurate technique with a sensitivity of 80–93%, specificity of 94–100% and an accuracy of 95–97% for the diagnosis of acute appendicitis.[15] Another technique for improving visualization of retrocecal appendix in obese or muscular patients is posterior manual compression of right lower quadrant in anterior or anteromedial direction using the left hand with simultaneous anterior graded compression by transducer. Turning the patient from supine position to left oblique lateral decubitus position also displaces cecum, terminal ileum and appendix medially on to the psoas muscle and reduces the depth of the lateral portion of the retrocecal area, thereby improving visualization of retrocecal appendix.[16]

The US criteria for a normal appendix are presence of a compressible, tubular, blind-ending structure filled with fluid, gas or feces, originating from the base of the cecum having a wall thickness of 2 mm or less and diameter of 6 mm or less. The sonographic diagnosis of acute appendicitis is based on one or more of the following: direct visualization of a concentrically layered, aperistaltic, noncompressible appendix with an anteroposterior diameter >6 mm, or echogenic incompressible periappendicular inflamed fat with or without an appendicolith **(Fig. 9)**. On color Doppler, increased flow signals in the appendiceal wall or periappendicular space allow confirmation of the diagnosis. Perforation should be suspected if there is loss of symmetry of the concentric layers of the wall or a right lower quadrant fluid collection without visualization of inflamed appendix. However, inconclusive US studies may be seen in a right lower quadrant phlegmon or abscess without a visible appendix, retrocecal inflamed appendix, cecal edema or terminal ileum thickening, distal or tip appendicitis with a normal proximal appendix, obesity and if there is pain limiting compression. A false-positive sonogram may be seen in Crohn's disease, cecal diverticulitis and salpingitis.

Helical CT using thin sections (4–5 mm) has a higher reported sensitivity of 90–100%, specificity of 91–99% and accuracy of 94–98% compared to US.[17] CT signs of appendicitis include visualization of an abnormal appendix with a distended lumen, thickened and enhancing wall or an appendicolith, periappendicular inflammatory changes in the form of fat stranding, phlegmon, fluid, abscess or adenopathy, cecal changes like circumferential mural thickening of cecum and terminal ileum, cecal apical thickening or the "arrow head" sign which results due to funneling of contrast medium on both sides of the inflamed cecal apex coming to a point at the occluded orifice of the appendix **(Figs. 10 and 11)**. As the "arrowhead" sign highlights extension of inflammation to the upper portion of cecum, it may identify patients who require more than standard ligation appendectomy. CT is also of special value in suggesting an alternative diagnosis in patients who do not have appendicitis. MRI is a good imaging modality in pregnant patients and pediatric population, in whom ionizing radiation is of high concern. MRI has demonstrated high specificity and sensitivity for appendicitis in pediatric and pregnant patients, with nearly 100% sensitivities reported for both populations.[18]

Acute Cholecystitis

Sonography is the primary imaging modality of choice for evaluating acute inflammatory conditions of the gallbladder. Acute cholecystitis is associated with gallstones in 90–96% of patients with a calculus causing cystic duct obstruction being the most common cause. Sensitive sonographic features are positive Murphy's sign (in 96% of patients with acute cholecystitis), calculi (in 95%) and a thickened gallbladder (GB) wall (in 73%).[19] However, these signs are not specific and may occur in other conditions such as chronic cholecystitis, pancreatitis, cirrhosis or hepatitis. Other sonographic signs include distension of the gallbladder (GB), edematous wall,

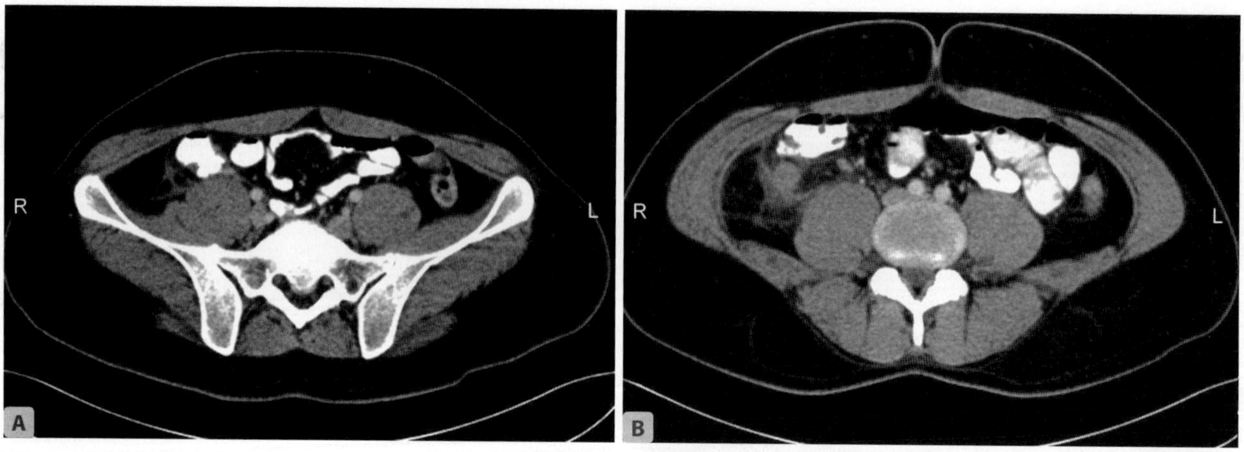

FIGS. 10A AND B: CECT abdomen, axial sections. (A) A thin streak of oral contrast is seen to enter the base of the appendix; (B) The appendix shows mural thickening with stranding in the surrounding fat in a case of acute appendicitis.

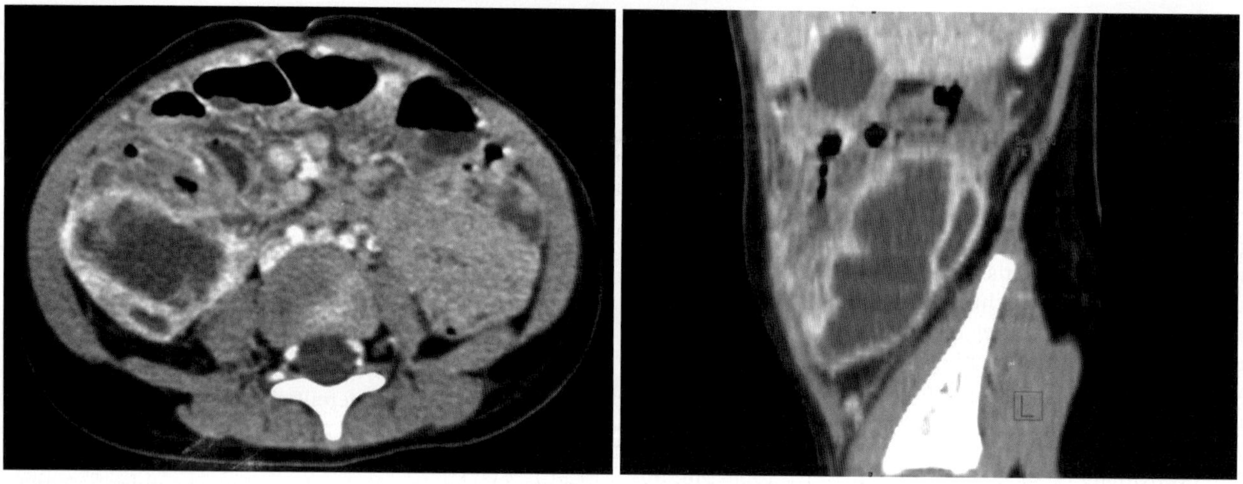

FIG. 11: Acute appendicitis: Axial and sagittal reconstructed CT images demonstrating a large, irregular collection with thick enhancing walls in the right iliac fossa posterior to the cecum which is displaced anteromedially. A tubular structure with enhancing walls is seen posterior to this collection representing the inflamed appendix.

mucosal irregularity, intramural gas and/or pericholecystic collection **(Fig. 12)**. Doppler sonography improves diagnostic confidence in acute cholecystitis by revealing mural hypervascularity **(Fig. 13)**.

The CT may be used as an adjunct to US if sonography is inconclusive, especially in acalculous cholecystitis or when complications such as perforation or emphysematous cholecystitis are suspected.[20] CT findings of acute cholecystitis include wall thickening, pericholecystic stranding, GB distension, pericholecystic fluid, subserosal edema, high attenuation bile and sloughed membranes, gas or septations within the gallbladder **(Fig. 14)**.[21] As the inflammatory response in calculous and acalculous cholecystitis is similar, the CT appearance of inflammation is similar in both. MRI can be a valuable complement to US and CT in demonstrating impacted calculi in the gallbladder neck or cystic duct which are often difficult to detect on US. Also, conditions causing acalculous cholecystitis like adenomyomatosis, gallbladder polyp, malignant neoplasm or other cancers can be depicted on MR.[22]

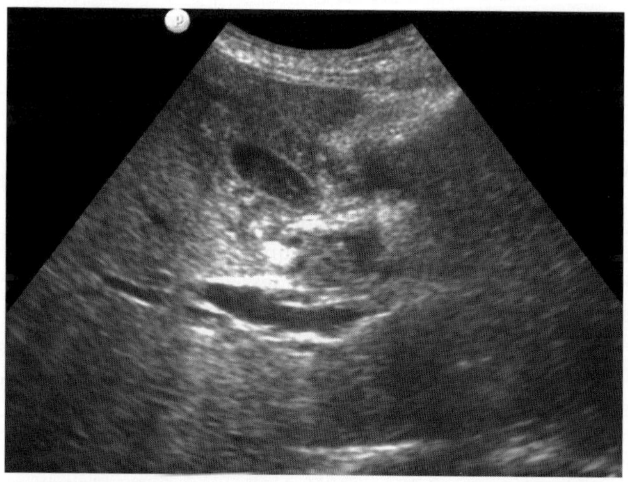

FIG. 12: Ultrasound image showing small calculi in the gallbladder with diffusely thickened walls in a case of acute cholecystitis. US Murphy's sign was positive.

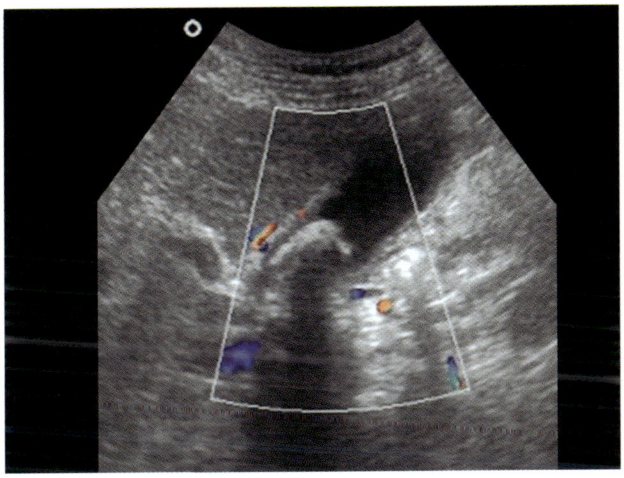

FIG. 13: Ultrasound (color Doppler) image showing cholelithiasis with increased vascularity in the gallbladder wall.

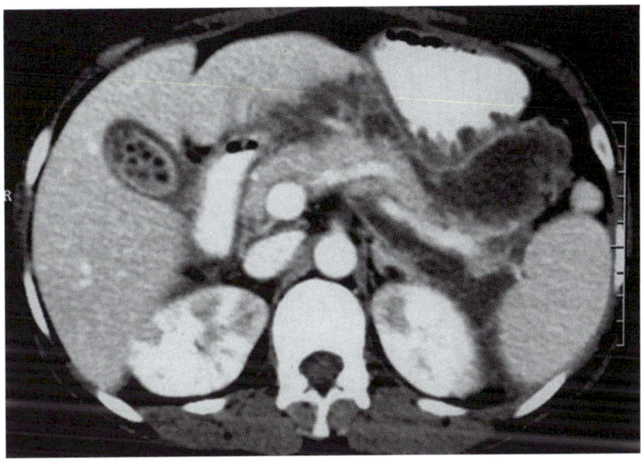

FIG. 14: Axial CECT abdomen. The gallbladder has thick, enhancing walls with a hypodense rim of pericholecystic fluid. The lumen is filled with high density bile resulting in the calculi appearing as filling defects. Note the loss of peripancreatic fat planes with a large collection in the lesser sac due to associated pancreatitis.

Complications of acute cholecystitis include the following:

- *Empyema*: It occurs when pus fills the distended and inflamed GB, typically in diabetic patients. On US and CT, pus resembles sludge. Heavily T2WI are sensitive in demonstrating purulent bile as a dependent hypointense layer relative to normal bile.
- *Gangrenous cholecystitis*: Gangrenous cholecystitis is an advanced, severe form of acute cholecystitis, seen more commonly in elderly men. It results from marked distension of the GB with resultant increase in tension in the wall. Associated inflammation leads to ischemic necrosis. US reveals heterogeneous or striated thickening of GB wall or intraluminal membranes representing desquamated mucosa. US findings typical of uncomplicated acute cholecystitis may be absent in this subset of patients. Gallbladder wall thickness may be <3 mm or Murphy's sign may be absent due to denervation of the GB wall.[23] CT features consist of intraluminal membranes, irregular wall, pericholecystic fluid/abscess and lack of mural enhancement.
- *Gallbladder perforation*: Gallbladder perforation is most often a complication of acute gangrenous cholecystitis. As blood supply is poor in the region of fundus, this is the most common site of perforation. Perforation can be classified into three types:
    a. Acute free perforation into peritoneal cavity,
    b. Subacute perforation with pericholecystic abscess, and
    c. Chronic perforation with a cholecystoenteric fistula.[24]
    Subacute perforations are the most common. Following perforation, US, CT and MR show complex pericholecystic fluid collections and the wall of GB can appear focally disrupted **(Fig. 15)**.[7]
- *Emphysematous cholecystitis*: Emphysematous cholecystitis is a rare form of acute cholecystitis seen in patients with diabetes and peripheral atherosclerotic disease. The majority of patients are between 50 and 70 years. US demonstrates intraluminal and intramural gas as highly echogenic foci. CT is the most sensitive and specific imaging modality to identify gas in the lumen or wall **(Fig. 16)**.[25]

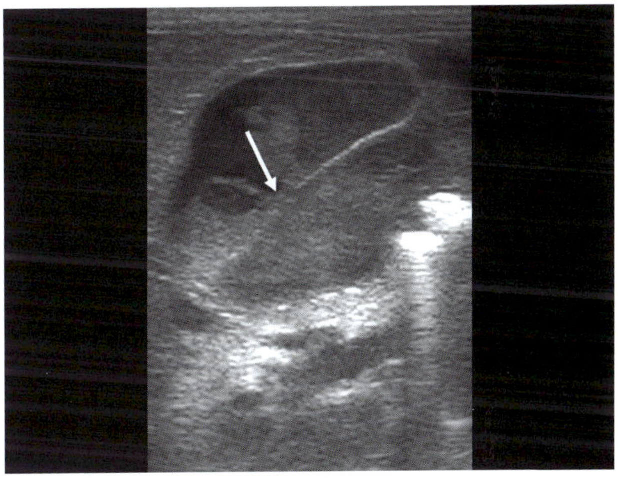

FIG. 15: Ultrasound image showing a rent in the gallbladder wall (arrow) with a large collection adjacent to the rent in a case of gallbladder perforation.

- *Hemorrhagic cholecystitis*: It can complicate acute calculous or acalculous cholecystitis, and the patient presents with acute biliary colic, jaundice, melena, and hematemesis.[25] It needs to be differentiated from other causes of gallbladder hemorrhage, which include trauma, tumors, and coagulopathy states. Ultrasound shows echogenic or heterogeneous material within the gallbladder lumen or wall, which are seen as high-attenuation contents on CT. MRI can be quite helpful in the diagnosis. Subacute blood products are generally hyperintense on both T1WI and T2WI because of the presence of extracellular methemoglobin.[26] Complications of hemorrhagic cholecystitis include gallbladder wall perforation and associated potentially life threatening hemoperitoneum.[26]

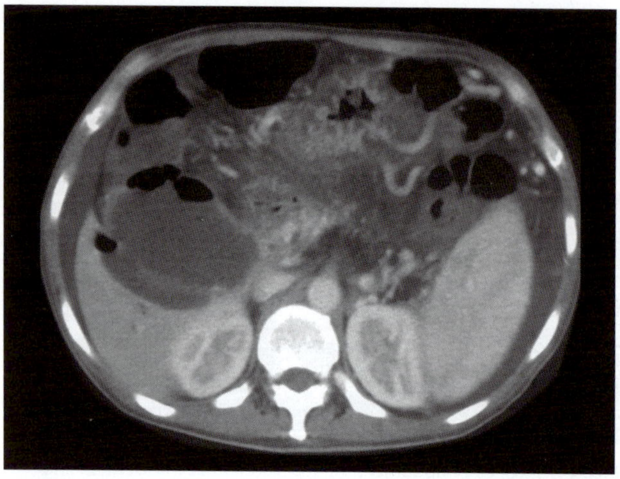

FIG. 16: Axial CECT image showing grossly distended gallbladder with intramural air foci suggestive of emphysematous cholecystitis.

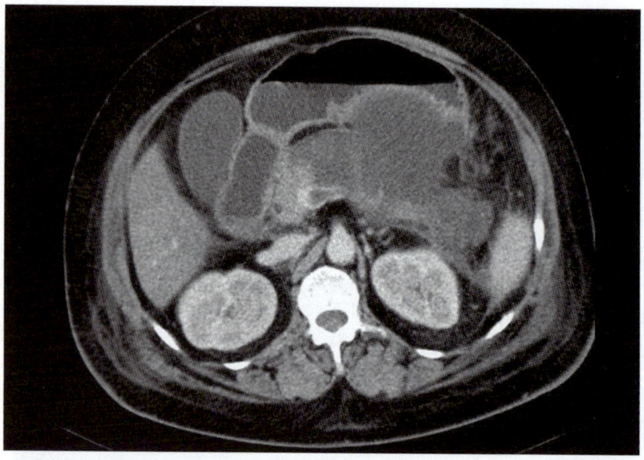

FIG. 17: Acute necrotizing pancreatitis grade E. The body and tail of the pancreas are hypodense with only a small amount of normally enhancing parenchyma seen in the head of pancreas. There are extra-pancreatic collections with a hypodense filling defect in the portal vein due to thrombosis (CTSI-10).

Acute Pancreatitis

Acute pancreatitis is an acute inflammatory process of the pancreas which may range in severity from a mild parenchymal edema to severe necrotizing pancreatitis with variable involvement of other regional tissues or remote organ systems. Most of the patients with the mild form of the disease have an uneventful recovery, however the cases with severe pancreatitis show significant mortality and morbidity with development of failure of various organ systems and require aggressive management.

The diagnosis of acute pancreatitis is usually made on clinical grounds supported by laboratory data. The role of imaging is to confirm the diagnosis, stage the severity of disease and detect complications such as infection, pseudocyst formation or vascular involvement. Ultrasound may reveal an enlarged, hypoechoic pancreas in the early stages with presence of peripancreatic fluid. It may also detect the presence of cholelithiasis or choledocholithiasis which is a major etiological factor for acute pancreatitis. It can also be used in the follow-up of acute fluid collections or pseudocysts particularly after percutaneous catheter drainage.

Contrast-enhanced CT is the modality of choice not only to confirm the diagnosis or detect extra-pancreatic intra-abdominal disease, but also to stage the severity of disease which is required for prognostication.[27] It is also highly accurate for the detection of necrosis and complications **(Fig. 17)**. The various grading systems, complications related to pancreatitis as well as pancreatic interventions will be dealt with in detail in a later chapter.

MR has also been reported to have similar accuracy to MDCT for the diagnosis of acute pancreatitis and assigning a severity index. The presence of hyperintensity in the pancreatic parenchyma on noncontrast T1 and T2 weighted images signifies the presence of hemorrhagic pancreatitis. Fat suppressed noncontrast sequences are used to detect hemorrhagic peripancreatic collections, both these situations signify a more severe form of pancreatitis.[28]

Intra-abdominal Abscess

A localized collection of pus can occur anywhere in the abdomen including the parenchyma of solid organs, in the peritoneal or extra-peritoneal spaces. Early detection, accurate localization and prompt drainage are the mainstay of successful management. US is an excellent modality for the detection of visceral abscesses and is also useful for screening for intraperitoneal abscesses, like in the post-operative patient.[29] Abscesses appear as a rounded, complex fluid collection with irregular walls, posterior acoustic enhancement, low level internal echoes, septations or debris **(Figs. 18A and B)**. A fluid-fluid level may be seen. At times, the abscess may have a solid appearance. Color Doppler demonstrates peripheral hypervascularity.

Computed tomography has a high sensitivity and specificity with an overall accuracy of 95% for the detection of intra-abdominal abscesses.[30] CT will show a low attenuation fluid collection with mass effect and peripheral rim enhancement with or without gas bubbles or an air-fluid level. MDCT allows accurate delineation of the complex anatomy which may exist in intra-abdominal collections and thus enables proper planning of a safe approach route for percutaneous catheter drainage **(Figs. 18A and B)**.

Intestinal Obstruction

Imaging studies such as US and CT are required to confirm the clinical diagnosis of obstruction (made on the basis of clinical findings and plain X-ray appearance), differentiate between mechanical obstruction and paralytic ileus and for determining the level and cause of mechanical obstruction. CT is also useful for detecting an obstruction not visualized on plain films, e.g. closed loop obstruction. More importantly, CT can detect complications like strangulation which require emergent surgery.

The CT diagnosis of bowel obstruction is based on the presence of dilated loops (small bowel >2.5 cm, large bowel

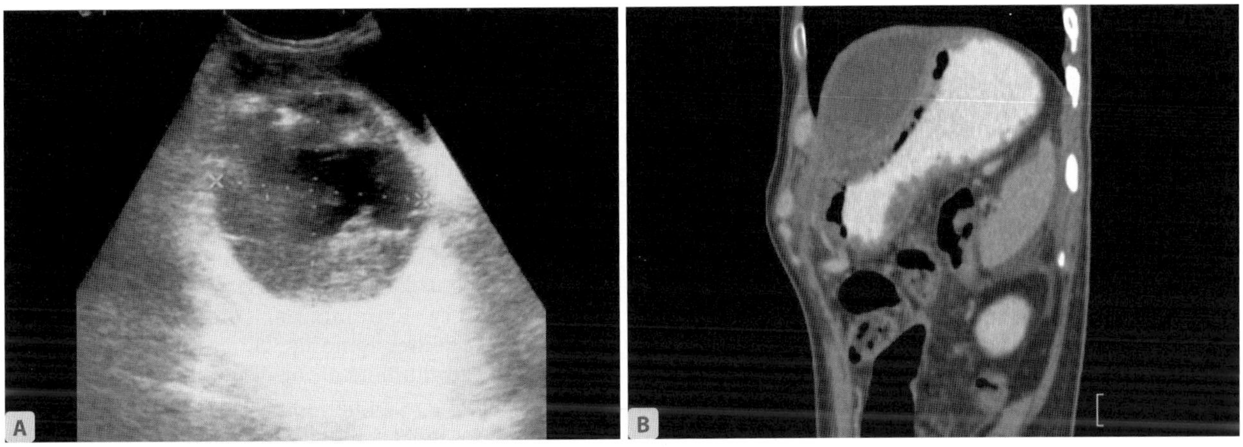

FIGS. 18A AND B: (A) The ultrasound of the pelvis shows a rounded fluid collection with internal echoes, debris and septations with posterior acoustic enhancement in a case of postoperative abdominal abscess; (B) Coronal MPVR image shows a large, left subphrenic, low-attenuation fluid collection elevating the left hemidiaphragm. The transpleural approach had to be employed for percutaneous drainage of this abscess.

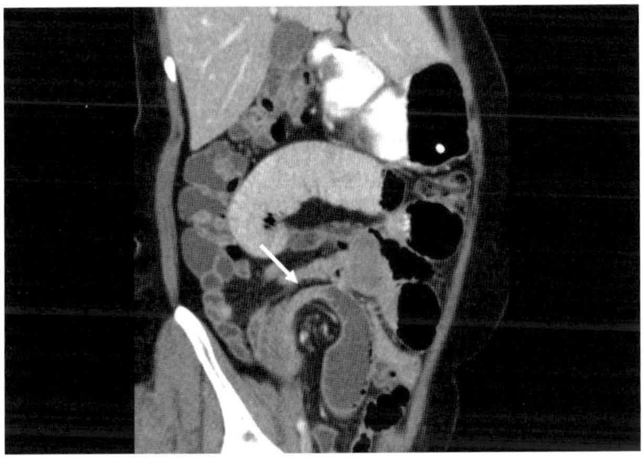

FIG. 19: Oblique MPR image showing abrupt angulation of an ileal loop with minimal mural thickening (arrow) at the site of postoperative adhesion in a case of small bowel obstruction.

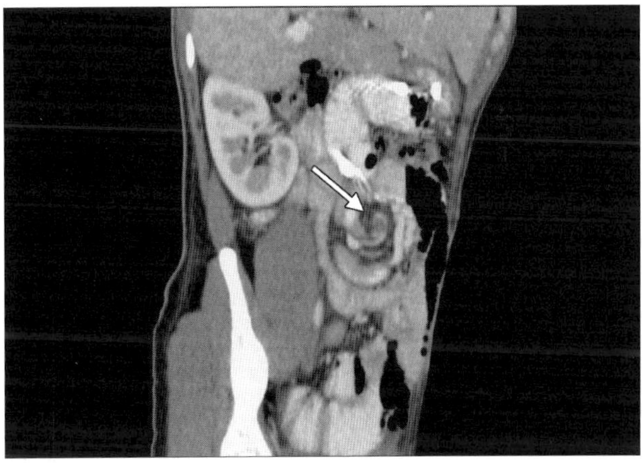

FIG. 20: Oblique MPR image showing midgut volvulus with presence of whirl sign (arrow).

>5 cm) with air-fluid levels proximal to a transition zone with collapsed distal bowel. Minimal mural thickening with enhancement may at times be seen at the transition zone in cases of adhesions **(Fig. 19)**.[31] The "small bowel feces" sign refers to the presence of gas bubbles mixed with particulate matter in dilated loops proximal to the site of obstruction. This is a less common but reliable indicator of mechanical obstruction. Gas filled loops, mesenteric vessels and fat may be seen in the inguinal canal or other sites of external hernias. Circumferential mural thickening of the dilated bowel loops with increased attenuation in the mesentery or bowel wall denotes the presence of strangulation. An internal hernia can be diagnosed if a cluster of dilated small bowel loops which appears to be enclosed in a sac is seen in an ectopic location (e.g. lesser sac or anterior to transverse colon) with crowding and twisting of the mesenteric vessels. A markedly dilated, fluid filled bowel segment with abrupt tapering ends denotes a closed loop obstruction. These show relatively little dilatation of the proximal bowel and are at greater risk for strangulation. Fixed radial distribution of several dilated small bowel loops with stretched and prominent mesenteric vessels converging towards the point of torsion (whirl sign) with mesenteric edema indicates a small bowel volvulus **(Fig. 20)**. A target appearance on cross-section with a bowel-within-bowel appearance on longitudinal scans suggests a diagnosis of intussusception. Mesenteric fat and vessels can be identified within the mass and the lead point if present **(Fig. 21)**. Enteroenteric intussusceptions without proximal dilatation that are less than 3.5 cm in length are probably not significant in adults. Intussusceptions involving the colon that are 4 cm in length or longer, have proximal dilatation or mural thickening should be carefully evaluated for an underlying neoplasm. Foreign bodies, gallstones and bezoars can all cause obstruction and can be readily identified on CT. CT has a sensitivity of 90–96%, specificity of 91–96% and overall accuracy of 90–95% for the diagnosis of high grade obstruction.[1,32] CT enterography with neutral oral contrast is also helpful in cases of partial small bowel obstruction demonstrating the exact site and the cause of obstruction **(Figs. 22A and B)**. It helps in improved visualization of mucosal lesions as compared with conventional CT.[33] Fast MRI has also been shown to be sensitive (95%), specific

(100%) and accurate (96%) in the setting of small bowel obstruction.[34]

Bowel Perforation

Gastrointestinal (GI) tract perforation can be caused by peptic ulcer disease, foreign body, appendicitis, bacterial enteritis, Crohn's disease, diverticulitis, bowel ischemia, obstruction or malignant neoplasms. Some studies have reported US to be a more sensitivity modality than plain radiography for the diagnosis of pneumoperitoneum.[35] Sonographic findings of perforated hollow viscus include demonstration of free air as echogenic spots or lines with posterior ring-down artifacts that shift with change in patient position, enhancement of the peritoneal stripe, echogenic free peritoneal fluid and decreased peristalsis.[36] When patient is in supine position, the reverberations are seen between anterior surface of left lobe of liver and anterior abdominal wall. Shifting phenomenon is seen on rolling the patient to left lateral position as free air rises to the highest portion of the right hypochondrium. Enhancement of peritoneal stripe refers to increased echogenicity and thickening of the peritoneal stripe due to free intraperitoneal air with associated dirty shadowing.

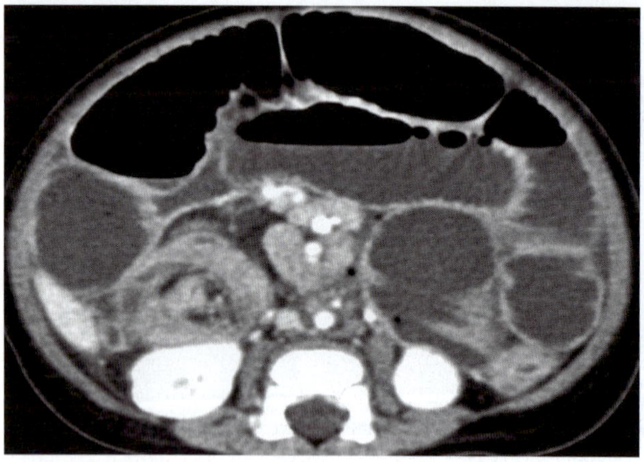

FIG. 21: Axial CECT section demonstrates a 4 × 5 cm, heterogeneous mass in the right lumbar region showing a target appearance with mesenteric fat and vessels within the lesion suggestive of intussusception. The proximal small bowel loops are dilated.

The CT is superior to both plain films and US for the detection of presence, cause and site of perforation. Preoperative localization of the site of perforation is beneficial for the surgeon, with the laparoscopic approach currently being used for most surgical procedures instead of open surgery. Extraluminal contrast extravasation, when seen, is pathognomonic. Other direct signs are the presence of extraluminal air or discontinuity of the bowel wall. Inflammatory changes may also be seen at the site of perforation. CT images should be assessed in wide window settings to distinguish free air from fat density. Careful analysis of anterior peritoneal surfaces of liver and mid-abdomen as well as of peritoneal folds should be done, so as not to overlook a small amount of extraluminal air. The site of colonic perforation may be predicted by the site of extraluminal contrast leakage, concentrated bubbles of air in close proximity to the bowel wall, focal interruption of bowel wall, segmental bowel wall thickening, ill-defined mass, adjacent fat stranding and extraluminal fluid **(Figs. 23A and B)**. A large amount of intraperitoneal air usually indicates gastroduodenal perforation, except for bowel perforation caused by obstruction or an endoscopic procedure.[37] The location of air also helps in determining the site of perforation. Air in the lesser sac can be seen in posterior perforation of stomach or duodenum, or less commonly, from perforation of transverse colon. Free air confined to the intra-hepatic ligamentum teres is commonly due to gastroduodenal perforations. Air trapped in the mesenteric folds is found in colon and small bowel perforation, but seldom in gastric perforation. Retroperitoneal air is caused by perforation of extraperitoneal sites of gastrointestinal tract, viz. descending and horizontal parts of duodenum, ascending and descending colon, sigmoid colon and rectum.

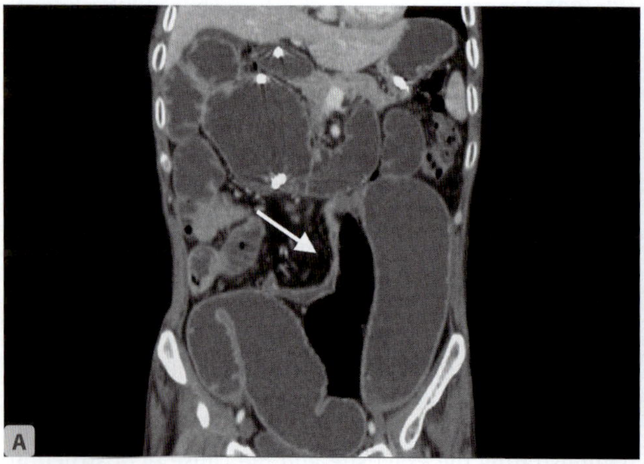

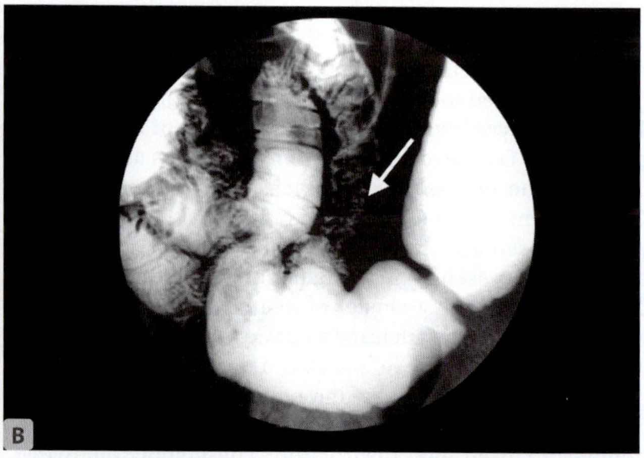

FIGS. 22A AND B: (A) CT enterography coronal MPR image showing a long segment distal ileal stricture (arrow) causing obstruction with dilatation of the proximal small bowel loops; (B) Barium enteroclysis done subsequently confirms the stricture (arrow) in a case of tuberculosis.

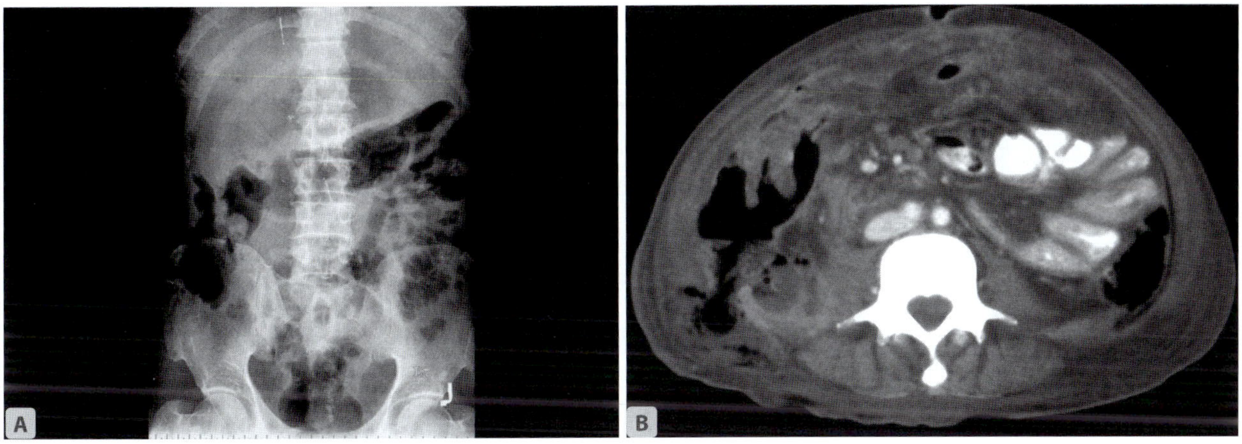

FIGS. 23A AND B: (A) Plain radiograph of the abdomen shows extraluminal, mottled air lucencies in the right iliac region denoting perforation of a hollow viscus; (B) Axial CECT section reveals an ill-defined mass involving the cecum with discontinuity of the lateral cecal wall. A large amount of extraluminal air is seen adjacent to the perforation with extension of inflammation into the right gluteal region and formation of an abscess. This was a case of carcinoma cecum with perforation.

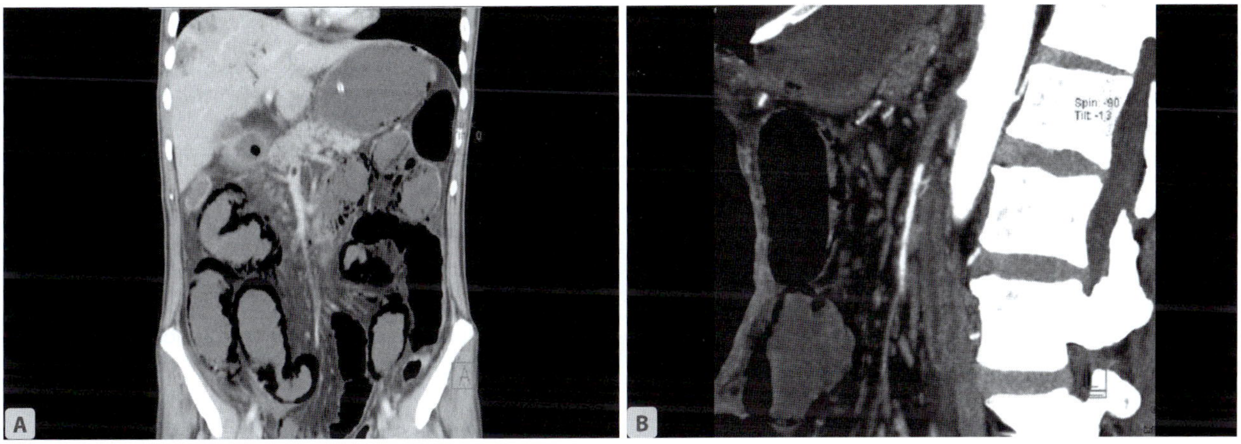

FIGS. 24A AND B: Mesenteric ischemia—CT angiography. (A) The small bowel loops are dilated with thinned-out walls and gross pneumatosis. Air is also seen in the mesenteric veins and the portal radicles in the liver. Note the irregular, nonenhancing hypodense areas in the periphery of the liver due to infarcts; (B) Sagittal MIP image demonstrates the occlusion of the proximal superior mesenteric artery.

Mesenteric Ischemia

Bowel ischemia or infarction is a common but complex disorder with a plethora of primary causes and a wide range of clinical and pathological manifestations. Acute mesenteric ischemia is therefore a diagnostic challenge particularly in view of its high mortality rate which ranges from 50% to 90% depending upon the cause and degree of bowel wall damage. Acute occlusion of the superior mesenteric artery (SMA) due to embolus is the most common cause of mesenteric ischemia accounting for nearly 50% of cases.[38] The manifestation may range from a self-limiting superficial ischemia involving the watershed zones to a diffuse ischemic injury to the entire bowel—"shock bowel" which requires immediate surgical intervention.[39] Plain films reveal the characteristic thick-walled dilated loops with thumb-printing in only 20–30% of cases.[40] Intramural air or portomesenteric air is also rarely visualized on the plain radiograph.

Multidector computed tomography (MDCT) angiography is the modality of choice for the evaluation of bowel ischemia with a sensitivity approaching that of angiography. The most common finding of mesenteric ischemia is bowel wall thickening though this feature strongly depends on the degree of bowel distension. In complete arterial occlusion, there can be absence of the normal enhancement of the bowel wall. Conversely, in nonocclusive ischemia there can be abnormal persistent mural enhancement. The target sign is seen when there is hyperenhancement of the mucosa and submucosa due to hyperemia and hyperperfusion with mural edema.

Luminal dilatation with air-fluid levels can be seen in 56–91% of cases. Pneumatosis and portomesenteric gas are less common but more specific findings of ischemia being present in 6–28% and 3–14% of cases respectively **(Figs. 24A and B)**.[38,39] The presence of pneumoperitoneum or focal peritonitis signifies perforation.

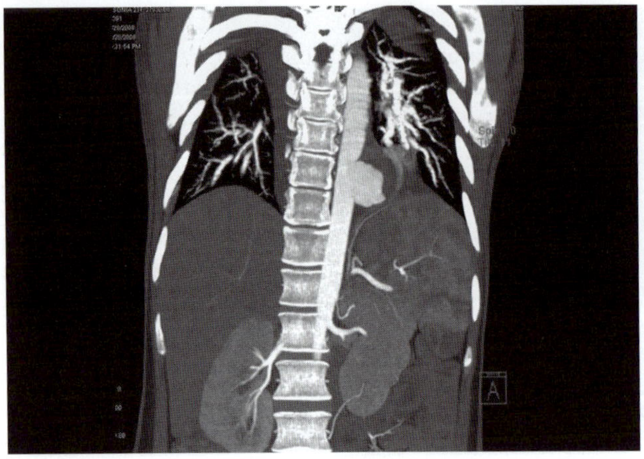

FIG. 25: CT angiography: MIP image shows an irregular, sac-like lobulated outpouching from the wall of the thoracoabdominal aorta due to a mycotic pseudoaneurysm in a case of infective endocarditis. There is associated thrombus as well as a peripheral rim of hyperdensity because of the surrounding hematoma.

Vascular Causes

Vascular conditions that may present as acute abdomen include rupture of an aortic aneurysm, spontaneous aortic occlusion, acute hemorrhage and hepatic or splenic vascular occlusion. Aneurysmal dilatation of the abdominal aorta is rare before the age of 50 with average age at the time of diagnosis being 65–70 years. Most abdominal aortic aneurysms are true aneurysms and occur below the level of renal arteries. An abdominal aortic aneurysm is defined as an aortic diameter of 3 cm or more while a diameter of 5.5 cm or more warrants urgent intervention.[41] Presence of a pulsatile mass and sudden hypotension in the clinical setting of acute pain abdomen suggests the diagnosis of a ruptured aortic aneurysm. Although US may detect the aneurysm as well as the associated thrombus and hematoma, frequently the entire aorta cannot be evaluated due to overlying bowel gas or body habitus. Multidetector CT is the modality of choice for evaluation of acute aortic syndrome. The most common finding of rupture of aortic aneurysm is a retroperitoneal hematoma adjacent to the aneurysm **(Fig. 25)**. Other CT features may include active extravasation of contrast, extension of periaortic blood into perirenal or pararenal spaces or the psoas muscle or peritoneal cavity. Signs predictive of impending rupture are:

- Draped aorta sign—seen with contained leak. The posterior wall of aorta cannot be defined due to close application and lateral 'draping' of the aneurysm around the adjacent vertebral bodies.[42]
- Increase in aneurysm size—a patient with a very large aneurysm (>7 cm diameter) who presents with acute aortic syndrome has a high likelihood of aneurysmal rupture. Also, a rate of enlargement of >10 mm/year warrants surgical repair.
- Thrombus-to-lumen ratio—this ratio decreases with increasing aneurysm size. A thick circumferential thrombus is protective against rupture.
- Focal discontinuity in intimal calcification.
- Hyperattenuating crescent sign due to hemorrhage in either the peripheral thrombus or aneurysm wall.

Acute abdominal hemorrhage may result due to ruptured aneurysm in a case of polyarteritis nodosa, ruptured tumor (usually renal cell carcinoma) or in a patient on anticoagulant therapy. Noncontrast CT demonstrates a hyperdense collection at the site of hemorrhage. MDCT angiography can accurately delineate the site and cause of hemorrhage.

Rare causes of acute abdomen include hepatic vein thrombosis (acute Budd-Chiari syndrome) and portal vein thrombosis. US in the acute phase may show liver enlargement, partial or complete inability to visualize hepatic veins, intraluminal hepatic vein echogenicity or thrombosis, marked narrowing of intrahepatic IVC and ascites. Color Doppler is the technique of choice for initial evaluation. Absence of flow or flow in an abnormal direction in all or part of the hepatic veins may be seen. CT and MR are complimentary techniques for definitive diagnosis which provide a more complete evaluation of the hepatic parenchyma, hepatic veins and IVC.

Pelvic Disease

The various entities that have to be additionally thought of while evaluating a young female in the reproductive age group presenting with acute abdomen are ruptured ectopic pregnancy, PID, twisted ovarian cyst and complications of early pregnancy, etc.

- Signs of a ruptured ectopic pregnancy on ultrasound include an inhomogeneous adnexal mass, pelvic fluid or hematoma, decidual reaction without intrauterine gestation sac, in the presence of a positive pregnancy test. Visualization of an echogenic adnexal ring separate from the ovary that has prominent peripheral flow on color Doppler is highly suggestive of ectopic gestation. Corpus luteum is a useful guide while looking for an ectopic pregnancy and is usually seen in the ipsilateral ovary in 70–85% cases.[43] Using transvaginal ultrasound, the live embryo can be detected in up to 17% of all ectopic pregnancies.
- Fibroids may present with acute pain if there is torsion or degeneration of a submucosal or subserosal fibroid. On imaging, uterine enlargement with a focal mass or contour deformity are seen. Degenerated fibroids may have a cystic appearance.
- Ovarian torsion usually occurs in children and is attributed to excessive mobility of the ovary. In adults, a cyst or mass, frequently a cystic teratoma, is present in the ovary undergoing torsion. Sonographic findings include an enlarged ovary with peripherally distributed follicles, an associated cyst or mass, with diminished or absent central venous flow on Doppler. On CT or MR, deviation of the uterus to the twisted side, obliteration of fat planes and an enlarged ovary displaced from its adnexal location is seen **(Fig. 26)**. Contrast enhanced CT may show surrounding enhancing blood vessels due to congestion.
- Hemorrhage into a corpus luteal or follicular cyst may manifest with abrupt onset of pelvic pain. If the cyst ruptures, associated hemoperitoneum can be life threatening. On imaging, hemorrhagic ovarian cysts can

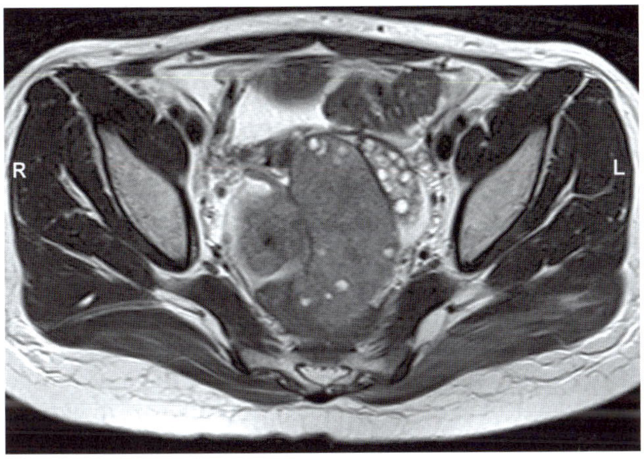

FIG. 26: Ovarian torsion: Axial MR T2WI shows an enlarged right ovary with peripheral follicles displaced into the midline. Note the adjacent normal left ovary.

mimic a variety of solid and mixed solid-cystic masses. A fluid-fluid level may be present. On CT, high attenuation components are usually seen due to hemorrhage.

- Pelvic inflammatory disease (PID) is among the common causes of acute pain in young women. In the early stage of PID, US may demonstrate a small amount of fluid in the cul-de-sac or endometrial canal. On CT, there may be stranding in the parapelvic fat, thickening of the uterosacral ligament and ovarian enlargement with oophoritis. In advanced stages, there is development of pyosalpinx or tubo-ovarian abscess.
- Ovarian vein thrombosis (OVT) should be suspected as a cause of abdominal pain in the postpartum period, in women with PID, recent abdominal surgery, malignancy or known hypercoagulable state. Pregnancy increases the risk for venous thrombosis due to stasis, alteration in coagulation factors and by nearly tripling the diameter of the ovarian veins. In 90% of cases, the right ovarian vein is involved due to dextrotorsion of the uterus.[44] Ovarian vein thrombosis (OVT) may be diagnosed by US, CT or MRI, however CT is the modality of choice and demonstrates a low attenuation thrombus in lumen of ovarian vein.[44]

MISCELLANEOUS

Diverticulitis

The tetrad of left lower quadrant pain and tenderness, fever and leukocytosis is the classic presentation of diverticulitis. Diverticular disease of the colon affects 65% of the Western population by the age of 65 years, and diverticulitis eventually develops in up to 25% of individuals with diverticulosis.[45] Findings on barium enema include diverticulae, muscular wall hypertrophy, intramural or extramural mass effect on the barium column, colonic obstruction or peritoneal extravasation of contrast material, such as with fistula or sinus tract formation. The full extent of peritoneal involvement cannot be estimated on barium examination, hence it has largely been replaced by CT for imaging of suspected diverticulitis. Findings on CT include diverticulae, muscular wall hypertrophy, symmetrical mural thickening >4 mm, pericolonic fat stranding, phlegmon, extraluminal gas bubbles, extravasation of contrast in case of perforation and paracolic abscess formation. Adequate distension and opacification of the colon by contrast material administered per-rectally is the cornerstone of an optimal CT evaluation and helps to distinguish true inflammatory wall thickening from apparent wall thickening due to incomplete luminal distension. The differential diagnosis includes carcinoma: presence of enlarged lymph nodes, mural thickening >1.5 cm and an abrupt change from normal to abnormal colon favors carcinoma over diverticulitis.[46]

Toxic Megacolon

Toxic megacolon is an acute transmural fulminant colitis which can occur as a complication of any colitis but is most commonly seen with ulcerative colitis (1.6–13% of cases). Plain radiographs show marked colonic dilatation (>8 cm) particularly of the transverse colon as this is the least dependent part of the large bowel in the supine position. The wall has a shaggy appearance with mucosal islands or pseudopolyps with absence of haustra due to profound inflammation and ulceration. There may be air-fluid levels and small bowel dilatation. CT shows the distended colon filled with air, fluid and blood with a distorted or absent haustral pattern and irregular, nodular wall.[47] There may be presence of intramural air or blood. The prognosis is poor in the presence of perforation and complications.

Acute Pyelonephritis

Acute pyelonephritis is the bacterial or fungal infection of the renal parenchyma and collecting system. Presenting features include flank pain, dysuria and high grade fever with rigors. On US, renal enlargement, decreased visualization of sinus fat secondary to compression, loss of corticomedullary differentiation, focal poorly marginated hypoechoic areas representing interstitial edema or complications like abscesses may be seen. Harmonic imaging and contrast—enhanced ultrasound can increase the conspicuity of renal parenchymal abnormalities in acute pyelonephritis.[48]

The CT is the imaging modality of choice and can reveal calculi, obstruction, renal enlargement, striated nephrogram, ill-defined, wedge-shaped areas of decreased attenuation radiating from the papillae to the cortical surface, abscess, thickening of Gerotas' fascia and perinephric stranding **(Fig. 27)**. Emphysematous pyelonephritis usually occurs in patients with poorly controlled diabetes with the most common infecting organism being *Escherichia coli*. Presence of air in the renal parenchyma is pathognomonic of this condition.

Acute Urinary Colic

Impacted ureteric stone is the most common cause of acute post-renal obstruction. US is useful for the detection of small/radiolucent calculi missed on plain films. Secondly, direct visualization of the effects of these calculi on the urinary tract is also possible. However, because pelvicaliectasis may be mild to negligible in acute obstruction, US may miss up to one-third of acute obstructions. Color Doppler US helps demonstrate absence of the normal urinary jet on the obstructed side. Unenhanced helical CT has emerged as an attractive modality in the diagnostic workup of urinary tract disease. NCCT KUB is performed rapidly, without patient preparation and without risk of contrast reaction. It can provide information about size, localization and chemical composition of the stone. In addition to direct stone visualization, secondary CT signs of urinary obstruction, including ureteral dilatation, perinephric or periureteric fat stranding, blurring of renal sinus fat and ureteral wall edema, are usually present to confirm the diagnosis even after recent stone passage.[49]

Acute Epiploic Appendagitis, Omental Infarction

Epiploic appendages are fat-containing peritoneal out-pouchings that arise from cecum to rectosigmoid junction, along the serosal surface of the colon. These are 0.5–5.0 cm long and contain fat and small vessels. Epiploic appendagitis is due to torsion of an epiploic appendage leading to venous occlusion and ischemia. It is usually associated with obesity, hernia and unaccustomed exercise. The condition manifests as acute left lower quadrant pain, predominantly in males in the 4th-5th decades of life. On US, a hyperechoic, incompressible mass delineated by a hypoechoic ring is seen at the point of maximum tenderness. The lesions are hyperechoic due to their fat content or hemorrhagic necrosis. CT features include an oval, fat attenuation lesion less than 5 cm in diameter that abuts the anterior or anterolateral serosal aspect of the colonic wall, surrounded by inflammatory changes.[50] A hyperattenuating rim corresponding to the hypoechoic ring on US is seen on CT due to swollen serosa covered by fibrinoleukocyte exudate.

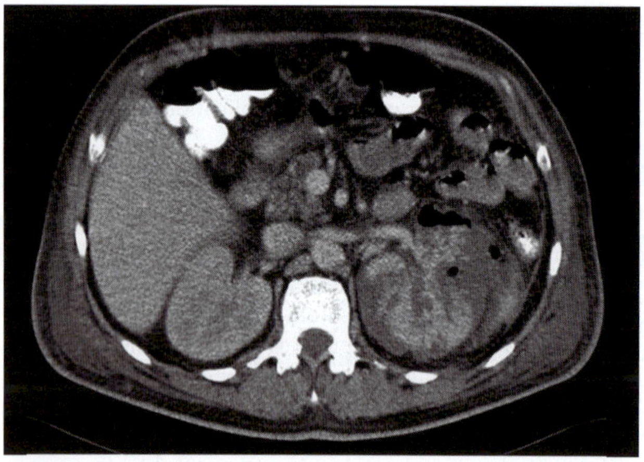

FIG. 27: Axial CT image shows multiple, irregular, linear, hypodense areas in the left kidney due to pyelonephritis. A hypodense area with an air-fluid level is seen in anterior cortex suggestive of renal abscess. In addition, perinephric collection with air is also visualized.

Omental infarction commonly involves the inferior aspect of right side of omentum. It is characteristically situated between the anterior abdominal wall and the transverse or ascending colon, corresponding in location to the greater omentum. Predisposing factors include obesity, strenuous activity, congestive heart failure, digitalis administration, recent abdominal surgery and abdominal trauma. Pain is localized to the right lower or upper quadrant and the presumptive diagnosis is usually appendicitis. Both US and CT show an ovoid, soft tissue mass just beneath the anterior abdominal wall. The infarcted omental fat is hyperechoic on ultrasound and appears heterogeneous with no enhancement on CT.

Although omental infarction may resemble acute epiploic appendagitis on CT, it lacks the hyperattenuating ring seen in the latter. Moreover, omental infarction is larger than epiploic appendagitis which is often less than 5 cm. Omental infarction is commonly located next to the cecum and ascending colon whereas acute epiloic appendagitis is usually located adjacent to sigmoid colon.[50]

Acute Abdomen in Neutropenic Patients

Neutropenic enterocolitis and acute graft versus host disease are common causes of acute abdominal pain in immunocompromised patients and patients with allogenic bone marrow transplants. Cecal wall thickening and involvement of the right side of the colon is the most common finding in neutropenic colitis **(Figs. 28A and B)** with the greatest degree of thickening being found in *Clostridium difficile* colitis.[51] In acute graft versus host disease, bowel wall thickening and abnormal mucosal enhancement are common, with small bowel being most commonly affected.[52]

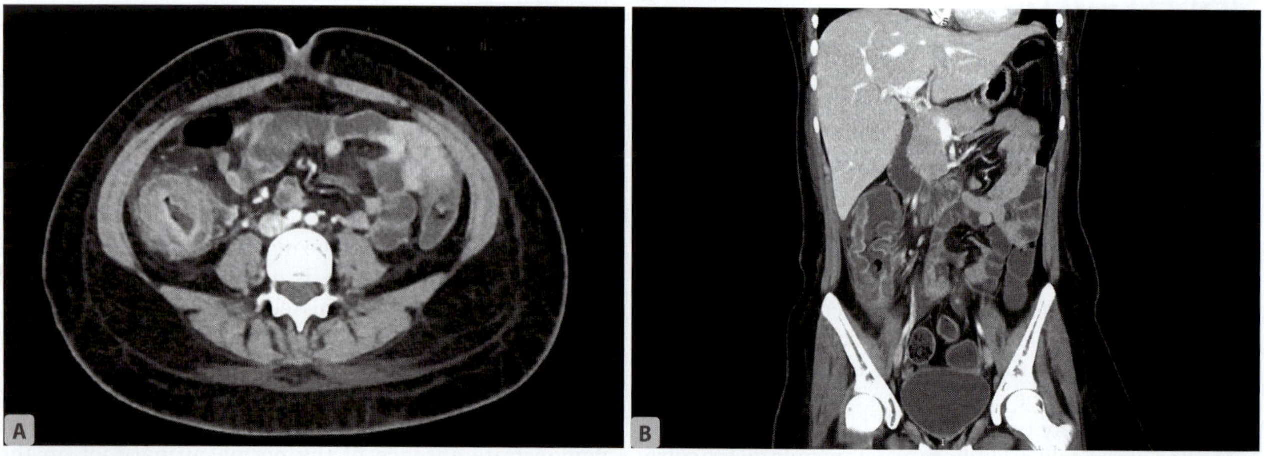

FIGS. 28A AND B: Neutropenic colitis: (A) Axial and (B) Coronal images demonstrate the gross mural thickening in the cecum and ascending colon.

REFERENCES

1. Gore RM, Thakrar KH, Wenzke DR, et al. The acute abdomen. In: Gore RM, Levine MS (Eds). Textbook of Gastrointestinal Radiology, 4th edition. Philadelphia: Elsevier-Saunders; 2015.pp.2255-69.
2. Field S, Morrisom I. The acute abdomen. In: Sutton D (Ed). Textbook of Radiology and Imaging, 7th edition. Edinburgh: Churchill Livingstone; 2003.pp.663-90.
3. de Bombal FT. Introduction. In: de Bombal FT (Ed). Diagnosis of acute abdominal pain, 2nd edition. Churchill Livingstone: Edinburgh, 1991.
4. Balthazar EJ, Chako AC. Computerized tomography in acute gastrointestinal disorders. Am J Gastroenterol. 1990;85:1445-52.
5. Macari M, Balthazar EJ. The acute right lower quadrant: CT evaluation. Radiol Clin N Am. 2003;41:1117-36.
6. Kundra V, Silverman P. Impact of mutlislice CT on imaging of acute abdominal disease. Radiol Clin N Am. 2003;41:1083-93.
7. Lomas DJ. Technical developments in bowel MRI. Eur Radiol. 2003;13:1058-71.
8. Mirvis SE, Young JWR, Keramati B, et al. Plain film evaluation of patients with abdominal pain: Are three radiographs necessary? AJR. 1986;147:501-3.
9. Morrison ID, McLaughlin P, Maher MM. Current status of imaging of the gastrointestinal tract: Imaging techniques and radiation issues. In: Adam A, Dixon AK, Gillard JH, Schaefer CL, Prokop CM (Eds). Grainger and Allison's diagnostic Radiology Edinburgh: Churchill Livingstone; 2015.pp.593-609.
10. Miller RE, Nelson SW. The roentgenological demonstration of tiny amounts of free intra-peritoneal gas: experimental and clinical studies. AJR. 1971;112:574-85.
11. Rubesin SE, Levine MS. Radiologic diagnosis of gastrointestinal perforation. Radiol Clin N Am. 2003;41:1095-115.
12. Messmer JM, Levine MS. Gas and soft tissue abnormalities. In: Gore RM, Levine MS (Eds). Textbook of gastrointestinal radiology, 4th edition. WB Saunders Company; 2015.pp.178-96.
13. Bongard F, Landers DV, Lewis F. Differential diagnosis of appendicitis and pelvic inflammatory disease. Am J Surg. 1985;150:90-6.
14. Rao PM, Rhea JT, Novelline RA, et al. Helical CT technique for the diagnosis of appendicitis: Prospective evaluation of a focused appendix CT examination. Radiology. 1997;140:139-44.
15. Gaitini D, Beck-Razi N, Mor-Yosef D, et al. Diagnosing acute appendicitis in adults: accuracy of color Doppler sonography and MDCT compared with surgery and clinical follow-up. AJR. 2008;190:1300-6.
16. Lee JH, Jeong YK, Park KB, et al. Operator dependent techniques for graded compression sonography to detect the appendix and diagnose acute appendicitis. AJR. 2005;184:91-7.
17. Poortman P, Lahle PNM, Schoemaker CMC, et al. Comparison of CT and sonography in the diagnosis of acute appendicitis: A blinded prospective study. AJR. 2003;181:1355-9.
18. Romero M, Buxbaum JL, Palmer SL. Magnetic Resonance Imaging of the gut: A primer for the luminal gastroenterologist. Am J Gastroenterol. 2014;109:497-509.
19. Uggowitzer M, Kugler C, Schramayer G, et al. Sonography of acute cholecystitis: comparison of color and power Doppler sonography in detecting a hypervascularized gallbladder wall. AJR. 1997;168:707-12.
20. Blankenberg F, Wirth R, Jeffry BR Jr, et al. Computed tomography as an adjunct to ultrasound in the diagnosis of acute a calculous cholecystitis. Gastrointestinal Radiol. 1991;16:149-53.
21. Fidler J, Paulson EK, Layfield L. CT evaluation of acute cholecystitis: Findings and usefulness in diagnosis. AJR. 1996;166:1085-8.
22. Watanabe Y, Nagayama M, Okumura A, et al. MR imaging of acute biliary disorders. Radiographics. 2007;27:477-95.
23. Bennett GL, Rusinek H, Lisi V, et al. CT findings in acute gangrenous cholecystitis. AJR. 2002;178:275-81.
24. Morris BS, Balpande PR, Morani AC, et al. The CT appearances of gallbladder perforation. BJR. 2007;80:898-90.
25. Gore RM, Yaghmai V, Newmark GM, et al. Imaging benign and malignant disease of the gallbladder. Radiol Clin North Am. 2002;40:1307-23.
26. Smith EA, Dillman JR, Elsayes KM, Menias CO, Bude RO. Cross-sectional imaging of acute and chronic gallbladder inflammatory disease. AJR. 2009;192:188-96.
27. Balthazar EJ, Ranson JHC, Naidich DP, Megibow AJ, Caccavak R, Cooper MM. Acute pancreatitis: prognostic value of CT. Radiology. 1985;156:767-72.
28. Stimac D, Miletic D, Radic M. The role of NEMRI in early assessment of acute pancreatitis. Am J Gastroenterol. 2007; 102(5):997-1104.
29. Joseph AEA, MacVicar D. Ultrasound in the diagnosis of abdominal abscess. Clin Radiol 1990;42:154-6.
30. Go HI, Baarslaq HJ, Vermeulen H, Laméris JS, Legemate DA. A comparative study to validate the use of ultrasonography and computed tomography in patients with post-operative intra-abdominal sepsis. Eur J Radiol. 2005;54(3):383-7.
31. Federle MP, Anne VS. Small bowel obstruction. In: Federle MP (Ed). Diagnostic Imaging—Abdomen, 1st edition Amirsys Inc, Utah, 2004.
32. Canon CL. Gastrointestinal Tract. In Lee JKT, Sagel SS, Stanley RJ, Heiken JP (Eds). Computed body tomography with MRI correlation, 4th edition Lippincott Williams and Wilkins, Philadelphia PA, 2006.
33. Ilangovan R, Burling D, George A, Gupta A, Marshall M, Taylor SA. CT enterography: review of technique and practical tips. BJR. 2012;85:876-86.
34. Beall DP, Fortman BJ, Lawler BC, et al. Imaging bowel obstruction: a comparison between fast magnetic resonance imaging and helical computed tomography. Clin Radiol. 2002;57(8):719-24.
35. Chen SC, Wang HP, Chen WJ, et al. Selective use of ultrasonography for the detection of pneumo-peritoneum. Acad Emerg Med. 2002;9:643-5.
36. Jones R. Recognition of pneumo-peritoneum using bedside ultrasound in critically ill patients presenting with acute abdominal pain. Am J Emerg Med. 2007;25:838-41.
37. Furukawa A, Sakoda M, Yamasaki M, et al. Gastrointestinal tract perforation: CT diagnosis of presence, site and cause. Abdom Imaging. 2005;30:524-34.
38. Rha SE, Ha HK, Lee S, et al. CT and MR imaging findings of bowel ischemia from various primary causes. Radiographics. 2000;20:29-42.
39. Wiesner W, Khurana B, Ji H, Ros PR. CT of acute bowel ischaemia. Radiology. 2003;226:635-50.
40. Ha HK, Rha SE, Kim AY, et al. CT and MR diagnosis of intestinal ischaemia. Seminars in US, CT and MRI. 2000;21(1):40-55.
41. Scott RA, Ashton HA, Kay DN. Abdominal aortic aneurysm in 4,237 screened patients: prevalence, development and management over 6 years. Br J Surg. 1991;78:1122-5.
42. Rakita D, Newatia A, Hines JJ, et al. Spectrum of CT findings in rupture and impending rupture of abdominal aortic aneurysms. Radiographics. 2007;27:497-507.
43. Condous G, Okaro E, Khalid A, et al. The accuracy of transvaginal ultrasonography for the diagnosis of ectopic pregnancy prior to surgery. Hum Reprod. 2005;20:1404-9.
44. Heavrin BS, Wrenn K. Ovarian vein thrombosis: A rare cause of abdominal pain outside the peripartum period. J Emerg Med. 2007;34:67-9.

45. Rao PM, Rhea JT, Novelline RA, et al. Helical CT with only colonic contrast material for diagnosing diverticulitis: Prospective evaluation of 150 patients. AJR. 1998;170:1445-9.
46. Chintapalli KN, Esola CC, Chopra S, et al. Pericolic mesenteric lymph nodes: An aid in distinguishing diverticulitis from cancer of the colon. AJR. 169:1253-55,1997.
47. Imbriaco M, Balthazar EJ. Toxic megacolon: role of CT in evaluation and detection of complications. Clin Imaging. 2001;25:349-54.
48. Kim B, Lim HK, Choi MH, Woo JY, Ryu J, Kim S, et al. Detection of parenchymal abnormalities in acute pyelonephritis by pulse inversion harmonic imaging with or without microbubble ultrasonographic contrast agent: Correlation with computed tomography. J Ultrasound Med. 2001;20:5-14.
49. Sourtzis S, Thibeau JF, Damry N, et al. Radiologic investigation of renal colic: unenhanced helical CT compared with excretory urography. AJR. 1999;172:1491-4.
50. Singh AK, Gervais DA, Halin PF, et al. Acute epiploic appendagitis and its mimics. Radiographics. 2005;25:1521-34.
51. Iain D, Kirkpatrick C, Greenberg HM. Gastrointestinal complications in the neutropenic patient: Characterization and differentiation with abdominal CT. Radiology. 2003;226: 668-74.
52. Kalantari BN, Mortelé KJ, Cantisani V, et al. CT features with pathologic correlation of acute gastrointestinal Graft-Versus-Host disease after bone marrow transplantation in adults. AJR. 2003;181:1621-5.

CHAPTER

116

Imaging in Abdominal Trauma

Atin Kumar, Shivanand Gamanagatti,
Chandrashekhara SH

INTRODUCTION

Blunt abdominal trauma in isolation accounts for 5% of trauma mortality and further contributes 15% to mortality as part of polytrauma.[1] Excessive bleeding accounts for 80–90% of acute deaths from abdominal injury. In recent years, advances in cross-sectional imaging coupled with image-guided interventional therapy have made significant contributions in enabling nonsurgical management of blunt abdominal trauma in hemodynamically stable patients.

A radiologist must have a detailed understanding of the patterns of injury, imaging appearance of traumatic injuries, assessment of hemodynamic status, and common image artifacts. The imaging evaluation must take place within the context of systematic and orderly resuscitation of the patient.

Abdominal trauma can be blunt or penetrating. Blunt trauma accounts for approximately two-thirds of abdominal injury patients. Motor vehicle accidents account for up to 80% of blunt trauma with the remainder being caused by falls, assault and industrial accidents. Penetrating injuries commonly result due to gunshot injuries and stab wounds.

The spleen, liver and kidneys are the most frequently injured organs in order of frequency followed by small bowel/ mesentry, bladder, colon, diaphragm, pancreas and major vessels. There are multiple organs involved simultaneously in many patients.[2]

Up to two-thirds of the abdominal trauma patients have a significant injury to other systems as well and these injuries may take precedence for both diagnosis and treatment.

Radiology plays an important role in the diagnosis and management of abdominal trauma patients. This has become even more relevant in the last two decades because there is an increasing trend towards conservative management of most solid abdominal organ trauma. The emergence of imaging as a strong marker for extent of injury has made the surgeons more comfortable with a trial of nonoperative management of these patients and has improved the outcome.

The various imaging modalities used and their current role is discussed below.

PLAIN RADIOGRAPHY

Plain radiography of abdomen is not routinely recommended in an abdominal trauma patient. It is insensitive for the detection of hemoperitoneum as intraperitoneal volume of greater than 800 cc is usually necessary for the demonstration of classic plain radiographic signs, e.g. "dog ear" or "bladder ear" sign when there is accumulation of intraperitoneal blood in the pouch of Douglas. According to Advanced Trauma Life Support (ATLS) guidelines, chest radiograph and pelvic radiographs are recommended as adjunct to primary survey and resuscitation of an abdominal trauma patient. The chest radiograph, besides being required for detecting chest injuries, can also detect pneumoperitoneum. It is possible with optimal radiographic technique to demonstrate as little as 1 cc of free air on an upright chest radiograph. However in this setting it is often not possible to obtain the radiograph in upright position The supine chest radiograph which is usually done is not that sensitive for detecting pneumoperitoneum. The pelvic radiographs are done to detect pelvic fractures in suspected pelvic injuries.

ULTRASONOGRAPHY

Sonography is commonly used for the initial assessment of abdominal trauma. Abdominal ultrasound in cases of major trauma is usually performed with a FAST (Focussed Assessment with Sonography in Trauma) examination. It provides a fast overview of the abdomen to detect free fluid which indicates hemoperitoneum and visceral organ injury in this setting. The FAST scan should be completed within few minutes with an aim to primarily search for free intraperitoneal fluid and screen organs for injury. While parenchymal organ injuries may be detected, search for such injuries should not delay the examination specially in the setting of suspicion of hemorrhage. Following standard views are recommended:

- Transverse view of epigastrium to detect pericardial fluid and injury to left lobe of liver.

- Longitudinal view of right upper quadrant for right lobe of liver, right kidney and Morison's pouch and perihepatic free fluid.
- Longitudinal view of left upper quadrant for spleen, left kidney and perisplenic free fluid.
- Longitudinal views of bilateral flanks to look for free fluid in paracolic gutters.
- Transverse and longitudinal views of suprapubic region for urinary bladder and free fluid in pelvis and pouch of Douglas.
- Bilateral longitudinal thoracic views for pleural effusion.

The reported sensitivity of FAST for detection of free intraperitoneal fluid ranges from 64% to 98% and specificity from 86% to 100%.[3] The false negative rate of FAST is on an average 15% for free fluid detection. Negative FAST should be interpreted as indicative of the absence of hemoperitoneum, not the absence of intra-abdominal injury. However, it should be remembered that the sensitivity of FAST for free fluid is less than that of CT. A negative FAST should be viewed with suspicion if the finding is not commensurate with the patient's clinical presentation. On the other hand, a positive FAST does not necessarily mandate laparotomy. Hemodynamically stable patients with positive FAST should have their injuries staged with CT, giving them the benefit of nonoperative management whenever possible. FAST is not reliable for assessment of the retroperitoneum.

The sensitivity of ultrasound for detection of liver injury ranges from 0.15 to 0.883 and it misses an average of 15% injuries to liver. The sensitivity for splenic injuries is reported to be between 37% and 85% with an average false negative rate of more than 50%. Sensitivity for renal and pancreatic injuries is less than of liver and spleen and even lesser for bowel and mesenteric injuries. The sensitivity for pericardial effusion is high (97–100%).[3] Hence, ultrasound as a modality to detect abdominal injuries is not recommended.

In a technically successful examination, hemoperitoneum **(Fig. 1)** is visualized as a lenticular collection in the subphrenic space, triangular in Morison's pouch and ovoid in the pelvis.

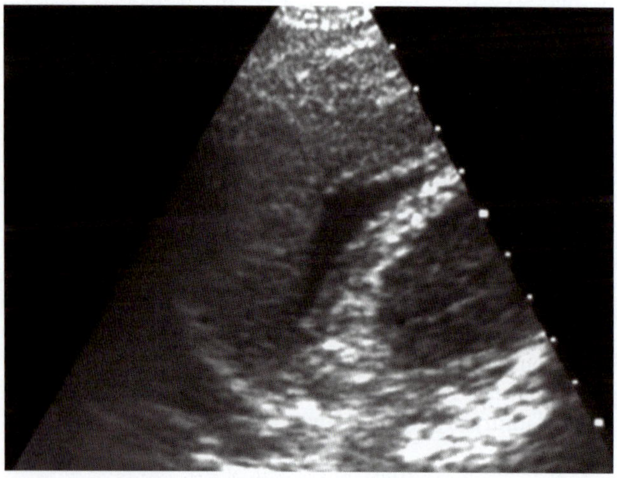

FIG. 1: Axial ultrasound image shows free fluid in hepatorenal pouch.

Recently contrast enhanced ultrasound (CEUS) has been used for improving the detection of solid abdominal organ injuries. It has been shown to detect hepatic, splenic and renal injuries including vascular injuries **(Figs. 2A to C)**. However, the assessment of bowel, mesentery and retroperitoneum is not possible. Hence, it can be used as an alternative to contrast-enhanced computed tomography (CECT) for use in low energy localized trauma in patients with contraindication to CT contrast. It may also be useful in follow-up of patients to monitor the organ injury especially in pediatric patients where radiation dose is a concern.[4]

Ultrasound has certain limitations as the technique is operator dependent and may be limited by excessive bowel gas (especially in post-traumatic paralytic ileus). It may also be limited by open wounds and bandages and by subcutaneous emphysema.

COMPUTED TOMOGRAPHY

Computed tomography (CT) is now firmly established as the principal imaging modality for diagnostic evaluation of abdominal trauma. It is useful in detecting otherwise occult injuries to both intra-abdominal and retroperitoneal structures and grading the severity of specific parenchymal injury. Associated injuries of head and chest, etc. can also be evaluated. According to American College of Radiology (ACR) guidelines, if the initial CT abdomen of a stable patient is negative, then the patient can be safely discharged from the emergency department without a period of observation.[5]

Computed Tomography Technique

Meticulous attention to scanning technique is essential. Scans should be done expeditiously and care should be taken to avoid artifacts and repeat scanning. Current MDCT scanners have significantly reduced the scan time with less motion artifacts besides providing excellent quality reconstructions in coronal and sagittal planes. Administration of intravenous iodinated contrast material is mandatory as it makes detection and location of parenchymal contusions and hematoma more conspicuous, identifies great vessels and provides information regarding integrity of organs or extent of the injury. MDCT protocols vary from institution to institution but typically involve imaging at sub-mm slice thickness, 60–70 seconds after initiating an injection of 100–120 mL of 300 mg/dL low osmolar intravenous contrast medium at 2.5–3.0 mL/second. This phase is best for parenchymal injury detection and is often the only phase done. Careful evaluation of the images is done on the console immediately after acquisition of this phase. If, there is evidence of a contained vascular injury (pseudoaneurysm or fistula) or active contrast extravasation, a localized repeat phase is taken immediately to confirm the same. If the scan shows renal injury then a delayed scan after 5–10 minutes during urographic phase is essential to detect collecting system injuries.[6] Some centers include an arterial phase (25–30 sec after start of contrast injection) to better delineate vascular injuries. However routine use of dual phase (arterial and venous) is not advocated due to concern of radiation. Presently arterial phase

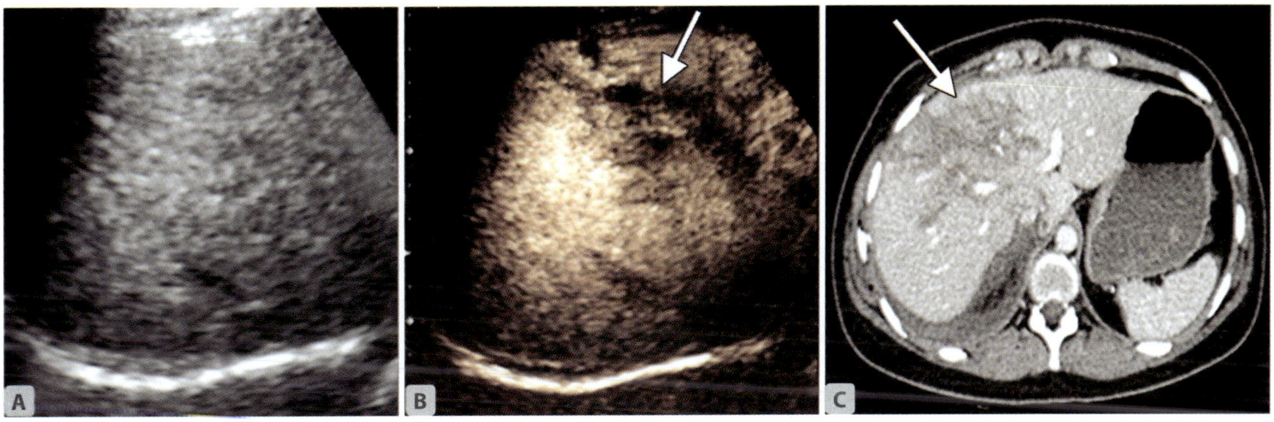

FIGS. 2A TO C: Contrast-enhanced ultrasound of right hypochondrium (B) shows the hypoechoic linear lacerations within the right lobe of the liver (arrow). These were not well appreciated on the grayscale ultrasound (A). CECT axial scan (C) also clearly shows multiple lacerations (arrow).

is obtained mainly in selected indications—pelvis radiograph showing displaced fracture of the pelvic ring and in patients with severe mechanisms of injury.

Computed tomography (CT) cystography may be done in specific situations like hematuria with no renal injury seen on CT or hematuria along with pelvic fracture.[2] It is done by instillation of approximately 300–400 mL of diluted (1:10) iodinated contrast into bladder via Foley's catheter or suprapubic catheter. A delayed phase with passive filling of urinary bladder by renal contrast excretion is not a substitute for the same.

Oral contrast is not administered in the setting of acute trauma in most trauma centers across the world.[2,6] It has a potential use for detecting bowel injuries by showing extravasated oral contrast. But, presence of pneumoperitoneum or pneumoretroperitoneum is an indirect marker for the same. Also usually there is not enough time available at hand to administer oral contrast. Rectal contrast is used occasionally in specific situations to detect colorectal injuries in patients with perineal lacerations and penetrating flank or back wounds.[6]

Viewing on bone window for detecting subtle fractures and upper sections with lung windows for unsuspected pneumothorax, lung contusion or free peritoneal gas should be done.

MAGNETIC RESONANCE IMAGING

Currently, magnetic resonance imaging (MRI) does not play much role in the initial evaluation of the acutely injured patient. MRCP may be useful in detecting biliary transection. MR imaging is useful only for niche indications in hemodynamically stable patients. It has been shown to be useful in detection of pancreatic injuries. The pancreatic parenchymal lacerations and contusions are sometimes better demonstrated on MRI than CT in the acute setting. However, CT remains the first modality for evaluation. If, there are equivocal findings on CT pertaining to pancreatic parenchymal injury, then MRI can subsequently be done to aid in the diagnosis. Moreover involvement of main pancreatic duct is also better characterized on MRI (and MRCP) which is important for deciding management.[7]

DIGITAL SUBTRACTION ANGIOGRAPHY

With recent trend towards nonoperative management of abdominal trauma patients, digital subtraction angiography (DSA) with embolization has been increasingly used in the management of post-traumatic hemorrhage. Angiographic embolization is indicated when CT shows evidence of vascular injury (pseudoaneurysm, arteriovenous fistula) and in active contrast extravasation as an alternative to surgery. It has also been used in controlling bleeding in patients with high grade (IV and V) liver and spleen injuries especially in hemodynamically stable patients with falling hematocrit.

IMAGING AND MANAGEMENT PROTOCOLS

When a patient of suspected abdominal trauma presents to the emergency department, the initial evaluation and assessment is done as per the ATLS guidelines. Chest and pelvic radiograph along with FAST ultrasound are considered as an adjunct of this primary survey and resuscitation. The subsequent management and further role of imaging is dependent upon the hemodynamic stability of the patient. As per the ACR guidelines/appropriateness criteria (first published in 1996 and subsequently updated in 2012)[6] the patients are divided into following categories:

Category A

Patients who remain hemodynamically unstable after initial evaluation and resuscitation. The further management and imaging protocol in this group is outlined in **Flowchart 1**.

Category B

Patients who are hemodynamically stable either at presentation or get stabilized after resuscitation. The imaging and management protocol in this group is outlined in **Flowchart 2**.

Category C

Patients of abdominal trauma who have hematuria. This group requires some modification of imaging workup which is outlined in **Flowchart 3**.

FLOWCHART 1: Hemodynamically unstable patient. Imaging and management protocol in Category A patients.

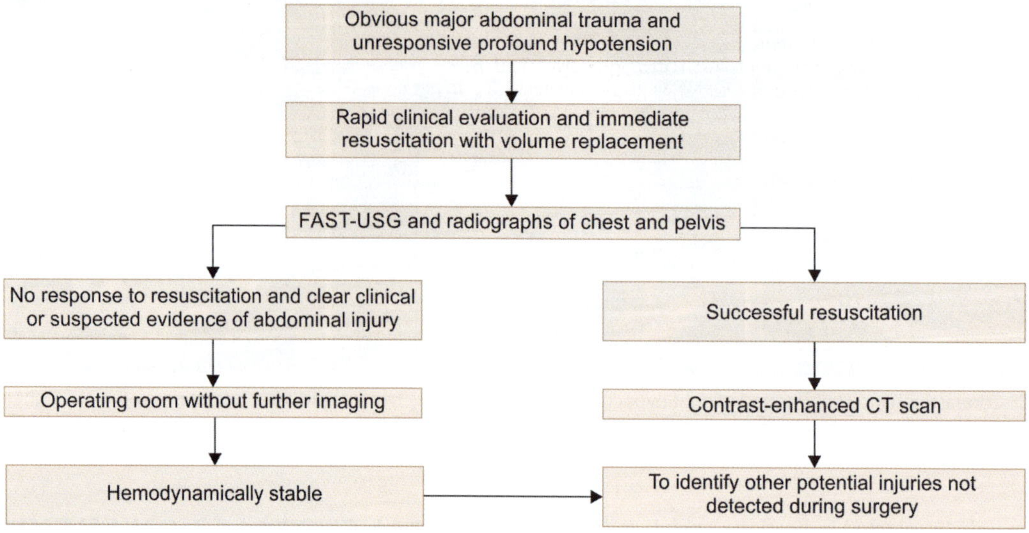

(FAST-USG: focused assessment with sonography for trauma-ultrasound)

FLOWCHART 2: Hemodynamically stable patient. Imaging and management protocol in Category B patients.

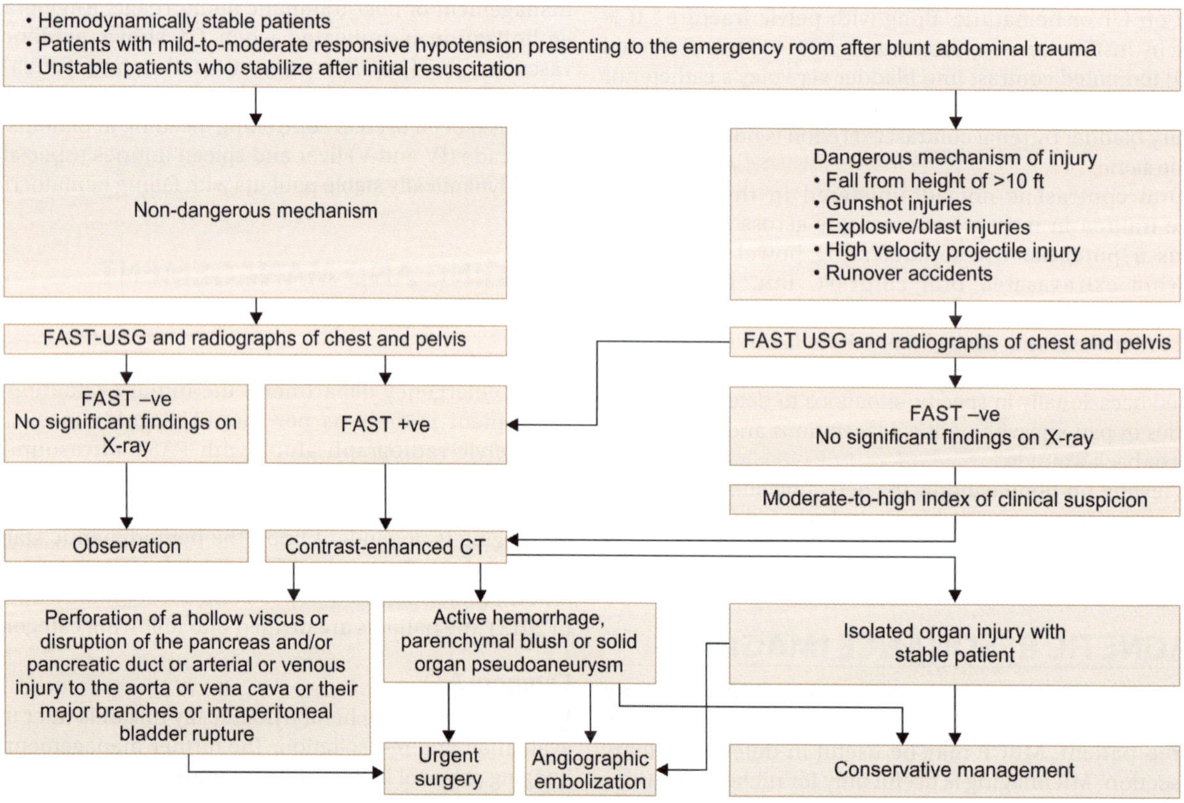

DIAGNOSTIC IMAGING

CT Signs in Blunt Abdominal Trauma

- *Hemoperitoneum:* Blood collects in the peritoneum following injury to the liver, spleen, bowel or mesentery. CT is sensitive in detecting intra-abdominal or pelvic hemorrhage. Non-clotted blood typically has an attenuation value of 30–45 HU whereas clotted blood has attenuation values between 45–70 HU. However a quarter of patients may have HU value less than 20 HU. Therefore hemoperitoneum may not be distinguishable from ascites, extravasated small intestinal fluid from bowel perforation or from intraperitoneal urine from

FLOWCHART 3: Suspected lower urinary tract injury. Imaging and management protocol in category C patients.

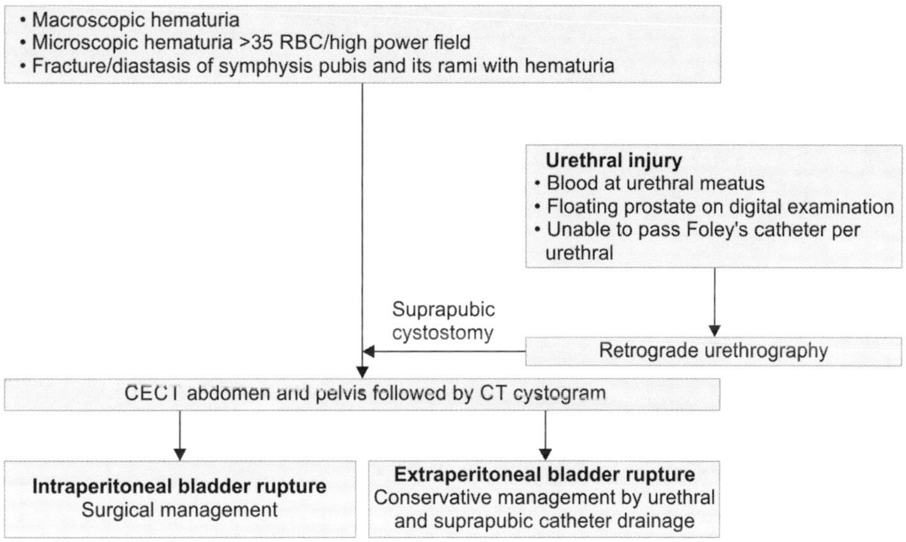

ruptured urinary bladder. Detection of fluid within the abdomen in a suspected patient of abdominal trauma is considered as hemoperitoneum unless proven otherwise. It should however be remembered that in women of child bearing age small amounts of intraperitoneal fluid may be a normal finding. Detection of fluid in each paracolic gutter indicates that at least 200 mL of blood must be present in each gutter. CT visualization of blood in the abdomen and pelvis corresponds with amounts greater than 500 mL.

- *Sentinel clot sign:* Clotted blood adjacent to the site of injury is of higher attenuation (45–70 HU) than unclotted blood which flows away **(Figs. 3A and B)**. When source of intraperitoneal bleed is not evident or in the situation of multiple organ injuries, the location of highest attenuating blood clot is a clue to the most likely source.
- *Interloop fluid:* Triangular fluid collection(s) between the leaves of mesentery are important indicators of bowel or mesenteric injury. Hemoperitoneum from liver or spleen injury typically does not form such collections, but instead tracks from the upper abdomen along the paracolic gutters into the pelvis. When interloop fluid is of low attenuation (<15 HU), bowel injury is suspected and when it is of high attenuation (>30 HU), mesenteric hematoma is likely.
- *Hemodynamic status:* There are a combination of CT findings which give valuable morphological information that correlates with the intravascular volume and cardiac output. Hypoperfusion complex is a gamut of visceral and vascular manifestations which signify the presence of clinical shock in the patient **(Figs. 4A to C)**. They are outlined in **Table 1**.[8]
- *Vascular injuries:* Vascular injuries are classified as free/uncontained and contained vascular injuries. The uncontained vascular injury is seen as active arterial contrast extravasation which is defined as leakage of intravascular contrast from vessel into surrounding extravascular tissues. The active contrast leak appears as a poorly marginated high attenuation contrast density (85–350 HU) seen outside the confines of a vessel **(Figs. 5A and B)**. It may be lobulated or may be spreading. It is usually surrounded by a hematoma. The extravasation appears more hyperdense than clotted blood which has HU values in the range of 45–70. On a repeat delayed scan, the active contrast leak can show change in shape (spreading). The attenuation may either increase or decrease. The contained vascular injuries (pseudoaneurysm or arteriovenous fistula) are seen as contrast outpouching which is usually rounded and well marginated **(Figs. 6A and B)**. It is typically of same attenuation as the adjacent major artery or aorta. On the delayed phase it does not change in shape and the attenuation parallels the attenuation of the adjacent artery or aorta. The vascular injuries must be actively looked for as they (especially uncontained) signify active arterial bleeding in the patient at the time of CT scanning. Detection of these injuries is often an indicator for surgical/angiographic intervention.
- *Pneumoperitoneum:* It is a sign of perforated hollow viscus, but may also occur following pneumothorax and mechanical ventilation. Small amount of air is easily detectable under the right hemidiaphragm on erect chest radiograph. CT is the most sensitive investigation for detection for free peritoneal air. In order not to miss small amounts of free air the images should be viewed on lung window settings. It may be detected on CT over the liver and anteriorly in the mid abdomen **(Fig. 7)**. Bubbles of free air may be trapped between the leaves of the mesentery or in the peritoneal recesses.
- *Contusion/hematoma:* The contusion/hematoma within the parenchyma of solid abdominal organs appears as focal, poorly marginated areas of low attenuation representing edema, hemorrhage and necrotic tissue **(Fig. 8)**. Subcapsular hematomas are characterized

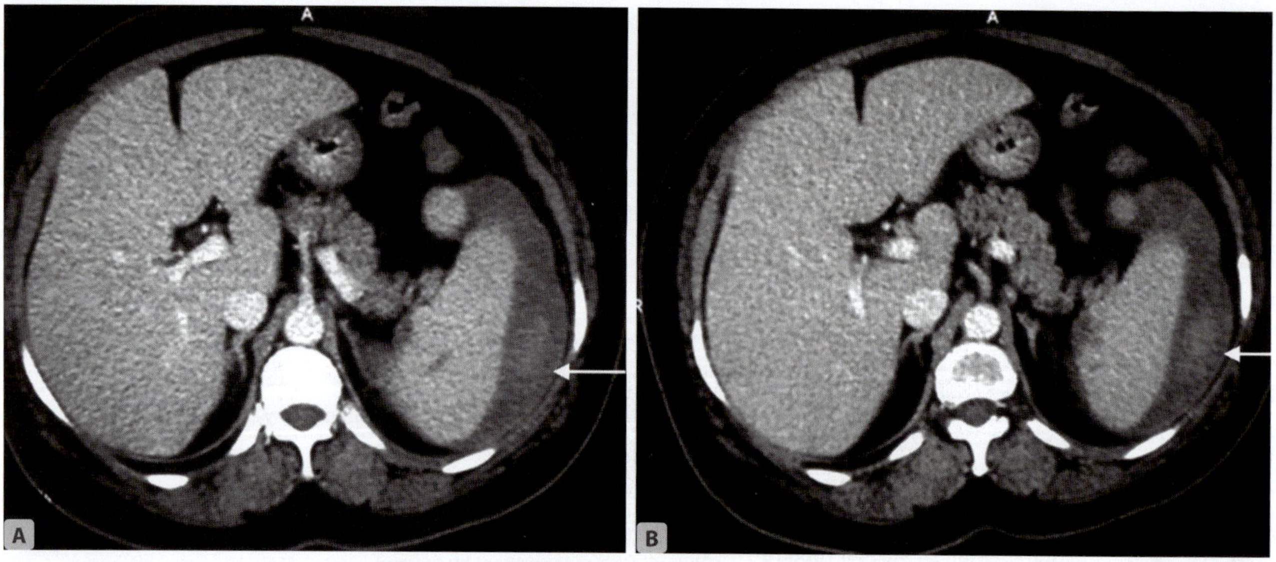

FIGS. 3A AND B: Axial CECT scans show hemoperitoneum in perisplenic region. Note the presence of higher density clotted blood adjacent to the spleen (arrows)—the 'sentinel clot sign'.

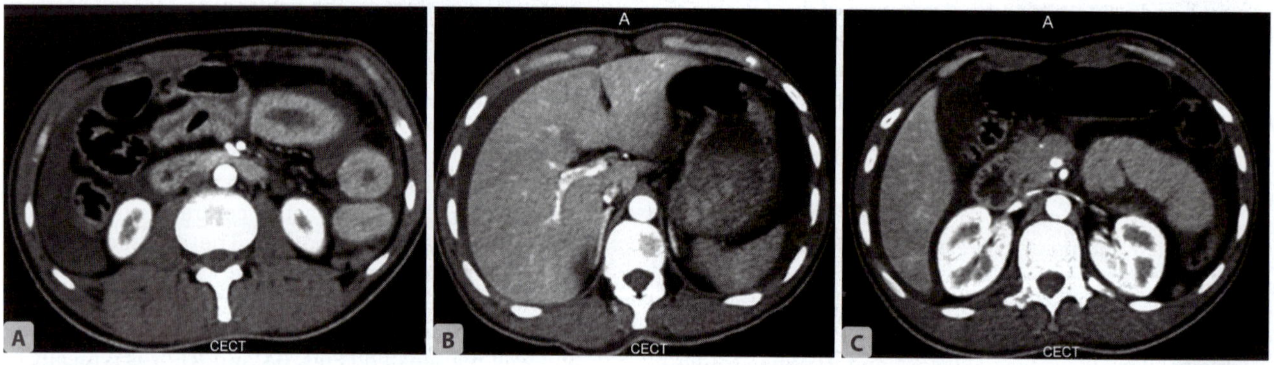

FIGS. 4A TO C: Hypoperfusion state (shock bowel). Axial CECT scan through midabdomen (A) shows diffuse thickening and hyperenhancement of jejunal loops. Note the presence of hemoperitoneum. Axial scan through adrenals (B) show hyperenhancing bilateral adrenal glands. Axial scan through kidneys (C) show flat IVC.

by their lenticular configuration and flattening of the adjacent parenchyma. The compression of underlying parenchyma helps to differentiate subcapsular location of hematoma from free intraperitoneal fluid or blood. Acute hematomas show increased density (40-60 HU) relative to the adjacent normal liver parenchyma at unenhanced CT.

- *Laceration:* Lacerations are seen as nonenhancing linear or branching areas usually at the periphery of the parenchyma **(Fig. 9)**. They are commonly multiple and may involve different areas including different segments. Lacerations decrease in size and number with time. When delayed phase images are taken, the lacerations appear to 'fill-in' from the periphery and become less visible.
- *Infarction/devascularization:* Infarct appears as a well-demarcated wedge-shaped area of low attenuation which remains unchanged on delayed images. It may decrease in size or remain unchanged on follow-up scans. Devascularization occurs secondary to vascular pedicle injury. The entire organ or a large segment does not show enhancement **(Fig. 10)**. Often the occluded major artery is also seen.

Computed Tomography Staging of Abdominal Injuries

Most of the organs in the abdomen are staged according to the American Association for Staging in Trauma (AAST) grading system. It is a surgical grading but can be very well correlated with CT. All organ injuries should be staged accordingly as it is an important marker for extent of injury and deciding further course of management. Majority of the injuries to the liver, spleen and kidneys can be managed nonoperatively. However, the higher grade injuries require a close observation and often surgical intervention.

TABLE 1: CT signs for hypoperfusion complex.

Vascular signs	***Visceral signs***
Diminished caliber of IVC: AP diameter less than 9 mm on 3 slices of intrahepatic IVC, at and 2 cm below renal veins	*Hollow visceral abnormalities*: • Increased bowel wall mucosal enhancement, gastric dilatation
Diminished caliber of aorta: AP diameter less than 1.3 cm, 2 cm above, at and below renal arteries	*Solid visceral abnormalities*: • Intense adrenal gland enhancement (greater than IVC) • Renal cortical enhancement (greater than that of aorta) • Dark spleen • Only pancreatic parenchymal enhancement

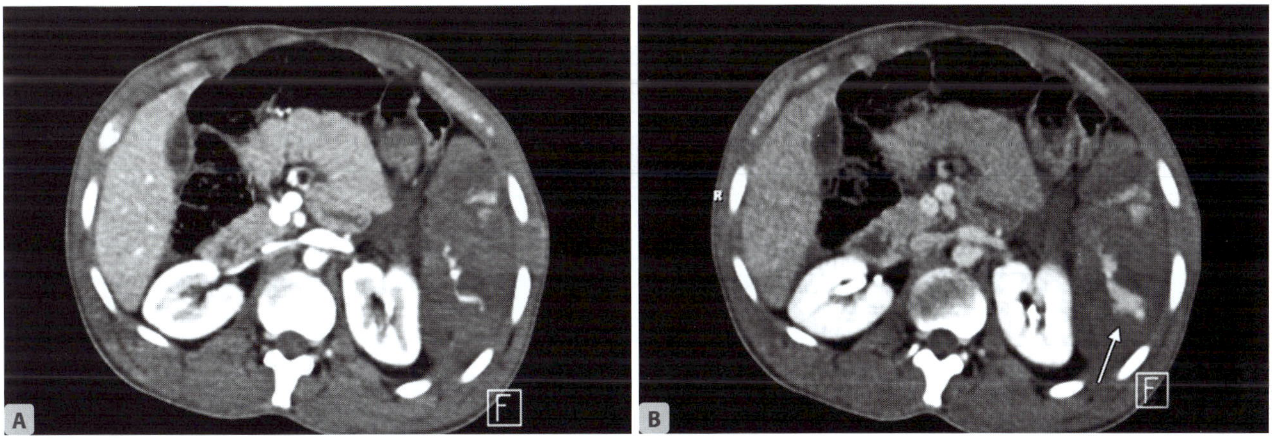

FIGS. 5A AND B: CECT abdomen axial image through the level of spleen (A) shows an irregular contrast density (arrow) in the region of splenic bed. The spleen is showing a large hematoma. The delayed image (B) acquired immediately after the first scan shows the contrast density to be spreading and changing in shape (arrow) confirming active contrast extravasation.

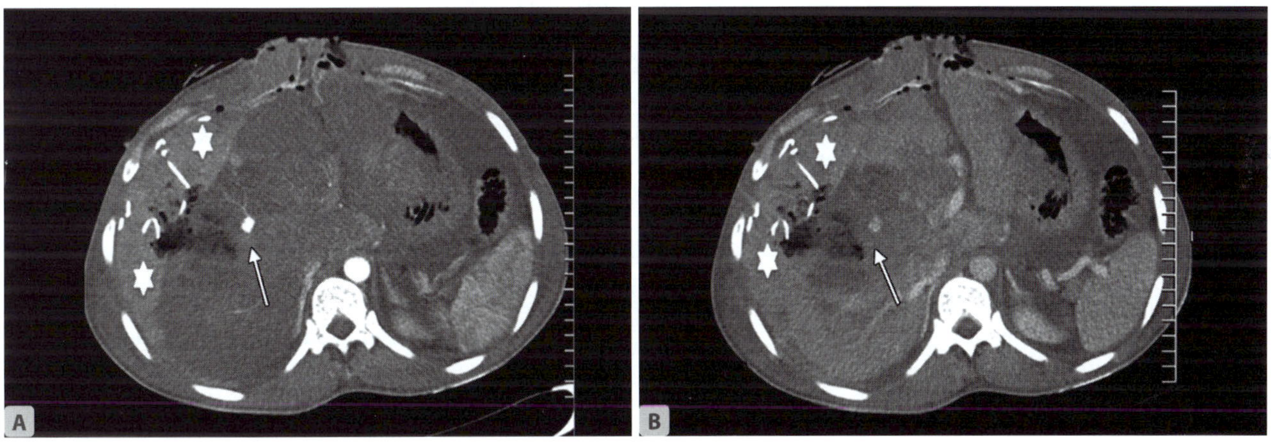

FIGS. 6A AND B: CECT abdomen axial image through the level of liver in a patient who underwent an urgent damage control surgery with perihepatic packing (A) shows a well-marginated, rounded-contrast density lesion (arrow) in the liver which is of same density as the aorta. On the delayed image (B) acquired immediately after the first scan, the lesion (arrow) maintains the same shape but shows decrease in attenuation paralleling the attenuation of the aorta. Note the presence of a large perihepatic hematoma (stars in A and B) with surgical packs.

Computed Tomography Signs for Operative/ Angiographic Intervention

As already discussed, most abdominal injuries are currently treated by nonoperative management. The surgical intervention is predominantly based on clinical condition of the patient. The CT grading aids the trauma surgeon to monitor the patient. The higher grade injury *per se* is not an indication for surgical intervention but are more likely to be associated with an unstable hemodynamic condition of the patient which may require surgery or angiography. However, there are few CT findings which when seen may warrant a surgical repair. These are:

- Pneumoperitoneum—signifies full thickness bowel injury (exclude other causes as described later)
- Pancreatic transection—with involvement of pancreatic duct
- Diaphragmatic injury

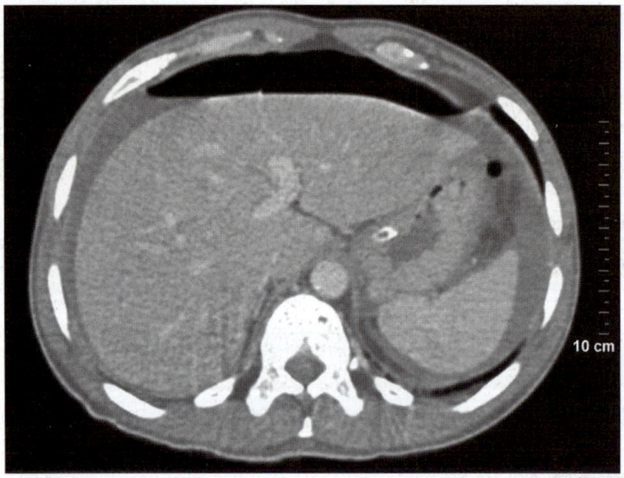

FIG. 7: Axial CECT scan through upper abdomen in lung window settings shows pneumoperitoneum anterior to liver.

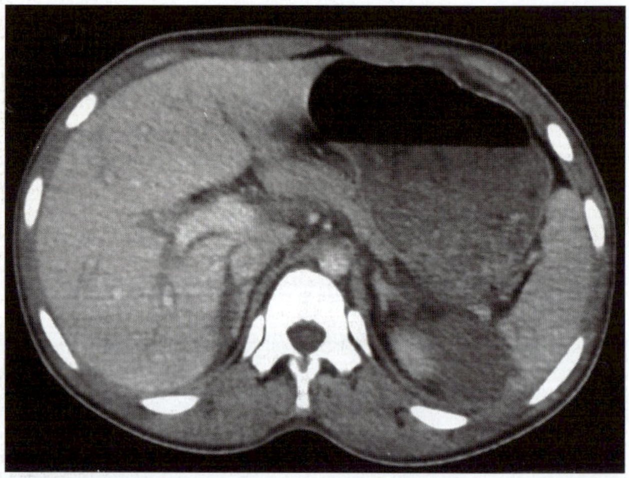

FIG. 8: Axial CECT scan through upper abdomen shows a splenic parenchymal hematoma.

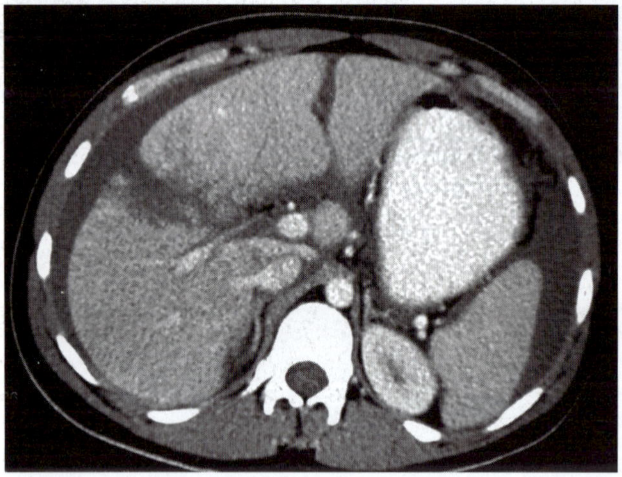

FIG. 9: Axial CECT scan shows a linear liver laceration

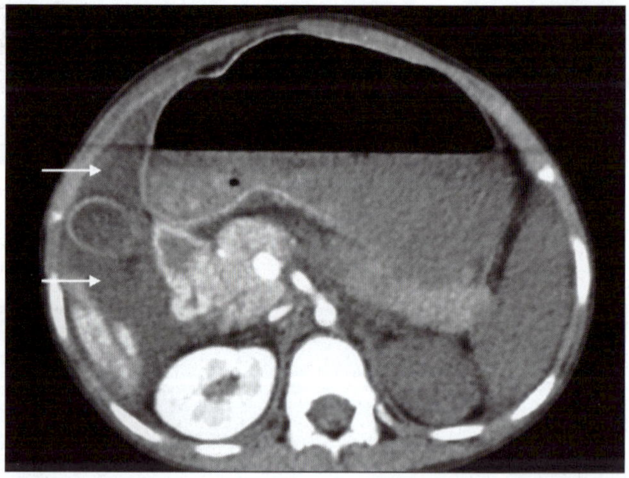

FIG. 10: Axial CECT scan shows nonenhancing and left kidney spleen (devascularized) (arrows).

- Intraperitoneal rupture of urinary bladder
- Mesenteric hematoma/vascular injury
- Renal pelvic injury.

The following CT features when seen are relative indications for either a surgical or angiographic intervention:

- Grade 4/5 liver injuries
- Grade 4/5 splenic injuries
- Vascular injuries—uncontained (active contrast extravasation) or contained (pseudoaneurysm or arteriovenous fistula).

SPLEEN

Spleen is the most commonly injured organ following blunt abdominal trauma. It is the most vascular organ of the body containing approximately 500–600 mL of blood. Although it may occur as an isolated injury, most patients with splenic trauma have associated intra-abdominal injuries.[9] The AAST splenic injury grading scale is depicted in **Table 2**.[10]

However, this AAST injury grading score is based on appearance of the spleen at surgery. CT may not be able to correctly show all the above features and hence there may be limitations in accurately grading the splenic injuries. Moreover the AAST grading does not take into account vascular injuries on CT. Marmery et al.[10] have proposed a modified splenic injury grading system taking into account the findings of active splenic hemorrhage and vascular injuries on CT. According to their modified grading system, active intraparenchymal and subcapsular splenic bleeding, splenic vascular injury (pseudoaneurysm or arteriovenous fistula) and shattered spleen should be classified as Grade IVa and active intraperitoneal bleeding as Grade IVb. There is no Grade V in their classification. It has now been well established that the presence of active hemorrhage and vascular injuries is predictive of the need for splenic artery transcatheter embolization or splenic surgery. The authors compared their modified grading with the AAST splenic injury grading scale and found it to be a better predictor for

TABLE 2: AAST organ injury scale for Spleen.

Grade*	***Description***
Grade I	*Hematoma:* Subcapsular, <10% surface area *Laceration:* Capsular tear, <1 cm in parenchymal depth
Grade II	*Hematoma:* Subcapsular, 10–50% surface area; intraparenchymal, <5 cm in diameter *Laceration:* Capsular tear, 1–3 cm in parenchymal depth, not involving a trabecular vessel
Grade III	*Hematoma:* Subcapsular, >50% surface area or expanding; ruptured subcapsular or parenchymal hematoma; intraparenchymal hematoma >5 cm or expanding *Laceration:* >3 cm in parenchymal depth, involving trabecular vessels
Grade IV	*Laceration:* Involving segmental or hilar vessels producing major devascularization (>25% of spleen)
Grade V	*Hematoma:* Completely shattered spleen *Laceration:* Hilar vascular injury that devascularizes spleen

*Advance one grade for multiple injuries up to grade III
(AAST: American Association for the Surgery of Trauma)

surgical or angiographic intervention in patients of splenic trauma (grade IV patients).

- Arterial phase, if obtained, shows vascular injuries better and they may sometimes be difficult to detect on venous phase alone.[9] However, it is important to evaluate spleen on portal venous phase of CT as heterogeneous enhancement in the arterial phase can simulate injury. If the arterial phase has not been obtained and the venous phase shows suspicion of a vascular injury then, as already stated above, another immediate delayed phase should be obtained. This will help to confirm vascular injury and also differentiate between contained and uncontained injury.
- Delayed phase may also be useful in differentiating a laceration from a splenic cleft.[9,11] When delayed phase images are taken, the lacerations appear to 'fill-in' from the periphery and become less visible. In contrast, splenic clefts remain unchanged in appearance on delayed phase images besides having smooth or rounded margins.

Splenic artery embolization (SAE) has now been established as an effective tool to aid in the nonsurgical management of splenic injuries. Currently grades 4 and 5 injuries **(Fig. 11)** and those showing vascular injuries (active leak or pseudoaneurysms) are indications for SAE **(Figs. 12A and B)**. Selected cases of grade III with large hemoperitoneum who may be transiently responding to resuscitative efforts can also benefit by SAE. The embolization aims to reduce the perfusion pressure to the spleen by blocking the arterial supply. However development of collaterals from pancreatic circulation prevents clinically significant infarction thereby preserving splenic function. SAE has been shown to have beneficial effect on hematocrit drop and fluid requirements of the patient besides decreasing the length of hospital stay.[12,13]

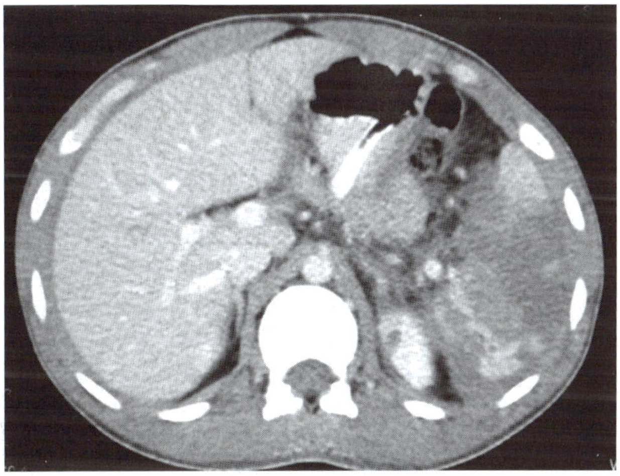

FIG. 11: Axial CECT scan through the spleen shows a shattered splenic parenchyma consistent with grade V injury.

LIVER AND BILIARY TRACT

The liver is the second most frequently injured solid abdominal organ after spleen.[2] The right lobe is injured more frequently and severely than the left and posterior segments are more frequently injured than anterior. As with spleen, CT is currently the diagnostic modality of choice for the evaluation of blunt liver trauma in hemodynamically stable patients. The AAST liver injury grading system is depicted in **Table 3.**[10]

- Majority (80%) of liver injuries cause hemoperitoneum. The finding of integrity of the liver capsule is important because it correlates with the amount of blood loss. Few specific features of liver injuries are discussed below. The subcapsular hematomas are located most commonly in the anterolateral aspect of right lobe of liver **(Figs. 13A and B)**.
- Laceration is the most common type of liver injury. They frequently course along the vascular planes (portal vein branches and hepatic veins) and fissures (ligamentum teres and venosum), which are anatomic weak zones. They can be classified as superficial (≤3 cm in depth) or deep (>3 cm).
- Periportal tracking is seen as low density areas along the portal vein branches. When accompanied by an adjacent parenchymal laceration, it indicates blood tracking along the periportal connective tissue **(Fig. 14)**.[14] It may also be secondary to distension of periportal lymphatic vessels due to increased central venous pressure of any cause

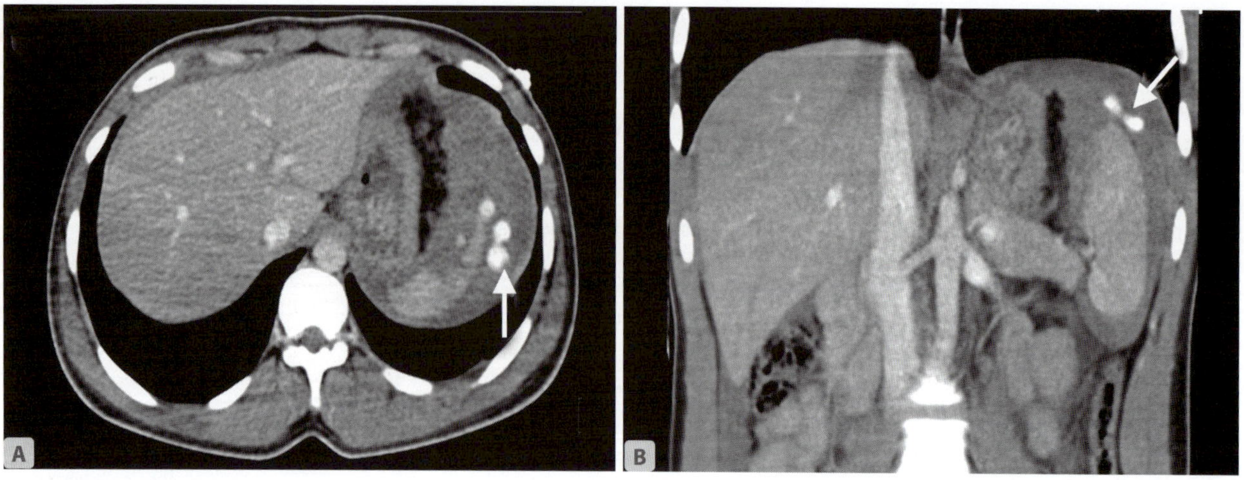

FIGS. 12A AND B: CECT axial (A) and coronal reformatted (B) images shows active contrast extravasation (arrows) from the spleen into peritoneum. The upper pole of the spleen shows a laceration. There is hemoperitoneum in perisplenic region.

TABLE 3: AAST organ injury scale for liver.

*Grade**	*Description*
Grade I	*Hematoma:* Subcapsular, <10% surface area *Laceration:* Capsular tear, <1 cm in parenchymal depth
Grade II	*Hematoma:* Subcapsular, 10–50 % surface area; intraparenchymal, <10 cm in diameter *Laceration:* 1–3 cm in parenchymal depth, <10 cm in length
Grade III	*Hematoma:* Subcapsular, >50% surface area or expanding; ruptured subcapsular or parenchymal hematoma; intraparenchymal hematoma >10 cm or expanding or ruptured *Laceration:* >3 cm in parenchymal depth
Grade IV	*Laceration:* Parenchymal disruption involving 25–75% hepatic lobe or 1–3 Couinaud segments
Grade V	*Laceration:* Parenchymal disruption involving >75% hepatic lobe or >3 Couinaud segments *Vascular:* Juxtahepatic venous injuries (i.e. central major hepatic veins or retrohepatic vena cava)
Grade VI	*Vascular:* Hepatic avulsion

*Advance one grade for multiple injuries up to grade III

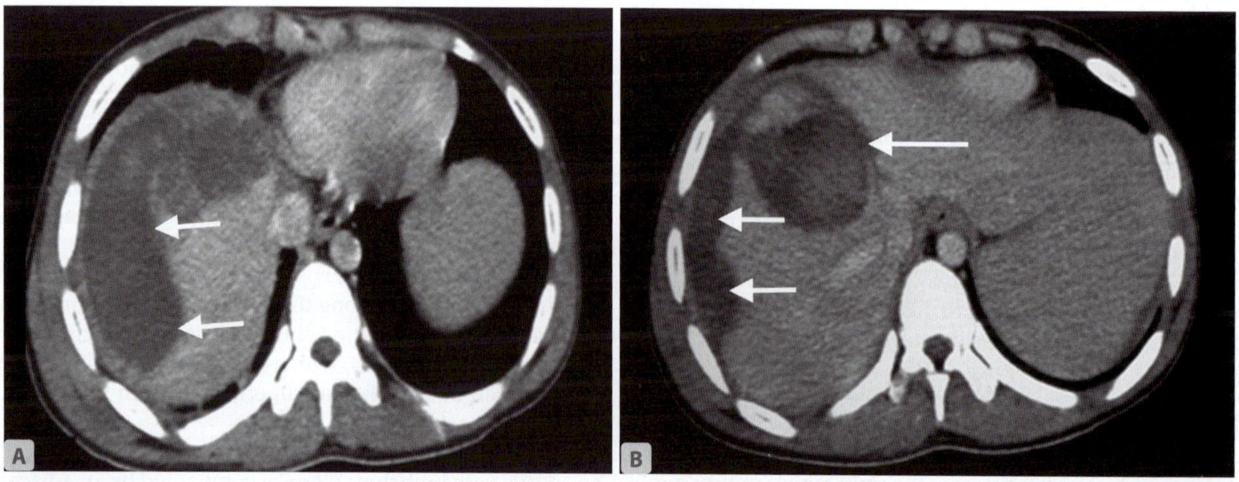

FIGS. 13A AND B: Axial CECT scans show a large subcapsular liver hematoma (small arrows in A and B) caused due to rupture of a parenchymal hematoma (long arrow in B).

most commonly following vigorous intravenous fluid replacement.

- Major hepatic venous injury should be suspected if CT shows lacerations or hematomas extending into one or more major hepatic veins or IVC. If detected, it is an indicator for surgical treatment.
- Uncommonly intrahepatic or subcapsular air may be seen up to 2 days after the injury, and it is attributed to necrosis rather than infection.
- Hemobilia is seen as high attenuating material in the gallbladder or biliary channels **(Figs. 15A and B)**. It is caused when persistent arterial hemorrhage elevates intrahepatic pressure leading to parenchymal necrosis and blood spilling into the biliary tree and gut.
- Intraperitoneal bile leak and peritonitis can occur secondary to disruption of biliary system by trauma. Bile leaks are seen as relatively low attenuation fluid collections as compared to hemoperitoneum. These may be intrahepatic or extrahepatic, diffuse, focal or encapsulated (biloma).[14]

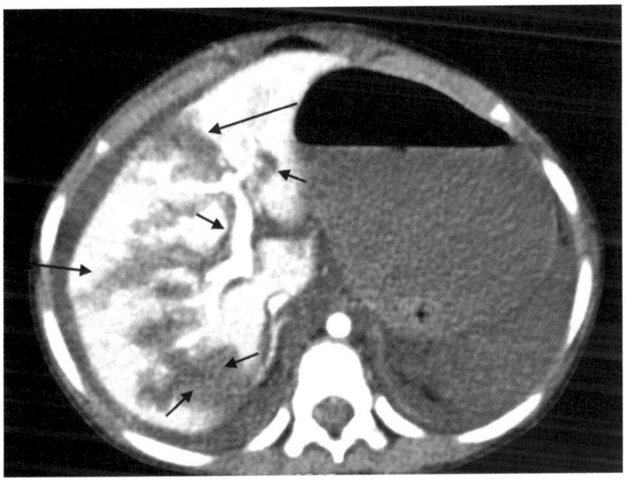

FIG. 14: Axial CECT scan though liver shows periportal fluid tracking (small arrows). The liver shows multiple lacerations (long arrows) and contusion.

With the current concept of nonsurgical conservative management being employed in majority of patients of liver injury including those with severe grades, there is increased frequency of delayed complications visualized on follow-up CT. These include:[14]

- *Delayed hemorrhage:* Secondary to rupture of pseudoaneurysm formed by a biloma or secondary to an initially minimal but expanding injury.
- *Hepatic artery pseudoaneurysm and hemobilia:* A pseudoaneurysm is formed when the arterial continuity is disrupted and blood extravasates into a parenchymal hematoma with formation of a fibrous tissue capsule. They appear as focal rounded enhancing lesions paralleling the attenuation of arterial blood in all phases. When the pseudoaneurysm ruptures into biliary system it leads to hemobilia and subsequent drainage into duodenum can lead to hematemesis or melena. These pseudoaneurysms should be treated early and angiographic embolization is the modality of choice.
- *Abscess:* Usually seen in follow-up of high grade liver injuries. It is visualized as fluid containing focal lesion with air bubbles or air-fluid levels. The treatment of choice is percutaneous catheter drainage.
- *Biliary complications:* Biliary leaks are usually self-limiting with no definitive treatment required. Hepatic scintigraphy and MRCP may be helpful in detecting bile leaks. Bile leak into a hematoma may cause necrosis of surrounding liver tissue leading to formation of biloma which on CT appears as low attenuating well circumscribed collection. Enlarging or symptomatic bilomas can be treated with percutaneous catheter drainage with or without ERCP guided endobiliary stent placement. Bile leak into peritoneal cavity leads to biliary peritonitis which may be suspected on CT if peritoneal thickening and enhancement is seen with increasing amount of low attenuation fluid.

Follow-up CT is usually not required in low grade injuries unless patient's clinical status demands so. However in high grade injuries (grades IV or V), due to increased incidence of delayed complications a follow-up ultrasound is usually

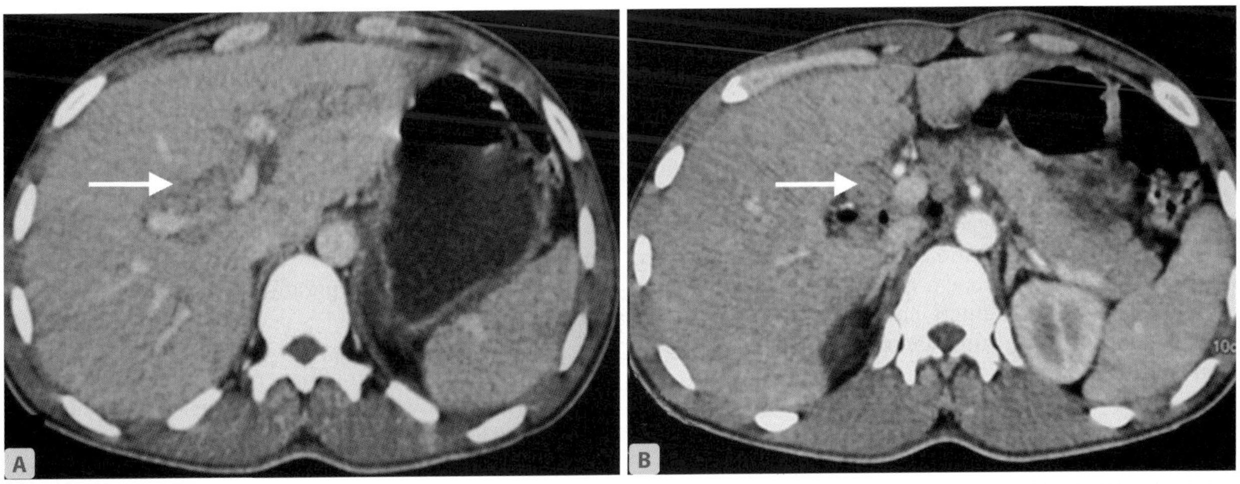

FIGS. 15A AND B: Axial CECT scans through upper abdomen show hyperdensity within intrahepatic bile ducts (arrow in A) and within the CBD (arrow in B) suggesting hemobilia.

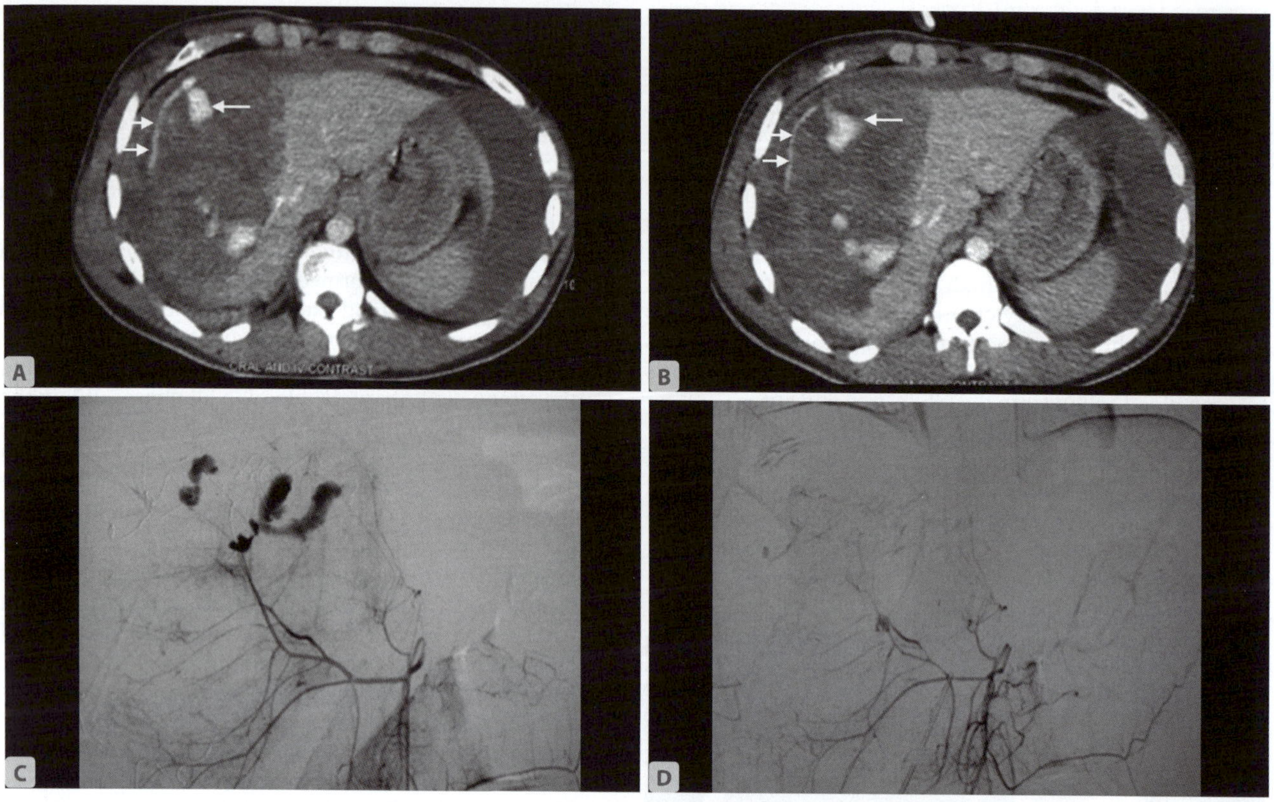

FIGS. 16A TO D: Axial CECT scans (A and B) show active contrast extravasation within liver parenchyma (arrows) extending into peritoneal space (small arrows). DSA image (C) of selective hepatic artery injection shows active contrast extravasation. Post coil embolization (D), the extravasation has stopped.

required and should be done between 7 days to 10 days after injury.[15] Contrast-enhanced ultrasound, if available, can improve the diagnostic accuracy. CT scan may be required in selected complicated cases.

Hepatic artery embolization (HAE) has also been increasingly used in the management of liver injuries.[15] It is indicated when CT shows presence of a vascular injury in the form of active contrast extravasation or pseudoaneurysm **(Figs. 16A to D)**. It can also be done prophylactically for grades 4 and 5 injuries and has been shown to decrease morbidity and mortality. The dual blood supply to the liver from hepatic artery and portal venous system helps in this regard wherein the hepatic artery or its branches can be sacrificed without much risk of infarction.

Gallbladder injuries are unusual. CT findings of ill-defined contour of gallbladder, wall thickening, intraluminal hemorrhage, or collapsed lumen, especially in the presence of pericholecystic fluid suggests primary gallbladder injury in patients with abdominal trauma. Injuries to the extrahepatic bile ducts are uncommon and occur at the points of fixations, i.e. where the hepatic ducts enter the liver and where common bile duct enters the pancreas. The diagnosis is most often made at surgery.

PANCREAS

The pancreas is the least commonly injured solid organ, accounting for 3–12% of all abdominal injuries.[16] This injury occurs after a sudden force that compresses the pancreatic neck against lumbar spine, e.g. in motor vehicle accidents in adults and bicycle accidents in children. Pancreatic injuries are difficult to diagnose. The presence of abdominal pain, leukocytosis and hyperamylasemia is nonspecific and frequently not present.

CT has been shown to have sensitivity and specificity of about 85% for detection of pancreatic injuries. The routine venous phase which is acquired for rest of the abdomen is often sufficient to diagnose pancreatic injuries. The injuries are classified according to the AAST grading for pancreatic injuries **(Table 4)**.[17] The following points are most relevant for clinical management:

TABLE 4: AAST organ injury scale for pancreas.

*Grade**	*Description of injury*
Grade I	Minor contusion without duct injury Superficial laceration without duct injury
Grade II	Major contusion without duct injury or tissue loss Major laceration without duct injury or tissue loss
Grade III	Distal transaction or parenchymal injury with duct injury
Grade IV	Proximal transaction or parenchymal injury involving ampulla
Grade V	Massive disruption of pancreatic head

*Advance one grade for multiple injuries up to grade III

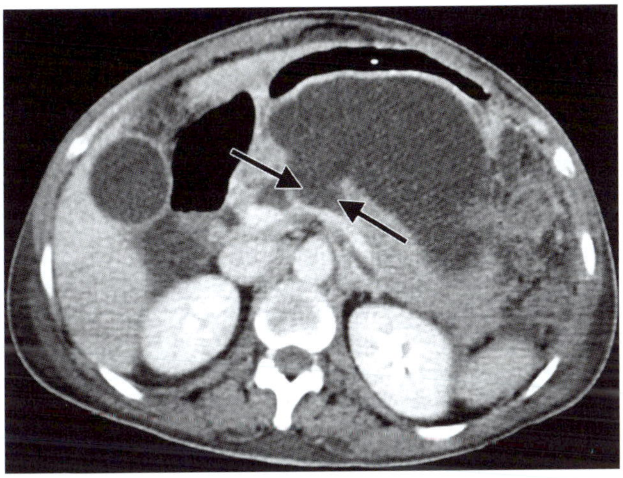

FIG. 17: Axial CECT scan through pancreas shows a laceration/transection involving neck/proximal body of pancreas (arrows) with a large collection seen anterior to pancreas.

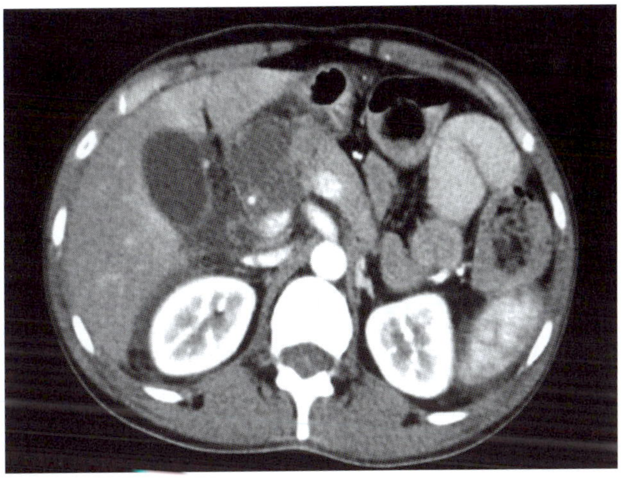

FIG. 18: Axial CECT scan shows a contusion involving the head of pancreas.

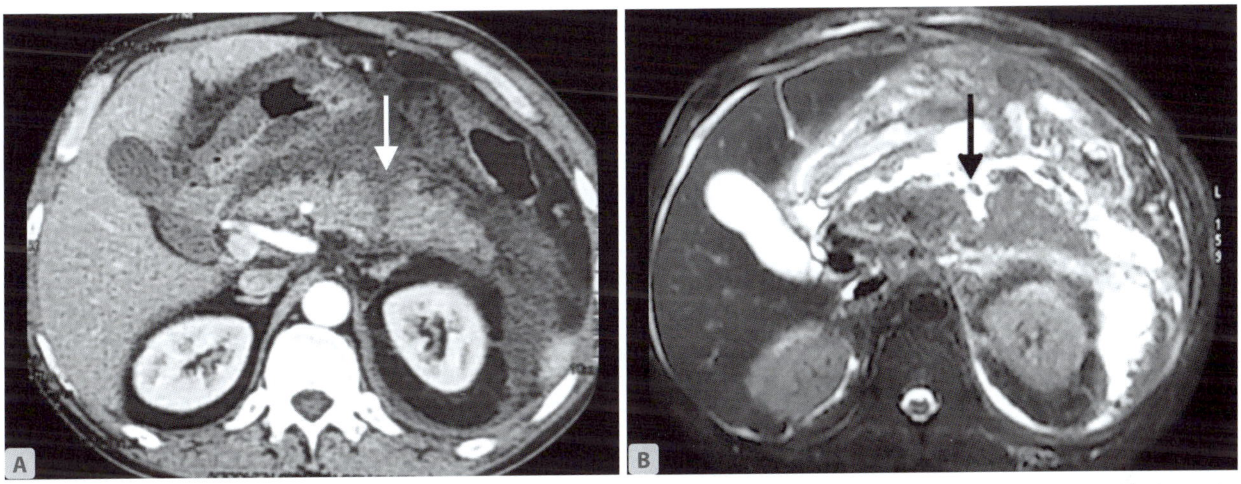

FIGS. 19A AND B: CECT axial scan (A) at level of pancreas shows a laceration (arrow) involving the distal body of the pancreas. The laceration extends to more than 50% of parenchymal depth, hence it is likely involving the main pancreatic duct. Note the surrounding inflammatory changes of pancreatitis. HASTE axial MRI image (B) at same level clearly shows the pancreatic laceration (arrow) with surrounding inflammatory changes.

- Presence of a laceration involving the pancreatic duct. However, the pancreatic duct may not often be seen. When a central laceration is seen extending for more than 50% of anteroposterior or craniocaudal width of the pancreatic parenchyma, then it is presumed to involve the main pancreatic duct. Hence, it is required to quantitate the depth of laceration as a percentage of parenchymal width.[16,18]
- *Location of the laceration:* It most commonly involves the region of pancreatic neck **(Fig. 17)**. Within the neck region, it is important to describe whether it is to the right or left of superior mesenteric artery (SMA). If the laceration (greater than 50%) or transection is seen to the right of SMA then it is managed by a Whipple's surgery. If it lies to the left of SMA, then a distal pancreatectomy is done.[18]
- Large lacerations and hematomas in the head of pancreas are managed with Whipple's surgery **(Fig. 18)**.
- Often the direct evidence of injury to pancreas is not visualized on CT especially when done within 24–48 hours of injury. Indirect CT signs of pancreatic injury include focal or diffuse enlargement of the gland, fluid in the peripancreatic fat, around the SMA, in the transverse mesocolon and lesser peritoneal sac, fluid separating pancreas from the splenic vein, and thickening of left anterior renal fascia. In a patient with suspected pancreatic injury in whom the initial CT scan shows a normal pancreas, a follow-up thin section CT scan within 24–48 hours of injury may show an injury not evident initially.

Recent studies have shown increasing role of MRI with MRCP in the diagnosis of pancreatic injuries. MRI has been shown to increase the diagnostic confidence for detection of parenchymal contusions and lacerations especially the involvement of the main pancreatic duct which is essential for planning treatment **(Figs. 19A and B)**.[5]

Endoscopic retrograde cholangiopancreatography (ERCP) may also be needed for confirmation but its role is mainly limited to pancreatic ductal stenting for treatment of ductal injury.

Major complications can result following pancreatic trauma, e.g. pancreatic fistula, intra-abdominal abscess, pseudocyst formation **(Fig. 20)**, hemorrhage, acute recurrent pancreatitis, etc.

URINARY TRACT

Urinary tract injuries are outside the purview of this book and will be described in detail in a forthcoming book in this series on 'Urogenital Imaging'.

Adrenal

With the increasing use of CT, adrenal injuries are now recognized as the most common retroperitoneal injury.[19] It is usually associated with injury to other organs especially liver and kidneys. Adrenal hemorrhage due to trauma is unilateral in more than 90% of cases and usually the right adrenal gland is involved. The mechanism of injury may be compression of the adrenal gland between the liver and spine. On CT, adrenal hematoma appears as round to oval homogeneous density mass (40–75 HU) that replaces all or a portion of the normal adrenal gland **(Figs. 21A and B)**. In addition there may be stranding of the periadrenal fat that extends to the upper pole of the kidney and apparent thickening of the ipsilateral diaphragmatic crus due to adjacent hemorrhage.[19] A post-traumatic cyst or calcification may be seen as a sequel on long-term follow-up. Adrenal hemorrhage is of little clinical significance, particularly when it is unilateral.[20] Rarely bilateral adrenal hemorrhage has been shown to precipitate adrenal insufficiency.[21]

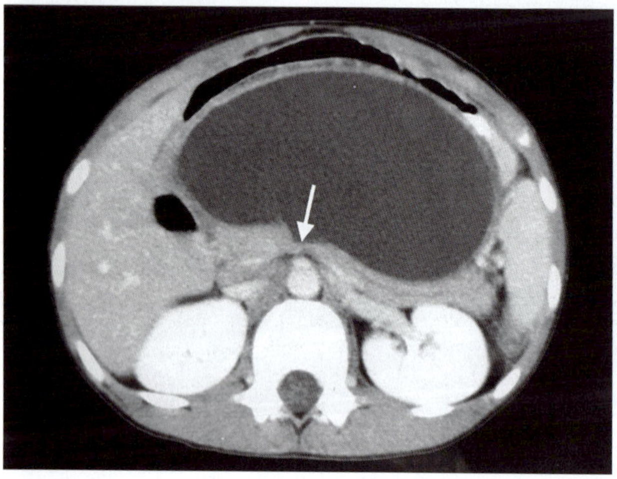

FIG. 20: Axial CECT scan at level of pancreas shows a large pseudocyst anterior to pancreas with a beak-shaped extension (arrow) in the neck of pancreas representing partial transection of pancreas.

HOLLOW VISCUS, OMENTAL AND MESENTERIC INJURY

The diagnosis of intestinal injury is one of the most difficult and controversial aspects of trauma care. The symptoms may be delayed for many hours. If not surgically repaired it may lead to bleeding and leakage of gastrointestinal contents into the peritoneal cavity or retroperitoneum, leading to peritonitis or sepsis. The plain radiographs of the abdomen are relatively insensitive in detecting bowel injury. Rupture of a hollow viscus may produce free air either in the peritoneal cavity or retroperitoneum. Additional findings of free intraperitoneal fluid may be seen. MDCT is the diagnostic modality of choice for detection of bowel and mesenteric injuries and has been shown to be more sensitive and specific than clinical examination, diagnostic peritoneal lavage and abdominal ultrasound.[22] The signs of bowel injury are frequently subtle. The most specific signs of bowel injury are:[22-24]

- Pneumoperitoneum or pneumoretroperitoneum,
- Extravasation of oral contrast material (if administered)
- Low attenuating fluid between loops
- Bowel wall discontinuity **(Figs. 22A to C)**.

Retroperitoneal air tends to localize near the site of injury, often accompanied by fluid, either blood or intestinal.

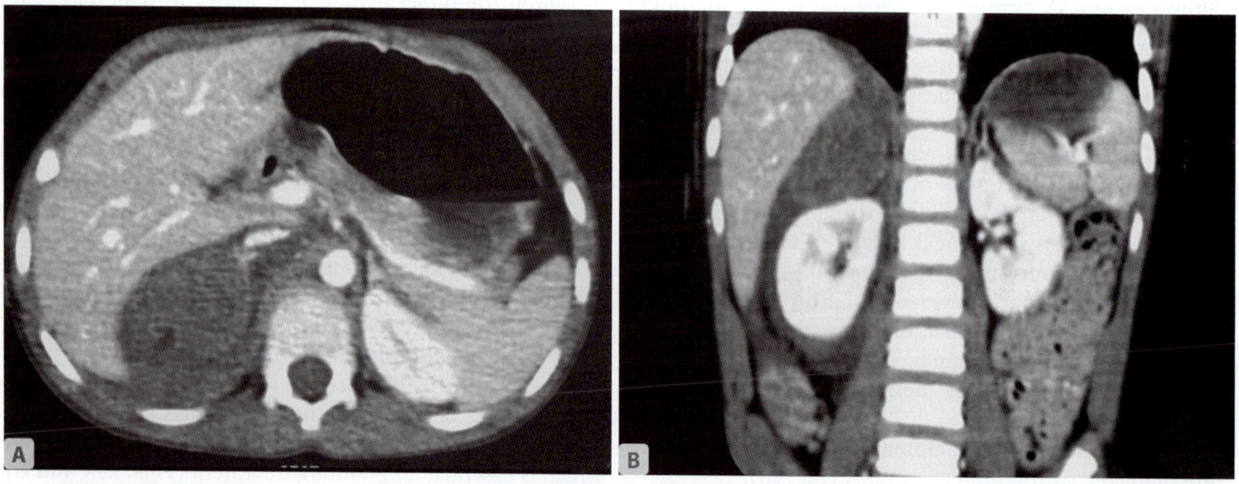

FIGS. 21A AND B: Axial (A) and coronal reformat (B) CECT scans show a right adrenal hematoma.

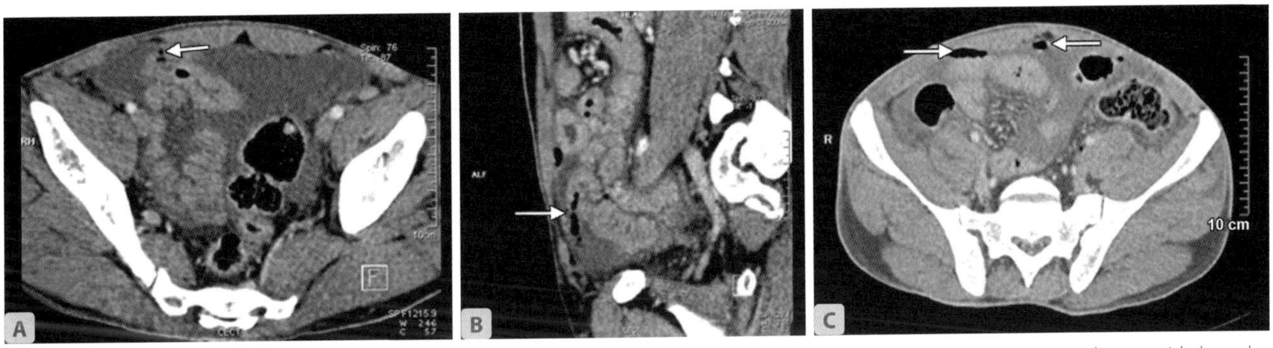

FIGS. 22A TO C: Axial (A) and sagittal reformat (B) images of CECT shows a focal defect in wall of ileum (arrows) with air extending outside bowel lumen. An axial section at a different level with changed window settings shows the presence of pneumoperitoneum (arrows).

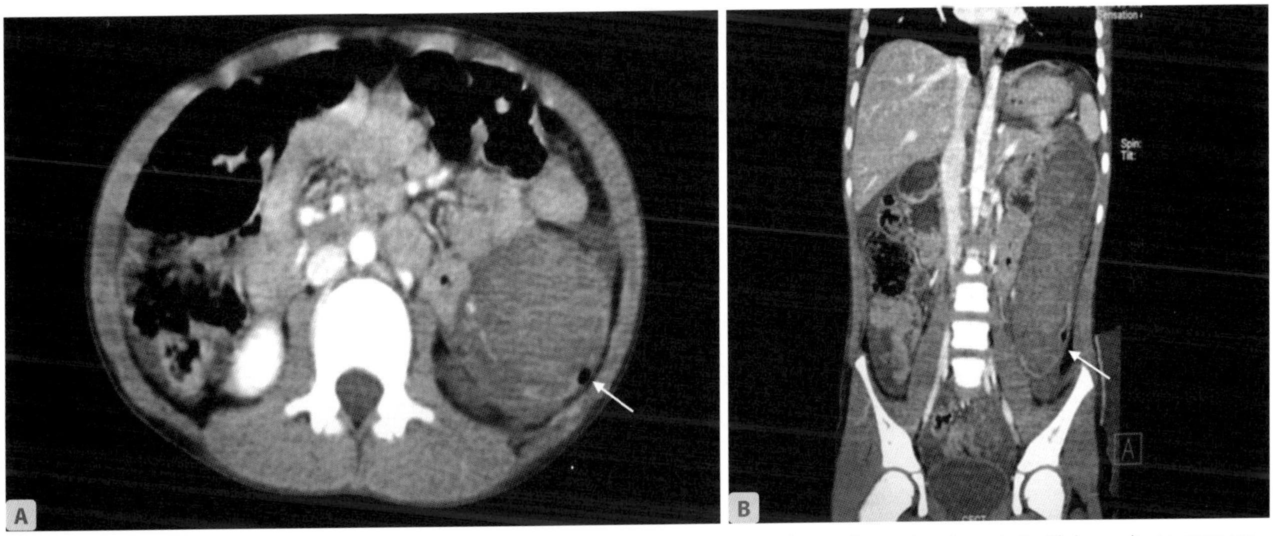

FIGS. 23A AND B: Axial (A) and coronal reformat (B) CECT scans of abdomen show entire descending colon distended with hyperdense contents representing hematoma with thinned out abnormally enhancing walls and air within the wall (arrow in A and B) suggesting colonic injury.

The presence of these signs usually mandates urgent laparotomy. All the above signs, though highly specific, are not as sensitive.[24] Also care must be taken to exclude other causes of extraluminal contrast (bladder injury) and extraluminal air (mechanical ventilation, pneumothorax, chest injury, peritoneal lavage prior to CT, Foley's catheter in a intraperitoneal bladder rupture). Another important consideration is 'pseudopneumoperitoneum' which leads to false positive diagnosis. It refers to trapped air between the parietal peritoneum and the abdominal wall. So, it is actually extraperitoneal, but can be confused as intraperitoneal on images. It is seen in patients with pneumothorax and pneumomediastinum especially on positive pressure ventilation where the air dissects and extends caudally beneath the abdominal wall. Careful evaluation of the CT images especially with coronal and sagittal reconstructions often helps in localizing this air to be extraperitoneal.

It should also be remembered that absence of pneumoperitoneum does not rule out bowel perforation. This can occur due to multiple causes like very early imaging post-trauma, spontaneous healing of perforation, paralytic ileus causing failure of gas to escape from intestine, or reabsorption of small quantity of gas through the peritoneal lining. Hence, other suggestive signs should also be looked for. Often the clinical signs on abdominal examination alone can warrant exploratory laparotomy.

Less specific signs of bowel injury include:[22-24]

- Peritoneal fluid without a known cause,
- Focal bowel wall thickening greater than 3 mm
- Mesenteric infiltration, thickening or hematoma
- Abnormal bowel wall enhancement **(Figs. 23A and B)**.

Patients manifesting these signs may have bowel perforation requiring surgery, a less severe bowel contusion or hematoma that may be managed without surgery or no bowel injury at all. It must be remembered that diffuse bowel wall thickening may also be noted in fluid overload or in hypoperfusion state (shock bowel) wherein it would have other accompanying features of hypoperfusion complex as detailed earlier in this chapter 8. There can be various abnormal patterns of bowel wall enhancement secondary to trauma:

- Increased enhancement as in hypoperfusion state (due to increased vascular permeability with interstitial leakage of contrast)

- Patchy and irregular enhancement due to wall injury
- Decreased or absent enhancement due to ischemia.

Blunt injuries to the stomach are uncommon. The second and third parts of duodenum are the most frequently injured portion of small bowel as they are fixed.[22] Duodenal hematoma has a characteristic appearance on CT scan. In the absence of duodenal perforation, focal thickening or high attenuating mass in the duodenal wall, possibly associated with retroperitoneal fluid, is suggestive of intramural hematoma. Blunt injuries of the small intestine are most commonly seen at the points of fixation (ligament of Treitz and terminal ileum) but may occur anywhere along the length of the small intestine. Blunt colonic injuries are rare.

The mesentery and omentum are most often associated with injuries elsewhere in the abdomen and pelvis. Avulsion of the superior mesenteric artery and vein occurs most commonly near their origin, because of shearing effect. Massive hemorrhage can result from rupture or tear of these vessels. Vascular thrombosis and occlusion by an intimal flap may also result from trauma. CT scan can be used to determine the extent and location of mesenteric injury.

Mesenteric injury has certain specific and nonspecific features on MDCT.[22,23] The specific CT features of mesenteric vascular injury are:

- Active contrast extravasation within mesentery
- Beaded appearance of mesenteric vessels
- Abrupt termination of mesenteric vessels.

The relatively nonspecific findings include:

- Mesenteric hematoma **(Fig. 24)**
- Mesenteric infiltration
- Bowel wall thickening
- Abnormal wall enhancement secondary to ischemia
- Increased fluid within the bowel lumen
- Pneumatosis intestinalis.

It must be remembered that some of these signs may also be seen in bowel injury alone without concomitant mesenteric injury.

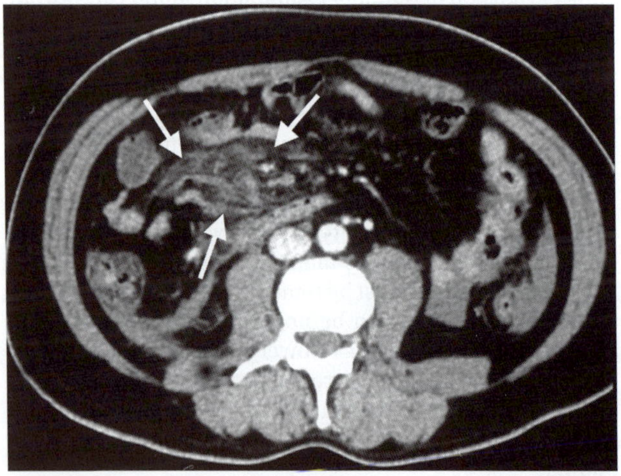

FIG. 24: Axial CECT scan through lower abdomen shows infiltration and hematoma (arrows) in mesenteric root representing mesenteric injury.

DIAPHRAGM

Diaphragmatic rupture and subsequent herniation of abdominal contents into thorax is nine times more common on left side than right due to the protective effect of the liver.[1] On the right side most injuries to the diaphragm go unrecognized during the acute phase. In the interval phase, the abdominal viscus may not have herniated or the patient may have acclimatized to the presence of abdominal contents in the thorax. In the later phase, obstruction or strangulation presents with severe abdominal or chest pain. The injury may also be evident at a later stage in those patients who were earlier on positive pressure ventilation and extubated later.

Chest radiograph may diagnose diaphragmatic rupture if the following specific signs are visualized:

- Visualization of bowel loops or solid masses above the diaphragm
- Loss of the normal diaphragmatic contour
- Detection of a nasogastric tube above the left hemidiaphragm.

The diagnosis may also be suspected on chest radiograph if a combination of following nonspecific signs is visualized:

- Indistinct or elevated hemidiaphragm **(Fig. 25A)**
- Pleural effusion
- Atelectasis with shift of the mediastinum to the contralateral side
- Hemothorax
- Pneumothorax
- Lower rib fractures.

Contrast studies (barium meal or enema) can be used to clearly delineate the herniation.

The advent of MDCT with multiplanar reconstructions has significantly improved the sensitivity of CT in detecting diaphragmatic injuries.[25] The various CT signs which are seen in diaphragmatic rupture are:

- Focal diaphragmatic discontinuity or elevation
- Focal diaphragmatic thickening (retraction)
- Herniated abdominal contents into thorax
- 'Collar' sign—narrowed waist of a herniated intra-abdominal organ due to compression at the neck (diaphragm tear)
- 'Dependent viscera' sign—herniated intra-abdominal contents abutting the posterior thoracic wall without intervening diaphragmatic slip **(Figs. 25A and B)**.

Amongst the above features the 'dependent viscera' sign and the 'collar' signs are reported to be 100% specific.[1] CT is unreliable in diagnosing diaphragmatic tears before herniation. MRI also has been reported to be highly sensitive in detecting diaphragmatic rupture.

RETROPERITONEUM

The most frequently injured retroperitoneal structures include the adrenals, pancreas, great vessels, gastrointestinal tract, genitourinary tract and musculoskeletal system.[1,2] Inability to account for blood loss either in the chest or abdomen in a patient with ongoing transfusion requirements should dictate angiographic investigation. The potential for simultaneous angiographic embolization of actively bleeding vessels is

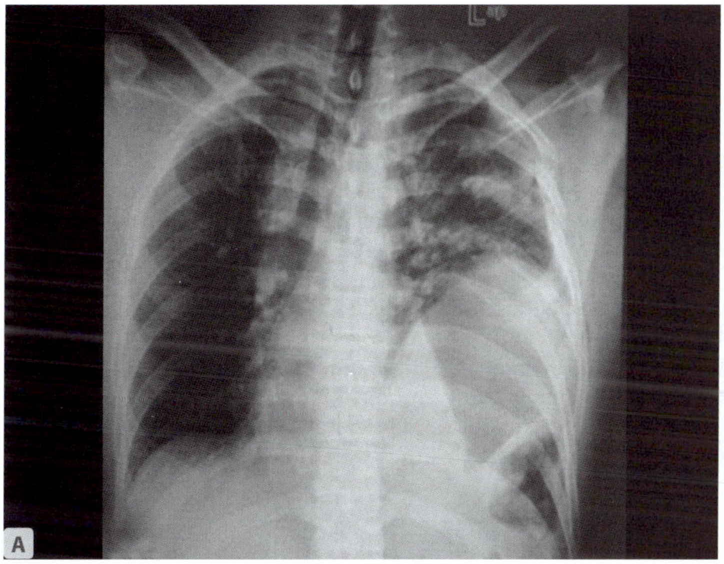

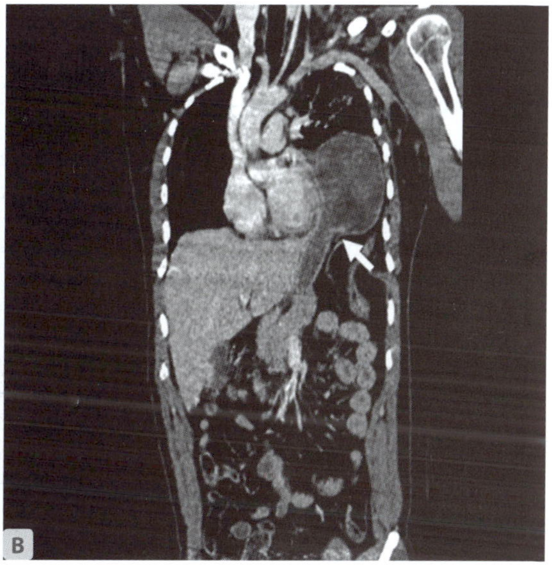

FIGS. 25A AND B: Chest radiograph PA view (A) shows opacity in left lower zone with smooth convex upper margin and air lucencies within. Coronal reformatted CECT image (B) shows clearly the diaphragmatic defect (arrow) with stomach herniating through it into the thorax.

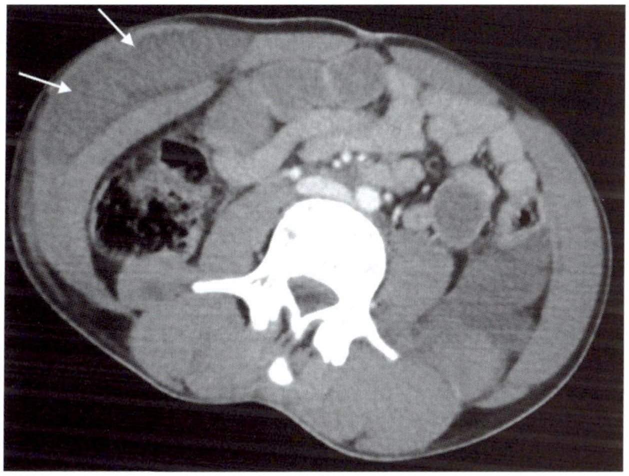

FIG. 26: Axial CECT scan through midabdomen shows a large abdominal wall hematoma (arrows).

well documented and may be lifesaving since opening the retroperitoneum to control bleeding is associated with high mortality.

ABDOMINAL WALL INJURY

Abdominal wall injuries are easily overlooked if not specifically looked for. Most common are bruises, which appear on CT as skin thickening and soft tissue infiltration of subcutaneous fat. Intramuscular hematomas may be seen **(Fig. 26)**. Tearing of lateral abdominal wall or rectus abdominis is an unusual occurrence that results in subcutaneous hematoma and occasionally bowel herniation. Morel Lavallee lesion representing internal degloving injury is seen on CT as separation of skin from the subcutaneous with intervening fluid collection.

PENETRATING ABDOMINAL TRAUMA

Traditionally, almost all stab and gunshot wounds to the abdomen used to undergo surgical exploration. With increasing interest in nonoperative management of penetrating injuries, CT has become important in evaluating extent of injury in selected hemodynamically stable patients. The most important information required by the surgeon is whether or not there is a breach of the peritoneum by the penetrating wound. If the wound is deep then it is important to look for solid organ laceration, bowel perforation, retroperitoneal hematoma, and hemoperitoneum. It is often difficult to detect small perforations of the bowel that result in only small amounts of peritoneal fluid on CT. In contrast to stab wounds, gunshot wounds are potentially complex injuries and depend upon the type of weapon, distance between the weapon and victim amongst others. CT is directly able to demonstrate the path of the bullet.

CONCLUSION

Diagnostic imaging technology has evolved considerably during the past decade and CT in particular has increased the sensitivity and specificity of imaging in abdominal trauma. Currently, CT is universally accepted as a valuable tool for evaluating hemodynamically stable patients. The value of CT in diagnosis of abdominal injuries can be optimized by using state of art MDCT scanners, maintaining adequate patient physiologic support and monitoring devices within the CT suite, using appropriate intravenous contrast, paying careful attention to CT technique and timely interpretation of CT images. However, CT must be considered as an adjunct to the clinical evaluation of the patient, which remains the most important criteria for guiding management of the patient with abdominal trauma. Increasing role of angioembolization in management of hepatic, splenic and pelvic injuries has widened the role of radiologist in successful nonsurgical management of these patients.

TAKE HOME KEY POINTS

- Chest and pelvic radiographs along with FAST ultrasound are done as initial investigations in all patients of suspected abdominal trauma.
- MDCT is done in patients for further evaluation depending upon the hemodynamic stability, mechanism of injury and findings of the initial radiological investigations.
- Role of radiologist is to detect and characterize the solid and visceral organ injuries and to grade them as per American Association for the Surgery of Trauma (AAST) grades.
- Most of the abdominal injuries are managed conservatively if the patient's condition remains hemodynamically stable.
- The few surgical indications which can be detected on CT should be carefully looked for and communicated to the surgeon. These include full thickness bowel injury, pancreatic transaction, intraperitoneal rupture of urinary bladder, diaphragmatic tear, mesenteric hematoma/ vascular injury and renal pelvic injury.
- Other CT findings which require close monitoring of patient and would often require a surgical or angiographic intervention also need to be specifically looked for. These include uncontained vascular injury (depicted by active arterial contrast extravasation), contained vascular injury (pseudoaneurysm or arteriovenous fistula) and high grade (4/5) liver and splenic injuries.
- Angiographic embolization procedures are frequently used to aid the nonoperative management of patients with vascular injuries and high grade liver and spleen injuries.

REFERENCES

1. Stanescu AL, Gross JA, Bittle M, Mann FA. Imaging of blunt abdominal trauma. Semin Roentgen. 2006;41(3):196-204.
2. Soto JA, Anderson SW. Multidetector CT of blunt abdominal trauma. Radiology. 2012;265(3):678-93.
3. Korner M, Krotz M, Degenhart C, Pfeifer KJ, Reiser MF, Linsenmaier U. Current role of emergency US in patients with major trauma. Radiographics. 2008;28:225-44.
4. Cokkinos D, Antypa E, Stefanidis K, et al. Contrast-enhanced ultrasound for imaging blunt abdominal trauma—indications, description of the technique and imaging review. Ultraschall in Med. 2012;33(1):60-67. *https://acsearch.acr.org/docs/69409/Narrative/*
5. Stuhlfaut JW, Lucey BC, Varghese JC, Soto JA. Blunt abdominal trauma: utility of 5-minute delayed CT with a reduced radiation dose. Radiology. 2006;238(2):473-9.
6. Panda A, Kumar A, Gamanagatti S, Bhalla AS, Sharma R, Kumar S, Mishra B. Evaluation of diagnostic utility of multidetector computed tomography and magnetic resonance imaging in blunt pancreatic trauma: a prospective study. Acta Radiol. 2015;56(4):387-96.
7. Prasad KR, Kumar A, Gamanagatti S, Chandrashekhara SH. CT in post-traumatic hypoperfusion complex: a pictorial review. Emerg Radiol. 2011;18(2):139-43.
8. Boscak A, Shanmuganathan K. Splenic Trauma: What is New? Radiologic Clinics of North America. 2012;50(1):105-22.
9. Moore EE, Cogbill TH, Jurkovich GJ, et al. Organ injury scaling: spleen and liver (1994 revision). J Trauma. 1995;38:323-4.
10. Marmery H, Shanmuganathan K, Alexander M, Mirvis S. Optimisation of selection for nonoperative management of blunt splenic injury: Comparison of MDCT grading systems. AJR. 2007;189:1421-7.
11. Gamanagatti S, Rangarajan K, Kumar A, Jineesh. Blunt abdominal trauma: imaging and intervention. Curr Probl Diagn Radiol. 2015;44(4):321-36.
12. Parihar ML, Kumar A, Gamanagatti S, Bhalla AS, Mishra B, Kumar S, et al. Role of splenic artery embolization in management of traumatic splenic injuries: a prospective study. Indian J Surg. 2013;75(5):361-7.
13. Yoon W, Jeong YY, Kim JK, Seo JJ, Lim HS, Shin SS, et al. CT in blunt liver trauma. Radiographics. 2005;25:87-104.
14. Kumar R, Kumar A, Baliyan V, Bhalla AS, Sharma R, Gupta A, Kumar S, Misra MC. Correlating MDCT liver injury grade and clinical outcome in patients without significant extrahepatic injury. Indian J Surg. 2016;78:275.
15. Melamud K, LeBedis CA, Soto JA. Imaging of pancreatic and duodenal trauma. Radiologic Clinics of North America. 2015;53(4)757-71.
16. Moore EE, Cogbill TH, Malangoni MA, et al. Organ injury scaling II: Pancreas, duodenum, small bowel, colon and rectum. J Trauma. 1990;30:1427.
17. Kumar A, Panda A, Gamanagatti S. Blunt pancreatic trauma: a persistent diagnostic conundrum? World J Radiol. 2016;8(2): 159-73.
18. To'o KJ, Duddalwar VA. Imaging of traumatic adrenal injury. Emerg Radiol. 2012;19:499.
19. Panda A, Kumar A, Gamanagatti S, Bhalla AS, Sharma R, Kumar S, Mishra B. Are traumatic bilateral adrenal injuries associated with higher morbidity and mortality?: a prospective observational study. J Trauma Manag Outcomes. 2015;9:6.
20. Francque SM, Schwagten VM, Ysebaert DK, et al. Bilateral adrenal hemorrhage and acute adrenal insufficiency in a blunt abdominal trauma: a case-report and literature review. Eur J Emerg Med. 2004;11:164-7.
21. Brofman N, Atri M, Epid D, Hanson JM, Grinblat L, Chughtai T, et al. Evaluation of bowel and mesenteric blunt trauma with multidetector CT. Radiographics. 2006;26:1119-26.
22. Iaselli F, Mazzei MA, Firetto C, et al. Bowel and mesenteric injuries from blunt abdominal trauma: a review. Radiol Med. 2015; 120:21.
23. Panda A, Kumar A, Gamanagatti S, Das R, Paliwal S, Gupta A, Kumar S. Can multidetector computed tomography detect the site of gastrointestinal tract injury in trauma?: a retrospective study. Diag Interv Radiol. 2016; 22...(ahead of print).
24. Panda A, Kumar A, Gamanagatti S, Patil A, Kumar S, Gupta A. Traumatic diaphragmatic injury: a review of CT signs and the difference between blunt and penetrating injury. Diagn Interv Radiol. 2014;20(2):121-8.
25. Barbiera F, Nicastro N, Finazzo M, et al. The role of MRI in traumatic rupture of the diaphragm. Our experience in three cases and review of the literature. Radiol Med. 2003;105(3): 188-94.

CHAPTER

117

Imaging of Peritoneum and Mesentery

Anju Garg, Anjali Prakash, Alpana Manchanda

The peritoneum is a thin, translucent, serous membrane made up of a single layer of mesothelial cells. It is supported by submesothelial connective tissue containing lymphatics, blood vessels, inflammatory cells like lymphocytes and plasma cells and a variable amount of fat. Just like the pleura, the peritoneum also has 2 layers—the *parietal peritoneum* lines the anterior, lateral and posterior walls of the peritoneal cavity and the *visceral peritoneum* which envelops the hollow and solid abdominal organs. Between these two layers lies the *peritoneal cavity*—a potential space containing a small amount of fluid which acts as a lubricant.[1] The peritoneal cavity is a closed continuous space in males, but in females, it communicates with the extraperitoneal compartment of the pelvis through the ostia of the fallopian tubes.[2]

EMBRYOLOGY

Knowledge of the developmental anatomy of the peritoneum, helps to understand the peritoneal ligaments, spaces and their relationship with the abdominal organs.The majority of the ligaments in the abdomen are formed from remnants of the ventral and dorsal mesenteries which suspend the primitive gut. The liver and its ligaments arise in the *ventral mesentery*. The anterior part of the ventral mesentery becomes the falciform, coronary and triangular ligaments and the posterior part of the ventral mesentery becomes the lesser omentum. The stomach, spleen and pancreatic tail and their ligaments develop in the *dorsal mesentery* of the foregut. At the level of spleen, the anterior part of the dorsal mesentery becomes the gastrosplenic ligament, and the posterior part of the dorsal mesentery becomes the splenorenal ligament **(Figs. 1A to C)**. Above the level of spleen the dorsal mesentery gives rise to gastrophrenic ligament and below the level of spleen it gives rise to the greater omentum (gastrocolic ligament).[3]

Below the level of the transverse colon, the ventral mesentery regresses while the dorsal mesentery forms the transverse mesocolon, small bowel mesentery and sigmoid mesocolon. During development, the duodenum, ascending and descending colon lose their mesenteries and become retroperitoneal.

ANATOMY OF THE PERITONEUM[4-7]

The peritoneum forms double layered folds, or ligaments, that interconnect the organs and viscera within the peritoneal cavity. The *peritoneal ligaments* are named according to the two major structures connected by them, e.g. splenorenal ligament or gastrohepatic ligament, etc. *Omentum* is a specialized ligament that attaches the stomach to other structures whereas *mesentery* is the ligament attaching the bowel to the posterior abdominal wall. These ligaments divide the peritoneal cavity into a number of compartments and recesses **(Figs. 2A and B)**.

The peritoneal ligaments carry vessels, nerves and lymphatics from the extraperitoneal spaces to the intraperitoneal organs. They act as boundaries for spread of pathological processes within the abdomen, but may also become conduits for spread of disease. They are not directly visible on cross sectional imaging but can be identified by either their typical position, organ relationships, or by the anatomical landmarks provided by their constituent vessels. They may become directly visible when they get thickened by edema, inflammation or neoplastic infiltration or when they are outlined by air or fluid in the peritoneal cavity. They can be grouped into:

- Ligaments of the stomach
- Ligaments of the liver and spleen
- Ligaments attached to the small bowel
- Ligaments attached to the large bowel
- Ligaments of the pelvis.

Ligaments of Stomach

The Peritoneal Ligaments of the Stomach Include Two Main Groups

Ligaments attached to the lesser curvature, the lesser omentum, and ligaments attached to the greater curvature which include gastrophrenic, gastrosplenic ligaments and the greater omentum.

Lesser Omentum

The lesser omentum is formed bythe gastrohepatic and hepatoduodenal ligaments **(Figs. 2A and B)**. *The*

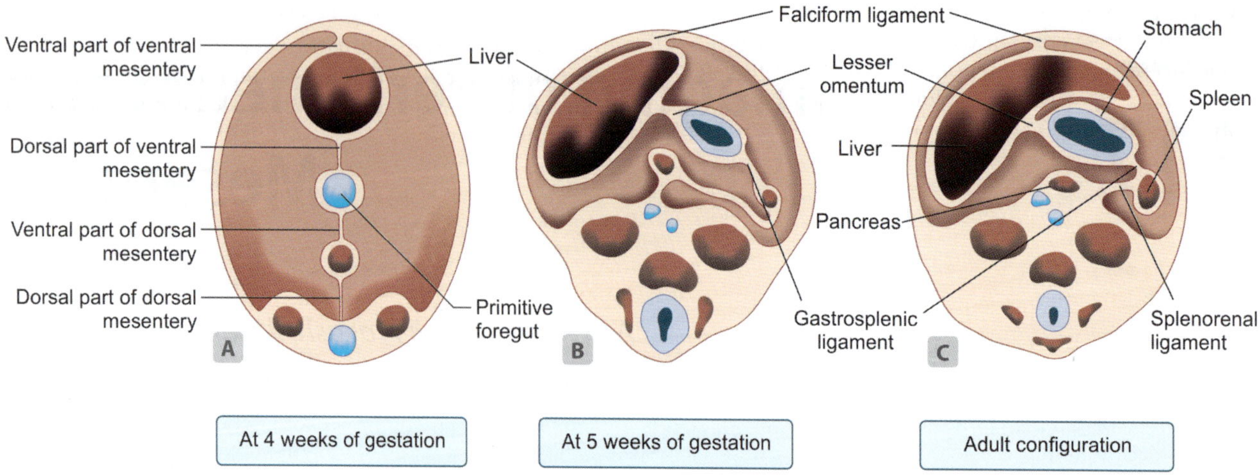

FIGS. 1A TO C: Embryologic development and rotation of the peritoneal structures to the eventual adult position. The ventral part of the ventral mesentery becomes the falciform ligament, the dorsal part of the ventral mesentery becomes the lesser omentum, the ventral part of the dorsal mesentery becomes the gastrosplenic ligament, and the dorsal part of the dorsal mesentery becomes the splenorenal ligament. The liver arises in the ventral mesentery, whereas the stomach, spleen and pancreatic tail develop in the dorsal mesentery. The liver fills and moves to the right side of the peritoneal cavity as it grows. The spleen moves to the left.

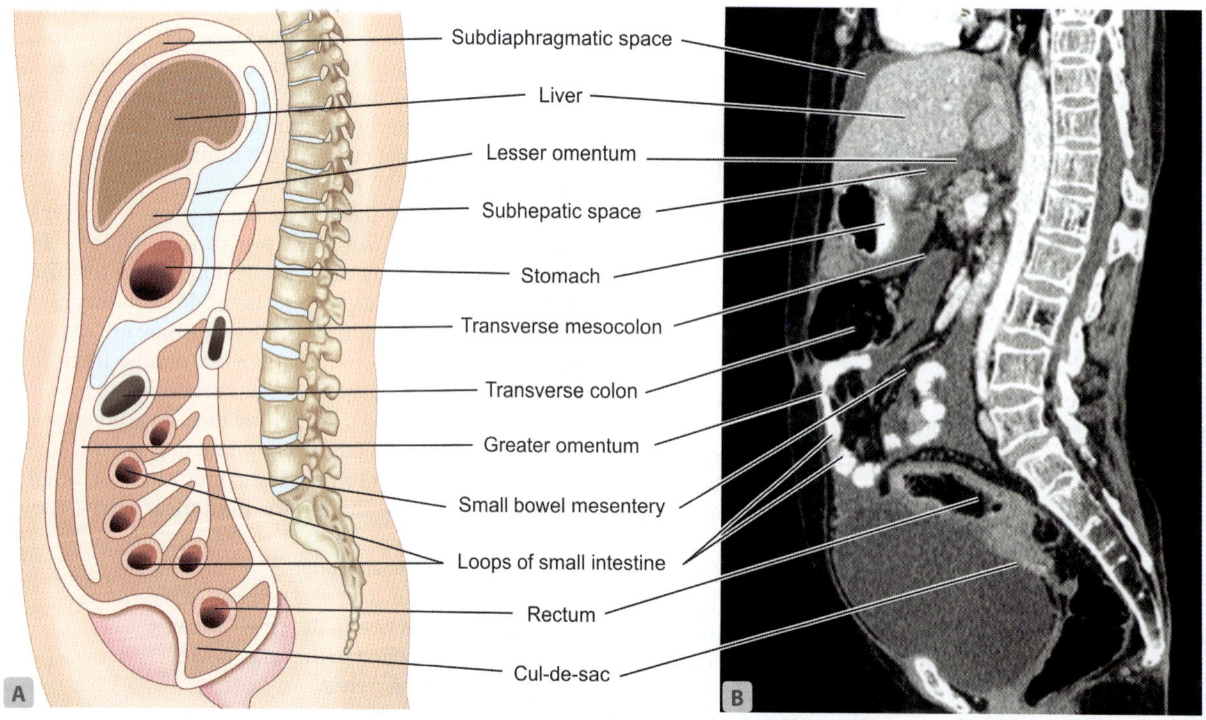

FIGS. 2A AND B: Sagittal illustration and corresponding sagittal CT scan in a patient with ascites, showing the peritoneal ligaments in the midline sagittal section.

gastrohepatic ligament (GHL) is attached to the lesser curve of the stomach and the visceral surface of the liver and contains the coronary vein and left gastric artery **(Figs. 3A and D)**. The GHL can be involved by pancreatitis or metastatic disease from oesophageal, gastric, and biliary tumors. It is also the site for coronary varices. The *hepatoduodenal ligament (HDL)* attaches the first part of the duodenum to the liver and contains the portal vein, hepatic artery, common hepatic ducts, and part of the cystic duct **(Fig. 3D)**. It is a common site for spread of biliary and gall bladder neoplasms.

Greater Omentum

It is also known as the *gastrocolic ligament* **(Figs. 2 and 3)**. It attaches to the greater curvature of the stomach and proximal part of duodenum. Its descending and ascending portion fuse to form a four layer vascular fatty apron which hangs down covering the small bowel. It has mostly fatty tissue with few gastroepiploic vessels. On CT, it is seen as a band of fatty tissue, just beneath the anterior abdominal wall and anterior to the stomach, transverse colon and small bowel. It is a mobile structure and has an important role in limiting spread of infections and confining injuries to the bowel. However, it is a common site of spread of metastatic peritoneal disease and is also commonly involved in tubercular peritonitis.

Gastrosplenic Ligament

It attaches the greater curvature of the stomach to the spleen and contains the short gastric and left gastroepiploic vessels and lymphatics **(Figs. 3A and D)**. It is a leftward continuation of the greater omentum and is also in continuity with the splenorenal and phrenicocolic ligaments. The gastrosplenic ligament is a frequent route for spread of pancreatitis-related fluid and the vessels form a collateral route of venous flow in cases of splenic vein thrombosis.

Gastrophrenic ligament is attached to the posterior surface of the stomach. The attachment of the gastrophrenic ligament lies in apposition with the diaphragm, and frequently with the upper portion of the left suprarenal gland.

Ligaments of the Liver and Spleen

The peritoneal ligaments of the liver include the suspensory ligaments of the liver and lesser omentum. The suspensory ligaments of the liver include the falciform, coronary and triangular ligaments. The peritoneal ligaments of spleen include gastrosplenic and lienorenal ligaments.

Triangular and Coronary Ligaments

These are peritoneal attachments between the liver and the parietal peritoneum. The triangular ligaments are formed by fusion of the coronary ligaments and outline the bare area of the liver. The right triangular ligament is long and separates the right subphrenic space from the right subhepatic space while the left triangular ligament is short and does not compartmentalize the left subphrenic space.

Falciform Ligament

It attaches the ventral surface of the liver to the anterior abdominal wall and contains the ligamentum teres, i.e. obliterated umbilical vein **(Fig. 3B)**. The recanalized paraumbilical vein is also found in the falciform ligament.

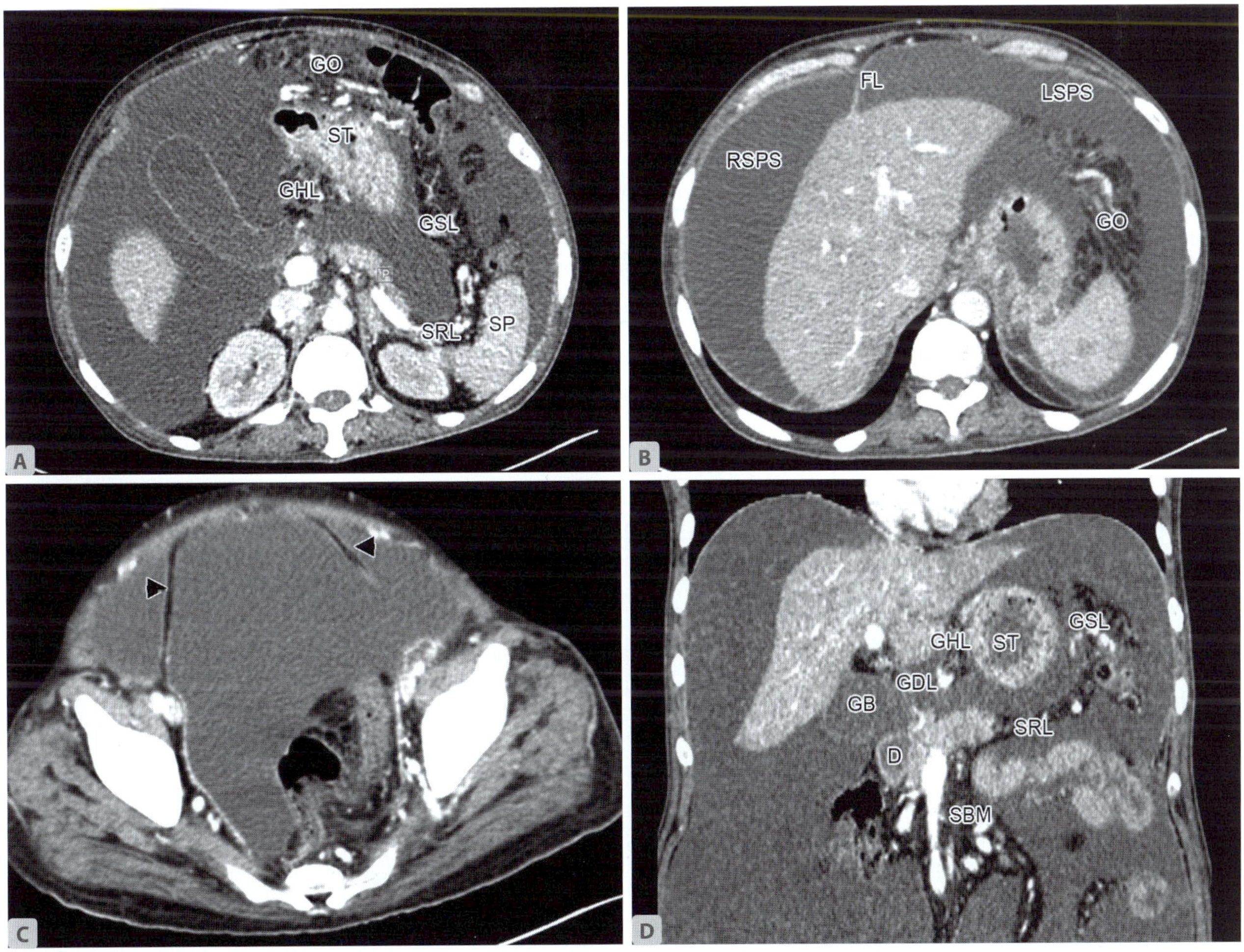

FIGS. 3A TO D: (A to C) Axial CECT and (D) Coronal scans showing the peritoneal ligaments in a 61-year-old man with peritoneal carcinomatosis with ascites, thickened enhancing peritoneum and omental nodularity. [FL: falciform ligament; GO: greater omentum; GHL: gastrohepatic ligament; GDL: gastroduodenal ligament; GSL: gastrospenic ligament; SRL: splenorenal ligament; SBM: small bowel mesentery; ST: stomach; SP: spleen; D: duodenum; RSPS: right subphrenic space; LSPS: left subphrenic space; and medial umbilical ligaments (arrowheads)].

It is an important site of peritoneal seeding of metastatic tumors which may be mistaken for hepatic metastases.

Splenorenal Ligament

It is the connecting peritoneal reflection between the spleen and the left kidney. It contains the tail of the pancreas, splenic vessels, and small vessels to the retroperitomeum. Tumor spread and systemic portal collaterals can develop in this space.

Ligaments Attached to Small Bowel

Small Bowel Mesentery

It is a broad fan-shaped peritoneal fold that attaches the jejunum and ileum to the retroperitoneum and contains branches of the superior mesenteric vessels, lymph nodes, nerves and varying amounts of fat **(Figs. 2 and 4)**. The root of the mesentery extends from the ligament of Trietz to the ileocecal valve, a length of approximately 15 cm, whereas the intestinal border is 6–8 meters long, and so the mesentery is thrown into a number of folds **(Figs. 4A and B)**.

The small bowel mesentery is commonly involved by metastatic disease and infectious processes of the peritoneum. Inflammation and tumor from the pancreatic body or jejunum can involve the small bowel mesentery directly or by way of neurovascular plexus or lymphatics. Rotational and fusion anomalies may lead to volvulus or internal hernias.

Ligaments Attached to Large Bowel

Transverse Mesocolon

It is a peritoneal fold that attaches the transverse colon to the anterior surface of the pancreas **(Figs. 2 and 5)**. It contains the middle colic vessels and lymph nodes. Local extension of pancreatic head cancers occurs along the transverse mesocolon.

Sigmoid Mesocolon

It is the peritoneal attachment of the sigmoid colon to the posterior pelvic wall **(Fig. 5C)**. It contains the hemorrhoidal and sigmoid vessels. It serves as a medial and caudal boundary for the spread of material from the left paracolic space. Acute diverticulitis, Crohn's disease and tumor of the sigmoid colon can involve the sigmoid mesocolon.

Phrenicocolic Ligament

It attaches the proximal descending colon to the left hemidiaphragm. It separates the supramesocolic compartment from the left paracolic gutter. Pancreatic disease can spread via this ligament to involve the splenic flexure of the colon.

Table 1 lists the peritoneal ligaments, their attachments, contents and the major pathological processes involving these ligaments.

Ligaments of the Pelvis

The *broad ligaments* extend from the uterus to the pelvic sidewalls and envelop the parametria, fallopian tubes, ovaries, uterine vessels and ureters. These ligaments can be involved by inflammatory and neoplastic processes affecting the uterus, ovaries and fallopian tubes.

Round ligaments are the anterior suspensory ligaments of the uterus. They run lateral to the deep inferior epigastric vessels, enter the inguinal canal and insert on the labia majora. They contain lymphatic channels.

There are two paired *lateral and medial umbilical ligaments* and *one median umbilical ligament* in the midline. The lateral folds are formed by reflection of the peritoneum over the deep inferior epigastric vessels, the medial folds are peritoneal reflections over the obliterated umbilical arteries and the median fold lies over the obliterated urachus **(*see* Fig. 3C)**.

PERITONEAL SPACES[4,5,7]

The peritoneal ligaments divide the peritoneal space into multiple compartments and recesses. On imaging these spaces are visualized only when they are distended with fluid or air. The transverse mesocolon divides the peritoneal

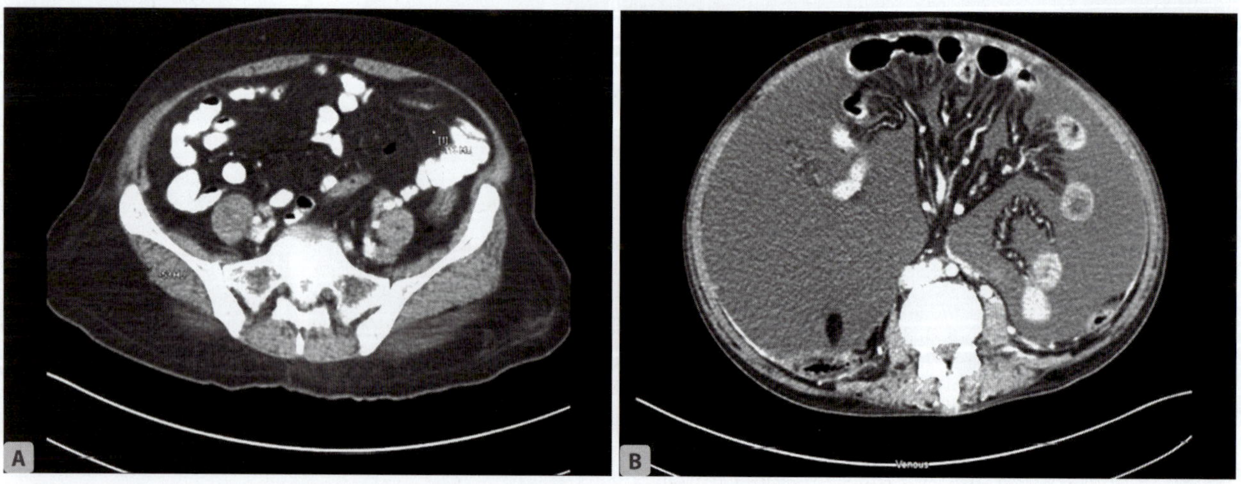

FIGS. 4A AND B: Axial CECT scans through abdomen in two different patients showing normal mesentery: (A) Mesentery is seen as diffuse fat density structure with mesenteric vessels within. The leaves of the mesentery cannot be made out separately; (B) In a patient with ascites, the leaves of the mesentery are separated by the ascitic fluid.

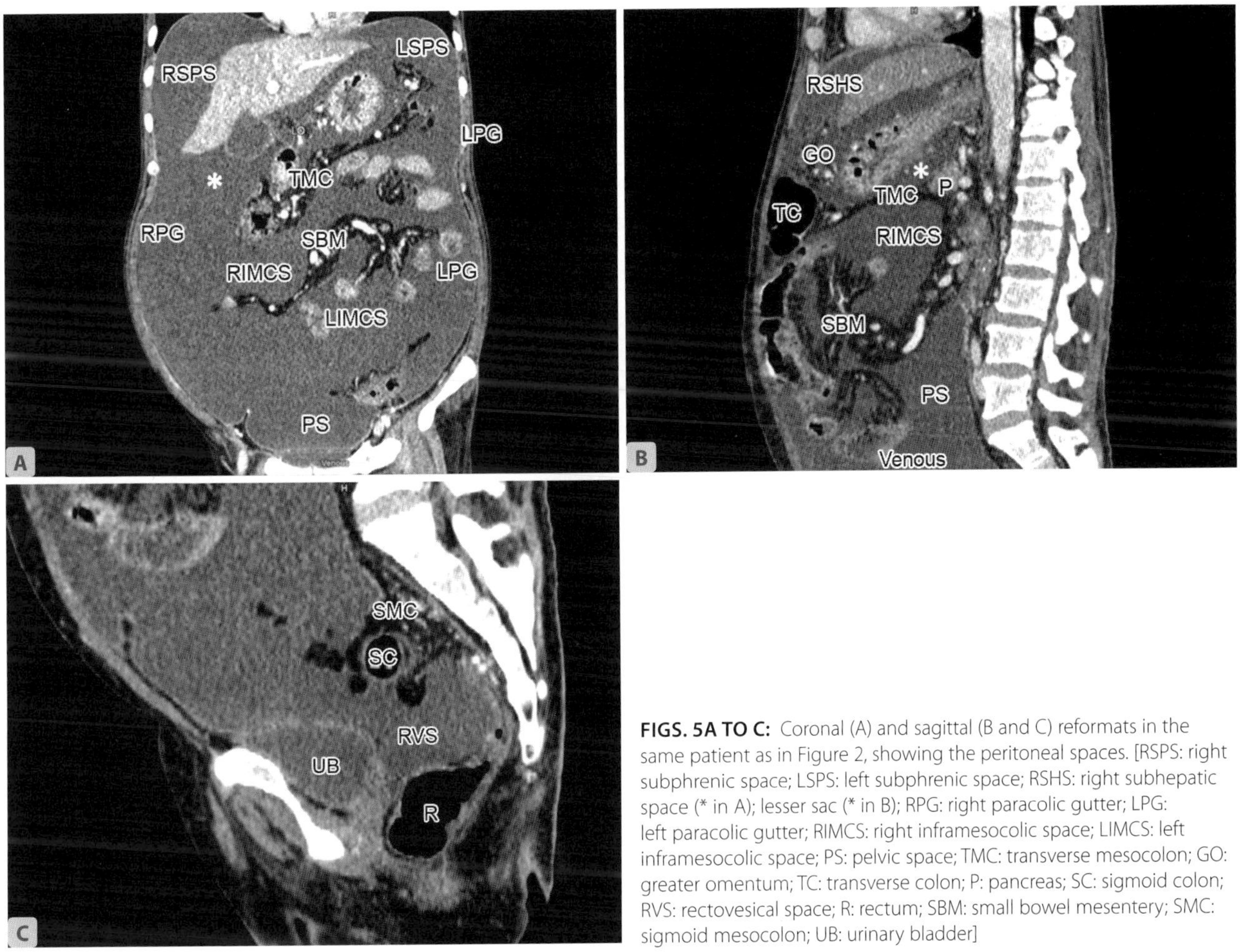

FIGS. 5A TO C: Coronal (A) and sagittal (B and C) reformats in the same patient as in Figure 2, showing the peritoneal spaces. [RSPS: right subphrenic space; LSPS: left subphrenic space; RSHS: right subhepatic space (* in A); lesser sac (* in B); RPG: right paracolic gutter; LPG: left paracolic gutter; RIMCS: right inframesocolic space; LIMCS: left inframesocolic space; PS: pelvic space; TMC: transverse mesocolon; GO: greater omentum; TC: transverse colon; P: pancreas; SC: sigmoid colon; RVS: rectovesical space; R: rectum; SBM: small bowel mesentery; SMC: sigmoid mesocolon; UB: urinary bladder]

cavity into the supramesocolic and the inframesocolic compartments.

Supramesocolic Space

It extends from the diaphragm to the transverse mesocolon. It includes the perihepatic spaces and the lesser sac. The perihepatic spaces consist of the subphrenic and subhepatic spaces which are right, left, anterior and posterior.

The *subphrenic space* lies adjacent to the lateral and superior portion of the liver, between the diaphragm and the abdominal wall. The right subphrenic space is limited medially by the falciform ligament, which separates it from the left subphrenic space **(Figs. 5A to C)**. Inferiorly it is continuous with the right subhepatic space and the right paracolic space. The left subphrenic space is located below and around the left lobe of liver and stomach. It is limited inferiorly by the phrenicocolic ligament.

The *right subhepatic space*, also known as the Morrison's pouch or hepatorenal space, lies adjacent to the gall bladder and duodenum, and extends posteriorly to the anterior surface of the right kidney **(Figs. 2 and 5)**. It is an important site of fluid collection as it is the most gravity dependant space. Medially it extends into the lesser sac through the foramen of Winslow. The *left subhepatic space* lies between the lateral segment of the left lobe of liver and the stomach.

The *lesser sac* also known as the *omental bursa*, lies behind the stomach, anterior to the pancreas **(Fig. 5)**. It is further subdivided by the reflection over the left gastric artery into 2 recesses—a smaller superior recess and a larger inferior recess. The *superior recess* surrounds the caudate lobe of the liver. It communicates with the subhepatic space through the foramen of Winslow that is located posterior to the free edge of the hepatoduodenal ligament. The larger *inferior recess* lies between the stomach and the anterior surface of the spleen and pancreas. Abnormalities of the pancreas, posterior wall of stomach, duodenum, caudate lobe and transverse colon may all extend into the lesser sac.

Inframesocolic Space

The right and left inframesocolic spaces are separated by the root of the mesentery. The *left inframesocolic space* is larger and communicates freely with the pelvic spaces. The *right inframesocolic space* is limited inferiorly by the attachment of the small bowel mesentery to the cecum and does not communicate with the pelvis **(Figs. 5A and B)**.

Paracolic Spaces

They lie lateral to the peritoneal reflections of the left and right side of the colon. The right space is larger and deeper than the

TABLE 1: Peritoneal ligaments, attachments, contents and major pathological processes which involve these ligaments.

Peritoneal ligaments	***Attachments***	***Contents***	***Other relevant information***
• *Ligaments of stomach and duodenum*: – Attached to lesser curvature ▪ Lesser omentum Gastrohepatic ligament	Lesser curvature of the stomach and the visceral surface of liver	Coronary vein and left gastric artery	• Can be involved by pancreatitis or metastatic disease from esophageal, gastric, and biliary tumors • Can be a site for coronary varices
– Hepatoduodenal ligament	First part of duodenum and liver	Portal vein, hepatic artery, common hepatic ducts, and part of the cystic duct	• Common site for spread of biliary and gallbladder neoplasms
– Attached to greater curvature ▪ Gastrosplenic ligament	Greater curvature of the stomach and spleen	Short gastric vessels	• Frequent route for subperitoneal spread of pancreatitis-related fluid
▪ Gastrophrenic ligament	Posterior surface of the stomach and diaphragm	Left inferior phrenic artery	
▪ Greater omentum	Greater curvature of the stomach and proximal part of duodenum	Fatty tissue with few gastro-epiploic vessels	• Common site of spread of metastatic peritoneal disease • Commonly involved in tubercular peritonitis • Important role in limiting spread of infections and confining injuries to bowel
• *Ligaments of liver and spleen*: – Triangular and coronary ligaments	Liver and the diaphragm	No vessels	• Right triangular ligament separates the right subphrenic space from the right subhepatic space • Left triangular ligament does not compartmentalize the left subphrenic space
– Falciform ligament	Ventral surface of the liver and the anterior abdominal wall	Ligamentum teres (obliterated umbilical vein) and recanalized paraumbilical vein	• Important site of peritoneal seeding of metastatic tumors
– Lesser omentum	As above		
– Ligaments of spleen ▪ Splenorenal ligament	Spleen and left kidney	Tail of the pancreas, splenic vessels, and small vessels to the retroperitoneum	• Systemic portal collaterals can develop in this space • Renal and splenic neoplasm can spread
▪ Gastrosplenic ligament	As above		
• *Ligaments attached to small bowel*: – Small bowel mesentery	Jejunum and ileum and the retroperitoneum (root of mesentery extends from the ligament of Trietz to ileocecal valve)	Branches of superior mesenteric vessels, lymph nodes, nerves and varying amounts of fat	• Commonly involved by metastatic disease and infectious processes of peritoneum • Rotational and fusion anomalies may lead to volvulus or internal hernias
• *Ligaments attached to large bowel*: – Transverse mesocolon	Transverse colon and the anterior surface of the pancreas	Middle colic vessels and lymph nodes	Local extension of pancreatic head cancer
– Sigmoid mesocolon	Sigmoid colon and the posterior pelvic wall	Hemorrhoidal and sigmoid vessels	Serves as medial and caudal boundary for spread of material from left paracolic space. Can be involved by acute diverticulitis, Crohn's disease and tumor of the sigmoid colon
– Phrenicocolic ligament	Proximal descending colon and the left hemidiaphragm		Separates the supramesocolic compartment from left paracolic gutter

left. It communicates freely with the right perihepatic space, whereas the left is partially limited by the phrenicocolic ligament. Both paracolic spaces communicate freely with the pelvic spaces **(Fig. 5A)**.

Pelvic Peritoneal Spaces

The pelvic cavity can be divided into the anterior and posterior paravesical spaces. The anterior paravesical space is divided by the medial umbilical folds, into lateral and medial compartments. On each side, the inferior epigastric artery divides the lateral pelvic compartments into lateral and medial inguinal fossae, the sites of direct and indirect inguinal hernias, respectively.

In males, the posterior paravesical space is subdivided into the *rectovesical* and *pararectal space* by the peritoneal coverings of the rectum and bladder. In females, peritoneal coverings of the uterus divide the rectovesical space into the *vesicouterine* and *rectouterine space* (cul-de-sac or pouch of Douglas). The rectouterine space is the most dependant portion of the pelvis in women while the rectovesical space is the most dependant portion of pelvis in men and these spaces are a common location for fluid, drop metastases and abscesses in women and men respectively **(Figs. 5A to C)**.[4]

PERITONEAL FLUID DYNAMICS

The peritoneal cavity contains a small amount of fluid—approximately 50–100 mL.[8] This fluid has a natural tendency to move inferiorly towards the pelvis due to gravity. However, due to the respiratory motion of the diaphragm, gravitational pull of the liver and peristalsis of bowel, there is an active flow of the peritoneal fluid laterally and upwards towards the diaphragm. It predominantly flows up the right paracolic gutter which is deeper and wider than the left to the subphrenic space where majority (about 90%) of the peritoneal fluid is cleared by the submesothelial lymphatics. These lymphatics are connected with lymphatics on the other side of the diaphragm. Thus, metabolic, infectious and neoplastic processes in the peritoneal cavity may pass through the diaphragm to the subdiaphragmatic lymph nodes.[9] Ascites and tumor cells may also pass through the lymphatics and produce an ipsilateral pleural effusion. As these lymphatics have unidirectional valves, pleural effusion cannot pass into the peritoneal cavity. There are some areas of fluid stasis in the peritoneal cavity namely ileocolic region, root of sigmoid mesentery and pouch of Douglas, which become important in harboring disease.

ASCITES

Ascites is the pathological accumulation of fluid in the peritoneal cavity. It can occur due to a large number of causes. Common causes are listed in **Table 2**. Ascitic fluid is traditionally characterized as either *transudate*—thin, with a low protein count and low specific gravity and *exudate*—high protein count and specific gravity. It has been seen that the serum-ascites albumin gradient is more accurate in classification of the causes of ascites.[10]

TABLE 2: Causes of ascites.

• *Hepatic*: - Cirrhosis, portal hypertension, Budd–Chiari syndrome, alcoholic hepatitis, fulminant hepatic failure
• *Cardiac*: - Congestive heart failure, constrictive pericarditis, cardiac tamponade
• *Renal*: - Nephrotic syndrome, renal failure
• Hypoalbuminemia
• *Infective peritonitis*: - Bacterial, tuberculosis, viral, fungal
• *Neoplasms*: - Primary neoplasms of abdominal organs—colon, pancreas, ovary, liver, etc. - Primary peritoneal malignancy - Metastatic peritoneal disease
• Trauma
• Blunt, penetrating or iatrogenic trauma to abdominal organs can lead to collection of blood, bile, chyle, urine, etc. depending on the organ involved

The imaging appearance of ascites depends on the amount of fluid, its contents and whether it is free flowing or loculated. In uncomplicated *transudative* ascites which is usually free flowing, the fluid tends to collect in dependant areas like pelvic cul-de-sac, Morrison's pouch and paracolic gutters in early stages. Due to the suction effect of the diaphragm, fluid also accumulates in the subphrenic spaces. Larger amounts of fluid will fill the entire peritoneal cavity and displace the small bowel loops centrally. The fluid collection is shaped by the surrounding structures, forms acute angles where fluid borders organs and does not deform the normal shape of adjacent organs. Complicated ascites, i.e. exudative or loculated ascites is associated with adhesions, malignancy or infection. Loculated ascites is noncompressible and has rounded margins with mass effect and frequently displaces adjacent structures.

Ultrasound is a sensitive modality for detection, quantification, localization and characterization of ascitic fluid. As little as 0.8 mm of fluid has been detected in the pouch of Douglas by transvaginal scanning.[11] US can also be very helpful in differentiating transudative from exudative ascites. In patients with transudative ascites, the US appearances are predominantly those of anechoic, mobile fluid. Features associated with exudative ascites due to inflammatory or malignant causes include loculated fluid collections, particulate ascites, septa, and matted bowel loops with interposed fluid. US can also help determine whether identified fluid is free or loculated, as free ascites moves when the patient changes position.

CT is most sensitive to small amounts of fluid in the peritoneum which collects preferentially in the dependent regions. The CT density of intraperitoneal fluid can give a clue to the underlying etiology, transudative ascites density is approximately that of water (–10 to +10 HU), whereas exudative ascites density is greater than 15 HU and increases with increasing protein content, hemoperitoneum density is higher still (~45 HU) and chylous fluid density is <0 HU. Enhancement of the peritoneum may be seen on CECT in infective and neoplastic ascites. As CT provides a more complete evaluation of the abdomen and pelvis than sonography, other intra- or extra-abdominal CT features may give further evidence to the origin of the ascites (e.g. features of heart failure, features of cirrhosis, peritoneal catheter *in situ*, etc).

It is often difficult to characterize the nature and underlying cause of peritoneal fluid collections on basis of imaging alone and a diagnostic paracentesis may be required to sample the fluid. US can be used to guide aspiration for diagnostic or therapeutic purpose.

PNEUMOPERITONEUM

Normally there is no free air within the peritoneal cavity. The most common cause of a pneumoperitoneum is due to rupture of an abdominal viscus. Other causes are—postoperative status, patient on peritoneal dialysis, rupture of a cyst in pneumatosis intestinalis etc. It is important to be able to recognize the signs of a pneumoperitoneum on various imaging modalities and to be able to differentiate a true pneumoperitoneum from a pseudopneumoperitoneum. This has been discussed in detail elsewhere in the book.

INTERNAL HERNIAS

Internal hernia is the protrusion of a viscus through a normal or abnormal aperture in the peritoneum or mesentery, within the confines of the peritoneal cavity. This aperture can be congenital or acquired, such as postsurgical, post-traumatic or even postinflammatory. Congenital hernias may occur through a normal aperture, e.g. foramen of Winslow, or abnormal defects which arise from anomalies of internal rotation and peritoneal attachment.

Based on the location, Meyers traditionally classified these hernias as paraduodenal (53%), pericecal (13%), foramen of Winslow (8%), transmesenteric and transmesocolic (8%), intersigmoid (6%), retroanastomotic (5%) and paravesical (7%—not a true internal hernia).[12] The most common internal hernias have been the paraduodenal hernias which are congenital hernias, however with the increasing surgical procedures being performed these days, the incidence of the acquired post-operative hernias is increasing.[13]

Clinically, internal hernias can have a variable presentation ranging from asymptomatic to mild colicky abdominal pain to acute intestinal obstruction. Imaging plays an important role in diagnosis as they are difficult to identify clinically. Imaging features on barium studies and CT include cluster of dilated/nondilated bowel loops in an abnormal location **(Figs. 6A and B)**, crowding of loops in a hernia sac and/or features of obstruction. CT may additionally show mesenteric vessel abnormalities as engorgement, twisting, or stretching of the vessels. **Table 3** lists the various hernias with their characteristic clinical and imaging findings.

PERITONEAL INFECTIONS AND INFLAMMATION

Peritonitis

Peritonitis is defined as a diffuse inflammation of the parietal and visceral peritoneum. It is most often caused by introduction of an infection into the otherwise sterile peritoneal environment through perforation of an abdominal viscus, but it may also result from other irritants, such as foreign bodies (such as talc or barium), bile from a perforated gallbladder or a lacerated liver, or gastric acid from a perforated ulcer. Gynecologic disease processes such as salpingitis may also cause peritonitis. Uncommonly, primary bacterial peritonitis may occur due to hematogenous spread of organisms in association with chronic liver or renal disease.

Clinically, patients may present with an acute or insidious onset of symptoms, limited and mild disease, or systemic and severe disease with septic shock. On imaging,

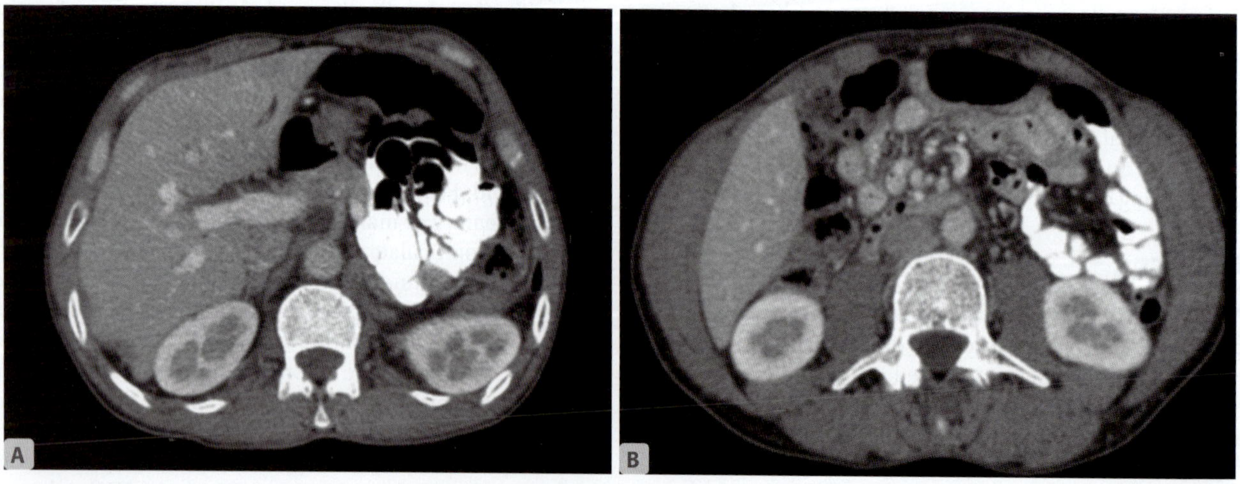

FIGS. 6A AND B: Left paraduodenal hernia in a 45-year-old man with chronic postprandial abdominal pain. Axial CECT image (A) shows a sac like mass of jejunal loops between stomach and pancreatic body. Section obtained at lower level (B) shows crowded and dilated mesenteric vessels.

TABLE 3: Internal hernias: Clinical and imaging features.

Type of hernia	*Congenital/Acquired site*	*Findings on plain radiographs and barium studies*	*CT findings*
Left paraduodenal	Congenital Through Landzert's fossa behind the fourth part of the duodenum	Cluster of jejunal loops in left hypochondrium, lateral to the 4th part of duodenum; may have mass effect indenting posterior wall of stomach or displacing transverse colon inferiorly	• Encapsulated cluster of dilated small-bowel loops between stomach and pancreas, behind pancreas itself, or between transverse colon and left adrenal gland • Inferior mesenteric vein displaced superoanteriorly in neck of hernia sac
Right paraduodenal	Congenital Through Waldeyer's fossa (representing a defect in the first part of the jejunal mesentery)	Clustered loops lateral and inferior to the 2nd part of duodenum; associated with nonrotation of small-bowel	• Encapsulated cluster of loops lateral and inferior to the 2nd part of duodenum; associated with small-bowel nonrotation • Superior mesenteric artery displaced anteriorly
Pericecal	Congenital/acquired Through a defect in the cecal mesentery and extending into the right paracolic gutter	Clustered small-bowel loops (usually distal ileal) posterior and lateral to the cecum in right paracolic gutter	Clustered small-bowel loops (usually distal ileum) posterior and lateral to the cecum in right paracolic gutter
Foramen of Winslow	Congenital Through Foramen of Winslow	Circumscribed loops medial and posterior to the stomach	Loops in the lesser sac between liver and inferior vena cava
Intersigmoid	Congenital/acquired Fossae/defects in and around sigmoid mesocolon	U- or C-shaped cluster of small bowel posterior and lateral to the sigmoid colon	U- or C-shaped cluster of small bowel posterior and lateral to the sigmoid colon
Transmesenteric	• Congenital in children through defect in small bowel mesentery • Acquired in adults associated with abdominal surgery	Variable, air within gastric remnant in postoperative cases; may simulate a left paraduodenal hernia	Small bowel lateral to colon; displaced omental fat with small bowel directly abutting abdominal wall
Retroanastomotic	Acquired Through a defect related to a surgical anastomosis	Variable	Variable

Source: Adapted from Martin LC, Markle EM, Thompson WM. Review of internal hernias: radiographic and clinical findings.[13]

there is presence of ascites which may be loculated or show presence of debris, septa or gas **(Fig. 7)**. US is superior to CT in demonstrating the nature of the ascitic fluid.[14] In association with ascites there is peritoneal and mesenteric thickening. The thickened peritoneum is seen to enhance on contrast administration, and is often smooth **(Fig. 8)**. In some cases evidence of the underlying primary pathology can be seen such as diverticulitis, appendiceal perforation, bowel ischemia, etc.

Peritoneal abscess is an infected fluid collection encapsulated by fibrinous exudate, omentum, and/or adjacent visceral organs. The majority of abscesses occur secondary to spread of infection from an adjacent infected organ or viscus, e.g. inflamed appendix, pancreatitis, diverticulitis, Crohn's disease, liver abscess, etc. Abscess formation may also occur as a complication of abdominal or pelvic surgery or penetrating trauma. The risk of abscess increases in cases of preoperative perforation of the hollow viscus, significant fecal contamination of the peritoneal cavity, bowel ischemia, as well as in the setting of immunosuppression.

Clinically patients present with fever, tachycardia, and symptoms localized to area of abscess, e.g. with a subphrenic collection, there may be shoulder tip pain, hiccups and unexplained pulmonary symptoms (pleural effusion, basal atelectasis). Sometimes clinical features may be minimal specially in immunocompromised patients.

The CT appearance of an abscess varies depending on its age. In early stages, it may appear as a mass with soft tissue attenuation values. As the liquefaction progresses, a central hypodense, nonenhancing area with a definable, enhancing wall is seen. Gas may be seen within the abscess cavity as multiple small bubbles or as an air fluid level **(Figs. 9 and 16B)**. Occasionally septations may be seen. There is thickening and obliteration of adjacent fat planes, mass effect on surrounding structures. Features of the predisposing cause of the abscess, e.g. acute appendicitis, Crohn's disease, or diverticulitis, etc. may be seen.

On US, an abscess is seen as a round or oval fluid collection with a well-defined irregular wall, with occasional internal septa or debris. Small pockets of air within the abscess cavity can be seen as echogenic foci with posterior reverberation artefact.[15] However, US detection of abscess is hampered by bowel gas, intra-abdominal fat, gas within the abscess cavity and in postoperative cases, there is limited availability of scanning surface. Thus, US has a low sensitivity in abscess detection. CT is the preferred modality and can confidently

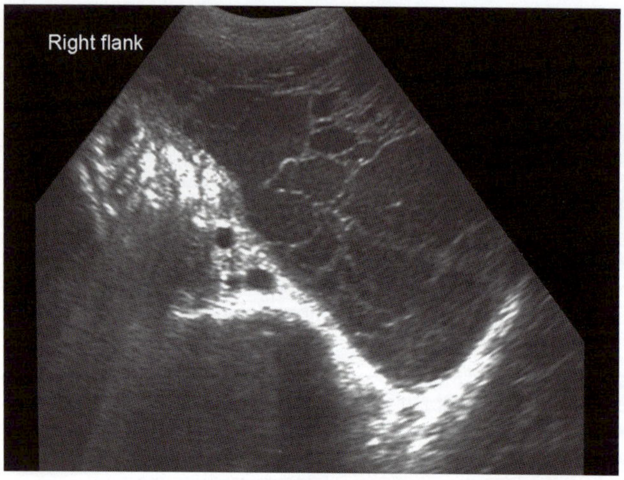

FIG. 7: Purulent peritonitis: Transverse US image through right flank shows ascites with peritoneal thickening and ascitic fluid. The fluid shows internal echoes characteristic of exudative nature and multiple septae within.

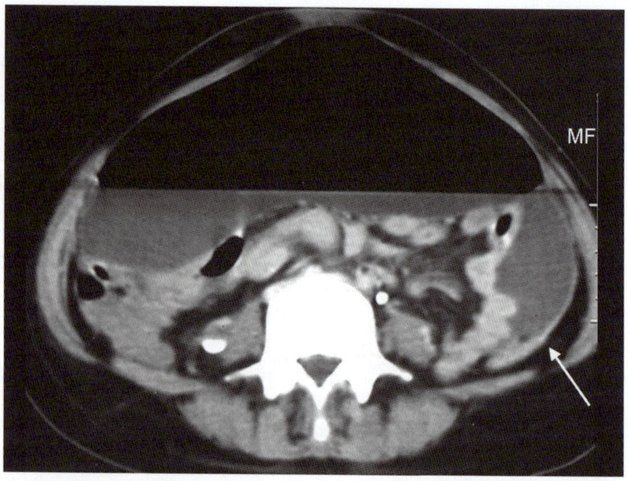

FIG. 8: Perforation peritonitis: CECT axial section through the abdomen, shows fluid in the peritoneal cavity with a large air fluid level. Smooth, enhancing, thickening of the peritoneal lining is seen (arrow).

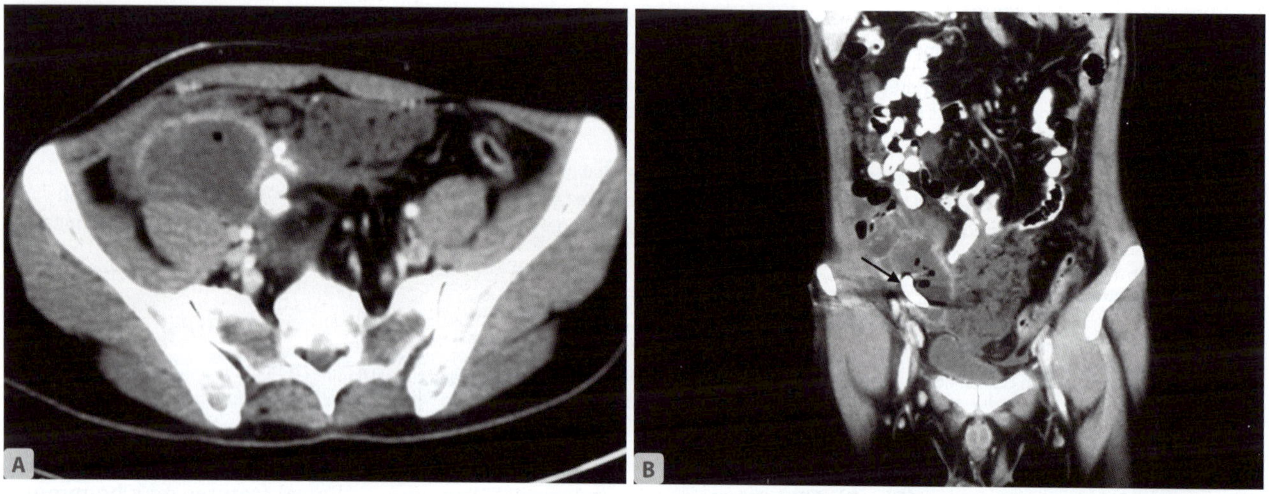

FIGS. 9A AND B: Appendicular abscess: CECT axial (A) and coronal scans (B) show a well defined hypodense collection with a thin peripheral enhancing rim in the right iliac fossa. Small gas bubbles are seen within the abscess. There is evidence of associated inflammatory changes in the adjacent fat. A drain can be seen in the abscess in (B) (arrow).

rule out intra-abdominal abscess if the CT examination is negative.

On MRI, abscesses are seen as well-defined fluid collection with low SI on T1W and high SI on T2W images. Adjacent inflammation can be seen as diffusely increased SI on T2W images.

Percutaneous aspiration is frequently required to confirm the presence of pus in a suspected abscess. Percutaneous drainage has become the widely accepted treatment for abdominal abscesses and can be done under US or CT guidance. US can be used for the follow-up evaluation of abscess under treatment.[7]

Tuberculous Peritonitis

The peritoneum and its reflections can also be commonly involved by tuberculosis. The mode of transmission may be hematogenous or lymphatic, reactivation of latent tuberculous foci in the peritoneum or peritoneal spill from tubercular salpingitis. Discharge of caseous material from diseased lymph nodes may also lead to tubercular peritonitis.

Classically, three forms of tuberculous peritonitis have been described.[16-18]

- *Wet ascitic type*: Seen in 90% cases characterized by large amount of free or loculated ascitic fluid. This may be accompanied by diffuse and smooth peritoneal thickening.
- *Fibrotic fixed type*: Characterized by mesenteric and omental thickening and matted bowel loops resembling masses, with formation of cocoon in some cases.
- *Dry or plastic type*: Predominant peritoneal and mesenteric thickening with caseous nodules, lymph node enlargement and dense adhesions.

Imaging Features

Tubercular infection diffusely involves the peritoneum, mesentery and omentum. *Free or loculated ascites* is seen in 30–100% cases and is demonstrated by both ultrasound and CT.[19-21]

Ultrasound may show fine, multiple, complete or incomplete mobile strands of fibrin and debris in the ascites **(Fig. 10A)**. Peritoneal thickening and tiny nodules are better visualized in presence of ascites on US. On CT, usually high density (25–45 HU) ascitic fluid due to high fibrin content and cellular debris is characteristic of TB.[22] However ascites may be near water density, representing an earlier transudative stage of immune reaction. Fat fluid level, a feature of chylous ascites with supportive evidence of mesenteric adenopathy has been described in tuberculosis.[23] CT fails to show the multiple, thin interlacing septa in most patients **(Figs. 11A to C)**. Smooth, slight peritoneal thickening and/or pronounced enhancement are seen in presence of ascites on CT in almost all cases. Enhancement of peritoneal lining in patients with tubercular ascites has been described on delayed contrast-enhanced MRI.

Mesenteric involvement is seen as linear striations, vascular engorgement, nodular lesions, increased density at the root of mesentery, mesenteric thickening and loss of normal mesenteric configuration. On US the mesentery becomes echogenic as a result of increased fat deposition due to lymphatic obstruction. Presence of enlarged lymph nodes adds to the diagnosis of early tuberculosis **(Figs. 10A to C)**. Mesenteric nodular lesions may present as micro (<5 mm) or macro (>5 mm) nodules. Mesenteric abscess may form as result of extension of caseous material from diseased lymph nodes. Fixed loops of bowel and mesentery standing out as spokes radiating out from the mesenteric root are described as ultrasound 'stellate' sign. CT demonstrates the thickened mesentery by its increased vascularity and thickened strands and tethering of bowel loops forming an abdominal mass **(Figs. 11 to 12)**. 'Club sandwich sign' or the 'sliced bread' appearance is due to localized or focal ascitis between radially oriented bowel due to local exudation from inflamed bowel or ruptured lymph nodes.

Omental thickening is a feature of both TB and peritoneal carcinomatosis and many different appearances 'nodular' 'smudged' or 'caked' have been described. The thickened omentum shows heterogeneous iso- to hyperintense signal on T2W sequences on MRI.[24] A marked degree of peritoneal enhancement is seen on enhanced CT and MRI **(Figs. 13 and 14)**. Sclerosing encapsulating peritonitis (abdominal cocoon) formation has also been described in tubercular involvement of peritoneum **(*see* Figs. 17A to D)**.

Associated features of intra-abdominal tuberculosis may also be present, such as thickening of the bowel wall, particularly the terminal ileum, focal abnormalities in the

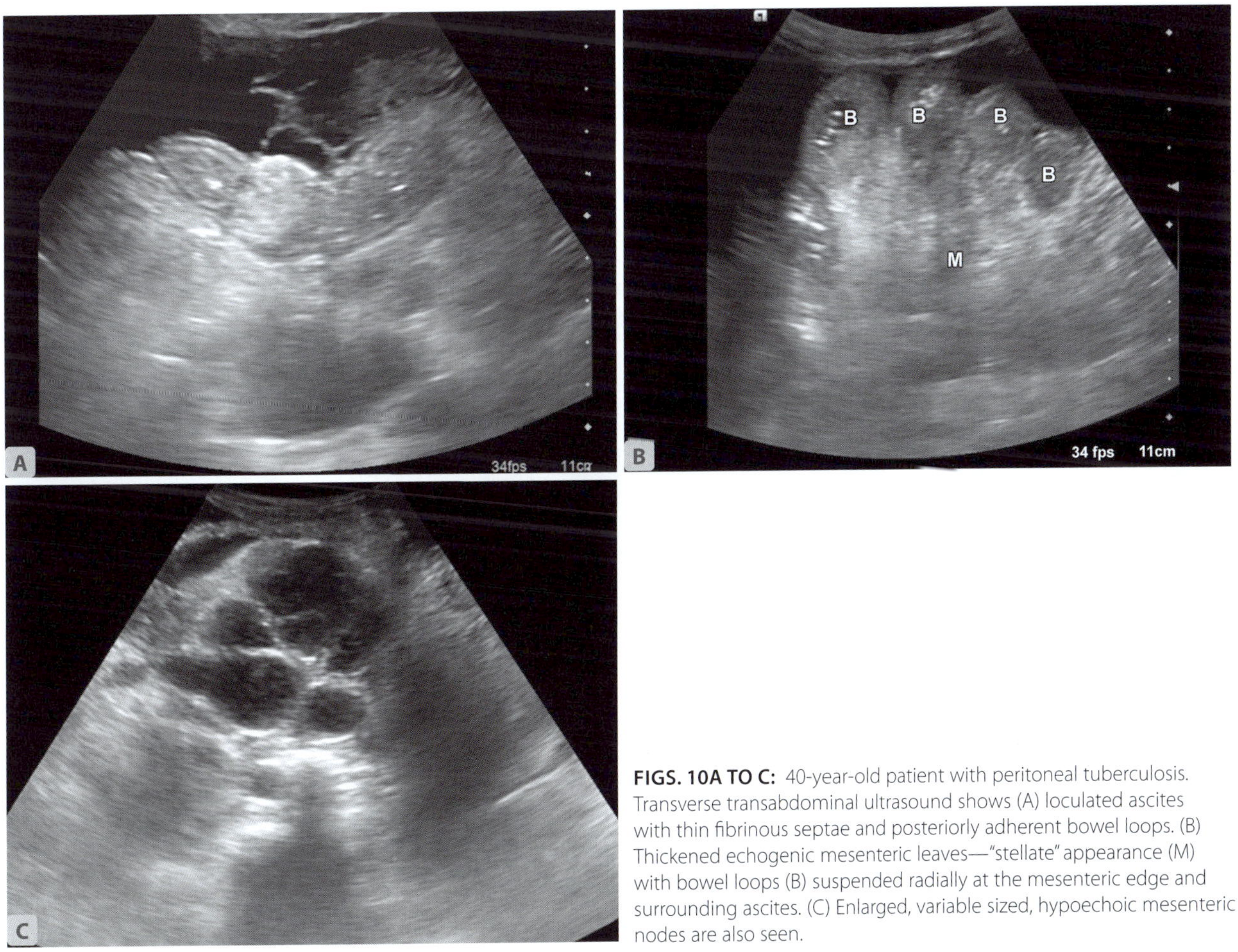

FIGS. 10A TO C: 40-year-old patient with peritoneal tuberculosis. Transverse transabdominal ultrasound shows (A) loculated ascites with thin fibrinous septae and posteriorly adherent bowel loops. (B) Thickened echogenic mesenteric leaves—"stellate" appearance (M) with bowel loops (B) suspended radially at the mesenteric edge and surrounding ascites. (C) Enlarged, variable sized, hypoechoic mesenteric nodes are also seen.

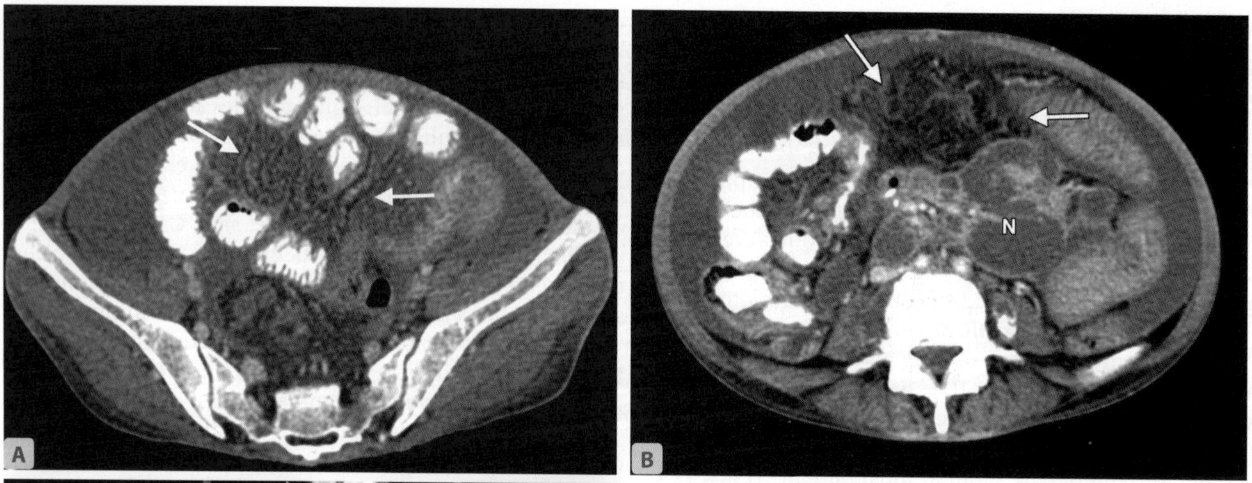

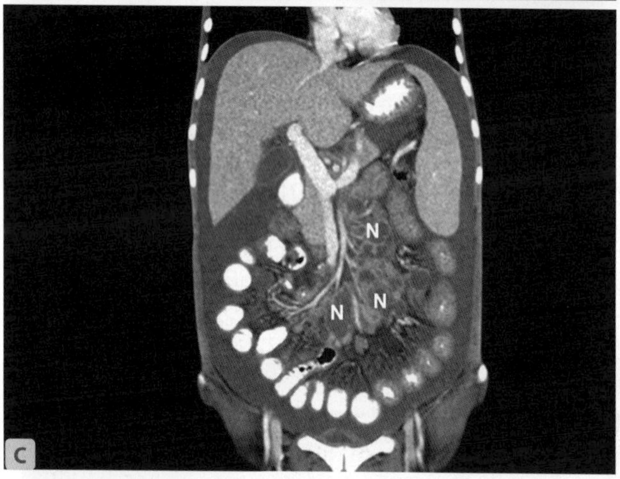

FIGS. 11A TO C: Peritoneal tuberculosis: CT of same patient as in Figure 10. Axial and coronal images show ascites; smooth, thickened, enhancing peritoneum; nodular, congested mesenteric and omental thickening (arrows) and multiple enlarged hypodense mesenteric nodes with peripheral enhancement (N).

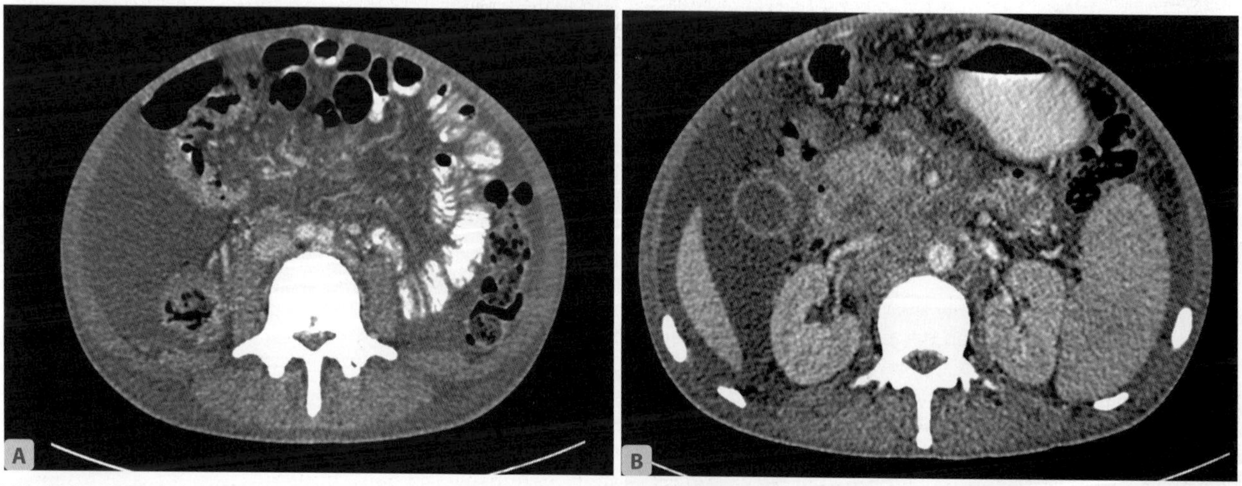

FIGS. 12A AND B: Tubercular peritonitis—wet ascitic type: CECT axial scans show the presence of ascites with small nodules and haziness in the mesentery and omentum (A); At a more cranial level (B), conglomerate caseous lymphadenopathy is seen in mesenteric and retroperitoneal regions.

liver or spleen due to granulomas and occasionally adrenal pathology. Notably the chest radiograph is abnormal in only 50% of patients with tuberculous peritonitis.[25]

The *differential diagnosis* of tubercular peritonitis constitutes peritoneal carcinomatosis, mesothelioma, peritonitis and rarely lymphoma. A marked overlap exists between the imaging appearances of tubercular peritonitis and peritoneal carcinomatosis. Features favoring carcinomatosis are nodular implants with irregular thickening. Irregularly thickened outer contour of the infiltrated peritoneum favors malignancy, whereas a thin omental line, suggestive of a fibrous wall covering the infiltrated omentum

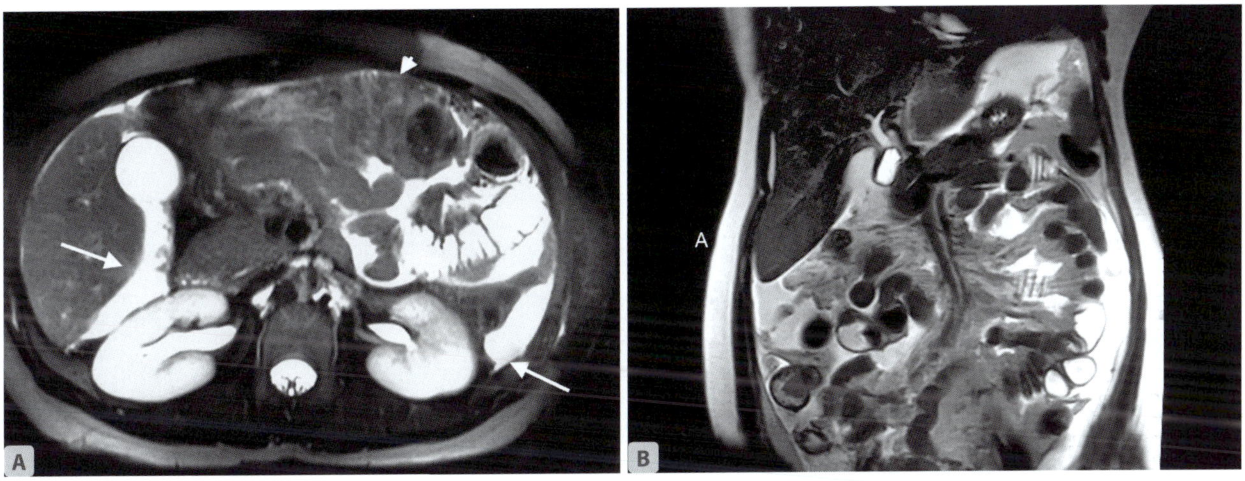

FIGS. 13A AND B: Peritoneal tuberculosis in 35-year-old woman with loss of weight and abdominal fullness for 1 month. (A) Axial T2W haste MR image shows presence of ascitic fluid in Morrison's pouch, left paracolic gutter (arrows) and in interloop regions. The omentum is thickened showing a heterogeneous soft tissue signal (arrowhead); (B) Coronal T2W haste MR image shows diffuse infiltration of the mesenteric fat by isointense soft tissue. Ascites is seen in the paracolic gutters and subhepatic space.

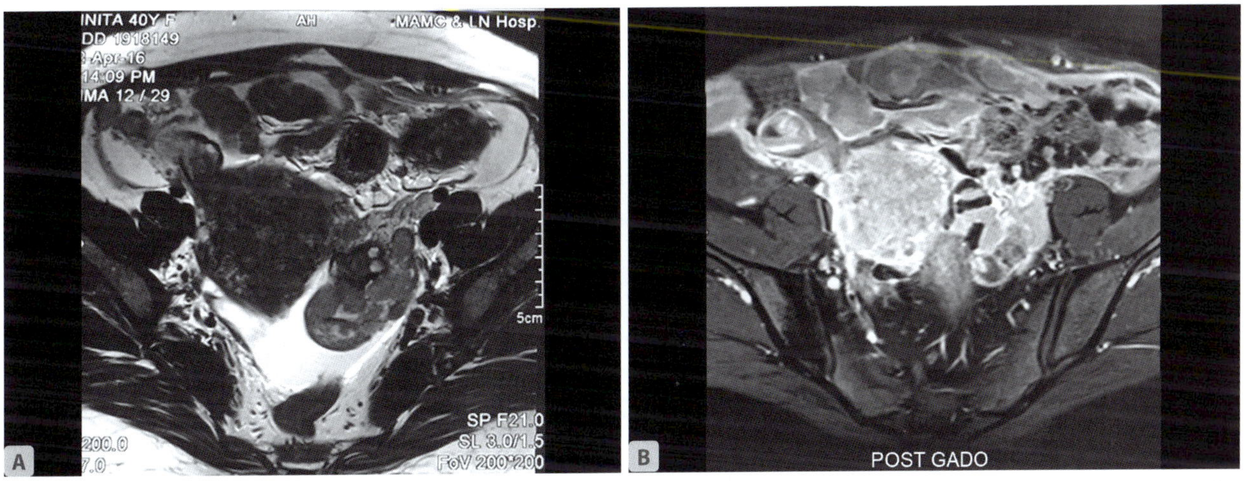

FIGS. 14A AND B: Peritoneal tuberculosis-same patient as in Figure 13: Axial T2W haste (A) and postcontrast (B) MR images show presence of ascites, clumped bowel loops, with thickened and enhancing serosa. Left tubo-ovarian was seen which also enhanced on the postcontrast scan. On laprotomy the bowel serosa and the adnexal mass were studded with multiple small granulomas, which were not identifiable individually on the MR images, but caused the intensely enhancing peritoneal lining.

is more common in tubercular peritonitis.[26,27] However, a clinical background of malignancy along with laboratory investigations are often required to differentiate between them. Peritoneal mesothelioma shows multifocal peritoneal thickening of either sheet or nodular type which can be up to 3 cm in thickness, omental or mesenteric soft tissue masses, thick rigid septae between peritoneal leaves and fixed bowel loops with disproportionately small amount of ascites to the degree of tumor dissemination.

PERITONEAL HYDATIDOSIS

Peritoneal hydatidosis is an uncommon manifestation of hydatid disease and is almost always secondary to hepatic disease. It occurs as a result of traumatic or surgical rupture of a hepatic or splenic hydatid cyst. However, spontaneous, asymptomatic microruptures of hepatic cysts into the peritoneal cavity are not uncommon leading to peritoneal seeding. Primary hydatidosis is a rare entity accounting for just 2% of all intra-abdominal hydatid disease.[28]

Clinical Picture

Most patients remain asymptomatic for years. Symptoms such as nonspecific pain, abdominal fullness, dyspepsia, anorexia, and vomiting arise due to enlarging abdominal cysts. Rupture of the cyst into the peritoneum may present as acute abdominal pain. Antigenic fluid released into the peritoneal cavity and absorbed into the circulation may present with acute allergic manifestations.[29]

Imaging Features

Hydatid cysts can be well seen on US, CT and MRI. Cysts may be multiple and located anywhere in the peritoneal cavity **(Figs. 15A to C)**. The imaging appearances of hydatid

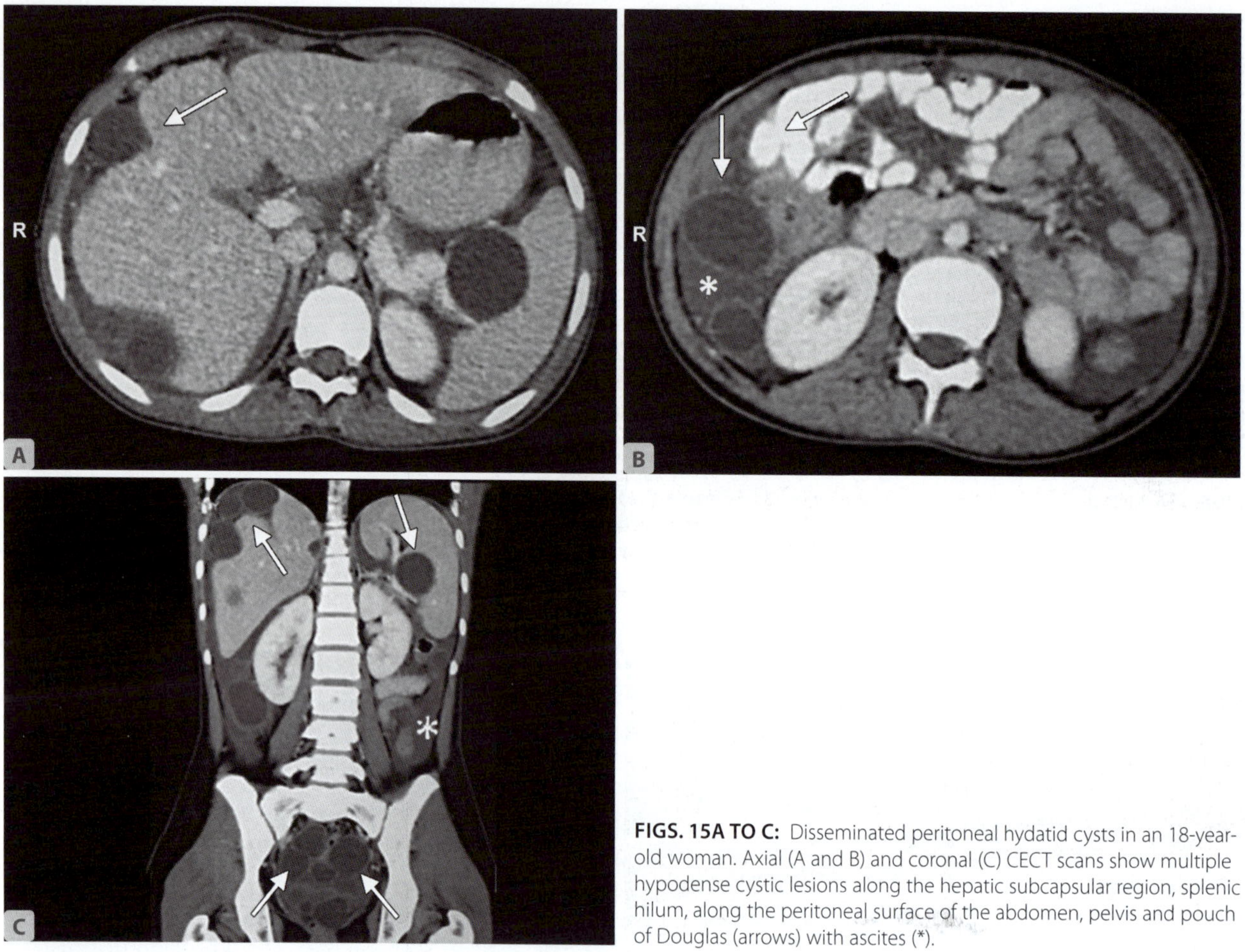

FIGS. 15A TO C: Disseminated peritoneal hydatid cysts in an 18-year-old woman. Axial (A and B) and coronal (C) CECT scans show multiple hypodense cystic lesions along the hepatic subcapsular region, splenic hilum, along the peritoneal surface of the abdomen, pelvis and pouch of Douglas (arrows) with ascites (*).

cysts are similar to those in hepatic disease. Sometimes, peritoneal hydatid disease occupy the entire peritoneal cavity, simulating a multiloculated mass which is known as encysted peritoneal hydatidosis.[28]

SECONDARY INFLAMMATORY PROCESSES

Inflammation of any part of the abdominal viscera may be accompanied by inflammatory change of the regional fatty tissue. This may progress to phlegmon formation, abscess or even generalized peritonitis. Appendicitis, diverticulitis, pancreatitis, inflammatory bowel disease, cholecystitis, etc. are conditions which commonly give rise to these localized inflammatory changes. They are best visualized on CT as soft tissue stranding of adjacent fat, fluid, phlegmon or abscess formation, sinus tracts and fistulas **(Figs. 16A and B)**.

Besides the above inflammatory changes, Crohn's disease may show other mesenteric abnormalities in the form of hypertrophied mesenteric fat (fibrofatty proliferation), engorged vasa recta (the comb's sign), and small mesenteric nodes. The presence of engorged vasa recta indicates active inflammation, whereas the fibrofatty proliferation can be seen even with quiescent disease.

Mesenteric edema is defined as diffuse increase in attenuation throughout the mesentery that obscures visualization of the blood vessels as they course through the mesentery, also termed as 'misty mesentery'. It may be secondary to various causes, including hypoalbuminemia, cirrhosis, nephrosis, heart failure, tricuspid disease, constrictive pericarditis, portal hypertension, portal vein thrombosis, mesenteric ischemia, vasculitis or trauma. On CT, mesenteric edema increases the density of the mesenteric fat from –100 to –160, which is similar to the density of subcutaneous fat, to values of –40 to –60.[30] On MRI, the mesentery shows abnormal signal. The mesenteric arteries and veins lose their sharp definition and are not clearly visualized as they course to the bowel. Associated ascites may be present and generalized subcutaneous and retroperitoneal fat haziness secondary to generalized edema can be seen. The extent and site of involvement gives a clue to the differential diagnosis.

SCLEROSING ENCAPSULATING PERITONITIS/ABDOMINAL COCOON

Sclerosing encapsulating peritonitis is a rare chronic inflammatory process of the peritoneum which is

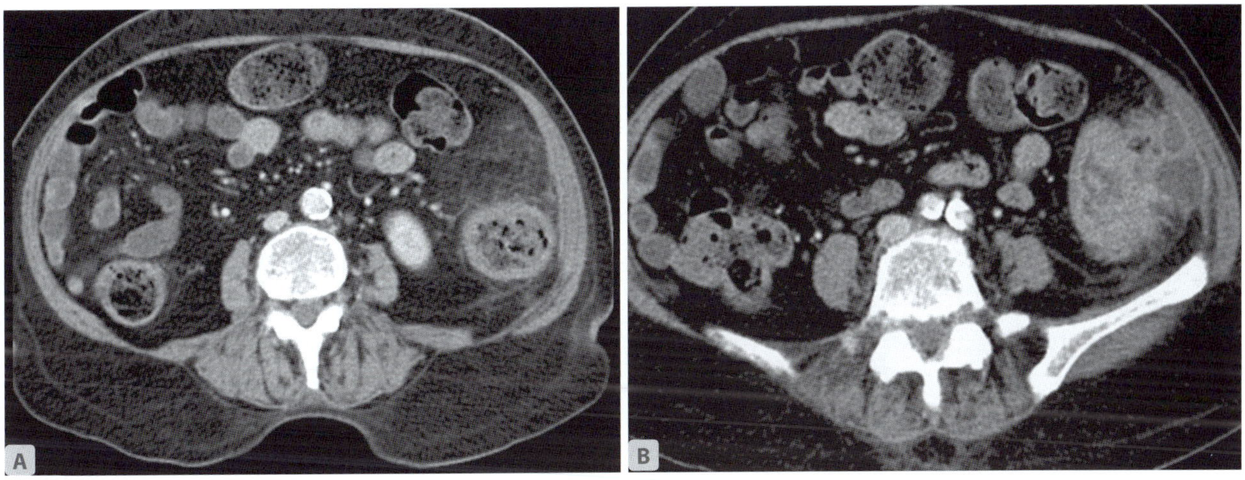

FIGS. 16A AND B: Acute diverticulitis showing local extension of inflammation: CECT axial scans (A) inflammatory fat stranding seen around the thickened segment of descending colon; (B) In another patient, there is formation of abscesses seen as rim enhancing hypodense masses in the left pericolonic region.

characterized by total or partial encasement of the small bowel within a thick fibrocollagenous membrane. Sclerosing encapsulating peritonitis (SEP) is most commonly associated with abdominal tuberculosis in our country. It can occur as a complication in patients who undergo continuous peritoneal dialysis. It has also been described in association with long-term β-blocker treatment, sarcoidosis, SLE, indwelling abdominal catheter, etc.[31] These conditions predispose patients to peritoneal irritation and inflammation which can lead to peritoneal fibroneogenesis. Sometimes no predisposing condition may be found for the SEP.

Clinically, patients may be asymptomatic or have abdominal distention, pain and vomiting that resolve spontaneously suggesting recurrent episodes of small bowel obstruction. A soft nontender mass may be felt at abdominal palpation. It is seen to be commoner in young adolescent girls.

Imaging Features

A barium meal follow-through study may show a conglomeration of multiple bowel loops that appear to adhere to each other with or without delayed passage of contrast material **(Fig. 17A)**. Characteristic sonographic findings include altered peristalsis, adherence of the bowel to the anterior abdominal wall and a membranous sac seen to encase the small bowel loops **(Fig. 17B)**. There is a concertina—like arrangement of small bowel loops with a narrow posterior base. The encapsulating membrane may be identified with high frequency linear probes.[32]

Contrast-enhanced computed tomography shows conglomeration of small-bowel loops in the central abdomen with a thick enhancing membrane surrounding the bowel, forming a saclike structure or a cocoon **(Figs. 17C and D)**. Small amount of fluid may be seen within the cocoon. Bowel loops may be of normal caliber or dilated. The fibrous membrane surrounding the bowel loops is best visualized on CT. CT also gives more accurate information on the degree of obstruction and the types of bowel loops involved. Multiple foci of linear calcification may develop or there can be diffuse peritoneal calcification.[33,34]

The most important differential diagnosis of SEP is from an internal hernia that also causes localized collection of small-bowel loops with symptoms of obstruction. However, there is no membrane like sac around the clustered small bowel loops in internal hernias. SEP may also be confused with congenital peritoneal encapsulation, which is characterized by a thin accessory peritoneal sac surrounding the small bowel.

SCLEROSING MESENTERITIS (MESENTERIC PANNICULITIS, MESENTERIC LIPODYSTROPHY, RETRACTILE MESENTERITIS)

Sclerosing mesenteritis is a rare, slowly progressive disorder characterized by nonspecific inflammation of the mesenteric fat. It usually involves the root of the small bowel mesentery, but may affect the transverse mesocolon, peripancreatic region, omentum, retroperitoneum or pelvis.[35]

Histologically, it has varying amounts of fibrosis, chronic inflammation, and fat necrosis. Depending on the predominant component it has been categorized into three subgroups:

1. Sclerosing/retractile mesenteritis when the fibrous component is dominant.
2. Mesenteric panniculitis when chronic inflammation predominates.
3. Mesenteric lipodystrophy, when fat necrosis is the predominant component.[36]

Although its exact cause remains unknown, various underlying possibilities have been suggested like prior surgery or trauma, ischemia, an autoimmune process or malignancy. An association with other idiopathic inflammatory disorders like retroperitoneal fibrosis, Reidel's thyroiditis, orbital pseudotumors and sclerosing cholangitis has been noted.

Clinical Picture

It occurs more commonly in males and the average age of presentation is around 60 years. Patients present with

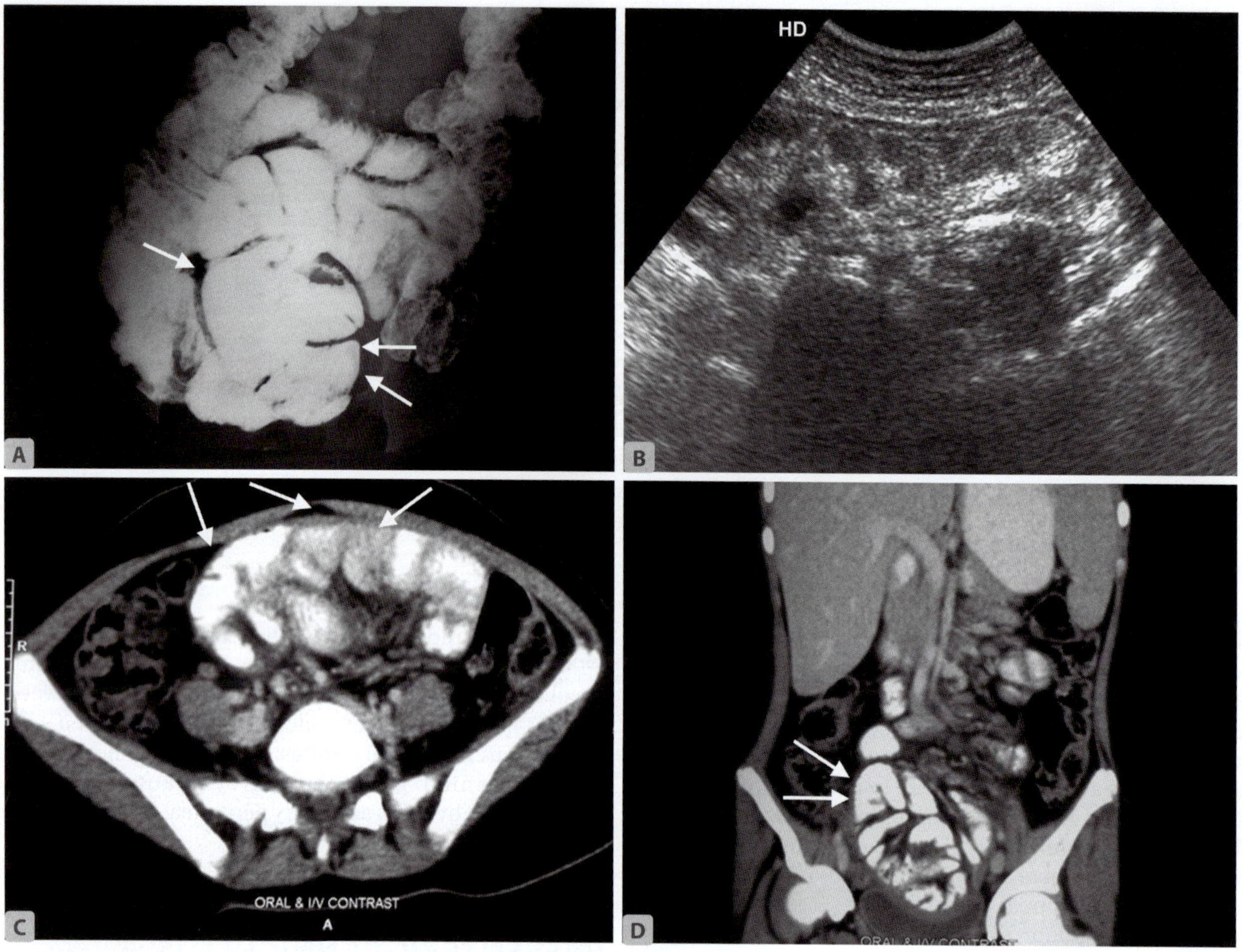

FIGS. 17A TO D: Sclerosing peritonitis. A 14-year-old girl with recurrent episodes of intestinal obstruction: (A) Barium meal follow through study shows clustered bowel loops in pelvis and lower abdomen (arrows); (B) Transverse US through lower abdomen show clumped bowel loops adherent to the anterior abdominal wall. An increased peristalsis was noted in the loops on real-time; Axial (C) and coronal (D) CECT scans show clumped small bowel loops in the lower abdomen with a thin surrounding membrane (arrows). Small mesenteric nodes are also seen.

abdominal pain, mass, obstructive symptoms or diarrhea or may even be completely asymptomatic.

Imaging Findings

The imaging findings reflect the underlying histology of the lesion. When the fibrous component is dominant, i.e. sclerosing type of mesenteritis, an infiltrative soft tissue mass with variable degree of enhancement is seen on CT. Central calcification or necrosis, radiating strands of soft tissue (desmoplastic reaction), small lymph nodes in the adjacent fat may all be seen **(Figs. 18A and B)**. There may be preservation of fat around the mesenteric vessels, a phenomenon that is referred to as the "fat ring sign".[37] On MRI, the signal intensity pattern is consistent with fibrosis, showing low signal intensity on both T1- and T2- weighted images. Sometimes a high signal on T2W image may be seen which correspons to myxomatous change or hypervascularity accompanying active proliferation of fibrosis. Secondary changes may be seen in the adjacent bowel as angulations by the fibrotic process in the mesentery, or edematous thickening due to obstruction of lymphatics and veins.[36]

In mesenteric panniculitis, CT may show subtle increase in attenuation with small nodes within it with no evidence of a mass. The term 'misty mesentery' may be used to describe this process as it is not specific for mesenteric panniculitis, but may also be seen in any infiltrating process in the mesentery like edema, hemorrhage, fibrosis or tumor. The 'fat-ring sign' can be seen in mesenteric panniculitis. A tumoral pseudocapsule, i.e. a peripheral band of soft tissue attenuation, appearing hypointense on T2W MR images, may sometimes be seen separating the normal mesentery from the inflammatory process.

Differential Diagnosis

Several conditions can mimic the CT appearance of sclerosing mesenteritis, including lymphoma, carcinoid tumor, carcinomatosis, primary mesenteric mesothelioma, and mesenteric edema.[38] Except for primary mesenteric mesothelioma, these conditions are considerably more common than sclerosing mesenteritis. Mesenteric panniculitis can be mimicked by mesenteric edema resulting from various conditions such as cirrhosis, hypoalbuminemia,

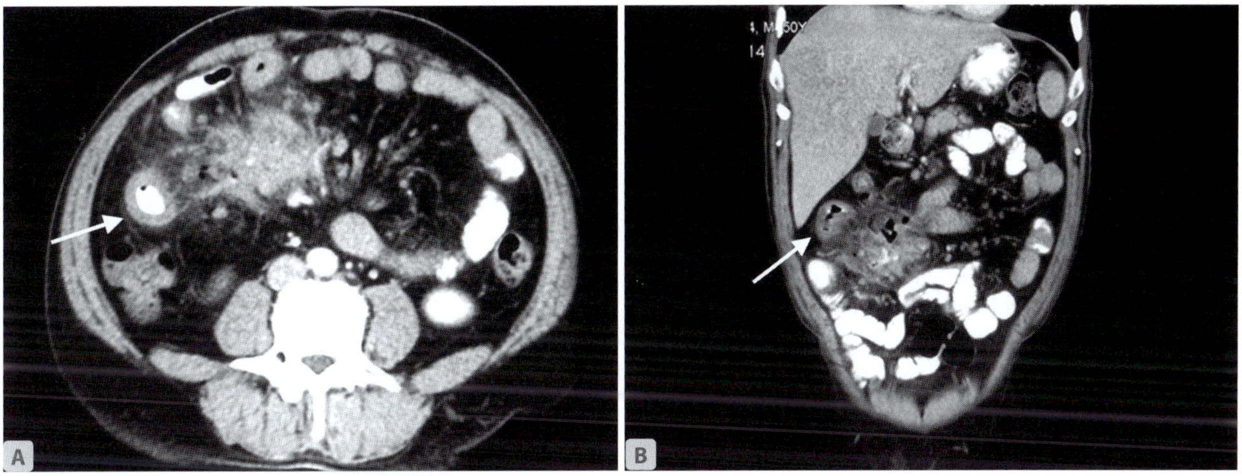

FIGS. 18A AND B: Sclerosing mesenteritis: Enhanced axial (A) and coronal (B) CT scans show an ill-defined soft tissue mesenteric mass with irregular, spiculated margins and thickening of adjacent jejunal loops (arrow). Small mesenteric lymph nodes are seen.

heart failure, portal or mesenteric vein thrombosis, and vasculitis. Trauma can also result in edema and hemorrhage in the mesentery. Mesenteric edema secondary to systemic disease is often diffuse and coexists with generalized subcutaneous edema and ascites, which will not be present in patients with sclerosing mesenteritis. Also, the clinical history will often be the clue to the correct diagnosis. A biopsy is necessary for diagnosis and although results of the biopsy may suggest the diagnosis, surgical excisional biopsy is often required for complete histologic analysis.

ACUTE EPIPLOIC APPENDAGITIS

Epiploic appendages are visceral peritoneal outpouchings that arise from the serosal surface of the colon, containing fat and blood vessels. Acute epiploic appendagitis occurs due to torsion or venous thrombosis of the vein, leading to ischemic or hemorrhagic infarction of epiploic appendages. It is seen to be associated with obesity and unaccustomed exercise.

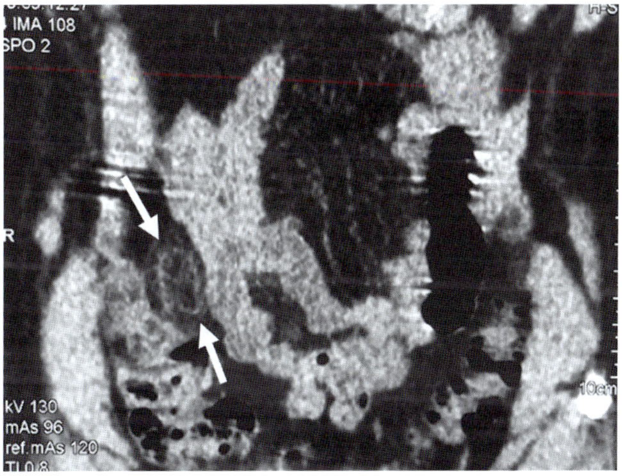

FIG. 19: Epiploic appendagitis: Coronal CECT shows a pericolic oval lesion of fat attenuation with a hyperdense rim (arrows). A central line seen within represents the thrombosed vein. There is associated inflammatory stranding seen in the adjacent fat.

Clinical Picture

Acute epiploic appendagitis occurs in the 4th to 5th decades of life, and is more common in males than females. Patients present with abdominal pain and rebound tenderness that correlates with the site of infarcted appendage. Clinical picture mimics that of acute appendicitis or diverticulitis. However, laboratory parameters are generally normal. Epiploic appendagitis is usually self limited and resolves spontaneously.

Imaging Features

On CT, the infarcted epiploic appendage is seen as a pericolic, oval to round lesion of fat attenuation with a hyperdense rim, less than 5 cm in size, surrounded by inflammatory changes. A central hyperattenuating dot or line may be seen corresponding to a thrombosed vessel **(Fig. 19)**. Mild reactive thickening of the adjacent colonic wall may be seen.[39] On ultrasound, a small, noncompressible hyperechoic mass surrounded by a hypoechoic rim, representing the inflamed visceral peritoneum, may be seen at the site of maximum tenderness. T1- and T2-weighted MR images show a focal lesion with the signal intensity of fat. Contrast-enhanced T1-weighted MR images show an enhancing rim around the oval fatty lesion.

The differential diagnosis of acute epiploic appendagitis presenting as an inflammatory fatty lesion associated with an acute abdomen include acute omental infarct, acute diverticulitis, sclerosing mesenteritis and occasionally a primary tumor or metastases that involve the mesocolon.[40]

OMENTAL INFARCTION

Omental infarction (OI) occurs due to vascular compromise, torsion or venous thrombosis, of the greater omentum. It can be primary or secondary. Primary omental infarction is generally right-sided and is related to the tenuous blood supply to the right edge of the greater omentum. Secondary omental infarction occurs due to vascular insult after trauma, surgery or inflammation of the greater omentum and it is located near the site of the initial insult. Unaccustomed exercise, straining or coughing can precipitate this condition.[40]

Clinical Findings

Primary OI is more common in children. Obesity is an important risk factor. Patients present with subacute onset of pain most often localized in the right upper or lower quadrant without any other gastrointestinal symptoms. There can be mild leucocytosis. Establishing a preoperative diagnosis of OI is difficult as it often mimics acute appendicitis or cholecystitis. The management is conservative.

Imaging Features

On CT, it appears as a fatty, large (>5 cm) encapsulated mass, with soft-tissue stranding adjacent to the ascending colon. Early or mild infarction may manifest as ill-defined, mild haziness. It is classically located between the anterior abdominal wall and the ascending or transverse colon **(Fig. 20)**. Swirling of vessels may be seen in omental torsion. At US, omental infarction may appear as a focal area of echogenic, noncompressible fat that corresponds to the site of focal tenderness.[40]

MESENTERIC LYMPHADENOPATHY

The mesentery contains multiple small lymph nodes which may get enlarged in a number of disease processes notably infective, inflammatory and neoplastic **(Table 4)**. Normal mesenteric lymph nodes may now be routinely identified at the mesenteric root and throughout the mesentery on US, CT and MRI, and are generally <5 mm in short axis diameter. The size of the nodes alone does not always reflect disease, the number and distribution of lymph nodes is also important. Lymph nodes greater than 6 mm in short axis diameter or a group of 3 or more clustered together in one anatomic location are taken as abnormal.[41,42]

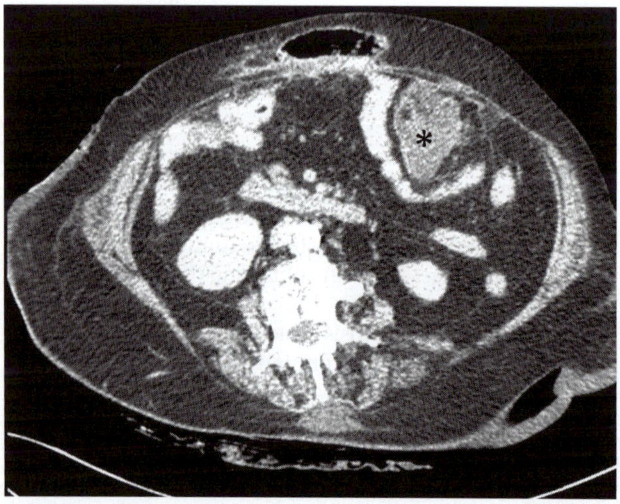

FIG. 20: Omental infarction: A 60-year-old patient with complaint of pain abdomen 6 days after undergoing abdominal surgery. CECT axial scan shows a hypodense, heterogeneous soft tissue mass with focal fatty areas within and adjacent fat stranding between the anterior abdominal wall and the transverse colon (*). A pocket of air is seen in the subcutaneous tissue due to dehiscence of the distal sutures.

Tuberculous Lymphadenitis

Lymphadenopathy in abdominal tuberculosis usually occurs in mesenteric, peripancreatic, periportal, and para-aortic groups of lymph nodes. It can occur through lymphatic spread, hematogenous route or direct spread from adjacent infected organs. The nodes may vary from increased number of normal-sized nodes to massive conglomerates with matting, the latter resulting from adhesions due to periadenitis. Pathologically tuberculous infection of a lymph node follows a spectrum from early exudative to caseous to late fibro-calcification phases.

On sonography, the lymph nodes are seen either as discrete or conglomerate masses. Enlarged nodes show central hypoechoic areas with a mixed heterogeneous echotexture, in contrast to homogeneously hypoechoic nodes seen in lymphoma **(*see* Fig. 10C)**. Heterogeneity of echo pattern in nodes of a single anatomic subgroup, prior to treatment is strongly suggestive of tuberculosis, rather than lymphoma. Larger areas of caseation may coalesce with adjacent nodes, resulting in larger collections. Lymph nodes may be adherent to intra-abdominal vasculature and a fibrous reaction surrounding clusters of nodes maybe seen as increase in background echogenicity.[43,44]

On CT the multicompartmental localization of nodes with relative sparing of the retroperitoneal compartment is the most characteristic feature of tuberculosis. On unenhanced

TABLE 4: Causes of mesenteric lymphadenopathy.

Infective processes: • Tuberculosis • Mesenteric adenitis syndrome • Celiac disease • Intestinal infection—Yersinia • Mycobacterium avium-intracellulare (MAC) infection • HIV • Whipple's disease
Inflammatory lesions: • Local inflammatory processes such as acute appendicitis, diverticulitis, pancreatitis, etc. • Crohn's disease • Mesenteric panniculitis • Connective tissue disorders—rheumatoid arthritis, scleroderma, SLE, etc. • Others
Neoplastic processes: • Lymphoma • Metastatic disease • Kaposi's sarcoma
Miscellaneous: • Castleman's disease • Sarcoidosis • Amyloidosis, etc.

scans, the nodes may display low attenuation values <30 HU or soft tissue attenuation values similar to muscle. Four different patterns of nodal enhancement have been described by Pombo et al.[45]

- Peripheral enhancement, the most frequent pattern, is characterized by peripheral rim enhancement, with or without low attenuation center. This pattern is seen in younger patients and reflects significant central liquefactive or caseous necrosis and a highly vascular perinodal inflammatory reaction which is relatively diagnostic for tuberculosis, although not pathognomic (***see* Figs. 11A to C**).
- Inhomogeneous enhancement is also a frequent manifestation of tubercular adenitis, due to intranodal granulomas and relatively less necrosis than in nodes that show peripheral enhancement (***see* Figs. 12A and B**).
- Homogeneous contrast enhancement represent a less frequent manifestation. These are indistinguishable from untreated lymphomatous nodes and are seen in patients with infection with mycobacterium avium intracellulare and AIDS.
- Nonenhancing nodes.

Magnetic resonance imaging shows majority of nodes to be hypointense on T1 and hyperintense on T2-weighted images when compared to abdominal muscle, with a few demonstrating a rim which is hypo- on T1W and hyperintense on T2W images. Minority of nodes are hypo- to isointense on both T1 and T2 weighted images. The varying signal intensity on T2W images is explained on the stage of evolution of the disease—the central T2 hyperintensity reflects caseous necrosis while central T2 hypointensity denotes presence of paramagnetic free radicles secreted from phagocytic cells. On contrast-enhanced images, different enhancement patterns, including peripheral, heterogeneous and less frequently homogeneous enhancement may be seen, similar to CT.[46,47]

With the institution of appropriate treatment, nodal masses tend to show a transient increase in size for 3–4 weeks followed by a gradual reduction in overall dimensions. Focal calcification may occur in nodal and omental masses and collections, which may be clustered along the periphery or may be central in location.

Tubercular adenitis may be confused with nodes of lymphoma and metastatic disease, and clinical and radiological differentiation may be difficult. Lymphoma nodes have a different anatomical distribution and near homogenous enhancement pattern prior to treatment. Caseation and calcification are highly suggestive of tubercular etiology.[48]

Lymph nodes with hypodense centers are also seen in metastatic malignancy, lymphoma after treatment, inflammatory conditions (such as Crohn's disease), pyogenic infection and Whipple's disease, however, other imaging findings and clinical features are helpful in diagnosis Lymphatic involvement is also a common feature in patients with AIDS. The nodes in these are usually located in mesenteric and retroperitoneal region. Nonenhanced low attenuation nodes may be seen in AIDS.

Primary Mesenteric Adenitis

Primary mesenteric adenitis consists of right-sided mesenteric adenopathy without any associated identifiable inflammatory process. Although it has been termed as primary, it is thought that the enlarged nodes arise from an infective process (e.g. *Yersinia sp*) causing a terminal ileitis that may or may not be seen on imaging.

Clinically patients present with nonspecific abdominal pain which maybe acute or chronic, often mimicking appendicitis. US and CT will show clustered, discrete, moderately enlarged nodes in the right lower quadrant with a short axis diameter of generally <10 mm. Occasionally, thickening of the terminal ileum may also be seen (**Figs. 21A and B**).[49]

This is a self limiting condition, which resolves on conservative treatment. The most important differential diagnosis is acute appendicitis, as enlarged reactive nodes may often be seen in the right lower quadrant in appendicitis.

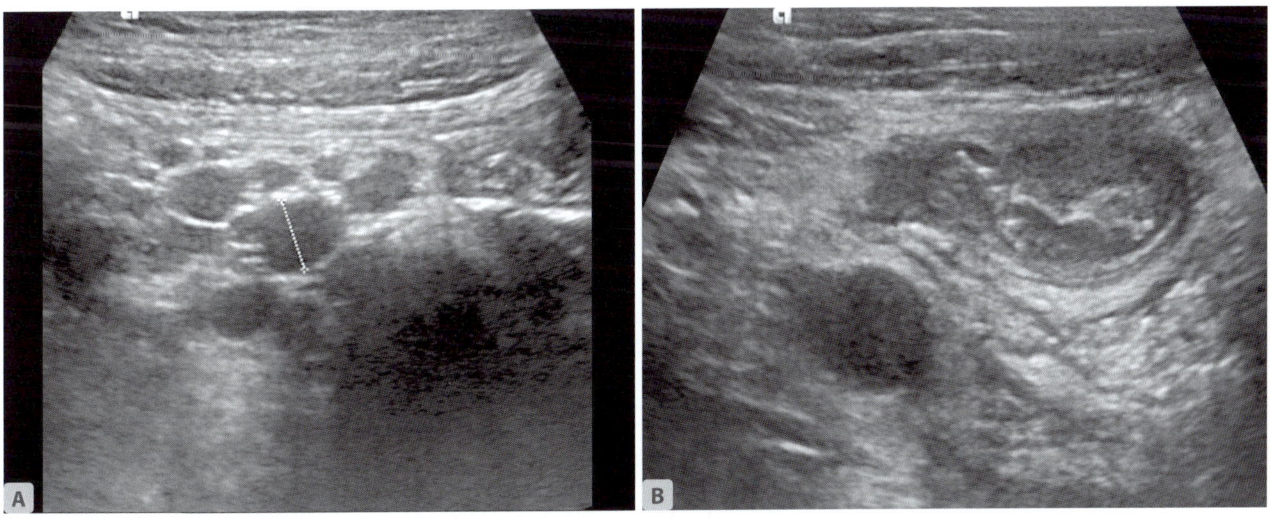

FIGS. 21A AND B: Mesenteric adenitis in a 10-year-old boy presenting with pain in right iliac fossa: (A) US shows multiple small nodes in the right iliac fossa; (B) A more caudal scan shows a thickened distal ileal loop.

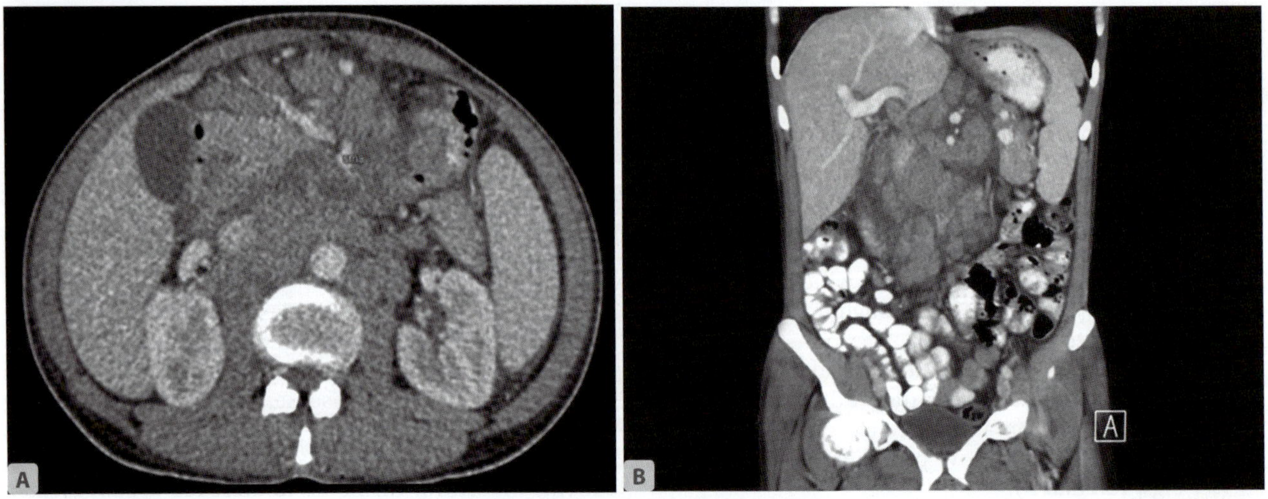

FIGS. 22A AND B: Lymphoma: CECT axial (A) and coronal (B) scans show multiple homogeneously enhancing mesenteric and retroperitoneal lymph nodes in a 45-year-old man with non-Hodgkin's lymphoma.

The identification of a normal appendix on imaging favors primary mesenteric adenitis.[50]

Neoplastic Lymphadenopathy

Lymphoma is the most common cause of neoplastic mesenteric lymph node enlargement. Non-Hodgkin's lymphoma involves the mesenteric nodes along with the retroperitoneal para-aortic nodes. Approximately 30–50% cases of NHL spread to the mesenteric nodes, commonly from the retroperitoneal nodes.[51] The enlarged nodes can show three patterns of involvement—in the mesenteric root, scattered throughout the peripheral mesentery or a mixed root-peripheral pattern **(Figs. 22A and B)**. In early cases, the lymph nodes may be small and discrete, but they progressively increase in size to form coalescent conglomerate masses. As they are soft tumors, they tend to grow around the vessels and the bowel without causing pressure effect. On CT images, lymphomatous nodes are seen as multiple round, mildly enhancing, homogeneous masses that often surround mesenteric arteries and veins. Pretreatment calcification is rare. Associated peritoneal and mesenteric involvement can be seen.[35]

Metastatic involvement of mesenteric nodes can occur from GI malignancies, however is rare from tumors of genitourinary or extrabdominal malignancies.

Kaposi's sarcoma is a low grade mesenchymal tumor seen in patients of AIDS involving the blood and lymphatic vessels. Mesenteric lymphadenopathy is seen as homogenously enhancing, large nodes, measuring 3–5 cm in short axis diameter. They may coalesce to form large masses. Associated lymphadenopathy may be seen in the porta hepatis, retroperitoneum and pelvis. Bowel, spleen and liver involvement may occur.[35]

PRIMARY PERITONEAL NEOPLASMS

The peritoneum can be involved by both, primary and secondary neoplastic disease, with metastatic involvement being much more common than primary tumors. Primary peritoneal tumors are defined as tumors with primary manifestation in the peritoneum in the absence of a visceral site of origin.[52]

They are uncommon lesions which arise from the mesothelial cells, submesothelial mesenchymal cells and uncommitted stem cells. As they share a common anatomic site of origin, they have similar clinical manifestations. Patients frequently present with abdominal discomfort and distention, gastrointestinal complaints, and, less commonly, pelvic pain or a palpable mass. **Table 5** lists the primary tumors that can involve the peritoneum.

PERITONEAL MALIGNANT MESOTHELIOMA

Malignant mesothelioma is an aggressive tumor arising from serous membranes of pleura, peritoneum, pericardium and tunica vaginalis. Peritoneal mesotheliomas account for 10–15% of all mesotheliomas.[53] They can be classified into two subtypes—the diffuse form which is highly aggressive and the localized or focal form which is amenable to surgery and has a good prognosis.

Clinical Picture

Similar to pleural mesotheliomas, peritoneal malignant mesotheliomas are also associated with asbestos exposure, and usually develop in individuals exposed to higher levels of asbestos, as compared to pleural mesotheliomas. The majority of malignant mesotheliomas occur in men, with a median age at presentation of 60 years, whereas in women, the mean age is 50 years.[54] Patients present with abdominal pain, abdominal distention, nausea, anorexia, and weight loss. Intestinal obstruction may occur with advanced disease.

Imaging Features

In the *diffuse* form of the disease, there is sheet-like thickening of the peritoneum, leading to an irregular and nodular

TABLE 5: List of primary tumors of peritoneum.
• Primary malignant mesothelioma
• Cystic mesothelioma
• Primary peritoneal serous carcinoma
• Desmoplastic small round cell tumor
• Desmoid tumor/Mesenteric fibromatosis
• Inflammatory myofibroblastic pseudotumor
• Primary peritoneal lymphoma
• *Benign mesenchymal tumors*: - Hemangioma - Lymphangioma - Lipoma - Leiomyoma - Nerve sheath tumor - Gastrointestinal stromal tumors (GIST) - Leiomyomatous pertonealis disseminata
• *Malignant mesenchymal tumors*: - Liposarcoma - Leiomyosarcoma - Fibrosarcoma - Angiosarcoma - Malignant fibrous histiocytoma - Synovial sarcoma - GIST - Nerve sheath tumors
• Others

thickening of the peritoneum. There is associated moderate amount of ascites and omental caking **(Fig. 23)**. In the *localized* form there are heterogeneous, solid intraperitoneal masses. The margins are often irregular. The ascites is small in amount and may be loculated. Local invasion can be seen into the abdominal wall, mesentery, liver, and other organs in both forms. Rarely calcification may occur. Mesenteric involvement can be seen as "pleated" or "stellate" appearance and sheet-like thickening can be seen to encase the small bowel loops in some cases. Generally, lymph node enlargement does not occur which is differentiating point from lymphomatosis and tubercular peritoneal involvement. Calcified pleural plaques and other asbestos-related changes such as pleural thickening and masses may be present within the chest.[55] CT radiographic findings of large tumor burden with significant bowel distortion or the presence of a small bowel obstruction is predictive of incomplete resectability. MRI imaging may quantify the extent of disease more accurately.

The role of positron emission tomography (PET) scan is not well-defined and may have some limited use in the detection of recurrent disease.[56] Biopsy is required to establish a diagnosis and can be performed under imaging guidance or surgically. Ascitic fluid cytology has a variable sensitivity of 32–76% with the major limitation being difficulty in distinguishing benign from malignant lesions.[57] Cytoreductive surgery (CRS) with hyperthermic intraperitoneal chemotherapy (HIPEC) have become the more widely adopted methods of treatment for peritoneal mesothelioma, however are associated with significant morbidity. Studies using novel molecular targets such as sphingosine kinase are under process to develop targeted therapies.[58]

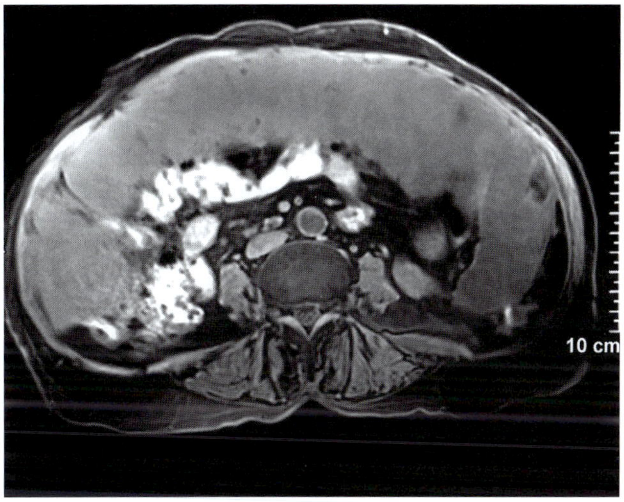

FIG. 23: Peritoneal mesothelioma: 57-year-old woman presenting with abdominal discomfort and distension. T2W MR image shows a thick characteristic 'omental cake' appearance.

Differential Diagnosis

The presence of peritoneal masses with or without ascites in the abdominal cavity is most suggestive of peritoneal carcinomatosis in the majority of patients. However, when a sheet like thickening is seen, the diagnosis of a primary mesothelioma must be kept in mind. Other differentials to be considered are tuberculous peritonitis—shows a smooth peritoneum with mild thickening and marked enhancement; lymphomatous peritonitis—which shows marked mesenteric and retroperitoneal lymphadenopathy; and sarcomatous peritonitis—which is characterized by heterogeneous, bulky, hypervascular masses with a variable amount of ascites.[7]

MULTICYSTIC MESOTHELIOMA/ PERITONEAL INCLUSION CYST/ MULTILOCULAR INCLUSION CYST

Multicystic mesothelioma is a benign, multilocular cystic tumor that most commonly arises from the pelvic surface of the peritoneum. There is an ongoing debate regarding the origin of this entity. It is considered by some authors to be a mesothelial neoplasm as it can recur locally and may rarely show malignant transformation, while others consider it to be non-neoplastic, reactive mesothelial proliferation.[59]

Clinical Features

It is most commonly seen in premenopausal women. It occurs much less commonly in men with an older age of presentation. Clinically, it can present with chronic or intermittent lower abdominal or pelvic pain, abdominal distension, tenderness, mass, and pressure symptoms like dyspareunia, urinary hesitancy, or constipation. It is very commonly associated with a history of prior abdominal surgery, endometriosis or PID which supports the reactive, non-neoplastic origin.

Imaging Features

Ultrasound is often the first modality in detection of these lesions. They are seen as large, multi-septated, cystic structures which are in close contact with the ovaries and uterus. They are frequently anechoic, but sometimes may show internal echoes due to debris or hemorrhage. The ovary may sometimes be completely surrounded by the cystic mesothelioma. Septations may be complete, incomplete, of varying thickness, and maybe nodular or polypoid **(Figs. 24A to C)**. Unilocular and multifocal cysts may also be seen. In men, multicystic mesothelioma typically arises from the peritoneal surface along the superior margin of the bladder or in the retrovesical space.[55]

CT and MRI are useful in defining the exact extent of the lesion and for identifying presence of multiple cysts. Large mutiseptated cyst with fluid attenuation can be seen on CT, while MR shows homogeneous fluid signal intensity that is hypointense on T1 and hyperintense on T2W images. The septations enhance with contrast administration.

Differential Diagnosis

Pseudomyxoma peritonei in the early stages, lymphangioma, complex loculated ascites, and cystic ovarian neoplasms can all be considered in the differential diagnosis of multicystic mesothelioma.

PRIMARY PERITONEAL SEROUS CARCINOMA

Primary peritoneal serous carcinoma is an epithelial tumor of the peritoneum, arising from the extraovarian mesothelium and is histologically similar to its ovarian counterpart. This tumor occurs in postmenopausal women and an association with BRCA1 gene has been demonstrated.[60]

Imaging Features

Ascites, peritoneal nodules and thickening, and omental nodules and masses are the most common cross-sectional imaging features of primary peritoneal serous carcinoma. A minority of patients have either no ascites or only a small amount at initial presentation. Calcifications within

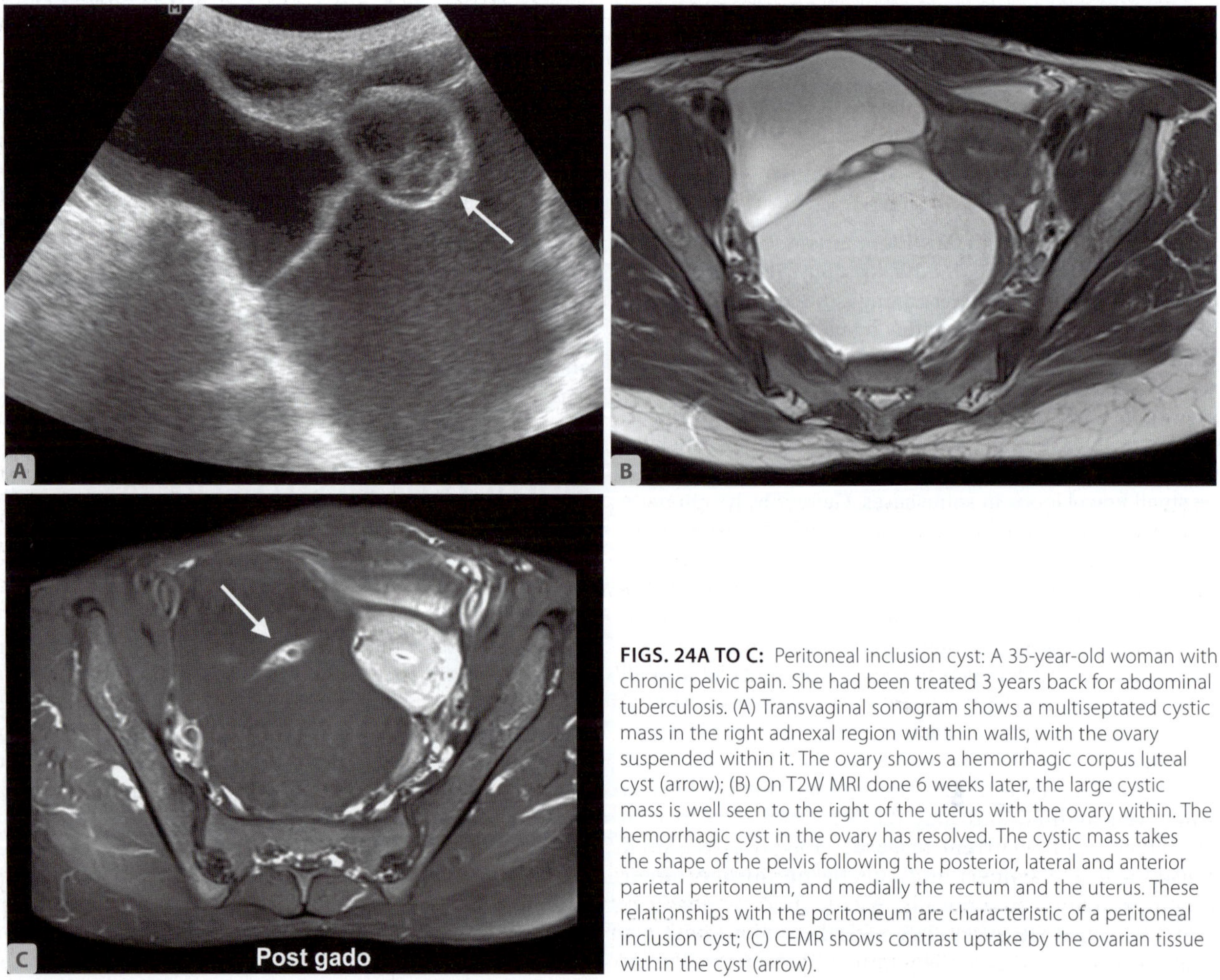

FIGS. 24A TO C: Peritoneal inclusion cyst: A 35-year-old woman with chronic pelvic pain. She had been treated 3 years back for abdominal tuberculosis. (A) Transvaginal sonogram shows a multiseptated cystic mass in the right adnexal region with thin walls, with the ovary suspended within it. The ovary shows a hemorrhagic corpus luteal cyst (arrow); (B) On T2W MRI done 6 weeks later, the large cystic mass is well seen to the right of the uterus with the ovary within. The hemorrhagic cyst in the ovary has resolved. The cystic mass takes the shape of the pelvis following the posterior, lateral and anterior parietal peritoneum, and medially the rectum and the uterus. These relationships with the peritoneum are characteristic of a peritoneal inclusion cyst; (C) CEMR shows contrast uptake by the ovarian tissue within the cyst (arrow).

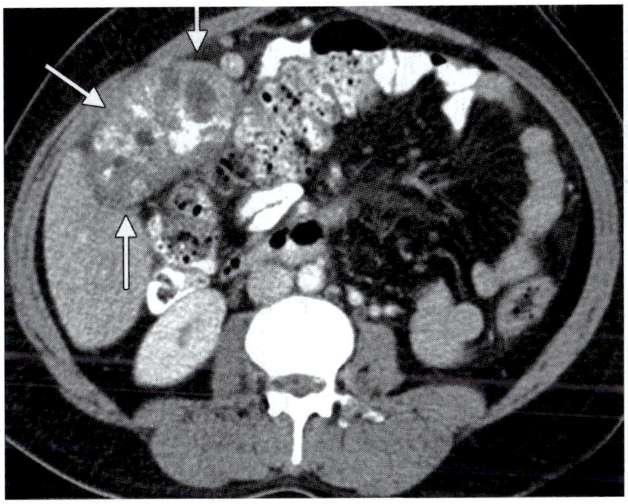

FIG. 25: Papillary serous carcinoma: A large well defined, enhancing, peritoneal mass is seen in the subhepatic region (arrows) with psammomatous calcification and few nonenhancing necrotic areas.

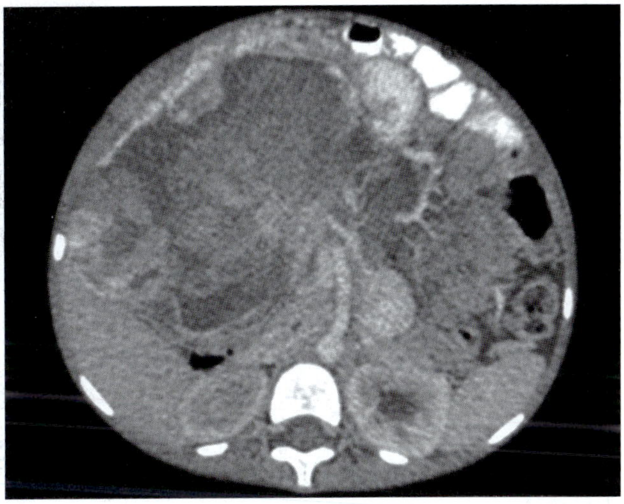

FIG. 26: Desmoplastic round cell tumor in a 15-year-old boy. CECT axial scan shows a large necrotic mass in the mesentery.

peritoneal and omental nodules representing psammoma bodies maybe seen in 30% cases **(Fig. 25)**.[55] The criteria for diagnosing primary peritoneal serous carcinoma are that:

- Both ovaries should be normal
- Involvement of extraovarian sites should be greater than involvement of ovarian surface
- Ovarian involvement should only be limited to surface epithelium.

However, histological confirmation is required to differentiate from metastatic ovarian disease and make a correct diagnosis.

DESMOPLASTIC SMALL ROUND CELL TUMOR

Desmoplastic small round cell tumor (DSRCT) is a rare aggressive malignancy occurring in adolescents and young adults. Histologically it is composed of small, round, blue cells, a group that includes Wilms tumor, neuroblastoma, Ewing sarcoma, primitive neuroectodermal tumor, and rhabdomyosarcoma. DSRCT most often develops as a primary tumor of the peritoneal cavity but can also arise in other sites including pleura, bone, testes, or salivary glands.[61]

Clinical Features

The mean age of presentation of DSRCT is of 22 years (range, 5–30 years) with a marked male preponderance. The most common signs at presentation are an intra-abdominal mass, abdominal pain and increased abdominal girth.[61]

Imaging Features

It is characterized by bulky, peritoneal masses in the omentum or paravesical region, which are heterogeneous, or have central low-attenuation areas on CT, suggestive of intratumoral necrosis or hemorrhage. The masses vary in size from 3 cm to 22 cm **(Fig. 26)**. When multiple masses are present, nearly all patients have a single dominant mass (>10 cm), usually in the retrovesical or retrouterine space. They may also show small, punctate calcifications. Ascites is frequently present. At MR imaging, the tumors are typically heterogeneous in signal intensity but predominantly hypointense on T1-weighted sequences and hyperintense on T2-weighted sequences. Imaging after intravenous administration of gadolinium shows heterogeneous enhancement. Lymph nodal metastases and hematogenous metastasis to the liver, lung, and bone may occur.[62]

DSRCT is FDG-avid with a mean standardized uptake value of 11.1 (range, 3.7–15.0) and FDG PET/CT has been shown to enable accurate detection of lesions with a sensitivity of 96.1% and specificity of 98.6%, but its role in assessment of treatment response and follow-up of DSRCT has not yet been defined.[63]

Well-differentiated papillary mesothelioma, adenomatoid tumor, primary peritoneal serous borderline tumor and solitary fibrous tumor are uncommon tumors of the peritoneum.

DESMOID TUMOR/MESENTERIC FIBROMATOSIS

Desmoids are locally aggressive fibrous tumors with a tendency to recur. Desmoids can be intra-abdominal, in the abdominal wall, or extra-abdominal. The mesentery is the most common site of involvement. Most cases are sporadic but approximately 10–15% occur in patients with familial adenomatous polyposis (FAP), particularly those with Gardener's syndrome. More than 80% of patients with FAP have a history of previous abdominal surgery, whereas only 10% of sporadic mesenteric fibromatosis have had abdominal surgery.[35]

Clinical Features

Desmoids may occur at any age but have a peak incidence in the third decade with a predilection for the female sex. Clinically, they may be asymptomatic or may present with abdominal pain or intestinal obstruction due to mass effect on the small or large bowel.[64]

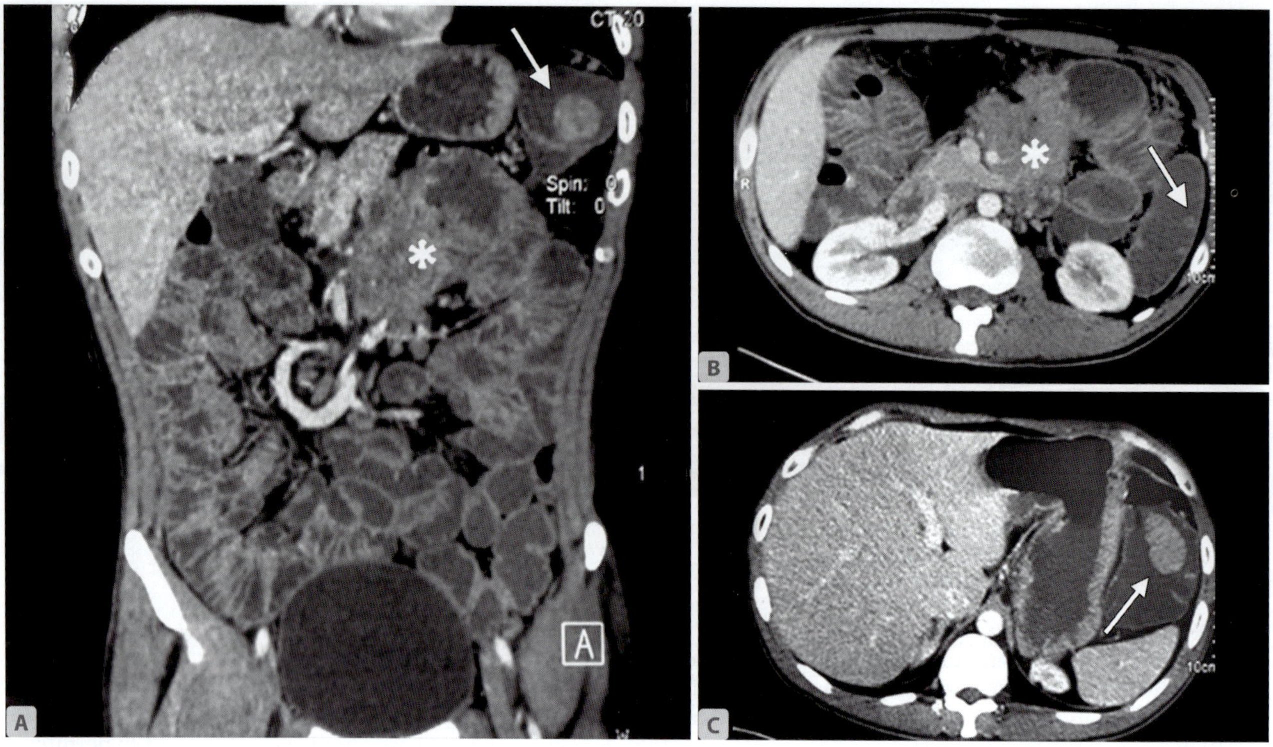

FIGS. 27A TO C: Desmoid tumor in a 31-year-old man with familial adenomatous polyposis: CECT coronal (A) and axial (B and C) scans show an irregular, heterogeneous mass with infiltrative margins in the mesentery (*). Multiple polypoid lesions can be seen in the large bowel (arrows).

Imaging Features

Focal masses with well-defined or infiltrative margins can be seen within the mesentery **(Figs. 27A to C)**. The internal features depend on the relative content of collagen and myxoid stroma within the tumor mass. On US, these tumors have variable echogenicity, appearing as masses of low, medium, or high echogenicity with smooth, defined margins. On CT, they can be seen as well-circumscribed homogeneous masses that may be isodense or hyperdense relative to muscle. Some cases show heterogeneous masses with infiltrative outer margins. Masses with high myxoid content may appear hypodense. On MRI, low to intermediate SI is seen on T1W images and intermediate SI on T2W images. Contrast enhancement is also variable as the myxoid component does not enhance. Some lesions that do not enhance on CT may show enhancement on MRI.[65]

Due to the close association with vital structures, resection of the tumor may not be possible, in which cases systemic therapy with or without surgical excision should be considered. FAP—associated mesenteric desmoids, are more likely to be unresectable or lead to significant morbidity, including perioperative hemorrhage, short-bowel syndrome, intestinal ischemia, obstruction, or fistula formation. Also, desmoid tumors have a tendency to recur, even after complete surgical resection. Therefore, conservative management has been recommended whenever possible, using analgesia and minimally invasive therapy as needed and recently, radiotherapy and chemotherapy have been used in the management of desmoid tumors.[66]

Differential Diagnosis

On the basis of imaging findings, desmoid tumors are difficult to differentiate from gastrointestinal stromal tumor and other malignant neoplasms of the mesentery, such as lymphoma, metastatic disease, and soft-tissue sarcoma. They may closely resemble lymphoma whenever the lesions manifest with well-defined margins, homogeneous attenuation, and involvement of adjacent small bowel segments. GISTs more commonly have areas of hemorrhage and necrosis, which are seen as focal areas of hypoattenuation.

INFLAMMATORY MYOFIBROBLASTIC PSEUDOTUMOR

Inflammatory myofibroblastic pseudotumor (IMP) is a rare solid tumor of mesenchymal origin, which may originate in virtually any anatomic site but is most often found in the lung, mesentery, and omentum. It was originally thought to be inflammatory or reactive in origin, but on the basis of more recent cytogenetic studies, it is now considered a neoplasm of intermediate biologic behavior.[67]

Clinical Features

This tumor is most commonly seen to affect children and young adults, with a slight tendency to occur more frequently in girls. The clinical symptoms are nonspecific and depend on the site of origin. The most common presenting symptom is abdominal pain due to mass effect. A minority of patients present with systemic signs and symptoms suggestive of infection.[68] Most inflammatory myofibroblastic tumors demonstrate benign behavior and are cured with resection.

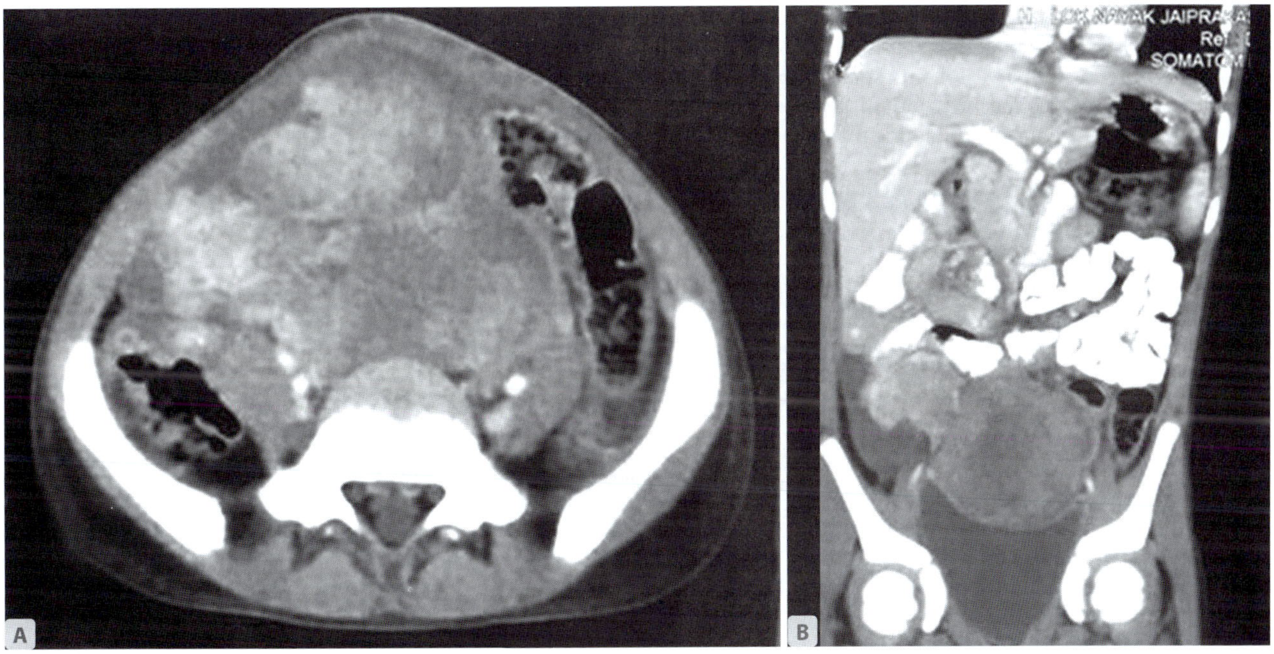

FIGS. 28A AND B: Inflammatory myofibroblastic tumor in a 7-year-old girl: CECT axial (A) and coronal (B) images show a large well circumscribed, multiloculated, heterogeneously enhancing mass in the lower abdomen displacing the bowel loops superiorly and laterally. Associated ascites is present.

Yet, a propensity for local recurrence and even multifocal regional recurrence has also been shown, particularly in the omentum and mesentery.

Imaging Features

At CT, inflammatory myofibroblastic pseudotumor typically manifests as a bulky, well-demarcated, homogeneous or heterogeneous, spherical or multilobulated mass **(Figs. 28A and B)**. A few cases may show central calcifications. Contrast enhancement is variable and includes early peripheral enhancement due to vascular tissue and delayed central enhancement of fibrotic components. Large tumors may demonstrate hypoattenuating, nonenhancing areas that represent central necrosis. These tumors rarely show aggressive growth patterns such as circumferential growth around vessels and extension into the bowel with mural infiltration and ulceration.[68,69]

At MR imaging, IMP is hypointense on T1-weighted images and hyperintense on T2-weighted images, although tumors with a great deal of fibrotic stroma may be dark on both T1- and T2-weighted images. On postcontrast scans, there is heterogeneous enhancement of the tumor mass. Delayed contrast enhancement of fibrotic components may be seen.[70] FDG-PET shows nonspecific increased uptake of radiotracer by inflammatory myofibroblastic tumor, similar to other malignancies.[71]

LEIOMYOMATOSIS PERTONEALIS DISSEMINATA/DIFFUSE PERITONEAL LEIOMYOMATOSIS

Leiomyomatosis peritonealis disseminata is a rare, benign disorder characterized by innumerable smooth muscle nodules throughout the peritoneal cavity. These nodules are derived from metaplasia of the submesothelial cells.

Clinical Features

Leiomyomatosis peritonealis disseminata is almost always seen in women. It may be associated with high estrogen states, caused by pregnancy and oral contraceptive use, but rarely may occur in postmenopausal women, and even in men.[72] It is often discovered incidentally during surgery or imaging examinations of women who have uterine leiomyomas. The clinical course is often benign, with spontaneous regression of the leiomyomas or regression can occur after withdrawal of hormonal stimulus. In rare cases, sarcomatous degeneration of the tumor nodules, may occur.[73]

Imaging Features

CT and MRI show numerous well-circumscribed, variable-sized solid masses in the peritoneal cavity. Heterogeneous attenuation is seen on CT. The masses enhance similarly to uterine leiomyomas. On MR imaging, the masses are isointense relative to muscle on T1-weighted sequences and low signal intensity on T2-weighted sequences with heterogeneous enhancement, similar to uterine leiomyomas, as seen on CT.[55]

MISCELLANEOUS MESENCHYMAL TUMORS

Mesenchymal tumors include benign entities such as leiomyoma, lipoma, neurofibroma and malignant tumors such as leiomyosarcoma, liposarcoma, fibrosarcoma, mesothelioma, and hemangiopericytoma. Imaging findings are nonspecific. Benign tumors are usually well ciurcumscribed and localized whereas malignant tumors have indistinct or infiltrative margins with invasion into surrounding structures. Lipomas and liposarcomas are more distinctive due to their characteristic features of fat containing masses.

LYMPHATIC MALFORMATION/ LYMPHANGIOMA

Lymphatic malformations (LMs) are rare nonmalignant masses consisting of fluid-filled channels or spaces thought to be caused by the abnormal development of the lymphatic system. Abdominal LMs occur most commonly in the mesentery, followed by the omentum, mesocolon, retroperitoneum and abdominal viscera.[74,75]

Clinical Features

Although LMs can occur at any age, they are seen more commonly in infants and young children.[75] Abdominal pain and distension are the common presenting features. Rarely, patients may present with acute abdominal pain due to complications like torsion, infarction or intestinal obstruction.

Imaging Features

LMs are thin-walled unilocular or multilocular cystic masses containing serous or chylous fluid. On US, these lymphatic malformations are seen as cystic, unilocular or multilocular masses with echogenecity varying from anechoic to hypoechoic depending on the internal content **(Figs. 29 and 30)**. CT shows enhancing cyst wall and internal septae with homogenous, low attenuation fluid content. The attenuation of the fluid may have negative values in the presence of chyle. MRI also shows similar findings with low signal intensity on T1W and high on T2W images. The presence of hemorrhage or infection in the cysts may change the CT attenuation or MR signal pattern. Calcification is uncommon.[74]

Differential Diagnosis

Large mesenteric lymphangiomas need to be differentiated from ascites. The presence of septa, compression of the adjacent intestinal loops and lack of fluid in the dependant peritoneal recesses helps to establish a diagnosis of lymphangioma. Other differentials to be considered are benign ovarian neoplasms and peritoneal inclusion cysts. Duplication cyst or mesothelial cyst are uncommon.

SECONDARY PERITONEAL NEOPLASMS

Secondary neoplasms are the most common malignancies involving the peritoneum. The dissemination of tumor cells within the peritoneal cavity can occur by several mechanisms: (a) intraperitoneal seeding, (b) direct invasion, (c) embolic hematogenous dissemination, and (d) lymphatic permeation.

Intraperitoneal seeding occurs most commonly from gastrointestinal and ovarian tumors due to intramural tumor growth and invasion through bowel wall or extension through the peritoneal lining of organs like ovary, pancreas or liver. Seeding can also occur due to iatrogenic spillage of tumor cells into the peritoneal cavity during biopsy or surgery. These tumor cells are carried by the peritoneal fluid and disseminated throughout the peritoneal cavity. They get preferentially deposited in the areas of fluid stasis, i.e. pouch of Douglas in women, rectovesical space in men, distal small bowel mesentery near the ileocecal junction, the sigmoid mesocolon, the right paracolic gutter, Morrison's pouch and the right subdiaphragmatic space **(Fig. 31)**[76] and these areas should be carefully examined in all cases when evaluating for metastic disease. Two unusual sites of peritoneal carcinomatosis are the umbilicus and the ovaries; such metastases are respectively called Sister Mary Joseph's nodule and Krukenberg tumors. Ovarian carcinoma is the most common tumor to spread by this mechanism. Gastric, pancreatic, colonic, biliary and endometrial tumors also spread through intraperitoneal seeding.

Direct Invasion

Intra-abdominal primary malignancies can directly invade into the leaves of mesentery along the mesenteric vessels or through ligamentous attachments to involve adjacent organs. Pancreatic, gastric, biliary, colonic, hepatic, splenic and

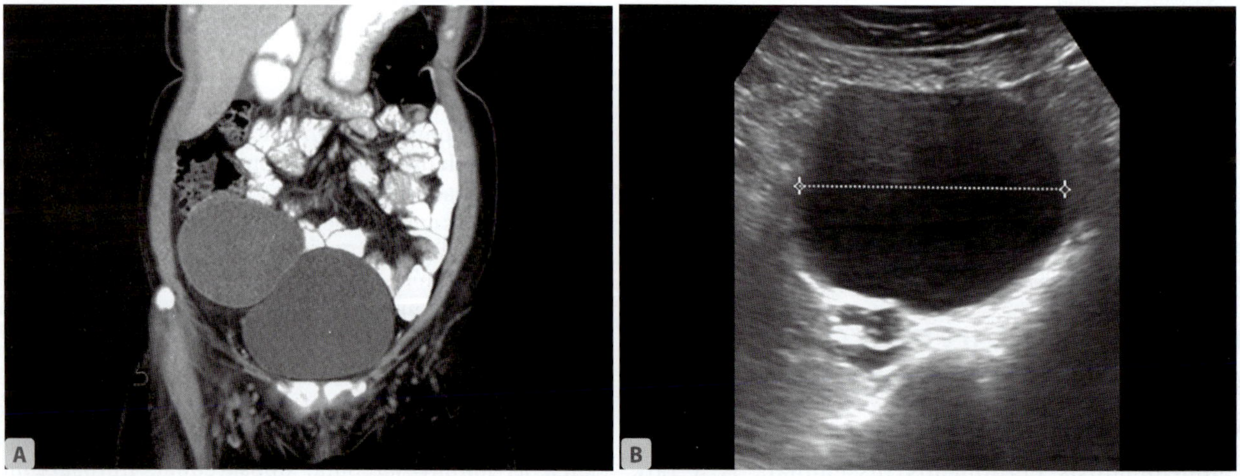

FIGS. 29A AND B: Mesenteric cyst in a 34-year-old woman with chronic pain in right iliac fossa. Coronal CT image (A) and US scan (B) show an anechoic, unilocular thin-walled cyst in the peritoneal fat.

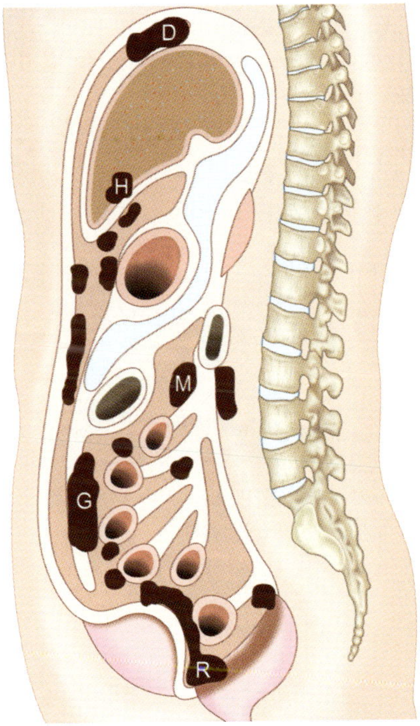

FIG. 31: Sagittal schematic illustration of the abdomen and pelvis showing common locations of peritoneal deposits. Commonly involved sites include greater omentum (G), rectouterine pouch (R), subdiaphragmatic region (D), subhepatic region (H) and small bowel mesentery (M).

ovarian tumors may spread in this way. Small bowel carcinoid tumor commonly invades the mesentery. Lymphoma and tumors arising from retroperitoneal structures may spread directly to the root of the small bowel mesentery along its retroperitoneal attachment.

Hematogenous Spread

Tumor emboli from malignant melanoma, lung or breast carcinoma and sarcomas may spread to the mesentery by hematogenous spread. These tumors usually involve the antimesenteric margins of the small bowel producing soft issue nodules that may cause bowel obstruction and/or intussusception.

Lymphatic Extension

Lymphatic dissemination plays a minor role in spread of gastrointestinal malignancies to the peritoneum, but it is the main pathway for spread of lymphomas to mesenteric lymph nodes. Chronic lymphocytic leukemia may also spread through the lymphatics and produce large mesenteric nodal masses which encase the branches of abdominal aorta-celiac trunk, superior and inferior mesenteric arteries without causing vascular compression.

PERITONEAL CARCINOMATOSIS

Peritoneal carcinomatosis is the malignant tumor seeding of the peritoneum with the most common primaries being the ovarian, gastric and colorectal malignancies. Other less

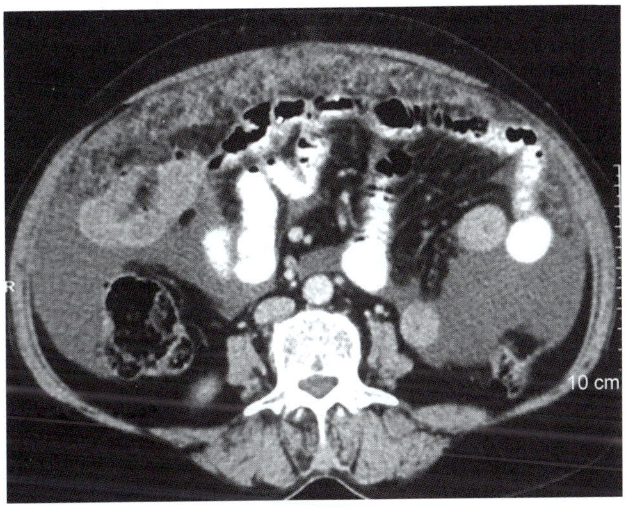

FIG. 32: Peritoneal carcinomatosis in a 65-year-old woman with ovarian malignancy. Enhanced axial CT scan shows thickening and nodular infiltration of the omentum with ascites.

common primary sites include pancreas, uterus, kidney, bladder and melanoma.

Patients with peritoneal carcinomatosis may be asymptomatic at the onset, but may progress to abdominal distension from ascites, or nausea, vomiting and abdominal pain from bowel obstruction.

Imaging Features

The classic feature of peritoneal carcinomatosis is *tumor nodules* studding the peritoneal surfaces. A fibrotic response can occur as the tumor grows along the peritoneal surface or invades into the subperitoneal tissues, replacing the omental fat with tumor and fibrosis which produces the gross appearance of *omental caking* **(Fig. 32)**. Peritoneal carcinomatosis can also exhibit a *sheet-like growth* pattern encircling and encasing intraperitoneal viscera producing an appearance similar to malignant mesothelioma. A variable amount of ascites may accompany the peritoneal seeding, but is not always present. Calcification can be seen in the peritoneal deposits from serous papillary ovarian carcinoma **(Figs. 33A to C)**, rarely gastric carcinomas, or in metastases after chemotherapy. Adenocarcinoma with abundant mucin and signet ring cell morphology is the most frequent tumor type seen on histopathology.

On US, the ascitic fluid seen in patients with peritoneal carcinomatosis may be anechoic or may contain echogenic particulate matter, which reflects proteinaceous exudate. Tumor nodules on peritoneal surfaces appear as hypoechoic nodules or sheet like masses **(Figs. 34A and B)**.[77] The omentum with tumor infiltration appears as an echogenic, plaque like structure either floating in the ascitic fluid or it may be adherent to the anterior abdominal wall or serosal surface of the bowel.

Multidetector computed tomography (MDCT) is the optimal technique for detecting the presence, location and extent of peritoneal carcinomatosis with reported overall diagnostic accuracy of 94%, specificity of 92% and sensitivities

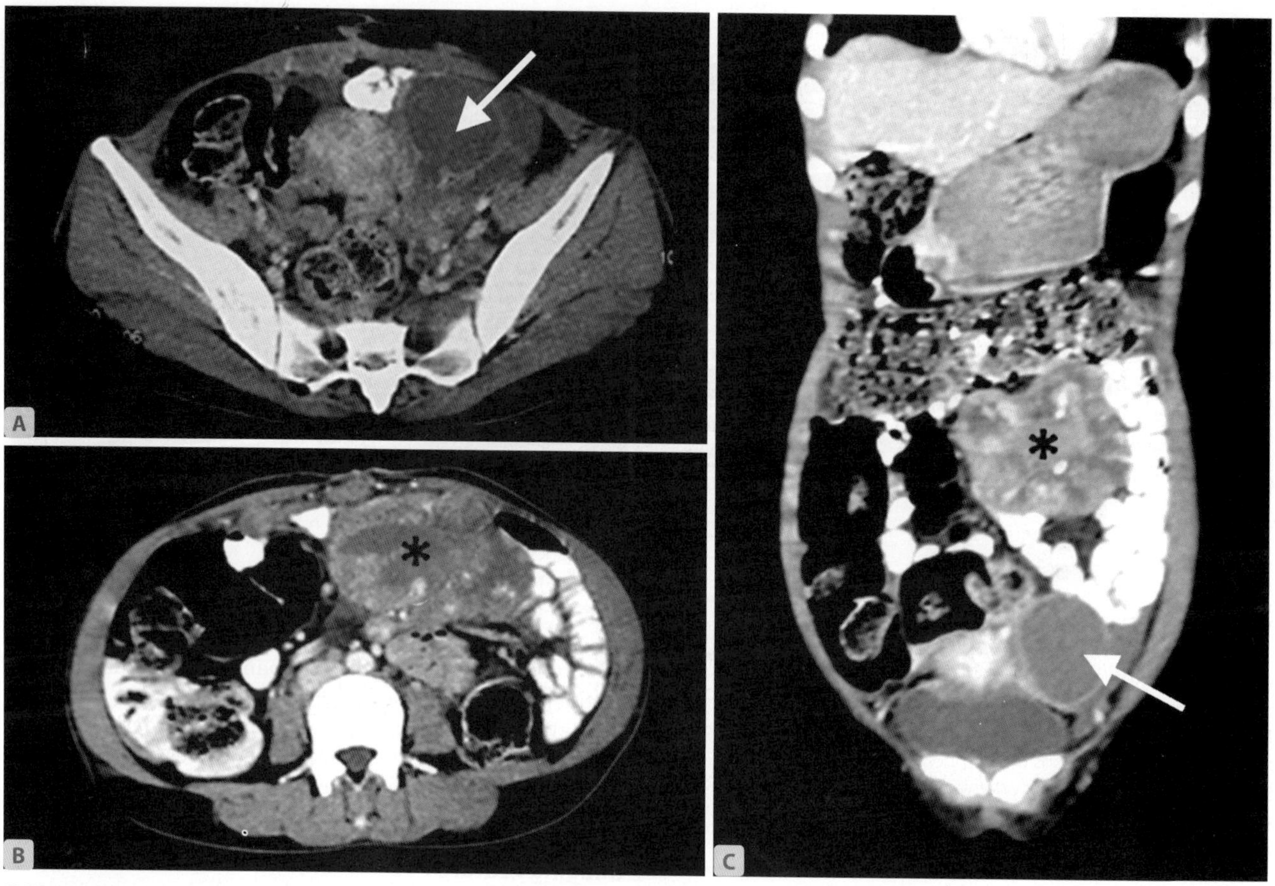

FIGS. 33A TO C: Peritoneal carcinomatosis from ovarian mucinous adenocarcinoma in a 45-year-old woman. Axial (A and B) coronal (C) CECT scans show a solid-cystic mass lesion in the left adnexa (arrow). There is an associated large heterogeneously enhancing solid mass lesion (*) in the mesentery with foci of calcification within.

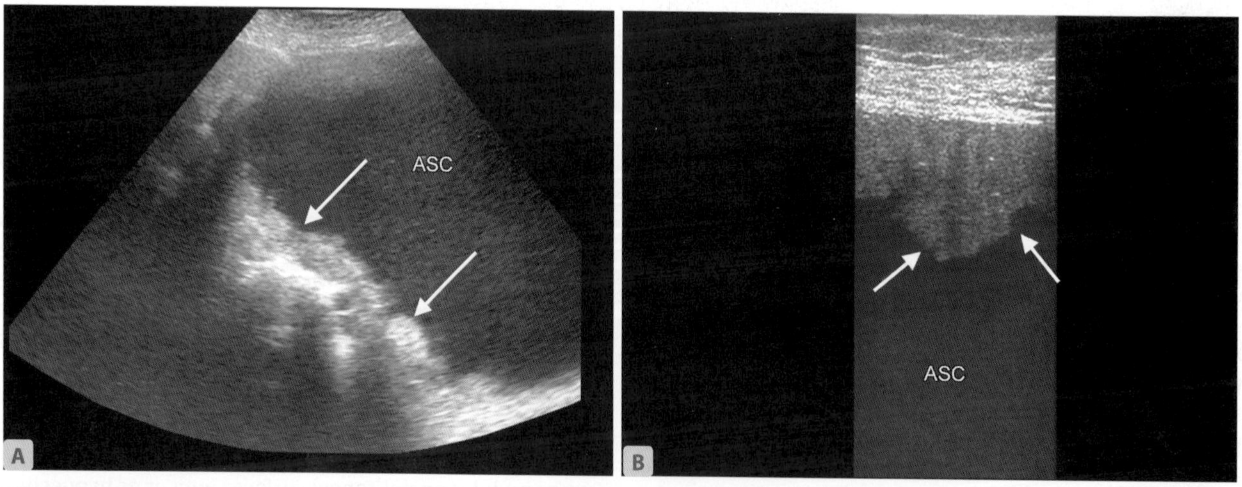

FIGS. 34A AND B: Peritoneal carcinomatosis with metastatic peritoneal deposits: (A) Transverse US image of right flank shows a large amount of ascites with fine internal echoes and multiple small peritoneal implants along the right paracolic gutter: (B) High frequency US image in a different patient shows an irregular solid hypoechoic mass projecting within the ascitic (ASC) fluid from the anterior peritoneal margin (arrows).

between 75% and 81%. However, CT sensitivities for detection of smaller nodules, less than 1 cm, is much lower.[78] The parietal peritoneum shows smooth, nodular or plaque like thickening which enhances on postcontrast scans **(Figs. 35A and B)**. As the tumor infiltrates the small bowel mesentery, it becomes stiff and loses its normal undulations. There is a characteristic straightening of the mesenteric vasculature producing a 'pleated' appearance on CT images. A 'stellate' pattern of mesenteric involvement may occur when the tumor infiltrates the perivascular spaces, causing the vessels

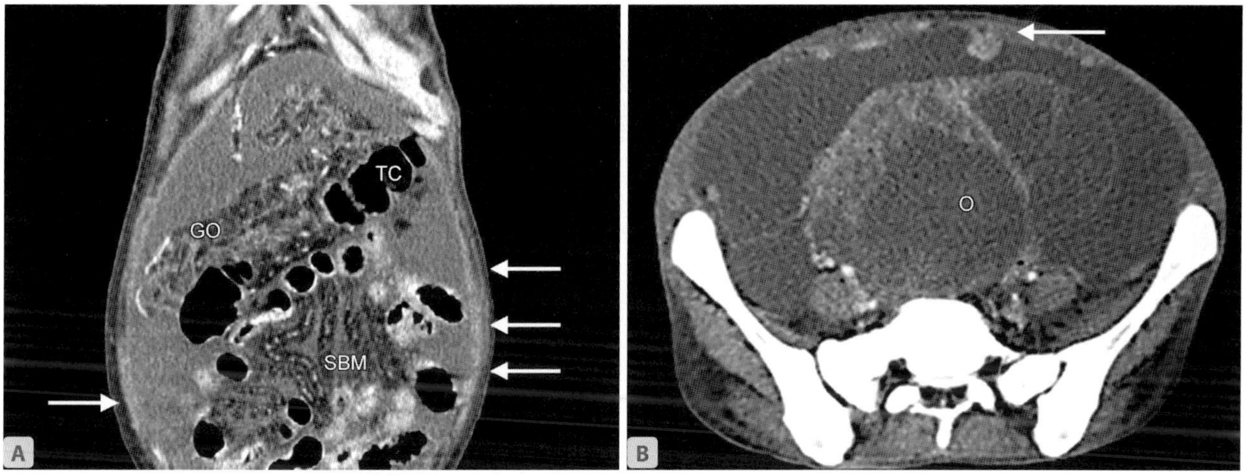

FIGS. 35A AND B: Peritoneal carcinomatosis in a 65-year-old woman with ovarian malignancy: Coronal (A) and axial (B) CECT scans show ascites with nodular enhancing peritoneum (arrows), thickened and nodular greater omentum (GO), and a stiffened small bowel mesentery (SBM); Ovarian mass (O).

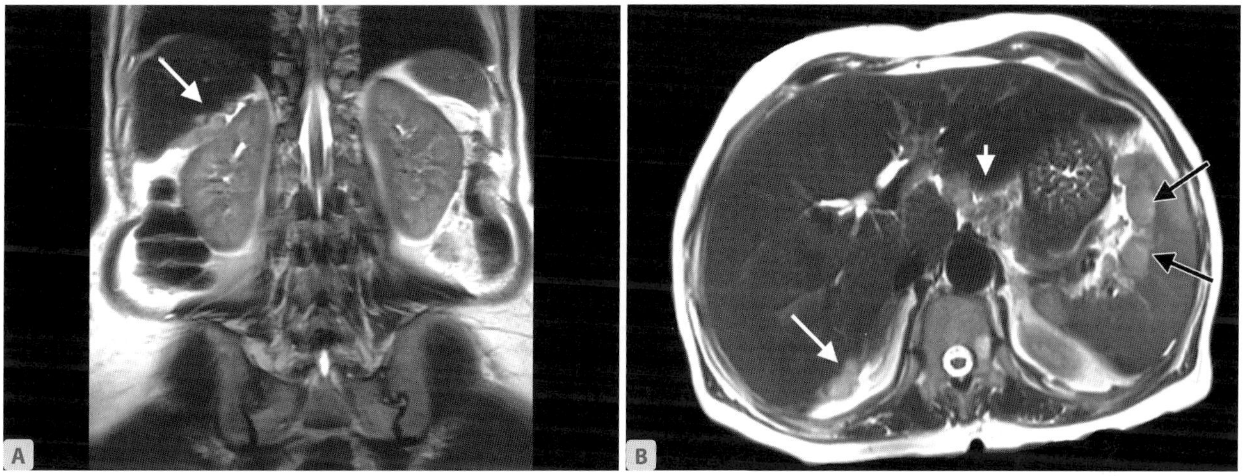

FIGS. 36A AND B: Peritoneal deposits: MR T2W images show multiple intermediate intensity nodular deposits in the Morrison's pouch (white arrows), gastrohepatic ligament (arrowhead) and perisplenic region (black arrows) in a case of colonic adenocarcinoma.

within the mesentery to appear denser than the surrounding fat and appears like stars in the sky on axial CT scans. Nodular or diffuse thickening can occur along the serosal surface of the bowel, leading to small bowel obstruction.[38]

Magnetic resonance imaging (MRI) can improve the detection of small peritoneal implants. These are best seen on contrast-enhanced T1-weighted images with fat suppression. Peritoneal carcinomatosis enhances slowly after intravenous administration of gadolinium and images should be obtained 5–10 minutes after injection. The normal peritoneum has an enhancement similar to that of liver. An abnormal enhancement should be suspected when peritoneum enhances more than liver or shows associated thickening, nodularity or mass. Typically, omental and mesenteric masses are of low T1-weighted and mixed T2-weighted signal intensity compared with surrounding soft tissues **(Figs. 36A and B)**. A combination of DWI and conventional sequences improves the accuracy for detection.[79]

Fluorodeoxyglucose (FDG) PET/CT is another promising modality for evaluation of peritoneal implants. Metastatic foci appear as round, oval, or globular areas of increased activity on FDG-PET.[80] One of the primary limitations of FDG PET/CT is that benign infectious or inflammatory peritoneal conditions may be FDG avid and therefore may mimic malignant peritoneal disease. Other sources of false-positive FDG PET/CT findings in the peritoneal cavity include physiologic bowel activity, motion artefact at the diaphragm, and urinary excretion of FDG.[81]

The evolution of cytoreductive surgery and hyperthermic intraperitoneal chemotherapy in the treatment of malignant peritoneal deposits has made it essential to have an extremely accurate preoperative assessment of the overall disease burden, and the exact sites of involvement in specific areas of the peritoneum. Analysis of imaging findings need to be done on a site to site basis, and presence, type and size of the deposits reported so as to be able decide on the feasibility and extent of surgery.[82]

TABLE 6: Main differentiating features between peritoneal carcinomatosis, lymphomatosis and sarcomatosis.

	Peritoneal carcinomatosis	*Peritoneal lymphomatosis*	*Peritoneal sarcomatosis*
Peritoneal lesions	Multiple small nodules	Bulky homogeneous masses	Bulky heterogeneous masses
Lymphadenopathy	Lymph nodes around primary mass	Diffuse enlarged lymph nodes	None
Ascites	++	+	+/–

Source: Cabral FC, Krajewski KM, Kim KW, et al. Peritoneal lymphomatosis: CT and PET/CT findings and how to differentiate between carcinomatosis and sarcomatosis[92]

Differential Diagnosis

There are several non-neoplastic and neoplastic conditions that may mimic peritoneal carcinomatosis on imaging. The most important differential is the involvement of the peritoneum by tuberculosis, which is very common in our country. The differentiating points have been discussed above. Other differentials include lymphomas, sarcomatous involvement of the peritoneum **(Table 6)** and primary peritoneal malignancies such as mesothelioma. Primary peritoneal mesothelioma may be indistinguishable from carcinomatosis when the predominant imaging findings are multifocal peritoneal nodules and omental involvement ranging from finely infiltrated fat to omental caking. A history of asbestos exposure favors mesothelioma.

PSEUDOMYXOMA PERITONEI

Pseudomyxoma peritonei (PMP) or 'jelly belly' is a specific type of peritoneal neoplasia resulting from peritoneal implants of columnar epithelium associated with progressive accumulation of mucinous ascites. It is most commonly seen with rupture of a benign or malignant mucin producing tumor of the appendix or ovary and occasionally pancreas, stomach, colon or urachus. The relationship between appendiceal and ovarian mucinous tumors has long been observed and a controversy exists as to whether in patients with pseudomyxoma peritonei and synchronous manifestation of ovarian and appendiceal tumors, the ovarian tumors are primary or secondary as the ovarian tumors are frequently seen to occur on the right side or are bilateral. Results of several clinical, histopathological and immunohistochemical studies strongly suggest that in these patients ovarian tumor deposits are almost always metastases of an appendiceal primary.[83,84]

Two types of pseudomyxoma have been described. *Disseminated peritoneal adenomucinosis* is a benign entity which spreads along the peritoneal surfaces, and does not invade the stroma. It is seen in association with low-grade mucinous carcinomas of appendix that penetrate or rupture into the peritoneal cavity. The second type is *peritoneal mucinous carcinomatosis*, which occurs from high grade mucinous carcinomas of the gastrointestinal tract, gallbladder, pancreas, or ovary, and its clinical course is often fatal.[85]

Clinical Features

It occurs more commonly in women than men. Patients typically complain of progressive abdominal pain, increasing abdominal girth, and weight loss. Small bowel obstruction can occur in later stages.

Imaging Features

On sonography, pseudomyxoma peritonei is seen as echogenic ascites, with nonmobile echoes in the ascitic fluid, in contrast to echoes seen with other exudative ascites. Echogenic septations within representing the margins of the mucinous nodules can be seen.[86,87]

Focal or sheet-like echogenic masses can occur due to involvement of omentum and parietal peritoneum. Scalloping of the visceral surfaces of the abdominal organs, specially liver and spleen, is an important hallmark of PMP. This scalloping represents indentations of the margins of organs due to extrinsic pressure of the intraperitoneal mucinous implants.[86]

On CT, the mucinous nodules are seen as hypodense areas filling the peritoneal cavity. Soft-tissue attenuation masses may be seen representing solid tumor elements, fibrosis, or compression of the mesentery and mucin. There may be curvilinear or amorphous calcifications. Scalloping of margins of liver and spleen is well visualized on CT **(Figs. 37A and B)**.

The regions of the appendix and ovaries should be closely evaluated in all newly diagnosed cases of PMP. However in many cases, it may be impossible to identify the originating appendiceal mucinous low-grade neoplasm or cystadenocarcinoma. It may be difficult to differentiate adenomucinosis from mucinous carcinomatosis as they have overlapping findings. Carcinomatosis tends to involve thorax more commonly. Pleural effusions, pleural masses, enlarged mesenteric or retroperitoneal lymph nodes, omental caking and invasion into parenchymal organs are characteristically seen. In contrast, adenomucinosis does not invade visceral organs or spread by lymphatic or hematogenous routes.[88]

PERITONEAL LYMPHOMATOSIS

Peritoneal lymphomatosis is defined as the intraperitoneal spread of lymphoma. Lymphomatous involvement of the peritoneum maybe a primary or secondary process. *Secondary* involvement is more common, and can occur from nodal or extranodal non-Hodgkin lymphomas, such as small B-cell lymphoma, diffuse large B-cell lymphoma, or Burkitt lymphoma. *Primary* lymphomas of the peritoneum, also called body cavity–based lymphomas or primary effusion lymphomas, are uncommon and nearly exclusively found in immunocompromised patients, most of whom are infected with the human immunodeficiency virus.[89]

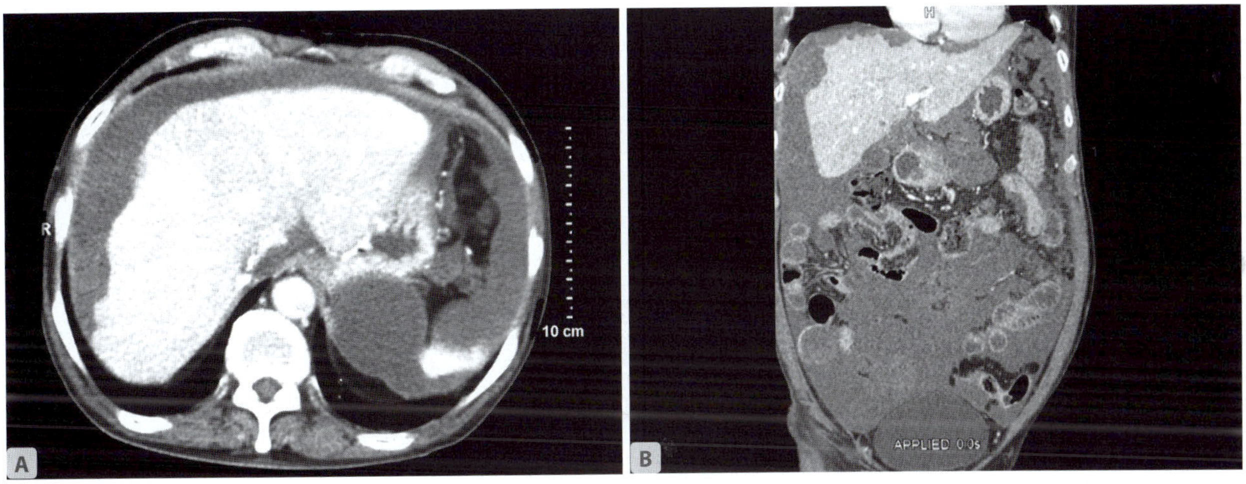

FIGS. 37A AND B: Pseudomyxoma peritonei from mucinous adenocarcinoma of appendix manifesting as increasing abdominal girth. Axial (A) and coronal (B) CECT scans show large locules of high density intraperitoneal fluid. Scalloping of the liver margins by the mucin locules can be very well seen.

Imaging Features

Diffuse thickening of peritoneal surfaces with multifocal nodules and masses that mimic peritoneal carcinomatosis can be seen. There can be associated ascites, peritoneal enhancement and thickening, omental caking, infiltration of the small bowel mesentery, and fine nodularity in the mesentery.[90] Enlarged lymph nodes, especially in the retrocrural region and in the small bowel mesentery are commonly seen in association with the mesenteric disease and should be a clue to the diagnosis. Associated GI involvement may also be seen in some cases.

In primary effusion lymphoma, the most common imaging manifestation is ascites without associated lymphadenopathy, organomegaly, or masses. In later stages, lymph node enlargement and nodular peritoneal thickening may occur, however, ascites remains the most predominant manifestation.[89,91]

The FDG-PET/CT has been shown to improve staging, evaluation of therapy response and earlier detection of recurrent disease in peritoneal lymphomatosis. FDG-PET/CT shows 2 patterns of glucose metabolism in peritoneal lymphomatosis—a nodular and a diffuse metabolic pattern. The FDG avidity in lymphoma is variable with aggressive and highly aggressive non-Hodgkin's lymphoma (NHL) and Hodgkin lymphomas showing high FDG avidity and indolent lymphomas showing an overall low-grade or no FDG uptake because of low metabolic activity. FDG-PET/CT not only has greater sensitivity than CT for depicting peritoneal involvement in subtle cases but it also has greater accuracy in identifying extranodal sites other than the peritoneum, even in the absence of CT findings. Due to its improved usefulness in distinguishing residual active lymphoma and benign fibrosis, FDG-PET/CT has been found valuable in assessment of treatment response.[92]

Sporadic Burkitt lymphoma is the most common form of NHL diagnosed in children younger than 15 years, accounting for 30–50% of cases.[93] It is a very aggressive B-cell lymphoma with a doubling time of only 24 hours, and thus needs to be diagnosed urgently. Burkitt lymphoma involving the peritoneum may appear as a large solitary mass or multiple abdominal masses **(Figs. 38A to C)**. Encasement of mesenteric vessels is a characteristic feature. Large tumors may show central necrosis. Associated peritoneal thickening or nodularity along the liver capsule and peritoneal reflections may be noted. Omental caking is not a feature of Burkitt lymphoma. Intrinsic involvement of the gastrointestinal tract is common, which is seen as bowel wall thickening or mural masses. Other solid organs like liver, spleen, kidneys and pancreas may be involved either intrinsically or by direct invasion by the peritoneal masses. Malignant ascites is found in 25% of cases of abdominal Burkitt lymphoma. Enlarged abdominal lymph nodes may be seen.[67]

Peritoneal lymphomatosis is treated nonsurgically, and often shows dramatic improvement with chemotherapy, and therefore its early and precise diagnosis is of utmost importance.

PERITONEAL SARCOMATOSIS

Peritoneal sarcomatosis or the disseminated intraperitoneal spread of sarcoma occurs most frequently from intra-abdominal sarcomas like malignant gastrointestinal stromal tumors (GIST), leiomyosarcomas or liposarcomas, by direct seeding of the peritoneal cavity. Metastases to peritoneum from extremity sarcomas are unusual and presumed to occur through the hematogenous route.

On imaging, peritoneal sarcomatosis may show focal, large soft-tissue masses, nodular infiltration, or confluent areas of increased attenuation within the mesentery and omentum **(Figs. 39A and B)**. Visceral deposits can occur and are seen as soft-tissue masses on serosal surfaces of the liver and spleen. Ascites is generally minimal and occurs late in the course of disease. GIST is the most common soft tissue sarcoma metastasizing to the peritoneum, seen in 21–45% cases of GISTs.[94,95]

The peritoneal deposits in GIST are seen as large, discrete masses with necrosis with heterogeneous enhancement. Less commonly, diffuse hypervascular peritoneal

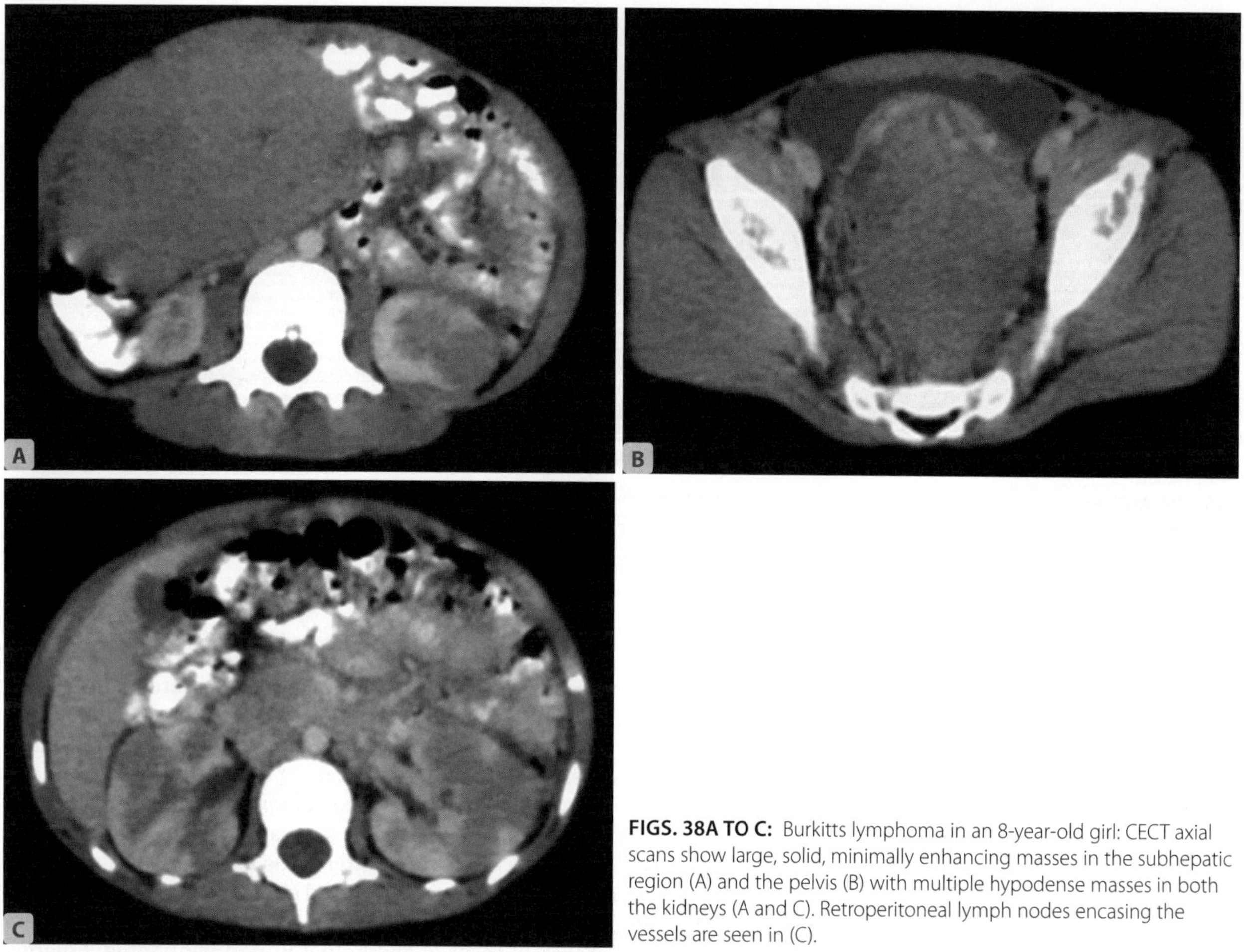

FIGS. 38A TO C: Burkitts lymphoma in an 8-year-old girl: CECT axial scans show large, solid, minimally enhancing masses in the subhepatic region (A) and the pelvis (B) with multiple hypodense masses in both the kidneys (A and C). Retroperitoneal lymph nodes encasing the vessels are seen in (C).

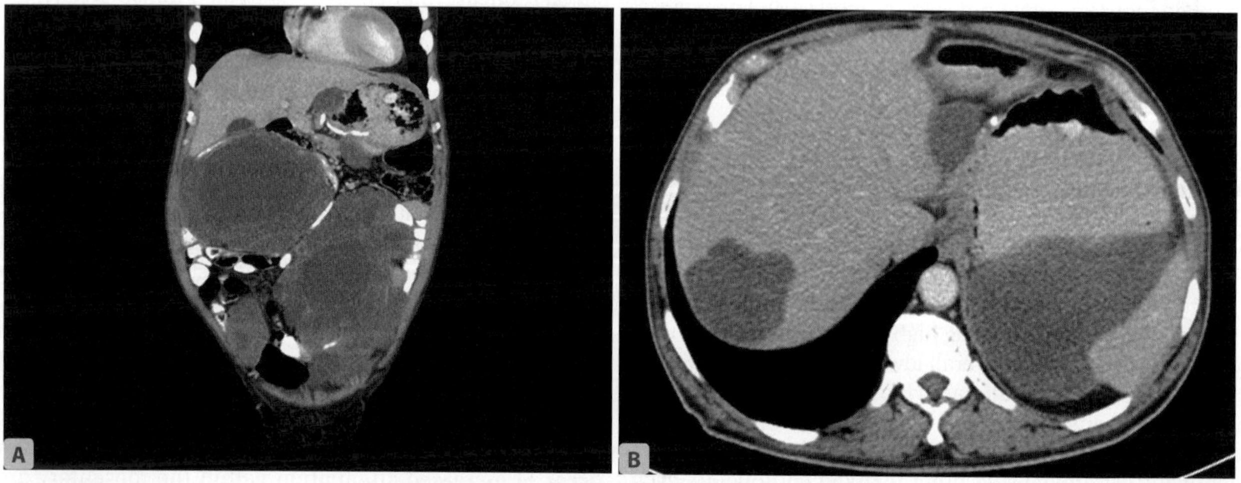

FIGS. 39A AND B: A 60-year-old man with gastrointestinal stromal tumor: Coronal (A) and axial (B) CECT images show bulky, heterogeneous peritoneal masses. Metastatic lesion seen in the liver on the axial scan (B). There is no evidence of ascites.

involvement may occur with omental 'cake' formation. The hypervasculature nature of the metastases may lead to GI bleeding and hemoperitoneum.[93]

The appearance of peritoneal sarcomatosis may show overlap with carcinomatosis and lymphomatosis, although bulky heterogeneous masses, hypervascularity, minimal ascites, and hemoperitoneum are more characteristic of sarcomatosis. **Table 6** lists the main differentiating features between peritoneal carcinomatosis, lymphomatosis and sarcomatosis.

MESENTERIC CARCINOID (NEUROENDOCRINE TUMOR)

The small intestine is the most common location for gastrointestinal carcinoid tumors. Independent of site of origin, aggressive carcinoid tumors typically spread to the mesentery, mesenteric lymph nodes, liver, ovaries, and spleen.

Approximately 40–80% of gastrointestinal carcinoids spread to the mesentery, either by direct extension or through the local lymphatics.[96] The primary intestinal mass is often small and difficult to detect, the mesenteric tumor is usually discovered first. Secondary involvement of the mesentery leads to a desmoplastic reaction incited by local release of serotonin and other vasoactive substances.

Imaging Features

CT/MR enterography is an appropriate imaging modality for evaluating patients suspected of having carcinoid tumors as it may show both the components of carcinoid tumor, the primary mural nodule and the secondary mesenteric mass.

Carcinoid tumor incites a strong desmoplastic reaction thought to be due to the effect of serotonin and other vasoactive peptides produced by the tumor. It is usually seen as a enhancing soft-tissue mass with linear bands radiating in the mesenteric fat **(Figs. 40A to C)**. Segmental thickening of adjacent bowel loops resulting from chronic ischemia or tumor infiltration as well as angulation can be seen. Dystrophic calcification may be seen in up to 40% of carcinoids on CT.[97] On MRI the lesions exhibit low T1 signal intensity, high T2 signal intensity and moderately intense gadolinium enhancement.[98] Functional imaging like octreotide scintigraphy and G-68 DOTANOC PET/CT play an important role in the diagnosis and management of these lesions.

CONCLUSION

Diseases of the peritoneum are common, but there is a considerable overlap in their imaging appearances. This often results in misinterpretation of the findings, and thus peritoneal diseases present a diagnostic challenge. With the appropriate clinical setting, CT and MRI substantially aid in the identification of peritoneal disease. Radiologists must be familiar with the anatomy of the peritoneal ligaments and spaces, and a knowledge of the various diseases that can involve the peritoneum, to provide an accurate interpretation of findings.

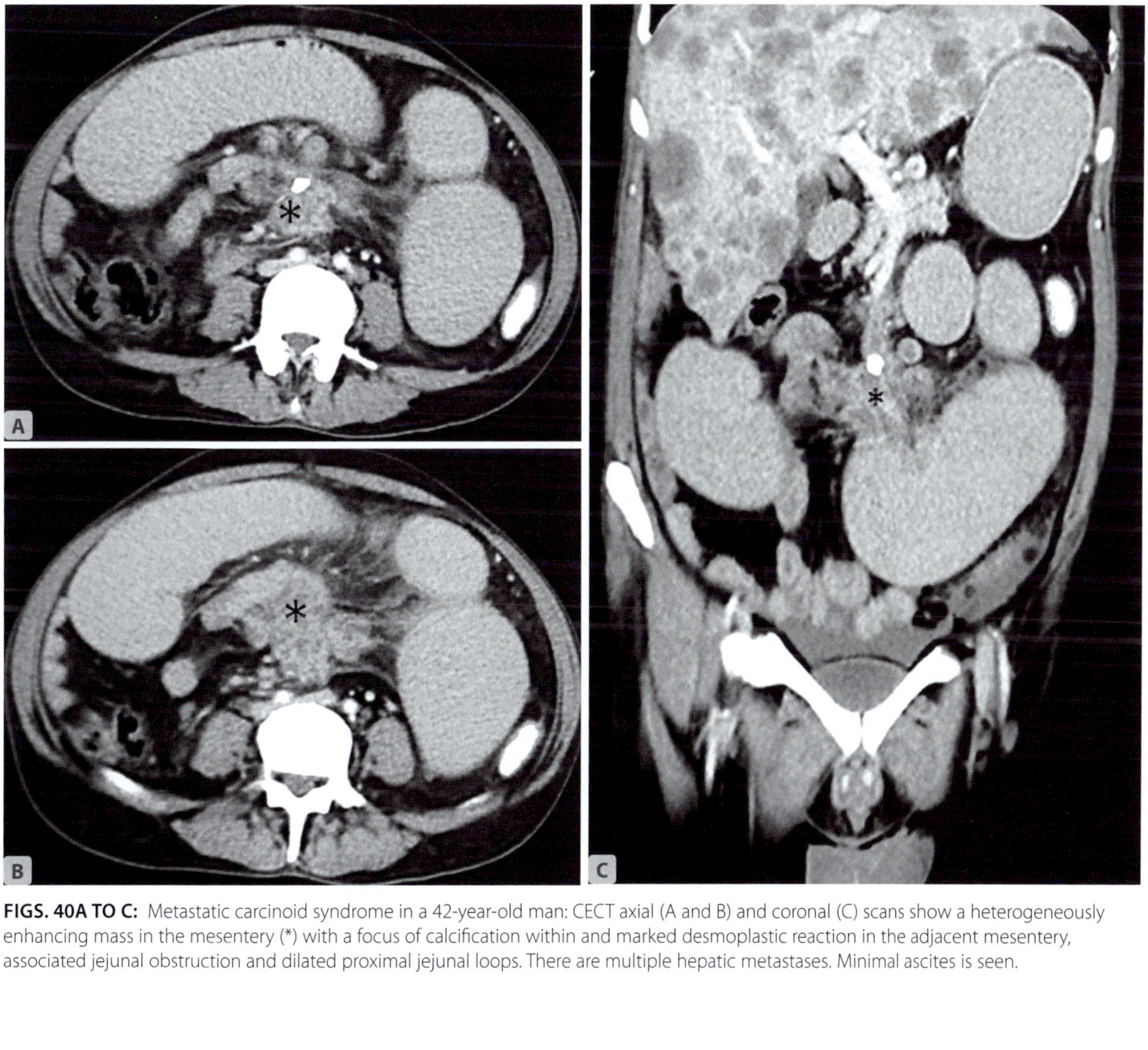

FIGS. 40A TO C: Metastatic carcinoid syndrome in a 42-year-old man: CECT axial (A and B) and coronal (C) scans show a heterogeneously enhancing mass in the mesentery (*) with a focus of calcification within and marked desmoplastic reaction in the adjacent mesentery, associated jejunal obstruction and dilated proximal jejunal loops. There are multiple hepatic metastases. Minimal ascites is seen.

REFERENCES

1. Kim S, Kim TU, Lee JW, et al. The perihepatic space: comprehensive anatomy and CT features of pathologic conditions. Radio Graphics. 2007;27(1):129-43.
2. Standring S. Gray's anatomy: the anatomical basis of clinical practice, Peritoneum and peritoneal cavity, 39th edition. Churchill Livingstone; 2004.
3. Le O. Patterns of peritoneal spread of tumor in the abdomen and pelvis. World J Radiol. 2013;5:106-12.
4. DeMeo JH, Fulcher AS, Austin RF. Anatomic CT demonstration of the peritoneal spaces, ligaments, and mesenteries: normal and pathologic processes. Radiographics. 1995;15(4):755-70.
5. Tirkes T, Sandrasegaran K, Patel AA, et al. Peritoneal and retroperitoneal anatomy and its relevance for cross-sectional imaging. Radiographics. 2012;32:437-51.
6. Sharma M, Rai P, Rameshbabu CS, et al. Imaging of peritoneal ligaments by endoscopic ultrasound. Endosc Ultrasound. 2015;4(1):15-27.
7. Haaga JR, Pickhardt PJ. Peritoneum. In: Haaga JR, Dogra VS, Frosting M, et al. (Eds). CT and NRI of the whole body, 5th edition. Philadelphia, PA: Mosby. 2009:1675-1730.
8. Turnage RH, Li BD, McDonald JC. Abdominal wall, umbilicus, peritoneum, mesenteries, omentum and retroperitoneum. In: Townsend CM, Beauchamp RD, Evers BM, Mattox KI (Eds). Sabiston Textbook of Surgery, 17th edition. Philadelphia, PA: Saunders; 2004.pp.1181-2.
9. Feldman GB, Knapp RC. Lymphatic drainage of the peritoneal cavity and its significance in ovarian cancer. Am J Obstet Gynecol. 1974;119:991-4.
10. Runyon BA, Montano AA, Akriviadis EA, et al. The serum-ascites albumin gradient is superior to the exudate-transudate concept in the differential diagnosis of ascites. Ann Intern Med. 1992;117(3):215-20.
11. Nicholas JE, Steinkampf MP. Detection of free peritoneal fluid by transvaginal sonography. J Clin Ultrasound. 1993;21:171-4.
12. Meyers MA. Dynamic radiology of the abdomen: normal and pathologic anatomy, 4th edition. New York, NY: Springer-Verlag; 1994.
13. Martin LC, Merkle EM, Thompson WM. Review of internal hernias: radiographic and Clinical findings AJR. 2006;186:703-17.
14. Edell SL, Gefter WB. Ultrasonic differentiation of types of ascitic fluid. Am J Roentgenol. 1979;133:111-4.
15. Gazelle GS, Mueller PR. Abdominal abscess: imaging and intervention. Radiol Clin North Am. 1994;32:913-32.
16. Batra A, Gulati MS, Sarma D, Paul SB. Sonographic appearances in abdominal tuberculosis. J Clin Ultrasound. 2000;28:233-45.
17. Leder RA, Low VHS. Tuberculosis of the abdomen. Radiol Clin North Am. 1995;33:691-705.
18. Burill J, Williams CJ, Bain G, et al. Tuberculosis: a radiological review. Radiographics. 2007;27:1255-73.
19. Hulnick DH, Megibow AJ, Nadiach DP, et al. Abdominal tuberculosis: CT evaluation. Radiology. 1985;157:199-204.
20. Lundstedt C, Nymon R, Brimsar J, et al. Imaging of abdominal tuberculosis. Abdominal manifestations in 112 patients. Acta Radiol. 1996;37:489-95.
21. Malik A, Saxena NC. Ultrasound in abdominal tuberculosis. Abdom Imaging. 2003;28(4):574-9.
22. Leder RA, Low VH. Tuberculosis of the abdomen. Radiol Clin North Am. 1995;33(4):691-705.
23. Anbarasu A, Upadhyaya A, Merchant SA, et al. Tuberculous chylous ascites: pathognomic CT findings. Abdom Imaging. 1997;22:50-1.
24. Joshi AR, Basantani AS, Patel TC. Role of CT and MRI in abdominal tuberculosis. Current Radiology Reports. 2014;2:66.
25. Healy JC, Reznek RH. The peritoneum, mesenteries and omenta: normal anatomy and pathological processes Eur Radiol. 1998;8:886-900.
26. Ha HK, Jung JM, Lee MS, et al. CT differentiation of tuberculous peritonitis and peritoneal carcinomatosis. Am J Roentgenol. 1996;167:743-8.
27. Rodriquez E, Pombo F. Peritoneal tuberculosis versus peritoneal carcinomatosis: distinction based on CT findings. J Comput Asst Tomogr. 1996;20(2):269-72.
28. Pedrosa I, Saíz A, Arrazola J, Ferreirós J Pedrosa CS. Hydatid disease: radiologic and pathologic features and complications. Radiographics. 2000;20(3):3795-817.
29. Acharya AN, Gupta S. Peritoneal hydatidosis: a review of seven cases. Tropical Gastroenterology. 2009;30(1):32-4.
30. Mindelzun RE, Brooke Jeffrey R, Lane MJ, Silverman PM. The misty mesentery on CT: differential diagnosis. AJR. 1996;167:61-5.
31. Demir MK, Akinci O, Onur E, et al. Case 108: sclerosing encapsulating peritonitis. Radiology. 2007;242(3):937-9.
32. Vijayaraghavan SB, Palanivelu C, Sendhilkumar K, Parthasarathi R. Abdominal cocoon: sonographic features. J Ultrasound Med. 2003;22:719-21.
33. Hur J, Kim KW, Park MS, Yu JS. Abdominal cocoon: preoperative diagnostic clues from radiologic imaging with pathologic correlation. Am J Roentgenol. 2004; 182:639-41.
34. Gupta S, Shirahatti RG, Anand J. CT findings of an abdominal cocoon. Am J Roentgenol. 2004;183(6):1658-60.
35. Auh YH, Kung S, Shih G. Mesentery. In: Haaga JR, Dogra VS, Frosting M, et al, (Eds). CT and MRI of the whole body, 5th edition. Philadelphia, PA: Mosby. 2009:1731-70.
36. Horton KM, Lawler LP, Fishman ER. CT Findings in Sclerosing Mesenteritis (Panniculitis): Spectrum of Disease. Radiographics. 2003;23:1561-7.
37. Valls C. Fat-ring sign in sclerosing mesenteritis. Am J Roentgenol. 2000;174:259-60.
38. Hamrick-Turner J, Chiechi M, Abbitt P, Ros P. Neoplastic and inflammatory processes of the peritoneum, omentum and mesentery: diagnosis with CT. Radiographics. 1992;12:1051-68.
39. Singh AK, Gervais DA, Hahn PF, Rhea J, Mueller PR. CT of acute appendagitis. Am J Roentgenol. 2004;183:1303-7.
40. Singh AK, Gervais DA, Hahn PF. Acute epiploic appendagitis and its mimics. Radiographics. 2005;25(6):1521-34.
41. Lucey BC, Stuhlfaut JW, Soto JA. Mesenteric lymph nodes: detection and significance on MDCT. Am J Roentgenol. 2005;184:41-4.
42. Lucey BC, Stuhlfaut JW, Soto JA. Mesenteric lymph nodes seen at imaging—causes and significance. Radiographics. 2005;25:351-65.
43. Jain R, Sawhney S, Bhargava DK, et al. Diagnosis of abdominal tuberculosis: sonographic findings in patients with early disease. AJR. 1995;165:1391-5.
44. Kedar RP, Shah PP, Shirde RS, et al. Sonographic findings in gastrointestinal and peritoneal tuberculosis. Clin Radiol. 1994;49:24-9.
45. Pombo F, Rodriquez E, Mato J, et al. Patterns of contrast enhancement of tuberculous lymph nodes demonstrated by CT. Clin Radiol. 1992;46:13-7.
46. De Backer AI, Mortele KJ, Deeren D, Vanschoubroeck IJ, De Keulenaer BL. Abdominal tuberculous lymphadenopathy: MRI features. Eur Radiol. 2005;15(10):2104-9.
47. Rocha ELD, Pedrassa BC, Bormann RL, et al. Abdominal tuberculosis: a radiological review with emphasis on CT and MRI findings. Radiol Bras. 2015;48(3):181-91.
48. Yang ZG, Min P, Sone S, et al. Tuberculosis versus lymphoma in the abdominal lymph nodes. Evaluation with contrast-enhanced CT. Am J Roentgenol. 1999;172:619-23.

49. Macari M, Hines J, Balthazar E, Megibow A. Mesenteric adenitis: CT diagnosis of primary versus secondary causes, incidence, and clinical significance in pediatric and adult patients. Am J Roentgenol. 2002;178:853-8.
50. Rao PM, Rhea JT, Novelline RA. CT diagnosis of mesenteric adenitis. Radiology. 1997;204:713-7.
51. Yenarkam P, Theni RF, Hanks D. Lymphoma of the mesentery. Radiology. 2007;242:628-31.
52. Mok SC, Schorge JO, Welch WR, Hendrickson MR, Kempson RL. Peritoneal tumors. In: Tavassoli FA, Devilee P (Eds). Pathology and genetics of tumours of the breast and female genital organs. Lyon, France: IARC. 2003;197-202.
53. Boffetta P. Epidemiology of peritoneal mesothelioma: a review. Ann Oncol. 2007;18:985-990.
54. Churg A, Cagle PT, Roggli VL. Tumors of the serosal membranes. Silver Spring, Md: ARP; 2006.
55. Levy AD, Arnáiz J, Shaw JC, Sobin LH. From the archives of the AFIP: primary peritoneal tumors—imaging features with pathologic correlation. Radiographics. 2008;28:583-607.
56. Cao Q, Lu M, Heath J, Hausner PF, Alexander HR, Dilsizian V, Chen W. 18F-FDG PET/CT in a recurrent diffuse malignant peritoneal mesothelioma. Clin Nucl Med. 2012;37:492-4.
57. Turner KM, Varghese S, Alexander HR. Surgery for peritoneal mesothelioma. Curr Treat Options Oncol. 2011;12:189-200.
58. Raza A, Huang WC, Takabe K. Advances in the management of peritoneal mesothelioma. World J Gastroenterol. 2014;7: 20(33):11700-12.
59. Ross MJ, Welch WR, Scully RE. Multilocular peritoneal inclusion cysts (so-called cystic mesotheliomas). Cancer. 1989;64:1336-46.
60. McLaughlin P, Flippone A, Maher MM. Neoplastic diseases of Peritoneum and Mesentery. AJR. 2013;200:W400-w420.
61. Zhang J, Xu H, Ren F, Yang Y, Chen B, Zhang F. Analysis of clinicopathological features and prognostic factors of desmoplastic small round cell tumor. Pathol Oncol Res. 2014;20(1):161-8.
62. Arora VC, Price AP, Fleming S, et al. Characteristic imaging features of desmoplastic small round cell tumor. Pediatr Radiol. 2013;43(1):93-102.
63. Magnan H, Abramson SJ, Price AP, et al. Positron emission tomography for response assessment in desmoplastic small round cell tumor. J Pediatr Hematol Oncol. 2013;35(5): e190-3.
64. Casillas J, Sais GJ, Greve JL, Iparraguirre MC, Morillo G. Imaging of intra- and extraabdominal desmoid tumors. Radiographics. 1991;11:959-68.
65. Azizi I, Bali M, Belkacem A, et al. MRI Features of mesenteric desmoids tumors in familial adenomatous polyposis. AJR. 2005;184:1128-35.
66. Shinagare AB, Ramaiya NH, Jagannathan JP, et al. A to Z of desmoids tumours. Am J Roentgenol. 201;197(6):W1008-14.
67. Chung EM, Biko DM, Arzamendi AM, et al. Solid tumours of the peritoneum, omentum, and mesentery in children: radiologic-pathologic correlation: from the radiologic pathology archives. Radiographics. 2015;35:521-46.
68. Aptel S, Gervaise A, Fairise A, et al. Abdominal inflammatory myofibroblastic tumour. Diagn Interv Imaging. 2012;93(5): 410-2.
69. Narla LD, Newman B, Spottswood SS, Narla S, Kolli R. Inflammatory pseudotumor. Radiographics. 2003;23(3): 719-29.
70. Sedlic T, Scali EP, Lee WK, Verma S, Chang SD. Inflammatory pseudotumors in the abdomen and pelvis: a pictorial essay. Can Assoc Radiol J. 2014;65(1):52-9.
71. Dong A, Wang Y, Dong H, et al. Inflammatory myofibroblastic tumor: FDG PET/CT findings with pathologic correlation. Clin Nucl Med. 2014;39(2):113-21.
72. Lausen I, Jensen OJ, Andersen E, Lindahl F. Disseminated peritoneal leiomyomatosis with malignant change in a male. Virchows Arch A Pathol Anat Histopathol. 1990;417:173-5.
73. Fulcher AS, Szucs RA. Leiomyomatosis peritonealis disseminata complicated by sarcomatous transformation and ovarian torsion: presentation of two cases and review of the literature. Abdom Imaging. 1998;23:640-4.
74. Levy AD, Cantisani V, Miettinen M. Abdominal lymphangiomas: imaging features with pathologic correlation. Am J Roentgenol. 2004;182:1485-91.
75. Merrot T, Chaumoitre K, Simeoni-Alias J, Alessandrini P, Guys JM, Panuel M. Abdominal cystic lymphangiomas in children. Clinical, diagnostic and therapeutic aspects: apropos of 21 cases. Ann Chir. 1999;53:494-9.
76. Meyers MA. Intraperitoneal spread of malignancies. In: Meyers MA (Ed). Dynamic Radiology of the Abdomen: Normal and Pathologic Anatomy, 5th edition. New York/London: Springer. 2000.pp. 131-263.
77. Hanbridge AE, Lynch D, Wilson SR. US of the peritoneum. Radiographics. 2003;23/3:663-83.
78. Marin D, Catalano C, Baski M, et al. 64-section multi-detector row CT in the preoperative diagnosis of peritoneal carcinomatosis: Correlation with histopathological findings. Abdom Imaging. 2010;35:694-700.
79. Iafrate F, Ciolina M, Sammartino P, et al. Peritoneal carcinomatosis: imaging with 64-MDCT and 3T MRI with diffusion-weighted imaging. Abdom Imaging. 2012;37:616-27.
80. Soussan M, Des Guetz G, Barrau V, et al. Comparison of FDG-PET/CT and MR with diffusion-weighted imaging for assessing peritoneal carcinomatosis from gastrointestinal malignancy. Eur Radiol. 2012;22:1479-87.
81. Anthony MP, Khong PL, Zhang J. Spectrum of 18F-FDG PET/CT appearances in peritoneal disease. AJR. 2009;193:1646.
82. Tentes KA, Courcoutsakis N, Prasopoulos P. Combined cytoreductive surgery and perioperative intraperitoneal chemotherapy for the treatment of advanced ovarian cancer—clinical and therapeutic perspectives. In: Samir F (Ed). Ovarian Cancer—Clinical and Therapeutic Perspectives. New York: InTech; 2012.pp.143-67.
83. Seidman JD, Elsayed AM, Sobin LH, Tavassoli FA. Association of mucinous tumors of the ovary and appendix: a clinicopathologic study of 25 cases. Am J Surg Pathol. 1993;17:22-34.
84. Young RH, Gilks CB, Scully RE. Mucinous tumors of the appendix associated with mucinous tumors of the ovary and pseudomyxoma peritonei: a clinicopathological analysis of 22 cases supporting an origin in the appendix. Am J Surg Pathol. 1991;15:415-29.
85. Ronnett BM, Zahn CM, Kurman RJ, Kass ME, et al. Disseminated peritoneal adenomucinosis and peritoneal mucinouscarcinomatosis: a clinicopathologic analysis of 109 cases with emphasis on distinguishing pathologic features, site of origin, prognosis, and relationship to "pseudomyxoma peritonei." Am J Surg Pathol. 1995;19:1390-408.
86. Seshul MB, Coulam CM. Pseudomyxoma peritonei: Computed tomography and sonography. Am J Roentgenol. 1981;136:803-6.
87. Yeh HC, Shafir MK, Slater G, Meyer RJ, Cohen BA, Geller SA. Ultrasonography and computed tomography in pseudomyxoma peritonei. Radiology. 1984;153:507-10.
88. Bechtold RE, Chen MY, Loggie BW, Jackson SL, Geisinger K. CT appearance of disseminated peritoneal adenomucinosis. Abdom Imaging. 2001;26:406-10.
89. Levy AD, Shaw JC, Sobin LH. Secondary tumours and tumour-like lesions of the peritoneal cavity: imaging features with pathologic correlation. Radiographics. 2009;29:347-73.

90. Kim Y, Cho O, Song S, Lee H, Rhim H, Koh B. Peritoneal lymphomatosis: CT findings. Abdom Imaging. 1998;23:87-90.
91. Ferrozzi F, Tognini G, Mulonzia NW, Bova D, et al. Primary effusion lymphomas in AIDS: CT findings in two cases. Eur Radiol. 2001;11:623-5.
92. Cabral FC, Krajewski KM, Kim KW, et al. Peritoneal lymphomatosis: CT and PET/CT findings and how to differentiate between carcinomatosis and sarcomatosis. Cancer Imaging. 2013:13(2):162-70.
93. Swerdlow SH. International Agency for Research on Cancer, World Health Organization. WHO classification of tumours of haematopoietic and lymphoid tissues. Lyon, France: International Agency for Research on Cancer, 2008.
94. Katz SC, DeMatteo RP. Gastrointestinal stromal tumors and leiomyosarcoma. J Surg Oncol. 2008;97:350-9.
95. Burkill GJ, Badran M, Thomas JM. Malignant gastrointestinal stromal tumor: distribution, imaging features, and pattern of metastatic spread. Radiology. 2003;226:527-32.
96. Sheth S, Horton KM, Garland MR, Fishman EK. Mesenteric neoplasms: CT appearances of primary and secondary tumors and differential diagnosis. Radiographics. 2003;23:457-73.
97. Levy AD, Sobin LH. From the archives of the AFIP: Gastrointestinal carcinoids: Imaging features with clinicopathologic comparison. Radiographics. 2007;27:237-57.
98. Elsayes KM, Staveteig PT, Narra VR, et al. MRI of the peritoneum: spectrum of abnormalities. Am J Roentgenol. 2006;186:1368-79.

CHAPTER

118

Imaging of Spleen

Mukesh Kumar Yadav, Priyanka Naranje, Ekta Dhamija

INTRODUCTION AND ANATOMY

The spleen is an encapsulated organ located intraperitoneally in the left subdiaphragmatic region of the abdomen. Multiple ligaments support the spleen in its normal position. The important ones are gastrosplenic ligament and lienorenal ligament. Others are phrenicosplenic, splenocolic, pancreaticosplenic, phrenocolic, and pancreaticocolic ligaments. The capsule is penetrated at the hilus located anteromedially, by the splenic artery, splenic vein, lymphatics, and nerves. Within the spleen, the branches of arteries, veins, nerves, and lymphatics form a trabecular network.

The parenchyma of spleen has a unique arrangement of white pulp (25%) and red pulp (75%).[1] Splenic cords and vascular sinuses containing predominantly erythrocytes constitute the red pulp, whereas lymphatic tissue, macrophages and lymphocytes compose the white pulp area of spleen. Some of the normal variations in enhancement pattern of spleen seen on contrast-enhanced computed tomography (CT) as well as gadolinium enhanced magnetic resonance imaging (MRI) are attributed to this unique anatomy of the spleen.

The spleen arises from aggregations of mesenchymal tissue between the layers of the dorsal mesogastrium during the fifth gestational week giving a lobulated pattern of the fetal spleen. The principal function of the embryonic spleen is erythropoiesis, which increases from the first to mid-second trimester and subsequently reduces. In the later life, spleen filters the damaged or aged red blood cells, bacteria, antigen-coated cells and foreign particles. The spleen comprises the largest functional mass of lymphoid tissue in the body. It consumes the circulating platelets when there is splenomegaly and also functions as reservoir for platelets, releasing them in response to epinephrine.[1]

IMAGING MODALITIES

Plain Abdominal Radiographs

A plain radiograph of the abdomen normally shows the spleen below the left hemidiaphragm in upper quadrant, lateral to gastric bubble and superior to colon. Excessive gaseous distension of bowel loops may obscure the splenic density. Enlarged spleen will be seen as soft tissue opacity displacing the stomach medially and colonic gas inferiorly **(Fig. 1)**. Curvilinear or chunky calcifications may be identified on plain radiographs in the region of spleen in cases of calcified hydatid cyst, calcified wall of splenic artery aneurysms or calcified granulomas.

Ultrasonography (USG)

Sonography is a nonionizing, radiation free, noninvasive and inexpensive modality for evaluating the spleen. It is frequently the initial investigation tool used for suspected splenic pathology. Sonography is used for evaluating splenic size, shape, location, and multiplicity, especially in children. Characterization of focal splenic lesions, splenic size evaluation in portal hypertension and cases of extrahepatic portal venous obstruction (EHPVO) along with assessment of perisplenic collaterals, splenic vein assessment in cases of pancreatitis, identification of splenic

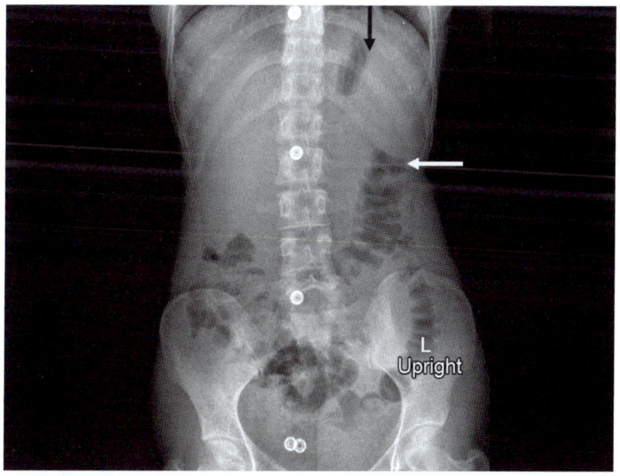

FIG. 1: Plain radiograph of abdomen shows indentation of splenic flexure (inferiorly) and greater curvature of stomach by soft tissue in left upper abdomen due to splenomegaly.

arterial aneurysms, preoperative work-up and postoperative follow-up of cases requiring splenectomy and as a guidance tool for various interventions such as fine needle aspiration cytology (FNAC), biopsies or drainages, are other common indications for using ultrasound for spleen. Sonography is ideally suited to study the internal architecture of a focal mass within the spleen, and distinguish a solid from a cystic lesion. Diffuse splenic involvement in infections like tuberculosis, fungal infections or in sarcoidosis or in cases of lymphoma, ultrasound may reveal the abnormality better than computed tomography **(Figs. 2A and B)**. Some lesions are known to have characteristic sonographic morphology and this modality helps to narrow the differential diagnosis and triage patients for further imaging work-up. The major drawback of this technique is that it is highly operator dependent. The details of sonographic features of different pathologies will be discussed subsequently. Role of focused assessment of spleen in trauma (FAST) by USG cannot be over emphasized and is covered in the chapter on Abdominal Trauma.

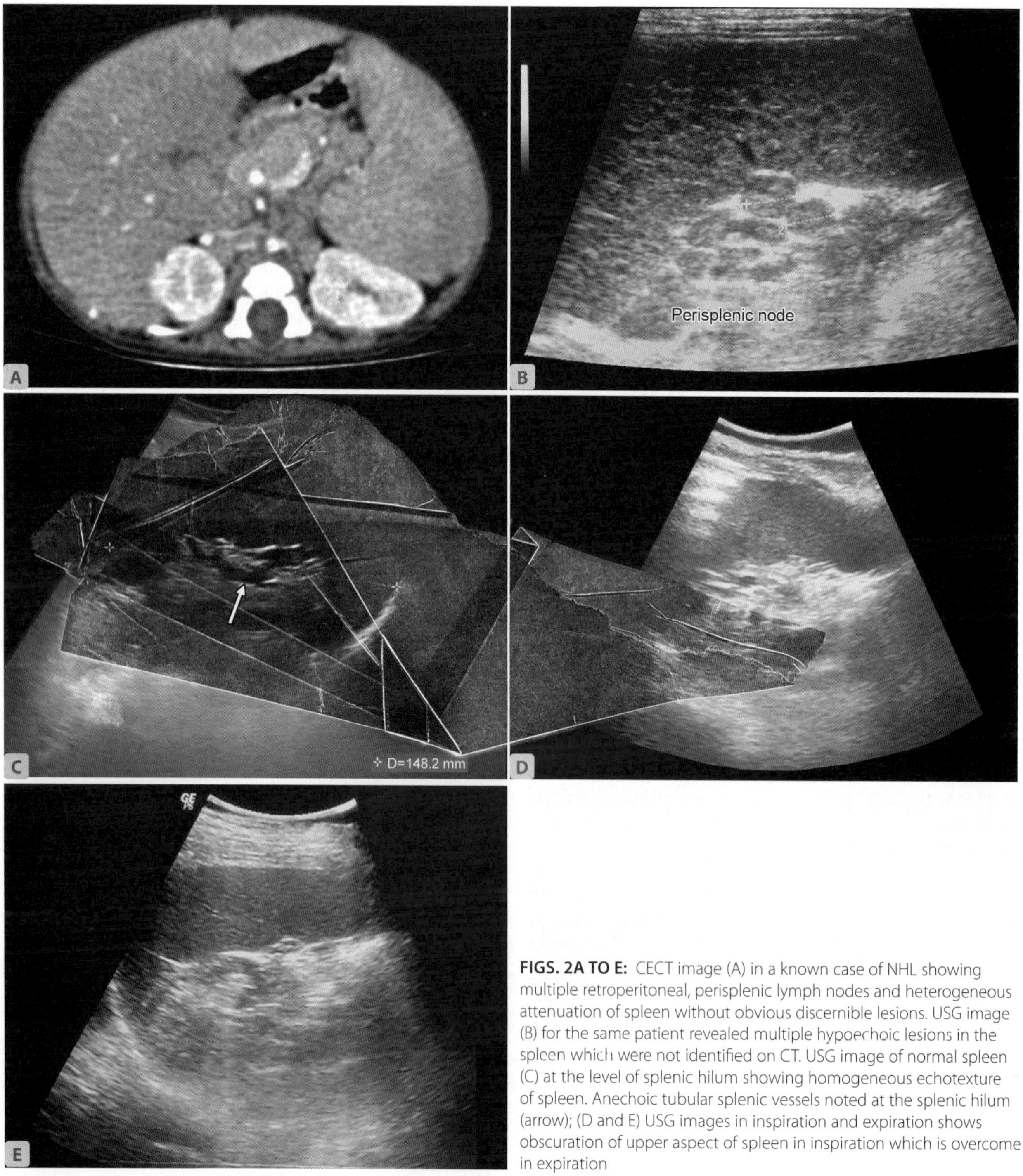

FIGS. 2A TO E: CECT image (A) in a known case of NHL showing multiple retroperitoneal, perisplenic lymph nodes and heterogeneous attenuation of spleen without obvious discernible lesions. USG image (B) for the same patient revealed multiple hypoechoic lesions in the spleen which were not identified on CT. USG image of normal spleen (C) at the level of splenic hilum showing homogeneous echotexture of spleen. Anechoic tubular splenic vessels noted at the splenic hilum (arrow); (D and E) USG images in inspiration and expiration shows obscuration of upper aspect of spleen in inspiration which is overcome in expiration

Technique

The spleen is usually scanned in the supine or right decubitus position with a 3.5–5 MHz convex array transducer in the sagittal and oblique planes as well as transversely, mostly from an intercostal approach in suspended deep inspiration and end expiration. Sometimes due to deep inspiration, the lateral margin of the left lung obscures the visualization of spleen **(Fig. 2D)**. In such situation, either scanning in expiration **(Fig. 2E)** or scanning with a small foot print probe in intercostal space may be helpful. An attempt is made to localize the splenic hilum, which represents the mid portion of the spleen, and the scanning is done taking a swipe posterior and anterior to the visualized hilum. Color Doppler is useful to assess the splenic hilar vein and artery at the hilum.

On ultrasonography, normal spleen shows a homogeneous echotexture **(Fig. 2C)**. Its echogenicity is a little more than that of the kidneys **(Fig. 3)** and is isoechoic to slightly hyperechoic compared to the liver. Tubular anechoic tortuous structures on gray-scale at the hilum of spleen are the splenic vessels **(Fig. 2C)** and intrasplenic vessels are visualized on color Doppler imaging.

Elasticity of the spleen can be measured with the real-time elastography, which measures the stiffness of parenchyma and it can be utilized as a marker for portal hypertension in patients with chronic liver disease.[2]

Few studies on contrast-enhanced ultrasound (CEUS) have described its utility in spleen.[3-5] The European Federation of Societies for Ultrasound in Medicine and Biology (EFSUMB) Guidelines and Recommendations on the Clinical Practice of CEUS, updated in 2011, recommend several indications where CEUS may be utilized in the spleen.[6] These are:

1. To characterize inhomogeneity of splenic parenchyma or to characterize suspected lesions on conventional US
2. To characterize accessory spleens or splenosis
3. To confirm suspected splenic infarction
4. To detect malignant splenic lesions in oncologic patients when CT and/or MRI and PET are contraindicated or inconclusive
5. To evaluate the spleen in selected patients following trauma.

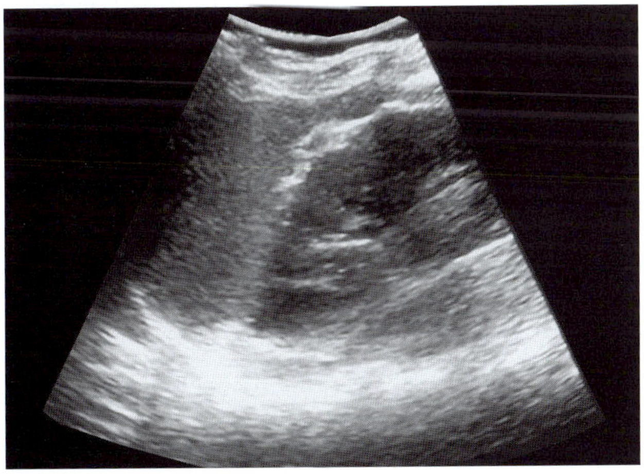

FIG. 3: USG images showing normal splenic echotexture as slightly more than the adjacent left kidney.

Computed Tomography

On a non-contrast CT (NCCT), a normal spleen reveals a homogeneous attenuation which is higher than the liver by 1–18 Hounsfield Unit (HU).[7] Normal HU of spleen is 40–60 HU. Splenic artery follows a tortuous course normally and splenic vein shows a straighter course and is usually located posterior to pancreatic body and tail.

For identification and characterization of focal lesion in the spleen or in trauma setting, contrast-enhanced computed tomography is frequently required.

Most often transient inhomogeneous splenic attenuation patterns are identified during the first minute of contrast-enhanced CT, particularly with rapid intravenous injection of iodinated contrast media.[8] This is a normal flow phenomenon and must not be misinterpreted as an indication of focal abnormality. It is thought to be due to different blood flow rates through the cords of red pulp[9] and white pulp. As the internal architecture of the spleen develops, this phenomenon gets more evident in children older than 1 year. Frequently described heterogeneity patterns include: (1) archiform pattern, consisting of ring-like or zebra-stripe bands of alternating low and high attenuation (commonest pattern) **(Figs. 4A and B)**; (2) diffuse, mottled areas of heterogeneity; and (3) focal areas of low density.[8] More homogeneous splenic enhancement is seen about approximately 70 seconds after commencement of the contrast injection. This heterogeneous splenic enhancement pattern can obscure pathologic lesions. With increasing age, the heterogeneous pattern is less often seen and in adults, several other factors may be responsible for the heterogeneous splenic enhancement, such as the liver disease, portal vein thrombosis, and congestive heart failure.[10]

CT angiography is performed for the detection of splenic artery aneurysms. Multiplanar reformation (MPR), maximum intensity projections (MIP) and volume rendered (VR) imaging help for complete morphological assessment of these aneurysms.

Magnetic Resonance Imaging

Magnetic resonance imaging (MRI) offers major advantages due to its high contrast resolution, lack of ionizing radiation and multiplanar capability. Technical advances in MR hardware and software have allowed the introduction of faster pulse sequences with significantly reduced motion artifacts that previously posed limitations to abdominal MR imaging. Indications for performing MRI for splenic pathology are mainly as a problem solving technique for focal splenic lesions or tumors, proliferative lymphatic diseases or in iron deposition conditions.

On MRI, normal adult spleen is T2 hyperintense relative to the liver **(Figs. 5A to D)**. On T1-weighted images (T1WI), the normal spleen shows lower signal intensity (SI) than that of liver and slightly greater SI than that of muscle. Such a signal intensity of spleen is attributed to large fractional heme content, which results in long T1 and T2 relaxation times.[11] However, in a neonate, due to the immaturity of the white pulp, the spleen is T1 as well as T2 hypo to isointense compared to the liver **(Figs. 6A and B)**. After 8 months of age as white pulp matures, the spleen becomes hyperintense on T2-weighted image (T2WI) relative to the liver and it maintains

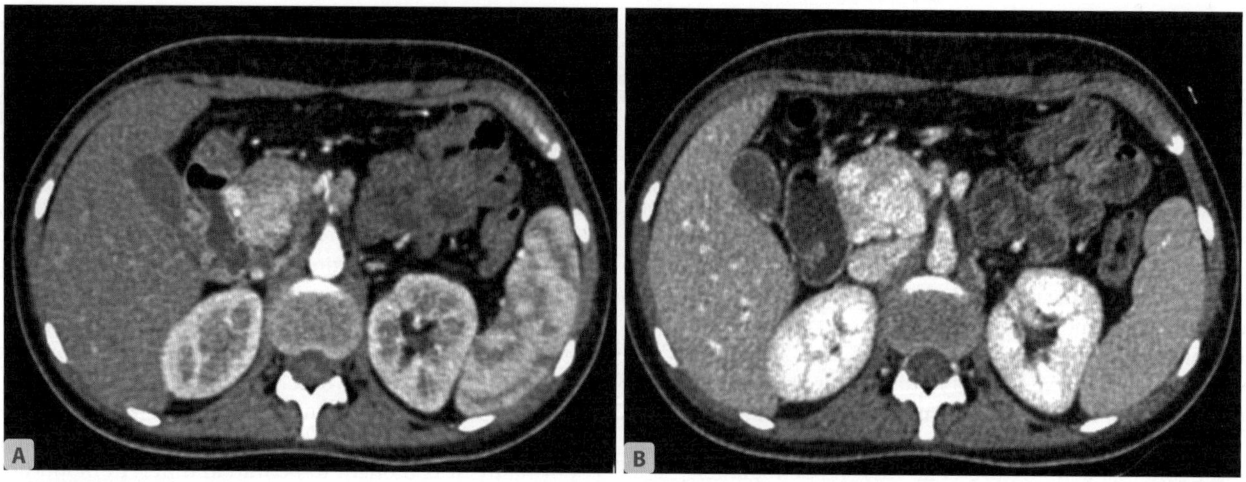

FIGS. 4A AND B: Contrast-enhanced CT images in arterial phase (A) showing normal Zebra-stripe/archiform enhancement pattern and venous phase (B) showing homogeneous enhancement.

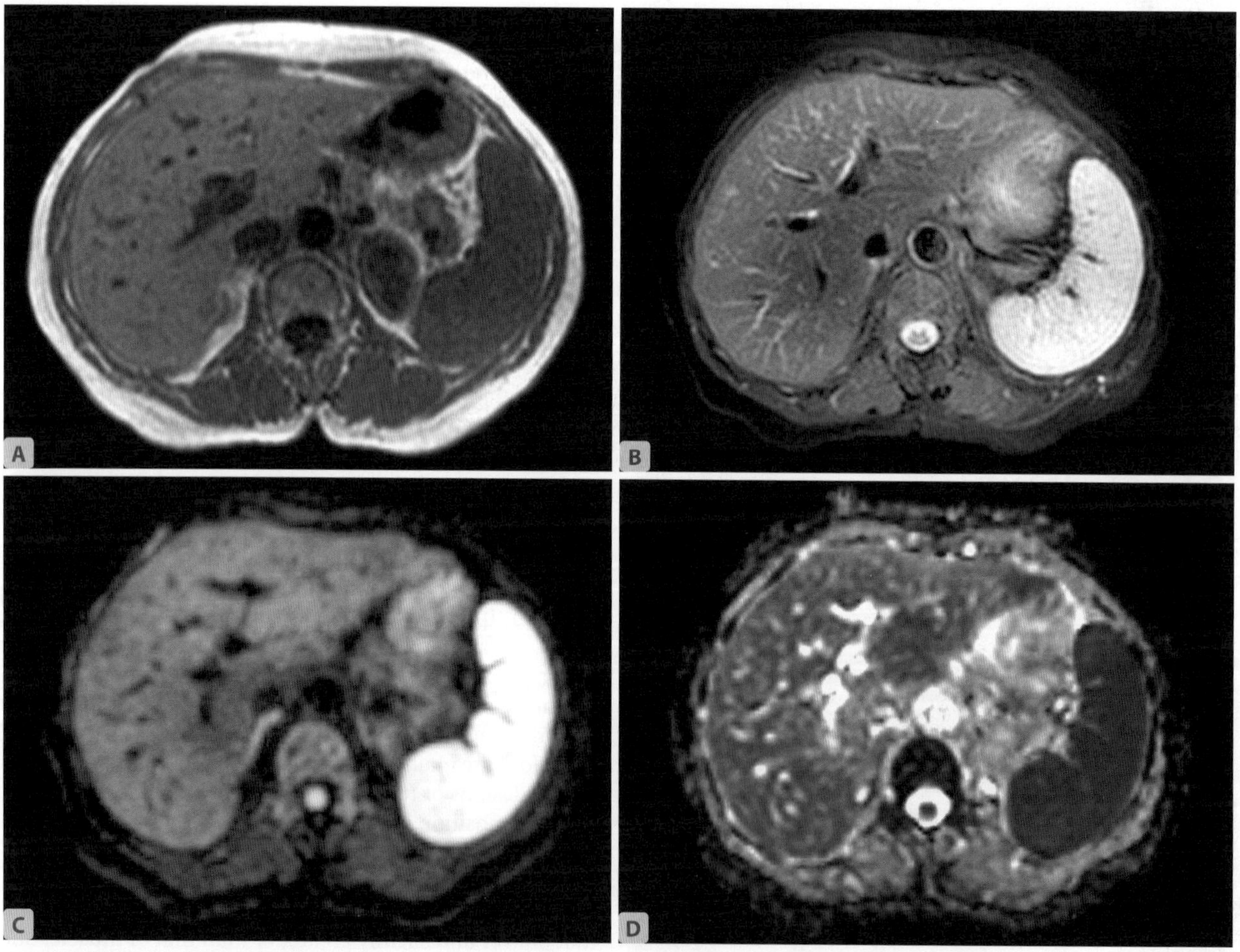

FIGS. 5A TO D: Axial T1WI (A), T2WI (B), DWI-b 1000 (C), and ADC map (D) showing T1 hypointensity, T2 hyperintensity and restricted diffusion on DWI and ADC maps of normal spleen.

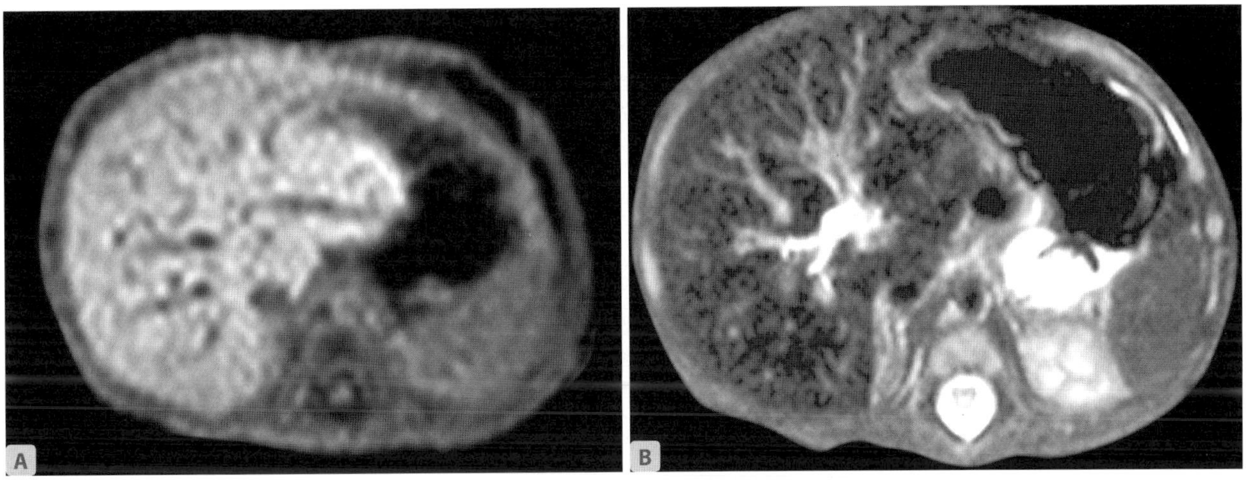

FIGS. 6A AND B: MRI T1WI (A) and T2WI (B) images showing normal hypointense spleen in a neonate.

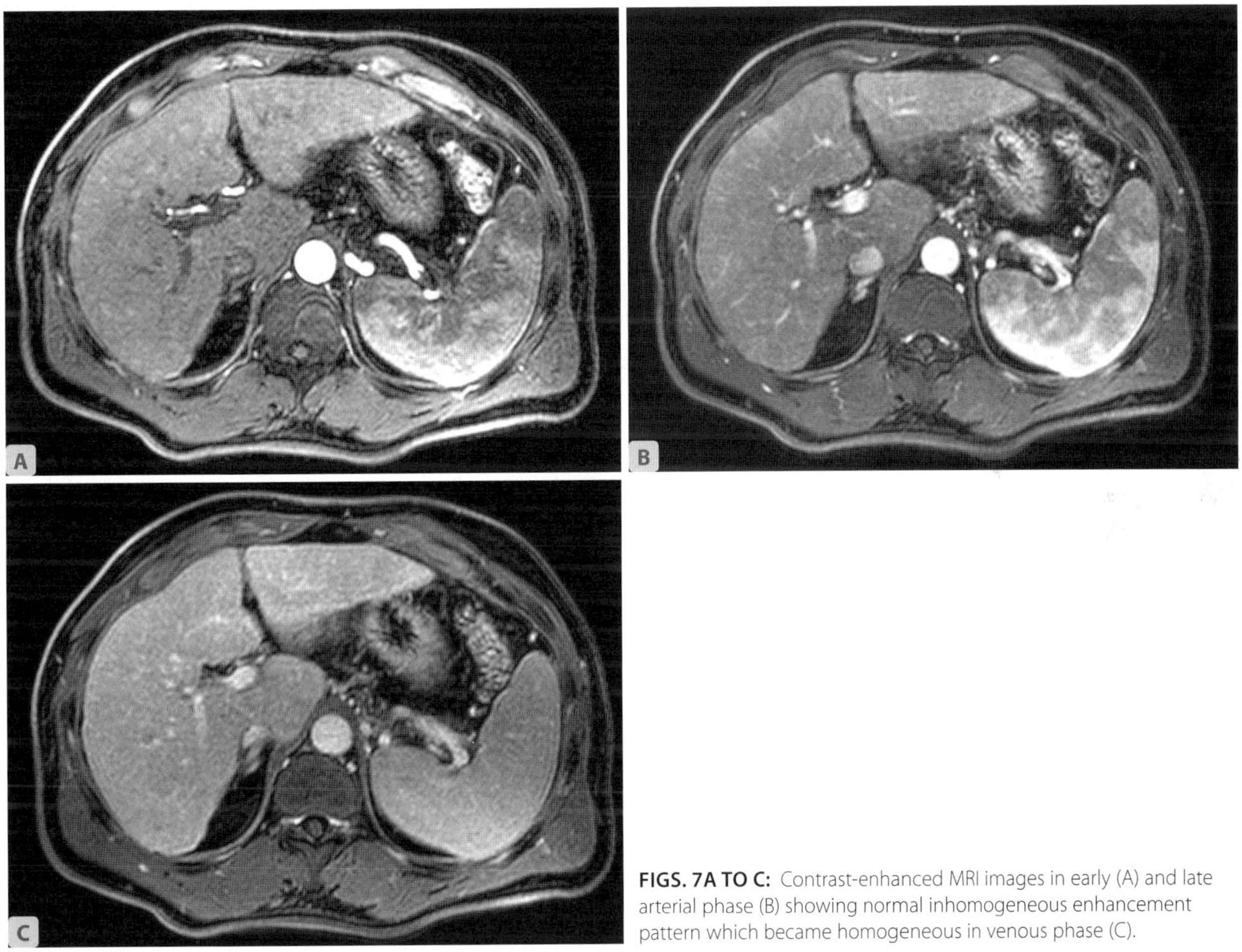

FIGS. 7A TO C: Contrast-enhanced MRI images in early (A) and late arterial phase (B) showing normal inhomogeneous enhancement pattern which became homogeneous in venous phase (C).

this appearance through adulthood.[12] On diffusion-weighted imaging, the spleen shows physiologically restricted diffusion **(Figs. 5A to D)**.[13]

Dynamic gadolinium-enhanced MR imaging has potential advantages over conventional MR imaging of the spleen because it can potentially provide differential contrast enhancement between splenic lesions and normal splenic tissue with greater contrast resolution compared with CT. Heterogeneous enhancement patterns of the normal spleen, seen commonly with early phase contrast-enhanced CT scans, are also seen with dynamic contrast-enhanced MRI **(Figs. 7A to C)**.

Scintigraphy

Scintigraphic splenic imaging involves the use of technetium-99m-labeled sulfur colloid. The tracer is taken up by the reticuloendothelial system and hence is helpful for the assessment of splenic congenital anomalies, e.g. splenic ectopia, accessory spleen, splenic hamartoma, etc.

Positron Emission Tomography/Computed Tomography (PET/CT)

It plays a role in evaluation of staging for lymphoma. Involvement of the spleen can be more accurately assessed using ^{18}F- FDG PET or fused PET/CT.[14]

Angiography

The high quality of images provided by cross-sectional imaging techniques has led to a dramatic change in the indications for splenic artery angiography. This technique is now seldom used for diagnostic purpose; however, it is widely used for vascular interventions for the management of splenic artery aneurysms and traumatic splenic injuries. CT angiography and MR angiography offer excellent visualization of the spleen and its vessels for diagnostic purposes.

SPLENIC SIZE

On USG, the measurement of splenic length is done by measuring maximum distance on a longitudinal coronal view obtained at the level of splenic hilum, between the most inferolateral and the most superomedial points **(Fig. 2C)**. CT and MRI also readily allow for more standardized and reproducible measurement. Splenic volume can be readily measured with CT or MRI.

Normal splenic size in children and adolescents vary according to age and the upper limit of normal at various age range are given in **Table 1**. In normal adult, the spleen measures approximately 12 cm in length, 4 cm in thickness and 7 cm in anteroposterior (AP) diameter. However, due to high variability in the shape of the spleen, these measurements are not very useful in evaluating splenic size. A more precise approach for the estimation of splenic volume is the splenic index, a product of length, width and thickness of the spleen, expressed in centimeters **(Figs. 8A to C)**. Length is determined by summing the number of contiguous sections on which the spleen is visible or simpler is to measure the craniocaudal length in coronal reconstruction. Width is the longest AP splenic diameter in an axial image. Thickness is measured between the inner and outer borders of the spleen, at the level of the splenic hilum (normal splenic index is 120–480 cm^3).[15]

NORMAL VARIANTS/DEVELOPMENTAL ANOMALIES

Various developmental anomalies are seen resulting from deficient fusion of separate splenic masses of the dorsal mesogastrium during embryogenesis. These include complete agenesis, persistent lobulations **(Fig. 9)**, clefts **(Figs. 10A and B)**, notches, isolated small splenunculi and polysplenia.

Splenunculus/Accessory Spleen

Accessory spleen is the most frequent congenital abnormality of the spleen. They can be found virtually anywhere in the abdomen **(Figs. 11A and B)**, but the most common sites are hilus and vascular pedicle of the spleen, around tail of the pancreas, along the greater curvature of the stomach, greater omentum, mesentery, near left ovary or left testicle and in the pouch of Douglas.[17] Splenunculi are found in 10–44% of autopsies.[18] They are usually found incidentally on imaging done for unrelated reasons and generally require no treatment. The clinical significance of accessory spleen is that after splenectomy, the accessory spleen may dramatically enlarge and cause recurrence of symptoms if splenectomy was done for some hematologic or other disorders. Intrapancreatic location of accessory splenic tissue is also described, which may, if

TABLE 1: Spleen length in children and adolescents.*[16]

Group	No.	10th percentile	Median	90th percentile	Upper limit
0–3 months	28	3.3	4.5	5.8	6.0
3–6 months	13	4.9	5.3	6.4	6.5
6–12 months	17	5.2	6.2	6.8	7.0
1–2 years	12	5.4	6.9	7.5	8.0
2–4 years	24	6.4	7.4	8.6	9.0
4–6 years	39	6.9	7.8	8.8	9.5
6–8 years	21	7.0	8.2	9.6	10.0
8–10 years	16	7.9	9.2	10.5	11.0
10–12 years	17	8.6	9.9	10.9	11.5
12–15 years	26	8.7	10.1	11.4	12.0
15–20 years (male)	5	9.0	10.0	11.7	12.0
15–20 years (female)	12	10.1	11.2	12.6	13.0

*All measurements are in centimeters.

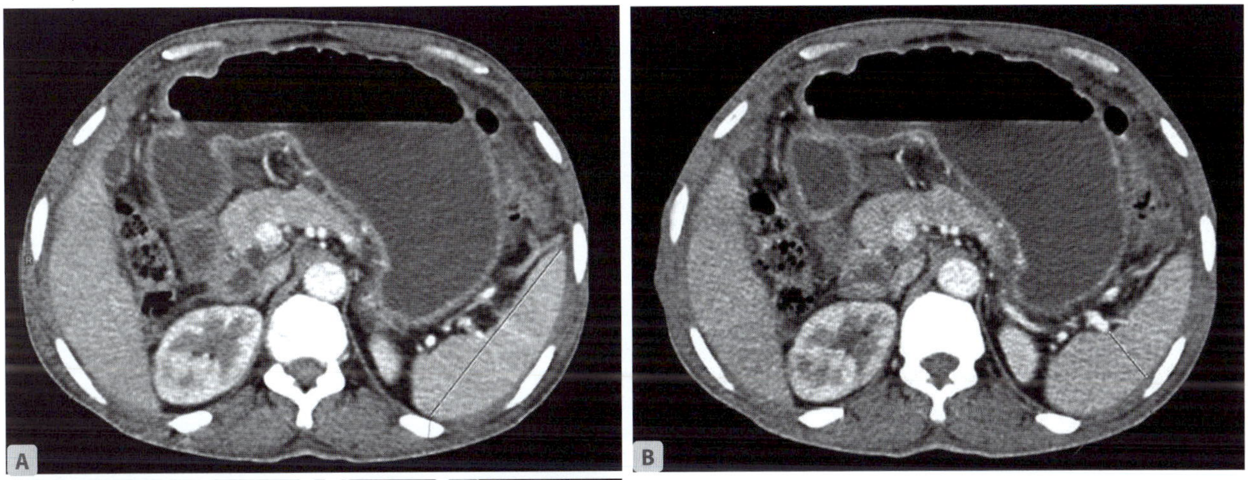

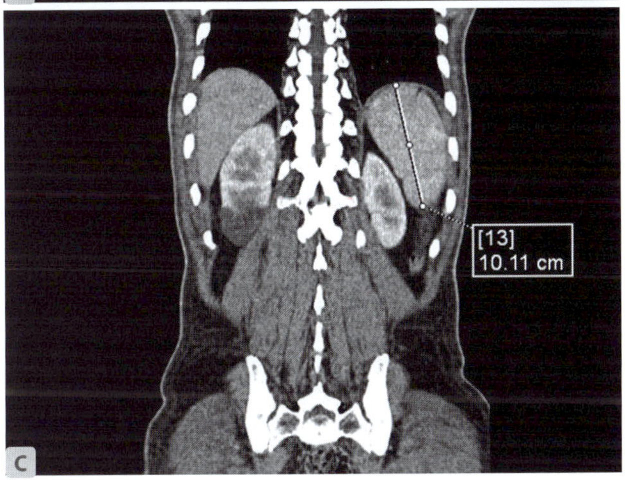

FIGS. 8A TO C: Axial (A and B) and coronal (C) CECT images showing the technique of measuring the width (A), thickness (B) and length (C) of spleen for the calculation of splenic index which is 302 cm^3 (normal) for the index case shown.

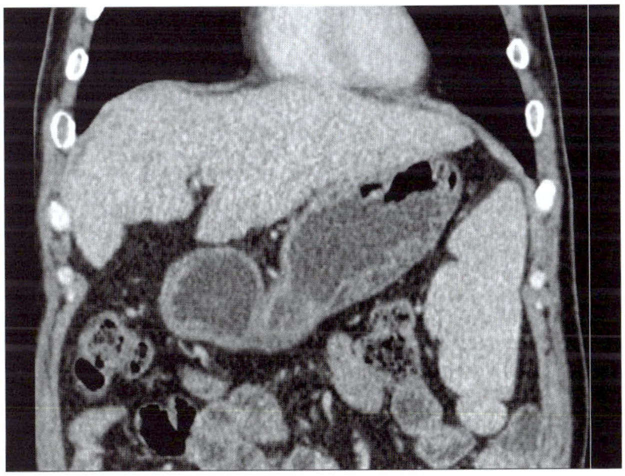

FIG. 9: Contrast-enhanced CT images (coronal reformat) showing prominent lobules of splenic tissue on medial and inferior aspect of spleen (suggesting persistence of fetal lobulations).

missed at surgery, be a cause of recurrence of the symptoms **(Figs. 11C and D)**. It enhances markedly in the arterial phase and is a rare differential diagnosis for neuroendocrine tumor of the pancreas. Splenunculi are usually six or fewer in number and they have histological features same as primary organ and has blood supply from a branch of the splenic artery.[17] They rarely exceed 2 cm in diameter and can be confused with splenic hilar or peripancreatic lymph nodes. Splenunculi can be identified on imaging modalities such as ultrasound, CT, or MRI, as of same attenuation or signal intensity as that of normal spleen **(Figs. 11E and F)** both before as well as after intravenous administration of contrast material but when there is doubt 99mTc sulfur colloid liver-spleen scan is definitive.

Ectopic splenic tissue can also be found due to acquired causes such as trauma (splenosis).

Wandering Spleen

Spleen changing its position within the abdomen due to ligamentous laxity, traumatic injury, maldevelopment of suspensory ligaments is referred to as wandering spleen. It may present as mobile unexplained mass in abdomen or may present with acute pain abdomen if torsion occurs.

It is thought to result from congenital abnormal fusion of the posterior mesogastrium.[19] Incidence of wandering spleen is higher in multiparous women. On imaging, the changing position of the spleen can be determined on USG. CT **(Figs. 12A and B)** also can depict the same and in case of torsion may show a 'whorled appearance' of splenic pedicle. Splenic infarcts, ascites, pancreatic tail necrosis can also be identified.

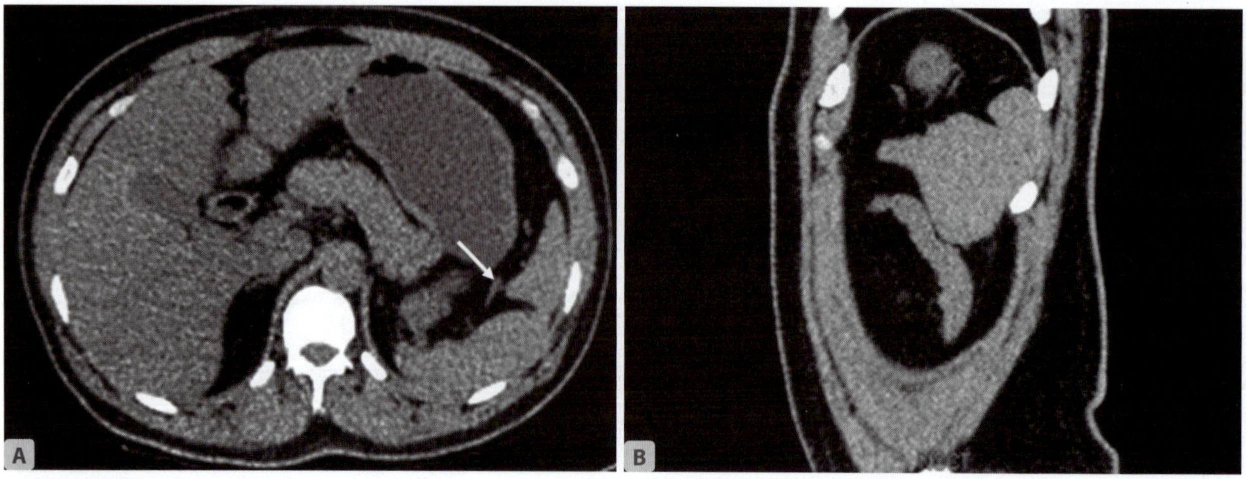

FIGS. 10A AND B: Non-contrast CT images [axial (A) and sagittal (B) reformat] showing splenic cleft (arrow). These may be confused with laceration in case of history of trauma.

Polysplenia

Presence of multiple splenules is known as polysplenia. It is seen in association with left-sided atrial isomerism syndrome and is more common in females than males. Patients with polysplenia may be asymptomatic or symptoms may occur due to congenital heart disease, biliary atresia or intestinal malrotation. On imaging, numerous small splenic masses are seen in the left **(Fig. 13)** or right hypochondrium.

Asplenia

Congenital absence of spleen is termed asplenia and it is seen in association with situs ambiguous. The condition is more common in males and association with congenital heart diseases is seen in 99–100% of the patients.[20]

CYSTIC LESIONS OF SPLEEN

The cystic lesions of the spleen can be primary (true) or secondary (pseudocyst) cysts, depending on the whether there is cellular or fibrous lining respectively.[21]

Primary cysts are divided into parasitic and non-parasitic. Primary non-parasitic cysts may be of epithelial origin (congenital cysts), such as epidermoid, dermoid, or transitional cell cysts, or of endothelial origin, such as lymphatic malformations and hemangiomas. Primary parasitic cysts include echinococcal cysts. Secondary/false or pseudocysts may form secondary to trauma, hematoma, infarction-degeneration or inflammation.

Congenital Cysts

Congenital or epithelial splenic cysts such as epidermoid, dermoid, or transitional cell cysts, account for about 25% of primary cysts of the spleen.[21] They are usually solitary, but can be multiple and are commonly seen in pediatric population and young adults. The exact etiopathogenesis of congenital splenic cysts is unknown. In general, these cysts are asymptomatic. Symptoms develop due to increase in size, trauma, hemorrhage, rupture or infection of the cyst.

When symptomatic, surgery in the form of partial or total splenectomy is the treatment of choice.

On USG, these cysts are generally anechoic, or may show fine internal echoes. CT shows splenic cysts as being characteristically spherical and well-defined lesions **(Figs. 14A to C)**. Attenuation value of near water and a thin or imperceptible nonenhancing wall are other features of a congenital cyst.[22] Internal debris, hemorrhage and peripheral calcifications of the cyst wall may give a more complex picture.

Epidermoid cyst **(Figs. 14D to G)** has a complex imaging appearance due to epithelial peripheral trabeculations causing thickening and irregularity of the posterior wall and due to presence of internal blood clots.

False Cyst (Pseudocyst)

False cysts/pseudocysts are lined by dense fibrous tissue which is often calcified and have no epithelial lining, and account for approximately 75% of the cysts of the spleen.[21] Trauma, infarction or infection are common causes. The most apparent etiologic factor is trauma. The majority of these cysts are solitary and asymptomatic. Cyst contains mostly blood and necrotic debris. It is often not possible to differentiate between primary and secondary cysts based on radiological appearance alone. Patient's history and clinical presentation may sometimes help to narrow the differential diagnosis.

Echinococcal Cyst

Splenic involvement by hydatid disease is uncommon. It can be seen in endemic areas. Clinical findings are nonspecific and patient may present with abdominal pain, fever and splenomegaly.

Ultrasonography demonstrates a cystic lesion which is either anechoic or with internal debris, membranes, daughter cysts or calcification depending upon the stage of cyst growth.

The three layers of hydatid cyst consist of the following:

1. The outer pericyst, composed of modified host cells that form a dense and fibrous protective zone.

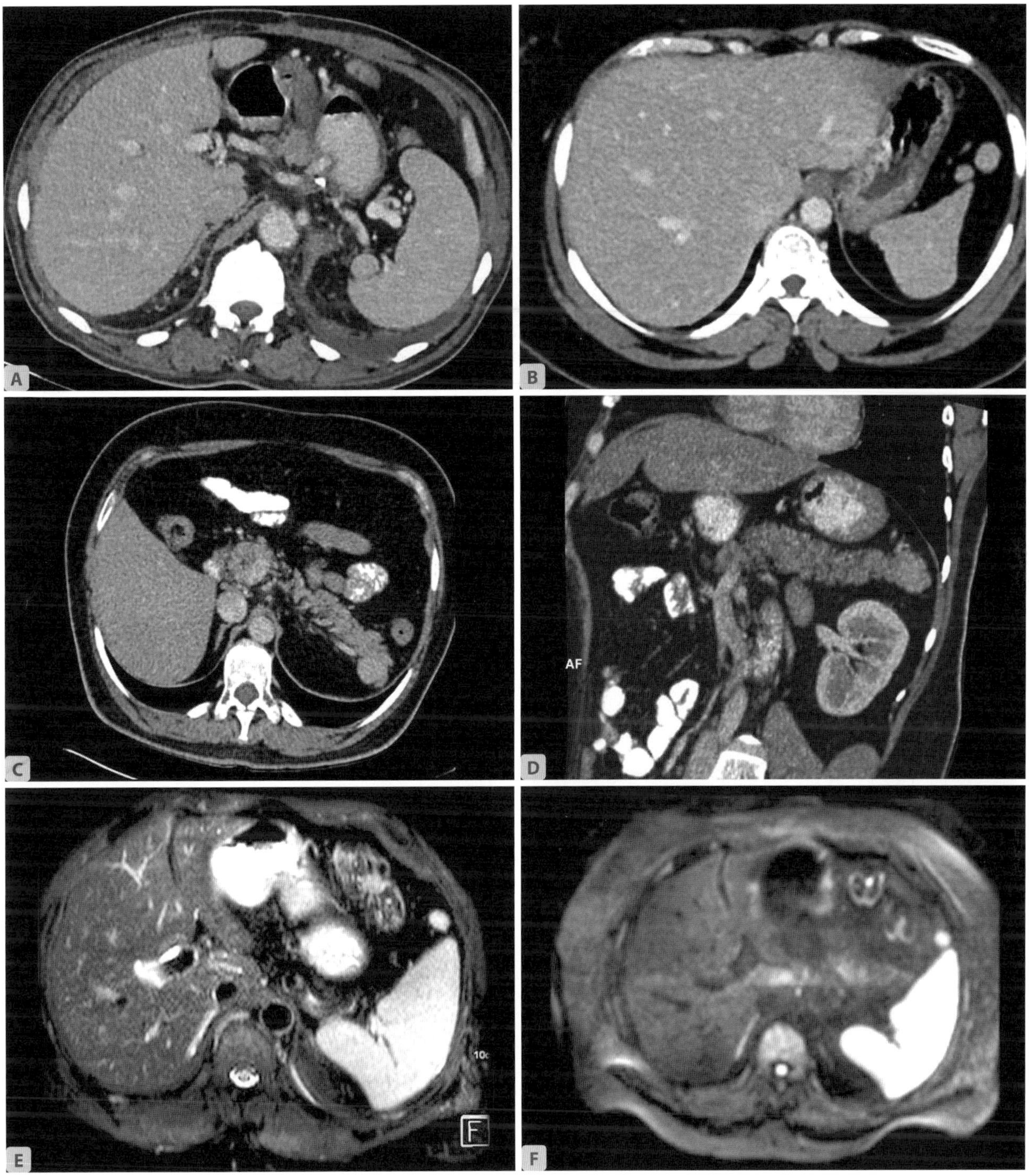

FIGS. 11A TO F: Axial contrast-enhanced CT images showing small rounded nodular well-defined structures having same enhancement as spleen at hilum (A), near pole (B) and within pancreatic parenchyma (C and D). Axial T2WI MRI image (E) and b-1000 diffusion-weighted image (F) reveals splenunculus showing similar T2 hyperintensity and restricted diffusion respectively as adjacent normal spleen.

2. Middle laminated layer, which is also referred to as ectocyst, allows passage of nutrients.
3. Inner germinal layer, where the scolices (the larval stage of the parasite) and the laminated membrane are produced. The true wall of the cyst is formed by this inner most germinal layer.

Daughter cysts are small spherical vesicles formed from rest of the germinal layer and contain the protoscolices. Cyst fluid secreted by the germinal layer is antigenic and may also contain scolices. When vesicles rupture within the cyst, scolices are mixed with cyst fluid and form white sediment known as hydatid sand.

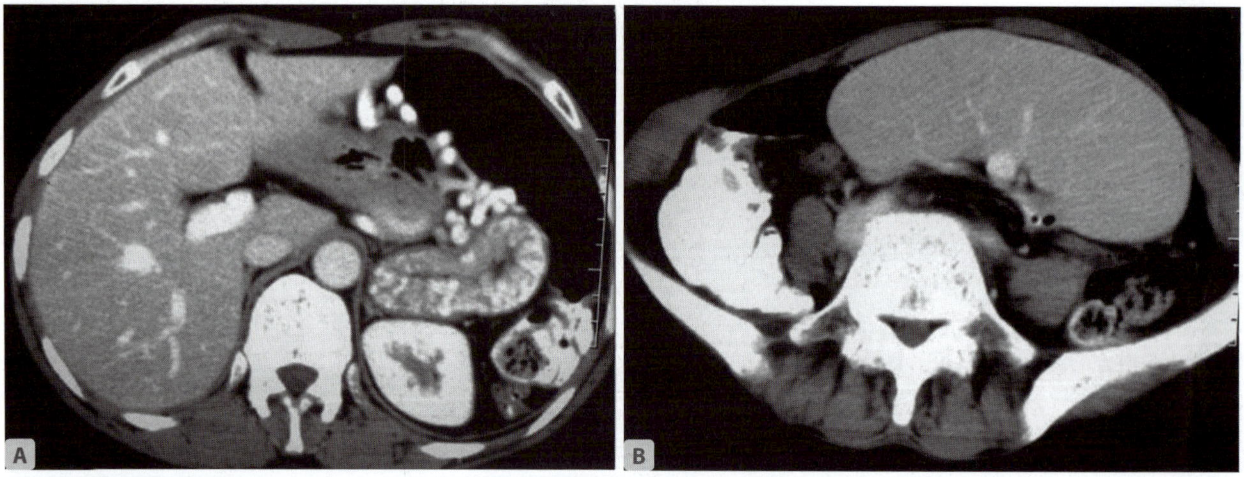

FIGS. 12A AND B: Axial contrast-enhanced CT showing absence of spleen in left upper abdomen (A) with centrally and inferiorly located spleen in lower abdomen (B). Follow-up USG revealed changing positions of spleen (not shown).

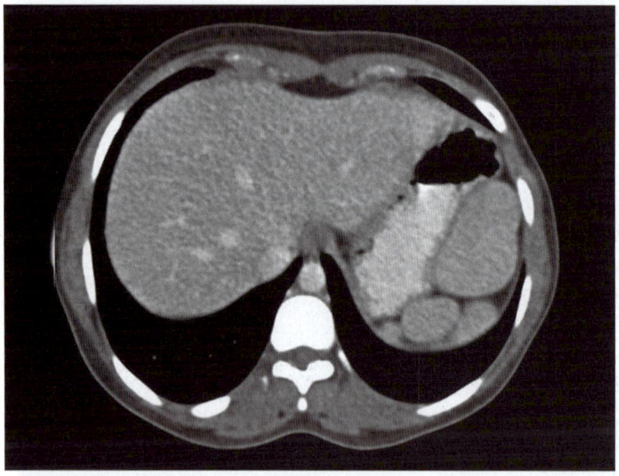

FIG. 13: Axial contrast-enhanced CT showing multiple small splenic masses in left subphrenic region suggestive of polysplenia.

Imaging features on USG, CT or MRI depend on stage of growth of the cyst, i.e. whether it is unilocular, have daughter vesicles, partially calcified or completely calcified signifying a dead parasite.

The ultrasonographic appearance of hydatid cysts are:

i. A well-defined anechoic cyst **(Fig. 15C)**.
ii. A well-defined anechoic cyst with hydatid sand.
iii. Detachment of the endocyst from pericyst resulting in "floating membranes" within the cavity.
iv. The honeycomb pattern due to presence of daughter cysts.
v. Calcification of either cyst wall or internal matrix. Partial calcification of the cyst does not always indicate the death of the parasite, nevertheless, densely calcified cysts may be assumed to be inactive.

Infected hydatid may give an appearance of abscess with thick irregular walls and internal debris and lose its characteristic sonographic appearance.

The CT scans show the cyst as a well-defined, round or oval cystic mass of near water density **(Figs. 15A to E)**. A multilocular appearance may be seen with the presence of multiple low attenuating daughter cysts. Detached membranes can be seen as curvilinear increased attenuation areas within the cyst. Homogeneous higher attenuation within the lesion is frequently encountered and may occur secondary to the formation of daughter cysts or as a result of the collection of dense debris (hydatid sand) within the cyst. Enhancement of internal septations may be seen with contrast administration. Calcification of cyst wall or internal septa is easily detected at CT.

Splenic hydatid cysts are T1-hypointense and T2-hyperintense on MRI. Collagen makes the pericyst appear T1 and T2 hypointense and this low signal intensity rim on T2WI has been proposed as a characteristic sign of hydatid cyst. MR also demonstrates daughter cysts as hypo to isointense on T1WI and isointense on T2WI relative to hyperintense hydatid fluid of the mother cyst. The floating membranes appear as low intensity structures within the degenerating cyst. Intraparenchymal rupture of the cyst appears as a defect in the low intensity rim. Thick calcifications may produce a signal void on MR imaging, however, are better demonstrated by CT.

INFECTIOUS DISEASES OF SPLEEN

Involvement of the spleen in systemic infectious processes is commonly seen in immunocompromised patients, and the prevalence has increased as a result of the increased use of steroids and chemotherapeutic agents and human immunodeficiency virus (HIV) infection.[11] Bacteria, fungi, and *Mycobacterium tuberculosis* are frequent agents. Splenic involvement can also occur in immune-competent hosts with cat scratch disease, granulomatous diseases such as histoplasmosis, parasitic diseases such as hydatid cyst, and viral infections. Nonspecific splenomegaly can be seen in viral infections and enteric fever.

Splenic abscesses are localized collection of pus and they are found in 0.14–0.7% of autopsy cases.[23] It may be solitary, multiple, or multilocular. USG shows single or multiple hypoechoic to frankly anechoic lesions. Larger lesion may

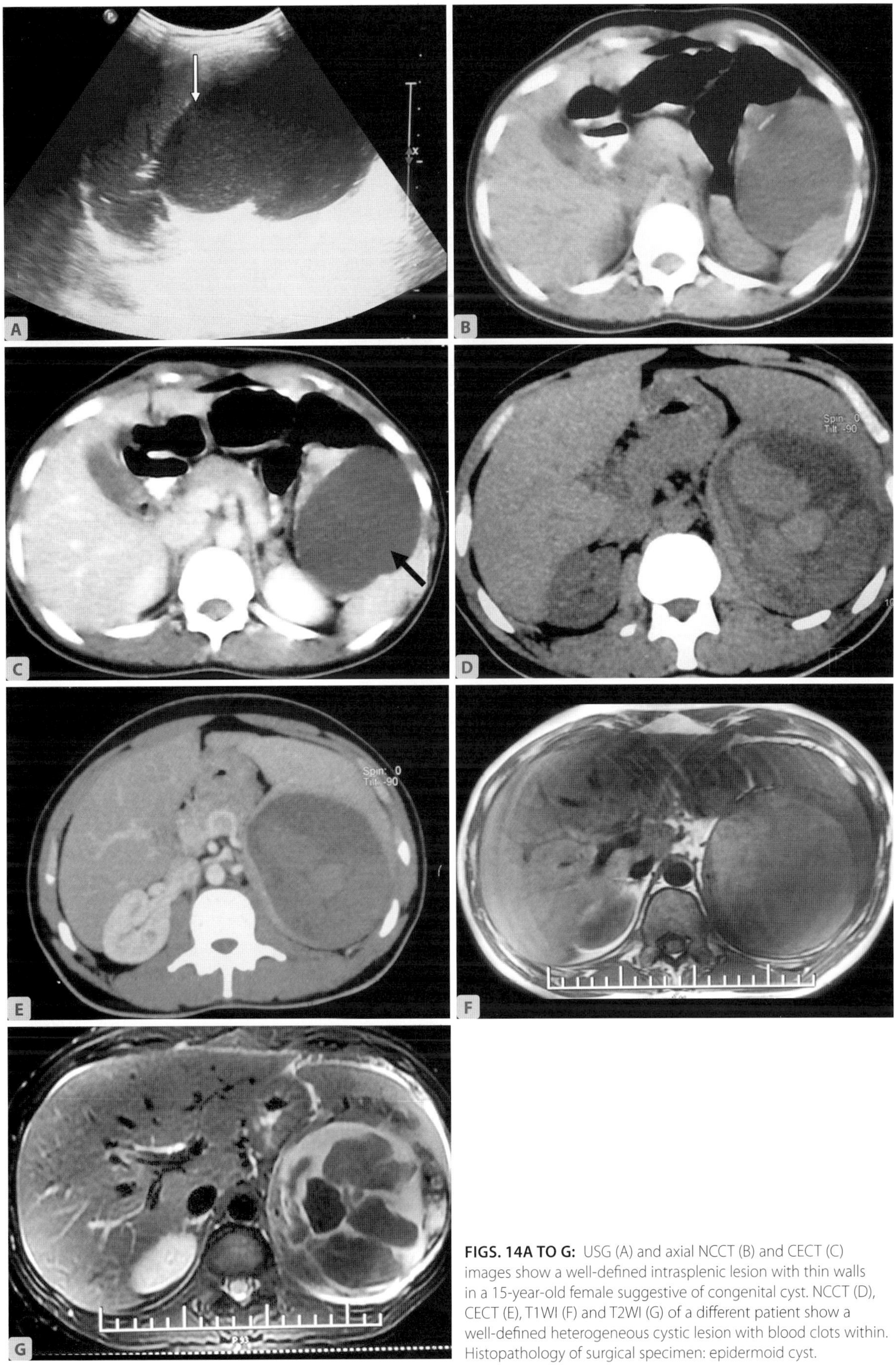

FIGS. 14A TO G: USG (A) and axial NCCT (B) and CECT (C) images show a well-defined intrasplenic lesion with thin walls in a 15-year-old female suggestive of congenital cyst. NCCT (D), CECT (E), T1WI (F) and T2WI (G) of a different patient show a well-defined heterogeneous cystic lesion with blood clots within. Histopathology of surgical specimen: epidermoid cyst.

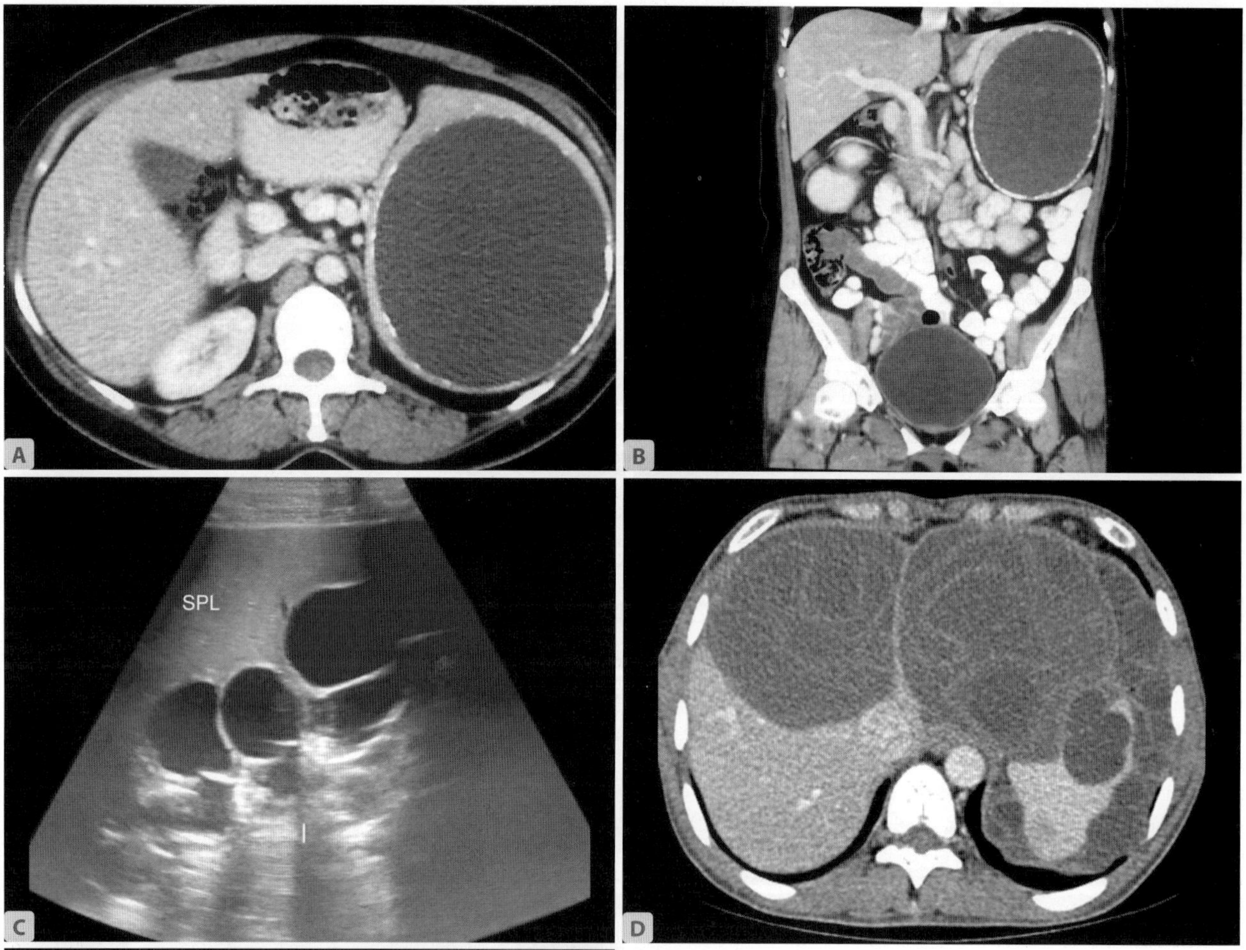

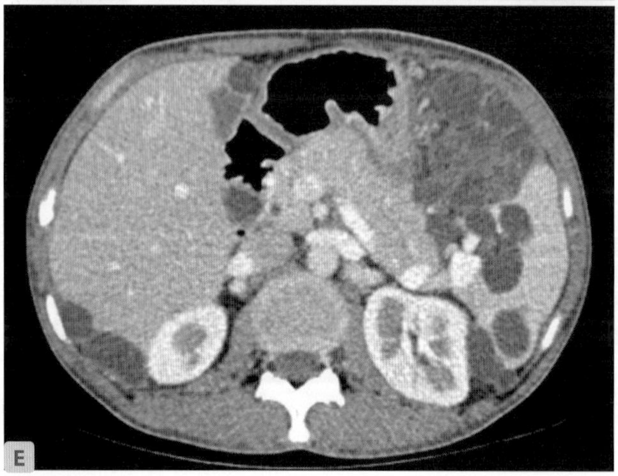

FIGS. 15A TO E: Axial (A) and coronal reformatted (B) CECT images showing well-defined unilocular cyst within spleen parenchyma. There is discontinuous peripheral calcification. At surgery, it was found to be a hydatid cyst. USG image (C) and axial CECT images (D and E) in a case of disseminated hydatidosis with liver, splenic and peritoneal involvement.

show internal echoes or septations. On CT and MR, the abscess appears as a lesion of fluid attenuation or signal intensity respectively and show peripheral enhancement on contrast administration when the capsule develops **(Figs. 16A and B)**.

Bacterial causes of splenic abscess include infection with aerobic organisms, commonly *Staphylococcus, Streptococcus, Escherichia coli* and *Salmonella*. The route of infection is mainly hematogenous (75%), penetrating trauma (15%) and prior splenic infarction (10%).[21] The factors leading to involvement of the spleen are metastatic infection (bacterial endocarditis, sepsis), contiguous infection (pancreatitis, periphrenic abscess), embolic noninfection events causing ischemia and superadded infection, trauma and immunodeficiency.[24]

On CT and MRI, the lesion shows thick, irregular, dense peripheral enhancing rim with internal nonenhancing area. Sometimes, air foci may also be seen within the bacterial abscesses. Peripheral enhancement of the wall of the abscess on a venous phase CT is less often seen than in liver abscesses.

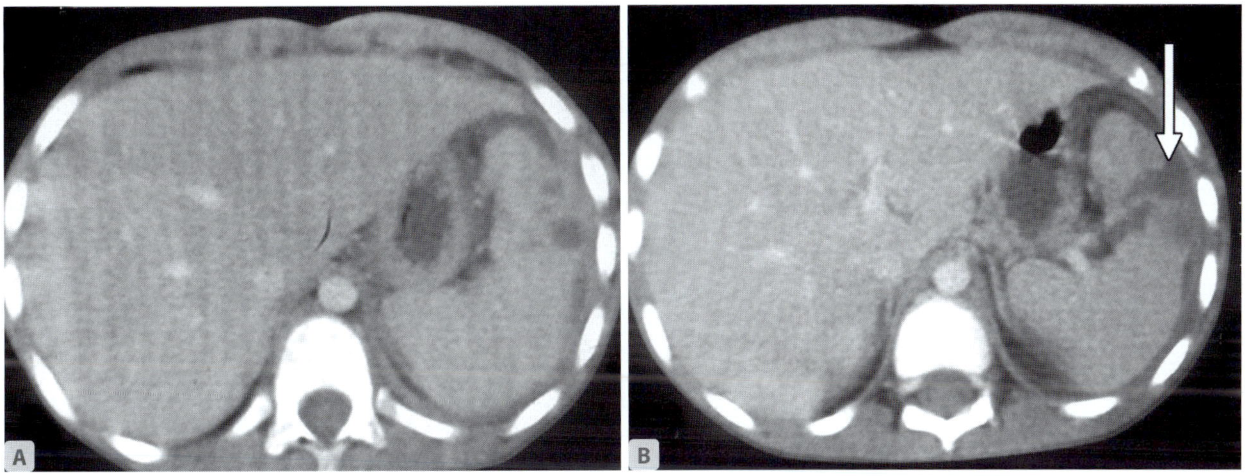

FIGS. 16A AND B: Axial CECT images (A and B) showing multiple small peripherally enhancing lesions in spleen suggestive of abscesses. Presence of perisplenic fluid (arrow) indicates rupture.

Post-gadolinium MRI is more sensitive to depict the rim enhancement.

Fungal abscesses are mainly seen in immunocompromised patients including post solid organ transplantation, patients on chemotherapy for malignancy or leukemia and children with immunodeficiency, such as chronic granulomatous disease. *Candida albicans, Aspergillus fumigatus,* and *Cryptococcus neoformans* are the commonly encountered fungi. Fungal infection of the spleen are mostly due to hematogenous spread and form microabscesses in the splenic parenchyma which may not be detectable on imaging at times even in the presence of disseminated infection and may only present with diffuse splenomegaly. When visible on CT, fungal abscesses are seen as multiple well-defined small hypoattenuating lesions and vary from few millimeters to 2 cm in size. Rim enhancement is usually not seen. Occasionally, CT may demonstrate a wheel within a wheel pattern/bulls-eye (e.g. Candidial infection) or a central focus of higher attenuation corresponding to ultrasound findings (echoic lesion with central hypoechoic nidus due to necrosis containing fungal elements). Histoplasmosis of the spleen demonstrates multiple scattered hypointense lesions on both T1 and T2WI on MRI **(Figs. 17A to D)**. Old granulomas can be calcified.

Splenic involvement is seen in 80–100% of autopsies of disseminated Tuberculosis since it has a rich network of reticuloendothelial cells.[25] Three forms of splenic involvement include splenomegaly, micronodular/miliary or macronodular form. USG may show normal spleen or mild heterogeneous echotexture whereas CT may demonstrate multiple low-density intrasplenic foci with nodules that range from 0.5 mm to 2.0 mm in diameter in the micronodular form of disease **(Figs. 18A to D)**. Macronodular form manifests as solitary or multifocal 1–3 cm sized lesions which are hypodense on CT **(Figs. 19A to F)**, and sometimes show peripheral rim of enhancement and may demonstrate calcification. MRI features vary depending on the stage of evolution of tuberculomas. A tuberculoma with central caseous necrosis appears as a centrally nonenhancing lesion with peripheral enhancement and this is one of their typical features. Such caseous necrosis might show hypointensity or hyperintensity on T2WI. The reason for the variable signal on T2WI is not clearly understood; however, internal hypointensity could suggest more solid caseation **(Fig. 19C)**.[26] Lesions with no central caseous necrosis may demonstrate gradual peripheral enhancement with complete fill-in of the lesions. Other imaging findings may be abdominal lymphadenopathy with low central attenuation, high-attenuation ascites with nodular peritoneal thickening, hepatomegaly, and pleural effusion. Other organ involvement or presence of necrotic lymph nodes makes a diagnosis of tuberculosis more certain.

It is difficult to distinguish between tubercular, pyogenic and disseminated fungal infections as well as leukemic and lymphomatous infiltration. Fine needle aspiration cytology (FNAC) from splenic focal lesions is required to reach a definitive diagnosis if there is no other focus of tuberculosis or in case of non-responders to treatment.

Splenic Infarcts

Splenic infarcts are a relatively common entity. It is usually secondary to arterial occlusion. The various recognized causes of spleen infarct are arterial embolism, massive splenomegaly secondary to myeloproliferative disorders or hematological malignancies, storage disorders, lymphoma, portal hypertension, torsion, infectious mononucleosis, etc. Imaging findings of splenic infarct depend upon the 'age of infarct'. On USG, it is seen as an ill-defined hypoechoic area in acute phase which progressively becomes more well defined. In later stage, secondary to fibrosis and calcification it may appear as hyperechoic area also. Splenic rupture and superimposed infection are complications seen in the areas of infarction.[9]

CT is the imaging investigation of choice for evaluation of splenic infarcts. Imaging should be performed in portal venous phase images, which reveal better depiction of the infarcted areas.

On CT, various imaging findings are described for infarcts. There are multiple, heterogeneous areas of patchy

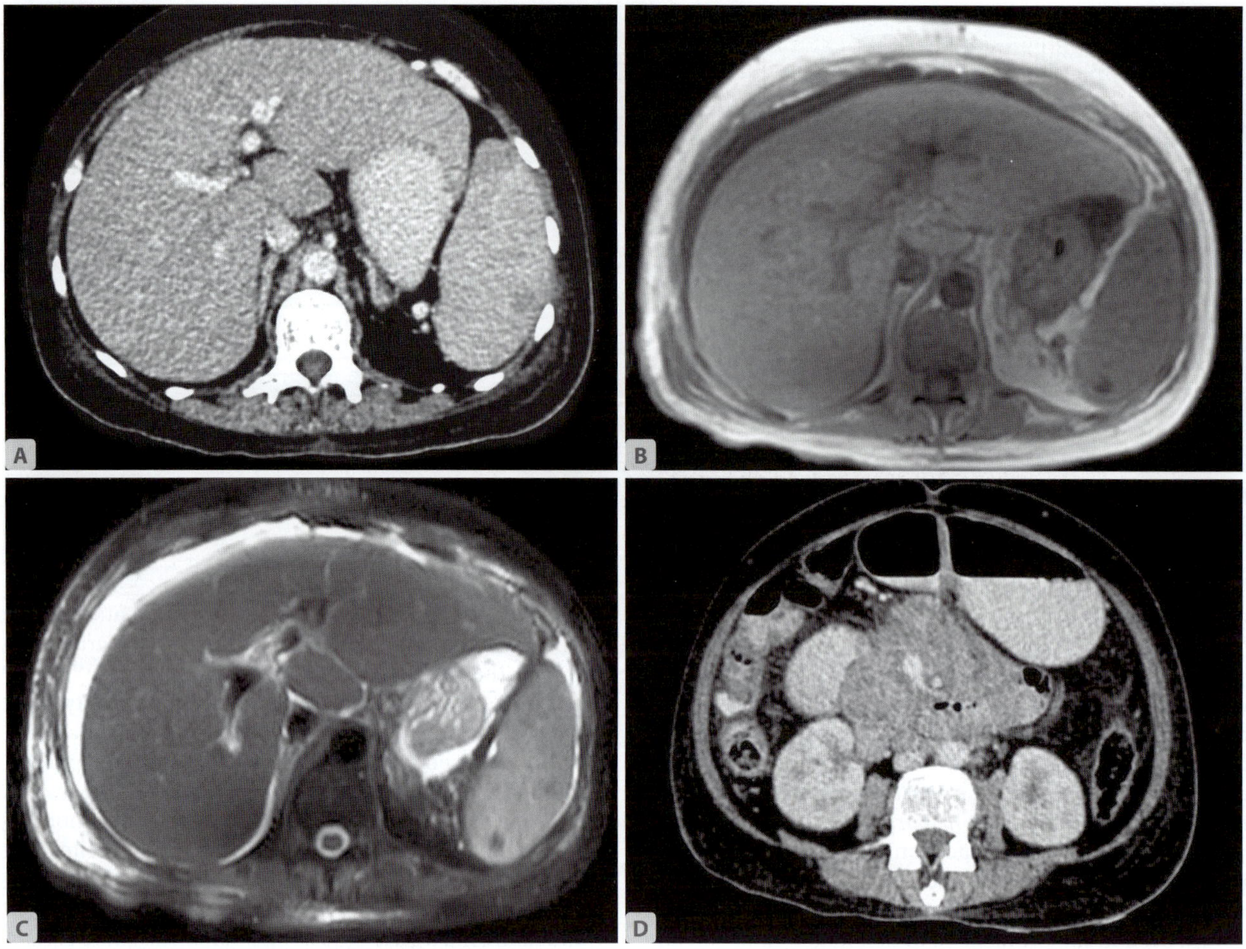

FIGS. 17A TO D: Axial CECT image (A) showing ill-defined focal lesions in spleen. Axial T1WI (B) and T2WI (C) shows hypointense lesions on both sequences. Axial CECT image (D) showing multiple lymph nodes with necrosis—Biopsy proven histoplasmosis.

enhancement in acute phase. Typical peripheral, wedge-shaped nonenhancing or hypoenhancing area is seen with further progression with time **(Fig. 20A)**. Entire splenic parenchyma may not be enhancing, e.g. in splenic torsion. With time, the infarcted area may decrease and sometimes may vanish entirely or may remain as a cystic lesion (pseudocyst).

The MRI shows various signal intensity in splenic infarct based on its chronicity and composition. If infarct is hemorrhagic, it may appear as hyperintense on T1 as well as T2WI. Chronic infarcts will be relatively well defined; wedge shaped and usually have hypointense signal on T1WI and hyperintense signal on T2WI **(Figs. 20A to H)**.[27]

Trauma

Please refer to chapter on Abdominal Trauma for full discussion of splenic trauma.

Splenic Rupture

Splenic rupture most commonly occurs secondary to significant trauma. However, there are many uncommon cause of splenic rupture other than trauma.[28] This condition of atraumatic splenic rupture has been variously described as 'spontaneous', 'pathological' or 'occult' splenic rupture. Practically, it refers to rupture of spleen in the absence of any perceivable significant injury to spleen. Various causes of atraumatic splenic rupture are malaria, leukemia, lymphomas, secondary to pancreatitis, congestive splenomegaly, amyloidosis, infectious mononucleosis or splenic abscess, etc.

Exact pathogenesis of truly idiopathic splenic rupture (with causes unknown) is still not clear. Majority of these patients have associated splenomegaly. Imaging findings associated with splenic rupture are commonly similar to cases of post-traumatic splenic rupture, however, the incidence of splenomegaly is more common in these atraumatic patients. On USG, fluid with internal echoes is seen in perisplenic area and peritoneal cavity. Other findings may be subcapsular hematoma and hypoechoic splenic laceration. CECT will depict similar findings **(Figs. 21A and B)**. On arterial phase CT images, sometimes areas of active extravasation may be seen which signifies ongoing active bleed. MRI may be helpful in deciding the 'age' of hematoma. Majority of these patients are treated by surgery.

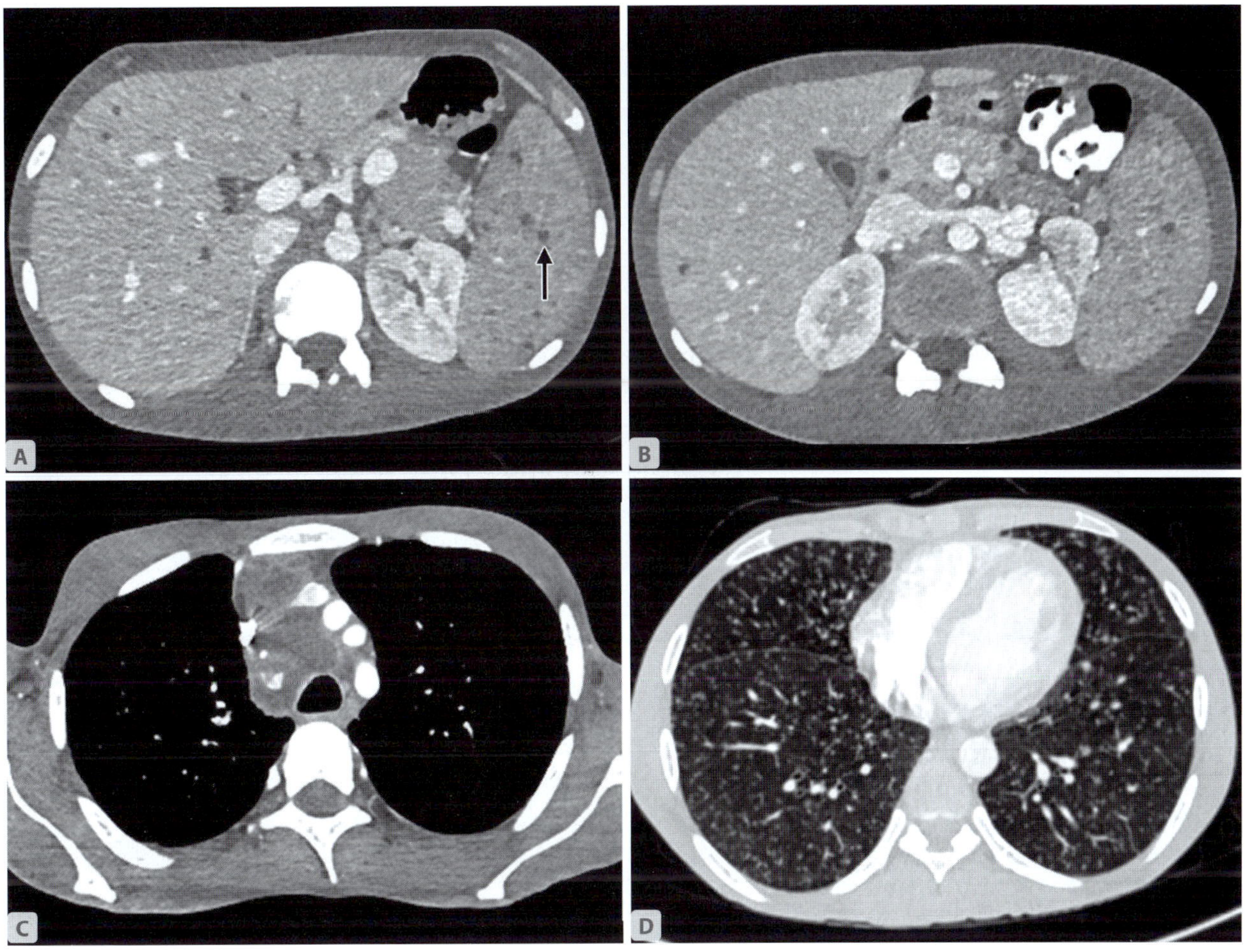

FIGS. 18A TO D: Axial CECT images (A and B) of 20-year-male patient with disseminated tuberculosis showing multiple diffusely scattered tiny hypodense lesions in spleen (arrow). Similar lesions also noted in liver and pancreas. Mediastinal (C) and lung window images (D) showing necrotic lymph nodes and miliary nodules respectively.

SPLENIC NEOPLASMS

Splenic neoplasms can be divided into benign and malignant neoplasms. Among the benign lesions, hemangioma, lymphangioma, hamartoma, littoral cell angioma, peliosis and inflammatory pseudotumors are common. Among the malignant lesions, metastasis, lymphoma and angiosarcoma are common entities.

Benign Neoplasms

Hemangioma

Hemangioma is the most common benign primary neoplasm of spleen with prevalence ranging from 0.3–14%.[29] Most hemangiomas are small in size and detected incidentally on imaging. When large, it may present with pain in left hypochondrium with presence of palpable non tender mass. Splenic hemangiomatosis may occur in cases with generalized angiomatosis, like Klippel-Trenaunay syndrome.[30] Spontaneous rupture may occur in 25% of the patients having large hemangiomas.[31]

On USG, they are seen as echogenic solid or cystic lesions which are iso to hypodense on unenhanced CT. Hemangioma can be capillary and cavernous on histology. The cavernous hemangiomas have solid isodense component which show enhancement on contrast administration while cystic component remains hypodense **(Fig. 22)**. Peripheral punctuate calcification may be seen on CT. On MRI, the lesions are hyperintense relative to spleen on T2WI and hypo-to isointense on T1WI. After injection of gadolinium, three patterns of enhancement have been described: (a) immediate homogeneous enhancement which persists, (b) early peripheral enhancement with delayed uniform enhancement, and (c) peripheral enhancement which progresses centripetally with presence of enhancing central fibrous scar.[32]

Lymphangioma

Lymphangioma is a congenital malformation of lymphatic system that occurs most commonly in neck, mediastinum and retroperitoneum; rarely affecting the spleen.[33] Splenic lymphangiomas are asymptomatic in majority of patients and detected incidentally. Spleen may be normal in size or enlarged and shows presence of predominantly cystic masses. These lesions are seen as anechoic to hypoechoic

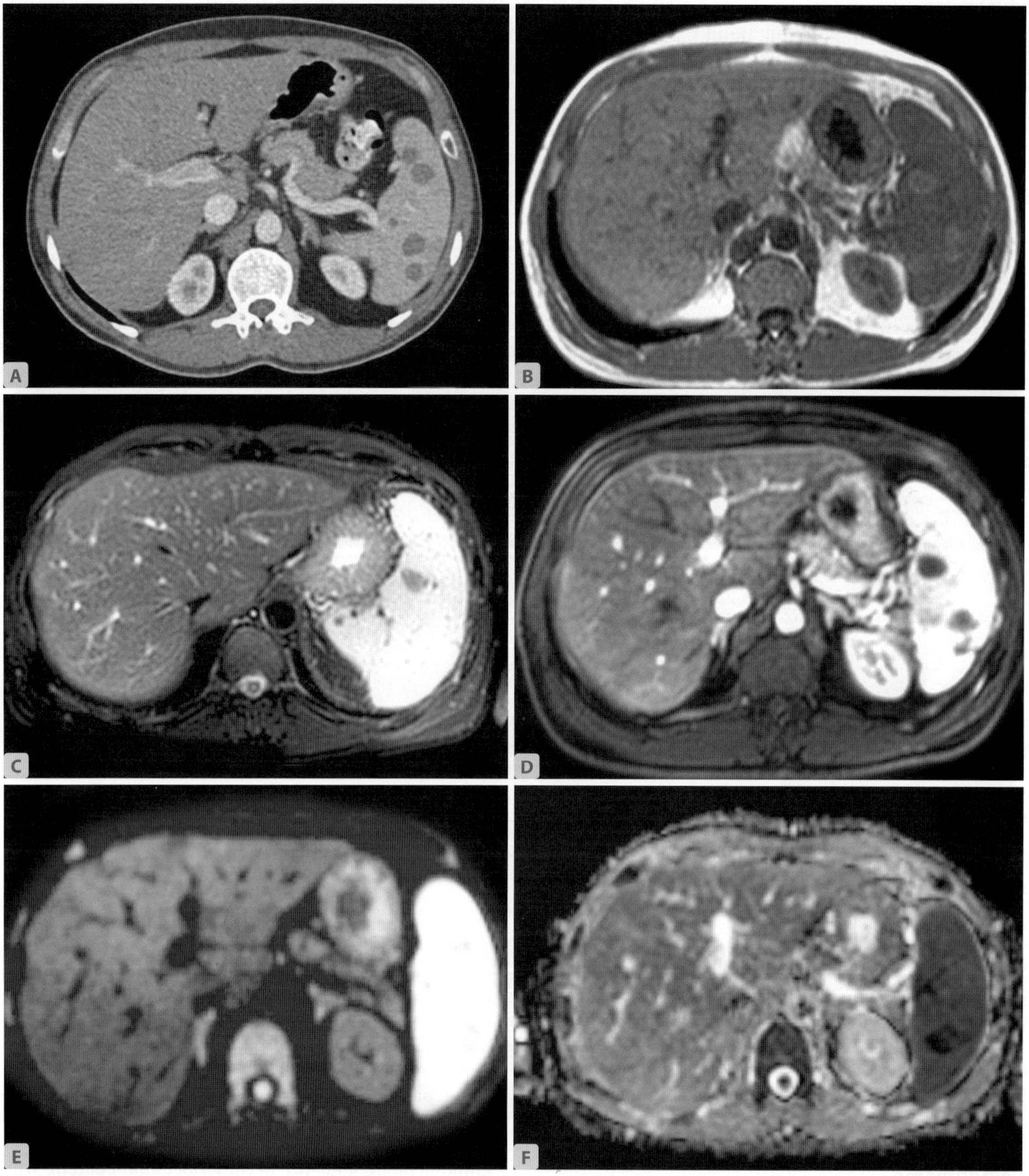

FIGS. 19A TO F: Axial CECT (A) image showing multiple large hypodense lesions in spleen. T1WI (B), T2WI (C), Postcontrast T1WI (D), DWI (E) ADC map (F) MRI images of patient with macronodular form of tuberculosis (FNAC proven).

well defined intrasplenic cysts on USG and hypodense lesions on CT; with few showing fine internal septations **(Figs. 23A and B)** or echogenic debris within. Thin calcification may be seen along the periphery.[34] The signal intensity on MRI corresponds to simple fluid; however, the cysts containing hemorrhage and proteinaceous material demonstrate high signal intensity on T1WI.[35]

Hamartoma

Splenic hamartoma is rare benign neoplasm, which is composed of malformed red pulp elements without organized lymphoid follicles. Incidence in autopsy series is estimated to be 0.024–0.13%.[36] Most patients have no symptoms and the lesion is detected incidentally.

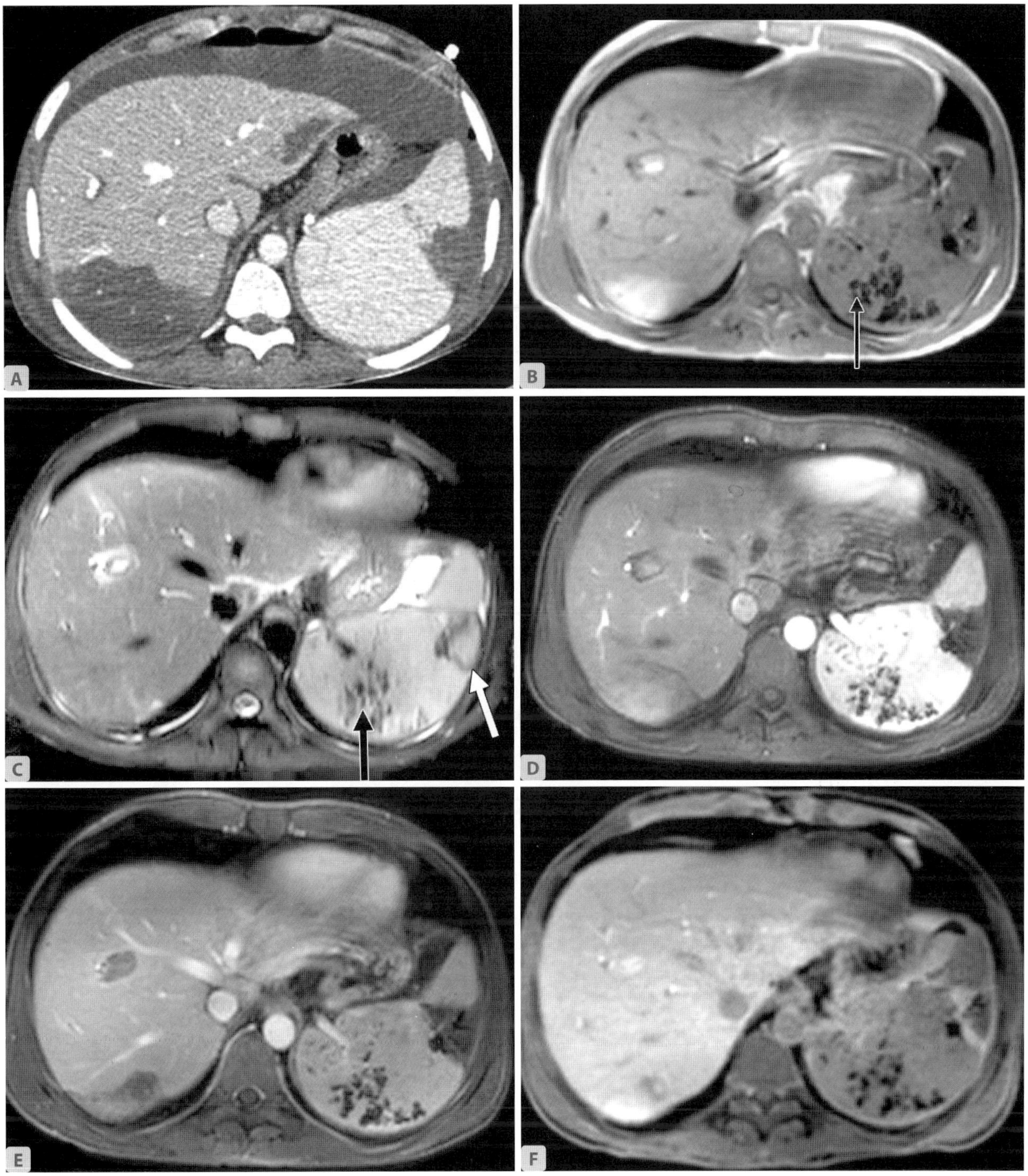

FIGS. 20A TO F *Continued*

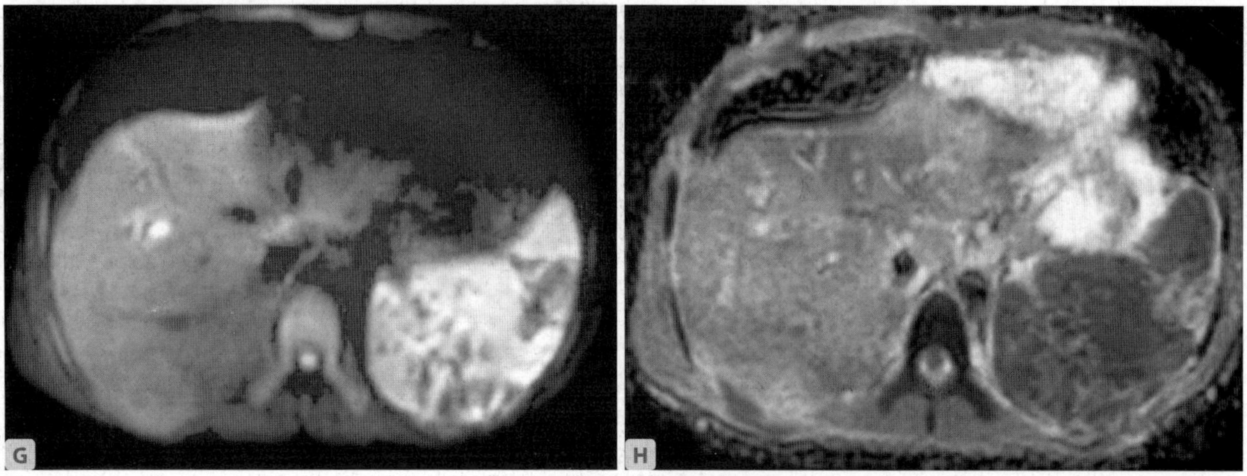

FIGS. 20A TO H: Contrast-enhanced CT scan (A) showing peripheral wedge-shaped hypodensity in spleen suggestive of infarct. Incidentally liver infarct is also seen. T1WI (hyperintense) (B) and T2WI (C) (hyperintense with hypointense rim) respectively showing peripheral wedge-shaped altered signal intensity (white arrow). Multiple T1 and T2 hypointense Gamna-Gandy bodies are also noted (black arrow). Arterial (D) venous (E) and delayed (F) MR images showing nonenhancing area with peripheral enhancement on delayed phase. DWI (G) and ADC map (H) showing no restriction (suggestive of chronic infarct—3 months).

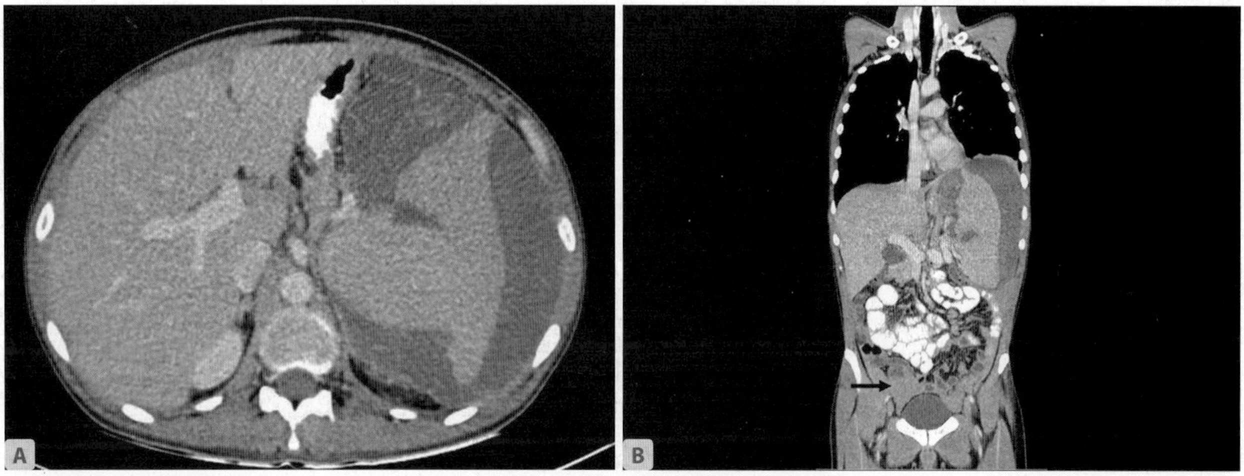

FIGS. 21A AND B: Axial (A) and coronal-reformatted (B) CECT images showing laceration in the medial margin of an enlarged spleen with perisplenic hematoma and hemoperitoneum (arrow) in a patient with high-grade fever and splenomegaly. No history of trauma was present suggestive of spontaneous splenic rupture.

On USG, it is depicted as solid mass with homogeneous or heterogeneous echopattern showing intense vascularity on color Doppler owing to presence of red pulp within it. CT scan reveals homogeneous or heterogeneous low density or isodense masses causing contour deformity with or without presence of calcification and fatty component within. Persistent enhancement in delayed images has also been documented due to stagnation of contrast within the sinusoids of red pulp.[37] The lesion shows variable signal intensity on MRI depending upon the amount of fibrous content within it. The non-fibrous hamartoma is isointense on T1WI and hyperintense on T2WI and fibrous hamartoma shows iso to hyperintense signal on T1 and hypointense signal on T2WI. However, both variants show mild early enhancement after IV contrast and uniform enhancement on delayed phase.[38]

Littoral Cell Angioma

Littoral cell angioma (LCA) is a very rare neoplasm arising from cells lining the sinuses of splenic red pulp, the Littoral cells. It may be asymptomatic or may present with anemia or splenomegaly. Sonography reveals splenomegaly with heterogeneous echotexture and presence of multiple nodules which are of low or iso attenuation on non-contrast CT and demonstrate minimal delayed enhancement on post-contrast CT.[39] MRI depicts markedly hypointense signal on T1WI and T2WI due to presence of hemosiderin within the lesions.[32]

Peliosis

Peliosis is an uncommon condition, which is characterized by presence of blood filled spaces within the splenic parenchyma. It may occur in isolation or along with peliosis hepatis. Usually asymptomatic; rupture of the hemorrhagic cyst leading to intraperitoneal hemorrhage has been described. It may appear as echogenic or heteroechoic mass lesion in the left upper quadrant on USG which shows rapid enhancement on contrast-enhanced USG without any centripetal enhancement.[40] Non-contrast CT demonstrates hypodense lesions with fine internal septations which enhance significantly on contrast administration. Variable signal intensity is seen on MRI owing to blood products at different stages. Fluid-fluid level may be visualized within these cysts due to hematocrit effect.[41] Based on these imaging features, the differential diagnosis would include hemangiomatosis, angiosarcoma and lymphangioma.

Inflammatory Pseudotumor

Inflammatory pseudotumors, also known as inflammatory myofibroblastic tumor, are basically myofibroblastic neoplasms which result from unusual inflammatory response to any injury or infection. They may present with features of mass effect on surrounding structures or may remain asymptomatic. Imaging features include well circumscribed mass on USG with hetero or homogeneous enhancement on CT and there may be calcification within or a central scar which does not show enhancement. Diagnosis solely based on imaging is difficult and is mostly established after surgery.[35,39]

The other tumors like hemangioendothelioma, hemangiopericytoma, fibroma, lipoma, angiofibromas are extremely rare.

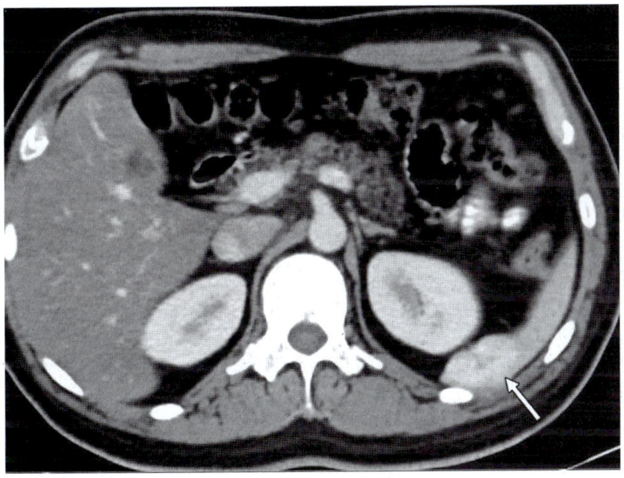

FIG. 22: Axial CECT showing an enhancing lesion in lower pole of spleen suggestive of hemangioma. Incidentally a metastatic lesion is seen in segment 5 of liver.

Malignant Neoplasms

Lymphoma

Spleen is affected in many hematological malignancies like lymphoma, leukemia, plasma cell malignancies; most common being Diffuse large B-cell lymphoma type of non-Hodgkin's lymphoma (NHL).[42] Hodgkin's lymphoma (HD) also involves the spleen in one third of patients when it is considered as nodal disease in contrast to NHL in which its infiltration is considered to be extranodal.[43] The lymphomatous involvement of spleen may be primary or secondary. Primary splenic lymphoma is rare, constituting approximately 1–2% of all lymphomas. DLBCL is the most common type in such patients[44] and magnetic resonance imaging (MRI).

On imaging, four patterns have been described: (a) homogeneous splenomegaly without any focal lesion; (b) diffuse infiltration with miliary lesions (less than 5 mm); (c) multiple focal nodular lesions (1-10 cm); and (d) large solitary mass. Li, et al. documented single large mass as the most common pattern.[44] Diffuse involvement may occur in normal sized spleen **(Fig. 25A)** and mild-to-moderate enlargement may represent reactive splenomegaly in 30% of cases.[45] However, marked splenomegaly almost always suggests infiltration.[46] Diffuse involvement of spleen is commonly seen in Hodgkin's disease due to predominant involvement of periarteriolar lymphoid sheath.[42,47] The nodules appear hypoechoic on ultrasound and hypoenhancing on contrast-enhanced CT **(Figs. 24A and B)**.[48] On MRI, the lesions are

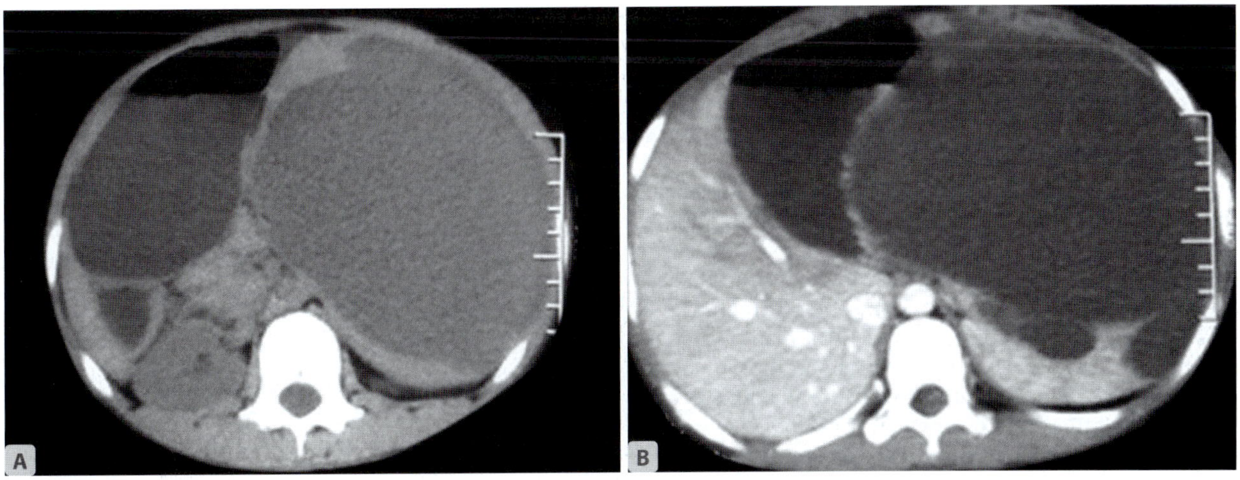

FIGS. 23A AND B: Axial NCCT (A) and CECT (B) images showing intrasplenic hypodense lesion with septations in a case of lymphangioma.

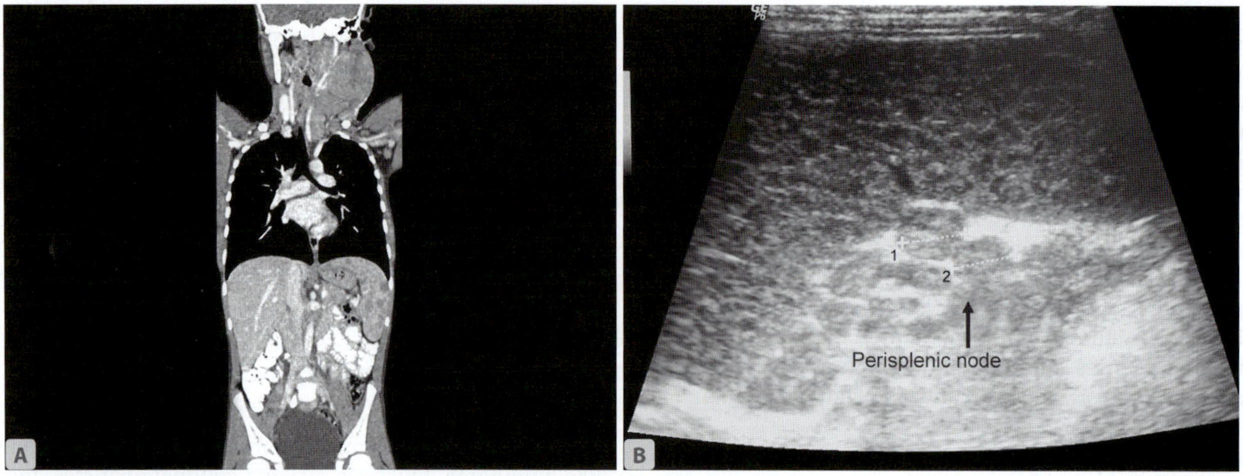

FIGS. 24A AND B: Coronal reformatted CECT image (A) showing bulky cervical lymphadenopathy and multiple lesions seen in the spleen in a case of Hodgkin's lymphoma. USG image (B) in a different patient of NHL showing multiple small hypoechoic nodular lesions diffusely distributed in the splenic parenchyma. Note is made of multiple homogeneous, non-necrotic perisplenic lymph nodes (arrow).

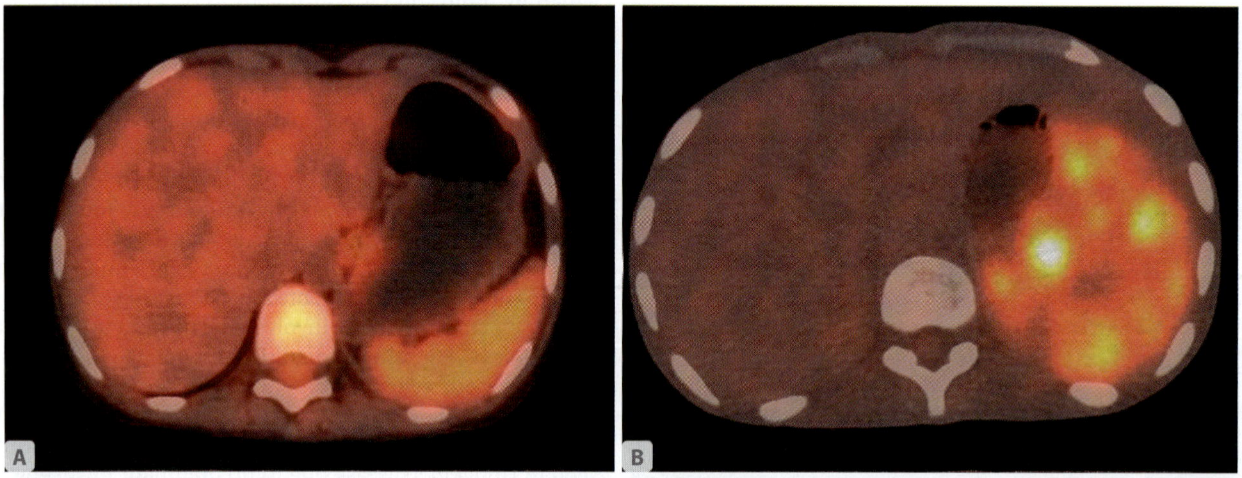

FIGS. 25A AND B: ^{18}F FDG PET-CT image showing diffuse involvement (A) and focal nodules (B) in patient of NHL as areas of avid uptake of FDG.

hyperintense on T2WI, iso to hypointense on T1WI and show reduced enhancement on contrast administration.[11]

^{18}FDG PET/CT is considered superior to CT in staging and restaging of lymphoma by virtue of detecting FDG avid normal sized nodes and detection of extranodal sites like liver, spleen **(Figs. 25A and B)** and bone marrow.[43] Sensitivity and specificity of CT, PET and PET/CT have been reported to be 91% and 96%, 75% and 99%, and 100% and 95%, respectively in a series of 111 patients.[49] Hence, for the staging of patients with FDG-avid, potentially curable lymphomas (e.g. diffuse large B-cell lymphoma and Hodgkin disease), PET is recommended routinely to delineate the disease extent more accurately and monitor response to therapy.[43] In lymphoma patients, the post-therapy inflammatory changes may persist for up to 2 weeks after chemotherapy alone and for up to 2–3 months or longer after radiation therapy or chemoradiotherapy. Thus to avoid false positive results, PET scans should not be performed for at least 3 weeks, and preferably 6–8 weeks, after completion of therapy.[50,51]

Angiosarcoma

Splenic angiosarcoma is a rare and aggressive neoplasm, which arises from the splenic vascular endothelium and the mesothelial cells of the sinusoids.[52] It is considered to be the most common primary non-lymphoid neoplasm of spleen with an estimated annual incidence of 0.14–0.25 cases per million persons.[53] The exact etiopathogenesis is unknown; although, it has been postulated that the benign splenic tumors such as hemangioma and lymphangioma may act as precursors. It presents with upper abdominal pain in 80% of patients and anemia in 75–81%.[52] Angiosarcoma of spleen is a fatal neoplasm and may present as splenic rupture in 13–32% of cases.[53] It is associated with high rate of metastases at the time of presentation (69–100%); liver being the most common site followed by lungs, lymph nodes and bone.[54] Early diagnosis and splenectomy is the treatment of choice with less defined role of chemoradiotherapy. Despite prompt measures, it has a dismal prognosis.

There is limited literature available on the imaging features of angiosarcoma in the form of anecdotal case reports and few case series. Splenomegaly with heterogeneous mass is seen in 60% cases on all imaging modalities.[55] On ultrasound, it appears as solid-cystic mass in an enlarged spleen with mixed echogenicity. CT demonstrates single or multiple masses, which show mixed attenuation and ill-defined margins. Nonenhancing areas represent necrosis and active contrast blush is seen in the areas of active bleeding. Areas of active hemorrhage appear hyperdense on non-contrast CT and the lesions may show peripheral enhancement after contrast administration.[55] On MRI, the nodules are hypointense on T1 and T2WI relative to splenic parenchyma; however, hyperintense signal may be seen due to presence of hemorrhage or necrosis within. Chronic hemorrhage leading to hemosiderin deposition causes reduction in signal intensity. The pattern of contrast enhancement includes peripheral nodular enhancement with nonenhancing areas due to necrosis or hemorrhage.[55]

Metastases

Splenic metastases occur mostly in the setting of multisystem metastatic disease. The prevalence ranges from 1.3% to 7.1%, reported in autopsy series.[56] It has been postulated that the relative lower incidence of splenic metastases is due to innate hostile environment for malignant invasion, the reticuloendothelial system inhibiting tumor cell seeding and lack of afferent lymphatics.[57] Agha Mohammadi, et al. reported gynecological malignancy to be the most common primary neoplasm followed by colorectal, lung and gastric cancer associated with splenic metastases.[58] The lesions are hypodense on imaging with majority being lobulated, well-defined, nonenhancing nodules on CT **(Figs. 26A to C)**.[59] On MRI, the lesions typically appear as hyperintense on T2WI and hypo- to isointense on T1WI.[11]

SPLENIC INTERVENTIONS FNAC AND BIOPSY OF SPLEEN

Fine needle aspiration cytology (FNAC) of spleen is a relatively safe procedure. Common indications of performing FNAC in spleen are infectious diseases, sarcoidosis and neoplastic conditions like metastases. Uncommonly, FNAC is also performed to rule out storage disorders, amyloidosis, hemophagocytic syndrome and primary splenic benign and malignant diseases. In India because of very high prevalence of tuberculosis, focal splenic lesions even in patients of a known malignancy may be infective in nature. This is a relatively common clinical scenario for performing FNAC to differentiate these two possibilities.

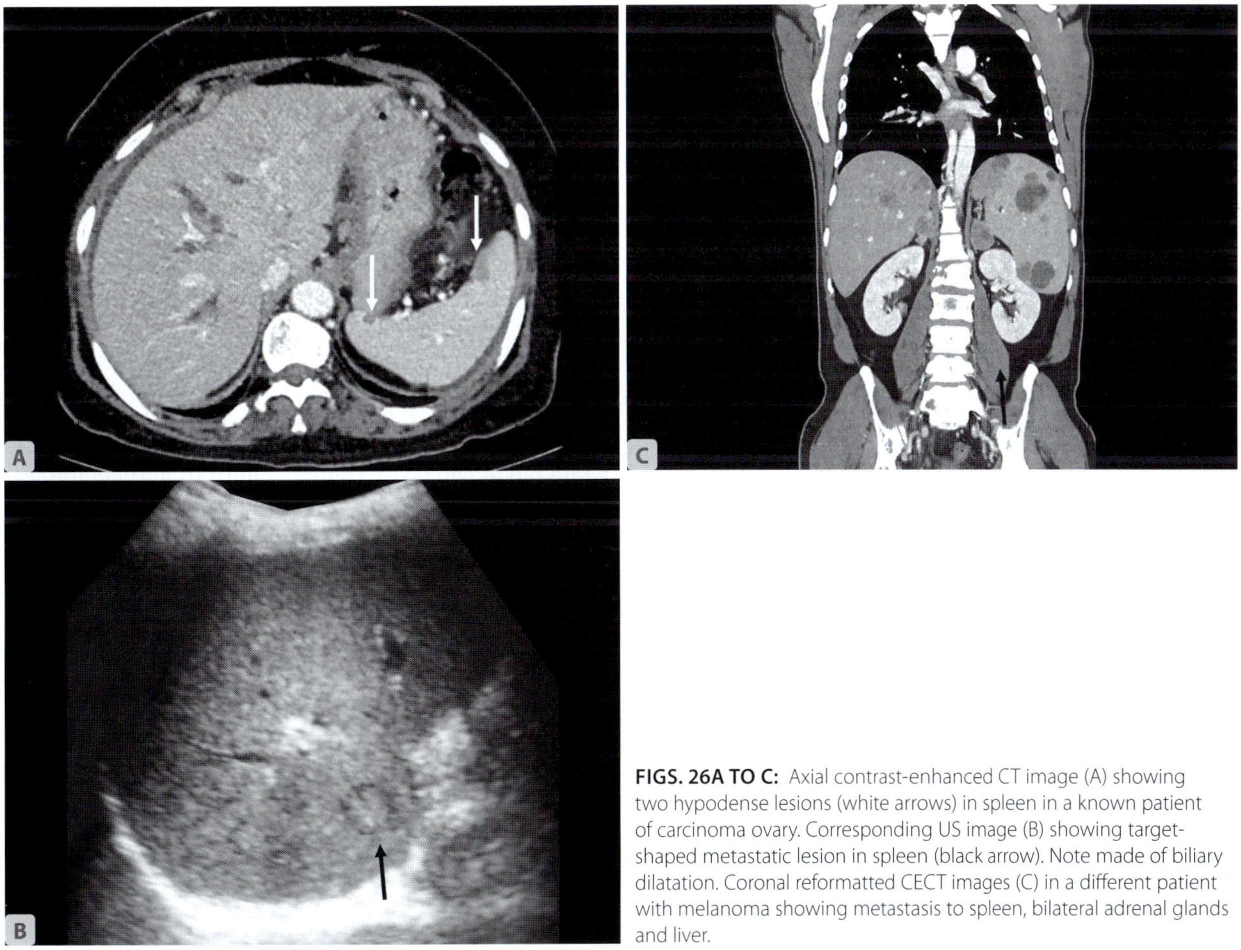

FIGS. 26A TO C: Axial contrast-enhanced CT image (A) showing two hypodense lesions (white arrows) in spleen in a known patient of carcinoma ovary. Corresponding US image (B) showing target-shaped metastatic lesion in spleen (black arrow). Note made of biliary dilatation. Coronal reformatted CECT images (C) in a different patient with melanoma showing metastasis to spleen, bilateral adrenal glands and liver.

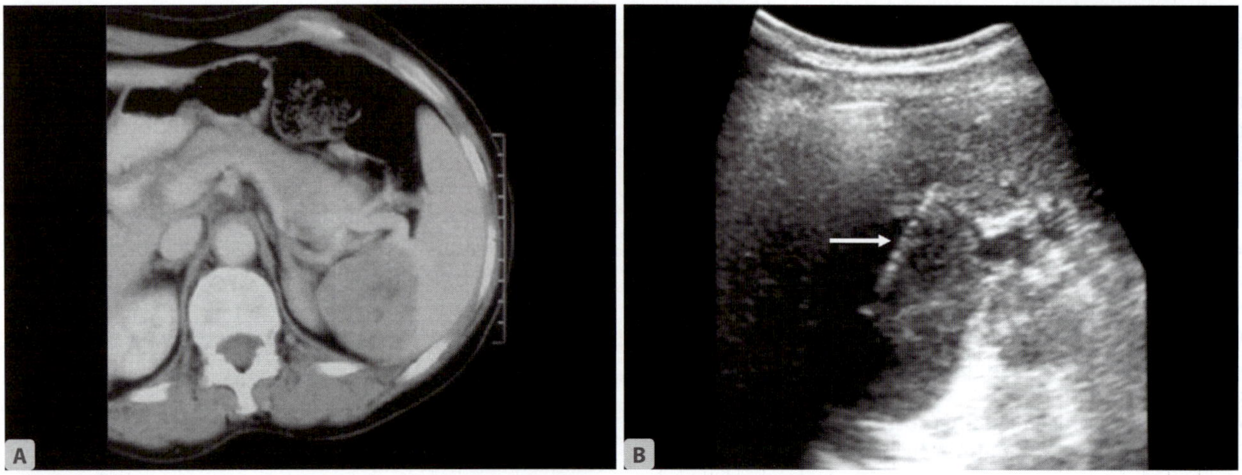

FIGS. 27A AND B: Axial CECT image (A) showing focal hypodense mass lesion in spleen. USG-guided FNAC procedure (B) showing echogenic needle in situ (arrow). FNAC was reported as NHL.

There is a reluctance to do guided interventions in spleen because of potential risk of hemorrhage that may necessitate urgent splenectomy. However, with the use of thinner gauge biopsy needles for splenic biopsy, the risk of complication is similar to risk associated with other large organ biopsies.[60]

Major indications of performing FNAC or biopsy in spleen are to evaluate a solid or cystic lesion or to evaluate splenomegaly of uncertain etiology. Most common indication for splenic biopsy is suspicion of lymphoma or presence of splenic lesion in a patient who is already known to have some primary malignancy apart from spleen.[61,62]

A significant percentage of patients of lymphomas (HD as well as NHL) have involvement of the spleen.[61] Another important consideration is that splenic involvement in lymphoma has got prognostic importance and overall treatment of the patient changes according to whether spleen is involved or not.

It is important to consider the fact that if metastasis is also present at some other site in addition to spleen, then it is advisable to obtain biopsy from these accessible sites.[63]

Whenever chances of bleeding are high, e.g. in presence of coagulopathy, it is advisable to obtain FNAC rather than core biopsy. FNAC is normally performed with 20–23 G Chiba needle **(Figs. 27A and B)**, which has safer profile compared to core biopsy which is done with 14–18 G needles. However, it is important to note that FNAC is not useful in evaluation of lymphoma because the obtained sample is usually insufficient to further subtype lymphomas. With the advent of specific targeted chemotherapeutic agents of different subtypes of lymphoma, it is essential to provide larger tissues to pathologist for subtyping, which directly results in better selection of chemotherapeutic regimen. Additional samples are taken for flow cytometry if lymphoma is one of the clinical possibilities.

Contraindications for splenic biopsy or drainage are uncorrectable coagulopathy, lack of safe access route and uncooperative patient. For biopsy, minimal caliber needle should be chosen which can give sufficient diagnostic yield so as to decrease chances of post-procedural bleed. It is advisable to traverse some normal splenic tissue before obtaining access to the target lesion in spleen to help decrease bleeding by way of tamponade effect. Frequent hemodynamic monitoring and placing the patient in left lateral decubitus is advisable.

Drainage

Drainage of splenic abscess is done uncommonly for tubercular, fungal or bacterial abscesses which are more common in patient with altered immunity status.[64]

The success rate of percutaneous drainage for splenic abscess is more than 80%[63,65,66] with reduced success in presence of loculations and multiple internal septations. Usually collections less than 3 cm^3 can be managed by single time needle aspiration only.[67] If lesion is bigger than 3 cm^3 then drainage is usually considered. Seldinger techniques as well as tandem trocar techniques, both are feasible for splenic drainage. Normally, 8–10 F pigtail catheters are selected, however, if on initial aspiration thick pus is aspirated it should be drained with bigger pigtail catheter (e.g. 12–14 F). Intermittent (every 8 hour) flushing of the catheter with 10 mL of saline helps in improving the patency of catheters. If the drainage from catheter drops to less than 10 mL/24 h, white blood cell (WBC) counts return to normal and fever subsides, then catheter removal should be planned. Repeat USG screening is useful before removing catheter to rule put significant residual collection.

Ultrasonography guidance is better than CT for evaluating internal architecture of fluid collection/abscess in spleen as the thin internal septations are better seen on USG.

Splenic Artery Aneurysm and Intervention

In abdomen, only aorta and iliac artery aneurysms are more common sites of aneurysm than splenic artery.[68] With more frequent use of USG and CT, incidental splenic artery aneurysms are also seen more commonly.[69] The difference between true aneurysm and pseudoaneurysm is with respect to the adventitial layer of the wall; which is present in true aneurysm but absent in pseudoaneurysm. The exact etiopathogenesis of true aneurysm are not yet completely elucidated. The clinical settings in which it is seen include atherosclerosis, pregnancy, portal hypertension, cirrhosis and post liver transplant.[70-72] Inflammatory and infectious conditions, collagen vascular diseases, arterial fibrodysplasia are other conditions, which are associated with it. In pancreatitits, release of proteolytic enzymes may cause weakening of the wall of splenic artery with consequent pseudoaneurysm formation. Other causes of pseudoaneurysms are iatrogenic or accidental trauma and postoperative causes.[73]

A large majority of unruptured splenic artery aneurysms are clinically silent.[70] In contrast, ruptured splenic artery aneurysms are almost always symptomatic with pain abdomen, intestinal hemorrhage and hemodynamic instability as presenting features. Rupture rate has been described as approximately 2–3%.[74,75] Liver transplantation, pregnancy and portal hypertension are associated with increased frequency of rupture.[76] CECT scan is the most commonly used modality for diagnosing splenic artery aneurysms and pseudoaneurysms however, the gold standard for diagnosing these conditions still remains direct catheter angiography. If CECT is utilized, a meticulous evaluation of arterial phase images is vital which reveals a well-defined rounded intensely enhancing outpouching from the splenic artery **(Figs. 28A and B)** or its branch. Other findings which may be seen are presence of calcification in its wall, mural thrombosis in peripheral part of the aneurysm or extravasation of contrast in its vicinity or within the lumen of adjacent bowel loops. If aneurysm is large, it may be seen on USG or color Doppler **(Fig. 28C)**, however small aneurysms may be missed on USG/Doppler as frequently there is poor sonographic window in presence of pancreatitis and postoperative changes.

The treatment strategies for splenic artery aneurysm and pseudoaneurysms are quite different. If patient is symptomatic then treatment of splenic artery aneurysm should be done.[70] For asymptomatic patients, treatment should be contemplated for certain high risk factors like pregnant women, patients of cirrhosis, hypertension and liver transplantation.[77] Treatment is also recommended for asymptomatic aneurysms larger than 2 cm in those patients with life expectancy more than 2 years and having reasonable operative risk.[68,70]

The modality of treatment depends on many factors like clinical condition of the patient, location of aneurysm and operative risks associated in given scenario. Elective surgery is associated with more than 0.5% mortality rate; hence, patient selection and treatment modality selection are of paramount importance.[76] Previously, surgical treatment for proximal and middle splenic artery used to be simple excision with ligation of proximal and distal stumps; in which

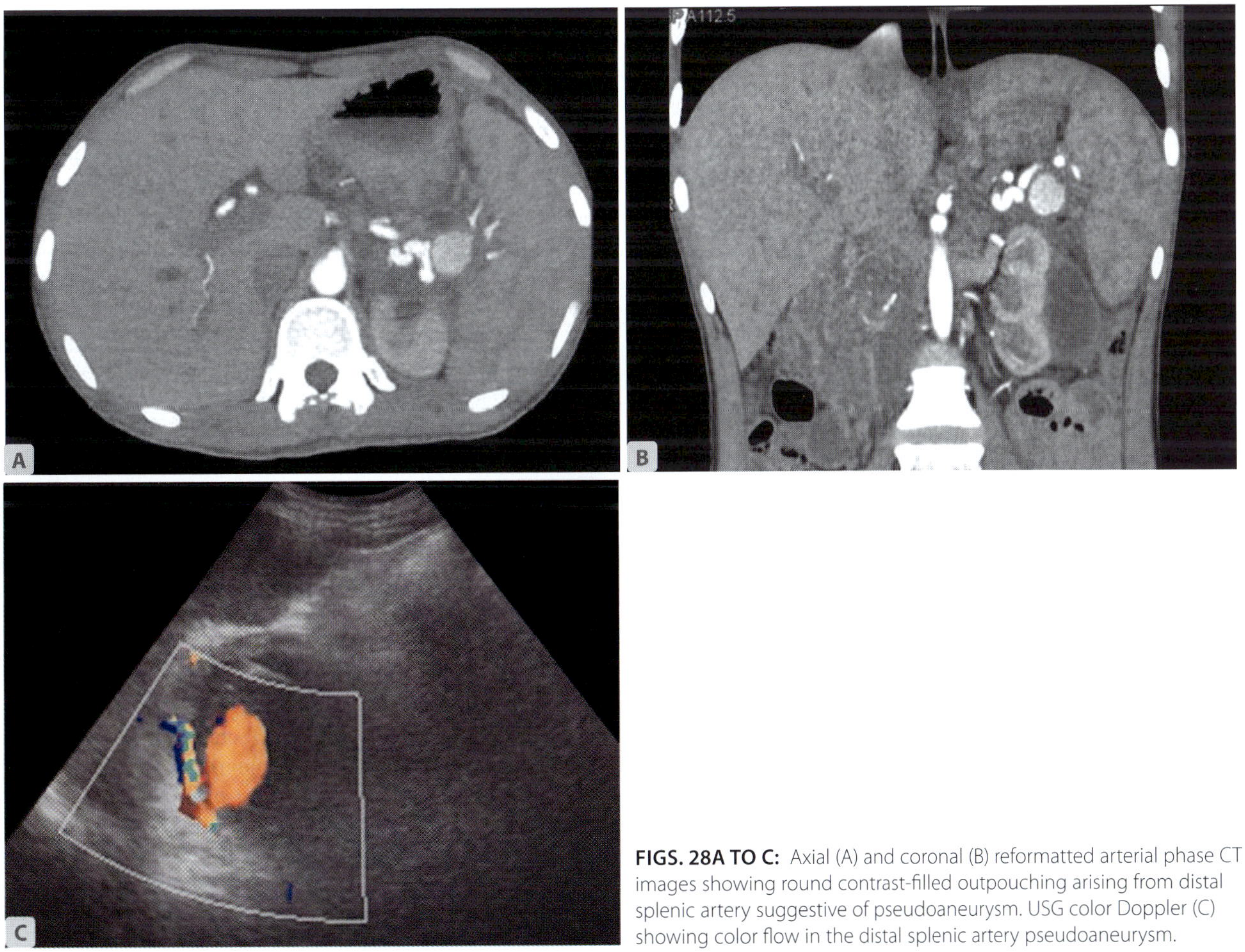

FIGS. 28A TO C: Axial (A) and coronal (B) reformatted arterial phase CT images showing round contrast-filled outpouching arising from distal splenic artery suggestive of pseudoaneurysm. USG color Doppler (C) showing color flow in the distal splenic artery pseudoaneurysm.

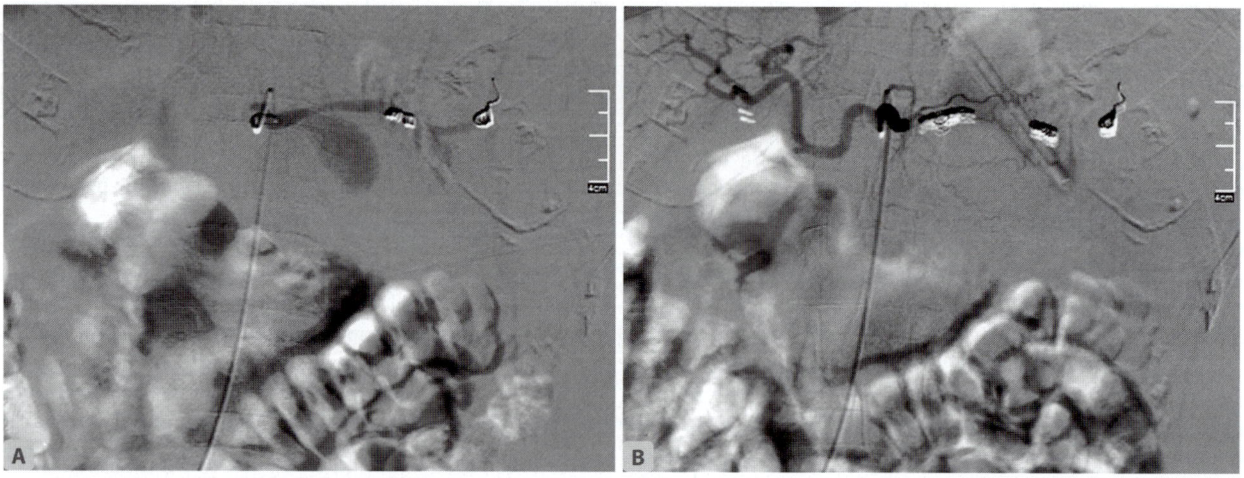

FIGS. 29A AND B: Angiogram (A) showing aneurysm in proximal part of splenic artery. Coils have been placed distal to splenic artery aneurysm. Incidentally, a coil is seen migrated in the distal most part of splenic artery. Coils have been placed proximal to aneurysm also to 'trap' the aneurysm (B).

case short gastric arteries may help to preserve splenic supply through collaterization. Surgical treatment for distally located aneurysms is splenectomy.[77]

Endovascular repair of splenic artery aneurysm is more efficacious than open surgical treatment in short-term follow-up with lesser perioperative mortality. However, late complications and reintervention rate is more with endovascular repair as compared to open surgical repair.[78] Endovascular repair has also been found to be more cost effective for treatment of splenic artery aneurysms.[79] Acceptable success rates have been achieved with endovascular techniques using embolization with coils **(Figs. 29A and B)** and gel foam.[80]

Splenic artery embolization has also been used successfully for treatment of hypersplenism.[81]

Occasionally use of percutaneous thrombin has been shown to be successful if the patients are not good candidates for endovascular treatment.[82,83]

Miscellaneous Conditions

Sarcoidosis

Splenic involvement in sarcoidosis is much less common than lungs, mediastinum and eyes. However, when involved it may be seen on CT as multiple hypodense nodules in spleen, which may vary in shape and size. If the nodules increase with time these may also look like confluent masses. These nodules and masses are hypodense and show less enhancement as compared to splenic parenchyma.[84] On MRI, these show hypointense signal on T1 and T2WI as compared to background parenchyma with hypoenhancement on early arterial phase.[85] These nodules may show enhancement on delayed phase images **(Figs. 30A to E)**. Other common finding is hepatosplenomegaly.

Gamna Gandy Bodies

Histologically, these are small siderotic nodules which contain hemosiderin, calcium and fibrosis. These are commonly seen in clinical setting of portal hypertension.[86] Other conditions in which these are seen include portal vein or splenic vein thrombosis and hemolytic anemias. They are best seen on MRI as hypointense foci in all sequences **(Figs. 31A to D)**.[87] Their usual size is from few millimeters to up to one centimeter.

Gaucher's Disease

Gaucher's disease occurs due to deficiency of lysosomal enzyme glucocerebrosidase. This disease affects the skeleton, spleen and liver most dominantly. Majority of times the patient is already diagnosed before they reach the radiology department. Skeletal involvement is in form of osteopenia, osteoporosis and fractures. Spleen may be massively enlarged with frequent findings of focal lesions and infarcts. On CT, these focal lesions are hypodense and enhance less as compared to splenic parenchyma. On MRI, most of these lesions are hyperintense on T2WI although occasionally they may be hypointense on T2WI also. These are hypointense on T1WI with hypoenhancement as compared to splenic parenchyma.[88] Liver enlargement is less striking as compared to splenic enlargement.

Hemochromatosis

Hemochromatosis may be primary (due to increased absorption from GIT) or secondary (due to increased extravscular hemolysis). In primary form, liver involvement is much more as compared to spleen and in secondary form, the spleen is predominantly involved. The usual imaging feature on CT, is presence of increased attenuation involving these organs. On MRI these involved organs show decreased signal on T2WI due to susceptibility artifacts because of presence of iron in visceral organs.[89,90] Spleen is also hypointense on T2WI however the involvement of liver is much more in primary forms **(Fig. 32)**. Conversely spleen is more profoundly hypointense than liver if the etiology is secondary hemochromatosis. MR using gradient echo sequences is also used to quantify liver iron load in an attempt to avoid the need of repeated biopsies.

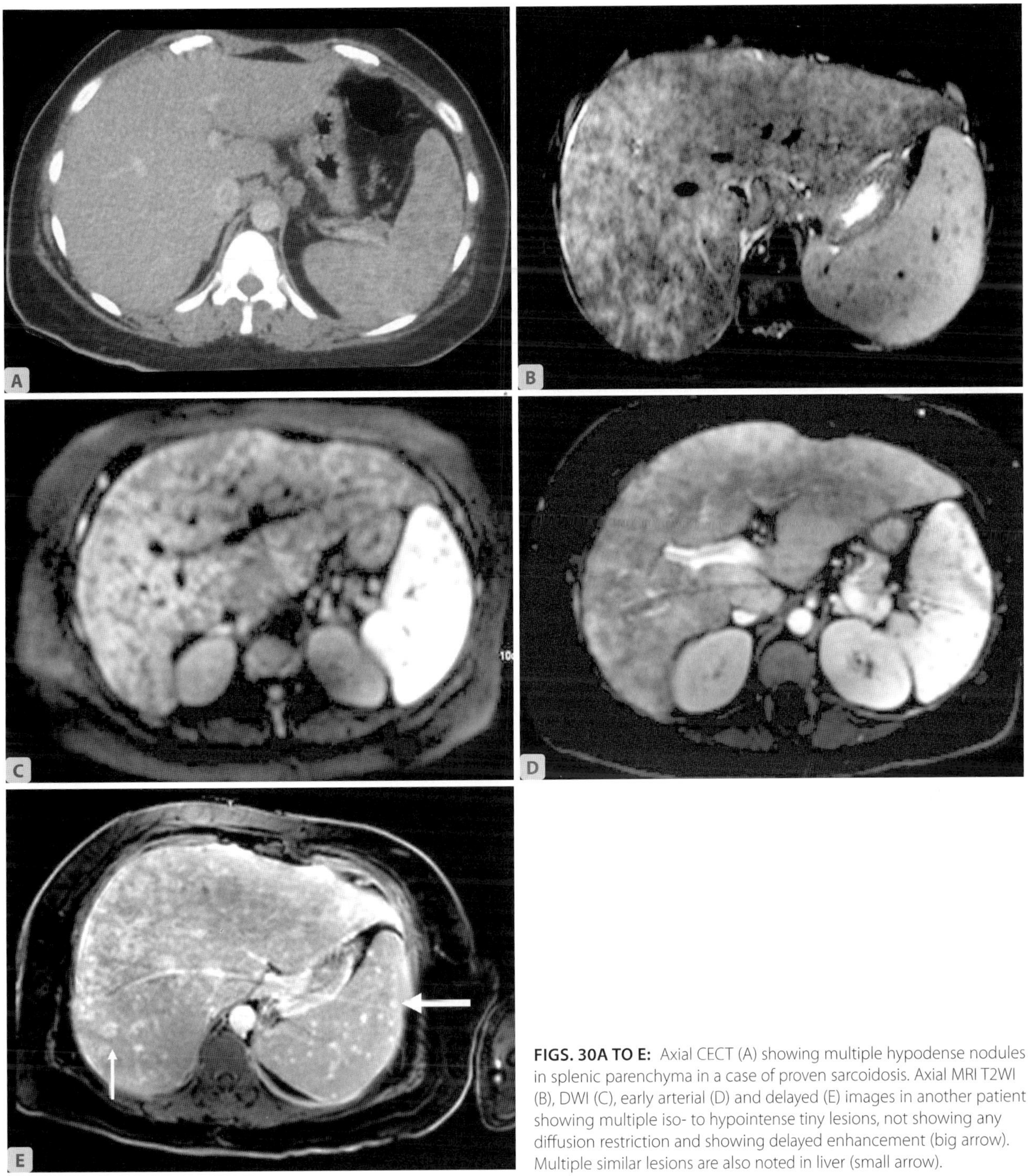

FIGS. 30A TO E: Axial CECT (A) showing multiple hypodense nodules in splenic parenchyma in a case of proven sarcoidosis. Axial MRI T2WI (B), DWI (C), early arterial (D) and delayed (E) images in another patient showing multiple iso- to hypointense tiny lesions, not showing any diffusion restriction and showing delayed enhancement (big arrow). Multiple similar lesions are also noted in liver (small arrow).

Amyloidosis

Pathologically in amyloidosis, there is abnormal accumulation of some fibrillar material in extracellular matrix in a wide variety of tissues in body. Based on the biochemical property of this fibrillar material, it can be divided into primary type (type AL, monoclonal proliferation) and secondary type (AA type, secondary to chronic inflammatory diseases). Both of these types can involve the spleen which may be diffuse (more commonly) or focal. Splenomegaly is quite uncommon.[91] Various imaging features are focal tumor like lesions,[92] diffuse low attenuation[91] and decreased enhancement. Occasionally, extensive focal splenic calcification has also been described in splenic involvement of amyloidosis.[93] On MRI, decreased signal on T2WI has been described.[94]

In conclusion, spleen is affected by a wide variety of disorders ranging from developmental abnormalities to storage disorders, infective, vascular and neoplastic

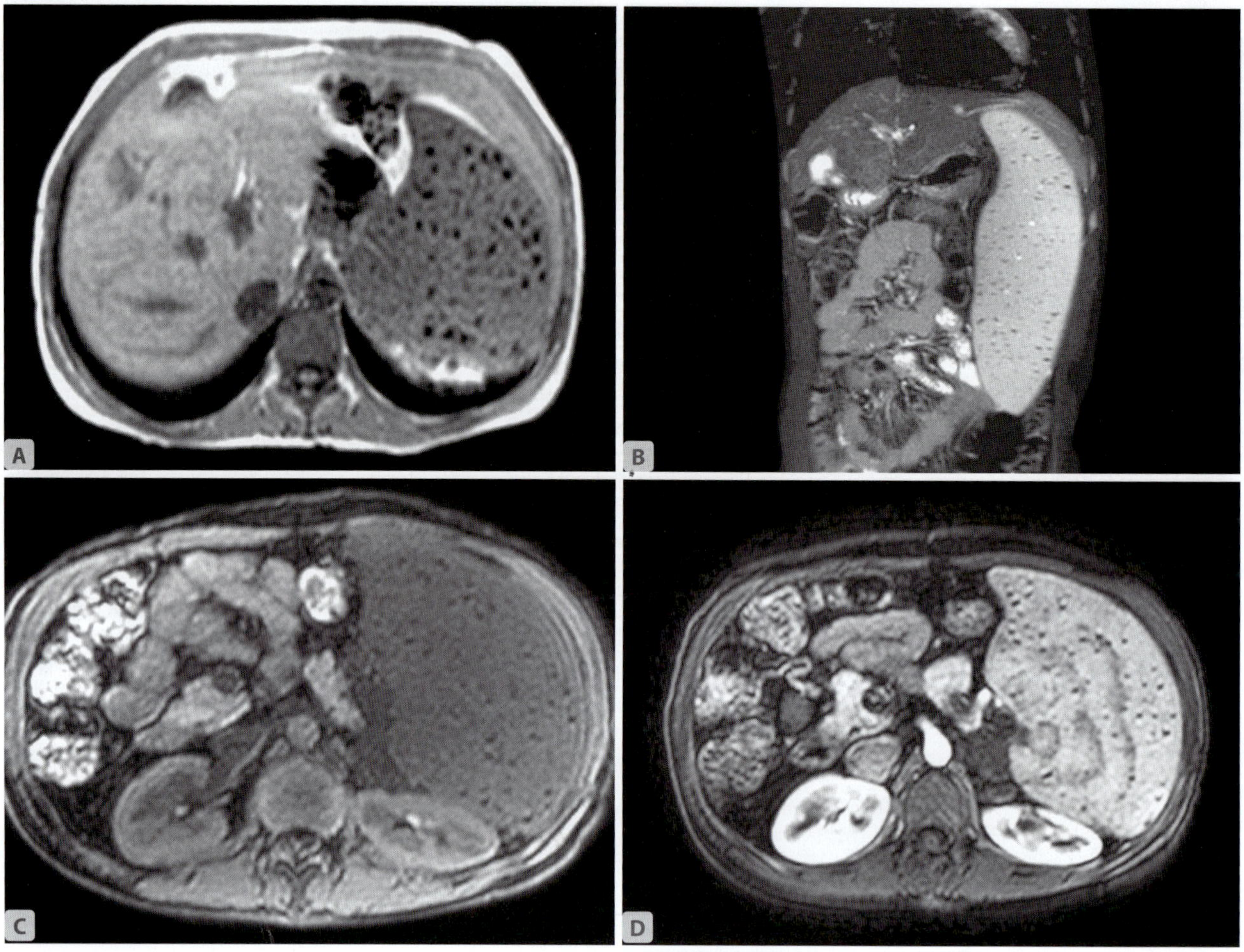

FIGS. 31A TO D: Axial T1WI (A), coronal T2WI (B), T1FS non-contrast (C) and post-contrast (D) MR images showing numerous hypointense tiny focal lesions in enlarged spleen on all sequences with no enhancement on postcontrast images suggestive of Gamna-Gandy bodies in a patient with portal hypertension.

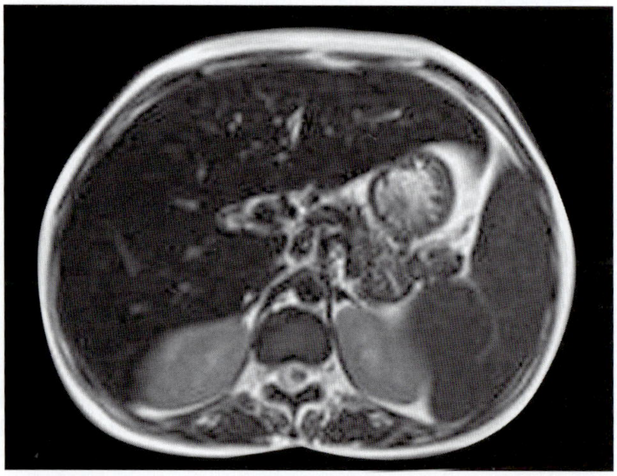

FIG. 32: Axial T2WI showing diffuse hypointense signal in spleen in a case of hemolytic anemia.

pathologies. A thorough knowledge of available imaging modalities and judicious utilization of these is necessary for optimal patient care. USG and CT are the most commonly used imaging modalities for evaluation of splenic disorders. MRI can be used as a problem solving tool. FNAC, biopsy and splenic artery embolization are major interventions performed, which need meticulous planning using these imaging modalities. FNAC with or without cell block is a safe and useful procedure for diagnosis of focal splenic lesions, especially granulomatous diseases such as tuberculosis.

ACKNOWLEDGMENTS

Dr Raju Sharma, Dr Shivanand Gamanagatti and Dr Manisha Jana.

REFERENCES

1. Chadburn A. The spleen: anatomy and anatomical function. Semin Hematol. 2000;37(1 Suppl 1):13-21.
2. Hirooka M, Ochi H, Koizumi Y, Kisaka Y, Abe M, Ikeda Y, et al. Splenic elasticity measured with real-time tissue elastography is a marker of portal hypertension. Radiology. 2011;261(3):960-8.
3. Grzelak P, Augsburg L, Majos A, Stefanczyk L, Gorski P, Piotrowski W, et al. Diagnostic potential of contrast-enhanced ultrasound (CEUS) in the assessment of spleen and liver granulomas in the course of sarcoidosis. Pneumonol Alergol Pol. 2013;81(5):424-8.
4. Omar A, Freeman S. Contrast-enhanced ultrasound of the spleen. Ultrasound. 2016;24(1):41-9.
5. Miele V, Piccolo CL, Galluzzo M, Ianniello S, Sessa B, Trinci M. Contrast-enhanced ultrasound (CEUS) in blunt abdominal trauma. Br J Radiol. 2016;89(1061):20150823.
6. Piscaglia F, Nolsoe C, Dietrich CF, Cosgrove DO, Gilja OH, Bachmann Nielsen M, et al. The EFSUMB Guidelines and Recommendations on the Clinical Practice of Contrast Enhanced Ultrasound (CEUS): update 2011 on non-hepatic applications. Ultraschall Med. 2012;33(1):33-59.
7. Park YS, Park SH, Lee SS, Kim DY, Shin YM, Lee W, et al. Biopsy-proven nonsteatotic liver in adults: estimation of reference range for difference in attenuation between the liver and the spleen at nonenhanced CT. Radiology. 2011;258(3):760-6.
8. Donnelly LF, Foss JN, Frush DP, Bisset GS 3rd. Heterogeneous splenic enhancement patterns on spiral CT images in children: minimizing misinterpretation. Radiology. 1999;210(2):493-7.
9. Rabushka LS, Kawashima A, Fishman EK. Imaging of the spleen: CT with supplemental MR examination. Radiographics. 1994;14(2):307-32.
10. Urban BA, Fishman EK. Helical CT of the spleen. AJR. 1998;170(4):997-1003.
11. Elsayes KM, Narra VR, Mukundan G, Lewis JS Jr, Menias CO, Heiken JP. MR imaging of the spleen: spectrum of abnormalities. Radiographics. 2005;25(4):967-82.
12. Donnelly LF, Emery KH, Bove KE, Bissett GS 3rd. Normal changes in the MR appearance of the spleen during early childhood. AJR. 1996;166(3):635-9.
13. Yoshikawa T, Kawamitsu H, Mitchell DG, Ohno Y, Ku Y, Seo Y, et al. ADC measurement of abdominal organs and lesions using parallel imaging technique. AJR. 2006;187(6):1521-30.
14. Rini JN, Leonidas JC, Tomas MB, Palestro CJ. 18F-FDG PET versus CT for evaluating the spleen during initial staging of lymphoma. J Nucl Med. 2003;44(7):1072-4.
15. Spleen. In: Lee JKT, Sagel SS, Stanley RJ, Heiken JP (eds). Computed Body Tomography with MRI Correlation, 4th edn. Philadelphia: Lippincott Williams and Wilkins; 2006.
16. Rosenberg HK, Markowitz RI, Kolberg H, Park C, Hubbard A, Bellah RD. Normal splenic size in infants and children: sonographic measurements. AJR. 1991;157(1):119-21.
17. Radu CC, Mutiu G, Pop O. Accessory spleen. Rom J Morphol Embryol. 2014;55(3 Suppl):1243-6.
18. al-Ahmadi M, Brundage S, Brody F, Jacobs L, Sackier JM. Splenosis of the mesoappendix: case report and review of the literature. J R Coll Surg Edinb. 1998;43(3):200-2.
19. Costello P, Kane RA, Oster J, Clouse ME. Focal splenic disease demonstrated by ultrasound and computed tomography. J Can Assoc Radiol. 1985;36(1):22-8.
20. Fulcher AS, Turner MA. Abdominal manifestations of situs anomalies in adults. Radiographics. 2002;22(6):1439-56.
21. Zech CJ, Bartolozzi C, Baron R, Reiser MF (eds). Multislice-CT of the Abdomen. Springer. Verlag Berlin Heidelberg, 2012.
22. Dachman AH, Ros PR, Murari PJ, Olmsted WW, Lichtenstein JE. Nonparasitic splenic cysts: a report of 52 cases with radiologic-pathologic correlation. AJR. 1986;147(3):537-42.
23. Al-Hajjar N, Graur F, Hassan AB, Molnar G. Splenic abscesses. Rom J Gastroenterol. 2002;11(1):57-9.
24. Ooi LL, Leong SS. Splenic abscesses from 1987 to 1995. Am J Surg. 1997;174(1):87-93.
25. Tirumani SH, Ojili V, Gunabushanam G, Shanbhogue AK, Nagar A, Fasih N, et al. Imaging of tuberculosis of the abdominal viscera: beyond the intestines. J Clin Imaging Sci. 2013;3:17.
26. Murata Y, Yamada I, Sumiya Y, Shichijo Y, Suzuki Y. Abdominal macronodular tuberculomas: MR findings. J Comput Assist Tomogr. 1996;20(4):643-6.
27. Ito K, Mitchell DG, Honjo K, Fujita T, Uchisako H, Matsumoto T, et al. MR imaging of acquired abnormalities of the spleen. AJR. 1997;168(3):697-702.
28. Renzulli P, Hostettler A, Schoepfer AM, Gloor B, Candinas D. Systematic review of atraumatic splenic rupture. Br J Surg. 2009;96(10):1114-21.
29. Husni EA. The clinical course of splenic hemangioma with emphasis on spontaneous rupture. Arch Surg. 1961;83:681-8.
30. Louis TH, Sanders JM, Stephenson JS, Harbour LN, Ford KL 3rd. Splenic hemangiomatosis. Proc (Bayl Univ Med Cent). 2011;24(4):356-8.
31. Shinde J, Pandit S, Kolte S, Singh SP. Laparoscopic splenectomy for haemangioma of the spleen. J Minim Access Surg. 2014; 10(1):42-4.
32. Abbott RM, Levy AD, Aguilera NS, Gorospe L, Thompson WM. From the archives of the AFIP: primary vascular neoplasms of the spleen: radiologic-pathologic correlation. Radiographics. 2004;24(4):1137-63.
33. Yang F, Chen WX. Splenic lymphangioma that manifested as a solid-cystic mass: a case report. World J Gastroenterol. 2013;19(5):781-3.
34. Ioannidis I, Kahn AG. Splenic lymphangioma. Arch Pathol Lab Med. 2015;139(2):278-82.
35. Kaza RK, Azar S, Al-Hawary MM, Francis IR. Primary and secondary neoplasms of the spleen. Cancer Imaging. 2010;10: 173-82.
36. Lam KY, Yip KH, Peh WC. Splenic vascular lesions: unusual features and a review of the literature. Aust NZJ Surg. 1999; 69(6):422-5.
37. Ohtomo K, Fukuda H, Mori K, Minami M, Itai Y, Inoue Y. CT and MR appearances of splenic hamartoma. J Comput Assist Tomogr. 1992;16(3):425-8.
38. Yu RS, Zhang SZ, Hua JM. Imaging findings of splenic hamartoma. World J Gastroenterol. 2004;10(17):2613-5.
39. Giovagnoni A, Giorgi C, Goteri G. Tumours of the spleen. Cancer Imaging. 2005;5:73-7.
40. Davidson J, Tung K. Splenic peliosis: an unusual entity. Br J Radiol. 2010;83(990):e126-8.
41. Maves CK, Caron KH, Bisset GS 3rd, Agarwal R. Splenic and hepatic peliosis: MR findings. AJR. 1992;158(1):75-6.
42. Saboo SS, Krajewski KM, O'Regan KN, Giardino A, Brown JR, Ramaiya N, et al. Spleen in haematological malignancies: spectrum of imaging findings. Br J Radiol. 2012;85(1009):81-92.
43. Paes FM, Kalkanis DG, Sideras PA, Serafini AN. FDG PET/CT of extranodal involvement in non-Hodgkin lymphoma and Hodgkin disease. Radiographics. 2010;30(1):269-91.
44. Li M, Zhang L, Wu N, Huang W, Lv N. Imaging findings of primary splenic lymphoma: a review of 17 cases in which diagnosis was made at splenectomy. PLoS One. 2013;8(11):e80264.

45. Fishman EK, Kuhlman JE, Jones RJ. CT of lymphoma: spectrum of disease. Radiographics. 1991;11(4):647-69.
46. Guermazi A, Brice P, de Kerviler EE, Ferme C, Hennequin C, Meignin V, et al. Extranodal Hodgkin disease: spectrum of disease. Radiographics. 2001;21(1):161-79.
47. Bhatia K, Sahdev A, Reznek RH. Lymphoma of the spleen. Semin Ultrasound CT MR. 2007;28(1):12-20.
48. Manzella A, Borba-Filho P, D'Ippolito G, Farias M. Abdominal manifestations of lymphoma: spectrum of imaging features. ISRN Radiol. 2013;2013:483069.
49. de Jong PA, van Ufford HM, Baarslag HJ, de Haas MJ, Wittebol SH, Quekel LG, et al. CT and 18F-FDG PET for noninvasive detection of splenic involvement in patients with malignant lymphoma. AJR. 2009;192(3):745-53.
50. Cheson BD, Pfistner B, Juweid ME, Gascoyne RD, Specht L, Horning SJ, et al. Revised response criteria for malignant lymphoma. J Clin Oncol. 2007;25(5):579-86.
51. Juweid ME, Stroobants S, Hoekstra OS, Mottaghy FM, Dietlein M, Guermazi A, et al. Use of positron emission tomography for response assessment of lymphoma: consensus of the Imaging Subcommittee of International Harmonization Project in Lymphoma. J Clin Oncol. 2007;25(5):571-8.
52. Hamid KS, Rodriguez JA, Lairmore TC. Primary splenic angiosarcoma. JSLS. 2010;14(3):431-5.
53. Badiani R, Schaller G, Jain K, Swamy R, Gupta S. Angiosarcoma of the spleen presenting as spontaneous splenic rupture: A rare case report and review of the literature. Int J Surg Case Rep. 2013;4(9):765-7.
54. Manouras A, Giannopoulos P, Toufektzian L, Markogiannakis H, Lagoudianakis EE, Papadima A, et al. Splenic rupture as the presenting manifestation of primary splenic angiosarcoma in a teenage woman: a case report. J Med Case Rep. 2008;2:133.
55. Thompson WM, Levy AD, Aguilera NS, Gorospe L, Abbott RM. Angiosarcoma of the spleen: imaging characteristics in 12 patients. Radiology. 2005;235(1):106-15.
56. Comperat E, Bardier-Dupas A, Camparo P, Capron F, Charlotte F. Splenic metastases: clinicopathologic presentation, differential diagnosis, and pathogenesis. Arch Pathol Lab Med. 2007;131(6):965-9.
57. Showalter SL, Hager E, Yeo CJ. Metastatic disease to the pancreas and spleen. Semin Oncol. 2008;35(2):160-71.
58. Agha-Mohammadi S, Calne RY. Solitary splenic metastasis: case report and review of the literature. Am J Clin Oncol. 2001; 24(3):306-10.
59. Senturk S, Karcaaltincaba M, Akata D. CT diagnosis of intrasplenic metastasis from ovarian carcinoma. Eur J Radiol. 2012;81(6): 1094-9.
60. McInnes MD, Kielar AZ, Macdonald DB. Percutaneous image-guided biopsy of the spleen: systematic review and meta-analysis of the complication rate and diagnostic accuracy. Radiology. 2011;260(3):699-708.
61. Tam A, Krishnamurthy S, Pillsbury EP, Ensor JE, Gupta S, Murthy R, et al. Percutaneous image-guided splenic biopsy in the oncology patient: an audit of 156 consecutive cases. J Vasc Interv Radiol. 2008;19(1):80-7.
62. Lucey BC, Boland GW, Maher MM, Hahn PF, Gervais DA, Mueller PR. Percutaneous nonvascular splenic intervention: a 10-year review. AJR. 2002;179(6):1591-6.
63. Kang M, Kalra N, Gulati M, Lal A, Kochhar R, Rajwanshi A. Image guided percutaneous splenic interventions. Eur J Radiol. 2007;64(1):140-6.
64. Kamaya A, Weinstein S, Desser TS. Multiple lesions of the spleen: differential diagnosis of cystic and solid lesions. Semin Ultrasound CT MR. 2006;27(5):389-403.
65. Thanos L, Dailiana T, Papaioannou G, Nikita A, Koutrouvelis H, Kelekis DA. Percutaneous CT-guided drainage of splenic abscess. AJR. 2002;179(3):629-32.
66. Singh AK, Shankar S, Gervais DA, Hahn PF, Mueller PR. Image-guided percutaneous splenic interventions. Radiographics. 2012;32(2):523-34.
67. Sammon J, Twomey M, Crush L, Maher MM, O'Connor OJ. Image-guided percutaneous splenic biopsy and drainage. Semin Intervent Radiol. 2012;29(4):301-10.
68. Trastek VF, Pairolero PC, Joyce JW, Hollier LH, Bernatz PE. Splenic artery aneurysms. Surgery. 1982;91(6):694-9.
69. Rokke O, Sondenaa K, Amundsen S, Bjerke-Larssen T, Jensen D. The diagnosis and management of splanchnic artery aneurysms. Scand J Gastroenterol. 1996;31(8):737-43.
70. Abbas MA, Stone WM, Fowl RJ, Gloviczki P, Oldenburg WA, Pairolero PC, et al. Splenic artery aneurysms: two decades experience at Mayo clinic. Ann Vasc Surg. 2002;16(4):442-9.
71. Lee PC, Rhee RY, Gordon RY, Fung JJ, Webster MW. Management of splenic artery aneurysms: the significance of portal and essential hypertension. J Am Coll Surg. 1999;189(5):483-90.
72. Selo-Ojeme DO, Welch CC. Review: spontaneous rupture of splenic artery aneurysm in pregnancy. Eur J Obstet Gynecol Reprod Biol. 2003;109(2):124-7.
73. Tessier DJ, Stone WM, Fowl RJ, Abbas MA, Andrews JC, Bower TC, et al. Clinical features and management of splenic artery pseudoaneurysm: case series and cumulative review of literature. J Vasc Surg. 2003;38(5):969-74.
74. Stanley JC, Wakefield TW, Graham LM, Whitehouse WM Jr, Zelenock GB, Lindenauer SM. Clinical importance and management of splanchnic artery aneurysms. J Vasc Surg. 1986;3(5):836-40.
75. Trastek VF, Pairolero PC, Bernatz PE. Splenic artery aneurysms. World J Surg. 1985;9(3):378-83.
76. Mattar SG, Lumsden AB. The management of splenic artery aneurysms: experience with 23 cases. Am J Surg. 1995;169(6): 580-4.
77. de Perrot M, Buhler L, Schneider PA, Mentha G, Morel P. Do aneurysms and pseudoaneurysms of the splenic artery require different surgical strategy? Hepatogastroenterology. 1999;46(27): 2028-32.
78. Hogendoorn W, Lavida A, Hunink MG, Moll FL, Geroulakos G, Muhs BE, et al. Open repair, endovascular repair, and conservative management of true splenic artery aneurysms. J Vasc Surg. 2014;60(6):1667-76 e1.
79. Hogendoorn W, Lavida A, Hunink MG, Moll FL, Geroulakos G, Muhs BE, et al. Cost-effectiveness of endovascular repair, open repair, and conservative management of splenic artery aneurysms. J Vasc Surg. 2015;61(6):1432-40.
80. Guillon R, Garcier JM, Abergel A, Mofid R, Garcia V, Chahid T, et al. Management of splenic artery aneurysms and false aneurysms with endovascular treatment in 12 patients. Cardiovasc Intervent Radiol. 2003;26(3):256-60.
81. Gu JJ, He XH, Li WT, Ji J, Peng WJ, Li GD, et al. Safety and efficacy of splenic artery coil embolization for hypersplenism in liver cirrhosis. Acta Radiol. 2012;53(8):862-7.
82. Puri S, Nicholson AA, Breen DJ. Percutaneous thrombin injection for the treatment of a post-pancreatitis pseudoaneurysm. Eur Radiol. 2003;13(Suppl 4):L79-82.
83. Krueger K, Zaehringer M, Lackner K. Percutaneous treatment of a splenic artery pseudoaneurysm by thrombin injection. J Vasc Interv Radiol. 2005;16(7):1023-5.
84. Hoeffel C, Bokemeyer C, Hoeffel JC, Gaucher H, Galanski M, Fornes P. CT hepatic and splenic appearances with sarcoidosis. Eur J Radiol. 1996;23(2):94-6.

85. Torres GM, Terry NL, Mergo PJ, Ros PR. MR imaging of the spleen. Magn Reson Imaging Clin N Am. 1995;3(1):39-50.
86. Minami M, Itai Y, Ohtomo K, Ohnishi S, Niki T, Kokubo T, et al. Siderotic nodules in the spleen: MR imaging of portal hypertension. Radiology. 1989;172(3):681-4.
87. Sagoh T, Itoh K, Togashi K, Shibata T, Nishimura K, Minami S, et al. Gamna-Gandy bodies of the spleen: evaluation with MR imaging. Radiology. 1989;172(3):685-7.
88. Hill SC, Damaska BM, Ling A, Patterson K, Di Bisceglie AM, Brady RO, et al. Gaucher disease: abdominal MR imaging findings in 46 patients. Radiology. 1992;184(2):561-6.
89. Housman JF, Chezmar JL, Nelson RC. Magnetic resonance imaging in hemochromatosis: extrahepatic iron deposition. Gastrointest Radiol. 1989;14(1):59-60.
90. Long JA Jr, Doppman JL, Nienhus AW, Mills SR. Computed tomographic analysis of beta-thalassemic syndromes with hemochromatosis: pathologic findings with clinical and laboratory correlations. J Comput Assist Tomogr. 1980;4(2): 159-65.
91. Kim SH, Han JK, Lee KH, Won HJ, Kim KW, Kim JS, et al. Abdominal amyloidosis: spectrum of radiological findings. Clin Radiol. 2003;58(8):610-20.
92. Liu TY, Chen SC, Wang LY, Chuang WL, Chang WY, Liu CS. Systemic amyloidosis presenting as splenic tumor. Gastrointest Radiol. 1991;16(2):137-8.
93. Kennan NM, Evans C. Case report: hepatic and splenic calcification due to amyloid. Clin Radiol. 1991;44(1):60-1.
94. Monzawa S, Tsukamoto T, Omata K, Hosoda K, Araki T, Sugimura K. A case with primary amyloidosis of the liver and spleen: radiologic findings. Eur J Radiol. 2002;41(3):237-41.

CHAPTER

119

Imaging of the Postoperative Abdomen

Mandeep Kang, Ujjwal Gorsi, Anmol Bhatia

INTRODUCTION

Recent advances in the understanding of the pathophysiology of disease processes has led to improved medical as well as surgical management. There have been substantial advances in the technique and type of surgical procedures being performed with an increasing trend towards minimally invasive techniques. This in turn has led to an increasing number of requests for radiological investigations for the evaluation of postoperative patients. These include the detection of complications both in the early (less than 4 weeks) and late phases (more than 4 weeks) as well as disease recurrence. To be able to recognize these complications, the radiologist needs to be familiar with the normal postoperative appearances of the surgery that has been performed as well as the complications that can occur after the procedure. It becomes critical here to be able to differentiate between what are the expected postoperative changes (relative to the temporal profile) and what findings constitute pathology, which in-turn can alter patient management.

In this chapter, we will address the basics of imaging of the postoperative abdomen, the general complications which may occur, the normal postoperative anatomy as well as specific complications which are peculiar to certain commonly performed surgical procedures.

IMAGING MODALITIES

Plain X-rays of the abdomen are commonly asked for in the immediate postoperative period and are useful for the detection of pneumoperitoneum, ileus or intestinal obstruction. Ultrasonography is often asked for to detect fluid collections or abscess or to look for biliary radicle dilatation after biliary procedures. The presence of surgical dressings on the abdominal wall and pneumoperitoneum or ileus in the immediate postoperative period limit its usefulness.[1] However, its portability as well as the use of non-ionizing radiation is of advantage particularly when children or young women have to undergo repeated imaging.

Helical CT is now the modality of choice for the radiological evaluation of the postoperative patient. Rapid acquisition is of advantage when critically sick patients need to be imaged. The ability to reconstruct multiplanar images is useful when complex postoperative anatomy has to be evaluated.

CT PROTOCOL

Positive water-soluble iodinated oral contrast should be used in most postoperative examinations, particularly when anastomotic leakage has to be ruled out. Any leakage of the water-soluble contrast into the peritoneal cavity will not have any deleterious effect on the patient. Oral contrast is also most useful for differentiating distended bowel loops from extraluminal fluid collections. Sick patients may not be able to tolerate larger volumes, administering between 500 to 1000 mL of oral contrast should be enough to achieve an optimal diagnostic study. If plain radiographs of the abdomen reveal evidence of bowel obstruction, oral contrast can be avoided as the fluid in the dilated bowel loops provides a natural contrast. If suspected bowel ischemia or acute gastrointestinal bleeding is the clinical indication for the CT scan, one should perform a biphasic CECT with negative oral contrast. In both these clinical scenarios, performing dual energy CT is of benefit, both from the point of view of reducing the patient's radiation dose as well as improving the diagnostic accuracy. By using dual energy CT and generating virtual non-enhanced images, one can omit the pre-contrast acquisition which is generally performed to detect presence of hyperattenuation signifying bleed in the bowel lumen.[2] Subtle differences in the enhancement of ischemic bowel loops become more conspicuous with the use of iodine maps or quantitative measurements of the iodine content in the wall of the bowel.[3] Rectal contrast should be used particularly following colorectal surgery.

Intravenous iodinated contrast should be used in all patients, unless there is a specific contraindication such as deranged renal parameters or history of allergy to contrast. Besides the clinical scenarios mentioned previously where one should acquire a biphasic CECT, a single portal venous phase acquisition is adequate. The anatomical coverage should be from the domes of the diaphragm to the public symphysis, even if the surgery has been performed in the upper abdomen or pelvis. This is because both the compartments are interconnected and fluid may track along anatomical pathways from one to the other.[4] Secondly many new pathways come into existence because of defects in the mesentery created due to the surgical procedure and so fluid may track to a location remote from the surgical bed.

NORMAL RADIOLOGICAL FINDINGS IN THE POSTOPERATIVE ABDOMEN

Some amount of changes will occur following surgery which do not represent complications but are due to the procedure itself. Soft tissue stranding or patchy increased density will be seen in the subcutaneous fat around the incision site and in the intra-abdominal fat around the operative site. When the surgical procedure has involved significant handling of the bowel loops, these can show mural thickening or ileus **(Fig. 1)**. Subcutaneous emphysema may be seen in the anterior abdominal wall which may be extensive following laparoscopic procedures.[5]

Presence of free intraperitoneal air can pose a diagnostic dilemma to the radiologist as it can be due to the procedure itself or represent a complication such as an anastomotic leak or development of infection. Detection of pneumoperitoneum on plain radiographs formed the basis of initial literature. CT shows a much higher sensitivity for the detection of free intraperitoneal air in comparison to plain radiographs (87% on day 3 on CT versus 53% on X-ray).[6] Pneumoperitoneum is reported to be present in up to 44% of CT scans performed on the third postoperative day, decreasing with time to 30% of cases between days 14 and 18 following surgery. The volume does not usually exceed 10 mL but larger volumes up to 40 mL may be seen in some patients.[7]

Laparoscopic surgery involves insufflation of carbon dioxide to create an artificial pneumoperitoneum. Carbon dioxide is more rapidly absorbed than nitrogen which is the main component of room air. Therefore, the amount of postoperative free intraperitoneal air is less with laparoscopic surgeries in comparison to open surgeries and is expected to be completely resorbed by 48 hours. It may however be seen up to the 9th postoperative day on plain X-rays[8] and up to 2 weeks on CT.[5] Presence of pneumoperitoneum more than 7–10 days following open surgery and more than two days after laparoscopic surgery is a cause for concern. Individual cases normally require clinicoradiological correlation. If there is still a doubt, one can consider follow-up radiological evaluation as any increase in the volume of pneumoperitoneum over time is definitely due to a complication.[9] One must also remember that surgical drains or percutaneous catheter *in situ* also lead to free intraperitoneal air and their presence must be kept in mind while interpreting the significance of the pneumoperitoneum.

A picture of generalized fluid retention may be seen in the postoperative period as a result of hypoproteinemia, fluid retention and fluid overload. This is more commonly seen in patients with comorbidities, particularly, renal or cardiac problems. This may result in a "Wet" patient with combinations of pleural effusion, mild ascities and edema of the mesenteric or subcutaneous fat **(Fig. 2)**.[9] Due to the surgical procedure, there is some accumulation of blood, lymph and intraperitoneal fluid in the operative bed. These appear radiologically as unencapsulated, crescentric collections which do not anatomically displace any surrounding structures. These are generally absorbed spontaneously.[10] There may be mild peritoneal enhancement **(Fig. 3)**. Due to the decreased diaphragmatic excursion secondary to the pain associated with movement of the abdominal wall, some degree of bilateral basal passive atelectasis of the lungs is also expected in the immediate postoperative period.

Hemostatic compounds may be used by the surgeons to control intraoperative bleeding. The most commonly used is Surgicel, made of oxidized regenerated cellulose which may be left behind in the abdomen as it is bioabsorbable. On CT, it appears hypodense with a bubbly appearance, containing multiple gas foci which may be peripheral, located in the operative bed **(Fig. 4)**. This may be mistaken for an abscess, however Surgicel will not show any enhancement following contrast.[11]

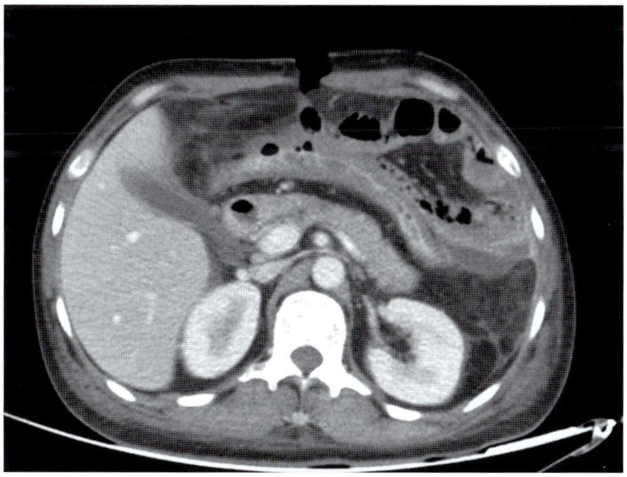

FIG. 1: A 42-year-old male underwent right hemicolectomy for carcinoma ascending colon. CECT axial image on postoperative day 4 shows diffuse mural thickening of the small bowel loops due to edema.

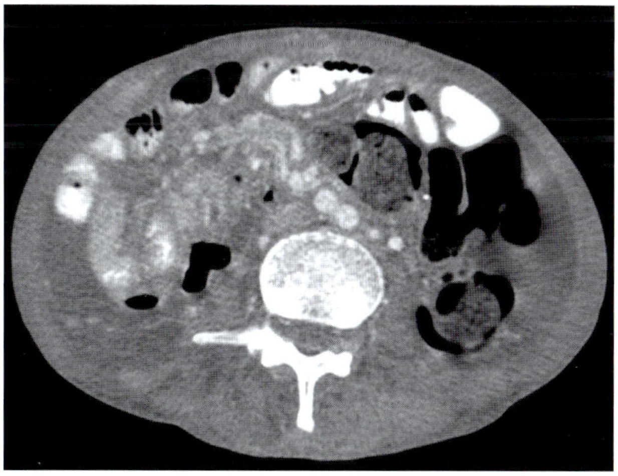

FIG. 2: A 53-year-old male underwent palliative distal gastrectomy with feeding jejunostomy for carcinoma distal stomach. CECT axial image on day 8 shows ascites with diffuse increased density of the mesentery with generalized edema of the subcutaneous fat.

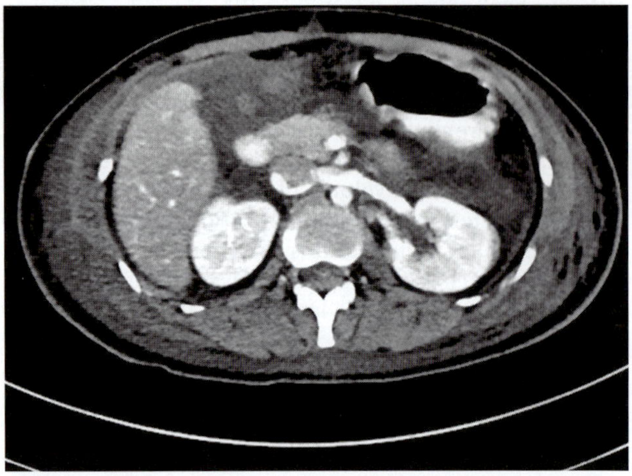

FIG. 3: A 28-year-old female postlaparoscopic cholecystectomy. CECT on day 4 following surgery shows mild peritoneal enhancement with fluid in the gallbladder fossa.

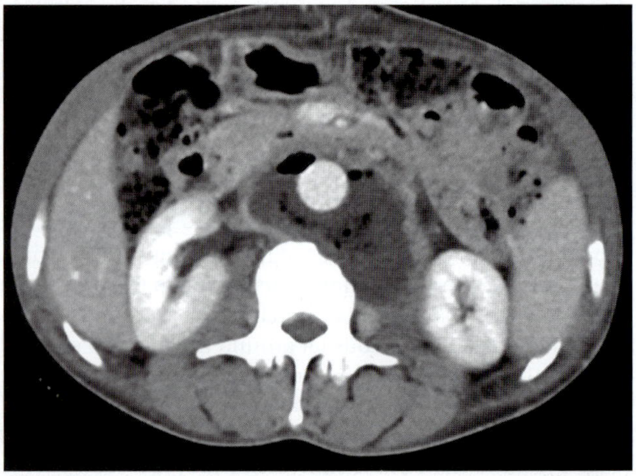

FIG. 4: A 70-year-old male underwent aortic aneurysm repair with graft placement. CECT axial image on postoperative day 3 shows surgicel as a hypodense area with a bubbly appearance surrounding the graft with air foci.

POSTOPERATIVE COMPLICATIONS

Postsurgical complications are common as they are part of the inherent risk of the procedure. In the immediate post-operative period, they are commonly related to infections or the surgical technique. Later complications may occur due to the altered anatomy, or recurrence of the primary disease process.

Anastomotic Leak

Anastomotic leaks are common to all reconstructive gastrointestinal surgeries and have an incidence of 1–5% after upper gastrointestinal surgeries and of 5–10% following colon resections.[12] They are associated with a high mortality (up to 50%) and morbidity and therefore require prompt recognition and early treatment.[10] Leaks occur at the anastomotic margins due to devascularization leading to necrosis, and therefore usually manifest clinically within the first fortnight following the surgery. Clinical symptoms are usually of sudden onset and consist of fever, which may show spikes, intense abdominal pain with guarding and rebound tenderness, tachycardia and rising leukocyte counts. Fluoroscopic gastrointestinal studies using water soluble iodinated contrast have been shown to be useful for the detection and localization of leaks,[4,10] however helical CT with its multiplanar reformation capability is a better modality. It has been reported to confirm clinically suspected leaks in 48–100% of cases.[13] The hallmark of an anastomotic leak is extraluminal extravasation of oral or rectal contrast with air in the operative bed **(Fig. 5)**. At times oral contrast may not have had time to reach the anastomotic site due to the associated ileus. In this case, presence of loculated fluid with excess of extraluminal air in the surgical bed should raise the possibility of leak **(Figs. 6A and B)**.[14] At times, one can also seen disruption of the staple line at the anastomotic site.

Postoperative Abscess

Postoperative intra-abdominal abscesses are a serious complication associated with high morbidity and mortality rates of 10–40%.[10] They usually occur due to anastomotic leaks, in association with wound infections or operative contamination. Enteric pathogens such as *Klebsiella, E. Coli,* and *Proteus* are the usual causative organisms. Helical CT is reported to have a high accuracy of more than 90% for the detection of intra-abdominal abscesses.[10,15,16] On CT, these appear as a low attenuation fluid collection, spherical or ovoid in shape, which is usually well defined. They usually show a peripheral enhancing rim. Air foci, air-fluid levels or septations may be seen at times. There may be mass effect with distortion or displacement of adjacent structures. The abscess may be located in the surgical bed or at a remote location due to spread of inflammation along anatomical pathways in the peritoneal cavity or along the surgically created non-anatomic pathways and spaces.[4,10] As an example, the gastrosplenic and gastrocolic ligaments are transected during gastrectomy while the gastrohepatic ligament is partially transected. This creates a communication between the lesser sac, left sub-phrenic, gastrosplenic and gastrohepatic spaces. Hence, an anastomotic leak may cause a fluid collection or abscess in this newly created compartment with spread to the left sub-phrenic space **(Figs. 7A and B)**. Abscesses in the left subphrenic space usually have associated left pleural effusion and basal consolidation.[17] Inter-loop abscesses may be accompanied by paralytic ileus.[10]

Image-guided percutaneous catheter drainage is the preferred management option, and therefore, the initial CT report should mention the suitability for safe drainage of the abscess, especially regarding the location and access route. The true internal character of the abscess may not be evident on CT. Ultrasonography and MR are better at determining the degree of liquefaction and presence of septations which in-turn help predict whether this particular abscess will respond to percutaneous catheter drainage alone or will surgical intervention be required.[9,18] Percutaneous catheter drainage is also less likely to succeed, if the abscess is due to an anastomic leak, or if there is a fistulous communication with the bowel.[9,10]

Postoperative Bleeding

Another serious complication of abdominal surgery is hemorrhage which may be due to inadvertent vessel or organ injury, inadequate hemostasis or vascular ligation.

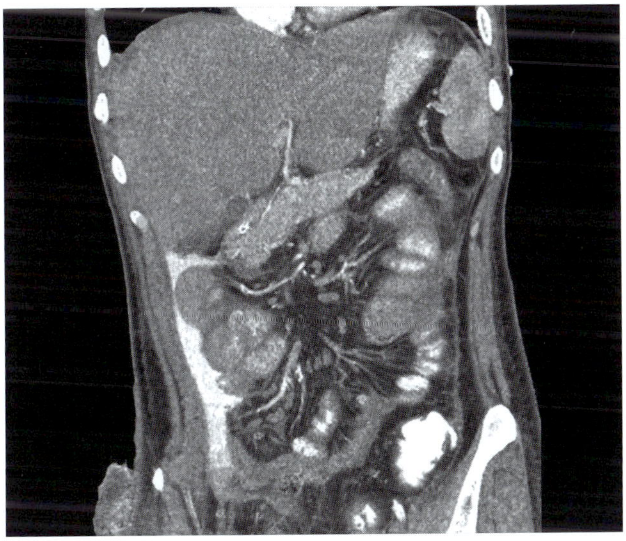

FIG. 5: A 27-year-old female underwent subtotal colectomy with endileostomy for a perforation at the hepatic flexure. Presented on day 3 following surgery with fever and pain abdomen. Coronal MPR demonstrates extraluminal oral contrast due to anastomotic leak.

In addition, in patients with obstructive jaundice or hepatic dysfunction, deficiency of vitamin K or coagulation factor may cause a hemorrhagic diathesis leading to this postoperative complication. Clinically, the patients present with signs of blood loss with falling hematocrit, tachycardia and hypotension. The surgical drains (if placed) may reveal bloody fluid or there may be oozing of blood through the incision site.[4,10,17] As mentioned previously, a biphasic CT scan should be done with negative oral contrast as intraluminal high attenuation can be masked by the positive oral contrast. A bleeding vessel may at times be seen on the CT showing active extravasation of the intravenous contrast **(Figs. 8 and 9)**. These patients may be managed by endovascular embolization. Acute hematomas are hyperdense on CT with attenuation values between 20–60 HU with a layered appearance, with gradual decrease in density over time as hemoglobin is removed from the clot **(Fig. 10)**. Chronic hematomas have fluid attenuation and may be indistinguishable from other fluid collections. There can be mass effect on the adjacent structures depending upon their location and size. Postoperative hematomas involving the solid organs (spleen, liver or kidneys) are usually confined by the organ capsule. Therefore, they appear as crescentric collections in the subcapsular space with variable compression of the underlying parenchyma.

Anterior abdominal wall hematomas can occur due to injury to perforators in the subcutaneous fat during the placement of trocars in laparoscopic surgery. High attenuation collections in the subcutaneous fat with thickening of the abdominal wall muscles which appear hyperdense will be visualized on CT **(Fig. 11)**.[5]

Anastomotic Strictures

Hold-up in the passage of contrast across the anastomotic sites on fluoroscopic examinations done in the immediate

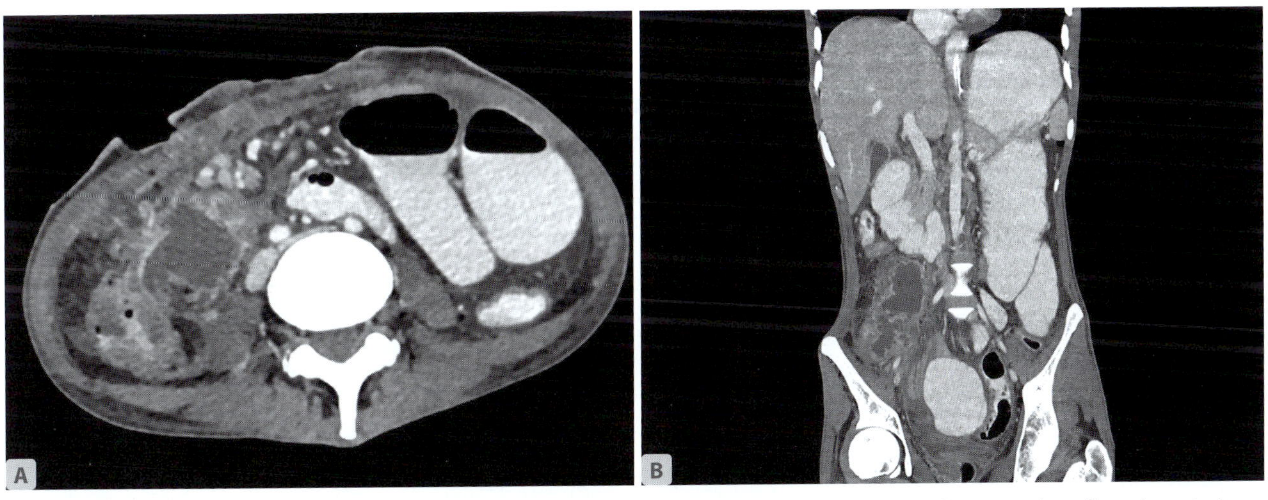

FIGS. 6A AND B: A 26-year-old female underwent ileal resection for bowel gangrene with end jejunostomy. Postrestoration of bowel continuity with jejunocolic anastomosis, presented on day 4 with high-grade fever and abdominal distension. (A) Axial CECT image shows a multiloculated collection with surrounding stranding adjacent to the anastomotic site. The ascending colon shows diffuse mural thickening. Note the thickening of the anterior abdominal wall with separation of the layers and few specks of air. (B) Coronal reconstructed image shows grossly dilated proximal jejunal loops.

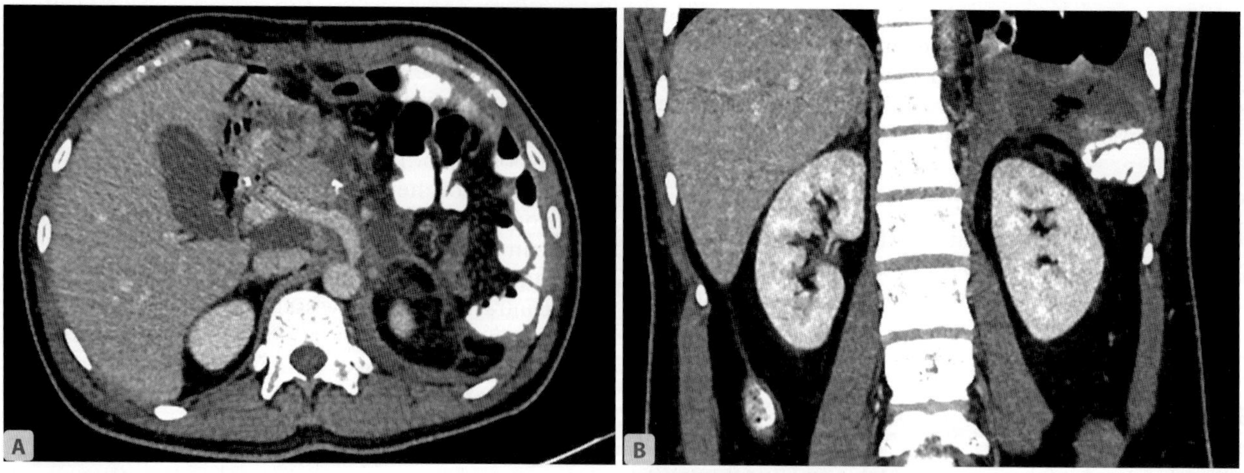

FIGS. 7A AND B: A 47-year-old male with gastric GIST underwent a total gastrectomy, distal pancreatectomy and splenectomy. Patient developed spiking fever on 7th postoperative day. (A) Axial CECT image shows small amount of fluid and fat stranding in the operative bed; (B) Coronal MPR demonstrates a fluid collection with specks of air and thick-enhancing rim in the left subphrenic space.

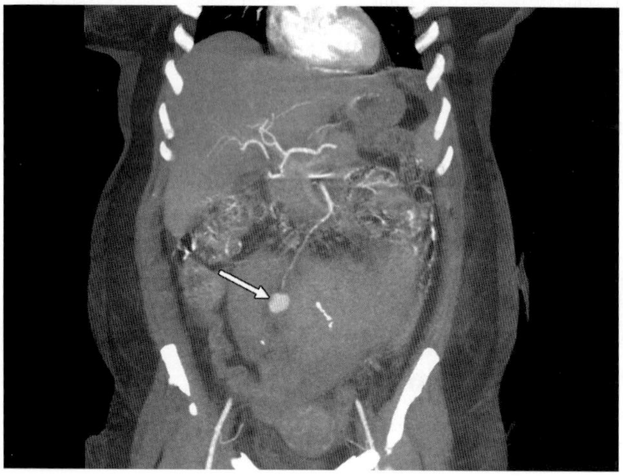

FIG. 8: A 56-year-old female underwent resection with end-to-end anastomosis for bowel gangrene. Presented with bleeding from main wound on fourth postoperative day. CT angiography coronal MIP image shows a 23 × 20 mm pseudoaneurysm arising from a branch of the superior mesenteric artery with surrounding hematoma.

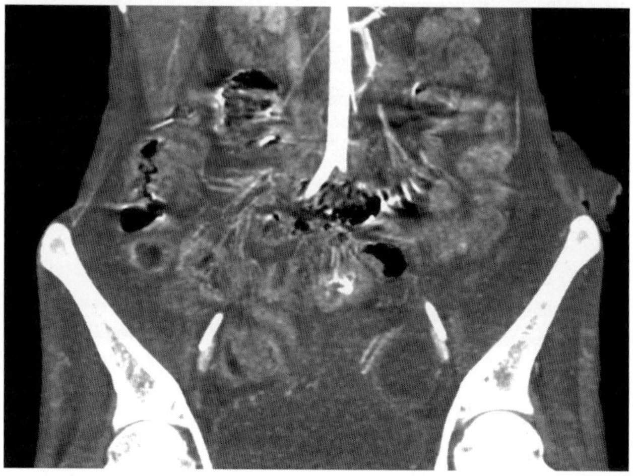

FIG. 9: A 32-year-old female who had undergone a right hemicolectomy for abdominal tuberculosis developed an enterocutaneous fistula. Presented with history of bleeding from site of fistula. CT angiography MIP image demonstrates high attenuation in the bowel lumen due to active extravasation of contrast from a branch of the superior mesenteric artery.

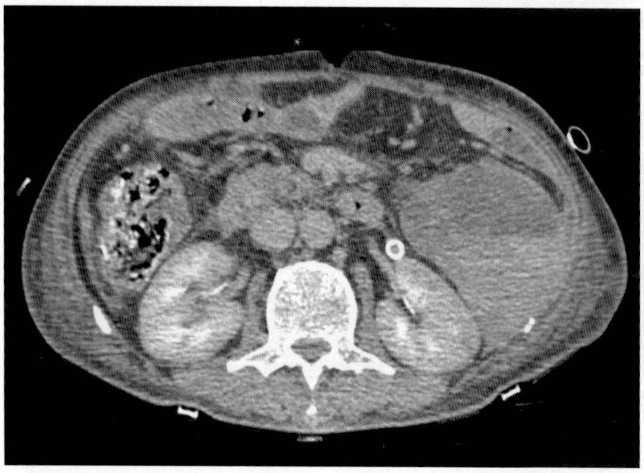

FIG. 10: A 42-year-old male underwent distal pancreatectomy with splenectomy. CECT axial image on postoperative day 4 shows a large hyperdense collection in the right lumbar region with a layered appearance consistent with acute hematoma.

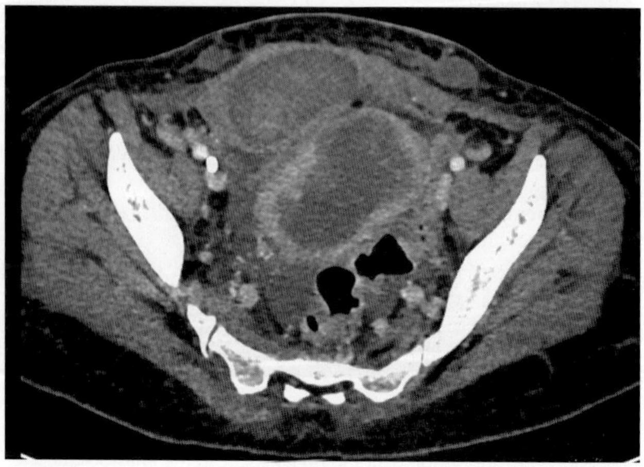

FIG. 11: A 22-year-old female underwent a cesarean section with development of postoperative sepsis. CECT on day 14 demonstrates a large hypodense collection in the right rectus sheath with few internal hyperdensities consistent with hematoma.

postoperative period is generally due to edema and resolves spontaneously over time. Nevertheless, anastomotic strictures may develop following surgical procedures due to ischemia and are more common when there has been an anastomotic leak. These can usually be managed with balloon dilatation, if an endoscopic approach is available.[19]

Postoperative Bowel Obstruction

Postoperative ileus is commonly seen in the early phase following abdominal surgery and may be due to excessive handling of the bowel loops during the procedure. It may later be a manifestation of inter-loop abscesses. Plain radiographs show mild dilatation of the small bowel loops. On CT, the small bowel is distended with fluid and air with no obvious transition point.[10] At times, there may be accompanying dilatation of the ascending and transverse colon extending till the splenic flexure with collapse of the distal colon. This is said to be due to the increase in the intra-abdominal pressure resulting in collapse of the left colon which lies in a dependent position posteriorly **(Fig. 12)**.[20] Small bowel mechanical obstruction can occur in the postoperative period due to the formation of adhesions, internal hernias or incisional or port site hernias, volvulus, strictures or tumor recurrence. Adhesions can occur in more than 90% of patients who have undergone major abdominal surgery.[21] Internal hernias can occur when the surgical procedure has involved creating defects in the mesentery or mesocolon, for example following Roux-en-Y gastrojejunostomy.[19] Typical radiological features include dilated proximal small loops with collapsed loops distal to the transition zone. There may be particulate feculent matter seen in the small bowel loop just proximal to the point of obstruction known as the "small bowel feces" sign **(Fig. 13)**.[22] An abrupt transition with no identifiable cause is likely due to adhesions **(Fig. 14)**. A cluster of dilated loops may be seen in cases of internal hernias or volvulus. The mesenteric vessels may be engorged and demonstrate the "swirl" sign as the mesentery is pulled into an abnormal location.

One must carefully look for signs of ischemia in the obstructed loop as the management of the patient may be radically altered, if present. In brief, these include mural thickening which can give a stratified appearance, abnormal enhancement of the involved segment of bowel and soft tissue stranding or fluid in the subtending mesentery. The presence of pneumatosis in the involved segment of bowel or gas in the portal venous radicles are signs of irreversible ischemia.[23]

Large bowel obstruction is less common in the postoperative period but can lead to marked dilatation of

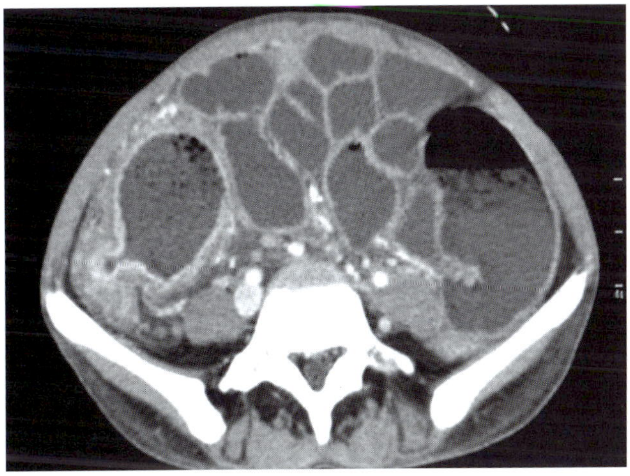

FIG. 13: A 38-year-male underwent a total colectomy with end ileostomy for ulcerative colitis. Presented with mechanical bowel obstruction two months after the surgery. CECT axial image shows gross dilatation of a small bowel loop with mottled air lucencies—the "small bowel feces" sign.

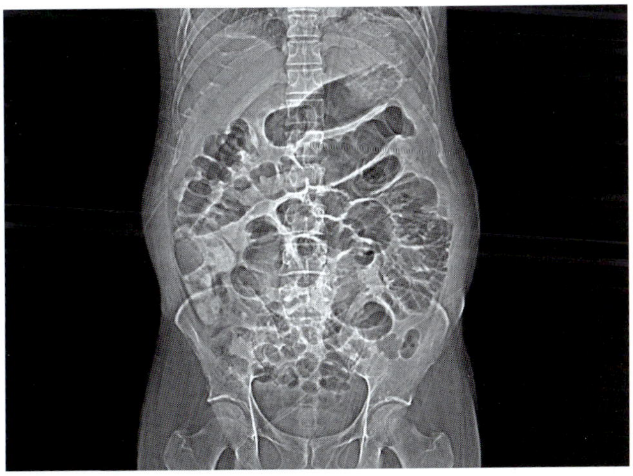

FIG. 12: A 38-year-old female developed abdominal distension on the second postoperative day following open cholecystectomy. Scout film prior to CT shows moderately dilated small bowel loops with dilatation of the ascending and descending colon and collapsed distal colon due to ileus.

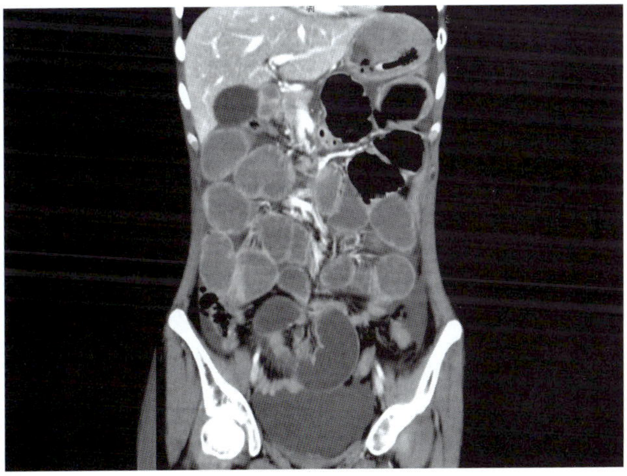

FIG. 14: A 35-year-old female postdistal pancreatectomy with splenectomy with abdominal distension and no passage of flatus. CECT reconstructed coronal image shows the dilated fluid-filled jejunal loops with an abrupt transition point beyond which the loops are collapsed. No obvious mass or stricture is seen at the transition zone, the cause of obstruction is most likely due to adhesions.

the colon. As the cecum is the most distensible segment of the colon, it bears the brunt of the dilatation. In the presence of a competent ileocecal valve, thereby preventing decompression into the small bowel, there is a grave risk of cecal ischemia as well as perforation.[9]

Wound Complications

On CT, the surgical incision site can be easily recognized as an area of increased attenuation in the subcutaneous fat and muscles of the abdominal wall. Wound infection develops in about 5–10% of patients who undergo abdominal surgery generally due to contamination by anaerobic organisms.[10] The resultant inflammation can lead to necrosis and pus accumulation at the incision site, with the potential adverse sequelae of wound dehiscence, necrotizing fasciitis, incisional hernia formation, peritonitis and systemic sepsis. Various risk factors associated with increased incidence of wound infections include elderly patients, obesity, tobacco, drugs or alcohol abuse, and presence of comorbidities. The risk also depends upon the kind of surgery performed with abdominoperineal resections having a higher incidence.[26]

CT scan can detect the presence of wound infection even before it becomes clinically apparent as small collections of fluid and air in the subcutaneous fat and muscles of the abdominal wall at and around the incision site **(Fig. 15)**.[4,10] Unless this condition is recognized early and treated promptly, it can lead on to frank abscess formation and ultimately separation of the fascia at the incision and wound dehiscence. On CT, one needs to meticulously evaluate all the layers of the abdominal wall around the incision site, including the anterior and posterior fascial sheaths for evidence of any separation which portends dehiscence.[27]

Incisional Hernia

Despite improvements in surgical techniques, incisional hernias develop in about 3–30% of cases[24,28] with the incidence

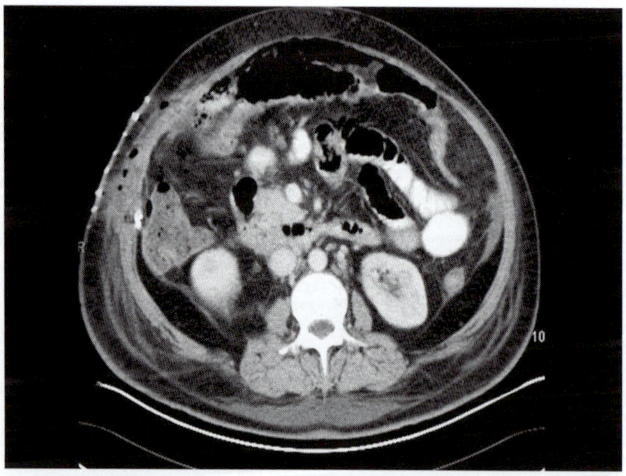

FIG. 15: A 41-year-old female underwent extended cholecystectomy for carcinoma gallbladder. Postoperative day 14 CECT shows thickening of the layers of the anterior abdominal wall at the incision site with multiple foci of air suggestive of wound infection.

rising in the presence of wound infection.[29] It is also more common when median or paramedian vertical incisions are used in comparison to horizontal incisions as vertical incisions transect the muscular fibers rather than dissect along them. These transected muscles are rendered more prone to disruption in the presence of increased abdominal pressure.[10,30] Most incisional hernias develop within the first year following surgery but may manifest clinically much later. Clinical examination usually suffices to reach the diagnosis, however in the presence of obesity or a thick keloid, the abdominal wall defect may not be palpable. Secondly, the omentum is usually the initial content of the hernia and may not be palpable, if the sac has dissected between the layers of the abdominal wall. In this clinical setting, a CT may be asked for in order to find a cause for the patients symptoms and will establish the correct diagnosis.[24-26] Once bowel loops also herniate into the sac, they can get incarcerated and obstructed.

CT scans will show a defect in the layers of the abdominal wall with protrusion of omentum, a loop of small bowel or mesentery through it into the subcutaneous fat. Presence of stranding in the fat, small fluid collections or mural thickening of the herniated bowel loop are early changes that suggest strangulation.[25] Herniation may also occur at port sites following laparoscopy with a reported incidence of 0.5% with a higher risk associated with the use of trocars over 12 mm and large diameter ports.[5] Parastomal herniation may also occur along ileostomy or colostomy sites **(Figs. 16A and B)**.[10]

Retained Surgical Foreign Material

Unintended retention of a surgical material in a patient poses a serious risk of complications for the patient and lays the surgical team open for a malpractice suit. Usual operating theater procedures include repeated counts of all surgical material being used to prevent this complication, but it still occurs though the exact incidence is not known. Reports reveal that surgical sponges are the most often retained foreign object followed by instruments.[31] Septic or aseptic complications result due to the retained foreign object (RFO). If the RFO remains sterile, fibrosis occurs due to a foreign body response leading to adhesions or fistula formation. Retained surgical swabs are referred to as gossypibomas or textilomas and appear on CT as well-defined soft tissue masses with a whorled texture and multiple internal foci of air **(Figs. 17A and B)**. Enhancement of the rim is seen following intravenous contrast. It is helpful to identify the wavy radiopaque markers which are now incorporated into most surgical sponges[9,32] which may be better appreciated on the scout image rather than the axial images. In the setting of infection, there is abscess formation with a loculated fluid collection often showing a thick enhancing rim. On MR imaging, retained sponges show an intermediate signal intensity on T1-weighted images similar to skeletal muscle. Internal high signal intensity fluid may be seen on T2-weighted images with low signal intensity structures having a whorled appearance.[31]

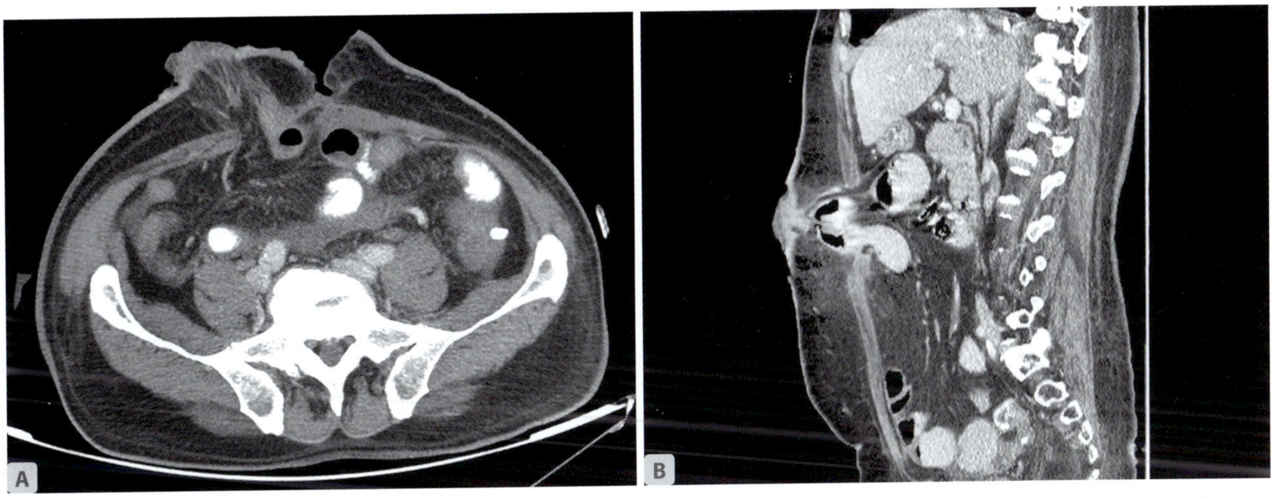

FIGS. 16A AND B: (A) Axial CECT image of a 78-year-old male showing a small parastomal hernia containing mainly omental fat and vessels; (B) Coronal MPR image of a 43-year-old female with a transverse colostomy with a large parastomal hernial sac containing small bowel loops.

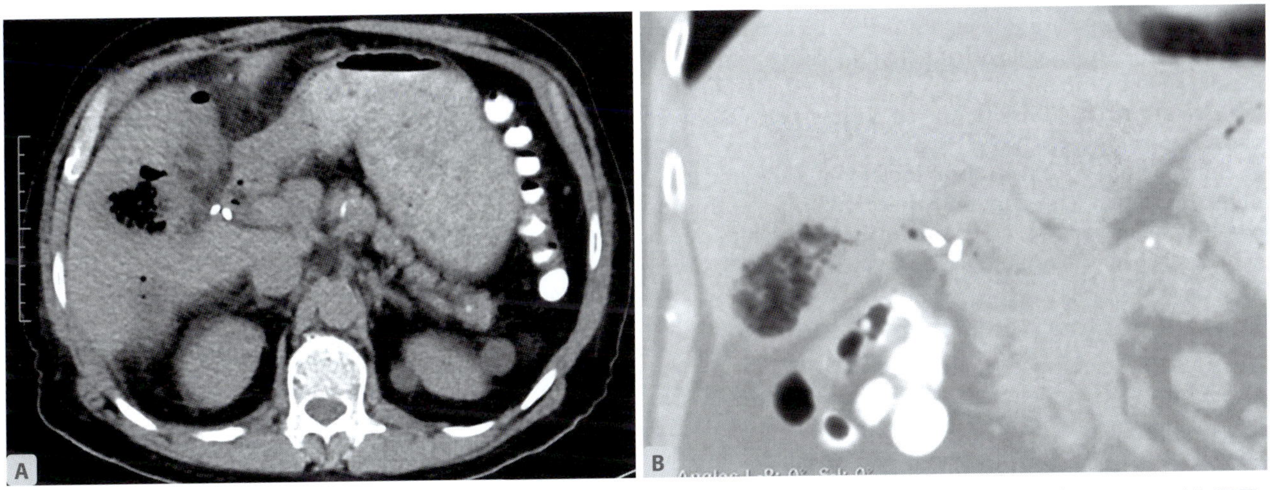

FIGS. 17A AND B: A 28-year-old female complained of intermittent right hypochondrial pain following a laparoscopic cholecystectomy. (A) CECT axial image shows an ill-defined hypodense area with multiple air foci adjacent to the surgical clips consistent with gossypiboma; (B) The internal whorled appearance is better appreciated on viewing at lung window settings.

NORMAL POSTOPERATIVE ANATOMY AND COMPLICATIONS SPECIFIC TO PROCEDURE

It is beyond the scope of this chapter to discuss the normal postoperative anatomy of the myriad surgical procedures performed in the abdomen. This chapter will limit itself to discussing some of the most commonly performed surgical procedures.

Esophageal Surgeries

Esophageal resections are commonly performed for malignancy but may also be performed for benign strictures refractory to balloon dilatation. The Ivor Lewis esophagectomy involves resection of the diseased part of the mid and distal esophagus, and mobilization of the stomach which is then placed vertically inside the mediastinum after fashioning it into a tubular structure by resection of the greater curvature. This is then anastomosed with the esophagus in an end-to end or end-to-side manner. In case of disease involving the upper esophagus a neck dissection is also done and the esophagogastric anastomotic is created in the neck. These are usually accompanied with a pyloroplasty to drain the stomach as the vagus nerve is sacrificed during the procedure.[33]

Upper gastrointestinal contrast studies are routinely performed between 5–10 days postoperatively to look for any anastomotic leak before the patient is allowed oral intake. Water-soluble non-ionic contrast is preferred as it does not carry the risk of chemical pneumonia in case of aspiration.[34] Many authors advocate the use of repeating the study with dilute barium in case the first study is negative in order to increase the sensitivity.[35,36] A plain radiograph should be obtained prior to administering contrast so that any subtle difference in density in pleural effusions can be detected which denote leak. It also aids in differentiating between a small leak and a surgical clip. CT may be done, if the contrast study is negative but the patient is unwell and improves the sensitivity for the detection of anastomotic leaks.[36]

Major complications occur in about 20% of patients which can be grouped into general complications of a thoracotomy such as pneumonia, atelectasis and respiratory failure or specific to the esophageal surgery. There can be vascular injury leading to a hemothorax or injury to the thoracic duct leading to a chylothorax but the most common complication is an anastomotic leak which carries significant morbidity and mortality. The leak usually occurs early in the postoperative period (2–3 days) due to technical failure of the anastomoses. Leaks occurring later at around 3–7 days are usually due to ischemia of the anastomotic margins. The leak may occur from the esophagogastrectomy, from the margins of the stomach where the greater curvature has been resected or from the pyloroplasty, hence all these sites need to be carefully examined. A leak can lead to formation of an esophago-bronchial or esophagopleural fistula, mediastinitis and sepsis **(Fig. 18)**. These patients are also at increased risk for the subsequent development of strictures.[37]

Imaging has a similar role to look for anastomotic leaks following bypass procedures where colonic, jejunal or myocutaneous flaps are used. A more dreaded complication is ischemia of the conduit which is diagnosed endoscopically.

Surgeries of the Stomach and Duodenum

Gastric resections are commonly performed surgical procedures for malignancies involving the stomach or complicated peptic ulcer disease. In the Billroth I partial gastrectomy, the distal stomach is resected and an anastomosis created between the duodenum and proximal stomach. The Billroth II/Polya partial gastrectomy involves resection of the distal stomach, closure of the duodenal stump and creation of a gastrojejunostomy in an antecolic or retrocolic position. In a Roux-en-Y procedure, the bowel continuity after distal gastrectomy is restored through construction of a Roux loop. Direct anastomoses of the distal esophagus with a jejunal Roux loop is performed following total gastrectomy. A contrast fluoroscopic study is usually performed using water soluble contrast in the immediate postoperative period to rule out leakage. However, the study can detect subclinical leaks in 7% of cases which do not require any further surgical intervention. The study may also return false negative results with leaks identified on subsequent endoscopy.[38] Hence, some surgeons reserve the contrast study to cases where there is a clinical suspicion of leak. The afferent limb may not opacify with oral contrast, hence a CT examination should be done in case of clinical suspicion of duodenal stump blow-out. It may show complex, air/fluid collections in the region of the duodenal stump which can be identified by the surgical staples line **(Figs. 19A and B)**. Collections may also be seen in the subhepatic or peripancreatic spaces.[17]

The afferent loop may get obstructed due to adhesion or twisting of the bowel at the gastroenterostomy site. Acute obstruction can cause duodenal stump blow-out and is an emergent situation. CT can demonstrate the dilated, fluid-filled loop passing posterior to the superior mesenteric vessels to the left side. Obstruction to the outflow of bile usually results in associated dilatation of the biliary tree.[39]

Tumor recurrence becomes a more common cause for obstructive symptoms developing later in the time course after the surgery. CT is the imaging modality of choice in this situation and should be carefully evaluated for recurrence in the surgical bed or anastomotic site and any evidence of spread of disease to the lymph nodes, liver or peritoneum.[40] If the initial malignancy was a gastrointestinal stromal tumor, addition of an arterial phase to the imaging protocol is of benefit as these tumours are typically hypervascular.

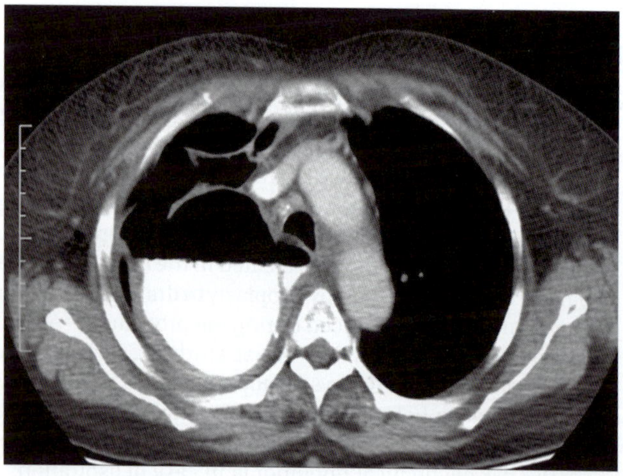

FIG. 18: A 42-year-old male underwent thoracoscopic assisted esophagectomy for carcinoma. Presented with complaints of chest pain, dyspnea and had tachycardia. CECT axial image demonstrates a leak from the esophagogastric anastomotic site with formation of a esophagopleural fistula.

Bariatric Surgery

Morbid obesity has shown an alarming increasing trend in its prevalence even in India over the last few years and has now reached epidemic proportions. A BMI over 25 kg/m^2 is considered overweight internationally. However, updated guidelines released by the Indian Council of Medical Research and the Ministry of Health and Family Welfare in 2012 considers a BMI over 23 kg/m^2 as overweight. This is due to a genetic tendency of Indians towards abdominal obesity with its attendant risk of life style diseases. Despite the morbidly obese forming a high-risk group, surgery for weight loss is offered to these patients as it reduces the long-term associated morbidity and improves life expectancy.[41]

Two kinds of procedures are used: malabsorptive procedures wherein the length of the absorptive surface is reduced by bypassing a segment of the small bowel. These are seldom used in isolation these days due to significant associated complications. Restrictive procedures aim to reduce the capacity of the stomach in order to induce early satiety. These include sleeve gastrectomy, vertical gastroplasty and laparoscopic adjustable gastric banding

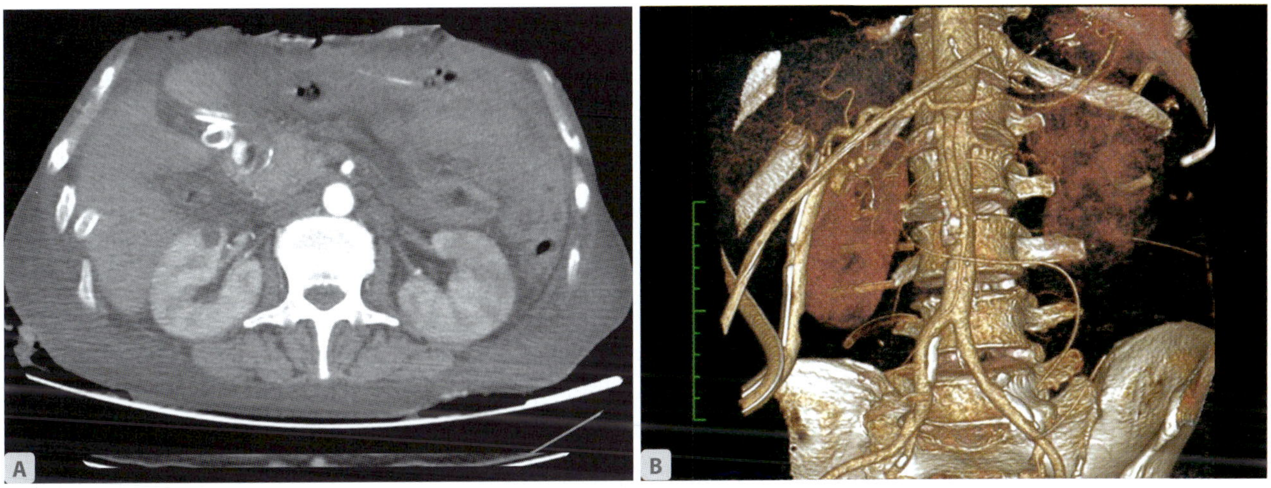

FIGS. 19A AND B: A 57-year-old male with gastric carcinoma, status postgastrectomy and Billroth II gastrojejunostomy. Had duodenal stump blow-out which was being managed conservatively with placement of a subhepatic drain. Now presented with bloody discharge from the drain. CT angiography (A) axial image shows active extravasation of intravenous contrast with pooling in the duodenum adjacent to the surgical drain; (B) Coronal volume-rendered image shows pseudoaneurysms arising from the gastroduodenal artery, probably due to leak of the pancreatic enzymes from the duodenal stump.

(LAGB). The Roux-en-Y gastric bypass (RYGB) and biliopancreatic diversion are combination procedures with both restrictive and malabsorptive components. Sleeve gastrectomy involves creating a narrow gastric tube along the lesser curvature by resecting 70–85% of the stomach along the greater curvature. In LAGB, an inflatable band is placed just below the gastroesophageal junction, thereby creating a small gastric pouch. The band is connected to a port in the anterior abdominal wall through which the volume of the band can be adjusted and therefore the degree of restriction. In the RYGB, a small gastric pouch is created in its proximal part and anastomosed to a Roux loop. The rest of the stomach and duodenum forms the biliopancreatic limb which is also anastomosed to the Roux loop. The length of the Roux loop determines the degree of malabsorption with more distal loops having more malabsorptive effect.[42]

Early in the postoperative period, a contrast fluoroscopic examination is usually performed to rule out anastomotic leaks. Following sleeve gastrectomy, most of the leaks occur from the proximal end, close to the gastroesophageal junction. CT is required for evaluation of the biliopancreatic limb in RYGB procedures. It is also the best modality for investigating a patient with suspected efferent loop obstruction, which may be due to adhesions, strictures, internal hernias or incisional hernias. Three types of internal hernias can occur following RYGB procedures:

a. Through the defect created in the transverse mesocolon when a retrocolic anastomosis has been created. Multiple, dilated small bowel loops will be seen superior to the transverse mesocolon, rather than the single anastomotic Roux loop on CT.
b. Through the defect created in the small bowel mesentery due to the jejunojejunostomy. In this case, a cluster of loops will be seen located beneath the anterior abdominal wall with absence of any intervening omental fat. The colon may be centrally displaced.
c. Through the defect in the mesentery posterior to the Roux loop (Peterson type).[43] Characteristically, there will be a cluster of small bowel loops in the left upper abdomen with shift of the superior mesenteric vessels to the left.

The gastric band placed in LAGB may migrate away from the gastroesophageal junction. The usual orientation of the balloon is at 45°, with migration it takes up a more vertical or horizontal position ("O" sign), which will be evident on plain radiographs.[44] A contrast swallow will confirm dilated stomach above the band. If the migration remains unrecognized or untreated, it may lead to gastric necrosis.

Small Bowel

Surgeries on the small bowel are commonly performed for resection of diseased segments or resections of segments which are required to be used as a conduit elsewhere. As mentioned earlier, the most common immediate postoperative complication is an anastomotic leak which is best evaluated by a CT after oral intravenous contrast. Delayed complications such as intestinal obstruction or recurrence of disease are usually evaluated with a combination of fluoroscopic contrast studies and cross-sectional imaging such as CT or MR enteroclysis or enterography.

Blind Pouch Syndrome

Side-to-side small bowel anastomoses or incorrectly performed end-to-side anastomoses can result in the formation of a blind pouch which is an enlarged, blind-ended, aperistaltic small bowel loop. These usually manifest late after surgery with features of malabsorption or due to complications such as perforation or bleeding. A dynamic investigation such as fluoroscopic enteroclysis will demonstrate the preferential filling of the blind pouch with dilatation of the loop. CT will demonstrate a saccular structure filled with oral contrast in close relation to surgical clips/staples.

Ileal Pouch-Anal Anastomoses (IPAA)

A total proctocolectomy is the definitive treatment for patients with ulcerative colitis or familiar adenomatous polyposis (FAP). This is followed by creation of an ileal pouch which is anastomosed to the anal canal, thus maintaining continence by preserving the anal sphincter. The ileal reservoir is created from the terminal ileum in a J, S or W manner of which the J-shape is the most commonly performed.[45] The pouch is usually allowed to heal by performing a proximal temporary ileostomy with restoration of the bowel continuity after 8-12 weeks. Routine fluoroscopic contrast studies are performed before closure of the ileostomy to rule out any leaks. CT may be done, if there is clinical suspicion of an abscess or obstruction.

Pouchitis is a non-specific inflammation of the pouch with uncertain etiology which can affect upto half the patients. The usual clinical presentation is with diarrhea, bleeding and tenesmus. The radiologic features are non-specific with dilatation of the pouch, mural thickening, mucosal enhancement and stranding in the surrounding fat.[46]

Large Bowel

Various kinds of resections of the large bowel are performed for both benign and malignant diseases. The right hemicolectomy involves resection of the right colon and terminal ileum with an ileotransverse colon anastomosis. In the extended right hemicolectomy, the transverse colon is also resected to varying extents. In a left hemicolectomy, the left colon including the splenic flexure and proximal sigmoid colon are resected. A Hartmann's procedure involves closing off of the rectum and sigmoid colon after a diverting colostomy after distal colectomy when a primary anastomosis is not considered safe. This rectal stump can later be reattached to the distal colon. At times, instead of closing off the stump, a distal mucous fistula is created by bringing the stump upto the anterior abdominal wall. Anterior resection consists of resecting the sigmoid colon and varying part of the rectum with a colorectal anastomosis. When the upper rectum is resected above the peritoneal reflection, it is termed a high anterior resection while in the low or extended low anterior resection, the middle or distal rectum are also resected. Abdominoperineal excision of the rectum involves resection of the anal canal as well. Restorative proctocolectomy involves resection of the entire colon and rectum with formation of an ileal pouch.

Some surgeons routinely ask for fluoroscopic contrast studies to rule out anastomotic leaks. These are most often posterior in location after procedures involving the rectum and may cause anterior displacement of the rectum (3-5 cm from the anterior sacral margin). The patient must be fluoroscoped again after being asked to void as some leaks may become evident only after emptying the rectum.[25]

CT may be asked for in the early postoperative period, if there is clinical suspicion of an anastomotic leak, abscess, fistula or bowel obstruction. Rectal contrast should always be administered prior to the scan. The "double rectum" sign has been described in rectal anastomotic leaks. This is due to the anteriorly displaced rectum with a fluid collection in the presacral space due to the leak **(Figs. 20A to C)**.[25,47] Other signs of leaks are frank extravasation of the rectal contrast, air within or outside the bowel wall, fluid collections, disruption of the staple line and pneumoperitoneum.

Diversion Colitis

Once the temporary colostomy has to be taken down with restoration of bowel continuity, a fluoroscopic contrast study is normally asked for by the surgeon prior to closure. The unused segment often appears nondistensible with diffuse mucosal nodularity or even punctuate ulcerations. The exact etiology is unclear, however, the colon returns to normal once the bowel continuity is restored with resumption of the fecal stream through it.[25]

HEPATOBILIARY SURGERIES

Curative liver surgeries are performed for many benign and malignant liver diseases. The type of surgery depends on the nature and location of the disease and expertise of the surgeon.[48] Most common indications for liver resections are malignancies such as colorectal metastasis, hepatocellular carcinoma (without underlying cirrhosis), neuroendocrine metastasis, cholangiocarcinoma, benign diseases such as hepatic adenomas, symptomatic cysts, intrahepatic biliary calculi and traumatic hepatic lacerations.[49]

Surgical Procedures

Hepatectomies are divided into anatomical and non-anatomical resections. Anatomical resections involve removing contiguous hepatic segments whereas non-anatomical resections are wedge resections which are usually small and peripheral. A standardized nomenclature for anatomical resections has been proposed by the Brisbane 2000 Terminology of Hepatic Anatomy and Resection.[50] Right hepatectomy involves resection of segments 5, 6, 7, and 8, that is, removing the entire liver parenchyma to the right of the middle hepatic vein. Extended right hepatectomy involves additional resection of segment 4 in addition to right lobe. Left hepatectomy involves resection of segments 2, 3, and 4, that is, resection of liver parenchyma to the left of the middle hepatic vein. Extended left hepatectomy involves additional resection of segments 5 and 8. Monosegmentectomy is resection of a single segment, whereas bisegmentectomy involves resection of two contiguous segments. Nonanatomical resections are suitable for small peripheral lesions.[48]

Normal Postoperative Imaging Features

Small fluid collections, hematomas or bilomas can be routinely observed in the early postoperative period and generally regress over a period of few weeks. In addition metallic surgical clips, extra-luminal gas accumulation, and pleural effusions are also routine findings on imaging. Thrombosis of the portal branch stump can also be seen in the early postoperative period. In addition, a linear band of low attenuation may be observed adjacent to the resection margins. This finding is transient and is possibly due to accumulation of bile or blood, or devascularized parenchyma.[48]

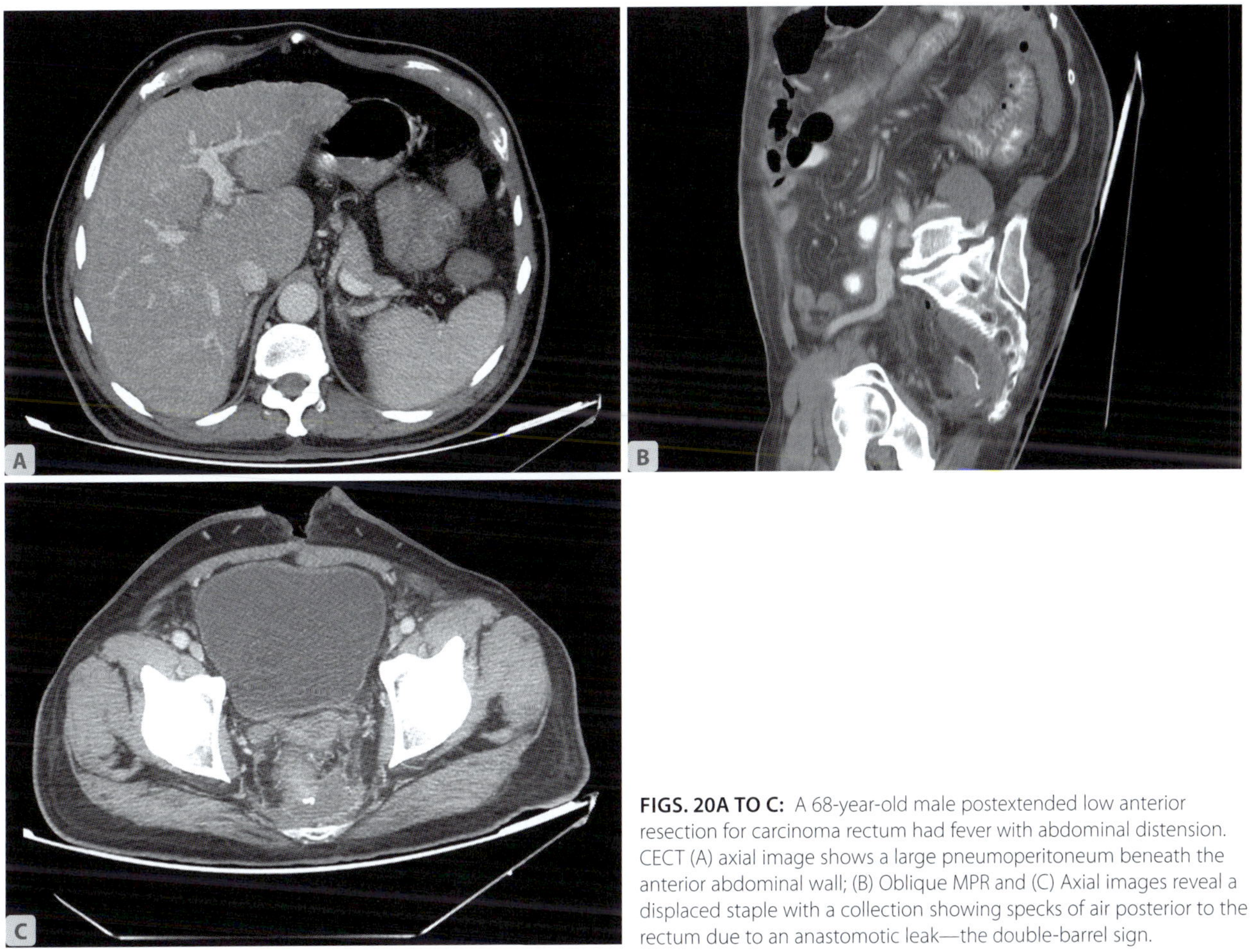

FIGS. 20A TO C: A 68-year-old male postextended low anterior resection for carcinoma rectum had fever with abdominal distension. CECT (A) axial image shows a large pneumoperitoneum beneath the anterior abdominal wall; (B) Oblique MPR and (C) Axial images reveal a displaced staple with a collection showing specks of air posterior to the rectum due to an anastomotic leak—the double-barrel sign.

Late Postoperative Period

The volume of the remaining liver rapidly increases up to 100% during 6 months to 1 year; with up to 60% in the first 7 days following the surgery.[51,52] After right hepatectomy, the left and caudate lobes hypertrophy and shift to the right. There is upward displacement of the right kidney, hepatic flexure, and small bowel loops with posterior displacement of the IVC. After left hepatectomy, there is hypertrophy of right and caudate lobes, right kidney is usually displaced caudally and stomach or colon occupy the left hepatic fossa. Transient splenic enlargement during initial 6 months after liver resection may be observed.[53]

EARLY POSTOPERATIVE COMPLICATIONS

The most frequent early postoperative complications are fluid collections, vascular thrombosis and biliary injuries. Fluid collections are usually adjacent to resection margins, and correspond to seromas, hematomas (50%), bilomas (25%), or infected collections (25%).[48]

Vascular Thrombosis

Thrombosis of a single hepatic vein is frequently seen after liver resections and is usually partial and seen close to the resection margins. Portal vein and hepatic artery thrombosis are rare, with segmental portal thrombosis more frequently observed than thrombosis of the main portal vein **(Fig. 21)**.[48]

Biliary Injuries

Biliary injuries can be bile leaks and biliary obstruction. Bile leak after hepatic surgery may originate from the site of a biliary-enteric anastomosis, or may be related to the removal of an external drainage tube, or to intraoperative bile duct injury.[54] Ultrasonography and MDCT may show fluid collections at the resection margin. MRCP may be used to identify the location and the nature of the leak.[54]

Biliary obstruction results from postoperative fibrosis at the bile duct stump or inadvertent bile duct ligation. It is most frequently seen after biliary-enteric anastomosis, with obstruction of the Roux-en-Y loop.[55] Multidetector computed tomography (MDCT) will show dilated biliary tree with dilated fluid-filled Roux-en-Y loop.[48]

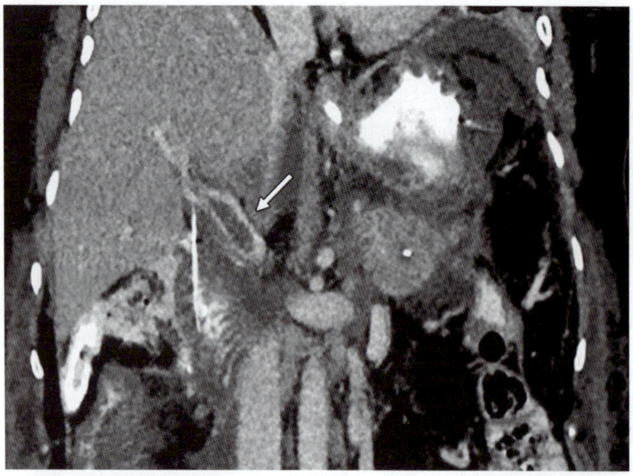

FIG. 21: A 61-year-old male underwent a left hepatectomy. CECT coronal MPR reveals a thrombus as a hypodense filling defect in the main portal vein (arrow).

Intraoperative Diaphragmatic Injury

Diaphragmatic injuries are very rare and mostly seen after right hepatectomy. Right pleural effusion with increased pleural enhancement may be seen on MDCT. They may present with early small bowel obstruction, if the bowel herniates through the diaphragmatic defect.[48]

LATE POSTOPERATIVE COMPLICATIONS

Late complications after hepatic resection are disease recurrence and ischemic cholangitis. Follow-up MDCT or MR are performed depending on the nature of the resected hepatic tumor for the detection of tumor recurrence. Presence of segmental or subsegmental bile duct dilatation although nonspecific, may be suggestive of disease recurrence, even in the absence of a visible focal lesion.[48]

Ischemic cholangitis may occur after liver resection within several months to several years in cases of intraoperative arterial injury. The clinical presentation is nonspecific with jaundice and fever. Magnetic resonance cholangiopancreatography (MRCP) is the modality of choice and may show irregular and multiple bile duct stenoses with intra-hepatic bile duct dilatations.[48]

Laparoscopic Cholecystectomy

Laparoscopic cholecystectomy is the preferred procedure for patients with symptomatic gallstones. However, complications after laparoscopic cholecystectomy especially bile duct injuries, have been reported to be more common in comparison to open surgery.[56] USG, CT, ERCP, MRCP and radionuclide imaging have a role to play in evaluating the postoperative patient.[57-59] These investigations are complementary and the primary imaging technique to be used will depend on the clinical problem faced and availability.

Normal Appearances after Laparoscopic Cholecystectomy

- A small amount of fluid in the surgical bed is a common finding postoperatively during the first week. These fluid collections have no distinct or well-demarcated borders on CT.[60]
- Increased density in the abdominal wall fat at the site of the laparoscopic ports and small amounts of free pelvic fluid may also be seen.[61]
- The diameter of the CBD may increase post-cholecystectomy, with a maximal diameter of 13 mm identified.[62] When biliary dilatation is identified on postoperative imaging, correlation with preoperative imaging and current clinical features and biochemistry is required.

Complications

Major complications after cholecystectomy can be divided into biliary, vascular, and laparoscopic complications. Biliary complications include bile duct injury, biliary obstruction, and dropped stones.

Biliary Injury

Bile leakage secondary to bile duct injury is the most common complication of laparoscopic cholecystectomy.[63] Most leaks occur from the cystic duct stump. Some common mechanisms for the leak include dislodgement of clips from the cystic duct stump, laceration, transection or thermal injuries of the duct.[64] The initial assessment in these patients is usually with sonography or MDCT which may show peri-hepatic fluid. Hepatobiliary scintigraphy is a less commonly used method of evaluating patients with suspected bile duct injury, however, it has been claimed to be more sensitive and specific than sonography or CT in detecting bile leaks.[65] Although it is an invasive procedure, ERCP is useful as it can show the exact site of leak and successfully treat the leak using internal stents. Endoscopic retrograde cholangiopancreatogram (ERCP) is more likely to be successful, if the injury to the duct is < 5 mm, the injury is extra-hepatic, and there is no associated abscess or biloma.[66] Open surgery may be required, if the leak persists. MRCP is a non-invasive way of assessing the anatomy of bile ducts. The use of mangafodipir trisodium, a contrast agent that is primarily excreted via bile helps to both diagnose a bile leak and identify the source of the leak.[67]

Biliary Obstruction

Retained gallstones, misplaced surgical clips, fibrosis due to inflammation from adjacent clips, and thermal injury from cautery devices are causes of biliary obstruction **(Fig. 22)**.[66] Patients present with progressive postoperative obstructive jaundice. Ultrasound and MRCP detect duct dilatation and exclude CBD stones. ERCP is useful in confirming the diagnosis and may be therapeutic.

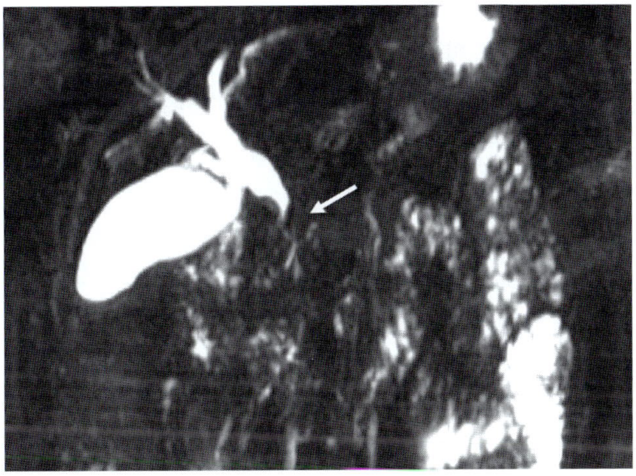

FIG. 22: A 25-year-old female underwent a laparoscopic cholecystectomy for gallstone disease. She presented with obstructive jaundice 6 months later. MRCP-MIP image shows a stricture (arrow) in the lower end of the CBD.

Stone Retention

Stone retention is an important complication of laparoscopic cholecystectomy, with an incidence between 1.1% and 7%.[68] Factors which predispose to retained stones are a long cystic duct pedicle and incomplete excision of gallbladder due to adhesions. Similarly, since the CBD is not explored during laparoscopic cholecystectomy, a gallbladder stone can migrate into the CBD in patients with patulous cystic duct when the gallbladder is pulled in a cephalad direction during cholecystectomy, causing biliary obstruction. In patients with suspected stone retention, MRCP is helpful in depicting these stones, while ERCP is both diagnostic and therapeutic.[64]

Dropped Gallstones

Spillage of gallstones occurs due to inadvertent entry into the gallbladder during dissection or at the time of gallbladder extraction through the port site. The majority of "dropped" gallstones are found in the right upper quadrant, but they may migrate to dependent areas (right paracolic gutter or pelvis).[69] Most remain asymptomatic, however, significant complications can occur since they cause a local foreign body reaction.[70] Abscess formation is the most common complication resulting from "dropped" stones and may develop months later following cholecystectomy.[69]

Vascular Injury

Injury to blood vessels during trocar insertion is responsible for peri or postoperative hemorrhage.[71] During dissection of Calot's triangle, the right hepatic artery is the most common vessel to be injured followed by the portal vein **(Figs. 23A to C)**.[70] Hepatic artery ligation may lead to the development of a delayed ischemic cholangiopathy. MRCP may show irregular ductal dilatation and stenosis.

Pancreatic Surgeries

Pancreatic resection surgeries for the tumors and chronic pancreatitis include Whipple and Beger's procedures as well as central and distal pancreatectomy, while drainage procedures include Puestow and Frey's operations.[72] Information regarding the type of surgery the patient has undergone as well as the interval between surgery and imaging is important for interpretation of postoperative scans.

Whipples Procedure

This procedure involves resection of pancreatic head, jejunum, gastric antrum, and duodenum, followed by hepaticojejunostomy (HJ), pancreaticojejunostomy (PJ), and duodenojejunostomy (DJ) or gastrojejunostomy (GJ). The normal postoperative findings include the presence of these different anastomoses.[72] Following pancreatic head resection, the splenomesenteric venous junction and superior mesenteric vein will be seen to the right of the residual pancreatic parenchyma and in close proximity to the inferior vena cava posteriorly.

Beger's Procedure

It involves resection of the pancreatic head with preservation of duodenum. PJ is done at two locations of the Roux-en-Y limb following pancreatic head removal. A sleeve of the pancreatic parenchyma is left behind along with duodenum ensuring the preservation of blood supply of the duodenum.[72]

Puestow Procedure

It consists of side-to-side longitudinal PJ with MPD draining directly into a loop of jejunum. The Roux-en-Y loop following this surgery lies immediately anterior to pancreatic body or tail.[72]

Frey's Procedure

It includes partial resection of pancreatic head and a longitudinal PJ, with an intact biliary duct.[72]

Central Pancreatectomy

Part of the pancreatic body or neck is resected, followed by a Roux-en-Y PJ to the remaining pancreatic tissue in the distal part. The distal end of the pancreas, may, however be anastomosed to the stomach. The proximal cut end is sutured, and the Roux-en-Y bowel is seen at the level of the splenoportal confluence, separating apart the pancreatic head from its body and tail.

Distal Pancreatectomy

The pancreatic parenchyma lying to the left of SMV is resected, and the cut end is sutured to prevent pancreatic juice leakage. The pancreas thereby ends abruptly, and the surgical bed will not have any bowel related to the pancreas, stomach or duodenum, as against in the above described surgeries. As the blood supply to the tail of pancreas comes mostly from splenic artery branches, splenectomy becomes necessary at times along with distal pancreatectomy.

NORMAL POSTOPERATIVE FINDINGS

Several normal postoperative CT and MRI findings may be misdiagnosed as the disease process, hence, knowledge of normal postoperative appearances is highly essential.

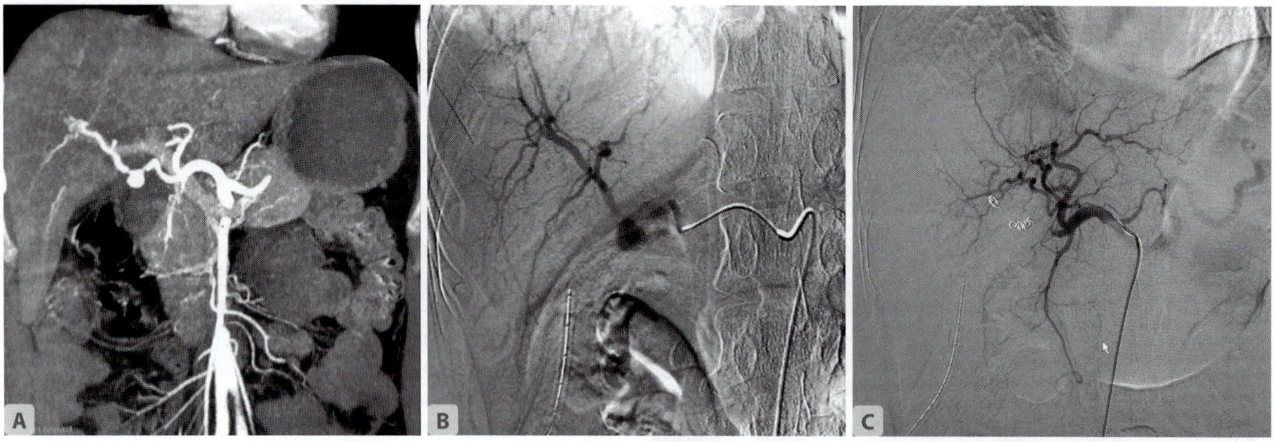

FIGS. 23A TO C: A 32-year-old female had a laparoscopic cholecystectomy following which she developed hemobilia and malena. (A) CT angiography coronal MIP image shows a large pseudoaneurysm arising from the right hepatic artery; (B) Selective right hepatic artery angiogram confirms the CT angiography findings; (C) Check angiogram postsuccessful endovascular coiling demonstrates no filling of the aneurysm.

- Pneumobilia (tends to persist) and periportal hepatic edema (usually resolves within a month) are universally seen. Air may be seen in the MPD also as a normal finding. However, pneumobilia should not be seen following surgeries in which there are no biliary anastomoses.[72]
- The afferent loop of bowel following Frey procedure which drains the biliary ducts and pancreas may be thick and edematous for the first three weeks following surgery, and should not be misdiagnosed as hemorrhage or ischemia.[72]
- Roux loop following the Puestow procedure lies between the body of the pancreas and stomach in the lesser sac, and may be falsely diagnosed to be a pancreatic mass or internal hernia.[72] The use of positive oral contrast for distending the bowel and changing the patient from a supine to a lateral decubitus position during CT, characteristic location as well as course of the Roux loop, and the presence of valvulae conniventes help in preventing a misdiagnosis.[73]
- Transient fluid collections in the surgical bed are common in the first month following surgery. The presence of air foci within these collections does not necessarily indicate infection but should raise the suspicion of a pancreatic fistula.[74-76]
- Reactive lymphadenopathy (nodes up to 1.5 cm in the short axis diameter) is seen up to two months after the surgery and regresses on follow-up imaging.[77]
- Perivascular cuffing around the celiac artery and its branches, and superior mesenteric artery is seen for up to 6 weeks following Whipple and Beger's procedures. This cuffing is inflammatory in nature in patients having negative surgical margins and should not be wrongly diagnosed as tumor recurrence. Follow-up imaging becomes necessary to distinguish between the perivascular cuffing and disease recurrence.
- Mild pancreatic duct dilation (1–2 mm in comparison to preoperative imaging) is an expected postoperative appearance, and does not correlate with subsequent pancreatitis.[72]
- There may be a cavity detected in the head of the pancreas after Frey's procedure, which may be falsely diagnosed as a pancreatic pseudocyst or cystic neoplasm.[72] This cavity usually decreases with time.

COMPLICATIONS

Minor complications are relatively more frequent (seen in 28–29% patients), as against major complications that may require surgical intervention or vascular embolization (seen in 11% patients).[72]

- *Delayed gastric emptying:* Seen in upto 50% of patients during the early postoperative course following pylorus preserving pancreatoduodenectomy.[78,79] Gastric outlet obstruction may also be seen due to narrowing of the gastric outlet.
- *Arterial complications:* Splenic artery and common hepatic artery pseudoaneurysms are known to occur after pancreatic surgery. Stenosis in the celiac artery can also be seen following pancreatic surgery, but is treated only when there are symptoms attributable to it, as isolated vessel stenosis is usually asymptomatic due to presence of rich collaterals between the celiac and SMA.
- *Thrombosis of portal vein and splenic infarction:* Due to postoperative pancreatitis or as a result of iatrogenic injury.
- *Pancreatic fistula and postoperative pancreatitis:* Detection of amylase-rich fluid after the 10th postoperative day in the drainage tube kept in the surgical bed raises the suspicion of a PJ fistula **(Fig. 24)**.[72]
- Extrahepatic CBD dilatation of >10 mm is abnormal and is likely due to ischemia of the distal CBD.[72]

CONCLUSION

A knowledge of the normal postoperative appearance following abdominal surgery is essential for the accurate interpretation of postoperative imaging. A two-way communication between the radiologist and his clinical colleagues is required so that the radiologist is aware of the exact nature of the procedure the patient has undergone. Helical CT with its multiplanar capability is the modality of choice for the detection and characterization of postoperative complications.

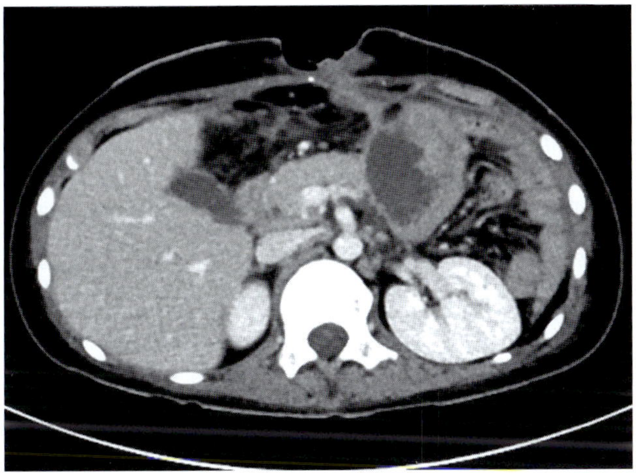

FIG. 24: A 38-year-old male underwent a distal pancreatectomy, gastrectomy and splenectomy for a desmoid tumor of the tail of pancreas. Presented with history of watery discharge from incision site. CECT axial image shows an irregular collection with thick enhancing wall in the region of the tail of pancreas with a fistulous track seen extending anteriorly to the anterior abdominal wall.

REFERENCES

1. Bader FG, SchrÖder M, Kujath P, Muhl E, Bruch HP, Eckmann C. Diffuse post-operative peritonitis: value of diagnostic parameters and impact of early indication for relaparotomy. Eur J Med Res. 2009;14(11):491-6.
2. Sun H, Xue HD, Wang YN, et al. Dual-source dual-energy computed tomography angiography for active gastrointestinal bleeding: a preliminary study. Clin Radiol. 2013;68(2):139-47.
3. Fulwadhva UP, Wortman JR, Sodickson AD. Use of dual-energy CT and iodine maps in the evaluation of bowel disease. Radiographics. 2016;36:393-406.
4. Ghahremani GG, Gore RM. CT diagnosis of post-operative abdominal complications. Radiol Clin North Am. 1989;27: 787-803.
5. Hindman NM, Kang S, Parikh MS. Common post-operative findings unique to laparoscopic surgery. Radiographics 2014;34:119-38.
6. Earls JP, Dachman AH, Colon E, Garrett MG, Molloy M. Prevalence and duration of postoperative pneumoperitoneum: sensitivity of CT vs left lateral decubitus radiography. AJR. 1993;161(4):781-5.
7. Gayer G, Jonas T, Apter S, et al. Postoperative pneumoperitoneum as detected by CT: prevalence, duration, and relevant factors affecting its possible significance. Abdom Imaging. 2000;25(3):301-5.
8. Hope WW, Herriford BT, Norton HJ, et al. Duration and clinical significance of radiographically detected "free air" after laparoscopic nephrectomy. Surg Laparosc Endosc Percut Tech. 2009;19(5):415-8.
9. Chalmers AG, Macafee D, Tolan DJM, Brittenden J. Introduction to the postsurgical abdomen. In: Brittenden J, Tolan DJM (Eds). Radiology of the post surgical abdomen. London: Springer-Verlag. 2012.pp.1-40.
10. Gore RM, Berlin JW, Yaghmai V, et al. CT diagnosis of post-operative complications. Semin Ultrasound CT MR. 2004;25(3):207-21.
11. Young ST, Paulson EK, McCam RC, Baker ME. Appearance of oxidised cellulose (Surgicel) on postoperative CT scans: similarity to postoperative abscess. AJR. 1993;160(2):275-7.
12. Bertelsen CA, Andreasen AH, Jørgensen T, Harling H. Danish Colorectal Cancer Group. Anastomotic leakage after anterior resection for rectal cancer: risk factors. Colorectal Dis. 2010; 12(1):37-43.
13. Nicksa GA, Dring RV, Johnson KH, Sardella WV, Vignati PV, Cohen JL. Anastomotic leaks: what is the best diagnostic imaging study? Dis Colon Rectum. 2007;50(2):197-203.
14. Power N, Atri M, Ryan S, Haddad R, Smith A. CT assessment of anastomotic bowel leak. Clin Radiol. 2007;62(1):37-42.
15. Burke C, Maura M, Molina PL. Interventional computed tomography. In: Lee J, Sagel SS, Stanley RJ (Eds). Computed Body Tomography. Philadelphia: Lippincott Williams & Wilkins; 2006. pp.95-144.
16. Kambadakone A, Mueller PR. Abdominal abscesses. In: Gore RM, Levine MS (Eds). Textbook of Gastrointestinal Radiology, 4th edn. Philadelphia: Elsevier-Saunders; 2015.pp.1254-78.
17. Kim KW, Choi BI, Han JK, et al. Postoperative anatomic and pathologic findings at CT following gastrectomy. Radiographics. 2002;22:323-36.
18. Kumar RR, Kim JT, Haukoos JS, et al. Factors affecting the successful management of intra-abdominal abscesses with antibiotics and the need for percutaneous drainage. Dis Colon Rectum. 2006;49:183-9.
19. Tolan DJM, Harris KM, Prasad D, Mehta SP. The stomach and duodenum. In: Brittenden J, Tolan DJM (Eds). Radiology of the post surgical abdomen. London: Springer-Verlag; 2012.pp.72-124.
20. Frager D, Rovno HD, Baer JW, Bashist B, Friedman M. Prospective evaluation of colonic obstruction with computed tomography. Abdom Imaging. 1998;23(2):141-6.
21. Dükstra FR, Niewenhuizen M, Reijinen MMPT, et al. Recent clinical developments in pathophysiology, epidemiology, diagnosis and treatment of intra-abdominal adhesions. Scand J Gastroenterol. 2000;232:52-9.
22. Berl S, Dawkins A, DiSantis D. The small bowel feces sign. Abdom Radiol. 2016;41(4):794-5.
23. Elsayes KM, Menias CO, Smullen TL, Platt JF. Closed-loop small bowel obstruction: diagnostic patterns by multidetector computed tomography. J Comput Assist Tomogr. 2007;31:697-701.
24. Ghahremani GG, Jimenez MA, Rosenfeld M, Rochester D. CT diagnosis of occult incisional hernias. AJR. 1987;148(1):139-42.
25. Weinstein S, Osei-Bonsu S, Aslam R, Yee J. Multidetector CT of the postoperative colon: Review of normal appearances and common complications. Radiographics. 2013;33:515-32.
26. Ogilvie JW, Ricciardi R. Complications of perineal surgery. Clin Colon Rectal Surg. 2009;22(1):51-9.
27. Smith-Behn J, Arnold M, Might J. Use of computerized tomography of the abdominal wall in the diagnosis of partial post-operative wound dehiscence. Postgrad Med J. 1986;62(732): 947-8.

28. Zhang L. Incidence of abdominal incisional hernia in developing country: a retrospective cohort study. Int J Clin Exp Med. 2015;8(8):13649-52.
29. Itatsu K, Yokoyama Y, Sugawara G, et al. Incidence and risk factors for incisional hernia after abdominal surgery. Br J Surg. 2014;101(11):1439-47.
30. Brown SR, Goodfellow PB. Transverse versus midline incisions for abdominal surgery. Cochrane Database Syst Rev. 2005:CD005199.
31. Gayer G, Lubner MG, Bhalla S, Pickhardt PJ. Imaging of abdominal and pelvic surgical and postprocedural foreign bodies. Radiol Clin North Am. 2014;52:991-1027.
32. Manzella A, Filho PB, Albuquerque E, Farias F, Kaercher J. Imaging of gossypibomas: pictorial review. AJR. 2009;193:S94-101.
33. Orrigner MB. Tumors, injuries and miscellaneous conditions of the esophagus. In: Greenfield LJ, Mulholland MW, Oldham KT, et al (Eds). Surgery: Scientific Principles and Practice. Philadelphia: Lippincott Williams & Wilkins; 2001.pp.692-735.
34. Tolan DJM, Harris KM, Prasad D, Mehta SP. The esophagus. In: Brittenden J, Tolan DJM (Eds). Radiology of the post surgical abdomen. London: Springer-Verlag; 2012.pp.41-71.
35. Swanson JO, Levine MS, Redfern RO, Rubesin SE. Usefulness of high density barium for detection of leaks after esophagogastrectomy, total gastrectomy and total laryngectomy. AJR. 2003;181:415-20.
36. Upponi S, Ganeshan A, D'Costa H, et al. Radiological detection of post-oesophagectomy anastomotic leak: a comparison between multidetector CT and fluoroscopy. Br J Radiol. 2008;81:545-8.
37. Rubesin SE. Postoperative esophagus. In: Gore RM, Levine MS (Eds). Textbook of Gastrointestinal Radiology, 4th edn. Philadelphia: Elsevier-Saunders; 2015.pp.449-61.
38. Lamb PJ, Griffin SM, Chandrashekar MV, Richardson DL, Karat D, Hayes N. Prospective study of routine contrast radiology after total gastrectomy. Br J Surg. 2004;91:1015-9.
39. Gayer G, Barsuk D, Hertz M, Apter S, Zissin R. CT diagnosis of afferent loop syndrome. Clin Radiol. 2002;57:835-9.
40. Tolan DJM, Harris KM, Prasad D, Mehta SP. The stomach and duodenum. In: Brittenden J, Tolan DJM (Eds). Radiology of the post surgical abdomen. London: Springer-Verlag; 2012. pp.72-126.
41. Carucci LR. Postoperative stomach and duodenum. In: Gore RM, Levine MS (Eds). Textbook of Gastrointestinal Radiology, 4th edn. Philadelphia: Elsevier-Saunders; 2015.pp.630-56.
42. Quigley S, Colledge J, Mukherjee S, Patel K. Bariatric surgery: a review of normal post-operative anatomy and complications. Clin Radiol. 2011;66(10):903-14.
43. Blachar A, Federle MP. Gastrointestinal complications of laparoscopic Roun-en-Y gastric bypass surgery in patients who are morbidly obese: Findings on radiography and CT. AJR. 2002;179:1437-42.
44. Pieroni S, Sommer EA, Hito R, et al. The "O" sign: a simple and helpful tool in the diagnosis of laparoscopic adjustable gastric band slippage. AJR. 2010;195:137-41.
45. Sandrasegaran K, Maglinte DD, Rajesh A, et al. CT findings for postsurgical blind pouch of small bowel. AJR. 2006;186:110-3.
46. Broder JC, Tkacz JN, Anderson SW, Soto JA, Gupta A. Ileal pouch-anal anastomosis surgery: imaging and intervention for post-operative complications. Radiographics. 2010;30(1):221-33.
47. Macklin CS, Brittenden J, Jayne D, Tolan DJM. The colon. In: Brittenden J, Tolan DJM (Eds). Radiology of the post surgical abdomen. London: Springer-Verlag; 2012.pp.255-93.
48. Mulé S, Colosio A, Cazejust J, Kianmanesh R, Soyer P, Hoeffel C. Imaging of the postoperative liver: review of normal appearances and common complications. Abdom Imaging. 2015;40(7): 2761-76.
49. Guthrie JA, Salahudeen HM, Lodge JPA. The liver. In: Brittenden J, Tolan DJM (Eds). Radiology of the post surgical abdomen. London: Springer-Verlag; 2012.pp.187-226.
50. Terminology Committee of the International Hepato-Pancreato-Biliary Association. Terminology of liver anatomy and resections. HPB (Oxford). 2000;2:333-9.
51. Kele PG, de Boer M, van der Jagt EJ, Lisman T, Porte RJ. Early hepatic regeneration index and completeness of regeneration at 6 months after partial hepatectomy. Br J Surg. 2012;99(8):1113-9.
52. Zappa M, Dondero F, Sibert A, et al. Liver regeneration at day 7 after right hepatectomy: global and segmental volume trianalysis by using CT. Radiology. 2009;252(2):426-32.
53. Petrovai G, Truant S, Langlois C, et al. Mechanisms of splenic hypertrophy following hepatic resection. HPB (Oxford). 2013;15(12):919-27.
54. Hoeffel C, Azizi L, Lewin M, et al. Normal and pathologic features of the postoperative biliary tract at 3D MR cholangiopancreatography and MR imaging. Radiographics. 2006;26(6):1603-20.
55. Boraschi P, Donati F. Biliary-enteric anastomoses: spectrum of findings on Gd-EOB-DTPA-enhanced MR cholangiography. Abdom Imaging. 2013;38(6):1351-9.
56. Kaman L, Sanyal S, Behera A, Singh R, Katariya RN. Comparison of major bile duct injuries following laparoscopic cholecystectomy and open cholecystectomy. ANZ J Surg. 2006; 76(9):788-91.
57. Z'graggen K, Wehrli H, Metzger A, Buehler M, Frei E, Klaiber C. Complications of laparoscopic cholecystectomy in Switzerland: a prospective 3-year study of 10,174 patients. Swiss Association of Laparoscopic and Thoracoscopic Surgery. Surg Endosc. 1998;12:1303-10.
58. Hjelmqvist B. Complications of laparoscopic cholecystectomy as recorded in the Swedish laparoscopy registry. Eur J Surg Suppl. 2000;585:18-21.
59. Gorsi U, Gupta P, Kalra N, Kang M, Singh R, Gupta R, et al. Multidetector computed tomography evaluation of post cholecystectomy complications: A tertiary care centre experience. Trop Gastroenterol. 2015;36(4):236-43.
60. Quinn SF, Sangster W, Standage B, Schuman E, Gross G. Biliary complications related to laparoscopic cholecystectomies: Radiologic diagnosis and management. Surg Laparosc Endosc Percutan Tech. 1992;2(4):279-86.
61. Moran J, Del Grosso E, Wills JS, Hagy JA, Baker R. Laparoscopic cholecystectomy: imaging of complications and normal postoperative CT appearance. Abdom Imaging. 1994;19:143-6.
62. Feng B, Song Q. Does the common bile duct dilate after cholecystectomy? Sonographic evaluation in 234 patients. AJR. 1995;183:1559-66.
63. Lohan D, Walsh S, McLoughlin R, Murphy J. Imaging of the complications of laparoscopic cholecystectomy. Eur Radiol. 2005;15(5):904-12.
64. Desai NS, Khandelwal A, Virmani V, Kwatra NS, Ricci JA, Saboo SS. Imaging in laparoscopic cholecystectomy: what a radiologist needs to know. Eur J Radiol. 2014;83(6):867-79.
65. Tripathi M, Chandrashekar N, Kumar R, et al. Hepatobiliary scintigraphy: an effective tool in the management of bile leak following laparoscopic cholecystectomy. Clin Imaging. 2004;28:40-43.
66. McGahan JP, Stein M. Complications of laparoscopic cholecystectomy: imaging and intervention. AJR. 1995;165: 1089-97.
67. Park M, Kim KW, Yu JS, et al. Early biliary complications of laparoscopic cholecystectomy: evaluation on T2-weighted MR cholangiography in conjunction with mangafodipir trisodium–enhanced 3D T1-weighted MR cholangiography. AJR. 2004;183:1559-66.
68. Glenn F. Retained calculi within the biliary ductal system. Ann Surg. 1974;179(5):528-39.
69. Jagadesham VP, Sheridan M, Lodge JPA, Brittenden J. The biliary tree. In: Brittenden J, Tolan DJM (Eds). Radiology of the post surgical abdomen. London: Springer-Verlag; 2012.pp.153-85.

70. Thurley PD, Dhingsa R. Laparoscopic cholecystectomy: postoperative imaging. AJR. 2008;191:794-801.
71. Shamiyeh A, Wayand W. Laparoscopic cholecystectomy: early and late complications and their treatment. Langenbecks Arch Surg. 2004;389:164-71.
72. Sandrasegaran K, Maglinte DD, Howard TJ, Lappas JC. Surgery for Chronic Pancreatitis: cross-sectional imaging of postoperative anatomy and complications. AJR. 2005;184: 1118-27.
73. Yamauchi FI, Ortega CD, Blasbalg R, Rocha MS, Jukemura J, Cerri GG. Multidetector CT evaluation of the postoperative pancreas. Radiographics. 2012;32:743-64.
74. Coombs RJ, Zeiss J, Howard JM, Thomford NR, Merrick HW. CT of the abdomen after the Whipple procedure: value in depicting postoperative anatomy, surgical complications, and tumor recurrence. AJR. 1990;154:1011-4.
75. Hashimoto M, Koga M, Ishiyama K, et al. CT features of pancreatic fistula after pancreaticoduodenectomy. AJR. 2007;188:W323-7.
76. Hashimoto N, Yasuda C, Ohyanagi H. Pancreatic fistula after pancreatic head resection: incidence, significance and management. Hepatogastroenterology. 2003;50:1658-60.
77. Cullen JJ, Sarr MG, Ilstrup DM. Pancreatic anastomotic leak after pancreaticoduodenectomy: incidence, significance, and management. Am J Surg. 1994;168:295-8.
78. Mortelé KJ, Lemmerling M, de Hemptinne B, de Vos M, de Bock G, Kunnen M. Postoperative findings following the Whipple procedure: determination of prevalence and morphologic abdominal CT features. Eur Radiol. 2000;10:123-8.
79. Riediger H, Makowiec F, Schareck WD, Hopt UT, Adam U. Delayed gastric emptying after pylorus preserving pancreatoduodenectomy is strongly related to other postoperative complications. J Gastrointest Surg. 2003;7:758-65.

CHAPTER

120

Portal Hypertension: Imaging and Intervention

Shivanand Gamanagatti,
Kumble S Madhusudhan

IMAGING OF PORTAL HYPERTENSION

INTRODUCTION

It is defined as increase in portal pressure above the normal range of 6–10 mm Hg or pressure gradient >5 mm Hg between portal and hepatic veins, as evaluated by hepatic vein cannulation. Portal hypertension is considered clinically significant, when the pressure gradient is more than 10–12 mm Hg.[1]

Portal hypertension is of hemodynamic importance, since it leads to range of complications such as gastrointestinal hemorrhage, ascites, portal-systemic encephalopathy, hepatorenal syndrome, hepatopulmonary syndrome, and spontaneous bacterial peritonitis.[2,3]

CAUSES OF PORTAL HYPERTENSION[4]

Causes of portal hypertension are divided into prehepatic, intrahepatic, and posthepatic causes **(Table 1)**.

ANATOMY OF PORTAL SYSTEM[5]

The liver has two sources of blood supply, 70% of blood flow is via the portal vein and remaining 30% is via hepatic artery. Portal blood is poorly oxygenated and has high content of chemicals absorbed from the gut, whereas hepatic arterial blood is rich in oxygen. Portal and hepatic blood merge within the portal sinusoids, which drain into hepatic veins and then to the systemic venous system, i.e. inferior vena cava (IVC).

The portal vein is formed by the confluence of the superior mesenteric vein (SMV) and splenic vein (SV) posterior to the neck of pancreas. It courses superiorly and laterally to enter the liver at the porta. Other tributaries include inferior mesenteric vein (IMV) and right and left gastric veins, which drain into portal circulation **(Fig. 1)**.

Work-up[6,7]

Laboratory Studies

Aimed at identifying the causes of cirrhosis (the most common cause of portal hypertension), Studies include **(Table 2)**.

Imaging Studies

- Duplex-Doppler ultrasonography[8-11]
- Ultrasound (US) is used as screening modality for evaluating portal hypertension, since it is a safe and cost-effective method. It helps in identifying the patency of portal vein, direction of portal flow (hepatopetal or hepatofugal), also helps in diagnosing cavernoma formation of main portal vein, splanchnic vein thrombosis.
    - *Limitations of US include*:
        - Reproducibility of findings is challenging.
        - Portal hemodynamics affected by several variables such as circadian rhythm, meals and medications.
        - Substantial inter-observer and intra-observer discrepancy.

TABLE 1: Causes of portal hypertension.

Prehepatic causes	*Intrahepatic causes*	*Posthepatic causes*
Caused by obstruction of the portal, splenic, or superior mesenteric veins. • Portal vein thrombosis/extrahepatic portal vein obstruction • Congenital origin, such as aplasia or hypoplasia • Infection, such as pylephlebitis • Splanchnic arteriovenous fistula	Caused by intrinsic diseases of the parenchyma • Cirrhosis due to various causes • Congenital hepatic fibrosis • Noncirrhotic portal fibrosis/Idiopathic portal hypertension	Caused by diseases obstructing the blood outflow from the liver • Budd-Chiari syndrome • Veno-occlusive disorder

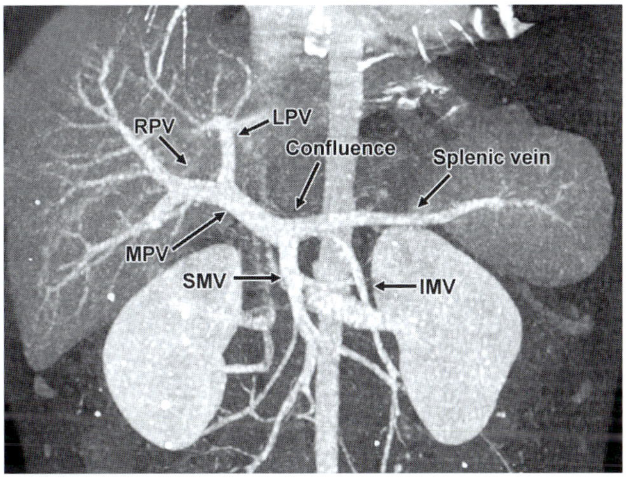

FIG. 1: Coronal 3D MIP image of CT portography showing anatomy of splenoportal axis. (SMV: superior mesenteric vein; IMV: inferior mesenteric vein; MPV: main portal vein; RPV: right branch of portal vein; LPV: left branch of portal vein)

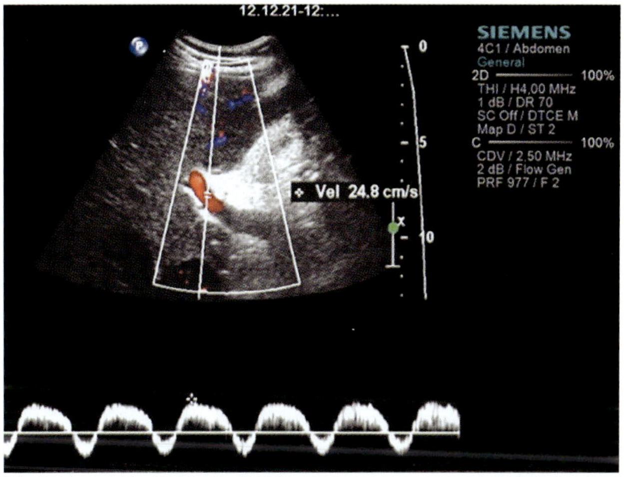

FIG. 2: Ultrasound Doppler image showing typical waveform of main portal vein exhibiting continuous hepatopetal (antegrade) flow with undulation due to respiratory and cardiac variation.

TABLE 2: Laboratory studies for the work-up of cirrhosis.
• Liver function tests
• Prothrombin time
• Albumin
• Viral hepatitis serologies
• Platelet count
• Antinuclear antibody, antimitochondrial antibody, anti-smooth muscle antibody
• Iron indices
• Alpha-1 antitrypsin deficiency
• Ceruloplasmin alone or along with 24 h urinary copper in selective cases

Normal Doppler Findings of Portal Vein

The portal vein has a typical Doppler waveform and exhibits continuous hepatopetal (antegrade) flow. The normal flow velocity range is 15–18 cm/sec. Mild undulation due to respiratory and cardiac variation in the waveform is a common finding **(Fig. 2)**.

Technique of Doppler of Portal System

Doppler evaluation of splenoportal axis can be extremely challenging, due to the altered anatomy, blood flow conditions, bowel gas and the type of the changes that happen in a diseased liver. Doppler examination should be performed following overnight fasting, because bowel gas may interfere with evaluation of superior mesenteric vein and retroperitoneal collaterals.

Checklist of typical Doppler evaluation of splenoportal axis **(Figs. 3A to F)** consists of looking at the:

- Patency of hepatic veins
- Patency of IVC
- Liver size and echo-texture, any space occupying lesion
- Patency of splenoportal axis (MPV/splenic vein/SMV)
- Diameter of SPA (dilated/normal)
- Direction of flow (hepatopetal/hepatofugal)
- Respiratory variation of portal blood flow (present or absent)
- Collaterals (intrahepatic/extrahepatic)
- Splenic size (normal/enlarged)
- Ascites (present or absent)
- Patency of left renal vein.

Challenges of Doppler evaluation include:

- Acquiring a suitable angle of insonation
- Altered depth of the vessels
- Slow flow velocities due to disease process
- Amount of tissue movement due to respiration

In portal hypertension, a Doppler signal demonstrates a low frequency shift and low amplitude, and also, there is an increase in noise from tissue movement. Hence, it is very important to optimize the imaging parameters and sonographic technique to increase the frequency shift and to increase the signal amplitude.

Optimization of Sonographic Technique

Angle of Insonation

Single most useful adjustment that improves the Doppler signal quality is to decrease the angle of insonation. Ideally, the angle of insonation should be less than 60°. In routine clinical practice, it is difficult to achieve this angle due to restrictions related to vessel position, body habitus, ribs and gas.

Useful modifications for improving the angle include:

- Roll the patient into left lateral decubitus position to move the liver away from the ribs and move bowel gas
- Use a small footprint phased array transducer to visualize vessels through intercostal space.

Color Frequency

Current ultrasound machines come with transducers having multiple Doppler frequencies. This offers, the sonographer a chance to increase the frequency shift or increase the

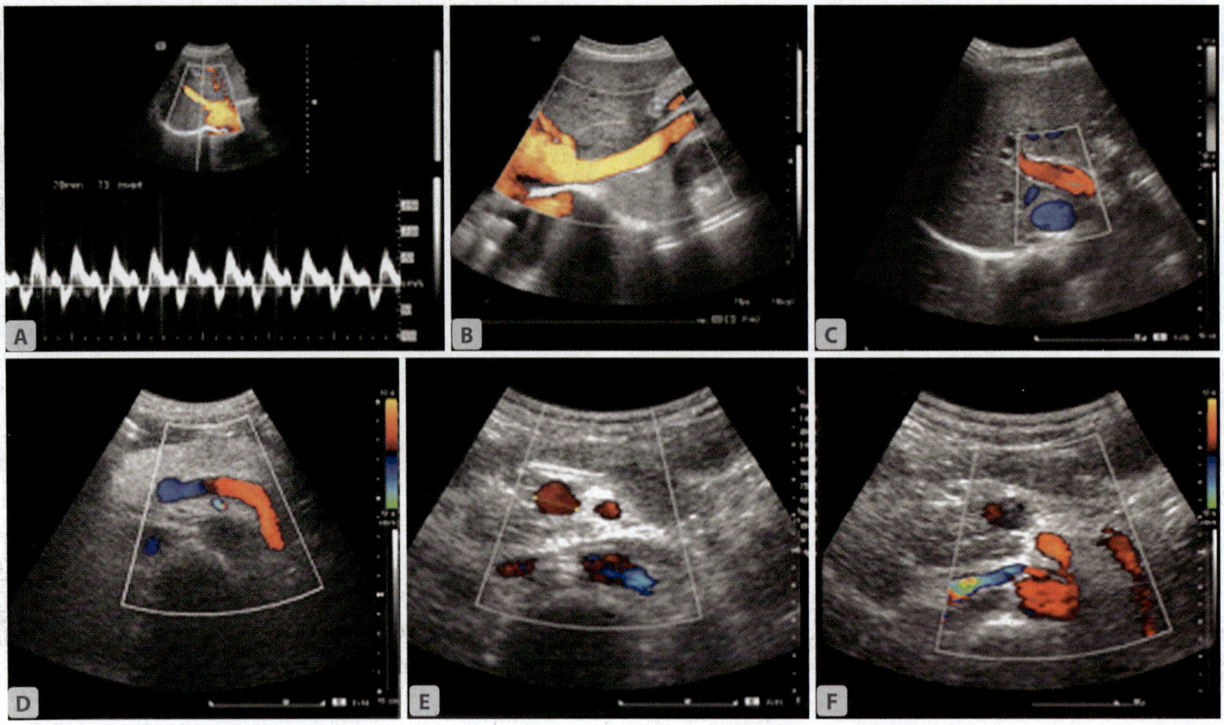

FIGS. 3A TO F: Power Doppler images showing normal Doppler findings to look at during scanning in setting of portal hypertension. (A) Patency of hepatic vein; (B) Patency of IVC; (C) Patency of MPV; (D) Patency of splenic vein; (E) Patency of SMV; (F) Patency of left renal vein (LRV).

amplitude of the returning echoes depending on conditions within the body.

A higher incident frequency will produce a greater frequency shift but subject to higher rates of attenuation thereby decreasing penetration and reducing signal amplitude. Hence, when scanning deep abdominal vessels a lower frequency shift should be used to overcome problems of poor penetration.

Optimization of the Received Signal

The scale or pulse repetition frequency (PRF) needs to be set appropriately in order to optimize the display of Doppler signal received. In cirrhosis, blood flow states are very low, hence the scale (PRF) should be set low enough to display these small frequency shifts.

One can use the zoom facility that significantly improve resolution and frame rate by reconfiguring the beam forming for a smaller field of view.

Respiration

Smart use of respiration can be very helpful. Performing Doppler in arrested inspiration may hamper the detection of flow as the increase in intra-abdominal pressure can halt or even reverse the flow in diseased portal venous system. Hence, scanning should be done with arrested expiration or gentle respiration even if flow is not seen.

Presets

It is recommended to use vendor presets as a starting point and also it is advocated that each department generate a dedicated presets for abdominal vascular studies.

Pathophysiology of Doppler Findings in Portal Hypertension

Cirrhosis is a mixture of fibrosis and regeneration that alters the normal liver architecture. Cirrhosis leads to obstruction to blood flow in distal sinusoids due to perisinusoidal collagen deposition and fibrosis. This obstruction reduces flow from the portal veins and hepatic artery into the hepatic veins. This increases arterial resistance and leads to an increase in arterial flow into the portal vein via existing and new anastomoses that result from the fibrotic scarring. The net result of this obstruction to venous outflow and increase in arterial to portal vein flow manifests as increase in portal vein pressure, drainage of blood away from the liver (hepatofugal flow) via collateral pathways.

Ultrasound Criteria for Detecting Portal Hypertension

Portal Vein Diameter

Portal vein diameter is a luminal measurement made at the level where the portal vein enters porta. A portal vein diameter of 13 mm or more is abnormal and an indicator of portal hypertension. While it has good specificity, it has a sensitivity of only about 40% **(Fig. 4)**.

This lack of sensitivity is due to collateral pathways, which partially decompress the system. Portal vein size normally varies with respiration and loss of this variation can also be used to identify portal hypertension. Less than 20% variation in diameter with respiration is reported as having 80% sensitivity and 100% specificity.

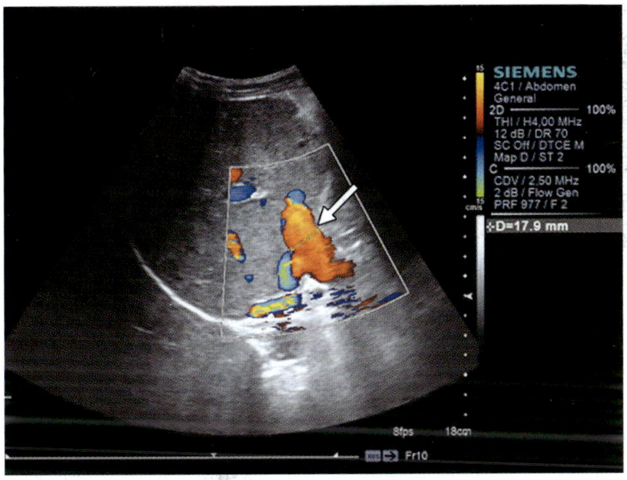

FIG. 4: Doppler ultrasound image showing dilated main portal vein (arrow) in a cirrhotic patient, which measures 17.9 mm at porta.

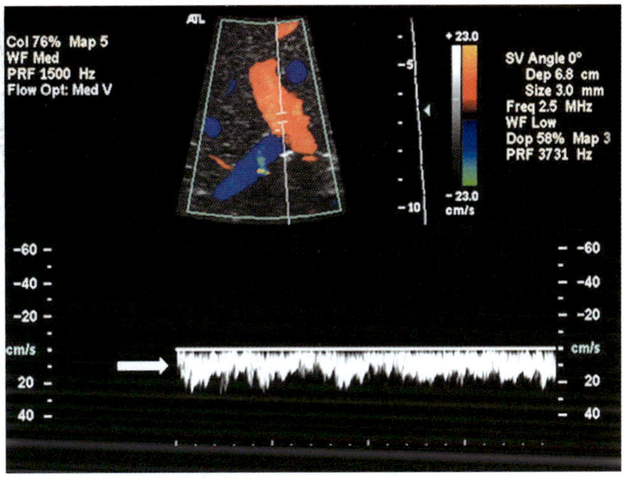

FIG. 5: Doppler ultrasound image showing dilated main portal vein with reversal of flow (arrow) on spectral waveform suggestive of hepatofugal flow.

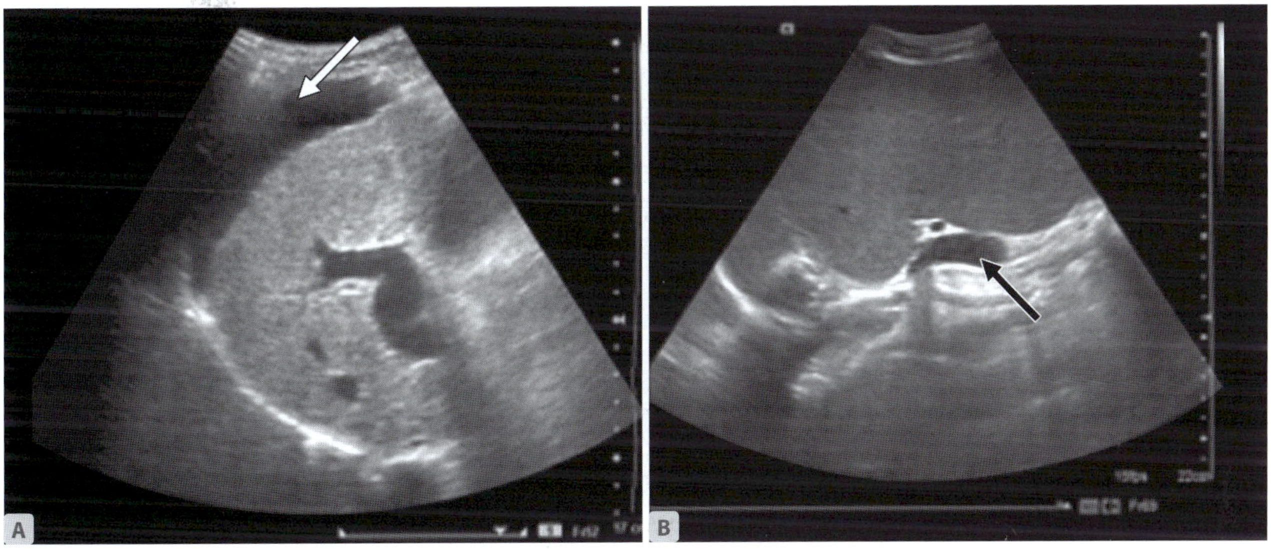

FIGS. 6A AND B: Ultrasound images of a cirrhotic patient showing shrunken liver with nodular surface, dilated splenoportal axis, splenomegaly (black arrow) and ascites (white arrow).

Although this is a sensitive test for portal hypertension, in practice obtaining reliable and reproducible measurements can be difficult as many of these patients have poor ultrasound access and limited ability to comply with directions.

Flow Reversal or Hepatofugal Flow

This is relatively uncommon in the portal vein and is a poor marker for portal hypertension being seen in only 1–8% of cases of portal hypertension **(Fig. 5)**. When present, it is usually associated with a reduction in vein diameter. It is highly dependent on the severity of the disease and the location of collaterals (if a paraumbilical collateral exists forward flow is usually maintained because the shunt is beyond the level of the portal vein).

Splenomegaly and Ascites

Splenomegaly develops in most, but not all cases, of portal hypertension however is of little use due to the large number of alternative causes **(Figs. 6A and B)**.

Ascites is not usually caused by uncomplicated portal hypertension. It is often secondary to underlying liver diseases with liver cell failure and is insensitive, as it tends to be a late complication.

Portosystemic Venous Collaterals

Collaterals have up to 90% sensitivity and excellent specificity for portal hypertension. Paraumbilical collaterals have a specificity of 100% for portal hypertension. Collaterals have predictable locations making them a very practical sign for the diagnosis of portal hypertension. Clues to their presence and location can also be found from changes in the flow patterns in the portal venous system.

The collaterals most frequently detected with ultrasound are the **(Figs. 7A to F)**:

- Paraumbilical
- Splenorenal
- Gastroesophageal.

Other, less common collaterals, such as mesenteric and pericholecystic **(Figs. 7A to F)**, may also be found.

Computed Tomography[12,13]

Computed tomography (CT) is not the prime diagnostic tool in patients with portal hypertension, usually done as second line technique to ultrasound with color Doppler imaging. Main limitation of CT scan include, unable to provide information about flow direction, portal flow rates or pressure gradients and radiation issue. CT findings practically depend upon morphologic changes rather than flow dynamic changes.

Indications for CT, in patients with known portal hypertension:

- To demonstrate the main collateral pathways
- To identify possible causes for portal hypertension
- To identify and characterize focal lesions like hepatocellular carcinoma (HCC).

Examination Technique

Multidetector computed tomography (MDCT) permits improved timing of contrast injection, excellent outlining of collateral pathways and better detection of accompanying liver lesions in patients with portal hypertension.

Scan parameters and protocols with respect to different MDCT scanners are mentioned in **Table 3**.

The amount of contrast to be used differs depending upon the iodine strength in contrast medium. If the iodine

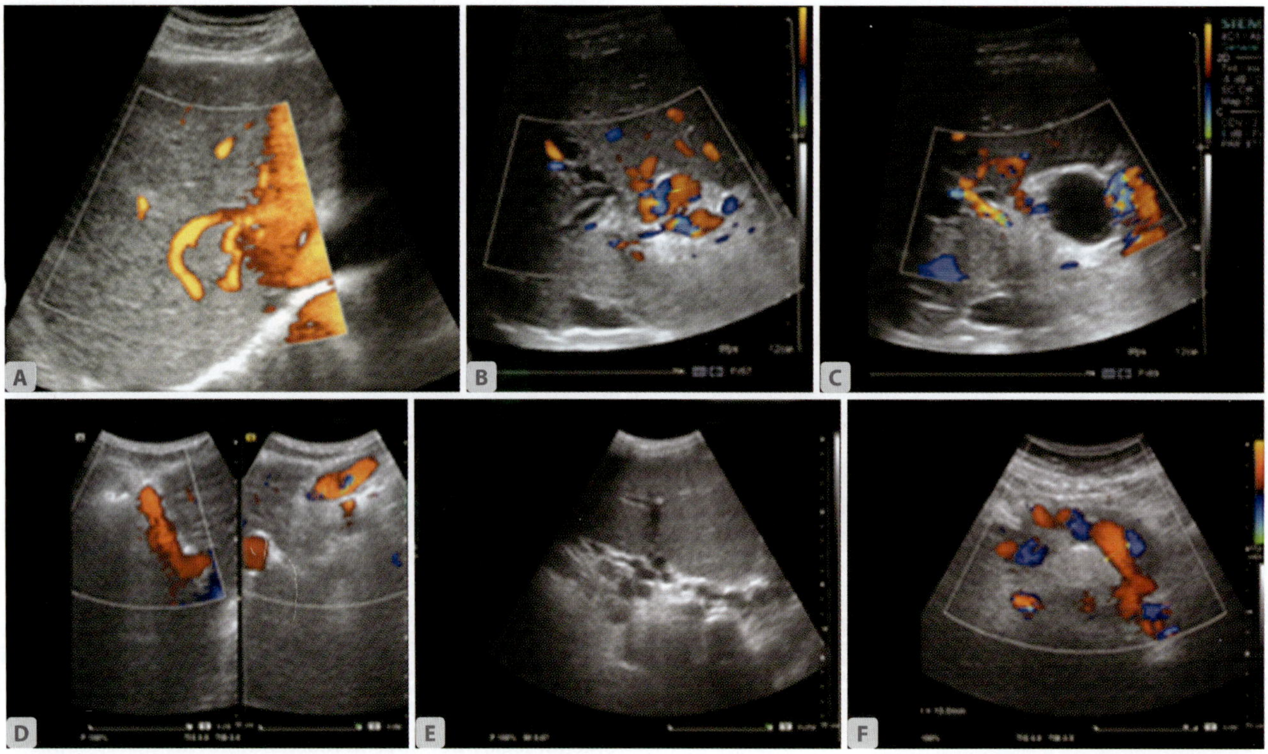

FIGS. 7A TO F: Doppler ultrasound images showing collaterals in various location; intrahepatic veno-venous collaterals (A), at porta (B), pericholecystic (C), paraumbilical (D), lienorenal location (E) and mesenteric location (F).

TABLE 3: Scan parameters and protocols with respect to different MDCT scanners.

Parameter	*4 channel*	*16 channel*	*64 channel*
Detector collimation (mm)	4 × 1.25	16 × 0.625	64 × 0.6
Slice thickness (mm)			
Arterial phase	1.25	1	1
Venous phase	1.25	1	1
Arterial delay	Bolus tracking/automated trigger Empirical delay: 25–30 s		
Venous delay	65–70 s	60 s	50–60 s

strength is 300 mg/mL, recommended amount is the range of 120–150 cc, whereas if iodine strength is 370 mg/mL, then amount only 80–100 cc. Also as a standard for liver imaging using MDCT, nonionic contrast medium is used with injection rate of 4–5 cc/sec, using pressure injector. Therefore, it is important to customize the injection rate protocols and amount of contrast used depending upon the higher or lower iodine concentration contrast media.

Oral Contrast

The positive oral contrast interferes with evaluation of varices. Hence, it is suggested to use water as a negative contrast agent that helps in better depiction of varices. Patients are advised to take about 1–1.5 L water, 30 minutes before the start of CT examination; to distend the stomach and the proximal bowel loops.

Precontrast scans are generally not required; however, in patients with suspected HCC or hypervascularized liver lesions, may be useful if hemorrhage or calcifications are suspected. In case of dual energy scanner, virtual non-contrast images can be obtained from the arterial phase data without subjecting the patient to additional radiation for obtaining the unenhanced scan.

For optimal visualization of splenoportal axis, scanning should start 45–50 sec following contrast injection. In patients with portal hypertension, this time delay has to be increased up to 65–70 sec, because of slower opacification of the portal branches.

For suspected HCC, a multiphasic technique should be used with injection of 100 mL of contrast at a flow rate of 4–5 mL/s using a power injector.

Display Technique[13]

CT images are usually assessed based upon axial sections. In patients with portal hypertension because of development of complex collateral pathways further assessment using interactive cine display is very helpful and will resolve most of the fundamental diagnostic information.

In certain cases, multiplanar reformats (MPRs)/ volume-rendering techniques (VRTs) and in particular, thin slab maximum intensity projection (MIP) are valuable in better understanding of the collateral pathways **(Figs. 8A and B)**.

Magnetic Resonance Imaging[14-16]

- Provides morphologic information comparable to CT scan when ultrasound findings are inadequate.
- MRI angiography also helps in localizing and defining the extent of the presence of portosystemic collaterals **(Figs. 9A to D)**.
- Special MR techniques (like Phase contrast) also offer quantitative information about portal venous flow.

Magnetic resonance portography has few benefits over other imaging techniques used for evaluation of portal hypertension. Doppler ultrasonography is an inexpensive and noninvasive, provides quantitative information on portal blood flow, but it is operator dependent and may be unproductive when a proper acoustic window is not available. CT portography can demonstrate the portal venous system in a short time, but this technique is associated with ionizing radiation and requires administration of large amount of contrast material.

MR Technique

Nonenhanced MR angiography using time-of-flight (TOF) and phase-contrast (PC) techniques can demonstrate portal venous system, but is limited by its long data acquisition time, motion and flow artifact, and in-plane saturation.

However, contrast enhanced MR portography overcomes flow artifacts and saturation effects. MR portograms reconstructed by maximum-intensity projection post-processing technique and source images, provide detailed information about the portal venous system **(Figs. 9A to D)**.

MR Protocol

MR imaging is performed with a 1.5-T superconducting magnetic unit using a torso-phased array coil. A 3D fast spoiled gradient recalled pulse sequence with minimum repetition time and echo time should be used. An optimized slab volume is placed in axial plane on coronal localizer extending from dome of diaphragm to inferior part of kidneys and the acquisition is performed during a single breath-hold period of 13–15 sec. An intravenous bolus of 0.2 mmol/kg of gadolinium is injected either using pressure injector or manually. Gadolinium injection was immediately followed by a 15-mL saline flush. Three repetitive acquisitions (performed within separate breath-hold of 13–15 sec) for portal venous phase imaging are obtained after a delay of 45–50 sec after start of contrast injection.

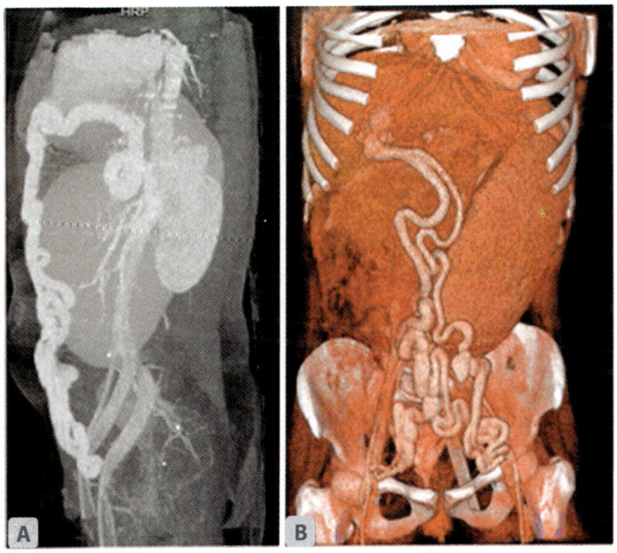

FIGS. 8A AND B: Thin slab MIP (Maximum Intensity Projection) (A) and VRT (Volume Rendered Technique) (B) images showing dilated tortuous paraumbilical vein, showing advantages of these techniques in understanding of the collateral pathways.

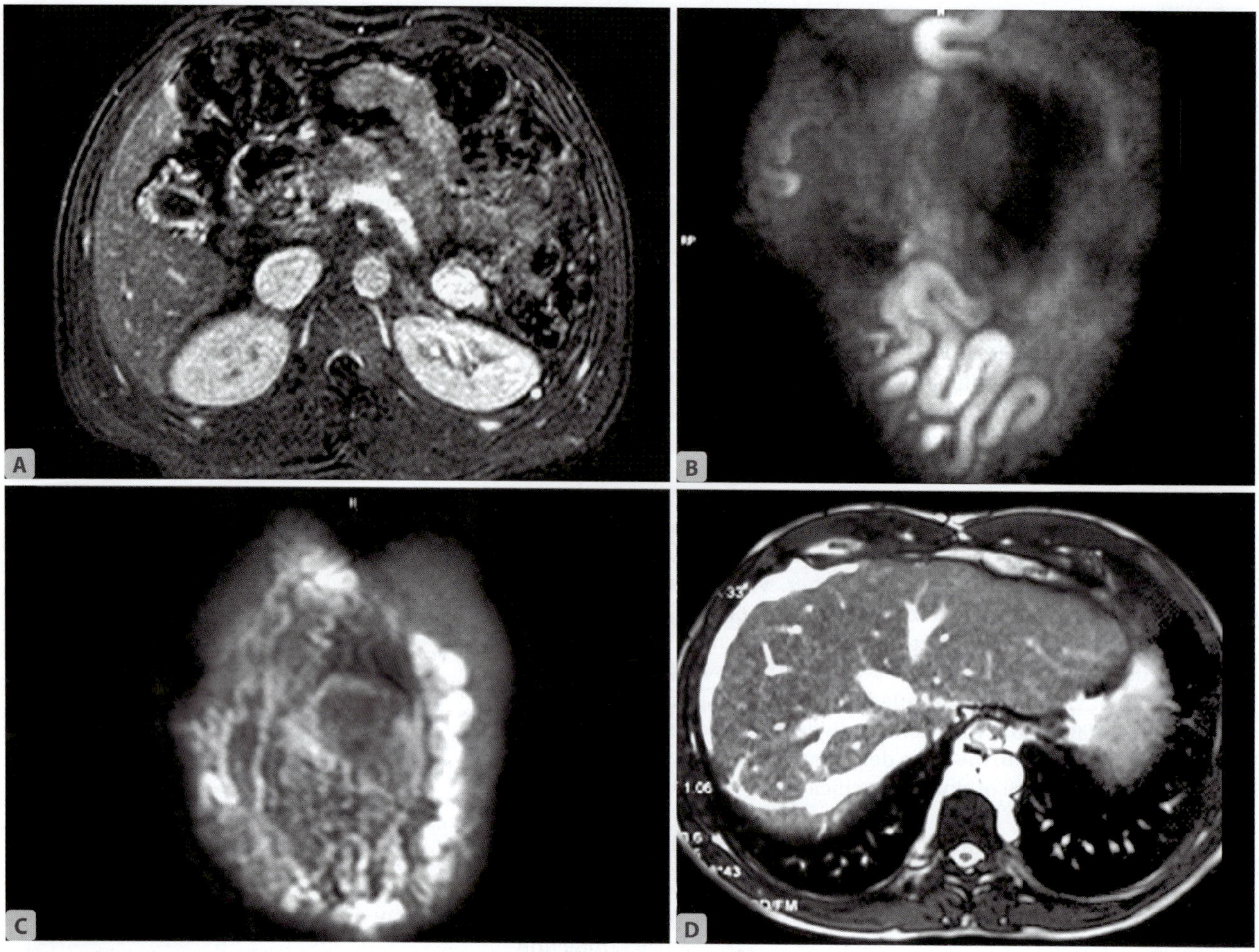

FIGS. 9A TO D: MR Images showing various collateral pathways; pericholecystic (A), paraumbilical (B), abdominal wall (C) and intrahepatic venovenous collaterals (D).

HEMODYNAMIC MEASUREMENT OF PORTAL PRESSURE[17]

Procedures (Figs. 10A and B)

- Portal pressure measurement by direct puncture of portal vein is not generally done due to invasive nature and also there is high risk of associated anesthetic and bleeding complications.
- However, most commonly indirect pressure measurement that closely matches the direct portal pressure is used, which is popularly known as hepatic venous pressure gradient (HVPG) measurement.
- In this procedure, through transfemoral route or more commonly through transjugular route, a Swan Ganz balloon catheter is placed into the right hepatic vein and free hepatic venous pressure (FHVP) is measured without inflating the balloon.
- In next step, the balloon is inflated using either diluted contrast or room air, occluding the hepatic vein outflow completely and occluded hepatic venous pressure or wedged hepatic venous pressure (WHVP) is measured **(Figs. 10A and B)**.
- The wedged pressure value minus free venous pressure value gives hepatic venous pressure measurement (HVPG).

Interpretation (Table 4)

- Normal hepatic vein pressure gradient (HVPG) is <5 mm Hg.
- Complications of portal hypertension such as variceal bleeding, ascites, or hepatorenal syndrome are seen when HVPG exceeds 10 mm Hg.
- If there is HVPG <10 mm Hg and complications of portal hypertension are present, then one should suspect non-cirrhotic portal hypertension.

MORPHOLOGIC SIGNS OF PORTAL HYPERTENSION

Divided into Direct and Associated Signs

Direct Signs include, dilatation of splenoportal axis, i.e. main portal vein diameter >13 mm, splenic vein diameter >10 mm **(Figs. 11A and B)**. If there are adequate venous collaterals, SPA may not show significant dilatation.

Collateral Pathways[18,19]

In healthy human, congenitally originated connections exists between portal and systemic circulation **(Table 5)**. In the setting of portal hypertension, these connections get dilated

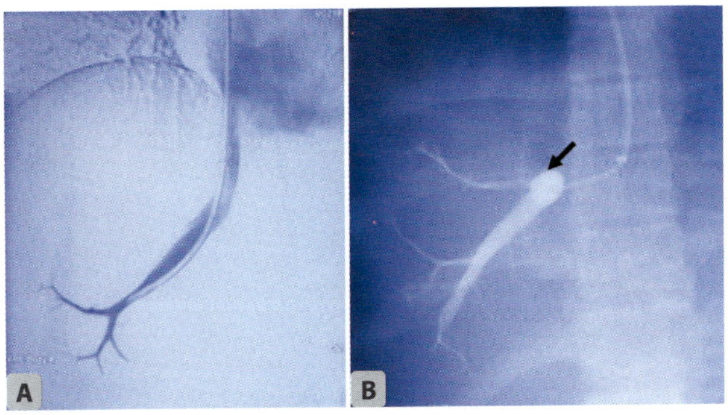

FIGS. 10A AND B: DSA spot images showing steps of HVPG measurement; Cannulation of the right hepatic vein (A) for measuring the free hepatic venous pressure (FHVP) followed by inflation of balloon catheter (B) (arrow) and measuring the wedged hepatic venous pressure (WHVP).

TABLE 4: Interpretation of HVPG findings.

Cause	*FHVP*	*WHVP*	*HVPG*
Prehepatic	Normal	Normal	Normal
Hepatic pre-sinusoidal	Normal	Normal to ↑	Normal to ↑
Sinusoidal	Normal	↑↑	↑↑
Post-sinusoidal	Normal	↑↑	↑↑
Post-hepatic	↑↑	↑↑	Normal to ↑

(FHVP: free hepatic vein pressure; HVPG: hepatic vein pressure gradient; WHVP: wedged hepatic vein pressure)

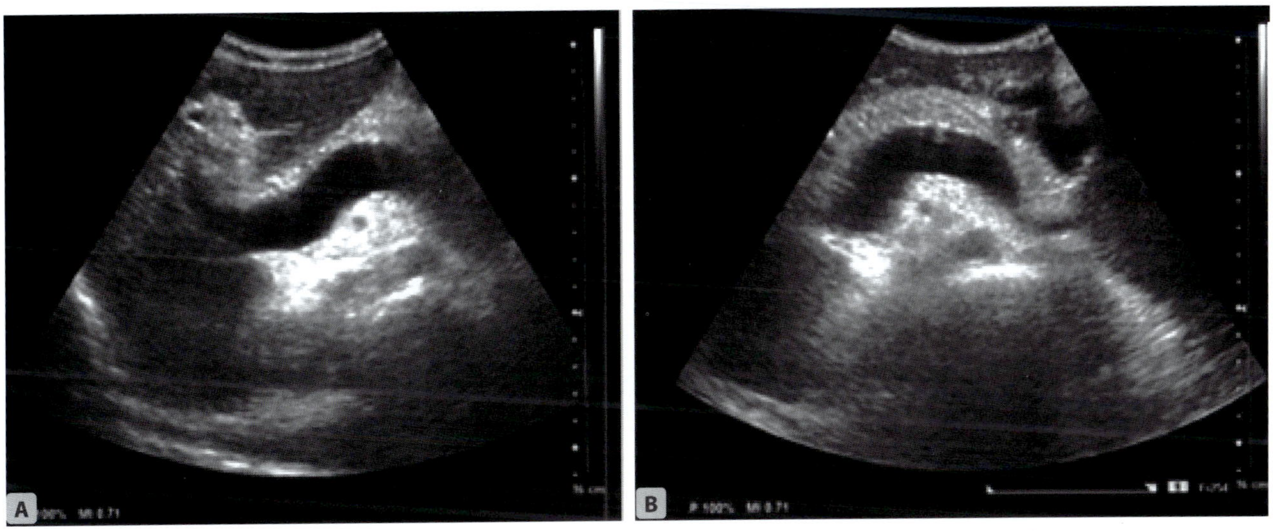

FIGS. 11A AND B: Ultrasound images showing dilated entire splenoportal axis. (A) Dilated MPV; and (B) Dilated splenic vein.

TABLE 5: Normal portosystemic communications **(Figs. 12A to D).**

Lower esophagus	*Left gastric vein*	*Esophageal veins*
Rectum and anal canal	Superior rectal vein	Middle and inferior rectal vein
Umbilicus	Paraumbilical veins	Superior and inferior epigastric veins
Bare area of liver	Portal vein branches	Inferior phrenic vein
Retroperitoneum	Tributaries of splenic, pancreatic and colic veins	Renal, suprarenal, gonadal and paravertebral veins

TABLE 6: Gastroesophageal and ectopic varices **(Figs. 13 and 14).**

Gastroesophageal varices	*Ectopic varices*
Esophageal	Duodenal
Paraesophageal	Jejunoileal
Gastric and perigastric	Colonic Pancreatic Mesenteric Vesical Pericholecystic Retroperitoneal Rectal/perirectal

leading to formation of varices at various sites within the body.

These varices are divided into two groups **(Table 6)**:

1. Gastroesophageal varices
2. Ectopic varices

In long-term, these varices develop large spontaneous shunts **(Table 7)**, which are categorized into intrahepatic, transhepatic and extrahepatic shunts.

VARICES

Esophageal and Paraesophageal Varices

The most common varices encountered in portal hypertension are esophageal varices (50%). Esophageal varices are located within the wall of the lower esophagus, whereas paraesophageal varices are located outside the esophageal wall. These are the most common varices to bleed

TABLE 7: Spontaneous shunts **(Figs. 15A to C)**.

Intrahepatic	*Transhepatic*	*Extrahepatic*
Rare	Recanalized paraumbilical vein	Gastrorenal Splenorenal Gastrocaval

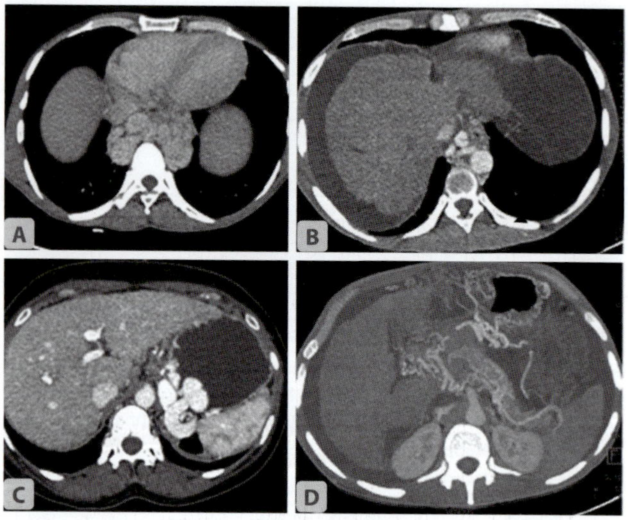

FIGS. 13A TO D: Axial CT images showing various gastroesophageal varices: Paraesophageal (A), Esophageal (B), Fundal (C) and Perigastric (D) locations.

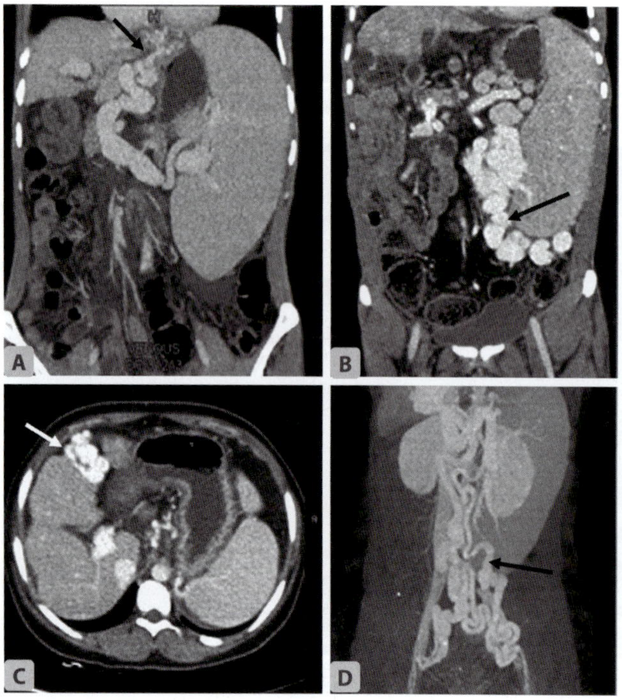

FIGS. 12A TO D: CT images showing various normal portosystemic communications; at lower end of esophagus (A), in retroperitoneum (B) and at umbilicus (paraumbilical veins) (C and D).

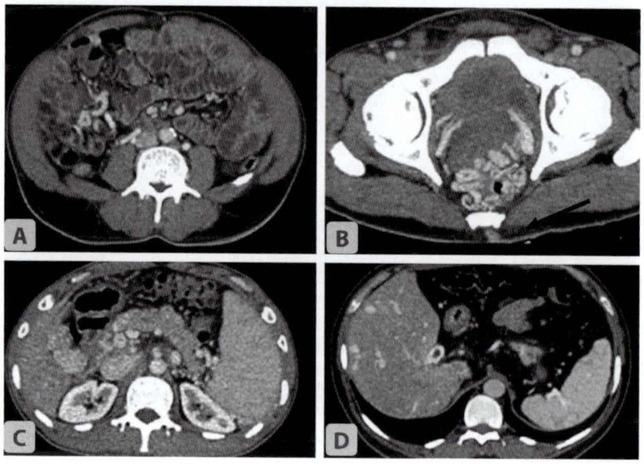

FIGS. 14A TO D: Axial CT images showing ectopic varices; colonic (A), rectal (B), pericholecystic (C) and pericholedochal locations (D).

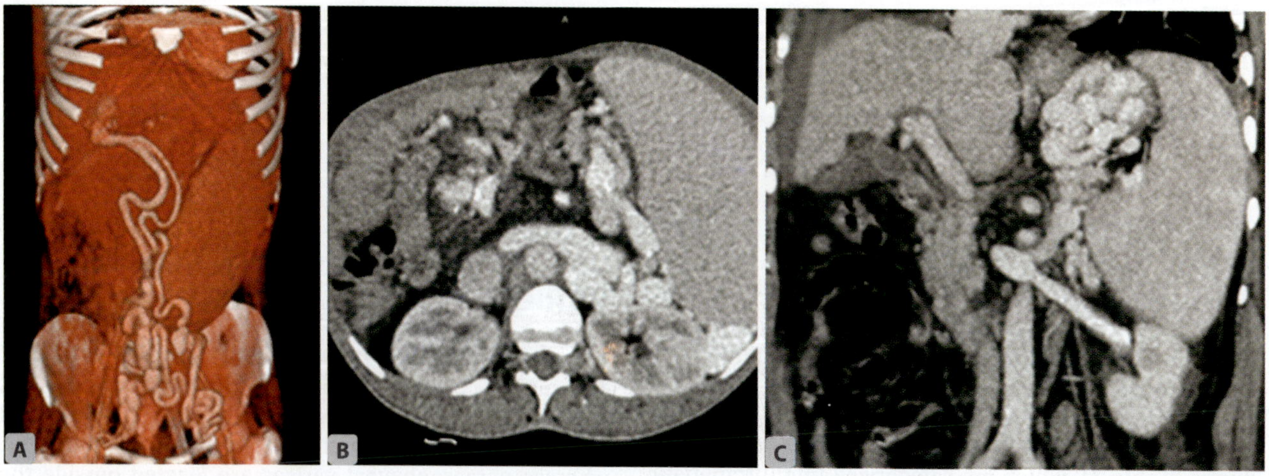

FIGS. 15A TO C: CT images showing spontaneous shunts; recanalized paraumbilical (Transhepatic shunt) (A), splenorenal (B), and gastrorenal (C) shunts.

in portal hypertension due to high pressure and high volume of blood that they carry and account for high mortality due to spontaneous hemorrhage.

Gastric and Perigastric Varices

Gastric varices are less common than esophageal varices (5–33%), drain either into the left renal vein through spontaneous gastrorenal shunt or directly into the IVC through a spontaneous gastrocaval shunt. Risk of bleeding is low as compared to esophageal varices but the severity of bleeding is much higher due to their large size.

Ectopic Varices

They account for 2–5% of variceal bleeding, have a 4-fold increased risk of bleeding as compared to esophageal varices and associated with high mortality rate. These varices are difficult to treat and there is no established standard treatment. When hemorrhage arises from these ectopic varices, it is challenging to control by any method, and the bleeding may be potentially lethal.

Associated Findings

The most important associated findings in portal hypertension are splenomegaly and ascites. Other associated findings are small bowel edema, thickening of the gallbladder wall, increased density within mesenteric fat (misty mesentery) and omentum. In addition, patients with PHT especially those with hypersplenism have an increased incidence of splenic artery true aneurysms due to hyperkinetic circulation, which may be seen as incidental finding on imaging.

Splenomegaly

Splenomegaly develops in most, but not all cases, of portal hypertension however is of little use due to the large number of alternative causes. The size of the spleen does not correlate with degree of portal hypertension. Also, if splenomegaly is absent, portal hypertension cannot be ruled out. Siderotic Gamna-Gandy nodules that represent small foci of perifollicular and trabecular hemorrhage may be seen as multiple faint hyperechoic foci on ultrasound or multiple faint calcifications on CT. They are seen as multiple low signal foci 3–8 mm in size on gradient echo sequences of MR images **(Figs. 16A and B)**.

Ascites is not usually caused by uncomplicated portal hypertension. It is often secondary to underlying liver diseases with liver cell failure and increase in sinusoidal pressure leading to an increase in fluid in the space of Disse with resultant ascites. In prehepatic PHT, liver function remains normal and ascites is minimal.

SPECIFIC SITUATIONS

Intrahepatic Portal Hypertension

Cirrhosis of Liver

Imaging features are described under diffuse liver diseases chapter.

Sonography can differentiate intrahepatic from extrahepatic portal hypertension in majority of cases and can also detect the presence of splenomegaly and ascites. Evaluation of the liver by ultrasound may reveal changes of cirrhosis such as coarsened echo texture with or without altered echogenicity, nodularity of liver surface, presence of regenerating nodules and reduction in the number of visible portal or hepatic veins. Reduction of liver size with a combination of segmental hypertrophy and atrophy in the form of caudate to right lobe ratio >0.65 and reduction of the transverse diameter of segment IV.

Noncirrhotic Portal Hypertension

NCPH includes a spectrum of diseases of diverse causes **(Table 8)**.

The most common causes of noncirrhotic portal hypertension (NCPH) are noncirrhotic portal fibrosis (NCPF) and extrahepatic portal vein obstruction (EHPVO). These constitute 1/3rd of all cases of portal hypertension (PHT) in India.[20,21]

The fundamental cause in both NCPF and EHPVO is thought to be vascular origin. However, the exact etiopathogenesis of the two conditions is not known, but

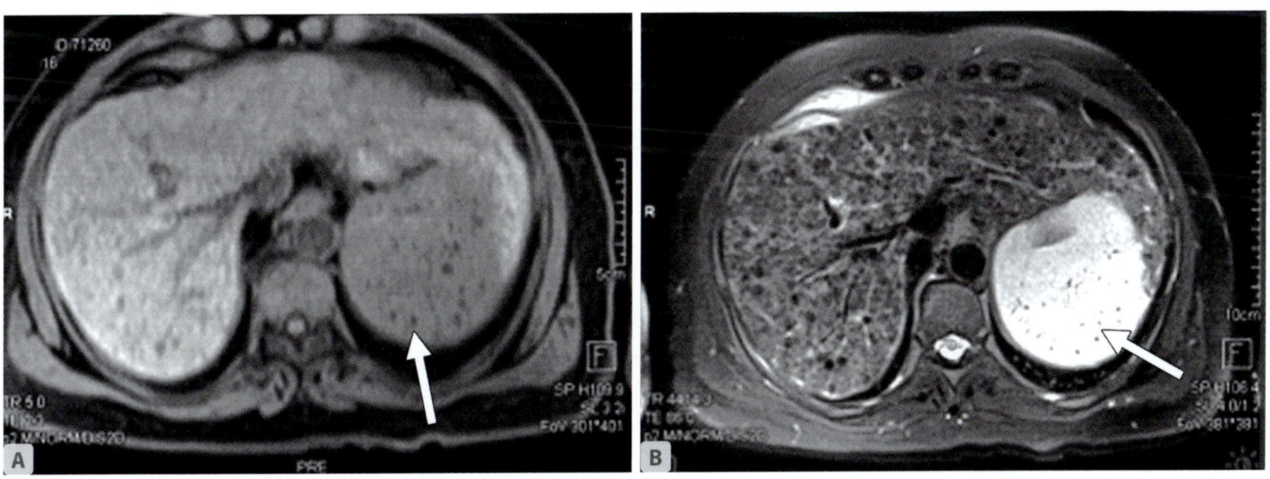

FIGS. 16A AND B: Axial T1W and T2W MR images (A and B) showing multiple low signal intensity foci (arrow) scattered in enlarged spleen in a cirrhotic patient.

TABLE 8: Causes of noncirrhotic portal hypertension.

- Extrahepatic portal venous obstruction (EHPVO)
- Noncirrhotic portal fibrosis (NCPF) or idiopathic portal hypertension (IPH)
- Nodular regenerative hyperplasia
- Partial nodular transformation
- Congenital hepatic fibrosis
- Schistosomiasis
- Peliosis hepatitis

TABLE 9: Guidelines for the diagnosis of NCPF.

- Presence of splenomegaly
- Normal liver function tests
- Varices on upper GI endoscopy
- Patent portal and hepatic veins on Doppler
- Normal or mildly elevated wedged hepatic venous pressure (WHVP); and markedly elevated intrasplenic and portal vein pressure
- No evidence of cirrhosis on liver biopsy

FLOWCHART 1: Etiopathogenesis of extrahepatic portal venous obstruction and noncirrhotic portal fibrosis.

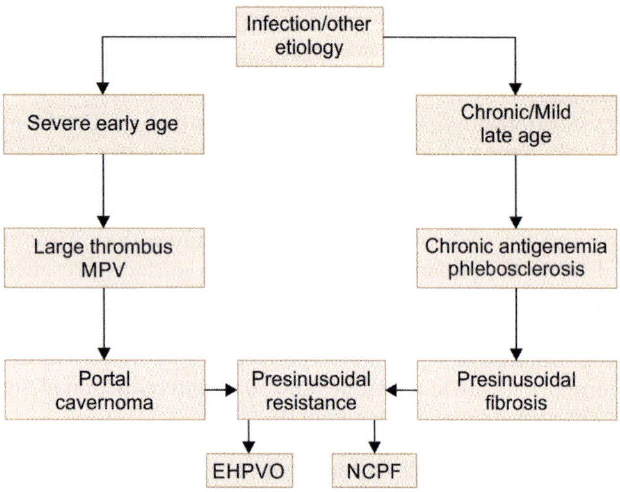

(EHPVO: extrahepatic portal venous obstruction; MPV: main portal vein; NCPF: noncirrhotic portal fibrosis)

a common pathway with different outcomes has been advocated and is depicted in **Flowchart 1**.

Basically, in a genetically susceptible patient, a trigger point such as infection or prothrombotic episode can incite thrombosis in portal system.

In EHPVO, a major thrombotic event in early life leads to occlusion of main portal vein with resultant cavernoma formation.

Where as in NCPF, repeated events of microthrombi in later life leads to occlusion of small and medium sized venous cannels with resultant presinusoidal fibrosis.

Noncirrhotic Portal Fibrosis

This condition was first described by Banti in late 19th century and was originally identified in India as an etiological factor of portal hypertension in mid-20th century.

NCPF is a seen in patients during their 3rd–4th decade of life and especially more common in individuals of low socioeconomic background.[20,21]

There are well-established guidelines for making diagnosis of NCPF **(Table 9)**.

Imaging findings include normal size liver with normal echogenicity, splenomegaly, patent hepatic veins, dilated splenoportal axis and presence of varices **(Figs. 17A to D)**. Few specific ultrasound findings are also described (which are difficult to document), such as echogenic thick-walled portal branches, narrowing or cuff of peripheral portal vein branches classically described as "withered tree" appearance.[21,22]

Management

Prognosis is generally excellent in NCPF, since, liver functions are well-preserved. Main concern is usually prevention/control of variceal bleeding which is the major cause of death in these patients.

PREHEPATIC CAUSES

Extrahepatic Portal Vein Obstruction[23,24]

Definition

Extrahepatic portal vein obstruction (EHPVO), an important cause of upper GI bleeding in pediatric age group, caused by thrombotic event in early life resulting in cavernoma formation.

The disease process may involve only the main portal vein and its branches at porta, or may extend to involve the splenic vein and upper portion of the superior mesenteric vein. Splenoportal confluence is the most common site to get involved in this disease process; whereas entire SPA is involved in only 10% of cases.

The etiopathogenesis of EHPVO is not known in nearly 50% of patients. Possible causes include, neonatal sepsis, omphalitis, umbilical vein catheterization, dehydration, multiple exchange transfusions, and hypercoagulable states.

These patients may present anywhere between 6 weeks to adulthood with well-controlled variceal bleeding and massive splenomegaly. Generally, LFTs are normal in young patients with EHPVO. Infrequently, these patients may present with jaundice due to portal biliopathy. Hemodynamically, wedged HVPG is normal since the block is (presinusoidal hepatic), however direct intrasplenic pressure is significantly increased in these patients.

Portal biliopathy refers biliary abnormalities (Intrahepatic/extrahepatic) either due to compression of bile ducts by prominent paracholedochal and epicholedochal varices or due to ischemic injury (stricture formation) **(Fig. 18)**. Although imaging biliary abnormalities have been described in 80–100% of cases, but only a few patients present with jaundice or pain.[25]

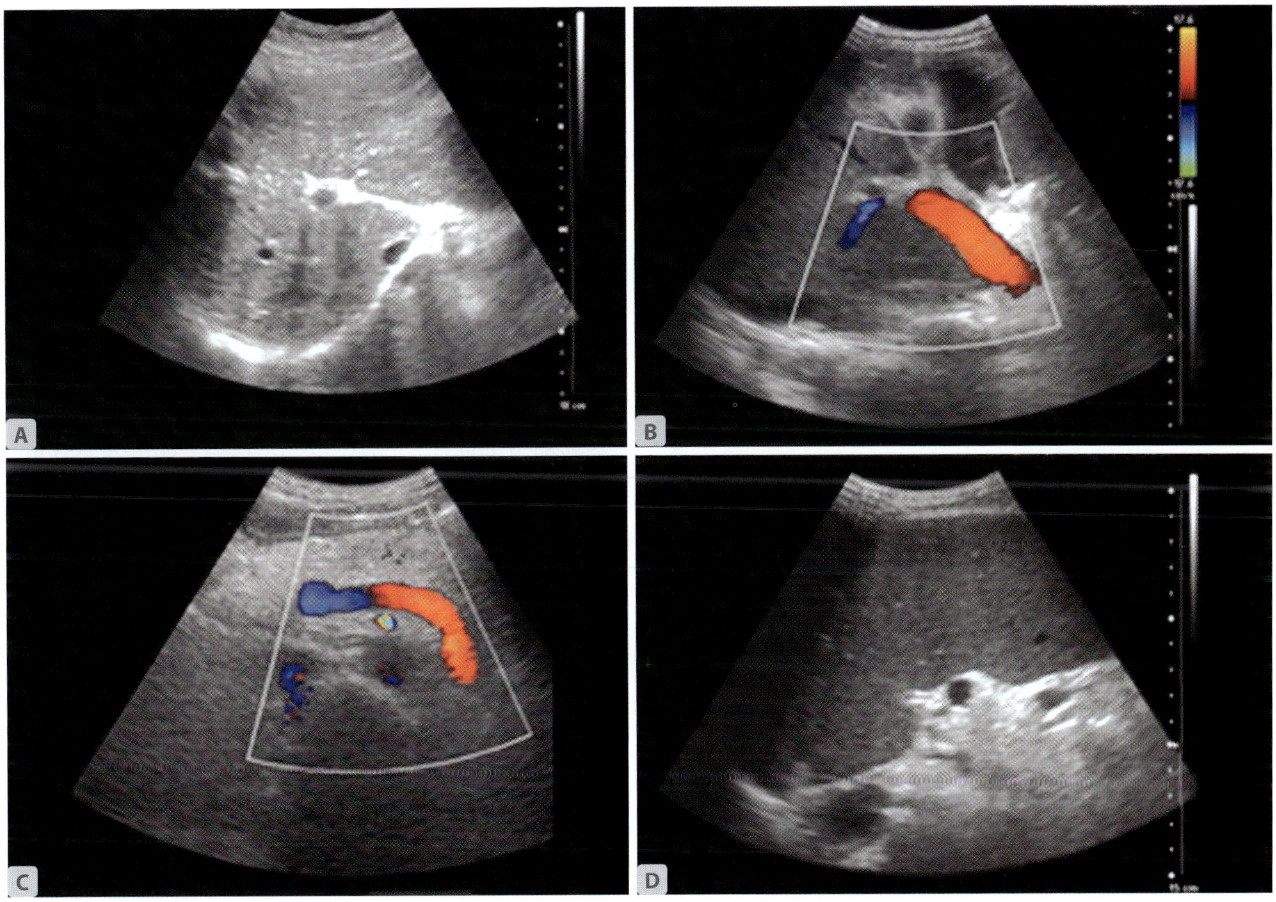

FIGS. 17A TO D: Ultrasound and Doppler images of noncirrhotic portal fibrosis (NCPF) patient showing normal size liver with normal echotexture (A), dilated MPV (B), splenic vein (C) and splenomegaly (D).

Imaging Modalities

Currently the ultrasonography with Doppler is best imaging modality to evaluate EHPVO patients **(Fig. 18)**. Invasive, direct splenoportography provides information about the portal venous system to identify the site of obstruction, extent of disease and extent of collateral circulation, however this procedure is obsolete these days **(Fig. 19)**. The more advanced techniques like computed tomographic portography and MR portography of the upper abdomen, are performed only if Doppler is of suboptimal quality **(Figs. 20A to D)**.

Imaging Findings

Main portal vein is replaced by echogenic fibrosis and multiple collaterals around the porta classically described as cavernoma formation **(Figs. 21A and B)**. Sometime, one may see recanalized portal vein or dominant collateral at porta. CT/MR portography are used as problem solving modalities when Doppler findings are inconclusive.

Treatment and Prognosis

Prognosis is generally good in EHPVO, since, liver functions are well-preserved. Main concern is usually prevention/control of variceal bleeding which is the major cause of death in these patients. Endoscopic therapy is the first line of treatment for variceal bleeding. However, surgery is reserved for patients with variceal bleeding who fail to respond to endoscopic management. Other indications for surgery include, patients with ectopic variceal bleeding, portal biliopathy and growth retardation.

Portal Vein Thrombosis[24,26,27]

Cirrhosis is an important risk for development of splanchnic vein thrombosis in cirrhotic patients, either due to development of portal venous hypertension or stasis of blood flow in portal circulation.

Other risk factors for development of acute portal vein include, infectious disease (e.g. sepsis, cholangitis, and pancreatitis), neoplasms, hypercoagulable states and surgery.

Contrast-enhanced CT/CT portal venography can exhibit a filling defect occludes the portal vein lumen either partially or completely **(Figs. 22A and B)**. Indirect signs include presence of cavernous transformation of the portal vein and the presence of portosystemic collateral vessels.

It is important to differentiate bland thrombus from malignant thrombus in cirrhotic patients. Bland thrombus will not enhance on post-contrast studies and will not distend the lumen **(Figs. 22A and B)**. Whereas malignant

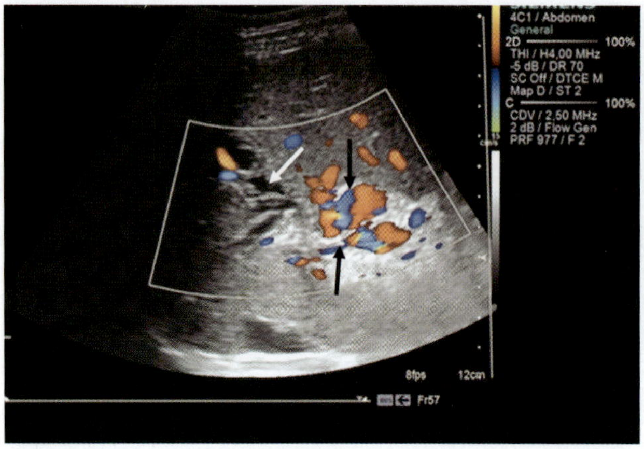

FIG. 18: Doppler ultrasound image showing multiple collaterals at porta (black arrow) replacing the main portal vein (MPV) with dilatation of intrahepatic biliary radicles suggestive of portal biliopathy (white arrow).

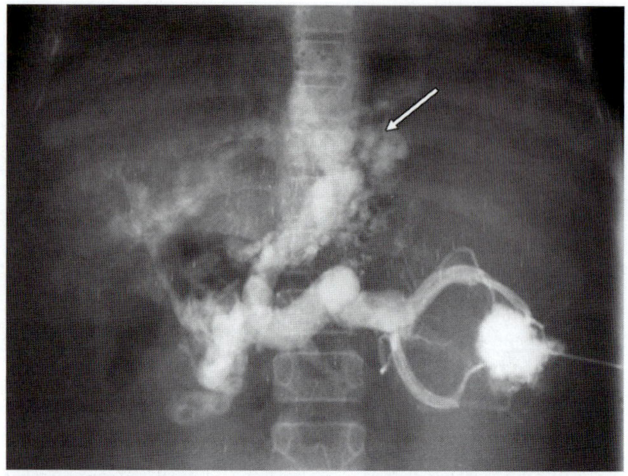

FIG. 19: Spot image of direct splenoportography showing patent and dilated splenoportal axis with varices supplied by the left gastric vein (arrow).

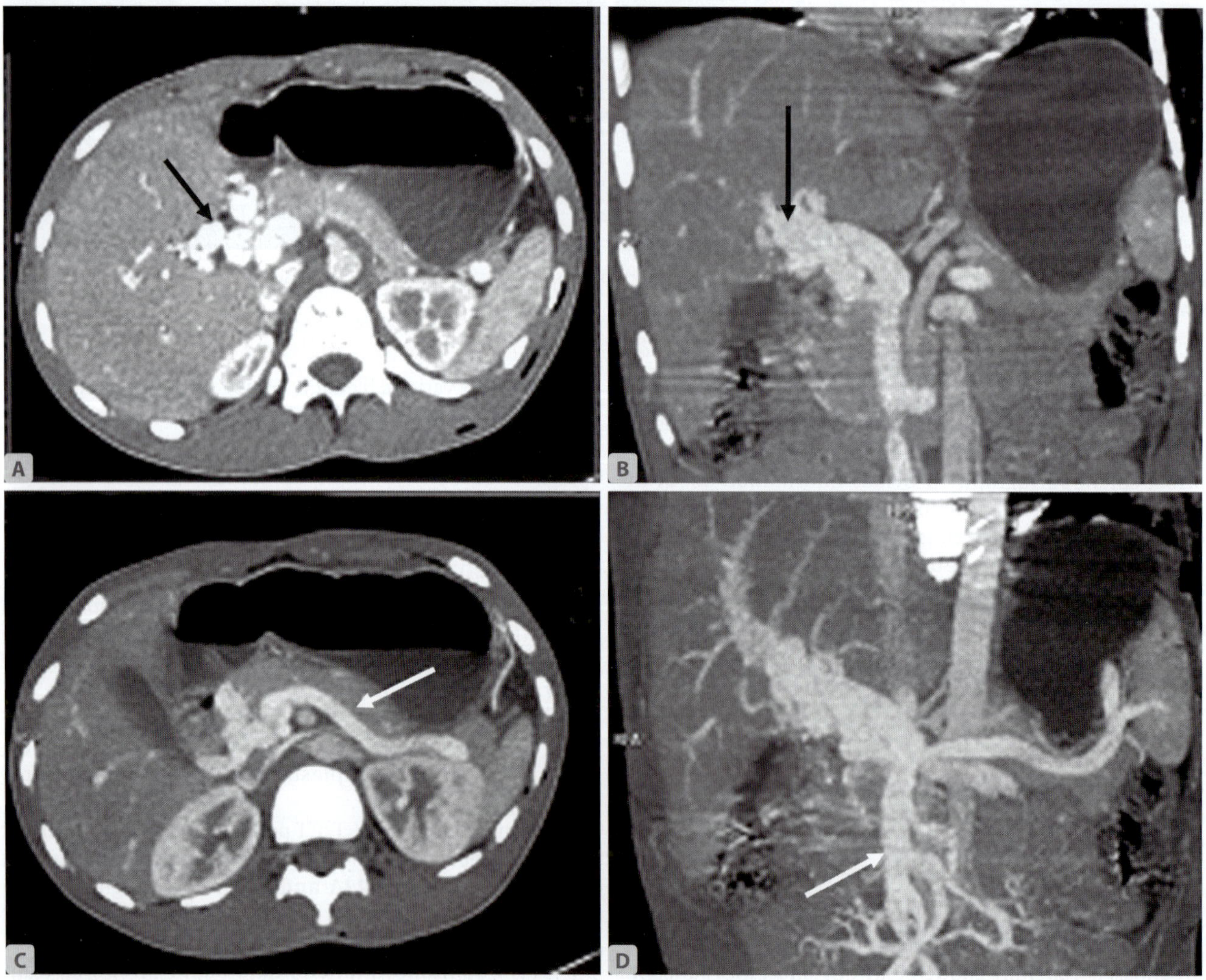

FIGS. 20A TO D: CT portography images showing multiple collaterals at porta (arrow) (A and B) replacing the main portal vein (MPV) with patent splenic (C) (arrow) and superior mesenteric vein (D) (arrow).

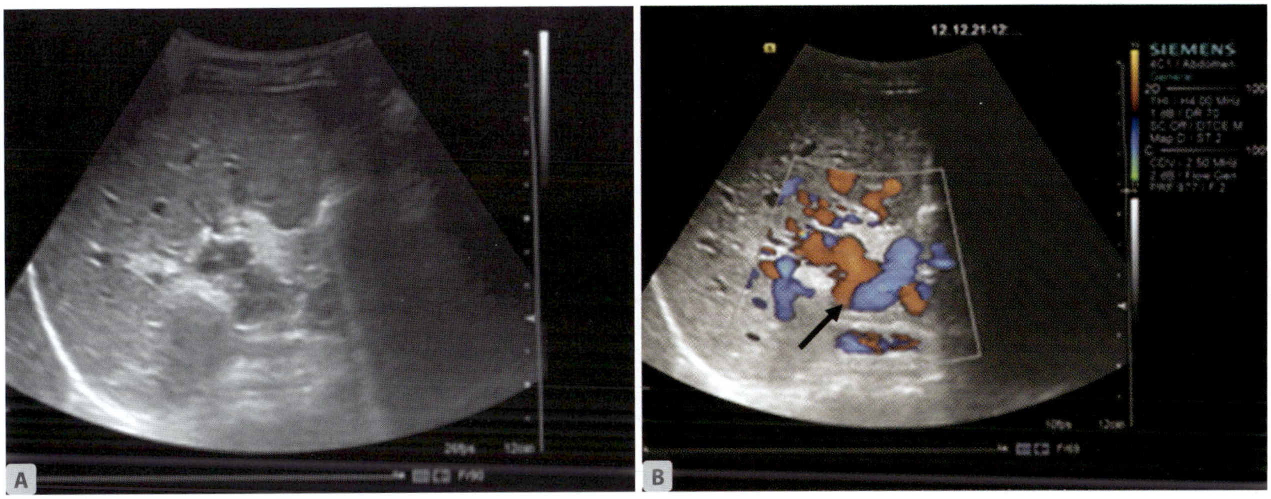

FIGS. 21A AND B: Doppler ultrasound images showing multiple collaterals at porta replacing the main portal vein (B) (arrow) with small size liver having normal echotexture (A).

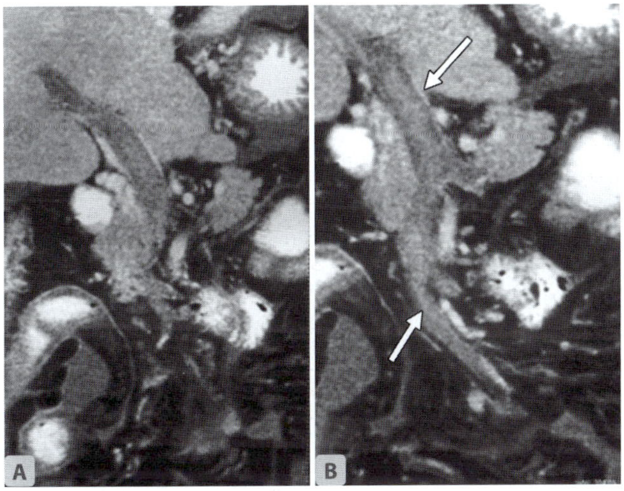

FIGS. 22A AND B: Coronal thin slab MIP image showing long segment non-enhancing filling defect (A) within the main portal vein extending into superior mesenteric vein (B) (arrows).

thrombus, distends the lumen and shows enhancement similar to primary lesion, classically described as "Threads-streaks" **(Figs. 23A and B)**. Malignant lesion shows diffusion restriction on diffusion-weighted MR imaging.

Left-sided Portal Hypertension

Left sided portal hypertension (LSPH) is a special form of portal hypertension that occurs due to obstruction of the splenic vein in isolation and presents with bleeding from isolated gastric varices. The main cause of LSPH is splenic vein thrombosis and pancreatic disease is the most common etiology. This entity is usually thought in situation of gastrointestinal bleeding with normal liver function and unexplained splenomegaly. At times, LSPH may be difficult to diagnose on both endoscopically and radiologically. On imaging, there is thrombosis or severe attenuation of splenic vein with extensive collaterals all around the stomach **(Figs. 24A and B)**. If repeated gastric variceal bleeding complicates this condition, splenectomy is considered.[28]

Splanchnic Arterioportal Fistula

Arterioportal fistula (APF) is rare, occurring mainly from a ruptured pseudoaneurysm communicating with portal system either due to iatrogenic cause or due to penetrating trauma. This entity is encountered increasingly, due to rising numbers of percutaneous transhepatic procedures. The predominant symptoms are due to complications of portal hypertension, most commonly variceal bleeding. Angiography remains the gold standard **(Figs. 25A to C)**. However, duplex ultrasonography is a useful screening tool. CT angiography helps in pretreatment planning such as artery involved, level of communication, diameter of communication and to see the extent of varices.

In broad, surgery is the treatment of choice for large extrahepatic fistula, whereas embolization is ideal for intrahepatic fistulas and small extrahepatic fistula. Embolization is also beneficial for patients with comorbidities who carry high risk of surgical mortality. Main goal of treatment is to occlude the fistula and maintain the arterial flow.[29]

Posthepatic Causes

Budd-Chiari Syndrome

Imaging findings and interventions are described in detail in separate chapter.

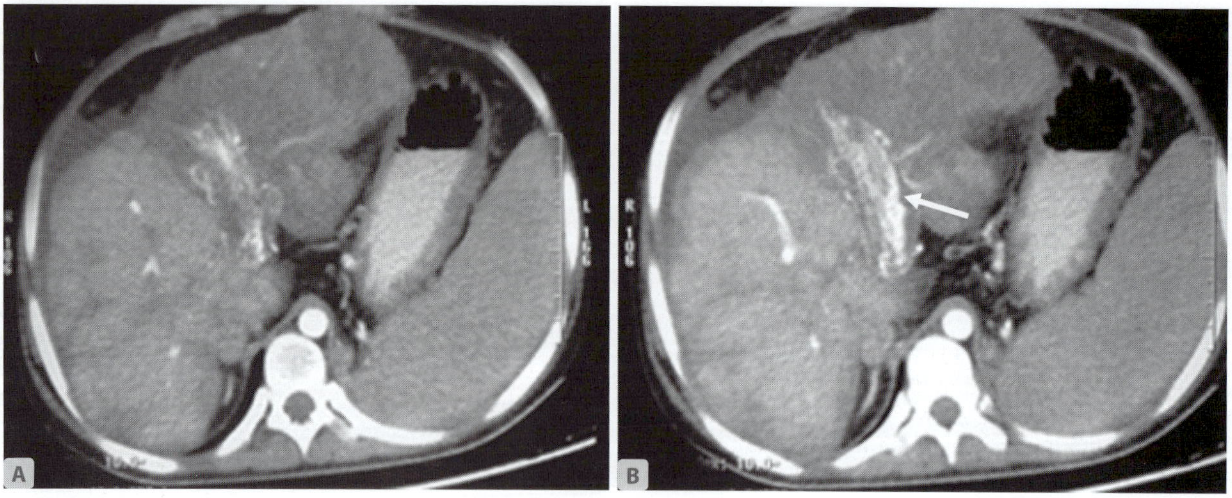

FIGS. 23A AND B: Axial CT images in arterial phase showing large infiltrative mass in left lobe of liver (A) with enhancing tumor thrombus in left portal vein (B) giving streaks and thread appearance (arrow).

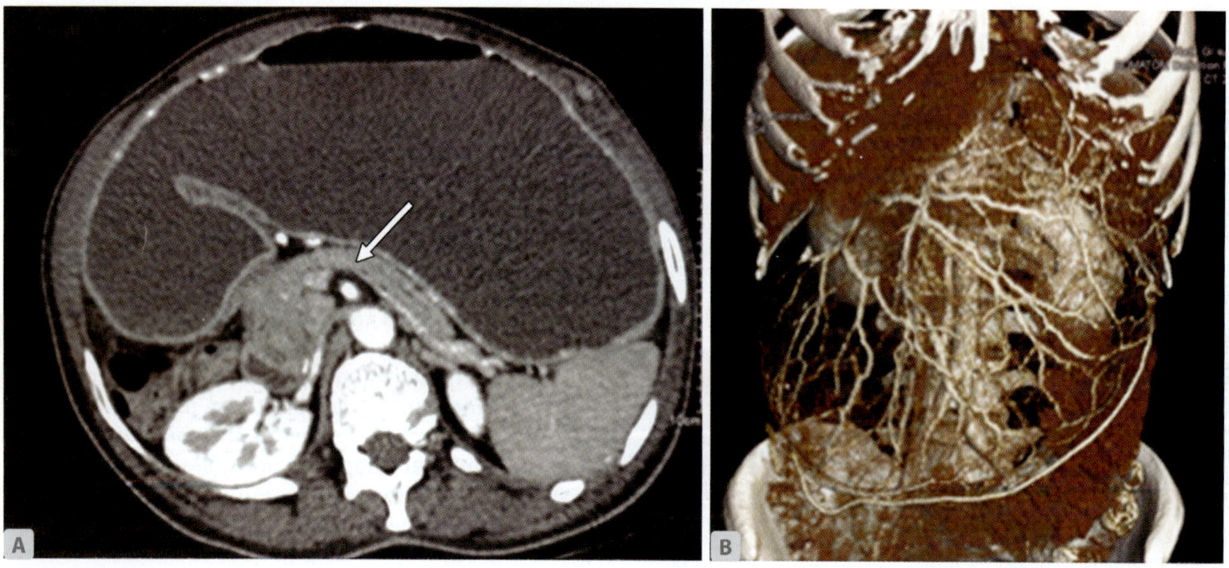

FIGS. 24A AND B: Axial CT (A) and coronal VRT (B) images showing severely attenuated and splenic vein (arrow) and is replaced by extensive collaterals around the stomach (B).

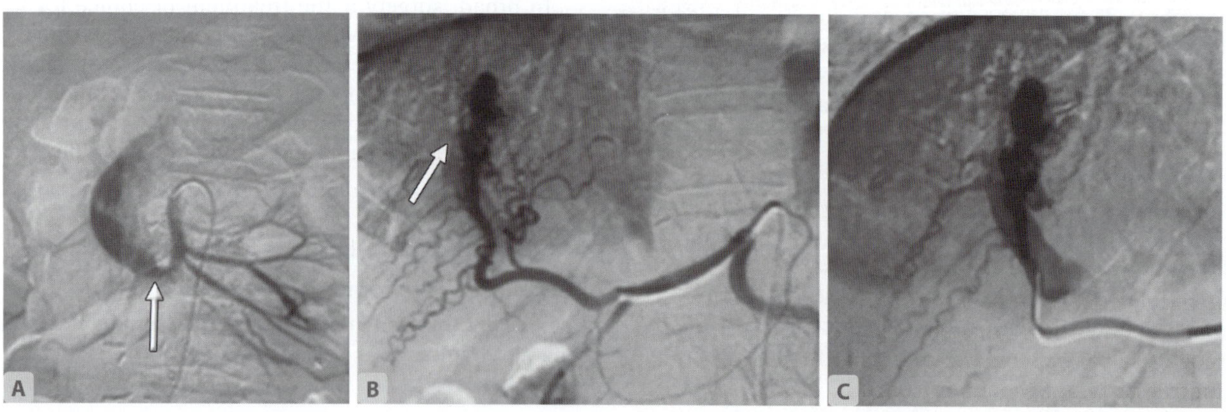

FIGS. 25A TO C: DSA spot images (A to C) showing fistulous communication between superior mesenteric artery and superior mesenteric vein (A) (arrow). Fistulous communication between right hepatic artery and right portal vein suggestive of arterioportal fistula (B and C) (arrow) as a prehepatic causes of portal hypertension.

RADIOLOGICAL INTERVENTIONS IN PORTAL HYPERTENSION

INTRODUCTION

The role of radiologists in the management of portal hypertension (PHT) had been confined to its diagnosis and treatment planning. However, with the advancements in the field of interventional radiology various minimally invasive techniques have evolved in the management of portal hypertension and its complications such as recanalization techniques, shunt creation and variceal bleeding control. Thus, with these technical advances, there is a shift in role of radiologist from diagnosis to the management of portal hypertension.

The management of portal hypertension and its complications requires multi-modality approach including medical and endoscopic management and surgical and nonsurgical (minimally invasive radiological techniques) methods to reduce portal pressure. Surgical methods carry significant morbidity and mortality in these groups of patients.

Interventions in Portal Hypertension

Primary aim is to reduce the portal pressure and thereby reduce the complications related to PHT such as variceal bleed, ascites, hydrothorax, and hepatorenal syndrome.

Secondary aim (In cases where it is difficult to bring down the portal pressure) is to deal with the complications of PHT such as esophageal and gastric varices, refractory ascites and encephalopathy.

The radiologic interventions in PHT are broadly categorized in **Table 10**.

Transjugular Intrahepatic Portosystemic Shunts

Transjugular intrahepatic portosystemic shunts (TIPS) involve the creation of a low resistance conduit between the portal vein and hepatic vein by deploying an intrahepatic stent. The procedure is done under fluoroscopic and ultrasound guidance, under conscious sedation or general anesthesia depending upon patients' condition. Prophylactic antibiotics may be given and coagulation defects have to be corrected prior to the procedure.

TABLE 10: Radiologic interventions in portal hypertension.

Interventions in portal hypertension
Interventions that reduce portal blood pressure: • Transjugular intrahepatic portosystemic shunts (TIPS) • Recanalization of hepatic venous outflow • Partial splenic embolization • Recanalization of occluded/thrombosed portal veins or tributaries • Occlusion of arterioportal shunts (congenital/acquired) • Revision of occluded surgical or radiological shunts
Interventions to control the symptoms of PHT: • Percutaneous transhepatic variceal embolization • Balloon-occluded retrograded transvenous obliteration of gastric varices (BRTO)
Occlusion of surgical or radiologic shunts in refractory encephalopathy

Technique

The procedure starts with puncture of right internal jugular vein for venous access under sonographic guidance. A 10F long vascular sheath is placed across the right heart into the inferior vena cava. Initial cavogram is obtained to look for the status of inferior vena cava and the ostium of hepatic vein. Diagnostic angiographic catheter is then introduced into one of the hepatic veins (preferably right hepatic vein). At this stage, baseline hepatic vein wedge pressure is obtained using balloon catheter occluding the hepatic vein outflow. After getting access into right hepatic vein, this catheter is exchanged with a long metallic cannula with 7F vascular sheath over the metallic guidewire. This metallic cannula is then wedged against the hepatic vein wall close to the ostium and gentle contrast study is done to look for retrograde visualization of intrahepatic portal vein branches. USG or direct transhepatic portography may also be used to visualize the portal vein and branches in difficult cases with distorted anatomy. Then using a combination of coaxial system of 16G metallic cannula with 7F sheath and 21G Chiba needle with 4F catheter, hepatic parenchyma is entered through hepatic vein wall. Using either fluoroscopic landmark of portal vein or USG guidance, access into the portal vein is done using 21G Chiba needle with 4F catheter loaded over it. This is the most critical step of TIPS that, utmost care should be taken not to breach the liver capsule to prevent life-threatening intraperitoneal bleed. The preferable site of portal vein puncture is at the portal vein bifurcation or within 2 cm of portal vein bifurcation. Once portal vein access is obtained, portogram is obtained to look for splenoportal axis anatomy and variceal status. The parenchymal tract is dilated using angiographic balloon catheters (diameter 8–10 mm) and specially designed TIPS stent (uncovered segment in portal vein and covered segment in hepatic parenchyma and hepatic vein) is deployed to maintain the patency of the tract. PTFE (polytetrafluoroethylene)-covered stents are preferred over bare stents as they showed improved long-term patency of the shunt and prevent porto-biliary fistula.[30-32] Customized TIPS stent graft has a small uncovered part (2 cm), which is to be kept in the portal vein to promote good inflow and avoid portal vein thrombosis **(Figs. 26A to E)**.

The established indication for TIPS is in the management of patients with cirrhosis and portal hypertension complicated by recurrent/refractory variceal bleeding and refractory ascites. Refractory acutely bleeding varices and complicated chronic/acute Budd-Chiari syndrome are among the optional indications **(Table 11)**.[33]

Absolute contraindications for TIPS placement include congestive cardiac failure, severe pulmonary hypertension, unrelieved biliary obstruction, pre-existing hepatic encephalopathy, etc. **(Table 12)**.[34]

Variceal bleeding is a major cause of death in cirrhotic patients and correlates with portal hypertension.

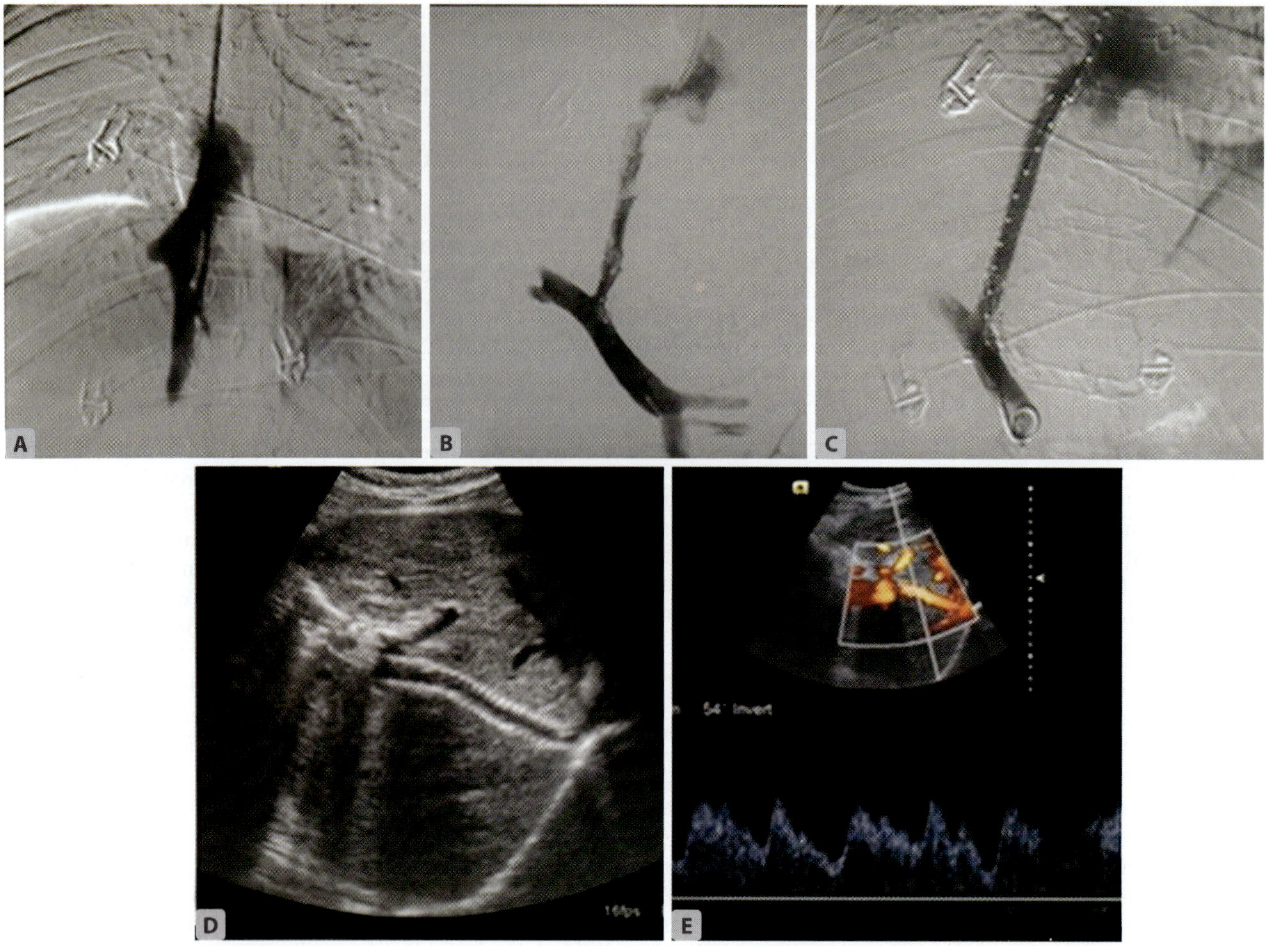

FIGS. 26A TO E: TIPS performed in a cirrhotic patient with uncontrollable variceal bleeding. (A) Initial cavogram showing normal caliber IVC and hepatic vein; (B) A parenchymal tract is made from the hepatic vein to the portal vein; (C) Post-TIPS venogram showing freeflow of contrast through the stent graft; (D and E) USG and color Doppler showing TIPS stent with optimal flow.

TABLE 11: Indications for TIPS.

- Refractory cirrhotic ascites
- Refractory acutely bleeding varices
- Portal hypertensive gastropathy
- Bleeding gastric varices
- Refractory hepatic hydrothorax
- Hepatorenal syndrome
- Budd-Chiari syndrome
- Veno-occlusive disease
- Hepatopulmonary syndrome

TABLE 12: Contraindications of TIPS.

Absolute
- Right-sided heart failure
- Biliary tract obstruction
- Uncontrolled infection
- Pulmonary hypertension
- Chronic recurrent disabling hepatic encephalopathy
- Hepatocellular carcinoma involving hepatic veins

Relative
- Severe liver failure (Pugh score >12)
- Portal vein thrombosis
- Multiple hepatic cysts

Many studies have demonstrated the efficacy of TIPS in controlling and preventing massive life-threatening variceal hemorrhage. It is recommended to reduce the HVPG below 12 mm Hg in controlling variceal bleeding. TIPS is also beneficial in preventing bleeding from hypertensive gastropathy.[34]

Refractory ascites reflects severe portal hypertension and advanced liver dysfunction and is associated with very poor outcome and survival. TIPS will decrease the need for repeated large volume paracentesis in patients with refractory ascites. However, in view of poor functional status of such patients and the higher risk of hepatic encephalopathy, TIPS is recommended for those who are intolerant to repeated paracentesis. Similarly in cases of refractory hepatic hydrothorax, TIPS is only recommended to those whose effusion is not controlled by diuretics and sodium restriction. In cases of Budd-Chiari syndrome TIPS or direct intrahepatic portosystemic shunt (DIPS) is recommended in cases with moderate severity and those who failed to respond to anticoagulation.[33]

Complications of TIPS

Immediate complications are procedure related; such as hematoma, arrhythmia, stent displacement, bilhemia and shunt thrombosis. Uncommon life-threatening complications include hemoperitoneum, cardiac failure, liver ischemia and sepsis. Chronic complications include congestive cardiac failure, portal vein thrombosis, chronic recurrent encephalopathy, TIPSitis and TIPS dysfunction. TIPS dysfunction is defined as loss of decompression of portal system due to occlusion or stenosis of the shunt. The best indicator of it is reappearance of symptoms such as variceal bleeding and ascites and can be demonstrated by imaging.

Recanalization of Hepatic Venous Outflow (Budd-Chiari Syndrome)

Budd-Chiari syndrome is a heterogeneous group of disorders characterized by hepatic venous obstruction at the level of hepatic veins, inferior vena cava (IVC) or right atrium. Hepatic venous outflow increases sinusoidal pressure, portal hypertension and decreased liver perfusion which in turn leads to progressive liver failure. The manifestations can range from fulminant acute liver failure to chronic liver disease depends on factors such as extent and acuteness of obstruction and adequacy of remaining collateral circulation. The etiology of obstruction in western population is primarily thrombosis (bland or tumor). Membranous web like obstruction of hepatic veins and IVC is seen commonly in Asian population.

Medical therapy including anticoagulation for preventing recurrence and extension of thrombosis and measures to control ascites and gastrointestinal bleeding has poor long term outcomes. Surgical options in BCS include creation of a portosystemic shunt and liver transplant. Portosystemic surgical shunts can only partially decompress the portal system and feasibility liver transplant depends largely on availability of donor.

Percutaneous techniques in BCS include transluminal balloon angioplasty of hepatic veins and or IVC and stent placement. Percutaneous interventions can restore physiologic hepatic venous outflow and help in resolution of venous congestion, improvement in hepatic function and arresting hepatic destruction. Hepatic venous recanalization techniques are feasible if the occlusion is short segment with large patent segment.

Transjugular approach is preferred for approaching the hepatic veins. Once the hepatic venous ostium is accessed, attempt is made to negotiate a guidewire across the stenosis followed by balloon angioplasty of the narrowed segment. Transjugular approach may fail in cases with tight stenosis at the ostium. Percutaneous transhepatic approach is preferred is such cases which involves USG-guided puncture of patent segment of hepatic veins and negotiating the guidewire across stenosis into the IVC. The guidewire is then snared through the transjugular route and procedure is completed by transjugular route to avoid making larger tracts in the liver. Successful angioplasty is seen as freeflow of contrast across the stenosis, reduction in pressure gradients and collapse of intrahepatic venovenous collaterals **(Figs. 27A to C)**. Metallic stents are deployed in cases of insufficient response and rapid re-stenosis following balloon angioplasty **(Figs. 28A to F)**. Good medium-term outcome is noted following angioplasty provided adequate anticoagulation is maintained.[35,36]

Inferior vena cava stenosis secondary to liver congestion in BCS get resolved after successful venous decompression procedures. However, primary caval stenosis that occludes hepatic venous outflow has to be addressed by IVC angioplasty. IVC angioplasty is performed by femoral or jugular approach **(Figs. 29A to D)**. Caval stenting is needed if angioplasty fails.

Long segment occlusion of hepatic veins is difficult to reopen and have higher chances of re-occlusion and this subgroup of patients require creation of a portosystemic shunt. TIPS and DIPS are being increasingly performed in such scenario with gratifying results.[37,38]

Partial Splenic Embolization

Partial splenic embolization (PSE) is performed to decrease portal venous inflow, thereby decreasing the portal

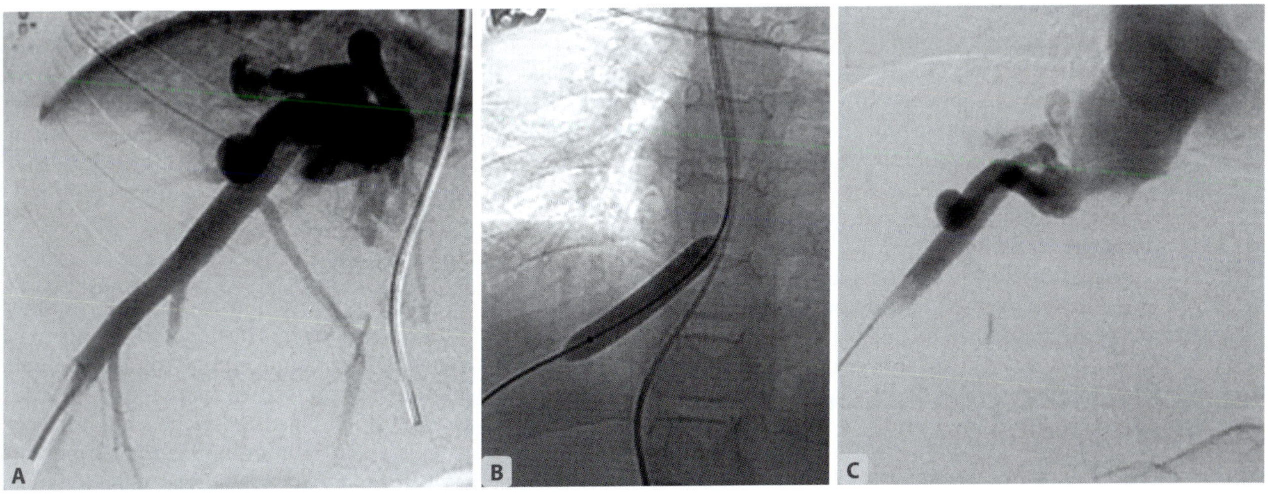

FIGS. 27A TO C: Hepatic vein angioplasty in a patient with Budd-Chiarri syndrome. (A) Hepatic venogram (percutaneous approach) shows complete occlusion at the ostium with multiple venous collaterals; (B) Balloon angioplasty of the stenosed ostium; (C) Postangioplasty hepatic venogram showing freeflow of contrast into IVC.

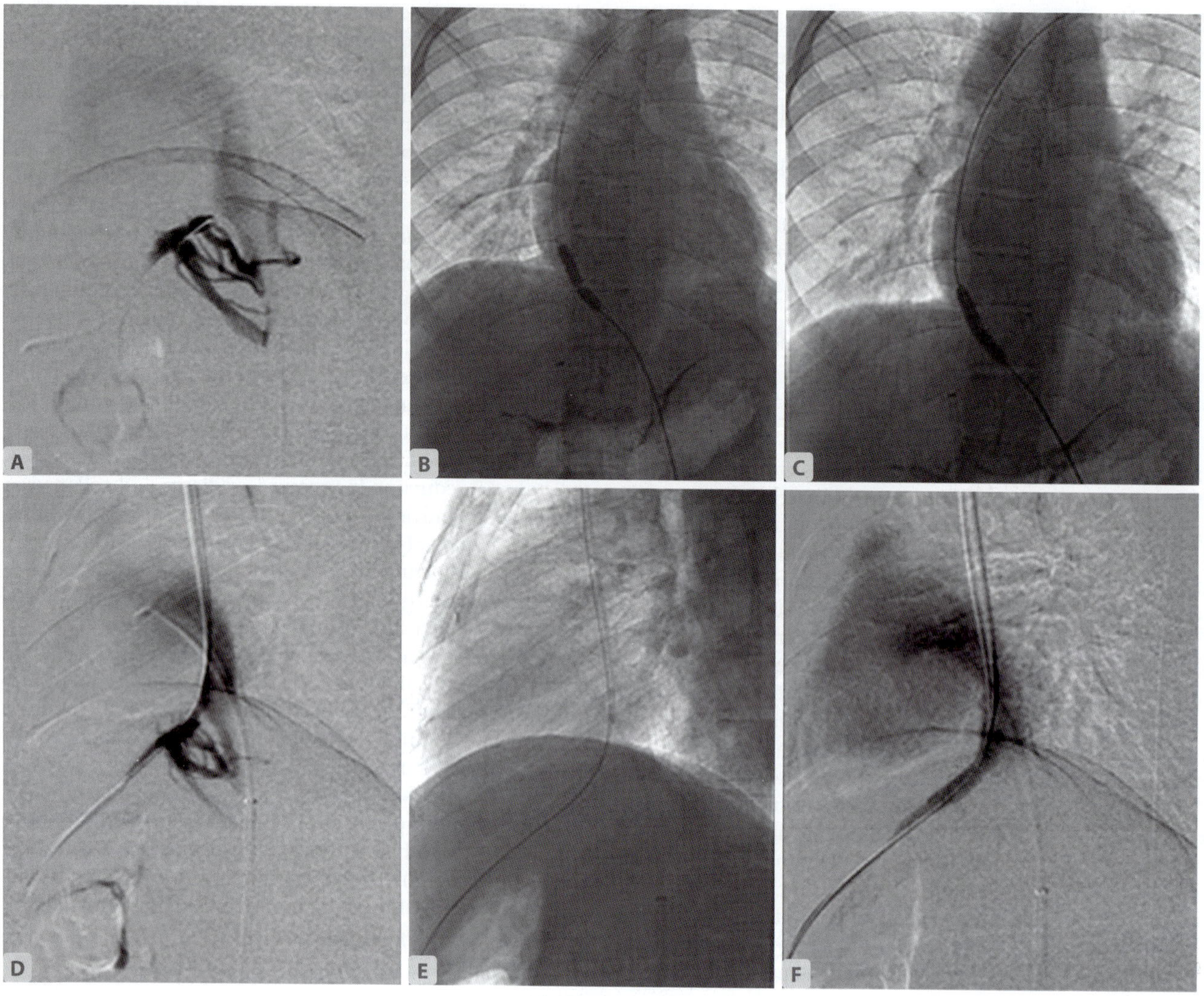

FIGS. 28A TO F: Hepatic vein stenting. (A) Hepatic venogram showing stenosis at ostium with multiple collaterals; (B and C) Balloon angioplasty; (D) Postangioplasty showing residual stenosis with persistent collaterals; (E and F) Stent deployment and subsequent study showing freeflow of contrast with disappearance of collaterals.

pressure. It is performed by super-selective catheterization of splenic arterial branches and embolization using polyvinyl alcohol particles **(Figs. 30A to D)**. PSE is efficacious in reducing the episodes of variceal bleeding. It also helps in decreasing splenic size and in improving hematologic parameters and hepatic protein synthesis.[39] PSE is an safe, simple and effective alternative for splenectomy in hypersplenism.[40] It causes partial necrosis of splenic parenchyma with minimal risk of complications such as liver abscess and sepsis. Splenic artery embolization can also be used in management of bleeding gastric varices secondary to splenic vein thrombosis.[41]

Recanalization of Occluded/Thrombosed Portal Veins or Tributaries

Portal hypertension can be caused by obstruction of portal vein or its tributaries. It can be due to inflammatory stenosis, bland thrombus or due to tumor infiltration. In both benign and malignant conditions, patients present with variceal bleeding, ascites or abdominal pain. These symptoms can be relieved by recanalization occluded vessels, which can be achieved by angioplasty and stenting through transjugular, transhepatic or transsplenic route.[42,43] Anastomotic strictures of portal vein can also be treated by angioplasty **(Figs. 31A to D)**.

Occlusion of Arterioportal Shunts (Congenital/Acquired)

Arterioportal shunts can cause portal hypertension by increased portal flow. Etiology of arterioportal shunts may be congenital malformation, trauma, tumors, aneurysms and surgery or hepatic interventions. Such patients may rarely present with gastrointestinal bleeding, ascites, heart failure and splenomegaly. Transarterial embolization of feeding arteries by coils, glue or other closure devises depending on the size of the fistula is the preferred treatment in such cases **(Figs. 32A to D)**.[44]

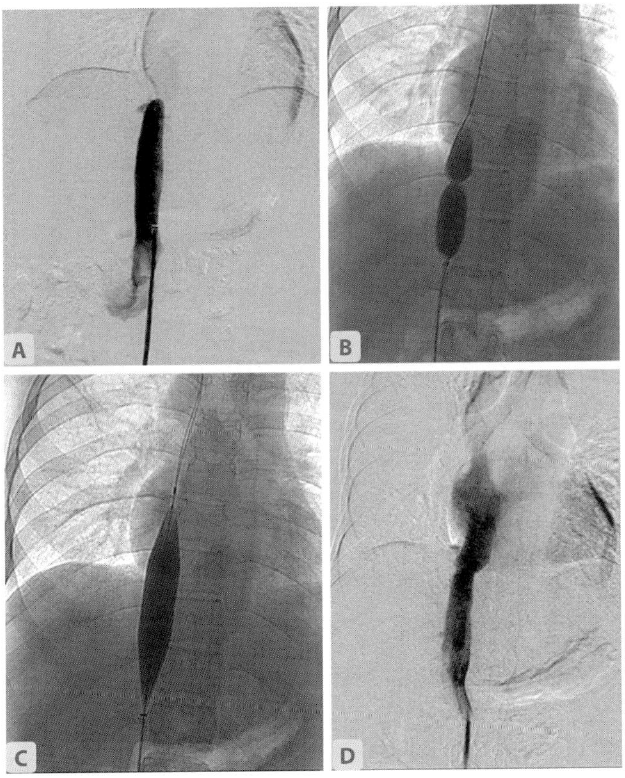

FIGS. 29A TO D: IVC angioplasty. (A) Cavogram showing total occlusion below cavo-atrial junction; (B and C) Angioplasty using balloon catheter; (D) Postangioplasty cavogram showing freeflow of contrast into right atrium.

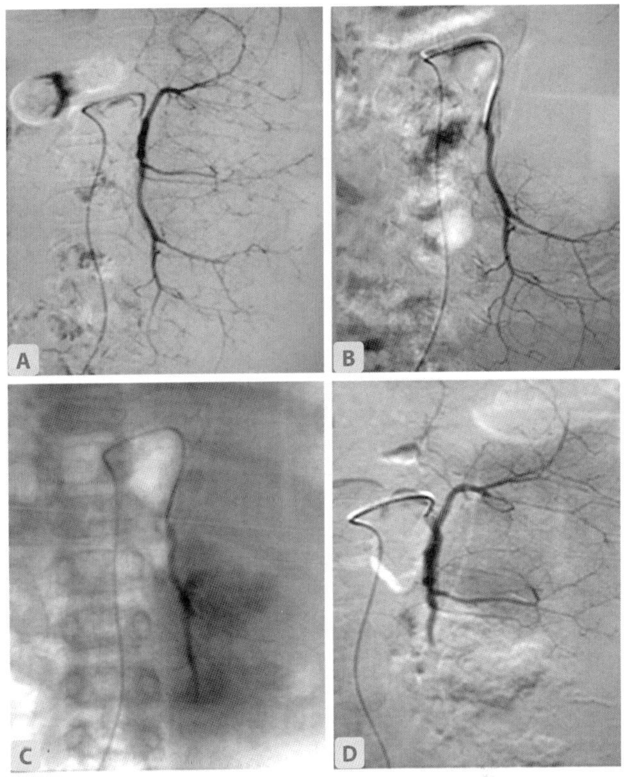

FIGS. 30A TO D: Partial splenic embolization in a patient with hypersplenism. (A) Splenic arteriogram showing parenchymal branches; (B) Selective run of lower branch of splenic artery; (C) Embolization of lower part of spleen using PVA particles; (D) Postembolization study showing decreased perfusion in lower part.

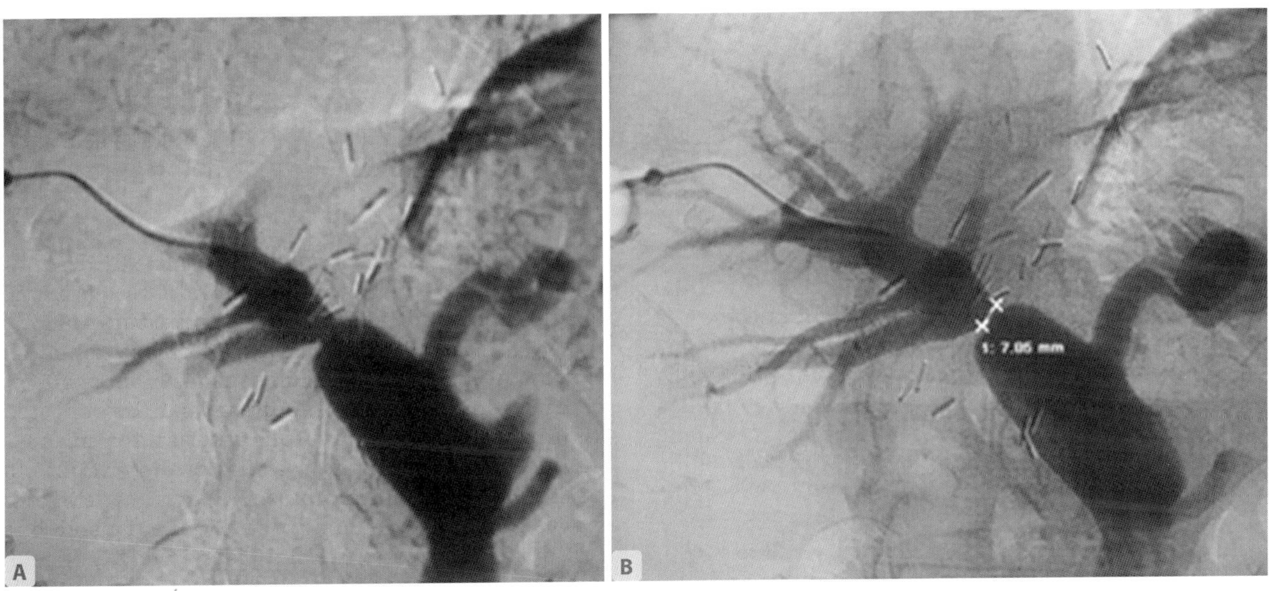

FIGS. 31A TO D: *Continued*

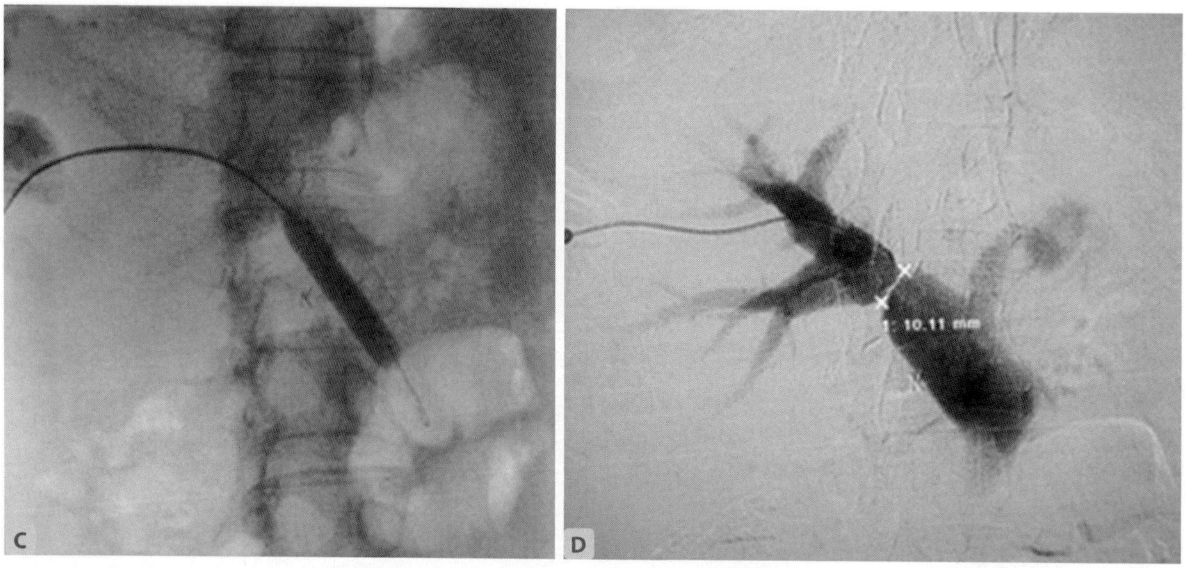

FIGS. 31A TO D: Recanalization of anastomotic stricture of portal vein. (A and B) Portogram showing stricture at anastomotic site; (C) Balloon dilatation of the stricture; (D) Postangioplasty run showing improvement in stricture.

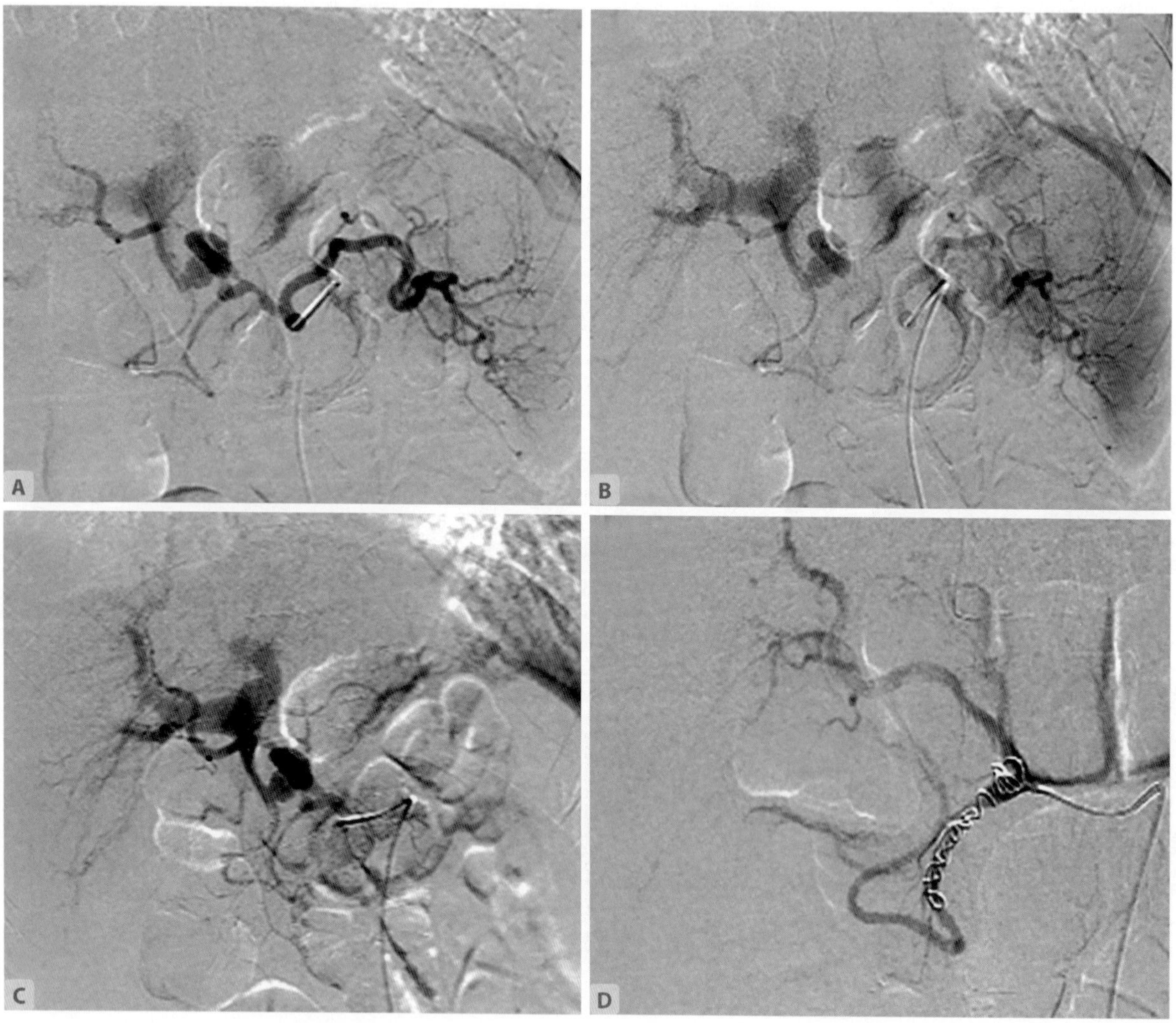

FIGS. 32A TO D: Occlusion of arterioportal shunts. (A and B) Celiac angiogram showing pseudoaneurysm of gastroduodenal artery communicating with portal vein; (C) Selective hepatic angiogram prior to embolization showing pseudoaneurysm; (D) Postembolization study showing complete isolation of pseudoaneurysm and disappearance of abnormal shunt.

Revision of Occluded Surgical or Radiological Shunts

Surgically created portosystemic shunts for portal hypertension may be complicated by thrombosis and occlusion. Surgical treatment of such cases is difficult and carries a high morbidity. Occluded leno-renal shunts and mesocaval shunts can be successfully recanalized by endovascular route **(Figs. 33A to E)**.[45,46]

Percutaneous Transhepatic (or Trans-splenic) Variceal Embolization

Percutaneous transhepatic variceal embolization was introduced as technique to manage bleeding esophago-gastric varices by Lunderquist and Vang in 1974.[47] Subsequent studies had shown excellent immediate success rate of 70–90%. Recurrent bleeding rate of 30–65% was noted in those studies since the procedure alone do not address

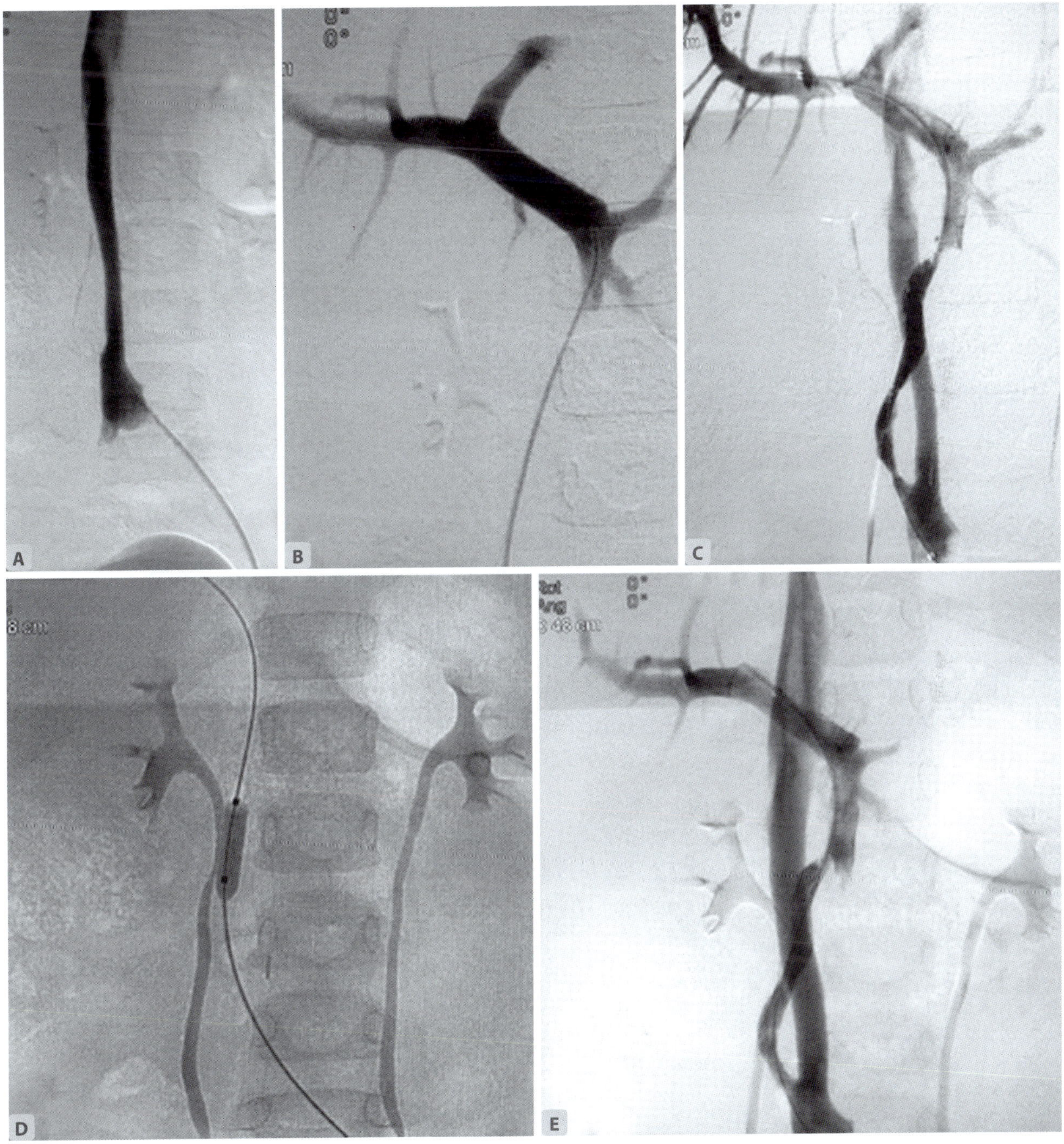

FIGS. 33A TO E: Mesocaval shunt revision. (A) Cavogram showing normal IVC; (B and C) Portogram done after advancing the catheter into portal vein through mesocaval shunt showing stenosis in the shunt; (D) Balloon dilatation of stenosis; (E) Subsequent portogram showing improved flow of contrast through the shunt.

the basic issues of portal hypertension and hepatic insufficiency.[48-52] Subsequently the procedure was recommended in acute settings when the variceal bleeding was not controlled by endoscopic sclerotherapy, vasopressin infusion and balloon tamponade.[53] It can also be used in the management of bleeding gastric varices, which are difficult to localize by endoscopy.[54,55]

The technique starts with percutaneous transhepatic puncture of the intrahepatic branch of portal vein with ultrasound or fluoroguidance and advancement of catheter into the splenic vein. Diagnostic splenoportography is then performed to delineate the feeding veins, varices and draining veins. The common veins feeding the gastric varices are the left gastric, short gastric and posterior gastric veins. Subsequently, the feeding vein is selectively catheterized and venography is performed to assess the size of the varices, velocity of flow and the size of gastrorenal shunt. On the basis of these data variceal sclerotherapy is performed with cyanoacrylate mixed with lipiodol. In cases with large gastrorenal shunts with rapid venous drainage, the gastrorenal shunts has to be occluded with angiographic balloon catheter prior to sclerotherapy. The track in the hepatic parenchyma is embolized using gelfoam and steel coils at the end of the procedure **(Figs. 34A to D)**.

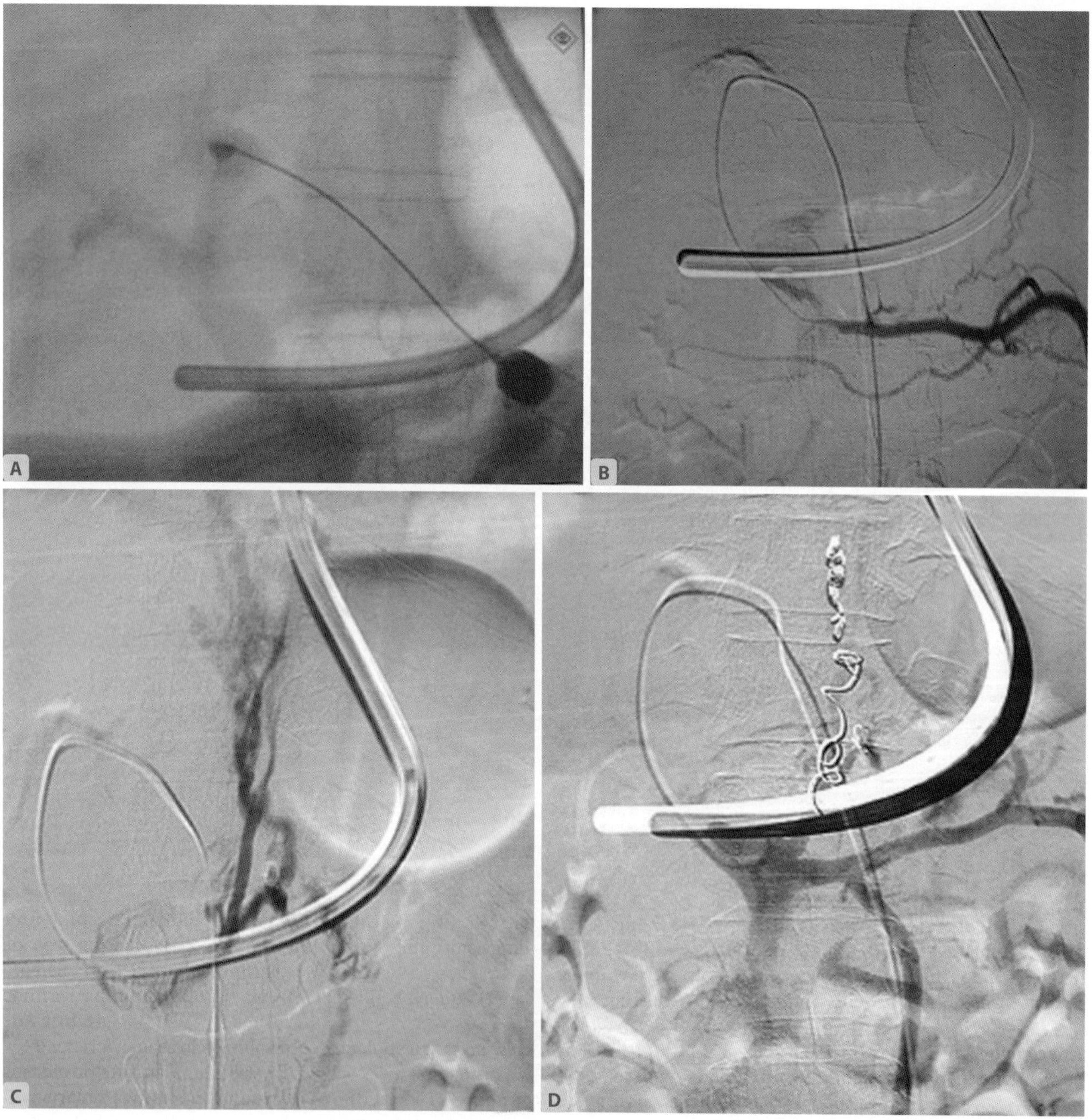

FIGS. 34A TO D: Percutaneous transhepatic variceal embolization. (A and B) Percutaneous transhepatic portogram showing portal vein and branches; (C) Selective angiogram of coronary vein is showing gastric varices; (D) Feeding vein is occluded by deploying stainless steel coils.

Variceal embolization can also be done with transsplenic route in which the access into portal system is through splenic vein and rest of the procedure being same. The transsplenic route is especially helpful in cases with pre-existing portal vein thrombosis.[56]

Balloon-occluded Retrograded Transvenous Obliteration of Gastric Varices (BRTO)

Patients of portal hypertension are often complicated by bleeding from esophagogastric varices. Although less common, gastric variceal rupture often leads to profuse bleeding and are difficult to manage with endoscopic and surgical technique.[57] BRTO is a novel technique in the management of gastric varices with major gastrosystemic shunts. It involves obliteration of gastric varices using sclerosants after occluding the communicating shunts with angiographic balloon catheter.

Contrast-enhanced computed tomography (CECT) of the abdomen is commonly performed for planning the procedure. The diameter of major shunts is assessed using CECT to calculate the size of balloon catheter which can occlude it. Gastrorenal shunt is commonly encountered. Other shunts such as gastrocaval and gastro-pericardiophrenic are also rarely seen.

The procedure is commonly performed with an access through right femoral vein. After cannulating the left renal vein, guidewire is advanced into left adrenal vein which is a common channel to gastrorenal shunt. Along the guidewire the balloon catheter is advanced into the shunt and inflated so as to block the shunt. Contrast study through the catheter is done to see the opacification of gastric varices. Some of

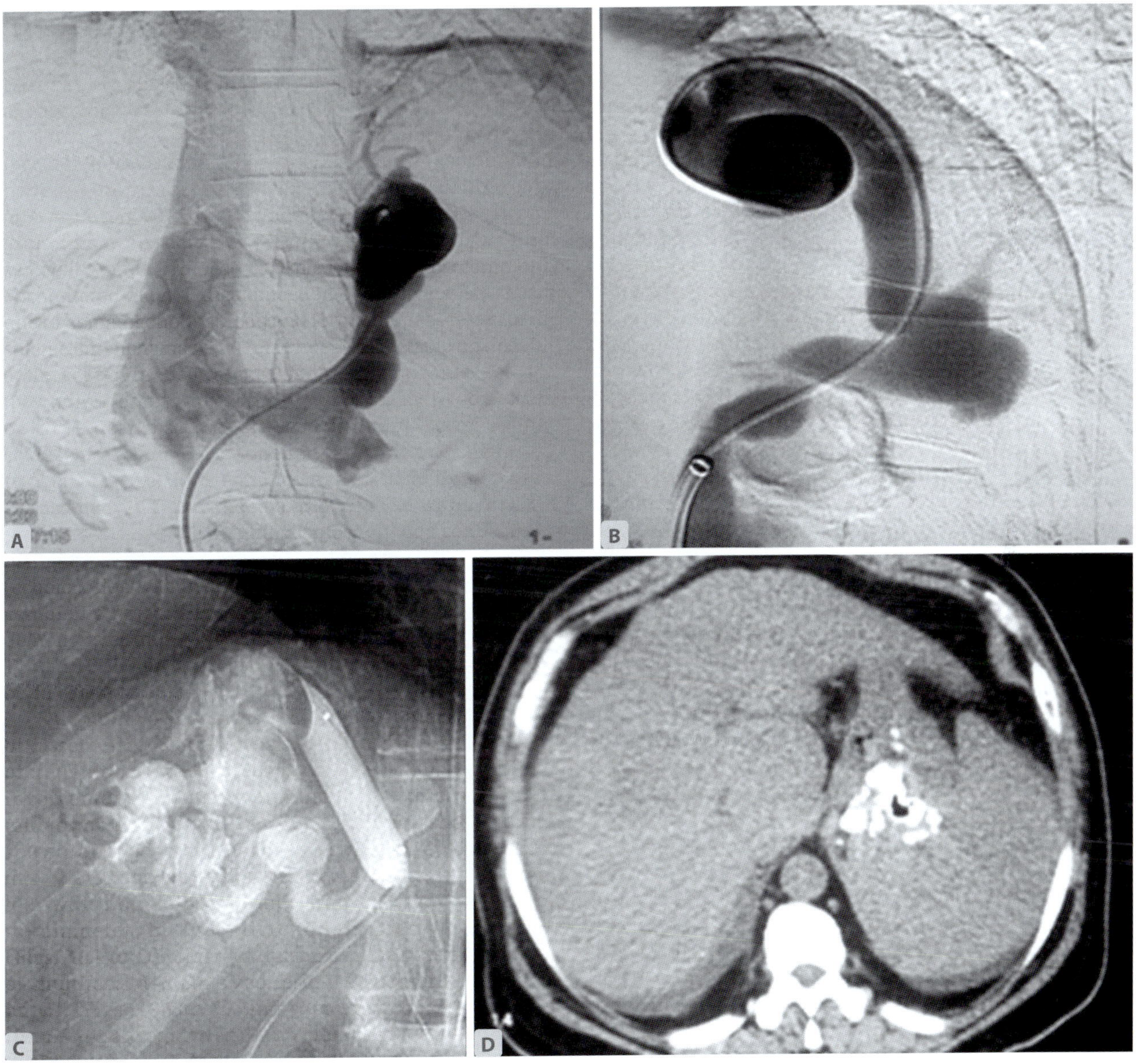

FIGS. 35A TO D: Balloon-occluded retrograded transvenous obliteration of gastric varices (BRTO). (A and B) Fundic gastric varices are approached through large gastrorenal collaterals of left renal vein; (C) Sclerosing agent (STS) mixed with lipiodol is injected into the varices with the balloon inflated and kept for about 3 hours; (D) Follow-up NCCT scan is showing lipiodol cast formation within the varices in fundal region of stomach.

the varices may show leaking collaterals which can be dealt by deploying microcoils or gelfoam pledgets after selective catheterization. Subsequently, the sclerosant mixed with contrast (e.g. 5% ethanolamine oleate with lipiodol or sodium tetradecyl sulfate with contrast medium like iomeron) is injected into the varices through the balloon catheter. The angiographic balloon is kept inflated for a variable time ranging from 1 hours to 24 hours for adequate thrombosis to occur in the varices. After a period of time to allow thrombi formation, the hemolyzed blood with the remaining sclerosant is aspirated and balloon is deflated and catheter removed. If freeflow of blood is seen in aspirate, supplemental dose of sclerosant can be injected. Amount of sclerosant and duration of application is up to the discretion of the radiologist and it varies with the size and extent of varices. Rarely varices may show multiple shunts and balloon occlusion of all the shunts would be required in such cases. CT scan is performed after 2–4 days for immediate response. Follow-up with CT or endoscopy every 3–6 months is done depending on different patient factors **(Figs. 35A to D)**.

Since the introduction of the technique by Kanagawa et al, BRTO has been widely performed as a minimally invasive technique to manage gastric fundal varices.[58] The technique has an excellent efficacy of 81–100% and relapse rate of 0–10% reported in literature.[59-64] Complications reported include technique related errors like coil migration, balloon malposition and extension of thrombus outside the varices. Renal failure secondary to hemolysis is a known complication with the use of ethanolamine oleate and can be prevented by administration of haptoglobin. Development of ascites,

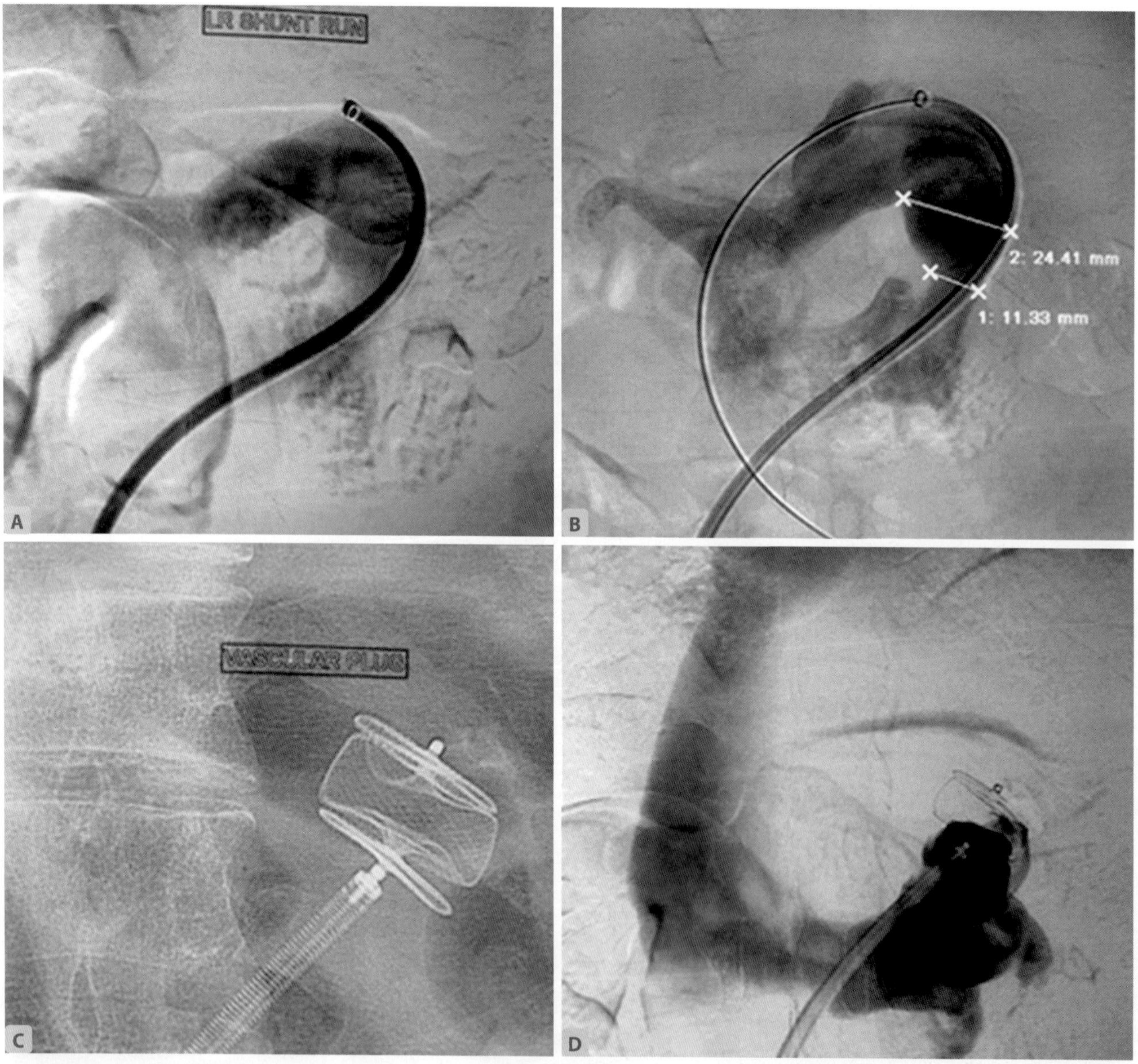

FIGS. 36A TO D: Occlusion of surgical shunts in refractory encephalopathy. (A and B) The surgically created lienorenal shunt for the extrahepatic portal vein obstruction (EHPVO) was accessed through left renal vein. Contrast study showing the large patent shunt, diameter is approximately 11 mm; (C) Deployed vascular plug (16 mm diameter) at the level of shunt close to the renal vein; (D) Post-shunt closure contrast showing complete closure of the shunt and patent left renal vein.

pleural effusion, hepatic encephalopathy and worsening of esophageal varices are also observed in occasional patients depending on their preprocedure functional status.[64]

Occlusion of Surgical or Radiologic Shunts in Refractory Encephalopathy

In occasional patients of advanced cirrhosis the surgical porto-systemic shunts (or TIPS) can cause or aggravate hepatic encephalopathy. In such scenarios, therapeutic occlusion of the shunts can be achieved by surgical or endovascular route. Endovascular route is preferred because of its minimally invasive nature favored in a sick patient. Using endovascular approach different occlusion devices are used depending on the size of shunt vessels. Large lumen shunts are closed with larger devices such as Amplatzer vascular plugs **(Figs. 36A to D)**.

REFERENCES

1. Kumar A, Sharma P, Sarin SK. Hepatic venous pressure gradient measurement: time to learn! Indian J Gastroenterol. 2008;27(2):74-80.
2. Peck-Radosavljevic M, Trauner M, Schreiber F. Austrian Society of Gastroenterology and Hepatology. Austrian consensus on the definition and treatment of portal hypertension and its complications. Endoscopy. 2005;37(7):667-73. Review.
3. Sanyal AJ, Bosch J, Blei A, Arroyo V. Portal hypertension and its complications. Gastroenterology. 2008;134(6):1715-28.
4. DeLeve LD, Valla DC, Garcia-Tsao G. American Association for the Study Liver Diseases. Vascular disorders of the liver. Hepatology. 2009;49(5):1729-64.
5. Schmidt S, Demartines N, Soler L, Schnyder P, Denys A. Portal vein normal anatomy and variants: implication for liver surgery and portal vein embolization. Semin Intervent Radiol. 2008;25(2):86-91. doi: 10.1055/s-2008-1076688.
6. Brůha R, Petrtýl J. Evaluation and treatment of portal hypertension. Cas Lek Cesk. 2016;155(2):22-6.
7. Procopet B, Cristea VM, Robic MA, Grigorescu M, Agachi PS, Metivier S, et al. Serum tests, liver stiffness and artificial neural networks for diagnosing cirrhosis and portal hypertension. Dig Liver Dis. 2015;47(5):411-6.
8. Zwiebel WJ. Sonographic diagnosis of hepatic vascular disorders. Semin Ultrasound CT MR. 1995;16(1):34-47.
9. Görg C, Riera-Knorrenschild J, Dietrich J. Colour Doppler ultrasound flow patterns in the portal venous system. Br J Radiol. 2002;75;919-29.
10. Kruskal JB, Newman PA, Sammons LG, Kane RA. Optimizing Doppler and colour flow US: application to hepatic sonography. Radiographics. 2004;24:657-75.
11. Wachsberg RH, Bahramipour P, Sofocleus CT, Barone A. Hepatofugal flow in the portal system: pathophysiology, imaging findings and diagnostic pitfalls. Radiographics. 2002;22:123-40.
12. Kang HK, Jeong YY, Choi JH, Choi S, Chung TW, Seo JJ, et al. Three-dimensional multi-detector row CT portal venography in the evaluation of portosystemic collateral vessels in liver cirrhosis. Radiographics. 2002;22(5):1053-61. Review.
13. Calhoun PS, Kuszyk BS, Heath DG, Carley JC, Fishman EK. Three-dimensional volume rendering of spiral CT data: theory and method. Radiographics. 1999;19:745-64.
14. Prince MR, Grist TM, Debatin JF (Eds). Portal Venous System. 3D Contrast MR Angiography, 3rd edn. New York: Springer-Verlag; 2003.pp.171-84.
15. Leyendecker JR, Rivera E, Washburn WK, Johnson SP, Diffin DC, Eason JD. MR angiography of the portal venous system: techniques, interpretation, and clinical applications. Radiographics. 1997;17:1425-43.
16. Kim HC, Bae SH, Choi CS, Kim EA, Kim IJ, Cho SY, Yun KS. MR portography. J Korean Radiol Soc. 1994;31(6):1121-5.
17. Bosch J, Abraldes JG, Berzigotti A, García-Pagan JC. The clinical use of HVPG measurements in chronic liver disease. Nat Rev Gastroenterol Hepatol. 2009;6(10):573-82.
18. Sharma M, Rameshbabu CS. Collateral pathways in portal hypertension. J Clin Experimen Hepatol. 2012;2(4):338-52.
19. Arora A, Rajesh S, Meenakshi YS, Sureka B, Bansal K, Sarin SK. Spectrum of hepatofugal collateral pathways in portal hypertension: an illustrated radiological review. Insights into Imaging. 2015;6(5):559-72. doi:10.1007/s13244-015-0419-8.
20. Bissonnette J, Rautou PE, Valla DC. Idiopathic non-cirrhotic portal hypertension: An update. Presse Med. 2015;44(10):1009-15.
21. Arora A, Sarin SK. Multimodality imaging of obliterative portal venopathy: what every radiologist should know. Br J Radiol. 2015;88(1046):20140653.
22. Sarin SK, Kumar A, Chawla YK, Baijal SS, Dhiman RK, et al. Members of the APASL Working Party on Portal Hypertension. Noncirrhotic portal fibrosis/idiopathic portal hypertension: APASL recommendations for diagnosis and treatment. Hepatol Int. 2007;1(3):398-413.
23. Arora A, Sarin SK. Multimodality imaging of primary extrahepatic portal vein obstruction (EHPVO): what every radiologist should know. Br J Radiol. 2015;88:1052.
24. Rajesh S, Mukund A, Arora A. Imaging diagnosis of splanchnic venous thrombosis. Gastroenterol Res Pract. 2015;2015:101029.
25. Baskan O, Erol C, Sahingoz Y. Portal biliopathy, magnetic resonance imaging and magnetic resonance cholangiopancreatography findings: a case series. Gastroenterol Rep (Oxf). 2016;4(1):68-72.
26. Chawla YK, Bodh V. Portal vein thrombosis. J Clin Exp Hepatol. 2015;5(1):22-40.
27. Yerdel MA, Gunson B, Mirza D, et al. Portal vein thrombosis in adults undergoing liver transplantation: risk factors, screening, management, and outcome. Transplantation. 2000;69(9):1873-81.
28. Köklü S, Coban S, Yüksel O, Arhan M. Left-sided portal hypertension. Dig Dis Sci. 2007;52(5):1141-9. Epub 2007 Mar 24. Review.
29. Lumsden AB1, Allen RC, Sreeram S, Atta H, Salam A. Hepatic arterioportal fistula. Am Surg. 1993;59(11):722-6.
30. Angermayr B, Cejna M, Koenig F, Karnel F, Hackl F, Gangl A, et al. Survival in patients undergoing transjugular intrahepatic portosystemic shunt: ePTFE-covered stentgrafts versus bare stents. Hepatol Baltim Md. 2003;38(4):1043-50.
31. Bureau C, Pagan JCG, Layrargues GP, Metivier S, Bellot P, Perreault P, et al. Patency of stents covered with polytetrafluoroethylene in patients treated by transjugular intrahepatic portosystemic shunts: long-term results of a randomized multicentre study. Liver Int Off J Int Assoc Study Liver. 2007;27(6):742-7.
32. Cejna M, Peck-Radosavljevic M, Thurnher SA, Hittmair K, Schoder M, Lammer J. Creation of transjugular intrahepatic portosystemic shunts with stent-grafts: initial experiences with a polytetrafluoroethylene-covered nitinol endoprosthesis. Radiology. 2001;221(2):437-46.
33. Boyer TD, Haskal ZJ, American Association for the Study of Liver Diseases. The role of transjugular intrahepatic portosystemic shunt in the management of portal hypertension. Hepatol Baltim Md. 2005;41(2):386-400.

34. Boyer TD. Transjugular intrahepatic portosystemic shunt: current status. Gastroenterology. 2003;124(6):1700-10.
35. Fisher N, McCafferty I, Dolapci M, Wali M, Buckels J, Olliff S, et al. Managing Budd-Chiari syndrome: a retrospective review of percutaneous hepatic vein angioplasty and surgical shunting. Gut. 1999;44(4):568-74.
36. Cura M, Haskal Z, Lopera J. Diagnostic and interventional radiology for Budd-Chiari syndrome. Radiogr Rev Publ Radiol Soc North Am Inc. 2009;29(3):669-81.
37. Michl P, Bilzer M, Waggershauser T, Gülberg V, Rau HG, Reiser M, et al. Successful treatment of chronic Budd-Chiari syndrome with a transjugular intrahepatic portosystemic shunt. J Hepatol. 2000;32(3):516-20.
38. Ochs A, Sellinger M, Haag K, Nöldge G, Herbst EW, Walter E, et al. Transjugular intrahepatic portosystemic stent-shunt (TIPS) in the treatment of Budd-Chiari syndrome. J Hepatol. 1993;18(2):217-25.
39. Koconis KG, Singh H, Soares G. Partial splenic embolization in the treatment of patients with portal hypertension: a review of the english language literature. J Vasc Interv Radiol. 2007;18(4):463-81.
40. Alwmark A, Bengmark S, Gullstrand P, Joelsson B, Lunderquist A, Owman T. Evaluation of splenic embolization in patients with portal hypertension and hypersplenism. Ann Surg. 1982;196(5):518-24.
41. Saugel B, Gaa J, Phillip V, Schmid RM, Huber W. Splenic artery embolization in a woman with bleeding gastric varices and splenic vein thrombosis: a case report. J Med Case Reports. 2010;4(1):247.
42. Yamakado K, Nakatsuka A, Tanaka N, Fujii A, Isaji S, Kawarada Y, et al. Portal venous stent placement in patients with pancreatic and biliary neoplasms invading portal veins and causing portal hypertension: initial experience. Radiology. 2001;220(1):150-6.
43. Shan H, Xiao X-S, Huang M-S, Ouyang Q, Jiang Z-B. Portal venous stent placement for treatment of portal hypertension caused by benign main portal vein stenosis. World J Gastroenterol. 2005;11(21):3315-8.
44. Vauthey JN, Tomczak RJ, Helmberger T, Gertsch P, Forsmark C, Caridi J, et al. The arterioportal fistula syndrome: clinicopathologic features, diagnosis, and therapy. Gastroenterology. 1997;113(4): 1390-401.
45. López-Medina A, Peiró J, Gonzalez de Garay M, Antoñana MA, Sustacha J, Grande D. Treatment of occluded distal splenorenal shunts with endovascular stents: a report of two cases. Cardiovasc Intervent Radiol. 2001;24(3):194-7.
46. Lorenz JM, Funaki B, Denison G. Balloon dilatation of a distal splenorenal shunt in a child. AJR. 2005;184(6):1915-6.
47. Lunderquist A, Vang J. Transhepatic catheterization and obliteration of the coronary vein in patients with portal hypertension and esophageal varices. N Engl J Med. 1974; 291(13):646-9.
48. Bengmark S, Börjesson B, Hoevels J, Joelsson B, Lunderquist A, Owman T. Obliteration of esophageal varices by PTP: a follow-up of 43 patients. Ann Surg. 1979;190(4):549-54.
49. Benner KG, Keeffe EB, Keller FS, Rösch J. Clinical outcome after percutaneous transhepatic obliteration of esophageal varices. Gastroenterology. 1983;85(1):146-53.
50. Lunderquist A, Börjesson B, Owman T, Bengmark S. Isobutyl 2-cyanoacrylate (bucrylate) in obliteration of gastric coronary vein and esophageal varices. AJR. 1978;130(1):1-6.
51. Smith-Laing G, Scott J, Long RG, Dick R, Sherlock S. Role of percutaneous transhepatic obliteration of varices in the management of hemorrhage from gastroesophageal varices. Gastroenterology. 1981;80(5 pt 1):1031-6.
52. L'Herminé C, Chastanet P, Delemazure O, Bonnière PL, Durieu JP, Paris JC. Percutaneous transhepatic embolization of gastroesophageal varices: results in 400 patients. AJR. 1989;152(4): 755-60.
53. Sos TA. Transhepatic portal venous embolization of varices: pros and cons. Radiology. 1983;148(2):569-70.
54. Kwak HS, Han YM. Percutaneous transportal sclerotherapy with N-butyl-2-cyanoacrylate for gastric varices: technique and clinical efficacy. Korean J Radiol Off J Korean Radiol Soc. 2008;9(6):526-33.
55. Tian X, Wang Q, Zhang C, Liu F, Cui Y, Liu F, et al. Modified percutaneous transhepatic variceal embolization with 2-octylcyanoacrylate for bleeding gastric varices: long-term follow-up outcomes. AJR. 2011;197(2):502-9.
56. Gong GQ, Wang XL, Wang JH, Yan ZP, Cheng JM, Qian S, et al. Percutaneous transsplenic embolization of esophageal and gastro-fundal varices in 18 patients. World J Gastroenterol. 2001;7(6):880-3.
57. Sarin SK, Lahoti D, Saxena SP, Murthy NS, Makwana UK. Prevalence, classification and natural history of gastric varices: a long-term follow-up study in 568 portal hypertension patients. Hepatol Baltim Md. 1992;16(6):1343-9.
58. Kanagawa H, Mima S, Kouyama H, Gotoh K, Uchida T, Okuda K. Treatment of gastric fundal varices by balloon-occluded retrograde transvenous obliteration. J Gastroenterol Hepatol. 1996;11(1):51-8.
59. Hirota S, Matsumoto S, Tomita M, Sako M, Kono M. Retrograde transvenous obliteration of gastric varices. Radiology. 1999;211(2):349-56.
60. Matsumoto A, Hamamoto N, Nomura T, Hongou Y, Arisaka Y, Morikawa H, et al. Balloon-occluded retrograde transvenous obliteration of high risk gastric fundal varices. Am J Gastroenterol. 1999;94(3):643-9.
61. Koito K, Namieno T, Nagakawa T, Morita K. Balloon-occluded retrograde transvenous obliteration for gastric varices with gastrorenal or gastrocaval collaterals. AJR. 1996;167(5):1317-20.
62. Kiyosue H, Mori H, Matsumoto S, Yamada Y, Hori Y, Okino Y. Transcatheter obliteration of gastric varices: Part 2. Strategy and techniques based on hemodynamic features. Radiogr Rev Publ Radiol Soc North Am Inc. 2003;23(4):921-37; discussion 937.
63. Ninoi T, Nishida N, Kaminou T, Sakai Y, Kitayama T, Hamuro M, et al. Balloon-occluded retrograde transvenous obliteration of gastric varices with gastrorenal shunt: long-term follow-up in 78 patients. AJR. 2005;184(4):1340-6.
64. Arai H, Abe T, Takagi H, Mori M. Efficacy of balloon-occluded retrograde transvenous obliteration, percutaneous transhepatic obliteration and combined techniques for the management of gastric fundal varices. World J Gastroenterol. 2006;12(24):3866-73.

CHAPTER

121

Percutaneous Nonvascular Gastrointestinal Tract Interventions

Shivanand Gamanagatti, Deep Narayan Srivastava, Chandrashekhara SH

In the treatment of patients suffering from gastrointestinal tract diseases various therapeutic interventional techniques have been developed using percutaneous routes. These are:

- Percutaneous gastrostomy
- Percutaneous jejunostomy
- Esophageal stenting
- Gastroduodenal stenting
- Colorectal stenting
- Percutaneous enterocutaneous fistula closure.

PERCUTANEOUS GASTROSTOMY

Its procedure is used to provide nutritional support for patients with swallowing disorders. Enteral feeding is preferred in those with adequate small-bowel function to absorb sufficient water, electrolytes, and nutrients from a normal or elemental diet.[1-3]

Enteral feeding may be can be provided through various tubes placed either through nose or percutaneously. Nasogastric tube placement either blind approach or fluoroscopic approach is naive technique; also patients poorly tolerate this intubation when considered for long duration.[4] Nasogastric or nasojejunal tubes are usually used for short term duration.

For long-term feeding, tubes are placed directly into the stomach or jejunum percutaneously by fluoroscopic/endoscopic/surgical gastrostomy or jejunostomy technique.

Surgical gastrostomy involves an abdominal incision usually performed under general anesthesia and is associated with significant morbidity; Majority of patients undergoing some form of enteral feeding are poorly nourished, hence surgical wound may not heal properly leading to seepage and morbidity.[5,6]

Gauderer et al. described the percutaneous endoscopic gastrostomy (PEG) technique in 1980.[7] In PEG, the stomach is punctured percutaneously and, with the aid of a gastroscope, a string is brought up out of the patient through the mouth. The feeding tube is attached to the string and is pulled downward into the stomach and out through the anterior gastric and abdominal wall. PEG has fewer complications than surgery as it is performed under IV sedation instead of general anesthesia.

Percutaneous transgastric jejunostomy, another alternative to surgery, is a method that uses the Seldinger technique. In this technique, under image guidance a feeding tube is placed in the stomach and sometime up to the jejunum.[8-10]

Indications

Nutritional support: For patients with swallowing disorders, like abnormal peristalsis associated with cerebrovascular accidents, anoxic brain damage, degenerative central nervous system disease, trauma, and neurosurgery. It can be used to provide enteral nutritional support for patients with anorexia nervosa, severe depression, and advanced malignancy.

Decompression of the stomach or small intestine patients with chronic small-bowel obstruction may benefit from drainage with large-bore (24- to 28-French) gastrostomy tubes, which obviates long-term nasogastric suction. This indication is more common in patients with chronic intestinal obstruction secondary to carcinomatosis.

Other Indications

Innovative use of percutaneous gastrostomy has been reported in few unusual clinical settings, like retrograde dilatation of a gastroplasty stoma constructed for weight reduction in morbidly obese patients, to divert bile into the duodenum in patients with an external biliary drainage catheter where attempts to internalize the catheter are unsuccessful and in prolonged ileus after major surgery.

Contraindications

In cases of massive ascites, gastric varices, total gastrectomy and abnormal coagulation parameters.

Hardwares

The procedure requires following hardwares:

- 18G needle
- Suture anchoring set
- J guidewire 0.038 inch
- Superstiff guidewire
- Gastrostomy tube (18-24F).

Technique (Figs. 1A to E)

Preprocedure preparation includes overnight fasting. Procedure is performed under local anesthesia. If the nasogastric tube is already in place or else under fluoroscopic guidance a 5F angiographic catheter is passed into the stomach, after administration of 40 mg butylscopolamine (Buscopan), the stomach is totally distended with 750–1200 mL atmospheric air so that anterior wall of the stomach abuts the abdominal wall. Then, puncture is made halfway between the greater and lesser curvatures of the stomach at the junction of the upper 2/3rd and lower 1/3rd (to avoid the arterial injury) with an 18 G needle, preferably in lateral projection. Following gastric puncture, iodinated contrast medium is injected to see the precise needle location. Once satisfied with needle position, T-fastener present (preloaded) inside the needle is subsequently pushed into the gastric lumen (Cope gastrointestinal suture anchor set; Cook, Bloomington, MA) by using the stiff guidewire that comes with suture anchor set. The needle is then withdrawn out of the stomach leaving the T-faster in place. Now, T-fastener is retracted tightly so that the anterior wall of stomach closely approximates the abdominal wall and T-faster is then sutured to the abdominal wall. The stiff guidewire is still inside the stomach and the stomach wall is retracted to the anterior abdominal wall with suture anchor, the tract is dilated over the guidewire serially using Seldinger technique. Preferably larger bore catheter like 18F–20F Malecot catheter or loop forming pigtail catheter is inserted as gastrostomy tube. Next day, iodinated contrast study is done, prior to start of feeding.

Sutured T-fasteners are mostly removed after 10–15 days, to fall inside the stomach lumen.[11,12]

Technical Difficulty

- Different angiographic catheters can be used to negotiate through the stomach and duodenum.
- In difficult situations, gastric puncturing can be done under CT guidance.
- If access is lost after tract dilatation, patient may complain of gastric leak. It is advisable to give antibiotic and supportive care.[13]

Complications

- *Minor complications:*
  - Pain, fever
  - Wound contamination
  - Pericatheter seepage
  - Tube dislodgement

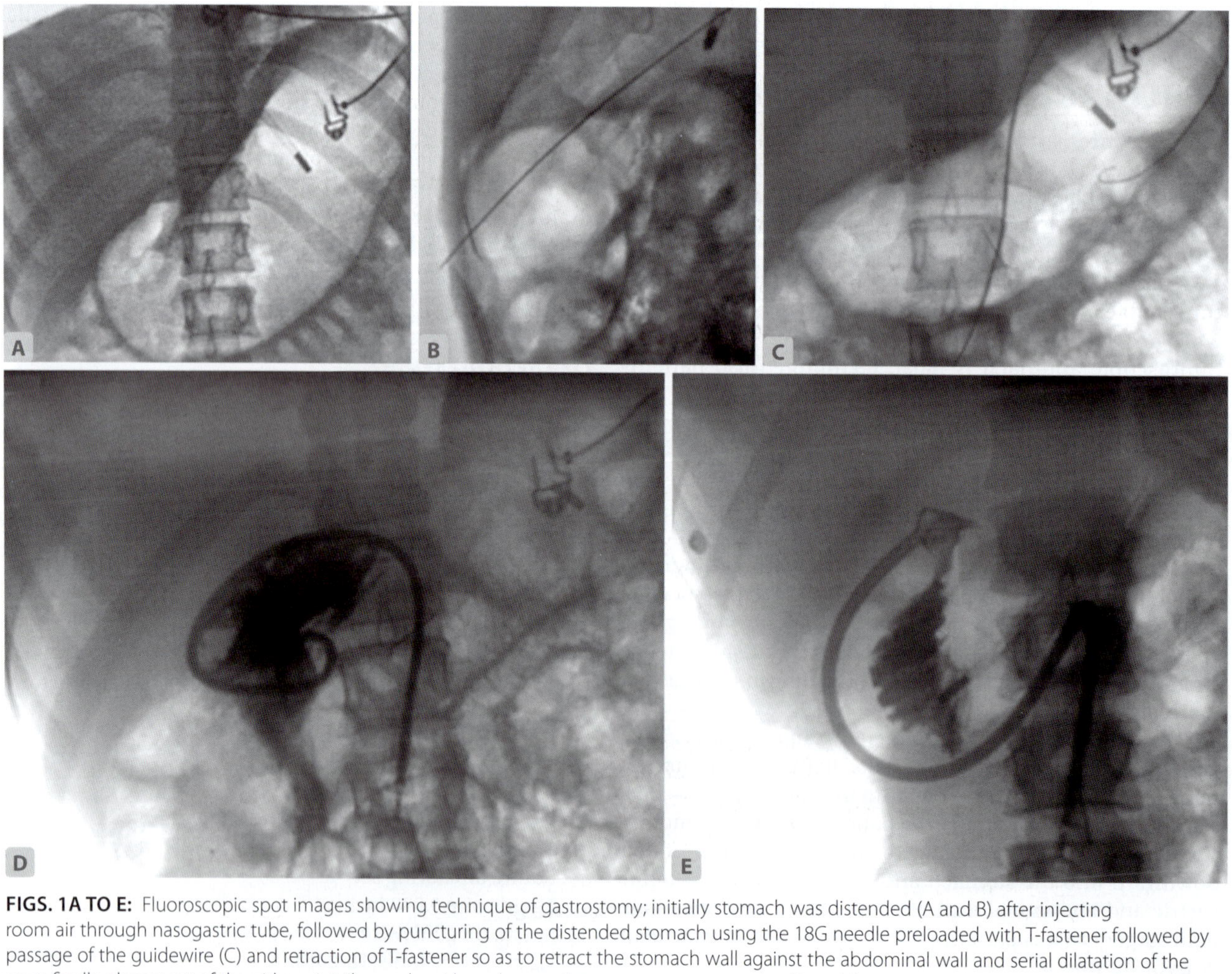

FIGS. 1A TO E: Fluoroscopic spot images showing technique of gastrostomy; initially stomach was distended (A and B) after injecting room air through nasogastric tube, followed by puncturing of the distended stomach using the 18G needle preloaded with T-fastener followed by passage of the guidewire (C) and retraction of T-fastener so as to retract the stomach wall against the abdominal wall and serial dilatation of the tract, finally placement of the either pigtail or malecot large bore catheter as gastrostomy tube (D and E).

- *Major complications:*
  - Hemorrhage requiring blood transfusion or other intervention
  - Peritonitis
  - Aspiration pneumonitis

Feeding through percutaneous gastrostomy is associated with gastroesophageal reflux and aspiration in some patients. It is better to advance the tube beyond duodenal cap into jejunum.

Tips to Avoid Complications[14]

- Puncturing site should be proper to avoid arterial injury.
- Prior oral barium would help to opacify colon; help to deliniate colon and stomach.
- Keeping the stomach fully distended during procedure
- Ascites if present need to be drained prior to the procedure.

PERCUTANEOUS JEJUNOSTOMY

Gray, described the fluoroscopic percutaneous jejunostomy in 1987 and was later revised by Coleman in 1990.[15,16]

Main concern of this procedure is technical difficulties like:

- Puncture of the mobile and collapsed jejunum
- Difficulty in supporting the location of the jejunum during the catheter placement.

Ultrasound or CT guidance can be used to puncture the jejunum, thus avoiding the colon. Care has to be taken not to transverse more than one jejuna loop.

Indications

In cases, where percutaneous gastrostomy is not be possible due to unfavorable position of the stomach or because of previous partial or total gastrectomy.

Other indications included diversion of success from a leaking anastomosis after esophagectomy and access to a limb of a Roux-en-Y anastomosis to facilitate biliary interventions.

Technique (Figs. 2A to D)

General preparation should include overnight fasting and, whenever possible, insertion of a nasogastric tube. Interposition of colon or liver between the stomach and the anterior abdominal wall should routinely be excluded by both sonographic and fluoroscopic assessment of the upper abdomen. Procedure is performed under local anesthesia.

A 120 cm long, jejunal tube is used to catheterize the duodenum or proximal jejunum through the nose. After administration of 40 mg butylscopolamine (Buscopan), the proximal jejunum was opacified with dilute, iodinated, aqueous contrast material and distended. Using the 18G needle preloaded with suture anchor set (Cope gastrointestinal suture anchor set; Cook, Bloomington, MA), one of the jejunal loop which is close to anterior abdominal wall is punctured under fluoroscopy and ultrasound. Following bowel puncture, iodinated contrast medium is injected to see the precise needle location **(*see* Figs. 1A to E)**. Once needle position is confirmed inside the bowel lumen, rest of the steps is similar to gastrostomy technique as described above (vide supra). Next day, iodinated contrast study is done, prior to start of feeding. Sutured T-fasteners are mostly removed after 10–15 days, to fall inside the jejunal lumen.[1-3]

Complications

Are same as in case of percutaneous gastrostomy.

ESOPHAGEAL STENTING

The palliation of esophageal cancer was first described by Celestin in 1959, through a plastic stent inserted at laparotomy.[17] Whereas endoscopic esophageal plastic stent insertion was described by Atkinson in 1970.[18] Endoscopic placement of esophageal metallic stent was first introduced in 1983 by Frimberger.[19]

Indications

The main purpose of esophageal stenting is restoring oral feeding and improve quality of life. Stents are used primarily in patients with advanced or inoperable malignant esophageal obstruction and in those patients in whom surgery is contraindicated.

Other indications are:

- Anastomotic tumor recurrence following surgery
- Malignant esophageal fistula
- Primary or secondary tumors within the mediastinum causing extrinsic esophageal compression
- Esophageal perforation (iatrogenic/traumatic)
- *Benign esophageal strictures:* As a last option, if the patient condition is high risk for surgery. Benign esophageal strictures are caustic ingestion, esophageal surgery, radiotherapy, etc. Esophageal stenting is indicated in refractory benign stenosis after 5 repeated endoscopic dilations and for long stenosis (>2 cm).[20] Uncovered metallic stents should be avoided in benign strictures due to risk of incarceration.

Types of Stents

- Metallic—Nitinol stents
- Partially covered stents—better embedding and achoring
- Fully covered stents—chances of migration are high; used for benign conditions
- Uncovered self-expandable metallic stent (SEMS)—tumor ingrowth is major problem.

Stent Designs

Esophageal stents are available in covered and uncovered forms. The covered stents are coated with plastic lining either from inside or outside.

The main benefit of uncovered stent is less chances of migration, particularly through the gastroesophageal (GE) junction. But they have high chances of blockage due to tumor in-growth. Current practice of esophageal stenting is to use covered stent in setting of esophageal cancer. Majority of esophageal stents are placed under endoscopic guidance.

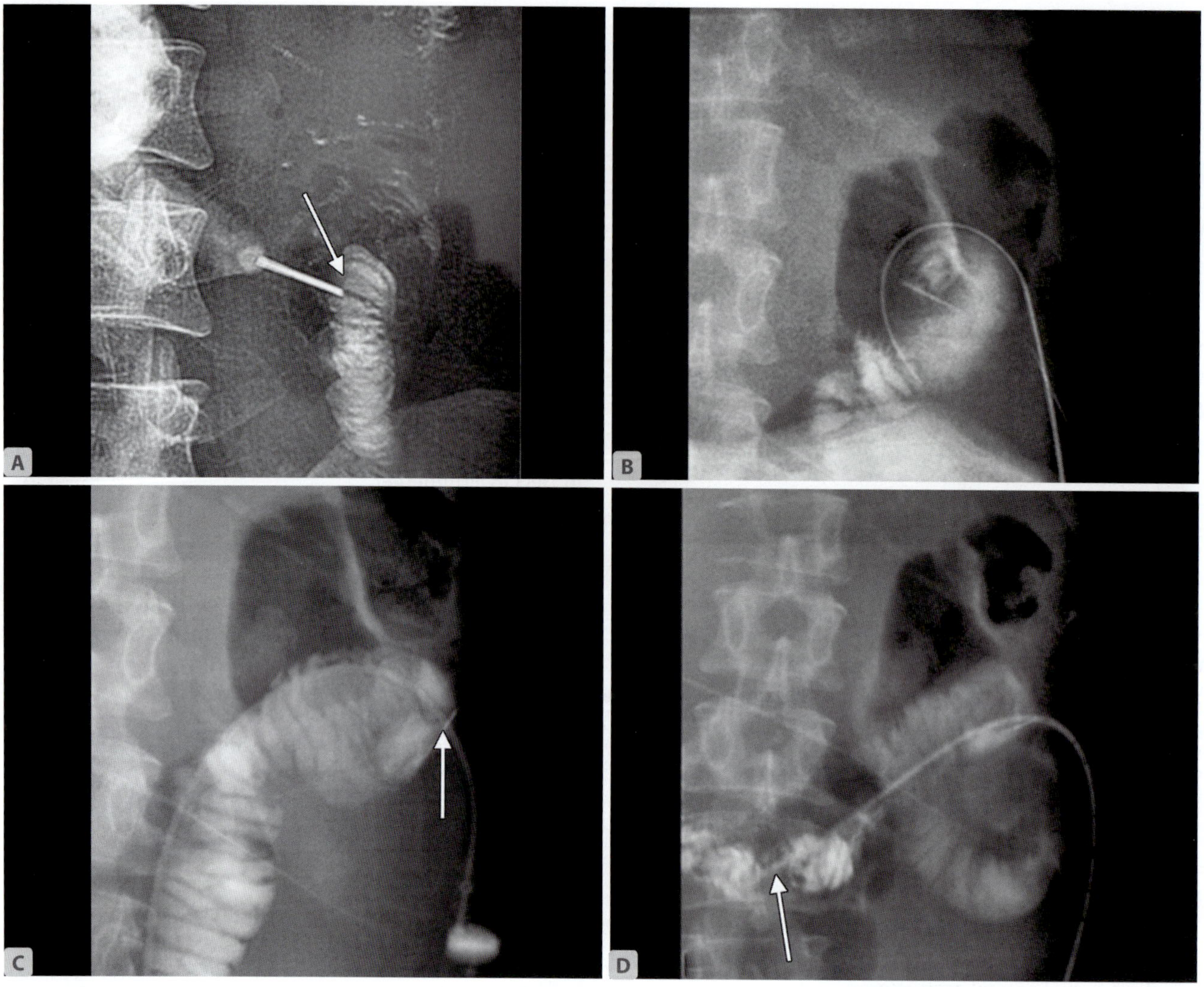

FIGS. 2A TO D: Technique of percutaneous jejunostomy. Jejunal loop is punctured and the correct needle position is checked by contrast injection (A) (arrow). The T-fastener mounted in the needle is then pushed into the jejunum using the stiff guidewire that comes with suture anchor set (B). The needle is withdrawn and the T-fastener retracted and sutured to the abdominal wall (C) (arrow). The tract is dilated over the guidewire serially using Seldinger technique till the desired size of catheter to be inserted (D) (arrow).

However, esophageal stenting is also performed under fluoroscopic guidance, which allows accurate positioning. In market, various types of esophageal stents are available **(Fig. 3)**.[21]

Stent Selection

Across the GE junction, it is desirable to use an uncovered stent (Flamingo/Gianturco stent), to reduce the chances of stent migration. When stent is placed across GE junction, majority of patients will develop reflux and may lead to aspiration. Hence, it is recommended to use medicines prophylactically to reduce reflux symptoms.

Currently, anti-reflux stents (Gianturco, FerX-Ella and Choo stents) are also available to place stents across the GE junction, which prevent GE reflux.

For treating stricture located high, close to cricopharynx, more flexible stent (Ultraflex) should be used. However, it is important to remember that, patient will complain of foreign body sensation, if the stent is placed across the cricopharynx.

They also have increased risks of perforation, proximal migration, and poor tolerance.[20] For the management of refractory benign stricture, retrievable stents are recommended.

Technique (Figs. 4 and 5)

Before the start of the procedure, patient is given thin barium suspension for fluoroscopic study to localize the abnormal segment and length of stricture. Once abnormal segment is localized, it is important to desensitize the pharyngeal mucosa prior to the procedure by local anesthesia using lidocaine aerosol spray. Under fluoroscopy, combination of a diagnostic angiographic catheter and a hydrophilic guidewire is introduced, attempt is made to cross the strictured segment. Once the strictured segment is crossed, the hydrophilic guidewire is exchanged with stiff metallic

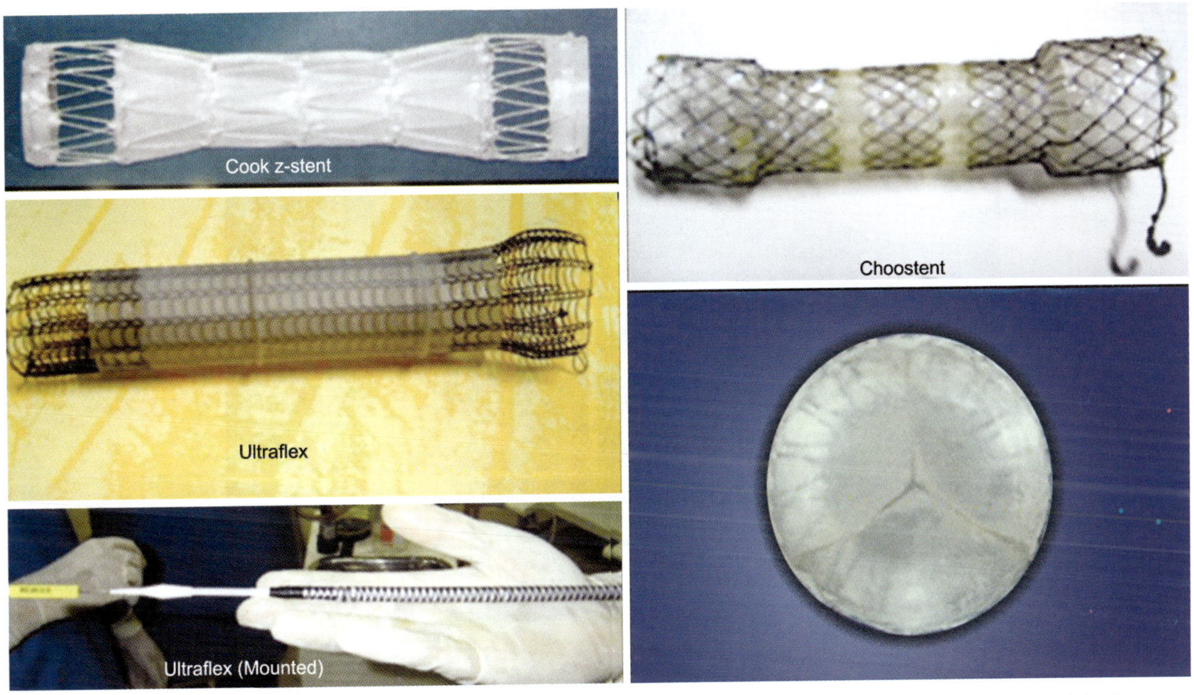

FIG. 3: Various designs of stents: Gianturco-Z stent (Cook). This is made from stainless steel and a polyethylene covering with barbs on the outside or uncoated flared ends to prevent migration. Ultraflex (Boston Scientific Ltd). This stent is made from a knitted Nitinol mesh and is available in both uncovered and covered. It has the weakest radial force but greater flexibility. These stents may be best for tortuous and upper third strictures. *Choostent (Diagmed):* This is a polyurethane-covered stent made from Nitinol and has a retrievable attached thread. These stents also come with an internal distal anti-reflux valve.

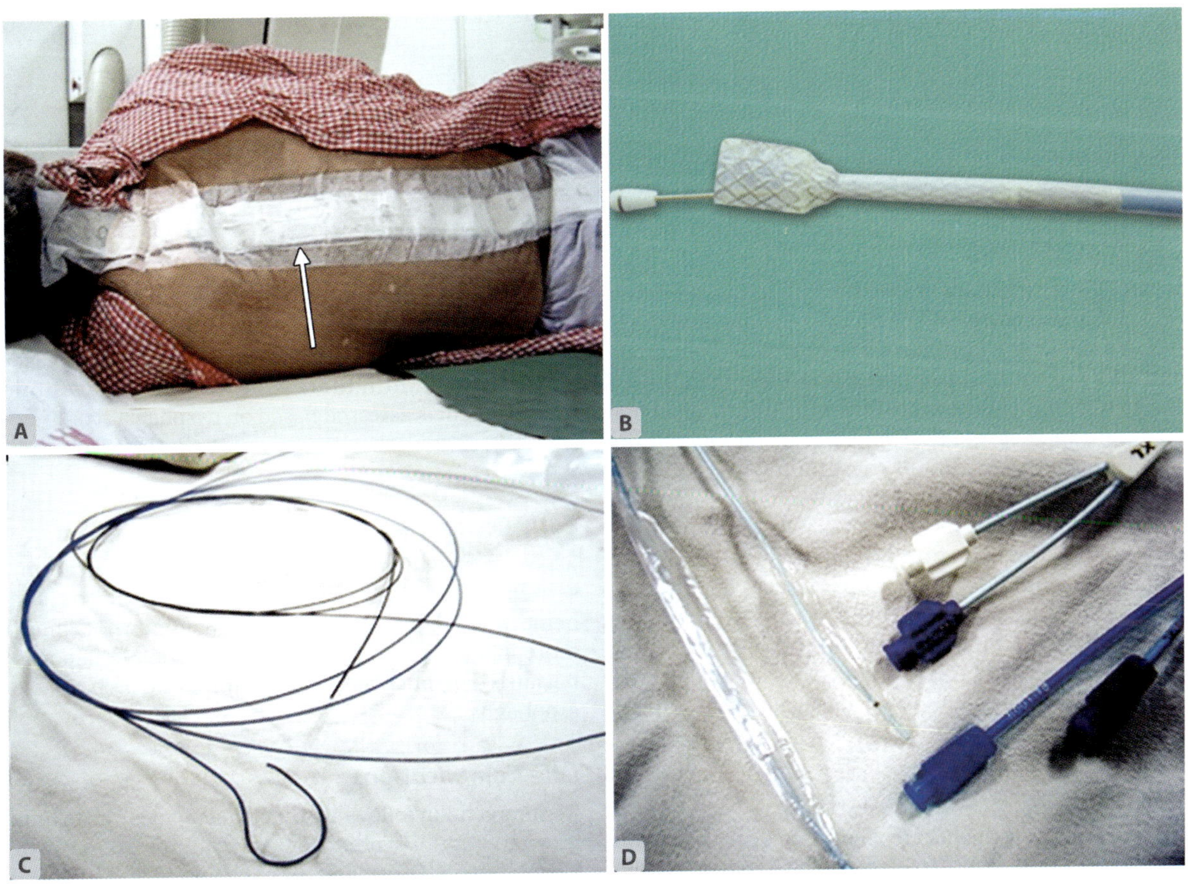

FIGS. 4A TO D: The preparation of esophageal stenting. Metallic marker pasted over the back of the patient (A) (arrow). Delivery system loaded with self-expandable fully covered metallic stent (partially released). (B) Metallic and terumo guidewire; (C) and Balloon catheter (D).

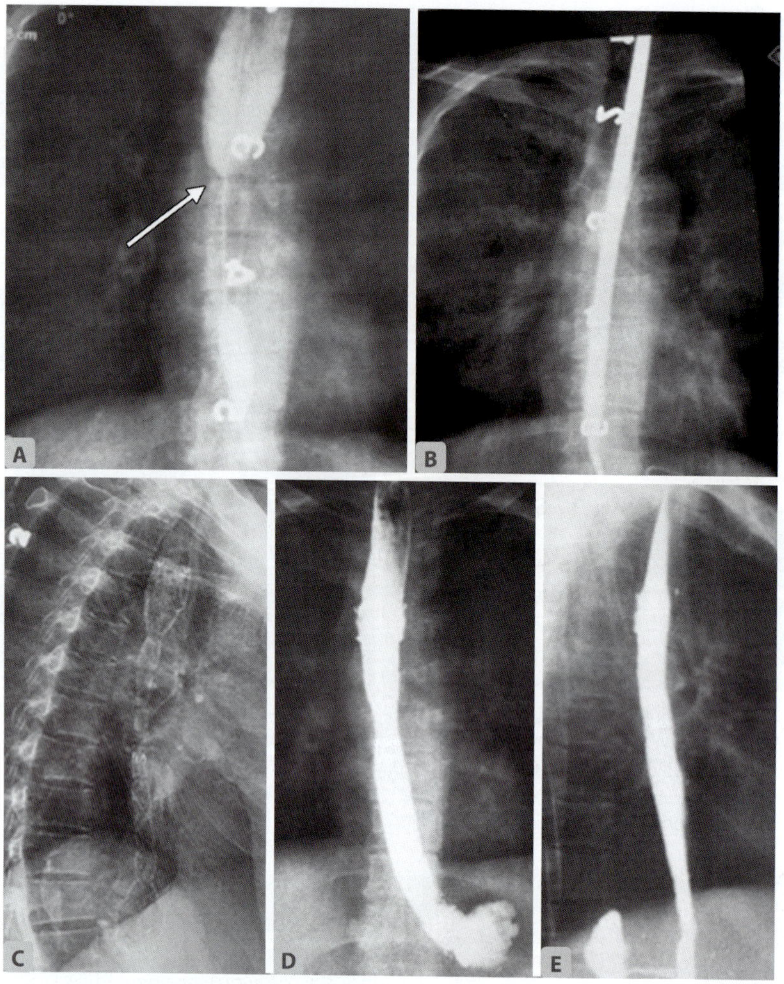

FIGS. 5A TO E: Technique of esophageal stenting. Barium swallow shows irregular narrowing in mid third of thoracic esophagus with proximal hold up of barium column (A) (Arrow). Dilatation of the stricture with bougie (B). Completely deployed Choostent seen in situ (*Note:* Lead markers placed on the patient's back for exact localization of stricture) (C). Esophagogram showing freeflow of contrast across the stent (D and E).

guidewire. Then strictured segment is dilated using either balloon catheter or surgical bougie over the metallic guide wire. Based the length of abnormal segment on preliminary barium study, a covered stent usually 4–5 cm longer than strictured segment is selected to cover the entire abnormal segment and to keep the proximal and distal ends of the stents in normal segments of the esophagus **(Fig. 3B)**. Prior to insertion of stent, delivery system is lubricated with lidocaine jelly. Then delivery system is negotiated over the metallic guidewire and appropriately placed across the abnormal segment under fluoroscopy. Stent is deployed by uncovering the outer sheath of delivery system, while holding the pusher handle in place. Once the stent is positioned, the delivery system and metallic guidewire are withdrawn. Patient is given thin barium suspension again to confirm the stent location and patency.[22]

Postprocedure Care

After the procedure, patients are allowed to take clear fluids and kept on a soft diet for few days, then shifted to a semi-solid diet. Progressive change in diet is recommended after stent placement. It is imperative to tell the patients not to take grassy, unprepared vegetables and meat.

Patients are evaluated immediately after stent placement and every month thereafter. Patient's symptomatic improvement is assessed based on dysphagia score.

Complications

Early Complications

Early chest pain is the major-minor complication, that settles with analgesics. Major complications such as hemorrhage and perforation are uncommon. Bleeding occur more in stents extending above the level of the aortic arch because left subclavian artery and aortic arch are close to esophagus.[20]

Late Complications

Re-intervention following stent placement is due to tumor in-growth with uncovered stents and tumor over growth with covered stents. Other late complications include hemorrhage, stent migration and stent fracture.

Guidelines for Esophageal Stenting

- Uncovered stents are selected for gastroesophageal junction strictures and covered stents for non-gastroesophageal junction strictures.
- Covered stents should be used for esophageal fistulas.[14]
- SEMS are used commonly for palliation of dysphagia in advanced esophageal carcinoma.
- Partially covered stents are used for malignant esophageal fistula and strictures caused by villous tumors.
- Plastic stents can be used for benign strictures and removed after 4–16 weeks to prevent epithelial hypertrophy and stent incarceration.
- Plastic stent delivery system is wider and stiffer than SEMS. Hence, dilatation before stent insertion may increase the complication rates.
- Antireflux stents have similar efficacy of SEMS with benefit in gastroesophageal reflux.
- Combined stent and brachytherapy is a safe palliative option in patients with inoperable advanced esophageal carcinoma.[20]

MDCT in Esophageal Stent Evaluation

- Stent evaluation using CT is usually performed using water as oral contrast. Positive contrast material is used to evaluate perforation, fistula and collections
- Noncontrast CT scan evaluates stent position, location and stent fractures.
- MDCT can identify the complications such as:
  - Esophageal perforation, seen as periesophageal air pockets, adjacent collection and leakage of oral contrast.
  - Stent leakage, stent fracture, tracheal compression by the stent and stent migration.[20]
- MDCT also helps in identifying tumor overgrowth (tumor growth at either ends of the stent) and tumor ingrowth (through the struts of uncovered stent) as a long-term complications or as progression of disease process.

GASTRODUODENAL STENTING

Patients with cancers of stomach/duodenum usually present with symptoms of gastric outlet obstruction such as nausea, vomiting, electrolyte discrepancy, under nutrition, and signs of dehydration.[23]

Patients with unresectable tumors/poor surgical candidates are offered palliative treatment to relieve symptoms of gastric outlet obstruction by placement of stenting across the gastroduodenal area. The ideal gastroduodenal stent should possess enough radial and axial force with good flexibility to overcome tortuosity.[24]

Indications

- Gastric, duodenal malignant obstructions caused by unresectable tumors either by primary tumors or by secondary involvement by the cancers of adjacent organs such as gallbladder and pancreas.
- Patients with tumor recurrence who had surgical anastomosis and present with symptoms of gastric outlet obstruction.[25]
- *Benign gastroduodenal strictures:* As a last option, if the patient condition is high risk for surgery.

Contraindications

- Presence of perforation
- Additional distal or multisegment intestinal obstruction due to extensive peritoneal carcinomatosis.

Available Devices

Unlike esophageal stenting, uncovered stents are more suitable for malignant gastroduodenal strictures compared to covered stents due to less chances of migration and longer patency.[26,27]

Various stent designs available in the market, however, more commonly used stents is Wall stent **(Fig. 2)**, because of its flexibility to overcome the tortuosity and good radial force. One of the main concern of this stent is fore-shortening after deployment to the extent of 40–50%.

Endoscopic versus Fluoroscopic Placement

Routinely, endoscopic approach is used for placing the gastroduodenal stents. However, fluoroscopic approach can also be used with nearly similar technical success rate.[28] Technical failure rates is low (<5%), usually due to unable to cross the stricture.

Precise stent positioning is better done under fluoroscopy rather than endoscope alone. There are reports in literature who reported higher technical rate with fluoroscopic guidance than with endoscopic approach.[29,30]

Technique (Figs. 6A to D)

Oral contrast study, using either iodinated or thin barium suspension), is performed prior to the stenting to look for location and length of abnormal segment. Because of long-standing obstruction the stomach hugely distended and stretched out, that makes procedure difficult due to buckling of the catheter system inside the stomach.

Hence, nasogastric suction is recommended prior to stent placement that not only assist manipulation of deliver system and also helps in preventing aspiration during the procedure.

Technique of gastroduodenal stenting is similar to esophageal stenting as described above. Initial pharyngeal anesthesia is done using lidocaine spray, followed by negotiating the stricture using catheter and hydrophilic guidewire combination. Once the stricture is crossed, hydrophilic guidewire is exchanged with superstiff metallic guidewire usually of 260-300 cm. Then stent of appropriate size based on preliminary contrast study is advanced over the metallic guidewire. Technique of stent deployment is similar to esophageal stenting. In case of difficulty in negotiating delivery system across the stomach, right lateral decubitus positioning helps by unfolding the tortuous anatomy.

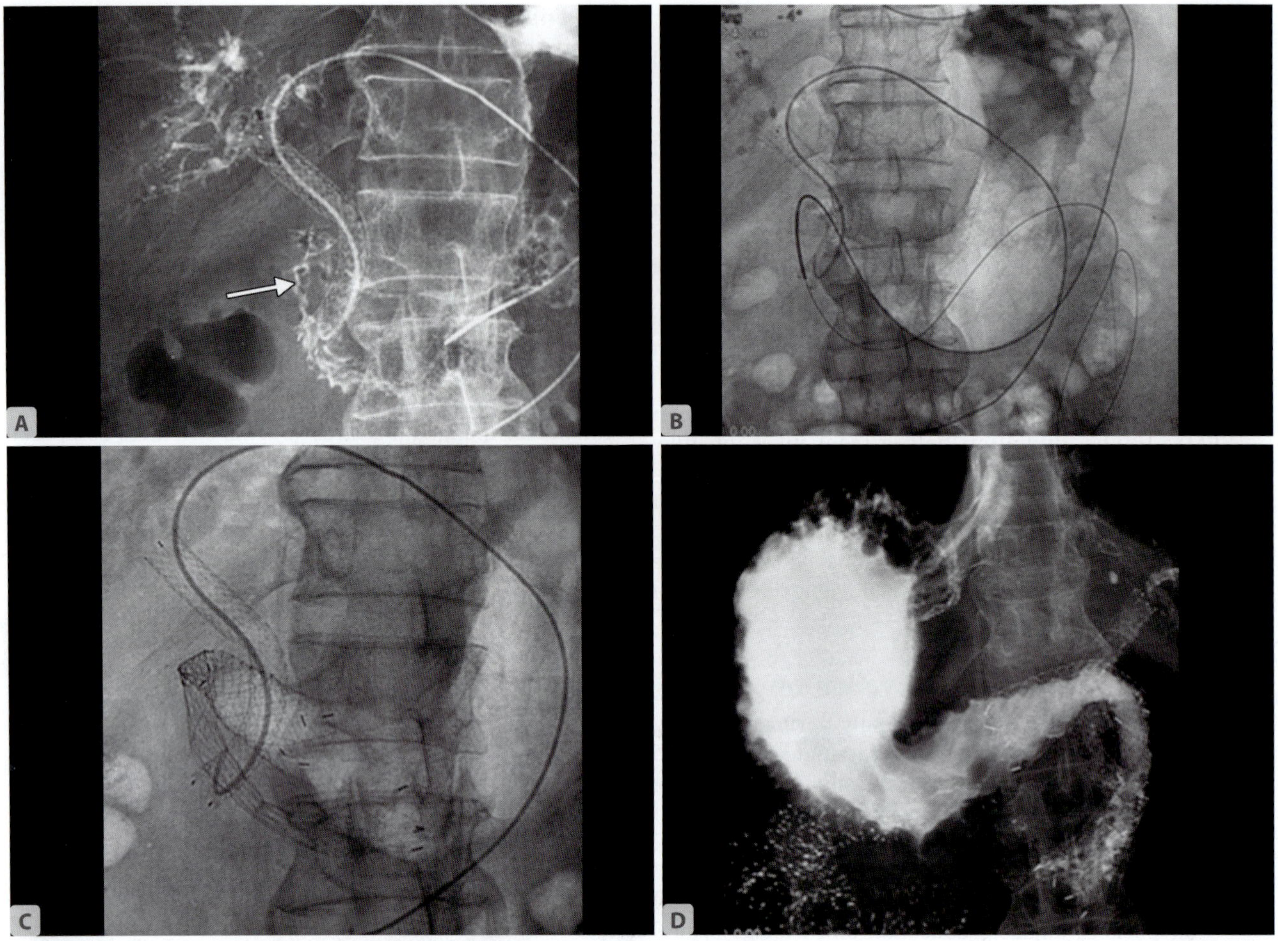

FIGS. 6A TO D: Technique of duodenal stenting. Contrast study showing narrowing of D2 segment, proximal to ampulla (A) (arrow), Guidewire negotiated across the stricture (B), Completely deployed Wall stent seen in situ (C) and barium study showing freeflow of contrast across the stent (D).

It is recommended to "overstent" the stricture segment to include at least 2 cm distal and 2 cm proximal normal segments to prevent recurrence of obstruction by tumor ingrowth. Usually, stents are not dilated using balloon after stent placement, since these stents mostly expand over next few days.[31]

In difficult situations like simultaneous biliary and duodenal stenting, it is better to do prior biliary decompression through percutaneous transhepatic approach.[26] Newly designed duodenal metal stent, which has central unfixed structure helps in tackling the problems of biliary and duodenal stenting. [32]

Postprocedure Care

A follow-up upper gastrointestinal study is usually performed the next day to look for patency and location. Postprocedure instructions to the patient are similar to esophageal stenting.

Clinical success of the procedure is usually assessed by relief of symptoms of gastrointestinal obstruction. Clinical failure rate is nearly 10% inspite of technical success is usually due to distal obstruction.[33,34]

Guidelines for Duodenal Stents[20]

- Self-expandable metallic stent (SEMS) are standard of care for malignant duodenal stenosis, when surgery is not possible.
- No clear guidelines for the duodenal stenting in benign strictures.
- Biliary decompression is done prior to duodenal stenting in case of biliary dilatation.[26]

MDCT in Duodenal Stent Evaluation[20]

- Stent evaluation using CT is usually performed using water as oral contrast.
- Oral positive contrast material is used in suspected cases of perforation, fistula and collection.
- Perforation is seen as retroperitoneal or intraperitoneal free air on CT. The free gas at distal tip of stent should raise the suspicion of perforation.
- Stent fracture is seen as buckling of stent and may be associated with incomplete or complete duodenal obstruction.
- Multidetector computed tomography (MDCT) also helps in finding out the cause for post-stent duodenal bleed.

Complications

Complications are infrequent and potential complications include pain, perforation, migration, hemorrhage and food impaction. Post stent chemotherapy reduce the chances of tumor in growth and prolong the patency, but increase the rate of stent migration.[26,35] Migration is rare with uncovered stents.

COLORECTAL STENTING

Indications

The primary indications for colorectal stenting include:[33]

- Colorectal stenting is done as temporary procedure to decompress the colon in patients with an acute obstruction who have potentially resectable malignancy to allow bowel preparation followed by surgical resection.
- More commonly, long-term stenting is done as palliative procedure to relieve symptoms of colonic obstruction in patients with unresectable malignancy.

Contraindications

- Clinical or radiologic evidence of perforation
- More proximal lesions within the colon.

Technical Considerations

Various stent designs available in the market, however, more commonly used colonic stents are Wall stent, Ultraflex stent, and Memotherm stent.[36-39]

Stenting can be performed either endoscopic route or fluoroscopic route or combined.

Prior to the procedure, water-soluble contrast enema is performed to look for location and length of abnormal segment. Based upon the contrast study findings the suitable device can be selected.

Technique of stent placement is similar to esophageal or gastroduodenal stenting, first step is to cross the strictured segment using catheter-guidewire combination. Once the stricture is crossed, hydrophilic guidewire is exchanged with superstiff metallic guidewire usually of 260–300 cm. Then stent of appropriate size based on preliminary contrast study is advanced over the metallic guidewire. Technique of stent deployment is similar to esophageal/gastroduodenal stenting.

It is recommended to "overstent" the stricture segment to include at least 2 cm distal and 2 cm proximal normal segments to prevent recurrence of obstruction by tumor ingrowth. Long lesions may require two stents.[33]

Postprocedure Follow-up

A water-soluble contrast enema study is done following the procedure look for patency and leakage.

Patients with unresectable malignancy are kept on placed on a low-residue diet and advised to take lubricant laxative to prevent probability of stent obstruction.

Complications

Complications are rare and are usually minor such as pain and temporary bleeding, which do not require any treatment. Major complications include perforation, persistent hemorrhage, stent migration, and restenosis.[26]

Guidelines for Colonic Stents

- Uncovered self-expanding metallic stents are used in colonic stenting
- Colonic stenting is used as palliative procedure for malignant colonic stenosis
- Colonic stenting can also be used as bridge to surgery to relieve obstruction.
- It is associated with less stoma rate, lesser complications, shorter hospital stay and less morbidity.
- The role of SEMS in benign colonic stenosis is controversial. They have limited role in diverticular disease and radiation-induced stenosis.[20]

MDCT in Colonic Stent Evaluation[20]

- Stent evaluation using CT is usually performed using water as oral contrast.
- It helps in evaluating site of obstruction and number of sites of colonic obstruction. Colonic stenting is not preferred in multiple sites of obstruction.
- CT helps to rule out perforation both before and after colonic stenting. Colonic perforation may be seen as pneumoperitoneum and adjacent fluid collection.
- CT may show marked colonic edema suggesting colonic ischemia in patients with post stent colonic dilatation.
- During follow-up scans, tumor ingrowth within stenting can be demonstrated on CT.

PERCUTANEOUS ENTEROCUTANEOUS FISTULA CLOSURE WITH N-BUTYL-2-CYANOACRYLATE

Enterocutaneous fistulae usually occur as complications of complex alimentary tract surgery but may also arise spontaneously in patients with inflammatory bowel disease or after trauma or radiation therapy.[40,41] Gastrointestinal fistula are classified into high output and low output fistulas, based on amount of output from fistula per day. Most fistulae that originate in the duodenum, jejunum, and ileum are classed as high-output and may drain as much as 4,000 mL of intestinal contents per day.

The problems posed by such fistula include massive losses of fluid, electrolytes, and nutrients are formidable and, frequently, management is complicated by the presence of one or more intra-abdominal abscesses. Currently, most authors recommend a trial of conservative management before surgical therapy is attempted; accurate fluid and electrolyte replacement and prevention of malnutrition are combined with attempts to reduce the drainage of intestinal contents by nasogastric intestinal intubation.[41-44] Although this approach is occasionally successful, both the quantity and quality of bowel effluent and the presence of ongoing infection usually prevent the development of a mature, fibrous, external tract and spontaneous closure.

Radiologic involvement in the care of patients with enterocutaneous fistulae has largely been limited to opacification of the fistulous tract and identification of the morbid anatomy.[45] However, recent technical advances in interventional radiology techniques have made the treatment of low output fistula closure more practically feasible. The glues have been used successfully in the closure of fistulas in various locations such as pancreas, biliary and gastrointestinal.[46,47]

Mechanism of Action of the Glue (N-butyl-2-cyanoacrylate)

Glue polymerizes and produces a cast immediately, when it comes in contact with body fluids. Usually it is used in endovascular or surgical procedures. Mild inflammatory reaction is seen within 24 hours. By end of one week, inflammatory reaction is minimal.[48]

Prerequisites

- Fistula should be low output
- The fistulous tract should be short in length (longer the tract lesser the chances of success)
- Tract should be linear, nonbranching
- No associated abscess cavity
- Nonepithelialized tract (if the tract is epithelialized, it is traumatized the tract to make the surface raw).

Technical Consideration

Percutaneous closure of fistulous tract is performed as an outpatient procedure and no anesthesia is required.

Preparation

Before the procedure, it is advisable to administer intravenous antibiotics covering gram-negative gastrointestinal flora. The potency (i.e. "stickiness") of glue requires dilution prior to its use. Dilution of glue is usually done by mixing with lipiodol that delays polymerization and improves visibility during injection under fluoroscopy.

Various combination of dilution (range: 1:1 to 1:3) has been suggested. If the mixture is too strong that causes premature polymerization and catheter occlusion whereas very dilute mixture increases the risk of distal embolization. 5% dextrose solution is used to flush the catheter and to prevent the risk of polymerization inside the catheter.

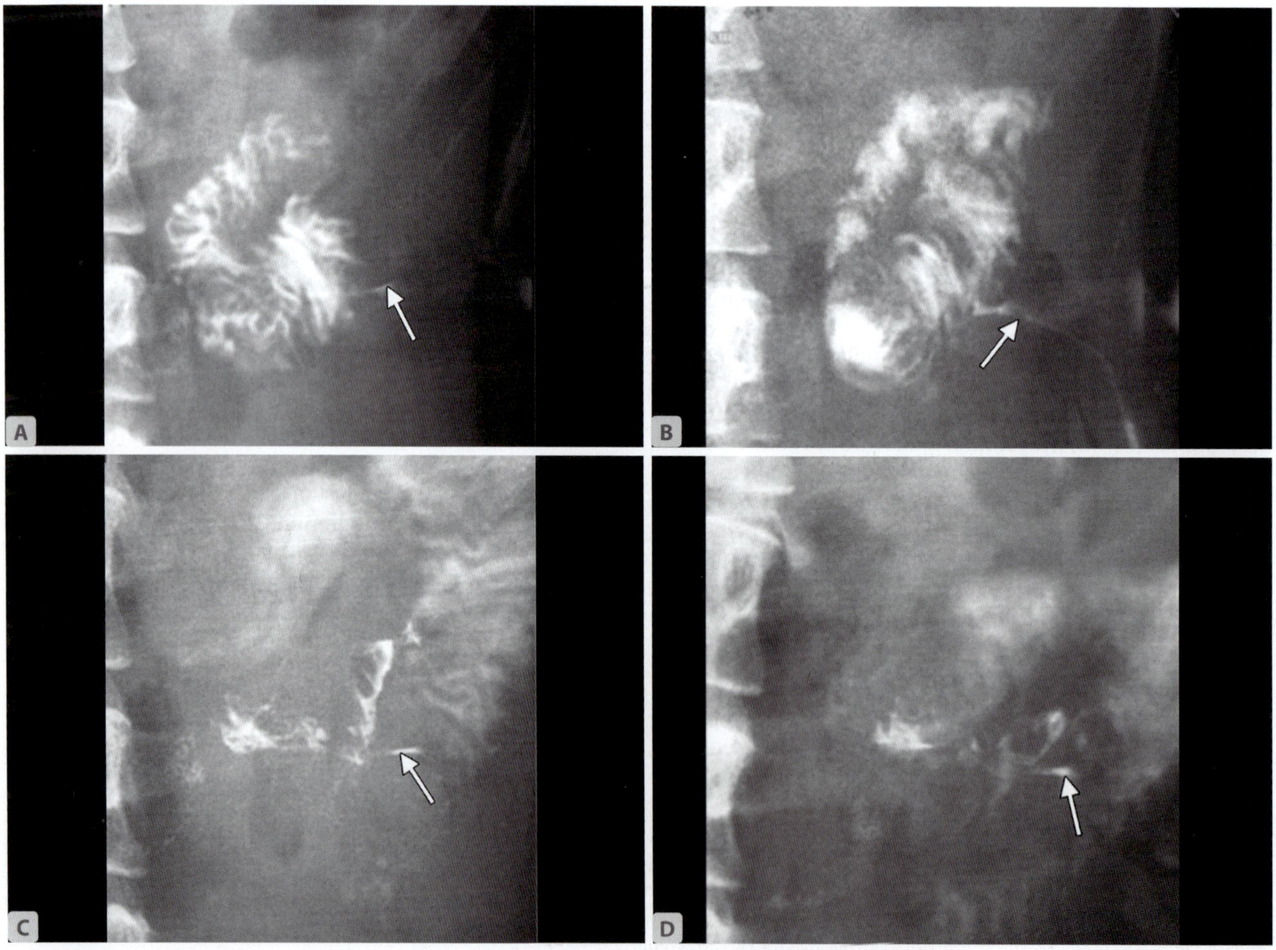

FIGS. 7A TO D: Technique of enterocutaneous fistula closure with glue. Contrast study to show outline and length of the fistulous tract (arrow) (A and B). Following glue injection, the cast of glue outlining the fistulous tract is seen (arrow) (C and D). The tract was completely obliterated on follow-up.

Technique (Figs. 7A to D)

After obtaining the contrast fistulogram study, the fistulous tract is catheterized either with angiographic catheter (4F) or using venflon (18–20G). The catheter should be advanced close the inner opening of fistula. After flushing the catheter with 50% dextrose solution, the diluted glue preparation (1:1 or 1:2) is injected, starting from inside and gradually withdrawing the catheter outside, while continuously injecting the glue.

After the procedure, recatheterization of the tract is not done; otherwise the glue may get dislodged. If the fistula has not closed, another session of glue injection is tried. Sometime we may need 3–4 session to close the tract depending upon the length, diameter and degree of epithelialization of the tract.

REFERENCES

1. Yang ZQ, Shin JH, Song HY, Kwon JH, Kim JW, Kim KR, Kim JH. Fluoroscopically guided percutaneous jejunostomy: outcomes in 25 consecutive patients. Clin Radiol. 2007;62(11):1061-5; discussion 1066-8. Epub 2007 Sep 4.
2. van Overhagen H, Ludviksson MA, Laméris JS, Zwamborn AW, Tilanus HW, Dees J, Hansen BE. US and fluoroscopic-guided percutaneous jejunostomy: experience in 49 patients. J Vasc Interv Radiol. 2000;11(1):101-6.
3. Cope C, Davis AG, Baum RA, Haskal ZJ, Soulen MC, Shlansky-Goldberg RD. Direct percutaneous jejunostomy: techniques and applications—ten years experience. Radiology. 1998;209(3):747-54.
4. Miller KS, Tomlinson JR, Sahn SA. Pleuropulmonary complications of enteral tube feedings, two case reports: review of the literature and recommendations. Chest. 1985;88:230-3.
5. Wasiljew BK, Ujiki GT, Beal JM. Feeding gastrostomy: complications and mortality. Am J Surg. 1982;143:194-5.
6. Shellito PC, Malt RA. Tube gastrostomy: technique and complications. Ann Surg. 1985;201:180-95.
7. Gauderer WL, Ponsky JL, Izant AJ. Gastrostomy without laparotomy: percutaneous endoscopic technique. J Pediatr Surg. 1980;15:872-5.
8. Ho CS. Percutaneous gastrostomy for jejunal feeding. Radiology. 1983;149:595-6.
9. Tao HH, Gillies AR. Percutaneous feeding gastrostomy. AJR. 1983;141:793-4.
10. Wills JS, Oglesby JT. Percutaneous gastrostomy. Radiology. 1983;149:449-53.
11. Brown AS, Mueller PA, Ferrucci JT. Controlled percutaneous gastrostomy: nylon T-fastener for fixation of the anterior gastric wall. Radiology. 1986;158:543-5.
12. Cope C. Suture anchor for visceral drainage. AJR. 1980;135:402-3.
13. Kessel D, Robertson I. Interventional Radiology: A survival guide, 3rd edn. Churchil Livingstone Elsevier; 2011.pp.325-30.
14. Kaufman JA, Michael JL (Eds.). The requisites: Vascular and interventional radiology, 2nd edn. Elsevier Saunders, Philadelphia, PA; 2014.pp.425-50.
15. Celestin LR. Permanent intubation in inoperative cancer of the esophagus and cardia. Ann R Coll Surg Eng. 1959;25:165-70.
16. Atkinson M, Ferguson R. Fibre-optic endoscopic palliative intubation of inoperable oesophogastric neoplasms. BMJ. 1997;1:266-7.
17. Gray RR, Ho CS, Yee A, et al. Direct percutaneous jejunostomy. AJR. 1987;149:931-2.
18. Coleman CC, Coons HG, Cope C, et al. Percutaneous enterostomy with the Cope suture anchor. Radiology. 1990;174: 889-91.
19. Frimberger E. Expanding spiral: a new type of prosthesis for the palliative treatment of malignant oesophageal stenosis. Endoscopy. 1983;15:213-4.
20. Malgras B, Lo Dico R, Pautrat K, et al. Gastrointestinal stenting: Current status and imaging features. Diagn Interv Imaging. 2015;96(6):593-606.
21. Lee SH. The role of oesophageal stenting in the non-surgical management of oesophageal strictures. Br J Radiol. 2001;74(886):891-900. Review.
22. Neyaz Z, Srivastava DN, Thulkar S, Bandhu S, Gamanagatti S, Julka PK, Chattopadhyaya TK. Radiological evaluation of covered self-expandable metallic stents used for palliation in patients with malignant esophageal strictures. Acta Radiol. 2007;48(2):156-64.
23. Patton JT, Carter R. Endoscopic stenting for recurrent malignant gastric outlet obstruction. Br J Surg. 1997;84:865-6.
24. Wei Zhong Zhou, Zheng Qiang Yan. Stenting for malignant gastric outlet obstruction: Current status. Gastrointest Interv. 2014;3:65-8.
25. Klose KJ. Nitinol prostheses for the treatment of inoperable malignant esophageal obstruction. J Vasc Intervent Radiol. 1994;5:899-904.
26. Shi D, Qiu Xm, Feng Ty. Current status of metal stents for malignant gastro-Duodenal obstruction. J Gastroint Dig Syst. 2013;3:140. doi: 10.4172/2161-069X.1000140.
27. Woo SM, Kim DH, Lee WJ, Park KW, Park SJ, et al. Comparison of uncovered and covered stents for the treatment of malignant duodenal obstruction caused by pancreaticobiliary cancer. Surg Endosc. 2013;27:2031-9.
28. Spinelli P, Cerrai FG, Dal Fante M. Endoscopic treatment of upper gastrointestinal tract malignancies. Endoscopy. 1993;25:675-8.
29. de Baere T, Harry G, Ducreaux M, et al. Self-expanding metallic stents as palliative treatment of malignant gastroduodenal stenosis. AJR. 1997;169:1079-83.
30. Pinto IT. Malignant gastric and duodenal stenosis: palliation by peroral implantation of a self-expanding metallic stent. Cardiovasc Intervent Radiol. 1997;20:431-4.
31. Lopera JE, Brazzini A, Gonzales A, Castaneda-Zuniga WR. Gastroduodenal stent placement: current status. Radiographics. 2004;24(6):1561-73. Review.
32. Moon JH, Choi HJ, Ko BM, Koo HC, Hong SJ, et al. Combined endoscopic stent-in-stent placement for malignant biliary and duodenal obstruction by using a new duodenal metal stent (with videos). Gastrointest Endosc. 2009;70:772-7.
33. Mauro MA, Koehler RE, Baron TH. Advances in gastrointestinal interventions: the treatment of gastroduodenal and colorectal obstructions with metallic stent. Radiology. 2000;215:659-69.
34. Kaw M, Singh S, Gagneja H, Azad P. Role of self-expandable metal stents in the palliation of malignant duodenal obstruction. Surg Endosc. 2003;17:646-50.
35. Park CI, Kim JH, Lee YC, Jahng J, Youn YH, et al. What is the ideal stent as initial intervention for malignant gastric outlet obstruction? Dig Liver Dis. 2013;45:33-7.
36. Rey JF, Romanczyk T, Greff M. Metal stents for palliation of rectal carcinoma: a preliminary report of 12 patients. Endoscopy. 1995;27:501-4.
37. Spinelli P, Dal Fante M, Mancini A. Rectal metal stents for palliation of colorectal malignant stenosis. Bildgebung. 1993;60(Suppl 1):48-50.

38. Mainar A, Tejero E, Maynar M, et al. Colorectal obstruction: treatment with metallic stents. Radiology. 1996;198:761-4.
39. Saida Y, Sumiyama Y, Nagao J, et al. Stent endoprosthesis for obstructing colorectal cancers. Dis Colon Rectum. 1996;39:552-5.
40. Edmunds LH Jr. Williams GM, Welch CE. External fistulas arising from the gastrointestinal tract. Ann Surg. 1960; 152:445-71.
41. Fischer JE. The management of high out-put intestinal fistulas. Adv Surg. 1975;9:139-76.
42. Reber HA, Roberts C, Way LW, Dunphy JE. Management of external gastrointestinal fistulas. Ann Surg. 1978;188:460-7.
43. Blackett RL, Hill GL. Postoperative external small bowel fistulas: a study of a consecutive series of patients treated with intravenous hyperalimentation. Br J Surg. 1978;65:775-8.
44. Soeter PB, Ebeid AM, Fischer JE. Review of 404 patients with gastrointestinal fistulas. Ann Surg. 1979;190:189-202.
45. Miller WT, Sullivan MA. Roentgenologic demonstration of sinus tracts and fistulae. AJR. 1969;107:812-7.
46. Lee YC, Na HG, Suh JH, et al. Three cases of fistulae arising from gastrointestinal tract treated with endoscopic injection of histoacryl. Endoscopy. 2001;33:184-6.
47. Seewald S, Brand B, Omar S, et al. Endoscopic sealing of pancreatic fistula by using N-butyl-2-cyanoacrylate. Gastrointest Endosc. 2004;59:463-70.
48. Suga T, Akamatsu T, Kawamura Y, et al. Actual behaviour of N-butyl- 2-cyanoacrylate (histoacryl) in a blood vessel: a model of the varix. Endoscopy. 2002;34:73-7.

AIIMS-MAMC-PGI's

Comprehensive Textbook of

DIAGNOSTIC RADIOLOGY

AIIMS-MAMC-PGI's

Comprehensive Textbook of DIAGNOSTIC RADIOLOGY

Third Edition

VOLUME 3

- Chest and Cardiovascular Imaging
- Musculoskeletal and Breast Imaging

Editors

Anju Garg MD
Director Professor and Head
Department of Radiodiagnosis
Maulana Azad Medical College
New Delhi, India

Manavjit Singh Sandhu MD FICR CCST (UK)
Professor and Head
Department of Radiodiagnosis
Postgraduate Institute of
Medical Education and Research
Chandigarh, India

Arun Kumar Gupta MD FAMS
Professor and Head
Department of Radiodiagnosis
All India Institute of Medical Sciences
New Delhi, India

JAYPEE

JAYPEE BROTHERS MEDICAL PUBLISHERS
The Health Sciences Publisher
New Delhi | London

Jaypee Brothers Medical Publishers (P) Ltd

Headquarter

Jaypee Brothers Medical Publishers (P) Ltd
4838/24, Ansari Road, Daryaganj
New Delhi 110 002, India
Phone: +91-11-43574357
Fax: +91-11-43574314
Email: jaypee@jaypeebrothers.com

Overseas Office

J.P. Medical Ltd
83 Victoria Street, London
SW1H 0HW (UK)
Phone: +44 20 3170 8910
Fax: +44 (0)20 3008 6180
Email: info@jpmedpub.com

Website: www.jaypeebrothers.com
Website: www.jaypeedigital.com

Inquiries for bulk sales may be solicited at: jaypee@jaypeebrothers.com

AIIMS-MAMC-PGI's Comprehensive Textbook of Diagnostic Radiology, ***Third Edition (Volumes 1 to 4)* /** *Arun Kumar Gupta, Anju Garg, Manavjit Singh Sandhu*

First Edition: 2016
Second Edition: 2019
Third Edition: 2021
Reprint: **2024**

ISBN: 978-93-90595-55-6

Printed at: Sanat Printers

ASSOCIATE EDITORS

VOLUME 1

Section 1: Genitourinary Imaging

Gaurav Shanker Pradhan DMRD DNB
Director Professor
Department of Radiodiagnosis
Maulana Azad Medical College
New Delhi, India

Alpana Manchanda MD
Director Professor
Department of Radiodiagnosis
Maulana Azad Medical College
New Delhi, India

Sapna Singh MD DNB MNAMS
Professor
Department of Radiodiagnosis
Maulana Azad Medical College
New Delhi, India

Section 2: Advances in Imaging Technology

Sanjay Sharma MD DNB MNAMS FRCR FICR
Professor
Department of Radiodiagnosis
(RP Center division)
All India Institute of Medical Sciences
New Delhi, India

Atin Kumar MD DNB MNAMS FICR
Professor
Department of Radiodiagnosis
(Trauma Centre Division)
All India Institute of Medical Sciences
New Delhi, India

Shivanand Gamanagatti MD MNAMS FICR
Professor
Department of Radiodiagnosis
(Trauma Centre Division)
All India Institute of Medical Sciences
New Delhi, India

VOLUME 2

Section 3: Paediatric Imaging

Ashu Seith Bhalla MD MAMS FICR
Professor
Department of Radiodiagnosis
All India Institute of Medical Sciences
New Delhi, India

Manisha Jana MD DNB FRCR
Additional Professor
Department of Radiodiagnosis
All India Institute of Medical Sciences
New Delhi, India

Devasenathipathy Kandasamy MD DNB FRCR
Additional Professor
Department of Radiodiagnosis
All India Institute of Medical Sciences
New Delhi, India

Priyanka Naranje MD DNB MNAMS
Associate Professor
Department of Radiodiagnosis
All India Institute of Medical Sciences
New Delhi, India

Section 4: Gastrointestinal and Hepatobiliary Imaging

Deep Narayan Srivastava MD MBA FAMS FICR
Professor
Department of Radiodiagnosis
All India Institute of Medical Sciences
New Delhi, India

Raju Sharma MD MAMS FICR
Professor
Department of Radiodiagnosis
All India Institute of Medical Sciences
New Delhi, India

VOLUME 3

Section 5: Chest and Cardiovascular Imaging

Sanjiv Sharma MD
Professor and Head
Department of Cardiovascular Radiology and Endovascular Interventions
CN Centre
All India Institute of Medical Sciences
New Delhi, India

Rashmi Dixit MD
Director Professor
Department of Radiodiagnosis
Maulana Azad Medical College
New Delhi, India

Section 6: Musculoskeletal and Breast Imaging

Mahesh Prakash MD MAMS FIACM FICR
Professor
Department of Radiodiagnosis
Postgraduate Institute of Medical Education and Research
Chandigarh, India

Anindita Sinha MD MAMS
Additional Professor
Department of Radiodiagnosis
Postgraduate Institute of Medical Education and Research
Chandigarh, India

VOLUME 4

Section 7: Neuroradiology Including Head and Neck Imaging

Paramjeet Singh MD FICR
Professor
Department of Radiodiagnosis
Postgraduate Institute of Medical Education and Research
Chandigarh, India

Shailesh B Gaikwad MD FNAMS CCST
Professor and Head
Department of Neuroimaging and Interventional Neuroradiology (CN Centre)
All India Institute of Medical Sciences
New Delhi, India

Vivek Gupta MD DM
Former Professor
Department of Radiodiagnosis
Postgraduate Institute of Medical Education and Research
Chandigarh, India

Ajay Garg MD
Professor
Department of Neuroimaging and Interventional Neuroradiology (CN Centre)
All India Institute of Medical Sciences
New Delhi, India

CONTRIBUTORS

Ajay Garg MD (Radiodiagnosis) Eur Dip in Neuroradiology (EDiNR) Eur Dip in Pediatric Neuroradiology (EDiPNR)
Professor, Department of Neuroimaging and Interventional Neuroradiology
CN Centre
All India Institute of Medical Sciences
New Delhi, India

Ajay Gulati MD MAMS
Additional Professor
Department of Radiodiagnosis
Postgraduate Institute of Medical Education and Research, Chandigarh, India

Ajay Kumar MD
Professor
Department of Radiodiagnosis
Postgraduate Institute of Medical Education and Research, Chandigarh, India

Akshay Kumar Saxena MD DNB FICR
Professor
Department of Radiodiagnosis
Postgraduate Institute of Medical Education and Research, Chandigarh, India

Alpana Manchanda MD
Director Professor
Department of Radiodiagnosis
Maulana Azad Medical College
New Delhi, India

Anil Kumar Pandey MSc PhD
Associate Professor (Medical Physics)
Department of Nuclear Medicine and PET
All India Institute of Medical Sciences
New Delhi, India

Anindita Sinha MD MAMS
Additional Professor
Department of Radiodiagnosis
Postgraduate Institute of Medical Education and Research
Chandigarh, India

Anjali Prakash DMRD DNB MNAMS
Director Professor
Department of Radiodiagnosis
Maulana Azad Medical College
New Delhi, India

Anju Garg MD
Director Professor and Head
Department of Radiodiagnosis
Maulana Azad Medical College
New Delhi, India

Ankur Goyal MD DNB MNAMS
Associate Professor
Department of Radiodiagnosis
All India Institute of Medical Sciences
New Delhi, India

Anmol Bhatia MD FPGI (Paediatric Radiology)
Assistant Professor
Department of Radiodiagnosis and Imaging
Postgraduate Institute of Medical Education and Research
Chandigarh, India

Anuj Prabhakar DNB DM (Neuroradiology)
Assistant Professor
Postgraduate Institute of Medical Education and Research
Chandigarh, India

Anupam Lal MD
Professor
Department of Radiodiagnosis
Postgraduate Institute of Medical Education and Research
Chandigarh, India

Arun Kumar Gupta MD FAMS
Professor and Head
Department of Radiodiagnosis
All India Institute of Medical Sciences
New Delhi, India

Ashu Seith Bhalla MD MAMS FICR
Professor
Department of Radiodiagnosis
All India Institute of Medical Sciences
New Delhi, India

Atin Kumar MD DNB MNAMS FICR
Professor
Department of Radiodiagnosis
(Trauma Center Division)
All India Institute of Medical Sciences
New Delhi, India

Chandan J Das MD DNB MAMS FICR FRCP
Additional Professor
Department of Radiodiagnosis
All India Institute of Medical Sciences
New Delhi, India

Chandrashekhara SH MD DNB MNAMS
Additional Professor
Department of Radiodiagnosis
Dr BRA Institute—Rotary Cancer Hospital
All India Institute of Medical Sciences
New Delhi, India

Chirag Kamal Ahuja MD DM (Neuroradiology)
Associate Professor
Department of Radiodiagnosis and Imaging
Postgraduate Institute of Medical Education and Research
Chandigarh, India

Deep Narayan Srivastava MD MBA FAMS FICR
Professor
Department of Radiodiagnosis
All India Institute of Medical Sciences
New Delhi, India

Devasenathipathy Kandasamy MD DNB FRCR
Additional Professor
Department of Radiodiagnosis
All India Institute of Medical Sciences
New Delhi, India

Ekta Dhamija MD
Associate Professor
Department of Radiodiagnosis
Dr BRA Institute—Rotary Cancer Hospital
All India Institute of Medical Sciences
New Delhi, India

Gaurav Shanker Pradhan DMRD DNB
Director Professor
Department of Radiodiagnosis
Maulana Azad Medical College
New Delhi, India

Gita Devi MD DNB
Assistant Professor
Department of Radiodiagnosis
Postgraduate Institute of Medical Education and Research
Chandigarh, India

Gurpreet Singh Gulati MD
Former Professor
Department of Cardiac Radiology
Cardio-Thoracic Sciences Centre
All India Institute of Medical Sciences
New Delhi, India

Harish Bhujade MD FVIR
Assistant Professor
Department of Radiodiagnosis
Postgraduate Institute of Medical Education and Research
Chandigarh, India

Jyoti Kumar MD DNB MNAMS FICR
Professor
Department of Radiodiagnosis
Maulana Azad Medical College
New Delhi, India

Kartik Ganga MD
Fellow
Department of Cardiovascular Radiology and Endovascular Interventions
All India Institute of Medical Sciences
New Delhi, India

Kirti Gupta MD, Neuropathology Fellowship (St Jude, USA)
Professor
Department of Histopathology
Postgraduate Institute of Medical Education and Research
Chandigarh, India

Kumble S Madhusudhan MD FRCR MAMS
Additional Professor
Department of Radiodiagnosis
All India Institute of Medical Sciences
New Delhi, India

Kushaljit Singh Sodhi MD PhD MAMS FICR
Professor
Department of Radiodiagnosis
Postgraduate Institute of Medical Education and Research
Chandigarh, India

Madhavi Tripathi MD DNB (Nuclear Medicine)
Additional Professor
Department of Nuclear Medicine and PET
All India Institute of Medical Sciences
New Delhi, India

Madhusudhan KS MD MAMS FRCR
Additional Professor
Department of Radiodiagnosis
All India Institute of Medical Sciences
New Delhi, India

Mahesh Prakash MD MAMS FIACM FICR
Professor
Department of Radiodiagnosis
Postgraduate Institute of Medical Education and Research
Chandigarh, India

Manavjit Singh Sandhu MD FICR CCST (UK)
Professor and Head
Department of Radiodiagnosis
Postgraduate Institute of Medical Education and Research
Chandigarh, India

Mandeep Garg MD FRCR
Professor
Department of Radiodiagnosis
Postgraduate Institute of Medical Education and Research
Chandigarh, India

Mandeep Kang MD MAMS FICR
Professor
Department of Radiodiagnosis
Postgraduate Institute of Medical Education and Research
Chandigarh, India

Manisha Jana MD DNB FRCR
Additional Professor
Department of Radiodiagnosis
All India Institute of Medical Sciences
New Delhi, India

Manish Modi MD DM
Professor
Department of Neurology
Postgraduate Institute of Medical Education and Research
Chandigarh, India

Manphool Singhal MD DNB MAMS FICR (India) FSCCT (USA) CMR-fellowship (London) CMR-Certification (SCMR USA and ESCVI France)
Additional Professor
Department of Radiodiagnosis
Postgraduate Institute of Medical Education and Research
Chandigarh, India

Mukesh Kumar Yadav (MD Radiodiagnosis)
Formerly Associate Professor
PGIMER, Chandigarh
Associate Professor
Department of Radiodiagnosis
All India Institute of Medical Sciences (IRCH)
New Delhi, India

Naveen Kalra MD FICR MAMS
Professor
Department of Radiodiagnosis
Postgraduate Institute of Medical Education and Research
Chandigarh, India

Nidhi Prabhakar MD DNB
Senior Research Associate
Department of Radiodiagnosis
Postgraduate Institute of Medical Education and Research
Chandigarh, India

Niraj N Pandey DM
Assistant Professor
Department of Cardiovascular Radiology and Endovascular Interventions
CN Centre
All India Institute of Medical Sciences
New Delhi, India

Niranjan Khandelwal MD Dip NBE FICR FAMS
Former Head
Department of Radiodiagnosis
Postgraduate Institute of Medical Education and Research
Chandigarh, India

Pankaj Gupta MD DNB
Assistant Professor
Department of Radiodiagnosis and Imaging
Postgraduate Institute of Medical Education and Research
Chandigarh, India

Paramjeet Singh MD FICR
Professor
Department of Radiodiagnosis
Postgraduate Institute of Medical Education and Research
Chandigarh, India

Pratik Kumar PhD (AIIMS) Dip RP (BARC)
Professor, Medical Physics Unit
BRA Institute Rotary Cancer Hospital
AIIMS, New Delhi, India

Priya Jagia MD DNB
Professor
Department of Cardiovascular Radiology and Endovascular Interventions
All India Institute of Medical Sciences
New Delhi, India

Priyanka Naranje MD DNB MNAMS
Associate Professor
Department of Radiodiagnosis
All India Institute of Medical Sciences
New Delhi, India

Punit Sharma MD
Former Senior Resident
Department of Nuclear Medicine
All India Institute of Medical Sciences
New Delhi, India

Radhika Batra MD DNB
Associate Professor
Department of Radiodiagnosis
Maulana Azad Medical College
New Delhi, India

Rajat Jain MD DNB FRCR FICR MNAMS
Assistant Professor
Department of Radiodiagnosis
Maulana Azad Medical College
New Delhi, India

Raju Sharma MD MAMS FICR
Professor
Department of Radiodiagnosis
All India Institute of Medical Sciences
New Delhi, India

Rakesh Kumar DRM DNB PhD
Professor and Head
Diagnostic Nuclear Medicine Division
Department of Nuclear Medicine and PET
All India Institute of Medical Sciences
New Delhi, India

Rakesh Kumar Vasishta MD FRCPath
Former Professor and Head
Department of Histopathology
Postgraduate Institute of Medical Education and Research
Chandigarh, India

Rashmi Dixit MD
Director Professor
Department of Radiodiagnosis
Maulana Azad Medical College
New Delhi, India

Sameer Vyas MD DM MAMS (Neuroradiology)
Additional Professor
Department of Radiodiagnosis
Postgraduate Institute of Medical Education and Research
Chandigarh, India

Sanjay Sharma MD DNB MNAMS FRCR FICR
Professor
Department of Radiodiagnosis
(Division at Rajendra Prasad Center for Ophthalmic Sciences)
All India Institute of Medical Sciences
New Delhi, India

Sanjeev Kumar MD
Associate Professor
Department of Cardiovascular Radiology and Endovascular Interventions
All India Institute of Medical Sciences
New Delhi, India

Sanjiv Sharma MD
Professor and Head
Department of Cardiovascular Radiology and Endovascular Interventions
CN Centre
All India Institute of Medical Sciences
New Delhi, India

Sapna Singh MD DNB MNAMS
Professor
Department of Radiodiagnosis
Maulana Azad Medical College
New Delhi, India

Satyam DNB MNAMS
Specialist
Department of Radiodiagnosis
Lok Nayak Hospital and Associated
Maulana Azad Medical College
New Delhi, India

Shailesh B Gaikwad MD FNAMS CCST
Professor and Head
Department of Neuroimaging and Interventional Neuroradiology
CN Centre
All India Institute of Medical Sciences
New Delhi, India

Shamim Ahmed Shamim MD (Nuclear Medicine)
Associate Professor
Department of Nuclear Medicine
All India Institute of Medical Sciences
New Delhi, India

Shashi Bala Paul PhD MAMS
Senior Scientist
Department of Radiodiagnosis
All India Institute of Medical Sciences
New Delhi, India

Shivanand Gamanagatti MD MNAMS FICR
Professor
Department of Radiodiagnosis
(Trauma Center Division)
All India Institute of Medical Sciences
New Delhi, India

Smita Manchanda MD DNB MNAMS
Associate Professor
Department of Radiodiagnosis
All India Institute of Medical Sciences
New Delhi, India

Smriti Hari MD MAMS
Professor
Department of Radiodiagnosis
All India Institute of Medical Sciences
New Delhi, India

Sreedhara BC MD FVIR
Assistant Professor
Department of Radiodiagnosis
Postgraduate Institute of Medical Education and Research
Chandigarh, India

Subrat Kumar Acharya DM FNASc
FASc FNA JC Bose Fellow
Former Professor and Head
Department of Gastroenterology
All India Institute of Medical Sciences
New Delhi, India

Sudesh Prabhakar MD DM
Former Professor and Head
Department of Neurology
Postgraduate Institute of Medical Education and Research
Chandigarh, India

Sudha Suri MD
Emeritus Professor
Department of Radiodiagnosis
Postgraduate Institute of Medical Education and Research
Chandigarh, India

Surabhi Vyas MD DNB MNAMS
Additional Professor
Department of Radiodiagnosis
All India Institute of Medical Sciences
New Delhi, India

Swati Gupta MD DNB FRCR
Associate Professor
Department of Radiodiagnosis
Maulana Azad Medical College
New Delhi, India

Tulika Singh MD
Additional Professor
Department of Radiodiagnosis
Postgraduate Institute of Medical Education and Research
Chandigarh, India

Ujjwal Gorsi (MD Radiodiagnosis)
Associate Professor
Department of Radiodiagnosis
Postgraduate Institute of Medical Education and Research
Chandigarh, India

Uma Debi MD
Associate Professor
Department of Radiodiagnosis
Postgraduate Institute of Medical Education and Research
Chandigarh, India

Veenu Singla MD
Professor
Department of Radiodiagnosis
Postgraduate Institute of Medical Education and Research
Chandigarh, India

Vikas Bhatia MD DNB
DM (Neuroradiology)
Assistant Professor
Department of Radiodiagnosis
Postgraduate Institute of Medical Education and Research
Chandigarh, India

Vineeta Ojha MD DNB
DM Senior Resident
Department of Cardiovascular Radiology and Endovascular Interventions
All India Institute of Medical Sciences
New Delhi, India

Virendra Jain MD FRCR
Former Senior Resident
Department of Radiodiagnosis
Maulana Azad Medical College
New Delhi, India

Vivek Gupta MD DM
Former Professor
Department of Radiodiagnosis
Postgraduate Institute of Medical Education and Research
Chandigarh, India

PREFACE TO THE THIRD EDITION

In 1996, a unique venture was jointly initiated by the faculty of Radiodiagnosis, All India Institute of Medical Sciences (AIIMS), New Delhi; Maulana Azad Medical College (MAMC), New Delhi; and Postgraduate Institute of Medical Education and Research (PGIMER), Chandigarh, India, to organize continuing medical education (CME) programs based on a series of imaging courses. An integral part of this endeavour was publishing books covering all organ systems. The aim was to provide state-of-the-art knowledge for postgraduate students as well as the practicing radiologists along with establishing a uniform pattern of teaching in radiology across the country.

The first series of seven imaging courses was successfully completed in the year 2000. A second series of these courses was then initiated in the year 2002 and was completed in 2004. This was also highly successful. The third series of seven extremely popular and successful courses covering all the organ systems and advances in physics was started in 2008 and was completed in 2013. The fourth series started in 2016 and was completed successfuly in 2020.

Every course in each of the series has resulted in publication of a book. These books have been very popular amongst residents as well as among practicing radiologists.

Considering the popularity of these books, the editors, along with publishers, M/s Jaypee Brothers Medical Publishers (P) Ltd, New Delhi, India, had decided to combine the individual course books into three volumes— *"AIIMS-MAMC-PGI's Comprehensive Textbook of Diagnostic Radiology"*. Its first edition was released in 2016.

In keeping pace with newer developments in the field of diagnostic radiology and in order to cater to the contemporary needs of users, the second edition of *"AIIMS-MAMC-PGI's Comprehensive Textbook of Diagnostic Radiology"* was presented in 2019 after a gap of three years. It was anticipated that with such a complete coverage of all the subjects, the users will not have to refer to any other book during their routine learning of diagnostic radiology.

However by the time fourth AIIMS MAMC PGI Imaging course series was near completion in early 2021, it was felt that there is a very strong need for updating of second edition along with addition of new chapters in view of rapid advancement of knowledge in the last few years. So third edition was planned. It was also agreed that in view of increasing size of individual course books and to keep the size of individual volumes of the Textbook handy and managable the whole textbook should be divided into four volumes from its current three volumes.

We are sure that residents and radiologists will find these comprehensive four volumes easy to handle and very useful in day-to-day practice.

We are once again grateful to all the contributors from the three apex academic institutions of India, i.e. AIIMS, New Delhi; MAMC, New Delhi; and PGIMER, Chandigarh, India.

We are thankful to M/s Jaypee Brothers Medical Publishers (P) Ltd, for helping us to make our dream come true.

Arun Kumar Gupta
Anju Garg
Manavjit Singh Sandhu

PREFACE TO THE FIRST EDITION

In 1996, a unique venture was jointly initiated by the faculty of radiodiagnosis at All India Institute of Medical Sciences, Maulana Azad Medical College, New Delhi, and Postgraduate Institute of Medical Education and Research, Chandigarh, India, to organize continuing medical education programs based on a series of imaging courses. An integral part of this endeavor was publishing books covering all organ systems. The aim was to provide state of the art knowledge for postgraduate students as well as the practicing radiologists along with establishing a uniform pattern of teaching in radiology across the country.

The first series of seven imaging courses was successfully completed in the year 2000. A second series of these courses was then initiated in the year 2002 and was completed in 2004. This was also highly successful.

With the great success of the second series, we, the current editors, decided to start a third series of these courses in 2008. Seven extremely popular and successful courses covering all the organ systems and advances in physics were completed in 2013.

Every course in each of the three series have resulted in publication of a book. These books have been very popular amongst residents as well as among practicing radiologists.

Considering the popularity of these books, we, the three current editors, along with publishers M/s Jaypee Brothers Medical Publishers (P) Ltd., decided to combine the individual books published so far into a *"AIIMS-MAMC-PGI's Comprehensive Textbook of Diagnostic Radiology"* with three volumes.

We are very happy to see the end result of this great effort.

We are sure that residents and radiologists will find these comprehensive three volumes easy to handle and very useful in day-to-day practice.

We are once again grateful to all the contributors from the three apex academic institutions of India, i.e. AIIMS, MAMC, New Delhi and PGIMER, Chandigarh, India.

We are thankful to M/s Jaypee Brothers Medical Publishers (P) Ltd., for helping us to make our dream come true.

Niranjan Khandelwal
Veena Chowdhury
Arun Kumar Gupta

ACKNOWLEDGMENTS

We would like to put on record our deep appreciation and gratitude:

To Professors Manorama Berry, Sudha Suri and Veena Chowdhury (Past Editors) the three pioneers who in 1996 took a bold initiative and started a unique teaching course now popularly known as AIIMS-MAMC-PGI's imaging course. By October 2020, four series, each series comprising of seven courses, have been completed. This course series has become extremely popular and every course is followed by the publication of a book which too is highly appreciated and popular.

To Professors Sima Mukhopadhyay, Sushma Vashisht and Niranjan Khandelwal who have been the Editors of past series and who contributed to organizing the earlier courses in their capacity as Heads of Departments.

To all the Associate Editors of the different course books who put in immense effort to bring the books out on time.

To all the Authors who contributed chapters without whom we could not have collected such an outstanding content of teaching and academic material.

To our respective hospitals for giving us the privilege and unique opportunity to work, which enabled us to amass data from patients and document images of diverse diseases that provide the reader with a wide spectrum of knowledge.

Our sincere and grateful thanks to Shri Jitendar P Vij (Group Chairman), Mr Ankit Vij (Managing Director), Mr MS Mani (Group President), Dr Richa Saxena (Associate Director-Professional Publishing), Ms Nedup Denka Bhutia (Development Editor) and Other staffs of M/s Jaypee Brothers Medical Publishers (P) Ltd, New Delhi, India, for their untiring coordination efforts in the production of this book.

We are very proud indeed at the culmination of two decades of these course series, to compile and present them together in the form of these four volumes of *"AIIMS-MAMC-PGI's Comprehensive Textbook of Diagnostic Radiology".*

Arun Kumar Gupta
Anju Garg
Manavjit Singh Sandhu

CONTENTS

VOLUME 1

Section 1: Genitourinary Imaging

VOLUME 2

Section 3: Paediatric Imaging

Section 4: Gastrointestinal and Hepatobiliary Imaging

VOLUME 3

Section 5: Chest and Cardiovascular Imaging

Section 6: Musculoskeletal and Breast Imaging

VOLUME 4

Section 7: Neuroradiology Including Head and Neck Imaging

SECTION

5

Chest and Cardiovascular Imaging

CHAPTER

122

Chest Radiography and Sonography: Techniques and Anatomy

Mahesh Prakash, Manavjit Singh Sandhu

INTRODUCTION

Chest radiography is the most commonly performed radiological investigation around the world, and it forms an integral part of the routine study of individual case along with and as important as physical examination and laboratory investigations. The Chest radiograph nearly constitutes 50–60% of the total workload of the radiology department of any large or small general hospital. The cornerstone of the radiological diagnosis of the chest diseases is chest radiograph. All other radiological procedures including bronchography, computed tomography (CT) and magnetic resonance imaging (MRI) are strictly ancillary.[1]

Sonography of chest is relatively newer method to evaluate the diseases of thorax particularly useful for pleural and chest wall abnormalities and some pathologies of lungs The techniques and normal anatomy as demonstrated on plain chest radiographs and ultrasound have been discussed herewith.

CONVENTIONAL CHEST RADIOGRAPHY

Conventional film screen radiography using kV range of 50–85 depending on patient's build is the standard and most commonly used technique for chest evaluation. The benefits of this technique include low cost, high- spatial resolution, operation simplicity and dependability. The important factors that influence the contrast in the radiograph include kilovoltage, shape of sensitometric curve of film, exposure parameters and conditions of film processing. At low kV, the difference in attenuation by soft tissue and bone or air and bone is large, resulting in high contrast. Calcified lesions, pleural plaque, pulmonary nodules are well delineated in low kV radiograph. However, some of the limitations of conventional chest radiograph are given here:

- There is poor visibility of mediastinum, retrocardiac and subphrenic areas when lungs are well seen
- Lungs may be obscured by high contrast of bones
- Inadequate detail of airway and lung apices.

TECHNICAL ADVANCES

Following technical advances have been developed over the years to overcome limitation of the conventional chest radiograph:

- High kV technique
- New screen film combinations
- Beam equalization radiography
- Digital chest radiography.

High kV Technique

In this technique, we use more than 120 kV. The coefficient of X-ray absorption of bone and soft tissue approach each other at high kV and thus the lungs are not obscured by bones. It has better penetration of the mediastinum which provides more details of airway. Short exposure time with high kV allows less scatter radiation to reach intensifying screens and results in sharp details of structures within the lungs. However, high kV results in greater scatter radiation as compared to conventional radiography. Use of an air gap of 6 inches is required to reduce scatter radiation.[2]

New Screen Film Combinations

Fine details on radiograph is principally determined by screen film system. Generally, medium-speed system is preferred which provides better visualization of small vessels, fissures and depiction of abnormalities. The major advance in screen film system has been the introduction of faster rare earth phosphor screen and development of wide latitude film. The improved light emission from rare earth phosphor over traditional calcium tungstate crystal screen results in short exposure time and thus sharp image.

Another important development is the introduction of asymmetric screen film system, the asymmetric zero crossover screen film system. It was introduced by Eastman Kodak in 1990 called insight thoracic imaging system.[3] This uses different emulsion on either side of film base and different front and back intensifying screens. In addition, layers of absorbing dye in the film base prevent crossover of light between two emulsions so that both screen film combinations operate independently. The front side has high resolution screen and high-contrast film emulsion. This combination optimizes visualization of fine details in lungs. The back side consists of high speed screen and film emulsion with low maximum density. This combination provides adequate visualization of high attenuating areas, e.g. mediastinum without overpenetration of lungs. Patient dose reduction up to 30% has been reported.[4]

Dupont in 1993 introduced an ultravision screen film system. In this system, screens use a high density rare earth phosphor (yttrium tantalate) which emits ultraviolet light that diffuses substantially less than the lower energy wave length visible light. The film emulsion used is symmetric.

These combinations of film screen system have provided increased information that can be recorded and displayed. The asymmetric system is slightly superior particularly for visualization of mediastinal and retro-diaphragmatic structures. The improved image sharpness achieved with these systems potentially can improve visualization of subtle parenchymal abnormalities.

Beam Equalization Radiography

Screen film system provides acceptable image-contrast of chest radiograph in most situations. However, the relatively narrow range of film sensitivity limits image contrast in poorly penetrated areas of chest. The technique of beam equalization radiography refers to varying the intensity of X-ray beam passing through various parts of chest so as to produce a chest radiograph with uniform density of areas with extremely variable attenuation differences on the same film. This can be achieved by two methods:

1. Interposing a customized filter unique to the patient that would attenuate the beam over the lungs and allow increased radiation exposure over the mediastinum.
2. Modulation of exposure for each part of the chest by electronic feedback system.

The first one lacks practicality, the latter one is the principle used in technique of beam equalization radiography that utilizes screen film receptors by increasing X-ray exposure in the thicker, denser part of chest while keeping the lung exposure unchanged, thereby reducing the dynamic range of intensities that ultimately reach the image recorder.[5,6]

Oldelft from Netherlands introduced in 1986 the Advanced Multiple Beam Equalization Radiography (AMBER) which is the only commercially available system for chest radiography. This system has horizontal X-ray fan beam which is divided into 20 adjacent beam segments, each of which is independently controlled by its own intensity modulator located in front of X-ray tube and corresponding exposure detector between patient and image recorder. As the fan beam scans the patient, the detector array measures local X-ray intensity passing through the patient and an electronic feedback mechanism dynamically adjusts each of beam modulators such that dense areas are imaged at higher exposure levels. This increases signal to noise ratio in the denser areas of chest and shifts the background film optical density in these areas onto higher contrast portion of H and D curve.

The advantages of this technique are as follows:

- Better delineation of mediastinum, retrocardiac and retrodiaphragmatic areas
- Improved visualization of lung apices in lateral view.

The reported disadvantage of AMBER are as follows:

- Decreased contrast between consolidation and normal lung
- Edge artefacts occur where there are abrupt changes in radiolucency, e.g. lung heart interface, lung diaphragm interface
- Dark halo around the heart may simulate pneumomediastinum
- Active imaging areas are limited to upright 14″ × 17″ orientation so it is not possible to acquire transverse image of chest
- Exposure parameter to be set manually
- Difficulty in comparing the radiograph of patient with previous one using conventional technique
- This system can not be used on bed side and for patient on stretcher
- Radiation dose is about 50% more than conventional chest radiograph.

The experience till date is not clearly indicative of the justification of additional expense even though images are more informative and this seems to have limited its popularity in clinical use.

Digital Chest Radiography

Advances in electronics and computer technology, over the past decades, have led to development of digital radiography or computed radiography system. This is different from conventional film-based analog system where the film is in direct contact with intensifying screen and there is no storage of information as digits in computer. In digital radiography, image detection can be completely separated from image display. The data of image is stored in the computer and can be retrieved, displayed, quantified, manipulated and hardcopied whenever required.[6]

Digital system using phosphor technique in which the entire receptor is exposed by conventional radiography equipment was introduced by Fuji in 1980 and is the most widely used technique for general digital radiography. This technique is based on reusable imaging plate coated with photostimulable phosphor material. When exposed to X-ray, a portion of X-rays is absorbed as to release stored energy as light and intensity of light measured and digitized. The resultant digital image is then preprocessed for contrast and spatial resolution before display. Imaging plate is ready for reuse after exposure to room light.

Introduction of selenium detector system is an important development in digital chest radiography. Unlike storage phosphor detector, which requires laser stimulation for image acquisition, selenium-based detectors capture image information as charge pattern and thus image can be read directly, eliminating image noise.[7,8] Also selenium is more efficient in detection of X-rays.

Flat panel detectors are relatively new development in the technology. Depending on the material, there are two types of flat panel detectors, indirect type uses a phosphor screen like cesium iodide to convert the X-ray to light photons. Direct flat panel detectors use instead a photoconductive layer, most commonly amorphous selenium, that converts X-ray energy directly to charge. By using flat panel detectors, patient dose can be reduced without degradation of image quality and multiple images can be acquired in a short time.[9,10]

Dual energy imaging is a new technique which utilizes a receptor with two layers, each of which records different energy components of X-ray beam and is possible for a computer to analyze and separate the components of dual energy in order to display both soft tissue and bone images of the same radiograph.[6] Dual energy imaging is one of the few areas in which digital radiography has proved of diagnostic advantage over conventional chest radiography.

Temporal subtraction imaging is used to improve the visual assessment of chest radiograph. This technique aims to selectively enhance areas of internal change by subtracting the patient's previous radiograph from the current one. Studies have shown that temporal subtraction improves the visual perception of subtle abnormalities such as pulmonary nodules, infiltrative opacities and diffuse lung disease.[11,12]

Digital tomosynthesis is a technique that has evolved from conventional tomography and solves many of the problems associated with conventional tomography. Digital tomosynthesis can produce an unlimited number of section images at arbitrary depths from single set of acquisition images. This technique is another method for improving detection of subtle lesions, such as pulmonary nodules.[13,14]

Digital Radiography and Chest

Major advantage of digital radiography lies in the control of display of optical density of radiographs in portable chest X-ray examination with dynamic range and control processing. It improves visibility of tubes and lines superimposed on the mediastinum. Although it may not offer any significant advantage over conventional film screen system, digital radiography improves visibility of normal lung structures, thus one has to be careful in distinguishing prominent blood vessels from interstitial disease. To avoid this misinterpretation, mild-to-moderate edge enhancement is required for better visualization of interstitial disease. Because of smaller size of digital radiograph, there is a definite learning curve to adjust to digital radiograph and one may have to interpret the film from a closer distance.

Numerous observe performance studies have shown that digital radiography can equal conventional film radiography in virtually any specific task. However, for this, post-processing of the digital image is required to match the digital radiograph to the task. A problem inherent in all forms of digital manipulation is that enhancement of the image for one purpose, degrades it for another.

There have been conflicting reports about whether digital chest radiography can be satisfactorily interpreted on high-resolution television monitors, as distinct from laser printed films. Recent studies suggest that 2K × 2K monitors may be adequate for making primary diagnosis on digital chest radiograph.

RADIOGRAPHIC PROJECTIONS

Posteroanterior View

The most satisfactory and standard radiographic view for evaluation of the chest is posteroanterior (PA) view with patient standing **(Fig. 1)**. Visualization of lungs is excellent because of inherent contrast of the tissues of the thorax.

The diagnostic accuracy of chest disease is partly related to the quality of radiographic images. It is incumbent on all radiologists to ensure that images on which their diagnostic impression is based are of the highest quality. Careful attention to several variables is necessary to ensure such quality.

Patient Positioning

Positioning must be such that the X-ray beam is properly centered, the patient's body is not rotated, and the scapulas are rotated sufficiently anteriorly so that they are projected away from the lungs. On properly centered radiographs, the medial ends of the clavicles are projected equidistant from the margins of the vertebral column.

Patient Respiration

Respiration must be fully suspended, preferably at total lung capacity (TLC). It has been shown that in erect chest radiographs, normal subjects routinely inhale to approximately 95% of TLC without coaxing;[15] thus, such radiographs can be of value in estimating lung volume, and by comparison with subsequent radiographs in appreciating an increase or decrease in volume as a result of disease.

Film Exposure

Exposure factors should be such that the resultant radiograph permits faint visualization of the thoracic spine and the

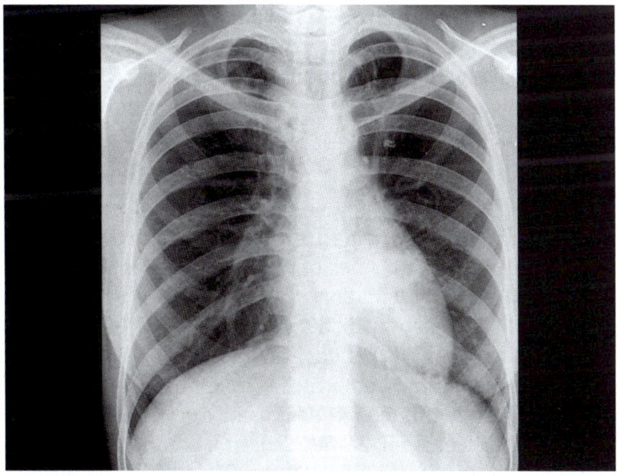

FIG. 1: Normal chest X-ray: Posteroanterior view in standing position.

intervertebral disks on the PA radiograph so that lung markings behind the heart are clearly visible. Exposure should be as short as possible, consistent with the production of adequate contrast. Unfortunately, all too frequently technical factors are such that optimal radiographic density is achieved over the lungs generally but without adequate exposure of the mediastinum or the left side of the heart, a tendency that seriously limits radiological interpretation, moderate overexposure can be easily compensated for by bright illumination; underexposure on the other hand cannot be compensated for by any viewing technique and since it prevents visualization of vital areas of the thorax, should not be tolerated in any circumstances. With perseverance, it is always possible to overcome problems of underexposure.

For a PA chest radiograph, the mean radiation dose at skin entrance should not exceed 0.3 mGy per exposure and the exposure time should not exceed 40 msec.[16] An optimally exposed radiograph presents the lung at a mid-gray level (average optical density, 1.6–1.9). (Optical density is a measurement of the ability of the film to stop light (film blackness), and it is equal to the logarithm of light incident on the film over light transmitted by the film ($D = \log I_O/I_t$).

The focal film distance should be at least 180 cm (72 inches) to minimize magnification (Focal film distance is the distance between the focal spot of the X-ray tube and the radiograph).[16]

Kilovoltage

A high kilovoltage technique appropriate to the film speed should be used;[10] for PA and lateral chest radiographs, the recommended kVp is 115–150 kVp. Since the coefficients of X-ray absorption of bone and soft tissue approximate each other in the higher kilovoltage ranges, radiographic visibility of the bony thorax is reduced with only slight change in the overall visibility of lung structures. Furthermore, the mediastinum is better penetrated, thereby permitting visibility of lung behind the heart and the many mediastinal lines and interfaces whose identification is so important to the overall assessment of both the mediastinum and lungs. This technique can produce chest radiographs superior in all respects to those obtained with other techniques in addition to better penetration of the mediastinum. High kilovoltage also results in lower radiation exposure than does lower kilovoltage. The only drawback of the high kilovoltage techniques is the diminished visibility of calcium that results from the lower coefficient of X-ray absorption; however this shortcoming has not proved troublesome in practice.

Grids and Filters

When using a grid, at least a 10:1 aluminum interspace grid with a minimum of 103 lines per inch recommended by the American College of Radiology.[16] An alternative option uses an air gap technique in which a space of 15 cm (6 inches) is interposed between the patient and the X-ray.[17] Since the air gap reduces radiation scatter by distance dispersion, no grid is required. When this technique is used, a constant focal film distance of 10 feet is recommended. In a comparative study of air gap and grid techniques, it was shown that the former can provide contrast equal to those obtained with grids[18] of the various combinations of distances possible. A focal distance of 10 feet with an air gap of 6 inches provides a good compromise. Patient exposure with an air gap technique was comparable to a no-grid, no-air gap technique and was less than that obtained with a grid.

Lateral View

The lateral view is the most important supplement to standard PA chest radiograph since much of the lung and mediastinum is hidden on the PA film. Right or left lateral view, depending on the area of interest closer to the film is obtained. The lateral view helps in localization of different lobes and segments and often this is the only view that will provide this information.[19] Important observations on lateral film of the chest include the clear spaces, vertebral translucency and outline of diaphragms. There are two spaces of increased translucency where both lungs lie closest. These are retrosternal and retrocardiac areas. Retrosternal space normally measures less than 3 cm at its widest point. Vertebral bodies normally are progressively more translucent caudally because of increase in the volume of aerated lung overlying the spine. Both diaphragms are visible throughout their length except the left anteriorly where it merges with the heart **(Fig. 2)**. The diaphragm of the side closer to the film is also more sharply defined. The ribs of the side away from the film appear wider.

Anteroposterior View

This is sometimes the only projection that is possible in very sick patients and usually it is obtained in wards and ICUs with portable X-ray machines. The quality is usually poor. In this view, the scapulae cannot be projected out of the lung fields. The ribs and clavicle are more horizontal and the heart is magnified as compared to the PA view **(Fig. 3)**. Anteroposterior (AP) view is, sometimes, very helpful in deciding whether a small questionable pulmonary opacity on the PA view is genuine, by altering its relationship to the overlying ribs and vascular shadows.[20] It is also useful in differentiating free and loculated pleural fluid.

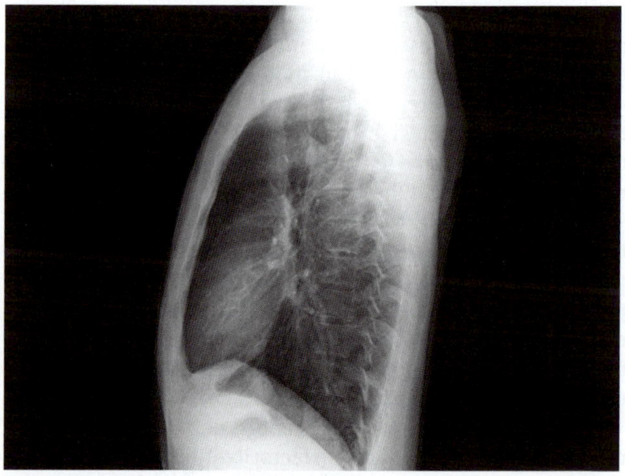

FIG. 2: Right lateral X-ray of normal chest.

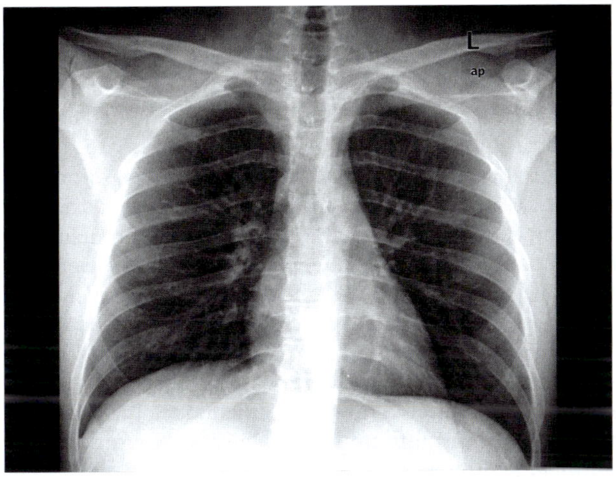

FIG. 3: Anteroposterior view of chest: The clavicle and ribs are more horizontal in position.

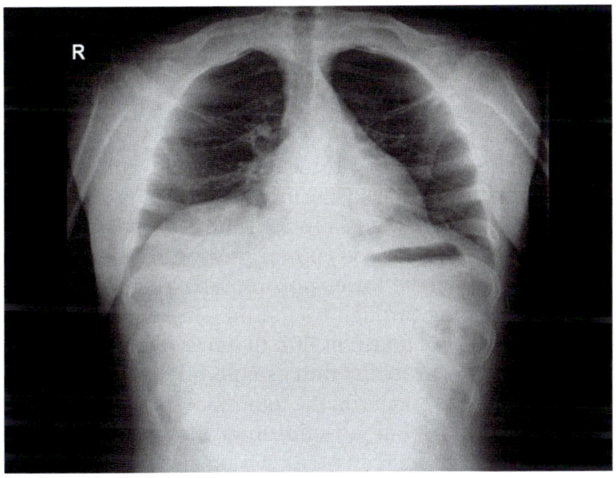

FIG. 4: Lordotic view of chest: The clavicles are projected superior to apex.

Decubitus View

The cross-table lateral decubitus views are helpful in determining the confines of the cavity and demonstrating small pneumothorax or pleural effusions. The dependent hemidiaphragm normally rises considerably in this view.

Lordotic View

This view is obtained either with patient leaning backward in lordotic position or, more commonly, with cranial tilt of the X-ray tube. It is particularly useful for clear demonstration of lung apices. It is important in confirming middle lobe and lingular abnormalities. The clavicles are projected above the lung fields and anterior and posterior parts of the ribs usually overlap each other **(Fig. 4)**. The lower chest is highly distorted in this view.

Oblique View

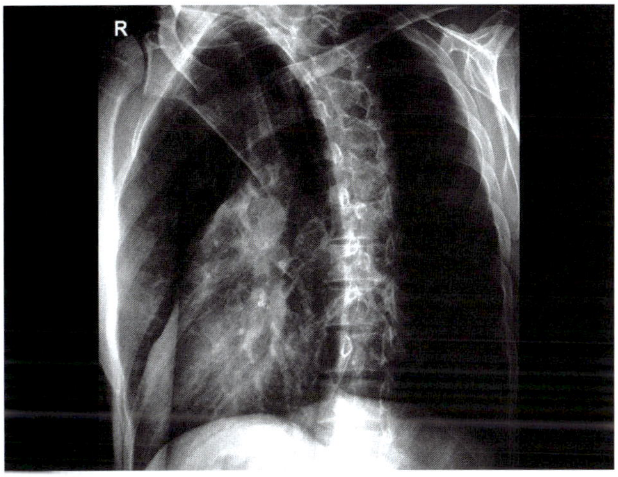

FIG. 5: Right oblique view of normal chest.

Right or left posterior oblique views are obtained with degree of obliquity best determined with fluoroscopy. These are preferred to lateral views in case of bilateral disease, since the superimposition of two lungs is significantly obviated **(Fig. 5)**. The left posteroanterior oblique view is particularly useful for better demonstration of trachea and its divisions.

SPECIAL RADIOGRAPHIC TECHNIQUES

Inspiratory–Expiratory Radiography

Comparison of radiographs exposed in full inspiration and maximal expiration may supply useful information in two specific situations. The main indication is the investigation of air trapping, either general or local. The former is exemplified by asthma or emphysema. In both these abnormalities, diaphragmatic excursion is reduced symmetrically and lung density changes little between expiratory and inspiratory radiographs to demonstrate these features convincingly, expiration must be forced and preferably timed. When air trapping is local as in bronchial obstruction or lobar emphysema, the expiratory radiograph reveals decreased ipsilateral diaphragmatic elevation, a shift of the mediastinum toward the contra- lateral hemithorax and relative absence of density change involves bronchopulmonary segments.

The second indication for expiratory–inspiratory radiography is when pneumothorax is suspected and the visceral pleural line is not visible on the standard inspiratory radiograph or the findings are equivocal. In these situations, a film taken in full expiration may show the line more clearly.

Valsalva and Müller Maneuvers

The Valsalva and Müller maneuvers respectively consisting of forced expiration and inspiration against a closed glottis may aid in determining the vascular or solid nature of intrathoracic masses. A change in size indicates a vascular lesion. Lack of change in size, however, is not helpful, because it may occur with solid lesions or with insufficient effort. Although potentially helpful, these maneuvers are seldom used in clinical practice.

Bedside/Portable Radiography

The number of requests for radiographic examination of the chest with a mobile apparatus at a patient bedside has increased enormously since its introduction owing partly to the growth of intensive care units (ICUs) and partly to the introduction of complex cardiovascular surgical procedures that require close postoperative surveillance.

Such radiographs are almost invariably technically inferior to those obtained in the standard manner in the radiology department itself. This inferior quality derives from multiple factors, some of which are uncontrollable (e.g. the patient's supine position, a short focal film distance and the restricted ability of many such patients to suspend respiration or to achieve full inspiration). Other factors, however, including the technical ones used in the exposure, are subject to control.[21] Frequently, these radiographs are overexposed or underexposed, sometimes, to a degree that limits or even precludes recognition of the subtle changes that are so important in the radiologist either accepting an inferior product or arranging a repeat examination, with associated patient discomfort, increased radiation exposure and increased cost. Some of these problems can be minimized by using a wide latitude screen film combination. An alternative technique that is rapidly replacing the screen film combination for bedside radiographs is digital radiography, since it allows satisfactory images to be obtained over a wide range of X-ray exposures.

From the various studies in the literature, it seems reasonable to conclude that daily routine chest radiographs are indicated in ICU patients with acute cardiac or pulmonary problems, in patients receiving mechanical ventilation, patients admitted for cardiac monitoring, or ICU patients admitted because of extrathoracic disease. Chest radiographs are recommended after insertion of endotracheal tubes, central venous lines, chest tubes and intra-aortic balloons.[22-24]

NORMAL ANATOMY ON CHEST X-RAY

The normal Roentgen anatomy of the chest as seen on chest radiographs can be described in following headings:

Trachea

Trachea is a straight tube, midline in the upper part and deviates slightly to the right around the aortic knuckle. It shortens and deviates more to right on expiration. Its caliber is even with decreasing translucency as it is traced caudally. On plain chest radiograph, the upper limits of coronal diameters in adults are 21 mm (in females) and 25 mm (in males); sagittal diameters are 23 mm (in females) and 27 mm (in males).[25] The right tracheal margin (right paratracheal stripe) can be traced down to the right main bronchus. It is 4 mm or less in thickness and measured above the azygos vein.[26] The left paratracheal line is rarely visualized. After the age of 40 years, calcification of the cartilage rings of the trachea is a common finding.[27] The enlarged azygos vein, which lies in the angle between the right main bronchus and trachea, may be normally seen as a round opacity in the tracheobronchial angle in the supine chest film.

Tracheobronchial Divisions

The trachea divides into right and left main bronchus usually at D5 or D6 level in adults. The left main bronchus is longer and has more acute angle with trachea as compared to right main bronchus.

The right main bronchus divides into upper lobe bronchus and bronchus intermedius. The upper lobe bronchus divides into apical, posterior and anterior segmental bronchi. The bronchus intermedius divides into middle and lower lobe bronchi. Middle lobe bronchus has medial and lateral branches. The lower lobe bronchus has five branches: each for superior, anterior, lateral, posterior and medial basal segments of lower lobe. Absence of middle lobe on left side modifies the bronchial division on left side. The left main bronchus divides into upper and lower lobe bronchi. The upper lobe bronchus has two divisions: the upper division divides into apicoposterior and anterior branches to supply upper lobe, the lower division supplies the lingula with superior and inferior branches. The lower lobe bronchus on left side divides similar to the right side except the absence of separate medial basal branch. Major tracheobronchial divisions are illustrated in **Figures 6A and B**.

Lungs

The lungs are divided into three lobes on the right side and two lobes on the left side by the interlobar fissures. The major (oblique) fissures on both sides are similar. It runs obliquely forwards and downwards (upper portion facing forward and laterally and the lower portion facing backward and medially), passing through the hilum. On a lateral view, it starts at the level of fourth or fifth thoracic vertebra to reach the diaphragm 5 cm behind the costophrenic angle on the left and just behind the angle on the right side[28] **(Fig. 7)**.

The right lung has an additional fissure, the minor (horizontal) fissure. It can be drawn on chest PA film from right hilum to the sixth rib in axillary line **(Fig. 8)**. It separates the middle lobe from right upper lobe. There are some accessory fissures, which are occasionally seen. The azygos lobe fissure, so called because it contains the azygos vein on right and hemiazygos vein on left within its lower margin, is commonly seen on the right side with an incidence on 0.4%.[28] It appears as a hairline with slight lateral convexity running across the right upper zone to end in a comma-like expansion (azygos vein) near the hilum. The azygos lobe is the area of the lung medial to the azygos fissure. The left-sided horizontal fissure, similar to the minor fissure on the right, separates the lingular from the other upper lobe segments. The superior accessory fissure separates the apical from the basal segments of the lower lobes. The inferior accessory fissure separates the medial basal from the other basal segments.

Bronchopulmonary Segments

Bronchopulmonary segments of individual lobes are based on the subdivisions of lobar bronchi. These segments represent the volume of the lung, which is supplied by an integral and relatively constant segmental bronchus and blood vessels. The boundaries between various segments are complex and with the rare exception of accessory fissure, the segments are not

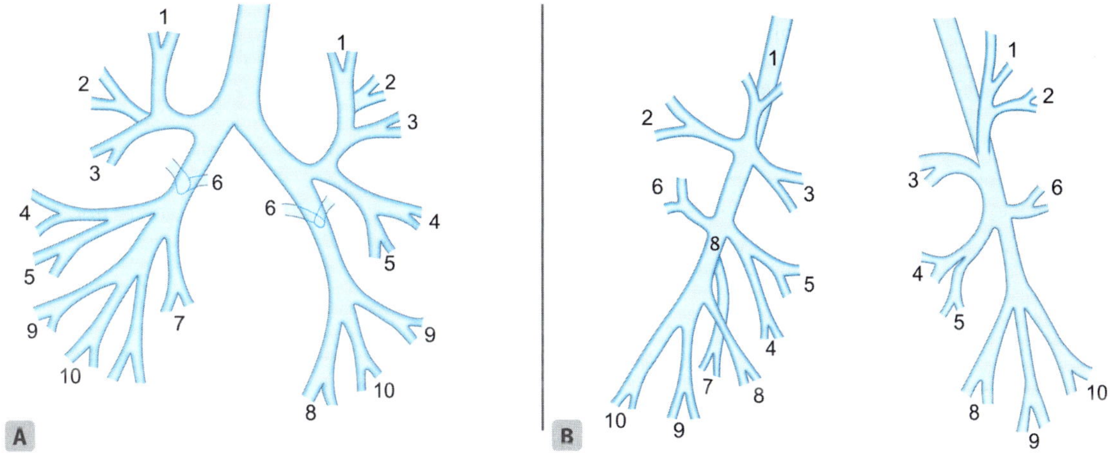

FIGS. 6A AND B: Diagrammatic representation of major tracheobronchial division as seen on frontal (A) and lateral (B) orientation. (1. Apical; 2. Posterior; 3. Anterior segments of upper lobe; 4. Lateral segment of middle lobe/superior lingula; 5. Medial segment of middle lobe/inferior lingula; 6. Superior; 7. Medial basal; 8. Anterior basal; 9. Lateral basal; and 10. Posterior basal segments of lower lobe).

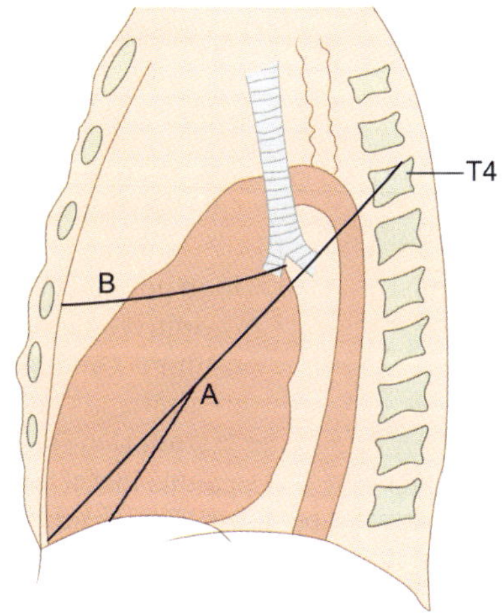

FIG. 7: Line diagram on lateral chest X-ray showing position of major (line A) and minor fissure (line B).

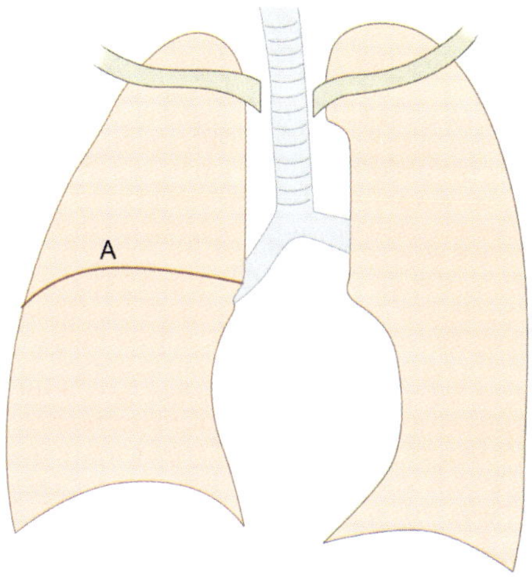

FIG. 8: Line diagram on chest X-ray (PA view) showing position of minor fissure (line A).

divided by septae. Although many pathological process may predominate in one segment or another, these usually never confirm precisely to whole of just one segment since collateral air drift occurs across segmental boundaries. However, information of segmental involvement in disease process is particularly important to surgeons since these segments can be removed separately. These bronchopulmonary segments are designated as per the divisions of segmental bronchi. There is a lot of overlap of bronchopulmonary segments on a PA view of chest but they project separately on a lateral view. Their approximate location, as seen on frontal and lateral radiographs, is illustrated **(Figs. 9A to D)**.

The radiographic density of the two lungs is symmetrical on a well-taken PA film. If the patient is rotated, the hemithorax closer to the film appears more radiodense. Both PA and lateral views are necessary to localise a lesion in one or more of the pulmonary segments. Since the normal bronchi are not visualised in the peripheral lung fields, it is difficult to make out the boundary of different pulmonary segments on plain radiographs of the chest.

Hilum and Pulmonary Vasculature

The structures contributing to the formation of the hilum are the pulmonary arteries and their main branches, upper lobe pulmonary veins, the major bronchi and lymph glands. Of all the structures in the hilum, only the pulmonary arteries and upper lobe veins significantly contribute to the hilar shadows on a plain radiograph. Normal lymph nodes are not seen. The left hilum is usually 0.5–2 cm higher than the right. Both hila are of equal density and size with a concave lateral border on PA film.

The diameter of the normal descending branch of right pulmonary artery is between 10–16 mm in males and 9–15 mm in females. The course of the pulmonary vessels can be described by dividing them into three zones depending upon their positions in the lungs, i.e. hilar, mid lung and peripheral.

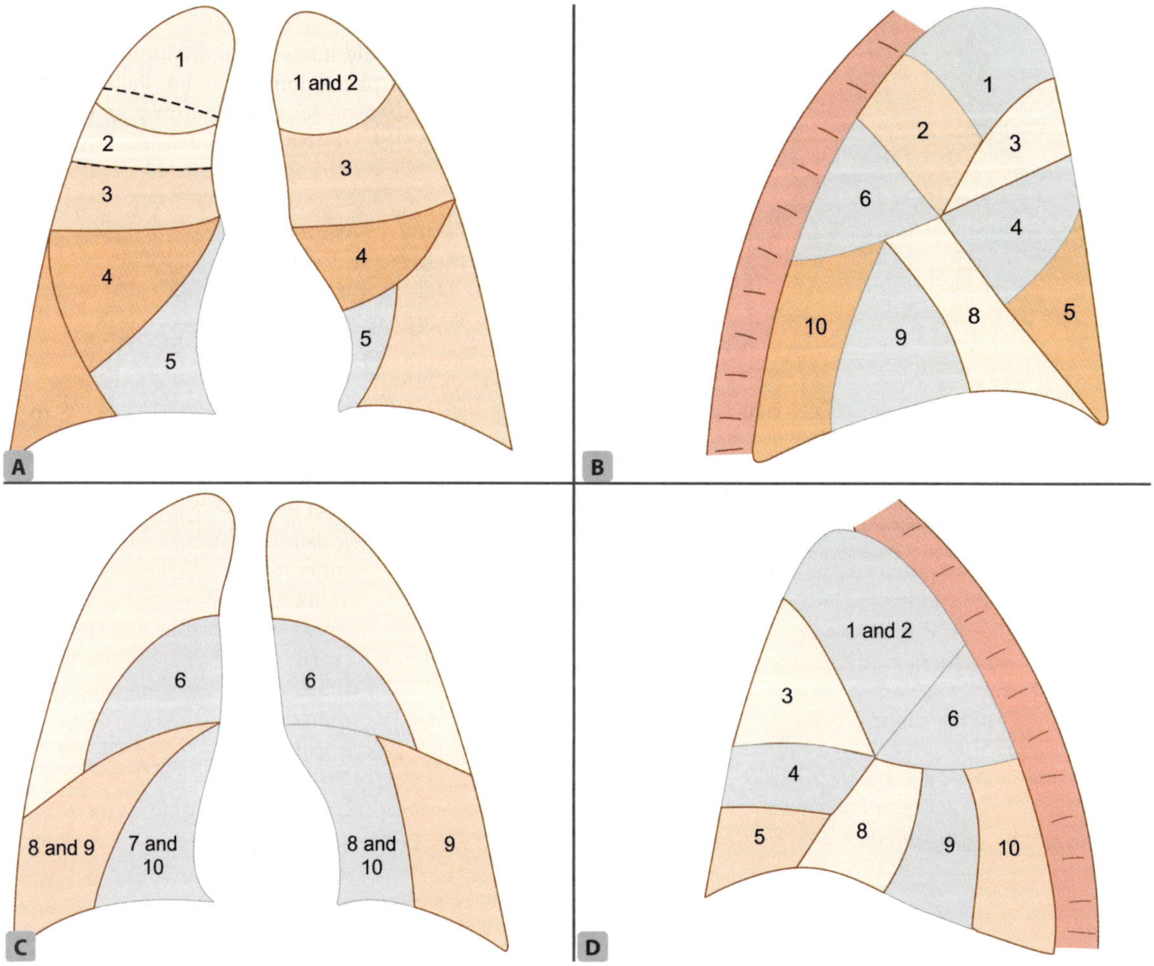

FIGS. 9A TO D: Line diagram showing approximate locations of various bronchopulmonary segments. (A) Upper and middle lobe/lingula on PA projection; (B) Lower lobe on PA projection; (C) Right lung on lateral projection; (D) Left lung on lateral projection (The segments numbers as per Figure in 6).

Mid-lung vessels extend from hilum up to 2 cm from the chest wall. Peripheral vessels are present in other 2 cm of the lung fields and these are rarely seen on a normal chest radiograph. The pulmonary veins have fewer branches and are straighter. The distinction between intrapulmonary arteries and veins is difficult and seldom useful so that they are collectively referred to as pulmonary vasculature. The pulmonary vessels taper gradually as they proceed peripherally. On erect PA chest radiographs, the upper zone vessels are comparatively narrower than lower zone vessels because of the effect of gravity. The bronchial vessels are normally not seen on chest radiograph.

Pleura

Normal pleura is not visible on chest radiographs. The mediastinal surface of the pleura can occasionally be demonstrated near the midline in a well-penetrated chest radiograph.

Mediastinum

It is a space lying between two lungs. It is bounded by sternum anteriorly, dorsal spine posteriorly and pleural sacs on both sides. The borders of the heart and mediastinum are clearly defined except where the heart is in contact with the left hemidiaphragm. The bracheocephalic (innominate) vessels, superior vena cava and right atrium form the right mediastinal border. Rarely a dilated aorta may also contribute. The left border is formed by left subclavian artery, aortic knuckle, left atrial appendage and left ventricle.

The radiological division of the mediastinum can be ascertained on a lateral chest radiograph by two imaginary lines **(Fig. 10)**. The first line is drawn from the diaphragm upward along the posterior border of heart and anterior border of the trachea into the neck. A second line is drawn connecting a point on each thoracic vertebra, 1 cm behind their anterior borders. The anterior mediastinum is in front of the first line, the middle mediastinum is between the two lines and the posterior mediastinum is behind the second line.

The anterior mediastinum contains thymus, heart with pericardium, great vessels and occasionally, aberrant thyroid. Middle mediastinum contains trachea and esophagus. Nerve roots and descending thoracic aorta are the main contents of posterior mediastinum. Normal lymph nodes and adipose

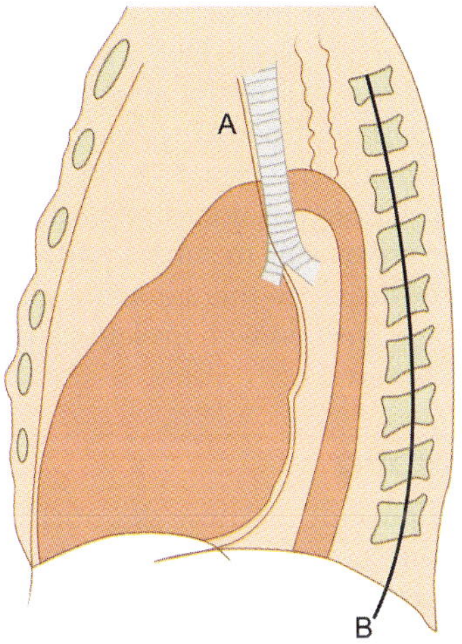

FIG. 10: Line diagram on lateral radiograph of chest showing division of mediastinum by A and B lines.

tissue is seen in all divisions of mediastinum. Conventional PA and lateral views of the chest are the first radiological investigation in any suspected mediastinal abnormality. However, a lesion may not be detected if it is not large enough to cause contour abnormality in the lung-mediastinum interphase.

In neonates and young children, the normal thymus is seen as a triangular sail-shaped structure with well-defined borders, sometimes, wavy in outline. Its borders project from one or both sides of the mediastinum.

Mediastinal Lines and Interfaces

As the two lungs approximate anteriorly, four layers of pleura and anterior mediastinum separate them forming a septum called as anterior junctional line. On PA film this line is oriented from upper right to lower left of the sternum. Similarly, posterior junctional line is produced by the posterior approximation of the lungs behind the esophagus and anterior to spine. On PA film, the posterior junctional line usually projects through the air column of trachea. Adjacent to the vertebral bodies runs the para- spinal lines. Azygoesophageal recess is formed by contact of right lower lobe with esophagus and azygos vein. The recess is frequently identified on a well-penetrated PA film as an interface that extends from the diaphragm below to the azygos arch above. Typically, it is seen as a continuous arch concave to the right. It may be straight in young adults.[28] The paraspinal lines are usually 1–2 mm wide on PA film.

Heart

Normally two thirds of the cardiac shadow lies to the left of the midline and one-third to the right. In normal individuals, the transverse diameter of the heart on PA film is usually in the range of 11.5–15.5 cm. It is less than 11.5 cm in about 5% of people and only rarely exceeds 15.5 cm in heavy, stocky individuals. Assessment of cardiac size by determining cardiothoracic ratio is more useful. Cardiothoracic ratio of 50% is accepted widely as the upper limit of normal, however, it exceeds 50% in at least 10% of normal individuals.[29] The cardiothoracic ratio may be up to 60% in neonates.[30]

Diaphragm

In most individuals, it has a smooth dome shape. The peak or the highest point of the dome is medial. Flattening of the dome can be measured on PA view by dropping a perpendicular from midpoint of the dome to the line connecting costophrenic and cardiophrenic angles of the same side. The distance is normally greater than 1.5 cm.[31] In approximately 90% of normal individuals, the right hemidiaphragm is 1.5–2.5 cm higher than the left. In rest, either the domes are at the same level or the right diaphragm may be at the slightly higher level. The discrepancy in the levels of the diaphragms is related to the position of the cardiac apex and not to the position of the liver. A difference greater than 3 cm in the levels of two hemidiaphragms is significant.[32]

Sonography of Chest

Ultrasound of the chest is rapidly emerging valuable method in diagnosis of various thoracic diseases including pleural, chest wall and peripheral lung parenchymal pathologies.[33] The ultrasound examination of chest is very useful in critical care unit at bedside where standard radiography can be suboptimal due to various factors.[34] Other than diagnostic use, ultrasound can be used for guidance for FNAC/biopsy and placement of intercostal drainage tubes. The chances of successful thoracentesis increase when ultrasound used as guidance compared with physical examination.[35]

Ultrasound has several advantages, including its wide availability, better portability, absence of radiation, real time imaging and dynamic properties. The limitations of ultrasound are low resolution images and operator dependence.

The major indications of chest ultrasound are:

- Evaluation of pleural pathologies (effusion, hemothorax, empyema, pleural thickening, calcification, pleural mass, etc.)
- Diagnosis of pneumothorax
- Evaluation of opaque hemithorax
- Assesment of chest wall diseases (like neoplasms, hematoma, abscess, rib fracture)
- Assesment of diaphragmatic mobility
- To differentiate subpulmonic effusion with subphrenic collection
- Evaluation of peripheral lung parenchymal pathologies (consolidation, collapse, abscess and tumors)
- Evaluation of mediastinum (anterior mediastinal mass, lymphadenopathy, IVC thrombosis and pericardial effusion)
- Guidance for interventional procedures.

Ultrasound Technique

Appropriate ultrasound probe, proper patient positioning and placement of probe, are the important factors to get better result while doing chest ultrasound. Ultrasound of chest can be performed with any modern ultrasound machine equipped with curvilinear (3–5 MHZ) and high-resolution linear array probe (5–13 MHz). Curvilinear transducers convex shape has a wider field of view and provides visualization of deeper structures. Initially quick look of chest wall, pleura and lung can be done by curvilinear probe and once abnormality detected then detailed depiction of lesion should be done by high-resolution linear probe.[33,36] The lesion can be assessed by both grayscale and color Doppler imaging. Before doing chest ultrasound, it is important to review previous imaging including chest X-ray to localize the area of interest. It is useful to increase the rib space to facilitate the exam by asking the patient to elevate his/her arm above the head.[33]

USG gelly should be placed on the patient's skin to provide smooth slide to probe and airless interface. Scanning should be done in quite respiration to know the normal lung movement. The detailed assessment of lesion should be done in breath-hold particularly when using color Doppler. The various useful positions/methods are given below:

- *Sitting position:* Posterior chest is best imaged with patient sitting upright and putting probe in the intercostal space **(Fig. 11)**. It is useful to detect pleural effusion which gravitates to dependent position.
- *Lateral decubitus position:* The anterior and lateral chest may be assessed in the lateral decubitus position **(Fig. 12)**.
- *Suprasternal and parasternal position:* It is useful to evaluate superior and anterior mediastinum **(Fig. 13)**.
- *Supraclavicular access:* It allows the visualization of apex of lung and brachial plexus **(Fig. 14)**.
- *Subcostal position:* It is useful to examine diaphragm
- *Subxiphoid position:* Good to evaluate pericardial effusion and cardiac chambers **(Figs. 15A and B)**.

Changing to various positions may be difficult to critically ill patients who are usually in supine position with multiple leads/support devices.[37] In this situation, ultrasound should be done in supine position with ipsilateral hand put to chest towards opposite side.

Normal Anatomy

It is utmost important to know the normal sonographic appearance of the chest components for the diagnosis of any abnormality and interventional guidance.

Chest Wall and Pleura

The normal chest wall and pleura shows characteristic features on ultrasound.[38-39] There is, series of layers representing intercostal muscles which are hypoechoic and

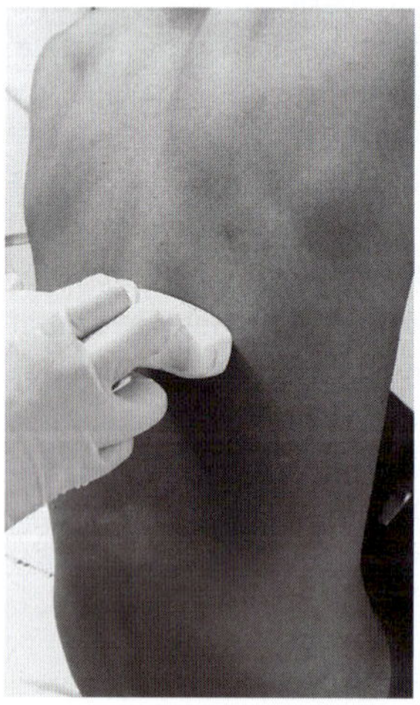

FIG. 11: Ultrasound probe and patient position for the examination of posterolateral chest wall.

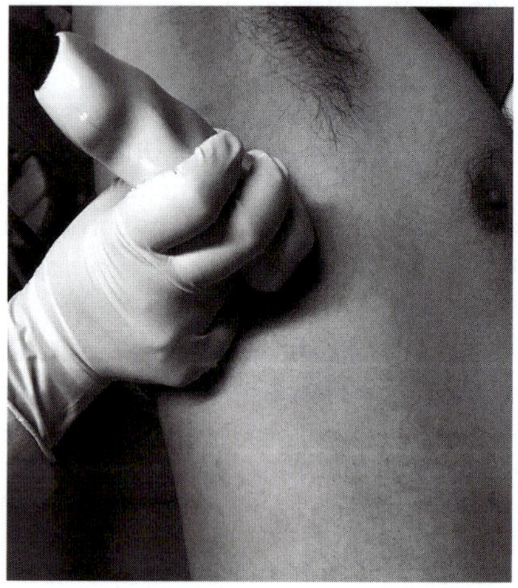

FIG. 12: Anterolateral chest ultrasound in decubitus position.

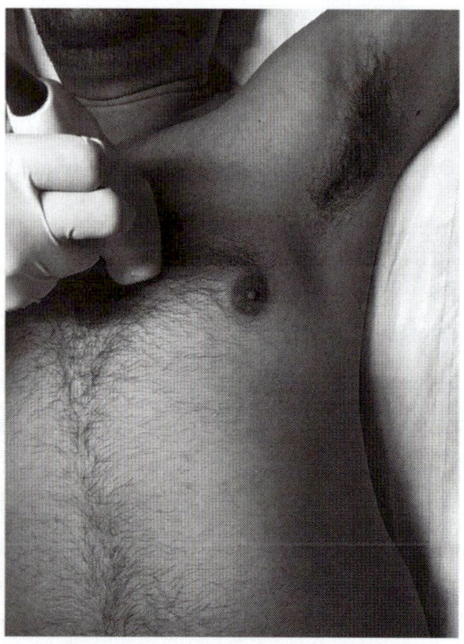

FIG. 13: Parasternal positioning of probe to evaluate anterior mediastinum, pleura and heart.

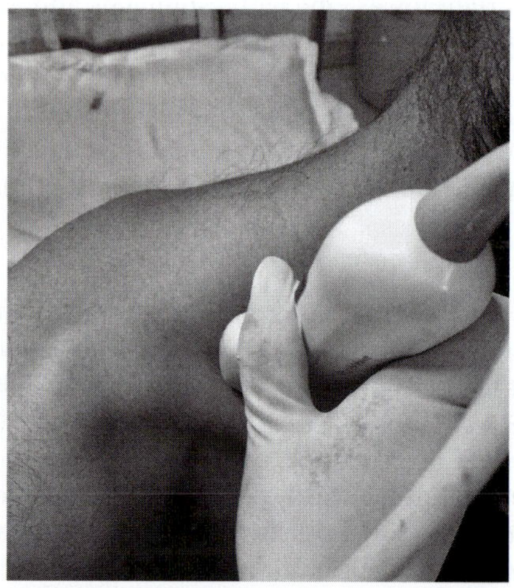

FIG. 14: Evaluation of lung apex by putting probe in supraclavicular location.

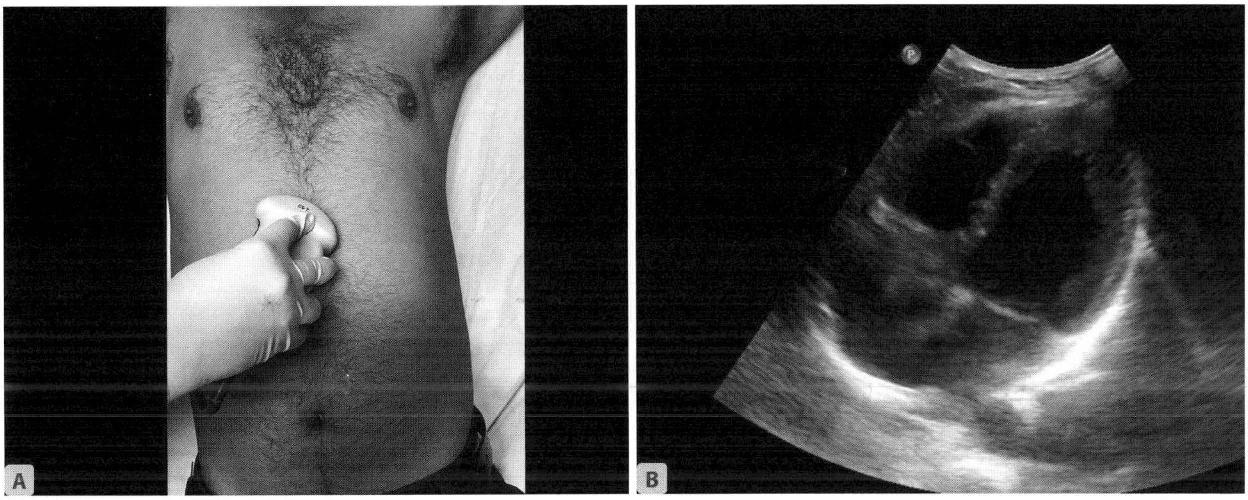

FIGS. 15A AND B Subxiphoid position of ultrasound probe (A) and corresponding USG image (B).

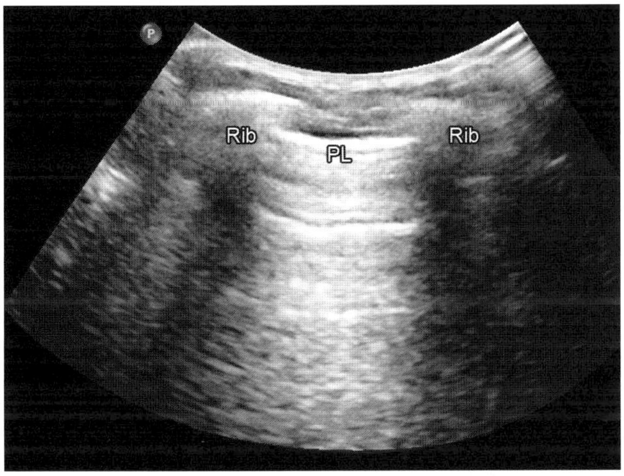

FIG. 16: Grayscale image of thoracic ultrasound by curvilinear convex probe showing wide view of components of thorax. Note made of acoustic shadowing of ribs and echogenic pleural line (pl).

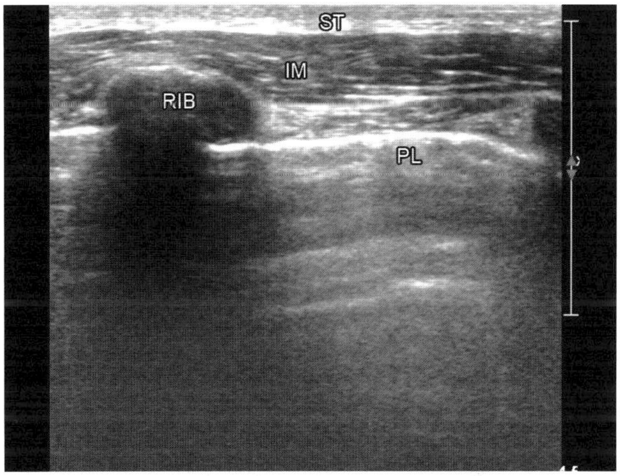

FIG. 17: Grayscale image by high-resolution linear ultrasound probe shows better visualization of structures of chest. (ST: subcutaneous tissue; IM: intercostal muscles; PL: pleural line).

fascia seen as echogenic structure. Below the chest wall, the ribs appear curvilinear echogenic continuous structure with posterior acoustic shadowing **(Fig. 16)**. Posterior to rib, the pleura appears as thick approximately 2 mm echogenic line when imaged with 3-5 MHZ curvilinear probe. The high-resolution linear ultrasound probe is needed to differentiate parietal and visceral pleura which are seen echogenic lines deep to ribs **(Fig. 17)**. Both the layers of pleura can be seen sliding over each other during real time USG imaging.

Diaphragm

The diaphragm is seen as approximately 1-2 mm thick echogenic line which shows movement during respiration. Usually the diaphragm is located inferior to 9th rib when patient is in sitting position. Apart from the location of diaphragm subdiaphragmatic recesses should be evaluated **(Fig. 18).**

Lung

The lung is air-filled and cannot be visualized deep to pleural lung interface. There are gross changes of acoustic impedance at this interface leading to horizontal artefacts which are seen as echogenic parallel lines. Additionally, comet tail artefacts which are vertically oriented can be seen in normal healthy individual **(Fig. 19)**. These artefacts are usually seen at the level of just above the diaphragm.

Heart

Identification of heart is important when planning for thoracentesis in left anterolateral aspect for safe puncture. The imaging features of heart on ultrasound depend upon axis and position of probe.

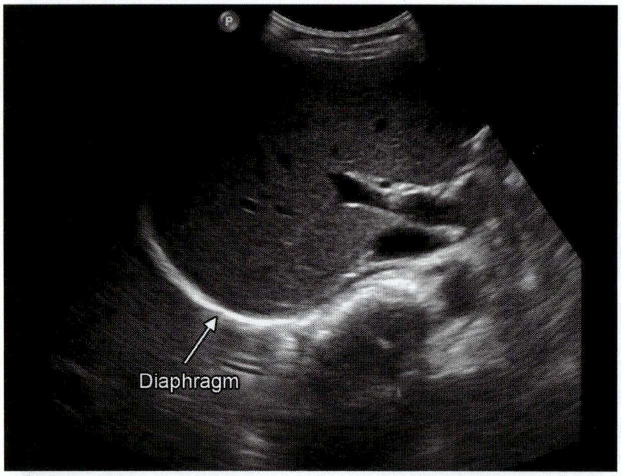

FIG. 18: Subcostal view ultrasound image shows echogenic (arrow) diaphragm.

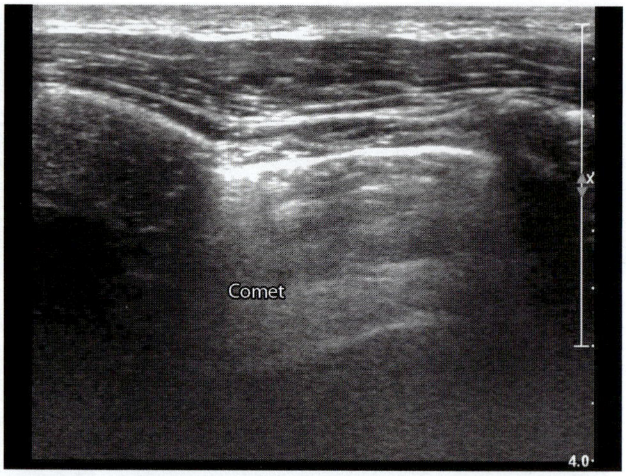

FIG. 19: Ultrasound image by linear probe shows comet-tail artefacts.

CONCLUSION

Chest radiography still remains the first investigation in the diagnosis of various chest diseases. Knowledge of normal anatomy has utmost importance in proper diagnosis of disease process on chest X-ray. Conventional radiograph may have technical limitation in some situations like critically ill patients in ICU; however, recent advances in electronics and computer technology have resulted in development of digital imaging which improves diagnostic quality of chest imaging.

Sonography of chest is emerging technique to evaluate the pathologies of chest which requires proper understanding of the techniques and anatomy of chest components.

ACKNOWLEDGMENT

We acknowledge the help of Dr Harish Bhujade for drawing line diagrams (***see* Figs. 7, 8 and 10**).

REFERENCES

1. Fraser RS, Muller NL, Colman N, et al. The normal lung. In: Fraser RS, Muller NL, Colman N, Pare PD (Eds). Diagnosis of Diseases of Chest (4th edition). Philadelphia: WB Saunders Co; 1999.
2. MacMohan H, Vyborny C. Technical advances in chest radiography. AJR. 1994;163:1049-59.
3. Bunch PC. Performance characteristic of asymmetric zero-crossover screen film system. SPIE Proc Med Imaging IV. 1992;1653:46-65.
4. Swension SJ, Grey JE, Brown LR, et al. A new asymmetric screen film combination for conventional chest radiology: evaluation of 50 patients. AJR. 1993;160:483-6.
5. Chotas HG, Floyd CE JR, Ravin CE. Film-based chest radiography: AMBER vs asymmetric screen film system. AJR. 1993;161:743-7.
6. Hansell DM. Technical consideration. In: Peter Armstrong, Alam G, Wilson, Paul Dee, David M Hansell (Eds). Imaging of diseases of chest (2nd edition). Mosby. 1995.pp.1-14.
7. Neitzei U, Maack I, Gunther-Kohfahl S. Image quality of digital chest radiography system based on selenium detector. Med Phys. 1994;21:509-16.
8. Chotas HG, Floyd CE JR, Ravin CE. Memory artifact related to selenium-based digital radiography system. Radiology. 1997;203:881-3.
9. Samei E, Flynn MJ. An experimental comparison of detector performance for direct and indirect digital radiography system. Med Phys. 2003;30:608-22.
10. Samei E. Performance of digital radiography detectors: factors affecting sharpness and noise. In: Samei E, Flynn MJ (Eds). Syllabus: categorical course in diagnostic radiology physics-advances in digital radiography. Oak Brook, Ill: Radiological Society of North America. 2003.pp.49-61.
11. Abe H, MacMahon H. Engelmann R, et al. Computer-aided diagnosis in chest radiography: results of large scale observer tests at the 1996–2001 RSNA scientific assemblies. Radiographics. 2003;23:255-65.
12. Okazaki H, Nakamura K, Watanabe H, et al. Improved detection of long cancer arising in diffuse lung diseases on chest radiographs using temporal subtraction. Acad Radiol. 2004;11:498-505.
13. Dobbins JT 3rd. Godfrey DJ. Digital X-ray tomosynthesis: current state of the art and clinical potential. Phys Med Biol. 2003;48:R65-106.
14. Godfrey DJ, McAdams HP, Dobbins JT 3rd. Optimization of the matrix inversion tomosynthesis (MITS) impulse response and modulation transfer function characteristics for chest imaging. Med Phys. 2006;33:655-67.
15. Crapo RA, Montague T, Armstrong J. Inspiratory lung volume achieved on routine chest films. Invest Radiol. 1979;14:137.
16. American College of Radiology: ACR standard for the performance of pediatric and adult chest radiography. American College of Radiology, Reston VA; 1997.p.27.
17. Jackson Fl. The air gap and improvement, and an improvement by anteroposterior positioning for chest roentgenography. Am J Roentgenol. 1964;92:688.
18. Trout RD, Kelly JP, Larson VL. A comparison of air gap and grid in roentgenography of the chest. Am J Roentgenol. 1975;120:404.
19. Felson B. The Roentgen work-up. In: Felson B (Ed). Chest Roentgenology. Philadelphia: WB Saunders Co; 1988.

20. Flower CDR, Armstrong P. Techniques. In: Graingern RG, Allison D (Eds). Diagnostic Radiology, 3rd edition. New York: Churchill Livingstone. 1997.p.201.
21. Wandtke JC. Bedside chest radiography. Radiology. 1994;190:1.
22. Fong Y, Whalen G, Hariri RJ, et al. Utility of routine chest radiographs in the surgical intensive care unit. Arch Surg. 1995;130:764.
23. Gray P, Sullivan G, Ostryzniuk P, et al. Value of postprocedural chest radiographs in the adult intensive care unit. Crit Care Med. 1992;20:1513.
24. Hill JR, Horner PE, Primack SL. ICU Imaging. Clin Chest Med. 2008;29(1):59-76,vi.
25. Breatnach E, Abbott GC, Fraser RE. Dimensions of the normal human trachea. AJR. 1984;142:903-6.
26. Savoca CJ, Austin JHM, Goldberg HI. The right paratracheal stripe. Radiology. 1977;122:295.
27. Murfitt J. The normal chest: Methods of investigation and differential diagnosis. In: Sutton D (Ed). Textbook of Radiology and Medical Imaging, 4th edition. Churchill Livingstone. 1987;2:326-67.
28. Mukherjee S, Gupta R. Imaging in chest diseases. In: Pande JN (Ed). Respiratory Medicine in the Tropics, 1st edition. Delhi, Oxford University Press. 1998.p.90.
29. Muller NL. The normal chest. In: Muller NL, Fraser RS, Colman NC (Eds). Radiologic Diagnosis of Diseases of the Chest (1st edition) Philadelphia: WB Saunders Company: 2001.
30. Edwards DK, Higgins CB, Gilpin EA. The cardiothoracic ratio in newborn infants. AJR.1981;136:136.
31. Lennon FA: Simon 6. The height of the diaphragm in the chest radiographs of normal subjects. Br J Radiol. 1965;38:937.
32. Flower CDR, Verschakelan JA. The diaphragm. In: Grainger RG, Allison D (Eds). Diagnostic Radiology, 3rd edition. New York: Churchill Livingstone. 1997. p. 270.
33. Koh DM, Burke S, Davies N, Padley SP. Transthoracic US of the chest: clinical uses and applications. Radiographics. 2002; 22(1):e1.
34. Yu CJ, Yang PC, Chang DB, Luh KT. Diagnostic and therapeutic use of chest sonography: value in critically ill patients. Am J Roentgenol. 1992;159:695-701.
35. Weingardt JP, Guico RR, Nemcek AA Jr, et al. Ultrasound findings following failed, clinically directed thoracenteses. J Clin Ultrasound. 1994;22:419.
36. Havelock T, Teoh R, Laws D, et al. Pleural procedures and thoracic ultrasound: British Thoracic Society Pleural Disease Guideline 2010. Thorax 2010; 65 Suppl 2:ii61-76.
37. Feller-Kopman D. Ultrasound-guided thoracentesis. Chest. 2006;129:1709.
38. Diacon AH, Theron J, Bolliger CT. Transthoracic ultrasound for the pulmonologist. Curr Opin Pulm Med. 2005;11:307.
39. Tsai TH, Yang PC. Ultrasound in the diagnosis and management of pleural disease. Curr Opin Pulm Med. 2003;9:282.

CHAPTER

123

MDCT and MRI Thorax: Techniques and Normal Anatomy

Rashmi Dixit, Anjali Prakash, Alpana Manchanda

Imaging evaluation of thoracic disease invariably begins with a chest radiograph. Cross-sectional imaging is indicated not only for detailed evaluation of abnormalities seen on the radiograph but also to detect occult lesions not apparent on the radiograph especially when there is strong clinical suspicion of thoracic disease. Multidetector computed tomography (MDCT) remains the imaging method most widely used for the study of thoracic diseases due to its high spatial and temporal resolution, ease of performance and widespread availability. MR largely remains a problem-solving modality with emerging applications.

MDCT THORAX

CT TECHNOLOGY

Spiral CT systems introduced in the 1990s represented a significant advancement in CT technology allowing volumetric data acquisition as opposed to the discontinuous data acquisition in conventional CT.[1] In 1998, the first multidetector CT scanners ware introduced allowing simultaneous acquisition of four slices (or sections) with gantry rotation times which were as low as 0.55 s.[1] These scanners resulted in improvement in acquisition speed, Z-axis coverage, temporal and spatial resolution over the single slice spiral or helical CT scanners. Thus high-resolution, single-breath-hold imaging of the entire thorax became feasible.

Thereon MDCT technology has developed at a breath-taking pace, with increasing detector rows and decreasing tube rotation times. Currently, scanners with 128 and more active detector rows and gantry rotation times as low as 0.33–0.25 second per rotation are available. These scanners are able to scan the entire thorax in 2–3 seconds dramatically reducing motion artefacts.[1,2]

The best temporal resolution that is achievable in a single-source CT scan is half the rotation time of the scanner as this is the minimum data needed for image reconstruction close to the isocenter. With gantry rotation time of 0.3 s. The best possible temporal resolution is 125–150 ms. In recent years, further increase in spatial and temporal resolution has been made possible by the use of either wide area detectors or dual source CT systems.[2]

An area detector is a CT detector that is wide enough in the Z-axis to cover an entire organ such as the heart, kidney or brain without table movement. There are two CT systems providing a16 cm coverage at isocentre. One with a collimation of 256 × 0.625 mm and 0.28 s rotation time and the other with 320 × 0.5 mm collimation and 0.27 s rotation time. These CT systems are useful for cardiac imaging as they cover the entire heart in a single axial scan without table movement avoiding the stair step or banding artefacts which may be seen with CT systems with lower detector coverage range. MDCT systems with lower detector range provide a Z coverage of up to 8 cm at isocentre so 2–4 image stacks, acquired in 2–4 consecutive heart beats are put together for volume coverage of the heart. These may be shifted or blurred with respect to each other due to insufficient temporal resolution or variation in cardiac motion from one cycle to next resulting in stair step or banding artefacts. However, on the flip side, all images acquired with an area detector may be affected by arrhythmias or ectopic beats during acquisition. Area detector systems have the ability to acquire dynamic volume data by scanning the same anatomic range repeatedly without table movement. This is useful for perfusion scanning of pulmonary nodules.[2]

Dual source CT (DSCT) systems use two X-ray tubes and detector systems positioned at 90° to each other which can simultaneously acquire data at the same Z-position. Dual source CT systems allow a significant improvement of temporal resolution to below 100 ms.[3] The third generation DSCT scanners acquire 2 × 192 slices with gantry rotation time of 0.25 s. Due to two X-ray tubes the best temporal resolution achievable in these CT systems is quarter of a gantry rotation as the two 90º segments acquired can be put together to give the required minimum 180º of scan data at the isocenter achieving temporal resolution of 0.66 s. Thus with dual source CT scanners, the entire thorax can be scanned within 0.3 s, almost eliminating respiratory and even cardiac motion artefacts.[1,4] They also allow a reduction in contrast dose.

DSCT systems with ECG triggering are useful for coronary imaging in one heart beat at very low dose. They are also excellent for comprehensive evaluation of acute chest pain or triple rule out studies and planning of trans aortic valve replacement (TAVR) procedures by providing adequate visualization of coronary arteries, aorta and iliac arteries.[5,6] The challenges with DSCT systems include cross-scattered radiation which, if not corrected, can produce artefacts and reduce contrast to noise ratio (CNR), and the limited scan field of view (SFOV) of the second detector. This was increased from 25 cm in the first generation to 35.5 cm in the third generation.[2] DSCT systems also provide dual energy applications which are discussed later.

CT ACQUISITION AND RECONSTRUCTION PROTOCOLS

Routinely, scans are acquired in the supine position in full inspiration to fully expand the lungs. This optimizes the contrast between the aerated lung and other normal high attenuation structures (e.g. vessels) and various abnormalities. Full inspiration also minimizes the occurrence of transient atelectasis which can be confounding at times. Scanning is generally done with thin collimation while images are reconstructed at a thickness slightly greater than the collimation to reduce noise in the reconstructed image. For example, in a 64 detector row scanner, the collimation is 64 × 0.625 or 64 × 0.5 (depending on vendor) while images can be reconstructed at 1, 3 and 5 mm thickness from the same data set.

The clinical indication dictates the choice of reconstruction. While 1 mm sections provide higher spatial resolution, a 3 mm thick slice has a better signal to noise ratio for the same acquisition dose. Thin section reconstructions are used for volumetric assessment and characterization of pulmonary nodules, pulmonary embolism and for evaluation of interstitial lung disease. Thin sections with 20–25% overlap are also used for 3D reconstructions. Thicker 3–5 mm sections are generally adequate for assessment of mediastinal masses, lung cancer staging, quick review and for archiving.[1,2,7]

Use of Iodinated Contrast Medium

Most thoracic CT examinations, except HRCT scans, are routinely performed with intravenous contrast. The aim of contrast administration is to opacify organs and delineate vessels within the area of interest. For most indications like lung cancer staging, evaluation of mediastinal masses or lymphadenopathy, a small-to-moderate amount of contrast medium, i.e. 60–120 mL of 300 mg I/mL at a slow injection rate of 1.5–3 mL/s with a long injection duration and scan delay of about 25 s produces adequate opacification of thoracic vessels. The contrast injection should ideally end about 5s before the MDCT acquisition and should be followed by a saline flush to reduce perivenous artefacts and improve the contrast bolus. A caudocranial direction of acquisition also minimizes perivenous artefacts.[7,8]

Window Settings and Reconstruction Algorithms[1,7]

Organs in the thorax have a wide range of densities or HU values ranging from –800 for the aerated lungs to +700 for the osseous structures like the ribs. A single window setting would be unable to represent these. A minimum of two-window settings are required, one to display the lung parenchyma and another to display the soft tissue structures of the mediastinum. Although the exact window settings may vary between institutions a window width of 300–500 HU and center of +40 HU is used for the mediastinum; while for the lungs, a wide window of 1200–1500. HU with a center of –600 HU is more appropriate. For evaluation of osseous structures, bone window settings at a window width of around 1500 and center of 450 are used in addition.

The choice of window settings is important as it can affect the approximate size of normal structures and pathology. The most accurate size measurement is done when the window level is half-way between the density of the structure to be measured and density of the surrounding tissue. Thus, the diameter of a pulmonary nodule will be underestimated if measured at soft tissue settings appropriate for the mediastinum. The smaller structures e.g. peripheral pulmonary vessels are more affected by inappropriate window settings than larger structures. Some authors recommend the use of specific window setting for certain conditions like use of wide window settings (600 HU – WW and 100–150 HU for window level) while interpreting routine CT scans of the chest to improve detection of unsuspected pulmonary embolism. Specific window settings have also been described for evaluation of airways and emphysema.

Each manufacturer provides several **reconstruction algorithms** to optimize visualization of various structures. The high frequency algorithm provides the best visualization of lung architecture while a standard smooth algorithm gives best soft tissue resolution and lowest noise for the mediastinum.

HIGH-RESOLUTION COMPUTED TOMOGRAPHY

High-resolution computed tomography (HRCT) is the use of thin section CT images (0.625–1.5 mm) with high spatial frequency reconstruction algorithm to detect and characterize diseases of pulmonary parenchyma and small airways.

Before the advent of multidetector CT routine CT chest and HRCT were strongly differentiated. The traditional HRCT protocol consisted of thin section CT obtained with 1 mm slice thickness at intervals of 10 or even 20 mm and reconstructed using high spatial frequency algorithms. The logic behind this protocol was that analysis of a diffuse parenchymal process did not require continuous coverage. The other reason being that the relatively higher doses required to achieve excellent signal to noise ratio and image quality did not result in an exponential increase in patient dose with discontinuous scanning. With the current MDCT scanners, each CT chest is an HRCT as the whole chest can be covered with narrow detector width of 0.5–1.25 mm and images reconstructed at 1–1.5 mm thickness with a high spatial frequency algorithm—the two essential factors that constitute an HRCT. Thus, in the past few years, discontinuous HRCT acquisition has been largely replaced by volumetric HRCT.[1,7,9] The factors responsible are:

- Volumetric HRCT can now be done at acceptable dose levels and doses have declined further with the use of reconstruction techniques such as iterative reconstruction. Discontinuous HRCT with 10 mm gap resulted in a dose of 0.7 mSv. Volumetric HRCT with 3D modulation and iterative noise reconstruction results in doses as low as 1.5–3 mSv as opposed to up to 7 mSv with volumetric HRCT in its early days. Hence increased dose is no longer a major concern.

- Volumetric scan allows easier and more precise delineation of disease distribution and comparison in follow-up studies.
- Subtle focal disease can also be detected which may be missed on the discontinuous scan. This may be especially useful when the diagnosis of ILD vs focal lung disease is not apparent clinically.

Modifications in Scanning Technique for HRCT[7,10,11]

Intravenous contrast is not required and, in fact, should be avoided as it may cause fallacious parenchymal opacification and interfere with interpretation.

Images are usually obtained in the **supine position in full inspiration** like routine scanning. In the normal lung effects of gravity on blood flow and gas volume, as well as some non-gravity, dependent effects can result in increase in attenuation and vessel size from anterior to posterior portion of the lung and may produce appearances similar to subpleural lines or atelectasis. In the **prone position**, these hydrostatic densities will disappear while true pathology will persist. The older publications with scans obtained on slower scanners with discontinuous technique reported the utility of prone scans in around 20% patients. This, however, is not the case with the current fast scanning technique. Prone scanning may be useful in a few selected patients with questionable subtle disease in dorsobasal area only, which would be critical in deciding the presence or absence of early disease, e.g. in a patient with asbestosis.

Addition of **expiratory scans** may be useful in the detection of focal or diffuse air trapping. In most cases with clinically significant small airway disease, mosaic attenuation may be visible on inspiratory scans, though much less conspicuous than expiratory scans. Diseases of the larger airways such as tracheobronchomalacia, however, will not be detected if only end inspiratory images are obtained.

High-quality HRCT examinations provide a spatial resolution of 0.5 mm and due to the high contrast within the lung parenchyma even structures as small as 0.2 mm can be seen well. Certain **modifications in reconstruction techniques** are important for achieving this:

- Use of **thin collimation** of 1 mm slice improves resolution and allows detection of important morphological features such as septal thickening, dilatation of airways, detection of small nodules, etc. However, a slice thickness below 1 mm does not result in any significant improvement in spatial resolution while increasing image noise.
- Application of **high-spatial frequency reconstruction algorithm**: Standard reconstruction algorithms result in smoothening of the image by reducing visible image noise and increasing the contrast resolution. High-spatial frequency or 'sharp' high-resolution algorithms reduce image smoothening and increase spatial resolution. Tissue interfaces and anatomic margins, e.g. the pleura, fissures or septae appear sharper and small vessels and bronchi are better seen **(Figs. 1A and B)**.
- Use of a **suitably small FOV** decreases pixel size and thus increases spatial resolution. The field of view should be adjusted to the outer cortex of the ribs—this ensures that the field is restricted to the size of the lungs while no portion of the lung is cut-off. This results in a spatial resolution of 0.5–0.3 mm. Sometimes, targeted reconstruction of a particular lung or lobe may be done to further increase the spatial resolution for evaluation of minute abnormalities. However, here the resolution is limited by the intrinsic resolution of the detectors. Targeted reconstruction is generally a matter of personal preference and there is no definitive literature recommending its use.

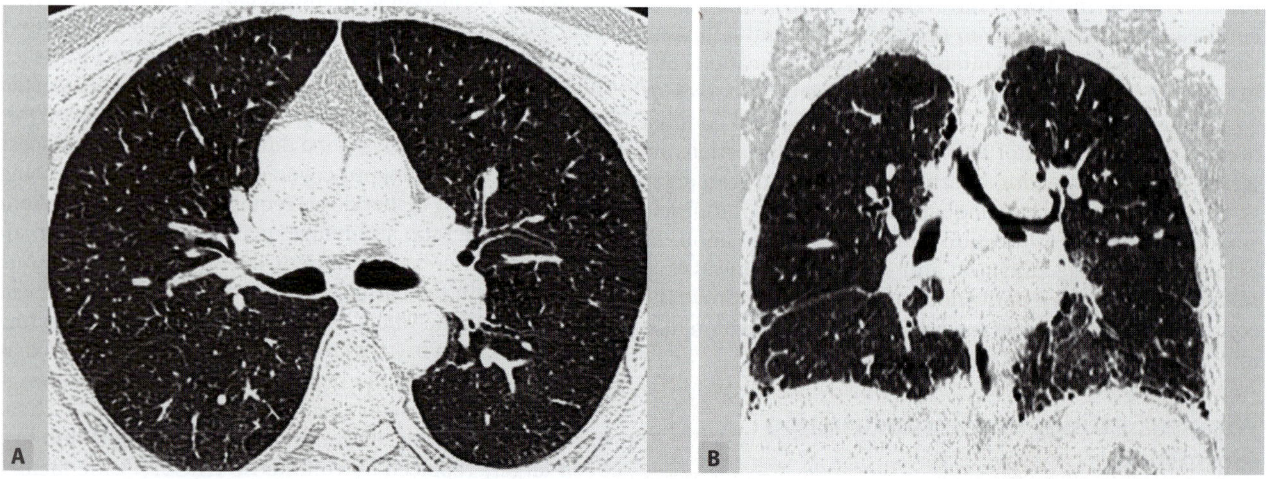

FIGS. 1A AND B: Normal HRCT. (A) 1 mm axial section from a volumetric spiral acquisition on a 128 slice MDCT scanner shows small vessels and bronchi in exquisite detail; (B) Coronal reconstruction in another patient shows the apicobasal gradient of interstitial lung disease.

ACQUISITION PROTOCOL AND CONTRAST OPACIFICATION FOR CT PULMONARY ANGIOGRAPHY[1,8,12]

The major factor to be considered for the technical success of a CT pulmonary angiography (CTPA) examination is excellent opacification of pulmonary vessels. The attenuation within the pulmonary arteries should be at least 250 HU to allow detection of filling defects and thrombi. A caudocranial acquisition is preferred as with this the basal portion will not show motion artefacts even in severely dyspneic patients. This is a common region for pulmonary emboli to lodge. Caudocranial acquisition also reduces perivenous streak artefacts. With the older generation of scanners which took about 20–25 s to scan the thorax 120–140 mL of 350–380 mg/mL iodine was required however with the latest MDCT scanners injected volume and iodine dose can be reduced markedly and 50 mL of contrast may be sufficient **(Figs. 2A and B)**. Scanners with capability of scanning at 70 kV are now available where the dose of iodine may be reduced to as low as 20 ml. In order to reduce radiation and optimize the contrast dose during CTPA the following should be done:

- Reduce KV from the routine 120 kV to 100 kV or even 80 kV if patient weighs less than 65 kg to take advantage of the K-edge absorption of iodine.
- Optimize flow rates to patient physiology, e.g. for old patients with possible altered left ventricular function, flow rate of 3 mL/s with high iodine concentration of 350–400 mg/mL is needed while in a young patient or a pregnant patient, a much higher flow rate of 5–6 mL/s will be required.[12]
- Calculate the correct contrast volume required: the acquisition time should be noted by setting the acquisition box in the scout. For a 128 slice scanner this is about 2 s. Acquisition time is added to time for breath-hold instruction (generally 5 s) and a reserve time of 5s which equals 12 s (2+5+5) in this case. Using a flow rate of 4 cc/s total volume can be calculated as total time × flow rate (12 × 4 = 48 cc) for perfect vessel opacification. Scan should be triggered by bolus-tracking ROI in the main pulmonary artery with a trigger threshold of 80–120 HU.
- Holding of breath in deep inspiration or Valsalva maneuver is to be avoided to prevent **transient interruption of contrast medium**. This results in poor opacification of the pulmonary artery while the SVC and aorta are well opacified. Various mechanisms have been proposed for this, which include increased venous return of unopacified blood from IVC to right atrium resulting in poor opacification of pulmonary arteries. Opening of patent foramen ovale due to Valsalva maneuver is thought to be the other reason. Hence the patient should be asked simply to hold his breath and not to take a deep inspiration during acquisition.

EVALUATION OF THE AORTA AND CORONARY ARTERIES

Evaluation of the aorta and coronary arteries is discussed elsewhere in this book, however, ECG gating is mandatory for coronary artery evaluation and can also help to eliminate confusing artefacts at the aortic root in patients with suspected dissection.

EVALUATION OF PULMONARY VEINS

Evaluation of pulmonary veins may be indicated in suspected stenosis after radiofrequency catheter ablation treatment of chronic atrial fibrillation. A preprocedure CT is also indicated to map variant venous anatomy to enhance success rate of the procedure and to exclude atrial thrombi which are an absolute contra-indication for the procedure. This requires 70–85 mL of 300–370 mg I/mL contrast to be administrated at 4–5 mL/s, acquisition being triggered by bolus tracking ROI placed in the left atrium. ECG gating is not routinely required as the atria move much less compared with coronary arteries with cardiac motion and the pulmonary veins are much larger structures.[13]

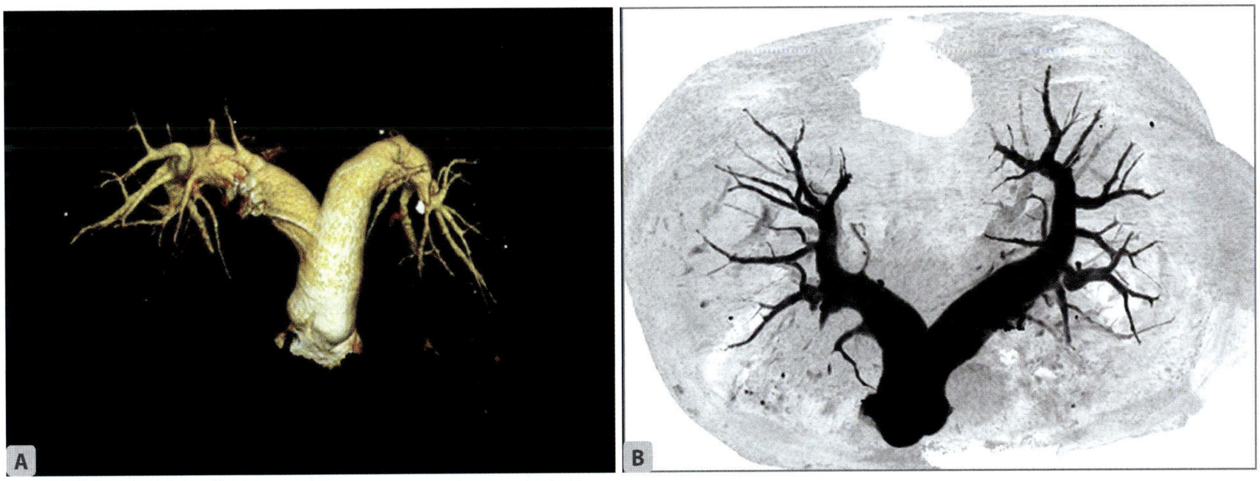

FIGS. 2A AND B: Normal CT pulmonary angiogram: Volume rendered (A) and MIP imaging displayed in the negative or angiographic mode (B) obtained with 30 mL of 350 mg I/mL contrast.

EXTENDED CHEST PAIN PROTOCOL OR TRIPLE RULE OUT CT

In this case, the aim of contrast injection is to achieve opacification of the aorta, coronary arteries and pulmonary arteries simultaneously. 130–160 mL of 300–370 mg I/mL contrast medium is injected between 4–5 mL/s with bolus tracking in the ascending aorta. ECG gating is used to freeze cardiac motion of the coronaries and aortic root. The acquisition is done in the caudocranial direction to minimize streak artefacts from the SVC.[14]

POST-PROCESSING TECHNIQUES[1,11,15,16]

The goal of true isotropic imaging, i.e. each voxel with equal dimensions in all 3 axes was achieved with the introduction of modern MDCT scanners. This allows high-quality 2D and 3D reconstructions, converting CT from a 2D imaging modality to a volumetric or 3D imaging technique. Although, axial images remain critical to establish the diagnosis, these reconstructions are extremely useful for display of airways (including complex congenital abnormalities) vascular structures and distribution of pulmonary disease. Isotropic imaging has also helped the development of computer-aided detection and diagnosis programs. They increase diagnostic confidence, allow preprocedural planning for surgery or bronchoscopy and improve communication with clinicians and patients.

Multiplanar and Curved Multiplanar Reconstruction or Curved Planar Reconstruction (MPR and CMPR)

These are 2D post-processing techniques that can be used to obtain images in coronal, sagittal, oblique or even curved planes by reordering of voxels into a single voxel thick tomographic section, excluding the voxels outside the imaging plane **(Fig. 3)**. They allow viewing of a structure or abnormality in alternative planes, hence are useful when there are interpretative difficulties on axial sections. MPRs are useful for evaluation of large airways, vascular structures and to distinguish periarterialor peribronchial lesions from endoluminal ones. They are especially valuable for determining the craniocaudal length of airway stenosis which may be underestimated on axial images alone. They also allow accurate delineation of structures that run oblique to the axial imaging plane. Demonstration of centrilobular emphysema is facilitated as well. Coronal reformation helps to display of the distribution of parenchymal lung disease, e.g. the craniocaudal gradient in interstitial lung disease. Sagittal images can sharply delineate fissures and help to assess transfissural extension of disease.

Maximum Intensity Projection

Maximum intensity projection (MIPS) is a 3D reconstruction technique in which a ray is passed through the dataset and only pixels above a certain assigned value are used reducing the data to a single plane. (This lacks depth information). Slabs

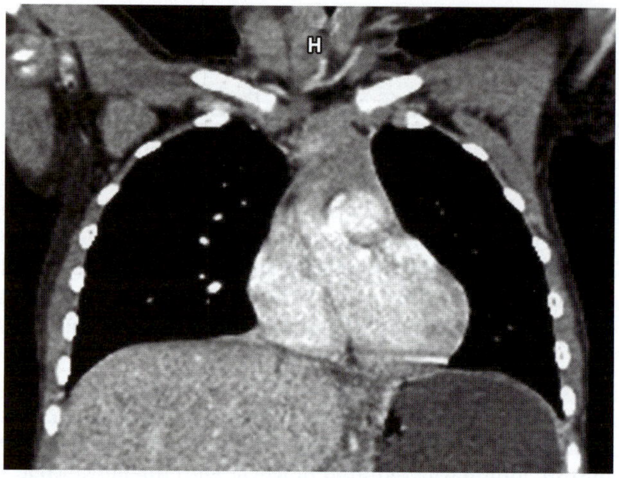

FIG. 3: Coronal multiplanar reconstruction at mediastinal window setting depicting the normal cardiac chambers.

of 5–10 mm for thin MIPS or the entire dateset may be used for thick MIPS. In the thorax, it is used mainly for vascular imaging and for evaluation of small pulmonary nodules where it may help to distinguish small nodules from vessels and in precise delineation of nodule distribution **(Figs. 4A and B)**. In patients with mosaic attenuation, it can help in differentiation of ground-glass attenuation (normal vascular diameter) and mosaic perfusion (altered vascular diameter).

Minimum Intensity Projection (MinIP)

This is similar to MIP hut only data below a certain value is displayed. It is useful to increase the conspicuity of low attenuation areas such as emphysema, air trapping or cystic changes **(Fig. 5)**. It is also useful for detection of ground-glass and linear attenuation patterns. Some authors have also found it useful to distinguish between bronchiectasis and honeycombing and for demonstrating bronchopleural fistula.

Shaded Surface Display

Shaded surface display (SSD) is a 3D surface-rendering technique that defines surface of tissue but does not provide any internal details. It is used in evaluation of airway abnormalities.

Volume-rendering

This is a unique 3D post-processing technique which displays depth information and 3D spatial relationships. A histogram representation of the entire dataset is done based on attenuation values. Voxels that are only partially filled with density of interest are also included. This is then manipulated to display internal and external perspective. The CT attenuation data can be mapped to brightness, color and opacity to display a particular structure of interest. Volume-rendered imagings can provide invaluable information because they preserve the 3D interrelationships of data. This is used extensively in the thorax for angiographic examinations and airway

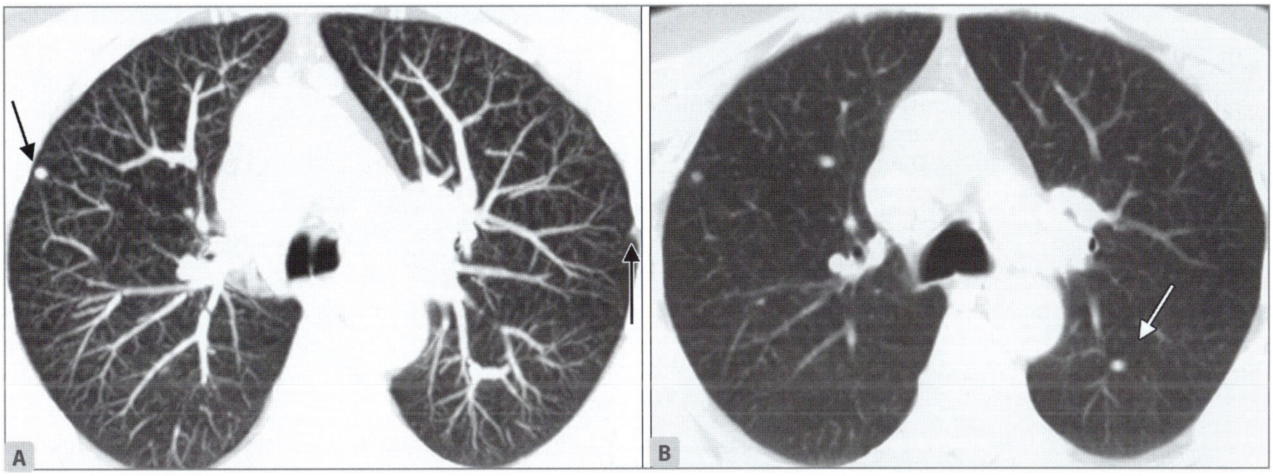

FIGS. 4A AND B: Axial MIP image at lung window settings (A) showing small nodules in the subpleural location on both sides (arrows) which are easily discerned from vessels. Note that one lesion that appears to be a small nodule in the apical segment of left lower lobe (arrow) on the 3 mm axial CT section (B) is actually a vessel on the MIP image.

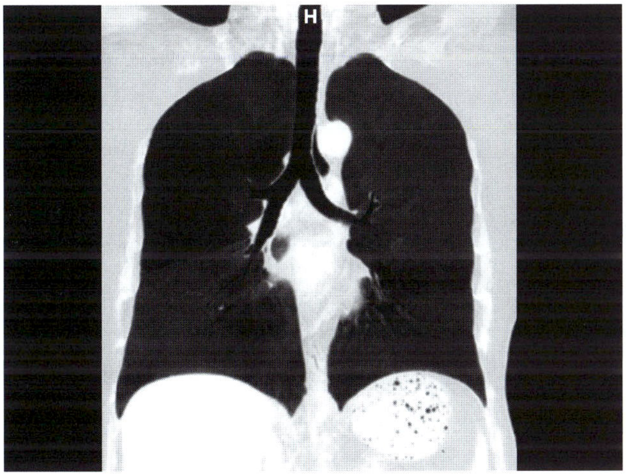

FIG. 5: Coronal MinIP image demonstrating not only the trachea, carina and central bronchi but also the smaller segmental bronchi.

evaluation allowing evaluation of both central and peripheral airways and chest wall abnormalities **(Figs. 6A and B)**. Volume-rendering (VR) technique is extremely useful for evaluation of aneurysms and pseudoaneurysms, dissection, vascular slings and anomalous vessels. These images are valuable for preoperative planning. Imaging of the chest wall and thoracic cage benefits from VR because of the extremely complex anatomy of this region with a number of overlapping structures such as the shoulder girdle.

Virtual Bronchoscopy

Virtual endoscopic images of the airway are produced akin to bronchoscopy using surface and volume-rendering techniques. The major advantage over conventional bronchoscopy is the ability to visualize the airway distal to an obstructing lesion **(Figs. 7A and B)**.

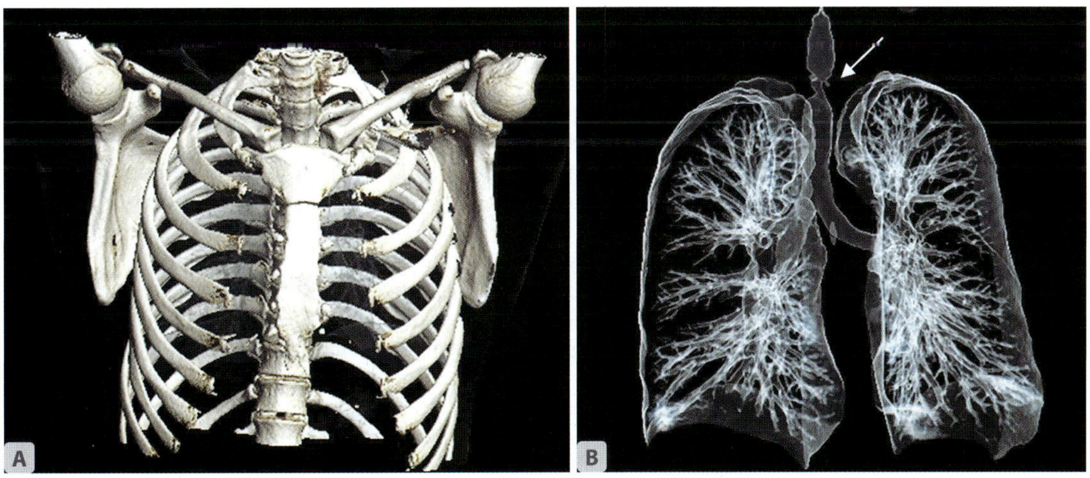

FIGS. 6A AND B: VRT images demonstrating the complex interrelationship between thoracic structures forming the thoracic cage (A) VRT image (transparency rendering) to show the central and peripheral airways. Note the area of narrowing in the trachea (arrow).

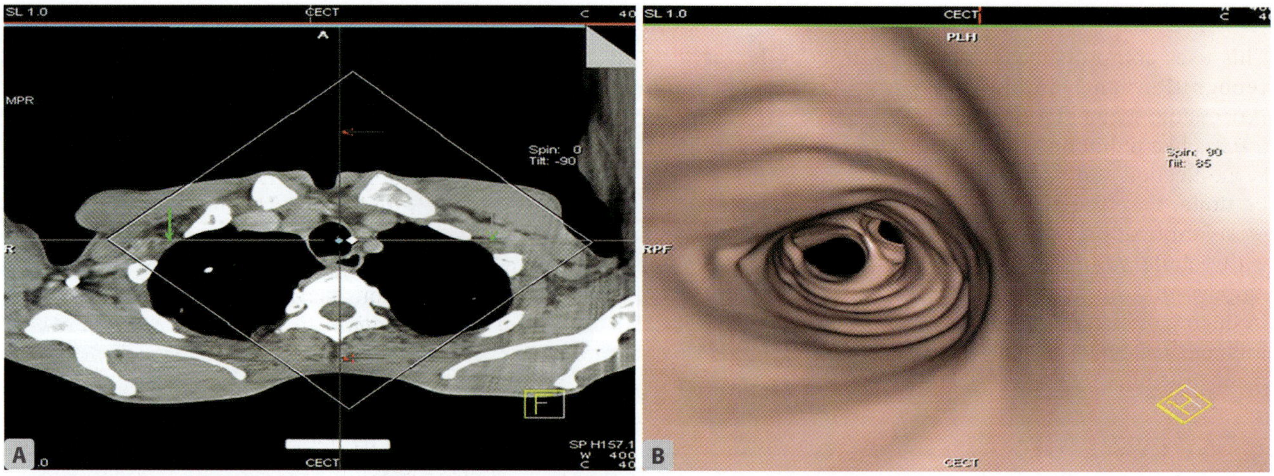

FIGS. 7A AND B: Virtual bronchoscopy image along with a source image showing the normal inner surface of trachea and the carina.

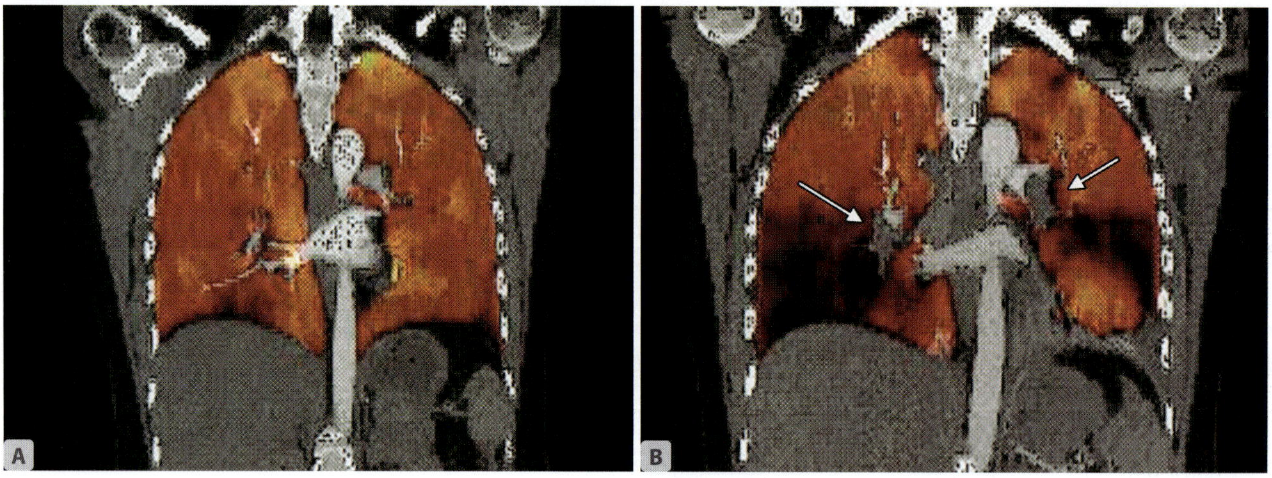

FIGS. 8A AND B: (A) Normal lung perfusion with DE acquisition displayed in a coronal format; (B) Large wedge-shaped perfusion detects due to pulmonary emboli in another patient (arrows).

ADVANCED APPLICATIONS

Dual Energy CT: Thoracic Applications[1]

Dual energy (DE) CT allows differentiation of materials due to their different attenuation properties at different photon energies.[1] DECT requires simultaneous acquisition of data at two different kilo-Voltages, generally 100 kVp and 140 kVp. This can be achieved using a dual-source CT scanner with two X-ray tubes positioned at 90º to each other operating at two different kVs (Siemens) or a single-source CT with rapid KVs switching (GE) or a dual layer detector with different detectors absorbing different energies (Phillips). Recently, one vendor (Siemens) has introduced a single source twin beam dual energy CT which uses two filters one of tin (Sn) and the other gold (Au) to split a 120 Kv beam into a high-energy and low-energy beam respectively allowing DE acquisition.

Thoracic applications are based on the fact that the need for pre- and post-contrast images is eliminated and the computation of pseudomonoenergetic images. This avoids respiratory misregistration and reduces dose. For pulmonary nodule characterization, the generation of virtual noncontrast images thus allows exact enhancement to be measured. Iodine only maps of the lung parenchyma can also be generated to get a map of pulmonary blood volume and lung perfusion. This can help detect perfusion defects in acute and chronic thromboembolism providing a new functional aspect independent of thrombus visualization **(Figs. 8A and B)**.[17]

4D Scanning[18,19]

Dynamic 4D images to gain functional information on breathing mechanism can be obtained using physiologic respiratory triggers. Retrospective gating can be done using a cine mode where the table is still in one breathing cycle and then it is moved to cover a subsequent portion of lung. All the pieces of each respiratory phase are then put together to create a volume data set of the lung or tracheobronchial tree. The other technique is continuous acquisition of the whole chest in free shallow breathing. These can be acquired at low dose protocols with iterative reconstruction algorithms so that the radiation dose is not higher than an average low dose CT. Prospective gating similar to cardiac step and shoot is also becoming available.

Computer-aided Detection

This uses computer-based software for complex pattern recognition and employs a combination of image processing, segmentation and pattern classifiers to identify lesions like pulmonary nodules or emboli. Nodule volume quantification and quantification of pulmonary emboli can be done. Emphysema quantification has also been done by quantification of parenchymal lung density choosing a threshold value (usually below –950 HU) to identify emphysema. However, variation can occur due to differences in degree of inspiration, between contrast-enhanced and noncontrast scans and probably with the use of iterative reconstructions.[1,7,18,19]

DOSE CONSIDERATIONS AND DOSE REDUCTION TECHNIQUES IN THORACIC CT[1,2,20]

In the past few decades, the utilization of CT for diagnostic purposes has increased exponentially raising concerns related to radiation exposure. Complicating this further is the fact that radiation exposure is higher with MDCT scanners as compared with a single slice scanners. This is because with multidetector CT the dose profile is trapezoidal along the Z-axis and only the central or umbral portion of the beam contributes to the image while the penumbral dose is wasted (also referred to as **over beaming) (Fig. 9)** In a single slice CT, on the other hand, in the entire dose contributes to image formation. However, the relative contribution of the penumbral region decreases as the number of simultaneously acquired slices increase thus a 128 slice CT results in less wasted radiation than a 4 slice CT. Gaps between detector elements in MDCT are another reason for decreased geometric efficiency and wasted dose as the photons falling in these regions do not contribute to image formation. Another problem with helical scanners is **over ranging**, i.e. irradiation beyond the imaged length is necessary in helical scanning for reconstruction of first and last images. This is larger with wider Z beam collimation (or larger number of detectors) offsetting improvement in dose efficiency of over beaming for shorter scan lengths. Modern CT systems now have **dynamic collimation diaphragms** such that the collimator opens asymmetrically at the beginning and end of an acquisition to eliminate radiation of tissues outside the range reducing this problem.

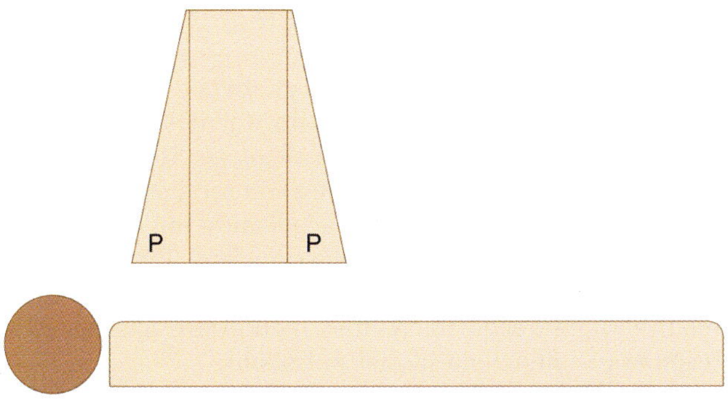

FIG. 9: Line diagram to show the trapezoidal dose profile along the Z-axis. The area outside the rectangle (P) on both sides represents the penumbra.

Dose Reduction Strategies

The first and foremost step in dose reduction is assessment of need. No CT should be performed without a valid indication and each study should be tailored to answer the specific clinical question at hand. Several technological advancements and modifications in technique can result in significant dose reduction. These are:

- *Tube current modulation using automatic exposure control or AEC*: Essentially, there are three methods available. Patient size-based modulation, Z-axis AEC and angular or X-Y-axis AEC. For patient size AEC, the appropriate current is selected by the system for the given patient size. Scanners assess the X-ray absorption profile over the patient's thorax during the topogram or scout acquisition and automatically choose the lowest tube potential for the patient and selected protocol. In the Z-axis or longitudinal modulation, the tube current is adjusted as the patient attenuation changes in the longitudinal direction or Z axis to ensure a constant image quality at each anatomical level. The angular tube current modulation adjusts the tube current as the tube rotates around the patient to compensate for attenuation changes as the view angle changes. The tube current is reduced at angles that are of less diagnostic importance. In most modern scanners automatic tube current modulation (A TCM) adapts the tube current in all 3 X-Y-Z-axes according to patient weight and can result in significant dose reduction while maintaining image quality.

  There are, however, two important considerations: determination of an acceptable level of image noise (this is generally preset by the manufacturer) and optimal patient position. The patient should be positioned centrally on the CT table ideally close to the isocenter prior to acquisition. This is because the use of automatic dose nodulation software in patients who are off the isocenter by as little as 3 mm may result in a 30% higher dose.
- *Tube current reduction in low dose examinations*: A 50% reduction in the tube current can reduce the effective radiation dose to half the original level. Several studies have demonstrated that the tube current time product or mAS may be reduced to levels as low as 40–70 mAS in chest CT without significantly affecting image quality since the lung is a high contrast organ. Most of these have been studies to detect pulmonary nodules in a screening setting. Some authors have demonstrated that common patterns of pulmonary diseases such as solid nodules, air space consolidation, airway and pleural diseases could be adequately demonstrated at 120 kV/40 mAS protocol using thin slices, high spatial frequency reconstruction kernel and standard filtered back projection (FBP) reconstruction. However ground-glass opacities and interstitial opacities require higher tube current or iterative noise reconstruction.
- *Tube potential reduction or low KV examinations*: The standard chest protocol is usually acquired at 120 kV, A low tube potential of 70–80 kV is useful in children and

small adults due to the lower X-ray absorption profile. A tube potential of 80–100 kVp is also beneficial in adults when the area of interest is enhanced by iodinated contrast as for the thoracic aorta or pulmonary arteries. This is because the X-ray attenuation of iodine increases with the use of lower kV due to the K edge of iodine at 33 KeV. The X-ray attenuation of soft tissue depends only weakly on tube potential hence the contrast of vessels and tissue that take up iodinated contrast increases with respect to surrounding tissue increasing the contrast to noise ratio or CNR at the same dose. This effect can be utilized to either reduce radiation dose to patient or reduce the amount of iodinated contrast administered. A trade off while decreasing tube potential or voltage is that the mAs has to thus be significantly increased. Because of the lack of tube power reserves low kV scanning was limited to children and small patients. Recently new X-ray tubes with increased mA reserves and increased power at low kV have been introduced (VECTRON Siemens) which can extend this advantage to adults and obese patients. This may reduce radiation dose by as much as 52%. Technologies that automatically adapt the tube voltage to the size and shape of the patient keeping in mind the power reserves of the tube are also available. This automatic tube voltage selection may reduce radiation dose in CT chest angiographies by as much at 38% compared to 120 KV protocol.

- *Use of a higher pitch*: Pitch is defined as table feed per rotation divided by the total width of the collimated beam. Using a higher table speed for a given collimation can significantly reduce patient dose if all other acquisition parameters are same. An important factor to take into account however is that in some modern scanners, e.g. Siemens and Phillips, an increase in table feed is automatically compensated by an increase in tube current to maintain the same effective tube current time product or **mAS effective** (defined as mAS/pitch). With these scanners an increase in pitch merely reduces examination time and not radiation dose. However, this may be very useful in sick, uncooperative patients in avoiding repeat examinations.
- *Use of filters*: These are of two types:
  - Beam shaping filters: Filters such as bowtie filters reduce ray intensity in the peripheral parts reducing radiation dose, especially skin radiation dose.
  - Spectral shaping: Spectral shaping by using a tin filter in the prepatient tube collimator box can significantly reduce patient dose in noncontrast lung examinations. The filter makes the beam 'harder' removing lower energy photons which would be absorbed in the patient without contributing to the image. This provision is available in the third generation dual source CT system. Low dose CT with spectral shaping and iterative reconstruction can reduce patient dose in quantitative lung CT and non-enhanced CT chest for pulmonary nodule detection to as low as 0.06 mSv when using 100 kv. This effect is however not valid for contrast-enhanced examinations as increased X-ray absorption of iodine at lower energies over compensates this. It also needs to be determined how well subtle features of lung parenchyma can be evaluated at such low doses.
- The length of coverage should be carefully planned so as not to extend the beyond the area of interest.
- Newer detector systems such as the solid state detectors have much higher detector efficiency than the conventional ionisation chamber-based detectors helping to reduce radiation dose.
- *Patient shielding*: Use of lead or lead free shields to protect areas outside the scan zone may help to reduce radiation exposure (e.g. thyroid and gonads). However, the use of bismuth breast shields to reduce radiation exposure to breast tissue during chest CT is not recommended as this increases image noise and artefacts. A similar breast dose reduction can be achieved by the methods already mentioned, such as tube current modulation.
- Newer reconstruction techniques: Newer reconstruction techniques that have become available can also help to reduce exposure indirectly as they help to reduce image noise making it possible to obtain diagnostic images with low dose examinations. CT images were traditionally reconstructed using the **filtered back projection (FBP)** technique. However, this requires a large amount of X-ray data to produce diagnostic quality images. The introduction of **iterative reconstruction (IR)** techniques into routine CT, made possible by the increased computational power of computers greatly enhances image resolution and reduces noise. In FBP increased spatial resolution is directly correlated with increased image noise while IR allows for decoupling of spatial resolution and image noise to a certain extent. (It maintains or enhances spatial resolution for high contrast objects while reducing noise in low-contrast areas). The first generations IR algorithms were image based IR, the second generation statistical weight based while the latest third-generation IR algorithms are model-based IR. It is reported that with the use of iterative reconstruction radiation dose could be reduced to less than 2 mSv for contrast-enhanced chest CT and to sub-mSv levels for noncontrast CT chest.
- Prospective ECG gating rather than retrospective gating for ECG gated examinations also reduces radiation exposure.

MAGNETIC RESONANCE IMAGING

The superior soft tissue contrast of MRI over CT ensures better tissue characterization in the evaluation of mediastinal masses, chest wall and diaphragm. In these areas, MRI already has an established role in diagnosis. However, most often it is performed subsequent to a CT examination not only due to the latter's faster image acquisition but also greater acceptance and familiarity among clinicians. The challenges to magnetic resonance imaging of the chest are due to its relatively longer acquisition times, motion artefacts related to respiratory motion and cardiac pulsations.

MR imaging of the lung especially is a very challenging field. This is because about 70% of the lung consists of air-filled spaces. Protons are localized within the tissues of the lung or blood vessels accounting for only 30% of the volume.

The healthy lung thus has a tissue proton density which is about ten times lower than other tissues producing a signal that is 10 times weaker than other tissues even under perfect conditions.[21] The generation of MR signal from even these protons is hampered by two factors: the lung has countless air tissue interfaces which have very different magnetic properties leading to susceptibility artefacts with resultant loss of signal in structures such as alveolar septae and the pulsatile nature of blood flow. These problems are further compounded by artefacts due to respiratory and cardiac motion making lung one of the most difficult organs to image on MR. The susceptibility differences result in rapid dephasing of spins in gradient echo imaging hence pulse sequences with very short echo times (TE <1–2 ms) are required. The magnetic field inhomogeneity increases with field strength hence even shorter TE's would be required for 3T systems offsetting the expected increase in SNR.[21]

Recently, there have been several advances in hardware and pulse design helping to overcome several of these limitations—such as multichannel MR systems, powerful gradients, parallel imaging, very short echo times, ultrafast turbo spin echo acquisitions, etc. These along with improved technology for k space sampling and development of contrast agents for perfusion and ventilation studies have put MR on the threshold of a radiation free alternative to CT in some clinical situations.[22-24]

TECHNICAL CONSIDERATIONS

Magnet Strength and Coils

For MRI of the thorax scanners with **a field strength** of 1.5 T and full parallel imaging capability are recommended. Chest MRI at 3T is more challenging because though theoretically, there should be an increase in SNR, this is offset by the faster signal decay due to susceptibility artefacts in the lungs. There are changes in relaxation times, increased magnetic field inhomogenity and increased SAR with 3T imaging hence modifications are required for imaging of the mediastinum, as well. The latest generation of MR scanners do provide some pretailored sequences for thoracic imaging allowing good quality images on 3T. Although field strength lower then 1.5 T has some potential advantages with respect to lung field homogeneity it requires signal averaging to improve SNR making imaging times unacceptably long.[21]

Along with the **spine coil** integrated in the table receive only **phased array body coils** are used over the chest. These increase SNR and allow parallel imaging reducing acquisition time. The coverage must be adequate in the craniocaudal and anteroposterior direction.[25]

Respiratory Motion

The availability of fast imaging sequences on modern scanners has ensured that most sequences can be acquired in less than 20 seconds. Thus, it is advisable to acquire images during a single breath hold or as a multibreath hold sequence. This minimizes blur associated with respiratory motion and is better than triggered or navigator sequences. The success of breath hold imaging can be significantly increased provided breath holding is rehearsed with the patient before lying down and the patient is informed about the frequency and duration of breath hold. If breath hold difficulty is anticipated, a MR compatible 2L nasal cannula oxygen can be provided to improve breath hold.[26] In patients who are unable to hold breath and for longer sequences synchronization of the image acquisition to the respiratory cycle is done. This can be done using respiratory or spirometric triggering or gating using external hardware such as pneumatic bellows or the signal of lung itself. Another method is to use navigator echoes to detect the motion of the diaphragm directly via MRI which can be used for retrospective gating of scans during free breathing.[21]

Cardiac Gating

Cardiac gating is useful to freeze cardiac motion for evaluation of cardiac and paracardiac lesions. ECG gating is preferred to peripheral gating because it freezes cardiac motion more reliably, eliminating pulsatility artefacts.[26]

PROTOCOL AND SEQUENCES

A basic protocol consists of noncontrast breath hold T1- and T2-weighted sequences without fat saturation. Gadolinium-based contrast agents are required for a number of indications such as evaluation of mediastinal and lung masses or pulmonary nodules, chest wall masses, pleural pathology, lung perfusion and evaluation of vasculature. A set of precontrast TIW images are acquired without fat saturation to facilitate detection of mediastinal nodes or masses surrounded by fat while postcontrast images are acquired with fat saturation. This may be done using the DIXON technique for a more homogeneous fat saturation near the neck. Identical parameters should be used for pre and post-contrast images when evaluating enhancement.[21,25] The postcontrast images can be acquired as a single post contrast T1W fat saturated sequence or as a dynamic contrast-enhanced examination (DCE) where multiple fast. 3D-T1W-GRE acquisitions are done after intravenous contrast.

Advantages of the dynamic technique include ability to show rate of enhancement over time, eliminating guess work about when maximal vascular or lesion enhancement will occur. The pattern of enhancement may help to increase specificity of diagnosis. In addition because exactly the same imaging parameters are used in the pre- and postcontrast acquisition, it is possible to measure relative ROI assessment of lesion hyperintensity and to subtract postcontrast images from precontrast which is very useful to assess enhancement in T1W hyperintense lesions.

The details of sequences used in MRI are summarized in **Table 1**. These sequences are obtained in the standard axial, coronal and sagittal planes. Additional planes may be used to optimize lesion characterization, e.g. to better characterize mediastinal or chest wall invasion acquisition can be planned to get images perpendicular or parallel to the site of invasion.

TABLE 1: Sequences for lung and mediastinal MRI.[21,25,27,28]

S. No.		Sequence	Vendor Acronym	Characteristics/Advantages	Uses
1.	3D T1W GRE	GRE with parallel imaging/ slice interpolation	VIBE / THRIVE / LAVA	Covers entire thorax/lung in single breath hold at 5 mm slices	Pulmonary nodules masses
		With fat saturation (use Dixon for more homogeneous fat suppression)		Postcontrast imaging dynamic acquisition possible	• Airways • Dynamic for lung nodules • Dynamic lung volume • Tumor mobility for RT planning
		Heavily T1W 3D GRE	Flash 3D/FFE/SPGR	High spatial resolution for angiography (1.2 x 1 mm)	High resolution pulmonary angiography
		3D–GRE with echo sharing	TWIST/TRICKS/TRAK, etc.	Low spatial but high temporal resolution (<1–5 ms)	Lung perfusion and multiphase angiography
2.	Fast spin-echo T2W	Half fourier acquisition single shot TSE	HASTE/half scan FSE/½ NEXFSE	• Single/multibreath hold acquisition to cover entire chest • Low spatial, high temporal resolution • High SAR makes use at 3 T challenging	• Pulmonary infiltrates, bronchiectasis • Bronchial wall thickening
		• Rotating phase encoding • Central K space over sampling and inherent motion correction	BLADE/PROPELLOR/ Multivane	• Multibreath hold with moderate spatial resolution • Less motion artefacts from respiration and cardiac motion	• Pulmonary nodules and masses • Lymphadenopathy
		Conventional high resolution T2W/TSE	TSE/FSE	• Respiratory triggered acquisition during shallow breathing	Increased sharpness of lung pleural interphase
			Fat saturated FSE/BLADE, etc.		• Lymphadenopathy • Excellent for bone metastasis
3.	T2W GRE	Balanced steady state free precession (GRE)	True FISP/SSFE/FIESTA, etc.	*At short TR contrast is proportional to T2/T1*: • Single breath hold/free breathing Excellent anatomic information and soft tissue contrast Cine imaging possible *Disadvantages*: • High SAR • Susceptible to off resonance and field inhomogeneities resulting in banding artefacts especially at 3 T	• Effective for imaging blood and mucus (due to their long T2) • Differentiate masses/nodes vs vessels due to bright blood appearance • Respiratory mechanics diaphragmatic excursion • Relative tumor motion to assess mediastinal/chest wall invasion

Contd...

Contd...

TABLE 1: Sequences for lung and mediastinal MRI.[21,25,27,28]

S. No.		Sequence	Vendor Acronym	Characteristics/Advantages	Uses
			3D – bSSFP		Quick contrast free pulmonary angiogram Evaluation of pulmonary embolism without contrast
4.	STIR			Respiratory triggered sequence	Lymph node, bone metastases, lung nodule detection
5.	DWI (3 'b' values)	EPI		Respiratory triggered	Benign vs malignant pulmonary nodule/ masses, COPD
6.	Dual echo 2D GRE (T1 SPGR) In-opposed phase imaging (chemical shift)*		Turbo FLASH/FSPGR/TSE	Single breath hold imaging possible Detects microscopic fat	Useful for thymic hyperplasia vs neoplasm. Pulmonary hamartoma
7.	Double IR T2 cardiac gated		Double IR FSE 2/FSE 2/UFSE 2	Cardiac gated respiratory gated/breath hold	Exquisite anatomical information of mediastinal structures and cardiac chambers
8.	Double IR T1 cardiac gated		Double IR prep TSE T1/FSE 1/ SFSE T1	Fat saturation can be added	Exquisite anatomical information of mediastinal structures and cardiac chambers

*Some authors have reported that in and out of phase images from precontrast 3D–T1 SPGR with Dixon technique can provide similar information as a separate in—opposed phase sequence saving time.[21]

(bFFE: balanced fast field echo (gradient echo sequence with steady state acquisition: (Philips); BLADE: brand name/not an acronym (rotating phase encoding sequence; Siemens); FFE: fast field echo (gradient echo sequence synonymous to FLASH; (Toshiba, Philips); FIESTA: fast imaging employing steady-state acquisition (gradient echo sequence with steady state acquisition; GE); FLASH: fast low-angle shot (GE; Siemens); FSE: fast spin-echo (sequence; GE, Hitachi, Toshiba); GRE: gradient echo (gradient echo sequence); Half scan: Half Fourier acquisition technique (Philips, Hitachi); HASTE: half-Fourier short turbo spin echo (sequence; Siemens); LAVA: liver acquisition with volume acceleration (a 3D gradient echo sequence with volume interpolation and RF fast saturation (GE); MRA: magnetic resonance angiography; Multi Vane: Brand name/not an acronym (rotating phase encoding sequence; Philips); SPGR: spoiled gradient echo recalled (sequence synonymous to FLASH; GE); SSFP: steady state free precession (gradient echo sequence with steady state acquisition); STIR: short tau inversion recovery sequence; THRIVE: T1 high-resolution isotropic volume excitation (a 3D gradient echo sequence with volume interpolation and RF fat saturation; Philips); TRAK: time-resolved angiography using keyhole (a temporally resolved 3D gradient echo sequence with temporal resolution (3D+T) achieved by echo sharing; Philips); TRICKS: time-resolved imaging of contrast Kinetics (a temporally resolved 3D gradient echo sequence with temporal resolution (3D+T) achieved by echo sharing; GE Philips; True FISP: True fast imaging with steady-state precession (gradient echo sequence with steady-state acquisition; Siemens); True SSFP: true steady state free precession (gradient echo sequence with steady state acquisition; Toshiba); TWIST: time-resolved angiography with stochastic trajectories (temporally resolved 3D gradient echo sequence with temporal resolution (3D+t) achieved by echo sharing' Siemens); VIBE: volumetric interpolated breath-hold examination (a 3D gradient echo sequence with volume interpolation and RF fat saturation; Siemens).

MR PULMONARY ANGIOGRAPHY

Heavily T1W 3D GRE FLASH/SPGR/FFE) sequences are used to obtain high resolution breath hold pulmonary angiograms. The shortest possible TR and TE is used with modest parallel imaging. Contrast is usually given via a pressure injector in a dose of 0.2 mL/kg body weight at 2–3 mL followed by a saline flush of 20 mL at 5 mL/sec. The acquisition is optimized to peak vascular enhancement using a test bolus or care bolus technique.

Alternatively a time resolved 3D sequence with echo sharing such as TRICKS/TREAT/TWIST can be used after intravenous injection of gadolinium, the so called "4D MRA" (3D over time). Acquisition times of 1.5 sec or less are possible so that multiple data sets in arterial and venous phases can be acquired **(Figs. 10A to D)**. The postcontrast images are subtracted from the precontrast images to enhance visualization of vasculature.[21,28]

MR PERFUSION IMAGING

MR perfusion of the lung or mediastinum is feasible using a time resolved low spatial resolution version of the time resolved pulmonary angiography sequence. With parallel imaging and view sharing spatial resolution can be enhanced. At a temporal resolution of <1s per 3D data set, this allows generation of passage kinetics curves and parametric maps of regional blood flow and blood volume. The contrast dose needed for a perfusion study is lower than that needed for a pulmonary angiography at 0.05 mL/kg followed by a 20 mL saline flush at 5 mL/sec. Generation of fully quantitative map of pulmonary blood volume PBV, pulmonary blood flow PBF and transit time (MTT) requires a deconvolution with arterial input function (AIF) measured in the larger arteries **(Figs. 11A and B)**. This may be challenging due to lack of linearity between local tissue contrast agent concentration and MR signal intensity. MR perfusion can provide information not just on presence or absence of perfusion but also on the time course of perfusion or capillary filling time. Delayed filling presumably via collaterals can be identified. Pulmonary hemodynamics and blood flow can also be analyzed using techniques developed for cardiac MRI.

Noncontrast methods proposed for assessing pulmonary perfusion include **arterial spin labeling techniques (ASL)**. Although several different variants of this have been proposed, they largely remain experimental.

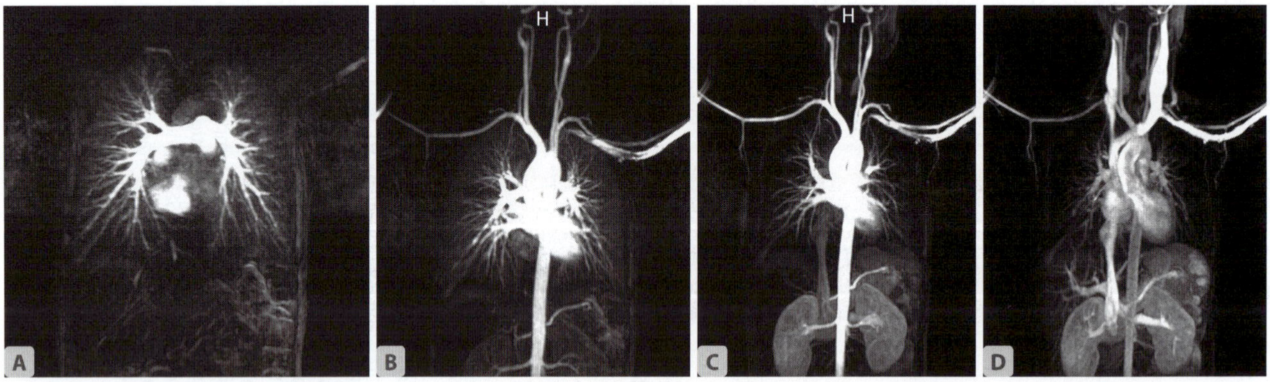

FIGS. 10A TO D: Multiphasic pulmonary angiogram using TWIST on a 3 T magnet. Note all the phases from the pulmonary opacification in the first image (A) to venous in the last image (D).

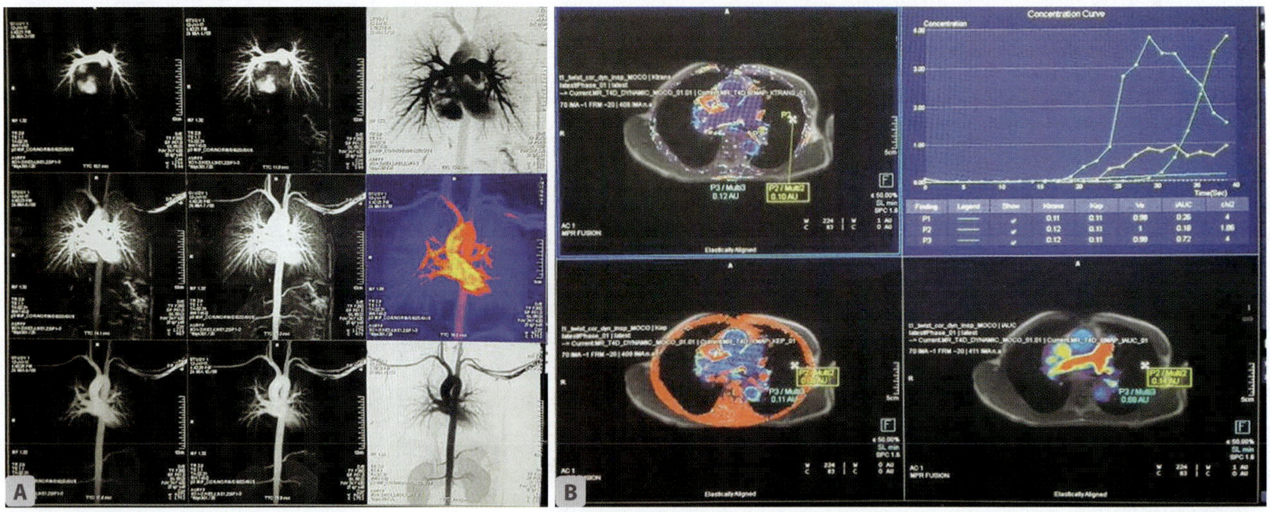

FIGS. 11A AND B: Multiphasic MR acquisition with generation of qualitative perfusion maps (A) and quantitative perfusion curves; (B) The yellow curve represents the pulmonary perfusion.

OTHER ADVANCED/NEWER IMAGING TECHNIQUES

Ultrashort Echo Time Imaging

Ultrashort echo time (UTE) sequences that use radial K space sampling have recently become available. These shorten echo times to below 1 ms. At these very short TE (≤100 ms) the short T2 of the lung is less problematic and images with parenchymal sensitivity are possible. The resolution of these images is below the routine images, however they do make possible proton density contrast which allows visualization of parenchymal lung disease hitherto impossible with MRI.

Novel Contrast Methods and Ventilation MR

Ventilation is the second important aspect of gas exchange in the lung. 4D-MRI can visualize breathing motion and analyze lung volumes which have demonstrated excellent agreement with spirometric studies.

Direct visualization of lung ventilation can be done using hyperpolarized noble gases, sulfur hexafluoride or oxygen inhalation. Oxygen is paramagnetic, when the patient breathes in pure oxygen instead of air, it shortens the T1 of blood, plasma and tissue in the lungs resulting in an increase in signal. This can be used to generate parametric maps with ventilation and perfusion weighting. Hyperpolarized noble gases like Xe-129 and He-3 can also be used to give high signal to noise images of lung ventilation. These techniques, however largely remain experimental.

CLINICAL APPLICATIONS OF MR THORAX

There are a number of emerging areas of thoracic imaging (besides cardiac applications) where MRI can play a significant role depending on the availability of expertise.

Mediastinum

MR can help to better characterize mediastinal abnormalities and masses. It is superior to CT in distinguishing solid from cystic masses, presence of hemorrhage and can help to detect both microscopic and macroscopic fat within the lesion. The detection of microscopic fat by chemical shift MR can help to distinguish between thymic hyperplasia (which has microscopic fat) from tumor (which lacks microscopic fat). Dynamic contrast enhancement patterns and low ADC values have been used to distinguish between benign and malignant lesions. Due to superior demonstration of fat planes and cine imaging capability MR can help to more accurately demonstrate lesion invasiveness, its relationship to critical vascular structures and discernment of mediastinal from paramediastinal lesions. Mediastinal and hilar nodes can be easily detected without the use of contrast however calcified nodes are difficult to detect.

Pulmonary Embolism and Pulmonary Hypertension

In a meta-analysis gadolinium enhanced MRA has a reported sensitivity varying from 77–100% and specificity of 95–98%.[30] The sensitivity is reported to be 100% for central and lobar arteries while it falls to 40% for subsegmental branches. MRA with MR perfusion has been shown to be highly accurate (98%) for detection of embolism with the perfusion sequence having a sensitivity of 100% and specificity 91%.[29,31] MR imaging using a combination of MRA and perfusion sequence allows differentiation between idiopathic pulmonary artery hypertension and secondary pulmonary artery hypertension due to thromboembolic disease. The latter shows features of segmental perfusion defects besides vascular change while the idiopathic variety shows a more diffuse and patchy perfusion pattern.[24,32] Even more importantly MR allows assessment of right ventricular dilatation, hypertrophy and estimation of cardiac strain and pulmonary artery pressures.[23]

Lung Cancer

In lung cancer imaging MR has a role in evaluation of Pancoast's tumors where it is reported to be more accurate than CT in demonstrating blood vessel and brachial plexus involvement. It is superior to CT for demonstrating pericardial, heart, mediastinal, vessel and chest wall involvement and may be indicated in specific situations as a problem-solving tool. MR may also be useful to distinguish between a central mass and postobstructive atelectasis, the latter showing higher signal intensity on T2W images, the central mass also shows lower ADC values than atelectasis **(Figs. 12A to D)**.[23,24]

Detection and Characterization of Pulmonary Nodule

MRI and CT have been reported to be equally accurate in distinguishing between benign and malignant pulmonary nodules in a recent meta-analysis.[32,33] For nodule detection noncontrast MR has significantly lower sensitivity (82.5%) as compared to MDCT (97%) but in detection of malignant nodules, there is no significant difference between the two techniques **(Figs. 13A and B)**. Nodules smaller than 5 mm are difficult to detect on MR. Malignant nodules have been reported to show lower ADC values than benign nodules. Enhancement characteristics can also be assessed using contrast-enhanced dynamic MR sequence. In and opposed phase imaging have been used to demonstrate microscopic fat in pulmonary hamartoma.[34]

Pneumonitis

In children with suspected pneumonitis MR can detect thoracic abnormalities such as consolidation, ill-defined nodules and effusions.[23,27] In a recent study, rapid lung MR has been reported to be comparable to MDCT in detecting thoracic abnormalities in pediatric patients with suspected pulmonary infection.[35] MR may be used in the follow up of pulmonary infections in order to reduce radiation exposure associated with CT.

Emphysema and Chronic Obstructive Pulmonary Disease

Researchers have attempted to use ventilation MR using He-3 to grade and characterise chronic obstructive pulmonary disease (COPD) with large wedge shaped or lobar defects

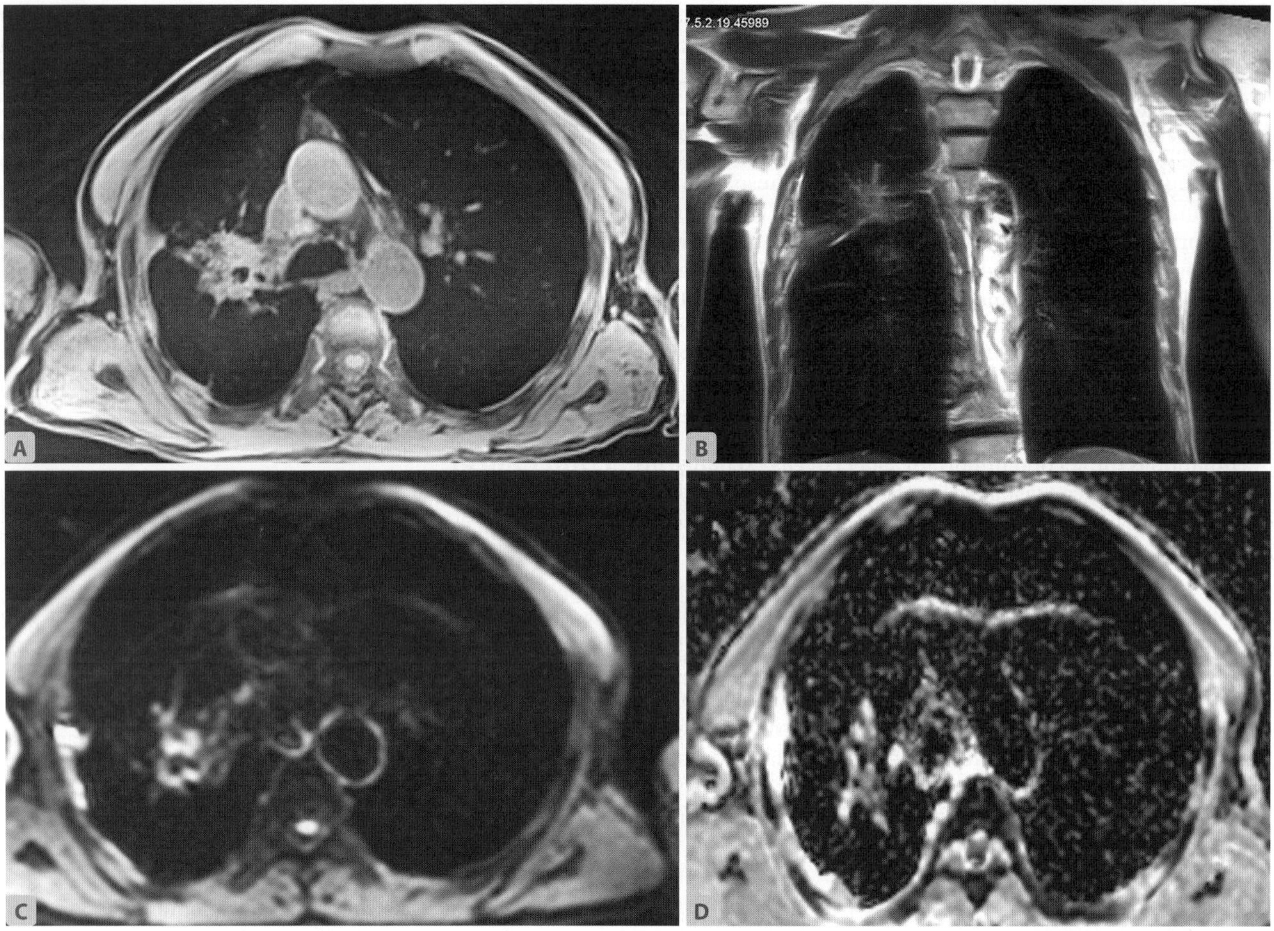

FIGS. 12A TO D: Axial T1(A) and coronal T2W (B) images in a case of lung cancer show a spiculated mass obstructing the right upper lobe bronchus with a pleural tail. DWI and ADC Map (C and D). Note the areas of diffusion restriction within the mass and in the pleura suggesting pleural spread.

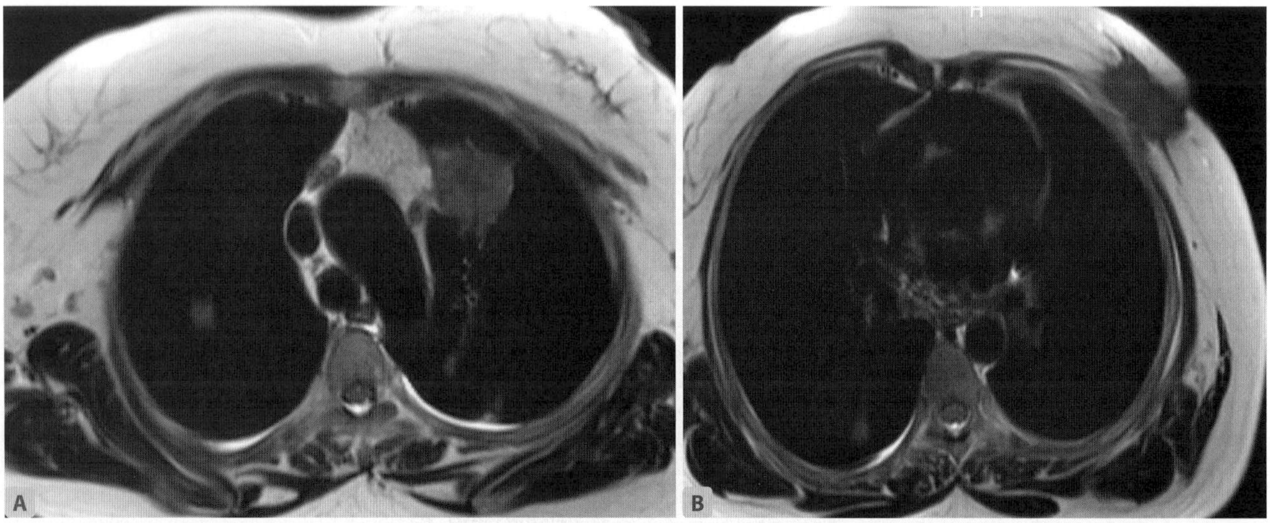

FIGS. 13A AND B: Axial T2W (HASTE) MR images show multiple lung metastases that appear hyperintense to skeletal muscle in a patient with carcinoma breast. Note the mass lesion in the right breast.

being typical of advanced COPD. Alveolar filling time can be calculated using dynamic imaging of ventilation kinetics and alveolar size estimation may be done using ADC. MR perfusion can show perfusion defects correlating with severity due to hypoxic vasoconstriction. It can also evaluate diaphragmatic motion and dynamic lung volumes which are often altered in these patients.[23,27]

Cystic Fibrosis

Since patients with cystic fibrosis are young at presentation and require multiple examinations for follow-up MR-has been suggested as a tool for follow-up imaging. MR has been reported to be comparable to CT in detecting morphological lung changes while it is superior to CT in assessment of functional alterations. It is possible to visualize bronchiectasis, bronchial wall thickening, mucus plugging, air fluid levels and consolidation on MR. Functional assessment includes evaluation of respiratory mechanics, lung perfusion, blood flow and pulmonary ventilation using hyperpolarized gases for MRI.[22,24,27]

Interstitial Lung Disease

Three essential applications of MR have been suggested in literature—assessment of morphological changes and patterns, evaluation of inflammatory disease activity and effect of morphological changes on functional parameters. Consolidation, fibrotic changes, nodules, reticulation, etc. can be detected due to the increased T2W signal although subtle changes in subpleural region are difficult to detect. Post-contrast T1W images which increase the signal of the lung have been used to assess honeycombing. Dynamic MR and differences in T2W signal have been used to distinguish between active inflammation from fibrosis **(Figs. 14A and B)**.[27]

Pleura, Chest Wall and Diaphragm

MR can easily demonstrate pleural effusion, deposits and plaques of asbestosis. It is superior to CT in distinguishing pleural effusion from thickening and discernment of pleural invasion by tumours. Calcifications, a sign of benignity are however not well seen. MR is routinely used for evaluating chest wall masses to demonstrate the exact extent and invasion by the mass. MR can also be used to evaluate diaphragmatic pathologies like eventration, hernia and paralysis **(Figs. 15A to D)**.[25,27]

NORMAL ANATOMY

MEDIASTINUM

Normal mediastinal anatomy can be evaluated by analyzing CT or MR images at certain predefined anatomical levels due their characteristic appearance and landmarks.

Axial Sections (Cranial to Caudal)

Thoracic Inlet (Junction of Neck and Thorax)

Most mediastinal structures are vascular at this level. The internal jugular veins join the subclavian veins to from the brachiocephalic veins posterior to the clavicular heads. These veins are the most anterior and lateral vessels at this level. Medially lie the two common carotid arteries-while just posteriorly are the two subclavian arteries. The SCA cross over the first rib to exit the mediastinum and enter the axilla. The esophagus lies posterior or posterolateral to the trachea **(Fig. 16A)**.

Left Brachiocephalic Vein Level

The left brachiocephalic vein crosses the midline just beneath the manubrium to join the vertically oriented right brachiocephalic vein to form the superior vena cava. Between the brachiocephalic vein and the trachea are the three major branches of the arch of aorta—the innominate artery which is nearly midline, the left common carotid artery which is slightly to the left and posterior and the left subclavian artery which is the most posterior and lateral vessel in close contact with the left upper lobe **(Fig. 16B)**.

Aortic Arch Level

The aortic arch traverses obliquely from right to left and anterior to posterior to left side anteriorly posteriorly just

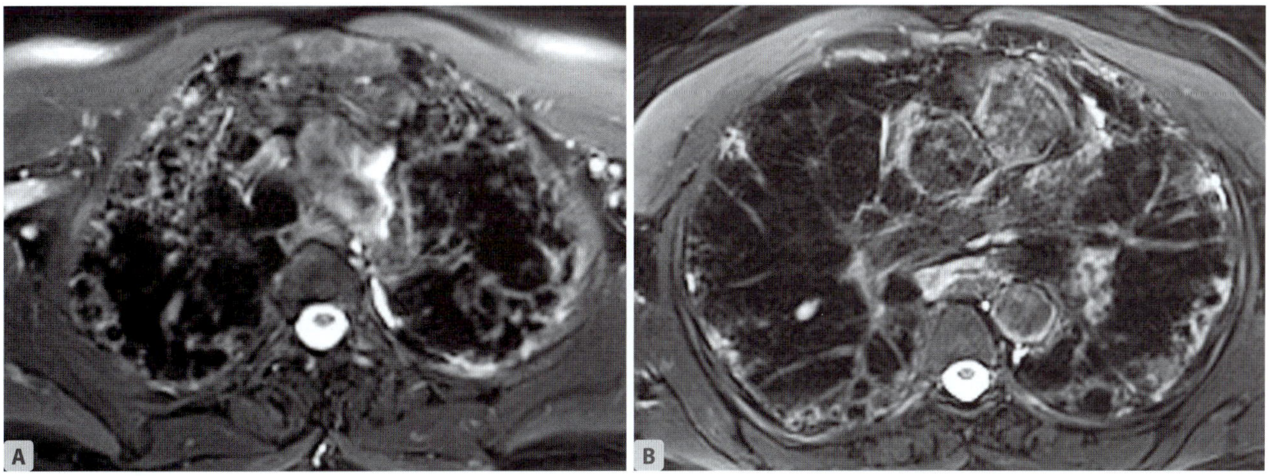

FIGS. 14A AND B: T2W images (FSE BLADE with fat saturation) show honeycombing in the subpleural regions of both lungs. Note some areas show higher signal, than the rest on the T2W images suggesting active inflammation according to some researchers.

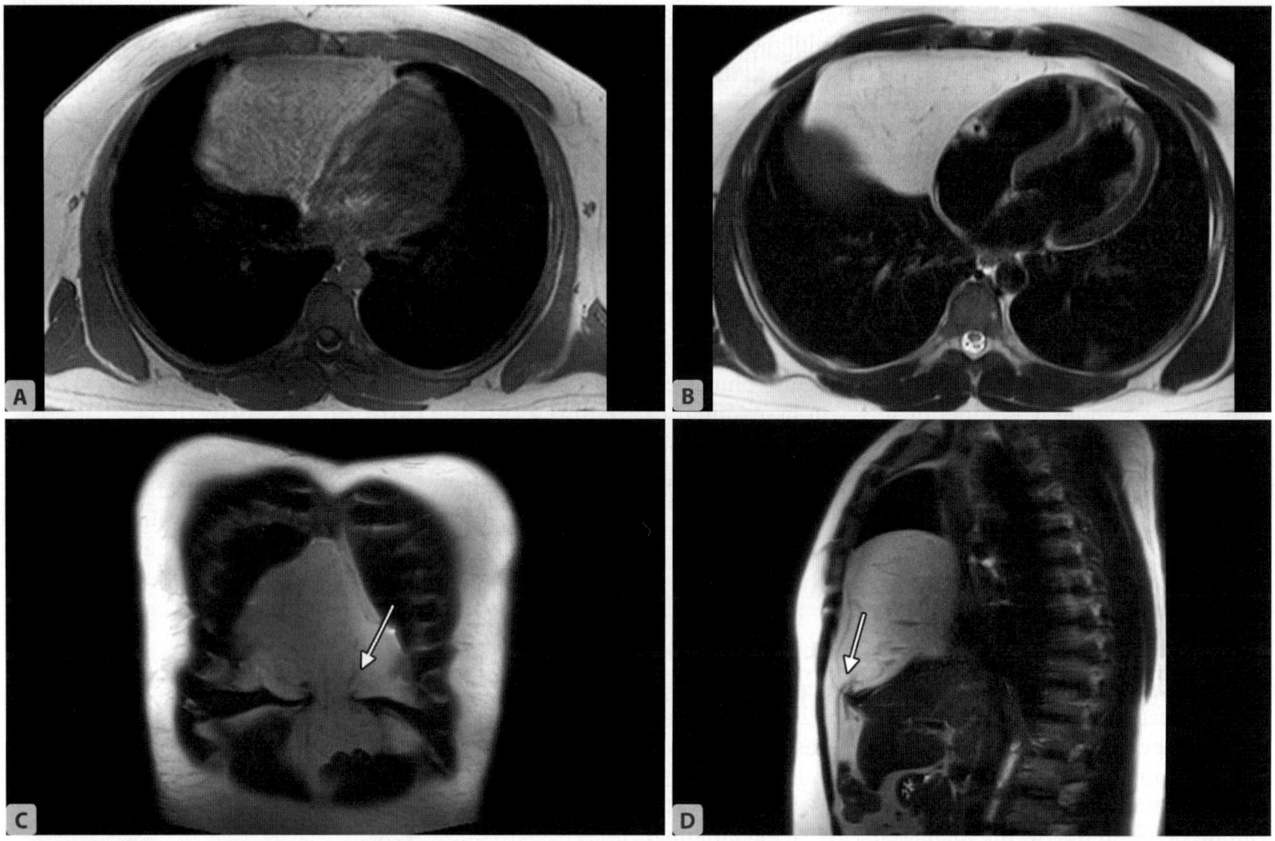

FIGS. 15A TO D: Axial T1W FLASH (A) and T2W HASTE (B) in a case of Morgagni's hernia show a paracardiac mass with signal identical to subcutaneous fat. The diaphragmatic discontinuity (arrows) through which the omentum is herniating into the thorax is well seen on the coronal and sagittal HASTE images (C and D).

anterior to the trachea. The superior vena cava is seen in cross section adjacent to the anterior portion of the arch to the right side of trachea. The space posterior to the SVC, anterior to the trachea and lateral to the transverse aorta is the pretracheal space or anterior paratracheal space. Anterior to the great vessels and brachiocephalic veins is prevascular space. Both these spaces contain fat and small lymph nodes. Posterior or posterolateral to the trachea and anterior to the spine is esophagus **(Fig. 16C)**.

Azygos Arch-aortopulmonary Window Level

The azygos vein arches anteriorly from its location just anterior and slightly to the right of the spine to join the SVC. The entire arch may not be visible in a single section and occasionally this is poorly opacified leading to confusion with lymphadenopathy. The ascending aorta lies anterior to the trachea and descending aorta on the left posterolateral aspect of trachea. The ascending aorta in larger than the descending aorta measuring about 3.5 cm in mean diameter while the descending measures about 2.5 cm (this varies with age and sex). The aortopulmonary window is also seen at this level as a fat filled space. It is located between the inferior aspect of aortic arch superiorly and the superior aspect left pulmonary artery inferiorly. The contents of this important space include lymph nodes, left recurrent laryngeal nerve and the ligamentum arteriosum. The esophagus is seen anterior to the spine and posterior to trachea **(Fig. 16D)**.

Left Pulmonary Artery Level

The left pulmonary artery (LPA) is seen at a superior level compared to the main pulmonary artery and is located anterolateral to the left main bronchus at the level of carina. The left superior pulmonary veins are located just lateral to the posterior LPA. The right upper lobe bronchus can be seen arising from the right main bronchus at the level of carina. The right upper lobe pulmonary artery also called truncus anterior lies anterior to the right upper lobe bronchus. To the right of the esophagus lies the azygos vein. The hemi azygos vein lies to the left of the spine and parallels the course of the azygos vein. Along the posterior aspect of ascending aorta and anterior to the carina is a crescentic extension of the pericardium—the superior pericardial recess. It may contain a small amount of fluid or extend to more cephalad location and must not be confused with a lymph node or mass. Demonstrating continuity with the superior pericardial recess on contiguous sections can help to establish the true nature of a high riding pericardial recess **(Fig. 16E)**.

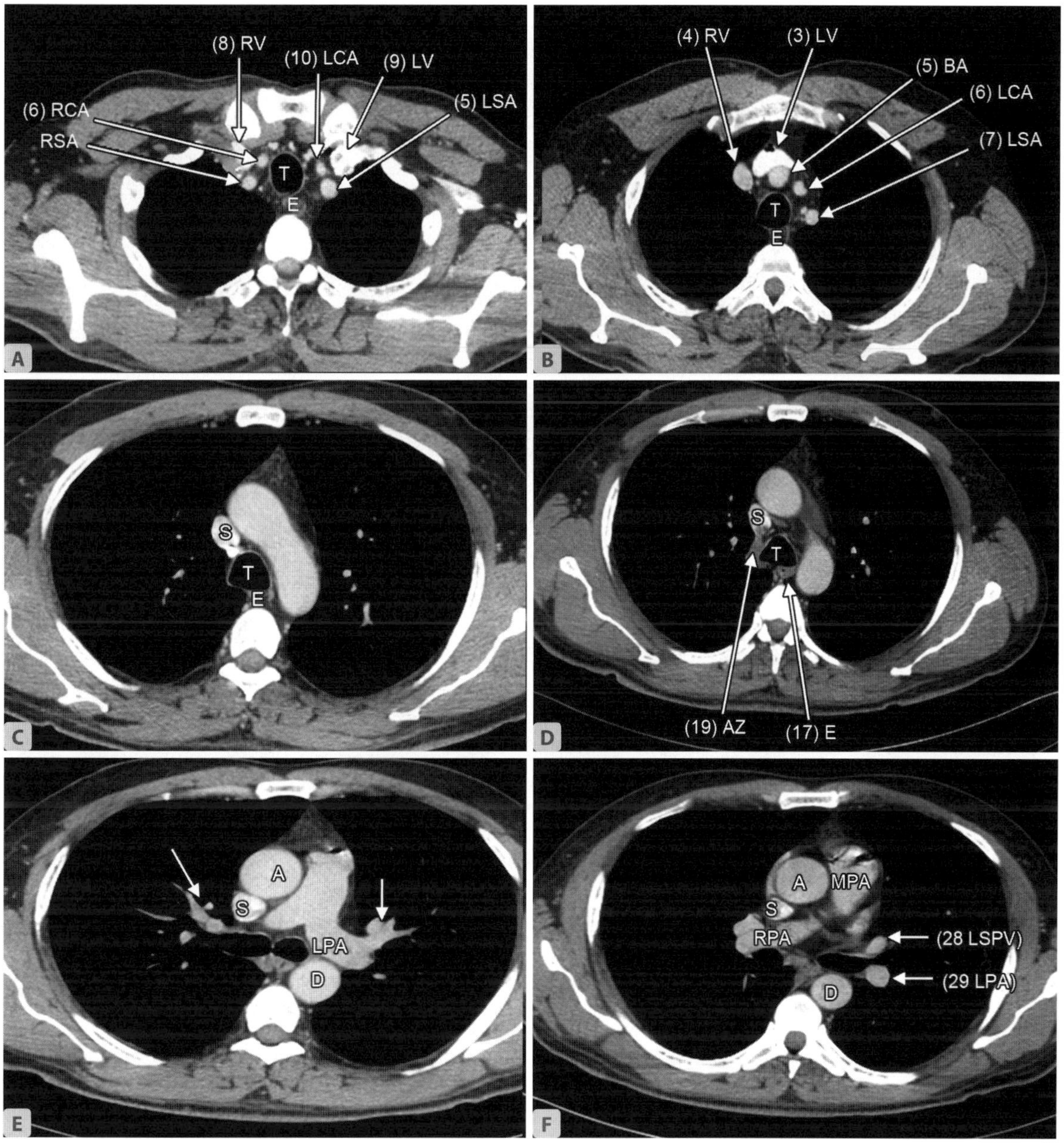

FIGS. 16A TO F: (A) Thoracic inlet level: The trachea (T) and esophagus (E) in midline. RV, Right brachiocephalic vein; RSA, right subclavian artery; RCA, right common carotid artery; LV, left brachiocephalic vein; LSA, left subclavian artery; LCA, left common carotid artery; (B) Left brachiocephalic vein level: Trachea (T), and esophagus (E); left subclavian artery (LSA); left common carotid artery (LCC); the right brachiocephalic vein (BRV) and left brachiocephalic veins (BLV) are anterior to the right brachiocephalic artery (BA); (C) Aortic arch level: The superior vena cava (S) and aortic arch lie anterior to the trachea (T) and esophagus (E). Anterior to the arch is the thymus, which has undergone fatty replacement; (D) Azygos arch-aortopulmonary window level: E, esophagus; T, trachea; the azygos vein (AZ) arches from a posterior position beside the esophagus to join the superior vena cava (S) crossing over the right upper lobe bronchus. The aortopulmonary window is between the ascending and descending aorta; (E) Left pulmonary artery level: To the left of the left pulmonary artery (LPA) lie the left superior pulmonary vein (zigzag arrow). The ascending (A) and descending (D) aorta and superior vena cava maintain their relative positions from the level above. The truncus anterior (TA), or right upper lobe pulmonary artery, is anterior to the right upper lobe bronchus. (arrow); (F) Right pulmonary artery level: S, superior vena cava; D, descending aorta; A, ascending aorta. The left superior pulmonary vein (LSPV) is anterior to the left main bronchus, and left pulmonary artery is posterior. The main pulmonary artery (MPA) divides into right pulmonary artery (RPA) and left pulmonary artery, which is more superior and not visible.

Right Pulmonary Artery Level

The main pulmonary artery (MPA) is situated anterior and to the left of ascending aorta. The right pulmonary artery courses posteriorly from the MPA between the SVC anteriorly and bronchus intermedius posteriorly. The right superior pulmonary vein lies to the right of the intrapulmonary portion of RPA. Anterior to the left main and upper lobe bronchus lies the left superior pulmonary vein while posteriorly is the left lower lobe pulmonary artery **(Fig. 16F)**.

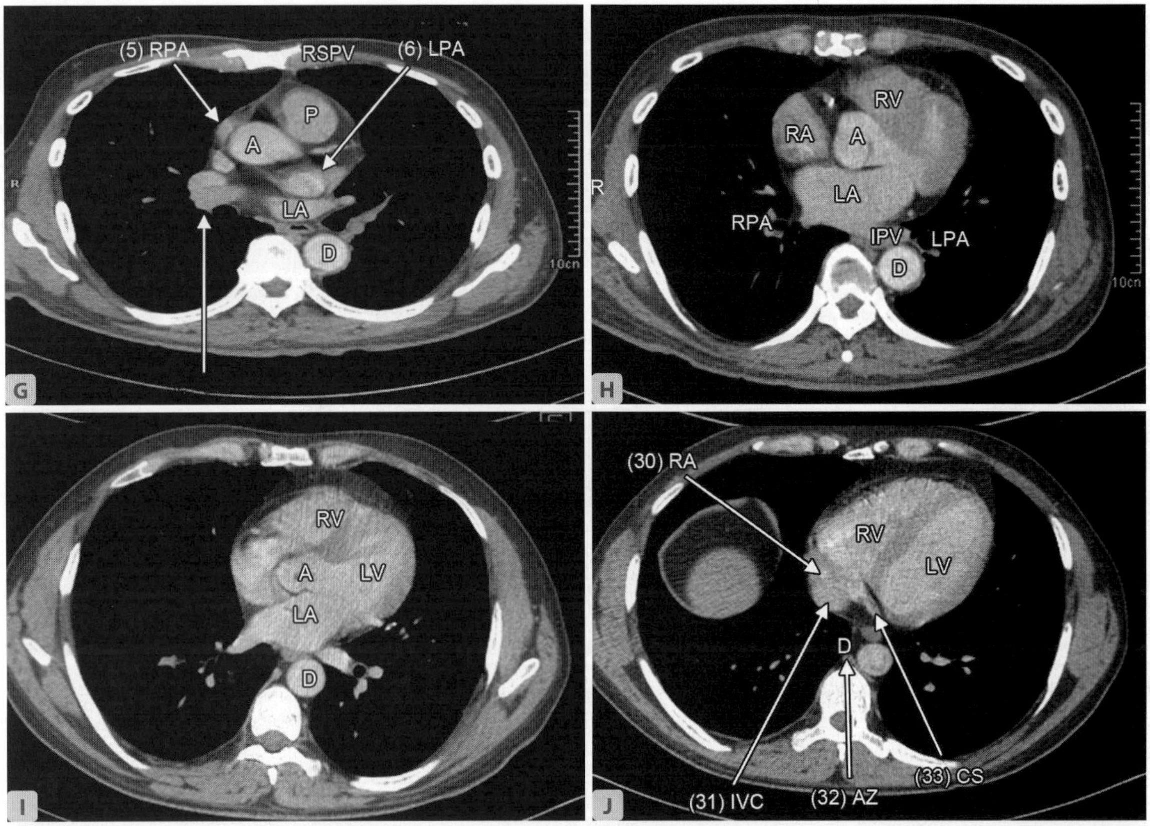

FIGS. 16G TO J: (G) Left atrial level: D, descending aorta; the right atrial appendage is anterior to the superior vena cava (S) and adjacent to the ascending aorta (A). The left atrial appendage is situated anterior and to the left of the left atrium, adjacent to the main pulmonary artery (P). The left atrium (LA) is the most superior and posterior chamber of the heart. Superior pulmonary veins enter the anterosuperior portion of the left atrium. (H) Left atrial level (at a caudal level). A, aortic root; D, descending aorta; IPV, left inferior pulmonary vein; LA, left atrium; LPA, left lower lobe pulmonary arteries; RA, right atrium; RPA, right lower lobe pulmonary artery; RV, right ventricle; (I) Four chamber level. A, aortic root; D, descending aorta; LA, left atrium; LV, lateral ventricle; RA, right atrium; RV, right ventricle; (J) Three chamber level: The left atrium is more cranial to this level and is not visible. The three visualized chambers are the right atrium (RA) with the IVC draining into it, right ventricle (RV), and left ventricle (LV). The coronary sinus (CS) is between the inferior vena cava (I) and the left ventricle. AZ, azygos vein; D, descending aorta.

Left Atrial Level

In the upper sections, the right atrial appendage is situated anterior to the superior vena cava. It curves around the ascending aorta which is situated almost in the center of the mediastinum. The pulmonary artery out flow tract is located is located anterior and to the left of aorta. Posterior and to the left of the pulmonary artery outflow tract is the left atrial appendage (LAA)—roughly triangular in shape. The left main coronary artery courses in the fat between the LAA and aortic root. The right superior pulmonary veins drain into the left atrium just posterior to the superior vena cava **(Figs. 16G and H)**.

Four Chamber Level

All four cardiac chambers can be identified at this level. The left atrium is located posteriorly and is the most cranial of the chambers. On the posterolateral aspect inferior pulmonary veins can be seen entering the LA. The right atrium is situated anterior and to the right of the left atrium, which communicates with the right ventricle (RV) situated anteriorly and slightly to the left of RA. Just posterior and to the left of the RV lies the left ventricle. The right coronary artery may be seen in the right atrioventricular groove, the left circumflex in the left atrioventricular and left anterior descending coronary artery in the interventricular groove between the RV and LV **(Fig. 16I)**.

Three Chamber Level

At this level the left atrium, which has a more cephalad position is not visible. The right ventricle is seen just beneath the sternum, the left ventricle lying to the left posterolateral aspect. The right atrium is located posterior and to the right of right ventricle. The inferior vena cava opens into the inferior aspect of right atrium. Between the IVC and the left ventricle the coronary sinus can be seen opening into the right atrium **(Fig. 16J)**.

The normal axial anatomy on MRI can be seen in **Figures 17 and 18.**

Coronal and Sagittal Planes

These planes can be extremely useful for assessing the relationship between the mediastinal structures and their

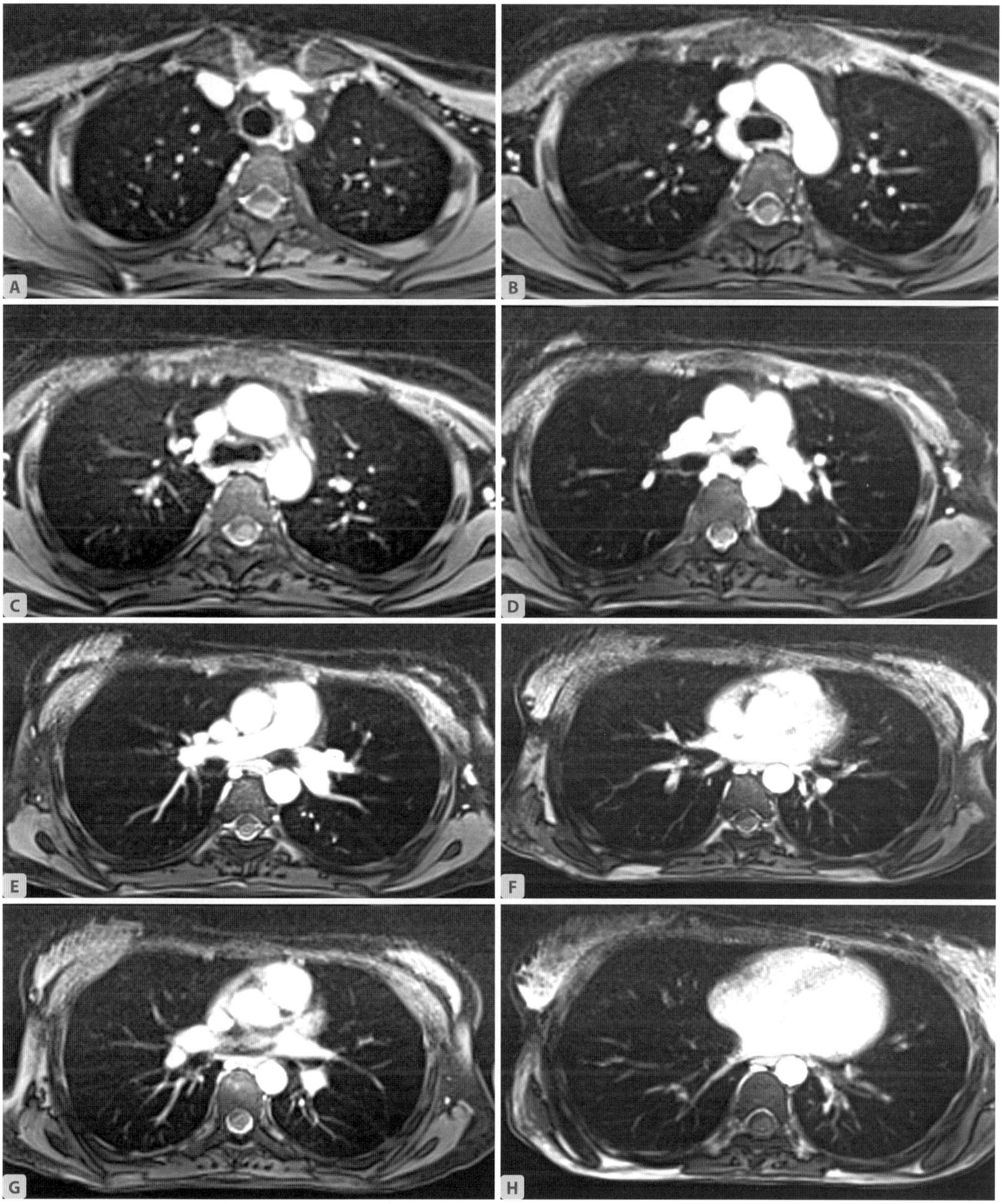

FIGS. 17A TO H: Postcontrast T1w (VIBE) images: Normal mediastinal anatomy on MR.

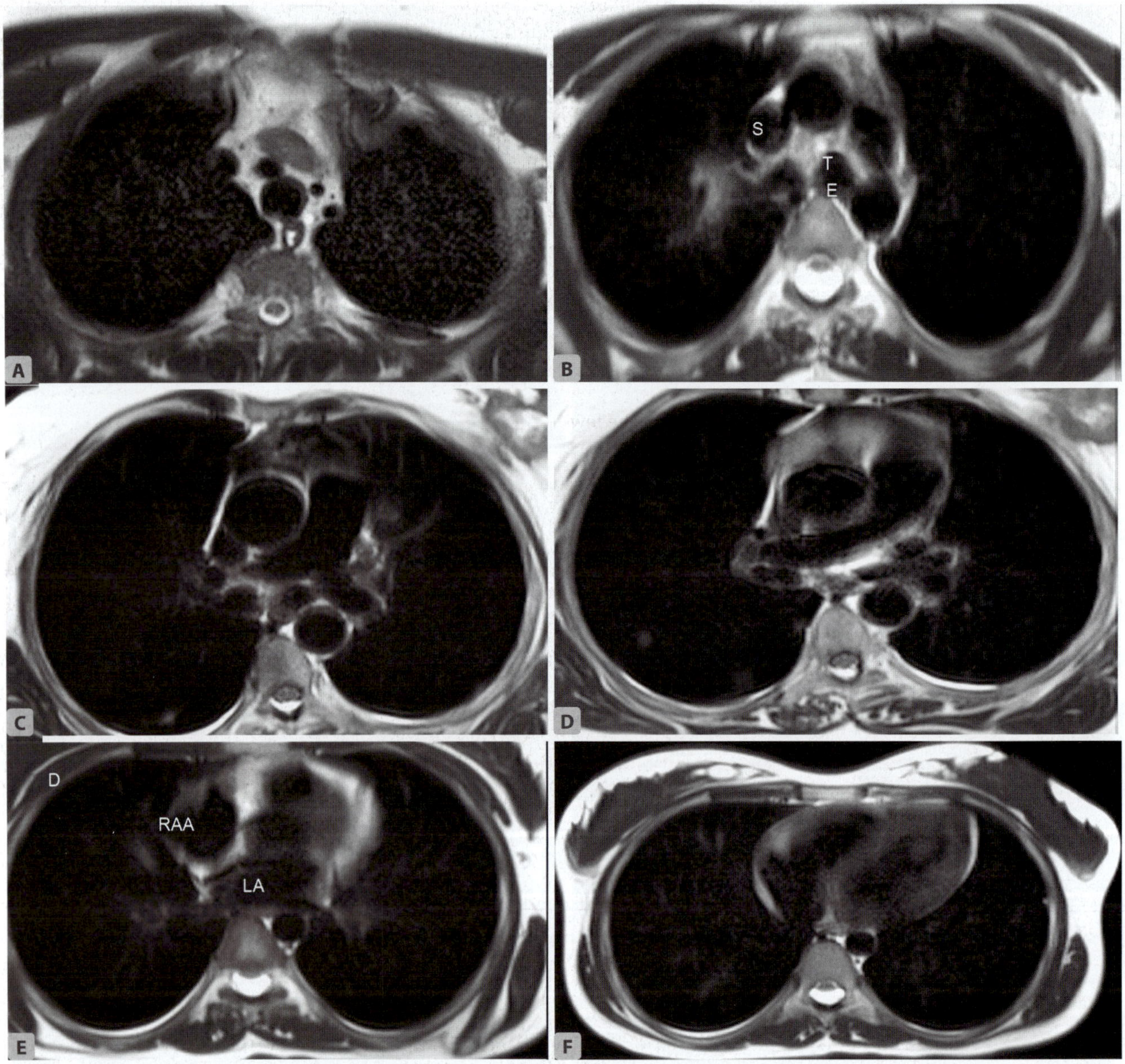

FIGS. 18A TO F: Representative HASTE axial images showing the normal mediastinal anatomy.

relationship with pathology. The anatomy is depicted in **Figures 19 and 20**.

Thymus

The thymus is situated anterior to the aorta and the pulmonary artery or right ventricular outflow tract in the prevascular space. It is usually best seen on a section through the aortic arch or great vessels. In children before puberty most of the mediastinum anterior to the great vessels is filled by the thymus. The size of the gland varies so much in this age group that it is not possible to decide if the gland is normal based on measurements alone, approximate symmetry is the norm. In addition, the normal gland appears to be moulded by the anterior chest wall and the great vessels **(Fig. 21)**. The size of the gland decreases with age. The average thickness of each lobe on CT decreases from 8–9 mm at 20 years to 5–6 mm at 50 years with the maximum thickness of each lobe being upto 15 mm.[1] The measurements are slightly greater on MRI probably because MR demonstrates thymic tissue replaced by fat as well. The craniocaudal measurements are 5–7 cm as measured on sagittal MR images. The density of the gland also changes from soft tissue attenuation prior to puberty to gradual fatty replacement so that above 40 years the attenuation is near, identified to fat making the gland indistinguishable from surrounding fat. Some streaky or modular densities may be seen representing residual thymic parenchyma. On T1W MR images the thymus has a signal similar to that of muscle and lower than that of mediastinal fat, with increasing age the signal of the gland increases approaching that of mediastinal fat. On T2W images the

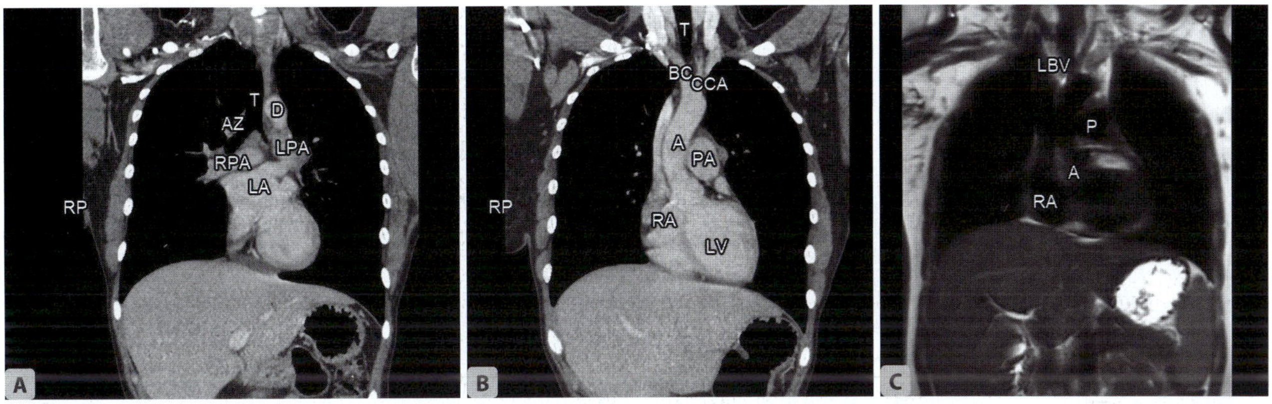

FIGS. 19A TO C: Coronal plane—CT at the level of carina (A) and at aortic outflow tract level (B) and corresponding MR (C). (A: aorta; LB: left brachiocephalic vein; LV: left ventricle; PA: pulmonary artery; RA: right atrium; LPA: left pulmonary artery; RPA: right pulmonary artery; D: descending aorta).

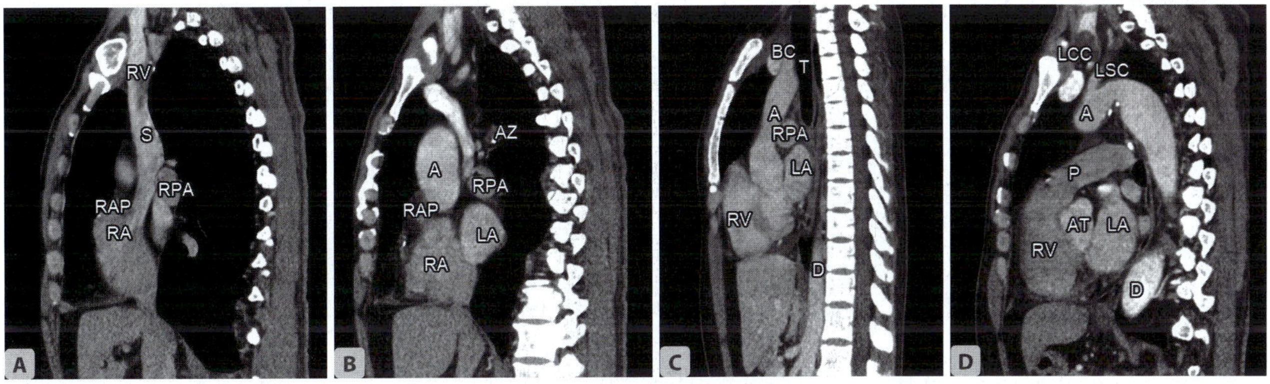

FIGS. 20A TO D: CT images. (A) Sagittal plane—superior vena cava level. RA, right atrium; RAP, right atrial appendage; RPA, right pulmonary artery; RV, right brachiocephalic vein; S, superior vena cava; (B) Sagittal plane—right atrial level. A, ascending aorta; AZ, azygos vein; LA, left atrium; RA, right atrium; RPA, right pulmonary artery; T, trachea; (C) Sagittal plane—aortic outflow tract level. A, ascending aorta; BC, brachiocephalic artery; D, Descending aorta; LA, left atrium; RPA, right pulmonary artery; RV, right ventricle; (D) Sagittal plane—pulmonary artery outflow tract level. A, ascending aorta; AT, aortic outflow tract; D, descending aorta; LA, left atrium; LCC, left common carotid artery; LSC, left subclavian artery; P, pulmonary artery (outflow tract); RV, right ventricle.

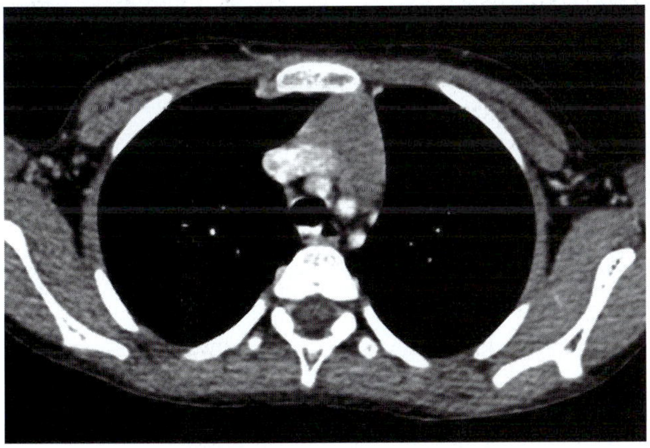

FIG. 21: Axial CT: Normal thymus in a 7-year-old boy seen as a triangular homogeneous soft tissue density anterior to the great vessels.

signal intensity differences are minimal and do not change with age **(Figs. 22A and B)**.

Lymph Nodes

Lymph nodes are distributed throughout the mediastinum. Normal lymph nodes are less that 10 mm in diameter in 95% cases. The remainder with a few exceptions being less than 15 mm. Retrocrural nodes (behind diaphragmatic crura) paraspinal nodes and those in the region of brachiocephalic veins are usually 6 mm or less. On the other hand, nodes in the aortopulmonary window, pretracheal, lower paratracheal and subcarinal compartment are often 6–10 mm in diameter. The nomenclature of mediastinal nodes should be in accordance with the international lymph node map in the TNM classification of lung cancer given by International Association for Study of Lung Cancer (IASLC).

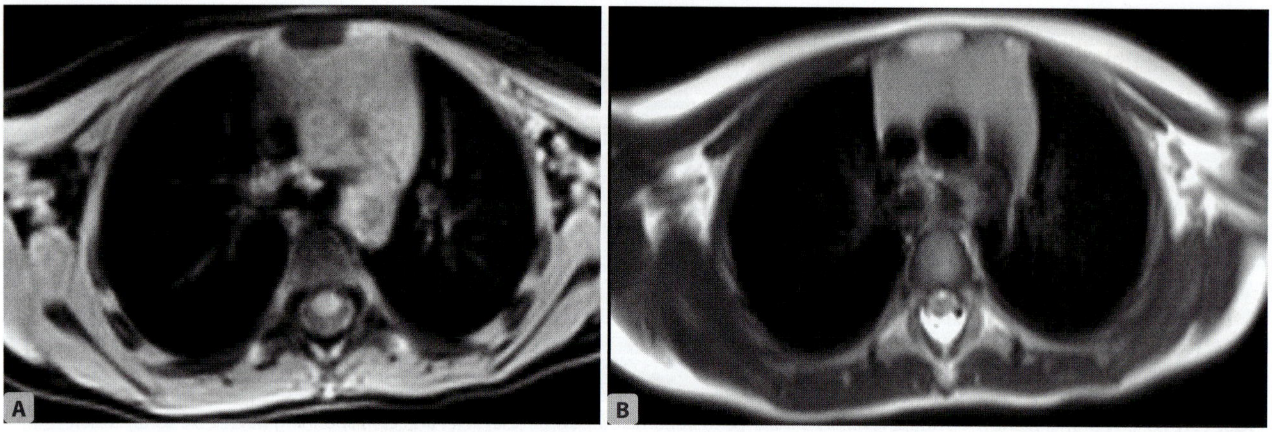

FIGS. 22A AND B: T1W FS (A) and T2W MR (B) images in a five-year-old demonstrate the thymus in the prevascular space appearing homogeneously isointense to skeletal muscle on T1 and hyperintense to skeletal muscle on T2.

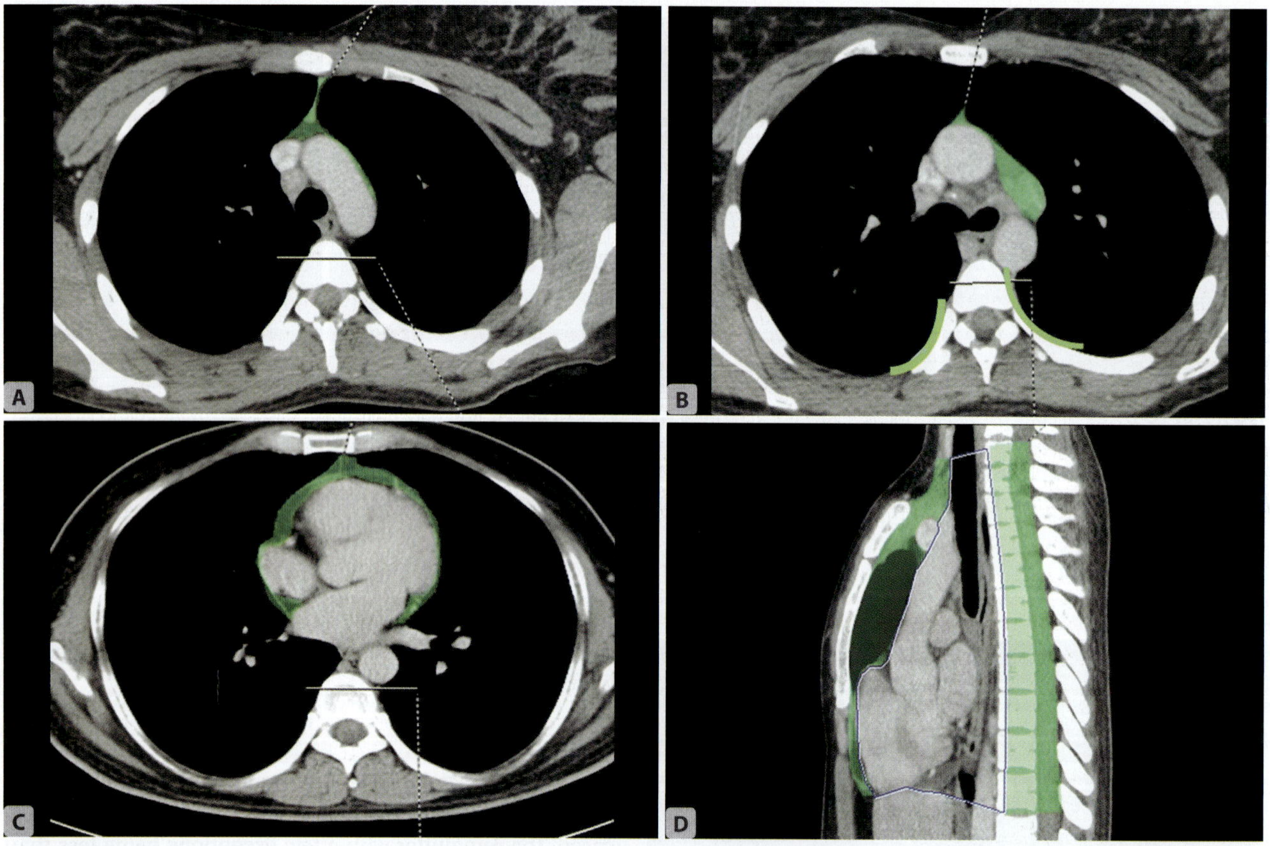

FIGS. 23A TO D: Axial and sagittal CT sections showing the mediastinal divisions according to the ITMIG classification. The prevascular space is depicted in green anteriorly. The horizontal line 1 cm behind the anterior vertebral imaging is the demarcation between the visceral and posterior mediastinal or paravertebral region which is again shaded in green.

Mediastinal Divisions on Cross-sectional Imaging[36,37]

Recently International Thymic Malignancy Interest Group (ITMIG) has introduced a new definition of mediastinal compartments to be adopted as a new standard with cross-sectional imaging. The three compartments as per this system are: (1) prevascular or anterior, (2) visceral or middle, (3) paravertebral or posterior **(Figs. 23A to D)**. The boundaries and contents of these are listed in **Table 2**.

TRACHEOBRONCHIAL TREE[38,39]

The trachea is seen as a thin-walled air containing structure on axial CT scans lying anterior to the dorsal spine and esophagus. It is round or oval in shape with a slightly flattened

TABLE 2: International Thymic Malignancy Interest Group (ITMIG) classification of mediastinal compartments on cross-sectional imaging.

Compartment	Boundaries	Major contents
Prevascular	• *Anteriorly*: Sternum • *Posteriorly*: Anterior aspect of the pericardium as it wraps around the heart in a curvilinear manner • *Superiorly*: Thoracic inlet* • *Inferiorly*: Diaphragm • *Laterally*: Parietal mediastinal pleura	• Thymus • Lymph nodes • Left brachiocephalic vein • Fat
Visceral	• *Anteriorly*: Posterior boundary of the prevascular compartment • *Posteriorly*: Vertical line connecting a point on each thoracic vertebral body 1 cm posterior to its anterior margin** • *Superiorly*: Thoracic inlet • *Inferiorly*: Diaphragm	• Trachea, carina, esophagus, lymph nodes • Heart, ascending aorta, aortic arch, descending thoracic aorta, SVC intrapericardial pulmonary arteries, thoracic duct
Paravertebral	• *Anteriorly*: Posterior boundary of the visceral compartment • *Posteriorly*: Vertical line against the posterior margin of the chest wall at the lateral margin of the transverse process of the thoracic spine	• Thoracic spine • Paravertebral soft tissues

*The thoracic inlet is a thin plane demarcated by superior border of manubrium anteriorly, body of 1st thoracic vertebra posterosuperiorly and 1st ribs and their costal cartilages on each side.

** This line was chosen as the posterior boundary of the visceral compartment and the anterior boundary of the paravertebral compartment as most abnormalities in the posterior compartment are neurogenic masses that arise from the dorsal root ganglia/neurons adjacent to the intervertebral foramina.

posterior margin in about 25% patients. On expiratory scans, the posterior margin of the intrathoracic becomes more concave.

The normal dimensions of the trachea vary with the sex of the patient. In males, it ranges from 13 to 27 mm in transverse dimension and 13–27 mm in sagittal plane while in females the corresponding measurements are 10–21 mm and 10–23 mm. The tracheal index (coronal diameter in mm/ sagittal diameter in mm) is approximately 1. Due to the angled course of the trachea a true perpendicular cross-section of its lumen is not obtained on axial CT images. The tracheal wall measures 3 mm in thickness. The posterior wall being thinner than the anterior wall. The cartilage within the anterior and lateral walls may appear slightly hyperdense as compared to surrounding soft tissue and fat. The cartilages may calcify in the elderly.

The trachea divides into the right and left main bronchi at carina. The right and left man bronchi course obliquely in the axial plane and are well seen on multiplanar reconstructions. On axial CT sections bronchi are seen as ring structures in cross-section while they appear as tubular structures when horizontally oriented.

The right upper lobe bronchus has a horizontal course and is seen just at or below the carina arising from the lateral aspect of right main bronchus. The anterior and posterior divisions of this, being horizontal in their proximal part are seen as tubular structures. The middle lobe bronchus arises from the anterior aspect of right main bronchus and is seen as a tubular structure due to its horizontal course. It divides into the medial and lateral segmental bronchi. At nearly the same level, the apical segmental bronchus of the lower lobe can be seen coursing posteriorly in the horizontal plane. The rest of the lower lobe bronchi are seen in cross-section below this level as they have a vertical course. The lung closely abuts the posterior aspect of the right main bronchus and the bronchus intermedius so that their posterior walls are clearly delineated as a thin stripe on axial CT images.

On the left side, the left upper lobe bronchus arises at a lower level than the right upper lobe bronchus with a horizontal course. The lingular bronchus courses anteriorly in the horizontal plane after arising from the upper lobe bronchus. The lower lobe bronchi have a roughly similar course as on **Figures 24A to F**.

LUNG SEGMENTS, FISSURES AND PLEURA[1,38,39]

Fissures are poorly seen on routine axial CT sections as avascular areas or broad bands as they represent subpleural regions with relative paucity of vessels. On HRCT sections, they are well seen as thin white lines and may be better appreciated on multiplanar reconstructions. **(Figs. 25A and B)**. The individual lung lobes and segments can be identified by their position within the hemithorax and their relationship to the segmental bronchi and fissures Segmental anatomy on CT is shown in **Figures 26A to D**. The normal pleura and extrapleural spaces are not visible.

CONCLUSION

The increasing, almost universal use of CT for thoracic imaging and emerging applications of MR imaging makes it imperative that one is aware of the advancements, strengths and limitations of these techniques so that they can be tailored to answer the clinical question at hand while minimizing radiation exposure.

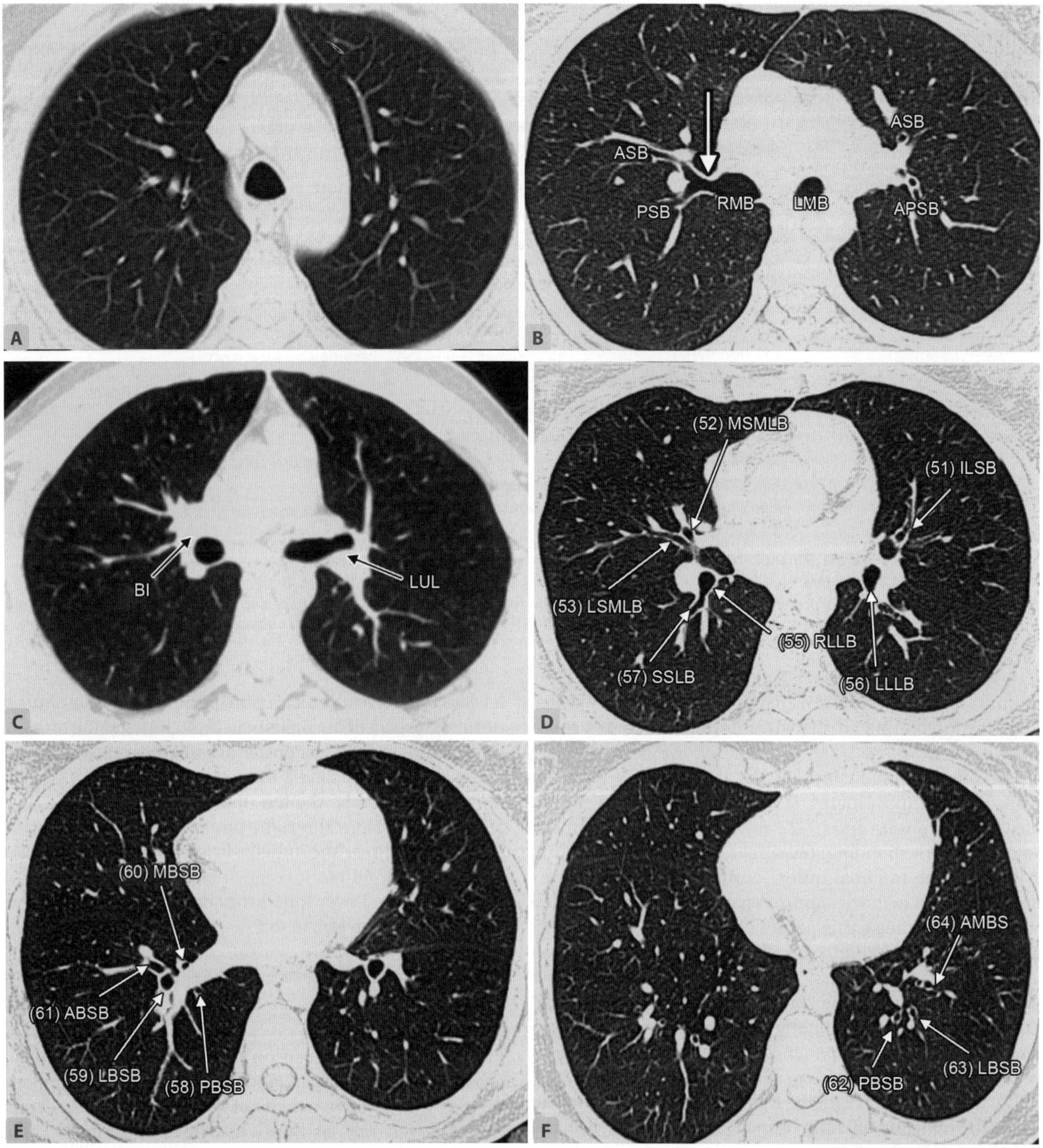

FIGS. 24A TO F: (A) Bronchial anatomy as seen on CT section just above the carina shows apical and apicoposterior segmental bronchi in cross-sections on right and left side respectively; (B) Section at the level of carina shows right and left main bronchi, right upper lobe bronchus I (arrow) and its division into anterior and posterior segmental bronchi; (C) Section just below carina shows bronchus intermedius on right side and left upper lobe bronchus arising from left main bronchus; (D) On the left side, lingular branch of upper lobe bronchus is seen. On right side, middle lobe bronchus and its divisions into medial and lateral segmental bronchi. The superior segmental bronchi of both lower lobes are also seen coursing posteriorly (E and F) Section at further caudal level shows major lower lobe segmental bronchi on both sides.

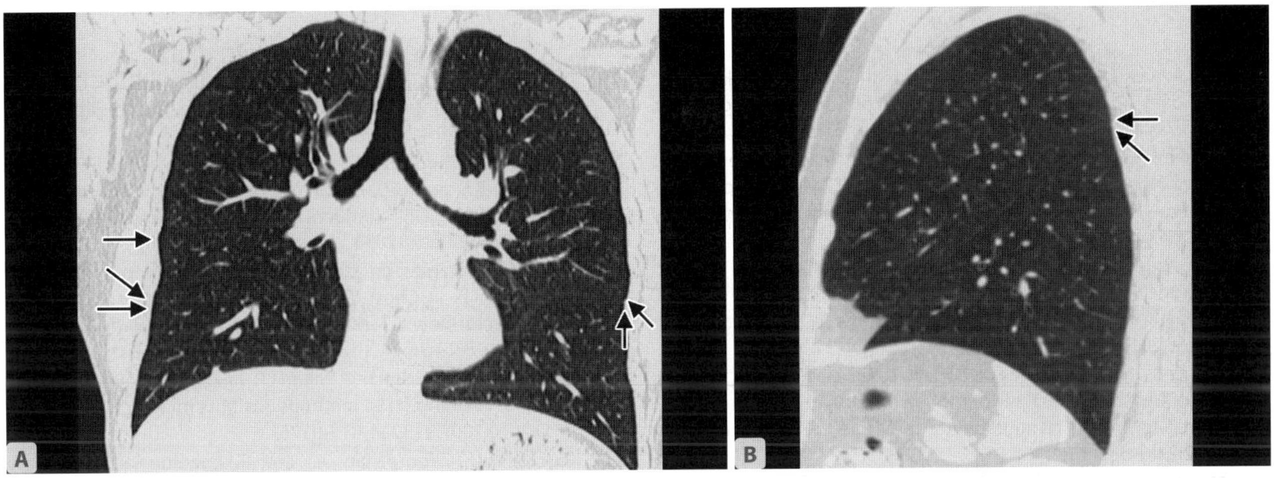

FIGS. 25A AND B: Coronal and sagittal CT sections in lung window showing the oblique fissures on both sides and the horizontal fissure on the right side (double and single arrows respectively).

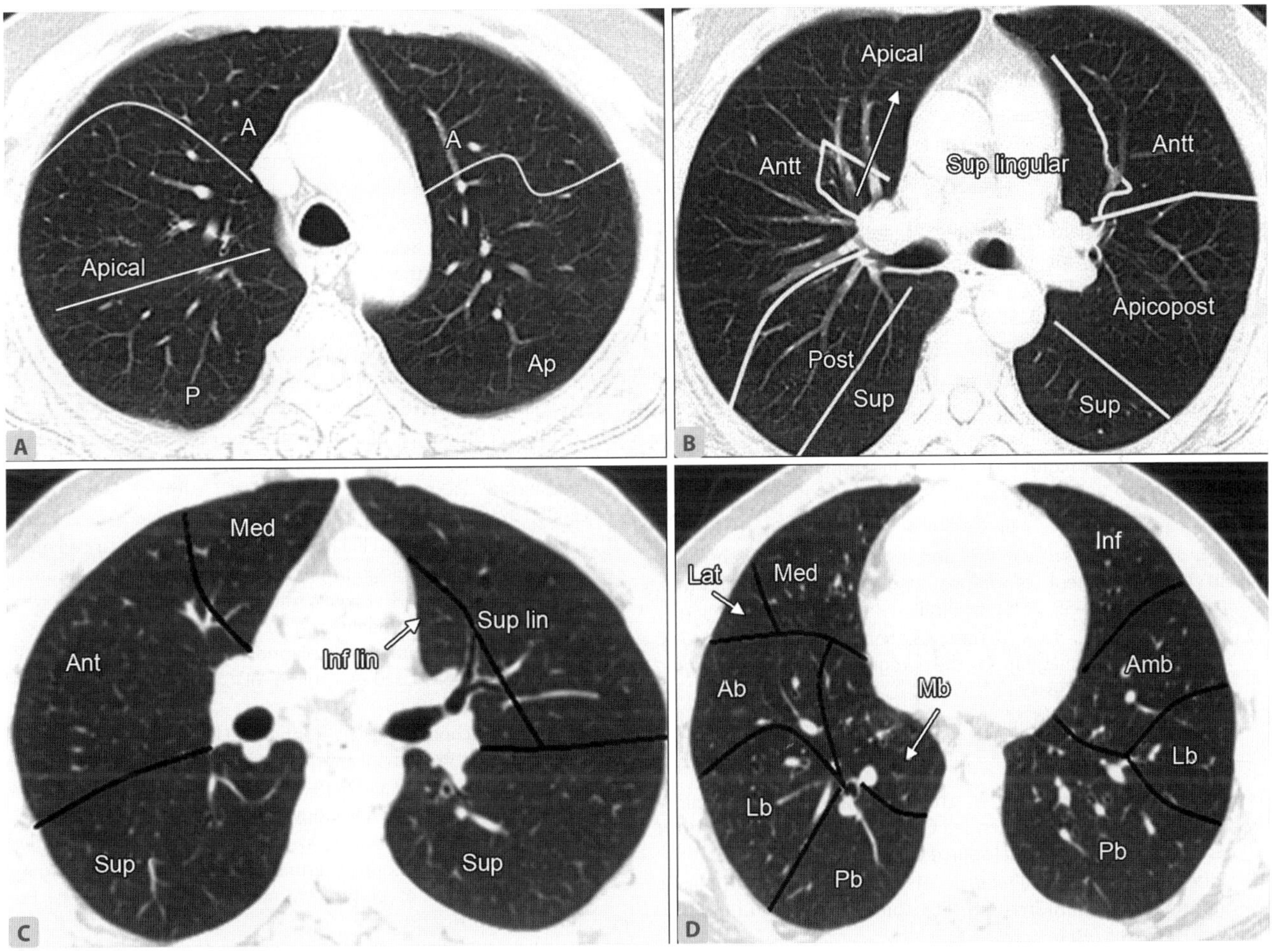

FIGS. 26A TO D: Normal segmental lung anatomy. (A) Section at the level of aortic arch; (B) Left pulmonary artery level; (C) Right pulmonary artery level; (D) Cardiac ventricular level. Apical: Apical segment of right upper lobe (S_1); P: Posterior segment of right upper lobe (S_2); Apicopost: Apicoposterior segment of left upper lobe (S_1+S_2); A: Anterior segment of right upper lobe (S_3); Lat: Lateral segment of right middle lobe (S_4); superior lingular segment (S_4); Med: medial segment of right middle lobe (S_5); Inf: inferior lingular segment of left upper lobe (S_5); Sup: Superior segment of right or left lower lobe (S_6); Mb: Medial segment of right lower lobe (S_7); Ab: Anterior segment of right lower lobe (S_8). Amb: Anteromedial segment of left lower lobe (S_7+S_8); Lb: lateral segment of right or left lower lobe (S_9); Pb: Posterior segment of right or left lower lobe (S_{10}).

REFERENCES

1. Nair A, Aziz ZA and Hansell DM. Techniques in Thoracic Imaging. In: Adam A, Dixon AK, Gillard JH, Prokol S (Eds). Grangier and Alison's Diagnostic Radiology. 6th edition. 2015;149-83.
2. Thomas FG, Bernhard. CT technology for Imaging the Thorax: State of the Art. In: Schoepf UJ, Meinel FG (Eds). Multidetector-Row CT of the Thorax, Medical Radiology, 2nd edition, Springer, 2016;3-28. DOI 10.1007/978-3-319-30355-0_1
3. Hutt A, Tacelli N, Faivre JB, Flohr T, Duhamel A, Remy J, et al. Is bronchial wall imaging affected by temporal resolution? comparative evaluation at 140 and 75 ms in 90 patients. Eur Radiol. 2016;26(2):469–77.
4. Schulz B, Jacobi V, Beeres M, Bodelle B, Gruber T, Lee C, Bauer R, et al. Quantitative analysis of motion artifacts in high-pitch dual-source computed tomography of the thorax. J Thorac Imaging. 2012;27(6):382–6.
5. Morsbach F, Gordic S, Desbiolles L, Husarik D, Frauenfelder T, Schmidt B, et al. Performance of turbo high-pitch dual-source CT for coronary CT angiography: first ex vivo and patient experience. Eur Radiol. 2014;24(8):1889–95.
6. Wuest W, Anders K, Schuhbaeck A, May MS, Gauss S, Marwan M, et al. Dual source multidetector CT-angiography before Transcatheter Aortic Valve Implantation (TAVI) using a high-pitch spiral acquisition mode. Eur Radiol. 2012;22(1):51–8.
7. Tack D, Appiah V. Acquisition Protocol for Thoracic CT. In: Schoepf UJ, Meinel FG (Eds). In Multidetector-Row CT of the Thorax. Medical Radiology. 2nd edition. 2016;59-68. DOI 10.1007/978-3-319-30355-0_4.
8. Dominik F, Richard HL. Contrast Medium Injection Technique. In: Schoepf UJ, Meinel FG (Eds). In Multidetector-Row CT of the Thorax, Medical Radiology, 2nd edition. 2016;37-57. DOI 10.1007/978-3-319-30355-0_3
9. Mayo JR, Webb WR, Gould R, Stein MG, Bass I, Gamsu G, et al. High-resolution CT of the lungs: an optimal approach. Radiology. 1987;163(2):507–10.
10. Murata K, Khan A, Herman PG. Pulmonary parenchymal disease: evaluation with high-resolution CT. In: Nishino M, Boiselle PM, Copeland JF, et al. (Eds). Radiology. 2004;170:629–35.
11. Beigelman-Aubry C, Hill C, Guibal A, Savatovsky J, Grenier PA. Multi-detector row CT and postprocessing techniques in the assessment of diffuse lung disease. Radiographics. 2005;25(6):1639–52. 25/6/1639 [pii].
12. Litmanovich DE, Tack D, Lee KS, Shahrzad M, Bankier AA. Cardiothoracic imaging in the pregnant patient. J Thorac Imaging. 2014;29:38-49.
13. Harald B, Heuschmid M, Andreas F. Kopp-Tubingen .Vascular: Pulmonary Veins. In: Medizin S, Heidelberg V (Eds). Dual source CT imaging. 2008;140-50.
14. Thorsten RCJ, Konstantin N, Christoph BR, Becker R. Munich-Grosshadern Vascular: Extended Chest Pain Protocol. In: Medizin S, Heidelberg V (Eds). Dual source CT imaging. 2008;130-9.
15. Eibel R, Türk T, Kulinna C, et al. Value of multiplanar reformations (MPR) in multi-slice spiral CT of the lung. Rofo. 2001;173(1):57–64.
16. Eibel R, Türk TR, Kulinna C, et al. Multidetector row CT of the lungs: multiplanar reconstructions and maximum intensity projections for the detection of pulmonary nodules. Rofo. 2001;173(9):815–21.
17. Kuettner A, Anders K, Lell M–Nuremberg E. Dual Energy: Virtual Non Contrast in Dual source CT imaging. Springer Medizin Veriag Heidelberg. 2008;242-51.
18. Dinkel J, Hintze C, Rochet N, Thieke C, Biederer J. Computed tomography of the lungs. A step into the fourth dimension. Radiologe. 2009;49(8):698–704.
19. Wielputz MO, Bardarova D, Weinheimer O, Kauczor HU, Eichinger M, Jobst BJ, et al. Variation of densitometry on computed tomography in COPD –influence of different software tools. PLoS One; 2014;9(11), e112898
20. Paul NS. Strategies for Dose Reduction and Improvement of image Quality in Chest CT. In: Schoepf UJ, Meinel FG (Eds). In Multidetector-Row CT of the Thorax, Medical Radiology, 2nd edition. 2016;29-36. DOI 10.1007/978-3-319-30355-0_2
21. Wild JM, Marshal H, Bock M, Schad LR, Jakob PM, Molinary MPF, et al. MRI of the lung (1/3): methods. Insights imaging. 2012;3:345-53. DOI 10.1007/s13244-012-0176x.
22. Kauczor HU, Zaporozhan JL, Ley S. Imaging of pulmonary pathologies. Focus on Magnetic Resonance Imaging. Proc Am Thorac Soc. 2009;6:458-63
23. Hochhegger B, de Souza VVS, Marchiori E, Irion KL, Souza Jr AS, Junor JE, et al. Chest magnetic resonance imaging: a protocol suggestion. Radiol Bras. 2015;48(6):373-80.
24. Henzler T, Bindert GS, Schoenberg SO, Fink C. Diffusion and perfusion MRI of the lung and mediastinum. Eur J Radiol. 2010;76:329-36.
25. Christine UL, White DB, Sykes AMG. Establishing a Chest MRI practice and its Clinical Application: Our Insight and Protocols. Published online 2014, doi: 10.4103/2156-7514.129288
26. Ackman JB. MR imaging of mediastinal masses, Magn Reson Imaging Clin Normal Am. 2015;23:141-64.
27. Mirasadraee JBS, Beer M, Molinary F, Hintze C, Bauman G, Both M, et al. MRI of the lung (3/3)-current application and future perspectives. Insights Imaging. 2012;3:373-86. DOI 10.1007/s13244-011-0142-z
28. Biderer J, Beer M, Hirsch W, Wild J, Fabel M, Puderbach M, Van Beek EJR. MRI of the lung (2/3). Why.... when...... how?. Insights Imaging. 2012;3:355-71. DOI 10.1007/s13244-011-0146-8.
29. Kluge A, Luboldt W, Bachmann G. Acute pulmonary embolism to the subsegmental level: diagnostic accuracy of three MRI techniques compared with 16-MDCT. Am J Roentgenol. 2006;187:W7-14.
30. Stein PD, Woodard PK, Hull Rd, et al. Gadolinium-enhanced magnetic resonance angiography for detection of acute pulmonary embolism: an in-depth review. Chest. 2003;124:2324-8
31. Kluge A, Loboldt W, Bachmann G. Acute pulmonary embolism to the subsegmental level: diagnostic accuracy of three MRI techniques compared with 16-MDCT. Am J Roentgenol. 2006;187(1):W7-14.
32. Nikolaou K, Schoenberg SO, Attenberger U, Scheidhler J, Dietrich O, Kuehn B, et al. Pulmonary arterial hypertension: diagnosis with fast perfusion MR imaging and high-spatial-resolution MR angiography-preliminary experience. Radiology. 2005;236:694-703.
33. Koyama H, Ohno Y, Kono A, et al. Quantitative and qualitative assessment of non-contrast-enhanced pulmonary MR imaging for management of pulmonary nodules in 161 subjects. Eur Radiol. 2008;18:2120-31.
34. Hochhegger B, Marchiori E, Dos Reis DQ, et al. Chemical-shift MRI of pulmonary hamartoma: initial experience using a modified technique to assess nodules fat. Am J Roentgenol. 2012;199:W331-4.
35. Sodhi KS, Khandelwal N, Saxena AK, Singh M, Aggarwal R, Bhatia A, et al. Rapid lung MRI in children with pulmonary infections: time to change our diagnostic algorithms J. Magn. Reson imaging. 2016;43:1196-206.

36. Carter BW, Benveniste MF, Madan R, Godoy MC, de Groot PM, Truong MT, et al. ITMIG Classification of Mediastinal Compartments and Multidisciplinary Approach to Mediastinal Masses. Radiographics. 2017;37(2):413-36.
37. Carter BW, Tomiyama N, Bhora FY, et al. A Modern definition of mediastinal compartments. J Thorac Oncol. 2014;9(9 suppl 2): S97-101.
38. Mukherjee S, Gupta R. Imaging in chest disease. In: Pande JN (Ed). Respiratory Medicine in the Tropics, 1st edition. Delhi, Oxford University Press, 90, 1988.
39. Amstrong P. The normal chest. In: Grainger RG, Allison D (Eds). Diagnostic Radiology, 3rd edition. New York: Churchill Livingstone, 207, 1997;1114-88.

CHAPTER

124

Basic Radiographic Pattern of Lung Diseases

Gaurav Shanker Pradhan, Radhika Batra, Rashmi Dixit, Alpana Manchanda

Plain film radiography is the first and most frequently used radiological investigation in the diagnostic workup of chest ailments. Chest radiographs are one of the oldest noninvasive methods for identifying abnormalities in the chest.[1] Evaluation of a chest radiograph requires careful observation and a good understanding of chest anatomy. Many common clinical conditions can be evaluated with a chest radiograph for example pneumonia, pleural effusion, pneumothorax, rib fractures, pulmonary edema, etc. It is a quick, inexpensive and widely available investigation making it particularly useful in the emergency setting.

PATTERN RECOGNITION

Felson[2,3] popularized a pattern recognition approach to pulmonary disease, on the basis of classifying lung diseases as either alveolar or interstitial. An alternative approach to pattern recognition is the description of an abnormal radiograph and a differential diagnosis based on the radiographic features of the disease, rather than on its presumed histologic appearance. This system was endorsed by Felson[4] in 1989, who believed that it may be easier for radiologists to determine the correct diagnosis by describing the appearance of the radiograph, rather than by attempting to suggest the histology of the lesion. The basic radiographic signs as they indicate the fundamental nature of pulmonary disease are subdivided into three major sections:[5]

1. Increased radiographic density
2. Decreased radiographic density
3. Diseases of the pleura.

The basic difference in evaluating a chest radiograph as compared to high-resolution computed tomography (HRCT) chest is that on radiographs the diagnosis depends on the appearance of disease as opposed to HRCT images where diagnosis is virtually at histologic levels. A pulmonary opacity is defined as an area that preferentially attenuates the X-ray beam and therefore appears more opaque than the surrounding area.[6] There are various patterns of pulmonary opacities such as airspace opacities, atelectasis, nodules, ring shadows, linear and bandlike opacities and reticulonodular opacities.

Airspace Disease

Airspace Opacity

A small nodular opacity measuring about 4 to 10 mm in the alveoli may be the first radiological evidence of parenchymal pathology on chest radiograph **(Fig. 1)**. There can also be presence of remnant air in the alveoli and bronchioles seen as tiny radiolucencies within the nodule. The lucencies have been referred to as air alveolograms, although they do not correspond to alveoli **(Box 1)**.

Coalescence

Rapid dissemination of fluid through the collateral pathways of the lung into adjacent airspaces results in ill-defined margins of air space opacities. Asymmetric involvement of the lung results in an irregular area of consolidation with ill-defined margins **(Fig. 2)**.

Distribution Characteristics

Rapid spread of fluid or infection results in early coalescence of airspace opacities leading to widespread consolidation which is characteristically non-segmental in distribution, seen typically in pyogenic infections. Lack of segmental distribution is also seen with acute pulmonary edema. This is in stark contrast to segmental distribution observed in diseases spread through tracheobronchial route like aspiration pneumonias or those through hematogenous route like infarcts. The area of lung involvement in aspiration pneumonias depends on the patient's position at the time of aspiration.

Only certain diseases and not others appear to respect acinar boundaries. This is likely due to the viscosity of the consolidating medium. The inflammatory edema caused by some organisms, e.g. *Streptococcus pneumoniae*, is of low viscosity and therefore spreads rapidly via interalveolar pores, whereas that of others, such as *Mycobacterium tuberculosis*, may be of sufficient viscosity to prevent such ready dissemination.

Margination

The edge characteristics of airspace processes show poor margination. An example of the phenomenon is the

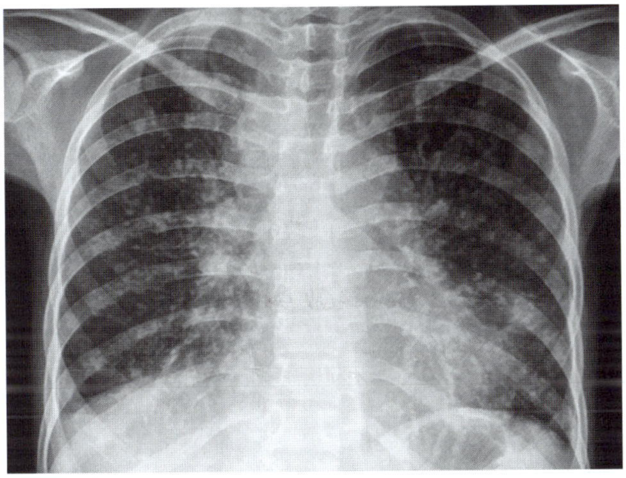

FIG. 1: Multiple nodular airspace opacities in bilateral lungs with areas of coalescence in left lower zone.

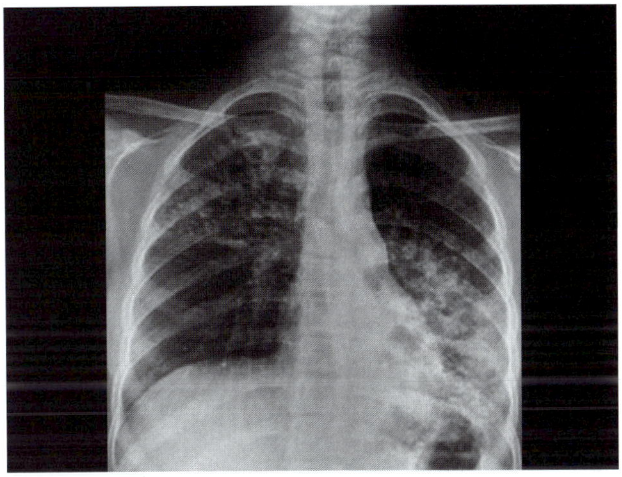

FIG. 2: Confluent airspace opacities in right upper, bilateral mid and left lower zones with areas of breakdown in left retrocardiac region.

Box 1: Causes of multifocal airspace opacification on chest radiograph.

- Infective pneumonia
- Eosinophilic pneumonia
- Organizing pneumonia
- Pulmonary edema
- Infarction due to pulmonary emboli
- Connective tissue disorders
- Alveolar proteinosis
- Pulmonary hemorrhage
- *Neoplasms*: Bronchoalveolar carcinoma, lymphoma, lymphangitis carcinomatosa
- Sarcoidosis
- Silicosis, coal workers' pneumoconiosis

"butterfly" or "bat's wing" appearance of acute airspace edema or hemorrhage **(Fig. 3)**. However, in acute diplococcal or *Klebsiella pneumoniae*, as the infection is propogated by centrifugal spread, the advancing margin of consolidation is sometimes smooth and sharply defined **(Fig. 4)**. When consolidation extends up to a pleural surface it may appear lobar.

Air Bronchogram

Presence of remnant air within the bronchi and its branches within the parenchymal opacity gives the radiologically important "air-bronchogram" sign. These bronchi stand out in contrast to opacified lung due to fluid or tissue filled alveolar spaces. It is important to remember that for air-bronchogram to be present, the bronchi need to be patent. The parenchyma may be airless when its air has been replaced by liquid or tissue (consolidation) or when it has been absorbed and not replaced (atelectasis). This sign originally described by Fleischner in 1927, was named the air bronchogram sign by Felson. It is most frequently encountered in pneumonia and pulmonary edema. Bronchoalveolar carcinoma, lymphoma, alveolar hemorrhage, fibrosis due to radiation and sarcoidosis can also present with this sign. In some diseases like pulmonary infarction, air bronchogram may be only temporary because of early filling of airway by blood or exudate.

Time Factor

The airspace opacification persisting for prolonged periods of time usually indicates persistent pathologies like infection and neoplasm (bronchoalveolar carcinoma and lymphoma) as opposed to rapidly clearing or evolving opacities as seen in pulmonary edema, which clear with treatment of underlying heart failure.

Atelectasis

Air space opacity with resorption of air with no significant air replacement results in loss of lung volume. This is referred to as atelectasis or collapse. The natural tendency of the lung to collapse is opposed by the recoil of the chest wall outwards caused by the contraction of inspiratory muscles and diaphragm. Atelectasis can result due to mechanisms that interfere directly or indirectly with lung expansion. It can be divided into six types: resorptive, adhesive, compressive, passive, cicatrization and gravity dependent.[7]

When the lung is compressed by any space occupying lesion in the thorax such as pneumothorax, pleural effusion or a mass lesion in the pleural cavity, compressive atelectasis results. The distinction between compressive and passive atelectasis is not well defined, any space occupying lesion in the thorax may compress the lung or lead to passive retraction of the lung.

The most common form of atelectasis is caused by the resorption of gas from the alveoli.[5] When there is partial or total obstruction to flow of air from tracheobronchial tree to the alveoli, with inadequate air filling by collateral pathways, resorption atelectasis results. The lung becomes devoid of air within 24 hours of bronchial obstruction. Resorption atelectasis occurs rapidly when the patient is breathing pure oxygen as it is quickly absorbed from the alveoli. Mucous impaction in subsegmental bronchus and bronchiolitis

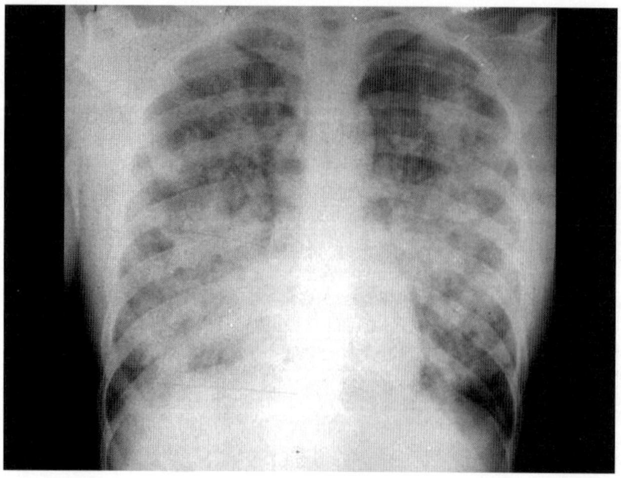

FIG. 3: Chest radiograph showing multiple patchy airspace opacities in bilateral lung fields giving rise to "Bat's wing" appearance in a case of pulmonary edema.

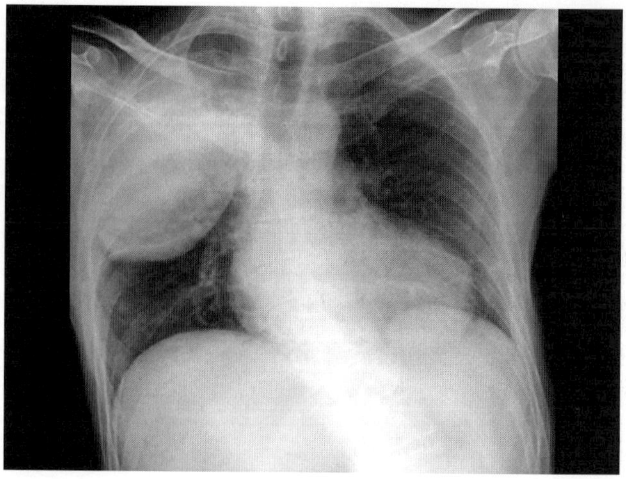

FIG. 4: Bulging fissure sign in *Klebsiella pneumoniae.*

obliterans due to repeated infections in early life can result in resorption atelectasis. It is also seen commonly after surgery and general anesthesia.[8]

When the compliance of the lung decreases because of it being diseased due to fibrosis, cicatrization atelectasis can develop. It is often associated with bronchiectasis. Cicatrization atelectasis can be seen with many conditions like idiopathic pulmonary fibrosis, sarcoidosis, chronic tubercular and fungal infections and collagen vascular diseases.

When there is deficiency of alveolar surfactant along with other coexistent factors, then even in the presence of a patent airway, atelectasis can occur. This is referred to as "non-obstructive" atelectasis or adhesive atelectasis. It is characteristically seen in respiratory distress syndrome of the newborn. It may also be seen in acute respiratory distress syndrome (ARDS), acute radiation pneumonitis and in postoperative patients.[8]

Gravity dependent atelectasis can occur in bedridden patients with shallow breathing. Gravity dependent alterations in alveolar volume may aggravate atelectasis in dependent parts of the lung.

'Plate like atelectasis' are the common linear opacities seen on a chest radiograph. These are usually 1 to 3 mm in thickness, 4 to 10 cm in length and are seen in the mid and lower lung zones. These shadows may be horizontal or oblique, single or multiple, unilateral or bilateral. These linear opacities are associated with diseases that limit diaphragmatic excursion, a frequent contributing factor being intra-abdominal disease (such as inflammatory conditions, ascites, etc.).

Direct and Indirect Signs of Collapse

The signs of lobar atelectasis are seen due to the opacity of a given lobe and the volume loss that results.[9-11] There can be direct and indirect signs. Direct evidence of presence of collapse can be inferred by displacement of lobar fissures which is the most reliable sign. Crowding of vessels and bronchi in a lobe can help in diagnosis if displacement of fissures is not apparent. Increased density of an atelectatic part of the lung usually becomes apparent when the collapse is almost complete.

Other indirect signs that may help us to suspect underlying collapse include elevation of part of diaphragm or hemidiaphragm usually seen in lower lobe collapse, whereas upper lobe collapse may be inferred by tracheal or upper mediastinal displacement. Lower lobe collapse may also be associated with cardiac displacement **(Fig. 5)**. Hilar displacement may also point to underlying collapse of lung. This is usually more evident with upper lobe collapse than with lower lobe collapse **(Fig. 6)**. Reduction of intercostal spaces with resultant rib crowding may occasionally be seen with chronic processes and old collapse. A change in the site of a parenchymal lesion, as seen after comparison with previous images, may result from atelectasis and is referred to as the **"shifting granuloma sign"**.

Compensatory hyperinflation of adjoining lung can also be seen with collapsed lung. The hyperinflation may occur over a prolonged period of time and may involve adjacent lobe or entire lung. There is resultant mediastinal displacement with paucity and spread out vascular markings when compared to contralateral lung. When a large portion of a lung becomes atelectatic, the tendency is greater for overinflation to involve the contralateral lung; this may progress to the stage in which the opposite lung displaces the mediastinum either generally or locally **(Fig. 7)**.

Local displacements occur in the three areas of the mediastinum, where the two lungs are separated only by loose connective tissue: (1) the anterior mediastinal compartment, at the level of the first three or four costal cartilages, limited anteriorly by the sternum and posteriorly by the great vessels; (2) the posterosuperior mediastinum, at the level of the third to fifth thoracic vertebrae, limited anteriorly by the esophagus and trachea and posteriorly by the vertebral column; and (3) the posteroinferior mediastinum, limited anteriorly by the heart and posteriorly by the vertebral column and aorta.

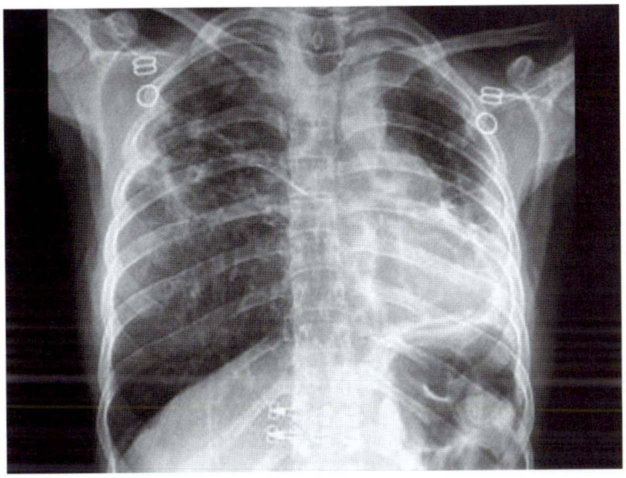

FIG. 5: Left lower lobe collapse with elevated left hemidiaphragm and ipsilateral mediastinal shift alongwith nodular and few fibrotic opacities in right lung field.

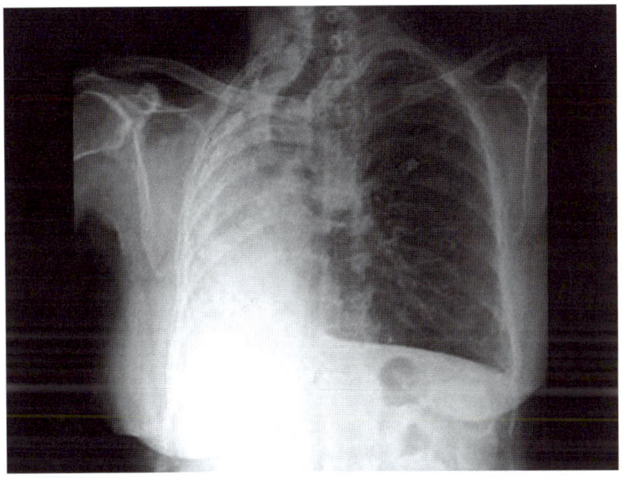

FIG. 7: Opaque right hemithorax with ipsilateral tracheomediastinal shift and compensatory hyperinflation of left lung—Complete right lung collapse.

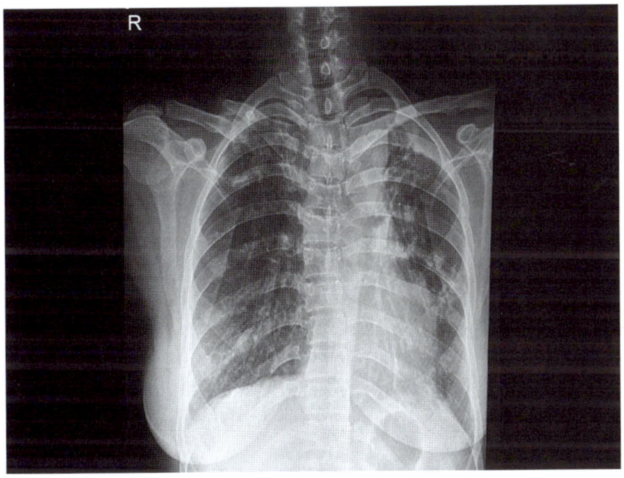

FIG. 6: Left upper lobe collapse with mild ipsilateral tracheal shift, pulled up left hilum and juxtaphrenic peak of left hemidiaphragm.

Lobar Atelectasis

Right upper lobe collapse—As the right upper lobe collapses, the lateral end of the horizontal fissure moves upwards and medially towards the superior mediastinum and the anterior end moves upwards towards the apex. The upper half of the oblique fissure moves anteriorly **(Figs. 8A and B)**.[12] Other radiographic findings associated with right upper lobe collapse include increased density in the upper thorax, silhouetting of the upper mediastinum, mediastinal widening, ipsilateral tracheal shift, elevated hilum, outward rotation of hilum or bronchus and juxtaphrenic peak **(Fig. 9)**. The "**Golden's S sign"** is seen with right upper lobe collapse due to a centrally located mass **(Fig. 10)**. The superiorly displaced, lateral and concave aspect of the "S" is formed by the minor fissure, while the inferiorly and medially located convex part is formed by the margin of the mass.[13]

Right middle lobe collapse: It is seen as an increased density of the lung silhouetting the right heart border and the minor fissure is invisible. In this condition, the horizontal fissure and lower half of the oblique fissure move towards each other **(Figs. 11A and B)**.

Left upper lobe collapse: Left upper lobe collapse is seen as a hazy opacity in upper, mid and sometimes lower zones. Pulmonary vessels in the hyperinflated lower lobe are seen through the haze. On the lateral radiograph, it is seen as an elongated opacity extending from the paex and reaching the diaphragm. In left upper lobe collapse, there is vertical positioning and anterior and medial displacement of the major fissure **(Figs. 12A and B)**. Migration of the superior segment of the left lower lobe superiorly and anteriorly between the arch of the aorta and the collapsed lobe causes a crescent-shaped radiolucency around the aortic arch which is known as the **"Luftsichel sign" (Fig. 13)**.[14]

Lower lobe collapse: In lower lobe collapse, there is posterior and medial displacement of the oblique fissure. It is seen as a triangular density in the retrocardiac location on a frontal radiograph, downward displacement of the hilum is seen **(Figs. 14 and 15)**.[15] The lower lobe pulmonary artery is also obscured on the frontal radiographs. The diaphragmatic contour is obscured and shift of the heart or mediastinum becomes apparent **(Fig. 16)**. The **"flat waist sign"**[16] can be seen with left lower lobe collapse where there is straightening of the left heart margin, aorta and pulmonary artery. With severe left lower lobe collapse the outline of the superior aortic knuckle may not be seen. On the lateral radiograph, lower lobe collapse may cause partial obscuration of the hemidiaphragm in its posterior aspect and the vertebral column appears to be progressively dense inferiorly.

Interstitial Pattern

Pulmonary interstitium encompasses support tissues within the lung and includes alveolar epithelium, pulmonary capillary endothelium, perivascular and perilymphatic tissues. It can be divided into the axial, parenchymal and peripheral interstitial spaces. The axial interstitial space is

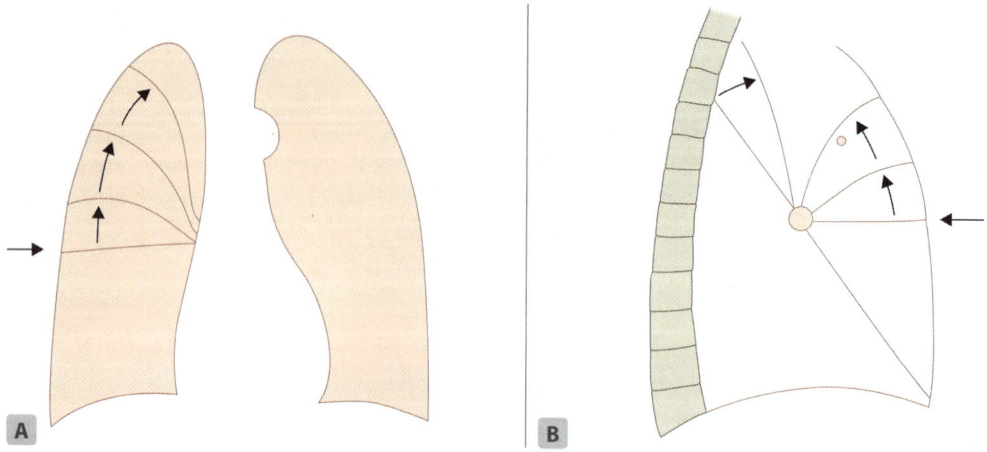

FIGS. 8A AND B: Right upper lobe collapse PA (A) and lateral (B) views: Horizontal fissure is drawn upward and curves towards the apex and mediastinum on PA view. On the lateral view there is upward displacement of the horizontal fissure with forward displacement of the oblique fissure above the hilum.

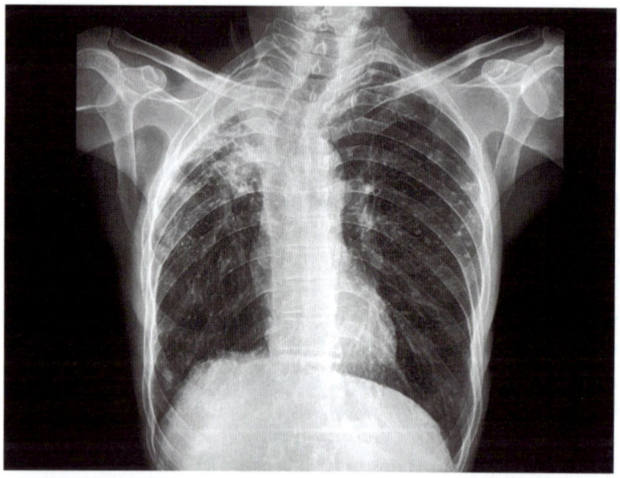

FIG. 9: Right upper lobe collapse with ipsilateral tracheal shift and pulled up right hilum. Multiple nodular calcific opacities are seen in bilateral lungs.

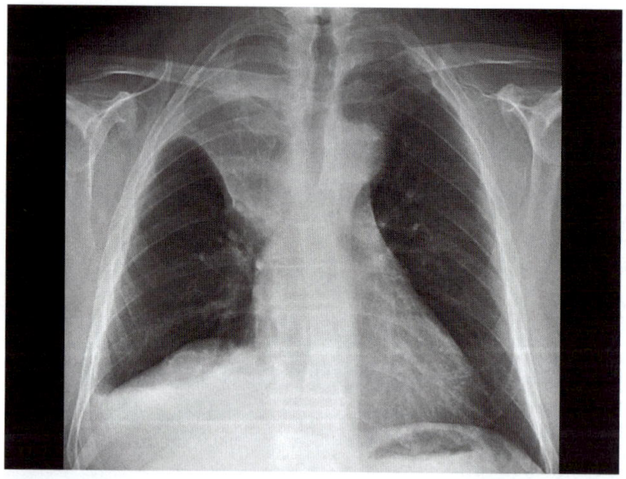

FIG. 10: Golden S-sign—centrally located mass causing right upper lobe collapse.

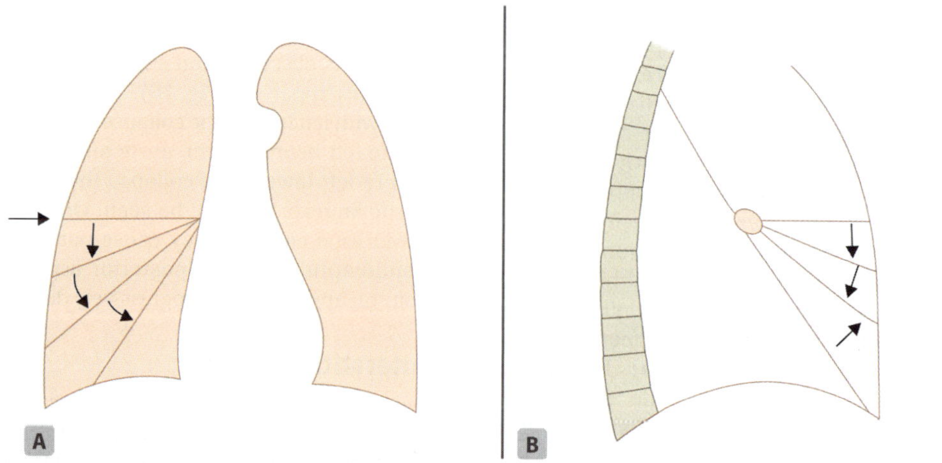

FIGS. 11A AND B: Right middle lobe collapse PA (A) and lateral (B) views: The horizontal fissure is displaced downwards on both views, on the lateral view there is forward displacement of the lower part of the oblique fissure.

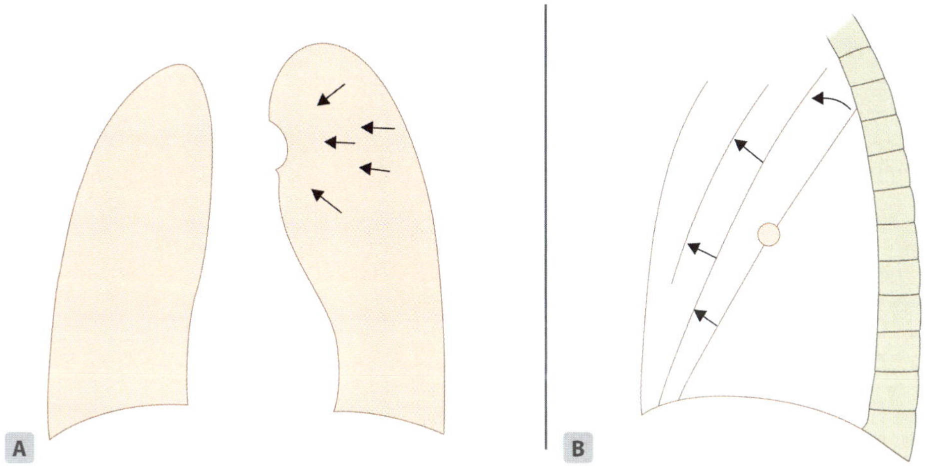

FIGS. 12A AND B: Left upper lobe collapse on PA (A) and lateral (B) views: Increased density is seen with increasing severity of collapse on PA view. The fissure moves forward on lateral view.

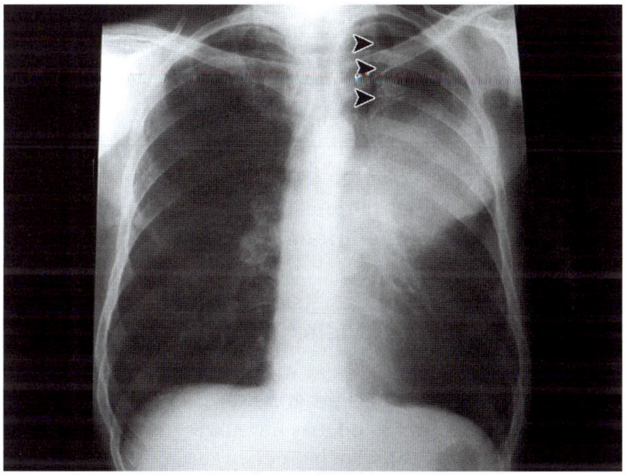

FIG. 13: Luftsichel sign: Crescent of hyperlucency seen in para-aortic location in left upper lobe collapse.

constituted by sheath of loose connective tissue around the bronchovascular bundles, the blood vessels, nerves and lymphatics lie in this space. Parenchymal interstitial space is a small space in the walls of the alveoli. Peripheral interstitial space is adjacent to the pleura. The interstitial involvement can be in the form of reticular, nodular, reticulonodular and linear opacities. Inhomogeneous radiographic density can result because of primarily interstitial involvement. It is important to remember that alveolar air may be less but is not significantly compromised in interstitial disease and volume loss is not a feature of interstitial involvement as opposed to diseases with alveolar involvement.

Reticular Pattern

Reticular involvement is characterized by the development of thickening of interstitium around air containing cystic spaces. It can be further subdivided as fine, medium or coarse depending on the size. Fine reticulation implies a slender

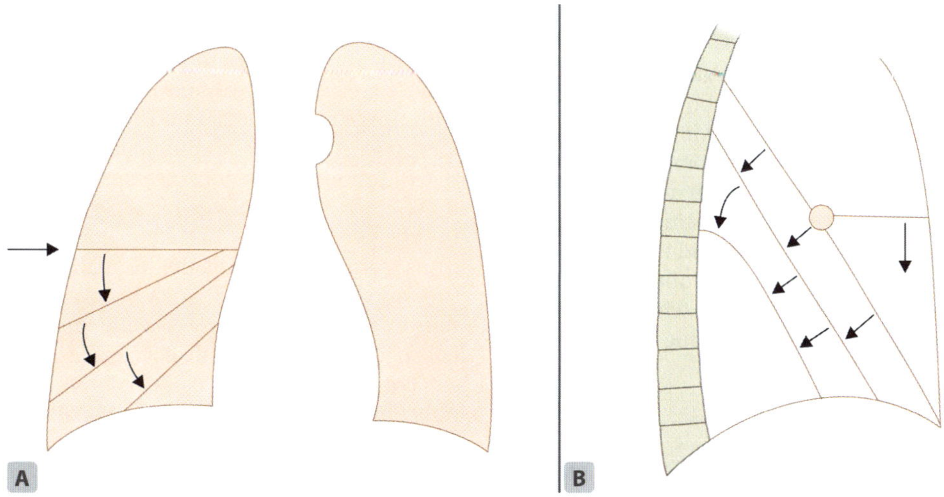

FIGS. 14A AND B: Right lower lobe collapse on PA (A) and lateral (B) views: Downward displacement of horizontal fissure is noted on PA view. The oblique fissure is displaced backwards on lateral view.

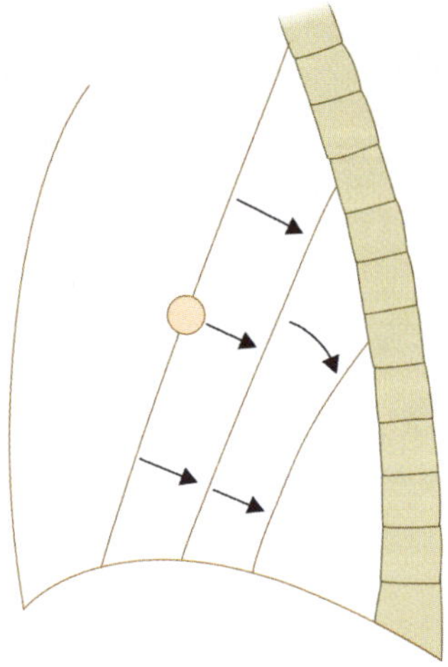

FIG. 15: Left lower lobe collapse on lateral view: No fissure is seen on the PA projection. Lateral view shows the oblique fissure to be displaced posteriorly.

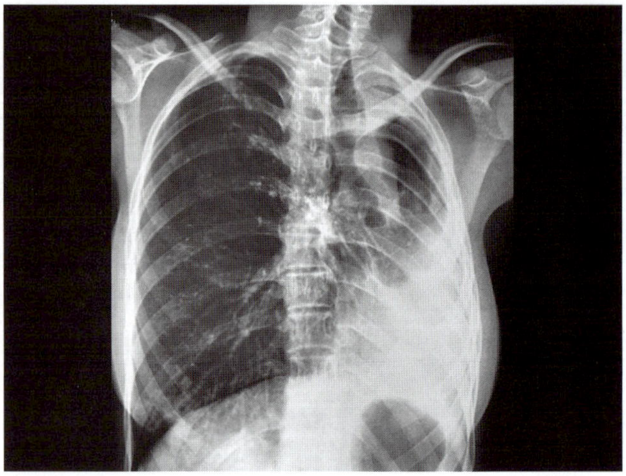

FIG. 16: Near complete collapse of the left lung with ipsilateral tracheomediastinal shift, obscured cardiac margins and left hemidiaphragm. Compensatory hyperinflation of right lung is seen which appears hyperlucent, few calcified granulomas are also seen in right lung.

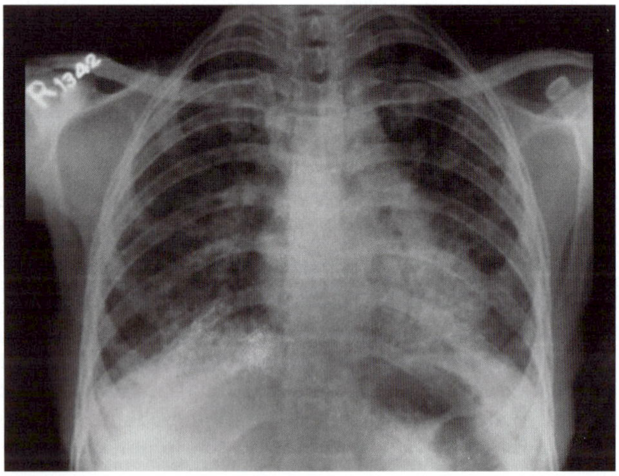

FIG. 17: Chest radiograph showing coarse reticular pattern in a patient with Idiopathic pulmonary fibrosis.

delicate mesh giving rise to ground-glass type of opacity. Medium reticular opacities enclose around 3 to 10 mm size of air spaces, whilst coarse reticulation encompass large cystic spaces of 1 cm or more. Honeycombing can result as a result of both medium and coarse reticulation and is seen in many conditions afflicting lung interstitium like fibrosing alveolitis, systemic sclerosis, rheumatoid lung, sarcoidosis, etc. **(Figs. 17 and 18)**. There is upper lobe predilection in sarcoidosis and eosinophilic granuloma while most of other disease entities displaying honeycombing have lower lobe preponderance.

Nodular Pattern

Formation of various sized nodules in the interstitium can also occur. These nodules can be of varying sizes but are rounded and usually homogeneous in density. The sizes may vary from micronodular (less than 1 mm), small (1-3 mm), medium (3-5 mm) to large (more than 5 mm). Miliary tuberculosis is a classic example of widespread nodular interstitial involvement occurring as a result of blood-borne spread **(Fig. 19)**. Similar appearance can also result in other conditions like miliary carcinomatosis, sarcoidosis and inhalational diseases like silicosis **(Box 2)**.

Reticular as well as Nodular Pattern

Reticular pattern may coexist with nodular pattern due to disease etiology as well as progression. The disease may be interstitial to begin with and may have both nodular as well as reticular components as can be seen in sarcoidosis **(Box 3)**.

Combination of Airspace Opacities and Interstitial Pattern

Combined involvement of alveolar and interstitial compartments is commonly seen histologically. A similar pattern may be evident radiographically.[17] The disease affecting one compartment may spread to adjoining area with progression of disease. The disease may be interstitial to start with as seen with pulmonary edema, but with further rise of pulmonary venous pressures there is outpouring of fluid in alveolar spaces giving fluffy appearances. Similarly, in infective processes like staphylococcal pneumonias the disease initially involves the bronchial walls with resultant inflammation referred to as bronchiolitis. This leads to narrowing of smaller airways with consequent collapse and consolidation involving alveolar spaces.

This combination is also characteristic of certain infectious diseases of the lung—*Pneumocystis jirovecii* and cytomegalovirus. These two infections are characterized by diffuse interstitial pneumonitis, the disease then spreads into parenchymal airspaces, producing widespread alveolar consolidation **(Fig. 20)**. So, the diseases frequently coexist in interstitial as well as alveolar compartment.

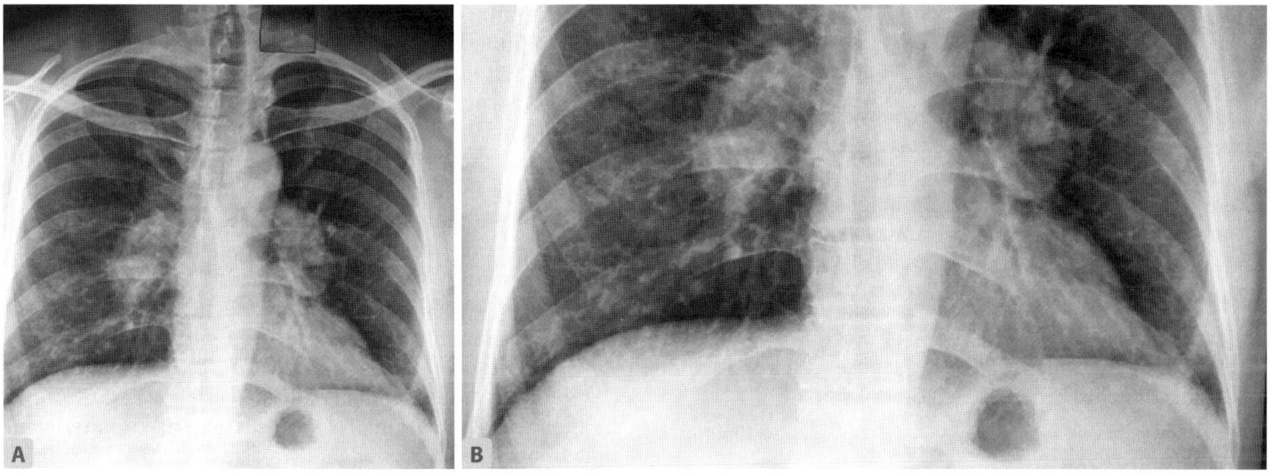

FIGS. 18A AND B: Bilateral hilar lymphadenopathy and reticular opacities in bilateral lower zones in a case of sarcoidosis.

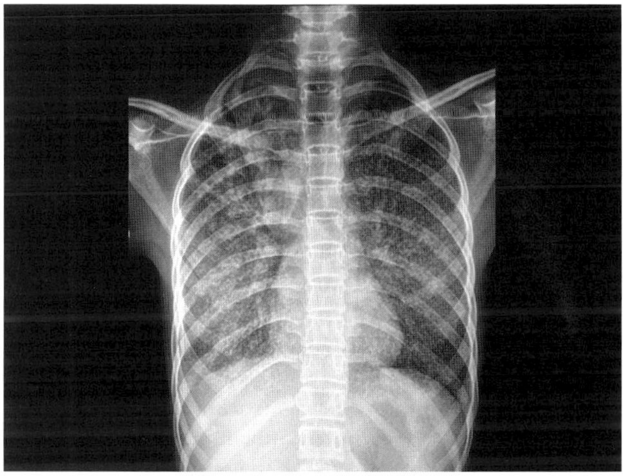

FIG. 19: Multiple small nodules seen scattered in bilateral lungs suggestive of miliary tuberculosis, subsegmental collapse of right upper lobe is noted.

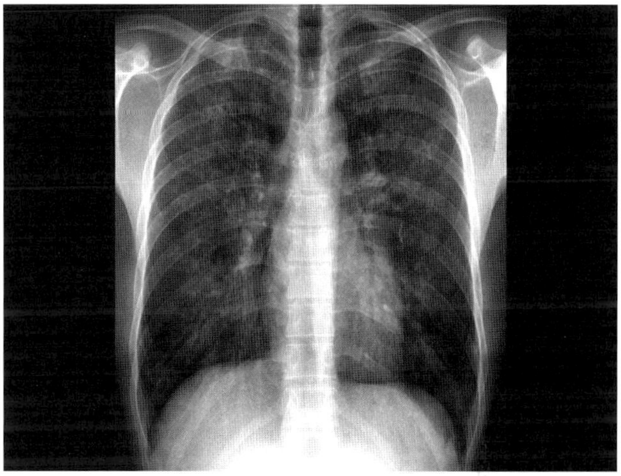

FIG. 20: *Pneumocystis jirovecii* pneumonia (PJP) showing reticular interstitial pulmonary pattern with few areas of airspace opacification, changes are more marked in perihilar location.

Box 2: Causes of miliary pattern on chest radiographs.

- Miliary tuberculosis
- Histoplasmosis
- Coccidioidomycosis
- Cryptococcosis
- Nocardiosis
- Viral infections
- Sarcoidosis
- Silicosis
- Siderosis
- Berylliosis
- Metastases
- Amyloidosis
- Alveolar microlithiasis

Box 3: Causes of reticulonodular opacities in bilateral lungs on chest radiography.

- Idiopathic pulmonary fibrosis
- Rheumatic lung disease
- Scleroderma, systemic lupus erythematosus
- Hypersensitivity pneumonitis
- Pneumoconiosis (Coal workers' pneumoconiosis, silicosis, asbestosis)
- Sarcoidosis
- Amyloidosis
- Mycoplasma, viral pneumonia
- Pulmonary edema
- Lymphangitic spread of carcinoma
- Hemosiderosis
- Lymphoid interstitial pneumonitis

Ring Shadows

Ring shadows can be seen in many conditions on chest radiography such as congenital causes including sequestered segment, bronchogenic cysts; infectious causes like bacterial abscesses, tuberculosis and *Pneumocystis jirovecii* pneumonia; connective tissue diseases like rheumatoid nodules, Wegener granulomatosis; neoplasms and bronchiectasis **(Fig. 21)**. The lesions may be single or multiple and of varying sizes.

Line and Band Shadows

Linear opacities with a diameter of more than 5 mm are referred to as band shadows whereas those with a diameter of less than 5 mm are called line shadows.[6]

Parenchymal Scarring

Linear shadows can be seen in a segment of lung that was the site of infectious disease and has healed through fibrosis. This may be seen in cases of healed upper lobe postprimary tuberculosis. It can also be seen in healed pulmonary infarction resulting in fibrous scarring secondary to lung necrosis . These linear shadows always extend to a pleural surface and this may be caused in part by an indrawing of the pleura by the scar.

Mucoid Impaction

Branching bandlike opacities pointing towards the hilum can be seen due to mucoid impaction and give rise to the "gloved finger" shadow. These are characteristically seen in allergic bronchopulmonary aspergillosis but can also be seen in many obstructive conditions like bronchial carcinoid, carcinoma lung, metastases, bronchial atresia, foreign body aspiration and benign strictures.

Septal Lines

Interstitial thickening involving the interlobular septae and bronchovascular bundle can lead to the development of primarily linear opacities.

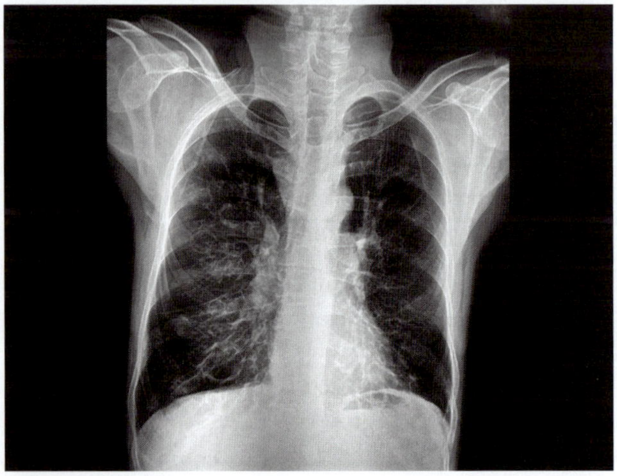

FIG. 21: Chest radiograph showing multiple ring shadows in bilateral lungs (right > left), with some showing thickened walls in a case of cystic bronchiectasis.

Kerley first described septal lines on chest radiographs in cases of pulmonary edema.[18] They were named A, B and C lines as their anatomical basis was uncertain. Septal lines is a more appropriate term as increased fluid or tissue in the interstitium can result in linear opacities called Kerley B lines or rarely Kerley A or C lines **(Box 4)**.[19]

Kerley B lines are horizontal, peripheral nonbranching fine lines less than 2 cm long, seen typically at lung bases. These linear opacities are less than 1 mm thick, and lie roughly perpendicular to the pleural surface. They are commonly seen as a result of interstitial edema secondary to increase of pulmonary venous pressures, as in rheumatic heart disease and left ventricular failure **(Fig. 22)**.

Kerley A and C lines are rare. Overlapping of Kerley B lines especially near pleural surfaces give rise to interlacing network of fine linear opacities referred to as Kerley C lines. Kerley A lines on the other hand, are slightly thicker than Kerley B lines and about 6 cm long, coursing from pleural interfaces to the lung hilum.

The Kerley B lines may be reversible in early stage of interstitial edema, with treatment of underlying cardiac pathology. However, these lines would persist if interstitial tissue pathology is irreversible, like in lymphangitic carcinomatosis, pneumoconiosis.

Tubular Shadows (Bronchial Wall Shadows)

The air column of the trachea, main bronchi, right intermediate bronchus, and left lower lobe bronchus is normally visible on well-exposed radiographs. Where these structures are in contact with aircontaining parenchyma their walls are also visible, their thickness being sufficient to cast a radiographic shadow. When tubular shadows are identified outside the hilar limits they constitute a definite sign of disease. Tubular shadows are doubleline shadows that may be parallel or slightly tapered as they proceed distally, and always follow the bronchovascular distribution.

Bronchiectasis is the most common cause of tubular shadows. The width of the air column separating them depends upon the severity of the bronchial dilatation. Since chronic bronchiectasis is often associated with atelectasis, multiple tubular shadows may be crowded together.

Tubular shadows may also be seen in the lungs of children with bronchial asthma. The tubular shadows seen in chronic bronchitis have been attributed to the accompanying bronchiectasis. Bronchial wall thickening may also be seen in pulmonary edema and in cases with neoplastic infiltration of the peribronchial tissues.

Box 4: Causes of septal lines on chest radiograph.

- Pulmonary edema
- Lymphangitis carcinomatosa
- Malignant lymphoma
- Sarcoidosis
- Pneumoconiosis
- Lymphoid interstitial pneumonitis
- Idiopathic pulmonary hemorrhage (late stages)

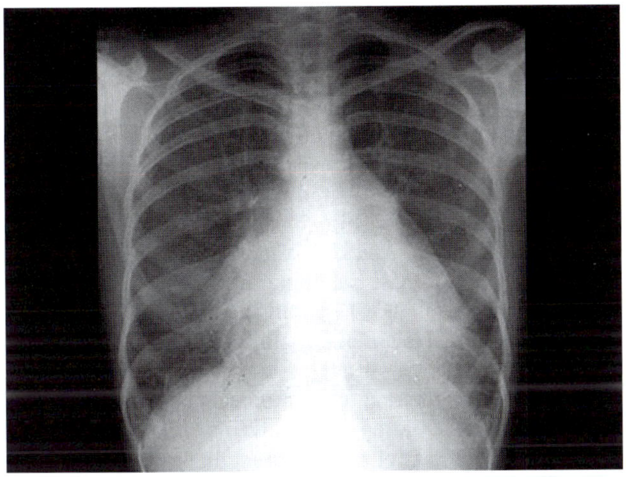

FIG. 22: Septal (Kerley B) lines seen in a case of mitral valve disease.

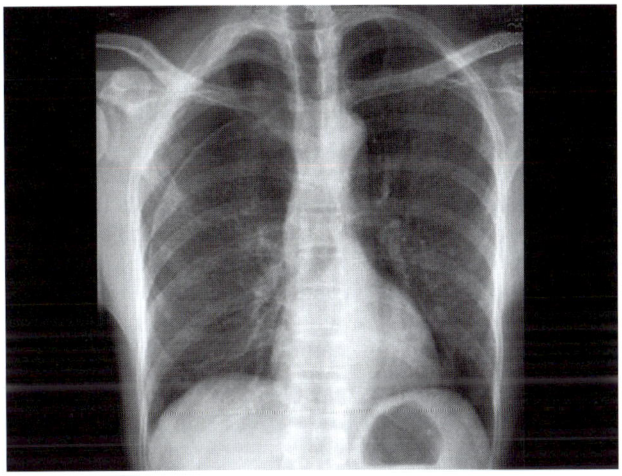

FIG. 23: Right-sided pneumothorax with passive atelectasis of right lung. Visceral pleural line is seen. Fractures of third to sixth ribs on right side.

Line Shadows of Pleural Origin

In addition to the normal interlobar fissure lines, some line shadows that originate in the pleura indicate direct or indirect signs of disease. For example, with loss of lower lobe volume, the upper portion of the major fissure sweeps downward and medially and becomes visible on frontal radiograph as an obliquely-oriented shadow extending inferiorly and laterally from the lateral aspect of mediastinum above the hilum. Thickening of an interlobar fissure is caused more often by pleural edema than by pleural effusion. Since the pleural connective tissue layer is continuous with the interlobular septa, edema fluid also collects in the subpleural space. It not only thickens the interlobar fissures but also widens the pleural layer along the lung's convex surface.

The visceral pleural line is seen in pneumothorax **(Fig. 23)**. The double pleural line seen along either side of the mediastinum in cases of mediastinal emphysema is created by the combined thickness of parietal and visceral pleura displaced laterally by mediastinal gas.

Several other signs may aid in determining the nature of a pathologic process within the lungs.[5] To assess and interpret the ongoing process caused as a result of underlying disease, it is important to take into account ancillary findings that might prove contributory in the better understanding of the disease. These include position of fissures and hila on the chest radiograph and the characteristics of the lesion itself.

Position of Fissures and Hila

Frequently, displacement of the interlobar fissures and hila towards an area of increased density point to the presence of disease nearby like lung collapse **(Fig. 24)**. Displacement away from a lesion may be rarely seen because of volume expansion as in Friedlander's pneumonia (*Klebsiella*) where bulging fissure can be seen. This is due to the abundant exudates produced by the organism. It may also be seen with *Streptococcus pneumoniae, Mycobacterium tuberculosis* and plague pneumonia. Expansion of a lobe may also be seen with acute lung abscess, when air trapping by a check valve mechanism in the communicating airway distends the abscess cavity.

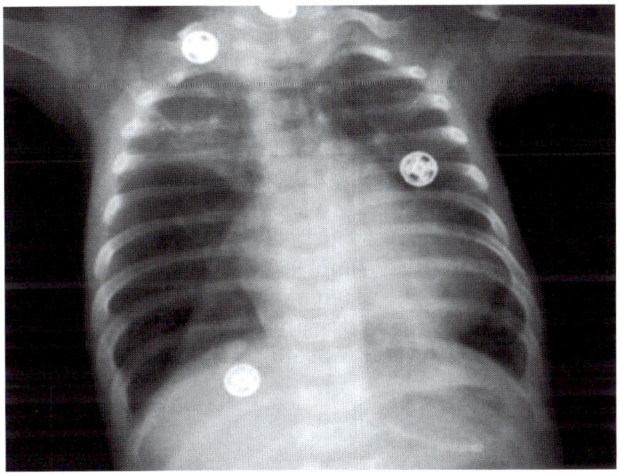

FIG. 24: Right upper lobe atelectasis showing increased density with upper displacement of transverse fissure. Atelectasis of posterior basal segment of right lower lobe.

The interlobar fissures are an efficient barrier to the interlobar spread of parenchymal disease. A few diseases have a propensity for crossing pleural boundaries which is commonly seen with mycotic or actinomycotic infection of the lungs. In the latter, the organisms pass across visceral and parietal pleural layers and they may form abscesses leading to osteomyelitis in the chest wall.

Characteristics of the Lesion Itself

Single or Multiple

Primary malignant tumor of lung is characteristically solitary while metastatic disease frequently presents with multiple lesions. Pyemic abscesses are also multiple because of hematogenous spread.

Border

The smoothness of contour suggests benign disease and nodularity or lobulation indicates malignancy. A sharply defined contour is seen with acute airspace pneumonia that has extended to an interlobar pleural surface **(Figs. 25A and B)**, its margin is less distinct if it is formed by a spreading zone of confluent acinar lesions. A mass originating from the pleural space or extrapleurally, displaces the pleura and underlying lung inward such that the angle formed by the margins of the mass and the chest wall is obtuse. An intrapulmonary mass tends to be more sharply defined and forms an acute angle with the surrounding lung parenchyma.

Cavitation

A cavity is a gas-filled space, seen as a lucency or low-attenuation area, within pulmonary consolidation, a mass, or a nodule.[20] It sometimes contains a fluid level. Pulmonary cavities are mostly caused by tissue necrosis and expulsion of necrotic material into the bronchial tree **(Fig. 26)**. Rupture of a bronchogenic cyst or an *Echinococcus* cyst are exceptions where contents were originally fluid; as is infection of an existing cystic space, such as a bulla.

Wall thickness of the cavity, especially at its thickest part, can point to underlying disease process as being benign or malignant. Malignant lesions show a thick, nodular wall whereas benign lesions tend to have a thin, smooth wall. Nearly 85% of cavities with a wall measuring more than 15 mm in its thickest portion are malignant. If the thickest part of the wall is less than 5 mm, 95% are benign.[8] Presence of internal contents like aspergilloma, blood clot or floating membranes as seen with ruptured echinococcal disease giving rise to the **"water lily sign"** help in narrowing down the differential diagnosis.

Calcification

Presence of parenchymal lung calcification is a helpful indicator, usually pointing towards a benign process. Deposition of calcium in dead or non-vital tissue is referred to as dystrophic calcification, as is commonly seen in India in tubercular afflictions of the lung. Rarely calcification or ossification may occur in healthy lung as in metastasis from osteosarcoma. This is referred to as metastatic calcification.

Dystrophic calcification is fairly common in Ghon's focus as well as healed or old pulmonary tuberculosis and it may be solitary **(Fig. 27)**, localized or widespread **(Fig. 28)**. Popcorn or speckled calcification can also be seen in benign hamartomas. Calcification may be seen in other infective processes like histoplasmosis, post-chickenpox sequelae and miscellaneous conditions like arteriovenous malformations (phleboliths). Multiple ossific densities due to repeated hemorrhage can often be seen in patients of mitral stenosis. In patients with alveolar microlithiasis and hyperparathyroidism cloudlike punctate calcification of the lung is seen.[21,22]

Irregular calcification in lymph nodes is frequently encountered in healing or healed tubercular infections. Rarely calcification results not in the substance but around the margins resulting in what is described as 'Egg shell' calcification **(Fig. 29)**. This is seen in occupational lung diseases like silicosis and coal workers pneumoconiosis.

Calcification of the pleura may occur and may be seen as a focal plaque of calcification or a long and broad sheet of calcification involving the visceral pleura. This can follow blood, purulent collections in the pleural cavity or tuberculous effusion. Rarely, parietal pleural calcification may be seen, typically involving diaphragmatic pleura as in asbestosis.

Physiological calcification of the tracheobronchial tree may occur in old age, seen more commonly in women. In younger patients however, it may point to an underlying hypercalcemic state. Costal cartilage calcification is also commonly seen on chest radiographs. Vascular calcifications may be evident along the aorta and coronary arteries. Main pulmonary arterial wall may occasionally show calcification in chronic pulmonary arterial hypertension.

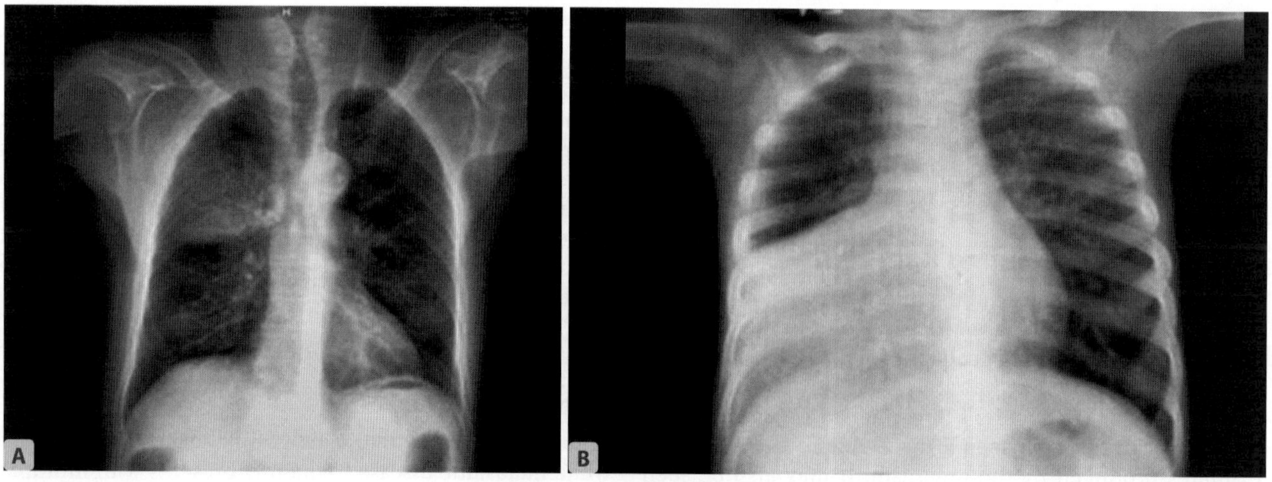

FIGS. 25A AND B: (A) Consolidation involving right upper lobe with poorly defined upper border; (B) Consolidation of right middle and lower lobes with smooth and sharply marginated upper border by the horizontal fissure. The right cardiac border and dome of diaphragm are silhouetted.

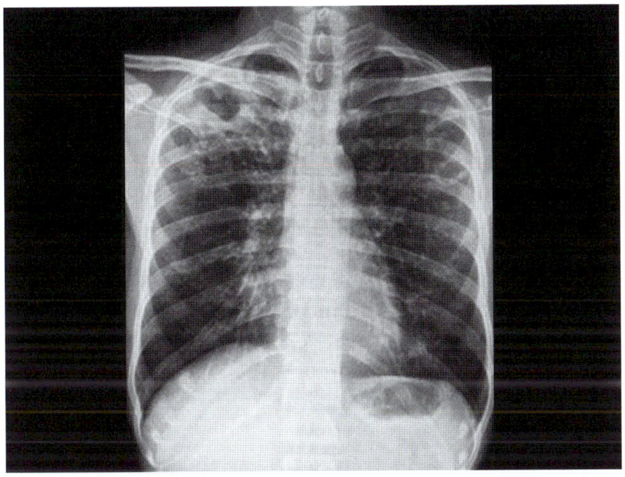

FIG. 26: Cavity in right upper lobe with surrounding consolidation. Multiple nodular opacities seen in bilateral upper and left mid zones.

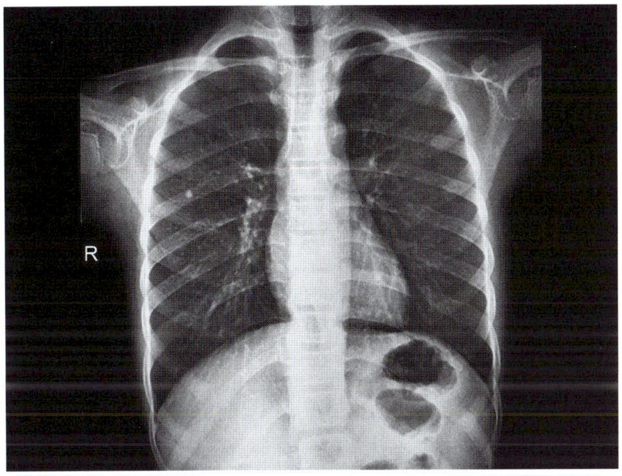

FIG. 27: Calcified granuloma in right mid zone.

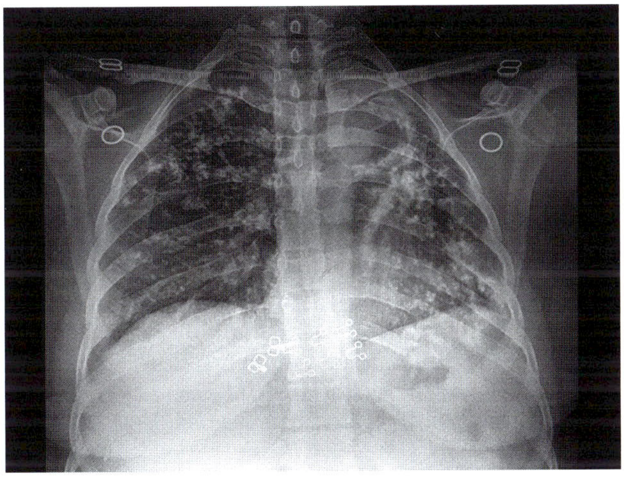

FIG. 28: Multiple calcified nodular opacities in bilateral lung fields with volume loss of left lung and an area of cavitation in left upper zone.

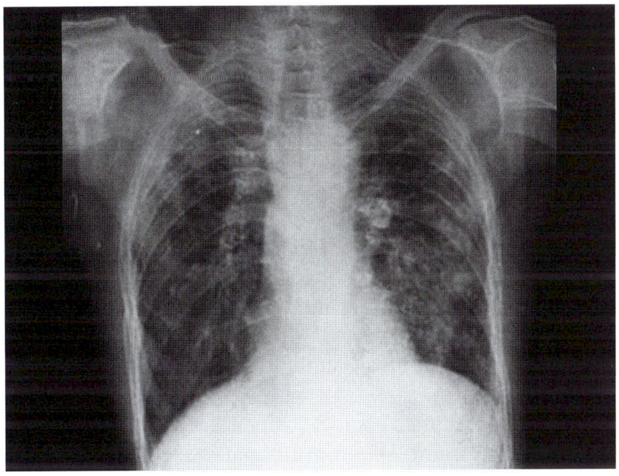

FIG. 29: In a case of sarcoidosis, chest radiograph shows multiple reticulonodular opacities and egg-shell calcifications in the hilar lymph nodes.

Anatomical Basis of Disease

The site of involvement by a particular disease process in the lungs is influenced by certain physiological factors. The ventilation: perfusion ratio is different throughout the lung, primarily because of the influence of gravity. Gravity largely establishes the distribution of disease in aspiration pneumonia. The upper lobes are involved if aspiration occurs when the patient is supine, their posterior portions more frequently than the anterior. If the patient is erect, involvement of the lower lobes predominates. Aspiration occurs more readily into the right than left lung because the right main bronchus is more in line with the trachea.

Blood-borne diseases predominate at the lung bases due to the greater perfusion of the lung bases in the upright patient. The hemodynamics of blood flow within the lungs causes embolic phenomena to also produce a peripheral distribution of disease. Pulmonary infarction occurs much more frequently in lower lobes than in upper lobes. Metastatic lesions occur more frequently in lower lobes. In bedridden patients, metastatic deposits do not show the usual anatomic bias and may predominate in upper zones. Pulmonary sequestration occurs almost exclusively in the lower lobes, most commonly in the posterior basal segment and on the left side than the right. The groundglass opacity and reticulation of asbestosis shows basal distribution. Chronic idiopathic interstitial fibrosis and interstitial fibrosis of progressive systemic sclerosis are also predominantly basal in distribution.

Primary pulmonary carcinoma has an unexplained predilection for upper lung zones. The decrease in perfusion of the well-ventilated lung apices causes the apices to have a higher partial pressure of oxygen (pO_2) than the remainder of the lungs. The predilection of tuberculosis for the lung apices has been attributed to this difference in oxygen pressures. Upper lobe predilection is shown by silicosis, sarcoidosis, eosinophilic granuloma, and the conglomerate shadows of complicated silicosis and coal workers' pneumoconiosis.

The Silhouette Sign

This sign was described by Felson and helps in the localization and at times recognition of pulmonary disease. "An intrathoracic lesion touching a border of the heart, aorta or diaphragm will obliterate that border on the roentgenogram. An intrathoracic lesion not anatomically contiguous with a border of one of these structures will not obliterate that border". The sign is produced when the juxtaposed borders are of similar density. On a frontal radiograph, obscuration of specific contours indicate abnormalities in specific lobes, for instance if right superior mediastinum (superior vena cava) is obscured, the pathology is in the right upper lobe. Right heart border is obscured in right middle lobe involvement **(Fig. 30)** and right hemidiaphragm is obscured in right lower lobe involvement. The left superior mediastinum (aortic arch) is obscured in left upper lobe pathology, the left heart border in lingular involvement and the left hemidiaphragm or descending aorta in left lower lobe disease.[8]

The **"hilum overlay sign"** was described by Felson and helps in determining whether an opacity is within the hilum or anterior or posterior to it **(Fig. 31)**. If the opacity is situated within the hilum it will be obscured by the opacity from the proximal pulmonary artery and will appear inseparable from hilar structures. If hilar vessels are clearly seen through an opacity then it can be situated anterior or posterior to the hilum.[23]

Increased hilar size and density is seen with pulmonary artery enlargement. When pulmonary vessels are seen to converge on the lateral aspect of the hilum, it is referred to as the **"hilum convergence sign"** and is suggestive of vascular dilatation as the cause of hilar enlargement. The hilar angle shows its normal concave appearance.[8]

The **"cervicothoracic sign"** is used to differentiate between an anterior and posterior mass in the superior mediastinum. A posterior mediastinal mass is surrounded by lung tissue from all sides as the posterior part of the lung extends superior to the clavicle at the level of the thoracic inlet. Anterior mediastinal masses show ill-defined superior margins due to their anatomical contact with the soft tissues of the neck, either at or below the clavicle.[24]

DECREASED DENSITY ON CHEST RADIOGRAPH

Diffuse increase in transradiancy of both lungs is seen in airway disease, constrictive bronchiolitis, asthma, emphysema, right to lung cardiac shunts like tetralogy of Fallot, Eisenmenger physiology or severe peripheral pulmonary arterial stenoses.

A focal increase in transradiancy can be seen in emphysema and bullous diseases, cysts, pneumatoceles and cavities. A bulla appears as a rounded focal lucency, 1 cm or more in diameter and is bounded by a thin wall. Multiple bullae may often be seen and are associated with other signs of pulmonary emphysema.[20] A cyst appears as a round parenchymal lucency with a well-defined interface with normal lung. Cysts have variable wall thickness but are usually thin-walled (2 mm) and occur without associated pulmonary emphysema. Cysts in the lung usually contain air but occasionally contain fluid or solid material.[20] Air cysts that develop following infections are known as "pneumatoceles" and are seen following *Pneumocystis jirovecii* or staphylococcal pneumonia **(Figs. 32A and B)** and hydrocarbon fluid aspiration.[6] Cavities are gas-filled areas of the lung within a nodule, mass or area of consolidation.

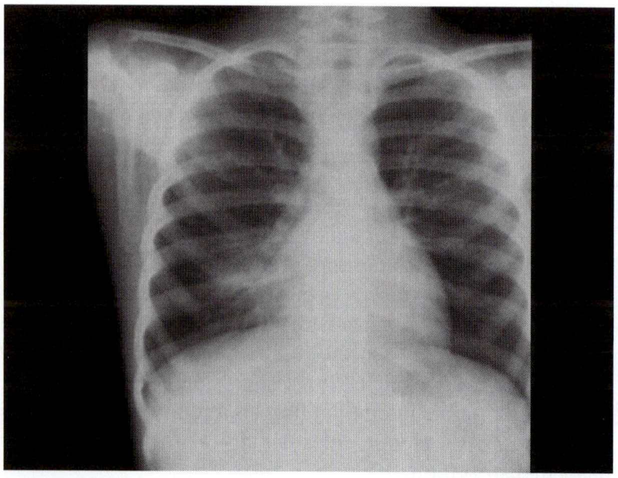

FIG. 30: "Silhouette sign"—right middle lobe consolidation obscuring the right cardiac border.

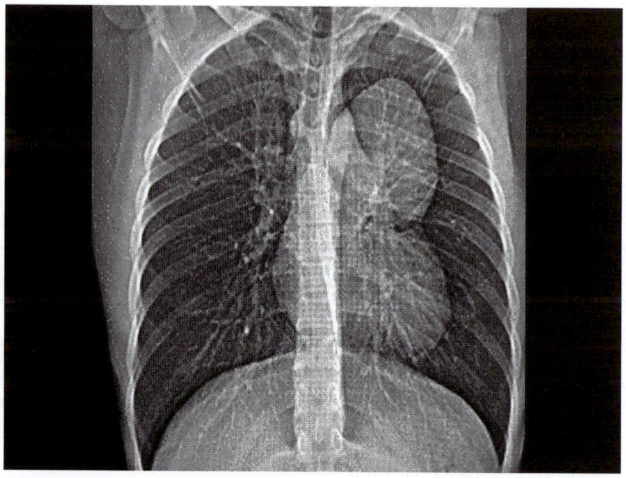

FIG. 31: Hilum overlay sign in anterior mediastinal mass, the hilar vessels are seen through the lesion.

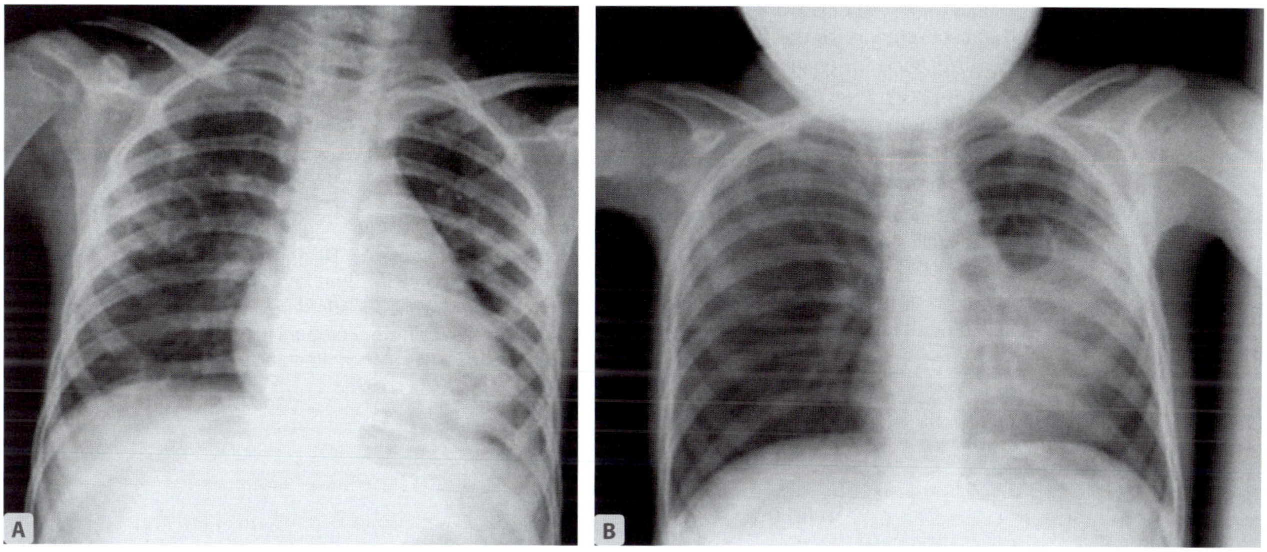

FIGS. 32A AND B: (A) Pneumatoceles in right lung field; (B) resolving staphylococcal pneumonia in left lung with pneumatocele.

Unilateral hyperlucent lung can be seen with thoracic wall and soft tissue abnormalities, diminished perfusion of lung, compensatory hyperinflation of lung associated with collapse **(Fig. 33)** and foreign body impaction with obstructive emphysema.[6] Decrease in pulmonary blood volume may be associated with congenital defects like agenesis or hypoplasia of pulmonary arteries or acquired reasons such as thromboembolism.[25]

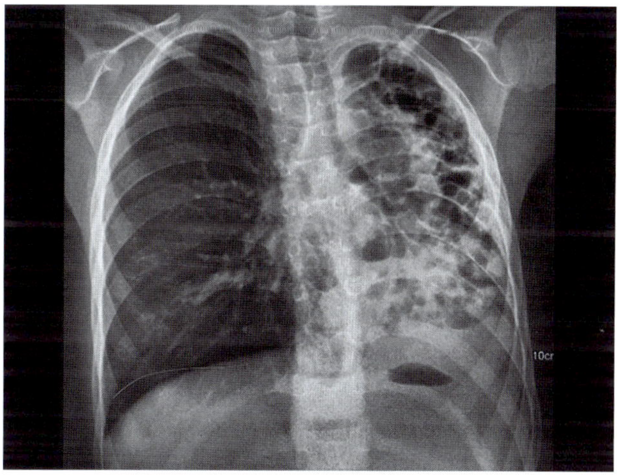

FIG. 33: Multiple cystic bronchiectatic opacities in left lung field with volume loss on left side and compensatory hyperinflation of right lung which appears hyperlucent.

CONCLUSION

Chest radiography is an integral part of the diagnostic work-up of patients with respiratory disease. The natural contrast of the air containing pulmonary tissue provides a window which allows radiographic evaluation of diseases involving the lungs, tracheobronchial tree, and pleura. Computed tomography serves as an important adjunct to the plain film for the purposes of diagnosis and characterization of parenchymal lung disease.[26]

REFERENCES

1. Chest X-ray interpretation: Not just black and white. Pezzotti, William MSN, RN, ACNP-BC, CEN. Nursing. 2014;44:(1) p. 40-7.
2. Felson B. The roentgen diagnosis of disseminated pulmonary alveolar diseases. Semin Roentgenol. 1967;2:321.
3. Felson B. Chest Roentgenology. Philadelphia: WB Saunders, 1973.
4. Felson B. A new look at pattern recognition of diffuse pulmonary diseases. Am J Roentgenol. 1979;133:183-9.
5. Fraser RG, Pare JAP, Pare PD, et al. Diagnosis of Diseases of the Chest (3rd edn). Vol I: WB Saunders, 1988.
6. Hansell DM. Imaging of Diseases of the chest. 5th edition. St. Louis: Mosby Elsevier, 2009.
7. Collins J. Chest Radiology: The Essentials. 3rd edition. Philadelphia: Wolters Kluwer, 2015.
8. Webb WR. Thoracic Imaging: Pulmonary and Cardiovascular Radiology. 2nd edition. Philadelphia: Wolters Kluwer, 2010.
9. Woodring JH, Reed JC. Types and mechanisms of pulmonary atelectasis. J Thorac Imaging. 1996;11:92-108.
10. Proto AV, Tocino I. Radiographic manifestations of lobar collapse. Semin Roentgenol. 1980;15:117-73.
11. Woodring JH, Reed JC. Radiographic manifestations of lobar atelectasis. J Thorac Imaging. 1996;11:109-44.
12. Sutton D. Textbook of Radiology & Imaging. 7th edition. Edinburgh: Churchill Livingstone, 2009.
13. Golden R. The effect of bronchostenosis upon the roentgen-ray shadows in carcinoma of the bronchus. Am J Roentgenol. 1925;13:21-30.
14. Oktay Algın, Gökhan Gökalp, Uğur Topa. Signs in chest imaging. Diagn Interv Radiol. 2011;17:18-29.
15. Adam Grainger & Allison's Diagnostic Radiology, 6th edition. Philadelphia: Elsevier, 2014.

16. Kattan KR, Wlot JF. Cardiac rotation in left lower lobe collapse. 'The flat waist sign.' Radiology. 1976;118:275-9.
17. Felson B. A new look at pattern recognition of diffuse pulmonary disease. Am J Roentgenol. 1979;133:83.
18. Kerley P. Radiology in heart disease. BMJ. 1933;2:594-7.
19. Trapnell DH. The differential diagnosis of linear shadows in chest radiographs. Radiol Clin North Am. 1973;11:77-92.
20. Hansell DM, Bankier AA, MacMohan H, McLoud TC, Muller NL, Remy J. Fleischner Society: Glossary of Terms for Thoracic Imaging. Radiology. 2008; 246:697-722.
21. Brown K, Mund DF, Aberle DR, et al. Intrathoracic calcifications: radiographic features and differential diagnoses. Radio. Graphics 1994;14:1247-61.
22. Chai JL, Patz EF Jr. CT of the lung: patterns of calcification and other high-attenuation abnormalities. Am J Roentgenol. 1994;162:1063-6.
23. Felson B, Felson H. Localization of intrathoracic lesions by means of the posteroanterior roentgenogram; The silhouette sign. Radiology. 1950;55:363-74.
24. Kumaresh A, Kumar M, Dev B , Gorantla R, Venkata Sai PM, Thanasekaraan V. Back to Basics—'Must Know' Classical Signs in Thoracic Radiology. J Clin Imaging Sci. 2015;5:43.
25. Altinsoy B, Altintas N. Diagnostic approach to unilateral hyperlucent lung. JRSM Short Rep. 2011;2:95.
26. Kuhlman JE. Nonneoplastic Parenchymal Lung Disease. In: Haaga, Lanzieri, Sartoris, Zerhouni (Eds). Computed Tomography and Magnetic Resonance Imaging of the Whole Body, 3rd edition. Mosby, Vol I; 1998.

CHAPTER

125

Basic Patterns of Lung Disease on CT

Alpana Manchanda, Satyam, Gaurav Shanker Pradhan, Jyoti Kumar

Computed tomography (CT) of the chest, especially high resolution computed tomography (HRCT) is the radiological imaging technique which best depicts changes in lung structure and is widely used for evaluating a variety of focal and diffuse lung disease. HRCT is superior to plain chest radiography in the detection and characterization of abnormalities due to the inability of plain radiographs to resolve small differences in lung density.

A CT "pattern" refers to a nonspecific finding or collection of findings suggesting one or more specific disease processes.[1] Various HRCT findings when taken together can represent typical patterns. The patterns, in conjunction with the anatomical distribution of findings along with clinical findings can narrow the differential diagnosis of diffuse lung disease, and in many cases indicate the correct diagnosis.[2]

HIGH RESOLUTION CT PATTERNS OF LUNG DISEASE

In order to successfully interpret the high resolution CT scan findings, it is important to follow a systematic approach with understanding of pathologic presentations of disease on HRCT.[3]

HRCT scan findings can broadly be classified into two groups:

1. Those manifesting as increased lung opacity
2. Those manifesting as decreased lung opacity

HRCT disease patterns, manifesting both as increased as well as decreased lung opacity can be further sub-classified to simplify and thereby aid in differential diagnosis. At times, findings of increased and decreased lung opacity may be present on the same imaging study, suggestive of presence of two or more diseases or in certain cases be due to a pathologic process that manifests with both an infiltrative or obstructive process.

HIGH RESOLUTION CT SCAN FINDINGS MANIFESTING AS INCREASED LUNG OPACITY

HRCT scan findings manifesting as increased lung opacity can be further subclassified into the following abnormalities or patterns:

- Nodular pattern
- Linear and reticular pattern
- Ground-glass opacity
- Consolidation

Nodular Pattern: Nodules and Nodular Opacities

A number of diseases of the lung are characterized by multiple nodules as the primary abnormality. The term 'nodule' is used to describe a pulmonary opacity which is nearly circular, discrete, sharply defined or ill-defined ranging in size from 2 mm to 30 mm.[3] Nodules are usually further characterized according to their size, (uniform or variable) margin (sharply or poorly defined) density (solid or soft tissue vs sub-solid or ground-glass density), number and location. A small nodule is one which measures less than 1 cm, while a nodule 1 cm or larger in diameter is considered as a large nodule.[4]

The term 'micronodule' has been used by some authors to describe a very small, discrete, round, focal opacity. A variety of diameters have been used in the past to define a micronodule that is those with a diameter less than 7 mm, 5 mm, or 3 mm.[4]

The Nomenclature Committee of the Fleischner Society has recommended that the term micronodule be reserved for nodules less than 3 mm in diameter.[5] However, in patients of multinodular lung disease, the nodules are often of various sizes and except for miliary disease one does not usually come across cases characterized only by micronodules.

A nodular pattern is characterized on chest radiographs by innumerable, small, rounded opacities that are discrete and range from to 2 mm to 10 mm.[5] These are widespread but not necessarily uniformly distributed. On CT, the nodular pattern may be classified according to the three anatomic distribution of nodules, i.e. centrilobular, lymphatic or random, which will be discussed later.

The detection of pulmonary nodules on CT depends on their size, profusion, density and CT technique. Scan acquisition with narrow collimation is superior to thick section acquisition for detecting very small nodules as there is less partial volume effect which can average out the attenuation of tiny nodules.[6] The depiction of minute nodules on CT can be improved by the use of maximum intensity projection reconstructions of contiguous thin sections acquired by volumetric CT **(Figs. 1A and B)**.[7]

The HRCT evaluation of a patient with nodular lung disease is based on several findings and patterns.[8] These are:

- The craniocaudal distribution of nodules
- The appearance and attenuation of nodules
- The specific distribution of the nodules relative to lung structures.

The craniocaudal distribution of nodules helps in the differential diagnosis of nodular lung disease as certain diseases such as sarcoidosis and other granulomatous diseases are seen predominantly in the upper lobes while others such as hematogenous metastases tend to be lower lobe predominant **(Figs. 2A and B)**.

However, the craniocaudal distribution of nodules should not be considered in isolation and should be used in combination with other findings. Some diseases may show overlap between the distributions (upper or lower lobe) and there may be variability among patients with the same disease.

The appearance of nodules may help to ascertain whether they are of interstitial or air space (alveolar) origin. Interstitial nodules are usually well-defined, of soft tissue (solid) attenuation and obscure the edge of vessels or other structures they are in contact with. Airspace nodules are typically ill-defined, and can be of homogeneous soft tissue attenuation (solid) or hazy and less dense than the vessels called ground-glass opacity (GGO). The following tables enumerate the differential diagnosis of multinodular lung disease based on sharpness of nodule margin **(Table 1)** and nodule attenuation **(Table 2)**.

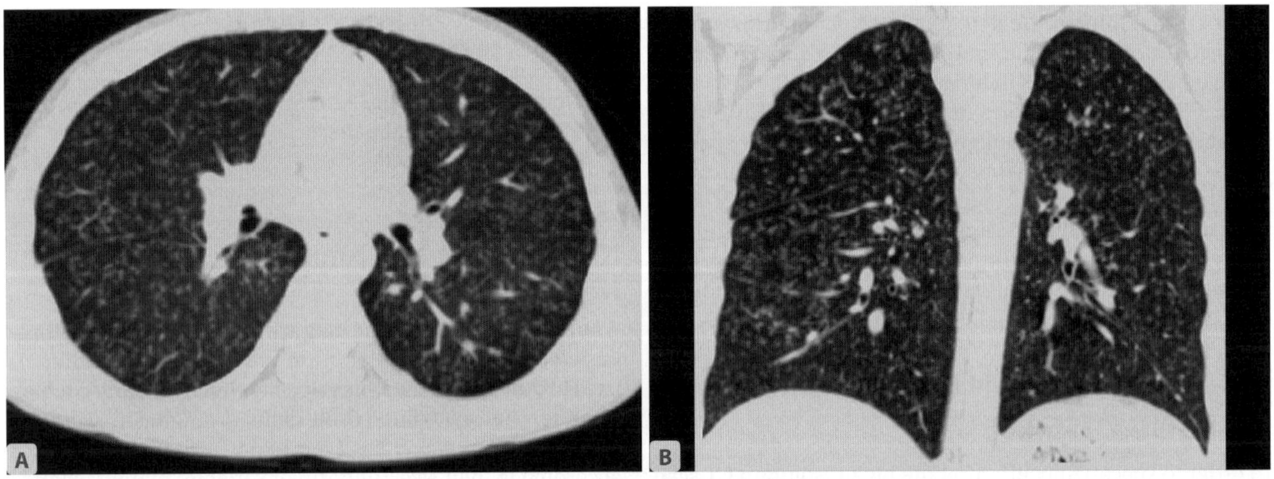

FIGS. 1A AND B: (A) Axial CT shows multiple, small, sharply defined nodules uniformly distributed in bilateral lung parenchyma; (B) Coronal reformatted CT MIP reconstruction delineates the miliary nodules better in bilateral lung fields.

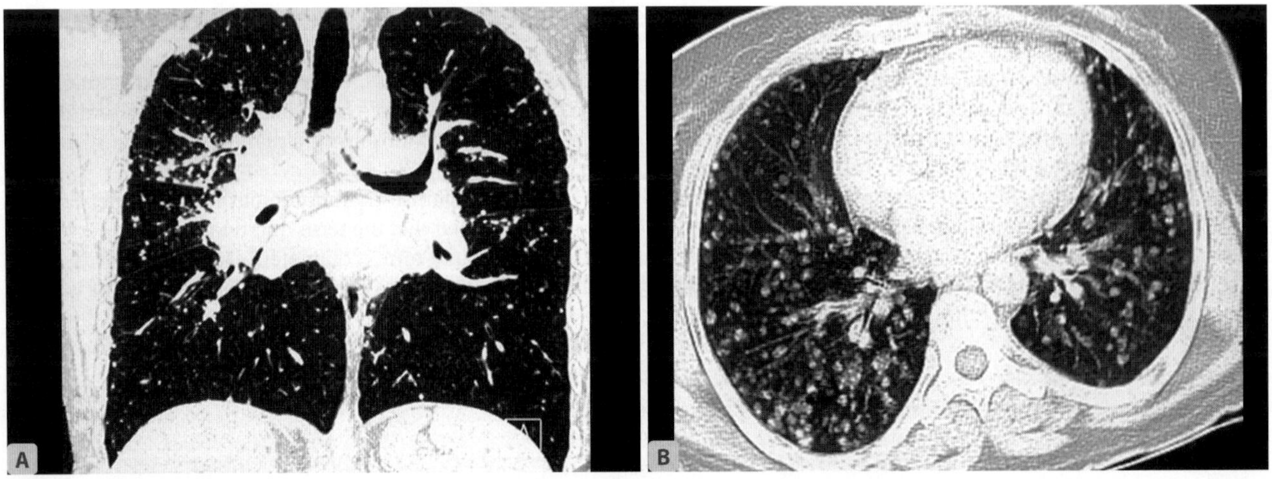

FIGS. 2A AND B: (A) Coronal MPR shows typical micronodules of sarcoidosis predominantly in bilateral upper lobes in perilymphatic distribution; (B) Axial CT shows multiple sharply defined random nodular opacities due to hematogenous metastasis.

TABLE 1: Differential diagnosis of nodular lung disease based on the sharpness of nodule margin.

Usually well-defined margins	Usually ill-defined margins	Either well or ill-defined margins
• Sarcoidosis • Metastases • Miliary infection (tubercular, fungal/viral)	• Hypersensitivity pneumonitis • Respiratory bronchiolitis • Follicular bronchiolitis	• Langerhans cell histiocytosis • Lymphoid interstitial pneumonia • Pneumoconioses
Amyloidosis	Infection (bacterial, fungal or viral)	
	Organizing pneumonia	
	Invasive mucinous adenocarcinoma (previously bronchioloalveolar carcinoma)	
	Aspiration	
	Pulmonary edema	
	Pulmonary hemorrhage	
	Metastatic calcification	

TABLE 2: Differential diagnosis of lung nodules based on nodule attenuation.

Usually solid	Usually GGO	Either solid or GGO
Sarcoidosis	Hypersensitivity pneumonitis	Lymphoid interstitial pneumonia
Metastases	Respiratory bronchiolitis	Pneumoconioses
Miliary infections	Follicular bronchiolitis	Bronchopneumonia
Amyloidosis	Pulmonary edema	Invasive mucinous adenocarcinoma
Langerhans cell histiocytosis	Pulmonary hemorrhage	Organizing pneumonia
	Metastatic calcification	Aspiration

Differentiating lung nodules into interstitial and airspace nodules on HRCT scan is not always accurate as many diffuse lung diseases involve both the interstitial and airspace compartments histologically. Also, there are many exceptions to the rule. For example, hypersensitivity pneumonitis (HP) which is an interstitial lung disease is characterized by very indistinct nodules **(Fig. 3)**.

In the assessment of diffuse nodular disease, *the anatomic distribution of nodules* relative to the secondary pulmonary lobule is diagnostic value on HRCT scans as it provides a focused differential diagnosis and is reflective of the pathophysiology of the underlying disease.

There are three specific distributions of small nodules in the secondary pulmonary lobule which can be distinguished on HRCT:

(A) Perilymphatic or lymphatic distribution, (B) Random, (C) Centrilobular distribution **(Figs. 4A to D)** are the representative schematic diagrams showing normal anatomy of the secondary pulmonary lobule and the various distribution patterns of nodules at the level of secondary pulmonary lobule. Recognizing one of these three distributions is fundamental to the HRCT interpretation of nodular lung disease and HRCT is found to be 90–95% accurate in determining the pattern present and formulating the correct differential diagnosis.[6]

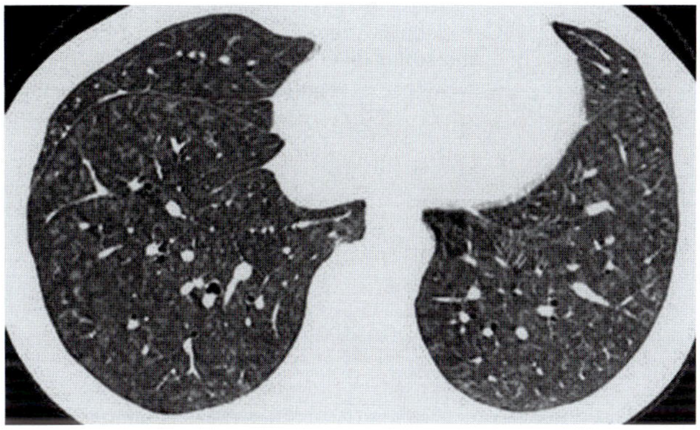

FIG. 3: Axial HRCT shows poorly defined ground-glass nodular opacities scattered in bilateral lower lobes in hypersensitivity pneumonitis.

Perilymphatic or Lymphatic Nodules

Diseases with perilymphatic distribution of nodules are characterized by involvement or spread through the pulmonary lymphatics.

Pulmonary lymphatics are normally found within the visceral pleura, the interlobular septa and along the veins and bronchovascular bundles. Hence, diseases which involve the lymphatics may produce nodules in relation to these structures.

The most common diseases which show a perilymphatic distribution are given in **Table 3**.

On HRCT and histologically, perilymphatic nodules are seen in one or more of the four locations:

i. *Peribronchovascular nodules* are seen individually or in clusters adjacent to large bronchi and vessels in the central lung regions, giving a nodular appearance to the walls of bronchi and arteries. There are most typically seen in sarcoidosis **(Fig. 5)**.
ii. *Subpleural nodules* are easily recognized beneath the pleural surfaces and adjacent to the interlobular fissures. Confluent subpleural nodules can result in the appearance of pseudoplaques. Subpleural nodules have been seen in around 80% of patients with silicosis or CWP and at least 50% of patients with sarcoidosis and also common with lymphangitic spread of carcinoma **(Fig. 6)**.[4]
iii. *Interlobular septal nodules* give the appearance of 'beaded' septa or nodular septal thickening. These are most frequent in patients of lymphangitic spread of carcinoma **(Figs. 7A and B)**.
iv. *Centrilobular peribronchovascular nodules* are also seen in relation to small airway and vessels in centrilobular location (center of pulmonary lobules), giving a beaded appearance to the centrilobular artery.

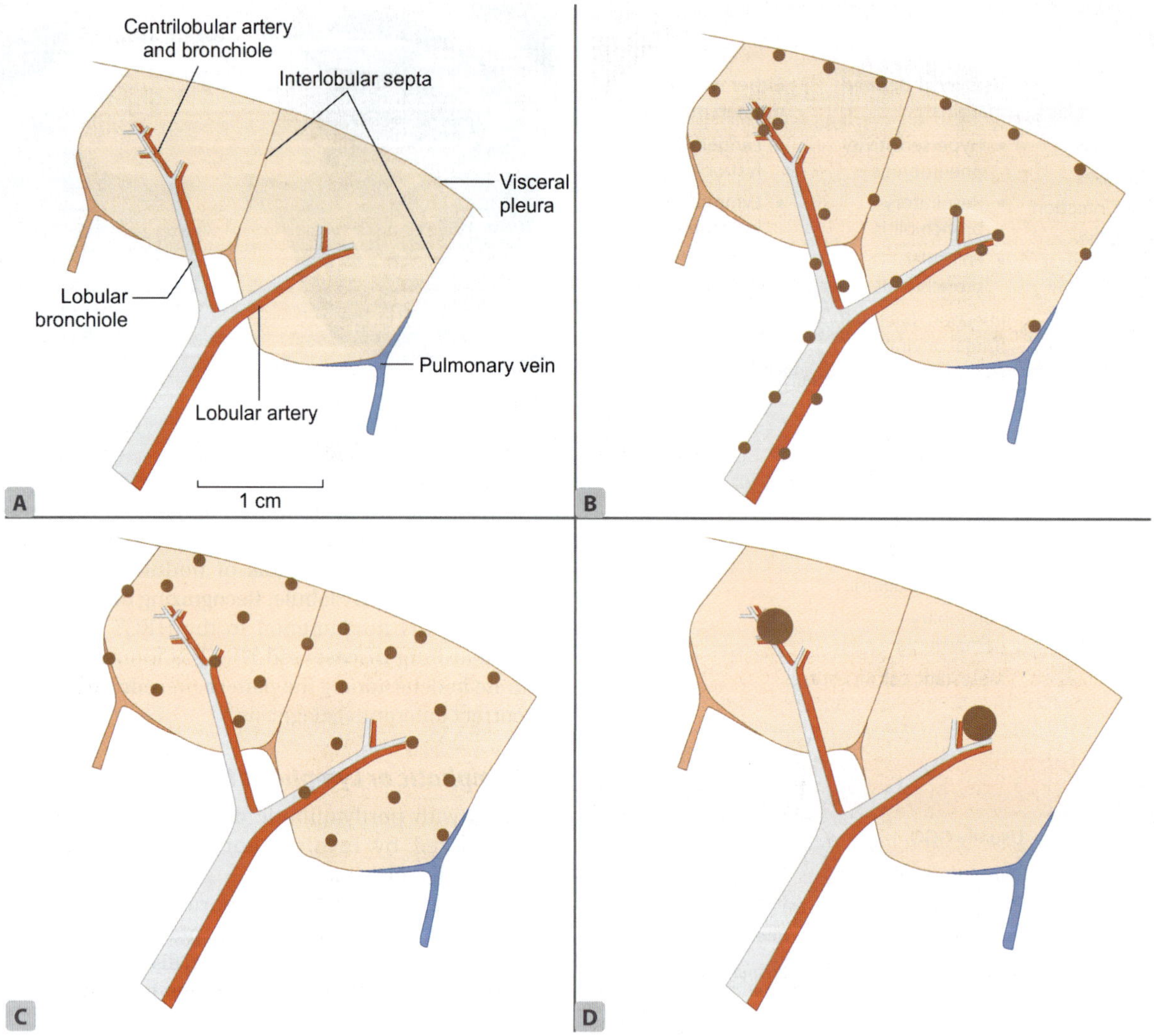

FIGS. 4A TO D: Schematic representations of distribution of nodules at the level of the secondary pulmonary lobule. (A) Normal anatomy of the secondary pulmonary lobule; (B) Perilymphatic distribution of nodules; (C) Random distribution of nodules; (D) Centrilobular distribution of nodules.

TABLE 3: Differential diagnosis of perilymphatic nodules.[8]

- Sarcoidosis (common)
- Lymphangitic carcinomatosis
- Pneumoconioses—silicosis, coal-workers pneumoconiosis (CWP), beryllosis, talc, rare earth
- Lymphoid interstitial pneumonia (rare)
- Amyloidosis (rare)

A combination of two of the above four possible sites has been described to be usually sufficient of perilymphatic nodules for diagnosis.[4] As perilymphatic nodules occur only in relation to these specific locations, the distribution of the nodules is patchy, with both normal and abnormal areas of lung regions seen on HRCT **(Table 4)**.[8]

Random Nodules

Random nodules show a diffuse and homogeneous distribution with no particular distribution relative to the secondary pulmonary lobule. The nodules are seen in contact with interlobular septa, visceral pleural surfaces and in the center of the pulmonary lobule. In contrast to perilymphatic nodules which show a patchy distribution, random nodules are usually distributed uniformly throughout the lung parenchyma in a bilateral symmetric manner.[3] **Table 5** lists the differential diagnosis of random nodules.

Random nodules are smooth, sharply marginated and usually of soft tissue attenuation. A random pattern is most common in those diseases which show a hematogenous spread such as metastatic nodules. Metastatic nodules may show a basilar predominance due to a preferential blood flow to the lung base. Individual nodules may show a 'feeding vessel sign' consistent with their hematogenous origin **(Fig. 8)**. Metastatic nodules may be surrounded by a 'halo' of ground-glass attenuation which is typically seen in hemorrhagic metastasis such as due to choriocarcinoma.[9] In some patients with metastases, features of lymphangitic spread may be seen on HRCT along with metastatic nodules.

The size of the nodules may be useful in determining the most likely diagnosis. Metastatic nodules tend to be larger

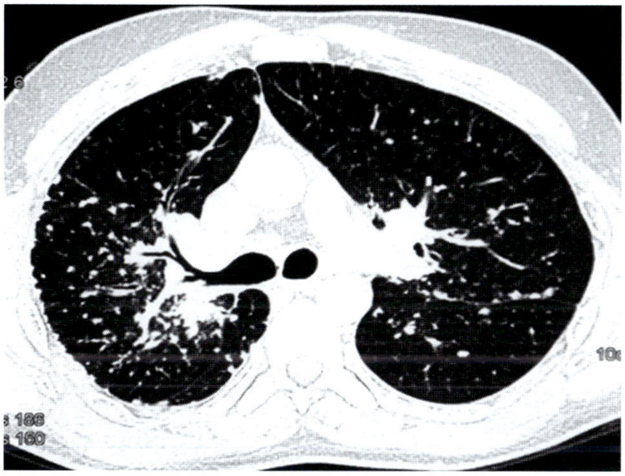

FIG. 5: Nodular interlobular septal thickening. Multiple granulomas in sarcoidosis in peribronchovascular, subpleural and centrilobular interstitium more marked in right upper lobe.

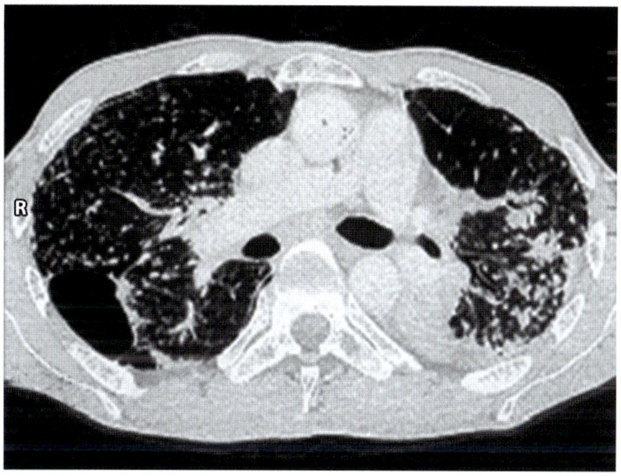

FIG. 6: Perilymphatic distribution of nodules in silicosis. Axial HRCT shows multiple small discrete and confluent micronodules in centrilobular and subpleural regions without tree in bud morphology. These are bilateral, symmetrical with upper lobe predominance. Subpleural bulla is noted on right side.

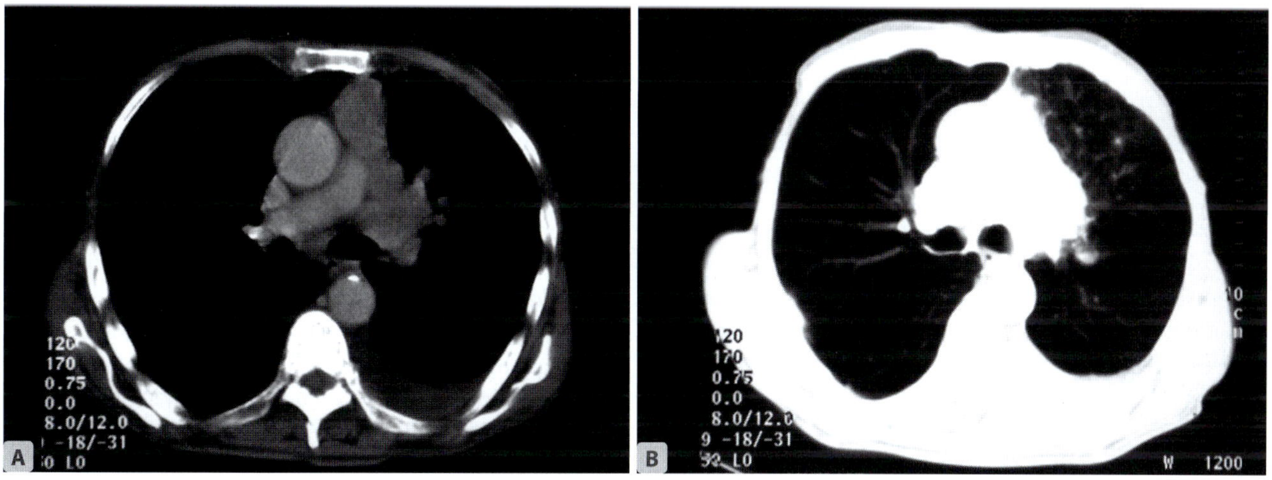

FIGS. 7A AND B: Lymphangitis carcinomatosis. Axial CT: (A) Mediastinal window shows a left suprahilar mass involving the left main bronchus, encasing the left main pulmonary artery with left pleural effusion; (B) Lung window depicts nodular interlobular septal thickening in the adjacent lung parenchyma.

TABLE 4: Typical pattern of involvement of the perilymphatic interstitium of some common diseases showing perilymphatic nodules.

	Sarcoidosis	Silicosis	Lymphangitic spread of carcinoma
Site	• Upper lobe predominance • Diffuse distribution/lower lobe involvement also seen	May be diffuse but in mild disease may be seen in upper lobes	Upper or lower lobes or diffuse
Perilymphatic interstitium most commonly involved by nodules on HRCT	• Along central bronchi and vessels • In relation to major fissures	Centrilobular and subpleural in location	• Within thickened peribronchovascular interstitium, interlobular septa • Subpleural nodules less profuse
Size of nodules	Few mm to 1 cm	2–5 mm	Seen as beaded appearance of septum
Appearance of nodules	Usually well-defined	Well-defined	Septal thickening smooth/nodular
Lung involvement	Patchy and asymmetric distribution of nodules	More evenly distributed Typical bilateral and symmetrical nodules	Variable-unilateral, patchy, bilateral or symmetric

TABLE 5: Differential diagnosis of random nodules.

- Hematogenous metastases
- Miliary tuberculosis
- Miliary fungal infections (coccidiomycosis, histoplasmosis)
- Disseminated viral infection
- Silicosis or coal-workers pneumoconioses (may occasionally appear random)
- Langerhans cell histiocytosis

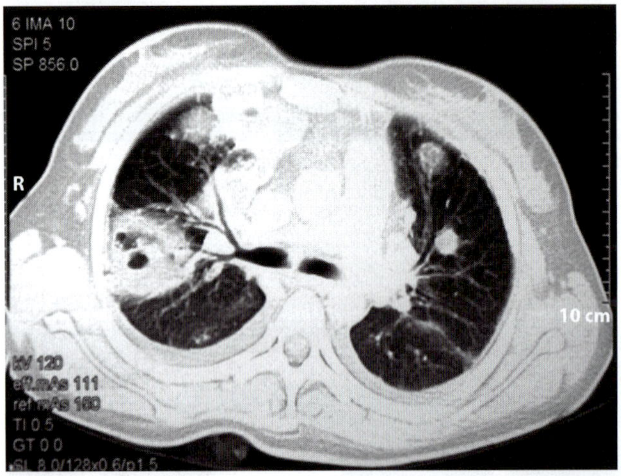

FIG. 8: Feeding vessel sign. Axial CT shows multiple variable sized nodules in angiocentric distribution scattered in bilateral lungs fields. Some of nodules show cavitation within.

(range from a few millimeters to greater than 1 cm in size) and are frequently similar in size. While tiny well-defined nodules of a few millimeter are commonly due to miliary tuberculosis. Miliary tuberculosis may show an upper lobe predominance as the organism grows best where there is high oxygen tension which is present in the upper lobes. However, considerable overlap may be seen in the size of nodules that each disease produces. Miliary tuberculosis can result in nodules larger than 5 mm size.[8]

A number of malignancies can result in a miliary pattern which can render the differential diagnosis to be difficult. This includes tumors such a renal cell carcinoma, head and neck cancer and testicular tumors which have their primary venous drainage in the lungs. In contrast, larger, less profuse metastatic nodules tend to be adenocarcinomas, typically originating from the lung, breast or the gastrointestinal tract. Less commonly, multiple cavitary nodules may be identified in patients with septic emboli, metastasis usually of squamous cell histology, Wegener's granulomatosis, rheumatoid lung disease, invasive fungal infections and pulmonary vasculitides **(Fig. 9)**.[1,9] Multiple irregular nodules in a bronchovascular distribution are characteristic of lymphoproliferative disorders, lymphoma, leukemia and Kaposi's sarcoma. When associated with thin walled cysts, randomly distributed nodules are suggestive of Langerhans cell histiocytosis.

When numerous, nodules in patients with sarcoidosis, Langerhans cell histiocytosis or silicosis may appear to be randomly and diffusely distributed and may be difficult

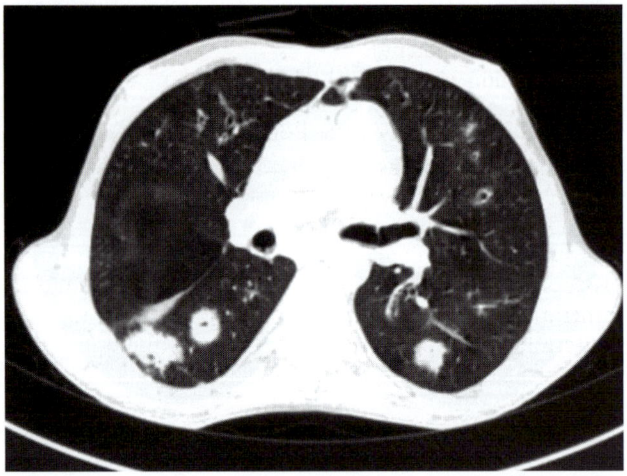

FIG. 9: Cavitating nodules. Axial CT in a patient of rheumatic heart disease reveals multiple nodules in bilateral lower lobes with central hypodensity consistent with septic emboli.

to distinguish from the nodules of miliary infection or metastasis.[4]

Correlation with clinical history is important in the differential diagnosis of the nodular pattern. If patient has a known malignancy, the nodular pattern is diagnostic of hematogenous spread. If signs of infection such as fever or elevated counts are present, miliary tuberculosis or fungal infection is likely. However, it should be remembered that in the elderly or debilitated patients, miliary tuberculosis may be associated with very few symptoms.[8]

Centrilobular Nodules

Centrilobular nodules are distributed in the center of the secondary pulmonary lobule which contain the branches of the terminal bronchioles, their accompanying pulmonary arteries and supporting connective tissue with lymph vessels. Hence, centrilobular opacities can result from bronchiolar and peribronchiolar disease as well as from vascular and perivascular diseases.[2] They may be due to either interstitial or airspace abnormalities and may be dense (solid) or of ground-glass density and may range from a few mm to about a cm in size. They may be ill-defined or well-defined depending on the underlying disease process.

On HRCT, centrilobular nodular opacities show characteristic distributions which distinguishes them from other patterns. These are:

- The most peripheral centrilobular nodules show sparing of the visceral pleural surface. This is because the most peripheral pulmonary lobules are 5 to 10 mm from the pleural surfaces.
- The nodules appear evenly spaced from one another which is due to the similar size of the pulmonary lobules.[4,8]

Differential Diagnosis of Centrilobular Nodules

The differential diagnosis of centrilobular nodules depends on many findings:

- *Attenuation of centrilobular nodules:* (i) Ground-glass opacity (GGO), or (ii) Homogeneous soft tissue attenuation.

- *The overall distribution of nodules:* (Whether diffuse/symmetrical/patchy).
- Association with tree-in-bud (TIB) pattern.

Ground-glass Opacity Centrilobular Nodules

Centrilobular nodules of ground-glass opacity may be seen as a result of airway disease or vascular disease, with ground-glass opacity centrilobular nodules due to airway disease being more common of the two. They typically reflect processes which produce peribronchiolar inflammation, infiltration or fibrosis without dense consolidation or obliteration of alveoli. **Flowchart 1** depicts the differential diagnosis of GGO centrilobular nodules.

Soft Tissue Attenuation Centrilobular Nodules

Centrilobular nodules of homogeneous soft tissue attenuation are characterized by inflammation or infiltration with consolidation of peribronchiolar alveoli or dense peribronchiolar fibrosis. There may be bronchiolar filling or impaction **(Fig. 11)** and the entire lobule may be involved with disease progression.[8] The differential diagnosis includes disease processes such as bronchopneumonia **(Fig. 12)**, aspiration **(Fig. 13)** and tumor, invasive adenocarcinoma (previously known as bronchioalveolar carcinoma).

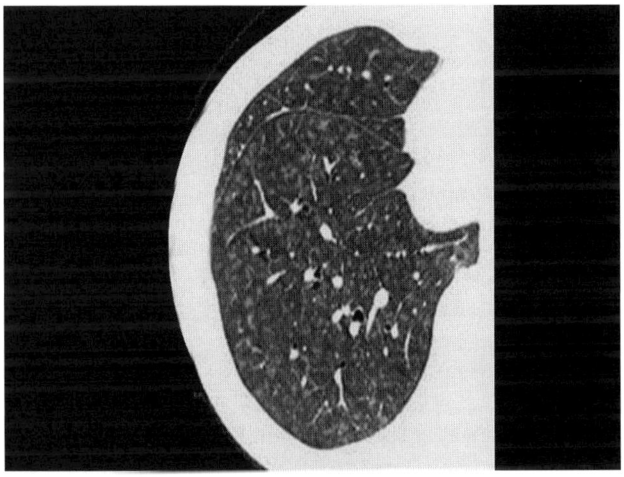

FIG. 10: Magnified axial HRCT image of right lung depicting diffuse ill-defined GGO nodules in subacute hypersensitivity pneumonitis.

FLOWCHART 1: Differential diagnosis of ground-glass opacity centrilobular nodules.[8]

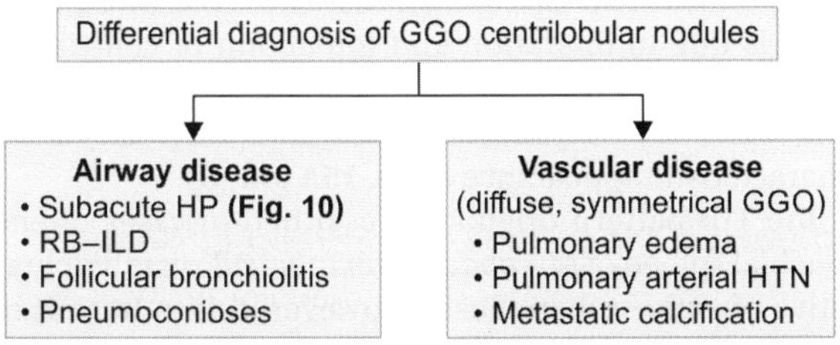

(HP: hypersensitivity pneumonitis; RB-ILD: respiratory bronchiolitis interstitial lung disease; GGO: ground-glass opacity; HTN: hypertension)

Table 6 enumerates the differential diagnosis of soft tissue attenuation centrilobular nodules with their salient features.

Distribution of Centrilobular Nodules in Differential Diagnosis

When formulating a differential diagnosis of centrilobular nodules, the overall distribution of centrilobular nodules, whether diffuse, symmetrical or patchy should be taken in conjunction with nodule attenuation (ground-glass or soft tissue attenuation). **Table 7** enumerates the differential diagnoses of centrilobular nodules based on overall distribution.[8]

"Tree-in-Bud" Pattern

Once nodules are characterized as being primarily centrilobular in distribution,further assessment is required to determine whether they have a "tree in bud" configuration or not.

"Tree-in-bud" (TIB) opacities are nearly always the result of inspissated secretions lodged within centrilobular

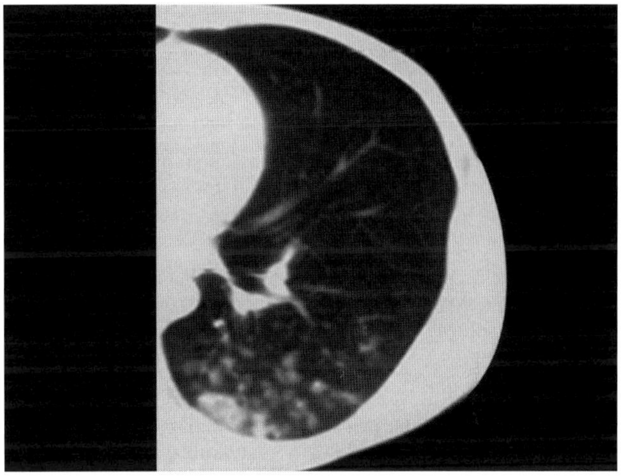

FIG. 11: Soft tissue centrilobular nodules. Axial CT image of left lung shows peripheral branching nodular opacities consistent with bronchiolar impaction.

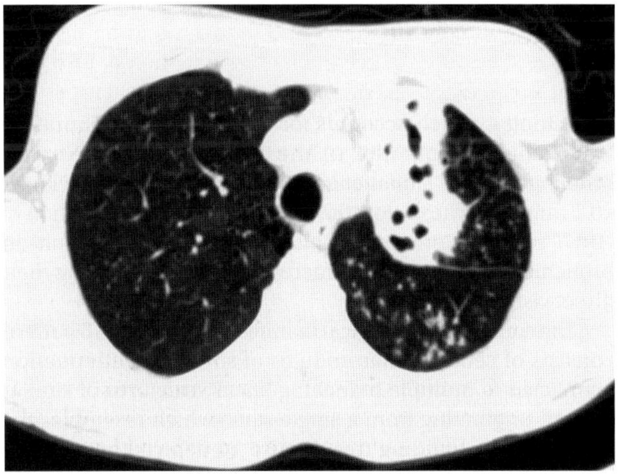

FIG. 12: Airspace nodules in bronchopneumonia. Axial CT reveals ill-defined soft tissue nodules in left lower lobe with collapse—consolidation of left upper lobe.

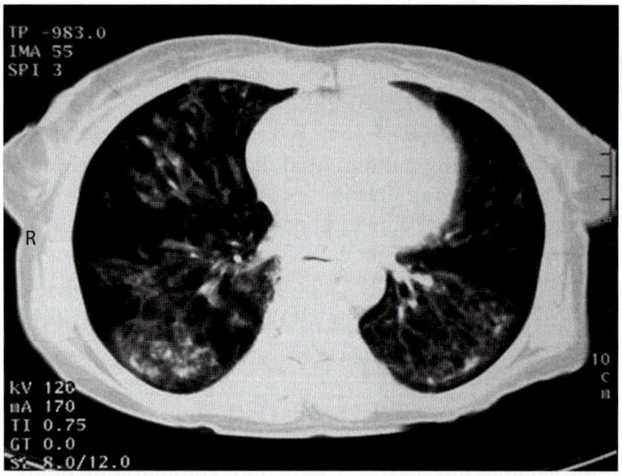

FIG. 13: Axial CT shows multiple discrete and confluent centrilobular nodules predominantly in bilateral lower lobes in aspiration pneumonitis.

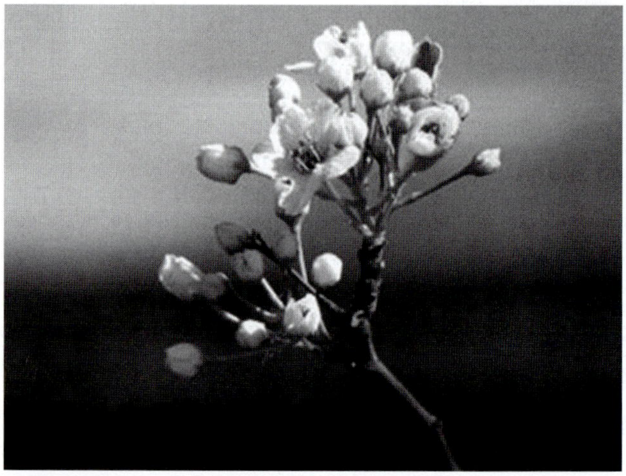

FIG. 14: Photographic representation of "tree-in-bud" pattern.

TABLE 6: Differential diagnosis of soft tissue attenuation centrilobular nodules.

Soft tissue attenuation centrilobular nodules	Salient features
• *Bronchopneumonia* resulting from endobronchial spread of infection—bacterial, mycobacterial, fungal, viral	• Most common cause • *Acute symptoms:* Nodules are focal, multifocal or patchy
• *Endobronchial spread of tumor* invasive mucinous adenocarcinoma (formerly BAC)	• Multifocal or patchy nodules ± larger areas of consolidation or GGO • Multiple lobes and both lungs may be involved
• Langerhans cell histiocytosis	• Early disease, centrilobular nodules in peribronchovascular distribution
• *Vascular diseases* (pulmonary edema, pulmonary hemorrhage)	• ± GGO or soft tissue attenuation nodules

TABLE 7: Differential diagnosis of centrilobular nodules based on distribution.

Distribution of centrilobular nodules	Differential diagnosis
Diffuse distribution	• Hypersensitivity pneumonitis (HP) • Respiratory bronchiolitis (RB or RB–ILD) • Follicular bronchiolitis • Atypical/viral infection • Pneumoconiosis • Pulmonary edema • Pulmonary hemorrhage • Pulmoary arterial hypertension
Upper or mid lung predominance	• HP • RB or RB–ILD • Langerhans histiocytosis • Pneumoconiosis
Lower lobe distribution	• Aspiration • Endobronchial spread
Patchy distribution	• Endobronchial infection (bacterial mycobacterial, fungal) • Invasive mucinous adenocarcinoma • Aspiration

bronchioles, which accounts for a branching configuration when coursing parallel to the CT scan plane. Normal bronchioles have a diameter of < 1 mm and a wall thickness <0.1 mm which are below the limit of the spatial resolution of HRCT scan. The presence of inspissated secretions results in bronchiolar distension and increased density, allowing their direct visualization.[9]

The common radiological manifestation of the TIB pattern consists of centrilobular nodules of soft tissue attenuation connected to multiple branching linear structures of similar caliber, originating from a single stalk, which resembles the branches of a budding tree. **Figure 14** depicts the 'tree-in-bud' pattern.

On HRCT, the TIB pattern is well recognized by the presence multiple V or Y shaped branching linear opacities 1-2 mm in thickness and 1-2 cm in length, often associated with small nodules at the tips of their branches. The HRCT finding of TIB is due to dilatation and impaction of centrilobular bronchioles by pus or mucus (branches) associated with small region of peribronchiolar inflammation (buds) and has a characteristic appearance **(Figs. 15A and B)**.[8]

The TIB pattern originally described in cases of endobronchial spread of *Mycobacterium tuberculosis* is highly suggestive of active tuberculosis. However, this pattern is now recognized as a CT manifestation of many diverse entities. **Table 8** enumerates the differential diagnosis of "tree-in-bud" pattern.[10]

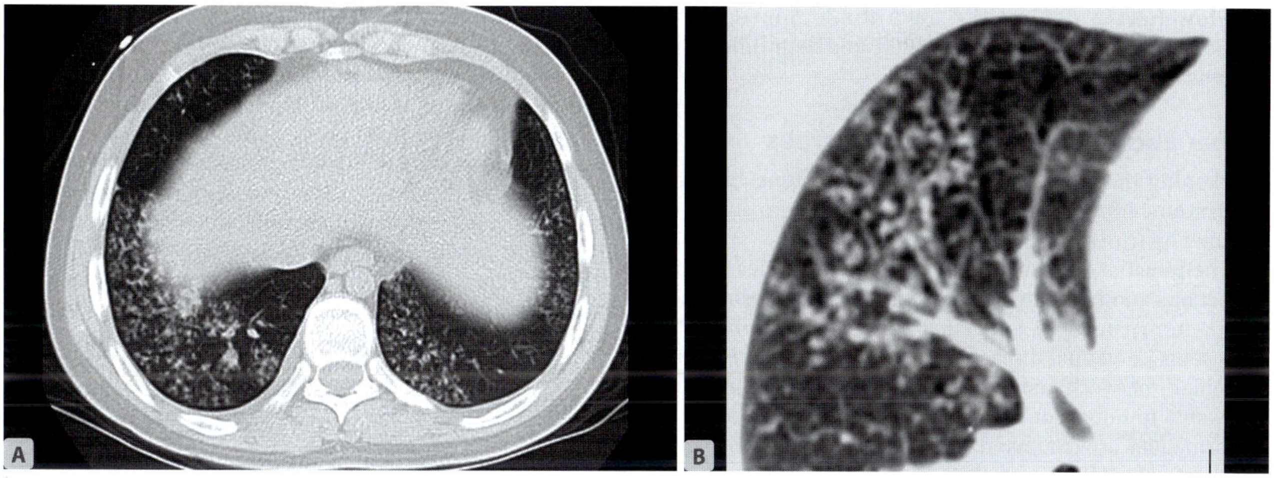

FIGS. 15A AND B: Tree-in-bud (TIB) pattern (A) Axial CT showing peripheral poorly defined small (2–4 mm) centrilobular nodules and branching linear opacities of similar caliber originating from a single stalk (TIB) pattern in bilateral lower lobes; (B) Magnified image depicting TIB pattern.

TABLE 8: Differential diagnosis of "tree-in-bud" pattern.

Infections
• Bacterial infections (*Staph. aureus, H. influenzae*)
• Mycobacterial infection (*M. tuberculosis*, MAIC)
• Fungal infections (airway invasive Aspergillosis)
• Viral infection (CMV, RSV)
Infectious variants (congenital/immunological/ idiopathic)
• Cystic fibrosis
• Kartagener's syndrome
• Allergic bronchopulmonary aspergillosis (ABPA)
• Obliterative bronchiolitis
• Panbronchiolitis
Aspiration
Inhalation

(MAIC: *Mycobacterium avium intracellulare*; CMV: cytomegalovirus; RSV: respiratory syncytial virus).

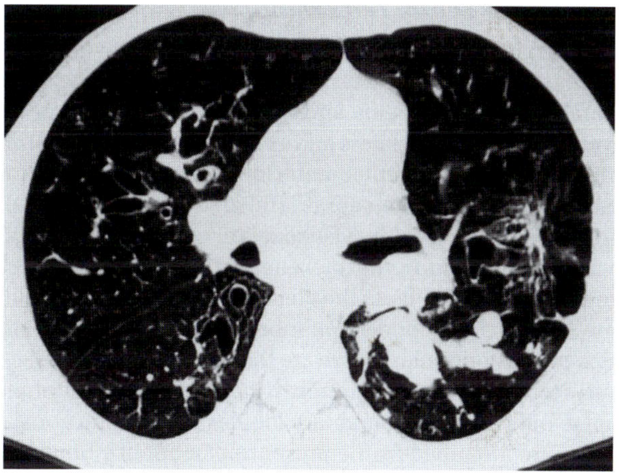

FIG. 16: Axial CT shows central bronchiectasis in bilateral lung fields with mucus filled bronchi in left lower lobe with centrilobular nodules in adjacent lung: Allergic bronchopulmonary aspergillosis.

The "tree-in-bud" pattern is most common due to infection with involvement of the small peripheral airways. It is not specific with regard to the type of infection, though bacterial and mycobacterial infections are seen most frequently. Bronchiectasis or bronchial wall thickening may be present depending on the cause or duration of the infection. In contrast, the non-infections causes of "tree in bud" pattern are relatively less common and include follicular bronchiolitis (usually in patients of connective tissue disease), mucoid impaction in asthma and allergic bronchopulmonary aspergillosis **(Fig. 16)**.[8]

Diagnostic Approach to Nodular Lung Disease

Differentiation of the three patterns of nodules (perilymphatic, random and centrilobular) on HRCT is essential to be able to formulate an appropriate differential diagnosis. It is important to keep the following points in mind when identifying the pattern of nodules:

- Subpleural nodules are present in both perilymphatic and random patterns, but should not be present in patients with centrilobular nodules. If the distribution is not clear, then one should pay attenuation to the fissures and peripheral subpleural interstitium to determine if the nodules are present there.
- A diffuse distribution is typical of a random pattern, while a patchy distribution is typical of perilymphatic nodules. Centrilobular nodules may be either diffuse or patchy in distribution, depending on the underlying cause. For example, hypersensitivity pneumonitis (HP) is often diffuse while endobronchial spread of infection is typically patchy.
- When centrilobular nodules are present, one must ascertain the presence of "tree in bud" pattern. Infection is very likely when a "tree in bud" pattern is present, and when not present, the differential diagnosis depends on the attenuation and distribution of nodules.

Flowchart 2 depicts the algorithmic approach for distribution of small nodules on HRCT and their differential diagnosis.[8]

Linear and Reticular Pattern Opacities

Thickening of interstitial fiber network of lung by fluid, infiltration, fibrous tissue leads to increase in linear or reticular opacities on HRCT.

The reticular pattern consists of linear opacities that intersect one another at right angles, producing a mesh or net-like pattern.[3] On HRCT a reticular pattern almost invariably represents interstitial disease. It is a purely descriptive term (reticular - network) ranging from thickening of the interlobular septa to honeycomb lung destruction.[5] These reticular abnormalities are characterized into the following recognizable pattern on HRCT scan:[11]

- Interlobular septal thickening
- Honeycombing
- Intralobular interstitial thickening.

Interlobular Septal Thickening

Interlobular septa form the borders of the secondary pulmonary lobule. They comprise of connective tissue and contain pulmonary veins and lymphatics. These septa are around 0.1 mm in thickness and 1-2 cm in length. It is normal to find interlobular septae anteriorly or along mediastinal pleural surfaces.[3] The septae are seen when abnormally thickened, leading to the visualization of numerous septae. In the peripheral lung, the thickened septa of 1-2 cm in length are seen perpendicular to the pleural surface and may outline part or all of the secondary pulmonary lobule. On HRCT, the thickened interlobular septae are the counter part of Kerley B lines seen on chest radiographs.[12] The thickened interlobular septae outlining the pulmonary lobules appear polygonal in shape, are identified by the presence of a dot like branching centrilobular artery in the center. This characteristic relationship is valuable in identifying these structures on HRCT.

The terms septal lines or septal thickening may be used to describe interlobular septal thickening. Apart from interstitial lung disease, thickened interlobular septa may be seen in normal elderly patients and smokers.[11]

It should be kept in mind that the differential diagnosis of septal thickening is limited when it is seen as an isolated or predominant abnormality. Septal thickening can be characterized as smooth, nodular or irregular in morphology in different pathologic processes and recognizing this morphologic pattern is useful in differential diagnosis.[8,11]

Smooth septal thickening is present when the septae are thicker than normal and otherwise appears normal and are well-visualized on HRCT. It is usually a manifestation of pulmonary edema or lymphangitic spread of tumor with fluid or tumor infiltrating the lymphatics located within the septa. Irrespective of the cause, smooth interlobular septal thickening is often associated with smooth peribronchovascular and subpleural interstitial thickening which is most easily seen as thickening of fissures.[11]

In *pulmonary edema*, the smooth interlobular septal thickening may be diffuse and bilaterally symmetrical with basal predominance. Often the thickened septa are more defined in the apical and upper lobes as the interlobular septae are best developed in this region **(Fig. 17)**.[11]

Septal thickening in *lymphangitic spread of tumor* may be either smooth or nodular, with smooth thickening being more common. The abnormality may be unilateral or bilateral, asymmetric, patchy, having upper or lower lobe involvement. Both pulmonary and extra-pulmonary tumors (from breast, stomach, pancreas and prostate) can result in lymphangitic spread of tumor.[2,8]

Nodular septal thickening is most commonly seen in patients with sarcoidosis or lymphangitic spread of tumor **(Fig. 18)**. It reflects the lymphatic involvement within the septa, with the nodules representing clusters of granulomas or tumor nodules. In both conditions the nodules are seen in perilymphatic distribution.[13]

Sarcoidosis is often associated with architectural distortion which reflects the underlying pulmonary fibrosis. While lymphangitic spread of carcinoma is a non-fibrosing process which does not produce any architectural distortion.

Irregular interlobular septal thickening is usually seen in fibrotic lung disease with architectural distortion associated

FLOWCHART 2: Algorithm of distribution and differentials of multiple small nodules on HRCT.

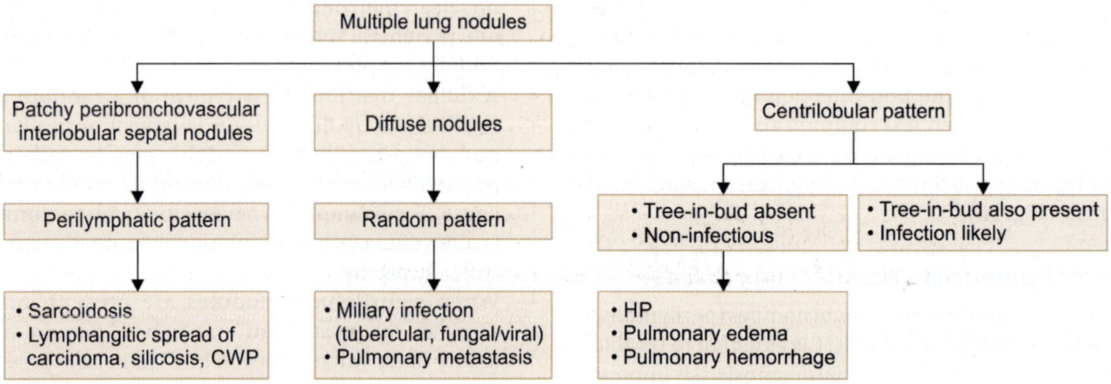

(HRCT: high-resolution computed tomography; HP: hypersensitivity pneumonitis; CWP: coal workers' pneumoconiosis)

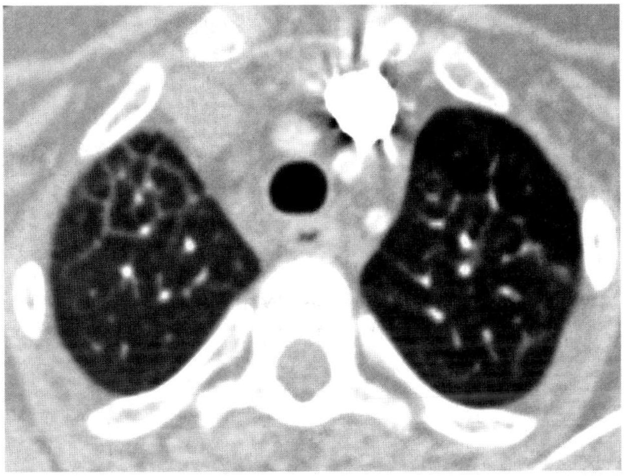

FIG. 17: Smooth interlobular septal thickening. Axial CT shows diffuse smooth interlobular septal thickening outlining pulmonary lobules with ground-glass opacity in bilateral upper lobes in a patient with pulmonary edema.

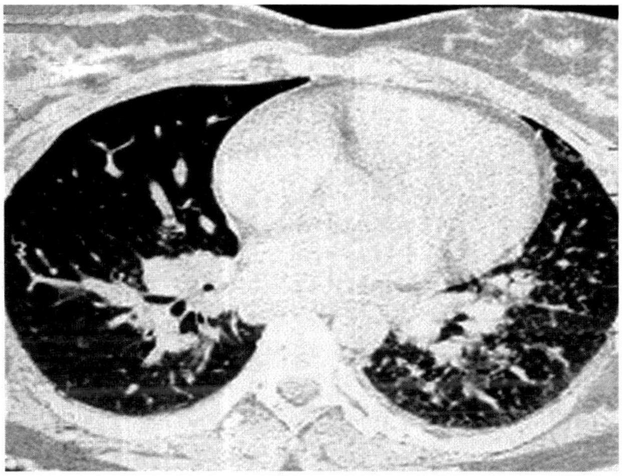

FIG. 18: Perilymphatic distribution of nodules in sarcoidosis. Axial HRCT shows multiple small nodules scattered in centrilobular, peribronchovascular and perilymphatic distribution. Micronodular beading is seen along major fissures.

with fibrosis resulting in the septa to become jagged in appearance. On HRCT, other findings such as honeycombing, traction bronchiectasis are of importance in reaching a differential diagnosis **(Fig. 19)**.[13]

Flowchart 3 illustrates the algorithmic approach to the differential diagnosis of interlobular septal thickening when it is a predominant abnormality.[3,11]

Honeycombing

Presence of honeycombing is the most specific HRCT sign of fibrosis, appearing as air-filled cystic spaces. This will be discussed later under the HRCT findings manifesting as decreased lung opacity.

Intralobular Interstitial Thickening

The intralobular interstitium refers to the interstitial network that supports the structures of the pulmonary lobules and does not include the interlobular septa. It is normally not visible on HRCT. It comprises mainly of the fine network of very thin connective tissue fibers within the alveolar walls or the parenchymal interstitium.[1]

Intralobular interstitial thickening is an early sign of fibrosis. It is a non-specific finding and may be associated with interstitial infiltration or inflammation in the absence of fibrosis. The term 'intralobular lines' is used to describe the presence of intralobular interstitial thickening. These lines are less than 5 mm long and form a fine lace like network and usually do not conform to the lobular anatomy. They are seen in all types of fibrotic lung disease, especially idiopathic pulmonary fibrosis usual interstitial pneumonia (UIP), nonspecific interstitial pneumonia (NSIP), pulmonary disease associated with collagen vascular diseases.

Intralobular interstitial thickening are usually associated with other features of lung fibrosis such as architectural distortion or tractional bronchiectasis. The term tractional bronchiectasis refers to the bronchial dilatation occurring

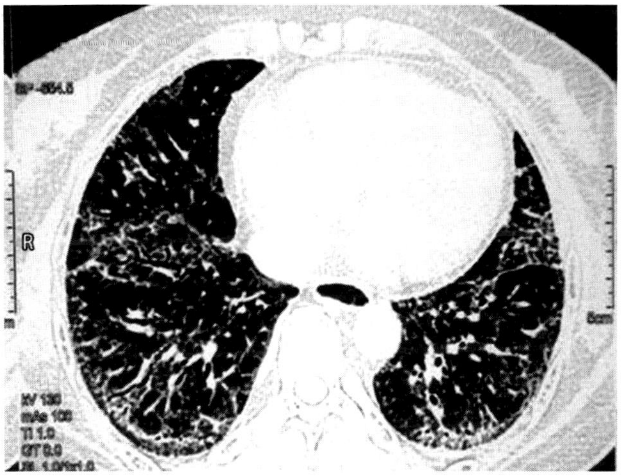

FIG. 19: Irregular interlobular septal thickening. Axial HRCT showing intralobular, interlobular and subpleural interstitial thickening involving bilateral lower lobes with traction bronchiectasis.

as a result of interstitial fibrosis, whereby the bronchi appear irregular, but are not associated with any radiological evidence of bronchial inflammation, i.e. bronchial wall thickening or mucus impactions.

Intralobular interstitial thickening may also be seen in other idiopathic interstitial pneumonias, pulmonary infections (viral pneumonias), pulmonary edema, pulmonary hemorrhage and lymphangitic carcinomatosis.

Irregular reticulation: Irregular reticulation is a non-specific finding and is said to be present when normal reticular opacities do not represent any of the other two patterns, i.e. interlobular septal thickening and honeycombing. They are known by various names like parenchymal bands and subpleural lesions. The presence of irregular reticulation is moderately specific for fibrosis.

FLOWCHART 3: Algorithmic approach to differential diagnosis of interlobular septal thickening.

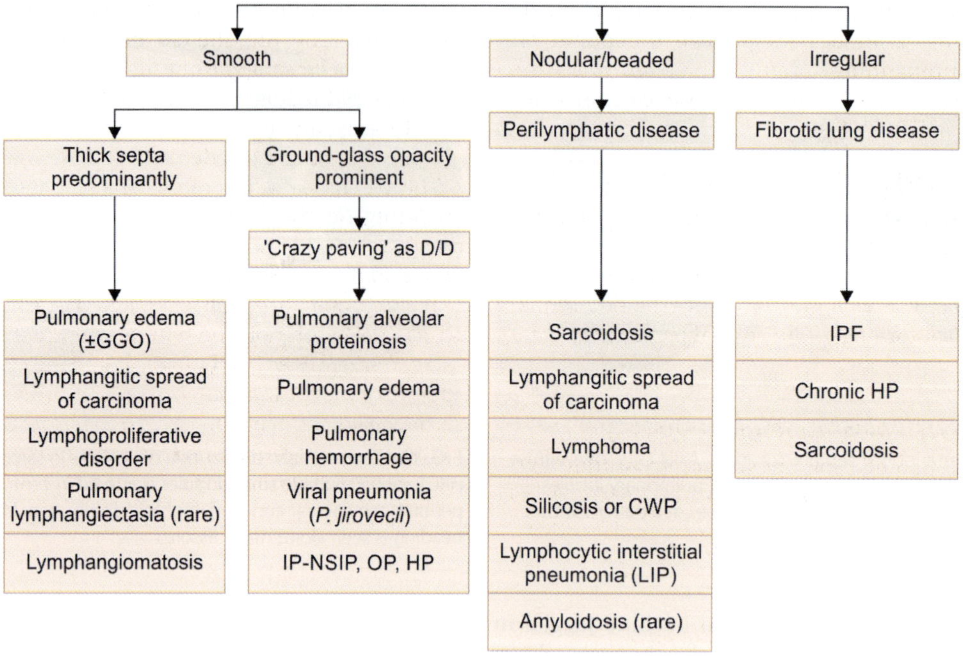

(D/D: differential diagnosis; GGO: ground-glass opacity; NSIP: nonspecific interstitial pneumonia; OP: organizing pneumonia; HP: hypersensitivity pneumonitis; CWP: coal workers' pneumoconiosis; IPF: idiopathic pulmonary fibrosis)

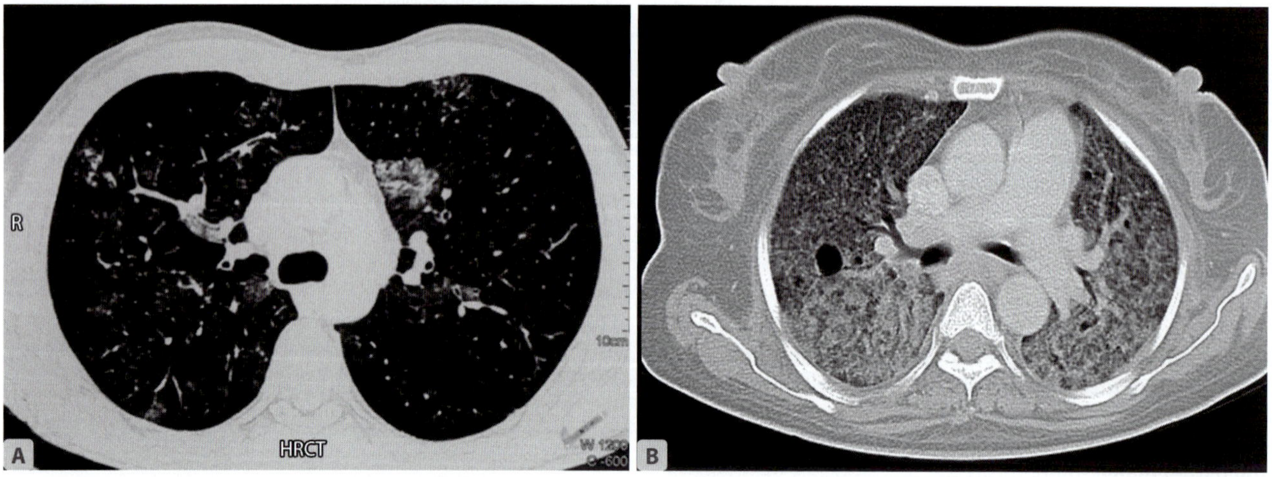

FIGS. 20A AND B: (A) Axial HRCT chest in a 40-year-old male with recurrent episode of cough, wheeze and blood eosinophilia reveal multiple patchy areas of transient GGO in bilateral lung fields which resolved following antihelminthic therapy—Loeffier syndrome; (B) Axial HRCT of *Pneumocystis jirovecii* infection in an HIV patient in the form of symmetric diffuse ground-glass opacity associated with cyst in right lung.

Ground-glass Opacity

Ground-glass opacity (CGO) refers to the hazy increase in lung attenuation that does not obscure the underlying vessels or bronchial margins. It is a common but non-specific finding on HRCT. Ground-glass opacity results from volume averaging of morphological abnormalities that are too small to be clearly resolved by HRCT. It may reflect the presence of air space disease, interstitial disease, or a combination of both. It may be a manifestation of lung infiltration, active inflammation, or fibrosis and may also result from atelectasis.

Ground-glass opacity is a subjective finding on HRCT and may be difficult to recognize if it is minimal or involves the entire lung diffusely. However, it is mostly patchy or geographic in distribution, effecting some areas of lung and sparing other regions, thereby making it easier to recognize **(Figs. 20A and B)**. In cases where the presence of GGO is equivocal, comparing the attenuation of the lung parenchyma with air in the bronchi may be helpful. In normal individuals the density difference is marginal, while with GGO the airways appear "too black" within an area of lung (the 'black bronchus' sign).

Ground-glass opacity is a significant finding on HRCT and its presence indicates an ongoing active and potentially treatable/reversible disease. Its significance depends on the patient symptomatology (acute versus chronic), the distribution of GGO on HRCT, and the presence or absence of other findings on HRCT **(Fig. 21)**.

Differential Diagnosis of Ground-glass Opacity

A large number of diseases can show GGO on HRCT. Knowing the duration of patients' symptoms (acute, subacute or chronic) is fundamental to the differential diagnosis with this HRCT appearance. **Tables 9 and 10** depict the differential diagnosis of GGO according to the clinical presentation and distribution.[14]

Pitfalls in Diagnosis of Ground-glass Opacity

There are several potential pitfalls in the recognition and diagnosis of GGO which a radiologist must be aware so as to avoid misdiagnosis of the same. GGO may be spuriously diagnosed on HRCT in the following circumstances:

- In pediatric patients
- HRCT performed with thick collimation
- 'Dependent density' in the posterior lung in supine scanning which clears on prone scan
- Expiratory scans may mimic the appearance of GGO due to reduced amount of air in the alveoli on expiration.
- In scans showing patchy emphysema or other causes of hyperlucency such as airways obstruction and air trapping, normal lung regions can mimic the appearance of ground-glass opacity by appearing relatively dense which can be distinguished on expiratory scan.

Consolidation

Consolidation is characterized by abnormal dense opacification of the lung parenchyma with obscuration of the underlying vessels. It may be alveolar or interstitial in origin, though most commonly the alveolar air is replaced by fluid, cells, tissue or pus. Consolidation is detected both on plain radiography and CT, and may be visualized earlier on CT than plain radiographs.[6] HRCT provides useful diagnostic information regarding the distribution and characteristics of consolidated lung. But, the rate of change of consolidation should always be sought from serial chest radiographs. For example, rapid radiographic resolution in hours rather than days of diffuse lung opacification of acute onset is highly suggestive of pulmonary edema or hemorrhage.

The CT appearances of air space consolidation differ depending on the degree of involvement. The earliest findings consists of poorly marginated small nodules called acinar nodules approximately 7 mm in diameter which occur when single acini are replaced by fluid or tissue **(Figs. 22A and B)**. These are not true nodules and represent clusters of single acini filled with fluid, inflammatory cells or blood, depending on the disease process. With involvement of adjacent acini, the acinar nodules coalesce and may progress to lobular, subsegmental, segmental, lobar or multilobar areas of consolidation **(Figs. 23A and B)**. Unlike ground-

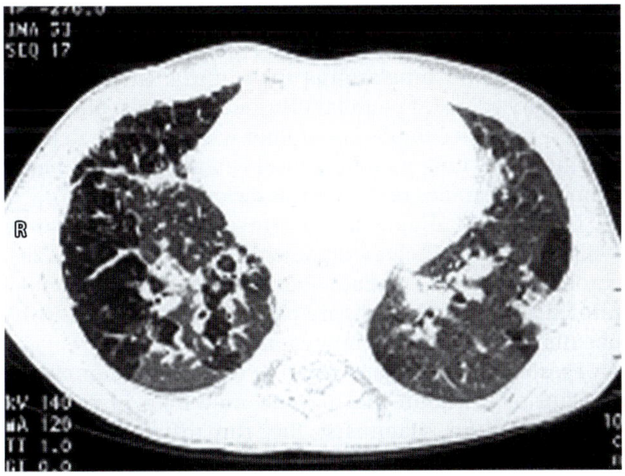

FIG. 21: Acute hypersensitivity pneumonitis. Axial HRCT shows extensive areas of ground-glass attenuation in bilateral lung fields.

TABLE 9: Differential diagnosis of GGO on the basis of clinical presentation.

Acute presentation

• Pulmonary edema
• Pulmonary hemorrhage
• All types of pneumonias (especially atypical pneumonia)
  – *Pneumocystis jirovecii*
  – Viral—cytomegalovirus (CMV)
  – Mycoplasma
  – Acute interstitial pneumonitis
  – Acute eosinophilic pneumonia
• Hypersensitivity pneumonitis
• Aspiration

Subacute or chronic presentation
• Nonspecific interstitial pneumonia (NSIP) • Pneumonia associated with collagen vascular disease • Desquamative interstitial pneumonia (DIP) • Respiratory bronchiolitis interstitial lung disease (RB–ILD) • Hypersensitivity pneumonitis (HP) • Organizing pneumonia (OP) • Chronic eosinophilic pneumonia • Chronic/recurrent aspiration • Adenocarcinoma *in situ* (formerly BAC) • Pulmonary alveolar proteinosis (PAP)

TABLE 10: Differential diagnosis of GGO on the basis of distribution.

Distribution of GGO	Causes
• Peripheral and subpleural	NSIP, DIP, OP
• Patchy and geographic	HP, OP, eosinophilic pneumonia
• Peribronchovascular	Sarcoid, OP, eosinophilic pneumonia
• Diffuse and extensive	HP

(GGO: ground-glass opacity; NSIP: nonspecific interstitial pneumonia; DIP: desquamative interstitial pneumonia; OP: organizing pneumonia; HP: hypersensitivity pneumonitis)

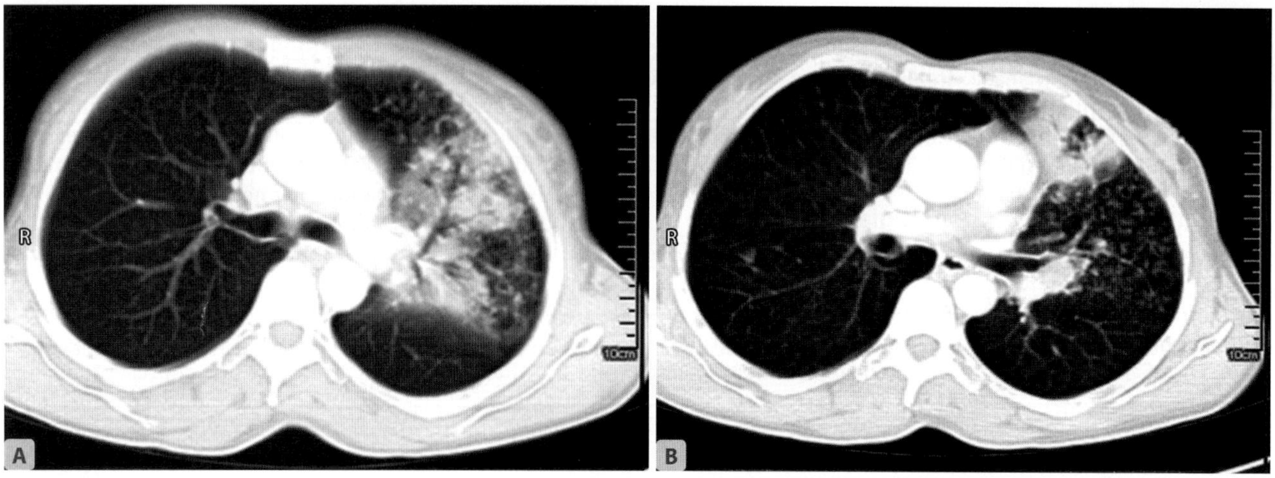

FIGS. 22A AND B: Axial CT shows consolidation with air bronchogram and adjacent airspace nodules in left upper lobe.

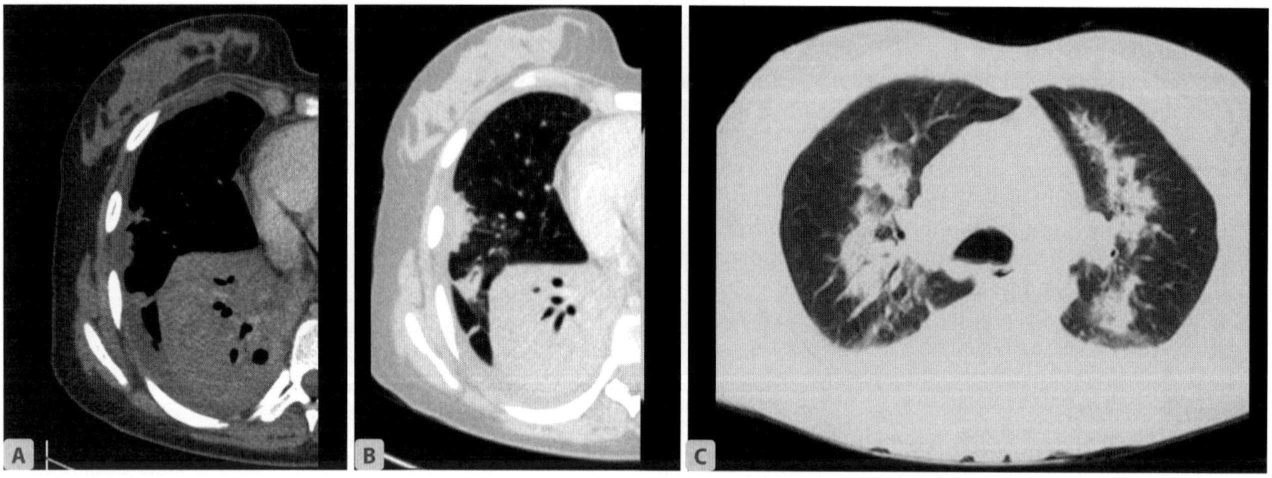

FIGS. 23A TO C: (A and B) Axial CT shows consolidation with air bronchogram in right lower lobe with subpleural smaller areas of consolidation and mild pleural effusion; (C) CT shows perihilar 'batwing' consolidation in pulmonary edema, with peripheral sparing.

glass opacity, on HRCT, consolidation results in an increase in lung opacity with underlying vessels being obscured. Air bronchogram are usually seen if the bronchi are patent.[15]

Differential Diagnosis

The differential diagnosis of consolidation overlaps considerably with ground-glass opacity. **Table 11** enumerates the differential diagnosis of consolidation with their salient features.[14]

The differential diagnosis of consolidation depends mainly on:

a. Duration of symptoms
b. Distribution of consolidation

Consolidation presenting in an acute condition is mostly seen in pneumonias and aspiration. The various causative organisms of pneumonia result in different patterns of parenchymal opacification on HRCT. Aspiration may be focal or patchy and typically involves the lower lobes and posterior upper lobes.

Perihilar "bat-wing" consolidation with sparing of the periphery of the lung is typical of pulmonary edema **(Fig. 23C)**. This pattern may also be seen with pulmonary hemorrhage, pneumonia such as *Pneumocystis jirovecii* pneumonia and inhalational lung injury. In patients of pulmonary edema, a perihilar distribution is most often seen when a rapid accumulation of fluid has occurred. Relative sparing of the lung periphery has been attributed to better lymphatic clearance of fluid in this region.[16]

Differential diagnosis of consolidation of chronic symptomatology include organizing pneumonia **(Fig. 24)**, chronic eosinophilic pneumonia, invasive adenocarcinoma, sarcoidosis, lymphoma, lipoid pneumonia, hypersensitivity pneumonitis, pulmonary infarction.[14,17]

Presence of focal consolidation within single or cluster of acini or a tree-in-bud pattern may help in reducing the differential diagnosis. But the differentiation of adenocarcinoma and organizing pneumonia may rarely be made with certainly on HRCT appearance alone and a tissue diagnosis is usually required.

TABLE 11: Differential diagnosis of consolidation.

Differential diagnosis	Salient features
Acute consolidation	
Pneumonia (bacterial, mycobacterial, fungal, viral)	Patchy, nodular, lobular or diffuse, depending on the organism
AIP, ARDS	Patchy or diffuse
Pulmonary edema	Diffuse, GGO more common
Pulmonary hemorrhage	Patchy or diffuse, GGO more common
Acute eosinophilic pneumonia	Diffuse GGO more common
Radiation pneumonitis	Extent usually corresponds to radiation port
Subacute/Chronic consolidation	
Organizing pneumonia (OP)	Mostly peripheral, may be mass like or reversed halo in some
Chronic eosinophilic pneumonia	Patchy or nodular, peripheral, resembles OP
Invasive mucinous adenocarcinoma	Diffuse, patchy or nodular
Nonspecific interstitial pneumonia (NSIP)	Patchy, subpleural GGO more common
Hypersensitivity pneumonitis (HP)	Patchy, GGO more common
Lipoid pneumonia	Patchy or lobular, low attenuation consolidation
Lymphoma	Focal, patchy or mass like in peribronchovascular distribution
Sarcoidosis	Patchy or mass like confluence of very small granulomas
Alveolar proteinosis	GGO more common, patchy or diffuse
Pulmonary infarction	Wedge-shaped, pleural-based

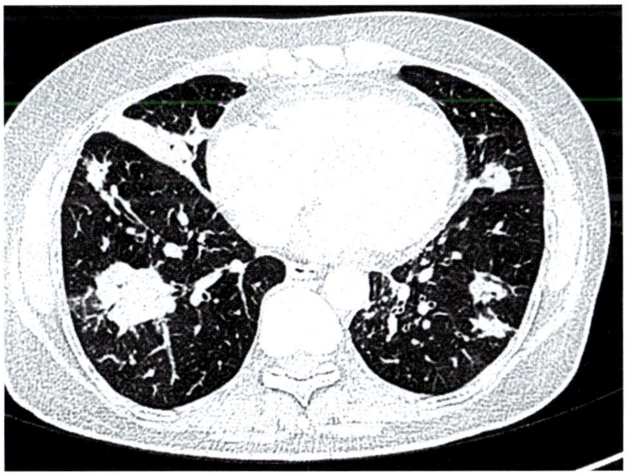

FIG. 24: Organizing pneumonia. Axial HRCT shows multiple focal consolidations with air bronchogram in peribronchial regions with surrounding GGO.

HIGH RESOLUTION CT SCAN FINDINGS MANIFESTING AS DECREASED LUNG OPACITY

Area of Decreased Attenuation with Walls

Various abnormalities associated with reduced attenuation in this sub-group include bronchiectasis, honeycombing, lung cysts, cystic lung disease and pneumatocele.

Bronchiectasis

Bronchiectasis is a chronic condition characterised by irreversible dilatation of the bronchi, usually associated with inflammation which occur secondary to bronchial obstruction, bronchial wall damage or parenchymal fibrosis.[18]

High Resolution CT Findings of Bronchiectasis

Bronchial dilatation is the most specific finding of bronchiectasis and is considered when the broncho-arterial ratio exceeds one . However, this may normally be seen in the elderly, people living in high attitude or in asthmatics. When bronchial dilatation is marked, the cross section appearance of the bronchus and artery together appears as a ring and is termed as the "signet ring" sign.

Lack of bronchial tapering: This is the earliest sign of bronchiectasis and is easiest to detect when the bronchus is seen in longitudinal section.

Visualization of peripheral airway: Normal airways are not visualized within 1 cm of the costal pleura. If visualized, then are considered abnormal and indicative of bronchiectasis. Airways may be seen within 1 cm of mediastinal pleura, but should not abut the mediastinal pleura.[3]

Mucoid impaction: Dilated bronchi when filled with fluid or mucous are easily appreciated on HRCT. They appear as gloved finger, V or Y shaped branching densities.

When oriented perpendicular to the scan slice, fluid or mucus filled dilated bronchi are visualized as nodular opacities. CT also demonstrates any atelectasis or hyperinflation distal to the impacted bronchi.

Types of Bronchiectasis

On the basis of morphological appearance on HRCT or pathology, bronchiectasis is classified into three types in increasing order of severity.

a. *Cylindrical or tubular bronchiectasis* is the mildest form which consist of uniformly dilated bronchi with smooth wall thickening **(Fig. 25A)**. They are often associated with chronic airway infections.[19,20]
b. *Varicose bronchiectasis:* In varicose bronchiectasis the bronchial lumen is characterized by alternating area of luminal dilatation and narrowing giving a beaded appearance with irregular or nodular wall thickening **(Fig. 25B)**. This is commonly seen in cystic fibrosis and allergic bronchopulmonary aspergillosis.[19,20]
c. *Cystic bronchiectasis:* Cystic or saccular bronchiectasis is the most severe form of bronchiectasis where the dilated

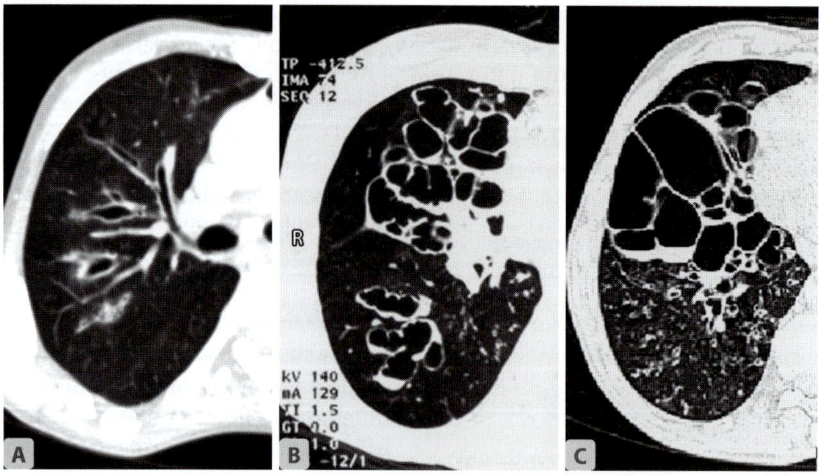

FIGS. 25A TO C: (A) Axial CT shows cylindrical bronchiectasis with bronchial wall thickening in right upper lobe with mucoid impaction in terminal bronchioles; (B) Varicose bronchiectasis with air-fluid levels in right lung; (C) Cystic bronchiectasis with air fluid levels and mucoid impaction in right lung.

bronchi terminate as a cluster of thin walled air-filled cysts **(Fig. 25C)**.[19] Air fluid levels may be present in the dependent portion of the dilated cystic bronchi. Cystic bronchiectasis often reflects an early childhood infection, is often patchy in distribution, and may be lobar.

More than one type of bronchiectasis may be seen in the same patient.

The radiologist has an important role in the detection and characterization, bronchiectasis and should be able to differentiate bronchiectasis from motion artifact (most commonly from cardiac pulsation in the middle and lingular lobes) and bronchial dilatation in acute lung disease.[19] CT has limited ability to determine the cause of bronchiectasis, but the distribution and pattern of disease can help suggest the most likely cause as given in **Table 12**.[15,21]

TABLE 12: Distribution and pattern of bronchiectasis.

Distribution and pattern of bronchiectasis	Likely etiology
Bilateral upper lobe bronchiectasis Cystic fibrosis Allergic broncho-pulmonary aspergillosis	Bilateral symmetrical, central, upper lobe predominance Bilateral asymmetrical, central bronchiectasis, cylindrical or varicose type with mucoid impaction
Unilateral upper lobe distrbution	Most common with tuberculosis
Lower lobe distribution	Most common secondary to childhood viral infection
Right middle lobe and lingular distribution	Bronchiectatic form of atypical mycobacterial infection, immotile cilia syndrome, hypogammaglobinemia

Honeycomb Cysts

Honeycomb cysts are characterized by air containing space having thick walls that are lined by bronchiolar epithelium and fibrous walls. Pathologically honeycombing represents interstitial fibrosis with lung destruction and dilatation of peripheral air spaces and is the most specific HRCT sign of fibrosis. In patients with extensive disease (fibrosis), the stacked appearance of cysts resembles a 'honeycomb', hence the term honeycomb cysts.

Honeycombing produces a characteristic appearance on HRCT. Several HRCT findings must be present to make a confident diagnosis of honeycomb cysts, which are:

- Peripheral subpleural location of the cysts
- A layer or cluster of cysts which share walls
- Cysts are of air attenuation and appear lucent as compared to the normal lung parenchyma
- They range in size from few mm to 1 cm
- The cysts have clearly definable fibrous walls of 1-3 mm in thickness. This finding helps in distinguishing honeycombing from paraseptal emphysema or areas of subpleural air trapping **(Fig. 26)**
- The cysts appear as empty black holes with no vessels, bronchi or septations within the cysts
- The cysts of honeycombing do not branch. Branching cystic structures are likely to represent traction bronchiectasis
- Honeycomb cysts are associated with other signs of lung fibrosis such as architectural distortion, traction bronchiectasis, irregular reticulation and volume loss in the same lung region.

Significance of Honeycombing

Honeycombing on HRCT usually represents usual interstitial pneumonia (UIP) with the most common cause being idiopathic pulmonary fibrosis (IPF). The presence of lower lobe, subpleural honeycombing in such patients strongly suggests usual interstitial pneumonia—idiopathic pulmonary fibrosis (IPF) and obviates the need for surgical lung biopsy **(Figs. 27A to C)**.[3] However, number of other diseases show honeycombing on HRCT. **Table 13** gives the differential diagnosis of honeycombing on HRCT.

The honeycombing in these conditions may be indistinguishable on HRCT and require correlation with clinical, exposure or drug history to suggest the appropriate diagnosis.

Pitfalls in Diagnosis of Honeycombing

Paraseptal emphysema by virtue of its subpleural location may resemble honeycombing. But, there are several differentiating features between the two which are tabulated in **Table 14**.

Cystic Lung Disease

Lung disease may be characterized by cystic air spaces or lung cysts. Lung cysts are used to describe clearly defined air containing spaces that is 1 cm or more with a definable epithelial or fibrous usually less than 3 mm thick wall.

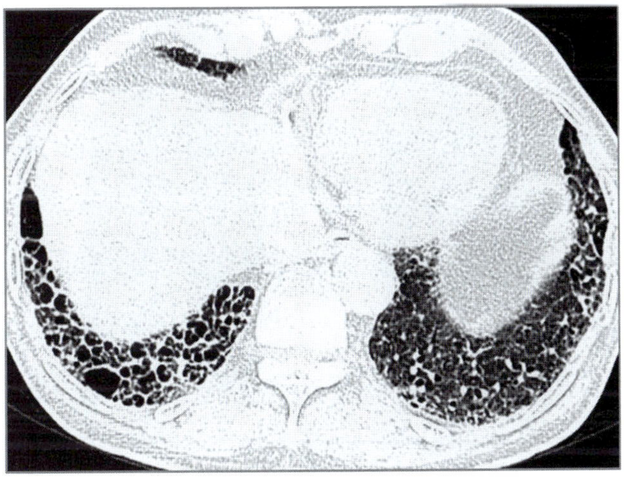

FIG. 26: HRCT image shows honeycomb cysts with predominance in right basal and subpleural region. The cysts are variable sized shows well-defined thick walls and occur in several layers.

Although the precise mechanism of cystic change is not understood, a check valve mechanism has been advocated in the pathologies of some cysts.[15] On chest radiography, multiple cysts may not be identifiable and result in delicate reticular pattern due to the superimposition of their walls. **Table 15** gives the differential diagnosis of conditions characterized by lung cysts.[6] HRCT is often helpful in suggesting a diagnosis on the basis of their size, wall characteristics and distribution of the cysts.

Langerhans Cell Histiocytosis

It is a multiorgan disease with pulmonary involvement seen mostly in ages between 20 to 40 years in cigarette smokers. The predominant HRCT findings consists of cysts and nodules.

TABLE 13: Differential diagnosis of honeycombing.

- Idiopathic pulmonary fibrosis
- Connective tissue disease (rheumatoid arthritis most common)
- Drug-related fibrosis
- Cyclophosphamide (common), nitrofurantoin
- Asbestosis

TABLE 14: Differentiating features of honeycombing and paraseptal emphysema.

Features	Honeycombing	Paraseptal emphysema
Layers	Cysts of one or more layer	Single layer only
Wall thickness	Thick walled	Very thin wall
Size	Small (few mm to 1 cm)	Large (up to several cm)
Distribution	Lower lobes	Upper lobes
Associated features	Traction bronchiectasis, irregular reticulation	± centrilobular emphysema
Overall lung volume	Volume loss	Increased

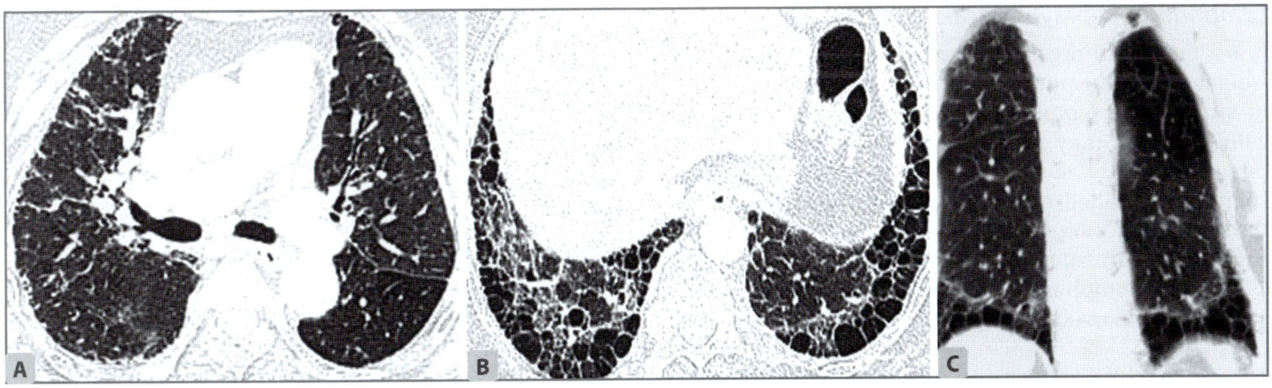

FIGS. 27A TO C: (A) Axial HRCT at the level of upper lobe bronchus shows mild septal thickening in bilateral lung parenchyma; (B) Axial HRCT through lung bases reveals extensive reticulation and honeycombing with lower lobe and posterior, peripheral predominance; (C) Coronal MPR image reveals an apicobasal gradient of abnormalities typical of UIP pattern.

TABLE 15: Differential diagnosis of lung cysts.

- Langerhans cell histiocytosis (LCH)
- Lymphangioleiomyomatosis (LAM)
- Lymphoid interstitial pneumonia (LIP)
- *P. jirovecii* pneumonia
- Cavitating form of bronchoalveolar carcinoma
- Tracheobronchial papillomatosis
- Birt-Hogg-Dube syndrome
- Sarcoidosis
- Hypersensitivity pneumonitis (subacute)
- Elderly healthy individuals (>75 years)

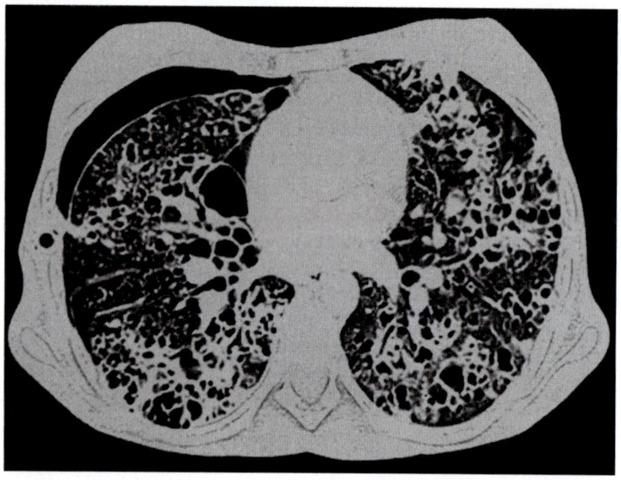

FIG. 28: Axial HRCT shows multiple thick wall cysts of varying sizes in bilateral lung parenchyma. A large thin wall cyst suggestive of bulla is seen along the right mediastinal pleura with associated pneumothorax: Langerhans cells histiocytosis.

The cysts are of irregular or bizarre shape, thin or thick walled may be of unequal sizes and show a predominant upper lung zone distribution with relative sparing of costophrenic sulci **(Fig. 28)**. Serial CT scan shows the natural history of the disease with nodules which cavitate, become cystic air spaces and finally coalesce.[22]

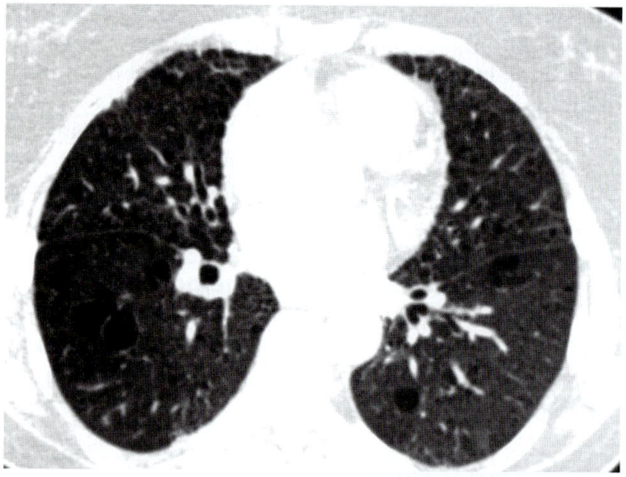

FIG. 29: Axial HRCT in early lymphangioleiomyomatosis shows subtle thin-walled cysts interspersed with normal lung parenchyma predominantly in lower lobes.

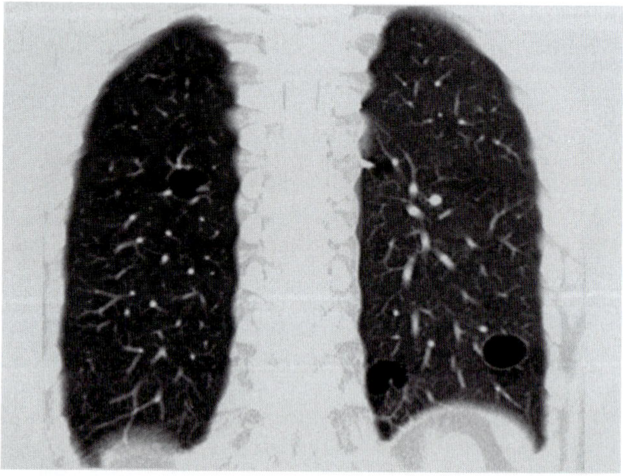

FIG. 30: Coronal MPR showing multiple bilateral thin-walled cysts (LIP) in a 40-year-old female of Sjögren syndrome having dyspnea on exertion.

Lymphangioleiomyomatosis (LAM)

It is a rare multi-organ disease that is almost exclusive to women of child bearing age and characterized by infiltration of airways and lymphatics by immature smooth muscle cells. Patients may present with dyspnea or recurrent pneumothorax. The typical HRCT pattern is of multiple, round, thin walled cysts which are diffusely distributed throughout the lungs, with involvement of the costophrenic sulci, the intervening lung parenchyma appears normal **(Fig. 29)**. Lymphangioleiomyomatosis (LAM) is not associated with nodules but pleural effusions are common.[22]

Lymphoid Interstitial Pneumonia

Lymphoid interstitial pneumonia (LIP) is a part of spectrum of pulmonary lymphoproliferative disorders characterized on HRCT by diffuse ground-glass opacities and ill-defined centrilobular nodules. Multiple thin walled cysts may be seen in the patients with LIP **(Fig. 30)**. They are usually associated with a history of connective tissue disease, especially Sjögren syndrome and immunosuppression. The cysts are less numerous in number than the cysts occurring in patients with histiocytosis or LAM. In patients with LIP, the cysts are seen mainly in the lower lobes with vessels often associated with wall of cysts.[20]

Incidental Lung Cysts

Randomly scattered thin wall cysts have been seen as a normal finding in 25% of elderly patients older than 75 years on HRCT. The cysts ranging from 5 mm to 22 mm have been seen in all lobes in asymptomatic non-smoking individuals, likely to represent part of the aging process.[22]

DECREASED LUNG OPACITY WITHOUT DISCERNIBLE WALL

Emphysema

Emphysema is the permanent, abnormal enlargement of air spaces distal to the terminal bronchiole and is accompanied by destruction of the walls of the involved air spaces. It is the end result of several different processes such as cigarette smoking, enzyme deficiency and drug abuse. Emphysema result in focal areas of very low attenuation without well-defined walls which can be accurately diagnosed on HRCT.[23]

Emphysema is categorized according to the part of the secondary pulmonary lobule involved into the following types:

- Centrilobular emphysema
- Panlobular emphysema
- Paraseptal emphysema

Table 16 depicts the differences between the three types of emphysema.

Centrilobular emphysema (CLE) seen most commonly in the upper lobes manifests as multiple small areas of low attenuation without a perceptible wall, producing a punched out appearance. A centrilobular artery is often visible within the center of these lucencies **(Fig. 31)**. This appearance is diagnostic of CLE and biopsy is not required for diagnosis if the patient has a smoking history. HRCT is often more sensitive than pulmonary function tests and is able to detect very early stage of centrilobular emphysema.[24]

Panlobular emphysema (PLE) is histopathologically characterized by complete destruction of the secondary pulmonary lobule and shows either diffuse or lobar distribution. On HRCT, it is seen as generalized lung lucency with attenuated small vessels with increased lung volume.[22]

Paraseptal emphysema (PSE) preferentially destroys the distal portion of the pulmonary acinus, hence, findings on HRCT are characteristically peripheral in distribution. On HRCT, paraseptal emphysema typically appears as air attenuation cysts seen in a single layer in the subpleural lung adjacent to the mediastinum and fissure **(Fig. 32)**. The cysts of PSE are outlined by a thin, discrete wall which may correspond to interlobular septa. As they are associated with smoking, they are often seen with centrilobular emphysema.

TABLE 16: Comparison of different types of emphysema.

Type of emphysema	Causes	Distribution	HRCT appearance
Centrilobular	Cigarette smoking	Upper lobes, central	Focal lucencies without visible walls
Panlobular	Alpha-1 antitrypsin deficiency, cigarette smoking	Lower lobes, diffuse	Generalized increase in lung lucency
Paraseptal	Cigarette smoking or idiopathic	Subpleural	Focal round, well-defined lucencies in a single layer with thin walls

Bullous Emphysema

The term is used to refer to emphysema that is associated with large bullae. They occur most commonly in patients of paraseptal and centrilobular emphysema. A bulla is defined as a sharply defined area of emphysema that measures more than 1 cm in diameter. Walls of bulla appear as thin, hair-like on HRCT. **Flowchart 4** gives the algorithmic approach to cystic airspaces.

HRCT Findings Manifesting as Inhomogeneous Lung Opacity

Mosaic Attenuation Pattern

Inhomogeneous lung attenuation or mosaic attenuation pattern is a common finding on HRCT due to a wide range of

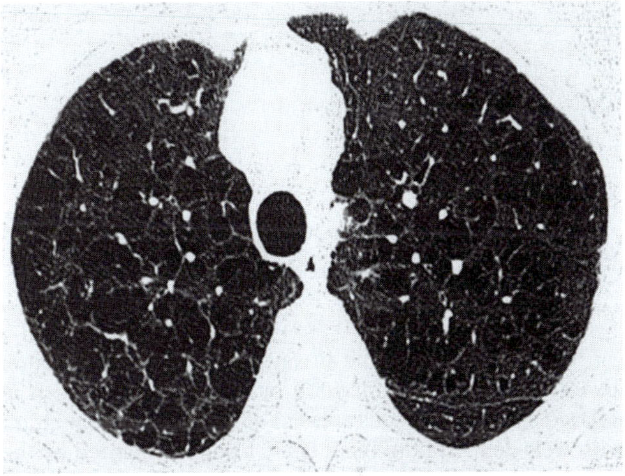

FIG. 31: Axial HRCT shows numerous small low-attenuation areas with ill-defined borders evenly distributed in bilateral upper lobes in centrilobular emphysema.

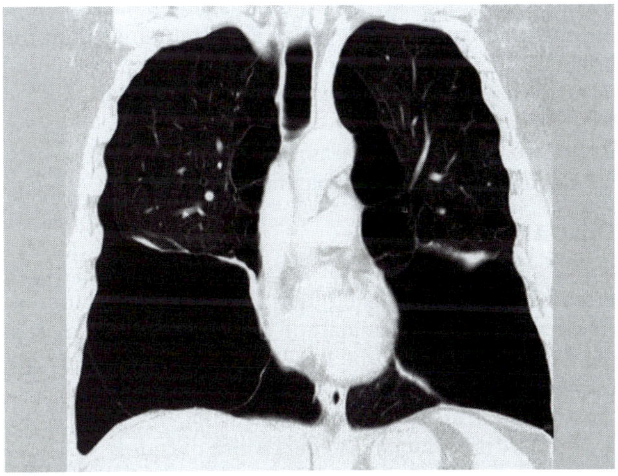

FIG. 32: Coronal MPR CT chest shows single layer of subpleural areas of low attenuation marginated by interlobular septa in bilateral upper zones along mediastinal pleural surface consistent with paraseptal emphysema. Large subpleural bullae in bilateral lower zones and small centriacinar emphysematous spaces are seen in bilateral upper and mid zones. A small pneumothorax is seen along the right lateral chest wall.

FLOWCHART 4: Algorithmic approach to the diagnosis of cystic airspaces.

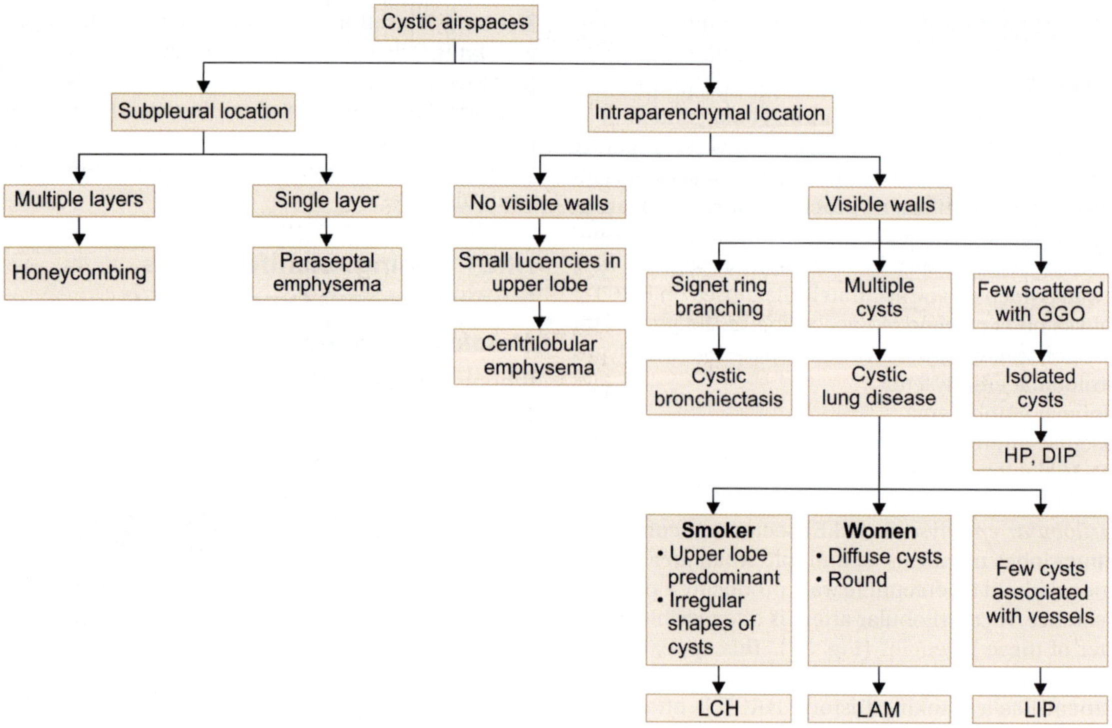

(GGO: ground-glass opacity; LCH: Langerhans cell histiocytosis; LAM: lymphangioleiomyomatosis; LIP: lymphoid interstitial pneumonia)

causes that can involve the airways, pulmonary vasculature, alveoli and interstitium alone or in combination.[25] It is defined as heterogeneous areas of differing lung attenuation with well-defined borders. It is a CT pattern defined by the Fleischner society glossary as a "patchwork of regions of differing attenuation seen on CT of the lung" **(Fig. 33)**.[5] This pattern is a challenge for the radiologist to decide which are abnormal regions of lung, those of low attenuation or those of high attenuation or both. Non-uniform distribution of disease gives a mosaic pattern on imaging. Mosaic pattern of lung attenuation is the preferred terminology than the original terms of mosaic oligemia and perfusion and is caused by three categories of disease:[26]

1. Small airways disease
2. Pulmonary vascular disease
3. Infiltrative lung disease (parenchymal disease).

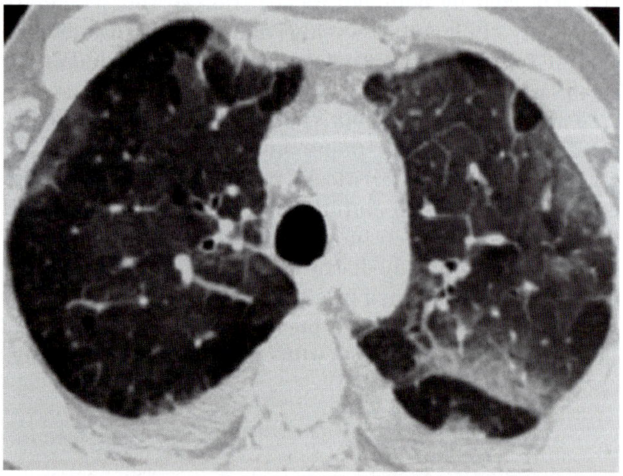

FIG. 33: Axial HRCT chest shows multiple geographic areas of GGO with low-attenuation areas showing reduced caliber of vessels within: Mosaic attenuation pattern.

Small Airways Disease

Small airways are non-cartilaginous airways less than 2 mm in diameter, located from the eighth generation of airways down to the terminal and respiratory bronchioles. In the normal population, the small airways are not visible, but may be visible due to underlying disease.

Small airways disease can be classified as:

a. Primary bronchiolar disorders which includes:
   - Constrictive bronchiolitis
   - Cellular bronchiolitis
   - Diffuse panbronchiolitis
   - Respiratory bronchiolitis
   - Follicular bronchiolitis.

b. Bronchiolar involvement in diffuse interstitial lung disease, such as hypersensitivity pneumonitis.

c. Bronchiolar involvement in large airway disease, such as bronchiectasis or asthma.

Obstruction of small airways due to small airways inflammation is a common pathologic process and is usually reversible. In contrast; in constrictive bronchiolitis, the submucosal and peribronchiolar fibrosis leads to irreversible obstruction of the small airways **(Figs. 34A and B)**.

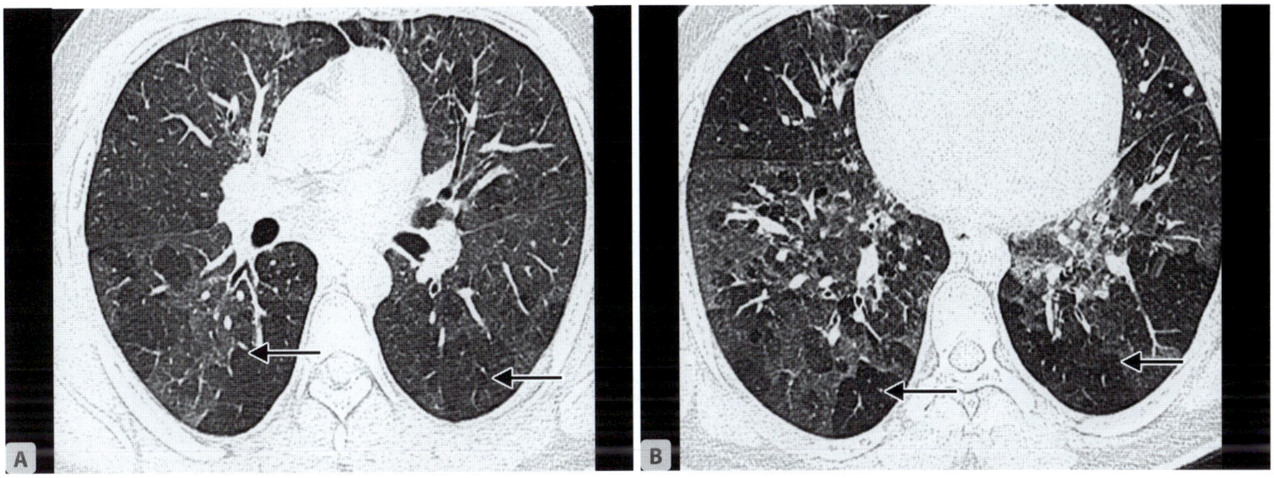

FIGS. 34A AND B: Mosaic attenuation. (A) Axial HRCT inspiratory scan showing patchy areas of mosaic attenuation seen as focal areas of reduced lung density with decreased vessel size within (arrows) along with normal appearing denser lung regions. Corresponding expiratory scan (B) Shows persistent lucency in same areas (arrows in B) confirming air trapping: Constrictive bronchiolitis in a patient of rheumatoid arthritis.

Pathophysiology of Mosaic Attenuation in Small Airways Disease

Airway obstruction in small airways disease leads to hypoxia of underventilated lung resulting in reflux vasoconstriction and air-trapping which is reflected on HRCT as areas of decreased lung attenuation with reduced caliber of vessels as compared to normal lung. There is redistribution of blood flow to the uninvolved areas, which results in increase in attenuation and decrease in volume of the normally ventilated lung.

On CT scan, there are certain direct signs and indirect signs of small airways disease:

- Direct signs—thickened peripheral airways, dilatation of peripheral airways
- Indirect signs—air trapping, subsegmental atelectasis, mosaic lung attenuation, centrilobular nodules and tree in bud opacities.

The radiologist needs to look at the following structures on CT chest to ascertain the underlying cause of mosaic attenuation pattern:

i. *Peripheral vessels:* If these are smaller in the areas of decreased lung attenuation, then, it is either a vascular cause or small airways disease and not parenchymal disease (appearing on HRCT as GGO, reticular or reticulonodular opacities).

ii. *Heart and pulmonary vasculature:* Amongst the pulmonary vascular causes, mosaic attenuation is most commonly seen in pulmonary hypertension and pulmonary thromboembolism. In pulmonary hypertension, enlargement of the pulmonary trunk is suggestive of vascular cause of mosaic attenuation and right ventricular enlargement and hypertrophy seen on CT. In patients with left ventricular and/or left atrial dilatation, pulmonary edema may be the cause of mosaic appearance especially if interlobular septal thickening is present.

   In pulmonary hypertension, the mosaic attenuation often manifests as scattered areas of low attenuation confined to the secondary pulmonary lobules **(Figs. 35A and B)**. While in pulmonary thromboembolism, the mosaicism is confined to segmental or subsegmantal distribution in the vascular distribution of thrombi.

iii. *Small airways:* Abnormally dilated or thick-walled airways in the lucent areas confirms small airways disease. In addition, presence of centilobular nodules along with mosaicism on CT is the clue to injury to small airways.

iv. *Parenchymal changes:* Mosaic attenuation pattern can be produced by interstitial lung disease (parenchymal disease) characterized by GGO, interlobular septal thickening. It may be seen in conditions, such as *P. jirovecii* pneumonia, diffuse alveolar hemorrhage, pulmonary edema, hypersensitivity pneumonitis or organizing pneumonia wherein areas of higher attenuation represent the interstitial process and areas of lower attenuation represent the normal lung.

v. *Air trapping:* Air trapping on expiratory HRCT is the best clue to the diagnosis of small airways disease. It refers to the regions of lung which do not show increase in attenuation or show little change in cross sectional area on expiration.

Pitfalls in Classification[27]

- Areas of air trapping can be seen in normal patients and some degree of heterogeneity in lung parenchyma is seen on expiratory scan. One should inspect the posterior wall of trachea on CT scan. In case of acquisition during expiratory scan, the posterior wall of trachea shows bowing.
- Presence of air trapping excludes primary parenchymal disease unless there is suspicion of HP which has mixed features of both parenchymal and small airway disease.
- Rarely air trapping can occur in pulmonary vascular disease.

Flowchart 5 gives the algorithmic approach to mosaic attenuation pattern.

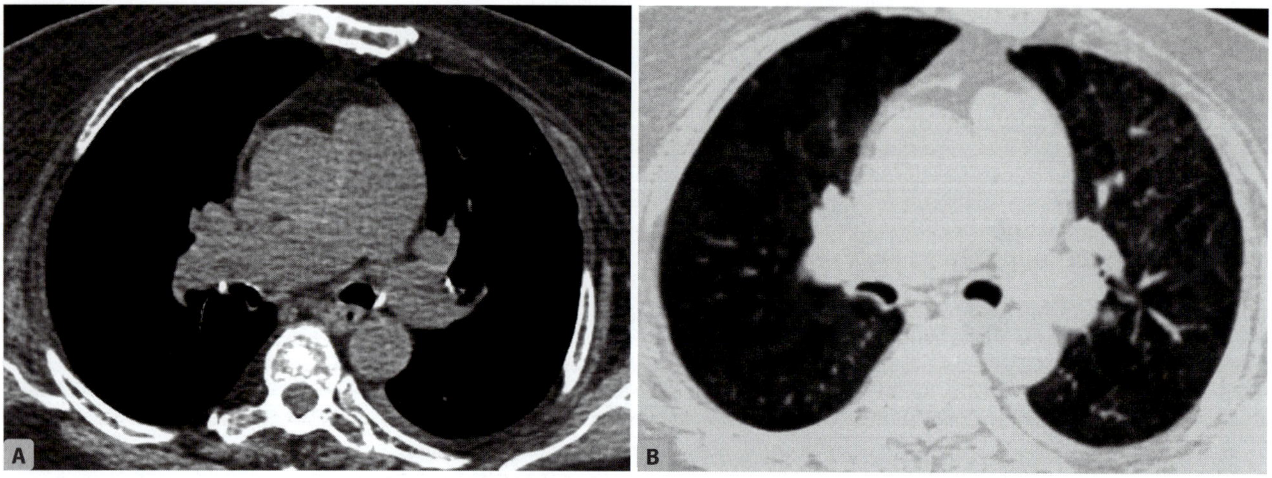

FIGS. 35A AND B: CT chest mediastinal window. (A) reveals dilated main pulmonary artery in patient of pulmonary artery hypertension; (B) lung window image reveals areas of mosaic attenuation in bilateral lung fields.

FLOWCHART 5: Algorithmic approach to inhomogeneous lung opacity mosaic attenuation pattern.

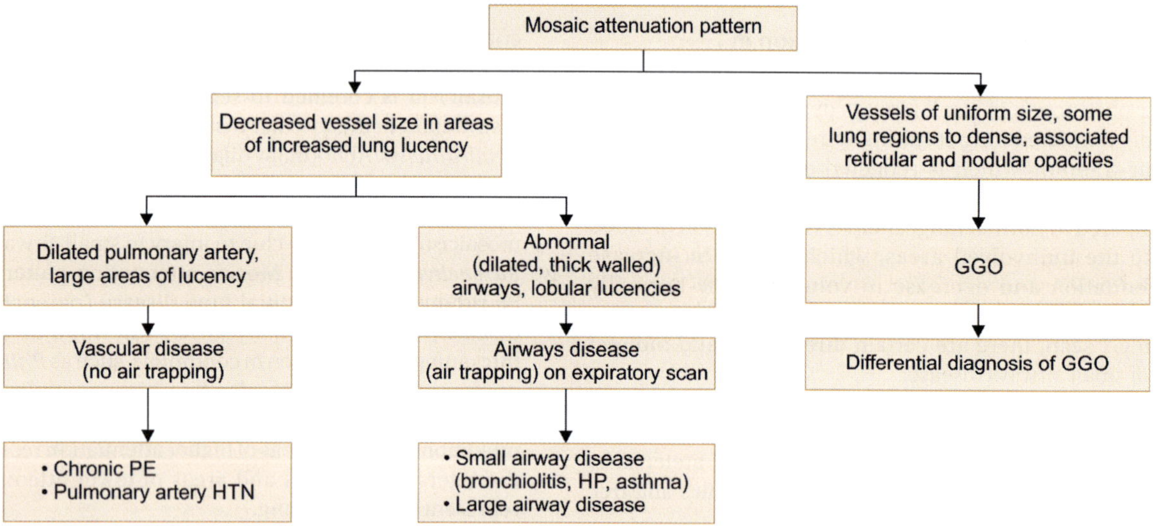

(GGO: ground-glass opacity; PE: pulmonary embolism; HTN: hypertension; HP: hypersensitivity pneumonitis)

CONCLUSION

Lung disease can produce recognizable alteration in parenchymal anatomy on CT resulting in various patterns and distributions of abnormalities. However, the various patterns described are not always isolated findings on CT. They commonly occur in combination with other patterns and findings. Use of an organized algorithmic approach in conjunction with clinical data is essential in the evaluation of CT patterns of lung disease so as to formulate a differential diagnosis or reach a specific diagnosis.

REFERENCES

1. Collins J. CT signs and pattern of lung disease. RCNA. 2001;39(6):1115-35.
2. Elicker B, Pereira C, Webb R, et al. High resolution computed tomographic pattern of diffuse interstitial lung disease with clinical and pathological correlation. J Bras Pneumol. 2008;34(9):715-44.
3. Gotway MB, Reddy GP, Webb WR, et al. High-resolution CT of the lung: pattern of disease and differential diagnosis. Radiol Clin N Am. 2005.pp.513-42.
4. Webb RW, Muller NL, Naidich DP. HRCT findings: Nodules and nodular opacities in High resolution CT of the lung, 5th edition, Wolter Kluwer; 2015.pp.106-39.
5. Hansell DM, Bankier AA, McMohan H, et al. Fleischner society-glossary of terms for thoracic imaging. Radiology. 2008;246: 697-722.
6. Hansell DM, Lynch DA, McAdams HP, et al. Basic HRCT pattern of lung disease in imaging of diseases of the chest. Mosby Elsevier; 2010.pp.153-204.

7. Remy JH, Remy J, Artaud D, et al. Diffuse infiltrative lung disease: clinical value of sliding. thin slab maximum intensity projection CT scans in the detection of mild micronodular pattern. Radiology. 1996;200:333-9.
8. Elicker BM, Webb RW. Nodular lung disease in fundamentals of high-resolution lung CT: Common findings, common patterns, common diseases, and differential diagnosis, 1st edition, Wolter Kluwer; 2013.pp.37-54.
9. Raoof S, Amchentsev A, Vlahos I, et al. Pictoral Essay: Multinodular disease: a high resolution CT scan diagnostic Algorithm. Chest. 2006;129(3):805-15.
10. Rossi SE, Franquet T, Volpacchio M, et al. Tree-in-bud pattern at thin-section CT of the lungs: radiologic-Pathologic Overview. Radiographics. 2005;25:789-801.
11. Webb RW, Muller NL, Naidich DP. HRCT findings: linear and reticular opacities in high resolution CT of the lung, 5th edition Wolters Kluwer; 2015.pp.74-105.
12. Collins J, Stern EJ. Signs and patterns of lung disease in chest radiology. The Essentials, 3rd Edition, Wolters Kluwer, 2015. pp.17-37.
13. Elicker BM, Webb RW. Reticular opacities in fundamentals of high-resolution lung CT: Common findings, common patterns, common diseases, and differential diagnosis, 1st edition, Wolters Kluwer; 2013. pp.17-36.
14. Webb RW, Muller NL, Naidich DP. HRCT findings: Parenchymal opacification in high resolution CT of the lung, 5th edition Wolter Kluwer. 2015. pp. 140-65.
15. Frauquet T. Non-neoplastic parenchymal lung disease in CT and MRI of the whole body. In: Hagga JR, Dogra VS, Forsting M, Gilkeson RC, Ha HK, Sundaram M (Eds). Volume 1, 5th edition, Mosby, Elsevier; 2009. pp. 863-926.
16. Pawa S. Basic patterns of lung disease in diagnostic radiology with chest and cardiovascular imaging. In: Chowdhury V, Gupta AK, Khandelwal N (Eds). Jaypee Brothers Medical Publishers, 3rd edition; 2010. pp. 28-59.
17. Elicker BM, Webb RW. Increased lung attenuation: Ground-glass opacity and consolidation in fundamentals of high-resolution lung CT: Common findings, common patterns, common diseases and differential diagnosis. 1st edition, Wolters Kluwer; 2013. pp. 59-70.
18. Grenier PA, Aubry CB. Airway disease and chronic airway obstruction in Grainger and Allson's Diagnostic Radiology: A Textbook of Medical Imaging, 6th edition, Churchill Livingstone, Elsevier; 2015. pp. 267-97.
19. Javidan NC, Bhalla S. Bronchiectasis. Radiol Clin N Am. 2009;47:289-306.
20. Webb RW, Muller NL, Naidich DP. HRCT findings: Air filled cystic lesions in high resolution CT of the lung, 5th edition, Wolters Kluwer. 2015.pp.165-86.
21. Cartier Y, Kavanagh PV, Johkoh T, et al. Bronchiectasis: Accuracy of high resolution CT in the differentiation of specific diseases. AJR. 1999;173:47-52.
22. Beddy P, Babar J, Devraj A. A practical approach to cystic lung disease on HRCT insights Imaging. 2011;2(1):1-7.
23. Webb RW, Muller NL, Naidich DP. HRCT findings: Decreased lung attenuation in high resolution CT of the lung. 5th edition, Wolters Kluwer; 2015. pp. 187-205.
24. Elicker BM, Webb RW. Decreased lung attenuation: Emphysema, mosaic perfusion and cystic lung disease in fundamentals of high-resolution lung CT: Common findings, common patterns, common diseases and differential diagnosis, 1st edition, Wolter Kluwer; 2013. pp. 71-82.
25. Kligerman SJ, Henry T, Lin CT, et al. Mosaic attenuation: etiology, methods of differentiation, and pitfalls. Radiographics. 2015;35:1360-80.
26. Stern EJ, Swensen SJ, Hartman TE, et al. CT mosaic pattern of lung attenuation: distinguishing different causes. AJR. 1995;165:813-6.
27. Ridge CA, Bankier AA, Eisenberg RL. Mosaic attenuation. AJR. 2011;197:W970-7.

CHAPTER

126

Imaging of Pulmonary Tuberculosis

Mandeep Garg, Anmol Bhatia, Naveen Kalra

INTRODUCTION

Tuberculosis (TB) is caused by *Mycobacterium tuberculosis,* and is responsible for significant morbidity and mortality, particularly in the countries of developing world.[1] As per the World Health Organization (WHO) data, in 2012 national programs on TB notified around 6.1 million cases of TB, 5.4 million of these being new cases. Of these, 2.5 million were sputum positive, 1.9 million were sputum negative, and 0.8 million were of extrapulmonary TB (EPTB); case type was not known in rest of the cases. India alone accounted for 26% of total cases of TB worldwide in 2012. TB causes significant mortality in Indian population, and kills two people every 3 min, and nearly a thousand persons every day.[2]

The disease course and clinical-radiological presentation is dependent upon and altered by nature of interaction between the mycobacteria and response by the body of the host. Due to variation of immune response of the body in some of the patient population, like immunocompromised and aging population, it is common to see various atypical clinical-radiological presentations. Also, the changing panorama where there tuberculosis can be encountered, as well as the resurgence of the disease around the world, and the changing clinical-radiological spectrum of the disease, justify the persistence of the concern in the radiology community to assess the imaging findings in pulmonary tuberculosis.

TB can affect any organ system, although the lungs are the commonest and often the initial organs to be involved. In the chest, after the lungs TB commonly affects the lymph nodes followed by pleura. The lymph nodes and pleural involvement are included under EPTB.[2]

CHANGING CONCEPTS OF RADIOLOGIC MANIFESTATIONS OF PULMONARY TB

The notion that the "clinical, pathologic, and radiologic findings of reactivation form of TB are quite different from those seen in primary form" has been challenged based on research related to DNA fingerprinting.[3] It has been found that samples from patients who are infected with epidemiologically different strains of TB have different restriction fragment length polymorphism (RFLP) patterns, while patients infected with epidemiologically similar strains have similar RFLP patterns. Therefore, the cases in which the samples have similar or related genotypes have usually been recently transmitted. Vis-à-vis, cases in which the isolates have different genotypes represent reactivation form of TB.[4]

A preliminary study on DNA fingerprinting showed that the radiologic findings are usually similar in patients having a primary or postprimary TB.[5] Therefore, period from contracting the infection to clinically obvious disease will not reliably predict the radiologic findings. The immune response of the patient is the sole forecaster of radiologic findings; with severely immunocompromized patients showing features of primary form, whereas immunocompetent patients showing propensity for the reactivation form of TB.[5]

ROLE OF IMAGING IN PULMONARY TUBERCULOSIS

- Making a diagnosis.
- Evaluating the treatment response and residual disease activity.
- Detecting the complications and sequelae.

RADIOLOGICAL PATTERNS OF PULMONARY TB

Radiological patterns may be considered under the following groups:

- Typical radiological patterns of primary TB.
- Postprimary TB or phtysis.
- Patterns encountered both in primary and/or post primary forms.
- Complications and sequelae of TB.
- Atypical patterns.

Typical Radiological Patterns of Primary TB

Four entities are known to occur in primary pulmonary TB: gangliopulmonary pattern; miliary pattern; tuberculous pleuritis; and involvement of tracheobronchial airway. The gangliopulmonary TB is seen only in primary TB while others are seen in both primary and postprimary TB. Gangliopulmonary form is characterized by the presence of enlarged lymph nodes in mediastinum and/or hila, with relatively less involvement of parenchyma (Ghon focus). This form preferentially occurs in children, and hence is known as "childhood-type TB". In areas where there is a low incidence of the disease, except for nonindigenous pediatric population, it has a high incidence of occurence in adults and older age groups.[6] Right paratracheal and hilar lymph nodes are the most commonly enlarged nodes seen in primary TB, although involvement of various other nodal stations in different combinations can be seen. The prevalence of lymph nodal enlargement decreases with increasing age.[7] On CECT, tuberculous nodes that are greater than 2 cm show central areas of low attenuation suggestive of caseous necrosis and peripheral rim enhancement **(Figs. 1A and B)**. In approximately two-thirds cases of primary TB in pediatric population, parenchymal lesions are encountered on the ipsilateral side of enlarged lymph nodes.[7] Lesions in parenchyma are typically located in the peripheral lung fields involving the subpleural locations.

The gangliopulmonary form of TB is usually self-limiting, with immunocompetent individuals usually remaining asymptomatic. Sometimes, the lone radiological finding is Ranke complex which includes both the parenchymal lesion (Ghon focus) and affected lymph nodes **(Fig. 2)**. The course in Gangliopulmonary form may be complicated in form of lymph node perforating in the bronchus, retro-obstructive pneumonia, and/or atelectasis (known as epituberculosis). Retro-obstructive pneumonia may evolve into a fibrotic lesion which may or may not be calcified. Destruction of the parenchyma of the lung result in fibrosis associated with traction bronchiectasis. In adults, the primary infection mostly causes parenchymal consolidation without lymphadenopathy **(Fig. 3)**. Cavitatory form is rarely encountered in children.

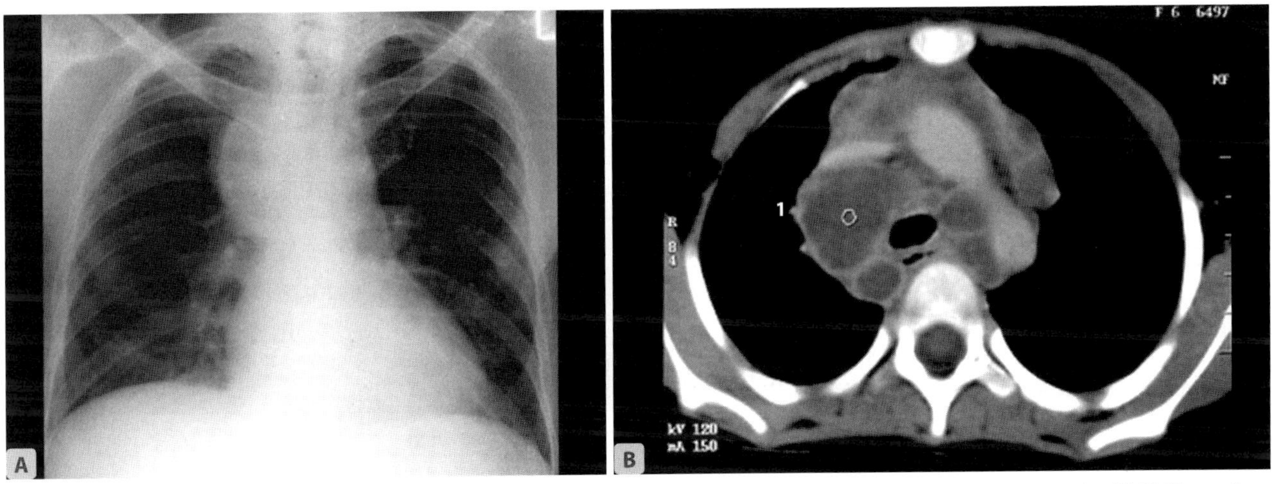

FIGS. 1A AND B: Tuberculous mediastinal lymphadenopathy. (A) Chest radiograph shows right paratracheal lymphadenopathy; (B) CECT reveals low density center with peripheral rim enhancement of the node. Similar but smaller nodes are also seen in the posterior mediastinum.

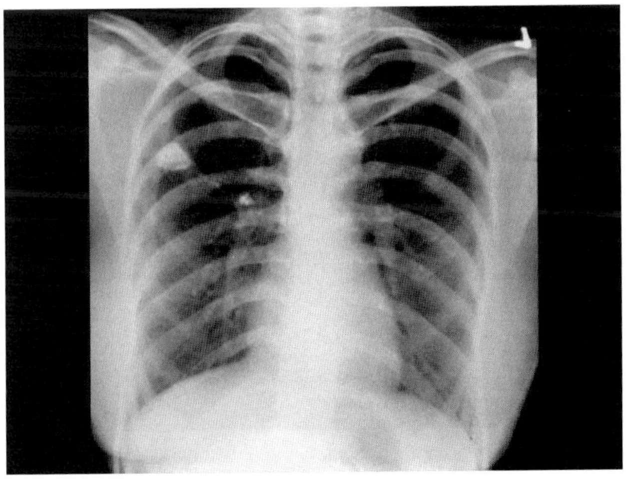

FIG. 2: Ranke complex. Chest radiograph shows a calcified lesion in the right upper zone along with calcification of the right hilar node and of the intervening lymphatic channel.

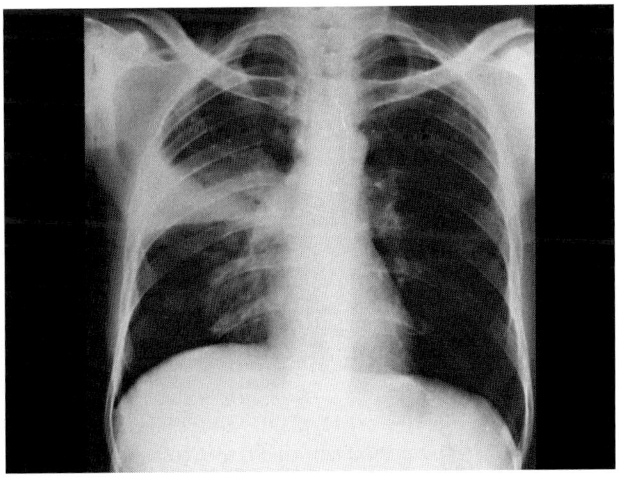

FIG. 3: Primary tuberculosis in a 40-year-old male. Chest radiograph shows multilobar consolidation of the right lung affecting the upper and lower lobes without lymphadenopathy.

Postprimary TB or Phtysis

This form evolves and progresses depending upon the status of acquired immunity, due to reactivation of residual dormant infective focus. It is mostly, but not always, a disease affecting adult population.[8] In pediatric population, it mostly occurs in adolescent children, particularly in girls at menarche.[7] This form of TB is characterized by caseous necrosis undergoing liquefaction, progressive lung destruction associated with fibrosis and formation of cavities. The lesions are typically located in the upper lobes (apicoposterior segments) and with a relative less degree of involvement of the lower lobes (superior segments). The areas of caseous necrosis undergoing liquefaction later on communicate with the adjacent airways resulting in formation of cavities **(Figs. 4A and B)**. The findings include parenchymal infiltrates in apicoposterior locations, cavities, pleural effusion, fibrotic areas causing lung parenchyma destruction, pulling up of hila/fissures, traction bronchiectasis, and pleural adhesions.[9] Cavitation may be seen in 40% cases in postprimary form radiographically. There may be thin and smooth walls as well as thick and nodular walls of the cavities. Air-fluid levels can be seen in 10% of cases with cavities,[10] which may because of superimposed infection by bacteria or fungus. Bronchogenic spread is characterized by multiple, ill-defined nodules, having a lobar/segmental distribution, typically involving lower lung zones.[11] HRCT typically shows 2- to 4-mm sized nodules which are centrilobular in distribution presenting as sharply marginated branching structures within and around terminal and respiratory bronchioles giving "tree-in-bud" appearance **(Fig. 5)**.[12] Cicatrization atelectasis is a common finding following postprimary TB which presents as atelectatic changes in the upper lobe, retracted hilum, lower lobe compensatory hyperinflation, and ipsilateral tracheomediastinal shift. This may also be associated with pleural thickening in the apices along with fibrosis, proliferation of extrapleural soft tissues and subpleural atelectatic changes on CT.[13]

Radiological Patterns Seen in Both Primary and/or Postprimary TB

Miliary TB

Miliary TB results from the hematogenous spread of the infection in lungs and other organs, resulting in innumerable tiny granulomas. Initially, skiagrams may be normal in up to 25–40% of patients.[14] CT helps in demonstration of the miliary nodules before they become perceptible on radiographs **(Figs. 6A and B)**. It shows a combination of both sharply as well as poorly defined, diffusely distributed 1- to 4-mm nodules in a random fashion commonly associated with thickening of the interstitium (both interlobular and intralobular septae).[15] A typical "snowstorm" appearance on Chest X-ray suggesting an evolution to adult respiratory distress syndrome has also been reported.[16] The second most common finding on HRCT in cases of miliary tuberculosis includes ground-

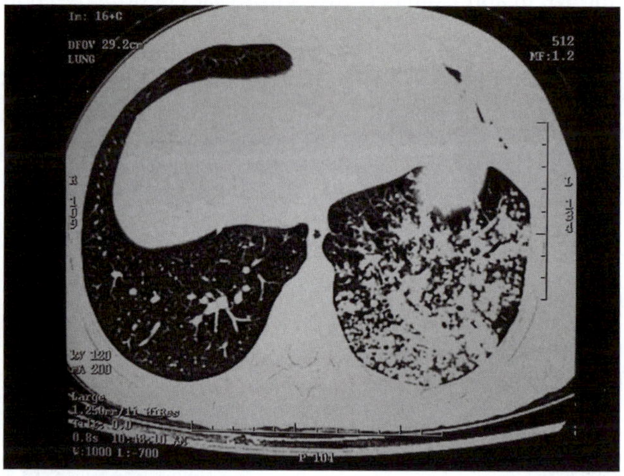

FIG. 5: Endobronchial spread depicted on HRCT. There is presence of extensive bronchiolar and alveolar ductal lesions with a typical 'tree-in-bud appearance in the right lower lobe.

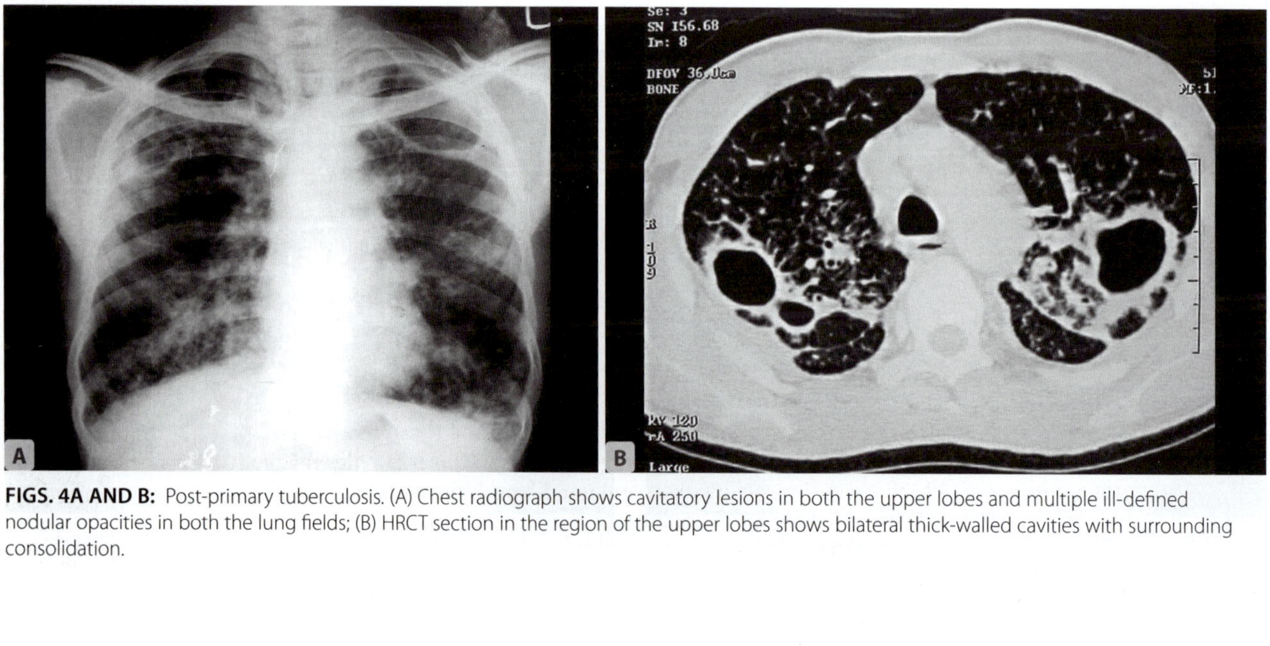

FIGS. 4A AND B: Post-primary tuberculosis. (A) Chest radiograph shows cavitatory lesions in both the upper lobes and multiple ill-defined nodular opacities in both the lung fields; (B) HRCT section in the region of the upper lobes shows bilateral thick-walled cavities with surrounding consolidation.

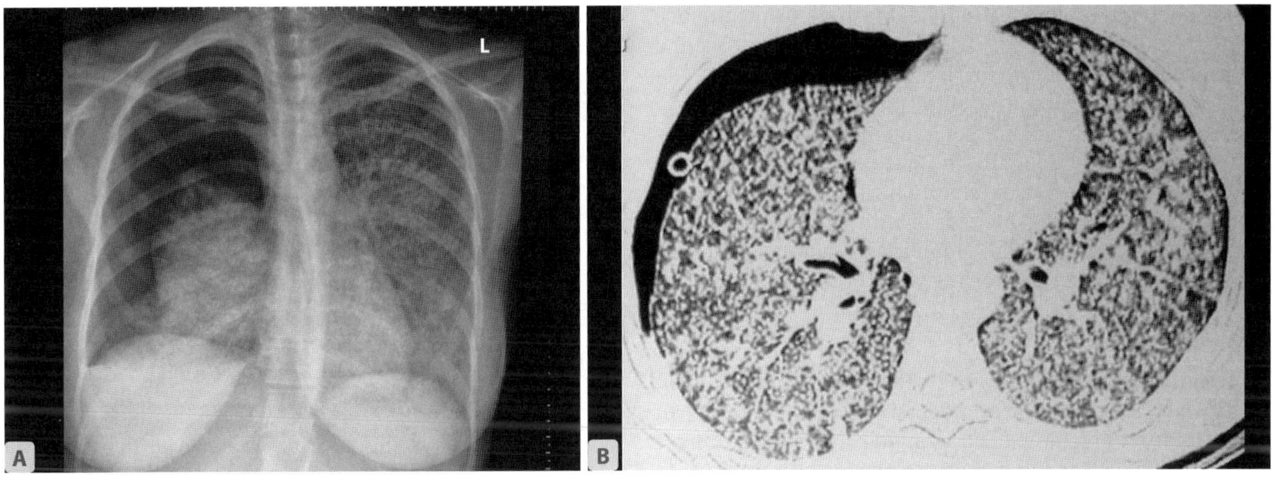

FIGS. 6A AND B: Miliary tuberculosis. (A) Chest radiograph shows diffuse fine micronodular opacities in both lungs. (B) HRCT demonstrates peribronchiolar and perivascular nodules with airspace consolidation in the superior segment of left lower lobe.

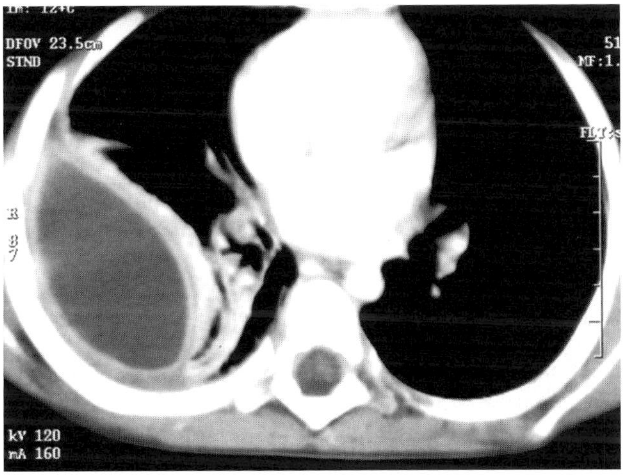

FIG. 7: Empyema. CECT chest depicting right pleural effusion with enhancing visceral and parietal pleura giving split-pleura sign.

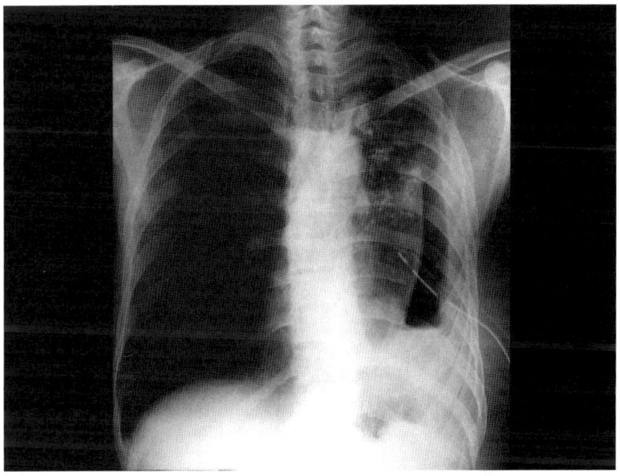

FIG. 8: Bronchopleural fistula in a patient with non-resolving hydropneumothorax on intercostals tube drainage. Chest radiograph shows left pleural effusion with an air-fluid level and partial atlectasis of the left lung.

glass opacities which represent small granulomas below the resolution of HRCT superimposed on exudative changes of the lung.[17]

Exudative Pleuritis

Pleural cavity may be involved from a caseating granuloma in parenchyma adjacent to pleural, or through hematogenous route. It is usually seen along with parenchymal and/or lymphadenopathy. It may however be seen sometimes in as the only radiologic finding 5% of adult patients suggesting primary TB.[18] CECT in shows smooth thickening with enhancement of parietal and visceral pleura resulting in split-pleura sign **(Fig. 7)**. Tuberculous pleurisy when localized results tuberculous empyema, which sometimes ruptures outside forming a subcutaneous abscess, called as empyema necessitans. Diffuse pleural thickening without any effusion suggests fibrothorax, and indicates disease inactivity. Pleural collection when communicates with the bronchial tree results in development of bronchopleural fistula and an air fluid level within **(Fig. 8)**. Diagnosis of bronchopleural fistula is suggested clinically by copious amount of sputum production by the patient, and radiologically by appearance of hydro pneumothorax with changing air-fluid level as well as involvement of contralateral side. CT may demonstrate the communication between the collection in pleural cavity and bronchi or lung parenchyma.[19]

Tracheobronchial TB

Tracheobronchial TB is known to occur in 2–4% of patients of pulmonary TB.[20] It usually results from a perforation of enlarged lymph nodes into a bronchus,[21,22] although it may also result from lymphatic and hematogenous dissemination. The ulcerogranulomatous lesions in the involved submucosa; and granulomatous polypoidal growths are seen which result in fibrotic stenoses after healing, and later on postobstructive bronchiectasis **(Fig. 9)**. The acute form of tracheobronchial TB manifests as smooth or irregular thickening of the walls resulting in circumferential bronchial narrowing.[23] Encasement by the enlarged enhancing mediastinal nodes is also commonly seen in the active stage. Cicatricial bronchostenosis may occur lately following the healing of the focal infection involving the walls of bronchi. Chronic fibrotic stage shows circumferential symmetric thickening of the wall resulting in concentric narrowing of the bronchus.[24]

Tuberculoma

Tuberculomas are usually the sequelae of healed form of primary TB, but can be seen in 3–6% of patients of postprimary tuberculosis as the only or the main finding.[25] These can be multiple or solitary, varying in size from 0.4 to 5 cm **(Figs. 10A and B)**. The possible pathogenesis resulting in tuberculoma formation include roundening of a contracted healing tubercular lesion, or a healed filled-in cavity.[25] Most of the tuberculomas remain static in size. Calcification is seen to occur in 20–30% cases in a diffuse or a nodular fashion.[26]

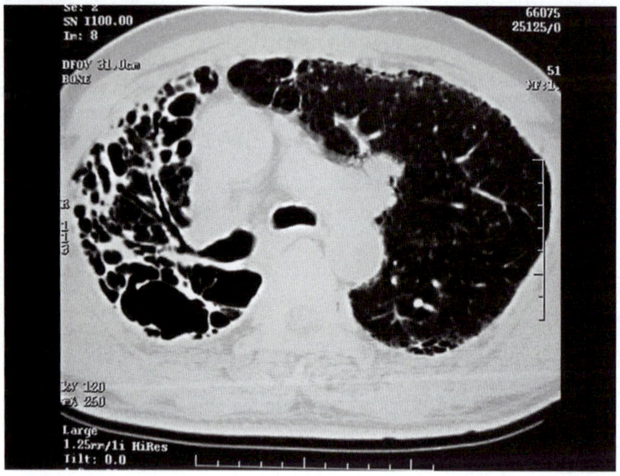

FIG. 9: Bronchiectasis. HRCT shows traction bronchiectasis in the right upper lobe.

Complications and Sequelae of Pulmonary TB

A tuberculous cavity can be invaded by *Aspergillus* species resulting in an "aspergilloma" which consists of a bunch of entangled hyphae knotted together with cellular fragments and mucus. Thickening of the walls of the cavity or of the adjacent pleural lining are early radiographic findings seen suggesting the invasion of tubercular cavity. Radiographs show a nodular radioopacity or a mass which is separated from the adjacent wall by a crescent-shaped area of radiolucency or air **(Figs. 11A and B)**.[27]

Tuberculosis may predispose to the malignancy by local mechanism which is known as scar cancer, or there may be co-existence of TB and carcinoma. Malignancy may also cause tubercular reactivation, both by compromising the patient's immunity, and by erosion into an encapsulated focus. Hence, any predominant or an enlarging nodule on follow up imaging should raise a suspicion for coexisting carcinoma in tuberculosis patients.[28]

In the areas of active foci, pulmonary arteries and veins may demonstrate findings of vasculitis and/or thrombosis. There may be increased tortuousity of the bronchial arteries which commonly are hypertrophied in patients having bronchiectasis associated with TB or may be in parenchymal TB only **(Figs. 12A and B)**. Rasmussen aneurysm results when a tubercular cavity erodes the branch of pulmonary artery in the surrounding parenchyma **(Fig. 13)**.[29]

Broncholithiasis is an uncommon complication, and is a result of erosion of a calcified node in peribronchial location into the adjacent bronchus. CT shows a lymph node in endobronchial or peribronchial location which causes bronchial obstruction resulting in focal hyperinflation, atelectasis, obstructive pneumonitis, bronchiectasis, and branching opacities (obstructive bronchoceles).[30]

Esophageal involvement by TB from adjacent lymph nodes result in formation of strictures, fistulae between esophagus and mediastinum or airway, and traction diverticulae.[31]

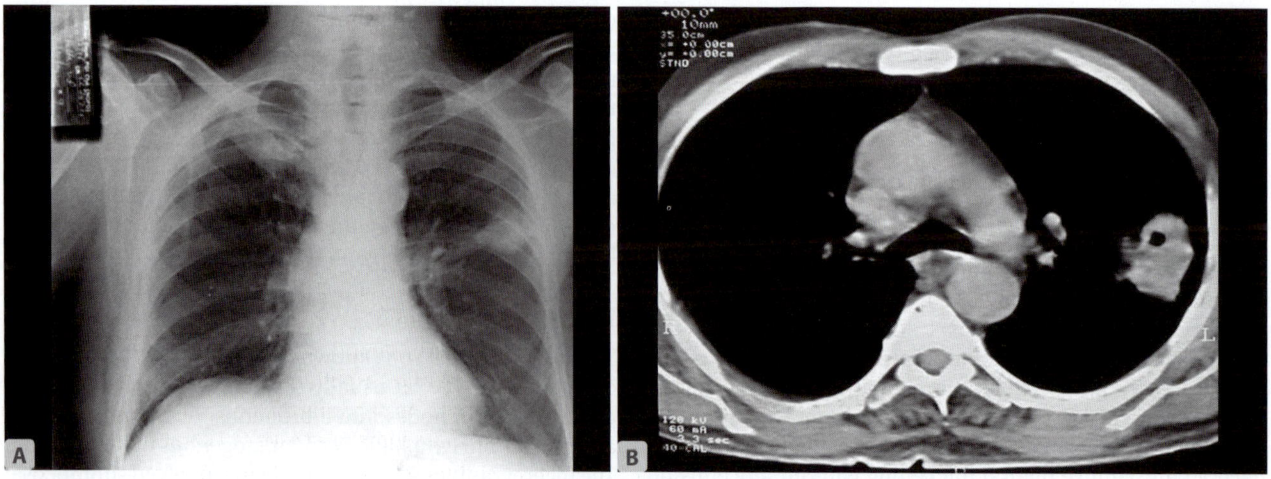

FIGS. 10A AND B: Tuberculoma. (A) Chest radiograph shows a pulmonary nodule in the left middle zone; (B) CECT of the chest shows eccentric cavitation of the nodule. CT-guided aspiration revealed caseous material positive for Mycobacterium tuberculosis.

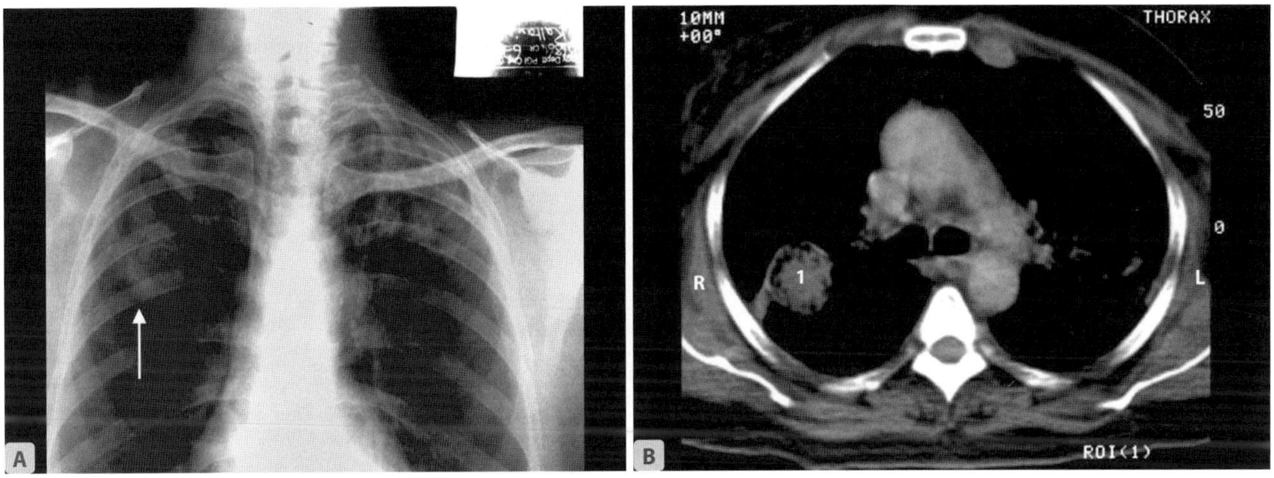

FIGS. 11A AND B: Mycetoma in a cavity. (A) Chest radiograph shows a cavity in the right upper lobe with a nodular lesion inside (arrow); (B) CECT of chest showing soft tissue filling the cavity with an air crescent anteriorly.

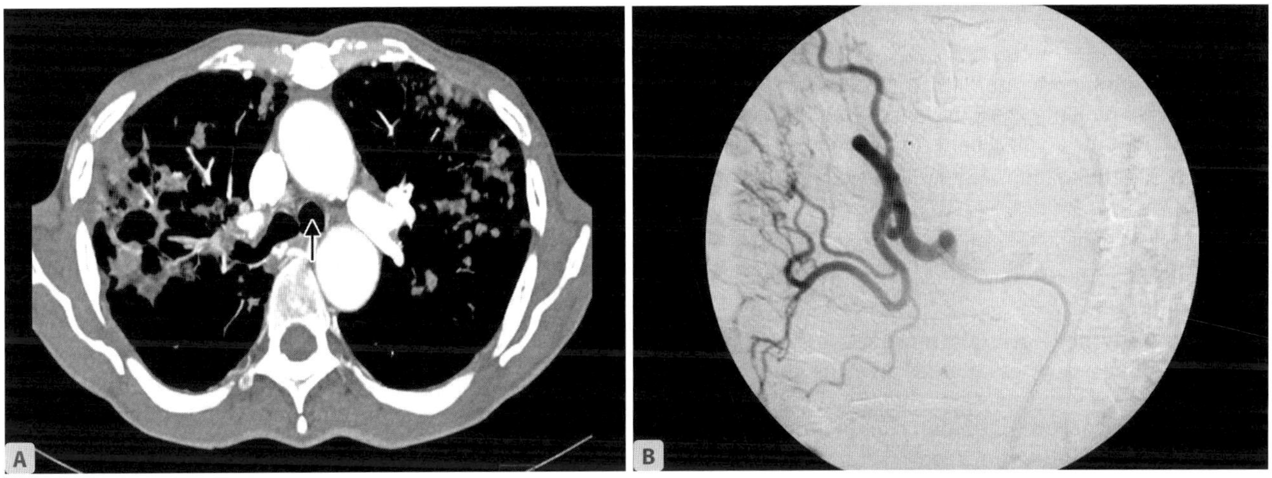

FIGS. 12A AND B: A 62-year-old man with pulmonary TB having massive hemoptysis. (A) Axial CECT image shows ostium of the enlarged right bronchial artery (arrow). Bilateral consolidation and multiple nodules are seen in both lungs. (B) Selective right bronchial angiogram shows enlarged and tortuous right bronchial artery.

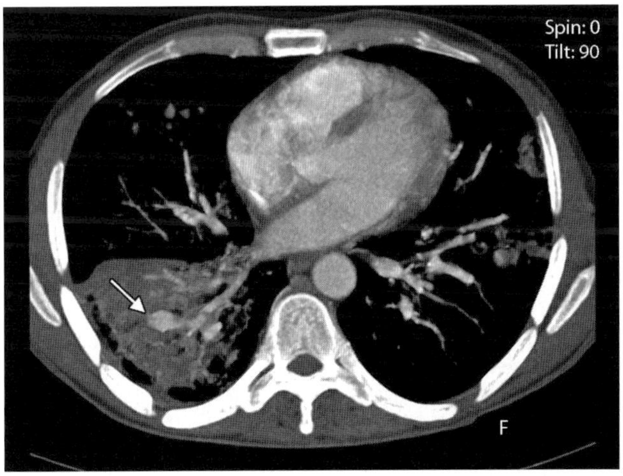

FIG. 13: Rasmussen aneurysm. Axial 10 mm MIP image in a patient with massive hemoptysis showing pseudoaneurysm arising from the branch of right pulmonary artery (arrow).

Tuberculous pericarditis is seen to occur in 1% of cases of TB. It may result from the direct invasion of enlarged lymph nodes into the pericardium or by miliary spread of the infection. Pericardial thickening (with or without effusion) along with enlarged lymph nodes is seen on CT. Constrictive pericarditis characterized by fibrous or calcified pericardial thickening measuring >3 mm is seen as a delayed complication 10% of patients of tuberculous pericarditis **(Figs. 14A and B)**.[25]

Pneumothorax is seen in around 5% of cases of postprimary form, usually in severe cavitatory form of disease. It indicates severe and widespread lung involvement, and the inception of empyema and bronchopleural fistula.

Fibrosing mediastinitis in TB is an unusual complication which progresses slowly without obvious clinical symptoms. The findings on CT in fibrosing mediastinitis include a hilar or a mediastinal mass showing coarse calcification, narrowing of tracheobronchial tree, encasement of pulmonary and other mediastinal vasculature, sometimes presenting as a superior vena cava syndrome.[32]

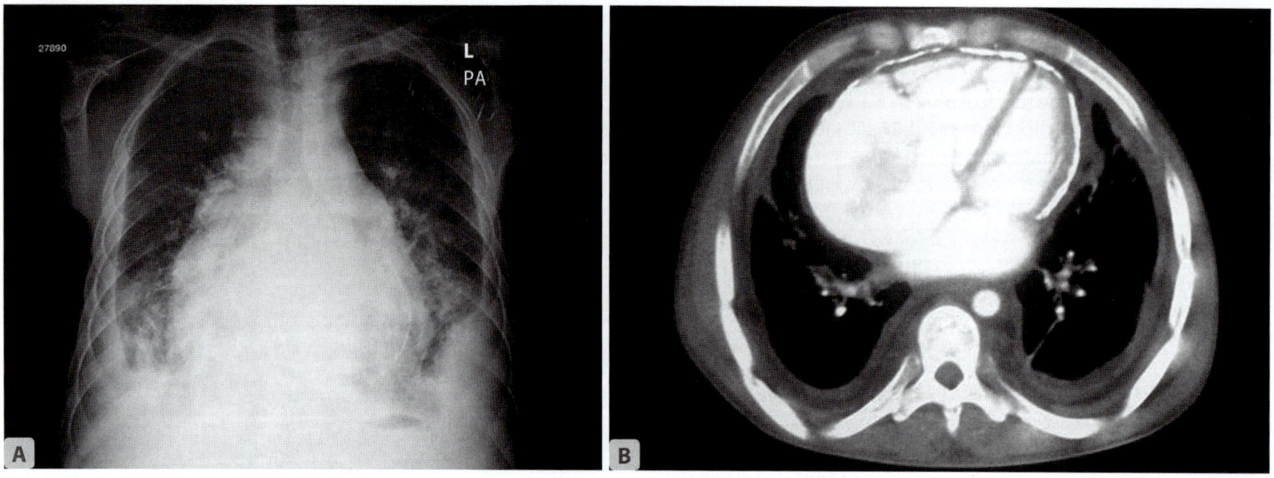

FIGS. 14A AND B: Tuberculous pericarditis. (A) Chest radiograph depicting curvilinear pericardial calcification over left heart border. (B) Axial CECT section showing thickened and calcified pericardium. Also noted is bilateral pleural effusion.

Atypical Patterns

These are usually encountered in elderly and immunocompromised patients. Various factors which may alter the pathogenesis of the atypical patterns include:

- Deficient cellular immunity resulting in reactivation of TB (typical pattern)
- Reinfection or second primary infection can happen[33]
- Elderly subjects getting contracted by the disease for the first time.

A shift from the usual trail (reactivation) to an unusual trail is seen in cases where there is an exogenic reinfection or a second primary infection, thereby the presentation similar to what occurs in pediatric population.[34,35] These atypical radiographic findings like anterioinfiltrates, lymphadenopathy and exudative pleuritis can result in wrong initial diagnosis and thus delayed treatment.

MRI in Pulmonary Tuberculosis

Several recent technical advances have helped MRI to overcome its main limitations (low proton density and low SNR) for characterization of pulmonary pathologies. MRI as a radiation free modality can be used for follow-up of the already known lesions in young patients to reduce radiation exposure.[36-38] MRI has been shown equivalent to CT for detection of lymph nodes, lung cavitation and pleural effusion having a sensitivity and specificity of 100%. Sensitivity and specificity of MRI has been shown to be up to 88.2% and 95.7% respectively for the detection of nodules in pulmonary tuberculosis, while a specificity of 92.9% and sensitivity of 100% for detection of consolidation.[39] However, high cost and limited availability are its main limitations.

PET/CT in Tuberculosis

PET/CT has a high sensitivity in detecting malignancies, infections and various inflammatory lesions. Hence, it has a potential role to play in the diagnostic algorithm and managing the patients of PUO.[40,41] However, due to high incidence of TB in Indian population, large number of false positive cases are commonly seen in patients on PET/CT during oncologic work-up. Hence, although PET/CT may not be very specific in tuberculosis, it can have a crucial role in assessment of suspected or known cases of TB. One approach which can increase the diagnostic accuracy for detection of TB involves use of combine F-18 FDG and C-11 acetate in combination. Amongst these two, C-11 acetate is taken up by malignant lesions but not by infective/inflammatory lesions.[42] FDG PET/CT can help in determining the activity in the lesions, thereby guiding for sampling from foci showing activity, detect occult foci at other places, as well as evaluate the response to treatment. Furthermore, new, radiotracers with more specificity, like antituberculous drug molecules labeled with positron emitters may help in differentiating TB from malignancies and other infective/inflammatory processes.

REFERENCES

1. Harkirat S, Anand SS, Indrajit IK, et al. Pictorial essay: PET/CT in tuberculosis. Indian J Radiol Imaging. 2009:18;141-7.
2. Bhalla AS, Goyal A, Guleria R, Gupta AK. Chest tuberculosis: Radiological review and imaging recommendations. Indian J Radiol Imaging. 2015;25:213-25.
3. Jeong YJ, Lee KS. Pulmonary tuberculosis: Up-to-date imaging and management. AJR. 2008;191:834-44.
4. Alland D, Kalkut GE, Moss AR, et al. Transmission of tuberculosis in New York City: An analysis by DNA fingerprinting and conventional epidemiologic methods. N Engl J Med. 1994; 330:1710-6.
5. Geng E, Kreiswirth B, Burzynski J, et al. Clinical and radiographic correlates of primary and reactivation tuberculosis: a molecular epide miology study. JAMA. 2005;293:2740-5.
6. Gyselen A, Uydebroeck M, Weyler J Epidemiologie. In: Demedts M, Gyselen A, Van den Brande P (Eds). Tuberculosis. Een blijvende uitdaging. Garant, Leuven-Apeldoorn. 1992; pp 17–30.
7. Leung AN, Muller NL, Pineda PR, et al. Primary tuberculosis in childhood: radiographic manifestations. Radiology. 1992;182: 87-91.

8. Lamont AC, Cremin BJ, Pelteret RM. Radiologic patterns of pulmonary tuberculosis in the paediatric age group. Paediatr Radiol. 1986;16:2-7.
9. Palmer PE. Pulmonary tuberculosis: usual and unusual radiographic presentations. Semin Roentgenol. 1979;14:204-42.
10. Woodring JH, Vandiviere HM, Fried AM, et al. Update: radiographic features of pulmonary tuberculosis. Am J Roentgenol. 1986;146:497-506.
11. Hadlock FP, Park SK, Awe RJ, et al. Unusual radiographic findings in adult pulmonary tuberculosis. Am J Roentgenol. 1980:134:1015-8.
12. Im JG, Itoh H, Shim YS, et al. Pulmonary tuberculosis: CT findings—early active disease and sequential change with antituberculous therapy. Radiology. 1993;186:653-60.
13. Im JG, Webb WR, Han MC, et al:. Apical opacity associated with pulmonary tuberculosis: high-resolution CT findings. Radiology. 1991;178:727-31.
14. Kwong JS, Carignan S, Kang EY, et al. Miliary tuberculosis. diagnostic accuracy of chest radiography. Chest. 1996; 110:339-42.
15. Leung AN. Pulmonary tuberculosis: the essentials. Radiology. 1999;210:307-22.
16. Piqueras AR, Marruecos L, Artigas A, et al. Miliary tuberculosis and adult respiratory distress syndrome. Intensive Care Med. 1987;13:175-82.
17. Hong SH, Im JG, Lee JS, et al. High resolution CT findings of miliary tuberculosis. J Comput Assist Tomogr. 1998;22:220-4.
18. Choyke PL, Sostman HD, Curtis AM, et al. Adult-onset pulmonary tuberculosis. Radiology. 1983;148:357-62.
19. Westcott JL, Volpe JP. Peripheral bronchopleural fistula: CT evaluation in 20 patients with pneumonia, empyema or postoperative air leak. Radiology. 196:175-81.
20. Lee KS, Kim YH, Kim WS, et al. Endobronchial tuberculosis: CT features. J Comput Assist Tomogr. 1991;15:424-8.
21. Auerbach O. Tuberculosis of the trachea and the major bronchi. Am Rev Tuberc. 1949;60:604-20.
22. Smith L, Schillaci R, Sarlin R. Endobronchial tuberculosis. Serial fiberoptic bronchoscopy and natural history. Chest. 1987;91: 644-7.
23. Moon WK, Im JG, Yeon KM, et al. Tuberculosis of central airways: CT findings of active and fibrotic disease. Am J Roentgenol. 1997;169:649-53.
24. Kim Y, Song KS, Goo JM, et al. Thoracic sequelae and complications of tuberculosis. Radiographics. 2001;21:839-58.
25. Sochocky S. Tuberculoma of the lung. Am Rev Tuberc. 1958;78: 403-10.
26. Lee KS, Song KS, Lim TH, et al. Adult-onset pulmonary tuberculosis: findings on chest radiographs and CT scans. Am J Roentgenol. 1993;160:753-8.
27. Fraser RS. Pulmonary aspergillosis: pathologic and pathogenetic features. Pathol Annu. 1993;28:231-77.
28. Snider GL, Placi B. The relationship between pulmonary tuberculosis and bronchogenic carcinoma: a topographic study. Am Rev Respir Dis. 1969;99: 229-36.
29. Santelli ED, Katz DS, Goldschmidt AM, et al. Embolization of multiple Rasmussen aneurysms as a treatment of hemoptysis. Radiology. 1994;193: 396-8.
30. Adler O, Peleg H. Computed tomography in diagnosis of broncholithiasis. Eur J Radiol. 1987;7:211-2.
31. Fraser RS, Muller NL, Colman N, et al. Diagnosis of diseases of the chest. Saunders, Philadelphia. 1999;pp 798-873.
32. Lee JY, Kim Y, Lee KS, et al. Tuberculous fibrosing mediastinitis: radiological findings. Am J Roentgenol. 1996;167:1598-9.
33. Stead WW, Lofgren JP, Warren E, et al. Tuberculosis as an endemic and nosocomial infection among the elderly in nursing homes. N Engl J Med. 1985; 312:1483-7.
34. Korzeniewska-Kosela M, Krysl J, Muller N, et al. Tuberculosis in young adults and the elderly: a prospective comparison study. Chest. 1994;106:28-32.
35. Umeki S. Comparison of younger and elderly patients with pulmonary tuberculosis. Respiration. 1989; 55:75-83.
36. Sodhi KS, Khandelwal N, Saxena AK, et al. Rapid lung MRI: Paradigm shift in evaluation of febrile neutropenia in children with leukemia: a pilot study. Leuk Lymphoma. 2016;57:70-5.
37. Sodhi KS, Khandelwal N, Saxena AK, et al. Rapid lung MRI in children with pulmonary infections: Time to change our diagnostic algorithms. J Magn Reson Imaging. 2016;43:1196-206.
38. Sodhi KS, Bhatia A, Khandelwal N. Rapid lung magnetic resonance imaging in children with pulmonary infection. Pediatr Radiol. 2017 May;47(6):764-5.
39. Sodhi KS, Sharma M, Saxena AK, et al. MRI in Thoracic Tuberculosis of Children. Indian J Pediatr. 2017 Jun; 10. doi: 10.1007/s12098-017-2392-3. [Epub ahead of print]
40. Meller J, Altenvoerde G, Lehmann K, et al. Fever of unknown origin—prospective comparison of 18FDG-imaging with a double head coincidence camera (DHCC) and Ga-67 citrate SPECT. Eur J Nuc Med. 2001; 28:OS387.
41. Meller J, Sahlmann CO, Scheel AK. 18F-PET and PET/CT in fever of unknown origin. J Nuc Med. 2007;48:35-45.
42. Liu RS, Shei HR, Feng CF. Combined 18F-FDG and 11C acetate PET imaging in diagnosis of pulmonary tuberculosis. J Nuc Med. 2002;43:127.

CHAPTER

127

Nontubercular Pulmonary Infections

Anju Garg, Swati Gupta, Jyoti Kumar

INTRODUCTION

Pulmonary infections or pneumonia are an important cause of morbidity and mortality especially in our country. Inflammatory disease of the lung may be referred to as either pneumonia or pneumonitis. Although these terms are used interchangeably, pneumonia usually implies an infection by pathogenic organisms whereas pneumonitis refers to a non-infective inflammatory process involving the alveolar wall.[1]

Community-acquired pneumonia (CAP) is an infection of the alveoli, distal airways and interstitium of the lungs that occurs outside of hospitals. ***Hospital- acquired pneumonia (HAP)*** is defined as a pneumonia not incubating at the time of hospital admission and occurring 48 hours or more after admission. ***Ventilator-acquired pneumonia (VAP)*** is defined as a pneumonia occurring more than 48 hours after endotracheal intubation. The term ***health care-associated pneumonia (HCAP)*** was introduced to include an already ill population of nursing-home residents, patients in long-term care, patients undergoing same-day procedures, patients receiving home or hospital based intravenous therapy, and patients undergoing dialysis. However, it has recently been removed by the 2016 Clinical Practice Guidelines of the Infectious Diseases Society of America and the American Thoracic Society.[2]

Patients with pneumonia commonly present with cough (with or without sputum), fever—often with chills, dyspnea and pleuritic chest pain. On physical examination, there may be tachypnea, with bronchial breath sounds and crepts on auscultation. In addition to these clinical features, an infiltrate on the chest radiograph or other imaging technique, with or without supporting microbiological data, is required for the diagnosis of pneumonia. The specific organism causing the infection can be established with certainty only in approximately 50% of patients, despite intensive laboratory investigation.

Although the specific diagnosis requires a microbiological workup, the radiologist plays a very important role in the workup of a suspected case of pulmonary infection. The radiologist can establish the presence of disease, localise and define the extent of disease, suggest an etiological diagnosis, recognize any underlying pathology, assess the response to treatment and establish the presence of complications.

IMAGING MODALITIES

Chest radiography and computed tomography (CT) are the most useful imaging modalities available for evaluation of a patient with known or suspected pulmonary infection.

A **chest radiograph** (posteroanterior view) is the basic and most useful imaging tool to establish the presence of pneumonia, determine its location and extent, and monitor its response to therapy. Further, the chest radiograph can suggest an etiological agent, prognosis, associated conditions, complications (cavitation, abscess formation, pneumothorax, pleural effusion), alternative diagnoses and sometimes guide invasive diagnostic procedures. Patients who are hospitalized for suspected pulmonary infection, but have negative chest radiography findings, should be presumptively treated with antibiotics and imaging repeated in 24–48 hours, as chest radiographs can be negative early in the course of the disease.

Computed tomography (CT) is not recommended for the initial evaluation of patients with pneumonia, but is recommended when there is a strong clinical suspicion of pneumonia that is accompanied by normal, ambiguous or non-specific radiography. It is a useful adjunct to conventional radiography in complicated cases or in patients in whom the response to treatment is unexpectedly slow. In these cases, the role of CT is to further characterize the complex pneumonias, look for complications and detect underlying disease within the lung or mediastinum. It also plays an important role in differentiating lung abscess from empyema.

Ultrasonography (US): In recent years, ultrasound has been used as an additional modality both, in the diagnosis, and follow up of patients with pneumonia.[3] Multiple studies have compared the findings in pneumonia on lung ultrasound (LUS) with chest radiography, and have shown that LUS is at least equivalent, if not superior to chest radiography.[4] Its use is specially recommended in the emergency setting, bedridden patients and in pregnant women and children because of its lack of ionizing radiation, portability (it can be done at the bedside) and repeatability.[5] It can also give quantitative and qualitative information about pleural fluid collections and serve as a guide for aspiration in cases of pulmonary infections.

Magnetic resonance imaging (MRI): With the recent advances in MRI, resulting in faster and shorter protocols, it has become possible to use MRI to diagnose pulmonary infection and its complications. MRI has been found to have a sensitivity and specificity equal to that of CT in the detection of pneumonia, with a better accuracy than chest radiographs. The major advantage of MRI is the lack of ionising radiation and therefore, it can be used as a non radiation alternative in children and pregnant patients. Challenges that remain are the need for sedation/anaesthesia in paediatric patients, cost and motion artefacts.[6,7]

RADIOGRAPHIC PATTERN

Pneumonias can be categorized according to their radiographic appearances. Although widely used, this categorization may have limited value because the same organism may produce several patterns and because patterns often overlap in an individual patient.

In **lobar/airspace pneumonia** the infective organism reaches the acini leading to a rapid production of abundant edema fluid with minimal cellular reaction. There is an initial peripheral localization but as the fluid increases in amount, it flows from alveolus to alveolus limited only by pleural boundaries, leading to a confluent involvement of the lung parenchyma.[8] Airspace disease is typically due to bacterial infection; however, some viruses can also cause this pattern.

On chest radiographs the classical appearance is a homogeneous non-segmental consolidation Eventually, the pneumonia may involve the whole lobe, but usually symptoms develop before the entire lobe is consolidated and antibiotic therapy, if started, halts the process. The consolidation is usually confined to one lobe, although multilobar involvement is not uncommon. Because the airways are not primarily affected, there is little or no volume loss and visible air bronchograms are common **(Fig. 1A)**.

On ultrasound, consolidated lung appears similar in echogenicity to liver or spleen—"hepatization" of the lung. Multiple bright dot-like structures and branching linear structures can be seen within the consolidated lung which represent scattered residual air in alveoli and bronchi—the "sonographic air bronchogram" **(Fig. 1B)**. These air bronchograms may show centrifugal movement with breathing.[9] Consolidation can be differentiated from atelectasis on the basis of this movement—the "dynamic air bronchogram". According to a recent study, dynamic air bronchograms have a 97% positive predictive value for pneumonia.[10]

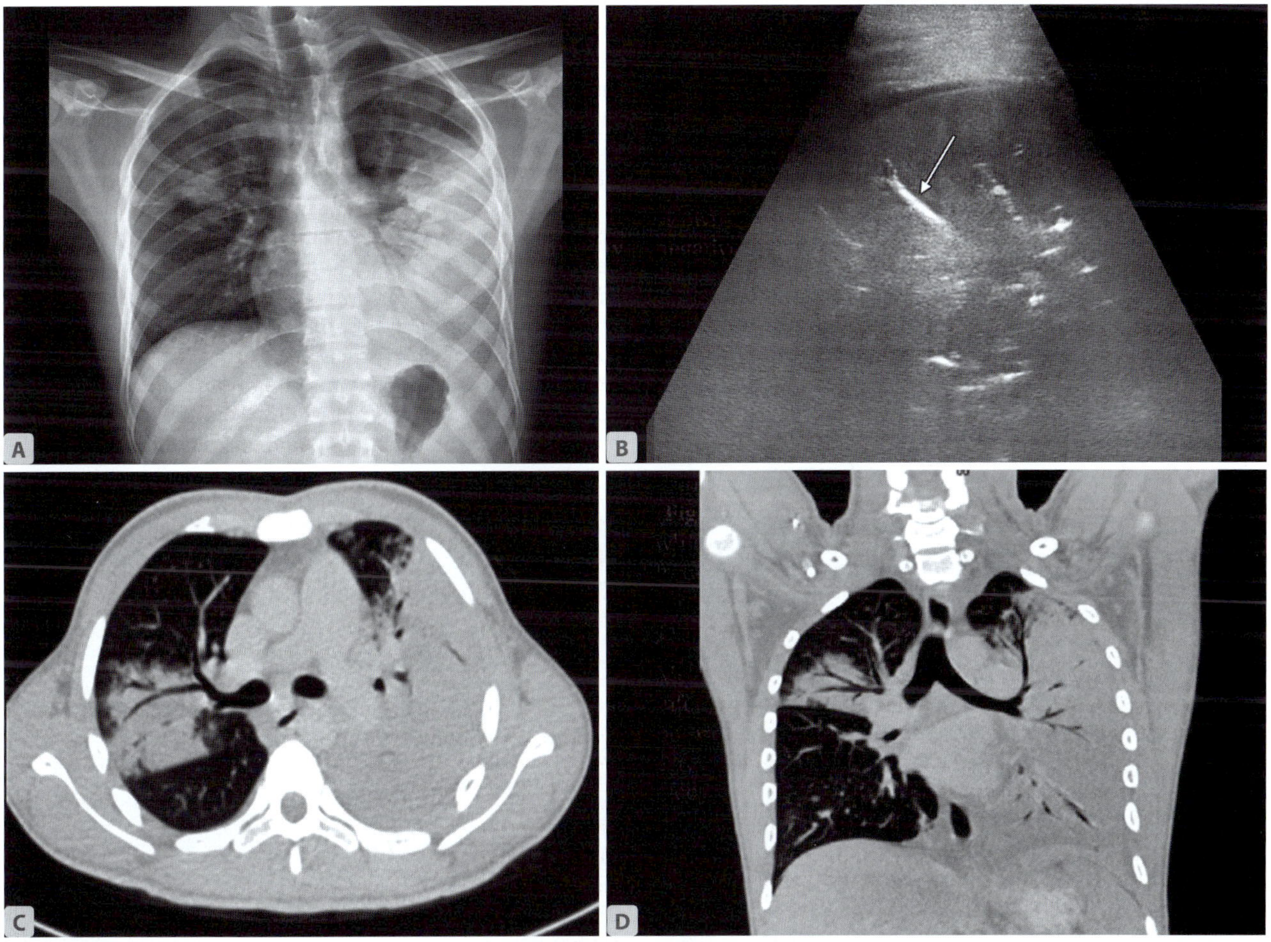

FIGS. 1A TO D: Airspace pneumonia: Chest radiograph (A) shows a homogeneous opacity in right mid zone, left mid and lower zone with air bronchogram within. Ultrasound image (B) showing lung parenchyma resembling liver (hepatization) with linear echogenic structure within representing air in bronchi—the sonographic air bronchogram (arrow). CT scan at lung window settings axial (C) and coronal reformat (D) shows airspace consolidation in the left lower lobe and right upper lobe with air bronchogram. Consolidation in right upper lobe is limited by major fissure.

On CT, airspace consolidation localizes in the middle and outer zones of the lungs and is seen as dense opacification with air bronchograms or air bronchiolograms. Areas of ground-glass attenuation may be seen around this denser airspace consolidation **(Figs. 1C and D)**.[11]

Lobar pneumonia must be distinguished from atelectasis and pleural involvement. Secondary causes of pneumonia like pulmonary edema, hemorrhage, or obstructed bronchi should be looked for. In lower lobes involvement aspiration pneumonia should be considered in appropriate clinical context. Non-infective causes of lobar pattern include acute interstitial pneumonia, radiation pneumonia, pulmonary alveolar proteinosis, organizing pneumonia, adenocarcinoma in situ (formerly bronchoalveolar carcinoma), and lymphoma.[12]

In **bronchopneumonia**, it is the mucosal surfaces of the bronchi and bronchioles that are affected, rather than the terminal airspace. There is development of a peribronchiolar focus of infection, which subsequently spreads along the intralobular airway to the alveolus, and then from one alveolus to another, until the pulmonary lobule is partially or totally involved. A bronchopneumonia pattern is most commonly due to infection by staphylococcal or gram-negative organisms; anaerobic organisms may also cause this pattern of involvement.[13]

On chest radiographs, mild bronchopneumonia results in peribronchial thickening and poorly defined airspace opacities. More severe disease results in inhomogeneous, patchy, poorly defined opacities with absence of air bronchograms. The process is diffuse, as several foci of disease are often seeded at the same time, and frequently both lungs are involved **(Fig. 2)**. It is often difficult to make a radiographic distinction between lobar pneumonia and confluent bronchopneumonia.[13] On CT, consolidation which involves the terminal and respiratory bronchioles and adjacent alveoli results in poorly defined centrilobular nodular opacities measuring between 4 to 10 mm in diameter. When the infection extends to involve the entire secondary lobule, lobular distribution of airspace consolidation is seen **(Fig. 3)**.[11] This pattern can also be seen in adenocarcinoma *in situ* (formerly bronchoalveolar carcinoma), hyperesoniphilic syndrome and lymphoma which can present as multifocal alveolar consolidation. In chronic cases, differential diagnoses include lipoid pneumonia, pulmonary alveolar proteinosis or radiation pneumonitis.[12]

In **interstitial pneumonia,** the infection results in diffuse edema of the airway walls along with inflammatory cellular infiltration which extends from the peri-bronchial tissues into the interlobular septa. The usual causes of acute interstitial pneumonia are viral or *Mycoplasma pneumoniae* infection.

The chest radiographs show generalized hyperaeration, widespread peribronchial thickening, increased reticular markings or small ill-defined nodules **(Fig. 4)**. On CT, the lesions are seen to be distributed in the central zone of the lung as well as middle and outer zones. There is thickening of bronchial walls, centrilobular shadows, acinar and lobular shadows **(Fig. 5)**. A predominantly ground-glass pattern may be seen.[11]

A **spherical or round pneumonia** is a well-circumscribed rounded consolidation, often pneumococcal in origin, which mimics a mass lesion.[14] It is seen more commonly in children and in the posterior segment of the lower lobes. It is thought to represent an early manifestation of the infectious focus that has spread centrifugally. An alternative theory is that round pneumonia occurs in children, because of underdeveloped pores of Kohn and the absence of canals of Lambert, which limits spread of the organism and results in a focal, round mass seen on radiographs and CT scans. As adults have fully developed canals of Lambert, this theory can also explain why round pneumonia is seen less often in adults.[15]

On chest radiographs, the appearance of a round pneumonia can vary from a small dense mass, to a large ill-defined rounded opacity **(Fig. 6)**. Margins may be smooth, irregular, lobulated, or even occasionally spiculated.[16] Air bronchograms can be seen in some cases but they are not specific for an infective process.

On CT scans, round pneumonia is seen as a heterogeneous mass of soft tissue attenuation that can have spicules, air bronchograms, pleural thickening and satellite lesions. The

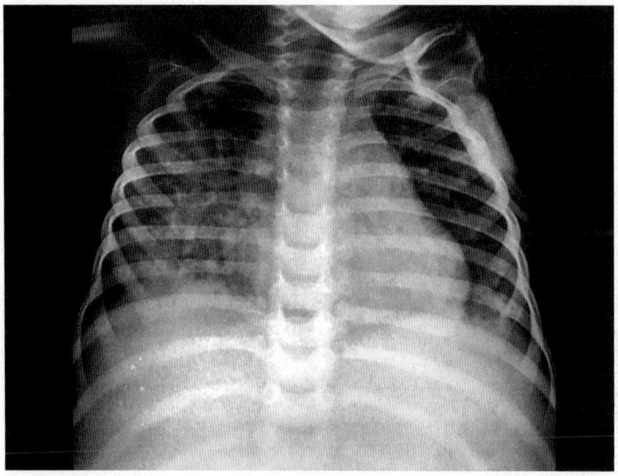

FIG. 2: Bronchopneumonia: Chest radiograph shows patchy opacities in right mid zone and bilateral lower zones.

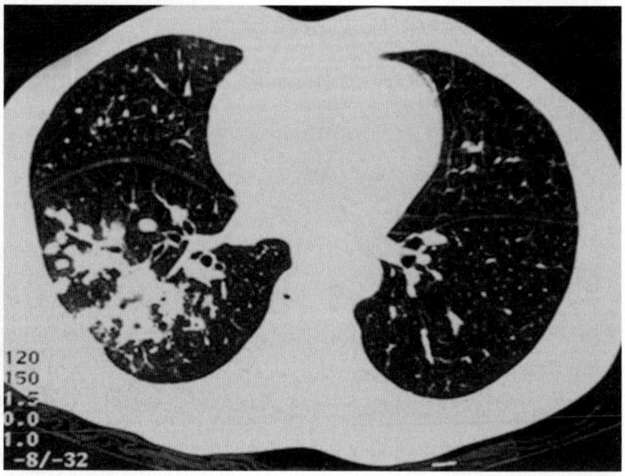

FIG. 3: Bronchopneumonia. CT scan shows acinar and centrilobular nodules along with lobular consolidation in right lower lobe.

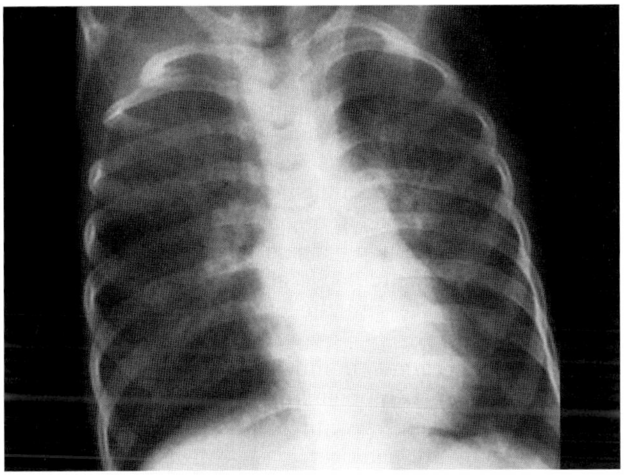

FIG. 4: Interstitial viral pneumonia: Chest radiograph showing bilateral poorly defined linear and nodular shadowing radiating from the hila with hyperinflated lung fields.

last two findings are found to be the most useful for diagnosis, while the presence or absence of air bronchograms does not help in distinguishing between malignancy and round pneumonia. Comparison with prior recent radiographs and short-term (3-7 days) interval follow-up are very useful in establishing the correct diagnosis.[14,16]

A **nodular pattern** may sometimes be seen as presence of random nodules in the lung parenchyma, which can occur due to hematogenous spread of disease **(Figs. 7A and B)** or granulomatous infection. Miliary TB, septic emboli, varicella zoster and some fungal infections can show a nodular pattern of lung infection.

In practice, these patterns may be of limited use as the radiological appearance may be indeterminate, the pathological and radiological classification can be varied and the pattern produced by various organisms is often inconstant.[17]

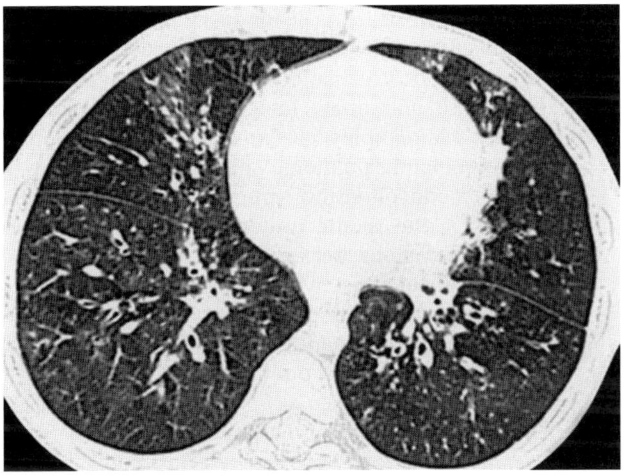

FIG. 5: Interstitial pattern of pneumonia: CT scan in a case of viral pneumonia shows focal areas of ground-glass attenuation with peribronchial thickening and centrilobular nodules.

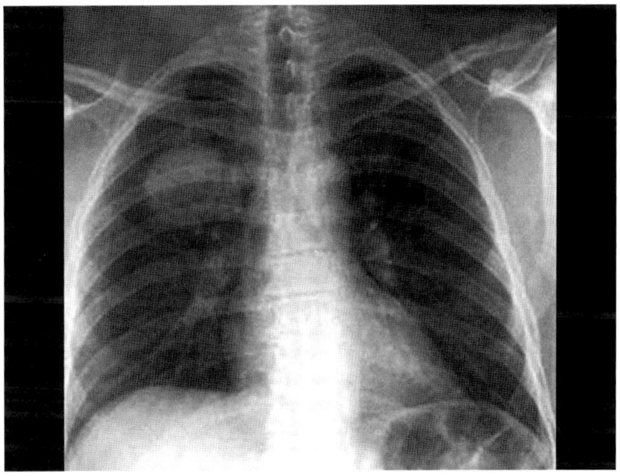

FIG. 6: Round pneumonia: Chest radiograph shows a rounded opacity in the right upper lobe containing an air bronchogram.

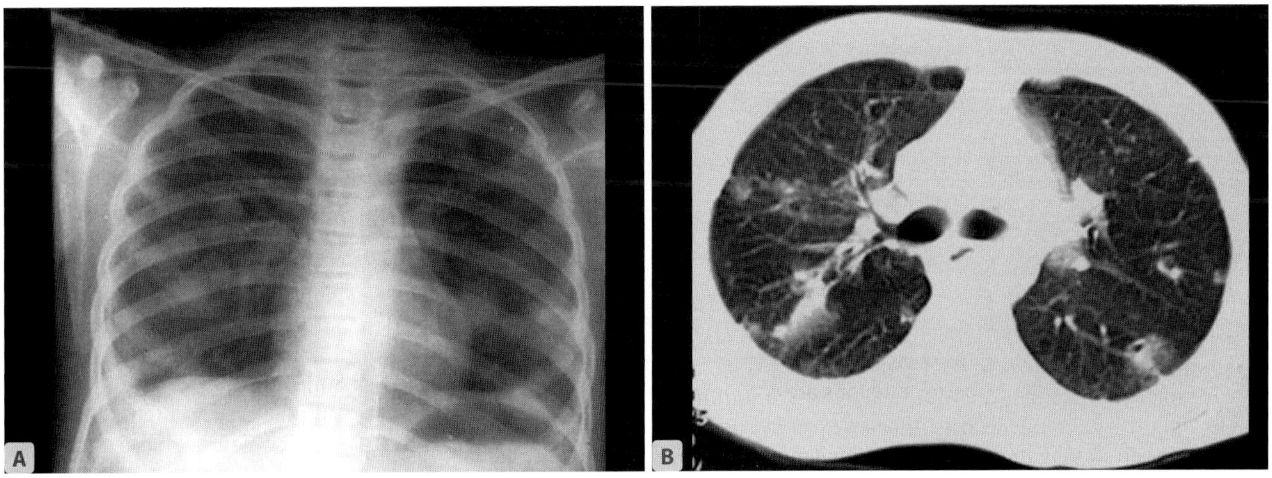

FIGS. 7A AND B: (A) Septic emboli seen as multiple nodular opacities scattered in both lung fields on a chest radiograph. (B) CT scan shows multiple nodular densities scattered in both lung fields, showing the "feeding vessel" sign. Few of the nodules show evidence of cavitation.

ETIOPATHOGENESIS OF PULMONARY INFECTIONS

The radiological manifestations of pneumonia are based on the etiopathological factors.[18] The type of pneumonic pattern and the consequent radiographic pattern is dependent on **(Table 1)**:

- The specific inherent properties of the organism, i.e. its virulence, its site of action and its mode of action, e.g. the staphylococcal bacteria cause marked destruction and abscess formation; *Klebsiella* leads to a more productive type of inflammation; a fungal or tubercular infection evokes a granulomatous response, etc.
- The route of entry of the organism has a significant influence on the radiographic appearance of the resulting pneumonia.
  - *Via the tracheobronchial tree:* By inhalation or aspiration. Inhalation, the most common route of entry of microorganisms, is in the form of droplet nuclei. The organisms reach the lower respiratory tract where they form a focus of infection and depending on the virulence, amount of inoculum and the state of the local and systemic defences of the host they can cause inflammation. The pneumonia caused by this route can be airspace, lobular or interstitial pneumonia.
  - *Via the blood vessels:* This kind of spread normally occurs in conjunction with an extrapulmonary source of infection which causes septicemia which in turn localizes in the lung. Radiographically, this is a random, patchy distribution with increased involvement of the basal segments due to preferential gravity related blood flow.
  - *Via direct spread* from infective lesions in the chest wall, across the diaphragm and from the mediastinum. The disease is usually localized to an area contiguous to the source and generally leads to formation of an abscess.
- Certain host factors also alter the classical appearance of a given pneumonia due to specific organism and should be evaluated to help narrow the radiographic differential diagnosis.

TABLE 1: Factors affecting pathogenesis of pneumonia.

Inherent properties of the organism	• Virulence • Site of action • Mode of action
Route of entry	• Via tracheobronchial route • Via the blood vessels • Via direct spread
Host factors	• Age • Immune status • Underlying lung disease • Systemic conditions • Aspiration pneumonia
Environmental factors	• Community acquired pneumonia • Nosocomial pneumonia • Infections in returned travellers

  - *Age:* In newborns, infection can be congenital or acquired.[19] Congenital infection is generally viral if due to transplacental spread. The acquired type is more often bacterial. Children are prone to respiratory infections with bronchiolitis and pneumonia as the common manifestations and are usually caused by viruses. In young adults, most pneumonias are viral or mycoplasmal in origin while pneumococcal is the most common bacterial infection. In middle age and beyond, streptococcal pneumonias become the leading cause and the incidence of non-bacterial pneumonia drops.[19]
  - *Immune status:* Immunosuppressed patients are unusually susceptible to infection with common pathogens and several microorganisms which are normally not pathogenic, e.g. *Pneumocystis jiroveci*, cytomegalovirus, etc. Differentiation between pneumonia, drug reaction, and parenchymal changes of pulmonary disease is difficult and often needs other investigations.
  - *Underlying lung disease:* A decrease in local resistance or a local obstruction leads to increased incidence of infection, e.g. bronchiectasis, sequestrated lung or chronic obstructive diseases. In emphysematous lungs, the pulmonary infection can often assume bizarre radiographic patterns due to the distorted emphysematous pulmonary parenchyma.[20]

    The consolidation appears to have multiple cavities due to the underlying low attenuation emphysematous areas giving rise to a "swiss cheese appearance" **(Figs. 8A to C)**. These pseudocavities and pseudohoneycombing should be differentiated from true cavities and honeycombing. Resolution is often delayed in pneumonias associated with pulmonary emphysema.[21]
  - *Systemic conditions:* Diseases associated with increased lung infections are poor nutrition, diabetes, alcoholism, connective tissue disorders, malignancy and AIDS.
  - *Aspiration pneumonia:* Occurs in patients with impaired consciousness, chronic debilitating diseases, structural abnormalities of the pharynx and esophagus, neuromuscular disorders, impaired swallowing mechanisms, indwelling tracheal or esophageal/gastric tubes and in postoperative patients, due to inhalation of bacteria, food, gastric contents, etc. leading to parenchymal inflammation or edema. It has several different pathophysiological aspects—bacterial pneumonia caused by the oral flora, chemical pneumonitis by gastric acid or exogenous lipids such as paraffin liquid and granulomatous reaction to foreign bodies. It occurs in the gravity dependent portions of the lung, so in recumbent patient it involves the posterior segment of the upper lobes and the superior segment of the lower lobes whereas in an erect patient, aspiration is more likely to involve bilateral basal segments, middle lobe, and lingular lobe. On imaging, it is often seen as a bronchopneumonia or bronchiolitis pattern **(Figs. 9A and B)**. Aspirated material may sometimes

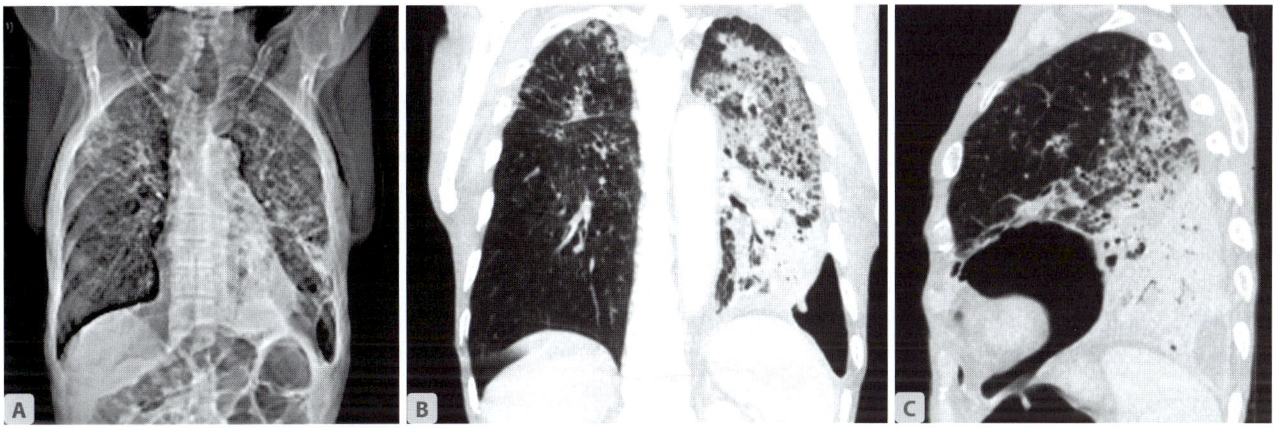

FIGS. 8A TO C: Chest radiograph (A) shows bilateral patchy opacities with a loculated left pneumothorax in a 60-year-old patient with emphysematous lungs. Coronal (B) and sagittal (C) CECT images show dense consolidation with air bronchogram in the left lower lobe, segmental consolidation in left upper lobe showing multiple small cysts within (Swiss cheese appearance), due to underlying centriacinar emphysematous changes with an associated small left pneumothorax. Few ground-glass opacities and apical nodular opacities seen in right lung.

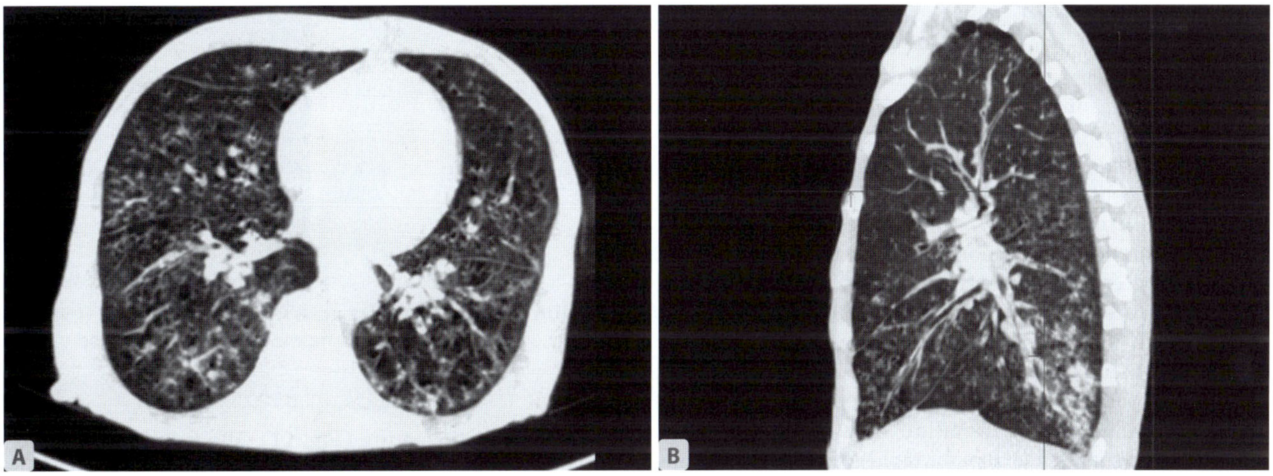

FIGS. 9A AND B: Axial (A) and sagittal (B) aspiration pneumonia: In a patient with carcinoma tongue, multiple confluent centriacinar opacities seen in posterior aspect of bilateral lower lobes and posterior segment of upper lobes, consequent to aspiration.

be seen in the bronchial lumen. A lung abscess may also be seen in bacterial aspiration.[22]

- *Environmental factors*:
  - *Community acquired infections (CAP):* Refers to pneumonia that develops in people in the community rather than in a hospital, nursing home, or assisted-living facility. The etiological causes of community acquired pneumonia are listed in **Table 2.**[23]
  - *Nosocomial infections (HAP and VAP):* It is paradoxical but true that pneumonia is more likely to occur in patients who are admitted to a hospital. This is because of the ease with which hospital strains of staphylococci and gram-negative bacilli can be acquired from other patients, hospital staff or inhalation therapy machines. Also, the frequent use of antibiotics in hospitalized patients suppresses the growth of normal respiratory flora, greatly increasing the susceptibility of treated patients to infection.[19] Causal organisms depend on onset of disease and host conditions **(Table 3)**.[24] A variety of radiographic patterns are seen, including airspace, interstitial and mixed compounding the problem. It is often difficult to distinguish atelectasis from hospital-acquired pneumonia, and the two may co-exist, although

TABLE 2: Common causative organisms of community acquired pneumonia.[23]

Bacteria	• *Streptococcus pneumoniae* • *Staphylococcus aureus* • *Chlamydia pneumoniae* • *Mycoplasma pneumoniae* • *Haemophilus influenzae* • *Klebsiella pneumoniae* • *Streptococcus pyogenes* • *Legionella pneumophilia*
Viruses	• Influenza virus • Respiratory syncytial virus • Adenovirus

TABLE 3: Causative organisms of nosocomial pneumonia.[24]

	Early onset (within 48–72 hours)	Late onset (>72 hours)
Hospital-acquired pneumonia	• *Haemophilus influenzae* • *Streptococcus pneumoniae* • Methicillin-sensitive *Staphylococcus aureus* (MSSA) • *Enterobacteriaceae (Klebsiella, Escherichia coli, Serratia)* • Anaerobes • *Legionella*	• Organisms same as in early onset hospital-acquired pneumonia • *Pseudomonas aeruginosa* • Methicillin-resistant *Staphylococcus aureus* (MRSA)
Ventilator-acquired pneumonia	• *Streptococcus pneumoniae* • *Haemophilus influenzae* • MSSA • Enterobacteriaceae	• Enterobacteraciae • *Pseudomonas aeruginosa* • MRSA • *Acinetobacter* species

atelectasis often develops rapidly and may resolve rapidly.[25] The incidence of pneumonia in ventilated patients (VAP) can be as high as 20% with a high mortality rate.

Diagnosing pneumonia in ventilated or post-operative patients can be difficult. Portable chest radiography may not show basal consolidation in approximately one-fourth of patients following abdominal surgery.[26]

Pneumonia, edema, acute respiratory distress syndrome (ARDS), drug toxicity, atelectasis, infarction and hemorrhage have overlapping signs, so a confident diagnosis based on radiographic features alone is often impossible.[25,27] In patients with ARDS, CT may reveal areas of cavitation or empyema, not seen on chest radiographs and are suggestive of coexisting infection.[28] The use of ultrasound in correlation with clinical findings makes it an ideal tool for rapid diagnosis, especially in situations with unstable patients.

c. *Infections in returned international traveller:* Some pathogens are related to specific regions and locations. Travel to these regions may result in contracting travel related pulmonary diseases. Risk depends upon travel destination, activities undertaken and length of stay. High degree of clinical suspicion is of paramount importance in early diagnosis.[29]

SPECIFIC PNEUMONIAS

Bacterial Infections

Pneumococcal Pneumonia

Pneumococcal pneumonia is caused by *Streptococcus pneumoniae*. It is the commonest community acquired pneumonia and can occur at any age. The clinical presentation is in form of abrupt onset of fever, chills, cough and chest pain, often associated with bloody or rusty sputum. The organism tends to affect the terminal airways first and then disseminates to the surrounding segments giving rise to the classical unilateral airspace pneumonia **(Figs. 1 and 10)**. An air bronchogram is commonly present and this

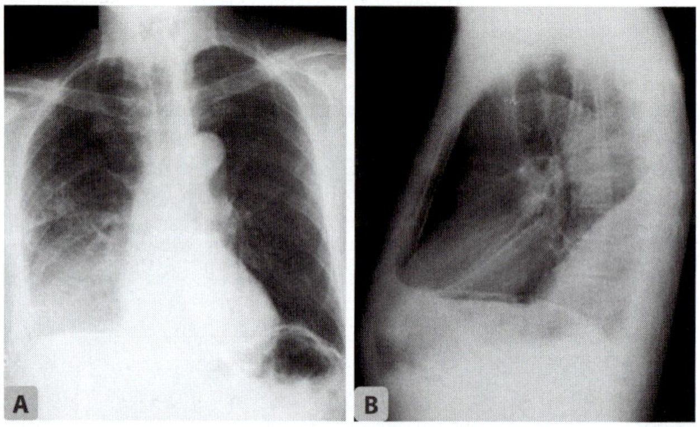

FIGS. 10A AND B: Chest radiographs PA view (A) and lateral view (B) Pneumococcal pneumonia involving the entire right lower lobe.

is a characteristic feature **(Fig. 11)**. The volume of the lobe usually remains unchanged. Classically, it causes a lobar pattern of consolidation but may sometimes even have a bronchopneumonic or interstitial pattern.[30] Occasionally, early during the disease, a spherical or round pneumonia may be seen, particularly in children. One study that investigated the radiographic appearance in 81 inpatients with culture documented pneumococcal pneumonia, demonstrated a lobar pattern of consolidation in 81% of patients. Lobar consolidation was focal in 48% and multifocal in 33%. A bronchopneumonic pattern was seen in 19% cases.[31]

Associated small pleural effusions may sometimes be seen, but empyema and cavitation are distinctly unusual. A very rare complication is pulmonary gangrene. Uncomplicated infection usually shows complete radiographic clearance within 10–14 days of appropriate treatment. The presence of multilobar disease is associated with increased morbidity and mortality.

Staphylococcal Pneumonia

It is caused by *Staphylococcus aureus*. The infection follows aspiration of organisms from the upper respiratory tract, occurring particularly in hospitalized patients. Staphylococcal pneumonia may be community acquired, particularly in infants and elderly individuals, often complicating

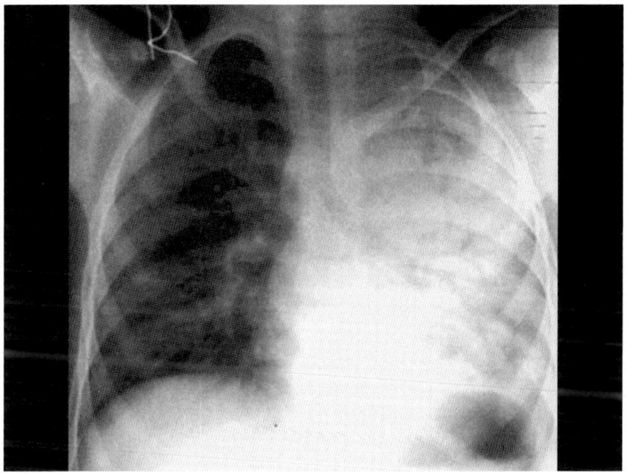

FIG. 11: Pneumococcal pneumonia involving almost the entire left lung with air bronchogram seen within.

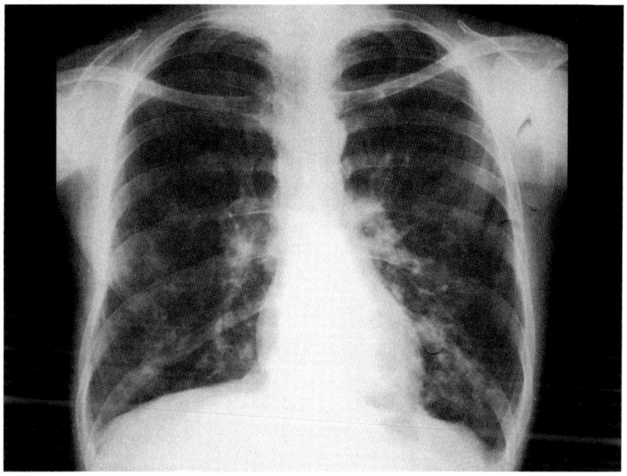

FIG. 12: Staphylococcal pneumonia showing patchy opacities in bilateral lung fields on background of emphysema.

influenza. Infection can also occur because of staphylococcal bacteremia.

The chest radiograph typically shows a bronchopneumonic pattern, initially involving the lower zones **(Figs. 2 and 12)**. The consolidation can spread rapidly and become confluent, resembling lobar pneumonia. Volume loss, early and large effusions, empyema and abscess formation are common **(Figs. 13A to D)**. Resolution is generally slower than pneumococcal infections and residual fibrosis can occur. Pneumatoceles **(Figs. 14A to C)** are more common in childhood than in adulthood, and may lead to pneumothorax.[32]

Septicemic staphylococcal infection occurs by hematogenous spread from endocarditis, thrombophlebitis or staphylococcal infection of indwelling catheters. It is also seen in drug addicts and immunocompromised patients. The usual radiographic and CT appearance is that of multiple pulmonary opacities **(Figs. 7 and 15)**. CT often shows more lesions than plain radiographs. The opacities may be of varying sizes, generally round (sometimes wedge-shaped or irregular), often show cavitation and have a lower zone predominance.[33] The "feeding vessel" sign i.e. a direct vessel leading up to the opacity can be seen on CT **(Figs. 15B and C)**. Accompanying pleural effusion and empyema are common features.

Gram-negative Pneumonias

These are caused by a great variety of organisms, the most important being the Enterobacteriaceae (notably *Klebsiella, Enterobacter, Escherichia coli* and *Proteus mirabilis*), *Pseudomonas aeruginosa, Acinetobacter* and *Haemophilus influenzae.* They are the most important cause of nosocomial infections and a major cause of morbidity and mortality in the hospital set-up. Very often, the affected patients have a known predisposing factor such as chronic obstructive pulmonary disease, a major medical condition like diabetes or history of recent surgery.

The organisms most commonly enter the lungs by aspiration, but pneumonia following inhalation of bacteria or spread by bloodstream is also occasionally seen. Aspiration is particularly important because the carriage of gram-negative organisms in the upper respiratory tract is greatly increased in debilitated patients in hospital.[17] The radiographic pattern is entirely nonspecific and ranges from small ill-defined nodules to patchy consolidation which may become confluent and resemble lobar pneumonia. Lower lobes tend to be predominantly affected; upper and middle lobe involvement may be seen in 50% of cases. Cavitation, pleural effusions and empyema are quite commonly associated **(Figs. 16 and 17)**.

The pneumonia caused by *Klebsiella pneumoniae* (also known as Friedlander's pneumonia) differs from other gram-negative pneumonias in that it is not uncommonly acquired outside the hospital and usually affects people with chronic debilitating illnesses or alcoholism. The symptoms include high fever, toxemia and resemble those of severe pneumococcal pneumonia. On chest radiography, the consolidations are also like those seen with *S. pneumoniae* pneumonia, i.e. a lobar pneumonia pattern. *Klebsiella pneumonia* has a tendency for the formation of voluminous inflammatory exudates leading to lobar expansion with resulting bulging of interlobar fissures **(Fig. 18)**, a greater tendency for abscess and cavity formation which are frequently multiple and large, and also a greater frequency of pleural effusion and empyema.[34]

Anaerobic Pneumonias

Most anaerobic lung infections result from aspiration of infected oral contents and obvious periodontal disease may be present in most patients.[20] Predisposing factors such as a recent episode of altered consciousness, dysphagia or alcoholism are frequent. The infection may be acute but is commonly subacute or chronic with prominent systemic symptoms and an indolent course. Anaerobic pneumonias are caused by a variety of organisms that are normally found in the oropharynx but which are abnormally aspirated into the lung including species of *Bacteroides, Clostridium, Fusobacterium, Peptococcus,* etc.[35]

Following aspiration, the chest radiograph is frequently normal initially. The appearance of abnormality is delayed for

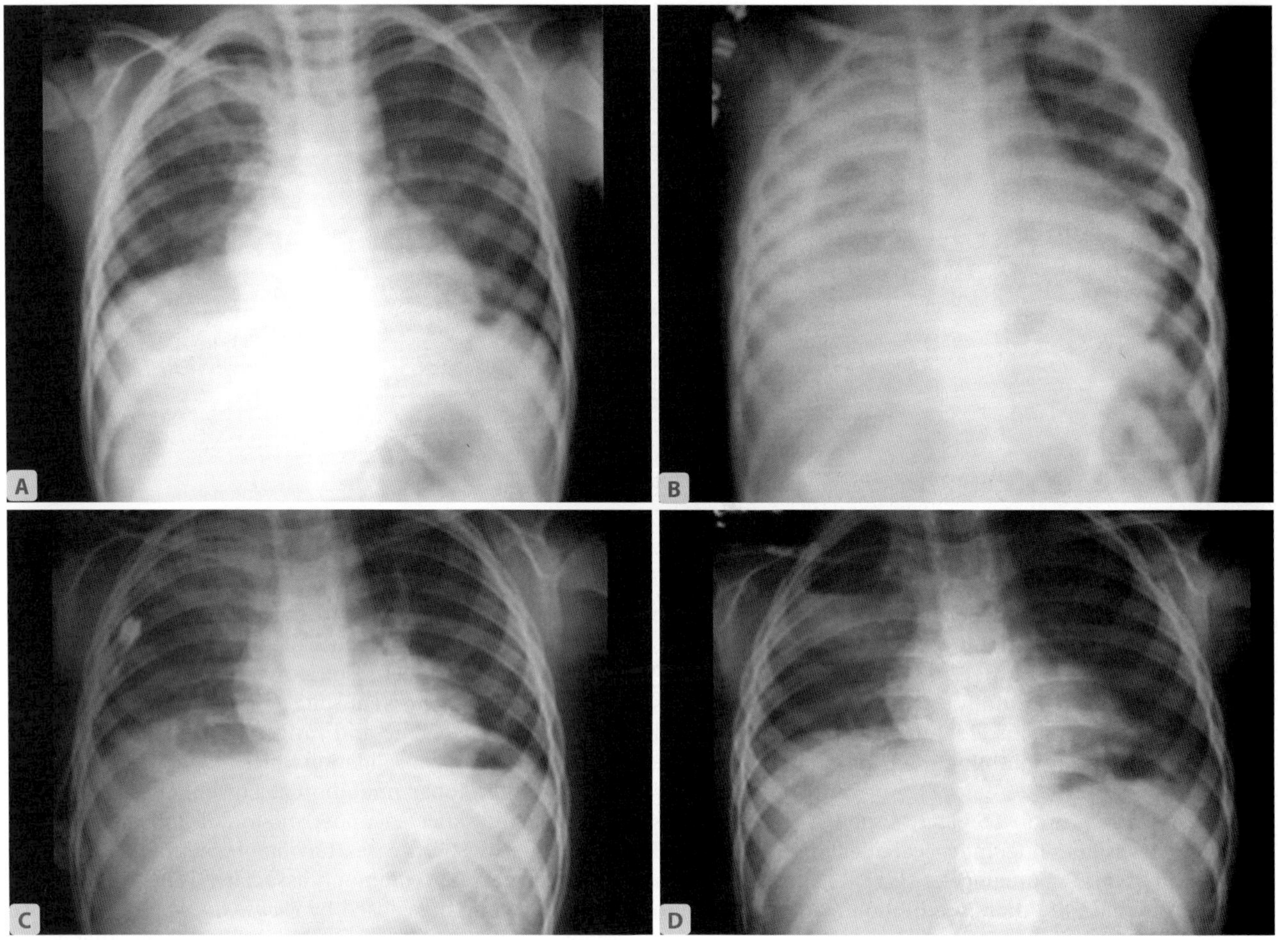

FIGS. 13A TO D: Serial chest radiographs of a 5-year-old child with a complicated staphylococcal pneumonia. (A) Areas of patchy consolidation in the right lung with evidence of volume loss. (B) 3 days later—complete opacification of right hemithorax was seen. A chest tube was inserted which drained pus. (C) Chest radiograph taken 2 days after chest tube insertion shows almost complete clearing of the empyema, however, there is an increase in the underlying patchy consolidation in right upper zone. (D) An abscess has developed in the right upper lobe.

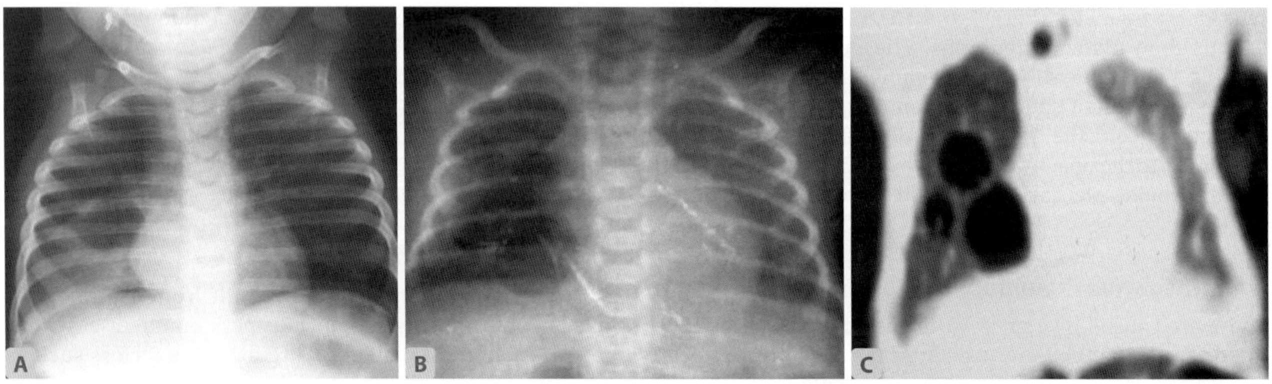

FIGS. 14A TO C: Chest radiograph (A) shows pneumatocele formation in a right lower lobe consolidation due to staphylococcal pneumonia. Chest radiograph (B) and CT scan—coronal reconstruction (C) in another infant showing multiple residual pneumatoceles following an episode of staphylococcal pneumonia.

24 to 72 hours. Three types of radiographic appearances may be seen—pulmonary parenchymal infection, pneumonia with cavitation or a discrete lung abscess, each of which may be associated with empyema. These pneumonias commonly involve the superior and posterobasal segments of the lower lobe and/or posterior segment of upper lobe due to drainage of infected material from the mouth into these segments as the patient lies on his back (gravitational pneumonia). Involvement may be unilateral or bilateral. Heterogeneous opacities may be seen in the involved lobes. Multiple cavities

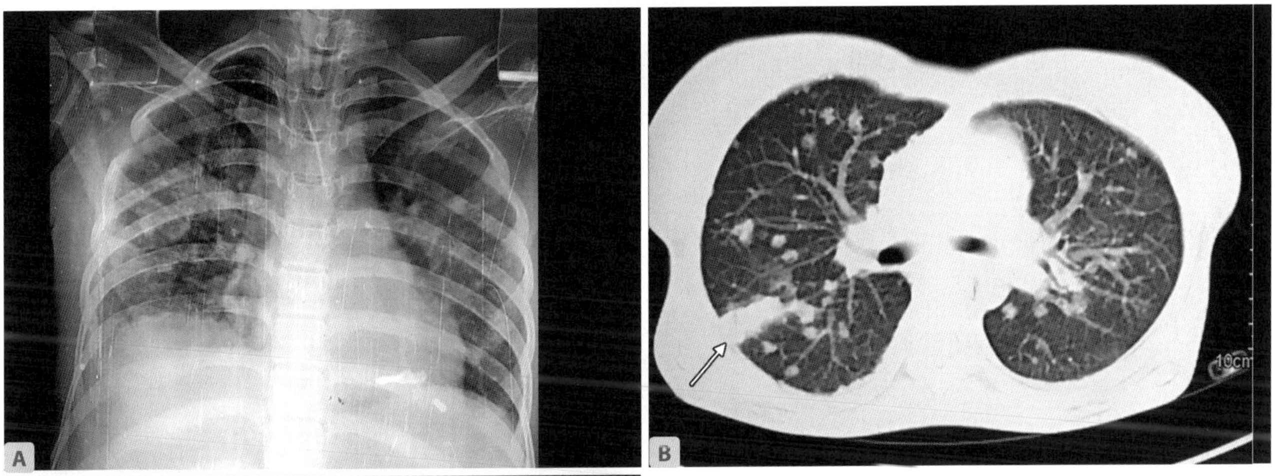

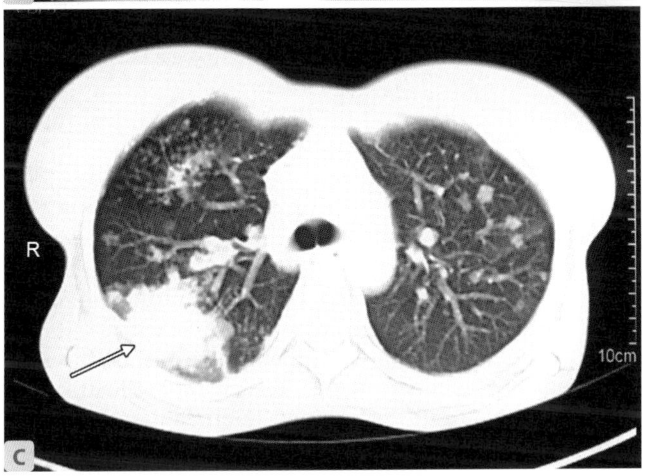

FIGS. 15A TO C: Septic emboli: An 18-year-old girl developed fever and cough in postoperative period. Chest radiograph (A) and CT (B and C) show multiple rounded opacities with few showing the feeding vessel sign, small area of peripheral consolidation (arrows in B and C).

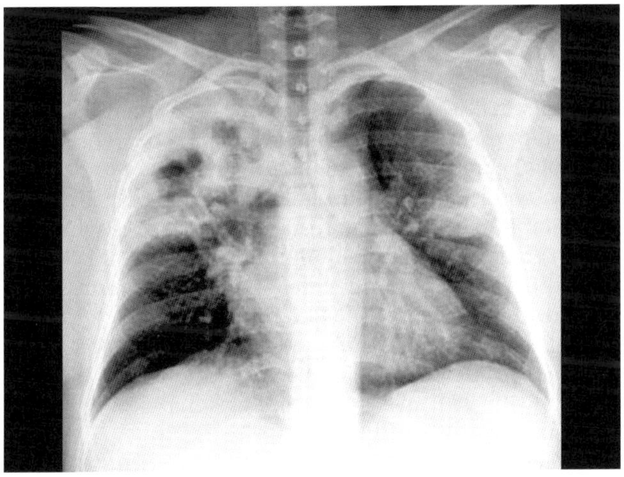

FIG. 16: Bilateral consolidation with extensive cavitation in the right upper lobe caused by gram-negative bacteria in a hospital setting.

may be seen within the area of consolidation due to severe lung necrosis or formation of lung abscess.

The other manifestation of an anaerobic lung infection is a focal cavitary mass with very little surrounding consolidation—the so called 'primary lung abscess'. The abscess may vary in size from 2 to 12 cm and characteristically has a thick, irregular wall **(Figs. 19 and 20)**. Hilar or mediastinal lymphadenopathy may accompany the lung abscess and such cases may closely resemble lung carcinoma.[36] Empyema is a common complication; may be large and may occur with or without radiographic evidence of pneumonia.[37]

Atypical Pneumonias

Atypical pneumonia or "walking pneumonia" is caused by atypical bacteria like *Mycoplasma pneumoniae, Chlamydophila pneumoniae* and *Legionella pneumophilia*. Some viral and fungal pathogens may also give rise to atypical pneumonia. Atypical community-acquired pneumonia (CAP) is characterized by prodromal upper airway symptoms, low grade fever, myalgias, dry cough and headache. There may also be associated extrapulmonary manifestations like diarrhea, abdominal pain, arthritis, facial rash etc. As the symptoms differ from those of typical pneumonia and are generally milder, they have been termed as atypical pneumonias. The importance of the atypical pneumonias is not related to their frequency (approximately 15% of CAPs), but to difficulties in their diagnosis, and their non-response to beta-lactam therapy.

Mycoplasma pneumonia is caused by *Mycoplasma pneumoniae* which is the smallest free-living organism,

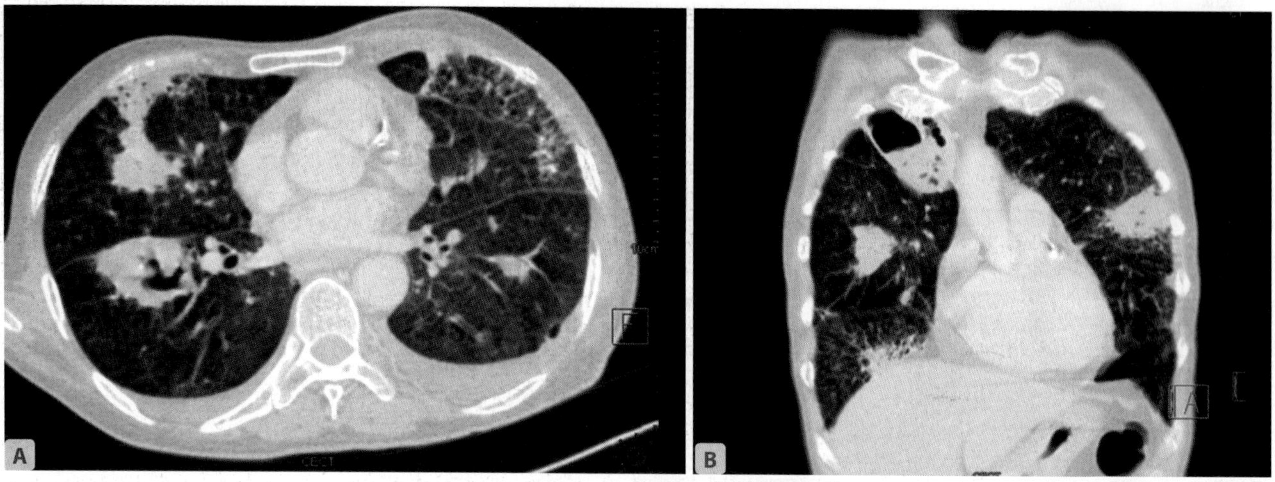

FIGS. 17A AND B: Axial (A) and coronal (B) CT showing multifocal areas of consolidation, bilateral ground-glass opacities and bilateral pleural effusions in a 65-year-old patient with *Pseudomonas* pneumonia in a hospital setting. Cavitation is seen in some of the consolidated areas.

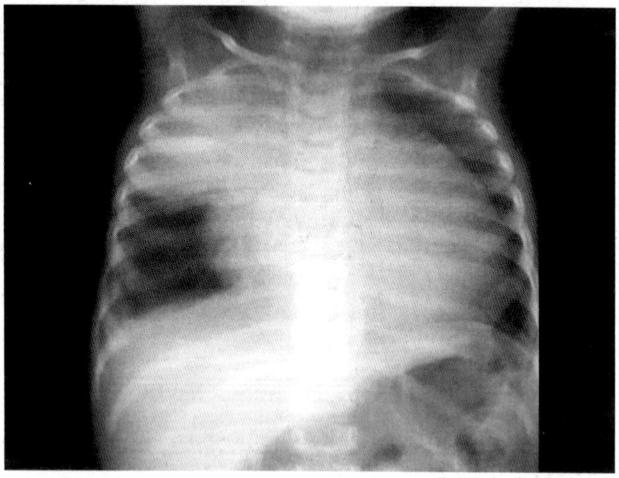

FIG. 18: Bulging fissure seen as downward convexity of the horizontal fissure in a case of consolidation of the right upper lobe with associated pleural effusion.

sharing some similarities with bacteria. It is a major non-bacterial cause of community-acquired pneumonias in the 20–40 year age group. Spread is via droplets, and the symptoms resemble a viral rather than a bacterial infection. The definitive diagnosis is serological and therefore, delayed and often retrospective. The radiological findings are very variable; the most common pattern is unilateral lower lobe involvement, beginning as a patchy/nodular, peribronchial consolidation that progresses to become sublobar or lobar and homogeneous **(Figs. 21A to C)**.[18] Sometimes the initial features are those of an interstitial process with small, irregular nodules and linear shadows.[38] Slow progression of this pattern to that of a typical consolidation is very suggestive of a mycoplasmal infection. Pleural effusion generally does not occur, and cavitation is rare. Nodal enlargement is common in children and is an unusual, but recognized, finding in adults. The CT findings consist of centrilobular nodules and branching linear opacities in a patchy distribution, thickening of the bronchovascular bundles and areas of lobular or segmental consolidation.[39]

Chlamydia pneumonia is caused by *Chlamydophila pneumoniae* and is a common cause of community-acquired pneumonia. It often affects children and young adults. The radiographic findings are non-specific with overlap of features with pneumonias from other organisms. The most common radiographic finding is airspace consolidation with interstitial infiltrates, combined interstitial and airspace infiltrates and pleural effusion.[40]

Legionella pneumonia is also known as Legionnaires' disease. It is caused by infection with any *Legionella* species, most commonly by *Legionella pneumophila*. It is seen more often in middle-aged and older adults, smokers, and those with chronic illnesses or a weak immune system. Infection occurs due to inhalation of airborne microscopic sources of contaminated water. It can be more severe than the other atypical pneumonias. The radiographic appearances may often lag behind the clinical picture and deterioration can be seen on imaging despite clinical improvement. The early radiographic and CT manifestations are nonspecific and similar to those found in community-acquired pneumonia from other bacterial origin. The chest radiograph shows asymmetric air space consolidation, more in middle and lower zones. Pleural effusion and mediastinal lymphadenopathy may be seen in a few cases. On CT, there is lobar or multilobar consolidation with adjacent ground-glass haze.[41,42]

Actinomycosis

Although previously grouped with the mycosis, *Actinomyces Israeli is* now regarded as a branching bacteria. It causes infection of the lung by aspiration or direct extension from abdomen or cervicofascial disease. The organism produces proteolytic enzymes that allow the infection to cross fascial planes. Therefore, the pneumonia readily spreads to pleura, producing empyema, and may spread extrapleurally to give rise to abscesses and sinus tracks in the chest wall, bones of the thorax, pericardium and mediastinum.[43] The

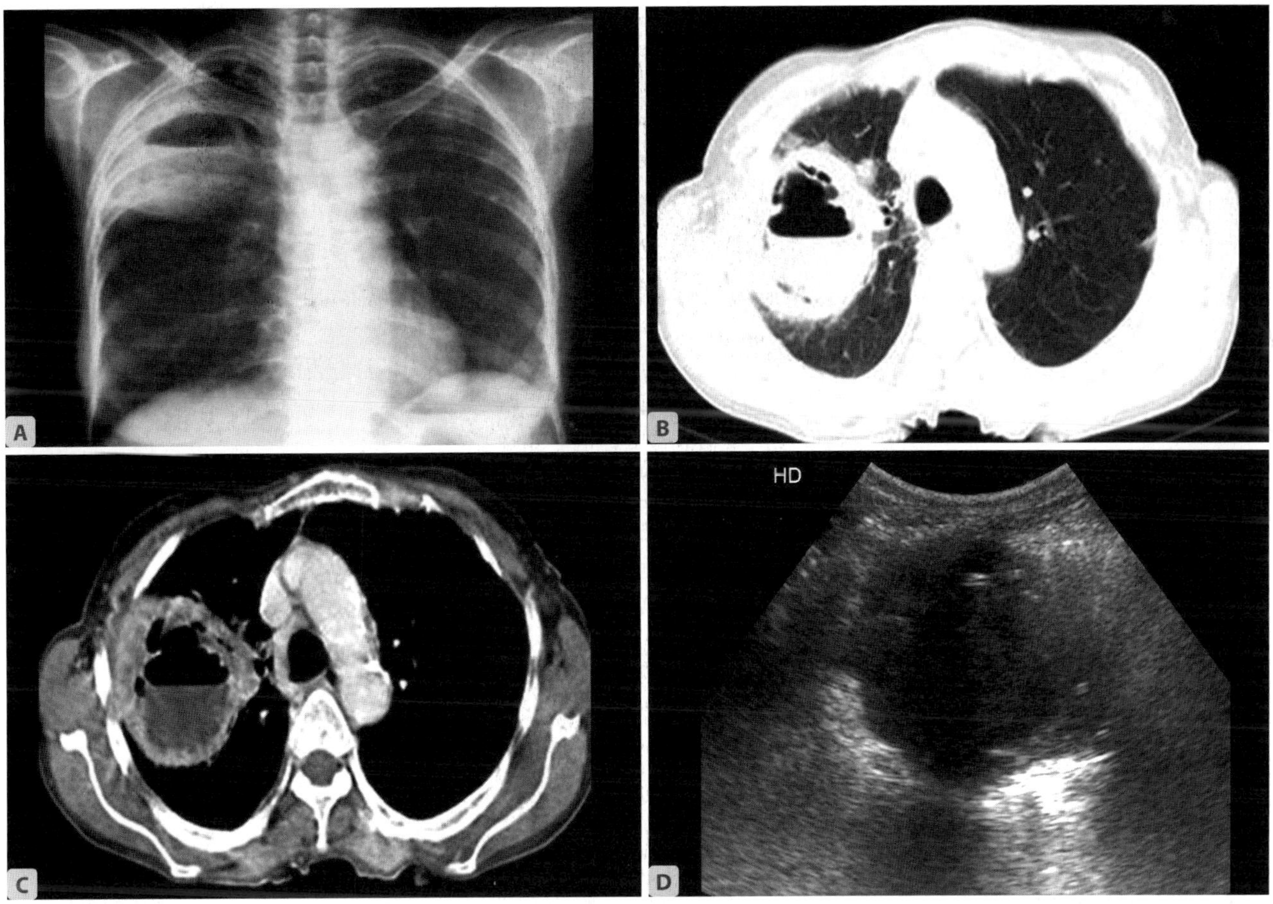

FIGS. 19A TO D: Anaerobic lung abscess in an alcoholic patient with poor orodental hygiene—Chest radiograph (A) CT scan at lung window settings (B) and mediastinal window settings (C). Lung abscess is seen in posterior segment of the right upper lobe with thick irregular walls. Ultrasound image (D) shows the abscess as an irregularly walled lesion with anechoic contents. This abscess was aspirated under US guidance.

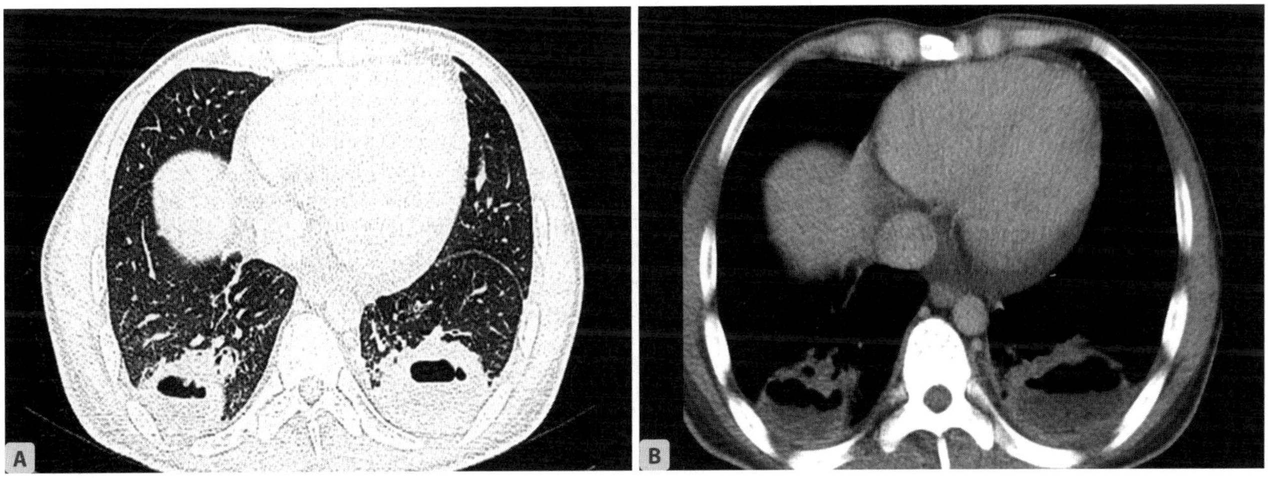

FIGS. 20A AND B: In a patient on ventilator, CT scan with lung window (A) and mediastinal window (B) settings, shows bilateral thick-walled abscesses seen in the posterior aspects of both lower lobes.

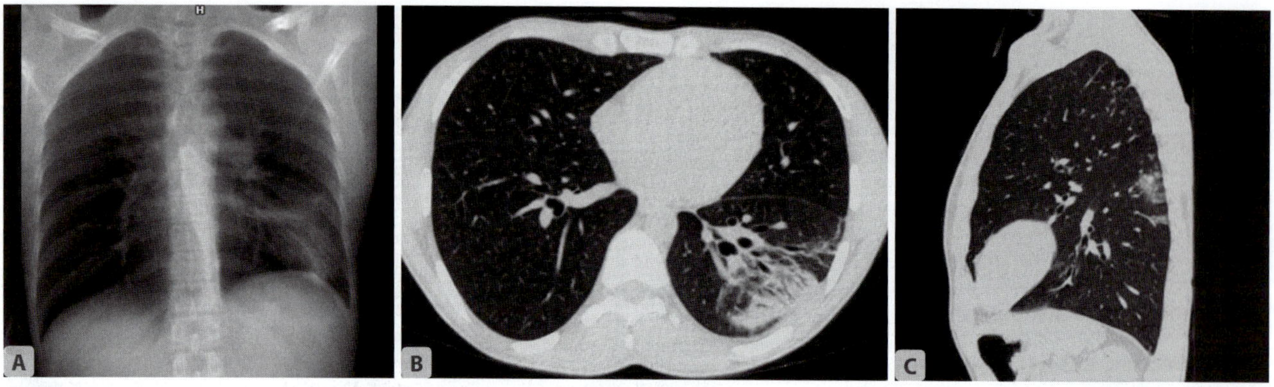

FIGS. 21A TO C: *Mycoplasma pneumoniae*: Chest radiograph (A) shows a homogeneous opacity in left lower zone. CT scan at lung window settings axial (B) and sagittal reformat (C) shows a peripherally based airspace consolidation in the left lower lobe with air bronchogram.

chest radiograph usually shows an area of non-segmental airspace consolidation, commonly in the periphery of the lung and with a predilection for the lower lobes. If therapy is not instituted, an abscess may develop and infection may extend into the pleura. Pleural involvement manifests as pleural effusion, pleural thickening, or empyema formation but is seldom associated with large accumulations of fluid. Rib involvement causes lytic destruction with periostitis. Actinomycosis may also present as a mass which may cavitate.[44] On CT, the typical findings are those of chronic low attenuation areas (representing actinomycotic or sulfur granules) with peripheral enhancement (representing granulation tissue in wall of abscess) and adjacent pleural thickening. CT can demonstrate chest wall, pleural, mediastinal and spinal invasion to advantage.[45] Associated mediastinal lymphadenopathy may be present.

Viral Infections

Viruses are a major cause of respiratory tract infection in the community, particularly in children. The usual mode of spread is by transmission by droplets. In infants and young children who are immunocompetent, respiratory syncytial virus, parainfluenza virus, adenovirus and influenza virus are the most common cause offenders, whereas in adults, influenza type A and B and adenovirus are more common.[46] Immunocompromised patients are susceptible to CMV and other herpes viruses.[47]

Viruses result in several forms of lower respiratory infections, which include tracheobronchitis, bronchiolitis, and pneumonia. The pneumonia usually begins in the distal bronchi and bronchioles and giving rise to the interstitial pattern of involvement. Parenchymal involvement initially involves the lung adjacent to the terminal and respiratory bronchioles, but spread throughout the lobule can occur. In elderly patients, rapidly progressive pneumonia may occur, with diffuse alveolar damage leading to a hemorrhagic pulmonary edema.

The imaging findings of viral pneumonias do not usually allow the diagnosis of a specific viral infection. Clinical features such as patient age, immune status, time of year, illness in other family members, community outbreaks; onset, severity and duration of symptoms, and the presence of a rash remain important aids in diagnosing viral pneumonia.

Chest radiograph shows reticular opacities that are often bilateral and diffuse in distribution. The associated bronchiolitis leads to hyperinflation of the lung fields **(Figs. 4 and 22)**. Presence of hilar lymphadenopathy is variable; it is common in measles pneumonia and infectious mononucleosis but rare with other viral pneumonias. Pleural effusions are not a prominent feature, although small ones do not negate the diagnosis. CT scan may show poorly defined airspace nodules (4–10 mm diameter), patchy areas of peribronchial ground-glass opacity and consolidation along with hyperinflation **(Figs. 5 and 22C)**. The combination of CT findings varies somewhat between the individual viral pneumonias and has been summarized in **Table 4**.

The progressive form of the pneumonia shows large areas of homogeneous or patchy, unilateral or bilateral airspace consolidation or poorly defined centrilobular nodules.[48]

Influenza and Parainfluenza Virus

Infections with influenza virus occur in epidemics, pandemics or sporadically. Influenza subtypes A and B are most commonly responsible for the severe outbreaks associated with pneumonia.

Swine Flu is caused by a strain of human influenza A (H1N1) virus which originated in Mexico in 2009 and spread to more than 190 countries, including India. In June 2009, the World Health Organisation had declared it a level 6 (highest level) pandemic. The virus causes a wide spectrum of respiratory illnesses, which range from mild febrile illness to severe respiratory distress.[49] Symptoms include fever, dry cough, myalgia and headache. The predominant radiological pattern in H1N1 pneumonia is bilateral ground-glass opacities and alveolar consolidation. The opacities are usually in the mid zone and bases in the chest radiograph, while on the CT they are mainly peripheral and peribronchovascular in distribution, with diffuse zonal involvement.[50] Pneumonia is more common in the very young, those over 65 years of age, in late pregnancy and in those with underlying disease. Pleural effusion is rare.[48]

An acute form of pneumonia with rapid progression, shows fast confluence of the consolidation caused by the diffuse alveolar damage, which may be homogeneous or irregular, unilateral or bilateral, giving rise to an ARDS type of picture **(Figs. 23 and 24)**.

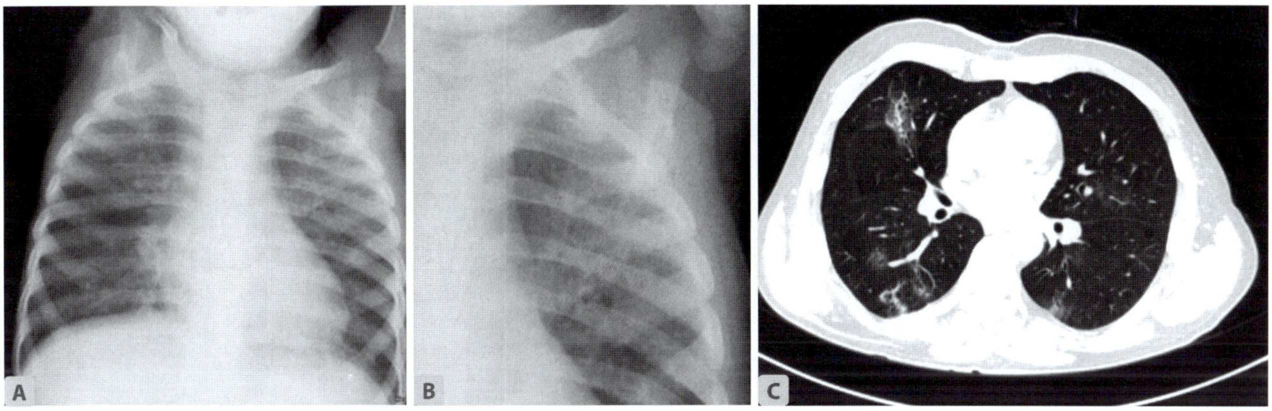

FIGS. 22A TO C: Viral pneumonia: Chest radiograph (A) with magnified view of left upper zone (B) shows hyperinflated lung fields with linear streaky opacities representing peribronchial thickening, nodular opacities. (C) Axial CT shows bilateral multifocal peripheral regions of ground-glass opacities in a case of non-specific viral pneumonia.

TABLE 4: Summary of CT findings in viral pneumonias.[46]

Cause of pneumonia	Centrilobular nodules	Ground-glass attenuation with lobular distribution	Segmental consoliation	Thickened interloular septa	Diffuse ground-glass attenuation
Influenza virus	+++	+++	+	---	+
Measles virus	++	+	+	---	+
Hantavirus	---	---	++	+	+++
Adenovirus	++	+	+++	---	---
Herpes simplex virus	+	+++	+++	---	+
Varicella-zoster virus	+++	+	---	---	---
Cytomegalovirus	++	++	+	+	++
Epstein-Barr virus	+	+	+	---	+

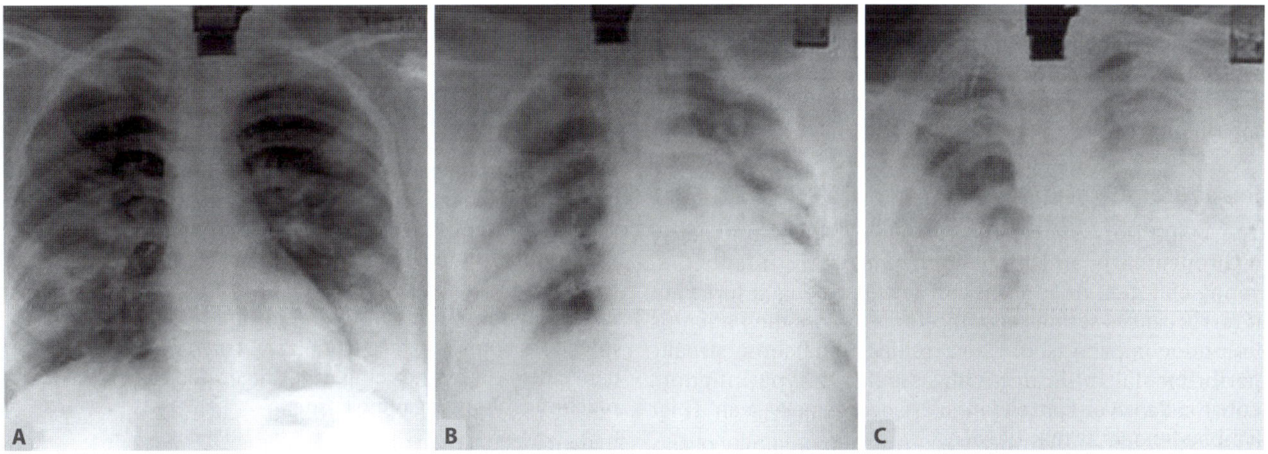

FIGS. 23A TO C: Serial radiographs of a 22-year-old female with swine flu. (A) At presentation areas of ill-defined consolidation seen in the lower zones. (B) Three days later, there is an increase in the consolidation. (C) A further 3 days later, there is extensive bilateral airspace consolidation like that seen in ARDS.

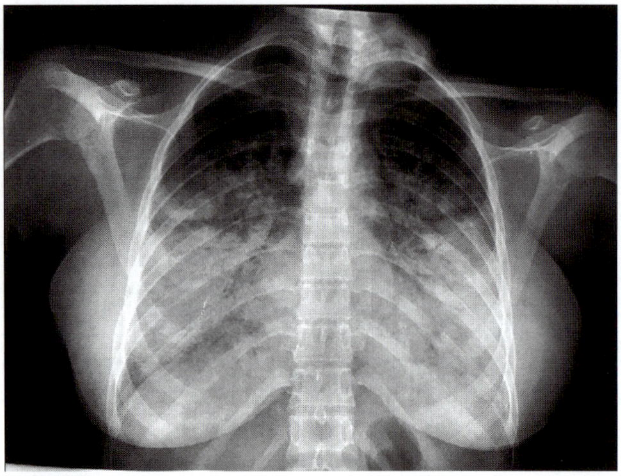

FIG. 24: Swine Flu: Confluent fluffy opacities due to alveolar consolidation in bilateral mid and lower zones in a young girl with swine flu.

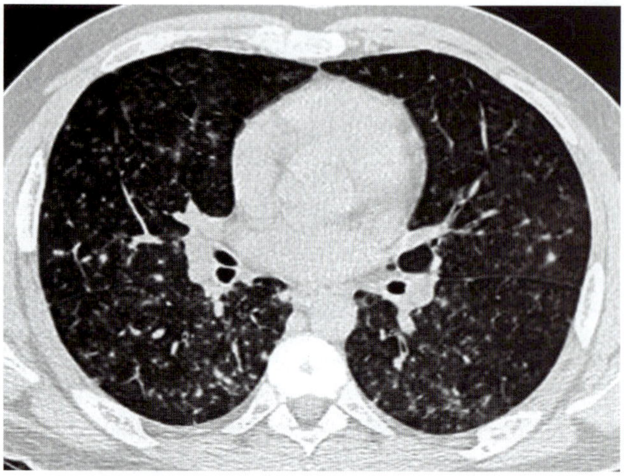

FIG. 25: Varicella pneumonia: Axial CT scan showing multiple nodular opacities scattered in bilateral lung parenchyma.

Avian influenza or "bird flu" is caused by the H5N1 subtype of the influenza A virus. Human infection occurs as a result of close contact with infected birds, usually poultry or their products. Chest radiograph commonly shows multifocal consolidations. On CT, the most common findings consist of focal, multifocal, diffuse ground-glass opacities or areas of consolidation. Centrilobular nodules can be seen. There may be associated pseudocavitation, pneumatocele formation and lymphadenopathy.[51]

Severe Acute Respiratory Syndrome

Severe acute respiratory syndrome (SARS) is caused by a coronavirus, the SARS-associated coronavirus (SARS-CoV). It was recognized as a global threat in March 2003, after first appearing in Southern China in November 2002. It leads to a systemic infection clinically manifesting as a progressive pneumonia. Chest radiograph and CT show focal unilateral or bilateral areas of ground-glass opacities and/or consolidation. The areas of ground-glass opacity may be associated with thickening of the intralobular and interlobular septae.[17]

Respiratory Syncytial Virus

The respiratory syncytial virus (RSV) is a major cause of bronchiolitis and bronchopneumonia in infants and young children. In adults it can cause prolonged fever but it rarely causes serious complications, unless the patient is immunocompromised. Chest radiographs show streaky peribronchial infiltrates with associated hyperinflation. Lobar collapse or consolidation are occasionally seen. Hilar lymphadenopathy may be seen.

Varicella

Varicella pneumonia occurs more commonly in adults than in children. It has a specific radiographic appearance of multiple small, discrete acinar nodules scattered throughout both lung fields **(Fig. 25)**. Hilar lymph node enlargement may be present. HRCT findings mirror the radiographic abnormalities, but smaller nodules (1–10 mm) can be identified, few of them have a halo of ground-glass opacification representing hemorrhage. The nodules usually resolve in a week but may persist for months and in 2% of patients they may calcify.[17]

Adenovirus

The common cold virus—may sometimes cause pneumonia in epidemics. Radiographically, widespread scattered patchy/confluent opacities occur which are peribronchial in distribution. Hilar lymphadenopathy may occur. The infection can be highly damaging particularly if acute infection occurs before 2 years of age, causing bronchiectasis, obliterative bronchiolitis and in some cases Swyer-James/McLeod's syndrome.[52]

Fungal Infections

Fungi can be divided into two major groups according to the pathogenesis of infection: (1) Opportunistic invaders; (2) Primary pathogens.

1. Opportunistic invaders: These fungi invade debilitated or immunocompromised individuals and those with a pre-existing, diseased and scarred lung parenchyma. These include species like *Aspergillus, Candida,* and *Cryptococcus.*[13] In contrast to the primary pathogens, these organisms can be found throughout the world and usually are ubiquitous in the environment. In addition to saprophytic and invasive infection, some fungi (particularly *Aspergillus* species) can cause disease by inducing an exaggerated hypersensitivity reaction without invading tissue.

Aspergillosis

Aspergillus infections of the lung are caused by *Aspergillus fumigatus* which are ubiquitous fungi found throughout nature and may result in disease in susceptible hosts when inhaled. The pathogenesis of *Aspergillus* infection varies with quality and virulence of the inhaled organism and the status of the host defence mechanisms. Four varieties of pulmonary aspergillosis have traditionally been described.[53]

a. Aspergilloma—a saprophytic non-invasive infection of a pre-existing cavity.
b. Allergic aspergillosis—including allergic bronchopulmonary aspergillosis (ABPA) and hypersensitivity pneumonitis caused by hypersensitivity to fungus.
c. Semi-invasive aspergillosis or chronic necrotizing aspergillosis a form of infection seen in patients with mild immunological suppression.
d. Invasive aspergillosis—an infection in immunocompromised hosts, which is invariably fatal without treatment.

Aspergilloma: Aspergilloma, also known as mycetoma is a ball of coalescent mycelial hyphae that typically colonize pre-existing chronic cavities. The pre-disposing causes can range from tuberculosis, sarcoidosis, cavities in rheumatoid lung or ankylosing spondylitis, etc. In most of the cases reported from India, there was a history of tuberculosis in the past or during detection.[54] Common clinical manifestations include cough and expectoration. Hemoptysis is frequent and has been reported in at least half of the cases. The mechanism of the bleeding is unknown; it has been attributed to friction between the fungus ball and the hypervascular wall, to endotoxins liberated from the fungus, and to a type 3 reaction in the cavity wall.[55]

On chest radiographs, an aspergilloma is seen as a round to oval mass of soft tissue density lying within a pre-existing cavity. As most of the pre-existing cavities colonised by the fungus are due to tuberculosis, mycetomas are most often found in the upper lobes or in the superior segment of the lower lobes. Typically, there is an airspace separating the fungus ball from the wall of the cavity resulting in a distinctive "air crescent sign" **(Fig. 26A)**. The air crescent sign is not specific to mycetoma formation, as it can also be seen in patients with blood clot within a pre-existing cavity, necrotic carcinoma, ruptured hydatid cyst and lung abscess with necrosis. If the mycetoma completely fills the cavity, it may obliterate the air crescent. The fungus ball is usually mobile within the cavity and this mobility can be demonstrated on a decubitus chest radiograph **(Fig. 26B)**. Thickening of a cavity wall may be an early sign of *Aspergillus* infection.

CT demonstrates to advantage the finding of a mobile intracavitary mass characteristic of aspergilloma. The fungus ball is a sponge like mass that contains irregular airspaces. The air crescent sign and the wall of the pre-existing cavity are well seen and fungal strands bridging the fungus ball and cavity wall may be seen **(Fig. 27)**. Mobility can be readily demonstrated by turning the patient although it is rarely necessary as the diagnosis is obvious in most cases. Occasionally, flecks of calcification may be seen within the mycetoma.[56]

Allergic aspergillosis is a result of hypersensitivity reaction that produces allergic bronchopulmonary aspergillosis (ABPA) or less commonly an extrinsic allergic pneumonitis, a Loeffler-like syndrome. The common symptoms of ABPA are cough, wheezing and associated allergic symptoms and radiographic findings include central bronchiectasis and mucoid impaction seen typically as branching opacities, usually central and in an upper lobe distribution—the "gloved finger sign". These opacities are commonly transient and recurrent but may occasionally remain unchanged

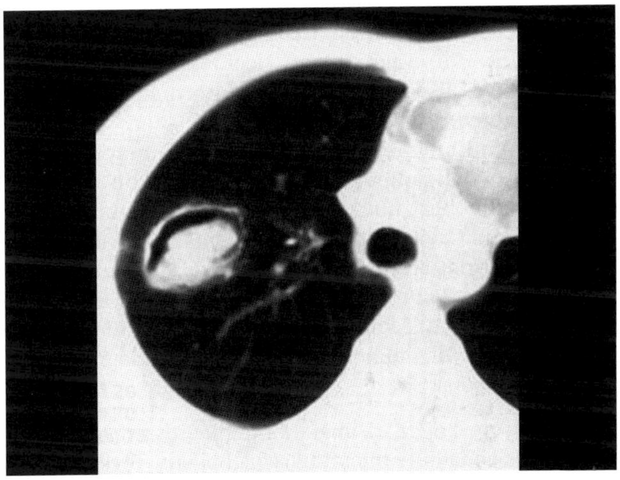

FIG. 27: Aspergilloma: CT shows the fungus ball lying in dependent portion of the cavity with a characteristic air-crescent sign.

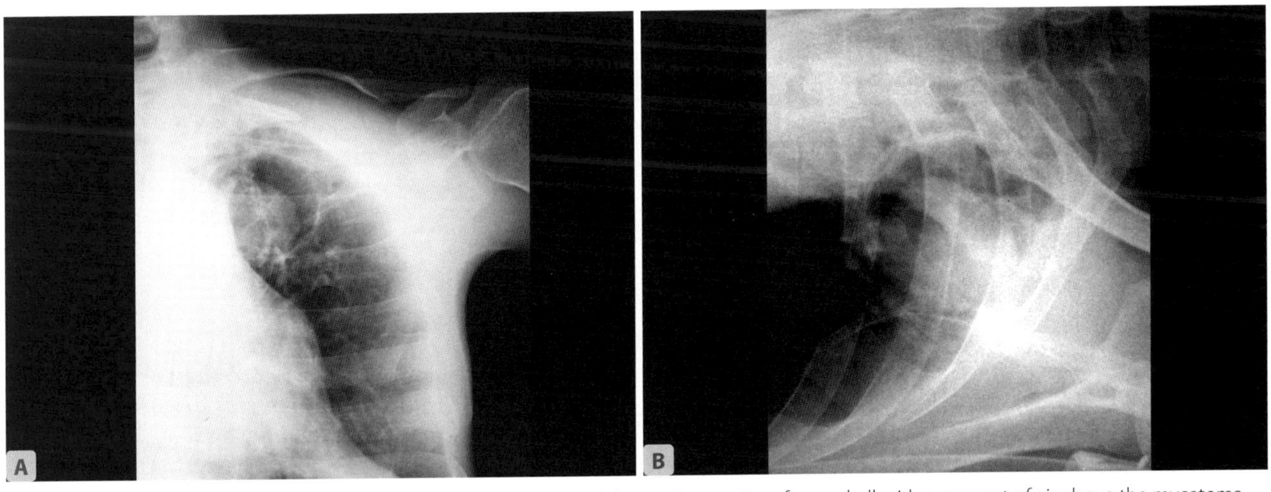

FIGS. 26A AND B: Frontal chest radiograph (A) shows a cavity containing an intracavitary fungus ball with a crescent of air above the mycetoma. Lateral decubitus view (B) shows the fungus ball lying in the dependant part of cavity suggesting movement of the mycetoma within the cavity.

or even grow overtime. CT shows the bronchiectasis and mucoid impaction very well **(Figs. 28 and 29)**.[57] The central distribution of bronchiectasis suggests the diagnosis of ABPA, even though it is not specific for the diagnosis. The findings of ABPA overlap with other entities such as cystic fibrosis or post infectious bronchiectasis.

Hypersensitivity pneumonitis can occur with *Aspergillus* inhalation. It is seen on chest radiographs as a ground-glass opacity and/or diffuse small nodules. Sometimes recurrent transient opacities superimposed on a fine micronodular pattern may be seen.[58] Diffuse, small centrilobular nodules of ground-glass attenuation are seen on CT, which are characteristic of subacute hypersensitivity pneumonitis. Chronic hypersensitivity pneumonitis demonstrates traction bronchiectasis and interstitial thickening often associated with areas of ground-glass opacity and mosaic perfusion. The major differential diagnosis is idiopathic pulmonary fibrosis.[58]

Semi-invasive and *invasive aspergillosis* will be dealt in detail in a later chapter.

Cryptococcosis

Cryptococcosis is caused by the fungus *Cryptococcus neoformans*. Although it can occur as pulmonary or disseminated disease in otherwise normal individuals, cryptococcosis is more frequently seen to affect immunocompromised patients. In the immunocompetent individuals, the radiographic findings can be single or multiple pulmonary nodules or areas of segmental or lobar consolidation. Cavitation and pleural effusion are rare. Hilar and mediastinal lymphadenopathy may be seen. Rarely a disseminated pattern of bronchopneumonia may be seen. Many patients with cryptococcal pneumonia have no symptoms and the pulmonary lesions seen radiographically heal spontaneously.[34]

2. Primary pathogens: Fungi that frequently infect healthy individuals constitute the primary pathogens. These include species like *Histoplasma, Coccidioides, Blastomyces*, and *Paracoccidioides*. They are natural inhabitants of North and South America and are not commonly found in the Indian subcontinent.[54,59]

Histoplasmosis

It is caused by the fungus *Histoplasma capsulatum* which is found in moist soil and in bird excreta in many parts of the world, but human infection is only seen with more frequency in parts of North America.[17] The radiographic picture closely resembles tuberculosis. In both, there is necrosis of pulmonary tissue followed by fibrosis and contraction. Parenchymal and/or nodal calcification is commonly seen. Other manifestations can be pulmonary granulomas or small nodules scattered in both lung fields resembling military tuberculosis. An uncommon late manifestation of histoplasmosis is a fibrosing mediastinitis which can be well evaluated by CT.[17]

Coccidioidomycosis

It is caused by the fungus *Coccidioides immitis* and found principally in endemic areas in southwestern United States

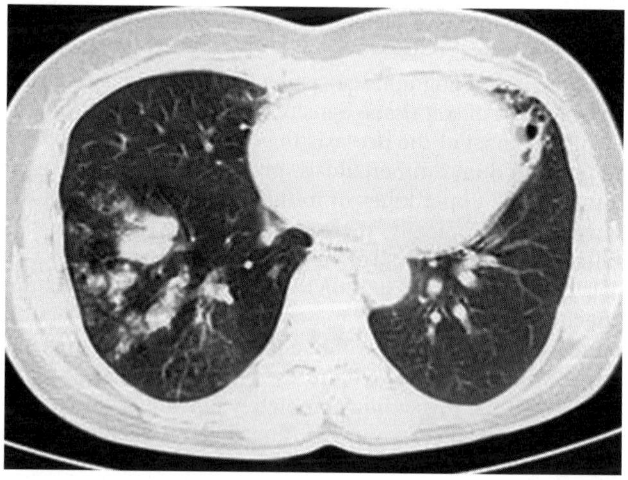

FIG. 29: CT scan in ABPA showing the characteristic "gloved finger" sign of mucoid-filled dilated bronchi in right lower lobe.

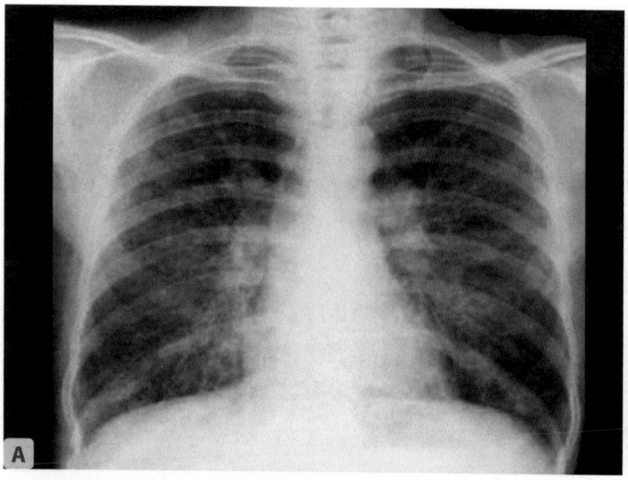

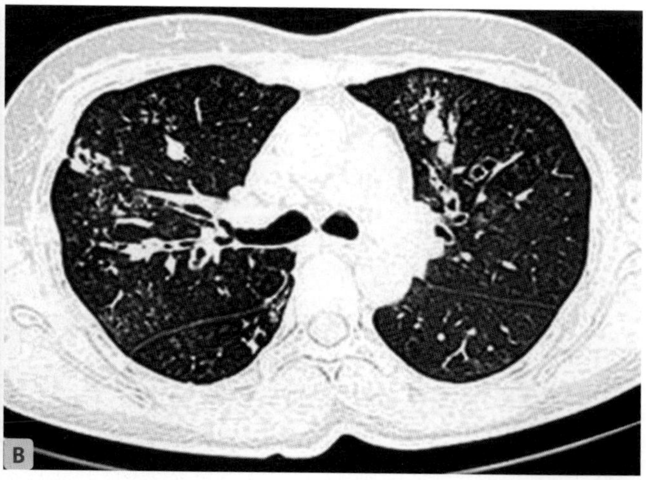

FIGS. 28A AND B: Allergic bronchopulmonary aspergillosis (ABPA): Chest radiograph (A) and HRCT scan (B) showing bronchial thickening, central bronchiectasis and mucoid impaction within dilated bronchi and bronchioles in bilateral lung fields.

and northern Mexico. The most common radiological manifestation of primary coccidioidomycosis is a single or multiple foci of airspace consolidation. Thin walled cavities, pleural effusion and mediastinal lymphadenopathy may rarely be seen. Most patients of primary coccidioidomycosis recover within 3 weeks. Patients with persisting radiographic abnormalities after 6–8 weeks are considered to have chronic pulmonary coccidioidomycosis. The radiologic manifestations include lung nodules, cavities and rarely bronchiectasis and scarring. Apical fibrocavitary disease with lobar contraction, bronchiectasis and rarely calcification may resemble reactivation tuberculosis.[34]

Parasitic Infections

Protozoal Infections

Pleuropulmonary amebiasis is usually secondary to liver involvement.[60,61] Pleural effusion and lower lobe consolidation may be present contiguous to an amebic abscess in the liver or sub-diaphragmatic space, just as they may accompany any other suppurative process in these sites. Changes can occur at the base of either lung, because of the relationship of the liver to the diaphragm, but are much more frequent on the right. An amebic liver abscess may extend through the diaphragm into the pleural cavity, giving rise to an empyema. If it extends into the lung, it can cause pneumonia or a lung abscess.[62]

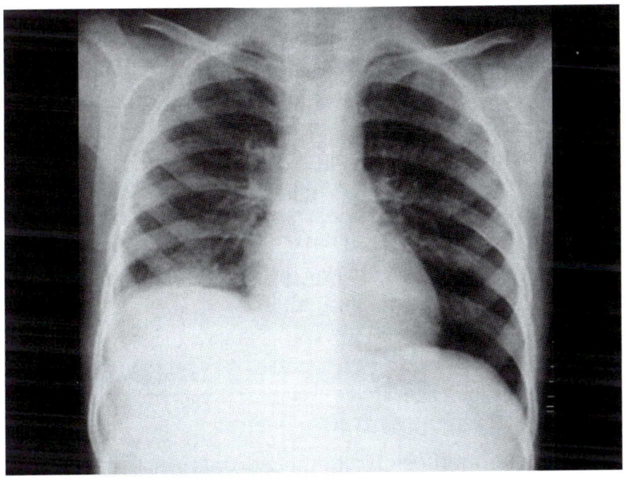

FIG. 30: Chest radiograph shows elevation of right dome of diaphragm with associated pleural effusion and basal consolidation. Ultrasound showed a subdiaphragmatic liver abscess.

Chest radiographs may show an elevated hemidiaphragm, pleural effusion and/or thickening and basal atelectasis **(Fig. 30)**. If the abscess ruptures through the diaphragm, basal consolidation with cavitation may be seen. Fistulas may develop to airways, pericardium or rarely skin. The diagnosis can be established by ultrasound, CT or MRI and serological tests **(Figs. 31A to C)**.

Metazoal Infestations

Roundworm, hookworm and strongyloides infections: Many parasitic worms including Ascaris, Taenia, Ankylostoma, and Strongyloides pass through the lungs as part of their life cycle. In most instances, no pulmonary complications occur with any of these worms, but in a few patients, an allergic reaction takes place in the lung parenchyma, which manifests itself radiographically as dense migratory pulmonary consolidations without recognizable segmental distribution **(Fig. 32)**.[34,63] Blood and sputum eosinophilia are often present and the entity is therefore included as one of the causes of Loeffler's syndrome.[64]

Filariasis

The most common filarial worm to cause pulmonary manifestations is *Wuchereria bancrofti* which is responsible for elephantiasis. *W. bancrofti* can cause tropical eosinophilia, which is a syndrome consisting of cough, wheezing and severe blood eosinophilia. It is believed to occur due to an immunologic response to microfilariae rather than to a direct infection. The chest radiograph either be normal or may show widespread fine nodular or reticulonodular shadowing, closely resembling military tuberculosis. Occasionally, localized consolidation may be seen.[65]

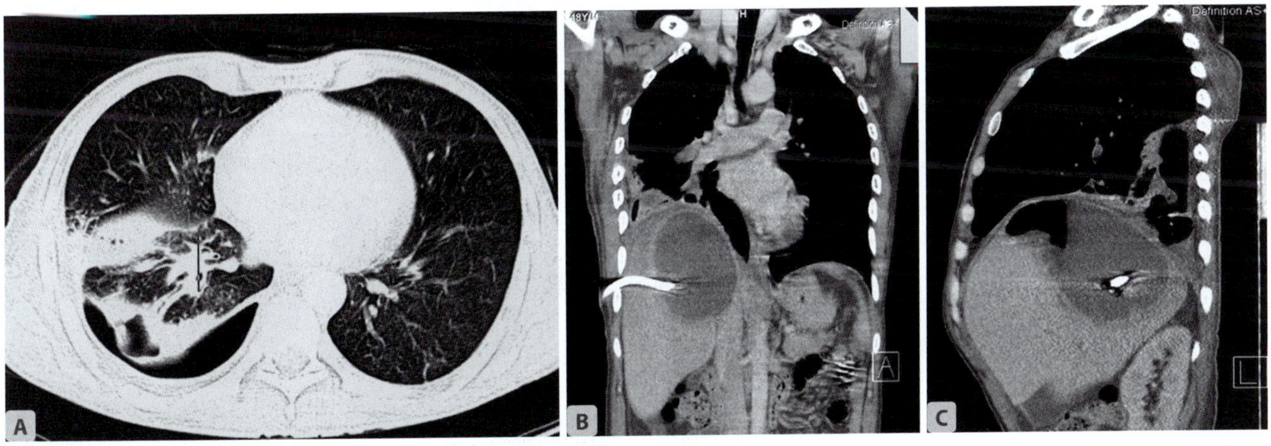

FIGS. 31A TO C: Pleuropulmonary amebiasis: CECT axial-lung window (A), coronal (B) and sagittal (C). Mediastinal window: A large abscess in the liver with a drain in situ, with a loculated pyopneumothorax and focal basal consolidation suggestive of an amebic liver abscess which has ruptured through the diaphragm.

Echinococcus Infection/Hydatid Disease

Echinococcus infection is caused by a tapeworm *Echinococcus granulosus*. Humans are actually accidental hosts and acquire the infection by ingesting ova from fomites or contaminated water and by direct contact with dogs. Larvae develop in the host's duodenum, enter the bloodstream and travel to the end organs. Liver is the most common organ involved, followed by the lung. Cysts develop around this parasite in the end organs. The cyst wall consists of 3 layers: an outermost layer or the "pericyst" is a fibrotic capsule formed by the compression of the adjacent lung tissue. The cyst itself has a thin wall composed of 2 adherent layers, an outer ectocyst and an inner delicate lining—the endocyst. Multiple cysts are seen in approximately one third of patients and are bilateral in 20%.[66]

Unruptured pulmonary cysts are generally asymptomatic and may be discovered incidentally on a routine chest film. They are homogeneous, roughly spherical or oval, sharply demarcated mass lesions, ranging in size from 1–10 cm and occur more commonly in mid and lower zones **(Fig. 33A)**. CT scan shows the masses to be cystic in nature with a well-defined enhancing wall **(Fig. 33B)**. The internal contents are of water density and daughter cysts when present, are curved septations within the main cyst. The cysts are relatively pliant and mould to adjacent structures, resulting in indentation, lobulation and flattening. Calcification, which is a common feature of hydatid cysts in the liver, is very rare in lung cysts. Approximately, two-thirds of the cysts rupture. Cyst rupture may occur into the surrounding lung, airways or pleural space. If the pericyst ruptures, with the two inner layers remaining intact, air dissects between the pericyst and ectocyst giving rise to a crescent or meniscus sign. If there is disruption of the inner layers, a complex cavitatory lesion results which may show any of the following features like air fluid level, a floating membrane—water-lily sign **(Figs. 34A to C)**, a double wall, an essentially dry cyst with crumpled membranes lying at its bottom **(Fig. 35)**, or an empty cyst.[67] All these signs are particularly well seen on CT.[68] CT may also show air bubbles or blebs in the wall of a hydatid cyst which are specific for detection of rupture.[69] Secondary infection of a hydatid cyst may produce a lung abscess with or without surrounding consolidation. Rupture into the pleural space causes an effusion or if there is an additional airway communication, a hydropneumothorax.

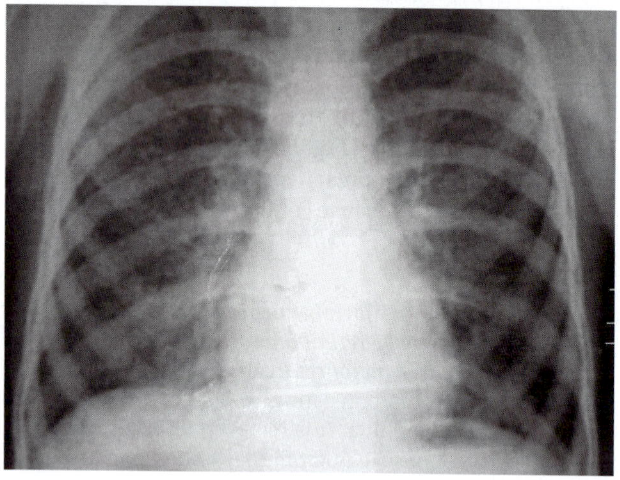

FIG. 32: Tropical eosinophilia: Chest radiograph shows diffuse nodular opacities in a child presenting with cough with a TLC of 40,000 cells/cc with 75% eosinophils.

MRI can display complex cysts contents well and the cyst membrane, whether collapsed or not, is clearly seen as a low intensity curvilinear structure on both T1W and T2W sequences. MRI and MDCT reconstructions may be particularly helpful in revealing the exact location of a hydatid cyst in relation to the diaphragm.[70,71]

COMPLICATIONS OF PNEUMONIA

Pleural Effusion and Empyema

Parapneumonic effusions complicate the course of 20–60% of patients hospitalized with bacterial pneumonia.[72] Effusions are quite common in staphylococcal and gram-negative

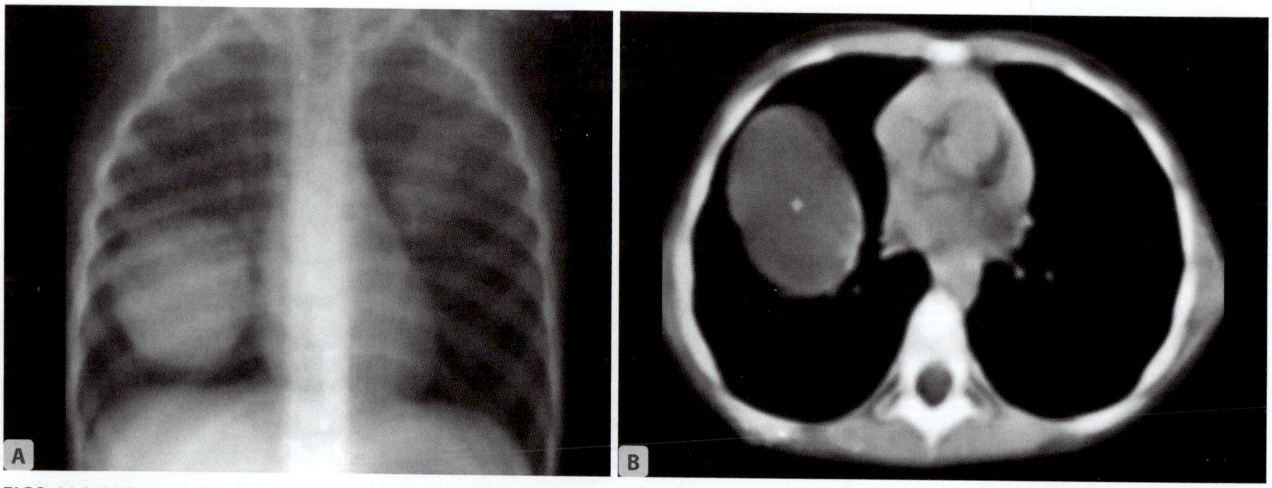

FIGS. 33A AND B: Hydatid cyst: Chest radiograph (A) shows a well-defined slightly lobulated mass in right lower zone and another oval shaped mass in left upper zone. CT scan (B) through the lower mass shows a homogeneous fluid density cyst.

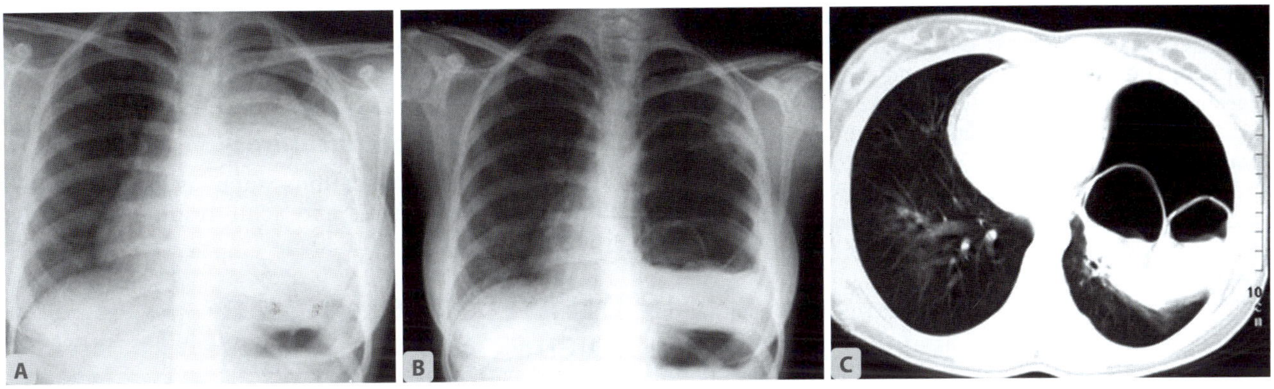

FIGS. 34A TO C: Chest radiograph (A) shows an unusually large unruptured hydatid cyst in left lung field, displacing the mediastinum to the right. After rupture, chest radiograph (B) and CT scan (C) show air-fluid level within the cyst with floating membranes—Water-lily sign.

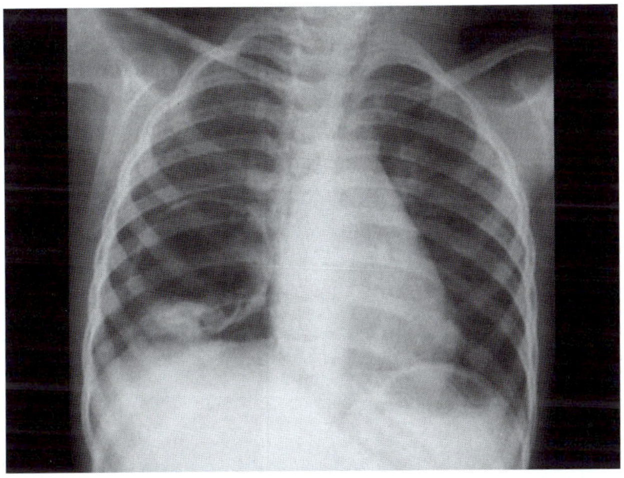

FIG. 35: Chest radiograph shows ruptured hydatid cyst with crumpled membranes lying at the bottom of the cyst.

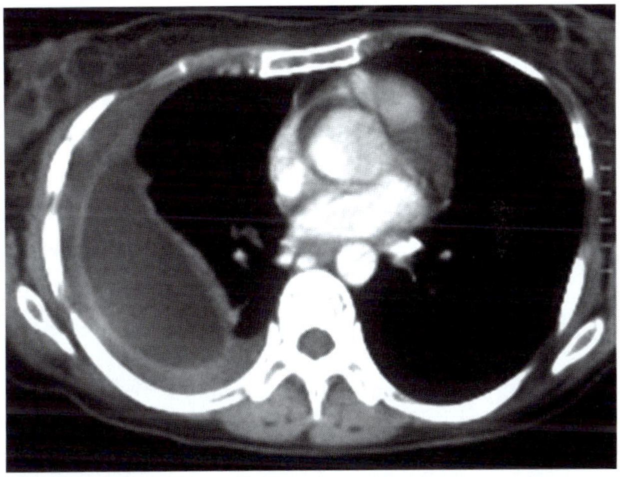

FIG. 36: CT scan in a case of empyema showing a homogeneous lenticular-shaped fluid collection based on the chest wall enclosed within thick enhancing pleura—split pleura sign.

pneumonias, much less common in pneumococcal pneumonias and distinctly unusual in viral and mycoplasmal infections.

Parapneumonic effusion progresses to empyema formation in 5–10% of patients, resolution occurs in the rest with antibiotic therapy. Progression to empyema in debilitated and elderly patients increases morbidity and likelihood of mortality.

The choice of modality for evaluation of effusion depends on the clinical context. Blunting of costo phrenic angle occurs in a chest radiograph with pleural fluid up to 200–500 mL.[73] Ultrasound is useful for detecting small amount of fluid (as little as 5 mL), loculations and viscosity.[74] On the other hand, CT allows detailed evaluation of complex fluid collections **(Fig. 36)**.

Hydropneumothorax

The appearance of gas in the pleural space together with fluid is usually iatrogenic in origin. It may be associated with a bronchopleural fistula casued by rupture of a pneumatocele or abscess, and is seen particularly with *S.aureus*, gram-negative and anaerobic infections.

Pneumatoceles

Pneumatoceles commonly follow staphylococcal infections in children (not so common in adults). They are thin-walled cavities of variable sizes **(Fig. 14)**. They are formed due to check valve obstruction between the lumen of a small bronchus and adjacent interstitium. They can resolve completely or persist for months in which case they are of no clinical significance unless they cause pressure on adjacent structures.

Bronchiectasis

Bronchiectasis commonly occurs during the acute phase of pneumonia but resolves as the inflammation subsides.[75] Occasionally this can persist and act as source of hemoptysis or recurrent infections.

Pulmonary Abscess, Necrotizing Pneumonia and Pulmonary Gangrene

These conditions present a continuum caused by microbial infections, predominantly anaerobic microbes.[76] *Abscess* occurs due to cavitation secondary to necrosis in a variety of bacterial pneumonias, particularly those caused by *S. aureus*, gram-negative bacteria and anaerobes. Cavitation is also seen in amebic, fungal and metazoal infections, but it is rare with viral and mycoplasmal pneumonias. Abscesses that fail to establish airway communication do not cavitate and are undetected on chest radiographs, being isodense with surrounding consolidated lung. However, they can be seen on CT because of the low attenuation centre within the abscess **(Figs. 37A and B)**.

Necrotizing pneumonia is characterized by consolidation combined with peripheral necrosis and formation of multiple small cavities. In the continuum, necrotising pneumonia lies between lung abscess and pulmonary gangrene **(Figs. 38A to C)**.[77,78]

Pulmonary gangrene occurs due to progressive devitalization of pulmonary parenchyma. It is characterized by sloughing of a pulmonary segment or lobe as a consequence of thrombosis in branches of pulmonary and bronchial arteries supplying the necrotic area.[79] CECT shows obliteration of the pulmonary artery supply to the segment or lobe which has large cavities and necrotic parenchyma.[77]

Differential diagnosis of necrotizing pulmonary infections includes infected bullae, pleural empyemas and lung tumors.[76]

Miscellaneous Complications

Miscellaneous complications such as osteomyelitis, obliterative bronchiolitis and acute respiratory distress syndrome can occur.

DELAYED RESOLUTION OF PNEUMONIA

Non-resolving or slowly resolving pneumonia (NRP) refers to persistence of radiographic abnormalities beyond the expected time course and affects 10–20% patients hospitalized with community acquired pneumonia (CAP).[80]

It has been defined as either less than 50% clearing at 2 weeks or less than complete clearing after 4 weeks inspite of antibiotic therapy for a minimum period of 10 days.[81]

The various causes that can lead to non-resolving pneumonia are listed in **Table 5**.[82] Causes may be pathogen

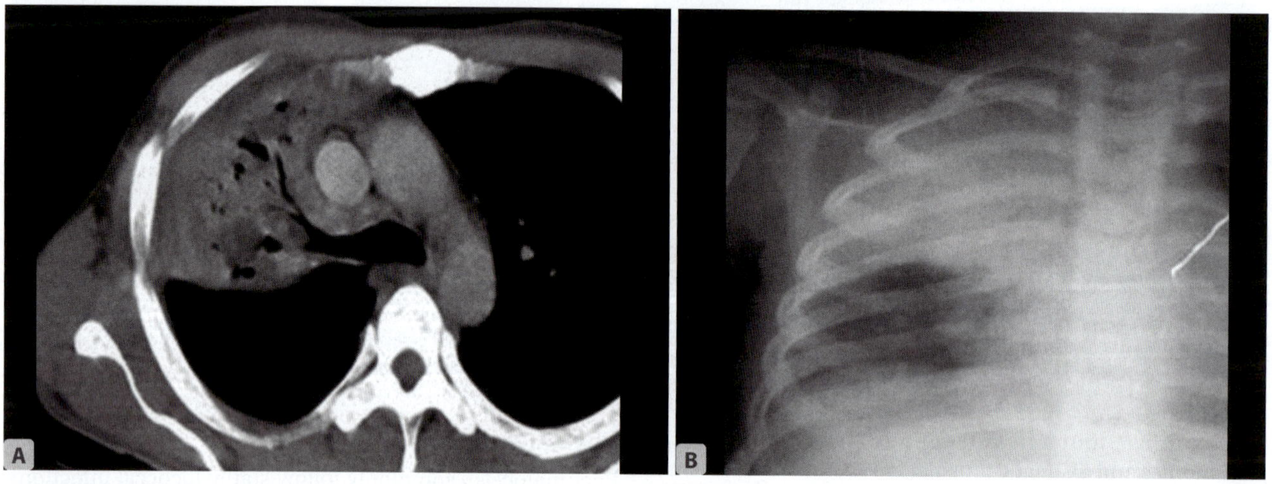

FIGS. 37A AND B: CT scan (A) demonstrates dense consolidation in the right upper lobe containing a focal region of low attenuation and gas consistent with necrosis and abscess formation not appreciated on chest radiograph (B).

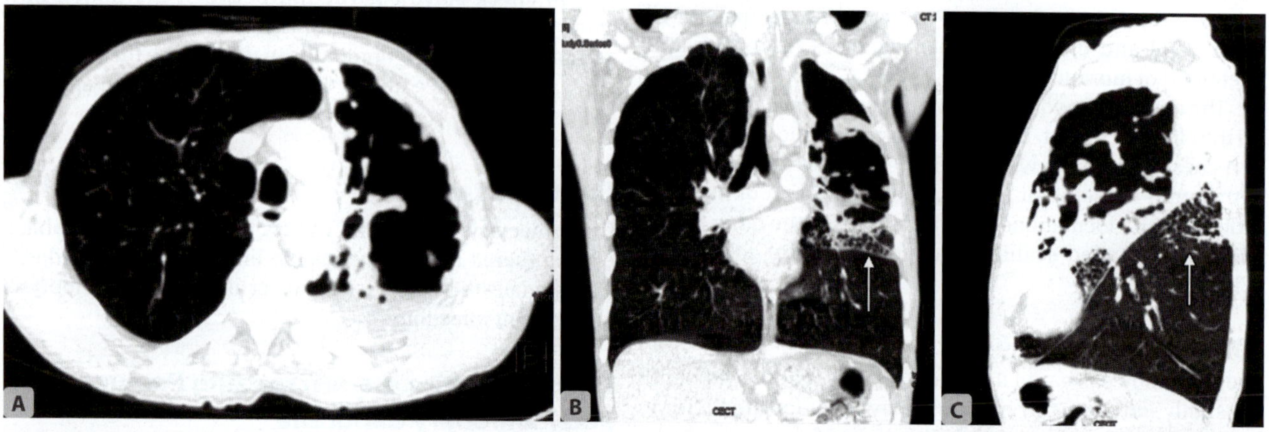

FIGS. 38A TO C: Necrotizing pneumonia: Axial (A), Coronal (B) and Sagittal (C) CECT in a 65-year-old patient with emphysema shows consolidation of left upper lobe with marked destruction of the lung parenchyma with an air-fluid level. Adjacent areas of consolidation show small cysts within due to centriacinar emphysema (arrows in B and C).

TABLE 5: Causes of non-resolving pneumonia.

Factors	Causes
Pathogen-related	• Atypical organism • Resistant organism • Uncommon organism • Nosocomial infection
Host-related	• Severity of initial illness • Presence of comorbidities • Immunosuppressed state • Metastatic infection
Presence of complications	• Para-pneumonic effusion/empyema • Abscess • Gangrene
Non-infectious disease	• Neoplastic disorders (adenocarcinoma *in situ*, lymphoma, lymphangitis carcinomatosis, etc.) • Pulmonary embolism • Systemic vasculitis (Wegner's granulomatosis) • Connective tissue disorders • Drug-induced disorders (amodiarone, nitrofurantoin, methotrexate, etc.) • Cryptogenic organizing pneumonia • Eosinophilic pneumonia • Congestive cardiac failure

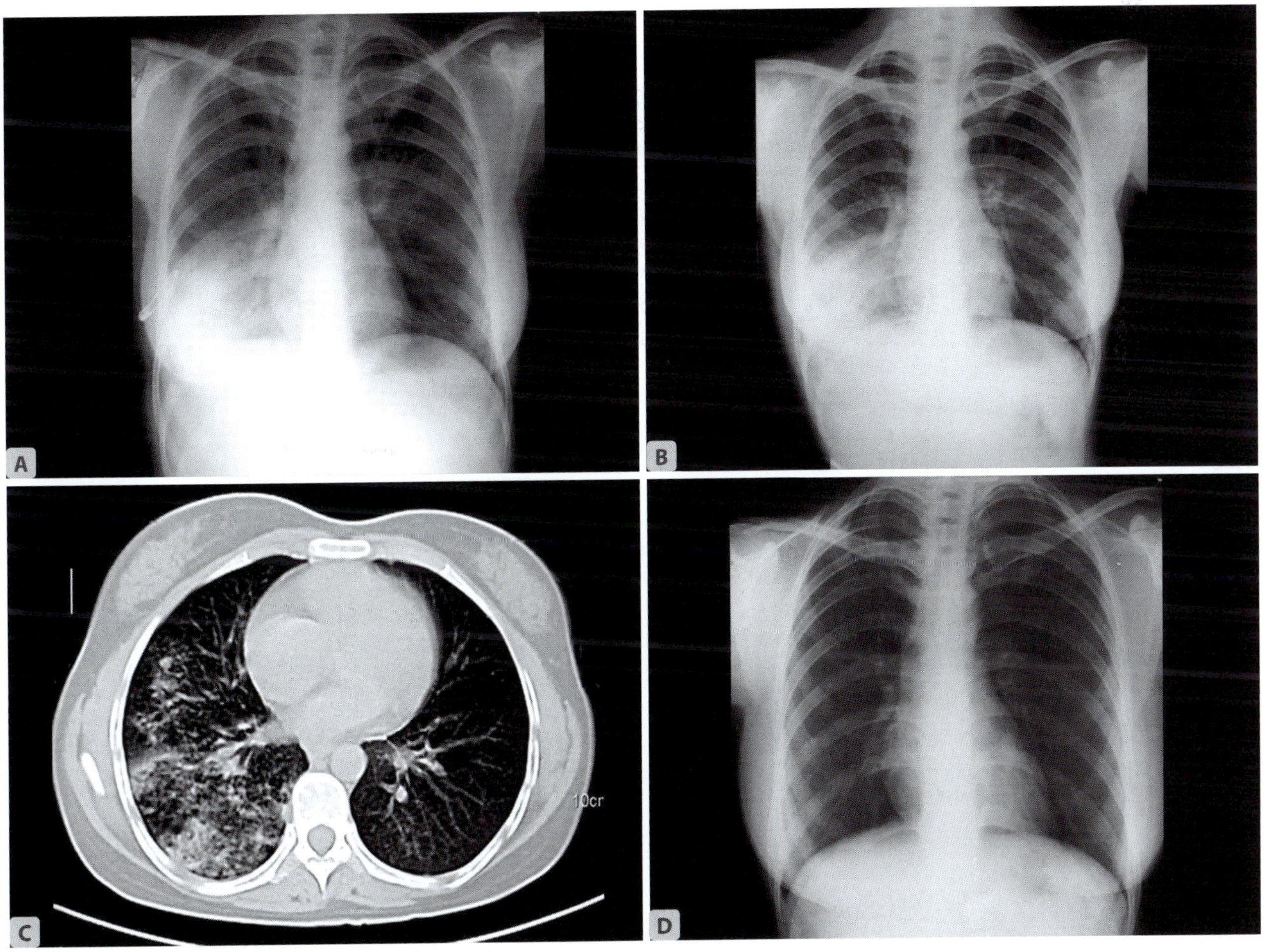

FIGS. 39A TO D: Non-resolving pneumonia: Chest radiograph (A) in a young 25-year-old girl with high-grade fever and cough, shows a right lower zone consolidation, which shows only partial clearance even after a prolonged course of antibiotics on chest radiograph (B) after 5 weeks. CT (C) showed multiple focal lobular alveolar and tree-in–bud opacities. ATT was started. Chest radiograph (D) after 4 weeks of ATT shows complete resolution.

related or host related. The presence of complications is another cause of delayed resolution of pneumonia. Non-infectious diseases or "pneumonia mimics" as enumerated in the table can be misdiagnosed as pneumonia and thus be another reason for delayed resolution. In our country, tuberculosis is one of the most common cause for a non-resolving pneumonia **(Figs. 39A to D)**.[83]

Further evaluation in the form of CT chest, microbiological tests for etiological agent, bronchoscopy, biopsy and other tests specific to the suspected organisms/disease are required for these patients.

Diagnostic Algorithm in Patients Suspected with Pneumonia

An imaging algorithm for diagnosis of pneumonia has been suggested in **Flowchart 1**. In patients with mild disease, empirical treatment usually suffices, whereas in patients with severe disease, an aggressive approach is sometimes needed for identification of specific causative organism. Demonstration of the pathogen can be done by examination of stained smears of sputum, pleural fluid, by culture of respiratory secretions, blood or other biological material. Interventional procedures like transthoracic needle biopsy done, ultrasound or CT guidance are a reliable and cost-effective means to obtain material for culture.[84]

In cases with underlying co-morbidities or immunosuppressed state of the host, specific treatment may be initiated accordingly. In cases of complicated pneumonia CT can assist in identify in the complication and hence aid management. If the disease is suspected to be a "pneumonia minic", specific and ancillary test may be needed to reach a conclusive diagnosis.

CONCLUSION

Chest radiography is the imaging technique of choice in evaluating patients with suspected pneumonia because of its low radiation dose, low cost, and wide accessibility. In daily practice, radiographs are used to confirm the clinical diagnosis of pneumonia, characterize the extent and severity of disease, search for complications, monitor the response to therapy, and examine for possible alternative or additional diagnoses. The radiographic pattern needs to be correlated with the clinical background to suggest an etiological diagnosis summarized in **Table 6**. CT scan has the advantage of superior contrast resolution and cross-sectional display which is helpful in the analysis of complex or slowly resolving cases, particularly when radiographic evidence of associated conditions and complications is equivocal.

FLOWCHART 1: Clinicoradiological algorithm for diagnosis of pneumonia.

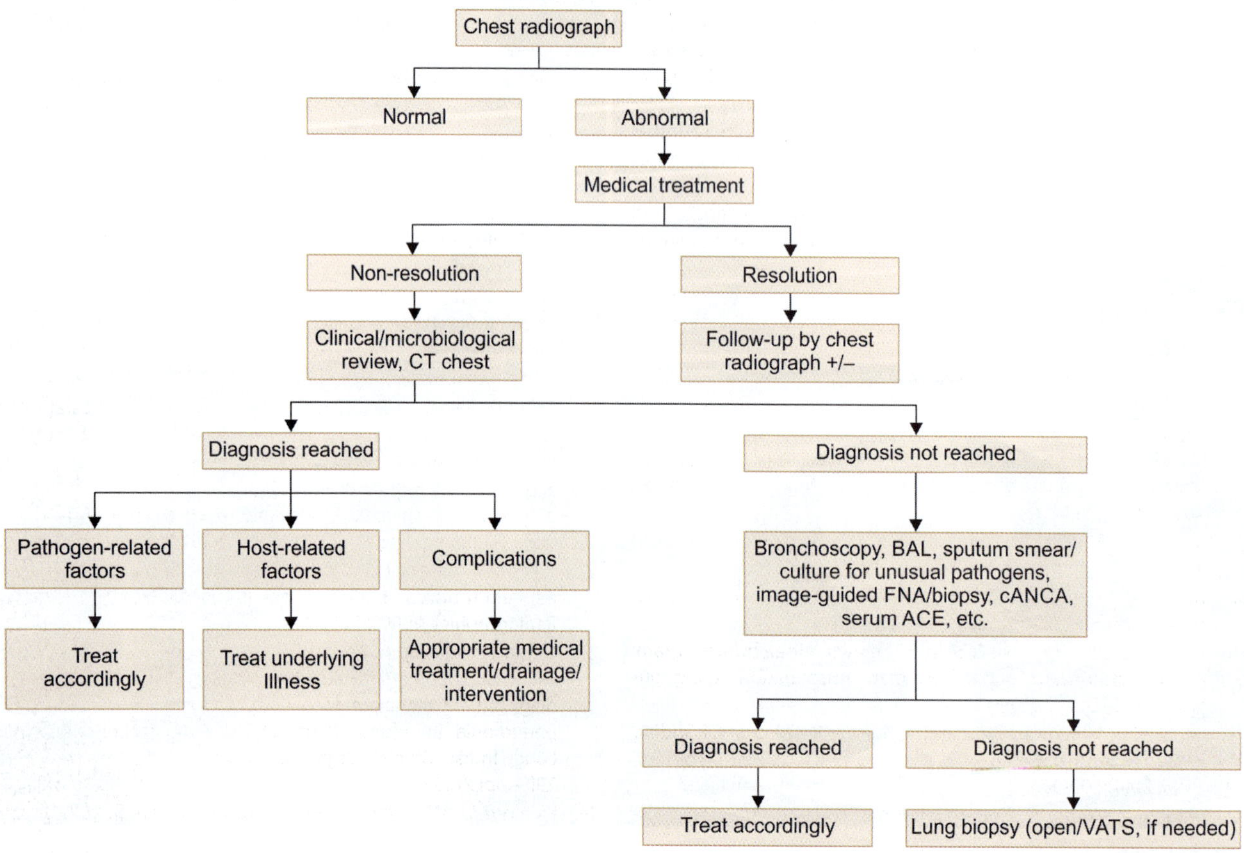

(BAL: bronchoalveolar lavage; cANCA: cytoplasmic antineutrophil cytoplasmic antibodies; ACE: angiotensin-converting enzyme; VATS: video-assisted thoracoscopic surgery)

TABLE 6: Summary of clinical and radiographic clues to the etiological diagnosis of pneumonia.[84]

Radiographic findings	Clinical circumstance	Organism
Segmental consolidation	Community-acquired	*S. pneumoniae, M. pneumoniae*
Lobar consolidation	Community-acquired diabetes	*S. pneumoniae* (2/3 of community-acquired pneumonias), *K. pneumoniae* Gram-negative bacilli
Round pneumonia	Community-acquired	*S. pneumoniae*
Bronchopneumonia	Hospital-acquired	*P. aeruginosa, S. aureus,* streptococci, gram- negative bacilli, anaerobes, *M. pneumoniae,* aspiration
Interstitial pneumonia	Community-acquired	Virus, *M. pneumoniae*
Cavitation/necrosis	Aspiration COPD	*S. aureus,* Gram-negative bacilli, anaerobes, *Actinomycosis, M. tuberculosis, Aspergillus*
Multiple cavitatory nodules	Drug addict, septicemia	*S. aureus*
Pneumatoceles	Postinfluenza	*S. aureus*
Empyema	Complication of pneumonia	*S. pneumoniae, S. aureus,* Gram-negative bacilli, *M. tuberculosis*
Chest wall invasion	Alcoholic	Actinomycosis, *M. tuberculosis,* fungi
Lymphadenopathy		*M. pneumoniae, M. tuberculosis*

REFERENCES

1. Padley SPG, Rubens MB. Pulmonary infections. In: David Sutton (Ed). Textbook of Radiology and Imaging. Edinburgh: Churchill Livingstone. 2003;1:131-60.
2. Kalil AC, Metersky ML, Klompas M, et al. Management of adults with hospital-acquired and ventilator-associated pneumonia: 2016 Clinical Practice Guidelines by the Infectious Diseases Society of America and the American Thoracic Society. Clin Infect Dis. 2016;63(5):e61-111.
3. Alkhayat KF, Hasan M, Alam-Eldeen. Value of chest ultrasound in diagnosis of community acquired pneumonia. Egyptian Journal of Chest Diseases and Tuberculosis. 2014;63(4):1047-51.
4. Schenck EJ, Rajwani K. Ultrasound in the diagnosis and management of pneumonia. Current Opinion in Infectious Diseases. 2016;29(2):223-8.
5. Pereda MA, Chavez MA, Hooper-Miele CA, et al. Lung ultrasound for the diagnosis of pneumonia in children: A meta-analysis. Pediatrics. 2015;135(4):715-22.
6. Sodhi KS, Khandelwal N, Saxena AK, et al. Rapid lung MRI in children with pulmonary infections: Time to change our diagnostic algorithms. J Magn Reson Imaging. 2016;43: 1196-1206.
7. Liszewski M, Görkem S, Sodhi K, Lee E. Lung magnetic resonance imaging for pneumonia in children. Pediatric Radiology. 2017;47(11):1420-30.
8. Spencer H. The bacterial pneumonias. Pathology of the lung, 4th edn. Oxford: Pergamon Press. 1985. pp. 167-212.
9. Blaivas M. Lung Ultrasound in Evaluation of Pneumonia. Journal of Ultrasound Medicine. 2012;31:823.
10. Liechtenstein D, Meziere G, Seitz J. The dynamic air bronchogram: A lung ultrasound sign of alveolar consolidation ruling out atelectasis. Chest. 2009;135(6):1421-5.
11. Tanaka N, Matsumoto T, Kuramitsu T. High Resolution CT finding in Community-acquired Pneumonia. J Comput Assist Tomogr. 1996; 20(4):600-08.
12. Beigelman-Aubry C, Godet C, Caumes E. Lung infections: The radiologist's perspective. Diagn Intervent Imaging. 2012;93: 431-40.
13. ER Heitzman. The radiological diagnosis of pneumonia in the adult: A commentary. Semin in Roentgenology. 1989;XXIV(4):212-17.
14. Rose RW, Ward BH. Spherical pneumonias in children simulating pulmonary and mediastinal masses. Radiology. 1973;106: 179-82.
15. Wang N. Anatomy. In: Dial DH, Hammar SP (Eds). Pulmonary Pathology. New York: Springer Verlag. 1988;17-40.
16. Wagner AL, Szabunio M, Hazlett KS, et al. Radiologic manifestations of round pneumonia in adults. AJR. 1998;170: 723-26.
17. Goodman PC, Wilson AG, Armstrong P, et al. Pulmonary Infections in Adults. In: Grainger RG, Allison D, et al (Eds). Diagnostic Radiology, Edinburgh: Churchill Livingstone. 2001;377-417.
18. Scanlon GT, Unger JD. The Radiology of Bacterial and Viral Pneumonias. RCNA. 1973;11(2):317-38.
19. Smith CB, Overall JC. Clinical and epidemiologic clues to the diagnosis of respiratory infections. RCNA. 1973;11(2):261-78.
20. Fein AM, Feinsilver SH, Niederman MS. Atypical manifestations of pneumonia in the elderly. Clin Chest Med. 1991;12:319.
21. Nambu A, Ozawa K, Kobayashi N, et al. Imaging of community-acquired pneumonia: Roles of imaging examinations, imaging diagnosis of specific pathogens and discrimination from noninfectious diseases. World J Radiol. 2014;6(10):779 93.
22. Franquet T, Giménez A, Rosón N, Torrubia S, Sabaté JM, Pérez C. Aspiration diseases: findings, pitfalls, and differential diagnosis. Radiographics. 2000;20:673-85.
23. Gupta D, Agarwal R, Aggarwal AN, Singh N, Mishra N, Khilnani GC, et al. Pneumonia Guidelines Working Group. Guidelines for diagnosis and management of community-and hospital-acquired pneumonia in adults: Joint ICS/NCCP (I) recommendations. Lung India: Official Organ of Indian Chest Society. 2012; 29(Suppl 2):S27.
24. Kieninger AN, Lipsett PA. Hospital-acquired pneumonia: pathophysiology, diagnosis, and treatment. Surg Clin North Am. 2009,89(2):439–61. ix 10.1016/j.suc.2008.11.001.

25. Rubin SA, Winer-Muram HT, Ellis JV. Diagnostic imaging of pneumonia and its complications in the critically ill patients. Clin Chest Med. 1995;16;45.
26. Beydon L, Saada M, Liu N, et al. Can portable chest X-ray examination accurately diagnose basal consolidation after abdominal surgery? A comparison with CT scan. Chest. 1994;106:221-35.
27. Winer-Muram HT, Rubin SA, Ellis JV, et al. Pneumonia and ARDS patients receiving mechanical ventilation: Diagnostic accuracy of chest radiography. Radiology. 1993;188:479.
28. Winer-Muram HT, Steiner RM, Gurney JW: Ventilator- associated pneumonia in patients with adult respiratory distress syndrome: CT evaluation. Radiology. 1998;208:193.
29. A Trimble, V Moffat, AM Collins. Pulmonary infections in the returned traveller. Pneumonia. 2017;9:1
30. Kantor HG. The many radiologic faces of pneumococcal pneumonia. AJR. 1981;137:1213.
31. Shah RM, Gupta S, Angeid-Backman E, et al. Pneumococcal pneumonia in patients requiring hospitalization: Effects of bacteremia and HIV seropositivity on radiographic appearance. AJR. 2000;175(6):1533-36.
32. Macfarlane J, Rose D. Radiographic features of staphylococcal pneumonia in adults and children. Thorax. 1996;51:539-40.
33. Naraqi S, McDonnel G. Haematogenous staphylococcal pneumonia secondary to soft tissue infection. Chest. 1981;79: 173-75.
34. Armstrong P. Bacterial pneumonia. In: Hansell DM, Armstrong P, Lynch DA, et al (Eds). Imaging of Diseases of Chest. Philadelphia: Mosby. 2005. pp. 183-276.
35. Bartlett JG, Finegold SM. Anaerobic infections of the lung and pleural space. Am Rev Respir Dis. 1974;110:56-77.
36. Groskin SA, Panicek DM, Ewing DK, et al. Bacterial lung abscess: A review of the radiographic and clinical features of 50 cases. J Thoracic Imaging. 1991;6:62-7.
37. Landay MJ, Christensen EE, Bynum LJ, et al. Anaerobic pleural and pulmonary infections. AJR. 1980;134;233.
38. Putnam CE, Curtis AM, Aimeone JF, et al. *Mycoplasma pneumonia*: Clinical and roentgenographic patterns. Radiology. 1975; 124:417.
39. Reittner P, Muller NL, Heyneman L, et al. *Mycoplasma pneumoniae* pneumonia: Radiographic and high resolution CT features in 28 patients. AJR. 2000;174:37-41.
40. Traver RD, Shawn DT, Heitkamp DE, et al. Radiology of community-acquired pneumonia. RCNA. 2005;43:497-512.
41. Poirier R, Rodrigue J, Villeneuve J, et al. Early radiographic and tomographic manifestations of Legionnaire's disease. Can Assoc Radiol J. Published online May 4, 2017.
42. Kim KW, Goo JM, Lee HJ, et al. Chest computed tomographic findings and clinical features of legionella pneumonia. J Comput Assist Tomogr. 2007;31 (6): 950-5.
43. Mabeza GF, Macfarlane J. Pulmonary actinomycosis. Eur Respir J. 2003;21:545-51.
44. Frank P, Strickland B. Pulmonary actinomycosis. Br J Radiol. 1974;47:373-78.
45. Cheon JE, Im JG, Kim MH, et al. Thoracic actionomycosis: CT findings. Radiology. 1998;209:229-33.
46. Greenberg SB. Viral pneumonia. Infect Dis Clin North Am. 1991;5:603-21.
47. Waite S, Jeudy J, White CS. Acute lung infections in normal and immunocompromised hosts. RCNA. 2006;44:295-315.
48. Kim EA, Lee KS, Primack SL, et al. Viral pneumonias in adults: radiologic and pathologic findings. Radiographics. 2002;22:S137-49.
49. Chowell G, Bertozzi SM, Colchero MA, et al. Severe respiratory disease concurrent with the circulation of H1N1 influenza. N Engl J Med. 2009;361(7):674–9.
50. Abdelsalam M, Diab HS, Ragab Y. Radiologoical findings in patients with H1N1 influenza pneumonia. Egyptian Journal of Chest diseases and Tuberculosis. 2016;65(1):135-42.
51. Qureshi NR, Hien TT, Farrar J, et al. The radiologic manifestations of H5N1 avian influenza. J Thorac Imaging. 2006;21(4):259-64.
52. Teper AM, Kofman CD, Maffey AF, et al. Lung function in infants with chronic pulmonary disease after severe adenoviral illness. J Pediatr. 1999;134:730-33.
53. Gotway MB, Dawn SK, Caoili EM, et al. The radiologic spectrum of pulmonary Aspergillus infections. JCAT. 2002;26(2):159-73.
54. Panda BN. Fungal infections of lungs: The emerging scenario. Indian J Tuberculosis. 2004;51:63-69.
55. Johnson J. Pulmonary aspergillosis. Semin Respir Med. 1987;9: 87-199.
56. Roberts CM, Citron KM, Strickland B. Intrathoracic aspergilloma. Role of CT in diagnosis and treatment. Radiology 1987;165:123-28.
57. Neeld DA, Goodman LR, Gurney JW, et al. Computerized tomography in the evaluation of allergic bronchopulmonary aspergillosis. Am Rev Respir Dis. 1990;142:1200-05.
58. Patel RA, Sellami D, Gotway MB, et al. Hypersensitivity pneumonitis: Spectrum of imaging findings. JCAT. 2000; 24:965-70.
59. Fraser RS, Pare JAP, Eraser RG, Pare PD. Infectious Diseases of Lungs in Synopsis of Diseases of Chest (2nd edn). WB Saunders and Co; Philadelphia. 1994;332-54.
60. Wilson ES. Pleuropulmonary amebiasis. AJR. 1971;111:518- 24.
61. Kinura K, Stoopen M, Reeder MM, et al. Amebiasis: Modern diagnostic imaging with pathological and clinical correlation. Semin Roentgenol. 1997;32:250-75.
62. Shamsuzzaman SM, Haschiguchi Y. Thoracic amebiasis. Clin Chest Med. 2002;23:479-92.
63. Bean W. Recognition of ascariasis by routine chest or abdomen roentgenograms. AJR. 1965;94:379-84.
64. Gelpi AP, Mustafa A. Ascaiasis pneumonia. Am J Med. 1968;44:377-89.
65. Udwadia E. Tropical eosinophilia. Prog Respir Res. 1975;7:35-155.
66. Beggs I. The radiology of hydatid disease. AJR. 1985;145:639-48.
67. Von Sinner WN. Radiographic, CT and MRI spectrum of hydatid disease of chest: A pictorial essay. Eur Radiol. 1993;3:62-70.
68. Kervancioglu R, Bayram M, Elbeyli L. CT and MRI spectrum of hydatid disease. Acta Radiol. 1999;40:510-14.
69. Kokturk O, Ozturk C, Diren B, et al. Air bubble: A new diagnostic CT sign of perforated pulmonary hydatid cyst. Eur Radiol. 1999;9:1321-23.
70. Von Sinner WN. New diagnostic signs in hydatid disease; radiography, ultrasound, CT and MRI correlated to pathology. Em J Radiol. 1991;12:150-59.
71. Prieto A, Diaz A, Calvo J, et al. MR imaging of pulmonary hydatid disease. Eur J radiol. 1996;23:85-87.
72. Heffner JE. Infection of the pleural space. Clinics in Chest Medicine. 1999;20(3):607-20.
73. Blackmore CC Black WC, Dallas RV, et al. Pleural fluid volume estimation: A chest radiograph prediction rule. Acta Radiol. 1996;3:103.
74. Hirsh JH, Rogers JV, Mack LA. Real-time sonography of pleural opacities. AJR. 1981;136:297.
75. Nelson SW, Christoforidis AJ. Reversible bronchiectasis. Radiology. 1958;71:375.
76. Poole PS, Stark HE, Stark P. Necrotizing pneumonia, pulmonary abscess, and lung gangrene: multiple pathways to lung parenchymal destruction. Contemporary Diagnostic Radiology. 2011;34(13):1-6.

77. Reimel BA, Krishnadasen B, Cuschieri J, Klein MB, Gross J, Karmy-Jones R. Surgical management of acute necrotizing lung infections. Can Respir J. 2006;13:369–73. [PMC free article] [PubMed]
78. Penner C, Maycher B, Long R. Pulmonary gangrene: A complication of bacterial pneumonia. Chest. 1994;105:567-73. [PubMed]
79. Curry CA, Fish aEK, Buckley JA. Pulmonary gangrene: Radiological and pathologic correlation. South Med J. 1998;91:957–60. [PubMed]
80. Finich S, Chalmers JD. Brief clinical review: Non-responding pneumonia. EMJ Respir. 2014;2:104-11.
81. Kirtland SH, Winterbauer RH. Slowly resolving chronic and recurrent pneumonia. Clin Chest Med. 1991;12:303-18.
82. Kuru T, Lynch JP. Nonresolving or slowly resolving pneumonia. Clin Chest Med. 1999;20:623-51.
83. Jayaprakash B, Varkey V, Anithakumari K. Etiology and clinical outcome of non-resolving pneumonia in a tertiary care centre. J Assoc Physicians India. 2012;60:98-101.
84. Franquet T. Imaging of Pneumonia: Trends and algorithms. Eur Respir J. 2001;18:196-208.

CHAPTER

128

Pulmonary Manifestations in Immunocompromised Host

Mandeep Kang, Pankaj Gupta

INTRODUCTION

Immunocompromised hosts constitute a special group of patients who are predisposed to infections by both opportunistic and non-opportunistic organisms.[1] The number of individuals who are immunocompromised is growing steadily, not only because of the continuing human immunodeficiency virus/acquired immunodeficiency syndrome (HIV/AIDS) epidemic, but also due to the growing incidence of various kinds of malignancies and the increasing number of patients undergoing solid organ or bone marrow transplants. Pulmonary infections are a major cause of mortality and morbidity in this group of patients.[2-4] Diagnostic possibilities include infections (opportunistic or routine), hemorrhage, spread of underlying malignancy, chemotherapy or radiotherapy induced lung changes and conditions not directly related to the underlying disease process such as congestive heart failure or pulmonary embolism, therefore the development of a pulmonary infiltrate on the chest radiograph is an ominous sign which poses a considerable diagnostic challenge.[5]

This chapter will separately address two groups of patients which are: HIV/AIDS patients and non-HIV immunocompromised patients who have hematological malignancy or have recieved solid organ or hematopoietic stem cell transplantation.

HIV/AIDS

The epidemic of HIV and AIDS has affected the entire world. According to the World Health Organization (WHO) and Joint United Nations program on HIV/AIDS, it was estimated in 2007 that there are around 33 million people living with HIV infection throughout the world. Around twenty-five million deaths have occurred due to AIDS with opportunistic pulmonary infections accounting for a majority of these.[6] Pulmonary infections will occur in nearly all patients with HIV infection during the course of their illness at some time. HIV infection is associated with an increased risk for lung complications due to alterations in the host defenses in the lung, such as muco-ciliary functional abnormalities and impairment in the immune response to pathogens.[7] In the past several years, there have been various trends noted in the demographics as well as treatment of HIV patients, which have had an important impact on the incidence of various pulmonary complications.[3,8] A change in the epidemiology with higher rates of infection in women and children and lower rates of infection in intravenous drug abusers (IVDA) and homosexual or bisexual men has been reported. IVDA are far more likely to suffer recurrent *Staphylococcus aureus* infections, aspiration pneumonia, lung abscess, septic emboli and tuberculosis (TB). In IVDAs, the rates of bacterial pneumonia are more than twice of any other risk group, regardless of the CD4+ lymphocyte count. Tuberculosis is much more common in Africa and South-East Asia, and globally, is the major cause of mortality (13% according to estimates by the World Health Organization).[9] Kaposi's sarcoma (KS) is seen almost exclusively in homosexual males. In the subset of the patient population who have acquired the HIV infection through sexual contact, *Cytomegalovirus* (CMV) infection is seen more commonly.

With the introduction in 1989 of trimethoprim sulfamethoxazole (TMP-SMX) prophylaxis, there has been a marked reduction in the frequency of *Pneumocystis jeroveci pneumonia* (PCP), however opportunistic infections by atypical mycobacteria and CMV have increased in incidence.[8]

The introduction of combination antiretroviral therapy (ART) which effectively suppresses viral replication, has resulted in decreased viral loads and increased CD4+ lymphocyte counts thereby dramatically reducing the HIV-associated morbidity and mortality. Conversely, immune restoration which occurs with initiation of HAART has been associated with new clinical syndromes known variously as reversal syndrome, immune reconstitution syndrome or paradoxical response.[9]

Systematic Approach to Imaging Diagnosis

A systematic approach should be employed for the radiological evaluation of HIV/AIDS patients. The chest radiograph should be carefully analyzed for the pattern of abnormality.[10] This should then be integrated with the available demographic, clinical and laboratory information for interpretation. The clinical presentation of the patient is of vital importance as diseases which present acutely or in a more insidious fashion may demonstrate an identical pattern on the chest radiograph. Awareness of the CD4+ lymphocyte count is of critical importance as it predicts the vulnerability of the patient to specific opportunistic infections and malignancies.

CD4+ count less than 200 cells/mm^3 marks clinical AIDS in a HIV positive patient. If CD4+ counts are higher than 500 cells/mm^3, there is an increased risk of infection with virulent pathogens leading to recurrent community acquired bacterial pneumonias and reactivation TB. When the CD4+ counts are between 200 and 499 cells/mm^3, lymphoproliferative disorders and primary lung carcinoma are seen in addition to the above infections. PCP and disseminated TB occur with increasing frequency with a count less than 200/mm^3, however, the greatest risk of PCP is seen below a count of 100/mm^3. At profound levels of immune depression with CD4+ counts below 50 cells/mm^3, viral pneumonias (commonly CMV), atypical mycobacterial infection and disseminated fungal infections have a markedly increased frequency.[7,11]

Imaging Methods

After a thorough history and complete physical examination, the next steps in the evaluation of a symptomatic patient are a chest radiograph, sputum and various blood examinations. If the radiographic and clinical findings are nonspecific or unrevealing, computed tomography (CT) of the chest and fiberoptic bronchoscopy (FOB) with bronchoalveolar lavage (BAL) are the usual next steps. The indications for CT include: (i) evaluation of symptomatic patients with normal chest radiographs, (ii) characterization of abnormalities detected on the chest radiograph, (iii) assessment for complications of pneumonia such as development of empyema or lung abscess, (iv) staging AIDS related malignancies and (v) planning and guiding biopsy procedures. Computed tomography has been shown to be highly sensitive for the detection of disease and fairly specific in its characterization. Most importantly, a normal CT chest virtually rules out a pneumonia as the site of infection.[12,13] Bronchoalveolar lavage and transbronchial lung biopsy (TBLB) have been shown to have a high diagnostic yield for the diagnosis of both PCP and CMV infections.[14]

Radiological Pattern Approach to Diagnosis

A useful approach in the evaluation of a symptomatic patient is to identify the radiological pattern and correlate the differential diagnosis of the specific pattern with the clinical findings and CD4+ counts.

Normal Chest Radiograph

Chest radiographs may be normal in 10–39% of patients with proven PCP at initial presentation **(Figs. 1A and B)**.[3,4,8] About 6 to 17% of AIDS patients with pulmonary TB with positive sputum may also have normal radiographs.

Ground-glass Opacities

Ground-glass opacity (GGO) on high-resolution CT (HRCT) in a patient with HIV/AIDS is highly sensitive for the diagnosis of PCP and may be seen in 92% of patients **(Figs. 1A and B)**. Viral infections such as CMV or herpes may also present with GGO and tend to occur with severe degrees of immune depression. Lymphocytic interstitial pneumonia may also give rise to patchy GGO. In children, PCP presents at a much lower age (4–5 months) in comparison to lymphocytic interstitial pneumonitis (LIP). In comparison to children infected with PCP, children suffering from LIP generally tend to be older and less acutely ill.[16]

Consolidation

Focal segmental or lobar air space consolidation most likely represents a community acquired bacterial pneumonia. Multiple areas of consolidation may be seen in TB or bacterial pneumonias with unusual organisms such as *Nocardia* or *Rhodococcus*.[3,8]

Multiple Pulmonary Nodules

A miliary pattern characterized by 1–3 mm nodules diffusely scattered in the lung parenchyma most commonly represents

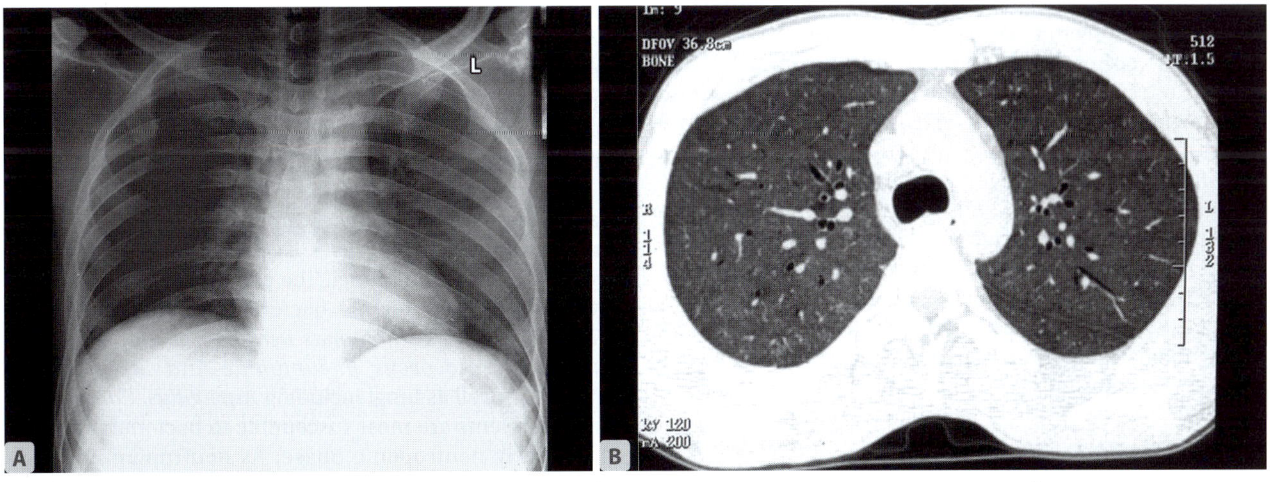

FIGS. 1A AND B: A 30-year-old HIV positive male with dry cough. (A) Chest radiograph is normal; (B) HRCT chest show disuse GGOs. Bronchoalveolar lavage demonstrated *Pneumocystis*.

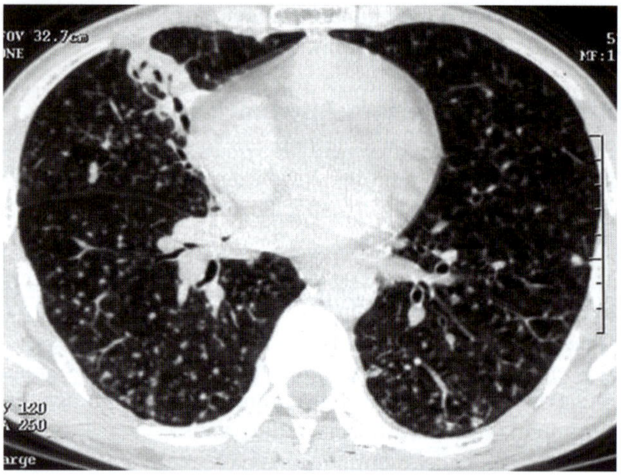

FIG. 2: A 23-year-old HIV positive male with fever and cough. High resolution CT chest show multiple, 1–2 mm miliary nodules randomly scattered in the pulmonary parenchyma. Note the sub-segmental atelectasis in the RML with bronchiectasis. Sputum was positive for acid-fast bacilli.

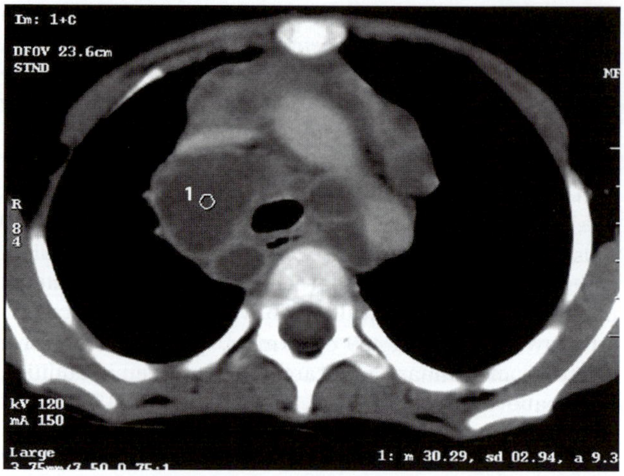

FIG. 3: A 40-year-old HIV positive female with fever and cough. Contrast-enhanced CT chest shows conglomerate, hypodense lymph nodes with rim enhancement in the pre- and paratracheal regions in a case of TB.

mycobacterial infection **(Fig. 2)**. In endemic areas, disseminated fungal infections such as *Histoplasma* and *Coccidioidomycosis* maybe the causative organisms. Larger nodules (<1 cm) associated with a reticular pattern are seen with CMV infections. *Cryptococcus* may also present with a reticulonodular pattern or as discrete nodules. Multiple subpleural nodules of 1–2 cm size with cavitation favor septic emboli. Larger nodules, associated with wedge-shaped, pleural based opacities are seen in invasive *aspergillosis*. These nodules may frequently show a 'halo' of surrounding GGO. Tuberculosis or atypical mycobacteria may also present with large nodules which are typically poorly marginated. Lymphoma may also present with large nodules as may metastases. The nodules in KS are typically clustered along the bronchovascular bundles.[3,7,8,11] A solitary pulmonary nodule with spiculated margins may represent a primary bronchogenic carcinoma.

Lymphadenopathy

The most common cause of hilar and/or mediastinal lymphadenopathy in a patient with AIDS are mycobacterial infections, either TB or atypical mycobacteria.[17] These lymph nodes classically show low density centers with rim enhancement post-contrast **(Fig. 3)**. Conversely, lymph nodes in KS and bacillary angiomatosis show intense enhancement reflecting their hypervascular nature. Mediastinal nodes with punctate calcifications are seen in disseminated *Pneumocystis* infection. Calcification may also be seen in the liver, kidneys and spleen in this situation. Unlike lymphoma in an immunocompetent host, lymphoma in an AIDS patient does not predominantly involve the lymph nodes, mediastinal or hilar lymphadenopathy is seen in only up to 25% of cases.

Pleural Effusion

The radiographic features of pleural effusion are generally unhelpful in narrowing the differential diagnosis. Large or massive pleural effusions with predominantly lymphocytes on cytology are due to TB, while hemorrhagic fluid is suggestive of Kaposi's sarcoma (KS).

NON-HIV IMMUNOCOMPROMISED HOSTS

The number of non-HIV immunocompromised patients has significantly increased in the last two decades due to increase in the number of patients receiving solid organ or hematopoietic stem cell transplants, advances in cytotoxic therapy for various malignancies and immunosuppressive therapy.[18]

Organ transplantation is the most important treatment in end stage liver, kidney, heart and lung diseases. The immunosuppression caused by the anti-rejection medications render the solid organ transplant recipient vulnerable to a wide variety of infections causing significant mortality and morbidity. This group of patients is at further risk of pneumonia for several reasons which are as follows: (i) prolonged hospitalization, (ii) endotracheal tube injury to the trachea, and (iii) impaired clearance of respiratory secretions due to anesthesia and diminished cough. Lung transplant recipients are also at increased risk due to denervation of the lung and surgically impaired mucociliary transport.[4]

Cytotoxic chemotherapy causes neutropenia. As the granulocyte count declines, the risk of infections increases and the patient becomes susceptible to infections by pyogenic bacteria and fungi. The common organisms in the setting of neutropenia are bacteria including *Escherichia coli, Klebsiella, Pseudomonas aeruginosa, Staphylococcus aureus, Streptococcus pneumoniae* and *Streptococcus viridians* as well as fungi including *Aspergillus, Candida* and *Mucor*. Patients are most susceptible to bacterial infections in the early neutropenic phase. As neutropenia persists, fungal infections become more common.[3,18] Chemotherapy also causes defects in the humoral immunity which are associated with infections with encapsulated bacteria such as *Streptococcus pneumoniae* and Gram negative organisms such as *Haemophilus influenzae, Neisseria meningitidis* and *Pseudomonas aeruginosa*.[2]

Cellular immunity mediated by T-lymphocytes is affected in patients undergoing chemotherapy and solid organ transplant recipients. Defects in cellular immunity renders the patient susceptible to more unusual pathogens, including viruses (CMV, *varicella, herpes zoster*), protozoa, fungi (*Pneumocystis jirovecii, Aspergillus, Cryptococcus, Histoplasma*) and bacteria (*Legionella, Nocardia asteroides*).

Following solid organ transplant, in the first 4 weeks, infections are usually caused by nosocomial bacteria, or fungi in patients with prolonged neutropenia. At one to three months post-transplant, opportunistic pathogens such as PCP or CMV increase in frequency. One-half to all of the seronegative patients who receive a graft from a seropositive donor suffer from primary CMV infection. In the late post-transplant phase (>3 months), PCP remains a concern but mycobacteria and nocardia should also be considered.[13,18,19] After 6 months, the degree of immunosuppression required to prevent graft rejection dictates the frequency of infections.

In immunocompromised patients with hematological malignancies, the pulmonary involvement occurs in many ways, viz. (i) infection (ii) recurrence of the underlying hematological disease, (iii) adverse reaction to drugs, (iv) unrelated processes such as pulmonary emboli and (v) combination of the above mentioned processes. One-third of patients with hematological malignancies suffer a combination of at least two processes such as pneumonia caused by two different pathogens or a drug related pulmonary complication occurring along with infection. A reasonable differential diagnosis may be considered if one is aware of the host defenses that get compromised. Suppression in the number of granulocytes, B-lymphocytes, or T-lymphocytes is the most common pattern of impairment, though multiple types of cells may be frequently affected. A critical reduction in the number of each of these cell types predisposes to infection by a particular group of organisms. In these patients, most pulmonary complications, including drug-induced pulmonary disease and pulmonary emboli, are associated with fever that mimics infection. Noninfectious causes comprise one-fourth of the pulmonary complications.[20] With improved survival the late effects of treatment like second malignancy are becoming more common. Lately, due to better regimens, the incidence of radiation related complications have decreased.

Hematopoietic stem cell transplantation (HSCT) is now the treatment of choice for malignant diseases such as leukemias, aplastic anemia and congenital immunodeficiency syndromes. Pulmonary complications in these patients can be divided into two broad categories, i.e. HSCT nonspecific and HSCT specific complications. Hematopoietic stem cell transplantation specific pulmonary complications may develop in approximately half of transplant recipients.[21] Stem cells for HSCT may be obtained from patients own blood (autologous), related or unrelated donors (allogeneic), or may be obtained from peripheral blood, bone marrow or cord blood.[22] Complications related to the allogeneic HSCT are due to the toxicity of the conditioning regimen that includes chemotherapy with or without radiation.[23]

Imaging Approach

Chest radiographs remain the basic imaging investigation for the diagnosis of suspected pulmonary infection. However, early in the course of disease, chest radiographs maybe normal. Computed tomography has a higher sensitivity and allows diagnosis in the setting of a normal chest radiograph in patients with a high clinical suspicion for pneumonia. In a study by Heussel et al. 60% of pulmonary infections in febrile neutropenia were diagnosed by CT scans 5 days before radiographic abnormalities became evident.[24]

BACTERIAL INFECTIONS

Bacterial infections are responsible for most infections in HIV positive patients, having surpassed PCP. *S. pneumoniae* and *H. influenzae* account for most episodes of community acquired pneumonia in the general population. Recent hospitalization, antibiotic or steroid therapy are the predisposing factors for *Pseudomonas* infection. Unusual organisms such as *Rhodococcus* or *Bartonella* can also infect patients with AIDS. The radiological pattern of bacterial pneumonia does not differ from an immune intact host and consists of single or multiple sites of consolidation in a segmental or lobar distribution **(Figs. 4A and B)**. However, bilateral patchy opacities may be seen with certain organisms such as *Pseudomonas*. In contrast to immune intact individuals, there is a higher propensity for bilateral and multilobar disease in immunocompromised patients with a tendency for rapid progression as well as development of local and systemic complications, including cavitation, abscess formation and bacteremia. Pleural effusions may also occur.

In IVDAs, *Staphylococcus aureus* and Gram negative bacteria are common causes of generalized sepsis with secondary pneumonia. Septic embolic appear as multiple, bilateral, 1–2 cm nodules which frequently cavitate and are more numerous in the lower lobes.

Nocardia infection may be seen in solid organ transplant recipients in the late post-transplant phase (more than 1 year post heart-lung transplant).[4,25] It is also seen in diabetics and patients receiving steroid therapy. It most commonly appears as a solitary nodule or nodular infiltrate with cavitation. Pleural effusion occurs in up to 50% of cases.

Pyogenic airways diseases viz. infectious bronchitis, bronchiolitis and bronchiectasis has increased in frequency in HIV positive patients. Chest radiographic findings in extensive bronchiolitis present an interstitial pattern with reticulonodular opacities distributed in a symmetrical fashion which mimics PCP. On CT, small nodular and branching Y-and V- shaped centrilobular opacities (tree-in-bud appearance) are seen which represent bronchioles impacted with inflammatory secretions **(Fig. 5)**. Similar imaging findings may be noted in viral and mycobacterial infections.

Bronchiectasis is commonly seen in association with HIV infection. It is thought to be a complication of prior lung infections. However, it has also been described in patients

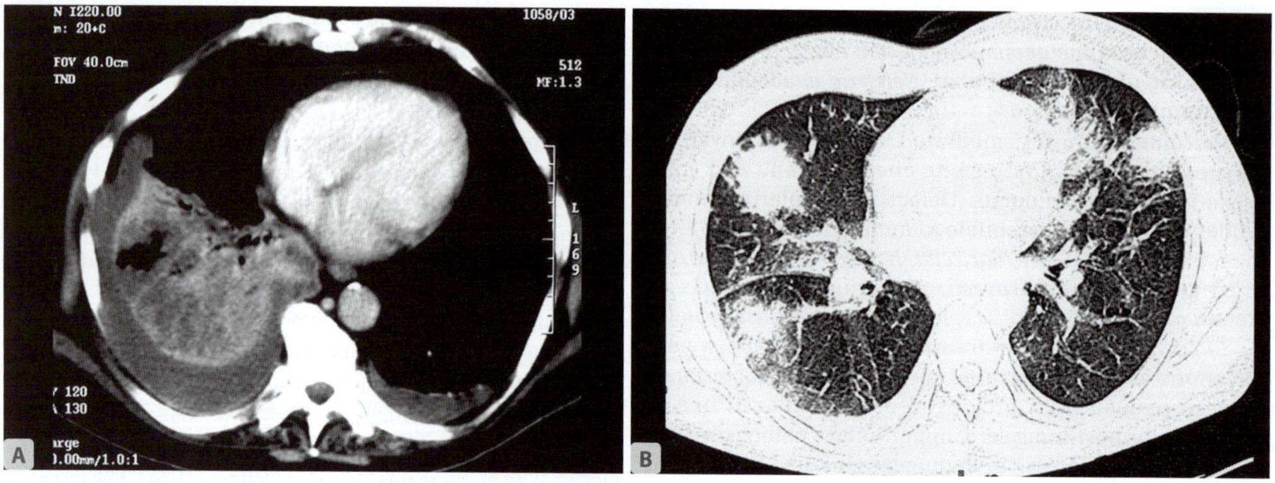

FIGS. 4A AND B: Bacterial pneumonia. (A) Airspace consolidation with air bronchograms and eccentric cavitation with associated pleural effusion; (B) Multifocal, bilateral, patchy airspace consolidation. Sputum culture revealed *Pseudomonas aeruginosa*.

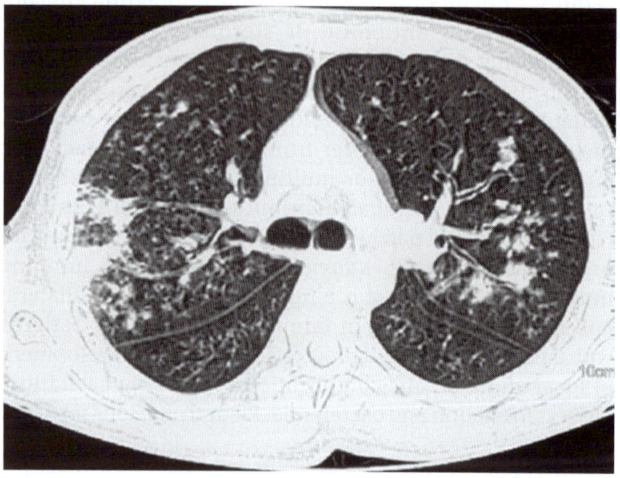

FIG. 5: A 50-year-old male post-chemotherapy presented with fever and dyspnea. High-resolution CT chest shows multifocal, patchy consolidation with centrilobular nodules and tree-in-bud appearance. Sputum was positive for *Streptococcus viridans*.

without history of previous infections and may represent an accelerated form of lung injury.[7]

Bacterial pneumonia affect 20–50% of HSCT recipients in the neutropenic phase.[26] Gram-negative organisms from the oral mucosa or gastrointestinal tract have been typically associated. However, more recently, Gram-positive organisms such as *Staphylococcus aureus* and coagulase negative *Staphylococcus* represent 60–70% of infections. The radiographic appearances include consolidation, ground-glass opacity, centrilobular, acinar and lobular opacities.

PNEUMOCYSTIS JIROVECII PNEUMONIA

Pneumocystis jirovecii is classified as a fungus and is an opportunistic eukaryote.[27] The incidence of *pneumocystis jirovecii* pneumonia (PCP) has decreased secondary to improved prophylaxis regimens and combined ART, however it still remains one of the most common AIDS defining illnesses as well as the most common cause of serious pulmonary infections in HIV positive patients.[3,27] In fact, at least one episode of infection with PCP will occur in most (more than 70%) of the patients with HIV/AIDS during the course of their illness. PCP occurs twice as frequently in homosexual males versus IVDAs. Also it affects males at twice the frequency of females. Although it can occur at any level of immune depression, it typically occurs at CD4+ counts below 200 cells/mm^3.

PCP has been reported in 33% of heart-lung transplant recipients, 3–10% of heart transplant, 0–11% of liver transplant and 6–14% of kidney transplant recipients. However, prophylaxis with TMP-SMX has dramatically reduced the incidence of PCP. The infection can occur at any time following solid organ transplant but commonly occurs in the 4th–6th month post-transplant and carries a mortality rate of 47%.[4,15]

PCP also affects patients with hematological malignancies undergoing intensive chemotherapy or HSCT. Its incidence is reported to be less than 10% in patients receiving HSCT.[6]

Clinically, affected patients present with a low-grade fever, dry cough and dyspnea. The initial symptoms may be subtle in HIV infected patients and be present even up to several weeks before diagnosis. This is in contrast to PCP in non-HIV patients in whom the presentation is more acute.[28] *Pneumocystis jirovecii* pneumonia classically presents on a chest radiograph with a bilateral, peri-hilar or diffuse, symmetric, interstitial pattern which may be ground-glass, reticular or granular in appearance. These opacities may progress to air space consolidation. The typical appearance on HRCT is extensive GGOs which histopathologically correspond to the presence of intra-alveolar exudates comprising fluid, debris and organisms **(Fig. 6)**. The ground-glass attenuation shows a patchy or geographical distribution with sparing of the subpleural regions. There may be a mosaic pattern with involved secondary lobules seen adjacent to uninvolved lung **(Figs. 7A and B)**. The parenchymal opacities have a predilection for the upper lobes which was earlier thought to be due to prophylaxis with aerosolized pentamidines. However, this upper lobe predominance is still prevalent in the present era of TMP-SMX prophylaxis. Thickening of the interlobular septal lines occurs in the subacute phase of the disease. Thin-walled cystic lesions may develop at any time during the course of the illness with an incidence of 10–34%. Cystic PCP is associated with a 35% risk for spontaneous pneumothoraces which are often refractory to treatment and may require surgical intervention. Although the radiographic abnormalities may clear within two weeks of therapy, it is not uncommon to see residual fibrosis or irregular cystic spaces.

Some patients may develop clinical symptoms and signs over months to years which is referred to as chronic PCP. This appears radiographically as thickened septal lines with honeycombing and traction bronchiectasis.[3,4,7,8] Rare presentations of PCP (5–10%) include focal lobar consolidation, nodules, mediastinal lymphadenopathy, bronchiectasis or pleural effusion.

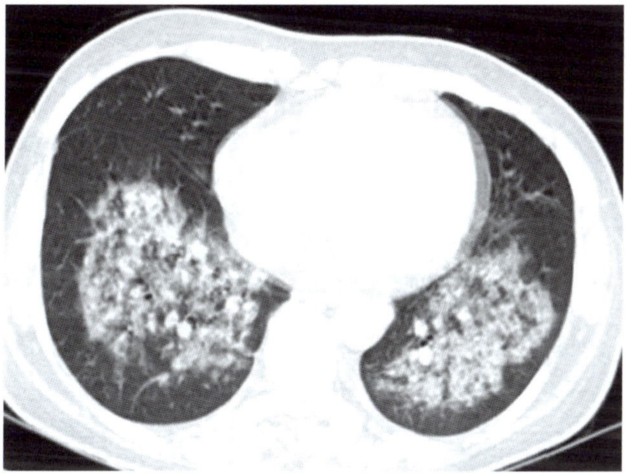

FIG. 6: A 45-year-old HIV positive lady presented with cough and dyspnea. High resolution CT chest shows typical, diffuse GGOs with subpleural sparing in both lower lobes in a case of *Pneumocystis* pneumonia.

MYCOBACTERIAL INFECTIONS

HIV/AIDS Patients

It has been estimated that there is a 50–200 fold increased risk of contracting TB by a HIV positive individual as compared to the general population in non-endemic areas. This risk increases for IVDAs and patients in endemic areas such as India and sub-Saharan Africa. Tuberculosis may accelerate the progression of AIDS. Prompt diagnosis and treatment are therefore critical. Tuberculosis may affect patients with HIV infection at any stage, however, the imaging findings are determined by the level of immune suppression. Early in the course of disease, when the CD4+ counts are >200 cells/mm^3, it usually manifests with the traditional pattern of reactivation TB with upper lobe opacities with cavitation and nodular bronchogenic spread **(Fig. 8)**. Pleural effusions are common. In severely immunocompromised individuals (CD4+ <200 cells/mm^3), the imaging appearance is reminiscent of primary TB with parenchymal consolidation and mediastinal lymphadenopathy which typically shows low attenuation centers with peripheral rim enhancement. A miliary pattern is also common. Atypical findings may be seen including diffuse infiltrates, multiple nodules, frequent middle and lower lobe involvement or even normal chest radiographs (14–20%). Compared to immunocompetent hosts, AIDS patients infected with TB are more likely to present with extra-pulmonary involvement (genitourinary system, bone marrow, central nervous system and lymph nodes) or systemic dissemination **(Fig. 9)**. These manifestations increase with increasing degrees of immune compromise: 70% of AIDS patients show extrathoracic disease when the CD4+ counts are <100 cells/ mm^3 as compared to 44% when CD4+ count is >300 cells/ mm^3. Almost half of the patients with extra-pulmonary involvement will show a miliary

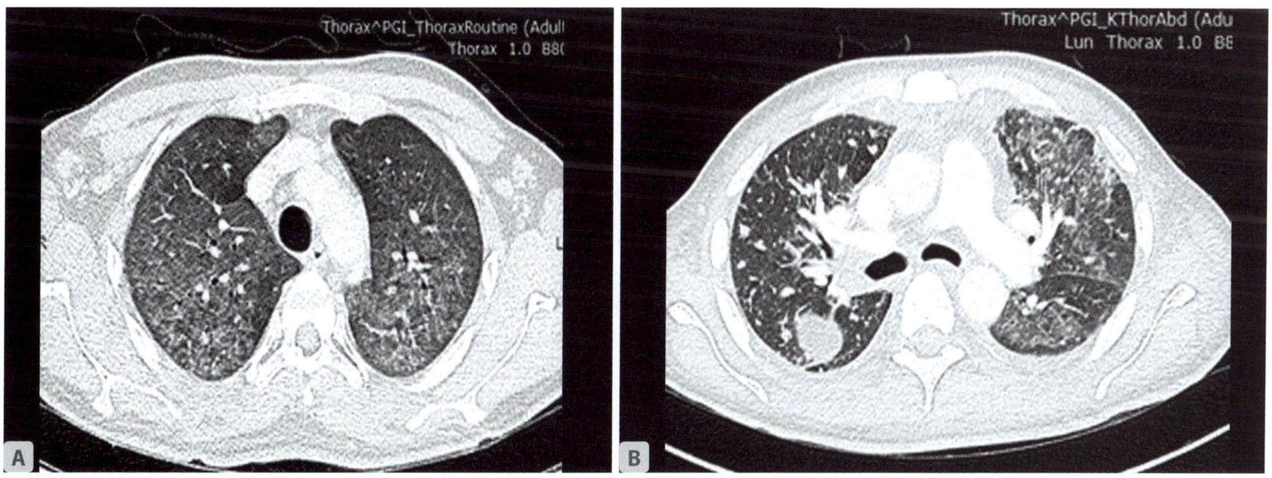

FIGS. 7A AND B: (A) A 30-year-old HIV positive male with dry cough of insidious onset. High resolution CT chest reveals diffuse GGOs with interstitial septal thickening giving a crazy paving appearance; (B) A 42-year-old HIV positive male with dry cough and low-grade fever. HRCT chest demonstrates involvement of the secondary lobules with sparing of adjacent lobules in the left lung. Note the nodules and focal consolidation in the right lung. Bronchoalveolar lavage demonstrated *Pneumocystis* in both the patients.

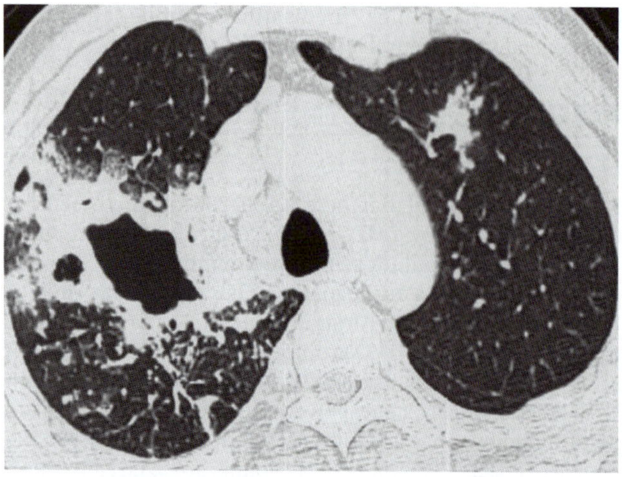

FIG. 8: A 32-year-old HIV positive lady presented with fever and productive cough. High resolution CT chest shows patchy, multifocal areas of consolidation with cavitation. Sputum was positive for acid-fast bacilli.

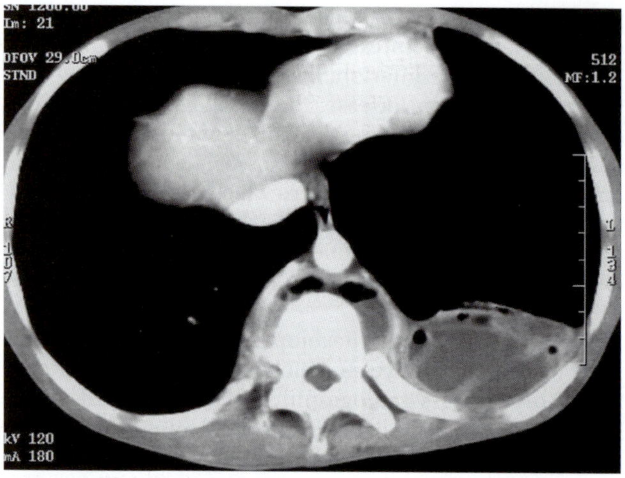

FIG. 9: A 23-year-old HIV positive male presented with fever, cough and back pain. Contrast-enhanced CT chest shows pre- and paraspinal fluid collections with multiple septae and enhancing walls due to spinal TB, miliary nodules were seen in the lungs.

pattern in the lungs.[29] Tuberculosis can involve the central airways with stenosis and wall thickening. Involvement of the lower airways manifests as bronchiectasis or tree-in-bud appearance.

In patients who are put on ART, there may be worsening or appearance of new lymphadenopathy, lung parenchymal opacities or pleural effusion accompanied by fever. This is referred to as the immune reconstitution or the paradoxical syndrome. Patients who are severely symptomatic may benefit from steroid therapy.

Atypical mycobacterial infections are usually caused by *Mycobacterium avium intracellulare* (MAI) and less frequently by *Mycobacterium kansasii*. These usually occur when the CD4+ count is <50 cells/mm^3. *Mycobacterium avium intracellulare* infection commonly presents as disseminated disease with the gastrointestinal tract being the normal portal of entry. Imaging features are ill-defined nodules, multifocal consolidation, and cavities. Mediastinal lymphadenopathy may occur. The chest radiograph may be normal in roughly 20% of cases. *M. kansasii* commonly presents as focal alveolar consolidation.

The reversal syndrome has been recently described in HIV patients with MAI who are started on ART. This manifests as an acute febrile episode associated with new or enlarging lymphadenopathy.

HIV Negative Immunocompromised Patients

Solid organ transplant recipients are at increased risk of contracting TB with 50–100 times the incidence in the general population in the west. However, studies from India have reported a higher incidence, reflecting the endemic nature of the disease.[30] The infection may appear at any time after the surgery ranging from 1–96 months following transplant. Steroids and other anti-rejection medications affect cell-mediated immunity which is the primary means of controlling and eradicating mycobacterial infections. There is a high (40–64%) incidence of disseminated disease with pulmonary

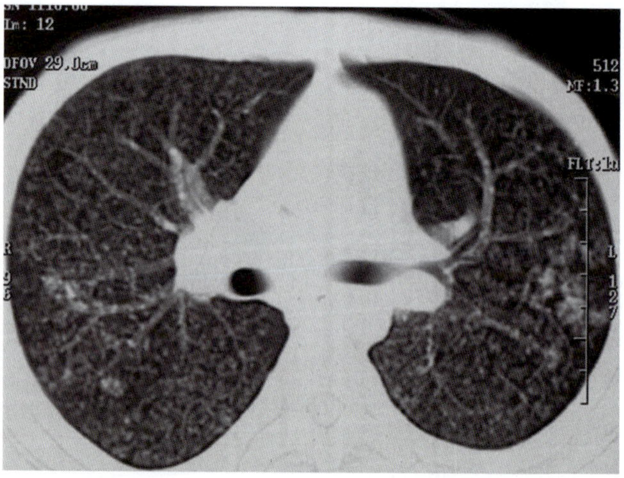

FIG. 10: A 35-year-old renal transplant recipient presented with fever three months after transplant surgery. High resolution CT chest shows multiple, 1–3 mm, randomly distributed nodules in both lungs with tree-in-bud appearance at places. Sputum was positive for acid-fast bacilli.

infection seen in approximately 40% of cases. The rate of progression is also faster than in the general population with higher morbidity and mortality.

The imaging appearance consists of cavitary upper lobe opacities in about one-third of patients. Another third demonstrate a miliary pattern **(Fig. 10)**. The rest may show a solitary lower lobe opacity, large nodule or pleural effusion. Lymphadenopathy is uncommon (3.5%).

Nontubercular mycobacterial infection is usually with MAI or *M. kansasii*. These account for a higher fraction of mycobacterial infections in the transplant recipient: 25–43% of mycobacterial infections as compared to 5–10% in the general population. These usually present as multiple, moderate sized pulmonary nodules. Miliary nodules may be seen and are associated with a high mortality.

VIRAL INFECTIONS

Respiratory viral infections are commonly seen in HIV/AIDS patients with CD4+ counts <50 cells/mm^3. Cytomegalovirus is the most common viral pathogen with a reported incidence of up to 90% in advanced HIV disease.

The herpes group of viruses are the predominant viral pathogens in solid organ transplant recipients. Since these are most often reactivation infections of dormant organisms residing in the host or the transplant organ, they occur in the first few months post-transplant.

Although cytomegalovirus infection affects almost two-third of allogeneic HSCT recipients, CMV pneumonia develops in less than one-third of patients.[21] It typically occurs in the early phase and is associated with a high mortality rate of up to 85%. Infection with CMV is associated with increased susceptibility to bacterial, fungal and protozoal superinfections, increased risk of rejection and overall mortality.

The imaging appearance of CMV pneumonitis is classically that of diffuse ground-glass or patchy interstitial opacities resembling PCP. With severe infection, diffuse alveolar infiltrates may appear which mimic adult respiratory distress syndrome. Pulmonary nodules may be seen in about two-thirds of cases **(Fig. 11)**. Airway disease which manifests as bronchiectasis, bronchial wall thickening and bronchiolitis may be seen in a third of cases.

Herpes simplex (HSV-1, HSV-2) pneumonia is uncommon with a reported incidence of 0.8–10% in solid organ transplant recipients and 0.2% in AIDS patients.[3,4] The chest radiograph will demonstrate multifocal or diffuse consolidation. *Varicella zoster* is also a reactivation infection in the solid organ transplant recipient and usually manifests as disseminated disease. 5–15 mm, diffuse, ill-defined, nodular densities with fuzzy outlines are seen on chest radiographs.

Adenovirus and *respiratory syncitial virus* are common causes of viral community acquired pneumonia. Radiographs may show interstitial opacities, alveolar consolidation, nodules or pleural effusion.

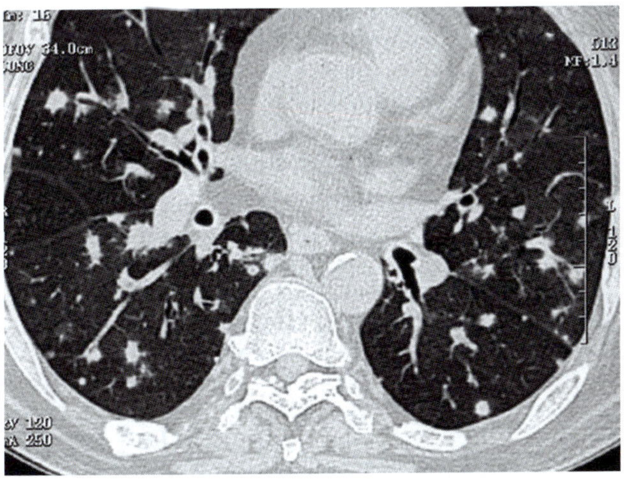

FIG. 11: A 42-year-old HIV positive male with fever. High resolution CT chest shows multiple, 5–8 mm nodules randomly distributed in both the lungs. Bronchoalveolar lavage showed CMV. Later autopsy confirmed cytoplasmic inclusion bodies.

FUNGAL INFECTIONS

Fungal pneumonias characteristically develop in patients who are neutropenic (from cytotoxic drugs and transplant recipients) or on corticosteroid therapy. The infecting organisms fall into two categories which are as follows: those that occur exclusively in immunocompromised hosts such as *Aspergillus, Candida* and *Mucor* species and endemic fungi with increased virulence in immunocompromised hosts such as *Histoplasma, Coccidioides, Cryptococcus* and *Blastomyces* species. Invasive aspergillosis and disseminated candidiasis are the most common agents, accounting for 80% of fungal infections in solid organ transplant recipients. Most will occur (80%) within two months post-transplant. The incidence varies from 5% in kidney transplant to 40% among liver transplant patients.

Fungal pneumonias are relatively uncommon in AIDS occurring in less than 5% of patients with the most common pathogen being *Cryptococcus*. The incidence of *Aspergillus* infection is increasing and almost exclusively occurs in AIDS patients who are neutropenic due to drugs such as zidovudine or ganciclovir or on steroids. Affected individuals are generally in an advanced stage of immune depression with CD4+ counts <50/mm^3. Although meningitis is the most common manifestation of *Cryptococcus* infections, active pulmonary infection is present in 40% of patients with cryptococcosis.

Fungal pneumonias are also common in patients undergoing chemotherapy for hematological malignancies during and following HSCT. Neutropenia is the most important risk factor.[28] Most common pathogen is *Aspergillus,* while *Mucor, Candida,* and *Cryptococcus* may also occur. *Aspergillus* infection has the greatest propensity to occur when the peripheral white cell count falls to less than 1,000/mm^3.

The radiographic abnormalities in angio-invasive aspergillosis consist of nodular or wedge-shaped opacities, frequently abutting the pleural surfaces. These often cavitate reflecting the angioinvasive nature of the fungus and may show central low density areas or the air crescent sign **(Fig. 12)**. The CT "halo" sign refers to GGOs surrounding a nodular opacity representing a rim of hemorrhage due to thrombosis within the adjacent vessels caused by the fungus and is an early sign of disease **(Fig. 13)**.[31] Although considered to be characteristic of angio-invasive aspergillus, the "halo" sign may also be seen with *Mucor, Candida,* CMV infections and Wegener's granulomatosis.[32] The "air-crescent" sign is seen when there is resorption of the necrotic tissue by returning neutrophils and is therefore is a relatively late sign, representing recovery from the infection.[33] Necrotizing tracheobronchial aspergillosis may be present in 10–30% of patients and may be seen on CT as nodular tracheal or bronchial wall thickening, or non-specific findings of bronchopneumonia.

Pulmonary mucormycosis may be seen in 0.2% of transplant recipients and is clinically and radiologically indistinguishable from *Aspergillus* infection. Pulmonary infection with *Candida* is rare, usually occurring as part of a disseminated infection. The radiologic appearances are nonspecific and consist of diffuse air-space consolidation or single or multiple, nodular infiltrates resembling *Aspergillus*.

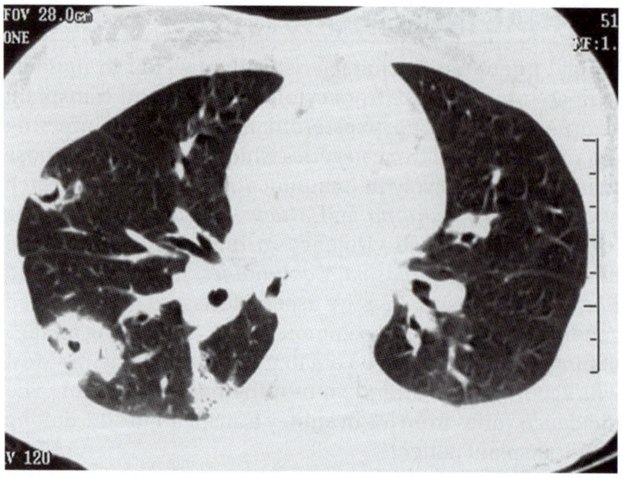

FIG. 12: A 28-year-old male presented with fever and chest pain following chemotherapy. High resolution CT chest shows multiple nodules with cavitations and air-crescent sign with wedge-shaped areas of consolidation. Computed tomography guided fine needle aspiration cytology revealed *Aspergillus*.

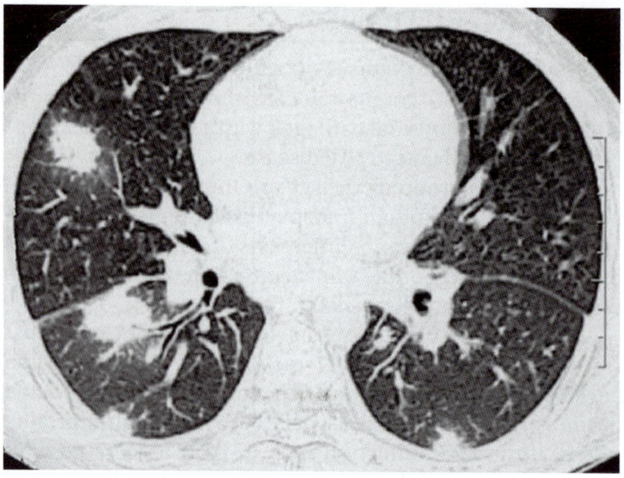

FIG. 13: A 40-year-old male (post-renal transplant) presented with fever and dyspnea. High resolution CT chest demonstrates multiple, bilateral, large nodules with surrounding ground-glass attenuation—the CT halo sign. Bronchoalveolar lavage revealed *Aspergillus*.

Single or multiple, well-defined nodules with or without cavitation is the common radiological appearance of infection with *Cryptococcus*. Adenopathy and pleural effusion may be present. Atypical findings include diffuse pulmonary infiltrates, miliary nodules and areas of ground-glass haze.

Radiographic features in histoplasmosis include diffuse small nodules (usually <3 mm in size), miliary nodules or larger nodules around 1cm in size. Small pleural effusions and mediastinal lymphadenopathy may be seen. Chest radiographs may be normal in 35–50% of patients. In patients with coccidiomycosis, diffuse, small, nodular opacities are the most common radiographic manifestation. Thin-walled cavities which are characteristically seen in immunocompetent individuals are uncommon in the immune compromised host. Reports of infection with blastomycosis are rare. Pulmonary findings include focal alveolar infiltrates or bilateral patchy or nodular opacities.

NONINFECTIOUS MANIFESTATIONS OF AIDS

Kaposi's Sarcoma

Kaposi's sarcoma (KS) is a malignancy which almost exclusively occurs in bisexual and homosexual males with AIDS. It is also known to affect certain ethnic groups. Its incidence is decreasing in recent years due to greater awareness of safe sex habits and the introduction of ART.[33] The CD4+ counts in patients with KS are generally <100 cells/mm^3.

Kaposi's sarcoma is a multisystem disease that affects the skin, lymph nodes, lungs and the gastrointestinal tract. Characteristic findings of pulmonary KS are nodular thickening along the bronchovascular bundles, growing from the perihilar region to the periphery. The nodules may become coalescent, leading to dense air-space consolidation. Pleural effusion occurs in 30–89% of cases and may be unilateral or bilateral. Mediastinal lymphadenopathy is uncommon but when present, demonstrates characteristic enhancement following intravenous iodinated contrast.[34]

On MR, KS lesions demonstrate increased signal intensity on T1 weighted images, markedly reduced signal intensity on T2 weighted images with intense enhancement following gadolinium administration. On nuclear scanning, KS lesions are thallium avid, however, in contrast to infectious conditions they do not take up gallium, thereby allowing differentiation between the two conditions.

Lymphoma

Acquired immunodeficiency syndrome related lymphoma occurs in AIDS patients at an advanced stage of immune depression when CD4+ counts are <50 cells/mm^3. Most cases consist of non-Hodgkin's lymphoma, usually of high grade with an aggressive nature. Intrathoracic involvement is seen in 10% of cases and is typically extra-nodal. Pleural effusions are the most common radiographic abnormality. Diffuse, well-defined nodules, focal consolidation or mediastinal lymphadenopathy may also be seen.

Lymphocystic Interstitial Pneumonitis

Lymphocystic interstitial pneumonitis is a lymphoproliferative disorder characterized by infiltration of the pulmonary interstitium by lymphocytes, histiocytes and plasma cells. It is much more common in the pediatric population. The radiographic appearance consists of a diffuse, micronodular, interstitial pattern. On HRCT, the most common finding is of GGOs along with poorly defined centrilobular nodules. Cystic air spaces and interstial thickening may also be seen.

Post-transplant Lymphoproliferative Disorder

Post-transplant lymphoproliferative disorder is a spectrum of lymphoproliferative abnormalities ranging from a benign febrile illness with lymphadenopathy to a rapidly fatal malignant lymphoma. This may develop in 1–10% of transplant patients. The Epstein-Barr virus appears to be causally related to the development of PTLD. With current immunosuppressive regimes, the peak incidence of PTLD is in the third month following transplant.

Radiographically, PTLD manifests as one or multiple, uniform, non-enhancing masses in large organs including the lung, liver, kidney, bowel and brain. Lymphadenopathy may be seen in 15–37% of cases, either in isolation or in association with the organ masses. Endobronchial masses resulting in atelectasis have also been reported.[17]

NONINFECTIOUS MANIFESTATIONS IN HSCT

Noninfectious lung injury has emerged as a major cause of morbidity and mortality due to decline in infectious complications due to the widespread use of prophylactic broad spectrum antibiotics. The frequency of noninfectious complications is similar in allogeneic and autologous HSCT.[36] Definitive diagnosis of noninfectious complications is challenging as the clinical manifestations overlap with those of the infections and the difficulty in obtaining a histological diagnosis. Imaging studies particularly HRCT play a major role in the management of these patients. Noninfectious complications usually follow a time-line due to the underlying immunological status of the host. The neutropenic phase following HSCT lasts from 2 to 3 weeks. After allogeneic HSCT, the immunosuppressive phase continues for 1 year. This is divided into an early (up to 100 days) and a late phase which continues for one year or more.[37]

PRE-ENGRAFTMENT PERIOD

Noninfectious complications that occur during neutropenic (also known as pre-engraftment period) include idiopathic pulmonary syndrome (IPS), pulmonary edema, diffuse alveolar hemorrhage (DAH), and periengraftment respiratory distress syndrome (PERDS).[38]

Idiopathic Pulmonary Syndrome

It is defined as a diffuse lung injury without an infectious cause. Predisposing factors are pre-transplant chemotherapy and total body irradiation. It carries a high mortality. It progresses from an acute exudative to a subacute proliferative to a chronic fibrotic phase. HRCT findings are those of diffuse alveolar damage manifesting as focal or diffuse ground-glass opacity with density gradient towards the dependant regions. Consolidation is less common. Chronic phase is characterized by traction bronchiectasis and honeycombing. HRCT findings are thus nonspecific and IPS remains a diagnosis of exclusion.[39,40]

Pulmonary Edema

It is a common complication with a rapid onset, usually occurring in the 2nd or 3rd week after HSCT. Underlying mechanisms include GVHD, cardiac or renal dysfunction secondary to chemotherapy regimens, pulmonary vasculature hyperpermeability induced by total body irradiation, sepsis, cyclosporine A or fluid overload.[3,23.] CXR suggests a diagnosis when there are diffuse interstitial markings, peribronchial cuffing, perihilar haziness, ground-glass appearance and vascular prominence. HRCT features include perihilar ground-glass opacity or consolidation, thickening of interlobular septa, enlargement of pulmonary vessels and pleural effusions **(Fig. 14)**.

Diffuse Alveolar Hemorrhage

Diffuse alveolar hemorrhage (DAH) is the commonest noninfectious pulmonary complication in leukemia.[35] Around 20% of HSCT patients may develop DAH in the neutropenic phase.[21] The manifestations of DAH are secondary to pulmonary vessel damage by acute GVHD, pre-transplantation chemotherapy or total body irradiation. Clinical presentation is nonspecific, mild hemoptysis occurs in about two-third of the patients; frank hemoptysis is rare.[34] It carries a high mortality rate of about 80%. Early diagnosis and prompt steroid therapy improves survival. Bronchoalveolar lavage (BAL) may aid the diagnosis by demonstrating hemosiderin laden macrophages. Radiological findings are nonspecific. HRCT findings include widespread ground-glass opacity or consolidation with interlobular septal thickening (crazy-paving appearance) **(Fig. 15)**. The peripheral lungs are spared.

Peri-engraftment Respiratory Distress Syndrome

Peri-engraftment respiratory distress syndrome (PERDS) presents with diffuse capillary leak, cutaneous rash, and fever that occurs during the engraftment and neutrophil recovery phases. It is thought to result from proinflammatory cytokines released during engraftment. Autologous HSCT has a greater incidence of this complication. The HRCT findings of interlobular septal thickening with bilateral ground-glass opacities and perihilar or peribronchial

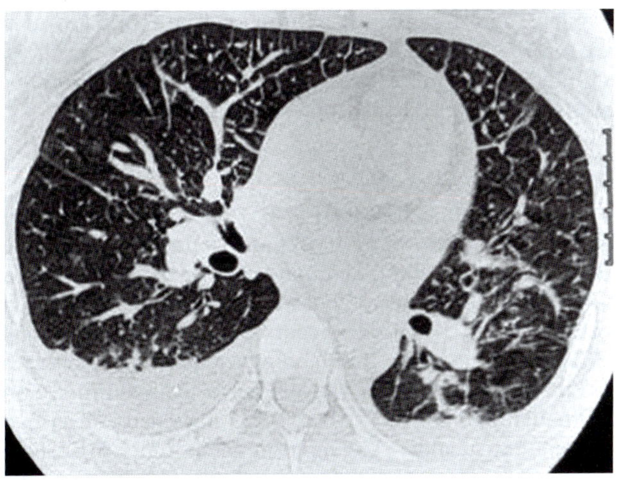

FIG. 14: A 38-year-old female following HSCT developed breathlessness. HRCT shows perihilar ground-glass opacity, thickening of interlobular septa, enlargement of pulmonary vessels and pleural effusion suggestive of pulmonary edema.

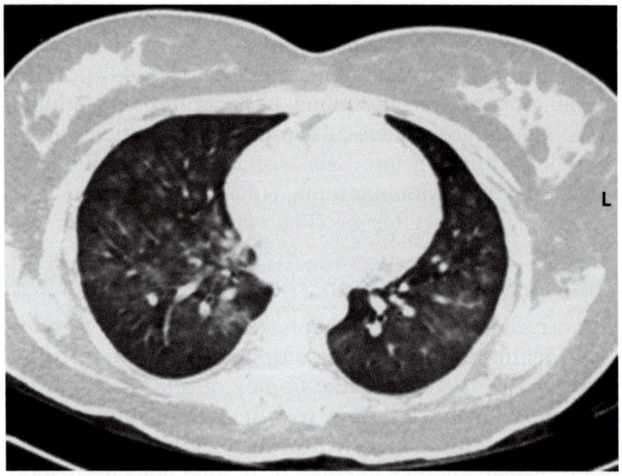

FIG. 15: A 28-year-old female with leukemia following HSCT complained of streaky hemoptysis. HRCT chest shows diffuse GGOs due to diffuse alveolar hemorrhage.

consolidation and pleural effusions are indistinguishable from that of pulmonary edema and acute respiratory distress syndrome.[38]

EARLY POST-TRANSPLANT PERIOD

During the early post-transplant period (30 to 100 days after HSCT), the neutrophil count has recovered. Impaired cellular and humoral immunity however persists. Reconstitution of the immune system leads to a reduction in the frequency of infectious complications as well. Noninfectious pulmonary complications during this period include acute GVHD, acute radiation injury and rarely, pulmonary cytolytic thrombi.

Drug-induced Lung Injury

Drug-induced lung injury occurs in around 10% patients with hematopoietic stem cell transplant. There are variable patterns of injury including nonspecific interstitial pneumonia, hypersensitivity pneumonitis, diffuse alveolar damage, and organizing pneumonia. The HRCT features are nonspecific and include diffuse ground-glass opacities, subpleural or peribronchial consolidation, centrilobular nodules and interlobular septal thickening.[38]

Acute GVHD

Graft versus host disease (GVHD) is a major cause of morbidity and mortality in patients following allogeneic HSCT and is secondary to immune reaction of the donor cells to the host tissues. Autologous transplant are not associated with acute GVHD. GVHD occurs in 20–75% of allogeneic HSCT recipients. Skin, liver, and gastrointestinal system are the primary targets. Lung involvement is uncommon and a broad spectrum of GVHD changes have been described histopathologically—ranging from acute injury to chronic irreversible damage.[41] HRCT demonstrates nonspecific changes including diffuse interstitial and alveolar opacities that mimic pulmonary edema.

Acute Radiation Pneumonitis

This complication occurs in patients who receive radiation therapy for intrathoracic lymphoma. Most patients are asymptomatic. More-over with modern techniques of radiation, the radiation related acute toxicity has reduced. The early stage changes (8-12 weeks after completion) are characterized by cellular infiltration composed predominantly of macrophages. On imaging, there is patchy consolidation in the radiation field that may coalesce to form a relatively sharp border conforming to the radiation portal. The late stage (6–24 months after completion) is characterized by fibrotic changes which appear on CT as parenchymal distortion and traction bronchiectases.[38]

Pulmonary Cytolytic Thrombi

Like GVHD, this is a rare pulmonary complication that occurs exclusively in allogeneic HSCT recipients. In fact, it may be a manifestation of GVHD. Children are primarily affected. A median onset of 72 days after HSCT has been reported.[38] Pathologically, there are intravascular thromboemboli composed of necrotic basophilic debris occluding the small and medium pulmonary vessels leading to surrounding alveolar hemorrhage or infarct. Multiple bilateral pulmonary nodules with surrounding ground-glass opacities are seen on HRCT.

LATE PULMONARY COMPLICATIONS

Late complications occur 3 months after HSCT. During this period, noninfectious causes are more common.[23] The most common complication during this period is chronic GVHD manifesting either as bronchiolitis obliterans, organizing pneumonia, or non-classifiable interstitial pneumonia. Air-leak syndrome (ALS), post-transplant lymphoproliferative disorder (PTLD), pulmonary veno-occlusive disease (PVOD), and pleuroparenchymal fibroelastosis are less frequently encountered complications.

Chronic GVHD

It occurs only in patients with allogeneic HSCT secondary to immune-mediated reaction of the donor T-lymphocytes against the host tissues.[41] Lung involvement is common unlike acute GVHD. It manifests either as organizing pneumonia (reversible with favorable prognosis) or bronchiolitis obliterans (irreversible).

Bronchiolitis Obliterans

It occurs most commonly in allogeneic HSCT for leukemia or aplastic anemia. About 10% of patients who develop chronic GVHD develop bronchiolitis obliterans. Factors that increase the risk include immunosuppression with methotrexate, chemotherapy or irradiation prior to HSCT and low serum immunoglobulins after HSCT. Pathologically, there is constrictive bronchiolitis with submucosal and peribronchiolar fibrosis. HRCT findings are best demonstrated on expiratory CT and include air trapping, mosaic perfusion and bronchial dilatation.[42]

Bronchiolitis Obliterans Organizing Pneumonia

The pathological hallmark is granulation tissue in the lumen of alveolar ducts and bronchioles followed by fibroblastic proliferation. HRCT findings include patchy, bilateral, multifocal areas of ground-glass opacity or consolidation in a peribronchial or subpleural distribution. Areas of consolidation tend to be multifocal, bilateral, peripheral and lower lobe predominant **(Fig. 16)**.[43]

Air-leak Syndrome

Air-leak Syndrome (ALS) is characterized by spontaneous pneumothorax, pneumomediastinum, pulmonary interstitial emphysema or subcutaneous emphysema in HSCT recipients. Typically, patients with ALS have chronic GVHD and bronchiolitis obliterans syndrome. On HRCT, the diagnosis of pneumothorax, pneumomediastinum and subcutaneous emphysema is straightforward; however, changes of interstitial emphysema are subtle and appear as linear lucencies along the bronchovascular bundles. Findings of bronchiolitis obliterans will also usually be evident.[44]

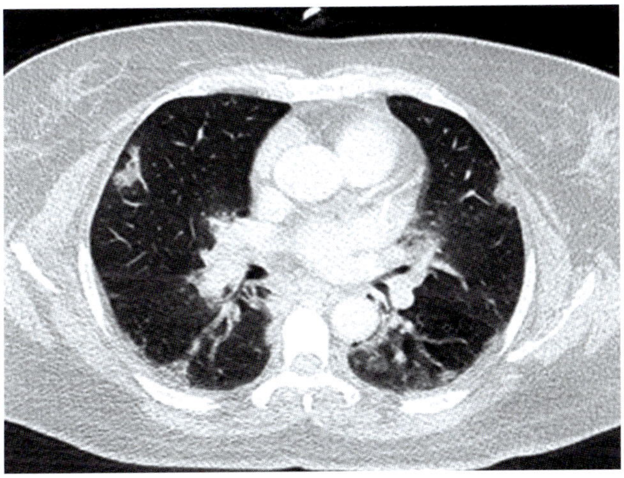

FIG. 16: A 47-year-old female with chronic myeloid leukemia. HRCT shows patchy, bilateral areas of ground-glass opacity and consolidation in a subpleural distribution. TBLB confirmed the diagnosis as BOOP.

Pulmonary Veno-occlusive Disease

Pulmonary veno-occlusive disease (PVOD) is a rare complication that may be encountered following either autologous or allogeneic HSCT.[45] The diagnosis is based on a triad of pulmonary edema, pulmonary hypertension and normal pulmonary artery occlusion pressure. HRCT demonstrates main pulmonary artery dilatation, ground-glass opacities and smooth interlobular septal thickening.

Pleuroparenchymal Fibroelastosis

Pleuroparenchymal fibroelastosis is a rare complication with upper lobe involvement characterized by fibrotic thickening of the pleura and fibroelastosis of the subpleural parenchyma.[46]

CONCLUSION

Pulmonary infections are the most common complications in patients with HIV/AIDS patients and solid organ transplant/ HSCT recipients and account for significant morbidity and mortality. It is important for the radiologist to demand and utilize all available clinical information such as signs and symptoms, degree of immunosuppression, risk factor for HIV infection and time period since solid organ or HSC transplant. In most cases, the clinical and chest radiograph findings are sufficient for confident diagnosis. However, chest radiographs may be normal or demonstrate subtle or nonspecific findings. Chest CT plays an important role in identifying the presence of disease and may specifically diagnose many conditions. Equally important, a negative HRCT chest virtually excludes active infectious disease.

REFERENCES

1. Afessa B, Green B. Bacterial pneumonia In hospitalized patients with HIV infection. Chest. 2000;117(4):1017-22.
2. Aronchick JM. Pulmonary infections in cancer and bone marrow transplant patients. Semin Roentgenol. 2000;35(2):140-51.
3. Daniel DM. Pulmonary infections in HIV/AIDS. Semin Roentgenol. 2000;35(2):124-39.
4. Miller WT. Pulmonary infections in patients who have received solid organ transplants. Semin Roentgenol. 2000;35(2):152-70.
5. Moore EH. Diffuse lung disease in the current spectrum of immunocompromised hosts (non-AIDS). Radiol Clin N Am. 1991;29(5):983-97.
6. World Health Organization/Joint United Nations programme on HIV/AIDS. Report on the global AIDS epidemic, 2008. *http:/ www. unaids.org*.
7. Beck JM. The immune-compromised host: HIV infection. Proc Am Thorac Soc. 2005;2:423-7.
8. Boiselle PM, Aviram G, Fishman JE. Update on lung disease in AIDS. Semin Roentgenol. 2002;37(1):54-71.
9. Grubb JR, Moorman AC, Baker RK, Masur H. The changing spectrum of pulmonary disease in patients with HIV infection on antiretroviral therapy. AIDS. 2006;20:1095-107.
10. Huang L, Crothers K. HIV-associated opportunistic pneumonias. Respirology. 2009;14:474-85.
11. Castaner E, Gallardo X, Mata JM, Esteba L. Radiologic approach to the diagnosis of infectious pulmonary diseases in patients infected with the human immunodeficiency virus. Eur J Radiol. 2004;51:114-29.
12. Jasmer RM, Edinburgh KJ, Thompson A, Gotway MB, Creasman JM, et al. Chest. 2000;117:1023-30.
13. Kang E, Staples CA, McGuinness G, Primack SL, Muller NL. Detection and differential diagnosis of pulmonary infections and tumors in patients with AIDS: Value of chest radiography versus CT. Am J Roentgenol. 1996;166:15-9.
14. Hartman TE, Primack SL, Muller NL, et al. Diagnosis of thoracic complications in AIDS: Accuracy of CT. Am J Roentgenol. 1994;162:547-53.

15. Shorr AF, Susla GM, O'Grady NP. Pulmonary infiltrates in the non-HIV infected immunocompromised patient: Etiologies, diagnostic strategies and outcomes. Chest. 2004;125:260-71.
16. Kuhlman JE. Pneumocystic infections: The radiologist's perspective. Radiology. 1996;198:623-35.
17. Greenberg SD, Frager D, Suster B, Walker S, Stavropoulos C, et al. Active pulmonary tuberculosis in patients with AIDS: Spectrum of radiographic findings. Radiology. 1994;193:115-9.
18. George R, Andronikou S, Theron S, du Plessis J, Hayes M, et al. Pulmonary infections in HIV-positive children. Pediatr Radiol. 2009;39:545-54.
19. Carignan S, Staples CA, Muller NL. Intrathoracic lymphoproliferative disorders in the immunocompromised host. J Thoracic Imaging. 1995;197:53-8.
20. Franquet T. High resolution computed tomography (HRCT) of lung infections in non-AIDS immunocompromised patients. Eur Radiol. 2006;16:707-18.
21. Mesurolle B, Tanaka N, Kosiuk J, Mignon F, Choquet S. The treated thorax in patients with hematological malignancies. In: Guermazi A (Ed). Radiogical imaging in hematological malignancies. Medical Radiology, Diagnostic Imaging. 1st edn. Berlin, Hiedelberg, Gemany. Springer-Verlag. 2004; pp. 443-72.
22. Rosenow EC, Wilson WR, Cockerill FR. Pulmonary disease in the immunocompromised host. I Mayo Clin Proc. 1985; 60(7):473-87.
23. Worthy SA, Flint JD, Muller NL. Pulmonary complications after bone marrow transplantation: High resolution CT and pathological findings. Radiographics. 1997;17:1359-71.
24. Hows JM. Status of umbilical cord blood transplantation in the year 2001. J Clin Pathol. 2001;54:428-34.
25. Mesurolle B, Tanaka N, Kosiuk J, Mignon F, Choquet S. The treated thorax in patients with hematological malignancies. In: Guermazi A (Ed). Radiogical Imaging in Hematological Malignancies. Medical Radiology, Diagnostic Imaging. 1st edition. Berlin, Hiedelberg, Gemany. Springer-Verlag; 2004.pp. 443-72.
26. Heussel CP, Kanczor HU, Heussel GU, et al. Pneumonia in febrile neutropenic patients and in bone marrow and blood stem cell transplant recipients: use of high resolution computed tomography. J Clin Oncol. 1999;17:796-805.
27. Huang L, Cattamanchi A, Davis L, den Boon S, Kovacs J, et al. HIV-associated *Pneumocystis* pneumonia. Proc Am Thorac Soc 2010;8:294-300.
28. Kramer MR, Marshall SE, Starnes VA, et al. Infectious complications in heart lung transplantation: Analysis of 200 episodes. Arch Intern Med. 1993;153:2010-6.
29. Spalgais S, Jaiswal A, Puri M, Sarin R, Agarwal U. Clinical profile and diagnosis of extra-pulmonary TB in HIV infected patients: routine abdominal ultrasonography increases detection of abdominal tuberculosis. Indian J Tuberc. 2013;60(3):147-53.
30. Soubani AO, Miller KB, Hassoun PN. Pulmonary complications of bone marrow transplantation. Chest. 1996;109:1066-77.
31. Gulati M, Kaur R, Jha V, et al. High resolution CT in renal transplant patients with suspected pulmonary infections. Acta Radiologica. 2000;41:1-6
32. Park YS, Seo JB, Lee YK, et al. Radiological and clinical findings of pulmonary aspergillosis following solid organ transplant. Clin Radiol. 2008;63:673-80.
33. La Ferla L, Pinzone MR, Nunnari G, Martellotta F, Lleshi A, Tirelli U, et al. Kaposi's sarcoma in HIV-positive patients: the state of art in the HAART-era. Eur Rev Med Pharmacol Sci. 2013;17(17):2354-65.
34. Davis SD, Henschke CI, Chamides BK, Westcott JL. Intrathoracic Kaposi sarcoma in AIDS patients: radiographic-pathologic correlation. Radiology. 1987;163(2):495-500.
35. Hildebrand FL Jr. Rosenow EC, Habermann TM, et al. Pulmonary complications of leukemia. Chest. 1990;98: 1233-9.
36. Brodoefel H, Faul C, Salih H, Vogel W, Fenchel M, Horger M. Therapy-related noninfectious complications in patients with hematologic malignancies: high-resolution computed tomography findings. J Thorac Imaging. 2013;28(1):W5–W1.
37. Tyndall A. Successes and failures of stem cell transplantation in autoimmune diseases. Hematology Am Soc Hematol Educ Program. 2011;(1):280-84.
38. Franquet T, Müller NL, Lee KS, Giménez A, Flint JD. High-resolution CT and pathologic findings of noninfectious pulmonary complications after hematopoietic stem cell transplantation. Am J Roentgenol. 2005;184(2):629-37.
39. Kantrow SP, Hackman RC, Boeckh M, Myerson D, Crawford SW. Idiopathic pneumonia syndrome: changing spectrum of lung injury after marrow transplantation. Transplantation. 1997;63 (8):1079-86.
40. Panoskaltsis-Mortari A, Griese M, Madtes DK, et al. An official American Thoracic Society research statement: noninfectious lung injury after hematopoietic stem cell transplantation—idiopathic pneumonia syndrome. Am J Respir Crit Care Med. 2011;183(9):1262-79.
41. Yousem SA. The histological spectrum of pulmonary graft-versus-host disease in bone marrow transplant recipients. Hum Pathol. 1995;26(6):668-75.
42. Ooi GC, Peh WC, Ip M. High-resolution computed tomography of bronchiolitis obliterans syndrome after bone marrow transplantation. Respiration. 1998;65(3):187-91.
43. Yoshihara S, Yanik G, Cooke KR, Mineishi S. Bronchiolitis obliterans syndrome (BOS), bronchiolitis obliterans organizing pneumonia (BOOP), and other late-onset noninfectious pulmonary complications following allogeneic hematopoietic stem cell transplantation. Biol Blood Marrow Transplant. 2007;13(7):749-59.
44. Franquet T, Rodríguez S, Hernández JM, et al. Air-leak syndromes in hematopoietic stem cell transplant recipients with chronic GVHD: high-resolution CT findings. J Thorac Imaging. 2007;22 (4):335-40.
45. Mandel J, Mark EJ, Hales CA. Pulmonary veno-occlusive disease. Am J Respir Crit Care Med. 2000;162(5):1964-73.
46. Frankel SK, Cool CD, Lynch DA, Brown KK. Idiopathic pleuroparenchymal fibroelastosis: description of a novel clinicopathologic entity. Chest. 2004;126(6):2007-13.

CHAPTER

129

Pattern Approach to Interstitial Lung Disease and Imaging of Idiopathic Interstitial Pneumonias

Mandeep Garg, Uma Debi

Interstitial lung diseases (ILDs) are defined as a group of diffuse lung parenchymal diseases which result from damage to the lung parenchyma caused by different degrees of inflammation and fibrosis.[1] It refers to variable patterns/ diseases characterized histologically by inflammatory infiltrate in the interstitium with variable degree of fibrosis. Correlation of clinical, radiological and pathologic features is often required to reach a correct diagnosis of ILD. According to the updated American Thoracic Society–European Respiratory Society classification, idiopathic interstitial pneumonias (IIPs) are ILDs of unknown etiology sharing common clinical features and can be categorized into (a) "chronic fibrosing IIPs" [idiopathic pulmonary fibrosis (IPF) and idiopathic nonspecific interstitial pneumonia (NSIP)], (b) "smoking-related IIPs" [respiratory bronchiolitis associated interstitial lung disease (RB-ILD) and desquamative interstitial pneumonia (DIP)], and (c) "acute or subacute IIPs" (cryptogenic organizing pneumonia (COP) and acute interstitial pneumonia (AIP)) and (d) "rare IIPs" [lymphoid interstitial pneumonia (LIP) and idiopathic pleura-parenchymal fibro-elastosis (IPPFE)] **(Table 1)**. In addition, another category "unclassifiable IIPs" has been proposed, which includes IIPs in which final diagnosis is not possible.[2]

IMAGING

Plain Radiography

It is an important part of initial imaging. During imaging interstitial pneumonias, the goals of chest radiograph interpretation are to determine the pattern of lung disease, recognize any change in lung volume and to determine any other accompanying abnormalities **(Fig. 1)**.

High Resolution Computed Tomography

High resolution computed tomography (HRCT) is required for evaluating the morphology and density of lung abnormalities and their location in relation to secondary pulmonary lobule. HRCT is much better than routine CT for this purpose. Previously sequential HRCT was performed in supine position with 1–2 cm spacing and 1 mm slice thickness. But this method is nearly obsolete now expect for follow-up imaging as it gives involves less radiation exposure to the patient. The development of multidetector CT scanners, capable of rapidly imaging the thorax using an isotropic technique has enabled another way in which HRCT scan may be obtained. HRCT scan can be obtained from thin-section (1–2 mm) reconstruction of volumetric data obtained by using multidetector CT, narrow detector width and with image reconstruction with a high spatial frequency algorithm. Expiratory scans should be performed in patients with obstructive disease at three or more levels. Prone scans may be needed to differentiate dependent densities from early changes of ILD.

ANATOMY OF THE SECONDARY PULMONARY LOBULE (MILLER'S)[3]

The secondary pulmonary lobule is the smallest unit of lung structure, which is demarcated by septae of connective tissue. It is the smallest unit of the lung, which is visible on HRCT scan **(Fig. 2)**. The secondary pulmonary lobule is a polyhedron that depicts the smallest lung unit, which measures approximately 1–2 cm on one side and contains a few terminal bronchioles, which ultimately supply 5–15 pulmonary acini. Terminal bronchiole and centrilobular artery are present at the center of a secondary pulmonary lobule and pulmonary veins and lymphatics are present in the periphery. The interlobular septa in the periphery contain connective tissue, venules, and lymphatics. On HRCT, centrilobular artery and intralobular acinar arteries supplying a secondary pulmonary lobule can be discerned, while normal bronchioles supplying it cannot be. Centrilobular arteries measure approximately 1 mm in diameter. Intralobular acinar arteries measure approximately 0.5 mm in diameter. Normal bronchiole supplying a secondary pulmonary lobule measure approximately 1 mm in diameter with wall thickness of approximately 0.15 mm, which is beyond the resolution of HRCT. However, abnormal thickening of the interlobular and intralobular septa, axial interstitium surrounding the bronchovascular bundles and subpleural peripheral interstitium should always be identified on HRCT.

TABLE 1: Radiological features and differential diagnosis of the idiopathic interstitial pneumonias (IIPs).[2]

IIP Group and clinical radiologic pathologic diagnosis	HRCT patterns	Typical HRCT distribution	Typical HRCT findings	HRCT differential diagnosis
Chronic fibrosing IIPs				
Idiopathic pulmonary fibrosis	Usual interstitial pneumonia	Peripheral, subpleural, basal	Reticular opacities, honeycombing, traction bronchiectasis, architectural distortion	Collagen vascular disease, hypersensitivity pneumonitis, asbestosis, sarcoidosis
Idiopathic nonspecific interstitial pneumonia	Nonspecific interstitial pneumonia	Peripheral, basal, symmetric	GGO, irregular lines, traction bronchiectasis, consolidation	Usual interstitial pneumonia, cryptogenic organizing pneumonia, desquamative interstitial pneumonia, hypersensitivity pneumonitis
Smoking IIPs				
Desquamative interstitial pneumonia	Desquamative interstitial pneumonia	Lower zone, peripheral predominance in most cases	GGO, reticular lines, cysts	Respiratory bronchiolitis—interstitial lung disease, nonspecific interstitial pneumonia, hypersensitivity pneumonitis
Respiratory bronchiolitis-associated interstitial lung disease	Respiratory bronchiolitis	Upper lung predominant	Centrilobular nodules, bronchial wall thickening, patchy GGO	Nonspecific interstitial pneumonia, desquamative interstitial pneumonia, hypersensitivity pneumonitis
Acute or Subacute IIPs				
Cryptogenic organizing pneumonia	organizing pneumonia	subpleural or peribronchial	Patchy consolidation or nodules, perilobular pattern reverse halo sign	Infection, aspiration pneumonia, eosinophilic pneumonia, nonspecific interstitial pneumonia, vasculitis, sarcoidosis, mucinous adenocarcinoma, lymphoma
Acute interstitial pneumonia	Diffuse alveolar damage	Bilateral or patchy	Consolidation, GGO, later traction bronchiectasis	Hydrostatic edema, pulmonary hemorrhage, acute eosinophilic pneumonia
Rare IIPs				
Lymphoid interstitial pneumonia	Lymphoid interstitial pneumonia	Lower lung predominant	GGO, centrilobular nodules, septal and bronchovascular thickening, thin-walled cysts	Nonspecific interstitial Pneumonia, sarcoidosis, Langerhans cell histiocytosis, lymphangioleiomyomatosis
Idiopathic pleura parenchymal fibro-elastosis	Idiopathic pleural parenchymal fibroelastosis	Peripheral, upper lung predominant	Pleural thickening, subpleural fibrotic changes or consolidation	Sarcoidosis, pneumoconiosis, postinfective pulmonary fibrosis, connective tissue disease, hypersensitivity pneumonitis

The correct diagnosis of interstitial lung disease on HRCT depends on evaluating the morphology and density of the lung abnormalities and their distribution in relationship to the secondary pulmonary lobule. Lung abnormalities are first classified into four categories—increased lung attenuation, decreased lung attenuation, linear and reticular opacities, and nodules and nodular opacities.

Increased Lung Attenuation

It is classified into ground-glass opacity (GGO), consolidation, alveolar microlithiasis, metastatic calcification and granulomatous diseases (tuberculosis, silicosis, sarcoidosis). GGO is defined as mild increase in lung opacity, which does not cause obscuration of underlying vessel **(Fig. 3)**. It suggests an active or acute disease. Consolidation is defined as increased lung opacity, which causes obscuration of underlying vascular markings **(Fig. 4)**. Air bronchogram is characteristic finding seen in consolidation.

Decreased Lung Attenuation

It is categorized into mosaic perfusion, honeycombing, bronchiectasis, emphysema, pneumatoceles and lung cysts.

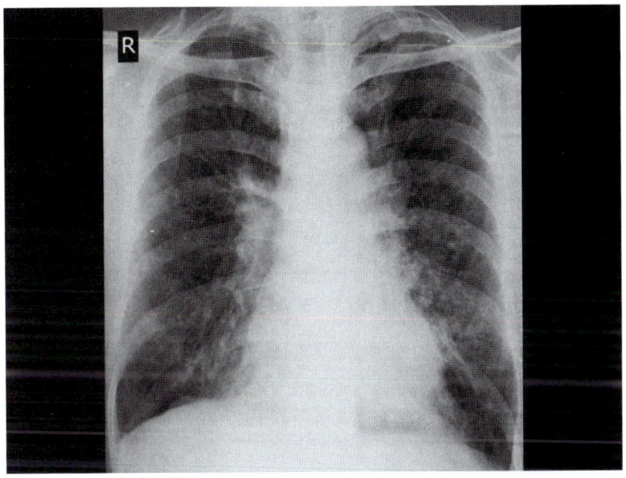

FIG. 1: Frontal chest radiograph posteroanterior view reveals reticulonodular opacities in bilateral lower lobes.

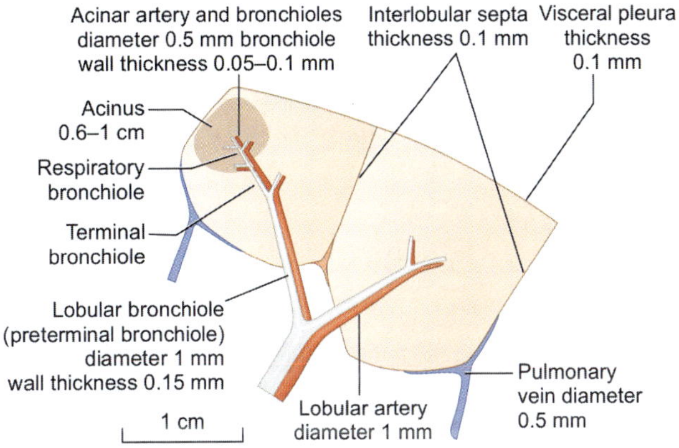

FIG. 2: Anatomy and dimensions of secondary lobule and pulmonary acinus. Two secondary pulmonary lobules in the lung periphery are illustrated along with the dimensions of their components.

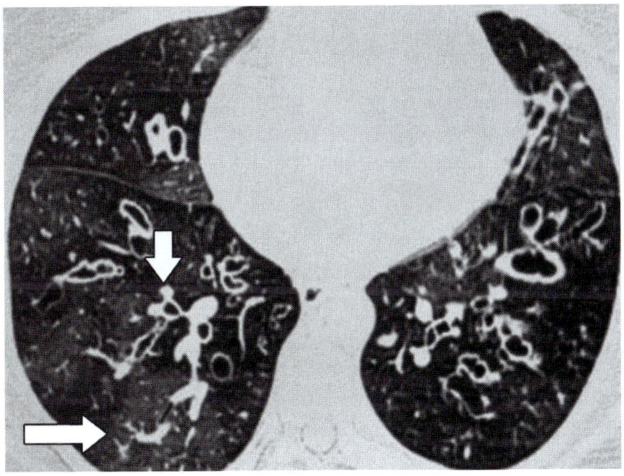

FIG. 3: Axial HRCT chest shows patchy areas of ground-glass opacity (long arrow) in bilateral lungs with varicose bronchiectasis, bronchial wall thickening and signet ring sign (short arrow).

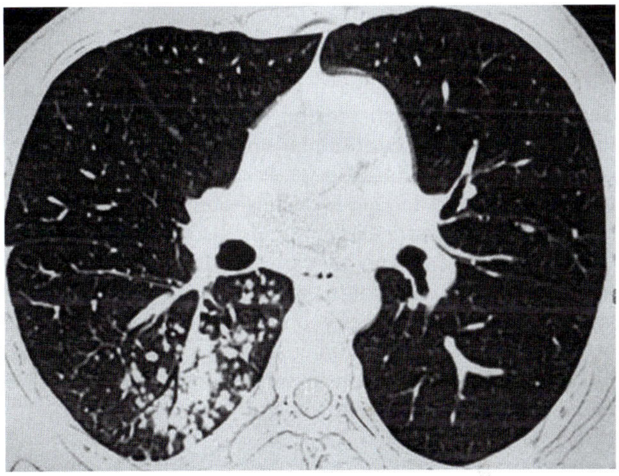

FIG. 4: Axial HRCT chest shows patchy areas of consolidation with air bronchogram in right lower lobe surrounded by multiple centrilobular nodules.

Mosaic perfusion pattern is obtained due to differential attenuation of areas of lungs, caused due to differences in lung perfusion, either due to pulmonary vascular disease or airway disease. The pulmonary arteries are reduced in size in the lucent lung fields, which helps to distinguish mosaic perfusion from GGO **(Fig. 5)**. Honeycombing can be defined as clustered cystic airspaces, which have clearly definable walls and are most commonly seen in peripheral and subpleural lung **(Fig. 6)**. Bronchiectasis is localized, abnormal dilatation of bronchial tree usually segmental and subsegmental bronchi, which occurs as a result of airway inflammation, infections or impaired mucociliary clearance **(Fig. 3)**. Emphysema is known as irreversible abnormal enlargement and destruction of airspaces distal to terminal bronchiole **(Fig. 7)**. Lung cysts are well defined, thin walled (approximately 1–3 mm) air containing lesions. Multiple lung cysts are seen in diseases like lymphangioleiomyomatosis, Langerhans cell histiocytosis and lymphoid interstitial pneumonias.

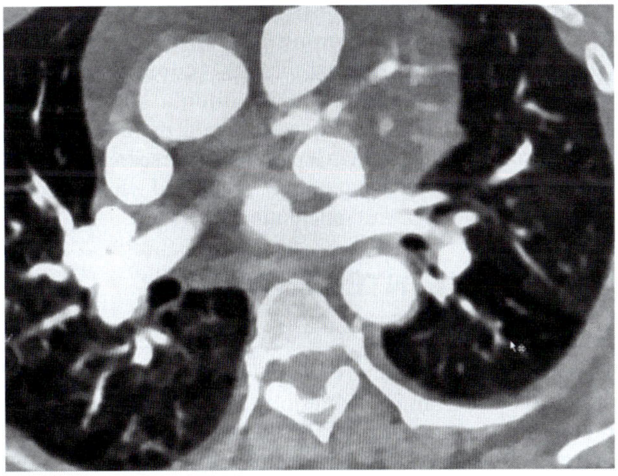

FIG. 5: Axial HRCT chest shows areas of mosaic perfusion in bilateral lungs.

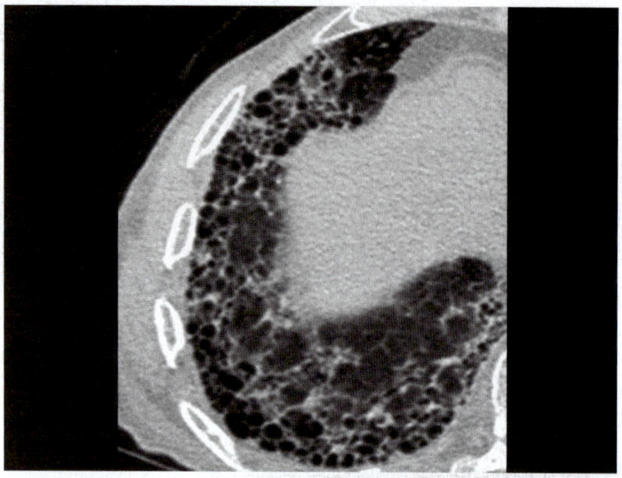

FIG. 6: Axial HRCT chest shows honeycombing consisting of multilayered thin-walled cyst.

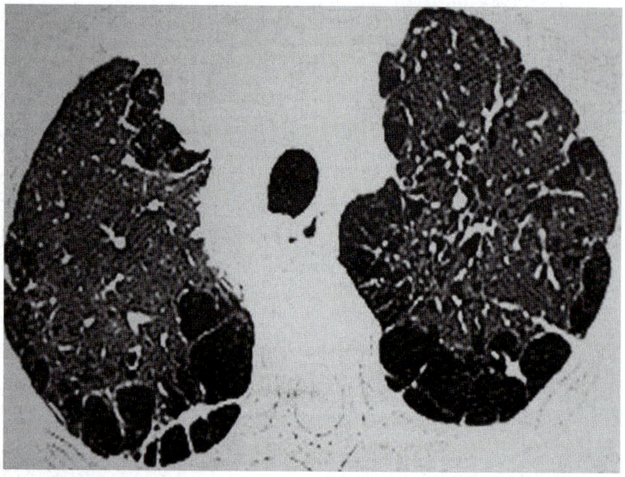

FIG. 7: Axial HRCT chest shows centriacinar and paraseptal emphysematous changes in bilateral upper lobes.

Nodules and Nodular Opacities

HRCT classifies nodules into 3 categories depending on location, i.e. which portion of secondary pulmonary lobule is involved. Centrilobular nodules involve terminal/ respiratory bronchioles **(Fig. 4)**. Perilymphatic nodules are seen in subpleural and peribronchovascular region. Random nodules have no particular anatomic distribution. Common causes of centrilobular nodules are infectious airway diseases, hypersensitivity pneumonitis and respiratory bronchiolitis. Perilymphatic nodules are seen in sarcoidosis, lymphangitic carcinomatosis, silicosis and coal worker pneumoconiosis. Random nodules are seen in tuberculosis, angioinvasive fungal infections and hematogenous metastasis.

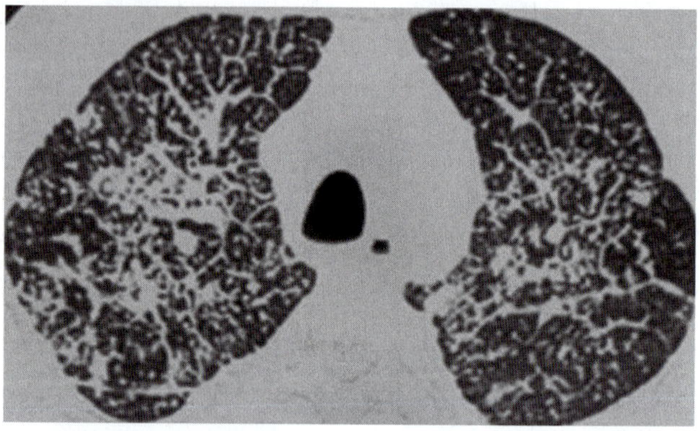

FIG. 8: Axial HRCT chest shows intralobular and interlobular septal thickening in bilateral upper lobes.

Linear and Reticular Opacities

These are categorized into intralobular septal thickening**,** interlobular septal thickening **(Fig. 8)**, parenchymal bands, peribronchovascular interstitial thickening and subpleural lines. Intralobular septal thickening is seen in IPF, chronic hypersensitivity pneumonitis, NSIP and asbestosis. Interlobular septal thickening is seen in lymphangitis carcinomatosis, LIP, IPF, sarcoidosis, pulmonary edema, silicosis, CWP, pneumocystis pneumonia. Parenchymal bands are linear opacities, which are several millimeters thick and approximately 2–5 cm in length. They are seen in patients with fibrosis. Crazy paving pattern is formed when there is concurrence of GGO with reticulations.

IDIOPATHIC INTERSTITIAL PNEUMONIAS

The final diagnosis of an IIP's should always be a consensus diagnosis made after evaluation by the chest physician, radiologist, and pathologist. The diagnosis may be altered as more details emerge from the patient's history, fine needle aspiration cytology, biopsy, bronchoalveolar lavage, or post-surgery lung histopathology. Lung damage similar to that seen in IIPs is also seen in diseases like connective tissue disorders, asbestosis, chronic hypersensitivity pneumonitis and drug reaction. The term idiopathic is used, when the cause of lung damage is not known and other known etiologies of lung damage have been excluded.

CHRONIC FIBROSING IDIOPATHIC INTERSTITIAL PNEUMONIAS

Idiopathic Pulmonary Fibrosis

Idiopathic pulmonary fibrosis (IPF) is a chronic fibrosing form of IIP, which is associated with the radiological or histopathological pattern of usual interstitial pneumonia (UIP). It occurs predominantly in older adult population and is associated with median survival of less than 5 years. The term IPF is used when other recognized causes of ILD have been excluded and there is UIP pattern seen on HRCT. IPF particularly excludes IIPs such as NSIP and DIP.[4] IPF is the most common ILD accounting for 25–50% of diffuse lung diseases. According to the current guidelines of American Thoracic Society and European Respiratory Society, an algorithm has been devised on the basis of which three levels of certainty can be assigned for UIP on the basis of HRCT findings (UIP, possible UIP, and inconsistent with UIP).[5]

Radiologic Features

Chest radiograph: Almost all patients of IPF who present with symptoms, have abnormal chest radiograph findings. The most common chest radiograph pattern is peripheral reticular opacities, which are predominant in the lower zones and are sometimes associated with honeycombing and volume loss of lower zones. Chest radiographs may sometimes also be normal.

HRCT: The diagnosis of UIP is usually made on the basis of clinical and imaging features, because of the high diagnostic accuracy of HRCT for cases of UIP.[4] Those cases without a confident HRCT diagnosis may require a biopsy. Characteristic HRCT features of UIP include reticular lines, traction bronchiectasis and bronchiolectasis, and honeycombing which are predominant in lower lobes and subpleural, peripheral lung. They may be associated with lower lobe volume loss **(Figs. 9A and B)**. GGO is much less common. Architectural distortion due to lung fibrosis is often seen. The HRCT findings of GGOs which occur in association with reticular opacities and traction bronchiectasis, always indicates lung fibrosis. Patients with preponderant reticular opacities or honeycombing on HRCT, usually progress despite being given treatment.[6]

Nonspecific Interstitial Pneumonia

Nonspecific interstitial pneumonia (NSIP) is less common than UIP. The mean age of patients at onset is about 40–50 years.[7] Onset of NSIP is gradual, but some patients may have subacute onset. Patients usually present with symptoms of breathlessness and cough. Histologic and radiologic findings of NSIP can be found in patients with drug-induced lung diseases, collagen vascular diseases and hypersensitivity pneumonitis. Hence, when HRCT pattern of NSIP is seen, these etiologies should be ruled out. In addition, HRCT features similar to those seen in NSIP may be seen in patients of organizing pneumonia, UIP and DIP and surgical biopsy may sometimes be required to differentiate them.

NSIP is further classified into two types: fibrotic or cellular subtypes. Fibrotic NSIP is more common than cellular subtype. On histology, interstitial thickening is mainly due to fibrosis with mild inflammation. In cellular NSIP, thickening of interstitium is due to infiltration by plasma cells and lymphocytes. Cellular NSIP has a better prognosis and usually shows response to corticosteroids.[8] It is sometimes difficult to differentiate fibrotic NSIP and UIP on histology. While fibrotic NSIP shows temporal homogeneity, UIP shows heterogeneity with collagen and fibroblastic foci, representing old and active disease together. This may aid in differentiating the two.[9]

Radiologic Features

Chest radiograph: NSIP shows infiltrates in bilateral lungs which are more common in lower zones.

HRCT features: The predominant HRCT finding of NSIP is GGO, which is usually bilateral, symmetric and preponderant in lower lobes and peripheral lung. Pathologically, GGO corresponds to homogeneous interstitial inflammation.[10] Irregular linear or reticular opacities are seen which may be associated with traction bronchiectasis or bronchiolectasis **(Figs. 10A and B)**. Honeycombing is rarely seen. Other occasional findings include nodules, pleural effusion, and hilar or meditational lymphadneopathy.

SMOKING-RELATED INTERSTITIAL PNEUMONIAS

RB, RB-ILD and DIP are currently thought of as a continuum of smoking-related lung diseases. There is similarity in their clinical, radiological and histological findings.[2] RB is asymptomatic and is detected at autopsy. RB-ILD is the term used when RB is associated with pulmonary symptoms or radiological findings. DIP represents the worst of this spectrum, in which imaging and histologic findings are more extensive.

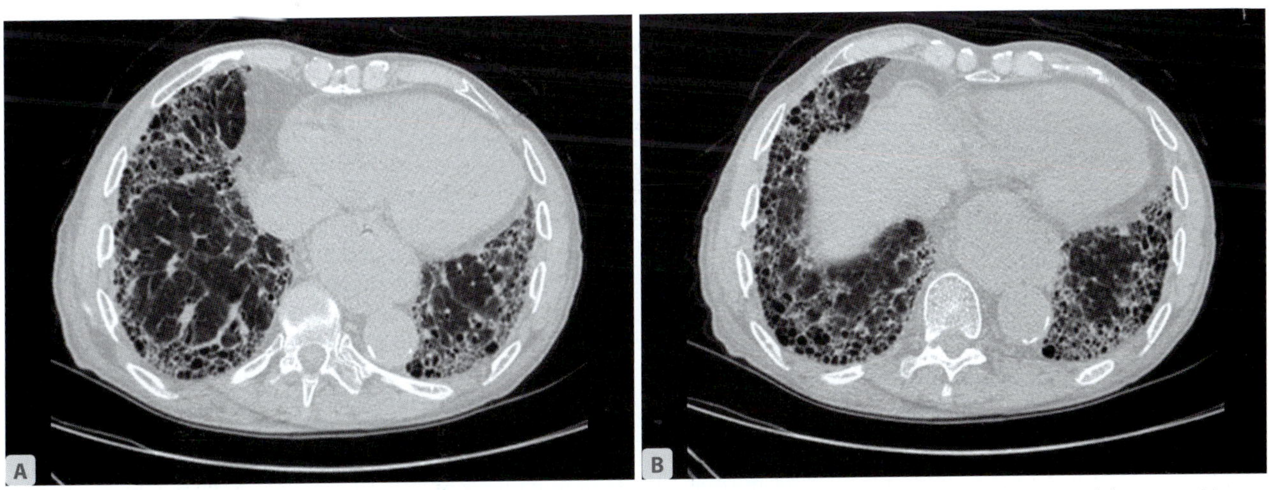

FIGS. 9A AND B: Idiopathic pulmonary fibrosis (IPF): Axial HRCT chest shows intralobular and interlobular septal thickening with honeycombing and tractional bronchiectasis more pronounced in bilateral lower lobes.

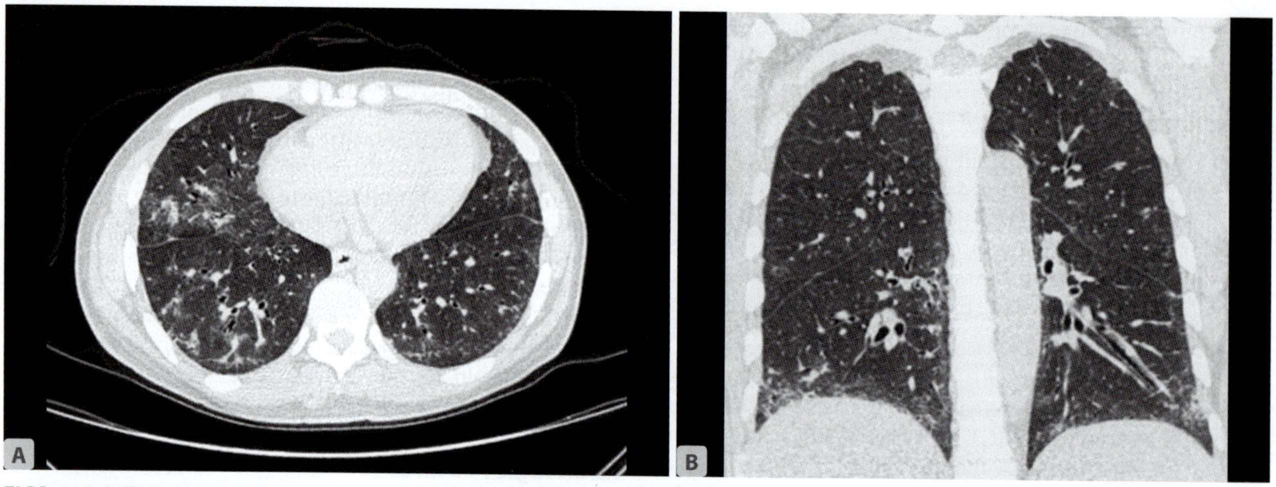

FIGS. 10A AND B: Nonspecific interstitial pneumonia (NSIP): Axial and coronal HRCT chest shows bilateral patchy areas of ground-glass opacity and subpleural reticulations with mild-traction bronchiectasis in bilateral lower lobes. Fissural nodularity and fibronodular lesions seen are also seen in bilateral upper lobes and RML.

Respiratory Bronchiolitis-associated Interstitial Lung Disease

Both RB and RB-ILD on histology show pigmented macrophages within first and second order respiratory bronchioles.[11] In RB-ILD, the degree of abnormality is generally more.[12] The course of this disease following smoking cessation generally improves.[13]

Radiologic Features

Chest radiograph: The most common abnormality in RB-ILD, on chest radiograph is thickening of the central or peripheral airway walls, which is seen in approximately 76% of patients. Ground-glass opacity is seen in 57% of patients.[14]

HRCT features: The common findings of RB-ILD include centrilobular nodules, patchy GGOs, and thickening of the central or peripheral airway walls **(Fig. 11)**. RB-ILD can be usually diagnosed in smokers with these HRCT findings, without the aid of lung biopsy.[5] The HRCT features of hypersensitivity pneumonitis may overlap with those of RB and RB-ILD. However, the centrilobular nodules, mosaic attenuation, air trapping and GGO found in hypersensitivity pneumonitis are usually more extensive. Additionally, almost all patients with hypersensitivity pneumonitis are nonsmokers.

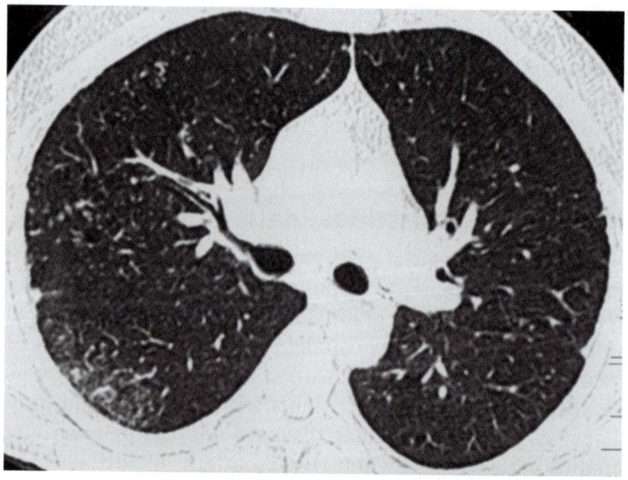

FIG. 11: Respiratory bronchiolitis-interstitial lung disease (RB- ILD): Axial HRCT chest shows multiple ill-defined nodules in a chronic smoker with RB-ILD.

Desquamative Interstitial Pneumonia

DIP is an uncommon interstitial pneumonia. It overlaps with RB-ILD in that the quality of the pigment-laden macrophages is identical, but their distribution and extent differ, with pigment-laden macrophages being more diffuse and extensive in desquamative interstitial pneumonia.[2]

Radiologic Features

Chest radiograph: Chest radiograph may be normal in approximately 3–22% of cases of DIP. On chest radiograph, findings that can be seen are diffuse patchy GGOs, with predominance in lower zones and in periphery.[15]

HRCT: The most common and characteristic finding of DIP is GGOs, which are present on HRCT in all cases of DIP **(Fig. 12)**. This occurs due to the homogeneous accumulation of intra-alveolar macrophages and alveolar septal thickening. Mid and lower lobes predominance with peripheral distribution is seen in most of the cases. Reticular opacities are sometimes present. Well-defined and thin-walled cysts may be seen. The GGOs usually resolve with treatment. The main imaging difference between RB-ILD and DIP is the distribution of disease, which is predominantly centrilobular in RB-ILD and diffuse in DIP. Centrilobular nodules are uncommonly seen in patients of DIP. GGOs are usually patchier, less well defined, and less extensive in RB-ILD.

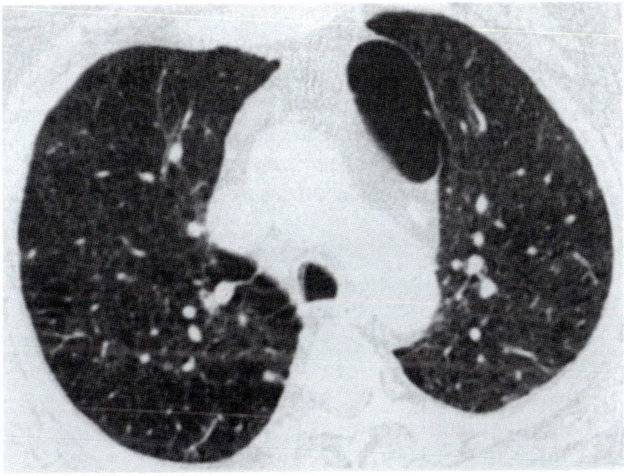

FIG. 12: Desquamative interstitial pneumonia (DIP): Axial HRCT chest shows diffuse ill-defined bilateral symmetrical ground-glass opacification. Centrilobular emphysema with large left-sided bulla is also noted in this 45 years old heavy smoker.

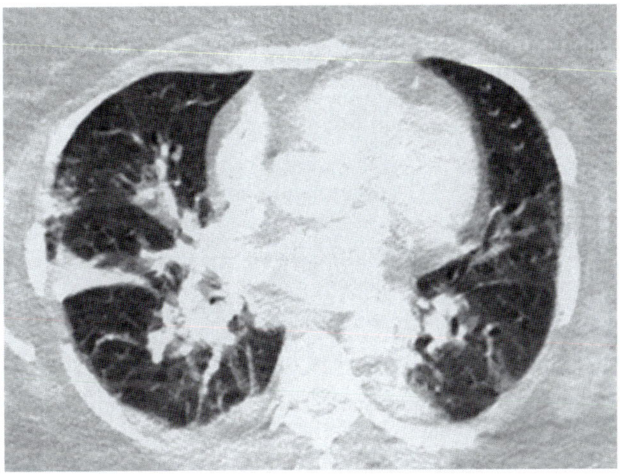

FIG. 13: Cryptogenic organizing pneumonia (COP): Axial HRCT chest shows bilateral ill-defined ground-glass opacities with patchy areas of consolidation in bilateral upper lobes.

ACUTE AND SUBACUTE INTERSTITIAL PNEUMONIAS

Cryptogenic Organizing Pneumonia

Cryptogenic organizing pneumonia (COP) was previously referred to as bronchiolitis obliterans organizing pneumonia. However, cryptogenic organizing pneumonia is the preferred term because organizing pneumonia is the predominant feature and is responsible for the physiologic abnormalities and radiologic findings.

Radiologic Features

Chest radiograph: The most common chest radiograph findings in COP are unilateral or bilateral areas of consolidation.

HRCT: HRCT typically shows patchy, possibly migratory, unilateral or bilateral areas of consolidation or/and GGOs in a peribronchovascular or subpleural location **(Fig. 13)**. Air bronchograms with mild cylindrical bronchial dilatation may be frequently seen in areas of consolidation. Pleural effusions may uncommonly occur.[16] Nodules are seen in 30% of cases. They are usually small and present predominantly along the bronchovascular bundles. Reticular opacities may be sometimes present and signify histologic evidence of fibrosis.

Acute Interstitial Pneumonia

AIP is a type of interstitial pneumonia that progresses rapidly. On histology, there is presence of diffuse alveolar damage (DAD). The term acute interstitial pneumonia is used when there is DAD of unknown origin. Patients with AIP often have a clinical prodrome suggesting viral upper respiratory tract infection. Patients have hypoxemia which rapidly progresses to respiratory failure, with mortality rate of 50% or more. Treatment is generally supportive and mechanical ventilation is usually required.

Radiologic Features

Chest radiograph: The chest radiograph shows patchy/ diffuse areas of air space opacities bilaterally **(Fig. 14A)**.

HRCT: AIP is characterized by three stages, early exudative phase, subacute proliferative phase and chronic fibrotic phase. The first exudative phase of AIP, shows bilateral patchy GGOs with areas of focal sparing, often with consolidation in the dependent part of lungs **(Figs. 14B and C)**. While the later fibrotic stage of AIP shows distortion of bronchovascular bundles and traction bronchiectasis. AIP can progress to severe fibrosis with areas of honeycombing.[2] Few patients who survive this disease show progressive resolution of the areas of GGO and consolidation. On later HRCT scans, areas of hypoattenuation, reticular pattern, traction bronchiectasis and associated architectural distortion occurring predominantly in the nondependent part of lungs can be seen.

RARE INTERSTITIAL PNEUMONIAS

The recently created category of rare IIPs includes idiopathic LIP and IPPFE.[2]

Lymphoid Interstitial Pneumonia

LIP is a lymphoproliferative disorder, in which there is infiltration of lung interstitium predominantly by lymphocytes. The incidence of idiopathic LIP is low. LIP is most frequently associated with Sjögren's syndrome, autoimmune thyroid diseases, AIDS, and Castleman syndrome.

Radiologic Features

Chest radiograph: It is neither sensitive nor specific. Findings include bilateral basal reticular opacities and ill-defined nodules.[17]

HRCT: The predominant HRCT findings are usually GGO and perivascular cysts **(Fig. 15)**, sometimes leading to misdiagnosis

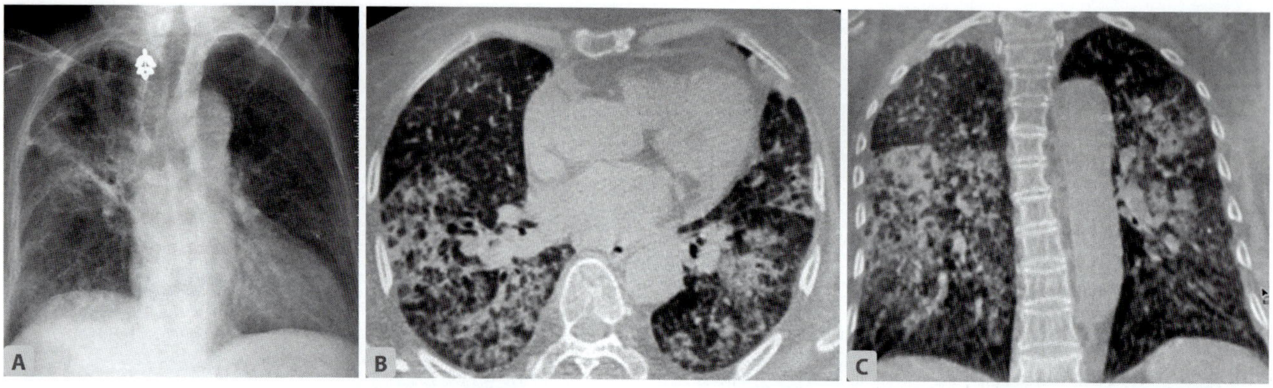

FIGS. 14A TO C: Acute interstitial pneumonia (AIP). (A) Frontal chest radiograph posteroanterior view reveals bilateral airspace opacification with air bronchograms, with sparing of the costophrenic angles; (B and C) Axial and coronal HRCT shows bilateral diffuse ground-glass opacity and consolidation of the dependent lung.

of lymphangioleiomyomatosis. However, cysts related to LIP usually predominate in the lower lungs and around bronchi and vessels, in contrast to the diffuse distribution of cysts in lymphangioleiomyomatosis. Peribronchovascular and interlobular septae thickening are also seen frequently in cases of LIP. Centrilobular nodules may also be seen. Rarely, perivascular honeycombing can be seen.[18,19]

Idiopathic Pulmonary Fibroelastosis

This rare condition of IPPEE is diagnosed when there is upper-lobe predominant fibrosis involving the subpleural lung parenchyma and pleura. On histologic evaluation, intra-alveolar fibrosis is present and the fibrosis is elastotic.[20] Recurrent infections have been noted in half of patients. HRCT in patients with IPPFE is characterized by dense subpleural consolidation in the upper lobes. In addition, areas of traction bronchiectasis and architectural distortion may be seen.[21]

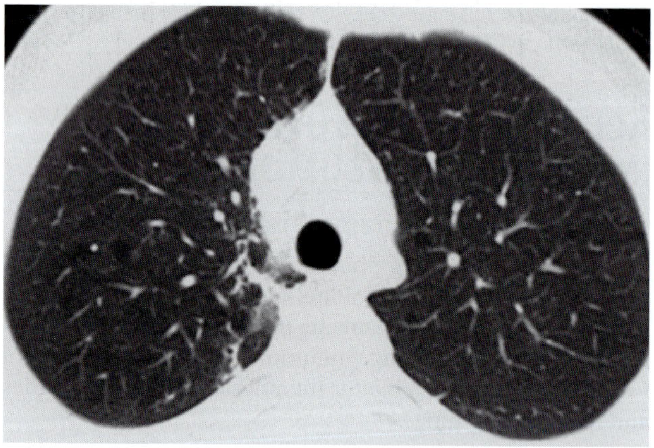

FIG. 15: Lymphoid interstitial pneumonia (LIP): Axial HRCT chest shows few thin wall perivascular cysts in bilateral lungs in a patient with AIDS and LIP.

REFERENCES

1. American Thoracic Society/European Respiratory Society international multidisciplinary consensus classification of the idiopathic interstitial pneumonias. This joint statement of the American Thoracic Society (ATS), and the European Respiratory Society (ERS) was adopted by the ATS board of directors, June 2001 and by the ERS Executive Committee, June 2001. Am J Respir Crit Care Med. 2002;165(2):277-304.
2. Sverzellati N, Lynch DA, Hansell DM, et al. American Thoracic Society—European Respiratory Society Classification of the Idiopathic Interstitial Pneumonias: Advances in Knowledge since 2002. RadioGraphics. 2015;35:1849-72.
3. Hobbs S, Lynch D. The Idiopathic Interstitial Pneumonias: An Update and Review. Radiol Clin N Am. 2014;52:105-20.
4. American Thoracic Society. Idiopathic pulmonary fibrosis: Diagnosis and treatment—International Consensus Statement: American Thoracic Society (ATS), and the European Respiratory Society (ERS). Am J Respir Crit Care Med. 2000;161:646-64.
5. Mueller-Mang C, Grosse C, Schmid K, et al. What Every Radiologist Should Know about Idiopathic Interstitial Pneumonias? RadioGraphics. 2007;27:595-615.
6. Travis WD, Matsui K, Moss J, et al. Idiopathic nonspecific interstitial pneumonia: prognostic significance of cellular and fibrosing patterns—survival comparison with usual interstitial pneumonia and desquamative interstitial pneumonia. Am J Surg Pathol. 2000;24:19-33.
7. Flaherty KR, Thwaite EL, Kazerooni EA, et al. Radiological versus histological diagnosis in UIP and NSIP: survival implications. Thorax. 2003;58:143-8.
8. Ferguson EC, Berkowitz EA. Lung CT: Part 2, The Interstitial Pneumonias—Clinical, Histologic, and CT Manifestations AJR. 2012;199:W464-76.
9. Remy-Jardin M, Remy J, Gosselin B, et al. Lung parenchymal changes secondary to cigarette smoking: pathologic-CT correlations. Radiology. 1993;186(3):643-51.
10. Holt RM, Schmidt RA, Godwin JD, et al. High resolution CT in respiratory bronchiolitis-associated interstitial lung disease. J Comput Assist Tomogr. 1993;17(1):46-50.
11. Vassallo R, Ryu JH. Tobacco smoke-related diffuse lung diseases. Semin Respir Crit Care Med. 2008;29(6): 643-50.
12. Portnoy J, Veraldi KL, Schwarz MI, et al. Respiratory bronchiolitis-interstitial lung disease: longterm outcome. Chest. 2007;131(3):664-71.
13. An Official American Thoracic Society/European Respiratory Society Statement: Update of the International Multidisciplinary

Classification of the Idiopathic Interstitial Pneumonias William D. Travis, Ulrich Costabel, David M. Hansell Am J Respir Crit Care Med. 2013;6(188):733-48.
14. Dalphin JC, Debieuvre D, Pernet D, et al. Prevalence and risk factors for chronic bronchitis and farmer's lung in French dairy farmers. Br J Ind Med. 1993;50(10):941-4.
15. Lynch DA, Travis WD, Müller NL, et al. Idiopathic interstitial pneumonias: CT features. Radiology. 2005;236:10-21.
16. Lee JS, Lynch DA, Sharma S, et al. Organizing pneumonia: prognostic implication of high-resolution computed tomography features. J Comput Assist Tomogr. 2003;27(2):260-5.
17. Johkoh T, Muller NL, Pickford HA, et al. Lymphocytic interstitial pneumonia: thin-section CT findings in 22 patients. Radiology. 1999;212(2):567-72.
18. Ichikawa Y, Kinoshita M, Koga T, et al. Lung cyst formation in lymphocytic interstitial pneumonia: CT features. J Comput Assist Tomogr. 1994;18(5):745-8.
19. Becker CD, Gil J, Padilla ML. Idiopathic pleura parenchymal fibro elastosis: an unrecognized or misdiagnosed entity? Mod Pathol. 2008;21(6):784-7.
20. Frankel SK, Cool CD, Lynch DA, et al. Idiopathic pleura parenchymal fibroelastosis: description of a novel clinico-pathologic entity. Chest. 2004;126(6):2007-13.
21. Reddy TL, Tominaga M, Hansell DM, et al. Pleuroparenchymal fibroelastosis: a spectrum of histopathological and imaging phenotypes. Eur Respir J. 2012;40(2):377-85.

CHAPTER

130

Imaging of Interstitial Lung Disease of Known Etiology

Smriti Hari, Surabhi Vyas, Sanjay Sharma, Deep Narayan Srivastava

INTRODUCTION

Interstitial lung diseases (ILDs) are a group of disorders characterized by diffuse parenchymal lung abnormalities and clinically present with dyspnea, restrictive pulmonary function, and impaired gas exchange. The etiological cause is sometimes not known. The consensus statement on interstitial pneumonias classifies interstitial lung diseases into idiopathic interstitial pneumonias and those secondary to a known cause viz.[1]:

- Connective tissue diseases
- Granulomatous diseases (sarcoidosis)
- Infections
- Exposure related
- Miscellaneous.

The revised joint statement by American Thoracic Society/European Respiratory Society (2013) emphasised a multidisciplinary approach towards clinical, imaging and histopathological findings of ILDs and reclassified the Idiopathic interstitial pneumonias (IIP) in the following broad groups:[2]

1. Chronic fibrosing IIPs—idiopathic pulmonary fibrosis, idiopathic non-specific interstitial pneumonia
2. Smoking related IIPs—respiratory bronchiolitis, desquamative interstitial pneumonia
3. Acute or subacute IIPs—cryptogenic organising pneumonia and acute interstitial pneumonia
4. Rare IIPs—idiopathic pleuroparenchymal fibroelastosis, lymphoid interstitial pneumonia
5. Unclassifiable IIPs.

Although ILDs more commonly affect adults, some entities like Langerhans cell histiocytosis (LCH) hypersensitivity pneumonitis (HP), and idiopathic interstitial pneumonias (IIPs) are seen in children as well.[3] Diagnosis is based on history, clinical examination, pulmonary function tests, imaging in the form of chest radiographs and computed tomography and occasionally histopathology from lung biopsy.

In this chapter, we shall discuss the major imaging modalities, imaging nomenclature, followed by ILDs due to known cause and the idiopathic interstitial pneumonias.

PLAIN RADIOGRAPHY

The radiological diagnostic approach to ILDs classically begins with chest X-ray evaluation, which is done as a PA radiograph, though radiography is not sensitive in detecting changes associated with ILDs. In assessing diffuse lung disease, radiography may help in indicating:

1. Pattern of lung disease
2. Lung volume abnormalities
3. Additional findings like lymphadenopathy, pleural thickening/effusion, cardiomegaly, soft tissue or musculoskeletal involvement
4. Interval changes from previous imaging.

Common patterns seen on radiography include nodular pattern reticular pattern airspace disease, or a combination of these. Most commonly, a reticulonodular pattern is encountered.

- Nodular pattern is found in sarcoidosis, silicosis, coal worker's pneumoconiosis (CWP), miliary tuberculosis or fungal infection, berylliosis, and Langerhans cell histiocytosis (LCH).
- A reticular pattern is seen in idiopathic pulmonary fibrosis (IPF), asbestosis, collagen vascular disease, and chronic hypersensitivity pneumonitis.
- Airspace filling is the dominant pattern in cryptogenic organizing pneumonia (COP), eosinophilic pneumonia, alveolar proteinosis, vasculitis, and so called "alveolar sarcoidosis."

Volume loss:

- Involving the upper lobes—sarcoidosis, silicosis, chronic hypersensitivity pneumonitis, CWP, ankylosing spondylitis, radiation pneumonitis.
- Involving the lower lobes—asbestosis, IPF, and collagen vascular disease
- Lung volumes are preserved in LAM and LCH.

Mediastinal lymphadenopathy: It can occur with sarcoidosis or progressive systemic sclerosis (PSS). Pleural effusion points to rheumatoid disease, lupus erythematosus, or LAM.

Pleural plaques indicate asbestos exposure and the possibility that basal fibrosis could represent asbestosis.

Comparison with old radiographs can help to distinguish interstitial diseases—which typically run a subacute or chronic course—from acute diseases, such as infection or edema. It is also important in assessing progression and response to treatment.

However, chest radiography has substantial limitations viz.:

- Obscuration and overlap of various lung zones
- Limited contrast resolution, which impairs sensitivity to subtle alterations in lung density (e.g. ground-glass opacity or emphysema)
- Superimposition of the interstitial opacities within the lung which makes it difficult to characterize their shape and distribution.

Chest radiograph may be normal in 10–15% of proven infiltrative lung disease and may simulate changes of paraseptal emphysema and small-airway disease or may show non-specific findings.[4]

HIGH-RESOLUTION CT

High-resolution CT (HRCT) is routinely used in the assessment of ILD with the following common indications:

- Confirming presence, pattern, distribution, activity of disease
- Response assessment
- The selection site and type of biopsy
- Follow-up of on medical treatment
- Evaluation of associated conditions like emphysema, bronchiectasis, and bronchiolitis.

Details of the technique of HRCT have already been discussed in other chapters.

Anatomy of Secondary Pulmonary Lobule

- Secondary pulmonary lobule is the smallest anatomical unit of the lung visible on HRCT which on histology is the smallest area of lung parenchyma surrounded by connective tissue septa **(Fig. 1)**.[5] These septa, being 0.1 mm thick are only occasionally visible on HRCT.
- The secondary pulmonary lobule is shaped like a polyhedron measuring approximately 1 to 2.5 cm on a side containing few terminal bronchioles, which supply 3 to 12 acini. Pulmonary arterioles accompany the bronchioles.
- The interlobular septa contain connective tissue, venules, and lymphatics. Thickening of the interlobular and intralobular septae, peribronchovascular interstitium and subpleural interstitium is well identified on HRCT.
- Terminal bronchioles supplying a secondary lobule are not seen on HRCT.

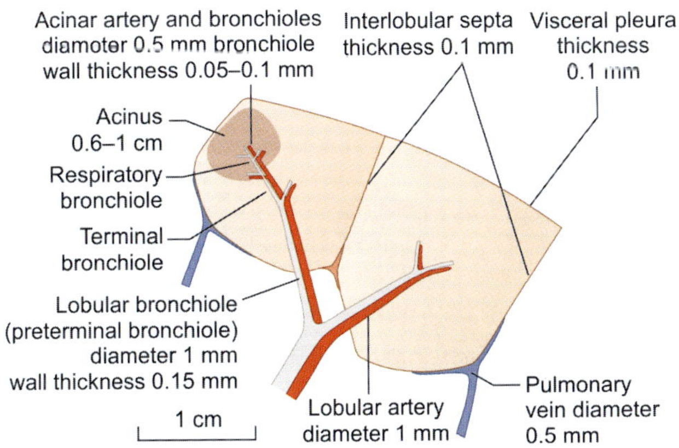

FIG. 1: Anatomy of secondary lobule and pulmonary acinus. Two adjacent secondary pulmonary lobules with their measurements and components.

CT interpretation in ILD takes in account the morphology, density and distribution of the lung abnormalities with respect to the secondary pulmonary lobule.

A glossary of terms that is used in HRCT interpretation is provided by the Fleischner Society and are summarized below:[6]

Air-trapping: Abnormal retention of gas within a lung or lung units following expiration.

Consolidation: An increase in lung opacity that results in obscuration of blood vessels.

Cyst: A clearly-marginated lucency with a wall that contains air, and no residual lung tissue. Emphysema is another cause of lucency in the lung, but an emphysematous space lacks clear margins and may contain some tissue strands, including blood vessels.

Ground-glass opacity: A hazy increase in lung opacity (compared with the density of normal lung) not associated with obscuration of underlying vessels.

Honeycombing: Cystic spaces ranging from several millimeters to several centimeters in diameter, characterized by thick, clearly definable fibrous walls, which typically are lined by bronchiolar epithelium.

Interlobular interstitial thickening: Abnormal thickening of the interlobular septae.

Intralobular interstitial thickening: Thickening of the intralobular interstitium, resulting in a fine reticular appearance to the lung parenchyma.

Nodule: A discrete, round, small opacity, ranging from 1 mm to 3 cm.

Reticulation: A network of linear strands of thickened interstitium.

Traction bronchiectasis: Bronchial dilation and irregularity occurring in patients who have pulmonary fibrosis, because of traction by fibrous tissue on the bronchial wall.

SARCOIDOSIS

Sarcoidosis is a chronic, multisystem disease of unknown etiology characterized pathologically by the presence of noncaseating granulomas.

- Commonly affects young and middle aged patients, females>males.
- Signs and symptoms—nonspecific, include fatigue, weight loss, and less commonly fever. About 50% of patients remain asymptomatic. Pulmonary manifestations[7] occur in 90% of the patients, in the form of symmetrically enlarged bilateral hilar and mediastinal lymph nodes, with or without lung parenchymal involvement.

There are five stages of intrathoracic abnormalities on radiography:[8]

Stage 0: Normal chest radiograph
Stage 1: Mediastinal and hilar lymphadenopathy
Stage 2: Lymphadenopathy with pulmonary parenchymal lesions
Stage 3: Pulmonary parenchymal lesions in the absence of hilar lymphadenopathy
Stage 4: Significant lung fibrosis with architectural distortion or bullae.

The main utility of this staging system is in predicting outcome.[9] However, interobserver concordance is the major limitation.

Imaging Features

Chest radiography—Hilar adenopathy is easily recognized on radiographs **(Fig. 2)**. Garland triad/1-2-3 sign/ Pawnbrokers sign, is the characteristic nodal involvement at the right paratracheal and bilateral hilar groups which may be identified on radiography.

CT-HRCT is the modality of choice:

- It is superior for demonstrating subtle mediastinal lymphadenopathy in the right paratracheal, aorto-pulmonary window and subcarinal region. In contrast to tubercular adenopathy, enlarged sarcoidosis lymph nodes tend to remain discrete, maintain their shape and do not have central necrosis. Sometimes, the nodes are calcified which may be amorphous, punctate, popcorn like, or eggshell-like peripheral.
- On HRCT, nodules are seen at initial evaluation in 90 to 100% of patients who have parenchymal abnormalities. They are small (5–10 mm), well-defined nodules **(Fig. 3)** occurring in a perilymphatic distribution in relation to the bronchovascular interstitium, pleural surfaces, interlobular septa, and interlobar fissures, predominantly in the upper and mid lungs. Miliary nodules may also occur. In about 15–25% of the patients, coalescing granulomas form large mass-like nodules (1–4 cm in diameter), the so-called 'alveolar sarcoid pattern **(Figs. 4A and B)**.[10] When there are discrete nodules surrounding these confluent masses, it is termed as the "Galaxy sign". Unlike metastasis, these nodules are poorly defined and may contain air bronchogram within. Cavitating nodules are rare in sarcoidosis. The presence of cavitary disease should prompt exclusion of other conditions, such as vasculitis, tuberculosis, and necrotizing sarcoidosis.[11]
- Roughly 20% of the patients develop pulmonary fibrosis (Stage 4 disease): Conglomerated parahilar masses distorting bronchi and vessels **(Figs. 5A and B)**, traction bronchiectasis, septal thickening and honeycombing. The conglomerate masses near the hila with surrounding cicatricial emphysema resemble progressive massive fibrosis in complicated silicosis. Extensive calcification may be present within fibrotic granulomas.
- Airway involvement in the form of air trapping, mosaic attenuation and bronchial stenosis are non-specific findings, yet not uncommon.

Radionuclide scanning: Historically gallium scanning was performed for activity assessment, with limited specificity.[18] FDG-PET is used now-a-days for disease activity, location, and for prebiopsy planning.[12]

MRI has a role in evaluation of cardiac involvement of sarcoidosis.

CONNECTIVE TISSUE DISEASE (CTD) ASSOCIATED INTERSTITIAL LUNG DISEASE

Interstitial lung disease is re-frequently seen in patients with various collagen vascular diseases like systemic lupus erythematosus, rheumatoid arthritis, progressive systemic sclerosis, polymyositis and dermatomyositis, Sjögren syndrome and mixed connective tissue disease. At histopathologic examination, interstitial lung diseases associated with collagen vascular disease are diverse and include usual interstitial pneumonia, nonspecific interstitial

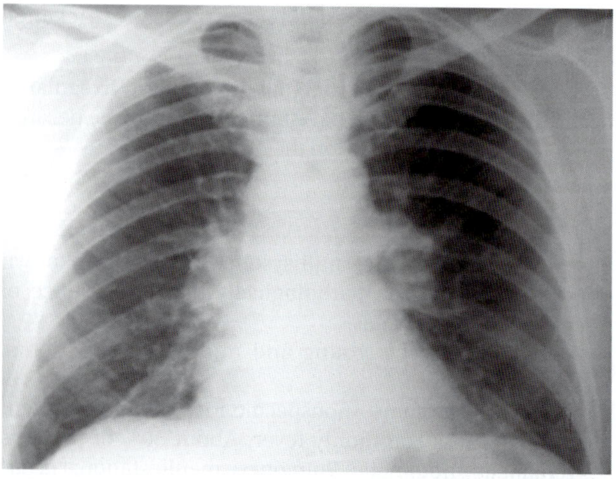

FIG. 2: Sarcoidosis: Frontal chest radiograph shows bulky, bilateral hilar lymphadenopathy.

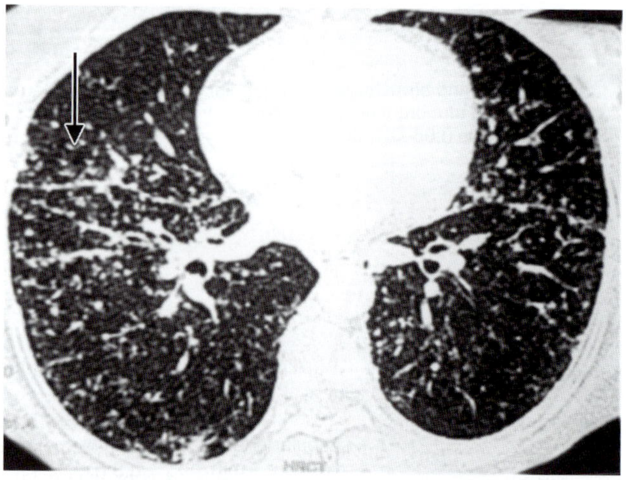

FIG. 3: Sarcoidosis: Axial HRCT shows numerous micronodules in subpleural, centrilobular and peribronchovascular distribution. Micronodular beading seen along the right major fissure (arrow).

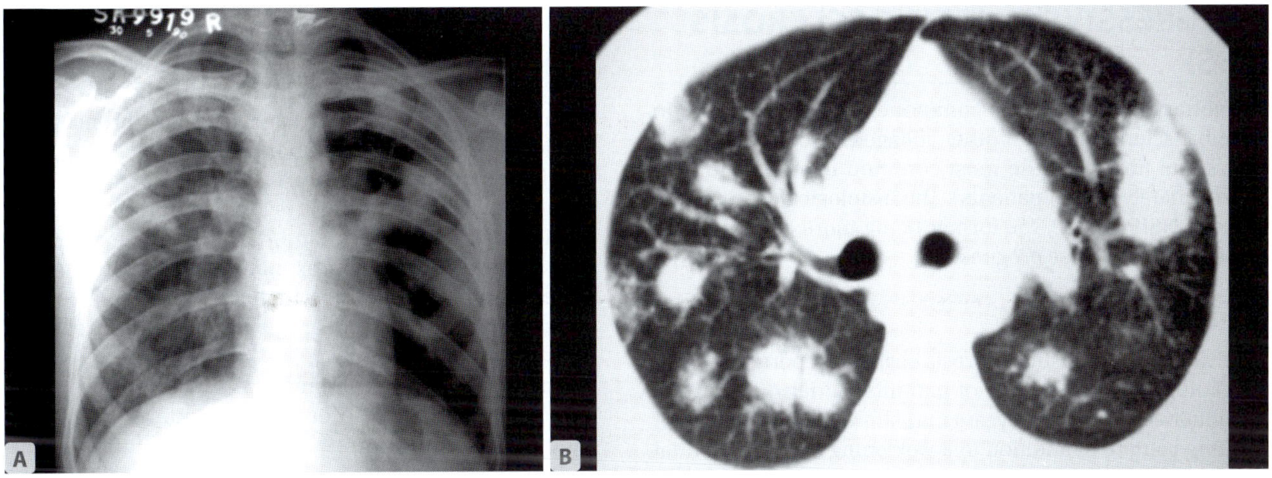

FIGS. 4A AND B: Alveolar sarcoidosis. (A) Frontal radiograph shows bulky hilar adenopathy and multiple lung nodules in bilateral upper and mid zones. (B) Axial CECT in the same patient shows well-defined, irregular parenchymal nodules indicating alveolar sarcoidosis.

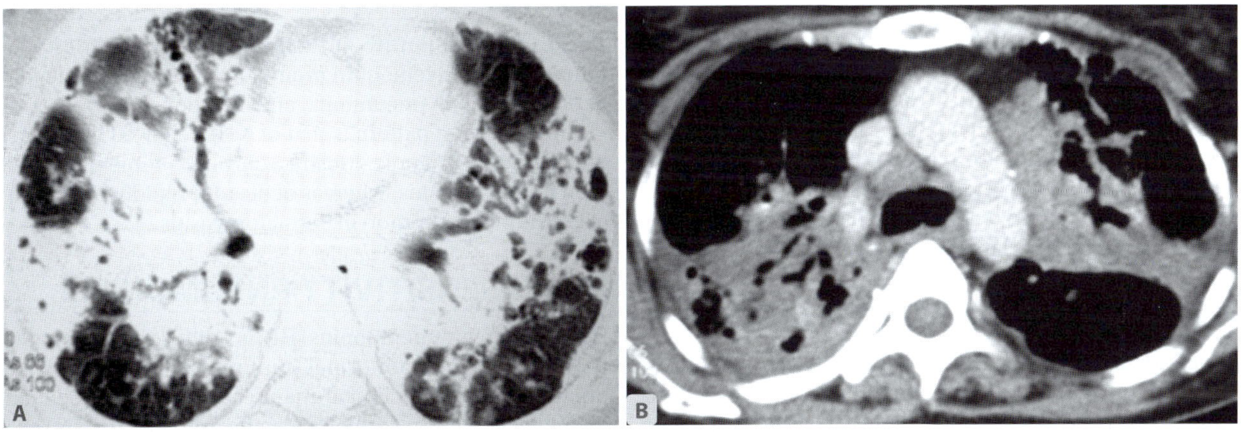

FIGS. 5A AND B: Sarcoidosis. (A) CECT chest (lung window) shows extensive, parahilar fibrotic masses with traction bronchiectasis, findings that indicate stage 4 disease; (B) CECT chest (mediastinal window) shows large fibrotic lesions, mediastinal adenopathy and irregularly thickened pleura.

pneumonia, COP, diffuse alveolar damage, lymphocytic interstitial pneumonia, and apical fibrosis.[13] The radiologic and pathological findings of CTD-ILD are identical to their idiopathic counterparts. HRCT has proved to be very sensitive in the detection and characterization of various histopathologically confirmed interstitial lung diseases in patients with collagen vascular diseases.

RHEUMATOID ARTHRITIS (RA) ASSOCIATED INTERSTITIAL LUNG DISEASE

About 5–40% of patients of rheumatoid arthritis (RA) have respiratory system involvement, including interstitial pneumonitis and fibrosis, rheumatoid (necrobiotic) nodules, COP, obliterative bronchiolitis, follicular bronchiolitis, and pleural effusion.[14] Interstitial pneumonitis and fibrosis are the most common pulmonary manifestations of rheumatoid arthritis with the later present in almost 5% of patients or radiography and 30–40% on HRCT.

Imaging Features

- UIP is the most common pattern of RA related ILD, with fine reticular pattern in early disease on radiography, with involvement of the lower lung zones. With disease progression, these reticulations become coarser and more diffuse in distribution. Honeycombing may also be seen in advanced disease. Similar to the findings at radiography, the predominant abnormality at HRCT consists of irregular linear opacities caused by a combination of thickening of interlobular and intralobular septa. Honeycombing is seen, most markedly near the diaphragm.
- NSIP is seen as the second most common pattern, with ground-glass opacities and microcyst formation.
- Acute interstitial pneumonia and organising pneumonia are less commonly seen patterns in RA-ILD.
- Drug-induced ILD may complicate the imaging appearance of RA-ILD with differentiation between the two possible on studying the temporal relationship only. Methotrexate is the most common causative agent.[15]

PROGRESSIVE SYSTEMIC SCLEROSIS (PSS)

Pulmonary involvement is commoner and more severe in systemic sclerosis than in other collagen vascular disease.[16] Interstitial fibrosis is the most common manifestation (in approximately 80% of patients). The histological features are those of NSIP or UIP, the former being more common and associated with worse prognosis.

Imaging Features

- Evidence of interstitial fibrosis has been reported at chest radiography in 20–65% of patients. Serial radiographs obtained over several years may show progressive loss of lung volume in addition to a worsening of the interstitial disease.
- HRCT frequently shows evidence of interstitial pneumonitis and fibrosis in patients who have normal or equivocal radiographic findings and may be used for monitoring the disease overtime. The abnormalities have a predominantly peripheral and posterior distribution **(Figs. 6A and B)**. The most common abnormalities that are seen on CT are peripheral and basal ground-glass opacities and fibrosis (often with subpleural sparing), pleural or pericardial effusion, esophageal dilatation, mediastinal lymphadenopathy, and sometimes pulmonary arterial dilatation that reflects pulmonary hypertension. Organizing pneumonia is a less commonly seen pattern in PSS-ILD.

SYSTEMIC LUPUS ERYTHEMATOSUS

Pulmonary manifestations of systemic lupus erythematosus (SLE) may be acute (pulmonary hemorrhage, acute lupus pneumonitis, and pulmonary edema), subacute (pleural effusion and thickening) and chronic (interstitial pneumonitis and fibrosis) manifestations. The most common radiologic abnormality is pleural effusion (25–35%). Pericardial effusion is seen in approximately 20% of patients and pulmonary parenchymal involvement in 20%.

Imaging Features

- Ground-glass attenuation and consolidation on HRCT may be due to interstitial pneumonitis/fibrosis, acute lupus pneumonitis, hemorrhage, or, rarely, bronchiolitis obliterans organizing pneumonia (BOOP).
- Reticular pattern mainly involves the lower lung zones on radiography, and is seen in only about 3% of patients. On the other hand, HRCT may demonstrate the abnormalities in approximately 30% of patients. The interstitial abnormalities include interlobular septal thickening, irregular linear hyperattenuating areas and architectural distortion.
- Honeycombing is uncommon.
- Infections may occur secondarily, including community-acquired pneumonias, atypical pneumonia and tuberculosis.

POLYMYOSITIS AND DERMATOMYOSITIS

These are idiopathic inflammatory myopathies with pulmonary involvement in around 40% patients in the form of ILD, aspiration pneumonia, and infections.

The common pattern is that of NSIP followed by UIP and organizing pneumonia. Mostly a chronic, indolent course is seen in polymyositis, whereas acute and rapidly progressive course is more common in dermatomyositis.

HYPERSENSITIVITY PNEUMONITIS

Hypersensitivity pneumonitis (HP) is a diffuse granulomatous ILD caused by an abnormal immune response to various organic dusts. The clinical manifestations, radiologic and histological patterns are nonspecific and may be similar to other interstitial and small airway diseases.[17] A high index of suspicion, detailed exposure and occupational history is paramount in making the diagnosis. Still the causative antigen may remain unidentifiable in up to 40% of histologically proven cases of HP.[18]

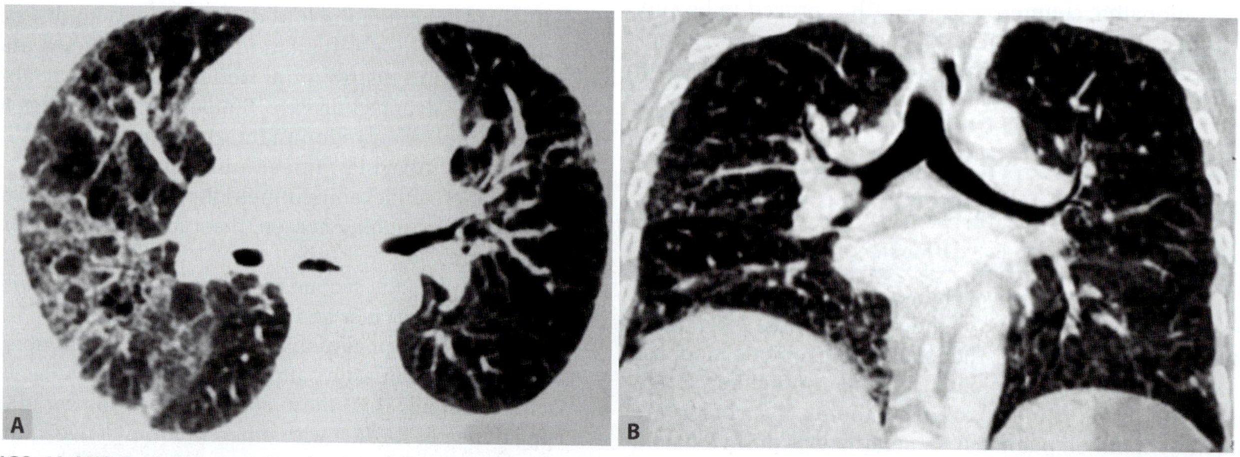

FIGS. 6A AND B: Progressive systemic sclerosis associated ILD. (A) Axial HRCT shows fine intralobular and interlobular septal thickening and ground-glass opacification in NSIP pattern. (B) Coronal multiplanar reconstruction shows the predominantly basal distribution of the patchy ground-glass opacities.

Imaging Features

The radiologic findings vary with the stage of the disease. HP manifests in three phases: Acute, subacute, and chronic. Early in the course of the acute stage, the chest X-ray may be normal. Later, bilateral, patchy areas of consolidation appear, which may be diffuse or in the lower lung zones. Most characteristic findings during the subacute stage are multiple ground-glass opacities and poorly defined centrilobular nodules. These abnormalities frequently resolve if the antigenic exposure is stopped. If exposure is continued or repeated, the diffuse nodular or ground-glass pattern is replaced by a reticular pattern characteristic of interstitial fibrosis.

HRCT

- Acute and subacute stages—the predominant abnormalities on HRCT are patchy or diffuse bilateral ground-glass opacities **(Figs. 7A and B)** superimposed on poorly defined small centrilobular nodules in the middle and lower lung zones.
- The ground-glass opacities may be concentrated in the centers of the secondary pulmonary lobules with sparing of the periphery. Another frequent finding in patients with subacute disease is the presence of localized areas of decreased attenuation and vascularity. Such areas have a striking lobular distribution and show evidence of air trapping on expiratory images.
- The HRCT differential diagnosis include DIP, alveolar proteinosis, lymphoid interstitial pneumonia (LIP) and respiratory bronchiolitis-associated interstitial diseases.
- Chronic HP shows reticulation, traction bronchiectasis and architectural distortion due to fibrosis with background changes of subacute HP. The reticulation may be random or subpleural and peribronchovascular in distribution. In a few cases, there is subpleural honeycombing resembling idiopathic pulmonary fibrosis, however the areas of air trapping and centrilobular nodules are rarely seen in idiopathic pulmonary fibrosis.[19]

SILICOSIS AND COAL WORKERS' PNEUMOCONIOSIS

Silicosis and coal worker's pneumoconiosis are ILDs related to exposure of dust-containing crystallized silicon dioxide and coal dust. A positive inhalational history with characteristic findings on imaging are often sufficient to make the diagnosis.

Imaging Features

HRCT—Small (2–5 mm), perihilar and dorsal lung zones centrilobular nodules with upper lobe predominance **(Fig. 8)**.[20] Miliary distribution can be rarely seen in these patients. Calcified lymphadenopathy (hilar and mediastinal) is common, sometimes with characteristic egg-shell calcifications.

- The nodules in silicosis patients tend to coalesce and initially form clusters, and later form large conglomerate masses, i.e. progressive massive fibrosis (PMF) **(Fig. 9)**. Conglomerate masses are seen more in apical and posterior segments of the upper lobes.
- Associated peripheral parenchymal distortion with paracicatricial emphysema is common. PMF is typically bilateral and often symmetric. PMF lesions may uncommonly be calcified or show central cavitation which may result from ischemic necrosis or tuberculosis.
- On imaging, coal worker's pneumoconiosis and silicosis show overlapping features. The radiographic pattern of

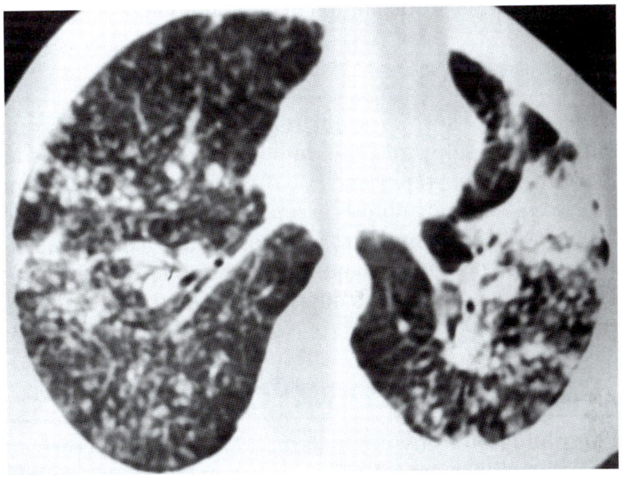

FIG. 8: Silicosis: Axial HRCT shows clusters of 5 mm of centrilobular and subpleural micronodules in a foundry worker with silicosis. Some of the nodules are seen aggregating into PMF masses.

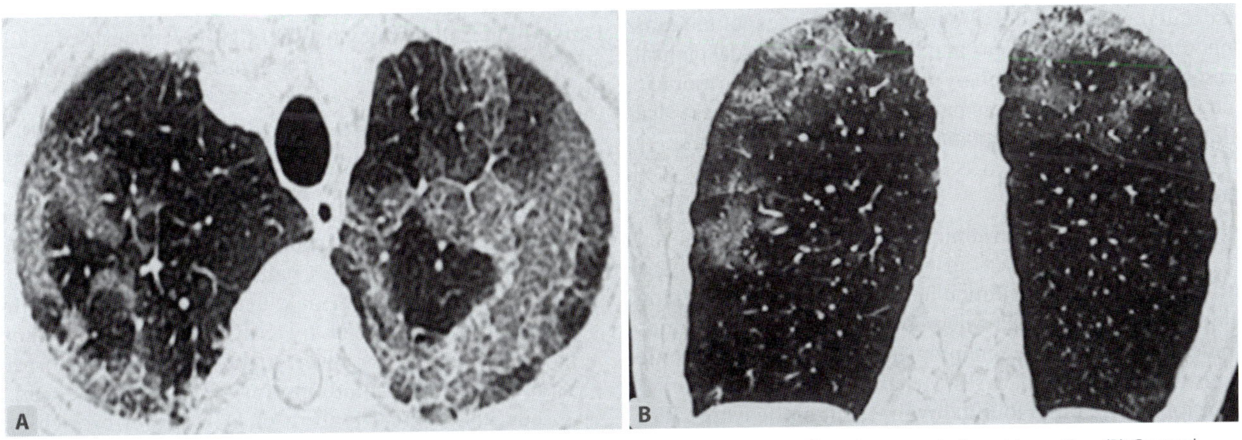

FIGS. 7A AND B: Acute hypersensitivity pneumonitis. (A) Axial HRCT shows extensive areas of patchy ground-glass attenuation; (B) Coronal multiplanar reconstruction shows the predominantly upper lobar distribution of the patchy ground-glass opacities.

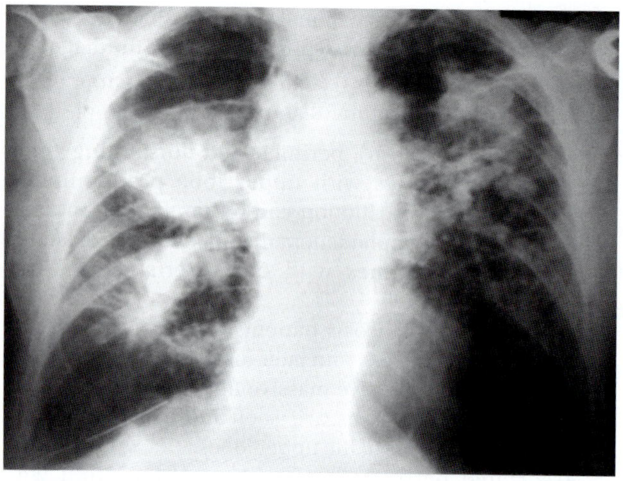

FIG. 9: Advanced Silicosis with PMF: Frontal chest radiograph shows large, parahilar fibrotic masses with surrounding cicatricial emphysema. As PMF progresses the number of nodules decreases because of their aggregation into fibrotic lesions.

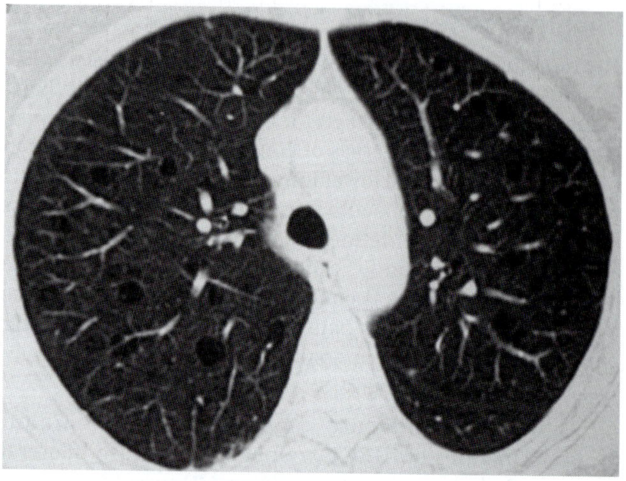

FIG. 10: Axial HRCT shows early LAM with subtle thin-walled cysts interspersed with normal lung parenchyma.

simple coal worker's pneumoconiosis include small 1–5 mm round ill-defined/granular nodules. Eggshell calcification is uncommon in the condition.[21]

ASBESTOSIS

Asbestos exposure is seen in miners, millers, persons employed in shipyards, and building trades. Asbestosis at plain chest radiography and HRCT is indistinguishable from other causes of lung fibrosis except when pleural plaques are visible, which then indicates asbestosis as the likely cause. In the absence of pleural plaques, the pattern of fibrosis alone in asbestosis is difficult to differentiate from UIP from other causes.

LYMPHANGIOLEIOMYOMATOSIS

Lymphangioleiomyomatosis (LAM) is characterized pathologically by interstitial proliferation of atypical smooth muscle and is a rare disease. Peribronchiolar proliferation causes distal air trapping and air-cyst formation.[22] It can occur in isolation or in association with tuberous sclerosis. It is restricted to women of childbearing age, and is not associated with smoking. Progressive dyspnea, spontaneous pneumothorax, chylothorax and hemoptysis are usual clinical presentations. Extrapulmonary manifestations include thoracic and abdominal lymphadenopathy, chylous ascites, pericardial effusion, renal angiomyolipomas, and lymphangiomatosis.

Imaging Features

Pleural and parenchymal abnormalities are clearly visualized on chest radiography in around 70% of the patients. A bilateral, symmetrical reticular pattern is seen involving all lung zones to a similar degree (80%) or the lower zones predominantly in the remaining 20% patients. Cysts can be identified in 50–60% of cases. Hyperinflation and expiratory air trapping are often found. Involvement of the lymphatics may cause obstruction and accumulation of chylous pleural effusions in 10–20%. Recurrent pneumothorax is a frequent complication (30–40%), due to spontaneous rupture of the thin-walled cysts.

- HRCT features of LAM are characteristic in the form of uniformly distributed multiple thin-walled cysts of 2 mm to 5 cm size, with intervening normal lung parenchyma **(Fig. 10)**. The wall thickness of the cysts is variable up to few millimeters.
- The main differential diagnosis on HRCT is LCH. However, the cysts in LCH typically involve the middle and upper lung zones, with sparing of the lung bases. In addition most patients with LCH also have nodules, a finding that is seen rarely in LAM. The presence of pleural effusion further helps to distinguish the cystic lung disease in LAM from LCH.

LANGERHANS CELL HISTIOCYTOSIS

Langerhans cell histiocytosis (LCH) refers to a group of diseases mostly affecting children with unknown etiology, in which Langerhans cell accumulate in one or more body systems like bone, lung, pituitary gland, mucous membranes, skin, lymph nodes, and liver. On the other hand, pulmonary Langerhans cell histiocytosis (PLCH) is a disease of adults affecting the lung, usually in isolation or less commonly in other organ systems.[23]

- Up to 100% of PLCH patients are current or former smokers and there is a slight male predominance. The peak is at 20–40 years of age.
- Extrapulmonary manifestations of PLCH (bone lesions, diabetes insipidus, and skin lesions) may occur in 5–15% of patients. About 20–25% patients are asymptomatic.
- Dry cough and dyspnea are common presenting complaints, followed by constitutional symptoms, such as weight loss, fever, night sweats, and anorexia. Spontaneous pneumothorax may occasionally be seen.
- A key histological feature of LCH is peribronchiolar nodules containing Langerhans cells and inflammatory

cells in the early stages. With time, these nodules become fibrotic causing stellate peribronchiolar scars.
- Cessation of smoking is sufficient for stabilization of symptoms in most patients. Medical therapy includes corticosteroids which are the mainstay. Chemotherapeutic drugs such as vinblastine, methotrexate, and cyclophosphamide may be used in non-responders and in multi-organ involvement.

Imaging Features

Chest radiographs—show nodular or reticulonodular opacities predominantly in the upper lungs.[22]
- Costophrenic angles are spared.
- Lung volumes are preserved.
- With disease progression, cystic changes and bullae develop in the upper lungs and lung volumes increases.

HRCT—show characteristic findings of nodules and cysts predominating in the upper and mid lungs, with sparing of the bases. Early in the disease, peribronchiolar centrilobular nodules of 1 to 5 mm diameter predominate.
- With disease evolution, thick- or thin-walled cysts (usually less than 10 mm in diameter) are identified in 80% of the patients **(Figs. 11A and B)**. These cysts may be round, lobulated, irregular or bizarre in shape, often with normal intervening parenchyma. Rupture of cysts into the pleural space causes episodic pneumothorax. Longitudinal HRCT studies have shown progression of solid nodules to cavitary nodules to thick-walled cysts, and finally thin-walled cysts.[23]
- In patients showing isolated nodular disease on HRCT, the differential diagnosis includes sarcoidosis, silicosis, metastatic disease, and tuberculosis. The distribution in the upper and mid lungs and the centrilobular nature of the nodules in PLCH may in differentiation. Cystic changes may simulate the appearance of LAM; however, the cysts in LAM occur throughout the lung without sparing the lung bases and nodules are rarely seen. In both conditions, lung volumes are preserved and pneumothorax can occur.

The natural history of LCH is variable and unpredictable. Approximately, 50% of patients may have partial or complete clearing of radiologic abnormalities with symptom resolution. Follow-up CT scans may show regression of nodules, whereas any cysts that have formed are permanent. In 30–40% of patients, persisting symptoms are variable severity; scarring supervenes which results in reticulation, thickening of the cyst walls, and architectural distortion. In 10–20% patients, recurrent pneumothorax or progressive respiratory failure with cor-pulmonale occurs.

PULMONARY ALVEOLAR PROTEINOSIS

Pulmonary alveolar proteinosis (PAP) is a rare disease characterized by accumulation of abnormal proteinaceous material in the alveoli, causing hypoxemia, restrictive lung disease and a radiological appearance like pulmonary edema. Idiopathic PAP accounts for up to 90% of cases. Secondary PAP (5–10% of cases) is seen in patients with industrial inhalational exposure to silica particles, cement dust, aluminum dust, titanium dioxide, nitrogen dioxide, and fiberglass; underlying hematologic malignancy; or immunodeficiency disorders like cytotoxic or immunosuppressive therapy and human immuno-deficiency virus infection.

Imaging Features

Chest radiography: Bilateral central and symmetric lung opacities, with relative sparing of the apices and costophrenic angles.
- Less commonly, radiographs show multifocal asymmetric opacities or extensive diffuse consolidation without any clear zonal predominance. Opacities may be ground-glass, reticular/reticulonodular, to consolidation with air bronchogram. Although the radiographic appearance of PAP may suggest pulmonary interstitial edema, pleural effusion and cardiomegaly are absent.
- There is often a discordance between marked radiographic abnormalities in the presence of more benign clinical symptoms (clinicoradiologic discrepancy).[24]

HRCT—bilateral, symmetric alveolar consolidation or ground-glass opacity, in a perihilar or hilar distribution. Geographic ground-glass attenuation, sharply demarcated from the surrounding normal parenchyma, with superimposed polygonal shape intra- and interlobular septal thickening **(Fig. 12)** creates the 'crazy paving' appearance.[25] The crazy paving appearance for alveolar proteinosis, although highly sensitive, is not specific.

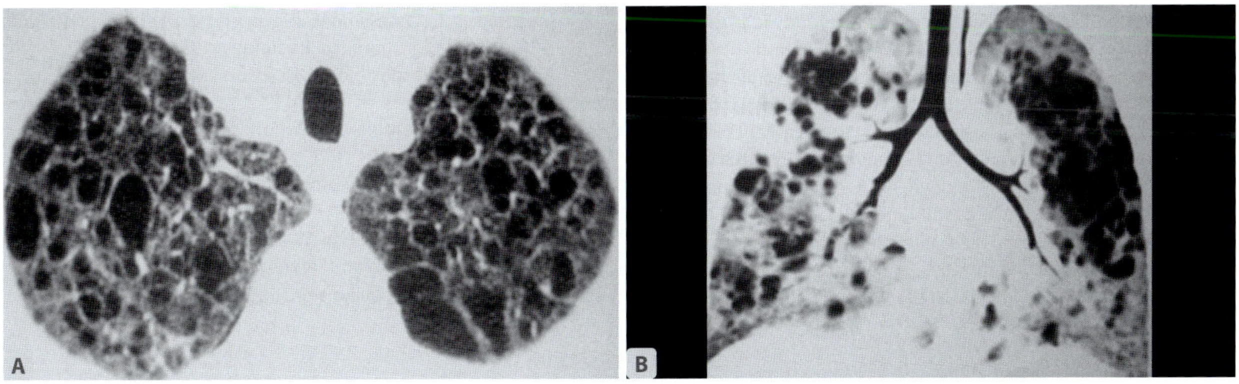

FIGS. 11A AND B: (A) Axial HRCT shows multiple, varying sized thick-walled cysts diffusely involving bilateral lungs; (B) Coronal multiplanar reconstruction shows the relative sparing of the bilateral lung bases.

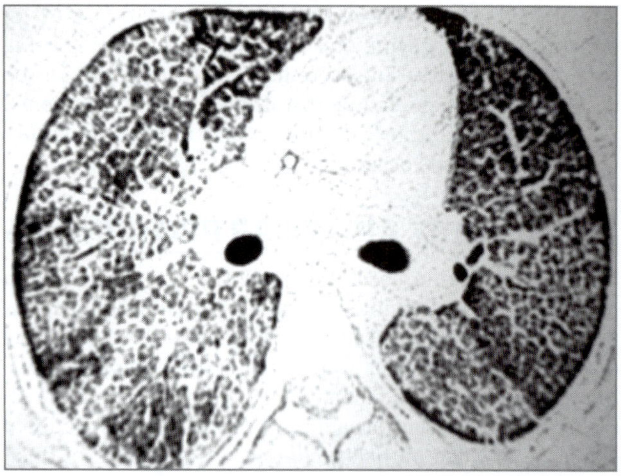

FIG. 12: Pulmonary alveolar proteinosis (PAP): Axial HRCT shows classic findings of "crazy paving"; geographic ground-glass attenuation superimposed with thickening of interstitium producing polygonal opacities.

- The radiological differential diagnosis includes diffuse alveolar damage superimposed on UIP, acute interstitial pneumonia, acute respiratory distress syndrome and bronchoalveolar carcinoma.

Sequential therapeutic whole-lung lavage is the main treatment in idiopathic PAP, which involves the use of saline solution and chest percussion to remove the lipo proteinaceous material from pulmonary alveoli. Post-therapeutic whole-lung lavage CT may reveal resolution of ground-glass opacity, however, the septal lines may still persist.

CONCLUSION

A whole gamut of conditions in the wide group of interstitial lung disease due to a known cause have similar clinical presentation. A meticulous history with regards to the offending allergens if any with thorough biochemical evaluation helps in narrowing down the diagnosis. A multidisciplinary approach with radiologist, pulmonary physician and pathologist is desired to achieve optimum care for such patients.

REFERENCES

1. American Thoracic Society/European Respiratory Society International Multidisciplinary Consensus Classification of the Idiopathic Interstitial Pneumonias. Am J Respir Crit Care Med. 2002;165:277-304.
2. Travis WD, Costabel U, Hansell DM, et al. An official American Thoracic Society/European Respiratory Society statement: Update of the international multidisciplinary classification of the idiopathic interstitial pneumonias. Am J Respir Crit Care Med. 2013;188(6):733-48.
3. Bokulic RE, Hilman BC. Interstitial lung disease in children. Pediatr Clin North Am. 1994; 41:543-67.
4. Epler GR, McLoud TC, Gaensler EA, et al. Normal chest roentgenograms in chronic diffuse. Infiltrative lung disease. N Engl J Med. 1978;298(17):934-9.
5. Webb WR. High-revolution CT of the lung parenchyma. Radiol Clin North Am. 1989;27:1085-97.
6. Hansell DM, Bankier AA, MacMahon H, et al. Remy J Fleischner Society: glossary of terms for thoracic imaging. Radiology. 2008;246(3):697-722.
7. Webb WR, Muller NL, Naidich DP. Standardized terms for high-resolution computed tomography of the lung: A proposed glossary. J Thorac Imaging. 1993;8:167-75.
8. Lynch JP, Kazerooni EA, Gay SE. Pulmonary sarcoidosis. Clin Chest Med. 1997;18:755-85.
9. James DG, Neville E, Siltzbach LE. A worldwide review of sarcoidosis. Ann NY Acad Sci. 1976;278:321-34.
10. Koyama T, Ueda H, Togashi K, et al. Radiologic manifestations of sarcoidosis in various organs. Radiographics. 2004;24(1):87-104.
11. Ichikawa Y, Fujimoto K, Shiraishi T, et al. Primary cavitary sarcoidosis: High-resolution CT findings. Am J Roentgenol. 1994;163(3):745.
12. New Silva M, Nunes H, Valeyre D, Sverzellati N. Imaging of Sarcoidosis. Clin Rev Allergy Immunol. 2015; 49(1):45-53.
13. Kim EA, Lee KS, Johkoh T, et al. Interstitial lung diseases associated with collagen vascular diseases: radiologic and histopathologic findings. Radiographics. 2002;22 Spec No: S151-65.
14. Tanaka N, Kim JS, Newell JD, et al. Rheumatoid arthritis-related lung diseases: CT findings. Radiology. 2004;232 (1):81-91.
15. Vyas Surabhi. Connective tissue disorders and related interstitial lung disease: Imaging. In: Bhalla AS, Jana M (Eds). Imaging of interstitial lung diseases, Clinicoradiological series. 2017. The Health Sciences Publishers. P. 81-96.
16. Goldin JG, Lynch DA, Strollo DC, et al. Scleroderma Lung Study Research Group. High-resolution CT scan findings in patients with symptomatic scleroderma-related interstitial lung disease. Chest. 2008;134(2):358-67.
17. Glazer CS, Rose CS, Lynch DA. Clinical and radiologic manifestations of hypersensitivity pneumonitis. J Thorac Imaging. 2002;17:261-72.
18. Silva CI, Churg A, Müller NL. Hypersensitivity pneumonitis: spectrum of high-resolution CT and pathologic findings. Am J Roentgenol. 2007;188 (2):334-44.
19. CI, Müller NL, Lynch DA, Curran-Everett D, et al. Chronic hypersensitivity pneumonitis: Differentiation from idiopathic pulmonary fibrosis and nonspecific interstitial pneumonia by using thin-section CT. Radiology. 2008;246 (1):288-97.
20. Begin R, Ostiguy G, Fillion R, et al. Computed tomography scan in the early detection of silicosis. Am Rev Respir Dis. 1991;144: 697-705.
21. Remy-Jardin M, Degreef JM, Beuscart R, et al. Coal worker's pneumoconiosis: CT assessment in exposed workers and correlation with radiographic findings. Radiology. 1990;177:363-71.
22. Abbott GF, Rosado-de-Christenson ML, Frazier AA, et al. From the archives of the AFIP: Lymphangioleiomyomatosis: Radiologic-pathologic correlation. Radiographics. 2005;25 (3): 803-28.
23. Tazi A. Adult pulmonary Langerhans' cell histiocytosis. Eur Respir J. 2006;27 (6):1272-85.
24. Holbert JM, Costello P, Li W, et al. CT features of pulmonary alveolar proteinosis. Am J Roentgenol. 2001;176:1287-94.
25. Lee CH. The crazy-paving sign. Radiology 2007;243;905-6.

CHAPTER

131

Miscellaneous Interstitial Lung Diseases

Ashu Seith Bhalla, Manisha Jana

INTRODUCTION

This chapter includes a wide range of diffuse lung diseases (DLDs), not covered in the previous chapters. Some of them are interstitial lung diseases (ILDs), whereas some are diseases mimicking ILD. Since description of all of these is beyond the scope of this chapter, a pattern approach on High-resolution computed tomography (HRCT) will be followed. Uncommon DLDs presenting with ground-glass opacity (GGO), septal thickening and nodules is covered. This is followed by discussion of 'cystic lung diseases'.

DIFFUSE LUNG DISEASES PRESENTING WITH GROUND-GLASS OPACITY

Commoner DLDs presenting with a predominant GGO pattern have been discussed in detail in earlier capters. **Table 1** enlists less frequent etiologies.

INFECTIONS

Interstitial pneumonia[1,2] may appear as ill defined areas of GGOs. Severity can range from mild forms to those causing respiratory failure. A few more severe specific forms are described here.

TABLE 1: Uncommon DLDs presenting with GGO pattern.

Infections	• Interstitial pneumonia • Viral pneumonia • *Mycoplasma pneumoniae* • *Pneumocystis jirovecii*
Others	• Eosinophilic lung diseases • Lipoid pneumonia • Acute respiratory distress syndrome (ARDS) • Diffuse alveolar hemorrhage (DAH) • Pulmonary alveolar proteinosis (PAP)

Severe Acute Respiratory Syndrome

Severe acute respiratory syndrome (SARS) is an acute respiratory disorder caused by coronavirus. The pathology is alveolar damage and airspace edema.[3] Usual presenting symptoms are high-grade fever, dry cough and dyspnea usually within 10 days after SARS exposure. Chest radiograph reveals unifocal or multifocal consolidation. HRCT can show either GGO, consolidation or crazy paving appearance. The findings can either be unilateral or bilateral.

Swine Influenza (H1N1)

It is caused by Swine-origin influenza A (H1N1) virus. The pathology is a diffuse alveolar damage. Patients present with dry cough and dyspnea usually following a prodromal period of 2–7 days. Swine influenza is usually a mild disease but can be complicated by acute respiratory distress syndrome or secondary pneumonia. On HRCT, the predominant findings can be unilateral or bilateral GGO. Consolidations can be peribronchovascular or subpleural consolidations.

Mycoplasma Pneumoniae

It is a common cause of community-acquired pneumonia in children and young adults, caused by *Mycoplasma pneumoniae* (walking pneumonia). Usual presenting symptoms are fever and productive cough, nonspecific complaints, fatigue and myalgia. Chest radiograph can show diffuse reticulonodular opacities, peribronchial thickening or even frank consolidation. HRCT findings include centrilobular nodules, peribronchovascular and interlobular septal thickening, lobular or segmental consolidation **(Figs. 1A and B)**.

Pneumocystis jirovecii Pneumonia

This is the most common cause of opportunistic infection in HIV- infected patients. The causative organism is an atypical fungus *Pneumocystis jiroveci.* The clinical features depend on the immune status of the patient. While it presents as an

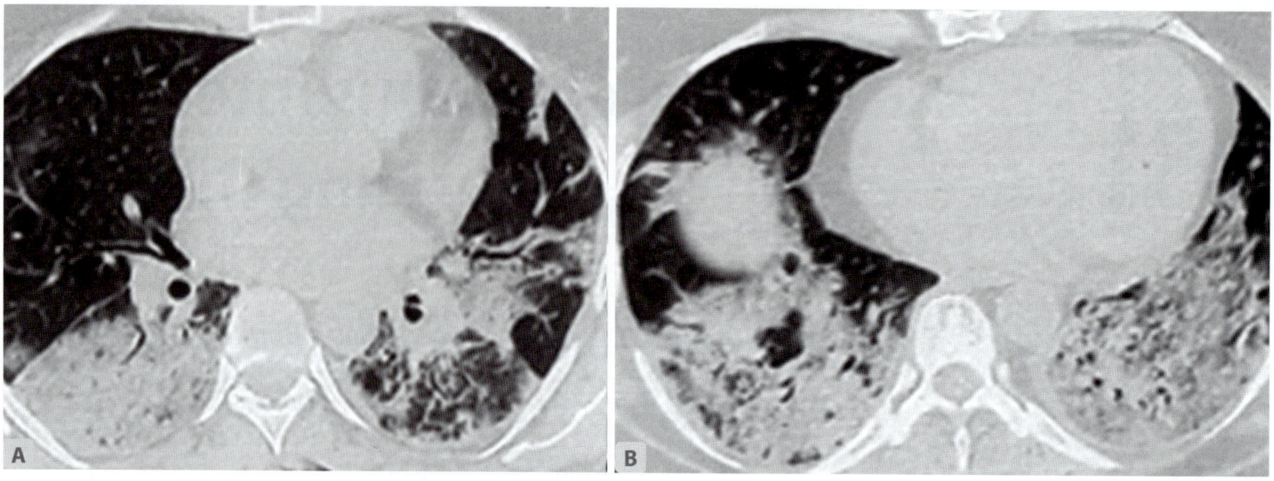

FIGS. 1A AND B: *Mycoplasma pneumoniae*: HRCT images reveal multifocal patchy consolidation in dependent locations.

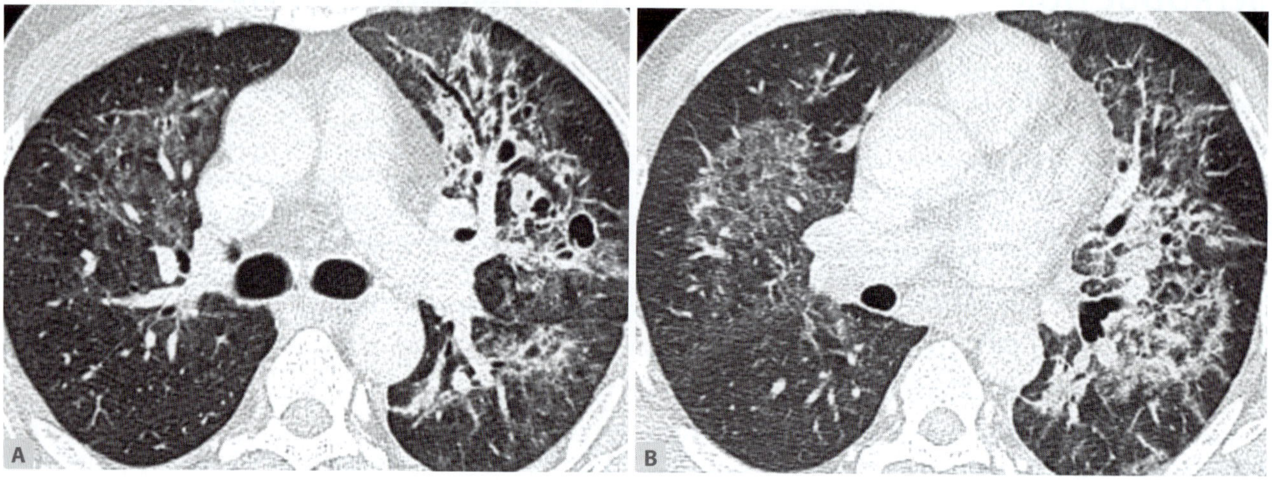

FIGS. 2A AND B: Subacute *Pneumocystis jirovecii* pneumonia: CT reveals central perihilar GGO with superimposed septal thickening and thin-walled cysts.

acute illness with severe hypoxia and respiratory failure in an immunocompetent individual; the symptoms are more gradual in onset in HIV-infected patient. It is common in patients with a CD4 count <100.

Chest radiograph reveals a bilaterally symmetric perihilar reticulonodular pattern; which can progress to consolidation subsequently. HRCT reveals bilateral symmetric perihilar groundglass opacities **(Figs. 2A and B)**. In subacute stage of the disease, consolidation with septal thickening produces a 'crazy paving' pattern. Thin walled varying sized cysts can also develop in subacute stages; which can rupture and lead to spontaneous pneumothorax/pneumomediastinum.

ACUTE RESPIRATORY DISTRESS SYNDROME

Acute respiratory distress syndrome (ARDS) is a diffuse alveolar damage resulting from variety of insults and requiring mechanical ventilation. The pathology is diffuse alveolar damage, increased capillary and alveolar permeability, leading to edema (interstitial and alveolar), followed by a phase of fibrosis. Three clinical phases are recognized-acute, subacute and chronic.[4,5]

Acute (Exudative) Phase

This is seen in the initial 7 days following insult. The chest radiograph can be normal in the first 24 hours. Over the next 2–3 days—extensive, bilateral air space opacification/consolidation ("White lung") can develop. The consolidation can be patchy and multifocal. Radiographic criteria for diagnosis of ARDS include bilateral opacities (consistent with pulmonary edema), findings not explainable by pleural effusion, lung collapse or nodules. CT findings can appear by 12 hours. HRCT findings include GGO and consolidation having a diffuse or patchy distribution. Usually there is an apico-basal gradient, with more opacification of the lung bases.

Subacute (Proliferative) Phase

It is between one and two weeks, when there is conversion of alveolar exudates into cellular granulation tissue. Imaging in subacute phase shows an increasing consolidation in early phase, followed by appearance of interlobular septal thickening, "crazy paving pattern" and bronchiectasis and bronchiolectasis **(Figs. 3A and B)**.

Chronic (Fibrotic) Phase

It is seen two weeks or more following injury. Diffuse parenchymal fibrosis and architectural distortion ensue. HRCT reveals fibrosis, bronchiectasis, bronchiolectasis with distortion of airways and volume loss with bullae formation. Morphological changes may persist in survivors even when imaged months after the acute episode.

HYDROSTATIC PULMONARY EDEMA

Hydrostatic pulmonary edema is seen in cardiac failure or fluid overload due to accumulation of fluid in the extravascular compartment of the lung. There are two pathological phases—interstitial edema and alveolar filling.

Chest radiograph shows enlargement of upper lobe pulmonary veins (due to diversion of blood flow) in early phase. Later on airspace opacities with central/parahilar (batwing distribution) develop. CT reveals diffuse/patchy and parahilar GGO and smooth interlobular septal thickening **(Figs. 4A and B)**. Hydrostatic pulmonary edema has a preponderance towards involvement of the dependent areas; which differentiates it from increased permeability edema; which has more subpleural and peripheral distribution. Peribronchovascular interstitial thickening can appear as bronchial wall thickening or prominence of pulmonary vessels. In cardiogenic pulmonary edema, pulmonary arteries and veins appear dilated. Transudative pleural effusion is commonly seen.

DIFFUSE ALVEOLAR HEMORRHAGE

Diffuse alveolar hemorrhage (DAH) can be secondary to various causes, including coagulation disorders, collagen vascular disorders and vasculitis.[6] The isiopathic form is termed idiopathic pulmonary hemorrahge (IPH). The clinical presentation is variable; hemoptysis and anemia are some of the presenting symptoms. On pathology, three different

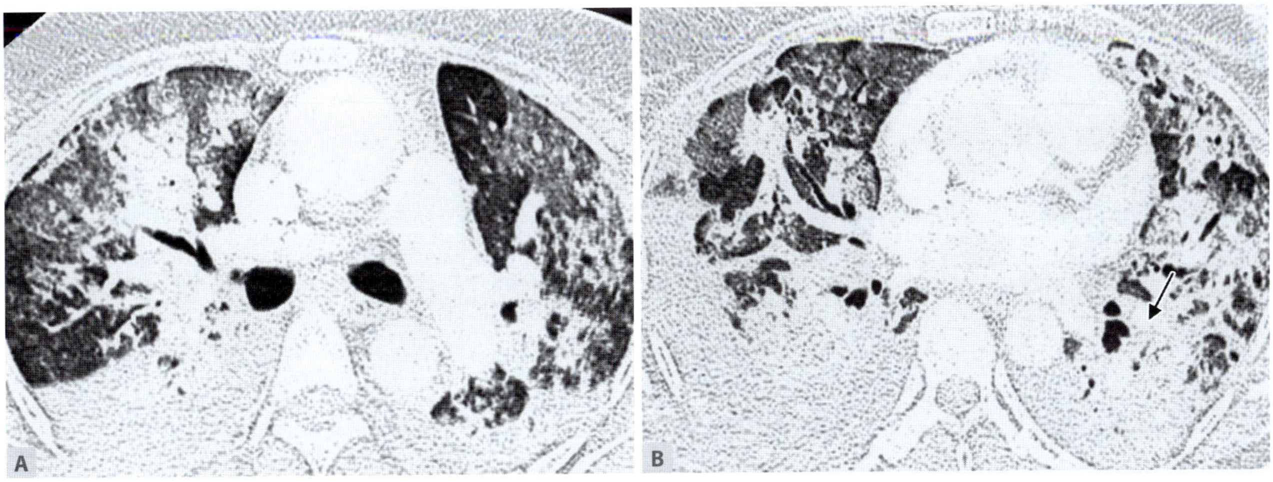

FIGS. 3A AND B: Acute respiratory distress syndrome in subacute phase. HRCT images reveal multifocal nonsegmental patchy consolidation and GGO with superimposed septal thickening (arrow). Bilateral pleural effusion is also present.

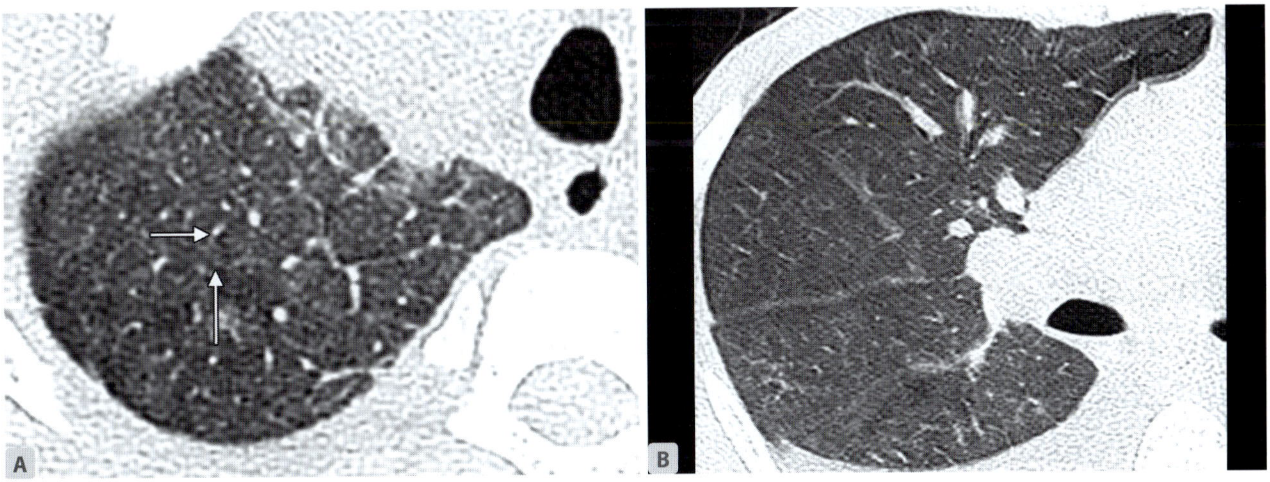

FIGS. 4A AND B: Hydrostatic pulmonary edema: HRCT images reveal smooth septal thickening (arrow), fissural thickening and right pleural effusion.

patterns have been described—associated with pulmonary capillaritis, bland alveolar hemorrhage with no vasculitis and diffuse alveolar damage (DAD) related DAH. HRCT reveals bilateral GGO/consolidation having a lobular appearance and more involvement of dependent areas **(Figs. 5A and B)**. In most cause, the pulmonary changes are reversible, except in those with DAD.

EOSINOPHILIC LUNG DISEASE

Eosinophilic lung disease comprises of varied disease entities, which are characterized by pulmonary manifestations and eosinophilia (peripheral or tissue eosinophilia).[7] On the basis of etiolgy, they can be classified as—eosinophilic lung diseases of unknown cause, eosinophilic lung diseases of known cause and eosinophilic vasculitis. On the basis of clinical presentation, the folloing subtypes are describe.

Acute Eosinophilic Pneumonia (Figs. 6A and B)

It presents with fever and respiratory distress which shows immediate response to steroids. Usually there are >25% eosinophils in bronchoalveolar lavage (BAL) fluid. HRCT findings include bilateral patchy GGO and septal thickening. Ill-defined nodules and consolidation are other unusual findings.

Chronic Eosinophilic Pneumonia

It usually affects middle aged women, has an insidious onset and mild eosinophilia. HRCT shows GGO, peripheral nonsegmental consolidation with a upper lobe predominance.

Idiopathic Hypereosinophilic Syndrome

In contrast, usually affects males in their 30 s and presents with multiorgan dysfunction. There is persistent eosinophilia without any demonstrable allergic or parasitic cause. HRCT shows a focal or diffuse nonlobar distribution of nodules, perinodular GGO and patchy GGO.

Other forms of eosinophilic lung disease include tropical pulmonary eosinophilia (TPE) which presents with ill-defined nodules, and eosinophilic bronchitis presenting with features of small airway disease.

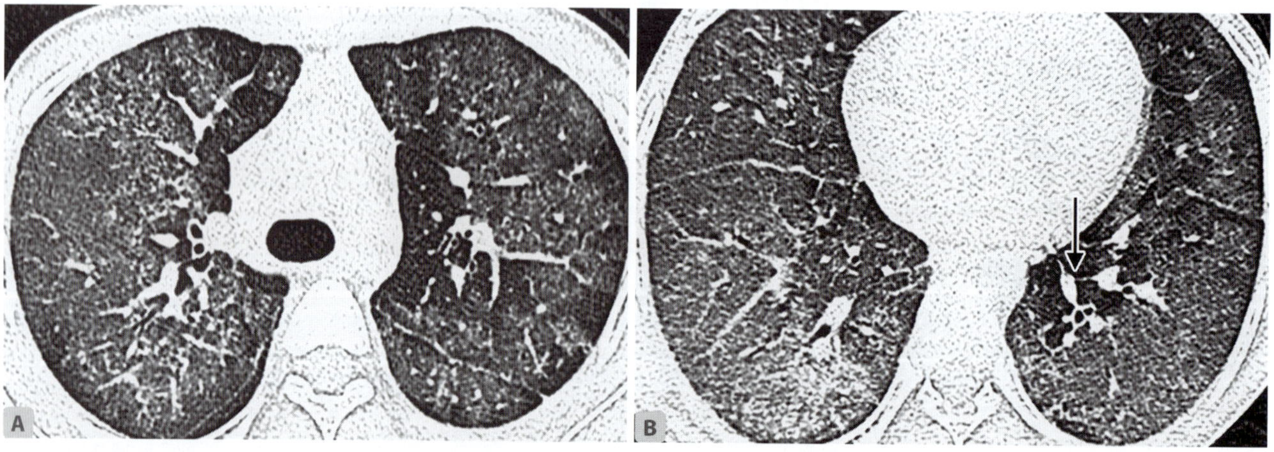

FIGS. 5A AND B: Diffuse alveolar hemorrhage in a 15-year-old male patient with anemia. HRCT images show diffuse GGO and septal thickening with sparing of lung bases and the periphery. Note the lobular sparing (arrow).

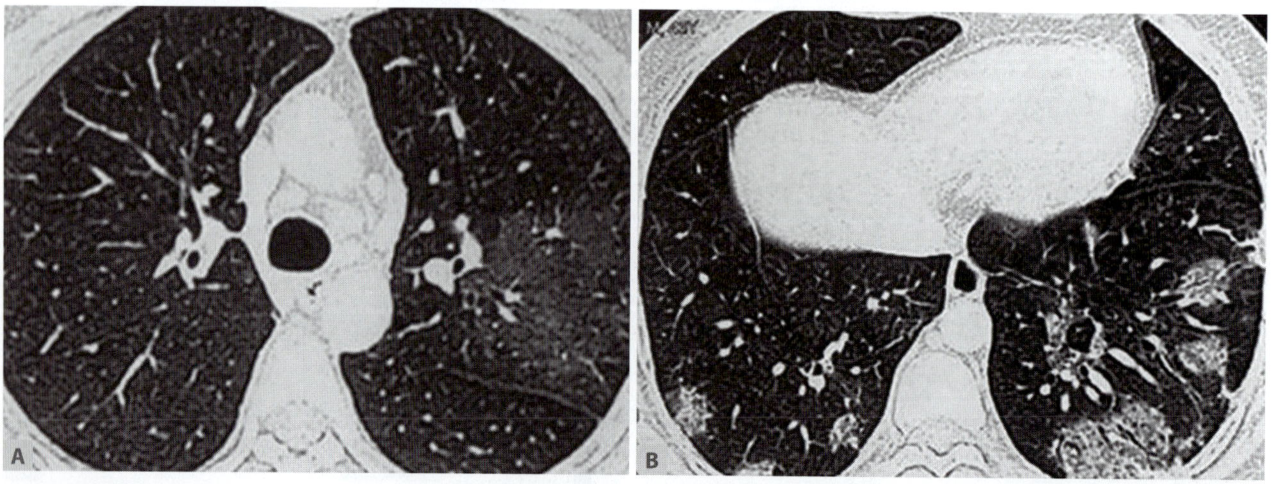

FIGS. 6A AND B: Acute eosinophilic pneumonia in a 30-year-old male with acute onset cough. HRCT images reveal bilateral peripheral ground-glass opacities.

LIPOID PNEUMONIA

Lipoid pneumonia is characterized by the alveolar accumulation of lipids.[8-10] It can be of three main types depending on the source and the presentation—exogenous acute, exogenous chronic and endogenous forms.

Acute Exogenous Lipoid Pneumonia

It is caused by inhalation/aspiration of large quantity of animal fats/mineral or vegetable oils. The radiological manifestations develop within 30 minutes to 24 hours. The findings include bilateral segmental or lobar GGO/consolidation; having a middle and lower lobe preponderance. Ill-defined nodules, pneumatoceles, pleural effusions are uncommon findings.

Chronic Exogenous Lipoid Pneumonia

It is cause by recurrent episodes of aspiration/inhalation. On imaging, segmental GGO/consolidation with a peribronchovascular distribution can be seen in the lower lobes. Other associated imaging findings are septal thickening or fibrosis. Sometimes the consolidation shows a mass like appearance with fat attenuation within **(Figs. 7A to D)**.

Endogenous Lipoid Pneumonia

It is caused by bronchial obstruction or chronic pulmonary infection causing accumulation of fat within intra-alveolar macrophages. In contrast to the exogenous form; endogenous "cholesterol pneumonia" usually does not show any fat attenuation on CT. It presents as a consolidation distal to a central obstructing lesion. The diagnosis is histopathologic.

PULMONARY ALVEOLAR PROTEINOSIS

Pulmonary alveolar proteinosis (PAP) is characterized by the alveolar accumulation of surfactant-like proteins.[11] It can be of three types—congenital, idiopathic (primary) and secondary: Secondary PAP is seen in patients of hematological malignancies, dust/metal exposure, chemotherapy or infection and responds well to treatment of the predisposing cause. Congenital form results from inherited disorders of surfactant proteins. Patients with PAP can have variable symptoms. They can either be asymptomatic, or can even present with an insidious onset of dyspnea, dry cough and easy fatigability.

Chest radiograph reveals bilateral symmetric or patchy airspace opacification. HRCT shows the 'crazy paving pattern', caused by GGO and septal thickening **(Figs. 8A and B)**.[11] The involvement of the lungs is usually patchy, with geographic/lobular sparing. Differential diagnoses include—pulmonary hemorrhage, pulmonary edema, radiation exposure, drug induced, inhalation disorders, mucinous carcinoma, and storage disorders in children.

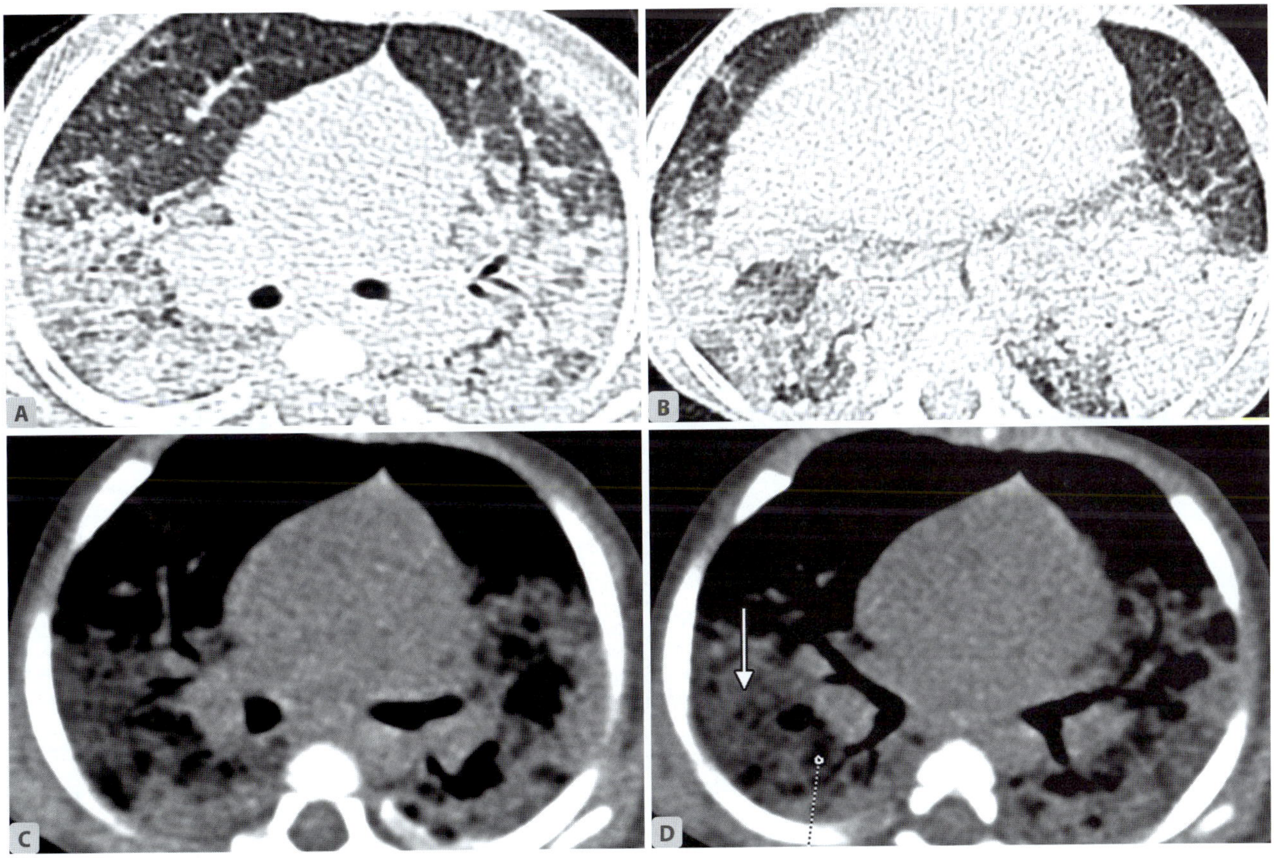

FIGS. 7A TO D: Exogenous lipoid pneumonia in a 7-year-old male child. HRCT images (A and B) reveal bilateral dense consolidation in dependent location. Soft tissue window images (C and D) reveal low attenuation areas within the areas of consolidation (arrow).

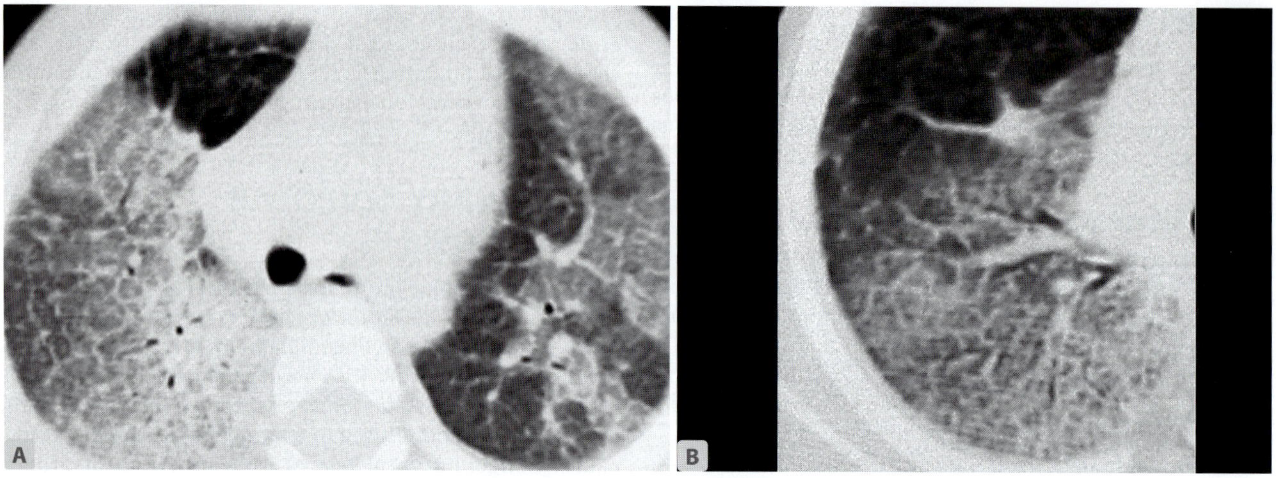

FIGS. 8A AND B: Pulmonary alveolar proteinosis pattern in storage disorder in a 6-year-old girl. CT images reveal diffuse 'crazy paving' pattern.

TABLE 2: Uncommon DLDs with predominant septal thickening.

Infections	• Atypical pneumonia—mycoplasma • *Pneumocystis jirovecii* pneumonia (PJP) • Severe acute respiratory syndrome (SARS)
Neoplastic	• Lymphangitis carcinomatosa • Lymphoma • Pulmonary leukostasis • Kaposi's sarcoma
Vascular	• Hydrostatic pulmonary edema • Acute respiratory distress syndrome (ARDS) • Pulmonary veno-occlusive disease (PVOD) • Pulmonary capillary hemangiomatosis (PCH)
Others	• Pulmonary alveolar proteinosis (PAP) • Diffuse alveolar septal amyloidosis • Diffuse alveolar hemorrhage (DAH)

SEPTAL THICKENING PREDOMINANT DIFFUSE LUNG DISEASES

Uncommon DLDs presenting with septal thickening are listed in **Table 2**.

Lymphangitis carcinomatosa, Kaposi's sarcoma and lymphoma are covered elsewhere in this book.

PULMONARY LEUKOSTASIS

Pulmonary leukostasis is a complication observed in acute myeloid leukemia M4 (myelomonocytic type). When white blood cell count exceeds one lac/μL, leukemic cells start accumulating within the small vessels of lungs, heart, brain and testis; and clog these small vessels. The clinical and radiographic findings are often discordant.[12,13] Chest radiograph can either be normal even in the presence of severe dyspnea; or may show alveolar or interstitial opacities. CT may reveal thickened bronchovascular bundles and segmental ground-glass opacities **(Figs. 9A and B)**.

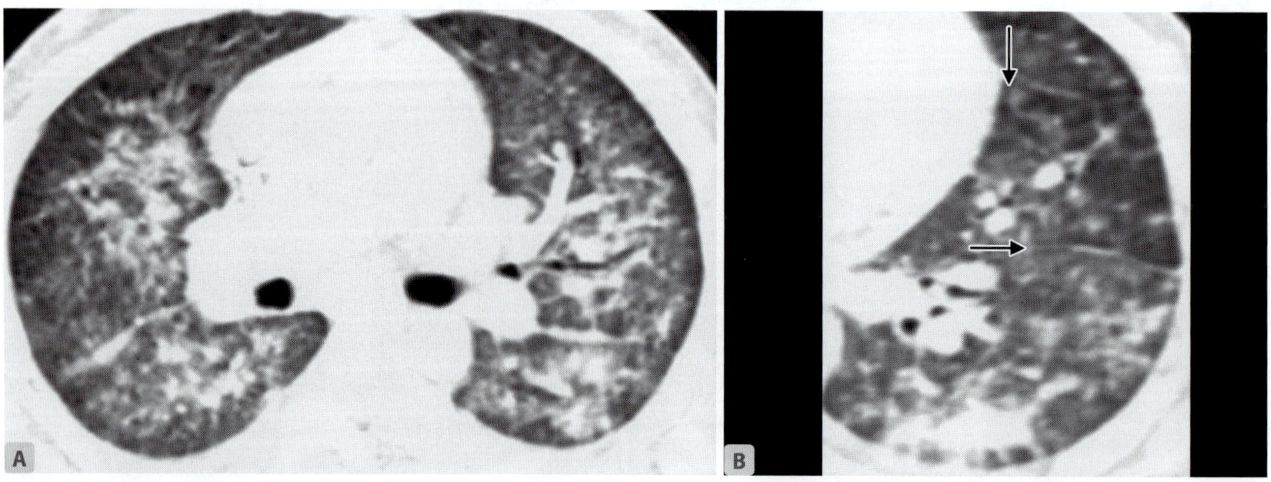

FIGS. 9A AND B: A 38-year-old male patient with AML having leukocytosis. CT reveals diffuse GGO, patchy consolidation and smooth septal thickening (arrow).

PULMONARY VENO-OCCLUSIVE DISEASE AND PULMONARY CAPILLARY HEMANGIOMATOSIS

Pulmonary veno-occlusive disease (PVOD) and pulmonary capillary hemangiomatosis (PCH) are rare disorders characterized by severe pulmonary arterial hypertension with normal pulmonary artery occlusion pressure and signs of pulmonary edema.[14-18] Although both are causes of pulmonary arterial hypertension the pathology in PVOD lies at the post-capillary level. There is fibrous occlusion of pulmonary venules. In PCH the problem lies at the capillary level [proliferation of alveolar capillaries (PCH)]. Definitive diagnosis is made on surgical lung biopsy.

The clinical features of both these entities include dyspnea on exertion, chronic cough, cyanosis, syncope and chest pain. In addition, hemoptysis is seen in PCH. The imaging findings **(Table 3)** are often quite characteristic **(Figs. 10A and B)**, in an appropriate clinical setting.

Diagnosing these entities on imaging in crucial; as administration of vasodilators on a presumptive clinical diagnosis of primary pulmonary hypertension can cause pulmonary edema in case of PVOD/PCH.

PULMONARY AMYLOIDOSIS

Amyloidosis is characterized by the abnormal extracellular deposition of proteins. Thoracic involvement can be localized or a part of systemic disease. Three main patterns of pulmonary involvement are described—nodular parenchymal, diffuse alveolar septal and airway/tracheo-bronchial amyloidosis.[19]

Diffuse Alveolar Septal Amyloidosis

It is usually associated with systemic involvement; and presents with cough and dyspnea. The prognosis is poor; and progression to pulmonary hypertension and respiratory failure may ensue. Chest radiograph reveals well-defined small nodules and reticular opacities. HRCT findings **(Fig. 11)** include well-defined, small nodules, smooth septal thickening, bilateral basal consolidations, areas of punctate calcifications and occasional cysts and traction bronchiectasis.

TABLE 3: Clinical and imaging findings of PVOD and PCH.

	PVOD	PCH
Gender predilection	M = F	F > M
Hemoptysis	Uncommon	Common symptom
HRCT	Dilated main pulmonary artery Smooth septal thickening Patchy ground-glass opacities Uncommon findings—multiple small nodules, consolidation in dependent lungs	Dilated main pulmonary artery Bilateral ill-defined ground-glass centrilobular nodules
Hemorrhagic pleural effusion	Uncommon	Common

(PVOD: pulmonary veno-occlusive disease; PCH: pulmonary capillary hemangiomatosis; HRCT: high resolution computed tomography)

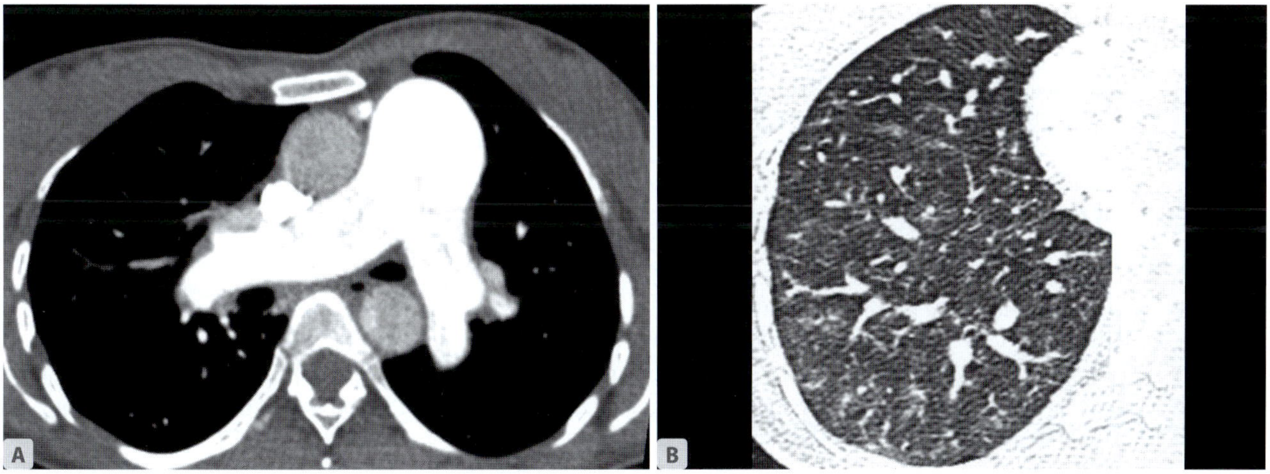

FIGS. 10A AND B: Pulmonary capillary hemangiomatosis in a 33-year-old lady with hemoptysis and PAH. CT reveals a dilated main pulmonary artery (A). HRCT image (B) reveals diffuse ground-glass nodules in the lungs.

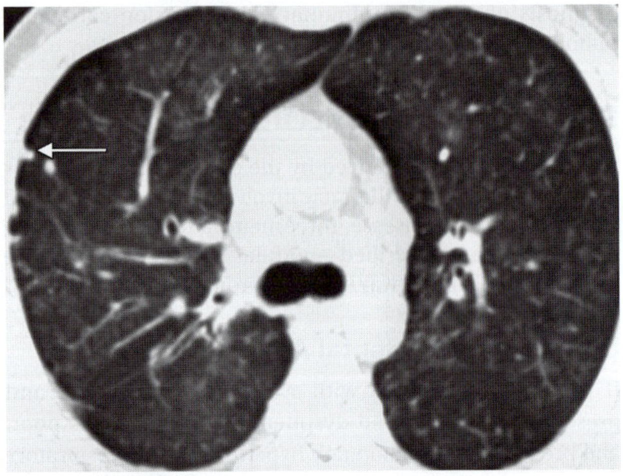

FIG. 11: Pulmonary amyloidosis: CT image reveals multiple small nodules, bronchovascular thickening, patchy GGO and peripheral bigger and well-defined subpleural nodules (arrow).

TABLE 4: Uncommon ILDs presenting with nodules.

Centrilobular	Random	Perilymphatic
• Viral pneumonia, *Haemophilus, Chlamydia, Mycoplasma* • PCH	• Pulmonary nodular amyloidosis	• Lymphangitis carcinomatosa • LIP • Amyloidosis

(ILDs: interstitial lung diseases; PCH: pulmonary capillary hemangiomatosis; LIP: lymphocytic interstitial pneumonia)

TABLE 5: DLDs presenting with cysts.

Cystic DLDs	Mimics of lung cysts
Pulmonary Langerhans' cell histiocytosis	Emphysema
Lymphangioleiomyomatosis (LAM)	Bronchiectasis
Tuberous sclerosis	Honeycombing
Birt-Hogg-Dubé (BHD) syndrome	
Cysts associated with other DLDs—LIP, DIP, PJP, any fibrosing ILD	

(DLDs: diffuse lung diseases; LIP: lymphocytic interstitial pneumonia; DIP: desquamative interstitial pneumonia; PJP: *pneumocystis jirovecii* pneumonia)

DIFFUSE LUNG DISEASES PRESENTING WITH NODULES

Many diffuse lung diseases have a predominantly nodular pattern. These disorders have been discussed elsewhere in this book/previously in this chapter **(Table 4)**.

DIFFUSE LUNG DISEASES PRESENTING WITH CYSTS

Lung cysts are defined as small air containing lesions in lungs. Cystic lung diseases **(Table 5)** refer to a pattern where lung cysts are the predominant finding. These need to be differentiated from honeycombing, emphysema and cystic bronchiectasis.

EMPHYSEMA

Emphysema is caused by permanent dilatation of the airspace distal to the terminal bronchioles with associated destruction of the alveolar wall. Three main types of emphysema are—centrilobular, panlobular and paraseptal.

Centrilobular Emphysema

It is the most common type, seen usually in smokers and affects lobules around the central respiratory bronchioles. HRCT reveals well-defined round lucencies in centrilobular portion of secondary pulmonary lobule. Borders of secondary pulmonary lobule are preserved.[20] Apices and lower lobe superior segments are usually more involved. CT is more superior to chest radiography to detect early disease.

Panlobular Emphysema

It is associated with α1-antitrypsin deficiency. Panlobular pattern can also be seen in advanced smoking-related emphysema and emphysema related to intravenous drug abuse. It affects the whole secondary lobule and on imaging seen as generalized diffuse decrease in CT attenuation, mainly in the lower lobe.

Paraseptal Emphysema

In paraseptal emphysema the destruction pattern is located in the periphery of the lung adjacent to the pleura or along the interlobular septa. Upper lung zones are more affected. On CT paraseptal emphysema is seen as small subpleural lucencies arranged as single tier of "cystic" spaces. Large emphysematous bullae may be seen and can cause pneumothorax.

COMBINED PULMONARY FIBROSIS AND EMPHYSEMA

Combined pulmonary fibrosis and emphysema (*CPFE*) is a relatively new entity, which is characterized by upper-lobe emphysema and lower-lobe fibrosis. On pulmonary function tests the typical findings include preserved lung volume and severely diminished capacity of gas exchange (DLco). Smoking, connective tissue disorders and mineral dust exposure are labelled as a few risk factors of this disease. It usually presents with symptoms of exertional dyspnea; and frequently complicated by pulmonary hypertension, acute lung injury and lung cancer. The prognosis is poor. This entity is defined radiographically by the presence of classic features of emphysema in the upper lobes and pulmonary fibrosis (mainly IPF/UIP) in the lower lobes. HRCT **(Figs. 12A to D)** shows upper-lobe centrilobular and/or paraseptal emphysema with multiple bullae and lower-lobe honeycombing with subpleural reticular opacities and traction bronchiectasis, and sometimes ground-glass opacities.[21,22]

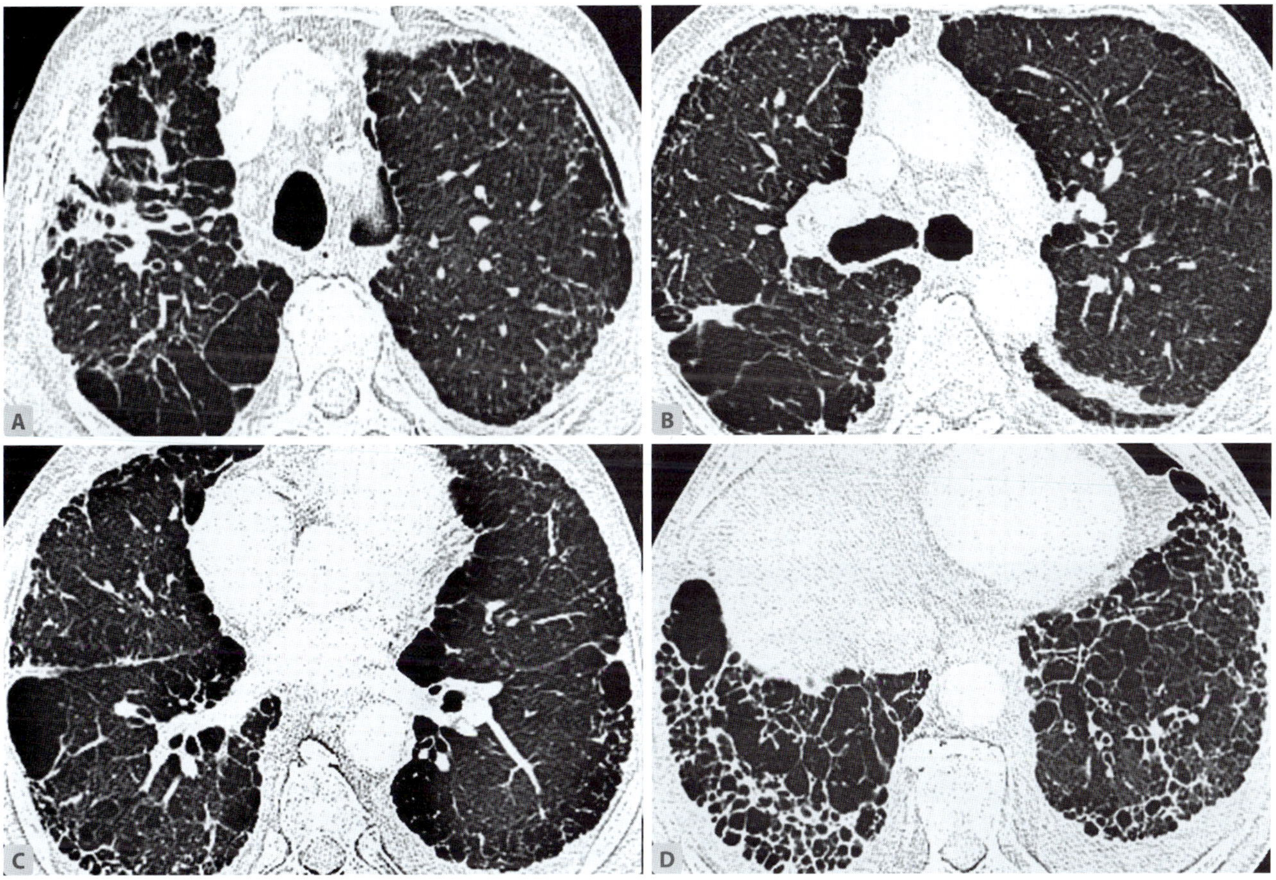

FIGS. 12A TO D: Combined pulmonary fibrosis and emphysema: HRCT images reveal upper-lobe centrilobular and/or paraseptal emphysema and lower-lobe honeycombing with subpleural reticular opacities.

PULMONARY LANGERHANS' CELL HISTIOCYTOSIS

Pulmonary Langerhans' cell histiocytosis[23-25] is preferred term for isolated pulmonary involvement; occurs most commonly in young adult smokers. The clinical features include dyspnea, nonproductive cough, fatigue, chest pain, weight loss or spontaneous pneumothorax. In children pulmonary LCH is usually seen as a part of multisystem involvement.

Imaging

Chest radiograph reveals bilateral diffuse symmetrical reticulonudolar opacities, which are predominantly distributed in upper zones. The lung volume is usually preserved. Small irregular-shaped nodules are seen in early disease; which later on cavitates and result in pneumothorax.

CT findings **(Figs. 13A to C)** depend on the stage of the disease. In early disease multiple small (1-10 mm in size), irregular-shaped nodules are seen. They have a distribution in centrilobular, peribronchial and peribronchiolar location. The nodules and cavitate. Cystic pattern dominates in later stage. These cysts are irregular, small (1-3 cm) and sometimes bizarre shaped. Nodules and cysts usually seen in upper/mid lung zone. The cysts can rupture and produce spontaneous pneumothorax (in 10-15%). When LCH is confined to the lungs, the prognosis is good.

LYMPHANGIOLEIOMYOMATOSIS

Lymphangioleiomyomatosis (LAM) is a disorder caused by abnormal smooth muscle and lymphatic proliferation. It can present either as sporadic form, or syndromic form (associated with tuberous sclerosis). In proven cases of tuberous sclerosis, about 30-40% patients can have LAM. Patients of tuberous sclerosis with LAM may not have the classical imaging triad of tuberous sclerosis (epilepsy, mental retardation and adenoma sebaceum). Sporadic form of LAM is commoner than syndromic form; and is seen almost exclusively in women of child-bearing age. Syndromic LAM can affect both males and females; although incidence is higher in females.

The pulmonary imaging findings of sporadic and syndromic LAM are similar. Chest radiograph may reveal bilateral reticular shadows with preserved lung volumes. HRCT **(Figs. 14A and B)** shows the presence of thin walled cysts uniformly distributed in lungs, and chylous pleural effusion. The parenchymal cysts are usually thin walled (less than 2 mm in size), uniform in size, randomly

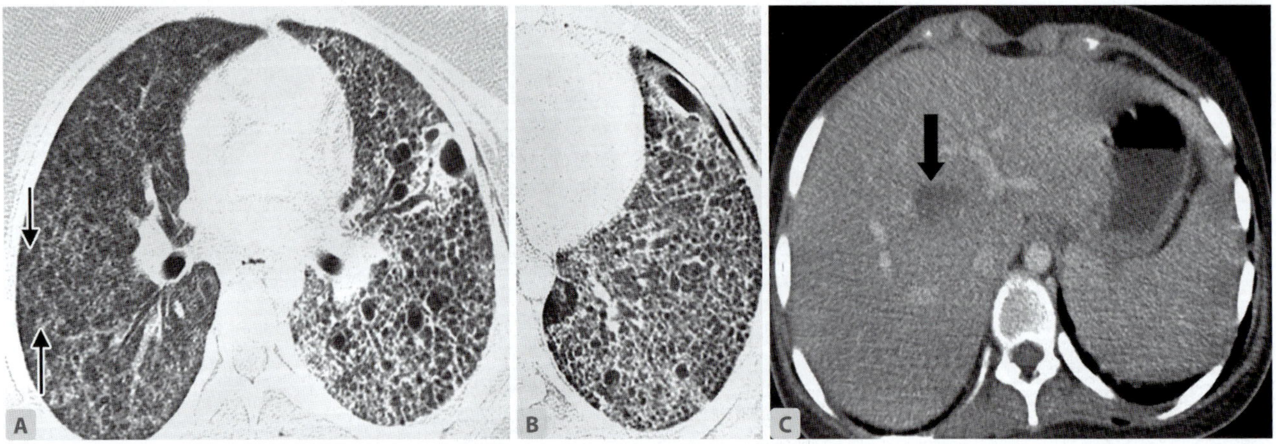

FIGS. 13A TO C: Langerhans' cell histiocytosis in a 16-year-old girl. HRCT images (A and B) reveal multiple irregular parenchymal nodules (arrow) in right lung and multiple cysts in left lung. Note left-sided pneumothorax. Soft tissue image (C) reveals focal a small hypodense liver lesion (block arrow).

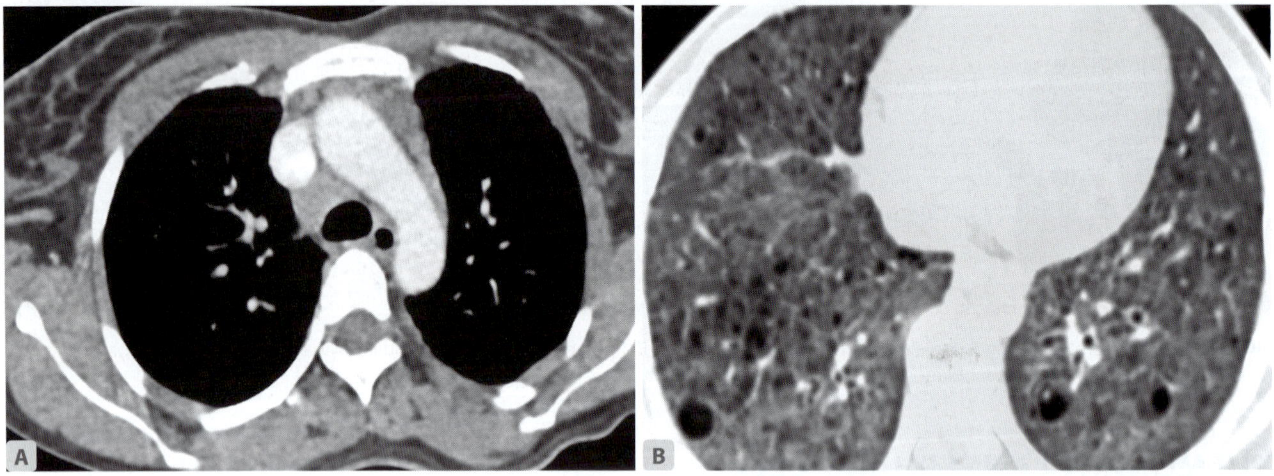

FIGS. 14A AND B: Lymphangioleiomyomatosis in a 30-year-old lady. Axial soft tissue window image (A) reveals mediastinal lymphadenopathy. HRCT image (B) reveals diffuse ground-glass opacities in both lungs; with scattered thin-walled cysts.

distributed without zonal predominance. The intervening lung parenchyma is usually normal. Rupture of cysts may cause pneumothorax; recurrence of pneumothorax is quite common. Hilar and mediastinal lymphadenopathy and pericardial effusion are other imaging findings.

Differential Diagnosis

LCH cysts are more irregular, bizzare shaped; intervening lung often abnormal, systemic manifestations commonly associated with pediatric LCH. LAM is a disease which is charecaterized by proliferation of peribronchovascular smooth muscle casuing air trapping and subsequent development of cysts.

TUBEROUS SCLEROSIS

Tuberous sclerosis is a genetic disorder having an autosomal-dominant inheritance. It affects multiple systems and the classic triad comprises of epilepsy, mental retardation and facial angiofibroma (adenoma sebaceum). While the disease equally affect men and women; pulmonary involvement is more commonly observed in females.

HRCT findings of tuberous sclerosis similar to those of those of LAM. Multiple uniformly distributed cysts and few small nodules (multifocal micronodular pneumocyte hyperplasia) may seen. Chylous pleural effusions usually not seen in tuberous sclerosis as compared to LAM.

BIRT-HOGG-DUBÉ SYNDROME

Birt-Hogg-Dubé (BHD) syndrome is a multisystem disease[26-28] caused by a deletion mutation on the FLCN gene (chromosome 17). The disease affects multiple organ systems, abnormalities include cutaneous angiofibromas, perifollicular fibromas, acrochordons, fibrofolliculomas; and renal masses. On imaging, multiple lung cysts are seen, along with multiple bilateral renal tumors (renal cell carcinoma, oncocytoma). Multiple lung cysts and secondary spontaneous pneumothoraces. CT reveals multiple small cysts **(Figs. 15A to D)** are located in lower zones, subpleural location. The cysts may be septated when they become large).

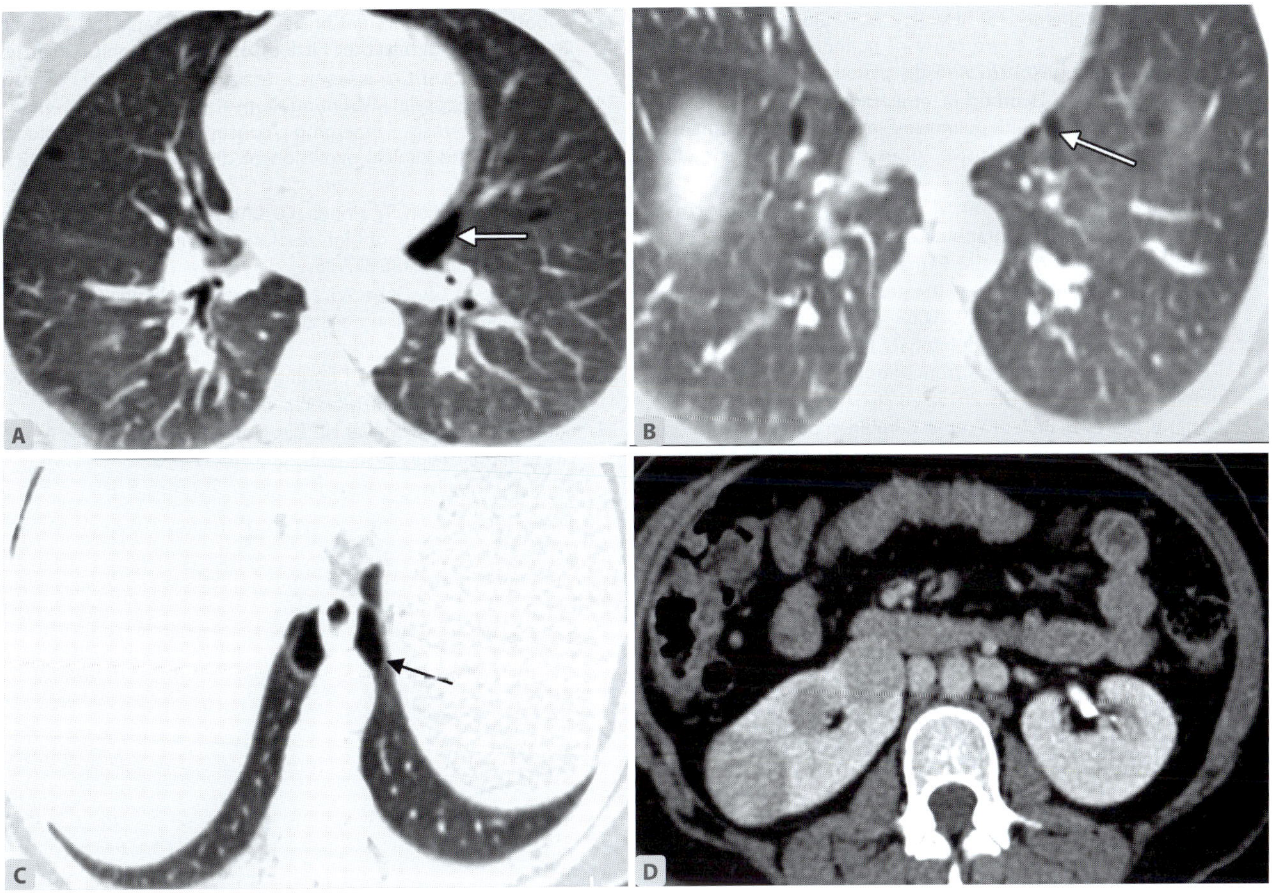

FIGS. 15A TO D: Birt-Hogg-Dubé syndrome in a 39-year-old lady. Note the thin-walled cysts in subpleural locations (arrows) and multiple solid enhancing right renal masses.

CONCLUSION

Diffuse lung disease is a complex disease with various etiologies; sometimes without any identifiable cause. While reaching a precise diagnosis requires a team effort and combination of clinical, laboratory and radiological findings; adoption of a pattern approach on HRCT can help the radiologist to narrow down the differential diagnoses.

REFERENCES

1. Franquet T. Imaging of pulmonary viral pneumonia. Radiology. 2011;260:1.
2. Kim EA, Lee KS, Primack SL, et al. Viral pneumonias in adults: radiologic and pathologic findings. Radiographics. 2002;22 (Spec Issue):S137-49.
3. Cheung OY, Chan JW, Ng CK, et al. The spectrum of pathological changes in severe acute respiratory syndrome (SARS). Histopathology. 2004;45(2):119-24.
4. Chiumello D, Froio S, Bouhemad B, et al. Clinical review: Lung imaging in acute respiratory distress syndrome patients—an update. Crit Care. 2013;17(6):243.
5. Ashbaugh DG, Bigelow DB, Petty TL, et al. Acute respiratory distress in adults. Lancet. 1967;2:319-23.
6. Pnimack SL, Miller RR, Nestor L. Diffuse pulmonary hemorrhage: Clinical, pathologic, and imaging features. AJR. 1995;164:295-300.
7. Jeong YJ, et al. Eosinophilic lung diseases: A clinical, radiologic, and pathologic overview. Radiographics. 2007;27:617-39.
8. Betancourt SL, et al. Lipoid pneumonia: Spectrum of clinical and radiologic manifestations. AJR. 2010;194:103-9.
9. Gaerte SC, et al. Fat-containing lesions of the chest. Radiographics. 2002;22:S61-78.
10. Tamura A, Hebisawa A, Fukushima K. lipoid pneumonia in lung cancer: radiographic and pathologic features. J Clin Oncol. 1998;28:492-6.
11. Holbert MJ, Costello P, Li W, et al. CT features of pulmonary alveolar proteinosis. AJR. 2001;176:1287-94.
12. van Buchem MA, Wondergem JH, Kool LJ, et al. Pulmonary leukostasis: radiologic-pathologic study. Radiology. 1987;165(3): 739-41.
13. Tanaka N, Matsumoto T, Miura G, et al. HRCT findings of chest complications in patients with leukemia. Eur Radiol. 2002;12(6):1512-22.
14. Frazier AA, Franks TJ, Mohammed TLH, et al. Pulmonary veno-occlusive disease and pulmonary capillary hemangiomatosis. Radiographics. 2007;27:867-82.
15. Mandel J, Mark EJ, Hales CA. Pulmonary veno-occlusive disease. Am J Respir Crit Care Med. 2000;162:1964-73.
16. Ito K, Ichiki T, Ohi K, et al. Pulmonary capillary hemangiomatosis with severe pulmonary hypertension. Circ J. 2003;67:793-5.

17. Masur Y, Remberger K, Hoefer M. Pulmonary capillary hemangiomatosis as a rare cause of pulmonary hypertension. Pathol Res Pract. 1996;192:290-5; discussion 296-9.
18. Dufour B, Maitre S, Humbert M, et al. High-resolution CT of the chest in four patients with pulmonary capillary hemangiomatosis or pulmonary veno-occlusive disease. Am J Roentgenol. 1998;171:1321-4.
19. Czeyda-Pommersheim F, et al. Amyloidosis: Modern cross-sectional imaging. Radiographics. 2015;35:1381-92.
20. Washko GR, Hunninghake GM, Fernandez IE, et al. Lung volumes and emphysema in smokers with interstitial lung abnormalities. N Engl J Med. 2011;364(10):897-906.
21. Lin H, Jiang S. Combined pulmonary fibrosis and emphysema (CPFE): an entity different from emphysema or pulmonary fibrosis alone. J Thorac Dis. 2015;7(4):767-79.
22. Cottin V, Nunes H, Brillet PY, et al. Combined pulmonary fibrosis and emphysema: a distinct underrecognised entity. Eur Respir J. 2005;26:586-93.
23. Abbott GF, Rosado-de-Christenson ML, Franks TJ, et al. Pulmonary Langerhans cell histiocytosis. Radiographics. 2004;24: 821-41.
24. Sundar KM, Gosselin MV, Chung HL, et al. Pulmonary Langerhans cell histiocytosis: emerging concepts in pathobiology, radiology, and clinical evolution of disease. Chest. 2003;123: 1673-83.
25. KoyamaM, Johkoh T, Honda O. Chronic cystic lung disease: diagnostic accuracy of high-resolution CT in 92 patients. Am J Roentgenol. 2003;180:827-35.
26. Birt AR, Hogg GR, Dube WJ. Hereditary multiple fibrofolliculomas with trichodiscomas and acrochordons. Arch Dermatol. 1977;113: 1674-7.
27. Prachi P, et al. Thoracic CT findings in Birt-Higg-Dubé syndrome. Am J Roentgenol. 2011;196:349-52.
28. Souza CA, Finley R, Müller NL. Birt-Hogg-Dubé Syndrome: A rare cause of pulmonary cysts. AJR. 2005;185:1237-9.

CHAPTER

132

Mediastinum

Raju Sharma, Kumble S Madhusudhan, Arun Kumar Gupta

INTRODUCTION

Mediastinum is the space between the mediastinal pleura, extending from the thoracic inlet to the diaphragm, bounded anteriorly by the sternum and posteriorly by the paravertebral gutters and the ribs. There are no anatomical divisions or fascial planes that divide this space into compartments, and hence pathology from one compartment can spread to another and large masses are often multicompartmental. The division into radiographic compartments is done solely for the purpose of narrowing the differential diagnosis. This can be done by many methods, none of which are perfect.[1,2]

DIVISIONS OF THE MEDIASTINUM

Mediastinum is anatomically divided into superior and inferior compartments by a line extending from manubriosternal junction to lower margin of 4th dorsal vertebral body. The inferior compartment is further divided into anterior, middle and posterior mediastinum.[3] Felson modified this classification to include only three compartments, without any superior/inferior division.[4] This division into anterior, middle and posterior mediastinum is based on the lateral chest radiograph, by two lines drawn from thoracic inlet to diaphragm. The first line is drawn along the anterior margin of trachea and posterior margin of cardiac silhouette and the second line is drawn along the points 1 cm posterior to anterior margin of vertebral bodies. Many other classifications are also available in literature. However, these classifications are arbitrary and theoretical. Since most of the lesions of the mediastinum are detected on cross-sectional imaging, a CT or MRI based classification would be more appropriate. In 2014, Japanese Association for Research on Thymus (JART) defined CT based classification of mediastinum into four compartments.[5] This was later modified by the International Thymic Malignancy Interest Group (ITMIG), thus introducing new definitions and standards.[6,7] This divides the mediastinum into prevascular (anterior), visceral (middle) and paravertebral (posterior) compartments **(Table 1)**. All compartments extend superiorly from thoracic inlet to diaphragm inferiorly. This division has anatomical correlation, better distinguishes diseases and is less complicated.

IMAGING MODALITIES

The imaging modalities available to the radiologist to evaluate the mediastinum include chest radiograph, computed tomography (CT), sonography, magnetic resonance imaging (MRI), and positron emission tomography (PET). Occasionally barium swallow, digital subtraction angiography and scintigraphy are also used. The main role of imaging is in localization and characterization of the lesions. Further it also helps in staging of the tumors, assessing the surgical resectability and in guiding radiological interventions such as aspiration, biopsy and drainage.

Chest Radiograph

Chest radiograph is usually the initial modality used for evaluation of a mediastinal mass. Many mediastinal masses are discovered incidentally on chest radiographs done for other indications. Evaluation of a suspected mediastinal mass on a chest radiograph begins with the attempt to determine if the mass is mediastinal or pulmonary and then to place it in the appropriate mediastinal compartment.

A mediastinal mass on chest radiograph is usually sharply marginated with broad base towards the mediastinum. Its medial margin is not defined as it forms an obtuse angle with mediastinum. In contrast to this, intrapulmonary mass is often poorly defined, margins are spiculated, nodular or irregular, and it makes an acute angle with the mediastinum. Presence of air bronchogram within the mass lesion further points to intra-pulmonary location. Also bilaterality of the lesion and bone destruction of adjoining vertebra, rib or sternum favor mediastinal lesion.

Once the location in mediastinum is confirmed, the differential diagnosis of mediastinal mass starts with a classification scheme adopted by Felson. The mediastinum is conventionally divided into anterior, middle and posterior compartments on a lateral chest radiograph using two imaginary lines—the first line drawn along anterior border

TABLE 1: Classification of mediastinal compartments.			
Classification of compartments	**Borders**	**Contents**	**Pathologies**
Prevascular	Posterior margin of sternum to anterior margin of pericardium	• Thymus • Fat • Lymph nodes • Left brachiocephalic vein	• Thymic—cysts, hyperplasia, carcinoma, thymoma, neuroendocrine tumor • Germ cell tumors • Lymph nodal—lymphoma, metastatic • Thyroid/parathyroid lesions
Visceral	Anterior aspect of pericardium to line along 1 cm posterior to anterior vertebral margins	• Nonvascular—trachea, carina, esophagus, lymph nodes • Vascular—heart, ascending thoracic aorta, aortic arch, descending thoracic aorta, superior vena cava, intrapericardial pulmonary arteries, thoracic duct	• Lymph nodal—lymphoma, metastatic • Tracheal lesions • Esophageal lesions • Duplication cysts • Vascular—cardiac, pericardial, great vessels
Para-vertebral	Posterior limit of visceral compartment to vertical line against the posterior margin of the chest wall at the lateral margin of the transverse process of the thoracic spine	• Thoracic spine • Paravertebral soft tissues	• Neurogenic tumors • Infection—discitis, osteomyelitis • Trauma—hematoma • Extramedullary hematopoiesis

of trachea to back of the heart extending to the diaphragm and a second line joining a point 1.0 cm behind the anterior margin of the dorsal vertebrae **(Fig. 1)**. Space anterior to first line is anterior mediastinum, between first and second line is middle mediastinum and posterior to second line is posterior mediastinum.[1]

Meticulous evaluation of frontal chest radiograph should be done for presence of silhouette sign, cervicothoracic or thoracoabdominal sign, effect of the mass on adjacent structures (e.g. trachea, paraspinal lines, ribs), the hilum overlay and convergence signs. These signs in combination are often more useful for localizing a mediastinal mass to different compartments rather than lateral chest radiograph.

The silhouette sign is useful for localizing a mediastinal mass to a particular compartment. It states that an intrathoracic opacity, if in anatomic contact with a border of the heart, the aorta, or the diaphragm will obliterate that border. This sign helps in locating the mediastinal mass lesion to appropriate compartment. An anterior mediastinal mass obliterates cardiac border **(Fig. 2)** and ascending aorta or overlaps aortic knuckle. A posterior mediastinal mass obliterates descending aorta and aortic knuckle but overlaps ascending aorta. A posterior mediastinal mass is often associated with adjacent rib or vertebral involvement. The hilum convergence sign states that when the vessels are seen converging to the opacity, it is an enlarged pulmonary artery but if the vessels are going through the opacity it is a mediastinal mass. The cervicothoracic sign says that when an opacity is seen extending above the clavicle with a clear margin, it is located in the posterior mediastinum and is entirely within the thorax. However, if the margins of this opacity disappear as it nears the clavicle, the mass is cervicothoracic, i.e. partly in the thorax and partly in the neck.

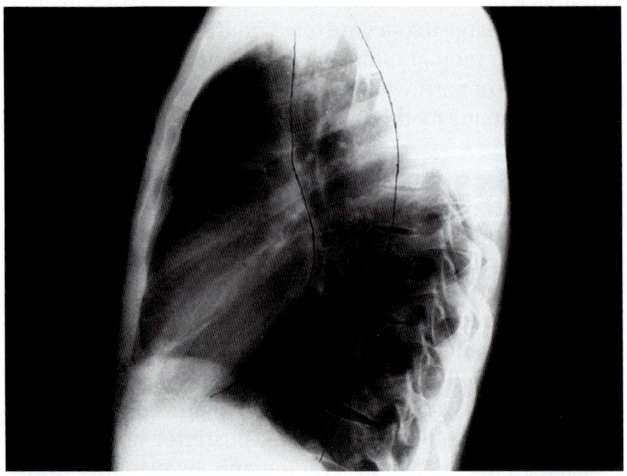

FIG. 1: Lateral radiograph showing the two lines that are drawn to divide the mediastinum into compartments. The first line is drawn along anterior border of trachea to back of the heart extending to the diaphragm and a second line joining a point 1.0 cm behind the anterior margin of the dorsal vertebrae. Space anterior to first line is anterior mediastinum, between first and second is middle and posterior to second line is posterior medisatinum.

Computed Tomography (CT)

CT is the most often and widely used imaging modality for the evaluation of mediastinal masses. It is also the gold standard modality according to ITMIG. Although conventional radiographs can show recognizable abnormalities in many patients with mediastinal pathology, radiographs are limited in their sensitivity and ability to delineate the extent of mediastinal abnormalities and the relationship of masses to specific mediastinal structures. Multidetector CT provides

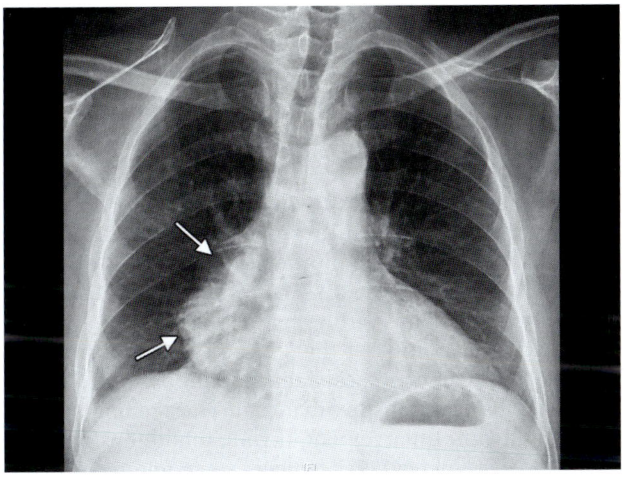

FIG. 2: Chest radiograph (PA view) showing a homogeneous mass in the right hemithorax (arrows) with broad base toward mediastinum and silhouetting the right cardiac margin suggesting anterior mediastinal mass. Hilum can be seen through the mass.

excellent spatial resolution and helps identify normal mediastinal structures, opacified vessels, and vascular abnormalities and is often able to characterize masses based on their morphology (homogeneous or heterogeneous, cystic areas, calcification, fat components, enhancement pattern) and precisely localize them and assess their extent. The thin sections acquired allow multiplanar reconstructions which give an excellent depiction of anatomy.

The indications for mediastinal CT can be divided into two broad categories: First, CT is commonly used to characterize a mediastinal abnormality suspected or diagnosed on plain chest radiographs. When a mediastinal contour abnormality is visible on plain films, CT should generally be the next imaging procedure performed. Secondly, CT is the most common imaging modality used to evaluate the mediastinum in patients who have normal chest radiographs yet there is a clinical reason to suspect mediastinal disease. For example, in the diagnostic workup of pyrexia of unknown origin to detect lymphadenopathy which could be due to tuberculosis, sarcoidosis or lymphoma. CT is done in patients with myasthenia gravis to detect thymic hyperplasia or thymoma, even when the chest radiograph is normal.[1,2]

Magnetic Resonance Imaging

The clinical indications for mediastinal MRI are increasing with the availability of better scanners and faster and new sequences. It is helpful in the differentiation of solid from cystic masses, for demonstration of septations in cystic masses and distinguishing benign cysts from cystic tumors. Primary uses of MRI include the evaluation of posterior mediastinal or paravertebral masses and neurogenic tumors, to detect neural foraminal and/or intraspinal extension and in differentiating thymic hyperplasia from thymoma.[8,9] It is also useful in the diagnosis of mediastinal abnormalities that are suspected to be vascular. In many other instances, however, MRI is best reserved as a secondary or problem-solving tool, in patients who have equivocal or confusing CT findings, or in whom specific anatomic information is required, which is less clearly demonstrated using CT. In such cases, a limited number of MR images can be helpful. MR provides multiple paradigms for lesion characterization, such as the T1 and T2 signal, presence or absence of diffusion restriction, etc. Recently the cine sequence has been reported to be useful in assessing invasion of surrounding mediastinal vessels and pericardium. In addition, it can be used as an alternative to CT in patients in whom iodinated contrast cannot be given or radiation risk has to be avoided. Another emerging role of MR is in the field of response assessment of tumors to chemoradiotherapy where it can be an alternative to PET-CT.

However, if MRI provides information that is merely equivalent to that given by CT, then CT is usually the more appropriate modality. It is more widely available, is less expensive, faster and is more suitable for imaging sick patients. However, CT and MRI are not competitive, but play a complementary role for many clinical problems.

DIFFERENTIAL DIAGNOSIS OF MEDIASTINAL MASSES

The most common lesions in anterior mediastinum include four Ts: Thymoma, Thyroid lesion, Teratoma and Terrible lymphoma. The key structures in middle mediastinum are lymph nodes, tracheobronchial tree and esophagus. Metastatic disease commonly affects lymph nodes in anterior and middle mediastinum. Posterior mediastinal masses are generally neurogenic tumors.[1,2,10]

The differential diagnosis of a mediastinal mass on CT is usually based on several findings, including its location and identification of the structure from which it is arising; whether it is single or multifocal (involving several different areas or lymph node groups), or diffuse; its size and shape and its attenuation (fatty, fluid, soft tissue, or a combination of these); the presence of calcification—its character and amount; and its enhancement following administration of contrast agents.

Rather than using the conventional compartment model, on CT, it is more appropriate to base the differential diagnosis of a mediastinal mass on directly observing the tissue or structure from which the mass is arising (e.g. lymph nodes, thymus, thyroid, parathyroid, trachea, esophagus, vertebral column). If this is not possible, then localizing the mass to specific regions of the mediastinum (e.g. prevascular space, pretracheal space, subcarinal space, anterior cardiophrenic angle, etc.) can be valuable in differential diagnosis. The differential diagnosis of masses arising in the prevascular area includes thymoma and other thymic tumors, cysts, lymphoma and other lymph node masses, germ-cell tumors, thyroid masses, parathyroid masses, fatty masses, and lymphangioma. The differential diagnosis of cardiophrenic angle mass includes pericardial cyst, fat pad, Morgagni hernia and occasionally thymoma and lymph node mass.[10] However, it is also important to remember that, although many pathologic processes have a typical location or locations, most can be seen in any part of the mediastinum.

The attenuation of mediastinal masses is also of primary importance in their differential diagnosis. Masses can be categorized as having fatty, low or high attenuation.

Masses with fat attenuation value are composed primarily of or partially containing fat or lipid-rich tissues. These include lipomatosis and fat pads, thymolipoma, teratoma, lymphangioma and hemangioma, lipoma, liposarcoma, hernias, etc. Low-attenuation masses are usually cystic or fluid filled or contain some lipid. These include a variety of congenital or acquired cysts (bronchogenic, esophageal duplication, neurenteric, pericardial, and thymic); necrotic neoplasms, including lymphoma, cystic thymoma, germ-cell tumors, and lymph node metastases; lymphangioma and hemangioma; neurogenic tumors; thoracic meningocele and fluid collections, such as mediastinal abscess.[11-13]

High-attenuation masses generally contain calcium, have high iodine content, or are related to the presence of fresh blood. They include calcified lymph nodes secondary to granulomatous infection, sarcoidosis, silicosis, partially calcified primary neoplasms, including germ-cell tumors, thymoma, and neurogenic tumors, calcified goiter, calcified vascular lesions, goiter with high iodine content, and mediastinal hematoma.

The pattern of enhancement also aids in the differential diagnosis. Enhancing masses are highly vascular and include substernal thyroid and parathyroid glands, carcinoid tumors, hemangiomas, paraganglioma, Castleman disease, and a variety of partially necrotic, inflammatory, and neoplastic lesions in which some rim enhancement is visible.[2,14]

ANTERIOR MEDIASTINUM

Lesions of Thymus

Normal thymus is a bilobed triangular gland **(Fig. 3)** in the anterior mediastinum. Its size and morphology vary with age. In newborn, it is large and the size decreases with age. Normal thymus shows homogeneous attenuation on CT. Focal contour abnormality, heterogeneous attenuation on CT or signal intensity on MRI suggest thymic mass lesion.

CT remains the technique of choice following a standard chest radiograph when thymic lesion is suspected. Thymic enlargement is usually caused by tumor, most common being thymoma. Other lesions include thymolipoma, malignant lymphoma and carcinoid. Occasionally, thymic enlargement is caused by a thymic cyst and rarely by hyperplasia or infection.

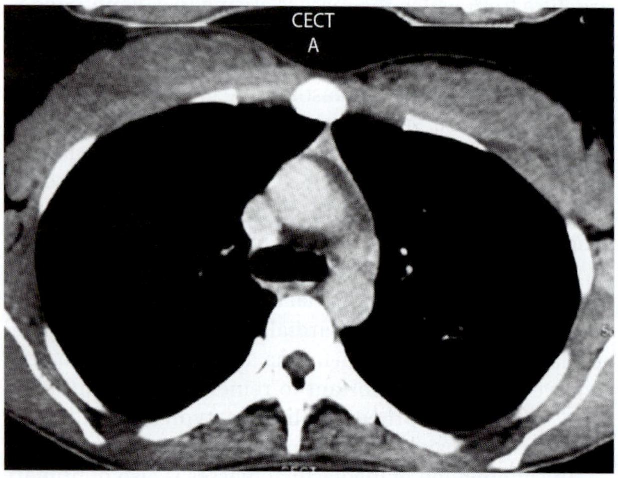

FIG. 3: Normal thymus: Axial CT scan showing the normal triangular configuration of the thymus gland in a young adult.

Thymic Rebound

Thymic rebound refers to thymic enlargement following atrophy from severe illness, steroid treatment or chemotherapy. This phenomenon is most marked in children, but it has also been seen in young adults. Following involution, the thymus grows back to its baseline volume within several months of the stressful episode. In about 12–25% patients it may exceed the baseline volume by 50%.[2] Because CT is more sensitive than plain chest radiographs for detecting thymic enlargement, thymic rebound is detected with greater frequency when patients are monitored with CT. CT or MRI show symmetrically enlarged but normal in shape and smooth outline of the gland with CT density and MR signal intensity being similar to normal thymic tissue.

In most patients with extrathoracic malignancies, thymic rebound is unlikely to cause concern or diagnostic confusion. Practically, thymic rebound is most problematic when it is seen in patients with malignant lymphoma who have been treated using chemotherapy. When an enlarged thymus is seen in such patients, it can be difficult to distinguish thymic rebound from recurrent lymphoma. However, when a patient with lymphoma shows thymic enlargement as an isolated finding after treatment with no adenopathy being visible, it is reasonable to follow the patient with the presumption that thymic rebound is responsible. However, in equivocal cases, chemical shift MRI and PET may be used to distinguish thymic hyperplasia from lymphoma. Thymic hyperplasia shows a signal drop on the opposed phase image whereas thymic tumors will not.[15] Diffusion weighted MRI can also be useful in distinguishing rebound hyperplasia from lymphoma because of the marked restriction of diffusion seen in the latter.

Thymic Hyperplasia

This is present in more than 50% of patients with myasthenia gravis. It is also seen in thyrotoxicosis, systemic lupus erythematosis, polyarteritis nodosa, Addison's disease, Hashimoto's thyroiditis. It is not recognized on chest radiograph; CT and MRI may show enlargement of both lobes but the normal shape of the gland is maintained and density and signal characteristics are same as normal thymus. In difficult cases, assessment may be done with chemical shift MRI due to the presence of interspersed fat within the thymic tissue.[15] Biopsy or surgery is rarely necessary. The normal thymus and thymic hyperplasia in the adult patient shows loss of signal on the opposed phase image due to the presence of microscopic fat **(Figs. 4A and B)**. A chemical shift ratio (thymus SI (OP)/muscle SI (OP)/thymus SI (IP)/muscle SI (OP) has been found reliable. A CSR of 0.7 or less is suggestive of thymic hyperplasia whereas a CSI of 1 or more is suggestive of thymic tumor. This is not reliable in the pediatric patient as there may be insufficient amount of fat and the signal drop may not be seen. Normal thymic tissue and thymic hyperplasia can be avid on FDG PET-CT and this should not

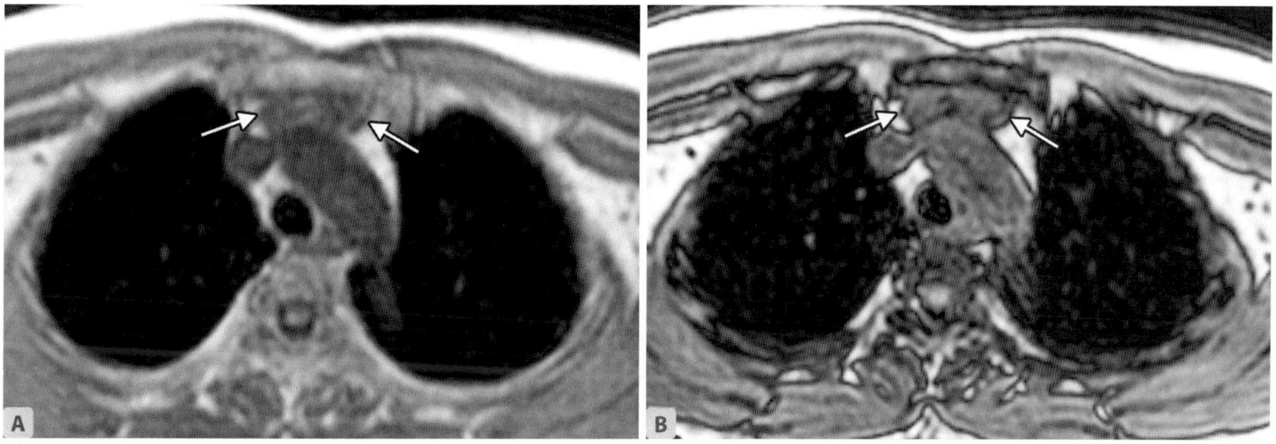

FIGS. 4A AND B: Thymic hyperplasia: Axial T1-weighted MR images with TE – 4.6 ms (in phase; A) and TE – 2.3 ms (in opposed phase; B) showing small lesion in the anterior mediastinum (arrows). The lesion showed a mean signal intensity of 448 in in-phase and 267 in opposed-phase, suggestive of thymic hyperplasia.

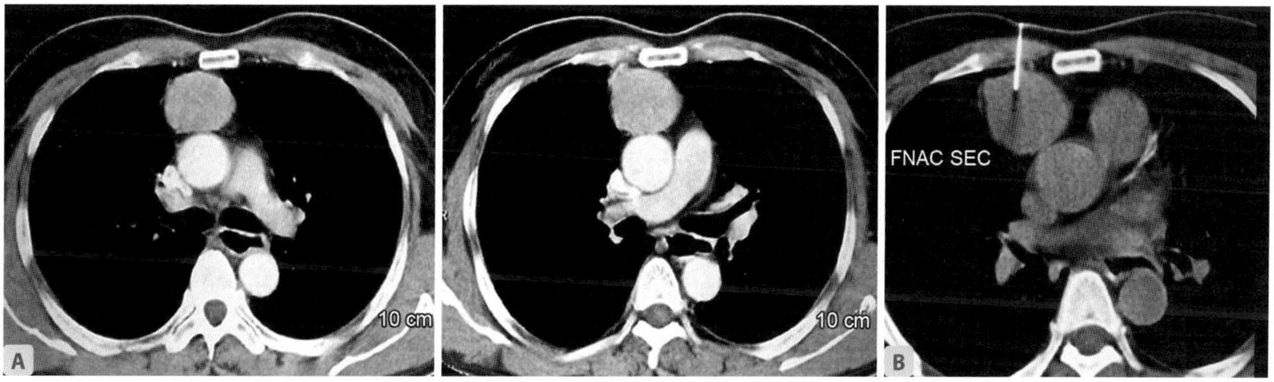

FIGS. 5A AND B: Thymoma: Contrast-enhanced (CE) CT (A) of a patient with myasthenia gravis showing a well-defined mass anterior to the ascending aorta suggestive of thymoma. CT-guided biopsy is seen in Figure B.

be mistaken as malignancy. Correlation with the CT and MR morphology can help in resolving this pitfall.

Thymoma

Thymoma is comprised of epithelial cells and lymphocytes, the proportion of each varies. It may be benign or malignant, but there is no distinction histologically, and therefore, the term invasive thymoma is used to describe a tumor which has spread beyond the capsule. Approximately 15–40% of thymomas are invasive.

Most are discovered between 40 years and 50 years of age, and there is no sex predilection. It is frequently associated with autoimmune disease, most commonly myasthenia gravis. About 35–40% of patients with thymoma have myasthenia gravis while 10–23% patients with myasthenia gravis have thymoma. Red blood cell aplasia is seen in 21–50% of patients and hypogammaglobulinemia in about 10% of patients.[16]

Most thymomas occur in anterior mediastinum, usually located anterior to ascending aorta, above the right ventricular outflow tract and main pulmonary artery, projects into hemithorax, less commonly extend on either side of the midline. Thymoma may project from anterior mediastinum to adjacent middle and posterior mediastinum. Thymoma is seen as a spherical mass, characteristically arising from one lobe of the thymus, with smooth or lobulated outline, often silhouetting vascular or cardiac border. Thymomas are usually small and often obscured by surrounding mediastinal vessels and hence are difficult to see on chest radiograph.

CT is the most sensitive technique for detection of thymoma and lesions as small as 1 cm can be detected. The characteristic CT features include focal asymmetrical homogeneous soft tissue density mass, oval round or lobulated mass with sharply demarcated outline **(Figs. 5A and B)**, focal areas of calcification seen in nearly 25% and uniform contrast enhancement. Necrosis and hemorrhage may occur in one third of patients. It may appear cystic with discrete nodular components.

On MRI thymoma shows low to intermediate signal intensity on T1W and high signal intensity on T2W image. Heterogeneous signal intensity due to septation, cystic change or hemorrhage is common. MRI is indicated in patients with invasive thymoma to look for vascular invasion when there is contraindication to use intravenous contrast for CT examination.

The features that suggest invasive thymoma **(Figs. 6A to D)** on CT or MRI include poorly defined or infiltrative/lobulated

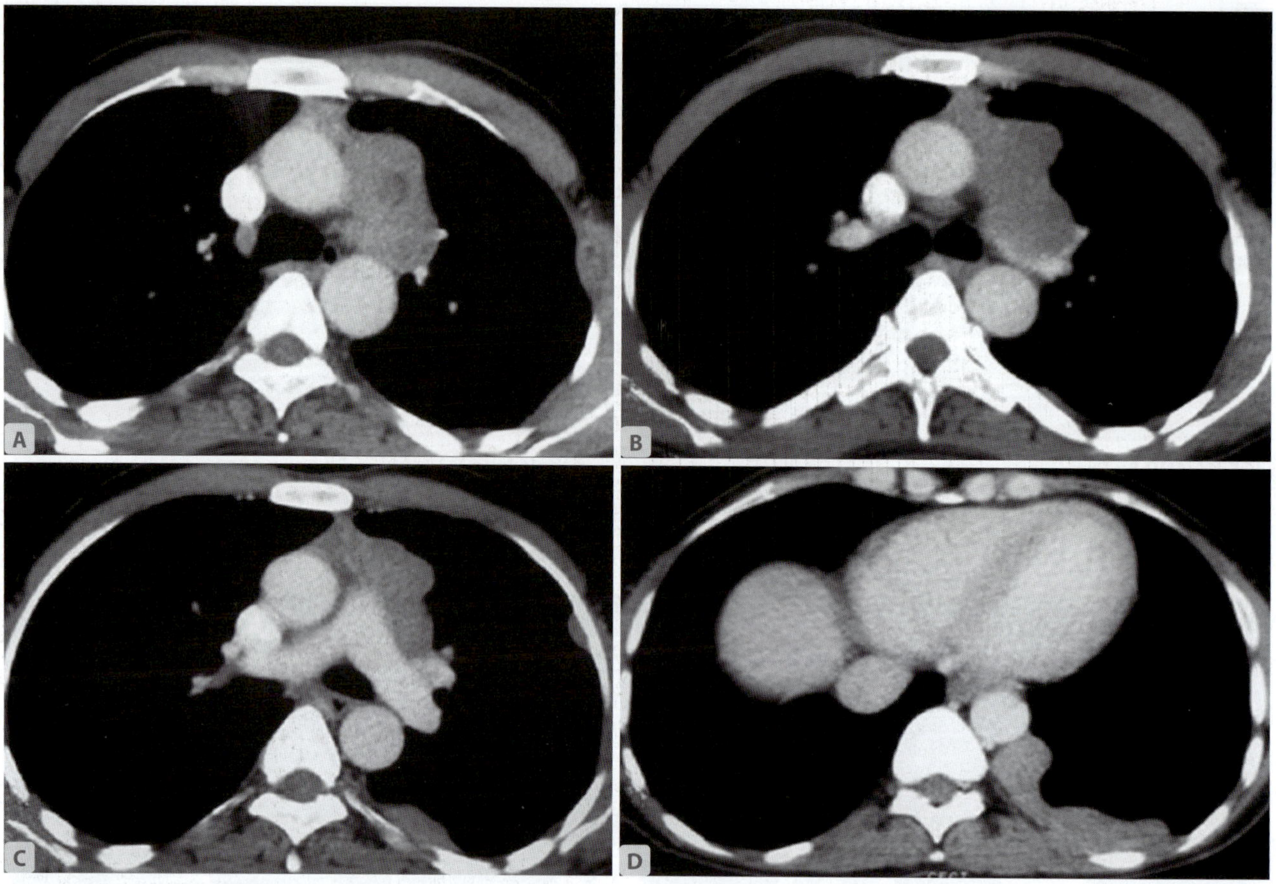

FIGS. 6A TO D: Invasive thymoma. CECT showing lobulated anterior mediastinal mass (A and B) with ill-defined fat plane with the ascending aorta and pulmonary artery. Nodular pleural metastases are also seen (C and D) suggestive of invasive thymoma.

margins, presence of cystic or necrotic areas, multiple calcific foci, definite vascular or chest wall invasion, irregular interface with adjacent lung or evidence of spread to ipsilateral pleura. Pleural spread may manifest either as discrete pleural nodules at a distance from the primary lesion **(Figs. 6A to D)** or as a sheet of neoplastic tissue extending from the primary lesion often mimicking pleural mesothelioma. Pleural effusion is uncommon despite frequent occurrence of pleural metastasis.[17-19]

The staging system proposed by Masaoka[18] is generally used to stage thymomas. The principal features of this staging system are as follows:

- Stage I: Tumor capsule is intact
- Stage II: Invasion of the tumor capsule or surrounding fat or mediastinal pleura
- Stage III: Invasion of surrounding organs (pericardium, great vessels, or lung)
- Stage IVa: Pleural or pericardial implants
- Stage IVb: Hematogenous or lymphogenous metastases

Thymic epithelial neoplasms were initially classified as (i) thymoma (benign tumor without invasion), (ii) invasive thymoma (benign tumor with invasion) and (iii) thymic carcinoma (malignant histology). Of all these, thymic carcinoma has the poorest prognosis with 5-year survival as low as 30%.[20] Differentiation of invasive thymoma from thymic carcinoma on imaging is difficult. World Health Organization (WHO) has classified thymomas based on histology to maintain uniformity.[21] This is shown in **Table 2**.

Thymolipoma

This is a rare benign tumor seen in any age group, which is composed of mixture of mature fat and normal looking or involuted thymic tissue.[22] It usually grows to a large size, and being pliable it moulds itself to adjacent mediastinum and diaphragm. It is often detected incidentally as a mediastinal mass or mimics cardiomegaly or lobar collapse on chest radiograph. It may change in shape or position on decubitus views.

CT shows presence of fat, thymic tissue and fibrous septae running through the lesion **(Figs. 7A and B)**. Calcification may be present. MRI shows imaging characteristics of fatty mass, i.e. increased signal intensity on both T1W and T2W images. Low signal intensity strands may be seen coursing through the lesion, representing residual fibrous stroma or thymic tissue.

Thymic Carcinoid

This is a rare tumor, thought to arise from thymic cells of neuroendocrine origin. Approximately 40% of patients have Cushing' syndrome as a result of tumor secretion of adrenocorticotropic hormone, and up to 20% have been associated with multiple endocrine neoplasia (MEN)

TABLE 2: WHO classification (4th edition) of thymoma.

Type	Histological description	Frequency (%)	Association with myasthenia gravis (%)	Prognosis
Type A	Spindle cell or medullary thymoma	4–7	17	Excellent 15-year survival in up to 100%
Type AB	Mixed thymoma	28–34	16	Good; 15-year survival 90%
Type B1	Predominantly cortical or lymphocyte rich thymoma	9–20	57	Good; 15-year survival 90%
Type B2	Cortical thymoma	20–36	71	Moderate; 20-year survival 60%
Type B3	Well-differentiated thymic carcinoma, epithelial thymoma or squamoid thymoma	10–14	46	Moderate; 20-year survival 40%
Type C	Heterogeneous thymic carcinoma	--	--	Poor; 10-year survival 28%

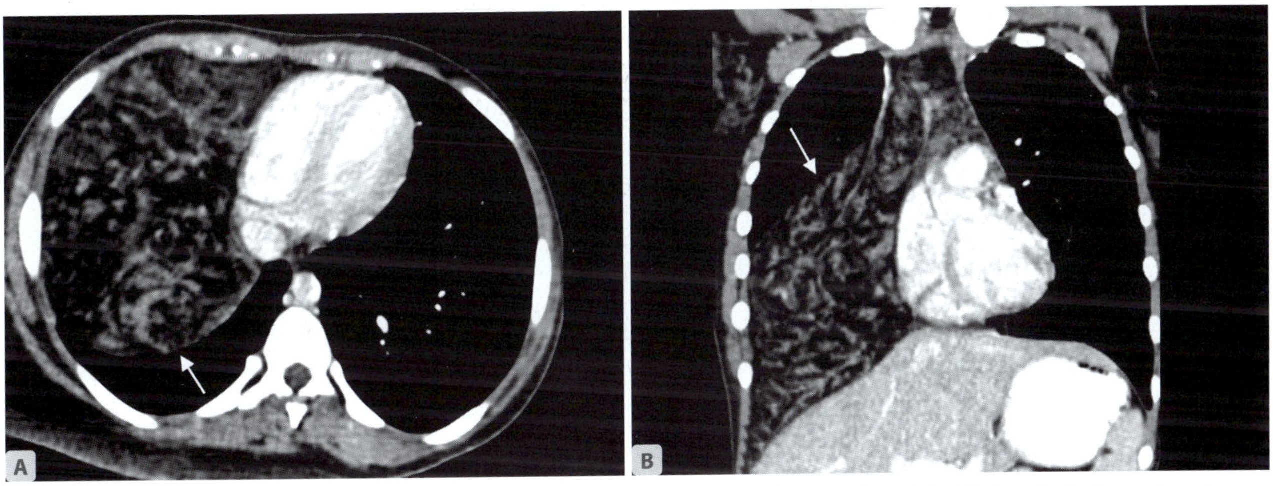

FIGS. 7A AND B: Thymolipoma: Axial (A) and coronal (B) contrast-enhanced CT images showing a large right-sided mediastinal mass (arrow) containing fat and soft tissue density, suggesting thymolipoma.

syndromes I and II. They can be small, not detected on CT or MRI, or may be large **(Figs. 8A to C)** and aggressive with metastasis to distant site. This tumor is more aggressive than thymoma, often presenting in an advanced stage, and superior vena cava obstruction is more common with thymic carcinoid than with thymoma. Regional lymph node metastases and distant metastases may be seen, which may include blastic bone lesions. CT features are indistinguishable from invasive thymoma. The chest radiograph may be normal. Therefore, CT or MRI should be done to look for a thymic mass in a patient with unexplained Cushing's syndrome. Octreotide radionuclide imaging or PET may be valuable in imaging these tumors.[2]

Thymic Lymphoma

Hodgkin's disease has a predilection for involving the thymus gland in conjunction with lymph node involvement. It occurs in about one third of the patients either at the initial presentation or during relapse. This presents either as generalized thymic enlargement or as single or multiple focal masses along with mediastinal lymphadenopathy. Non-Hodgkin lymphoma (NHL) much less commonly involves the thymus. On CT and MRI the appearance of thymic mass mimics thymoma. The possibility of thymic lymphoma should be considered whenever a thymic mass is seen in combination with mediastinal lymphadenopathy. FDG PET-CT is more accurate than CT in the diagnosis of lymphomatous involvement in the mediastinum and thus is useful in staging of the disease.[7]

Thymic Cyst

Thymic cysts can be either congenital or acquired. They account for 1% of anterior mediastinal masses. Acquired thymic cysts are generally associated with inflammation and have been reported following radiation therapy for lymphoma, in association with thymic tumors, and following thoracotomy. Congenital thymic cysts are usually unilocular, have a thin wall, and contain clear fluid. Acquired thymic cysts are often multilocular. Multilocular thymic cysts have been seen in children with HIV infection. The attenuation of

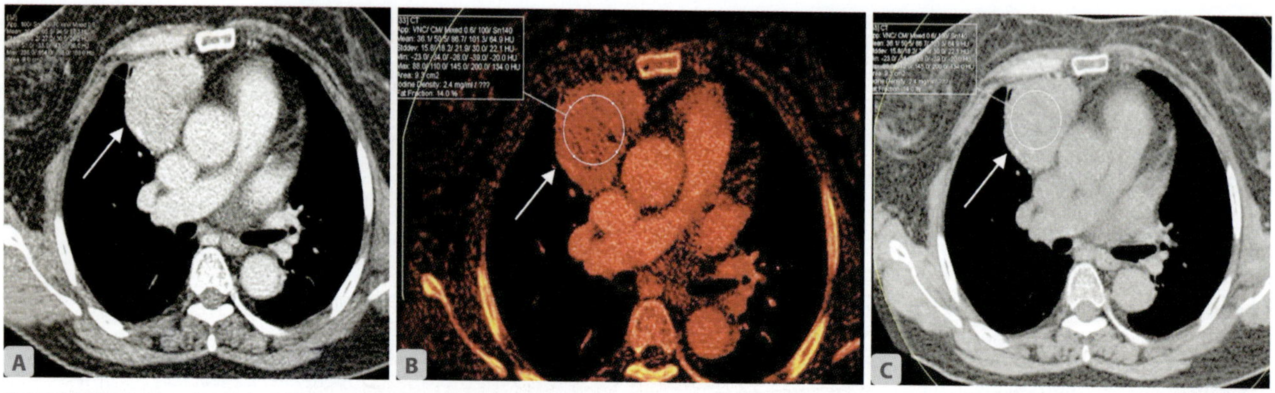

FIGS. 8A TO C: Thymic carcinoid: Monoenergetic (A), iodine (B) and virtual non-contrast (C) axial CT scans performed on dual energy scanner shows a homogeneously enhancing mass in the anterior mediastinum (arrow).

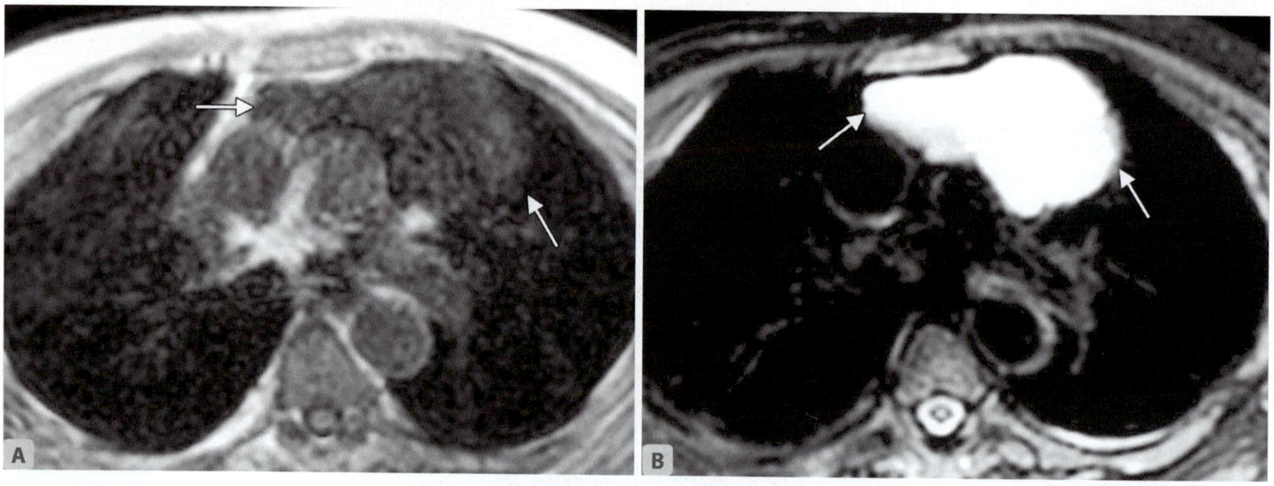

FIGS. 9A AND B: Thymic cyst. Axial T1-weighted (A) and T2-weighted (B) MR images showing a well-defined lesion in the anterior mediastinum (arrows) appearing hypointense on T1W and hyperintense on T2W, suggestive of a cyst.

thymic cysts is usually that of water but can be higher or lower depending on the presence of hemorrhage or lipid deposits. Calcification of the cyst wall can also be seen.

On chest radiograph, thymic cyst is seen as any other nonlobulated thymic mass with or without calcification of the wall. Ultrasonography demonstrates cystic nature of the mass. CT shows a thin walled, non-enhancing water density lesion. MRI shows typical characteristic of fluid i.e. low signal intensity on T1W and uniform high signal intensity T2W images with no restriction on the diffusion weighted image **(Figs. 9A and B)**. The cyst will show high signal intensity in both T1W and T2W images in the presence of hemorrhage. A thymic cyst with features of multiloculation, heterogeneous attenuation with thick wall and association of soft tissue component must be sampled or resected to exclude malignancy (cystic thymoma). Thymic cyst should be diagnosed with caution as cystic regions can be seen in a variety of thymic tumors, including thymoma and lymphoma.[1,2]

Germ-cell Tumors

These tumors are derived from the primitive embryonic germ cell layers, and account for 15–20% of mediastinal masses. They arise from cell rests within or in intimate contact with the thymus. They are classified as teratoma, seminoma, and nonseminomatous germ-cell tumor which include embryonal carcinoma, endodermal sinus tumor, choriocarcinoma and tumors with mixtures of these cell types. Mediastinum is the most common extragonadal primary site of these lesions. Malignant germ-cell tumors secrete beta human chorionic gondotropin and alpha-fetoprotein in 90% cases which can be used as markers to diagnose and monitor the tumor.[23-25] Serum lactate dehydrogenase may also be elevated, but it is less specific and may be elevated in other tumors like lymphoma.

Teratomas are the most common germ-cell tumors and are classified as mature, immature and malignant. Mature cystic teratomas are referred to as dermoid cyst which consists of predominantly ectodermal elements, such as skin, sebaceous material, hair and calcification. Benign teratoma contains elements of more than one of the three germinal layers. Mature teratomas and dermoid cysts account for majority of these lesions. They are seen at all ages, more common in adolescents and young adults, with females slightly outnumbering males. These are mostly asymptomatic and diagnosed incidentally. Occasionally, patient may present with symptoms due to local compression, rupture or infection.[2,23]

These lesions are usually seen as round or lobulated well defined mass, mainly to one side of the midline, located in anterior mediastinum, in front of the root of the aorta and main pulmonary artery. Calcification, ossification or even teeth and sometimes fat can be seen on chest radiograph.

On CT, these lesions are well encapsulated, may show curvilinear calcification of the wall and rim enhancement following intravenous contrast injection. The internal contents are inhomogeneous with variable density of water, fat and soft tissue **(Figs. 10 and 11)**. Presence of amorphous calcification, malformed teeth or bone, layering of fat and fluid within the mass confirms the diagnosis. Local invasion is the only criteria to suggest malignancy. The features of irregular outline of the mass with infiltration of the

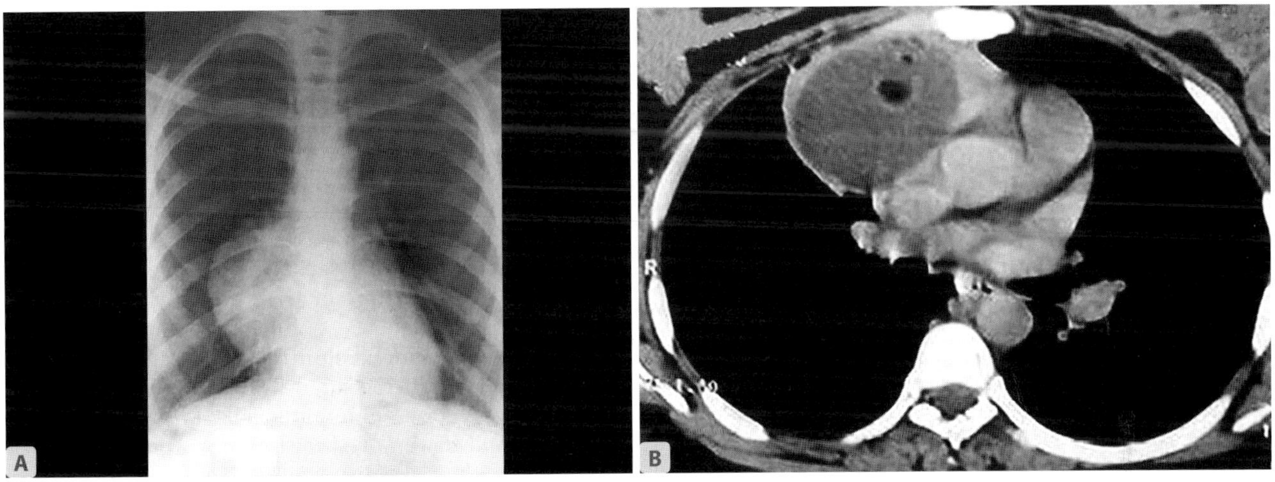

FIGS. 10A AND B: Teratoma: Chest radiograph (A) showing a large mediastinal mass in right paracardiac location obliterating the right heart border, suggesting its anterior location. Axial CT (B) shows a large well-encapsulated low-attenuating mass, with fat attenuation within it suggestive of teratoma.

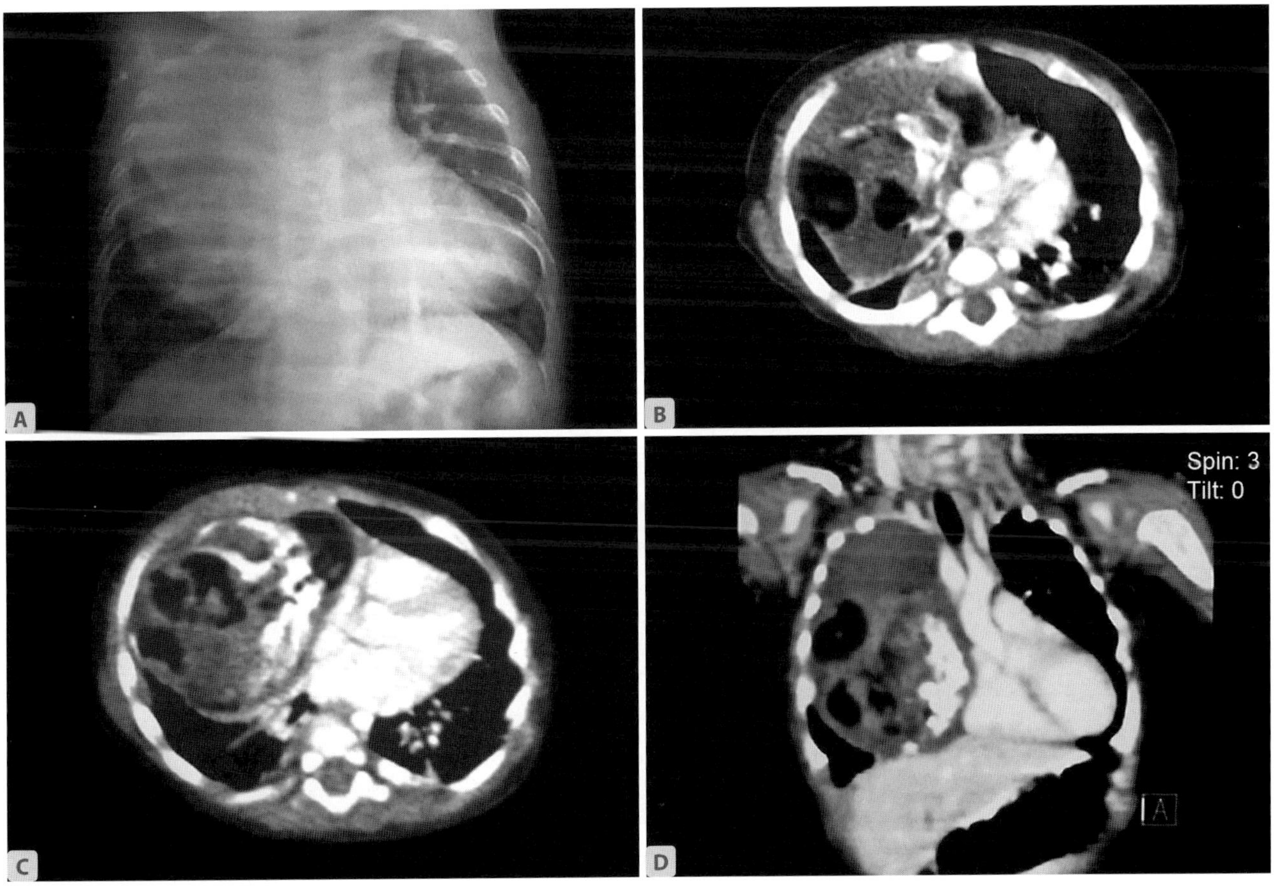

FIGS. 11A TO D: Teratoma: Chest radiograph (A) of a 3-month-old child showing a large mediastinal mass with foci of calcification, and contralateral mediastinal shift. Axial CT (B and C) and coronal reformatted image (D) show a large right-sided low-attenuating mass with calcification and fat within it. *Diagnosis:* Teratoma.

mediastinal fat, compression or invasion of the mediastinal vessels or airways on CT suggest malignant teratoma.[23-25] On MRI, fatty component shows hyperintense signal on T1 and T2 weighted images and shows chemical shift artefact. Cystic teratoma appears hyperintense on T2 weighted images with peripheral rim contrast enhancement. Occasionally, teratomas may rupture into the pleural space or in to the lung when the appearance becomes heterogeneous with poorly defined fat planes and spiculation mimicking malignant germ-cell tumors.[26] A fat fluid level in the pleural effusion has also been reported.

Malignant germ-cell tumors are usually seen in young adults, more common in men than in women, mostly in 3rd and 4th decades. They appear as irregular soft tissue mass, often with central areas of cystic degeneration or necrosis and even intratumoral calcification. They can invade the adjacent mediastinal fat, pleura or pericardium resembling CT or MR appearance of invasive thymoma or lymphoma. The only distinguishing feature is absence of transpleural droplet spread. Presence of lung metastases may help distinguish it from lymphoma.

Seminomas occur almost entirely in men with mean age at presentation of 29 years. They present as large smooth or lobulated, homogeneous soft tissue masses with obliteration of fat planes. They are sensitive to radiation and chemotherapy.

Nonseminomatous germ-cell tumors are seen as irregular, ill-defined heterogeneous masses on CT, with necrosis, hemorrhage and cystic areas. They have a poor prognosis and are associated with elevated levels of alfa fetoprotein.

Thyroid Mass

An intrathoracic thyroid mass is usually a multinodular colloid goiter or adenoma but occasionally may be a carcinoma. It is usually a downward extension of neck mass, the continuity between mediastinal mass and thyroid gland in the neck is an important diagnostic feature on chest radiograph and CT. An isolated thyroid mass in the mediastinum, arising from heterotropic thyroid tissue without any connection with thyroid in the neck is extremely rare. CT scan of the lower neck should always be done in the evaluation of mediastinal masses, especially those in the upper thorax.

On chest radiograph, this is seen as a well-defined spherical or lobular mass which may displace and compress trachea at the level of the thoracic inlet **(Figs. 12A to C)**. Dense amorphous calcification is seen on radiograph in 25% cases.

CT shows well-defined mass in the paratracheal region, continuous with thyroid gland in the neck with relatively high attenuation on non contrast CT which enhances homogeneously with intravenous contrast. Focal areas of calcification are seen in up to 75% cases, and low density areas may also be seen. The mass extends anterior to the trachea in 75% cases.[1,2] On MRI, signal intensity similar to muscle on T1W while heterogeneous increased signal intensity on T2W image is seen. However, it is not possible to distinguish adenoma from carcinoma from signal intensity. Radionuclide imaging is a sensitive and specific method of confirming thyroid nature of an intrathoracic mass, but is often unnecessary.

CT plays an important role in the preoperative assessment of substernal goiters. The surgical approach to these lesions depends on precise anatomic localization. Intrathoracic goiters should be removed for symptomatic relief as well as to reduce the risk consequent to acute hemorrhage or inflammation. Although anterior substernal goiters usually can be removed through a routine cervical incision, posterior mediastinal goitres may need a thoracotomy or a combined cervicothoracic incision depending on the size of the lesion.

Parathyroid Adenoma

Ten percent of parathyroid glands are ectopic in location. Two-thirds of these are present in the anterior mediastinum and are closely connected with thymus. Likelihood of an ectopic adenoma increases in postoperative patients who continue to have persistent hyperparathyroidism. Adenoma is usually homogeneous in density, often less than 2.0 cm in diameter and is difficult to distinguish from thymic remnant or lymph node on CT **(Figs. 13A and B)**. It may show cystic areas due to necrosis and hemorrhage. MRI shows intermediate

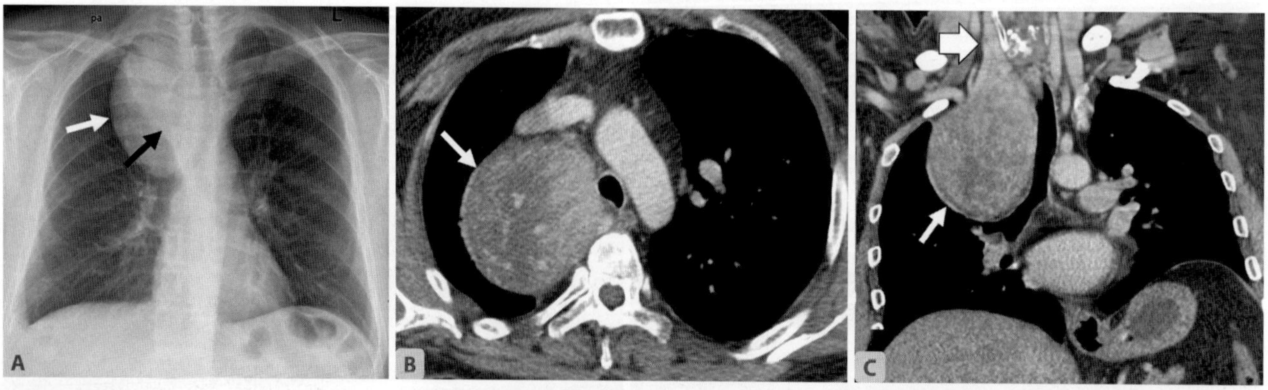

FIGS. 12A TO C: Thyroid mass. (A) Chest radiograph showing a right-sided mediastinal based mass (white arrow), indenting the trachea and not silhouetting the brachiocephalic vessel outline (black arrow) suggesting middle mediastinal location. Axial (B) and coronal (C) CT images showing heterogeneously enhancing mass in the middle mediastinum. Coronal image shows continuity with the right lobe of thyroid gland in the neck (block arrow) suggesting thyroid origin.

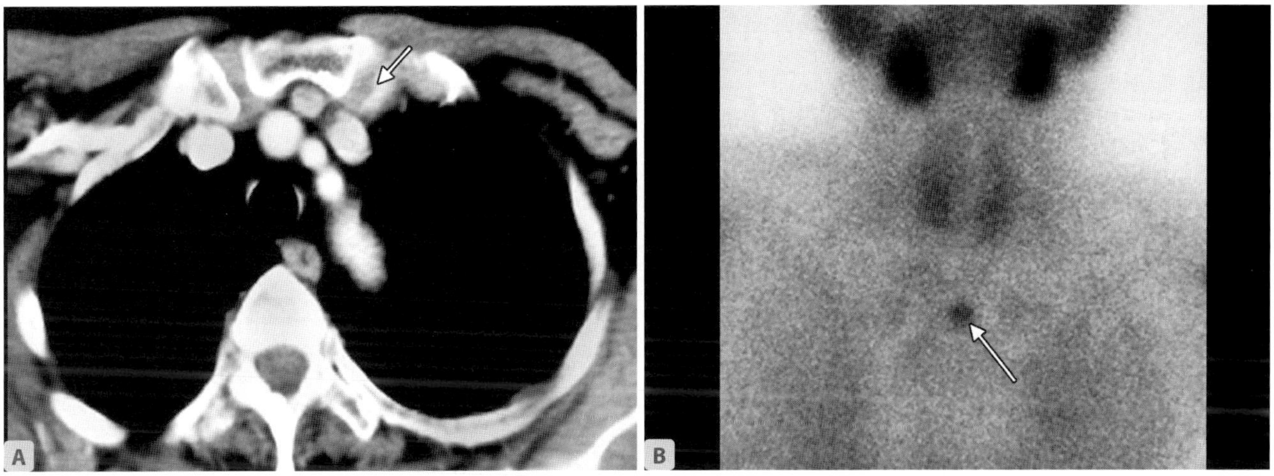

FIGS. 13A AND B: Parathyroid adenoma: Axial CECT (A) in a patient with hyperparathyroidism shows a small anterior mediastinal mass just behind the sternum. ^{99m}Tc Sestamibi scan (B) shows a small focus of increased uptake in the mediastinum confirming the diagnosis of an ectopic parathyroid adenoma.

signal intensity on T1W and marked hyperintensity on T2W image. Sestamibi radionuclide imaging is a sensitive technique to detect ectopic parathyroid adenomas **(Figs. 13A and B)**. Combined use of ^{99}mTcMIBI and MRI has been shown to be 89% sensitive and 95% specific for preoperative localization.[2,27] 4D multidetector CT is a recent advancement in the imaging of parathyroid lesions and is more sensitive than other imaging modalities.[28] The adenoma characteristically shows enhancement in the arterial phase with washout in the venous phase. A 'polar vessel' which may be a feeding artery or draining vein may also be seen in a hypervascular tumor.

Lymphangioma (Cystic Hygroma)

Lymphangioma is a rare benign lesion of lymphatic origin and represents 0.7–4.5% of mediastinal tumors; most are present at birth and are detected in the first 2 years of life. They are most common in the neck (75%) and axilla (20%). About 10% of cervical lymphangiomas extend into the mediastinum, but less than 5% of lymphangiomas are limited to the mediastinum itself.

They result from congenital malformation of the lymphatic system consisting of lymph channels and cystic lymph spaces lined by endothelium, containing clear or straw colored fluid. It grows slowly and commonly compresses surrounding tissues. It is a round, smooth mass with homogeneous attenuation value, sometimes lower than water. Septation is a common feature on CT, septae being thin or thick which enhance with intravenous contrast. MRI confirms the cystic nature of the lesion.

Patients may be asymptomatic because the mass is soft and yielding, but compression of mediastinal structures can result in chest pain, cough, or dyspnea. Because of a tendency for local growth, surgery is recommended. Lymphangioma can be seen in adults, with or without a history of incomplete resection as a child.

They are classified as capillary, cavernous, or cystic (hygroma), depending on the size of the lymph channels they contain. In adults, lymphangiomas are most common in the anterior (28–37%) or superior (16–36%) mediastinum but are also seen in the middle and posterior mediastinum. They can be quite large, ranging up to 30 cm in diameter.[2]

The imaging appearance of a lymphangioma is related to its type (i.e. cystic, cavernous, or capillary). On CT, cystic lymphangioma usually appears homogeneous and near to water in attenuation, but they can be of higher attenuation **(Figs. 14A to D)**. Lymphangioma may be variably composed of a combination of fluid, solid tissue, and fat; calcification is rare. Although they are usually well circumscribed and localized, they may appear to envelop mediastinal structures and insinuate between them. Lymphangioma may be associated with vascular malformations that are easily identifiable following the administration of intravenous contrast. Lymphangiomas composed of capillary-sized, thin-walled channels may appear as solid masses.

On MRI, heterogeneous signal is typical, with increased signal on T2-weighted images reflecting their fluid content. MR may also show an enhancing, multicystic, and multiseptated appearance; this suggests the presence of cavernous lymphangioma.

Other Vascular Tumors

Hemangiomas, hemangioendothelioma and hemangiopericytoma are other vascular tumors that occur in the mediastinum. Hemangiopericytoma is now considered identical to solitary fibrous tumor and the former term has been removed from the WHO classification.[29] Preoperative diagnosis of these entities is difficult. Mediastinal hemangiomas are most common in young patients, and about 75% present before the age of 35 years. Hemangiomas most commonly arise in the anterior and posterior mediastinum and may extend into the neck.

On CT, they are often heterogeneous in attenuation on unenhanced scans, and may occasionally show foci of fatty attenuation. Enhancement may be dense, multifocal or diffuse, and central or peripheral. Central enhancement is thought to be suggestive of this tumor. Phleboliths, thought to be pathognomonic, are visible in up to 10% of cases on plain radiographs. On CT, punctate calcifications are visible in

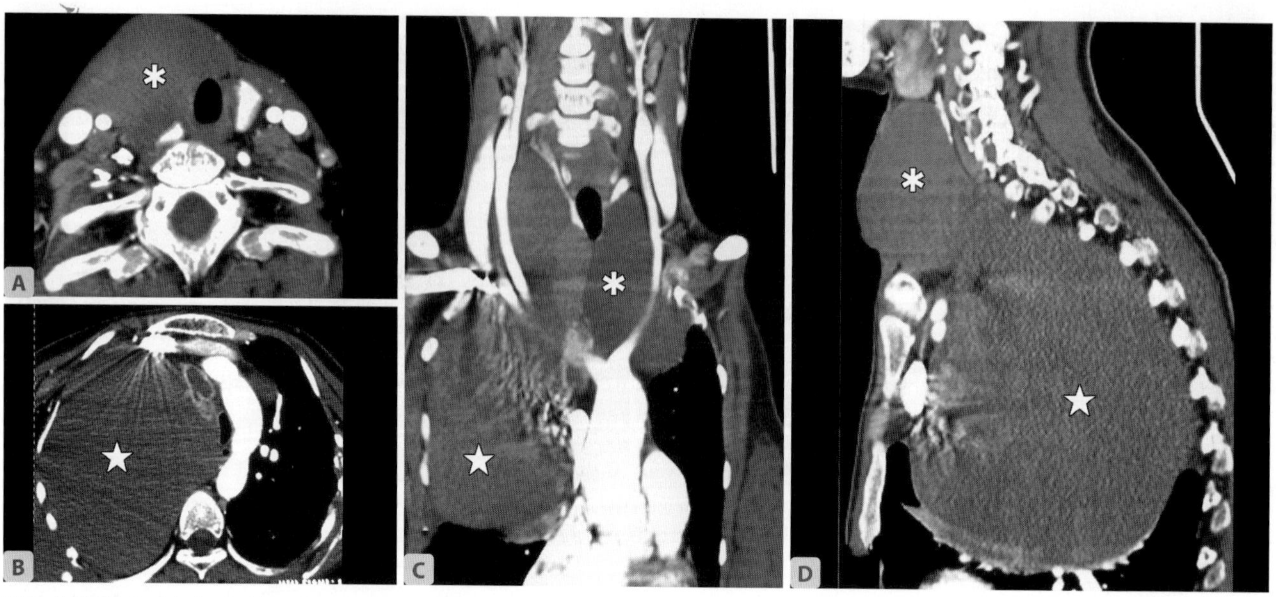

FIGS. 14A TO D: Mediastinal lymphangioma: Axial (A and B), coronal (C) and sagittal (D) contrast-enhanced CT scans showing a cystic lesion in the neck region (asterisk) with a large component in the mediastinum (star).

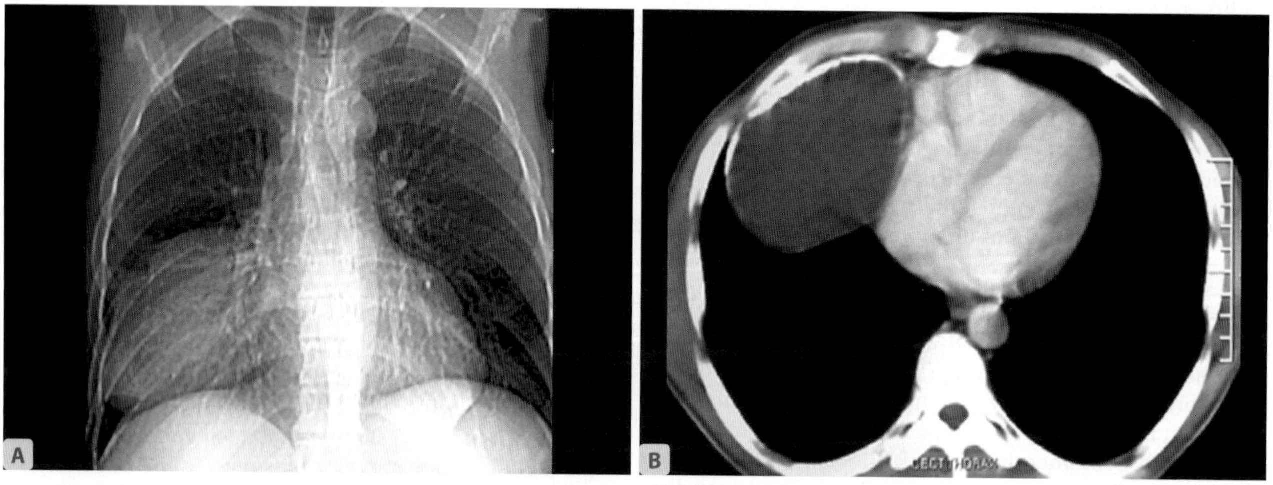

FIGS. 15A AND B: Pericardial cyst: Chest radiograph (A) showing a large right cardiophrenic angle mass; CECT (B) shows a fluid attenuating non-enhancing mass with peripheral rim calcification in right paracardiac location suggesting a diagnosis of pleuropericardial cyst.

21% and phleboliths are visible in 7%. Hemangiopericytoma may appear on CT as a large, well-circumscribed, enhancing mass. It may have a predominance in the superior mediastinum.[1,2,14]

Pericardial Cyst

Pericardial or pleuropericardial cyst results from a defect in the embryogenesis of the celomic cavity. Their walls are composed of connective tissue and a single layer of mesothelial cells. Approximately 90% of pericardial cysts are in contact with the diaphragm, heart or chest wall. About 65% occur in the right cardiophrenic angle and 25% in the left cardiophrenic angle; 10 percent are seen at higher levels. They can be seen as high as the pericardial recesses at the level of the proximal aorta and pulmonary arteries. True cysts contains all layers of pericardium and do not communicate with pericardial space. They are usually asymptomatic and often an incidental finding on chest radiograph. CT is the diagnostic modality of choice and reveals their cystic nature **(Figs. 15A and B)**. They are sharply marginated, fluid attenuating lesions although pericardial cysts with high CT attenuation numbers have been reported.[2] Pericardial cysts are not always round and may assume different shapes when studied at different times. When small, they may sometimes be confused with enlarged cardiophrenic angle lymph nodes. Ultrasonography demonstrates cystic nature of the lesion. On MRI, they are hypontense on T1W and brightly hyperintense on T2W images. Hyperintense signal on T1W may be seen in case of proteinaceous contents. No contrast enhancement is usually seen. Peripheral calcification may be seen on CT due to repeated infection.[30]

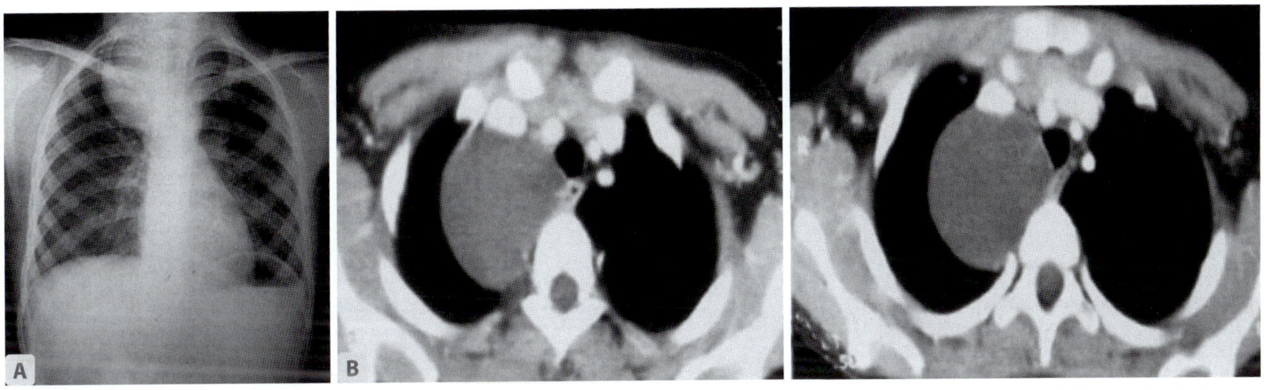

FIGS. 16A AND B: Bronchogenic cyst: Chest radiograph (A) showing a large right paratracheal mediastinal mass. Axial CT (B) shows a fluid-attenuating transcompartmental mass closely related to the trachea suggesting the diagnosis of a bronchogenic cyst.

MIDDLE MEDIASTINUM

Most developmental mediastinal cysts occur in the middle mediastinum and include bronchogenic, esophageal duplication and neuroenteric cysts. The distinction between these cysts may not be always clear and therefore, are classified as foregut cysts because these originate from embryologic foregut. A mediastinal cyst containing cartilage is bronchogenic, one with gastric epithelium is enteric while with seromucinous glands is probably respiratory in origin.[31]

Bronchogenic Cyst

It arises from abnormal budding of the ventral foregut and is histologically lined with ciliated respiratory epithelium, cartilage, smooth muscle, fibrous tissue and mucous glands. The common location is near carina or along right paratracheal wall. More than half of the patients present with symptoms like dyspnea, wheeze due to mass effect. The remaining are detected incidentally.

On chest radiograph, it is seen as well defined mass usually in close proximity to the major airways. CT shows well-defined mass with smooth or lobular outline, uniformly thin wall and fluid density **(Figs. 16A and B)**. Sometimes, it may show high density because of proteinaceous contents, mucin or hemorrhage. MRI features vary according to the cyst contents: uniform low signal intensity on T1W and high signal intensity on T2W similar to water, uniform high signal intensity on T1W and T2W images from proteinaceous contents and variable signal intensity in presence of hemorrhage. Post contrast, there is enhancement of cyst wall without internal enhancement.

Esophageal Duplication Cyst

It is a rare foregut malformation which may be indistinguishable from bronchogenic cyst, except for its location in close proximity to the esophagus. It is composed of a muscular coat and mucosa that resembles esophagus, stomach or small intestine. It occurs within the esophageal wall or may be adherent to the wall, but does not communicate with its lumen. It is spherical or tubular, usually located distally along the lateral aspect of the esophagus and has a thick wall.

Barium swallow examination may demonstrate extrinsic or intramural compression. CT shows spherical or tubular mass in close proximity to esophageal wall **(Figs. 17A to D)**, usually homogeneous with water density but may have soft tissue attenuation in presence of proteinaceous material or intracystic hemorrhage. MRI shows variable signal intensity on T1W image depending on intracystic contents and increased signal intensity on T2W image. The wall of the lesion is thick due to the presence of all the layers. Lesions accessible by ultrasonography (abutting chest wall) may show typical 'gut signature' of the wall (alternating hypoechoic and hyperechoic layers). This may be visualized on endoscopic ultrasound also. The cysts may contain ectopic gastric mucosa and ^{99m}Tc sodium pertechnetate may be useful in their diagnosis.

Neurenteric Cyst

It is a foregut cyst often associated with vertebral anomalies. It results from incomplete separation of the notochord (ectoderm) from foregut (endoderm) during early embryogenesis resulting in persistent communication between them. The cyst is lined by gastrointestinal mucosa and connected to the meninges through a midline defect in one or more vertebral bodies. Ectopic gastric mucosa may be seen in 60% cases.[30] The vertebral anomalies include hemivertebra, sagittal cleft of the vertebral body, butterfly vertebra and spina bifida. Neurenteric cysts occur in middle or posterior mediastinum, usually located above the level of carina. CT and MRI features are similar to those seen in other foregut cysts **(Figs. 18A to C)**. MRI is useful for optimally demonstrating extent of spinal abnormality and degree of intraspinal involvement.[13] Air-fluid level or air foci may be seen when there is communication with esophageal lumen.

Esophageal Lesions

A detailed discussion of esophageal pathology is beyond the scope of this chapter. Dilated esophagus as seen in achalasia, esophageal diverticuli, smooth muscle tumors (leiomyoma and leiomyosarcoma) of the esophagus and hiatus hernia may present as a mediastinal mass. Longitudinally oriented right sided mediastinal mass with air densities and food residue

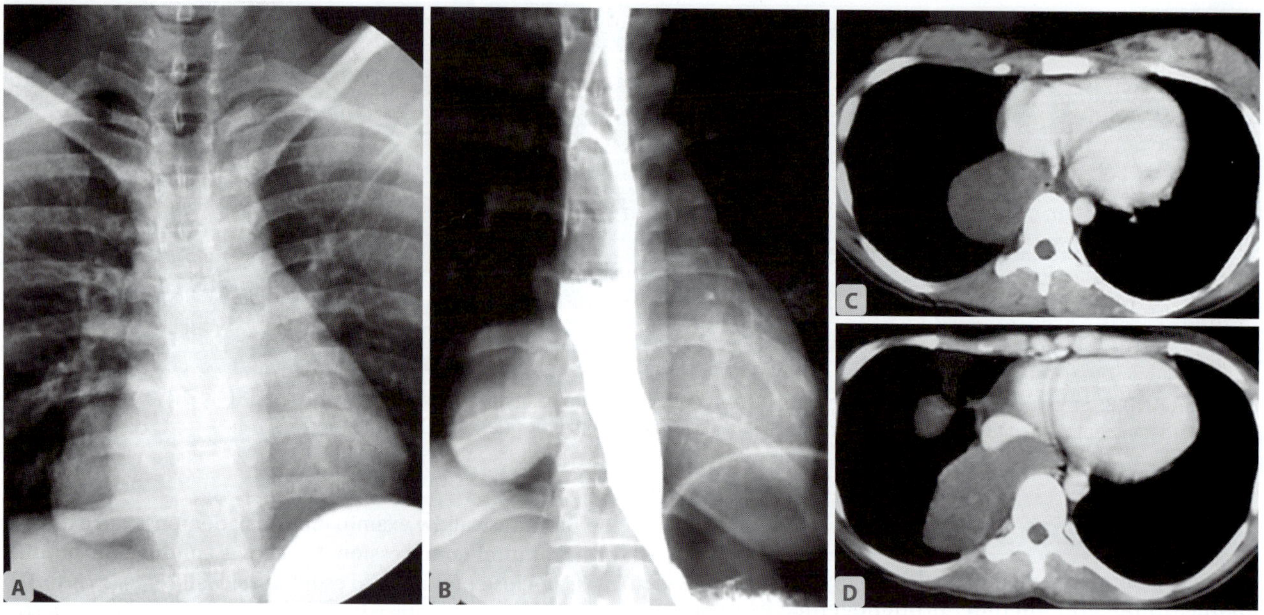

FIGS. 17A TO D: Esophageal duplication cyst: Coned down radiograph (A) showing a right paracardiac mass which is not silhouetting the cardiac border. Barium swallow (B) shows no communication of the esophagus with this mass. Axial CECT scans (C and D) show a fluid density mass intimately related to the esophagus, causing anterior displacement of the inferior vena cava. *Diagnosis:* Esophageal duplication cyst.

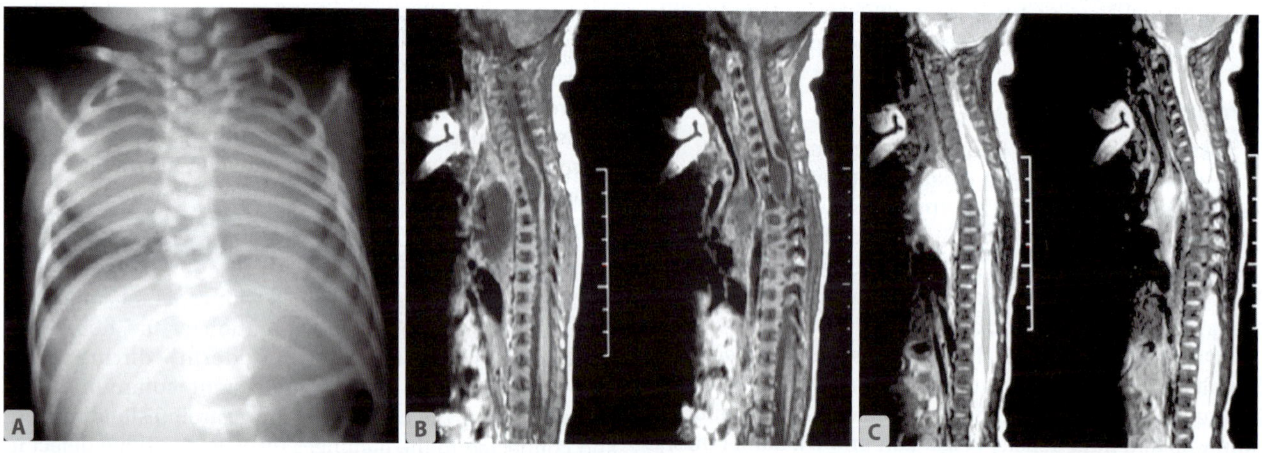

FIGS. 18A TO C: Neuroenteric cyst: Chest radiograph (A) shows a mediastinal mass, with congenital vertebral anomalies and scoliosis of dorsal spine. T1W (B) and T2W (C) sagittal images show a prevertebral mass with intraspinal extension which is hypointense on T1 and bright on the T2W image. *Diagnosis:* Neuroenteric cyst.

is suggestive of a dilated esophagus on a chest radiograph **(Figs. 19A and B)**. CT and barium swallow assist in making a specific diagnosis.

POSTERIOR MEDIASTINUM

The most common lesion in this location is neurogenic tumor, accounting for almost 90% of posterior mediastinal masses.[1,2]

Neurogenic Tumors

These tumors are classified in the following three groups:

- Tumors arising from nerve sheath include neurofibroma, schwannoma, malignant tumor of nerve sheath
- Tumors arising from sympathetic ganglia include ganglioneuroma, ganglioneuroblastoma and neuro-blastoma
- Tumors originating from neuroectodermal cells located in relation to the autonomic nervous system include paraganglioma and pheochromocytoma.

Peripheral Nerve Tumors

These tumors are commonly seen in adults, and have no sex predilection. Most of these tumors are asymptomatic and often seen incidentally on chest radiograph. They usually arise from intercostal nerves close to the spine, near the junction of vertebral body with adjacent rib and may extend through neural foramina into spinal canal (dumb-bell tumor).

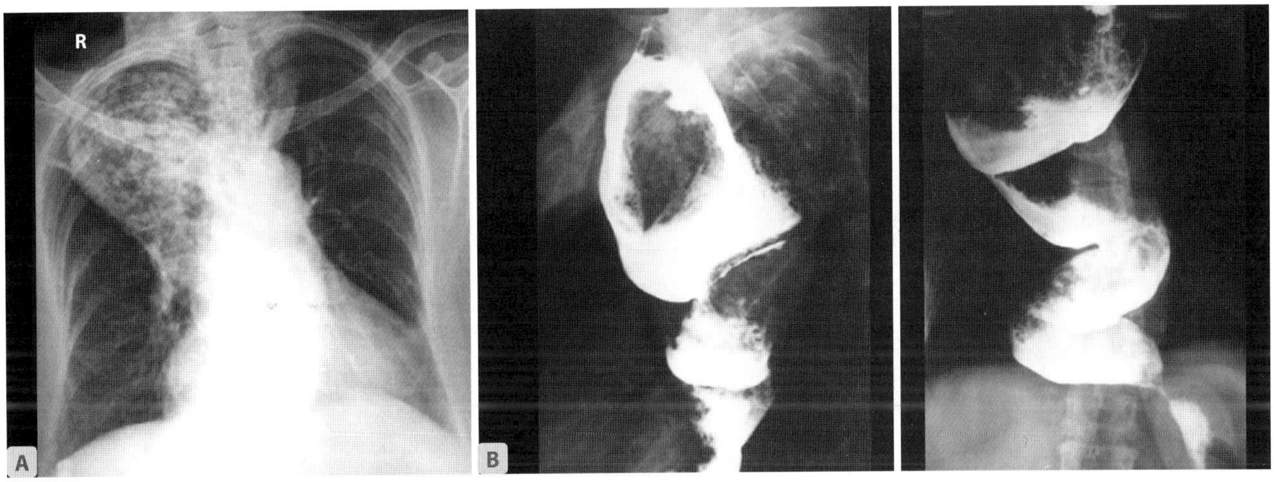

FIGS. 19A AND B: Achalasia cardia: Chest radiograph (A) shows a large right-sided mediastinal mass with air lucencies within it. Barium swallow (B) shows a grossly dilated sigmoid esophagus with a smooth narrowing at the lower end suggestive of achalasia cardia.

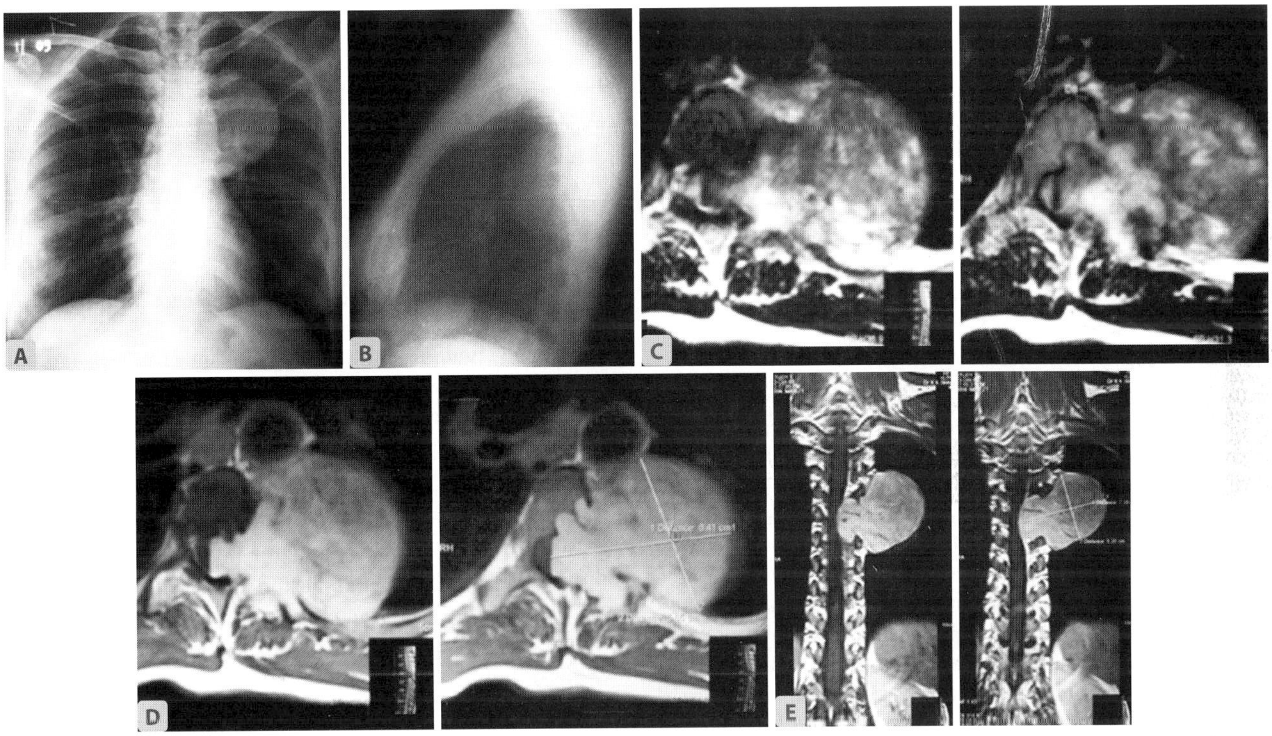

FIGS. 20A TO E: Neurogenic tumor: Chest radiograph frontal (A) and lateral (B) projection showing a posterior mediastinal mass. T2W (C) and post-gadolinium T1W axial (D) and coronal (E) images show an enhancing posterior mediastinal mass with intraspinal extension. The mass shows heterogeneous signal on T2W scan. *Diagnosis:* Nerve sheath tumor.

Neurofibromas are unencapsulated tumors which result from proliferation of all nerve elements, including Schwann cells, nerve fibers and fibroblasts. They grow by diffusely expanding the parent nerve. More than 1/3rd of patients with neurofibromas may have neurofibromatosis type I (von Recklinghausen's disease). The plexiform neurofibroma infiltrates along the nerve trunk or plexuses. Schwannomas are encapsulated, arise from the nerve sheath, from Antoni A or B tissues. They grow eccentrically, along parent nerve and cause symptoms by compressing the nerve. They usually contain areas of cystic degeneration, hemorrhage and calcification.

Chest radiograph shows a well-defined posterior mediastinal mass **(Figs. 20A to E)** which may show pressure deformity of adjacent rib or vertebra, scalloped edge with preservation of cortex, thin and splayed apart ribs, widened intervertebral foramina or scoliosis of spine. They follow the axis of the involved nerve, commonly extending horizontally along the intercostal nerves.

CT shows a homogeneous density mass which enhances with intravenous contrast. Calcification is rare. Schwannoma on noncontrast CT shows low attenuation because of high amount of lipid content and cystic degeneration. Intraspinal involvement is better defined on MRI than on CT.

Neurofibroma shows variable signal intensity on T1W with characteristic target pattern consisting of higher signal intensity peripherally and low signal intensity centrally on T2W image. It enhances with gadolinium. Schwannoma shows inhomogeneous high signal intensity throughout the lesion on T2W corresponding to cystic degeneration and low to intermediate signal intensity on T1W image. The combination of coronal and axial imaging planes is a great advantage of MRI **(Figs. 20A to E)** and its ability to show spinal cord and its surrounding cerebrospinal fluid without the need of intrathecal contrast makes MRI, the imaging procedure of choice.[2,8,9] Two MRI signs have been described in the literature for neurogenic tumors. 'Fascicular sign', typically seen in schwannoma, indicates multiple fascicular bundles and is seen on T2W sequence as multiple ring-like lesions with central hypointensity. The 'target sign', seen more commonly in neurofibroma, appears as central hypointensity with peripheral hyperintensity within the tumor on T2W images.

Plexiform neurofibroma usually shows low attenuating infiltrative mass along the nerve on CT and low signal intensity on T1W and T2W images because of fibrous nature of the tumor. Malignant tumor tends to have poorly defined margins which may show bone destruction. Sudden increase in size of pre-existing mass or development of heterogeneous signal intensity on MRI because of necrosis and hemorrhage, suggests malignancy. FDG PET-CT is useful in differentiating benign from malignant neurogenic tumors with SUV_{max} less than 2.5 suggesting benignity and more than 3.5 suggesting malignancy.[32]

Tumors from Sympathetic Ganglia

These include ganglioneuroma, ganglioneuroblastoma and neuroblastoma. Ganglioneuroma is a benign tumor, neuroblastoma is at the malignant end of the spectrum, while ganglioneuroblastoma is an intermediate form. These tumors are essentially tumors of childhood. The mediastinum is the second most common site for these tumors, the adrenal being the most common site.

These tumors are well-defined with smooth or lobulated outline located in the posterior mediastinum. Ganglineuroma and ganglioneuroblastoma usually extend vertically over three to five vertebrae lateral to the spine, may show broad base on the spine and cause pressure erosion of adjacent vertebra. CT shows homogeneous attenuation whereas MRI shows homogeneous and intermediate signal intensity on both T1W and T2W images.

Almost 10% of neuroblastoma may show stippled calcification that can be seen on chest radiograph. Evidence of widespread local invasion with tendency to cross midline, is characteristic of neuroblastoma. CT shows paraspinal mass with heterogeneous soft tissue attenuation because of hemorrhage, necrosis, cystic degeneration and calcification. MRI shows heterogeneous signal intensity on all pulse sequences and heterogeneous enhancement with gadolinium.[2,9]

Metaiodobenzylguanidine (MIBG) scintigraphy is useful for imaging neuroblastoma, especially to assess the extent of disease. However up to 30% neuroblastomas are not MIBG avid.

Paraganglioma

Paraganglioma (chemodectoma) is a rare tumor originating from neuroectodermal cells located in relation to the autonomic nervous system, especially in the region of the aortopulmonary window and the posterior mediastinum.

Paraganglioma appears as round, extremely vascular soft tissue mass that enhances markedly on contrast-enhanced CT. It is hypointense on T1W and hyperintense on T2W images, with flow voids within, indicating hypervascular nature.

Arteriography demonstrates large feeding vessels, pathologic vessels and intense tumor blush. MIBG scintigraphy shows increased activity and is a good technique to demonstrate paragangliomas.

MRI has largely replaced CT as an initial imaging modality in the evaluation of patients with suspected neurogenic tumors. Unfortunately, MRI is no more specific than CT in differentiating benign from malignant lesions.

Lateral Thoracic Meningocele

This is an anomalous herniation of spinal meninges through the intervertebral foramina. It usually (in 85%) occurs in association with neurofibromatosis type I. Patients present with back pain, neurological and/or respiratory symptoms. It is seen as well-defined paravertebral mass, scalloping and deforming adjacent ribs and vertebral body. Enlargement of intervertebral foramina is an important diagnostic feature. Kyphoscoliosis is often present. The features are indistinguishable from a dumb-bell nerve root tumor.

CT shows well circumscribed paraspinal mass of water attenuation, because bulk of it consists of cerebrospinal fluid. MRI shows low signal intensity on T1W and high signal intensity on T2W image, similar to CSF signal and it does not enhance with gadolinium.

Paraspinal Infection

Vertebral osteomyelitis can result in paraspinal abscess which may present as a mass lesion. The common causative organism in India is *Mycobacterium tuberculosis*, others being *Staphylococcus aureus* and anaerobic organisms. Plain radiograph of the dorsal spine may show narrowing of disk space with destruction of two or more contiguous vertebrae. CT shows heterogeneous attenuation of soft tissue density with rim enhancement with intravenous contrast. MRI shows low signal intensity on T1W and high signal intensity on T2W images. MRI with gadolinium defines the extent of inflammatory process better. MRI is preferred to CT because of its ability to see disc space, bone destruction, spinal canal and its contents.

Extramedullary Hemopoiesis

Extramedullary hemopoiesis is a compensatory mechanism for chronic anemias due to bone marrow dysfunction. Rarely, it causes paravertebral soft tissue masses typically bilaterally, along lower thoracic vertebrae, secondary to severe hemolytic anemia, particularly thalassemia and sickle cell disease. The best diagnostic clue is the presence of multiple lobulated posterior mediastinal masses with vertebral bodies which have prominent trabeculae. CT and MRI show fat density within the masses and there is no bony erosion. They show significant contrast enhancement. The masses are usually asymptomatic but neurological deficit may occur due to intraspinal extension. In difficult cases, marrow scanning may be done with ^{99m}Tc sulfur colloid and SPECT/CT to detect hemopoietic tissue and thus may avoid the need of biopsy.[7] The differential diagnosis includes nerve sheath tumors, varices, lymphoma and lateral thoracic meningocele.

Mediastinal Varices

Abnormal dilatation of veins in the mediastinum may occur in the setting of portal hypertension and obstruction of superior vena cava (downhill varices). They are seen as serpiginous enhancing vascular channels in or around the esophagus, in the portal venous phase. However, on a non-enhanced CT or arterial phase CT, they are unopacified and can mimic asymmetric thickening of esophageal wall, hiatus hernia or any mediastinal mass. On MRI they are seen as serpiginous flow voids on both T1W and T2W images.[2]

MULTICOMPARTMENT MEDIASTINAL MASSES/LESIONS

Mediastinal Lymphadenopathy

Mediastinal lymphadenopathy can occur in any mediastinal compartment **(Figs. 21 and 22)** but is more commonly seen in anterior or middle mediastinum. It can occur due to infection, neoplasm, sarcoidosis or reactive hyperplasia.[33,34]

It has been observed that most lymph nodes with a short axis diameter of more than 2.0 cm can be seen as mediastinal widening if they are present in the right paratracheal, aortopulmonary window and hilar region. Pretracheal, left paratracheal, subcarinal nodes may not be visible on chest radiograph even if they are larger than 2.0 cm. Right paratracheal lymphadenopathy is seen as uniform or lobular widening of right tracheal stripe, convexity of superior vena cava outline and increased density of superior vena cava almost equal to density of aortic arch. Left paratracheal nodes can cause recognizable mediastinal widening only when they enlarge to an extent as to project beyond the vascular pedicle. Nodes in the aortopulmonary area when enlarged significantly

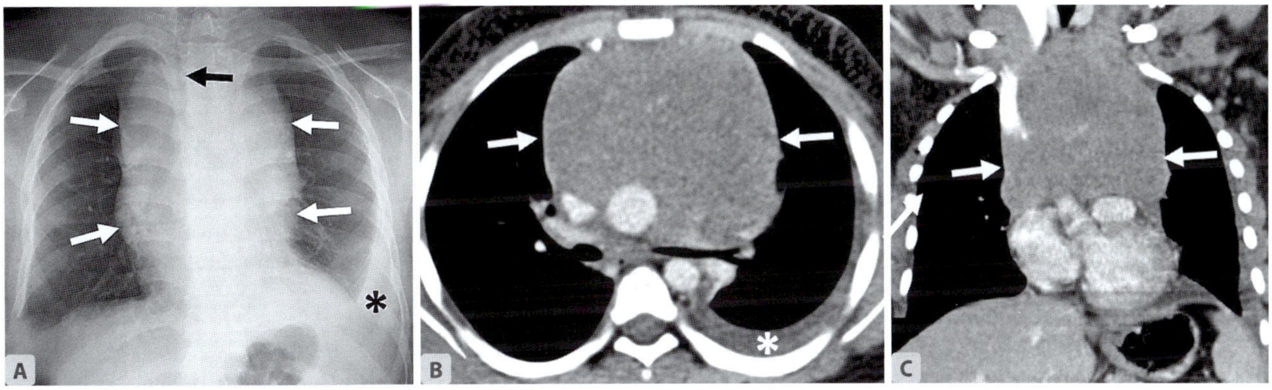

FIGS. 21A TO C: Mediastinal lymphoma. (A) Chest radiograph of a 20-year-old male presenting with respiratory distress showing mediastinal-based mass extending on either side of midline (white arrows), compressing and displacing the trachea (black arrow) and silhouetting cardiac margins suggesting anterior location. Left pleural effusion is noted (asterisk). Axial (B) and Coronal (C) CT images showing a homogeneous anterior mediastinal mass (arrows) and left pleural effusion (asterisk in B).

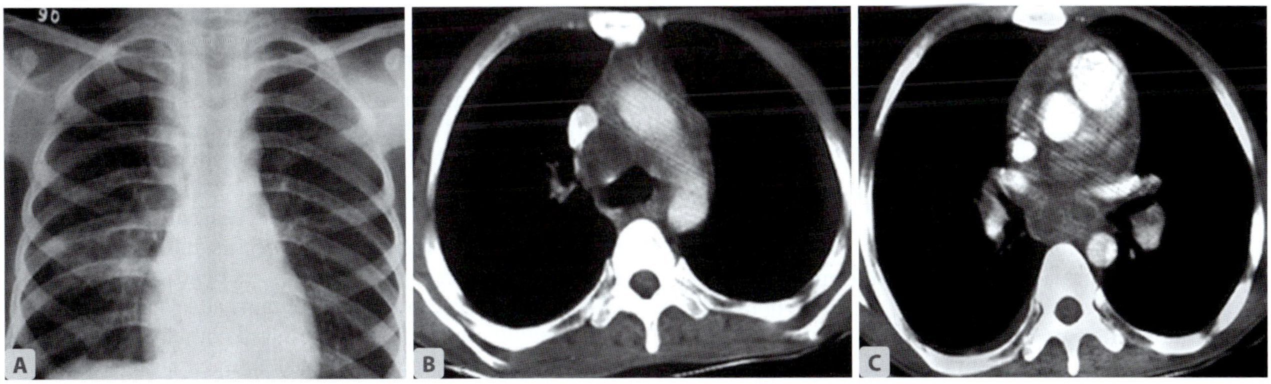

FIGS. 22A TO C: Tuberculosis: Chest radiograph (A) shows a right paratracheal mass with right middle lobe consolidation in a young boy presenting with pyrexia of unknown origin. Axial CECT scans (B and C) show necrotic lymph nodes with peripheral enhancement in right paratracheal and subcarinal location. Biopsy: Tuberculosis.

can cause a bulge in the angle between the aortic arch and main pulmonary artery. Subcarinal lymphadenopathy can be assessed by convex bulge of azygoesophageal line, increased opacity and lack of visibility of the medial wall of right main stem bronchus and bronchus intermedius, also may simulate appearance of left atrial enlargement. Posterior mediastinal lymph node enlargement causes localized displacement of the paraspinal and paraesophageal line. The features of hilar lymphadenopathy are overall hilar enlargement, lobular outline or round mass in the area of the hilum that does not contain major vessels.[2]

Lymph node enlargement on CT can be assessed by measurement of short axis diameter. Nodes less than 10 mm in short axis diameter are normal within 95th percentile. Nodes between 10 and 15 mm in short axis diameter may occur in subcarinal and tracheobronchial region in 5–7% of normal subjects. The CT features of lymph node enlargement are increase in size of individual nodes, focal bulge or lobulation of the interface between the mediastinum and lung, invasion of surrounding mediastinal fat, coalescence of nodes to form large mass or diffuse soft tissue density of the mediastinum obliterating fat planes. Hilar node enlargement on CT can be determined by presence of round soft tissue density which is too large to be blood vessel or nonenhancing mass larger than 5.0 mm in short axis diameter. Contrast-enhanced CT is necessary to distinguish between vascular structures and soft tissue mass. MRI is particularly useful when use of intravenous contrast is contraindicated to differentiate soft tissue signal intensity of lymph node enlargement against the signal void of air and of fast flowing blood on spin echo images.

Lymph node calcification is commonly seen in infective pathology like tuberculosis and fungal infection, may also be seen in other conditions namely sarcoidosis, pneumoconiosis, Castlemann's disease but rarely seen in neoplastic disease. Common patterns of calcification are coarse, irregularly distributed clumps within the node or homogeneous calcification of entire node. Peripheral ring like calcification of node, known as eggshell calcification is characteristic of sarcoidosis or in patients exposed to dust while working in coal or metal mines.

Low density areas within enlarged node due to necrosis are commonly seen in tuberculosis **(Figs. 22A to C)**. This may also be seen in fungal disease, infections in immunocompromised patients, and metastases particularly from testicular tumors.

Mild-to-moderate contrast enhancement is nonspecific, seen in tuberculosis, fungal disease, sarcoidosis or neoplasm. Low density area due to necrosis with peripheral rim enhancement is a characteristic feature of tubercular infection. Marked contrast enhancement is seen in metastatic disease, particularly from melanoma or primary in kidney or thyroid. Diffuse uniform enhancement is seen in Castleman's disease, a rare condition.[34]

CT and MRI provide comparable information; however, the distinct disadvantage of MRI is its inability to demonstrate calcification. Hilar node enlargement is easier to recognize on MRI, which is seen as distinct round or oval density with relatively high signal intensity against the background of signal void of air from bronchi and lungs.

Based on the morphology, site of involvement, presence of calcification, presence of associated lung or pleural pathology, it is possible to offer reasonable etiological diagnosis of lymphadenopathy.

Tuberculosis

Central low density with peripheral rim enhancement, loss of perinodal fat planes, obliteration of azygoesophageal recess suggest tuberculosis **(Figs. 22A to C)**. Associated area of pulmonary consolidation may or may not be present. On healing, the nodes usually become small with dense calcification.

Sarcoidosis

Discrete homogeneous enlargement, no necrosis, well-defined fat planes, classical site of involvement being bilateral hilar and right paratracheal in nearly two third of the patients are characteristic features.

Lymphoma

Anterior mediastinal and paratracheal nodes are more frequently involved **(Figs. 21A to C)**, lymphadenopathy is usually bilateral but asymmetrical. Isolated hilar node enlargement is rare and hilar adenopathy is usually seen along with mediastinal lymphadenopathy. Confluent mass of lymph nodes with irregular areas of necrosis, obliteration of fat planes encasement of vessels are specific features. Superior vena cava thrombosis, invasion of surrounding structures, pleural effusion, consolidation are commonly present.

Metastasis

There is no particular pattern or site of involvement of lymph nodes. However, invasion of pleura, pericardium or chest wall suggests metastasis.

Vascular Lesions

Various vascular abnormalities and anomalies can simulate mediastinal mass. These include right sided or double aortic arch, persistent left SVC or vertical vein, aberrant subclavian artery, dilatation of pulmonary artery, SVC, azygous and hemiazygous system, aortic aneurysm or dissection, SVC syndrome and mediastinal varix. Contrast-enhanced CT or MRI are essential for confirmation of diagnosis.

Aortic Aneurysm

Aortic aneurysms may present as mediastinal widening. This entity is discussed in detail in the chapter on aortic imaging. The most common site of thoracic aortic aneurysm is descending aorta, followed by aortic arch, ascending aorta being the least common. Aneurysm can be of two types: true aneurysm and pseudoaneurysm. True aneurysm occurs due to degeneration of elastic fibers of media. Due to loss of structural support, vessel dilates. True aneurysm contains all layers of the vessel wall. Pseudoaneurysm is the result of contained perforation of the vessel wall. Almost 70% of all thoracic aortic aneurysms are due to atherosclerosis, other causes include trauma, fungal infection and syphilis. The morphologic types are fusiform, saccular, dissecting or false. By definition a diameter more than 4.0 cm is taken as fusiform aneurysm.[2]

The common radiological features on chest radiograph are mediastinal widening/mass or enlarged segment of aorta with peripheral curvilinear calcification. Displacement and less frequently compression of esophagus, trachea and bronchi may be seen. Erosion of vertebrae or ribs may occur but is uncommon. Curvilinear or plaque like calcification is better seen on CT. Most of these aneurysms have lining thrombus with calcification. CT has excellent spatial resolution and both aortic wall and its associated complications are well seen. The availability of MDCT has improved diagnostic accuracy and reduced examination time. MRI is an excellent modality for assessing size and shape of aneurysm, demonstrating relationship of aneurysm to branch vessels and compression effects. MRI combines the strength of echocardiography, angiography and CT. Using spin echo and dynamic imaging techniques, combined with large FOV, MRI can fully characterize thoracic aneurysm and its complications.

Aortic Dissection

Spontaneous aortic dissection results from repeated trauma to the media, often in a patient with persistent hypertension, with development of intramural hematoma, localized to the media. As the hematoma evolves into a seroma, a rent can occur in the overlying intima, with subsequent establishment of a false lumen tracking down the media that communicates with true aortic lumen, also called dissecting aneurysm. The false lumen is usually between the inner one third and outer two-thirds of media. The dissection can extend in both antegrade and retrograde fashion. The dissecting channel usually spirals so that the false lumen lies anterior and to the right in ascending aorta, posterior and to the left in descending aorta. Cystic medial necrosis, Marfan's syndrome, hypertension are important predisposing factors.[1,2]

The chest radiograph is often abnormal but the findings are nonspecific. Superior mediastinal widening with distinctly undulating appearance of aorta, progressive change in aortic configuration on sequential radiographs, unexplained discrepancy between caliber of ascending and descending aorta suggest aortic dissection. The most specific sign is 1.0 cm or more displacement of aortic calcification inside the aortic contour on sequential chest radiographs. This sign is however, seen in a small percentage of patients.

CT and MRI are used to image aortic dissection. A detailed discussion of the imaging findings is given in the chapter on imaging the aorta. Transthoracic and transesophageal ultrasonography are proving increasingly useful in the diagnosis of aortic dissection.

Superior Vena Cava Obstruction

The most common cause of superior vena cava obstruction is compression and invasion by bronchogenic carcinoma either by primary tumor or lymphadenopathy. Other causes are metastatic disease, lymphoma, mediastinal fibrosis. The dilated collaterals, enlargement of azygous vein, and widened superior mediastinum can be seen on chest radiograph.

Contrast-enhanced CT is an excellent technique to show narrowing, filling defects in cava and collaterals besides providing information about the cause of obstruction. MRI also provides similar information with added advantage of multiplanar imaging and no need of contrast. The limitation of MRI is its inability to demonstrate calcification, an important feature in the diagnosis of granulomatous mediastinal fibrosis.

Abnormalities of the Mediastinal Fat

Mediastinal Lipomatosis

This is a benign condition in which exuberant deposition of unencapsulated fat occurs in the mediastinum. The etiology includes obesity, exogenous steroids, and Cushing's syndrome. The most common location is superior mediastinum, and it may be associated with enlarged epicardial and pericardial fat pad. The cardiophrenic fat pad may resemble a mass. Massive fat collection may be seen throughout the mediastinum in mediastinal lipomatosis. Chest radiograph may show smooth mediastinal widening without tracheal compression or displacement. The fat shows uniform low density on CT in the range of –70 to –130 HU, no soft tissue component or enhancement and it usually does not compress or invade adjacent structures.[2] MRI shows homogeneous hyperintense signal on T1W and T2W images with signal suppression on fat-saturated images.

Lipoma

This mediastinal tumor of fatty origin is uncommon, comprising less than 1% of all mediastinal masses. Benign as well as malignant fatty tumor appear as well-defined round or oval mass on chest radiograph. It is usually soft and moulds to the mediastinal contour, mimicking cardiomegaly. CT and MRI show uniform fat containing lesion with few strands of soft tissue within. Some liposarcomas may show inhomogeneous fat density with predominant soft tissue attenuation.

Herniation of Abdominal Fat

Herniation of omental fat through the esophageal hiatus, foramen of Morgagni or foramen of Bochdalek presents as focal fatty mass in the mediastinum. Bowel loops, liver, spleen and kidney may herniate into the thorax. Herniation through foramen of Morgagni almost always occurs on right side in the anterior mediastinum simulating cardiophrenic angle mass **(Figs. 23 and 24)**. Herniation through foramen of Bochdalek occurs often on the left side in posterior mediastinum presenting as diaphragmatic hump close to the spine. Diagnosis can be made on chest radiograph because of the characteristic location. Fat density with fine linear densities within, representing omental vessels on CT differentiates omental hernia from lipoma. Similarly on MRI **(Figs. 24 and 25)**, high signal intensity on T1W and moderately high signal intensity on T2W image (the characteristics of fat on MRI) with low intensity linear areas representing blood vessels, provide a specific diagnosis.

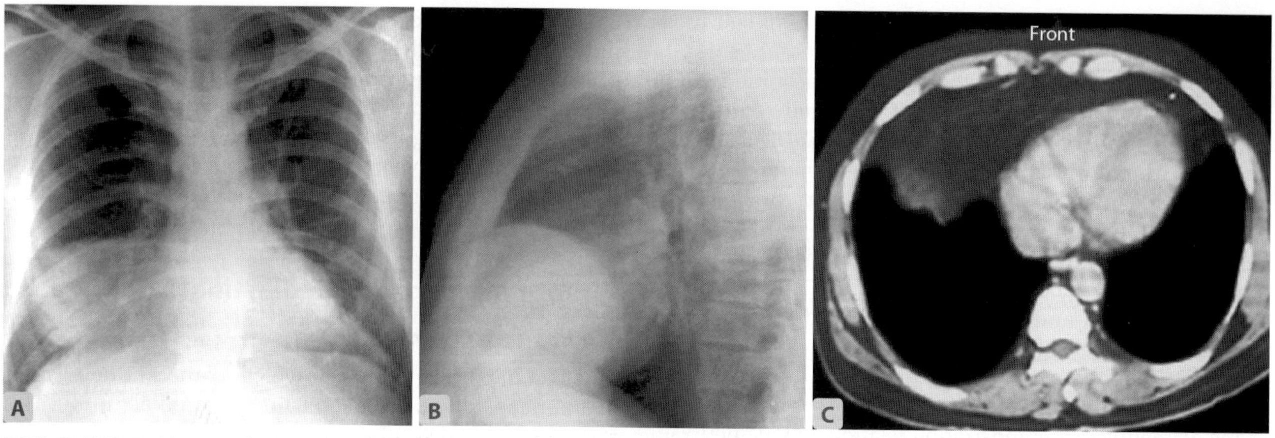

FIGS. 23A TO C: Morgagni hernia: Chest radiograph frontal (A) and lateral (B) projection showing an anteriorly located right cardiophrenic angle mass. Axial CECT (C) shows a fatty attenuating mass in this location, which shows vessels running through it. Diagnosis: Morgagni hernia containing omental fat.

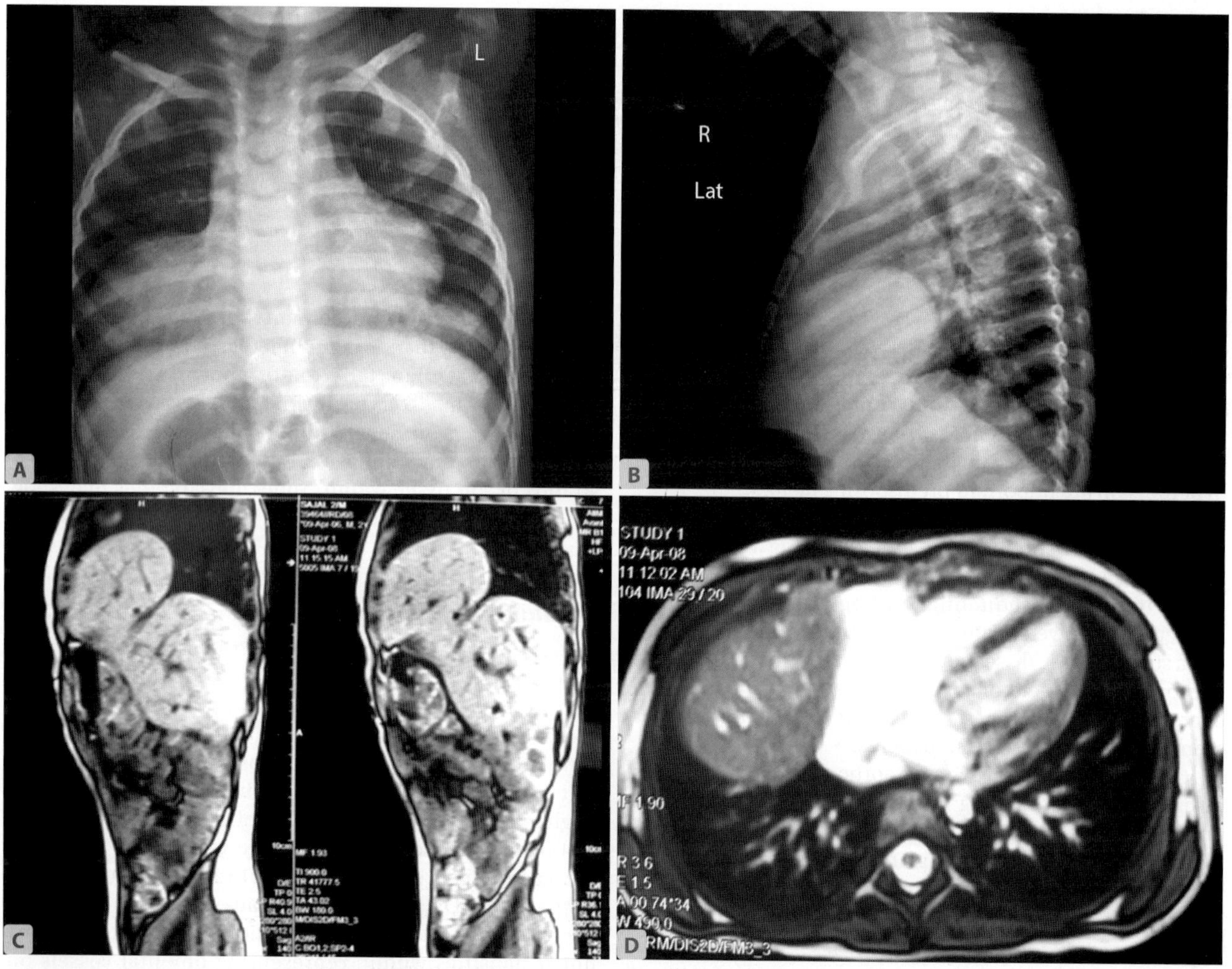

FIGS. 24A TO D: Morgagni hernia: Chest radiograph frontal (A) and lateral (B) projection showing an anteriorly located right cardiophrenic angle mass (C). T1W sagittal and T2W axial (D) MRI scans confirm the herniated liver in a Morgagni hernia.

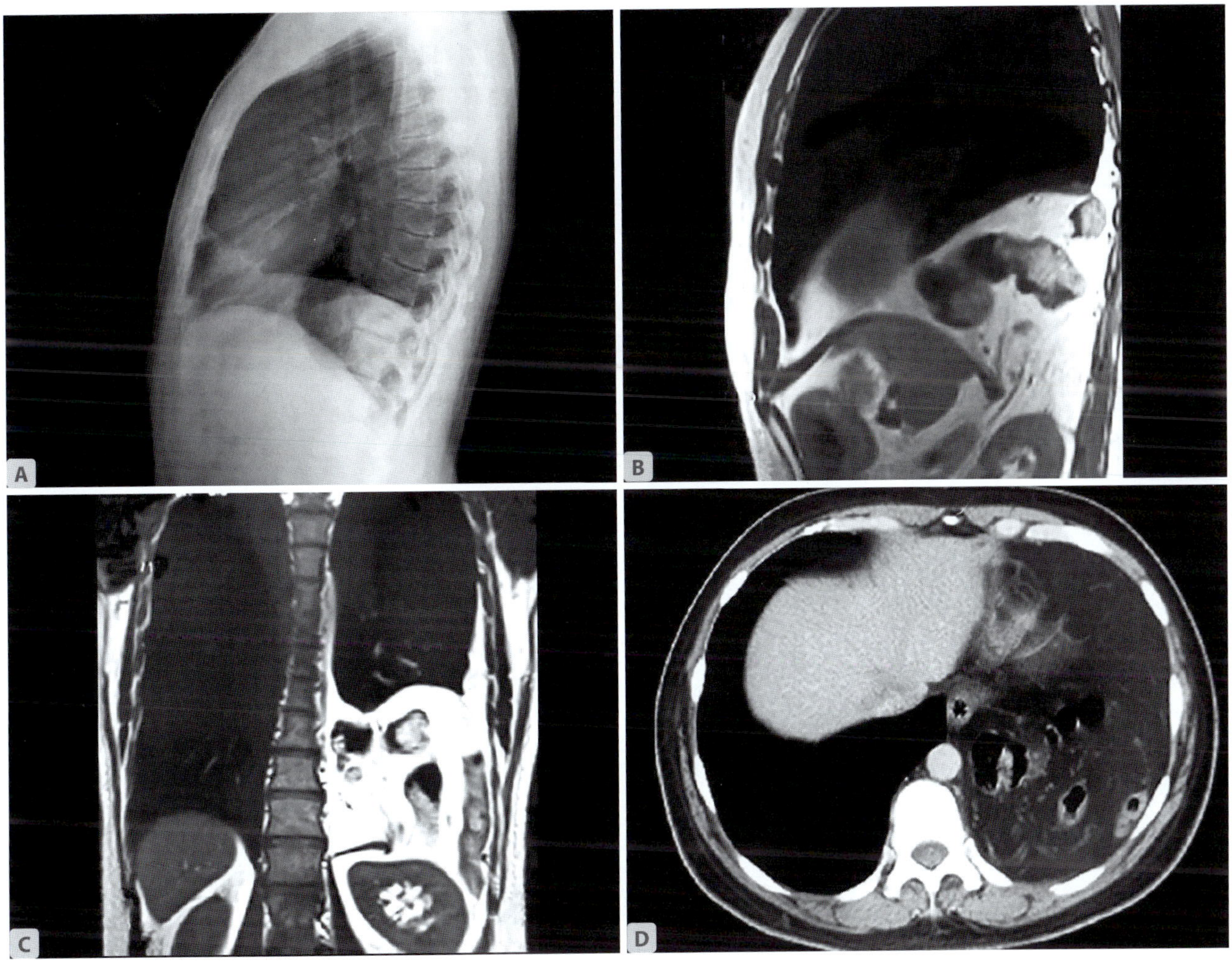

FIGS. 25A TO D: Bockdalek hernia: Chest radiograph (A) in lateral projection shows an apparent elevation of the left dome of diaphragm. Axial CT (B) shows fat and bowel loops in the left hemithorax. Coronal (C) and sagittal (D) T1W MR scans show herniation of mesenteric fat and bowel loops through a defect in the posterior part of the left dome suggestive of a Bockdalek hernia.

MISCELLANEOUS LESIONS OF THE MEDIASTINUM

Mediastinal Hemorrhage

Trauma to the aorta or one of its major arteries is a frequent cause of mediastinal hemorrhage. The other causes include dissecting aneurysm, rupture of the aneurysm, patient having bleeding diathesis or on anticoagulant therapy.

Chest radiograph shows mediastinal widening. The blood may track along extrapleural space over the lung apices producing apical capping. It may rupture into pleural cavity or track into lung along perivascular, peribronchial sheath producing changes resembling pulmonary edema. Noncontrast CT shows streaky soft densities interspersed through mediastinal fat and high density associated with fresh hematoma **(Figs. 26A to C)**. The appearance of hemorrhage on MRI depends on the duration of bleed. In the acute phase, there is low signal intensity on T1W and high signal intensity on T2W images. As the days pass, signal intensity on T1W images increases and in subacute phase, both T1W and T2W images show high signal intensity. In chronic phase, signal intensity depends on the amount of water in the hemorrhage and degree of conversion from methemoglobin to ferritin and hemosiderin.[1,2]

Pneumomediastinum

Common causes include blunt chest trauma, asthma, mechanical ventilation, esophageal perforation, etc. Features of pneumomediastinum on chest radiograph are air outlining the left heart border, air dissecting under and medial to thymus outlining it distinctly, extrapleural tracking along upper surface of diaphragm, air between heart and diaphragm producing continuous diaphragm sign. Dissection of air along tissue planes overlying the mediastinal blood vessels, major airways or esophagus is better seen on lateral chest radiograph than in frontal view.

CT is more sensitive than chest radiograph, and shows streaky air densities in the mediastinal fat and around tubular structures like trachea and esophagus **(Figs. 27A and B)**.

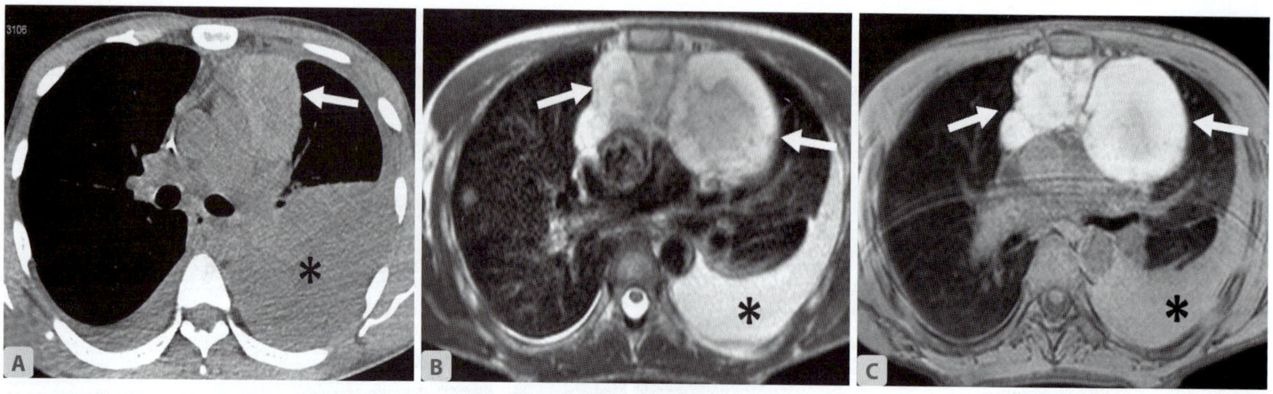

FIGS. 26A TO C: Mediastinal hematoma. (A) Axial noncontrast CT image showing hyperdense hematoma in the anterior mediastinum (arrow) with left pleural effusion (asterisk); (B and C) Axial T2-weighted (B) and T1-weighted fat saturated (C) MR images showing anterior mediastinal hematoma (arrows) appearing hyperintense on both sequences. Left pleural effusion is noted (asterisk).

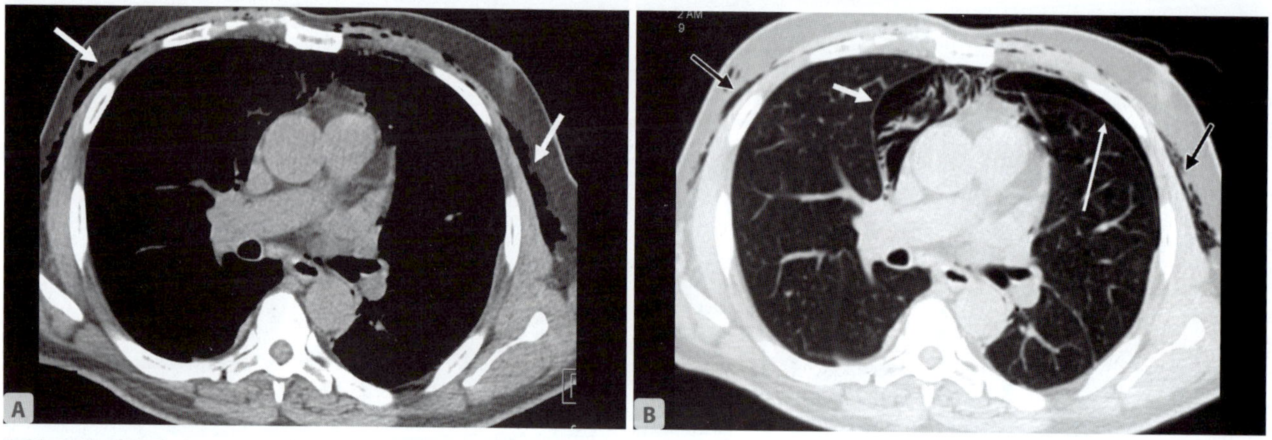

FIGS. 27A AND B: Pneumomediastinum. (A) Axial CT scan in mediastinal window shows air in chest wall (white arrows) suggesting surgical emphysema. Mediastinal air cannot be appreciated; (B) Lung window at the same level shows the pneumomediastinum clearly (white short arrow) along with left pneumothorax (long thin white arrow) and surgical emphysema (black arrows).

CT may also give a clue about the cause of pneumomediastinum. Differential diagnosis includes pneumothorax and pneumopericardium.[2]

Acute Mediastinitis

Acute mediastinal infections are uncommon and usually related to surgery, esophageal perforation, or spread of infection from adjacent regions. Infections may present as diffuse mediastinitis or mediastinal abscess, depending on their extent. Diffuse mediastinitis has a relatively poor prognosis. Chest radiograph may show mediastinal widening, pneumomediastinum, pleural effusion, localized fluid collection and abscess formation. CT shows obliteration of fat planes and air bubbles in the mediastinum. The features seen on chest radiograph are better defined on CT.

CT is superior and the findings in mediastinitis include diffuse or streaky infiltration of mediastinal fat, localized fluid collections, pleural or pericardial effusion, lymph node enlargement, and compression of mediastinal structures.[1] Gas bubbles in the mediastinum, with or without associated fluid collections, are seen in up to half of cases, and are an important finding. A localized fluid collection with an air-fluid level and an enhancing wall is suggestive of a mediastinal abscess. There may be a coexisting empyema or subphrenic abscess. Although most of the times diagnosis may be made on imaging, occasionally percutaneous image guided aspiration may be necessary.

Fibrosing Mediastinitis

Tuberculosis, histoplasmosis and radiation therapy are important causes of fibrosing mediastinitis. An idiopathic variety which is autoimmune in origin occurring in association with retroperitoneal fibrosis and orbital pseudotumor is also reported. Radiological features depend on the site and degree of lymphadenopathy and chest radiograph may show severity of obstructive phenomenon. Unilateral or bilateral hilar or mediastinal lymphadenopathy, often asymmetrical and mostly in superior mediastinum, narrowing of trachea and major bronchi, pulmonary oligemia due to narrowing of pulmonary artery are commonly present. Pulmonary consolidation resulting from bronchial, venous or lymphatic obstruction

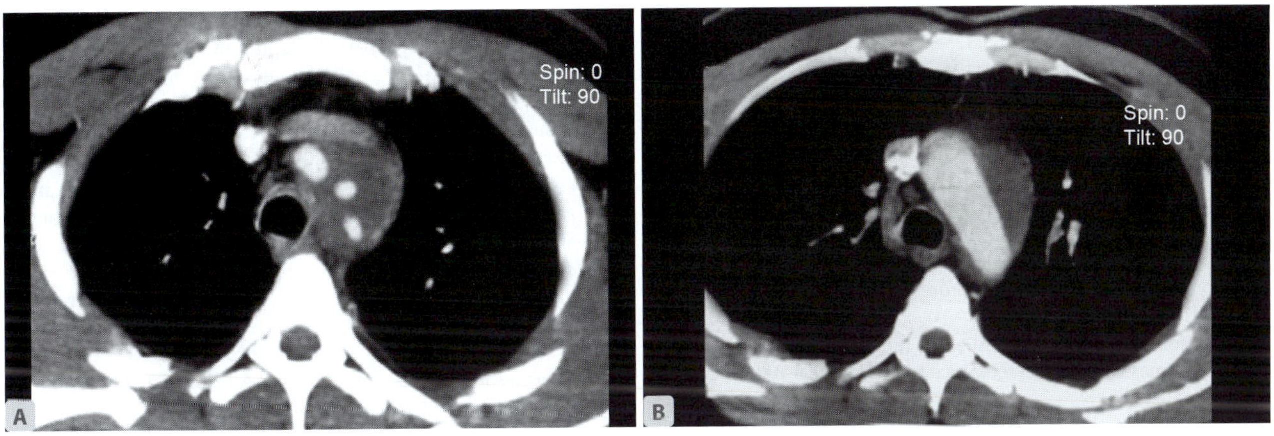

FIGS. 28A AND B: Mediastinal fibrosis. Axial CECT (A and B) showing a plaque-like soft tissue infiltrating the mediastinum and encasing the brachiocephalic trunk, left common carotid and the left subclavian artery. *Diagnosis:* Mediastinal fibrosis.

may be seen. CT features are lymphadenopathy with or without calcification, narrowing of airways, venous or arterial compression, collateral venous pathways, and obliteration of fat planes.

CT can diagnose and assess the severity of mediastinal fibrosis. Two distinct patterns of mediastinal involvement may be seen. A focal pattern present in 82% of cases is seen as a localized mass or masses of soft tissue attenuation, usually in the right paratracheal or subcarinal regions or hila, which frequently show calcification. A diffuse pattern of involvement is seen in 18% of cases and manifest as a diffusely infiltrating **(Figs. 28A and B)**, noncalcified mass, affecting multiple mediastinal compartments. In the presence of fibrosing mediastinitis, discrete enlarged lymph nodes cannot be identified.[2]

On T1-weighted MR images, fibrosing mediastinitis is typically seen as a heterogeneous, infiltrative mass of intermediate signal intensity. Its appearance on T2-weighted MR images is variable; regions of both increased and markedly decreased signal intensity are frequently seen in the same or in different parts of the mediastinum. Decreased signal intensity on T2-weighted images probably indicates the presence of calcification or fibrous tissue and hyperintense areas indicate more active inflammation. After the administration of Gd-DTPA, the mediastinal masses usually show heterogeneous enhancement. MRI is particularly valuable in assessing vascular patency without the need for intravenous contrast media. FDG-PET may show uptake in areas of active inflammation.

CONCLUSION

A wide spectrum of pathology can affect the mediastinum, and the radiologist plays a vital role in the clinical work up of mediastinal lesions. Many different classifications are available for mediastinal compartments primarily based on the radiograph with only the more recent one suggested by ITMIG being based on CT. Chest radiograph and CT are the primary imaging modalities and are invaluable for characterization and extent evaluation. MRI is used as a problem solving tool and can help differentiate atypical cysts from solid masses, distinguish thymic hyperplasia from thymoma and for the evaluation of posterior mediastinal lesions. The location of a lesion within the different mediastinal compartments and its imaging appearance help arrive at a precise diagnosis.

REFERENCES

1. Fraser R, et al. Fraser and Pare's Diagnosis of diseases of the chest, 4th edn. Philadelphia: WB Saunders.
2. Naidich, et al. Computed Tomography and Magnetic Resonance of the Thorax, 4th Edn. Lippincott Williams and Wilkins; 2007.
3. Gray's anatomy: Williams PL, Warwick R, Dyson M, Bannister LH. Splanchnology. In: Gray's anatomy. 37th edn. New York, NY: Churchill Livingstone; 1989.pp.1245-475.
4. Felson B. The mediastinum. Semin Roentgenol. 1969;4:41-58.
5. Fujimoto K, Hara M, Tomiyama N, Kusumoto M, Sakai F, Fujii Y. Proposal for a new mediastinal compartment classification of transverse plane images according to the Japanese Association for Research on the Thymus (JART) General Rules for the Study of Mediastinal Tumors. Oncol Rep. 2014;31(2):565-72.
6. Carter BW, Tomiyama N, Bhora FY, et al. A modern definition of mediastinal compartments. J Thorac Oncol. 2014;9(9 suppl 2): S97-101.
7. Carter BW, Benveniste MF, Madan R, Godoy MC, de Groot PM, Truong MT, Rosado-de-Christenson ML, Marom EM. ITMIG Classification of Mediastinal Compartments and Multidisciplinary Approach to Mediastinal Masses. Radiographics. 2017;37(2):413-36.
8. Webb WR, Sostman HD. MR imaging of thoracic diseases: clinical uses. Radiology. 1992;182:621-30.
9. Erasmus JJ, McAdams HP, Donnelly LF, Spritzer CE. MR imaging of mediastinal masses. Magn Reson Imaging Clin North Am. 2000;8:59-89.
10. Laurent F, Latrabe V, Lecesne R, et al. Mediastinal masses: diagnostic approach. Eur Radiol. 1998;8:1148-59.
11. Jeung MY, Gasser B, Gangi A, et al. Imaging of cystic masses of the mediastinum. Radiographics. 2002;22(spec no):S79-93.
12. Kim JH, Goo JM, Lee HJ, et al. Cystic tumors in the anterior mediastinum. Radiologic-pathological correlation. J Comput Assist Tomogr. 2003;27:714-23.

13. Merten DF. Diagnostic imaging of mediastinal masses in children. Am J Roentgenol. 1992;158:825-32.
14. Macchiarini P, Ostertag H. Uncommon primary mediastinal tumors. Lancet Oncol. 2004;5:107-18.
15. Inaoka T, Takahashi K, Mineta M, et al. Thymic hyperplasia and thymus gland tumors: Differentiation with chemical shift MR imaging. Radiology. 2007;243(3):869-76.
16. Strollo DC, Rosado-de-Christenson ML. Tumors of the thymus. J Thorac Imaging. 1999;14:152-71.
17. Tomiyama N, Muller NL, Ellis SJ, et al. Invasive and noninvasive thymoma: distinctive CT features. J Comput Assist Tomogr. 2001;25:388-93.
18. Masaoka A, Monden Y, Nakahara K, Tanioka T. Follow-up study of thymomas with special reference to their clinical stages. Cancer. 1981;48:2485-92.
19. Jeong YJ, et al. Does CT of thymic epithelial tumors enable us to distinguish histologic subtypes and predict prognosis? Am J Roentgenol. 2004;183(2):283-9.
20. Azizad S, Sannananja B, Restrepo CS. Solid tumors of the mediastinum in adults. Semin ultrasound CT MRI. 2016; 37:196-211.
21. Marx A, Ströbel P, Badve SS, et al. ITMIG consensus statement on the use of the WHO histological classification of thymoma and thymic carcinoma: refined definitions, histological criteria, and reporting. J Thorac Oncol. 2014; 9(5):596-611.
22. Nishino Mizuki, Simon K, et al: The thymus: A comprehensive review. Radiographics. 2006;26:335-48.
23. Moeller KH, Rosado-de-Christenson ML, Templeton PA. Mediastinal mature teratoma: imaging features. Am J Roentgenol. 1997; 169:985-90.
24. Rosado-de-Christenson ML, Templeton PA, Moran CA. Mediastinal germ-cell tumors: radiologic and pathologic correlation. Radiographics. 1992;12:1013-30.
25. Drevelegas A, Palladas P, Scordalaki A. Mediastinal germ cell tumors: a radiologic-pathologic review. Eur Radiol. 2001;11: 1925-32.
26. Madhusudhan KS, Sharma R, Gadodia A, Kumar A. Spontaneous rupture of benign mediastinal teratoma: a report of two cases. Indian J Med Pediatr Oncol. 2012; 33(2):123-5.
27. Perez-Monte JE, Brown ML, Shah AN, et al. Parathyroid adenomas: accurate detection and localization with Tc-99m sestamibi SPECT. Radiology. 1996;201:85-91.
28. Kukar M, Platz TA, Schaffner TJ, et al. The use of modified four-dimensional computed tomography in patients with primary hyperparathyroidism: an argument for the abandonment of routine sestamibi single-positron emission computed tomography (SPECT). Ann Surg Oncol. 2015;22 (1):139-45.
29. Jo VY, Fletcher CD. WHO classification of soft tissue tumours: an update based on the 2013, 4th edition. Pathology. 2014;46(2): 95-104.
30. Vargas D, Suby-Long T, Restrepo CS. Cystic lesions of the mediastinum. Semin Ultrasound CT MRI. 2016;37:212-22.
31. Kim Y, Lee KS, Yoo JH, et al. Middle mediastinal lesions: imaging findings and pathological correlation. Eur J Radiol. 2000;35: 30-8.
32. Warbey VS, Ferner RE, Dunn JT, Calonje E, O'Doherty MJ. [18F] FDG PET/CT in the diagnosis of malignant peripheral nerve sheath tumours in neurofibromatosis type-1. Eur J Nucl Med Mol Imaging. 2009;36(5):751–7.
33. Kazama T, Faria SC, Varavithya V, et al. FDG PET in the evaluation of treatment for lymphoma: clinical usefulness and pitfalls. Radiographics. 2005;25:191-207.
34. Ko SF, et al. Imaging Spectrum of Castleman's Disease. Am J Roengenol. 2004;182(3):769-75.

CHAPTER

133

Imaging of Solitary Pulmonary Nodule

Sapna Singh, Anju Garg, Anjali Prakash

INTRODUCTION

A solitary pulmonary nodule (SPN) is defined as a well-defined round or oval lesion less than 3 cm in size surrounded at least partially by the lung parenchyma **(Figs. 1A and B)**. Lesions larger than 3 cm are called masses. There is no lymphadenopathy, atelectasis or pneumonia associated with SPN **(Figs. 2A and B)**.[1,2] However, practically, there is a lot of overlap between the two terms, SPN and mass, and many times are used interchangeably.

Differentiation between benign and malignant SPNs forms the goal of imaging. This differentiation is important because the overall mortality associated with lung cancer is about 85% and about 20 % of lung cancers are discovered in the form of SPN.[3] SPN is seen in about 0.2% of chest radiographs.[4]

SPURIOUS SPN

Pleural based and chest wall lesions, nipple shadow, skin nodules like neurofibroma, artifacts may be the causes of spurious SPNs, however oblique views, repeat radiographs or even CT at times may help to differentiate these from a true SPN **(Figs. 3A to C)**.

MORPHOLOGICAL CHARACTERISTICS OF SPN

Of the malignant lesions, adenocarcinoma is the most common carcinoma to give rise to a SPN though all the histological types may present as intrapulmonary nodules.[5,6] Of the benign nodules, granulomas and intrapulmonary lymph nodes account for 80% while hamartomas account for about 10% of the nodules.[6] Morphological characteristics of the nodule such as shape, size, margin, etc. have been used to differentiate between benign and malignant nodules.

Size

The larger the lesion, the more likely it is to be malignant **(Table 1)**. For a SPN to be detected on chest radiographs, it should be at least 9 mm in diameter while CT detects smaller

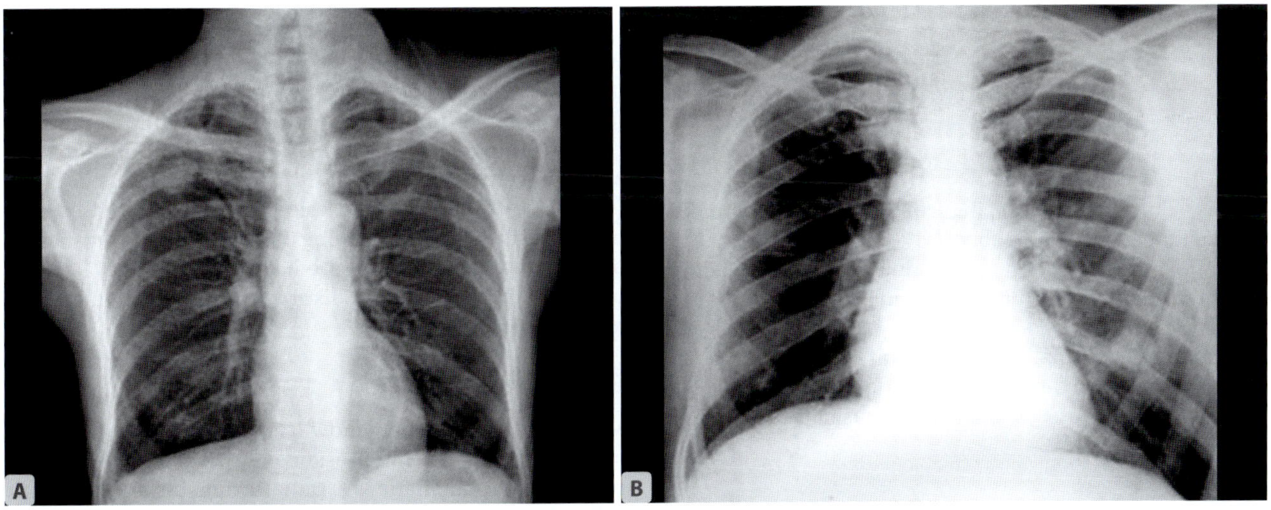

FIGS. 1A AND B: Chest radiographs in two patients showing a well-defined spherical lesion less than 3 cm in diameter surrounded by lung and not associated with lymphadenopathy, atelectasis or pneumonia. The lesions are seen in the right upper zone in one (A) and in the left lower zone in the other (B)—Solitary pulmonary nodules.

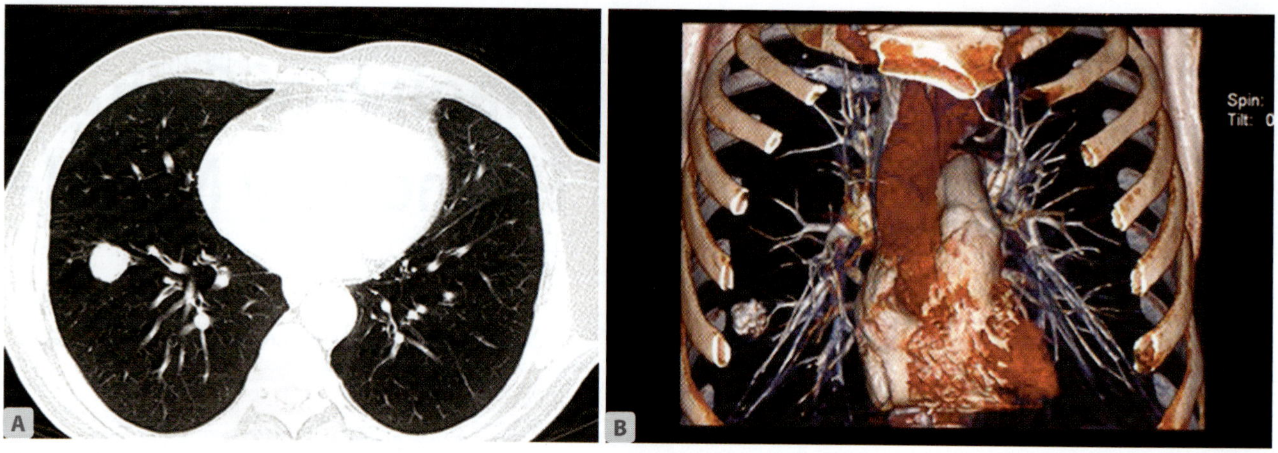

FIGS. 2A AND B: CT scan (A) in patient with suspected pulmonary embolism reveals an incidental SPN in the right lower lobe. VRT pulmonary angiogram image (B) showing the normal vasculature with the nodule in the lower lobe.

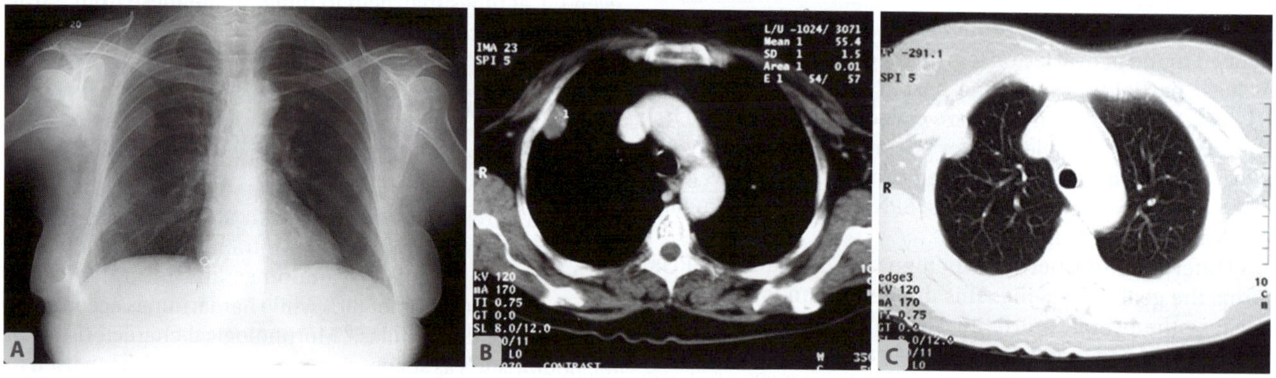

FIGS. 3A TO C: Chest radiograph (A) revealing a solitary nodule in the right lung. CT mediastinal window (B) and lung parenchymal window settings (C) reveal the lesion to be clearly pleural based—A case of pleural fibroma mimicking SPN.

TABLE 1: Likelihood of malignancy related to nodule diameter.[9]

Diameter	Malignancy rate
<1 cm	35%
1–2 cm	50%
2–3 cm	80%
>3 cm	97%

lesions.[7] For a nodule ranging from 0.5-1 cm in diameter, the likelihood of cancer is about 35%, for nodules 1.0–2.0 cm in diameter it is 50%, and for a nodule more than 2.0 cm in diameter, the likelihood of it being malignant is 85% **(Figs. 4A and B)**.[8,9]

Though a very small lesion can turn out to be malignant, lesions larger than 3 cm in diameter are more likely to be malignant while those less than 1 cm are usually benign **(Figs. 5A and B)**.[8,9]

Shape

Benign lesions are usually round/oval with smooth margins, for example, hamartomas. Malignant lesions, on the other hand, tend to be irregular in shape, notched and lobulated **(Figs. 6A to C)**. Lobulation and notching are more indicative of a malignant lesion than a benign lesion.[10] A linear or angular shape may be seen in scars/atelectasis.

Location

About 70% of lung cancers are located in the right upper lobe, the right lung being a more common site for malignancy than the left lung.[11-13] While squamous cell carcinoma is more likely to be centrally located, adenocarcinoma is usually peripheral in location **(Figs. 7A to C)**.[14] Metastatic lesions usually involve the outer one third and bases of the lungs. *Location*, however, cannot be used as an independent predictor of malignancy because benign nodules are equally distributed throughout the upper and lower lobes.[15]

Edge Characteristics

Malignant lesions often show irregularity, spiculation and lobulation **(Fig. 8)**. The presence of spiculation is a strong predictor of malignancy. A radial extension of malignant cells, along the interlobular septa, lymphatics, small airways or blood vessels is the cause for the spiculation and has been likened to the spokes of a wheel or "corona radiata" or

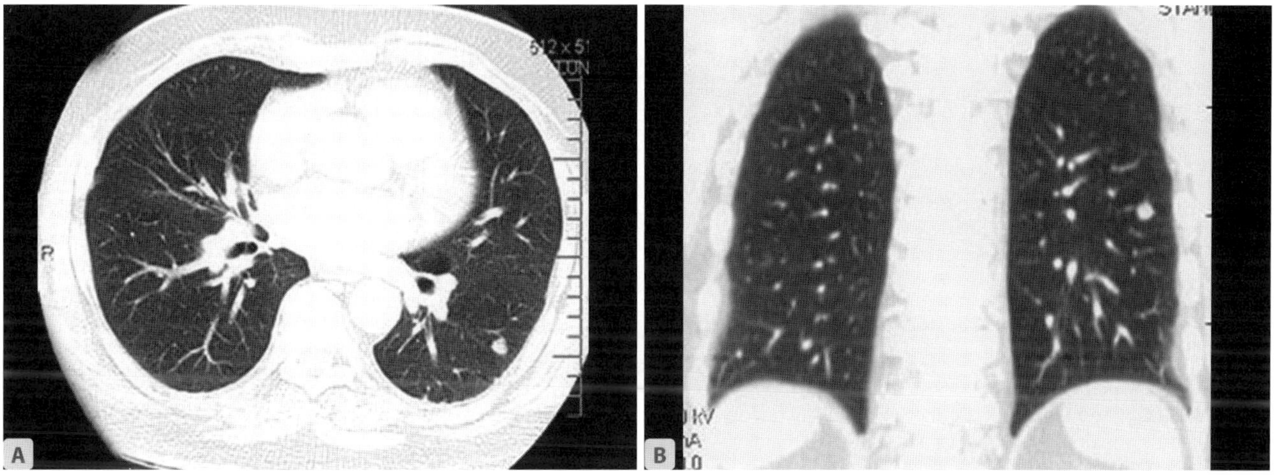

FIGS. 4A AND B: Chest CT scans showing a smooth, sharply marginated, rounded nodule in the left lower lobe with no evidence of calcification/ cavitation. The small size of the lesion (<1 cm) makes malignancy less likely—Benign SPN/granuloma.

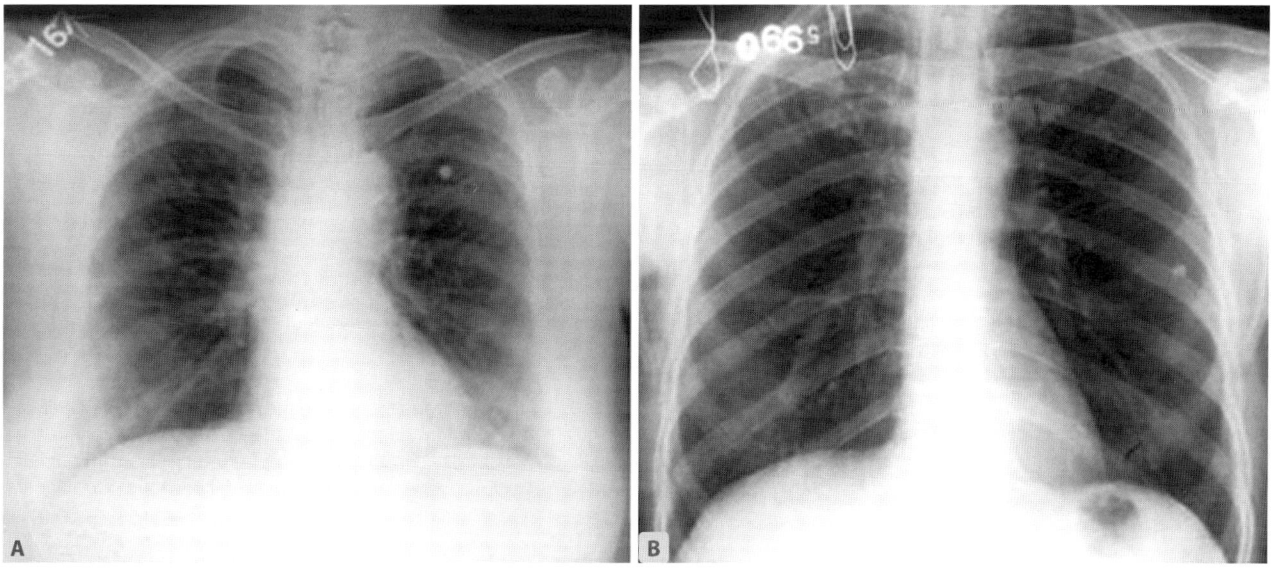

FIGS. 5A AND B: Chest radiographs in two cases showing well-defined nodules <1 cm clearly seen on plain radiographs due to being calcified—Benign SPNs/calcified granulomas.

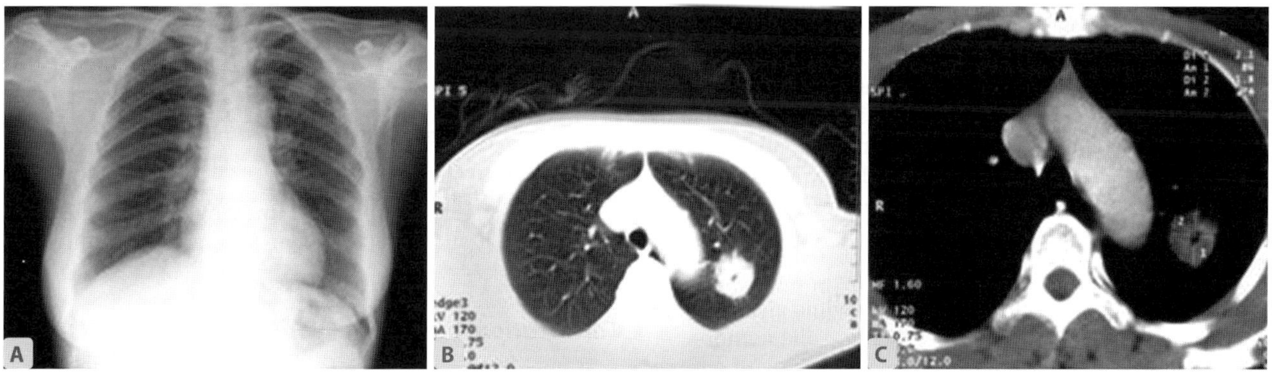

FIGS. 6A TO C: Chest radiograph (A) showing a nodule in the left upper lobe. The lesion is classified as a nodule because it is relatively well-defined, surrounded by lung, roughly spherical in shape and less than 3 cm in size. CT scan (B) showing the edge of the nodule to be ill-defined and lobulated with pleural tails extending to the pleural surface. The lesion measures 2.3 x 1.8 cm in size and shows evidence of central cavitation (C). The larger the nodule (>2 cm) the more likely it is malignant—Adenocarcinoma lung.

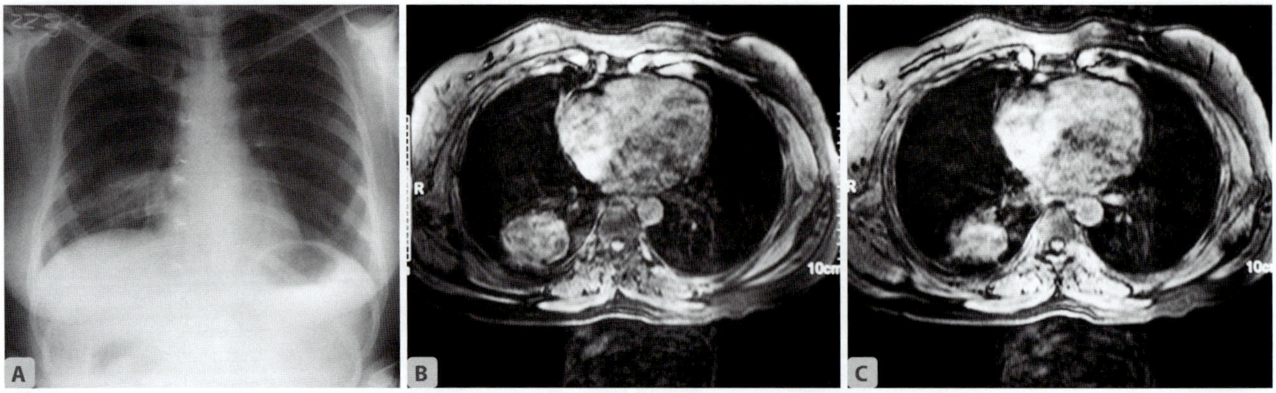

FIGS. 7A TO C: Chest radiograph (A) showing a solitary nodule in the right lower lobe. MR images in the same case (B and C) showing the large nodule in the right lung, it has irregular and spiculated margins—Adenocarcinoma manifesting as a peripheral SPN.

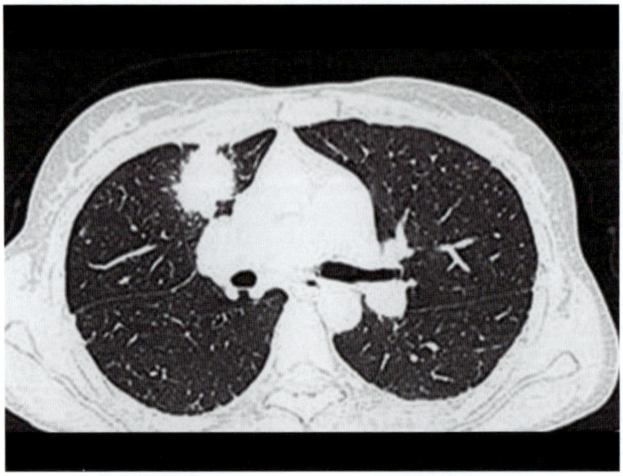

FIG. 8: CT scan showing a nodule in the right upper lobe. The nodule shows lobulations and evidence of notching. Edge irregularity and spiculation is clearly seen.

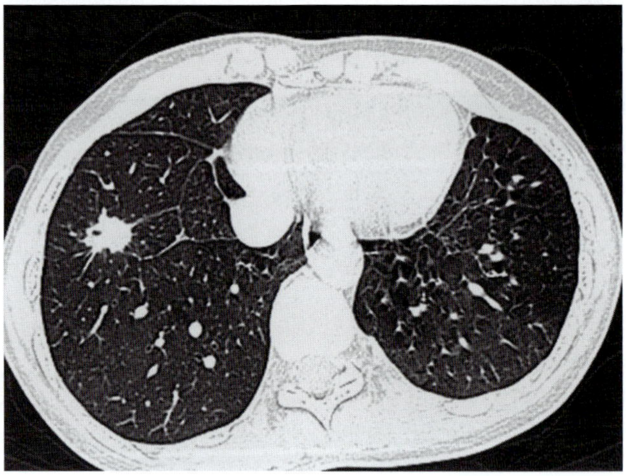

FIG. 9: CT chest showing a nodule in the right upper lobe with irregular, spiculated margins termed the "sunburst appearance" or corona radiata. Multiple pleural tails are seen extending from the mass to the pleural surface. A small eccentric cavitation is noted—Bronchogenic carcinoma.

"corona maligna" or the "sunburst appearance" **(Fig. 9)**.[16-18] In patients with adenocarcinoma and adenocarcinoma in situ (bronchioloalveolar carcinoma) it reflects the presence of fibrosis surrounding the tumor.[19] The fibrosis usually reflects a desmoplastic reaction and not a pre-existing lung fibrosis. Carcinoma can show the presence of a "pleural tail" or a "pleural tag" in which a thin linear opacity is seen extending from the edge of the lung nodule to the pleural surface. The presence of spiculation is more indicative of the lesion being malignant rather than pleural tail as pleural tail may also be seen with lesions which are benign such as granulomatous disease like tuberculosis.[20,21]

Presence of a Halo

Ground-glass opacity surrounding the nodule gives a "halo sign" to the nodule.[22] This peripheral non-solid component surrounding a nodule should not be confused with corona radiata.

Halo sign is seen in[23]:

- Invasive aspergillosis
- Adenocarcinoma
- Adenocarcinoma in situ (formerly Bronchioloalveolar carcinoma)
- Pulmonary hemorrhage

In lesions such as aspergillosis, the halo sign represents hemorrhage, while in malignancies it represents the lepidic spread of tumor.

INTERNAL CHARACTERISTICS

Calcification

Calcification is an important imaging feature that can be used to distinguish between benign and malignant SPNs.

Calcification in a Benign Nodule (Figs. 10A to D)

- Concentric rings of calcification (target calcification)
- Conglomerate foci of calcification involving a large part of the nodule (popcorn calcification)
- Homogeneous calcification/uniform calcification
- Dense central (bull's eye) calcification.

When any of these patterns is seen, the probability of the lesion being benign is almost 100%[24] **(Figs. 11A and B)**. Popcorn calcification is virtually diagnostic of cartilage containing tumors such as hamartomas **(Figs. 12A to C)**. Concentric (laminated) and uniform calcifications are suggestive of a calcified tuberculous or fungal granuloma.

Indeterminate Calcification

Eccentric calcification may be seen in a benign lesion which gets calcified in an eccentric fashion or when a benign calcified lesion is engulfed by a malignant lesion. Stippled/ punctate calcification may be seen in both benign and malignant lesions and is thus classified as indeterminate.[25]

Calcification in a Malignant Nodule

A malignant nodule may show calcification which is diffuse and amorphous or psammomatous (in case of metastasis from mucin secreting tumors from the colon or ovary) or dystrophic (in areas of tumor necrosis).[25,26] Centrally located calcification in a spiculated SPN also suggests malignancy.[27]

Fat

The presence of fat (-40 to -120 HU) within a lesion is virtually diagnostic of a hamartoma **(Fig. 13)**. Other lesions that may show fat include lipoid pneumonia, lipoma and metastatic liposarcoma.[28]

Cavitation

Both benign and malignant SPNs can cavitate. A thick irregular cavity with wall thickness greater than 16 mm is likely to be malignant. About 95% of the nodules with wall thickness less than 5 mm are benign.[29] About 75% of the cavities with wall thickness 5–15 mm are benign. Cavitation usually occurs in squamous cell carcinoma, large cell carcinoma and adenocarcinoma while small cell cancers rarely show cavitation.

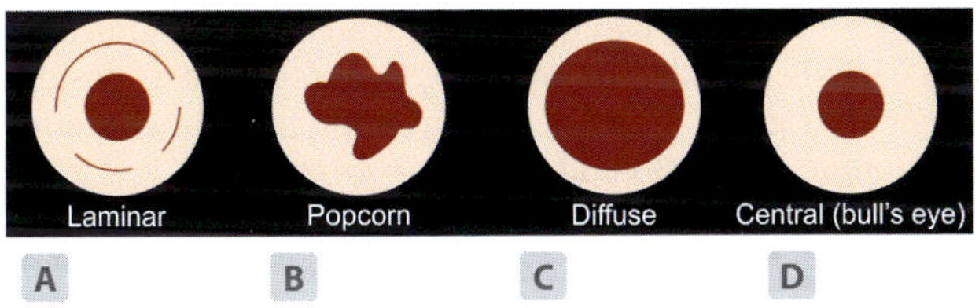

FIGS. 10A TO D: Calcification in benign module.

Air Bronchiolograms and Pseudocavitation

Air bronchiologram or bubble like lucencies or pseudocavitation may simulate cavities and are more commonly seen in malignant nodules (29%) than in benign nodules (6%).[30-32] Pseudocavitation results from sparing of alveoli and bronchi by tumor infiltration in malignant lesions.

Air Crescent Sign

An "air crescent" or "air meniscus" sign results from a peripheral halo of air between the intracavitatory mass and the cavity wall **(Figs. 14A and B)**. The commonest cause is a fungal ball, i.e. aspergilloma/mycetoma. Other causes include blood clot in a cavity, cavitatory carcinoma, complicated hydatid disease, Rasmussen's aneurysm, mucous plug in bronchiectasis and pulmonary gangrene.

Air-fluid Level

Presence of an air-fluid level within a lesion favours benignity such as a lung abscess or an infected cyst **(Figs. 15A to C)**. Intracavitatory hemorrhage or superinfection may rarely give rise to an air fluid level in cavitatory carcinoma.

OTHER CHARACTERISTICS OF SPN

Satellite Nodules

The presence of small nodules adjacent to a large nodule or mass favors a benign lesion such as tuberculosis and sarcoidosis. A cluster of small nodules seen within a segment or subsegment of the lung, 3–15 mm in diameter usually indicates a granulomatous process **(Figs. 16A and B)**. In sarcoidosis, the term "galaxy-sign" refers to the presence of multiple satellite nodules.

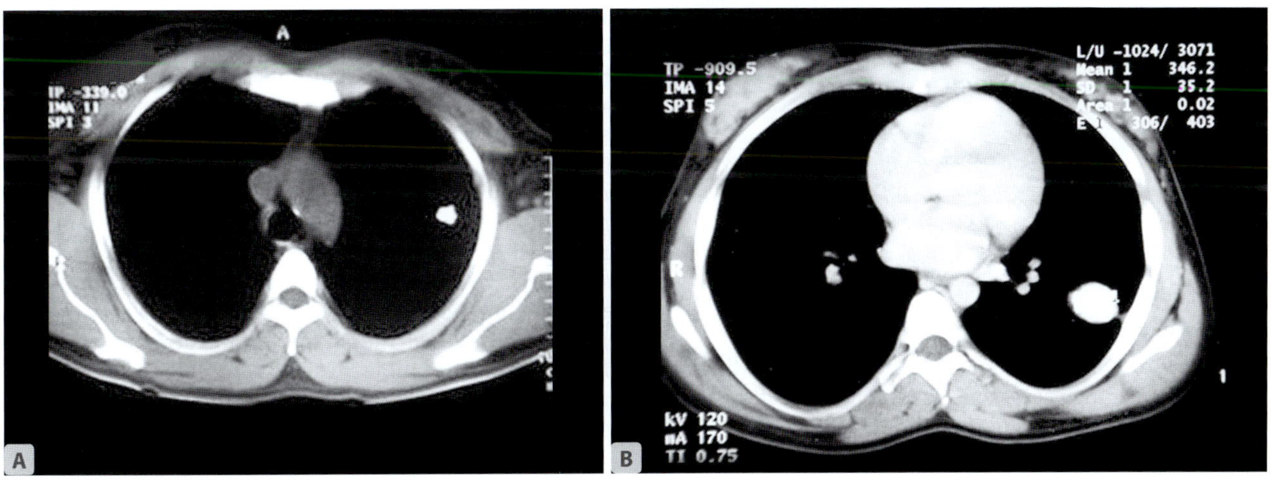

FIGS. 11A AND B: CT scans showing uniform homogeneous calcification in two cases of tuberculomas.

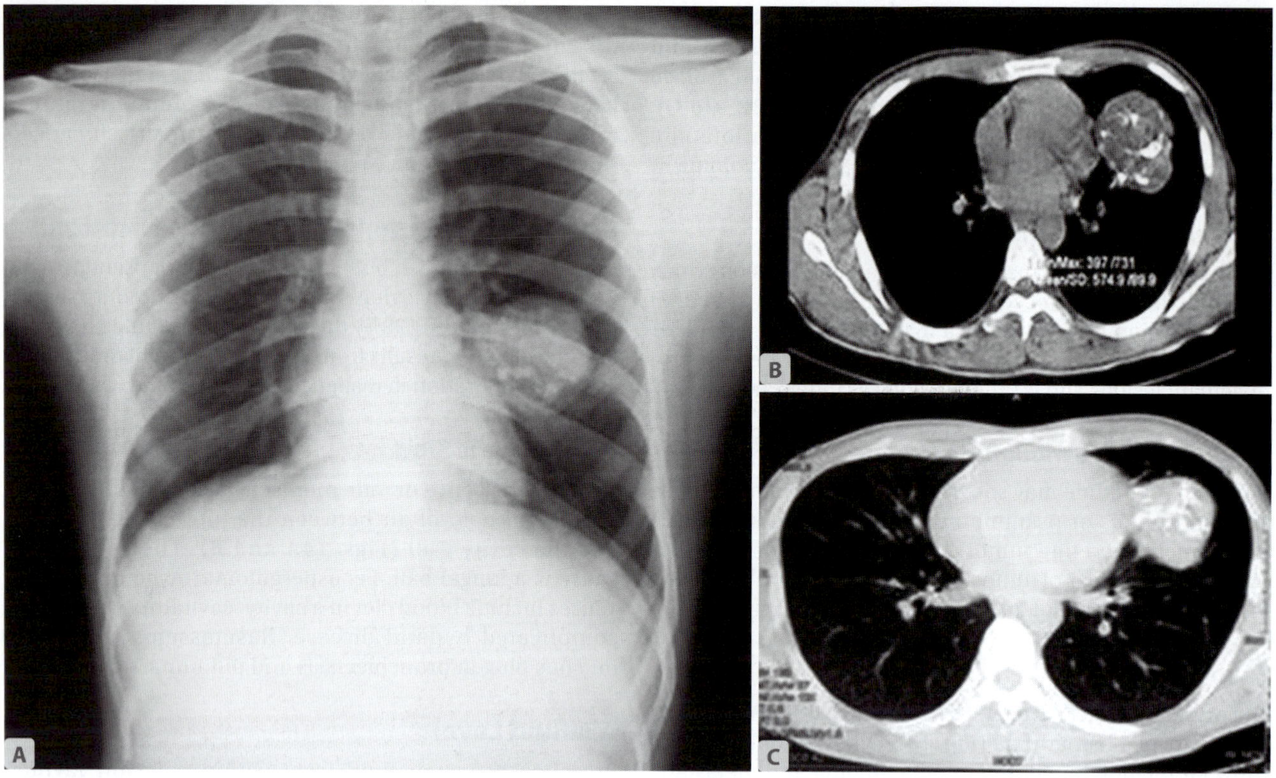

FIGS. 12A TO C: Chest radiograph (A) showing a large solitary nodule in the left lung with dense nodular foci of calcification within s/o characteristic popcorn calcification/central cartilage calcification. Noncontrast CT scan mediastinal window (B) showing a 3 x 3 cm nodule containing overlapping, randomly distributed small rings of calcification or the popcorn calcification and lung parenchymal window settings (C) reveal the nodule to be round in shape and sharply marginated—Pulmonary hamartoma.

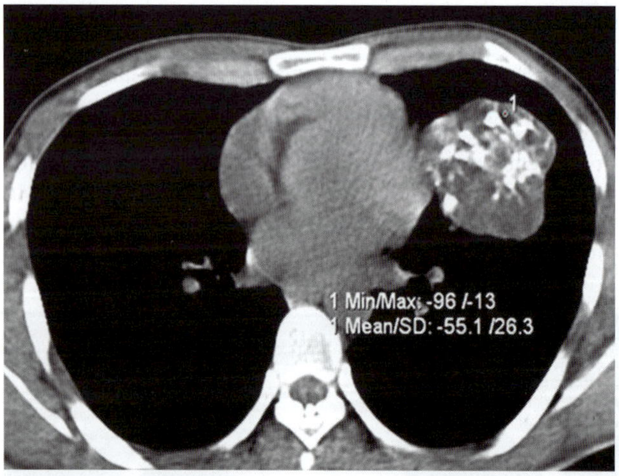

FIG. 13: Noncontrast CT scan showing foci of fat or negative attenuation (–50 to –100 HU) within the nodule in the left lung consistent with pulmonary hamartoma.

Feeding Vessel Sign

This refers to a small pulmonary artery directly leading to a nodule. A "feeding vessel sign" is seen in metastasis, septic emboli, arteriovenous fistula or infarct **(Fig. 17)**.[33,34]

Positive Bronchus Sign

When a bronchial carcinoma infiltrates around but does not occlude an adjacent bronchus it gives rise to a "positive bronchus sign".[35] This is seen as a patent bronchus entering the nodule **(Figs. 18A and B)**.

NODULE ATTENUATION

CT density of the nodule has been used to characterize nodules as benign or malignant based on the density measurement. Siegelman and co-workers suggested that a CT number above 164 HU represents benignity. Proto and Thomas gave a different cut off value of 200 HU above which the lesions could be diagnosed as benign.[36] The limitation of using cut-off value is that 6–7% of bronchial carcinomas may contain some type of calcification giving high value of CT density.[37] CT densitometry is not recommended for nodules greater than 3 cm, those with irregular or spiculated borders or those showing a growth rate compatible with bronchial carcinoma. To overcome these problems, Zerhouni used a reference phantom to provide a standard for density. The phantom simulated the shape, dimensions and density of the thorax at multiple levels to resemble the conditions under which SPN was measured.[38] If more than 10% of the voxels in the patient's nodule were higher in density than in

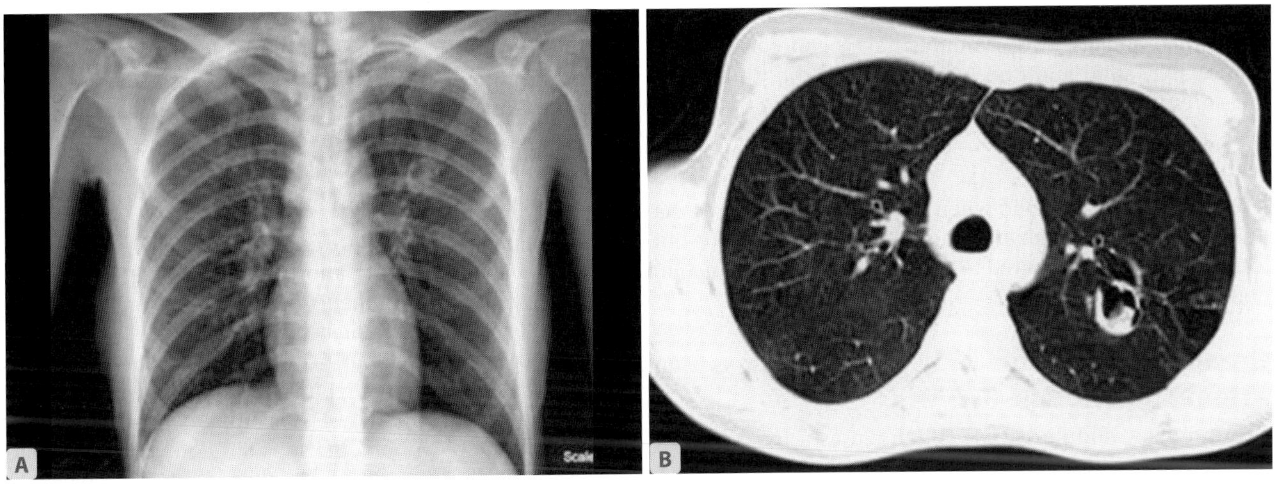

FIGS. 14A AND B: Chest radiograph (A) showing a small solitary lesion in the left upper lobe with a crescent of air between the intracavitatory mass and the cavity wall giving rise to the "air crescent" or air meniscus sign. CT scan (B) showing the same—Aspergilloma/mycetoma.

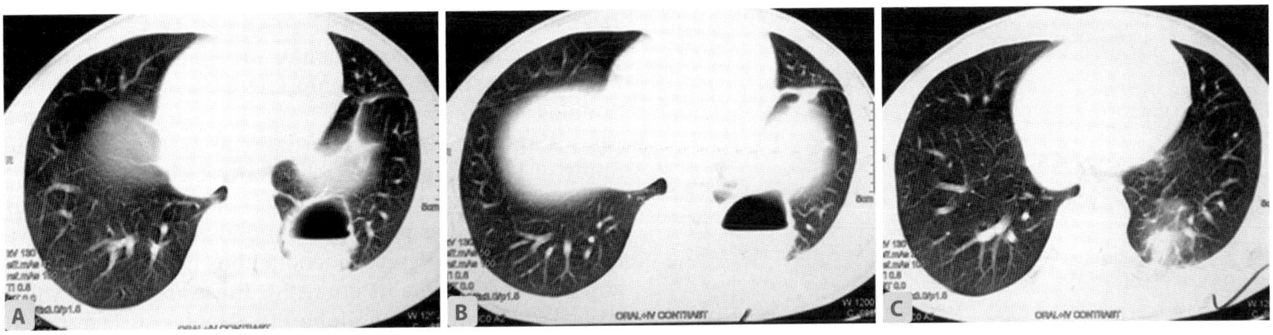

FIGS. 15A TO C: CT scans in a case showing a well-defined cavity with an air-fluid level with wall thickness <5 mm and surrounding consolidation—Lung abscess.

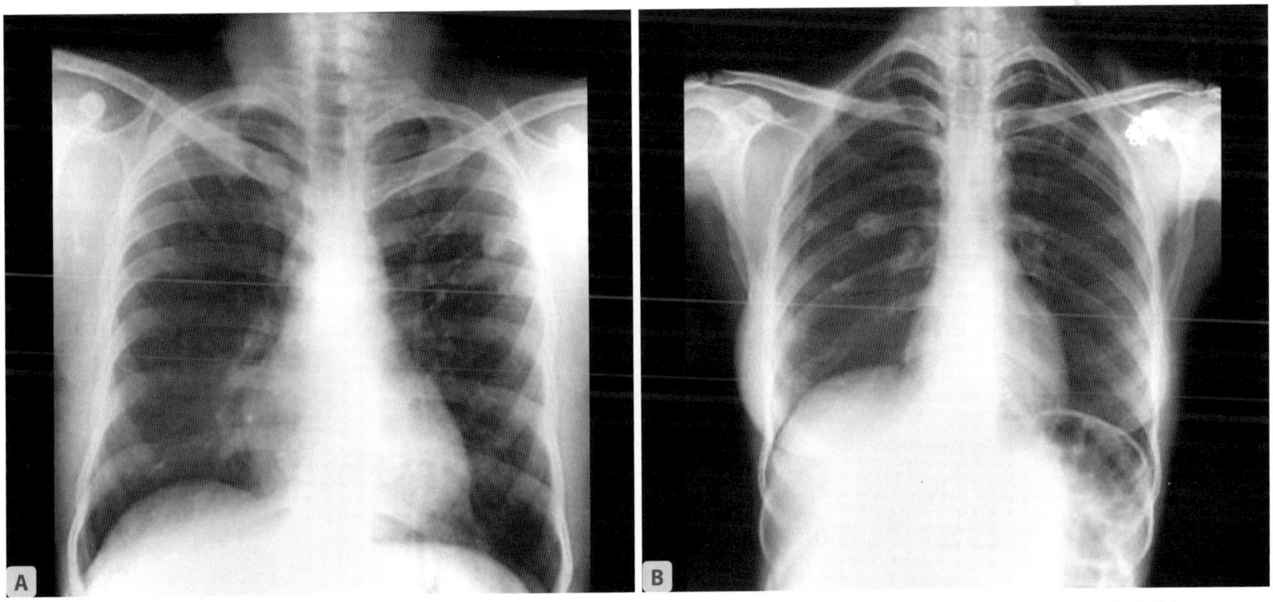

FIGS. 16A AND B: Chest radiograph in two cases showing a calcified tuberculoma with multiple small nodules adjacent to it in the left lung in one case (A) and the right lung in the other (B)—Satellite nodules predicting a benign disease.

the phantom nodule, the lesion was considered to be above the critical density level. Nodules have been classified as solid, partly solid and non-solid based on the CT density measurements.[39]

Solid Nodule

A lesion is said to be solid when it completely obscures the underlying lung parenchyma. This is the commonest type but less malignant as compared to the partly solid and non-solid nodules.[40,41]

Ground-glass Nodule (GGN)/Ground-glass Attenuation Nodule (GGAN)

Ground-glass nodule (GGN) is defined as a focal area of increased lung attenuation through which the pulmonary vessels and bronchial structures, that is, the lung parenchyma structures can be observed.[42] Contiguous thin CT sections (1 mm) should be performed to establish lesions as true GGNs whenever possible to avoid the pitfall of interpreting them as solid or subsolid nodules.[43] Use of thick sections precludes accurate nodule characterization due to volume averaging.

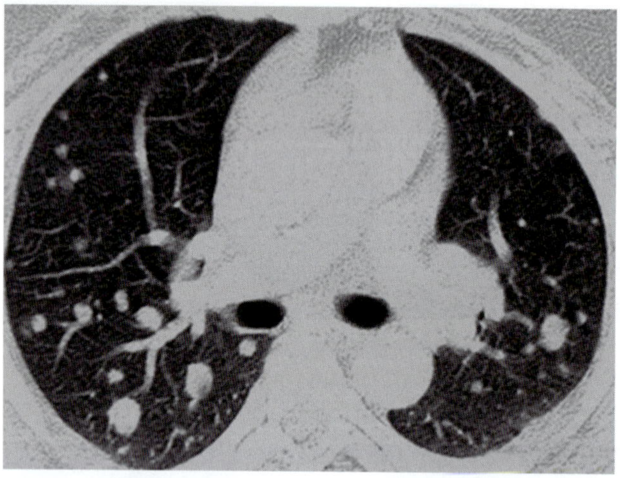

FIG. 17: CT scan in a case of hematogenous pulmonary metastases showing small pulmonary arteries directly feeding the nodules—"Feeding vessel sign".

Subsolid Nodules (SSNs)

This term includes both pure and part solid GGNs **(Figs. 19A and B)**. It is important to know the percentage of ground-glass versus solid components of subsolid lesions as greater the solid component, greater the chance of the lesion being an invasive adenocarcinoma with a poorer prognosis.

The incidence of malignancy in subsolid nodules has been estimated to be about 34% in comparison to the 7% seen in solid nodules.[44] Among the subsolid nodules, partly solid nodules have the highest rate of malignancy (63%) while pure ground-glass nodules have an incidence of 18%.[44]

Association of Nodule Attenuation with Adenocarcinoma

Adenocarcinoma which accounts for about 50% of all lung cancers presents more commonly as a solitary subsolid nodule (SSN) than the other histologic types of carcinoma. According to the IASLC (International Association for the Study of Lung Cancer), ATS (American Thoracic Society) and European Respiratory Society (ERS), adenocarcinomas can be classified as preinvasive and invasive.[45] Preinvasive lesions comprise atypical adenomatous hyperplasia (AAH) and adenocarcinoma in situ (AIS). These are lesions which typically exhibit growth along the alveolar surface called lepidic growth.[46] Atypical adenomatous hyperplasia (AAH) is a lesion which is purely ground-glass in attenuation and usually less than 1 cm in size.[47] Adenocarcinoma in situ (AIS) is a lesion with ground-glass attenuation and less than 3 cm in size. The invasive lesions include minimally invasive carcinoma (MIC) and invasive adenocarcinoma. Minimally invasive carcinoma (MIC) is defined as a lesion that shows a predominant lepidic growth with no necrosis, no lymphatic,

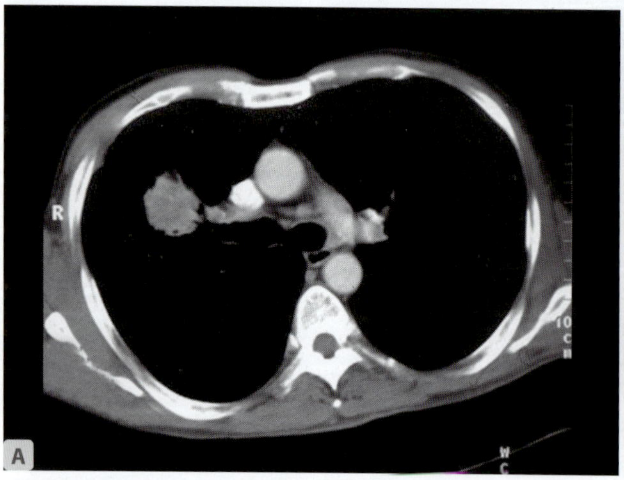

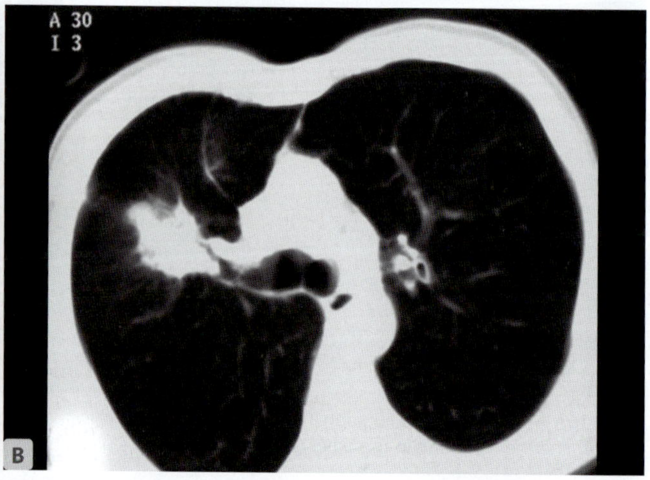

FIGS. 18A AND B: CT scans of the chest showing a pulmonary lesion abutting and narrowing the right upper lobe bronchus without completely occluding it. The positive bronchus sign in bronchogenic carcinoma.

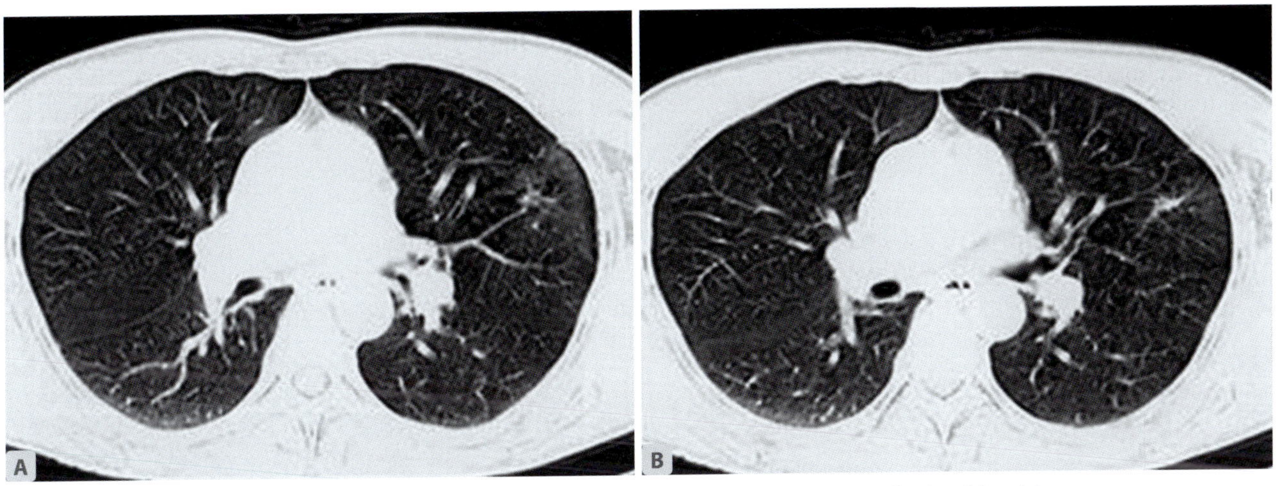

FIGS. 19A AND B: CT scans show an ill-defined central nodule along with ground-glass attenuation—Partly solid nodule.

TABLE 2: Correlation of the histological patterns with CT features of subsolid nodules.[45,46]

2011 IASLC, ATS and ERS classification	CT features
• Atypical adenomatous hyperplasia (AAH) • Adenocarcinoma in situ (AIS)	• GGAN • GGAN with a possible solid component
• Minimally invasive adenocarcinoma (MIA) • Lepidic predominant adenocarcinoma • Invasive adenocarcinoma	• GGAN, partly solid nodule • Partly solid nodule, solid nodule • Partly solid nodule with a solid component, solid nodule

vascular or pleural invasion, is less than 3 cm in size with an invasive component not more than 5 mm in any location.[45,46] MIA may be seen as ground-glass attenuation(GGAN) or partly solid nodule (PSN) on CT.[48] Classification of invasive adenocarcinoma as having a lepidic, acinar, papillary, micropapillary or solid pattern is based on the histological features. The MIA, AIS and lepidic forms may have both mucinous and non-mucinous forms **(Table 2)**. The term bronchioloalveolar carcinoma is now an obsolete term and should be called adenocarcinoma *in situ*.[49,50]

The solid component of a SSN is important as it predicts the prognosis of the patient, the solid component representing the invasive foci of adenocarcinoma. A direct correlation has been reported between presence of solid component, the size of the solid component and increasing attenuation with the invasiveness or aggressiveness of a subsolid nodule.[49,50] The higher the attenuation value of the subsolid nodule, the greater is the degree of invasion.

ASSESSMENT OF MALIGNANT POTENTIAL OF A SPN

Nodule Growth

An important criterion to differentiate between benign and malignant nodules is nodule growth. Previously, assessment of the size was done by measuring the maximum dimensions on posteroanterior and lateral radiography and also by matching circular standards printed on transparency with that of the nodule margin. However, such measurements are inaccurate. Nodule growth is also assessed by a volume doubling time (VDT) defined as the time in which the volume of a nodule becomes double. As the most common shape is spherical, the volume is calculated using the equation $4\pi r$.[3] A 26% increase in diameter is taken as a doubling in volume based on

$$VDT = [t \times \log 2]/\log (V_t/V_o)$$

Where V_o is the initial volume and V_t is the volume at time t.[51]

This formula is based on an exponential model of nodule growth, i.e. a 5 mm nodule will reach a diameter of 20.3 mm in 12 months if the doubling time (DT) is 60 days but will reach a diameter of only 7.1 mm in 12 months, if the doubling time is 240 days. Also the 26% increase in axial diameter taken as the volume doubling time is difficult to assess in case of nodules less than or equal to 5 mm in size because 5 mm nodule which doubles its volume increases in diameter by 1.25 mm only.[52] It has been seen that two-dimensional measurements obtained with electronic calipers are unreliable as compared to the three-dimensional measurements.

The volume doubling time (VDT) for malignant SPNs is rarely less than a month or more than a year (range 20–400 days).[53] Nodules with a doubling time less than 20 days and more than 400 days are considered benign. Also stability of nodule size over 2 years (730 days) has been considered to suggest benignity.[54] The radiologic pathologic correlation of partly solid and pure ground-glass attenuation nodule with the histologic spectrum of adenocarcinoma has been described.[55] It has been seen that small purely ground-glass

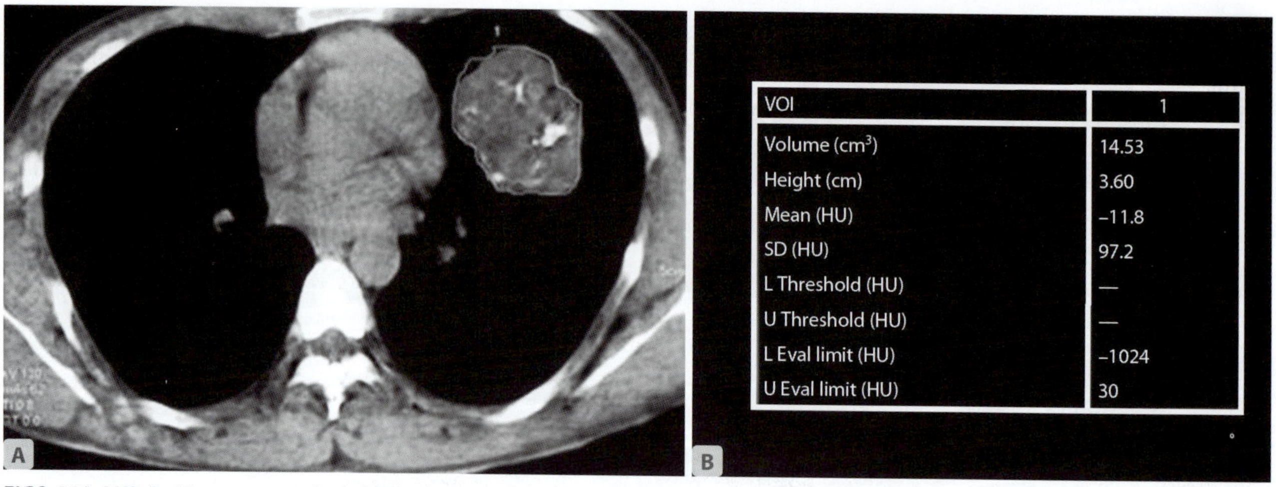

FIGS. 20A AND B: Measurement of volume in a case of pulmonary hamartoma. The volume of the nodule is measured on each axial section and then summed to obtain the total nodule volume (B).

opacity (nonsolid) nodules with malignant histologic features may have a mean volume DT of about 2 years while it is about 6 months for the solid cancers.[56] Subsolid nodules that have a higher likelihood of malignancy have a volume doubling time between the two extremes. Carcinoids and adenocarcinomas in situ may remain stable for more than two years. Therefore, the dictum that 2 year stability indicates a benign process should be used with caution.[57] Longer follow up is advisable for ground-glass nodules which have a longer doubling time.

Three-dimensional Volume Quantification

Three dimensional volume quantification utilizes the entire CT data to calculate nodule volume **(Figs. 20A and B)**.[58] Volume quantification method is able to detect smaller differences in nodule size than the two dimensional method. In order to separate/segment out the nodules from the lung parenchyma, threshold method is used, which takes into account the voxel attenuation above and below a particular threshold as nodule or parenchyma.[58,59] It is important to include the ground-glass component of a subsolid nodule in volume determination as ground-glass component has a high incidence of malignancy.[60] In the case of subsolid nodules, growth may occur in the form of an increase in size, an increase in attenuation, appearance of a solid component or increase in the size of the solid component. For optimal CT evaluation of subsolid pulmonary nodules, it is essential to obtain thin section CT.[61] Measurement of attenuation values on serial CT examinations is less variable than measurements of volume and diameter.[62] For these nodules, an increase in mass is calculated which is the product of mean volume and attenuation.

Computer-aided Diagnosis

The volume and morphology of nodules can be assessed by computer-aided diagnosis (CAD) that can act as a second reader. Identification of the nodule, size of the nodule, morphology and internal architecture of the nodule can all be studied with CAD. Differentiation of nodules with uniform attenuation from those with inhomogeneous attenuation called texture analysis can be undertaken with the help of computer-aided technique.[63] An association between nodule characteristics and rate of malignancy is also facilitated through this technique.

Image Registration

The follow up of the pulmonary nodules emphasizes the need for image registration techniques. Image registration entails superimposing image data or determining the spatial alignment between different images from the same modality at different points in times (intra-modality registration) or between different imaging modalities, such as CT, MR PET (intermodality registration). To correlate a nodule accurately on CT study with its matching counterpart on a subsequent CT, global registration of the thorax and the local registration of nodules and smaller structures need to be performed. An interactive system enables easy identification of corresponding structures on initial and subsequent CT studies, recording of nodules and their characteristics including volume and storage of image results for future analysis and documentation.[64]

Nodule Enhancement

Enhancement of the nodule can be assessed on CT to differentiate between benign and malignant solid SPNs.[65] Enhancement pattern can be studied by administration of iodinated contrast material intravenously (300 mg/mL at 2 mL/sec) with a pressure injector. The protocol consists of 3 mm images of the nodule at 1, 2, 3 and 4 minutes after contrast injection.[66,67] Enhancement value is obtained by subtraction of the precontrast value from the peak enhancement. Measurements should be done on mediastinal window and the region of interest (ROI) should be so placed as to cover 70% of the diameter of the nodule **(Figs. 21A to C)**. A cut-off value of 15 HU for enhancement has been found to have a sensitivity of 98% and specificity of 58% for benignity with benign lesions showing enhancement

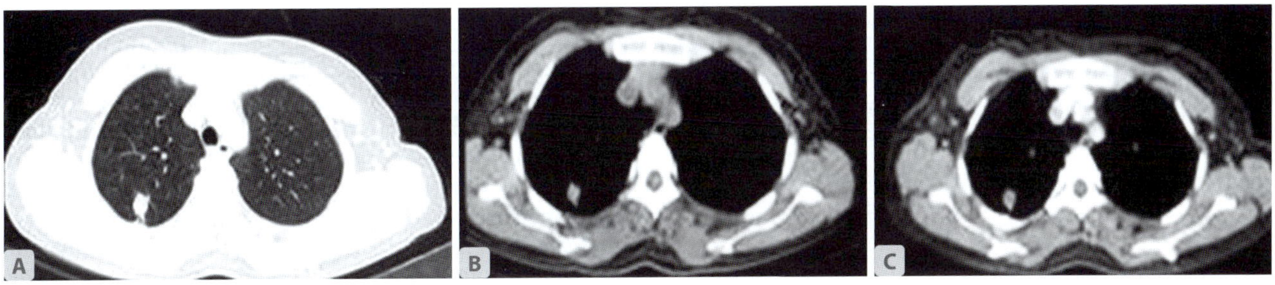

FIGS. 21A TO C: Lung parenchymal window settings on chest CT (A) showing a small (<1 cm) smooth rounded lesion with a small pleural tail in the right upper lobe. Noncontrast and contrast-enhanced scans with mediastinal window settings (B and C) showing no enhancement of the lesion on the postcontrast scans—Benign lesion/tuberculoma.

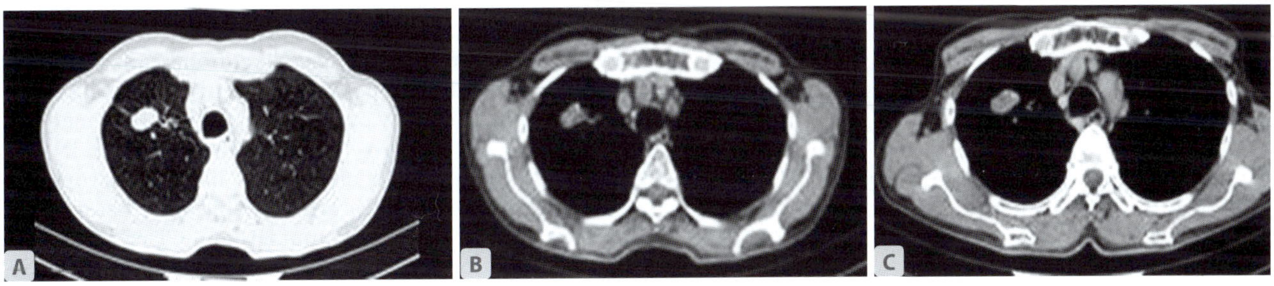

FIGS. 22A TO C: Lung parenchymal window settings (A) showing a small (1 cm) solitary lesion in the right upper lobe. The lesion is irregularly marginated with spiculated contour and multiple pleural tails. Noncontrast and contrast-enhanced scans with mediastinal window settings (B and C) reveal significant enhancement >15 HU on the postcontrast scans—Malignant lesion.

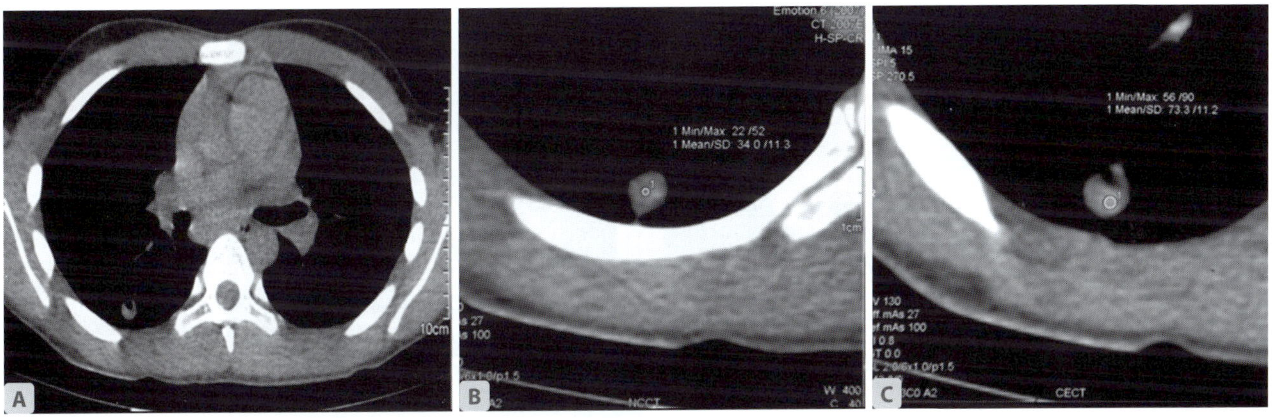

FIGS. 23A TO C: (A) CT scan image showing a lesion <1 cm in size in the right lower lobe with an eccentric cavitation. Pre- (B) and postcontrast (C) images reveal an enhancement of 34 HU (56-22 HU) suggestive of a malignant nodule.

<15 HU.[68] An enhancement of more than 20 HU is indicative of tumor neovascularity or malignancy **(Figs. 22A to C)**. The limitation of this technique includes its use in lesions smaller than 2 cm as larger lesions would have areas of necrosis and placement of cursor would be a problem. This technique is more applicable for lesions which are relatively spherical in shape and relatively homogeneous in attenuation with no large areas of necrosis, fat, calcification or cavitation **(Figs. 23A to C)**. Also, benign vascular tumors and granulomas show enhancement leading to a considerable overlap.[69] An analysis of combined wash-in and wash-out characteristics (studied at 15 minute delay) gives a more precise evaluation of the nodule enhancement.

For benign nodules:
- Wash in <25 HU
- Wash in ≥25 HU with a washout ≥31 HU
- Wash in ≥25 HU and a persistent enhancement without a washout.

For malignant nodules:[70]
- Wash in ≥25 HU
- Washout of 5–31 HU (not more than 31 HU).

The arterial supply of a nodule is via the bronchial arteries while the washout is via the bronchial veins. In the case of malignancy, a retarded flow in the intravascular and interstitial space accounts for contrast retention.[71] In the case of benign nodules, this washout takes place through relatively straight vessels and active lymphatic flow resulting in a significant washout. A persistent enhancement when seen in a benign nodule occurs due to the presence of fibrosis in the nodule, the fibrotic portion of the nodule retaining contrast for a long time without washout.

TABLE 3: LRs for selected radiologic features of nodules and patient characteristics.[76-78]

Feature or characteristic	LR
Spiculated margin	5.54
>3 cm	5.23
>70 years	4.16
Malignant growth rate	3.40
Smoker	2.27
Upper lobe location	1.22
<1 cm	0.52
Smooth margins	0.30
30–39 years	0.24
Never smoked	0.19
20–29 years	0.05
Benign calcification	0.01
Benign growth rate	0.01

Bayesian Analysis

The risk factor of the patients should be evaluated when a SPN is considered to be indeterminate in the initial examination. Age is an important factor in the evaluation with lung cancer being uncommon in patients younger than 40 years and being rare in those below 35 years of age (<1% of all cases).[72] The risk of developing cancer in male smokers is about 10 times than in non-smokers and the risk is related to the degree and duration of cigarette smoking.[73,74]A history of cancer in first degree relative, occupational exposure, exposure to asbestos, radon and uranium are other risk factors for the development of lung carcinoma.[75]

Bayesian analysis can be useful in the evaluation of these indeterminate solitary pulmonary nodules by allowing more precise determination of the probability of malignancy (pCa). Bayesian analysis uses likelihood ratio (LRs) for numerous radiological findings and clinical features associated with solitary pulmonary nodules to estimate pCa **(Table 3)**.

In a new Bayesian model that has been proposed, certain morphological features like edge have been added, criteria such as VDT, minimum HU and CT enhancement have been introduced as predictive features. The new model is an important update on Bayesian analysis and allows for a better differentiation between benign and malignant entities. [79]

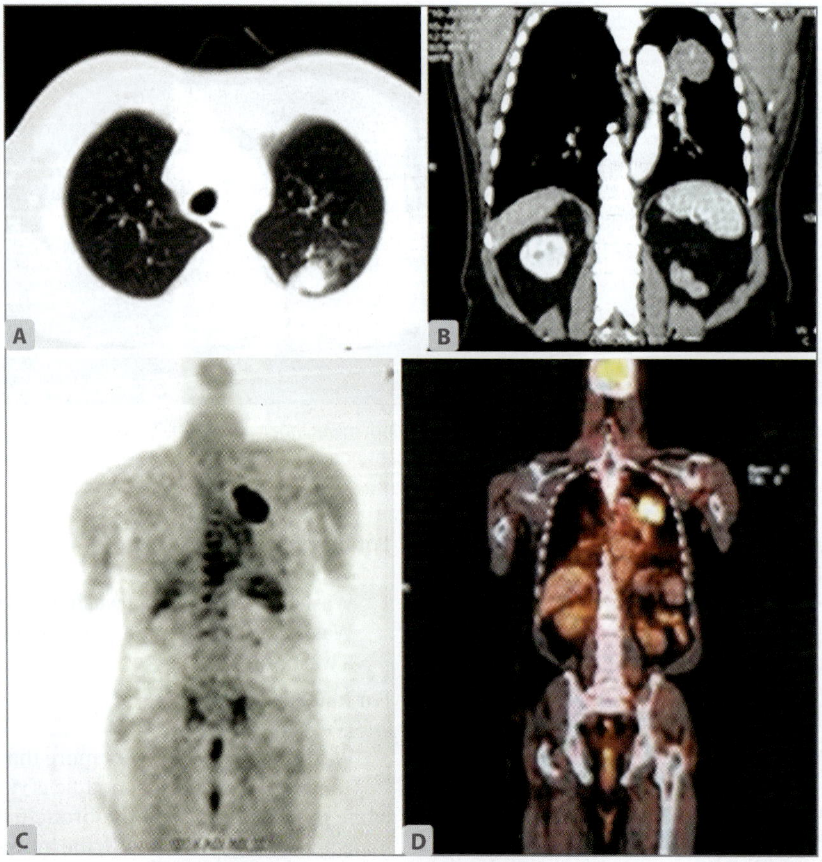

FIGS. 24A TO D: CT chest axial and MPR images (A and B) showing an irregularly marginated lesion with surrounding halo in the left upper lobe. FDG PET scans (C and D) in the patient showing an increased uptake and accumulation of FDG in the nodule—malignant lesion/bronchogenic carcinoma.

Fluorodeoxyglucose Positron Emission Tomography

Nodule metabolism can be evaluated by functional imaging with fluorine 18 (^{18}F)- labelled fluorodeoxyglucose (FDG) positron emission tomography (PET). The technique is a measure of glucose metabolism and aids in the differentiation of benign and malignant nodules[80] **(Figs. 24A to D)**. A standardized uptake value (SUV) of more than 2.5 is usually seen in malignancy while a value less than 2.5 is seen in benign lesions. PET has a sensitivity and specificity of about 90% for detecting malignant nodules which are larger than 10 mm in diameter, but this high sensitivity and specificity is applicable to solid nodules. In the case of partly solid nodule (PSN) and ground-glass attenuation nodule (GGAN) FDG uptake cannot be used to reliably distinguish between benign and malignant lesions. PET has been found to have a sensitivity as low as 10% and specificity of about 20% for evaluating ground-glass opacities.[81] Also, FDG PET can give false negative results in the case of carcinoid tumors, mucinous adenocarcinomas and adenocarcinomas in situ and false positive results in the case of inflammation and infection.[82,83] There may be a respiratory mismatch between CT and PET images leading to an underestimation of the SUV with resultant false negative result. It has been suggested that a respiratory averaged CT, i.e. CT cine images obtained over different portions of the respiratory cycle rather than a mid-expiratory CT improves SUV quantification.

Transthoracic Needle Aspiration Biopsy (TNAB)

For a SPN with a high clinical suspicion of malignancy, surgical resection is the best option if the lesion is operable as needle biopsy does not alter management. If the biopsy result is positive, resection has to be done, a negative result does not exclude malignancy and has to be followed by resection if there is a high clinical suspicion of malignancy as the sensitivity of this technique is about 60% for lesions less than 2 cm in diameter **(Figs. 25A to D)**. The diagnostic yield further falls to 51% for GGO dominant lesions.[84] Thus, needle biopsy is usually indicated for inoperable SPN to confirm the histology. As compared to bronchoscopy, the complication rate of TNAB is high. Complications include pneumothorax and hemorrhage seen in about 5–30% of cases.[85]

Fiberoptic Bronchoscopy

Fiberoptic bronchoscopy (FOB) with transbronchial biopsy and washing has a limited role in evaluating SPN. Although transbronchial biopsy is accurate for assessing endobronchial lesions, the yield for peripheral nodules is less than 60 percent and is only 25 to 30 percent for a SPN smaller than 2 cm. The sensitivity of FOB is best when a bronchus leads directly to or is seen within the SPN (the positive bronchus sign).[35]

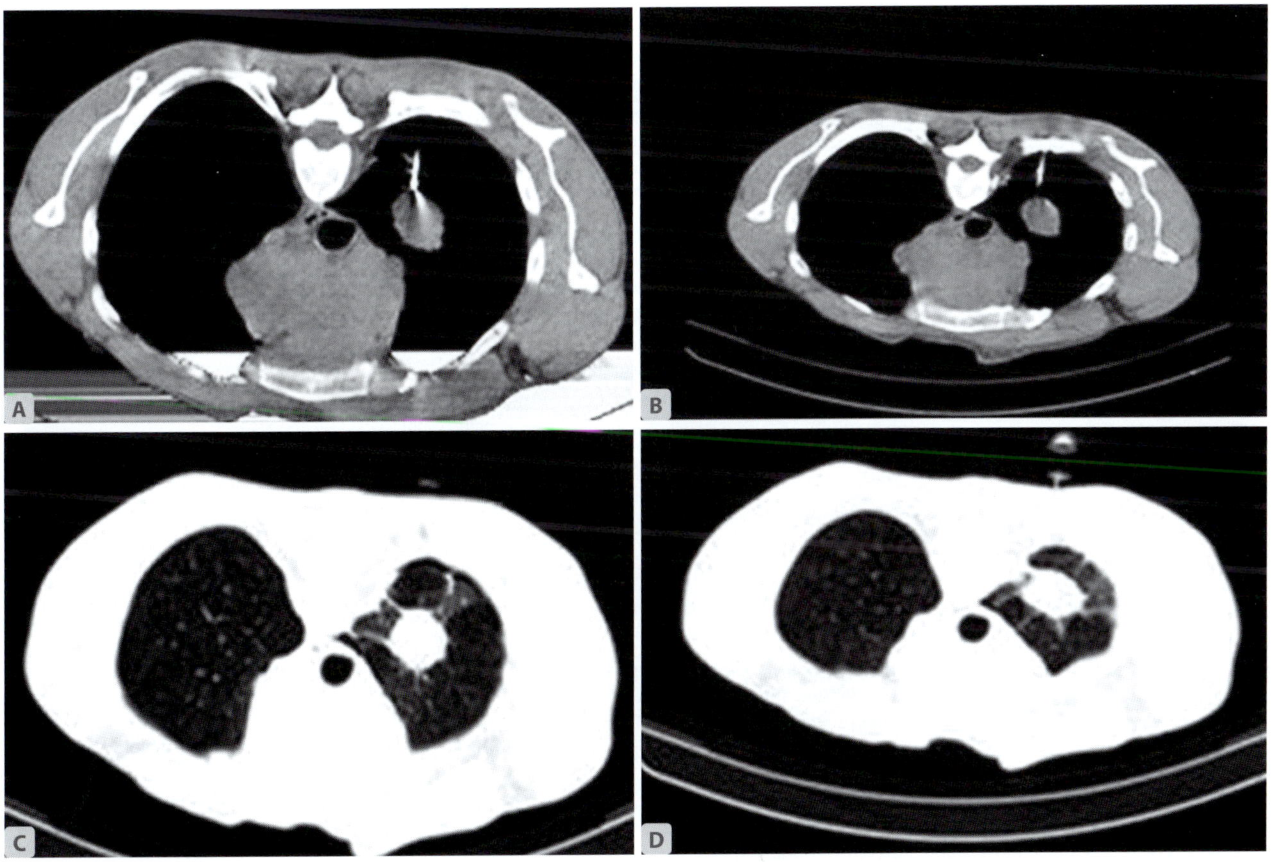

FIGS. 25A TO D: Transthoracic needle aspiration in a case of a nodule in the right lung with needle in situ (A and B) in prone position. The nodule is irregularly marginated with evidence of corona radiata and multiple pleural tails (C and D)—Bronchogenic carcinoma.

NEWER IMAGING TECHNIQUES FOR THE EVALUATION OF SPN

Dynamic MR Imaging

Blood patterns and tissue perfusion have been studied by dynamic MR imaging in liver, brain and breast. This technique can be used to characterize SPNs as well.[86] Signal intensity time curves are generated following intravenous injection of gadolinium and maximum relative enhancement ratio and shape of enhancement can be calculated from these. A ratio >0.15 indicates a malignant SPN, a ratio <0.80 indicates benign lesion and ratio between 0.8 and 0.15 usually indicates active infection. These MR indices are useful for differentiating between benign and malignant SPNs.[87,88]

Diffusion-weighted MRI Imaging

MRI has an inherent advantage in terms of tissue characterization. Tissue contrast attained using diffusion weighted imaging (DWI) is different from that obtained using conventional MR sequences. In a study by Satoh, et al difference between benign and malignant was based on a DWI scale graded from 1 to 5. These were: 1) nearly no signal intensity as seen in an almost normal lung; 2) signal intensity between 1 and 3; 3) Signal intensity almost equal to the spinal cord at thoracic spine; 4) higher signal than spinal cord; 5) much higher signal than that of the spinal cord. A score of 3 (a nodule with signal intensity equal to that of the spinal cord) was considered the threshold for differentiation between benign and malignant pulmonary nodules in their study.[89] Lower ADC values for malignant lesions has been reported helping in their characterization.

Dual Energy CT in the Evaluation of SPN

Angiogenesis of malignant nodules leads to a stronger enhancement of malignant tumors on CT. Iodine is the main ingredient of contrast medium and directly reflects blood flow. Iodine concentration maps can assess the vasculature and relative vascularity of pulmonary nodule. By single

TABLE 4: Fleischner Society 2017 guidelines for management of incidentally detected pulmonary nodules in adults.*[95]

A: Solid nodules

Nodule type	**Size**			**Comments**
	<6 mm (<100 mm^3)	6–8 mm (100–250 mm^3)	>8 mm (>250 mm^3)	
Single:				
• Low risk	No routine follow-up	CT at 6–12 months, then consider CT at 18–24 months	Consider CT, PET/CT, or tissue sampling at 3 months	Nodules <6 mm do not require routine follow-up, but certain patients at high risk with suspicious nodule morphology, upper lobe location, or both may warrant 12-month follow-up
• High risk	Optional CT at 12 months	CT at 6–12 months, then CT at 18–24 months	Consider CT, PET/CT, or tissue sampling at 3 months	Nodules <6 mm do not require routine follow-up, but certain patients at high risk with suspicious nodule morphology, upper lobe location, or both may warrant 12-month follow-up
Multiple:				
• Low risk	No routine follow-up	CT at 3–6 months, then consider CT at 18–24 months	CT at 3–6 months, then consider CT at 18–24 months	Use most suspicious nodule as guide to management. Follow-up intervals may vary according to size and risk.
• High risk	Optional CT at 12 months	CT at 3–6 months, then at 18–24 months	CT at 3–6 months, then at 18–24 months	Use most suspicious nodule as guide to management. Follow-up intervals may vary according to size and risk

B: Subsolid nodules

Nodule type	**Size**		**Comments**
	<6 mm (<100 mm^3)	≥6 mm (>100 mm^3)	
Single:			
• Ground-glass	No routine follow-up	CT at 6–12 months to confirm persistence, then CT every 2 years until 5 years	In certain suspicious nodules <6 mm, consider follow-up at 2 and 4 years. If solid component(s) or growth develops, consider resection.
• Part solid	No routine follow-up	CT at 3–6 months to confirm persistence. If unchanged and solid component remains 6 mm, annual CT should be performed for 5 years	In practice, part-solid nodules cannot be defined as such until ≥6 mm, and nodules <6 mm do not usually require follow-up. Persistent part-solid nodules with solid components ≥6 mm should be considered highly suspicious
Multiple:	CT at 3–6 months. If stable, consider CT at 2 and 4 years	CT at 3–6 months. Subsequent management based on the most suspicious nodule(s)	Multiple <6 mm pure ground-glass nodules are usually benign, but consider follow-up in selected patients at high risk at 2 and 4 years

*These are the new guidelines given by the Fleischner Society 2017 for incidentally detected pulmonary nodules in adult patients <35 years of age.[95]

scanning after contrast injection, the degree of enhancement can be obtained without an additional non-enhanced scan. Iodine concentration in malignant nodules has been found to be significantly higher than benign nodules, thus allowing for the differentiation between benign and malignant nodules.[90] Owing to its material decomposition ability, DECT allows differentiation of calcification from enhanced tissue.

MANAGEMENT OF A SOLITARY PULMONARY NODULE

Following the Fleischner Society Guidelines of solid nodules in 2005[91] and the subsolid nodules in 2013[92–94] several modifications have taken place leading to the new guidelines of the Fleischner Society in 2017 **(Table 4)**.

The Fleischner Society guidelines are not for:

I. Patients with known primary cancer
II. Immunocompromised patients who are at risk of infection
III. Those at risk for metastasis
IV. Children and adults younger than 35 years

Management in these groups should be based on the specific clinical situation and on a case-by-case basis.

Changes in the revised guidelines include:

1. The minimum threshold of the nodule for follow-up has been increased to 6 mm rather than 5 mm.
2. Follow-up intervals have been given a range rather than a precise time period.
3. The guidelines for solid and semisolid nodules are now included in one single table with specific recommendations for multiple nodules.

For multiple nodules, the subsequent management is based on suspicious nodule which may not be the largest nodule. Pure GGNs more than 10 mm, part solid GGN with solid component larger than 5 mm, bubbly appearance of reticulation, atypical subsolid nodules with spiculation should be interpreted with high degree of suspicion.

It has been recommended that thin CT sections of the thorax (≤1 mm) should be performed to enable accurate characterization of the small pulmonary nodules. Sagittal and coronal reconstruction should always be obtained. A low radiation dose technique is recommended for follow up CT scans with the use of dose modulation and iterative reconstruction techniques to reduce radiation. According to the ACR recommendations for screening CT, the CT dose index volume (CTDI vol) should not be more than 3 mGy.[96]

It is also recommended that the average of the long and short axis diameters rather than the maximum transverse diameter should be taken as it yields better results. All measurements should be rounded to the nearest mm rather than fractional millimeter measurements. It is stated that volumetric measurements can be performed instead of linear measurements with volume of 100 and 250 mm^3 corresponding to the 6 and 8 mm thresholds. Volumetric measurements should be performed with identical software versions.[95]

The differential diagnosis of a SPN is given in **Table 5**.

TABLE 5: Differential diagnosis of solitary pulmonary nodule.[97]

• **Malignant neoplasm:** - Carcinoma (squamous cell, small cell, adenocarcinoma, bronchioloalveolar carcinoma) - Lymphoma - Carcinoid - Pulmonary metastasis (colon, melanoma, renal cell, breast, osteosarcoma)
• **Benign neoplasm and neoplasm-like condition:** - Hamartoma - Chondroma - Fibroma
• **Infective causes:** - Round pneumonia - Abscess - Granuloma (fungal, mycobacterial)
• **Noninfectious inflammatory:** - Sarcoidosis - Rheumatoid arthritis - Amyloidosis - Wegener's granulomatosis
• **Airway and inhalational disease:** - Mucoid impaction (mucous plug) - Bronchial atresia - Cystic fibrosis - Conglomerate mass or progressive massive fibrosis (e.g., silicosis) - Lipoid pneumonia
• **Vascular lesions:** - Pulmonary artery aneurysm - Hematoma - Infarct - Arteriovenous malformation (AVM)
• **Congenital lesions:** - Sequestration - Bronchogenic cyst - Bronchial atresia
• **Idiopathic/Miscellaneous:** - Amyloidosis - Fluid filled bulla - Round atelectasis

MORPHOLOGICAL CHARACTERISTICS IN SPECIFIC LESIONS

Lung Malignancies

About 20% of lung cancers present as SPNs **(Figs. 26A and B)**. The most common type presenting as a nodule is adenocarcinoma. Bronchogenic carcinoma will show irregular, spiculated margins with absence of calcification. However, presence of calcification does not completely

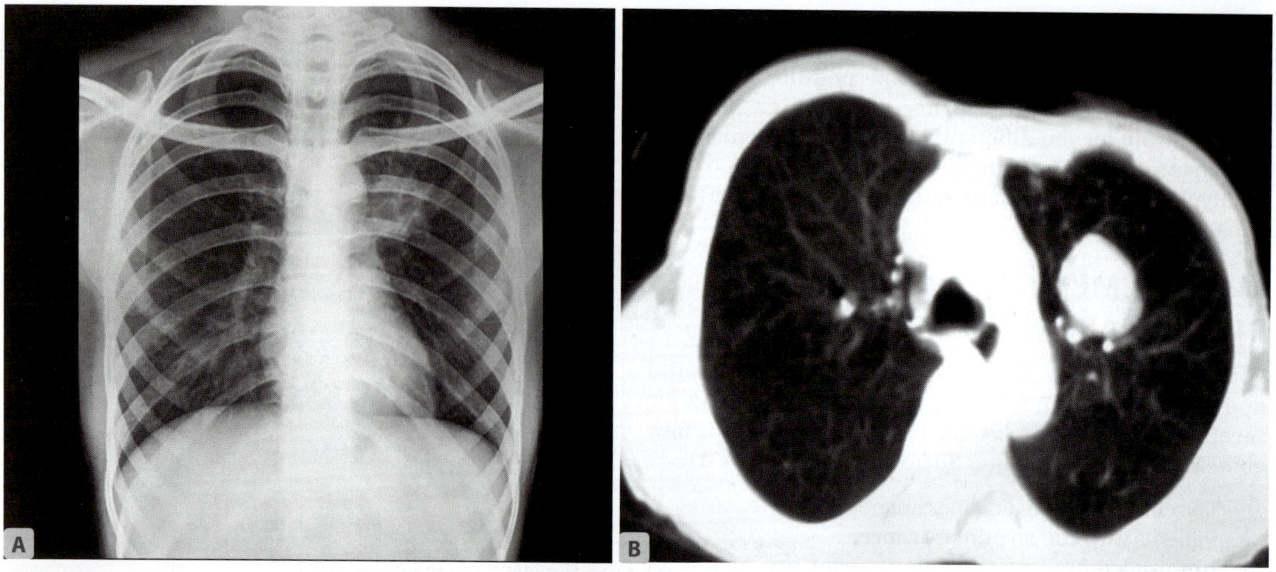

FIGS. 26A AND B: Chest radiograph shows a large nodule with irregular margins in the left upper lobe. Larger the lesion the more likely it is to be malignant—Bronchogenic carcinoma.

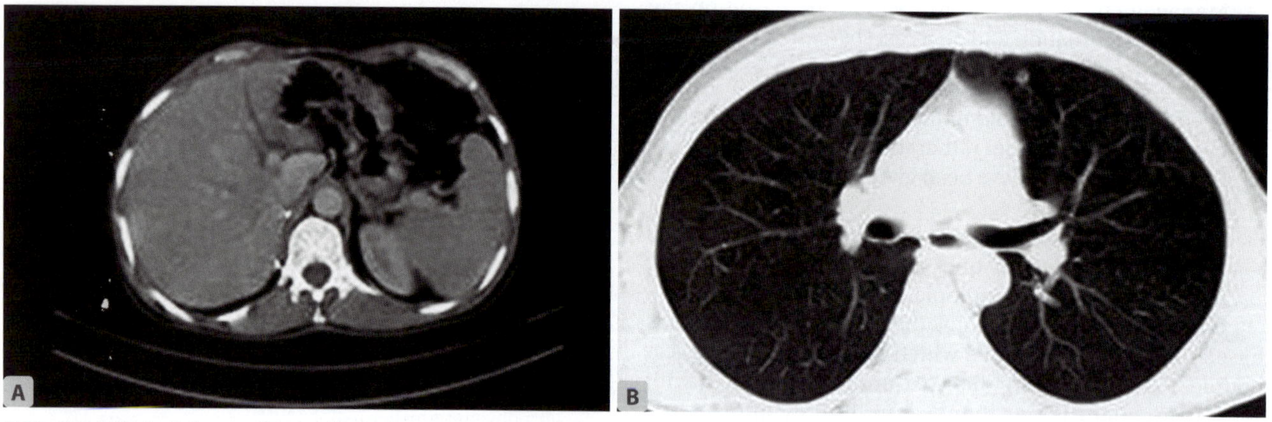

FIGS. 27A AND B: Follow-up CT scan (A) in a postoperative case of right renal cell carcinoma showing a small, smoothly marginated round solitary lesion in the left lung. The lesion is seen at the tip of a small artery (feeding vessel sign) (B)—Solitary metastasis in renal cell carcinoma.

rule out malignancy as cancers may develop in a scar or granuloma which shows pre-existing calcification. The pre-existing calcification is usually of the stippled or eccentric type and occupies less than 10% of the nodule.

Metastasis

Though metastatic nodules are usually multiple, rarely these may present as solitary pulmonary nodule. Carcinoma of the colon, melanoma and carcinomas of the kidney and testicle may present with solitary metastasis **(Figs. 27A and B)**.

The metastatic nodules are usually sharply marginated though local invasion and surrounding hemorrhage may lead to the nodules being poorly defined. Metastatic lesions are predominantly seen in the lung bases because of greater blood flow. "Feeding vessel sign" may be seen in these nodules owing to a hematogenous origin because these nodules are usually seen at the tips of small arteries.[98]

Carcinoid Tumor

These account for 10–20% of SPNs. These are neuroendocrine tumors and two forms have been described: typical and atypical. Typical carcinoids account for 85–90% of these lesions and occur in the main, lobar or segmental bronchi in a central location. The atypical ones usually have a peripheral location with a worse prognosis than the typical variety.[99] Carcinoids can be intraluminal or extraluminal and are seen as well-defined, lobulated, round or notched with a smooth edge. Spiculation is rarely seen. Curvilinear or multiple nodular calcification may be seen. Rarely, dense ossification may be seen within the lesion.

A triad of:

- Well defined, lobulated round lesion
- Location adjacent to bronchial bifurcation
- Eccentric calcification

Is highly suggestive of bronchial carcinoid **(Figs. 28A to C)**.[100]

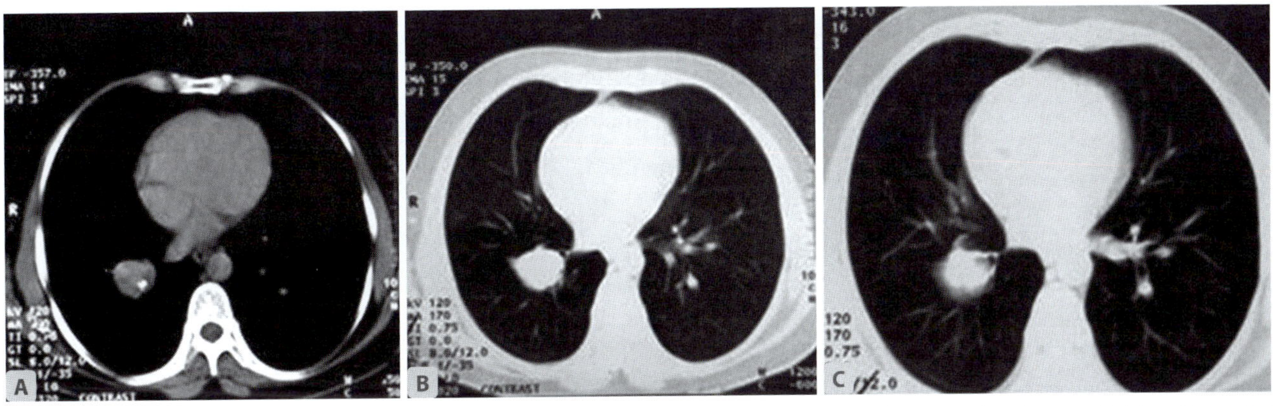

FIGS. 28A TO C: CT sections showing a well-defined rounded lesion in the right lung lying centrally in a perihilar location/vicinity of bronchial bifurcation with eccentric calcification noted within (A). Lung window shows the lesion to have a smooth edge with minimal lobulations (B). The right lower lobe bronchus shows the characteristic widening as it approaches the tumor (C)—Bronchial carcinoid.

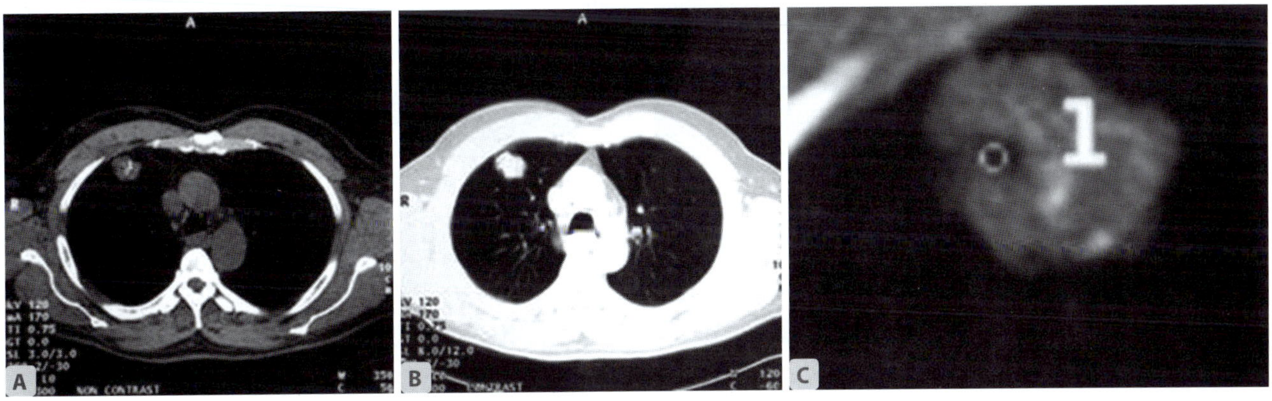

FIGS. 29A TO C: CT chest mediastinal (A) and lung parenchymal (B) window settings revealing a well-defined nodular lesion in the right upper lobe. The lesion shows fat attenuation (negative attenuation) values within. Magnified view of the lesion (C) showing the fat clearly and small specks of calcification in the lesion—Pulmonary hamartoma.

Lymphoma

Both Hodgkin's and non-Hodgkin's lymphoma involves the lung in about 10–15% cases and is characterized by single/multiple nodules, masses or consolidation which may cavitate. Associated hilar and mediastinal adenopathy is usually present.[101]

Benign Neoplasms

Pulmonary Hamartoma

It is a benign pulmonary mass composed of cartilage, myxomatous connective tissue, fat, marrow, bone, smooth muscle in different amounts. 90% of the hamartomas have a peripheral location. These are seen as well-defined, round or lobulated nodules with a characteristic "popcorn calcification" owing to the cartilaginous and osseous component.[102] CT detects fat as areas with negative attenuation values. The presence of fat and calcification within a well-defined nodule is virtually diagnostic of a pulmonary hamartoma **(Figs. 29A to C)**.[103]

Other Benign Tumors

These may arise from epithelial or mesenchymal tissue. Carney's triad is a condition comprising of multiple pulmonary chondromas, extra-adrenal paragangliomas and gastric epitheloid leiomyosarcoma. This condition is seen in women less than 35 years of age, the presence of multiple cartilage tumors in the lung should warrant a search for the other tumors which are more lethal than chondromas.[104]

Infective Causes

Granuloma

The most common cause of granuloma is tubercular though other causes include histoplasmosis, cryptococcosis, coccidioidomycosis. These are seen as a solitary nodule 1–3 cm in diameter with a well-defined smooth regular margin and often showing calcification **(Figs. 30A to C)**. The patterns of calcification seen in a granuloma include amorphous, punctate, fleck-like or laminar, often subpleural in location, granulomas rarely show cavitation. Cavitation when seen should suggest reactivation.

Hydatid Cyst

Caused by Echinococcus granulosus, the hydatid cyst is seen as a sharply demarcated, well-defined round or oval lesion with a homogeneous soft tissue density on radiographs **(Figs. 31A and B)**. The cysts occur more

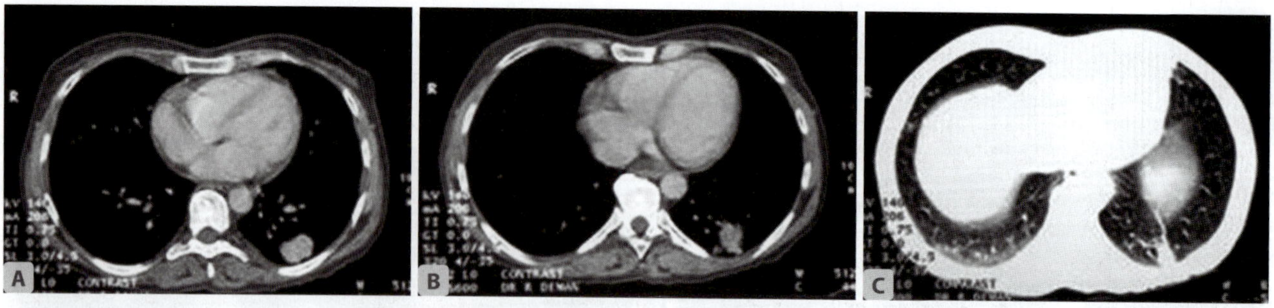

FIGS. 30A TO C: CT scans showing a single well-defined lesion 2 cm in size located subpleurally with no evidence of cavitation (A). The lesion shows evidence of multiple fibrotic strands around it (B and C)—Tuberculoma.

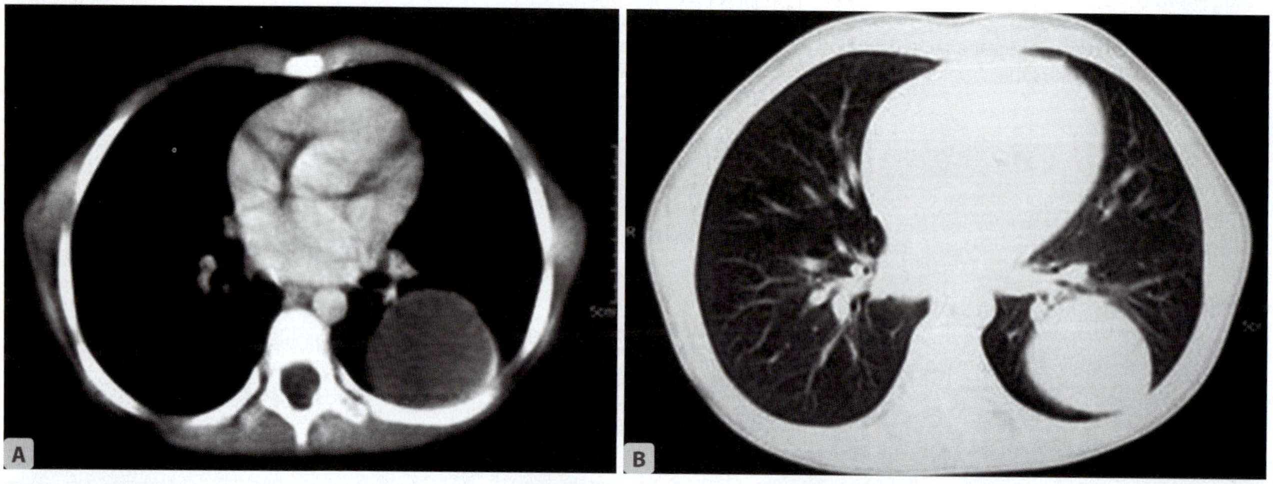

FIGS. 31A AND B: CT scan chest mediastinal (A) and lung windows (B) showing an oval, sharply marginated homogeneous fluid density cystic lesion in the left lower lobe—Hydatid cyst.

commonly in mid and lower lobes. An air-fluid level, water lily sign and rising sun sign are seen in cases of rupture of the hydatid cyst.

Mycetoma/Fungal Ball

A mycetoma results from saphrophytic invasion of a pre-existing cavity. The causes of the cavity in the majority of the cases is tubercular, but sarcoidosis, bronchiectasis, bulla, histoplasmosis, etc. may also result in a cavity in which the fungal mass develops. Matting of the aspergillus hyphae results in a fungal ball/mycetoma seen as a intracavitory mass in the upper lobe or superior segment of lower lobe usually. "Air-crescent sign" (air between the wall of the cavity and the fungal ball) is usually seen and is a diagnostic imaging finding **(Figs. 32A and B)**. CT shows a sponge like appearance of the mass with irregular air spaces.

Round Pneumonia

Round pneumonias are more commonly seen in children in cases of Streptococcus infection. Other causative organisms include K.pneumoniae, S.aureus, M.tuberculosis and fungi. On imaging round pneumonia appears as a focal round wedge shaped opacity in a peripheral location typically in the posterior lower lobe **(Figs. 33A and B)**. These have a predominant posterior distribution owing to the supine sleeping position of children while the gravity dependent passage of bacteria loaded fluid into the most dependent bronchus accounts for the lower lobe distribution. The underdeveloped pores of Kohn and the absence of canals of Lambert in children accounts for the sharp margins of the round pneumonia in contrast to the ill-defined margins of pneumonia seen in adults.[105] The centrifugal pattern of spread of the inflammation results in the lesion margin being sharply demarcated from the unaffected lung parenchyma **(Figs. 34A to C)**.

Lung Abscess

The etiology can be pyogenic, anaerobic bacteria or mycobacterial. Radiographs show an abscess as an ill-defined opacity with surrounding consolidation. An air-fluid level is seen in cases of communication with the bronchus. Contrast enhancement CT shows the abscess as a hypodense lesion with thick enhancing walls, shaggy margins and an air fluid level **(Figs. 35A to C)**.

Inflammatory Nodules

Rheumatoid Nodules

These are an uncommon manifestation of rheumatoid arthritis, may be seen as solitary or multiple nodules in the lung parenchyma.[106]

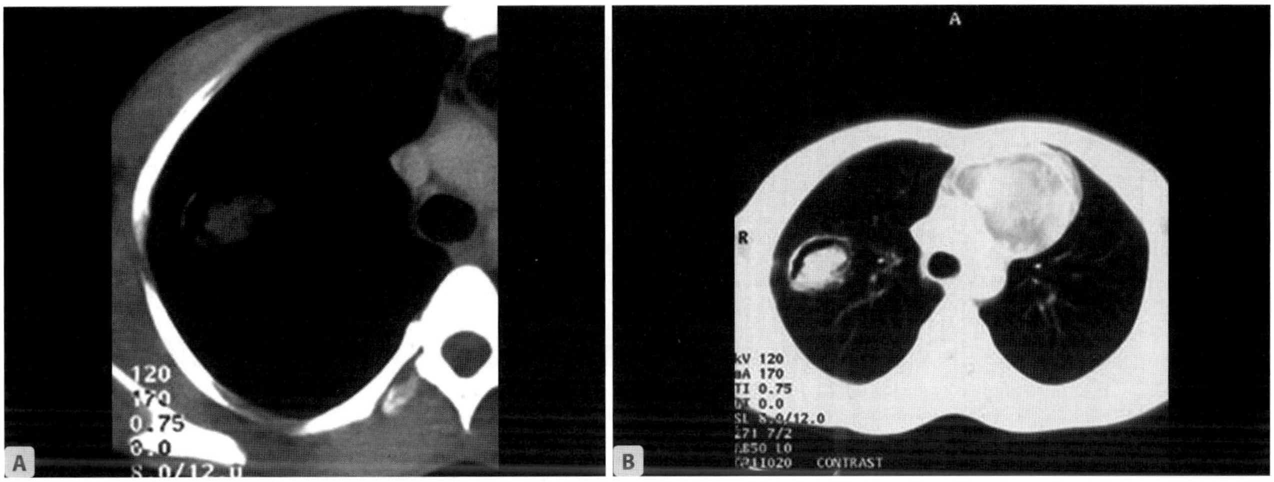

FIGS. 32A AND B: CT sections of the chest mediastinal and lung windows (A and B) showing the "air meniscus sign" seen as air crescent between the mass and the cavity in the right lung—Mycetoma.

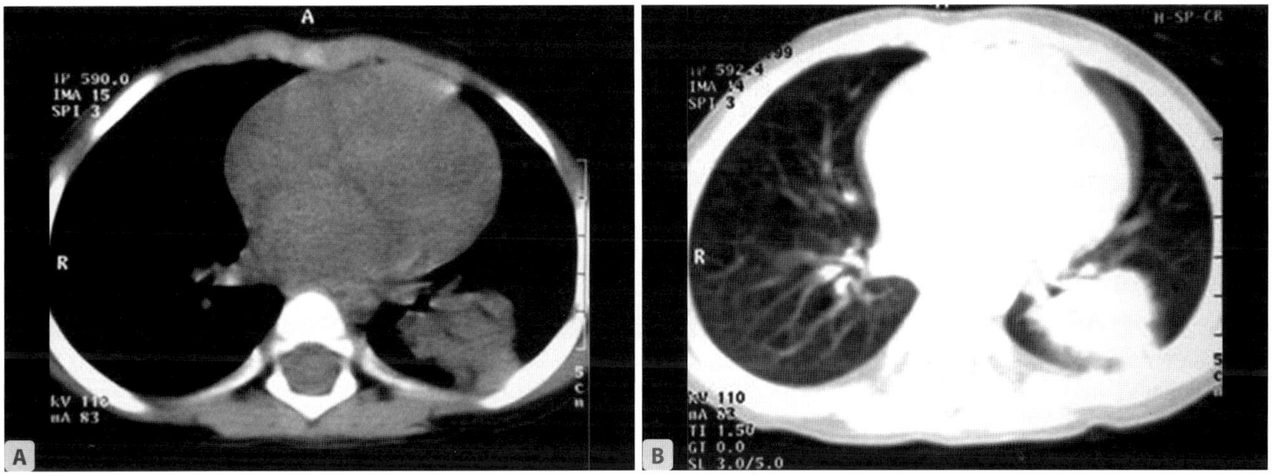

FIGS. 33A AND B: CT scan in a 2-year-old child showing a peripherally located wedge-shaped opacity with air bronchogram within the left lower lobe located posteriorly. The opacity is based against a focally thickened pleura—Round pneumonia.

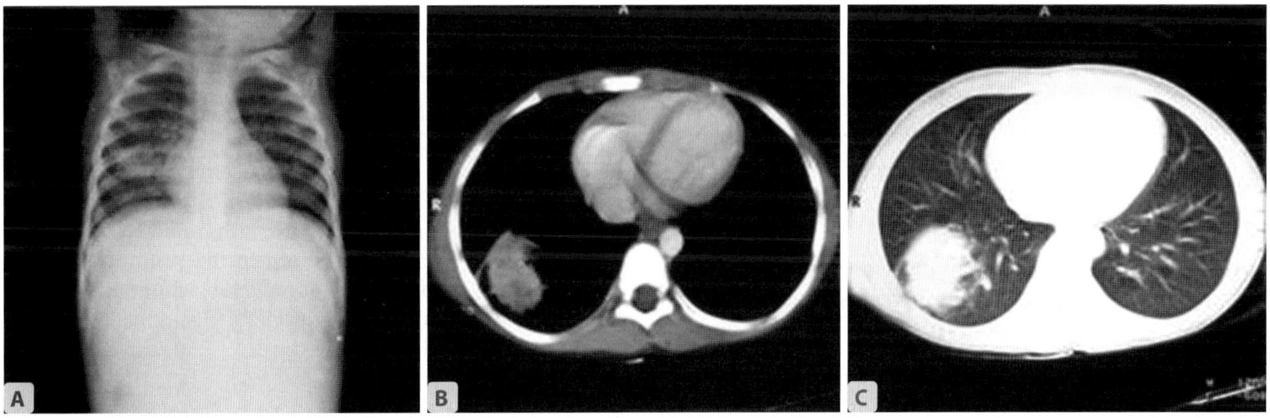

FIGS. 34A TO C: Chest radiograph (A) in a child showing a focal round nodule in the right lung. CT sections (B and C) showing an area of spherical consolidation in the right lower lobe with associated pleural thickening—Round pneumonia.

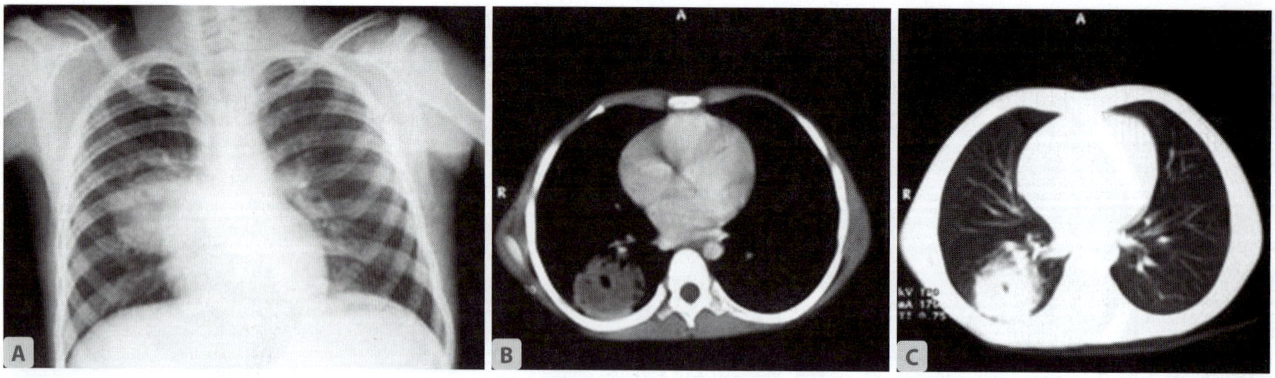

FIGS. 35A TO C: Chest radiograph (A) showing a focal round lesion in the right lung. A small air loculus is seen within. CT sections (B and C) showing a low attenuation lesion (i.e. fluid attenuation) lesion with enhancing wall. Multiple air loculi are seen in the center and in the periphery of the lesion (B). The margins are mildly irregular with surrounding consolidation (C)—Lung abscess.

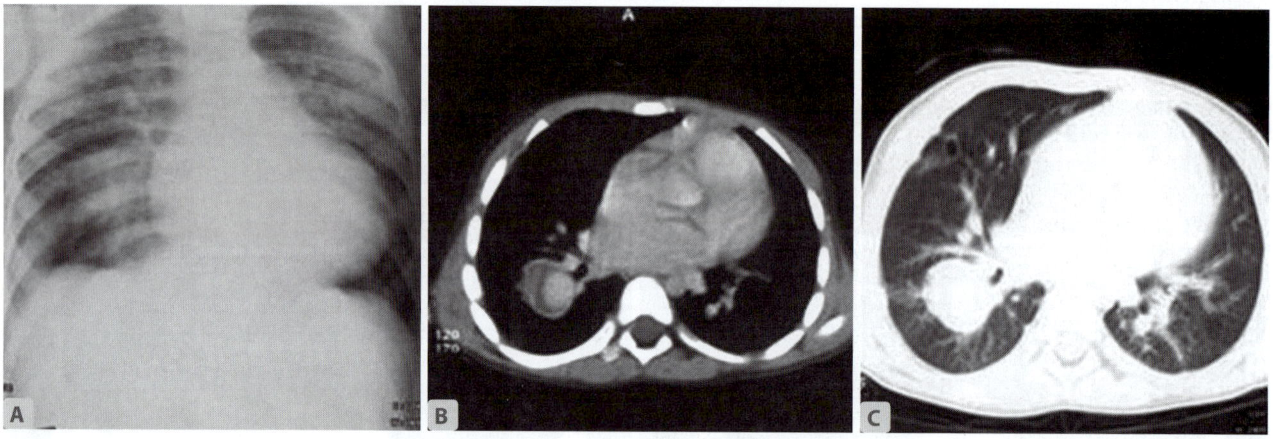

FIGS. 36A TO C: Chest radiograph (A) showing a sharply marginated solitary lesion located centrally in a perihilar location in the right lung (A). CT sections (B and C) showing an enhancing nodule in relation to a right interlobar pulmonary artery. A crescentic hypodensity is seen in the periphery of the lesion symptom of thrombus—Pulmonary artery aneurysm.

Airway or Inhalational Disease

Lipoid Pneumonia

Lipoid pneumonia is seen as an ill-defined nodule or mass in posterior lower lobe. Exogenous variety of lipoid pneumonia results from chronic aspiration of fat while the endogenous form occurs due to accumulation of lipid rich cellular debris distal to bronchial obstruction.

Vascular Lesions

Pulmonary Artery Aneurysm

Pulmonary artery aneurysm can present as a lung nodule.[107] Rasmussen aneurysm is seen in tuberculosis and is a mycotic aneurysm developing in the infectious cavity. Contrast-enhanced CT is diagnostic as the aneurysm is seen as a densely opacified nodular lesion in relation to lobar, segmental or smaller arteries **(Figs. 36A to C)**.

Pulmonary Vein Varix

A varix can result from a congenital defect of the wall, mitral valvular diseases or elevated pulmonary venous pressure. Radiologically, a pulmonary varix is seen as a round or oval density adjacent to the left atrium. Usually asymptomatic, a pulmonary varix can enlarge in response to high atrial pressure with resultant rupture and hemorrhage.

Arteriovenous Malformation

Arteriovenous malformation (AVM) is characterized by an enlarged artery feeding the nodule and a draining vein. Radiographs reveal the AVM as a well circumscribed nodule with a lobular outline, usually seen in the lower lobe, in a subpleural location. Contrast-enhanced CT reveals rapid enhancement and washout in the pulmonary AVM corresponding to the opacification and washout of the main pulmonary artery and right ventricle.[108]

Pulmonary Infarction

A pulmonary infarct is seen as a wedge-shaped opacity in contact with the pleural surface known as Hampton's hump **(Figs. 37A and B)**. A halo sign due to adjacent hemorrhage or low attenuating areas due to necrosis may be seen. On contrast administration, feeding vessels may be seen and

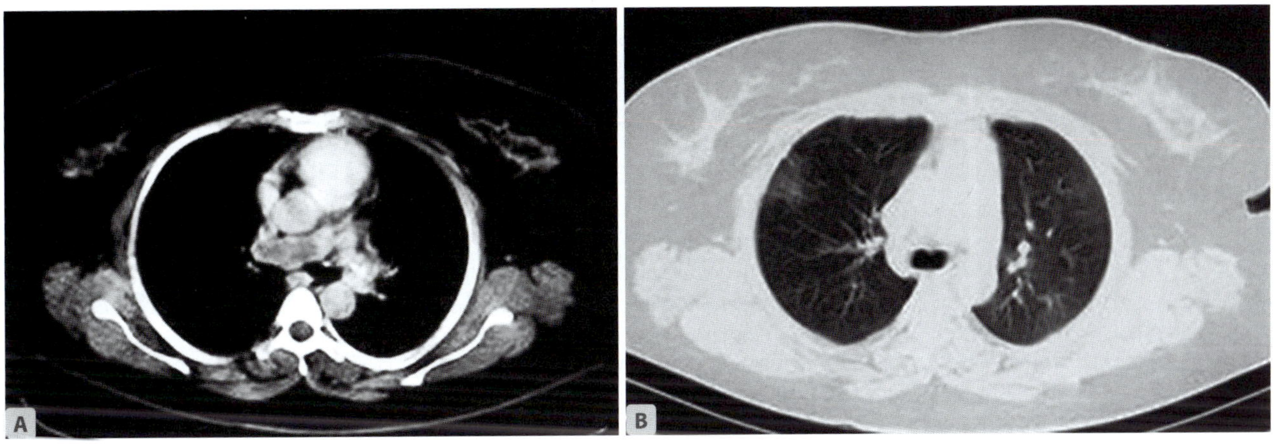

FIGS. 37A AND B: Contrast-enhanced CT (A) in a case of DVT showing a filling defect in the right pulmonary artery suggestive of thrombus. Lung parenchyma (B) shows a wedge-shaped pleural based opacity with surrounding halo symptoms of Hampton's hump in the right lung—Pulmonary infarction.

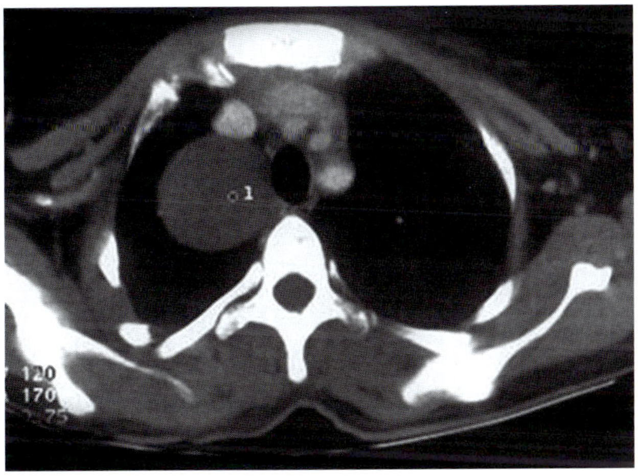

FIG. 38: CT scan showing a well-circumscribed cystic density lesion adjacent to the trachea on the right side. The cyst wall is thin and smooth—Bronchogenic cyst.

the periphery of the infarct may enhance owing to collateral flow. Cavitation of a pulmonary infarct occurs with infection of the bland infarct or with septic emboli. Pulmonary infarcts decrease in their size slowly over months what has been described as the "melting sign".[109]

Congenital Lesions

Pulmonary Bronchogenic Cyst

A bronchogenic cyst results from abnormal development of the lung bud. On the radiographs, it is seen as a well-circumscribed mass in a perihilar or subcarinal location. The fluid in the cyst can be serous, viscous and gelatinous or hemorrhagic. An air fluid level may be seen if the cyst is infected.

On CT, a variable density of the cyst ranging from water to soft tissue may be seen. The wall of the cyst is usually thin and smooth **(Fig. 38)**.

Sequestration

A disorganized area of pulmonary parenchyma without normal pulmonary arterial or bronchial communication is called sequestrated lung. It is of two types intralobar and extralobar. Intralobar, the more common form, occurs usually in the posterior basal segment of the left lower lobe adjacent to the diaphragm **(Figs. 39A to D)**.[110] The intralobar form has a normal pulmonary venous drainage and infections are common in this form. The extralobar variety is more commonly associated with other congenital anomalies, has its own pleural covering and is separate with a systemic venous drainage.

Miscellaneous

Round Atelectasis

Round atelectasis is a type of chronic atelectasis resembling a mass lesion. It is most often associated with asbestos related pleural disease but it may occur in association with other conditions like tuberculosis, other infections, Dressler syndrome and mesothelioma. According to one of the suggested mechanisms, the common event is pleural thickening and pleural exudates with the resultant effusion causing passive atelectasis of the adjacent lung. Fibrinous adhesions develop between the pleural surface of the atelectatic lung and the adjacent parietal pleura. Another explanation is that as the pleural fibrosis matures, it retracts causing infolding and atelectasis of the lung parenchyma.[111]

On imaging, round atelectasis is seen as a peripheral opacity which is oval or wedge shaped. It is based against a thickened pleura with the edge pointing towards the hilum being ill-defined and irregular. Distortion, displacement of the blood vessels and bronchi which appear pulled towards the lesion forms a characteristic imaging appearance called the "comet tail" or "crow feet" appearance **(Figs. 40A to C)**. Air bronchograms and calcification may be seen.[112] Round atelectasis may show contrast enhancement. Though mostly static, it may shrink and rarely resolve spontaneously.

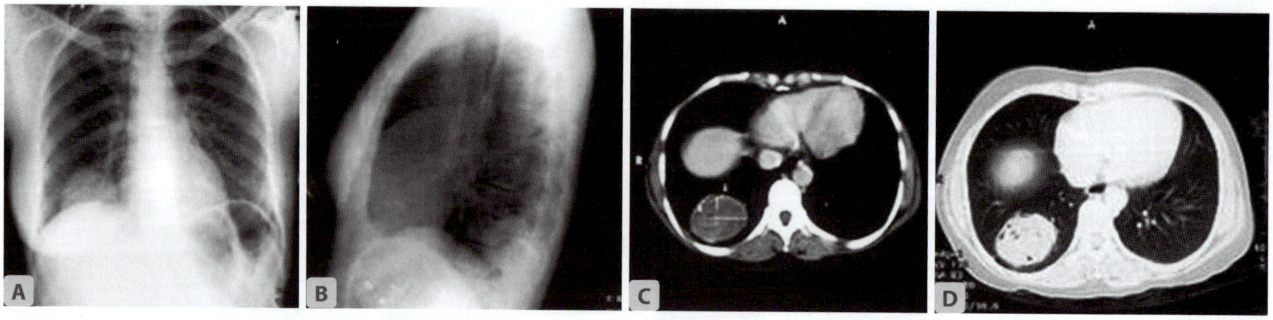

FIGS. 39A TO D: Chest radiograph frontal (A) and lateral projection (B) in a 35-year-female with recurrent chest infections showing a well-defined sharply marginated lesion in the posterior basal segment of the right lower lobe. CT sections (C and D) showing a hypodense well-circumscribed lesion with multiple air foci suggesting communication with adjacent bronchi due to infection—Pulmonary intralobar sequestration.

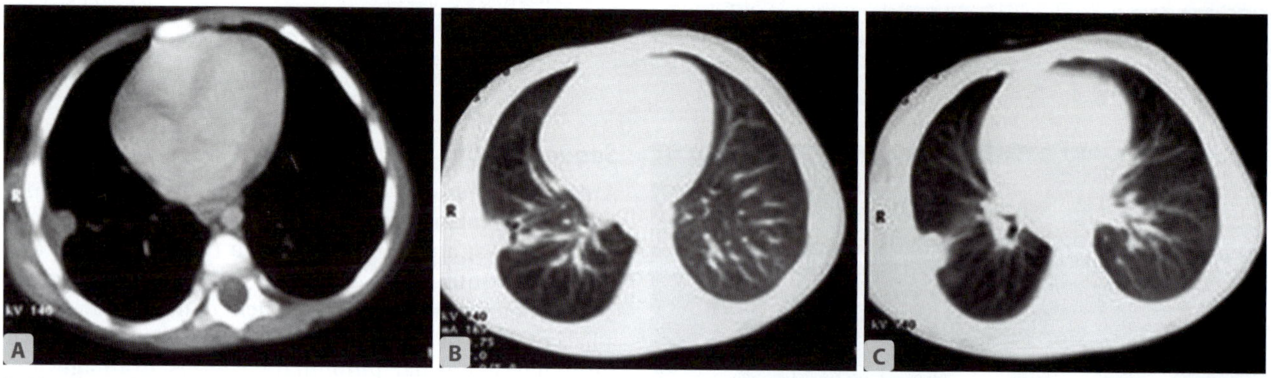

FIGS. 40A TO C: CT sections showing a peripherally located wedge-shaped opacity against thickened pleura (A). There is distortion and displacement of vessels adjacent to the opacity. The vessels are more numerous than normal in this portion (B) and have a characteristic curvilinear configuration (C)—Round atelectasis.

CONCLUSION

The workup and management of patients with SPNs relies on the imaging features and the clinical findings with the aim to differentiate benign lesions from small malignant tumors. One should strive not only to identify small malignant tumors where resection results in high survival rates, but also spare patients with benign disease from unnecessary surgery.

REFERENCES

1. Midthun DE, Swensen SJ, Jett JR. Approach to the solitary pulmonary nodule. Mayo Clin Proc. 1993;68:378-85.
2. Tuddenham WJ. Glossary of terms for thoracic radiology: recommendations of the Nomenclature Committee of the Fleischner Society. AJR. 1984;143:509-17.
3. Lillington GA, Caskey CI. Evaluation and management of solitary and multiple pulmonary nodules. Clin Chest Med. 1993;14: 111-9.
4. Holin SM, Dwork RE, Glaser S, et al. Solitary pulmonary nodules found in a community wide chest roentgenographic survey. Am Rev Tuberc. 1959;79:427-39.
5. Austin JH, Garg K, Aberle D, et al. Radiologic implications of the 2011 classification of adenocarcinoma of the lung. Radiology. 2013;266:62-71.
6. Beigelman-Aubry C, Hill C, Grenier PA. Management of an incidentally discovered pulmonary nodule. Eur Radiol. 2007;17:449-66.
7. Kundel HL. Predictive value and threshold detectability of lung tumors. Radiology. 1981;139(1):25-9.
8. Zerhouni EA, Stitik FP, Siegelman SS, et al. CT of the pulmonary nodule: a cooperative study. Radiology. 1986; 160(2):319-27.
9. Webb WR. Radiologic evaluation of the solitary pulmonary nodule. AJR. 1990;154:701-8.
10. Volterrani L, Vegni V, Pieraccini MGC, et al. Small solitary pulmonary nodule and high resolution CT: a preliminary report. Eur Radiol. 1995;5:443-7.
11. Garland LH. Bronchial carcinomas: lobar distribution of lesions in 250 cases. Calif Med. 1961;94:7-8.
12. Swensen SJ, Viggiano RW, Midthun DE, et al. Lung nodule enhancement at CT: multicentre study. Radiology. 2000;214:73-80.
13. Winer Muram HT, Jennings SG, Tarver RD, et al. Volumetric growth rate of stage I lung cancer prior to treatment: serial CT scanning. Radiology. 2002;223:798-805.
14. Quinn D, Gianlupi A, Broste S. The changing radiographic presentation of bronchogenic carcinoma with reference to cell types. Chest. 1996;110:1474-9.
15. Swensen SJ, Silverstein MD, Ilstrup DM. The probability of malignancy in solitary pulmonary nodules: application to small radiographically in determinate nodules. Arch Int Med. 1997;157:849-55.
16. Heitzman ER, Markarian B, Raasch BN, et al. Pathways of tumor spread through the lung: radiologic correlations with anatomy and pathology. Radiology 1982;144:3-14.

17. Zwirewich CV, Vedal S, Miller RR, et al. Solitary pulmonary nodule: High resolution CT and radiologic pathologic correlation. Radiology 1991;179:469-76.
18. Khan A, Herman PG, Vorwerk P, et al. Solitary pulmonary nodule: comparison of classification with standard, thin section and reference phantom CT. Radiology. 1991;179:477- 81.
19. Huston J III, Muhm JR. Solitary pulmonary opacities: plain tomography. Radiology. 1987;163:481-5.
20. Hill CA. "Tail" signs associated with pulmonary lesions: critical rappraisal. AJR. 1982;139:311-6.
21. Chen SW, Price J. Focal organizing pneumonia mimicking small peripheral adenocarcinoma on CT scans. Australas Radiol. 1998;42:360-3.
22. Gaeta M, Blandino A, Scribano E, et al. Computed tomography halo sign in pulmonary nodules: frequency and diagnostic value. J Thorac Imaging. 1999;14:109-13.
23. Primack SL, Hartman TE, Lee KS, et al. Pulmonary nodules and the CT halo sign. Radiology 1994;190:513-5.
24. Berger WG, Erly WK, Krupiniski EA, et al. The solitary pulmonary nodule on chest radiography: can we really tell if the nodule is calcified? AJR. 2001;176:201-4.
25. Grewal RG, Austin JH. CT demonstration of calcification in carcinoma of the lung. J Comput Assist Tomogr. 1994;18: 867-71.
26. Mahoney MC, Shipley RT, Corcoran HL, et al. CT demonstration of calcification in carcinoma of the lung. AJR. 1990;154:255-8.
27. Swensen SJ, Morin RL, et al. CT reconstruction algorithm selection in the evaluation of solitary pulmonary nodules. J Comput Assist Tomogr. 1995;19:932-5.
28. Ko JP, Naidich DP. Lung nodule detection and characterization with multislice CT. Radiol Clin North Am. 2003;41:575-97.
29. Woodring JH, Fried AM. Significance of wall thickness in solitary cavities of the lung: A follow up study. AJR. 1983;140:473-4.
30. Lee Ks, Kim Y. Han J, et al. Bronchioloalveolar carcinoma: clinical, histopathologic and radiologic findings. Radio- graphics 1997;17:1345-57.
31. Kuriyama K, Tateishi R, Doi O, et al. Prevalence of air bronchograms in small peripheral carcinomas of the lung on thin section CT: Comparison with benign tumors. AJR. 1991;156:921-4.
32. Kuii M, Templeton PA, White CS, et al. Evaluation of the air bronchogram sign on CT in solitary pulmonary lesions. J Comput Assist Tomogr. 1996;20(6):983-6
33. Milne EN, Zerhouni EA. Blood supply of pulmonary metastases. J Thorac Imaging. 1987;2:15-23.
34. Mori K, Saitou Y, Tominaga K, et al. Small nodular lesions in the lung periphery: new approach to diagnosis with CT. Radiology. 1990;177:843-9.
35. Singh SP. The positive bronchus sign. Radiology. 1998;209:251-2.
36. Proto AV, Thomas SR. Pulmonary nodules studied by computed tomography. Radiology. 1985;156:149-53
37. Goldstein MS, Rush M, Johnson P, et al. A calcified adenocarcinoma of the lung with very high CT numbers. Radiology. 1984;150:785-6.
38. Zerhouni EA, Boukadoum M, Siddiky MA, et al. A standard phantom for quantitative CT analysis of pulmonary nodules. Radiology. 1983;149:767-73.
39. Heneschke CI, Yankelevitz DF, Mirtcheva R, et al. CT screening for lung cancer: frequency and significance of part solid and non-solid nodules. AJR. 2002;178:1053-7.
40. Li F, Sone S, Abe H, et al. Malignant versus benign nodules at CT screening for lung cancer: Comparison of thin section CT findings. Radiology. 2004;233:793-8.
41. Libby DM, Smith JP, Altorki NK, et al. Managing the small pulmonary nodule discovered by CT. Chest. 2004;125:1522-9.
42. Godoy MCB, Naidich DP. Overview and strategic management of subsolid pulmonary nodules. J Thorac Imaging. 2012;27:240-8.
43. Park CM, Goo JM, Lee HJ, et al. Nodular ground glass opacity at thin section CT: histologic correlation and evaluation of change at follow-up. Radiographics. 2007;27:391-408.
44. Kim H, Park CM, Koh JM, et al. Pulmonary subsolid nodules: what radiologists need to know about imaging features and management strategy. Diagn Interv Radiol. 2014;20:47-57.
45. Honda T, Kondo T, Murakami S et al. Radiologic implications of the 2011 classification of adenocarcinoma of the lung. Radiology. 2013;266(1):62-71.
46. Travis WD, Brambilla E, Noguchi M, et al. Diagnosis of lung adenocarcinoma in resected specimens, implication of the 2011 International Association for the study of Lung Cancer/American Thoracic Society/European Respiratory Society classification. Arch Pathol Lab Med. 2013;137(5):685-705.
47. Park CM, Goo JM, Lee HJ, et al. CT findings of atypical adenomatous hyperplasia in the lung . Korean J Radiol. 2006;7(2):80-6.
48. Goo JM, Park CM, Lee HJ. Ground glass nodules on CT as imaging biomarkers in the management of lung adenocarcinoma. Am J Roentgenol. 2011;196:533-43.
49. Tsutani Y, Miyata Y, Nakayama H et al. Prognostic significance of using solid versus whole tumour size on high resolution computed tomography for predicting pathologic malignant grade of tumours in clinical stage IA of lung adenocarcinoma: a multicentric study. J Thorac Cardiovasc Surg. 2012;143(3): 607-12.
50. Truong MJ, Ko JP, Rosi SE et al. Update in the evaluation of the solitary pulmonary nodule. Radiographics. 2014;34:1658-79.
51. Soubani AO. The evaluation and management of solitary pulmonary nodule. Postgrad Med J. 2008;84:459-66.
52. Wang YX, Gong JS, Suzuki K, et al. Evidence based imaging strategies for solitary pulmonary nodule. J Thorac Dis. 2014;6(7):872-87.
53. Collins VP, Loeffler RK, Twey H. Observations on growth rates in human tumors. AJR. 1956;76:988-1000.
54. Dunnick NR, Parker BR, Castellino RA. Differentiation of benign and malignant pulmonary nodules by growth rate. Radiology. 1962;79:221-32.
55. Godoy MC, Naidisch DP, Subsolid pulmonary nodules and the spectrum of peripheral adenocarcinomas of the lung: recommended interim guidelines for assessment and management. Radiology. 2009;253:606-22.
56. Aoki T, Nakata H, Watanabe H, et al. Evolution of peripheral lung adenocarcinomas: CT findings correlated with histology and tumour doubling time. Am J Roentgenol. 2000;174:763-8.
57. Yankelevitz DF, Heneschke CI. Does 2 year stability imply that pulmonary nodules are benign? AJR. 1997;168:325-8.
58. Revel MP, Lefort C, Bissery A, et al. Pulmonary nodules: preliminary experience with three dimensional evaluation. Radiology. 2004;231:459-66.
59. Kim H, Park CM, Woo S, et al. Pure and part solid pulmonary ground glass nodules: measurement variability of volume and mass in nodules with a solid portion less than or equal to 5 mm. Radiology. 2013;269:585-93.
60. Petrou M, Quint LE, Nan B, et al. Pulmonary nodule volumetric measurement variability as a function of CT slice thickness and nodule morphology. AJR. 2007;188:306-12.
61. Zhang L, Yankelevitz PF, Carter D, et al. Internal growth of non-solid lung nodules: radiologic-pathologic correlation. Radiology. 2012;255:199-206.
62. de Hoop B, Gietema H, Vande Vorst S, et al. Pulmonary ground glass nodules: increase in mass as an early indicator of growth. Radiology. 2010;255:199-206.
63. Girvin F, Ko JP. Pulmonary Nodules: Detection, Assessment and CAD. AJR. 2008;191:1057-69.

64. Wormanns D, Kohl G, Klotz E, et al. Volumetric measurements of pulmonary nodules at multi-row detector CT: in vivo reproducibility. Eur Radiol. 2004;14:86-92.
65. Littleton JT, Durizch ML, Moeller G, et al. Pulmonary masses: contrast enhancement. Radiol. 1990;177:861-71.
66. Zhang M, Kono M. Solitary pulmonary nodules: Evaluation of blood flow patterns with dynamic CT. Radiol. 1997;205:471-8.
67. Yamashita K, Matsunobe S, Tsuda T, et al. Solitary pulmonary nodule: Preliminary study of evaluation with incremental dynamic CT. Radiol. 1995;194:399-405.
68. Swensen SJ, Brown LR, Colby TV, et al. Lung nodule enhancement at CT: Prospective findings. Radiol. 1996;201:447-55.
69. Murayama S, Murakami J, Hashimoto S, et al. Noncalcified pulmonary tuberculomas: CT enhancement patterns with histological correlation. J Thorac Imaging. 1995;10:91-5.
70. Jeong YJ, Lee KS, Jeong SY, et al. Solitary Pulmonary Nodule: Characterization with Combined wash in and washout features at Dynamic Multi detector Row CT. Radiol. 2005;237:675-83.
71. Yi CA, Lee KS, Kim EA, et al. Solitary pulmonary nodules: dynamic enhanced multi detector row CT study and comparison with vascular endothelial growth factor and microvessel density. Radiol. 2004;233:191-9.
72. Gadgeel SM, Ramalingam S, Cummmings G, et al. Lung cancer in patients <50 years of age: the experience of an academic multidisciplinary program. Chest. 1999;115:1232-6.
73. Guyatt GH, Newhouse MD. Are active and passive smoking harmful? Determination of causation. Chest. 1985;88:445-51.
74. Bach PB, Kaltan M, Thornquist MD, et al. Variations in lung cancer risk among smokers. J Natl Canc Inst. 2003;95:470-8.
75. Lee PN. Relation between exposure to asbestos and smoking jointly and the risk of lung cancer. Occup Environ Med. 2001;58:145-53.
76. Erasmus JJ, Mc Adams HP, Connolly JE. Solitary pulmonary nodules: Part-II. Evaluation of the indeterminate nodule. Radiographics. 2000;20:59-66.
77. Gurney JW, Lyddon DM, Mckay JA. Determining the likelihood of malignancy in solitary pulmonary nodules with Bayesian analysis Part II. Application. Radiology. 1993;186: 415-32.
78. Black WC, Armstrong P. Communicating the significance of radiologic test results: the likelihood ratio. AJR. 1986;147:1313-8.
79. Soardi GA, Perandini S, Molton M, et al. Assessing probability of malignancy in solid solitary pulmonary nodules with a new Bayesian calculator: improving diagnostic accuracy by means of expanded and updated features. Eur Radiol. DOI 10.1007/s00330-014-3396-2.
80. Sim YT, Poon FW. Imaging of solitary pulmonary nodule: a clinical review. Quant Imaging Med Surg. 2013;3:316-26.
81. Nomori H, Wattanbe K, Ohtsuka T, et al. Evaluation of F-18 fluorodeoxyglucose (FDG) PET scanning for pulmonary nodules less than 3 cm in diameter with special reference to CT images. Lung Cancer. 2004;45:19-27.
82. Lowe VJ, Fletcher JW, Gobar C, et al. Prospective investigation of PET in lung nodules (PIOPILN), J Clin Oncol. 1998;16:1075-84.
83. Huber KF, Buonocore E, Gould HR, et al. Differentiating benign from malignant lung lesions using quantitative parameters of FDG PET images. Clin Nucl Med. 1996;21:941-49.
84. Shimizu K, Ikeda N, Tuboi M, et al. Percutaneous Ct guided fine needle aspiration for lung cancer smaller than 2 cm and revealed by ground-glass opacity at CT. Lung Cancer. 2006;51(2): 173-9.
85. Moore EH. Needle aspiration lung biopsy: A comprehensive approach to complication reduction. J Thorac Imaging. 1997;12:259-71.
86. Ohno Y, Hatabu H, Takenaka D, et al. Solitary pulmonary nodules: potential role of dynamic MR imaging in management: initial experiences. Radiol. 2002;224:503-11.
87. Kono M, Adachi S, Kusumoto M, et al. Clinical utility of Gd– DTPA-enhanced magnetic resonance imaging in lung cancer. J Thorac Imaging. 1993;8:18-26.
88. Guckel C, Schnabel K, Deimling M, et al. Solitary pulmonary nodules: MR evaluation of enhancement patterns with contrast enhanced dynamic snapshot gradient echo imaging. Radiol. 1996;200:681-6.
89. Satoh S, Kitazume Y, Ohdama S. Can malignant and benign pulmonary nodules be differentiated with diffusion weighted MRI? AJR. 2008;191:464-70.
90. Chae EJ, Song JW, Seo JB, et al. Clinical utility of Dual. Energy CT in the evaluation of solitary pulmonary nodules: Initial Experience. Radiology. 2008;249(2):671-81.
91. MacMohan MB, Austin JHM, Gamsu G, et al. Guidelines for management of small pulmonary nodules detected on CT scans: a statement from the Fleischner Society. Radiology. 2005;237:395-400.
92. Patel VK, Naik SK, Naidich DP, et al. A practical approach to the diagnosis and management of solitary pulmonary nodules: part 2-pretest probability and algorithm. Chest. 2013;143(3): 840-6.
93. Naidich Dp, Bankier AA, McMohan H, et al. Recommendations for the management of subsolid pulmonary nodules detected at CT: a statement from the Fleischner Society. Radiol. 2013;266: 304-17.
94. Vasquez M, Carter D, Brambilla E, et al. Solitary and multiple resected adenocarcinomas after CT screening for lung cancer: histopathologic features and their prognostic implications. Lung Cancer. 2009;64(2):148-54.
95. MacMahon H, Naidich DP, Goo JM et al, Guidelines for management of incidental pulmonary nodules detected on CT images: from the Fleischner Society 2017. Radiology. 2017 Jul;284(1):228-43. doi: 10.1148/radiol.2017161659. Epub 2017 Feb 23.
96. Kazerooni EA, Armstrong M, Amorosa JK, et al. ACR CT accreditation program and lung cancer screening program designation. J Am Coll Radiol. 2016;13(2 Suppl):R 30-34.
97. Armstrong P. Basic patterns in lung disease. In: Hansell DM, Armstrong P, Lynch DA, McAdams HP, (Eds). Imaging of Disease of the Chest. Philadelphia: Mosby. 2005;69-141.
98. Hirakata K, Nakata H, Haratake J. Appearance of pulmonary metastases on high resolution CT scans. Comparison with histopathologic findings from autopsy specimens. AJR. 1993;161:37-43.
99. Choplin RH, Kawanmoto EH, Dyer RB, et al. Atypical carcinoid of the lung: Radiographic features. AJR. 1986;146:665-8.
100. Muller NL, Miller RR. Neuroendocrine carcinomas of the lung. Seminar Roentgenol 1990;25:96-104.
101. Au V, Leung AN. Radiologic manifestations of lymphoma in the thorax. AJR. 1997;168:93-8.
102. Gjevre JA, Myers JL, Prakash UB. Pulmonary hamartomas. Mayo Clin Proc. 1996;71:14-20.
103. Siegelman SS, Khouri NF, Scott WW, et al. Pulmonary hamartoma: CT findings. Radiol. 1986;160:313-7.
104. Carney JA. The triad of gastric epitheloid leiomyosarcoma pulmonary chondroma and functioning extra adrenal paraganglioma: a five year review. Medicine (Baltimore). 1983;62: 159-69.
105. Celebi S, Hacimustafaoglu M. Round pneumonia in children. Ind J Paed. 2008;75:523-5.

106. Cortet B, Flipo RM, Remy Jordin M, et al. Use of high resolution computed tomography of the lungs in patients with rheumatoid arthritis. Ann Rheum Dis. 1995;54:815-9.
107. Ferratti GR, Thony F, Link KM, et al. False aneurysm of the pulmonary artery induced by a Swan Ganz catheter: Clinical presentation and radiologic management. AJR. 1996;167:941-5.
108. Spear BS, Sully L, Lewis CT. Pulmonary arteriovenous fistula presenting as spontaneous hemothorax. Thorax. 1975;30:355-6.
109. Burkill GJ, Bell JR, Padley SP. Survey on the use of pulmonary scintigraphy, spiral CT and conventional pulmonary angiography for suspected pulmonary embolism in the British Isles. Clin Radiol. 1999;54:807-10.
110. Frazier AA, Rosado de Christenson ML, Stoker JT, et al. Intralobar sequestration: Radiologic pathologic correlation. Radiographics. 1997;17:725-45.
111. Carvalho PM, Carr DH. Computed tomography of folded lung. Clin Radiol. 1990;41:86-91.
112. O' Donovan PB, Schenk M, Lim K, et al. Evaluation of the reliability of computed tomographic criteria used in the diagnosis of round atelectasis. J Thoracic Imaging. 1997;12:54-8.

CHAPTER

134

Imaging of Pulmonary Neoplasms

Priyanka Naranje, Mukesh Kumar Yadav, Chandan J Das, Arun Kumar Gupta

INTRODUCTION

Lung cancer is amongst the most common and most lethal cancers around the world. It represents about 13% of the new cancer cases and up to 28% of the cancer deaths.[1] It is the most common cancer in males in India with age averaged incidence ranging from 3.6 to 18.9 per 100,000 per year in different parts of the country.[2] Overall 5 years survival with this cancer is less than 15%. Most lung cancers are directly attributed to smoking. Reported highest incidence in smokers is 362 cases per 100,000 per year while the same in non-smokers is up to 21 cases only.[3] Passive smoking increases the risk of lung cancer by up to 30%. Exposure to nickel, cobalt, asbestos, radiation, pesticides also increases the risk of lung cancer. Lung is also the most common site of metastatic involvement from other extrathoracic malignancies; 20–54% of extrathoracic malignancies have pulmonary metastatic disease.[3] Synchronous and metachronous second lung malignancy occurs in about 2% of patients with lung cancer.[4]

A wide variety of imaging techniques are currently available for detection, diagnosis, and management of pulmonary neoplasms. Chest radiography is the primary imaging modality for detection of lung nodules and masses. Computed tomography (CT) and Positron emission tomography (PET) are most commonly used imaging modalities for further characterization, to define extent and along with non radiological modalities; for pre-treatment staging of the lung malignancies. Imaging is also required to assess the response to nonsurgical treatment and for follow-up in treated patients. MRI has evolving role in evaluation of lung malignancies and is occasionally used as a problem solving modality and in assessment of treatment response.

WHO CLASSIFICATION[5]

Pulmonary neoplasms are classified pathologically according to 4th edition of WHO Classification 2015 which provides a standardized terminology for lung cancer **(Table 1)**. Previous classification of 2004 was based on resection specimens. In the present era, the therapeutic decisions are based on specific histologic and genetic characteristics of the tumor. Hence, in the 2015 classification system, whenever possible, *immunohistochemistry* is recommended for all cytology or biopsy or even resected specimens. For example, epidermal growth factor (EGFR) mutations, anaplastic lymphoma kinase (ALK) rearrangements and ROS1 are found in adenocarcinoma and these are effective targets for specific drugs such as EGFR tyrosine kinase inhibitors (Erlotinib, Gefitinib) or ALK inhibitors (crizotinib) in patients with advanced lung adenocarcinoma. Similarly, a pneumocyte marker such as thyroid transcription factor (TTF)-1 is desired to address primary versus metastatic adenocarcinoma.

CLINICAL FEATURES

Depending on the location, extent, size and histopathology of the tumor, various clinical manifestations are seen. Systemic symptoms of weight loss, anorexia and fever are common. Cough and hemoptysis are the most common clinical features of lung cancers. Hemoptysis may be streaky or massive at the presentation. Central tumors may present with wheeze and recurrent pneumonia due to bronchial obstruction. Advanced lung tumors with locoregional invasion of the pleura, chest wall or mediastinum may manifest with chest pain, brachial plexus neuropathy, Horner syndrome, phrenic or recurrent laryngeal nerve palsy, dysphagia or SVC obstruction. Besides, there are several paraneoplastic syndromes that may be associated with lung cancer such as Eaton-Lambart syndrome, subacute cerebellar degeneration, encephalomyelopathy, Cushing syndrome, hypertrophic pulmonary osteoarthropathy, etc. Some small peripheral lung cancers may be asymptomatic and only be detected incidentally or on screening. Signs and symptoms due to metastasis could be bone pain, neurologic symptoms or pathological fracture.

TABLE 1: 2015 WHO classification of lung tumors.

Histologic type and subtypes
Epithelial tumors
• *Adenocarcinoma*:
– Lepidic, acinar, papillary, micropapillary, solid, colloid, fetal, enteric
– Invasive mucinous adenocarcinoma
– Minimally invasive adenocarcinoma
▪ Nonmucinous
▪ Mucinous
– *Preinvasive lesions*:
▪ Atypical adenomatous hyperplasia
▪ Adenocarcinoma *in situ* (formerly called BAC)
• *Squamous cell carcinoma*:
– Keratinizing, nonkeratinizing, basaloid
– Preinvasive lesion
▪ Squamous cell carcinoma *in situ*
• *Neuroendocrine tumors*:
– Small cell carcinoma
– Large cell neuroendocrine carcinoma
– *Carcinoid tumors*:
▪ Typical carcinoid tumor
▪ Atypical carcinoid tumor
– *Preinvasive lesion*:
▪ Diffuse idiopathic pulmonary neuroendocrine cell hyperplasia (DIPNECH)
• Large cell carcinoma
• Adenosquamous carcinoma
• *Sarcomatoid carcinomas*:
– Pleomorphic carcinoma
– Spindle cell carcinoma
– Giant cell carcinoma
– Carcinosarcoma
– Pulmonary blastoma
• *Other and unclassified carcinomas*:
– Lymphoepithelioma-like carcinoma
– NUT carcinoma
• *Salivary gland-type tumors*:
– Mucoepidermoid carcinoma
– Adenoid cystic carcinoma
– Epithelial-myoepithelial carcinoma
– Pleomorphic adenoma
• *Papillomas*:
– Squamous
– Glandular
– Mixed
• *Adenomas*:
– Sclerosing pneumocytoma
– Alveolar adenoma
– Papillary adenoma
– Mucinous cystadenoma
– Mucous gland adenoma

Continued

Continued

Mesenchymal tumors
• Pulmonary hamartoma
• Chondroma
• PEComatous tumors
• Lymphangioleiomyomatosis
• Congenital peribronchial myofibroblastic tumor
• Diffuse pulmonary lymphangiomatosis
Inflammatory myofibroblastic tumor
Epithelioid hemangioendothelioma
Pleuropulmonary blastoma
Synovial sarcoma
Pulmonary artery intimal sarcoma
Lymphohistiocytic tumors
Extranodal MALT lymphoma
Diffuse large cell lymphoma
Lymphomatoid granulomatosis
Pulmonary Langerhans cell histiocytosis
Erdheim–Chester disease
Tumors of ectopic origin
Germ cell tumors (Teratoma)
Intrapulmonary thymoma
Melanoma
Meningioma NOS
Metastatic tumors

Source: This table is reproduced from the 2015 WHO Classification by Travis et al.[5]

IMAGING MODALITIES

Conventional chest radiography and cross-sectional imaging techniques such as computed tomography (CT), magnetic resonance imaging (MRI) and PET-CT play a role in the detection, diagnosis, and management of pulmonary parenchymal neoplasms. Ultrasonography(US) including CEUS has specific utility in guided sampling of the peripheral based lung tumors.[6]

Chest radiography (PA view) is the primary modality for *detection* of the lung cancer **(Fig. 1A)**.[7] Any solitary pulmonary nodule (rounded opacity <3 cm) or mass (opacity > 3 cm with any shape/margins) in an adult may be a lung cancer unless it is proved otherwise.

CT is more accurate for detection of abnormality and it is a modality of choice for characterization of pulmonary neoplasms.[7] CT forms an integral imaging technique for staging the lung cancers. Advanced CT techniques such as dynamic perfusion CT,[8] dual energy CT[9] and dual-energy spectral CT imaging[10] as well as software based texture analysis[11] are new methods under evaluation for the characterization of lung tumors and help in distinguishing benign from malignant lesions. A routine CT protocol for the evaluation of suspected lung cancer should consist of a contrast-enhanced CT (CECT) of chest and upper abdomen including liver and adrenals.

PET provides functional information and hence it is generally more precise for overall evaluation of the disease extent. PET is not useful in T staging as its resolution is inferior and CECT is sufficient for this purpose. FDG uptake is also variable in tumors like invasive mucinous adenocarcinoma, carcinoid and small cell lung cancer and this may result in high false negative results on PET.[12,13] Conversely, false positive results may be seen in benign conditions like tuberculosis and sarcoidosis.[14]

PET is recommended as a single test for comprehensive preoperative evaluation of local and distant disease spread, with overall staging accuracy of more than 90%.[15] It is especially useful for mediastinal lymph node staging, differentiating benign from malignant pleural effusions[16] and detection of bone metastases.[17] In some patients, inflammatory lymph nodes may show PET uptake and cause false positive PET results. Similarly, because of the resolution issue, lymph nodes smaller than 5 mm cannot be reliably evaluated on PETCT.[18]

PET is also useful in monitoring of patients undergoing nonsurgical management. Modern conformal radiotherapy techniques require accurate delineation of the tumor volume for the treatment plans. PET-CT is now preferred for radiotherapy planning as it can differentiate the viable tumor from adjacent necrotic tissues or consolidations and hence, more accurate than CT based planning.[19] This characteristic of PETCT is also useful for planning image guided biopsies from viable area of the tumor.

For the assessment of response to chemotherapy, SUV monitoring is also more accurate and correlates better with patient survival than the RESIST size criteria used for conventional imaging techniques.[20] PET-CT is also useful to detect recurrences in treated patients, as it is more accurate in differentiating post-treatment changes from recurrences. However, radiation changes can sometimes show FDG uptake. To avoid false positive results, PET should be deferred until six months after the radiotherapy.

Magnetic Resonance Imaging[21]

Owing to the recent advances made in overcoming the challenges in MR acquisition of lung, current status of MRI is increasing in detection, characterization of pulmonary nodules, TNM staging and tumor response assessments. DWI as well as dynamic contrast-enhanced MRI have shown to be useful in distinguishing benign and malignant lung nodules. Using a cutoff ADC value of 1.1×10^{-3} mm^2/s, a sensitivity of 70% and specificity of 97% using a b value of 1000 s/mm^2 was seen in one study.[22] DWI can be used for early assessment of tumor response post chemotherapy **(Figs. 1B to E).**

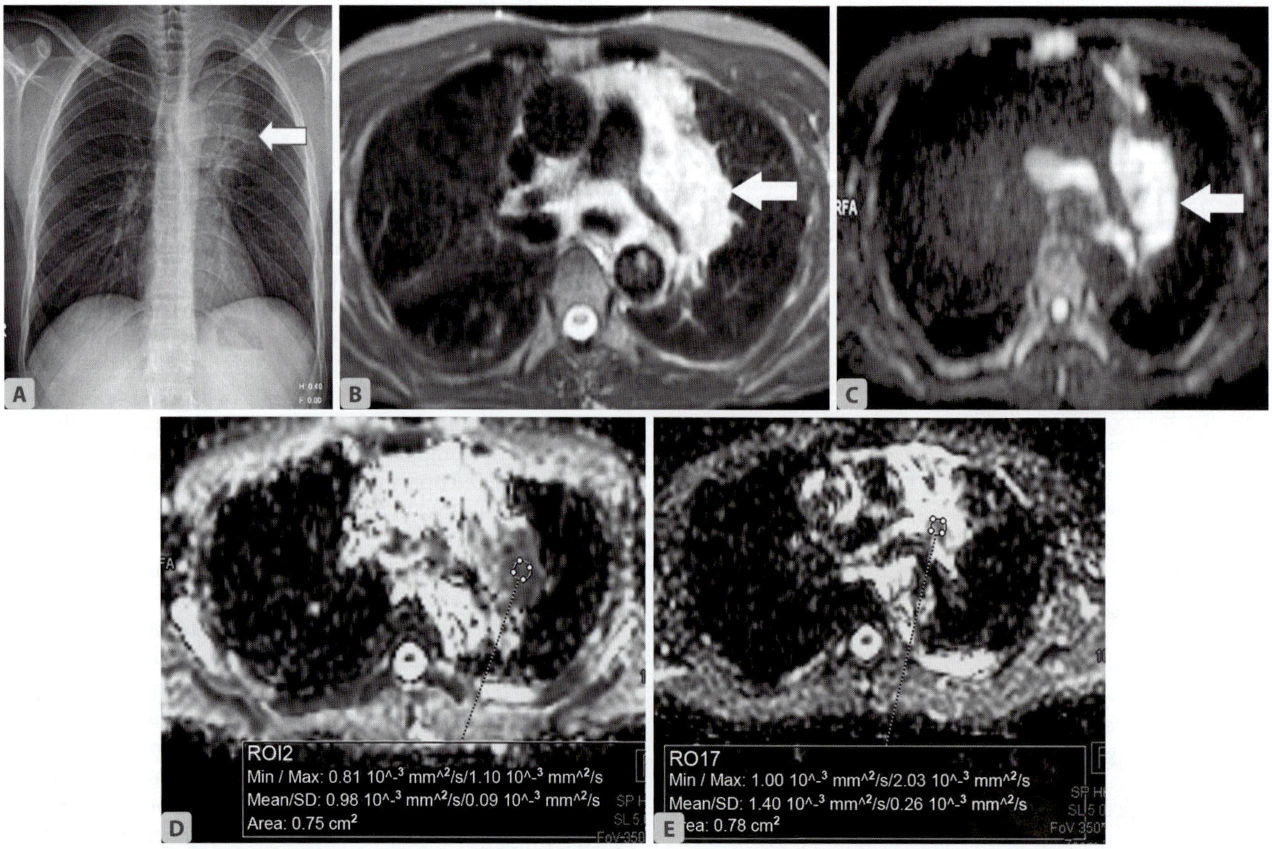

FIGS. 1A TO E: Diffusion weighted MRI in carcinoma lung. (A) Frontal chest radiograph showing mass in the left upper lobe extending in region of aortopulmonary window in a case of adenocarcinoma; (B) STIR axial image shows hyperintense mass in left upper lobe with mediastinal invasion; (C) Prechemotherapy DWI at b-1000 value, shows hyperintense signal in the region of mass with hypointense signal on corresponding ADC map; (D) ADC map shows a value of 0.98×10^{-3} mm^2/s suggestive of restricted diffusion; (E) Post-chemotherapy there is reduction in the size of the tumor with increase in the ADC value suggestive of good response to chemotherapy.

Similarly, there are various dynamic MRI techniques for distinguishing malignant nodules from benign nodules, with reported sensitivities ranging from 94% to 100%, specificities from 70% to 96%, and accuracies >88%.[23,24] MRI useful for brachial plexus involvement in superior sulcus tumors and assessment of chest wall, diaphragmatic pleura, great vessel and cardiac involvement.

IMAGING FEATURES

Imaging features of the lung cancer are discussed under following headings: Peripheral tumors and central tumors.

Peripheral Tumors

Peripheral tumors are those arising beyond the segmental bronchi. Most commonly presents as nodule or mass with following characteristics.

Shape: Majority are spherical or oval in shape **(Fig. 2A)**. Superior sulcus tumors may resemble apical pleural thickening **(Fig. 2B)**.

Margins: May be well defined or ill defined. Uneven rate of growth in different parts of the tumor may produce lobulations **(Fig. 3A)**. One or more strands may be seen extending from the main mass into surrounding lung giving rise to spiculated appearance which is termed as 'corona radiata' **(Fig. 3A)**. Spiculations represent either tumor extension or desmoplastic reaction to the tumor. Spiculated margin is a useful sign to differentiate lung cancer from benign pulmonary nodules, although it may be rarely seen in granuloma and organizing pneumonia as well. A sharply defined spherical smooth edged nodule due to a carcinoma is rare. Sometimes, one or more linear strands may extend from a peripheral mass to the pleura known as 'pleural tail' **(Fig. 3B)**. It can be seen in both benign and malignant

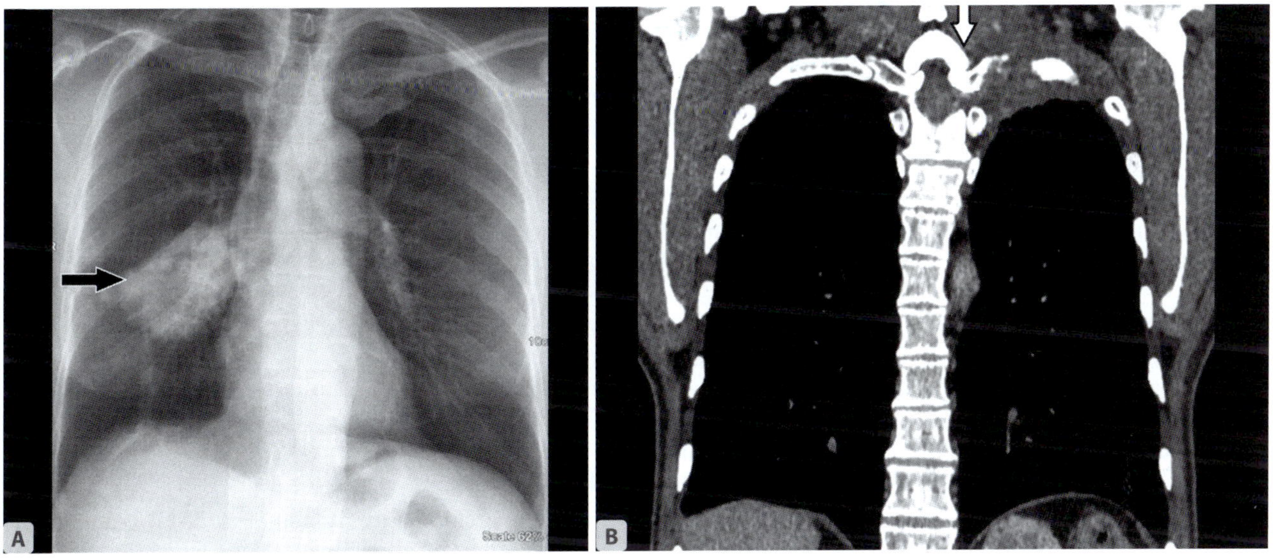

FIGS. 2A AND B: (A) Frontal chest radiograph showing an oval-shaped mass (black arrow) in right parahilar location in a case of squamous cell carcinoma; (B) Coronal CT image showing plaque-like thickening in the left apical region with adjacent rib erosion (white arrow) suggestive of superior sulcus tumor.

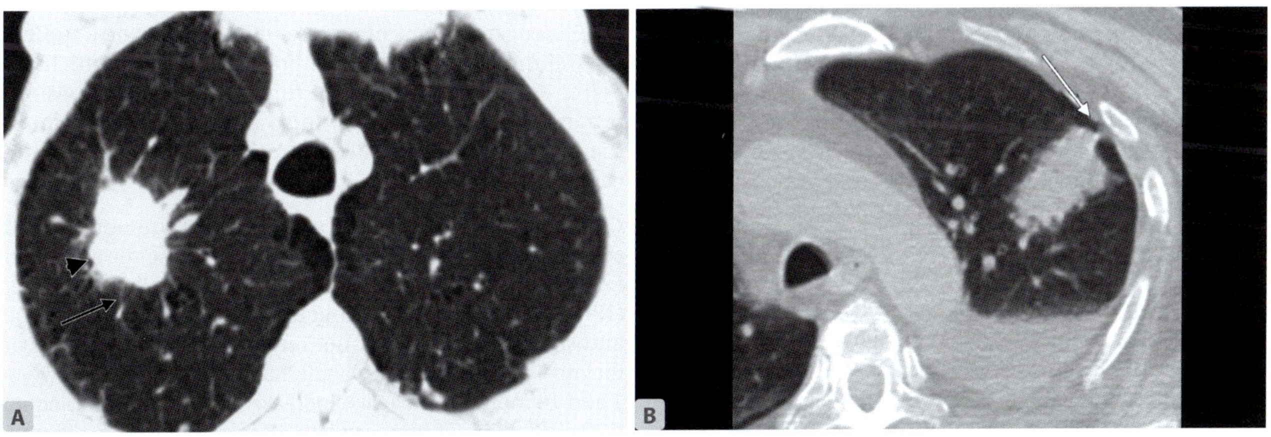

FIGS. 3A AND B: Corona radiata. (A) Axial CT image in a case of adenocarcinoma showing mass with multiple spiculations (arrow) as well as lobulations (arrowhead); (B) A small pleural tail is seen extending from the mass to pleura (arrow).

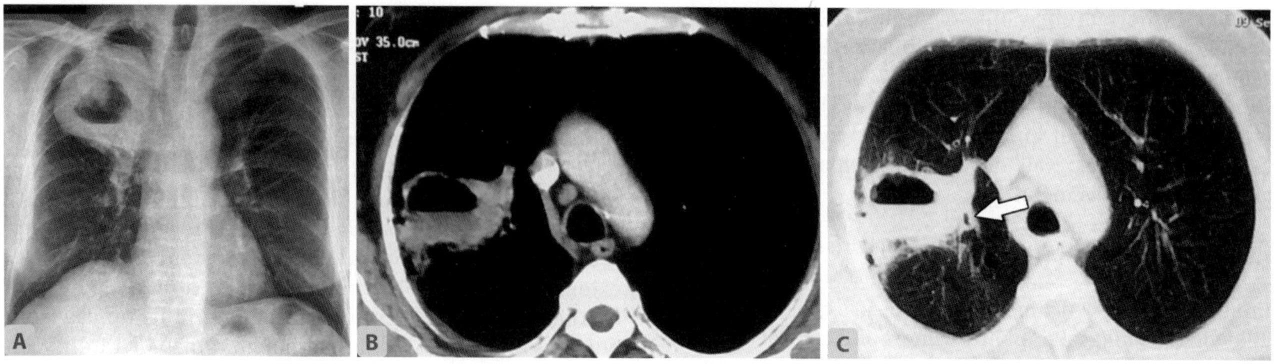

FIGS. 4A TO C: Squamous cell carcinoma. (A) Chest radiograph shows large cavitary lesion in right upper lobe with thick nodular walls and an air-fluid level; (B and C) CT scan of same patient shows right upper lobe cavity with irregular and nodular enhancing wall thickening with air fluid level. There is abrupt cutoff of bronchus at the tumor margin (arrow).

lesions and hence is not helpful in differentiating between the two.

Cavitation: Best seen on CT. Most commonly seen in squamous cell carcinoma histology, however may be seen in any type of lung cancer. The wall of the cavity is usually >8 mm thick, may be smooth or more commonly is irregular and nodular **(Figs. 4A to C)**. Fluid levels may be seen within the cavity. It develops due to central necrosis, liquifection and emptying of the contents in the airways. Rarely, the cavity is seen as an air crescent, similar to the fungal ball. This appearance is caused by the air around an intracavitary tumor.

Calcification: Calcifications are rarely seen in lung cancers on chest radiographs; however, CT may demonstrate it in 6–10% patients.[25] These represent either preexisting granulomatous calcifications engulfed by the tumor or dystrophic calcifications developed in the areas of tumor necrosis. The dystrophic tumor calcification is usually amorphous **(Fig. 5)** or cloudy in appearance and located centrally while engulfed calcifications tend to be located at the periphery of the tumor. Tumor calcification may be seen in any type of bronchogenic carcinoma and there is no predilection for any specific histological subtype.[26]

Consolidation pattern: Atypical presentation can be tumors with entirely ill-defined margins resembling consolidation/pneumonia on chest radiographs **(Figs. 6A and B)**, e.g. lepidic predominant adenocarcinoma [formally called bronchiolo-alveolar carcinoma (BAC)], invasive mucinous adenocarcinoma (formally called mucinous BAC). Persistent or recurrent consolidation at same site, air bronchograms, bubble-like lucencies or pseudocavitation, expansion of the consolidated lobe, Golden S sign, dilated fluid-filled bronchi are the features on CT/CXR suspicious of malignancy.

Ground-glass attenuation nodule: A feature of adenocarcinoma in situ, atypical adenomatous hyperplasia or minimally invasive adenocarcinoma which may present as pure ground-glass nodule **(Fig. 6C)** or part solid nodule and these tend to be slow growing tumors with better prognosis.[27] GGO surrounding a solid tumor may represent hemorrhage or inflammation or edema.

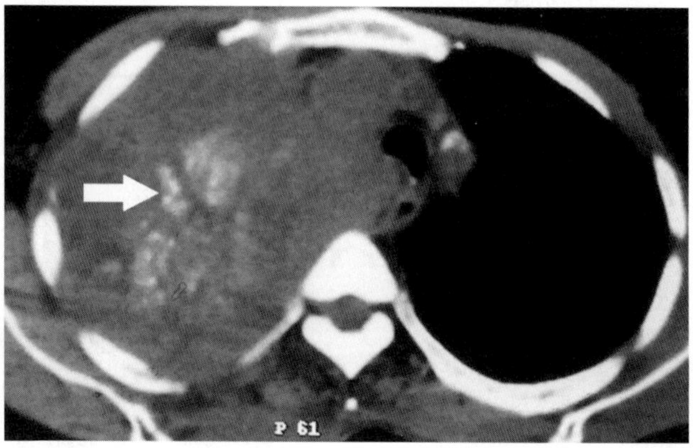

FIG. 5: Calcifications in lung cancer: NCCT shows large lung mass with fine, amorphous tumoral calcifications in a case of squamous cell carcinoma.

Other Findings

Bronchial carcinoma in segmental or distal bronchi may cause retention of mucoid secretions which is known as bronchocele or mucocele. On chest radiographs, these appear as tubular/oval densities with their stem pointing towards the hilum.

An abrupt cutoff of the bronchus at the tumor margin is highly suggestive of squamous cell carcinoma **(Fig. 4C)**.

Pancoast tumors may present as asymmetric apical pleural thickening with or without rib erosions which are better delineated on CT. Old tubercular fibrosis does not predispose to lung cancer. In so called scar carcinomas, the fibrous reaction follows, rather than precedes the carcinoma.

Growth rate: The round or oval shape of the opacity and slow growth on serial radiographs should raise the suspicion for malignancy. Growth rate of non-small cell lung cancer (NSCLC) is highly variable and related to histological subtype and smoking history, but not the presence of symptoms at diagnosis.[28] Lung cancers usually have doubling time between 1 and 18 months and a 26% increase in the diameter is equal to the doubling of tumor volume. Most lung cancers double in volume in 4 to 8 months, however, invasive mucinous adenocarcinomas tend to grow more slowly, and may even

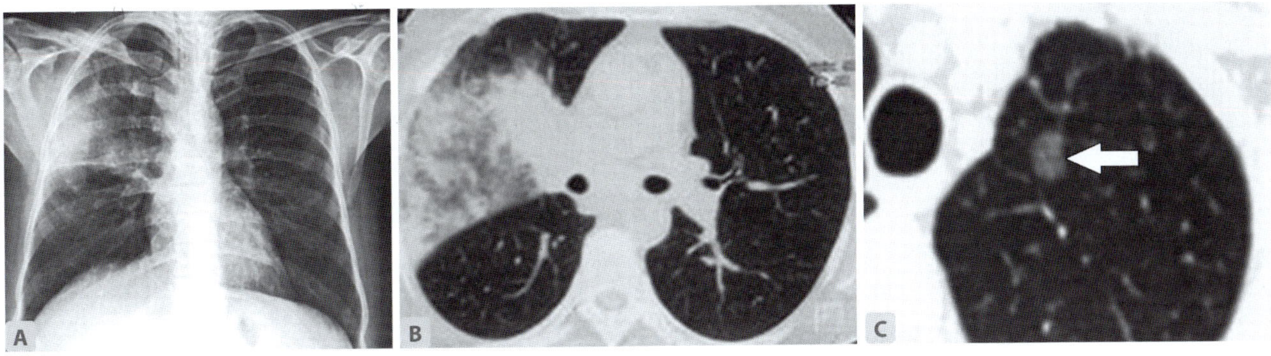

FIGS. 6A TO C: Lung cancer seen as non-resolving pneumonia. (A) Chest radiograph shows an airspace opacity in right upper lobe; (B) Corresponding CT shows consolidation and ground-glass opacity in right upper lobe. Endobronchial biopsy confirmed lepidic predominant adenocarcinoma; (C) Adenocarcinoma in situ presenting as focal ground-glass nodule in a different patient.

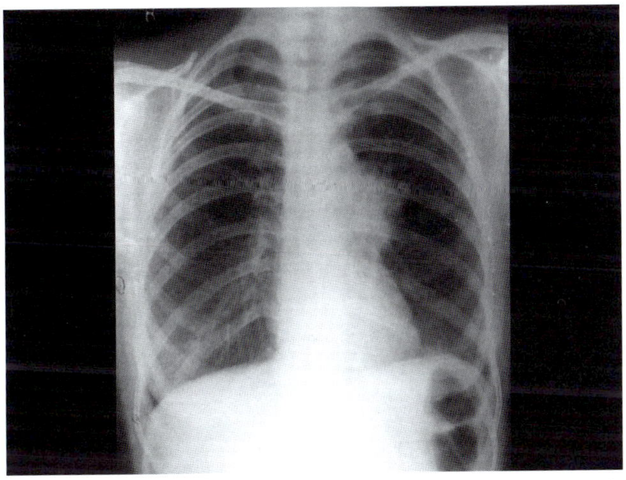

FIG. 7: Central lung cancer: Frontal chest radiograph shows increased density and enlargement of left hilum. Associated elevation of left hemidiaphragm is suggestive of mediastinal invasion and phrenic nerve palsy.

metastasize. Significant growth may be detected in as early as 2 months in smokers.

Central Tumors

Chest Radiograph Findings

Hilar enlargement: The cardinal imaging finding of a central tumor on chest radiograph is presence of hilar enlargement with or without distal collapse/consolidation of the lung. The hilar enlargement may be due to central tumor itself, enlarged lymph nodes, consolidation or combination of these **(Fig. 7)**.

Dense hilum sign: Sometimes, a small mass overlying the hilum may produce only an asymmetrically increased density of the hilum and this should raise a suspicion of tumor and a CECT is indicated.

Distal collapse: It is seen as homogeneous pulmonary opacity with volume loss, confined to one lobe. Air bronchogram however, is usually absent **(Figs. 8A to D)**. Displacement of the fissure towards the collapsed lung. 'Golden S sign' in right upper lobe collapse occurs due to central mass limiting the expected movement of the fissure and hence the medial aspect of fissure shows bulging contour. If there is retention of mucous in the collapsed lung bronchi, it may not lead to volume loss and rather an enlarged lobe 'drowned lung' may be visualized.

Consolidation: Inhomogeneous opacity persistent or recurrent in same lobe should raise a suspicion of central obstructing mass.

CECT Findings

Central lung cancers are seen as minimally enhancing soft tissue masses whereas distal collapse shows significant enhancement. Distended fluid filled bronchi may be seen as fluid bronchogram within the enhancing collapsed lung distal to the mass. Such an appearance should prompt a bronchoscopy, even when tumor is not visualized on CT. Delineation of the tumor separately from distal collapse consolidation cannot always be made on CT **(Figs. 8B and C)**. This may pose a difficulty in the confident initial diagnosis of lung cancer on CT. PETCT can demonstrate the central mass with FDG uptake separate from collapse. Accurate tumor delineation is an important requirement for radiotherapy planning. Dynamic perfusion CT can help distinguishing between tumor mass and collapsed lung as well as demonstrate viable tumor tissue separate from necrotic non-viable area, thereby guiding proper CT guided needle placement for biopsy **(Figs. 9A to D)**.

RADIOLOGICAL CHARACTERISTICS BY CELL TYPE

Amongst the common subtypes of the lung cancers, adenocarcinoma accounts for 38.5% of the cases, squamous cell carcinoma 20%, small cell carcinoma 15% and large cell carcinoma 2.9% of cases.[29]

Adenocarcinoma

Adenocarcinomas are typically peripherally located tumor. These can either present as a localized ground-glass opacity or as solid nodule or mass. They are usually less than

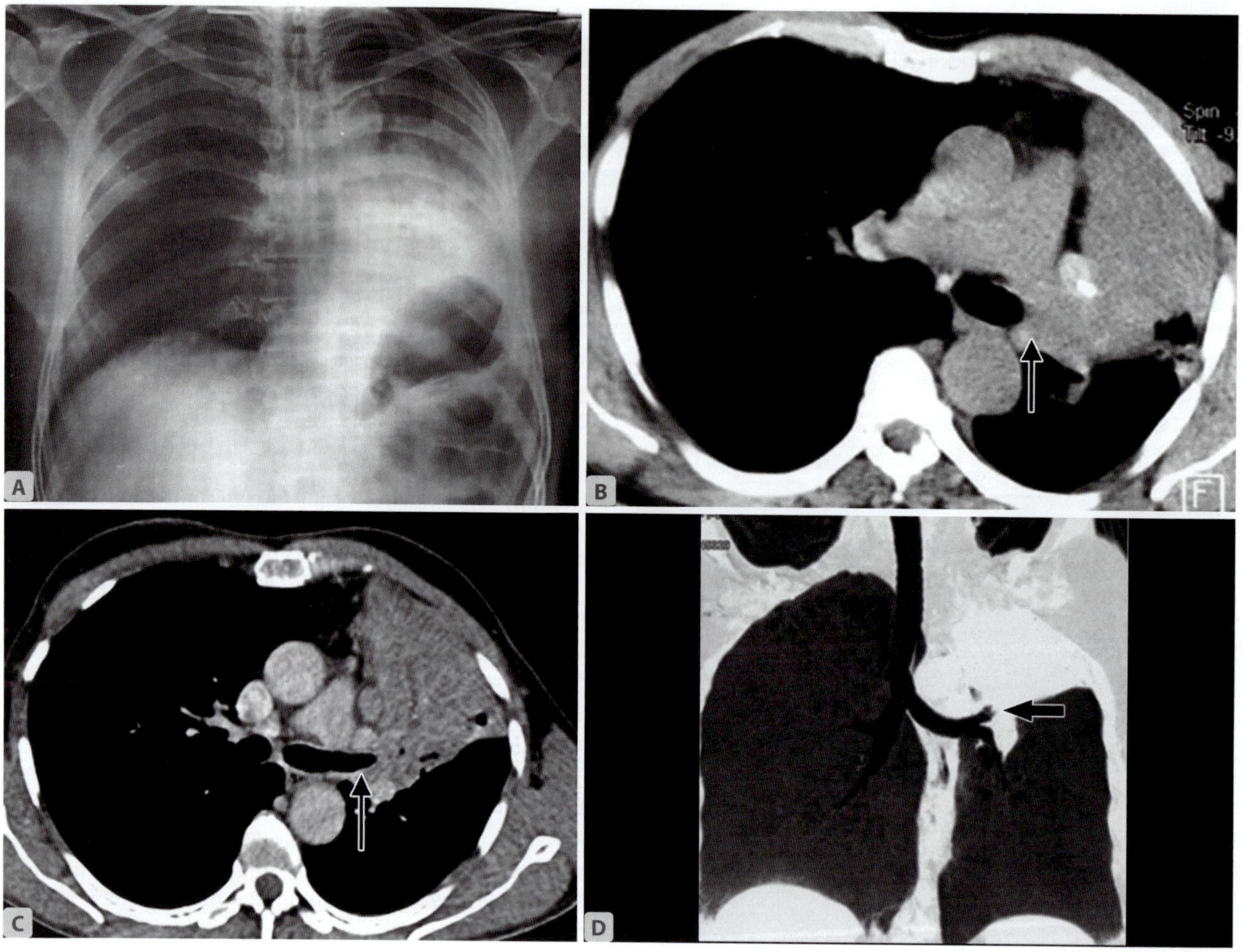

FIGS. 8A TO D: Central lung cancer with lobar collapse. (A) Chest radiograph shows signs of collapse of the left upper lobe with ipsilateral mediastinal shift; (B) Corresponding CT shows ill-defined mass occluding the left upper lobe bronchus (arrow) with distal collapsed lung. Endobronchial biopsy revealed squamous cell carcinoma; (C) CT scan of another patient showing cutoff of left upper lobe bronchus (arrow), left upper lobe collapse with no identifiable tumor. Bronchoscopy and biopsy confirmed squamous cell carcinoma; (D) Minimum intensity projection image in same patient, shows cutoff of the bronchus (arrow).

4 cm in diameter and cavitation is rare (seen in only 4–6% lesions).[30] Adenocarcinomas are frequently associated with enlarged hilar and mediastinal lymph nodes, though not as massive as seen in small cell carcinomas. Pleural effusion is a feature of adenocarcinoma.

Invasive mucinous adenocarcinoma: Formally known as mucinous bronchioloalveolar carcinoma (BAC). It may present as a peripheral single pulmonary nodule/mass or multicentric or diffuse disease **(Figs. 10A and B)** or a localized parenchymal consolidation form in decreasing order of incidence. Characteristic bubble-like lucencies can be identified on CT within the mass.[30] Sometimes, air bronchograms and cavitation may also be seen. Hilar and mediastinal lymphadenopathy is uncommon.

Squamous Cell Carcinoma

These are more often centrally located within the lung and may attain greater size. Cavitation is seen in up to 82% cases.[30] Being central obstructive lesions, these tumors frequently produce segmental or lobar lung collapse **(Figs. 8B and C)**.

Small Cell Lung Cancer

This tumor is characterized by a high growth fraction and rapid doubling time. It represents the most malignant form of the neuroendocrine carcinomas of the lung. It is associated with poor prognosis as 60–70% of patients present with metastatic disease at the time of diagnosis.[31] These tumors most often present with massive enlarged mediastinal or hilar lymphadenopathy **(Figs. 11A and B)**. A large noncontiguous centrally located mass can be seen within the lung parenchyma and it rarely cavitates. Mediastinal invasion is common and seen in upto 68 % of cases[31] on CT. Sometimes only conglomerate mediastinal nodal mass may be present without detection of primary lung tumor.

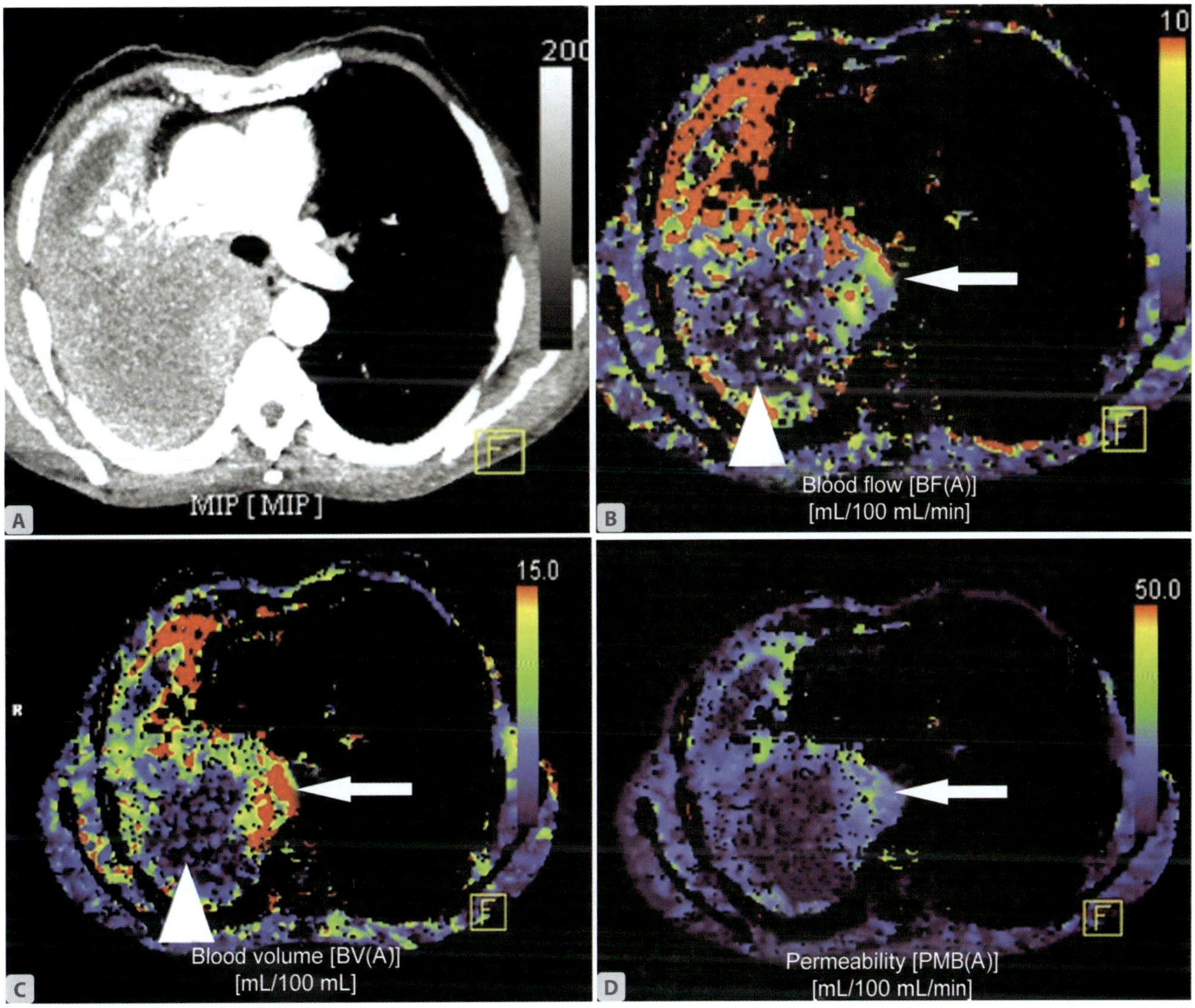

FIGS. 9A TO D: Dynamic perfusion CT lung. (A) MIP CT image shows heterogeneous mass in right lung and viable tumor tissue could not be confidently identified. CT perfusion blood flow color coded image (B) and blood volume image (C) shows increased blood flow and blood volume (areas depicted in red/yellow color) in the medial aspect of the mass suggestive of viable tumor tissue (white arrows). Minimal blood flow and volume in the central and lateral aspect of the mass suggesting necrosis (arrowhead); (D) Permeability image shows mildly increased permeability in medial aspect of the mass (arrow). CT-guided biopsy revealed adenocarcinoma.

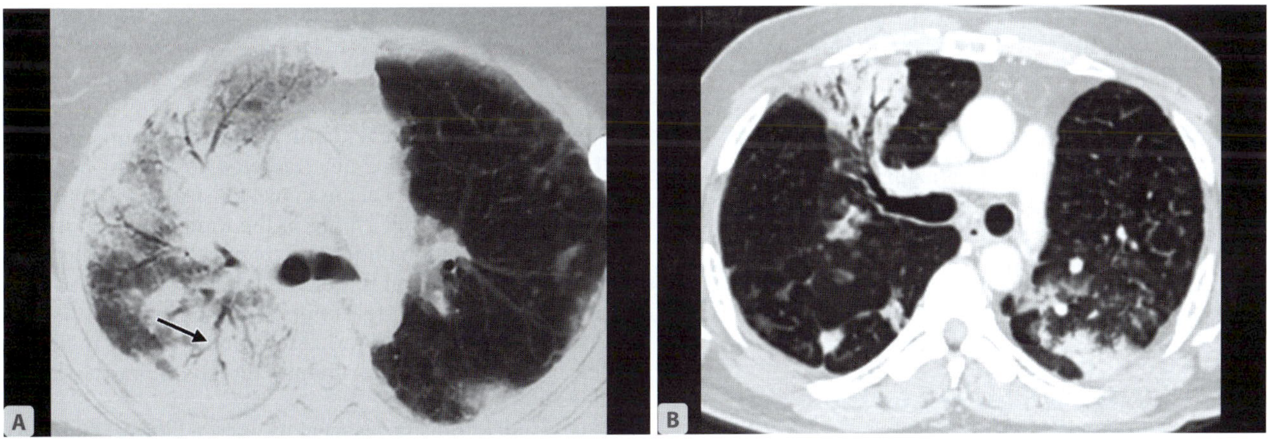

FIGS. 10A AND B: Invasive mucinous adenocarcinoma (formally known as invasive bronchoalveolar carcinoma). (A) CT shows pneumonic form of the cancer with extensive airspace opacities with characteristic stretching and narrowing of the bronchi (arrow) due to mass effect of the tumor; (B) Another patient showing multicentric pattern of disease.

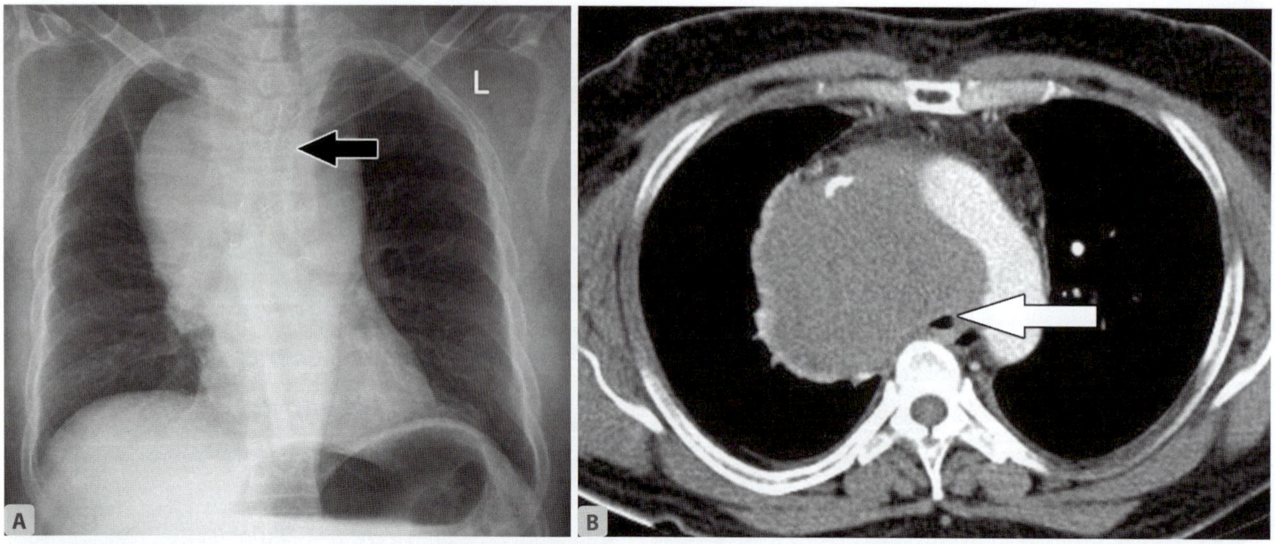

FIGS. 11A AND B: Small-cell carcinoma presenting as mediastinal mass. (A) Chest radiograph showing large mediastinal mass. A tracheal stent is seen as the mass was causing severe narrowing of the tracheal lumen; (B) Preprocedural CT shows large mediastinal lymphadenopathy with compression of SVC and trachea (arrow). No separate mass could be identified within the lungs.

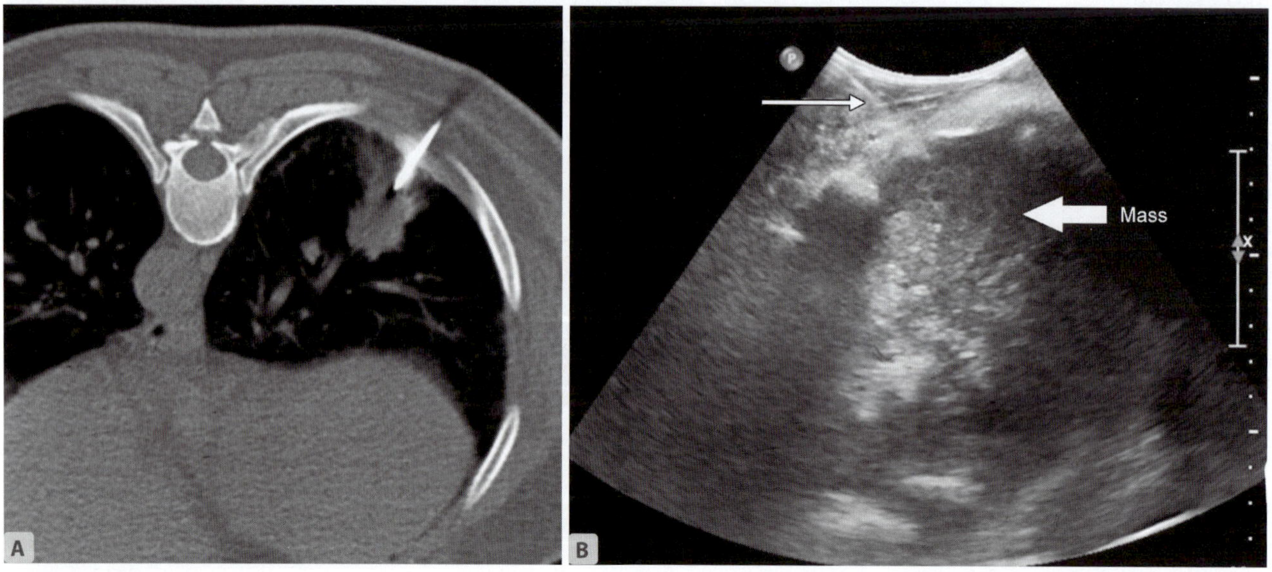

FIGS. 12A AND B: CT and USG guided biopsy of lung mass. (A) Prone CT image showing a coaxial needle in situ within a peripheral lung mass through which multiple biopsy cores were taken which revealed adenocarcinoma; (B) USG image of a large peripheral lung mass showing needle advanced through intercostal space (thin arrow) within the mass (thick arrow). Biopsy revealed squamous cell carcinoma.

Large Cell Carcinoma

It is a poorly differentiated non small cell carcinoma and is diagnosed in the absence of histopathologic features for adenocarcinoma or squamous cell carcinoma and presence of a large cell morphology. These are high grade tumors with rapid growth rate and tend to metastasize early to the mediastinum and brain.

SAMPLING FOR SUSPECTED LUNG CANCER

In a suspected lung cancer, if patient is producing sputum, the cytology assessment can often establish the diagnosis of malignancy. However, since the inception of 2015 WHO classification and new targeted treatment options, immunohistochemistry of the small biopsies or even cytology is indicated for further typing of the tumor. Bronchoscopy is used for evaluation and biopsy of most lung cancers. It is most useful for central tumors and diagnostic yield ranges from 81–90% for visible tumors.[32] Peripheral lesions can also be sampled using indirect bronchoscopic methods such as lavage, brushes, biopsy forceps or radial EBUS guided biopsy.[33]

CT-guided transthoracic FNAC or core biopsy **(Fig. 12A)** is accurate for the tumors not amenable to bronchoscopic visualization. However, non-diagnostic or nonspecific benign results are not reliable and repeat biopsy must be performed in these situations. Major complications include pneumothorax, hemotharax, hemoptysis, infection and air embolism. Peripheral lung tumors can be accessed under ultrasound guidance **(Fig. 12B)** and in case of necrotic tumors, a contrast enhance ultrasound may be used to differentiate between active areas and nonviable areas before sampling thereby increasing the accuracy of core needle biopsy.[6] CT or ultrasound guided biopsies are useful to obtain samples from metastatic sites of the lung cancer. In some patients with resectable disease on imaging, preoperative lymph node staging may be performed with mediastinoscopy and lymph node sampling and sometimes, with endoscopic or endobronchial ultrasound guided FNAC of mediastinal lymph nodes. Pleural effusions require thoracocentesis to determine if these are malignant. Video assisted thoracoscopic surgery (VATS) is frequently used for diagnosis, staging and occasionally, resection of the lung cancer.

STAGING OF LUNG CANCER

The TNM system remains the best prognosticator of lung cancer outcome and guides the treatment strategies. The 8th edition of Union for International Cancer Control and the American Joint Committee on Cancer (UICC/AJCC) TNM staging system of lung cancer[34] is recently published in January 2017 based on the recommendations of International Association for Study of Lung cancer (IASCL) **(Tables 2 and 3)**. This system is used to stage NSCLC, SCLC and bronchial carcinoids.

Imaging Modalities for the Staging of Lung Cancers

Chest radiographs and thin section CECT of the thorax and upper abdomen including liver and adrenals as well as supraclavicular areas are the basic imaging required for staging of the lung cancer. Multiplanar reconstructions are essential for the assessment of relationship of tumor with the fissure, adjacent cardiovascular structures and exact localization prior to surgery. CT is the primary modality to assess the resectability of the tumor and for assessing the treatment options. However, the accuracy of the CT staging is poor when compared with surgico-pathological staging.[35] For tumor size measurement, the largest long-axis diameter must be measured using multiplanar reformation. Performance of CT alone for T staging is significantly lower than PET-CT, and precise T stages are provided in 68% and 86% respectively.[36] PET-CT is recommended gold standard for N staging of the lung cancer as CT, though highly sensitive for detection of lymph nodes, has low specificity for lymph node characterization into benign or malignant.[36] Also, CT data should be analyzed in conjunction with other modalities such as bone scan or PETCT for accurate M staging.

TABLE 2: TNM descriptors.

T	Primary tumor
Tx	Cannot be assessed; Tumor in sputum/bronchial washings not in imaging/bronchoscopy
T0	No evidence
Tis	Carcinoma in situ
T1	≤3 cm surrounded by lung/visceral pleura, not involving main bronchus
T1a(mi)	Minimally invasive adenocarcinoma
T1a	≤1 cm
T1b	>1 to ≤2 cm
T1c	>2 to ≤3 cm
T2	>3 to ≤5 cm or Involves main bronchus without carina involvement or Visceral pleural invasion or Atelectasis/postobstructive pneumonitis extending to hilum
T2a	>3 to ≤4 cm
T2b	>4 to ≤5 cm
T3	>5 to ≤7 cm or Separate tumor in same lobe or Direct invasion of chest wall (includes parietal pleura and superior sulcus)/parietal pericardium/phrenic nerve
T4	>7 cm or Separate tumor in different lobe of ipsilateral lung or Invasion of heart/great vessels/diaphragm/ Mediastinum/trachea/carina/esophagus/ recurrent laryngeal nerve/vertebral body
N	Regional lymph node
Nx	Cannot be assessed
N0	No involvement
N1	Ipsilateral peribronchial and/or hilar nodes and intrapulmonary nodes
N2	Ipsilateral mediastinal and/or subcarinal nodes
N3	Contralateral mediastinal or hilar; ipsilateral/contralateral scalene/supraclavicular
M	Distant metastasis
M0	No distant metastasis
M1	Distant metastasis is present
M1a	Tumor (s) in contralateral lung; pleural/ pericardial nodule/malignant effusion
M1b	Single extrathoracic metastasis
M1c	Multiple extrathoracic metastases, in one/more organs

Salient Points

T Staging

- It includes measuring tumor size (largest long-axis diameter), invasion into adjacent structures and identification of satellite/separate nodule.
- It may be difficult to assess exact size of the tumor in presence of a postobstructive atelectasis/pneumonia and such lesion are considered T2.
- T1 and T2 tumors are most amenable for curative surgical resection. Parietal extension (T3) (rib bone

lysis, extrapleural extension) is not a contraindication for surgery and some candidates may benefit from surgical intervention. Though conventionally T4 tumors are unresectable, some cases of T4 tumors may also be eligible for surgery (after a multidisciplinary discussion).[36]

Tracheobronchial Invasion

On CT, the bronchial invasion (T2) or tracheal invasion (T4) is seen as fixed smooth/nodular thickening of their wall. A bronchoscopic correlation is indicated whenever CT detects this finding.

Mediastinal Invasion

- Parietal pericardium/phrenic nerve involvement—T3
- Invasion of heart/great vessels/diaphragm/mediastinum/trachea/carina/esophagus/recurrent laryngeal nerve/vertebral body are categorized under T4.
- On CT/MRI, criteria for vascular invasion include complete circumferential encasement of a vessel **(Figs. 13A and B)** or presence of an intravascular enhancing focus of tumor. Loss of fat planes with the adjacent tissue may not represent actual invasion and such tumors may also be amenable for resection.

TABLE 3: Stage groups.

		N0	N1	N2	N3
	T1a	IA1	IIB	IIIA	IIIB
	T1b	IA2	IIB	IIIA	IIIB
T1M0	T1c	IA3	IIB	IIIA	IIIB
	T2a	IB	IIB	IIIA	IIIB
	T2b	IIA	IIB	IIIA	IIIB
T2M0					
T3M0		IIB	IIIA	IIIB	IIIC
T4M0		IIIA	IIIA	IIIB	IIIC
	M1a	IVA	IVA	IVA	IVA
	M1b	IVA	IVA	IVA	IVA
TxM1	M1c	IVB	IVB	IVB	IVB

- If contact of the mass with the mediastinal vessel is more than 3 cm or more than 90 degree or there is parietal stiffness of the vessels, then it can be suggested as nonresectable; however, these findings needs surgical confirmation and hence a patient should not be deferred surgery on the basis of these imaging findings.
- Involvement of pulmonary veins or left atrium would be seen as hypodense filling defects within the intensely enhancing vessel/atrial chamber and it is categorized into T4 stage.

Pleural Invasion

- Crossing of the fissure by the mass classifies it into T2 **(Fig. 14A)**
- Involvement of parietal pleura makes it T3 lesion
- Distant or non-contiguous nodular pleural thickening—metastatic
- On CT, presence of definite pleural invasion is attributed when there is extension of tumor into the soft tissues beyond the pleura or associated rib bone lysis. Loss of extrapleural fat plane is also a sign of pleural invasion **(Fig. 14B)**. Mere presence of pleural effusion or contact with the pleura are not the signs for pleural invasion and diagnostic pleural fluid aspiration for malignant cytology or VATS guided pleural biopsy should be done to confirm the pleural involvement if it affects the therapy planning.

Chest Wall Invasion

Presence of extrapleural tumor tissue or extension into the ribs confirms the chest wall invasion and these are categorized as T3 lesions **(Figs. 15A and B)**.

MRI and PET-CT may be required for better delineation of chest wall invasion **(Fig. 15C)** as well as in cases of diaphragmatic involvement.

If a pancoast's tumor demonstrates involvement thoracic nerve roots, then it is a T3 stage. If it involves subcalvian vessels, vertebra, shows intraspinal extension **(Fig. 15D)** or involvement of lower cervical nerve roots (C8 and above) or cords of the brachial plexus, then T stage for such tumors would be classified as T4.

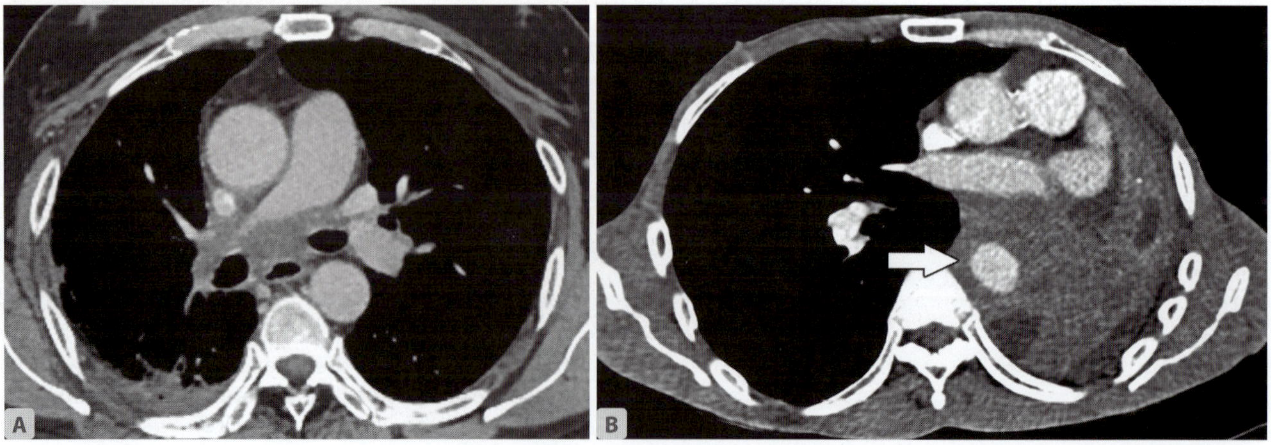

FIGS. 13A AND B: T4 tumors. (A) Central mass causing narrowing and circumferential involvement of right pulmonary artery suggestive of invasion; (B) Large left lung mass with circumferential invasion of aorta (arrow).

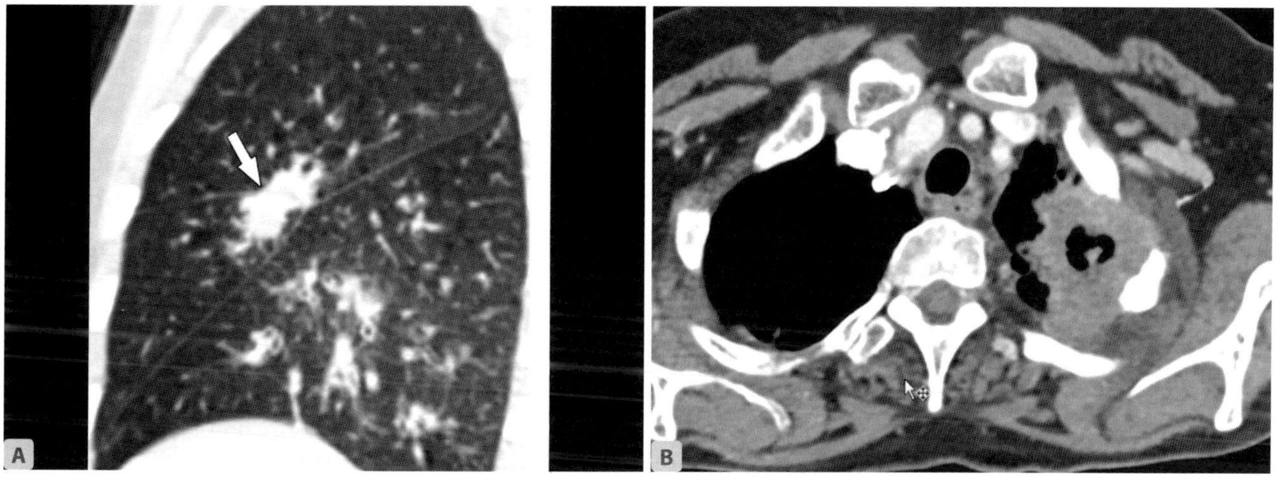

FIGS. 14A AND B: Invasion of fissure. (A) Sagittal CT image shows crossing of the horizontal fissure by a spiculated mass sign of invasion and T2 tumor; (B) Tumor is abutting the pleura with loss of extrapleural fat plane—A sign of chest wall invasion.

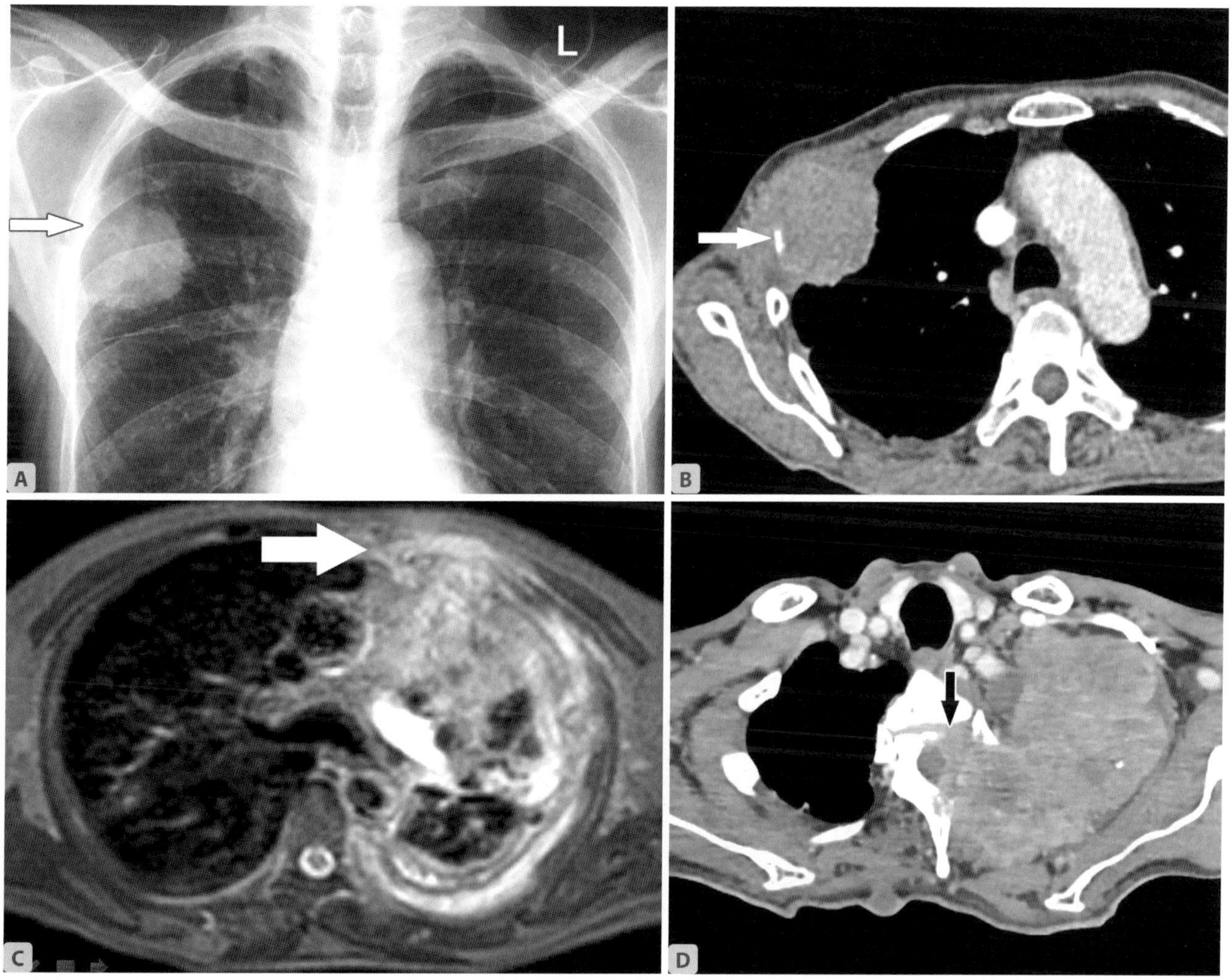

FIGS. 15A TO D: Chest wall invasion. (A) Frontal chest radiograph showing peripheral mass with nonvisualization of anterior end of second and third ribs; (B) CT shows a large right lung mass with contiguous invasion of the chest wall with rib destruction and extrathoracic soft tissue component (arrow); (C) Axial STIR MRI shows extension of the left upper lobe mass into the anterior chest wall muscles infiltrating the deep fibers of pectoralis muscle; (D) Intraspinal extension of left pancoast's tumor makes it T4 lesion.

Satellite Nodules

Tumor with separate nodules in the same lobe is classified as T3.
Tumor with an ipsilateral nodule in another lobe—T4
Tumor with a nodule contralateral to the primary tumor—M1.

CT is highly sensitive to detect the nodules however lacks specificity. However, presence of separate nodule in same lobe as that of tumor is an indicator of poor prognosis and usually represents tumor nodule.

Lymphangitic Carcinomatosis

This finding *has not been addressed* in TNM staging criteria; however it is important to identify this because presence of diffuse or more than one lobe involvement by lymphangitis carcinomatosis (LC) is a contraindication to surgery. Still, if same lobe as that of tumor is affected then it is not a contraindication.

On CT, it appears as nodular peribronchovascular and septal thickening which represents the perilymphatic extension of tumor nodules **(Fig. 16)**.

N Staging

On CECT, a hilar lymph node of more than 7 mm and mediastinal lymph node of more than 10 mm are considered involved. However, some studies have shown 40% normal sized lymph nodes up to 7 mm to be metastatic (such findings more commonly found in adenocarcinomas).

It should be reported according to 1 to 14 mediastinal lymph nodal stations described by IASLC.[37]

PET-CT is the gold standard for N staging with a high negative predictive value (>90%).[36]

M Staging

- *M1a:* Intrathoracic metastasis—pleural or pericardial nodules, contralateral lung nodule, malignant pleural/pericardial effusion **(Fig. 17)**.
- *M1b:* Single metastatic lesion in an extrathoracic organ/ non-regional lymph node.
- *M1c:* Multiple metastasis.

Most common organs involved by metastasis include brain, bones, liver and adrenals **(Fig. 18)**. Liver is most commonly involved in small cell lung cancers and sometimes in cases of diffuse metastasis CT may not demonstrate any nodular lesions. Adrenal incidentalomas and metastasis may not be differentiated based on single phase CT alone and may require further imaging in the form of MRI/PETCT and at times even sampling. On CECT, peripheral irregular enhancement of the nodule with central necrotic area is highly suggestive of adrenal metastasis over an adenoma. CT and PET-CT are adequate in demonstration of the metastatic lesions, and histological confirmation should be done in most of the cases.

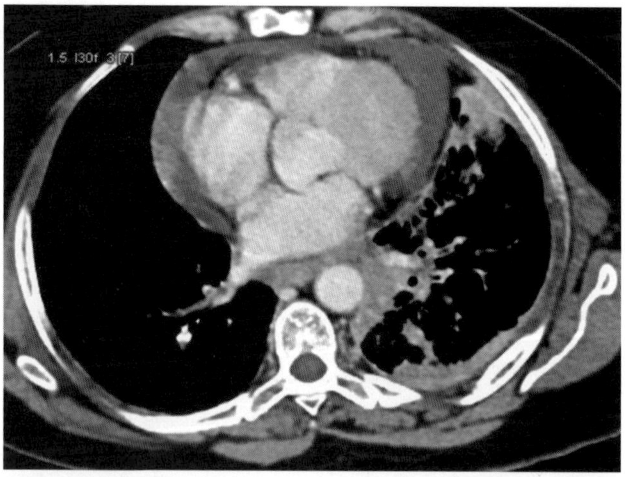

FIG. 17: Malignant pericardial and pleural effusion: CT axial image showing irregular left pleural thickening and mild pericardial effusion in a case of lung adenocarcinoma.

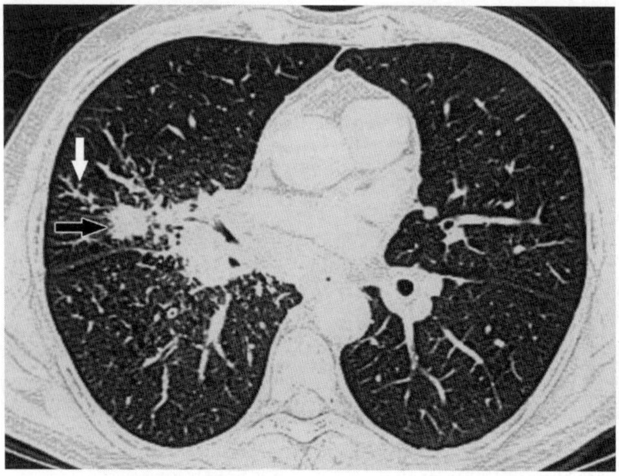

FIG. 16: Lymphangitis carcinomatosis: HRCT image showing a spiculated mass (black arrow) in right parahilar region adjacent peribronchovascular thickening and nodules (white arrow), also extending in right lower lobe.

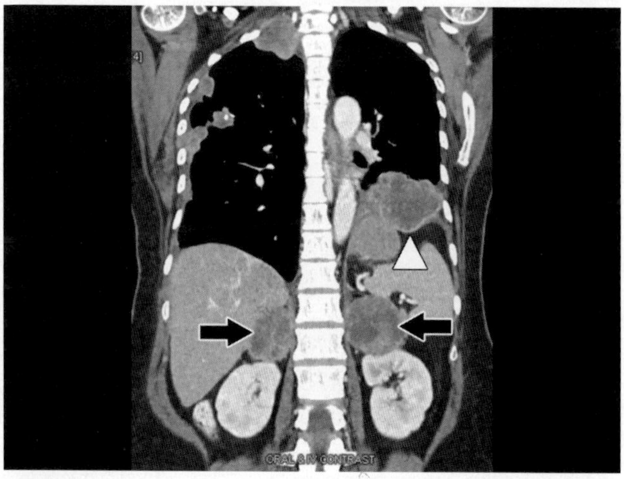

FIG. 18: Adrenal metastasis in disseminated adenocarcinoma lung (right apical tumor). Coronal CT image showing heterogeneous enhancing masses in bilateral suprarenal locations suggestive of adrenal metastasis (arrows). Note is also made of left invasive diaphragmatic metastatic deposit (arrowhead).

The CT report must always contain the TNM staging. If there is doubt about the correct T, N or M category then one should assign a lower category as well as stage.

TREATMENT OF LUNG CANCER

If detected in early stage, surgery remains mainstay of treatment for lung carcinoma in the form of either lobectomy, bilobectomy or pneumonectomy. Well defined lesions, away from fissures and no contiguous organ infiltration are the ideal lesions for surgery. However, tumors near carina, chest wall infiltration, or early mediastinal invasion can also be operated if there is no lymphadenopathy or metastatic lesions. Sleeve resection of tracheobronchial tree, chest wall reconstruction etc. are the adjunctive procedures in addition to primary surgery for such difficult lesions. A vast number of these patients will also be receiving chemo or radiotherapy or both. Involvement of trachea, pulmonary artery, aorta become contraindication for surgery. Hence involvement of these structures should be clearly documented in radiological reports.

Chemotherapy for carcinoma lung is different for different histological type of malignancy (squamous, adeno or small cell etc). The choice of chemotherapeutic agents also vary depending upon the presence or absence of many specific receptors, e.g. epidermal growth factor receptor (EGFR). Main therapeutic agents are cisplatin, etoposide, or gemcitabine, etc.[3] For some large (not disseminated) tumors chemotherapy may shrink the tumor to make it surgically resectable in follow-up period.

Conventionally for the cytotoxic drugs given for treatment of lung malignancies, Response Evaluation Criteria in Solid Tumors (RECIST) criteria are used for evaluating treatment response. It is suggested to read the recent RECIST criteria described by Eisenhauer EA et al.[38] and use this for assessing tumor response. However, for some newer (non-cytotoxic) chemotherapeutic agents the conventional RECIST criteria are not suitable as these drugs don't cause reduction in size. For these drugs newer evaluation criteria are being followed in randomized controlled trials (RCTs) which incorporate other imaging features like decrease in enhancement, increasing necrotic component etc. For such lesions even presence of few new lesions and initial increase in size of lesions are not strictly considered as progressive disease.

Patients with more advanced stage malignancies with invasion of major mediastinal structure or contralateral lymph nodes are usually offered supportive and palliative radiotherapy. There are many newer techniques to deliver radiotherapy in a more focused way to only the diseased area and avoiding adjacent normal lung thereby reducing radiation induced damage to the surrounding organs. These modalities are image guided radiotherapy (IGRT), intensity modulated radiation therapy (IMRT), conformational 3D radiotherapy and respiratory gated 4D CT techniques, etc.[39] Heart, esophagus and spinal cord are few of the more radiosensitive organs which need to be preserved more diligently and hence it is important on the part of the reporting radiologist to clearly define involvement of these structures by the neoplastic lesions so that during RT planning the treating radiotherapist is better equipped to avoid injury to these structures.

Radiofrequency ablation (RFA) is another option for those patients who have limited diseases but surgically unfit due to medical comorbidities.[40-43] Excellent results can be achieved for tumors less than 3–4 cm sizes. The complications of RFA can be pneumothorax, hemoptysis, pleural effusion, lung abscess etc. Another potential use of RFA is for treatment of isolated metastatic lesion in adrenal gland.[44]

SCREENING FOR LUNG CANCER

Screening for lung cancers was started based on the premise that if detected in early stage (stage 1 A) there is high survival rates for 5 years in these patients. In many previous randomized clinical trials (RCTs) which used chest X ray and/or sputum cytology for screening in chronic smokers, there was detection of many early stage cancers, however, there was no proven benefit regarding mortality rates.[45]

More recently many RCTs are going on in US and Europe (e.g. Mayo CT screening project, PLCO (Prostate, Lung, Colorectal and Ovary) and Early Lung Cancer Action Project (ELCAP) using low dose CT protocol (25–30 mAs). As CT is more efficient in detecting smaller nodules as compared to chest X-rays, the likelihood of detection of lung malignancies at earlier stages is more with CT as a screening tool. Few of these studies have evaluated the parameters and concluded that screening with CT for lung malignancies in high risk patient profile (age 55–80 and chronic smokers) provides significant decrease in mortality rates. Many of the societies have recommended that screening should be done in all elderly smokers (55/60 to 80 years) who smoke >30 pack cigarette per year. They have recommended strict criteria regarding definition of nodules, reporting format as well as guidelines for pathological evaluation and the treatment algorithms for such detected lesions in screening programs. The nodules detected during screening are typically smaller in size and represent less advance malignancies. Majority of these lesions will ultimately prove to be benign. High false positivity for these nodules to be cancers is a particular disadvantage. This problem is even more severe in areas with high prevalence of granulomatous diseases, e.g. in India. Careful evaluation of all the characteristics of these screening detected nodules is necessary to reduce the number of unnecessary biopsy or thoractomy. A nodule which is smaller than 10 mm is usually followed and subjected to biopsy when it shows suspicious growth pattern for malignancy. For larger lesions PET and CT guided biopsies are performed.

Till now there is no state sponsored lung screening program in India. This is partly attributed to high prevalence of granulomatous disease (TB) in our country in which imaging findings may mimic early cancers resulting in significant anxiety and resultant more invasive tests to prove the exact nature of these nodules; and partly due to lack of availability of sufficient imaging, pathology as well as surgical services which have got overburdened from various other diseases utilizing the already existing meager health care resources.

FOLLOW-UP IMAGING

Follow-up imaging for lung malignancies is done to detect treatment response. If patient has been treated with surgery and complete resection was feasible, then follow up imaging is done to detect recurrence and metastatic lesions. If patient has been treated with chemotherapeutic agents then follow-up imaging is done to detect early response. This helps in deciding whether to continue with same treatment regime or should change it early to try other regimens. With few newer non-cytotoxic chemotherapeutic agents the clinical question of interest is to find whether there is progression or not. If no progression is there, then the same agent will be continued for further treatment otherwise a decision will be taken to change the agent quite early in course of treatment. Similarly imaging is also done to detect complications due to treatments. If patient is asymptomatic then chest X ray and clinical examination are sufficient. There is no standard protocol to follow these patients on CT, some centers do not prefer any follow up if patient is asymptomatic while other centers prefer every six monthly follow up.[46,47] Other expected changes are pleural thickening , crowding of ribs, ipsilateral mediastinal shift, etc.

Radiologists should be familiar with expected changes in imaging after some treatment. In the initial phase after lobectomy, there is presence of postoperative cavity with air fluid level **(Figs. 19A to C)**. The pneumothorax may be large in initial phase of postoperative time. In due course of time the cavity disappears with absorption of fluid and compensatory hyperinflation of the residual lobes.

Post-radiotherapy changes are seen as acute or chronic changes. In acute radiation pneumonitis there is appearance of ground-glass opacities within three months of completion in the radiation portal area. In chronic phase other changes are seen like consolidation, fibrosis, bronchiectasis or volume loss. The area of involvement shrinks with passage of time. The changes of radiation pneumonitis need to be differentiated from infective etiology. Infections usually conform to lobar or segmental anatomy; on the contrary the radiation changes conforms to the radiation field and may even cross fissures. However, for proper evaluation of these postradiation changes the radiologist should have complete information regarding the radiation field, type of radiation technique used e.g. IGRT, IMRT or conformal RT.[48,49] Small pericardial or pleural effusions are quite common after radiation therapy and they usually develop up to initial 9 months and resolve themselves by 12–16 months.

Other changes seen in post treatment period are drug toxicity and infections both of which may give similar radiological appearance. One of the commonly given drug, Geftinib, causes interstitial pulmonary fibrosis.[50] Almost all chemotherapeutic agents given in patients with NSCLC can cause lung fibrosis. The main imaging findings are ground-glass opacity, fibrosis and interstitial opacities.

RECURRENT LUNG CANCER

In lung cancer patients who have been treated, recurrences are more common at distant site as compared to the loco regional site.[47] The imaging findings in recurrence are usually similar to original tumors. The main imaging features of recurrent lesions are either developing mass or lymphadenopathy. Other features suspicious of recurrence are increasing hydropneumothorax in post-pneumonectomy patients, or appearance of a new air fluid level. Because of significant distortion of normal bronchial anatomy following lobectomy and post radiotherapy fibrotic changes, interpretation of CT examination in these patients become particularly challenging. Still there are few features which make one suspicious of recurrence are, emergence of new pulmonary nodule, or new bronchial stenosis, new or increasing soft tissue at hilum or enlarging mediastinal or hilar lymph nodes.[50] Similarly new appearance of pleural effusion after 6 months of radiotherapy also is a suspicious finding which needs aspiration to exclude recurrent lesion. In the areas of postradiation pneumonitis, new opacification of previously dilated and patent bronchi is also an important clue for recurrence of the disease.[51] When recurrence is suspected, PET is the most sensitive modality to diagnose the recurrence.

RARE LUNG MALIGNANCIES

Other uncommon lung malignancies are sarcomas and pulmonary blastomas. Few of these sarcomas are quite benign in course of disease, e.g. endobronchial fibrosarcoma

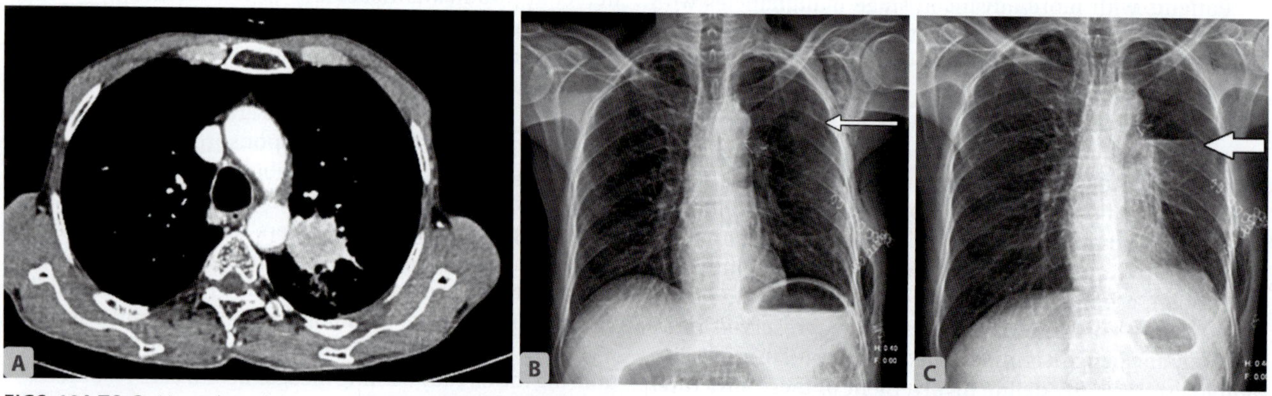

FIGS. 19A TO C: Normal postlobectomy appearance. (A) CT shows a stage IIA lobulated mass for which a left upper lobectomy was done; (B) Chest radiograph shows mild pneumothorax on postoperative day 4; (C) Postoperative day 14 radiograph shows air-fluid level in the pleural cavity in left upper zone which is normal finding after lobectomy.

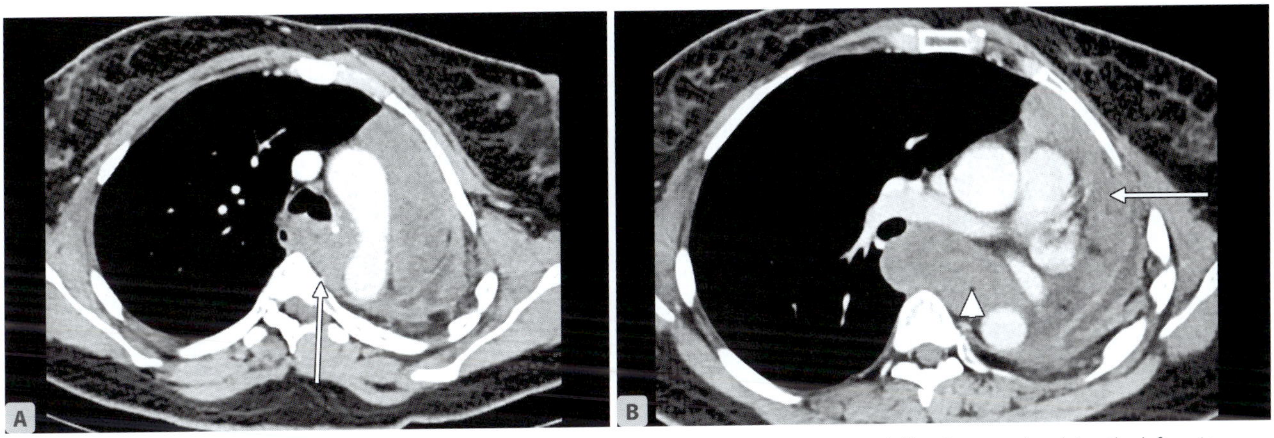

FIGS. 20A AND B: Myxoid sarcoma: Axial CT images of a 34-year-old female showing heterogeneous infiltrating mass involving the left main bronchus (arrowhead) with contiguous mediastinal extension (arrows) and complete collapse of left lung. Endobronchial biopsy was suggestive of myxoid sarcoma.

and leiomyosarcoma. Other sarcomas which are quite aggressive in clinical behavior are rhabdomyosarcoma, osteosarcoma, chondrosarcoma, angiosarcoma and malignant fibrous histiocytoma, myxoid sarcoma, etc **(Figs. 20A and B)**. Sometimes there are sarcomatous component in non-small cell lung carcinoma (NSCLC) which are classified as carcinosarcoma, which have imaging appearance similar to non-small cell lung cancer (NSCLC). Out of these the angiosarcomas have a characteristic enhancement on CT as well as MRI.[52] Kaposi sarcoma are common in AIDS patients which show multiple nodular flame shaped opacities or linear peribronchial opacities . Other findings associated with Kaposi sarcoma are ground-glass opacities secondary to hemorrhage, lymphadenopathy or pleural effusion.[53] Pulmonary blastomas are usually found in children with solid masses having extensive cystic changes. Another separate entity pleuropulmonary blastoma show solid cystic masses which may mimic congenital lung lesion like cystic adenomatoid malformation or sequestration.[54]

Pulmonary blastoma arises from germ cell and classified under carcinosarcoma. These are usually found in children and young adults. On imaging, these are seen as single or multiple peripheral solid lung masses with cystic changes, cavitation and occasionally, calcifications.[55] Pleuropulmonary blastoma is a separate entity seen in early childhood. These arise from primitive blastomatous tissues and develop in pre-existing congenital lung lesions like cystic adenomatoid malformation, sequestration or bronchogenic cysts. On imaging, these are seen as cystic-solid masses.[54]

PULMONARY LYMPHOMA

Primary Pulmonary Lymphoma

Most primary pulmonary lymphomas commonly arises from mucosa-associated lymphoid tissue commonly called MALT lymphoma, comprising up to 90% of cases although it is a fairly rare disease. Rest of the pulmonary lymphomas include diffuse large B-cell non-Hodgkin's lymphoma (NHL) followed by Hodgkin lymphoma (HL) usually from direct extension of mediastinal disease to involve parenchyma.[56,57]

There is lymphangitic spread at the periphery of these lesions leading to invasion of the adjacent pleura, vessels, and airways.[58] Main imaging findings on CT include nodules, masses, and/or nodular/mass like areas of ground-glass attenuation or consolidation (CT angiogram sign) with air bronchograms around bronchovascular distribution, hilar and mediastinal lymphadenopathy. Pleural effusion is uncommonly seen. They appear FDG avid in PET/CT scan in 50% cases. Patients tend to present around the 6th decade former or active smokers and has been associated with multiple autoimmune diseases such as Sjögren syndrome, rheumatoid arthritis, common variable immunodeficiency, concurrent lymphoid interstitial pneumonitis (LIP), chronic inflammation from smoking, and infections such as HIV and hepatitis C.[58,59]

The imaging picture on CT can be mimicked by sarcoidosis as it tends to show peribronchovascular distribution. Similarly polyangiitis (formerly Wegener granulomatosis), perilymphatic spread of metastatic disease and infection showing peribronchial consolidation can mimic MALT lymphoma. Clinical presentation and laboratory parameters can be helpful in narrowing the differential diagnosis.

Diagnosis is made usually by transbronchial, CT-guided percutaneous transthoracic biopsy or at times with a surgical biopsy. Immunohistochemical studies are required for definitive diagnosis to confirm a monoclonal B-cell population, which is positive for pan–B-cell antigens like CD19, CD20 and PAX-5.[5,60]

Treatment is usually with chemotherapy or immunotherapy (rituximab) with options of surgery and radiation therapy for localized disease. MALT lymphoma tends to recur in the lung in up to 50% cases within the first years after diagnosis. Although regional involvement of hilar lymph nodes does not affect prognosis, but presence pleural effusion or amyloid within the tumor signifies poorer prognosis.[57,60]

Secondary Pulmonary Lymphoma (SPL)

All the different forms of lymphoma may secondarily involve the lungs, but the mature B-cell neoplasms are the most

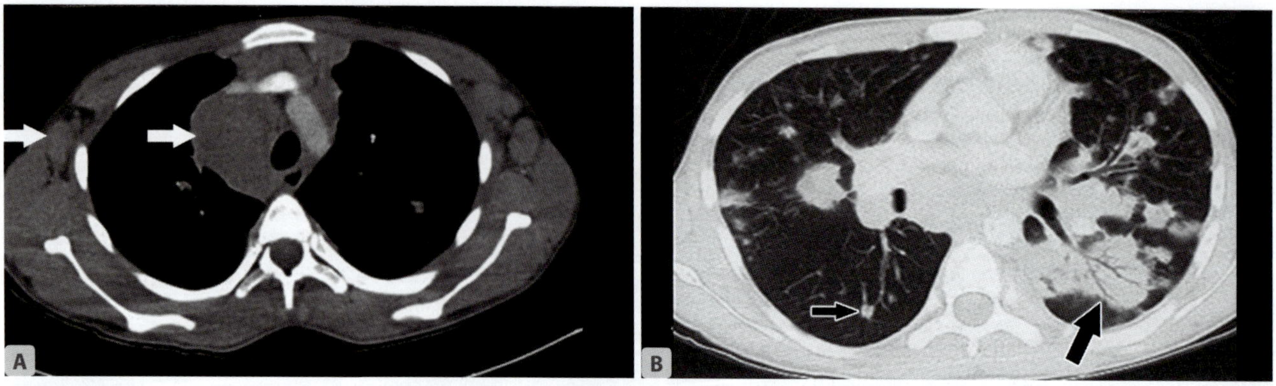

FIGS. 21A AND B: Secondary pulmonary involvement by lymphoma (nodular form). (A) Axial CT image mediastinal window shows homogeneous enlarged lymph nodes in mediastinum and bilateral axillae in a case of non-Hodgkin's lymphoma; (B) Multiple irregular lung nodules with air bronchograms (arrows) are seen in both lungs suggestive of lymphomatous involvement.

frequent. Although a greater proportion of patients with HL rather than NHL have lung involvement, more NHL SPL is seen in clinical practice because NHL is more prevalent. Lymphomatous involvement of the lung itself is often asymptomatic and non-specific. However, B-symptoms of HL more often related to the presence of mediastinal lymphadenopathy.

Imaging findings are varied and nonspecific and include nodules <1 cm in diameter, solitary or multiple, mass/mass-like consolidation, bronchovascular thickening mimicking lymphangitis carcinomatosa, air bronchograms (NHL > HL) **(Figs. 21A and B)**. Mediastinal lymphadenopathy with nodules/masses with or without air bronchograms are the commonest HRCT features.[61,62] In HL, there is contiguous spread of the disease from the adenopathy to involve parenchyma whereas isolated lung disease without mediastinal involvement can occur in NHL.

Acquired Immune Deficiency Syndrome-Related Lymphoma (ARL)

Lymphoma is the second most common tumor occurring in patients with AIDS, after Kaposi's sarcoma. Most patients are symptomatic, presenting with cough and shortness of breath. This subset of patients usually develops aggressive B-cell lymphomas.[63]

Imaging findings include well-defined pulmonary nodules (0.5–5 cm) with or without cavitation or a large solitary pulmonary nodule/mass (2–5 cm), Pleural effusions is commonest thoracic manifestation followed by pericardial effusions, consolidation and/or ground-glass opacity. Combinations of nodules, effusions, adenopathy in a HIV positive patient is highly suggestive of ARL.[64]

Post-transplantation Lymphoproliferative Disorder

The post-transplantation lymphoproliferative disorder (PTLD) is a lymphoid/plasmacytic proliferation that occurs following solid organ or hematopoietic stem cell transplantation, manifesting as a spectrum of disorders ranging from polyclonal benign proliferations to monoclonal and monomorphic aggressive lymphomas.

The etiology of PTLD is thought to be closely associated with EBV infection. PTLD is seen in less than 2% of all transplant cases and there is a clear association with the specific organ transplanted, with the highest incidence in lung transplantation (6–9%), followed by heart, liver and renal transplant. The majority of cases of PTLD occur within 2 years of transplantation, but it may be seen as early as 60 days post-transplant.[65]

The clinical presentation is variable and includes fever, lymphadenopathy, and abdominal pain with diarrhea, a mononucleosis-like syndrome and weight loss.

B-cell NHL is the most common type of lymphoma associated with PTLD. The most common imaging findings of PTLD are well defined usually multiple nodules (size range 0.3–5 cm), "halo sign" around nodules, patchy/focal consolidation or ground-glass opacity, more peribronchial/subpleural than diffuse distribution of nodules and lymphadenopathy.[66,67]

PULMONARY NEUROENDOCRINE NEOPLASMS

Pulmonary neuroendocrine neoplasms constitute approximately 20–25% of all invasive primary lung cancers. World Health Organization (WHO) in 2015 has grouped pulmonary neuroendocrine neoplasms into three histologic grades: Typical carcinoid as low-grade malignant neoplasm, atypical carcinoid as intermediate grade, and large cell neuroendocrine carcinoma (LCNEC) and small cell lung carcinoma (SCLC) as high-grade malignancies.[68,69]

Carcinoid Tumors

The respiratory tract is the second most common location after gastrointestinal tract, accounting for 20–30% of carcinoids.[70] They are indolent neoplasms with the potential to metastasize. Typical carcinoid is the least aggressive carcinoid type whereas atypical carcinoid is a more aggressive with 57% of affected patients present with lymph node metastases.[71]

Typical carcinoid is defined as a well-differentiated neoplasm with neuroendocrine histologic features, measuring 5 mm or more, exhibiting less than two mitoses per 10 high-power fields (HPF) or 2 mm^2, and no necrosis. The carcinoid is classified as atypical carcinoid when there are two to 10 mitoses per 10 HPF or necrosis, which is often punctate.[68] Most carcinoids are vascular lesions, and 30% of cases exhibit calcification.[72]

Most affected patients are adults although carcinoid is the most common malignant primary lung neoplasm till young adulthood.[71]

Most patients with centrally located neoplasms, present with symptoms like recurrent infections, cough, haemoptysis, and wheezing whereas peripheral tumors are asymptomatic and hence detected late.[69] Patients may present with Cushing syndrome and Carcinoid syndrome particularly patients with liver metastases. Carcinoid syndrome is characterized by skin flushing, bronchoconstriction, intractable diarrhoea, and right-sided heart disease.[73]

Imaging Findings

Carcinoids show a centrally located (hilar or perihilar), well-defined solitary 2–5 cm nodule more common in occur in the right lung (60%).[74] Atypical carcinoid tends to be larger and more peripheral than typical carcinoid.[75] Consider atypical carcinoid rather than typical carcinoid in older patients with well-defined peripheral nodule or central mass associated with lymph node or distant metastases. Multidetector CT demonstrates soft-tissue nodule located adjacent to airway[76] and may be completely endoluminal **(Figs. 22A and B)**, partially endoluminal, or may abut the airway. Positive "bronchus sign" demonstrating bronchus leading directly to the tumor may suggest the diagnosis. CT may demonstrate variable degrees of tumor enhancement differentiating it from adjacent atelectasis **(Figs. 22A and B)** or consolidation.[74] Calcification may be seen. CT is also useful for detection of lymphadenopathy and metastases in the liver, bone, or adrenal glands.[77]

MR imaging usually shows lesions with high T2 and STIR (short inversion time inversion-recovery) signal intensity and intense enhancement during the systemic circulatory phase.[77] Indium 111 octreotide or lanreotide (short- and long-acting somatostatin analogs) scintigraphy can be useful for localization of occult tumors.[71] 68 Gallium DOTANOC scan is currently used to image the primary as well as lymph node metastasis (more sensitive investigation).[78]

The diagnosis of carcinoid tumor requires microscopic evaluation of tissue, which can be obtained with bronchoscopy or CT guided biopsy or thoracotomy.[76]

Large Cell Neuroendocrine Carcinoma

The LCNEC is defined as a high-grade non-SCLC with neuroendocrine histologic features, more than 10 mitoses per 10 HPF (median, 70 mitoses per 10 HPF), and necrosis. Most patients with LCNEC are heavy smoker male, with a mean age of 65 years (range, 44–82 years). Presenting symptoms are like other lung masses whereas paraneoplastic syndromes are rare.[69] The diagnosis of LCNEC is by surgical lung biopsy.

Imaging Findings

At imaging, LCNEC typically manifests as a large (13 to 92 mm), peripheral mass indistinguishable from other lung cancers and typically exhibits well-defined lobular margins.[79] Approximately one-fifth of LCNECs are centrally located and may be associated with pressure symptoms.[80] Necrosis, heterogeneous or peripheral enhancement, calcification, hilar and mediastinal lymphadenopathy.

Small Cell Lung Carcinoma

SCLC is the most common neuroendocrine lung neoplasm, representing 15–20% of invasive lung malignancies.[68]

SCLC is characterized by its small cell size, scant cytoplasm, finely granular nuclear chromatin, absent or faint nucleoli, extremely high mitotic rates (>10 mitoses per 10 HPF; median, 80 mitoses per 10 HPF), and extensive necrosis. The diagnosis is often established by image-guided or bronchoscopy biopsy. A panel of immunohistochemical stains including CD56, TTF-1, and Ki-67 is typically used to differentiate SCLC from other lung masses. The Ki-67 proliferation index is most helpful in separating SCLC from

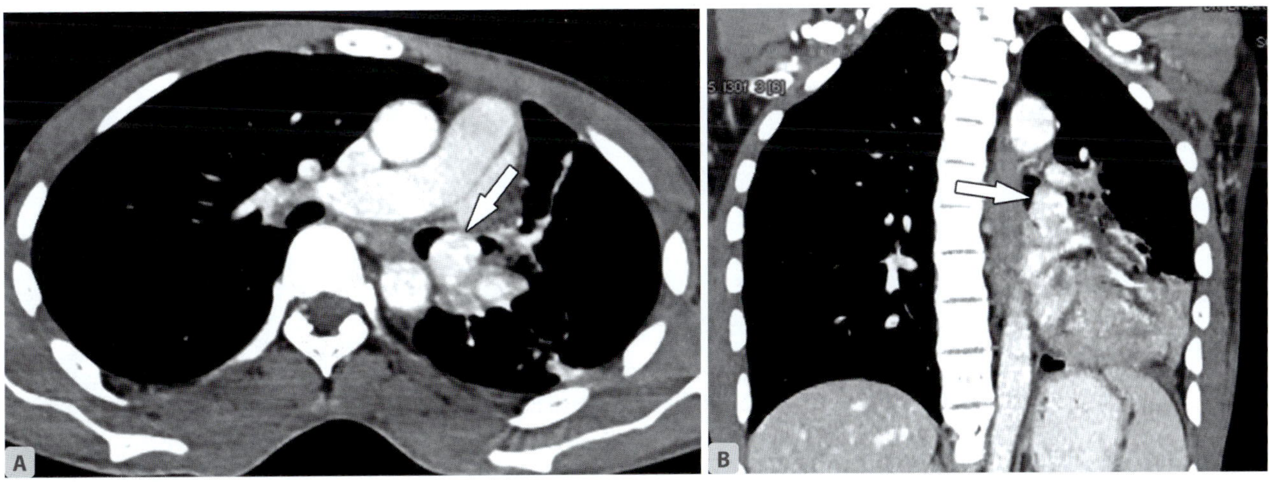

FIGS. 22A AND B: Typical carcinoid. (A and B) Intensely enhancing endoluminal nodule is seen in left main and lower lobe bronchus (arrows) with partial collapse of left lower lobe.

carcinoids.[69] SCLC occurs almost exclusively in smokers, and affected patients present with cough, hemoptysis, chest pain, and dyspnea. Constitutional symptoms, symptoms related to SVC invasion or extrapulmonary metastases. Patients with SCLC may also present with endocrine and nonendocrine paraneoplastic syndromes like SIADH and, Cushing syndrome, Eaton-Lambert syndrome, and encephalomyelitis.

Imaging Findings

On CT, SCLC typically manifests as a large central or mediastinal mass which are combination of the primary and associated lymphadenopathy. Bronchus cut-off sign, calcifications and pleural effusion may be present. The primary tumor may not be visible at times due to mediastinal lymphadenopathy.[81] Encasement or invasion of mediastinal structures, pleural effusion, pericardial thickening, pleural nodules, and metastases to the liver, adrenal glands, and bones may be seen.[81]

Diffuse Idiopathic Pulmonary Neuroendocrine Cell Hyperplasia (DIPNECH)

It is a preinvasive lesion of neuroendocrine group of tumors. On CT, it may present as mosaic attenuation secondary to expiratory air-trapping due to proliferation of neuroendocrine cells within bronchial/bronchiolar epithelium. Sometimes, it may manifest as multiple lung nodules or tumorlets (<5 mm).[82]

PULMONARY METASTASES

The lung metastasis is extremely common due to its high blood or lymphatics supply and through hematogenous and lymphatic routes. Lymphangitis carcinomatosis is a special form of lung metastasis where lymphatics in interlobular septa are clogged with tumor cells and appear nodular thickening of sepate on HRCT images. Most common cancers that metastasize to lungs include breast, colon, kidney, uterus, and head and neck are the most common primary sites with a pulmonary metastasis.[83] Cancers like choriocarcinoma, osteosarcoma, testicular tumor, melanoma, Ewing tumor, and thyroid carcinoma also frequently metastasize to the lung.[84] The early diagnosis of pulmonary metastases is crucial for treatment planning as well as for prognostication. MDCT is the most common imaging modality used for detection of possible pulmonary metastases. Typically, metastases appear well circumscribed soft tissue attenuation, rounded lesions, more often in the periphery of the lung of variable size, a feature which is of some use in distinguishing them from a granuloma.[85] A prominent pulmonary vessel (feeding vessel sign) can be seen heading into a metastasis **(Fig. 23A)**. The usual radiologic findings of a pulmonary metastasis include multiple peripherally located round variable-sized nodules (hematogenous metastasis) and diffuse thickening of the interstitium (lymphangitic carcinomatosis).[84] Among cases of multiple nodules detected with CT, 73% were reported to be pulmonary metastases.[86] The unusual radiologic features include cavitation **(Fig. 23B)** (squamous cell carcinoma, most often from the head and neck or from the lung), hemorrhage around the metastatic nodules (choriocarcinoma, angiosarcoma) **(Fig. 23C)**, pneumothorax (osteosarcoma), calcification (osteosarcoma **(Figs. 24A to C)**, chondrosarcoma, papillary thyroid carcinoma), air-space pattern, tumor embolism, endobronchial metastasis, solitary mass, dilated vessels within a mass, and sterilized metastasis. Innumerable small metastases (miliary pattern) may be seen in malignant melanoma, osteosarcoma, renal cell carcinoma, thyroid carcinoma and trophoblastic disease. Conversely, a pulmonary metastasis may be single in colorectal carcinoma, malignant melanoma, skeletal sarcoma and testicular carcinoma.[85] Adenocarcinoma metastases, rather than displace or destroy adjacent lung parenchyma, may grow in a lepidic fashion (spread along alveolar walls) resulting in pneumonia-like consolidation/air bronchograms.

PULMONARY HAMARTOMA

Hamartoma is the most common, slowly growing benign mesenchymal pulmonary neoplasm and represents about 6% of SPN detected on a CXR.[87] It consists of connective tissue elements such as fat, calcification, muscle, lymphatics. On CT, hamartomas typically manifest as well-circumscribed peripheral solitary pulmonary nodules or masses with smooth or lobular borders **(Fig. 25)**. About 10% are central

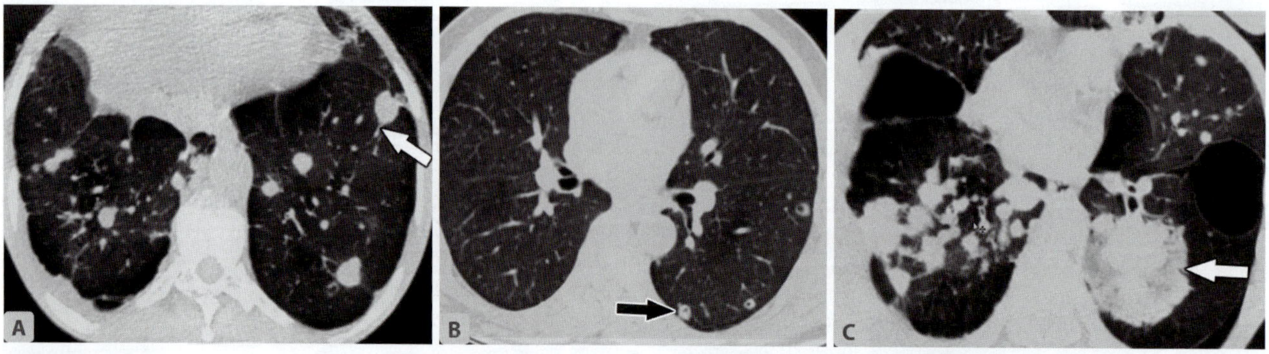

FIGS. 23A TO C: Pulmonary metastases. (A) CT lung window shows multiple well-defined nodules predominantly in peripheral lung with feeding vessel sign (arrow); (B) Cavitory metastases: CT of the patient with supraglottic squamous cell cancer shows multiple lung metastases in left lung showing cavitation (arrow); (C) Hemorrhagic metastases: CT of the patient with renal cell carcinoma shows multiple lung masses with ground-glass opacities around them (arrow), secondary to hemorrhages.

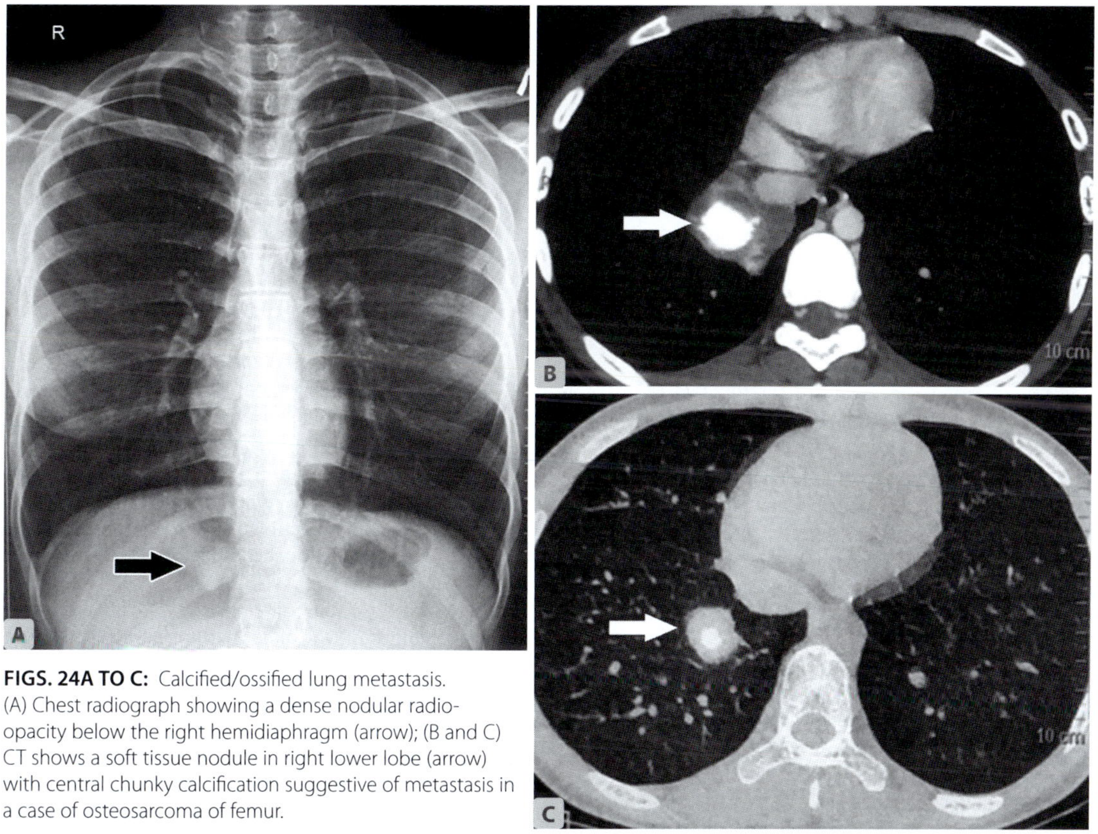

FIGS. 24A TO C: Calcified/ossified lung metastasis. (A) Chest radiograph showing a dense nodular radio-opacity below the right hemidiaphragm (arrow); (B and C) CT shows a soft tissue nodule in right lower lobe (arrow) with central chunky calcification suggestive of metastasis in a case of osteosarcoma of femur.

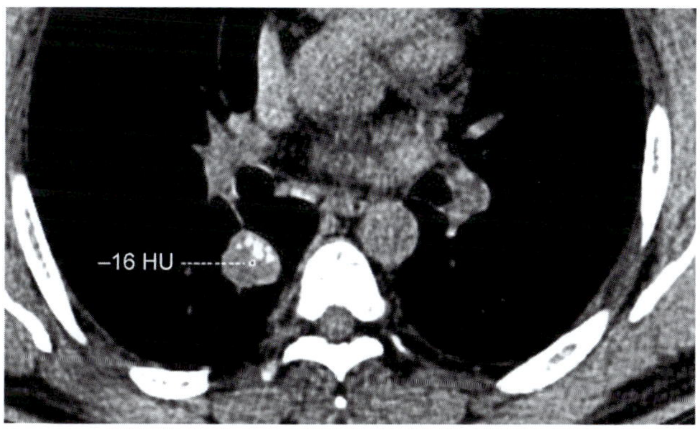

FIG. 25: Pulmonary hamartoma. A non-contrast CT axial image shows a well-defined nodule in peripheral aspect of right lower lobe with internal calcification and fat attenuation suggestive of a pulmonary hamartoma.

and endobronchial. Calcification is more common in larger lesions and is much better visualized on CT than on radiography. Although a characteristic popcorn pattern of calcification has been described, it is only present in 10–15% of cases. Internal fat, identified by Hounsfield units of -20 to -120 on CT, is present in 60% of cases. Identification of both internal fat and calcium is virtually diagnostic of a hamartoma. Following the administration of intravenous contrast, most lesions demonstrate heterogeneous enhancement.

CONCLUSION

In conclusion, imaging is an integral part of management protocol for pulmonary neoplasms. A thorough knowledge of available imaging modalities and judicious utilization of these is necessary for optimal patient care. Chest radiography and CT are most commonly used modalities. MRI can be used as a problem solving tool. Survival in carcinoma lung depends on stage; an early detection and diagnosis can help in achieving surgical cure. Here, the cross sectional imaging play a key role in the assessment of malignancy. CT, being less expensive and more widely available than MRI, is more likely to remain as a principal modality for evaluation of this disease. PET-CT helps for further characterization and assessment of extent of disease. It is important that radiologists are familiar with the new 8th TNM staging system for accurate assessment of prognosis and treatment planning. FNAC, biopsy and image guided ablations (e.g. RFA) for lung tumors are major interventions performed, which need meticulous planning using various imaging modalities.

REFERENCES

1. Siegel RL, Miller KD, Jemal A. Cancer Statistics, 2017. CA Cancer J Clin. 2017;67(1):7-30.
2. Time trends in cancer incidence rates 1982-2010 [Internet]. 2013.
3. Schrump DS GG, Kelsey CR. Non Small Cell Lung Cancer. In: DeVita VT LT, Rosenberg SA (Eds), 8th edition. Philadelphia: Lippincott Williams & Wilkins; 2008. p. 896-946.
4. Xue X, Liu Y, Pan L, et al. Diagnosis of multiple primary lung cancer: a systematic review. J Int Med Res. 2013;41(6):1779-87.
5. Travis WD, Brambilla E, Nicholson AG, et al. The 2015 World Health Organization Classification of Lung Tumors: Impact of Genetic, Clinical and Radiologic Advances Since the 2004 Classification. J Thorac Oncol. 2015;10(9):1243-60.
6. Dong Y, Mao F, Wang WP, et al. Value of Contrast-Enhanced Ultrasound in Guidance of Percutaneous Biopsy in Peripheral Pulmonary Lesions. Biomed Res Int. 2015;2015:531507.
7. Batra P, Brown K, Aberle DR, et al. Imaging techniques in the evaluation of pulmonary parenchymal neoplasms. Chest. 1992;101(1):239-43.
8. Tacelli N, Santangelo T, Scherpereel A, et al. Perfusion CT allows prediction of therapy response in non-small cell lung cancer treated with conventional and anti-angiogenic chemotherapy. Eur Radiol. 2013;23(8):2127-36.
9. Zhang LJ, Yang GF, Wu SY, et al. Dual-energy CT imaging of thoracic malignancies. Cancer Imaging. 2013;13:81-91.
10. Hou WS, Wu HW, Yin Y, et al. Differentiation of lung cancers from inflammatory masses with dual-energy spectral CT imaging. Acad Radiol. 2015;22(3):337-44.
11. Dennie C, Thornhill R, Sethi-Virmani V, et al. Role of quantitative computed tomography texture analysis in the differentiation of primary lung cancer and granulomatous nodules. Quant Imaging Med Surg. 2016;6(1):6-15.
12. Heyneman LE, Patz EF. PET imaging in patients with bronchio-loalveolar cell carcinoma. Lung Cancer. 2002;38(3):261-6.
13. Erasmus JJ, McAdams HP, Patz EF, et al. Evaluation of primary pulmonary carcinoid tumors using FDG PET. Am J Roentgenol. 1998;170(5):1369-73.
14. Chang JM, Lee HJ, Goo JM, et al. False positive and false negative FDG-PET scans in various thoracic diseases. Korean J Radiol. 2006;7(1):57-69.
15. Fischer B, Lassen U, Mortensen J, et al. Preoperative staging of lung cancer with combined PET-CT. N Engl J Med. 2009;361(1): 32-9.
16. Gupta NC, Rogers JS, Graeber GM, et al. Clinical role of F-18 fluorodeoxyglucose positron emission tomography imaging in patients with lung cancer and suspected malignant pleural effusion. Chest. 2002;122(6):1918-24.
17. Song JW, Oh YM, Shim TS, et at. Efficacy comparison between (18)F-FDG PET/CT and bone scintigraphy in detecting bony metastases of non-small-cell lung cancer. Lung Cancer. 2009;65(3):333-8.
18. Lardinois D, Weder W, Hany TF, et al. Staging of non-small-cell lung cancer with integrated positron-emission tomography and computed tomography. N Engl J Med. 2003;348(25):2500-7.
19. Greco C, Rosenzweig K, Cascini GL, et al. Current status of PET/CT for tumour volume definition in radiotherapy treatment planning for non-small cell lung cancer (NSCLC). Lung Cancer. 2007;57(2):125-34.
20. Hicks RJ. Role of 18F-FDG PET in assessment of response in non-small cell lung cancer. J Nucl Med. 2009;50(Suppl 1): 31S-42S.
21. Koyama H, Ohno Y, Seki S, et al. Magnetic resonance imaging for lung cancer. J Thorac Imaging. 2013;28(3):138-50.
22. Mori T, Nomori H, Ikeda K, et al. Diffusion-weighted magnetic resonance imaging for diagnosing malignant pulmonary nodules/masses: comparison with positron emission tomography. J Thorac Oncol. 2008;3(4):358-64.
23. Schaefer JF, Schneider V, Vollmar J, et al. Solitary pulmonary nodules: association between signal characteristics in dynamic contrast enhanced MRI and tumor angiogenesis. Lung Cancer. 2006;53(1):39-49.
24. Kono R, Fujimoto K, Terasaki H, et al. Dynamic MRI of solitary pulmonary nodules: comparison of enhancement patterns of malignant and benign small peripheral lung lesions. Am J Roentgenol. 2007;188(1):26-36.
25. Grewal RG, Austin JH. CT demonstration of calcification in carcinoma of the lung. J Comput Assist Tomogr. 1994;18(6):867-71.
26. Khan AN, Al-Jahdali HH, Allen CM, et al. The calcified lung nodule: What does it mean? Ann Thorac Med. 2010;5(2):67-79.
27. Aoki T, Tomoda Y, Watanabe H, et al. Peripheral lung adenocarcinoma: correlation of thin-section CT findings with histologic prognostic factors and survival. Radiology. 2001;220(3):803-9.
28. Mackintosh JA, Marshall HM, Yang IA, et al. A retrospective study of volume doubling time in surgically resected non-small cell lung cancer. Respirology. 2014;19(5):755-62.
29. Dela Cruz CS, Tanoue LT, Matthay RA. Lung cancer: epidemiology, etiology, and prevention. Clin Chest Med. 2011;32(4):605-44.
30. Hollings N, Shaw P. Diagnostic imaging of lung cancer. Eur Respir J. 2002;19(4):722-42.
31. Carter BW, Glisson BS, Truong MT, et al. Small cell lung carcinoma: staging, imaging, and treatment considerations. Radiographics. 2014;34(6):1707-21.
32. Acharya KV, Shenoy A, Holla R. Utility of Various Bronchoscopic Modalities in Lung Cancer Diagnosis. Asian Pac J Cancer Prev. 2017;18(7):1931-6.
33. Zhan P, Zhu QQ, Miu YY, et al. Comparison between endobronchial ultrasound-guided transbronchial biopsy and CT-guided transthoracic lung biopsy for the diagnosis of peripheral lung cancer: a systematic review and meta-analysis. Transl Lung Cancer Res. 2017;6(1):23-34.
34. Kay FU, Kandathil A, Batra K, et al. Revisions to the Tumor, Node, Metastasis Staging of lung Cancer: Rationale, Radiologic Findings and Clinical Implications, 8th edn. World J Radiol. 2017;9(6):269-79.
35. Lewis JW, Pearlberg JL, Beute GH, et al. Can computed tomography of the chest stage lung cancer? Yes and no. Ann Thorac Surg. 1990;49(4):591-5; discussion 5-6.
36. Beigelman-Aubry C, Dunet V, Brun AL. CT imaging in pre-therapeutic assessment of lung cancer. Diagn Interv Imaging. 2016;97(10):973-89.
37. Detterbeck FC, Boffa DJ, Kim AW, et al. The Lung Cancer Stage Classification. Chest, 8th edition. 2017;151(1):193-203.
38. Eisenhauer EA, Therasse P, Bogaerts J, et al. New response evaluation criteria in solid tumours: revised RECIST guideline (version 1.1). Eur J Cancer. 2009;45(2):228-47.
39. Ezhil M, Vedam S, Balter P, et al. Determination of patient-specific internal gross tumor volumes for lung cancer using four-dimensional computed tomography. Radiat Oncol. 2009;4:4.
40. Simon CJ, Dupuy DE, DiPetrillo TA, et al. Pulmonary radiofrequency ablation: long-term safety and efficacy in 153 patients. Radiology. 2007;243(1):268-75.
41. Sano Y, Kanazawa S, Gobara H, et al. Feasibility of percutaneous radiofrequency ablation for intrathoracic malignancies: a large single-center experience. Cancer. 2007;109(7):1397-405.

42. Lencioni R, Crocetti L, Cioni R, et al. Response to radiofrequency ablation of pulmonary tumours: a prospective, intention-to-treat, multicentre clinical trial (the RAPTURE study). Lancet Oncol. 2008;9(7):621-8.
43. Lanuti M, Sharma A, Digumarthy SR, et al. Radiofrequency ablation for treatment of medically inoperable stage I non-small cell lung cancer. J Thorac Cardiovasc Surg. 2009;137(1):160-6.
44. Mayo-Smith WW, Dupuy DE. Adrenal neoplasms: CT-guided radiofrequency ablation—preliminary results. Radiology. 2004;231(1):225-30.
45. Marcus PM, Bergstralh EJ, Fagerstrom RM, et al. Lung cancer mortality in the Mayo Lung Project: impact of extended follow-up. J Natl Cancer Inst. 2000;92(16):1308-16.
46. Younes RN, Gross JL, Deheinzelin D. Follow-up in lung cancer: how often and for what purpose? Chest. 1999;115(6):1494-9.
47. Bogot NR, Quint LE. Imaging of recurrent lung cancer. Cancer Imaging. 2004;4(2):61-7.
48. Koenig TR, Munden RF, Erasmus JJ, et al. Radiation injury of the lung after three-dimensional conformal radiation therapy. Am J Roentgenol. 2002;178(6):1383-8.
49. Aoki T, Nagata Y, Negoro Y, et al. Evaluation of lung injury after three-dimensional conformal stereotactic radiation therapy for solitary lung tumors: CT appearance. Radiology. 2004;230(1):101-8.
50. Munden RF, Swisher SS, Stevens CW, et al. Imaging of the patient with non-small cell lung cancer. Radiology. 2005;237(3):803-18.
51. Libshitz HI, Sheppard DG. Filling in of radiation therapy-induced bronchiectatic change: a reliable sign of locally recurrent lung cancer. Radiology. 1999;210(1):25-7.
52. Cox JE, Chiles C, Aquino SL, et al. Pulmonary artery sarcomas: a review of clinical and radiologic features. J Comput Assist Tomogr. 1997;21(5):750-5.
53. Bhatia K, Ellis S. Unusual lung tumours: an illustrated review of CT features suggestive of this diagnosis. Cancer Imaging. 2006;6:72-82.
54. Manivel JC, Priest JR, Watterson J, et al. Pleuropulmonary blastoma. The so-called pulmonary blastoma of childhood. Cancer. 1988;62(8):1516-26.
55. Weisbrod GL, Chamberlain DW, Tao LC. Pulmonary blastoma, report of three cases and a review of the literature. Can Assoc Radiol J. 1988;39(2):130-6.
56. Lee WK, Duddalwar VA, Rouse HC, et al. Extranodal lymphoma in the thorax: cross-sectional imaging findings. Clin Radiol. 2009;64(5):542-9.
57. Lee KS, Kim Y, Primack SL. Imaging of pulmonary lymphomas. Am J Roentgenol. 1997;168(2):339-45.
58. Kurtin PJ, Myers JL, Adlakha H, et al. Pathologic and clinical features of primary pulmonary extranodal marginal zone B-cell lymphoma of MALT type. Am J Surg Pathol. 2001;25(8):997-1008.
59. Huang H, Lu ZW, Jiang CG, et al. Clinical and prognostic characteristics of pulmonary mucosa-associated lymphoid tissue lymphoma: a retrospective analysis of 23 cases in a Chinese population. Chin Med J (Engl). 2011;124(7):1026-30.
60. Ahmed S, Kussick SJ, Siddiqui AK, et al. Bronchial-associated lymphoid tissue lymphoma: a clinical study of a rare disease. Eur J Cancer. 2004;40(9):1320-6.
61. Mentzer SJ, Reilly JJ, Skarin AT, et al. Patterns of lung involvement by malignant lymphoma. Surgery. 1993;113(5):507-14.
62. Lewis ER, Caskey CI, Fishman EK. Lymphoma of the lung: CT findings in 31 patients. Am J Roentgenol. 1991;156(4): 711-4.
63. Hamilton-Dutoit SJ, Pallesen G, Franzmann MB, et al. AIDS-related lymphoma. Histopathology, immunophenotype, and association with Epstein-Barr virus as demonstrated by in situ nucleic acid hybridization. Am J Pathol. 1991;138(1):149-63.
64. Blunt DM, Padley SP. Radiographic manifestations of AIDS related lymphoma in the thorax. Clin Radiol. 1995;50(9):607-12.
65. Bates WD, Gray DW, Dada MA, et al. Lymphoproliferative disorders in Oxford renal transplant recipients. J Clin Pathol. 2003;56(6):439-46.
66. Carignan S, Staples CA, Müller NL. Intrathoracic lymphoproliferative disorders in the immunocompromised patient: CT findings. Radiology. 1995;197(1):53-8.
67. Dodd GD, Ledesma-Medina J, Baron RL, et al. Posttransplant lymphoproliferative disorder: intrathoracic manifestations. Radiology. 1992;184(1):65-9.
68. Rekhtman N. Neuroendocrine tumors of the lung: an update. Arch Pathol Lab Med. 2010;134(11):1628-38.
69. Travis WD. Advances in neuroendocrine lung tumors. Ann Oncol. 2010;21 Suppl 7:vii65-71.
70. Pinchot SN, Holen K, Sippel RS, et al. Carcinoid tumors. Oncologist. 2008;13(12):1255-69.
71. Gustafsson BI, Kidd M, Chan A, et al. Bronchopulmonary neuroendocrine tumors. Cancer. 2008;113(1):5-21.
72. Jeung MY, Gasser B, Gangi A, et al. Bronchial carcinoid tumors of the thorax: spectrum of radiologic findings. Radiographics. 2002;22(2):351-65.
73. Fox DJ, Khattar RS. Carcinoid heart disease: presentation, diagnosis, and management. Heart. 2004;90(10):1224-8.
74. Chong S, Lee KS, Chung MJ, et al. Neuroendocrine tumors of the lung: clinical, pathologic, and imaging findings. Radiographics. 2006;26(1):41-57; discussion-8.
75. Soga J, Yakuwa Y. Bronchopulmonary carcinoids: An analysis of 1,875 reported cases with special reference to a comparison between typical carcinoids and atypical varieties. Ann Thorac Cardiovasc Surg. 1999;5(4):211-9.
76. Detterbeck FC. Management of carcinoid tumors. Ann Thorac Surg. 2010;89(3):998-1005.
77. Rosado de Christenson ML, Abbott GF, Kirejczyk WM, et al. Thoracic carcinoids: radiologic-pathologic correlation. Radiographics. 1999;19(3):707-36.
78. Caplin ME, Baudin E, Ferolla P, et al. Pulmonary neuroendocrine (carcinoid) tumors: European Neuroendocrine Tumor Society expert consensus and recommendations for best practice for typical and atypical pulmonary carcinoids. Ann Oncol. 2015;26(8):1604-20.
79. Jung KJ, Lee KS, Han J, et al. Large cell neuroendocrine carcinoma of the lung: clinical, CT, and pathologic findings in 11 patients. J Thorac Imaging. 2001;16(3):156-62.
80. Oshiro Y, Kusumoto M, Matsuno Y, et al. CT findings of surgically resected large cell neuroendocrine carcinoma of the lung in 38 patients. Am J Roentgenol. 2004;182(1):87-91.
81. Pearlberg JL, Sandler MA, Lewis JW, et al. Small-cell bronchogenic carcinoma: CT evaluation. Am J Roentgenol. 1988;150(2):265-8.
82. Benson RE, Rosado-de-Christenson ML, Martínez-Jiménez S, et al. Spectrum of pulmonary neuroendocrine proliferations and neoplasms. Radiographics. 2013;33(6):1631-49.
83. Coppage L, Shaw C, Curtis AM. Metastatic disease to the chest in patients with extrathoracic malignancy. J Thorac Imaging. 1987;2(4):24-37.
84. Libshitz HI, North LB. Pulmonary metastases. Radiol Clin North Am. 1982;20(3):437-51.
85. Collins J SE. Chest Radiology: The Essentials LWW Doody's all reviewed collection, illustrated ed: Lippincott Williams & Wilkins; 2008.
86. Padovani B, Mouroux J, Seksik L, et al. Chest wall invasion by bronchogenic carcinoma: evaluation with MR imaging. Radiology. 1993;187(1):33-8.
87. Gleeson T, Thiessen R, Hannigan A, et al. Pulmonary hamartomas: CT pixel analysis for fat attenuation using radiologic-pathologic correlation. J Med Imaging Radiat Oncol. 2013;57(5):534-43.

CHAPTER

135

Imaging of the Tracheobronchial Tree

Ashu Seith Bhalla, Smita Manchanda

INTRODUCTION

Airway is divided into the upper airway (above the thoracic inlet) and the lower airway (below the thoracic inlet). The lower airway is further divided into the large and small airways. This chapter focuses on the lower airways.

Large airways is a term used for airways which are >2 mm in diameter. This includes the:

- Central airway—trachea and main bronchi
- Peripheral airway—lobar, segmental, and proximal subsegmental bronchi.

Small airways refer to the distal airways, which are small in size (<2 mm in diameter) and lack cartilage and submucosal glands.

ROLE OF IMAGING (BOX 1)

Imaging plays a key role in diagnosis and planning management. The main role of imaging is to detect and localize the lesion (with respect to carina), delineate the exact length of the lesion (for stent placement as a therapeutic option), measure the degree of airway narrowing, and lastly to give a specific diagnosis, if possible. The current role of the various *imaging modalities* is detailed below.

IMAGING MODALITIES

Chest Radiograph

Plain frontal and lateral chest radiographs are useful in acute obstructions such as foreign body and aspiration. These may occasionally demonstrate large masses involving the central airways. Areas of severe narrowing may also be appreciated. The effects of airway disease on the lung, i.e. consolidation, atelectasis or hyperinflation is well seen on plain films. Signs of bronchiectasis are also well described on plain radiographs **(Fig. 1)**. However, largely radiographs are unable to provide enough information for diagnosis or preoperative planning of patients.

BOX 1: Role of imaging in evaluation of the tracheobronchial tree.

- Detection
- Localization—proximal and distal extent
- Etiology—extrinsic or intrinsic (mural or intraluminal)
- Length for abnormal segment
- Diffuse/focal
- Obstruction—fixed or dynamic
- Degree of narrowing
- Specific diagnosis, if possible

Systemic Evaluation on Chest Radiograph

Refer **Box 2**.

Digital Tomosynthesis

Digital tomosynthesis (DTS) is a new technique using digital radiography and flat-panel detectors, which is based on the principle of geometric tomography.[1] DTS images represent sections through the anatomy that are generated and reconstructed from a set of projection radiographs. Because it removes overlapping clutter, there is improved visualization of thoracic abnormalities compared to radiography and better coronal plane resolution

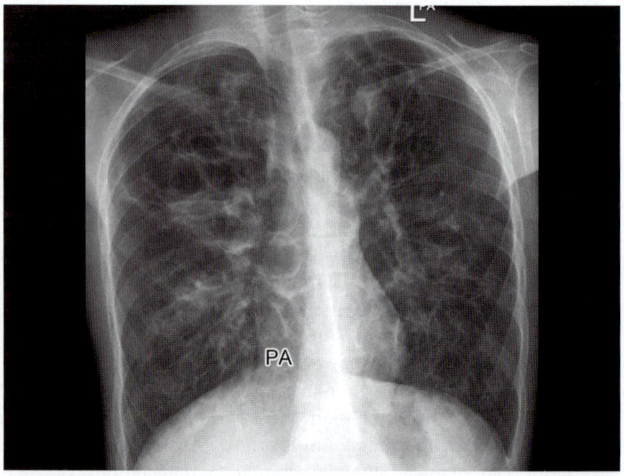

FIG. 1: Plain radiograph showing cystic lucencies and tram-track linear opacities in bilateral lung fields in a case of cystic fibrosis.

(Figs. 2A and B). The radiation dose to patients is less than that of chest CT.[2] The demonstration of the central airways is considered to be superior or equivalent compared with radiography.[1] In terms of airway evaluation this technique is useful in suspected cases of foreign body.

Multidetector Computed Tomography

Multidetector computed tomography (MDCT) is the investigation of choice for initial evaluation of suspected tracheobronchial tree pathology and for follow-up of these cases.[3] In the current generation of scanners, there is volumetric CT acquisition in a single breath hold and precise delineation of the entire tracheobronchial tree, including the distal airways can be done.[4]

Acquisition

Scans are routinely performed in deep inspiration in supine position. In a single breath hold of 6–8 seconds, the entire chest can be scanned without respiratory motion artifacts. Cardiac gating is not recommended and is not usually done.[3,5]

BOX 2: Systematic evaluation on chest radiograph.

- Tracheal caliber
- Mediastinal widening
- Asymmetric lung aeration
- Lung collapse/consolidation
- Length of tracheal narrowing
- Radiopaque foreign body
- Cardiac size
- Position of the aortic arch

Although visualization of airways per se does not require contrast administration, IV contrast may prove helpful in some conditions; for example, differentiating a central mass from atelectatic lung.

CT acquisition technique has been summarized in **Box 3**. Until recently axial imaging by CT scan was the accepted standard modality for diagnostic work-up for suspected airway pathology. However, MDCT has significantly enhanced the imaging of airways. The numerous reconstruction techniques have virtually revolutionized the way that CT images are viewed and interpreted.[4,6]

Of great concern is the potential of added risk resulting from increased radiation exposure especially when paired inspiratory-expiratory CT is performed. Cine imaging also has the potential for high radiation exposure.

The problem of additional radiation exposure can be reduced by routinely using reduced milliamperage whenever, feasible. This is especially true in young patients and those likely to require multiple follow-ups.

Diagnostic images of acceptable quality can be obtained with 80–100 mAs, and use as low as 40 mAs has been reported in thin patients. For the expiratory scans, a low-dose (30–40 mAs) technique should be used. Radiation exposure can be reduced further by using dose modulation techniques.

Acquisition in Special Situation (Tracheobronchomalacia)

There are various techniques described for the evaluation of tracheobronchomalacia; using either expiratory scans or coughing manuevers.[8] These include:

1. Paired end-inspiratory and end-expiratory MDCT: Scans at end inspiration and incremental scans at end expiration.

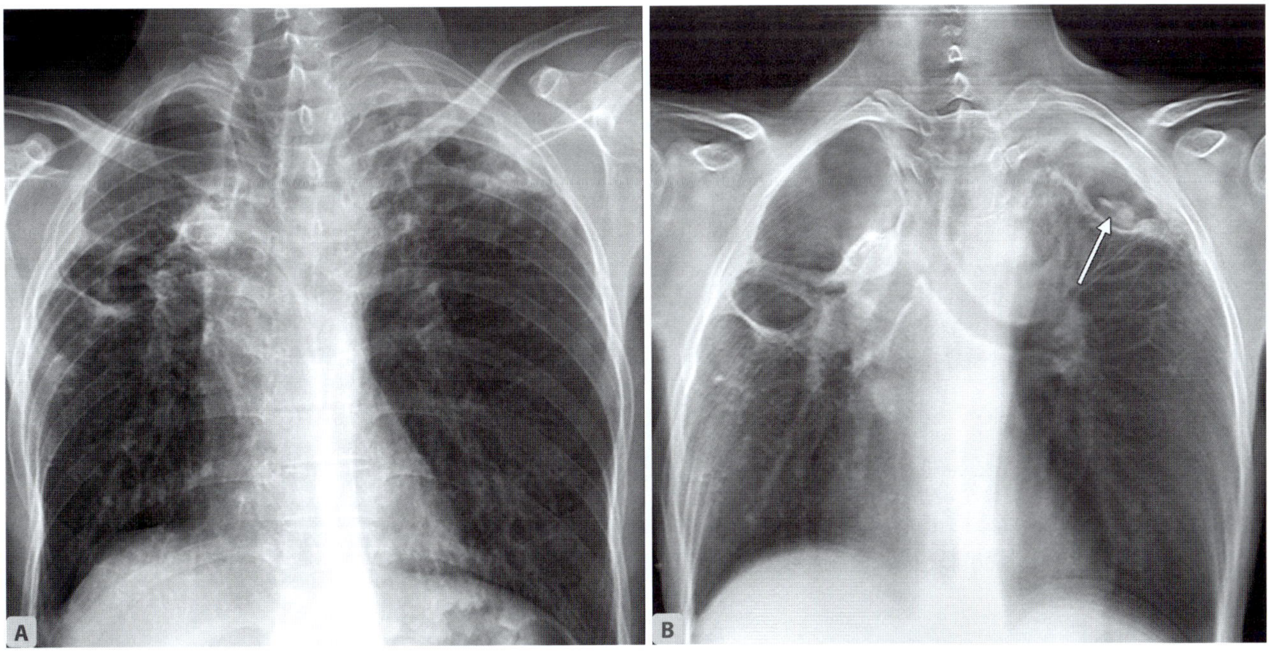

FIGS. 2A AND B: Digital tomosynthesis: Plain radiograph (A) reveals fibrocavitary lesions in bilateral upper lobes with suspicious fungal ball in left upper lobe cavity. DTS image (B) better depicts the central airways and fungal ball (arrow) as it removes overlapping clutter.

BOX 3: CT acquisition technique.[6,7]

- Tube potential and tube current appropriate to patient size
- Use of tube current modulation
- *Scan area*: From the lung apices to the costophrenic sulci
- *Position*:
  - At isocenter to minimize radiation dose and optimize image quality
  - Supine
  - Prone (in specific cases)
- *Phase*:
  - Deep inspiration
  - *Expiratory (end expiration)*:
    - To demonstrate air trapping
    - Obtained throughout the lung fields or at selected 3 to 5 levels
    - Low dose (30–40 mAs)
  - *Dynamic (paired inspiratory and expiratory)*: In cases of tracheobronchomalacia
- Thin overlapping 0.5–1 mm sections acquired
- *Field of view*:
  - *Scan FOV*: Appropriate to patient size at time of image
  - *Reconstructed FOV*: Limited to the lungs with optimal spatial resolution for each patient (lung window)
- *Data sets*:
  - 5 mm width every 5 mm reconstruction interval at lung and mediastinal window settings
  - 1 mm width at 10 mm interval high resolution scans
  - Thin reconstruction at 1–1.5 mm slice thickness
- Retention of the radiation dose report in the radiological record

(FOV: Field of view)

2. Paired end-inspiratory and dynamic expiratory MDCT: Scans at end inspiration and during expiration.
3. Cine MDCT combined with a coughing maneuver: Scans beginning at end inspiration which is followed by coughing movements.

Image Reconstruction

The various techniques available in MDCT scanners incude multiplanar reconstructions (MPRs), maximum intensity projections (MIPs), minimum intensity projections (minIPs) and internal rendering or virtual bronchoscopy (VB)[6,9-11] **(Figs. 3 and 4)**. The role of numerous reconstruction techniques is described in **Table 1**.

Quantitative CT Assessment of Airways

The lumen and area of airways can be measured quantitatively on CT images. With the use of MDCT scanners oblique reconstructions can be made in the axis and perpendicular to the axis of the airway.[12]

Box 4 summarizes the current role of MDCT in evaluation of airway pathology.

Endoscopic Ultrasound

Over the past decade, there has been a growing interest in the use of endoscopic ultrasound (EBUS) to diagnose to the central and peripheral lesions of tracheobronchial tree. EBUS has the unique capability to differentiate various layers of the bronchial wall.[13] Also pathologic changes both in and adjacent to airways can be assessed. Vessels can be readily identified and differentiated from lymph nodes. It has hence found a significant role in guided transbronchial needle

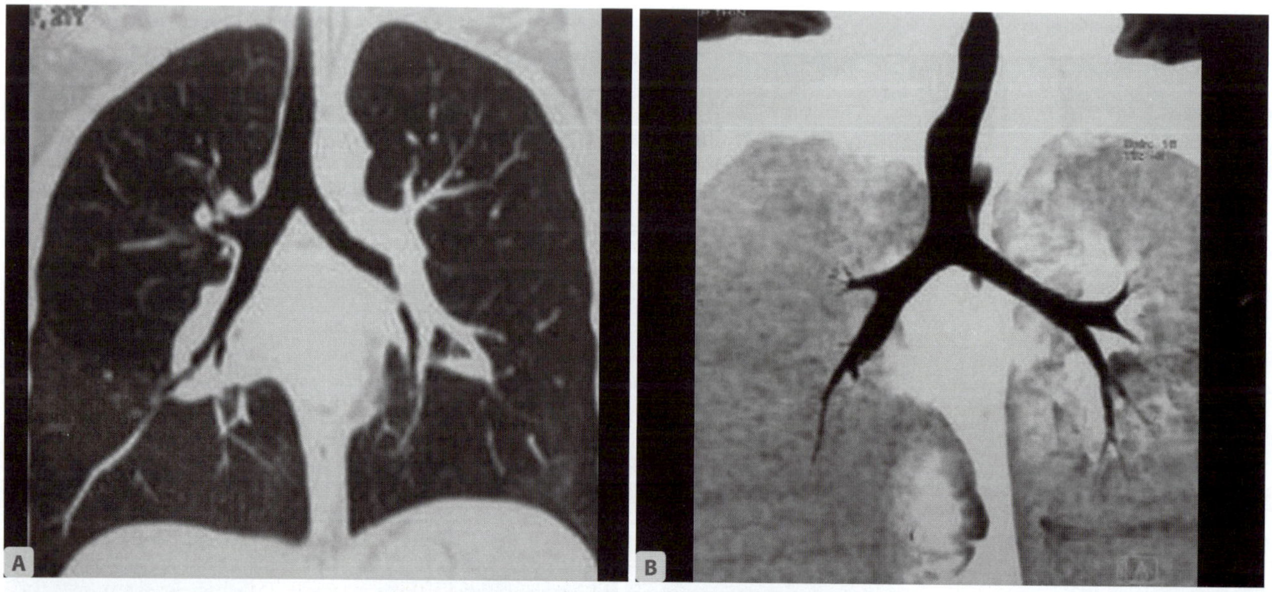

FIGS. 3A AND B: Coronal MPR (A) and coronal minIP (B) showing trachea, main bronchi and lobar bronchi.

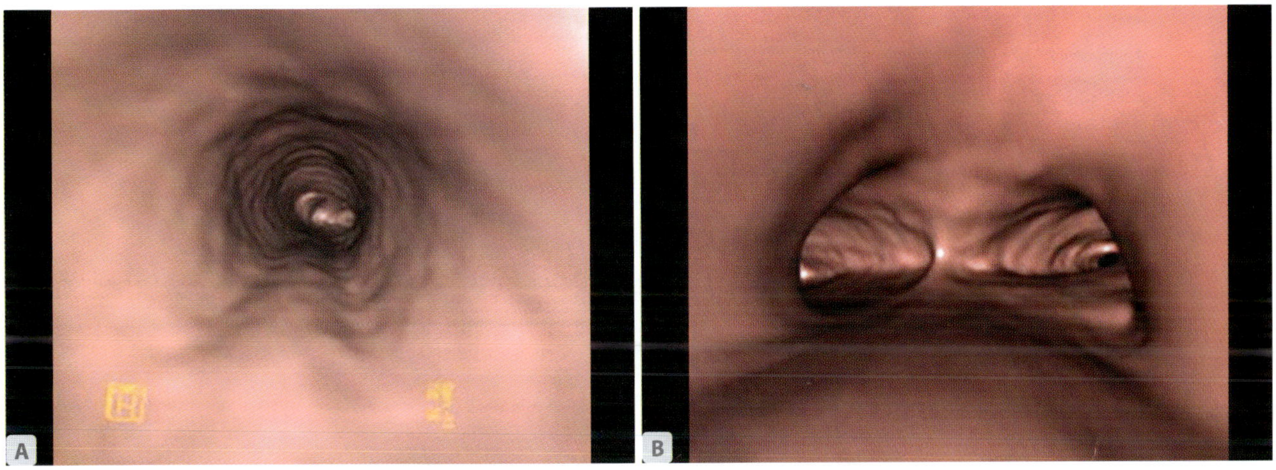

FIGS. 4A AND B: Virtual bronchoscopy images showing endoluminal view of normal trachea (A) and carina (B).

TABLE 1: CT reconstruction techniques (role in airway diseases).

Name	Technique	Role
MPR	• Multiplanar reconstruction • Evaluate in both mediastinal and lung window	• To visualize anatomical structures in reality • Airway stenosis • Resectability of bronchogenic carcinoma as well as hilar and mediastinal structures
minIP	• Minimum intensity projection • Thick slabs of 25–35 cm used to demonstrate entire TB tree	• Overall morphology of the tracheobronchial tree • Detecting airway stenosis (overestimates degree of narrowing) • Improved depiction of ground-glass pattern
MIP	Maximum intensity projection	• Improves detection of pulmonary nodules • Bronchiolar diseases, especially for patients with so-called tree-in-bud opacities • Size and location of vessels
VB	Virtual bronchoscopy	• Accurate reproduction of major endoluminal abnormalities • Assessment of airway stenoses • Unable to identify the causes of bronchial obstruction or detect mild stenosis, submucosal infiltration and superficial spreading tumors

BOX 4: Role of MDCT in evaluation of airway pathology.

- Workhorse of airway imaging
- Reconstructions definitely improve lesion evaluation compared to axial images alone
- MPR in both mediastinal and lung windows—length of stenosis
- VB does not have a distinct diagnostic utility, useful where fiberoptic bronchoscopy not available or not feasible
- minIP, volume rendered images useful in overall depiction of airway anatomy
- Excellent for congenital anomalies
- *Limitations of MDCT*:
  - Lesions smaller than 2–3 mm not detected
  - Difficult to differentiate between mucosal and submucosal lesions

(MPR: multiplanar reconstruction; VB: virtual bronchoscopy; minIP: minimum intensity projection; MDCT: multidetector computed tomography)

aspiration (TBNA) of mediastinal nodes currently, the major limitation of EBUS guided TBNA is its high cost, and the need for special configuration of endoscopic probes to provide consistent positioning adjacent to bronchial walls.[3]

Magnetic Resonance Imaging

Magnetic resonance imaging (MRI) provides adequate visualization of the tracheobronchial tree up to lobar bronchi.[14] This is best seen on the coronal T1 TSE sequence **(Fig. 5)**. Mediastinal and hilar masses are also well evaluated on MRI with the superior depiction of vascular or cardiac invasion. MRI has also been used to demonstrate air trapping. There is an increasing use in those requiring repeated imaging such as cystic fibrosis and allergic bronchopulmonary aspergillosis (ABPA). The presence of mucus with high T1 SI and low T2 SI has been found to be highly specific for the diagnosis of ABPA in cystic fibrosis **(Box 5)**.[15]

NORMAL AIRWAY ANATOMY

The trachea is a cartilaginous and fibromuscular tube extending from the inferior aspect of cricoid cartilage to the carina, measuring 10–12 cm in length. It is divided into intrathoracic and extrathoracic parts. It contains 16–22 cartilaginous rings, which are incomplete posteriorly. The posterior portion of the tracheal wall, lying between the open ends of the tracheal cartilages, is a thin fibromuscular membrane termed posterior tracheal membrane.[16]

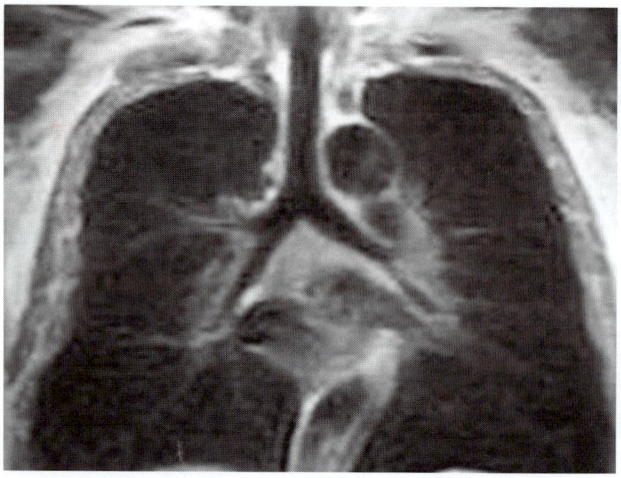

FIG. 5: MRI showing normal airway on T1W SE coronal image.

BOX 5: Suggested MRI protocol for central airway evaluation.

1. *T1-weighted gradient sequence*:
   - *With fat supression (pre- and postcontrast)*: Axial
   - *Without fat supression*: Axial, Coronal
2. *T2-weighted fast spin echo sequence*:
   - *With fat supression*: Axial
   - *Without fat supression*: Axial
3. *T2-weighted sequence HASTE*: Coronal
4. *Diffusion-weighted sequence*: Axial (b0, 400, 800) (in cases of masses)

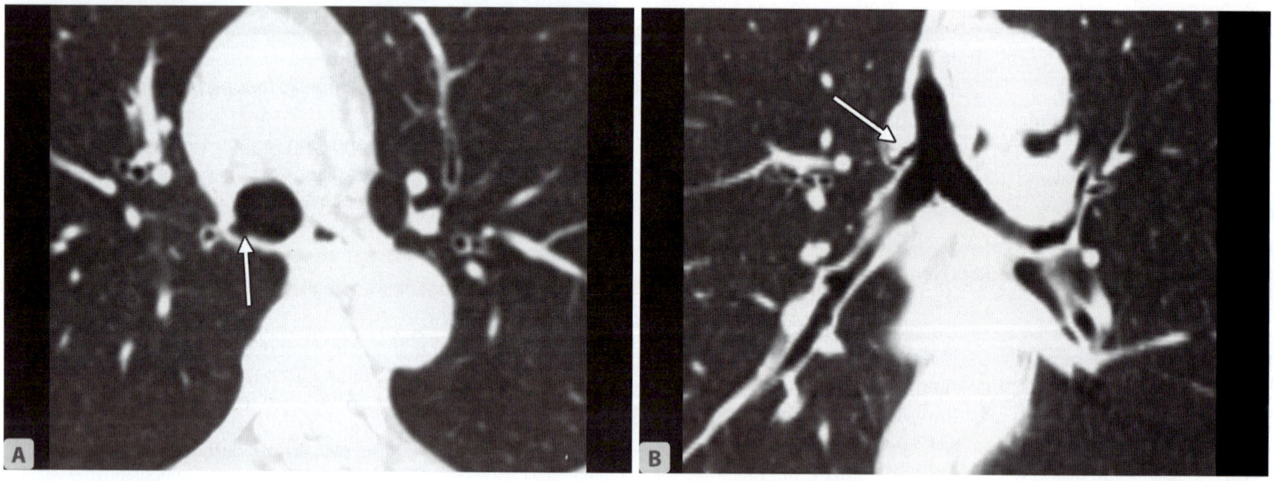

FIGS. 6A AND B: Tracheal bronchus: Axial (A) and coronal MPR (B) in lung window show the right upper lobe bronchus (arrow) arising directly from the trachea.

There is marked variability in the cross-sectional appearance of the trachea, which may appear rounded or oval (most common) or horseshoe-shaped trachea with flat posterior tracheal membrane (in about 25% of normal individuals).[16] Tracheal diameter can vary widely in anatomically normal persons. In men, tracheal diameter ranges from 13 to 25 mm (mean 19.5 mm) and in females it is slightly less, ranging from 10 to 21 m in the coronal plane (average 17.5 mm). In children variations in tracheal diameter at different levels can be as much as 20%. During forced expiration, there is invagination of the posterior tracheal membrane and the lumen becomes horseshoe shaped.

There is dichotomous branching with approximately 23 generations of branches from trachea to alveoli.

ANATOMIC VARIANTS

In adults, the most commonly encountered anomalies are either anomalous or supernumerary bronchi.[3] Other anomalies include agenesis, congenital bronchial atresia, bronchogenic cysts or even cogenital lobar obstruction. A clinically useful modified classification has been proposed by Wu et al. for these anomalies.[17]

1. *Anomalies arising from normal higher order bronchial divisions.* These include accessory superior segmental bronchi and axillary bronchi supplying lateral aspect of right upper lobe.
2. *Anomalies arising from sites typically lacking branches:* This group refers to tracheal bronchi, accessory cardiac bronchi and bridging bronchi.

   The most common amongst these is *the 'tracheal or pig bronchus'*, seen in up to 1–2% of normal individuals.[18] Tracheal bronchus arises on the right side exclusively, and on endoscopy may be confused with tracheal diverticula or tracheoceles. CT readily identifies these **(Figs. 6A and B)**

   The 'cardiac bronchus' usually arises from the bronchus intermedius, the origin being opposite and distal to origin of upper lobe bronchus **(Fig. 7)**. It is variable is size and in many cases is a blind ending stump; which does not aerate any lung parenchyma.

3. *Anomalies associated with abnormalities of situs.* In this category, reversal of the right- and left-sided airways is the most commonly encountered form. Less frequent anomalies include bronchial isomerism, in which pattern of airway branching and pulmonary location is identical in both the lungs.

TRACHEOBRONCHIAL TREE PATHOLOGIES

Pathologies affecting the tracheobronchial tree can be broadly considered in three categories—those affecting the central airways, the peripheral airways and others involving the small airways. The levels of lower airway pathologies are described in **Figure 8**.

CENTRAL AIRWAYS

Central airway obstruction can occur because of extrinsic or intrinsic causes (which are further divided into mural and intraluminal causes). These are detailed in **Table 2**.

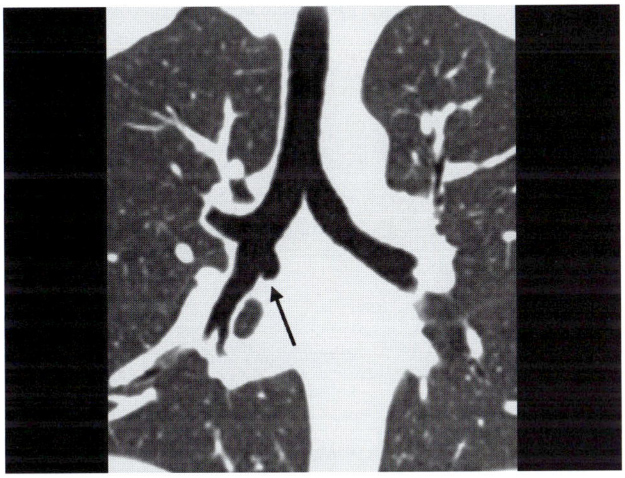

FIG. 7: Cardiac bronchus: Blind ending bronchial stump (arrow) arising medially from the bronchus intermedius.

EXTRINSIC

A diverse variety of mediastinal masses or mass like lesions can cause extrinsic compression of the airways. These have been described in detail elsewhere.

INTRINSIC MURAL

Congenital

Tracheobronchomalacia

Tracheobronchomalacia (TBM) is characterized by weakness of the tracheobronchial walls and/or supporting cartilage. This results in a dynamic obstruction of the airway because of excessive collapse during expiration.[8,19] CT diagnosis **(Figs. 10A to C)** can only be made in paired scans (end inspiration and expiratory scan/during coughing) as described above in CT acquisition. It may be congenital or acquired due to prior intubation, trauma, prolonged extrinsic compression **(Figs. 11A and B)**, infection or chronic inflammation.[20]

Tracheal Stenosis

Congenital subglottic or tracheal stenosis occurs because of incomplete recanalization of the laryngotracheal tube. The various types of congenital tracheal stenosis include hypoplasia, funnel-shaped and segmental stenosis.[21]

Inflammatory/Infective

Infections/Fibrotic Stricture

Inflammatory Tracheal Stenosis due to Tuberculosis

Tubercular stenosis **(Figs. 12A to E)** is an endobronchial complication of pulmonary tuberculosis that can develop acutely at the time of infection or can become manifest years later. Endobronchial tuberculosis has been reported in 10–37% of patients with pulmonary parenchymal tuberculosis.[22] Tuberculosis typically involves the distal trachea and proximal mainstem bronchi **(Figs. 13A and B)**; isolated tracheal disease is rare.[23] Granulation tissue formation and subsequent fibrosis involving the airway causes luminal

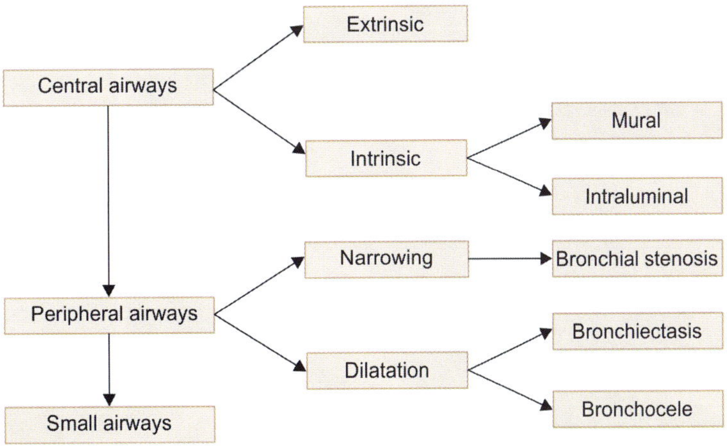

FIG. 8: Levels of lower airway pathologies.

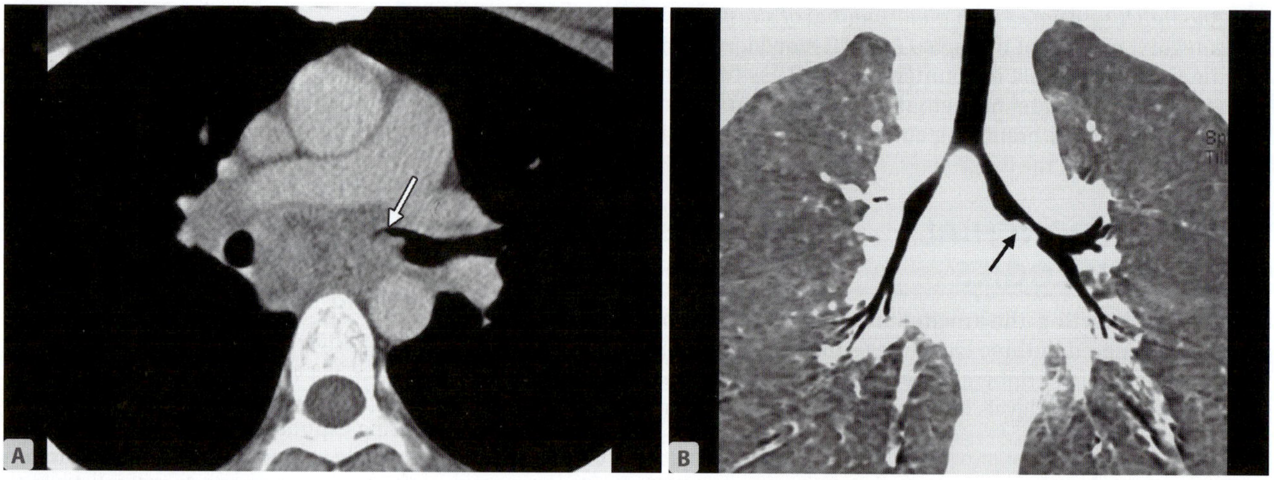

FIGS. 9A AND B: Extrinsic involvement by TB lymph nodes: Axial CT (A) and min IP (B) show necrotic subcarinal nodes extending into the left main bronchus (arrow).

TABLE 2: Etiology of central airway obstruction.

Etiology	Extrinsic	Intrinsic	
		Mural	Intraluminal
Congenital	• Vascular compression • Bronchopulmonary foregut malformations • Thoracic deformity • Vascular malformations	• Tracheobronchomalacia • Tracheal stenosis	
Inflammatory/ infective	• Lymph nodes **(Figs. 9A and B)** • Mediastinal abscess/cellulitis • Fibrosing mediastinitis	• Tuberculosis/fibrotic stricture • Vasculitis • Relapsing polychondritis • Post-intubation stricture • Sarcoidosis	• Granulation tissue • Broncholithiasis
Masses	• Lymphoma • Germ cell tumor • Vascular malformations		• Malignant tumors • Benign tumors
Miscellaneous		• Amyloidosis • Tracheopathia osteochondroplastica	• Mucus plugs • Foreign body • Clots

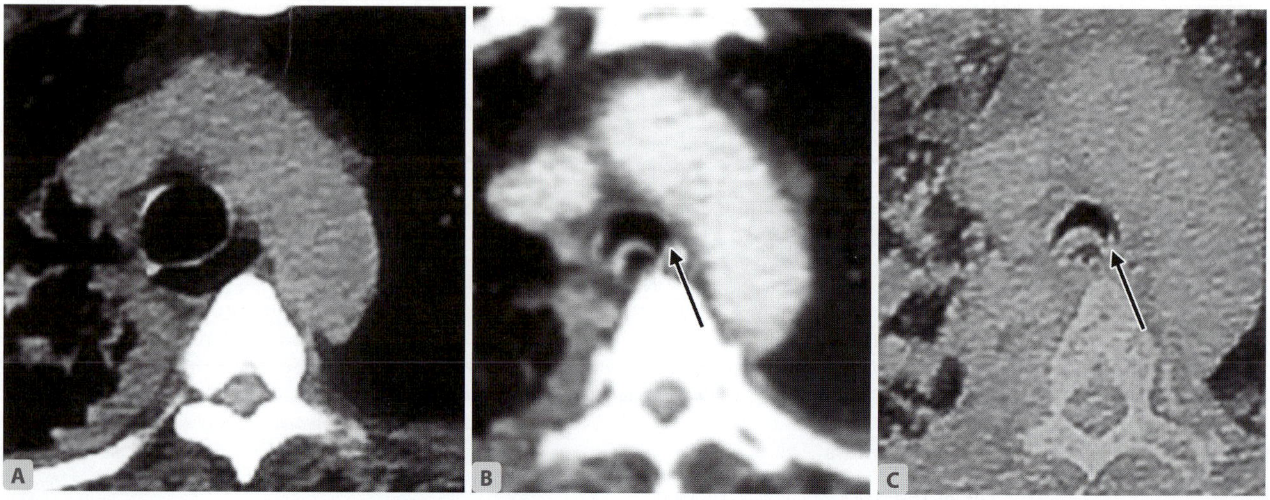

FIGS. 10A TO C: Tracheomalacia: Axial end-inspiration CT (A) shows normal appearance of trachea with collapse of the lumen during expiration (arrow in B and C).

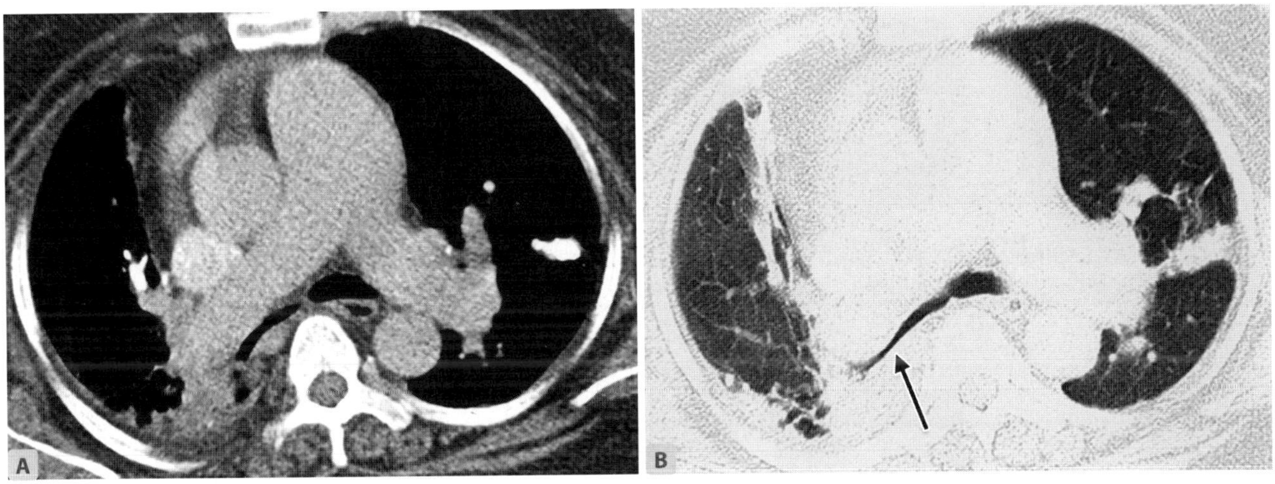

FIGS. 11A AND B: Bronchomalacia: Narrowing of the bronchus intermedius (arrow) because of chronic compression by enlarged pulmonary artery.

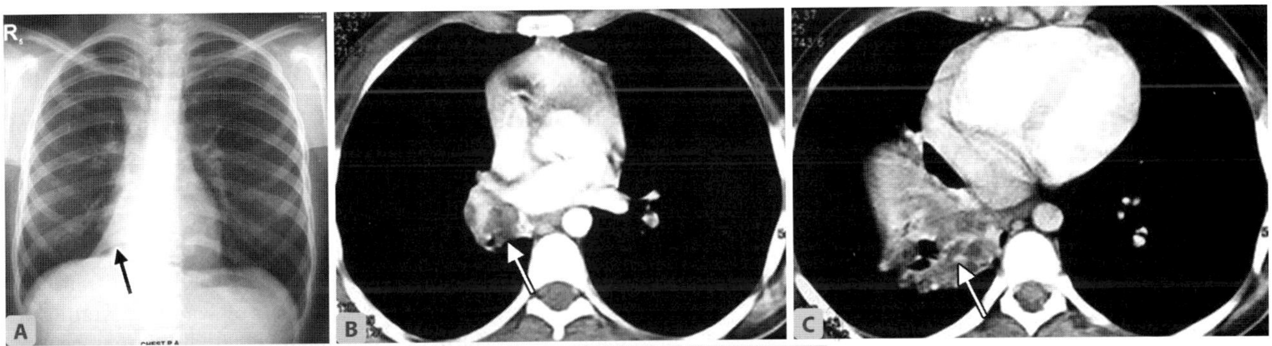

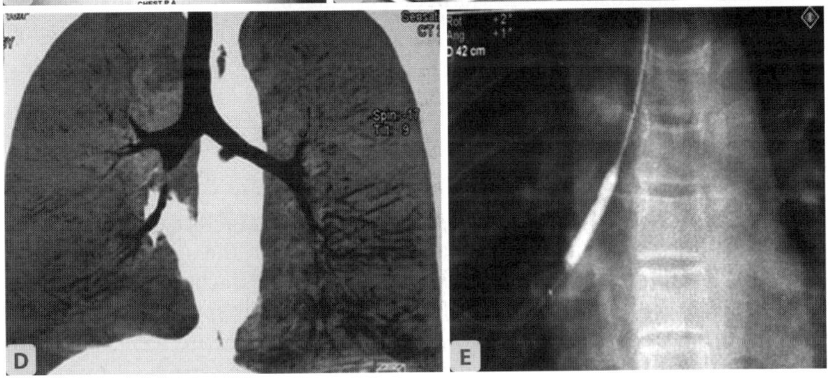

FIGS. 12A TO E: Tubercular stricture: Chest radiograph (A) of a 19 years old girl showing collapse of right lower lobe (black arrow). Axial CT (B and C) and coronal min-IP (D) demonstrates necrotic right hilar nodes (white arrows) narrowing the bronchus intermedius and lower lobe bronchus (black arrow). (E) balloon dilatation of the stricture was performed.

narrowing. Unlike active tuberculosis, which involves both mainstem bronchi equally, fibrotic TB usually involves the left main bronchus, perhaps because of its greater length. Evidence of associated mediastinal inflammation, in the form of enlarged mediastinal nodes or increased attenuation of mediastinal fat, may also be identified. CT findings are seldom specific. Findings that help differentiate tuberculosis from bronchogenic carcinoma include longer circumferential involvement and the absence of an intraluminal mass.[24] Focal infection may be responsible for tumor-like lesions when it produces granulation or endoluminal masses.

Fungal Infections (Aspergillosis)

Airway disease caused by Aspergillus takes many forms, including saprophytic colonization, tracheobronchitis, ulcerative tracheobronchitis with or without pseudomembrane formation, and necrotizing (invasive) aspergillosis,[25] the latter being further divided into acute and chronic airway invasive forms. Multifocal or diffuse tracheobronchial wall thickening, causing luminal narrowing is seen on CT.

Rhinoscleroma

Rhinoscleroma is an insidious infectious granulomatous disease caused by Klebsiella rhinoscleromatis.[26] The involvement is characteristically of the upper respiratory tract; trachea and proximal bronchi may occasionally be involved. CT findings include diffuse nodular tracheobronchial wall thickening, causing luminal narrowing with mediastinal or hilar lymphadenopathy.[27]

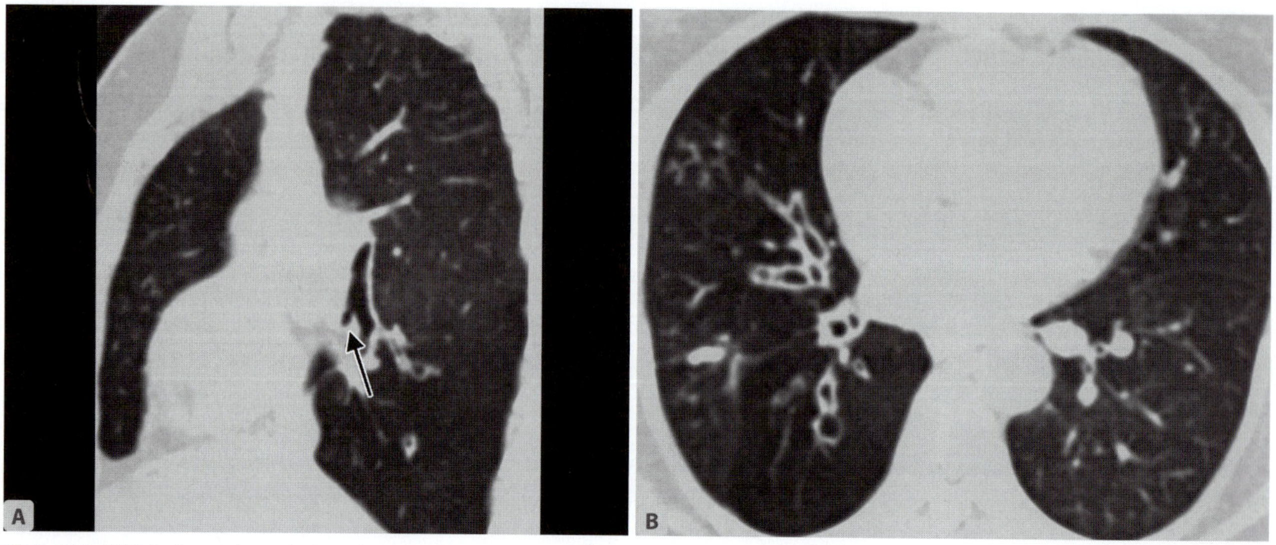

FIGS. 13A AND B: Post-tubercular bronchostenosis: Sagittal MPR (A) and axial CT (B) show narrowing of right middle lobe bronchus (arrow) with bronchiectatic changes in middle and lower lobes.

Vasculitis

Granulomatous Polyangitis (GPA)

Airway involvement in GPA includes bronchial stenosis, inflammation and pseudotumors.[28] Often, no correlation is seen between c-ANCA levels and the presence of tracheobronchial inflammation.

Relapsing Polychondritis

Relapsing polychondritis is a multisystem disease of unknown etiology characterized by recurrent inflammation of cartilage of nose, external ear, peripheral joints, larynx, trachea and bronchi.[29] It is commonly seen in the third and sixth decades with initial involvement of larynx and subglottic trachea. Distal trachea and bronchi may be involved as the disease progresses. An acute inflammatory infiltrate in the cartilage and perichondrial tissue is seen on pathology. CT findings include increased airway wall attenuation in association with smooth tracheal or bronchial wall thickening. The increased attenuation may appear as frank calcification in later stages. There is characteristic sparing of the posterior membranous portion of the trachea.[30]

Post-intubation Stenosis

Among acquired strictures, the most common cause is injury resulting from intubation. Although investigators have estimated that complications occur in up to 10–15% of patients after intubation and up to 40% patients with tracheostomies, the incidence of serious complications after intubation has decreased dramatically since the introduction of high-volume/low-pressure tubes.[31] The two principal sites for post-intubation stenoses are at the stoma or at the level of the endotracheal tube or tracheostomy tube balloon. Strictures result from pressure necrosis, which causes ischemia and subsequent scarring **(Figs. 14A to C)**. Other complications of intubation include tracheal rupture and tracheobrachiocephalic artery or tracheoesophageal fistulas. Stent placement remains one temporary option for treating such strictures, though optimal surgical technique is laryngotracheal resection and reconstruction.

Sarcoidosis

Tracheal involvement is rare and usually associated with laryngeal disease.[27] In sarcoidosis, airway involvement is usually in the form of bronchial involvement. It may be seen in up to 65% of patients with sarcoidosis on high resolution CT in the form of nodular or smooth wall thickening.[32]

Miscellaneous

Tracheopathia Osteoplastica

Tracheopathia osteoplastica is characterized by multiple small osteocartilaginous growths in the submucosa of the inner anterior and lateral walls of the trachea. Usually seen in asymptomatic elderly males. Multiple, small (1–5 mm sized) irregular nodules (occasionally calcified are seen protruding into the tracheal lumen on CT **(Figs. 15A to C)**.

Amyloidosis

Amyloidosis entails a number of entities characterized by deposition of an autologous fibrillar protein and associated protein derivatives in extracellular tissue. Amyloidosis can be either primary (frequently associated with multiple myeloma or Waldenstrom macroglobulinemia) or secondary (in the setting of chronic inflammatory diseases including TB, cystic fibrosis, bronchiectasis, etc.).Within the lung, three types of localized amyloidosis have been identified—tracheobronchial, nodular and diffuse septal amyloidosis.[33] Tracheobronchial amyloidosis is the most common form of respiratory system involvement in patients with localized amyloidosis. Clinical presentation depends on the part of airway involved. Patients with proximal subglottic or laryngeal involvement typically present with hoarseness and stridor,

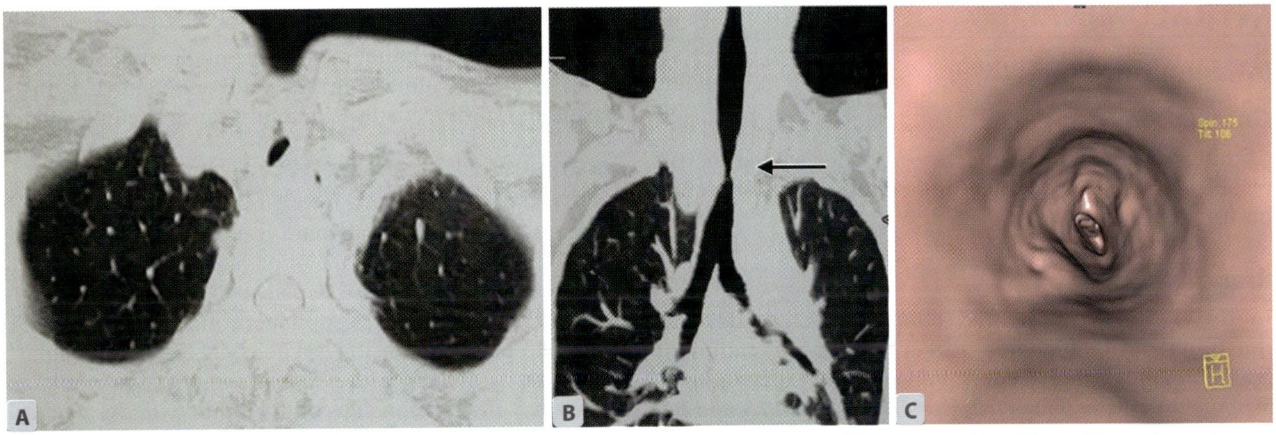

FIGS. 14A TO C: Post-intubation stenosis: Axial CT (A), coronal MPR (B) and VB (C) showing a tracheal stricture. Patient had a past history of prolonged intubation.

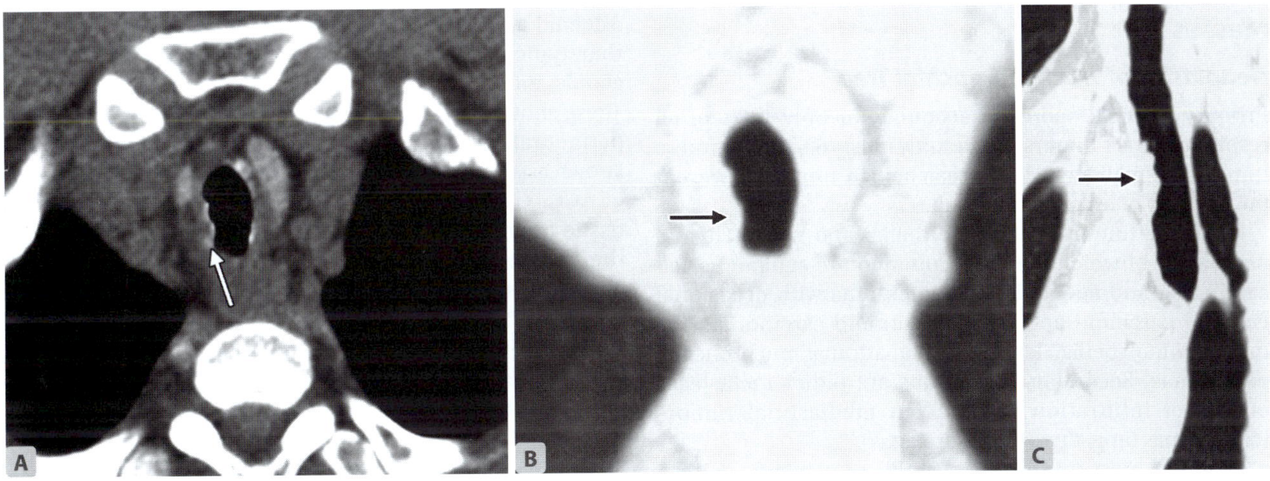

FIGS. 15A TO C: Tracheopathia osteoplastica: Axial CT (A and B) and sagittal MPR (C) showing multiple, small soft tissue nodules along the inner tracheal aspect with sparing of the posterior tracheal wall.

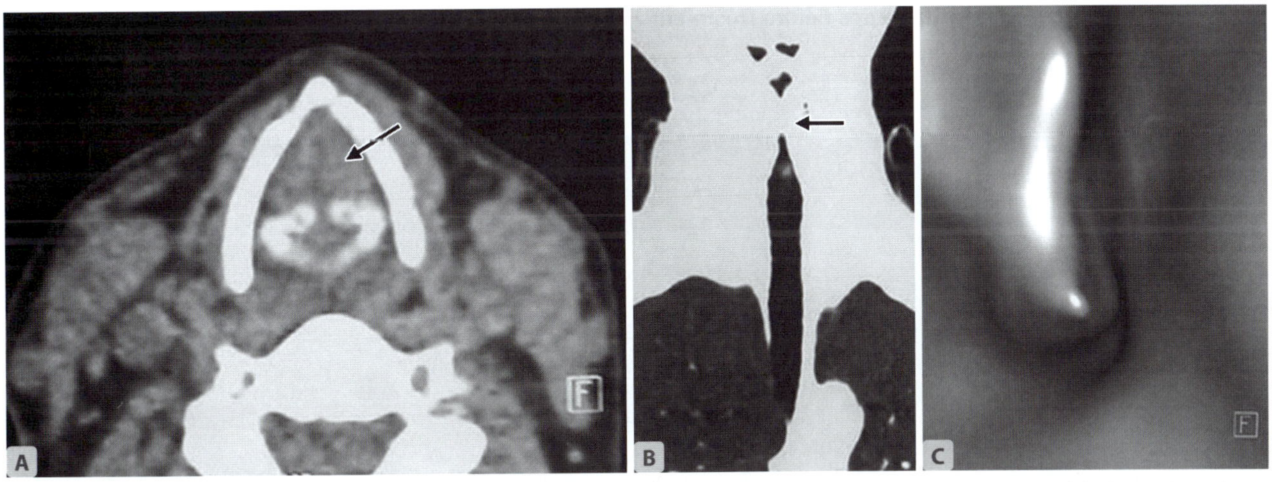

FIGS. 16A TO C: Amyloidosis: MDCT reveals diffuse wall thickening of the laryngeal wall and vocal cords with obliteration of the lumen (arrow).

distal trachea or mainstem bronchi involvement causes cough, wheezing, dyspnea.

CT images of tracheobronchial amyloidosis **(Figs. 16A to C)** appear as nodular thickening or focal mass partially or completely occluding airways; mimicking the appearance of benign or malignant tracheal neoplasms.[34] Mural calcifications are promiment features. In patients with recurrent infiltrates, bronchiectasis may develop.

INTRALUMINAL

Inflammatory/Infective

Granulation Tissue

Chronic inflammation of infective/noninfective nature can result in nonspecific granulation tissue forming bronchial obstructive lesions.

Broncholithiasis

In this condition, calcified lymph nodes erode into the tracheobronchial tree and it is a complication of granulomatous lymphadenitis. Patients may expectorate or aspirate the calcified material. On MDCT **(Figs. 17A and B)**, calcified focus is seen within the bronchial lumen without any mass. Peribronchial lymph node calcification may be seen and post-obstructive abnormalities are often associated.[3,35]

Masses

Neoplasms of Tracheobronchial Tree

Primary tracheal neoplasia accounts for only 1–2% of all respiratory tract tumors.[36] In adults, most (60–90%) of these tumors are malignant,[37] whereas benign tumors represent the majority of lesions in children.

Primary tumors include epithelial and mesenchymal neoplasms of which the most common are squamous cell carcinoma and adenoid cystic carcinoma with occasional cases of carcinoid and mucoepidermoid carcinoma. The most common benign lesions are hamartomas and bronchial papillomas. Secondary neoplasms are either metastases or, direct infiltration by adjacent mediastinal tumors (carcinomas lung, thyroid or esophagus).[36]

Clinical presentation is usually nonspecific with a significant overlap between the imaging appearances of benign and malignant lesions. The main role of imaging **(Figs. 18A to D)** is in delineation of tumor extent within the lumen, airway wall, and surrounding structures before treatment planning.

Malignant Tumors

Primary tracheal cancer is rare and seen commonly in middle aged/elderly males smokers. The prognosis of patients is poor, with the 5-year survival rate being 5–35%.[38]

Squamous Cell Carcinoma (SCC)

SCC is usually seen in smokers with up to one-third of the cases associated with other malignant lesions of the respiratory tract.[39] In approximately 10% of patients, these tumors are multifocal and extend into the mainstem bronchi or adjacent esophagus, resulting in esophagobronchial fistula.[39] CT **(Figs. 19A to C)** demonstrates a polypoid intraluminal mass of soft tissue density with irregular, smooth, or lobulated contours.[36] The relationships of the tumor with the tracheal wall vary from localized eccentric pedunculated lesions to circumferential invasion.

Adenoid Cystic Carcinoma

Adenoid cystic carcinoma (ACC) are low-grade malignancies that typically arise from the tracheobronchial mucous glands, most frequently on the posterolateral tracheal wall. These show a marked propensity for local, submucosal and perineural invasion. Unlike squamous call carcinoma, no known association exists between smoking and development of ACC. CT appearances **(Figs. 20A and B)** include soft-tissue attenuating intraluminal mass which may infiltrate the mediastinal fat or localized stenosis because of circumferential wall thickening.[40]

Mucoepidermoid Carcinoma

Mucoepidermoid carcinoma arises from the minor salivary glands lining the tracheobronchial tree.[41] Patients are less than 40 years old and usually present with obstructive airway symptoms. On CT, it is seen as a smooth, oval or lobulated, mildly enhancing endobronchial mass, often smoothly oval or lobulated.[42] Punctate calcifications are occasionally seen.

Malignancies of trachea or esophagus can also lead to the formation of acquired tracheoesophageal fistulas **(Figs. 21A and B)**.

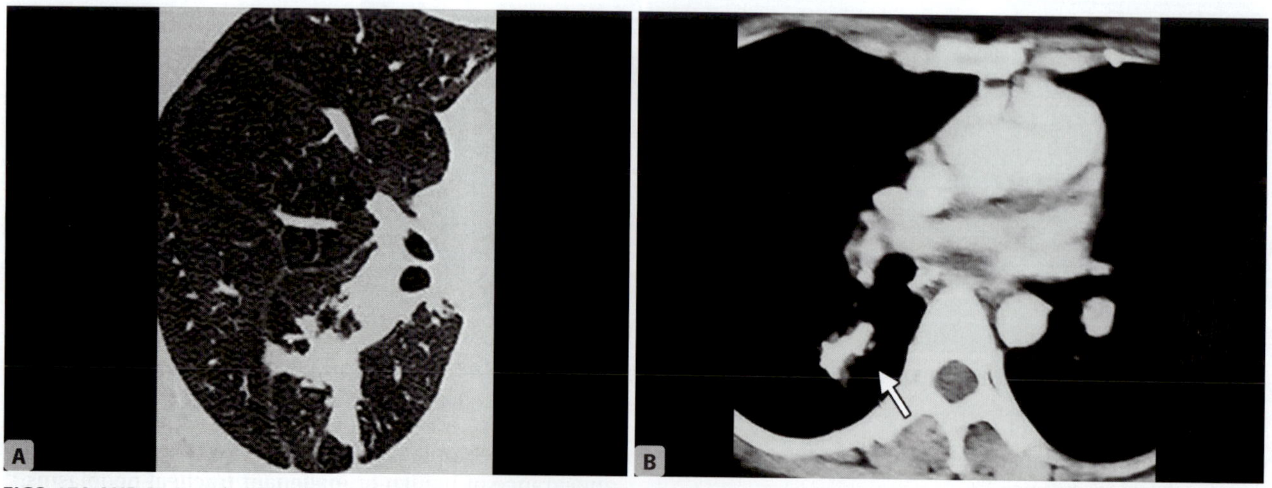

FIGS. 17A AND B: Broncholith: A branching tubular opacity is seen in the right lower lobe (A) of a 32-year-old woman with past history of tuberculosis. (B) On mediastinal window, the lesion is seen to be calcified (arrow).

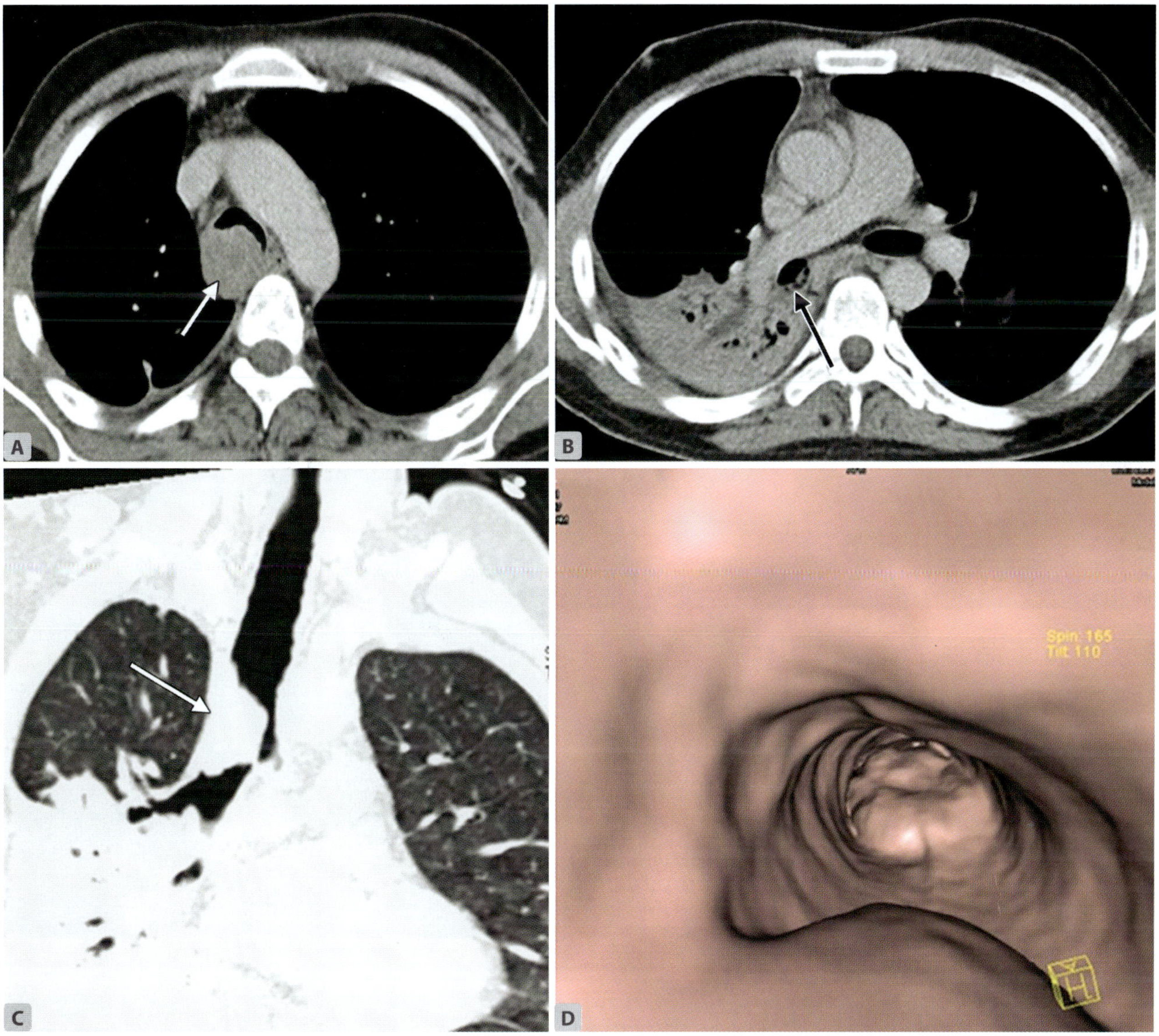

FIGS. 18A TO D: Tracheal mass: Axial CT (A and B), coronal MPR (C) and VB (D) showing a mass involving the trachea (white arrow). In addition, a low density lesion with air bubbles is seen in the right lower lobe with distal collapse suggestive of a mucous plug (black arrow in B).

Carcinoid Tumors

Carcinoid tumors are neuroendocrine tumors, which arise from bronchial, or bronchiolar epithelium. They present a histologic spectrum of low-grade to high-grade neoplasms, with the highest grades merging with small cell carcinoma.[3] Most endobronchial carcinoids are central in location arising in the main, lobar, or segmental bronchi. On CT **(Figs. 22 and 23)**, they appear as a hilar mass or an endobronchial lesion. Classical findings have been described, of a well-defined round or lobulated tumor causing narrowing of the adjacent airway, associated with eccentric calcifications.[43] These often show intense enhancement.

Endobronchial Metastases

Metastases to the bronchus can also present like an endobronchial mass. The metastases are usually from carcinoma breast, colon and kidney.

Benign Tumors

Benign tumors of the central airways are rare.[36] They can be of epithelial, mesenchymal, neural or composite origin. These tumors appear in clinical practice as the differential diagnosis of malignant lesions that are much more common.

Most common amongst these is the *squamous cell papilloma*. These most often occur in middle-aged male smokers, and typically involve the larynx or bronchi, tracheal involvement being uncommon. Involvement, when present, is limited to tracheal wall.[36] Papillomatosis is a condition associated with multiple papillomas. This condition typically affects children and young adults and is often limited to the larynx. It may involve the intrathoracic airways and also present with cavitating lung nodules and is referred to as *recurrent respiratory papillomatosis (RRP)* **(Figs. 24A and B)**. These lesions have a high propensity for recurrence and even malignant transformation.[44]

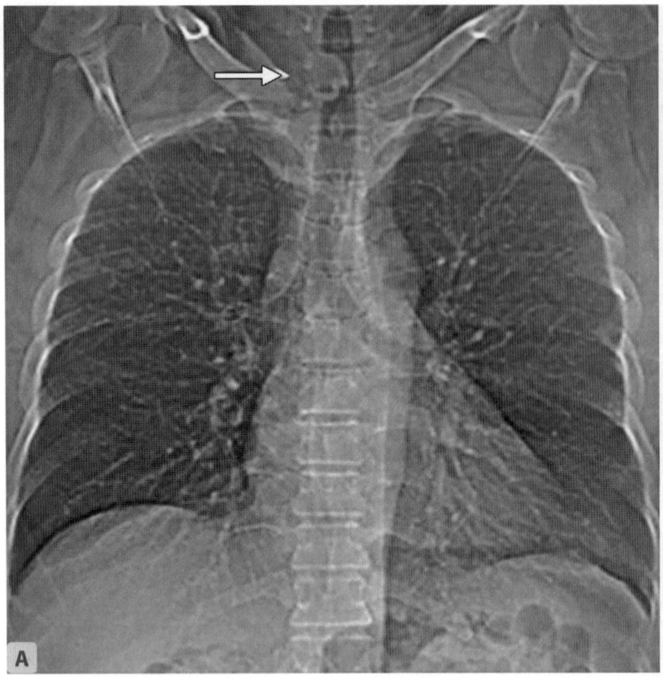

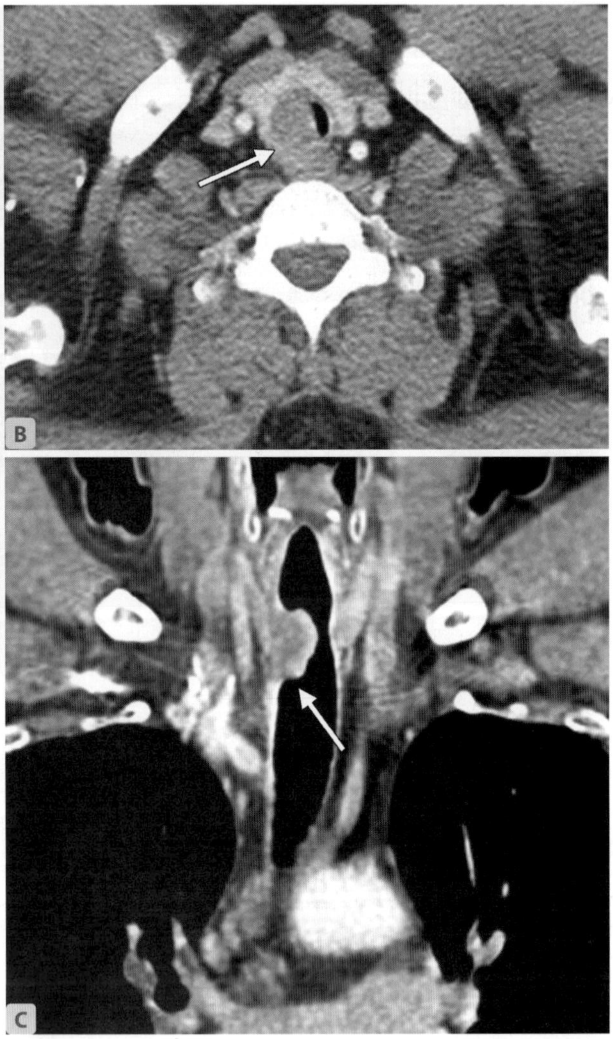

FIGS. 19A TO C: Tracheal squamous cell carcinoma: CT scout (A), axial contrast-enhanced image (B) and coronal MPR (C), reveal a polypoidal, lobulated tracheal mass (arrow) focally involving about 180° of the tracheal wall.

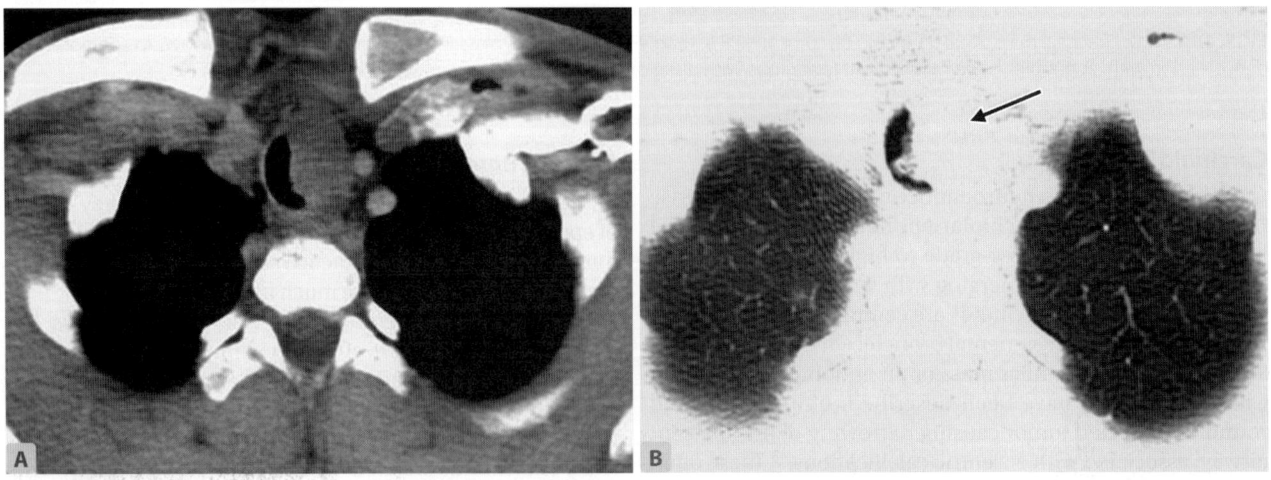

FIGS. 20A AND B: Tracheal adenoid cystic carcinoma: Axial contrast-enhanced CT in mediastinal window (A) and lung window (B) showing an irregular, soft tissue mass (arrow) with focal tracheal wall involvement. CT appearances of different tracheal tumors show significant overlap.

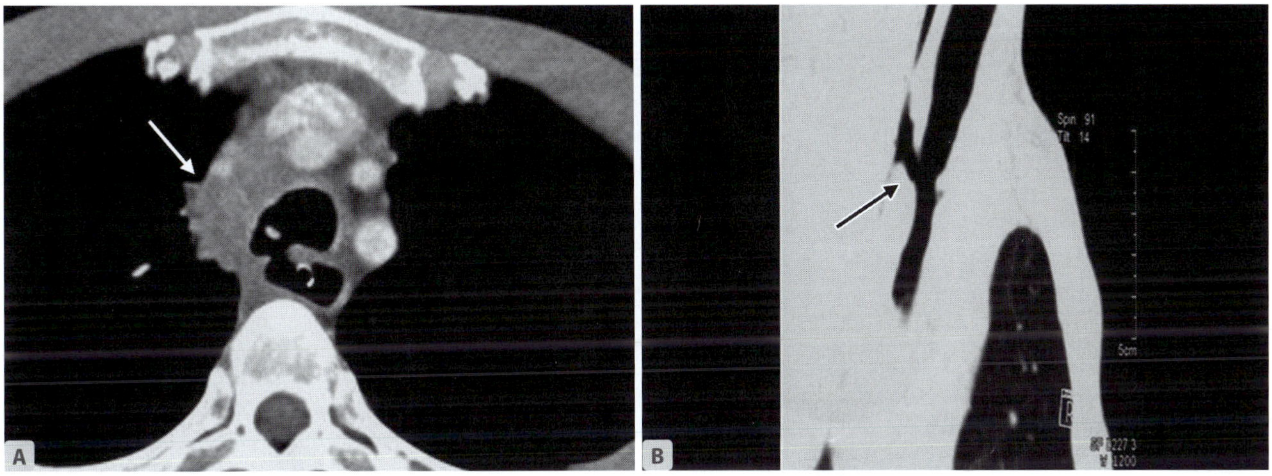

FIGS. 21A AND B: Tracheoesophageal fistula: Axial CECT (A) showing necrotic mediastinal nodes (white arrow) with a communication between trachea and esophagus. Sagittal MPR demonstrates the fistula (black arrow) well (B).

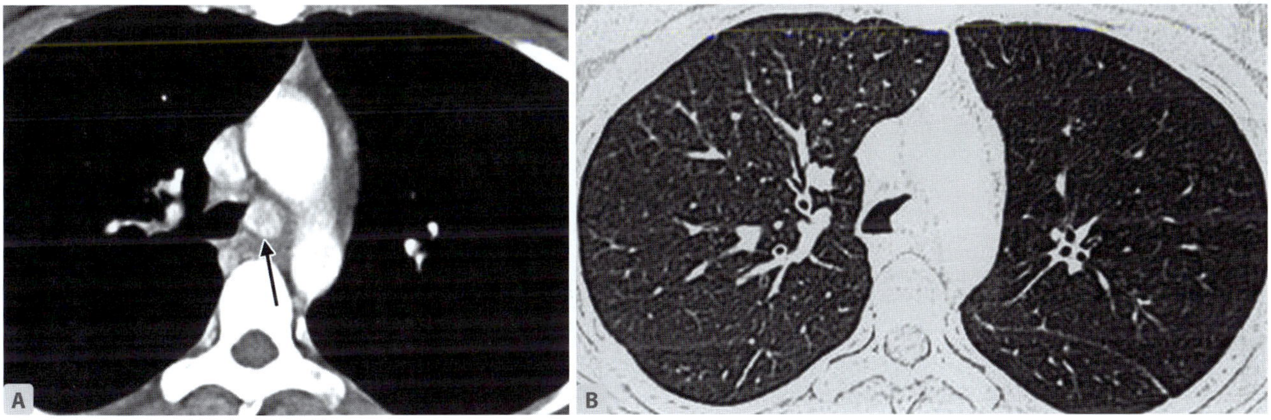

FIGS. 22A AND B: Carcinoid tumor: CT showing an intensely enhancing mass (arrow) involving the left main bronchus with hyperlucent left lung.

CT appearance may suggest the pathology of the neoplasm. Fat attenuation is seen in lipoma or hamartochondroma, while calcification may occur in hamartoma, chondroma or carcinoid. Presence of both fat and calcification suggests a hamartoma. High contrast-enhancement is seen in carcinoid, hemangioma, glomus tumor or fibroma.

MISCELLANEOUS

1. **Mucous plug/mucoid pseudotumor:** Mucus is the most common soft tissue mass within the airways. On CT scan **(Figs. 18 and 25)**, it is of low attenuation, non-enhancing, may contain small air bubbles and is not associated with cartilaginous ring disruption. Typically seen in the dependent portions of the airway it can move after coughing.
2. Other miscellaneous causes of focal airway narrowing include **foreign bodies (Figs. 26 and 27) and blood clot (Figs. 28A and B)**.

Prolonged increased intraluminal pressure can lead to the formation of acquired ***tracheal* (Figs. 29A and B) *and bronchial diverticula* (Fig. 30)**. Usually these are seen in COPD patients with chronic cough. Tracheal diverticulum is typically seen as an air filled outpouching from the right posterolateral tracheal wall.

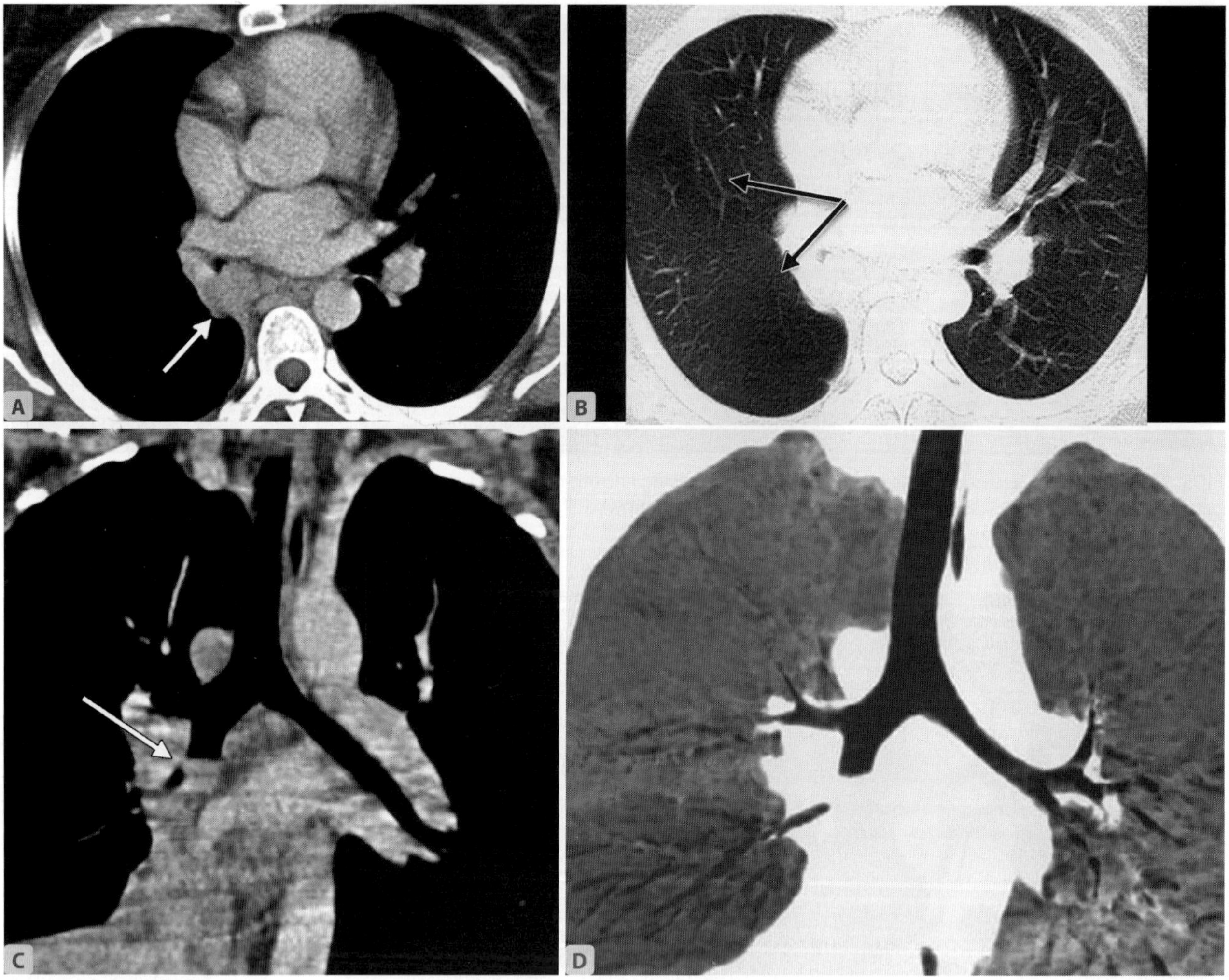

FIGS. 23A TO D: Carcinoid tumor. Axial CT (A and B), coronal MPR (C) and minIP (D) showing a lobulated mass (white arrow) involving the right bronchus intermedius with hyperlucent (black arrow) right middle and lower lobes. MinIP shows the craniocaudal extent of airway involvement the best.

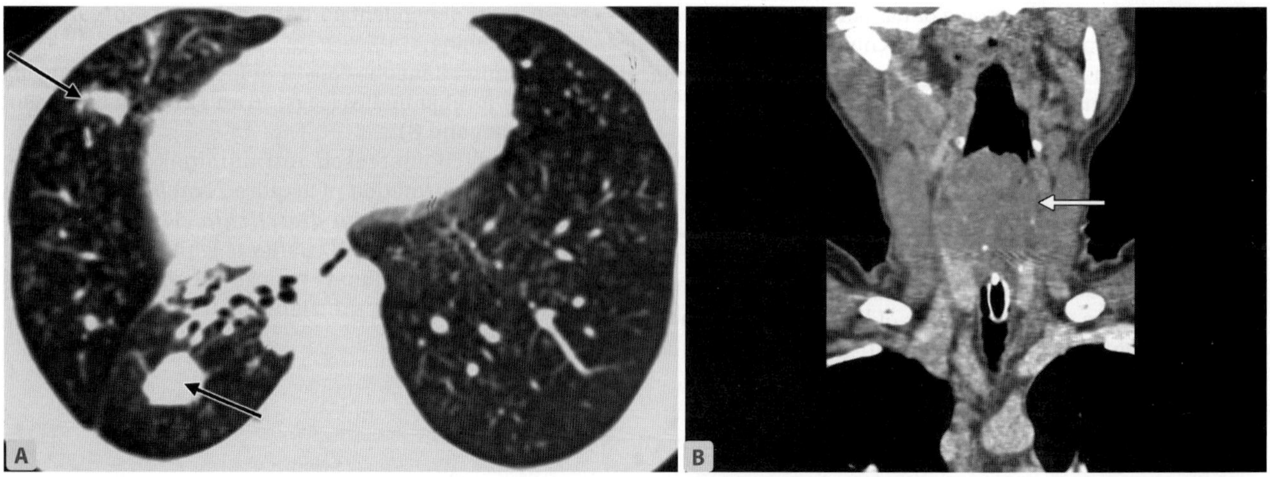

FIGS. 24A AND B: Recurrent respiratory papillomatosis: Multiple lung nodules (black arrow) and transglottic carcinoma (white arrow) in a young male with recurrent respiratory papillomatosis. The right lower lobe bronchiectasis is because of recurrent infections due to aspiration.

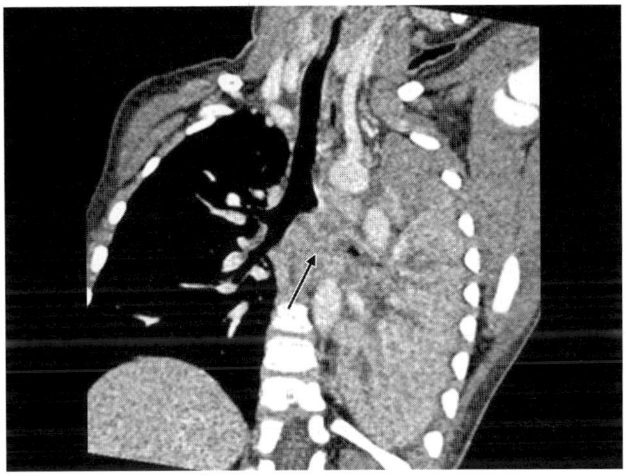

FIG. 25: Mucus plug: A fluid attenuating lesion is present in the left main bronchus (arrow) of an elderly male, with distal collapse of the left lung. These plugs can be successfully cleared bronchoscopically.

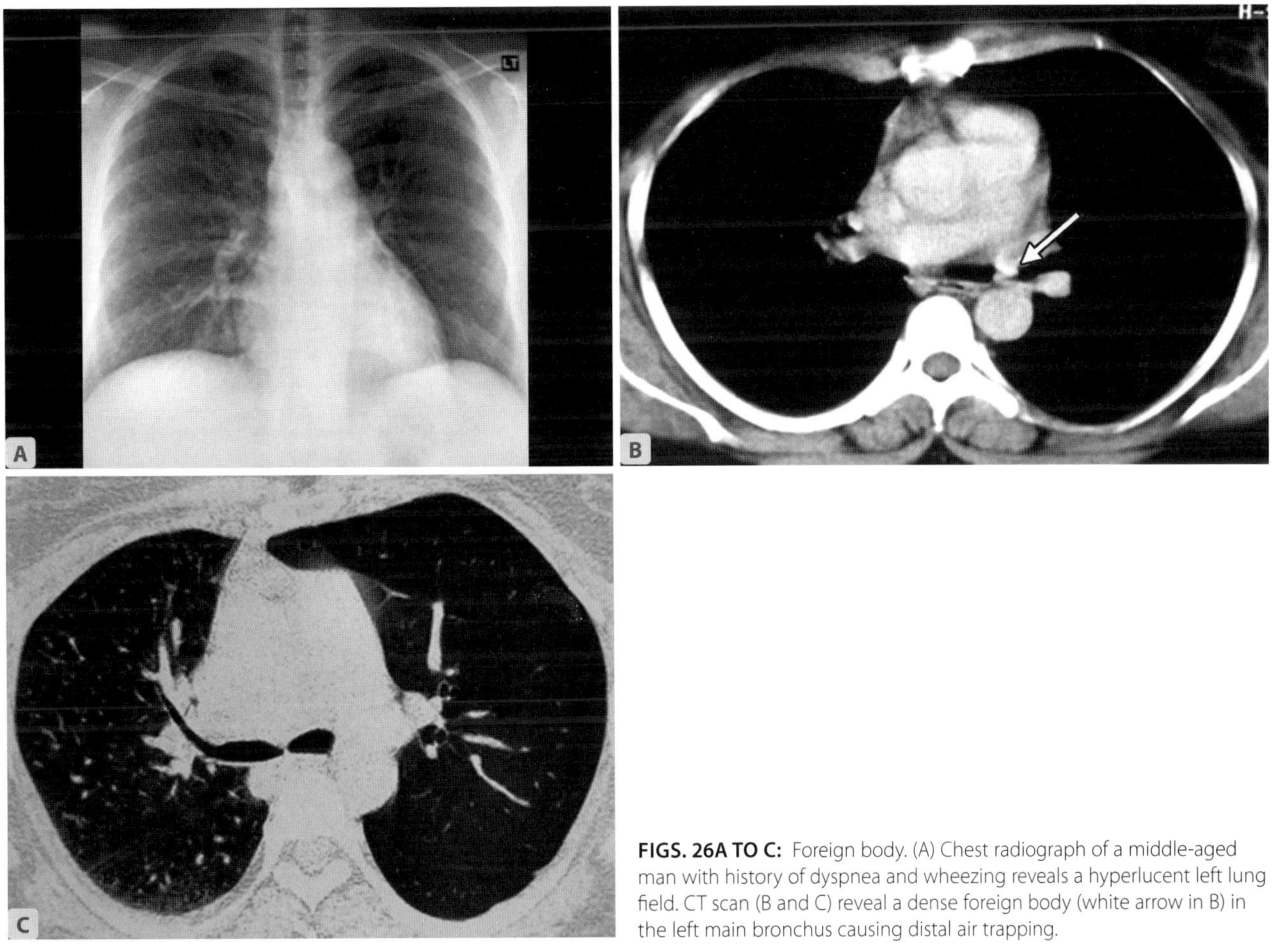

FIGS. 26A TO C: Foreign body. (A) Chest radiograph of a middle-aged man with history of dyspnea and wheezing reveals a hyperlucent left lung field. CT scan (B and C) reveal a dense foreign body (white arrow in B) in the left main bronchus causing distal air trapping.

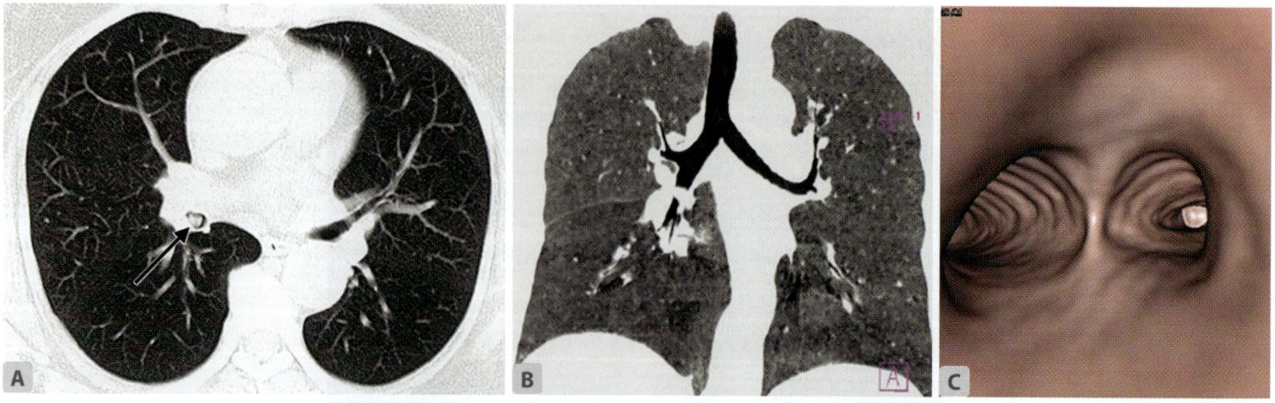

FIGS. 27A TO C: Foreign body: MDCT of a 65 years old woman with one week history of cough and breathlessness reveals a low density lesion in the bronchus intermedius with subtle lucency of the distal lung (A). The foreign body is well visualized on the minIP (B) and VB (C). The left-right orientation is reverse of an axial image on VB to simulate FB. Two days later, the patient coughed out a chickpea.

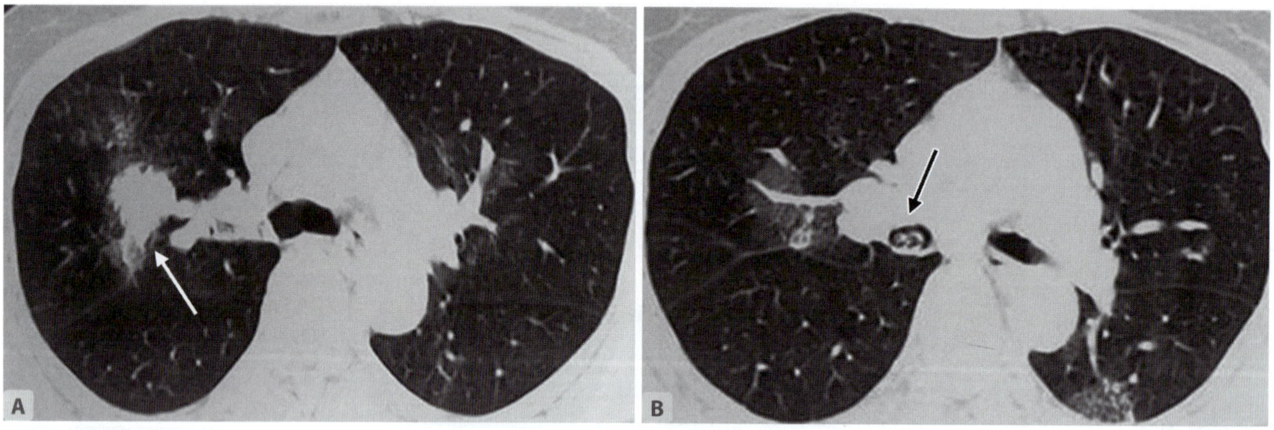

FIGS. 28A AND B: Blood clot: An elderly male presenting with hemoptysis. CT reveals a malignant mass in right upper lobe with surrounding hemorrhage (white arrow), and a blood clot (black arrow) in the right upper lobe bronchus. A blood clot resembles a mucous plug on imaging.

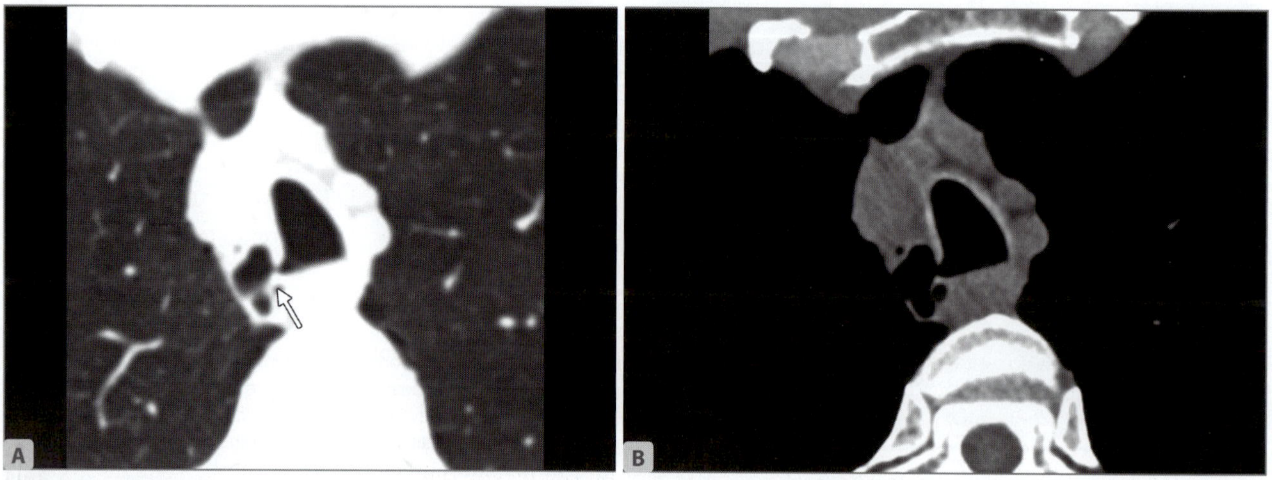

FIGS. 29A AND B: Tracheal diverticulum: Air-filled outpouching from the right posterolateral tracheal wall with small focal communication (arrow).

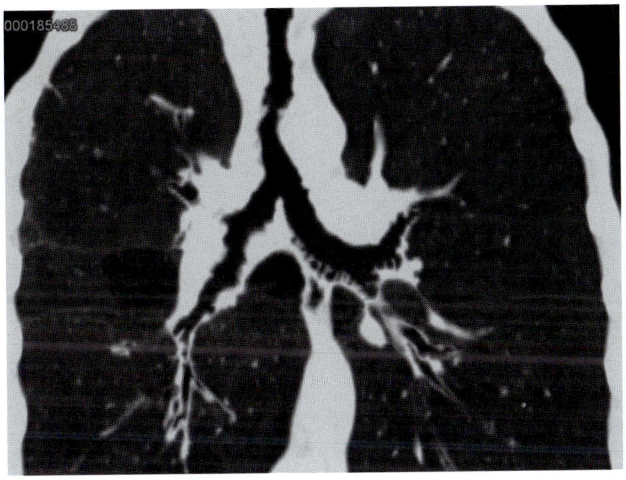

FIG. 30: Bronchial diverticulae. Multiple small diverticulae along the bilateral main and segmental bronchi with bronchial wall thickening and emphysematous changes in bilateral lung fields in a case of COPD.

PERIPHERAL AIRWAYS

BRONCHIECTASIS

Definition and Pathophysiology

Bronchiectasis is the localized, irreversible dilatation of the cartilage-containing airways or bronchi. It usually results from bronchial wall injury, bronchial lumen obstruction, and traction from adjacent fibrosis.[45] Obstruction and fibrosis are readily apparent on imaging. Bronchial wall injury and subsequent bronchiectasis can occur because of infection and, impaired host defense leading to recurrent infections, exaggerated immune response, congenital structural defects of the bronchial wall, and extrinsic insults damaging the airway wall.[46] Underlying mechanism of mucus plugging and superimposed bacterial colonization is common to these conditions.

Dilatation is classified by its gross appearance as tubular (cylindric), varicose, or cystic (saccular). These types are discussed in **Table 3** and shown in **Figures 31A to C**.

Clinical Features

Symptoms can be very nonspecific varying from mild cough or minimal dyspnea to chronic cough, abundant sputum production, progressive dyspnea, and repeated pulmonary infections. Chronic hypoxemia and hypercarbia can lead to digital clubbing, anemia, and weight loss. Other associated symptoms or manifestations include sinusitis, hemoptysis and pulmonary hypertension.[46]

Diagnosis is usually confirmed by spirometry and HRCT. The diagnostic workup may include a sweat electrolyte test, serum immunoglobulin levels, or serum *Aspergillus* antibody and precipitin, or even genetic testing according to the age of presentation and symptoms.

TABLE 3: Types of bronchiectasis.

Type of bronchiectasis	Luminal dilatation	Wall thickening
Cylindrical	Uniform	Smooth
Varicose	Alternating areas of dilatation and constriction (beaded appearance)	Irregular
Cystic	Uniform-dilated bronchus	Thick-walled bronchus terminates in a thick-walled cyst

Imaging Findings (Figs. 1 and 32)

The imaging findings on *conventional radiography* are due to the bronchial wall thickening and are detailed in **Table 4**.

HRCT is reliable to diagnose bronchiectasis. The key imaging features are due to bronchial dilatation and bronchial wall thickening and are detailed in **Table 5**. Bronchial wall thickening is seen in all cases of bronchiectasis, except those caused by congenital cartilage deficiency (William-Campbell syndrome, Mounier-Kuhn syndrome) or in allergic bronchopulmonary aspergillosis (ABPA).[46]

Etiology

The most common cause is postinfectious, followed by idiopathic bronchiectasis; bronchiectasis related to abnormal mucociliary clearance (cystic fibrosis and primary ciliary dyskinesia), and ABPA and systemic immunodeficiency.[47] Few of the common etiologies are discussed below.

Congenital Airway Wall Abnormality

There is abnormal physiologic clearing of mucoid excretions in congenital defects of cartilage, collagen, or other components of the bronchial wall. This pre-disposes to repeated infections and progressive bronchial dilatation.

Tracheobronchomegaly (Mounier-Kuhn Disease)

An uncommon disease presenting in males, in the fourth and fifth decades, it is believed to be congenital in origin. The common assocaitions include Ehlers-Danlos syndrome, Marfan syndrome, and generalized elastosis (cutis laxa). Tracheobronchomegaly is characterized by pathological thinning of the muscle, cartilage, and elastic tissue of the airway walls. There is increased distensibility of the tracheal and bronchial walls with uniform dilatation of the tracheal and bronchial lumina predisposing to recurrent infections in the dependent lungs. Tracheal diameter more than 3 cm in both coronal and sagittal planes with central bronchiectasis but without airway wall thickening is seen on CT **(Figs. 33A and B)**.[46]

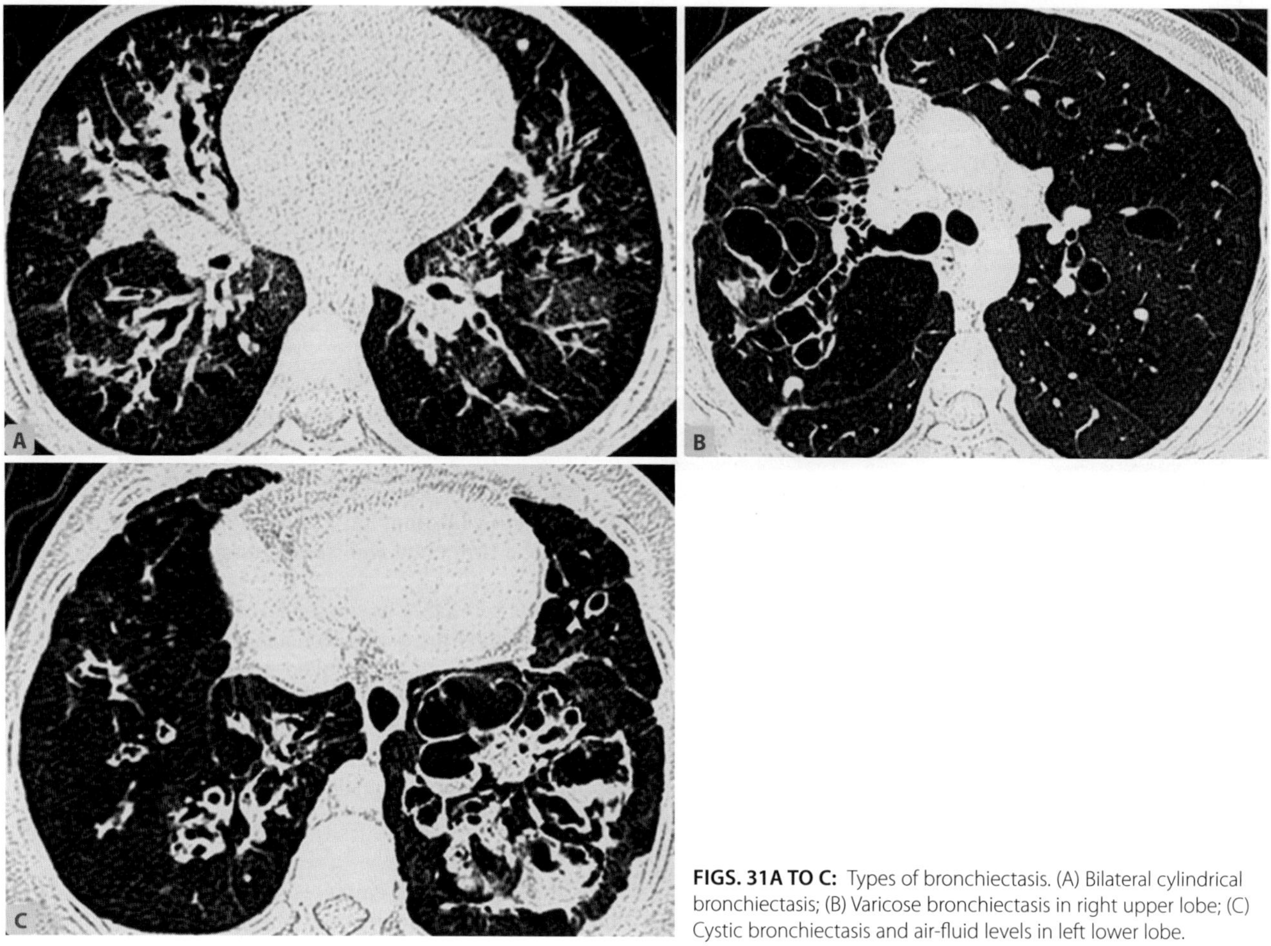

FIGS. 31A TO C: Types of bronchiectasis. (A) Bilateral cylindrical bronchiectasis; (B) Varicose bronchiectasis in right upper lobe; (C) Cystic bronchiectasis and air-fluid levels in left lower lobe.

Williams-Campbell Syndrome

Williams-Campbell syndrome is a rare disease characterized by defect in the cartilage of the fourth-, fifth-, and sixth-generation bronchi. It maybe congenital or acquired (likely as a sequelae of prior adenovirus (measles and pertussis) infections). On CT imaging there is cystic bronchiectasis distal to the third-generation bronchi with ballooning on inspiratory CT and collapse on expiratory phase.[48]

Congenital Bronchial Atresia

There is congenital focal obliteration of the lumen of a segmental bronchus. This results in focal bronchiectasis and air trapping more distally. Usually identified as an incidental finding on a chest radiograph as an ovoid, tubular, or branching density. CT **(Figs. 34A to C)** shows the characteristic bronchial, branching nature, and distal air trapping. It should be differentiated from an acquired mucocele which is caused by focal scarring of a segmental bronchus (infective) or from an endobronchial lesion.[49] In case of an acquired mucocele an endobronchial neoplasm should be excluded.

Acquired Wall Abnormalities

Inflammation of the bronchial wall because of chronic infections, inhalational injury, and cellular infiltration in the setting of graft versus host disease can cause damage to the bronchial wall.

Mucociliary Clearance Abnormalities

In cystic fibrosis, the consistency of mucus is abnormal whereas primary ciliary dyskinesia and immotile ciliary syndrome are characterized by abnormalities of the structure and function of the cilia of the airway epithelium. This leads to ineffective mucus clearance and secondary colonization of the airway lumina by bacteria and repeated episodes of infections. There is upper lobe involvement in cystic fibrosis whereas in primary and acquired ciliary dyskinesia the bronchiectasis is worse in the lower lungs.[46] Primary ciliary dyskinesia (PCD) or immotile ciliary syndrome is caused by a defect in structure and function of the airway cilia and causes progressive bronchiectasis. Kartagener syndrome **(Figs. 35A and B)** or triad (situs inversus, bronchiectasis, and sinusitis) is seen in half of the PCD patients.[50,51] Bronchiectasis in PCD is primarily in the lingular, middle and lower lobes of the lung.

Hyperimmune Response

Hyperimmune response to internal or external antigens with inflammation of the airway wall and subsequent

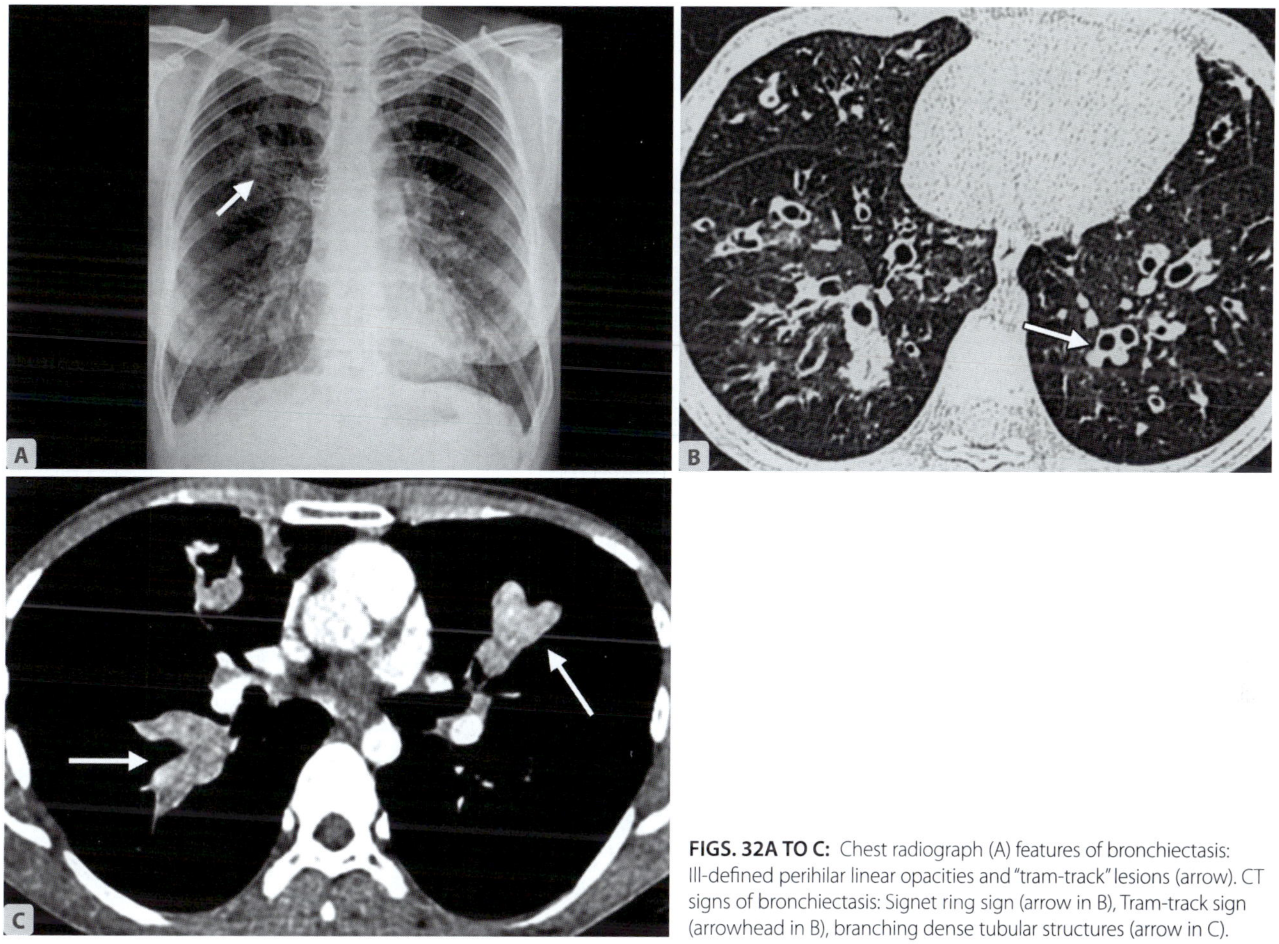

FIGS. 32A TO C: Chest radiograph (A) features of bronchiectasis: Ill-defined perihilar linear opacities and "tram-track" lesions (arrow). CT signs of bronchiectasis: Signet ring sign (arrow in B), Tram-track sign (arrowhead in B), branching dense tubular structures (arrow in C).

TABLE 4: Key radiographic features of bronchiectasis.

Imaging finding	Etiology
Ill-defined perihilar linear densities with indistinctness of the margins of the central pulmonary arteries	Bronchial wall thickening
Ill-defined ring shadows (bronchus seen end on)	Bronchial wall thickening
Tramlines or parallel lines along expected course of bronchi	Bronchial wall thickening in severe bronchiectasis
Elongated opacities ± calcified	Mucus plugging
Air-fluid levels in thick-walled cysts with surrounding consolidation	Superadded infection
Hyperinflation	Increased lung volume

TABLE 5: Key HRCT findings of bronchiectasis.

Imaging Finding	Etiology
Internal luminal diameter of one or more bronchi > diameter of adjacent artery	Bronchial dilatation
Lack of normal tapering of a bronchus	Bronchial dilatation
Visible bronchus abutting mediastinal pleura	Bronchial dilatation
Visible bronchus within 1 cm of pleura	Bronchial dilatation
Signet ring sign	Jewel: Artery abutting the Ring: Thick-walled dilated bronchus on axial view
Tram-track sign	Parallel, thickened walls of a dilated bronchus on a longitudinal section
Branching dense tubular structures	Mucus plugging of dilated bronchi and bronchioles
Centrilobular nodules, in a "tree-in-bud" pattern	Mucus-filled bronchiolectasis
Mosaic attenuation and air trapping	Coexisting constrictive bronchiolitis

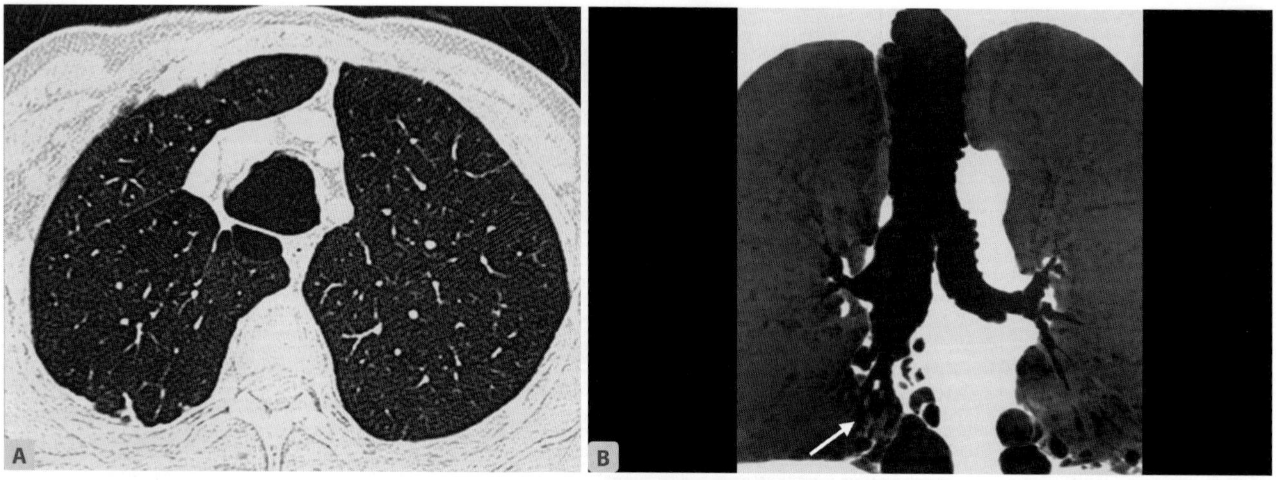

FIGS. 33A AND B: Mounier-Kuhn disease: CT reveals dilatation of the trachea and major bronchi. Bronchiectasis is seen in right lower lobe (arrow).

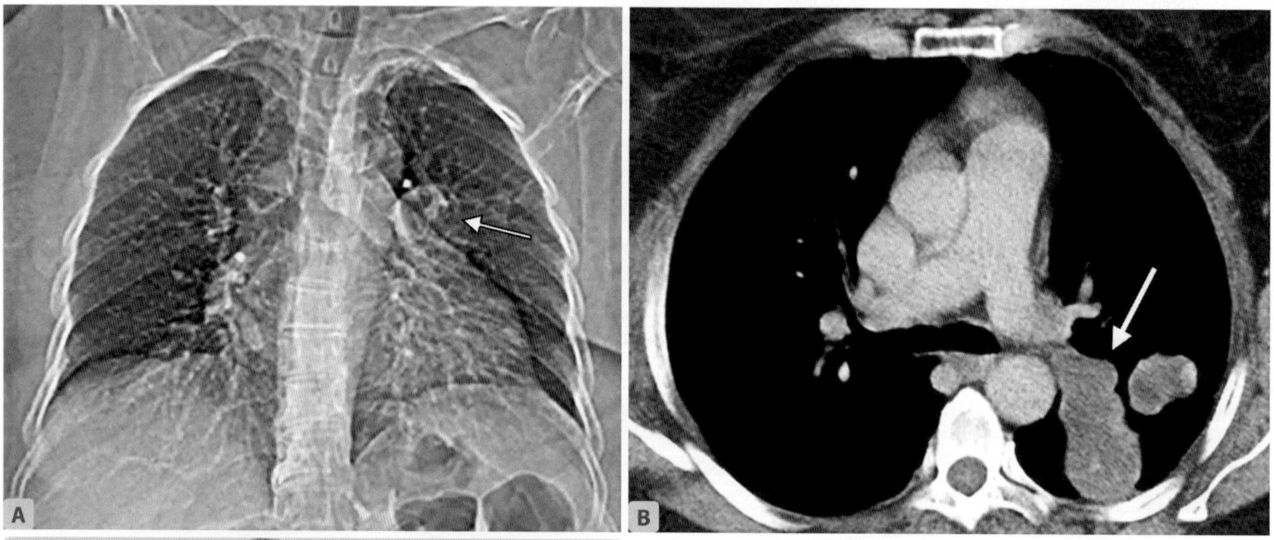

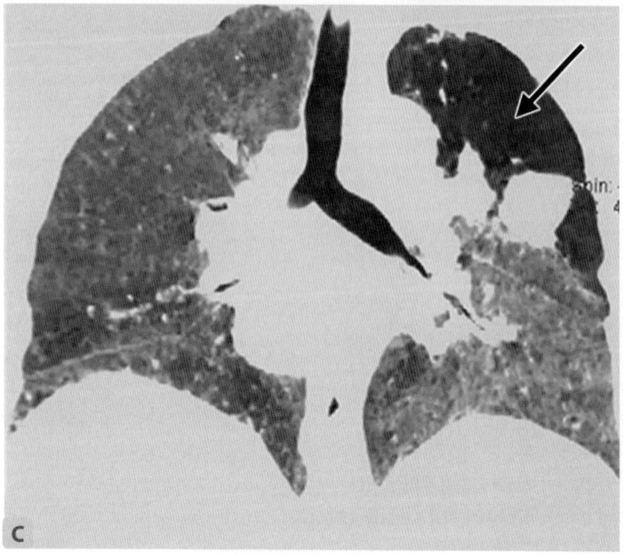

FIGS. 34A TO C: Congenital bronchial atresia: CT scout film (A) shows a well-defined left parahilar opacity (arrow). Mediastinal window (B) reveals a fluid-filled branching, tubular lesion (arrow) in the posterior segment of left upper lobe. MinIP (C) demonstrates the distal hyperinflation (arrow).

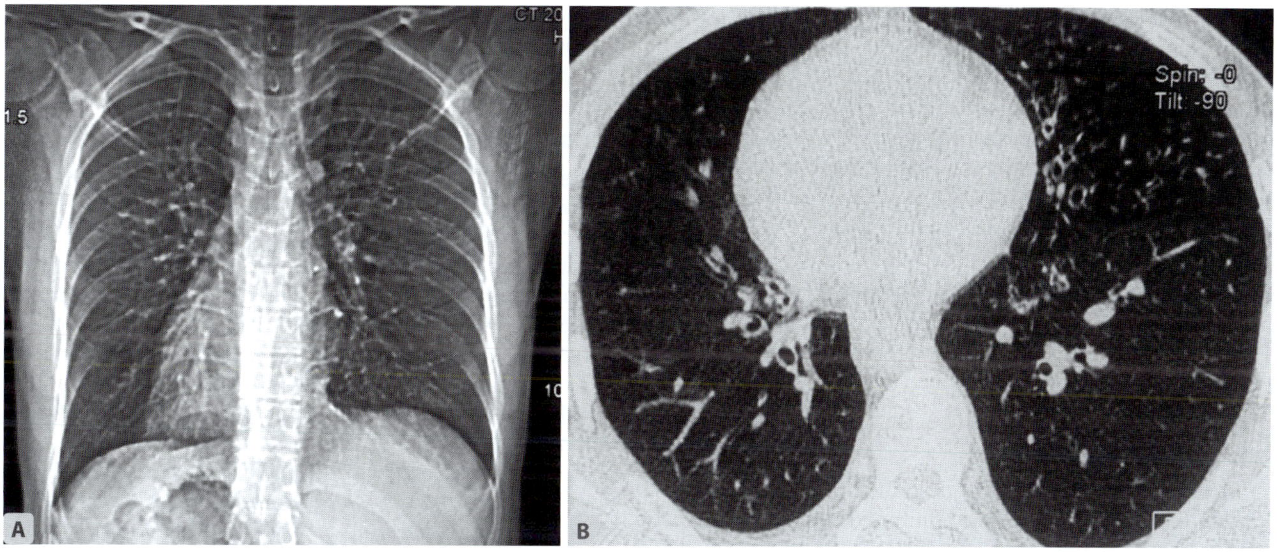

FIGS. 35A AND B: Kartagener syndrome: CT scout film (A) shows situs inversus. HRCT chest (B) reveals bilateral central bronchiectasis.

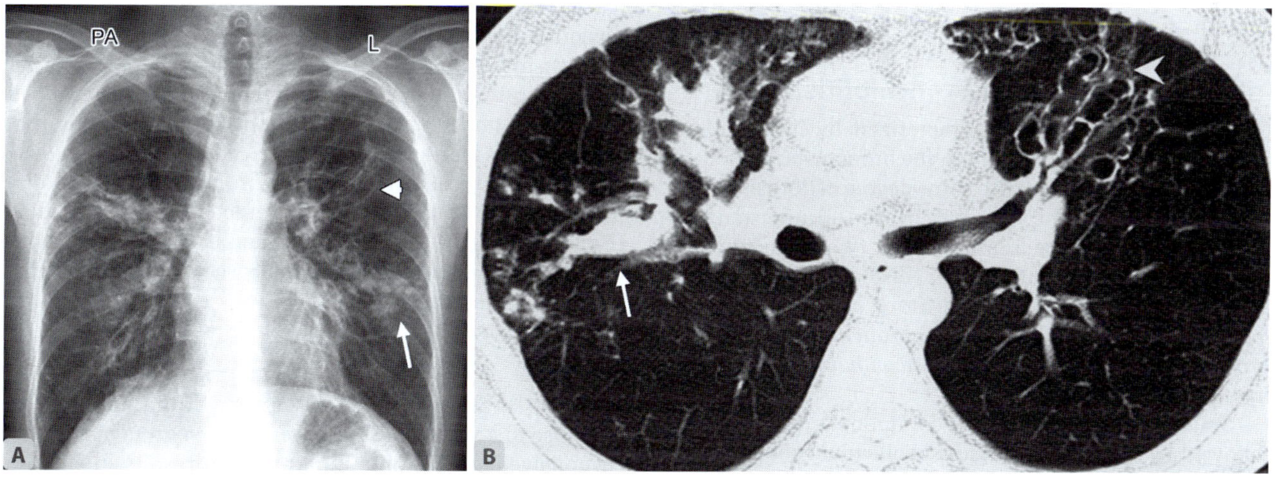

FIGS. 36A AND B: Allergic bronchopulmonary aspergillosis (ABPA): Chest radiograph (A) and CT scan (B) showing classical central, tubular bronchiectasis (arrowhead) with mucous plugging giving "finger-in-glove" appearance (arrow).

bronchiectasis can be seen in allergic bronchopulmonary aspergillosis, inflammatory bowel disease, rheumatoid arthritis, Sjögren disease and granulomatous polyangitis.

Allergic Bronchopulmonary Aspergillosis

Allergic bronchopulmonary aspergillosis (ABPA) is a hypersensitivity reaction to *Aspergillus fumigatus* antigens seen commonly in patients with atopic rhinitis, asthma, or CF. Patients present with fever, wheeze and expectoration of brown mucus plugs. Elevated serum IgE level, eosinophilia on peripheral blood smears, or positive skin reaction to *Aspergillus* antigen are seen on clinical evaluation. Mycelia can sometimes be identified in the expectorated mucus plugs. Imaging characteristically shows migratory consolidation early in the disease, usually involving the upper lobes. On HRCT **(Figs. 36A and B)**, there is central and upper lobe bronchiectasis, varicose or cystic subtypes. Inspissated mucus in the dilated central bronchi gives the classic finger in-glove appearance on the chest radiographs in more chronic cases.[46,50] There is atelectasis or hyperinflation of the lung distal to the impacted bronchi. In up to 20% of the patients, high-attenuation mucus may be seen.[52]

SMALL AIRWAYS

Small airway refers to the distal airways, which are small in size (<2 mm in diameter) and lack cartilage and submucosal glands. This includes the membranous (purely conducting) and respiratory bronchioles (conducting and gas exchange function). *Hence, the term bronchiolitis is used interchangeably with small airway disease (SAD).*

ROLE OF IMAGING IN EVALUATION OF SAD

CT is the mainstay of diagnosis as chest radiograph is often normal in early cases and also PFT derangements are evident only in advanced forms of the disease. The CT technique for evaluation of SAD has been described above **(Box 3)**.

CT SIGNS OF SMALL AIRWAY DISEASE

These include both direct and indirect signs and are detailed in **Table 6**.[53]

CLASSIFICATION

Bronchiolitis is a term used to describe bronchiolar inflammation of diverse causes. The combined radiopathological approach is a commonly accepted classification system. According to this classification, there are two major types of small airway diseases.[54,55]

1. Inflammatory/cellular bronchiolitis
2. Constrictive/fibrotic bronchiolitis

Inflammatory/Cellular Bronchiolitis

Cellular bronchiolitis is characterized by inflammatory cellular infiltrates involving both the bronchiolar lumen and walls, usually associated with some degree of fibrosis.

According to the clinical presentation, acute or chronic, and the predominant cell type, classification includes a number of specific etiologies, including—*infectious bronchiolitis, respiratory bronchiolitis (RB), follicular bronchiolitis, Asian panbronchiolitis, aspiration bronchiolitis; bronchiolitis associated with bronchiectasis and hypersensitivity pneumonitis.*

Smoking-related RB is the commonest of these forms followed by infectious diseases.[56] Follicular bronchiolitis is often of autoimmune etiology or associated with connective tissue disorders or immunodeficiency.

On imaging **(Box 6)** cellular bronchiolitis **(Fig. 37)** is characterized by the presence of centrilobular nodules, ground-glass nodules and bronchial wall thickening. RB **(Figs. 38A and B)** usually has fine nodules compared to infections where there is patchy distribution of larger and coarse nodules.

TABLE 6: CT signs of small airway disease.

Direct signs	Indirect signs
1. Centrilobular nodules with 'tree-in-bud' appearance (branching nodules; V or Y shaped) 2. Ground-glass opacities typically centrilobular or peribronchiolar in distribution 3. Bronchiolectasis (seen in chronic stages)	1. Air trapping (seen as areas of low attenuation, best on expiratory scans) 2. Atelectasis/collapse (less common)

BOX 6: HRCT features of cellular/inflammatory bronchiolitis.

- Centrilobular nodules with or without "tree-in-bud"
- Ground-glass nodules
- Bronchial wall thickening

Constrictive/Obliterative Bronchiolitis

Obliterative bronchiolitis is characterized by irreversible circumferential submucosal fibrosis, which results in bronchiolar narrowing or obliteration in the absence of surrounding parenchymal inflammation or intraluminal granulation tissue. This narrowing of bronchiolar lumen may be due to collagen deposition, fibrosis or scarring of bronchiolar wall/peribronchiolar area.[57,58]

Conditions associated with constrictive bronchiolitis include—*post-infectious (Swyer-James or Macleod syndrome), inhalation of toxic fumes, autoimmune/connective tissue diseases, drug related, chronic allograft rejection associated with heart-lung or lung transplantation and graft-versus-host disease associated with bone marrow transplantation and idiopathic.*

Obliterative bronchiolitis is most frequently post-infectious (often viral) or connective tissue disease related (commonest being rheumatoid arthritis). Acute exposure to noxious fumes can also result in this form of lung injury.

Post-infectious *McLeod/Swyer James syndrome*, earlier thought to be unilateral is not uncommonly bilateral. On imaging, a unilateral (or bilateral) hyperlucent lung that demonstrates air trapping is seen.

Radiographically in obliterative bronchiolitis, hyperinflation is frequently apparent. The characteristic HRCT finding **(Box 7 and Fig. 39)** is air trapping and bronchiectasis/bronchiolectasis may also be occasionally seen. However, centrilobular nodules are rare.[58,59]

Asthma

Asthma is characterized by airway inflammation in response to a variety of stimuli resulting in bronchial hyperresponsiveness. Chronic inflammation results in smooth muscle thickening, neovascularity and fibrosis, leading to

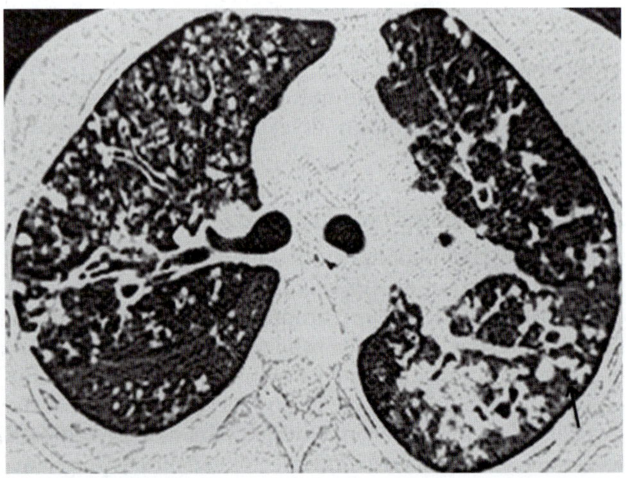

FIG. 37: Infectious bronchiolitis (tubercular): CT shows extensive "tree-in-bud" nodules (arrow) with bronchial wall thickening in bilateral lung fields.

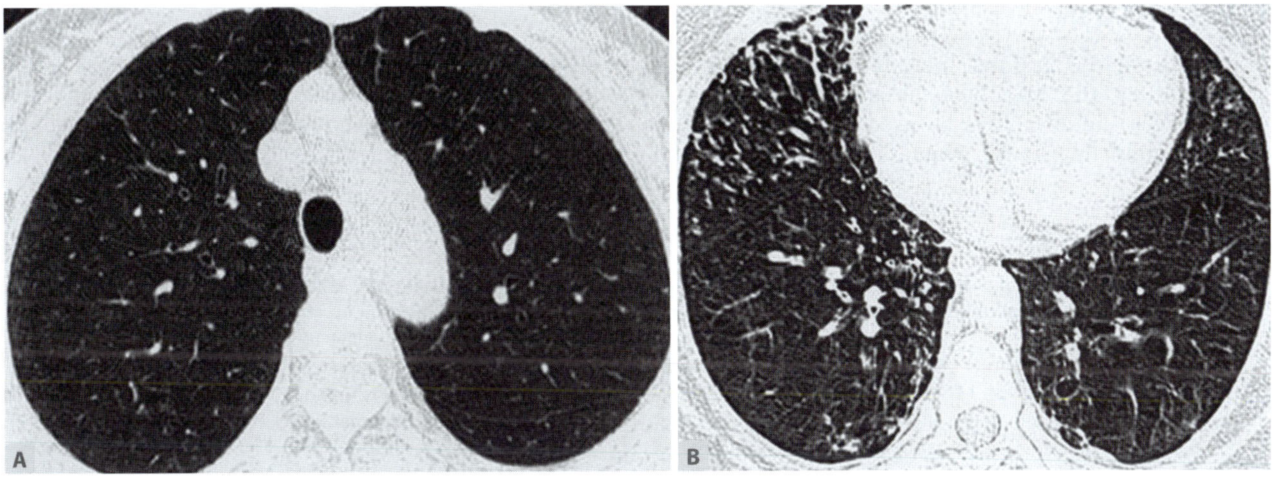

FIGS. 38A AND B: Respiratory bronchiolitis: CT scans of two different patients showing fine centrilobular nodules (A) with additional interstitial thickening in (B) (RB-ILD).

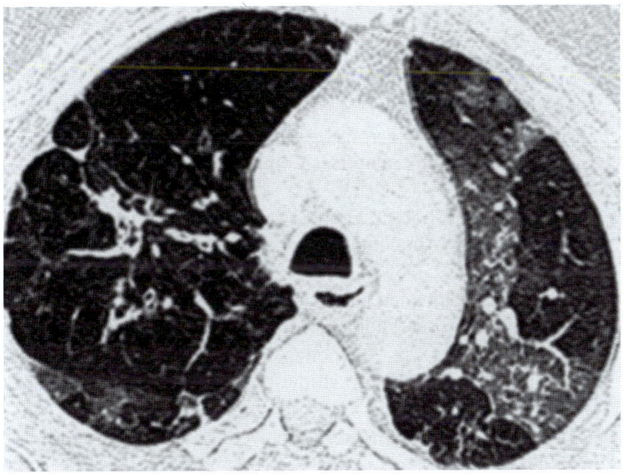

FIG. 39: Obliterative bronchiolitis: CT scan of 53-year-old patient with rheumatoid arthritis and dyspnea reveals bilateral areas of air trapping/ mosaic attenuation.

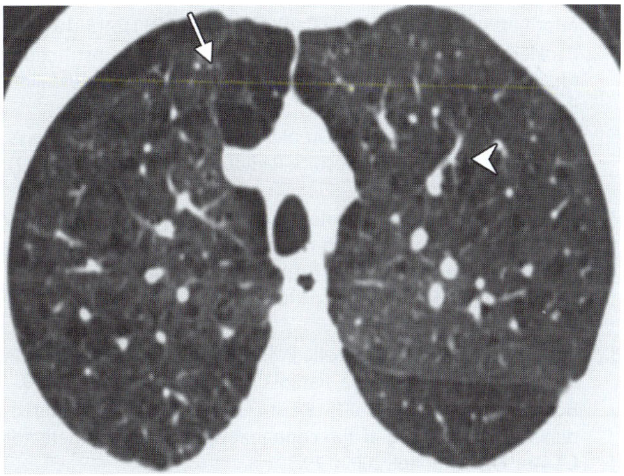

FIG. 40: Chronic obstructive pulmonary disease: CT scan of 35-year-old male smoker reveals paraseptal (arrow) and centrilobular (arrowhead) emphysema.

BOX 7: HRCT features of constrictive/obliterative bronchiolitis.

- Air trapping
- Bronchiectasis/bronchiolectasis
- Centrilobular nodules are rare

irreversible airway narrowing. Bronchiectasis may also result from chronic inflammation.

The clinical indications for CT in patients with asthma are limited and include identification of subtle radiographically occult airspace infection or treatable causes of airway inflammation, including ABPA and hypersensitivity pneumonitis and for documenting emphysema in smokers with asthma. CT may also be useful in excluding structural causes of localized wheezing, such as focal tracheal or mainstem bronchial lesions.

High-resolution CT findings in asthma include bronchial wall thickening, bronchial dilatation, and expiratory air trapping.[3,60]

CHRONIC OBSTRUCTIVE PULMONARY DISEASE

There is airflow limitation that is not fully reversible in chronic obstructive pulmonary disease (COPD) and is usually progressive. It results from variable mixture of airway obstruction (obstructive bronchiolitis) and parenchymal destruction (emphysema). Chronic bronchitis (clinical term) is characterized by presence of cough and sputum production for at least 3 months in each of two consecutive years. Pulmonary emphysema (pathologic term) is abnormal permanent enlargement of the air spaces distal to the terminal bronchiole, accompanied by the destruction of their walls. Expiratory scans well document the extent of central tracheobronchomalacia and peripheral small airway obstruction. There may be associated mild bronchiectasis. CT signs of small airways disease on CT are often present along with emphysematous changes **(Fig. 40)**.[61]

CONCLUSION

Tracheobronchial lesions include a wide range of abnormalities and MDCT is the modality of choice. Axial images should always be used with MPR and 3D reconstruction images for evaluating tracheobronchial disorders. MPR images are a useful adjunct and minIP gives good overview of airway. Virtual bronchoscopy can guide the bronchoscopist and may avoid bronchoscopy especially in children.

REFERENCES

1. Chou SSH, Kicska GA, Pipavath SN, et al. Digital Tomosynthesis of the chest: Current and Emerging Applications. Radiographics. 2014;34:359-72.
2. Dobbins JT 3rd, McAdams HP, Godfrey DJ, et al. Digital tomosynthesis of the chest. J Thorac Imaging. 2008;23(2):86-92.
3. Naidich DP, Webb WR, Muller NC, Vlahos L, Krinsky GA (Eds). "Airways" in Computed Tomography and Magnetic Resonance of the thorax, 4th edition. Lippincott Williams, and Wilkins, Philadephia, USA; 2007. pp. 453-556.
4. Sundarakumar DK, Bhalla AS, Sharma R, et al. Multidetector CT evaluation of central airways stenoses: Comparison of virtual bronchoscopy, minimal-intensity projection, and multiplanar reformatted images. Indian J Radiol Imaging. 2011;21(3):191-4.
5. Bankier AA, O'Donnell C, Boiselle PM. Respiratory instructions for CT examinations of the lungs: a hands on guideline. Radiographics. 2008;28:919-31.
6. Beigelman AC, Brillet PY, Grenier PA. MDCT of the Airways: Technique and Normal Results Radiol. Clin N Am. 2009;47(2): 185-201.
7. American College of Radiology. ACR–STR practice parameter for the performance of high-resolution computed tomography (HRCT) of the lungs in adults. https://www.acr.org/~/media/ACR/Documents/PGTS/guidelines/HRCT_Lungs.pdf. Accessed on July 27, 2017.
8. Lee EY, Litmanovich D, Boiselle PM. Multidetector CT. Evaluation of Tracheobronchomalacia. Radiol Clin N Am. 2009;47(2):261-9.
9. Boiselle PM, Reynolds KF, Ernst A. Multiplanar and three-dimensional imaging of the central airways with multidetector CT. Am J Roentgenol. 2002;179:301-8.
10. Hooper KD, et al. Mucosal details at CT virtual reality: Surface versus volume rendering. Radiology. 2000;214:517-22.
11. Boiselle PM, Lynch DA. Anatomical airway imaging methods. In: Boiselle PM, Lynch DA (Eds). CT of the airways. Totowa (NJ): Humana Press; 2008. pp. 75-94.
12. Fetita CI, Preteux F, Beigelman-Aubry C, et al. Pulmonary airways: 3D reconstruction from multislice CT and clinical investigation. IEEE Trans Med Imaging. 2004;23:1353-64.
13. Tanaka F, et al. Evaluation of tracheobronchial wall invasion using transbronchial ultrasonography (EBUS). Eur J Cardio Throac Surg. 2000;17:570-4.
14. Hochhegger B, et al. Chest magnetic resonance imaging: a protocol suggestion. Radiol Bras. 2015;48(6):373-80.
15. Dornes, et al. Allergic Bronchopulmonary aspergillosis in cystic fibrosis: MR Imaging of Airway Mucus Contrasts as a Tool for Diagnosis. Radiology. 2017. doi.org/10.1148/radiol.2017162350.
16. Gamsu G, Webb WR. Computed tomography of the trachea: Normal and abnormal. Am J Roentgenol. 1982;139:321-6.
17. Wu Ju, et al. Variant bronchial anatomy: CT appearance and classification. Am J Roentgenol. 1999;172:741-4.
18. Landing BH, Dixon LG. Congenital malformation and genetic disorders of the respiratory tract. Am Rev Respir Dis. 1979;120:151-85.
19. Fraser RS, Colman N, Müller NL, et al. Upper airway obstruction. In: Fraser RS, Colman N, Müller NL, Pare PD (Eds). Synopsis of diseases of the chest. 3rd edition. Philadelphia: BW Saunders; 2005. pp. 631-4.
20. Carden KA, Boiselle PM, Waltz DA, et al. Tracheomalacia and tracheobronchomalacia in children and adults: An in-depth review. Chest. 2005;127:984-1005.
21. Sundarakumar DK, Bhalla AS, Sharma R, et al. Multidetector computed tomography imaging of congenital anomalies of major airways: A pictorial essay. World J Radiol. 2011;3(12): 289-97.
22. Swensen SJ, Aughenbaugh GL, Douglas WW, et al. High-resolution CT of the lungs: Findings in various pulmonary diseases. Am J Roentgenol. 1992;159:971-2.
23. Arora A, Bhalla AS, Jana M, et al. Overview of airway involvement in tuberculosis. J Med Imaging Radiat Oncol. 2013;57: 576-581.
24. Moon WK, et al. Tuberculosis of the central airways: CT findings of active and fibrotic disease. Am J Roentgenol. 1997;169: 649-53.
25. Franquet T, et al. Necrotizing aspergillosis of large airways. CT findings in eight patients. J Comput Assist Tomogr. 2002;26: 342-5.
26. Yigla M, Ben-Izhak O, Oren I, et al. Laryngotracheobronchial involvement in a patient with nonendemic rhinoscleroma. Chest. 2000;117(6):1795-98.
27. Grenier PA, Beigelman AC, Brillet PY. Nonneoplastic Tracheal and Bronchial Stenoses. Radiol Clin N Am. 2009;47(2):243-60.
28. Cordier JF, et al. Pulmonary Wegener's granulomatosis. A clinical and imaging study of 77 cases. Chest 1990;97: 906-12.
29. Trentham DE, Le CH. Relapsing polychondritis. Ann Intern Med. 1998;129(2):114-22.
30. Behar JV, Choi YW, Hartman TA, et al. Relapsing polychondritis affecting the lower respiratory tract. Am J Roentgenol. 2002;178(1):173-7.
31. Stark P. Imaging of tracheobronchial injuries. J Thoracic Imaging. 1995;10:206-19.
32. Lenique F, Brauner MW, Grenier P, et al. CT assessment of bronchi in sarcoidosis: endoscopic and pathologic correlations. Radiology. 1995;194(2):419-23.
33. O'Regan A, et al. Tracheobronchial amyloidosis. The Boston University experience from 1984 to 1999. Medicine. 2000;79: 69-79.
34. Kim HY, et al. Localized amyloidosis of the respiratory system: CT features. J Comput Assist Tomogr. 1999;23:627-31.
35. Conces DJ, Tarver RD, Vix VA. Broncholithiasis: CT features in 15 patients. Am J Roentgenol. 1991;157:249-53.
36. McCarthy MJ, Rosado-de-Christenson ML. Tumors of the trachea. J Thorac Imaging. 1995;10(3):180-98.
37. Macchiarini P. Primary tracheal tumors. Lancet Oncol. 2006;7: 83-91.
38. Honings J, van Dijck JA, Verhagen AF, et al. Incidence and treatment of tracheal cancer: A nationwide study in the Netherlands. Ann Surg Oncol. 2007;14(2):968-76.
39. Grillo HC, Mathisen DJ, Wain JC. Management of tumors of the trachea. Oncology. 1992;6:61-7.
40. Kwak SH, Lee KS, Chung MJ, et al. Adenoid cystic carcinoma of the airways: Helical CT and histopathologic correlation. Am J Roentgenol. 2004;183(2):77-81.

41. Yousem SA, Hochholzer L. Mucoepidermoid tumors of the lung. Cancer. 1987;60(6):1346-52.
42. Kim TS, Lee KS, Han J, et al. Mucoepidermoid carcinoma of the tracheobronchial tree: Radiographic and CT findings in 12 patients. Radiology. 1999;212(3):643-8.
43. Naidich DP. CT/MR correlation in the evaluation of tracheobronchial neoplasia. Radiol Clin North Am. 1990;28:555-71.
44. Marchiori, et al. Laryngotracheobronchial papillomatosis: findings on computed tomography scans of the chest. J Bras Pneumol. 2008;34(12):1084-9.
45. Shoemark A, Ozerovitch L, Wilson R. Etiology in adult patients with bronchiectasis. Respir Med. 2007;191:1163-70.
46. Nejad CJ, Bhalla S. Bronchiectasis Radiol Clin N Am. 2009;47(2):88-306.
47. Muller NL, Fraser RS, Lee KS, et al. Diseases of the lung-radiologic and pathologic correlations. 1st edition (Chapter 15). Philadelphia: Lippincott Williams and Wilkins; 2003. pp. 280-1.
48. Hartman TE, Primack SL, Lee KS, et al. CT of bronchial and bronchiolar diseases. Radiographics. 1994;14:991-1003.
49. Kinsella D, Sissons G, Williams MP. The radiological imaging of bronchial atresia. Br J Radiol. 1992;65:681.
50. Martinez S, Heyneman LE, McAdams HP, et al. Mucoid impactions: Finger-in-glove sign and other CT and radiographic features. Radiographics. 2008;28:1369-82.
51. Brown DE, Pittman JE, Leigh MW, et al. Early lung disease in young children with primary ciliary dyskinesia. Pediatr Pulmonol. 2008;43:514-6.
52. Agarwal R, Khan A, Garg M, et al. Pictorial essay: Allergic bronchopulmonary aspergillosis. Indian J Radiol Imaging. 2011;21:242-52.
53. Jana M, Bhalla AS. Small Airway Disease: Imaging. In: Bhalla AS, Jana M. Imaging of interstitial lung diseases, 1st edition. Jaypee Brothers Medical Publishers (P) Ltd., 2017. pp. 331-41.
54. Pipavath SJ, Lynch DA, Cool C, et al. Radiologic and pathologic features of bronchiolitis. Am J Roentgenol. 2005;185(2):354-63 [review].
55. Pipavath SJ, Stern EJ. Imaging of Small Airway Disease (SAD) Radiol. Clin N Am. 2009;47(2):307-16.
56. Hansell DM, Nicholson AG. Smoking-related diffuse parenchymal lung disease: HRCT-pathologic correlation. Semin Respir Crit Care Med. 2003;24(4):377-92.
57. Myers JL, Colby TV. Pathologic manifestations of bronchiolitis, constrictive bronchiolitis, cryptogenic organizing pneumonia and diffuse panbronchiolitis. Clin Chest Med. 1993;14:611-22.
58. Edwards RM, Kisska G, Schmidt R, et al. Imaging of small airways and emphysema. Clin Chest Med. 2015;36:335-47.
59. Burgel PR, et al. Small airway diseases, excluding asthma and COPD: an overview. Eur Respir Rev. 2013;22:128,131-47.
60. Park CS, et al. Airway obstruction in asthmatic and healthy individuals: Inspiratory and expiratory thin-section CT findings. Radiology. 1997;203:361-7.
61. Zaporozhan JL, Kauczor HU. Imaging of Airways: Chronic Obstructive Pulmonary Disease. Radiol Clin N Am. 2009;47(2): 331-42.

CHAPTER

136

Intensive Care Chest Radiology

Akshay Kumar Saxena, Kushaljit Singh Sodhi, Nidhi Prabhakar

INTRODUCTION

Imaging of chest in patients of intensive care unit (ICU) is a challenging job. Rapid and accurate interpretation of radiological investigations in these patients can make significant contribution in management of these critically sick patients. Since most of these patients are on life support devices, portable chest radiography is the most commonly performed radiological investigation. This is supplemented by portable ultrasonography and computed tomography (CT) in selected patients.

CHEST RADIOGRAPH

A chest radiograph is the most commonly requested radiology examination in the ICU. It is an essential supplement to physical examination, which is difficult to properly perform in an ICU setting, as most of these patients are uncooperative, unconscious and intubated.[1] Chest radiography is an economically viable investigation that can be performed rapidly with ease at the bedside of a critically ill patient. It can help in the diagnosis of a number of cardiopulmonary diseases. It is also used to evaluate monitoring and support devices.[2] Usually, upright posteroanterior and lateral views are performed for chest radiography. However, in the ICU, an anteroposterior (AP) radiograph is most commonly performed using a portable X-ray unit (portable radiography). The American College of Radiology has described a number of recommendations for the use of portable radiography in an ICU. The indications described by them include placement of enteric tubes, endotracheal tubes, central venous catheter, Swan-Ganz catheter, any other life support device or to evaluate any change in clinical status of the patient. Routine daily radiograph is not advised.[3]

Interpretation of chest radiographs for patients admitted in the ICU is a difficult task as the X-ray is not usually of optimum quality. The portable radiograph is taken with the patient usually in supine position and there is inconsistency in the technique from day to day. Patients are often critically ill and are monitored and supported by various medical devices which makes it still more difficult to obtain a good quality chest radiograph. Digital radiography in place of conventional portable chest radiography has gained acceptance in most centers because of consistent film quality and wide latitude of exposure possible with this technique which decreases the need for repeat examinations.

ULTRASOUND

While portable radiography is the mainstay of imaging for ICU patients, other modalities have started making an impact in management of these patients. Rapid strides in technology have now made available good quality portable color Doppler machines. Bedside sonography and color Doppler are now being increasingly used as imaging supplements for ICU patients. The indications may be broadly categorized as diagnostic thoracic, diagnostic non-thoracic, echocardiography and interventional procedures including vascular catheterization.[4-8] The diagnostic performance of sonography is seen to approach that of CT and exceed chest radiography especially for indications such as pneumothorax, qualitative reporting of pleural fluids and demonstration of consolidation. Quantitative reporting of pleural fluids as well as evaluation of the causes of septal edema is also possible with sonography, however these need more collaborative research for optimization.[9]

COMPUTED TOMOGRAPHY

While computed tomography (CT) scan is known to provide superior diagnostic information for chest diseases, its use for patients admitted in ICU has remained limited. This is because the patients admitted in ICU are dependent on life support devices and their transportation to CT scan room is hazardous. However, recent studies unequivocally reveal the potential of CT scan in providing superior diagnostic information and having impact on patient management. CT scan has been shown to change the therapeutic decision of patients in more than half of the cases. CT scan is also invaluable in rapid assessment of cerebral complications in the ICU patients.[10,11] Role of CT scan in imaging patients of pulmonary thromboembolism is discussed in details elsewhere in this book.

IMAGING OF CARDIOPULMONARY COMPLICATIONS IN ICU PATIENTS

Common cardiopulmonary complications, which can be visualized on imaging in patients of ICU, are atelectasis, aspiration, pneumonia, hydrostatic pulmonary edema, adult respiratory distress syndrome (ARDS) and barotrauma. By careful attention to the imaging pattern, the timing of the changes and the clinical setting, these entities may be correctly diagnosed.

Atelectasis

The most common cause of pulmonary opacities in the ICU is atelectasis. Atelectasis is frequently seen in postoperative and intubated patients. It often appears quickly and changes quickly. If unresolved in several days, secondary infection should be suspected. The most common locations of atelectasis are the left lower lobe, right lower lobe and right upper lobe. It is usually subsegmental. Atelectasis is classified as obstructive, cicatricial, compressive or adhesive. Obstructive atelectasis, which occurs due to impaired mucociliary clearance, retained secretions and altered consciousness, is the most commonly seen type of atelectasis in an ICU setting. If only the distal airways are blocked, peripheral areas of atelectasis are seen with crowding of bronchi and air bronchograms. However, if larger airways are obstructed, air bronchograms may not be visualized. A common cause of large airway obstruction leading to acute lung collapse is mucus impaction **(Figs. 1A and B)**. If acute lobar collapse is seen without an air bronchogram within the atelectatic area, mucoid impaction is usually the cause. This predicts a favorable response after bronchoscopy. Compressive atelectasis is caused due to mass effect on lungs, pleural fluid being the most common cause. Cicatricial atelectasis occurs secondary to lung fibrosis. Adhesive atelectasis is seen in premature neonates, due to inadequate production of surfactant. On CT, atelectasis is seen as areas of collapse with evidence of volume loss, like crowding of airways and vessels. Lung atelectasis shows higher attenuation on postcontrast CT, as compared to areas of consolidation due to pneumonia. This can help in differentiating the two entities.[2]

Aspiration Pneumonitis

A depressed state of consciousness and a nasogastric tube, which disrupts the esophagogastric sphincter are the most frequent predisposing factors to aspiration pneumonia in an ICU patient. Aspiration can occur in spite of inflated cuff of endotracheal tube and has varying clinical presentation. Mild cases may not be clinically apparent while severe cases may cause respiratory distress. Aspirated contents may cause obstruction of airway, chemical pneumonitis or infective pneumonia.[12]

Chest radiography often shows patchy ground-glass or nodular opacities with areas of consolidation, in the dependent parts of the lungs (posterior segments of the upper lobes, and the superior, posterior basal segments of lower lobes).[2] These changes often occur within a few hours after aspiration and progress in the next 24–48 hours after which they regress. Persistence of opacities beyond this time is suggestive of aspiration pneumonia **(Fig. 2)**. On CT, patchy ground-glass opacities (GGOs), nodules and areas of consolidation in the dependent parts of lung are seen in cases

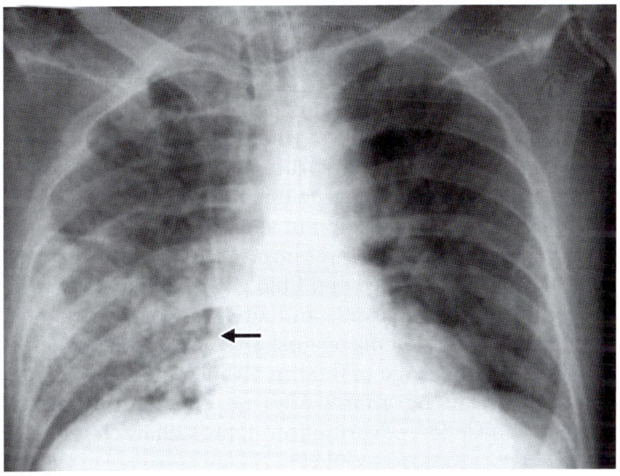

FIG. 2: Aspiration pneumonia: Chest radiograph showing patchy alveolar opacities predominantly involving the right lower zone (arrow).

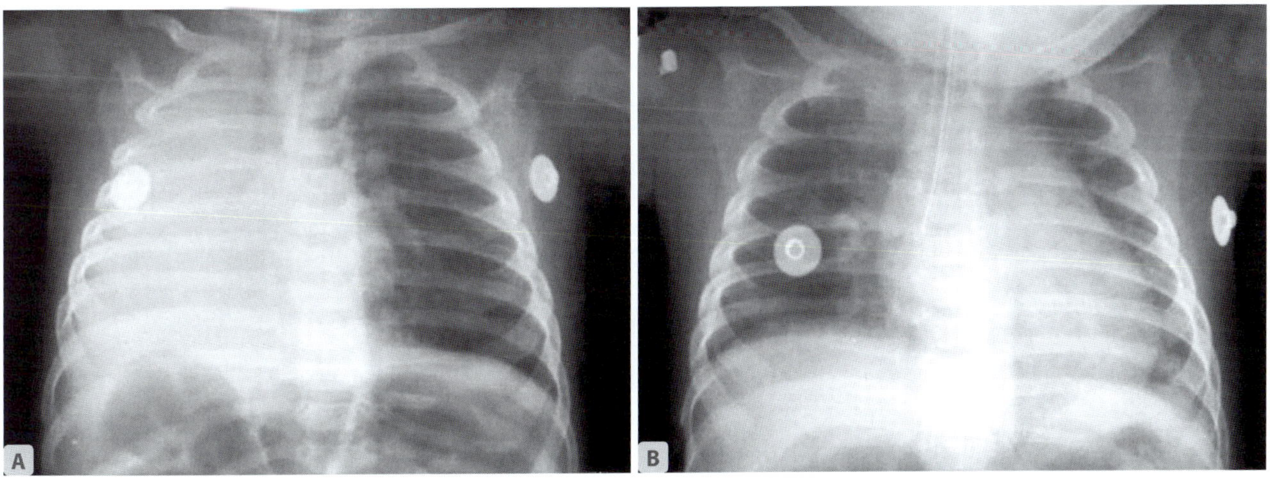

FIGS. 1A AND B: Atelectasis. (A) Chest radiograph of a child on mechanical ventilation reveals complete collapse of right lung; (B) Suction via the endotracheal tube followed by chest radiograph after few hours reveals re-expansion of the right lung.

of aspiration pneumonitis. *Tree-in-bud* pattern in dependent regions on CT scan is highly suggestive of aspiration.[12]

Pneumonia

Pulmonary infection is a major cause of morbidity and mortality in the ICU. Colonization of the upper airway is almost universal with prolonged hospitalization. The respirators and endotracheal tubes may act as a source and distributor of infected material. Aspiration is another risk factor for patients developing pneumonia.[12] This diagnosis is made when there is combination of fever, leukocytosis and sputum production, which is rich in white cell count and bacteria. Mixed anaerobic bacteria are the most common cause of pneumonia in the ICU. However, in the ventilated patients, aerobic gram-negative bacteria are also an important cause. Pneumonia is seen as areas of focal or multifocal consolidation on chest radiography and CT **(Figs. 3A and B)**. The infiltrates usually progress over several days, but their radiographic appearance is seldom as rapid as in atelectasis, aspiration or pulmonary edema.[2] Air bronchogram is usually seen. Lung infection secondary to septicemia may appear as nodules (which are peripheral and may be cavitatory) or wedge-shaped peripheral lesions on imaging.

Hydrostatic Pulmonary Edema

Hydrostatic pulmonary edema in an ICU patient may be due to various etiologies, which include renal failure, cardiac failure and overhydration.[12] The progression is often rapid and the response to therapy is equally rapid. The earliest change is congestion of vessels due to an increase in capillary hydrostatic pressure. As the pressure rises, lymphatics get congested and fluid gets accumulated in the interstitium around vessels and airways. This mechanism initially protects the lung against alveolar edema, which is caused due to leakage of fluid in alveoli. These sequences of changes can be appreciated on chest radiography. The first phase is 'redistribution' that is characterized by distension of upper lobar pulmonary veins. Subsequently, prominence of hila and loss of their definition is seen, followed by the appearance of septal lines (Kerley A and B) in lower lobes. Peribronchovascular thickening with hazy margins and thickening of interlobar fissures is seen in the later stage. Redistribution is only seen when there is chronic pulmonary venous hypertension. Cardiomegaly and pleural effusion are other findings seen on imaging.[13] Early alveolar edema is seen as diffuse poorly defined ground-glass opacities predominantly in perihilar and lower regions. This can progress to air space consolidation.

The diagnosis and management of hydrostatic pulmonary edema is commonly based on radiographic findings in appropriate clinical settings. However, recognizing the appearance of hydrostatic pulmonary edema on CT is also important, as edema may be seen on Chest CT done for other indications.[14] The HRCT findings include GGOs, smooth interlobular septal thickening, consolidation, increased vascular diameter, peribronchovasular thickening and pleural fluid **(Figs. 4A and B)**. The distribution of these findings is usually central and gravitational. In patients with an underlying disease such as emphysema, pulmonary edema can have atypical appearance and can mimic aspiration pneumonitis or pneumonia. Mitral regurgitation patients may have asymmetric pulmonary edema localized to right upper lobe.[2]

Noncardiogenic Pulmonary Edema

Noncardiogenic pulmonary edema is also called increased permeability edema. It is difficult to differentiate radiologically from the hydrostatic pulmonary edema and the two conditions may sometimes co-exist. The etiology of noncardiogenic pulmonary edema is diverse and includes thoracic (e.g. pneumonia, pulmonary contusion, aspiration, etc.) as well as extrathoracic pathologies (e.g. sepsis, shock, systemic inflammatory response syndrome, extra thoracic trauma, drug toxicity, etc.). Pathologically, there is diffuse alveolar damage secondary to the injury to alveolar capillaries

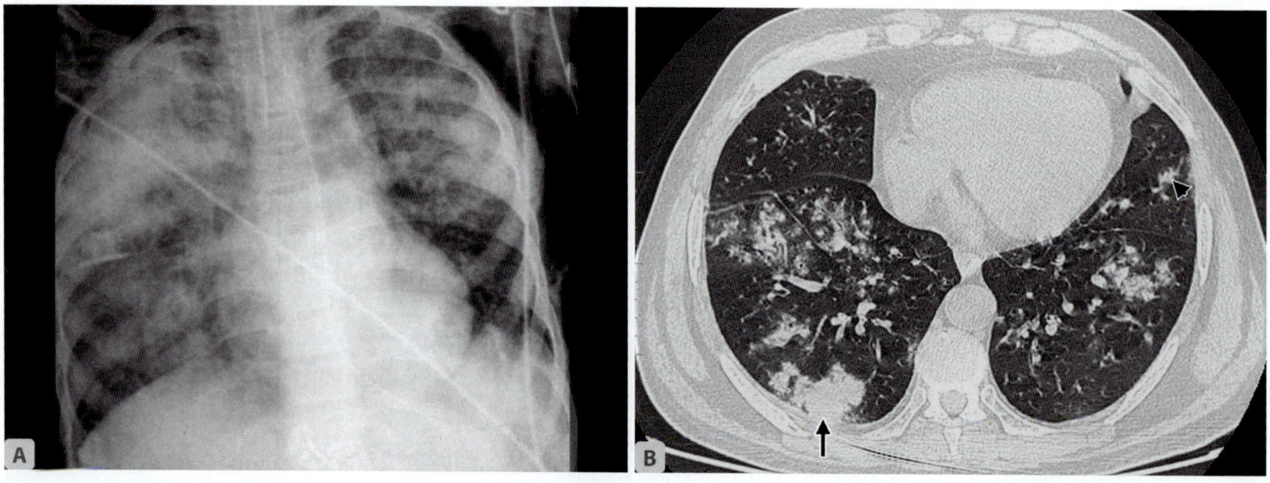

FIGS. 3A AND B: Pneumonia. (A) Chest radiograph in a 12-year-old male child shows patches of consolidation in both lungs suggestive of pneumonia. The patient was a diagnosed case of Bruton's disease; (B) CT chest in a 50-year old male patient shows multiple nodules (arrowhead) and areas of consolidation (arrow) in bilateral lungs suggestive of pneumonia.

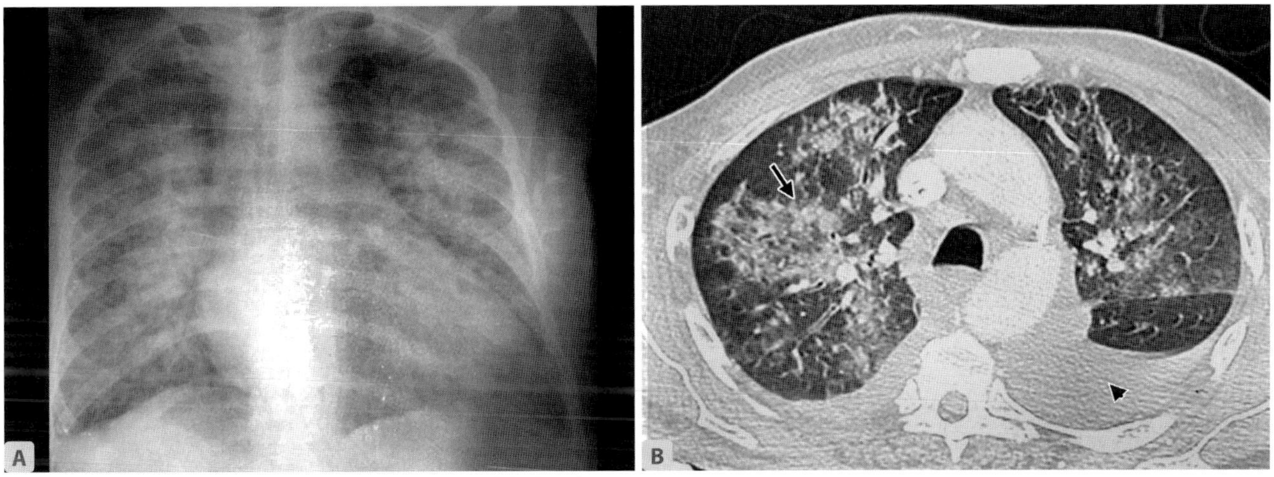

FIGS. 4A AND B: Hydrostatic pulmonary edema. (A) Chest radiograph of a postrenal transplant patient shows cardiomegaly and bilateral pulmonary consolidation with predominantly perihilar distribution; (B) CT chest in another chronic renal failure patient shows areas of ground-glass opacities and consolidation, predominantly in perihilar location (arrow) involving bilateral lungs suggestive of pulmonary edema. In addition, bilateral pleural effusion is seen (arrowhead).

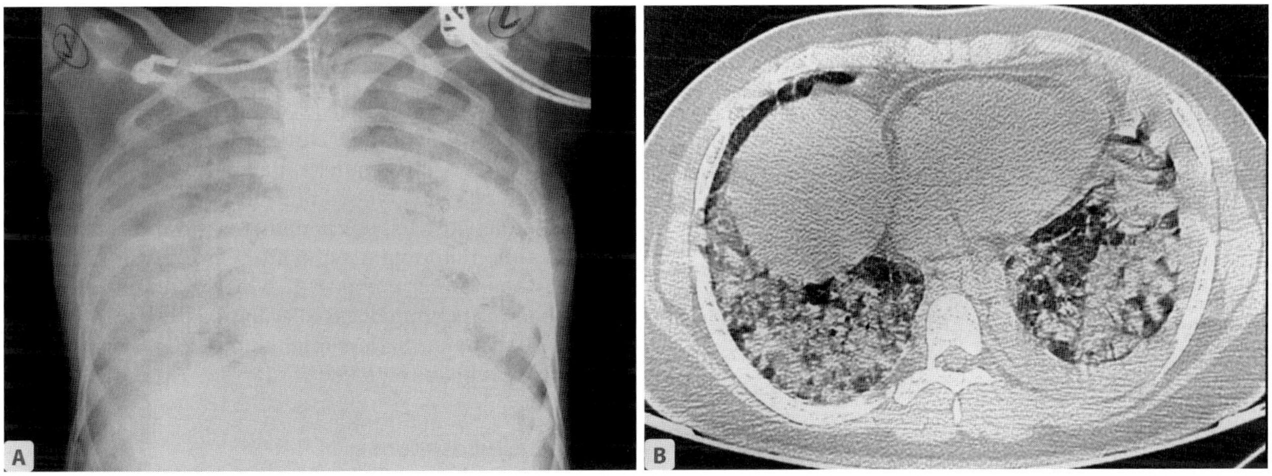

FIGS. 5A AND B: Acute respiratory distress syndrome. (A) Chest radiograph of a 7-year-old child shows bilateral diffuse airspace consolidation; (B) CT chest of a 25-year-old male, admitted in ICU and in sepsis, shows multiple areas of consolidation in bilateral lungs, predominant in the lower lobes due to ARDS. In addition, mild left empyema was noted.

and epithelium. The severe form of diffuse alveolar damage is ARDS. The 'Berlin definition' as created by ARDS definition task force, defined ARDS as respiratory failure (1) occurring within 1 week of a known clinical insult or new or worsening symptoms, (2) with opacities involving two or more quadrants on imaging (frontal radiograph or CT), (3) not attributable to cardiac failure or volume overload and (4) having arterial partial pressure of oxygen to fraction of inspired oxygen (Pa_2/FiO_2) ratio of less than 300 mm Hg. These levels were further classified as mild ARDS (200–300 mm Hg), moderate ARDS (100–200 mm Hg) or severe ARDS (less than 100 mm Hg). The term 'acute lung injury' is now no longer used and has been replaced by 'mild ARDS'.[15,16]

The course of ARDS is a continuum of findings, which is frequently classified into proliferative, exudative and fibrotic phases. The radiographic findings frequently lag behind the onset of respiratory failure and chest radiograph may not be helpful in first few hours of illness. Pulmonary opacities coalesce to cause diffuse pulmonary opacification on radiograph or CT **(Figs. 5A and B)**. These opacities can last for a variable duration (days to months), which depends on the cause, severity, treatment and presence of associated complications such as aspiration and/or pneumonia. Chest radiograph findings may resemble hydrostatic pulmonary edema, however, patchy, peripheral distribution is more common in noncardiogenic than cardiogenic pulmonary edema. Radiographic changes are also slow in ARDS. The heart size is frequently normal in ARDS as compared to hydrostatic pulmonary edema. When ARDS is caused by extrathoracic causes, more symmetric pattern of GGOs is predominant and when ARDS is secondary to thoracic diseases, asymmetric GGOs and consolidation patches predominant. The prevalence of fibrotic changes early in the disease predict bad prognosis. The most common finding in survivors of ARDS is anterior fibrotic opacities.[17]

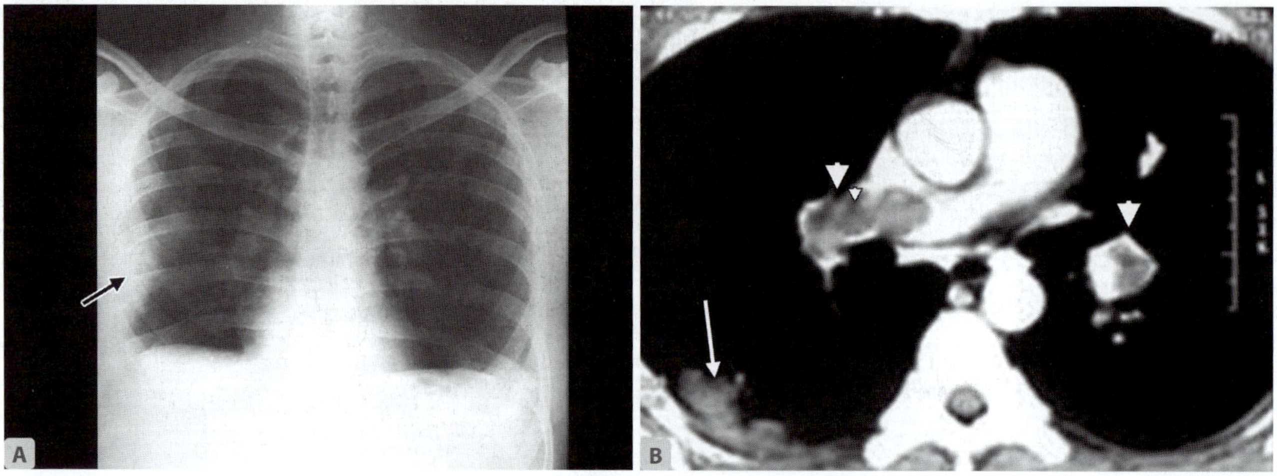

FIGS. 6A AND B: Pulmonary thromboembolism. (A) Chest radiograph of a 32-year-old male patient presenting with sudden onset shortness of breath. The right mid and lower zones show an ill-defined peripheral opacity (black arrow); (B) CT pulmonary angiography in the same patient shows thrombi in right and left main pulmonary arteries (white arrowheads). Infarction is seen in right lower lobe (arrow).

Pulmonary Embolism

In the critically-ill patient, there are numerous risk factors such as cardiac disease, obstructive airway disease, indwelling catheters, prolonged bed-rest, etc. which predispose the patient to pulmonary embolism. The diagnosis of pulmonary embolism can be very difficult when multiple factors can lead to respiratory distress. The most common chest radiographic findings are normal radiograph, pleural effusion, elevated hemidiaphragm, cardiac enlargement, pulmonary artery enlargement, peripheral consolidation and peripheral atelectasis **(Figs. 6A and B)**.[18] These radiographic signs are non-specific. In a patient with sudden onset respiratory distress, a normal radiograph is usually suggestive of pulmonary embolism. Ventilation perfusion scanning is of limited value in a critically ill patient as other accompanying conditions such as pneumonia, obstructive airways disease and pulmonary edema make definitive interpretation difficult in a majority of patients. Multidetector CT pulmonary angiography is emerging as imaging modality of choice for radiological evaluation of patients of pulmonary embolism. This topic is discussed in details elsewhere in this book.

Barotrauma

The term barotrauma refers to the deleterious effects of mechanical ventilation in the lungs. The most commonly recognized manifestation of barotrauma is the occurrence of extra-alveolar air collection due to airleak phenomenon. The overall incidence of barotrauma is approximately 3% in mechanically ventilated patients. Incidence varies depending on the presence of underlying lung diseases.[19]

Pulmonary Interstitial Emphysema

Pulmonary interstitial emphysema (PIE) occurs due to increased alveolar pressure causing rupture of alveolar wall followed by dissection of air along the pulmonary interstitium upto the hilum (Macklin effect).[20] The air can subsequently reach mediastinum and pleural cavity to cause pneumomediastinum and pneumothorax. Radiographic findings of PIE include multiple lung cysts of variable size, lucent lines, which are directed toward the hilum, air around large vessels, subpleural air, intraseptal air and subpleural cysts. However, these findings may be subtle and may not be detected on radiography in the absence of opacified lung parenchyma. On CT, perivascular and peribronchial cysts or air within interlobular septa are seen. The 'line and dot' sign has been described on CT, which is due to air in the interstitium. The bronchovascular bundles are seen as 'lines or dots' (depending on their orientation with respect to plane of the CT) within the air lucencies **(Figs. 7A and B)**.[21]

Pneumomediastinum

Pneumomediastinum signifies presence of extraluminal air in the mediastinum. When occurring due to barotrauma, it may be accompanied by PIE. The radiographic findings in pneumomediastinum depend on the visualization of normal anatomic structures, outlined by the air in the mediastinum. These signs include the thymic sail sign, "ring around the artery" sign, double bronchial wall sign, continuous diaphragm sign, tubular artery sign and extrapleural sign. It is sometimes difficult to distinguish pneumomediastinum from pneumopericardium and medial pneumothorax. False positive diagnosis of pneumomediastinum may be made due to Mach band effect, which manifests as apparent radiolucency adjacent to convex border structures. In addition, normal anatomic structures (e.g. anterior junction line, major fissure) may occasionally mimic pneumomediastinum.[22,23]

Pneumothorax

Pneumothorax resulting from barotrauma is the most common life-threatening emergency in patients supported by mechanical ventilation. It may or may not always be

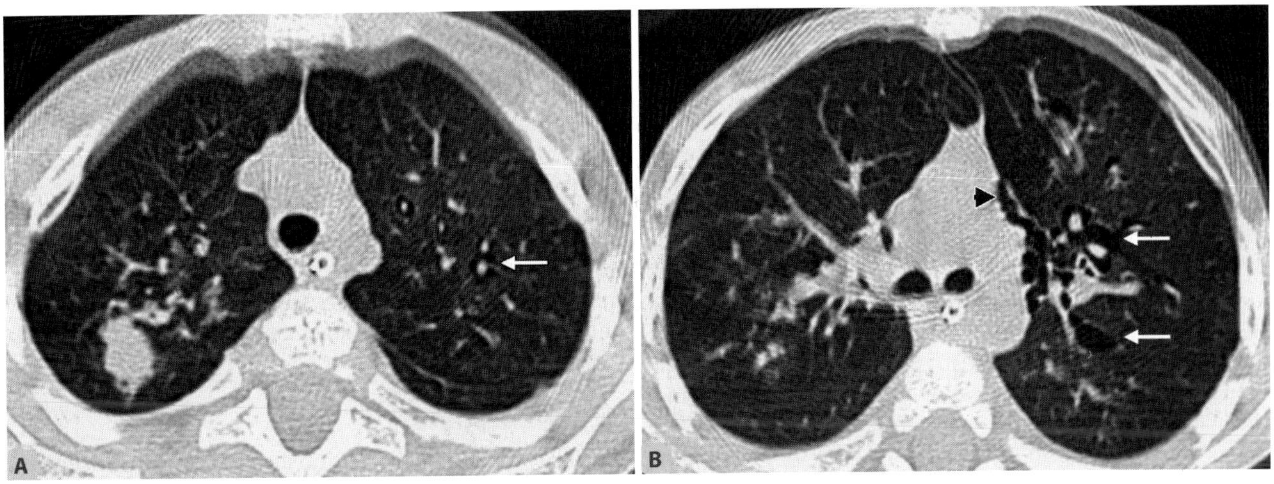

FIGS. 7A AND B: Pulmonary interstitial emphysema. (A and B) CT chest of a 7-month-old child showing air-filled cystic structures in pulmonary interstitium (arrows). The pulmonary vessels appear as line and dot-like structures within the interstitial air. These findings are suggestive of pulmonary interstitial emphysema. Pneumomediastinum (arrowhead) is also seen. In addition, few nodules and consolidation areas are seen in the right lung.

preceded by pneumomediastinum. The diagnosis of pneumothorax, although of great clinical significance, is many times missed on the X-rays. This is because apicolateral accumulation of air is rather uncommon in the supine films.[24] Air preferentially accumulates in the anteromedial and subpulmonic recesses in the supine position.[24] The anteromedial air collection may cause sharp outline of contiguous mediastinal structures. Subpulmonic pneumothorax presents as a relatively lucent area in the left or right upper abdominal quadrant. Sometimes, the only radiographic sign of subpulmonic pneumothorax is deep lateral costophrenic angle (deep sulcus sign).[25] The air can also collect in apicolateral, posteromedial, inter lobar fissures and inferior pulmonary ligament.[24] The position of air collection is also modified by underlying lung diseases.

Tension Pneumothorax

Tension pneumothorax develops when one-way valve is formed between the lung and pleural cavity. This leads to an increase in intrathoracic pressure, due to accumulation of air in the pleural cavity, during each respiratory cycle. Rapid progressive collapse of the ipsilateral lung and contralateral shift of mediastinum occurs. Venous return is obstructed, causing cardiac arrest.[26] Characteristic radiological features include flattening or inversion of dome of diaphragm and contralateral mediastinal shift **(Fig. 8)**.[12] Loculated tension pneumothorax is a complication of respiratory therapy in ARDS patients, in which there is accumulation of air, usually in an inferior subpulmonic or paracardiac location. This may occur even if there is a functioning ipsilateral chest tube. The only radiographic evidences of loculated tension pneumothorax may be subtle degree of mediastinal shift, slight flattening of the cardiac border and ipsilateral change of contour or depression of the diaphragm, which may be apparent only after comparison with previous radiographs. This loculated tension pneumothorax may lead to severe pulmonary and cardiovascular compromise even from a small volume of pleural air and rapid drainage is required.

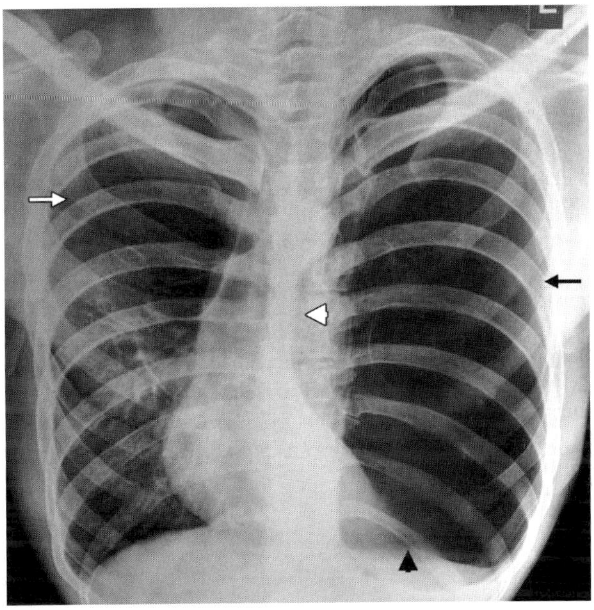

FIG. 8: Tension pneumothorax: Chest radiograph shows tension pneumothorax on the left side (black arrow) with complete collapse of left lung, flattening of the left diaphragm (black arrowhead) and contralateral mediastinal shift (white arrowhead). Large emphysematous bullae are seen on the right side in the upper zone (white arrow).

On few occasions, the diagnosis of tension pneumothorax in ARDS patient may only be apparent on CT scan.[27]

Subcutaneous Emphysema

From the mediastinum, air can travel along fascial planes into the subcutaneous tissues of the neck and chest wall and abdominal wall. The presence of air in the chest wall in patients receiving mechanical ventilation is often the first radiographic sign of barotrauma because the underlying pneumothorax may be impossible to detect in the supine portable radiograph.

IMAGING OF SUPPORT AND MONITORING APPARATUS

A number of medical devices are used in the care of patients in the ICU. A good knowledge of their normal positions and complications is of vital importance to the radiologist and critical care physician.

Endotracheal and Tracheostomy Tube

Endotracheal intubation is done to provide short-term ventilatory support. Following endotracheal intubation, a radiograph should be obtained to ensure proper endotracheal tube placement. The ideal location for the tube tip is the mid trachea approximately 4 +/– 1 cm above the carina, in neutral head position **(Figs. 9A and B)**. Flexion or extension of the neck can alter the position by as much as 2 cm caudally or cranially respectively. Tubes placed too high may lead to inadvertent extubation or damage to the larynx. Tubes placed too deeply may irritate the carina or enter the main bronchus (usually right side).[12] Apart from localizing the endotracheal tube tip, the chest radiograph may also show contralateral atelectasis and ipsilateral hyperinflation and features of barotrauma. Following repositioning of the tube, re-expansion of the contralateral lung may take several hours to days. Endotracheal balloon cuff should not be inflated beyond the diameter of the trachea else it can lead to rupture or tracheal stenosis (as chronic complication). Esophageal intubation is usually clinically apparent, and leads to introduction of large amounts of air in gastrointestinal tract.[2]

Tracheostomy is done to provide long-term ventilation support. The tip of tracheostomy tube should be approximately at T3 level. The tube's position does not change with flexion or extension. The diameter of the tracheostomy tube should be approximately 2/3rd of tracheal diameter and the cuff should not dilate the tracheal wall. Pneumomediastinum may be noted sometimes even after uncomplicated tracheostomy tube placement.[2]

Chest Tube

Chest tubes may be malpositioned in approximately 10% of cases. Chest tube side holes are seen as interruptions of tube's radiopaque line on chest radiography. All these side holes must be located within the pleural space. If the tube is inserted into the lung parenchyma, a lung contusion may occur. This is seen as a new opacity adjacent to the chest tube on either radiography or CT. Sometimes, malpositioned chest tubes can injure the heart, major blood vessels, diaphragm or upper abdominal organs.[2] Hence, critical assessment of chest tube placement should be done to differentiate correct placement from aberrant position.

Venous Catheter

The tip of the central venous line should be within the superior vena cava, beyond the venous valves, to decrease the risk of thrombosis **(Figs. 10A and B)**. Presence of catheter tip in the lower SVC or at cavoatrial junction is associated with reduced thrombosis around the catheter.[28] However, the tip should not be within the atria to avoid arrhythmias and cardiac perforation.

Aberrant positioning of the venous catheters intra-arterially (usually subclavian artery or common carotid artery) is usually apparent because it leads to bright red oxygenated blood flowing from the catheter. However, in patients of sepsis and hypotension, this may not be so apparent. On an anteroposterior radiograph, if the venous catheter is noted above the level of clavicles, subclavian artery placement should be suspected.

Pneumothorax following subclavian vein catheterization is not uncommon because of the proximity of the apical pleura to the subclavian vein. Another complication is extravascular fluid collections. Widening of the mediastinum following catheterization usually indicates mediastinal fluid or blood accumulation due to venous laceration or extravenous insertion of the catheter. Rapidly developing pleural effusion may also occur due to faulty position.

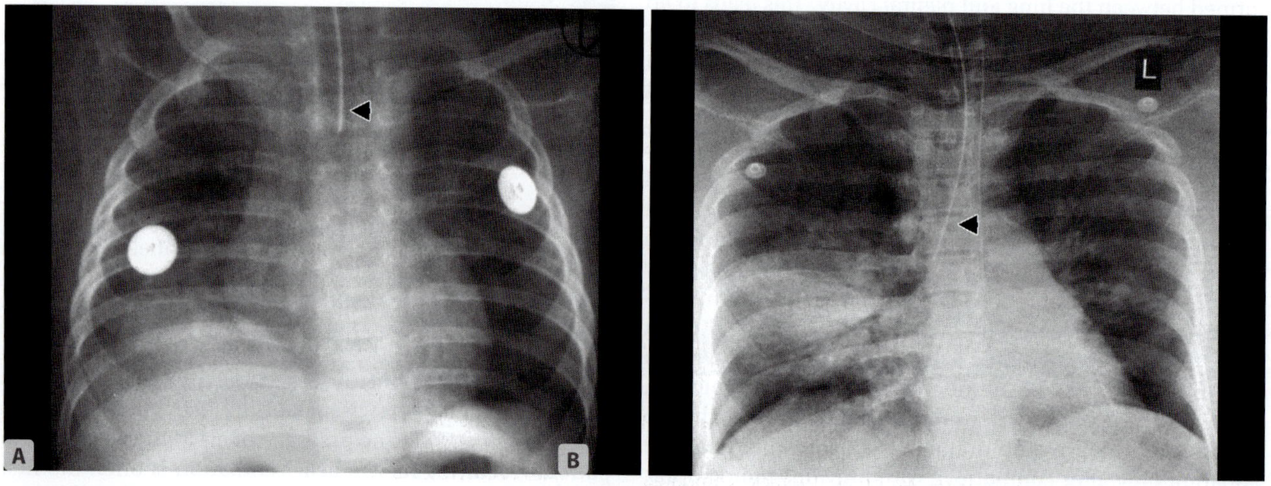

FIGS. 9A AND B: Endotracheal tube position: Chest radiographs showing (A) correct and (B) abnormal (right bronchial) positions of the endotracheal tube (arrowheads).

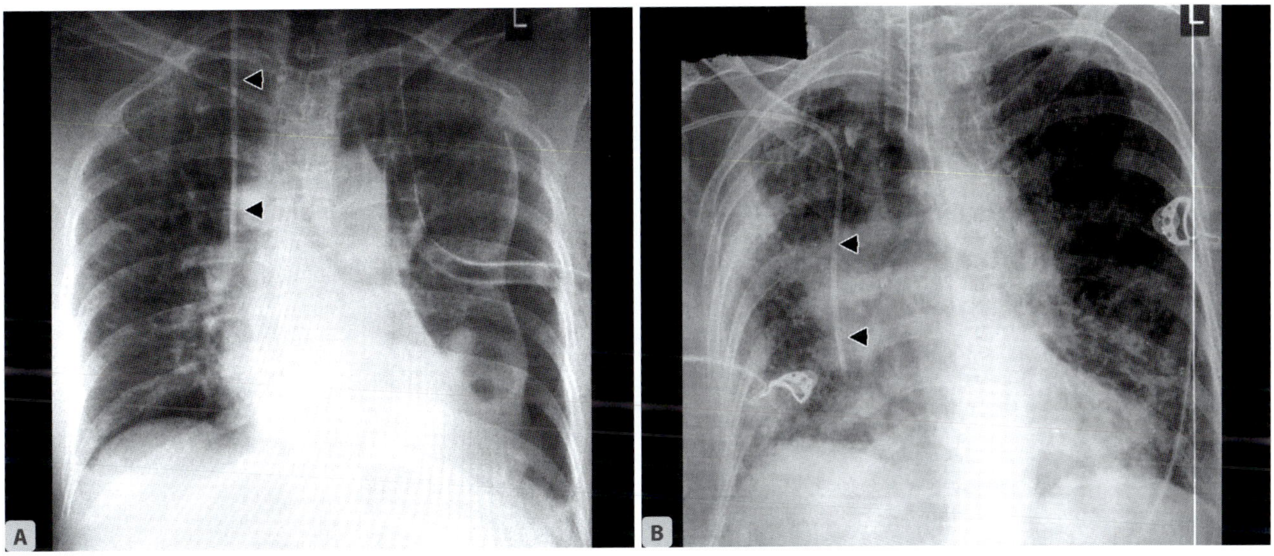

FIGS. 10A AND B: Central venous catheter position: Chest radiographs showing (A) correct and (B) deep positions of the venous catheters (arrowheads).

Swan-Ganz Catheter

The flow directed balloon-tipped Swan-Ganz catheter measures the pulmonary capillary wedge pressure, pulmonary artery pressure and cardiac output. The Swan-Ganz catheter tip should be either within the right main pulmonary artery, left main pulmonary artery or proximal interlobar pulmonary arteries. On the radiograph, the catheter should be seen in the main pulmonary artery and not extending beyond the major hilar vessels. This is because the pulmonary arteries narrow in caliber as they extend from the hila. Thus, distal location of catheter may result in arterial occlusion and rupture. The chest X-ray should be scrutinized for any knots, which may complicate catheter removal.[12] Other complications similar to those seen in venous catheter placement such as dysrhythmias, cardiac perforation, pneumothorax or hemothorax may be also seen.

REFERENCES

1. Rubinowitz AN, Siegel MD, Tocino I. Thoracic imaging in the ICU. Crit Care Clin. 2007;23(3):539-73.
2. Bentz MR, Primack SL. Intensive care unit imaging. Clin Chest Med. 2015;36(2):219-34.
3. Suh RD, Genshaft SJ, Kirsch J, et al. ACR Appropriateness Criteria® Intensive Care Unit Patients. J Thorac Imaging. 2015;30(6): W63-5.
4. Beaulieu Y, Marik PE. Bedside ultrasonography in the ICU: part 1. Chest. 2005;128:881-95.
5. Beaulieu Y, Marik PE. Bedside ultrasonography in the ICU: part 2. Chest. 2005;128:1766-81.
6. Guillory RK, Gunter OL. Ultrasound in the surgical intensive care unit. Curr Opin Crit Care. 2008;14:415-22.
7. Lichtenstein DA. Ultrasound in the management of thoracic disease. Crit Care Med. 2007;35(Suppl):S250-61.
8. Nicolaou S, Talsky A, Khashoggi K, et al. Ultrasound-guided interventional radiology in critical care. Crit Care Med. 2007;35(Suppl):S186-97.
9. Ashton-Cleary DT. Is thoracic ultrasound a viable alternative to conventional imaging in the critical care setting? Br J Anaesth. 2013;111(2):152-60.
10. Aliaga M, Forel JM, De Bourmont S, et al. Diagnostic yield and safety of CT scans in ICU. Intensive Care Med. 2015;41(3):436-43.
11. Dorenbeck U, Bein T, Strotzer M, et al. Thoracic computed tomography in intensive care patients: evaluation of clinical usefulness. Anasthesiol Intensivmed-Not fallmed Schmerzther. 2002;37:273-9.
12. Hill JR, Horner PE, Primack SL. ICU imaging. Clin Chest Med. 2008;29:59-76.
13. Cardinale L, Priola AM, Moretti F, et al. Effectiveness of chest radiography, lung ultrasound and thoracic computed tomography in the diagnosis of congestive heart failure. World J Radiol. 2014;6(6):230-7.
14. Storto ML, Kee ST, Golden JA, et al. Hydrostatic pulmonary edema: high-resolution CT findings. Am J Roentgenol. 1995;165:817-20.
15. ARDS Definition Task Force. Acute respiratory distress syndrome: the Berlin definition. JAMA. 2012;307(23):2526-33.
16. Sweeney RM, McAuley DF. Acute respiratory distress syndrome. Lancet. 2016;388(10058):2416-30.
17. Desai SR, Wells AU, Rubens MB, et al. Acute respiratory distress syndrome: CT abnormalities at long-term follow-up. Radiology. 1999;210:29-35.
18. Elliott CG, Goldhaber SZ, Visani L, et al. Chest radiographs in acute pulmonary embolism. Results from the International Cooperative Pulmonary Embolism Registry. Chest. 2000;118(1):33-8.
19. Anzueto A, Frutos-Vivar F, Esteban A, et al. Incidence, risk factors and outcome of barotrauma in mechanically ventilated patients. Intensive Care Med. 2004;30(4):612-9.
20. Wintermark M, Schnyder P. The Macklin effect: a frequent etiology for pneumomediastinum in severe blunt chest trauma. Chest. 2001;120:543-7.
21. Donnelly LF, Lucaya J, Ozelame V, et al. CT findings and temporal course of persistent pulmonary interstitial emphysema in neonates: a multiinstitutional study. Am J Roentgenol. 2003;80(4):1129-33.

22. Zylak CM, Standen JR, Barnes GR, et al. Pneumomediastinum revisited. Radiographics. 2000;20:1043-57.
23. Bejvan SM, Godwin JD. Pneumomediastinum: old signs and new signs. Am J Roentgenol. 1996;166:1041-8.
24. Tocino IM, Miller MH, Fairfax WR. Distribution of pneumothorax in the supine and semirecumbent critically ill adult. Am J Roentgenol. 1985;144:901-5.
25. Gordon R. The deep sulcus sign. Radiology. 1980;136:25-7.
26. Watts BL, Howell MA. Tension pneumothorax: a difficult diagnosis. Emerg Med J. 2001;18(4):319-20.
27. Gobien RP, Reines HD, Schabel SI. Localized tension pneumothorax: unrecognized form of barotrauma in adult respiratory distress syndrome. Radiology. 1982; 142:15-9.
28. Cadman A, Lawrance JA, Fitzsimmons L, et al. To clot or not to clot? That is the question in central venous catheters. Clin Radiol. 2004;59:349-55.

CHAPTER

137

Imaging in Thoracic Trauma

Atin Kumar, Shivanand Gamanagatti

INTRODUCTION

Thoracic injury is the third most common injury in the trauma patient after head and extremity injury. The mortality from thoracic injury with related complications ranges from 15–77% especially in the setting of multisystem trauma.[1] Thoracic injuries can potentially affect airway and breathing which are the two most important components responsible for early mortality in patients with torso trauma. The mode of injury can be blunt trauma or penetrating trauma. The chest wall remains intact in blunt trauma whereas its integrity is breached in penetrating trauma resulting in communication between the external environment and internal contents of the thorax, even if only transiently. Blunt trauma due to motor vehicle collision is the most common cause.

ROLE OF IMAGING

Imaging plays an important role in the diagnosis of the injuries due to thoracic trauma. After ensuring the hemodynamic stability of the patient, chest radiograph is obtained as the initial imaging evaluation during the primary survey.

The Chest Radiograph

It is usually obtained in the supine anteroposterior projection. It is a useful adjunct to rule out immediate life-threatening conditions like large pneumothorax, massive hemothorax, and hemomediastinum (mediastinal widening). Besides, it is also useful to detect lung injuries, osseous trauma and the position of various internal catheters, lines and tubes. However, it has multiple limitations including suboptimal patient positioning, magnification and distortion of mediastinum, overlap of soft tissue and lung parenchyma, inability to detect air-fluid level in the supine position besides being less sensitive in characterizing mediastinal and lung parenchymal injuries.

Ultrasound

Ultrasound of the chest is done as an extension of the Focussed Assessment with Sonography in Trauma (eFAST). This is also done alongwith the chest radiograph during the primary survey of the patient as part of initial evaluation and resuscitation. It is used to detect hemothorax, pneumothorax and hemopericardium. Pneumothorax is diagnosed on ultrasound by detecting loss of 'lung sliding sign'. When the chest is evaluated by ultrasound in a healthy patient, the parietal and visceral pleura are seen opposed to each other and appear as a bright echogenic line. This is the first air interface and acts as a barrier for the ultrasound beam. Beyond this line, the ultrasound beam is not able to penetrate and gets reflected back. Hence only reverberation artefacts and comet tail artefacts are seen deeper to this interface. With respiratory movements, the visceral pleura slides in a craniocaudal direction in relation to the parietal pleura. The ultrasound detects it as an inner bright echogenic line moving up and down. The reverberation artefacts and the comet tail artefacts also move with this line. This has been described as 'lung sliding sign'. When there is pneumothorax, the parietal and visceral pleura get separated by air. Now the ultrasound beam encounters air just after the parietal pleura and the first air interface is, therefore, the parietal pleura rather than visceral pleura. The beam is not able to penetrate beyond this and therefore the visceral pleura or the lung parenchyma which are deeper are not visualized. In this scenario, the echogenic bright line does not move with respiration as the air column in the pleural space is static. This leads to loss of 'lung sliding sign'. This is a marker of pneumothorax. It should be looked for in the most nondependent area like beneath the second intercostal space in parasternal location. The reverberation and the comet tail artefacts are also not well seen in pneumothorax.

Multidetector Computed Tomography

It is the modality of choice for detection of pulmonary, pleural, mediastinal and osseous abnormalities in the setting of thoracic trauma. However, it is done after the patient has been stablized hemodynamically. The current indications in patients of thoracic trauma include significant findings on a chest radiograph or eFAST, penetrating chest injury, suspicion of mediastinal vascular injury (aortic injury), significant osseous injuries on radiograph especially upper rib fractures or flail segments. It is also done in patients with dangerous mechanism of injury even when the chest radiograph and eFAST are normal. The CT is done as a part of torso imaging protocol combined with abdomen. At our center, we routinely do the CT chest in arterial phase to look for vascular injuries. A negative contrast CT examination virtually rules out any significant thoracic injury.

The following section describes the radiographic and CT findings of major lung parenchymal, pleural, mediastinal, diaphragmatic and chest wall injuries.

PULMONARY PARENCHYMAL INJURIES

Pulmonary Contusion

Pulmonary contusions are the most common cause of pulmonary opacifications in blunt chest trauma with a prevalence of 17–70%.[2] The causative force is direct injury to the lung parenchyma at the site of impact or in the opposite portion of the lung (contercoup injury). It represents a combination of parenchymal edema and hemorrhage secondary to alveolar membrane disruption. Patients may be asymptomatic (50%) or may have hemoptysis, fever, tachypnea, hypoxia and hypercarbia. The initial chest radiograph may be normal but the findings usually are evident within 6 hours. The contusions appears as unilateral or bilateral, ill-defined, focal or multifocal, patchy airspace opacity which is not confined by fissural boundaries (nonsegmental distribution). They are usually seen in the lung periphery adjacent to the site of lung trauma and frequently have associated bony injuries of ribs or spine except in pediatric patients where they often occur without overlying bony injuries. Lung bases are a preferred site due to increased basilar mobility. Air bronchograms are usually absent due to blood filling the airways. The maximal radiographic opacity is seen within 24–72 hours after which it gradually clears completely over the next 3–10 days.

CT is more sensitive than chest radiograph for detection of pulmonary contusions.[3] In CT also it appears as ill-defined areas of ground-glass opacity which readily cross pleural fissures **(Figs. 1A and B)**. The peripheral 1–2 mm of lung may show sparing especially in pediatric population.[4] Recently CT has been used to quantify the volume of contusion to predict the clinical course and outcome. Miller et al.[5] found contusion volume to be a direct predictor of subsequent development of acute respiratory distress syndrome (ARDS).

Pulmonary Laceration

Pulmonary laceration represents a tear of lung parenchyma secondary to penetrating injury, lung perforation from rib fractures or shearing forces caused by inertial deceleration. Clinically, it may manifest as hemoptysis. The lacerations are more common in children and young adults because of the greater flexibility of the chest wall causing higher likelihood of lung getting injured with blunt trauma.[6] They are not frequently identified on the initial chest radiograph because they get obscured by surrounding contusions. A chest CT is significantly more sensitive to detect and evaluate the extent of the pulmonary laceration than a conventional chest radiograph. Lacerations are usually ovoid. Radiologically, lacerations appear as ovoid lucent areas because of the elastic recoil of the lung with a thin rim of hyperdensity, representing a pseudomembrane. The laceration cavity may be filled with air (traumatic pneumatocele), blood (traumatic hematocele) or both with air and blood (traumatic hematopneumatocele). On CT, when air filled, they appear as localized air collections within areas of contusion **(Figs. 2A and B)**. After clearing of the adjacent lung contusion they are seen as thin-walled cysts filled with air or blood. The lacerations resolve slowly over a period of 3 weeks to a year. They may persist as a pulmonary nodule containing blood clots.

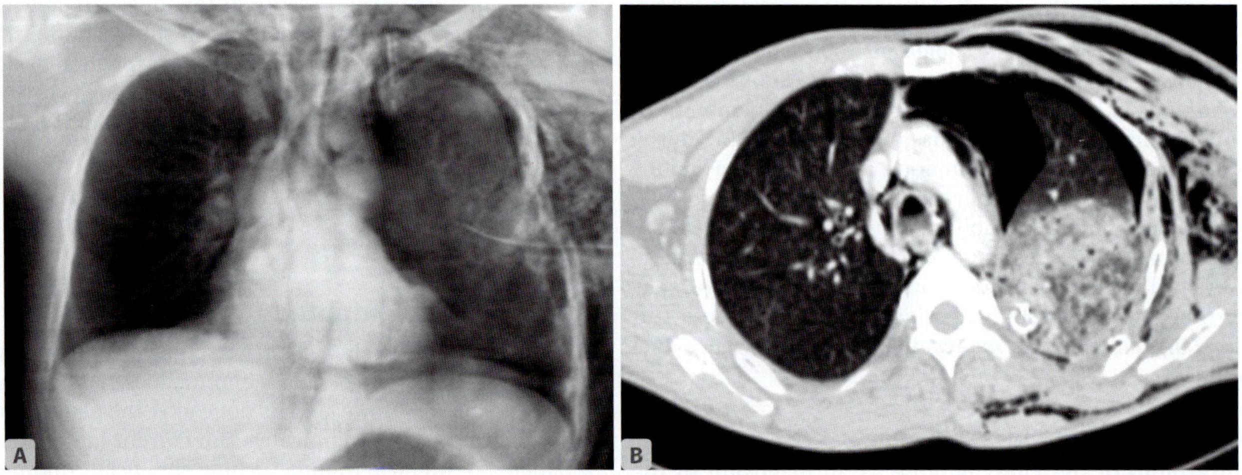

FIGS. 1A AND B: Pulmonary contusion: Thick coronal multiplanar reconstruction (A) and axial (B) CT images show homogeneous ground-glass density in left upper lobe of lung consistent with pulmonary contusion. Note presence of left pneumothorax and pneumomediastinum.

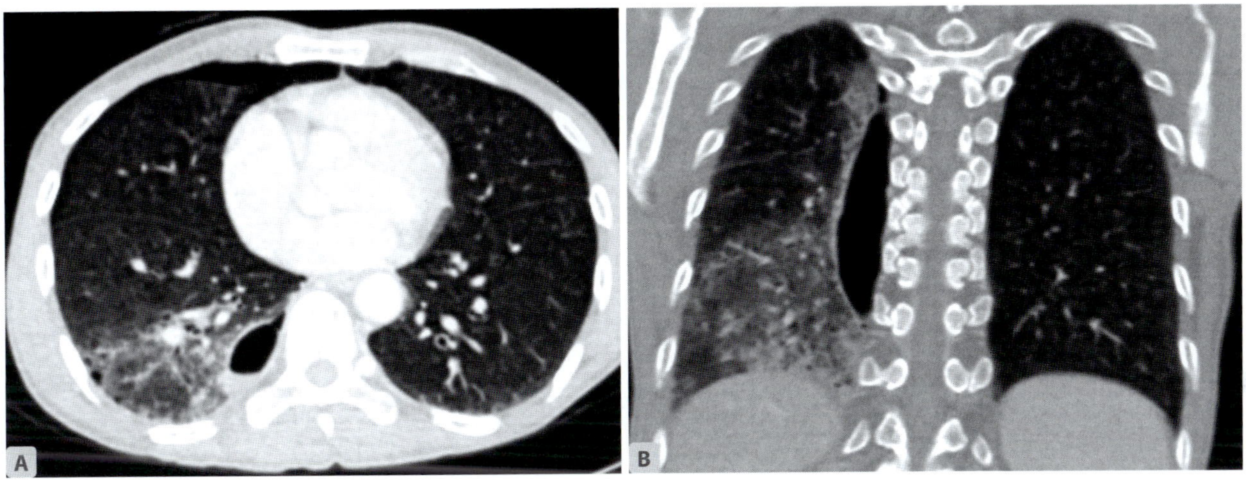

FIGS. 2A AND B: Pulmonary laceration: Axial (A) and coronal multiplanar reconstruction (B) CT images show an ovoid lesion with an air fluid level in paravertebral location of right lung representing laceration. Note the adjacent ground-glass density representing contusion and a small pneumothorax on right side.

Potential complications include infection leading to pulmonary abscess, increased size of laceration or development of bronchopleural fistula when the laceration communicates with a bronchus and pleural surface.[2,7] The abscess appears as thick-walled cavity with irregular inner margins and an air-fluid level. Bronchopleural fistula leads to persistent air leak which does not respond to chest tube placement. Abscess and bronchopleural fistula often require surgical or percutaneous drainage if the medical therapy fails.

Aspiration Pneumonitis

Aspiration pneumonitis is a frequent finding seen in post-traumatic patients especially those with head or maxillofacial injuries. It is important to differentiate aspiration pneumonitis from contusion because the management for the two entities is different. Aspiration produces "tree-in-bud" poorly defined centrilobular opacities usually in the dependent portions of the lung in contrast to contusions which appear as ill-defined areas of ground-glass opacity not respecting fissural boundaries with likely associated lacerations appearing as cysts **(Fig. 3)**. The CT "tree-in-bud" appearance of aspiration reflects aspirated material filling the distal small airways, whereas the confluent ground-glass opacity of contusion represents injury to the localized parenchymal area. The most frequently involved lung segments in aspiration include the superior and posterior basilar segments of the lower lobes and the posterior segments of the upper lobes. The classical "tree-in-bud" opacities are not easily visualized after few hours as they become confluent resulting in consolidative appearance except along the periphery where some isolated filled terminal bronchioles often persist.

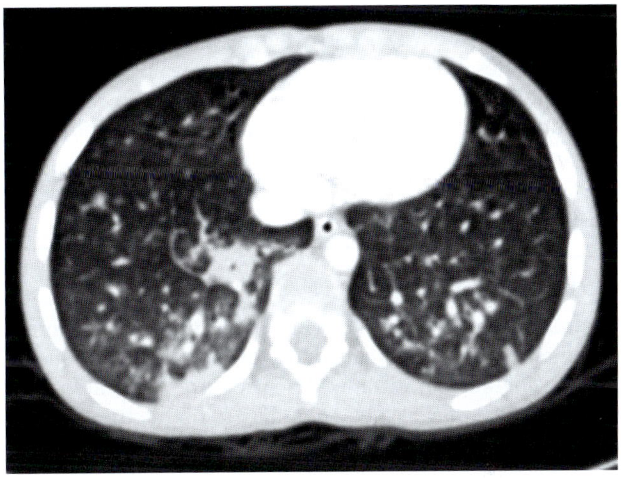

FIG. 3: Aspiration pneumonitis: Axial CT image shows poorly defined centrilobular nodules with some having 'tree-in-bud' configuration in the apical segment of right lower lobe.

Atelectasis

Lung collapse in the trauma patient can be separated broadly into the categories of obstructive, compressive, passive, and adhesive atelectasis. Obstructive atelectasis occurs due to obstruction of the airway by mucus plug, foreign body, blood or airway rupture. Compressive atelectasis occurs from mass effect of large contusions or traumatic lung cysts. Passive atelectasis occurs secondary to pneumothorax or hemothorax which disrupts the inherent elastic recoil properties of the lung **(Figs. 4A and B)**. It is the most common form seen in the setting of trauma. Adhesive atelectasis is caused by decreased surfactant production secondary to pulmonary contusion. Air bronchograms are often seen in all forms of atelectasis except from a central bronchial obstructive cause.

Radiologically atelectasis appears as a dense homogeneous opacity with signs of volume loss such as fissure deviation, bronchovascular crowding, ipsilateral hilar or mediastinal shift and elevated diaphragm. On contrast enhancement, the collapsed part shows greater enhancement due to crowded pulmonary vasculature compared to consolidation. These above findings help to differentiate atelectasis from contusion or consolidation.

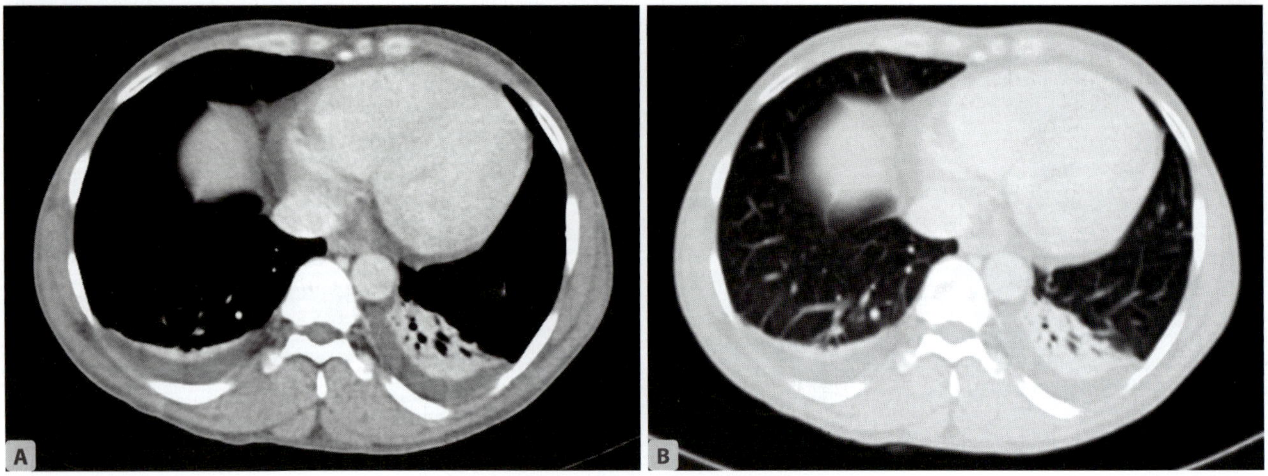

FIGS. 4A AND B: Atelectasis: Axial chest CT images in mediastinal (A) and lung (B) window shows passive atelectasis of left lower lobe segment with air bronchogram within secondary to pleural fluid. Also seen in right pleural fluid.

Traumatic Lung Herniation

This uncommon entity occurs when a pleura covered part of lung herniates through a defect in the chest wall.[2,6] it is usually associated with a rib fracture. It is important to recognize this condition because if left untreated the herniation may increase secondary to positive pressure ventilation.

PLEURAL INJURIES

Pneumothorax

Pneumothorax is seen in 30–40% of all blunt chest trauma patients.[2] It is usually caused by alveolar rupture due to sudden increase in intrathoracic pressure associated with pleural tear. It may also be secondary to rib fracture with rib piercing the pleura and the lung. The diagnosis is first made on a chest radiograph. However, 30–50% pneumothoraces are missed on the radiographs which are usually taken in supine position in the setting of trauma.[6] These can be seen on CT and are called as 'occult pneumothoraces'. In the supine position air collects anteriorly and medially in the anterior costophrenic sulcus. The signs of pneumothorax on a supine chest radiograph are described in **Box 1**.

On an upright chest radiograph pneumothorax is seen as thin, sharply defined line that represents the visceral pleura. Lung markings are not seen beyond this line. False positive cases may be due to skin folds, large bullae, overlying tubes and catheters, bedding, scapular margin mimicking the pneumothorax. The correct diagnosis can be made by an upright expiratory chest radiograph or CT.

As described earlier in this chapter, eFAST has been increasingly used to detect pneumothorax and has shown very high sensitivity in experienced hands. Loss of 'lung sliding sign' confirms pneumothorax.

The clinical significance of a small pneumothorax which remains undetected on the chest radiograph or the eFAST is very low and does not warrant further radiographs in additional views except if the patient is on ventilation where even a small pneumothorax can quickly become life-threatening due to positive pressure ventilation.

BOX 1: Signs of pneumothorax on supine chest radiograph.

- Abnormally increased lucency in the lower chest or upper abdomen **(Fig. 5)**
- The 'deep sulcus' sign—abnormally wide and deep costophrenic sulcus
- The 'double diaphragm' sign—when air outlines the dome and anterior insertion of diaphragm
- Sharply outlined diaphragmatic or cardiac border
- Depression of hemidiaphragm

CT is highly sensitive for detecting the pneumothoraces **(Fig. 6)**. Even evaluation of an abdominal CT often detects pneumothorax because of the tendency of the air to collect in the anterior costophrenic sulcus in the supine patient.

Chest tube placement is usually required in patients who are symptomatic, have >20% pneumothorax, in patients who are on ventilator or are likely to be put on ventilator or who have to undergo a lengthy operative procedure.

If the pneumothorax is persistent and does not completely respond to treatment including a chest tube placement, then malpositioned chest tube, tracheobronchial injury or a bronchopleural fistula needs to be ruled out on imaging.

Tension pneumothorax develops when the intrapleural pressure exceeds that of the atmosphere. This serious condition occurs when the pulmonary or bronchial injury acts as a one-way valve with air entering into pleural space without exit. This leads to pulmonary and cardiac compromise. It is a clinical diagnosis. However, there are signs to suggest tension pneumothorax on a radiograph **(Figs. 7A and B)**. These have been enumerated in **Box 2**.

If suspected, it warrants an immediate rapid decompression with a large bore needle followed by a chest tube placement.

Hemothorax

Hemothorax is seen in approximately 50% of patients of blunt thoracic trauma, especially those caused by penetrating trauma.[2] Source of bleeding is injury to pleura,

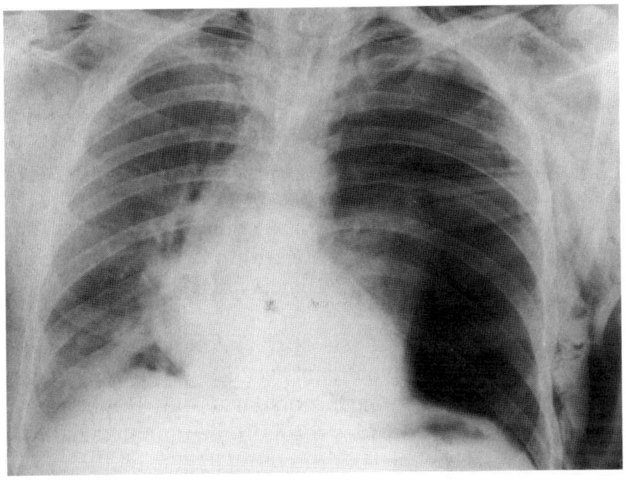

FIG. 5: Pneumothorax: Chest radiograph shows left-sided pneumothorax with clear visualization of lung border and deep sulcus sign. Also note subcutaneous emphysema along the pectoralis muscle.

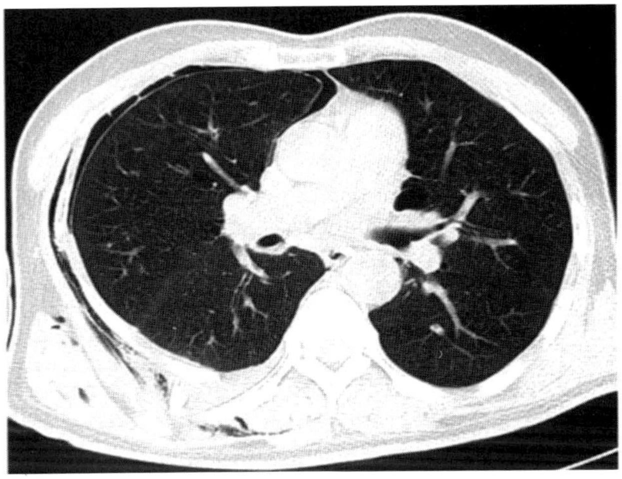

FIG. 6: Pneumothorax: Axial chest CT image shows minimal right sided pneumothorax. Rib fractures are seen posteriorly on right side.

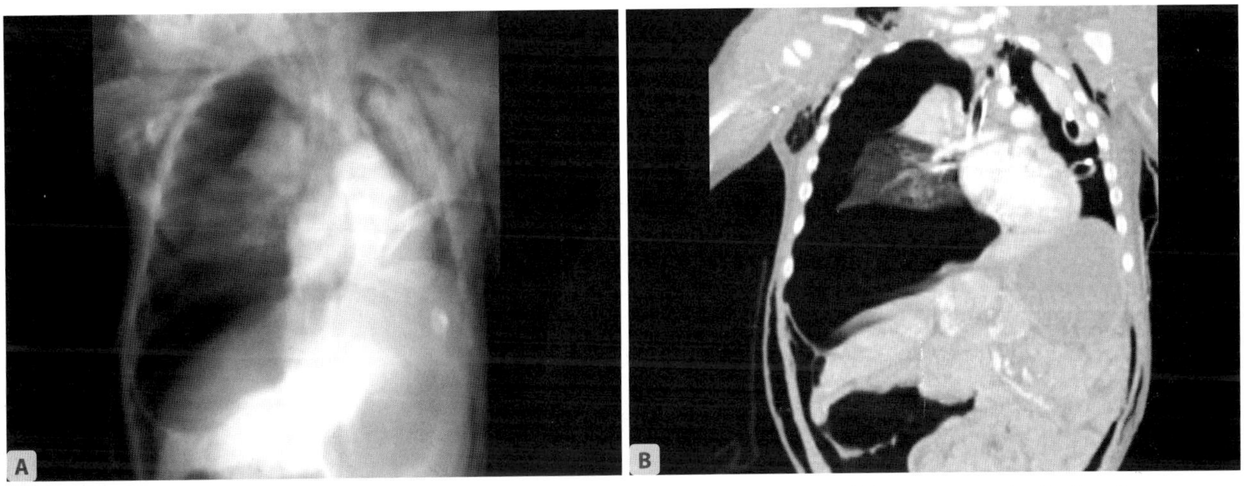

FIGS. 7A AND B: Tension pneumothorax: Coronal thick (a) and thin (B) multiplanar reconstruction CT images show right-sided tension pneumothorax with inversion of right diaphragm, collapsed left lung and mediastinal shift towards right.

BOX 2: Signs of tension pneumothorax on chest radiograph in addition to presence of pneumothorax.

- Widening of lateral diameter of thorax
- Contralateral mediastinal shift
- Flattening or inversion of ipsilateral diaphragm
- Collapsed lung in the hilar region
- Deep sulcus sign
- Widening of intercostal spaces

lung parenchyma, mediastinum, diaphragm or with injuries to liver and spleen with associated diaphragmatic injury. Decubitus chest radiograph can detect as less as 5 mL of fluid in pleural space whereas blunting of costophrenic angle is seen on upright radiograph when approximately 200 mL of fluid accumulates in the pleural space. Progressive increase leads to the 'meniscus' sign, i.e. concave upward sloping of the fluid in the costophrenic angle **(Fig. 8)**. An air-fluid level indicates hemopneumothorax. However, in the setting of trauma since most often it is the supine radiograph which is acquired, the hemothorax is seen as increased opacity of the ipsilateral hemithorax with mediastinal shift to contralateral side **(Figs. 9A and B)**. eFAST is used to detect hemothorax with high sensitivity.

CT is highly sensitive for small amounts of pleural fluid and is also helpful in its characterization. A Hounsfield unit (HU) value of 35–70 represents hemothorax whereas HU less than 15 typically is seen in sympathetic pleural effusion which is seen in patients with hepatic, splenic or pancreatic injuries.

Other uncommon causes of pleural fluid in the setting of trauma include chylothorax which may occur secondary to injury to the thoracic duct, bilious effusion which is caused by biliopleural fistula secondary to hepatic and diaphragmatic injury and urinothorax which occurs secondary to renopleural fistula.

However, any fluid detected in the pleural cavity at presentation in a post-traumatic patient is considered as hemothorax unless proven otherwise and managed accordingly.

Source of bleeding can be venous which is usually self-limiting or arterial which usually progresses on follow-up imaging. Arterial bleed may also be seen on CT as active contrast extravasation usually from an intercostal artery.

It is also important to note the placement of the chest tube on CT. A malpositioned tube impinging into mediastinum, displaced into fissure or outside the pleura or in the lung parenchyma should be communicated to the clinician **(Fig. 10)**. A chest tube in the fissure may adequately drain a pneumothorax but is less effective for a hemothorax.

INJURIES OF THE MEDIASTINUM

Tracheobronchial Injury

Tracheobronchial injuries are uncommon injuries occurring in 1–3% of blunt chest trauma and 2–9% of patients with penetrating chest trauma.[8] Penetrating injury accounts for 70% of tracheobronchial injuries and rest is from blunt trauma, iatrogenic from intubation or tracheostomy, foreign body aspiration, inhalation. Penetrating injuries most commonly involve the cervical part of trachea whereas blunt injury most commonly involves the intrathoracic part.[9] Right main stem bronchus is injured more commonly than the left side due to less protection from surrounding structures. The bronchial injuries usually occur within 2.5 cm of the carina whereas the tracheal injuries usually occur more than 2 cm above the carina.[10]

Clinically, the diagnosis of tracheobronchial injury is often delayed in many patients because the airway column is maintained by the peribronchial tissue. Tracheal and proximal bronchial injuries result in pneumomediastinum whereas distal bronchial injuries result in pneumothorax.

On chest radiograph, presence of significant pneumomediastinum, persistent pneumothorax and atelectasis with increasing subcutaneous emphysema despite adequate

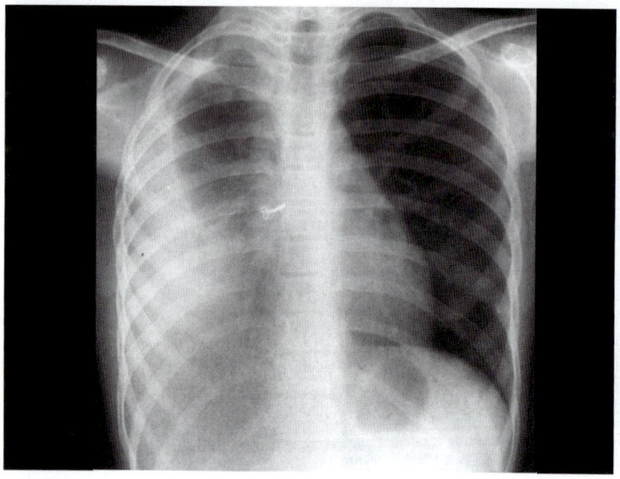

FIG. 8: Hemothorax: Chest radiograph in erect position shows right-sided pleural fluid with meniscus sign.

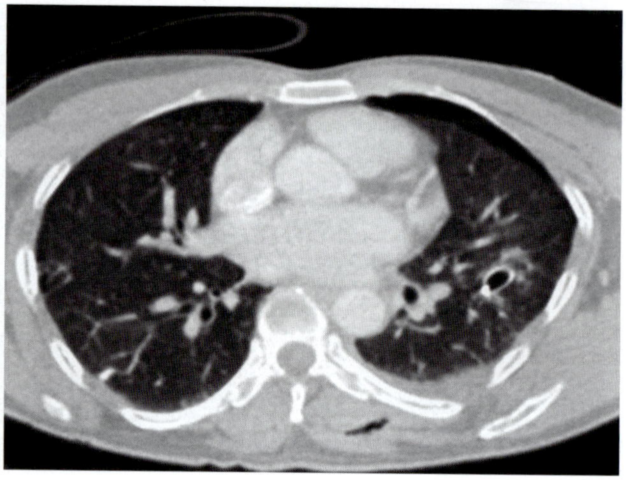

FIG. 10: Malpositioned chest tube: Axial CT image shows the tip of chest tube lying within lung parenchyma. Note small pneumothorax on left side.

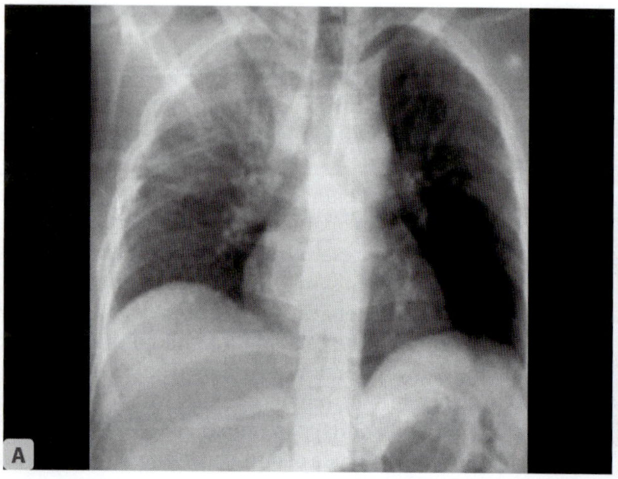

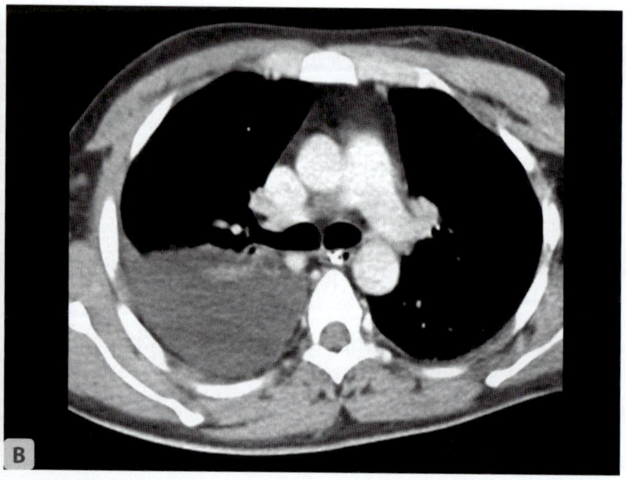

FIGS. 9A AND B: Hemothorax: CT thick coronal multiplanar reconstruction image (a) shows appearance of pleural fluid in supine patient appearing as diffuse haze of right hemithorax. CT axial image (b) shows moderate amount of right pleural fluid in dependent position. The fluid appears of high density signifying hemothorax.

chest tube placement should raise a doubt of airway injury. The classical radiological signs described for tracheobronchial injury are enumerated in **Box 3**.

CT with multiplanar reconstructions is superior to radiograph for detection of airway injury. The most direct sign on CT is demonstration of wall defect or deformity **(Figs. 11A and B)**. The tracheal lacerations are usually vertical and longitudinal and located at the junction of cartilaginous and membranous portion of the trachea whereas bronchial lacerations occur parallel to the cartilaginous rings. The indirect signs on imaging include an abnormal configuration of endotracheal balloon cuff, pneumomediastinum or pneumothorax and distal atelectasis. Multiplanar images with three-dimensional volumetric images as well as virtual bronchoscopy aid in the diagnosis of tracheobronchial injuries.

Esophageal Injury

Iatrogenic trauma due to endoscopic procedures is the most common cause for esophageal injury followed by penetrating trauma, toxic ingestions, emetic injury (Boerhaave's syndrome) and rarely blunt trauma. Early diagnosis and treatment is important as esophageal injury is associated with high morbidity and mortality. Radiological signs of esophageal perforation include cervical and mediastinal emphysema, pleural effusion, abnormal mediastinal contour due to leakage of fluid, hematoma or mediastinitis, leakage of oral contrast material into mediastinum or pleural space, and esophageal wall thickening. Mid to distal esophageal rupture causes right pleural effusion whereas lower esophageal or rupture of injury at gastroesophageal (GE) junction causes left pleural effusion. Contrast esophagography (radiographic or CT) followed by flexible esophagoscopy may be required to confirm and evaluate the site of injury **(Fig. 12)**.

Rarely, a traumatic tracheoesophageal, fistula may be formed. It is usually secondary to long-term use of an endotracheal or nasogastric tube.

BOX 3: Radiological signs of tracheobronchial injury.

- 'Double wall' sign—due to intramural air within the proximal airway[2]
- 'Fallen lung' sign—inferior falling of collapsed lung in the dependent portion due to complete disruption of the central airway
- 'Bayonet' sign—tapered air-filled bronchus[6]

Pneumomediastinum

Pneumomediastinum can be due to intrathoracic and extrathoracic sources. Intrathoracic sources include injury to lung, tracheobronchial tree or esophagus whereas extrathoracic sources include head and neck and anterior retroperitoneum. The mediastinum and retroperitoneum communicate through the aortic and esophageal hiatus and at sternocostal attachments of diaphragm.

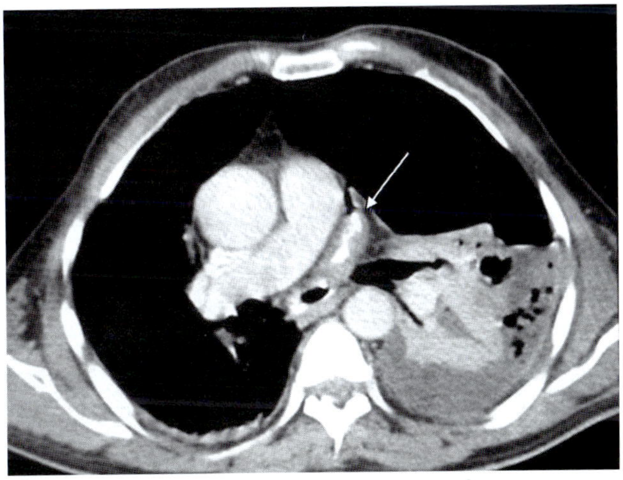

FIG. 12: Esophageal injury. Axial chest CT image shows leak of oral contrast (arrow) into mediastinum from a tear in the esophagus. Also seen is left pleural fluid with atelectasis of left lower lobe.

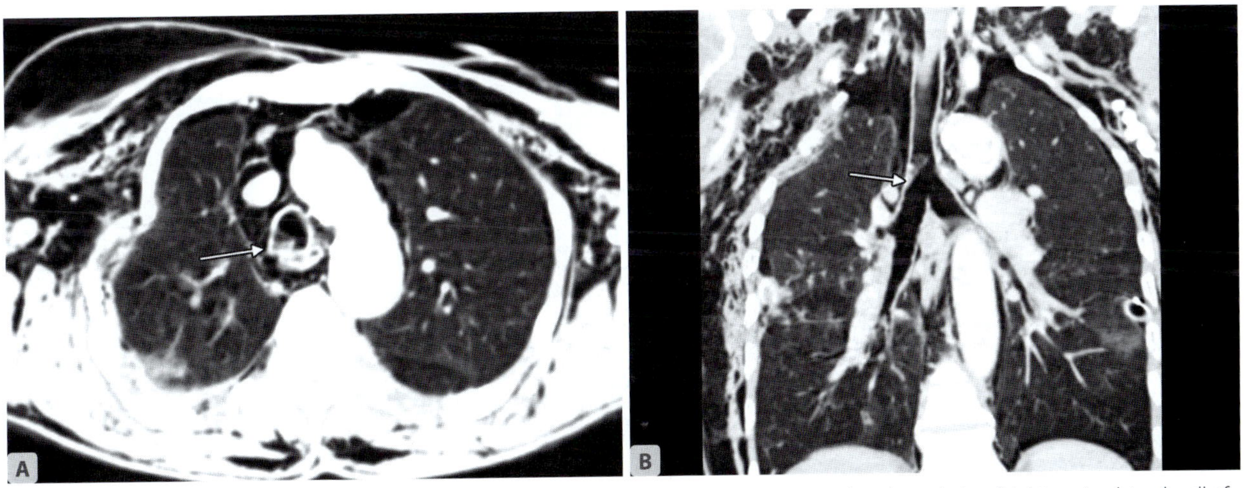

FIGS. 11A AND B: Tracheal injury: Axial (A) and coronal multiplanar reconstruction; (B) CT images show irregularity of right posterolateral wall of lower trachea (arrows) with formation of a luminal flap representing tracheal injury. Note the extensive pneumomediastinum and subcutaneous emphysema.

Pneumomediastinum is not itself a dangerous condition but a sign of potentially more serious other injuries.

The most common cause of pneumomediastinum is air from rupture of alveoli due to increased alveolar pressure secondary to trauma. The leaked air dissects along the bronchovascular sheath and spreads into mediastinum. This phenomenon is known as 'Macklin effect'. The pneumomediastinum may increase in size with positive pressure ventilation. The CT appearance of Macklin effect is that of streaks of air along the bronchovascular bundles (similar to that seen in pulmonary interstitial emphysema) along with pneumomediastinum.[9,11]

Pneumomediastinum is visualized on anteroposterior chest radiograph as a lucency bordered by a thin white pleural line coursing along the pericardium and lateral mediastinum **(Fig. 13)**. It needs to be differentiated from pneumopericardium and pneumothorax. Pneumopericardium appears as more ovoid in shape than linear and does not extend above the level of aortic arch respecting the boundaries of the pericardium. Also the pericardium can be visualized in pneumopericardium. Medial pneumothorax may mimic pneumomediastinum but is usually associated with rib fractures and other evidences of pneumothorax. Also visualization of apparent septae favors a pneumomediastinum. Repeating the imaging in decubitus position confirms the diagnosis as the mediastinal air does not change in location whereas pneumothorax and pneumopericardium would show change in location of air. The pneumomediastinum may dissect into neck and soft tissues on increasing in size. The radiographic signs of pneumomediastinum are described in **Box 4**.

False-positive pneumomediastinum may be caused by 'Mach effect', where a thin linear lucency outlines the dense opaque cardiac silhouette. This is due to visual perception of edge enhancement and occurs at the level of the retina.

CT is most sensitive modality for detecting small amount of pneumomediastinum **(Figs. 14A and B)**.

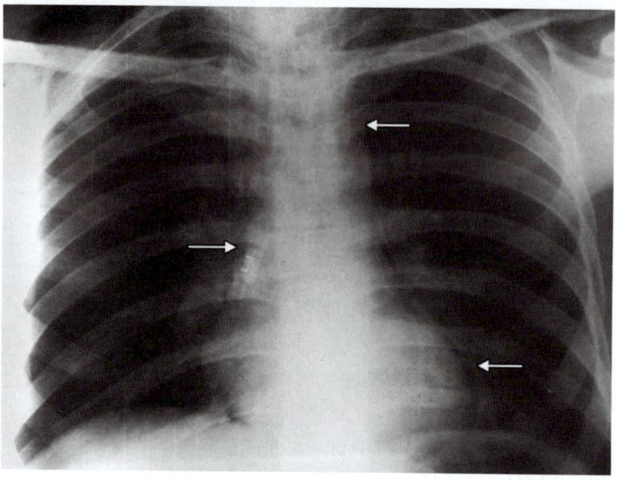

FIG. 13: Pneumomediastinum: Chest radiograph shows air outlining the mediastinum (arrows) on both sides. The air is seen above the level of aortic arch also (upper left arrow).

Vascular Injury

Traumatic aortic injury is an important cause of morbidity and mortality in patients with blunt thoracic trauma. Early

BOX 4: Radiological signs of pneumomediastinum.

- 'Double bronchial wall' sign—visualization of both sides of bronchial wall due to air accumulating adjacent to bronchial wall
- 'Continuous diaphragm' sign—visualization of entire diaphragm from medial to lateral due to air trapped posterior to the pericardium at base
- 'Tubular artery' sign—air outlining the medial side of aorta with lung air outlining the lateral side
- 'Ring around the artery' sign—air outlining the pulmonary artery
- Elevation of the thymus especially in children

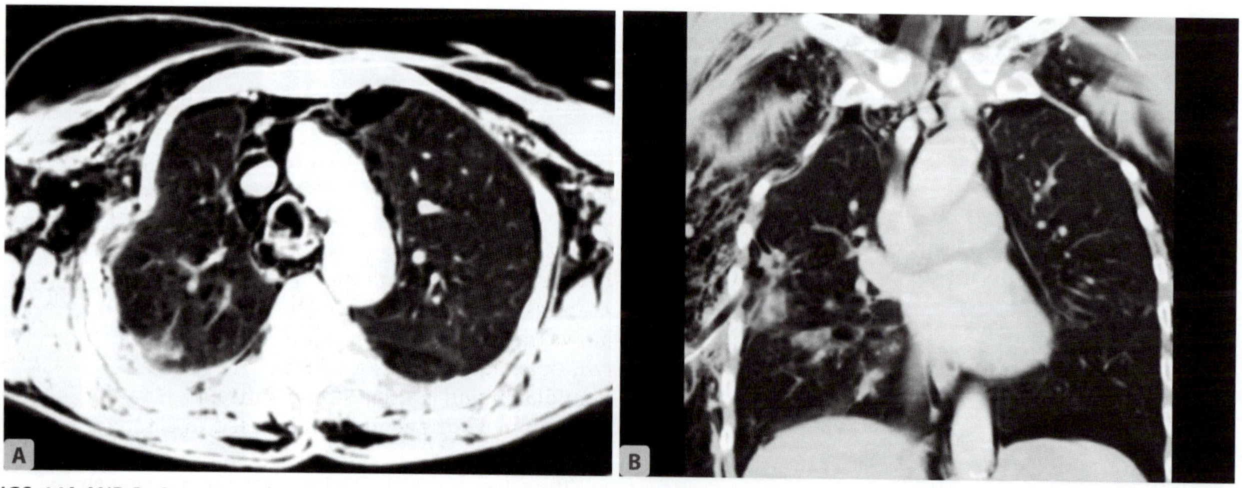

FIGS. 14A AND B: Pneumomediastinum: Axial (A) and coronal multiplanar reconstruction (B) CT images in a patient with tracheal injury (same patient as in **Figure 11**) shows extensive air in the mediastinum. The coronal image (B) shows the air to be present above the level of aortic arch and also tracking along the descending aorta inferiorly.

recognition and treatment is of utmost importance as early medical and definitive surgical treatment can improve survivability in these patients. The sites of aortic injury in descending order of frequency are—proximal descending aorta at isthmus (90–95%), ascending aorta including aortic root, aortic arch and distal descending aorta.[10,12] It causes mediastinal hemorrhage especially in the periaortic region due to bleeding from small veins in the area or from vasa vasorum of the aorta.

Plain chest radiograph is the first investigation after initial resuscitative efforts. The findings on chest radiograph for possible traumatic aortic injury are shown in **Box 5**.

Mediastinal widening has a high sensitivity (90–100%) for mediastinal hematoma and associated aortic injury but the specificity is low (60%). False-positive diagnosis may be due to variety of causes including supine position, expiratory film, atelectasis, pleural effusions or lung injuries obscuring mediastinal margins, mediastinal tumors and mediastinal hemorrhage due to nonaortic causes like spinal fracture or spinal ligamentous injury. A negative plain chest radiograph has high negative predictive value of 90%. It should, however, be noted that rarely the radiograph may also be normal in aortic injury especially in intimal injuries.

Multislice CT with CT angiography is now the investigation for choice for detecting aortic injury. It has replaced catheter angiography for screening for aortic injury. Catheter angiography is reserved for doubtful cases and for interventional treatment. The American College of Radiology (ACR) appropriateness criteria recommends using CT angiography for evaluation of all suspected cases of traumatic aortic injury.[13] CT has been reported to have sensitivity of 100% and specificity of 96% for diagnosing aortic injury.[7] The signs of aortic injury on CT are enumerated in **Box 6**.

BOX 5: Chest radiograph signs for possible aortic injury.

- Mediastinal widening
- Depression of the left mainstem bronchus
- Blurring of aortic contour
- Thickening of right or left paratracheal stripe
- Shift of trachea and nasogastric tube to the right
- Left hemothorax (effusion)
- Left apical pleural cap

BOX 6: Signs of traumatic aortic injury on CT.

- *Direct signs*:
  - Active contrast extravasation
  - Pseudoaneurysm formation
  - Abrupt change in aortic diameter caliper
  - Aortic dissection
  - Intimal flaps or filling defects **(Figs. 15A and B)**
  - Aortic wall irregularity
- *Indirect signs*:
  - Indistinctness of mediastinal fat planes
  - Mediastinal hematoma
  - Periaortic hematoma

Multiplanar reconstructions (MPR) with volume rendering, and virtual angioscopy have been shown to aid in the detection of small rents. Thinner collimations used in CT have allowed detection of 'minimal aortic injuries' which include small intramural hematomas, intimal flaps and intimal thrombus.

Non-aortic vascular injury may also occur in thoracic trauma. These include injury to aortic arch branches, internal mammary artery, pulmonary artery and venous injuries. The spectrum of injuries include intimal tears, dissection, pseudoaneurysm, partial or total occlusion and arteriovenous fistula.

Cardiac and Pericardial Injury

The diagnosis of blunt cardiac injury relies on a high degree of clinical suspicion. Elevated cardiac enzymes with alterations in ECG findings in the setting of blunt thoracic trauma should raise a doubt of cardiac injury. Transthoracic echocardiography is the most appropriate modality for evaluation of the cardiac injury. If it is equivocal, then transesophageal echocardiography or cardiac MRI can be used as problem-solving tool. If contrast CT of the thorax has been done for evaluation of thoracic trauma, cardiac and pericardial injury manifestations include pericardial effusion/hemopericardium, pneumopericardium, contrast extravasation into pericardium or a decreased area of myocardial enhancement **(Figs. 16A and B)**.

Pericardial injury is most commonly on left side of pericardium parallel to phrenic nerve followed by diaphragmatic surface of pericardium. A large pericardial tear can cause cardiac herniation and death.

INJURY OF DIAPHRAGM

Diaphragmatic rupture and subsequent herniation of abdominal contents into thorax is nine times more common on left side than right due to the protective effect of the liver. On the right side most injuries to the diaphragm go unrecognized during the acute phase. In the interval phase, the abdominal viscus may not have herniated or the patient may have acclimatized to the presence of abdominal contents in the thorax. In the later phase, obstruction or strangulation presents with severe abdominal or chest pain. The injury may also be evident at a later stage in those patients who were earlier on positive pressure ventilation and have now been extubated. Chest radiograph may reveal nonspecific findings that include an indistinct or elevated hemidiaphragm, pleural effusion, atelectasis with shift of the mediastinum to the contralateral side, hemothorax, pneumothorax or lower rib fractures. Specific findings are visualization of bowel loops or solid masses above the diaphragm and loss of the normal diaphragmatic contour. Detection of a nasogastric tube above the left hemidiaphragm is also a strong indicator. Contrast studies (barium meal or enema) can be used to clearly delineate the herniation.

The advent of MDCT with multiplanar reconstructions has significantly improved the sensitivity of CT in detecting diaphragmatic injuries. The various CT signs of diaphragmatic injury are given in **Box 7**.[14]

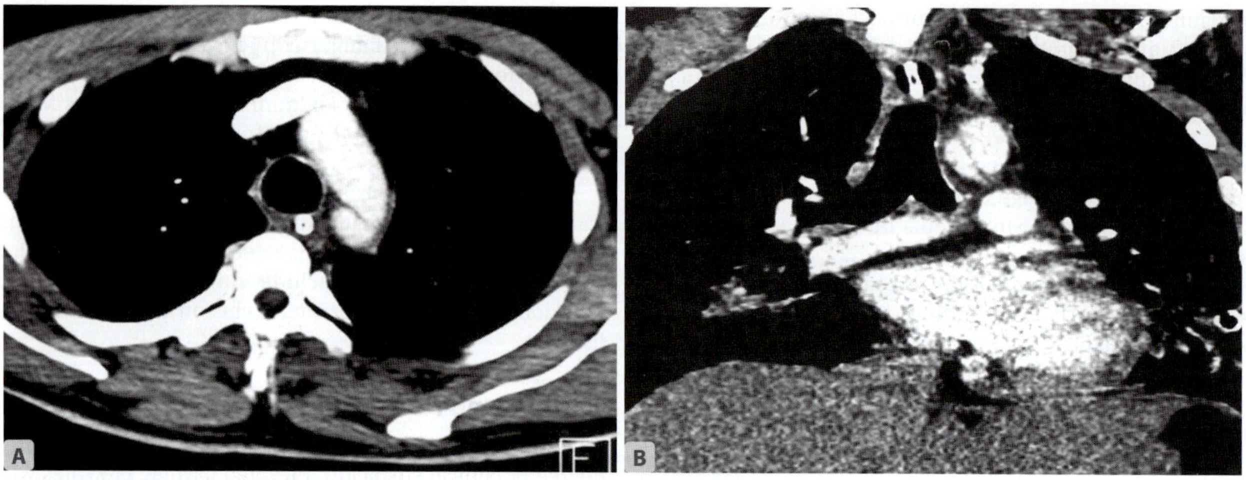

FIGS. 15A AND B: Aortic arch injury: Axial (A) and coronal MPR (B) CT images shows mild outpouching with an intimal flap in the aortic arch representing dissecting pseudoaneurysm.

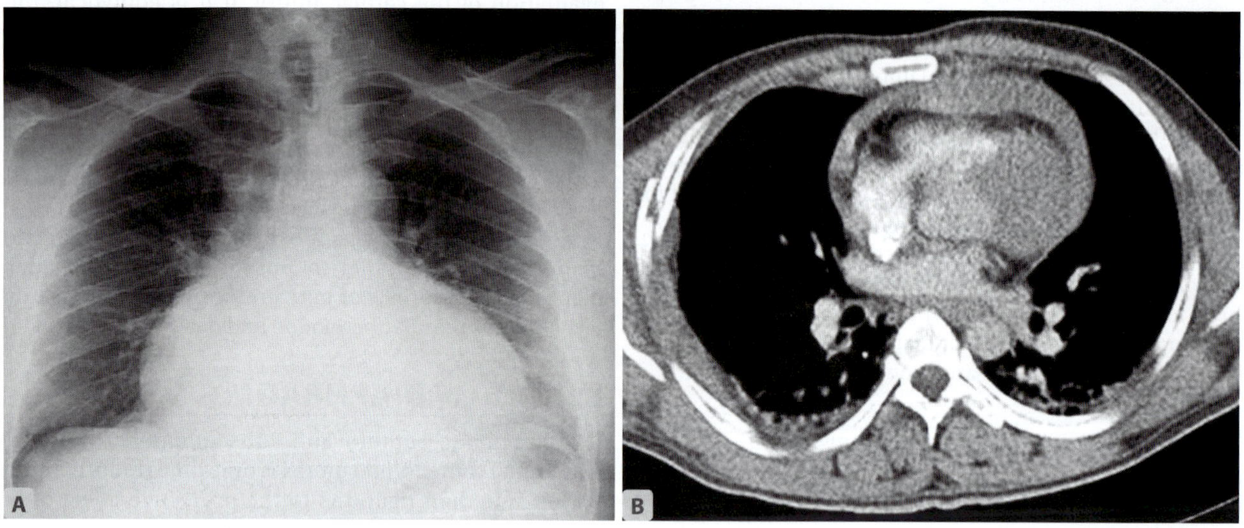

FIGS. 16A AND B: Hemopericardium: Chest radiograph (A) shows enlarged flask-shaped cardiac silhouette representing pericardial fluid. Axial CT image (B) in a different patient shows the hemopericardium. The patient was found to have ventricular wall injury perioperative.

BOX 7: Signs of diaphragmatic injury on CT.

- Focal diaphragmatic discontinuity or elevation
- Focal diaphragmatic thickening (retraction)
- Herniated abdominal contents into thorax
- 'Collar' sign
- 'Dependent viscera' sign

The 'collar' sign refers to the narrowed waist of a herniated intra-abdominal organ due to compression at the neck (diaphragm tear). In a healthy individual, the intra-abdominal organs such as spleen and stomach are seen to be separated by the costal margin by a layer of the diaphragm on cross-sectional imaging. However, if these organs have herniated through the diaphragm into the chest, then they appear to lie directly in contact with the posterior thoracic wall without the diaphragm intervening between them **(Figs. 17A and B)**. This has been described as the 'dependent viscera' sign. The 'dependent viscera' sign and the 'collar' signs are reported to be 100% specific.[15] MRI also has been reported to be highly sensitive in detecting diaphragmatic rupture.[16]

INJURY OF CHEST WALL

Rib fractures occur in approximately 50% of all blunt chest trauma and are the most common skeletal manifestation of injury. Isolated rib fractures are usually not clinically significant. However, multiple and bilateral rib fractures signify severe trauma and act as external manifestation of coexisting thoracic or abdominal injuries. Fractures of first three ribs occurs after severe trauma and is associated with injuries of brachial plexus or subclavian vessels. Fractures of lower three ribs is associated with intra-abdominal visceral organ injuries to kidney, spleen and liver. Further, due to the pain and immobility associated with rib fractures, the underlying lung is more prone to atelectasis and pneumonia.

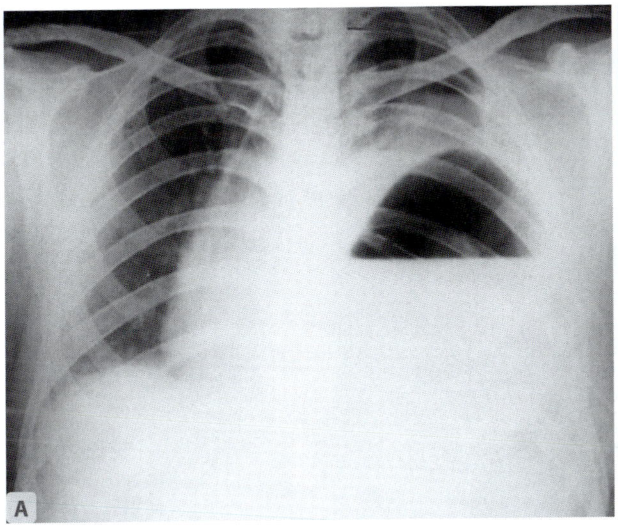

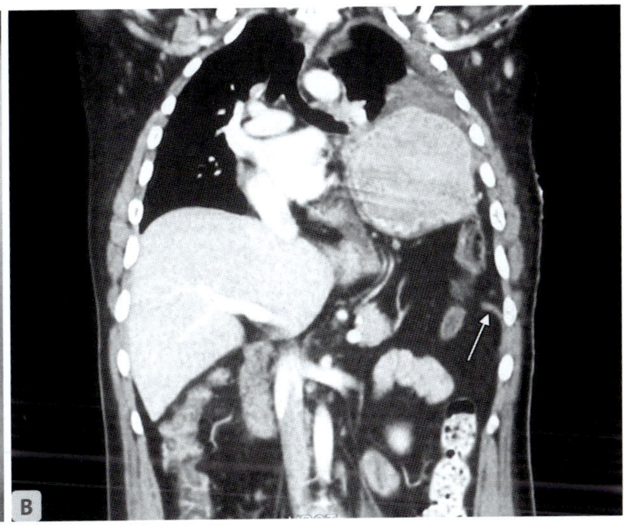

FIGS. 17A AND B: Diaphragmatic injury: Erect chest radiograph (A) shows indistinct left hemidiaphragm outline with large air-fluid level (of stomach) in left thoracic cavity with mediastinal shift towards right. Coronal MPR CT image (B) shows the left diaphragmatic hernia with thickened and retracted torn diaphragm (arrow).

Rarely traumatic lung herniation, as described previously, can also occur. Chest radiography is much less sensitive than CT in detecting rib fractures. CT with three-dimensional volume rendering best depicts the rib fractures.

Flail chest occurs when there are atleast two sites of fractures on each of three or more consecutive ribs creating a flail segment which moves paradoxically with respiratory motion **(Fig. 18)**. It signifies significant chest trauma and is associated with atelectasis and pneumonia and often requires ventilator support or surgical intervention.

Sternal fractures are uncommon. The fracture typically involves the manubrium or body. CT is most sensitive for detection followed by lateral chest radiograph **(Figs. 19A and B)**. A retrosternal hematoma may be seen. A significantly displaced sternal fracture may be associated with underlying cardiac injury.

Fractures of the clavicle are classified according to their location. Group 1 fractures are most common (80%) and involve the mid-part of clavicle; group 2 fractures (15%) involve the lateral third of clavicle; and group 3 fractures (5%) involve the medial third of the clavicle **(Figs. 20A and B)**. Most fractures are managed conservatively although the surgical rate for distal third fractures is more as they have high rate of nonunion.

Sternoclavicular dislocations can be anterior or posterior. Anterior dislocation of clavicle is more common. It is usually not associated with significant injuries and is managed conservatively. Posterior dislocation of clavicle at sternoclavicular joint is more serious as the clavicle can cause injury of trachea, esophagus and mediastinal blood vessels.

Scapular fractures are seen with severe trauma and are usually associated with vascular and neurological injuries. Most fractures occur at the body or neck of scapula. They are usually managed conservatively except for displaced glenoid intra-articular fractures and juxta-articular fractures which require surgical management. Rarely there may be scapulothoracic dissociation in which scapula is displaced laterally. Multiplanar CT reconstructions are best to visualize the fracture fragments.

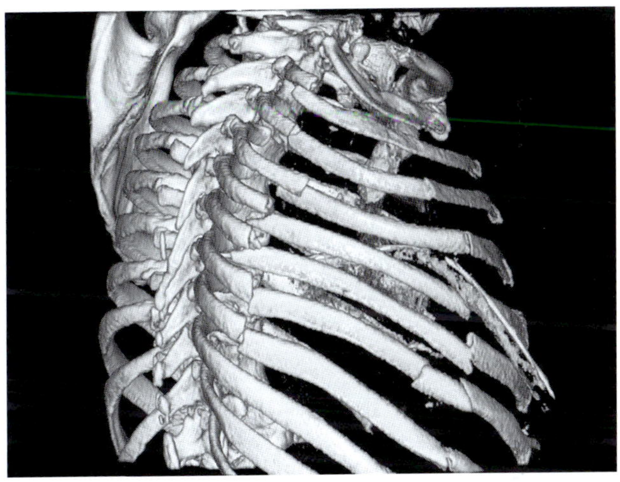

FIG. 18: Flail chest: Three-dimensional volume rendered CT image shows fractures of multiple ribs on right side with many ribs fractured at two places at lateral and posterior ends.

Spinal fractures may also be associated with thoracic trauma. The spinal fractures are easily seen on the multiplanar reconstructions of the CT done for chest. The fractures may be associated with significant neurological deficits in up to 60% of patients. MRI is indicated in patients with spinal trauma and associated neurological deficit for characterization of the spinal cord damage.

CONCLUSION

Diagnostic imaging quickly gives important information on extent and type of thoracic injuries from blunt and penetrating trauma. The chest radiograph is the 'first look' imaging modality and has a role in detecting some immediate

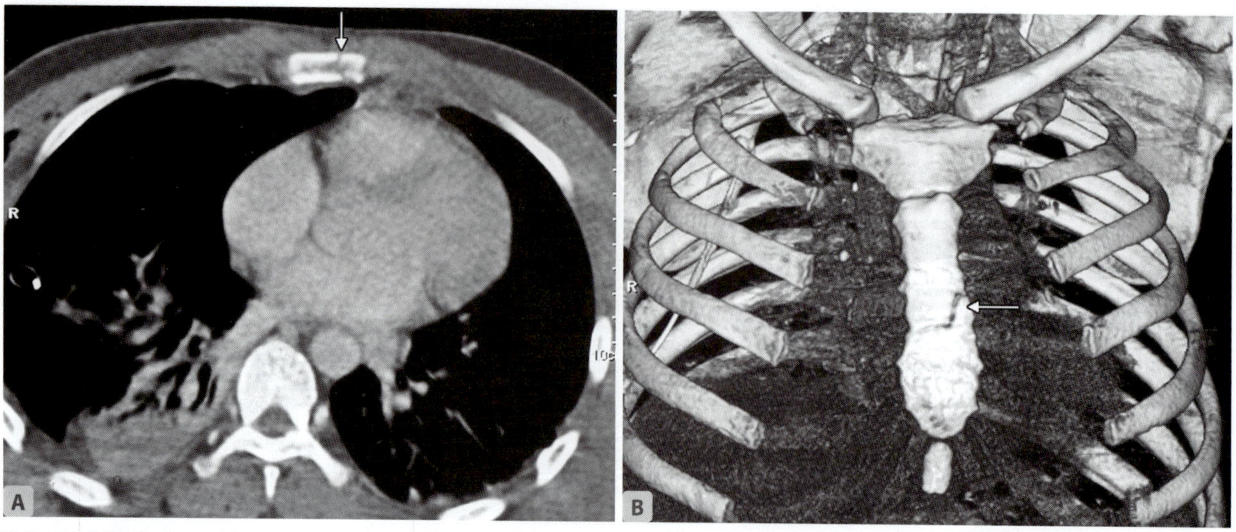

FIGS. 19A AND B: Sternal fracture: Axial (A) and volume rendered three-dimensional (B) CT images show fracture of mid body of sternum.

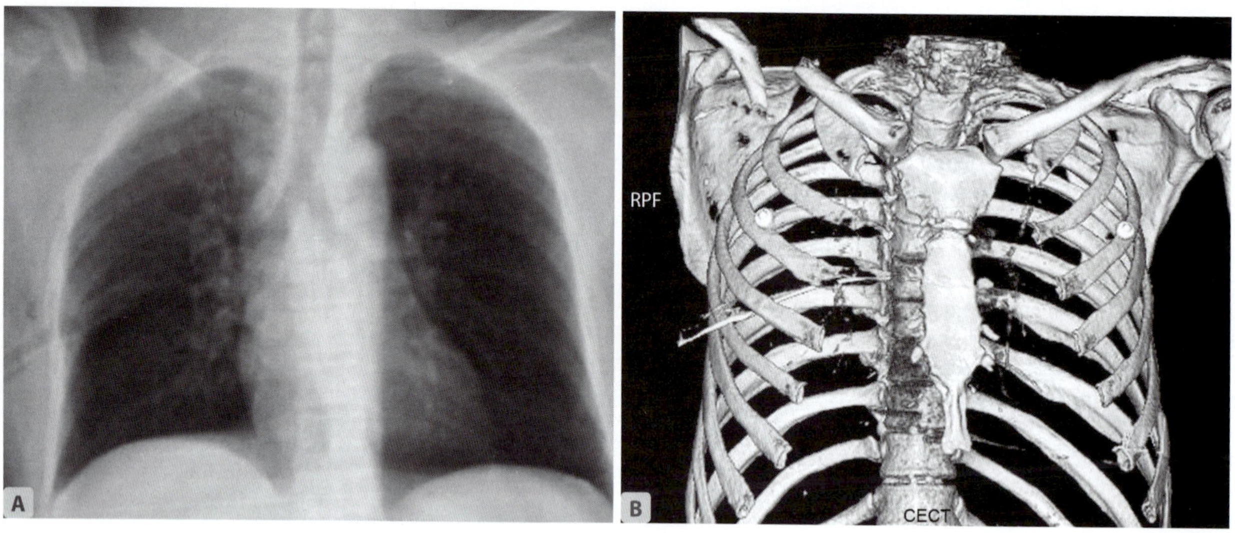

FIGS. 20A AND B: Clavicle fracture: Thick MPR (A) and volume-rendered three-dimensional (B) CT images show fracture of mid-part of right clavicle.

life-threatening conditions like tension pneumothorax and massive hemothorax. Ultrasound is also used as a first line investigation for detecting hemothorax, pneumothorax and hemopericardium. Multislice CT has become the definitive modality which detects and characterizes the full extent of spectrum of thoracic trauma. MRI does not have any significant role in the setting of acute trauma except for evaluation of spinal cord in spinal injuries.

REFERENCES

1. Lomoschitz FM, Eisenhuber E, Linnau KF, et al. Imaging of chest trauma: radiological patterns of injury and diagnostic algorithms. European Journal of Radiology. 2003;48:61-70.
2. Miller LA. Chest wall, lung, and pleural space trauma. Radiol Clin North Am. 2006;44:213-24.
3. Costantino M, Gosselin MV, Primack SL. The ABC's of thoracic trauma imaging. Semin Roentgenol. 2006;41(3):209-25.
4. Donnelly LF, Klosterman LA. Subpleural sparing: a CT finding of lung contusion in children. Radiology. 1997;204:385-7.
5. Miller PR, Croce MA, Bec TK, et al. ARDS after pulmonary contusion: accurate measurement of contusion volume identifies high-risk patients. J Trauma. 2001;51:223-30.
6. Kaewlai R, Avery LL, Asrani AV, et al. Multidetector CT of blunt thoracic trauma. Radiographics. 2008;28(6):1555-70.
7. Rivas LA, Fishman JE, Múnera F, et al. Multislice CT in thoracic trauma. Radiol Clin North Am. 2003;41(3):599-616.
8. Lee RB. Traumatic injury of the cervicothoracic trachea and major bronchi. Chest Surg Clin N Am. 1997;7:285-304.

9. Durso AM, Caban K, Munera F. Penetrating Thoracic Injury. Radiol Clin N Am. 2015;53:675-93.
10. Sangster GP, González-Beicos A, Carbo AI, et al. Blunt traumatic injuries of the lung parenchyma, pleura, thoracic wall, and intrathoracic airways: multidetector computer tomography imaging findings. Emerg Radiol. 2007;14:297-310.
11. Wintermark M, Wicky S, Schnyder P, et al. Blunt traumatic pneumomediastinum: using CT to reveal the Macklin effect. Am J Roentgenol. 1999;172:129-30.
12. Fishman JE. Imaging of blunt aortic and great vessel trauma. J Thorac Imaging. 2000;15:97-103.
13. Demehri S, Rybicki FJ, Desjardins B, et al. ACR Appropriateness Criteria: Blunt chest trauma—suspected aortic injury. Emerg Radiol. 2012;19:287-92.
14. Panda A, Kumar A, Gamanagatti S, et al. Traumatic diaphragmatic injury: a review of CT signs and the difference between blunt and penetrating injury. Diagn Interv Radiol. 2014;20(2):121-8.
15. Stanescu AL, Gross JA, Bittle M, et al. Imaging of blunt abdominal trauma. Semin Roentgen. 2006;41(3):196-204.
16. Barbiera F, Nicastro N, Finazzo M, et al. The role of MRI in traumatic rupture of the diaphragm. Our experience in three cases and review of the literature. Radiol Med. 2003;105(3):188-94.

CHAPTER

138

Imaging of Pleura

Anjali Prakash, Rashmi Dixit, Sapna Singh

INTRODUCTION

The pleura is a serous membrane of mesodermal origin that envelops the lungs, mediastinum, diaphragm and rib cage. It is composed of two layers—parietal and visceral. The lung is covered with visceral pleura, the parietal pleural covers the mediastinum, diaphragm and inner surface of thoracic cage. The layers are in continuity, both at the hilum and below, where they form the pulmonary ligament.

The parietal pleura is divided into costal pleura, diaphragmatic pleura, mediastinal and cervical pleura, based on its relationship to various regions of the thoracic cavity. The visceral and parietal pleural are separated by a potential space that normally contains only a few mL of fluid. As the thickness of the pleural space and its visceral and parietal pleura measures about 0.2–0.44 mm, it is only seen when parallel to the X-ray beam or outlined by air, extrapleural fat or fascia. This pleura is appreciated as:

1. The major, minor or accessory fissures, all of which (with the exception of azygous fissure) consists of two invaginated sheets of visceral pleura.
2. The junctional lines, which consists of four sheets of pleura (two parietal and two visceral), which are often more than a hairline thickness as both (particularly posterior) may contain fibrofatty tissue.

The vascular supply of the parietal pleural is from the systemic circulation, whereas the visceral pleural is supplied by branches of the pulmonary arteries and to a lesser extent by bronchial arteries. Lymphatic drainage of the visceral pleural is by a lymphatic plexus that covers the surface of the lung, just beneath the visceral pleural. This elaborate plexus connects to the bronchial lymphatics that drain centrally along the bronchovascular bundles to the pulmonary hilum. The parietal pleural is the primary drainage route for the pleural space and is lymphatically connected to the intercostal, internal mammary and mediastinal lymph node chains.

IMAGING MODALITIES

Chest radiograph is the initial screening radiological investigation when pleural disease or pulmonary disease is suspected. Chest frontal, lateral, decubitus views are helpful in detecting small amount of pleural effusion. Expiratory films may be required to visualize a small pneumothorax. The drawback is its limited ability to differentiate benign from malignant pleural disease. It is important to differentiate pleural from extrapleural disease and pulmonary disease.

Extrapleural masses usually displace the overlying parietal and visceral pleura resulting in an obtuse angle between the lesion and chest wall. Associated abnormalities include soft tissue mass or rib destruction. They are sharply marginated at the point they contact lung and displace pulmonary vessels away from them.

Pleural masses, arising from visceral or parietal pleura, usually remain confined to pleural space. The presence of an obtuse angle is common, unless the lesion is large. Large pleural lesions may have acute angle, where they meet the chest wall, although some pleural thickening is seen adjacent to them. Pleural lesions are also sharply marginated and displace pulmonary vessels away from them.

A peripherally placed pulmonary lesion will have acute angle with the pleural surface, unless there is pleural invasion, which could result is an obtuse angle. Pulmonary lesions are often ill defined along their inner aspect and may engulf, rather than displace vessels **(Table 1)**.

Ultrasonography is an efficient, 'point of care' imaging modality for evaluation of the chest wall and pleura because of the superficial location. It has low cost, bedside availability and involves no radiation. The indications and uses of chest ultrasound examination for pleural disease are:

- To clarify the nature of unknown pleural densities.
- To detect pleural effusion and to guide thoracocentesis and drainage, especially in minimal or loculated effusion.
- To differentiate subpulmonic effusion from subphrenic fluid accumulation.
- To detect pneumothorax in emergency setting.
- To localize pleural tumors/thickening and guide biopsy of the pleura.

Pleura is a superficial structure and hence seen with a high frequency linear tranducer applied directly over the chest—**the direct intercostal approach**. A sector probe (3.5 MHz) may be used for the lower aspect of pleura via the **abdominal approach**, with the liver and spleen providing an acoustic window. Normal pleura is identified just below the ribs and is seen on ultrasound as an echogenic line just beneath the chest wall **(Fig. 1)**. The air-filled lung covered by visceral pleura reflects the ultrasound beam producing the echogenic line that moves with respiration. This normal movement of lung surface is called '**gliding sign**'. This echogenic line represents the visceral pleura, with the parietal pleura appearing as a weakly echogenic, less distinct line, often obscured by artifacts. Using the abdominal approach, the diaphragm is seen as a bright curving echogenic line. An air-filled lung above it will cause specular reflection and mirror image reflection of liver or spleen on the left side **(Fig. 2)**. The presence of this mirror image implies presence of an air-filled lung and absence of pleural fluid above the diaphragm.

CT is the modality of choice in evaluating diseases of the pleura, especially pleural tumors. It is particularly helpful in determining chest wall, mediastinum and diaphragmatic involvement. CT allows differentiation of benign from malignant pleural disease except in very early disease. It can display anterior and paravertebral pleural plaques, areas not well seen on chest radiographs.

TABLE 1: Radiological differentiation of pleural, extrapleural and pulmonary lesion.

Features	Pulmonary	Pleural	Extrapleural
Incomplete border sign (radiograph)	Absent	Present	Present
Angle with chest wall	Acute	Obtuse	Obtuse
Epicenter	In lung	Along chest wall	Along chest wall
Pulmonary vasculature	Engulfs	Displace	Displace
Extrapleural fat displacement	-	Outwards	Inwards
Rib erosion	Unusual	Unusual	Usual

For complete evaluation of the pleural surfaces the patient is scanned contiguously from the thoracic inlet to the L3 level. Pleural enhancement is best demonstrated with a delayed scan time of 45–60 seconds.

On HRCT the pleura may be identified when it forms the fissures. Depending on its obliquity to the imaging plane, a fissure appears as a thin, high density line or band. On conventional CT, the fissure is appreciated as an avascular band. Peripherally on CT and HRCT, there is a thin line–the intercostal stripe separating the lung margin and the fat lying inside the internal intercostal muscle **(Fig. 3)**. This line (the lung chest wall interface) connects the inner aspect of the ribs and is 1–2 mm thick. It comprises the two layers of pleura.

Subparietal pleural fat: Separates parietal pleura from endothoracic fascia. This is very thin in most locations, but can be markedly thickened over the lateral or posterolateral ribs, resulting in extrapleural fat pads.

Endothoracic fascia: This fibroelastic fascia covers the surface of the intercostal muscles and intervening ribs, blends with the perichondrium and periosteum of the costal cartilages. Posteriorly, it is continous with the prevertebral fascia that covers the vertebral bodies and intervertebral discs.

MRI suffers from the drawback of a poor signal to noise ratio in lung, cardiac and respiratory motion artefacts and susceptibility artifacts at air tissue boundaries. However, it is sometimes used as a problem solving tool

Diffusion imaging (DWI) helps to non-invasively characterize various types of effusion. Diffusion weighted imaging can differentiate benign from pleural malignant disease with a cut-off ADC threshold being 1.52×10^{-3} mm^2/sec. This has a sensitivity of 71.4% and specificity of 100%. In cases where ADC is indeterminate, dynamic contrast-enhanced MRI improves the diagnostic confidence.[1]

MRI also plays an important role in the evaluation of extent of pleural neoplasm especially in areas like lung apices and diaphragm.

FDG-PET is complementary to CT in the evaluation of pleural tumors. It has an important role in staging pleural mesothelioma.

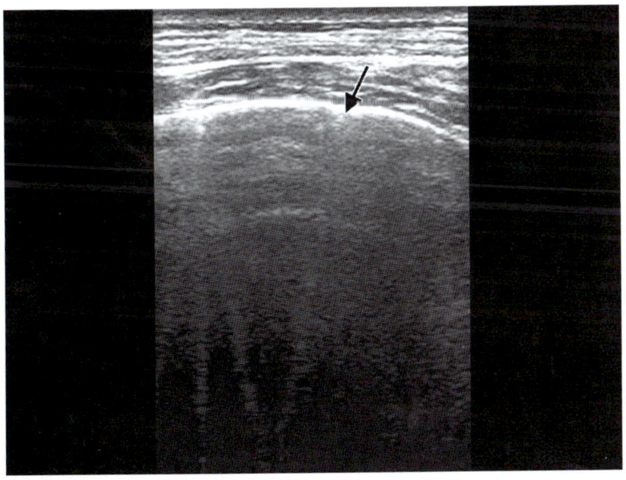

FIG. 1: Ultrasound chest direct intercostal approach: Echogenic line depicting the lung pleura interface.

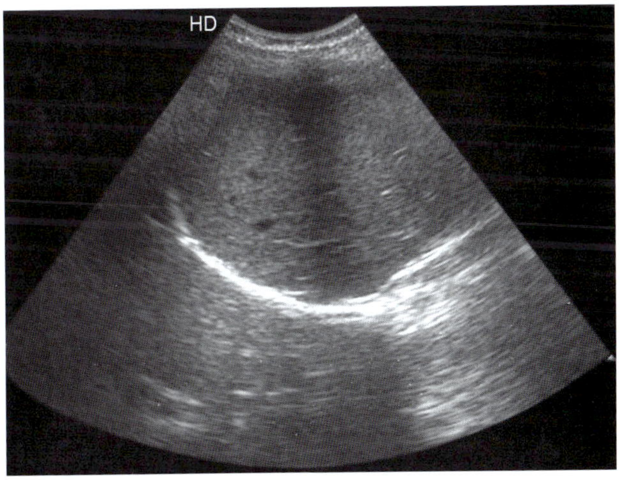

FIG. 2: Ultrasound chest-abdominal approach: Mirror image of liver seen above the diaphragm implying presence of air-filled lung.

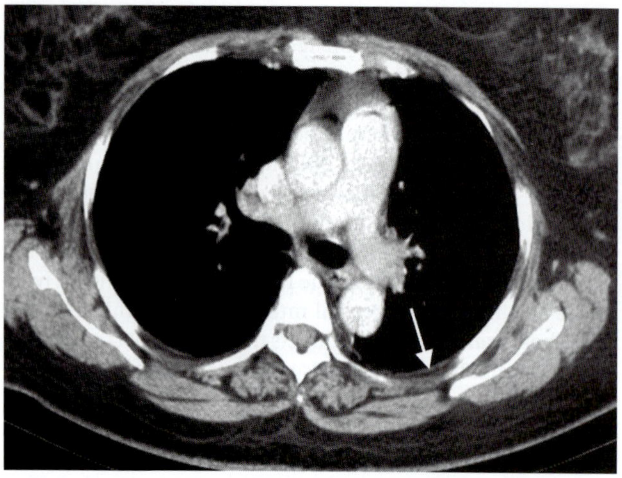

FIG. 3: CT: A thin white stripe (marked with arrow) between adjacent ribs represents the intercostal stripe, primarily representing the innermost intercostal muscle. This is anatomically absent in the paravertebral region.

PLEURAL PATHOLOGY

Pleura may be affected by the following pathologies which may be linked to each other:

- Effusion
- Pneumothorax
- Pleural thickening
- Tumor
- Tumor-like conditions

PLEURAL EFFUSION

Fluid moves across the capillary membranes of the visceral pleura into the pleural space and is then reabsorbed by the lymphatic system. Changes in capillary permeability, hydrostatic and oncotic pressure or lymphatic function affects the balance between the formation and resorption of pleural fluid leading to accumulation of fluid in the pleural space.

The pleural fluid may be transudate, exudate, blood or chyle. All types of pleural effusion are radiographically identical, though clinical and biochemical features may help limit the differential diagnosis. Most pleural effusion are classified as exudates or transudates based on their chemical composition which is usually defined by thoracocentesis. The criteria most commonly used to separate transudative from exudative effusion are known as **Light's criteria**.[2] Pleural fluid is considered an exudate if one or more of the following criteria are met.

1. A ratio of pleural fluid protein to serum protein higher than 0.5.
2. A ratio of pleural fluid lactate dehydrogenase (LDH) to serum LDH leval that exceeds 0.6.
3. A pleural fluid LDH level more than two-thirds the upper limit of normal serum LDH.

Exudative effusion reflects the presence of a pleural abnormality associated with increased permeability of pleural capillaries. These effusions have high protein content. Common causes of exudative effusion include pneumonia with parapneumonic effusion, empyema, TB, pleuritis, neoplasm, pulmonary embolism, drug reaction, etc.

Transudative effusion is unassociated with pleural disease. It usually results from systemic abnormalities causing an imbalance in the hydrostatic and osmotic forces governing pleural fluid formation. These are low in protein and are usually bilateral. Common causes include CHF, pericardial disease, liver cirrhosis, renal disease, and hypoalbuminemia.

Bilateral effusions are usually transudates as they are secondary to generalized causes such as hypoproteinema. Some bilateral effusions may be exudates, e.g. those associated with metastatic disease, lymphoma, rheumatoid disease, systemic lupus erythematosus (SLE). Right-sided effusions are typically associated with ascitis, heart failure and liver abscess. Effusions associated with pancreatitis, pericarditis, esophageal rupture and aortic dissection tend to be left sided.

Massive effusions are most commonly due to malignant disease, especially metastatic (lung or breast), but may also occur in heart failure, cirrhosis, tuberculosis, empyema and trauma.

Specific Causes of Pleural Effusion

Congestive Heart Failure

Congestive heart failure (CHF) is the most common cause of transudative effusion, though exudative effusions may also occur. Pleural fluid accumulates in CHF because pulmonary interstitial fluid (due to edema) crosses into the pleural space. Bilateral effusions are seen is 70% of cases, if unilateral, it is usually right sided. A large unilateral pleural effusion should suggest an alternative diagnosis.

Renal Disease

Pleural effusion is seen with renal disease due to various causes.

- Renal failure with overhydration may result in transudative effusion, usually bilateral.
- Nephrotic syndrome may causel transudative effusions due to increased hydrostatic pressure and hypoalbuminemia resulting in decreased oncotic pressure.
- Uremia may result in fibrinious pleuritis and a bloody exudative effusion that is often unilateral and large. Pleural thickening may also be seen.
- Hydronephrosis due to retroperitoneal lesion may result in ipsilateral pleural effusion—which is rich in creatinine.
- Effusion may result from peritoneal dialysis, fluid enters the pleural space via diaphragmatic defects.

Radiation (Therapeutic)

Approximately 5% of patients having chest radiation develop a small exudative pleural effusion. This is usually in association with radiation pneumonitis the effusion being on the same side as that of radiation, develops within 6 months of radiation. It resolves slowly with time.

Dressler's Syndrome

Occurs in a few patients post myocardial infarction or cardiac surgery. It occurs 2–3 weeks after the event and is associated with chest pain, fever, dyspnea. Radiographs show pleural effusion (85%) lung consolidation and pericardial effusion. It is thought to be an immunologically mediated response. They are usually bilateral, when unilateral, it is usually left sided.

Pulmonary Embolism

Pleural effusion occurs in 30% of patients with pulmonary embolism. Usually associated with infarction, exudates (75%) are more common than transudates.

Pericardial Disease

Pleural effusion is common in patients with inflammatory pericardial disease. They are left sided in 70%. In patients with constrictive pericarditis, effusions or CHF may result from elevated left or right sided venous pressure.

Meig's Syndrome

Pleural effusion with ascitis and ovarian fibroma is the classical triad of Meig's syndrome. Other ovarian tumors may show similar presentation. It may be exudative or transudative. Resection of the tumor results in resolution of pleural effusion and ascitis.

Pancreatitis

Pleural effusion is associated with acute and chronic pancreatitis. The effusion shows high amylase levels. In acute pancreatitis, exudative effusion is seen, mostly on left side. In chronic pancreatitis, effusions are large and indolent. The pleural effusion is probably secondary to fistula formation following ductal rupture.

Chylothorax may result from rupture of thoracic duct or of a prominent lymphatic channel. Lymph may also accumulate as a result of oozing from pleural lymphatics or due to passage of chylous ascitis via diaphragm. Chylous effusion is associated with neoplastic etiology in majority[3] of cases, seen in patients with lymphoma, metastatic neoplasm. Chylothorax also develops following thoracic surgery chest trauma, inflammatory mediastinal lymph node disease, and in some developmental anomalies like lymphangioma, lymphangioleiomyomatosis. Traumatic chylothorax resolves over time as the thoracic duct heals. Reduction in lymph flow may be helpful. Ligation of duct is curative.

Chylous effusion contains intestinal lymph (i.e. chyle), which is high in protein and fatty acids and is low in cholesterol. It looks milky on naked eye examination. Chylothorax does not have a low CT number despite presence of fat as it is rich in proteins. A chylous effusion can show high signal intensity on T1WI. **Pseudochylous or chyleform effusion** contains cholesterol, but not chyle. It may be seen in patients with chronic inflammatory disease like to TB, rheumatoid arthritis. Chylous effusions may remain chronic for years.

Hemothorax

It refers to pleural fluid having a hematocrit of over 50% of blood hematocrit. On CT, hemothorax results in fluid with high attenuation (mostly higher than 50 HU) containing a dense clot or a fluid-fluid level, with the densest fluid posteriorly. Most of cases are traumatic in origin, others may be spontaneous, including rupture of aneurysm/dissection, pulmonary or pleural neoplasm, coagulopathy. Treatment includes drainage. Organization of hemothorax results in fibrosis and calcification. A resolving exudative effusion or hemothorax may deposit a clot of fibrin within the pleural space termed as fibrin body or pleural mouse. These appear 1–2 cm in diameter, mimicking a solitary nodule, localized to pleural space and are sometimes seen to move with change in patient position. They resolve or may remain stable for years.

IMAGING IN PLEURAL EFFUSION

Plain Radiographs

The radiological signs of a pleural effusion depend on the posture of the patient and distribution of fluid which may be free or loculated. The pleural space extends inferiorly below the visible lung, in relation to the diaphragm and ribs. Small amount of pleural fluid is not visible on erect radiograph as it collects under the lung. These small **subpulmonic** effusions are detected by ultrasound or CT.

In an upright subject at least 175 mL of fluid must be present to result in blunting of the lateral costophrenic angle on the frontal radiograph and rarely as much as 500 mL may be present without blunting **(Fig. 4)**. On a lateral decubitus film, as little as 10 mL fluid may be seen.

The classical signs of pleural effusion include—homogeneous opacification of lower chest with obliteration of costophrenic angle and the hemidiaphragm. The upper margin of the opacity is concave to the lung and is higher laterally than medially. The highest point of the "meniscus" reflects the true level of fluid **(Fig. 5)**. This is because the X-ray beam traverses a greater thickness of fluid at the periphery due to circumferential configuration of the pleural space around the air containing lung. Above and medial to the meniscus, there is a hazy increase in opacity owing to fluid behind and in front of the lungs.

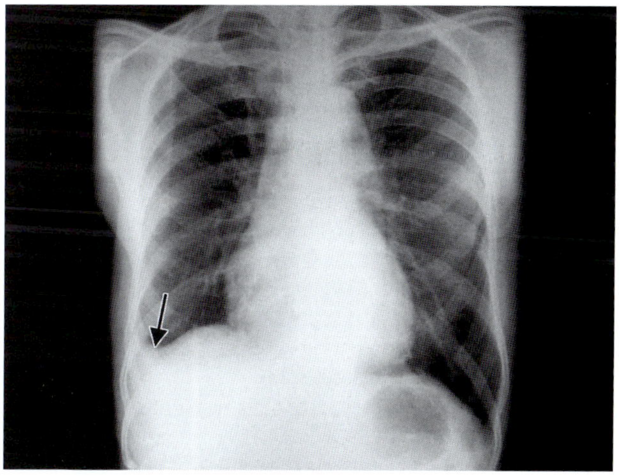

FIG. 4: X-ray chest PA view: Blunting of right costophrenic angle-pleural effusion.

Massive effusion can cause dense opacification of the hemithorax with contralateral mediastinal shift **(Figs. 6A to C) (Table 2)**. Shifted structures include the trachea, the heart, the azygoesophageal recess, producing a paravertebral retrocardiac density convex to the lung. Absence of mediastinal shift with a large effusion should raise the possibility of obstructive collapse of the ipsilateral lung or extensive pleural malignancy such as seen with mesothelioma or metastatic carcinoma.

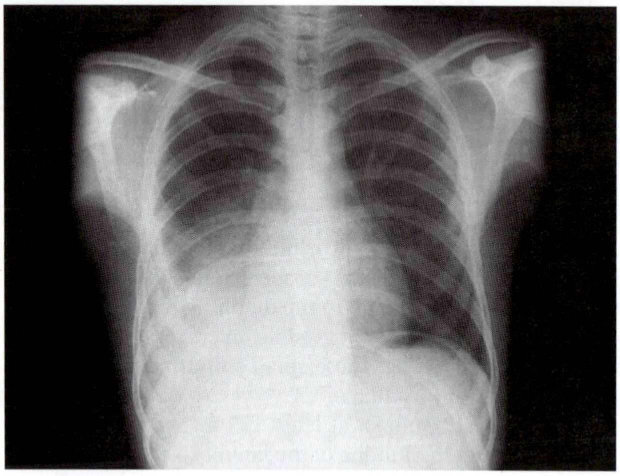

FIG. 5: X-ray chest PA view: Homogeneous opacification of right lower zone with obliteration of the right costophrenic angle and the hemidiaphragm. The upper margin of the opacity is concave and extends higher laterally "meniscus sign"—Pleural effusion.

TABLE 2: Causes of opaque hemithorax.
Pleural effusion
Consolidation
Collapse
Massive tumor
Fibrothorax
Pneumonectomy
Lung agenesis

Fluid entering into fissures may produce other opacities like middle lobe step or broad band with a curvilinear inner margin extending from midlung to chest wall, often becoming denser as it passes laterally.

On the frontal radiograph, fluid extending into the posterolateral major fissure typically results in an arcuate opacity, sharply defined medially and inferiorly. Fluid extending into the lateral aspect of the minor fissure and slightly separating the lobes, result in an opacity resembling a rose thorn (the thorn sign—**Fig. 7**).

As the lung is fixed medially, medial pleural fluid collections are usually smaller and more difficult to recognize. Medial fluid collection may be seen when effusions are large. More often, these accumulate in the posterior gutters, with thickening of the paravertebral stripe. The fluid collection may be triangular simulating lower lobe collapse.

Pleural fluid may accumulate in the subpulmonic space, allowing the lung base to float superiorly on a frontal radiograph. Subpulmonic effusion presents as a 'high hemi diaphragm' with an unusual contour that peaks more laterally **(Fig. 8)**. On the left side, 2 cm of separation of the lung base from the top of the stomach bubble is taken as an evidence of subpulmonic effusion, although distance may be variable. Most subpulmonic effusion are mobile with postural change. These are often transudates. On the lateral view, a subpulmonic effusion elevates the posterior lung, flattening its under surface, insinuates into the major fissure resulting in focal triangular thickening of the fissures, flattens the inferior contour of the lung anterior to the fissure which then angles sharply downward.

Fluid may accumulate between the lung and visceral pleura, a common finding in patients of heart failure. This is called 'lamellar effusion' and is not a true pleural effusion because it lies outside the pleural sac. It is a manifestation of waterlogged lung interstitium and is often accompanied by septal lines. Lamellar effusion is seen as vertical band of soft tissue density between the lung and chest wall above the

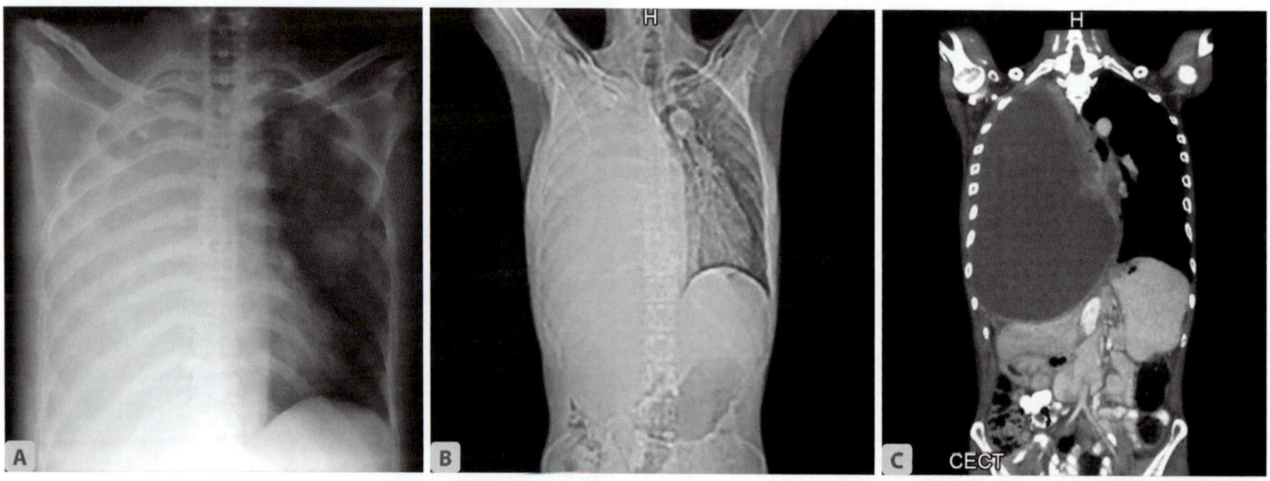

FIGS. 6A TO C: X-ray chest (A) Opaque hemithorax without shift of the mediastinum—scanogram (B) and coronal MPR (C) opaque hemithorax with shift of mediastinum and inversion of right hemidiaphragm in another patient.

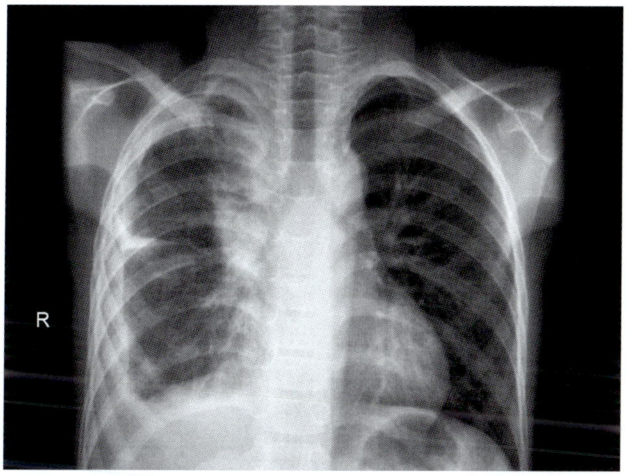

FIG. 7: Right pleural effusion is seen with associated mediastinal lymphadenopathy. Fluid is entering the minor fissure resembling a 'rose thorn'.

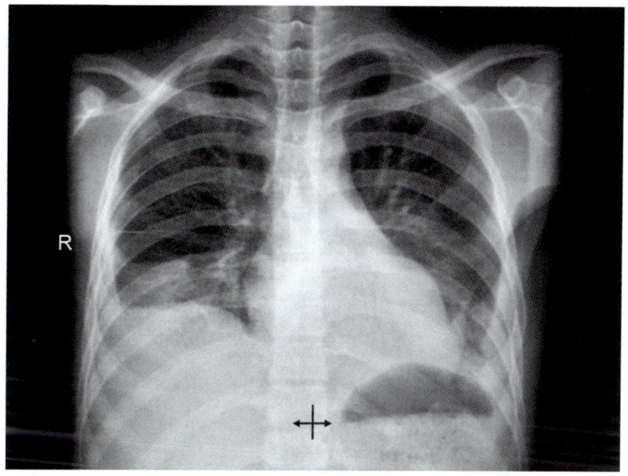

FIG. 8: Bilateral pleural effusion. Raised right hemidiaphragm with a lateralized apex suggestive of subpulmonic effusion.

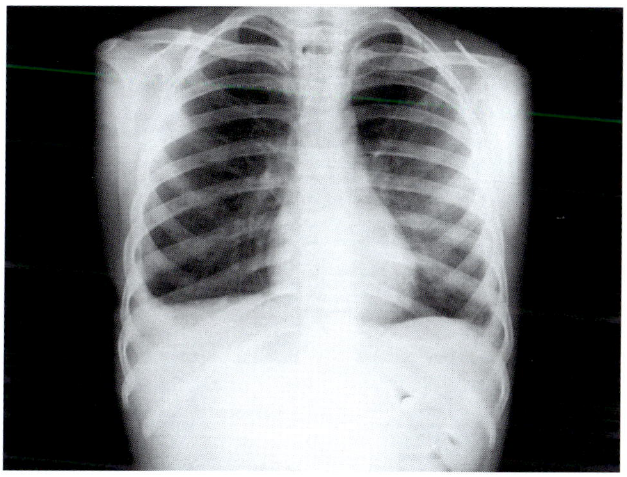

FIG. 9: Bilateral lamellar effusion with blunting of the costophrenic angles.

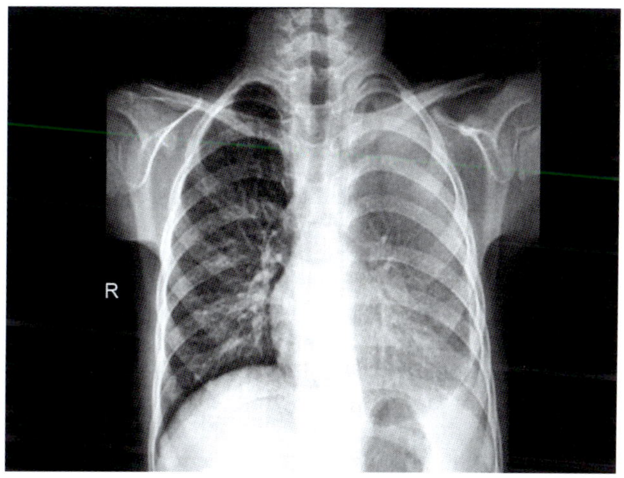

FIG. 10: X-ray chest: AP view (supine) shows a veil-like opacification of the left hemithorax with preserved vascular markings due to pleural effusion.

costophrenic angle, this remains fixed with postural change **(Fig. 9)**.

Supine and semi erect radiographs are less sensitive in showing pleural effusion. Signs of effusion on a supine radiograph are a hazy veil like opacity affecting the whole or lower part of hemithorax with preserved vascular opacities in the overlying lung **(Fig. 10)**. Additional signs include haziness of the diaphragmatic margins blunting of the costophrenic angle, a pleura apical cap which disappears in an upright film, thickening of the minor fissure and widening of the paraspinal interface. The lack of an air bronchogram and preserved vascular markings differentiate it from parenchymal disease such as pneumonia.

Loculated Pleural Fluid (Encysted/Encapsulated)

Fluid can loculate between visceral pleural layers in fissures or between visceral and parietal layers, usually against the chest wall. Loculated effusion usually occurs in association with exudative effusion, high in protein, such as those that occur in empyema, hemothorax or chylothorax.

The appearance of loculated pleural fluid on chest radiograph varies with its location and the radiographic projection used. It is sharply marginated when the surface is parallel to the X-ray beam and ill-defined when viewed en-face **(Figs. 11A and B)**. A collection loculated in the lateral pleural space will appear sharply marginated on the frontal radiograph and ill-defined on lateral film. For the effusion loculated anteriorly or posteriorly, the converse is true.

Fissural interlober loculation, seen particularly in heart failure produces the 'pseudotumor' or the 'phantom' tumor which can recur in the same place on repeated occasions. Pleural pseudotumors are transudates. Besides congestive cardiac failure these are seen with renal failure and in cirrhotic patients. In the presence of pleural effusion, the elastic recoil of the lung causes each lobe to retract toward the hilum. This widens the fissure and can draw fluid into the fissure even in nondependent locations. The middle lobe, because it is

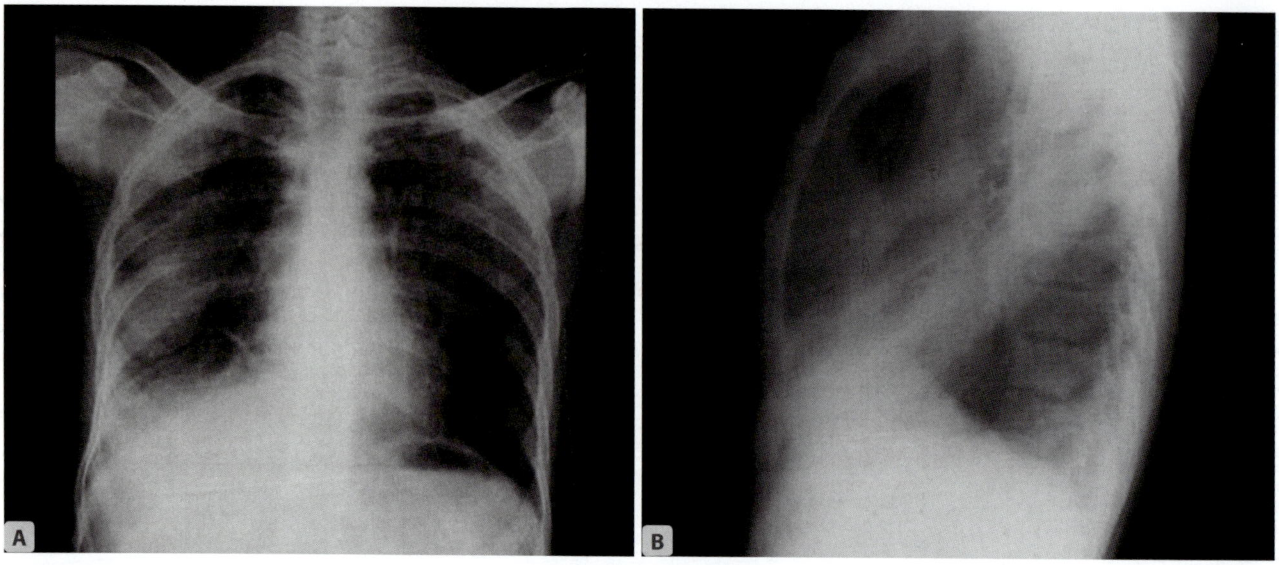

FIGS. 11A AND B: X-ray chest PA (A) and lateral (B)—opacities bilaterally with sharper medial margin and fading towards periphery-loculated fluid.

the smallest lobe, has the greatest tendency to retract, and therefore the minor fissure is the most likely fissure to have a pseudotumor.[4]

Viewed in the lateral view, it is sharply marginated and biconvex, with a tail passing through the fissure. The en-face appearance depends on the thickness of the effusion. If it is relatively thin, it may produce a vague area of radio-opacity. If it has a certain thickness, it may appear clear edged and mass like. Sometimes encysted fluid in the right lower oblique fissure may be confused with middle lobe collapse. Features that favor a collapsed, consolidated middle lobe collapse include non-homogeneity, a straight or concave border in the lateral view, and a wedgelike outline with the base reaching the sternum. The presence of a dependent pleural effusion aids in recognizing a pleural pseudotumor. Fluid collections are rounded or lenticular and may show a tapering triangular opacity or 'beak' at the point they merge with the fissure. Fluid collections in the minor fissure appear sharply marginated and lenticular on both frontal and lateral views. Collection in the major fissure may be ill defined on the frontal view.

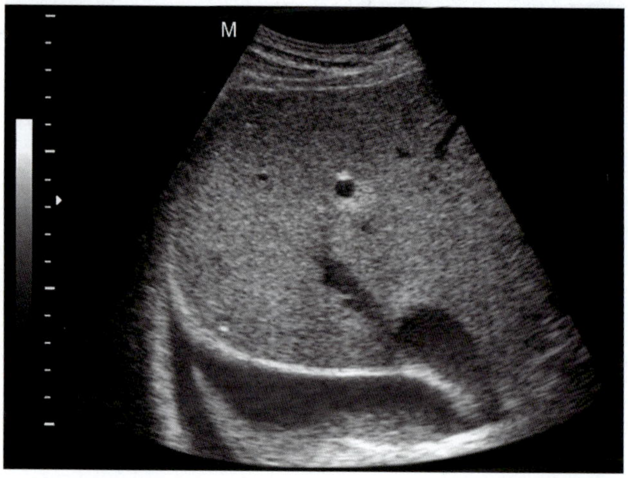

FIG. 12: Anechoic fluid in the right pleural space—seen on transabdominal ultrasound. Note absence of mirror image of liver.

Ultrasound of Pleural Effusion

Ultrasonography is extremely sensitive to the presence of fluid, detecting even small amounts accurately. It is helpful in detecting subpulmonic and subphrenic effusion by noting the position and movement of diaphragm. USG is also useful in opaque hemithorax, to differentiate solid from fluid lesion and is mandatory before performing a thoracocentesis of an opaque hemithorax.

The US image of pleural effusion is characterized by echo free space between the visceral and parietal pleura **(Fig. 12)**. Visceral pleura is identified by movement of echogenic line with breathing,parietal pleura is identified by its position approximately 1 cm deep to ribs. The rough estimate of the amount of fluid can be made by measuring the maximum perpendicular distance between the lung surface and chest wall. The patient is supine and measurement is done in full inspiration. A 20 mm width has a mean volume of 380 mL ± 130 mL, 40 mm width would correspond to 1000 ± 330 mL.[5]

The sonographic characteristics of effusion may be helpful in differentiating transudates from exudates.[6] Pleural fluid, especially when it is a transudate is echo-free, though occasionally an exudates may also be anechoic. Exudative and hemorrhage effusions may be echogenic, complex and septated **(Fig. 13)**. The septae may be profuse giving rise to honeycomb appearance. These may not be well-appreciated on CT and may pose difficulty in tube drainage. Other sonographic features may be helpful in assessing the nature of pleural effusion such as associated consolidation favors empyema, while pleural nodules favor malignancy.

Ultrasound can be used to distinguish between pleural fluid, solid pleural or extrapleural lesions and peripheral lung lesions. Features that help distinguish a fluid from a solid

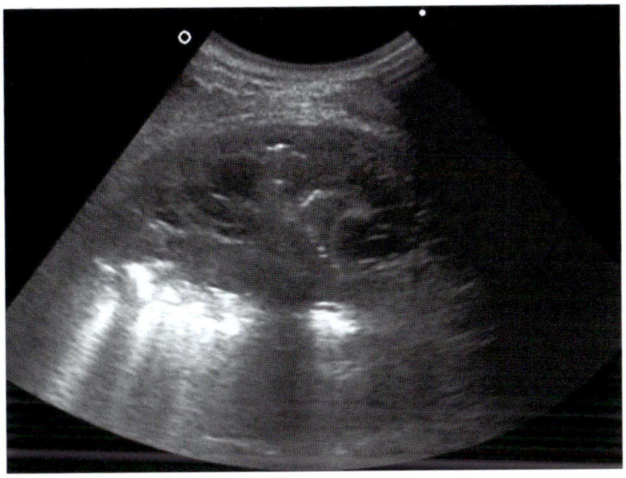

FIG. 13: USG chest shows multiseptated collection in the right pleural cavity.

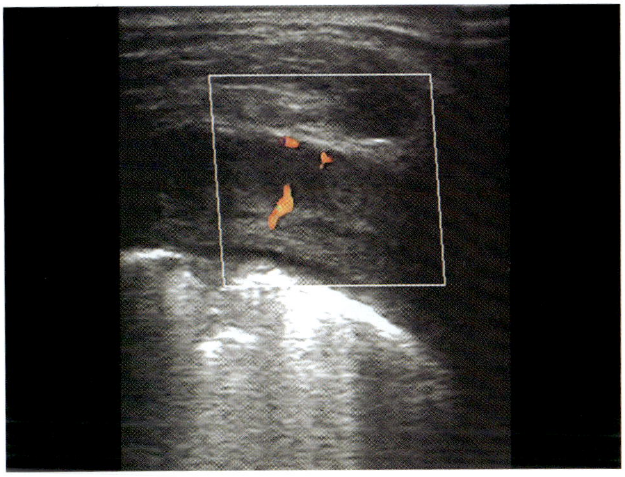

FIG. 14: Color Doppler depicting the "color fluid sign".

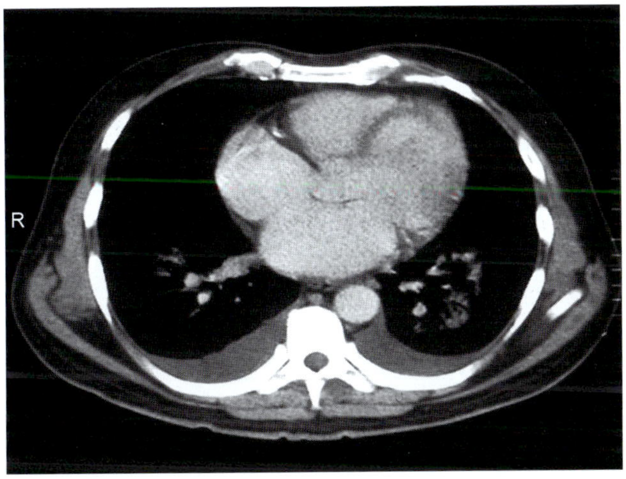

FIG. 15: CT-sickle-shaped opacity seen in dependent location—bilateral pleural effusion.

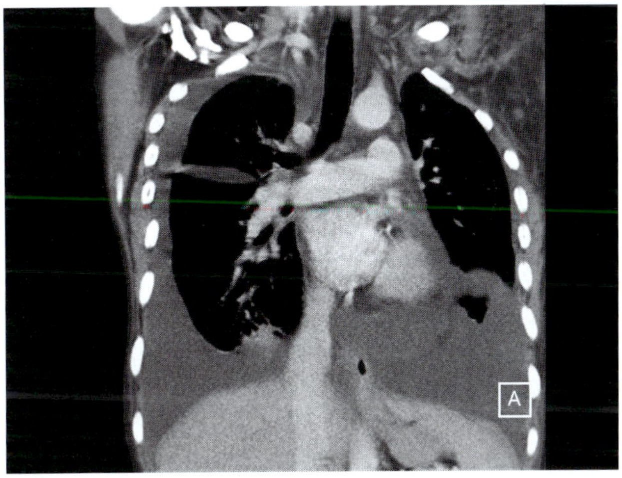

FIG. 16: Coronal MPR—bilateral pleural effusion, also tracking in the horizontal fissure.

echogenic lesion include changes in shape with breathing, presence of septa and fibrous strands and the movement of the components, induced by breathing. In peripheral lung lesions, the presence of fluid bronchograms and vessels on Doppler identify consolidation. Color Doppler signal in the fluid collection in the pleural space during respiratory or cardiac cycle is a pointer towards presence of fluid. Patients with pleural thickening do not show this sign **(Fig. 14)**.[7]

Computed Tomography of Pleural Effusion

CT is sensitive in detecting pleural fluid and can distinguish between free and loculated fluid, identifying the extent and location of the loculation. It also allows differentiation of pleural from parenchymal pathology and the evaluation of underlying lung disease. Pleural morphology such as thickening or masses may also be studied by CT.

A pleural effusion appears as a dependent, sickle shaped opacity with a lower CT number than any adjacent pleura thickening or mass **(Fig. 15)** Most pleural effusions are near water attenuation on CT, ranging up to 20–30 HU regardless of cause.CT attenuation numbers alone do not allow a reliable distinction between an exudate and a transudate.[8] Distinguishing between the two is important for clinical management. The differentiation has to be made on the basis of thoracocentesis. The appearance of parietal pleura on CECT is of value in predicting the nature of pleural fluid collection. Visibility of enhancement of the parietal pleura indicates that it is thickened (enhancing pleura is thickened pleura) the presence of thickened parietal pleura is indicative that the fluid is an exudates. This is seen in up to 60% of exudative effusions and its accuracy in predicting the presence of exudates is nearly 100%. If pleural thickening is not present, an associated effusion may be a transudate or exudate.

CT findings of fluid loculation include a localized collection, an elliptical or lenticular shape/rather than crescentric, a non-dependent location (i.e. anterior, lateral or posterolateral) **(Figs. 16 and 17)**. If air is present within a loculated effusion, multiple septations may be seen, resulting in multiple localized air collections or air-fluid levels.

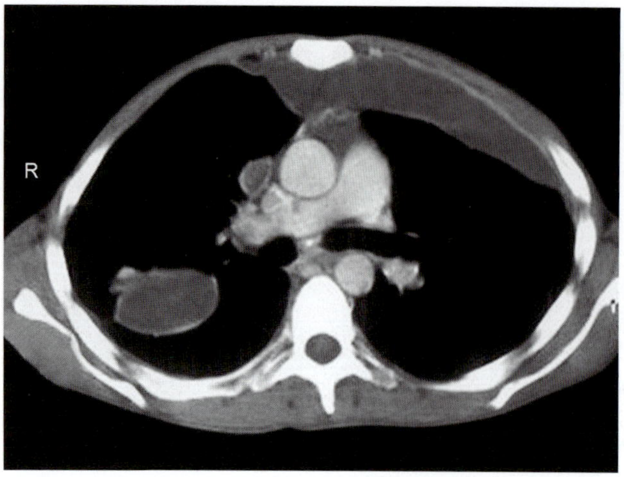

FIG. 17: CECT chest—loculated fluid along the chest wall anteriorly and horizontal fissure.

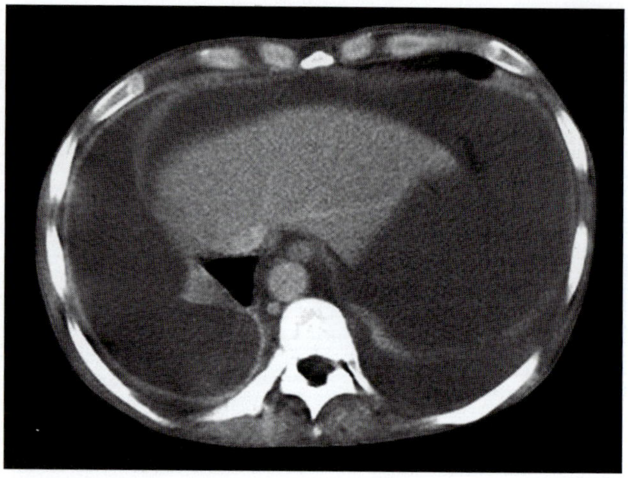

FIG. 18: Pleural effusion and ascitis in the same patient. Pleural fluid is seen medial and posterior and lateral to the crus of the diaphragm. Crus is displaced away from the vertebral body, better appreciated on the left side ascitis does the reverse. The displaced crus and diaphragm sign.

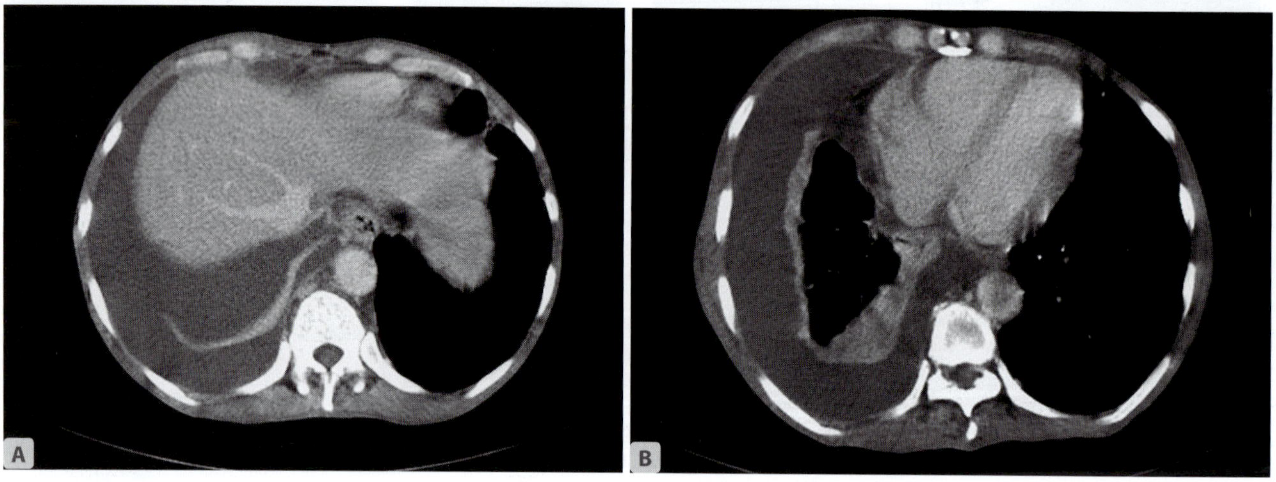

FIGS. 19A AND B: CT shows posterior edge of the right lower lobe as an arcuate density surrounded by fluid anteriorly and posteriorly resembling the diaphragm: (A) On sequential cephalad scan; (B) This is contiguous with the remainder of the lower lobe.

PLEURAL EFFUSION OR ASCITIS

Subpulmonic effusion and pleural fluid in the costophrenic angle can be seen below the lung bases on CT and mimic ascites. The parallel curvilinear configuration of the pleura and peritoneal cavities at the level of perihepatic and perisplenic recesses allows fluid in either cavity to appear as a crescentic collection displacing liver or spleen away from the adjacent chest wall. The two can be distinguished by certain signs.[9,10.]

1. **The 'displaced crus' sign**: Pleural fluid collections in the posterior costophrenic angle lie medial and posterior to the diaphragm and causes lateral displacement of the crus—away from adjacent vertebral body, ascitis does the reverse **(Fig. 18)**.
2. **The 'diaphragm sign'**: The most reliable sign to localize fluid is to identify its relationship to the diaphragm, if visible. The diaphragm is seen as uniform curvilinear structure of muscle density, fluid posterior or lateral to the diaphragm is pleural. A large pleural effusion will allow the lower lobe to float anteriorly and lose volume. On CT the posterior edge of the lower lobe, when surrounded by fluid, both anteriorly and posteriorly can appear to represent the diaphragm—pseudo- diaphragm **(Figs. 19A and B)**. On sequential scans at more cephalad levels, the density of atelectatic lower lobe becomes thicker, merges with the rest of lower lobe and often contains air-bronchograms.
3. **The 'bare area sign'**: Ascitic fluid is excluded from the bare area between coronary ligaments on the posterior aspect of the liver as the peritoneal space does not extend into this region.

   Pleural fluid can be seen in the entire posterior costophrenic sulcus **(Figs. 20A and B)**.
4. **The 'interface sign'**: Pleural fluid can be distinguished from ascitis by the clarity of the interface of the fluid

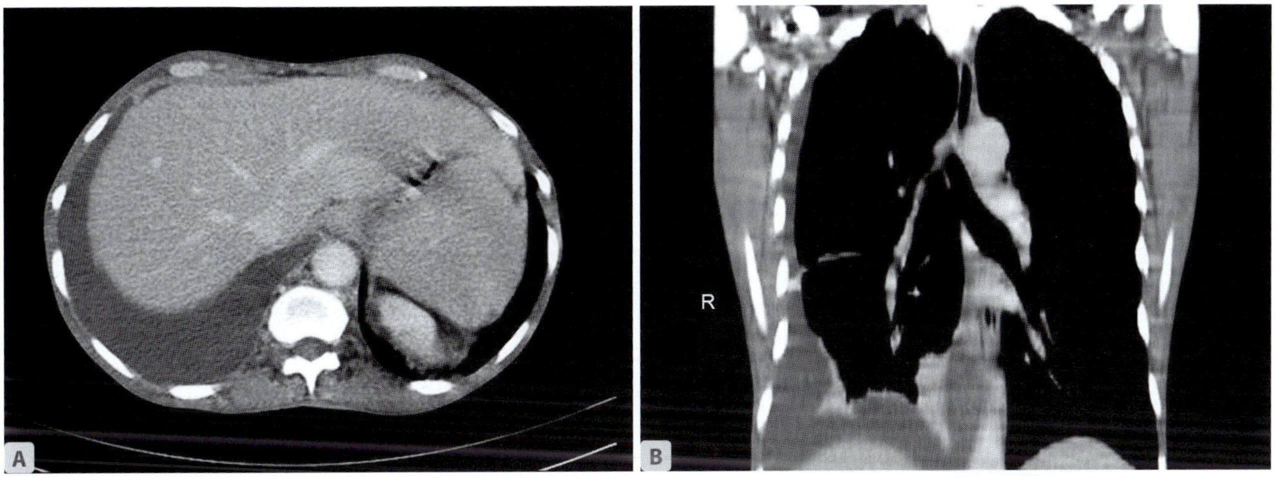

FIGS. 20A AND B: CT–axial (A), MPR (B), shows the pleural fluid occupying the entire posterior costophrenic sulcus, ascitis is excluded from this space due to lack of peritoneal reflection—bare area sign. Note that the interface with liver is hazy—interface sign.

with diaphragm. With pleural fluid, the interface is hazy, whereas with ascitis it is sharp.

MRI of Pleural Effusion

Pleural fluid has a low signal on T1 and a high signal on T2 weighted images. Exudates give a higher signal than transudates on T2WI. A chylous effusion shows signal intensity similar to subcutaneous fat on T1W images. In the sub acute and chronic stage hematomas show a bright signal on T1WI, surrounded by a dark rim caused by hemosiderin.

MRI may be used to differentiate transudates from exudates. A gradual enhancement on delayed images of malignant pleural effusions after intravenous administration of GD-DTPA, in patients with lung cancer has been reported. Signal enhancement of the pleura indicates the presence of exudates while absence of the same suggests transudate. Non-invasive characterization of pleural effusion by means of DWI with single shot EPI technique may obviate the need for thoracocentesis with its associated patient morbidity. Most transudative effusions are isointense, while exudative effusions are hyperintense on DWI with b factor of 500 and 1000 s/min **(Figs. 21A to E)**. The ADC of exudative effusion is significantly lower than those of transudative effusions. The higher the protein content of pleural fluid, the less is the diffusion. The cellular content of exudates may also contribute to ADC values. At a cut off value of 3.6×10^{-3} mm^2/s, ADC has a sensitivity of 71% and a specificity of 63% for differentiating transudative from exudative effisions.[11,12]

Parapneumonic Effusion with Empyema

Pleural fluid accumulates in approximately 40% of patients with pneumonia. This is diagnosed by thoracocentesis and culture of the aspirated fluid. The term 'parapneumonic' effusion is used and it is classified into three stages of empyema. Progression from one stage to another does not necessarily take place.[13-18]

Simple Parapneumonic Effusion (Exudative Stage)

Simple parapneumonic effusion results from increased permeability of the visceral pleura occurring in association with pulmonary inflammation in patients with pneumonia. Effusions in this stage are usually sterile exudates and have a normal glucose level (>40–60 mg/dL) and pH (>7. 2). They are usually dependent in location, do not show evidence of loculation, show a meniscus on plain radiographs and appear crescent shaped on CT. These usually resolve with antibiotic treatment of the pneumonia.

Empyema (Fibropurulent Stage)

The term empyema is used when a pleural effusion is infected, although the definition necessitates the presence of pus in the pleural space. Although most occur in association with pneumonia, approximately 10% are unassociated with obvious lung disease.

A large percentage of bacterial empyemas result from anaerobic infections. Common anerobic organisms include bacteroides, *Fusobacterium*. Common aerobic organisms are *Staphylococcus aureus*, *Streptococcus pneumoniae*, *Haemophilus influenzae*. Tuberculosis may also result in empyema.

Empyema is characterized by presence of infectious organisms in pleural fluid, increased white blood cells and polymorph nuclear cells, fibrin deposition along the pleural surfaces, a tendency for loculation, decreased glucose levels (<40 mg/dL) and (pH <7. 2) and increased LDH (>1000 IU/L).

In a patient who has pneumonia, presence of localized or loculated pleural effusion strongly suggests the presence of an empyema. On plain radiographs, empyemas often have a lenticular shape and tend to appear larger or better defined in one projection (e.g. frontal) than in other (e.g. lateral). On radiographs, an empyema containing air may be difficult to differentiate from a peripheral lung abscess abutting the chest wall. This distinction can be important to make because

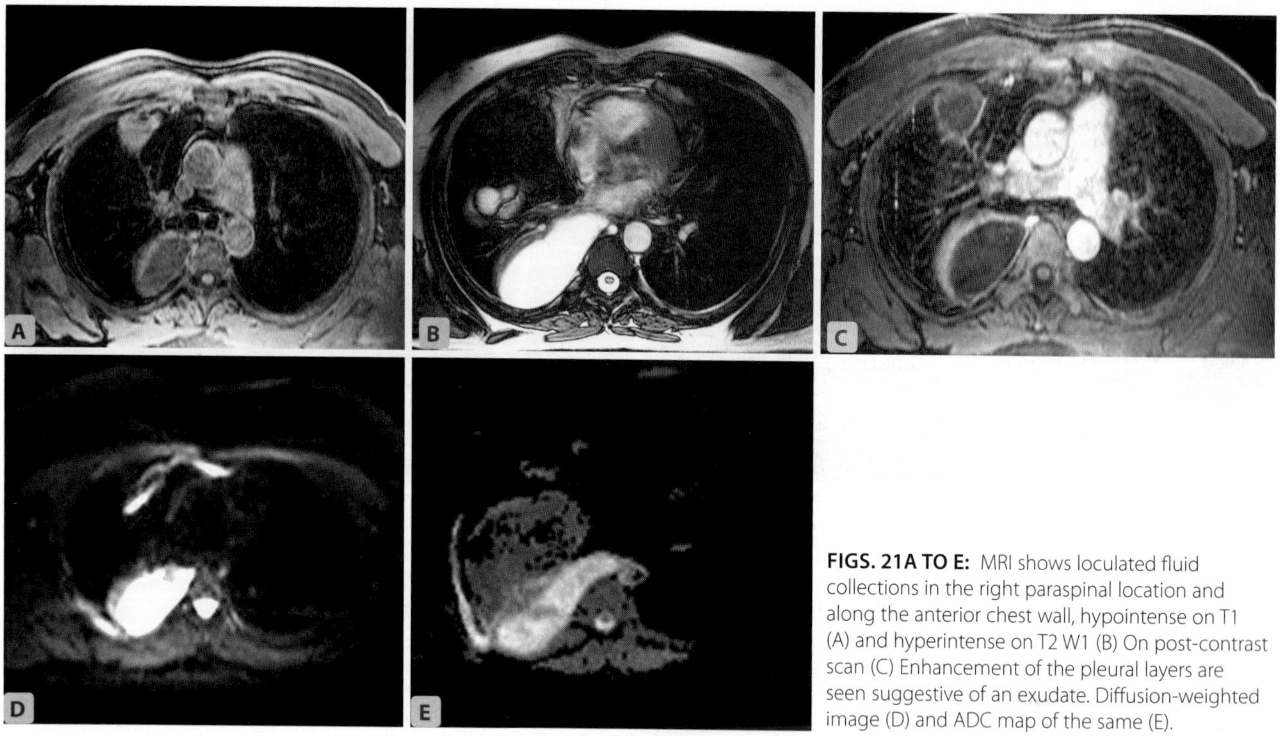

FIGS. 21A TO E: MRI shows loculated fluid collections in the right paraspinal location and along the anterior chest wall, hypointense on T1 (A) and hyperintense on T2 W1 (B) On post-contrast scan (C) Enhancement of the pleural layers are seen suggestive of an exudate. Diffusion-weighted image (D) and ADC map of the same (E).

empyemas are often treated by tube thoracostomy in addition to systemic antibiotics, whereas most lung abscesses require antibiotics alone.

CT shows characteristic findings of empyema. It is seen in a non-dependent location with an elliptical or lenticular shape, with a sharp demarcation from the adjacent lung; the enhancing visceral and parietal pleural surfaces split apart by the fluid collection giving the-'**split pleura sign**' **(Fig. 22)**.

Empyemas show the thickened pleural layers as smooth and of uniform thickness when enhanced by contrast or outlined by air. Empyemas compress and displace adjacent lung and vessals. In patients with parapneumonic effusion or empyema, extrapleural fat is commonly thickened. The extrapleural fat adjacent to empyema may show increased attenuation with edema of chest wall muscles **(Figs. 23 and 24)**. In contrast to empyemas, lung abscesses are round and poorly defined owing to surrounding pneumonia, have shaggy walls or irregular thickness and tend to obliterate bronchi and vessals **(Figs. 25 and 26)**. The differences between a peripherally located lung abscess and empyema are enumerated in **Table 3**. Malignant neoplasms may arise in the walls of chronic long-standing empyemas, mostly in tubercular cavities. Non-Hodgkin's lymphoma, mesothelioma and rarely sarcoma may occur.

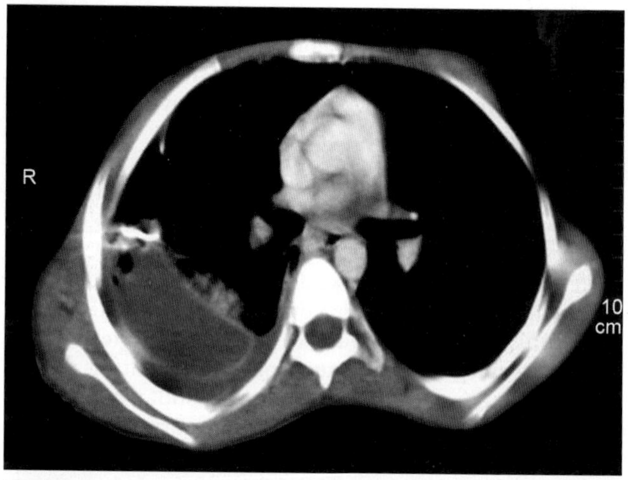

FIG. 22: Empyema CT show loculated collection in the hemithorax with enhancement of the visceral and parietal pleura—split pleura sign.

Organization Stage (Pleural Peel)

In patients with chronic empyema ingrowth of fibroblasts and organization can result in extensive pleural fibrosis and the development of an inelastic fibrotic pleural peel or fibrothorax. This can cause lung restriction and decreased lung volume—the trapped lung **(Fig. 27)**. Plain radiographs and CT show smooth pleural thickening. Extrapleural fat thickening is frequently visible on CT,separating the thickened parietal pleura from the intercostal muscle or rib. On CT a fibrothorax is defined as pleural thickening that extends >8 cm in craniocaudal direction, 5 cm laterally and with a thickness equal or more than 3 cm. Focal or extensive calcification is common with a tubercular etiology. Asbestos exposure related fibrothorax is usually bilateral and rarely calcified. An important finding in diagnosing pleural peel is reduction in the volume of the affected hemithorax **(Figs. 28A and B)**. A pleural peel may result from chronic pleural effusion and inflammation in the absence of infection, e. g. in cases of collagen vascular disease, uremia, etc.

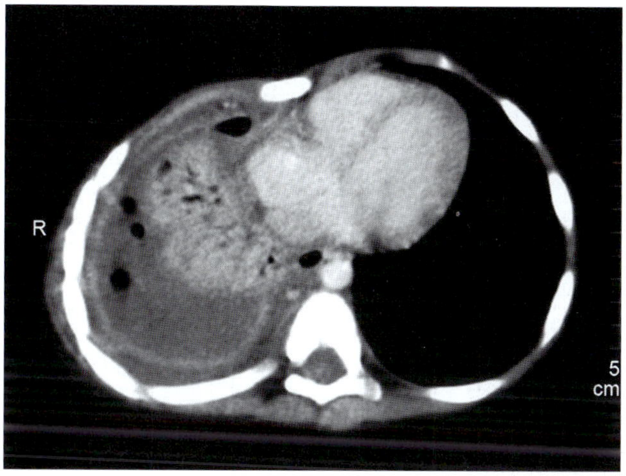

FIG. 23: Thickened enhancing pleura with proliferation of extrapleural fat on the right side. there are air loculi within the pleural cavity (post-intervention). Loss of volume with underlying consolidation is also noted.

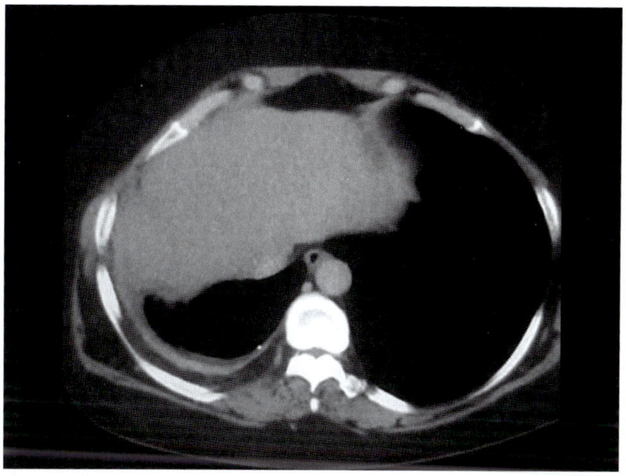

FIG. 24: CT—pleural thickening with proliferation of extrapleural fat.

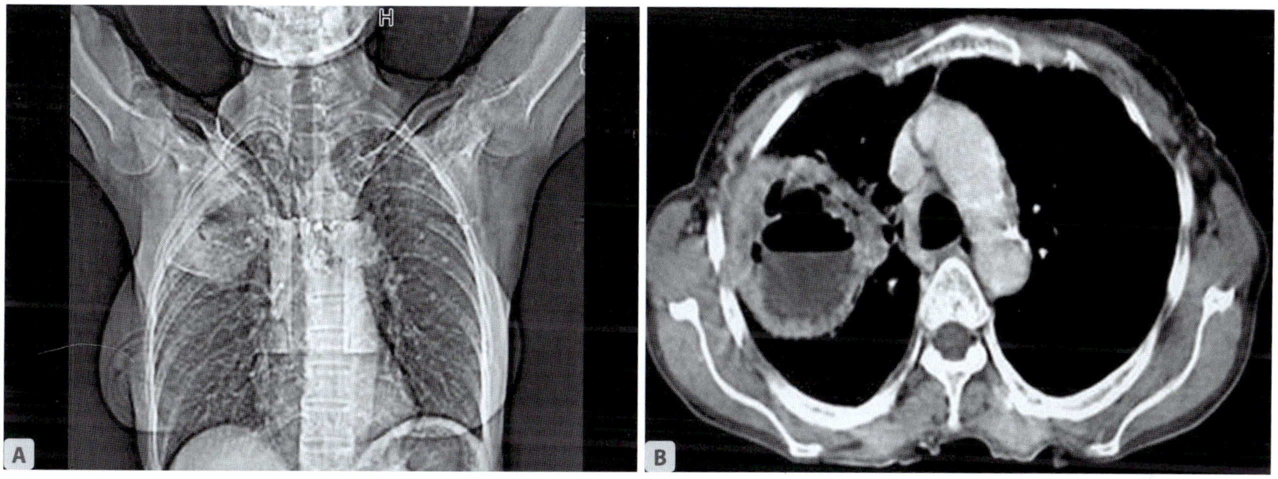

FIGS. 25A AND B: A large opacity with an air-fluid level with an acute angle with the chest wall with shaggy inner walls—lung abscess.

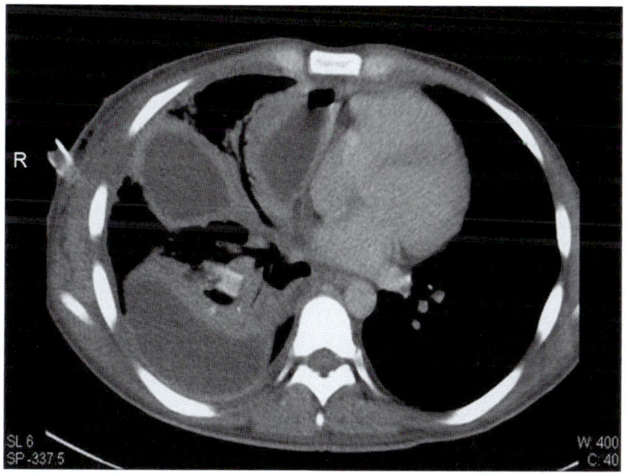

FIG. 26: CT chest—multiple loculated empyemas.

TABLE 3: Differences between empyema and lung abscess.

Empyema	Lung abscess
Lenticular shape	Round shape
Uniform enhancing wall	Non-uniform thick wall
Compression of adjacent lung	Non-compression of surrounding lung
Obtuse angle with chest wall	Acute angles with chest wall
Separation of pleural layers	—

Empyema Necessitans

Empyema can involve the chest wall directly and this is called empyema necessitatis or necessitans. Tuberculosis accounts for about 70% of these cases, other organisms like actinomycosis or nocardia have also been implicated. Extensive extrapleural fat thickening, edema and subcutaneous collections of pus can be seen on CT **(Figs. 29A and B)**.

Tube Drainage of Empyema

Drainage of empyema is required if there is:

- Thick pus on thoracocentesis
- Positive gram stain
- Positive pleural fluid culture
- Pleural fluid glucose <60 mg/dL
- Pleural fluid pH <7.2
- LDH >1000 IU/L
- No response to antibiotics

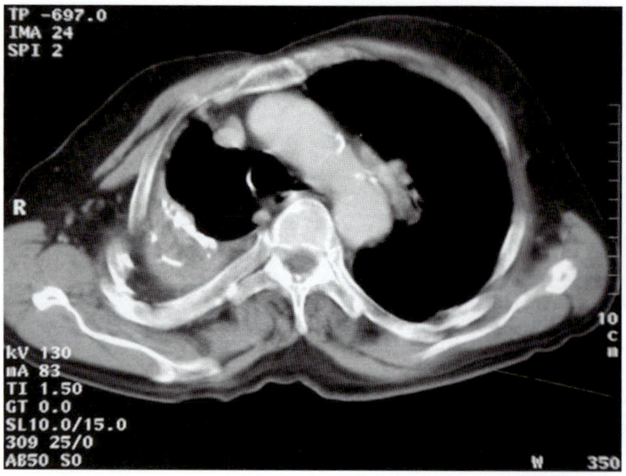

FIG. 27: CECT thorax: Calcified and thickened pleural layers on the right with a fluid collection between them and loss of volume indicative of fibrothorax—tubercular etiology.

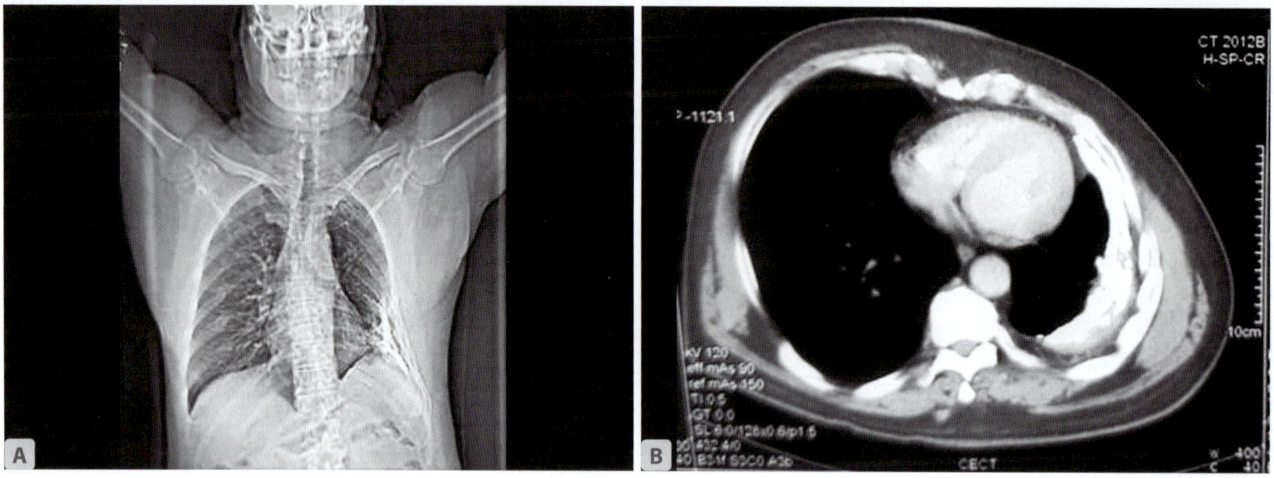

FIGS. 28A AND B: chest X-ray (A), CT (B): Loss of volume on the left with extensive pleural thickening with calcification—fibrothorax.

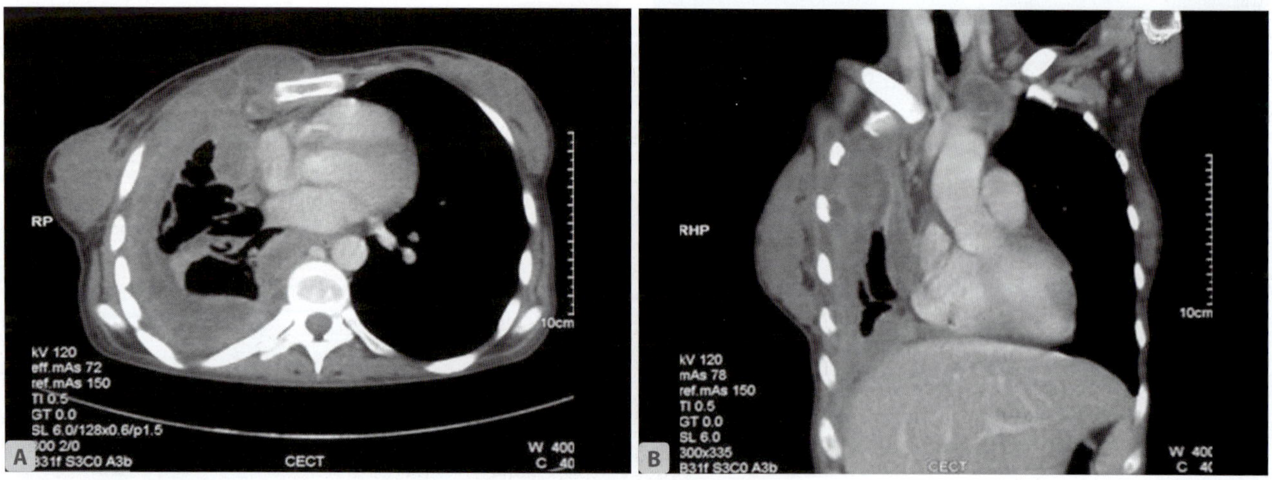

FIGS. 29A AND B: Empyema with direct extension into chest wall—empyema necessitans.

Multiple septations within an infected or reactive fluid may be broken down by instillation of fibrinolytic agents such as urokinase. Indications for decortication include persistent sepsis despite appropriate antibiotic therapy and drainage, persistent thick pleural rind that appears to be trapping the underlying lung. CT can be used to determine the adequacy of chest tube drainage, the thickness of the pleural rind, the presence of loculi, and the extent to which the lung is trapped.

After thoracocentesis of a large pleural effusion, the re-expanded lung shows edema which persists for a few days. The lung sometimes fails to expand fully and a pneumothorax may persist. This usually occurs in patients with malignancy and is known as **"trapped lung"**. Metastatic implants on the visceral pleural surface prevents the lung from expanding. A trapped lung can also occur in cases of chronic empyema when a rind of thickened visceral pleura encases and contracts the underlying lung, preventing re-expansion of the lung despite adequate drainage of the empyema fluid. The other cause of persistent pneumothorax or hydropneumothorax is a bronchopleural fistula.

BRONCHOPLEURAL FISTULA

Bronchopleural fistula (BPF) is a communication between the pleural cavity and the bronchial tree. A parenchymal pleural fistula (PPF) refers to a fistula between pleura and parenchyma lung. In both these conditions there is a pneumothorax not attributable to trauma. Bronchopleural fistula results from rupture of the visceral pleura with a direct communication with the airway. It may occur following trauma or surgery or in association with necrotizing infections—empyema, TB, septic embolus and infected pulmonary infarct. Gas within a pleural fluid collection, in absence of a recent thoracocentesis is a presumptive evidence of empyema and BPF. It differs from pneumothorax in that the communication with the pleural space is via airways rather than the distal air spaces **(Figs. 30A and B)**. MDCT can detect bronchopleural fistula with the same or superior sensitivity as bronchoscopy **(Fig. 31)**.[19]

Postsurgical BPF

Following an uncomplicated pneumonectomy, the residual space contains air and fluid and there is ipsilateral mediastinal shift and elevation of the hemidiaphragm. Over 2-4 months, there is gradual resorption of air and increasing fluid accumulation, followed by organization and progressive movement of the mediastinum and hemidiaphragm, leading to obliteration of the space. BPF arises as an early complication, usually develops 7–10 days later with clinical deterioration, pneumonia, hemopytsis and the sudden expectoration of fluid and a persistent large air leak from the pleural drain. The diagnosis is made radiologically by the following signs:

- Return of the mediastinum to the midline.
- Presence of increasing air and decreasing fluid in the pneumonectomy space.
- Contralateral aspiration pneumonitis. If less than the whole lung has been removed, the main radiological sign

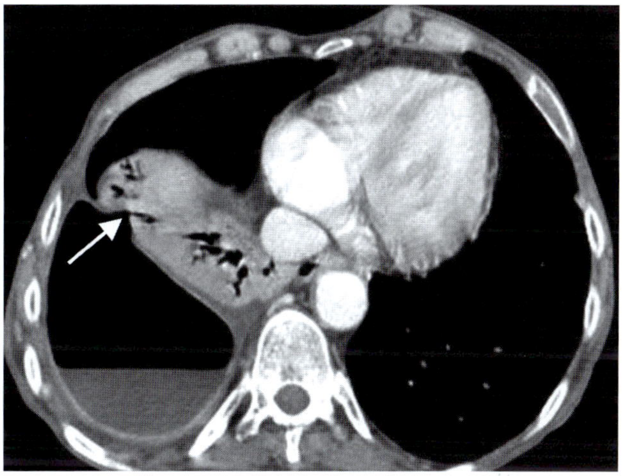

FIG. 31: CT chest-bronchus in communication with a hydropneumothorax—bronchopleural fistula.

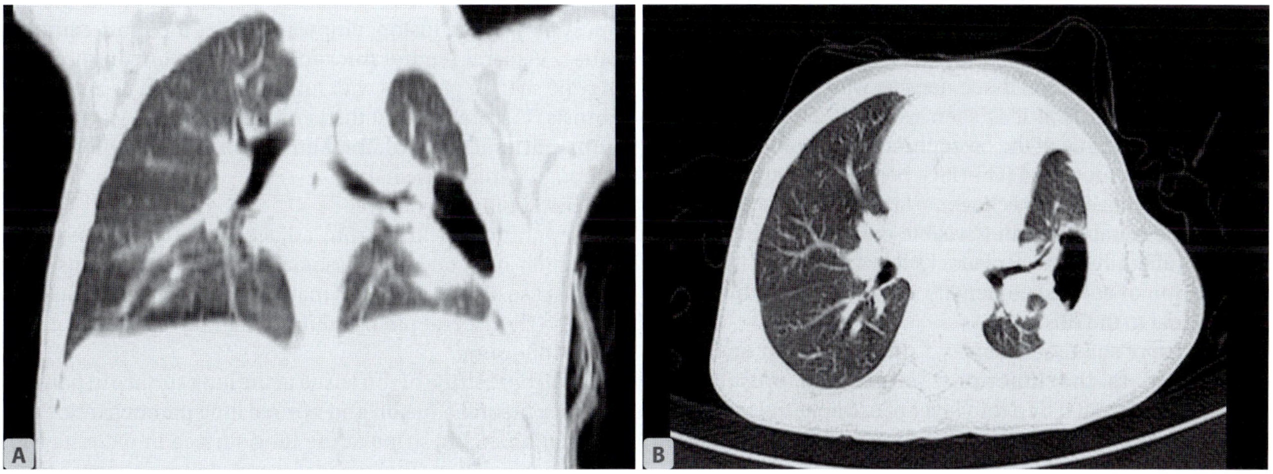

FIGS. 30A AND B: CT chest shows a loculated air containing space in the left pleural cavity that was not draining completely. A segmental bronchus is seen in close proximity to it—bronchopleural fistula.

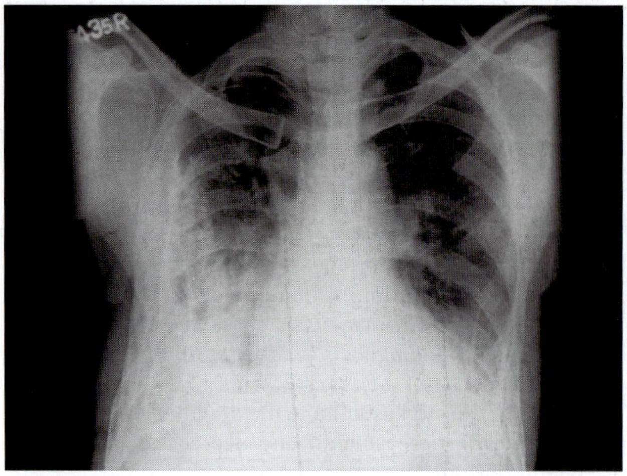

FIG. 32: Chest radiograph—diffuse pleural thickening bilaterally with calcification.

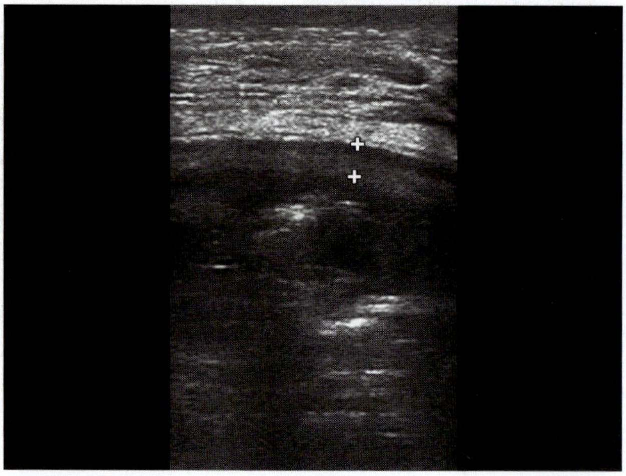

FIG. 33: Ultrasound chest—pleural thickening with minimal effusion.

is the sudden appearance of air-fluid level within the pleural space.

The delayed appearance of a fistula (>6 months after surgery) means tumor recurrence and is signaled by the appearance of air in the previously air free post-pneumonectomy space.

Infective BPF

This occurs in the setting of necrotizing pulmonary infection and is heralded by the appearance of an air-fluid level in the pleural cavity. The mimickers can be air introduced at thoracocentesis, pleuroesophageal fistula, herniated bowel and a subdiaphragmatic abscess.

PLEURAL THICKENING

Pleural thickening results as an end stage of infective or non-infective (e.g. asbestosis) processes. Generalized and gross pleural thickening is termed as **fibrothorax** and may cause significant ventilatory impairment.

On a chest radiograph pleural thickening appears as a fixed shadow of water density, most commonly located at the dependent parts of the pleural cavity **(Fig. 32)**. En profile it appears as a band of soft tissue density, with a sharp interface with the lung. Enface it is seen as an ill-defined veil like shadowing. Blunting of the costophrenic angle and tenting of the diaphragm are noted (On USG, benign pleural thickening is seen as homogeneous echogenic layer inside the chest wall **(Fig. 33)**. Pleural thickening, visible on radiographs and CT primarily affect the parietal pleura **(Table 4)**. On CT, it is seen as:

- A stripe of soft tissue density 1 mm more in thickness, internal to the ribs.
- A stripe of soft tissue density 1 mm or more in thickness, internal to the innermost intercostal muscle and separated from it by a thin layer of extrapleural fat.
- A distinct stripe in the paravertebral region 1 mm or more in thickness.
- Thickening of the normal extrapleural fat layer.

TABLE 4: Pleural thickening—criteria.
• A stripe of soft tissue density 1 mm more in thickness, internal to the ribs or innermost intercostal muscle
• A distinct stripe in the paravertebral region >1 mm thickness
• Thickening of the normal extrapleural fat layer

Diffuse pleural thickening may be seen unilaterally or bilaterally. The radiographic criteria used for diffuse pleural thickening are coverage of at least 25% of the total chest wall on a chest radiograph (50% if unilateral); and it must extend to a thickness of at least 5 mm in at least one site on the chest radiograph. [20]

CT criteria of diffuse pleural thickening includes, a continuous sheet of pleural thickening more than 5 cm wide, more than 8 cm in craniocaudal extent, and more than 3 mm thick.[21]

Visceral Pleural Thickening

This occurs almost always in association with parietal pleural thickening and effusion, empyema being the most common cause. Visceral pleural thickening alone is uncommon and may be seen in patients with lung disease, such as abscess or fibrosis. Visceral pleural thickening cannot be distinguished from parietal pleural thickening on chest radiographs, although it may appear as:

- Thickening of a fissure
- Separation of lung from adjacent ribs and chest wall, which may occur in association with contiguous lung disease. Both these signs may be seen in pleural effusions.

On CT, visceral pleural thickening may appear as either of the following:

- A distinct stripe of soft tissue at the lung surface in patients with pleural effusion and normal lung parenchyma.
- An enhancing stripe at the lung surface in patients with abnormal lung. Thickened visceral pleura enhances more than airless lung.

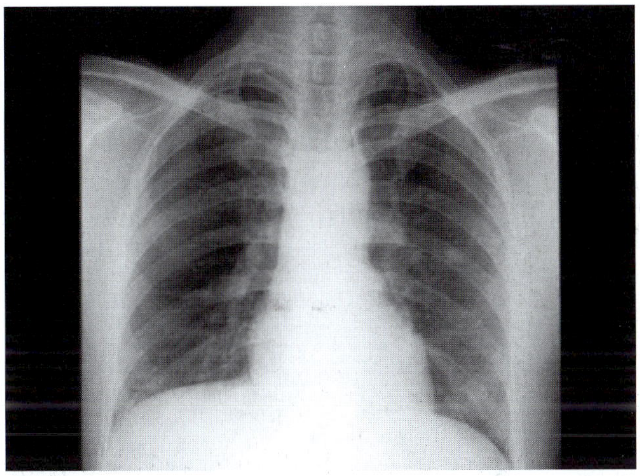

FIG. 34: Right pleural apical cap with soft opacities in left mid zone.

Pleural Apical Cap and Fibrous Thickening

Fibrous pleural thickening is common at the lung apex.[22] This may be secondary to tuberculosis or represent age related changes of unknown etiology. Apical caps may have a scalloped contour or be associated with tenting towards the lung **(Fig. 34)**. They can be unilateral or bilateral. Apical pleural caps need to be differentiated from companion shadows of upper ribs and from extrapleural fat.

Mimics of Pleural Thickening

Normal structures may mimic the findings of pleural thickening or effusion.

Normal fat pads: Normal extrapleural fat is most abundant over the posterolateral 4th–8th ribs and can be several mm thick that extend into the intercostal space. In contrast to pleural thickening or effusion, normal fat thickening is typically symmetrical, smooth in contour, low in attenuation and unassociated with costophrenic angle blunting. On CT, extrapleural fat appears very low in density.

The subcostalis and transversus thoracis muscles: These are not seen on chest radiograph. On CT, a 1 to 2 mm thick line is seen internal to one or more ribs, along the posterior chest wall at the level of heart, representing the subcostalis muscle. Anteriorly, at the level of heart, adjacent to lower sternum or xiphoid process, the transversus thoracis muscle is nearly always visible on CT, internal to the anterior ends of ribs or costal cartilages. These muscles are smooth, uniform in thickness and bilateral.

Paravertebral intercostal veins: They may sometimes be seen in the paravertebral regions. Continuity of these opacities with azygous or hemiazygous veins may be visible these do not indent the lung surface, as pleural thickening would.

PLEURA AND ASBESTOSIS[23,24]

Asbestos-related neoplastic and nonneoplastic diseases of the lungs and pleura range from pleural effusion and pleural plaques to lung cancer and malignant mesothelioma. Pleural effusions are typically hemorrhagic exudates of mixed cellularity but do not typically contain asbestos bodies.

Pleural plaques are the most common manifestation of asbestos inhalation and occur 20–30 years after first exposure. Pleural plaques are seen in 3–14% of dockyard workers and in 58% of insulation workers. The pathogenesis of plaques is uncertain, but is postulated that fibers reach the pleura via lymphatic channels and cause an inflammatory response, which in turn leads to hyaline fibrosis along the parietal pleural surface. They usually arise from the parietal pleura but may arise from the visceral pleura. Plaques are seen over the diaphragmatic dome and the undersurface of the lower posterolateral ribs. Diagnosis is usually by chest-X-ray. The diameter of the plaques can vary from several millimeters to 10 cm. Any pleural or pericardial surface can be affected, but asbestos-related pleural plaques are usually in the lower 2/3 of the thorax and are bilateral. Calcification most often affects the parietal and diaphragmatic pleura (virtually pathognomonic) and spares the costophrenic sulci and apices **(Figs. 35A and B)**. The size and number are variable. Calcification may be the only evidence of exposure. Dense pleural fibrosis surrounding the entire lung and >1 cm in thickness can also follow asbestos exposure. It results from thickening and fibrosis of visceral pleura, which leads to fusion with parietal pleura.

Patients with pleural plaques are asymptomatic, there is no risk of malignant degeneration, but patients with pleural plaques may have an increased risk of developing mesothelioma and bronchogenic carcinoma compared with a control population matched for exposure but without pleural plaques. The plaques are most useful as a marker of asbestos exposure.

ASBESTOSIS PSEUDOTUMOR (ROUND ATELECTASIS)

The pathogenesis is thought to be due to an inflammatory reaction and fibrosis in the superficial layer of pleura. As the fibrous tissue matures, it contracts, causing pleura to fold into the lung, which in turn causes the atelectasis.

Chest radiograph shows a rounded peripheral "mass" with or without lung distortion. The CT features are of a round or oval mass that abuts the pleura, a "comet tail" of bronchovascular structures going into the mass, and thickening of the adjacent pleura. USG may show an echogenic line that extends into the mass from the pleura, representing the scarred invaginated visceral pleura **(Figs. 36A and B)**.

MRI shows a curved low signal intensity line caused by thickened indentation of visceral pleura. The main differential is malignancy of the lung. Stability or shrinkage of the mass with time suggests benignancy, but biopsy may be required.

PLEURAL CALCIFICATION

This is seen following asbestos exposure, empyema, tuberculosis, hemothorax. In the later two conditions calcification is irregular and resembles a plaque **(Figs. 37A and B)** or sheet and is contained within thickened pleura.

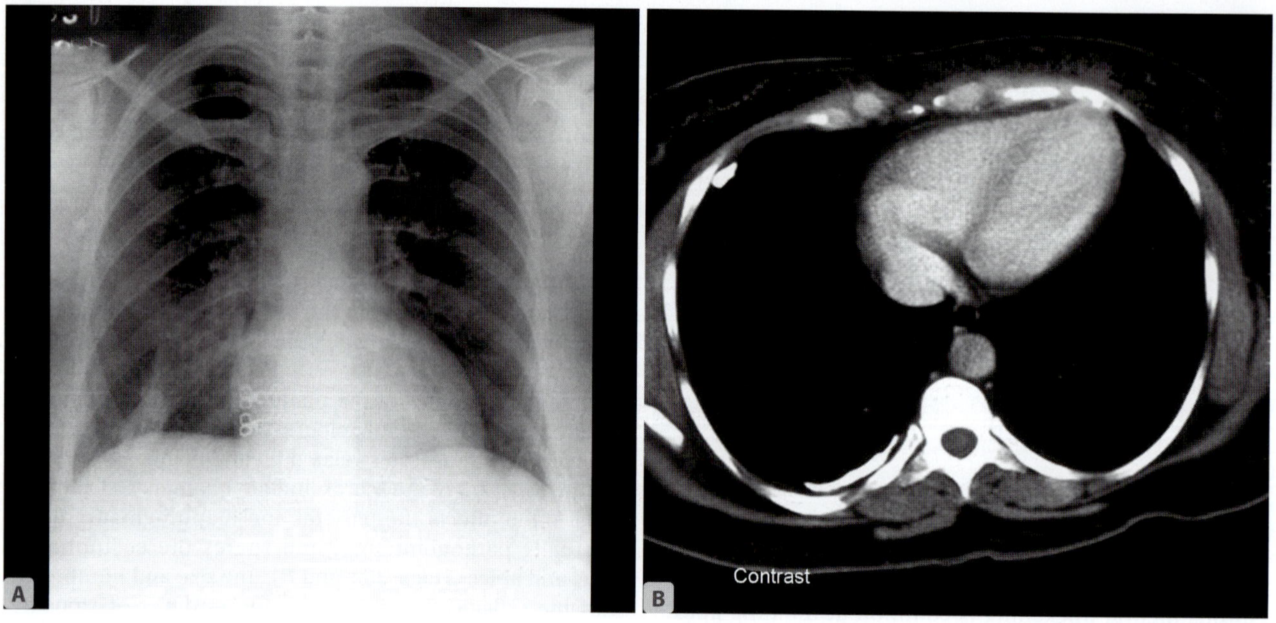

FIGS. 35A AND B: (A) X-ray chest—calcified pleural plaque on the right side; (B) CT chest—calcified pleural plaque seen in the right costal pleura and posteriorly along paraspinal gutter in a patient with history of asbestos exposure.

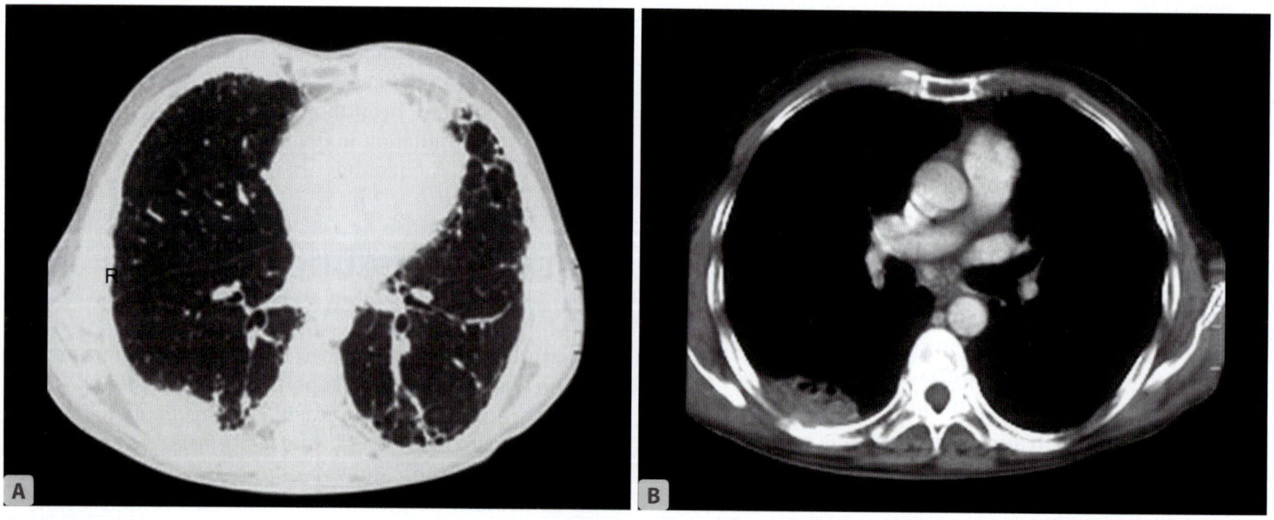

FIGS. 36A AND B: CT chest shows a peripherally based opacity on the right side with vessels curling up to it—round atelectasis.

It may occur anywhere but is most common in the lower posterior half of chest and is usually unilateral. Following tubercular empyema both parietal and visceral pleura may be calcified. These layers are separated by a soft tissue opacity that may contain fluid for many years.

PNEUMOTHORAX

Air within the pleural cavities is referred to as pneumothorax. It is classified as spontaneous or traumatic. The causes of pneumthorax are summarized in **Table 5**.

Spontaneous Pneumothorax

These are classified as primary or secondary.

Primary Spontaneous Pneumothorax

It occurs without an antecedent cause in an otherwise healthy patient. It often occurs at rest, as a result of rupture of an apical subpleural bulla. The peak incidence is in young patients (20–40 years), men (80%), tall and thin patients and smokers (90%). Pain is common and a small pleural effusion is present in 10–20% manifested as an air-fluid level. It may be asymptomatic and detected incidentally. These patients are at increased risk of another pneumothorax.

Secondary Spontaneous Pneumothorax

Occurs due to an underlying disease such as COPD, Langerhans histiocytosis. These are symptomatic and have a high recurrence rate.

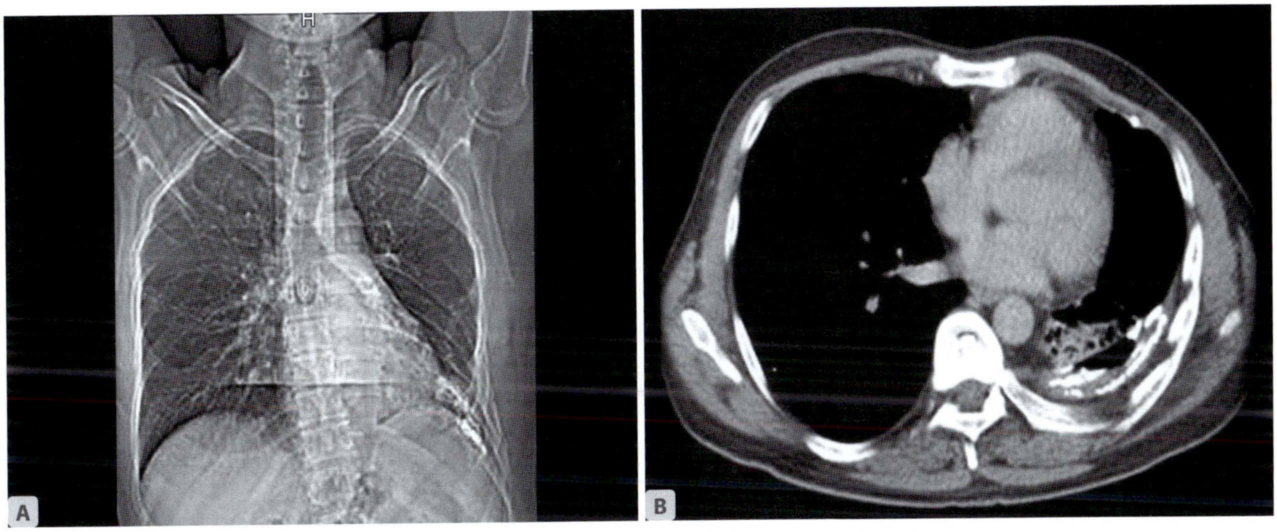

FIGS. 37A AND B: (A) Chest scanogram; (B) CT—pleural calcification with loss of volume—post-tubercular.

TABLE 5: Causes of pneumothorax in adult.
Spontaneous
• Primary spontaneous
Secondary spontaneous: – Airflow obstruction—asthma, COPD, cystic fibrosis – Pulmonary infection—cavitary pneumonia, tuberculosis, fungal disease, AIDS, pneumatocele – Pulmonary infarction – Neoplasm—metastatic sarcoma – Diffuse lung disease—histiocytosis X lymphangioleiomyomatosis – Endometriosis (catamenial pneumothorax)
Traumatic
• Non-iatrogenic—ruptured esophagus/trachea, closed chest trauma (± rib fracture), penetrating chest trauma
• Iatrogenic—thoracotomy/thoracocentesis, percutaneous biopsy, tracheostomy, central venous catheterization

Pneumothorax Ex-vacuo

It is a rare cause of secondary spontaneous pneumothorax, occurring in patients with acute lobar collapse due to bronchial obstruction. Sudden collapse results in rapid decrease in intrapleural pressure adjacent to the collapsed lobe. This leads to gas, entering the pleural space. The resulting pneumothorax is seen adjacent to the collapsed lung.

Traumatic Pneumothorax

It can be caused by chest trauma (penetrating/non-penetrating, accidental or iatrogenic) or in patients on mechanical ventilation. Pneumothoraces with mechanical ventilation (due to high ventilator pressures) occurs due to alveolar rupture leading to interstitial emphysema, pneumomediastinum and rupture of pneumomediastinum into pleural subpleural location. Traumatic pneumothorax requires chest tube drainage.

Catamenial Pneumothorax

Pneumothorax, coincident with menstruation is rare. The symptoms start within 48 hours of onset of menses. Air may reach the peritoneum via vagina, uterus or the fallopian tubes. From there it may enter the pleural space via defect or diaphragm, common on the right. Endometrial implants may enter the pleural space by the same route. Endometrial implants involve visceral space and peripheral lung; the breakdown may result in pneumothorax.

IMAGING FINDINGS OF PNEUMOTHORAX

Radiograph

In an ***upright patient*** air usually collects first above the lung apex. The presence of a visible visceral pleural line is a key to diagnosis. This is visible as a very thin line at the pleural space with an avascular space above or lateral to it and one in the lung below and medial to it **(Figs. 38 and 39)**. Air may enter the fissure, outlining its pleural surface. In absence of underlying lung disease or adhesions; the partially collapsed lung maintains its normal shape. Lung markings are not seen peripheral to the pleural line. The visibility of pneumothorax is accentuated on expiration as there is increase in volume. Expiratory film or decubitus view with suspected side uppermost may demonstrate a small pneumothorax. Skin folds, hair, clothing, etc. may mimic the walls of bulla and visceral pleural line of pneumothorax. Artefacts and skin folds can be distinguished from pneumothorax by extension of these beyond margin of chest cavity laterally located vessels. The margin of the skin fold is usually wider than the thin line of the visceral pleura. A repeat radiograph or an expiratory radiograph may be required in certain situation.

Distinction of a bulla from a pneumothorax is usually based on shape. Pneumothoraces are typically crescent shaped and taper towards the lung base. Bullae are rounded and have inner margin concave to the chest wall and do not

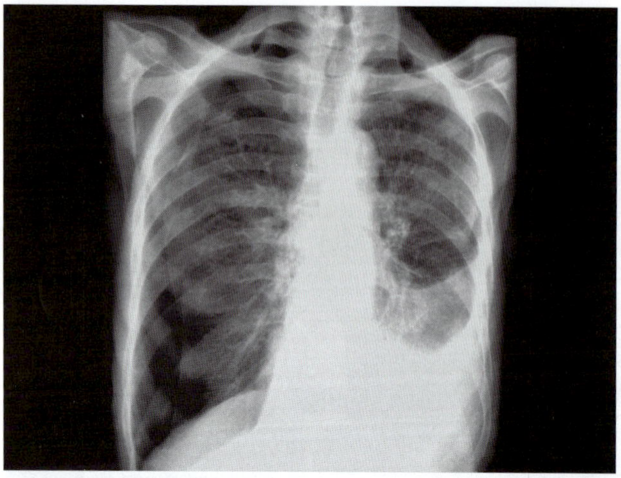

FIG. 38: Right-sided pneumothorax seen on chest skiagram as an avascular space, bounded by the visceral pleural line. Left pleural effusion is also seen.

conform to the costophrenic angle when they are at the lung base.

In ***supine patients***, free pneumothorax usually collects within the anterior pleural space. A visceral pleural line may be seen medially in some patients mimicking a pneumomediastinum. Pneumothorax in a supine patient may be inferred by the following:

- **Deep sulcus sign**: Costophrenic angle may appear abnormally deep and lucent because of air in the anterolateral pleural space **(Figs. 40 and 41)**.[25]
- **Increased lucency over the chest wall and abdomen**
- Visualization of the anterior costophrenic angle as an edge separate from the diaphragm, but parallel to it—**the double diaphragm sign.**
- **Increased sharpness of the hemi-diaphragm, cardiac border or mediastinum** (because it is outlined by air)
- A lumpy appearance at the cardiac apex, due to alteration in the shape of the epicardial fat pat.
- Air in the minor fissure.

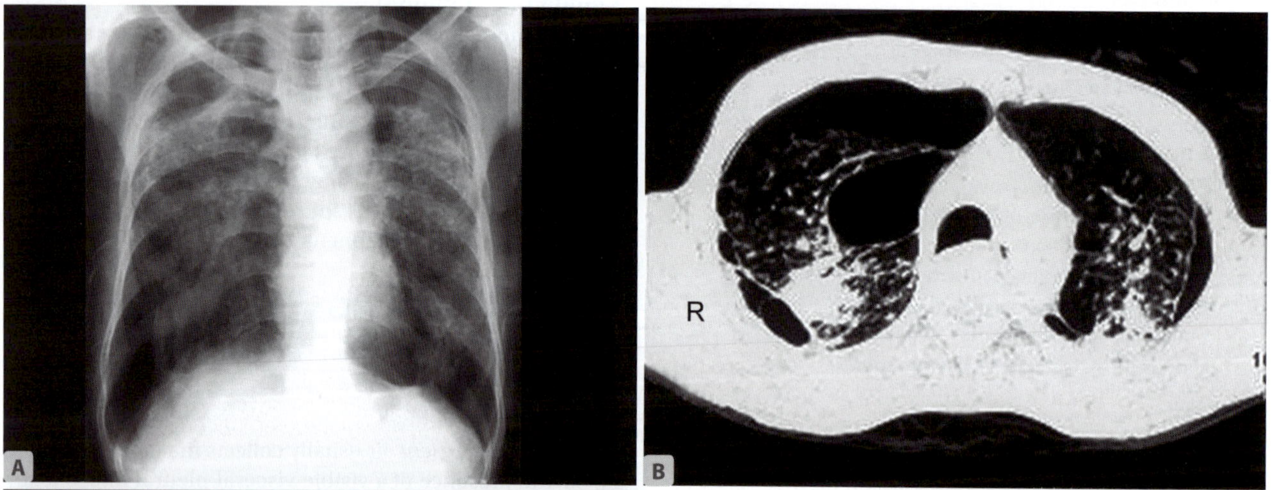

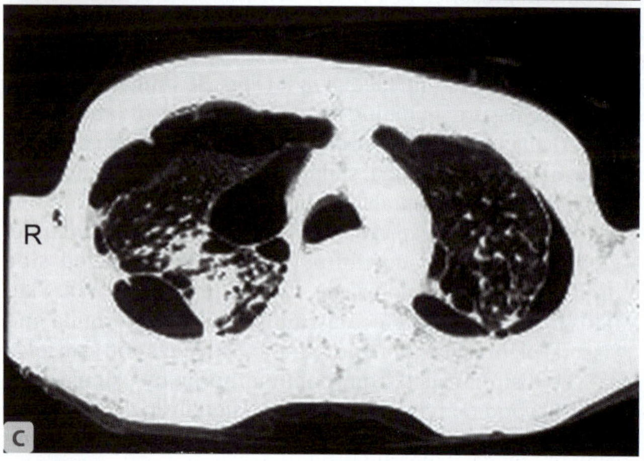

FIGS. 39A TO C: (A) Chest X-ray; (B and C) CT multiple pleural adhesions causing loculation of air—pneumothoraces in a case of silicosis.

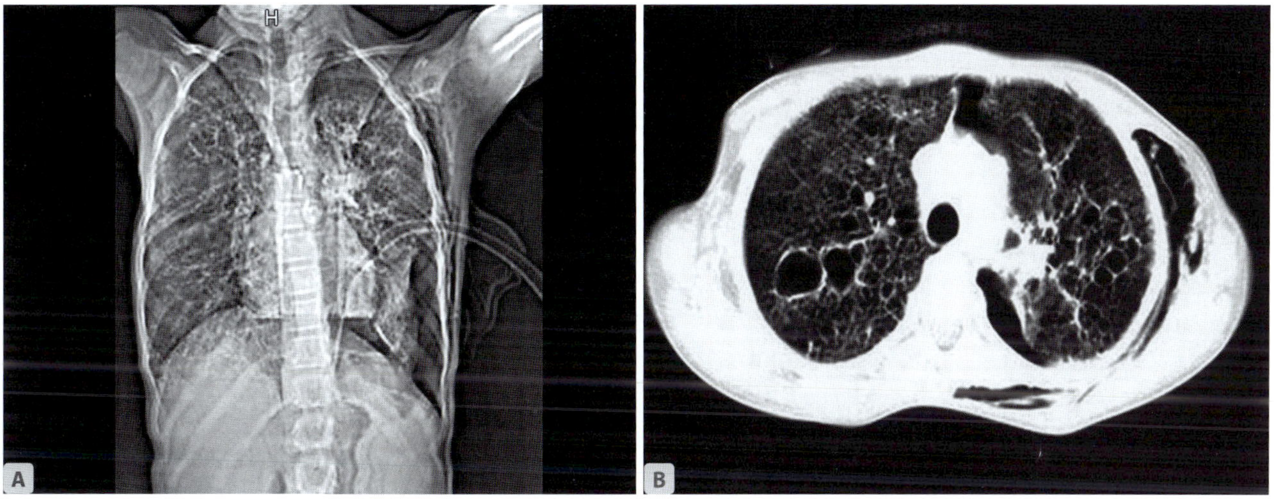

FIGS. 40A AND B: CT- topogram (A) demonstrates the deep costophrenic sulcus on the left and clarity of the left hemidiaphragm due to pneumothorax in a patient of lymhangioleiomyomatosis (B).

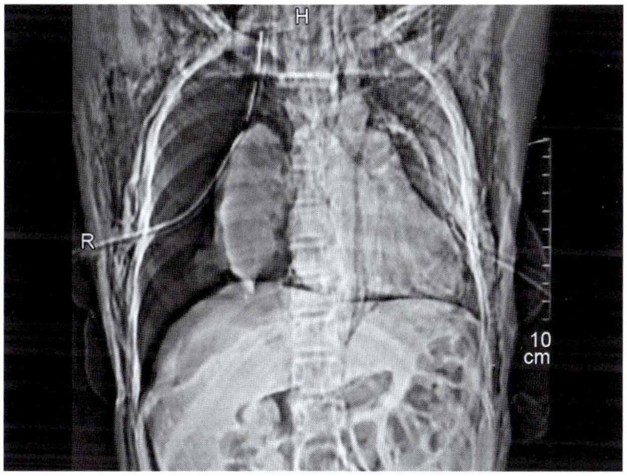

FIG. 41: Scanogram—traumatic pneumothorax. Note the clarity of the diaphragm and the deep costophrenic sulcus on the right side.

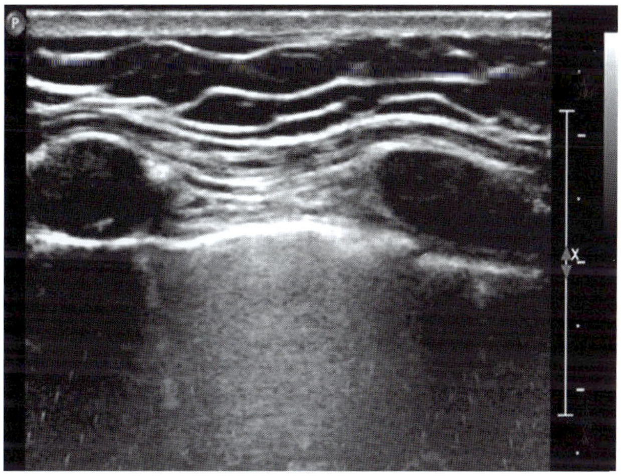

FIG. 42: Ultrasound chest transverse view intercostal approach—bright pleural line identified between two ribs-bat sign.

Ultrasonography in Pneumothorax

Ultrasound is now routinely used to detect pneumothorax in emergency settings. Standard lung views are now part of **E-Fast ultrasound (Extended - focussed assessment with Sonography in trauma)**.[26] Ultrasound has higher sensitivity than chest radiograph in the diagnosis of pneumothorax, especially in identifying occult pneumothoraces of traumatic origin.

Technique of Ultrasound to Detect Pneumothorax[27,28]

A high frequency linear probe is used for analysing superficial structure such as pleura. Patients are scanned in supine positions, with the probe placed on the anterior chest wall in a sagittal plane at the 2nd intercostal space in the mid clavicular line. Two adjacent ribs are indentified by posterior shadowing behind them and bright hyperechoic pleural line in between them. This is termed the **'bat sign' (Fig. 42)**. In the supine position air rises to least dependent part of chest which is anteriorly. In a normal lung the visceral pleura will glide in a to and fro pattern over the parietal pleura with respiration. This is seen on dynamic ultrasound as horizontal sliding movement of pleural line, best seen over apex of lung.

M-mode is also used to detect this sliding movement. M-mode cursor is placed over the pleural line. The chest wall above the pleural line forms horizontal—the 'waves' and sliding pleural line forms a granular pattern—the 'Sand'. The resultant image of motionless chest wall and sliding pleura is **seashore sign (Fig. 43)**.

Reverberation artifacts are also seen as hyperechoic vertical lines that extend from pleura to edge of screen without fading. These are seen due to acoustic impendence differences.

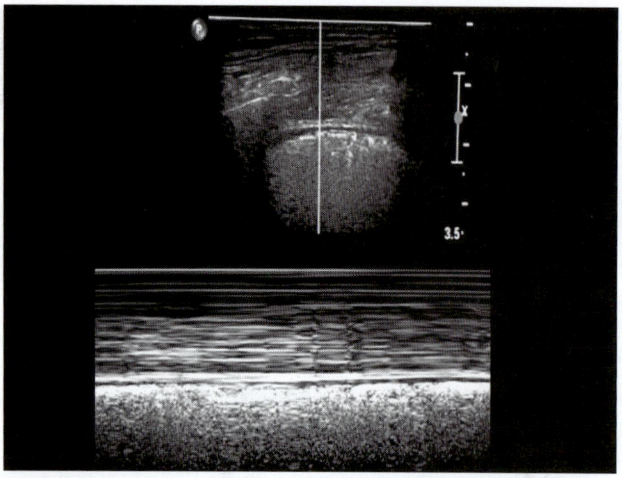

FIG. 43: M-mode—The chest wall above the pleural line forms horizontal—the'waves' and sliding pleural line forms a granular pattern—the 'Sand'-seashore sign.

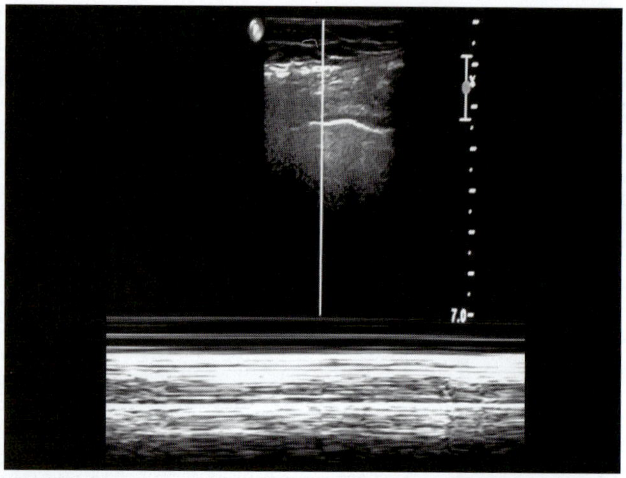

FIG. 44: M-mode tracing displays one pattern of parallel horizontal lines above and below the pleural line—'barcode sign' or the' stratosphere sign'.

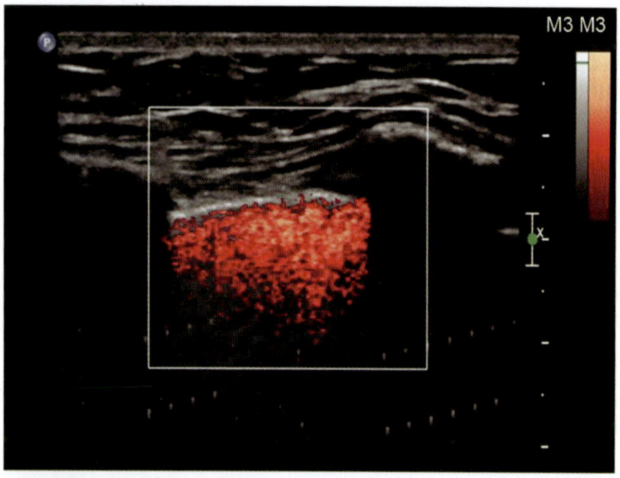

FIG. 45: Power Doppler—depicting normal sliding motion of lung. Absence of this sliding is seen in pneumothorax.

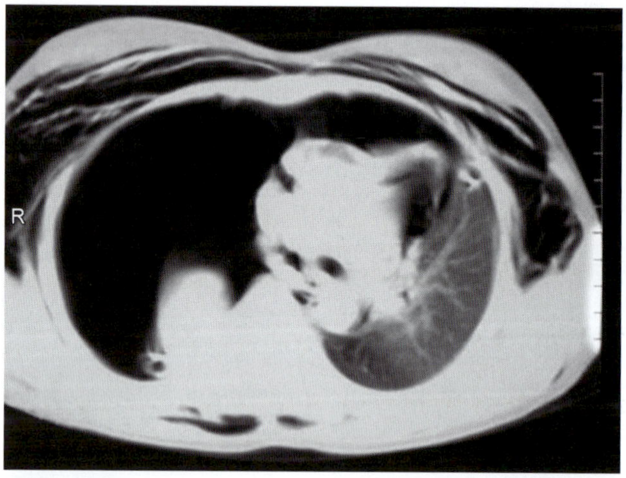

FIG. 46: Large right pneumothorax with passive collapse of the underlying lung, mediastinal shift to the opposite side. Extensive subcutaneous emphysema noted secondary to tube placement.

Sonographic Signs of Pneumothorax

- **Absence of lung sliding in presence of pneumothorax**, visualized pleura will not be identified and movement of pleural line will not be present.[29,30] The M-mode tracing will display one pattern of parallel horizontal lines above and below the pleural line. This is termed the **'barcode sign'** or the **'stratosphere sign'**. **(Fig. 44)** This is an important sign as it has a negative predictive value of almost 100%. Presence of sliding sign rules out pneumothorax. Absence of lung sliding may be seen in other conditions like adult respiratoy distress syndrome, pulmonary fibrosis, etc.

  Comet tail artifacts or B lines: These reverberation artifacts will be absent in pneumothorax. This is duc to presence of air which does not allow sound to propagate. The negative predictive value of this sign is 98–100%.
- **Lung point sign:**[30] This indicates the border of pneumothorax and is useful to assess the size of pneumothorax which has therapeutic implications. At this point sliding and non-sliding lung will be seen together. On M-mode alternate seashore and barcode pattern will be seen. The probe is slowly moved from anterior part to lateral or posterior chest to locate the lung point. The more lateral this point is, the bigger is the pneumothorax.
- **Power slide sign:**[31,32] Power Doppler is sometimes used to detect sliding movement. This requires the probe to be steady and patient motionless to avoid artefacts. Absence of sliding indicates pneumothorax **(Fig. 45)**.

Computed Tomography

CT is extremely sensitive to the presence of air in pleural cavity. Lung Window settings should be used to detect pneumothorax. A pneumothorax is imaged as air in the pleural space outside the lung and visceral pleura **(Fig. 46)**. CT can be used to distinguish bullae from a

TABLE 6: Tension pneumothorax.
Clinical diagnosis
Life threatening—immediate decompression required
Suggestive radiographic signs:
• Contralateral displacement of mediastinum
• Inferior displacement of the diaphragm
• Hyperlucent hemithorax
• Ipsilateral collapse

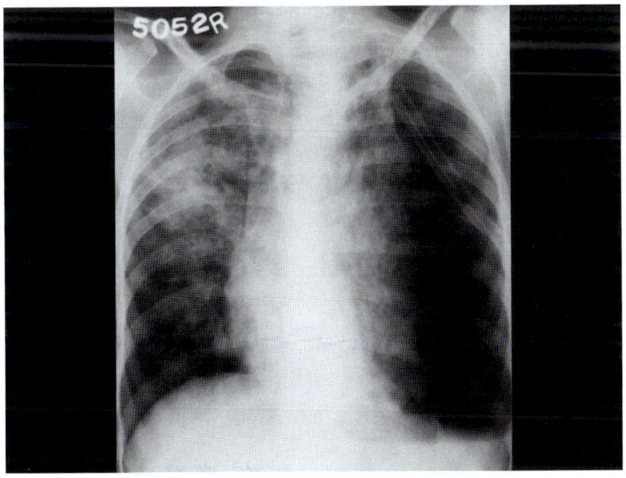

FIG. 47: X-ray chest—infiltrative opacities right uppper and mid zone, with left-sided pneumothorax—shift of the mediastinum to the right and flattening of left hemidiaphragm—tension pneumothorax.

pneumothorax. Differentiating a medial pneumothorax from a pneumomediastinum may be difficult.

Tension Pneumothorax

This is a life-threatening emergency. It occurs when the pressure in pleural air exceeds atmospheric pressure for a significant part of the respiratory cycle. Tension has an adverse effect on gas exchange and cardiovascular performance causing a rapid deterioration in the patient's condition. It is most often seen in mechanically ventilated patients or in patients of chest trauma.

Tension pneumothorax is difficult to diagnose on chest radiographs **(Table 6)**. Shift of mediastinum away from side of pneumothorax may be seen in any large pneumothorax **(Fig. 47)**. Combination of this with clinical symptom of circulatory compromise is diagnostic. Downward displacement or inversion of hemidiaphragm, is a reliable sign of tension especially in a ventilated patient in whom mediastinal shift is absent. The condition must be urgently treated by immediate decompression of the pleural space.

Size of Pneumothorax

A large pneumothorax may be differentiated from a small pneumothorax by the presence of a visible rim of more than 2 cm between lung margin and the chest wall at the level of the hilum. Pneumothorax may be calculated as percentage of the pleural space[33] as shown in **Figure 48**. A pneumothorax of >30% is generally considered to require treatment.

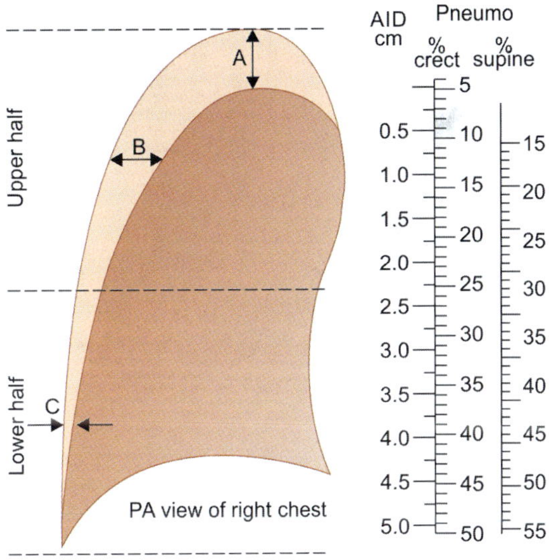

FIG. 48: Illustration depicting the calculation of size of pneumothorax. A = Maximum apical interpleural distance, B = interpleural distance at the midpoint of upper half of lung, C = interpleural distance at the midpoint of lower half of lung. Average interpleural distance AID = A+B+C/3 in cm.

PLEURAL NEOPLASM

The pleura may be involved by primary tumor or one of several metastatic neoplasms. **Metastatic disease is the most common pleural neoplasm.[34]**

Pleural neoplasm may present as pleural effusion or pleural thickening/mass.

Pleural Effusion

A malignant effusion is secondary to pleural involvement by tumor and contains malignant cells. Exudative effusion in patients with malignancy can reflect lymphatic or pulmonary venous obstructions by tumor or pneumonia. The most common causes are metastasis from lung cancer and breast cancer. Pleural fluid cytology is positive in 80–90% cases. Demonstration of tumor cells in pleural fluid is difficult but when present renders the primary disease as unresectable. Regardless of the cause, exudative effusions in a cancer patient requires treatment by drainage.

Pleural Thickening

Pleural thickening, in a patient of cancer with pleural effusion indicates the presence of exudates. Pleural thickening is seen in 30% of cancer patients. CT findings specific in diagnosing malignancy are:

1. Nodular pleural thickening.
2. Circumferential pleural thickening, surrounding the lung.
3. Mediastinal pleural thickening.

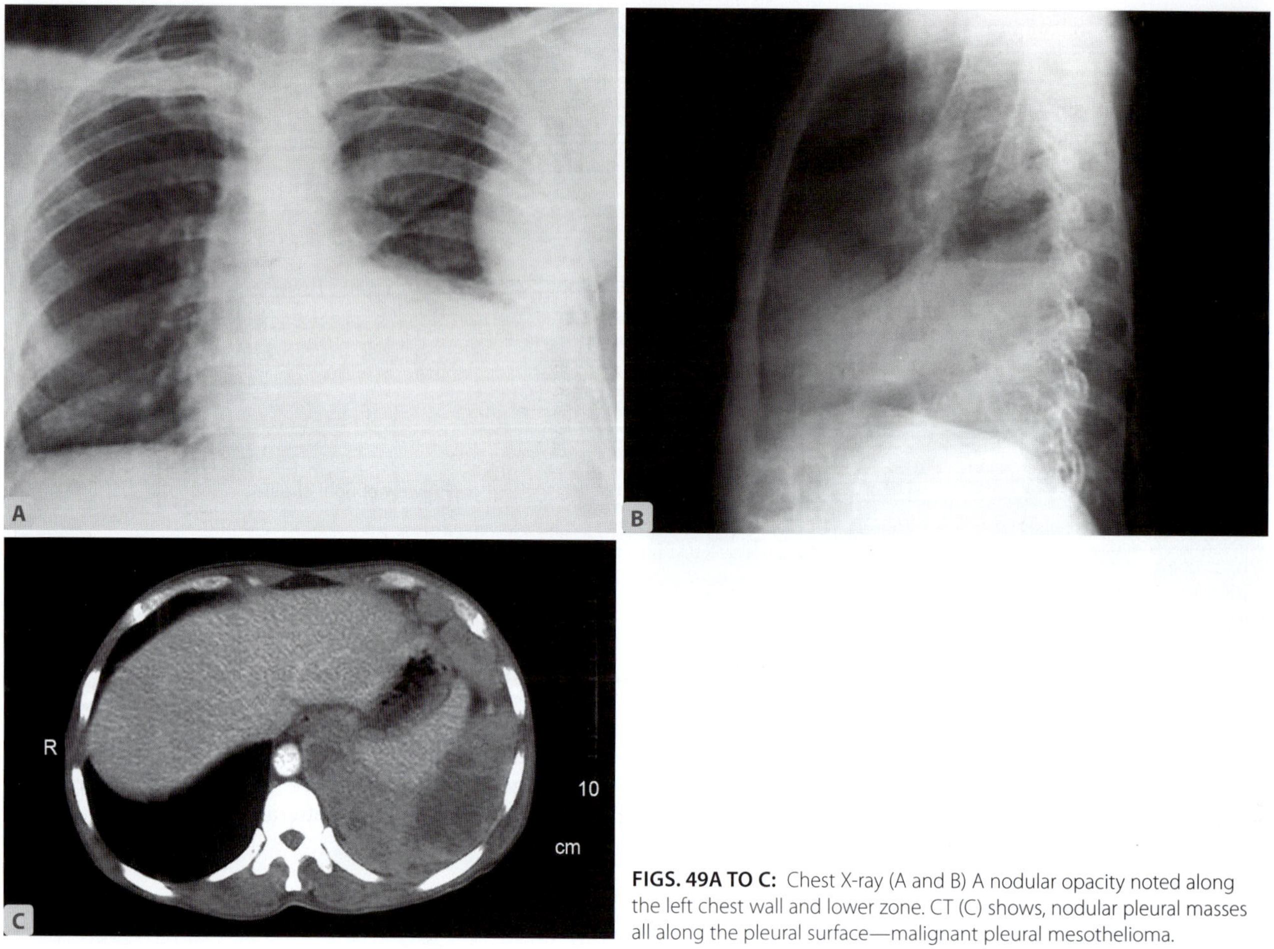

FIGS. 49A TO C: Chest X-ray (A and B) A nodular opacity noted along the left chest wall and lower zone. CT (C) shows, nodular pleural masses all along the pleural surface—malignant pleural mesothelioma.

MESOTHELIOMA (MALIGNANT PLEURAL MESOTHELIOMA)[35-37]

Malignant pleural mesothelioma (MPM) is the most common primary neoplasm of the pleura. It is a highly malignant aggressive neoplasm of mesothelial cell origin. It occurs mainly in the pleura or peritoneum, but may arise in the pericardium or tunica vaginalis testis. There is a strong association between development of this neoplasm and asbestos exposure, particularly crocidolite. Approximately 5–7% of asbestos workers will develop it. A latency period of 20 to 40 years between exposure and development of tumor is seen. Symptoms include chest pain, dyspnea and weight loss with mean age at presentation of 60 years. Mesothelioma arises in relation to parietal pleura. It is classified pathologically as epithelial (50%), sarcomatous (25%) or mixed (25%). The epithelial type has a slightly better prognosis and is associated with pleural effusion.

Mesothelioma is characterized morphologically by gross and nodular pleural thickening, which can involve fissures. Hemorrhagic pleural effusion often occurs. It spreads by local infiltration of the pleura. The tumor can invade both visceral and parietal pleura and frequently extends to adjacent structures, such as chest wall, mediastinum and diaphragm, lymph node spread or metastasis to different organs such as liver, lung and kidneys can occur. The overall survival is related to the extent of the primary tumor.

Radiographic Findings of MPM

The most common plain radiographic findings are unilateral pleural effusion (30–95%) and concentric or lobulated pleural thickening **(Figs. 49 to 51)**.

Solid pleural lesions may vary from focal masses to diffuse thickening surrounding and encasing the entire lung surface. Extension into the interlobar fissure is common occurring in 40–86% patients. Distinct pleural masses without effusion are identified in less than 25% of patients. Benign calcified or noncalcified plaques may be present. Because of pleural thickening and mediastinal infiltration, the involved hemithorax may be normal in volume, despite presence of large effusion **(the frozen mediastinum sign).** The hemithorax may be reduced in volume because of restriction of lung expansion.

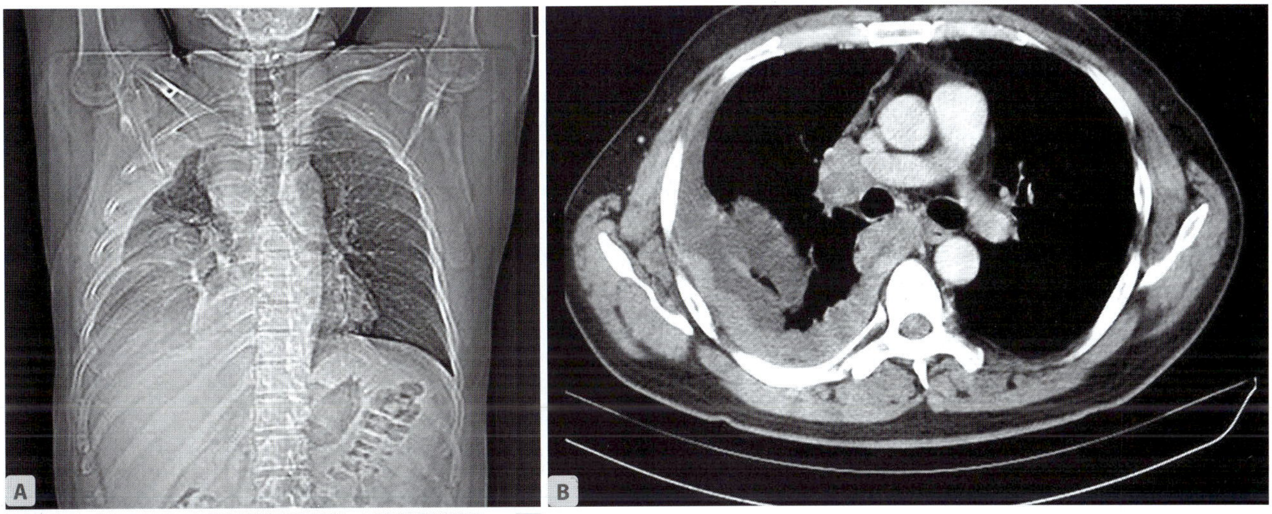

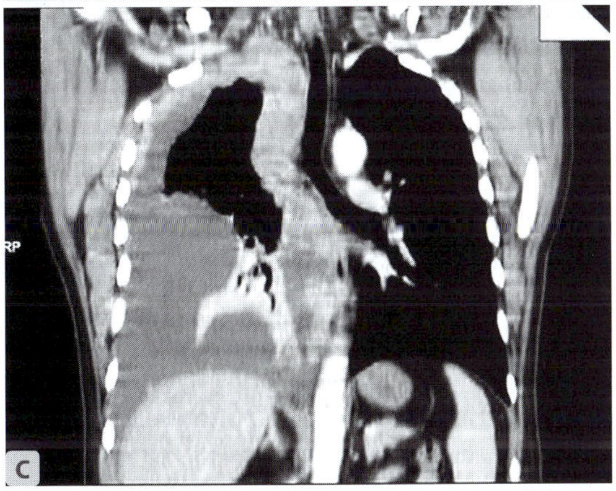

FIGS. 50A TO C: X-ray (A) CT chest (B and C)—circumferential and nodular enhancing pleural tumor with associated effusion. Extension into the mediastinal pleura and partial encasement of the right lung is suggestive of mesothelioma.

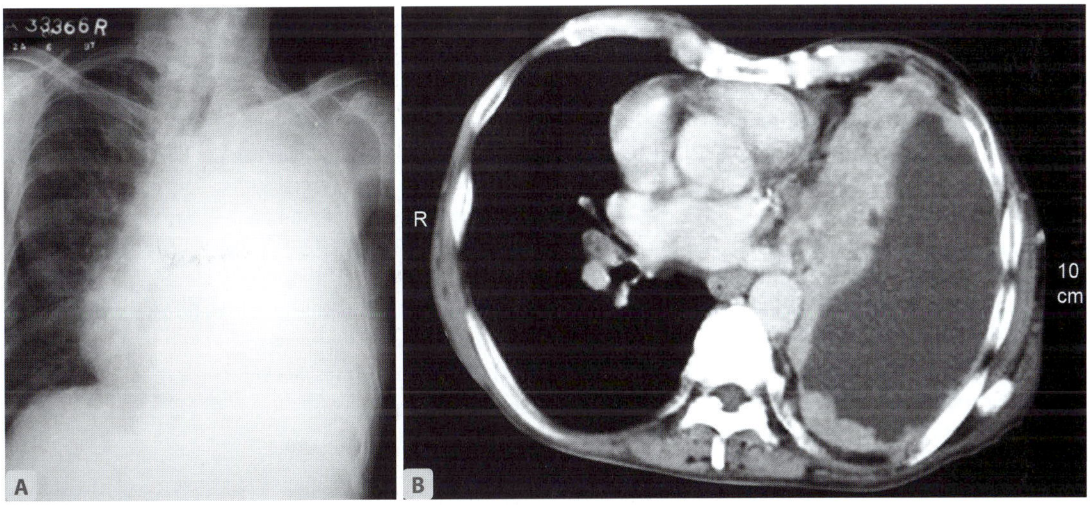

FIGS. 51A AND B: Chest X-ray (A)—opaque left hemithorax with shift of mediastinum to the right. CT scan (B) of the same patient shows nodular, thickened, enhancing pleura with associated effusion, malignant pleural mesothelioma.

Ultrasonography

Ultrasound will show pleural effusion and nodular soft tissue masses. The accuracy of US in detecting invasion of pleura and chest wall is high. US criteria of tumor invasion have been described. If the tumor is in contact with only visceral pleura it is UP1, if in contact with parietal pleura it is UP2 and with breech of pleura is UP3.

Computed Tomography

Computed tomography (CT) is the primary imaging modality for MPM. Major findings include nodular pleural thickening, unilateral pleural effusion,tumor invasion into the adjacent structures. Pleural thickening is circumferential/rind like with multiple nodules. Nodular concentric pleural thickening is highly suggestive of mesothelioma, rarely it may be thin and smooth. Calcified plaques are a sign of asbestos exposure; these are not a precursor to mesothelioma.

In early disease, pleural thickening may appear localized and discontinuous. As the disease progresses, pleural thickening becomes continuous, it increases in thickness and nodularity and the amount of fluid may decrease as pleural layers become fused.

In some cases, pleural effusion may be the only finding. The combination of an unexplained pleural effusion and pleural pain should raise the possibility of mesothelioma. Enhancement of the pleura after contrast administration can help differentiate tumor from adjacent fluid collections. Mesothelioma is visible most frequently along the lateral chest wall; mediastinal pleural thickening is seen with extensive disease. The abnormal hemithorax can appear contracted and fixed with little change in size during inspiration. Thickening of fissures, particularly the lower part of major fissures can reflect tumor infiltration or associated pleural effusion. Involvement of fissures is seen on CT in 85% of cases of mesothelioma.

The features that are helpful in distinguishing malignant from benign pleural disease are: Circumferential and nodular pleural thickening and mediastinal pleural thickening, parietal pleural thickening of >1 cm is not a helpful differentiating feature. Infiltration of adjacent structures like chest wall suggests malignancy. Some infectious process like tuberculosis can invade the chest wall, but do so at a single focus, rather than at multiple sites, as seen in malignant disease.

There is a TNM international staging system,proposed by the International Mesothelioma Interst Group for diffuse malignant pleural mesothelioma **(Table 7)**.[38] This new system emphasizes criteria that help in determining local tumor extension and regional lymph node status in an attempt to identify patients with potentially curable early disease (T1 a and b); those who may benefit from surgery without necessarily being cured (T2 and T3); and patients with extensive local tumor spread (T4), extensive regional node involvement, or distant metastases for whom surgery would provide no benefit. The system therefore stratifies patients into prognostic groups.

CT criteria of resectability include:

- Preservation of extrapleural fat planes
- Absence of extrapleural soft tissue masses
- Normal CT attenuation values of adjacent structures
- Smooth inferior diaphragmatic surface.

CT criteria of unresectability include:

- Invasion of extrapleural soft tissue or fat
- Infiltration, separation, displacement of ribs by tumor
- Bone destruction
- Tumor encasing the diaphragm.

CT remains suboptimal because enlarged nodes do not imply nodal involvement. CT can also lead to underestimation of the extent of disease in early chest wall involvement.

TABLE 7: International Mesothelioma Interest Group TNM staging system.

TNM
T – Tumour
TX: primary tumour cannot be assessed
T0: no evidence of primary tumour
T1a
• Potentially resectable
• Only parietal pleura
• No mediastinal pleural involvement
T1b
• Potentially resectable
• Parietal pleura and
• Scattered foci of mediastinal pleural involvement
T2
• Potentially resectable
• Parietal and visceral pleural involvement, and /or
• Pulmonary parenchymal involvement and/or
• Diaphragmatic muscle involvement
T3
• Potentially resectable
• Localized tumor extension into endothoracic fascia and/or
• Localized non-transmural involvement of pericardium and/or
• Localized extension into mediastinal fat
T4
• Unresectable
• Multiple foci of extension into chest wall +/– rib destruction and/or
• Extension through diaphragm into peritoneum and/or
• Extension into contralateral pleura and/or
• Extension into mediastinal organs and/or
• Extension through pericardium +/– direct extension into heart
N – Nodes
NX: nodes cannot be assessed
N0: no evidence of nodal involvement
N1: ipsilateral bronchopulmonary or hilar nodal involvement
N2: subcarinal or ipsilateral mediastinal/internal mammary nodes
N3: contralateral mediastinal/internal mammary nodes, or ipsilateral/contralateral supraclavicular nodes
M – Metastases
MX: presence of metastases cannot be assessed
M0: no evidence of metastases
M1: distant metastases present
Stage groupings
Stage IA: T1a, N0, M0
Stage IB: T1b, N0, M0
Stage II: T2, N0, M0
Stage III: T1 or 2, N1 or N2, M0 or T3, any N, M0
Stage IV: any T, any N, M1

Magnetic Resonance Imaging

Malignant mesothelioma has a slightly high signal intensity on T1WI, as compared to adjacent chest wall musculature, and moderately high signal intensity on T2WI. Mesotheliomas enhance on post gadolinium scans. Other findings include diffuse pleural thickening, pleural effusion and involvement of adjacent structures similar to CT.

MRI has been found to be superior to CT, in revealing invasion of the diaphragm, endothoracic fascia or solitary respectable focus of chest wall invasion. Diffusion MRI can also help to differentiate benign from malignant pleural disease. Presence of hyperintense pleural spots on high b value DW images called as "pleural pointillism" and has a sensitivity of 93% and a specificity of 79%.[39] The diagnostic accuracy of pleural pointillism is substantially better than that of mediastinal pleural thickness. Pleural pointillism can be used to provide guidance for biopsy or thoracoscopic evaluation. Perfusion MRI is a promising technique for assessment of perfusion, vascularity and permeability of tumors. Therapeutic effect of chemotherapy can be monitored with perfusion MRI.

Positron Emission Tomography

Functional imaging with FDG-PET has facilitated the non-invasive evaluation of tumor pathophysiology, metabolism and proliferation. Most mesotheliomas are FDG avid. Mesothelioma shows moderate to high FDG uptake involving areas of thickened pleura. Tumors at earlier stage tend to have focal or linear patterns of uptake, wheras the mixed and encasing patterns are indicative of more advanced disease. PET/CT increases the accuracy of overall staging and improves the selection of patients for extrapleural pneumonectomy as it detects more extensive disease and identifies occult distant metastasis.

The differential diagnosis of malignant mesothelioma includes benign causes of pleural thickening (such as post infection or diffuse pleural thickening) and metastatic adenocarcinoma. The lobulated outline, pleural effusion, or evidence of more advanced disease may help differentiate mesothelioma from diffuse pleural thickening.

Histologic or cytologic diagnosis is always required. Image guidance can be used to obtain the necessary tissue diagnosis, but spread along biopsy/drainage site is well documented, the differentiation between mesothelioma and metastatic adenocarcinoma is difficult even with biopsy. Immunohistochemistry and electron microscopy aid the diagnosis.

Pleural Metastasis

Metastatic disease accounts for the majority of pleural neoplasm. Approximately 40% of pleural metastases arise from lung carcinoma, 10% from lymphoma and remaining 30% from other primary sites. Several extrathoracic primary tumors like ovarian, uterine,gastrointestinal or pancreatic may metastasize to the pleura. In absence of a recognizable primary, metastatic adenocarcinoma is difficult to diagnose, because of histological similarity to malignant mesothelioma.

Invasive thymoma is an uncommon thoracic primary neoplasm with a propensity for pleural extension. This pleural implantation results in widespread pleural thickening and/or multiple discrete masses. It may be indistinguisble from mesothelioma, especially when anterior mediastinal component is small.

Malignant effusion is the most frequent manifestation of metastatic pleural disease and is often accompanied by solid tumor deposits of varying size **(Fig. 52)**. They may appear as solitary implant on the costal, diaphragmatic or mediastinal pleura or within the interlobar fissure.

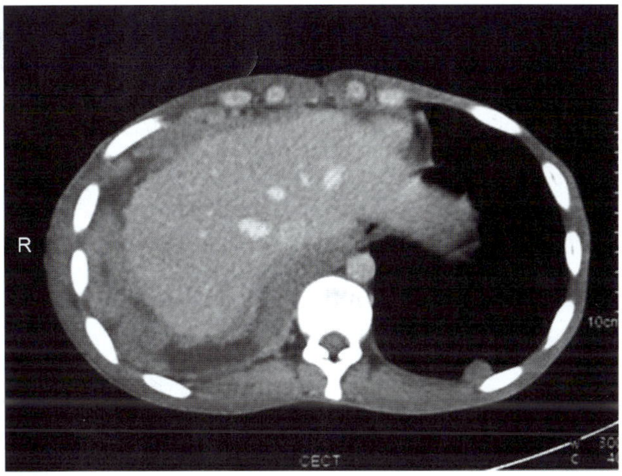

FIG. 52: CT multiple-enhancing pleural nodules—metastases.

Pleural Lymphoma

Involvement of pleura occurs in both Hodgkin and non-Hodgkin disease. Solid pleural lymphoma occurs as either a solitary nodule or as diffuse tumor infiltration. Associated exudative pleural effusion may be seen due to lymphatic obstruction and resolves with radiation. Marked thickening of extrapleural soft tissue may be seen with associated posterior mediastinal lymph node enlargement.

Localized Fibrous Tumor

Localized fibrous tumor (LFT) of the pleura was formerly known as benign mesothelioma, but it is not mesothelial in origin, and not always benign (30% are malignant).[40] About 50% of cases are encountered in patients in 6th–7th decade, with no gender predilection. It has no association with asbestos exposure. Patients are frequently asymptomatic, LFT is detected incidentally on chest radiographs. It can be associated with hypoglycemia (15%), chest pain or hypertrophic pulmonary osteoarthopathy (1/3rd of cases). These symptoms resolve with resection.

LFT arises from the visceral pleura in about 80%. They appear as solitary, well-circumscribed spherical ovoid, non-calcified lesions, contacting a pleural surface. The size ranges from less than 2 cm to 30 cm. They are often pedunculated and as a consequence may show change in position and shape during fluoroscopy.

LFT, when small has an obtuse angle at the pleural surface, when large angles can be acute. LFT can be seen within a fissure, mimicking appearance of loculated fluid. A "beak" or "thorn" sign is often seen on radiographs in patients with a LFT originating from or projecting into a fissure. Pleural effusion is not usually present.On CT, localized fibrous tumor appears as well-defined lobulated pleural mass **(Figs. 53A to C)**. Slight pleural thickening is usually visible adjacent to the mass. This is due to small amount of fluid accumulating at the pleural surface at the point of separation of visceral and parietal pleura by the mass. CT is useful in identifying masses arising from the interlobar fissure, which simulates a parenchymal lesion.On MR imaging, LFT may show low signal on both T1 and T2 weighted images or may have

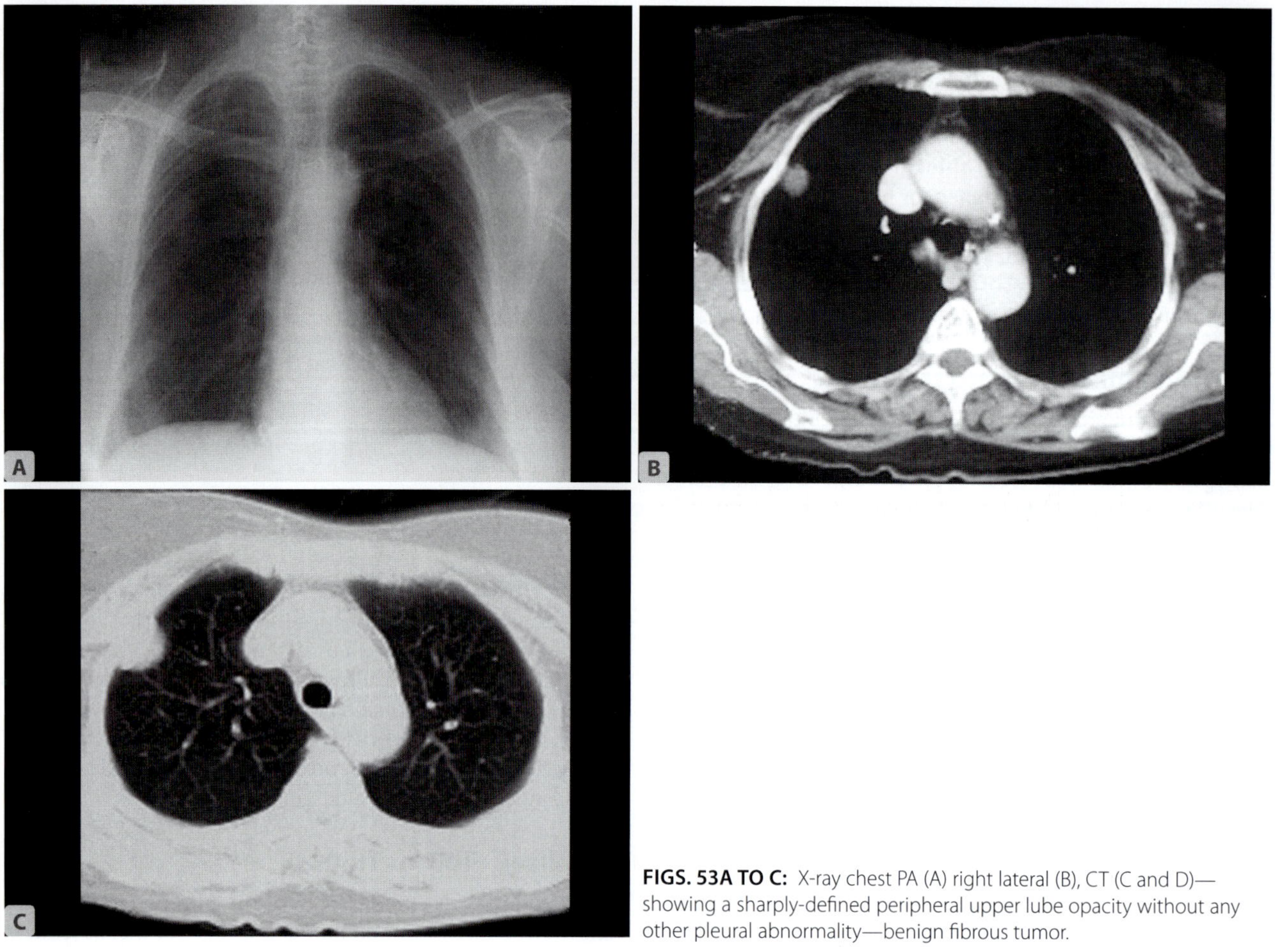

FIGS. 53A TO C: X-ray chest PA (A) right lateral (B), CT (C and D)—showing a sharply-defined peripheral upper lube opacity without any other pleural abnormality—benign fibrous tumor.

heterogeneous signal intensity reflecting the cellularity of these tumors. Surgical excision is the treatment with operative respectability being the most important predictor of clinical outcome.

TUMOR-LIKE CONDITIONS OF THE PLEURA

A tumor-like condition of the pleura is any non-neoplastic lesion of the pleura itself, or within the pleural space, that resembles a tumor.[3] These may be focal or diffuse. **Pleural plaque, thoracic splenosis, thoracic endometriosis** causing catamenial pneumothorax, and **pseudotumor** caused by pleural effusion are focal tumor-like conditions of the pleura. Diffuse tumor-like conditions of the pleura include diffuse pleural thickening and rare conditions such as **Erdheim-Chester disease** and **diffuse pulmonary lymphangiomatosis**. Erdheim-Chester disease is classified as non-Langerhans histiocytosis and is characterized by typical skeletal findings of femoral sclerosis, perirenal soft tissue halo. Diffuse pulmonary lymphangiomatosis is a rare condition, demonstrates diffuse pleural thickening, interlobular septal and peribronchovascular interstitial thickening, and mediastinal fat infiltration limited to the thorax.

REFERENCES

1. Coolen J, Keyzer FD, Nafteux P, et al. Malignant pleural disease: Diagnosis by using diffusion weight and dynamic contrast enhanced MR imaging initial experience. Radiology. 2012;263(3):884-92.
2. Parcel JM, Vives. Classic abbreviated and modified Light criteria; Chest. 1999;116:1833-6.
3. Sasson CS,Light RW.Chylothorax &pseudochylothorax. Clin Chest Med. 1985;6:163-71.
4. Walker CM, Takasugi JE, Chung JH, et al. Tumour like conditions of the pleura. Radiographics. 2012;32:971-85.
5. Eibenberger K, dock W, Ammann M, et al. Quantification of pleural effusions: Sonography versus radiography. Radiology. 1994;191:681-4.
6. Yang PC, Luh KT, Chang DB, et al. Value of sonography in determing the nature of pleural effusion: Analysis of 320 cases. Am J Roentgenol. 1992;159:29-33.

7. Wu RG, Yang PC, Kuo SH. "Fluid colour" sign-a useful indicator for discrimination between pleural thickening and pleural effusion. J Ultrasound Med. 1995;14(10):767-9.
8. Abramowitz Y, Simanovsky N, Goldstein MS, et al. Pleural effusion: Characterisation with CT attenuation values and CT appearance. AJR. 2009;192:618-23.
9. Halvorsen RA, Fedyshin PJ, Korobkin M, et al. Ascitis or pleural effusion? CT differentiation: four useful criteria. Radiographics. 1986;6:135-49.
10. Dwyer RA. The displaced crus: A sign for distinguishing between pleural fluid and ascitis on computed tomography. Comput Assist Tomog. 1978;2:598.
11. Baysal T, Bulut T, Gokirmak M. Diffusion weighted MR imaging of pleural fluid: Differentiation of transudative vs exudative pleural effusions. Eur Radiol. 2004;14:890-6.
12. Ivan N, Arsalan A, Akansel G, et al. Diffusion weighted MRI in the characterization of pleural effusions: Diag Interv Radiol. 2009;15(1):13-18.
13. Chen HJ, Yu YH, Tu CY, et al. Ultrasound in peripheral pulmonary air fluid lesions: Colour Doppler imaging as an aid in differentiating empyema and abscess. Chest. 2009;135(6):1426-32.
14. Kuhlman JE, Singha NK. Complex disease of the pleural space: Radiographic and CT evaluation. Radiographics. 1997;17:63-97.
15. Kuhlman JE. Complex disease of the pleural space: The 10 questions most frequently asked of the radiologist-new approaches to their answers with CT and MR imaging. Radiographics. 1997;17:1043-50.
16. Stark DD, Federle MP, Goodman PC, et al. Differentiating lung abscess and empyema: Radiography and computed tomography. Am J Roentgenol. 1983;141:163-67.
17. Leung AN, Muller NL, Miller RR. CT in differential diagnosis of diffuse pleural disease. Am J Roentgenol. 1990;154: 487-92.
18. Neff CC, vanSonnerberg E, Lawson DW, et al. CT follow-up of empyemas: Pleural peels resolve after percutaneous catheter drainage. Radiology. 1990;176:195-97.
19. Seo H, Kim TJ, Jin KN, et al. Multi-detector row computed tomographic evaluation of bronchopleural fistula: correlation with clinical, bronchoscopic and surgical findings. J Comput Assit Tomogr. 2010;34(1):13-8.
20. McLoud TC, Woods BO, Carrington CB, et al. Diffuse pleural thickening in the asbestos-exposed population. Am J Roentgenol. 1985;144:9-18.
21. Lynch DA, Gamsu G, Aberle DR. Conventional and high-resolution tomography in the diagnosis of asbestos-related diseases. Radiographics. 1989;9:523-51.
22. Renner RR, Pernice NJ. The apical cap: Semin Roentgenol. 1977;12:299-302.
23. Cugell DW, Kamp DW. Asbestos and the pleura—a review. Chest. 2004;125(3):1103-17.
24. Roach HD, Davies GJ, Attanoos R. Asbestos: when the dust settles an imaging review of asbestos-related disease. Radiographics. 2002;S167-84.
25. Gordon R. The deep sulcus sign. Radiology. 1980;136:25-7.
26. Kirkpatrick AW, Sirois M, Laupland KB, et al. Hand-held thoracic sonography for detecting post-traumatic pneumothoraces: The Extended Focussed Assessment with Sonography for Trauma (EFAST). J Trauma. 2004;57:288-95.
27. De Luca C, Valentino M, Rimondi M, et al. Use of chest sonography in acute care radiology. J Ultrasound. 2008;11:25-34.
28. Barillari A,Kiuru S. Detection of spontaneous pneumothorax with chest ultrasound in emergency department. Intern Emerg Med. 2010;1:253-5.
29. Lichtenstein DA, Menu Y. A Bedside ultrasound sign ruling out pneumothorax in the critically ill-lung sliding. Chest. 1995;108:1345-8.
30. Lichtenstein D, Meziere G, Biderman P. The lung point: An ultrasound sign specific to pneumothorax. Intensive care Med. 2000;26:1434-40.
31. Lichtenstein DA, Meziere G, Lascols N, et al. Ultrasound diagnosis of occult pneumothorax. Crit care Med. 2005;33:1231-8.
32. Cunnigham J, Kirkpatrick AW, Nicolaous, et al. Enhanced recognition of "lung sliding"with power colour Doppler imaging in the diagnosis of pneumothorax. J Trauma. 2002;52:769-71.
33. Choi BG, Park SH, Yun EH, et al. Pneumothorax size:correlation of supine anteroposterior with erect posteroanterior chest radiograph. Radiology. 1998;209: 567-9.
34. Dynes MC, White EM, Fry WA, et al. Imaging manifestations of pleural tumors. Radiographics. 1992;12:1191-201.
35. Wang ZJ, Reddy GB, Gotway MB, et al. Malignant pleural mesothelioma: Evaluation with CT, MR imaging and PET. Radiographics. 2004;24(1):105-19.
36. Yanamuro M, Gerbando VH, Gill RR, et al. Morphological and functional imaging of malignant pleural mesothelioma. Eur Radiol. 2007;64(3):355-66.
37. Nickell LT, Licchtenberger JP, Khorashadi L, et al. Multimodality imaging for characterisation, classification and staging of malignant pleural mesothelioma. Radiographics. 2014;34: 1692-706.
38. Rusch VW. A proposed new international TNM staging system for malignant pleural mesothelioma: from the International Mesothelioma Interest Group. Chest. 1995; 108(4):1122-8.
39. Coolen J, Keyzer FD, Nafleux P, et al. Malignant pleural mesothelioma: Visceral assessment by using pleural pointillism at diffusion weighted MR imaging. Radiology. 2015;274: 576-84
40. Rosado-de-christenson ML, Abbot GF, Mc Adams HP, et al. Localised fibrous tumours of the pleura. Radiographics. 2003;23(3):759-83.

CHAPTER

139

Imaging of the Diaphragm and Chest Wall

Ujjwal Gorsi, Sameer Vyas, Anupam Lal

EMBRYOLOGY AND ANATOMY

Diaphragm is a thin dome-shaped musculotendinous structure which serves two important functions: (1) it acts as a physical barrier between the thoracic and abdominal cavities, (2) It is the chief muscle of inspiration. Embryologically, it develops from septum transversum, pleuroperitoneal membranes, dorsal mesentery of the esophagus, and muscular body wall. Diaphragm develops during 4–12 weeks of embryogenesis.[1] The anteriorly placed septum transversum forms the central tendon of the diaphragm. Septum transversum fuses with pleura-peritoneal membranes and esophageal mesentery posteriorly and gets attached to the muscular body wall laterally to form diaphragm.

The peripheral muscular part of diaphragm arises from the margin of the thoracic outlet and is inserted into a trefoil-shaped central tendon. The muscular fibers arise from three sources and may be grouped into three parts, two slips from the back of the xiphoid (sternal part), muscle fibers arising circumferentially from inner surfaces of the cartilages and the adjacent parts of lower six ribs of each side interlocking with fibers of the transversus abdominis (costal part), and from the superior three lumbar vertebrae by the right and left crura (lumbar part) that unite anterior to the aortic hiatus to form the median arcuate ligament **(Fig. 1)**.[1,2] Lateral to the crura, the diaphragm arise from the arcuate ligaments (medial and lateral) which are the thickened fascia of the quadratus lumborum and psoas.The anterior muscle fibers are shorter than the posterior ones, which gives the diaphragm its characteristic dome-shaped configuration.

There are three openings in the normal diaphragm **(Fig. 2)**; aortic hiatus, esophageal hiatus and the hiatus for inferior vena cava (IVC). Aortic hiatus (osseoaponeurotic opening) is at level of 12th thoracic vertebra (T12). The aorta, thoracic duct, azygos and hemiazygos veins course through this hiatus. Decussation of the medial fibers of the right crus at level of T10 forms esophageal hiatus which gives passage to esophagus, vagus, sympathetic nerves and left gastric vessels. IVC hiatus is in the central tendon at level of T 8–9 and transmits IVC and branches of the right phrenic nerve.

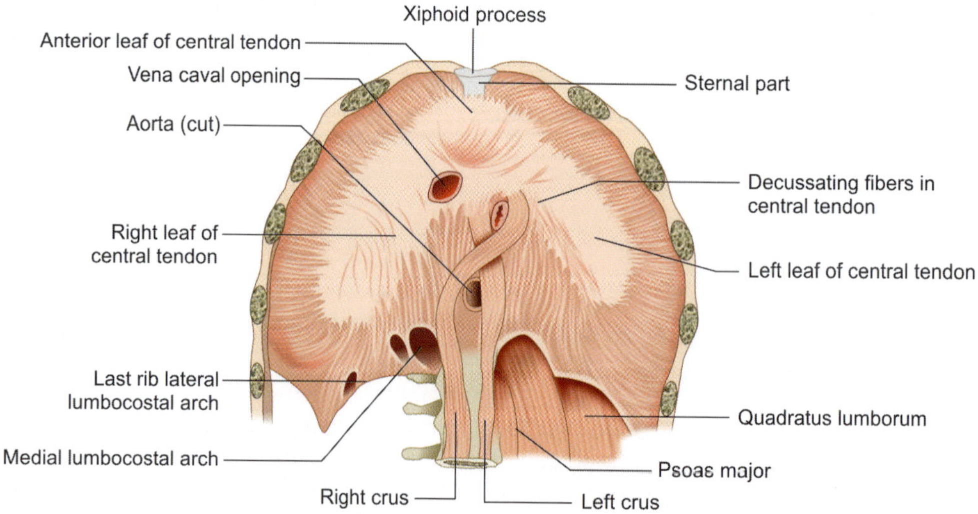

FIG. 1: Schematic diagram of diaphragm as viewed from abdominal aspect.

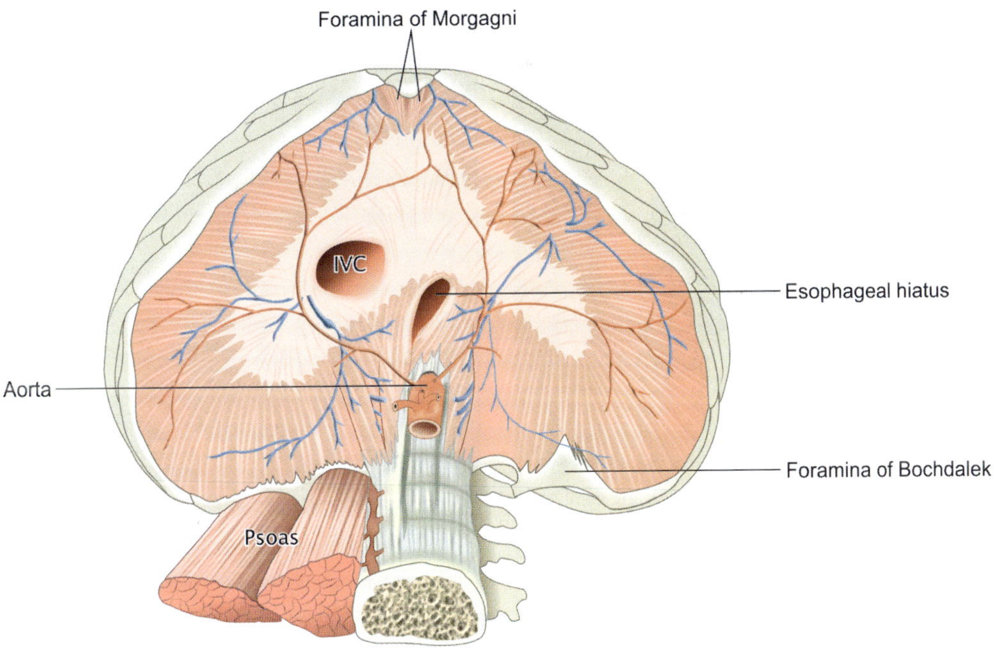

FIG. 2: Schematic diagram of diaphragm showing the hiatuses as viewed from its caudal aspect (IVC: inferior vena cava).

Nerve supply of the diaphragm is from left and right phrenic nerves, which arise from C3–C5 cervical nerves and have sensory as well as motor function.

FUNCTIONS

The main function of the diaphragm is to act as a muscle of respiration. It contracts along with sternocleidomastoid, scalene, and intercostal muscles which are the accessory muscles of respiration, during inspiration. This contraction causes expansion of thoracic cavity and reduces the intrathoracic pressure due to which air is drawn into the lungs. During expiration, along with elastic recoil of the lungs, diaphragm relaxes. The diaphragm, by increasing intra-abdominal pressure helps in urination, defecation and emesis. In addition diaphragm helps in preventing gastroesophageal reflux as it exerts external pressure at the esophageal opening.[1]

IMAGING MODALITIES

Imaging modalities for diaphragmatic disorders include plain radiography, fluoroscopy, ultrasonography, CT and MRI.

Plain Radiograph

Normal diaphragm is not separately identifiable on a chest X-ray. On a chest X-ray, usually the top of the abdominal cavity which normally represents the upper abdominal organs such as liver, stomach, spleen, or colon with the overlying diaphragm and is opaque on radiograph is spoken off as diaphragm. It is visualized as a distinct entity only if outlined by air on both the sides, i.e. on thoracic and abdominal sides **(Fig. 3)**. On inspiration, the domes of diaphragm are at the level of the sixth rib anteriorly and at or below the tenth rib posteriorly. The right hemidiaphragm is 1.5–2.5 cm higher than the left in most individuals. In about 9%, the two hemidiaphragm are at the same level, and the left hemidiaphragm is up to 1 cm higher than right in few normal individuals.[3] On lateral radiograph, both the domes project on each other. Right and left domes can be easily differentiated from each other by the fact that the anterior part of the left hemidiaphragm is mostly obscured by the heart, whereas the right dome can be seen in its entirety. On the left lateral view, the posterior part of the right dome projects under the left dome. The IVC stops at the right hemidiaphragm while stomach bubble or gas in splenic flexure is in close contact with the left hemidiaphragm. The distance between the dome of diaphragm and the top of the gastric air bubble of the left hemidiaphragm, is less than 1 cm in most of individuals (about 88%) and is best demonstrated in the lateral view.[2]

Fluoroscopy

The fluoroscopic sniff test is real time fluoroscopic assessment of motor function of diaphragm (excursion). It is commonly used in patients who have breathing difficulties following stroke or in patients who have suffered phrenic nerve palsy to look for absence of muscular contraction of the diaphragm during inspiration.[1]

Ultrasonography

Ultrasonography (USG) is cheap, portable, easily available, radiation risk free imaging modality. Structures above and below the diaphragm can be examined in real time using USG. Structural and functional components of the diaphragm can be assessed with USG even at the bedside. In

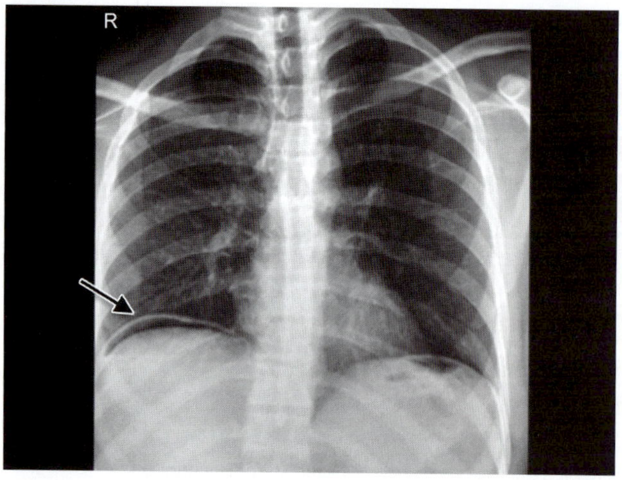

FIG. 3: Chest radiograph showing diaphragm (arrow) clearly identified because of pneumoperitoneum.

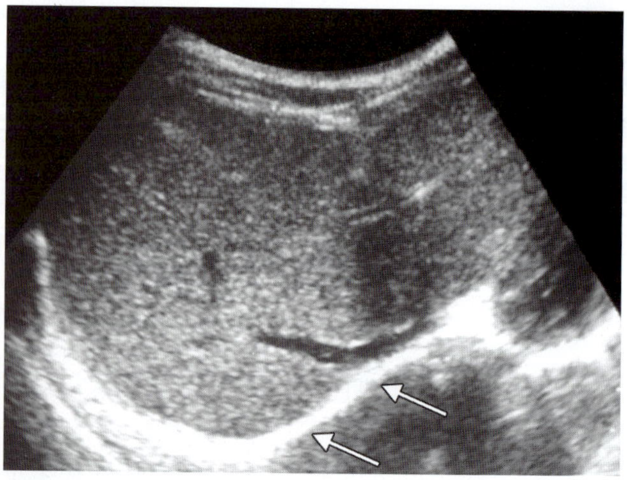

FIG. 4: The transverse ultrasound scan of right hemidiaphragm showing the diaphragm/lung interface as a thick curvilinear echogenic band (arrows). The triangular hypoechoic band between this and the liver is the peripheral muscular bundles of diaphragm.

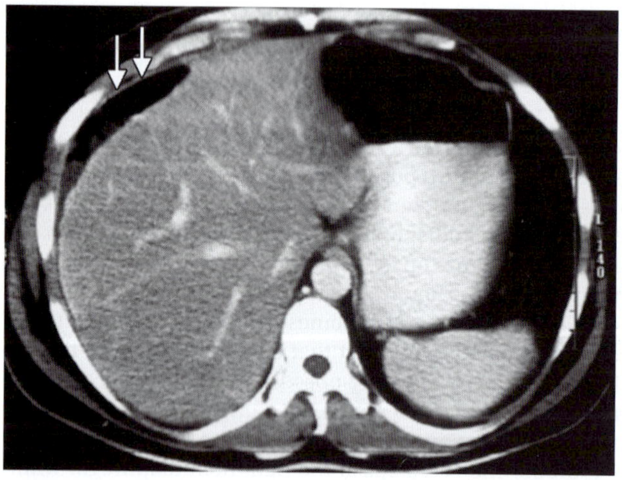

FIG. 5: Axial CT scan showing diaphragm (arrows) outlined by air present in the subphrenic abscess.

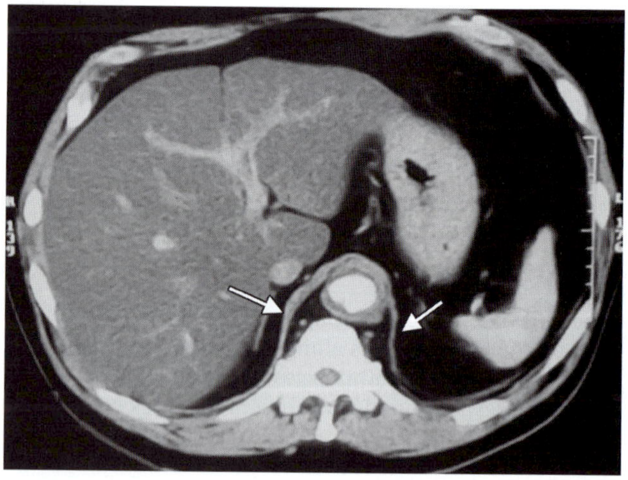

FIG. 6: Axial CT scan of abdomen showing diaphragmatic crura (arrows).

children and young adults, it is preferred imaging technique for interrogating the diaphragm. Ultrasound visualizes the lateral and posterior parts of the diaphragm, instead of anteriorly located central tendon, which is examined by fluoroscopy. Transhepatic and trans-splenic sector scanning is the most appropriate technique to visualize the diaphragm **(Fig. 4)**. Pleural disease can also be used as an acoustic window to study the lateral parts of the dome. The diaphragm itself is seen as a thin hypoechoic line. The interface between diaphragm and liver (or spleen) appears as a thin echogenic line. The interface between diaphragm and lung appears as a stronger and thicker echogenic band. The diaphragm can be clearly visualized on USG when pleural effusion and ascites are present at the same time. B mode USG can assess both echogenicity and thickness of the diaphragm where as M mode ultrasound by assessing a specific site over time can evaluate excursion, velocity, and response to phrenic nerve stimulation.[4]

Computed Tomography

The diaphragmatic disorders are usually difficult to assess with computed tomography (CT) in axial plane, because of the tangential course of the diaphragm to the imaging plane. However, with the arrival of the multidetector CT (MDCT) and use of multiplanar reconstructions various diaphragmatic pathologies and injuries can be easily demonstrated **(Fig. 5)**.[5] The costal part of the diaphragm is frequently seen as a stripe of soft tissue between the aerated lung above and fat below. The sternal part is sometimes visualized as linear soft tissue densities anterior to the heart. The crura appear as smooth linear densities that decussate ventral to the aorta at the cranial level and are located lateral to the aorta at the more caudal level **(Fig. 6)**. Crus of the diaphragm extend up to third lumbar vertebra on the right side and up to second lumbar vertebra on the left side. As the right crus extend far below the left it can be mistaken for a lymph node.

Magnetic Resonance Imaging

Coronal and sagittal MR images provide the best way to evaluate the relationship and involvement of the diaphragm to pathologic processes such as hernia, infection, and tumor.[6] MR can easily identify congenital, acquired and traumatic diaphragmatic hernias which commonly present as thoracic masses. In all MRI sequences, diaphragm has signal intensity which is lower than other skeletal muscles. It is excellent for demonstrating the extent and anatomic relationships of juxtadiaphragmatic tumors and can help to identify the location of peridiaphragmatic fluid collections. However, the respiratory motion may impair imaging of the normal diaphragm. In addition to morphologic abnormalities, MRI can be helpful in evaluating functional disorders of the diaphragm. With the advent of faster MR imaging, such as 'Gradient Recalled Echo' (GRE), it is possible to obtain sequential dynamic images of the diaphragm during real-time breathing, which can be viewed as cine loops.[6] This approach allows for the evaluation of diaphragmatic motion without the use of ionizing radiation. MRI allows quantitative evaluation, including the synchronicity, excursion, and velocity of motion of diaphragm.[7]

Radionuclide Scan

The role of radionuclide scans in assessing diaphragmatic pathology is limited. Most of the scans are performed for assessing diaphragmatic integrity in occult cases where the radiologic imaging is equivocal. Intraperitoneal injection of technetium sulfur colloid and subsequent scintigraphy has been shown to be a sensitive test for the diagnosis of diaphragmatic laceration. Radionuclide liver-spleen imaging with ^{99m}Tc sulfur colloid permits assessment of liver and splenic injuries and also their herniation into thorax in cases of traumatic diaphragmatic hernias.[8]

NORMAL VARIANTS

Scalloping

Appear as short curves of diaphragm which are convex upwards. It gives poly arcuate appearance and seen in approximately 5% individuals. They are commonly seen on the right side, and in patients with pulmonary emphysema or pneumothorax. Muscle slips: appear as small curved lines which are concave upwards and are common on the right side. They are commonly seen in tall, thin patients and in those with emphysema. Diaphragmatic humps and dromedary diaphragm: represents mild forms of eventration with incomplete muscularization of the hemidiaphragm but there is no muscle defect. They are commonly seen on right side and anteriorly.

Eventration

Eventration is a congenital anomaly with failure of muscular development of part or all of one or both hemidiaphragms. Total eventration of a hemidiaphragm is more common on the left side which is often associated with torsion or volvulus of the stomach **(Fig. 7)**. Partial eventration is more common on right side and frequently involves its anteromedial portion. On chest radiography, partial eventration is seen as a semioval or semicircular homogeneous opacity which has soft tissue density arising from the diaphragm.[2,3] On deep inspiration, eventration becomes more apparent as dorsal and lateral part of the diaphragm moves downward whereas convex segment may remain at the same level or shows upward movement. MDCT **(Fig. 8)**, USG and MRI may be required to differentiate eventration from mediastinal pericardial or pleural lesions. Differentiating an eventration involving a large part of a hemidiaphragm from a paralyzed hemidiaphragm and Morgagni hernia with herniation of liver or fat may not be easy at times. The paralyzed hemidiaphragm often has an adjacent area of atelectatic lung on chest X-ray whereas large eventration does not. This is due to the fact that an eventration still has some net inspiratory downward movement while a paralyzed hemidiaphragm has a paradoxical upward motion.

Accessory Diaphragm

It is partial duplication of a hemidiaphragm, almost always seen on the right side. It courses obliquely backward and upward and get attached along the third to seventh ribs. Part

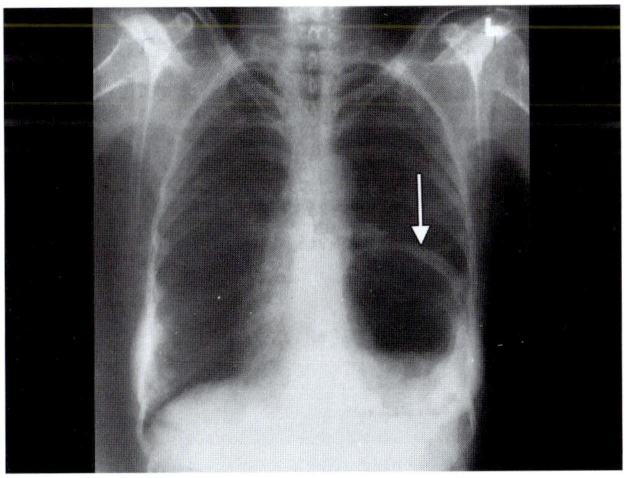

FIG. 7: Chest radiograph showing eventration of the left hemidiaphragm (arrow) with gastric volvulus.

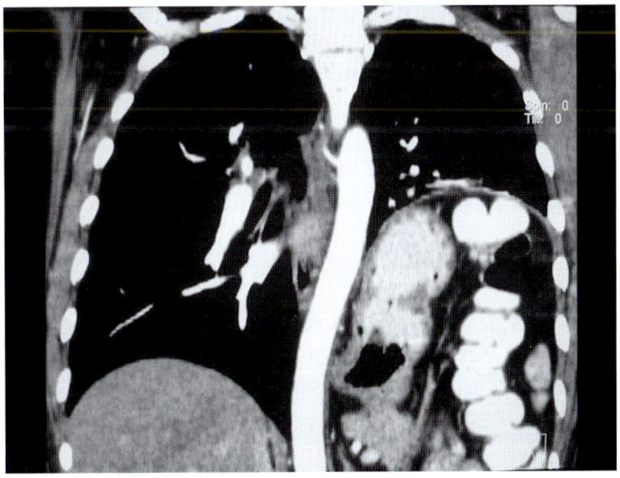

FIG. 8: Coronal reformats of multidetector CT showing eventration of the left hemidiaphragm with intrathoracic herniation of stomach and colon.

of the entire lower lobe is contained between the true and accessory hemidiaphragm. On the frontal view of the chest, the entire hemidiaphragm may be elevated and the heart and mediastinum are shifted to the affected right side. The adjacent right mediastinal margin is indistinct. On the lateral view, the accessory diaphragm appear as an oblique line rising posteriorly.[2]

Elevated Hemidiaphragm

Unilateral Elevation

Causes of a unilateral high hemidiaphragm are eventration, unilateral atelectasis, severe gastric distension, gross hepatomegaly, gross splenomegaly, obstructive emphysema of the contralateral lung, phrenic nerve palsy, subpulmonic effusion, subphrenic abscess, and ipsilateral pulmonary hypoplasia.[2,3]

Bilateral Elevation

Causes of a bilaterally high diaphragm are ascites, pregnancy, hepatosplenomegaly, large intra-abdominal tumors, poor inspiratory effort and causes of unilateral elevation present bilaterally.[2]

Low Lying Diaphragm

May be seen in cases of hyperinflated lungs, intrathoracic masses, and large pleural effusions.

Inversion of the Diaphragm

Represents reverse curvature of the diaphragm and can be partial or complete. It can occur with tension pneumothorax, large basal bulla, large pleural effusion or large tumors. The condition is usually seen on the left side as the right dome is somewhat protected by the underlying liver. An inverted diaphragm rises actively on inspiration and falls on expiration, resulting in paradoxical movement of the diaphragm and mediastinal shift toward the affected side during inspiration.

Peridiaphragmatic Collections

For localization of peridiaphragmatic collections, identification of the diaphragm is the key factor.[3] Accurate localization of a fluid collection in sub- or supradiaphragmatic location at times may be difficult on cross-sectional imaging. USG, CT and MRI are helpful in differentiating subdiaphragmatic (ascites) vs supradiaphragmatic (pleural) fluid **(Figs. 9 and 10)**.[9] On axial CT images, a number of CT signs are helpful in differentiating ascites from pleural effusion **(Table 1)**.

DIAPHRAGMATIC MOVEMENTS

Abnormal movement of the diaphragm during respiration is an important radiologic sign of diaphragmatic or juxtadiaphragmatic disease. Fluoroscopy, ultrasound and MRI may be employed for assessing diaphragmatic movements.[4,6] The normal amplitude of the motion ranges from 0.8 to 8 cm in normal, healthy, young adults. Most (77%) individuals may show asymmetry of diaphragmatic motion when observed on fluoroscopy, although the difference in excursion is usually less than 1 cm.[3] Minor asynchronous motion of the hemidiaphragm and even momentary minimal paradoxical movement may be seen. The dome also may move differently from the rest of the diaphragm. In the lateral decubitus position, the dependent hemidiaphragm rises higher than usual and its respiratory excursion is greatly exaggerated. Abnormal diaphragmatic movement can be classified into three types, paradoxical, complete or incomplete fixation. Paradoxical movement is the upward movement of the affected hemidiaphragm on inspiration instead of the normal descent; complete fixation is no movement of the affected hemidiaphragm during the respiratory cycle; and incomplete fixation is greatly decreased motion of the affected hemidiaphragm on respiration. These three types of abnormal movement can be seen in various conditions including paralysis, eventration, subphrenic abscess, traumatic diaphragmatic hernia, unilateral obstructive emphysema, and pneumothorax. Fluoroscopy and realtime ultrasonography are reliable in assessing diaphragmatic motion.

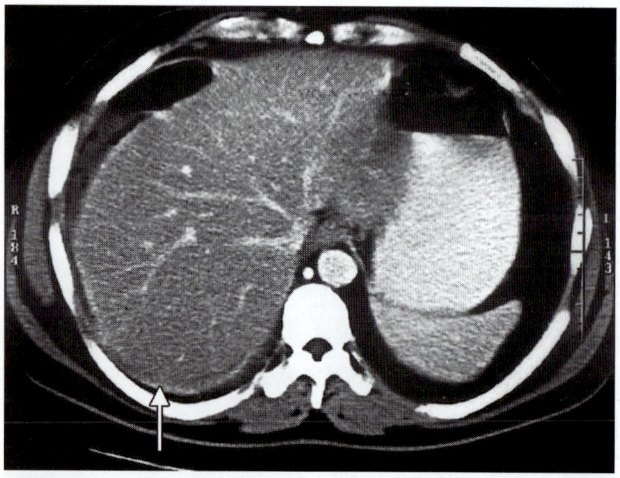

FIG. 9: Axial CT scan showing fluid collection anterior to the posterior aspect of the diaphragm (arrow) is subphrenic in location.

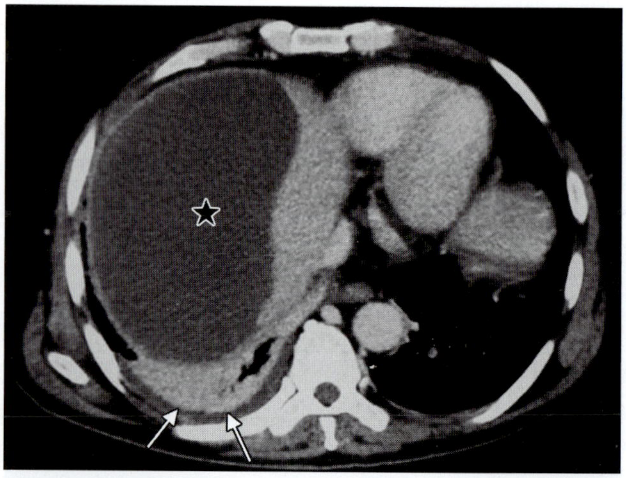

FIG. 10: Axial CT scan of the abdomen showing right pleural effusion (arrows) and subdiaphragmatic collection (star).

TABLE 1: Differences between ascites and pleural effusion on the basis of CT signs.

S. No.	Feature	Ascites	Pleural effusion
1.	Diaphragmatic circle	Center	Outside
2.	Displaced crus sign	Posteromedial	Anterolateral
3.	Bare area sign	Seen	Not seen
4.	Interface (abdominal viscera)	Sharp	Hazy
5.	Lung	Anterior	Surrounds
6.	Caudally	Increases	Decreases
7.	Cranially	Decreases	Increases

DIAPHRAGMATIC WEAKNESS AND PARALYSIS

Weakness or paralysis, of diaphragm may be due to central nervous causes or phrenic nerve involvement due to tumor invasion or thoracic surgery.[9] Paralysis of diaphragm is more often unilateral which is asymptomatic, and is found on imaging incidently. Bilateral diaphragmatic paralysis is mostly symptomatic, and may present with respiratory failure.

On chest radiograph, bilateral diaphragm paralysis is seen as the smooth elevation of the both hemidiaphragms and associated reduced volume of the lungs. The costovertebral and costophrenic sulci become narrow and deep. On lateral view, smooth elevation of diaphragmatic position may be better appreciated. At lung bases linear atelectasis may also be seen. In unilateral diaphragm paralysis, the left hemidiaphragm may lie at or above the right hemidiaphragm. If right hemidiaphragm is paralyzed, it lies more than the one interspace higher than the left side. A paralyzed hemidiaphragm is elevated entirely, including the posterior take off point, this feature helps in differentiating it from eventration. On fluoroscopic sniff test, if unilateral diaphragmatic weakness or paralysis is present, during quiet inspiration, deep inspiration, and sniffing weak side moves more slowly downwards (caudal) or paradoxically upwards (with paralysis).[9] The sniff test is not as useful in patients with bilateral paralysis. Ultrasonography and dynamic MRI are other modalities to assess weakness or paralysis of diaphragm.

DIAPHRAGMATIC HERNIAS

Abdominal viscera can herniate into the thoracic cavity through the diaphragmatic hiatus (sliding and paraesophageal hiatus hernia) or congenital defect (Bochdalek and Morgagni hernia).

Hiatal Hernia

It develops from a weakness or tear (rupture) of the phrenicoesophageal ligament. Sliding hiatus hernias are the most common type (99%) of diaphragmatic hernias. In sliding hernia, the gastroesophageal junction lies above the esophageal hiatus whereas in paraesophageal hernia, all or portion of the stomach herniates into the chest with gastroesophageal junction lying below the diaphragm.

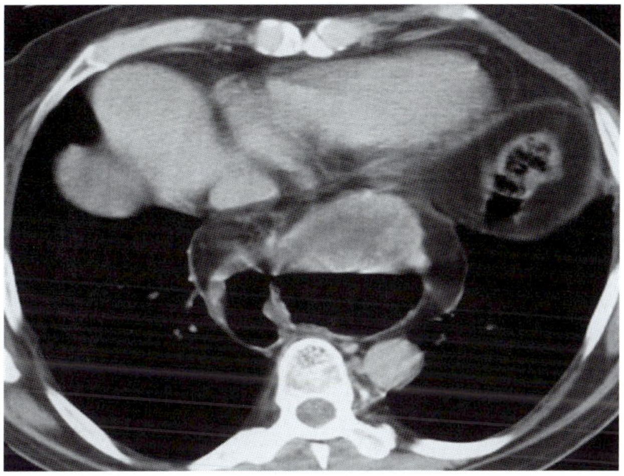

FIG. 11: Axial CT scan of upper abdomen showing large hiatus hernia.

They can be diagnosed by barium examination but cross-sectional imaging (CT, MRI) may show the size, site and content of the hernia. Sliding hernia is diagnosed on barium study when pouch of stomach protrudes more than 2 cm above the hiatus, or three or more gastric folds passing across the hiatus and on CT when the hiatus is wide with diaphragmatic crura separated by more than 15 mm **(Fig. 11)**. In paraesophageal (rolling) hernia, the stomach herniates through widened esophageal hiatus or occasionally through separate diaphragmatic gap to lie alongside the lower esophagus.

Between the eighth and tenth weeks of fetal life, the diaphragm forms and the pleuroperitoneal canals close, dividing the celomic cavity into the abdominal and thoracic cavities. During the same period, the gastrointestinal tract elongates into the umbilical pouch and rotates on its return to the abdominal cavity. The left pleuroperitoneal canal closes slightly later than the right. The interrelationship of these two important developmental events results in the clinical spectrum of diaphragmatic hernias: Bochdalek hernia (posterolateral defect), Morgagni hernia (retrosternal defect), and Intrapericardial hernia (defect of central tendon).

Bochdalek Hernia

It is the most common congenital hernia and involves the posterior defects in the diaphragm caused by defective fusion or maldevelopment of the pleuroperitoneal membranes. Stomach, bowel and even spleen or kidney may herniate into the left hemithorax. On the right side, part of the liver may be found above the diaphragm. Bochdalek hernia occurs in one in 2000–5000 births with involvevment of left hemidiaphragm in 80% of the cases.[10,11] The chest radiograph may show aerated intrathoracic bowel loops and shift of mediastinum to opposite side **(Figs. 12 and 13)**. On CT, Bochdalek hernia often presents as fatty or soft tissue density mass which abuts the posteromedial aspect of either side of diaphragm. With the advent of CT, however, many small asymptomatic defects are being detected in adults. On the lateral chest radiograph,these hernias are seen as a smooth bulge with epicenter approximately 4–5 cm anterior to posterior

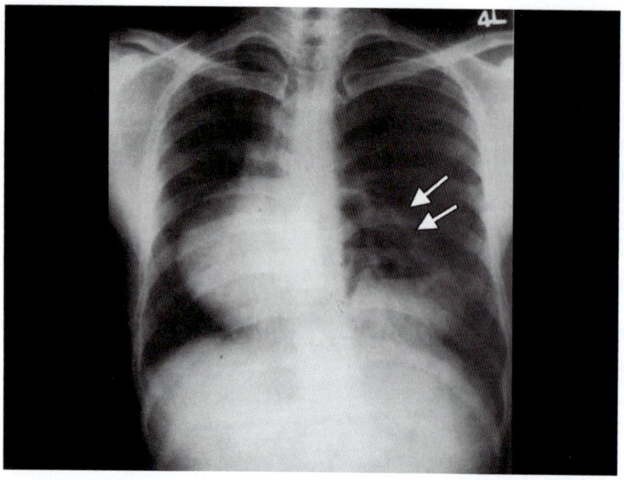

FIG. 12: Bochdalek hernia: Plain radiograph shows herniated bowel loops (arrows) into the thorax and right mediastinal shift.

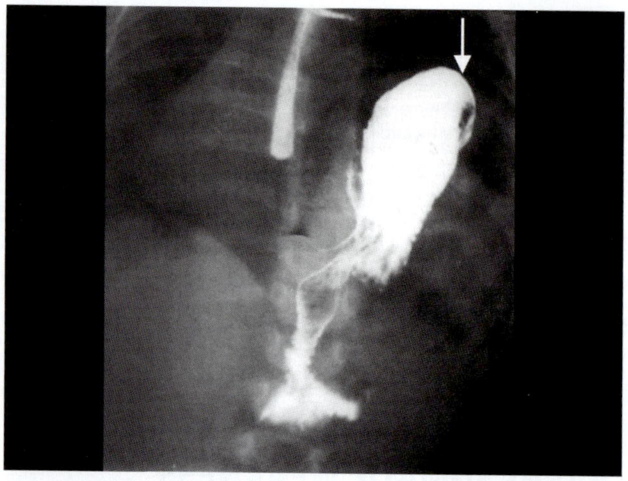

FIG. 13: Bochdalek hernia: Barium study showing herniation of stomach (arrow) into thorax.

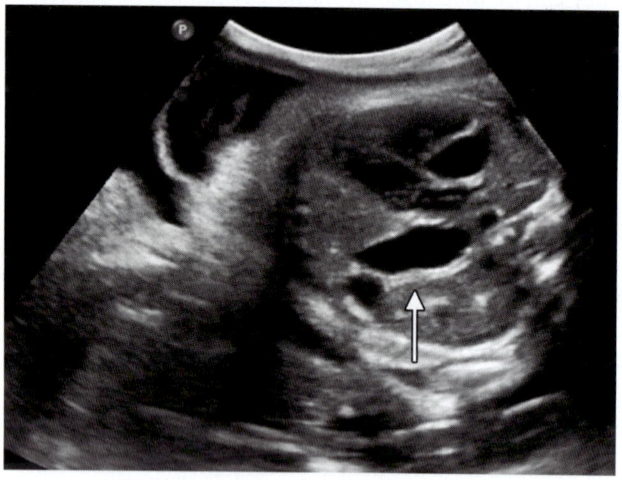

FIG. 14: Congenital diaphragmatic hernia: Antenatal ultrasound showing intrathoracic herniation of stomach (arrow).

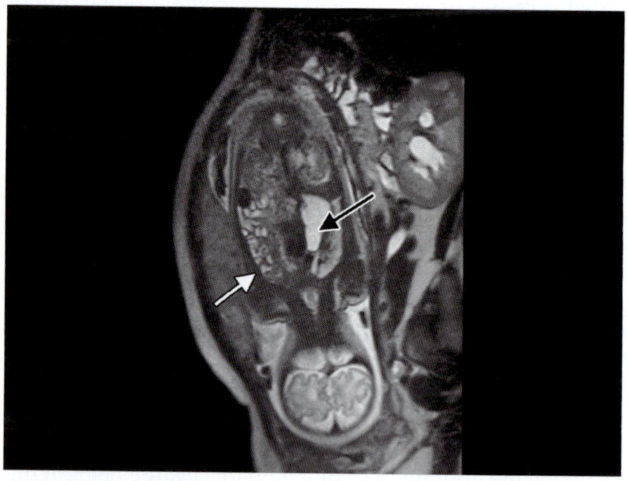

FIG. 15: Bilateral congenital diaphragmatic hernia: Antenatal T2-weighted MR image showing bilateral diaphragmatic hernia with intrathoracic herniation of stomach (black arrow) and bowel loops (white arrow).

costophrenic angle. Antenatal diagnosis of congenital diaphragmatic hernia on ultrasound is suspected when the fetal heart is displaced either by an intrathoracic solid mass (liver, kidney) or by a fluid filled structure (stomach, bowel) with decreased abdominal circumference **(Fig. 14)**.[10,11] MRI can also be extremely helpful modality to look for congenital diaphragmatic hernia **(Fig. 15)**. Pulmonary hypoplasia often results from compression of the fetal lung by the herniated viscera.

Morgagni Hernia

It is commonly seen in adults and is mostly asymptomatic. It is due to the failure of fusion between the fibrotendinous elements of the sternal part and costal part of developing diaphragm. In Morgagni hernia, peritoneum or abdominal contents pass upwards through foramen of Morgagni in retro or para-sternal location into the thoracic cavity. In Morgagni hernia, weak area is congenital however the herniation of the abdominal contents is often acquired and conditions causing increase intra-abdominal pressure like severe effort, obesity and trauma. Morgagni hernia is mostly right sided because the the left sided defects are covered by heart and pericardium. On chest radiograph, a Morgagni hernia containing fat or liver presents as a rounded density occupying the right anterior cardiophrenic angle. Herniated organs and diaphragm defect are better evaluated by CT and MRI **(Fig. 16)**.

Intrapericardial Hernia

It results from herniation of abdominal viscera into the pericardial sac through a defect of the central tendon of the diaphragm but is extremely rare.

DIAPHRAGMATIC INJURY

Both blunt and penetrating injuries can injure diaphragm. Diaphragmatic injuries are usually caused blunt trauma

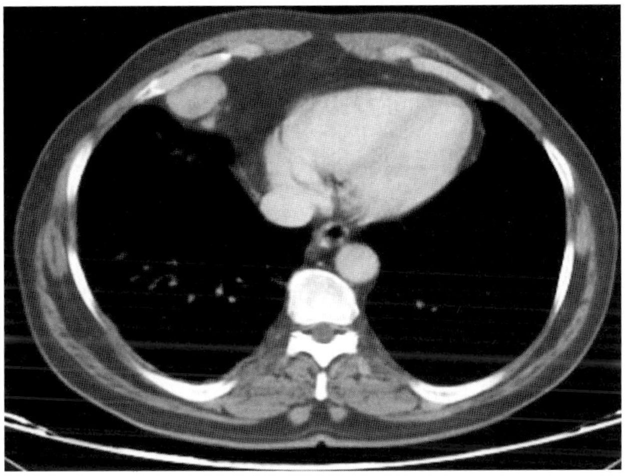

FIG. 16: Morgagni hernia: Axial CT scan of the abdomen showing fatty lesion with traversing vessels in right paracardiac region.

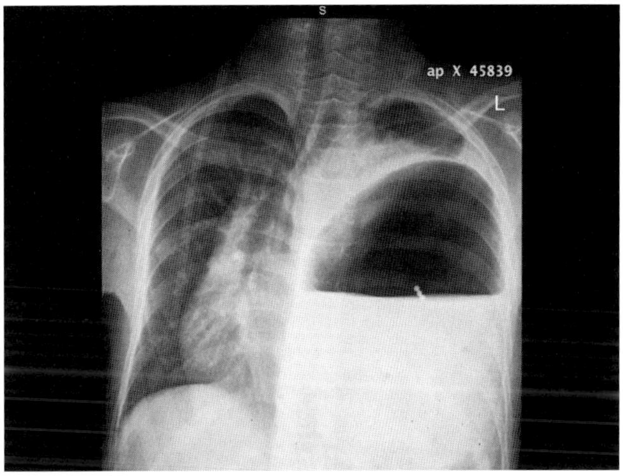

FIG. 17: Chest radiograph with left diaphragm tear showing intrathoracic herniation of the stomach with contralateral mediastinal shift.

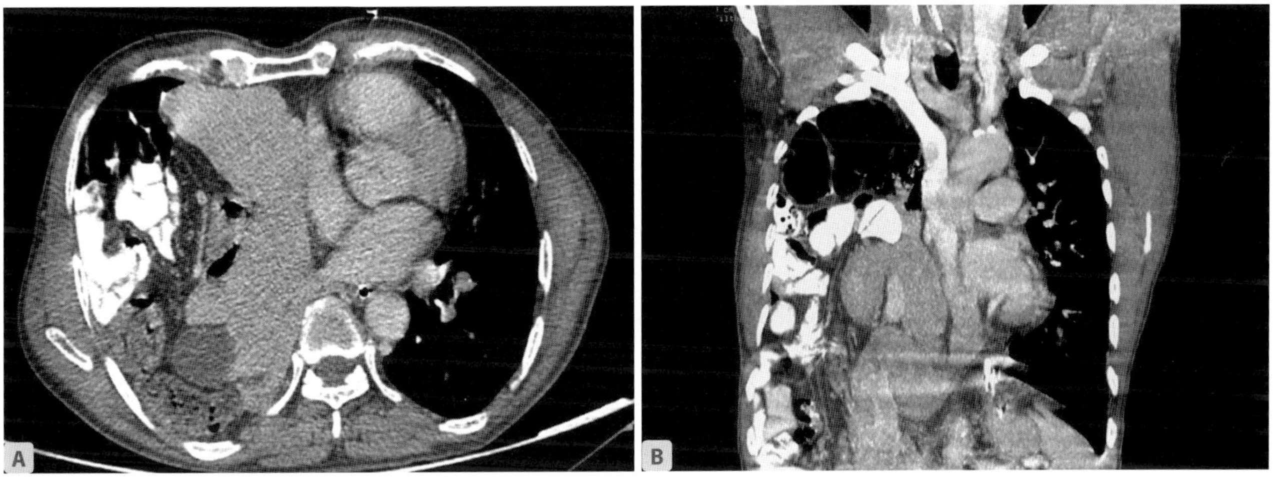

FIGS. 18A AND B: Traumatic right diaphragmatic hernia. (A) Axial and (B) coronal CECT sections show right diaphragmatic hernia with herniation of both hollow and solid viscera.

or penetrating injuries. They occur in 0.8–8% after blunt trauma.[12] The confusing clinical and radiographic findings can delay the diagnosis. Tear is left sided in 70–90% and right sided in 10–30% in blunt trauma patients. This is attributed to the protection offered by the liver. The stomach is the most commonly herniated organ, but bowel, spleen, liver and omentum can also herniate into the chest **(Fig. 17)**. The chest X-ray remains valuable in the acute phase for detection of diaphragmatic injuries, despite its technical limitations which include supine positioning, use of portable radiography and limited patient cooperation. Specific diagnostic findings of the injury include the following: asymmetry of a hemidiaphragm or changing hemidiaphragm levels, intrathoracic herniation of the hollow viscus which may be associated with focal constriction of the viscus at the site of the tear called collar sign. On left side, nasogastric tube may be seen above the hemidiaphragm.[6] Nonspecific X-ray finding are rib fractures, hemo- or pneumothorax, and atelectasis at the lung bases.

CT is usually the next imaging modality in trauma patients because of speed and global information provided. Multidetector CT (MDCT) with multiplanar reconstructions is very valuable diagnostic tool. MDCT features of the diaphragmatic trauma include direct visualization of injury, diaphragm thickening, segmental diaphragm non visualization, viscera herniation **(Figs. 18A and B)**, dependent viscera sign, the collar sign, and peridiaphragmatic active contrast extravasation.[12,13] Direct visualization of injury is often possible by depicting the free edge of the disrupted diaphragm. Isolated segmental nonvisualization of the diaphragm is highly sensitive but this sign must be used with caution when seen in isolation, especially in the elderly, in whom it can be a normal variant. Intrathoracic herniation of viscera has high specificity but have variable sensitivity. If an abdominal structure herniates through a diaphragm rent, the free edges of the diaphragm can constrict the herniated organ, and hence result in a "collar". The **collar sign (Fig. 19)** is an indication of intrathoracic herniation of abdominal contents even when its relative level does not clearly suggest so. When the diaphragm is torn, its constraints are released, and the viscera may lie "dependent" against

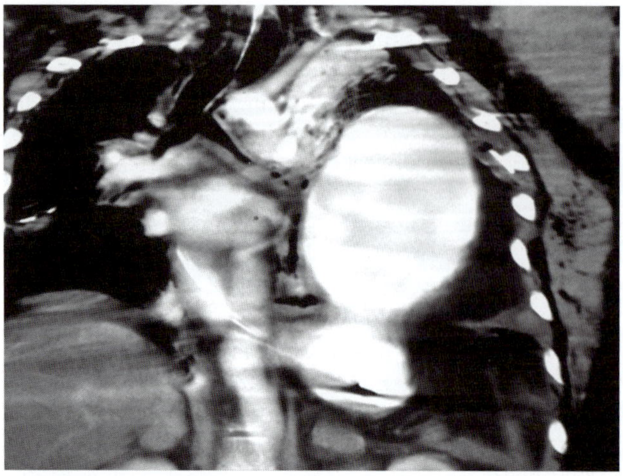

FIG. 19: Collar sign: MDCT with coronal reformation showing intrathoracic herniation of stomach through left diaphragmatic defect with constriction of stomach by the free edges of diaphragm at the site of herniation.

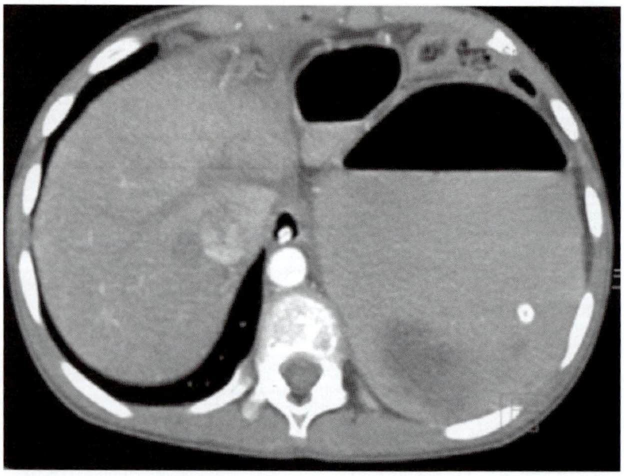

FIG. 20: Dependent viscera sign: CT axial sections showing intrathoracic herniation of the stomach through left diaphragmatic rupture and the stomach lying in a dependent position against the posterior ribs.

the posterior chest wall as compared to the normal intact diaphragm which prevents the upper abdominal viscera from contacting the chest wall **(Fig. 20)**. The diaphragm is considered abnormally thickened by subjective comparison with the contra lateral side or diaphragmatic crus thickness more than 10 mm. In the presence of injury, intramuscular hematoma or edema or muscle retraction accounts for the abnormally thick diaphragm.

MRI is helpful in equivocal cases of diaphragmatic injury. Direct coronal and sagittal imaging with respiratory and cardiac gating may allow confirmation or exclusion of the diagnosis. Diaphragmatic signal may be interrupted due to the laceration hence confirm a traumatic diaphragmatic injury. [13] Barium studies allow confirmation of herniated intestine or stomach but are limited to evaluation of the hollow viscera. Fluoroscopic demonstration of severely decreased motion is highly suggestive but not diagnostic of injury. USG signs include herniation of viscera, diaphragm disruption, diaphragm non-visualization, and absent diaphragm excursion during the respiratory cycle.

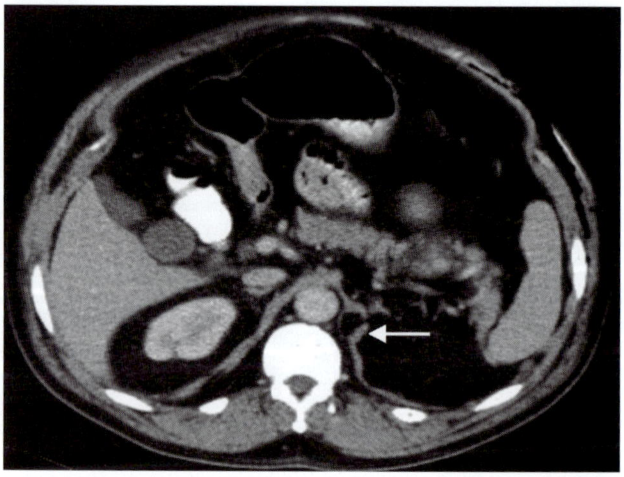

FIG. 21: Lipoma: CT axial sections showing well-marginated fat density lesion in the left crus of the diaphragm.

TUMORS OF THE DIAPHRAGM

Tumors of the diaphragm are rare. The most common benign solid tumor is a lipoma **(Fig. 21)**. Benign tumors of the diaphragm may be removed surgically if there is a doubt about the diagnosis or they are symptomatic. Fibroma, angiofibroma, neurofibroma and neurilemmoma are the other benign tumors. The most common primary malignant tumor of diaphragm is rhabdomyosarcoma.[14] Metastatic neoplasms of the diaphragm may be due to direct invasion from tumors of adjacent organs. These include tumors of the lung, liver, stomach, colon pancreas, adrenal or liver. Cystic lesions of the diaphragm can be acquired or congenital. The most common benign cystic lesions of the diaphragm are bronchogenic or mesothelial cysts.[14] Acquired cysts include simple, fibrous lined and post-traumatic cysts. Hydatid disease and tuberculosis rarely cause inflammatory mass of the diaphragm. The majority of patients present with pleuritic chest pain. Radiographically, a mass which abuts the diaphragm is seen. Imaging modalities like CT and MRI are provide a specific diagnosis and look for extent of the tumor.

CHEST WALL

The chest wall structures are grouped into soft tissue and bony structures on the basis of the radiographic appearances. The soft tissue structures include muscles of the chest wall, breasts, fat, nerves, blood and lymphatic vessels. The bony structures include ribs, costal cartilages, sternum, clavicles and spine. Chest wall may be affected by a variety of disorders affecting these constituents. Chest radiography may be the first imaging study to suggest the presence of a chest wall mass given its widespread availability and utilization. However, it is difficult to detect, localize and characterize these disorders by means of conventional radiography alone most of the times and cross-sectional imaging such as MDCT and MRI, helps in the evaluation of these disorders and sometimes allow definitive diagnosis.[15] MDCT and MRI help in knowing the extent and character of the diseases. CT helps in better depiction of small calcifications and bone destruction whereas MRI in marrow involvement and soft tissue extension. Multiplanar imaging and three-dimensional (3D) reconstructions can be achieved with both modalities. Ultrasound generally provides less detailed information as compared to CT and MRI however it can be very helpful at times in localizing the lesion. It also helps in differentiating cystic and solid lesions and can characterize cystic lesions. It also provides imaging guidance for aspiration and biopsy when cytological/histopathological diagnosis is required. 2-(fluorine-18) fluoro-2-deoxyd- glucose (FDG) positron emission tomography (PET)/CT is not performed commonly to evaluate chest wall tumors, because many primary and secondary malignancies may demonstrate increased FDG uptake. PET/CT may be used, however, to determine the presence and extent of metastatic disease and assess response to therapy.[16]

Diseaes affecting chest wall can be grouped into congenital and developmental anomalies, inflammatory and infectious diseases and various primary and secondary tumors.[15]

CONGENITAL AND DEVELOPMENTAL ANOMALIES

Funnel Chest (Pectus Excavatum or Depressed Sternum)

It is the most common congenital anomaly affecting sternum. In this deformity, sternum is depressed and on each side ribs extent beyond the sternum anteriorly. Postero-anterior radiograph shows shift of the heart to the left, straightening of the left heart border with prominence of the main pulmonary artery segment, loss of the descending aortic interface, and an increase in the opacity in the right cardio-phrenic angle **(Figs. 22A and B)**.[15] The extent of sternal depression is evaluated easily at lateral radiograph and the severity can be best quantified with CT. MDCT is usually reserved for the individuals in whom surgery is planned. Severity may be graded using the Haller index. Haller index is ratio of the maximum internal transverse diameter of the chest divided by the minimum anteroposterior diameter. An index of >3.25 require correction surgically. Haller index ranges from 1.9 to 2.7 in normal children.[17]

Pigeon Chest (Pectus Carinatum)

It is less common than pectus excavatum. It may be congenital or acquired. In this condition, there is convex anterior protrusion of the sternum and costochondral joints and results due to disproportionate overgrowth of the costochondral cartilages. It is considered cosmetic deformity only and may be associated with family history, connective tissue disease and scoliosis.[18]

Poland Syndrome

In this syndrome, there is partial or total absence of pectoralis major muscles with ipsilateral hand and arm anomalies (particularly syndactyly). Radiograph shows an area of hyperlucency on the affected side and abnormal axillary fold. CT and MRI shows the absence of the muscles and associated anomalies.[15]

Cervical Rib

Cervical rib commonly originates from the seventh cervical vertebra. Usually, it is found in approximately 0.5% of the general population. In 90% of the cases its asymptomatic. It is seen as supernumerary rib that articulates with cervical-type transverse process which is horizontal as compared to upward-sloping thoracic transverse process of thoracic vertebra. MDCT helps in showing relationship between vascular compression and bony deformity.

Clavicles

It may be hypoplastic in number of syndromes including cleidocranial dysplasia, Holt-Oram syndrome,

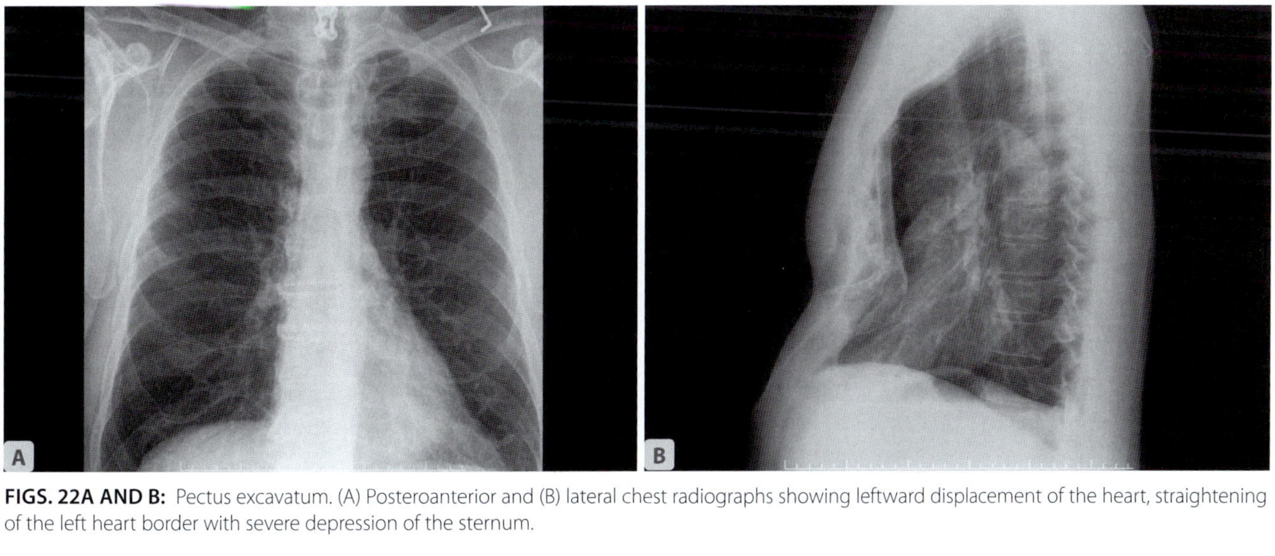

FIGS. 22A AND B: Pectus excavatum. (A) Posteroanterior and (B) lateral chest radiographs showing leftward displacement of the heart, straightening of the left heart border with severe depression of the sternum.

pelvic-shoulder dysplasia, some trisomy disorders and progeria.

INFLAMMATORY AND INFECTIOUS DISEASES

Primary infections of the chest wall are rare, and are more common in setting of trauma, immunosuppression and diabetes mellitus. They occur more commonly secondary to infectious processes in the lungs or to pleural empyema (empyema necessitatis). Other causes are hematogeneous spread or iatrogenic (median sternotomy for cardiac surgery).

Cellulitis and Necrotizing Fasciitis

Infections of chest wall soft tissues range from cellulitis to infections of deeper soft tissues, including myositis, osteomyelitis, abscess, and necrotizing fasciitis. Cellulitis often appears more extensive on MR imaging than on other imaging modalities because of MR imaging's sensitivity for tissue edema. Cellulitis is characterized by high T2 signal in subcutaneous soft tissues.[19] Necrotizing fasciitis is a serious septic condition more common in immunocompromised, alcoholic, or diabetic patients. It affects subcutaneous fat and the superficial fascia and should not involve the underlying muscles. MRI shows the complete extent of the involvement and CT may show gas formation. In pyomyositis, predominant involvement is of muscles and MRI is the best imaging modality to assess intramuscular necrosis.

Pyogenic Osteomyelitis

Osteomyelitis of the chest wall is frequently associated with periosteal elevation, loss of planes of soft tissue and adjacent soft tissue masses. Common causative organisms are *Staphylococcus aureus* and *Pseudomonas aeruginosa*. CT and MRI can clearly depict the abnormality **(Figs. 23A and B)**. Median sternotomy is the main surgical approach to variety of cardiothoracic procedures. Poststernotomy complications can occur in less than 5% of the cases and include sternal dehiscence, mediastinitis, and osteomyelitis. They manifest usually 1–2 weeks after surgery. CT is useful modality for detecting and localizing retrosternal abscess. Acute mediastinitis at CT show inflammatory tissue replacing mediastinal fat.

Tuberculosis

Chest wall involvement in tuberculosis is commonly due to hematogenous route. However, it may occur as contiguous spread from underlying pleural or pulmonary involvement. It presents as destruction of bone and or cartilage with associated soft tissue mass **(Figs. 24A and B)** which may show rim enhancement and calcifications.

Fungal Infections

Actinomycosis and *Aspergillosis* may infect the chest wall. Actinomycosis may present as sinuses, massive thickening of the soft tissue, wavy periostitis, and underlying rib destruction. *Aspergilosis* involving the chest wall is associated with pulmonary involvement and cause permeative osteolytic destruction of underlying ribs.[15]

TUMORS OF THE CHEST WALL

Chest wall tumors represent approximately 5% of thoracic tumors.[21] These tumors are typically divided into categories based on the site of origin and tissue composition (osseous or soft tissue) as well as whether they are benign or malignant.[16,20] Greater than 50% of chest wall tumors are malignant, and most of these malignancies represent direct invasion by or metastasis from adjacent tumors of the lung, breast, pleura, and mediastinum. The most common primary malignancies of the chest wall are sarcomas, 45% of which arise from soft tissue and 55% of which arise from bone. Once a chest wall mass has been identified, the next step is to determine whether it is malignant or benign. A large soft-tissue mass with invasion into adjacent osseous and/or soft-tissue structures is nearly always malignant.

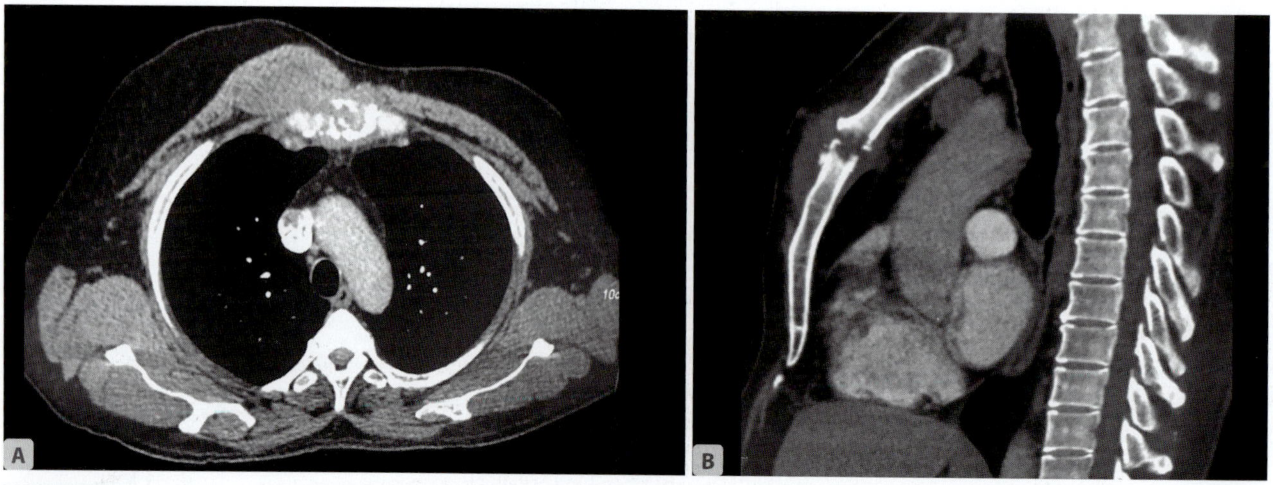

FIGS. 23A AND B: Sternal osteomyelitis. (A) Axial and (B) sagittal MDCT showing expansile lytic desctuction of sterum with associated soft tissue extending both anterior and posterior to sternum.

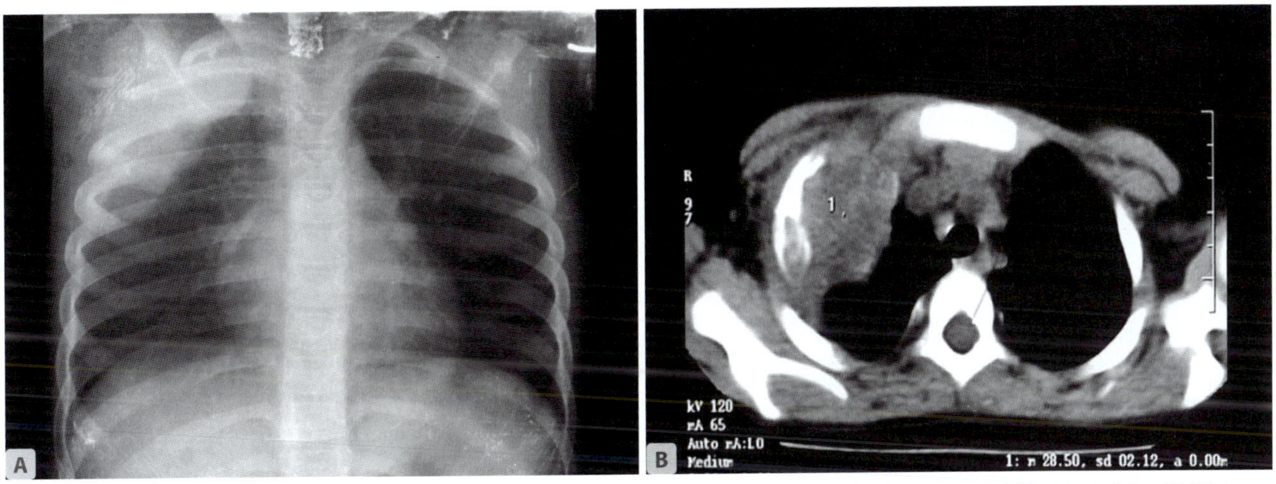

FIGS. 24A AND B: Chest wall tuberculosis. (A) Chest radiograph shows large right upper chest wall soft tissue with destruction of ribs; (B) CT shows expansion and destruction of rib with associated soft tissue. Aspiration from the soft tissue confirmed the lesion to be tubercular.

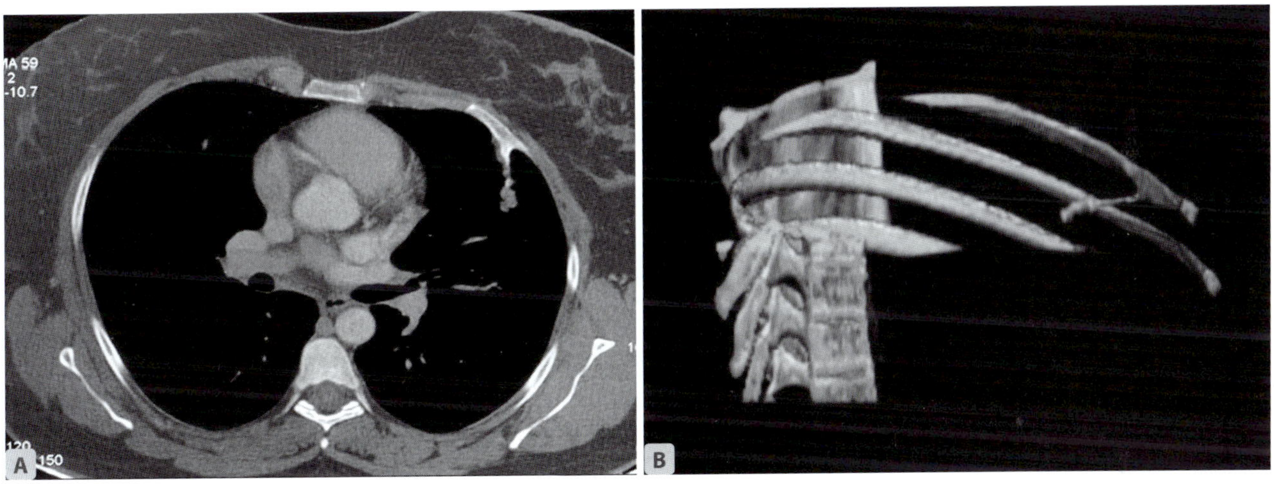

FIGS. 25A AND B: Osteochondroma. (A) Chest CT and (B) 3D bony reformat showing prick-like inward projecting intrathoracic osteochondroma with thickened overlying pleura.

Primary chondrosarcoma or osteosarcoma as well as their metastasis will show characteristic mineralization patter.[16] Benign osseous neoplasms do not result in extraosseous soft-tissue masses unlike their malignant counterpart and mostly exhibit nonaggressive radiological features.

Benign Osseous Tumors

Benign osseous tumors of the chest wall are less frequently encountered than malignant neoplasms. Most of these lesions are osseous or cartilaginous.

Fibrous Dysplasia

Present as fusiform enlargement with cortical thickening and increased trabeculation of involved bones. The ribs are commonly affected, followed by clavicle. This lesion appears lytic or mixed lesion with lytic regions and ground-glass matrix. Osseous erosion is generally not seen.

Osteochondroma

These tumors arise as aberrant growth of normal tissue. These tumors frequently involve costochondral junction of the ribs. Osteochondromas are pedunculated lesions arising from the surface of the bone **(Figs. 25A and B)**. Evaluation of the associated cartilaginous cap should be carefully evaluated, as caps measuring greater than 3 cm in children, greater than 2 cm in adults raises suspicion for malignant transformation.[22]

Aneurysmal Bone Cyst and Giant Cell Tumor

It may involve chest wall. In aneurysmal bone cyst (ABC), the most common sites of involvement is posterior elements of the spine whereas giant cell tumor involves sternum, clavicle and ribs.

Malignant Osseous Tumors

Malignant osseous tumors of the chest wall account for approximately 55% of all chest wall masses.[21] The most common primary malignancies include sarcomas, such as chondrosarcoma, osteosarcoma, the Ewing sarcoma family of tumors (ESFT) as well as multiple myeloma (MM) whereas metastatic disease and direct invasion from intrathoracic malignancies are the most frequent secondary causes.[20]

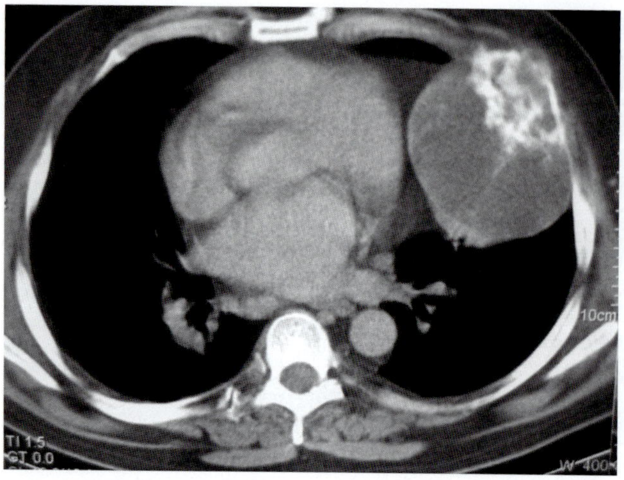

FIG. 26: Chondrosarcoma: Chest CT showing large expansile mass arising from the rib with matrix calcification and large associated soft tissue.

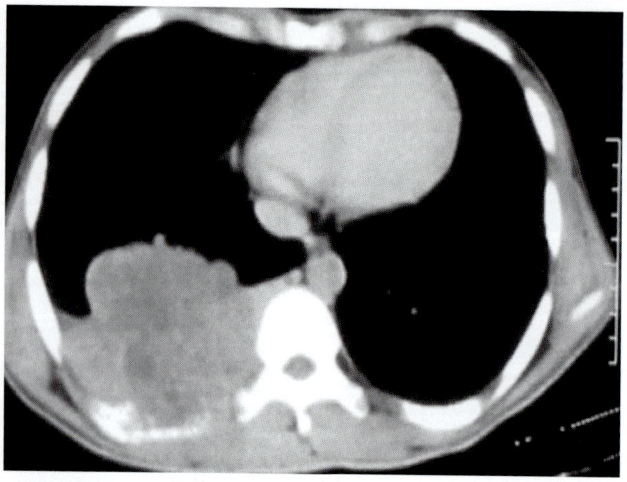

FIG. 27: Ewing sarcoma: Axial CT sections showing large heterogeneous chest wall lesion with erosion destruction of the posterior rib.

Chondrosarcomas

Chondrosarcoma is the most common malignant primary tumors of the chest wall. It frequently involves anterior chest wall originating from the costochondral arches or sternum **(Fig. 26)**.[23] Most of (90%) the tumors occur in the ribs, commonly along the upper five, adjacent to costal cartilage. These are primary lesions most of the times, however, approximately 10% arise from benign tumors which were preexistent. On chest radiograph bony destruction, irregular contours, and intratumoral mineralization are present. CT demonstrates well-defined, calcified soft-tissue masses with associated bony changes. MRI also shows characteristic features. On T1-weighted imaging, signal intensity of the lesion matches that of muscle signal intensity and on T2 weighted it is equal to or greater than that of fat and show heterogeneous enhancement post-contrast.

Osteosarcomas

Osteosarcomas account for 10–15% of malignant chest wall tumors. When osteosarcomas arise in a primary fashion from the chest wall, the most frequently affected structures include the ribs, clavicle, and scapula.[23] On T1-weighted images, the nonmineralized regions of osteosarcomas demonstrate variable signal intensity but are often hyperintense to muscle. On T2-weighted images, the nonmineralized regions demonstrate high signal intensity. Tumor mineralization is usually hypointense on both T1- and T2- weighted imaging. Heterogeneous enhancement after the administration of IV contrast is typical.[20]

Ewing Sarcoma

Ewing sarcoma of the chest wall presents either as a solitary mass or as multiple masses with an eccentric growth pattern. Ewing sarcoma can arise from rib, scapula, clavicle, or sternum but may originate from extra skeletal site.[23] These lesions commonly displace adjacent soft-tissue structures instead of encasement or invasion. They may arise in para-vertebral region and extend through the vertebral foramina. CT scans show a large ill-defined mass with an inhomogeneous enhancement caused by cystic degeneration. Mass lesion may be accompanied by calcification **(Fig. 27)**. These tumors generally have signal intensity equal to or greater than that of muscle on T1, in homogeneous high signal intensity on T2-weighted MR images and show marked enhancement. Small lesions are homogeneous where as large lesions have heterogeneous appearance with areas of necrosis and hemorrhage.

Multiple Myeloma

It may involve vertebral column, ribs, or clavicles and causes multiple osteolytic lesions with discrete margins. At MR imaging, lesions have low signal intensity on T1-weighted images on T2-weighted images have high signal intensity.

Soft Tissue Tumors

Malignant and benign soft tissue tumors of the chest wall are a heterogeneous group and can be divided into the following groups based on the tissue of origin: adipocytic, vascular, peripheral nerve sheath, fibroblastic–myofibroblastic, fibrohistiocytic, and cutaneous.[24]

Adipocytic

Lipoma

Lipomas are the most common soft tissue tumor and present as encapsulated masses composed of adipocytes that are similar to normal fatty tissue found within the chest wall. Lipoma has fat attenuation on MDCT, high signal intensity at T1-weighted imaging, and shows uniform signal loss at fat-suppressed MR imaging. Internal septations may be present and appear hypointense on T1-weighted images. After the administration of IV contrast, lipomas do not enhance, although internal septations may enhance when present.[24,25]

Liposarcoma

Liposarcomas are the second most common chest wall malignancy of soft tissue origin. These tumors constitute approximately 15% of all sarcomas, although only 10% of involve the chest wall.[23] Well-differentiated liposarcomas are typically composed of 50–75% adipose tissue, which results in high signal intensity on T1-weighted and low signal intensity on T2-weighted images. Depending on the volume of fat, it may be difficult to distinguish well-differentiated liposarcoma from lipoma. Features which suggest diagnosis of well differentiated liposarcoma are large tumors (size greater than 10 cm), thick internal septations, nodular regions of nonadipose tissue, and adipose tissue comprising less than 75% of the tumor.[26]

Vascular

Hemangioma and Angiosarcoma

Hemangiomas have high signal intensity at T2-weighted imaging, demonstrates variable amounts of internal fat at multidetector CT and T1-weighted MR imaging, and frequently contains phleboliths **(Figs. 28A to C)**.[16] In contrast, angiosarcoma are heterogeneous, lack internal fat, are aggressive and invade adjacent structures. These tumors may be associated with chronic lymphedema and may exhibit findings related to their origin (such as fibrous thickening, soft-tissue nodules, and fluid collections)adjacent to the chest wall musculature.[23]

Peripheral Nerve Sheath Tumors

Benign nerve sheath neoplasms such as neurofibroma and schwannoma appear as low-attenuating soft-tissue masses which contain fat or cystic components. The "target" sign which is characterized by central low signal intensity and peripheral high signal intensity on T2-weighted MR images and central enhancement following the intravenous administration of gadolinium-based contrast material, and the fascicular sign, characterized by heterogeneous low signal intensity with a ring-like pattern on T2-weighted MR images, are frequently visualized.[16] The "split fat" sign, characterized by fat attenuation around the soft-tissue mass at multidetector CT, also may be seen. These radiologic signs are typically absent in malignant peripheral nerve sheath tumors which, when compared with benign nerve sheath neoplasms, demonstrate greater heterogeneity and aggressive behavior and invasion into surrounding structures.[23]

Fibroblastic–Myofibroblastic

Fibromatosis also known as desmoid tumor has been reported to primarily arise from the chest wall in 10–28% of cases.[23] Fibromatosis typically manifests as an ill-defined mass that grows in an infiltrative manner. On MR imaging, lesions has relatively homogeneous low to intermediate signal intensity on T1-weighted images whereas they appear more heterogeneous on T2-weighted images, low signal intensity bands have been reported in fibromatosis, and likely represent dense collagen bundles. Although fibromatosis may demonstrate moderate to marked heterogeneous enhancement, the collagen bundles do not enhance.[20]

Fibrohistiocytic

Undifferentiated pleomorphic sarcoma (UPS), also called malignant fibrous histiocytoma, is classified as a fibrohistiocytic malignancy and represents the most common malignant soft tissue neoplasm of the chest wall in adults.[26] At MDCT, UPS appears as a soft-tissue mass that involves the deep fascia or skeletal muscle and enhances heterogeneously after intravenous contrast material administration **(Figs. 29A and B)**. Involvement of adjacent osseous structures is common. Internal mineralization can often be identified in the peripheral aspect of the lesion after treatment. UPS demonstrates low signal intensity and is isointense to muscle on T1-weighted MR images. On T2-weighted images, UPS has intermediate to high signal intensity and is iso- to hyperintense to fat.

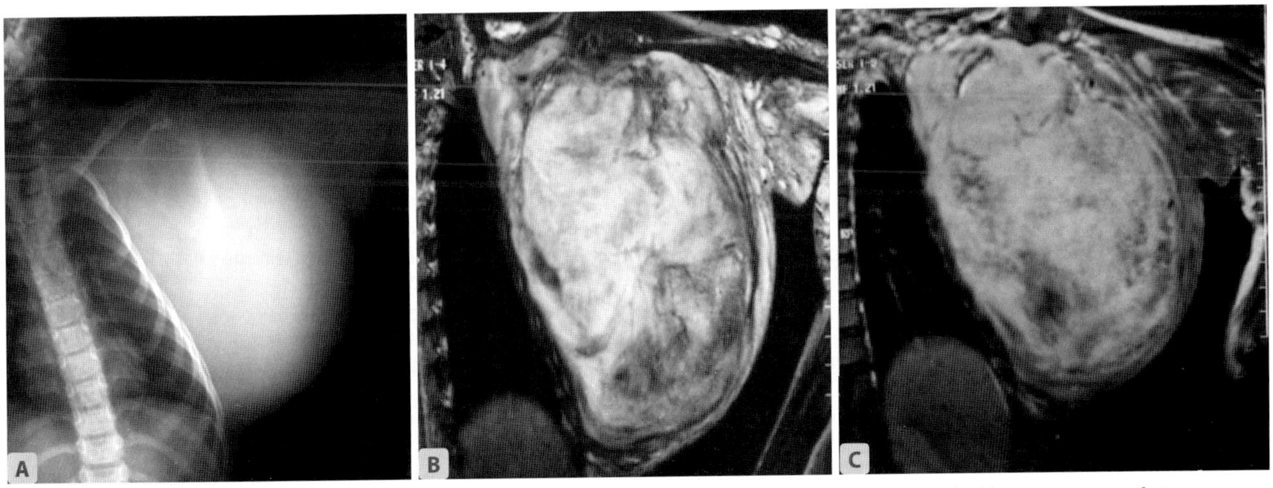

FIGS. 28A TO C: Child with large chest wall hemangioma. (A) Chest radiograph showing large well-circumscribed homogeneous soft tissue mass along lateral chest wall; (B) Coronal T2 and (C) postcontrast images showing heterogeneously enhancing chest wall lesion.

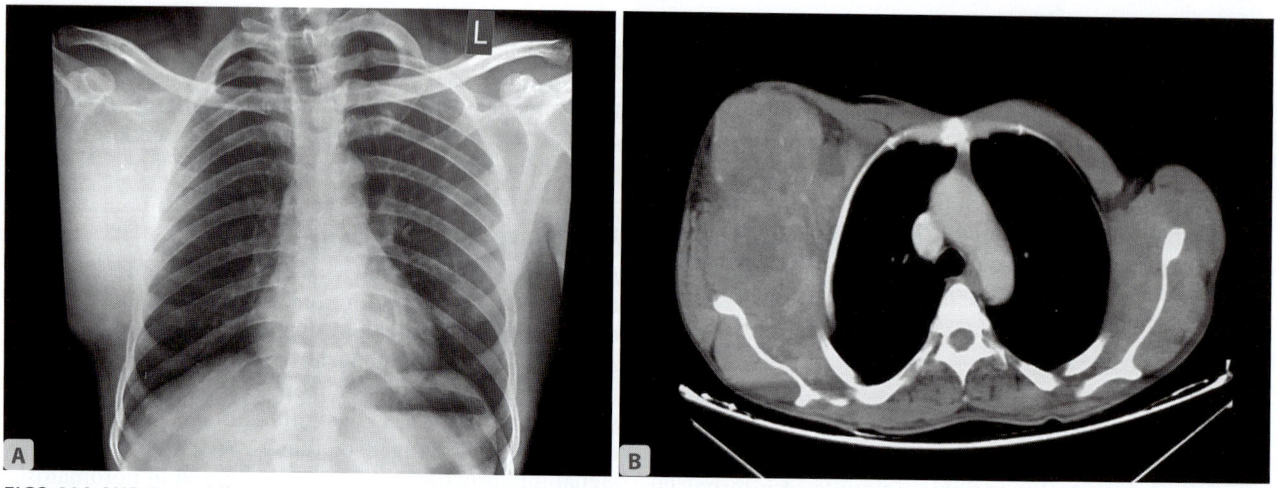

FIGS. 29A AND B: Undifferentiated pleomorphic sarcoma: (A) Chest radiograph showing large well-defined homogeneous mass along the right upper chest wall with no erosion or destruction of underlying bones; (B) CECT chest shows large heterogeneous soft tissue mass anterior to scapula with no bony involvement.

METASTATIC DISEASE

Osseous metastatic disease affecting the chestwall is typically encountered in the setting of extensive metastatic disease elsewhere in the body, but it may be seen early in association with aggressive primary malignancies. These lesions can manifest in many different ways, with some metastases demonstrating imaging characteristics specific to the primary malignancies from which they are derived. Soft-tissue metastatic disease typically is seen only in the setting of extensive metastatic disease elsewhere in the body, is considered an indicator of a poor prognosis.[16]

CHEST WALL INVASION BY THORACIC MALIGNANCY

The chest wall may be directly invaded by aggressive thoracic malignancies—typically lung cancer, breast cancer, pleural tumors, or mediastinal neoplasms. Although MR imaging and MDCT have been shown to have similar utility in the detecting chest wall invasion by lung cancer, MR imaging is considered to be superior due to better spatial resolution and soft tissue contrast.[16]

REFERENCES

1. Nason LK, Walker CM, McNeeley MF, et al. Imaging of the diaphragm: Anatomy and function. Radiographics. 2012; 32:E51-70.
2. Felson B: Chest Roentgenology. WB Saunders, Philadelphia. 1973.
3. Adam A, Dixon AK, Gillard JH, et al. Grainger and Allison's Diagnostic Radiology: A Textbook of Medical Imaging, 6th edition. Churchill Livingstone/Elsevier. 2014.
4. Sarwal A, Walker FO, Cartwright MS. Neuromuscular ultrasound for evaluation of the diaphragm. Muscle Nerve. 2013;47:319-29.
5. Shackleton KL, Stewart ET, Taylor AJ. Traumatic diaphragmatic injuries: spectrum of radiographic findings. Radiographics. 1998;18:49-59.
6. Gierada DS, Curtin JJ, Erickson SJ, et al. Diaphragmatic motion: fast gradient-recalled-echo MR imaging in healthy subjects. Radiology. 1995;194:879-4.
7. Kiryu S, Loring SH, Mori Y, et al. Quantitative analysis of the velocity and synchronicity of diaphragmatic motion: dynamic MRI in different postures. Magn Reson Imaging. 2006;24(10):1325-32.
8. May AK, Moore MM. Diagnosis of blunt rupture of the right hemidiaphragm by technetium scan. Am Surg. 1999;65:761-5.
9. Kharma N. Dysfunction of the diaphragm: Imaging as a diagnostic tool. Curr Opin Pulm Med. 2013;19(4):394-8.
10. Panicek D, Benson C, Gottlieb R, et al. The diaphragm: Anatomic, pathologic, and radiologic considerations. Radiographics. 1988;8(3):385-425.
11. Chavhan G, Babyn P, Cohen R, et al. Multimodality imaging of the pediatric diaphragm: Anatomy and pathologic conditions. Radiographics. 2010;30(7):1797-818.
12. Lochum S, Ludwig T, Walter F, et al. Imaging of the diaphtagmatic injury: a diagnostic challenge? Radiographics. 2002;22:S103-18.
13. Sliker CW. Imaging of diaphragmatic injuries. Radiol Clin N Am. 2006;44:199-211.
14. Kim MP, Hofstetter WL. Tumors of the diaphragm. Thorac Surg Clin. 2009;19:521-9
15. Jeung MY, Gangi A, Gasser B, et al. Imaging of chest wall disorders. Radiographics. 1999;19:617-37.
16. Carter BW, Benveniste MF, Betancourt SL, et al. Imaging evaluation of malignant chest wall neoplasms. Radiographics. 2016;36(5):1285-306.
17. Haller JA Jr, Kramer SS, Lietman SA. Use of CT scans in selection of patients for pectus excavatum surgery: a preliminary report. J Pediatr Surg. 1987;22:904-6.
18. Mak SM, Bhaludin BN, Naaseri S, et al. Imaging of congenital chest wall deformities. Br J Radiol. 2016;89(1061):20150595.
19. Lee TJ, Collins J. MR imaging evaluation of disorders of the chest wall. Magn Reson Imaging Clin N Am. 2008;16(2):355-79.
20. Carter BW, Gladish GW. MR imaging of chest wall tumors. Magn Reson Imaging Clin N Am. 2015;23(2):197-215.
21. Incarbone M, Pastorino U. Surgical treatment of chest wall tumors. World J Surg. 2001;25(2):218-30.

22. Zarqane H, Viala P, Dallaudière B, et al. Tumors of the rib. Diagn Interv Imaging. 2013;94(11):1095-108.
23. Tateishi U, Gladish GW, Kusumoto M, et al. Chest wall tumors: radiologic findings and pathologic correlation; Part 2. Malignant Tumors. Radiographics. 2003;23:1491-508.
24. Nam SJ, Kim S, Lim BJ, et al. Imaging of primary chest wall tumors with radiologic-pathologic correlation. Radiographics. 2011;31(3):749-70.
25. O'Sullivan P, O'Dwyer H, Flint J, et al. Soft tissue tumours and mass-like lesions of the chest wall: a pictorial review of CT and MR findings. Br J Radiol. 2007;80(955):574-80.
26. Kransdorf MJ, Bancroft LW, Peterson JJ, et al. Imaging of fatty tumors: distinction of lipoma and well differentiated liposarcoma. Radiology. 2002;224(1):99-104.

CHAPTER

140

Bronchial Artery Embolization

Ashu Seith Bhalla, Ankur Goyal

INTRODUCTION

Massive hemoptysis is an emergency; but even a small volume of hemoptysis can be life-threatening, especially in diseased lungs.[1,2] Lungs are supplied by two vascular systems; pulmonary arteries are involved in gas exchange and bronchial arteries provide oxygenated blood for nourishment.[3] Latter is a high-pressure circulation and is responsible for clinically significant hemoptysis in most of the cases.

Bronchial artery embolization (BAE) was first described by Remy et al. in 1974 as a measure to control hemoptysis.[4] Since then, the technique of BAE has evolved significantly and its clinical utility increased manifold. The procedure may be more aptly called *systemic artery embolization* because in addition to the bronchial arteries, the hypertrophied non-bronchial systemic collaterals are also embolized to control hemoptysis. A broader term of *endovascular embolization* would also include pulmonary arterial interventions to control hemoptysis. It is important to note that embolization is a palliative procedure and unless the causative disease is addressed, hemoptysis may recur.

PATIENT SELECTION

Hemoptysis is expectoration of blood, i.e. it originates from the respiratory tract. There is subjectivity in the literature regarding the grades of hemoptysis because the severity can be described in terms of volume of bleeding, duration of bleeding or its clinical impact. **Trivial hemoptysis** refers to blood-tinged sputum or few drops of blood. **Mild hemoptysis** means volume <100 mL/day or <50 mL/episode. **Moderate hemoptysis** refers to 100–300 mL/day or more than three bouts of at least 100 mL/day in a week. **Severe/Massive/Life-threatening hemoptysis** generally refers to either of the following:[2,5]

- Hemoptysis >300 mL/day.[1,2,6,7]
- Any volume hemoptysis leading to >1 g/dL drop in hemoglobin or >5% drop in hematocrit OR
- Any volume hemoptysis leading to respiratory failure ($SpaO_2$ <60%) OR
- Any volume hemoptysis leading to hypotension (systolic blood pressure <90 mm Hg).

Death from hemoptysis is rarely due to blood loss. Rather, it is the asphyxia caused from flooding of the airways and alveoli with blood, which is lethal.

MANAGEMENT APPROACH

For practical purposes, occasional blood-stained sputum can usually be managed conservatively but recurrent episodes of greater hemoptysis warrant intervention. Latter can be in the form of surgery or BAE. *BAE is the procedure of choice in patients with bilateral/extensive disease and in poor surgical risk patients.* In cases of episodic hemoptysis, BAE may be done electively in the quiescent phase to maximize the chances of technical success; rather than waiting for the patient to present in emergency. Massive hemoptysis is an emergency with high mortality and BAE is the management of choice in such a setting. Majority of the published literature on BAE includes patients with moderate-massive hemoptysis.

Surgery is the treatment of choice, if the pulmonary disease is localized and patients have adequate pulmonary reserve without comorbidities. Surgery is also indicated, if the hemoptysis is due to hydatid cyst, bronchial neoplasms or mediastinal vascular injuries.[1] *Even in surgical candidates, BAE has a role to reduce the intraoperative bleeding and especially if the patient presents in emergency department with massive hemoptysis.*

PATHOPHYSIOLOGY

In majority cases of non-cardiac hemoptysis, the source of bleeding is systemic circulation (bronchial arteries more commonly responsible than non-bronchial collaterals). This is because majority of the patients have chronic inflammatory lung disease. This leads to hypoxic vasoconstriction of the pulmonary arterioles in the areas of abnormality, which then incites hypertrophy of systemic arteries. These systemic arteries are recruited in order to participate in gas exchange through anastomoses with the pulmonary vascular system. The hypertrophic bronchial arteries are prone to rupture in the inflamed surroundings and since they are part of high pressure systemic circulation, this results in clinically significant hemoptysis.

In about 5% cases, the bleeding is from pulmonary vascular causes (pulmonary arterio-venous malformation, Rasmussen aneurysm, injury from Swan-Ganz catheter, etc.). Thus, most of the cases of significant hemoptysis result from systemic arterial source rather than pulmonary circulation.

INDICATIONS OF BAE

The common causes of hemoptysis requiring BAE are shown in **Table 1**.[2,8-10] and **Figures 1A to I** show examples of some of the common causes of hemoptysis.

It may be noted here that bronchial artery abnormalities are much less common in malignancies, whereas in infective/postinfective causes, these are usually hypertrophied. Thus, BAE is much more commonly done for non-neoplastic causes.[8,11] Majority of the published data on BAE is from Asia where TB (active disease/sequelae) is the most common cause of significant hemoptysis;[4,8-10,12-14] whereas sarcoidosis and cystic fibrosis are common indications in the west.[15,16] In addition, it is necessary to rule out cardiovascular (mitral stenosis, left heart failure, pulmonary embolism, aneurysm of aorta/pulmonary artery, iatrogenic injury by Swan-Ganz catheter) and systemic (bleeding diathesis, anticoagulation) causes of hemoptysis.

TABLE 1: Non-cardiac causes of significant hemoptysis.[7]

Post-tuberculosis (TB) sequelae: (fibrosis, bronchiectasis) ~30%	*Neoplasms:* Carcinoma, carcinoid, tracheobronchial lesions
Active TB: ~30%	*Vasculitis:* Granulomatosis with polyangiitis, Behçet's disease, SLE
Other inflammatory lung diseases: Bronchiectasis/bronchitis/ Aspergilloma/cystic fibrosis/ sarcoidosis/hydatid cyst	*Vascular causes:* Vascular malformations, post biopsy
Other lung infections: Non-tubercular infections, lung abscess	*Miscellaneous:* Pneumoconiosis, chronic obstructive pulmonary disease, and cryptogenic hemoptysis

PRE-PROCEDURE DIAGNOSTIC WORK-UP

The purpose of pre-procedure work-up is to identify the cause and site of hemoptysis. This would not only enable to exclude the cardiac and pulmonary vascular causes, but also to plan the embolization/surgical procedure. **Flowchart 1** depicts the diagnostic approach and management in a case with significant hemoptysis of pulmonary etiology.

Chest radiograph (CXR): Frequently performed as the first investigation and may be the only investigation feasible in emergency cases. Advantages include wide availability, low cost and can be done immediately. American College of Radiology (ACR) recommends a chest radiograph in the evaluation of all patients with hemoptysis, because it not only lateralizes the bleeding but may also identify the cause.[17] Radiographs are diagnostic in about 50% cases.[1]

Computed tomography (CT): Multidetector CT is the modality of choice for evaluation of hemoptysis. Contrast-enhanced CT (CECT) has the capability to detect airway, parenchymal as well as vascular causes of hemoptysis **(Figs. 1 and 2)**. CT bronchial angiography (CTBA) provides a vascular roadmap by delineating the hypertrophied bronchial and systemic arteries **(Figs. 2A to H)** while CT pulmonary angiography (CTPA) acquisition can delineate the rarer pulmonary vascular causes of hemoptysis. As per ACR recommendations, CTBA is the next most appropriate investigation in patients with significant hemoptysis.[17] This technique has the potential to reduce the procedure time as well as improve the outcomes of BAE (by identifying the ectopic and uncommon arterial supply preprocedural). CTA has been found to reduce the rate of vascular catheterization failure in elderly patients.[18] A combined CTA for simultaneous evaluation of both systemic and pulmonary circulations in a single acquisition would be ideal and can be done by employing varying rates and concentration of contrast injection **(Figs. 2A to H)**.[19]

Fiberoptic bronchoscopy (FB): FB and CTA are complementary in the evaluation of hemoptysis and both should be done prior to BAE, in the elective setting.[20] CT is more useful to identify the cause while bronchoscopy is more accurate in localizing the site of active bleed. This is especially useful in case there is multifocal/bilateral lung disease. Bronchoscopy has the advantage that it can identify the bleeding endobronchial lesions, enable sampling as well as local ablation procedures. Such lesions may not that well seen on CT and are usually not amenable to endovascular embolization. Furthermore, vasoconstrictive drugs can be administered locally to control bleeding. Intrabronchial antifungal agents can also be injected in cases of aspergilloma. The main problem in patients with massive hemoptysis is that blood/clots may fill up the bronchi and preclude further evaluation. Also, the feasibility of FB depends on the local availability as well as patient condition.

RELEVANT ARTERIAL ANATOMY

It is important to have a good understanding of the anatomy of the bronchial and commonly hypertrophied non-bronchial arteries so that the same may be communicated in the radiological report as well as guide management.

Bronchial Arteries

Bronchial arteries are systemic arteries which course along the branching of the major bronchi. This is a key finding which helps to distinguish (ectopic) bronchial arteries from non-bronchial systemic collaterals. The bronchial arteries supply the tracheobronchial tree (both intra- and extrapulmonary), regional lymph nodes, (visceral) pleura, esophagus, and vasa vasorum of aorta, pulmonary artery and vein.

Origin: Majority of the bronchial arteries are *orthotopic* i.e. arise from the descending thoracic aorta (DTA) between the superior border of T5 and inferior border of T6 vertebral levels **(Figs. 3A to H)**.[3] Angiographic landmark for the same is 1 cm above and below the crossing of left main bronchus over the

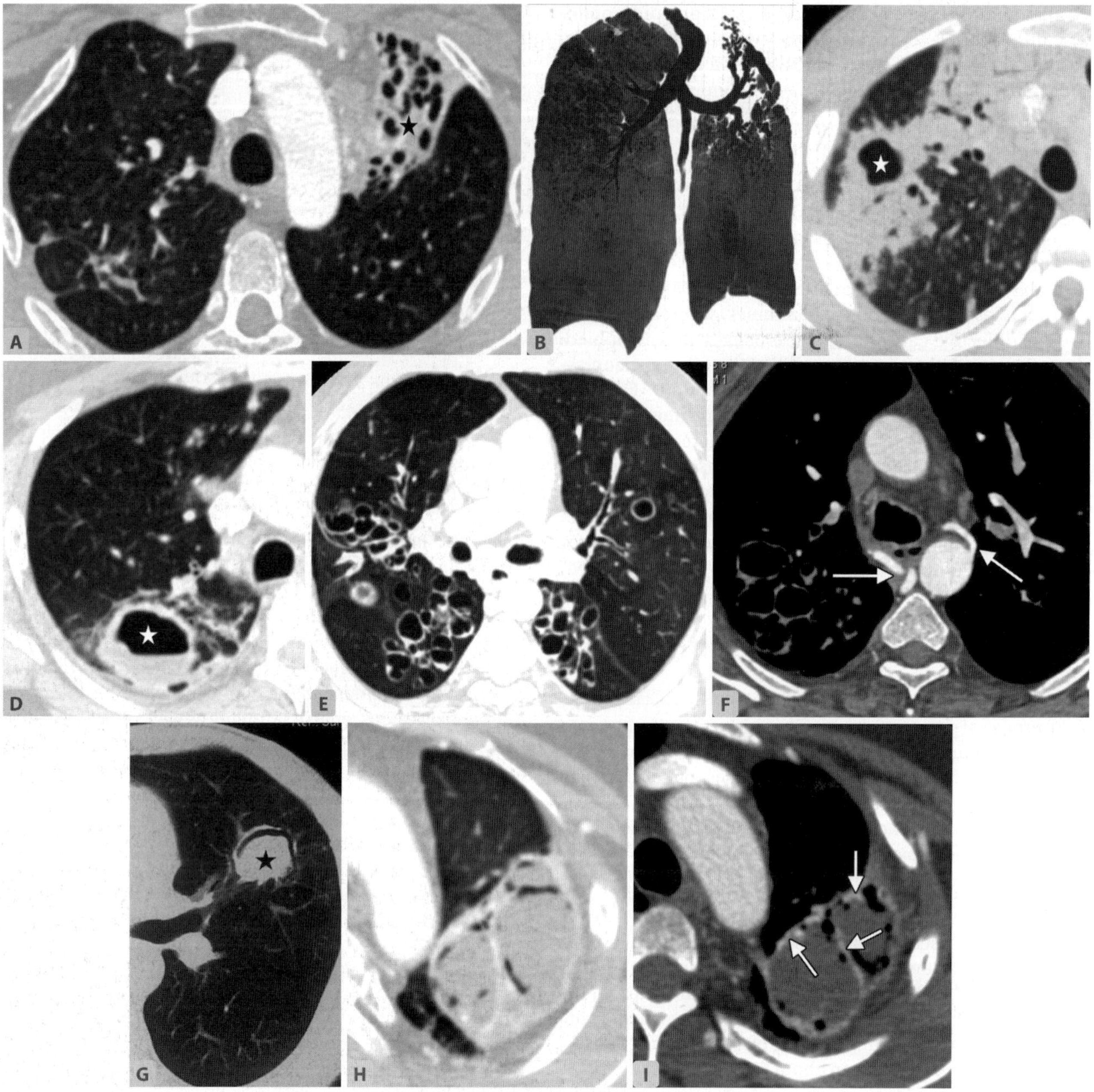

FIGS. 1A TO I: CT images showing common causes of hemoptysis. (A) TB sequelae (Fibrobronchiectasis and collapse left upper lobe (asterisk) and fibroparenchymal lesions right upper lobe); (B) Coronal MinIP image showing upper lobe predominant post TB fibrosis with bronchiectasis, volume loss and cavitation left upper lobe; (C) Active TB [thick-walled cavity right upper lobe (asterisk) with surrounding dense consolidation and centrilobular nodules]; (D) TB sequelae with superimposed pyogenic bacterial infection [Cavity (asterisk) with air-fluid level]; (E and F) Bilateral bronchiectasis with hypertrophied bronchial arteries (arrows); (G) Thin-walled cavity with aspergilloma (asterisk); (H and I) Chronic cavitary pulmonary aspergillosis with pleural thickening and vascularity in the walls of cavity (arrows).

DTA or just below the carina.[21] The frequency of orthotopic bronchial arteries varies depending on whether the study is based on CT, DSA or post-mortem; approximately 65% patients have orthotopic bronchial arteries.[3] If the origin is anywhere else from DTA or even from a branch of the aorta, but the course is parallel to the bronchial tree, then it is labeled as *ectopic* bronchial artery **(Figs. 4A to I)**. Practically, majority of the bronchial arteries arise from DTA between T4-T7 vertebral levels. Many variations can however occur, and ectopic bronchial arteries may arise from the inferior surface of aortic arch, internal mammary artery (IMA), thyrocervical and costocervical trunk, innominate artery, left subclavian artery and inferior thyroid artery, inferior phrenic artery or abdominal aorta.[22]

Cauldwell documented the variations in bronchial artery anatomy by describing nine patterns based on autopsy study of 150 cadavers.[23] Uflacker described 10 patterns of bronchial arterial anatomy based on angiography records of

FLOWCHART 1: Approach to a patient with hemoptysis.

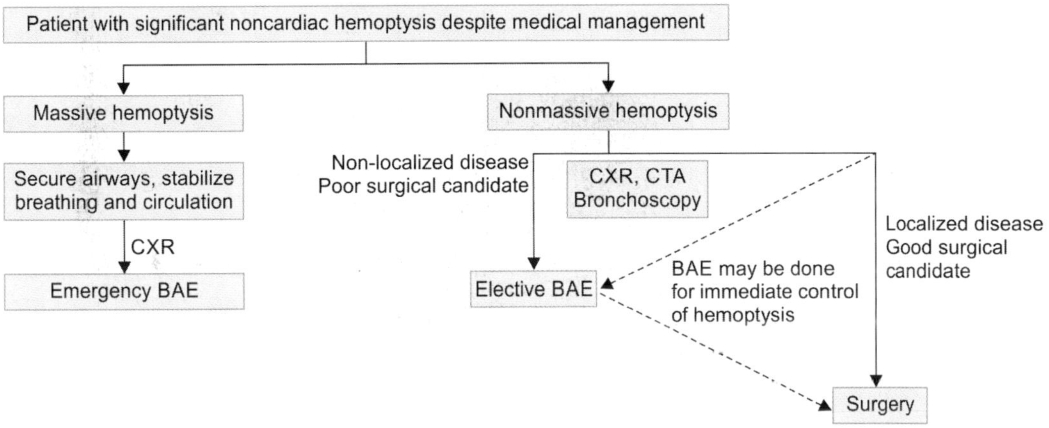

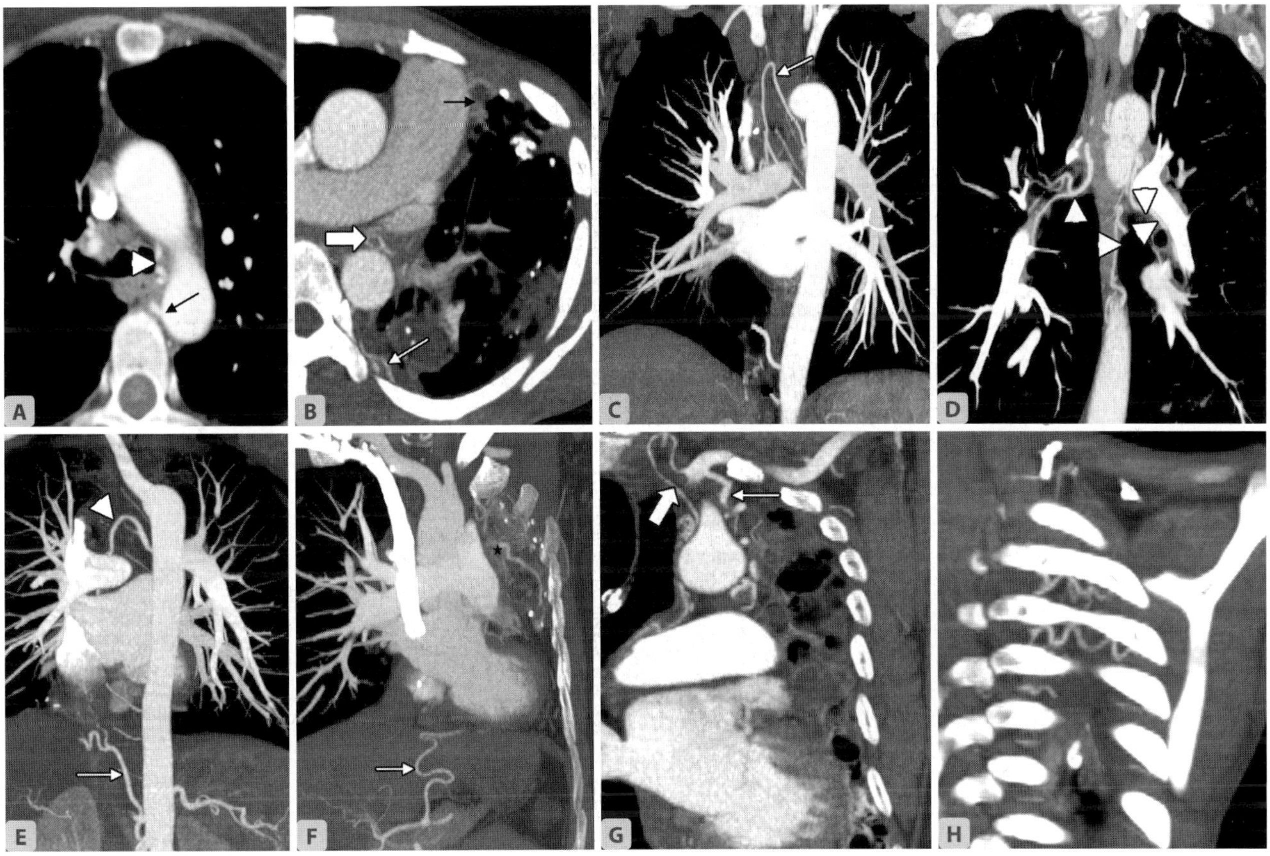

FIGS. 2A TO H: CT angiogram images showing hypertrophied bronchial arteries and NBSC. (A) RT-ICBT arises laterally from the descending aorta (black arrow). Left bronchial artery is seen around the left main bronchus (white arrowhead); (B) Left bronchial artery arises from anterior wall of aorta (solid white arrow). Also noted are NBSC from left internal mammary artery (black arrow) and tortuous left posterior intercostal artery (white thin arrow); (C) Combined CT angiogram coronal MIP image showing good opacification of both systemic and pulmonary arterial trees. The entire course of RT-ICBT is well seen (white arrow); (D) Multiple hypertrophied bronchial arteries (arrowheads); (E) Hypertrophied right bronchial (arrowhead) and inferior phrenic arteries (thin white arrow); (F) Hypertrophied left inferior phrenic artery (white arrow) and multiple chest wall collaterals (asterisk); (G) Coronal oblique MIP image depicts enlarged left costocervical trunk (solid white arrow) and internal mammary artery IMA (thin white arrow); (H) Tortuous hypertrophied left posterior intercostal arteries.

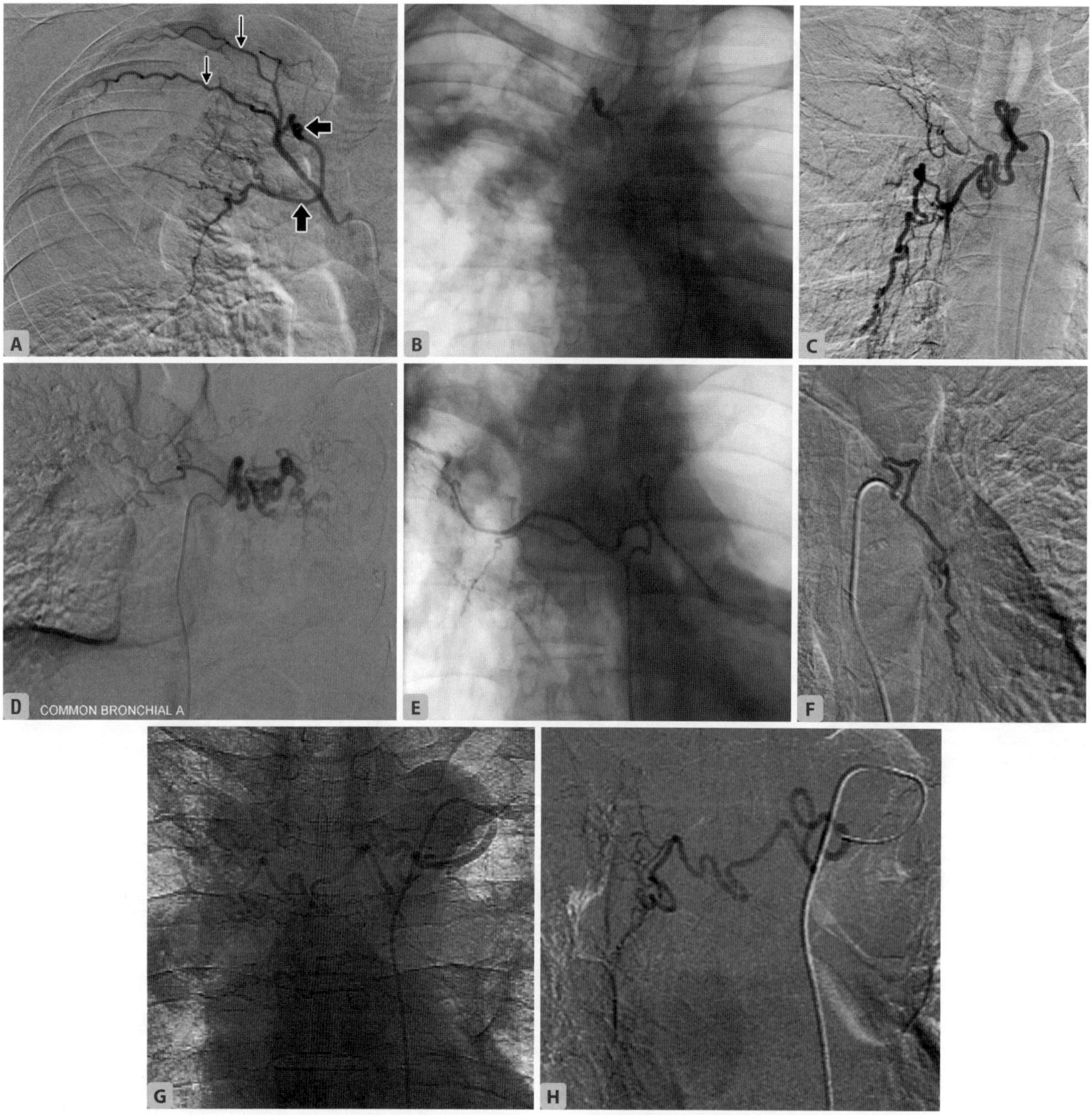

FIGS. 3A TO H: DSA images showing abnormal bronchial arteries. (A) Selective DSA run shows hypertrophied RT ICBT. The bronchial component is hypertrophied (solid black arrows) while the intercostal component is normal (thin black arrows), RB; (B) Stasis of contrast after superselective embolization; (C) Hypertrophied right bronchial artery; (D) Common bronchial artery with hypertrophied left component; (E) Common bronchial artery with right component more hypertrophied than left; (F) Hypertrophied left bronchial artery; (G) Ectopic right bronchial artery arising from the arch of aorta; (H) Superselective DSA run through microcatheter shows stable catheter position, just before embolization.

72 patients.[24] However, what is more relevant is the information regarding number and origin of the hypertrophied bronchial arteries and pattern approach is not that helpful.

Right side: There are usually two bronchial arteries supplying the right lung. The first arises from DTA as a common intercostobronchial trunk (ICBT) with the third right posterior intercostal artery, and has a posterolaterally lying orifice **(Figs. 2A to H)**. **Right ICBT** is the most consistently seen artery at DSA. The initial course is oblique and upwards and can be seen on CT in the retro-esophageal region. Then the trunk divides, with the bronchial component hooking down and paralleling the branching of RT bronchus while the intercostal component ascends up and then traverses horizontally along the inferior border of the rib **(Figs. 3A to H)**. The second artery is the **common bronchial (CB)** that arises from the anterior surface and supplies both lungs by dividing into right and left bronchial arteries **(Figs. 3A to H)**. Depending upon the parenchymal abnormality, one or both the branches may be hypertrophied.

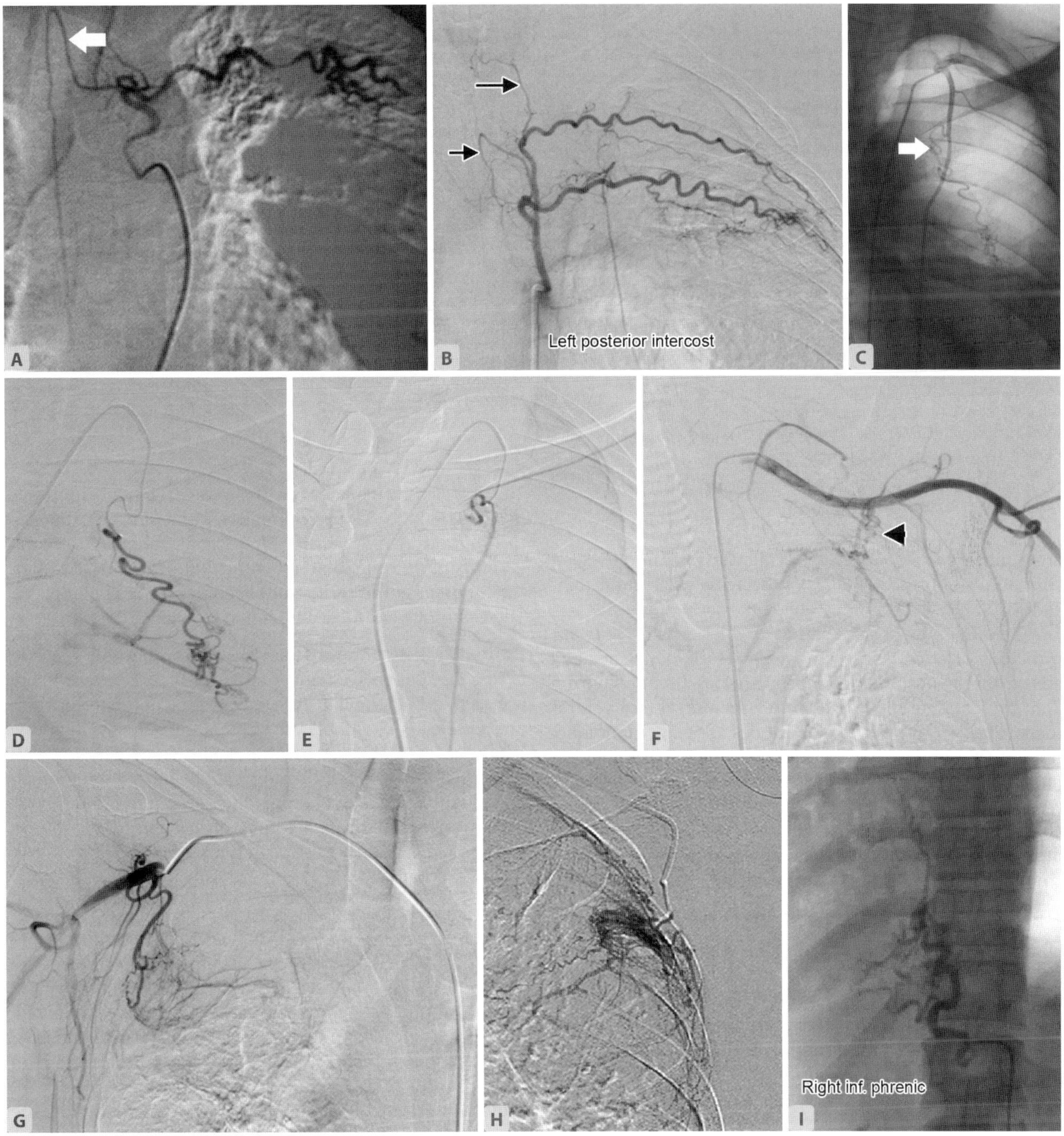

FIGS. 4A TO I: DSA images showing abnormal NBSC and communications with spinal artery. (A) Anterior medullary artery (solid white arrow) arising from left posterior intercostal artery; (B) Radicular arteries (thin black arrows) arising from left posterior intercostal artery; (C) Left subclavian artery (SCA) run shows abnormal branch arising from LT IMA; (D) Superselective catheterization of abnormal branch of LT IMA with stable catheter position and check run; (E) Postembolization run of the same; (F) Abnormal costocervical branch of second part of left SCA (arrowhead); (G) Abnormal pulmonary parenchymal blush from right superior thoracic artery (branch of first part of axillary artery); (H) Superselective catheterization of left superior thoracic artery; (I) Hypertrophied right inferior phrenic artery.

Left side: On the left side, a separate **left bronchial (LB)** artery is usually present, and arises from the anterior-left anterolateral surface of the aorta **(Figs. 2 and 3)**. Rarely the left bronchial artery may arise from the RT-ICB trunk but LB arising from left intercostal is not described.

On CT, bronchial arteries can be identified in the retroesophageal, retrotracheal, retrobronchial or aorto-pulmonary window locations **(Table 2) (Figs. 2A to H)**. Bronchial arteries can have communications with other systemic arteries. Most important of such communication is that of RT ICBT with anterior medullary artery that contributes to vascular supply of the spinal cord through anterior spinal artery. The **anterior medullary arteries** have a characteristic 'hairpin' configuration, and follow a vertical course parallel to the spinal cord[25] **(Figs. 4A to I)**. These arteries, when they originate from D9 to D12, may communicate with the great anterior medullary

TABLE 2: Tips to identify abnormal bronchial and systemic arteries (NBSC).

- RT ICBT arises from right lateral wall of aorta and courses behind the right main bronchus
- RB or right branch of CB arise anterolaterally from aorta and course anterior to the RT main bronchus
- LB arises from anterior wall of aorta and may course anterior or posterior to left main bronchus
- Ectopic LB/RB arising from the arch course anterior to the corresponding bronchus
- Internal mammary arteries are hypertrophied in case disease is localized to anterior segments of upper lobes, RT middle lobe or lingual
- Right posterior intercostal arteries arise posterolaterally and left posterior intercostal arteries arise posteriorly from the aorta
- Posterior intercostal arteries are hypertrophied in case of posterior or posterolateral lung involvement.
- Inflammatory lung disease close to the lateral chest wall may recruit collaterals from lateral thoracic artery.
- Inferior phrenic arteries may hypertrophy in basal lung disease.

artery (artery of Adamkiewicz). Other less commonly seen communications are with the subclavian artery and right coronary artery.[26,27]

The other type of spinal arteries which may be seen are *radicular arteries*. These are small vessels which usually arise from the posterior intercostal arteries, do not have the 'hairpin' configuration, and supply the dorsal and ventral roots **(Figs. 4A to I)**. Radicular arteries are more commonly seen at DSA and are not considered to be a contradiction to embolization. Medullary arteries, on the other hand, are rarely seen but may give rise to cord ischemia, if inadvertently embolized.[1] Nevertheless, it is advisable to go superselectively beyond the origin of any spinal artery to prevent ominous complications.

Non-bronchial Systemic Collaterals

Non-bronchial systemic collaterals (NBSC) enter the lung parenchyma through adjacent pleura or the pulmonary ligament, and have a course that does not parallel the bronchial tree. The CT features that suggest the presence of NBSC include pleural thickening and presence of chronic inflammatory disease in the lung apex or base. NBSC may arise from the following:[13,28,29]

- Intercostal arteries in case of peripheral lung/pleural inflammation **(Figs. 2 and 4)**
- Branches of subclavian and axillary arteries (internal mammary, lateral thoracic, costocervical and cervicothoracic) in case of apical/anterior paramidline lung disease **(Figs. 2 and 4)**
- Phrenic arteries in case of basal lung disease **(Figs. 2 and 4)**
- Rarely left gastric artery.

Normal bronchial arteries have a diameter of <1.5 mm at their origin, and 0.5 mm at the level of the entrance into a bronchopulmonary segment. Indicators of abnormal bronchial arteries are[6,12,30] enumerated in **Table 3 (Figs. 5A to E)**. Systemic collaterals going into abnormal lung parenchyma are considered abnormal irrespective of diameter.

TABLE 3: Criteria to identify abnormal bronchial and systemic arteries (NBSC).

- *Hypertrophy:* Diameter at ostium >2 mm
- Increased tortuosity
- Bronchial artery traceable upto corresponding hilum on CT
- *DSA features:*
  - Neo- and hypervascularity in the form of abnormal vascular blush, dense soft tissue staining/parenchymal blush **(Figs. 5A to E)**
  - Shunting into the pulmonary vascular system (arterial or venous) **(Figs. 5A to E)**
  - Extravasation of contrast into the alveoli or bronchial tree
  - Pseudoaneurysm
- Any non-bronchial systemic collateral supplying diseased lung parenchyma is deemed abnormal

TECHNIQUE OF BAE

The first priority in patients with life-threatening hemoptysis is to maintain the airway, optimize oxygenation and stabilize the hemodynamic status. Blood tests for coagulopathy (Prothrombin time, platelet count) and renal dysfunction (blood urea, serum creatinine) need to be done before BAE. The technique of BAE is outlined in **Flowchart 2**.

Route: Transfemoral arterial access is routinely used to access the bronchial circulation. Transbrachial/ transaxillary access may be helpful in case of increased aortic tortuosity[8,9] and to selectively catheterize branches of subclavian artery. A long arterial sheath (carotid sheath) may also be used in case of tortuosity of the aortic arch. In case pulmonary angiography needs to be done, then common femoral vein access is used. 6F sheath is commonly used in adults while in young children, 5F access sheath is used.

Thoracic aortogram: After securing a vascular sheath in the femoral artery, the next step is usually to take flush aortogram using 5F angiographic pigtail catheter (having multiple side holes). The loop of the pigtail catheter is formed in the proximal DTA. About 25–30 mL of ~80% diluted contrast (concentration ≥300 mg iodine/mL) is injected at flow rate of 18 mL/s (~650 psi pressure) and patient is asked to hold breath. The contrast run is acquired in digital subtraction angiography (DSA) mode (3 frames per second), AP projection with wide field of view (FOV) after coupling the contrast inflow with fluoroscopic DSA acquisition. The aim is to identify all the abnormal bronchial and non-bronchial systemic collaterals from DTA so as to facilitate selective catheterization of the same **(Figs. 6A to E)**. The limitation of flush aortogram is that the opacification of subclavian arteries is suboptimal. So, either take separate subclavian artery runs or take the pigtail loop upto proximal arch. Problem with the latter technique is that contrast will unnecessarily go into the head and neck arteries. Due to several limitations of aortogram, this step may be omitted, if a good quality CT bronchial angiogram is available.

Superselective catheterization: The bronchial arteries are usually hooked using angiographic catheters having more than one curve such as RDC (renal double curve)/cobra

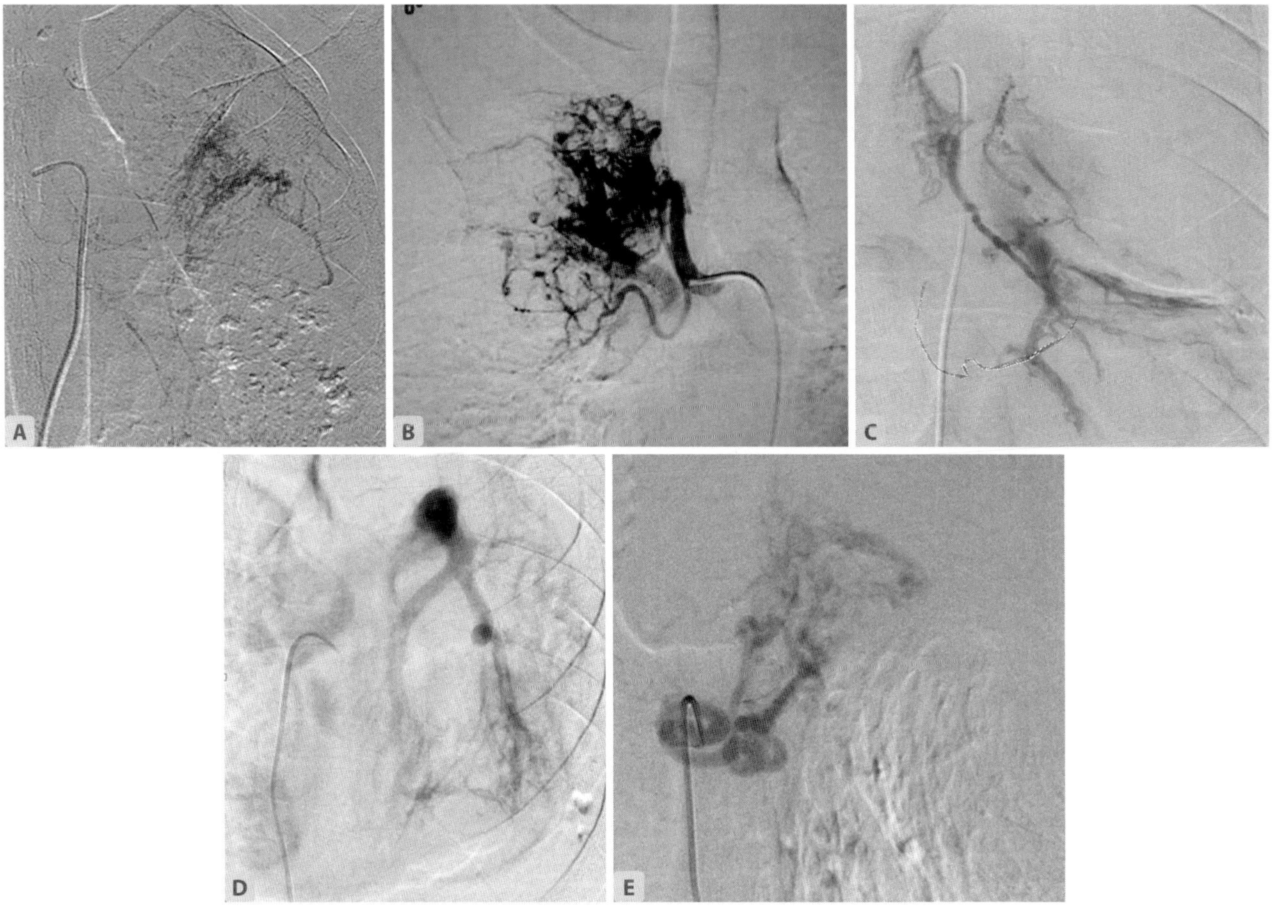

FIGS. 5A TO E: DSA features of abnormal bronchial arteries. (A) Abnormal parenchymal blush; (B) Hypertrophied right bronchial artery with dense vascular blush and shunting; (C) Vascular blush with shunting into pulmonary vein; (D) Delayed phase DSA run depicts shunting into pulmonary artery; (E) Hypertrophied tortuous left bronchial artery with pulmonary arterial shunting.

FLOWCHART 2: Basic steps in the procedure of bronchial artery embolization.

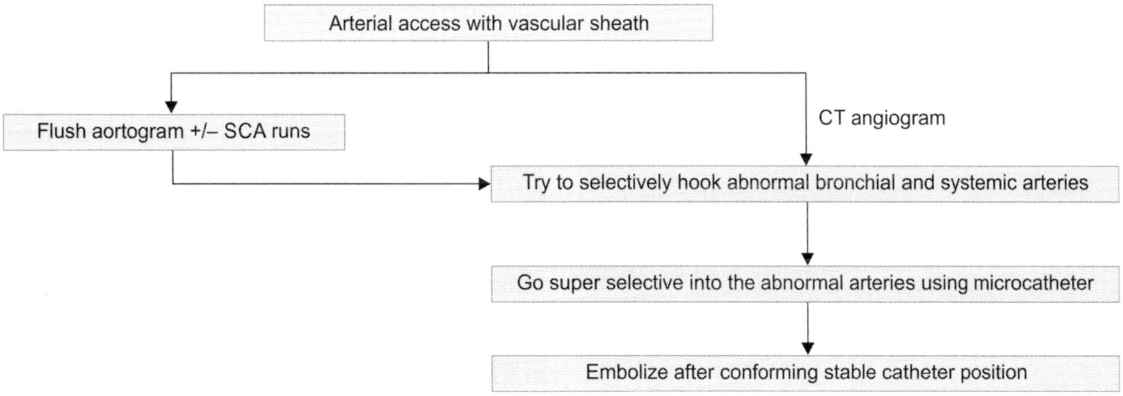

catheter **(Table 4)**. Reverse seeking catheter (like Simmons) may also be used, especially of there is sharp upward course from the origin. Once the artery is hooked, then check contrast run is taken. Using this roadmap, the main catheter is secured into the artery and then microcatheter (2.7Fr) is advanced through the main catheter (co-axial system). A multipurpose catheter or slip catheter may also be used to go selectively into the artery, by exchanging RDC/cobra over a long (~260 cm) guidewire.

In case of ICBT, attempt should be made to superselectively go into the bronchial component, unless the intercostal component is also abnormal **(Figs. 3A to H)**. Care must be taken to look for any contrast opacification of the anterior medullary artery **(Figs. 4A to I)**. Superselective catheterization by microcatheter enables delivery of embolizing agent specifically into the culprit branches with lesser risk of complications, and thus providing better patient care.[8-10,31] Care should be

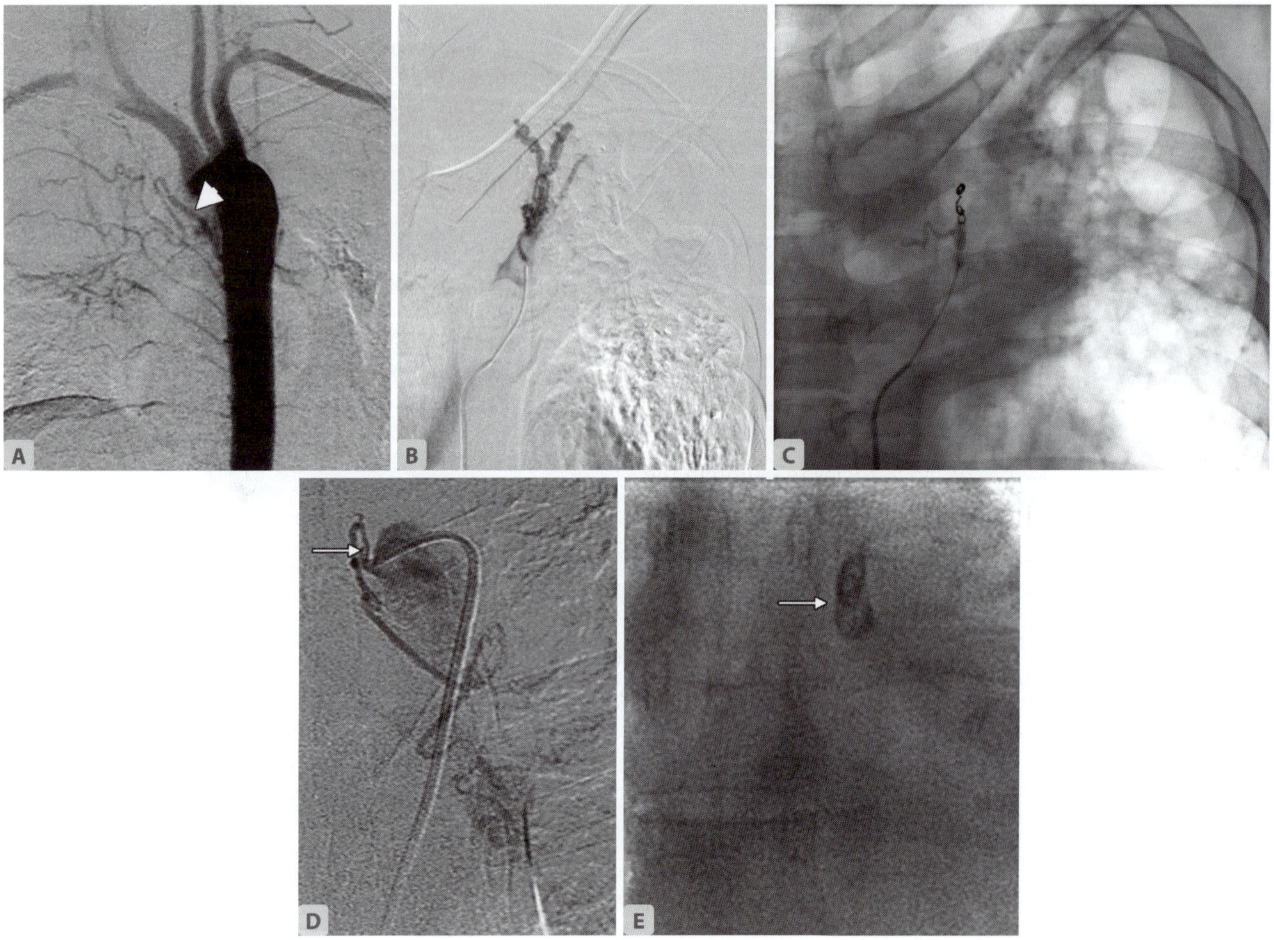

FIGS. 6A TO E: BAE technique and complications. (A) Flush aortogram shows hypertrophied RT-ICBT; (B) Superselective catheterization of left bronchial artery shows large shunt into the pulmonary vein; (C) Due to large size of the shunt and resultant potential of cerebral embolism, the shunt was blocked using microcoils; (D) DSA run shows shelf-like filling defect at the origin of ectopic left bronchial artery (suggesting dissection), caused by wire manipulation due to acute upward angulation; (E) Fluoroscopic spot image depicts contrast blob at the origin of this ectopic left bronchial artery (likely representing intramural hematoma in aortic wall).

TABLE 4: Commonly used catheters for selective cannulation.

Bronchial and intercostal arteries	RDC (double curve), Cobra (complex curve), Simmons (Reverse curve)
Subclavian artery and its branches	Picard, vertebral (Forward seeking simple curve angled-tip), headhunter (double curve)
Inferior phrenic artery	RDC, RC, Simmons

(RDC: renal double curve; RC: reverse curve)

taken not to create spasm or dissection while negotiating the smaller catheter.

Usually, the bronchial arteries are searched first, followed by any expected NBSC. Intercostal arteries can be searched by directing the RDC catheter posterolaterally for right-sided arteries and posteriorly for left posterior intercostal arteries. Subclavian artery branches are evaluated using Picard/vertebral catheter while phrenic may be hooked using RDC or RC catheter **(Table 4)**. The search for NBSC has been found to reduce the recurrence rates of hemoptysis.[7] A pre-procedural CTBA lays down the vascular roadmap for endovascular therapeutic interventions.

Again, attempt must be made to hook the hypertrophied branch of SCA using the main catheter and then go selectively into it using microcatheter **(Figs. 4A to I)**. If former is not feasible, then negotiation using microcatheter can be done after keeping the main catheter in subclavian artery itself, provided we use a large bore Tuohy-Borst sidearm adaptor (Y-connector). The latter allows for continuous flushing of the guiding catheter so as to avoid formation of thrombus in the dead space. Alternatively, a side hole can be created in a diagnostic catheter (at a distance from the tip), which can serve as an exit for microcatheter. This technique has been described to be helpful in the embolization of proximal subclavian arterial branches, when stable and selective position of the main catheter cannot be achieved.[32] In a similar fashion, catheters with pre-fabricated side holes can be used in difficult anatomical situations.[33] Before proceeding to the embolization of the target vessel, stability of the catheter tip and absence of backflow into the descending thoracic aorta should be confirmed by means of a test-injection using contrast medium.

Culprit arteries: The common culprit bronchial arteries in patients undergoing embolization are RB, RT-ICBT, CB, and LB (in descending order of frequency). Common NBSC are posterior intercostal and internal mammary arteries. Other branches of subclavian artery (like superior thoracic, lateral thoracic, costocervical and cervicothoracic), and inferior phrenic arteries may also be abnormal.

Embolizing agents: Particulate embolizing material are commonly used for BAE. Older literature describes use of gelatin sponge, but the current agent of choice is polyvinyl alcohol (PVA) particles. Gelatin sponge is readily available and inexpensive. Advantages of PVA over gelfoam include permanency of embolization (since gelatin sponge gets resorbed) and choice of different sizes **(Table 5)**. Gelfoam has the potential to cause more proximal embolization. Problems with PVA include tendency of the particles to clump in the microcatheter. Microspheres can overcome this problem because of hydrophilic nature and uniform size.[20] Commonly used size of PVA particles is 300–500 μ micron though use of all sizes from 150–1200 μ have been reported in literature. Particles smaller than 300 μ should ideally not be used because they can pass through the bronchopulmonary anastomoses and result in infarcts.[20] They may lead to occlusion of smaller branches resulting in bronchial or esophageal necrosis.[25]

Larger particles (500–700 μ) may be indicated in the presence of shunting. Shunting into pulmonary veins is potentially more dangerous than into the pulmonary arteries because of the risk of non-target systemic embolization. PVA/gelfoam is mixed with contrast and then injected under fluoroscopic guidance. It is important to monitor for slowing of flow and stasis so as to prevent any backflow/reflux of embolic material. 2 mL/1 mL syringes are routinely used for better precision. Intermittent contrast runs may be taken to look for any vascular anastomoses not previously visible. Always remember to empty the PVA column in the catheter before taking check runs.

PVA can also be used in conjunction with gelfoam. Former is used for distal embolization of the abnormal parenchymal bed and latter is typically used for proximal embolization. Recently, liquid embolic agents [glue, n-Butyl-2-cyanoacrylate (NBCA)] have been shown to result in better control of hemoptysis in case of bronchiectasis.[10] This has been attributed to lower rates of recanalization, compared with PVA. But use of glue calls for stable catheter position and need of greater expertise, owing to more chances of complications (distal necrosis, non-target complications due to reflux are more dangerous). Microcoils have been used uncommonly, and the chief indication is in case of pseudoaneurysms (provided microcatheter reaches upto the neck of the aneurysm) and large volume shunts **(Figs. 6A to E)**. Proximal coil embolization precludes repeat access in case of recurrence of hemoptysis due to distal collateralization.[34,35]

TABLE 5: Advantages and drawbacks of various embolizing agents.

Embolizing agent	Advantages	Drawbacks
PVA particles	• Relatively uniform size • Permanent • Different sizes available	• Tendency to clump • Costly
Microspheres	Better than PVA because do not clump	Costly
Gelfoam	Cheap, readily available	Heterogeneous particle size, temporary
Glue	• More permanent than PVA • Useful where significant shunting is there	Needs experienced hands and stable catheter position
Microcoils	• In case of pseudoaneurysms, markedly hyper-trophied artery with large volume shunt • To protect parent vessel in case superselective catherization not feasible	• Preclude future access • Expensive

Outcomes: The outcome of any interventional procedure is expressed in terms of technical as well as clinical success. The causes of technical and clinical failure of BAE have been listed in the **Table 6**. A pre-procedural CT angiogram enhances clinical success by depicting all the abnormal arteries. Few authors suggest a post-embolization flush aortogram to avoid missing a pathological vessel. The presence of NBSC is associated with higher rate of technical failures.[36]

Bronchial artery embolization is very effective in the treatment of acute hemoptysis. *Immediate clinical success* (significant reduction/cessation of hemoptysis within 24 hours of the procedure) is high (70-99%).[2] *Early recurrences* (within 1–3 months) suggest incomplete embolization, i.e. any abnormal vessel has been left untreated. This may be because of lack of complete search, ectopic origin or NBSC and too many hypertrophied arteries due to extensive collateralization. In latter scenario, it may be useful to split the embolization into two sessions, starting with the most abnormal arteries first, and bronchial arteries should be done prior to the NBSC.

TABLE 6: Causes of technical and clinical failure of BAE.

Causes of technical failure	Causes of clinical failure
• Patient not able to breath-hold/constantly coughing/expectorating. • Tortuous artery/acute angulation • Proximal/ostial narrowing • Aortic tortuosity may hamper stable catherization of subclavian artery branches • Failure to go beyond the origin of spinal cord branches	• Inability to embolize all culprit arteries • Presence of ectopic bronchial arteries • Pulmonary vascular causes

Late recurrences occur due to recanalization of previously treated arteries or new recruitment of non-bronchial systemic collaterals.[8,31,36,37] This occurs, if the underlying disease is not simultaneously controlled, thus emphasizing the need to address the underlying disease medically or surgically. Superimposed infection on background TB sequelae, chronic cavitary pulmonary aspergillosis, and development of multidrug resistance TB (MDR-TB) can contribute to recurrence of hemoptysis in previously treated cases.[31,37,38]

Recurrences at long-term follow-up can be as high as 52% and the probability of recurrence increases with time. The chances of rebleed are more with aspergillomas and with cavitary lung disease.[4,24,31,38,39] Recurrences can again be effectively controlled with BAE, and thus repeat sessions provide for long-term control of hemoptysis.[13,36,37] It has been noted that patients who remain hemoptysis free for 3 years post-BAE have excellent prognosis, but those who rebleed, tend to bleed again and again.[13,16] It may be noted here that BAE is a palliative procedure to control hemoptysis and does not treat the underlying cause. Thus, wherever feasible and considered safe, surgery may be considered for definitive treatment.[12,16]

COMPLICATIONS

The most common complication after BAE is (transient) *chest/back pain*, being reported in up to 34.5% of cases.[2] This is likely related to ischemia of embolized systemic branches, and can be severe when intercostal arteries are embolized. Dissection of the bronchial artery or subintimal perforation and wire manipulation may lead to sudden chest pain **(Figs. 6A to E)**. There may be dissection of the aorta as well while negotiating a smaller catheter into its branch **(Figs. 6A to E)**. In such cases, intravenous fluid should be immediately started and blood pressure should be maintained. Usually, these dissections are non-progressive, but further catheter/wire manipulation in the vicinity of the injured segment should be avoided. The second most common complication is *dysphagia*, caused by embolization of esophageal branches, with a reported occurrence from 0.7 to 18.2%.[12] Spontaneous resolution of symptoms usually occurs.

The most devastating complication is *spinal cord ischemia* that has been reported to occur in 1.4-6.5 percent of patients.[6,12] This may lead to transient or permanent paraplegia, and thus any doubt of spinal artery anastomosis should become a red-flag. The occurrence of this complication can be reduced by using a superselective embolization technique and by performing regular check angiograms before and after administration of embolic agents. *Post-embolization syndrome* may occur and patient may develop fever, leukocytosis and chest pain. This is however a self-limiting complication seen in upto 30% cases.[7,10,14,24,36] *Rare complications* include aortic and bronchial necrosis, bronchial stenosis, unilateral diaphragmatic paralysis, pulmonary infarction (especially in patients who have suffered pulmonary artery embolism), left main bronchial-esophageal fistula, and non-target embolization (colon, coronary, foot and cerebral circulation)[40-43] In addition, contrast-induced nephropathy, hypersensitivity reactions, and groin hematomas may also occur.

CONCLUSION

Bronchial artery embolization is the treatment of choice in acute hemoptysis and can be performed in both emergency as well as elective settings. Knowledge of bronchial and non-bronchial systemic circulation is mandatory to reduce complications and to increase technical success. It is imperative to identify hypertrophied bronchial arteries and other systemic collaterals on CTA to enable successful embolization. BAE is a safe and effective procedure and can be done repeatedly for recurrent hemoptysis as well.

KEY MESSAGES

- The common diseases leading to significant hemoptysis include TB (sequelae and active disease), bronchiectasis and aspergillomas.
- BAE is the procedure of choice for patients presenting in the emergency setting with massive hemoptysis. Also, it is the treatment of choice for immediate control of any amount of hemoptysis in nonsurgical candidates.
- CT angiogram provides a vascular roadmap and bronchoscopy helps in localizing the site of active bleed in diffuse lung disease.
- Superselective catheterization aids in reducing the complications.
- Embolizing agent of choice in BAE is PVA particles (300–500 μ). Larger particles may be used in case of vascular shunts.
- Reactivation TB, MDR-TB and CCPA patients are more prone to develop recurrence of hemoptysis.

REFERENCES

1. Yoon W, Kim JK, Kim YH, et al. Bronchial and nonbronchial systemic artery embolization for life-threatening hemoptysis: a comprehensive review. Radiogr Rev Publ Radiol Soc N Am Inc. 2002;22(6):1395-409.
2. Panda A, Bhalla AS, Goyal A. Bronchial artery embolization in hemoptysis: a systematic review. Diagn Interv Radiol Ank Turk. 2017;23(4):307-17.
3. Walker CM, Rosado-de-Christenson ML, et al. Bronchial arteries: anatomy, function, hypertrophy, and anomalies. Radiogr Rev Publ Radiol Soc N Am Inc. 2015;35(1):32-49.
4. Remy J, Voisin C, Dupuis C. Traitement des hemoptysies par embolization de la circulation systemique. Ann Radiol. 1974;17:5-16.
5. Hayakawa K, Tanaka F, Torizuka T, et al. Bronchial artery embolization for hemoptysis: immediate and long-term results. Cardiovasc Intervent Radiol. 1992;15(3):154-8; discussion 158-9.
6. Wong ML, Szkup P, Hopley MJ. Percutaneous embolotherapy for life-threatening hemoptysis. Chest. 2002;121(1):95-102.
7. Anuradha C, Shyamkumar NK, Vinu M, et al. Outcomes of bronchial artery embolization for life-threatening hemoptysis due to tuberculosis and post-tuberculosis sequelae. Diagn Interv Radiol Ank Turk. 2012;18(1):96-101.
8. Bhalla A, Kandasamy D, Veedu P, et al. A retrospective analysis of 334 cases of hemoptysis treated by bronchial artery embolization. Oman Med J. 2015;30(2):119-28.

9. Agmy GM, Wafy SM, Mohamed SAA, et al. Bronchial and Nonbronchial Systemic Artery Embolization in Management of Hemoptysis: experience with 348 Patients. Int Sch Res Not. 2013;2013:e263259.
10. Woo S, Yoon CJ, Chung JW, et al. Bronchial artery embolization to control hemoptysis: comparison of N-butyl-2-cyanoacrylate and polyvinyl alcohol particles. Radiology. 2013;269(2):594-602.
11. Swanson KL, Johnson CM, Prakash UBS, et al. Bronchial artery embolization: experience with 54 patients. Chest. 2002;121(3):789–95.
12. Ramakantan R, Bandekar VG, Gandhi MS, et al. Massive hemoptysis due to pulmonary tuberculosis: control with bronchial artery embolization. Radiology. 1996;200(3):691-4.
13. Yu-Tang Goh P, Lin M, Teo N, En Shen Wong D. Embolization for hemoptysis: a six-year review. Cardiovasc Intervent Radiol. 2002;25(1):17-25.
14. Shao H, Wu J, Wu Q, SUn X, et al. Bronchial artery embolization for hemoptysis: a retrospective observational study of 344 patients. Chin Med J Engl. 2015;128(1):58-62.
15. Tom LM, Palevsky HI, Holsclaw DS, et al. Recurrent bleeding, survival, and longitudinal pulmonary function following bronchial artery embolization for hemoptysis in a US adult population. J Vasc Interv Radiol. 2015;26(12):1806–13.e1.
16. Fruchter O, Schneer S, Rusanov V, et al. Bronchial artery embolization for massive hemoptysis: long-term follow-up. Asian Cardiovasc Thorac Ann. 2015;23(1):55-60.
17. Ketai LH, Mohammed T-LH, Kirsch J, et al. ACR appropriateness criteria® hemoptysis. J Thorac Imaging. 2014;29(3):W19-22.
18. Khalil A, Fartoukh M, Parrot A, et al. Impact of MDCT angiography on the management of patients with hemoptysis. Am J Roentgenol. 2010;195(3):772-8.
19. Meena P, Bhalla AS, Goyal A, et al. Comparison of contrast injection protocols for simultaneous optimal opacification of systemic and pulmonary arteries in CT angiography of patients with hemoptysis. In Boston, USA; 2017.
20. Sopko DR, Smith TP. Bronchial Artery Embolization for Hemoptysis. Semin Interv Radiol. 2011;28(1):48-62.
21. Tanomkiat W, Tanisaro K. Radiographic relationship of the origin of the bronchial arteries to the left main bronchus. J Thorac Imaging. 2003;18(1):27-33.
22. Sancho C, Escalante E, Domínguez J, et al. Embolization of bronchial arteries of anomalous origin. Cardiovasc Intervent Radiol. 1998;21(4):300-4.
23. Cauldwell EW, Siekert RG. The bronchial arteries: an anatomic study of 150 human cadavers. Surg Gynecol Obstet. 1948;86(4):395-412.
24. Uflacker R, Kaemmerer A, Picon PD, et al. Bronchial artery embolization in the management of hemoptysis: technical aspects and long-term results. Radiology. 1985;157(3):637-44.
25. Marshall TJ, Jackson JE. Vascular intervention in the thorax: bronchial artery embolization for haemoptysis. Eur Radiol. 1997;7(8):1221-7.
26. Furnari ML, Salerno S, Rabiolo A, et al. Bronchial to subclavian shunt in a CF patient. A potential pitfall for embolization. J Cyst Fibros Off J Eur Cyst Fibros Soc. 2003;2(4):217-9.
27. Van den Berg JC, Overtoom TT, De Valois JC. Case report: bronchial to coronary artery anastomosis: a potential hazard in bronchial artery embolization. Br J Radiol. 1996;69(822):570-2.
28. Keller FS, Rosch J, Loflin TG, et al. Nonbronchial systemic collateral arteries: significance in percutaneous embolotherapy for hemoptysis. Radiology. 1987;164(3):687-92.
29. Sellars N, Belli AM. Non-bronchial collateral supply from the left gastric artery in massive haemoptysis. Eur Radiol. 2001;11(1):76-9.
30. Zhang JS, Cui ZP, Wang MQ, Yang L. Bronchial arteriography and transcatheter embolization in the management of hemoptysis. Cardiovasc Intervent Radiol. 1994;17(5):276-9.
31. Shin BS, Jeon GS, Lee SA, et al. Bronchial artery embolisation for the management of haemoptysis in patients with pulmonary tuberculosis. Int J Tuberc Lung Dis Off J Int Union Tuberc Lung Dis. 2011;15(8):1093-8.
32. Won JH, Park SI, Park KJ, et al. Microcatheter placement through a side hole created in a 5-F catheter into proximal subclavian arterial branches causing hemoptysis. J Vasc Interv Radiol. 2004;15(8):881-4.
33. Miyayama S, Matsui O, Akakura Y, et al. Use of a catheter with a large side hole for selective catheterization of the inferior phrenic artery. J Vasc Interv Radiol. 2001;12(4):497-9.
34. Barben J, Robertson D, Olinsky A, et al. Bronchial artery embolization for hemoptysis in young patients with cystic fibrosis. Radiology. 2002;224(1):124-30.
35. Saluja S, Henderson KJ, White RI. Embolotherapy in the bronchial and pulmonary circulations. Radiol Clin North Am. 2000;38(2):425-48, ix.
36. Chan VL, So LK, Lam JY, et al. Major haemoptysis in Hong Kong: aetiologies, angiographic findings and outcomes of bronchial artery embolisation. Int J Tuberc Lung Dis. 2009;13(9):1167-73.
37. Lee S, Chan JW, Chan SC, et al. Bronchial artery embolisation can be equally safe and effective in the management of chronic recurrent haemoptysis. Hong Kong Med J Xianggang Yi Xue Za Zhi. 2008;14(1):14-20.
38. Hwang H-G, Lee H-S, Choi J-S, et al. Risk factors influencing rebleeding after bronchial artery embolization on the management of hemoptysis associated with pulmonary tuberculosis. Tuberc Respir Dis. 2013;74(3):111-9.
39. Yoo DH, Yoon CJ, Kang S-G, et al. Bronchial and nonbronchial systemic artery embolization in patients with major hemoptysis: safety and efficacy of N-butyl cyanoacrylate. Am J Roentgenol. 2011;196(2):W199-204.
40. Ivanick MJ, Thorwarth W, Donohue J, et al. Infarction of the left mainstem bronchus: a complication of bronchial artery embolization. Am J Roentgenol. 1983;141(3):535-7.
41. Girard P, Baldeyrou P, Lemoine G, et al. Left main-stem bronchial stenosis complicating bronchial artery embolization. Chest. 1990;97(5):1246-8.
42. Chapman SA, Holmes MD, Taylor DJ. Unilateral diaphragmatic paralysis following bronchial artery embolization for hemoptysis. Chest. 2000;118(1):269-70.
43. Munk PL, Morris DC, Nelems B. Left main bronchial-esophageal fistula: a complication of bronchial artery embolization. Cardiovasc Intervent Radiol. 1990;13(2):95-7.

CHAPTER

141

Diagnostic and Therapeutic Interventions in Chest

Naveen Kalra, Mandeep Kang, Anupam Lal, Ujjwal Gorsi

INTRODUCTION

A wide range of procedures used in the diagnosis and treatment of diseases of the chest constitute image-guided thoracic interventions. Percutaneous interventional procedures in the chest were actually in use before the advent of imaging. Leyden did the first transthoracic needle lung biopsy in 1882 to confirm pulmonary infections.[1] Lung biopsy continued to be used during the first half of the 20th century for confirming the microbiological diagnosis of infectious lobar consolidation. In 1964, the first fluoroscopically-guided bronchial brush biopsy was described.[2] Around the same time, the technique of transthoracic fine needle sampling in the chest was established by Nordenstrom.[3] Percutaneous mediastinal procedures were adopted on a routine basis after the advent of CT. Percutaneous drainage of fluid collections in the chest was introduced in the late seventies. Better catheter designs and refinement of embolic agents established bronchial artery embolization as an accepted technique in the next decade. Good results with minimally invasive treatment of superior vena cava (SVC) obstruction were achieved with the development of specialized stents. The commonly performed thoracic interventional radiological techniques will be discussed in this chapter. Bronchial artery embolization will be discussed in another chapter.

IMAGE GUIDANCE MODALITIES

Modalities used for image guidance include fluoroscopy, cross-sectional imaging (ultrasound, CT and MRI) or a combination of both. Uni- or biplanar fluoroscopy was the first imaging technique which was used for the guidance of percutaneous transthoracic needle biopsy (TNB) and percutaneous drainage of fluid collections. The advantages of fluoroscopy include its wide availability, familiarity to most radiologists and real-time control of the procedure. Fluoroscopy may be used in combination with ultrasound for adjusting the tip of catheters introduced into fluid collections. Ultrasound is used for image-guided biopsies of the chest wall, pleural lesions, pulmonary lesions with parietal contact or lesions in the anterior or superior mediastinum. Using this technique, the peripheral pulmonary lesions can be successfully biopsied with very high success rates which are more than 90%.[4] The ultrasound probe should be oriented parallel to the intercostal space as this facilitates the biopsy of the peripheral pulmonary lesions. Other procedures which can be done under ultrasound guidance include percutaneous aspiration and catheter drainage. The advantages of ultrasound guidance are real-time monitoring, lack of ionizing radiation, easy availability, portability and the ability to target non-necrotic part of the lesion. CT guidance provides anatomical display of all the thoracic structures in detail and ensures accurate placement of the needle and drainage catheter. It helps to determine the optimal percutaneous entry point so as to avoid transgression of the pleural fissure or puncture of bullae, large vessels, bronchi and the esophagus. Helical CT has not been found superior to sequential scanning.[5] CT fluoroscopy combines the advantages of both cross-sectional imaging and real-time control and is now widely available. High rates of technical success have been reported with sensitivity ranging from 89–95% and specificity of 100%.[6] Studies have shown that using intermittent 'quick check' CT fluoroscopy between needle advancements instead of continuous fluoroscopy can reduce the radiation exposure. Recently PET-CT is being used to guide biopsies by providing information about the abnormal metabolic activity of primary neoplasm and metastases. There is scanty literature on usage of MR guidance for thoracic interventions due to limited availability of this modality and the requirement of especially designed needles compatible with MR scanners.

NONVASCULAR INTERVENTIONS

The various percutaneous nonvascular image-guided thoracic interventions are transthoracic needle biopsy, diagnostic thoracocentesis, drainage of fluid collections, pleurodesis, pneumathorax/bulla drainage, lung abscess drainage, pericardial effusion drainage, treatment of secondary pulmonary aspergilloma, endoluminal tracheobronchial stenting and thermal ablation of pulmonary malignancy.

Transthoracic Needle Biopsy of Pulmonary Lesions

Indications

Transthoracic needle biopsy (TNB) is most commonly done for the diagnosis of a solitary pulmonary nodule (SPN). TNB is also used for confirming metastatic lung disease, staging of lung cancer or extrathoracic malignancy, and sampling of suspected focal infections.[7,8]

Patient Evaluation

Before biopsy, every effort should be made to establish the identity of the lesion using non-invasive methods including review of old chest radiographs and thin section CT for nodule characterization. Some clinicians use 'pulmonary nodule calculators' based on clinical and radiological risk factors to estimate pretest probability of malignancy. Coagulation parameters should be checked for all patients to exclude bleeding diathesis.

Contraindications

There are no absolute contraindications to TNB. However, percutaneous biopsy should be strictly avoided in suspected vascular lesion (e.g. arteriovenous malformation, pulmonary varix) and hydatid cyst. Bleeding diathesis should be corrected prior to the procedure. Severe pulmonary hypertension is a relative contraindication because of the danger of persistent pulmonary hemorrhage. Emphysematous bullae in the planned biopsy route increase the risk of pneumothorax and should be avoided if possible. Severe pulmonary disease, (FEV less than liter), contralateral pneumonectomy, ventilator dependence and patient's inability to cooperate or hold breath are relative contraindications.

Image Guidance

The choice of image guidance modality is dependent on the availability of various techniques, the skill and preference of the interventional radiologist, and the site, size and other characteristics of the lesion to be targeted. Fluoroscopy is particularly useful for biopsies of nodules in the lower third of the lungs, where large respiratory excursions occur. Orthogonal views of lung nodule and the needle obtained either with a rotating C-arm or a biplane fluoroscopy help confirm proper positioning of the needle tip within the lesion. CT guidance is useful for lesions that are adjacent to hilum or mediastinum (to avoid injury to adjacent vascular structures, bronchi and esophagus), for small lesions and the lesions not clearly seen on fluoroscopy **(Figs. 1A and B)**. The use of US guidance is limited to masses that are apical, juxtadiaphragmatic or adjacent to the chest wall **(Figs. 2 and 3)**. PET-CT guidance may improve the success rate of image-guided biopsies if the functional information obtained from the PET study is used to position the tip of the biopsy needle into the area of highest metabolism **(Figs. 4A to D)**. Endobronchial ultrasound (EBUS) guided biopsy is a safer technique than the percutaneous methods. However, it is expensive, not widely available and is primarily the domain of the interventional pulmonologist.

Biopsy Technique

A wide range of needles can be used for percutaneous biopsy procedure. Needles can be classified by their calibre or gauge tip configuration and the mechanism of sample acquisition. Needle sizes can either be smaller gauge (20–25 gauge) or larger gauge (14–19 gauge). Smaller gauge needles result in lesser bleeding and reduce other complications as well. Larger gauge needles on the other hand are easier to direct and provide better samples for cytology and histology. Needles have different angles and bevel of the tip. The Chiba and spinal needles have bevel angle of 25 and 30° respectively. Greene and Franseen needles have 90° tips. Needle tips can also be aspiration (non-cutting) and cutting types. Aspiration needles such as the Chiba, spinal and Greene needles provides cellular material for cytologic evaluation of malignancy. Cutting needle yield pieces of tissue for histologic

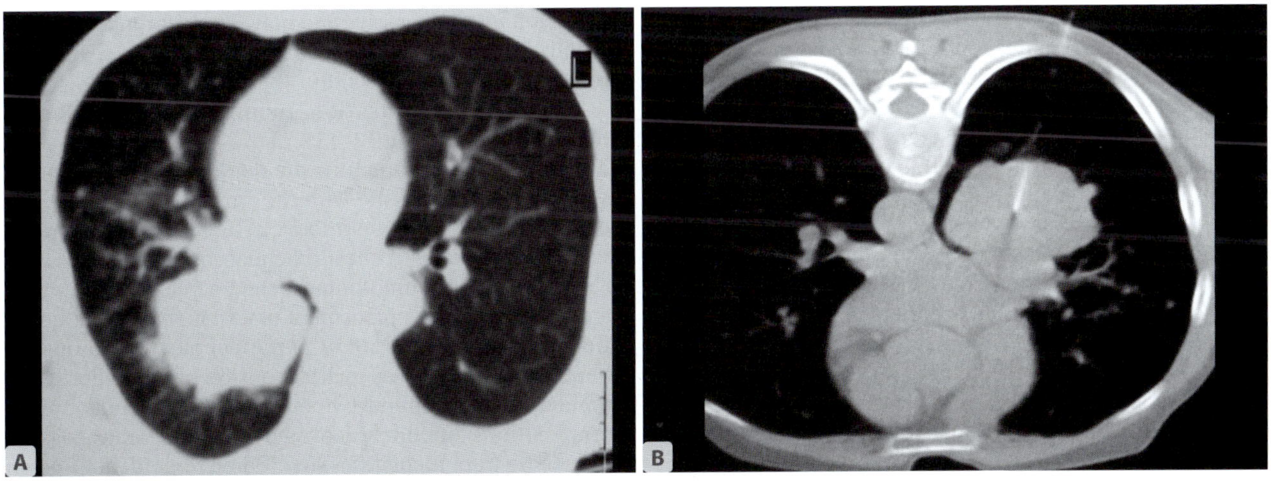

FIGS. 1A AND B: (A) Axial CT section of the chest at lung window settings shows a large mass with spiculated margins in the right hilar region; (B) Axial CT section of the chest in the prone position showing the needle in situ which has been placed in the mass after transgressing the lung parenchyma.

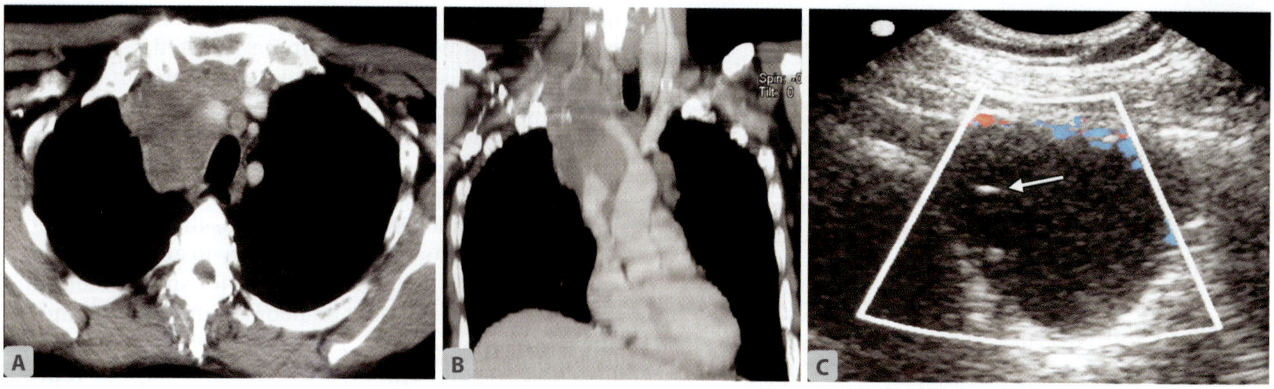

FIGS. 2A TO C: (A) Axial contrast-enhanced CT section shows an apical lung mass with loss of fat planes with the trachea and the brachiocephalic artery; (B) Coronal-reconstructed image showing the extent of the mass with lymph nodes in the neck region; (C) Color Doppler ultrasound showing the needle in situ (arrow). Doppler ultrasound ensures that there is no vessel in the course of the needle.

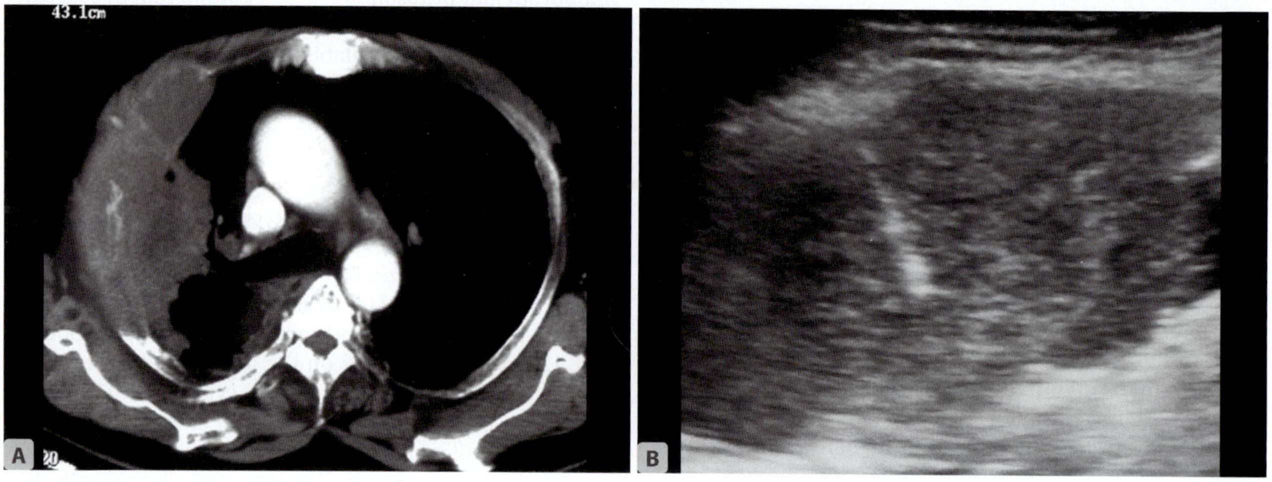

FIGS. 3A AND B: (A) Axial contrast-enhanced CT section shows a large peripheral mass with necrotic component in the right upper lobe with chest wall invasion and rib destruction; (B) Ultrasound image shows the entire extent of the needle which has been introduced percutaneously into the mass.

analysis and can be used for the diagnosis of benign lesions, lymphoreticular malignancies, and in hospitals where experienced cytopathologists are not available. Needles can also be classified as manual, spring-loaded or automated.

The biopsy can be done with the single needle technique or the coaxial technique. As a rough guide, large easily accessible lesions lend themselves to the single needle technique whereas smaller lesions or lesions that require lengthy imaging procedures for correct needle placement are more easily accessible by the coaxial system. In the coaxial technique, an 18 or 19 gauge needle is initially advanced to the proximal edge of the lesion. A 22 gauge needle is then advanced through the guide needle to obtain a fine needle aspirate for cytology or else, a 20 gauge cutting needle is used for obtaining a core biopsy. Post procedural chest radiographs, one immediately after the procedure and another 4 hours later are obtained to rule out pneumothorax.

Complications

The most common complication of percutaneous lung biopsy is bleeding (hemoptysis, chest wall, parenchymal) **(Fig. 5)**. Hemoptysis occurs in about 5% of patients.[8] Usually, it is minimal manifesting as blood stained sputum. Rarely, however, it may be massive and may require bronchial artery embolization, balloon occlusion of the affected segmental bronchus or surgical resection.

The most complication requiring intervention is pneumothorax seen in 12–45% of the patients.[9] Having the patient lie with the puncture site dependent approximates the visceral puncture site with the parietal pleural and can decrease the rate of pneumothorax. 2–15% of pneumothoraces require treatment with chest tube placement **(Fig. 6)**. Large or symptomatic pneumothoraces can be treated with image-guided percutaneous placement of a small caliber catheter. The reported fatality rate of percutaneous lung biopsy is about 0.02%. The causes include tension pneumothorax, air embolism and pulmonary hemorrhage. Other uncommon complications include vasovagal reaction, lobar torsion and needle tract metastases. According to guidelines given by the Society of Interventional Radiology, a higher overall complication rate of 10% is acceptable for lung biopsies compared to 2% for all other organ systems.[10]

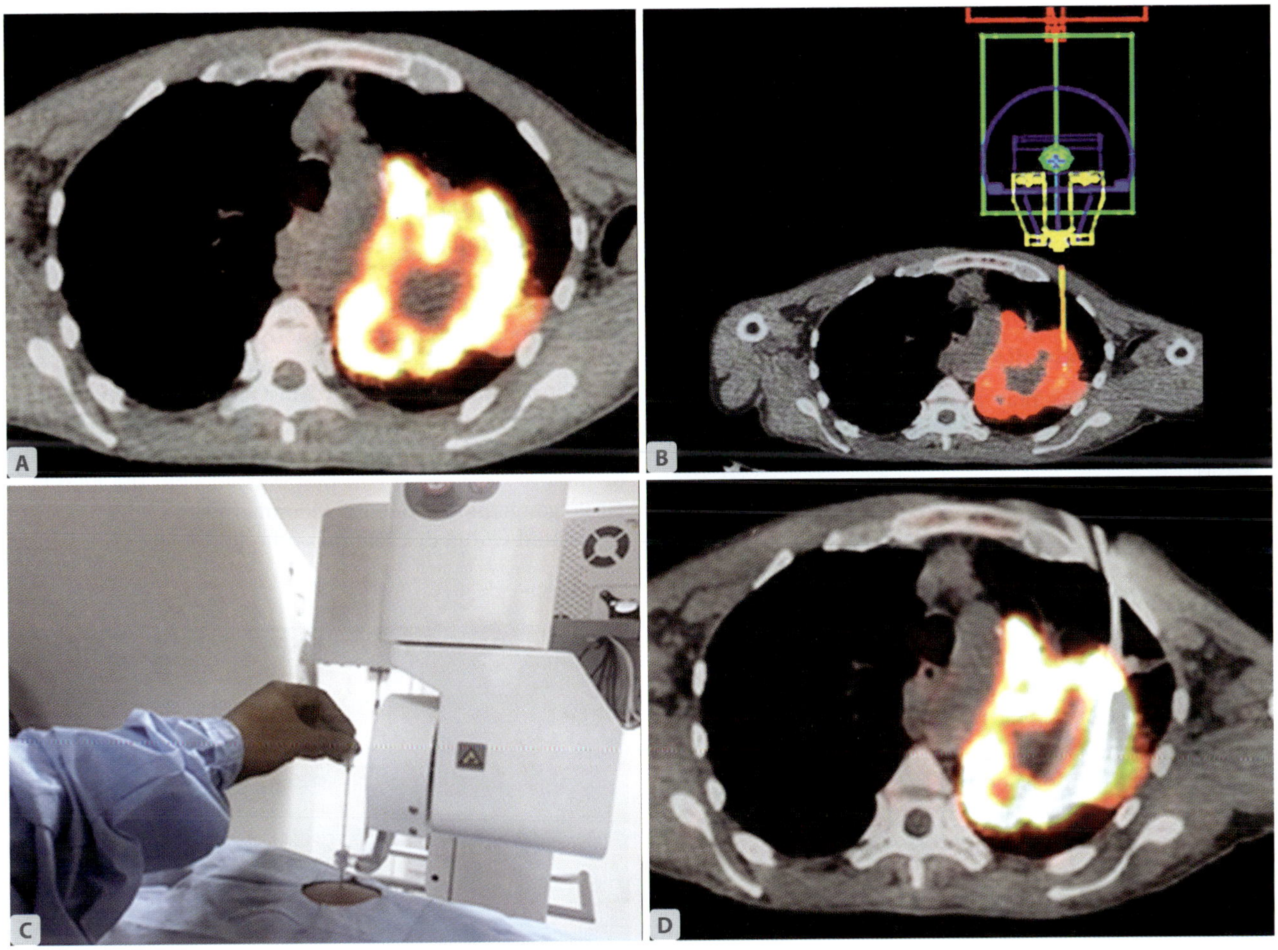

FIGS. 4A TO D: (A) Axial PET-CT functional image showing hypermetabolism in the periphery of the lesion in the left upper lobe of lung consistent with viable cells; (B) Planning of robotic arm-assisted trajectory for biopsy needle placement on robotic arm console; (C) Insertion of co-axial biopsy needle along the planned trajectory with the help of robotic arm needle navigation technique; (D) Check scan to confirm the tip of the semi-automated biopsy gun in the hypermetabolic region just before sampling.

Courtesy: Dr Rajender Kumar Basher and Dr BR Mittal, Department of Nuclear Medicine, PGIMER, Chandigarh.

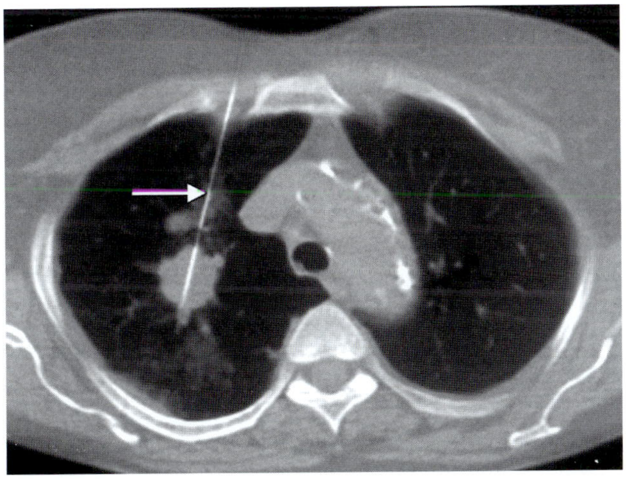

FIG. 5: Axial CT section shows a needle which has been placed in the lung nodule under CT guidance. There is presence of parenchymal hemorrhage along the needle tract (arrow).

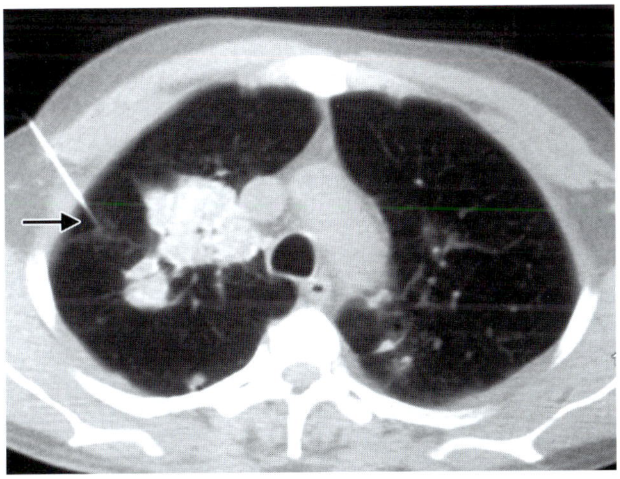

FIG. 6: Axial CT section shows presence of minimal pneumothorax at the site of needle entry. FNAC of the hilar mass was done under CT guidance in this patient (arrow). The pneumothorax was managed conservatively.

Results

Transthoracic needle biopsy of lung nodules is a relatively safe procedure with a high diagnostic yield. According to the guidelines for lung biopsy given by the Society of Interventional Radiology, an 85% success rate is acceptable.[10] TNB has an overall sensitivity of 70–100% in most series for the diagnosis of malignancy.[7,8] The yield for benign lesions, however is 50% or less since benign but non-specific results are not uncommon; this can be improved by performing both core biopsies and FNA of benign lesions.[11,12]

Transthoracic Needle Biopsy from Other Sites

Mediastinal masses may arise without any associated pulmonary mass and may represent metastatic disease. The best method of biopsy is determined by the location of the mass and its proximity to the vital structures. Biopsy of a mediastinal or hilar mass is usually performed under CT guidance as CT clearly shows the location of the mass and its relation to vital mediastinal structures, and allows selection of the optimal biopsy path. Ultrasound guidance can be used for large lesions which are in contact with the chest wall and where a safe acoustic window is available for lesion visualization and needle placement. Anterior mediastinal masses can be accessed by the parasternal **(Figs. 7A and B)**, suprasternal and trans-sternal **(Fig. 8)** approaches, while posterior mediastinal or subcarinal masses are accessed by the posterior paravertebral approach.[13-15] To avoid complications while using the parasternal approach, one should be aware of the anatomical location of internal mammary vessels. A direct mediastinal or extrapleural approach is preferred over a transpulmonary approach, as this reduces the risk of pneumothorax. Saline injection, 'salinoma,' can be used to widen the paravertebral or substernal extrapleural space for a direct mediastinal approach and is helpful in decreasing the incidence of post-biopsy pneumothorax.[16] A pleural space approach through an existing pleural effusion or an iatrogenically created pneumothorax has also been used for mediastinal biopsies.[17] According to the appropriateness criteria published by the American College of Radiology, nonradiologic mediastinal mass biopsy (bronchoscopically guided transbronchial FNA, transesophageal FNA, mediastinoscopy, thoracoscopy) may be safer and have higher yields compared to radiologic biopsy. However, the choices vary from institution to institution.

Percutaneous Needle Biopsy of the Pleura

Biopsies for diffuse disease are usually done without image guidance. Image-guided pleural biopsy is done for pleural masses or thickening with or without associated pleural fluid, small or loculated pleural effusions where thoracentesis has been nondiagnostic and where there are recurrent pleural effusions of unknown etiology. Most pleural biopsies are done using US guidance, although small pleural lesions require CT guidance for accurate needle placement. Solid masses or pleural thickening can be biopsied with the standard 16–20 gauge biopsy needle. Pleural effusions which are not associated with a discrete mass should be biopsied using a

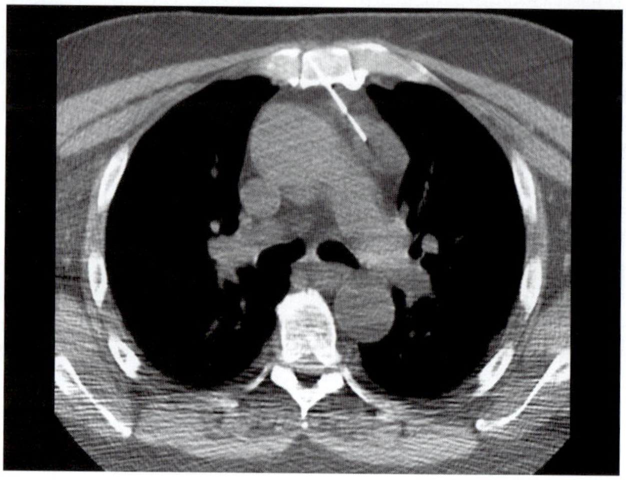

FIG. 8: CT-guided biopsy of the prevascular lymph node being done by the trans-sternal approach.

Courtesy: Dr Sanjay Gupta, MD Anderson Cancer Center, Houston, USA.

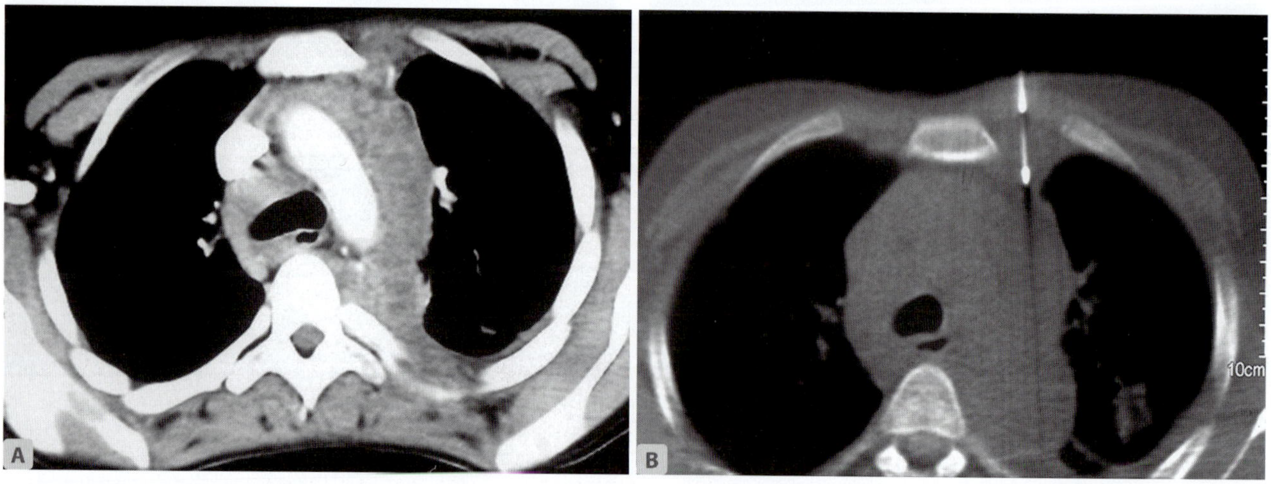

FIGS. 7A AND B: (A) Axial contrast-enhanced CT shows conglomerate lymph nodes in the prevascular and precarinal location; (B) CT-guided biopsy was done in this patient by the parasternal approach.

Cope needle system. Ultrasound guidance is able to localize even a small pleural effusion through which a core biopsy can be safely performed thus reducing the risk of pneumothorax. Complications such as pneumothorax, hemothorax, and laceration of diaphragm, liver or spleen have been reported in less than 1% of biopsies.[7]

Localization of a Nodule for Thoracoscopic Resection

Thoracoscopic resection has established itself as an effective method for diagnosing and treating a peripheral lung nodule that is near the visceral pleura. The radiologist can help by marking the lesion with a hook wire. The hook wire is inserted into the lesion through the guide needle of a coaxial system.[7]

Diagnostic Thoracocentesis

The most common indications for diagnostic thoracentesis are the evaluation of suspected infection or malignancy in the pleural space.[18,19] Sonographic guidance is used following a failed unguided thoracocentesis and when effusions are small or loculated. Using an aseptic technique an appropriate size needle (mostly 22 gauge; thicker up to 18 gauge for viscous collection) is inserted at a point where sonography shows the largest fluid dimension and the fluid is then aspirated. A post-procedure chest radiograph should be done to rule out a pneumothorax. Ultrasound guided diagnostic aspiration is successful in as many as 97% of cases.[20] The yield for cytological examination in documented malignant effusion has been reported to be approximately 50%. Pneumothorax rate is lower (0–3%) than that reported with blind aspiration (3–20%).[21]

Percutaneous Drainage of Pleural Space Fluid Collections

Image-guided percutaneous transthoracic catheter drainage of infected pleural collections is indicated in patients in whom diagnostic thoracocentesis shows frank pus, positive Gram stain on culture or a complicated parapneumonic effusion. Catheter drainage of pleural fluid is also performed for relief of symptoms (dyspnea, cough, pleuritic chest pain).

Empyema is an infected pleural collection caused by pneumonia, bronchiectasis, and/or trauma. Light[22] suggested three stages in the development of empyema. In the acute or exudative stage, although LDH and protein levels are raised, polymorphonuclear leukocytes, pH and glucose are normal. In this stage there is presence of a nonviscous, nonloculated effusion. Most of these collections resolve when appropriate antibiotic therapy is given. The subacute or fibrinopurulent stage is characterized by fall in pH (≤7.00) and glucose (≤40 mg/dL); at this stage, catheter drainage is usually required **(Figs. 9A to C)**. In the third or organizing stage, there is fibrin deposition and a pleural peel forms due to adhesion of visceral and parietal pleurae. In this stage, open thoracotomy and decortication is required for effective treatment.[19] Radiologic drainage is most effective in patients who have short duration of symptoms, free flowing or unilocular collections, absence of thick pleural peel and fluid that can be aspirated freely by needle insertion. Shankar et al.[23] found that radiologic drainage was more effective when on ultrasound the empyema was either anechoic or complex with diffusely distributed internal echoes and/or debris and no septations. On the other hand, empyemas which were complex and septated had a lower chance of successful percutaneous drainage. Postoperative empyemas, particularly those associated with bronchopleural fistula usually require open surgical procedure.

Most commonly, a combination of sonography and fluoroscopy is used for guidance. Fluoroscopy allows continuous monitoring of the course of needle, guidewire and catheter. Sonography is usually used for guidance of initial needle placement, and subsequent guidewire manipulations and catheter placement are performed under fluoroscopic guidance. For large collections, the entire procedure can be safely performed under sonographic control. CT is best used to drain loculated pleural collections, pleural fluid associated with underlying parenchymal fluid consolidation, and small less accessible collections.

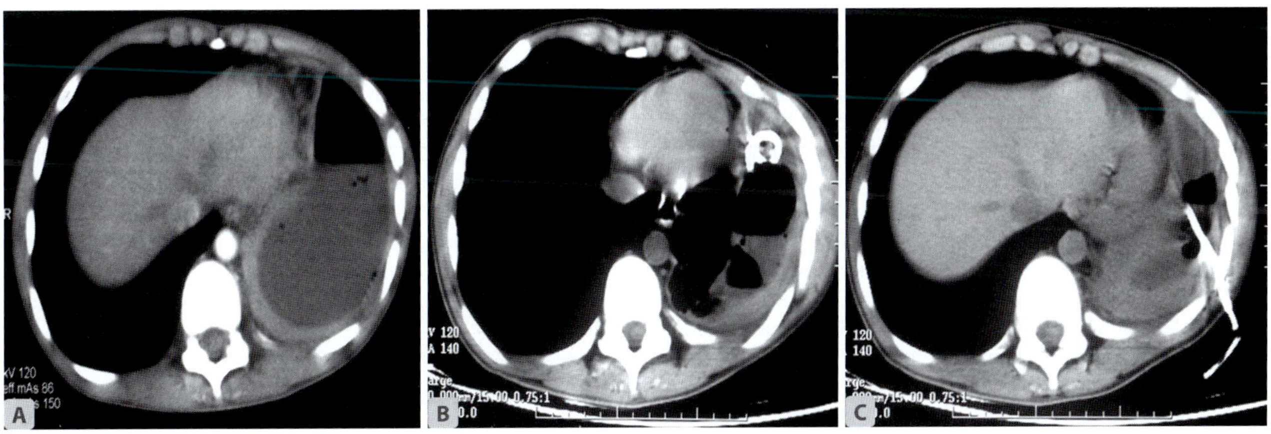

FIGS. 9A TO C: (A) Axial contrast-enhanced CT section showing a loculated collection with air-fluid level with enhancing pleura on the left side; (B and C) Axial CT sections done post-drainage show significant resolution of the collection after one week of drainage.

Catheters ranging in size from 8-30 French are introduced by the Seldinger or trocar techniques. The catheter is placed in the most dependent part of the collection and is immediately attached to a water-seal pleural drainage system with or without suction. The water-seal system not only allows a unidirectional flow but also permits visual observation of an air-leak. The patient is assessed daily for therapeutic response, amount of drainage, and catheter patency. Periodic imaging is required to assess size of the residual collection and lung re-expansion. Chest radiographs usually suffice for non-loculated collections, but CT scanning may be needed for assessing loculated collections. The drainage catheter is removed when the drainage output is less than 10 mL per day, the patient's fever and leukocyte counts have decreased and resolution of the pleural collection is documented on imaging.

Poor drainage of pleural fluid and inadequate lung re-expansion may be secondary to improperly positioned or kinked catheter, complex fluid collection, multiple separate locules, a bronchopleural fistula, or airway obstruction. Undrained non-communicating loculi may require additional catheters. Occasionally, repositioning of catheter or conversion to a large bore catheter may help enhance drainage. A wire advanced through the catheter can be used to disrupt septae in multiseptate collections. Intrapleural administration of fibrinolytic medication (streptokinase, urokinase, or more recently tissue plasminogen activator) may aid in septated or loculated collections. Intrapleural fibrinolytic administration helps dissolve viscous fibrinous material and septations that interfere with drainage. In one protocol, 2–4 mg of t-PA in 10–20 mL saline is injected every 8 hours for several days with clamping of the tube after each instillation.[24] The reported clinical success rate is 62–100%.

Retrospective studies of radiologically guided pleural drainage procedures have shown success rates of 72–88%, which compare favourably with success rates of 66–83% reported in surgical literature.[19] Complications including bleeding due to intercostal vessel injury, pneumothorax, bronchopleural fistula, re-expansion pulmonary edema, and bacteremia are uncommon, seen in less than 2% of cases.[18,19]

Pleural Sclerotherapy or Pleurodesis

Recurrent malignant effusions can be managed by instillation of a sclerosing agent into the pleural space. This induces chemical pleurodesis. The procedure is performed by placing a catheter in the pleural space. When the catheter output drops below 100 mL/day and chest imaging shows drainage of fluid and re-expansion of the lung, sclerotherapy is performed. There should be adequate apposition of the visceral and parietal layers of the pleura for sclerosis to be effective. The agents used for this procedure include tetracycline, doxycycline, minocycline, bleomycin, diluted sodium hydroxide and talc.[18,19] A 20–50 mL of 1-2% lidocaine can be instilled into the pleural space before the sclerotic agent for analgesia. Reported success rates range from 62–90%, and no particular agent has been shown to be superior.[18,19]

Pneumothorax Drainage

The indications for pneumothorax drainage are large volume of the air pocket (>25% of the volume of one hemithorax), an enlarging pneumothorax indicating persistent air leak, tension pneumothorax, a diseased contralateral lung or any sized pneumothorax associated with shortness of breath or severe chest pain.[18,19] Most pneumothoraces drainages can be performed using fluoroscopic guidance. However, CT guidance may be used for small and loculated air collections. The pneumothorax may be approached in two ways, either through the first or second intercostal space in the midclavicular line or through the 4th or 5th intercostal space in the anterior axillary line in females and in males with bulky pectoralis muscles. The anterior approach has the advantage of allowing easier positioning of the catheter tip in the lung apex. The lateral approach allows real-time visualization of the pneumothorax and catheter insertion is then easily performed. Catheters ranging in size from 6 to 16 French are used and are connected to an underwater seal drainage with suction or to a one-way flutter (Heimlich) valve. There is need to confirm the correct catheter placement and reduction in the pneumothorax by doing a chest radiograph immediately after the drainage. The catheter is removed when the lung remains expanded on a follow-up chest radiograph obtained 2 hours after clamping the tube and there is no evidence of air leak. Success rates range from 87 to 93% with majority of pneumothoraces resolving within 24–72 hours.

Lung Abscess Drainage

Lung abscess represents an infected collection of the lung parenchyma. Primary abscesses are the result of aspiration and are caused by anaerobic bacteria. Secondary abscesses arise from adjacent infection or by hematogenous spread (e.g. pneumonia, lung cyst, septic emboli). Majority of lung abscesses respond to antibiotics, postural drainage and bronchoscopic lavage. Image-guided percutaneous catheter drainage is used for the treatment of lung abscesses that fail to resolve with medical therapy. A CT scan is done to assess the presence of pleural involvement and to plan a safe transthoracic route for catheter placement. Fluoroscopy, US or CT guidance can be used for performing the procedure. One should avoid traversing normal lung because of the risk of hemorrhage and bronchopleural fistula formation with empyema. The catheter should transverse the abnormal lung to avoid pneumothorax and collapse of normal lung. The patient should be positioned to keep the opposite hemothorax nondependent in order to avoid the aspiration of the abscess contents into the normal lung. As lung abscess drainage represents a controlled bronchocutaneous fistula, the size of the drainage catheter should not be more than 12–14 French to avoid large air leaks. The catheter is removed once clinical assessment and chest radiographs indicate resolution of abscess. 73–100% patients show resolution of the abscess after 10–15 days of drainage. However, complete collapse of the cavity may take longer up to 4–5 weeks as abscesses have thick walls.[3]

Mediastinal Abscess Drainage

Mediastinal abscess is a life-threatening infection which occurs subsequent to thoracic surgery or endoscopy. Mediastinal abscesses not considered for surgical drainage can be successfully drained percutaneously or by a transesophageal approach.[25] Drainage is usually done under CT guidance by a parasternal or paraspinous approach to avoid the lung. The few reported series indicate a success rate of 83–100% but 30 days mortality is high.[3]

Pericardial Effusion Drainage

Pericardial effusions require drainage when they impair the diastolic filling of the ventricles. Large pericardial effusions are caused by renal failure, metabolic or immunologic diseases, infection and malignancy. Pericardial catheter drainage is done under ultrasound guidance using a subcostal or subxiphoid approach with or without fluoroscopy. Drainage can also be done under CT guidance by the left anterolateral approach.[26]

Pneumatocele and Bulla Drainage

Percutaneous drainage of an infected or tension pneumatocele or bulla has been performed.[27,28] However, an air-fluid level within a bulla does not indicate infection and a percutaneous diagnostic aspiration should precede catheter insertion in doubtful cases **(Figs. 10A to C)**.

Secondary Pulmonary Aspergilloma

Intracavitatory aspergilloma may present with life-threatening hemoptysis and require a surgical resection. However, open thoracotomy may be contraindicated in patients with severe underlying pulmonary pathology. In such patients, transthoracic instillation of amphotericin B has been described. This technique has a reported success rate of 50% for resolution of aspergilloma and 75–100% for acute control of hemoptysis.[29]

Endoluminal Tracheobronchial Stenting

Tracheobronchial airway obstruction can occur due to a malignant or benign cause. Although surgery is the treatment of choice, balloon dilatation or stenting may be done as a palliative treatment in patients who have short life expectancy or extensive airway stenosis. Balloon dilatation results in rapid improvement of the respiratory function. However, relief of symptoms is often short lasting. Stents can be placed under image guidance or bronchoscopic control or by using a combination of both modalities. Tracheobronchial stenting has been successfully done for symptom palliation in patients with inoperable bronchogenic cancer, esophageal or tracheal tumors and metastatic tumors causing extensive compression or submucosal disease or tracheoesophageal fistula. It has also been done in benign conditions like post-intubation or post-anastomatic stricture, tracheobronchomalacia, fibrosing mediastinitis, relapsing polychondritis and amyloidosis. Helical CT is used for precise measurement of the diameter of the stenosis and for determining the location of the stenosis. Two types of stents are used: silicone stents (Dumon, Dynamic and others) and metallic stents (balloon expandable stents like Palmaz and Strecker or SEMS, self-expandable stents such as Gianturco, Wallstent, Ultraflex). As some of these stents have poor visualization on conventional fluoroscopy, CT fluoroscopy guidance may be used to ensure precise and real-time control on stent deployment. Placement of stents leads to immediate and significant decrease in symptoms and respiratory function improvement in majority (80–95%) of patients. Complications of stent placement are early or late stent migration, infection, tracheobronchial fistula, deformation or breakage of stent and stent obstruction by secretions, granulations or tumor overgrowth.

THERMAL ABLATION OF LUNG LESIONS

The three most commonly used ablative techniques in the lung are radiofrequency ablation (RFA), microwave ablation (MWA) and cryoablation. These ablative techniques are used in the management of inoperable nonsmall cell lung cancer (NSCLC) and in selected patients with pulmonary metastases. Surgical resection is the gold standard for the treatment of stage I NSCLC. Unfortunately, only about one-third of patients are suitable for surgical resection due to various comorbidities or poor cardiopulmonary reserve. Dupuy et al. reported the first clinical experience of percutaneous RFA of lung lesions in the year 2000.[30] RFA is a minimally invasive thermal energy delivery system. It delivers a high frequency alternating current supplied by a radiofrequency generator through a needle electrode placed in the tumor. The application of an alternating current results in ionic

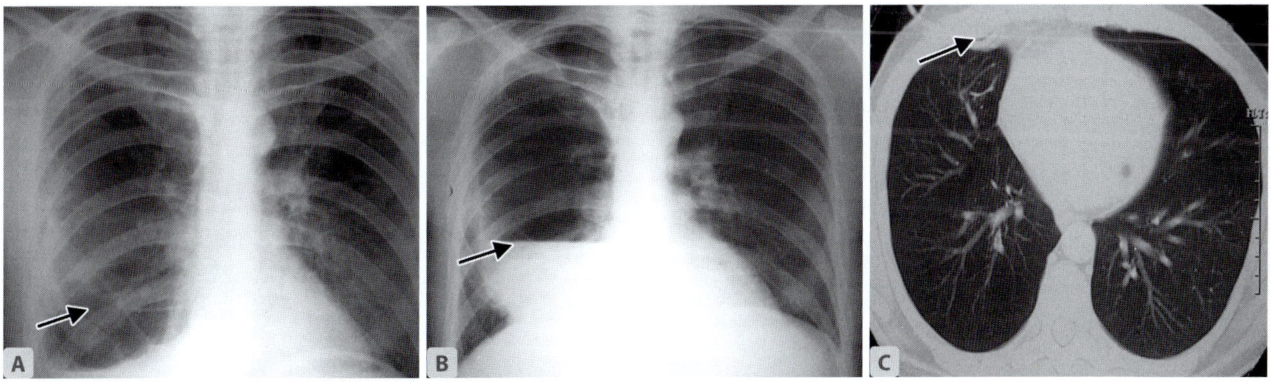

FIGS. 10A TO C: (A) Chest X-ray PA view shows multiple emphysematous bullae in the right mid and lower zones (arrow); (B) Chest X-ray PA view shows an air–fluid level in a large bulla in the right mid and lower zones (arrow) on follow-up; (C) Axial CT of the chest at lung window settings post-drainage shows the catheter in situ with resolution of the collection (arrow).

agitation and generation of frictional heat which ablates the tumor tissue. As air is a thermal insulator, the aerated lung has high electric impedance. Lung tumors are well suited for RFA as the surrounding normal lung parenchyma acts as an insulator for the heat energy delivered. Hence, less power input is required to achieve adequate ablation. By the same principle, pleural based lesions require more energy to treat and are associated with higher recurrence rates and complications. However, a longer approach traversing atleast 2 cm of aerated lung is recommended even for peripheral tumors to prevent air leak, chest pain and skin burns. When ablating lung tumors, tract cautery should be avoided to circumvent the risk of bronchopleural fistula formation.

The outcome of ablation is more promising in metastatic disease compared with primary malignancies and in lesions smaller than 3 cm in size. Most centers limit RFA to patients with five or fewer lesions and use 5 cm as the upper limit for size.[31] Contraindications for the procedure include lesions which are close to vessels (within 1 cm), poor lung function, presence of pacemaker and coagulopathy. The lesions are treated in a predetermined order, typically starting with the most dependent lesions as they may be obscured by blood from more anterior lesions as the treatment progresses **(Figs. 11A and B)**. CT done at this time shows the ablated lesion surrounded by ground-glass opacity (GGO). The treatment is considered technically complete when the entire tumor is surrounded by GGOs **(Figs. 12A and B)**. Complications of the procedure include pneumothorax, hemothorax, infective complications and tumor ablation syndrome. Symptoms of ablation syndrome include myalgia, fever and productive cough.

Follow-up imaging is done at 1 month and then at 3 months intervals for the first year. The criterion for complete resolution is reduction of the contrast enhancement compared with images taken before the procedure. A CT attenuation higher than 15 HU indicates disease persistence or relapse.[32] The postablation evolution of the lesion on imaging and histology is divided into three phases: early (<1 week), intermediate (1 week to 3 months) and late (>3 months) phases.[33] In the early phase, there are three layers of tissue seen on histology: an inner layer of thermal damage, a middle layer of alveolar congestion and an outer layer of congestion, hemorrhage and both damaged and viable cells. On CT the lesion is surrounded by an inner layer of GGO corresponding to the inner and middle layers on histology, and an outer thin, dense rim corresponding to the outer layer on histology. In the intermediate phase, there is granulation and fibrosis of the necrotic tissue. The size of the ablation zone may still exceed the size of the tumor in this phase. The benign periablational enhancement pattern still persists. In the late phase, the fibrous transformation is completed. The ablated area will be seen as fibrotic, nodular or cavitatory. CT done at this time should be taken as baseline examination in order to evaluate progression or recurrence. Even with PET-CT, an active lesion does not definitely represent tumor in the first three months.[34]

In the RAPTURE study (a prospective, intention-to-treat, multicenter trial), 106 patients (33 patients with primary disease, 73 patients with pulmonary metastases) with 183 lung tumors smaller than 3.5 cm were treated with RFA.[35] The study showed a 1-year overall complete response rate of 88% and a 2-year cancer-specific survival of 92% for primary disease. In another study of pulmonary metastases, RFA was found to be an effective treatment option for nodules less than 2 to 3 cm with a 4-year local efficacy of 89%.[36]

Microwave ablation is now becoming the favored technique for treating lung malignancies. It uses electromagnetic energy which is at a much higher frequency than RFA (300 MHz to 300 GHz). It delivers all the benefits of RFA and has several advantages.[37] The ablative zone is larger and is less susceptible to heat sink effect. The various benefits include consistently higher intratumoral temperatures, an improved convection profile, the capability of using multiple applicators, larger tumor ablation volumes and no need for grounding pads. Tumors smaller than 2 cm in maximal diameter are treated with a single applicator and tumors 2 cm or larger are treated with multiple antennae each powered by individual microwave generators. The reported cancer-specific 1-year survival is 83%, 2-year survival is 73% and 3-year survival is 61% for pulmonary tumors of mean size of 3.5 cm.[37]

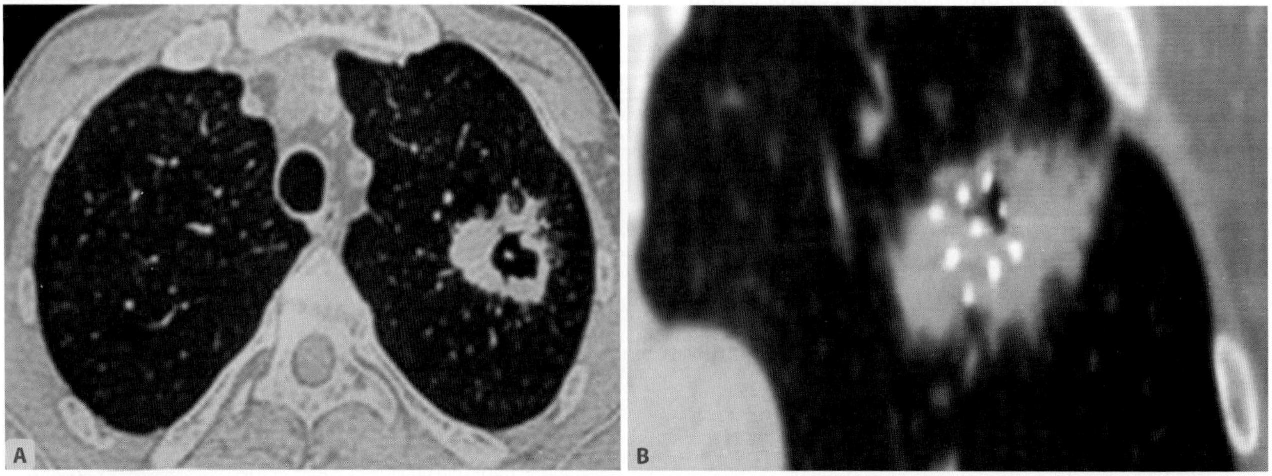

FIGS. 11A AND B: (A) Axial CT in the supine position at lung window settings shows a malignant cavitory nodule in the left upper lobe; (B) Coronal CT section during RF ablation shows the hyperattenuation with increase in the size of the nodule contributed by intraparenchymal hemorrhage.

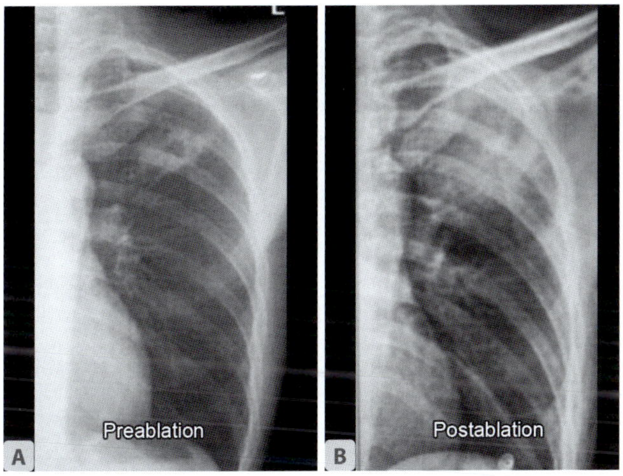

FIGS. 12A AND B: (A) Preablation chest X-ray showing cavitory lesion in left upper lobe; (B) Postablation chest X-ray showing a larger area of opacity due to the surrounding congestion and hemorrhage.

Cryoablation works on the principle of freeze-thaw-freeze cycle. Pressurized argon gas is used to generate temperatures of less than -40°C and helium is used to increase the temperature to 20°C. There is cell rupture, protein denaturation and microvascular thrombosis-induced ischemia. One can accurately visualize the ablation zone as an 'ice ball' on CT scan. Presently, cryoablation is considered safer than RFA and MWA for lung tumors near the chest wall or mediastinum. The newer cryoablation devices have the cautery option unlike the older equipment which decreases the risk of bleeding complications like pulmonary hemorrhage, hemoptysis and hemothorax.[38] However, the potential risk of a severe systemic adverse effect, i.e. cryoshock still remains.

VASCULAR INTERVENTIONS

The various vascular interventions are bronchial artery embolization, pulmonary artery embolization, superior vena cava (SVC) stenting and percutaneous vascular foreign body retrieval. Bronchial artery embolization will be discussed in another chapter.

Pulmonary Artery Embolization

Pulmonary artery embolization is done for pulmonary artery aneurysms and pulmonary arteriovenous malformations (PAVMs). Aneurysms and pseudoaneurysms of the pulmonary arteries have several causes. The main pulmonary artery may be dilated by left-to-right shunts or pulmonary artery hypertension. Post-stenotic dilatation following pulmonary valve disease may mimic an aneurysm. Central pulmonary artery aneurysms are caused by congenital disorders or vasculitis. Multiple aneurysms may be seen with infection (e.g. Rasmussen's aneurysms in tuberculosis, following septic emboli, necrotizing pneumonia, syphilis). Large pulmonary artery aneurysms present with hemoptysis, chest pain or dyspnea or may be seen as an incidental finding on CT or chest X-ray.

Pseudoaneurysms are usually seen in the right middle or lower lobe arteries. Distal arterial rupture with pseudoaneurysm formation is a rare complication of Swan-Ganz catheter placement. The patients present with hemoptysis or a lung mass on imaging studies. Transcatheter embolization of the parent artery with coils or vascular plugs is the treatment of choice and is usually successful.

PAVMs occur sporadically or in patients with hereditary hemorrhagic telangiectasia (HHT), also known as Osler-Weber-Rendu syndrome. PAVMs may also occur secondary to trauma. HHT is an autosomal dominant disorder in which there are telangiectasias of the mouth and telangiectasias or AVMs of the brain, gastrointestinal treat (GIT), liver and lungs. Pulmonary AVMs are seen in 20–50% of patients with HHT and 60% have multiple lesions. Many patients present with epistaxis.

The majority (90%) of AVMs are simple and have single segmental arterial supply. The rest are complex and have multiple segmental arterial supply. They are usually found in the lower lobes. The PAVMs are direct communications between pulmonary artery branches and veins and thus cause a right-to-left shunt. This results in dyspnea, fatigue, hemoptysis, stroke or brain abscess. The primary indication for embolization of PAVMs is prevention of neurologic complications.

CT angiography is done to identify all feeding arteries. Pulmonary embolotherapy is the treatment of choice.[39] Many devices have been used for occlusion including coils and detachable balloons or vascular plugs **(Figs. 13A to D)**. Coils should be 1–2 mm larger than the artery being embolized and should be deployed near the nidus of the malformations. In small feeding arteries (<5 mm in diameter), detachable balloons may be preferred due to the precision of placement. Embolization is successful in more than 90% of patients. A post-embolization syndrome with fever and chest pain is common. Complications occur in 10–20% of cases. Serious complications include paradoxical embolization of air or of the embolization device. All catheter and guide wire exchanges and coil introduction should be done 'under water' to avoid air embolism to the brain.

Endovascular Therapy of SVC Obstruction

The superior vena cava (SVC) may be obstructed as a result of luminal disease (thrombus or tumor), extrinsic compression (tumor or lymph node) or mural disease (intimal hyperplasia or tumor invasion). Fibrosing mediastinitis is a localized or diffuse infiltrative disease that may be idiopathic or may be caused by chronic infection. The SVC is involved in one-third of cases. Significant SVC or bilateral brachiocephalic vein stenosis or obstruction may lead to SVC syndrome. This is characterized by marked facial and neck swelling, bilateral arm swelling, cyanosis, shortness of breath, hoarseness and headache. Catheter directed therapy is considered only in patients with moderate to severe symptoms who fail to respond to less aggressive measures. SVC occlusion itself is rarely fatal and most patients die due to the underlying malignant disease. Therefore, the aim of treatment is only short-term palliation of symptoms. Long-term patency is required in

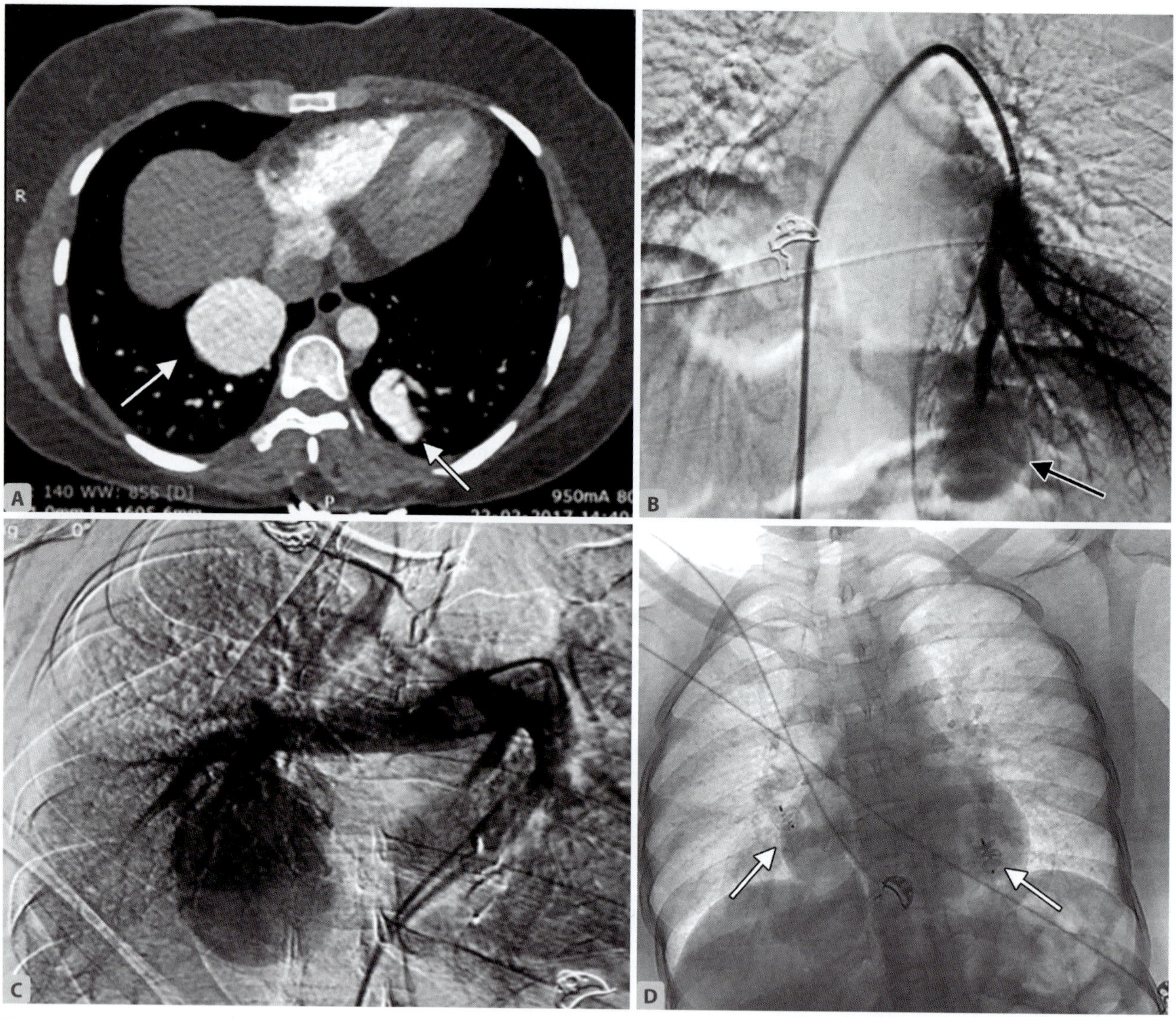

FIGS. 13A TO D: (A) Axial CECT showing pulmonary AVMs in lower lobes of both lungs (arrows); (B) Left pulmonary angiogram showing AVM in left lower lobe; (C) Right pulmonary angiogram showing large AVM in right lower lobe; (D) Post-embolization radiograph showing both vascular plugs (arrows).

patients with benign SVC obstruction. Intravascular stents are effective in both benign and malignant SVC obstruction. In patients with benign obstruction, PTA is done before stenting. It probes the degree of stenosis and localizes the level of maximum resistance within the stenosed segment. PTA is not done prior to stenting in malignant disease but should be done after stenting to establish optimal venous return. Relative contraindications to the procedure are preterminal patients with malignant disease, extensive chronic venous thrombosis, endoluminal tumor growth and upper limb paralysis. Complications include stent migration or misplacement, formation of *de novo* thrombosis and pulmonary embolism.

Percutaneous Vascular Foreign Body Retrieval

The percutaneous method of retrieval avoids thoracotomy and open heart surgery. The foreign bodies needing retrieval include lost central venous lines, Swan-Ganz catheters, ventriculoatrial shunts, port-a-caths, cardiac stimulator lines and pacemaker electrodes. Relative contraindications for retrieval are free-floating thrombus attached to the foreign body and chronic incorporation of the foreign body in a thrombus or vessel wall. The extraction is done by loop-snare technique, helical basket entrapment or the grasping forceps technique or a combination of the above. The reported success rate of closed percutaneous retrieval is >90%.[40]

CONCLUSION

There is a myriad of procedures that can be performed by the interventional radiologist in the chest. However there needs to be a close association between the radiologists, pulmonologists, oncologists, pathologists and thoracic surgeons to ensure the success of these procedures. The complication rate can also be kept low by following the prescribed guidelines for these interventions.

REFERENCES

1. Leyden OO. Uber infectiose pneumonie. Dtsch Med Wochenschr. 1883;9;52-5.
2. Hattori S, Matsuda M, Sugiyama T, et al. Cytologic diagnosis of early lung cancer: brushing method under X-ray television fluoroscopy. Dis Chest. 1964;45:129-42.
3. Ghaye B, Dondelinger RF. Imaging-guided thoracic interventions. Eur Respir J. 2001;17:507-28.
4. Middleton WD, Teefey SA, Dahiya N. Ultrasound-guided chest biopsies. Ultrasound Q. 2006;22:241-52.
5. Ghaye B, Dondelinger RF, Dewe W. Percutaneous CT-guided lung biopsy: sequential versus spiral scanning: A randomized prospective study. Eur Radiol. 1999;9:1317-20.
6. Gupta S. New techniques in image-guided percutaneous biopsy. Cardiovasc Intervent Radiol. 2004;27:91-104.
7. Tarver RD, Conces DJ Jr. Interventional chest radiology. Radiol Clin North Am. 1994;32:689-709.
8. Klein JS, Zarka MA. Transthoracic needle biopsy. Radiol Clin North Am. 2000;38:235-66.
9. Gupta S, Wallace MJ, Cardella JF, et al. Quality improvement guidelines for percutaneous needle biopsy. J Vasc Interv Radiol. 2010;21:969-75.
10. Cardella JF, Bakal CW, Bertino RE, et al. Quality improvement guidelines for image-guided percutaneous biopsy in adults. J Vasc Interv Radiol. 2003;14:S227-30.
11. Fraser RS. Transthoracic needle aspiration. The benign diagnosis. Arch Pathol Lab Med. 1991;115:751-61.
12. Greif J, Marmor S, Schwarz Y, et al. Percutaneous core needle biopsy vs. fine needle aspiration in diagnosing benign lung lesions. Acta Cytol. 1999;43:756-60.
13. Protopapas Z, Westcott JL. Transthoracic hilar and mediastinal biopsy. Radiol Clin North Am. 2000;38:281-91.
14. Gupta S, Gulati M, Rajwanshi A, et al. Sonographically guided fine-needle aspiration biopsy of superior mediastinal lesions by the suprasternal route. Am J Roentgenol. 1998;171:1303-06.
15. Gupta S, Wallace MJ, Morello FA Jr, et al. CT-guided percutaneous needle biopsy of intra-thoracic lesions by using the trans-sternal approach: Experience in 37 patients. Radiology. 2002;222: 57-62.
16. Langen HJ, Klose KC, Keulers P, et al. Artificial widening of the mediastinum to gain access for extra pleural biopsy: Clinical results. Radiology. 1995;196:703-06.
17. Bressler EL, Kirkham JA. Mediastinal masses: alternative approaches to CT-guided needle biopsy. Radiology. 1994; 191:391-96.
18. Boland GW, Lee MJ, Silverman S, et al. Interventional radiology of the pleural space. Clin Radiol. 1995;50:205-14.
19. Klein JS, Schultz S, Heffner JE. Interventional radiology of the chest: Image-guided percutaneous drainage of pleural effusions, lung abscess, and pneumothorax. Am J Roentgenol. 1995;164:581-8.
20. Silverman SG, Saini S, Mueller PR. Pleural interventions. Indications, techniques, and clinical applications. Radiol Clin North Am. 1989;27:1257-66.
21. Collins TR, Sahn SA. Thoracocentesis: Clinical value, complications, technical problems, and patent experience. Chest. 1987;91: 817-22.
22. Light RW. Parapneumonic effusions and empyema. Clin Chest Med. 1985;6:55-62.
23. Shankar S, Gulati M, Kang M, et al. Image-guided percutaneous drainage of thoracic empyema: Can sonography predict the outcome? Eur Radiol. 2000;10:495-99.
24. D' Agostino HB, Hurvitz D, Nall L, et al. Transcatheter fluid drainage. In: Valji K (Eds). Vascular and Interventional Radiology, Elsevier, 2006.pp.516-31.
25. Gobien RP, Stanley JH, Gobien BS, et al. Percutaneous catheter aspiration and drainage of suspected mediastinal abscesses. Radiology. 1984;151:69-71.
26. Szapiro D, Ghaye B, Dondelinger RF. Pericardial tamponade: CT-guided percutaneous drainage. J Interv Radiol. 1996;11:129-31.
27. Sewall LE. Franco AI, Wojtowycz MM, et al. Pneumatoceles causing respiratory compromise. Treatment by percutaneous decompression. Chest. 1993;103:1266-7.
28. Kalra N, Aiyappan SK, Jindal SL, et al. Image-guided percutaneous drainage of an emphysematous bulla with a fluid level. Indian J Radiol Imaging. 2010;20:34-6.
29. Giron J, Poey C, Fajadet P, et al. CT-guided percutaneous treatment of inoperable aspergillomas: A study of 40 cases. Eur J Radiol. 1998;28:235-42.
30. Dupuy DE, Zagoria RJ. Akerley W, et al. Percutaneous radiofrequency ablation of malignancies in the lung. Am J Roentgenol. 2000;174:57 59.
31. Roy AM, Bent C, Fotheringham T, et al. Radiofrequency ablation of lung lesions: Practical applications and tips. Curr Probl Diagn Radiol. 2009;38:44-52.
32. Akeboshi M, Yamakado K, Nakatsuka A, et al. Percutaneous radiofrequency ablation of lung neoplasms: Initial therapeutic response. J Vasc Interv Radiol. 2004;15:463-70.
33. Vogl TJ, Nour-Eldin NA, Albrecht MH, et al. Thermal ablation of lung tumors: Focus on microwave ablation. Rofo. 2017;189:828-43.
34. Bonichon F, Palussiere, Godbert Y, et al. Diagnostic accuracy of 18F-FDG PET/CT for assessing response to radiofrequency ablation treatment in lung metastases: A multicentric prospective study. Eur J Nucl Med Mol Imaging. 2013;40:1817-27.
35. Lencioni R, Crocetti L, Cioni R, et al. Response to radiofrequency ablation of pulmonary tumours: A prospective, intention-to-treat, multicentre clinical trial (the RAPTURE study). Lancet Oncol. 2008;9:621-28.
36. de Baere T, Auperin A, Deschamps F, et al. Radiofrequency ablation is a valid treatment option for lung metastases: experience in 566 patients with 1037 metastases. Ann Oncol. 2015;26:987-91.
37. Wolf FJ, Grand D, Machan JT, et al. Microwave ablation of lung malignancies: Effectiveness, CT findings, and safety in 50 patients. Radiology. 2008;247:871-9.
38. Lee KS, Erinjeri JP. Decision making in interventional oncology: Ablative options in the lung. Semin Intervent Radiol. 2017;34:176 81.
39. Mager JJ, Overtoom TT, Blauw H, et al. Embolotherapy of pulmonary arteriovenous malformation: Long-term results in 112 patients. J Vasc Interv Radiol. 2004;15:451-6.
40. Dondelinger RF, Lepoutre B, Kurdziel JC. Percutaneous vascular foreign body retrieval: experience of an 11 year period. Eur J Radiol. 1991;12:4-10.

CHAPTER

142

Chest X-ray Evaluation in Cardiac Disease

Sanjiv Sharma, Gurpreet Singh Gulati, Priya Jagia

INTRODUCTION

Chest radiography is an important imaging technique used for the assessment of heart disease.[1] A skilled interpretation of the chest radiograph may disclose important morphological changes and to some extent even indicate the functional status of the cardiovascular system. Despite the fact that it usually provides an indirect (inferential) information, and that other more specific imaging techniques for noninvasive cardiac imaging have now become available, the chest radiograph remains a widely available, economical and often the first examination performed in a patient with suspected cardiac disease. The size and shape of cardiac shadow can be determined and retained as a permanent record for future reference. A proper understanding of the normal anatomy is essential for correct interpretation of pathological states.

The evaluation of the chest radiograph must begin with the assessment of the situs. Normally, in the upper abdomen, the liver and the inferior vena cava (IVC) lie on the right side, and the gastric fundus and the spleen lie on the left side. The systemic venous atrium lies on the right side and opposite to the gastric fundus. This relationship is referred to as the "visceroatrial situs" meaning that the atrial situs almost always conforms to the situs of the upper abdomen, irrespective of the situs or position of the remainder of the heart. The right-sided bronchus is shorter, wider, and more vertically oriented than the left bronchus. The right lung is trilobed whereas the left lung is bilobed. This is referred to as the "bronchial situs". In addition, the ascending aorta is generally on the same side as the systemic venous atrium and opposite the side of the gastric fundus. The ipsilateral location of the ascending aorta and the gastric fundus is almost pathognomonic of corrected transposition of great vessels **(Fig. 1)**.

Situs solitus implies that the liver, IVC, right atrium, and right-sided bronchus are on the right side, and the gastric fundus, spleen, and left-sided bronchus are on the left side. The position of the cardiac apex is not directly related to the visceroatrial situs and may not correspond with it. In addition, other issues to be considered include atrioventricular and ventriculoarterial connections, the loop of the aorta (dextro or levo), and the relation of cardiac chambers to each other.

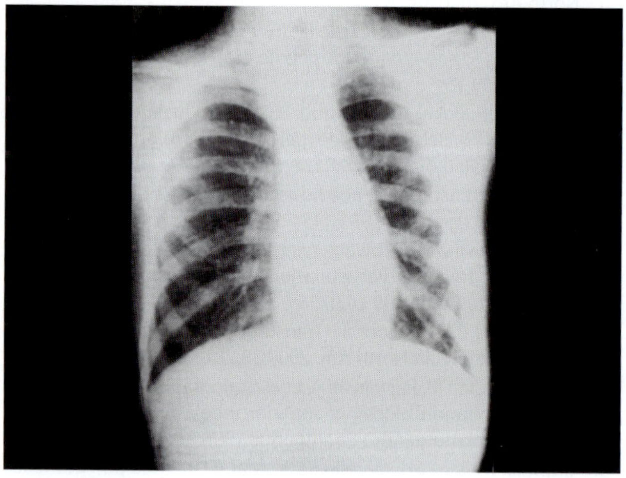

FIG. 1: Chest radiograph in a patient with corrected transposition of great vessels and pulmonary stenosis shows the absence of ascending aorta in the right upper cardiac border and a bulge along the left upper cardiac border obscuring the pulmonary conus. Peripheral pulmonary oligemia is also present.

CARDIAC SILHOUETTE

Cardiac Shape

Depending upon the build of the subjects, three types of shape are encountered in frontal projection. In hyposthenics, it is long and narrow, in hypersthenics, it is of transverse type, and in moderately built, it is oblique or globular in shape. In adults, 2/3rd of the heart lies on the left and 1/3rd on the right side of mid-line. In infants, the heart is of transverse or globular type, and the right heart is equal to the left. In infants and young children, there is enough thymic tissue to obscure the base of the heart and great vessels. By the age of 5–7 years, the globular infant heart attains the adult shape.

Cardiac Contour

Posteroanterior (PA) View

The right heart border consists of two segments. The upper segment is nearly vertical in normal young adults and is formed by the superior vena cava (SVC). The lower segment is usually convex and represents the lateral border of right atrium (RA) separated by a notch. In old age, the upper border may become convex due to the tendency of the aorta to dilate and elongate. The convexity represents the right lateral aspect of the ascending aorta. In hyposthenic subjects with a vertical heart, it is sometimes possible to see a small segment of the inferior vena cava (IVC) as a triangular shadow in the right cardiophrenic angle.

The left heart border can be divided into distinct segments. The uppermost is rounded and convex laterally and is formed by the posterior part of the transverse aortic arch, and is called the aortic knuckle or knob. Immediately below this, a flat or concave border is represented by the trunk of pulmonary artery and is called the pulmonary conus. Prominence of the conus is a normal variation in young females and children. A small concavity along the left heart border below the region of the pulmonary conus represents the region of the left atrial appendage. The lowest and largest segment of the left border is formed by the left ventricle (LV). This segment may be relatively straight in asthenics but is convex and rounded in hypersthenics. Diaphragmatic or inferior border is often not defined, but it may be seen in tall, asthenic-built subjects and is represented by the right ventricle (RV).

Right Anterior Oblique View

The anterior border from above downwards is formed by the transverse part of the arch of aorta, pulmonary trunk, RV and LV. The posterior border is formed by the left atrium (LA) above and RA below. The diaphragmatic surface is formed by the IVC, RA and RV.

Left Anterior Oblique View

The anterior border from above downwards consists of the innominate vein, SVC, ascending aorta, RA appendage and RV. The posterior border from above downwards includes a small part of LA and LV.

Lateral View

The anterior border is formed above by the RA appendage and below by the RV. The posterior border is formed above by LA and below by the LV.

Cardiac Size

The true size of the heart can only be assessed by orthodiagraphy with the help of an orthodiagraph. The method has now become obsolete. Conventional chest X-ray at a focus-film distance (FFD) of 6 feet provides some magnification and size of the heart is more than 1 cm greater in width than the orthodiagraphic measurements. If the FFD is doubled to about 12 feet, the measurements on the film are equal to those made on orthodiagraph. But this is not practical. Therefore, radiographic size at 6 feet is taken as a true representative size of the heart though there is some magnification.

Mathematical numerical cardiac measurement on chest radiograph has many variables, including age, sex, height, weight, race, occupation, phase of respiration, pulmonary and abdominal disease, which elevate or depress the diaphragm, and pose mathematical problems so that prediction tables are seldom used. The easiest method of measurement of cardiac size is to assess the transverse cardiothoracic ratio (CTR). This is the most adopted practical method though it is a rough estimate. This represents the ratio between the transverse cardiac diameter and the widest internal diameter of the thorax in PA view. The adult heart that measures more than half of the widest internal diameter of the chest is considered enlarged. In neonates, a ratio of up to 60%, and in infants, a ratio of up to 55% is taken as normal. The CTR may increase in the elderly probably due to infolding of the ribs which reduces the transverse thoracic diameter. Cardiomegaly has been graded as mild, moderate or severe by various authors based on the increase in the transverse diameter but these classifications are not widely used.

Cardiac Volume

Volume measurement is not done as a routine practice. It may be measured assuming the heart as an ellipsoid by the following formula:

$$V = l \times b \times d \times k \times m^3$$

V = Volume

l = Long or oblique diameter. This is drawn from the lowermost point of the heart on left side to the notch separating RA and right vascular shadow.

b = Broad diameter. It is obtained by joining the lower most point at the right cardiophrenic angle and uppermost point of the left vascular shadow.

d = AP diameter of the heart measured in lateral view. It is obtained by drawing a line from the point where the anterior border of the heart and sternum meet to the point of maximum convexity on the posterior surface of the heart.

m = Magnification factor

k = 0.63

Assessment of Chamber Enlargement

Right Atrium

When this is enlarged, the right heart border becomes more convex and also protrudes to the right away from the midline. The maximum convexity of right cardiac border >3 cm beyond right lateral vertebral border suggests RA enlargement. In early stages, only RA appendage fills the space between front of the heart and back of the sternum. The most reliable sign for the enlargement of the right atrium in the frontal chest radiograph is the increase in its height. In normal individuals, the distance between the top of the arch and the junction of the SVC and the right atrium is more than the distance between the latter and the right cardiophrenic angle. When the reverse happens, the right atrium is said to be enlarged **(Fig. 2)**.

Left Atrium

This chamber does not take part in the formation of any part of the cardiac border in frontal projection in normal subjects. It lies in the mid-line and in a posterior location. It usually enlarges posteriorly and to the right causing indentation and displacement of the esophagus posteriorly. With further

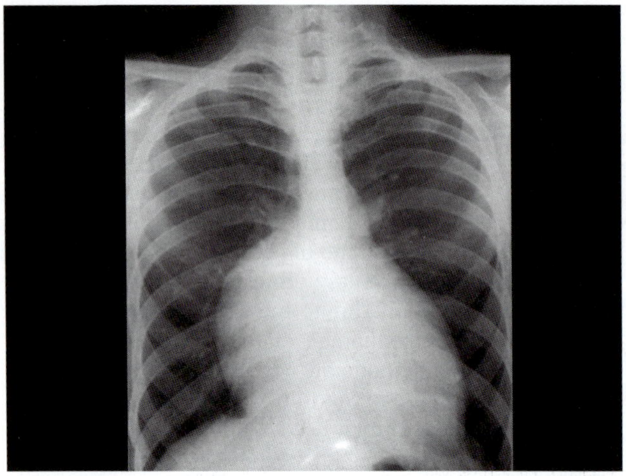

FIG. 2: Chest radiograph showing typical features of RA enlargement. Note that the height of the RA as seen by the distance between the junction of the SVC and RA, and the right cardiophrenic angle, is more than the distance between the top of the aortic arch and the junction of SVC and RA.

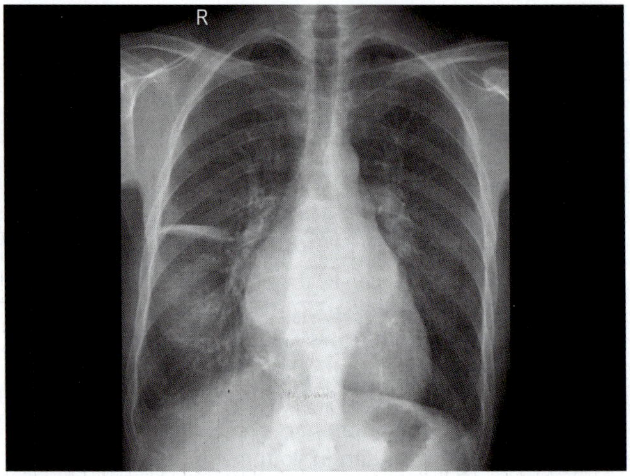

FIG. 3: Chest radiograph shows features of LA enlargement as seen by the double density in the mediastinum with widening of the carina. There is also evidence of bilateral hilar prominence with fluid in right fissure.

increase in size, enlargement is in all directions except anteriorly. The LA may project beyond the LV producing localized convexity of the left border of cardiac silhouette just below the PAS. The earliest evidence of LA enlargement is seen as lifting up of the left main bronchus. But, this is difficult to appreciate on the chest radiograph. Subsequently, the carinal angle widens. The normal carinal angle ranges between 51° and 71°. With LA enlargement, it becomes right or obtuse angled. When enlargement reaches this stage, the chamber is often large enough to produce an oval shaped, localized density on the right side and projecting outside the lower right cardiac border. This can be seen in frontal projection as a double density within the cardiac shadow on the right side **(Fig. 3)**. With massive enlargement, LA forms the right cardiac contour almost throughout except superiorly in the upper part where SVC forms the right heart border and inferiorly close to the diaphragm where the right atrium and, occasionally the IVC, form the right border. The enlarged LA can compress the left or occasionally the right bonchus and cause collapse, obstructive emphysema or rarely recurrent infection distal to the compressed lower lobe bronchus.

Left Ventricle

It enlarges to the left and posteriorly and only slightly to the right and anteriorly. Hypertrophy produces rounding of the cardiac apex whereas dilatation causes elongation either to the left or to the left and downwards, often combined with rounding of the apex **(Fig. 4)**. Rounding may also affect the left cardiac border when the LV gradually encroaches upon the pre-vertebral space. Left ventricular enlargement is best assessed in PA, LAO and lateral views.

Right Ventricle

It enlarges chiefly to the left and anteriorly . The outflow tract enlarges first and this is best seen in RAO and lateral views. When enlargement is significant, pulmonary conus becomes prominent in PA view. In some cases, the left border may be

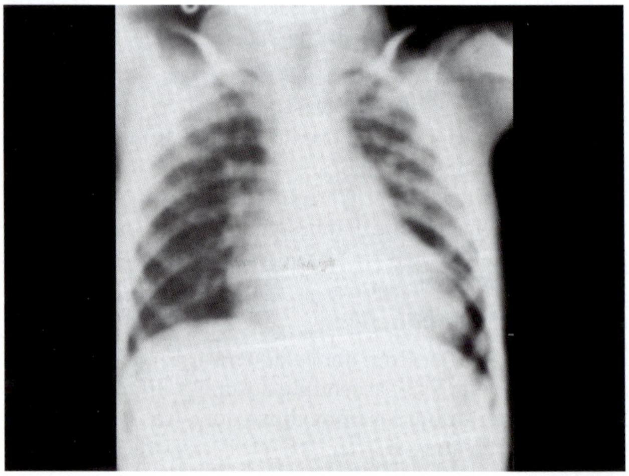

FIG. 4: Chest radiograph in a patient with a VSD shows LV enlargement, as evidenced by the concavity and elongation of the left cardiac border and rounding of the apex that is also shifted downwards and outwards.

formed by this ventricle and may cause rotation of LV to the left with elevation of the apex **(Fig. 5)**. In lateral view, there is encroachment upon the retrosternal space in the upper part. This rotation tends to swing the aorta to the right, so that the aortic knucle becomes less prominent.

Aorta

The normal ascending aorta does not contribute to the cardiac silhouette in frontal projection. When dilated and elongated in old age, it bulges to the right beyond the SVC to form the right upper border. The most posterior part of arch of the aorta forms the left upper cardiac border and is called the aortic knob or knuckle. In infants and young children, the aortic knob is not well seen. However, its position can be indirectly inferred by the extrinsic impression of the knuckle on the lateral margin of the air-filled trachea. The aortic

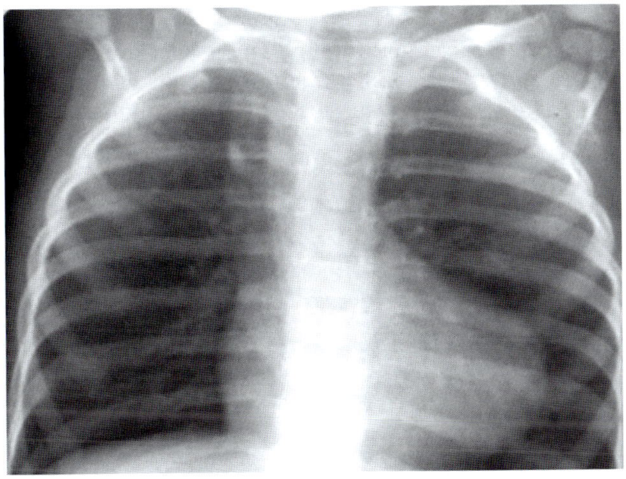

FIG. 5: Typical RV configuration is seen in this chest radiograph of a patient with TOF. There is elevation of the cardiac apex.

knuckle becomes more prominent, somewhat enlarged and may show curvilinear calcification in old age. The descending aorta can usually be seen as a straight line passing downwards and towards midline to the left of spine. The following should be looked for during the assessment of the aortic shadow:

- Is it a D-loop or L-loop?
- Is the aortic knuckle right or left sided?
- Is the aorta enlarged? If so, is there any disproportionate enlargement of the ascending or arch and descending aorta?
- Is there any calcification in the aorta? If so, its location (in the knuckle, descending thoracic or ascending aorta), pattern and extent.

Each of the above abnormalities has specific localizing value for the diagnosis.

PULMONARY VASCULATURE

Standard chest radiograph is a detailed record of the pulmonary vasculature. The pulmonary blood flow mirrors the pathophysiology of the heart since pulmonary blood vessels are clearly visualized on chest radiograph and the abnormal patterns of blood flow can be identified.[2]

Normal Radiographic Anatomy

The analysis of pulmonary vascularity begins at the hilum. Pulmonary circulation begins at the pulmonary valve. The left border of main pulmonary artery (MPA) forms the floor of pulmonary segment. The normal pulmonary segment (PAS) is concave or straight. The enlargement of MPA causes a convexity of the PAS. MPA bifurcates within the mediastinum into the right (RPA) and left (LPA) pulmonary arteries. The intrapulmonary branches parallel the bronchi, divide in an orderly manner, and gradually taper towards the periphery. The arteries and bronchial branches are approximately the same diameter at any particular level with the ratio of 1:2:1. The LPA and left hilum are 1 cm above the RPA. The course of the pulmonary arteries is interlobular and intersegmental. The veins are wider, less well defined and branch less often than the companion arteries. These are located medial to the companion artery in the upper zones, overlap each other in the mid-zone and are lateral to the artery in the lower zone. The pulmonary veins converge in to the left atrium (LA) 2–3 cm below the hilum. The pulmonary arteries radiate from the hila above the pulmonary venous confluence. It is often difficult to differentiate the artery from the vein due to variable arterial supply and venous drainage. In normal individuals, the pulmonary arteries and veins in outer 1/3rd of lung are too small to be seen in chest radiograph.

The right hilum is formed by the confluence of the shadows of the right upper lobe pulmonary vein and the right descending pulmonary artery (RDPA). These form a right angle. The width of the pulmonary vessels depends on the flow. Normal RDPA has a straight outer border. A convexity suggests an enlargement and concavity suggests a diminished size. In children, the ratio of RDPA to trachea is <1.0.[2] In adults, the normal transverse diameter of RDPA just above the origin of right middle lobe branch or 1.25 cm distal to the origin of right upper lobe branch is 10–16 mm in males and 9–15 mm in females in deep inspiration.[3] In erect position, blood flow is greater to the lower lobe because of gravity and differential intra-alveolar pressure. The lower lobe vessels are 2–3 times larger than the upper lobe vessels. In the erect chest radiograph, vessels in first intercostal space are <3 mm in diameter and those just above the diaphragm are up to 6 mm in diameter.

Increased Pulmonary Blood Flow (Pulmonary Plethora)

This is defined as an enlargement of vessels due to increased flow. The width of the pulmonary vessels depends on flow as long as the vascular reserve is not exceeded. Beyond this, the size depends on flow and pressure or pressure alone. Increased pulmonary flow can be caused by high output states, left to right (L-R) shunts, and admixture lesions. The pulmonary veins also enlarge as pulmonary arterial blood flow increases. Blood vessels become visible in the outer one-third of the lungs. In larger shunts, there is recruitment of upper lobe vessels, so that the differential flow between the upper and lower lobe vessels is lost. There is a fair correlation between vessel enlargement and shunt size. Shunts with QP:QS >2:1 can be reliably detected. Very large volume shunts can also cause pulmonary venous hypertension (PVH).

Gooding compared the diameter of the RDPA and trachea in children up to 14 years of age. The ratio in normal children at any age was close to one. About 90% had diameters within 2 mm of each other, with one-third having diameters of the RDPA that was less than that of the trachea. When a L-R shunt was present, the diameter of the RDPA was never less than that of the trachea.[4,5]

Radiological Signs of Plethora (Fig. 6)

- The presence of shunt vessels, end-on vessels more than two times the diameter of the accompanying bronchus.
- Prominent upper and lower zone vessels.
- En-face vessels below the tenth posterior rib.
- Prominent vessels below the crest of the diaphragm.
- RDPA diameter more than that of the trachea.
- > 6 vessels in peripheral one-third of the lungs.

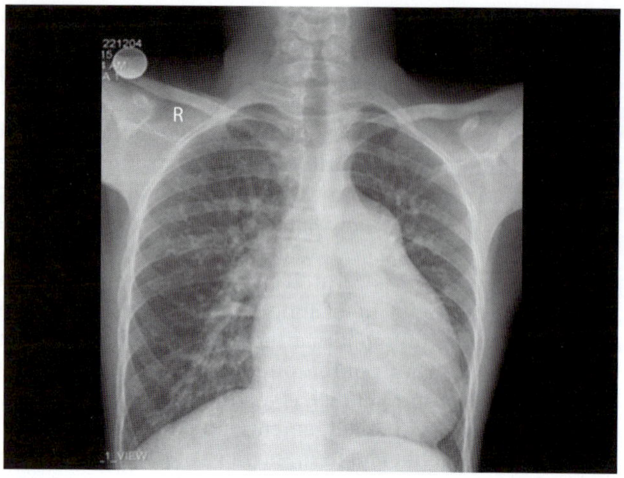

FIG. 6: Chest radiograph shows typical features of pulmonary plethora. Note the dilated pulmonary artery segment, increased caliber of the right descending pulmonary artery, and prominent end-on vessels in both lungs.

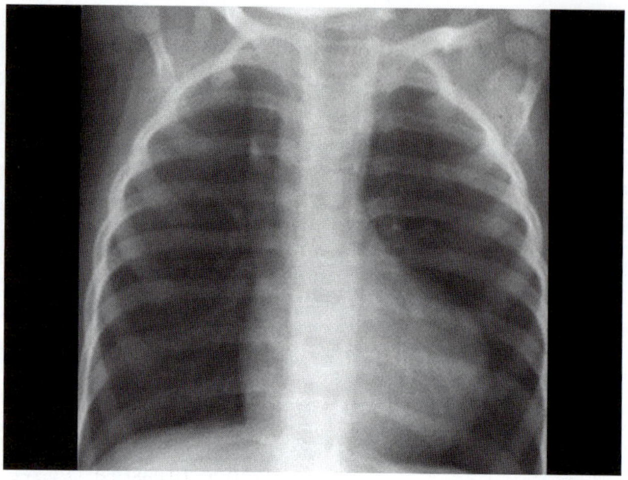

FIG. 7: Chest radiograph reveals typical oligemic lung fields. The hila are small in size, vascular markings are diminished in caliber, and the lungs appear hypertranslucent.

- RDPA >16 mm in diameter.
- Prominent hilar vessels on lateral view.
- In infants and children, generalised mottling may be seen. Plethora correlates with the size of L-R shunts better than the heart size.[6] With a normal or slightly increased heart size, QP:QS is >2:1 or 2:1 in 50%, with a larger heart, the shunt is >2:1 in at least 60% and with no plethora, the shunt is <2:1 in 100%. Assessment of plethora should not be based on measurements alone. However, measurements can be used in corroboration with a subjective impression.

Decreased Pulmonary Blood Flow (Pulmonary Oligemia)

It is difficult to diagnose pulmonary oligemia unless it is severe. Some normal persons may have small pulmonary vessels. Oligemia can be caused by pulmonary outflow tract obstruction and intracardiac right to left (R-L) shunts. The pulmonary arteries and veins are reduced in size, the central vessels become narrow, and peripheral arteries are not visible.

Radiological Signs (Fig. 7)

- Concave or absent MPA.
- Overall appearance of an over-penetrated film.
- Less than 4 vessels in peripheral one-third of the lungs.
- Small hilar, lobar, segmental vessels.
- Decreased size and density of hilar vessels on lateral chest radiograph in the presence of cyanosis is suggestive of pulmonary oligemia.
- Enlarged bronchial and other systemic collateral arteries are seen in pulmonary atresia with ventricular septal defect (VSD) and in tetralogy of Fallot (TOF). These are seen as small, tortuous, non-tapering and disorganized vascular markings not radiating from the hilum and also not conforming to known branching patterns of the pulmonary vessels. The hila are not enlarged.

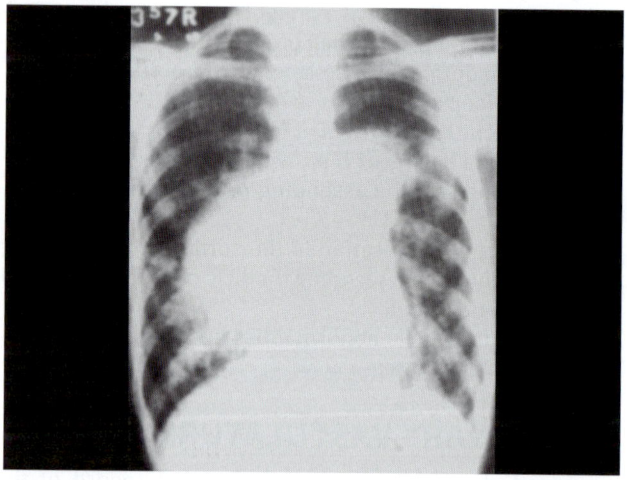

FIG. 8: A patient with primary PAH. The chest radiograph shows that the main pulmonary artery segment, and both pulmonary arteries are grossly dilated. There is a sharp transition between the centrally dilated hila and the vasculature of the peripheral lung fields.

Pulmonary Arterial Hypertension (Fig. 8)

This may be primary or secondary to PVH, long-standing L-R shunts, pulmonary thromboembolic disease, respiratory disease, high altitude, drugs, and pulmonary arterial occlusion. It is said to be present, if the mean pulmonary artery (PA) pressure is >20 mm Hg. The PAH is graded as mild, moderate and severe with the PAmean pressure ranging from 20–29, 30–49, and >50 mm Hg respectively. The central vessels from the MPA to the second order branching vessels dilate and peripheral (lobar) vessels constrict. The transition between centrally dilated and peripherally constricted vessels is more lateral in L-R shunts. The pruning of the pulmonary arteries is defined as more than a 50% loss of the vessel diameter at any degree branching and is suggestive of PAH. Chronic PAH leads to calcification of the MPA and proximal branches. The presence of calcification is pathognomonic of PAH. The severity of central dilatation has a rough correlation with the severity of PAH. In the lower pressure ranges, the ratio of the size of the hemithoracic diameter to the size of the MPA shows an approximate correlation with PA pressure. Hyperkinetic → PAH → versus → Eisenmenger → PAH → In hyperkinetic PAH, peripheral vessels increase in size and number, and cardiac enlargement is proportional to the amount of L-R shunt. In Eisenmenger PAH, peripheral vessels decrease, central vessels increase further in size, heart size decreases, and the right ventricle (RV) becomes more prominent.

Pulmonary Venous Hypertension

Pulmonary venous hypertension (PVH) is said to be present when the pulmonary capillary wedge pressure (PCWP) exceeds the normal range of 8–12 mm Hg. Progressive PVH produces changes reflecting the presence and severity of this disorder.

Stage 1: Redistribution/Cephalization of the Blood Flow (Fig. 9)

This may precede the clinical signs and symptoms. Thc venous pressure ranges from 13 to 19 mm Hg. The changes are characterized by constriction, blurring of lower zone vessels, effacement of hilar angle, and dilatation of upper lobe vessels. With increase in LA and PCW pressure, there is an increase in LA and PCW pressure. This results in an increase in the interstitial lung water and increased pulmonary lymphatic drainage, leading to "cuffing" of fluid around small bronchi. The increased interstitial water gravitates to dependent areas, causing increased interstitial pressure and vascular resistance at lung bases. Thus, blood is diverted to upper lobes leading to vascular redistribution. Exceptions to this pattern of redistribution are basal emphysema and pulmonary parenchymal diseases of the upper lobe.

Stage 2: Interstitial Edema (Fig. 10)

It is characterized by the presence of Kerley lines, peribronchial cuffing, background haze, septal and interstitial edema, and pleural effusion. The venous pressure ranges from 20 to 24 mm Hg.

Stage 3: Alveolar Edema (Fig. 11)

This occurs when the interstitial fluid accumulates at rates faster than it can be removed by the lymphatics. The venous pressure ranges from 25 mm Hg and above. Milking of edema fluid towards the hilum by the expanding lung imparts a "Bat's Wing appearance". However, a chronic lung disease and dependent posture may result in atypical patterns of edema. Pleural effusion occurs when pleural fluid formation by visceral pleura is faster than its absorption by the parietal pleura. This usually occurs when systemic venous pressure is also elevated, as in right heart failure. Several radiologic

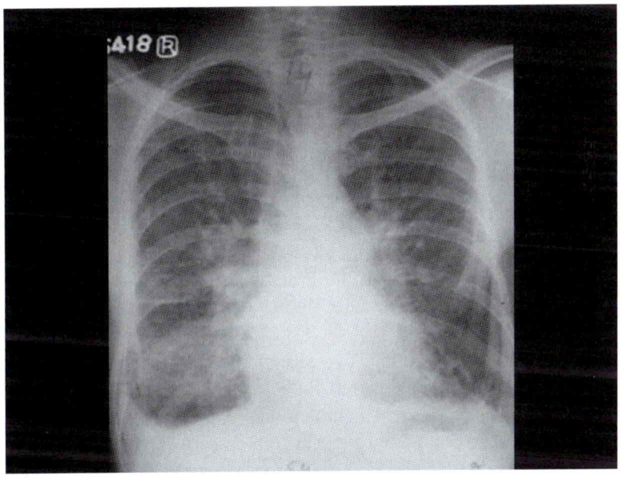

FIG. 10: Chest radiograph shows moderate (grade II) PVH in a case of MS. Kerley's B lines are present in both costophrenic angles.

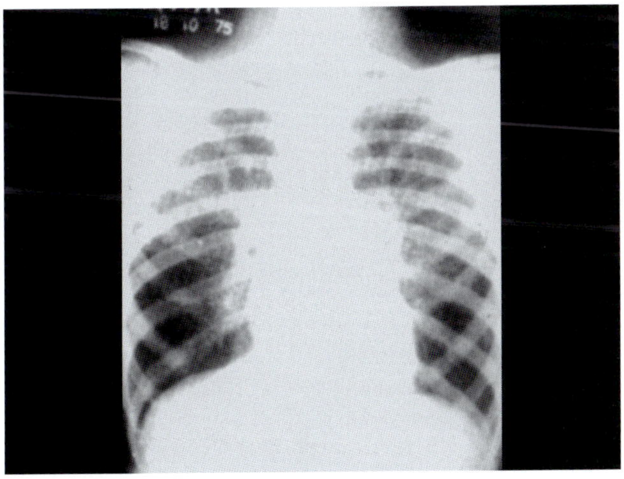

FIG. 9: Chest radiograph shows mild (grade I) PVH. There is cephalization of blood flow with increased caliber of the upper lobe vessels. Note that the patient has mitral stenosis, as evidenced by the enlargement of the LA and its appendage.

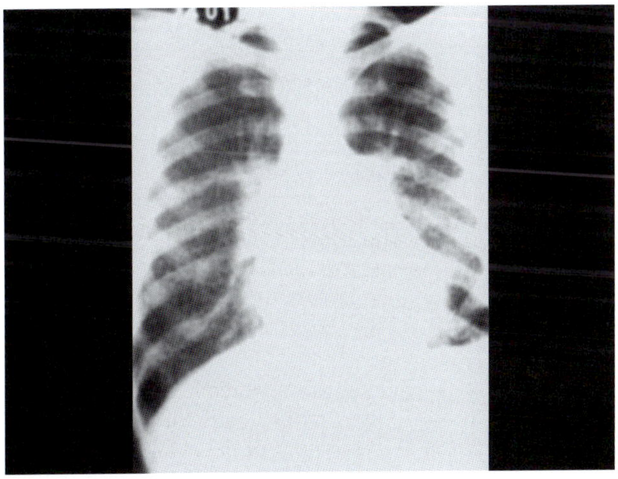

FIG. 11: Chest radiograph shows features of severe (grade III) PVH and PAH. In addition, there are miliary shadows in both lungs, due to the presence of secondary hemosiderosis.

findings have been correlated with the level of PCWP in patients with acute and chronic heart failure.

Asymmetrical Pulmonary Blood Flow (Fig. 12)

This is due to the presence of vessels in one lung that are smaller than the other:

- ***Localized decrease:*** Pulmonary thromboembolism, chronic obstructive airway disease (COAD), arteritis, segmental stenosis.
- ***Unilateral decrease:*** Pulmonary artery branch atresia/stenosis, hemi-truncus, TOF with unilateral pulmonary atresia.
- ***Unilateral increase:*** After shunt surgery (e.g. Blalock-Taussig shunt), Glenn shunt (on the side of shunt), PDA and anomalous origin of a pulmonary artery from the aorta.

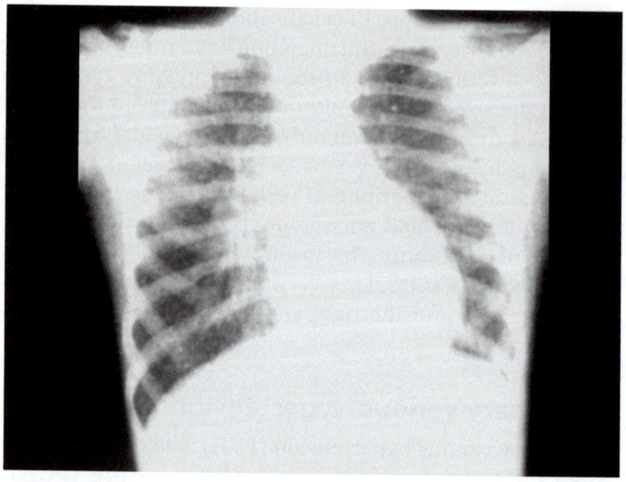

FIG. 12: This radiograph shows evidence of pleonemia, evidenced by the presence of increased vasculature on the right side and an inconspicuous left hilum with peripheral oligemia on this side.

Orientation of Pulmonary Outflow Tract

- *Towards left:* Valvular pulmonic stenosis
- *Towards right:* Transposition of great arteries

It is obvious from the above description that the chest radiograph is a mathematical record of the events produced by the cardiac disease. Its detailed, sequential interpretation provides important clues to the underlying heart disease and the functional impairment produced by it. The chest radiograph also serves as a useful method for follow-up after treatment in most cardiac conditions. Distinctive radiographic abnormalities in specific cardiac disorders will be dealt with in the following chapters.

REFERENCES

1. Radiology of the heart. In: Braunwald E (Ed). Heart Disease: A Textbook of Cardiovascular Medicine. WB Saunders, Philadelphia; 1992: pp. 204-324.
2. Coussement AM. Objective radiographic assessment of pulmonary vascularity in children. Radiology. 1973;109:649- 54.
3. Chang CH. The normal roentgenographic measurement of the right descending pulmonary artery in 1085 cases. AJR. 1962;87:929-35.
4. Roberts WC. Radiologic differentiation of common anomalies. In: Adult Congenital Heart Disease. 1988. pp. 191-219.
5. Moes CAF. Analysis of the chest in the neonate with congenital heart disease. RCNA. 1975;13:251-76.
6. Jefferson K, Rees R (Eds). Clinical Cardiac Radiology. Butterworth, London; 1980.

CHAPTER

143

Imaging Approach in Children with Congenital Heart Disease

Priya Jagia, Sanjiv Sharma, Gurpreet Singh Gulati, Sanjeev Kumar

INTRODUCTION

In children, severe congenital heart disease (CHD) is an important cause of mortality. Imaging is important to show the cardiac and vascular anatomy so that therapy can be planned. It is also useful in monitoring these children after surgery or endovascular interventions.

A correct diagnostic approach ensures that a functional diagnostic is made whereby correct decision in form of emergency surgery, endovascular intervention, medical therapy or just supportive measures can be arrived at. Approximately 75% cases of all CHD lesions either are not detected or do not have signs or symptoms warranting complete investigation in infants. Left-to-right shunts, even large, rarely present with serious respiratory or cardiac difficulty in first months of life, owing to high pulmonary vascular resistance.

There are nine congenital heart lesions, which account for most of the severe cyanotic heart disease in children. These can further be classified as follows, based upon pulmonary flow:

Group A: Lesions with decreased pulmonary blood flow:

1. Pulmonary atresia (PAt) or severe pulmonic stenosis (PS), with intact VSD.
2. Tricuspid atresia.
3. Pulmonary malformation of tricuspid valve.
4. Pulmonary atresia (or severe pulmonic stenosis) with VSD including tetralogy of Fallot (TOF).

Group B: Lesions with increased pulmonary blood flow:

1. Transposition of great arteries (TGA).
2. VSD with coarctation of aorta.

Group C: Lesions with severe pulmonary venous hypertension:

1. Total anomalous pulmonary venous return with obstruction (TAPVR).
2. Hypoplastic left heart (HLH).
3. Severe coarctation of aorta with intact ventricular septum.

PHYSICAL EXAMINATION

The conditions mentioned above might all cause cyanosis or respiratory distress or both in first few days of life itself. Patients with TGA, pulmonary atresia (or stenosis) and tricuspid atresia have marked cyanosis with minimal or no respiratory distress in neonatal period. On the other hand, respiratory distress is marked in TAPVR with obstruction and hypoplastic left heart syndrome with little cyanosis. In Ebstein's, child has cyanosis, tachypnea, pansystolic murmur and hepatomegaly which improves over first weeks of life.

RADIOLOGICAL APPROACH

Chest Radiograph

Chest radiograph is useful in the initial evaluation of a patient with a suspected CHD. It provides valuable information about the cardiac size, pulmonary vasculature, arterial and venous hypertension, the situs and the lungs. Echocardiography is a useful screening technique that allows real-time evaluation of each cardiac chamber in multiple orthogonal planes. It is noninvasive, easily available, provides a direct visualization of structural defects and also helps evaluate the attendant functional disturbances. The reports suggest that the results compare favorably with angiocardiography. Its major limitations include operator dependence and availability of a proper acoustic window. Recently, multi-slice computed tomography and magnetic resonance imaging are also being used in selected patients for optimal evaluation. Proper understanding of the imaging anatomy, image morphology in disease states, and the advantages and limitations of each technique is essential for its optimal utilization in a given patient or disease state.

A good quality chest radiograph still remains an important initial investigation for the evaluation of a patient with CHD. General principles in the interpretation of chest radiograph in CHD include a sequential evaluation of the cardiac size, chamber enlargement, aorta, status of pulmonary vasculature, assessment of the situs and other associated abnormalities. Chest radiographic abnormalities in various disease states are described below:

Left-to-Right (L-R) Shunt

Chest radiograph is useful in localizing the site of L-R shunts in CHD. If the aortic knuckle is enlarged, the shunt is extracardiac and if the aorta is normal, the shunt is intracardiac.

Large Aorta

If the aortic knuckle is enlarged disproportionate to the ascending aorta, the L-R shunt is caused by patent ductus arteriosus (PDA). The heart is usually normal or mildly enlarged with left ventricular (LV) configuration, aortic knuckle is obliterated or replaced by a bulge, pulmonary conus is enlarged, and lung vascularity is increased. In addition, pulmonary arterial hypertension (PAH) may be present. In a small group of patients, calcification may be present at the PDA site.

If the ascending aorta is enlarged disproportionate to the aortic knuckle, the L-R shunt is at the aortic root level. The causes include a ruptured aneurysm of the sinus of Valsalva, aortopulmonary window, and coronary arteriovenous fistula.

Ruptured aneurysm of the sinus of Valsalva (RSOV): The heart size is usually enlarged with a biventricular or LV configuration. An abnormal shadow of the aneurysm is usually present at the level of the aortic root. There may be curvilinear calcification in it. The aorta is enlarged with a disproportionate dilatation of the aortic root. The pulmonary conus is prominent and lung vascularity is increased. In addition, in symptomatic patients, some evidence of PVH is also present.

Usually, the right coronary sinus is involved and ruptures into the right ventricle. Simultaneous presence of pulmonary plethora and PVH is characteristic of an RSOV.

Aortopulmonary window: The heart size is usually enlarged with an LV configuration, there is disproportionate enlargement of the aortic root, pulmonary conus is prominent, lung vascularity is increased, and PAH is usually present.

Coronary arteriovenous fistula: The heart size is usually normal and there may be LV configuration. There is disproportionate enlargement of the aortic root, pulmonary conus is prominent and lung vascularity is normal or increased. Chest radiograph may be normal because the shunt is usually small.

Normal Aorta

Normal or apparently small aortic knuckle and inconspicuous ascending aortic shadow in a frontal chest radiograph in the presence of increased lung vascularity in a pink patient suggest an intracardiac L-R shunt. This shunt can be at pre- or post-tricuspid level.

Pre-tricuspid Shunt

The pre-tricuspid shunt is produced by an atrial septal defect or a partial anomalous pulmonary venous drainage.

Atrial septal defect (ASD): The heart size is usually normal. There may be mild cardiomegaly in approximately 25% of the patients. There is right atrial enlargement with right-sided configuration of the heart. Aortic shadow is normal in size with the ascending aortic shadow usually conspicuous by its absence in the upper right cardiac border. This sign is characteristic of an ASD. The heart appears to be shifted to the left and lung vascularity is increased. PAH may be present. The presence of associated anomalies may change this radiographic picture. Associated mitral valve disease should be suspected if LA/LA appendage is enlarged, PVH (especially if Kerley's lines) is present, or if the mitral valve is calcified. The association of ASD with mitral stenosis of rheumatic etiology is called "Lutembacher's syndrome". In patients over 40 years of age, a chest radiograph may show atypical features including the presence of LV configuration and distended upper lobe vessels due to left ventricular dysfunction which may be related to age, myocardial ischemia, or hypertensive heart disease.

Partial anomalous pulmonary venous drainage (PAPVD): This should be suspected if, in the presence of radiographic features of ASD, there is an abnormally enlarged shadow of superior vena cava (SVC) or an abnormally directed pulmonary vein is seen.

Post-tricuspid L-R Shunt

This results from the presence of a VSD. This is the most common form of acyanotic CHD. The findings on chest radiograph in VSD depend on the shunt size and the direction of predominant flow. In small <2:1 shunts, the chest radiograph may be normal. In presence of a large >2:1 shunt, the heart size is usually enlarged with a left or a biventricular configuration, and there is evidence of LA enlargement, a normal aorta, and increased lung vascularity. PAH may be present, In addition, there may be evidence of differential increase in lung vascularity in the right upper zone. In 3–5% of the patients, an associated right-sided aortic arch may be present.

Right-to-Left (R-L) Shunt

Although chest radiographic features of most of the following conditions can be characteristic, it is important to remember that typical features are not usually seen in most patients. As with L-R shunts, the size of the aortic shadow is important in the localization of R-L shunts.

Large Aorta with Decreased Lung Vascularity

Large aortic knuckle in the presence of cyanotic CHD and decreased vascularity is produced by tetralogy of Fallot (TOF), pulmonary atresia with VSD, tricuspid atresia, TGA with VSD and pulmonary stenosis (PS), double outlet right ventricle (DORV) with PS and allied conditions.

Tetralogy of Fallot: Etienne-Louis Fallot in 1888 described a tetralogy of defects, including pulmonary stenosis, a malaligned ventricular septal defect, overriding of the aorta and hypertrophy of the right ventricle. This is the most common form of cyanotic CHD in children. The pulmonic stenosis is usually infundibular in location. Additional valvular pulmonary stenosis and hypoplasia of the main pulmonary artery are also frequently present. The chest radiograph shows a characteristic picture produced by a normal heart size, RV configuration with an uplifted apex (coer-en sabot appearance), a large aortic knuckle, presence of pulmonary bay and pulmonary oligemia **(Fig. 1)**. A right-sided aortic arch is present in approximately 25% of the cases. In addition, characteristic criss-cross bronchial circulation may be present. Rarely, rib notching may be seen due to collateral flow. The heart size may be enlarged in the presence of tricuspid or pulmonary regurgitation, absent pulmonary valve, severe anemia, bacterial endocarditis, pulmonary atresia, or bacterial infections. Rarely, TOF may be associated with an absent pulmonary valve. This produces a pathognomonic appearance consisting of an enlarged heart, large central pulmonary arteries with peripheral oligemia in the setting of TOF. In addition, a host of lung abnormalities largely due to a defective bronchial cartilage and resultant tracheobronchomalacia may be associated. Occasionally, TOF may be associated with congenital absence of a pulmonary artery, left more commonly than right. When this happens, parenchymal lung abnormalities are frequently associated.

Pulmonary atresia with VSD: There is mild cardiomegaly RV configuration, a large aortic knuckle that frequently crosses the sternoclavicular joint into the neck, pulmonary bay, and peripheral oligemia. Aortic arch is right-sided in 30–40% patients. Bronchial collateral circulation is frequently present. Rib notching may be seen.

Tricuspid atresia: The chest radiographic picture depends on the relationship of great vessels, presence of PS, and the degree of RV hypoplasia. A typical picture is seen in only 15–20% of the cases and consists of a normal-sized or mildly enlarged heart, LV configuration, straight right heart border, some evidence of LA enlargement, enlarged aorta, pulmonary bay, and decreased vascularity, provided that there is PS and the great vessels are normally related **(Fig. 2)**. The aortic arch is right-sided in one-third of the cases. If the pulmonary arteries are not located in their normal position, an abnormal relationship of great vessels should be suspected. In the absence of PS, there is evidence of increased lung vascularity.

D-TGA, VSD and PS: A chest radiograph may superficially resemble TOF. The heart size is usually normal or may be mildly enlarged. The aortic knuckle is normal or the pedicle may appear narrow. Pulmonary artery segment is not present in the normal position and is located in a high and medial position. The lung fields are oligemic.

Small Aorta with Increased Vascularity

D-TGA: This is the second most common cause of cyanotic heart disease in infancy. It is caused by a ventriculoarterial abnormality in which the aorta originates from RV and PA from LV. The chest radiographic findings are characteristic, consisting of an enlarged heart, narrow pedicle, abnormally located pulmonary arteries, and increased lung vascularity.

The shape of the heart is typical and resembles an "egg-on-side" **(Fig. 3)**. There may be a differential increase in right lung vascularity, especially in the upper zone. This

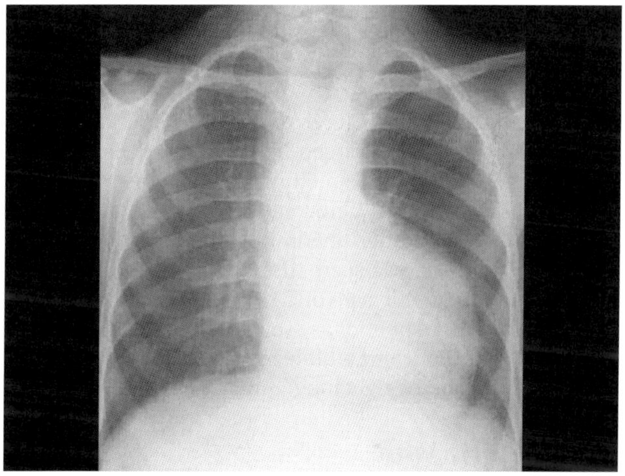

FIG. 2: Chest radiograph in tricuspid atresia. Note the straight heart border and right-sided aortic arch. Lung fields show peripheral oligemia.

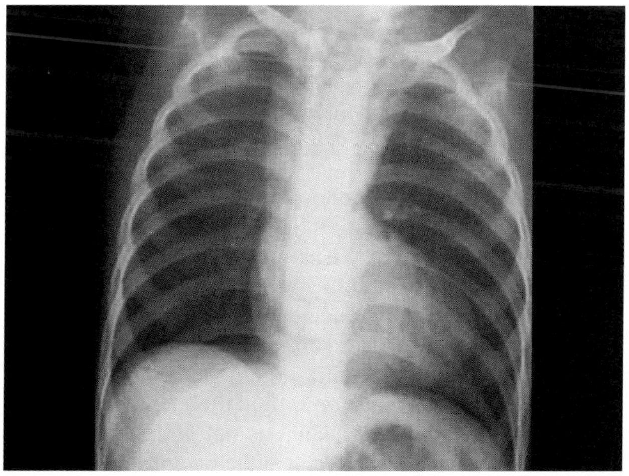

FIG. 1: Chest radiograph in tetralogy of Fallot. Cardiac size is normal with RV configuration. There is concave pulmonary bay and peripheral oligemia.

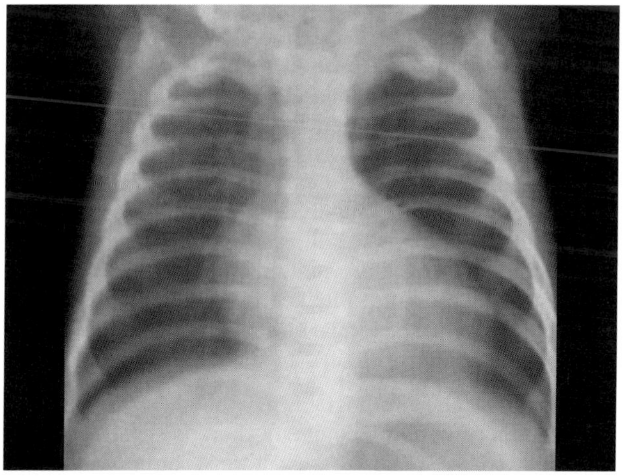

FIG. 3: Chest radiograph in transposition of great arteries. "Egg-shaped" heart is seen with narrow vascular pedicle.

pathognomonic picture is seen in patients in whom there is no evidence of PS. The typical chest radiograph findings are seen in about half the patients.

Large Pedicle with Increased Vascularity

This combination is seen in truncus arteriosus, total anomalous pulmonary venous drainage (TAPVC), and tricuspid atresia without PS.

Truncus arteriosus: The heart is usually enlarged, there is LV configuration, the aorta is enlarged, pulmonary artery is not in its usual position, and lung vascularity is increased. The abnormal location of the PA may produce a characteristic picture described as "comma or water-fall" sign. This is more often seen on the left side. The aortic arch is right sided in about 50% of the cases.

TAPVC: This may be divided into four main groups according to the site or sites of connection, supracardiac, cardiac, infracardiac and mixed. The chest radiographic picture depends on the type of TAPVC. In supracardiac type, which is also the most common, the heart is enlarged, the pedicle is wide with a classical "figure of 8 or Snowman's" appearance, produced by the dilated left vertical and left innominate veins and the right SVC. The left atrium is small and there is increased flow, as evidenced by pulmonary plethora. In cardiac or mixed types, the picture may be nonspecific and consists of cardiomegaly, normal or enlarged aorta, and increased lung vascularity. Shadow of an enlarged abnormal pulmonary vein may be seen. The scimitar sign is seen in the infra-diaphragmatic type of TAPVC and is caused by the drainage of the right pulmonary vein into the IVC, hepatic or portal vein. This syndrome is often associated with hypoplasia or sequestration of the right lung.

Normal Aorta with Decreased Lung Vascularity

This combination can be seen in patients with Ebstein's anomaly, and valvular PS in failure.

Ebstein's anomaly: This produces a characteristic radiographic picture. There is cardiomegaly, evidence of RA enlargement, sharp, well-delineated cardiac margins, as if drawn by a pencil, normal aorta and pulmonary oligemia. It can superficially resemble pericardial effusion, valvular PS in failure, tricuspid regurgitation caused by chronic rheumatic heart disease (RHD), dilated cardiomyopathy (DCM), and Uhl's anomaly. The pulmonary vascularity is important in differentiating these conditions. In pericardial effusion, the lung vasculature is normal and no specific chamber enlargement is present. In RHD, there is PVH and tell-tale signs of the underlying valvular disease are always present. In DCM, there is evidence of PVH. LA and LV may be enlarged.

Valvular PS: A chest radiograph may be normal except for a prominent pulmonary conus till there is severe PS with congestive failure. In such cases, there is cardiomegaly, RA enlargement, a normal aorta, prominent pulmonary conus produced by post-stenotic dilatation of MPA and LPA, and peripheral pulmonary oligemia.

Other Conditions

Coarctation of aorta: This refers to a narrowing of the distal aortic arch and/or proximal descending aorta due to a discrete membrane or narrowing of the aortic isthmus. Findings on chest radiograph depend on the age of the patient, location of the coarct, ventricular function, competence of the aortic valve and associated abnormalities. In an uncomplicated isolated coarctation, the heart size is usually normal. There may be left ventricular configuration. The classical feature of bilateral notching of the posterior and inferior margins of the 4th-8th ribs is usually not seen in the first decade of life. The coarct segment is usually located in the juxtaductal region. Occasionally, it can be postductal and rarely preductal. Postductal or juxtaductal coarctation produces typical radiographic features in the cardiac configuration, ribs and aorta. Rib notching is caused by the hypertrophied intercostal arteries that run along the posterior and inferior margins of the ribs. In juxtaductal coarct, the fourth to eight ribs are usually involved. Coarctation proximal to the origin of the left subclavian artery results in unilateral right-sided rib notching. If the coarctation is proximal to an aberrant right subclavian artery, unilateral notching of the left ribs occurs. Abnormal appearance of the aorta is seen in most patients. The ascending aorta is slightly dilated. *Figure-of-3* appearance of the descending aorta is characteristic but not commonly seen. The upper convexity is formed by the dilated subclavian artery and the lower convexity by the post-stenotic dilatation of the descending aorta. Usually, a prominent or a flat knuckle is seen. If there is associated left ventricular decompensation, then PVH may be present.

Thus, it is obvious that the chest radiograph provides useful diagnostic information in the patient with CHD. These appearances are relatively easy to familiarize with. This, coupled with the universal availability of this imaging technique, makes it ideally suited as the first diagnostic investigation in the patient with suspected CHD. It has the unique ability to assess the pulmonary vasculature and the associated or coincidental lung or spinal abnormalities. These reasons also make it well suited for utilization as a follow-up technique after surgical or non-surgical intervention.

MULTISLICE CARDIAC CT

With advances in cross-sectional imaging in form of multislice CT and MRI, chest X-ray is no longer relied upon to make the diagnosis.

In all cases, where echocardiography has failed to provide sufficient information. Cardiac CT or MR needs to be performed to delineate the cardiac and vascular anatomy. This not only helps decide the treatment modality but also helps in planning surgery, if decided upon, and also to follow-up the postoperative cases. Both cardiac CT and MR are capable of providing anatomic and functional assessment of heart. But MRI is time consuming, and therefore may require lengthy period of sedation, which is not desirable in small children. But it has the advantage of being non-invasive and not involving any ionizing radiation. Hence, it can be repeated without risk of radiation, as necessitated in postoperative patients for follow-up.

Multislice cardiac CT has the advantage of widespread availability and needs very short time for image acquisition. It has a higher spatial resolution as compared to MRI and also is better for evaluation of lung parenchyma. ECG-gated cardiac CT allows delineation of otherwise mobile small structures in heart and also helps to rule out associated coronary artery anomalies. In children, however, the risks of ionizing radiation and those inherent to contrast media must be kept in mind before subjecting them to CT.

Short-term sedation for CT is often necessary especially in small children. At our institute, we have a policy of performing the pediatric CT in presence of an anesthetist and the child is admitted for a short period after CT for observation.

Nonionic contrast is used with a dose of 2–3 mL/kg body weight of child, and in infants is administered intravenously at rate of 1.5–2 mL/sec.

We routinely use dual source CT scanner (Siemens Medical Solutions, Germany) for cardiac CT. For children, a body weight based low dose protocol is used to limit the radiation exposure. Tube voltage of 80 KV has also been recommended for this purpose.

The entire thorax is scanned in 4–5 seconds, and hence the need for breath-hold is more or less obviated. ECG gated CT scanning is advisable in cases with complex cardiac abnormality or when there is need to delineate an abnormal communication, so that motion artifacts are minimal. However, it is advisable to do ECG controlled tube current modulation whereby normal tube current is applied during motion-free diastole phase of cardiac cycle while much reduced current is applied during systole. An ECG gated study should only be performed when the advantages outweigh the risk of increased radiation in such study.

The scan delay is determined by bolus chase technique. In small children, the region of interest (ROI) is placed in right ventricle, if pulmonary arteries need to be evaluated and in LV, if aortic evaluation is required. Post-processing involves reconstruction of multiplanar reformation (MPR), maximum intensity projection (MIP) **(Fig. 4)** and volume-rendered (VRT) images **(Fig. 5)** on the dedicated workstation.

The greatest amount of anatomical delineation is obtained with MPR images.

CARDIAC MRI

As mentioned before, it gives excellent anatomical information without the use of ionizing radiation and contrast media **(Fig. 6)**. But it lacks the rapid acquisition of scans, and high spatial resolution offered by cardiac CT.

Small children need to anaesthetized prior to MRI. Use is made of small coil to cover chest of baby to provide highest signal to noise ratio.

For anatomic delineation, coronal, sagittal and axial nongated steady state free precession images covering the entire chest are taken. Vascular anatomy is best delineated by doing contrast-enhanced MR angiogram **(Fig. 7)**.

ECG gated cine images in short axis from base of ventricle to apex help assess cardiac function and measure ventricular volume. Cine imaging across desired vascular planes can be done, e.g. along ventricular outflow tract, to rule out any stenosis or regurgitations **(Figs. 8 and 9)**.

Velocity encoded phase-contrast cine images assess blood flow velocity and volume. Systemic to pulmonary blood flow ratio (Q_p/Q_s) can be calculated by measuring flow in pulmonary trunk and ascending aorta.

Pressure gradient (ΔP) across a stenosis can be calculated by measuring maximum poststenotic velocity (V_{max}) by using Bernoulli's equation:

$$\Delta P = 4\,(V_{max})^2$$

For cardiac tumors, ECG gated spin echo T1W and T2W sequences are performed before and after administration of gadolinium contrast.

Common indications for cardiac CT and MRI in children with CHD are:

- Evaluation of vascular and cardiac anatomy
- Arterial blood supply to lungs (PA anatomy, AP collaterals) **(Figs. 10A and B)**
- Aortic arch abnormalities (Coarctation, interrupted aortic arch, vascular rings)

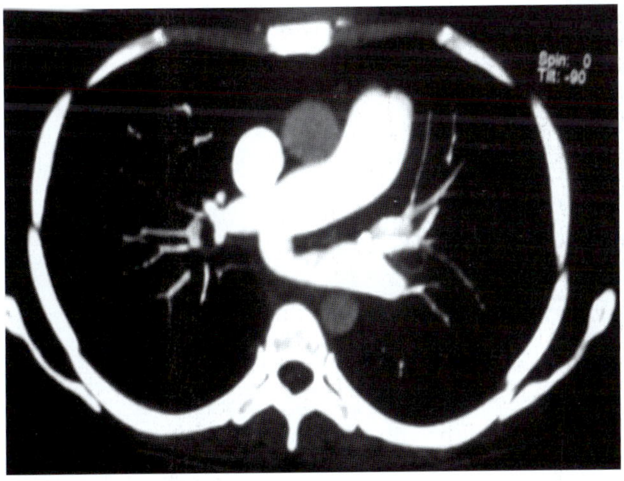

FIG. 4: LPA sling-axial CT image: MIP shows LPA arising from RPA and coursing behind trachea.

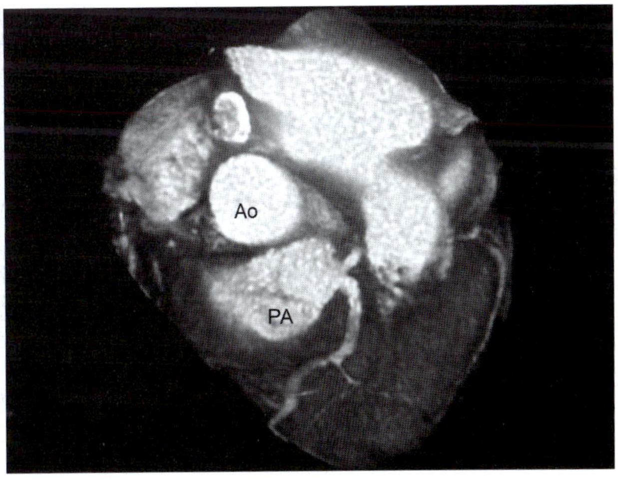

FIG. 5: Anomalous origin of left coronary artery from pulmonary artery (ALCAPA)—VRT image of coronary CT angiogram.

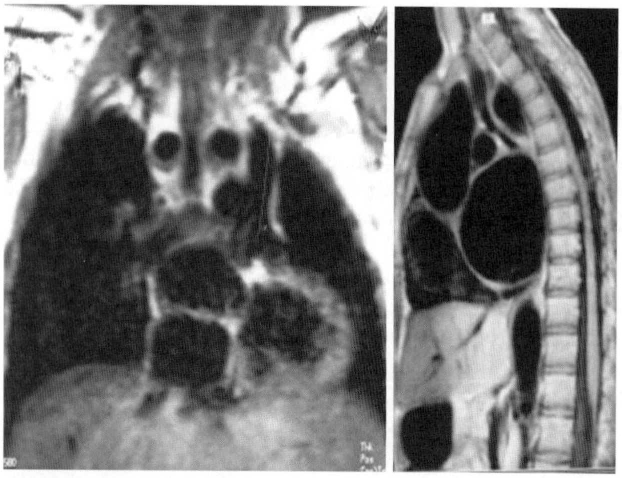

FIG. 6: Double aortic arch: Coronal and sagittal MRI-T1W image showing vascular structure on both sides of trachea.

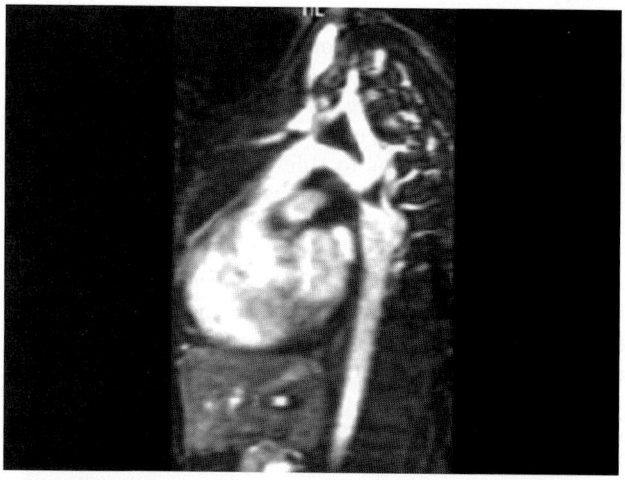

FIG. 7: Coarctation of aorta: Contrast-enhanced MR angiogram in oblique sagittal view shows coarctation just distal to left subclavian artery origin.

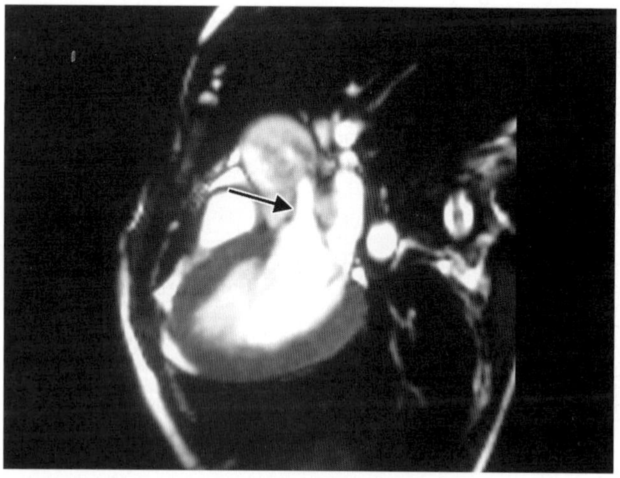

FIG. 8: Oblique sagittal cine MR image showing poststenotic jet in ascending aorta due to aortic stenosis.

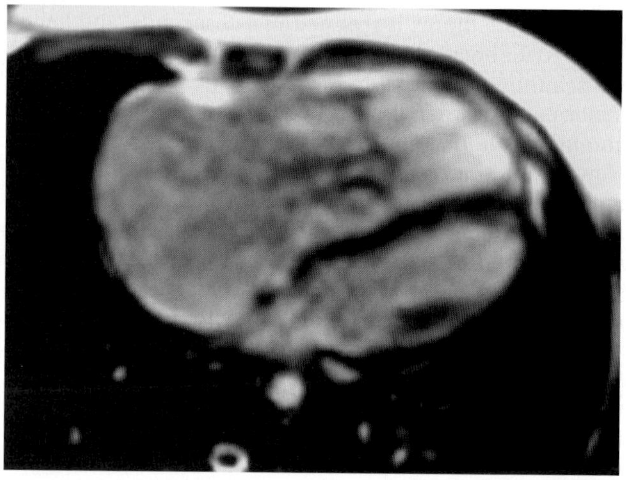

FIG. 9: Cine MR image in four-chamber view showing regurgitant jet in large RA in a case of Ebstein's anomaly, suggesting tricuspid regurgitation.

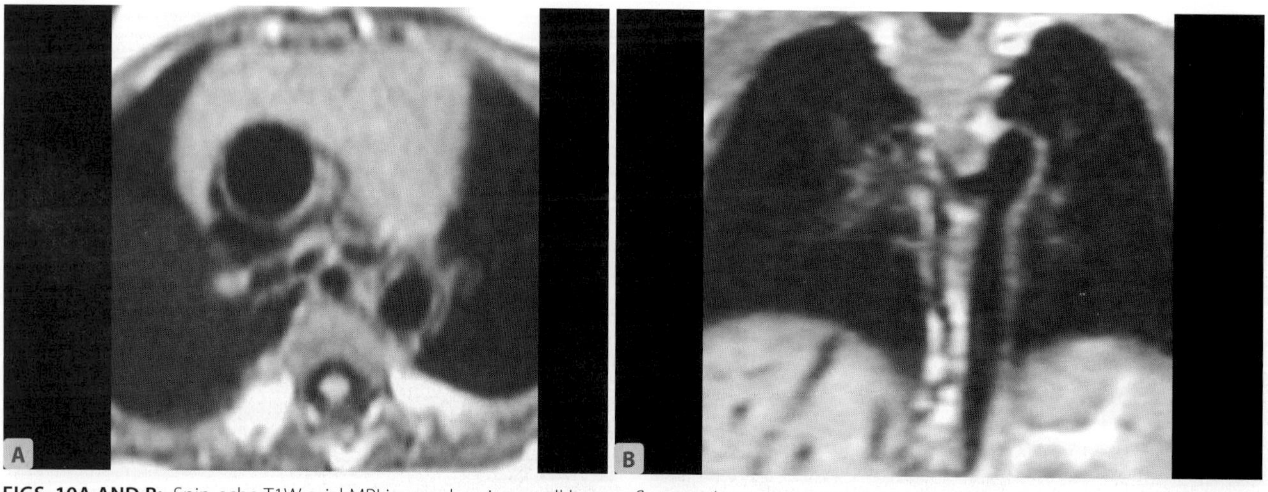

FIGS. 10A AND B: Spin-echo T1W axial MRI image showing small but confluent pulmonary arteries. Coronal image shows a large aortopulmonary collateral from descending thoracic aorta supplying right lung.

- Abnormal pulmonary venous drainage
- Abnormal coronary artery origin
- Quantification of ventricular volumes—in hypoplastic RV, hypoplastic LV
- Follow-up after surgery or intervention:
  - For shunt patency
  - Restenosis, aneurysm of aortic arch
  - For pulmonary artery stenosis
  - Valvular regurgitation, e.g. post-TOF repair
- Cardiac tumors.

Analyzing CT or MRI Images

The CT or MRI images need to be analyzed using a sequential segmental approach. This consists of following steps:

1. Determining cardiac sidedness (location of atrial chambers)
2. Identification of atria, ventricles and great arteries
3. Identification of venoatrial, atrioventricular and ventriculoarterial connections
4. Determination of cardiac position (in chest, apex orientation).

Anatomy

Cardiac sidedness is determined by position of morphological RA and this is independent of location of heart in chest, or position of ventricles and great vessels. In situs solitus, morphological RA lies to right of morphological LA.

Identifying atria is easy with the help of their respective appendages. Right atrial appendage is broad based and triangular while left atrial appendage has narrow base and is tongue shaped.

Ventricles have three parts—inlet, apex and outlet. Right ventricle shows atrioventricular discontinuity **(Fig. 11)** due to presence of supraventricular muscular crest. Right ventricle has tricuspid atrioventricular valve unlike bicuspid mitral valve of LV. Left ventricular trabeculae are fine while those is RV are few but coarse. Papillary muscles arising from septal surface, and moderator band crossing from septum to anterior papillary muscle are characteristic of RV.

Great arteries are identified by their branching pattern.

Bronchial branching pattern determines right or left sidedness. Right bronchus is superior to descending branch of RPA (epiarterial bronchus) while left bronchus traverses below the left upper pulmonary artery (hyparterial bronchus). The four pulmonary veins drain normally into left atrium.

The three systemic veins—superior and inferior vena cava and coronary sinus drain into right atrium.

Normal Connections

Venoatrial, atrioventricular and ventriculoarterial must be identified. Atrioventricular concordance and ventriculoarterial discordance is seen in complete transposition of great arteries. In corrected transposition of great arteries, there is both atrioventricular and ventriculoarterial discordance.

Extracardiac and intracardiac abnormalities must be identified. Extracardiac lesions include those associated with aorta (coarctation, PDA), Pulmonary arteries and veins (TAPVC, etc.).

Intracardiac lesions include atrial ventricular septal defects, conotruncal defects (truncus arteriosus, TOF), abnormal connections (single ventricles, d-TGA, C-TGA, double outlet RV).

Cardiac Tumors

Primary cardiac tumors are rare. MRI scores over CT in this entity because of its inherent tissue contrast. Gadolinium enhanced images help differentiate between tumor and thrombus. Cine imaging helps assess inflow or outflow obstruction and compression of adjacent vessels.

Follow-up after Surgery or after Endovascular Intervention

CT and MRI are useful to evaluate for:

- Patency of shunts/conduits and their caliber
- Complications such as aneurysms, restenosis, e.g. after aortic coarctation repair.

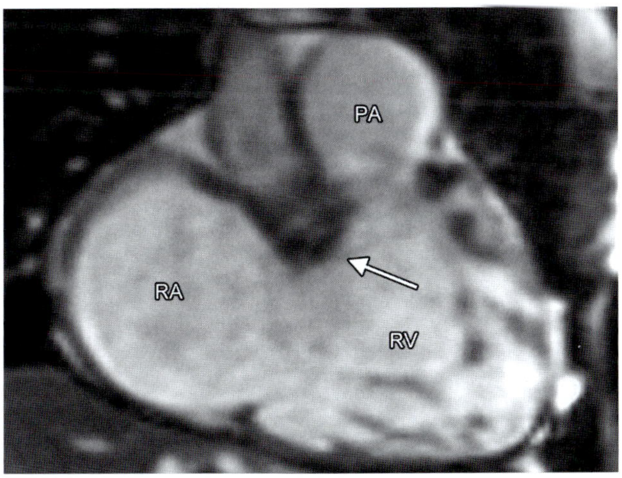

FIG. 11: MR image showing atrioventricular discontinuity in right ventricle due to supraventricular muscular crest (arrow), which is the distinguishing feature of RV.

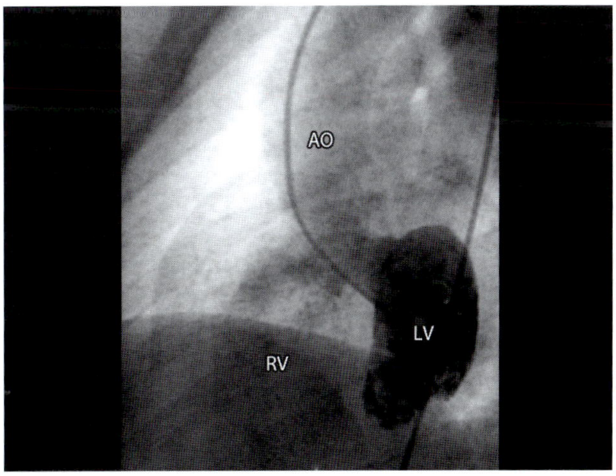

FIG. 12: Catheter angiogram image—injection through catheter in LV shows filling of RV by subaortic ventricular septal defect.

CARDIAC CATHETERIZATION

Cardiac catheterization and angiocardiography give physiologic and functional data besides revealing the morphology of the lesion **(Fig. 12)**. Though a detailed information of catheterization is beyond the scope of this chapter, there are certain things which must be kept in mind before taking up a child for this invasive procedure.

Firstly, the purpose of cath should clearly outweigh the risk of subjecting the ill child to this additional stress of contrast. The contrast must be limited to a maximum of 3 mL/kg body weight to ensure the safety of sick child.

With the advent of cardiac CT and MRI, cardiac catheterization is now limited to a few conditions where physiological information is required and pressure gradients need to be taken.

BIBLIOGRAPHY

1. Bıssoio RJ, Vincent WR. Diagnosis of congenital heart disease in first two weeks of life. California Med. 1969;110:200-6.
2. Chang CH. The normal roentgenographic measurement of the right descending pulmonary artery in 1085 cases. AJR. 1962;87:929-35.
3. Coussement AM. Objective radiographic assessment of pulmonary vascularity in children. Radiology. 1973;109:649- 54.
4. Elliot LP, Van Mierop LH, Gleason DC. Roentgenology of tricuspid atresia. Seminars in Roentgenol. 1968;3:399-409.
5. Elliott LP. Cardiac imaging in infants, children and adults, JB Lippincott Co., Philadelphia; 1991.
6. Flohr T, Stierstorfer K, Raupach R, et al. Performance evaluation of a 64-slice CT system with z-flying focal spot. Rofo. 2004;176:1803-10.
7. Goo HW, Park IS, Ko JK, et al. CT of congenital heart disease: normal anatomy and typical pathologic conditions. Radiographics. 2003;23:S147-65.
8. Gyepes MT, Vincent WR. Severe congenital heart disease in the neonatal period. AJR. 1972;490-500.
9. Jefferson K, Rees R. Clinical Cardiac Radiology, 2nd edn, Butterworth, London, 1980.
10. Kellenberger CJ, Yoo SJ, Buchel ER. Cardiovascular MR imaging in neonates and infants with congenital heart disease. Radiographics. 2007;27:5-18.
11. Leber AW, Knez A, von Ziegler F, et al. Quantification of obstructive and nonobstructive coronary lesions by 64-slice computed tomography: A comparative study with quantitative coronary angiography and intravascular ultrasound. J Am Coll Cardiol. 2005;46:147-54.
12. Leschka S, Alkadhi H, Plass A, et al. Accuracy of MSCT coronary angiography with 64-slice technology: first experience. Eur Heart J. 2005;26:1482-7.
13. Manghat NE, Morgan-Hughes GJ, Marshall AJ, et al. Multidetector row computed tomography: Imaging congenital coronary artery anomalies in adults. Heart. 2005;91:1515-22.
14. Moes CAF. Analysis of the chest in the neonate with congenital heart disease. RCNA. 1975;13:251-76.
15. Mollet NR, Cademartiri F, van Mieghem CA, et al. High-resolution spiral computed tomography coronary angiography in patients referred for diagnostic conventional coronary angiography. Circulation. 2005;112:2318-23.
16. Pugliese F, Mollet NR, Runza G, et al. Diagnostic angiography in patients with stable angina pectoris. Eur Radiol. 2006;16: 575-82.
17. Radiology of the heart. In: Braunwald E (Ed). Heart Disease: A Textbook of Cardiovascular Medicine. WB Saunders, Philadelphia; 204-34.
18. Raff GL, Gallagher MJ, O'Neill WW, et al. Diagnostic accuracy of noninvasive coronary angiography using 64-slice spiral computed tomography. J Am Coll Cardiol. 2005;46:552-7.
19. Roberts WC. Radiologic differentiation of common anomalies. In: Adult Congenital Heart Disease; 1988. pp. 191-219.
20. Sharma S. Proceedings of symposium and workshops in Cardiovascular and Interventional Radiology. Springer- Verlag, Singapore; 1997.
21. Tsai-Goodman B, Geva T, Odegard KC, et al. Clinical role, accuracy and technical aspects of cardiovascular magnetic resonance imaging in infants. Am J Cardiol. 2004;94(1):69-74.

CHAPTER

144

Imaging in Ischemic Heart Disease

Gurpreet Singh Gulati, Sanjiv Sharma, Priya Jagia

INTRODUCTION

Ischemic heart disease (IHD) continues to be the leading cause of mortality in the developed countries. The prevalence in India has risen markedly in recent years, especially in urban areas.[1] Current estimates suggest that by 2020, India will have the largest burden of cardiovascular disease in the world, the bulk of which will be comprised of IHD. An accurate and early detection of the disease is crucial for the optimal management and prognostication of these patients.

The various components of IHD that need evaluation on imaging include: presence, extent and localization of ischemia, presence and size of myocardial infarction (MI), myocardium at risk, guidance for revascularization and follow-up, and quantification of myocardial function. Several noninvasive techniques, both traditional and advanced, are available for this purpose. Conventional modalities include echocardiography (ECHO), nuclear imaging and angiography. Over the last 15 years, ischemia imaging with cardiac magnetic resonance (CMR) and multi-detector CT (MDCT) technology has evolved extensively. This review focuses upon the utility of these newer modalities for evaluation of IHD.

PATHOPHYSIOLOGY OF ISCHEMIC HEART DISEASE

Myocardial Ischemia

Stenoses of an epicardial coronary artery leads to reduced perfusion and correspondingly diminished myocardial oxygen delivery. However, at rest, the equilibrium between perfusion, metabolism, and contractile function can be maintained even in moderate to severe stenosis. Therefore, these stenoses are asymptomatic at rest and cannot be detected using perfusion studies at rest. At stress (induced pharmacologically or by physical exercise), there is a three- to four-fold increase in contractile function, accompanied by a four-fold increase in oxygen demand and perfusion. Whereas, the flow in normal coronary arteries can be increased by vasodilation (induced by using either dipyridamole or more commonly, adenosine), moderate and severe stenoses become flow limiting, resulting in perfusion deficits, wall motion abnormalities, and symptomatic angina.

Different stress tests are clinically used to detect myocardial ischemia. In the progression of ischemia, successive myocardial events occur, known as the cascade of ischemia.[2] Initially, hypoperfusion is only detectable in the subendocardium. Further reduction of the blood flow due to more severe stenosis leads to transmural perfusion deficits. Progression of ischemia leads to diastolic, followed by systolic wall motion abnormalities. These can be detected by dobutamine stress ECHO/CMR. Finally, electrocardiographic changes can be detected and typical symptomatic angina may occur. As perfusion abnormalities are the first step in this cascade of ischemia, direct visualization of these perfusion deficits seems to be the diagnostic test of first choice in patients with suspected CAD. Both CMR and nuclear imaging techniques can measure myocardial perfusion.

Myocardial Viability and Myocardial Infarction

Viability is continued cell life. A myocyte is viable while alive and nonviable once irreversible cellular damage and cell death occurs. By this definition, histology is the ultimate method for inspection of individual cells. Myocytes may be viable in the setting of severely reduced or absent contractile function, resulting from either acute or chronic reduction in perfusion. Differences between the acute and chronic settings in terms of the potential for contractile recovery of myocardium are related to the underlying mechanisms of myocyte dysfunction. A number of indirect methods have been used to detect presence of living myocytes for the purpose of in vivo assessment of myocardial viability. As a result, in clinical practice and research settings, viability has been defined in accordance with the method used to indirectly demonstrate the presence of living myocytes, leading to a number of clinical definitions of viability. For example: (1) recovery of contractile function following revascularization; (2) response to inotropic stimulation (e.g. dobutamine ECHO or dobutamine MRI); (3) presence of glucose metabolism (e.g. fluoro-2-deoxygluclose (FDG) positron emission tomography (PET)); 4) presence of active cellular transport mechanisms (e.g. Tl-201 Single photon emission computed tomography

(SPECT)); and presence of non-scarred (or more precisely, absence of scarred) myocardium (delayed enhanced MRI or DE-MRI).

Rationale for Ischemia and Viability Imaging

Although coronary artery luminal obstruction can be detected with catheter angiography or MDCT, assessment of myocardial perfusion helps to assess the functional relevance of the lesion. This is crucial to decide the need for revascularization, as coronary interventions should primarily be preformed where there is clinical evidence of myocardial ischemia associated with the coronary stenosis. Thus, even in patients with known intermediate stenosis of a coronary artery, there is frequently a need for stress testing to define whether the stenosis is hemodynamically significant. Also, there is a need to define the physiological significance of possible stenosis associated with highly calcified coronary arteries or in smaller stents that cannot be adequately resolved with current generation CT scanners.

Beyond establishment of a clinical diagnosis, an important value of stress perfusion imaging is in its ability to risk stratify patients. It is important to be able to separate low-risk group of patients from those at a high risk of sustaining subsequent cardiac events (cardiac death or MI), since it is towards the latter group that we direct our resources. This benefit of perfusion imaging has been well documented with nuclear cardiology techniques. A normal myocardial perfusion study is associated with a 0.3–1.0% annual risk of MI or cardiac-related death, in contradistinction to an abnormal study where the risk is five- to ten-fold.[3]

It is crucial to identify the myocardium that is viable and not infarcted. The presence of myocardial viability is especially important in patients with severe ventricular dysfunction, where the benefits of coronary revascularization may be questioned due to the increased risk of the procedure. Patients with viable areas clearly demonstrate survival benefit and improved quality of life after revascularization, as compared with those who do not.[4] The latter group may therefore be exposed to substantial operative risk without clear benefit.

IMAGING MODALITIES

Echocardiography

Echocardiography (ECHO) has emerged as the "workhorse" of cardiac imaging, since it is easily available, safe and quick and provides excellent information on morphology and function of nearly all cardiac structures. Stress ECHO has been shown to reliably demonstrate myocardial ischemia and helps to acquire prognostic data. There are two techniques for performing stress ECHO: (1) Detection of wall motion abnormalities induced with exercise/dobutamine; (2) Measurement of altered myocardial perfusion on contrast ECHO.[5] Myocardial contrast ECHO has been shown to be comparable to SPECT for the detection of CAD.[6] It is possible that the combination of stress perfusion and stress ECHO may improve accuracy of the technique.[7]

Limitations of ECHO include operator dependence with poor interobserver agreement. Also, an optimal acoustic window may not exist in every patient for detection of all wall motion abnormalities. The left ventricular apex, particularly in a large, hypocontractile left ventricle, may not be adequately assessed with this modality. In patients with MI, a mural thrombus may be difficult to distinguish from underlying myocardium on ECHO.

Nuclear Imaging

This is perhaps the most well established modality with a large body of literature available on its utility for detecting the presence of myocardial ischemia and infarction.

For detection of myocardial ischemia, the most common procedure is myocardial perfusion imaging (MPI) or single-photon emission computed tomography (SPECT). SPECT is a tomographic technique, providing 3-dimensional assessment of blood flow. Small amounts of radioactive material (including thallium-201, and the more recent available Tc-99m tetrofosmin and Tc-99m sestamibi) are injected intravenously and these tracers are taken up and retained in the heart tissue in proportion to regional blood supply. Usually, two scans are obtained after tracer injection, one at rest and one in which the agent is injected during exercise or medication-induced stress. Areas with reduced blood supply, either under resting conditions or following stress testing, indicate regions of scar or reversible perfusion alterations (ischemia), respectively. Additionally, an ECG-gated SPECT allows for assessment of LV function.

Positron-emission tomography (PET) has several technical advantages over SPECT, such as higher counting sensitivity, higher spatial resolution, and routine use of attenuation correction. PET (along with CMR) using metabolic tracers such as 18F-FDG (glucose analog), is currently regarded as the gold standard for tissue viability. Under normal conditions, fatty acids play a major role in the metabolism of the normoxic heart, while glucose becomes the major substrate for the myocardium under ischemic conditions. Therefore, PET imaging using metabolic tracers such as 18F-FDG enables detection of metabolic changes at the cellular level associated with ischemia. In clinical practice, 18F-FDG PET is often combined with flow tracers such as 13N-ammonia to assess myocardial perfusion. Although 18F-FDG PET imaging without flow tracer may work with reasonable sensitivity and specificity for detecting viable tissue, flow/metabolism combination would provide more comprehensive information on viability. The preserved or increased glucose utilization, and hence 18F-FDG uptake in hypoperfused and dysfunctional myocardium (flow metabolism mismatch) is regarded as a metabolic marker of cell survival and viability, whereas concordant reduction in both blood flow and 18F-FDG uptake is indicative of scar.

Limitations of nuclear imaging are discussed later, under "Evaluation of various components of IHD: Detection of myocardial ischemia".

Cardiovascular Magnetic Resonance Imaging (CMR)

During the past decade, significant advances have been made in the imaging speed, resolution, quality, and versatility of CMR. Reliable, reproducible CMR imaging can now be achieved as a result of advent of more rapid imaging acquisition along with breath-hold techniques, diaphragmatic navigator gating, and real-time imaging to counter the effects of respiratory motion. The availability of stress myocardial perfusion in mid 1990s, and steady state free precession (SSFP) imaging and DE-MRI at the start of the new millennium allows assessment of all aspects of ischemia, infarct and myocardial functional imaging in a single session of 45–50 min. There is growing evidence that CMR can be used at each step of the assessment of patients with IHD, from establishing the diagnosis to guiding the optimal therapeutic strategy through to risk stratification.

Other advantages of CMR are that it is operator independent and does not entail exposure to potentially nephrotoxic contrast or ionizing radiation. In the context of IHD, the high spatial resolution of CMR allows better detection of myocardial edema, subendocardial ischemia, subendocardial infarcts and microvascular obstruction.

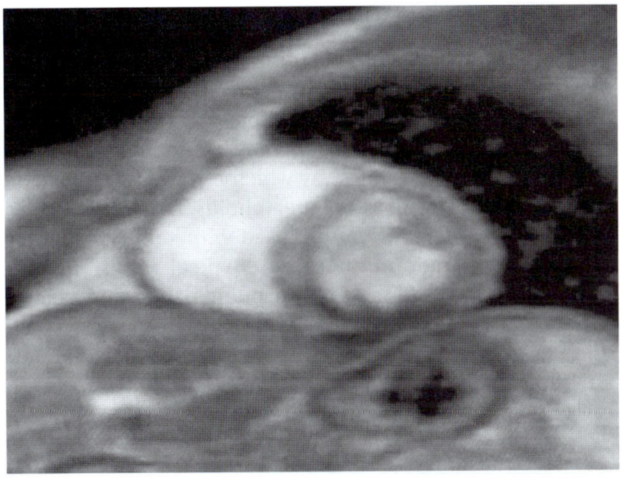

FIG. 1: Stress CMR perfusion—short axis image at the mid- ventricular level. There is a subendocardial perfusion defect (hypointensity) in the inferior wall, corresponding to right coronary artery (RCA) stenosis. The defect was not present at rest.

IMAGING SEQUENCES

Stress CMR

There are two CMR techniques for assessment of myocardial ischemia: dobutamine stress MR (DSMR) and perfusion CMR. DSMR has not yet gained wide acceptance in the clinical arena because of concerns relating to patient safety and monitoring inside the MR scanner. Additionally, from a pathophysiologic point of view, perfusion CMR should be more sensitive than DSMR since decreased perfusion is the first step of the ischemic cascade.

For optimal first pass perfusion studies, a series of T1 weighted images need to be obtained every heart beat or every other heart beat while a bolus of contrast passes through the heart and myocardium. Gadolinium (dosage varies between 0.025 and 0.15 mmol/kg) is the most widely used contrast agent for perfusion CMR. After localizer images, the vasodilator stress agent is started IV (most commonly adenosine, in a dose of 140 mg/kg/min for 5 minutes before injection of gadolinium). By 3 minutes of the infusion, adequate vasodilator stress is usually achieved to allow performance of stress perfusion imaging. T1 weighted sequences are then used to visualise the passage of gadolinium. Areas of myocardial hypoperfusion will appear as areas of decreased signal intensity **(Fig. 1)**. Typical perfusion deficits tend to follow the perfusion territories of the coronary artery, affect the distal segments first (with few exceptions), are subendocardial (except most severe cases), last for several heartbeats beyond the initial rapid upslope of myocardial enhancement, and are not present at rest (except in MI). One needs to be aware of the various artefacts (including the most common susceptibility artefacts) that can interfere with the interpretation of true deficits. Perfusion CMR analysis is based on the time-intensity curves and can be performed in a quantitative, semi-quantitative, or qualitative fashion.

CMR for Viability

The standard CMR technique for detection of myocardial viability is DE-MRI. This was introduced in the late 1990's and is being increasingly regarded as the gold-standard for

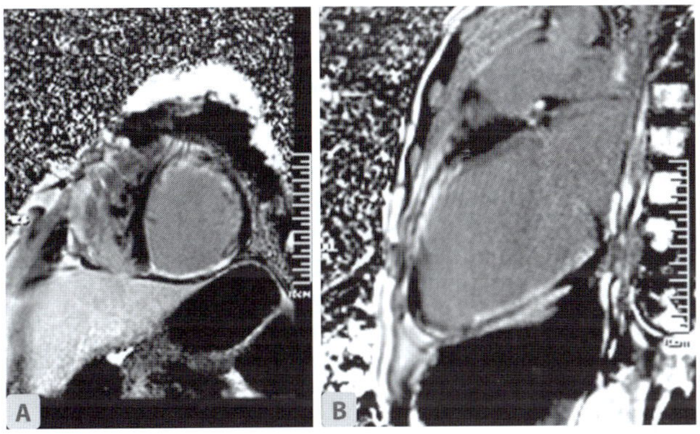

FIGS. 2A AND B: DE-MRI—short axis and vertical long axis views. There are transmural infarcts (hyperenhanced) in the anterior, anterolateral and anteroseptal segments (LAD territory), as well as in the inferior and inferolateral segments (RCA territory).

the detection of irreversibly damaged myocardium. The underlying concept is that infarcted tissue accumulates gadolinium and can be visualized as hyperenhanced or "bright" regions on T1-weighted images acquired at least 10 minutes after gadolinium injection **(Figs. 2A and B)**. Gadolinium is an inert extracellular contrast agent and the amount of contrast agent in a given tissue distribution volume determines the image signal intensity—the more contrast per distribution volume the higher the signal. In the normal myocardium, the tissue volume is predominantly intracellular. Because extracellular contrast media is excluded from this space by the intact sarcolemmal membrane, the volume of distribution of a contrast medium in normal myocardium is quite small (25% of water space), and one can consider viable myocytes as actively excluding contrast media. Therefore, the unifying mechanism for the hyperenhancement effect of nonviable myocardium may be regarded as being due to the absence of viable myocytes rather than any inherent properties that are specific for acutely necrotic tissue, collagenous scar, or other forms of nonviable tissue.

CMR for Myocardial Mass and Function

SSFP cine sequences provide high spatial resolution and a high contrast between the dark myocardium and the bright blood-pool and therefore are preferred for this purpose **(Figs. 3A and B)**: a stack of short-axis cine images (with a slice thickness of 8–12 mm) by which both ventricles can be covered without a gap in 1–2 breathholds. Either prospective or retrospective gating can be used with similar accuracy. The resulting section provides the typical volumetric and functional data for LV and RV including parameters such as EDV, ESV, SV, CO and filling rates. These calculations are done using the modified Simpson's rule. When both endo- and epicardial contours are drawn, ventricular mass and regional wall thickening can also be calculated.

OTHER USEFUL SEQUENCES

T2-weighted turbo spin echo sequences are used to detect increased water tissue content as an indirect measure of tissue inflammation or edema and can be useful in the differentiation between acute and chronic MI between myocarditis and CAD.

Multidetector Computed Tomography (MDCT)

This modality has developed tremendously over the last decade to emerge as an excellent non-invasive tool for demonstration of coronary artery anatomy. Key technical requirements for coronary MDCT are high temporal resolution (which minimizes motion artifacts and is achieved through fast gantry rotation), high spatial resolution [which enables detailed depiction of the coronary anatomy (both the wall and lumen) and is achieved through thin collimation], fast continuous coverage (which enables imaging of the entire heart in one comfortable breath-hold), and synchronization to the heartbeat (which enables imaging during a consistent cardiac phase and is achieved through ECG gating).

There are two methods for ECG-gating on MDCT. A retrospective ECG-gated MDCT obtains different image sets at different times in the cardiac cycle in a spiral mode. While individual time windows of end-systolic and end-diastolic phases are usually used for adequate visualization of the coronary arteries at times where they present minimal velocity, one can also reconstruct the data for all phases of the cardiac cycle from the same original dataset. It is thereby possible to generate dynamic cine sequences of the whole heart and to select oblique reformatted planes along standard anatomic axis of the heart. These reconstructed data provide high quality images for the assessment of heart anatomy and ventricular function. A disadvantage of retrospective gated MDCT scanning is the higher radiation exposure. To circumvent this limitation, prospective ECG triggering (a step-and-shoot sequential scanning method) may be used. Image acquisition is timed to coincide with a predefined point in the cardiac cycle. The advantages of prospective ECG-triggering are speed and a reduction in radiation dose. One disadvantage is the need for a regular heart rate and rhythm.

In a patient with an irregular heart rate, image acquisition can be triggered at the wrong point in the cardiac cycle, resulting in misregistration artifact. In addition, sequential scanning yields single trans-axial slices rather than volumetric data, and z-axis resolution is suboptimal.

Cardiac MDCT scan is usually begun by obtaining a calcium score, scanning from the level of the tracheal bifurcation to the bottom of the heart. Exceptions are patients being scanned following revascularization [coronary artery bypass surgery (CABG) or stent placement]. The calcium score not only provides independent prognostic information, it also helps in determining whether a patient is a good candidate for coronary MDCT. There is no recommended absolute threshold coronary calcium score that precludes coronary MDCT. However, in a patient with very dense calcification along the length of the coronary vessels and at multiple branch points, it is extremely difficult to interpret MDCT images. For the contrast MDCT, scan range is the same as the calcium score. Scan range is increased to include the top of the chest in patients scanned after CABG. The heart

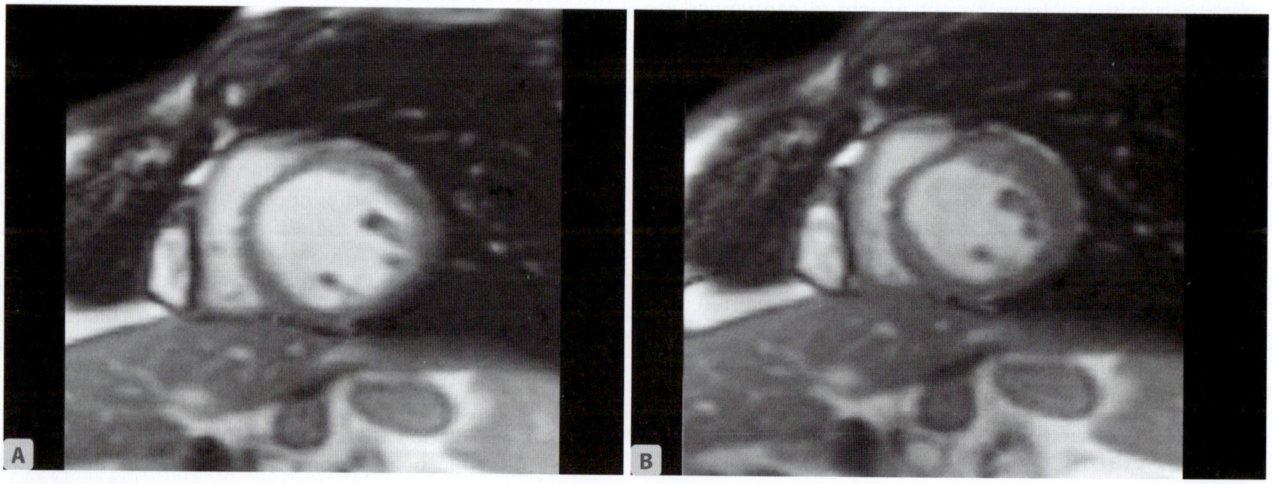

FIGS. 3A AND B: SSFP cine-CMR—short axis images in diastole (A) and systole (B). Thinning of myocardium is noted in the septal and anteroseptal segments (infarct in LAD territory). These segments do not thicken (akinesia) during systole. Also note reduced thickening (hypokinesia) in the inferolateral wall [left circumflex (LCx) artery territory].

is positioned at the isocenter, and images are reconstructed with a small field-of-view, to improve resolution. Contrast type, volume, rate, method of bolus (test or automatic bolus tracking) injection and scanner parameters vary depending on operator preference, particular vendor's equipment, scanner generation.

For 64 slice CT scanners, the patient's heart rate may need to be controlled. If the baseline heart rate exceeds 65 bpm, a beta-blocker—oral metoprolol 50 to 100 mg—45 minutes to 1 hour prior to the study is administered. If the rate still remains too high, IV metoprolol in 5-mg doses, up to a maximum of 20 mg may need to be given. It is important to use caution when administering beta-blockers to patients with asthma, severe aortic stenosis, atrio-ventricular block, or severe left ventricular dysfunction. With the higher temporal resolution available with dual source scanners, beta blockers are not usually indicated.

Up to the generation of scanners providing 16 slices per rotation, the ratio of non-conclusive studies was still in the range of 20 to 30% of the patients who had at least one coronary segment that could not be adequately evaluated despite the use of beta blockers. The advent of 64 slice scanners followed by new dual source and 256 (and 320) slice scanners have led to a quantum leap in temporal and spatial resolution with much higher performance allowing imaging patients with fast and irregular heart rates. Dual source scanners essentially double the speed of acquisition while maintaining the same spatial resolution of a 64-slice scanner.[8,9] With two X-ray beams and detectors rotating simultaneously on the same gantry, double the amount of data are acquired on each rotation. This increases the temporal resolution of the scan to 82 msec (1/4 gantry rotation time), which can be increased still further to 42 msec with multi-segment reconstruction. Furthermore, the ability of having each individual generator set to a different energy with different tissue penetration opens new perspectives in better tissue characterization that would potentially allow a better assessment of composition of vascular plaques. It is also possible using dual energy imaging to separate calcifications from contrast agent to generate images of the vascular lumens without interference from calcified plaques. Dual energy imaging has already been explored in peripheral vessels both for generating better calcium-free angiograms as well as assessing the tissue characteristics of vascular plaques. These techniques may also be applicable to coronary arteries in future.

Limitations of MDCT

- Need for a stable and well controlled heart rate
- Inadequate assessment of lesion severity
- Interference due to calcification in the vessel wall
- Need for iodinated contrast and radiation exposure.

The latter two aspects need to be weighed against the benefit of noninvasively depicting the coronary arteries. The risk of radiation exposure is more important in those cases in whom further functional nuclear assessment and, if necessary, invasive catheterization and interventions are required. With higher number of detectors (e.g. 64), images obtained with full spatial and temporal resolution over the complete heart cycle can easily deliver between 15 and 20 mSv. This is roughly double the radiation of conventional coronary angiogram that averages between 9 and 12 mSv.

There are various strategies to reduce radiation exposure. These include:

- Reducing dose to a level that is as low as reasonably achievable (the ALARA principle). The technologist can be instructed to only cover the area of the heart, instead of covering the whole chest. This can help reduce the exposure by half or more.
- Retrospective gating with pulsed radiation synchronous to the ECG that delivers lower radiation dose outside a selected window in diastolic phase. The radiation dose can be reduced significantly with ECG pulsing to approximately 10 mSv in men and 14 mSv in women.
- Lowering the tube voltage to 100 kV in patients with a normal body weight or body mass index.[10]
- Implementation of step-and-shoot cardiac CT is associated with an effective radiation dose of just 1–3 mSv.[11]
- A prospective gate window of 20% over diastole in patients with a heart rate around 60 bpm can reduce the total dose to the patient by 80%. At higher heart rates the reduction of dose may be less and still achieve 55–60% of dose reduction.

Recent publications have shown that by using prospective gating and proper imaging protocol, accurate images of the coronary arteries can be obtained at doses as low as 1 or 2 mSV.[12,13] With 256 detectors and higher, scanners can acquire full 3D images of the whole heart in a single rotation avoiding spiral averaging of multiple heart cycles. This can significantly reduce the dose down to 2.8 mSv with pulsed exposure over diastole and about 5 mSv for full dynamic assessment of LV function over the whole heart cycle.[14]

A more recent technical advance has been the introduction of a new dual source CT, generating 128 slices per detector system (instead of 64 slices per detector system in the earlier version). Besides having the fastest scanning speed for retrospective gating in spiral mode (43 cm/s) and highest temporal resolution (75 ms), the scanner operates at an extremely reduced radiation dose. For example, a spiral heart scan can be performed with less than 1 mSv, much lower than the annual radiation exposure from natural sources of 2–5 mSv.

EVALUATION OF VARIOUS COMPONENTS OF IHD

Coronary Artery Imaging

Conventional

X-ray angiography has the advantage of high spatial resolution (~ 0.3 mm) and temporal resolution (20 msec). However, it also has some important limitations: it is invasive, is a two-dimensional technique and does not provide any information about vessel wall structure or plaque morphology.

With CMR, despite the initial hype regarding its scope to image the coronary arteries, there are significant technical difficulties that preclude optimal coronary imaging: small vessel caliber, tortuous course, signal from surrounding epicardial fat and myocardium, near constant motion related to the cardiac and respiratory cycles and the fact that bulk of flow occurs in diastole (Which limits data acquisition time).

Coronary MDCT angiography produces high-quality images of the coronary arteries, in addition to defining their location and the extent of atherosclerotic involvement. Pooling of data from recent studies on accuracy of 64-slice CT and dual-source CT for the detection of coronary artery stenoses in patients with suspected CAD provided a sensitivity of 89% (95% CI 87–90), specificity of 96% (95% CI 96–97), and positive (PPV) and negative predictive values (NPV) of 78% (95% CI 76–80) and 98% (95% CI 98–99), respectively.[15-18] On average, 4.5% of segments (mainly distal segments or very small side branches) could not be evaluated. Importantly, the NPV was consistently high in all studies, indicating that the technique may be most suitable as a noninvasive tool to rule out significant CAD and avoid further imaging or invasive angiography **(Figs. 4A and B)**. Therefore, patients with low probability of CAD, with non-specific symptoms and/or non-conclusive functional tests such as exercise, stress ECHO or nuclear imaging are ideally suited for coronary MDCT.[19,20] Due to its ability to simultaneously assess the thoracic aorta, coronary arteries and the lungs, an ECG-gated MDCT of the chest may provide useful information in patients presenting with acute chest pain with intermediate probability for CAD and no enzyme or ECG changes **(Fig. 5)**. Hoffmann et al.[21] conducted a blinded, prospective study with 64-slice MDCT in this group of patients presenting to the emergency department. Among 103 consecutive patients, 14 patients were diagnosed clinically to have an acute coronary syndrome. Both the absence of significant coronary artery stenosis (73 of 103 patients) and non-stenotic coronary atherosclerotic plaque (41 of 103 patients) accurately predicted the absence of an acute coronary syndrome (NPV 100%). The PPV was rather low, indicating false-positive results in a considerable number of scans (47% for the detection of significant stenoses, 14/30 positive scans), and only a small percent age of patients with acute chest pain were actually included in the study (103 of 305 initially screened patients). Goldstein, et al.[22] randomized 197 patients with low-risk acute chest pain to an immediate 64-slice MDCT scan or 'standard of care' evaluation. CT was found to be safe, with no missed diagnosis of an acute coronary syndrome, faster (3.4 vs 15 hours until establishing the definitive diagnosis), and had lower cost ($1586 vs. 1872) compared with 'standard of care'.

MDCT is also suited for patients with intermediate probability for CAD where more traditional tests remain equivocal or in patients unable to exercise or undergo a stress test.

Coronary MDCT is also highly recommended for follow-up evaluation after CABG. Unlike invasive coronary angiograms, MDCT does not require accurate localization of ostia of venous grafts for selective contrast injections. Also, compared to native coronary arteries, grafts are larger in caliber, less mobile and away from heart. Pooled analysis of date from 180 patients showed the sensitivity, specificity, NPV and PPV of MDCT for graft stenosis/occlusion to be 97–100%, 95–100%, 92–99% and 99–100% respectively.[18]

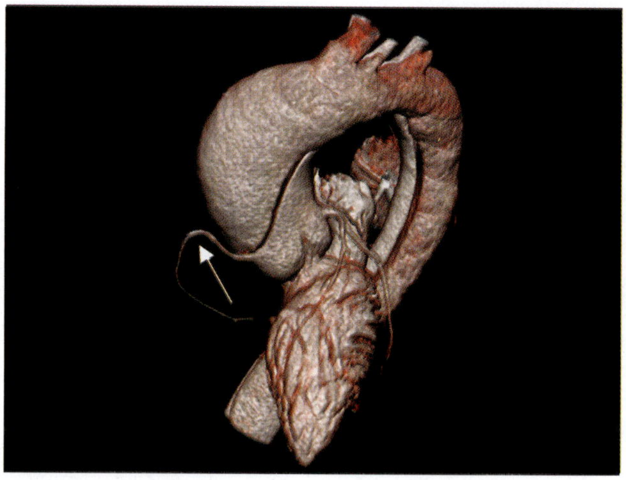

FIG. 5: ECG-gated thoracic MDCT in a patient presenting with acute chest pain, volume-rendered image. A type A aortic dissection, beginning in the aortic root and extending into the descending thoracic aorta, is seen. The RCA (arrow) is normal.

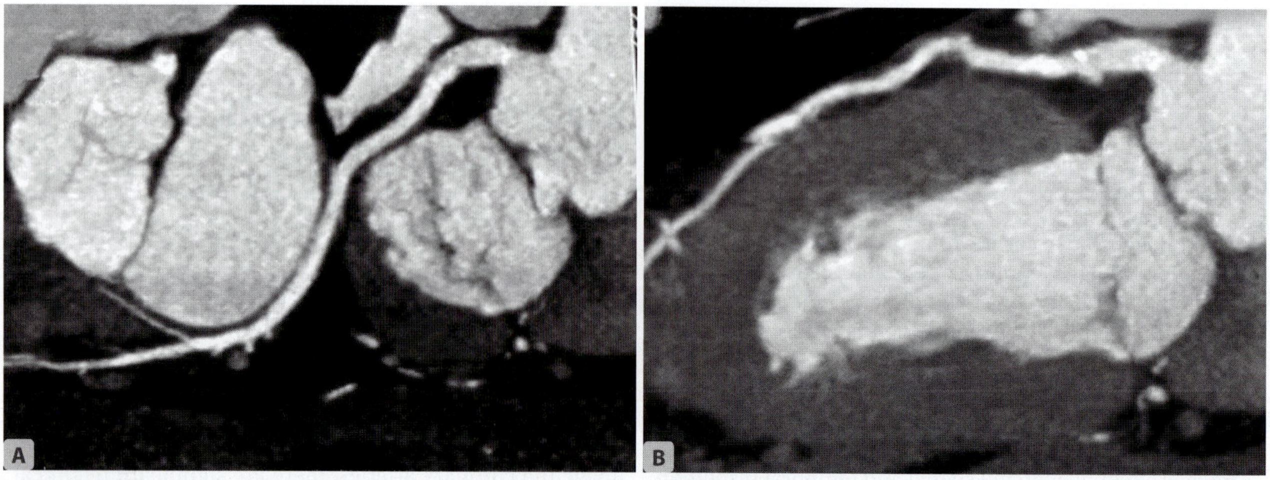

FIGS. 4A AND B: Coronary MDCT—curved multiplanar reconstructions along the RCA (A) and the LAD (B). There is no evidence of luminal obstruction (similar images were obtained for LCx), although calcified plaques are noted along the proximal and mid-LAD.

Only 0.7% of occluded and 6.4% of stenosed grafts were non-interpretable, proving MDCT to be an accurate and reliable test for detection of grafts stenosis as well as patency **(Figs. 6A and B)**. However, surgical metal clips may lead to artifacts that interfere with optimal visualization in some cases. Also, the native coronary artery visualization in CABG patients may not be adequate with MDCT due to extensive calcification.

Although in single, carefully selected cases (e.g. large diameter stents in a proximal vessel segment, low and stable heart rate, and absence of excessive image noise) coronary CT angiography may be a possibility to rule out in-stent restenosis, routine application of CT to assess patients with coronary stents is currently not recommended. Visualization of the stent lumen is often affected by artifacts, and especially the PPV is low.

For evaluation of the origin and course of aberrant coronary arteries, invasive angiography may be limited. Because of the three-dimensional nature of the data set, MDCT is very well suited to detect and define the anatomic course of coronary artery anomalies and their relationship to other cardiac and non-cardiac structures **(Figs. 7A and B)**. Numerous case reports and several research papers have demonstrated that the MDCT analysis of coronary anatomy in these patients is straight forward and very reliable with an accuracy close to 100%.[23,24]

Plaque Imaging

Calcified Plaque

Coronary calcium is a surrogate marker for the presence and amount of coronary atherosclerotic plaque. Both EBCT

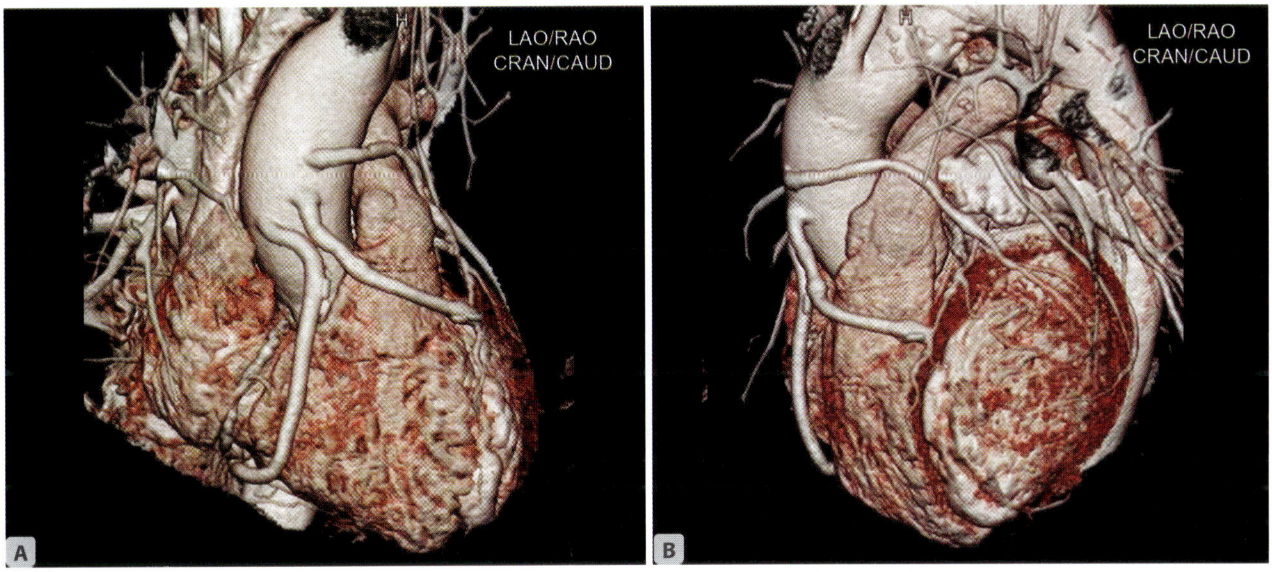

FIGS. 6A AND B: Coronary MDCT—postoperative CABG, volume-rendered images. There are three venous grafts, one each to the LAD, RCA and ramus intermedius. All grafts are patent.

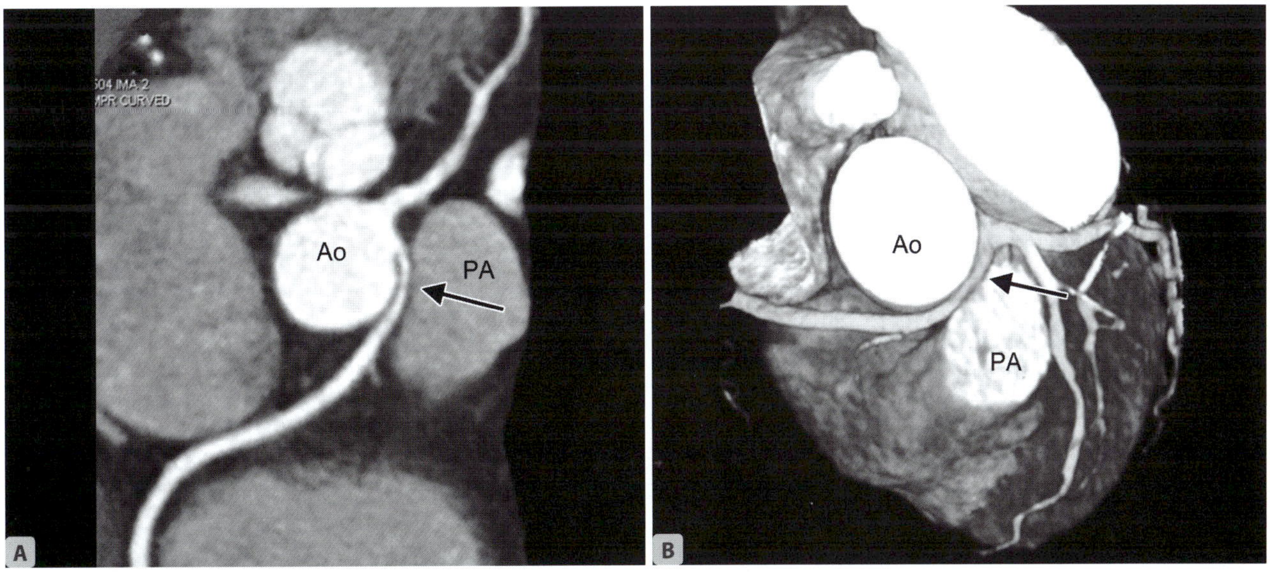

FIGS. 7A AND B: Coronary MDCT, curved multiplanar (A) and volume-rendered (B) images. The RCA (arrow) arises anomalously from the left coronary sinus, close to the origin of the left main coronary artery. It courses interarterially between the aorta (Ao) and pulmonary artery (PA).

and MDCT permit accurate detection and quantification of coronary artery calcium. The 'Agatston Score', which takes into account the area and the CT density of calcified lesions, is most frequently used to quantify the amount of coronary calcium in CT, and large population reference databases are available. With the exception of patients with renal failure, calcifications occur exclusively in the context of atherosclerotic lesions. The amount of coronary calcium correlates moderately closely to the overall atherosclerotic plaque burden.[25] On the other hand, not every atherosclerotic coronary plaque is calcified, and calcification is a sign of neither stability nor instability of an individual plaque.[26]

In several trials, the absence of coronary calcium ruled out the presence of significant coronary artery stenoses with high predictive value.[25,27] However, even pronounced coronary calcification is not necessarily associated with hemodynamically relevant luminal narrowing. Therefore, even the detection of large amounts of calcium does not indicate the presence of significant stenoses and it should not prompt invasive coronary angiography in otherwise asymptomatic individuals.

Numerous prospective trials have demonstrated that the presence of coronary calcium in asymptomatic individuals is a prognostic parameter with strong predictive power for future hard cardiac events. A beneficial contribution of coronary calcium assessment to risk stratification can however, be most likely expected in individuals who seem to be at intermediate risk for coronary events (1.0–2.0% annual risk) on the basis of traditional risk factor analysis. The incremental value of calcium scoring may necessitate intensifying lipid lowering therapy in these patients. Unselected 'screening' or patient self-referral is not recommended, and the value of calcium scoring in individuals with very low (<1.0% annual risk) or very high risk (>2.0% annual risk) is discussed controversially.[25,27-29]

Although the coronary calcium score has been found to be progressive over time, only very preliminary studies are available that have linked progression of coronary calcium to cardiac event rates. Results concerning the influence of lipid-lowering therapy on the progression of coronary calcium have been inhomogeneous. Currently, there is no indication for repeated coronary calcium score measurements.

Non-calcified Plaque

There is growing interest concerning the ability of contrast-enhanced MDCT coronary angiography to detect, quantify and characterize non-calcified plaque **(Fig. 8)**. Data on the accuracy of CT angiography to detect non-calcified plaque are limited to a small number of studies that have compared CT angiography with intravascular ultrasound (IVUS). Sensitivities for the detection of coronary segments with plaque were found to be 80–90% (which, however, was mostly based on the detection of calcified plaque). Correlation of plaque area ($r = 0.55$) and plaque volume ($r = 0.83$) between CT angiography and IVUS was found to be moderate, and inter-observer variability is high.[30-32] It has been shown that the extent of remodeling of coronary atherosclerotic lesions can be assessed by CT. Some data are available concerning plaque characterization by CT. On average, the CT attenuation within 'fibrous' plaques is higher than within 'lipid-rich' plaques (mean attenuation values of 91–116 vs 47–71 HU).[30] There is however, large variability of these measurements, which currently prevents accurate classification of non-calcified 'plaque types' by CT.

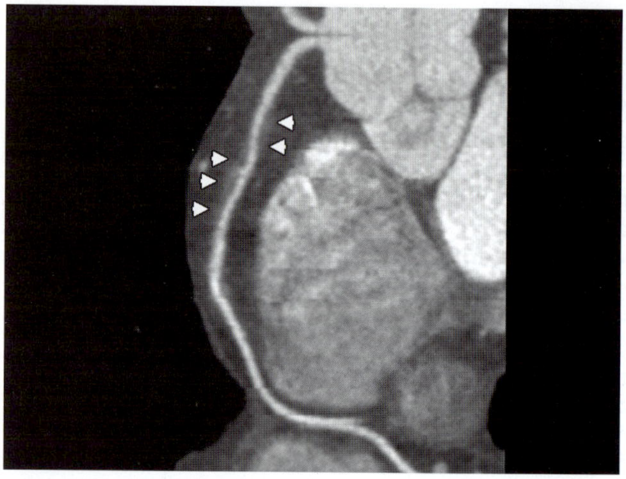

FIG. 8: Coronary MDCT—axial image. There is an non-calcified plaque (arrowheads) in the mid-RCA.

Preliminary retrospective, small studies have used CT to investigate plaque characteristics in patients after acute coronary syndromes in comparison with patients with stable angina. They reported a higher fraction of non-calcified plaque and more positive remodeling in patients with acute coronary syndromes and in lesions responsible for cardiac events. One study found a significantly higher prevalence of plaque with a CT attenuation <30 HU in lesions associated with acute coronary syndromes when compared with stable lesions.[33] One analysis of 100 patients who were followed for 16 months after coronary MDCT angiography demonstrated a higher cardiovascular event rate in patients with nonobstructive plaque detected by MDCT compared with individuals without any plaque.[34] These initial observations suggest that there may be a potential value of plaque imaging by MDCT coronary angiography for risk prediction.

Detection of Myocardial Ischemia

Stress perfusion nuclear imaging has several significant limitations: the test is quite lengthy, since it usually requires a stress and a rest study to be performed in separate sessions. In addition, conventional cardiac nuclear imaging has poor spatial resolution and lacks the ability to perform quantitative measurement of perfusion. It also suffers from attenuation artifacts. More importantly, it exposes patients to significant doses of ionizing radiation. Finally, nuclear imaging lacks specificity for detection of CAD. Therefore, alternatives for conventional perfusion nuclear imaging would be clearly desirable.

Although PET perfusion imaging can overcome many of these limitations,[35] its complexity and cost, and the requirement to have either a cyclotron or a rubidium generator on-site, have prevented widespread use of the technique. CMR has proven to be a more practical alternative for stress perfusion imaging. Since the physiological half-life of gadolinium-based contrast agents is short, it is possible to repeat a rest perfusion scan several minutes after the stress study.

There are several important differences between the mechanism by which these two modalities assess myocardial perfusion. With Thallium-201 or TC-99m sestamibi SPECT, the signal intensity in the myocardium depends on the myocardial blood flow and the amount of viable cells extracting the tracer into the intracellular space. Therefore, areas with decreased myocardial perfusion as well as areas with a reduced number of viable cells result in reduced tracer uptake. In contrast, the myocardial signal intensity on CMR images during first-pass perfusion of a paramagnetic contrast agent depends on myocardial blood flow, vascular permeability, and the size of the extracellular space. The viability of myocardial cells does not affect signal characteristics. Thus, reperfused but infarcted myocardium appears dark on SPECT images, whereas it may be isointense to normal myocardium on first-pass CMR at rest.

Theoretical advantages of CMR perfusion imaging over nuclear SPECT are its significantly higher spatial resolution, allowing detection of subendocardial ischemia; the possibility to combine evaluation of myocardial ischemia with evaluation of contractile function and myocardial viability all within 30 minutes; and most importantly, the absence of radiation exposure. Several single-center studies and two smaller multicenter trials have been performed for the clinical evaluation of CMR perfusion imaging. The results of 12 of these single-center and the two multicenter trials were summarized in a meta-analysis.[36] In a total of 1183 patients (after exclusion of 50 patients secondary to unsuccessful CMR studies), this technique was found to have a sensitivity of 91% [95% confidence interval (CI) 88–94%] and a specificity of 81% (95% CI 77–85%) for detection of coronary artery disease. The major limitation of all these trials was their small size. Furthermore, there remains a lot of uncertainty and variation among doses of contrast agents, scanner hardware, and perfusion sequences. This limited the generalization of the findings.

The MR-IMPACT study by Schwitter et al.[37] is the largest published study on perfusion CMR in comparison with other modalities, across multiple CMR vendors and operators. This prospective double-blind randomized study of 241 patients compared the effect of five different contrast doses on image quality and diagnostic accuracy of perfusion CMR. It also compared the diagnostic accuracy of perfusion CMR at the best dose vs SPECT for detection of significant CAD using catheter angiography as reference standard. Perfusion-CMR at the optimal contrast dose (0.1 mmol/kg) had similar performance as SPECT, if only the SPECT studies of the 42 patients with this dose were considered ($P = 0.12$); however, diagnostic performance of perfusion-CMR was better vs. the entire SPECT population ($P = 0.013$).

Ingkanisorn et al. evaluated the prognostic role of adenosine perfusion CMR on 135 patients presenting to the emergency department with troponin-negative chest pain.[38] The perfusion abnormalities had 100% sensitivity and 93% specificity as the single most accurate component of the CMR examination. Compared to conventional risk factors, presence of perfusion abnormalities was a stronger predictor of future cardiac events. In ROC (receiver operator characteristic) analysis, adenosine CMR was a more accurate predictor than cardiac risk factors ($P < 0.002$). A negative perfusion CMR predicted an excellent prognosis at 1 year follow-up.

Despite these enthusiastic prospects, it is important to understand that perfusion CMR does have important limitations and contraindications, which will prevent unrestricted use in every patient. Patients with devices such as pacemakers and AICDs cannot undergo CMR. This modality will also not be tolerated well by claustrophobic patients. Image quality is significantly hampered by arrhythmias. The optimal performance of the technique is also associated with a steep learning curve. Finally, gadolinium-based contrast media have been associated with the development of nephrogenic systemic sclerosis in patients with renal failure.

Myocardial Viability

Human studies demonstrate that delayed enhancement magnetic resonance imaging (DE-MRI) is effective in identifying the presence, location, and extent of MI in both the acute and chronic settings. Additionally, DE-MRI provides scar size measurements that are closely correlated with PET, and provides results superior to SPECT in patients with subendocardial infarctions. This advantage of DE-MRI stems from its high spatial resolution. With a standard implementation, a voxel 6 mm in a typical DE-MRI image would represent an infarction of 0.16 grams. This level of resolution is more than 40 times greater than with SPECT. Hence, even micro infarcts, which cannot be visualized with any other technique, can be seen with CMR.

Another advantage of DE-MRI over nuclear imaging is that it provides direct visualization of both non-viable as well as the viable myocardium. Concurrently, in the setting of acute MI, DE-MRI can differentiate between acute infarcts with necrotic myocytes and acute infarcts with necrotic myocytes and damaged microvasculature (the latter being termed as "no-reflow" phenomenon). Microvascular obstruction appears as a dark rim of hypoenhancement within the hyperenhanced infarcted myocardium. A SPECT or PET scan would have simply identified this as being non-viable due to reduced tracer activity. The detection of myocardial segments with profound microvascular damage has an important bearing on outcomes of revascularization and prognosis of patients following acute MI.[39]

Presence of mural thrombus can be missed on ECHO, but is reliably picked up on DE-MRI as a hypointense mass overlying the infarcted ventricular wall **(Fig. 9)**. MRI is the only technique that can consistently demonstrate thrombus in patients following MI.

Kim et al. demonstrated the importance of CMR in the evaluation of myocardial viability.[40] They analyzed 50 patients with ventricular dysfunction who underwent DE-MRI before and after revascularization. About 80% had some regions of hyperenhancement on the pre-intervention CMR, while 38% had abnormal contractility. The likelihood of wall motion improvement was strongly correlated to the transmural extent of hyperenhancement. In patients without hyperenhancement, 78% of segments showed improved contractility after revascularization, compared to only 1 of 58 segments improving if there was more than 75% transmural hyperenhancement. In patients with myocardial

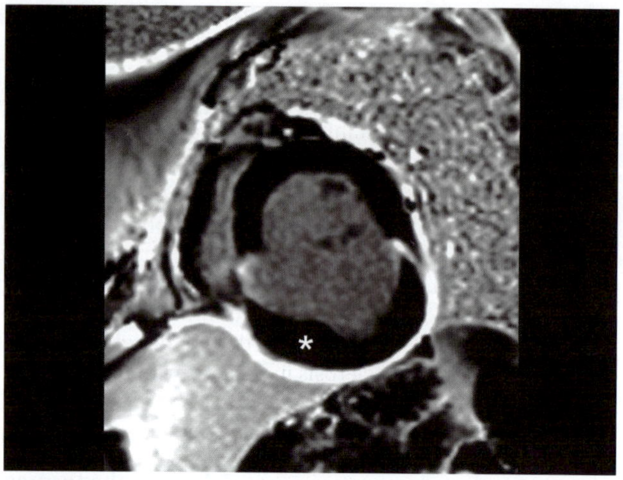

FIG. 9: DE-MRI—short axis view: There is a transmural infarct (hyperenhanced rim) in the inferior, inferoseptal and inferolateral segments (RCA territory). Overlying the infarct, there is a hypointense mural thrombus (*).

hyperenhancement involving 51 to 75% of the wall, only 10% of revascularized segments showed improved contractility. This was an extremely important study with great impact on the therapeutic management of patient with LV dysfunction and hibernating myocardium, since it meant that it was possible to target revascularization to vessel supplying blood to a territory where functional recovery can be reliably predicted. The ability of CE-CMR to discriminate between viable and non-viable myocardium in the same region has important implications in the understanding of myocardial thinning, resulting in a paradigm shift. Conventional understanding is that very thin myocardium (<5 mm) represents essentially transmural infarction and hence is unlikely to recover function following revascularization.[41] With DE-MRI, studies have shown that even thinned myocardium can recover function, sometimes dramatically, if it does not show late enhancement.[42]

The ability of DE-MRI to detect and characterize myocardial scar has been compared to SPECT and PET. Kuhl et al. compared DE-MRI with combined PET/SPECT in their assessment of reversible myocardial dysfunction in patients with chronic IHD.[43] Sensitivity and specificity for the prediction of functional recovery at follow-up was 97 and 68% for DE-MRI and 87 and 76% for PET/SPECT. The positive predictive value was identical for both techniques (73%). However, DE-MRI achieved a higher negative predictive value (93 vs 77%, respectively), indicating that it may be superior to PET/SPECT for the identification of segments unlikely to recover function after revascularization. Both methods had a similar yield in the prediction of global functional improvement. Wagner et al. studied patients with suspected or known CAD who underwent both DE-MRI and SPECT and the results were validated with an animal model.[44] For transmural infarcts, both studies had similar rate of detection. However, of the 181 segments that had subendocardial infarcts on CMR, 47% were missed by SPECT. On comparison with PET in patients with ischemic heart failure, Klein and their colleagues showed that DE-CMR was superior for detection of subendocardial infarction.[45] The results of these studies are not surprising, since CMR has a higher spatial resolution, as described above. Accordingly, CMR is the current gold standard for myocardial viability assessment.

Myocardial Function

Cine-CMR is a robust noninvasive technique for assessment of regional and global systolic function of both ventricles. The development of segmented k-space techniques allows for breath-held cine-MRI, making possible a rapid acquisition of the entire ventricles in short axis. Since ventricular volume estimations are made without any geometrical assumption, this method is particularly well suited for remodeled ventricles in patients with IHD. Regional function can be equally well studied by cine-MRI both qualitatively and quantitatively, as it represents the best technique in defining endo- and epicardial borders.[46] Further, myocardial tagging is a novel technique for assessing complex mechanism of myocardial contraction and to quantify myocardial strain. Recently, the application of myocardial tagging has been shown to improve the accuracy of dobutamine CMR in both the evaluation of viability and the detection of significant coronary stenosis.[47,48] Finally, MRI is also able to assess diastolic function with phase velocity mapping.

CMR has been shown to have better inter-study reproducibility compared with ECHO in normal subjects and patients.[49] For these reasons, CMR is considered the gold standard for assessment of ventricular function.

RECENT ADVANCES ON CT FOR ASSESSMENT OF CORONARY ARTERY STENOSIS

Over the last 5 years. there has been rapid advancement in CT technology, with increasing number of detectors and gantry rotation time. These have led to application of functional MDCT techniques for better evaluatoin of coronary artery disease. Two of these techniques are myocardial stress CT perfusion and CT-derived fractional flow reserve (CT-FFR). They are currently under research evaluation for guiding clinical management in appropriately selected patients with suspected ischemic heart disease. Briefly, CT perfusion is a myocardial perfusion imaging technique that measures the amount of iodine contrast present within the myocardium, allowing one to create an attenuation map of the left ventricle analogous to a single-photon emission CT (SPECT) perfusion map.[50] FFRCT, in contrast, is a computational fluid dynamics modeling technique that can be applied to a CT coronary angiography (CTCA) dataset for estimating lesion-specific functional information of a coronary stenosis without requiring any protocol modifications.[51] Both CT perfusion and FFRCT are complementary to CTCA and offer greater specificity and positive predictive value for detecting hemodynamically significant coronary artery disease (CAD) compared with anatomic imaging alone. The two strategies are particularly valuable in guiding clinical management for patients with moderate stenosis (50–70%) detected on CTCA and in special circumstances when the accuracy of CTCA is compromised, such as in patients with coronary stents and heavily calcified arteries. Data from the FAME (Fractional Flow Reserve Versus Angiography for Multivessel Evaluation)[52] and FAME 2 (Fractional Flow Reserve (FFR) Guided Percutaneous Coronary Intervention (PCI) Plus Optimal Medical Treatment (OMT) verses OMT)[53] trials have demonstrated that invasive fractional flow reserve ischemic-guided revascularization reduce major adverse cardiac events (MACE), whereas angiographic strategies alone are ineffective for guiding revascularization. Functional CT imaging in combination with CTCA offers an opportunity for comprehensive noninvasive evaluation of coronary anatomy and function within a single imaging session, leveraging both the strong negative predictive value of CTCA in low-to-intermediate-risk patients and the higher specificity and positive predictive value of CT perfusion and FFRCT in intermediate- to high-risk patients.

In appropriately selected patients, CT perfusion and FFRCT are ready for clinical use in light of their demonstrated added value across four key domains: (1) improvement in accuracy for hemodynamically significant CAD, (2) safety and improvement in patient outcomes, (3) reduction in healthcare costs, and (4) streamlined diagnostic workflow.

FUTURE DIRECTIONS

Continuing technical developments should increase the clinical value of cardiac MDCT and CMR still further. Novel CMR techniques combining high temporal and spatial resolution may make it possible to produce accurate coronary artery assessments. For imaging of atherosclerotic coronary plaques, dual-source MDCT or spectral CT technology may replace the current CT methods for plaque characterization that rely on Hounsfield units. CMR contrast agents are also being developed to identify vulnerable plaques, by targeting mediators of neovascularization or macrophages in inflamed plaques.[54,55]

Although MDCT has emerged as a reliable tool for coronary imaging, an abnormal scan does not necessarily predict ischemia. In fact, since MDCT and perfusion imaging provide different and complementary information, their sequential use or hybrid imaging may provide useful incremental information. Combining noninvasive imaging modalities for assessments of cardiac perfusion, coronary morphology and myocardial function (e.g. hybrid MDCT-CMR or hybrid PET-MDCT) will give new insights into the mechanisms of cardiovascular disease. In one study, hybrid PET/CT was evaluated in patients with suspected CAD, which yielded a sensitivity and specificity of 90 and 98%, respectively, for the detection of hemodynamically relevant coronary artery stenoses.[56] This approach promises to have a significant impact on clinical decision making.

Appropriateness Criteria for Use of Cardiac MDCT and CMR in the Investigation of IHD

According to the appropriateness criteria established by the American College of Cardiology,[57] the use of MDCT is considered appropriate (with a score between 7 and 9 on a scale of 1 to 9) for IHD in the following situations:

1. Detection of CAD in patient with chest pain with:
   - Intermediate pre-test probability of CAD
   - ECG uninterpretable or unable to exercise
2. Evaluation of suspected coronary anomalies
3. Evaluation of acute chest pain syndrome in patient with:
   - Intermediate pre-test probability of CAD
   - No ECG changes and serial enzyme negative
4. Detection of CAD in patients with chest pain syndrome with:
   - Uninterpretable or equivocal stress test (Exercise, perfusion or stress ECHO)

CMR is considered appropriate in the following conditions involving CAD patients:

1. DSMR and perfusion CMR for both the detection of CAD in symptomatic patients with intermediate pre-test probability of CAD and either uninterpretable ECG or unable to exercise, and for the risk assessment in patients with stenosis of unclear significance on coronary angiography
2. Coronary MR angiography for the evaluation of suspected coronary anomalies
3. LV function assessment in patients following myocardial infarction or heart failure with poor ECHO windows or in patients with discordant information from prior tests
4. Evaluation of myocarditis or MI with normal coronary arteries
5. DE-MRI to evaluate myocardial necrosis, including no-reflow regions, in post-acute MI; to establish the likelihood of recovery of function with revacularization or medical therapy and to evaluate viability when SPECT or dobutamine stress ECHO has provided equivocal or indeterminate results.

CONCLUSION

Noninvasive cardiac imaging is now central to the diagnosis and management of patients with known or suspected IHD. However, neither MDCT or CMR will ever replace any of the existing modalities. ECHO can be performed as a bedside examination, which is a considerable advantage for acutely ill patients. Cardiac catheterization offers the option of simultaneously performing coronary interventions. Among the newer modalities, the pretest likelihood of disease becomes the most important determinant of the initial test. If the likelihood is very low, no testing is needed. However, if the likelihood is low, recent data suggest that assessment of early atherosclerosis is likely to be the most useful and cost-effective test. In patients who have an intermediate likelihood of CAD, stress perfusion with nuclear imaging becomes highly valuable; however, MDCT may emerge as the initial test of choice. MPS would then be used if the MDCT is inconclusive or if there is a need to assess the functional significance of a stenosis defined by MDCT. MDCT however, is not yet widely available and is limited in patients with dense coronary calcification. In older patients with a high likelihood of CAD, MPS may be the initial test of choice, since a high proportion of these patients have too much coronary calcium to allow accurate assessment of the presence of coronary stenoses. PET/CT or SPECT/CT could emerge as important modalities combining the advantages of each modality. While CMR currently lags behind CTA for noninvasive coronary angiography, it has already emerged as a highly effective method for assessing ventricular function, myocardial mass, and myocardial viability, and there is increasing use of this approach for clinical rest and stress perfusion measurements.

REFERENCES

1. Ahmad N, Bhopal R. Is coronary heart disease rising in India? A systematic review based on ECG defined coronary heart disease. Heart. 2005;91:719-25.
2. Nesto RW, Kowalchuk GJ. The ischemic cascade: Temporal sequence of hemodynamic, electrocardiographic and symptomatic expressions of ischemia. Am J Cardiol. 1987;59:23C-30C.
3. Iskander S, Iskandrian AE. Risk assessment using single-photon emission computed tomographic technetium-99m sestamibi imaging. J Am Coll Cardiol. 1998;32:57.
4. Bonow RO. Identification of viable myocardium. Circulation. 1996;94:2674-80.
5. Smanio PE, Watson DD, Segalla DL, et al. Value of gating of technetium-99 m sestamibi single-photon emission computed tomographic imaging. J Am Coll Cardiol. 1997;30:1687-92.
6. Bax JJ, Van der Wall EE, De Roos A, et al. Clinical nuclear cardiology. In: Zaret BI, Beller GA (Eds). State-of-the-art and future directions. Philadelphia, Mosby; 2005. pp. 535-55.
7. Kaul S, Senior R, Dittrich H, et al. Detection of coronary artery disease with myocardial contrast echocardiography: Comparison with 99mTc-sestamibi single-photon emission computed tomography. Circulation.1997;96:785-92.
8. Matt D, Scheffel H, Leschka S, et al. Dual-source CT coronary angiography: Image quality, mean heart rate, and heart rate variability. AJR Am J Roentgenol. 2007;189(3):567-73.
9. Flohr TG, Schoepf UJ, Ohnesorge BM. Chasing the heart: New developments for cardiac CT. J Thorac Imaging. 2007;22(1):14-6.
10. Jakobs TF, Becker CR, Ohnesorge B, et al. Multislice helical CT of the heart with retrospective ECG gating: reduction of radiation exposure by ECG-controlled tube current modulation. Eur Radiol. 2002;12(5):1081-6.
11. Francone M, Di Castro E, Napoli A, et al. Dose reduction and image quality assessment in 64-detector row computed tomography of the coronary arteries using an automatic exposure control system. J Comput Assist Tomogr. 2008; 32(5):668-78.
12. Husmann L, Valenta I, Gaemperli O, et al. Feasibility of low-dose coronary CT angiography: first experience with prospective ECG-gating. Eur Heart J. 2008;29(2):191-7.
13. Husmann L, Valenta I, Kaufmann PA. Coronary angiography with low-dose computed tomography at 1.4 mSv Herz. 2008;33(1):75.
14. Kido T, Kurata A, Higashino H, et al. Cardiac imaging using 256-detector row four-dimensional CT: preliminary clinical report. Radiat Med. 2007;25(25):38-44.
15. Leber AW, Johnson T, Becker A, et al. Diagnostic accuracy of dual-source multislice CT-coronary angiography in patients with an intermediate pretest likelihood for coronary artery disease. Eur Heart J. 2007;28:2354-60.
16. Nikolaou K, Knez A, Rist C, et al. Accuracy of 64-MDCT in the diagnosis of ischemic heart disease. Am J Roentgenol. 2006;187:111-7.
17. Weustink AC, Meijboom WB, Mollet NR, et al. Reliable high-speed coronary computed tomography in symptomatic patients. J Am Coll Cardiol. 2007;50:786-94.
18. Schroeder S, Achenbach S, Bengel F, et al. Cardiac computed tomography: Indications, applications, limitations, and training requirements. Eur Heart J. 2008;29(4):531-56.
19. Pugliese F, Mollet NR, Runza G, et al. Diagnostic accuracy of non-invasive 64-slice CT coronary angiography in patients with stable angina pectoris. Eur Radiol. 2006;16(3):575-82.
20. Ohnesorge BM, Hofmann LK, Flohr TG, et al. CT for imaging coronary artery disease: Defining the paradigm for its application. Int J Cardiovasc Imaging. 2005;21(1):85-104.
21. Hoffmann U, Nagurney JT, Moselewski F, et al. Coronary multidetector computed tomography in the assessment of patients with acute chest pain. Circulation. 2006;114:2251-60.
22. Goldstein JA, Gallagher MJ, O'Neill WW, et al. A randomized controlled trial of multislice coronary computed tomography for evaluation of acute chest pain. J Am Coll Cardiol. 2007;49: 863-71.
23. Kim SY, Seo JB, Do KH, et al. Coronary artery anomalies: Classification and ECG-gated multidetector row CT findings with angiographic correlation. Radiographics. 2006;26:317-33.
24. Schmid M, Achenbach S, Ludwig J, et al. Visualization of coronary artery anomalies by contrast-enhanced multidetector row spiral computed tomography. Int J Cardiol. 2006;111:430-5.
25. Budoff MJ, Achenbach S, Blumenthal RS, et al. Assessment of coronary artery disease by cardiac computed tomography: A scientific statement from the American Heart Association Committee on Cardiovascular Imaging and Intervention, Council on Cardiovascular Radiology and Intervention, and Committee on Cardiac Imaging, Council on Clinical Cardiology. Circulation. 2006;114:1761-91.
26. Schmermund A, Erbel R. Unstable coronary plaque and its relation to coronary calcium. Circulation. 2001;104:1682-7.
27. Greenland P, Bonow RO, Brundage BH, et al. ACCF/AHA 2007 clinical expert consensus document on coronary artery calcium scoring by computed tomography in global cardiovascular risk assessment and in evaluation of patients with chest pain: A report of the American College of Cardiology Foundation Clinical Expert Consensus Task Force (ACCF/AHA Writing Committee to Update the 2000 Expert Consensus Document on Electron Beam Computed Tomography). Circulation. 2007;115:402-26.
28. De Backer G, Ambrosioni E, Borch-Johnsen K, et al. European guidelines on cardiovascular disease prevention in clinical practice. Third Joint Task Force of European and other Societies on Cardiovascular Disease Prevention in Clinical Practice (constituted by representatives of eight societies and by invited experts). Atherosclerosis. 2004;173:381-91.
29. Naghavi M, Falk E, Hecht HS, et al. From vulnerable plaque to vulnerable patient— part III: executive summary of the Screening for Heart Attack Prevention and Education (SHAPE) Task Force report. Am J Cardiol. 2006;98:2H-15H.
30. Leber AW, Becker A, Knez A, et al. Accuracy of 64-slice computed tomography to classify and quantify plaque volumes in the proximal coronary system: A comparative study using intravascular ultrasound. J Am Coll Cardiol. 2006;47:672-7.
31. Schoenhagen P, Tuzcu EM, Stillman AE, et al. Non-invasive assessment of plaque morphology and remodeling in mildly stenotic coronary segments: comparison of 16-slice computed tomography and intravascular ultrasound. Coron Artery Dis. 2003;14:459-62.

32. Moselewski F, Ropers D, Pohle K, et al. Comparison of measurement of cross-sectional coronary atherosclerotic plaque and vessel areas by 16-slice multidetector computed tomography versus intravascular ultrasound. Am J Cardiol. 2004;94:1294-7.
33. Motoyama S, Kondo T, Sarai M, et al. Multislice computed tomographic characteristics of coronary lesions in acute coronary syndromes. J Am Coll Cardiol. 2007;50:319-26.
34. Pundziute G, Schuijf JD, Jukema JW, et al. Prognostic value of multislice computed tomography coronary angiography in patients with known or suspected coronary artery disease. J Am Coll Cardiol. 2007;49:62-70.
35. Di Carli MF, Hachamovitch R. New technology for noninvasive evaluation of coronary artery disease. Circulation. 2007;115: 1464-80.
36. Nandalur KR, Dwamena BA, Choudhri AF, et al. Diagnostic performance of stress cardiac magnetic resonance imaging in the detection of coronary artery disease: a meta-analysis. J Am Coll Cardiol. 2007;50:1343-53.
37. Schwitter J, Wacker CM, van Rossum AC, et al. MR-IMPACT: comparison of perfusion-cardiac magnetic resonance with single-photon emission computed tomography for the detection of coronary artery disease in a multicentre, multivendor, randomized trial. Eur Heart J. 2008;29:480-9.
38. Ingkanisorn WP, Kwong RY, Bohme NS, et al. Prognosis of negative adenosine stress magnetic resonance in patients presenting to an emergency department with chest pain. J Am Coll Cardiol. 2006;47:1427-32.
39. Wu KC, Zerhouni EA, Judd RM, et al. Prognostic significance of microvascular obstruction by magnetic resonance imaging in patients with acute myocardial infarction. Circulation. 1998;97:765-72.
40. Kim RJ, Wu E, Rafael A, et al. The use of contrast-enhanced magnetic resonance imaging to identify reversible myocardial dysfunction. N Engl J Med. 2000;343:1445-53.
41. Cwajg JM, Cwajg E, Nagueh SF, et al. End-diastolic wall thickness as a predictor of recovery of function in myocardial hibernation: Relation to rest-redistribution T1-201 tomography and dobutamine stress echocardiography. J Am Coll Cardiol. 2000;35:1152-61.
42. John AS, Dreyfus GD, Pennell DJ. Images in cardiovascular medicine. Reversible wall thinning in hibernation predicted by cardiovascular magnetic resonance. Circulation. 2005;111:e24-e25.
43. Kühl HP, Lipke CS, Krombach GA, et al. Assessment of reversible myocardial dysfunction in chronic ischaemic heart disease: comparison of contrast-enhanced cardiovascular magnetic resonance and a combined positron emission tomography-single photon emission computed tomography imaging protocol. Eur Heart J. 2006;27(7):846-53.
44. Wagner A, Mahrholdt H, A Holly TA, et al. Contrast-enhanced MRI and routine single photon emission computed tomography (SPECT) perfusion imaging for detection of subendocardial myocardial infarcts: an imaging study. Lancet. 2003;361:374-9.
45. Klein C, Nekolla SG, Bengel FM, et al. Assessment of myocardial viability with contrast-enhanced magnetic resonance imaging: Comparison with positron emission tomography. Circulation. 2002;105:162-7.
46. Bellenger NG, Davies LC, Francio JM, et al. Reduction in sample size for studies of remodelling in heart failure by the use of cardiovascular magnetic resonance. J Cardiovasc Magn Reson. 2000;2:271-8.
47. Kramer CM, Malkowski MJ, Mankad S, et al. Magnetic resonance tagging and echocardiographic response to dobutamine and functional improvement after reperfused myocardial infarction. Am Heart J. 2002;143:1046-51.
48. Kuijpers D, Ho KY, van Dijkman PR, et al. Dobutamine cardiovascular magnetic resonance for the detection of myocardial ischemia with the use of myocardial tagging. Circulation. 2003;107: 1592-7.
49. Grothues F, Smith GC, Moon JCC, et al. Comparison of inter-study reproducibility of cardiovascular magnetic resonance with two-dimensional echocardiography in normal subjects and in-patients with heart failure or left ventricular hypertrophy. Am J Cardiol.2002;90:29-34.
50. Rochitte CE, George RT, Chen MY, et al. Computed tomography angiography and perfusion to assess coronary artery stenosis causing perfusion defects by single photon emission computed tomography: the CORE320 study. Eur Heart J. 2014;35: 1120-30.
51. Koo BK, Erglis A, Doh JH, et al. Diagnosis of ischemia-causing coronary stenoses by noninvasive fractional flow reserve computed from coronary computed tomographic angiograms. Results from the prospective multicenter DISCOVER FLOW (Diagnosis of Ischemia-Causing Stenoses Obtained Via Noninvasive Fractional Flow Reserve) study. J Am Coll Cardiol. 2011;58: 1989-97.
52. Tonino PA, De Bruyne B, Pijls NH, et al. Fractional flow reserve versus angiography for guiding percutaneous coronary intervention. N Engl J Med. 2009;360:213-24.
53. De Bruyne B, Fearon WF, Pijls NH, et al. Fractional flow reserve-guided PCI for stable coronary artery disease. N Engl J Med. 2014;371:1208-17.
54. Flohr TG, McCollough CH, Bruder H, et al. First performance evaluation of a dual-source CT (DSCT) system. Eur Radiol. 2006;16(2):256-68.
55. Johnson TR, Nikolaou K, Wintersperger BJ, et al. Dual-source CT cardiac imaging: Initial experience. Eur Radiol. 2006;16(7): 1409-15.
56. Namdar M, Hany TF, Koepfli P, et al. Integrated PET/CT for the assessment of coronary artery disease: a feasibility study. J Nucl Med. 2005;46:930-5.
57. Hendel RC, Patel MR, Kramer CM, et al. ACCF/ACR/SCCT/SCMR/ASNC/NASCI/SCAI/SIR 2006 appropriateness criteria for cardiac computed tomography and cardiac magnetic resonance imaging: a report of the American College of Cardiology Foundation Quality Strategic Directions Committee Appropriateness Criteria Working Group, American College of Radiology, Society of Cardiovascular Computed Tomography, Society for Cardiovascular Magnetic Resonance, American Society of Nuclear Cardiology, North American Society for Cardiac Imaging, Society for Cardiovascular Angiography and Interventions, and Society of Interventional Radiology. J Am Coll Cardiol. 2006;48(7):1475-97.

CHAPTER

145

Imaging in Cardiomyopathies

Priya Jagia, Gurpreet Singh Gulati, Sanjiv Sharma

INTRODUCTION

Cardiomyopathies (CMPs) comprise a spectrum of chronic progressive myocardial disorders which have distinct pattern of morphological, functional and electro- physiological changes. The expert consensus panel (2006) of the American Heart Association has proposed the following definition: "Cardiomyopathies are a heterogeneous group of diseases of the myocardium associated with mechanical and/or electrical dysfunction that usually (but not invariably) exhibit inappropriate ventricular hypertrophy or dilatation and are due to a variety of causes that frequently are genetic. Cardiomyopathies are either confined to the heart or are part of generalized systemic disorders, often leading to cardiovascular death or progressive heart failure-related disability".

CLASSIFICATION

Cardiomyopathies (CMPs) are broadly classified into: (1) Primary CMPs (genetic, nongenetic, acquired) comprise those few conditions that are either solely or predominantly confined to heart muscle. (2) Secondary CMPs are those group of conditions where the myocardial involvement occurs as part of a large number and heterogeneous variety of systemic disorders, usually affecting multiple organ systems.

This chapter will focus on those CMPs that can be diagnosed based upon the currently available imaging modalities. These include dilated, hypertrophic, restrictive, arrhythmogenic right ventricular and certain miscellaneous group of CMPs.

DIAGNOSTIC TECHNIQUES

It is important to detect exact cause of CMP as this determines the treatment and the patient survival. Echocardiography (ECHO) and radionuclide imaging alone cannot determine the exact etiology due to inadequate myocardial assessment (inferior spatial and contrast resolution and limited tissue characterization). Catheter angiography assesses only chamber lumen, with poor demonstration of myocardial changes. Also, significant overlap of features between CMPs frequently exists. Endomyocardial biopsy, though is the gold standard technique but has limitations in the form of sampling errors and poor sensitivity.

Cardiac multislice computed tomography (MSCT) can demonstrate ventricular function and some myocardial features. But **cardiac MR (CMR) is now considered the 'in vivo' gold standard imaging modality for the diagnosis and treatment monitoring of CMPs**. It provides high-resolution images of the heart in any desired plane without any radiation. Spin echo (SE) T1- and T2-weighted imaging allows for tissue characterization. Cine CMR helps assess cardiac morphology and function. Passage of gadolinium through the LV myocardium can be imaged during its first pass at rest and this provides important information about contrast kinetics of the myocardium. Delayed enhanced CMR (DE-CMR) helps to differentiate ischemic from nonischemic CMP. Late enhancement occurs in conditions where the extracellular volume is enlarged due to myocardial fibrosis, inflammation or edema. Delayed enhancement in non-ischemic myocardial disease does not correspond to any coronary artery territory and is often midwall rather than in subendocardial or transmural location.

All the various CMPs as described in this chapter are appropriate indications for performing a CMR examination, according to the recently published appropriateness criteria for CMR/cardiac CT.

DILATED CARDIOMYOPATHY

The anatomical abnormalities of dilated cardiomyopathy (DCM) include biatrial enlargement and increased size of the left (LV) and right (RV) ventricles **(Fig. 1)**. There may be pleural or pericardial effusion, SVC/IVC dilatation or ventricular thrombus. The functional abnormalities are in the form of segmental wall motion abnormalities or global dysfunction. Tagging sequences can help detect even subtle wall motion abnormalities mitral or tricuspid regurgitation, if present, can be well demonstrated on both ECG-gated CT and cine MR.

The pattern of enhancement in the myocardium can help differentiate LV dysfunction related to ischemia or nonischemic cardiomyopathy on CMR. Majority of DCM

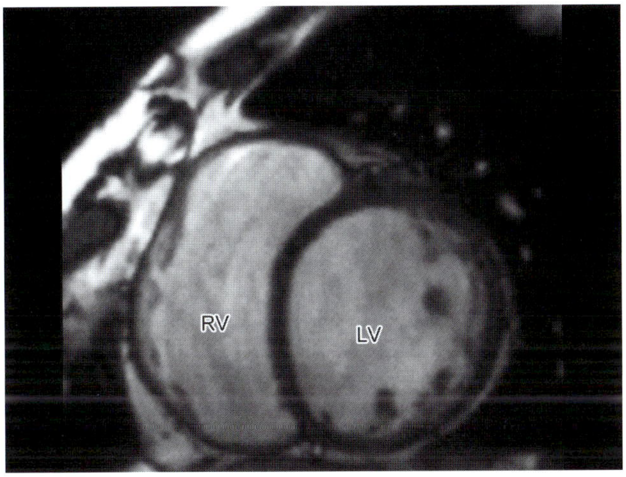

FIG. 1: Short axis image showing dilated right ventricle (RV) and left ventricle (LV) with thinned out walls in patient with dilated cardiomyopathy.

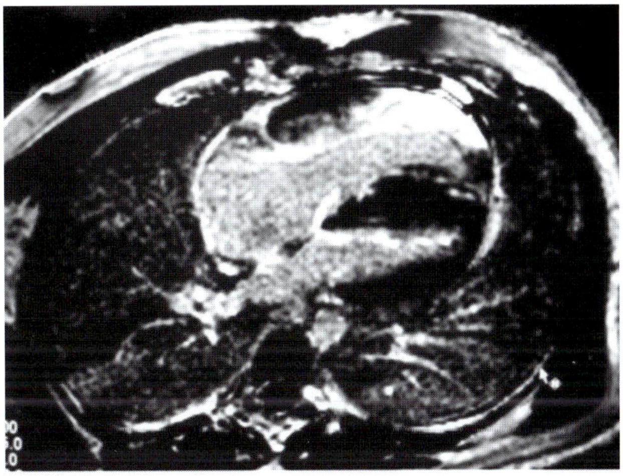

FIG. 2: Case of hypertrophic cardiomyopathy showing delayed dense enhancement in areas of hypertrophy in RV, interventricular septum and LV in this delayed enhanced four-chamber MR image.

patients do not show contrast uptake. But in some patients, the late enhancement is seen in midmyocardium in a noncoronary pattern, which is clearly distinguishable from coronary artery disease (CAD). CMR helps in quantifying the effects of therapy in these patients.

Hypertrophic Cardiomyopathy

Hypertrophic CMP is characterized by significant myocardial hypertrophy which may be symmetric or asymmetric, when it is regional in distribution.

Asymmetric hypertrophy at the LV apex may not be evaluated with echo. Cardiac CT and CMR define the site and extent of hypertrophy, especially at LV apex.

Cardiac function and flow dynamics of the outflow in cases of hypertrophic obstructive cardiomyopathy (HOCM), including systolic anterior motion of mitral valve, are well seen on cine-CMR and cardiac CT images. Precise planimetric measurements of the left ventricular outflow tract (LVOT) area during systole can also be determined on CMR. Myocardial tagging on CMR identifies regional myocardial strain and shear abnormalities. DE-CMR demonstrates a pattern of contrast uptake in the areas of hypertrophy **(Fig. 2)** or at the RV insertion points on the septum. Patients showing hyperenhancement are at increased risk of sudden cardiac death. Bello et al. showed that patients with late enhancement usually will not respond to heart failure drug therapy and will need an implantable defibrillator. The CMR can help monitor the functional and anatomical outcome of surgical and pharmacological septal ablation.

The CMR is useful to screen the relatives of probands also.

Restrictive Cardiomyopathy

The World Health Organization (WHO) defines restrictive cardiomyopathy (RCM) as a myocardial disease characterized by restrictive filling and reduced diastolic volume of either or both ventricles with normal or near-normal systolic function and wall thickness and it accounts for nearly 5% of all primary heart muscle disorders.

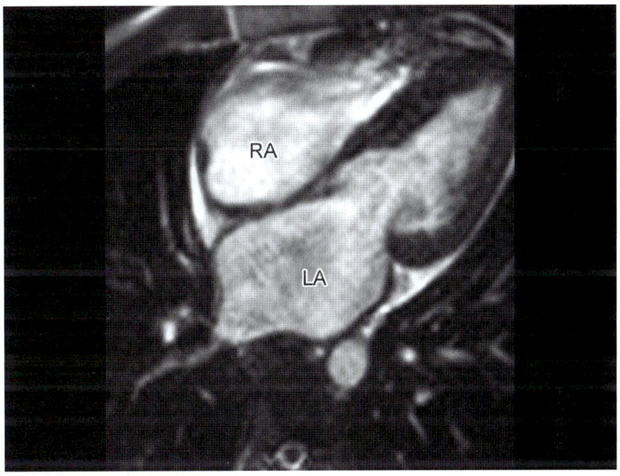

FIG. 3: Four-chamber spin-echo cardiac MRI showing typical biatrial enlargement with normal ventricular size in a patient with amyloidosis.

The RCM is identified on CT and MRI by normal LV size and normal or mildly impaired systolic function, abnormal severe diastolic ventricular function and biatrial enlargement **(Fig. 3)**. CMR can characterize tissue, identify anatomic alterations and can quantify myocardial mass, ventricular volumes and ejection fraction, thus making it a useful modality for investigating infiltrative or restrictive CMPs.

Common infiltrative disorders of the heart include amyloidosis, sarcoidosis, hemochromatosis (or siderotic CMP), and endomyocardial fibrosis. Rarer causes include storage disorders such as Anderson-Fabry disease and Gaucher's disease.

Amyloidosis

Cardiac amyloidosis is characterized by infiltration of interstitium with amyloid protein. Cardiac involvement is seen with most forms of amyloidosis, although it is most common and most often clinically significant with type AL amyloidosis (primary amyloidosis), often associated with multiple myeloma or other monoclonal gammopathies. It is the most common cause of RCM outside the tropics. In heart it leads to thickening of the left and right ventricular walls **(Fig. 4)**, sometimes associated with thickened atrial walls and the atrioventricular valves. On CT and CMR, the presence of these findings, in combination with pericardial and pleural effusions help to differentiate amyloidosis from hypertrophied myocardium. An increase in thickness of interatrial septum or posterior right atrial wall greater than 6 mm is quite specific for amyloid infiltration. There is a diffuse decrease in the myocardial signal intensity on both T1- and T2-weighted images. A ratio of myocardial to skeletal muscle signal intensity of < 1.0 at 20 ms TE is important feature of cardiac amyloidosis.

On DE-CMR, global contrast uptake **(Fig. 5)** is seen typically in the subendocardial location and does not match any specific coronary artery perfusion territory. Mahrholdt et al. reported that if more than 50% of LV myocardium nulls earlier than LV cavity and if this region is not in a coronary artery distribution territory, then the diagnosis of cardiac amyloidosis is highly likely. While performing the DE-CMR examination, the inversion time is shorter than normal and hence nulling occurs earlier. CMR can be used to follow-up the patients on drug therapy in amyloidosis.

Sarcoidosis

Heart is involved in about 25% of patients with sarcoidosis, but causes symptoms in only 5% of cases. An early diagnosis is important since early corticosteroid therapy can help prevent malignant arrhythmias, which can cause in sudden death. CMR is preferred since it shows characteristic abnormalities in cardiac sarcoidosis. In the acute phase, T2-weighted and early gadolinium enhanced images show focal areas of increased signal intensity. Confluent sarcoid granulomas show increased peripheral signal and low signal in the center on T2-weighted images **(Fig. 6)**. Focal myocardial thickening because of edema may be seen. Cine-CMR may show segmental wall motion abnormalities.

On DE-CMR, patchy or focal enhancement **(Fig. 7)** is seen which is often mid wall rather than subendocardial or transmural. The enhancement may be seen in the interventricular septum in basal region and sometimes in

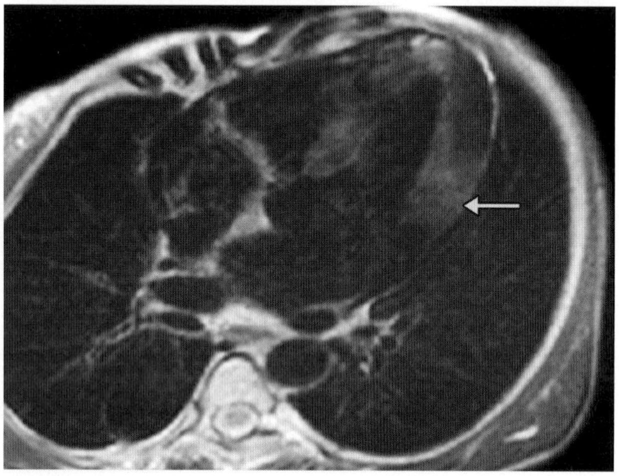

FIG. 4: Case of amyloidosis showing thickening of LV wall on T2W image.

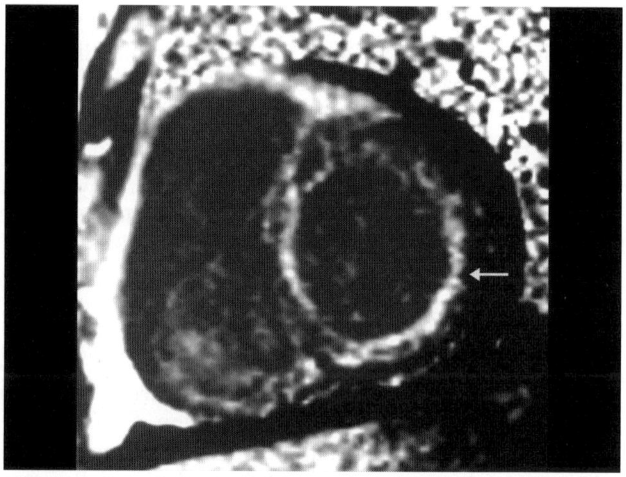

FIG. 5: Typical global subendocardial enhancement on DE-MRI image in short axis in amyloidosis.

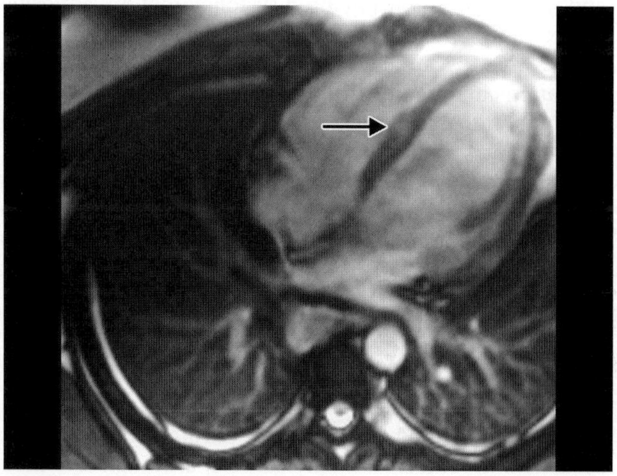

FIG. 6: T2W MR image showing a sarcoid granuloma in interventricular septum in four-chamber view.

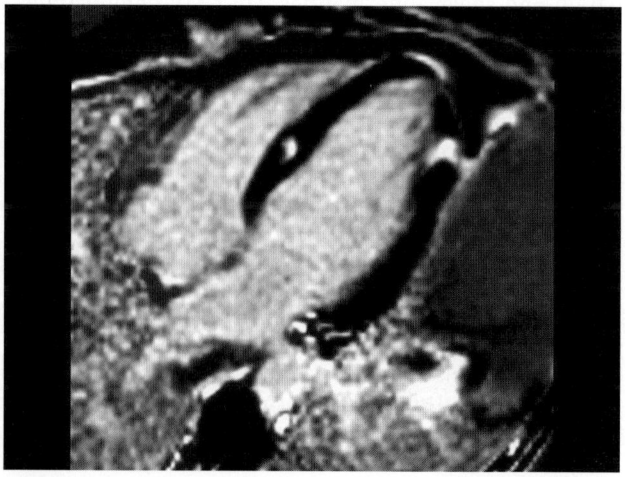

FIG. 7: Same case as in Figure 6—the granuloma shows enhancement on delayed contrast MRI.

the LV wall. Sometimes, papillary muscle and RV wall may be involved. In later stages, features of DCM are seen.

Follow-up CMR can be done to see absent gadolinium uptake. CMR may also show associated features like pericardial effusion, mediastinal adenopathy, etc.

Siderotic (or Iron Overload) Cardiomyopathy

This is seen in patients with hemochromatosis or in those with inherited severe anemias like thalassemia where multiple and regular blood transfusions are required. CMR offers a noninvasive method for detecting heart iron deposition which can cause heart failure and arrhythmias.

CMR reveals an extensive myocardial signal loss on T1- and T2-weighted images, a finding which is more prominent on the T2* images. Focal signal loss is seen in dysfunctional myocardium, associated with a dark liver, which is enough to confirm the diagnosis of systemic hemochromatosis.

Measurement of myocardial T2* on CMR has been found to correlate with LV dysfunction, and has been chemically validated through various studies. CMR has been used for evaluation of different chelation regimes in these patients.

Endomyocardial Fibrosis

Endomyocardial fibrosis (EMF) is characterized by extensive subendocardial fibrosis, apical thrombus formation and progressive diastolic dysfunction. This disease entity is a common cause of RCM in the tropics. It involves the RV more commonly than the LV. The etiology is unknown, though eosinophilia and immunopathological processes are thought to play a role in its pathogenesis.

The CMR findings in EMF include high signal intensity along the endocardium of the apex on T2-weighted sequences, an overlying nonenhancing thrombus, and a distinct high signal intensity plane separating the thrombus from the underlying myocardium on gradient echo cine sequences. Cine-CMR show mitral and tricuspid regurgitation and obliterated apices of the ventricles **(Fig. 8)**.

The DE-CMR shows subendocardial hyperenhancement of the apex, related to endocardial fibrosis **(Fig. 9)**.

Anderson-Fabry Disease

It is an X-linked disorder of lysosomal metabolism, with accumulation of glycosphingolipid in various tissues. In cardiac variant of anderson-fabry disease (AFD), myocardial hypertrophy is the main feature. This hypertrophy appears to be similar to that seen in HCM, but on DE-CMR helps it differentiate from hypertrophic cardiomyopathy (HCM) since the pattern of enhancement is different, with basal inferolateral wall being the commonest segment showing enhancement. Also unlike myocardial infarction, the subendocardium is commonly spared. Presence of myocardial scarring may imply that treatment with enzyme replacement therapy may be less effective at this stage, making a case for early initiation of this treatment before fibrosis has developed.

Tuberculosis

Myocardial tuberculosis is very rare, the reported autopsy incidence being 0.14–0.3%. Tuberculosis of the heart generally involves the pericardium and may result in constrictive pericarditis. Myocardial tuberculosis presenting as restrictive CMP is very unusual, with only 1 report till date. We have till now come across one case (not biopsy proven) of treated pulmonary tuberculosis presenting as restrictive CMP on ECHO. CMR showed diffuse myocardial thickening contiguous with the pericardial involvement and dilated atria. DE-CMR showed dense myocardial and pericardial enhancement.

Arrhythmogenic right ventricular dysplasia (ARVD): The ARVD has uncertain etiology and is marked by fibrosis and fatty replacement of the myocardium. It commonly involves the anterior wall of the right ventricle, in the so-called "triangle of dysplasia" (right ventricular subtricuspid area, the apex and the right ventricular infundibulum). It is more common in young males and has a familial occurrence. It leads to progressive right ventricular failure and dilatation, and is an important cause of sudden cardiac death due to ventricular arrhythmias. The diagnosis of ARVD is based on the presence of major and minor criteria encompassing genetic, electrocardiographic, pathophysiologic, and histopathologic

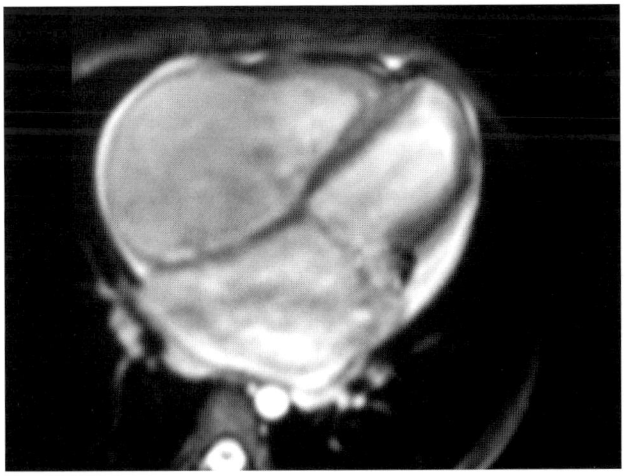

FIG. 8: Case of endomyocardial fibrosis showing obliteration of RV apex.

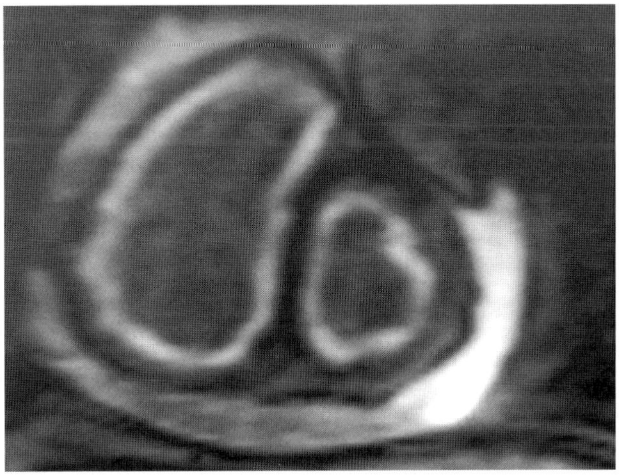

FIG. 9: Global subendocardial enhancement in this case of EMF suggesting gross fibrotic changes.

factors. To fulfill the appropriate criteria for ARVD, patients must have either two major criteria, one major and two minor criteria, or four minor criteria.

The traditional imaging modalities used to evaluate right ventricular abnormalities include conventional angiography, echocardiography and radionuclide angiography. However, all of them have low sensitivity and specificity for diagnosing ARVD, primarily because of their inability to accurately characterize structural and functional abnormalities of the right ventricle. Also, all these imaging modalities are limited by a lack of spatial resolution in diagnosing the typical fatty and fibrofatty changes of the right ventricular myocardium. Endomyocardial biopsy suffers from sampling errors, since involvement generally occurs in a segmental fashion and also because it most commonly involves the anterior right ventricular wall, whereas biopsy specimen is usually obtained from the septum.

Due to its high resolution, large field of view and ability to quantify RV abnormalities, CMR has emerged as the imaging modality of choice in investigating ARVD. T1-weighted spin-echo images show fatty infiltration as bright signal **(Figs. 10A and B)** with thinning of the RV wall and dysplastic trabecular structures. Cine CMR shows decreased global function, regional wall motion abnormalities or aneurysms. Delayed enhancement CMR may show hyperenhancement in regions of fibrofatty replacement and thus may be useful to guide endomyocardial biopsy.

The CMR can help measure intramyocardial fat and thus help monitor evolution of the disease. However, it should be remembered that significant fatty infiltration occurs in more than 50% of normal hearts in elderly people. Also in 15% of control subjects, some degree of intramyocardial fat is seen in anterior apex of right ventricle. So, focal wall motion abnormalities are considered to be a more reliable indicator of ARVD than presence of isolated intramyocardial fat.

Because first-degree relatives of individuals with ARVD have an increased chance of having the disease, with an increased risk of sudden death, CMR serves as an important tool for screening them for presence of preclinical disease.

Miscellaneous Myocardial Diseases

Left ventricular noncompaction: In this CMP, there is the persistence of deep intertrabecular recesses in communication with both the ventricular cavity and the coronary circulation. On imaging, the inner myocardial layer is spongy and less compacted compared to the outer compacted myocardium. Both CT and CMR image this differential compactness of the myocardium with superior spatial resolution, particularly in the ventricular apex where ECHO has inherent diagnostic limitations. The other common site of involvement is the lateral wall of the left ventricle. Lesser degrees of myocardial layering may also be seen in other CMPs. Peterson et al. reported that a noncompacted/compacted myocardium ratio of > 2.3 in diastole distinguished pathological noncompaction from other CMPs, with a specificity and negative predictive value of 99% each.

Takotsubo cardiomyopathy: The condition is likely thought to be due to stress related catecholamine upsurge causing cardiac dysfunction and is characterized by basal hypercontractile myocardium and a dyskinetic apex. Patients usually present with all clinical manifestations of an ST elevation myocardial infarction including chest pain, ECG changes and enzyme elevation. However, coronary angiography is normal. CMR is useful to show the reversible functional abnormalities as well as absence of any enhancement on DE-CMR, confirming noninfarcted myocardium.

Myocarditis: It is usually viral in origin and characterized by inflammation of the myocardium. Although spontaneous recovery is common, active myocarditis may occasionally lead to sudden death, and 5–10% of cases may progress to chronic dilated CMP.

Patchy involvement limits the use of myocardial biopsy for the diagnostic purposes. CT is not of much use in this entity. CMR may show focal areas of increased signal on T2-weighted images, representing active inflammation/edema. Both early and late gadolinium enhancement may be seen in areas of myocardial necrosis on histology. Cine CMR may show wall motion abnormalities. The late hyperenhancement is typically

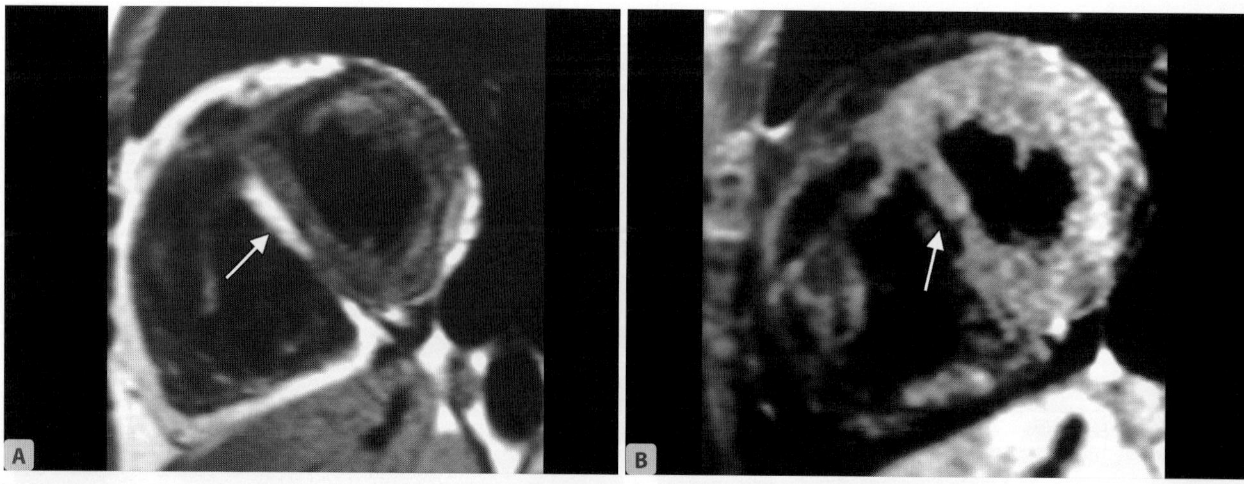

FIGS. 10A AND B: T1-weighted short axis image (A) showing bright signal along RV side in interventricular septum which nulls in fat-saturated images (B) confirming fatty infiltration.

subepicardial and has 'nonischemic' pattern of distribution. It is known to occur predominantly in lateral free wall.

CONCLUSION

Cardiomyopathies are a heterogeneous group of myocardial disorders associated with distinct anatomical, functional and electrophysiological alterations of the heart. Traditional imaging techniques are limited in their assessment of the myocardium. **Cardiac MR has emerged as the investigation of choice for imaging in CMPs** and is likely to be even better utilized once improved techniques for myocardial characterization and assessment of contrast kinetics evolve further.

BIBLIOGRAPHY

1. Anderson LJ, Holden S, Davis B, et al. Cardiovascular T2-star (T2*) magnetic resonance for the early diagnosis of myocardial iron overload. Eur Heart J. 2001;22:2171-99.
2. Aso H, Takeda K, Ito T, et al. Assessment of myocardial fibrosis in cardiomyopathic hamsters with gadolinium-DTPA enhanced magnetic resonance imaging. Invest Radiol. 1998;33:22-32.
3. Bali HK, Wahi S, Sharma BK, et al. Myocardial tuberculosis presenting as restrictive cardiomyopathy. Am Heart J. 1990;120:703-6.
4. Blake LM, Scheinman MM, Higgins CB. MR features of arrhythmogenic right ventricular dysplasia. Am J Roentgenol. 1994;162:809-12.
5. Bogaert J, Taylor AM, Van Kerkhove F, et al. Use of inversion recovery contrast-enhanced CMR for cardiac imaging: Spectrum of applications. Am J Roentgenol. 2004;182.609-15.
6. Dariusch H, Fleuchter S, Suselbeck T, et al. Delayed hyperenhancement in a case of Takotsubo cardiomyopathy. J Cardiovasc Magn Reson. 2005;7:845-7.
7. Eichstaedt H, Danne O, Langer M, et al. Regression of left ventricular hypertrophy under ramipril treatment investigated by nuclear magnetic resonance imaging. J Cardiovasc Pharmacol. 1989;13:75-80.
8. Fattori R, Rocchi G, Celletti F, et al. Contribution of magnetic resonance imaging in the differential diagnosis of cardiac amyloidosis and symmetric hypertrophic cardiomyopathy. Am Heart J. 1998;136:824-30.
9. Felker GM, Thompson RE, Hare JM, et al. Underlying causes and long-term survival in patients with initially unexplained cardiomyopathy. N Engl J Med. 2000;342:1077-84.
10. Friedrich MG, Strohm O, Schulz-Menger J, et al. Contrast enhanced, magnetic resonance imaging visualizes myocardial changes in the course of viral myocarditis. Circulation. 1998;97:1802-9.
11. Friedrich MG. Magnetic resonance imaging in cardiomyopathies. J Cardiovasc Magn Reson. 2000;2:67-82.
12. Gardin JM, Dabestani A, Glasgow GA, et al. Echocardiographic and Doppler β observations in obstructed and non-obstructed hypertrophic cardiomyopathy. Am J Cardiol. 1985;56:614-21.
13. Hendel RC, Kramer CM, Patel MR, et al. ACCF/ACR/ SCCT/SCMR/ ASNC/NASCI/SCAI/SIR appropriateness criteria for cardiac computed tomography and cardiac magnetic resonance imaging. J Am Coll Cardiol. 2006;48:1-23.
14. Kimura F, Sakai F, Sakomura Y, et al. Helical CT features of arrhythmogenic right ventricular cardiomyopathy. Radiographics. 2002;22:1111-24.
15. Kubo N, Morimoto S, Hiramitsu S, et al. Feasibility of diagnosing chronic myocarditis by endomyocardial biopsy. Heart Vessels. 1997;12:167-70.
16. Maceira AM, Joshi J, Prasad SK, et al. Cardiovascular magnetic resonance in cardiac amyloidosis. Circulation. 2005;111:186-93.
17. Mahrholdt H, Wagner A, Judd RM, et al. Delayed enhancement cardiovascular magnetic resonance assessment of nonischemic cardiomyopathies. Eur Heart J. 2005;26:1461-74.
18. Maron BJ, Towbin JA, Thiene G, et al. Contemporary definitions and classification of the cardiomyopathies: An American Heart Association Scientific Statement from the Council on Clinical Cardiology, Heart Failure and Transplantation Committee; Quality of Care and Outcomes Research and Functional Genomics and Translational Biology Interdisciplinary Working Groups; and Council on Epidemiology and Prevention. Circulation. 2006;113:1807-16.
19. McKenna WJ, Thiene G, Nava A, et al. Diagnosis of arrhythmogenic right ventricular dysplasia/cardiomyopathy. Task Force of the Working Group Myocardial and Pericardial Disease of the European Society of Cardiology and of the Scientific Council on Cardiomyopathies of the International Society and Federation of Cardiology. Br Heart J. 1994;71:215-8.
20. Ohneserge B, Flohr T, Becker C, et al. Cardiac imaging by means of ECG gated multisection spiral CT: Initial experience. Radiology. 2000;217:564-71.
21. Shimada T, Shimada K, Sakane T, et al. Diagnosis of cardiac sarcoidosis and evaluation of the effects of steroid therapy by gadolinium-DTPA-enhanced magnetic resonance imaging. Am J Med. 2001;110:520-7.
22. Varnava AM. Isolated left ventricular non-compaction: A distinct cardiomyopathy. Heart. 2001;86:599-600.
23. Vignaux O. Cardiac sarcoidosis: Spectrum of CMR features. Am J Roentgenol. 2005;184:249-54.
24. White RD, Obuchowski NA, Gunawardena S, et al. Left ventricular outflow tract obstruction in hypertrophic cardiomyopathy: Presurgical and postsurgical evaluation by computed tomography magnetic resonance imaging. Am J Card Imaging. 1996;10:1-13.

CHAPTER

146

Imaging Evaluation of Cardiac Masses

Gurpreet Singh Gulati, Priya Jagia, Sanjiv Sharma

INTRODUCTION

Cardiac masses comprise both the neoplastic and non-neoplastic lesions involving the heart. The latter group of lesions are more frequently encountered. Reaching an accurate diagnosis is important as management strategies vary depending upon the etiology. While non-neoplastic lesions usually respond well to conservative management, the neoplastic lesions often require surgical excision. Among the latter, defining the extra-cardiac extent of the lesion helps determine the treatment approach and prognosis. Additionally, it is necessary not to misinterpret normal cardiac structures and variants as cardiac masses.Hence, radiologists need to be familiar with the imaging appearances of various cardiac masses as well as normal structures and variants.

The advent and evolution of multidetector CT (MDCT) and MRI technology over the last 25 years has markedly improved our ability to evaluate and plan the optimal management of various pathological conditions of the heart. Prior to the availability of these modalities, the diagnosis of cardiac masses was difficult to make and often not possible antemortem. In this review, we discuss the clinical presentation, classification, modalities utilized for imaging along with the imaging features of various cardiac masses.

CLINICAL FEATURES

Cardiac masses are often detected incidentally on chest radiography or echocardiography (ECHO). Hence, a high degree of clinical suspicion is needed to make a reliable diagnosis. It should be noted, however, that symptoms related to cardiac masses are often non-specific and may not necessarily be cardiovascular in nature. At times, the presentation may even mimic a systemic illness. Often times, the symptoms are related to the anatomic location of the lesion rather than their histopathology. Therefore, a cardiac mass may be pathologically benign but may have a "malignant" clinical outcome. An example is a left atrial myxoma that may cause sudden cardiovascular collapse, if it obstructs the mitral valve, whereas an infiltrative malignant tumor may have a prolonged indolent course without producing any symptoms. Conduction disturbances (such as arrhythmia or heart block) and thromboembolic episodes may also be seen.

Imaging Techniques

An ideal imaging technique for cardiac masses should be able to provide holistic information regarding the nature, location, extent and hemodynamic abnormalities caused by the lesion. Importantly, it should be an accurate, operator-independent, reproducible, repeatable and a multi-planar technique with near isotropic resolution.

There is currently no single modality that possesses all the above characteristics. A multimodality approach is therefore, necessary in order to make an accurate and complete diagnosis.

Angiocardiography

Prior to the advent of non-invasive modalities, angiocardiography was the only modality available for detecting cardiac masses. Angiocardiography is however an indirect assessment based on the presence of a filling defect or a change in the luminal outline. It can often be misleading, and can easily miss small lesions and intramurally located masses. Further, it is invasive, and there is a real risk of embolization of dislodged tumor fragments during catheterization.

With the availability of non-invasive modalities that directly image the myocardium and can allow for tissue characterization, angiography is rarely indicated at present, and that too, in the following situations:

1. Suspicion of valvular or outflow tract obstruction by the mass, where catheterization may demonstrate a hemodynamically significant pressure gradient.
2. In vascular lesions, e.g. sinus of Valsalva (SOV) aneurysm or ventricular pseudoaneurysm.
3. Demonstration of coronary artery anatomy and tumor vascularity prior to surgery **(Fig. 1)**.
4. Performing endomyocardial biopsy for indeterminate lesions.

Both MRI and ECHO are capable of quantifying obstruction, MDCT can demonstrate coronary anatomy, while both MRI and MDCT can equally assess vascular

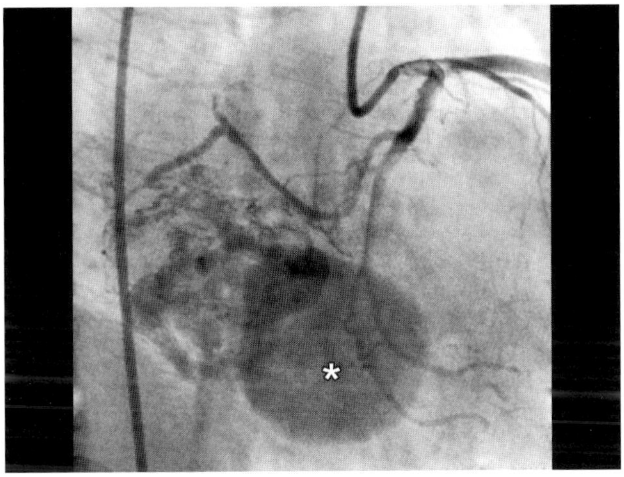

FIG. 1: Left coronary angiogram in a known case of right atrial myxoma. The atrial branches of the left circumflex artery are seen to supply a vascularized area within inter-atrial septum (representing the stalk) with an oval mobile mass (asterisk) that enhances immediately afterwards.

lesions. Therefore, angiography can easily be avoided for these indications.

Echocardiography

Transthoracic (TTE) is universally acknowledged as the screening modality of choice in patients with suspected cardiac masses. It is non-invasive, cheap, quick and widely available. It is capable of providing most of the required information regarding the lesion location, extent, mobility and hemodynamic consequences. It is especially useful for small, mobile lesions (e.g. valvular vegetation or tumor), since imaging is performed in real-time along multiple imaging planes. Image quality can also be substantially improved with use of tissue harmonic imaging. However, ECHO is operator-dependent, is suboptimal in patients with an inadequate acoustic window (obesity, emphysema or prior surgery), and may be limited in evaluation of lesions on right side of heart or those located away from chest wall. It is limited in assessing the extracardiac structures, which may be involved by intracardiac masses, or may themselves have a lesion that invades into the heart. Due to its limited ability for tissue characterization, ECHO is unreliable in suggesting the etiology, except in case of myxomas. Various authors have described an improved diagnostic yield of cardiac tumors with transesophageal echocardiography (TEE). This technique is superior to transthoracic echocardiography (TTE) for evaluation of small masses and lesions involving left atrium (LA), atrial appendage and inferior vena cava (IVC). TEE can detect the resolution or early recurrence of a tumor following medical or surgical therapy. However, this technique is invasive, complications may occur (related to the probe or drugs used) and some patients are not suited for the procedure (unstable angina, esophageal pathology or recent esophageal surgery).

Multidetector Computed Tomography

The development of multidetector computed tomography (MDCT) technology has dramatically improved the spatial and temporal resolution for cardiac imaging. Gating the cardiac images to the electrocardiogram (ECG) can be accomplished either by scanning or reconstructing raw data at the point of least cardiac motion. Due to its higher spatial resolution, MDCT is advantageous over MRI in that it generates three-dimensional images with nearly isotropic resolution. This allows for multiplanar reconstructions, which are useful for accurate demonstration of intra- and extra-cardiac masses, degree of myocardial or pericardial involvement, and associated lung abnormalities.[1,2] The volume rendered reconstructions provide a useful roadmap to the surgeon for tumor resection. Another distinct advantage of MDCT is its short image acquisition time. Current generation scanners also have large volume coverage with improved gantry rotation times, making these helpful in scanning unstable or pediatric patients. The latter often require deep sedation or even general anesthesia for doing MRI.

Compared to ECHO, MDCT has better soft tissue contrast and can definitively characterize fatty content and calcifications. While MDCT is as sensitive as MRI for detecting fatty content, it is superior to MRI for detecting calcification. The pattern of contrast enhancement on MDCT can also help to distinguish tumoral and non-tumoral masses to a certain extent. Overall however, MDCT is inferior to MRI for tissue characterization. A major advantage of MDCT over MRI and ECHO is its ability to assess coronary anatomy and rule out coronary artery disease, which make it a useful tool to evaluate older patients, who may require coronary artery bypass while undergoing surgical resection of cardiac tumors.

The major limitations to the routine use of MDCT include a relatively higher radiation dose, need for large volumes of intravenous contrast material and the high cost and limited availability of the technique. The former two limitations are however, being rapidly addressed by evolution in MDCT technology, leading to routine submillisevert scanning and low contrast requirements.

MRI

MRI has emerged as a useful tool for the detailed evaluation of cardiac masses, due to its ability to provide natural tissue contrast between flowing blood and surrounding structures, It is non-invasive, has a large field of view and allows for direct multiplanar imaging capability. It is better suited in suggesting the etiology, delineating the extent, relationship to adjacent structures, associated extracardiac lesions and presence of any hemodynamic effects. Tissue characterization ability is a distinct advantage of MRI over ECHO, allowing it to provide a tissue diagnosis in many cases. This is important since nearly half of all masses may be non-neoplastic and some of these may not even require surgical treatment. Also, many normal structures or variants that masquerade as mass lesions on ECHO can be resolved on MRI. MRI is particularly useful in detecting tumor recurrence, where ECHO may be of limited value due to a suboptimal acoustic window.

Compared to MDCT, MRI does not involve use of ionizing radiation or potentially nephrotoxic contrast (except for a small risk of causing nephrogenic systemic fibrosis with use of gadolinium in underlying severe renal insufficiency).

The major disadvantages of MRI include longer scanning period, susceptibility to motion artifacts, and requirement of a stable heart rate.

MR Imaging Sequences for Evaluation of Cardiac Masses

Conventional sequences may be limited in their diagnostic capability, due to presence of significant artifacts as a result of cardiac and respiratory motion, long examination times, and inadequate suppression of blood signal. Technical advances leading to newer imaging sequences have allowed for better spatial, contrast, and temporal resolution over the traditional imaging sequences. These have helped to enhance the capabilities of MRI in reliably diagnosing intracardiac masses.

Spin Echo (SE) Sequences

Compared to conventional SE imaging, segmented turbo (or fast) spin echo or single shot half-fourier spin echo (HASTE) sequences with double inversion recovery pulses lead to better suppression of blood signal, improving visualization of intracavitary masses.

Fat suppression techniques selectively saturate signal from fat and thus distinguish between high signal intensity (SI) lesions on the T1-weighted images (lipoma, exudative collection, thrombus).

Steady State Free Precession (SSFP) Sequences

Newer, faster, and short TE gradient echo sequences, with completely refocused gradients, (steady stage free precession or SSFP) provide excellent contrast-to-noise ratio. Due to their higher temporal resolution, mobile masses causing obstruction of a cardiac valve or the outflow tract of a ventricle, as well as the cardiac output and regurgitation volumes can be assessed using cine- SSFP MRI. The other advantages of SSFP techniques include better separation of myocardium from intracavitary blood, and reduction in examination time compared to SE acquisitions. The latter helps to optimize imaging in children and acute patients.

Contrast-enhanced Imaging

Myocardial perfusion and delayed enhanced imaging sequences are useful for evaluating the contrast enhancement characteristics of cardiac tumors.[3] Perfusion imaging can be useful to demonstrate increased tumor vascularity typical of malignant lesions such as angiosarcomas. Delayed enhanced imaging is useful to detect intramurally located lesions, distinguish tumors from thrombi, differentiate benign from malignant masses and identify areas of tissue necrosis. The usual dose of gadolinium used is 0.1 mmol per KBW.

Other Techniques

Myocardial tagging methods create a grid pattern on the myocardium and can thus help to differentiate contracting myocardial tissue from non-contractile tumor. This may help detect tumors of muscle consistency, such as rhabdomyomas. Phase-contrast imaging methods, being sensitive to slow flow, supplement SE techniques in distinguishing intra-cavitary mass lesions from a flow-related signal.

Classification (Table 1)

Cardiac tumors have a cumulative prevalence of 0.002–0.3% as determined in autopsy series.[4] Primary cardiac neoplasms include both benign and malignant histological types **(Table 1)**.[5] Importantly metastatic cardiac masses are nearly 20–40 times more prevalent than primary cardiac tumors. Secondary neoplasms can involve the heart by contiguous, hematogeneous, transvenous, or lymphatic spread. Non-tumorous masses include pathological conditions and various normal cardiac structures and variants that can present as a mass on imaging.

NEOPLASTIC LESIONS OF THE HEART

Primary

Benign Tumors

Myxoma: This is the most common benign tumor (50%) found in adults. These tumors usually present between the fourth and seventh decades of life. They arise from embryologic

TABLE 1: Classification of cardiac masses.

Tumors

- *Primary*:
  - *Benign*:
    - Myxoma
    - Lipoma
    - Papillary fibroelastoma
    - Fibroma
    - habdomyoma
    - Hemangioma
    - *Others*: Pheochromocytoma, lymphangioma, teratoma
  - *Malignant*:
    - Sarcoma
    - Lymphoma
    - Mesothelioma
  - *Secondary*:
    - Direct extension: Lung cancer, breast cancer, mediastinal lymphoma
    - Hematogenous: Malignant melanoma, lymphoma, leukemia
    - Transvenous: Renal and hepatic tumors
    - Lymph*atic:* Lymphoma, lung and breast carcinoma
  - Paracardiac and extracardiac tumors

Non-neoplastic lesions:

- Thrombus
- Sinus of valsalva aneurysm
- Atrial septal aneurysm
- Pericardial cyst
- *Infective*:
  - Valvular vegetation
  - Hydatid cyst
  - Tubercular

Normal structures and variants mimicking tumor

rests that get entrapped during the septation phase of cardiac embryogenesis. The classic triad of symptoms includes cardiac obstructive symptoms related to the obstruction of blood flow, embolic events, and constitutional symptoms such as fever, malaise and weight loss. Thromboembolic events occur in 35% of left-sided myxomas to the brain, kidney, spleen and extremities and 10% of right-sided myxomas to the lung. Friable and gelatinous myxomas are more likely to embolize than firm and fibrous lesions.[6] Pathologically, myxomas are gelatinous masses with calcification, necrosis and hemorrhage.

Approximately, 75% of myxomas are found in the LA, typically, in the interatrial septum in the region of the fossa ovalis; 20% of myxomas are located in the RA, and rare cases are found in the ventricles. Most lesions are sporadic. Carney's complex is an autosomal dominant disorder consisting of cardiac myxomas, hyperpigmented skin lesions and various extra-cardiac tumors.

The narrow stalk of myxomas may be difficult to appreciate on CT and MRI. The use of contrast-enhanced CT usually demonstrates the presence of a well-defined spherical or ovoid intracavitary mass, which typically has lobular contours and frequently calcified. Tumor attenuation is lower than that of the unopacified blood. The intravenous administration of contrast material helps better to define the lesion as a mass of low attenuation that is surrounded by enhancing intracardiac blood. Heterogeneity is a common feature of myxomas and is believed to reflect hemorrhage, necrosis, cyst formation, fibrosis or calcification.

Myxomas tend to show markedly increased signal intensity on the T2-weighted MR images. However, myxomas can show areas of decreased signal intensity due to presence of calcification or magnetic susceptibility artifacts caused by hemosiderin **(Fig. 2)**. Cine-MRI characteristically displays a mobile tumor which may prolapse through a cardiac valve. Contrast enhancement may be heterogeneous, and may be intense in highly vascular lesions.

Lipoma: They are the second most common benign cardiac tumors (10%), occur across a wide age range and are composed of mature adipose tissue.[7] Most lipomas are sporadic. Nearly 50% of lipomas arise subendocardially and the rest are epicardial or endomyocardial in location. The left ventricle (LV) and RA are the most frequently involved.

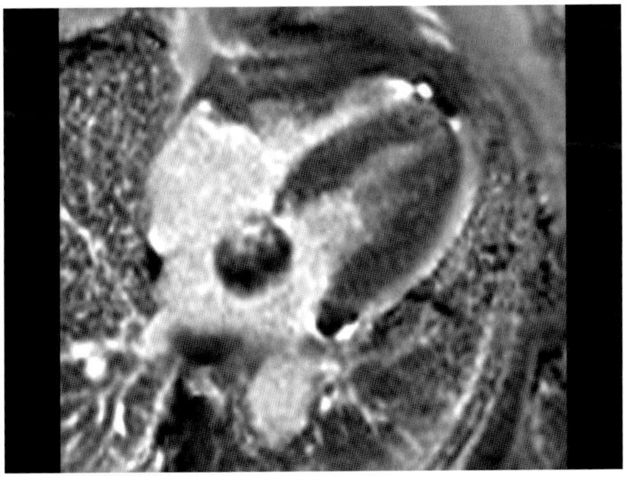

FIG. 2: late gadolinium enhancement MRI in 4-chamber view in a case of LA myxoma. The lesion is attached to the interatrial septum, and shows heterogeneous enhancement.

Both CT and MRI are highly specific and sensitive in the detection of lipomas. CT characteristically shows a homogeneous low density lesion of fatty attenuation. SE T1W MRI reveals a well circumscribed hyperintense lesion, whose SI is suppressed on fat-suppression technique. SI is slightly decreased on T2W images. As with soft-tissue lipomas, cardiac lipomas do not show enhancement with the administration of a contrast material.

Lipomatous hypertrophy of the interatrial septum (IAS), although not a true neoplasm, has been included in various reports of cardiac lipomas. This is defined as any fatty thickening of the IAS at the level of the fossa ovalis that exceed 2 cm in transverse dimension. It is seen in older, obese patients and is frequently associated with increased epicardial fat. It has a typical "dumb-bell" shape on imaging.

Papillary fibroelastoma: Papillary fibroelastomas are benign endocardial papillomas, composed of avascular fronds of connective tissue lined by endothelium. They comprise nearly 10% of all primary cardiac tumors. They usually affect the cardiac valves (more often the aortic and mitral valves) and account for approximately 75% of all cardiac valvular tumors.[8] Despite this predilection, these tumors are not known to cause valvular dysfunction. The tumor usually has a narrow stalk and is mobile.

Papillary fibroelastomas are usually not observed on CT or MR images as they are small (<1.5 cm in diameter) and are attached to the moving valves.[8] MR imaging typically demonstrates the presence of a mass on a valve leaflet or on the endocardial surface. These tumors can create turbulence in the blood flow, which might be demonstrated with the use of cine MR imaging.

Fibroma: Fibromas are neoplasms that mainly affect infants and children, being the second most common tumors found in this age group after rhabdomyomas. These occur with increased frequency in patients with Gorlin syndrome. Grossly, the lesions are solid tumors, composed of fibroblasts with intervening collagen tissue. They arise within the myocardium (most commonly in the LV) and can grow to a size that obliterates the cavity. Usually these tumors are large in size, but may be nodular and discrete or infiltrative. Due to the potential risk of sudden death due to arrhythmias, surgery is the preferred treatment even in asymptomatic cases.

The use of CT shows fibromas as homogeneous masses with soft-tissue attenuation, which may be either sharply marginated or infiltrative. Calcification is often observed.[9] On MRI, these tumors are normally homogeneously isointense to hypointense relative to the myocardium as seen on T1- and T2-weighted images due to a dense, fibrous nature. For the same reason, these tumors often show delayed enhancement on gadolinium-enhanced MRI **(Figs. 3A and B)**.[10]

Rhabdomyoma: Rhabdomyomas are the most common cardiac tumors in infancy and childhood. About 75% of neonatal primary tumors are rhabdomyomas. These tumors are often associated with tuberous sclerosis in up to 50% of cases.[11] Most patients are asymptomatic, and rhabdomyomas

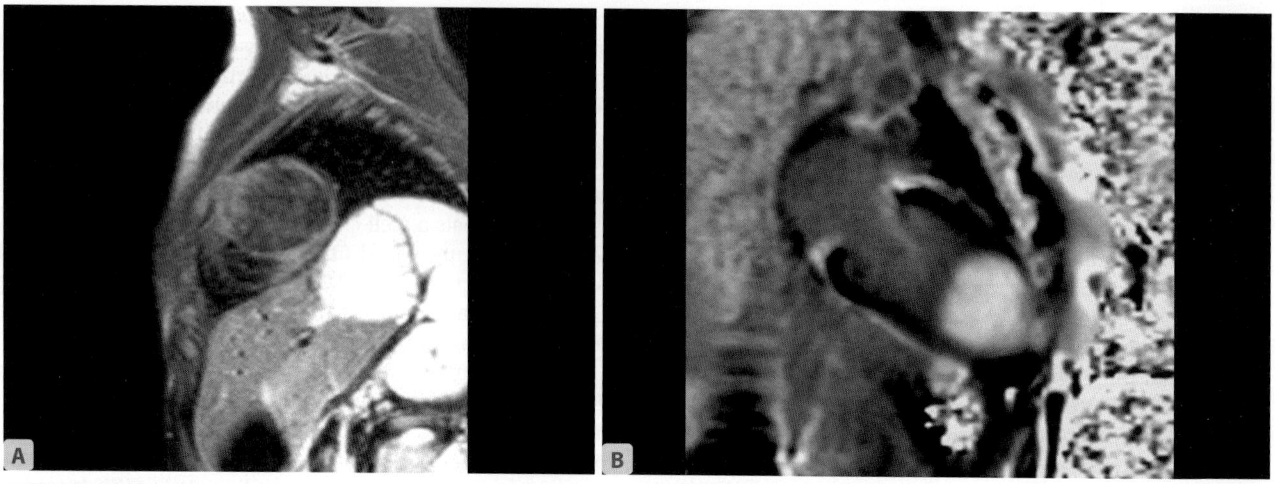

FIGS. 3A AND B: Short-axis SE T2W fat-suppressed (A) and VLA delayed enhanced (B) MRI in a case of LV fibroma. The lesion is hypo-intense to myocardium on T2W, and enhances homogeneously following contrast injection.

generally regress spontaneously. As such, these lesions are not considered as true neoplasms but as hamartomas.These tumors originate within the myocardium, typically in the ventricles, and multiple lesions may be present in up to 90% of cases.

Rhabdomyomas appear isointense to marginally hyperintense as compared with the myocardium as seen on T1-weighted images and hyperintense as seen on T2-weighted images. Contrast enhancement is similar to that of myocardium.

In a child, the presence of a solitary, calcified, ventricular mass favors a fibroma whereas multiple tumors located in both atria and ventricles with other features of tuberous sclerosis favor rhabdomyomas.

Hemangioma: These are tumors of vascular origin composed of either capillaries (capillary hemangiomas) or cavernous spaces (cavernous hemangiomas). They comprise 10% of primary benign tumors of the heart. The tumors can be solitary, either in LV or RV or the IVS, or multiple masses. They may be intramural or intracavitary in location with roughly an equal frequency.

Cardiac hemangiomas are heterogeneous as depicted on pre-contrast CT images and are intensely enhanced as seen on contrast-enhanced CT images. On MRI, due to the presence of slow flow, they have a heterogeneous intermediate- to-increased SI on T1W images and high SI on T2W images. Like CT, the tumors usually enhance well after gadolinium administration.[12]

Pheochromocytoma: Cardiac location is extremely rare, usually in the distribution of the cardiac paraganglia. Most often, they are seen in the LA, either the posterior wall or the roof. They may arise from the IAS or along coronary arteries, the latter making surgical excision exceedingly difficult.

The initial screening for extra-adrenal paragangliomas is usually with MIBG scanning. CT usually shows a circumscribed, heterogeneous, low attenuation mass that enhances strongly with contrast. On MRI, the tumor is iso- to hypo-intense on T1W images. Increased SI on T1W images may be due to hemorrhage. It is markedly hyperintense on T2W images. Intense enhancement is usually noted with gadolinium. Non-enhancing areas may represent necrosis within the lesion.

Lymphangioma: These are benign lymph containing neoplasms. Most lesions occur in children. They may be associated with other lymphovascular masses of the neck or the mediastinum. The most common location is in the pericardial spaces. These tumors may present with cardiac tamponade. CT features have not been described. MRI demonstrates an increased SI mass on T1W and T2W images.

Primary cardiac teratomas are other rare pericardial neoplasms seen in children.

Malignant Tumors

These comprise 25% of primary tumors of the heart. Secondary cardiac involvement by extra-cardiac malignancies is more common. Primary tumors are often asymptomatic till they become large. Even then, the symptoms can be non-specific. The lesions include sarcoma, lymphoma and mesothelioma.

Sarcoma

Angiosarcoma: The most common cardiac sarcomas are angiosarcomas that comprise 37% of all cases.[7] These lesions are malignant mesenchymal tumors that arise from endothelial cells lining the lymphatics or blood vessels. They usually present with right-sided heart failure or tamponade as the tumors tend to occur in the RA and involve the pericardium. Presentation is late, and there is often the presence of metastases at the time of diagnosis, particularly to the lung. These tumors have been reported to occur over a wide age range. They have a poor prognosis, with a mean survival of 6 months following presentation. Metastasis most frequently occurs to the lungs. There are two morphological subtypes of the tumor: A well-circumscribed intracavitary mass, or a diffusely infiltrative lesion of the myocardium.

CT often shows the presence of a low-attenuation mass in the right atrium, which might be irregular or nodular. There may pericardial effusion or thickening. Cardiac sarcomas may have heterogeneous signal intensity as seen on MR images, with areas of high signal intensity as seen on T2-weighted images representing the blood-filled spaces within the neoplasm. A papillary or "cauliflower" appearance can be observed as a specific MR feature of angiosarcoma, with a nodular area of high signal intensity interspersed within areas of intermediate signal intensity as seen on T1- and T2-weighted images. In cases with diffuse pericardial infiltration, some investigators have described linear enhancement along the vascular spaces as a "sunray" appearance.[13] Perfusion MRI shows early and increased contrast uptake within the tumor **(Figs. 4A and B)**. Delayed contrast enhancement is heterogeneous on both CT and MRI.

Hemangiopericytomas are rare cardiac sarcomas that are indistinguishable from angiosarcomas on imaging.

Other cardiac sarcomas: Although angiosarcomas are the most common cardiac sarcomas, all types of sarcomas, including undifferentiated sarcomas, malignant fibrous histiocytomas (MFHs), leiomyosarcomas, osteosarcomas, lymphosarcomas, myxosarcomas, neurogenic sarcomas, synovial sarcomas, neurofibrosarcomas, and Kaposi's sarcomas can affect the heart. Although most angiosarcomas occur in the RA, the other sarcomas affect the LA more frequently, which is an important differentiating feature.[7]

Malignant fibrous histiocytomas consist of primitive mesenchymal, fibroblastic, and histiocytic cells arranged in a storiform pattern.[14] The most common location of MFHs is the LA where the tumors are usually attached to the posterior wall.[14] Distinguishing MFHs from a benign cardiac tumor might be difficult on a clinical and imaging basis, but MFH is far more aggressive and has a greater propensity for recurrence and infiltration. MR imaging demonstrates the presence of MFH as a mass with a nonspecific signal intensity as seen on T1- and T2-weighted images. A MFH arises from the posterior wall of the LA and can extend into the pulmonary veins. This finding would not normally be expected with a myxoma.

Leiomyosarcomas are malignant tumors of smooth muscle origin. Primary cardiac involvement is extremely uncommon. Most lesions (75%) arise in the superior vena cava (SVC) or the IVC and extend to the heart. Intracardiac lesions usually arise in the LA and may invade the pericardium.

Myxosarcoma is a rare form of primary malignant tumors that is very difficult to differentiate from a myxoma. The ratio between the incidence of myxomas and myxosarcomas is approximately 100:0.8 and the prognoses of the two tumor types are very different.[15] Myxosarcomas have local recurrences, involving the pulmonary artery, pericardium or pleura and distant metastases, with the brain being the site most affected.[15]

Lymphoma: Primary cardiac lymphoma refers to the one involving only the heart or pericardium.[16] These tumors are extremely rare, with a reported incidence of 0.15 to 1%. Although cardiac spread of extracardiac non-Hodgkin's lymphoma is more common, there is a recent increase in the occurrence of the primary form due to its association with AIDS.

Pathologically, most primary tumors are diffuse large B-cell lymphomas. It most commonly arises in the RA but may involve any chamber. Sometimes, large pericardial effusion or thickening may be the only finding. Cardiac mass may be a polypoidal or an infiltrative intramural lesion. The latter may be diffuse form of infiltration of lymphoma cells in the myocardium, mimicking classic hypertrophic cardiomyopathy.

CT images show cardiac lymphomas as hypo- or iso-attenuated infiltrative soft tissue masses as compared with the myocardium, and the masses demonstrate heterogeneous enhancement after the administration of a contrast agent. On MRI, they usually appear as iso- to hypointense to cardiac muscle on both T1 and T2W images. They may be bright on T2W images. Contrast enhancement may be homogeneous, heterogeneous or minimal, with areas of low enhancement seen in the center of the lesion as compared with the periphery.

Pericardial mesothelioma: This most common primary pericardial neoplasm constitutes 15% of all malignant cardiac tumors. Unlike metastatic tumors to the pericardium, mesotheliomas are generally restricted to involvement of the pericardium without actually spreading to the cardiac chambers. There is no association with asbestos exposure.

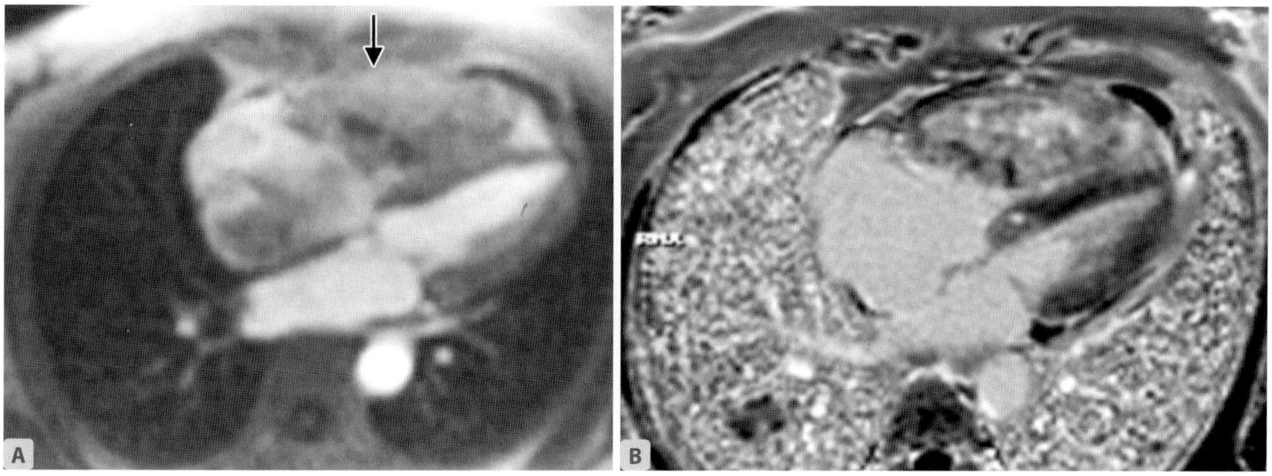

FIGS. 4A AND B: Rest-perfusion (A) and delayed enhanced (B) MRI in 4-chamber view, in a probable angiosarcoma of RV. There is early and increased contrast uptake in the lesion (arrow), that also shows heterogeneous enhancement on the delayed enhanced image.

Cross-sectional imaging helps to define the extent of the lesion and optimize the surgical approach. Contrast enhancement helps to differentiate the tumor from adjacent, normal myocardium. SI characteristics on MRI are nonspecific.

Secondary Neoplasms

Metastases to the heart are much more common than primary involvement, with an estimated ratio of 30:1.[17] In the presence of a malignant tumor, cardiac metastases are encountered in 11% of cases.[18] The tumors that most frequently metastasize to the heart are lung and breast cancers, melanomas and lymphomas.[18]

These lesions may involve the heart through direct extension or through hematogeneous, venous or lymphatic spread. Although imaging findings are not characteristic of any particular type of tumor, CT and particularly MRI is helpful in delineating the site and extent of cardiac and paracardiac involvement. The extent of involvement revealed by imaging may lead to a modification of the radiotherapy planning or the addition of chemotherapy.

The epicardium is the site most often affected by metastases.[17,18] Spread is mainly via a retrograde route through the mediastinal lymphatics, leading to implantation in the epicardial surface of the heart. Other tumors such as melanomas and sarcomas usually spread hematogeneously to the myocardium and epicardium through the coronary arteries, or less commonly, by the implantation of cancer cells through the vena cava.[18] Hematogeneous metastases in the heart and pericardium are normally accompanied by evidence of hematogeneous metastases in other organs. In particular, pulmonary metastases are usually present.[18]

Direct extension can occur with thymic, bronchial, breast and esophageal malignancies due to the proximity of the primary lesions to the heart. Invasion of the pericardium may be seen as interruption of the normal pericardial outline with nodular or diffuse pericardial thickening, hemorrhage, or effusion. Myocardial involvement is suspected when there is irregularity of the outline. Delayed enhanced MRI helps to demonstrate the extent of the cardiac invasion **(Figs. 5A and B)**. In addition, transvenous tumor spread relies on an extension of the tumor thrombus into the RA through the superior (lung cancers) or inferior vena cava (tumors from the kidney or liver) or an extension into the LA via the pulmonary veins. Both benign (uterine myoma, vessel wall leiomyoma) and malignant (hepatic, adrenal, renal and thyroid carcinoma) tumors can extend intracavally to the heart. This can cause caval or atrial occlusion. The tumor fragments may embolize distally with serious consequences. MRI is particularly suited to simultaneously demonstrate the primary site and its spread through the vena cava. This is helpful in planning the surgical treatment. Presence of intra-thrombus neovascularity on MRI may help to differentiate malignant from bland cavo-atrial thrombus.

Paracardiac and Extracardiac Tumors

These are mediastinal lesions that may extrinsically compress the cardiac structure or invade it. Anterior mediastinal masses include thymoma, thymolipoma, lymphoma, teratoma, terato-carcinoma and thyroid masses. Masses of neurogenic, airway (bronchogenic cyst or bronchial malignancy) or esophageal (carcinoma, duplication, leiomyoma) origin are the most common middle or posterior mediastinal lesions to about the heart. The direct orthogonal imaging capability of MRI makes it ideally suited to delineate the site of origin, extent and involvement of the heart by these tumors. CT and particularly MRI may localize the etiology by their ability to characterize tissue components. CT shows the presence of calcium and fat in germ cell tumors. On MRI, cystic lesions typically have a very high SI on the T2W images. High SI on T1W images may suggest high protein content, fat or hemorrhage within the lesion. Fat suppression techniques will distinguish fat, and GRE sequences will demonstrate hemosiderin deposits in chronic hemorrhage. Thymolipomas are anterior mediastinal lesions that usually conform to the shape of surrounding structures. CT and MRI

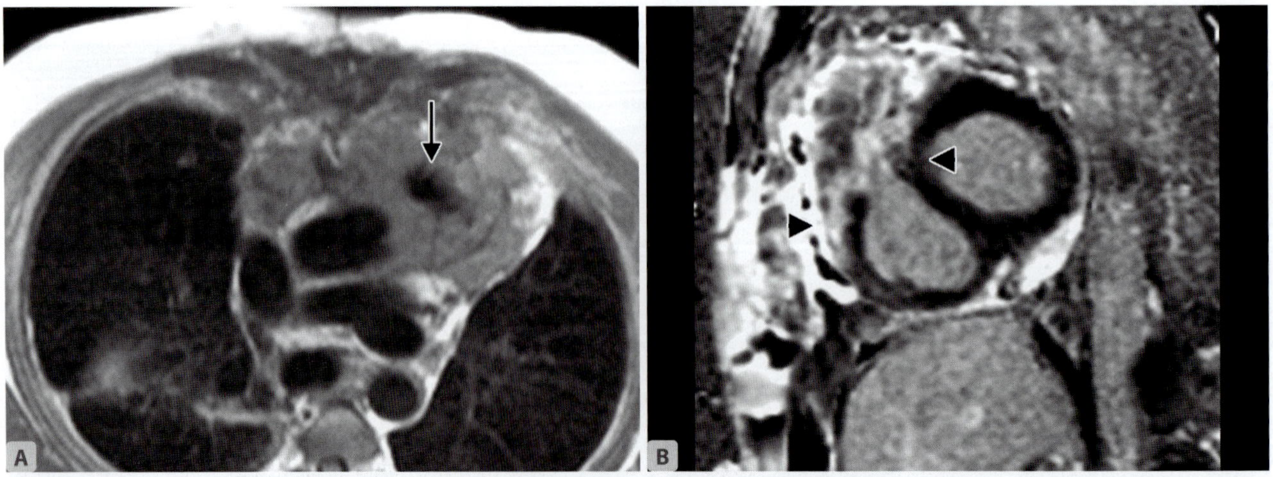

FIGS. 5A AND B: Axial SE T1W (A) and short-axis delayed enhanced (B) MRI images in a patient with anterior mediastinal tumor. The mass is seen to encase and infiltrate the right ventricular outflow tract (irregular outline, arrow)) and extends up to the ascending aorta. Delayed enhanced image shows the heterogeneous mass also involves the RV myocardium and the upper IVS (arrowheads).

characteristically display a mixture of fat and soft tissue within the lesion. Benign and invasive thymomas can, to some extent, be differentiated on MRI. The invasive thymomas tend to be more inhomogeneous, multinodular in appearance and less well-defined in outline.

NON-NEOPLASTIC LESIONS

Thrombus

Cardiac thrombi are more frequent than tumors and prompt recognition and appropriate treatment is important. Prior infarct (particularly in apical and interventricular septal location) and markedly depressed left ventricular systolic function predispose to thrombus formation in the left ventricular apical regions. These are most commonly and best diagnosed by transthoracic ECHO. Atrial fibrillation predisposes to thrombus formation in the LA appendage, whereas factors causing diastolic dysfunction (e.g. restrictive cardiomyopathy) or presence of mechanical valves, interatrial septal devices, and appendage occluder devices are other common factors leading to atrial thrombus formation that are best diagnosed by transesophageal ECHO. Thus presence of predisposing conditions along with a soft-tissue mass located in expected regions is the hallmark of echocardiographic diagnosis of intracardiac thrombi. Finding of a mass in the absence of predisposing conditions outlined above as well as of systemic hypercoagulable state make etiologic classification of a cardiac mass challenging by ECHO.

MRI, given its higher resolution, is able to better differentiate a cardiac mass based on its soft-tissue composition. Compared to ECHO, MRI has a higher sensitivity (90%) with a slightly higher specificity for detecting thrombus.[19,20] The signal intensity characteristics of a thrombus vary with MR imaging and are dependent on the age of the thrombus. An acute thrombus will appear bright as seen on both T1- and T2-weighted MR images, whereas a subacute thrombus will appear bright as seen on T1-weighted images with hypointense areas seen on T2-weighted images due to the paramagnetic effects of methemoglobin and shortening of the T2 relaxation times **(Figs. 6A and B)**. A chronic organized thrombus will exhibit hypointensity as seen on both T1- and T2- weighted images due to depleted water content.[20] Problems in differentiating thrombus and slowly flowing blood may frequently arise on SE MRI. GRE sequences are useful in this regard, since the thrombus always shows lower SI than blood. Also, on cine-GRE thrombus usually has a constant SI, whereas slowly moving blood continuously changes in SI. The other advantage of cine-GRE sequence is that it allows simultaneous assessment of the wall motion abnormalities. In cases where differentiation from tumor is difficult on MRI, imaging after administration of contrast with an inversion pulse to null normal myocardium may be useful (similar to the sequence for viability imaging, but imaging initiated at 3-5 minutes instead of waiting for at least 10 minutes). The thrombus should not show enhancement **(Figs. 6A and B)** whereas a tumor usually shows enhancement.[21] However, an organized thrombus may show some surface enhancement.

Aneurysm of Sinus of Valsalva

Sinus of valsalva (SOV) aneurysm is most commonly congenital in origin and caused by a deficiency of elastic tissue in the tunica media.[22] Rarely, it may be acquired secondary to aortic valve endocarditis or trauma. Most SOV aneurysms arise from the right and non-coronary sinuses. Unruptured SOV aneurysms are usually clinically silent and discovered serendipitously on ECHO as a vascular mass.[23,24] Rupture most often occurs into the RA or right ventricular outflow tract and may be a catastrophic event or present with rapid onset of heart failure caused by pronounced left to right shunting.

Although transesophageal ECHO is better for demonstration of site of communication of the aneurysm with a coronary sinus and its extension into a chamber wall (in case of unruptured aneurysms), it is an invasive technique and may be uncomfortable for the patient.

On CT, SOV aneurysm appears as a thin walled crescent shaped outpouching that is contiguous with the aortic root **(Figs. 7A and B)**. Occasionally, they are partially or

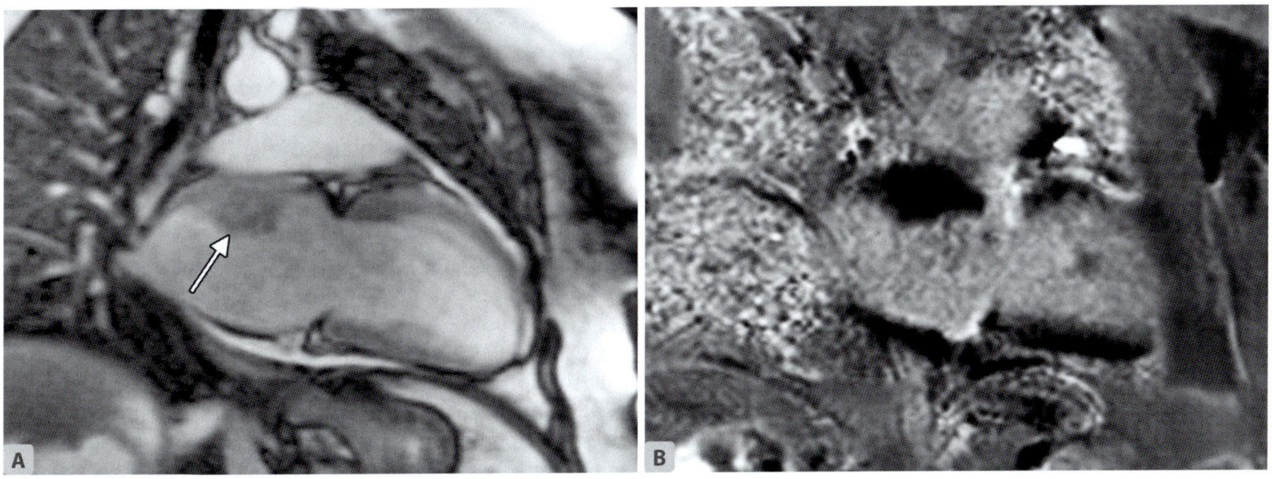

FIGS. 6A AND B: SSFP (A) and delayed enhanced (B) MRI in the vertical long-axis view, in a patient with mitral stenosis. There is a mural thrombus in the posterosuperior wall of the left atrium. The lesion does not enhance in the 10 minutes following contrast administration (B).

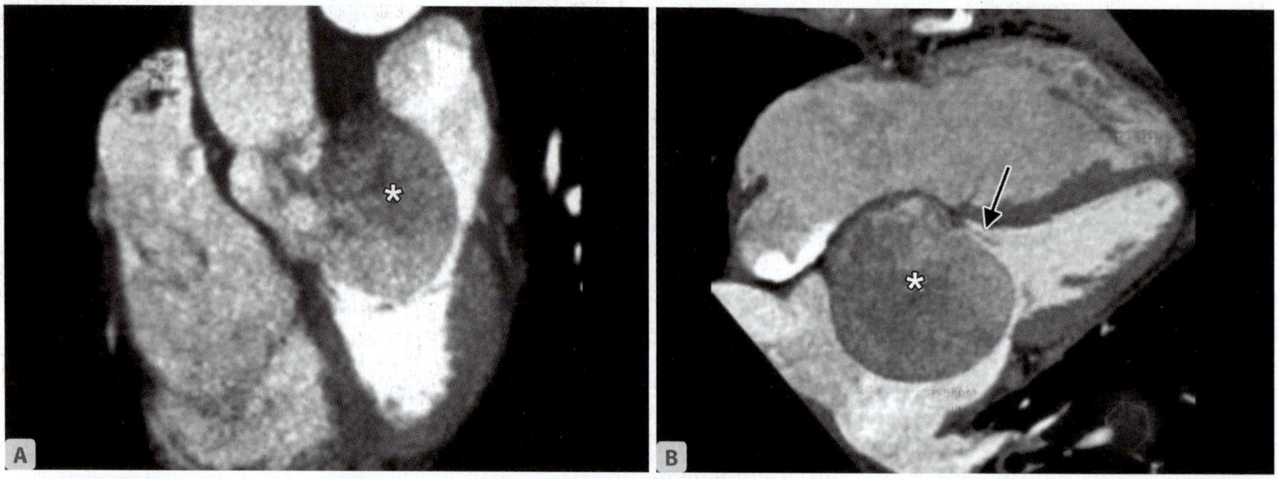

FIGS. 7A AND B: MDCT in a case of SOV aneurysm, sagittal (A) and 4-chamber (B) images. A round lesion (*) with heterogeneous enhancement in this early arterial phase (due to turbulent flow) arises from the aortic root and projects leftwards, posteriorly and inferiorly into LA. It also impinges on the mitral valve (arrow in Fig. B).

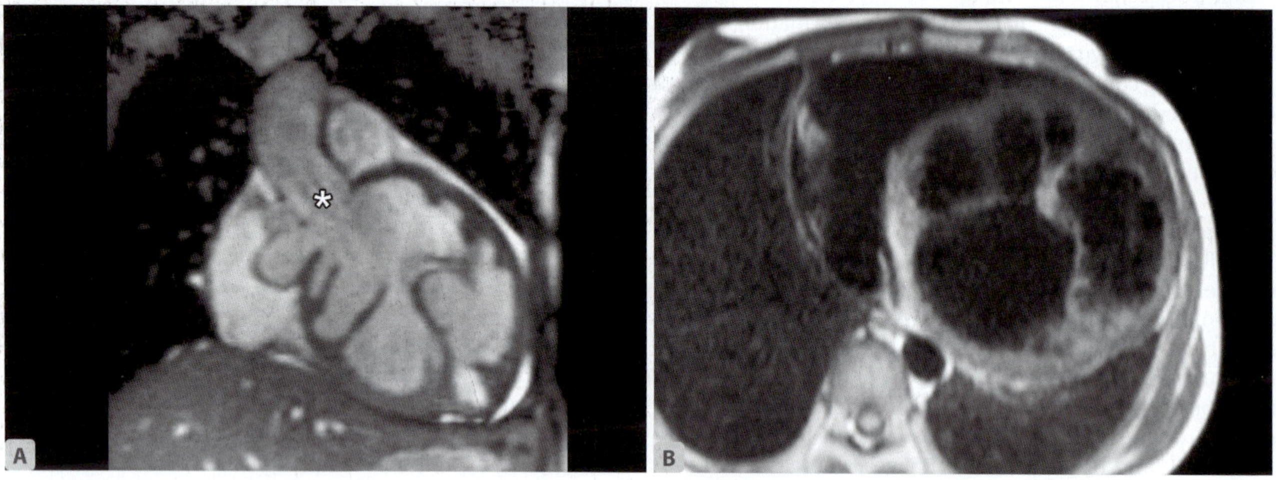

FIGS. 8A AND B: Coronal oblique SSFP (A) and axial SE T1W (B) MRI in a case of SOV aneurysm. The lesion arises from the aortic root (*), is multilobulated, and burrows into the interventricular septum. In (B), the lesion shows multiple large signal voids, consistent with its vascular nature.

completely thrombosed. MRI is very useful to confirm its vascular nature, by showing a signal void on SE sequences **(Figs. 8A and B)**. Both modalities are particularly useful for demonstrating extension into the adjacent cardiac chambers, valves and septum which can be difficult to fully evaluate with ECHO.

Atrial Septal Aneurysm

This is a localized protrusion of the primary component of the inter-atrial septum (IAS) through the fossa ovalis region, or a diffuse bulging of the entire septum into either of the atria. It may be associated with other congenital cardiac anomalies, or with acquired lesions that result in unequal pressures in the two atria. Due to thrombus formation in the concavity of the aneurysm, pulmonary or systemic embolic events may occur. Presence of an associated atrial septal defect may result in paradoxical embolism. Although, the diagnosis is usually made on ECHO, stagnant blood within aneurysm concavity may simulate a cystic tumor. Similar problems may result on SE MRI. Hence cine-SSFP MRI should be done and this shows blood flow within the aneurysm, as well as the mobility of the aneurysmal IAS.

Pleuropericardial Cyst

Though the most common pericardial mass lesion, these are very rare, the reported incidence being 1:100,000 of the general population. They are thought to be congenital in origin. The most common location is in the right cardiophrenic angle, although they may also be seen in left cardiophrenic angle and posterior mediastinum. Patients are usually asymptomatic, the lesion often being detected incidentally on imaging. Lesions are typically stable, and surgical excision is rarely required.

CT typically shows a well-marginated cyst of fluid attenuation **(Figs. 9A and B)**. There may or may not be a perceptible wall. MRI characteristically shows a well circumscribed, homogeneous paracardiac mass with iso- to hypointensity on T1W and hyperintensity on T2W images. Intracystic septae may be observed following paramagnetic contrast agent administration. The major role of MRI is

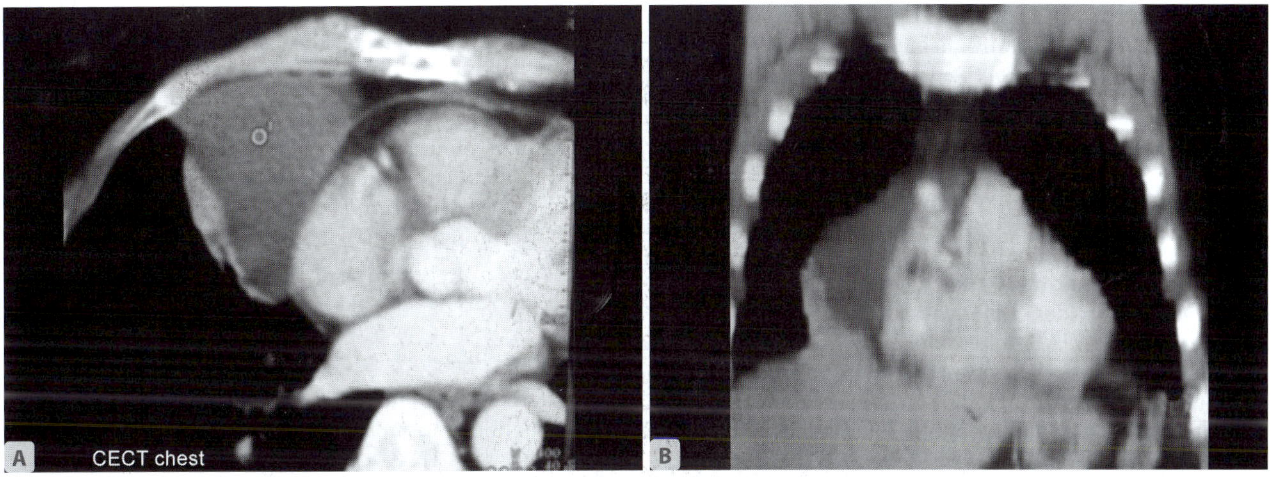

FIGS. 9A AND B: Axial (A) and coronal reformatted (B) contrast-enhanced CT images in pleuropericardial cyst. A well-marginated, fluid attenuation lesion with no rim enhancement is noted in its typical location (right cardiophrenic angle).

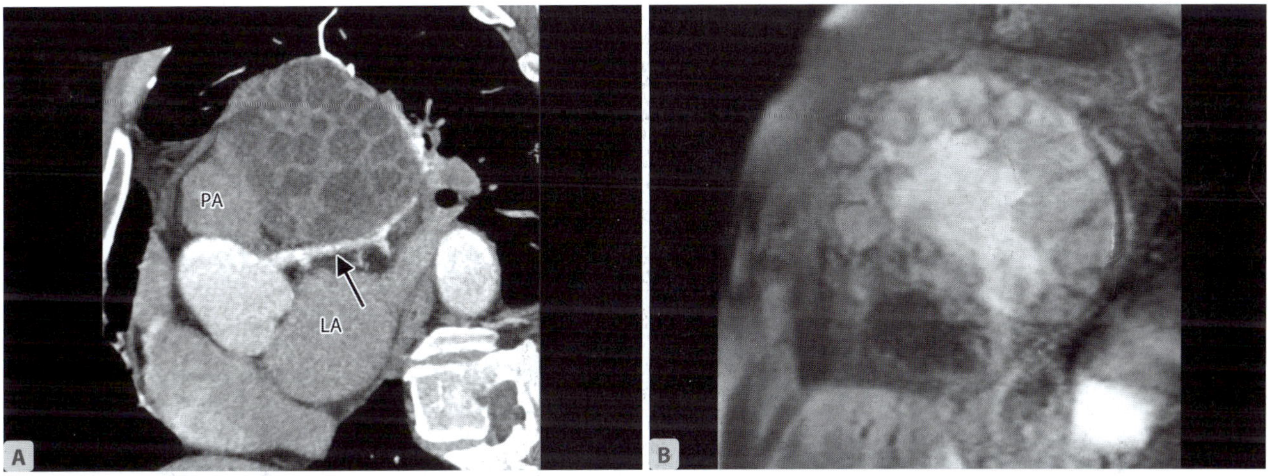

FIGS. 10A AND B: Short-axis MDCT (A) and short axis SE T2W (fat-suppressed) MRI (B) images in a patient with hydatid cyst. The lesion shows multiple daughter cysts and abuts the PA, LA and the left circumflex artery (arrow). In (B) the typical hypointense rim to the lesion is seen.

in differentiating pericardial cysts from other mediastinal masses and thus avoiding an inadvertent surgery.

Infective Lesions

Valvular Vegetation

Due to their inferior temporal resolution compared to ECHO, valvular vegetations are not visible on MDCT and MRI unless they are large. These modalities are mainly indicated for detection of extent of peri-valvular invasion, including abscess and/or fistula formation. Vegetations may be occasional findings when they appear as lesions intimately related to the valvular apparatus. Cine-SSFP MRI is useful to detect small lesions.

Hydatid Cyst

Cardiac hydatid cysts constitute 0.5–2% of all hydatid locations in the human body. The most common location is the LV (60%), followed by RV (10%), pericardium (7%), pulmonary artery (6%) and IVS (4%). Right sided lesions are seen to expand into the chamber cavity and subendocardially, while the left sided lesions more often grow subepicardially. The heart also can be secondarily affected by direct contact with hydatid cysts originating from the liver or the lung. These lesions are usually asymptomatic, and incidental detection is reported in 47% patients in one study. Symptomatic forms may compress the cardiac cavity or may rupture leading to anaphylaxis, tamponade or pericardial constriction.

Echocardiography, CT, and MRI can show the cystic nature of the mass and its relation to the cardiac chambers **(Figs. 10A and B)**. The cysts may be single or multiple, uniloculated or multiloculated, and thin or thick walled. More specific signs include calcification of the cyst wall, presence of daughter cysts and membrane detachment. CT best shows wall calcification. MRI depicts the exact anatomic location and nature of the internal and external structures and is the technique used for post-treatment follow-up. The appearance of a hydatid cyst on MRI is usually a characteristic oval lesion that is hypointense on T1-weighted images and hyperintense on T2-weighted images. MRI also demonstrates a thin low intensity peripheral rim on T2W images, reported to be a characteristic sign of a hydatid cyst **(Figs. 10A and B)**. This is thought to represent dense fibrous capsule from reactive host tissue.[24]

Tuberculoma

In tuberculosis, involvement of the heart apart from tuberculous pericarditis is extremely rare. The reported overall autopsy incidence of myocardial involvement ranges from 0.14 to 0.3%.[25,26] A tuberculoma, which is a mass like manifestation of the disease, is highly unusual and its description in the literature is confined to case reports.[26] The lesion most commonly involves the RA, close to SVC-RA junction or the RV. However, extensive infiltration of the myocardium, inseparable from pericardium and with the heart appearing literally "boxed in" has also been described. MRI usually demonstrates a homogeneous mass which is iso- to mildly hyperintense relative to the myocardium. The lesion is usually well defined with a sharp outline and without any flow voids. Delayed enhanced images may reveal homogeneous or heterogeneous enhancement. Lesions respond well to antitubercular therapy **(Figs. 11A and B)**.

VARIANT AND NORMAL ANATOMICAL STRUCTURES SIMULATING A CARDIAC MASS

Pericardium

The extension of the normal pericardial space into its various recesses and presence of small amounts of normally occurring pericardial fluid within them may lead to a false diagnosis of a pericardial or a vascular tumor. A typical example is a high extending superior pericardial recess that may simulate an enlarged lymph node, vascular tumor or an aortic dissection.

Left Atrium

The left atrial appendage is a tubular extension from the LA that is lined with thin, pectinate ridges, compared to the body of the LA that has a smooth endocardial outline. These ridges may be confused with thrombi. Also, other posterior mediastinal lesions such as cysts, esophageal tumors, and even a tortuous descending aorta may, at times, be misinterpreted as a LA mass. The multiplanar imaging capability of MDCT and MRI is useful in this regard to avoid a false-positive diagnosis.

Left Ventricle

False chordae and tendons are accessory structures that may appear as linear strands extending through the LV cavity, particularly on ECHO.

Right Atrium

The chiari network consists of fibrous strand-like structures arising from the region near the Eustachian valve and extending into the RA cavity. On MRI, these have a signal intensity (SI) similar to that of the mycocardium, and should not be misdiagnosed as a tumor or a thrombus. The crista terminalis is a prominent muscular ridge that runs along the posterior wall of the RA from the orifice of the SVC to that of the IVC. Embryologically, this represents the junction between the two parts of the RA that are derived from the sinus venosus and the embryologic atrium. It may present as a nodular mass on axial MDCT or MRI, but is resolved as a linear ridge on oblique coronal reconstructions.

Right Ventricle

The moderator band is a thin muscular band extending from the mid-portion of the IVS to the free wall of the RV across the cavity. It may enlarge and simulate a RV mass, particularly in patients with enlargement or hypertrophy. MDCT or

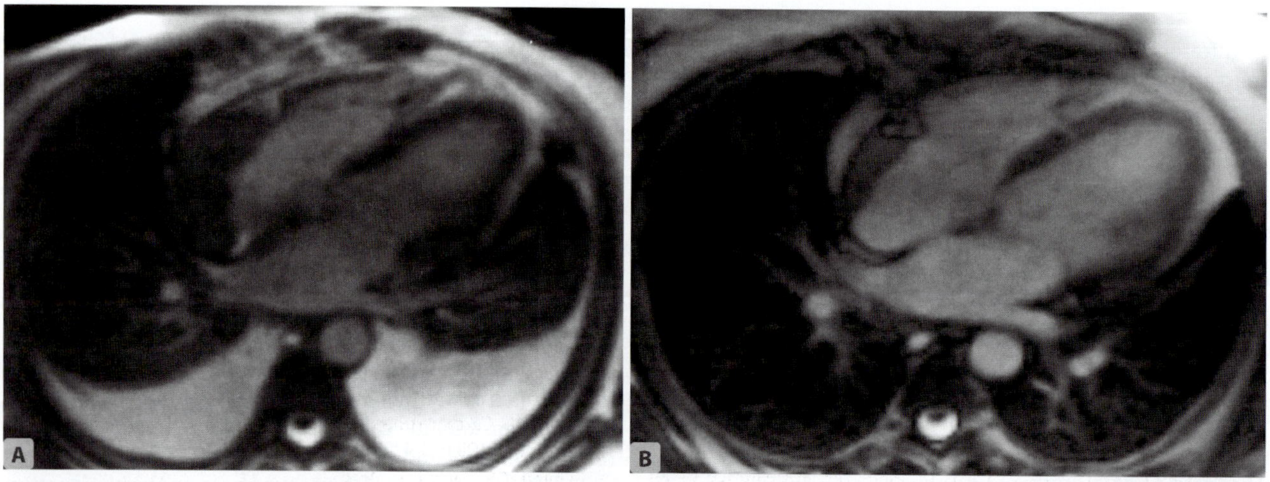

FIGS. 11A AND B: SSFP MRI in 4-chamber view in a case of RA tuberculoma, pre- (A) and 8 months post- (B) anti-tubercular therapy. There is a homogeneous, well-marginated right atrial mass that has significantly reduced in size following treatment. Pleural effusions have also disappeared.

MRI helps to delineate its points of attachment, with an attenuation/SI similar to that of the adjacent myocardium.

CONCLUSION

A high index of clinical suspicion supported by reliable non-invasive imaging is necessary to make a definite diagnosis of a cardiac mass lesion. It is imperative to differentiate between neoplastic, non-neoplastic and non-pathologic entities mimicking a mass, in order to avoid an inadvertent surgery. Although ECHO is universally accepted as the initial modality for evaluation of a suspected intracardiac mass, it has significant limitations. ECHO is the best modality, however, for valvular lesions.

MDCT is useful for vascular lesions, calcification and fat content, and for demonstration of coronary anatomy prior to surgery. It is also useful for staging malignant lesions. MDCT is distinctly superior to MRI in pediatric patients due to a significantly less scanning time. However, MDCT has significantly limited ability to characterize tissues compared to MRI.

Due to its superior contrast resolution and availability of multiple sequences (including perfusion and delayed enhancement), MRI is the ideal modality for complete evaluation of cardiac masses. It is capable of simultaneously assessing their nature, extent and hemodynamic consequences. MRI is particularly useful for differentiating thrombi from cardiac tumors. However, scanning time needs to be reduced by software modifications in order to improve image quality, obtain diagnostic images in small children and fast heart rates, and increase patient throughput. Adequate sedation remains a major requirement for a successful examination in a small child. This can be very difficult, at times. Despite these limitations, MRI is still the investigation of choice for providing a definitive diagnosis in a patient with a suspected cardiac mass. The higher signal-to-noise ratio of 3T MRI is expected to further improve the delineation of cardiac mass lesions with this modality.

REFERENCES

1. Kim EY, Choe YH, Sung K, et al. Multidetector CT and MR Imaging of Cardiac Tumors. Korean J Radiol. 2009;10(2):164-75.
2. Bogaert J. Cardiac masses. In: Bogaert J. Duerinckx AJ, Rademakers FE (Eds). Magnetic Resonance of the Heart and Great Vessels: Clinical applications. Chapter 10. Springer-Verlag, Berlin, Heidelberg, Germany. 2000:169-204.
3. Syed IS, Feng D, Harris SR, et al. MR imaging of cardiac masses. Magn Reson Imaging Clin N Am. 2008;16(2):137-64.
4. Sutsch G, Jenni R, von Segesser L, et al. Heart tumors: Incidence, distribution, diagnosis. Exemplified by 20,305 echocardiographies. Schweiz Med Wochenschr. 1991;121: 621-9.
5. McAllister Jr HA, Fenoglio Jr JJ. Tumors of the cardiovascular system. Atlas of tumor pathology, 2nd series. Fascicle 15 Washington DC, Armed Forces Institute of Pathology. 1978; 1-20:69-71.
6. Moriyama Y, Saigenji H, Shimokawa S, et al. The surgical treatment of 30 patients with cardiac myxomas: A comparison of clinical features according to morphological classification. Surg Today. 1994;24:596-8.
7. Burke A, Virmani R. Atlas of tumor pathology. Washington DC: Armed Forces Institute of Pathology. Tumors of the heart and great vessels. 1996;(3):79-90.
8. Edwards FH, Hale D, Cohen A, et al. Primary cardiac valve tumors. Ann Thorac Surg. 1991;52:1127-31.
9. Burke AP, Rosado-de-Christenson M, Templeton PA, et al. Cardiac fibroma: Clinicopathologic correlates and surgical treatment. J Thorac Cardiovasc Surg. 1994;108:862-70.
10. De Cobelli F, Esposito A, Mellone R, et al. Images in cardiovascular medicine. Late enhancement of a left ventricular cardiac fibroma assessed with gadolinium-enhanced cardiovascular magnetic resonance. Circulation. 2005;112:E242-3.
11. Webb DW, Thomas RD, Osborne JP. Cardiac rhabdomyomas and their association with tuberous sclerosis. Arch Dis Child. 1993;68:367-70.
12. Newell JD 2nd, Eckel C, Davis M, et al. MR appearance of an arteriovenous hemangioma of the interventricular septum. Cardiovasc Intervent Radiol. 1988;11:319-21.
13. Yahata S, Endo T, Honma H, et al. Sunray appearance on enhanced magnetic resonance image of cardiac angiosarcoma with pericardial obliteration. Am Heart J. 1994;127:468-71.
14. Okamoto K, Kato S, Katsuki S, et al. Malignant fibrous histiocytoma of the heart: Case report and review of 46 cases in the literature. Intern Med. 2001;40:1222-6.
15. Awamleh P, Alberca MT, Gamallo C, et al. Left atrium myxosarcoma: An exceptional cardiac malignant primary tumor. Clin Cardiol. 2007;30:306-8.
16. Cuotinsinger CR, Wilson J, Yoneda K. Primary cardiac lymphoma. Cancer. 1989;64:521-5.
17. Lam KY, Dickens P, Chan AC. Tumors of the heart. A 20 years' experience with a review of 12,485 consecutive autopsies. Arch Pathol Lab Med. 1993;117:1027-103.
18. Klatt EC, Heitz DR. Cardiac metastases. Cancer. 1990;65:1456-9.
19. Sechtem U, Theissen P, Heindel W, et al. Diagnosis of left ventricular thrombi by MRI and comparison with angio-cardiography, computed tomography and echocardiography. Am J Cardiol. 1989;64:1195-9.
20. Sparrow PJ, Kurian JB, Jones TR, et al. MR imaging of cardiac tumors. Radiographics. 2005;25:1255-76.
21. Mollet NR, Dymarkowski S, Volders W, et al. Visualization of ventricular thrombi with contrast-enhanced magnetic resonance imaging in patients with ischemic heart disease. Circulation. 2002;106:2873-6.
22. Sasson L, Katz MG, Ezri T, et al. Ruptured sinus of Valsalva aneurysm complicated by myocardial ischemia: Pathogenetic mechanisms. Cardiovasc Pathol. 2006;15:291-3.
23. Pepper C, Munsch C, Sivananthan M, et al. Unruptured aneurysm of the left sinus of Valsalva extending into the left ventricular outflow tract: presentation and imaging. Heart. 1998;80:190-3.
24. Dursun M, Terzibasioglu E, Yilmaz, R, et al. Cardiad hydatid disease: CT and MRI findings. AJR. 2008;190:226-32.
25. Rose AG. Cardiac tuberculosis: A study of 19 patients. Arch Pathol Lab Med. 1987;11:422-6.
26. Gulati GS, Singh S, Arepalli CD, et al. Superior vena caval obstruction after complete resolution of cardiac tuberculoma. Clin Rad. 2008;63:605-9.

CHAPTER

147

Imaging Diagnosis of Valvular Heart Disease

Priya Jagia, Sanjiv Sharma, Gurpreet Singh Gulati

INTRODUCTION

Valvular heart disease is one of the most common group of cardiac disorders, largely due to the high prevalence of rheumatic fever in India. This disease most commonly involves the mitral valve, followed by the aortic, tricuspid and pulmonary valves in this order. The resultant lesions can result in stenosis, incompetence or both in the involved valve.

The objectives of imaging in valvular disease irrespective of its etiology include:

- Diagnosis of the valvular disease: Qualitative as well as quantitative assessment of all valves,
- Assessment of the hemodynamic effects of valvular disease on the pulmonary vasculature and ventricular function,
- Detection of associated pulmonary pathologies as a complication or coincidental to heart disease, and
- Follow-up after treatment.

The recent advances in imaging techniques for non-invasive evaluation of the cardiac diseases have helped better delineate the anatomic location of the disease, and study the impact of the resultant structural abnormalities on the hemodynamic and functional consequences on the cardiovascular system. These have also gone a long way in an improved understanding of the natural history of the disease processes. Accurate diagnosis is now possible with nonmethods. Chest radiograph is useful in the initial evaluation of the patient. It provides valuable information about the cardiac size, pulmonary vasculature, arterial and venous hypertension, and the secondary changes in the lungs. Echocardiography is a useful screening technique that allows real-time evaluation of each cardiac chamber in multiple orthogonal planes. It is noninvasive, easily available, provides a direct visualization of cardiac valves and also helps evaluate the attendant functional disturbances on the cardiac chambers. The stenosis and regurgitation, as well as the resultant derangement of ventricular function, including the size of the chamber, wall thickness, size of valvular orifice, trans-stenotic pressure gradient or the regurgitant volume, can be reliably estimated by quantitative methods. The published reports suggest that the results compare favorably with the information obtained at cardiac catheterization and angiocardiography. Its major limitations include operator dependence and availability of a proper acoustic window. Now multislice computed tomography (MSCT) and cardiac magnetic resonance imaging (CMRI) are used in selected patients for optimal evaluation of the valvular heart disease and its hemodynamic consequences. Plain chest radiograph is useful in the initial evaluation of the patient. It helps aid the diagnosis and define the impact of the disease on the pulmonary vasculature. It is also useful in the assessment of the effect of treatment in a given patient. This technique is easily and widely available, and provides a reproducible and a permanent record of the patient. Therefore, it is widely used as the initial screening imaging technique in most patients. The chest radiographic abnormalities in various disease states are described here.

AORTIC VALVULAR DISEASE

The involvement of the aortic valve is characterized by LV hypertrophy in stenotic, and LV hypertrophy and dilatation in regurgitant lesions. The heart shows characteristic LV configuration in the form of rounding of cardiac apex, low apex and elongation of left border. Heart size is normal or minimally enlarged in stenotic lesions whereas it shows a moderate or severe enlargement in regurgitant lesions. Subtle cardiac enlargement in aortic stenosis is better detected on the lateral film and with volumetric measurements. Using the upper limit of normal (462 mL/m^2) for heart volume, LV enlargement confined to hypertrophy can only be detected with an accuracy of 79%. If one also takes into account other parameters of cardiac configuration, the false-negative rates are reduced to only 5%. The ascending aorta shows a typical post-stenotic dilatation in aortic stenosis (AS) whereas the dilatation is more diffuse and also involves the aortic knuckle in aortic regurgitation (AR). Aortic valve calcification is more frequently seen in AS with a bicuspid valve than in AS of rheumatic etiology. Calcification is best seen on fluoroscopy. The presence of calcification in the aortic valve is localized based on its characteristic location and movement. In presence of AR, the size of the heart roughly parallels the severity of regurgitation. Minimal LA enlargement and pulmonary venous hypertension (PVH) can be seen in aortic valve lesions. However, significant enlargement of LA indicates either an associated mitral valve involvement or left ventricular failure. A prominent LA appendage is virtually pathognomonic of rheumatic mitral valve disease. Frequently, AR and AS coexist **(Figs. 1 and 2)**.

MITRAL VALVULAR DISEASE

In mitral stenosis (MS), the heart size can be normal if assessed only by frontal projection. However, by volumetry, it is found to be enlarged in a majority of cases. Still a completely normal heart size can be seen in approximately 10% of the patients with critical MS **(Figs. 3 and 4)**. On the other hand, in mitral regurgitation (MR), the heart is generally enlarged with LV configuration and the size of the heart serves as a reliable indicator of the severity of MR. The radiographic picture can get modified in presence of TR **(Fig. 5)**, when there is a dominant enlargement of the right atrium with a less obvious PVH.

The hallmark of mitral valve disease is selective LA enlargement. Enlargement of the LA appendage (LAA) is pathognomonic of rheumatic etiology and can vary from a simple straightening of the left heart border to a large bulge in the typical site, immediately below the left main bronchus. Posteriorly, it can cause an indentation over the esophagus and may even deviate the middle descending aorta to the left (Bedford's sign). Rarely, LA or LAA may show calcification either in its wall or in the clot lining the wall. Valvular calcification, generally seen on fluoroscopy, strongly suggests a rheumatic etiology. In contrast, mitral annular calcification is often seen in age-related degenerative disease and in the postoperative patient after closed mitral valvotomy.

In MS, enlargement of LA may be mild or moderate but is rarely gross. In mitral regurgitation (MR), LA enlargement is usually gross or aneurysmal. In both MR as well as MS, the size of LA bears no correlation with the severity of the lesion as it is more dependent on the pliability of the atrial wall because of inflammation in rheumatic disease. The hemodynamic

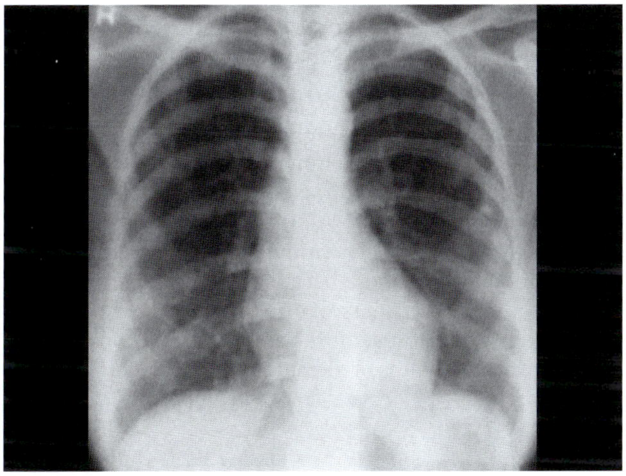

FIG. 1: Chest radiograph in a patient with valvular AS shows normal heart size, LV configuration, postdilatation of the ascending aorta and normal lung vasculature.

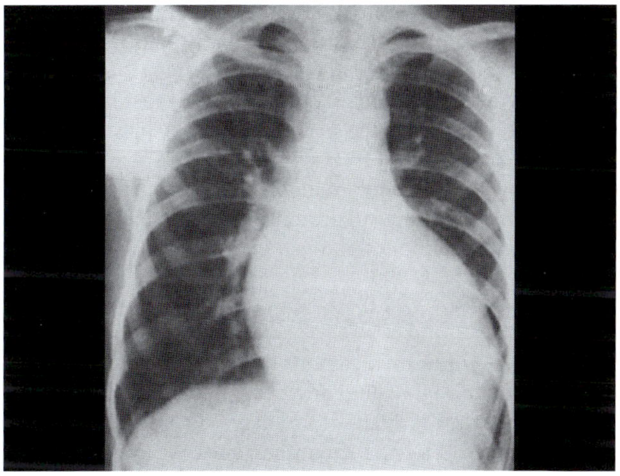

FIG. 2: Chest radiograph in a patient with AR shows a large heart, LV configuration, dilated aorta and mild PVH.

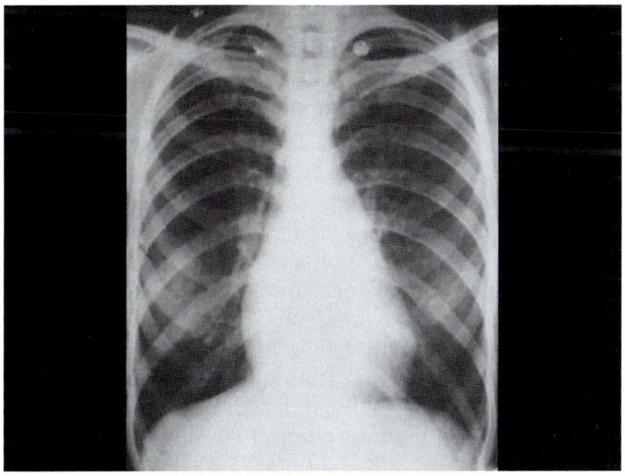

FIG. 3: Chest radiograph in a patient with MS shows normal heart size, LA enlargement and mild PVH.

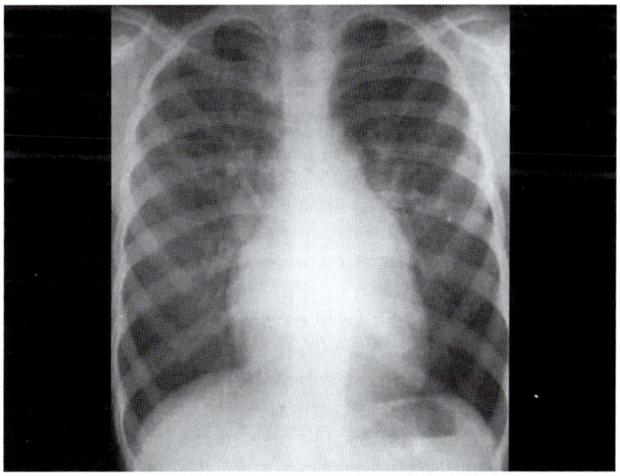

FIG. 4: Chest radiograph in a patient with MR shows a large heart, LV and LA enlargement, and mild PVH.

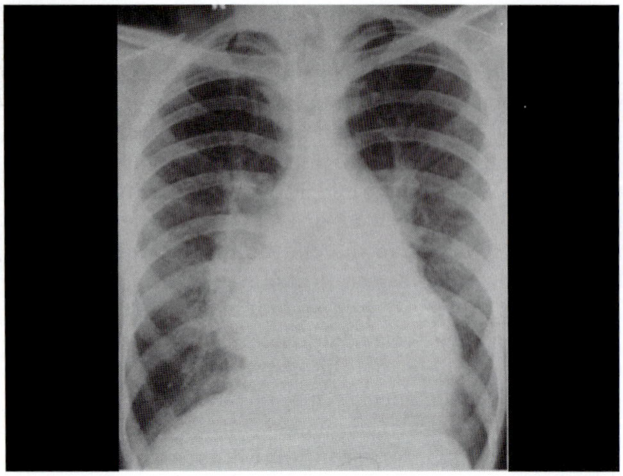

FIG. 5: Chest radiograph in a patient with MS and TR shows mild cardiomegaly, LA and RA enlargement and PVH.

changes in the pulmonary circulation are sensitive indicators of the severity of disease in MS. Frequently, the mitral valve has a combined lesion. In such situations, it is usually not possible to assess the severity of each lesion by chest radiography alone. However, a dominant MS can be suggested by small heart and LA relative to the severity of PVH. A large heart and LA with relatively mild PVH changes suggests a dominant MR. Similarly, a concomitant involvement of aortic valve and tricuspid valve can be suggested if there is prominence of ascending aorta or right atrium (RA) respectively.

TRICUSPID VALVULAR DISEASE

The most common involvement of tricuspid valve is in the form of a functional regurgitation secondary to RV dilatation caused by the underlying mitral valve disease. Rarely, it is directly involved by the rheumatic process and results in regurgitation or, less commonly, stenosis. The characteristic radiological feature is a large RA. This chamber is most difficult to assess by plain chest radiography, especially when the other chambers are also enlarged. The increase in the height of the RA relative to that of the vascular pedicle provides the most specific index of its enlargement.

HEMODYNAMIC EFFECTS ON PULMONARY VASCULATURE

Mitral valvular disease and, to a lesser extent, the aortic valvular disease is characterized by a rise in the LA pressure which in turn leads to a rise in pulmonary capillary wedge pressure (PCWP). Depending on the severity of PVH, a series of changes may be seen on the chest radiograph. These changes have been discussed earlier and have been shown to bear a rough correlation with the pressure values obtained at cardiac catheterization. Sustained PVH causes obstructive changes in the small pulmonary arteries leading to an increase in pulmonary vascular resistance. This can result in reactive or organic pulmonary arterial hypertension (PAH).

Thus, a chest radiograph, in addition to indicating specific hemodynamic disturbances, can also help in predicting the severity of valvular lesion like in MS where these changes roughly parallel the severity of the disease. The relative accuracy of different roentgen signs in predicting severe MS (area of 1.0 cm^2 or less) is as follows:

- Kerley B lines—96%.
- Combined venous and arterial abnormalities in the pulmonary vascular pattern—97%.
- LA enlargement producing >12 cm^2 posterior deviation of the esophagus—83%.
- Either 1 or 2 plus 3—100%.

Associated Pulmonary Pathologies

A plain chest radiograph is useful in assessing most abnormalities of the lungs in a patient with valvular heart disease. Various lung pathologies, if present, can simulate or aggravate the symptoms in these patients. These can be vital in deciding the management strategy. These include pulmonary tuberculosis, chronic airway obstructive disease, interstitial lung disease, and pneumonia among others. Rarely, a cardiac lesion itself causes a pulmonary complication like an enlarged LA causing lobar collapse, consolidation, bronchiectasis, or obstructive emphysema.

Effects of Treatment during Follow-up

It is necessary to monitor the effect of treatment on the cardiac and pulmonary changes. Since valvular heart diseases generally run a protracted course and most patients lead a near normal life after surgical or other intervention, their follow-up requires close monitoring. Echocardiogram is best suited for this purpose because it can precisely quantify the hemodynamic effects of the valvular lesions. Chest radiographs are also useful for a ready comparison of the heart size and the status of the pulmonary vasculature.

Heart Size

In regurgitant lesions of aortic and mitral valves, the heart size generally serves as a good indicator for the severity of the disease. Once the diagnosis has been established, the patient can be followed-up by monitoring the heart size. Similarly, a postoperative reduction in heart size serves as a good indicator of successful outcome.

Left Atrial Size

Reduction in the size of LA indicates a favorable outcome in cases of mitral valve replacement or balloon dilatation. Therefore, a quantitative assessment of left atrial size in such patients can offer an easy way to assess the progress of such patients. Few methods adopted in the past include grading of the size of the left atrium according to the indentation on the esophagus; or by measuring the size of LA either on the lateral view by measuring the distance from the anterior border of the right pulmonary artery to the anterior wall of the esophagus, or on the frontal view by measuring the distance from the mid-point of the curvilinear margin of the double density to the mid-point of the inferior wall of the left bronchus. A measurement of more than 7 cm is seen in approximately 90% patients with LA enlargement. Left atrial size may not change if there is severe rheumatic involvement of left atrial wall and resultant fibrosis. Such cases should be assessed by echocardiography.

Other Changes

There are a host of other changes that can indicate an improvement after successful intervention, especially in presence of mitral valve disease. Some examples include:

- Interstitial edema disappears within days while diminution in the size of upper zone vessel may take weeks or even months. Upper zone vessels do not usually return to normal.
- In patients with PAH, the dilated pulmonary trunk may return to normal with successful treatment.
- Presence of a flat or concave left midcardiac border on chest radiograph may be seen after a closed mitral valvotomy or following a thrombus in the appendage. However, this sign has a poor predictive value of the presence of the latter. Echocardiographic examination can easily detect this complication during the course of the disease. Overall, chest radiographs are widely available, quick and cost-effective in the imaging evaluation of a patient with valvular heart disease. However, because of undisputed advantages of echocardiography, information available from a chest radiograph should be complemented with echocardiography, wherever possible, for optimal patient management.

ECHOCARDIOGRAPHY

This technique is useful in the evaluation of stenosis and regurgitation of all cardiac valves, prosthetic valve function, and in patients with infective endocarditis. It provides valuable information regarding the diagnosis, valvular morphology, etiology of the disease, identification and quantification of lesions, detection and evaluation of associated abnormalities, delineation of cardiac size and ventricular function. This technique detects structural abnormalities of the valve, including fibrosis, calcification, thrombus, or vegetation, and abnormalities of valvular motion, including immobile, flail or prolapsing leaflets, or prosthetic valve dehiscence. A full evaluation provides prognostic as well as diagnostic information, allows for risk stratification, establishes the baseline data for subsequent examinations, and helps guide and evaluate the therapeutic approach. Echocardiography may obviate the need for cardiac catheterization in selected patients.

Valvular Stenosis

Two-dimensional and Doppler echocardiography reliably identify and quantitate the severity of the stenotic lesions. MS is accurately assessed by planimetry of transthoracic or transesophageal 2D images, Doppler measurement of trans-stenotic gradient, and estimation of valve area. Prognostic information is obtained from assessment of the hemodynamic response to exercise and/or delineation of morphological characteristics, which may help guide the selection of therapeutic interventions. Although tricuspid stenosis is readily detected and assessed hemodynamically, the accuracy of Doppler measurements is less well validated but still preferred over other methods. AS is accurately quantified by Doppler measurements of gradients and estimation of valve area. Pulmonary valve gradients are similarly quantified. While still experimental, contrast injection may allow more accurate recording of stenotic jet velocities and, therefore, transvalvular gradients.

Valvular Regurgitation

This is, perhaps, the most sensitive technique for detection of native valve regurgitation. Precise assessment of the severity of regurgitant lesions is difficult using any invasive or noninvasive technique, and no perfect method is, yet, available to judge the relative accuracy of a given technique. By far, angiography is the most widely used gold standard for this estimation. The results of echocardiography correlate well with it. Doppler methods for detection of regurgitation are similar for the native and prosthetic valves. Methods include assessment of regurgitant jet characteristics (length, height, area, and width), effective regurgitant orifice area, and measurement of regurgitant flow volumes. Doppler echocardiography is also an excellent technique for the re-evaluation of regurgitant lesions after surgery and in determination of the timing and method of operative intervention. In the evaluation of patients with mitral valve prolapse, this technique is useful for diagnosis and risk stratification, by identifying leaflet thickening and LV dilatation.

Infective Endocarditis

Echocardiography is useful for the detection and characterization of the hemodynamic and pathological consequences of infection, including valvular vegetations, regurgitant lesions, ventricular function, and associated abnormalities such as abscess, shunt and ruptured chordae. Controversy remains on the role of echocardiographic characteristics of vegetations in predicting embolization, although vegetation size, mobility, identification of the involved valve(s), and detection of myocardial involvement are important for risk stratification and prognosis.

Prosthetic Valves

Valve replacement carries a subsequent risk of valve degeneration, thrombosis, pannus formation, development of regurgitant or stenotic lesions and endocarditis. Obtaining baseline postoperative studies can be useful for comparison with future evaluation of changes in ventricular function and hemodynamics in response to surgery. Assessment of prosthetic valve stenosis is best performed by a combined echocardiography and Doppler technique. Estimation of prosthetic valve regurgitation is often hampered by prosthetic shadowing, particularly in the mitral position. The transesophageal approach may be useful in such cases. Contrast injection may enhance the spectral recording of both right-sided regurgitant velocities as well as the extent of the regurgitant jet.

CARDIAC MAGNETIC RESONANCE IMAGING

Cardiac magnetic resonance imaging (CMRI) offers a unique advantage of providing an observer independent, noninvasive technique for demonstration of pathological anatomy, quantification of global and regional function of both ventricles, flow disturbances across the stenotic valve, estimation of regurgitant volume, measurement of blood flows, and for assessing myocardial perfusion. Optimal cardiac imaging requires some form of physiological gating. Acquisition of signals without gating gives poor images because of loss of signal from moving structures and due to variable position of the heart structures in relation to image pixels when the data is acquired indiscriminately. The accuracy of MRI can be improved by using small voxels, thin slices and very short echo delay time. Cine MRI can be used for evaluation and monitoring of ventricular function, mass and wall stress in patients with valvular heart disease.

The CMRI has certain attributes that make it useful for imaging this body system. Firstly, there exists a natural contrast between the blood pool and the cardiovascular structures due to lack of signal from the flowing blood during spin-echo MRI, and bright signal from flowing blood in gradient-echo sequences. The differential blood signal is strikingly different from that of the myocardium, and hence, there is a good edge delineation of the endocardium. As a result, no additional contrast material is required for demarcation of the blood pool. This ensures that MRI remains a noninvasive imaging technique.

Secondly, there is a wide range of soft tissue contrast on MRI images that provides characterization of the myocardial tissue. This tissue characterization is improved by the use of paramagnetic contrast material.

Thirdly, the imaging can be done in any plane.

Lastly, cardiac MRI is also useful in giving us the functional and hemodynamic information besides giving morphological details. It can demonstrate valvular stenosis and regurgitation on cine images with poststenotic and regurgitant jets seen as flow voids on bright blood images. Quantification of flow and gradient across the valve can be done using phase contrast techniques and ventricular analysis. Phase contrast method is principally based on the phase shifts of moving spins in the magnetic field gradient. The extent of phase shifts of moving spins is proportional to the velocity along the velocity-encoding direction. Velocity-encoding is performed by using bipolar gradient pulses. Its direction can be selected in any orthogonal or oblique axis of the body. Velocity-encoding of blood flow in each pixel provides 2D quantitative velocity mapping of the vascular system. Once velocity across a vessel is obtained, gradient can be derived using formula $\Delta = 4 (V_{max})^2$.

Valve Leaflet Morphology

This can be seen with both black blood and steady-state free procession (SSFP) images **(Fig. 6)**.

Aortic valve leaflets can be seen on 2 chamber and 4 chamber views **(Figs. 7A and B)** while tricuspid valve's anatomy can be well seen on long axis and short axis views. Aortic valve area can be calculated by direct planimetry. For pulmonic valve, a double oblique view of right ventricular outflow tract is used as a guide to planimetric visualization of pulmonary valve.

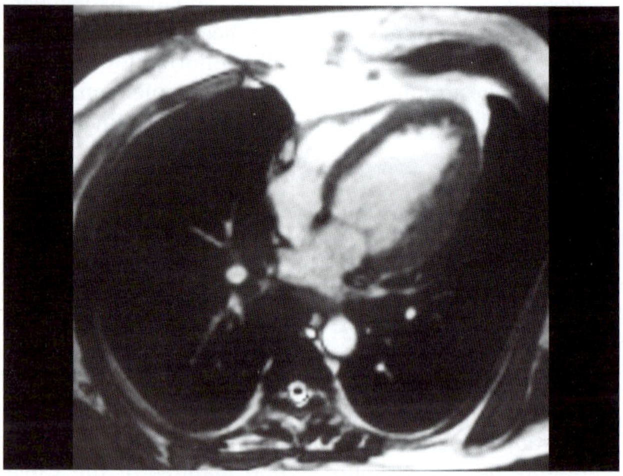

FIG. 6: Four-chamber SSFP MR image showing normal mitral valve in closed position.

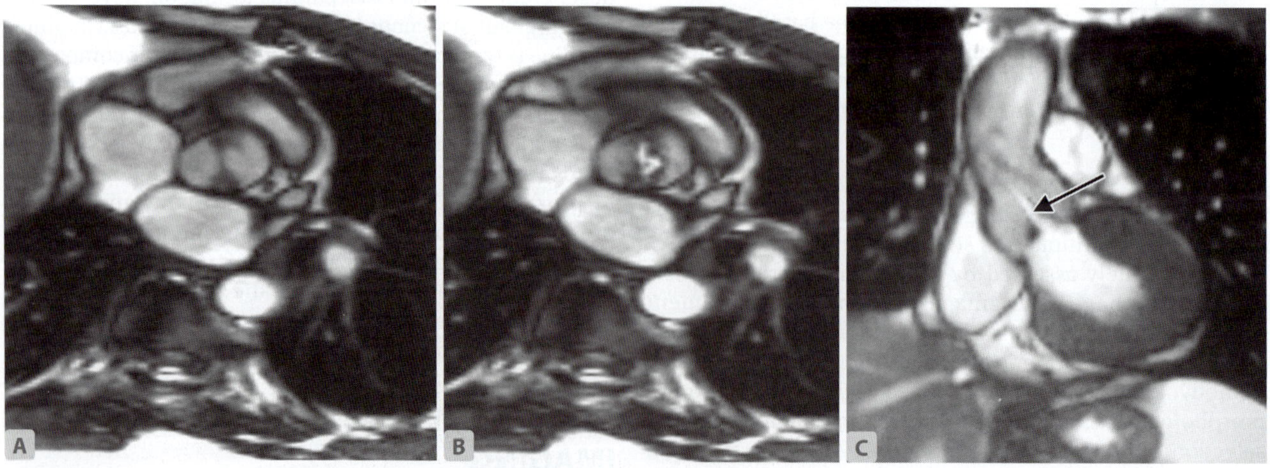

FIGS. 7A TO C: Bicuspid aortic valve seen in its short axis in diastole. (A) Aystole; (B) Planimetric measurement of aortic valve area can be done in the latter frame; (C) Oblique coronal view on cine bright blood MR image showing post-stenotic jet in ascending aorta in a patient with aortic valvular stenosis.

Valvular Stenosis

On cine images, leaflet movements appear to restricted and flow turbulence is seen in vessel/chamber in distal downstream **(Fig. 7C)**. For example, in valvular pulmonary stenosis, the turbulence and flow voids due to poststenotic jets are seen in main pulmonary artery.

Valvular Regurgitation

Signal void due to regurgitating blood is seen in the receiving chamber **(Fig. 8)**. Quantitative measurement of regurgitant volume can be done using volumetric or phase velocity methods or both. The difference between the end-diastolic and end-systolic volumes for a ventricle with a regurgitant valve includes both the forward stroke volume and the regurgitant volume. Because the forward or net stroke volume is equal to the volume ejected from the normal ventricle, the difference in stroke volumes between a regurgitant ventricle (e.g. LV with AR or MR) and normal ventricle (e.g. RV) is the regurgitant volume. The sum of the forward and regurgitant volume is called the total stroke volume of the regurgitant ventricle.

Phase-contrast techniques can be used to directly quantify the aortic and pulmonary regurgitation. For mitral and tricuspid regurgitation, a combined approach using phase contrast techniques and ventricular volume assessment is used. Velocity-encoded MRI is done to measure the systolic outflow from the LV at the level of the ascending aorta and diastolic inflow to LV at the level of the mitral annulus. The difference between the two is a measure of the volume of MR.

Valve Endocarditis and Tumors

Case reports have been published describing the use of MRI in evaluation of valve tumors. Cine images help identify the small valve vegetations and tumors. The regurgitation of valve, if present, can be also be quantified.

Prosthetic Valve

When prosthetic values are studied, they usually cause local signal loss and are not well seen. Early concerns regarding radio-frequency energy deposition and heating have, to date, been unfounded. Despite the increasing use of high gradient strengths for faster acquisition approaching close to physiological threshold for muscle and nerve stimulation limits set by FDA, there are no reports of MRI complications related to valve prosthesis. Valves that are strongly ferromagnetic (Starr-Edwards pre 6000 series valves), however, should not be scanned. Overall, MRI is well suited for the evaluation of a patient with valvular heart disease. A cooperative patient with a stable heart rate, that is not too fast or too slow and in normal sinus rhythm, is necessary for optimal image acquisition. Availability of the equipment, cost and familiarity of the operator and the treating physician will determine the optimal use of this modality.

COMPUTED TOMOGRAPHY

Multislice CT can, in single breath-hold, evaluate large volumes in orthogonal planes with a high signal-to-noise ratio. These features make imaging easier in children and in patients with any habitus.

The MSCT can identify cardiac calcification sensitively. It can be localized, characterized and quantified in the valves, chamber wall **(Fig. 9)**, pericardium and the coronary arteries. A negative MSCT used to assess coronary calcification has a strong negative predictive valve of 98% and excludes the need for coronary angiography in an elderly patient with valvular heart disease. Contrast enhancement is needed to evaluate the cardiac chambers and valves. CT can measure the cardiac chamber volume, wall thickness and myocardial mass. In addition, multi-slice CT can measure the cardiac output, ventricular mass and stroke volume. If only a single valve is regurgitating, the volume can be calculated by comparing RV and LV stroke volumes. ECG-gated CT images can help reconstruct cardiac motion throughout the cardiac cycle and the jets due to stenotic or regurgitant valves can be seen **(Fig. 10)**. With MSCT, it is possible to get stroke volumes and do ventricular analysis. CT is also useful in differentiating intracardiac thrombi from a tumor. Despite these advantages, the impact of CT techniques on valvular imaging is still evolving.

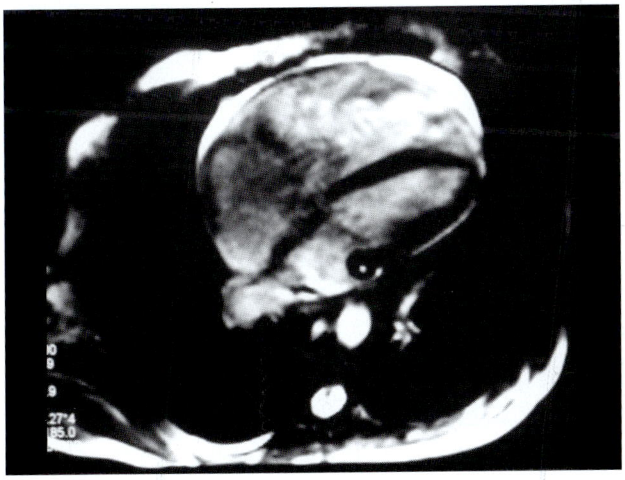

FIG. 8: Cine bright blood MR image in 4 chamber view showing jet due to tricuspid regurgitation, in right atrium.

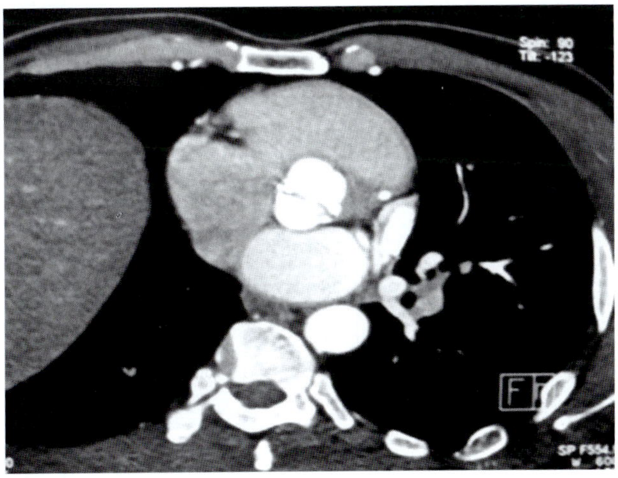

FIG. 9: Oblique axial CT image across the aortic valve showing bicuspid calcified valve.

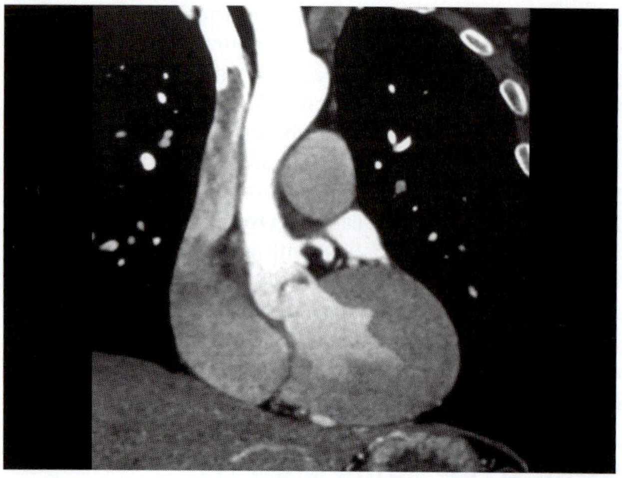

FIG. 10: Cine coronal image reconstructed from ECG-gated CT images shows doming of the bicuspid aortic valve in systole.

ANGIOCARDIOGRAPHY

In patients with valvular heart disease, cardiac catheterization provides data both confirmatory and complementary to noninvasive echocardiography and nuclear studies. Cardiac catheterization procedure includes pressure measurements in the cardiac chambers and the great vessels, oximetry in each chamber and resultant hemodynamic assessments, and angiography. Angiograms reveal typical diagnostic images in presence of stenotic **(Figs. 11 and 12)** and regurgitant **(Figs. 13 and 14)** lesions of all cardiac valves. The indications for angiocardiography are based on the assessment of risks versus benefits of the procedure. The availability and familiarity with noninvasive techniques, including echocardiography and MRI, has changed the indications of angiocardiography and all patients in whom surgical treatment is considered may not necessarily require angiography.

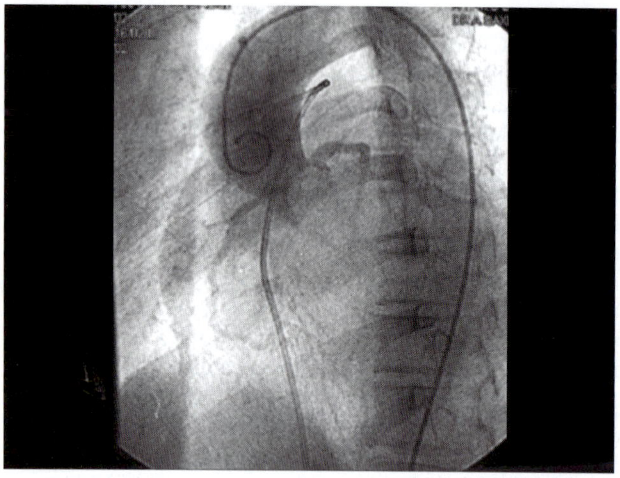

FIG. 11: Aortic root angiogram in the left anterior oblique (LAO) view in a patient with valvular AS shows doming of the aortic valve, restricted negative jet and poststenotic dilatation of the ascending aorta.

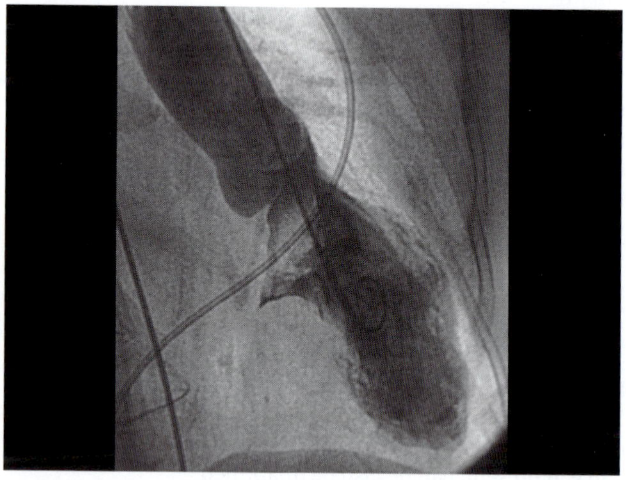

FIG. 12: LV angiogram in the right anterior oblique (RAO) view in a patient with MS shows doming of mitral valve, restricted negative bolus and no MR.

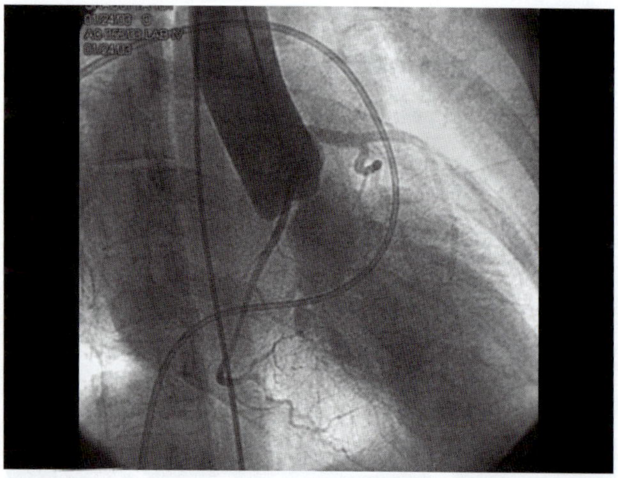

FIG. 13: Aortic root angiogram in the RAO view in a patient with severe AR shows opacification of the entire LV.

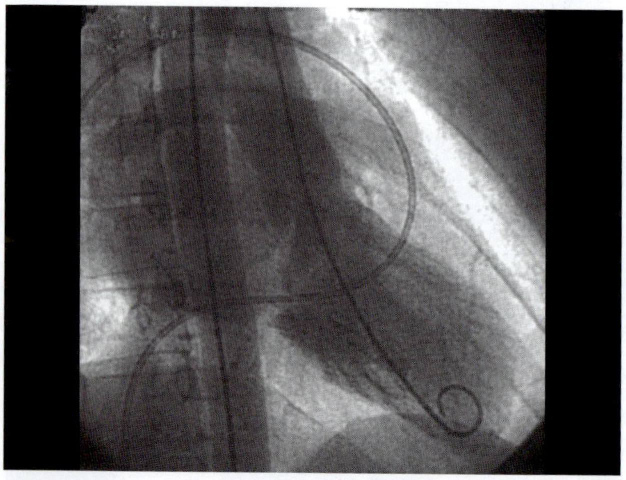

FIG. 14: LV angiogram in the RAO view in a patient with severe MR shows the opacification of the entire LV.

Whenever indicated, the overall benefits outweigh the risk of catheterization. At the present time, angiocardiography is not indicated in single valve pathologies in patients in whom coronary angiography is not required, and also in clear-cut double valve lesions in patients less than 40 years in age provided that the tricuspid valve is not involved. When performed, cardiac catheterization provides confirmation of the severity of valvular lesion, identifies associated coronary artery disease, quantifies the hemodynamic consequences of valvular lesions (such as pulmonary hypertension), and occasionally the acute hemodynamic response to pharmacological therapy. These may help select the optimal therapeutic strategy and define the risks of treatment. Valvular regurgitation may be assessed visually by determining the relative amount of the contrast medium that opacifies the chamber proximal to its injection. The estimation of regurgitation depends on the regurgitant volume as well as the size and contractility of the proximal chamber. In addition, cardiac catheterization is indicated whenever interventional catheter-directed treatment is planned.

CONCLUSION

A multimodality approach, using a combination of non-invasive techniques backed by a sound clinical assessment is usually adequate for the diagnosis and for defining the optimal management option in most patients. When choosing a given technique, it is important to keep in mind the availability, cost and familiarity of the operator and the other team members with its interpretation and pitfalls. Chest radiographs are useful for the initial evaluation and during follow-up after treatment in all patients. Echocardiography remains the mainstay for investigating these patients and planning their management strategy. Despite the fact that MRI and multislice CT are operator independent and are capable of providing excellent quality images along with information on the functional impairment caused by the valvular lesions in a noninvasive manner, their wider use in the diagnostic algorithm of these patients in most centers is still limited and investigational. Cardiac catheterization and angiography are indicated whenever coronary anatomy needs to be defined, in the evaluation of tricuspid involvement, in situations where a discrepancy between the clinical and imaging data exists and for interventional management of the lesions.

BIBLIOGRAPHY

1. Albers J, Nitsche T, Boese J, et al. Regurgitant jet evaluation using three-dimensional echocardiography and magnetic resonance. Ann Thorac Surg. 2004;78(1):96-102.
2. Cawley PJ, Maki JH, Otto CM. Cardiovascular magnetic resonance imaging for valvular heart disease: technique and validation. Circulation. 2009;119(3):468-78.
3. Chen JTT, Behar VS, Marris JJ, et al. Correlation of roentgen findings with hemodynamic data in pure mitral stenosis. AJR. 1968;102:280-92.
4. Chikos PM, Figley MM, Fisher L. Correlation between chest film and angiographic assessment of left ventricular size. AJR. 1977;128:367-73.
5. Higgins CB, Reinke RT, Jones NE, et al. Left atrial dimension on the frontal thoracic radiograph: a method for assessment left atrial enlargement. AJR. 1978;130:251-5.
6. Jefferson K, Rees S. Clinical Cardiac Radiology. Butterworths, London. 1973;230-9.
7. Kelley MR, Elliot LP, Schulman ST, et al. The significance of the dilated left atrial appendage in rheumatic heart disease. Circulation. 1976;54:146-53.
8. Murray JG, Brown AL, Anagnostov EA, et al. Widening of the tracheal bifurcation on chest radiographs: Value as a sign of left atrial enlargement. AJR. 1995;164:1089-92.
9. Newell JD, Higgins CB, Kelly MJ. Radiographic echocardiographic approach to acquired heart disease: Diagnosis and assessment of severity. Radiologic Clinics of North America. 1980;18: 387-409.
10. Pouleur AC, le Polain de Waroux JB, Pasquet A, et al. Aortic valve area assessment: Multidetector CT compared with cine MR imaging and transthoracic and transesophageal echocardiography. Radiology. 2007;244:745-54.
11. Raphael MJ. Cardiac radiology: techniques and normal appearances In: Grainger RG, Allison DJ (Eds). Diagnotic Radiology, An Anglo American Textbook of Imaging. Churchill Livingstone, Edinburgh, 1992; pp. 431-45.
12. Sharma S, Kumar MB, Aggarwal S, Reddy VM, Kaul U, Rajani M, Venugopal P. Chest radiographs are unreliable in predicting thrombi in the left atrium or its appendage in rheumatic mitral stenosis. Clin Radio. 1991;43:337-40.
13. Vogel-Claussen J, Pannu H, Spevak PJ, Fishman EK, Bluemke DA. Cardiac valve assessment with MR imaging and 64-section Multi-detector row CT. Radio Graphics. 2006;26(6):1769-84.
14. Westcott JL, Ferguson D. The right pulmonary artery-left atrial axis line. A method for measuring left atrial size on lateral chest radiographs. Radiology. 1976;118:265-74.

CHAPTER

148

Imaging of the Pericardium

Jyoti Kumar, Sapna Singh, Anju Garg, Gaurav Shanker Pradhan

INTRODUCTION

The initial approach to the evaluation of pericardial disease is usually performed with echocardiography and chest radiography. While echocardiography has its own advantages, namely high temporal and spatial resolution, easy availability, no involvement of ionizing radiation, it is usually limited by poor acoustic window, poor soft tissue characterization and operator variability. In addition, it can be very difficult to detect pericardial thickening or calcification.[1,2]

Computed tomography (CT) and magnetic resonance (MR) imaging techniques prove to be advantageous over echocardiography in the following respect: they provide excellent anatomic details, help in localizing pericardial pathology as well as depicting associated abnormalities of the lung and mediastinum. The advent of multidetector CT with its excellent temporal resolution helps us to image pericardium devoid of cardiac motion artifacts. Multiplanar reformats allow better visualization of pericardial pathology with easy communication to the referring physician.[3] A cinematic display of cardiac motion is now possible on CT with electrocardiography (ECG) gating and high resolution thin section images can be obtained. Increased sensitivity to detect calcification is another advantage of CT. MR imaging provides superior soft tissue characterization than CT and echocardiography. MR imaging can provide excellent display of cardiac motion in patients with regular heart rhythm.[3-6]

ANATOMY

The pericardium has an outer fibrous layer and an inner serous layer. The inner serosal layer is further composed of outer parietal and inner visceral layer. The outer parietal layer lines the inner surface of the fibrous pericardium and the inner visceral layer forms the epicardium.[7,8] Ligaments attach the outer pericardium to sternum and diaphragm. The serosal layer forms two complex sleeves as it reflects around major vessel. One of these sleeves enclose the aorta and pulmonary trunk and the other encloses the superior and inferior vena cava and the four pulmonary veins. These reflections form the sinuses and recesses **(Fig. 1)**. The transverse sinus is the channel in between these two sleeves around the arteries and veins and the oblique sinus is the channel behind the left atrium. The recesses are the blind ends of these sinuses **(Box 1)**. These sinuses and recesses can collect fluid within them in case of pericardial effusion. With the advent of MDCT, visualization of pericardial recesses without fluid accumulation is also possible with narrow collimation imaging.[8]

The normal pericardium can be seen as a thin line less than 2 mm in thickness.[7,9] On CT, it appears as a thin linear density surrounding the heart better visualized over the right ventricle **(Fig. 2A)**. It appears as a hypointense line on MR surrounded by epicardial fat on one side and mediastinal fat on the other side on T1-weighted, T2-weighted and gradient images **(Fig. 2B)**. Normally, up to 50 mL fluid may be present in the potential space created by two appossing serosal surfaces.[10]

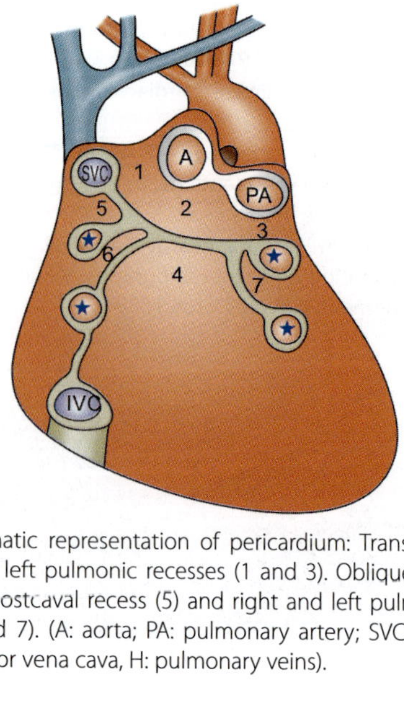

FIG. 1: Schematic representation of pericardium: Transverse sinus (2) with right and left pulmonic recesses (1 and 3). Oblique sinus (4) with its recesses—postcaval recess (5) and right and left pulmonary venous recesses (6 and 7). (A: aorta; PA: pulmonary artery; SVC: superior vena cava; IVC: inferior vena cava, H: pulmonary veins).

Transverse Sinus and Recesses

The transverse sinus lies behind the aorta and the main pulmonary artery and superior to the left atrium.

Superior Aortic Recess

The cranial most extent of this sinus is the superior aortic or superior pericardial recess. It can further be divided into posterior, right, and anterior portions depending on relationship with aorta. The posterior portion is seen as a crescentic fluid collection just posterior to the ascending aorta. It can be mistaken for a lymph node. The fluid in this posterior portion lies directly posterior to the aorta with no intervening fat. The crescent shape and fluid attenuation are other distinguishing features from lymph nodes. The anterior portion passes between the aorta and pulmonary artery, resulting in a triangular shape between them[8] **(Fig. 3A)**.

Inferior Aortic Recess

Inferiorly, the transverse sinus extends between the ascending aorta and the right atrium and forms the inferior aortic recess. This extends caudally till the level of the aortic valve annulus and lies anterior to the left atrium **(Figs. 4A and B)**.

Box 1: Sinuses and recesses of pericardium.

- *Transverse sinus*:
  - *Superior aortic sinus*:
    - Anterior triangular extension
    - Posterior crescentic extension
    - Right lateral extension
  - Inferior aortic recess
  - Right and left pulmonic recesses
- *Oblique sinus*:
  - Posterior pericardial recess
- *Recesses of pericardial cavity proper*:
  - Right and left pulmonary venous recesses
  - Postcaval recess

Right and Left Pulmonic Recesses

Laterally, the transverse sinus ends in right and left pulmonic recesses **(Figs. 3B to D)**. The former lies inferior to the right pulmonary artery. The left pulmonic recess lies below the left pulmonary artery. Below this lies the superior pulmonary vein. Fluid within these recesses can sometimes simulate lymph nodes.[8,11]

Oblique Sinus and Recess

The oblique sinus lies superior and posterior to the left atrium and posteromedial to the superior pulmonary veins **(Figs. 5A and B)**. It is separated from the transverse sinus by a pericardial reflection between the right and left superior pulmonary veins. Since this lies just anterior to the esophagus, fluid here may be mistaken for esophageal lesions and sometimes even as bronchogenic cysts.

The cranial reflection is the posterior pericardial recess. This extends behind the right pulmonary artery and medial to the bronchus intermedius **(Fig. 5A)**. Fluid within this recess can mimic peribronchial or subcarinal lymph nodes.[6,10]

Recesses of the Pericardial Cavity Proper

Right and Left Pulmonary Venous Recesses

The right and left pulmonary venous recesses are recesses of the pericardial cavity proper, located between the superior and inferior pulmonary veins on either side.

Fluid in these pulmonary venous recesses can be mistaken for bronchopulmonary lymph nodes. These may be distinguished by the fact that fluid lies both anterior and posterior to the veins whereas lymph nodes lie only on one side and may narrow the vein.[11]

Postcaval Recess

The postcaval recess is another small recess from the pericardial cavity proper, lying posterior to the superior vena cava (SVC) and to its right.[11]

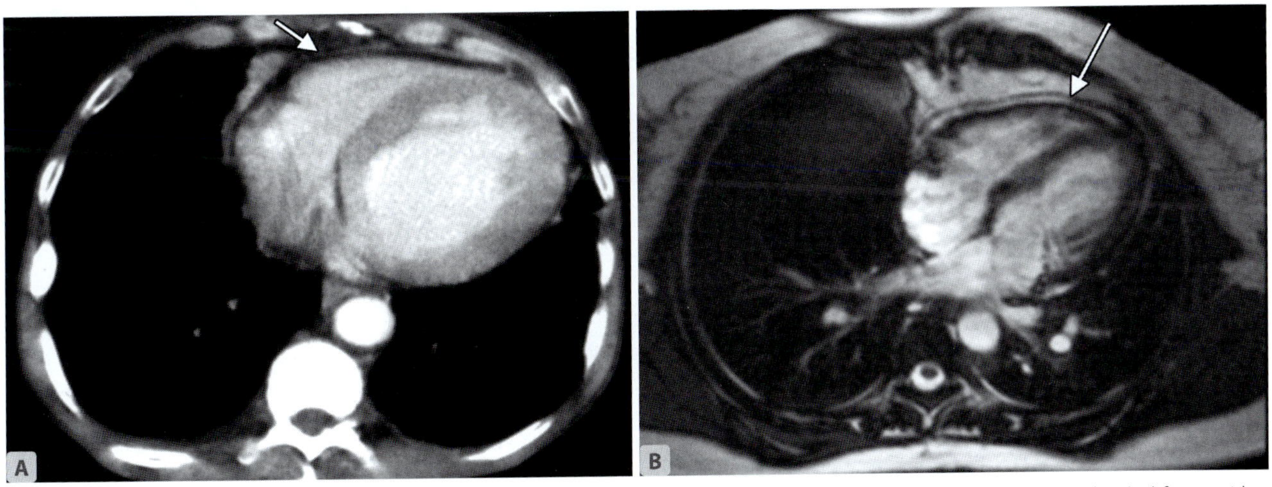

FIGS. 2A AND B: (A) Axial contrast-enhanced CT scan shows normal pericardium (arrow) outlined by epicardial fat and mediastinal fat on either side. Note made of subsegmental atelectasis in right lung; (B) Short axis cine gradient echo MR image shows normal pericardium as a thin curved line (arrow) surrounded by bright epicardial and mediastinal fat on either side.

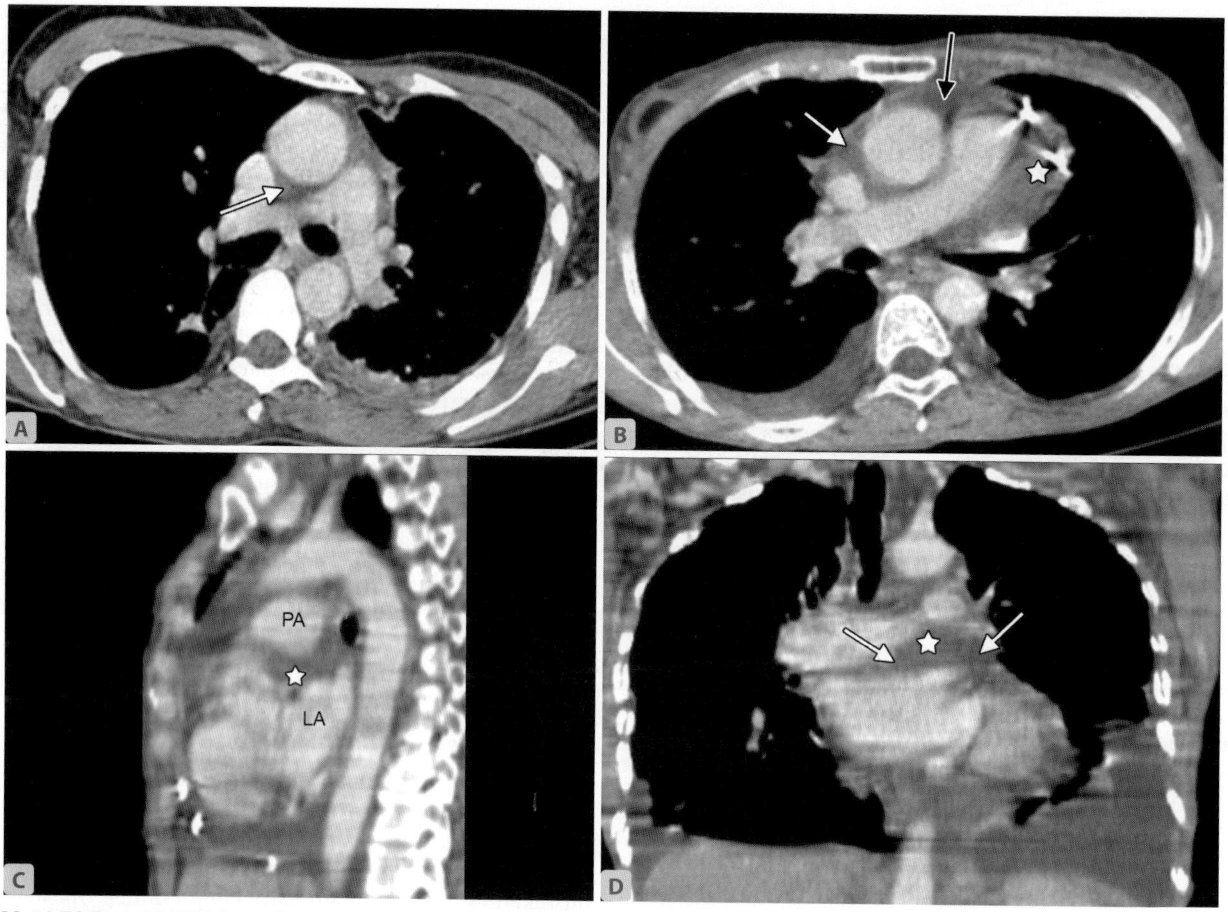

FIGS. 3A TO D: Axial CECT shows the posterior extension of the superior aortic recess posterior to the ascending aorta, as a crescentic fluid collection (arrow); (B) Axial CECT shows left pulmonic recess of the transverse sinus (star). Pericardial fluid is also seen in the anterior (black arrow) and right (white arrow) portions of the superior aortic recess. Note made of pericardial drainage catheter in situ; (C) Sagittal reformation shows the transverse sinus (star) between pulmonary artery (PA) and left atrium (LA). Note made of pericardial drainage catheter in situ; (D) Coronal reformation shows transverse sinus (star) along with right and left pulmonic recesses (arrows) at its right and left ends.

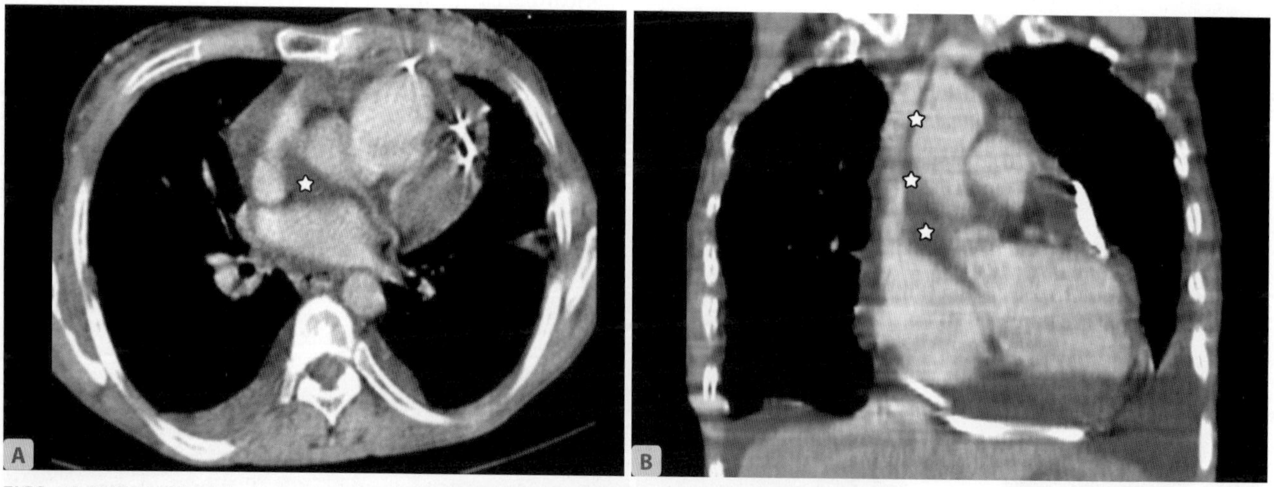

FIGS. 4A AND B: (A) Axial contrast-enhanced CT scan shows inferior aortic recess between the right atrium and aortic root (star). Note made of pericardial drainage catheter *in situ*; (B) Coronal reformation shows the vertical extent of the transverse sinus with its superior and inferior aortic recesses. (stars). Note made of pericardial drainage catheter *in situ*.

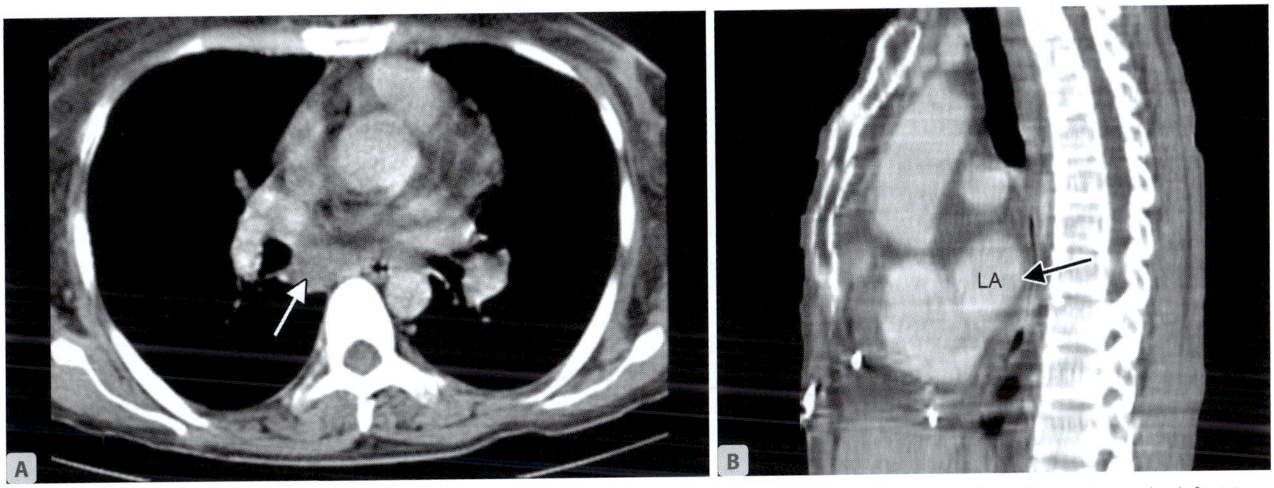

FIGS. 5A AND B: (A) Axial contrast-enhanced CT scan shows posterior pericardial recess of the oblique sinus (arrow) superior to the left atrium, medial to bronchus intermedius and posteromedial to the superior pulmonary veins; (B) Sagittal reformation shows the oblique sinus (arrow) between the left atrium anteriorly and the esophagus posteriorly.

PHYSIOLOGY

The pericardium supports the heart and cardiac function in the following major ways:[12]

- It fixes the heart within the anterior mediastinum protecting it from surrounding organs
- Its elasticity limits excessive dilatation of cardiac chambers in response to increased preload
- It equalizes compliance between right and left ventricle. When stroke volume of left ventricle is altered due to elevated systemic vascular resistance, it helps in adaptation of stroke volume of the right ventricle accordingly (ventricular coupling)
- The respiratory changes in intrathoracic pressure are directly transmitted to the pericardial cavity and then to the cardiac chambers. The effect is greater on the right ventricle than on the left because of its thinner wall.

CONGENITAL PERICARDIAL ANOMALIES

Pericardial Cysts (Box 2)

These are rare lesions which result from pinching off of a portion of pericardium. They can be found throughout the mediastinum but the most common location is the right anterior cardiophrenic angle. A pericardial cyst elsewhere in the mediastinum may be difficult to differentiate from a bronchogenic or thymic cyst.[6] When these pericardial cysts have a residual communication with the pericardial space, these are called pericardial diverticulae.[7] This communication may however be difficult to delineate. Although usually asymptomatic, few patients may have chest pain, dyspnea, cough, pneumothorax, or fever.[10,13] Another rarer presentation may be due to bronchial compression.

The pericardial cyst is usually sharply demarcated round or ovoid mass in the region of right cardiophrenic angle silhouetting the cardiac border. The cyst may have a pointed upper border as it droops down into the cardiophrenic region from higher up. On cross- sectional imaging, it is a well-defined unilocular, thin walled homogeneous nonenhancing mass contiguous with the pericardium. Ultrasound can depict the cystic lesion adjacent to pericardium. On CT, it has fluid attenuation and on MR imaging, it matches the signal characteristics of water. Presence of proteinaceous contents within the cyst can result in occasional high signal on T1 weighted images. An important feature is that the cyst changes in size or shape with respiration or body position.[10] Additionally, a pericardial cyst should not normally cause mass effect on the heart. The cysts may get infected and then show peripheral enhancement or mass effect, which is otherwise not seen. Symptomatic and complicated cysts may need to be resected.[3]

Box 2: Pericardial cyst.

- Rare congenital lesion
- Most common location is right cardiophrenic angle
- Typical imaging features—well-defined cyst with thin wall, no internal septations, low signal on T1W MR and high signal on T2W MR images
- Mass effect and enhancement not seen unless infected

CONGENITAL ABSENCE OF THE PERICARDIUM (BOX 3)

Compromise of the vascular supply to the pleuropericardial membrane results in congenital defects of the pericardium. Defect can be acquired after surgery or trauma also.[13]

Absence of the pericardium is rare. Absence of left pericardium is more common than complete absence.[3] Bilateral and isolated right sided defects are very rare. Pericardial defects are usually associated with defects in the parietal pleura through which lung can herniate. There may be other congenital anomalies along with pericardial defect which include cardiac anomalies (atrial septal defect, patent ductus arteriosus), and anomalies of the lung (bronchogenic cysts, pulmonary sequestration), chest wall (pectus excavatum) and diaphragm.[14] Patients are generally asymptomatic although vague chest pain can occur due to lack of fixation.[12-14] A focally deficient pericardium may allow a part of the heart to herniate through the hole. It most often involves the left atrial appendage. The left coronary artery may also be compressed by the herniation through this defect. This can rarely result in ischemia, especially during activity. In such situations, surgical closure or enlargement of the defect may be performed.[12]

In complete absence of left pericardium, left ventricle and pulmonary artery may be seen displaced to the left side on plain radiographs. The segments of the heart that make up the left heart border can be seen more distinctly. The medial and lateral borders of the main pulmonary artery are seen more clearly due to the absence of pericardium between the aorta and the pulmonary artery. In partial absence of the left pericardium, pulmonary artery or left atrial appendage may be prominent depending upon the location of pericardial defect.[13-15]

Box 3: Congenital absence of pericardium.

- Rare anomaly
- Left-sided absence commoner than complete absence
- *Radiographic findings*:
  - Left ventricle and pulmonary artery displaced to left
  - Main pulmonary artery borders distinctly seen
  - Pulmonary artery/left atrial appendage may be prominent in partial absence
- *CT/MR findings*:
  - Leftward shift of cardiac axis
  - Prominent atrial appendage
  - Lung seen interposed between aorta and main pulmonary artery

CT and MR may not depict the pericardium along its entirety. The pericardium may not be normally seen over the left atrial appendage and the left ventricle and should not be misinterpreted as pericardial defect.[7] The secondary signs, which include posterior and leftward shift of the cardiac axis, prominent atrial appendage and separation of the aorta and main pulmonary artery due to lung tissue interposition become more important features. Occasionally, lung tissue can be seen inferior to the heart, interposed between the heart and the diaphragm. The herniation may be intermittent; hence left lateral decubitus position of the patient can assist in diagnosing pericardial defects. Also, functional examination can pick up greater mobility of the cardiac apex which is otherwise essentially stationary in a normal cardiac cycle.[16]

PERICARDIAL EFFUSION

The various causes of pericardial effusion include heart failure, renal insufficiency, infection (bacterial, viral, tuberculous), neoplasm (carcinoma of the lung, breast, lymphoma, melanoma) and injury (trauma, myocardial infarction). Other causes may be hypothyroidism, connective tissue disorder, acquired immune deficiency syndrome (AIDS) or radiation pericarditis.[17]

The role of imaging is to confirm the presence and extent of fluid, to characterize the nature of fluid, to rule out pericardial inflammation, to determine its hemodynamic impact and to guide pericardiocentesis. Echocardiography is generally the first imaging modality to be used because of high sensitivity, specificity, easy availability and low cost **(Fig. 6A)**. Limited acoustic window may impair the utility of this modality in many cases. With exception of transesophageal echocardiography, it is not a reliable technique for estimating pericardial thickness and in assessment of loculated pericardial effusions. CT and MR provide a wider field of view and are superior in detecting the amount, nature and distribution of the fluid. Focal fluid accumulation may be seen posterolateral to the left ventricle and along the inferolateral wall of the right ventricle owing

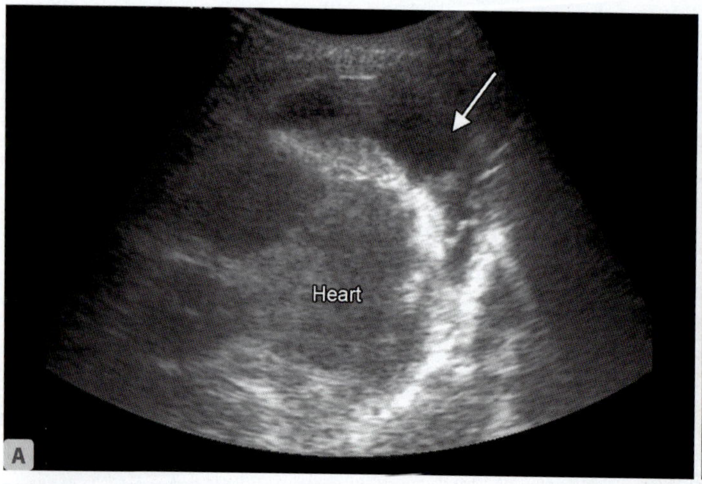

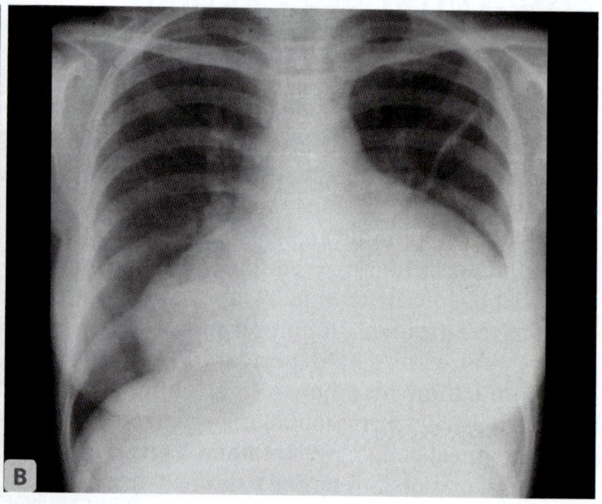

FIGS. 6A AND B: (A) Pericardial effusion: Ultrasound chest depicts fluid in the pericardial cavity (arrow); (B) Frontal chest radiograph shows enlarged 'flask'-shaped cardiac silhouette without specific chamber enlargement with bilateral hilum overlay sign. Both sides of the heart appear rounded and displaced laterally.

to their dependent locations. Superior pericardial recess is another common location of focal fluid accumulation.[12]

The size of a pericardial effusion may be semiquantitatively assessed by the thickness of fluid anterior to the right ventricle. Pericardial width of more than 4 mm may be regarded as abnormal. Using criteria established by echocardiography, a pericardial effusion may be quantified as small (<5 mm); moderate (5–10 mm); or large (>10 mm).[3,17,18] On a chest radiograph, pericardial effusion is suspected when there is diffuse cardiac silhouette enlargement without specific chamber enlargement. Filling of the retrosternal space, enlargement of normal cardiac borders, development of "flask" configuration and bilateral hilar overlay may be seen in larger effusions **(Fig. 6B)**. On the lateral projection, 'epicardial fat pad' sign is diagnostic of pericardial disease. This is positive when the anterior pericardial stripe, bordered by the epicardial fat and mediastinal fat on either side, is seen to be thicker than 2 mm. It may also be seen in the frontal view because of presence of abundant fat between the pericardium and pleura at the cardiac apex. This is seen as a radiolucent stripe internal to and parallel to the left lower cardiac border.[13] On a chest radiograph, pan chamber cardiac enlargement and large anterior mediastinal tumor may simulate pericardial effusion. On CT, the attenuation values of pericardial fluid are only of limited value. Serous effusions tend to have near-water attenuation values (<10 HU) **(Figs. 7A and B)**, while exudative effusions can range from 20 to 60 HU **(Figs. 7C and D)**. Chylopericardium can also present with low attenuation values but may be difficult to distinguish from transudative effusions. Acute hemopericardium can have attenuation values in the range of 60 to 80 HU, but if blood represents only a portion of the fluid, the attenuation values can then be similar to that of exudative effusions. Generally, 30 HU is a useful cut off between simple effusions and bloody or proteinaceous effusions.[7] It may sometimes be difficult to distinguish between pericardial effusion and thickening on CT which is better appreciated on echocardiography or MRI.

MR imaging may be performed to further characterize pericardial effusions. Transudates have a low signal intensity on T1-weighted images and high signal intensity on T2-weighted images and GRE cine images **(Figs. 8A and B)**. Exudates have a higher signal intensity on T1-weighted images and low signal intensity on T2 weighted images due to high cellularity and protein content within **(Figs. 9A and B)**. Hemopericardium is characterized by high signal on T1-weighted images and may be low signal on T2-weighted

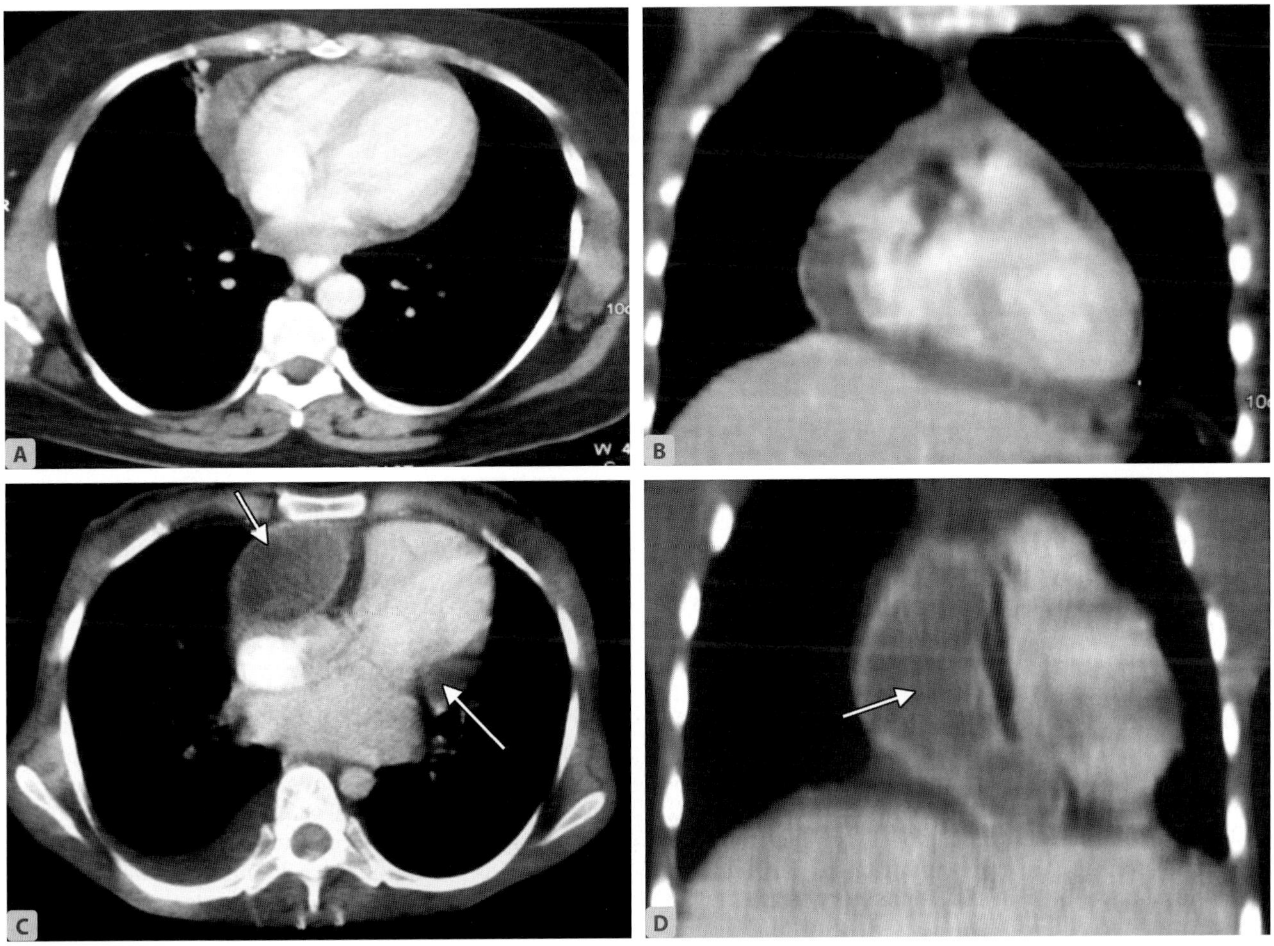

FIGS. 7A TO D: (A and B) Pericardial effusion: Axial CECT (A) and coronal reformation (B) show small simple pericardial effusion (HU = 10); (C and D) Exudative pericardial effusion: Axial CECT (C) and coronal reformation (D) shows high attenuation loculated effusion (HU = 45) (arrows) in atrioventricular groove in a case of tuberculous pericarditis.

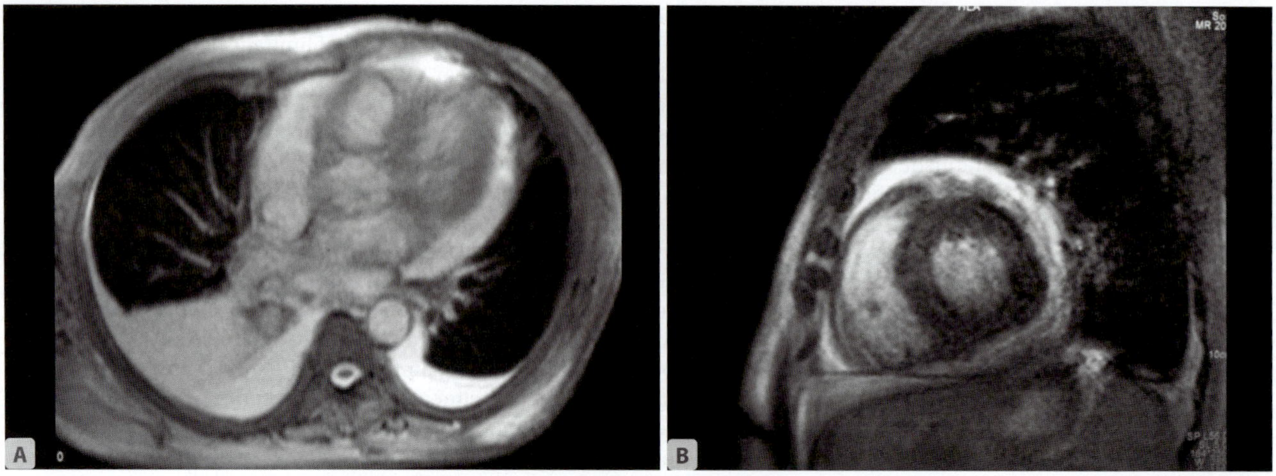

FIGS. 8A AND B: Pericardial effusion: Moderate simple effusion is seen on four-chamber (A) and short axis; (B) cine SSFP images. Bilateral pleural effusions are also seen.

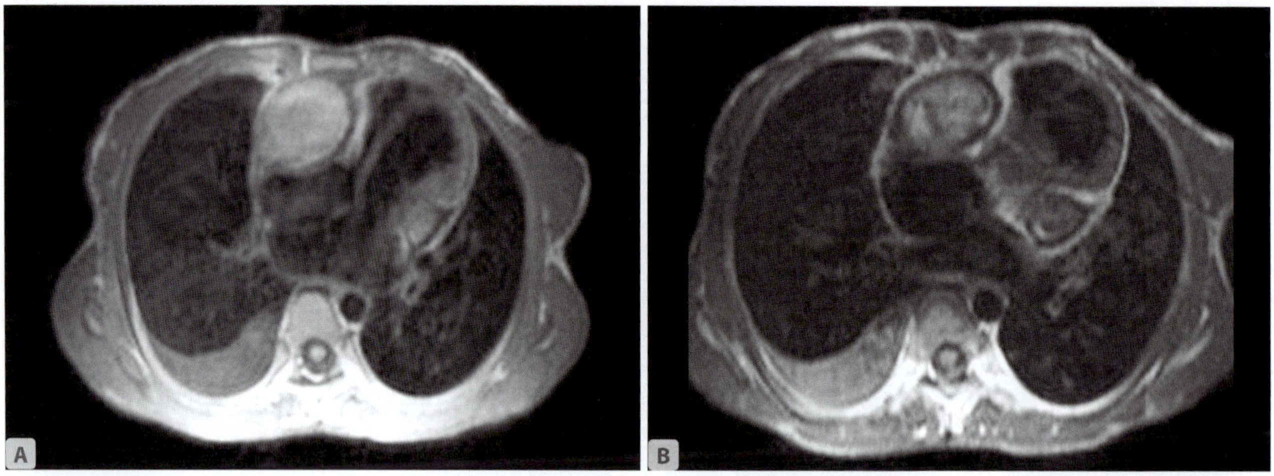

FIGS. 9A AND B: Exudative pericardial effusion (same case as in Fig. 8): Axial dark blood T1 and T2-weighted images show exudative effusion in the atrioventricular groove and associated pericardial thickening. It is seen as high signal intensity on T1-weighted images (A) with complex and inhomogeneous signal intensity on T2-weighted images (B). Note made of right pleural effusion.

images and GRE cine images. Hemorrhage or infection should be suspected on cine imaging when the effusion fluid is clearly complex and inhomogeneous, containing regions of different signal intensity.[19,20] The gradient images may better characterize a hemopericardium as they facilitate the visualization of fibrinous strands and presence of coagulated blood. The T1 and T2 signal intensity of a hemorrhagic pericardial effusion is dependent on the duration of the hematoma. However, certain artifacts like non-linear motion of pericardial fluid during cardiac motion may falsely cause high signal on T1-weighted spin-echo CMR even within a transudative effusion.[7,12] Effusion secondary to malignancy may have associated pericardial thickening and nodularity. MR is superior to CT in differentiating pericardial effusion from thickening. The high signal intensity on cine and T2-weighted images allows to clearly distinguishing between pericardial effusion and thickened pericardium which is low signal intensity on these sequences. In certain cases, double and triple IR sequences can aid in the differentiation between pericardial fluid and pericardial fat. Double IR images null the signal contribution of fluid, whereas triple IR images null the signal contribution of fat.[3] Delayed-enhancement imaging can demonstrate abnormal pericardial enhancement, indicative of inflammation or infection.[2]

CARDIAC TAMPONADE (BOX 4)

Slow accumulation of pericardial fluid may cause adaptive expansion of the pericardium with accumulation of up to 3 L of fluid without significant hemodynamic consequence.[21] However, in cases of rapid accumulation, as little as 100–200 mL of fluid may result in an effusion under tension or cardiac tamponade as pericardium has limited stretchability.[13] The resultant increased pericardial pressure is then transmitted to the cardiac chambers. Cardiac tamponade is a low cardiac output state due to excessive fluid in the pericardial space that compresses the heart. The diagnosis is generally made on clinical grounds and is confirmed by echocardiography

Box 4: Cardiac tamponade.

- Life-threatening condition requiring urgent intervention
- Causes include trauma, cardiac surgery, inflammation, pericardial neoplasm, aortic dissection
- Speed of fluid accumulation key determinant of symptoms
- Clinical diagnosis confirmed on echocardiography
- Role of CT and MR limited to atypical/chronic cases

Box 5: Nonconstrictive pericarditis.

- Inflammatory response of pericardium involving pericardial thickening and effusion
- Enhancement of pericardium can be seen
- Findings may be localized to part of pericardium
- No features of constriction

where RV free wall can show collapse during diastolic phase, right atrium depicts collapse during late diastole/systole, greater respiratory variations and distended hepatic veins and inferior vena cava due to back flow.

CT and MR have a limited role in the evaluation of acute cardiac tamponade; only long standing or less severe forms may sometimes be seen. CT and MRI may be helpful in non-emergent situations when echocardiographic findings are equivocal. The heart size, excluding the pericardial space is normal or decreased. This is contrary to restrictive cardiomyopathy and pericardial constriction in which the atria are typically enlarged.[2,3] The cavae and hepatic veins which are exterior to the pericardium dilate to accommodate back pooling of blood. Eventually, if pericardial pressure exceeds the ability of the circulation to fill the heart, the cardiac chambers especially right sided chambers collapse.[3]

Cine CT and MR imaging can show the dynamic features suggestive of tamponade. There is collapse of the right ventricular free wall in early diastole and collapse of the right atrial free wall in late diastole. This is because in early diastole less blood is present in the right ventricle than the right atrium, and so, the right ventricle has the least pressure to counteract the pressure of the pericardial effusion. In late diastole, the right atrium has less blood than the right ventricle, so the right atrium has less pressure. This collapse is especially evident during expiration which decreases right heart filling. Throughout the cardiac cycle there is enhanced intraventricular coupling from the taut pericardial space. This most often manifests as abnormal motion of the intraventricular septum. This is seen on cine images as septal rocking or sigmoid septum configuration. The diastolic dysfunction characteristic of tamponade is also well-evaluated on cine images.[3,7]

When cardiac tamponade is atypical, CT and MR may be better than echocardiography. In these unusual situations, the effusions tend to be loculated and exert mass effect on a part of the heart not well-visualized by transthoracic echocardiography, including the right atrium and left atrium.

Oftentimes, these effusions are malignant, postradiation, or postinfectious.[7]

PERICARDITIS

Nonconstrictive Pericarditis (Box 5)

Pericarditis is an inflammatory response of the pericardium which may be a result of various conditions, which include infections, uremia, rheumatic heart disease, systemic diseases like rheumatoid arthritis and sarcoidosis, postinfarction, malignancy and mediastinal irradiation. In about 30% of patients, it may be idiopathic.[12]

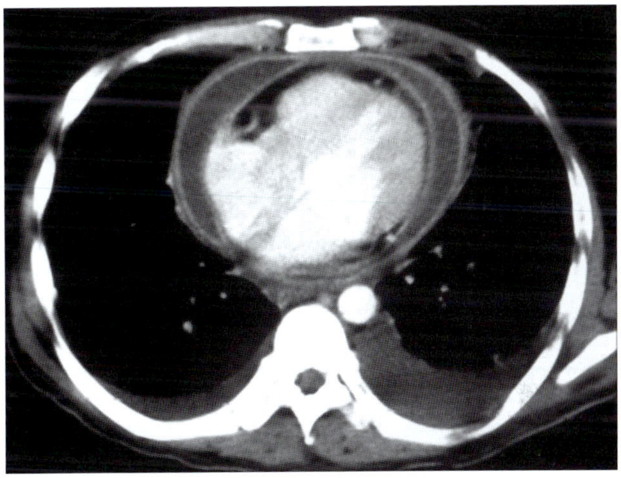

FIG. 10: Nonconstrictive pericarditis: Axial CECT shows enhancing thickened smooth pericardium with associated effusion in a known case of tuberculosis. Bilateral pleural effusions are also seen.

In acute pericarditis, the pericardium may develop a small effusion and become slightly thickened. On contrast-enhanced CT and MRI, acute pericarditis shows enhancement of the pericardium, which can show smooth thickening **(Fig. 10)**. Acute (nonfibrotic) pericarditis enhances in the early arterial phase of contrast administration in contrast to chronic (fibrotic) pericarditis, which enhances late.[21] Associated small effusion may be seen. There are accompanying inflammatory changes in the pericardial fat which may be increased or stranded. On CT imaging, it may sometimes be difficult to differentiate a small effusion from pericardial thickening which may be resolved on echocardiography. Also, care needs to be taken for assessment of pericardium in its entirety as the findings may only be localized.

In chronic inflammatory pericarditis, the effusion may increase or pericardium can get more thickened. The thickened pericardium shows enhancement and may show an irregular contour. This may progress to fibrosing pericarditis which is non-enhancing and shows low-signal intensity on MRI. The latter may or may not be associated with constriction.[3,22]

Constrictive Pericarditis (Box 6)

Constrictive pericarditis is a condition in which cardiac function is impaired by a thickened, rigid and often calcified pericardium. This results in diastolic dysfunction of the heart and subsequent right heart failure. Clinical symptoms and radiological concordance are required to make this diagnosis. It can clinically mimic restrictive cardiomyopathy, hepatic disease, and congestive heart failure. The distinction between constrictive pericarditis and restrictive cardiomyopathy is very important, since the former would benefit from pericardial stripping and the latter would not.

Box 6: Constrictive pericarditis.

- Reduced pericardial compliance leading to diastolic dysfunction
- Causes infection, radiation exposure, postoperative, etc.
- *Morphological findings*:
  - Pericardial thickening with calcification more over right ventricle
  - Unilateral/bilateral atrial enlargement
  - Dilated hepatic veins/IVC
  - Pleural effusion, ascites
  - Pericardial enhancement suggestive of residual inflammation
- *Findings on functional evaluation*:
  - Septal bounce on cine MR imaging
  - MR tagging technique—tag lines remain unbroken in case of pericardial lesions
- Dynamic MR imaging findings help distinguish constrictive pericarditis from restrictive cardiomyopathy

Constrictive pericarditis may be secondary to prior surgery, infection, trauma, radiation, uremia, connective tissue disorder, neoplasm or may be idiopathic.It is more often a sequelae to purulent and tuberculous pericarditis than viral amongst infectious causes.[23] Thickening may be localized involving only a portion of the pericardium, often overlying the right ventricle or may extend around the entire heart. The thickening is usually irregular. Calcified pericardium may be apparent on a chest radiograph **(Figs. 11A to D)**.

Both morphology and functional hemodynamic aspects are used to reach the diagnosis. CT and MR imaging findings center on the demonstration of global or focal thickened or calcified pericardium which is usually greater over the right ventricle, along with secondary morphologic signs of constriction. These include conical or tubular shape of either of the ventricles, sigmoid-shaped interventricular septum, enlargement of one or both atria, narrowing of one or both atrioventricular grooves and large inferior and superior vena cava in comparison with descending aorta[21,24,25] **(Fig. 12A)**. The diagnosis of pericardial constriction is absolutely certain if all these morphologic determinants are present. Any thickening of the pericardium more than a pencil-line is significant. Usually, pericardial thickness is greater than

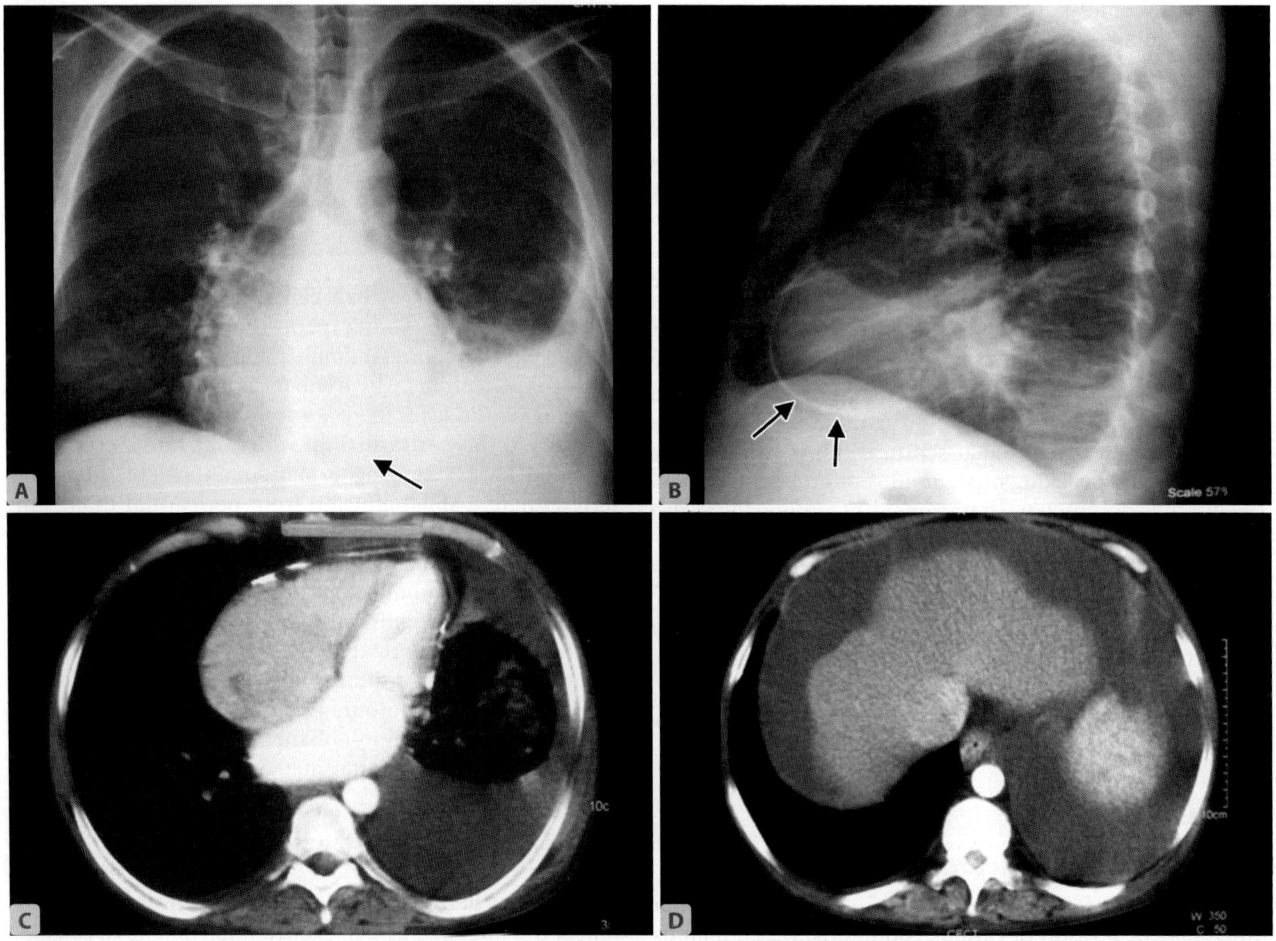

FIGS. 11A TO D: (A and B) Calcific constrictive pericarditis: In a patient with distant history of tuberculosis, posteroanterior (A) and lateral (B) chest radiographs demonstrate curvilinear calcification (arrows) along the lower left and diaphragmatic cardiac border; (C and D) Axial CECT shows global pericardial thickening with calcification. The ventricles are tubular shaped with dilated atria and IVC. Associated left pleural effusion and ascites noted. Liver appears congested with irregular outline suggestive of cardiac cirrhosis.

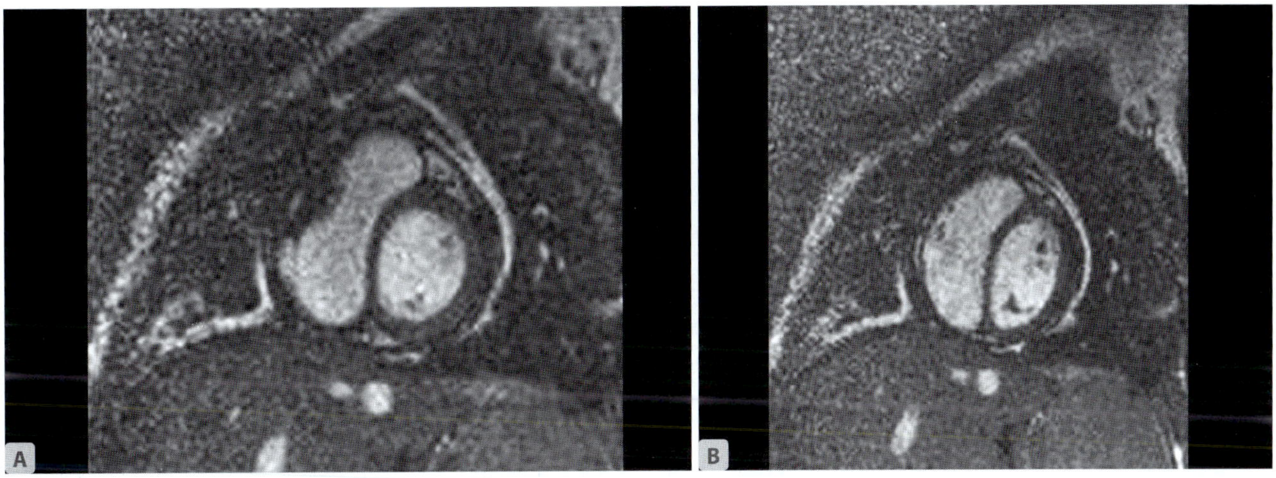

FIGS. 12A AND B: Short axis cine MR images in a patient with constrictive pericarditis in systole (A) and diastole (B) show straightening of the interventricular septum in diastole indicative of impaired right ventricular filling. Pericardium is focally thickened posterior to the left ventricle.

4 mm although there is no direct relationship between the extent of thickness of the pericardium and its hemodynamic significance.[21,26] In the end stage fibrosing forms of constrictive pericarditis, the pericardium usually does not enhance after contrast administration. However, pericardial enhancement, which indicates residual inflammation, may be seen on delayed postcontrast imaging (>70 seconds postcontrast). A small amount of pericardial effusion may also be seen. Calcification of the pericardium is better visualized on CT and strongly suggests constriction of tubercular etiology.[13] However, presence of constriction and calcification are not always related. Atrial dilatation may or may not be seen depending on whether the entire pericardium is abnormal or just the anterior part. This is an insensitive finding as patients with restrictive cardiomyopathy may also demonstrate atrial dilatation. Pleural effusions, hepatic congestion, and ascites may also be seen. Other radiological stigmata of chest tuberculosis should also be looked for. Other causes of pericardial calcification include viral, uremic pericarditis, collagen vascular disease, postoperative setting, radiation exposure and asbestosis. It should be remembered that the diagnosis of pericardial constriction is made only in the appropriate clinical setting.[27]

Since the diagnosis of constriction is ultimately that of altered physiology, cine imaging is a more direct means of confirming the diagnosis. The most sensitive and specific finding is the septal bounce, best appreciated in inspiration. In a study by Francone, et al. septal bounce was seen in 85% of patients with constrictive pericarditis and in no patients without constriction.[28] It is most pronounced at the beginning of inspiration. During inspiration, the negative intrathoracic pressure results in more rapid right heart filling than the left. In early diastole the pressure in the right ventricle is transiently higher than the left, causing the septum to bow leftward due to enhanced ventricular coupling **(Fig. 12B)**. In mid diastole the left ventricular pressure once again becomes higher, pushing the septum rightward, and in late diastole the pressures equalize. The result is shivering of the ventricular septum or septal bounce.[3] Tagging cardiac MR techniques may be of use to depict fibrotic adhesions of pericardial layers **(Figs. 13A to C)**.

Underlying myocardium also needs to be evaluated in these cases as the presence of the myocardial factor (myocardial atrophy or fibrosis) is a contraindication to pericardiectomy, because of the risk of acute dilatation or rupture of one or both cardiac chambers following surgery.[21] Imaging also aids in planning surgery. The presence of a fat plane between the myocardium and pericardium indicates easier dissection.[29]

There are atypical forms of constrictive pericarditis. *Effusive constrictive pericarditis* represents a combination of pericardial tamponade and constrictive pericarditis. This is seen most often following radiation therapy. The typical clinical setting is that pericardial effusion is identified in a patient with symptoms of heart failure and despite drainage of the effusion, the patient continues to have abnormal pericardial dynamics. *Inflammatory constrictive pericarditis* results due to constriction during acute and chronic pericarditis which may be transient. There is accompanying enhancement of pericardium. *Focal pericarditis* may result in constriction if present in strategic location. *Occult constrictive pericarditis* refers to presence of constriction only when there is volume overload and not on routine examination.

PNEUMOPERICARDIUM

Pneumopericardium may result from blunt or penetrating trauma. Other rarer causes may be infectious pericarditis or from a gastrointestinal fistula, increased intrathoracic pressure as in asthma or barotrauma, with adjacent lung infection/cancer, esophageal rupture, cocaine abuse or liver abscess rupture. Pneumopericardium following pneumothorax or pneumomediastinum usually indicates a disruption of the pericardium. On erect chest radiographs, it is seen as a radiolucent band around the heart ('halo sign') limited superiorly by the pericardial reflection at the root of great vessels **(Fig. 14)**. Air may be seen in the transverse pericardial sinus giving the 'transverse band of air' sign.

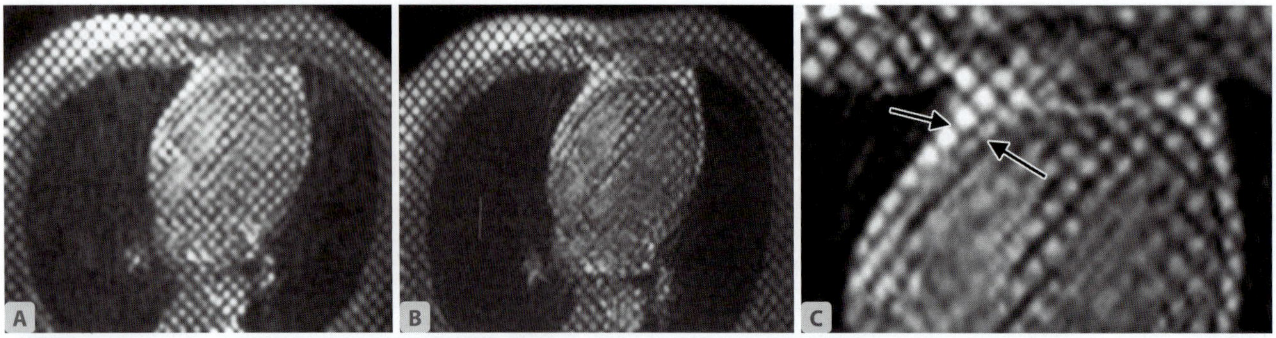

FIGS. 13A TO C: GRE tagging MR imaging in a healthy volunteer in axial plane. The continuity of the tags is lost during cardiac contraction because of shear motion between visceral and parietal layer of the pericardium [seen on the enlarged view (C)].

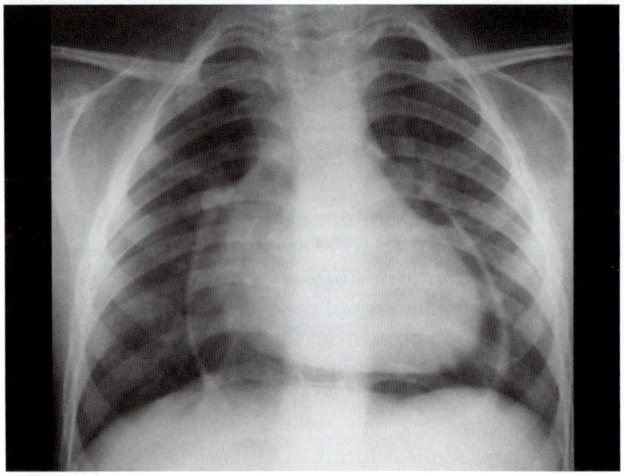

FIG. 14: Pneumopericardium. Posteroanterior chest radiograph shows radiolucent band of air surrounding the heart giving the 'halo sign'.

Lateral radiographs may show lucency of air behind the sternum and anterior to the base of heart and root of aorta ('triangle of air' sign).[30,31] In the setting of penetrating trauma, the presence of pneumopericardium should prompt investigation for potential cardiac laceration. Rarely, tension pneumopericardium may result in tamponade.[7] This may be seen as progressively decreasing cardiothoracic ratio. CT shows distension of SVC, IVC, hepatic veins, renal veins and periportal lymphedema.

PERICARDIAL TUMORS

Metastases (Box 7)

Metastases to the pericardium are more common than involvement of pericadium by primary tumors.

Metastases to the heart and pericardium have been reported at autopsy in 10–12% of patients with known primary malignancies.[10] Pericardial metastases may result from contiguous spread from lung or mediastinum. Other modes may be lymphatic, hematogenous or transvenous route. The common sources of pericardial metastases are lung and breast cancer. Leukemias, lymphomas and melanomas are the other malignancies that can spread to the pericardium.

BOX 7: Pericardial metastases.

- Metastases are commoner than primary pericardial tumors
- *Mode of spread to pericardium*:
  - Direct spread
  - Lymphatic
  - Hematogenous
  - Transvenous
- *Imaging findings include*:
  - Pericardial effusion
  - Pericardial thickening
  - Pericardial mass
- Hemorrhagic pericardial effusion adjacent to a lung/mediastinal mass is suggestive of pericardial invasion

Pericardial metastases when seen are a negative prognostic factor.

An effusion is the most common manifestation of metastatic pericardial disease. Pericardium can get irregularly thickened or a pericardial mass may be seen. To distinguish between inflammatory etiology and metastases (when effusion and thickening are the only findings), follow-up may be required. Pericardial invasion may be suggested when the pericardial line is not seen **(Figs. 15A and B)** and there is pericardial effusion. On MRI images, most deposits show low-signal on T1 and high-signal on T2- weighted images. Metastatic melanoma is an exception; high-signal intensity on T1-weighted images is virtually pathognomonic of this diagnosis.[2] The malignant tumor usually enhances significantly after the administration of contrast material.[6] Pericardium may remain intact adjacent to a primary mass. However, hemorrhagic effusion, seen as high-signal on spin echo MR images confirms the extension of the mass to the pericardium.[6,32] In a patient with a known primary tumor and pericardial effusion, other differential diagnoses are drug-induced and radiation-induced effusions.

Primary Pericardial Tumors

Primary pericardial tumors are rare. These include benign tumors (lipoma, benign teratoma, fibroma, and hemangioma) and malignant tumors (mesothelioma, lymphoma, sarcoma and liposarcoma, malignant teratoma). Although pericardial

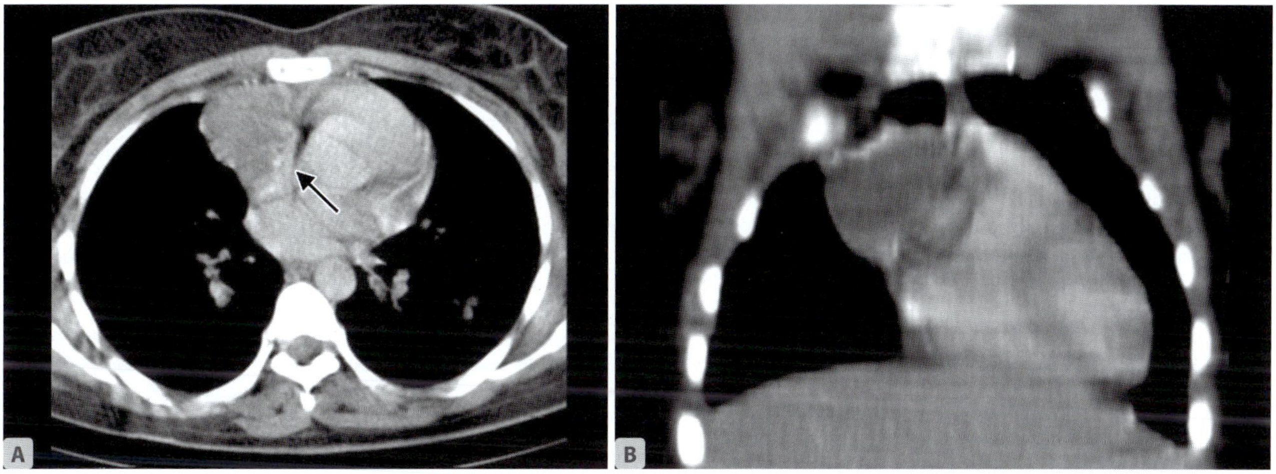

FIGS. 15A AND B: Axial CECT (A) and coronal reformation (arrow); (B) shows thymic carcinoma with direct invasion of the pericardium.

mesotheliomas are rare tumors accounting for less than 1% of all malignant mesotheliomas, they account for nearly half of primary pericardial tumors.[32]

Chest radiography in patients with pericardial mesothelioma typically demonstrates cardiac enlargement, evidence of pericardial effusion, an irregular cardiac contour or diffuse mediastinal enlargement. CT and MR may demonstrate hemorrhagic pericardial effusion accompanied by pericardial nodule or plaques. Lymphoma and sarcoma typically present with large masses accompanied by effusion.

Histopathology is usually necessary to achieve a definitive diagnosis of most pericardial tumors. The diagnosis of few tumors can be aided by specific signal and attenuation characteristics. Lipoma has low attenuation on CT images and high signal intensity on T1-weighted SE images. Presence of calcium or fat in a pericardial mass at CT suggests the diagnosis of a teratoma. Fibroma characteristically has low signal intensity on T2-weighted images with poor enhancement characteristics.[33,34]

Other entities that may simulate a pericardial mass are pericardial hematoma, coronary artery aneurysm and pericardial gossypiboma.[3,12] The signal characteristics of pericardial hematoma are age related. A coronary artery aneurysm should be suspected when a smooth enhancing mass is seen along the expected course of a coronary artery.[3] Pericardial gossypiboma should be considered in a patient with previous cardiac surgery.

CONCLUSION

Congenital disease, infection, injury, neoplasm may all affect the pericardium. Although echocardiography is often initially used to evaluate the pericardium, CT and MR are useful for further evaluation of the disease processes. With the advantages of a large field of view and high soft tissue contrast, these imaging modalities may help differentiate pericardial diseases, especially when echocardiography findings are equivocal.

REFERENCES

1. Gulati G, Sharma S, Kothari SS, et al. Comparison of echo and MRI in the imaging evaluation of intracardiac masses. Cardiovasc Intervent Radiol. 2004;27(5):459-69.
2. Grizzard JG, Ang GB. Magnetic resonance imaging of pericardial disease and cardiac masses. Magn Reson Imaging Clin N Am. 2007;15:579-607.
3. Misselt AJ, Harris SR, Glockner J, Feng D, Syed IS, Araoz PA: MR imaging of the pericardium. Magn Reson Imaging Clin N Am. 2008;16:185-99.
4. Budoff MJ, Achenbach S, Blumenthal RS, et al. Assessment of coronary artery disease by cardiac computed tomography: A scientific statement from the American Heart Association Committee on Cardiovascular Imaging and Intervention, Council on Cardiovascular Radiology and Intervention, and Committee on Cardiac Imaging, Council on Clinical Cardiology. Circulation. 2006;114(16):1761-91.
5. Coles DR, Smail MA, Negus IS, et al. Comparison of radiation doses from multislice computed tomography coronary angiography and conventional diagnostic angiography. J Am Coll Cardiol. 2006;47(9):1840-5.
6. Wang ZJ, Reddy GP, Gotway MB, Yeh BM, Hetts SW, Higgins CB. CT and MR imaging of pericardial disease. Radiographics. 2003;23:S167-80.
7. Lopez Costa I, Bhalla S. Computed tomography and magnetic resonance imaging of the pericardium. Semin Roentgenol. 2008;43(3):234-45.
8. Truong MT, Erasmus JJ, Gladish GW, Sabloff BS, Marom EM, et al. Anatomy of pericardial recesses on multidetector CT: Implications for oncologic imaging. Am J Roentgenol. 2003;181:1109-13.
9. Delille JP, Hernigou A, Sene V, et al. Maximal thickness of the normal human pericardium assessed by electron-beam computed tomography. Eur J Radiol. 1999;9:1183-89.
10. Oyama N, Oyama N, Komuro K, Nambu T, Manning W, Miyasaka K. Computed tomography and magnetic resonance imaging of the pericardium: anatomy and pathology. Magnetic Resonance in Medical Sciences. 2004;3(3):145-52.
11. Broderick LS, Brooks GN, Kuhlman JE. Anatomic pitfalls of the heart and pericardium. Radiographics. 2005;25:441-53.
12. Bogaert J, Francone M. Cardiovascular Magnetic resonance in pericardial diseases. J Cardiovasc Magn Reson. 2009;11(1);14.

13. O' Leary SM, Williams PL, Williams MP. et al. Imaging the pericardium: appearances on ECG-gated 64 detector row cardiac computed tomography. BJR. 2010;83:194-205.
14. Van Son JA, Danielson GK, Schaff HV, et al. Congenital partial and complete absence of the pericardium. Mayo Clin Proc. 1993;68(8):743-47.
15. Ellis K, Leeds NE, Himmelstein A. Congenital deficiencies in partial pericardium: Review with two new cases including successful diagnosis by plain roentgenography. Am J Roentgenol. 1959;82:125-37.
16. Psychidis-Papakyritsis P, de Roos A, Kroft LJM. Functional MRI of congenital absence of the pericardium. Am J Roentgenol. 2007;189:W312-W314.
17. Rajiah P. Cardiac MRI: Part 2, Pericardial disease. AJR. 2011; 197:W621-634.
18. Czum Jm, Silas AM, Althoen MC. Evaluation of the pericardium with CT and MR. ISRN cardiology 2014. http://dx.doi.org/10.1155/2014/174908.
19. Glockner JF. Imaging of pericardial disease. Magn Reson Imaging Clin N Am. 2003;11(1):149-62, vii.
20. Yared K, Baggish AL, Picard MH, Hoffmann U, Hang J. Multimodality imaging of pericardial disease. JACC Cardiovasc Imaging. 2010;3(6):650-60.
21. Rienmuller R, Groll R, Lipton MJ. CT and MR imaging of pericardial disease. Radiol Clin North Am. 2004;42(3):587-601.
22. Kim JS, Kim HH, Yoon Y. Imaging of pericardial diseases. Clinical Radiol. 2007;62:626-31.
23. Imazio M, Brucato A, Maestroni S, et al. Risk of constrictive pericarditis after acute pericardiectomy. Circulation. 2011;124(11): 1270-5.
24. Suh SY, Rha SW, Kim JW, et al. The usefulness of three-dimensional multidetector computed tomography to delineate pericardial calcification in constrictive pericarditis. Int J Cardiol. 2006;113:414-16.
25. Bogaert J, Francone M. Pericardial disease: Value of CT and MR imaging. Radiology. 2012;267(2):340-56.
26. Thavendiranathan P, Verhaert D, Wall MC, et al. Simultaneous right and left heart realtime, free-breathing CMR flow quantification indentifies constrictive physiology. JACC Cardiovasc Imaging. 2012;(1):15-24.
27. Verheart D, Gabriel RS, Johnston D, Lytle BW, Desai, MY Klein AL. The role of multimodality imaging in the management of pericardial disease. Circ Cardiovasc Imaging. 2010;3(3): 333-43.
28. Francone M, Dymarkowski S, Kalantzi M, et al. Realtime cine MRI of ventricular septal motion: A novel approach to assess ventricular coupling. J Magn Reson Imaging. 2005;21(3):305-9.
29. Westwood MA, Moon JC. Cardiovascular magnetic resonance for pericardial disease. Indian J Radiol Imaging. 2007;17(2): 133-36.
30. Ho ML, Gutierrez FR. Chest radiography in thoracic polytrauma. Am J Roentgenol. 2009;192:599-612.
31. Mirvis SE. Imaging of acute thoarcic injury: The advent of MDCT screening. Semin Ultrasound CT MRI. 2005;26:305-31.
32. Grebenc ML, Christenson MLR, Burke AP, et al. Primary cardiac and pericardial neoplasms: radiologic-pathologic correlation. Radiographics. 2000;20:1073.
33. Fussen S, De Boeck BW, Zellweger MJ, et al. Cardiovascular magnetic resonance imaging for diagnosis and clinical management of suspected cardiac masses and tumours. Eur Heart J. 2011;32(12):1551-60.
34. Hoffmann U, Globits S, Frank H. Cardiac and paracardiac masses: Current opinion on diagnostic evaluation by magnetic resonance imaging. Eur Heart J. 1998;19:553-63.

CHAPTER 149

Imaging and Interventions of Aorta

Manphool Singhal, Kartik Ganga, Sanjeev Kumar, Vivek Gupta, Niranjan Khandelwal

INTRODUCTION

The word 'Aorta' is derived from *Latin* word*:* aorta, and *Greek*: aorte which means "a strap to hang (something by)". This term was first used by Aristotle while describing the aorta: how it seems to be 'suspended' above the heart.[1] The function of the aorta has been documented since the ancient times of Bible and Talmud, where it was noted as one of three major vessels entering or leaving the heart, and how it's perforation was linked to death.[2]

The aorta is the largest artery in the body which carries oxygenated blood from left ventricle to various organs of the body. It also functions both as a conduit and a reservoir. Its viscoelastic and compliance properties are responsible for the laminar blood flow during systole, and modulate continued forward flow during diastole.[3]

Aorta is an elastic artery and its wall consists of:

- *Intima:* A thin endothelial layer
- *Media:* The thickest layer consisting of smooth muscles, collagen and elastic fibers.
- *Adventitia:* The outermost layer of collagen and elastic fibers also containing vasa vasorum, nerves and lymphatics.

SEGMENTATION ANATOMY OF AORTA

Aorta is divided into the following parts **(Figs. 1A and B)**:

- **Root:** Comprises of 3 aortic sinuses and extending from aortic valve to sinotubular junction where it becomes the ascending aorta.
- **Ascending aorta:** Extends from sinotubular junction to the origin of brachiocephalic artery.
- **Arch of aorta:** Extends from origin of brachiocephalic artery to the origin of left subclavian artery.
- **Descending aorta:** Extends beyond the origin of left subclavian artery till aortic bifurcation at L4 level into common iliac arteries. It is further divided into thoracic and abdominal portions by the diaphragm, where the aorta passes through the aortic hiatus at D12 level.

A normal narrowing may be present just distal to left subclavian artery and proximal to ligamentum arteriosum

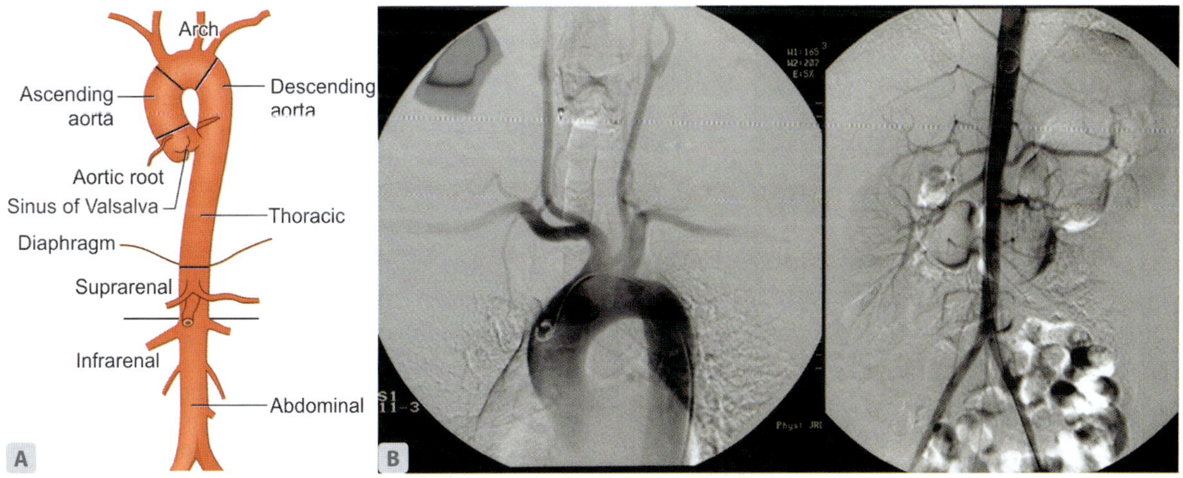

FIGS. 1A AND B: (A) Segmentation anatomy of aorta; (B) Normal angiographic anatomy: Arch and abdominal aortogram (DSA) shows normal branches.

called *isthmus*. Just beyond it, there may be a focal dilatation of the aorta, known as *aortic spindle*.

IMAGING OF AORTA: BASICS

Radiological evaluation of the anatomy and the pathology involving the aorta has undergone considerable refinement in recent years, which has been possible largely due to availability of multidetector CT (MDCT), dual source CT (DSCT) scanners and higher strength newer magnetic resonance imaging (MRI) and advanced software's. These modalities have largely replaced traditional contrast aortography.[4] Technological advances such as isotropic data acquisition with three-dimensional reconstruction capabilities, shorter acquisition times, improvement in processing and volume rendering have made it possible to visualize the aorta and its branches precisely. As a result, the role of catheter angiography is being restricted to special indications and to patients who may require catheter-based interventions.[5]

Angiographic Anatomy

The aorta is broadly divided into thoracic and abdominal aorta **(Figs. 1A and B)**. The thoracic aorta begins at the aortic root just cranial to the aortic valve as the ascending aorta. It courses superiorly and to the left uptil the origin of the right brachiocephalic trunk where the aortic arch begins. The aortic arch continues cranially and posteriorly and gives rise to the left common carotid and left subclavian arteries. At this point, the aorta turns caudally and posterior to form the descending thoracic aorta. A normal narrowing called the *isthmus* may be present just distal to the left subclavian artery and proximal to the ligamentum arteriosum. The isthmus is commonly present in younger individuals and may be focal or extended over a long distance with a mild dilatation beyond it. It may form a small diverticulum called the *ductus diverticulum* **(Fig. 2)**. The descending thoracic aorta continues caudally in the posterior mediastinum slightly on the left side, anterolateral to the spine and posterolateral to the esophagus. It passes through the diaphragmatic hiatus at D12 level where it continues in the retroperitoneum on the left side as the abdominal aorta up to the iliac bifurcation. With age, the aorta shows enlargement of its diameter and tends to follow a more tortuous course.

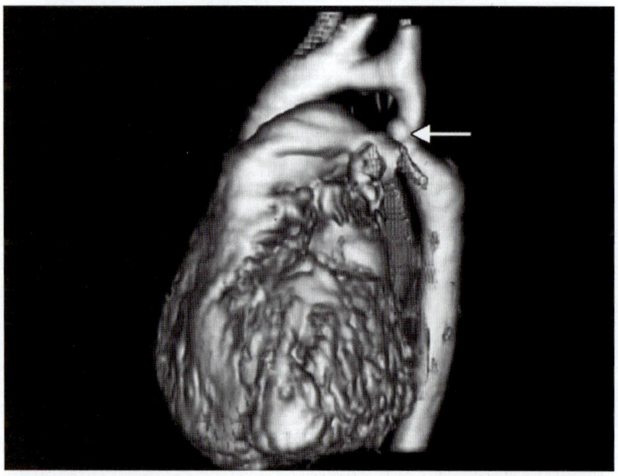

FIG. 2: Ductus diverticulum: CT angiogram (CTA) (Volume rendered-VR) shows isthmus and diverticulum (arrow).

The major branches which arise from the aorta are as follows:

- **Ascending aorta:** Right and left coronary arteries
- **Aortic arch:** Right brachiocephalic trunk (right subclavian and right common carotid artery), left common carotid artery and left subclavian artery
- **Descending thoracic aorta:**
  - Visceral branches: Pericardial branches, bronchial arteries (one on the right and two on the left side), mediastinal branches and phrenic branches.
  - Parietal branches: Intercostal arteries and subcostal arteries
- **Abdominal aorta:**
  - Ventral: Unpaired: celiac axis, superior mesenteric artery and inferior mesenteric artery
  - Lateral: Paired—inferior phrenic artery, middle suprarenal artery, renal artery, testicular or ovarian arteries
  - Dorsal: Lumbar (5-Paired), median sacral (unpaired)
  - Terminal: Common iliac arteries (paired).

The Measurement (Diameter) of Aorta

The aortic diameter varies with body size, sex and ageing. The average mean diameter is as follows:[6]

Aortic root	:	3.6 cm
Aortic arch	:	3.5 cm
Proximal descending aorta	:	2.6 cm
Distal descending aorta	:	2.4 cm
Abdominal aorta	:	2.0 cm

The ratio of ascending and descending aorta is 2.2 (young) and 1.2 (elderly). In adults, the aortic diameter increases by approximately 0.1 cm per decade.

Normal Anatomic Variations

There are various normal anatomic variations involving the arch, brachiocephalic vessels and visceral branching patterns of the abdominal aorta. The most common variation is the common origin of brachiocephalic trunk and left common carotid artery which is seen in approximately 20% of the population **(Fig. 3)**. In about 5% of the population, the left vertebral artery arises directly from the aorta **(Fig. 3)**. In 1%, there is a common origin of both common carotid arteries and a paired brachiocephalic trunk. Aortic arch anomalies include aberrant origin of the right subclavian artery as the last branch of the thoracic aorta just distal to left subclavian artery (1%), right-sided aortic arch (1%), and aberrant origin of left subclavian artery (1%), etc.[7]

The most common variant of the abdominal aorta involves the origin of the hepatic artery. The left lobe of liver may be supplied completely or partially by the left hepatic artery originating from the left gastric artery (25%). The "replaced origin" of the right hepatic artery from the superior mesenteric artery (SMA) may be seen in 10% of the population. Rarely, the common hepatic artery may take origin directly from

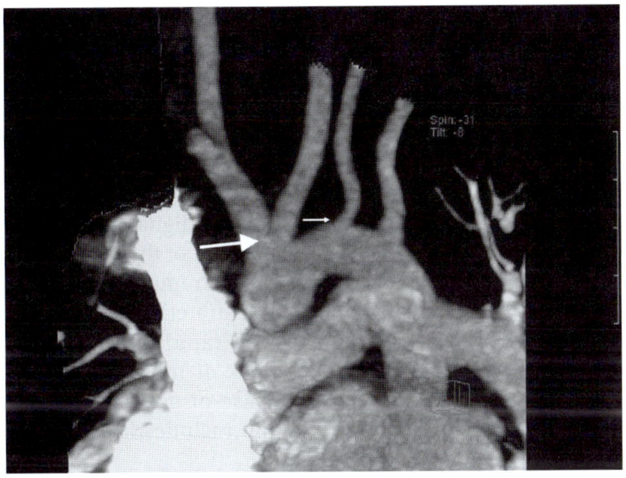

FIG. 3: MIP image of CTA showing common origin of right brachiocephalic and left common carotid arteries (thick arrow). Also seen is direct origin of the left vertebral artery from arch of aorta (thin arrow).

the SMA or the aorta or the celiac axis and SMA may have a common origin.[7]

IMAGING MODALITIES

- *Noninvasive:*
    - Ultrasound (US): Transthoracic echocardiography (TTE), duplex scanning, color Doppler (CD), transesophageal echocardiography (TEE) and intravascular ultrasound (IVUS).
    - Computed tomography (CT): MDCT or DSCT
    - MRI: Three-dimensional contrast-enhanced MR angiography (3D CE-MRA), bright blood (steady state free precession-SSFP) imaging, various black blood inversion sequences, a short tau inverse recovery (STIR) and phase contrast (PC) sequences for flow quantifications
    - Nuclear fusion imaging: Nuclear fusion imaging (PET) with 18-flurorodeoxyglucose (18F-FDG) with either CT or MRI has increasing role now in the evaluation of systemic vasculitis, in the detection of vascular inflammation, delineating disease extent as well as treatment response evaluation
- *Invasive:* Catheter angiography—conventional or digital. In addition, plain radiographs of the chest and/or abdomen, barium swallow, etc. may suggest aortic disease and may provide some clues for further imaging.

Ultrasound

Ultrasound whether TTE or abdominal duplex scanning is the first noninvasive imaging modality for evaluation of aortic diseases and has sufficient accuracy for the purpose of diagnosis as well as surveillance. Technological improvement including combination of B-mode with pulsed wave Doppler and color flow mapping have increased the utility of US in the diagnosis as well as follow-up of aortic diseases. It is cost effective and portable with no hazards of ionizing radiation. However, the quality of the examination may be affected by patient factors such as bowel gas, obesity and it is highly operator dependent.

TEE and IVUS are two major advances in US that have modified preoperative aortic imaging.

Transesophageal Echocardiography

It has overcome many of the limitations of TTE and has a high degree of accuracy in skilled hands. One of the main advantages of TEE, especially in unstable patients, is that the examination can be performed safely and quickly at the bed side.

High resolution imaging of the thoracic aorta is possible with TEE. A 5 MHz one or two phased array transducer is mounted on the top of a gastroscope which is manipulated in the esophagus to get high resolution images of the thoracic aorta. The high image quality is possible because of close proximity to the heart and great vessels, absence of interposed air/bone and excellent acoustic coupling of the transducer face with the esophageal mucosa. In thoracic aorta imaging, TEE provides excellent information except for a 1–3 cm segment of the distal ascending aorta or proximal arch which cannot be imaged because of tracheal air; this is known as the "blind-spot".[8]

The limitations are that it requires a great deal of the physician's skill and it is not possible in patients suffering from esophageal stricture/tumors.

Intravascular Ultrasound

It is a relatively new imaging modality, used mainly during coronary and peripheral interventions. It provides 2D, cross-sectional images of the vessel lumen with good resolution. It allows evaluation of plaque morphology, vessel walls, and perivascular structures. It has not been used widely in aortic evaluation but it has the potential to provide useful information.[9]

Computed Tomography

The advances in CT technology have broadened its use for screening, diagnosis, endovascular treatment planning or preoperative evaluation and post-treatment follow-up of aortic diseases. It is more commonly used than MRI because of fast acquisition, high temporal and spatial resolution, and provision for ECG-gating especially for assessment of ascending aorta.[10-12]

CT Angiography Technique

With the advent of MDCT and DSCT scanners entire aorta and its branches can be imaged in a single breath hold with excellent image quality without venous contamination.[10]

Present scanners allow acquisition with radiation optimization with high temporal resolution (73 milliseconds-128 DSCT). Newer techniques like prospective triggering, ECG-based tube current modulation, body adaptive automatic dose calculation(exposure), excellent image quality with lower tube kilovoltage (kVp) setting by iterative images reconstruction algorithms have revolutionized the vascular imaging like never before.[10,13-15]

For ascending aorta evaluation ECG gating is usually desirable especially when imaging Standford type A dissection and aneurysm for simultaneous evaluation of coronary arteries, and for planning transcatheter aortic valve implantation (TAVI).

A typical protocol for image acquisition of entire aorta on a 64 MDCT/128 DSCT (which we routinely use at our institution) is given below, which can be customized according to the area of interest (thoracic or abdominal aorta).

Area coverage: The scan should cover area 3 cm above the aortic arch till the level of femoral heads, to include the entire aorta and the origins of its major branches. The imaging till proximal femoral arteries is essential for planning of endovascular treatment.

Contrast injection protocol: Since, the aorta is a large artery, dilution of contrast occurs rapidly thus a high rate of injection is required. If possible dual head pressure injector with saline chase is recommended to minimize/avoid artifacts caused by the high-density contrast in the superior vena cava. Flow rate should be 3–4 mL/second and volume should be calculated as follows:

Flow rate × (scan time + scan delay)

This should be followed by saline chase with the same flow rate for 5–6 seconds.

Acquisition of data: Since, imaging is to be done when the contrast density is maximum in the lumen, 'bolus chase' technique is preferred over fixed time delay, with threshold of contrast density kept between 100–200 HU (at level of ascending aorta) to trigger the acquisition with delay of 4–5 seconds to achieve maximum luminal enhancement **(Table 1)**.[16,17]

Data analysis: Data thus acquired can be reconstructed in axial or 3D images [maximum intensity projections (MIP), shaded surface display (SSD) or volume rendered technique (VRT)]. The 3D depiction of the entire aorta depicts the entire extent of the pathology in a single image and any number of desired projections can be made. This can be done with either VRT or MIP technique **(Figs. 4A to C)**. When detailed evaluation of pathology is required thin MIP up to 0.5 mm can be made and evaluated.

The major advantages of CTA over a digital subtraction angiography of the aorta are visualization of the wall and its surrounding changes. Pathologies like intramural hematoma can be easily overlooked on digital substratction angiography (DSA). The other advantages being rapid imaging time, uniform arterial enhancement, lack of motion artifacts, identification of branch vessels, ease of use and it being less expensive. The major limitation includes lack of "flow quantification".

Magnetic Resonance Imaging and MR Angiography

Magnetic resonance angiography of the aorta offers certain advantages over CT angiography. Most important is that since it does not involve radiation, repeated examination can be done as required for follow-up, safely without any radiation concern.

One major advantage of MRI is that flow quantification and direction of flow can now be determined with advanced MR applications and MR angiography techniques.

Several techniques are available to image the aorta and can be broadly classified into:[11,12,18-22]

A. 3D contrast-enhanced MR angiography (3D CE-MRA)
B. White blood imaging—static and cine imaging
C. Black blood imaging—static imaging
D. Phase contrast (PC) sequences—for flow quantification.

TABLE 1: Scan protocol for 128 DSCT angiography of the entire aorta.

S. No.	CT coronary angiography scan parameters	Details of parameters
1.	Scan area	3 cm above the aortic arch till the level of femoral heads
2.	Data acquisition technique	Bolus tracking technique (region of interest in the ascending aorta with preset of 100 HU)
3.	Scan delay	5 seconds after achievement of 100 HU
4.	Kilovoltage	100–120 KV according to body habitus, sex and age
5.	Tube current	Automatic exposure control system-based tube current modulation
6.	Detector collimation	2 × 64 × 0.6 mm
7.	Slice acquisition	2 × 128 × 0.6 mm by means of a z-flying focal spot
8.	Gantry rotation time	280 milliseconds
9.	Temporal resolution	75 milliseconds
10.	Reconstructed slice thickness	0.75 mm with a reconstruction increment of 0.5 mm
11.	Image window	Soft-tissue convolution kernel (B26f)
12.	ECG gating *(for ascending aorta only)*	Retrospective ECG gating with tube current modulation
13.	Image post-processing	Images construction in multiplanar, maximum intensity projection and volume rendering along with axial data set

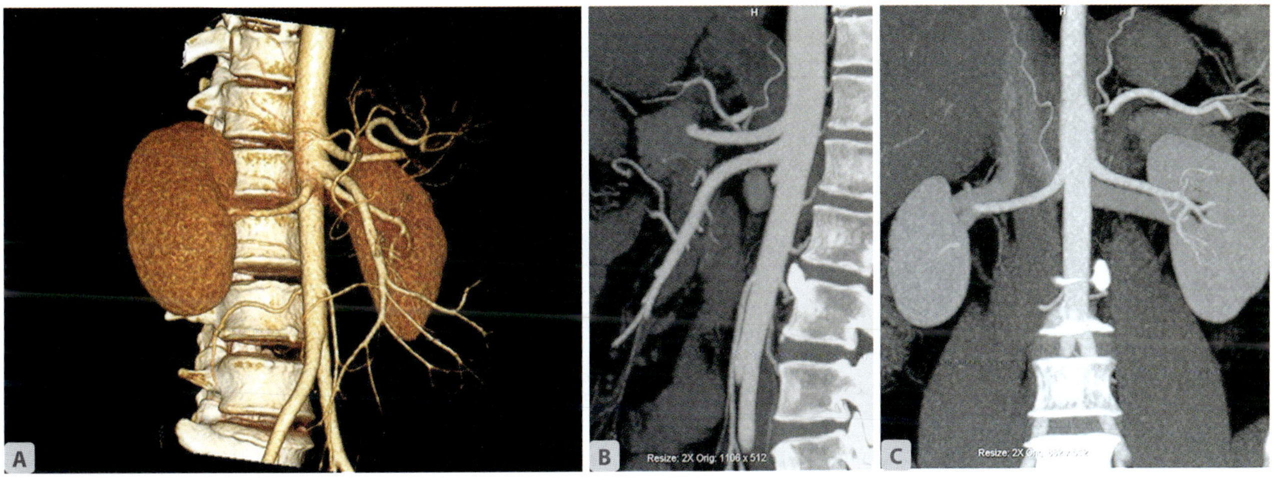

FIGS. 4A TO C: Normal abdominal CTA acquired on 128 DSCT: Volume rendering (A) and maximum intensity projection (B and C) projections showing major branches of aorta.

3D Contrast-enhanced MR Angiography (3D CE-MRA)

3D CE-MRA is gadolinium-enhanced 3D gradient echo (3D-GRE) where thin contiguous image partitions are obtained in a single breath-hold. It uses heavily T1-weighted 3D-GRE technique and is the work horse for evaluation of vascular abnormalities of primarily thoracic aorta **(Fig. 5)**. It allows post-processing just like CT angiography and techniques like MIP reformation, volume rendering and multiplanar reformation of the images can be generated for analysis.[11,12,23]

It is done with injection of gadolinium-based contrast agents (0.1 mmol/kg body weight) with a flow rate of 2–5 mL per second, followed by a saline flush of 20 mL injected at the same flow rate immediately after contrast administration. Scan can be started after a fixed time interval as determined by doing a test scan using a small amount of contrast or by MR fluoroscopy method when contrast reaches left ventricle.

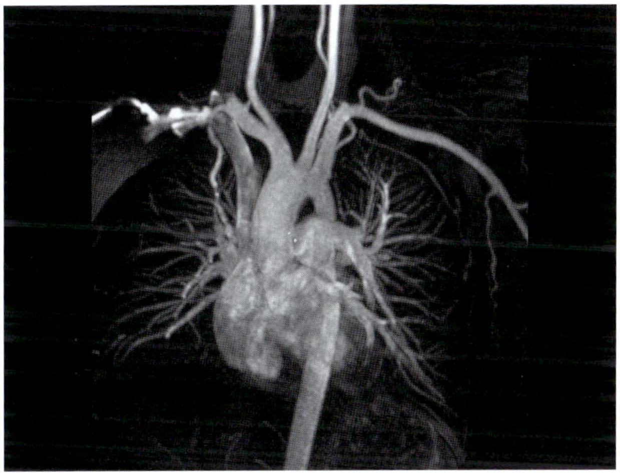

FIG. 5: 3D MIP image at 3T of contrast-enhanced MRA showing aortic arch, ascending and descending thoracic aorta and its major branches with high spatial resolution and without any artifacts.

Bright Blood Imaging

Bright blood imaging provides images with blood having hyperintense signal that works on steady-state free-precession (SSFP) sequence (FIESTA, TrueFISP). It is a short TE and TR sequence, which provides very high and homogeneous intraluminal signal even in cases of turbulent flow because this sequence depends mainly on a function of the T2/T1 ratio **(Figs. 6A to D)**.

SSFP images can be acquired in both breath-hold and free-breathing manners, either with or without ECG-gating and navigator/respiratory trigger. SSFP can provide rapid bright-blood images with high-contrast resolution. SSFP sequences can also be acquired in a cine mode, and have become the foundation for cine imaging. Advantages are the higher signal-to-noise ratio (SNR), shorter imaging duration, and freedom from the reliance on inflow effects for signal generation. This sequence has benefited from the application of parallel imaging techniques, allowing high temporal resolution, large filed of view (FOV) imaging of the thoracic aorta, and left ventricular outflow during acceptable breath-holds as low as 5–6 seconds. The inherently high blood signal achieved using SSFP throughout a cine acquisition period has been shown to aid evaluation of aortic mural and valvular characteristics and allowing exclusion of aortic dissection. SSFP is the most promising of the "bright-blood" noncontrast-enhanced MR angiography techniques.[20-22]

Black Blood Imaging

Black blood employs the inherent contrast between the rapidly flowing blood (flow void) and aortic wall to generate images so that aortic wall is well depicted. It can be obtained either with spin echo (either conventional or echo-train spin-echo techniques) or double inversion recovery sequences. Short tau inversion recovery (STIR) sequence is restricted for demonstration of wall edema.[11,20,21] Usually image acquisition is with ECG-gating, exploiting the contrast between rapidly flowing blood and the aortic wall **(Figs. 6A to D)**.

Black blood imaging is recommended when analysis of aortic wall pathology is desirable such as mural hematoma

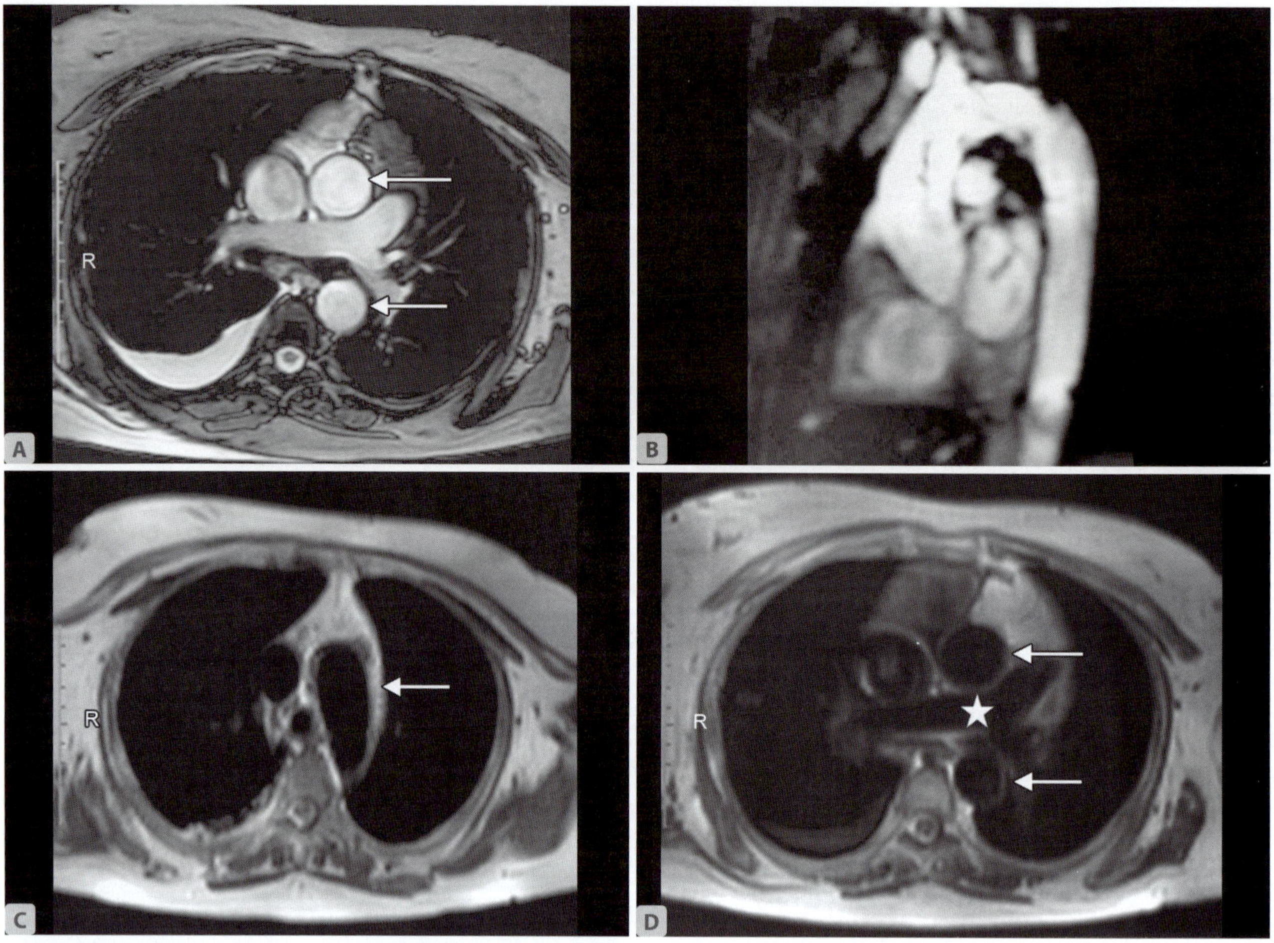

FIGS. 6A TO D: Axial (A) and "candy cane" view (B) SSFP images (bright blood images) at 3T through the thoracic aorta showing bright aortic lumen (arrows) due to sensitivity of the method to flowing blood; (C and D) Axial black blood double inversion recovery sequence images at 3T through the thoracic aorta showing dark aortic lumen with well-delineated arch (arrow in C), ascending and descending thoracic aorta (arrows in D) and pulmonary arteries (star in D).

and aortoarteritis. It may also be useful for the depiction of intraluminal abnormalities, such as dissection flaps and tumor thrombus.

Luminal signal void occurs because intravascular protons only produce signal if they are exposed to both a 90° excitation pulse and subsequent refocusing pulse while traveling through the image slice.[11,12] Therefore, low flow and entry/exit slice phenomena may produce high signal in the aortic lumen, artificially simulating wall disease, so before any conclusion is drawn all sequences and imaging planes need careful inspection and interpretation.

Phase Contrast (PC) Sequences

Quantification of aortic flow especially in aortic regurgitation, stenosis, congenital heart diseases and coarctation of aorta is required for management which is possible with PC sequences. It is based upon the principle that protons passing through a magnetic field gradient undergo a phase change in proportion to velocity, and this is utilized to measure the flow velocities within the aortic lumen during the entire cardiac cycle for measurement of forward flow, regurgitation and stenosis.[24-26]

18F-fluorodeoxyglucose (18F-FDG) with either CT or MRI

Fusion imaging of 18F-FDG PET with CT/MRI is now emerging as the modality of choice as it not only provides the anatomical imaging with high spatial resolution both also specific information about disease activity as 18F-FDG is a surrogate marker of increased activity of inflammatory cells. In specific it delineates extent of vascular inflammation and response to treatment in cases of aortitis. It also helps in selection of appropriate sites for biopsy—histopathologic confirmation of diagnosis.[27-29]

Catheter Angiography

It is the most definitive study in the evaluation of aortic disease. Both conventional angiography and DSA provide detailed anatomic information including aberrant origin of vessels. But DSA saves time, expenses on films and on contrast. The overlying bowel gas or osseous structures that obscure the area of interest is avoided. Contrast-related complications may be avoided by using CO_2 gas as contrast agent. Intravenous DSA, once the preferred noninvasive technique, has largely been discarded because of technical difficulties and poor contrast resolution. Nonetheless, it can be used in a limited way in acute settings like trauma. There has been progressive decrease in the size of catheter used from 6–7 French to 4–5 French, low flow rates and smaller arterial punctures with overall reduction in mortality and morbidity rate. All these factors have pushed the most invasive investigation to an outpatient procedure.[5]

Technique

A 5 or 6F arterial sheath is placed in the femoral or brachial artery by puncturing it with 18G puncture needle under strict aseptic precautions under local anesthesia: 2500 U of heparin is used normally for diagnostic studies. A 5F pigtail catheter is introduced over a 0.035"/0.032" guide wire in the ascending aorta (for arch study) 2.5 inches above the aortic valve or in the abdominal aorta (around T12) just above the origin of celiac axis. 25–30 cc of non-ionic contrast is injected at a flow rate of 12–14cc/sec through a power injector. A 45° LAO projection is taken for arch study and a straight AP and lateral views are taken for the abdominal aorta. Further studies like selective injection into branch vessels, lateral or oblique projection may be done depending upon the initial aortographic findings. After reviewing the entire study, the catheter and the arterial sheath are removed and pressure compression is applied at puncture site for 12–15 minutes till the bleeding stops.

Complications of Angiography

These are divided into three major categories: Reactions to contrast media, complications related to arterial puncture site and systemic complications related to arterial catheterization. A proper and carefully applied technique may reduce the complications rate to less than 0.1%.[30]

The contraindications of angiography include:

- Previous anaphylactic contrast reaction,
- Low cardiac output, and
- Anuria and bleeding diathesis.

INDICATIONS FOR IMAGING THE AORTA

Various diseases afflicting the aorta may warrant either noninvasive or invasive aortic imaging. The diseases can be classified as:

- *Congenital*:
  - Aortic arch anomalies
  - Coarctation
  - Aortic atresia
  - Aortic stenosis
- *Acquired*:
  - Aneurysms
  - Dissection
  - Aortitis
  - Trauma
  - Atherosclerosis.

CONGENITAL AORTIC ANOMALIES

Aortic Arch Anomalies

- Left aortic arch with aberrant origin of right subclavian artery **(Figs. 7A and B)**
- Right aortic arch
  - With mirror image branching
  - With aberrant origin of left subclavian artery
- Cervical arch
- Double aortic arch **(Figs. 8A and B)**

The detailed description and imaging findings are discussed in relevant chapters in this book.

Coarctation of Aorta

It is a congenital aortic narrowing in the region of the isthmus. It is more common in males (M:F = 4:1) and is rare in blacks. It is of two types:

1. Localized or adult or postductal or juxta-ductal type: It is the most common type where there is a short segment

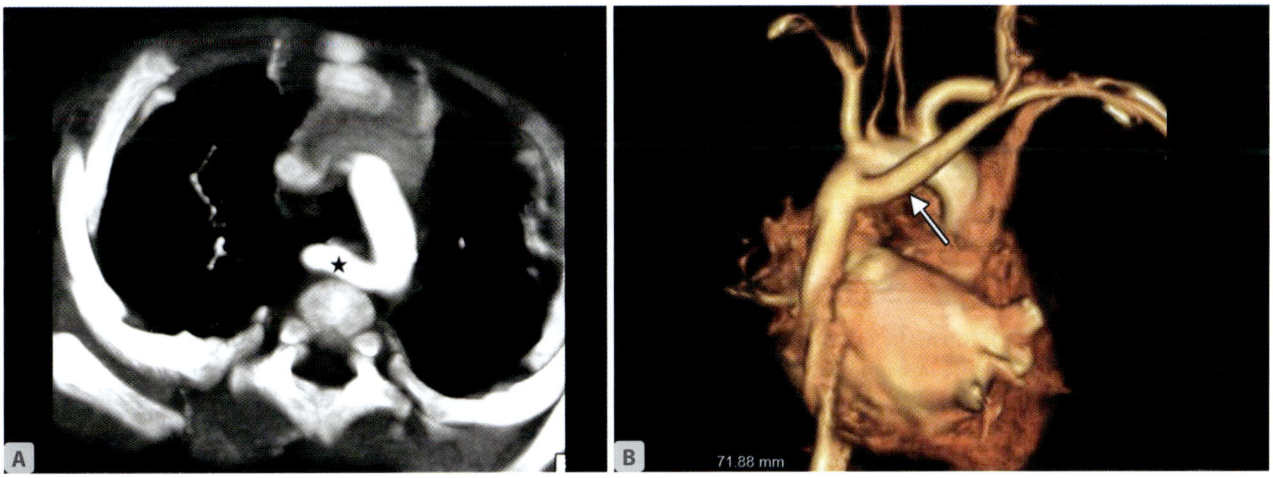

FIGS. 7A AND B: (A) MIP axial and (B) VR (posterior projection) shows aberrant origin of right subclavian artery (star and arrow) with retroesophageal course (star) from left-sided arch.

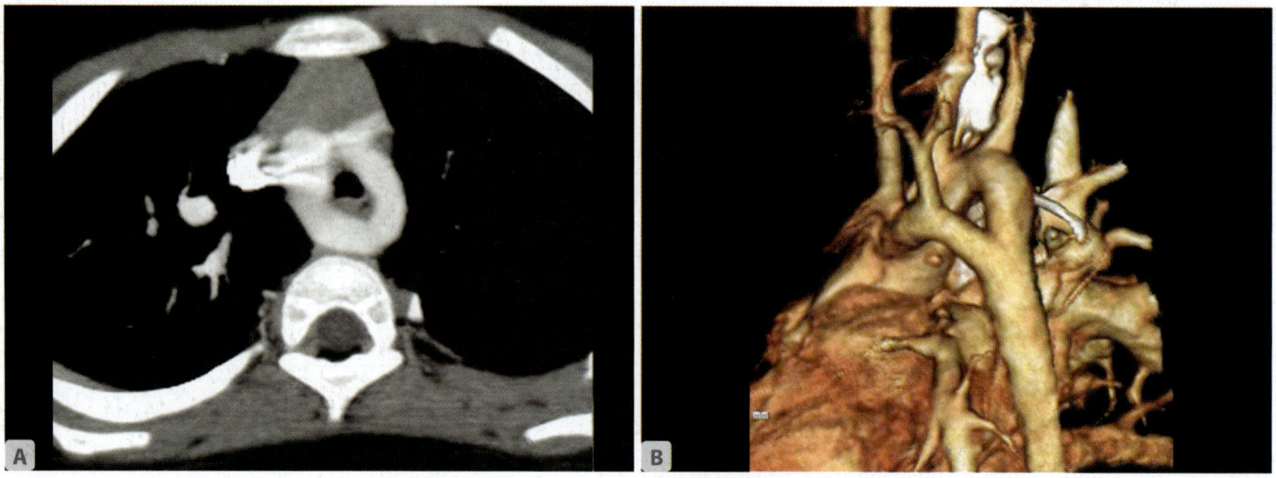

FIGS. 8A AND B: (A) MIP axial and (B) VR image (posterior projection) shows double aortic arch encircling trachea.

narrowing close to the ligamentum arteriosum. Coexistent cardiac anomalies are uncommon.

2. Tubular hypoplasia or infantile or preductal or diffuse type: There is hypoplasia of a long segment of the aortic arch after the origin of the brachiocephalic trunk. Coexistent cardiac anomalies are common.

Associated Anomalies

- Bicuspid aortic valve (25–50%)
- *Cardiac shunts*:
  - Patent ductus arteriosus (PDA) (33%)
  - Ventricular septal defect (VSD) (15%)
- Turner's syndrome (13–15%)
- Cerebral berry aneurysms (5–7%)

A review of the natural history of coarctation revealed that of those patients who survived infancy, 20% were dead before the age of 20 years, 50% by 32 years and 90% by 58 years.[31] Most common causes of death are due to cardiac failure, aortic rupture, infective endocarditis, intracerebral hemorrhage, etc.

Hemodynamics in Adults

The collateral circulation distal to the coarctation is through the subclavian arteries and its branches like internal mammary artery to intercostal arteries, scapular artery to anterior spinal artery and transverse cervical artery to lateral thoracic artery.

Radiological Findings

Conventional X-ray Chest

- Rib notching **(Table 2)**: It usually takes several years to develop. It is due to pressure erosion by the enlarged and tortuous intercostal arteries. It is typically bilateral but asymmetrical and is best seen on the inferior aspects of the posterior thirds of 4th to 9th ribs **(Fig. 9)**. It will be seen only on the left side if there is an aberrant origin of the right subclavian artery below the coarctation and only on the right side if there is involvement of the left subclavian artery in the coarctation.

TABLE 2: Causes of rib notching.

Aortic obstruction	**Pulmonary oligemia**
Coarctation	Fallot's tetralogy
Takayasu's arteritis	Pulmonary artery atresia
Thrombosis of abdominal aorta	Miscellaneous:
Subclavian artery obstruction	• Chronic SVC or IVC obstruction
Blalock-Taussig shunt	• Intercostal AV fistula
Takayasu's arteritis	• Fallot's tetralogy
Coarctation	• Pulmonary artery atresia

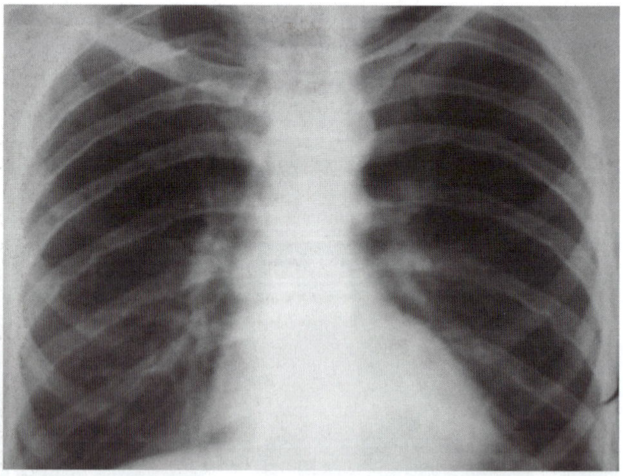

FIG. 9: Chest X-ray showing notching of posterior ribs bilaterally most prominent along inferior borders in a case of aortic coarctation.

- Left ventricular hypertrophy.
- *Figure of '3' appearance*: It is due to dilated left subclavian artery above the coarctation (CoA), a pinching at the site of CoA and the post-stenotic dilatation below.
- Small and flat aortic knuckle.

Angiography: It has been used for long to image CoA. A cardiac catheterization is also required to evaluate cardiac abnormalities and for the measurement of pressure gradient across the lesion. The CoA can usually be crossed from the femoral route but may require brachial artery catheterization in extreme stenosis. Multiple views are required in asymmetric lesions. The angiograms reveal the site, degree and size of the stenosis as well as the collateral circulation **(Figs. 10A to F)**.

Noninvasive Imaging

CTA, MRA and USG are often used in conjunction with angiography in the evaluation of coarctation. CT angiography can depict the morphology of the coarcted segment with good spatial resolution as well as status of aortic arch vessels and collaterals. However, it is not able to measure the gradient across the lesion, nor the direction of the flow. Still it is an important investigation for planning stent graft implantation and follow-up imaging after surgery **(Figs. 10A to F)**.

MRA now in addition to the anatomic details can give the information of the dynamics involved in the coarctation of aorta, noninvasively **(Fig. 11)**.

Phase-contrast velocity-encoded cine MR can give reliable information regarding flow velocity, flow volume and the pressure gradient across the stenosed segment. Also, it can give information regarding the collaterals and the direction of flow in them. Though this technique is promising, its use in routine clinical practise is limited because it also suffers from certain drawbacks like underestimation of flow volume and velocity and is also poor in small vessel assessment.

Management of Aortic Coarctation

Societal guidelines recommend that coarctation correction should be performed as early as possible (ideally as early as possible in childhood) to reduce the long-term morbidity and enhance survival.[32,33] The indications for corrective treatment are listed in **Box 1**. Percutaneous interventions and surgical correction are both acceptable options for coarctation repair. A multidisciplinary team (i.e. cardiologist, interventionists, and surgeons) with experience in treating patients with congenital heart disease should be involved in deciding the management protocol and is dependent on the morphology, age, associated cardiac lesions as well as the availability of either an experienced interventionist or surgeon. A suggested algorithmic approach to manage coarctation is given in **Flowchart 1**.

Balloon angioplasty may also be performed as a palliative procedure in very sick patients as part of a staged protocol for initial stabilization of the patient.

Pseudocoarctation is a condition that results from an elongation of the distal aortic arch which, as it is fixed at the arterial ligament, bulges backwards above and below

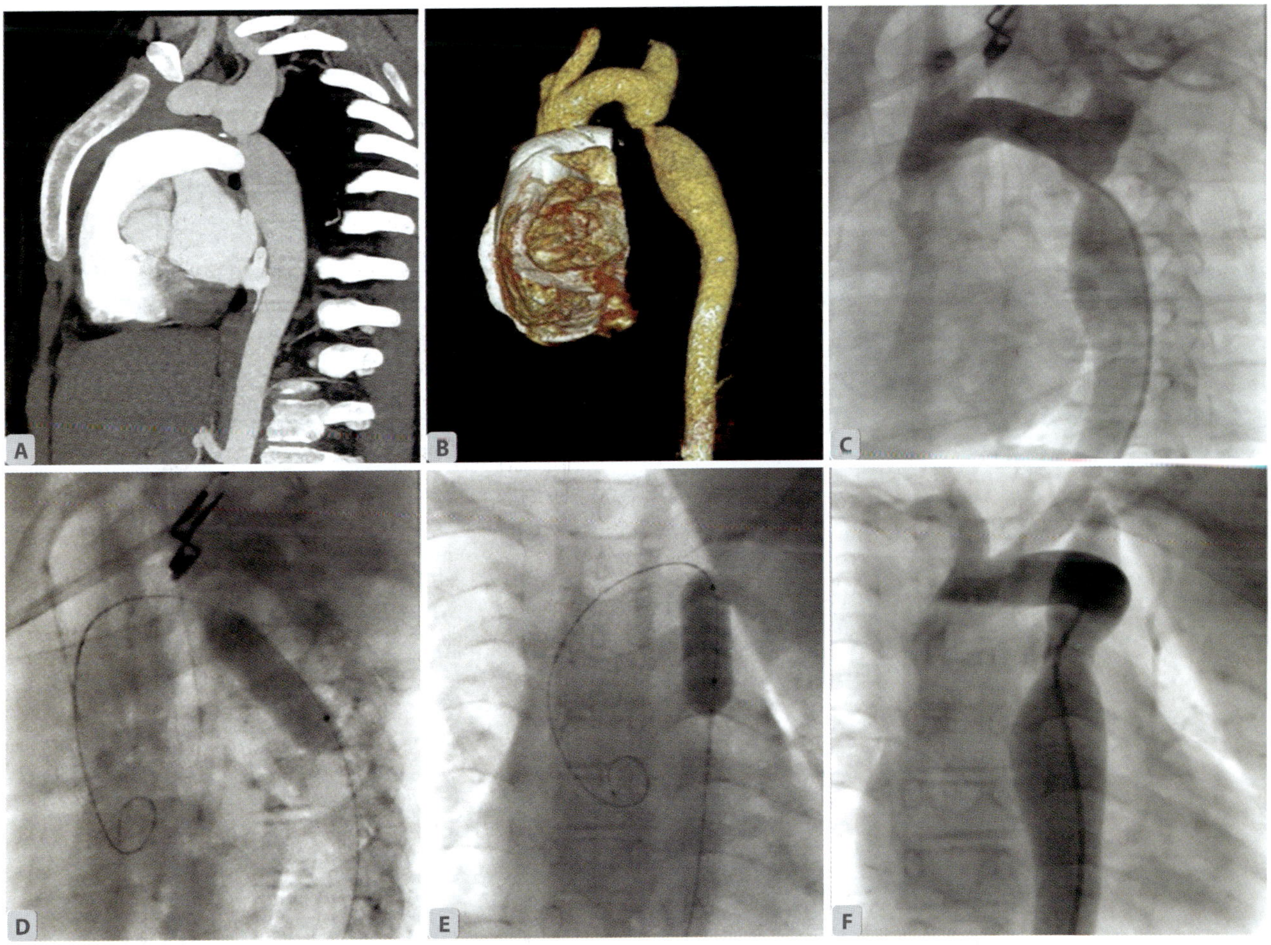

FIGS. 10A TO F: Balloon angioplasty of aortic coarctation. (A to C) Computed tomography and angiography showing coarctation of aorta; (D and E) Balloon angioplasty of the coarctation; (F) Postballoon angioplasty angiography showing significant reduction in severity of stenosis.

this point causing a 'double aortic' bulge. There is no hemodynamic obstruction. It may present as a mediastinal mass and the true nature can be demonstrated on CT or MRI.

Interrupted aortic arch is a rare condition in which a localized atresia of the arch occurs distal to the left subclavian artery (Type A: 42%), **(Figs. 12A to C)** distal to the left common carotid artery (Type B: 53%) or distal to the brachiocephalic trunk (Type C: 5%). It is usually associated with various cardiac anomalies such as PDA and VSD.

ACQUIRED AORTIC DISEASES

In this section, imaging in particular reference to endovascular and surgical management of aortic aneurysms, pathologies causing acute aortic syndrome, surveillance of aortic aneurysms is discussed in detail.

Imaging of common inflammatory aortitis like Takayasu and IgG4 related aortitis are also described. Infective or mycotic inflammatory pathologies have been included in the aneurysm section.

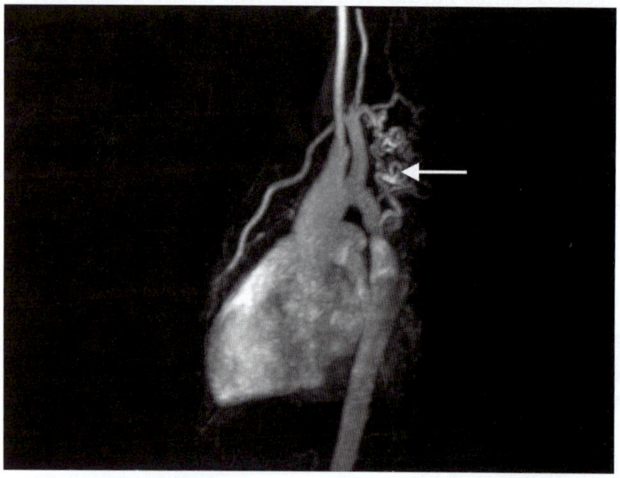

FIG. 11: MRA-MIP image lateral projection shows the coarctation, its length and the status of the aorta proximal and distal to it. Also note presence of collaterals seen on this MRA image (arrow).

Box 1: Indications for corrective treatment.

- Peak to peak (or maximum instantaneous) coarctation gradient ≥20 mm Hg
- Peak to peak coarctation gradient <20 mm Hg in the presence of significant coarctation with imaging evidence of significant collateral flow

AORTIC ANEURYSMS

An aneurysm is a localized or diffuse dilatation of an artery. Aneurysm is defined as a permanent focal dilatation of the artery having ≥ 50% increase in diameter compared with the expected normal diameter of the artery in question. Ectasia is arterial dilatation <150% of normal arterial diameter. Arteriomegaly is diffuse arterial dilatation involving several arterial segments, with an increase in diameter >50% in comparison with the expected normal arterial diameter.[34]

Incidence

The incidence of aortic aneurysm varies from 4% (60–70 years) to 11% (70 years and above) and is probably increasing. Patients with hypertension, coronary artery disease, peripheral vascular disease and those whose immediate family have aneurysms are at a higher risk of developing aortic aneurysms.

Classification

An aneurysm can be classified as:

- *True or false* **(Fig. 13)**: True aneurysms consist of all three layers of the arterial wall (intima, media, and adventitia) whereas false aneurysms are due to focal perforation of the aortic wall limited externally by the adventitia, perivascular connective tissue, or by hematoma.
- *Saccular or fusiform* **(Figs. 14A to D)**: Saccular aneurysms usually arise from a distinct portion of the aortic wall and have a mouth, while fusiform aneurysms involve the total circumference of an artery and have no distinctive mouth.
- *Congenital or acquired*: Acquired aneurysms are more frequent than congenital aneurysms.

FLOWCHART 1: Approach to treatment of coarctation of aorta.

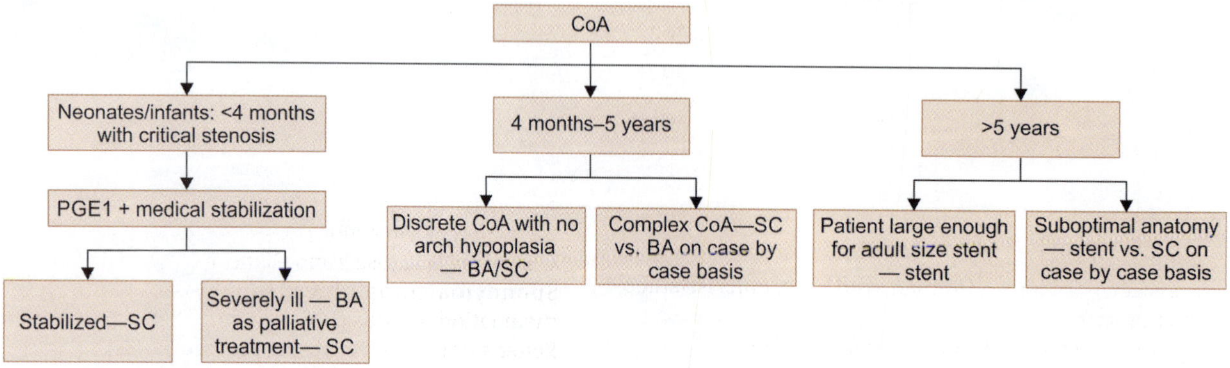

(CoA: coarctation; PGE1: prostaglandin E1; SC: surgical correction; BA: balloon angioplasty)

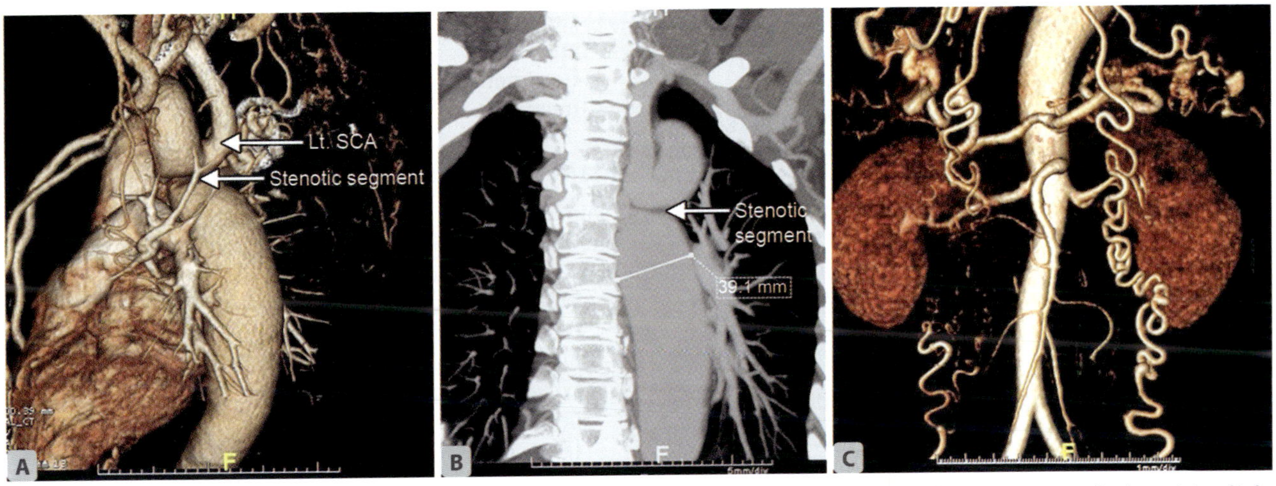

FIGS. 12A TO C: (A) CTA MIP image sagittal projection and (B) VR image show discontinuity of descending thoracic aorta just distal to origin of left subclavian artery; (C) Note extensive collaterals.

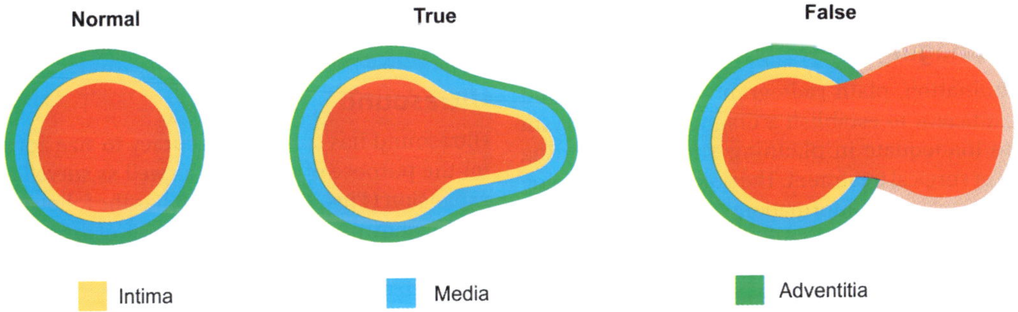

FIG. 13: Differentiation of true (covered by all layers) from false/pseudoaneurysm (arterialized periarterial hematoma).

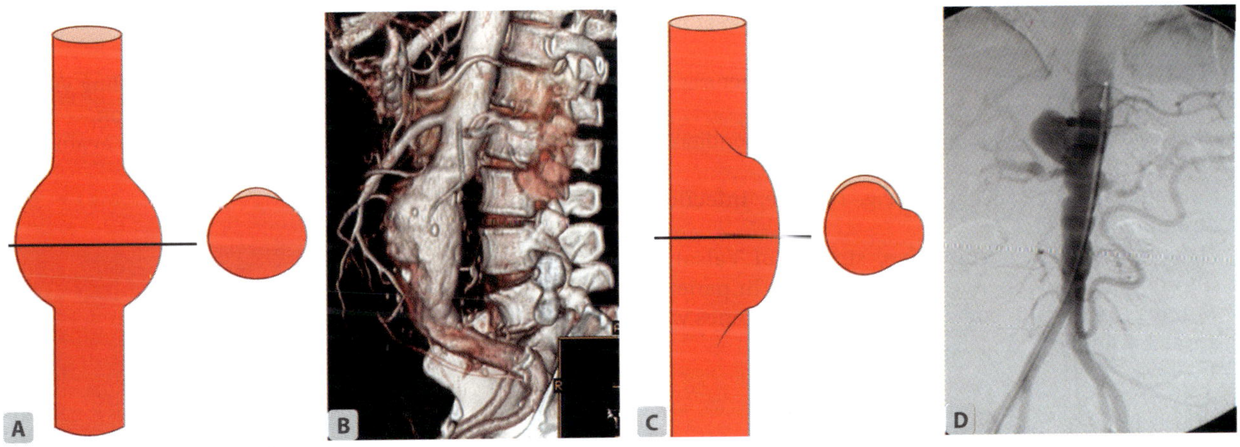

FIGS. 14A TO D: Images showing fusiform (A and B) saccular (C and D) aneurysms.

Etiology

- Atherosclerosis (70–80%)
- Cystic medial necrosis (Marfan syndrome, Ehlers-Danlos syndrome.)
- *Mycotic/infective (2–2.5%)—usually saccular*:
  - Tuberculosis (typically affects thoracic aorta),
  - Syphilis (90% affects ascending or arch of aorta)
  - Other infections (*Staphalococcus*, *Streptococcus*, salmonella infection)
- Vasculitis (Takayasu's and Giant cell arteritis)
- Spondyloarthropathies [Ankylosing spondylitis, rheumatiod arthritis (RA), psoriasis, Behcet's syndrome, Reiter's syndrome, Relapsing polychondritis]
- Post-traumatic (5–8%)—90% involving the isthmus and 8% in ascending aorta.

Growth Rates of Aneurysm

The mortality rate of untreated aortic aneurysms is unacceptably high and, once ruptured, it is almost 100%. Most aneurysms (80%) show progressive enlargement. The rate of growth is significantly greater for aneurysms of the descending aorta, at 1.9 mm per year, than those of the ascending aorta, at 0.7 mm per year.[35] Larger the aneurysm, more rapid is the growth. As the size (radius) of aneurysm increases, the wall tension increases, which tend to further increase the size of aneurysm *(Laplace law)*.

Risk of Rupture

Diameter of the aneurysm is the best predictor of rupture risk. Other parameters associated with increased risk are type of aneurysm (Saccular > Fusiform), wall stress, rate of expansion, family history, hypertension, smoking and gender (more common among females). Estimated annual rupture risk of abdominal aortic aneurysm (AAA) is tabulated in **Table 3**.[35,36]

Diagnostic Imaging

Physical examination, plain radiography and ultrasound are usually sufficient to establish a diagnosis of aneurysm but these are inadequate in planning and implementing endovascular or surgical treatment. The preoperative imaging must provide the following information:[10,11,37]

- Location, size, angulations, craniocaudal extension and type of aneurysm.
- The maximum diameter of any dilatation, measured from the external wall of the aorta, perpendicular to the true axis of flow, and the length of the abnormally dilated aorta.
- Integrity of the wall, presence of intramural hematoma, penetrating ulcer and associated thrombus.
- Involvement of visceral arteries or adjacent structures.
- Associated anatomic variations.
- Unrecognized intra-abdominal/intra-thoracic conditions, e.g. cholelithiasis.
- Complications of aneurysm, e.g. rupture, infection, thromboembolism.
- Measurements of aortic valve, sinuses of Valsalva, sinotubular junction, and ascending aorta in patients with presumed or documented genetic syndromes who are at risk for aortic root disease.
- Comments on coronary arteries for ascending aorta aneurysms.
- Comment on vascular access site for endovascular treatment.

TABLE 3: Rupture risk per year of AAA in relation to diameter of aneurysm.

AAA diameter (cm)	Rupture risk (%/year)
<4	0
4–5	0.5–5
5–6	3–15
6–7	10–20
7–8	20–40
>8	30–50

Plain Radiography

Plain radiography may suggest a diagnosis of aortic aneurysm but information essential for preoperative planning cannot be obtained. Findings include:

- Widening of mediastinum; in a standard supine chest radiography, if the mediastinum measures >8 cm, it is highly suggestive of thoracic aortic aneurysm **(Fig. 15)**
- Localized dilatation of ascending aorta/knuckle/descending aorta with or without curvilinear calcification, **(Figs. 16A and B)**
- Depressed left main bronchus, tracheal displacement, obliteration of aorto-pulmonary window, cardiomegaly (thoracic aortic aneurysm) **(Figs. 17A to C)**
- Mural calcification, displacement of adjacent organs of gastrointestinal tract (GIT), vertebral erosion (abdominal aortic aneurysm) **(Figs. 18A and B)**.

Ultrasound

Ultrasound has sufficient accuracy to size aortic aneurysms for the purpose of diagnosis as well as surveillance to detect expansion **(Figs. 19A and B)**. It has the following advantages:

- It confirms the clinical diagnosis of an aneurysm.
- It serves as a screening modality for follow-up of patients with aortic aneurysms, especially abdominal aortic aneurysms.
- It has a detection rate of 100% with size measurement within 4 mm of that obtained at surgery
- It is cost effective and portable.

The limitations of ultrasound are:

- It fails to provide reliable information regarding visceral artery involvement and craniocaudal extension.
- Obesity and intestinal gas hinder adequate evaluation, and

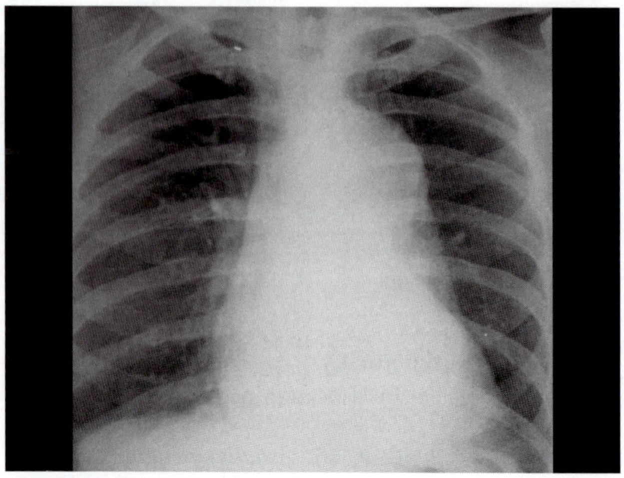

FIG. 15: Chest radiograph in a case of large thoracic aortic aneurysm showing mediastinal widening.

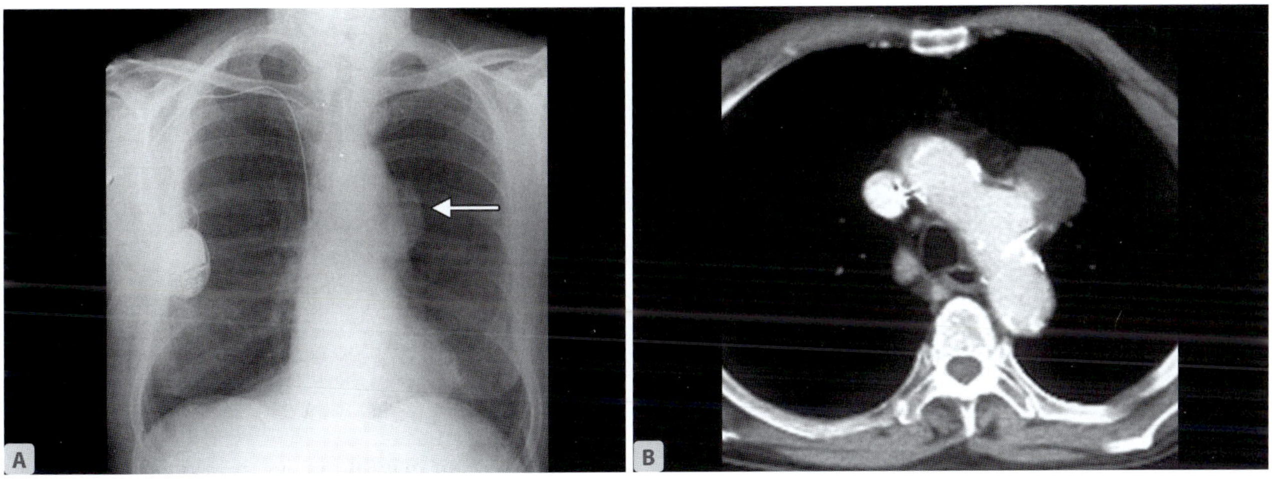

FIGS. 16A AND B: Chest radiograph in PA view shows prominent aortic kuncle (A), which on CTA (B) showed a peripherally thrombosed arch aneurysm with a penetrating ulcer.

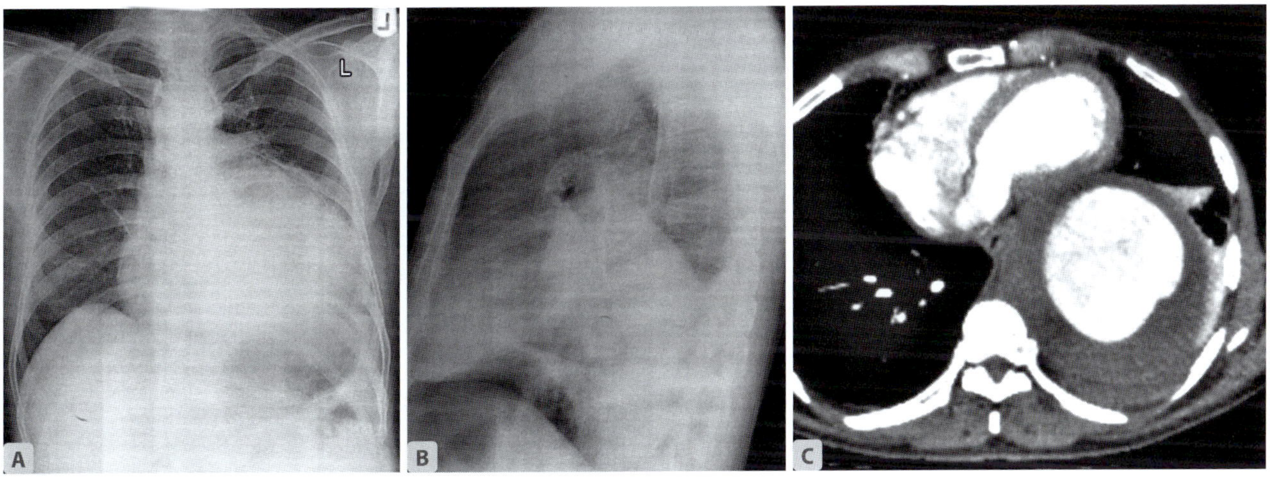

FIGS. 17A TO C: Chest radiograph in PA view shows cardiomegaly (A), which on lateral projection (B) shows a radio-opaque opacity overlying lower thoracic vertebra with loss of normal radiolucency. Subsequently on CTA (C) it was a large peripherally thrombosed DTA aneurysm.

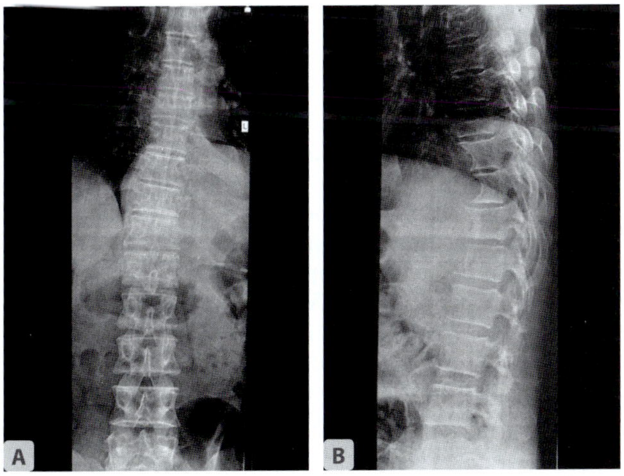

FIGS. 18A AND B: Front (A) and lateral thoracolumbar (B) spine radiograph shows a thoraco-abdominal mass-like lesion with well-defined lateral margins on both sides of spine. On lateral view anterior scalloping of lower dorsal vertebral bodies is prominently seen. On CTA it turned out to be a large mycotic aneurysm (refer Fig. 23).

- Expertise and experience is required for providing other essential morphological information.

Transoesophageal echocardiography (TEE) and intravascular ultrasound (IVUS) have limited role in the diagnosis, however it may further modify the preoperative planning in aortic aneurysms. IVUS helps in accurate measurement of the aneurysm for selection of stent grafts during endovascular repair and helps in prevention of type I endoleaks.

CT and MRI

CT and MRI are the modalities of choice for imaging of aorta, however CT is preferred over MRI because of shorter scanning time and high temporal and spatial resolution. MR angiography is usually recommended for post-treatment evaluation. Computed tomography permits one to choose an imaging plane in any arbitrary space orientation, measure the tortuous aorta in true cross-section and obtain an accurate diameter. Breath-held dynamic contrast-enhanced MRI also allows rapid acquisition of images in any plane, independent

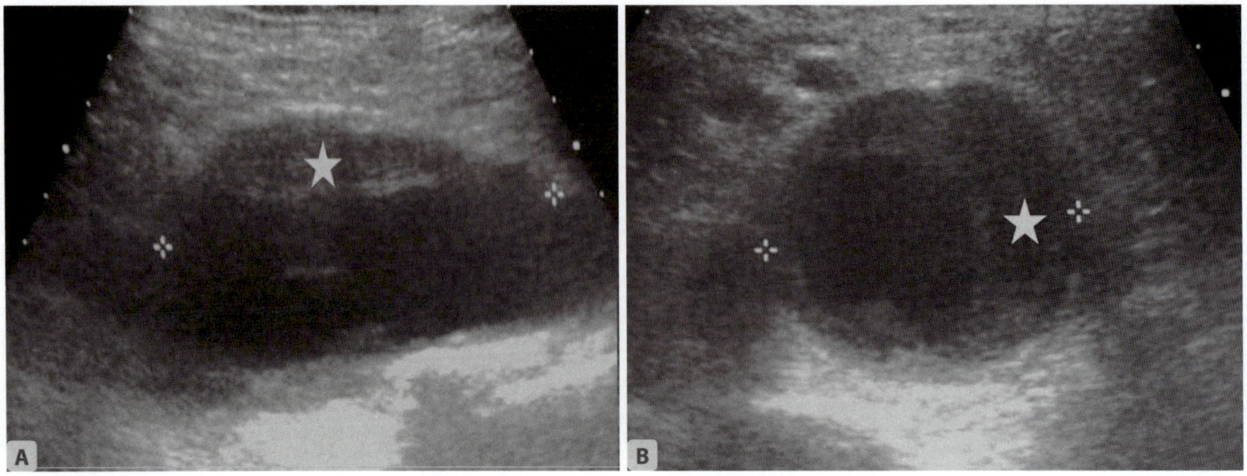

FIGS. 19A AND B: US abdomen longitudinal (A) and transverse (B) images show a peripherally thrombosed (along left lateral wall— stars) fusiform aneurysm of abdominal aorta.

of flow, however, disadvantages include non-visualization of calcifications and contraindications for MRI.[10-12,21,22,38]

In specific in cases of ascending arch aneurysm, ECG gated study should be considered for simultaneous evaluation of coronary arteries as significant CAD may be treated with by-pass grafts in one sitting.

Important Aneurysmal Features to be Assessed with CT or MRI[22,38,39]

- Proximal extent of the aneurysm whether it involves major vessels or aortic root. The surgical approach differs if there is involvement of major vessels **(Fig. 20)**.
- Distal extent of the aneurysm. Choice of the graft type depends on whether the aneurysm involves the common iliac vessels **(Figs. 21A to C)**.
- Congenital anomalies. The incidental anomalies like accessory renal artery or retroaortic/circumaortic left renal vein may warn an interventionist/surgeon to take due care during repair.
- *Etiology*: Based on imaging characteristics as whether it's inflammatory, mycotic or atherosclerotic (discussed in details later).

  Inflammatory aneurysm: It is variant of atherosclerotic aneurysm characterized by inflammatory and/or fibrotic changes in the periaortic regions **(Fig. 22)**. These changes are probably due to local autoallergic reaction to certain atherosclerotic plaque component. Aneurysmal repair is difficult in these patients because of fibrosis and involvement of important structures, e.g. ureter, GIT, vena cava, etc. CT or MRI demonstrates well-defined soft tissue mass with sharply defined margins surrounding the aneurysm in the anterolateral aspect with sparing of the posterior aspect. The contrast enhancement is variable. CT may rarely demonstrate infiltrative soft tissue mass with poorly defined margins or lobulated mass mimicking a pseudotumor. More details are enumerated in aortitis section.

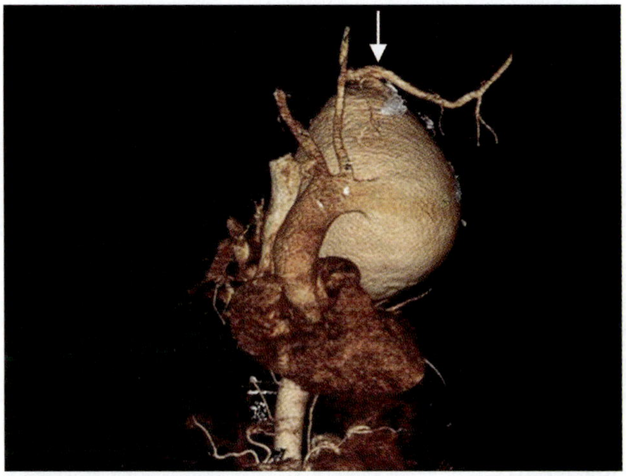

FIG. 20: Aortic Aneurysm: CTA-VR projection shows large saccular aneurysm arising from distal aortic arch and descending thoracic aorta. Note that this 64-slice VR projection clearly show origin of left subclavian artery from the aneurysmal sac (arrow) and sparing of right brachiocephalic and left common carotid.

  CT or MRI findings of mycotic aneurysm include **(Figs. 23A to C)**:
  - Saccular or irregular contour
  - Little or no mural calcification
  - Is adjacent to normal appearing aorta
  - Perianeurysmal fibrosis with or without air
- *Ruptured aneurysm*. CT or MRI demonstrates freshly hemorrhaged blood in the mediastinum/retroperitoneum and focal area of indistinctness in the aortic wall **(Figs. 24 to 26)**. The overall accuracy varies from 87–97%. Distinction between acute or chronic contained rupture is based on duration and severity of symptoms, the hematocrit and hemodynamic stability rather than on anatomic features demonstrated on CT/MRI.

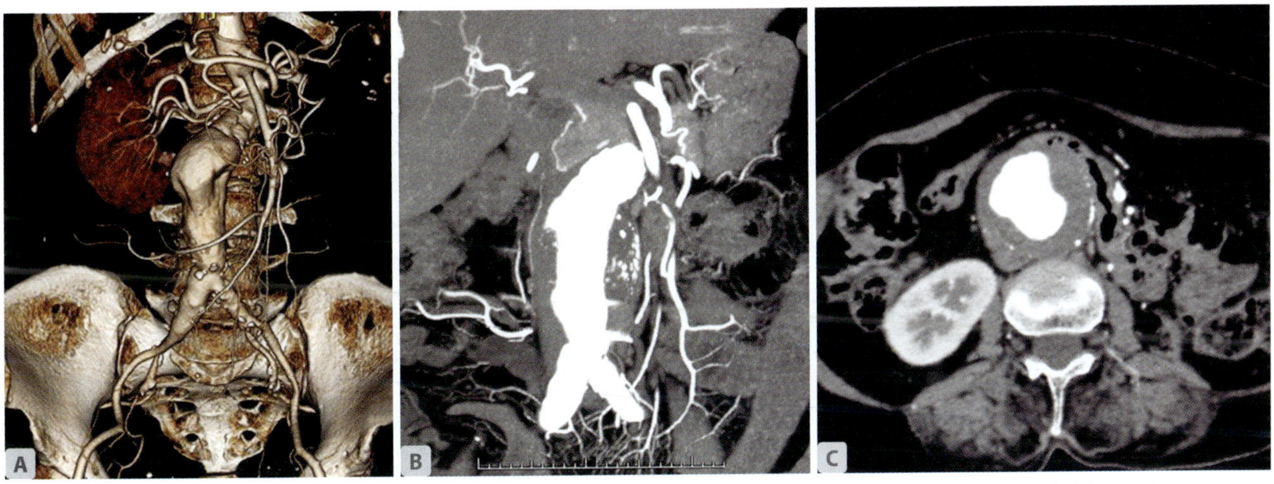

FIGS. 21A TO C: CTA-VR (A), MIP coronal (B) and axial (C) images demonstrate peripherally thrombosed fusiform infrarenal abdominal aortic aneurysm extending into both common iliac arteries.

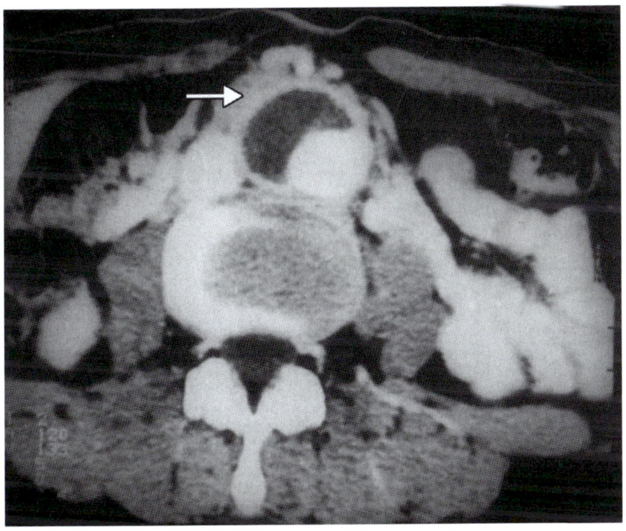

FIG. 22: Inflammatory aortic aneurysm: CECT shows a rind of soft tissue in right anterolateral aspect (arrow) of a partially thrombosed aneurysm (perianeurysmal fibrosis).

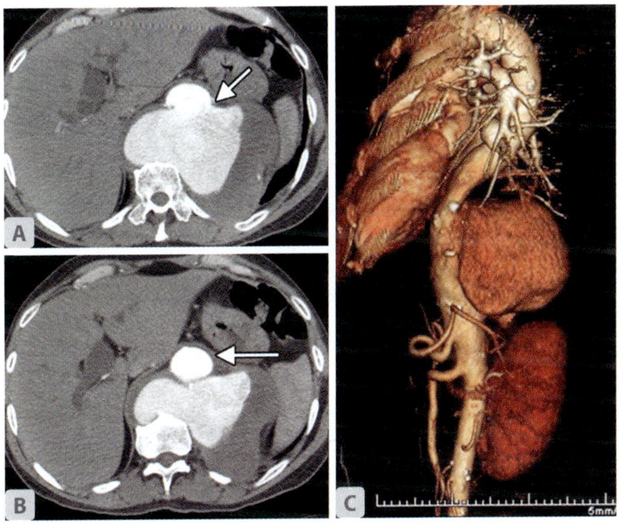

FIGS. 23A TO C: (A and B) CTA axial and (C) VR images show a large peripherally thrombosed juxta-diaphragmatic pseudoaneurysm (mycotic aneurysm) having lobulated outline with normal appearing anteriorly displaced aorta (thick arrow in B). Rent is posterior wall of aorta (thin arrow in A) is well seen. Note anterior scalloping of vertebral bodies (B). CTA pictures are of patient shown in Figure 18.

Catheter Angiography

Catheter angiography has limited role in diagnosis and follow-up aneurysms. However, with the advent of newer endovascular treatment methods, it has definitive role in preoperative evaluation and treatment planning of aortic aneurysms. It provides detailed arterial anatomy including aberrant origins, the location of the aneurysm relative to branch vessels and demonstrates occlusive lesions.

Surveillance of Small Abdominal Aortic Aneurysms

The risk of rupture of small (5 cm) AAA is low, and hence careful surveillance up to a diameter of 5.5 cm is safe, unless there is rapid expansion (1 cm/yea) or patient becomes symptomatic. Since benefits of early surgery over surveillance with later surgery are comparable, patient preference is important, especially for AAA 4.5–5.5 cm in diameter. The diameter of 5.5-cm appears to be an appropriate threshold for repair in an "average" patient based on the current evidences. For women, or AAA with greater than average rupture risk, elective repair at 4.5 cm to 5.0 cm is an appropriate threshold for repair.[40] Based on a recent individual-based meta-analysis of trials and observational studies with repeated AAA measurements over time, intervals of 3, 2, and 1 year(s) can be safely proposed for AAAs of 30–39, 40–44 and 45– 54 mm diameter, respectively, with a rupture risk of1% in men. Women with 45 mm AAA had a risk of rupture equivalent to men with a 55 mm AAA, so a lower intervention threshold, rather than shorter intervals of follow-up, may be considered.[41]

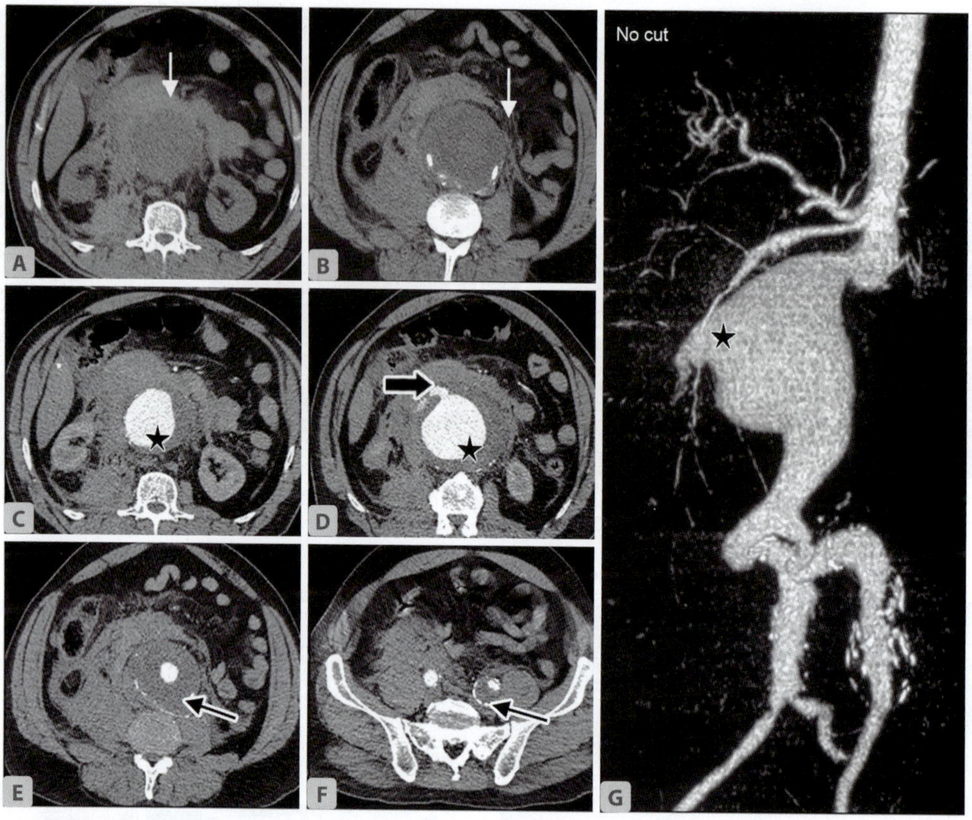

FIGS. 24A TO G: Noncontrast axial CT images (A and B), axial CTA (C to F) and VR (G) images shows fusiform infrarenal abdominal aortic aneurysm (black asterisk in C, D and G) with active contrast leak (block black arrow in D) associated hyperdense hematoma (black arrow in E and F) and associated significant periaortic stranding (white arrow in A and B). Patient expired on day 2 of admission and a diagnosis of IgG4 periaortitis was made on autopsy.

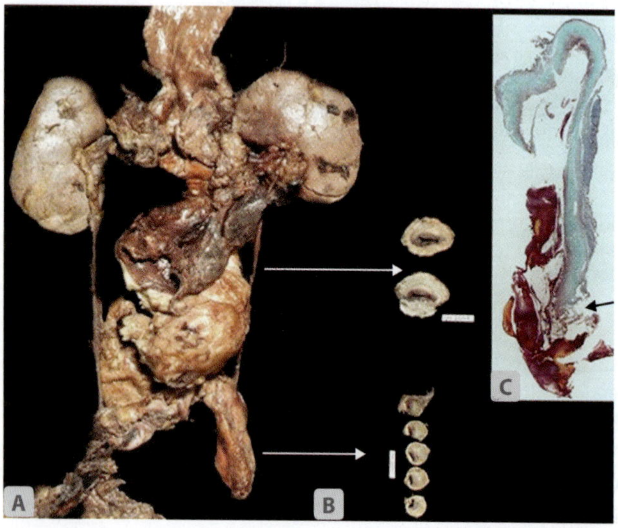

FIGS. 25A TO C: Autopsy specimen shows (A) gross specimen with evidence of blood collection in the area of aortic rupture confirmed (B and C) by cross-sections at the site of rupture and histopathology (arrow in C).

Courtesy: Professor Ritambra Nada, Department of Histopathology, PGIMER, Chandigarh, India.

Management of Aortic Aneurysms

Ascending Aortic and Arch Aneurysms

The treatment of ascending aortic and arch aneurysms remains surgical replacement. The extent of surgery depends on the status of the aortic valve, coronary arteries, and great vessels. Aortic valve replacement and complete arch replacement with re-implantation of the arch vessels may be required if the aortic valve is diseased or if the origins of the great vessels are involved. Hybrid debranching procedures as described in the section on dissection may be used in arch aneurysms where surgical grafts are placed to the great vessels from the ascending aorta followed by stent-graft placement across the arch from the ascending to the descending aorta.

Aneurysms of the Descending Thoracic Aorta

The relationship of the aneurysm to the arch vessels and the abdominal aortic visceral arteries determines the treatment. Involvement of these major aortic branches in the aneurysm increases the difficulty and morbidity of intervention. Complications of operative repair include a mortality rate of 5–10%, paraplegia due to spinal cord ischemia, renal failure, stroke and respiratory failure.[42]

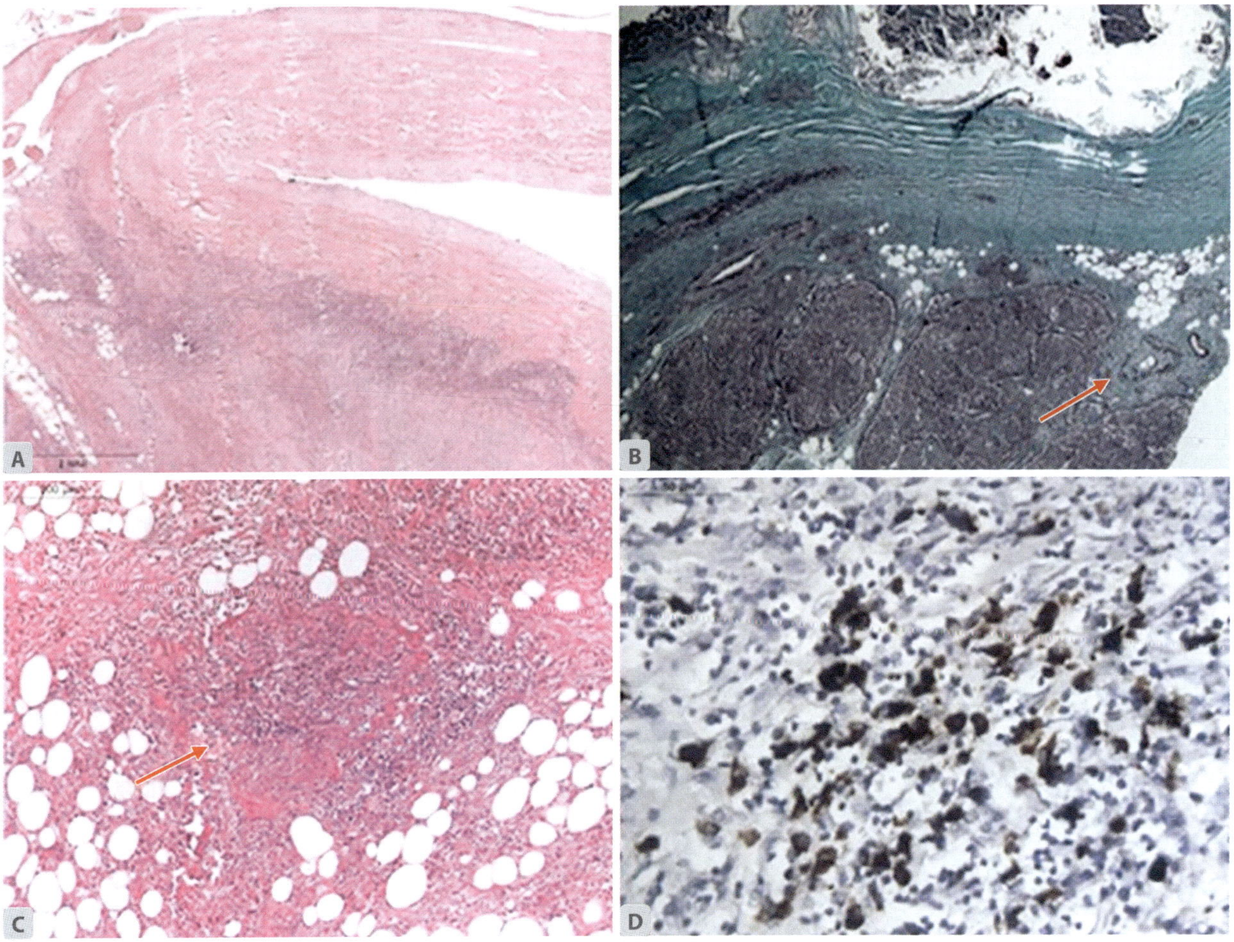

FIGS. 26A TO D: Photomicrograph shows (A) inflammatory periaortitis which had (B) evidence of fibrosis and venulitis (arrow). (C) shows obliterative venulitis (arrow) with immunohistochemistry (IHC) showing (D) IgG4 positive cells. Stains for CD3 CD 20 were negative (which are positive in aortoarteritis—not shown here).

Courtesy: Professor Ritambra Nada, Department of Histopathology, PGIMER, Chandigarh, India.

An attractive alternative to open surgical repair is endovascular repair where the anatomy is suited for stent graft placement. Stent-grafts function by depressurizing the aneurysm sac. Anatomical prerequisites and the procedure itself are similar to those described in the section on aortic dissection.

Stent-graft repair of thoracoabdominal aneurysms requires either a hybrid procedure with surgical debranching of the abdominal aortic branches followed by stent-graft placement, or branched stent-grafts **(Figs. 27A to D)**. Debranching procedures are major surgical interventions, which increases the morbidity and mortality of the procedure. Branched stent-grafts are less invasive for the patient but are complex time-consuming procedures with the expertise for such procedures being available in only certain tertiary care centers in India.

Multilayered flow modulator devices and stents are currently being developed for treatment of true fusiform aneurysm and holds promise for future application.[43]

Aneurysms of the Infrarenal Abdominal Aorta

Infrarenal AAA which fulfil the criteria for treatment **(Box 2)** may be treated by placement of a stent-graft or surgery. The mortality rate is 3–6% for elective surgery and 25–50% for emergent repair of a ruptured aneurysm making endovascular treatment attractive. Careful preprocedural planning **(Table 4)** is paramount as up to 37% of all patients may not be suitable candidate for endovascular aortic repair (EVAR).[44]

Patients must meet several anatomic criteria to be eligible for a stent graft **(*see* Table 4)**. Three types of stent graft configurations can be used to treat infrarenal AAA depending on the anatomic suitability. Most patients treated with current devices receive bifurcated stent-grafts as shown in **Figures 28A to F**. Other alternatives include aortounilateral iliac graft with surgical femoral-femoral bypass.[45] This type is used when the patient's anatomy is not suitable for a bifurcated graft. A single stent graft (similar to DTA stent graft) may also be used in rare situations where the proximal and distal landing zones are adequate.

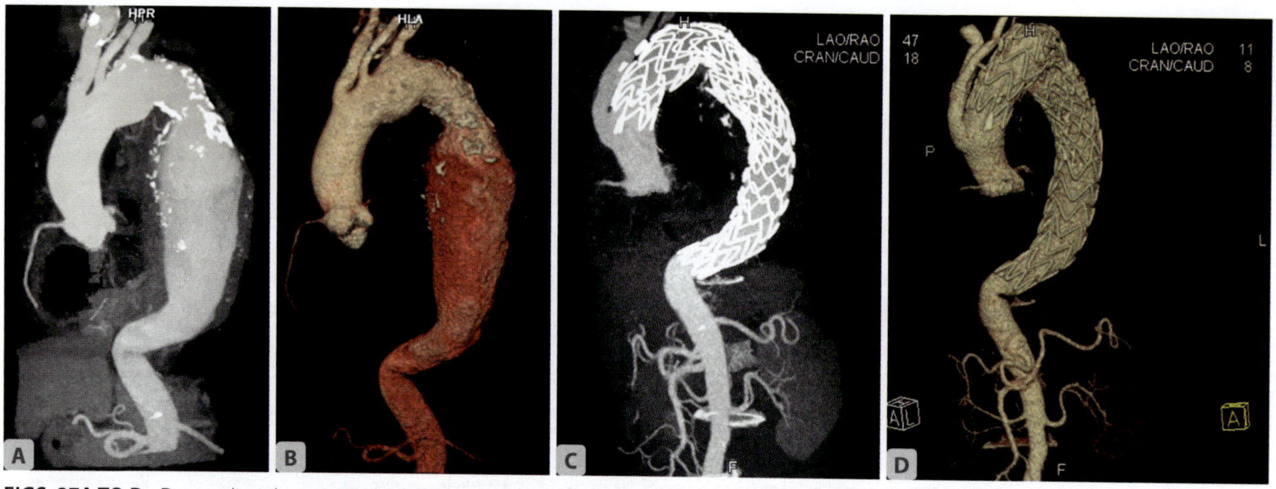

FIGS. 27A TO D: Descending thoracic aortic aneurysm treated with a stent graft after debranching to extend the proximal landing zone. (A and B) Oblique MIP and VRT computed tomography (CT) image showing the extent of the aneurysm; (C and D) CT of same patient 1 month after placement of a stent graft. The stent graft extends proximal and distal to the aneurysm with exclusion of the aneurysm sac. Transposed innominate artery to the ascending aorta is also noted.

Box 2: Indications for treatment of abdominal aortic aneurysms.

- AAA ≥5 cm diameter
- *Symptomatic aneurysms regardless of size*:
  - Contained-rupture AAA
  - Inflammatory AAA
- Rapidly expanding (>5 mm/yr) AAA
- High-risk for complication with open repair

TABLE 4: Eligibility criteria for interventional management of abdominal aortic aneurysm.

Criteria	Favorable	Unfavorable
Proximal aneurysm neck:		
• Diameter	<32 mm	>32 mm
• Length	>1.5 cm	<1.5 cm
• Angulation	<60°	>60°
• Morphological configuration	Cylindrical; Tapered	Reverse taper
• Calcification/thrombus	<90% circumference involved	>90% circumference involved
Aneurysm sac:		
• Residual lumen	>18 mm	<18 mm
• Distal aortic diameter	>20 mm	<20 mm
• Extension	CIA not involved	CIA involved
Ileofemoral vessels:		
• CIA diameter	<25 mm	>25 mm
• Landing zone length	>10 mm	<10 mm
• EIA diameter	>6 mm	<6 mm
• Tortuosity	<90°	>90°
• Calcification/thrombus	<50% circumference involved	>50% circumference involved

ACUTE AORTIC SYNDROME

Acute aortic syndromes (AAS) constitute a spectrum of conditions characterized by disruptions in the integrity of the aortic wall presenting with acute pain as the leading symptom in most cases. They include classic aortic dissection, intramural hematoma, penetrating aortic ulcer, and aortic aneurysm rupture **(Fig. 29)**. Because of the life-threatening nature of these conditions, prompt and accurate diagnosis is paramount. Misdiagnosis of these conditions, usually because of confusion with myocardial ischemia, can lead to undue mortality. Benign conditions or findings that can mimic AAS on imaging studies are aortitis, atheromatous plaque, prior surgery of aorta, pericardial recess, remnant of a non-patent PDA, streak and motion artifacts on CT, and periaortic fat and hemiazygos sheath.[38]

AORTIC DISSECTION

Aortic dissection is the most common acute emergency affecting the aorta, occurring 2 to 3 times more frequently than acute rupture of an aortic aneurysm. The peak incidence is in the 6th and 7th decades of life, men are affected more than women. The clinical presentation is with acute onset of chest pain, congestive heart failure, abdominal pain, or stroke. Approximately 15–20% may be asymptomatic and incidentally diagnosed. The predisposing conditions are hypertension (70–90%), pre-existing aortic diseases (Marfan syndrome, coarctation) or aortic valve disease, aortitis, family history of aortic diseases, history of cardiac surgery, cigarette smoking, direct blunt chest trauma and use of intravenous drugs. Though the exact pathogenesis is somewhat controversial, the most accepted theory for long is that the initial event is a tear in the intima which allows blood to enter the aortic wall creating a true and false lumen. The demonstration of intimal flap is thus essential to make the diagnosis. It is now recognized that degeneration of the media leads to rupture of

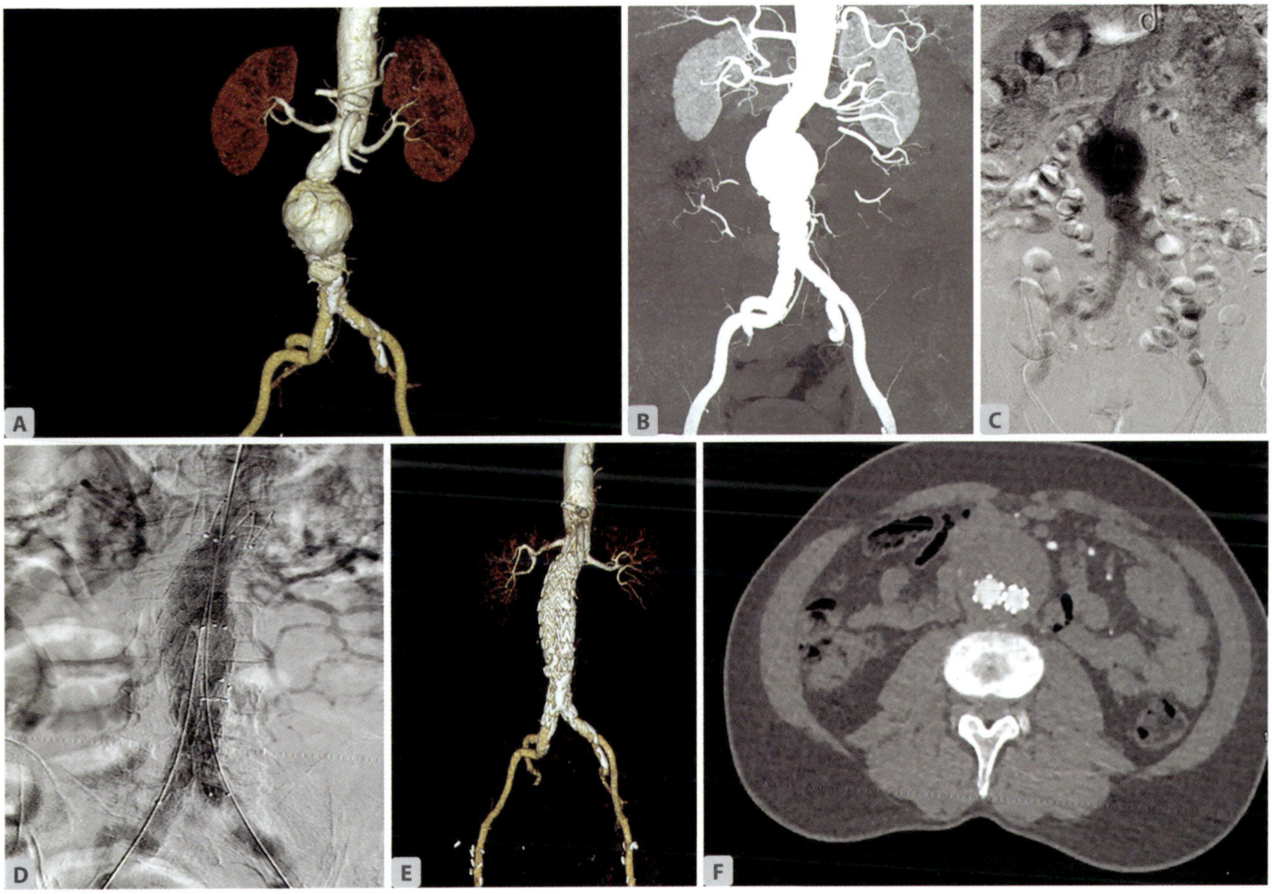

FIGS. 28A TO F: Infrarenal abdominal aortic aneurysm treated with a branched stent-graft: (A to C) VRT and MIP computed tomography images and aortogram showing a infrarenal abdominal aortic aneurysm; (D) Aortogram after deployment of stent graft shows exclusion of the aneurysm; (E) VRT computed tomography image of the same patient on 1 month follow-up; (F) Axial image showing good opacification of both limbs of the stent graft with aneurysm sac thrombosed.

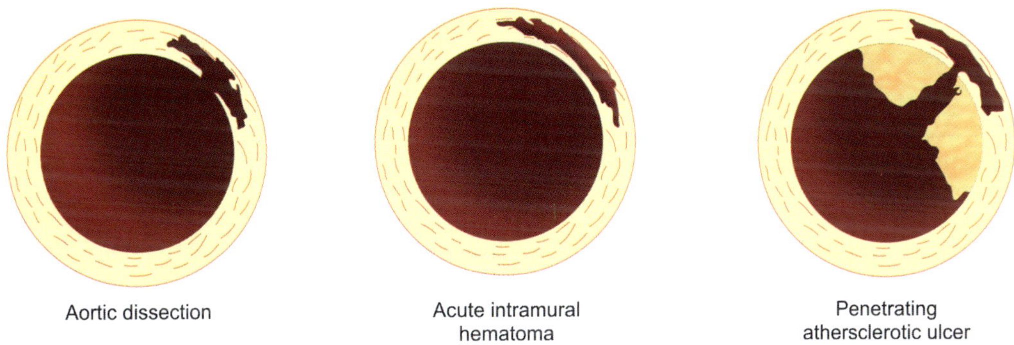

FIG. 29: Schematic diagrams demonstrating dissection, penetrating ulcer and intramural hematoma.

the vasa vasorum of the aortic wall which leads to dissecting hematoma between the media and adventitia which may or may not rupture through the intima into the aortic lumen. This explains the fact that no intimal tear is found at autopsy in a small number of cases of aortic dissection.[46]

Classification

The DeBakey classification categorized aortic dissections into:

- Type I (29–34%): Originates in the ascending aorta and extends to a variable distance beyond the aortic arch
- Type II (12–21%): Confined to ascending aorta
- Type III (50%): Originates distal to the left subclavian artery. It is subclassified into Type IIIA up to diaphragm and type IIIB: below diaphragm.

This classification has been replaced by 'Stanford classification' which takes into account of extent of dissection rather than location of entry site, and divided into type A (involving the ascending aorta) and type B (not involving the ascending aorta) **(Fig. 30)**. Approximately, 70% of dissections are type A and 30% are type B. Type A carries high mortality and morbidity and requires urgent intervention as compared

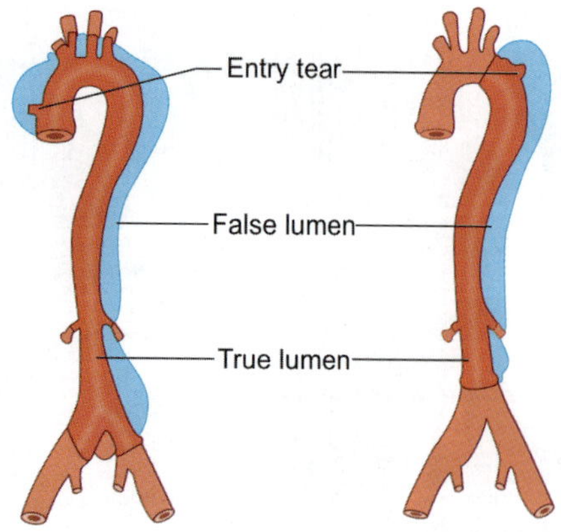

FIG. 30: Stanford types of dissections.

TABLE 5: Characteristics of Standford type A and type B aortic dissections.

Feature	Type A	Type B
Frequency (%)	65–70	30–35
Male:Female ratio	2:1	3:1
Average age (years)	50–55	60–70
Hypertension (%)	50	80
Atherosclerosis	+/–	+ +
Aortic insufficiency (%)	50	10
Intimal tear	Always present	Absent in 5–10%
Treatment	Urgent surgery	Usually conservative
Acute mortality (%)	90–95	35–50

to type B dissection, which is usually managed conservatively **(Table 5)**.[47]

IMAGING

The goal of imaging is not merely to detect presence and extent of AD but to define other important features:[38]

- Differentiation of true and false lumen
- Location of intimal tears
- Coronary artery ostia integrity (in type A)
- Aortic valve function
- +/– pleural or pericardial effusion.

There is no consensus as to which examination (s) should be used in the diagnosis of aortic dissections. The initial imaging should consist of a chest radiograph (CXR) and a transthoracic echocardiogram (TTE). Plain film findings include widening of the mediastinum and aortic contour, changes in aortic contour from prior examination(s), and displaced intimal calcification. However, a normal CXR does not exclude the diagnosis. TTE may show a pericardial effusion, adequately images the aortic valve and the aortic root but does not show the arch and descending aorta with confidence (blind spot). Transesophageal echocardiography (TEE) has overcome many of the limitations of TTE and has a high degree of accuracy in skilled hands. Onc of the main advantages of TEE, especially in unstable patients, is that the examination can be performed safely and quickly at the bed side, and can be used to monitor changes in-theater and in post-operative intensive care.

Computed Tomography

CT angiographic protocols typically begin with low-dose non-contrast CT to exclude the possibility of IMH, followed by contrast-enhanced ECG gated computed tomographic angiography. The coverage includes the entire thorax, abdomen, and pelvis to allow delineation of the extent of a flap and its extension into branch vessels and to evaluate for end-organ ischemia (e.g. bowel or kidneys), and possible extravasation **(Figs. 31 and 32)**.

The CT findings in aortic dissection include the following:

- *Precontrast images*:
  - Internal displacement of intimal calcification.
  - Visible intimal flap as a linear structure slightly higher in attenuation than surrounding blood.
  - High attenuation thrombosed false lumen, if acutely thrombosed.
  - Enlargement of long segment of the aorta
  - Pericardial, mediastinal and/or pleural hemorrhage, secondary to rupture.
- *Postcontrast images* **(Figs. 31 and 32):**
  - Contrast filled true and false lumen separated by intimal flap; false lumen typically seen in outer curvature of aorta.
  - Delayed enhancement of the false lumen because of slower flow.
  - Thrombosis of false lumen, with enhancement of only the true lumen.
  - Compression of true lumen by thrombosed false lumen.
  - Extension of dissection into branch vessels.
  - Ischemia/infarction of organs supplied by branch vessels from false lumen.

CT Signs of AD

Differentiation between true and false lumens of AD is important in planning of treatment with percutaneous endovascular grafts or surgical repair. It is critical to identify the lumen of origin of major branches such as coronary, carotid, renal and mesenteric arteries before treatment, as viscera supplied by false lumen are at risk when false lumen is spontaneously or surgically occluded **(Table 6)**.

The convex face of the intimal flap is usually towards the FL that surrounds the TL **(Figs. 31A to D)**. The FL usually has slower flow and a larger diameter and may contain thrombi. In Type A AD, the FL is usually located along the right anterolateral wall of the ascending aorta and extends distally, in a spiral fashion, along the left posterolateral wall of the descending aorta **(Figs. 32A to C)**. Slender linear areas of low attenuation may be observed in the FL, corresponding to incompletely dissected media, known as the 'Cobweb sign', a specific finding for identifying the FL. Discrimination between the FL and TL is utmost important to identify collaterals perfused exclusively by the FL, as well as when endovascular therapy is considered.[48]

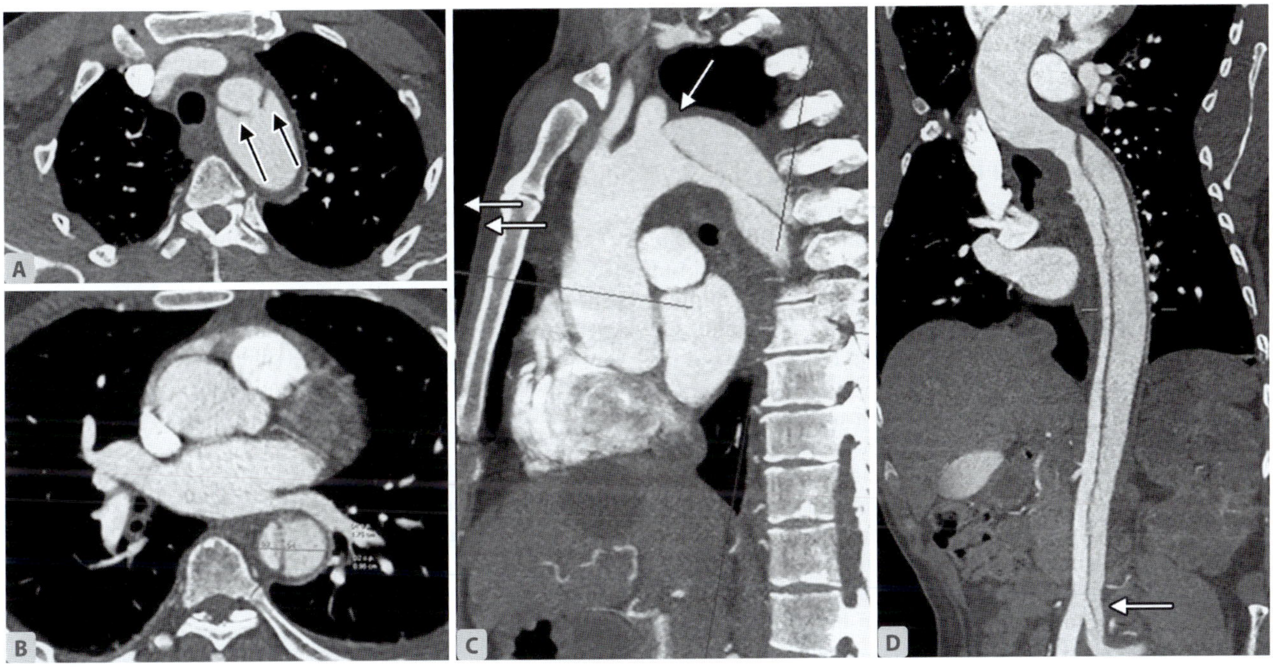

FIGS. 31A TO D: (A and B) CTA axial; (C) reconstructed sagittal and (D) stretched images shows type B dissection with entry point juxta-posed to the origin of left subclavian artery (arrows in A and C). Note "beak sign" with convex flap toward posterior false lumen (A). (D) Note extension of flap into the left common iliac artery.

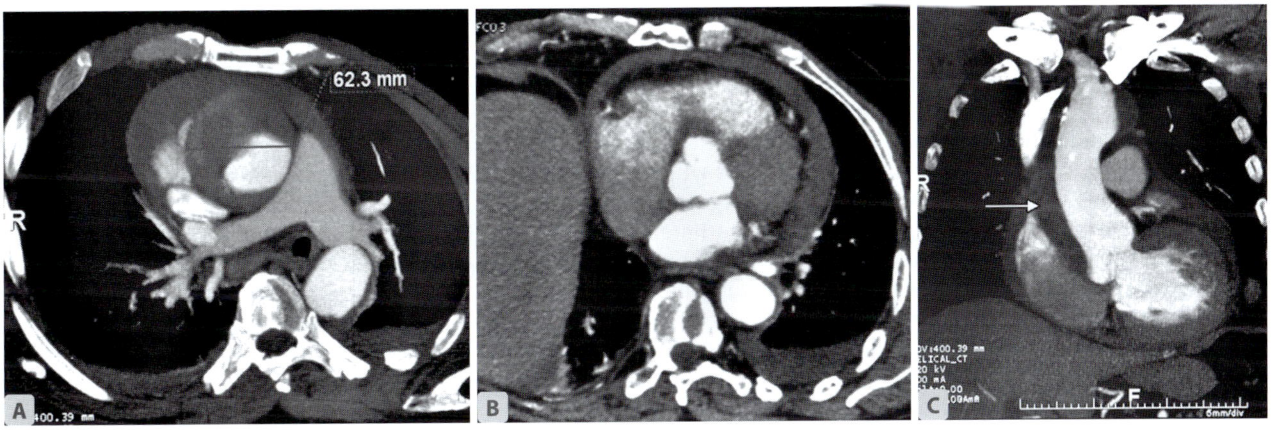

FIG. 32A TO C: (A and B) CTA axial and oblique coronal images showing type A dissection with thrombosis of false lumen (A and C) with rupture into pericardial and right pleural cavities (A to C).

TABLE 6: CT features for differentiating true from false lumen.

S. No.	Features	True lumen	False lumen
1.	Continuity of lumen with lumen of uninvolved portion of aorta (most reliable)	+	–
2.	Direction of free edges of the dissection flap at entrance tear	–	+
3.	Aortic Cobweb	–	+
4.	Outer wall calcification	+	–
5.	Beak sign	–	+
6.	Thrombosis	–/+	++
7.	Peak flow	Faster	Slower
8.	Size	Smaller and compressed	Larger and toward intimal concavity

If possible ECG-triggered CTA should be done for type A dissection for simultaneous evaluation of coronary arteries so that bypass grafts can be palced in one-sitting **(Figs. 33A and B)**.

Magnetic Resonance Imaging

It has been shown to be an effective alternative technique to CT for evaluation of aortic dissection with a reported sensitivity and specificity of 98%. MRI not only gives anatomical but also functional information required for treatment planning, however, because of ease of CT and its wider availability, CT is often the modality of investigation and MR is reserved for follow-up **(Figs. 34A and B)**.

Black blood imaging shows the intimal flap as thin linear structure in the aortic flow void. True lumen shows preservation of the flow void whereas the false lumen is seen as area of increased signal intensity because of turbulent flow.

Phase contrast images can be done to identify aortic insufficiency, intimal tear sites and to differentiate slow flow from thrombus in the false lumen. Combining black blood, bright blood with gadolinium-enhanced 3D MR angiography images can comprehensively give the required information.[19,24,38,49]

Aortography

It is highly accurate in the detection and evaluation of aortic dissection with diagnostic accuracy over 95%. The direct signs are identification of an intimal flap and a contrast filled true and false lumen. Indirect signs are aortic wall thickening, aortic regurgitation, compression of the true lumen, non-visualization of branch vessels and abnormal catheter position. False negative study may be seen when the false lumen is thrombosed, intimal flap not tangential to the X-ray beam, intimal tear proximal to the catheter and absence of intimal flap in some cases. Noninvasive imaging is more accurate in providing the diagnosis and therefore aortography is no longer used for the diagnosis of AD, except during coronary angiography or endovascular intervention.

Management of AD

Current classifications systems are not comprehensive at describing all the information pertinent to a surgeon/interventionist about the dissection. Information regarding chronicity of symptoms, location of primary entry tears, direction of flap extension (antegrade, retrograde, mixed), complications and patency of the false lumen are vital.

A mnemonic-based approach to the evaluation of aortic dissection was proposed by Dake et al.[50] The DISSECT classification system guides the radiologist through an assessment of six critical characteristics that facilitate a complete description of the most salient details that currently influence the selection of a treatment. The features of aortic dissection that are to be mentioned in the report are enumerated in **Table 7**.

Acute type A aortic dissection constitutes a surgical emergency since these patients are at high-risk for a life-threatening complication such as aortic regurgitation,

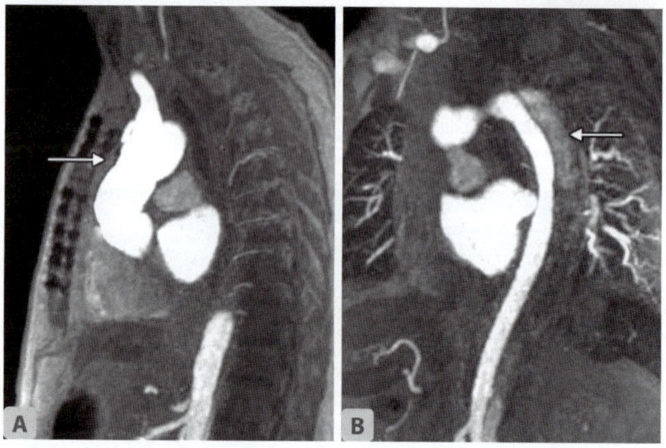

FIGS. 34A AND B: 3D CE-MRA oblique coronal views in a postoperative patient of type A dissection (post Bentall) show normally opacified ascending aorta (arrow in A) and faintly opacified false lumen (usually due to slow flow) in descending thoracic (arrow in B) and normally opacified true lumen.

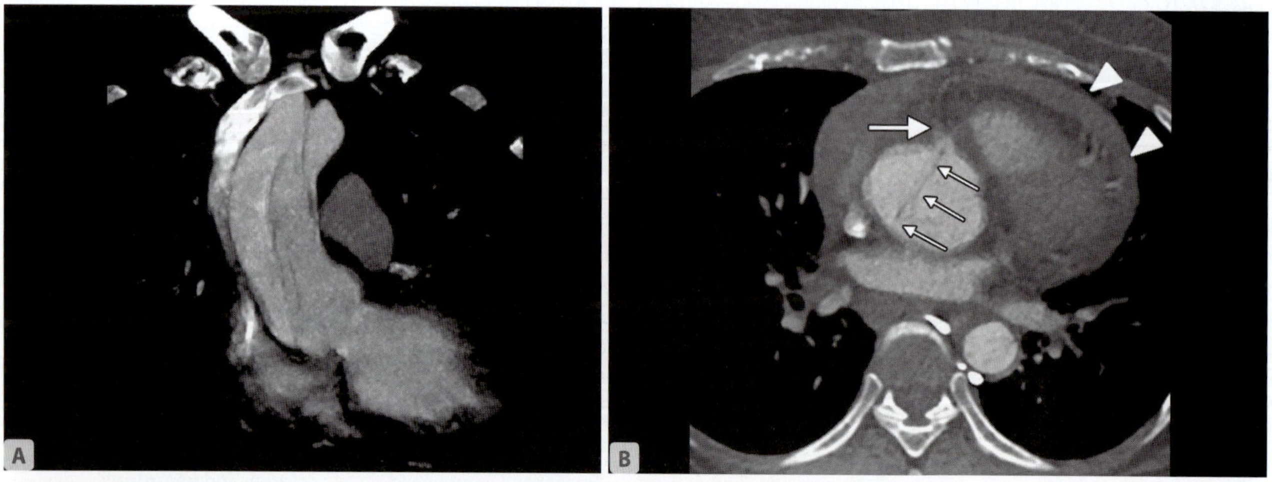

FIGS. 33A AND B: ECG –triggered CTA of ascending aorta oblique coronal and axial images show type A dissection (A and B) with intimal flap (thin arrows) extending into the ostia of right coronary artery (thick arrow). Note hemopericardium (arrowheads).

TABLE 7: DISSECT classification.

D—Duration of symptoms	• *Acute*: <2 weeks from onset of symptoms • *Subacute*: 2 weeks to 3 months after symptom onset • *Chronic*: >3 months from initial symptoms
I—Intimal tear location	Ascending aorta, aortic arch, descending aorta, abdominal aorta, unknown
S—Sizes	Maximum aortic diameter at any level
SE—Segmental extent	Proximal entry and distal re-entry tear locations
C—Complications	• Cardiac tamponade • Rupture • Branch vessel malperfusion • Static and/or dynamic branch involvement with accompanying stroke, paraplegia, coronary, mesenteric, visceral, renal, and/or extremity symptoms • Progression of aortic involvement with proximal or distal extension of dissection • Involvement of aortic valve in case of type A dissection • *Other*: - Uncontrollable hypertension - Uncontrollable clinical symptoms - Rapid false lumen dilation - Overall trans-aortic enlargement of >10 mm within the first 2 weeks of initial diagnosis
T—Thrombosis of false lumen	Patent, completely or partially thrombosed

cardiac tamponade, stroke, frank rupture and myocardial infarction. Medical management has a mortality of up to 50% as compared to the operative mortality of 7–36% in experienced centers.[51,52]

At certain advanced centers, a hybrid approach to the repair of type A aortic dissection, referred to as the "frozen elephant trunk repair," may be attempted. This involves combination of an open approach to surgically repair the ascending aorta, while deploying a stent-graft to manage the descending aorta.

Type B dissection is generally managed initially with best medical therapy as given in **Box 3**.

Intervention (surgical or endovascular) for descending thoracic aortic dissection is reserved for patients who develop complications as described in **Table 7**.

Type B aortic dissection with such complications is associated with mortality rates that can exceed 60%. Interventional management consists of placing a stent graft over the proximal entry tear which has been shown to acutely depressurize the false lumen and restore normal flow in the true lumen **(Fig. 35A to F)**.

The endograft should be sized to the estimated diameter of the true lumen, not the overall diameter of the dissected aorta. Successful stent-graft exclusion in the thoracic aorta, or any other aortic segment, necessitates at least 15-mm proximal and distal "landing zones" of non-diseased aorta to achieve fixation and seal. However, in case the proximal

Box 3: Best medical management for aortic dissection.

Four main management goals for type B dissection patients either with or without surgical/interventional management:

1. Antihypertensive drugs to minimize the aortic wall shear stress caused by increased blood pressure
2. Continued monitoring for high-risk clinical conditions/presence of complications which would require immediate treatment
3. Serial imaging to detect signs of progression, re-dissection, or aneurysm formation
4. Optimal pain management

landing zones are inadequate, there are strategies and techniques designed to "extend the landing zone". These techniques may be endovascular (use of branched stent graft, chimney, or snorkel technique) or surgical debranching techniques to extend the landing zones. These techniques are known as debranching techniques. Using the classification proposed by Criado et al.[53] landing zones can be classified into 5 types **(Fig. 36)**. The complexity of procedures required to lengthen the landing zones increases as the landing zone of stent graft extends more proximally.

An endovascular procedure with proximal landing zones at Zone 3 and 4 is an optimal situation and requires no extra step for aortic interventions. A proximal landing zone involving zone 2 would require either coverage (and occlusion) or transposition of the left subclavian artery (LSA). If the left common carotid artery (CCA) origin (Zone 1) is involved, transposition to the right CCA via a carotid-carotid bypass can be performed. If the disease involves the full entire aortic arch, coverage of the innominate artery (IA) would be required along with transposition of the IA and left CCA to the ascending aorta **(Figs. 37A to E)**. Alternatively, branched stent graft or chimney techniques can be used in these cases in centers where expertise is available.

When critical organ ischemia is not relieved by occlusion of the proximal entry tear with a stent graft, bare stents can be placed from the true lumen of the aorta into the true lumen of the branch vessel to restore flow.[54] Another minimally invasive option is percutaneous fenestration of the aortic flap. This intentionally causes creation of a large distal exit tear, which decompresses the false lumen and relieves the dynamic obstruction of the true lumen. This is usually done as a lifesaving or as an adjunctive procedure as mortality with fenestration alone can be high. One of the ways to create a fenestration is to cross the intimal flap with an intravascular ultrasound to guide the puncture. This fenestration may then be enlarged using angioplasty balloons.

Delivery systems for thoracic stent-grafts tend to be large, so assessment of the femoral arteries, iliac arteries and abdominal aorta is necessary when evaluating a patient for one of these procedures. Surgical placement of a temporary graft to the common iliac artery or distal aorta (termed a *conduit*) may be required to deliver the endograft in patients with small or diseased pelvic arteries.

Although type B complicated aortic dissection can be handled by stent graft placement, with various adjunctive techniques, total surgical repair may be needed for those whose anatomy cannot support a stent-graft.

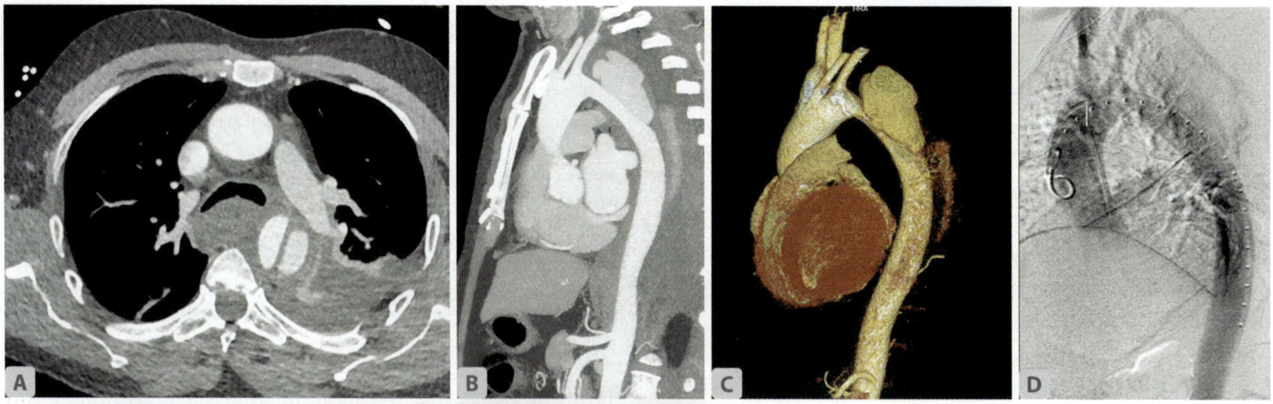
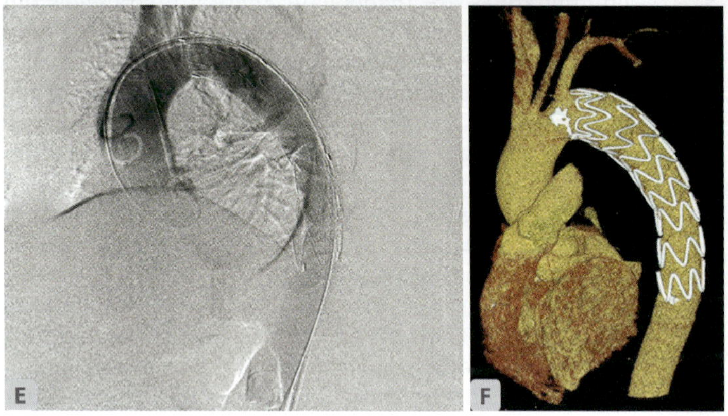

FIGS. 35A TO F: Stent-graft treatment of ruptured type B aortic dissection: (A and B) Axial, sagittal MIP and VRT images showing type B dissection with proximal tear distal to left subclavian artery; (C) Aortogram in the left anterior oblique projection with faint opacification of the false lumen as it fills more slowly than the true lumen; (D) Angiogram after a stent-graft placement over the entry tear in the true lumen of the descending thoracic aorta. The true lumen has a normal diameter and the false lumen is no longer opacified; (E and F) 1 month follow-up CT image showing stent *in situ*.

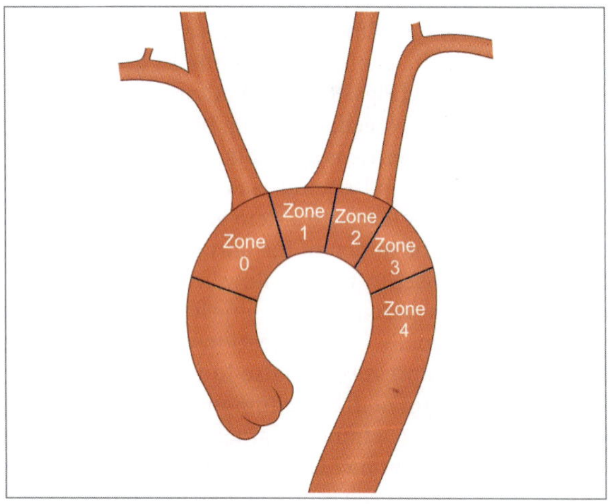

FIG. 36: Criado classification of aortic landing zones.

A summary of the prerequisites and challenges for interventional management is given in **Table 8**.

Endovascular intervention in patients with uncomplicated dissection may improve long-term outcomes by favorably influencing the dynamic relationship of the true and false lumen however, the results of multiple studies support a complication and patient-specific approach to type B dissection as the best treatment paradigm.

A suggested algorithmic approach to management of AD is given in **Flowchart 2**.

INTRAMURAL HEMATOMA

Intramural haematoma is diagnosed by the presence of a circular or crescent-shaped thickening of >5 mm of the aortic wall in the absence of detectable blood flow. It accounts for approximately 10 to 25% of AAS. IMH was first believed to be result of rupture of the vasa vasorum, allowing bleeding between the elastic lamina of the aortic media. However, recent findings suggest that at least some IMHs may be initiated by small intimal tears that are undetectable by current aortic imaging modalities and are often overlooked on gross inspection of the aorta at the time of surgery or autopsy.[55-58] IMH can be associated with several conditions, including spontaneous (''typical'') aortic dissection, penetrating ulcer, aortic trauma, and iatrogenic dissection (cardiac catheterization, cardiac surgery).

Imaging features of IMH are ***(Figs. 38A and B)****:*

- Focal aortic wall thickening (crescentic > concentric)
- Preserved luminal shape with smooth luminal border
- Absence of dissection flap and false lumen
- Echolucent regions may be present in the aortic wall
- Central displacement of intimal calcium.

Predictors of complication and surveillance:

Maximum aortic diameter (>40–50 mm), wall thickness(>10–12 mm) and associated periaortic hemorrhage or pleural effusion has been described as a predictor of progression. IMH may weaken the aortic wall and either progress outward with aortic expansion and/or rupture **(Figs. 39A to C)** or inward with disruption of the intima-

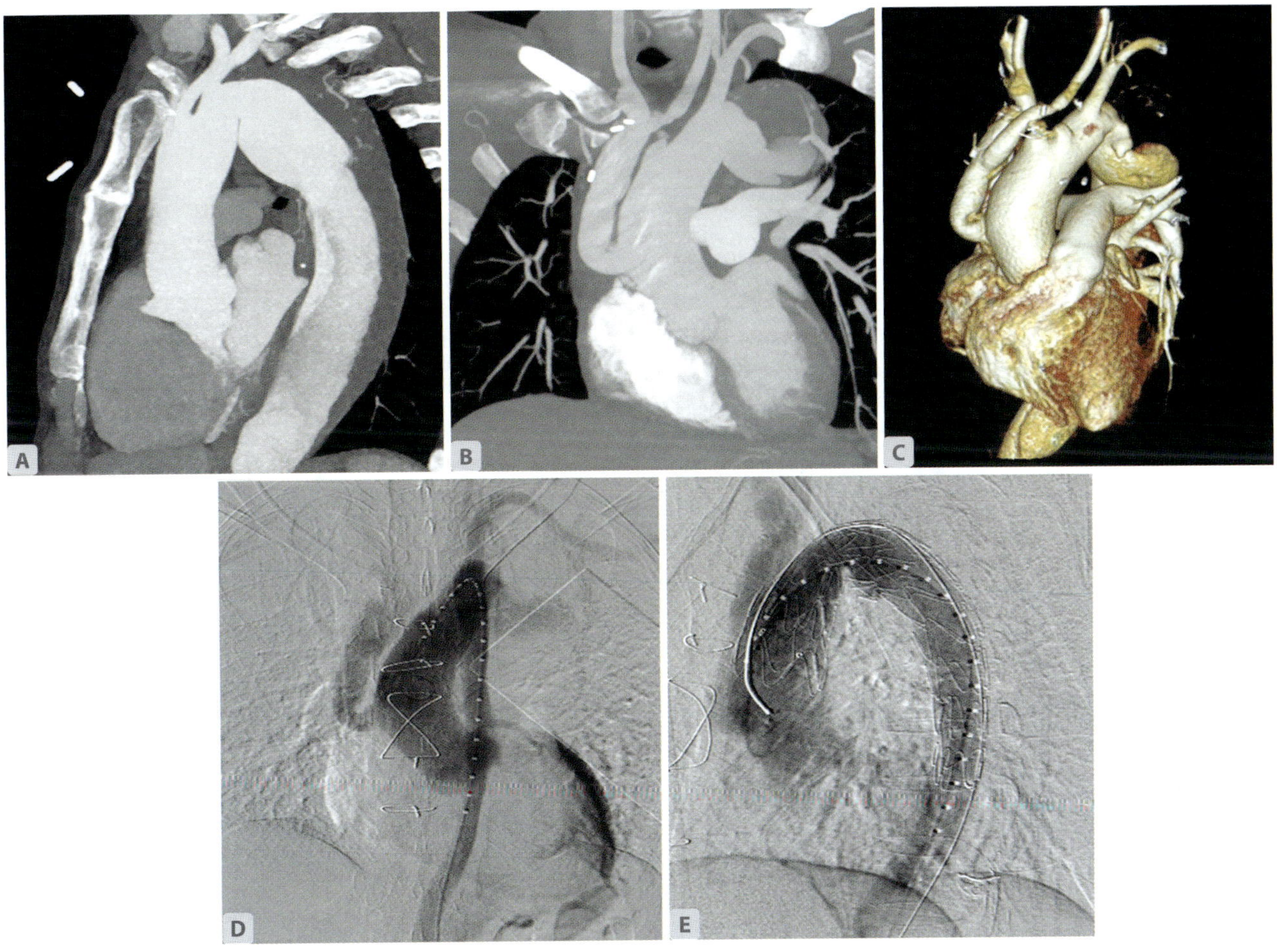

FIGS. 37A TO E: Stent-graft treatment with debranching technique of ruptured type B aortic dissection with unfavorable proximal landing zone anatomy. (A) Oblique sagittal image showing acute angulation of arch with proximal tear at the root of the left subclavian artery (not shown in image); (B to D) Oblique coronal, VRT images and aortogram showing innominate artery transposed to ascending aorta effectively "elongating the proximal landing zone". The left common carotid was transposed to the innominate artery; (E) Angiogram after a stent-graft placement over the entry tear in the true lumen of the descending thoracic aorta. The true lumen has a normal diameter and the false lumen is no longer opacified.

TABLE 8: Prerequisites for interventional management of dissection.

Proximal landing zone	• Atleast 1.5 cm normal aorta distal to left subclavian artery • If unavailable debranching procedures to extend the proximal landing zone
Distal landing zone	1.5–2 cm normal aorta above celiac artery
Landing zone diameters	Varies with device
Severe angulation of proximal or distal aorta	Longer landing zones needed which may necessitate debranching
Patency and caliber of pelvic arteries:	• Minimal external iliac/common femoral artery diameter required 7 mm • Smaller vessels may require direct access to common iliac artery or abdominal aorta via surgical conduit

media, resulting in typical aortic dissection. Therefore, serial imaging is necessary to rule out progression in patients who receive only medical treatment. Although there are no established guidelines for the optimal frequency and longitudinal duration for surveillance imaging of patients with IMH, Evangelista et al. on the basis of the significant dynamic evolution of IMH, recommended imaging at 1, 3, 6, 9, and 12 months from the time of diagnosis. Once stability has been documented, surveillance imaging may be annual.[59]

PENETRATING AORTIC ULCER

Penetrating aortic ulcer (PAU) is defined as ulceration of an aortic atherosclerotic plaque penetrating through the internal

FLOWCHART 2: Treatment strategy for dissection of aorta.

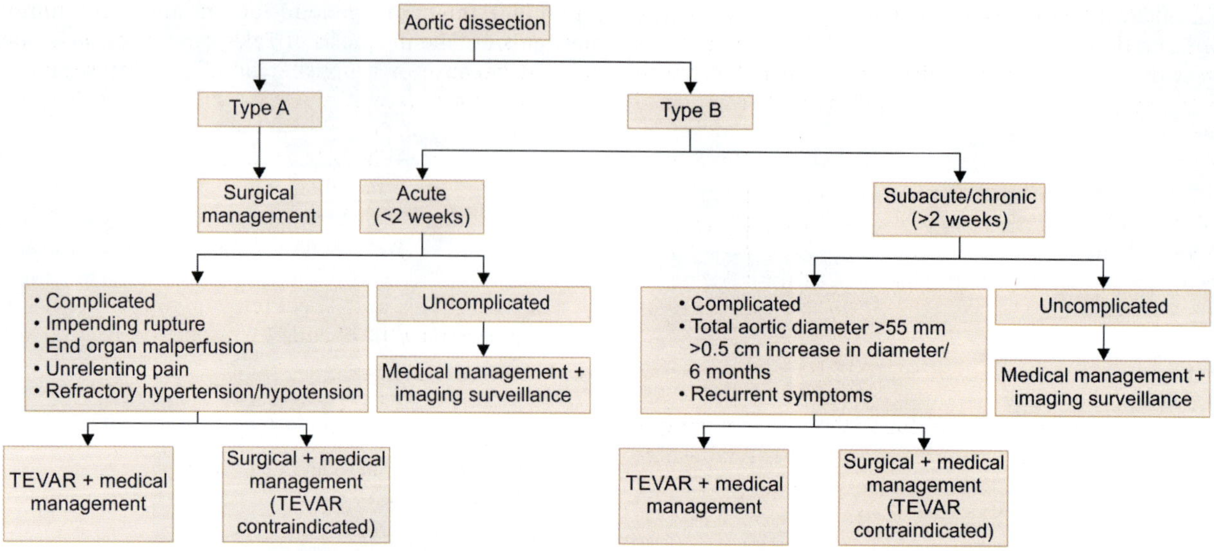

(TEVAR: thoracic endovascular aortic repair)

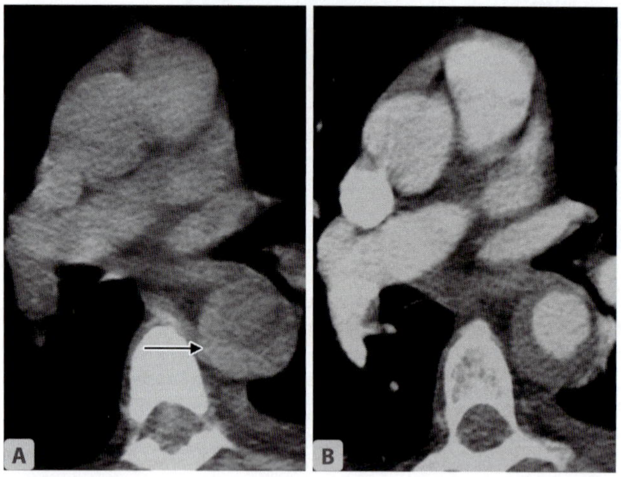

FIGS. 38A AND B: Noncontrast (a) axial and postcontrast CTA images show high density crescentic thickening along right posterolateral wall of distal descending thoracic aorta.

elastic lamina into the media.[60] These lesions represent 2 -7% of all AAS. Most common location of PAU is the middle and lower descending thoracic aorta, and less frequently noted in the aortic arch or abdominal aorta. Propagation of the ulcerative process may either lead to IMH, pseudoaneurysm, or even aortic rupture or an acute AD, and hence requires close follow-up.[61]

On noncontrast CT, PAU resembles an IMH. Contrast-enhanced CT is the technique of choice for diagnosis of PAU, which shows characteristic finding of localized ulceration, penetrating through the aortic intima into the aortic wall **(Figs. 39A to C)**. Focal thickening or high attenuation of the adjacent aortic wall suggests associated IMH. Limitation of MRI is that it is unable to detect displacement of intimal calcification, which frequently accompanies PAU.

Management of IMH and PAU

The management goals and treatment protocol for IMH and PAU are similar to type A and B AD. Surgery is advocated in

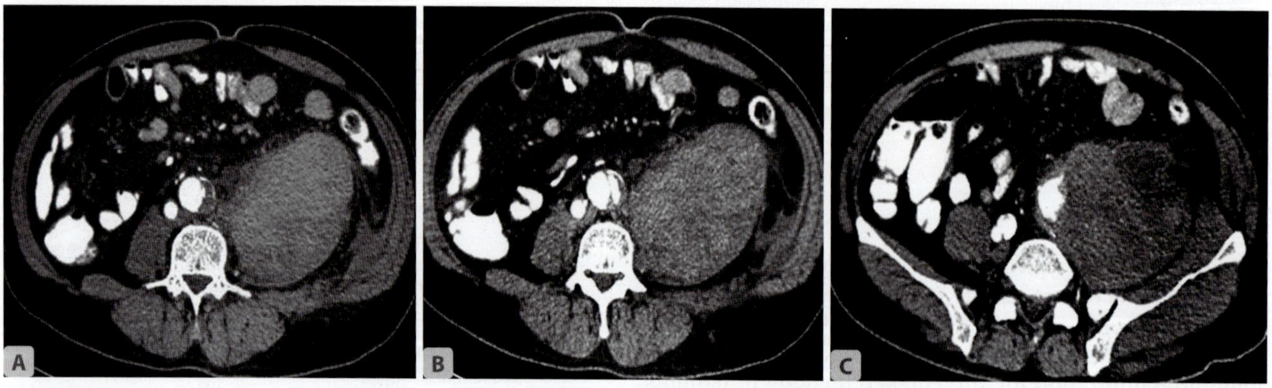

FIGS. 39A TO C: Serial CTA axial sections (craniocaudal) of distal abdominal aorta near bifurcation shows intramural hematoma along left lateral wall (A) penetrating ulcer (B) and rupture (C) leading to a large retroperitoneal hematoma (A to C).

patients with Type A IMH and ascending aortic ulcerations. Initial medical therapy is advocated in patients with type B IMH and descending thoracic aortic PAU. Some authors suggest that a symptomatic ulceration that is 20 mm in diameter or greater, or 10 mm in depth, should be managed aggressively.[62]

Complicated type B IMH with expansion of the hematoma, continued pain, development of hemorrhagic pleural effusion, or rupture requires more aggressive management with stent graft placement or surgery. The endovascular procedure is similar to that described for aortic dissection.

AORTITIS

Aortitis is an inflammatory condition of the aortic wall which can be infectious or noninfectious in origin. Imaging is required for assessment of aortitis and is crucial in establishing the diagnosis. CT, MRI and nuclear fusion imaging (PET CT/MRI) are the main imaging modalities for initial diagnosis and follow-up.[63,64]

Takayasu's Arteritis

Takayasu's arteritis (TA) is a necrotizing, obliterative and segmental primary large vessel panarteritis of unknown etiology that affects the aorta and its major branches including the pulmonary artery. It is most common in young Asian women and occurs about 10 times more commonly in women than in men. The etiologically factors implicated are previous tubercular infection, genetic factors and autoimmune mechanisms. The diagnosis of Takayasu's arteritis is often delayed because of a nonspecific clinical presentation. Ishikawa's criteria (sensitivity 60.4% and specificity 95%) and American College of Rheumatology criteria (sensitivity 77.4% and specificity 95%) have been widely used for diagnosis of this disease. Modified diagnostic criteria for Takayasu's arteritis by Sharma et al. have led to an early diagnosis of this condition thereby preventing high morbidity and mortality **(Table 9)**.[65,66]

The sensitivity and specificity using this modified diagnostic criteria is 92.5% and 95% respectively.

Incidence: 2.6 new cases/million/year
2.2% at autopsy

Pathology: TA is a T-cell-mediated panarterities which begins in adventitial vasa vasorum with inward progression. Destructive perivascular cuffing of vasa vasorum is followed by fibrosis and calcifications and leads to aneurysmal dilatations followed by stenosis of aorta and its branches. Arterial wall inflammation with adventitial mononuclear infiltration, multiple granulomas and perivascular cuffing of the vaso vasorum observed in early stages, followed by chronic fibrosis and wall calcification in later stages. Chronic necrotizing wall inflammation causes destruction of the media with resultant stenosis and/or aneurysm formations.[63,66-68]

TABLE 9: Modified diagnostic criteria for Takayasu's arteritis, Sharma et al.[65]

Three major criteria	
1. Left mid subclavian artery lesion	The most severe stenosis or occlusion present in the mid portion from the point 1 cm proximal to the vertebral artery orifice up to 3 cm distal to the orifice determined by angiography
2. Right mid subclavian artery lesion	The most severe stenosis or occlusion present in the mid portion from the right vertebral artery orifice to the point 3 cm distal to orifice determined by angiography
3. Characteristic signs and symptoms of at least one month duration	These include limb claudication, pulselessness or pulse differences in limbs, an unobtainable or significant blood pressure difference (>10 mm Hg systolic blood pressure difference in limb), fever, neck, pain, transient amaurosis, blurred vision, syncope, dyspnea or palpitations
Ten minor criteria	
1. High ESR	Unexplained persistent high ESR >20 mm/h (Westergren) at diagnosis or presence of the evidence in patients history
2. Carotid artery tenderness	Unilateral or bilateral tenderness of common carotid on palpation. Neck muscle tenderness is unacceptable
3. Hypertension	Persistent blood pressure >140/90 mm Hg brachial or >160/90 mm Hg popliteal
4. Aortic regurgitation or annuloaortic ectasia	• By auscultation or Doppler echocardiology or angiography • By angiography or two dimensional echocardiography
5. Pulmonary artery lesion	Lobar or segmental arterial occlusion or equivalent determined by angiography or perfusion scintigraphy, or presence of stenosis, aneurysm, luminal irregularity or any combination in pulmonary trunk or in unilateral or bilateral pulmonary arteries determined by angiography
6. Left mid common carotid lesion	Presence of the most severe stenosis or occlusion in the mid portion of 5 cm in length from the point 2 cm distal to its orifice determined by angiography
7. Distal brachiocephalic trunk lesion	Presence of the most severe stenosis or occlusion in the distal third determined by angiography
8. Descending thoracic aorta lesion	Narrowing, dilatation or aneurysm, luminal irregularity or any combination determined by angiography: tortuosity alone is unacceptable
9. Abdominal aorta lesion	Narrowing, dilatation or aneurysm, luminal irregularity or aneurysm combination
10. Coronary artery lesion	Documented on angiography below the age of 30 years in the absence of risk factors like hyperlipidemia or diabetes mellitus

Presence of two major or one major and two minor criteria or four minor criteria suggests a high probability of Takayasu's arteritis.

Types[69] (Fig. 40)

- **Type I** involves only the branches of the aortic arch.
- **Type IIa** involves the aorta only at its ascending portion and/or at the aortic arch. The branches of the aortic arch may be involved as well. The rest of the aorta is not affected.
- **Type IIb** affects the descending thoracic aorta with or without involvement of the ascending aorta or the aortic arch with its branches. The abdominal aorta is not involved.
- **Type III** is concomitant involvement of the descending thoracic aorta, the abdominal aorta, and/or the renal arteries. The ascending aorta and the aortic arch and its branches are not involved.
- **Type IV** involves only the abdominal aorta and/or the renal arteries.
- **Type V** is a generalized type, with combined features of the other types.

Note: Involvement of the coronary and pulmonary arteries should be indicated as C(+) or P(+), respectively.

The commonly involved arteries are left subclavian artery (50%), left common carotid (20%), brachiocephalic, renal arteries, celiac trunk, SMA and pulmonary arteries (50%).

Imaging Findings

Almost all the available imaging modalities have some role in diagnosis and follow-up of TA, however, currently CT, MRI and/or PET CT/MRI are the main imaging modalities. Role of conventional angiography in diagnosis of TA is almost obsolete and restricted for interventional procedures.[70]

Early/acute stage: The arterial wall thickening **(Fig. 41)** can be detected on CT or MRI (Fat-suppressed T1-weighted postcontrast MR images) as soft tissue thickening encircling the aorta (swollen intima) with circumferential peripheral contrast enhancement (inflamed media and adventitia. On T2-weighted sequences mural edema is depicted as high signal. Nuclear fusion imaging (PET) with 18-flurorodeoxyglucose (18F-FDG) with either CT or MRI is now emerging as the initial diagnosis and assessment of disease activity with high sensitivity of 60-90% and specificity of 88–100% as 18F-FDG is a surrogate marker of increased activity of inflammatory cells.[70,71-73]

Chronic stage: The disease is characterized by development of aneurysm and linear stenosis of descending and abdominal aorta. There may be long diffuse or short segmental irregular stenosis with occlusion of the major branches of the aorta near its origin **(Fig. 42)**. There may be skip lesions, abundant collateralization, saccular or fusiform aortic aneurysm (10–15%) **(Fig. 43)**.[74,75] These findings can be seen on conventional angiography, CT angiography or MR angiography. Cross-sectional imaging, in addition, shows arterial wall thickening, mural calcium deposition and full thickness calcification which is very suggestive of chronic phase of disease.[76,77]

Management of TA

Active TA is treated with steroids or immunosuppressants before revascularization as revascularization during the active phase can increase the risk of procedure-related complications, including restenosis and dissection.[78]

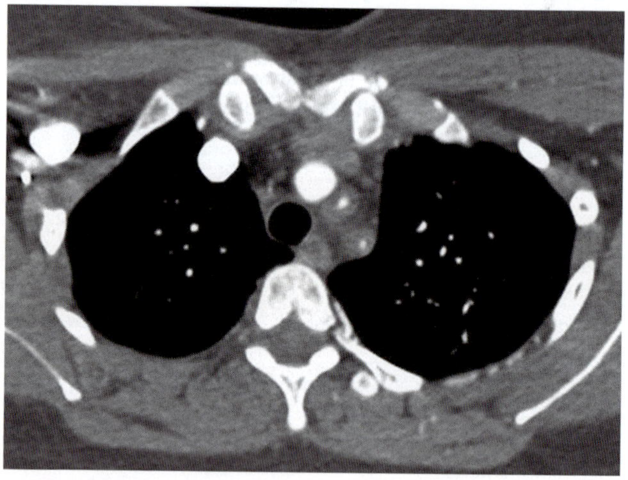

FIG. 41: Takayasu's arteritis: CTA source image showing circumferential mural thickening of the lateral common carotid and subclavian arteries.

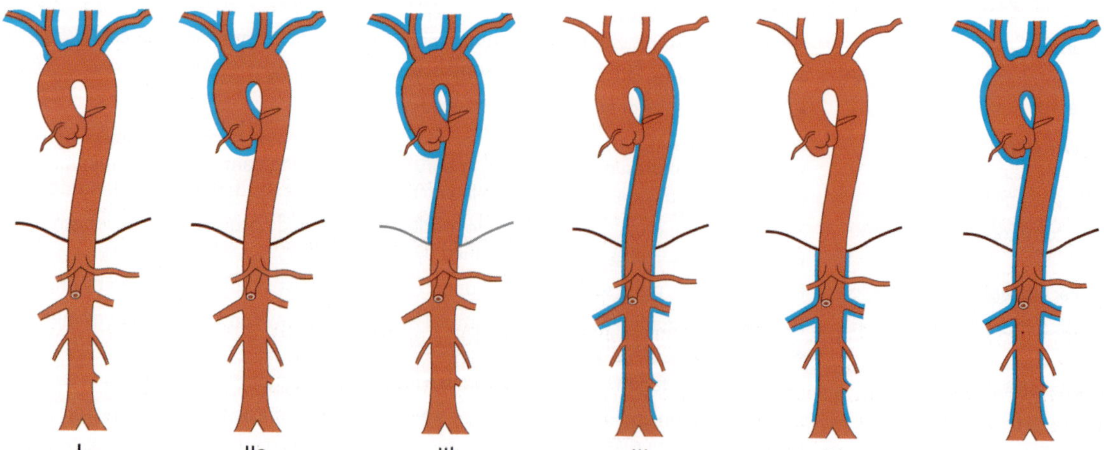

FIG. 40: Schematic diagrams show types of Takayasu's arteritis.

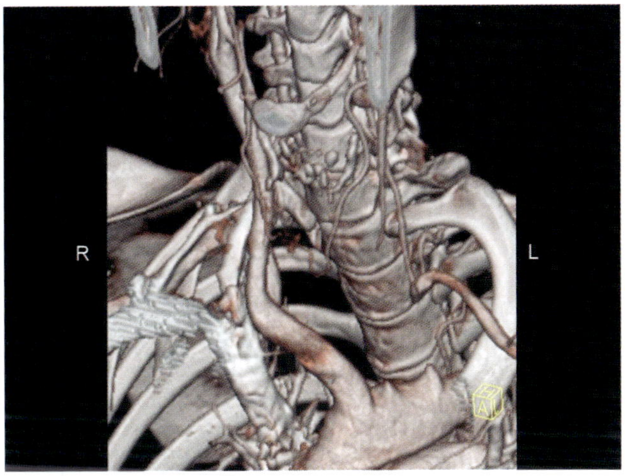

FIG. 42: Takayasu's arteritis: CTA VR image showing total occlusion of left common carotid and subclavian arteries just beyond their origins.

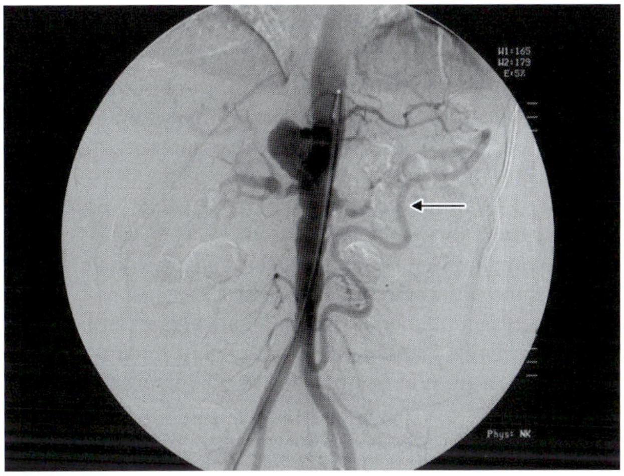

FIG. 43: Takayasu's arteritis: DSA shows aneurysmal dilatation of the abdominal aorta above renal arteries, irregular aortic contour, collaterals from IMA (arrow).

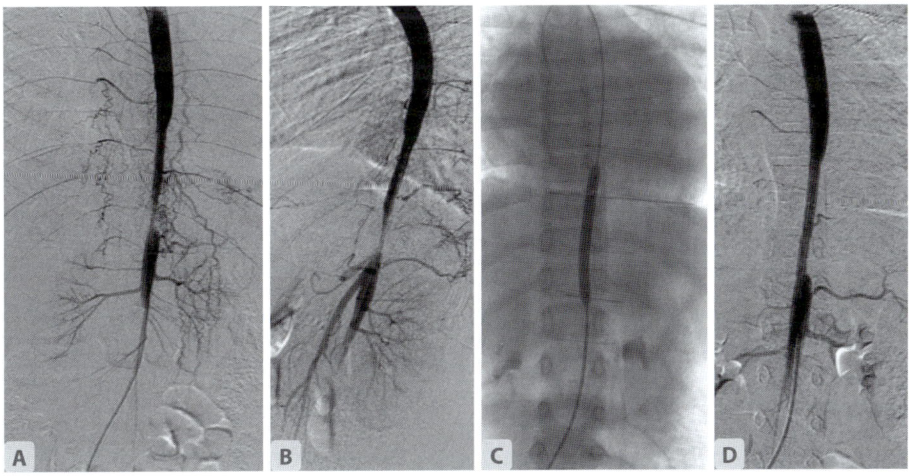

FIGS. 44A TO D: Balloon angioplasty in a patient of Takayasu's arteritis with heart failure: (A and B) Aortogram showing long segment tight stenosis of the juxta-diaphragmatic thoracic aorta; (C) Balloon angioplasty of the stenosed segment: (D) Postangioplasty aortogram showing significant reduction of degree of stenosis with reduction of the trans-stenotic gradient from 65 mm of Hg to 15 mm of Hg.

Occlusion/restenosis rate of transluminal angioplasty with or without stent implantation in active disease is reported to be as high as 71.4% after a follow-up of 1.3 years.

Symptomatic TA is treated with revascularization of the affected vessels. In general, surgical bypass or endovascular intervention should be avoided during the active phase of TA, unless the presence of an acute life-threatening condition outweighs the risk any intervention including restenosis and dissection.[78,79]

Even in life-threatening situations (hypertensive encephalopathy, flash pulmonary edema and congestive heart failure), endovascular treatment is the treatment modality that carries the lowest risk of morbidity and mortality to the patient and should be considered before open surgical therapy. This is due to the fact that, surgical procedures are complicated by graft reocclusion, anastomotic site aneurysm and increased morbidity. The progressive inflammatory nature of TA has is also a widespread problem limiting use of reconstructive surgery.

In the chronic fibrotic stage, the principle of treatment is revascularization either by surgery or balloon angioplasty. Balloon angioplasty is a relatively simple and cost-effective method for relief of stenotic lesions in patients with TA **(Figs. 44A to D)**. It avoids the risks of anesthesia and shortens the hospital stay. Percutaneous angioplasty yielded excellent results with success rates ranging from 81% to 100% and low morbidity and mortality.[78]

The problem with balloon angioplasty is recurrence of the stenosis, which is however, easily tackled by a secondary reintervention. Studies also reported improved results with primary stenting; however, stenting is better reserved for flow limiting dissections or persisting stenoses after balloon angioplasty. Moreover, the presence of long segment juxta diaphragmatic stenosis involving the origin of visceral arteries, often in a young child precludes the use of a stent. The risk of stent occlusion is also higher due to protracted nature of the disease with waxing and waning of disease activity.

Immunoglobulin G4 (IgG4)-related Aortitis

IgG4 related diseases are of unknown etiology which can affect any organ from head to toe. It is characterized by diffuse or focal tumor like lesions with lymphoplasmacytic infiltrate enriched with IgG4 positive plasma cells and fibrosis. They are often associated with elevated serum IgG4 levels. It predominantly affects males in their 4–6 decades however exact incidence is unknown. It is a great mimicker with varying differential diagnosis on imaging, ranging from inflammatory lesions to malignancy.[81]

Recognition of imaging findings can suggest a diagnosis, which can be confirmed on serology, and histopathology. This is of paramount importance as the disease responds to immunosuppressive therapy. On pathology the lymphoplasmacytic cells are IgG4 positive with negative CD3 and CD20 staining which are markers for T-cell and B-cell related inflammation respectively and are positive in aortoarteritis.

On imaging a soft tissue like mass is seen encasing aorta and its branches, typically without any luminal compromise unlike aortoarteritis. The soft tissue is hypodense on CT **(Figs. 45A and B)** and demonstrates varying signal intensity on MR depending on degree and stage of fibrosis.[82] Contrast enhancement can be variable depending upon degree of fibrosis.

In long-standing cases aneurysmal dilatation of abdominal aorta and extensive wall thickening with or without periaortic inflammatory extension can be seen.[83] Rupture though uncommon with IgG4-related disease may be seen **(*Refer* Figs. 24 to 26)**.

18F-FDG PET-CT and CT are useful in detecting inflammatory activity in the aneurysmal wall **(Figs. 46A to D)** and assessing treatment response.[84]

AORTIC TRAUMA

Traumatic injuries to the aorta may result from either blunt (nonpenetrating, indirect) or sharp (penetrating, direct) trauma. Penetrating trauma is usually caused by stab or bullet wounds that puncture the aortic wall. Rare causes include misplacement of spinal fixation screws and lacerations from spinal fractures. Blunt aortic injuries (BAIs) are far more common and the aortic wall is damaged from the inside to the outside, from the intima to the adventitia.

Traumatic transaction of the aorta is a common cause of death in high-speed accidents. Sudden deceleration causes torsion and a shearing stress at the isthmus where the aorta is relatively fixed. "Osseous pinch" effect is due to pinching of the aorta between the manubrium and medial end of clavicle anteriorly and spine posteriorly. It is due to this pinch that there is posterior displacement of the heart which generates aortic torsion.[85] About 90% of traumatic tears occur around the isthmus. The other sites include: aortic arch with avulsion of brachiocephalic trunk (4.5%), ascending aorta (1%) and descending aorta (2.5%). These patients often have multiple injuries and pose a considerable challenge for early and rapid imaging.

Grading of Aortic Injuries[86]

- *Grade 0*: Normal mediastinum and normal aorta
- *Grade I*: Abnormal mediastinum and normal aorta. About 5–10% of blunt trauma of chest may have isolated mediastinal hematoma
- *Grade II*: Minimal aortic injury (differential diagnosis of ductus arteriosus remnant or atherosclerosis)
- *Grade III*: Confined aortic injury
- *Grade IV*: Aortic disruption.

Imaging

The chest X-ray is a good screening tool for detection of mediastinal hemorrhage, but affords little as far as definitive diagnosis is concerned. An AP erect chest film with the patient leaning forward is ideal rather than a supine film with 90% sensitivity, 95% specificity and 95% negative predictive value.

The plain X-ray findings include widening of the superior mediastinum, an abnormal aortic contour, shift of the trachea to the right, inferior displacement of the left main bronchus, widening of left paravertebral stripe, etc.

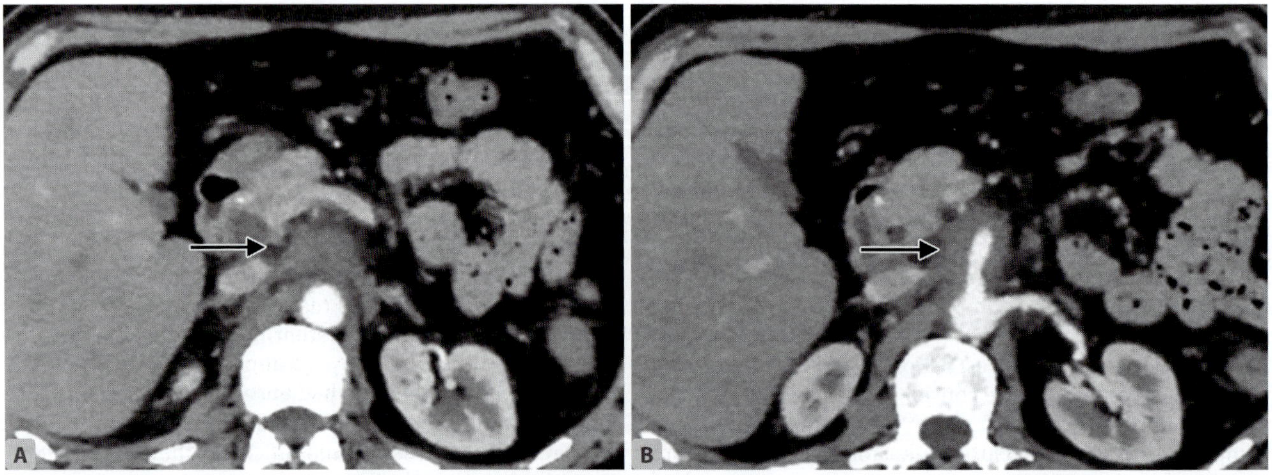

FIGS. 45A AND B: CTA axial images an ill-defined soft tissue is seen in preaortic location (arrow in A) which is encasing the celiac artery from its origin (arrow in B) without any luminal compromise.

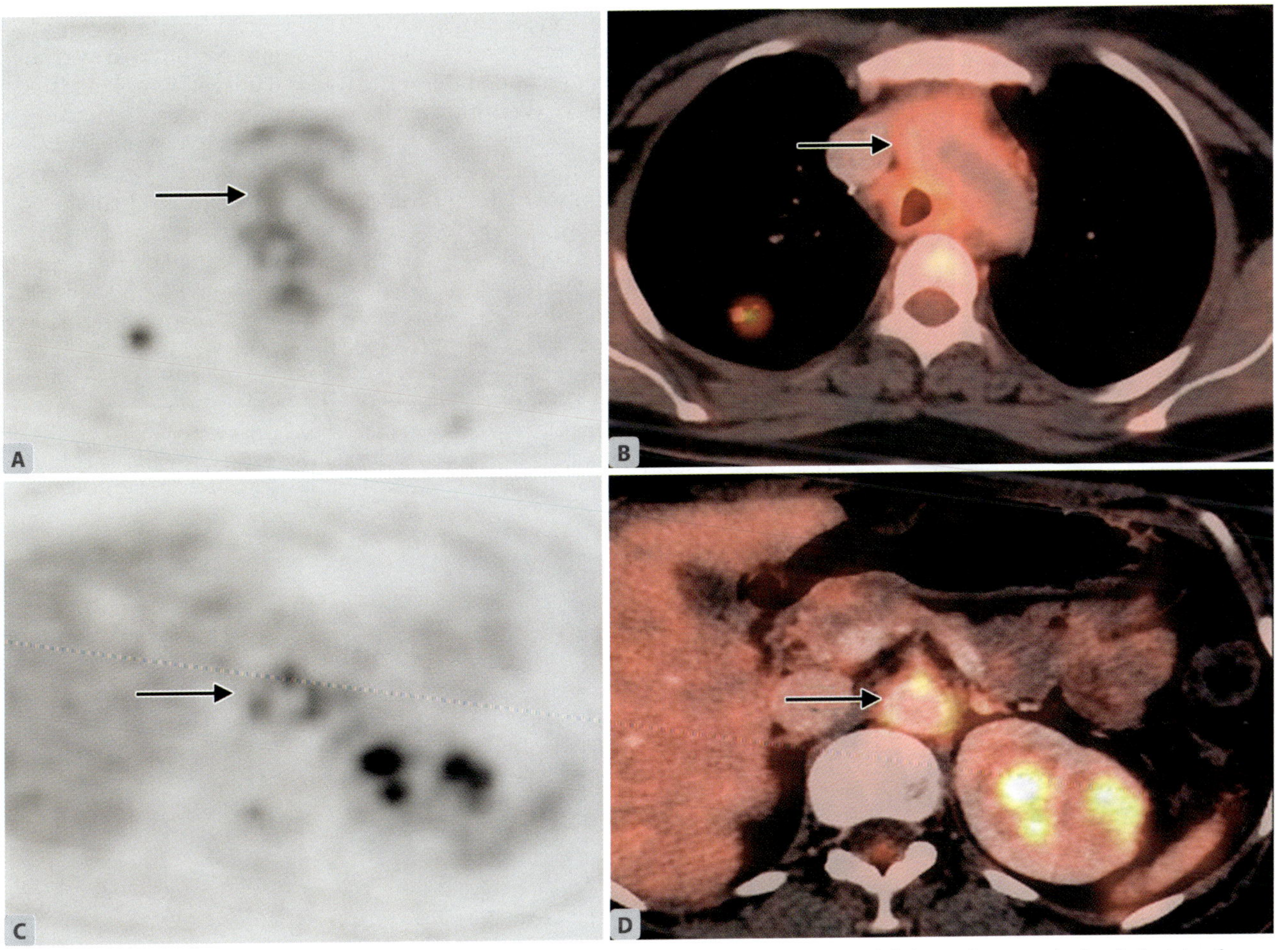

FIGS. 46A TO D: 18F-FDG PET and fused PET-CT images show increased activity in arch of aorta and abdominal aorta at the level of origin of celiac axis.

Courtesy: Dr Rajender Basher, Assistant Professor, Department of Nuclear Medicine, PGIMER, Chandigarh, India.

Computed Tomography

Plain CT may demonstrate mediastinal hematoma. CECT may show an abrupt change in aortic contour, intimal flap, pseudoaneurysm, pseudocoarctation and extravasation of contrast. CTA shows 96.2% sensitivity, 99.8% specificity and 99.7% accuracy for the diagnosis of aortic injury.

Magnetic Resonance Imaging

In an acute setting of multiple injuries, MR is not recommended.

Aortography

It is the definitive mode of diagnosis but in view of the high sensitivity of CT, aortography is indicated only in selected cases of chronic aortic trauma.

Management of Thoracic Aortic Injury

The initial management of the patient with a contained aortic transection is stabilization of vitals. Patients with multiple injuries can be managed medically for several days or weeks until an intervention can be performed. The conventional therapy of aortic transection was surgery but stent-grafts are increasingly used to treat TAI and now the current procedure of choice **(Figs. 47A to D)**. All patients with external aortic contour deformity should be treated with endovascular stent graft as soon as possible and atleast before hospital discharge.

Its advantages include that it can be performed quickly and percutaneously in the patients who would be at high-risk for open surgical repair and cardiopulmonary bypass. The challenges faced in this population are similar to the challenges faced in treating type B AD and may be overcome using similar techniques.

ATHEROSCLEROSIS

Atherosclerosis is the most common disease involving the aorta. The changes of atherosclerosis are seen in almost all people beyond middle age although they often remain asymptomatic. The abdominal aorta below the renal arteries is the most common site of atherosclerosis and most patients with aortoiliac occlusive disease also have associated femoral and distal arterial occlusions. Reconstruction of the aorta and the iliac arteries by thromboendarterectomy, shunts, stents or angioplasties is an extremely satisfactory therapy for

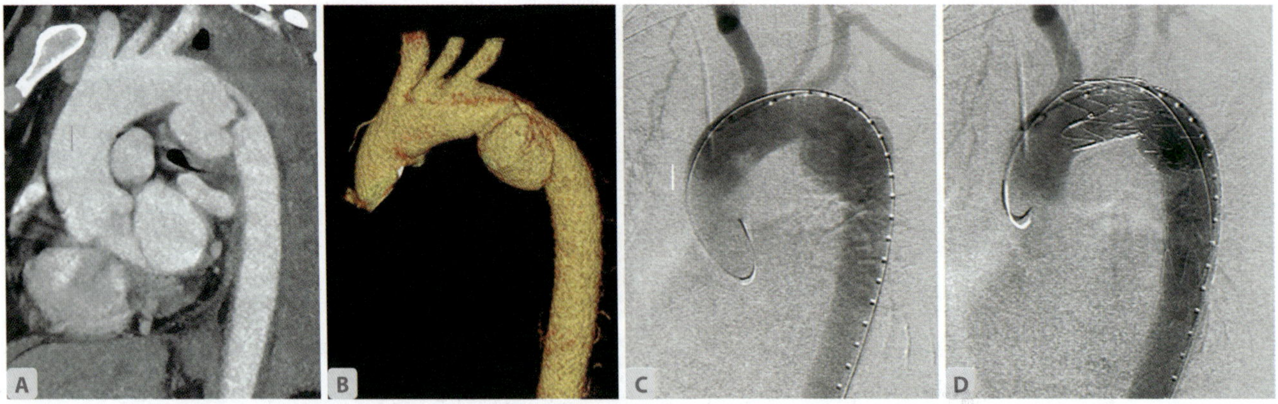

FIGS. 47A TO D: Stent-graft repair of traumatic aortic transection. (A and B) Computed tomography images showing transection with (A) pseudoaneurysm of the proximal descending thoracic aorta; (C) Angiogram prior to stent-graft placement shows in (A); (D) Angiogram following stent-graft placement. The pseudoaneurysm is excluded. Note that the left subclavian artery was sacrificed with its ostia covered by the stent graft.

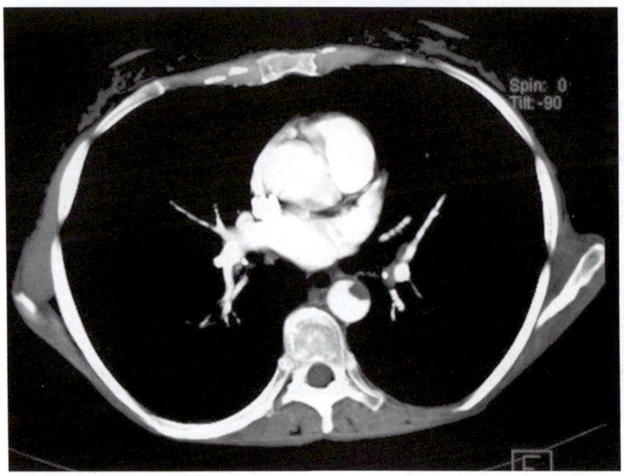

FIG. 48: Atheromatous aortic disease: CTA source image shows atheromatous plaque along anterolateral wall of aorta and projecting into the lumen.

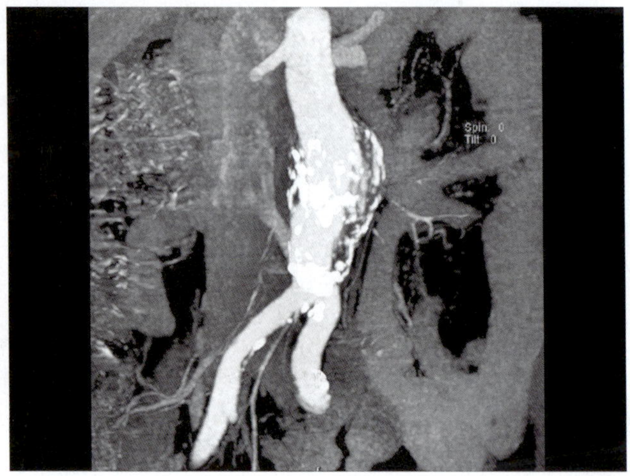

FIG. 49: Atheromatous aortic disease: large plaque with circumferential calcifications, aortic dilatation and mural thickening.

disabling arteriosclerosis obliterans of the aortoiliac system. CTA and DSA are the most effective imaging modalities for the demonstration of aorto iliac obstruction sites, distal run off vessels or collateral vessels and associated stenosis or occlusions of the major visceral arteries.

Pathology

Variable combination of changes of the intima of arteries with focal accumulation of lipids, complex carbohydrates, blood and blood products, fibrous tissue and calcium are the hallmark of atherosclerosis. The disease is divided into:

- Early changes: Fatty streak and gelatinous elevation reflected on imaging as "smooth plaque".
- Fibroatheromatous plaque: It is seen on imaging as irregular plaque, plaque ulceration, etc. **(Fig. 48)**.
- The complicated lesion: Hemorrhage in the plaque, fibrogenesis leading to irregularity and tortousity, weakening of the wall leading to aneurysm formation and calcification **(Fig. 49)**. Stenosis and occlusion may be due to combinations of plaque, fibrosis and calcification.

Imaging

The gross morphological changes can be seen on all imaging modalities. These signs are:[87]

- Diffuse narrowing of the vessels
- Irregular vascular contours and diameters
- Nicks, filling defects and calcifications along the vessel wall
- Spotty or ragged density of the opaque contrast column
- Vessels that are generally large or tortuous or both.
- Saccular dilatations and aneurysm
- Stenosis and or frank occlusion of a vessel (obliterative arteriosclerosis)

Cross-sectional imaging may show a greater degree of luminal compromise, intimal atherosclerosis, mural thrombus and the surgeons may palpate a greater hardening of vessel wall than is seen on catheter angiograms.

Occlusion of the Aorto-iliac System

It may be the terminal event in slowly progressive arteriosclerotic stenosis and may be tolerated without medical attention. The blood flow through a vessel may be relatively adequate until the vessel diameter is reduced to about 70%. Acute occlusion may occur following emboli from heart, atherosclerotic plaques or aneurysms.

Complete Occlusion of Aorta

It rarely extends upwards to involve the renal arteries but at surgery, the renal and other visceral arteries are frequently found to be partially involved **(Figs. 50A to D)**. Syphilis, aortic dissection and atherosclerosis have been reported to cause complete aortic occlusion. 'Leriche syndrome' is due to complete occlusion of the terminal part of abdominal aorta and bilateral common iliac arteries.

Collateral Pathways

In stenotic or occlusive disease extensive collateral pathways open up.

- *Visceral collateral network:* The SMA and IMA form the major visceral collateral circulation.
  - Aortic occlusion above IMA: The SMA acts as the main affluent vessel through the left branch of middle colic artery into left colic branch of the IMA (effluent vessel). The "meandering mesenteric artery" or "central anastomotic artery" represents this communication **(Fig. 51)**.
  - Aortic occlusion below IMA: The IMA acts as a key source of collateral circulation via retiform anastomosis between superior hemorrhoidal branches and middle and inferior hemorrhoidal branches of the internal iliac arteries which may reconstitute the external iliac artery.
- *Parietal collateral network:* The parietal vessels that may be seen to bridge aortic occlusions are the intercostals, subcostal, lumbar and median sacral branches of the aorta with iliolumbar, lateral sacral, superior gluteal and obturator branches of the internal iliac arteries, and deep iliac circumflex and medial and lateral circumflex branches of the external iliac and deep femoral arteries. Lumbar branches have anastomotic connections with iliolumbar and gluteal branches of the internal iliac artery. The epigastric arteries may form an important collateral circulation (Winslow's pathway), i.e. from the intercostals and internal mammary artery to the external iliac arteries through the epigastric arteries.

The indications for intervention in patients with occlusive disease of aorta are moderate to severe claudication, rest pain, acutely threatened limb and hemodynamically significant lesion proximal to a distal lesion for which revascularization is being attempted. Patients with mild claudication should undergo medical management with exercise therapy first. Surgical options including aortofemoral bypass, axillofemoral bypass, femoral-femoral bypass, and aortic endarterectomy are effective treatments but more morbid compared to endovascular approaches. Endovascular management includes balloon angioplasty with or without stenting. Stent placement is indicated for patients with obstructive dissection during balloon angioplasty, recanalization of total occlusions, or lesions that are likely to cause distal embolization. Stent-grafts may be used to exclude symptomatic ulcerated plaque, but otherwise currently have little role for aortic occlusive disease.

Postoperative Aorta

CTA or MRA is the preferred modality for evaluating postoperative aorta for demonstration of perigraft fluid

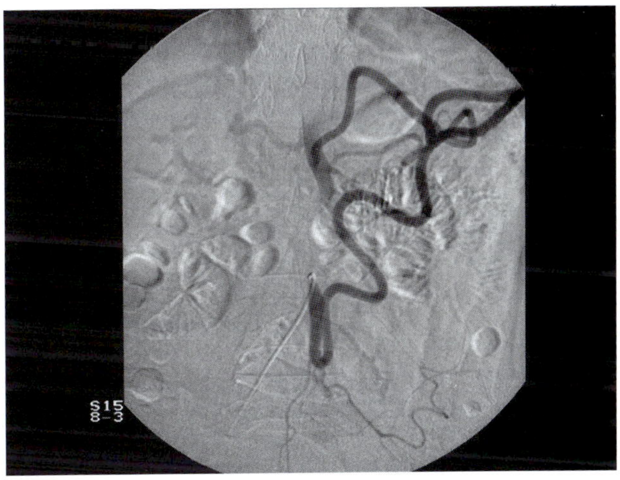

FIG. 51: Visceral collateral network: DSA shows IMA-SMA collateral network.

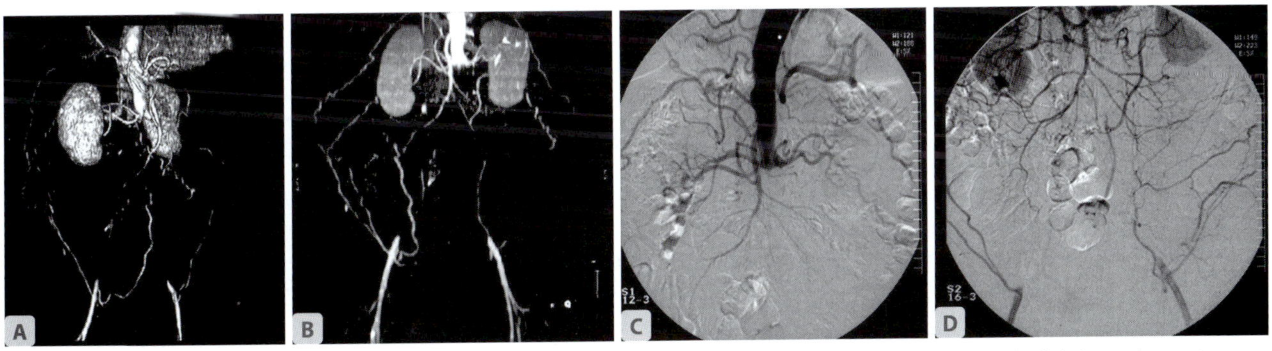

FIGS. 50A TO D: Atherosclerotic complete occlusion of aorta: CTA (A) and VR (B) MIP projections show complete block of abdominal aorta just distal to renal arteries with collaterals and run off to distal external iliac arteries. DSA (C and D) confirms the findings of CTA.

collection and acute hemorrhage. It is also more informative in the diagnosis of graft infection, aortoenteric fistula, anastomotic pseudoaneurysm. These modalities are also very helpful in evaluating the efficacy of endovascular treatment in aortic diseases.[88]

CONCLUSION

Noninvasive imaging of the aorta has almost replaced invasive aortography. US is a good screening modality to confirm or exclude aneurysm, dissection, atherosclerosis etc. but additional anatomic information needs to be obtained prior to an elective repair or endovascular treatment. TEE provides additional information for the thoracic aorta except in the area of the proximal arch (blind spot). Contrast-enhanced CT should be used routinely both for preoperative and postoperative assessment of aortic diseases. At a reasonable cost and low-risk to patients, CT and CT angiography can provide the diagnosis, operability, and anatomic definition including concomitant intra-thoracic or intra-abdominal abnormalities. The recent advances in MR hardware, sequences and computational ability pose a real challenge to all imaging techniques. MR can now provide all the information needed for evaluating aortic diseases, anatomic as well as functional and gadolinium enhanced 3D MRA may replace catheter angiography for both preoperative and postoperative evaluation. Angiography is indicated to answer specific questions posed by the results of clinical examination and/or CT or MR imaging or as a prerequisite to endovascular intervention. Knowledge of indication of treatment (medical vs. interventional) of different aortic pathologies is of paramount importance. Surgery has been traditionally used in management of these patients however with increasing expertise and development of hardware, endovascular techniques have become the first line of management in many of these aortic pathologies.

ACKNOWLEDGMENTS

Dr Sreedhar BC, Fellow Interventional Radiology, PGIMER, Chandigarh for his active support in literature search and preparation of manuscript, Dr Chirag Jain, Fellow Neuro-Radiology, PGIMER, Chandigarh for his contribution to art work, Professor Ritambra Nada, Department of Histopathology, PGIMER, Chandigarh for pathology specimens and slides, and Dr Rajender Basher, Assistant Professor, Department of Nuclear Medicine, PGIMER, Chandigarh for providing PET-CT images.

REFERENCES

1. Douglas H. "Aorta". Online Etymology Dictionary. Retrieved 9 October; 2017.
2. Rosner F. Medicine in the Bible and the Talmud: selections from classical Jewish sources (Augm. ed.). Hoboken, NJ: KTAV Pub. House.1995.pp.87-96.
3. Goldstein SA, Evangelista A, Abbara S. Multimodality imaging of diseases of the thoracic aorta in adults: from the American Society of Echocardiography and the European Association of Cardiovascular Imaging: endorsed by the Society of Cardiovascular Computed Tomography and Society for Cardiovascular Magnetic Resonance. J Am Soc Echocardiogr. 2015;28:119-82.
4. Wolf YG, Zarins CK. Noninvasive aortic imaging. In: Bruce L Gewetz (Ed.) Philadelphia. W.B. Saunders. 2000;1:34-40.
5. Rosenblum JD, Leef JA. Aortography. In: Bruce L Gewetz (ed.) Philadelphia. W.B. Saunders. 2000;1:41-50.
6. Lucarotti ME, Shaw E, Heather BP. Distribution of aortic diameter in a screened population. Br J Surg. 1992;79:641-2.
7. Jaffee RB. Radiographic manifestations of congenital anomalies of the aortic arch. RCNA. 1991;29:319-34.
8. Shinley BR. Transesophageal echocardiography in the diagnosis of aortic disease. Seminars in US, CT and MRI. 1993;14:106-16.
9. Benenati JF. Intravasclar ultrasound: the role in diagnostic and therapeutic procedures. RCNA. 1995;33:31-50.
10. Kumamaru KK, Hoppe BE, Richard T, et al. CT angiography: Current technology and clinical use. Radiol Clin North Am. 2010;48:213-35.
11. Rajiah P. CT and MRI in the Evaluation of Thoracic Aortic Diseases. International Journal of Vascular Medicine. 2013.pp.16.
12. Litmanovich D, Bankier AA, Cantin L, et al. CT and MRI in diseases of the aorta. Am J Roentgenol. 2009;193:928-40.
13. Gutstein A, Wolak A, Lee C, et al. Predicting success of prospective and retrospective gating with dual-source coronary computed tomography angiography: development of selection criteria and initial experience. Journal of Cardiovascular Computed Tomography. 2008;2:81-90.
14. Gies M, Kalender W A, Wolf H, et al. Dose reduction in CT by anatomically adapted tube current modulation. I. Simulation studies. Medical Physics. 1999:26;2235-47.
15. Leschka S, Stolzmann P, Schmid F T, et al. Low kilovoltage cardiac dual-source CT: attenuation, noise, and radiation dose. European Radiology. 2008;18:1809-17.
16. Macari M, Israel GM, Berman P, et al. Infrarenal abdominal aortic aneurysms at multi-detector row CT angiography: intravascular enhancement without a timing acquisition. Radiology. 2001;220:519-23.
17. Cademaritiri F, Mollet N, van der Lugt A, et al. Noninvasive 16-row multislice coronary angiography: usefulness of saline chaser. Eur Radiol. 2004;14:178-83.
18. Czum JM, Corse WR, Ho VB. MR angiography of the thoracic aorta. Magn Reson Imaging Clin N Am. 2005;13:41-64.
19. Sakamoto I, Sueyoshi E, Uetani M. MR Imaging of the Aorta. Radiol Clin N Am. 2007;45:485-97.
20. Amano Y, Takahama K, Kumita S. Non-contrast-enhanced MR angiography of the thoracic aorta using cardiac and navigator-gated magnetization-prepared three-dimensional steady-state free precession. J Magn Reson Imaging. 2008;27:504-9.
21. Gebker R, Gomaa O, Schnackenburg B, et al. Comparison of different MRI techniques for the assessment of thoracic aortic pathology: 3D contrast enhanced MR angiography, turbo spin echo and balanced steady state free precession. Int J Cardiovasc Imaging. 2007;23:747-56.
22. Galizia MS, Bolen MA, Flamm SD. MRI of the thoracic aorta. Applied Radiology. 2015.pp.22-6 (www.appliedradiology.com)
23. Prince MR, Yucel EK, Kaufman JA, et al. Dynamic gadolinium-enhanced three-dimensional abdominal MR arteriography. J Magn Reson Imaging.1993;3:877-81.
24. Russo V, Renzulli M, Buttazzi K, et al. Acquired diseases of the thoracic aorta: role of MRI and MRA. Eur Radiol. 2006;16:852-65.
25. Russo V, Renzulli M, Palombara CL, et al. Congenital diseases of the thoracic aorta: role of MRI and MRA. Eur Radiol. 2006;16: 676-84.

26. Hom JJ, Ordovas K, Reddy GP. Velocity-encoded cine MR imaging in aortic coarctation: functional assessment of hemodynamic events. Radiographics. 2008;28:407-16.
27. Lee YH, Choi SJ, Ji JD, et al. Diagnostic accuracy of 18F-FDG PET or PET/CT for large vessel vasculitis. Z Rheumatol. 2016;75:924-31.
28. Danve A, O Dell, J. The role of 18F-fluorodeoxyglucose positron emission tomography scanning in the diagnosis and management of systemic vasculitis. Int J Rheum Dis. 2015;18:714-24.
29. Glaudemans AW, de Vries EF, Galli F, et al. The Use of F-FDG-PET/CT for diagnosis and treatment monitoring of inflammatory and infectious diseases. Clin Dev Immunol. 2013;2013.623036.
30. Khandelwal N, Gupta S. Current concepts in imaging aortic aneurysms in Sanjiv Sharma (Ed). Recent advances in imaging and intervention in cardiovascular diseases. Singapore Springer. 1996;58-62.
31. Campbell M. Natural history of coarctation of aorta. Br Heart J. 1970;32:633-40.
32. Silversides CK, Marelli A, Beauchesne L, et al. Canadian Cardiovascular Society 2009 Consensus Conference on the management of adults with congenital heart disease: executive summary. Can J Cardiol. 2010;26:143-50.
33. Feltes TF, Bacha E, Beekman RH 3rd, et al. Indications for cardiac catheterization and intervention in pediatric cardiac disease: a scientific statement from the American Heart Association. Circulation. 2011;123:2607-52.
34. Hiratzka LF, Bakris GL, Beckman JA, et al. 2010 ACCF/AHA/AATS/ACR/ASA/SCA/SCAI/SIR/STS/SVM Guidelines for the diagnosis and management of patients with thoracic aortic disease. A report of the American College of Cardiology Foundation/American Heart Association Task Force on Practice Guidelines, American Association for Thoracic Surgery, American College of Radiology, American Stroke Association, Society of Cardiovascular Anesthesiologists, Society for Cardiovascular Angiography and Interventions, Society of Interventional Radiology, Society of Thoracic Surgeons, and Society for Vascular Medicine. J Am Coll Cardiol. 2010;55:e27-e129.
35. Davies RR, Goldstein LJ, Coady MA, et al. Yearly rupture or dissection rates for thoracic aortic aneurysms: simple prediction based on size. Ann Thorac Surg. 2002;73:17-27.
36. Brewster DC, Cronenwett JL, Hallett JW Jr, et al. Guidelines for the treatment of abdominal aortic aneurysms. Report of a subcommittee of the Joint Council of the American Association for Vascular Surgery and Society for Vascular Surgery. J Vasc Surg. 2003;37:1106.
37. LaRoy LL, Cormier PJ, Matalon TAS, et al. Imaging of abdominal aortic aneurysms. AJR. 1989;152:785-92.
38. Goldstein SA, Evangelista A, Abbara S, et al. Multimodality imaging of diseases of the thoracic aorta in adults: from the American Society of Echocardiography and the European Association of Cardiovascular Imaging: endorsed by the Society of Cardiovascular Computed Tomography and Society for Cardiovascular Magnetic Resonance. J Am Soc Echocardiogr. 2015;28:119-82.
39. Prince MR, Yucel EK, Kaufman JA, et al. Dynamic gadolinium-enhanced three-dimensional abdominal MR arteriography. J Magn Reson Imaging.1993;3:877-81.
40. Brewster DC, Cronenwett JL, Hallett JW Jr, et al. Guidelines for the treatment of abdominal aortic aneurysms. Report of a subcommittee of the Joint Council of the American Association for Vascular Surgery and Society for Vascular Surgery. J Vasc Surg. 2003;37:1106.
41. Bown MJ, Sweeting MJ, Brown LC, et al. Surveillance intervals for small abdominal aortic aneurysms: a meta-analysis. JAMA. 2013;309:806-13.
42. Walsh SR, Tang TY, Sadat U, et al. Endovascular stenting versus open surgery for thoracic aortic disease: systematic review and meta-analysis of perioperative results. J Vasc Surg. 2008;47:1094-8.
43. Zhang Y, Teng Z, Lu Q, et al. Management of complicated aortic aneurysms using multiple overlapping uncovered stents: mid-term outcome from a cohort study. Medicine (Baltimore). 2014;93:e209.
44. Sadat U, Boyle JR, Walsh SR, et al. Endovascular vs open repair of acute abdominal aortic aneurysms: a systematic review and meta-analysis. J Vasc Surg. 2008;48:227-36.
45. Kaufman JA, Geller SC, Brewster DC, et al. Endovascular repair of abdominal aortic aneurysms: current status and future directions. Am J Roentgenol. 2000;175:289-302.
46. William DM, Joshi A, Dake MD, et al. Aortic cobwebs: An anatomic marker identifying the false lumen in aortic dissection– imaging and pathologic correlation. Radiology. 1994;190:167-74.
47. Nienaber CA, vonKodolitsch Y, Nicholas V, et al. The diagnosis of thoracic aortic dissection by noninvasive imaging procedures. N Engl J Med. 1993;328:1-14.
48. LePage MA, Quint LE, Sonnad SS, et al. Aortic dissection: CT features that distinguish true lumen from false lumen. Am J Roentgenol. 2001;177:207-11.
49. Pereles FS, McCarthy RM, Baskaran V, et al. Thoracic aortic dissection and aneurysm: evaluation with nonenhanced true FISP MR angiography in less than 4 minutes. Radiology. 2002;223:270-4.
50. Dake MD, Thompson M, van Sambeek M, et al. DISSECT: a new mnemonic-based approach to the categorization of aortic dissection. Eur J Vasc Endovasc Surg. 2013;46:175-90.
51. Nienaber CA, Eagle KA. Aortic dissection: new frontiers in diagnosis and management: Part I: from etiology to diagnostic strategies. Circulation. 2003;108:628-35.
52. Hagan PG, Nienaber CA, Isselbacher EM, et al. The International Registry of Acute Aortic Dissection (IRAD): new insights into an old disease. JAMA. 2000;283:897-903.
53. Criado FJ, Barnatan MF, Rizk Y, et al. Technical strategies to expand stent-graft applicability in the aortic arch and proximal descending thoracic aorta. J Endovasc Ther. 2002;9(Suppl 2):II32-8.
54. Midulla M, Renaud A, Martinelli T, et al. Endovascular fenestration in aortic dissection with acute malperfusion syndrome: immediate and late follow-up. J Thorac Cardiovasc Surg. 2011;142:66-72.
55. Banning AP. Aortic intramural hematoma. N Engl J Med. 1997;337:1476-7.
56. Chao CP, Walker TG, Kalva SP. Natural history and CT appearances of aortic intramural hematoma. Radiographics. 2009;29:791-804.
57. O'Gara PT, DeSanctis RW. Acute aortic dissection and its variants. Toward a common diagnostic and therapeutic approach. Circulation. 1995;92:1376-8.
58. Park KH, Lim C, Choi JH, et al. Prevalence of aortic intimal defect in surgically treated acute type A intramural hematoma. Ann Thorac Surg. 2008;86:1494-500.
59. Evangelista A, Garcia-del-Castillo H, Gonzalez-Alujas T, et al. Diagnosis of ascending aortic dissection by transesophageal echocardiography: utility of Mmode in recognizing artifacts. J Am Coll Cardiol. 1996;27:102-7.
60. Bolger AF. Aortic intramural haematoma. Heart. 2008;94:1670-4.
61. Nathan DP, Boonn W, Lai E, et al. Presentation, complications, and natural history of penetrating atherosclerotic ulcer disease. J Vasc Surg. 2012;55:10-5.
62. Eggebrecht H, Plicht B, Kahlert P, et al. Intramural hematoma and penetrating ulcers: indications to endovascular treatment. Eur J Vasc Endovasc Surg. 2009;38:659-65.

63. Litmanovich DE, Yıldırım A, Bankier AA. Insights into imaging of aortitis. Insights Imaging. 2012;3:545-60.
64. Moyano JC, Magarolas MA, González EC, et al. Nonurgent aortic disease: clinical-radiological diagnosis of aortitis. Radiology. 2013;55:469-82.
65. Sharma BK, Siveski-Iliskovic N, Singal PK. Takayasu arteritis may be underdiagnosed in North America. Can J Cardiol. 1995;11: 311-6.
66. Sharma BR, Jain S, Suri S, et al. Diagnostic criteria for Takayasu arteritis. International Journal of Cardiology. 1996;54(S): 141-S147.
67. Restrepo CS, Ocazionez D, Suri R, et al. Aortitis: imaging spectrum of the infectious and inflammatory conditions of the aorta. Radiographics. 2011;31:435-51.
68. Kerr GS, Hallahan CW, Giordano J, et al. Takayasu arteritis. Ann Intern Med. 1994;120:919-29.
69. Gotway MB, Araoz PA, Macedo TA, et al. Imaging findings in Takayasu's arteritis. Am J Roentgenol. 2005;184:1945-50.
70. Matsunaga N, Hayashi R, Sakamoto I, et al. Takayasu's arteritis. Protean radiologic manifestations and diagnosis. Radiographics. 1997;17:579-91.
71. Gornik HL, Creager MA. Aortitis. Circulation. 2008;117:3039-305.
72. Kobayashi Y, Ishii K, Oda K, et al. Aortic wall inflammation due to Takayasu arteritis imaged with 18F-FDG PET coregistered with enhanced CT. J Nucl Med. 2005;46:917-22.
73. Meller J, Grabbe E, Becker W, et al. Value of F-18 FDG hybrid camera PET and MRI in early Takayasu aortitis. Eur Radiol. 2003;13:400-5.
74. Webb M, Chambers A, AL-N A, et al. The role of 18F-FDG PET in characterising disease activity in Takayasu arteritis. Eur J Nucl Med Mol Imaging. 2004;31:627-34.
75. Sharma S, Rajani M. Aortic occlusion in nonspecific aortoarteritis (Takayasu disease): incidence and spectrum of involvement. Australas Radiol. 1993;37:57-9.
76. Sharma S, Rajani M, Talwar KK. Angiographic morphology in nonspecific aortoarteritis (Takayasu's arteritis): a study of 126 patients from north India. Cardiovasc Intervent Radiol. 1992;15:160-5.
77. Sharma S, Sharma S, Taneja K, et al. Morphological mural changes in the aorta in non specific aortoarteritis (Takayasu's arteritis): assessment by intravascular ultrasound imaging. Clin Radiol. 1998;53:37-43.
78. Sharma S, Sharma S, Taneja K, et al. Morphologic mural changes in the aorta revealed by CT in patients with nonspecific aortoarteritis (Takayasu's arteritis). AJR. 1996;167:1321-5.
79. Keser G, Direskeneli H, Aksu K. Management of Takayasu arteritis: a systematic review. Rheumatology (Oxford). 2014;53:793-801.
80. Liang P, Tan-Ong M, Hoffman GS. Takayasu's arteritis: vascular interventions and outcomes. J Rheumatol. 2004;31:102-6
81. Hedgire SS, McDermott S, Borczuk D, et al. The spectrum of IgG4-related disease in the abdomen and pelvis. Am J Roentgenol. 2013;201:14-22.
82. Stone JH, Zen Y, Deshpande V. IgG4-related disease. N Engl J Med. 2012;366:539-51.
83. Kasashima S, Zen Y, Kawashima A, et al. Inflammatory abdominal aortic aneurysm: close relationship to IgG4-related periaortitis. Am J Surg Pathol. 2008;32:197-204.
84. Kasashima S, Zen Y. IgG4. IgG4-related inflammatory abdominal aortic aneurysm. Curr Opin Rheumatol. 2011;23:18-23.
85. Wintermark M, Wicky S, Schnyder P. Imaging of acute traumatic injuries of thoracic aorta. Eur Radiol. 2002;12:431-42.
86. Gavant ML. Helical CT grading of traumatic aortic injuries. RCNA. 1999;37:553-70.
87. Lipchick EO, Rogoff SM. The abnormal abdominal aorta: Arteriosclerosis and other diseases. In: Abrahams HL Little (Ed). Brown and Company, Boston. 1983;2:1057-78.
88. Sawhney R, Kerlan RR, Wall SD. Analysis of initial CT findings after endovascular repair of abdominal aortic aneurysms. Radiology. 2001;220:157-60.

CHAPTER

150

Imaging in Pulmonary Vascular Disease

Ujjwal Gorsi, Sanjeev Kumar, Kushaljit Singh Sodhi, Akshay Kumar Saxena

Pulmonary vascular diseases incorporate a large and distinctive group of pathologies which range from pulmonary thromboembolism to congenital malformations to vasculitides. The patient suffering from diseases of pulmonary vascular system can have a dramatic and acute onset of symptoms such as chest pain and dyspnea or an insidious onset and chronic course with symptoms ranging from fatigue, hypoxia dyspnea on exertion, and right heart failure.[1]

Imaging modalities available to evaluate diseases of the pulmonary vasculature include chest radiography (CXR), computed tomography (CT), magnetic resonance imaging (MRI), nuclear scintigraphy and transthoracic echocardiography (TIE).

ANATOMY

The pulmonary arteries carry deoxygenated blood from right ventricle to lungs and is primary circulation of the lungs other being bronchial circulation. Pulmonary arteries are low pressure system. The main pulmonary artery originates from the right ventricular (RV) outflow tract and divides into right and left branches before exiting the pericardium. Right and left pulmonary arteries give rise to lobar arteries and lobar arteries further divide into segmental and subsegmental arteries **(Figs. 1A and B)**.

The pulmonary veins are four in number: the right and left superior pulmonary veins and right and left inferior pulmonary veins in up to 70% individuals. Pulmonary veins bring oxygenated blood from lungs into left atrium. Right upper and middle lobes are drained by right superior pulmonary vein whereas left upper lobe and lingula are drained by left superior pulmonary vein. The lower lobes are drained by inferior pulmonary veins. Anatomic variations are seen in approximately 38% of the population.[2] On left side, a common trunk may be present which is formed by the union of superior and inferior pulmonary veins. On right side, atypical anatomic pattern is less common. Single or multiple accessory veins may be present with independent drainage in to left atrium. The central portions of the pulmonary veins which open into the left atrium are intra pericardial.[2]

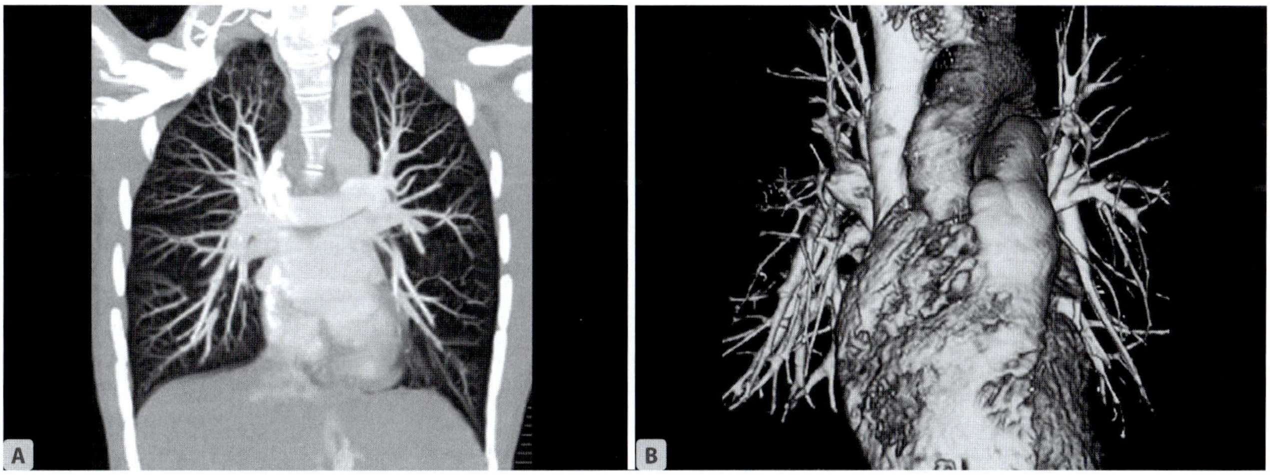

FIGS. 1A AND B: Normal pulmonary vasculature demonstrated on 64-row MDCT scanner. Coronal reconstruction using (A) maximum intensity projection and (B) volume-rendered technique demonstrate even the most peripheral pulmonary vessels with exquisite detail.

ACUTE PULMONARY EMBOLISM

Following coronary artery disease and stroke, pulmonary embolism (PE) is the third most common acute cardiovascular event disease.[3] PE commonly is the result of migration of deep vein thrombus from the lower limb veins. Diagnosis of acute pulmonary thromboembolism (PTE) has to be accurate and rapid as if left untreated outcome is dismal and needless treatment is associated with considerable morbidity. For both DVT and acute PE an annual incidence of 100–200 per 100,000 inhabitants has been reported.[4]

Clinical features of acute PE are nonspecific and often deceptive. It may remain asymptomatic or its first presentation can be sudden cardiac death. Hence imaging plays leading role in evaluation of patients suspected of having PE.

Massive PE is indicated by sustained systemic hypotension (systolic arterial pressure <90 mm Hg for at least 15 minutes which is not due to cause other than PE) symptoms and signs of shock and chest pain.[5] Clinical scores such as Wells[6] and Geneva scores[7] are important scores which allows assessment of clinical pre-test probability of acute PE. Electrocardiography (ECG), D-dimer, chest radiograph and compression ultrasound of lower limbs are the initial investigations. D-dimer has a high sensitivity and very high negative predictive value and is raised in venous thromboembolism. It is considered the most important laboratory screening test for PTE. Ninety percent of PE originate from DVT in a lower limb.[8] For symptomatic DVT, compression ultrasound of veins of lower limb has a high sensitivity (>90%) and specificity (95%).[4]

If a diagnosis of PE is suspected based on clinical findings and evaluation of D-dimer, in patients with symptoms and signs of DVT, compression ultrasound is indicated specially in pregnant patient with suspected PE.[5] Patients suspected of PE, in whom compression USG shows thrombus in lower limb veins, can be started on anticoagulant treatment without further testing.[9]

Imaging Techniques

Chest Radiography

Chest radiography is useful to exclude other causes of acute chest pain when acute PE is suspected. It is important to exclude pneumonia, pneumothorax, pericardial effusion aortic dissection, and free intraperitoneal air as symptoms because of these entities may mimic those due to PE. In addition ventilation perfusion scan interpretation is dependent on whether the chest radiograph is normal or abnormal.[10]

Although chest radiograph is the first investigation performed in patients of suspected pulmonary embolism, unfortunately the radiographic features of acute pulmonary embolism are rather nonspecific. Findings which may be seen are Hampton hump (peripheral, wedge-shaped consolidation with a rounded medial margin representing infarct), Westermark sign (oligemia of lung beyond the occluded vessel), Fleischner sign (prominent central pulmonary artery) plate like atelectasis, small pleural effusion and elevated ipsilateral hemidiaphragm **(Fig. 2)**.[11] Not all patients with PTE have positive finding on chest X-ray.

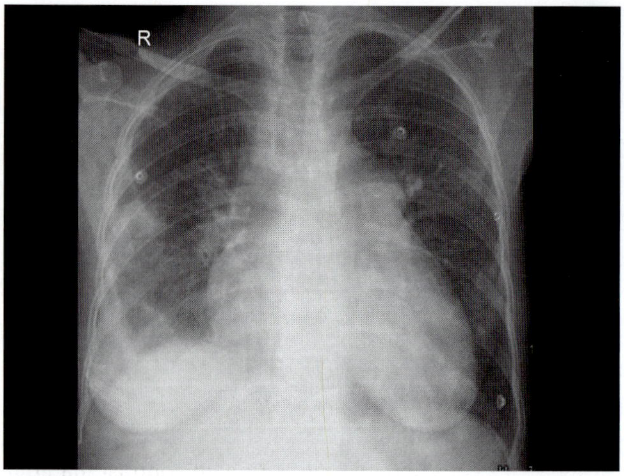

FIG. 2: Acute PE. Dilated central pulmonary artery with dilated right descending pulmonary artery proximally and acute cut-off. Dilated right-sided pleural effusion with peripheral wedge-shaped opacity in right middle zone symptoms of infarct.

Normal chest skiagrams have been reported in the presence of PTE in 12–30% of patients.

Echocardiography

Echocardiography is important as it can exclude significant abnormalities like right ventricular dysfunction. Thrombolytic therapy is often recommended for the patients who are hemodynamically stable and who have right ventricular dysfunction on echocardiography. In addition associated right atrial and right ventricular thrombus may also be diagnosed with echocardiography. It also estimates pulmonary artery pressure thus guiding the management in these patients. Transesophageal echocardiography can demonstrate pulmonary arteries better than TTE. Though it is invasive. TEE can directly visualize thrombus in right pulmonary artery.

CT Angiography

CT pulmonary angiography is standard for diagnosis of PE as it is accurate, safe and can be performed rapidly. It has replaced catheter angiography for diagnosing PE.[10] It is considered the best imaging modality for those with intermediate or high clinical risk for acute PE and those with abnormal D-dimer values. PIOPED II (Prospective Investigation of Pulmonary Embolism Diagnosis) studied the accuracy of CTPA with V/Q and conventional pulmonary angiography. Sensitivity of 83% and specificity of 96% was shown in patients with a high pretest probability[12] of PE.[12] However scanners used in 4-, 8-, and 16-row scanners used in the PIOPED II study were 4-, 8-.or 16- row scanners, with rapid evolution of multidetector computed tomography (MDCT) even greater accuracy is achieved. Another advantage of CTPA is ability to detect alternative causes for clinical symptoms mimicking PE[1] unlike V/Q scan and catheter angiography.

For CTPA 80 to 100 mL of nonionic iodinated contrast is injected intravenously at a rate of 4 mL/s from an antecubital vein. To time optimal contrast delivery to the pulmonary vessels at the time of imaging, test bolus and automated bolus tracking techniques are very helpful. Test bolus technique is especially useful in patients who have delayed opacification of the pulmonary arteries due to poor cardiac function. Although, caudal to cranial scanning is often used to reduce effect of respiratory motion at the lung bases where more emboli are seen and more diaphragmatic motion occurs, the availability of ultrafast MDCT usually obviates this modification. Thin collimation allows is volumetric 1-mm slice reconstruction helping in multiplanar reconstructions and detailed analysis.[1]

Dual-energy CT

With the implementation of multidetector CT scanners with two X-ray tubes (dual-source CT) and a single tube with two focal spots (dual-energy), both iodinated contrast material-enhanced and soft-tissue images from a single imaging examination can be obtained. This feature is useful in PE imaging as the area of perfused lung can be directly assessed and quantified in addition to the standard documentation of clot burden and presence of right heart strain.[13]

Dual-energy CT (DECT) permits functional data on lung perfusion (iodine distribution maps/lung perfusion blood volume [PBV] images). Which can quantitatively assess regional iodine density, a marker for pulmonary perfusion, and can be correlated to V/QSCAN or single photon-emission computed tomography (SPECT) V/QSCAN.[5,14] The diagnostic accuracy of iodine maps for occlusive acute PE is high but this is not the case for non-occlusive disease.[14] In addition dual-energy CT techniques has the potential to reduce contrast dose without compromising diagnostic capabilities.[15] Spectral CT can also be used to reduce both the iodine load and radiation dose to the patient. As shown by Szucs- Farkas et al. using a contrast injection of 75 mL (300 mg iodine per milliliter) and 80 kVp, images which were obtained were found to be equivalent to the standard dose of 100 mL (300 mg iodine per milliliter) and standard 100 kVp for diagnosing PE. The radiation dose was significantly less with this protocol (6.8 mSv for 100 kVp and 4.8 mSv for 80 kVp).[16]

Ventilation/Perfusion Scan

A ventilation/perfusion scan (V/Q scan) analyzes both the pulmonary blood flow and alveolar ventilation and is interpreted in correlation with a chest radiograph. It is an alternative test for patients who cannot undergo CTPA. The ability to detect PE on a V/Q scan can be improved by the addition of single-photon emission computed tomography imaging (SPECT imaging), which provides cross-sectional imaging of the lungs.[17] V/Q scans assess for perfusion defects without matched ventilation defects, the combination of which is suggestive of PE. V/Q scans are reported as normal, very low probability, low probability, intermediate probability, and high probability, on the basis of the number and sizes of unmatched defects as well as in correlation with the chest radiograph **(Figs. 3A and B)**. A normal V/Q scan indicates that chances of PE is <5% where as s high-probability V/Q scan indicates that chance of PE is >90%[18] where as the pretest probability of PE being present does not change with intermediate probability scan. In pregnant women, V/Q scan may be preferred rather than CTPA. The American Thoracic Society and the Society of Thoracic Radiology recommends that for pregnant women in whom PE is suspected but whose chest radiograph is normal, the V/Q scan should be performed. However, CTPA is to be carried out rather than a V/Q scan if abnormality is detected on chest radiograph.[19]

Magnetic Resonance Imaging

MRI has undergone significant technical improvement with large coverage, faster sequences, and ability to perform high-resolution MR pulmonary angiography (MRPA), lung perfusion imaging and functional studies. MRPA consists of a three-dimensional (3D) heavily weighted-T1 gradient echo MRI sequences acquired during first-pass perfusion following intravenous injection of gadolinium via an injector pump to visualize the pulmonary arteries. Noncontrast-enhanced MRPA can be performed using SSFP free-breathing real-time imaging technique with additional navigator-gating, which is used to obtain the images in the same phase without the need for breath-hold[20] **(Figs. 4A to D)** In acute PE MRPA is

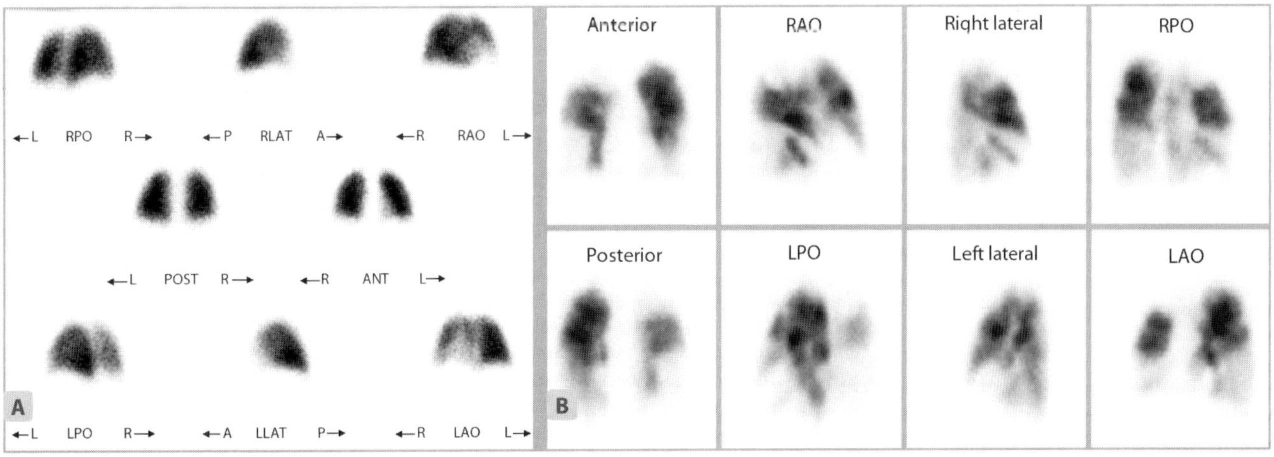

FIGS. 3A AND B: (A) Lung perfusion scan shows normal perfusion pattern; (B) Lung perfusion scan in another patient shows multiple large perfusion defects in both lungs, suggesting a high probability for pulmonary embolism.

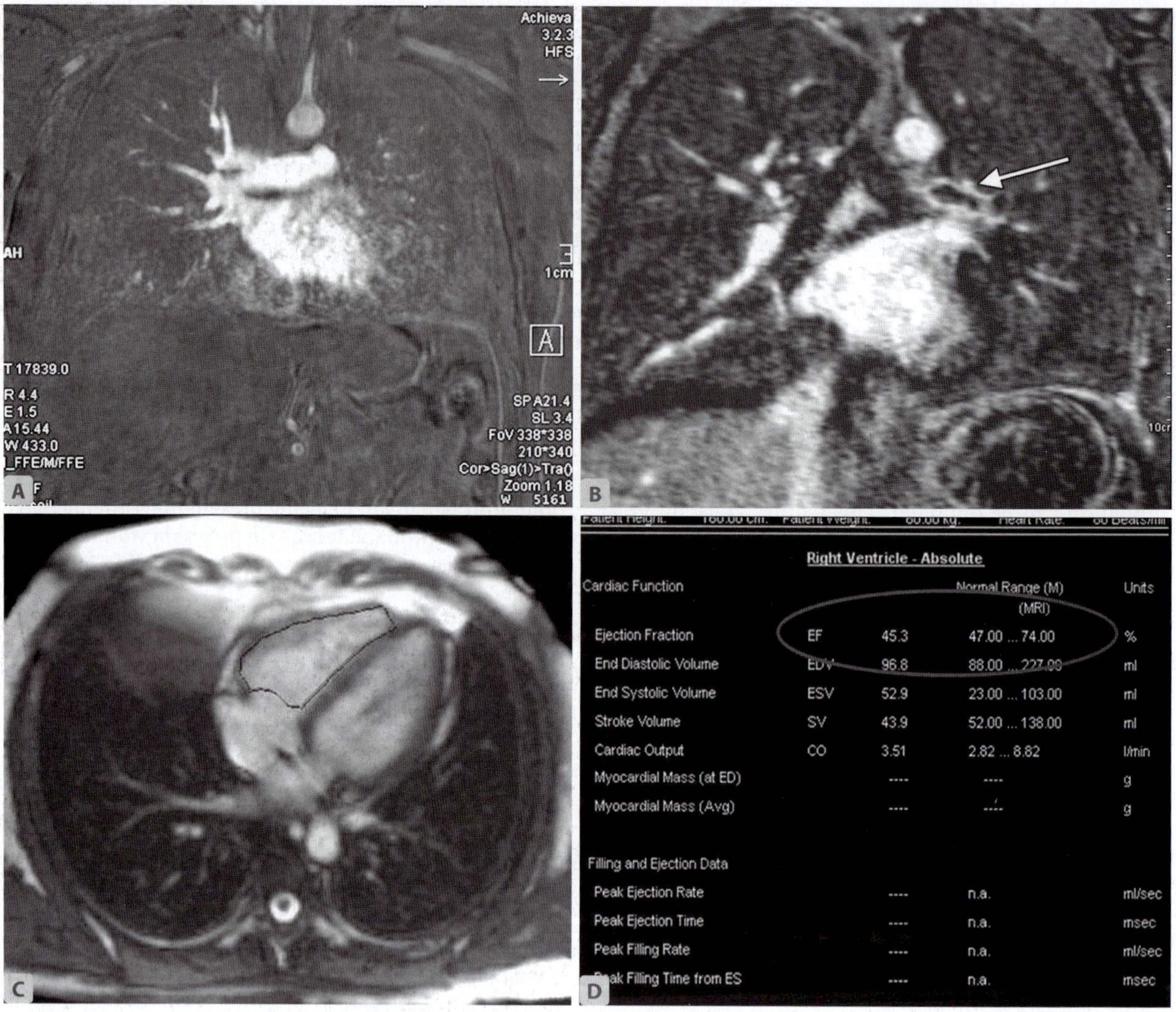

FIGS. 4A TO D: Acute pulmonary embolism: Coronal MRA images (A and B) showing acute thrombus in left pulmonary artery(arrow in B) with normal right pulmonary artery; (C) Cine steady-state free precession (SSFP) static image—calculation of RV function; (D) Argus values showing RV dysfunction with decreased EF (EF 43.55%) and mild strain.

not routinely used as CTPA is used routinely. PIOPED III study showed that a sensitivity of 78% and a specificity of 99% was achieved with MRPA when the studies were technically adequate a sensitivity of 92% and a specificity of 96% was shown when MRPA was performed along with MR venography. However, technically inadequate results were present in 52% of patients in this study. Conclusion from the study was that that MRPA should be considered only for patients for whom standard tests are contraindicated and only in those centers that routinely perform this study.[21]

Digital Subtraction Angiography

For the diagnosis of acute PE, CT angiography has largely replaced catheter angiography. Similar results are achiever with CTPA without the complications of catheter angiography noninvasively. Filling defect within main pulmonary arteries or their branches arteries or cut-off of a pulmonary artery branch is most accepted diagnostic sign of PTE[10] **(Fig. 5)**. Catheter angiography is now used only for therapeutic purposes including thrombolysis in setting of acute PE.

Imaging Features of Acute PE

CTPA is most common imaging modality used to image acute PE. Findings of acute PE on CTPA are described below though imaging features are similar on all angiographic studies.

Vascular Features

CTPA shows intravascular acute emboli with complete or partial vascular obstruction. In complete obstruction, the lumen is entirely occupied by thromboembolic material. Calibre of the vessel at the level of obstruction is either normal or enlarged as compared to chronic PTE **(Fig. 6)** In partial obstruction intraluminal central or eccentric filling defect are seen surrounded by contrast **(Figs. 7 and 8)**. The morphology of emboli varies according to whether the vessel is imaged in short axis ("rim" or "polo mint" sign) **(Fig. 9)** or long axis ("railway track" sign).[5] When analyzing small segmental branches for presence of emboli, in order to prevent obscuration of emboli by dense iodinated contrast, such window and level values should be chosen so that right heart structures such as trabeculations are visible.[1]

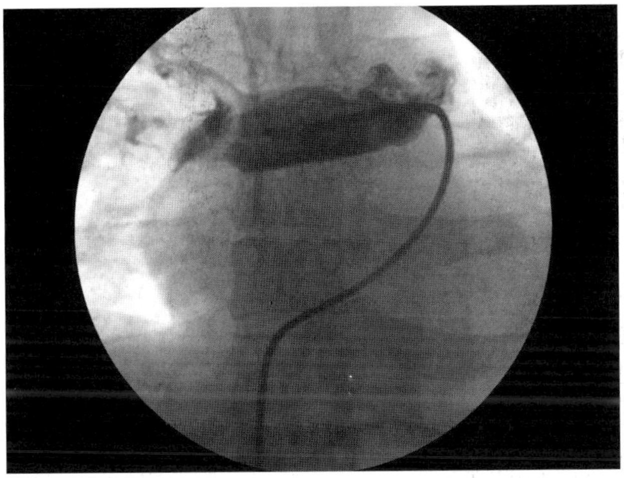

FIG. 5: Acute pulmonary embolism (PE): Catheter angiography of pulmonary artery confirming the filling defect in the right pulmonary artery typically forming concave margin suggestive of acute pulmonary embolism.

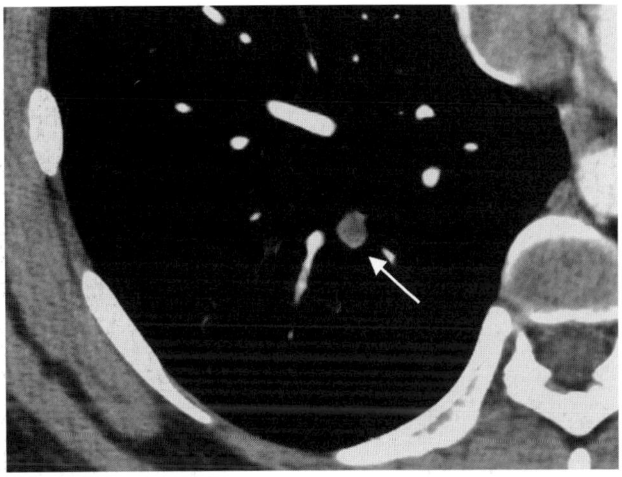

FIG. 6: Acute PE with complete obstruction. CTPA shows complete luminal occlusion with expanded vessel (arrow).

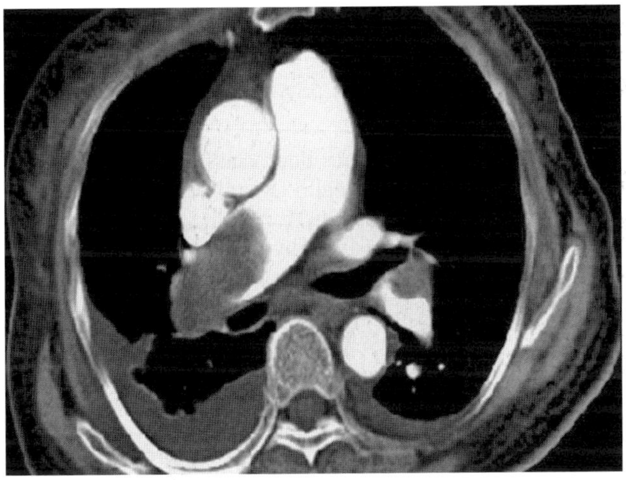

FIG. 7: Acute PE with partial obstruction: CTPA revealing filling defects in the right main pulmonary artery and left lower pulmonary artery branch with expansion of lumen symptoms of acute thrombus, as well as bilateral pleural effusion.

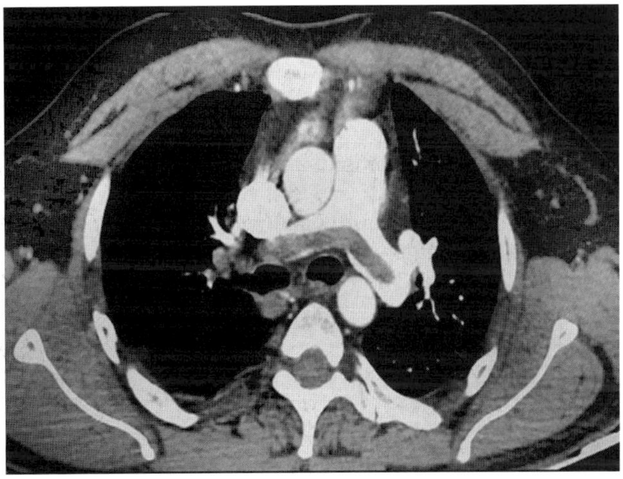

FIG. 8: Acute saddle pulmonary embolism: CTPA revealing a large pulmonary embolism that straddles the bifurcation of the pulmonary trunk extending into left and right pulmonary arteries.

Parenchymal Features

Complete occlusion of the artery causes the complete loss of perfusion with distal infarct which manifest as triangular subpleural consolidation or ground-glass opacity with fine reticular areas **(Fig. 10)**. When obstruction is partial, there is reduced flow rate (oligemia) which causes nonuniform arterial perfusion of the lung parenchyma with reduced vessel diameter patchy areas of low attenuation on CT or low signal on MRI (mosaic attenuation pattern). Atelectasis and pleural effusion may also be seen.

Cardiac Features

In acute PE, RV after load is rapidly increased as a result of obstruction to pulmonary arterial flow and the increase in PVR. Features of RV after load include dilatation of the right ventricle, bowing of the interventricular septum, dilatation of superior and inferior vena cava, dilatation of azygos vein, dilatation and reflux of contrast in the inferior vena cava and hepatic veins may also be present. Right ventricle dilatation is assessed commonly by RV/left ventricle (LV) ratio which can be calculated either on axial images or on a multiplanar reformatted four-chamber view. If the RV/LV ratio is >1.0 (on axial CT images) or >0.9 (on four-chamber view), RV dysfunction is suggetsted.[22] Artifacts that can limit assessment for acute PE on CTPA include flow artifacts which appear as transient interruption of the contrast column, image noise, motion and respiratory artifacts and partial volume averaging with surrounding structures.[1]

Non-thrombotic causes of PE are best evaluated with CT. These are rare as compared to venous thromboembolism. And include septic emboli, fat emboli, tumor emboli, venous air embolism, talc and cement embolism. Septic emboli contain microorganisms and appear as cavitatory nodules

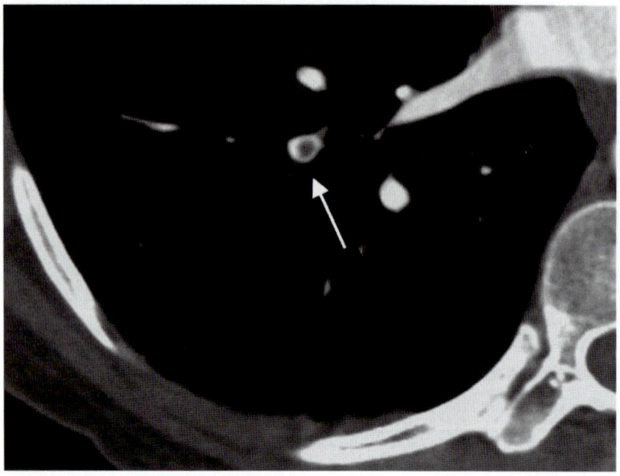

FIG. 9: Acute PE: Central filing defect in one of the branch of right lower lobar pulmonary artery (arrow) with contrast in periphery called as polo mint sign.

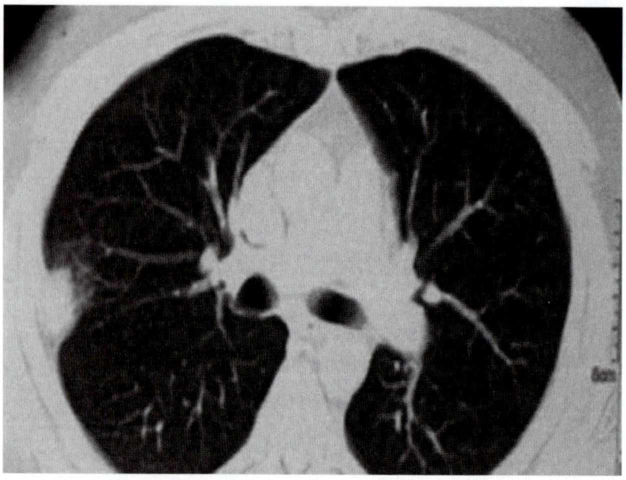

FIG. 10: Pulmonary infarct: CECT chest in a patient of acute PE shows characteristic peripheral wedge-shaped infarct.

usually multiple and bilateral. Tumor emboli expand the involved pulmonary arteries if smaller they may appear as patchy ground-glass opacity, or as tree-in-bud appearance. Hepatocellular carcinoma, renal cancer, prostate cancer, breast cancer and gastric malignancy are known for producing tumor emboli.

Cement emboli is embolism of polymethyl methacrylate, which can enter the external venous plexuses during vertebroplasty. Branching tubular hyperattenuating opacities are seen on radiography and CT. Talc embolism can happen in patients who grind and inject oral medications, such as amphetamines into their veins.[17]

CHRONIC THROMBOEMBOLIC DISEASE

Chronic thromboembolic disease (CTED) results due to incomplete resolution and recanalization of acute emboli. There occurs organization and endothelialization of thromboembolic material which may appear as laminated thrombi, single bands parallel to the vessel (shelves) or complex web-like network as well as complete vascular occlusions. The pathophysiological basis explaining transition from acute to chronic thromboembolism is uncertain; however, failed thrombolysis, a localized inflammatory response and localized endothelial dysfunction are thought to be responsible.[23] CTED can occur without or with chronic thromboembolic pulmonary hypertension (CTEPH). CTEPH shares many of the imaging features with other etiologies of pulmonary hypertension along with few features specific to chronic PTE. Imaging features of chronic PTE will be discussed in the section of pulmonary hypertension.

PULMONARY HYPERTENSION

Pulmonary hypertension (PH) is defined as a mean pulmonary artery pressure (mPAP) of 25 mm Hg or greater on right heart catheterization. A resting mean pulmonary arterial pressure of 20 mm Hg or less is normal. Symptoms of PH vary greatly and are nonspecific. Dyspnea, syncope, and fatigue can be clinical manifestation of pulmonary hypertension. Right ventricular failure and subsequent death may be the consequence of untreated pulmonary hypertension.[24]

Classification

Pulmonary hypertension has been classified into following five groups by the World Health Organization (WHO) based upon etiology.[25]

- *Group 1:* Pulmonary arterial hypertension (PAH)
- *Group 2:* Pulmonary hypertension which is secondary to to left heart disease
- *Group 3:* Chronic lung disease and/or hypoxemia leading to pulmonary hypertension
- *Group 4:* Chronic thromboembolic pulmonary hypertension
- *Group 5:* Pulmonary hypertension secondary to multifactorial mechanisms or unknown etiology

Causes of pulmonary arterial hypertension in Group 1 to 5.

- *Group 1:* Idiopathic PAH, heritable PAH, drug-induced PAH, PAH associated with CTD, HIV, portal hypertension, CHD and schistosomiasis.
  Pulmonary veno-occlusive disease (PVOD) and pulmonary capillary hemangiomatosis (PCH) are included in 1′ and persistent pulmonary hypertension of the newborn (PPHN) is designated as 1″ because these entities have unique features which are different from other causes of PAH.
- *Group 2:* Valvular heart diseases, LV systolic and diastolic dysfunction and cardiomyopathies may lead to pulmonary hypertension and they are included in this group.
- *Group 3:* Lung diseases like COPD, ILD, chronic exposure to high altitude and few developmental lung diseases may lead to pulmonary hypertension. PH secondary to these diseases is included in this group.
- *Group 4:* Chronic thromboembolic disease may be associated with pulmonary hypertension (CTPEH). PH secondary to chronic PE is included in group 4.
- *Group 5:* This group comprises pulmonary hypertension due to varied etiologies. PH secondary to hematologic

disorders (myeloproliferative disorders, splenectomy), systemic disorders (sarcoidosis, pulmonary Langerhans cell histiocytosis), metabolic disorders (glycogen storage disease, Gaucher disease, thyroid disorders), and other disorders (tumoral obstruction, fibrosing mediastinitis, chronic renal failure in patients undergoing dialysis) are included in this group.

Imaging Modalities

Imaging examinations that are useful in assessing of PH include chest radiography, transthoracic echocardiogram, CT/CTPA, MRI/MRA, ventilation perfusion scan and right heart catheterization. Many imaging features of PH are common irrespective of the etiologies on all imaging modalities which shall be discussed first. It will be followed by description of few features which are specific to a particular etiology.

Chest Radiography

As the symptoms and signs of PH are non-specific, chest radiography is usually the first imaging requested. In early course of the disease, chest radiography is usually normal but in advanced stage radiograph may show classic features of PH which include dilatation of central pulmonary arteries, dilated (15 mm in women and 16 mm in men) right interlobar artery, pruning of the peripheral arteries **(Fig. 11)**. On lateral radiograph, reduced retrosternal air space is easily appreciated which happens due to dilatation of right ventricle.[26] Radiograph may also show some of the causes of pulmonary hypertension, e.g. interstitial lung disease, emphysema and left-sided heart disease.

Transthoracic Echocardiogram

Transthoracic Doppler echocardiography is an investigation which is carried out routinely in patients suspected of having PH. Transthoracic Doppler echocardiogram can reveal the systolic pulmonary artery pressure. In patients with mild PH its accuracy and reliability is less.[17]

CT Pulmonary Angiography

The classic CTPA findings of pulmonary hypertension may be divided into three categories: Vascular, parenchymal and cardiac signs.

Vascular Signs

Main pulmonary artery is assessed at the level of its bifurcation, orthogonal to its long axis on axial sections. Sensitivity of 87%, specificity of 89% and positive predictive value of 97%, is achieved for the presence of pulmonary hypertension with a pulmonary artery diameter of 29 mm or more.[27] A segmental artery-to-bronchus diameter ratio of 1:1 or more in three or four lobes has a specificity of 100% for the presence of pulmonary hypertension.[27] A main pulmonary arterial diameter greater than that of the ascending aorta is also signifies presence of PH. This sign has a positive predictive value of 96% and specificity of 92%, especially in young patients who are less than 50 years old **(Fig. 12)**.[28]

Parenchymal Signs

Both lungs may show peripheral oligemia with areas of mosaic attenuation **(Fig. 13)**. Idiopathic pulmonary arterial hypertension[28] and pulmonary capillary hemangiomatosis may show centrilobular ground-glass nodules. Neovascularity is regarded as a manifestation of severe pulmonary hypertension.[29]

Cardiac Signs

Findings of adaptation of right ventricle as well as its failure may be appreciated. These include right ventricular hypertrophy, (wall thickness of more than 4 mm), straightening or leftward bowing of the interventricular septum, right ventricular dilatation **(Fig. 14)**, decreased right ventricular ejection fraction; dilatation of the inferior vena cava and hepatic veins; and pericardial effusion.[24,30]

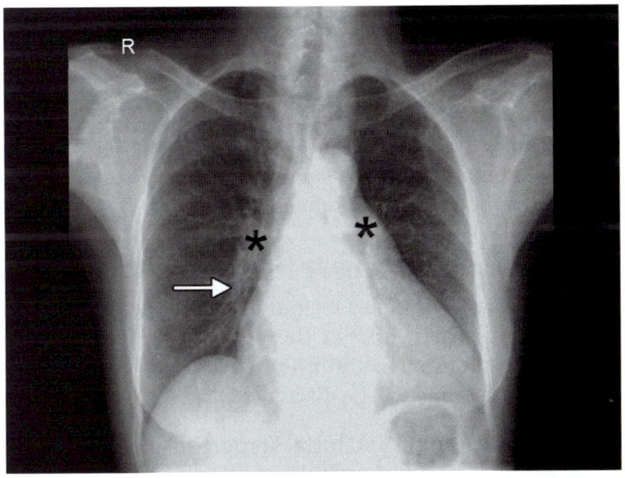

FIG. 11: Pulmonary hypertension: Posteroanterior chest radiograph showing dilated pulmonary arteries (stars), cardiomegaly, and rapid tapering (pruning) of right pulmonary artery (arrow). In addition, there is a decrease in the pulmonary vasculature in the periphery of the lung.

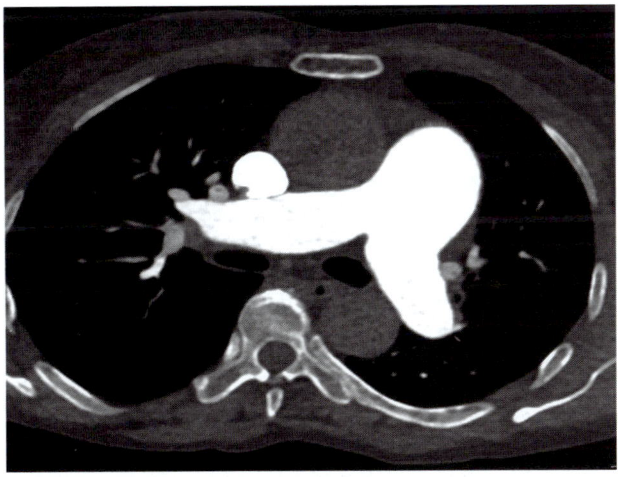

FIG. 12: Pulmonary hypertension: Pulmonary CT angiogram axial view shows dilated main, right and left pulmonary arteries consistent with the diagnosis of pulmonary hypertension.

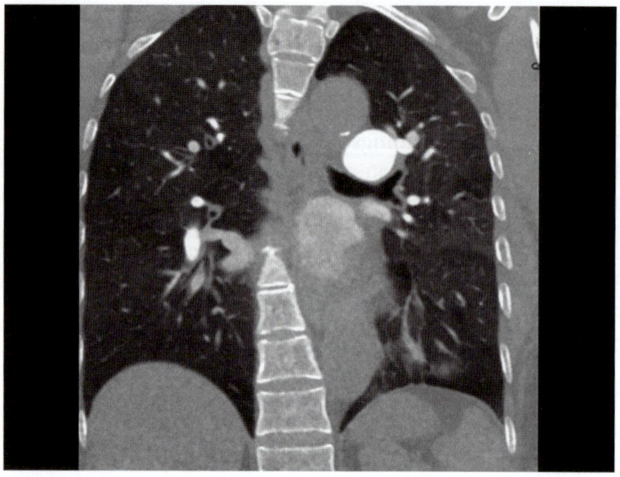

FIG. 13: Pulmonary hypertension: MDCT chest with coronal lung window showing multifocal areas of mosaic attenuation in bilateral lungs with peripheral oligemia.

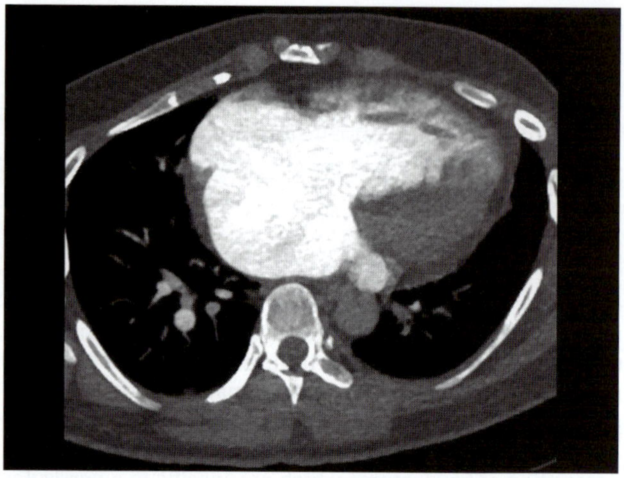

FIG. 14: Pulmonary hypertension: Contrast-enhanced computed tomography (CECT) chest shows cardiomegaly with dilatation of right atrium and right ventricle.

Ventilation/Perfusion Scanning

Ventilation/perfusion (V/Q) scanning is used as a screening in patients with pulmonary hypertension. Its primary role is to identify patients with CTEPH. Sensitivity of >96% and specificity of >90% is noted when scan is interpreted according to modified PIOPED (Prospective Investigation of Pulmonary Embolism Diagnosis) criteria. If the V/Q scan is normal or of low probability CTEPH can be excluded with a sensitivity of 90–100% and specificity of 94–100%.[31]

Cardiac MRI and Pulmonary MRA

Advantage of MR imaging, relative to other imaging modalities is ability to assess both anatomy and function. This is accomplished by MR angiography (MRA) sequences for pulmonary artery anatomy, MR flow sequences and perfusion for pulmonary blood flow quantification, and cardiac MR imaging sequences for cardiac morphology and function. Morphologic findings of PH are demonstrated by pulmonary MRA and cardiac MRI. These features include dilatation of central pulmonary arteries, pruning of peripheral vessels, right ventricular hypertrophy, dilation of right ventricle and straightening or leftward bowing of the interventricular septum. Patients who have PH are followed with MRI and MRA so that early changes of right ventricle dysfunction may be picked before becoming clinical significant. MRA and MR perfusion may be used to diagnose CTEPH.[24,32,33] MRI can assess reduced pulmonary artery dispensability and heterogeneous flow in the main pulmonary artery. Pulmonary artery dispensability, as defined by the relative change in the pulmonary artery area throughout the cardiac cycle may be decreased in PH and is associated with poor outcome in patients who have PH.[34]

Right ventricular size, function and wall motion can be assessed with MR cine imaging which is considered the gold standard for the same. Ventricular mass of both ventricles can be determined with cine imaging. These values are then used to calculate a ventricular mass index (right ventricular mass/left ventricular mass). A ventricular mass index which is >0.6 is considered compatible with PH.[24,35] Functional abnormalities which may result in a patient of PH include right ventricular hypokinesis and dysfunction, paradoxical movement of the interventricular septum, reduced ejection fraction and stroke volume and increased end-diastolic volume. MR imaging can demonstrate all these functional abnormalities.[24,33,34] Enhancement at the insertion points of the right ventricle into the interventricular septum is depicted by delayed contrast MRI. Flow sensitive MRI can quantify the severity of cardiac shunt (intra and extra).[24,36] Hemodynamic alterations such as abnormal proximal PA flow patterns, decreased wall shear stress, and increased tricuspid regurgitation velocities which develop in patients of PH can be assessed with 4-dimensional multidirectional flow MRI. An abnormal blood flow pattern which is characteristic present in PH is a vortex blood flow pattern in the proximal main pulmonary associated with early-onset systolic retrograde flow.[37-40]

Right Heart Catheterization and Pulmonary Angiography

Right heart catheterization (RHC) is considered the gold standard for the diagnosis of PAH. It is performed to confirm the diagnosis of PH and also helps in assessing the severity of PH.[24] Catheter pulmonary angiography is now used only if therapeutic procedure is planned.

Etiologies of Pulmonary Hypertension

There are many etiologies for pulmonary hypertension[25] as enumerated earlier. Few of these have specific imaging findings in addition to the findings compatible with PH discussed above and will be discussed.

Idiopathic Pulmonary Arterial Hypertension

Idiopathic pulmonary arterial hypertension is most common in women than men.[17] Both chest radiography and CT will show features of pulmonary hypertension already described. Centrilobular ground-glass attenuation which surrounds the enlarged and tortuous centrilobular arteries is a typical finding and may be appreciated on CT.[41] Rarely, small centrilobular nodules may also be noticed. Mosaic attenuation may be seen however its subtle as compared to the chronic PE.[41] CT may show pericardial effusion which is usually small.

Systemic-to-Pulmonary (Left-to-Right) Shunts

Left-to- right shunts such as atrial septal defect, ventricular septal defect and patent ductus arteriosus, increase the blood flow to pulmonary arteries. When pulmonary vascular resistance is similar or exceeds systemic vascular resistance Eisenmenger syndrome results with bidirectional or reversed flow in shunt. Eisenmenger syndrome may be associated with dilatation of the central pulmonary artery which may be massive, *in situ* thrombus formation with calcification may be noticed in Eisenmenger syndrome.[24,42]

Pulmonary Capillary Hemangiomatosis and Veno-Occlusive Disease

In PCH diffuse proliferation of capillaries occurs in the pulmonary interstitium with the obstruction of venules. CT in addition to features of pulmonary hypertension shows centrilobular ground-glass nodules, and interlobular septal thickening.[43] PVOD is caused by intimal fibrosis and thrombosis of pulmonary vein which leads to pulmonary venous hypertension followed by PH. CT will show pleural effusion and interlobular septal thickening in addition to enlarged pulmonary arteries. In PVOD, the left atrium is normal in size unlike left heart mitral valve disease. Mediastinal lymph node may be enlarged. Biopsy is required for the diagnosis of PCH and PVOD. Vasodilators are contraindicated in both of these diseases because they can precipitate pulmonary edema which may be fatal.[17,43]

PH Associated with Left Heart Disease

Mitral valve pathology can lead to PH. Reduced blood flow through the mitral valve backs up into the left atrium, and then into pulmonary veins followed by pulmonary arteries which results in PH. CT will show an enlarged left atrium, interlobular septal and an enlarged main pulmonary artery.[24]

Chronic Thromboembolic Disease

Not all the patients with acute PTE go on to develop hypertension. Approximately 4% of patients with acute pulmonary embolism develop chronic thromboembolic pulmonary hypertension. Patients with chronic thromboembolic pulmonary hypertension become symptomatic only when at least 60% of the pulmonary arterial bed is obstructed.[24] It is important to diagnose that chronic thromboembolic disease is a cause of pulmonary hypertension as it may be treated with pulmonary thromboendarterectomy. The CTPA findings of chronic thromboembolic pulmonary hypertension include parenchymal and vascular signs, which are highly suggestive of the cause. Vascular findings in CTEPH include complete obstruction, indicated by a tapered occluded vessel, eccentric narrowing of pulmonary arteries with segments of post-stenotic dilatation **(Fig. 15)**, partial filling defects, indicated by obtuse mural margins with the vessel wall **(Fig. 16)** partial filling defect, indicated by the presence of webs or bands and collateral systemic supply **(Fig. 17)**. Parenchymal findings in CTEPH include scars from prior pulmonary infarction mosaic pattern of perfusion, **(Figs. 18A and B)**, cylindrical bronchial airway dilatation and systemic perfusion of the peripheral pulmonary arterial bed.[24]

CTPA is useful modality in assessing whether patients are candidates for surgery or not. If the main, lobar, or proximal segmental arteries are involved, patients are considered for

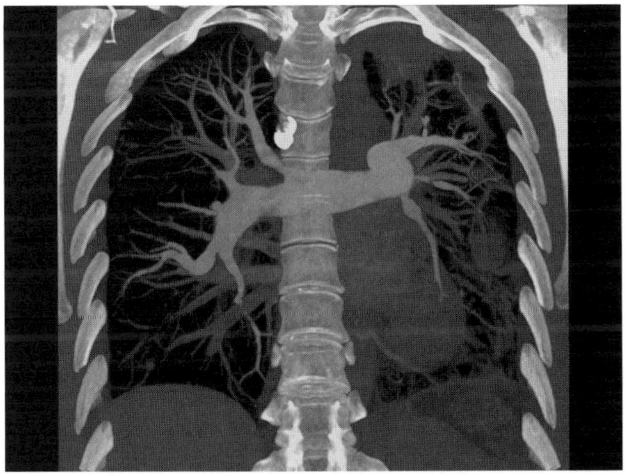

FIG. 15: Chronic thromboembolic pulmonary hypertension: CT pulmonary angiogram cornal reformatted image showing dilated central pulmonary arteries with eccentric narrowing of proximal right upper lobar pulmonary artery, posterior segmental branch of right lower, and left descending pulmonary artery with segment of post-stenotic dilatation (typical of chronic pulmonary thromboembolism), with relative oligemia in right middle and bilateral lower lobes.

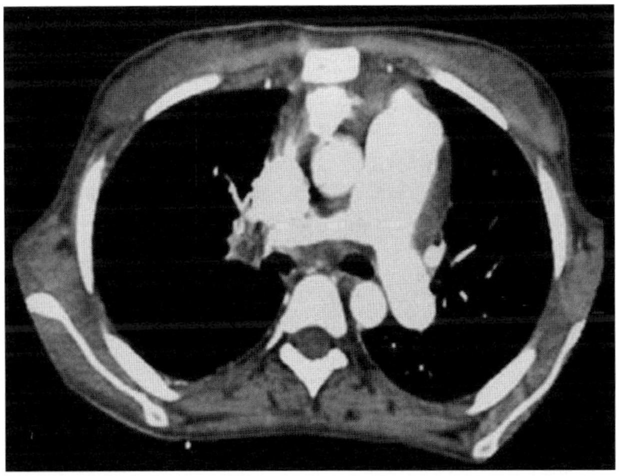

FIG. 16: Chronic pulmonary thromboembolism: Axial contrast-enhanced CT pulmonary angiography shows an attenuated right pulmonary artery with an eccentric thrombus, and irregular contours of intimal surface of main pulmonary artery and right pulmonary artery.

resection whereas if distal segments are involved medical treatment is considered.

VASCULITIS

Vasculitides affecting the pulmonary arteries can be classified by the size of vessel that is involved. Takayasu arteritis and Behcet disease involve large-size vessels such as the aorta, arch branches, and central pulmonary arteries. Vasculitides that involve medium (visceral arteries) and small vessels (arterioles, capillaries, and venules) include granulomatosis with polyangiitis (GPA), antibasement membrane disease (Goodpasture disease, Churg-Strauss syndrome (CSS), and microscopic polyangiitis.[17]

Takayasu Arteritis

Takayasu arteritis affect large elastic arteries. Young Asian women are most commonly affected. Disease usually involves aorta, arch branches. Involvement of pulmonary arteries may be seen in 50–80% of the patient population. In this disease, there is granulomatous inflammation of the arterial wall. Other histopathological features are proliferation of intima and fibrosis of the media and adventitia. These changes cause stenosis and occlusion of vessels, and may be associated with post-stenotic aneurysms. CT and MR show wall thickening of the aorta, aortic branches, and central pulmonary arteries early in the disease course **(Figs. 19A and B)** and stenosis, occlusion, and aneurysm formation later in the disease. Mural calcification can be seen on CT where as mural edema may be seen on MRI which is seen as high signal intensity on T2-weighted sequences on MR.[24,44]

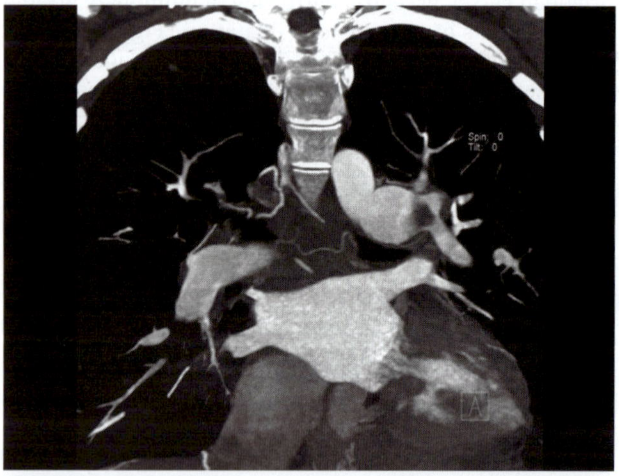

FIG. 17: Chronic pulmonary thrombolism: MDCT coronal reformation showing hypertrophied bronchial arteries.

Behçet Disease

Behcet disease is a multisystemic vasculitis which presents with uveitis, oral and genital ulcerations, and involvement of multiple organ systems. In the lungs, it involves large, medium, and small vessels. The aorta is the most commonly involved vessel, followed by pulmonary vessels. CT and MRI may show wall thickening of the involved vessels. In addition, there is pulmonary aneurysm formation, which are usually multiple and bilateral. These aneurysms occur almost exclusively in men. Areas of focal vasculitis and infarction may be seen which appear as wedge-shaped or rounded peripheral areas of consolidation.[44,45]

PULMONARY ARTERY ANEURYSMS AND PSEUDOANEURYSMS

Pulmonary artery aneurysms and pseudoaneurysms are uncommon but can have catastrophic consequences.

True Aneurysms

True aneurysms may be associated with connective tissue diseases such as Marfan's disease, Ehlers-Danlos syndrome, tuberous sclerosis, Behcet's disease and the Hughes-Stovin syndrome, in which both pulmonary artery aneurysms and pseudoaneurysms are seen that are typically central and at

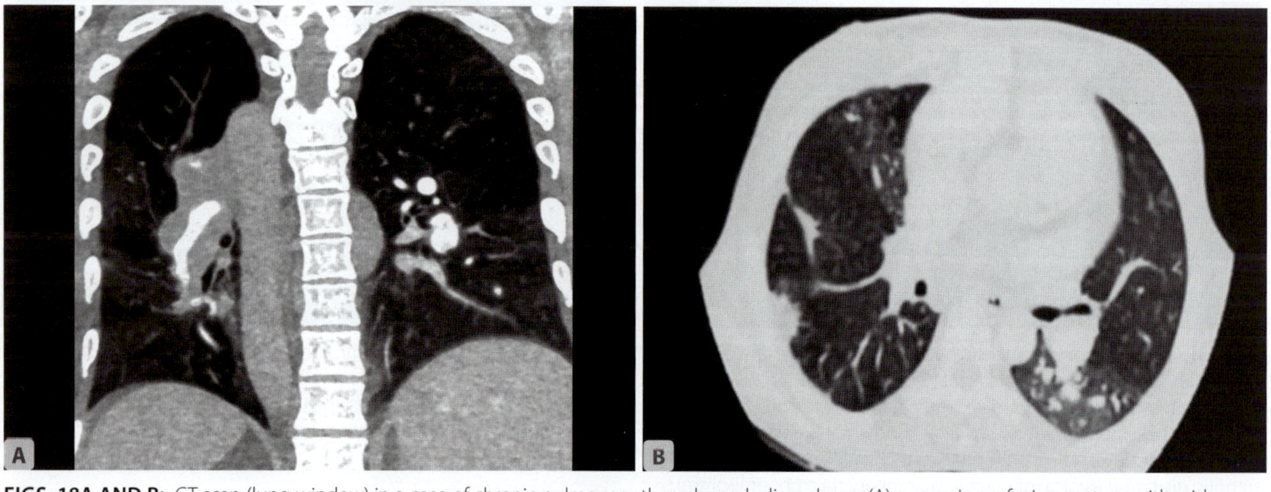

FIGS. 18A AND B: CT scan (lung window) in a case of chronic pulmonary thromboembolism shows (A) a mosaic perfusion pattern with wide regional variations in attenuation of the lung parenchyma and disparity in size of the segmental vessels. CT scan (B) in another patient shows mosaic attenuation with a peripheral parenchymal infarct and scar.

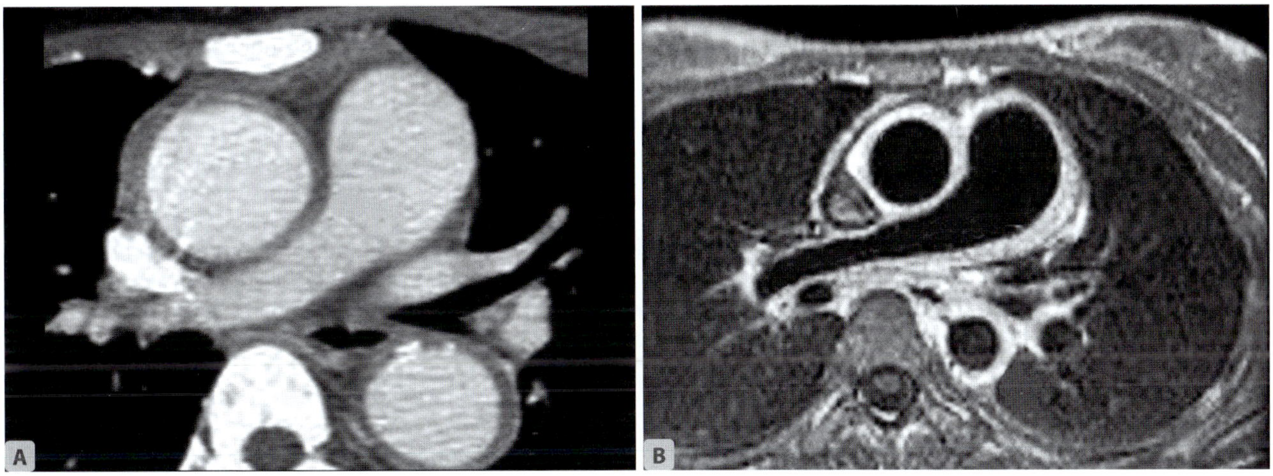

FIGS. 19A AND B: Takayasu arteritis—Involvement of aorta and pulmonary arteries: CT (A) shows thickening and enhancement of walls of aorta and pulmonary arteries. T2W MRI (B) shows thickening and edema of wall of aorta and pulmonary arteries.

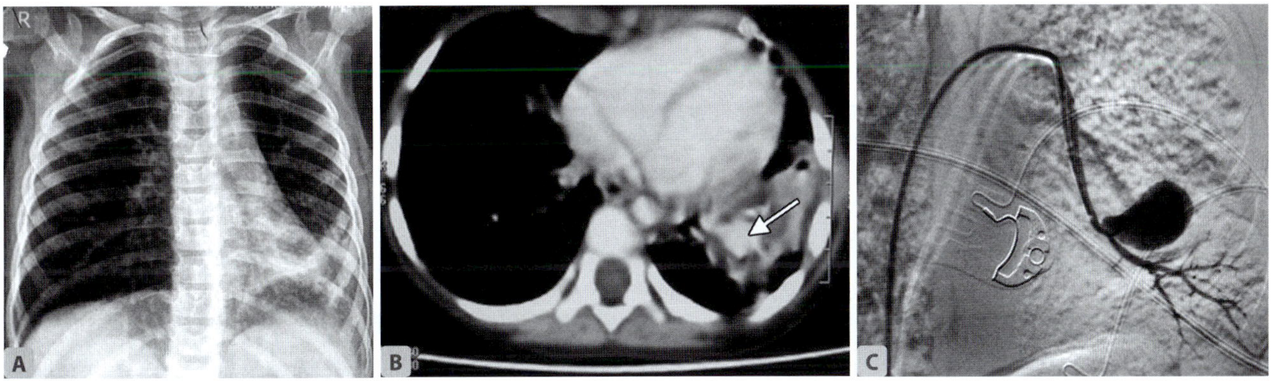

FIGS. 20A TO C: A four-year-child presented with fever and repeated episodes of hemoptysis. Radiograph (A) shows consolidation in left lower lobe . CECT chest (B) shows well-defined enhancing lesion (arrow) with in the necrotizing pneumonia consistent with the diagnosis of pseudoaneurysm. Catheter angiography of left lower lobar pulmonary artery (C) shows the pseudoaneurysm which was subsequently embolized using microcoils.

high-risk of spontaneous rupture. Some of the aneurysm can be idiopathic. Long-standing chronic thromboembolic pulmonary arterial hypertension, L-R shunts and pulmonary valve stenosis can cause dilatation of central pulmonary arteries which can be aneurysmal at times.[46,47]

Pseudoaneurysms

Pulmonary artery pseudoaneurysms are more common than true aneurysms. They may rupture spontaneously and require urgent management. They may be secondary to infections such as necrotizing pneumonia and tuberculosis (Rasmussen's aneurysms). Other etiologies include pulmonary arterial catheter trauma, e.g. Swan-Ganz catheters, septic pulmonary emboli, lung cancers and autoimmune vasculitides and penetrating trauma. Imaging findings of the underlying disease are usually apparent on radiograph and CT.[46,47] On plain chest radiography aneurysms and pseudoaneurysms may manifest as soft tissue nodule though they usually can not be diagnosed on radiography. On CECT, aneurysms and pseudoaneurysms show enhancement which matches the enhancement of adjacent pulmonary arterial branches **(Figs. 20A to C)**.[46,47]

PULMONARY ARTERIOVENOUS MALFORMATIONS

Pulmonary arteriovenous malformations (PAVMs) are arteriovenous (right-to-left) shunts between pulmonary artery and pulmonary vein with absence of intervening capillary bed. The site of shunt between the PA and PV is usually dilated and AVMs are more common in lower lung lobes. These can be congenital [e.g. in hereditary hemorrhagic telengectasia (HHT) syndrome] or acquired (e.g. traumatic, hepatopulmonary syndrome).[46,48] They can be solitary or multiple. Multiple bilateral AVMs are common in HHT syndrome. AVM can be simple when only a single feeder is present where as in complex AVMs, multiple feeding arteries are seen. Simple type of AVMs are commoner constituting 80–90% of pulmonary AVMs. Patients may be asymptomatic or may present with systemic oxygen desaturation, heart failure, ischemic or infectious emboli and hemorrhage (hemoptysis, hemothorax) due to rupture of the sac.[46,48]

On chest X-ray, AVM present as sharply defined lung nodules with one or more feeding artery and one or more draining vein.[46] CECT can demonstrate the number, size and site of these AVMs which is required before treatment by embolization **(Figs. 21A to E)**. Multiple bilateral AVMs are routinely found in HHT **(Figs. 22A and B)**. Catheter angiography is performed only for therapeutic purpose usually at the time of embolization.[46]

CONGENITAL ANOMALIES

A number of congenital anomalies can affect the pulmonary vasculature including proximal interruption of the pulmonary artery, pulmonary sling and partial anomalous pulmonary venous connection (PAPVC) syndrome. In proximal interruption of the pulmonary artery (right or left) is not present or terminates abruptly at the hilum. Collateral bronchial arteries supply the lung parenchyma. Cardiac defects are associated with interruption of the left pulmonary artery. Lateral chest radiograph will show the absence of the pulmonary artery and an ipsilateral small hemithorax. MRI/MRA or CT/CTPA will show these findings in details.[17,49] Pulmonary sling is formed when right pulmonary artery gives origin to left pulmonary artery which then courses between the trachea and the esophagus and supply the left lung. On chest radiography, the left pulmonary artery will appear as a nodular opacity posterior to the trachea. Both CT and MR will show the abnormal origin and the course of the left pulmonary artery.[17,49]

In PAPVC, an anomalous pulmonary vein drains into a systemic vein. On the left side, the left vertical vein will drain into either the left brachiocephalic vein or the coronary sinus. On the right side, an anomalous pulmonary vein may drain into coronary sinus, the azygos vein, superior vena cava or inferior vena cava. Scimitar syndrome refers to PAPVC to a systemic vein below the diaphragm, most commonly the inferior vena cava, which is associated with right pulmonary artery hypoplasia and a small right lung. Bronchial abnormalities, a horseshoe lung, sequestration, AVMs, and anomalous pulmonary systemic circulation may also be associated with scimitar syndrome. Radiography

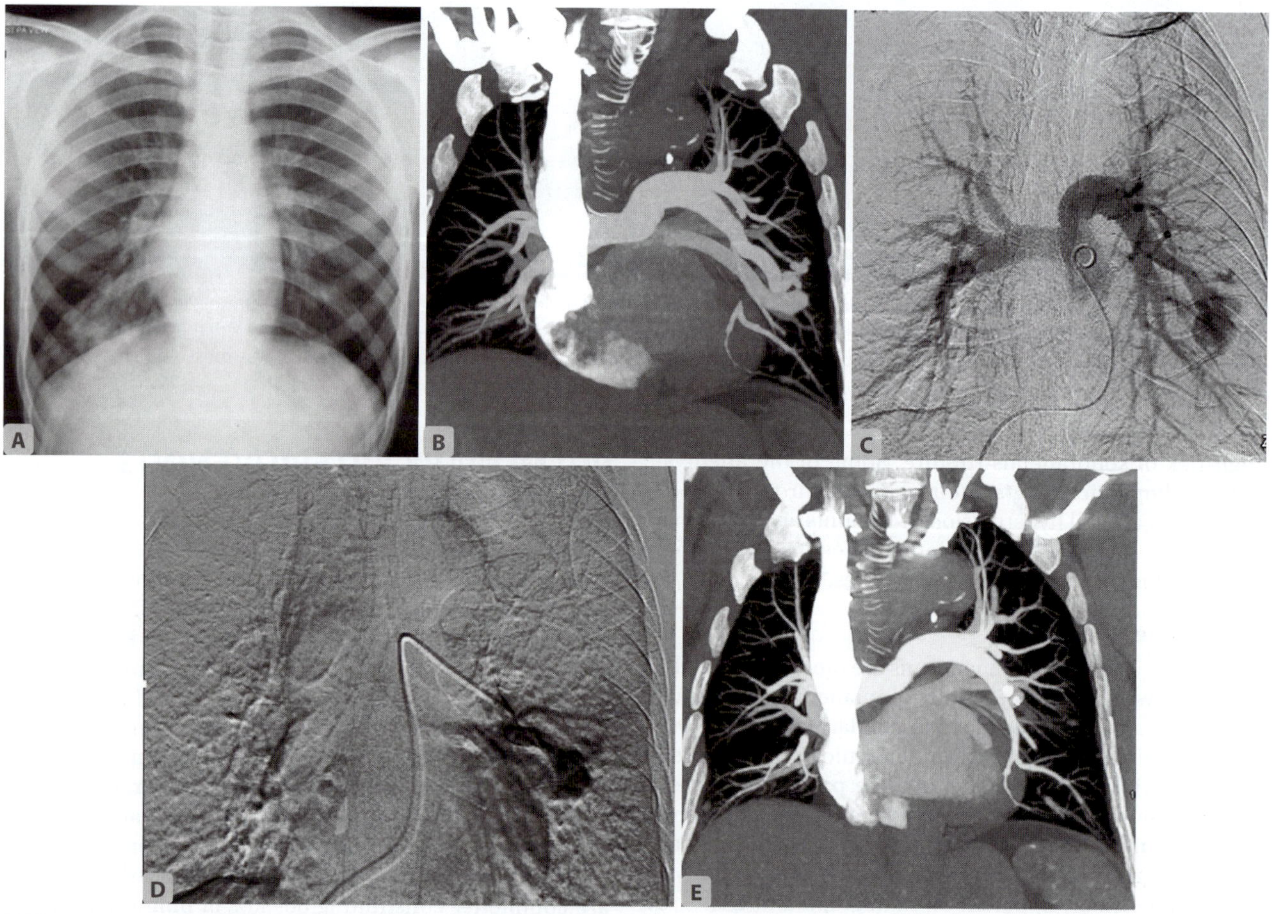

FIGS. 21A TO E: Solitary pulmonary arteriovenous malformation (AVM): Chest radiograph (A) shows solitary pulmonary AVM in right lower lobe with feeder vessel sign. Coronal CT pulmonary angiogram (B) in another patient showing solitary pulmonary AVM in left lateral basal segment with enlarged feeding artery and draining vein. Catheter pulmonary angiogram in main pulmonary artery (C) and on selective injection into feeding artery (D) showing similar findings as seen in DSA. Coronal CT pulmonary angiogram (E) postdeployment of vascular plug show no filling of pulmonary AVM.

shows a tubular opacity adjacent to the right atrium coursing toward the diaphragm in scimitar syndrome, which is better depicted on CT and MRI **(Figs. 23A to C)**.[2]

MALIGNANT TUMORS

Malignant neoplasms involving the pulmonary include pulmonary artery sarcoma (PAS), metastases, and direct invasion of pulmonary arteries and veins by adjacent malignancy such as lung cancer. Metastatic disease is most commonly seen. PAS is rare and can be undifferentiated sarcoma or leiomyosarcoma. It usually involves the main and the proximal pulmonary arteries. PAS mimics PE and appears as an intraluminal filling defect on CTPA and MRA that spans the entire lumen of the pulmonary artery and often causes its expansion **(Figs. 24A and B)**. Lesions may enhance with contrast, but this may be difficult to appreciate on CTPA. It can invade the adjacent lungs and the mediastinum. It may be hypermetabolic on PET-CT. Bland tumor thrombus may also be hypermetabolic on PET-CT; however, a maximum standard uptake value (SUV max) >2.25 is highly suggestive of tumor.[24,49,50]

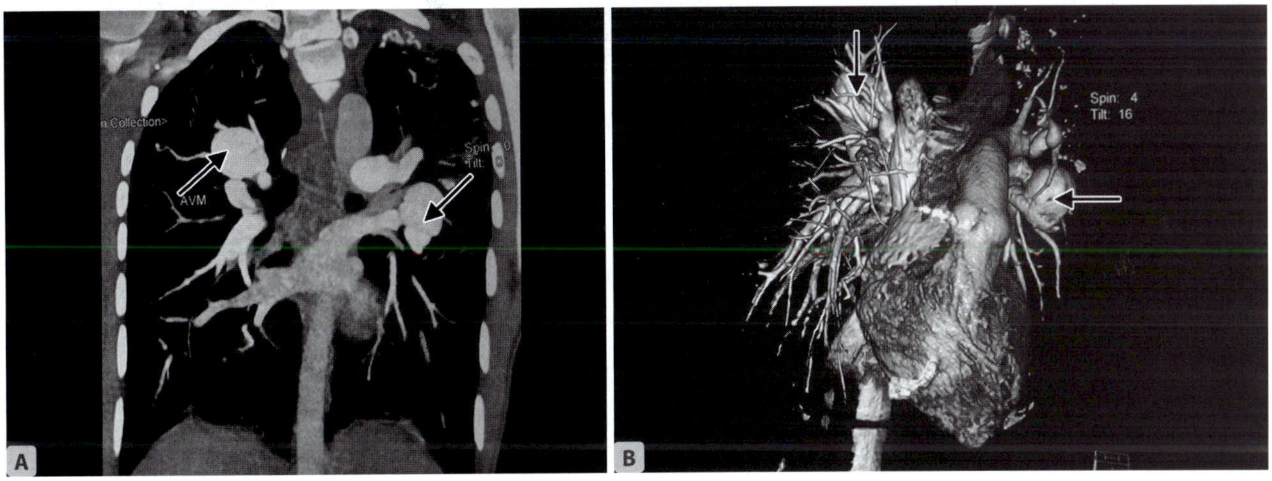

FIGS. 22A AND B: CT pulmonary angiogram—maximum intensity projection (A) and volume-rendered VR (B) images showing bilateral AVMs (arrows in A and B) in a patient of hereditary hemorrhagic telangiectasia.

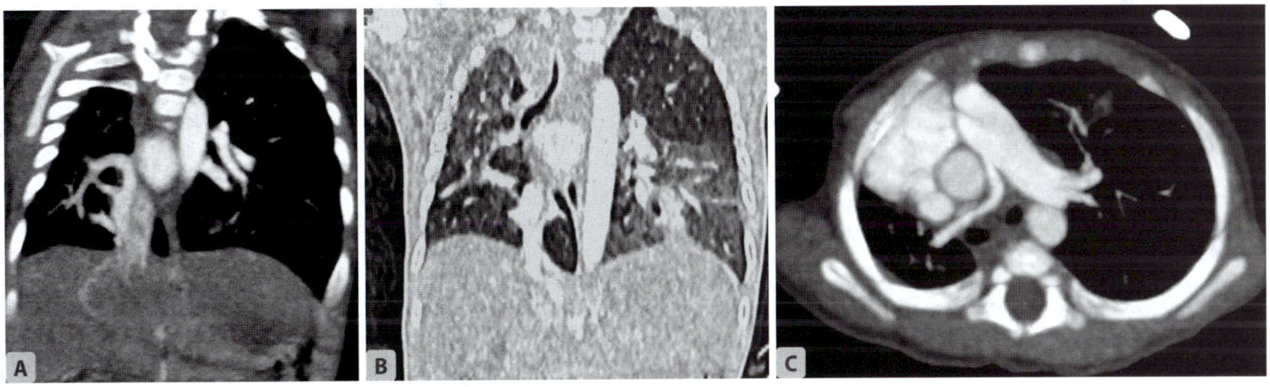

FIGS. 23A TO C: Scimitar syndrome: CT chest showing (A) abnormal drainage of right pulmonary veins into IVC; (B) Hypoplastic right lung with mosaic attenuation in bilateral lungs; (C) Hypoplastic right pulmonary artery.

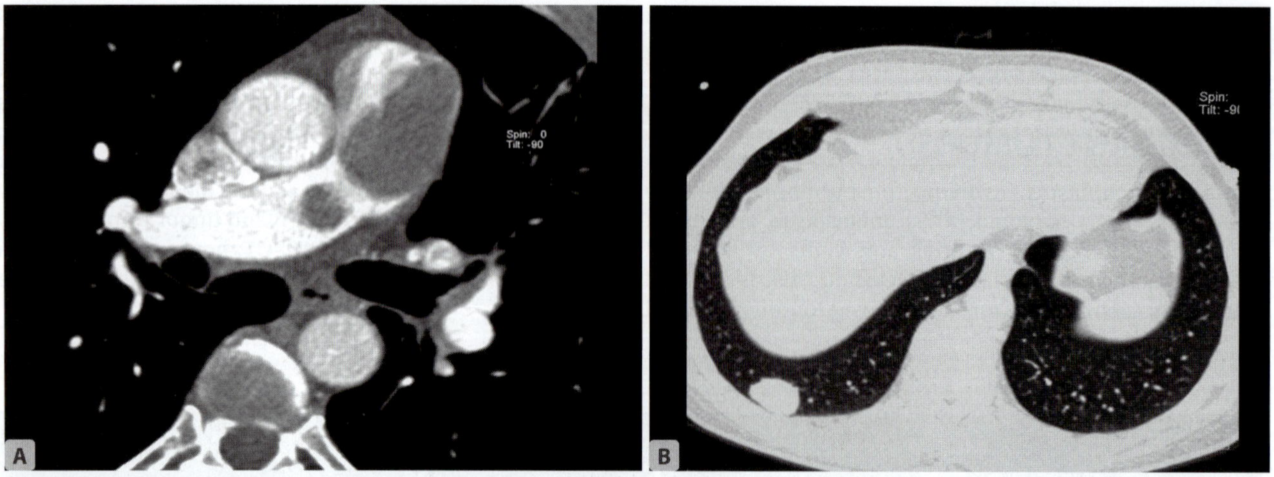

FIGS. 24A AND B: Pulmonary artery sarcoma: CT pulmonary angiogram (A) shows minimally enhancing main pulmonary artery mass with smaller similar lesion in right pulmonary artery. Lung section at a lower level (B) shows solitary metastasis in right lower lobe.

REFERENCES

1. Cummings KW, Bhalla S. Pulmonary vascular diseases. Clin Chest Med. 2015;36:235-48.
2. Porres DV, Morenza OP, Pallisa E, et al. Learning from the pulmonary veins. Radiographics. 2013;33:999-1022.
3. Goldhaber SZ, Bounameaux H. Pulmonary embolism and deep vein thrombosis. Lancet. 2012;379 (9828):1835-46.
4. Konstantinides SV. ESC guidelines on the diagnosis and management of acute pulmonary embolism. Eur Heart J. 2014;35(45):3145-6.
5. Ruggiero A, Screaton NJ. Imaging of acute and chronic thromboembolic disease: state of the art. Clin Radiol. 2017;72(5):375-88.
6. Wells PS, Anderson DR, Rodger M, et al. Derivation of a simple clinical model to categorize patients probability of pulmonary embolism: increasing the models utility with the SimpliRED D-dimer. Thromb Haemost. 2000;83(3):416-20.
7. Wicki J, Perneger TV, Junod AF, et al. Assessing clinical probability of pulmonary embolism in the emergency ward: a simple score. Arch Intern Med. 2001;161(1):92-7.
8. Sevitt S, Gallagher N. Venous thrombosis and pulmonary embolism: A clinico-pathological study in injured and burned patients. Br J Surg. 1961;48:475-89.
9. Le Gal G, Righini M, Sanchez O, et al. A positive compression ultrasonography of the lower limb veins is highly predictive of pulmonary embolism on computed tomography in suspected patients. Thromb Haemost. 2006;95(6):963-6.
10. Sista AK, Kuo WT, Schiebler M, Madoff DC. Stratification, imaging, and management of acute massive and submassive pulmonary embolism. Radiology. 2017;284(1):5-24.
11. Abdelaziz MM, Wali SO, Hamad MMA, et al. Pulmonary embolism: A diagnostic approach. Annals of Thorac Medicine. 2006;(1): 31-40.
12. Stein PD, Fowler SE, Goodman LR, et al. Multidetector computed tomography for acute pulmonary embolism. N Engl J Med. 2006;354(22):2317–27.
13. Fink C, Johnson TR, Michaely HJ, et al. Dual-energy CT angiography of the lung in patients with suspected pulmonary embolism: Initial results. Rofo. 2008;180(10):879-83.
14. Thieme SF, Becker CR, Hacker M, et al. Dual energy CT for the assessment of lung perfusion-correlation to scintigraphy. Eur J Radiol. 2008;68(3):369-74.
15. Delesalle MA, Pontana F, Duhamel A, et al. Spectral optimization of chest CT angiography with reduced iodine load: experience in 80 patients evaluated with dual-source, dual-energy CT. Radiology. 2013;267(1):256-66.
16. Szucs-Farkas Z, Christe A, Megyeri B, et al. Diagnostic accuracy of computed tomography pulmonary angiography with reduced radiation and contrast material dose: a prospective randomized clinical trial. Invest Radiol. 2014;49(4):201-8.
17. Sirajuddin A, François CJ, Kanne JP. Imaging studies for pulmonary vascular disease. Clinical Pulmonary Medicine. 2015;22(6): 307-21.
18. Bajc M, Albrechtsson U, Olsson CG, et al. Comparison of ventilation/perfusion scintigraphy and helical CT for diagnosis of pulmonary embolism; Strategy using clinical data and ancillary findings. Clin Physiol Funct Imaging. 2002;22:392-7.
19. Leung AN, Bull TM, Jaeschke R, et al. American Thoracic Society documents: an official American Thoracic Society/Society of Thoracic Radiology Clinical Practice Guideline—evaluation of suspected pulmonary embolism in pregnancy. Radiology. 2012;262:63546.
20. Kluge A, Luboldt W, Bachmann G. Acute pulmonary embolism to the subsegmental level: Diagnostic accuracy of three MRI techniques compared with 16-MDCT. Am J Roentgenol. 2006;187(1):W7-14.
21. Stein PD, Chenevert TL, Fowler SE, et al. Gadolinium-enhanced magnetic resonance angiography for pulmonary embolism: A multicentre prospective study (PIOPED III). Ann Intern Med. 2010;152(7):434-43. W142e433.
22. Furlan A, Aghayev A, Chang CC, et al. Short-term mortality in acute pulmonary embolism: Clot burden and signs of right heart dysfunction at CT pulmonary angiography. Radiology. 2012;265(1):283-93.
23. Lang IM, Pesavento R, Bonderman D, et al. Risk factors and basic mechanisms of chronic thromboembolic pulmonary hypertension: A current understanding. Eur Respir J. 2013;41(2):462-8.
24. Pena E, Dennie C, Veinot J, et al. Pulmonary hypertension: how the radioglogist can help. Radiographics. 2012;32:9-32.
25. Simonneau G, Gatzoulis MA, Adatia I, et al. Updated clinical classification of pulmonary hypertension. J Am Coll Cardiol. 2013;62:D34–41.

26. Fleischner FG. Pulmonary embolism. Clin Radiol. 1962;13: 169-82.
27. Tan RT, Kuzo R, Goodman LR, et al. Utility of CT scan evaluation for predicting pulmonary hypertension in patients with parenchymal lung disease. Medical College of Wisconsin Lung Transplant Group. Chest. 1998;113(5):1250-6.
28. Ng CS, Wells AU, Padley SPA. A CT sign of chronic pulmonary arterial hypertension: The ratio of main pulmonary artery to aortic diameter. J Thorac Imaging. 1999;14(4):270-8.
29. Sheehan R, Perloff JK, Fishbein MC, et al. Pulmonary neovascularity: A distinctive radiographic finding in Eisenmenger syndrome. Circulation. 2005;112(18):2778-85.
30. Van der Meer RW, Pattynama PM, van Strijen MJ, et al. Right ventricular dysfunction and pulmonary obstruction index at helical CT: Prediction of clinical outcome during 3-month follow-up in patients with acute pulmonary embolism. Radiology. 2005;235(3):798-803.
31. He J, Fang W, LV B, et al. Diagnosis of chronic thromboembolic pulmonary hypertension: Comparison of ventilation/perfusion scanning and multidetector computed tomography pulmonary angiography with pulmonary angiography. Nucl Med Commun. 2012;33:459-63.
32. Alassas K, Mergo P, Ibrahim el-S, et al. Cardiac MRI as a diagnostic tool in pulmonary hypertension. Future Cardiol. 2014;10: 17-30.
33. Schiebler ML, Bhalla S, Runo J, et al. Magnetic resonance and computed tomography imaging of the structural and functional changes of pulmonary arterial hypertension. J Thorac Imaging. 2013;28:178-93.
34. Swift AJ, Rajaram S, Condliffe R, et al. Pulmonary artery relative area change detects mild elevations in pulmonary vascular resistance and predicts adverse outcome in pulmonary hypertension. Invest Radiol. 2012;47:571-7.
35. Iwasawa T. Diagnosis and management of pulmonary arterial hypertension using MR imaging. Magn Reson Med Sci. 2013; 12:1-9.
36. Kondo C, Caputo GR, Masui T, et al. Pulmonary hypertension: pulmonary flow quantification and flow profile analysis with velocity-encoded cine MR imaging. Radiology. 1992;183: 751-8
37. Reiter G, Reiter U, Kovacs G, et al. Magnetic resonance-derived 3-dimensional blood flow patterns in the main pulmonary artery as a marker of pulmonary hypertension and a measure of elevated mean pulmonary arterial pressure. Circ Cardiovasc Imaging. 2008;1:23-30.
38. Barker AJ, Rolda´n-Alzate A, Entezari P, et al. Four-dimensional flow assessment of pulmonary artery flow and wall shear stress in adult pulmonary arterial hypertension: Results from two institutions. Magn Reson Med. 2015;73:1904-13.
39. Rolda´n-Alzate A, Frydrychowicz A, Johnson KM, et al. Noninvasive assessment of cardiac function and pulmonary vascular resistance in a canine model of acute thromboembolic pulmonary hypertension using 4D flow cardiovascular magnetic resonance. J Cardiovasc Magn Reson. 2014;13:16-23.
40. Odagiri K, Inui N, Miyakawa S, et al. Abnormal hemodynamics in the pulmonary artery seen on time-resolved 3-dimensional phase-contrast magnetic resonance imaging (4D-flow) in a young patient with idiopathic pulmonary artery hypertension. Circ J. 2014;78:1770-2.
41. Rich S, Pietra GG, Kieras K, et al. Primary pulmonary hypertension: radiographic and scintigraphic patterns of histologic subtypes. Ann Intern Med. 1986;105:499-502.
42. Perloff JK, Hart EM, Greaves SM, et al. Proximal pulmonary arterial and intrapulmonary radiologic features of Eisenmenger syndrome and primary pulmonary hypertension. Am J Cardiol. 2003;92(2):182-7.
43. Frazier AA, Franks TJ, Mohammed TL, et al. From the Archives of the AFIP: Pulmonary veno-occlusive disease and pulmonary capillary hemangiomatosis. Radiographics. 2007;27:867-82.
44. Castaner E, Alguersuari A, Gallardo X, et al. When to suspect pulmonary vasculitis: radiologic and clinical clues.Radiographics. 2010;30:33-53.
45. Hiller N, Liberman S, Chajek-Shaul T, et al. Thoracic manifestations of Behçet disease at CT. Radiographics. 2004;24:801-8.
46. Gill SS, Roddie ME, Shovlin CL, et al. Pulmonary arteriovenous malformations and their mimics. Clin Radiol. 2015;70:96-110.
47. Nguyen ET, Silva CI, Seely JM, et al. Pulmonary artery aneurysms and pseudoaneurysms in adults: Findings at CT and radiography. Am J Roentgenol. 2007;188:W126-34.
48. Shovlin CL, Jackson JE. Pulmonary arteriovenous malformations and other vascular abnormalities. In: Mason RJ, Broaddus VC, Martin T, et al (Eds). Murray and Nadel's Textbook of Respiratory Medicine, 5th edn. Philadelphia: Elsevier-Saunders. 2010.pp. 1261-82.
49. Castaner E, Gallardo X, Rimola J, et al. Congenital and acquired pulmonary artery anomalies in the adult: radiologic overview. Radiographics. 2006;26:349-71.
50. Lee EY, Khong PL. The value of 18 F-FDG PET/contrast enhanced CT in detection of tumor thrombus. Nuc Med. 2013;38: e60-5.

CHAPTER

151

Peripheral Vascular Diseases: Imaging and Interventions

Devasenathipathy Kandasamy, Shivanand Gamanagatti

INTRODUCTION

Peripheral vascular diseases (PVD) includes a wide spectrum of disease affecting the vessels of upper and lower extremity. The estimated prevalence of PVD increases with age which rises from 2.5% in the age group of 50–59 years to 14.5% in over 70 years of age.[1] Among the causes, atherosclerosis is by far the most common cause of PVD and commonly affects the lower limb. Atherosclerosis is the disease of the elderly, commonly affecting individuals more than 50 years of age. The common risk factors for developing atherosclerosis are smoking, diabetes mellitus, hyperlipidemia and hypertension. Other common nonatherosclerotic causes of PVD are Takayasu arteritis and Burgers disease, the former commonly affects the aortoiliac segment and the latter commonly affects the femoropopliteal and tibioperoneal circulation. PVD is less common in younger patients and common causes include trauma, thromboembolism and arteritis. Imaging plays an important role in the management of PVD because it is essential to know the arterial anatomy, extent and severity of pathology to choose the next appropriate step in management. Decades back, digital subtraction angiography (DSA) was the modality of choice for the diagnostic evaluation of PVD. However, in the current scenario, because of its invasiveness the role of DSA is usually limited to the endovascular interventional procedures. With the technological developments in Ultrasonography (USG), computed tomography (CT) and Magnetic resonance imaging (MRI) in the last few decades, the diagnostic evaluation of PVD has been taken over by these modalities.

Whenever PVD is suspected clinically, initial diagnostic evaluation is done using ankle-brachial index (ABI).[2] ABI is an effective method to detect significant stenosis and it is performed by measuring the systolic blood pressures at the level of ankle and arm in supine position. ABI less than 0.9 is suggestive of significant PAD in the lower extremity with the sensitivity and specificity of 79% and 96% respectively.[3] ABI between 0.9 and 1 is considered borderline. If there is extensive calcification of the arterial wall or reduced compliance of the vessel wall, ABI can be falsely elevated. Also ABI cannot assess the location and severity of the stenosis. Hence, ABI can be an effective screening method and further imaging is necessary for the detailed evaluation.

IMAGING MODALITIES

Digital Subtraction Angiography

Digital subtraction angiography used to be the diagnostic modality of choice decades ago which can show the arterial anatomy in great detail because of its superior spatial resolution compared to other modalities. It is a robust modality to show the flow dynamics across the lesion, distal run-off and it also provides an opportunity to perform interventional procedures in the same sitting. However, DSA has several limitations which eventually paved way to the newer modalities. It provides a 2D view of the vessels and hence the tortuosity and overlap can underestimate or overestimate the stenosis.[4] Other limitations of DSA are the need for invasive arterial access and associated complications, ionizing radiation and usage of iodinated contrast media.

Ultrasonography

Ultrasonography with color Doppler is another modality which can be of use in the evaluation of PVD. Apart from the grayscale (B mode), Doppler principle can be used to overlay color and generate graphical spectrum of the flow dynamics. It is safe, inexpensive, and widely available and can give functional information in the region of interest. Recent advances in the USG technology namely ultrafast Doppler made it possible to get spectral information in a large area rather than only from the sampling window. This technique allows the operator to get multiple spectral tracings over an area from a single data acquisition. Normal extremity artery shows a triphasic high resistance flow pattern with a preserved spectral window **(Figs. 1A to D)**. Whenever there is stenosis, B-mode USG shows vessel narrowing, the systolic flow rate across the stenosis increases and the flow changes from streamlined to turbulent **(Figs. 2A to C)**. This leads to increase in peak systolic velocity (PSV) which is the most sensitive parameter and spectral broadening causing

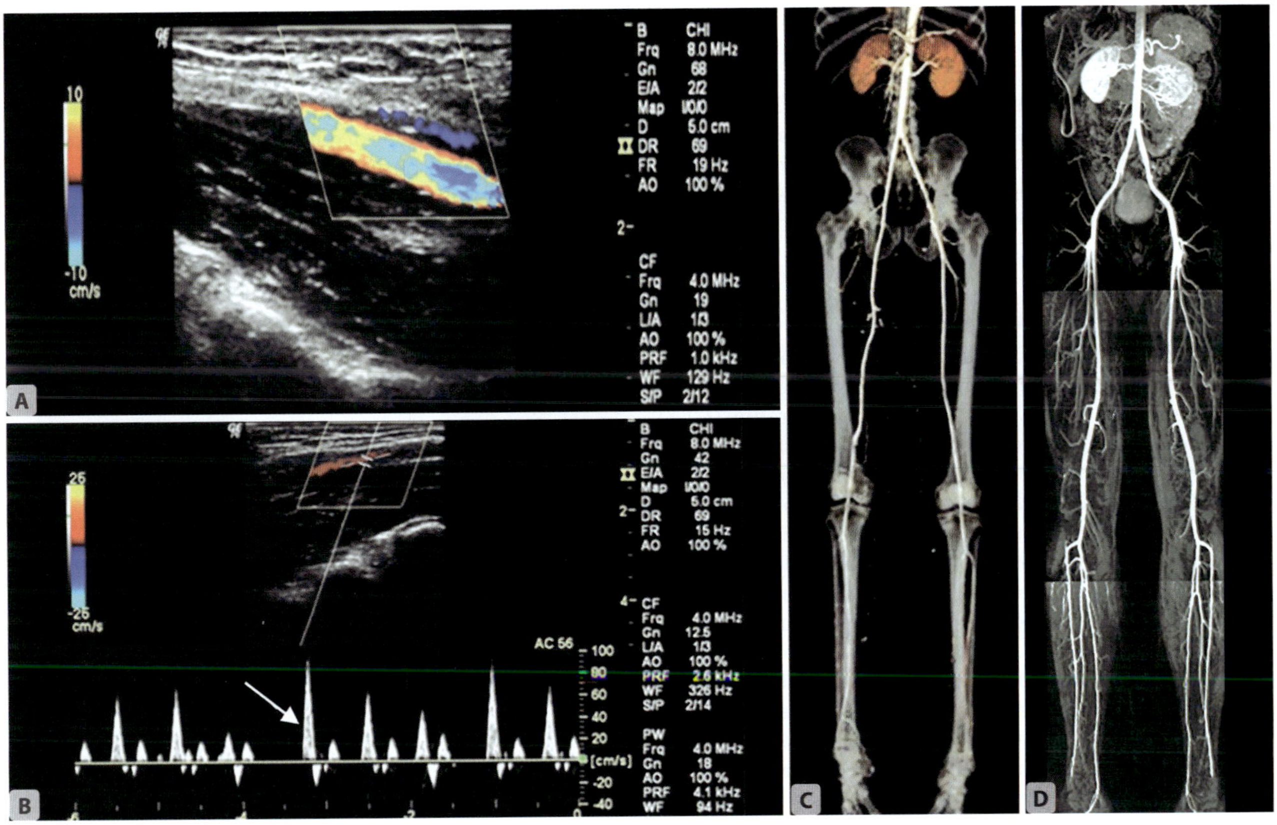

FIGS. 1A TO D: Normal lower extremity arteries on imaging. Color Doppler (A) with spectral tracing (B) of superficial femoral artery showing an uniform caliber artery which is showing typical triphasic flow pattern (arrow). Volume-rendered technique (VRT) image (C) showing normal appearance of abdominal aorta and bilateral lower limb arteries. The course, caliber and relationship of vessels with the bones are shown on the VRT image. Maximum intensity projection (MIP) image (D) acquired in three stations showing normal abdominal and lower extremity arteries.

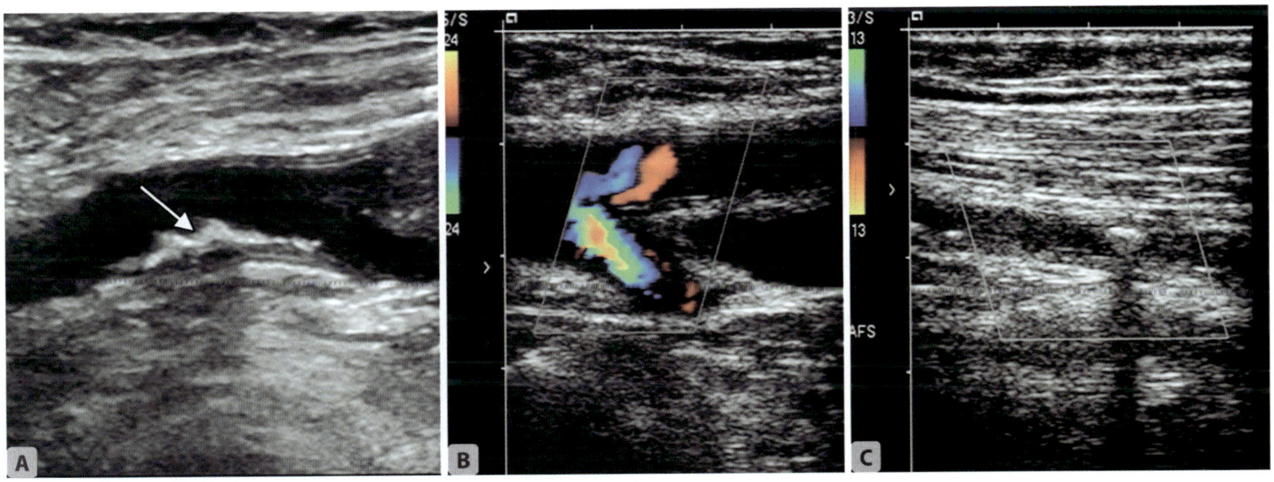

FIGS. 2A TO C: Arterial narrowing on color Doppler. B mode USG image (A) at the level of bifurcation of common femoral artery showing calcified plaques (arrow). Color Doppler image at the same level (B) and at the level of superficial femoral artery (C) showing no flow due to narrowing of the vessel.

obliteration of spectral window. To eliminate the variations in the PSV between vessel segments and patients, a ratio of PSV at the site of abnormality and at the normal proximal vessel is taken. The commonly used criteria to diagnose >50% stenosis is PSV ratio >2, PSV >200 cm/sec, color aliasing and spectral broadening.[5]

However, there are several shortcomings of color Doppler which made this modality less popular for the evaluation of PVD. The quality of the study depends on the operator, leading to moderate inter-observer agreement for the evaluation of aortoiliac and femoropopliteal segments.[6] The evaluation of aortoiliac segment is limited due to bowel gas and abdominal fat. The evaluation of infrapopliteal segments is usually challenging and time consuming. Because of the above reasons the complete evaluation of the entire arterial tree is not possible in many situations. Heavily calcified vessels cannot be evaluated using USG because of poor window. Another important limitation is that the sensitivity to detect the distal lesion in sequential stenosis is poor because of the change in arterial flow dynamics due to the proximal stenotic segment.

Computed Tomography

Computed tomography is currently one of the preferred modality to evaluate extremity arteries. The advent of multidetector CT has revolutionized CT angiography (CTA) leading to faster and high quality acquisition of images. Higher resolution compared to MRI and capability of 3D image generation are additional highlights. In the era of single slice CT scanners, optimal scanning of the entire extremity arterial tree in a single contrast injection was not possible. In the last decade due to the increase in the number of detector rows, more coverage per rotation of tube, faster rotation has made the evaluation of entire arterial tree from mid aorta till feet possible in the first pass of contrast (***see* Figs. 1A to D**). Faster scanning led to decrease in the contrast volume over years. With the current available scanning speed and lower dwelling time it is really critical to capture the peak enhancement of the arterial tree to obtain good quality images. The timing, rate of injection, contrast volume and the scanning speed of the scanner should be adjusted meticulously to avoid poor opacification of arteries. This is especially true in patients with stenosis or aneurysm where the blood flow is slow. The acquisition can be much faster than the leading edge of the contrast movement eventually resulting in scanning of unopacified arteries. Thus in the current generation scanners, there is a need to optimize the above said injector and scanner parameters to get the desired result. The typical scanning parameters are provided in **Table 1**.

Another factor which needs to be considered is the kVp of the scanning. Decrease in kVp increases the visualization of contrast and reduces radiation dose and thus 100–120 kVp scanning is recommended. Newer generation scanners have the capability of dual energy acquisition which opens up a wide range of applications such as accurate bone removal to generate high quality 3D images, automatic plaque characterization and removal which can give accurate stenosis measurements, reduction of streak artifacts and generation of optimum quality image sets with high contrast to noise ratio which has the potential to reduce radiation and contrast dose.

The 3D data of CT scan can be post processed to generate intuitive and clinically useful images. Maximum intensity projection (MIP) is a type of rendering in which the voxel with maximum value will be displayed from any point of view **(Figs. 3 and 4)**. The wall calcification and vessel contour are well-delineated on MIP and give an overview of the entire arterial tree. It can be used in two modes full-volume (thick) mode and sub-volume (thin) mode. Thin MIP is useful in depicting the inflow circulation (aortoiliac) so that the overlying abdominal visceral arteries are not visualized. Thick MIP is useful in showing the outflow circulation (femoropopliteal and tibioperoneal).

Curved planar reconstruction (CPR) is a specialized form of multiplanar reformat (MPR) in which the image can be reformatted in any curved plane. CPR is useful to visualize the entire length of artery in one image. It can also be used to create orthogonal axial images perpendicular to the axis of the artery so that the stenosis measurements can be done accurately even in the presence of calcified plaques.

Volume-rendering technique (VRT) is a post-processing technique which can give 3D perspective of the entire volume. It is useful to provide spatial relationships with the adjacent structures such as collaterals and bone which is immensely helpful for interventional radiologists and

TABLE 1: Typical injection protocol for CTA of lower extremity (for a 70 kg individual).

Contrast volume and rate	25 mL at 5 mL/s for 5 seconds followed by 120 mL at 4 mL/s for 30 seconds
Injection duration	35 seconds
Scanning time	40 seconds
Scanning delay after the arrival of contrast	3 seconds

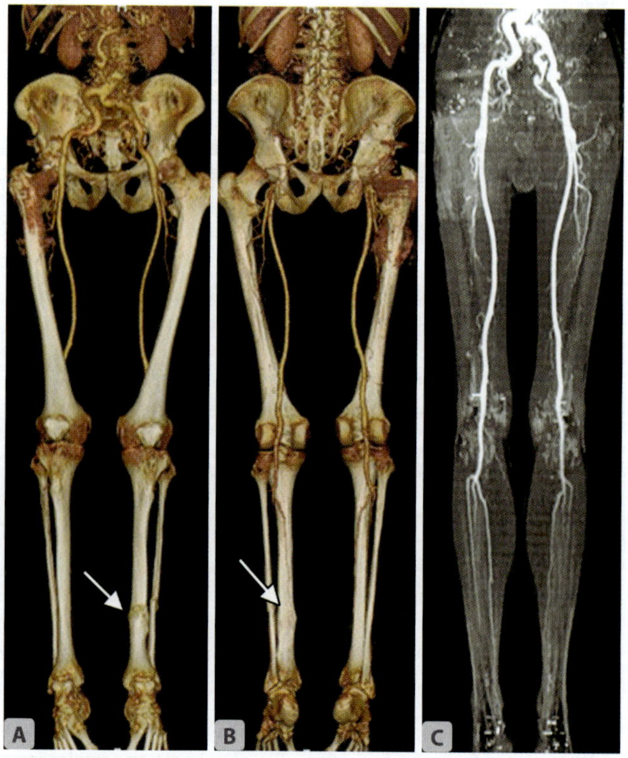

FIGS. 3A TO C: CTA—one stop shop technique in skeletal trauma. VRT images of CTA in front (A) and back (B) views showing fracture of both bones in the left leg (arrow). MIP image with bone removal of the same patient showing attenuated arteries in the left leg. CTA in this situation can provide information about the skeletal and soft tissue injuries apart from showing the detailed anatomy of the lower limb arterial tree.

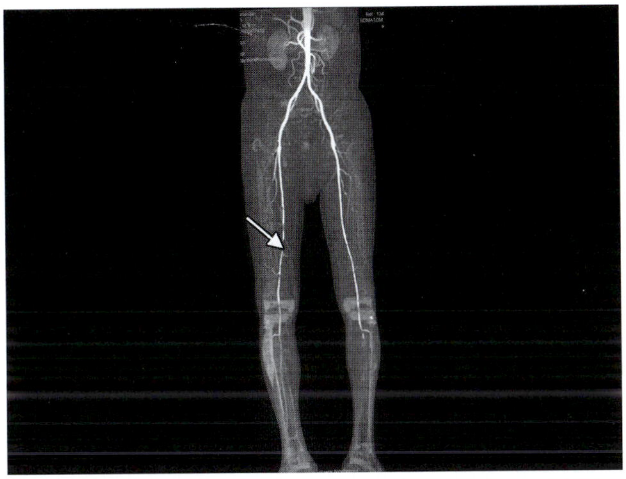

FIG. 4: Arterial narrowing on CTA: MIP image with bone removal of CTA data set showing short segment narrowing at the level of distal superficial femoral artery and good distal run-off. MIP image can provide an overview of the entire arterial tree on a single image based on the CTA data set which is otherwise huge.

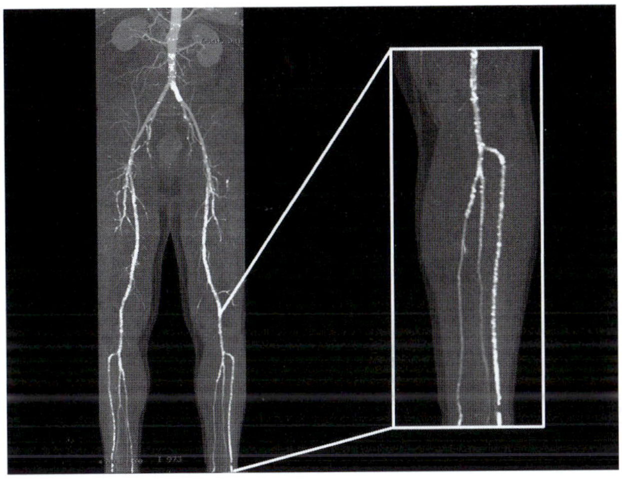

FIG. 5: Vessel wall calcification on CTA: MIP image of a CTA data set showing extensive vessel wall calcification involving the entire arterial tree. This is considered as a limitation of CTA in which the evaluation of vessel wall narrowing is known to be hampered by extensive calcifications.

surgeons **(Fig. 3)**. However, the distinction between the calcified plaque and vessel wall contour is not that well-visualized on VRT.

With the above post-processing methods especially the CPR along with axial images, stenosis can be easily categorized into mild (0–50%), moderate (50–70%) and severe (>70%).[7,8]

Magnetic Resonance Imaging

Magnetic resonance imaging has undergone several technological improvements over decades and with the current scanners it is possible to scan the entire arterial tree in a single injection of contrast. Advantage of MR angiography (MRA) as compared to CTA is that it can generate images without overlapping bones and calcified plaques without exposing the patient to ionizing radiation **(Figs. 1A to D, 5 and 6)**. Unique capability of MRI is that it can generate angiographic images without contrast media which comes handy in patients with chronic renal disease and patients with contraindication to contrast media. Because of superior background tissue suppression on 3 Tesla compared to 1.5 Tesla scanners, it is preferred for both contrast-enhanced MRA (CE-MRA) and non-contrast MRA studies.

CE-MRA is the most commonly performed, fast and robust MRA technique which depends on the T1 shortening effect of gadolinium-based contrast agents. Spatial resolution of CE-MRA is better than non-contrast MRA and artifacts are also less seen. CE-MRA sequence is a fast sequence with preferential filling of central k space which determines the contrast resolution of the image. Acquiring the entire lower extremity arteries without venous contamination is challenging. It is usually done in three stations namely aortoiliac, thigh and calf region and between the acquisitions the table has to move quickly to next station. This technique is called three station, moving table technique in which the contrast bolus is followed from aortoiliac to calf in the same order. Usually precontrast as well as post contrast volume sets are acquired and subtracted to obtain the MRA image.

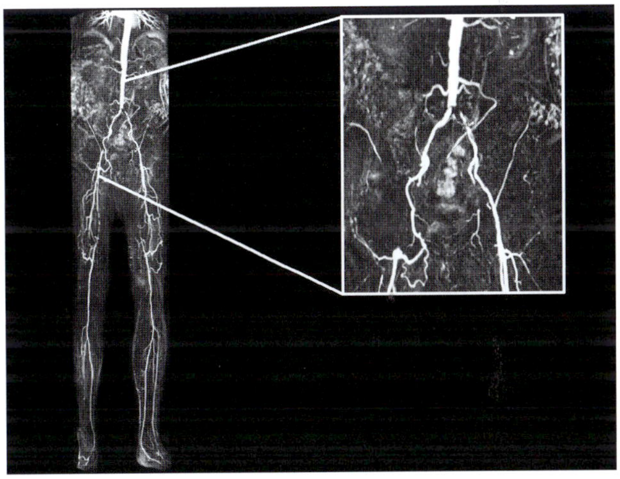

FIG. 6: Arterial narrowing on MRA: MIP image of MRA data set showing extensive atherosclerotic involvement of aorta and lower limb arteries. There is complete occlusion of bilateral common iliac arteries till superficial femoral arteries with good distal run-off. Extensive vessel wall calcifications do not hamper the vessel assessment on MRA which is an advantage over CTA.

This DSA like subtraction using precontrast mask provides good background tissue suppression and showing only the vessels. The aortoiliac station is usually done with breath holding to minimize motion blurring. However, this method can sometimes lead to venous contamination in the third station resulting in nondiagnostic studies **(Fig. 7)**. There are different approaches described to overcome the venous contamination including thigh compression cuffs and pillow under the knee to slow down the venous return, non-contrast MRA for the calf station and acquiring calf station in a separate contrast injection.[9] Another technique which can be used to overcome venous contamination in calf is by performing time resolved MRA which generates images in every 1–2 seconds to differentiate arteries from veins. If the

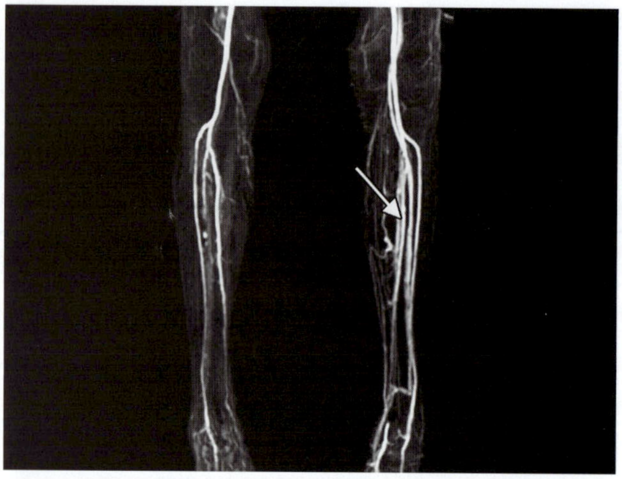

FIG. 7: Venous contamination in MRA: MIP image of MRA data set of bilateral legs showing venous contamination (arrow) in the left side. Venous contamination which usually occurs in the last station of data acquisition due to time delay can degrade the diagnostic quality of MRA.

data is acquired during the inflow of contrast, ringing artifacts will degrade the image quality. Thus, the image acquisition should be performed during the plateau phase of the arterial enhancement. Hence the timing of contrast injection and start of scanning are of paramount importance. Typically 0.2 mmol/kg body weight is the contrast dose used for lower limb MRA and it is injected at a rate of 2–2.5 mL/second followed by saline chase. One needs to be cautious in using contrast in patients with impaired renal function because they stand the risk of developing nephrogenic systemic fibrosis (NSF). The start of image acquisition can be either after an empirical delay or by performing a test bolus to know the arrival time of contrast or by MR fluoroscopic technique in which rapid real time images are taken and once the contrast arrival is ascertained, the MRA sequence is triggered manually.

There are various methods used to obtain non-contrast MRA in various parts of the body. Among those, time of flight (TOF), quiescent-interval single-shot (QISS) and fast spine echo (FSE) based gated subtraction MRA are commonly used for imaging extremity arteries especially if contrast injection is contraindicated. FSE-based subtraction technique suffers from motion which can degrade the image quality. However, it can be highly accurate if motion can be minimized. QISS MRA is another promising and robust method to evaluate extremity arteries which has been shown to have high sensitivity (85–97%) and specificity (95–98%) for the detection of significant stenosis compared to CE-MRA.[10–12]

IMAGING FEATURES CLINICAL ENTITIES

Atherosclerosis

Atherosclerosis is the most common cause of PVD affecting inflow or outflow circulation. Patients with significant aortoiliac disease present with buttock or thigh claudication and patients with femoropopliteal disease present with calf claudication. Isolated tibioperoneal circulation is a feature of diabetes in which patients usually present with calf and foot involvement. The role of imaging is to evaluate the location, arterial segment involved, length and severity of stenosis which is critical to decide on endovascular interventional therapy versus surgical therapy. Transatlantic Inter-society Consensus (TASC) Document on management of peripheral arterial disease (PAD) has categorized various stenotic lesions based on their length, severity and bilaterality into A, B, C and D and recommends the appropriate mode of treatment. The recommendations are shown in **Table 2**.

TABLE 2: TASC recommendations.

Type A lesions	Short length lesions—endovascular therapy is recommended
Type B lesions	Endovascular therapy is preferred unless other lesions in the same area necessitates surgical approach
Type C lesions	Generally longer lesions—surgical revascularization is recommended. Endovascular therapy, if the patient is a high-risk candidate for surgery
Type D lesions	Surgical revascularization is recommended in all

In patients with diabetes where there is extensive arterial wall calcifications especially in the tibioperoneal region, accurate evaluation of stenosis/occlusion may not be possible. MRA is a preferred imaging modality in these patients (***see* Fig. 5**).[13] With the emergence of dual energy CT, there is a potential to allow accurate distinction between arterial lumen and calcified plaque.

Atheroembolism and Thromboembolism

Atheroembolism is usually secondary to an ulcerative plaque in aortoiliac region leading to acute unilateral symptoms. The embolus usually occludes the smaller arteries of the leg. CTA can adequately evaluate the site of obstruction and also the probable source of embolus.

Thromboembolic events are generally from cardiac source, however paradoxical embolus from the systemic venous source is also a possibility. They are usually larger than atheroemboli and hence they occlude more proximal arteries in the femoropopliteal region. These patients need gated CTA of heart and thoracic aorta in addition to CTA of the extremity arteries to guide appropriate management.

Peripheral Arterial Aneurysm

Peripheral arterial aneurysms can co-exist with aortic aneurysm and they can be bilateral in almost 50% of patients.[14,15] Hence it is prudent to image the entire arterial tree from aorta till the toes. The size criteria for femoral artery aneurysm is >10 mm and popliteal artery is >7 mm.[16,17] Femoral artery aneurysms are usually secondary to trauma, arterial puncture or post bypass graft surgery. The initial evaluation is done using USG—color Doppler which can reliably diagnose the aneurysm and rule out other cystic lesions. The role of CTA is to provide more detailed visualization and detection of additional lesions.

Arteritis

Buergers disease and Takayasu arteritis are the most common arteritis affecting the extremity arteries. Other less common causes are giant cell arteritis, polyarteritis nodosa, Behcet's disease and Kawasaki disease. Buergers disease has strong association with smoking and usual age of presentation is around 40 years and they predominantly affect the small and medium-sized arteries (distal femoropopliteal and tibioperoneal circulation). Imaging studies show high-grade narrowing or complete occlusion of involved arteries with well-developed cork-screw collaterals because of slow progression of the disease.

Takayasu arteritis usually involves the large arteries such as arch vessels, aorta and iliac arteries with sparing of outflow circulation in the extremity. Young and middle aged females are usually affected. The role of imaging is to delineate the narrowing and assess the severity to direct appropriate management.

Popliteal Artery Entrapment Syndrome

It has 4 described types which is based on the extent of displacement of popliteal artery by the medial head of gastrocnemius muscle. The diagnosis can be made on USG in which narrowing can be demonstrated at the typical location and real time dynamic compression during dorsiflexion of foot can also be demonstrated. Similar findings can also be demonstrated on DSA.

Cystic Adventitial Disease

Cystic adventitial disease commonly affects the popliteal artery and seen in young patients. It leads to concentric or eccentric smooth narrowing of the involved segment. The underlying pathology is the mucin production in the adventitia of the arterial wall leading to narrowing. Although findings may be seen on USG, MRA is the modality of choice because of the ability to characterize mucin in the wall on T2-weighted images.

Imaging Strategy

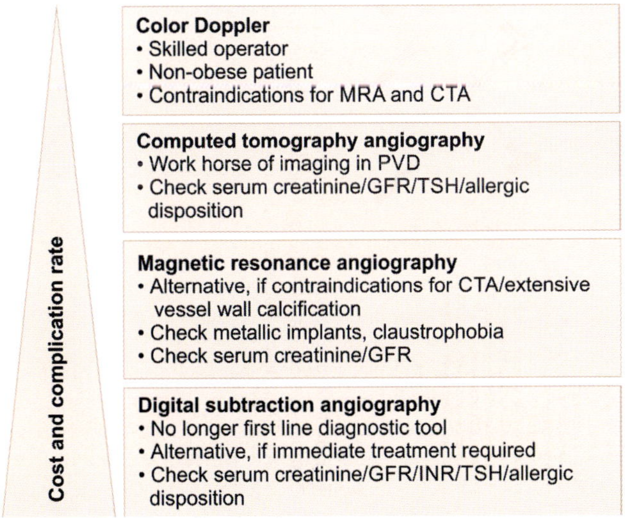

(PVD: peripheral vascular disease; GFR: glomerular filtration rate; TSH: thyroid stimulating hormone; MRA: magnetic resonance angiography; CTA: computed tomography angiography; INR: international normalized ratio)

Interventions

Endovascular treatment provides a lower risk substitute to conventional surgery in many patients with multiple comorbidities. Whenever possible, interventional treatments have become the first line of management in the treatment of PVD. Advances in interventional technology during the past few years have widened the choices for handling PVD percutaneously. The Inter-Society Consensus for the Management of Peripheral Arterial Disease (TASC) guidelines aimed to provide guidance on treatment decisions relating to the optimal revascularization strategy (endovascular versus surgical) based on the anatomic and clinical status of the patient **(Fig. 8)**.[18]

Noninvasive tests (ankle-brachial index) and arterial mapping (CT/MR angiography) done, prior to an endovascular treatment, help in localization of the disease and planning the procedure **(Figs. 9A and B)**.

Treatment Decision

The scheduling and necessity for revascularization depends upon the clinical settings. Three different clinical situations include:

1. Intermittent claudication
2. Critical limb ischemia
3. Acute limb ischemia

Most of the patients with intermittent claudication are managed by exercise and medical therapy. Interventional procedures are ascribed in circumstances, when these methods fail to improve quality of life and limb function.

In contrast, critical limb ischemia and acute limb ischemia impend the limb and warrants more imperative revascularization.

Types of Procedures

Balloon angioplasty and stenting are the key revascularization techniques. Latest advances in interventional treatments include, drug-eluting balloons, drug-eluting stents, plaque debulking devices (atherectomy) and devices for crossing tight chronic total occlusions.[19]

Results

In general, interventional therapies have better long-term durability for aortoiliac disease than femoral popliteal disease. Infrapopliteal revascularization has poor long-term results and is generally reserved for critical and acute limb ischemia.

Follow-up and Surveillance

Patients receiving any form of interventional revascularization measures need a planned surveillance strategy for follow-up care.

- Rigorous treatment of cardiovascular risk factors to avert myocardial infarction and stroke.
- Limb observation targets to identify restenosis and fresh disease elsewhere in the treated segments.

Technique of Angioplasty

Definition

Percutaneous transluminal angioplasty (PTA) refers to deliberate opening (dilatation) of a vascular stenosis or occlusion using a balloon catheter.

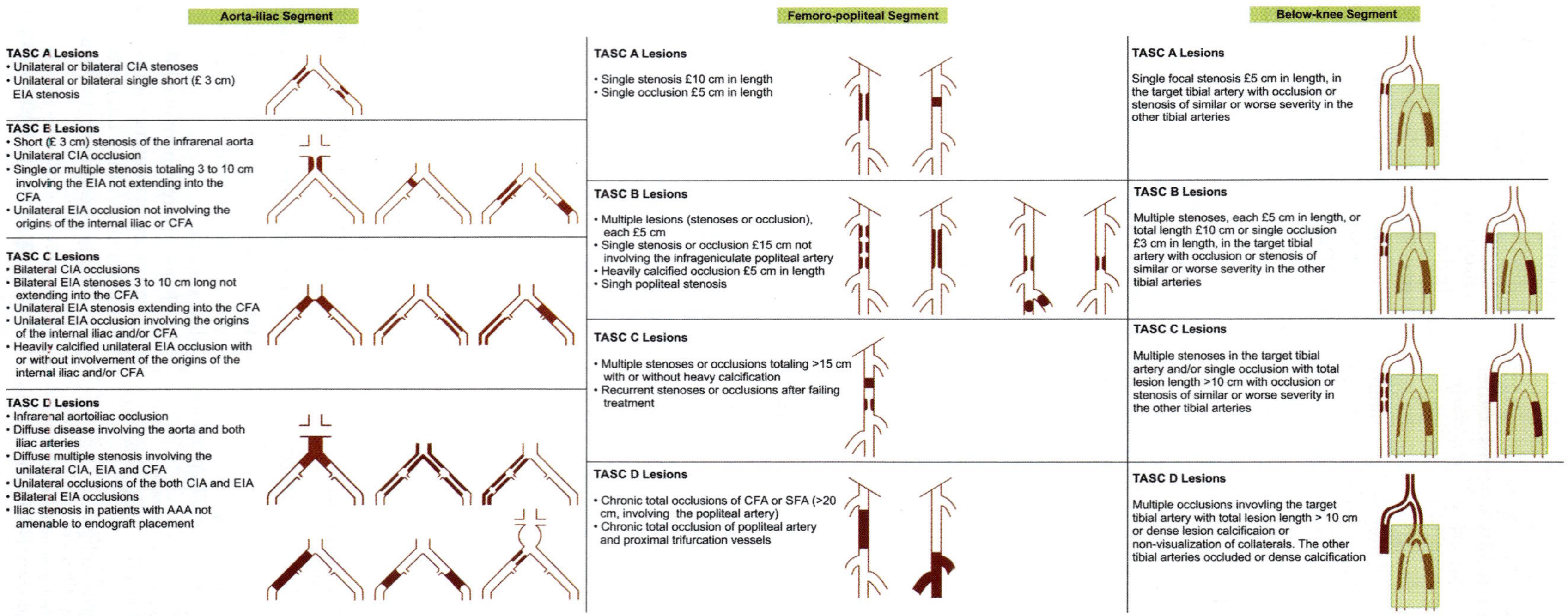

FIG. 8: TASC anatomic classification showing various patterns of disease based on extent of the disease at different segments of arterial tree. Used for treatment guidance regarding the optimal revascularization strategy (endovascular versus surgical) based on the complexity and location of the anatomic disease. (TASC: transatlantic inter-society consensus; CIA: common iliac artery; EIA: external iliac artery; CFA: common femoral artery; AAA: abdominal aortic aneurysm; SFA: superficial femoral artery).

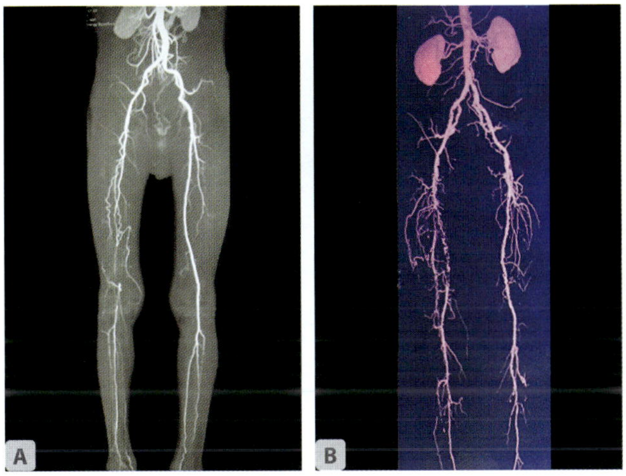

FIGS. 9A AND B: CT angiography (MIP and VRT) images of vascular mapping of bilateral lower limbs showing location of lesion and extent of the disease, important for planning the endovascular treatment.

Mode of Action of PTA

Angioplasty causes rupture of the atherosclerotic plaque and a limited split or dissection of the vessel wall.

The split might spread in the vessel wall either in circumferential or longitudinal direction. Also, it may spread deep into the internal elastic lamina or into the media, keeping adventitial layer intact. Concentric arterial narrowing have good response to PTA, since the plaque and the vascular wall layers are split in an even fashion, whereas eccentric vascular lesions respond poor to balloon dilatation due to recoil of the normal elastic wall.[20]

A cutting balloon has got non-compliant balloon with fine fins fixed longitudinally on the outer surface of the balloon. These fins are devised to cut a lesion during balloon inflation, permitting a simpler angioplasty at lower inflation pressures. Cutting balloons are recommended for stenoses resistant to standard angioplasty.[21]

Stenting

Vascular stents are designed to provide an internal support for the vascular lumen. Stents has got following advantages:

- Quick, consistent, and constant expansion of the luminal diameter.
- Trapping of the weak plaque material that may possibly embolize after angioplasty.
- Removal of elastic recoil after angioplasty.

Preprocedure Work-up

- A comprehensive clinical and medical history must be taken. History regarding claudication symptoms, pertinent past history of cardiac and renal disease, risk factors for vascular disease such as diabetes, smoking and hypercholesterolemia. Also, history of contrast allergy must be obtained.
- Take history about present-day medication. Some of the medications may need to be stopped or modified prior to the procedure, such as, oral anticoagulants, antiplatelets and insulin.
- Evaluate all the fresh imaging findings to choose the proper site and direction of vascular access, i.e. ipsilateral versus contralateral approach, antegrade versus retrograde puncture.
- Review the appearance of the lesion on imaging that will help to plan the appropriate management, i.e. angioplasty versus stenting. In general, short segment narrowing/ occlusions are likely to benefit satisfactorily to angioplasty.
- If there is renal dysfunction, IV hydration must be commenced a day prior to the procedure. Usage of iso-osmolar contrast agents is recommended.
- It is appropriate to discuss with the patient about treatment options (angioplasty versus surgery), results and the possible complications. Informed consent should be taken prior to the procedure.

Day of Procedure

- The patient reports to the vascular lab after fasting for 4–6 hours, however, clear fluids are allowed. The site of vascular access is cleaned and draped in a sterile manner.
- Close monitoring of the vital statistics (Pulse, BP, SPO_2) is done prior to the start of procedure and is continued till the procedure is completed.
- Patients are advised to start antiplatelet medicines (clopidogrel 75 mg/day, and aspirin 160 mg/day) 2 days prior to the procedure, which will help to diminish thrombotic events during the procedure.

Vascular Access

The site of vascular access is determined by the site of vascular lesion to be treated as determined by analysis of imaging studies prior to the start of procedure.

- For the lesions in iliac arteries (cranial to the inguinal ligament), an ipsilateral retrograde common femoral approach is preferred **(Fig. 10A)**.
- For the lesions caudal to the inguinal ligament:
  - Common femoral artery (CFA) and superficial femoral artery (SFA) till adductor canal level, cross over techniques from contralateral femoral artery **(Fig. 10B)**.
  - For distal SFA and beyond, the antegrade common femoral puncture is the preferred access route **(Fig. 10C)**.
- Other arterial access sites such as brachial artery **(Fig. 10D)**, the radial artery, the popliteal artery and the tibial arteries **(Figs. 10E and F)** may also be used to obtain vascular access.

Crossing of the Lesion[19]

- Appropriate size vascular sheath (preferably, 6F in common femoral access) is introduced into the access artery. If the contralateral approach is used, then crossover vascular sheath should be placed. The lesion is usually crossed using a combination of selective catheter and an atraumatic hydrophilic guidewire.
- Low molecular weight Heparin (3000–7000 IU) should be administered either in divided doses or as a single loading dose as per the institute practice.

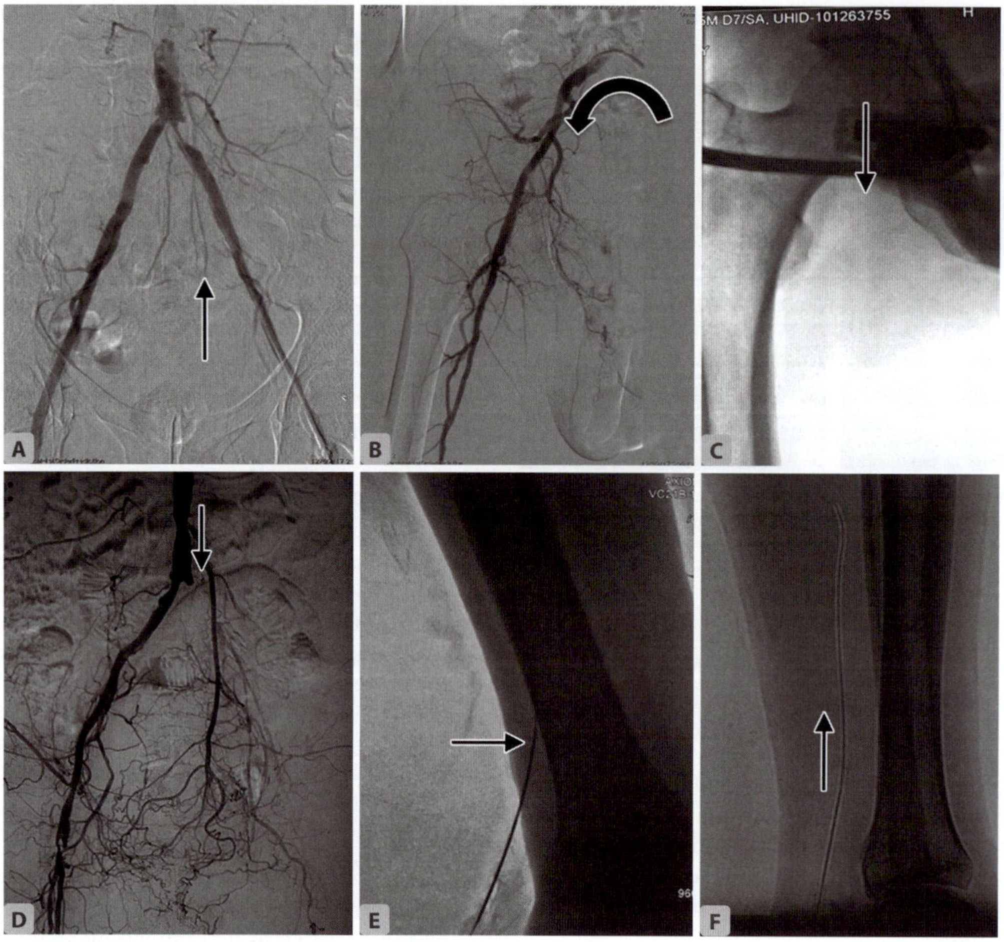

FIGS. 10A TO F: DSA spot images showing various types of vascular access. (A) Retrograde transfemoral approach; (B) Contralateral transfemoral access; (C) Antegrade transfemoral approach; (D) Brachial approach; (E) Anterior tibial approach; (F) Posterior tibial approach.

- After crossing the lesion with guidewire, the catheter is pushed over the guidewire and the guidewire is withdrawn. If the catheter tip is in true lumen, one should start seeing the free flow of blood coming from the catheter hub. It is always good idea to aspirate blood and/or inject contrast medium to check the catheter position within the lumen.
- It is always important to ensure that the guidewire is long enough (use exchange guidewire of 260 cm) for exchanging the selective catheter, the balloon catheter or stent delivery system.
- It is important to take care that the guidewire is of appropriate diameter, which is recommended for the lumen of the balloon catheter or stent delivery systems. For example, it is not feasible to introduce a stent delivery system devised for a 0.018-inch guidewire over a 0.035-inch guidewire.
- A choice of whether to treat the lesion by angioplasty alone or primary stenting could be made either prior to the start of procedure or after the initial angiographic images of the lesion location and appearance.
- Occasionally, choice of stenting is made, when angioplasty fails or makes the lesion worse.

Balloon Angioplasty (Figs. 11A to C and Table 3)

- A balloon catheter of suitable diameter and length must be chosen.
- Regarding balloon catheter size, there is a controversy whether to use oversized balloon or not in relation to the normal artery diameter. Most of the interventionists choose balloon catheters 10–20% larger than the native artery diameter.
- In case of uncertainty, it is a good idea to use a balloon catheter of lesser diameter than the artery as appreciated on a road map. This is to avoid selecting a balloon that is too big, which may cause vessel rupture.
- Many interventionists choose the balloon catheter diameter using the "Eyeball technique" based on their clinical experience of the estimated diameter of the vessel to be treated.
- Regarding the length of the balloon catheter, length must be sufficient to include the entire length of the lesion. If an undersized balloon is chosen for a considerably longer lesion, several dilatations may be needed to cover the full length of the lesion, which could be time consuming.

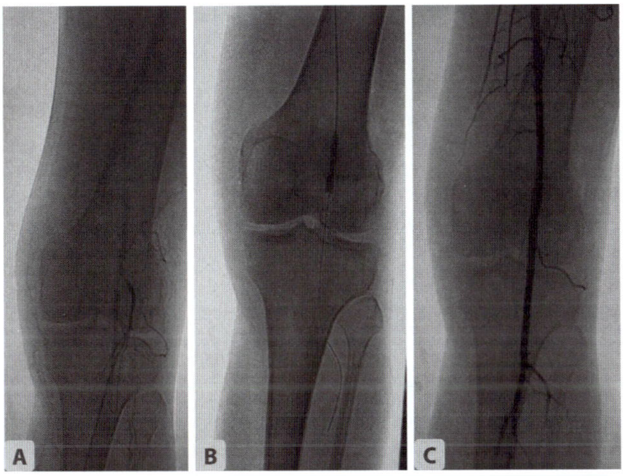

FIGS. 11A TO C: Image showing various steps of balloon angioplasty. Short segment occlusion of popliteal artery (A), crossed by the floppy end of hydrophilic guidewire followed by dilatation of the segment using balloon catheter (B). Final angiogram showing the opening of the occluded segment of popliteal artery (C).

- Proximal and distal radiopaque markers indicate the location of the balloon on the catheter.
- The balloon catheter is introduced over the guidewire under image guidance, steadily in smooth manner.
- Once the balloon is placed accurately across the lesion using the radiopaque markers as guidance, balloon catheter is slowly inflated using diluted iodinated contrast media.
- The inflation may be accomplished either by a 5 mL Luer-lock syringe or by mechanical inflation device having pressure measurement display.
- During balloon inflation, expansion starts from periphery of the balloon and extends gradually towards the middle as the lumen gets dilated. Frequently, the lesion creates a central waist on the balloon at the site of maximum resistance resulting in an hourglass configuration. The removal of the waist suggests effective dilatation of the stenosis.[22]
- There is no agreement about the ideal duration of balloon inflation. Balloon Inflation duration might range from a few seconds to a minute or more. However, the duration of balloon inflation does not matter in majority of cases.
- Usually, balloon dilatation is done from distal to proximal segments. At each station, after the balloon angioplasty, balloon should be fully deflated, so that it can be pulled easily to the next segment of narrowing.
- Pain is an important factor during balloon inflation and it should be closely observed. Generally, the balloon inflation produces some degree of pain due to stretching of the adventitia and this pain reduces following balloon deflation. However, when patient complains of continued pain following balloon deflation, one should suspect vessel rupture.
- Once, the entire length of stenotic/occluded segment is dilated, the balloon catheter should be withdrawn carefully, while keeping the guidewire across the site of angioplasty. It is very important to remember because by mistake if the guidewire is pulled out and the lesion entails additional management due to unsatisfactory outcome or a complication (such as rupture/dissection), it may not be possible to go across the freshly treated lesion that may end in technical failure or a limb-threatening complication.

TABLE 3: Recommended balloon catheter sizes.

Iliac segments	7–8 mm
Femoral segments	6 mm
Popliteal segment	4–5 mm
Below knee	2–3 mm

- Once the balloon catheter is removed over the guidewire, the vascular sheath should be aspirated for removal of the clots (if any) present inside the sheath and sheath is flushed with heparinized saline. Post-angioplasty angiogram must be obtained to assess the technical outcome and to look for complications (such as dissection/rupture/distal migration of ruptured plaque).
- Post-angioplasty angiogram should include the distal run of vessels (e.g. trifurcation and tibial vessels) along with angioplasty site to look for distal vessel occlusion due to distal migration of plaque material from angioplasty site.
- Once the angiogram looks acceptable, the guidewire and vascular sheath are removed. Manual compression is applied at the puncture site to achieve hemostasis.
- Sometimes, occlusion involves the origin of an artery (e.g. common iliac artery origin at the bifurcation), there is a hypothetical risk of creating an ostial stenosis of the contralateral vessel either by dissection or by dislodgment of plaque across the bifurcation. Hence, few interventionists ensure safety of the contralateral vessel by the placement of another balloon and is known as "kissing balloon technique" **(Figs. 12A and B)**. This is debatable and several interventionists do not advocate the use of this technique for treating ostial lesions at bifurcations.
- Similarly, if stenting has to be done for the lesion at bifurcation due to unsatisfactory angioplasty result, some operators choose to place a stent in the contralateral artery based on similar justification and is called as kissing stent technique **(Figs. 13A to C)**.[19,22]

How to Decide the Endpoint?

The angioplasty site must be cautiously assessed on the check angiogram to guarantee that the vessel is effectively opened with residual stenosis <30% as measured by pressure measurement using manometers. Another simple way of deciding the endpoint without pressure measurement is looking at the angiogram for disappearance of collaterals across the angioplasty site.

Subintimal Angioplasty (Figs. 14A to D)[23]

- In case of true lumen angioplasty, narrowing is negotiated by passing a guidewire through the true lumen of the vessel.

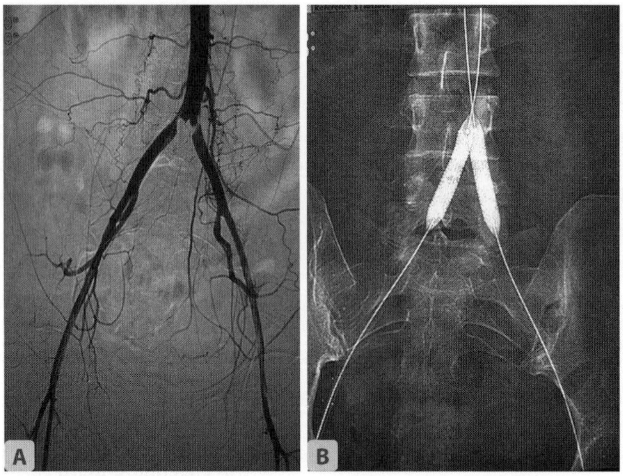

FIGS. 12A AND B: Kissing balloon technique: Digital subtraction angiography spot images showing (A) Ostial stenosis of bilateral iliac artery; (B) Managed by kissing balloon technique.

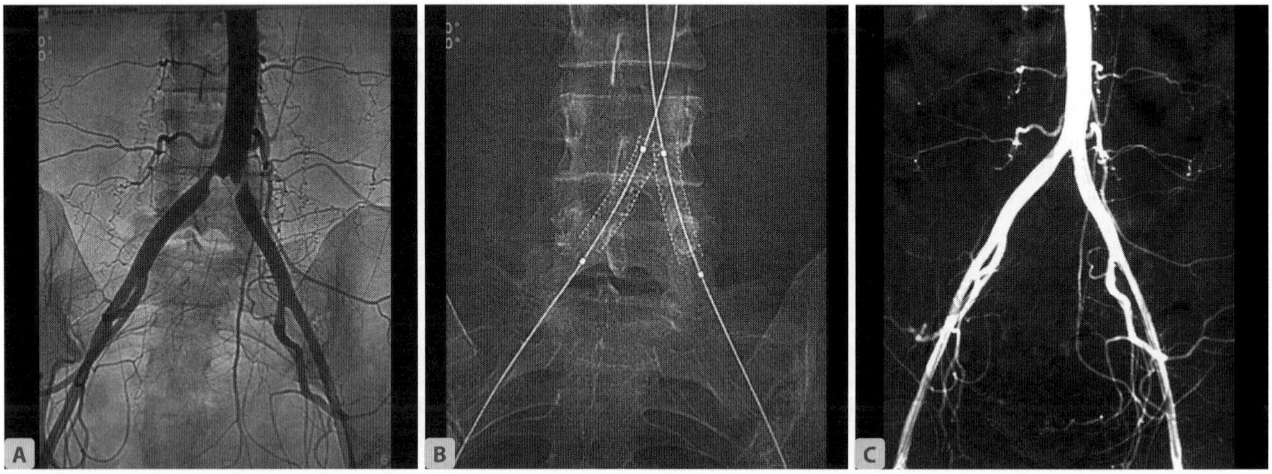

FIGS. 13A TO C: Digital subtraction angiography images showing kissing stent technique in the management of bilateral iliac ostial stenosis.

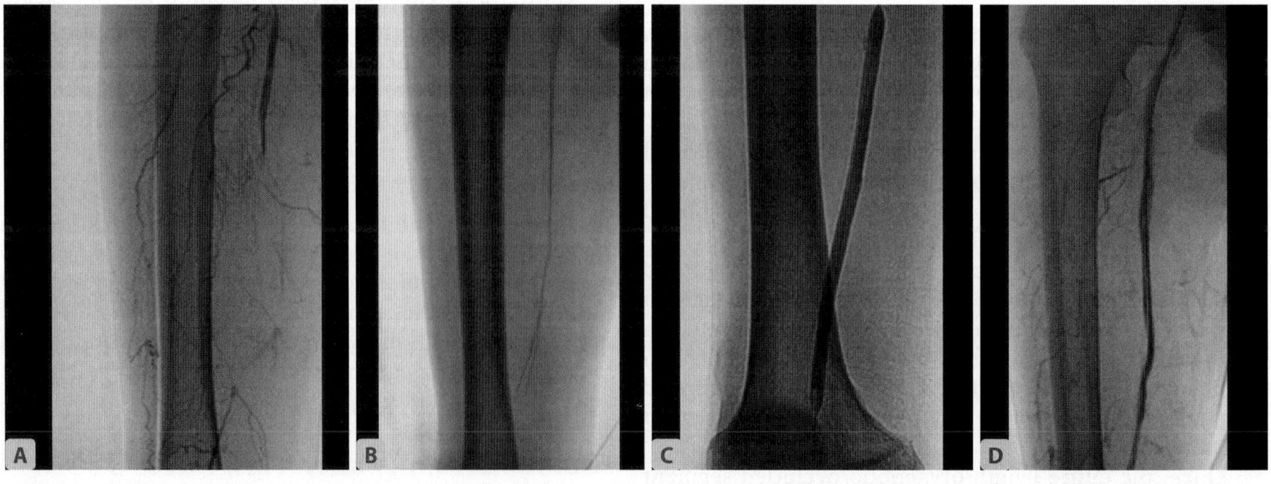

FIGS. 14A TO D: Digital subtraction angiography spots images showing technique of subintimal angioplasty (A). Long segment occlusion of superficial femoral artery, which was crossed by a loop of floppy end of hydrophilic guidewire into the subintimal space (B) and subsequently dilated by balloon catheter (C). Final angiogram showing the opening of the occluded segment of superficial femoral artery (D).

- Whereas in case of chronic tight occlusions, guidewire is intentionally negotiated through the wall of vessel (usually the subintimal space) rather than true lumen, and is known as subintimal angioplasty or also known as percutaneous intentional extraluminal recanalization (PIER).
- *Benefit of subintimal angioplasty:* Since we are doing angioplasty of the subintimal space, it provides a lumen that is free of atherosclerotic plaques as compared to true lumen angioplasty.
- In this procedure, combination of angled catheter (such as Picard catheter) and J-tip hydrophilic catheter is used for intentional passage of the guidewire into subintimal space. Just proximal to the site of occlusion, this catheter and guidewire combination is brought and forcibly pushed against the site of occlusion. During this forcible attempt to cross the occlusion, a loop of guidewire is created. This loop has to be advanced further, so that this loop dissects the intima and enter the subintimal space. Once, the loop enters the subintimal space, catheter and guidewire are progressively advanced distally till the entire segment of occlusion is traversed.
- When the loop has crossed past the distal limit of the occlusion, pull the guidewire to shorten the length of the loop. Now push the guidewire forward by rapid backward and forwards movements, so that guidewire re-enters the true lumen.
- Re-entry into the true lumen is complemented by sudden loss of resistance to passage of the guidewire
- If the catheter tip is in true lumen, one should start seeing the free flow of blood coming from the catheter hub. It is always good idea to aspirate blood and/or inject contrast medium to check the catheter position within the lumen.
- Once the guidewire position within true lumen is confirmed after re-entry, the dissection plane is dilated with an angioplasty balloon of a suitable size.[23,24]

Stents[19,22,25]

- There are two types of stenting technique and the prevailing indications for stenting differ depending upon the site of lesion.
- Types of stenting: Primary and secondary stenting.
- In primary stenting, stenting is done without preceding angioplasty. It is encouraged/suggested in few locations, such as stenosis involving ostium (renal artery stenosis, iliac artery stenosis) and malignant venous obstruction.
- In secondary stenting, stenting is done after the angioplasty especially when angioplasty results are poor due to elastic recoiling of wall or due to flow limiting dissection at angioplasty site.
- Stents may comprise of only metal known as bare metal stent or may comprise of a metallic stent covered with graft material, which is known as a stent-graft.
- Another method of classifying stents as balloon expandable and self-expandable, is based on their method of deployment.
- Balloon-expandable stents are valuable at sites where stent has to be deployed with highest accuracy (i.e. ostial lesions) **(Figs. 15A to D)**.
- As compared to balloon expandable stents, self-expanding stents have smaller profiles, are more flexible and are available in longer lengths. Hence, these are used for treating long segment tortuous occlusions like SFA occlusions **(Figs. 16A to C)**.
- Occasionally, self-expanding stents may require additional dilatation using balloon catheter of the equal diameter after deployment to assist their expansion to their full diameter. This is not required in case of balloon expandable stent, since they are deployed by balloon dilatation.

Complications[19,22]

Procedure-related complications (peri-procedural or post-procedural) are not uncommon and are commonly seen in elderly patients with diffuse disease and other comorbidities.[25]

The most common complications are puncture site complications such as hematoma and pseudoaneurysm formation which are easily managed by manual compression. Occasionally, pseudoaneurysm needs to be managed by thrombin injection **(Figs. 17A to F)**.

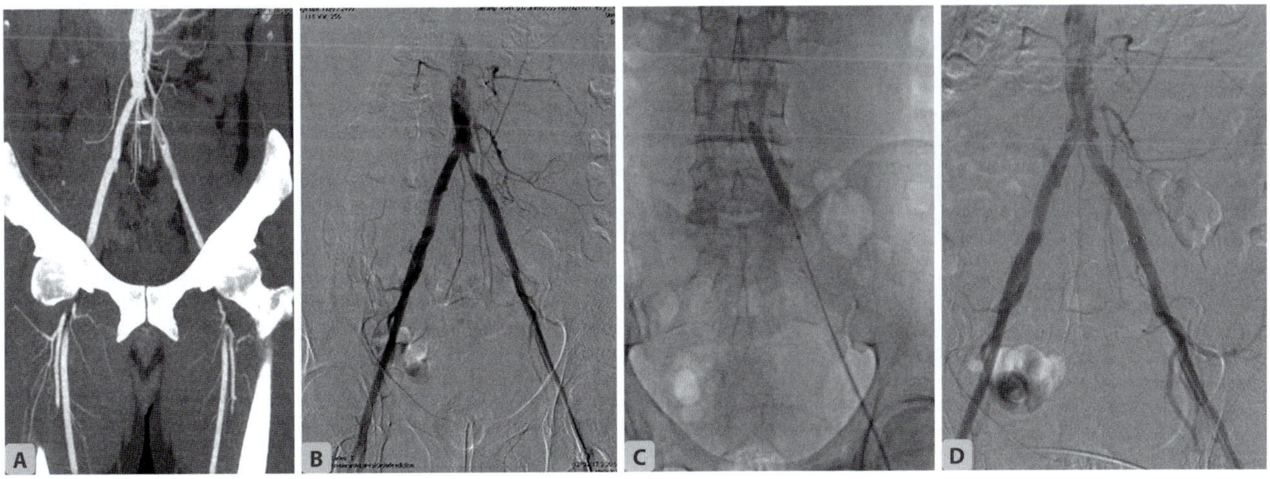

FIGS. 15A TO D: Images showing technique common iliac stenting using balloon mounted stent. Short segment occlusion of left common iliac artery involving the ostium (A and B), was initially crossed with floppy end of hydrophilic guidewire and subsequently managed by balloon mounted stent (C). Final angiogram showing the opening of the occluded segment of common iliac artery (D).

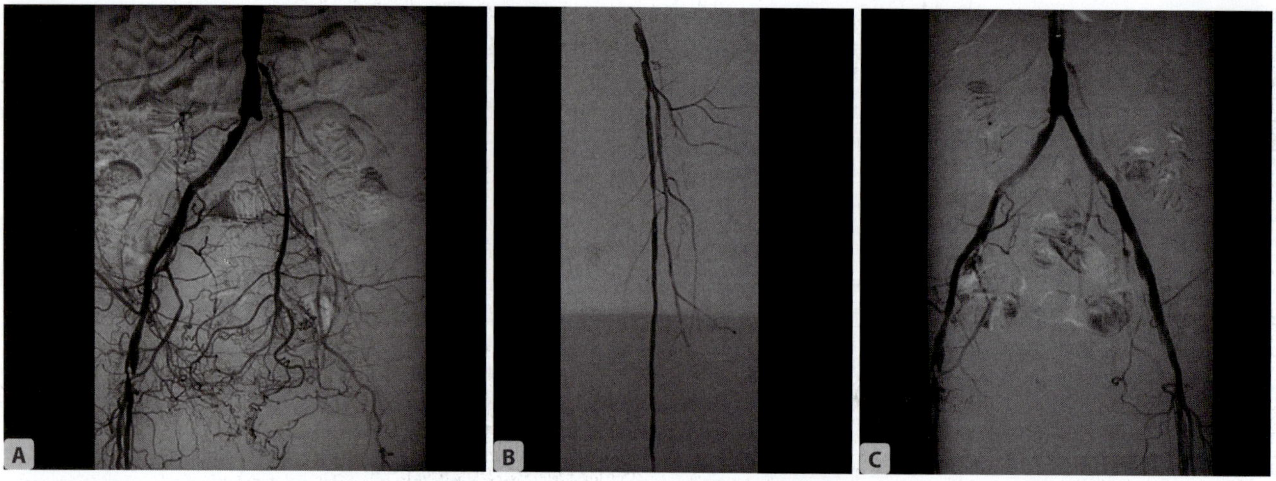

FIGS. 16A TO C: TASC type D lesion of left iliac segment managed by self-expandable stent. Long segment occlusion involving the left common iliac and external iliac arteries (A), with reformation of left common femoral and superficial femoral artery by collaterals (B), was subsequently managed by placing overlapping self-expandable stents across the occluded segment. Final angiogram showing the opening of the occluded entire segment of iliac artery (C).

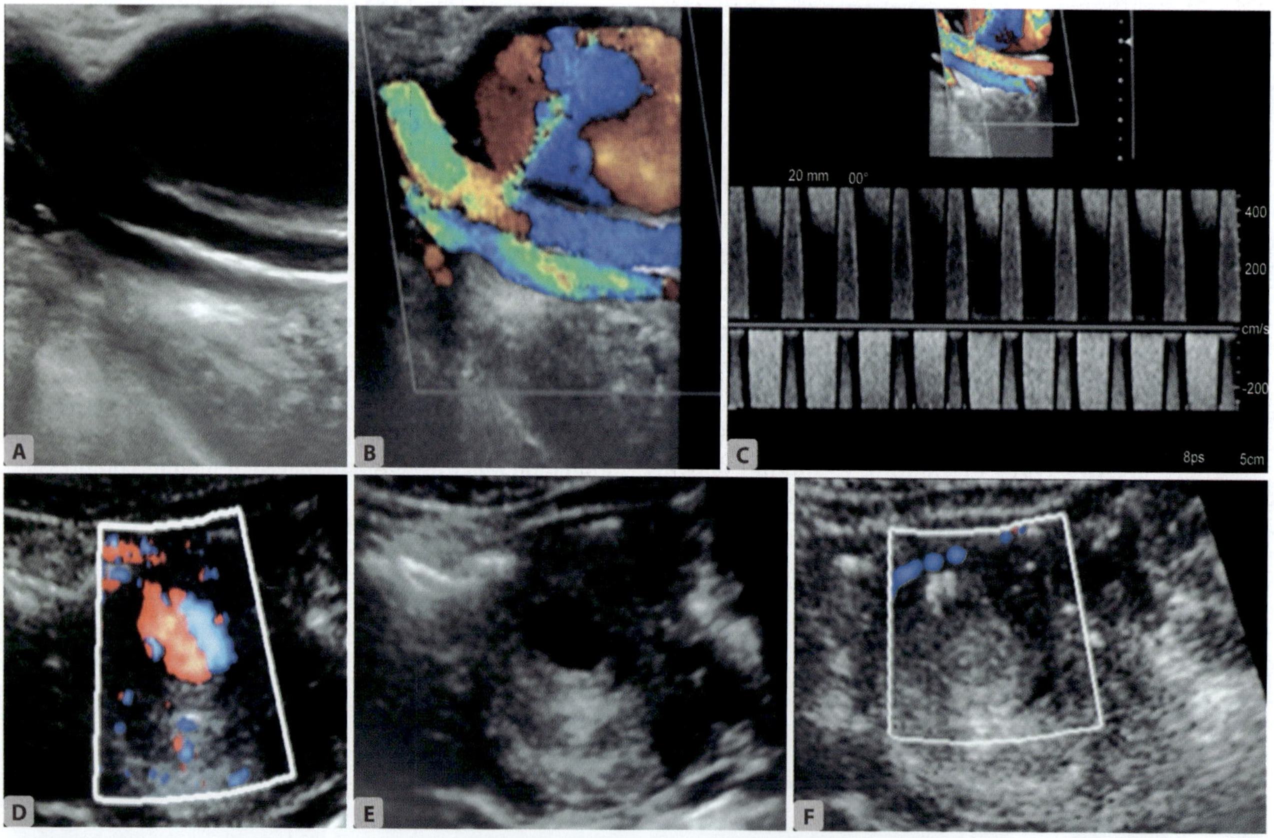

FIGS. 17A TO F: Post-angioplasty pseudoaneurysm complication management: Sonography with color Doppler images showing narrow neck pseudoaneurysm arising from the common femoral artery at the puncture site (A and B), with Yin-Yang spectral wave form at the neck of pseudoaneurysm (C), which was subsequently managed by percutaneous thrombin injection into the pseudoaneurysm and achieving complete thrombosis of the pseudoaneurysm (D to F).

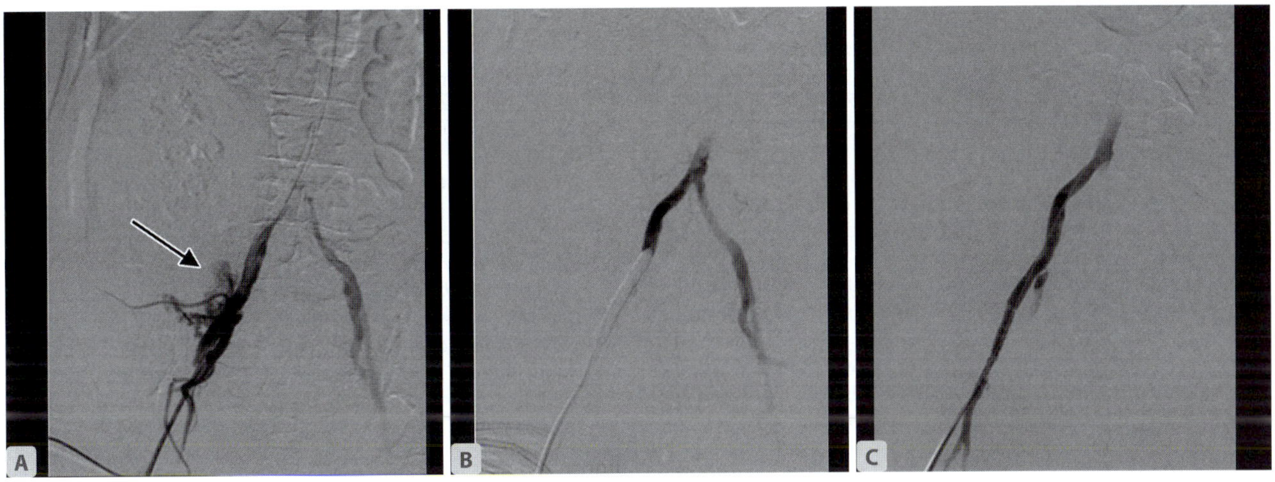

FIGS. 18A TO C: Post angioplasty complication of arterial rupture: DSA spot images showing rupture of the external iliac artery (arrow) following balloon angioplasty (A), which was subsequently managed balloon re-inflation for 10 minutes across the rupture site (B). Final angiogram showing the sealing of the ruptures site, maintaining the patency of external iliac artery (C).

The most serious complications include arterial rupture and distal plaque embolization.

Arterial Rupture

- It is the most serious complications and is seen <1% cases. If the rupture occurs in the periphery (infrainguinal), it is usually self-limiting and bleeding is controlled by local tamponade effect of the surrounding soft tissues. However, if the arterial rupture occurs above the inguinal ligament, it may be fatal because there is no tamponade effect by the surrounding area. If the patient complaints of severe pain, which continues even after balloon deflation and is accompanied by hypotension and tachycardia, one should suspect vascular rupture.
- Vascular ruptures below the inguinal ligament are usually self-limiting and require no specific treatment except for manual compression. Whereas arterial rupture above inguinal ligament needs immediate attention. Instant balloon re-inflation at the site of rupture to stop bleeding, followed by either placement of stent-graft across the rupture or shift the patient to operation theater for surgical repair **(Figs. 18A to C)**.

Distal Plaque Embolization

- Distal plaque embolization is another serious complication, which may lead to acute limb ischemia, tissue necrosis and amputation of limb. Certain amount of distal embolization occurs in most of the angioplasty procedures, however the volume of plaque embolization is high in iliac angioplasty.
- There is no specific treatment for this complication. Proper technique and careful patient selection are critical to circumvent this complication.

Stent-related Complications

- Stent migration during placement
- Stent fracture

Restenosis

Restenosis may occur following angioplasty alone or may occur within stents (in-stent restenosis). This restenosis may be due to disease progression or due to neo intimal hyperplasia. This restenosis is managed either by repeat angioplasty or repeat stenting.

Teaching Points

- Doppler sonography is used as screening modality in suspected peripheral vascular disease.
- CT angiography or MR angiography is needed to define disease extent and planning the treatment.
- Endovascular treatments offer low-risk alternative to surgery in majority of the patients.
- Angioplasty and stenting are the two most widely used treatment options.
- Antegrade access is generally preferable to contralateral access for infrainguinal lesions. Never withdraw the guidewire back across the lesion before the procedure is finished.
- Always check the run-off vessels at the end of the procedure for distal embolization.
- Stents are usually indicated if angioplasty results are unsatisfactory.
- Primary placement of stent is indicated in selected cases such as iliac artery occlusions and ostial renal artery stenoses.
- Proper patient selection and technique are two most important factors, which can prevent most of the complications.

REFERENCES

1. Selvin E, Erlinger TP. Prevalence of and risk factors for peripheral arterial disease in the United States: results from the National Health and Nutrition Examination Survey, 1999-2000. Circulation. 2004;110(6):738-43.
2. Pollak AW, Norton PT, Kramer CM. Multimodality imaging of lower extremity peripheral arterial disease: Current role and future directions. Circ Cardiovasc Imaging. 2012;5(6): 797-807.
3. Lijmer JG, Hunink MG, van den Dungen JJ, et al. ROC analysis of noninvasive tests for peripheral arterial disease. Ultrasound Med Biol. 1996;22(4):391-8.
4. Ota H, Takase K, Rikimaru H, et al. Quantitative vascular measurements in arterial occlusive disease. Radiographics. 2005;25(5):1141-58.
5. 2011 ACCF/AHA Focused Update of the Guideline for the Management of Patients With Peripheral Artery Disease (Updating the 2005 Guideline). J Am Coll Cardiol. 2011;58(19):2020-45.
6. Ubbink DT, Fidler M, Legemate DA. Interobserver variability in aortoiliac and femoropopliteal duplex scanning. J Vasc Surg. 2001;33(3):540-5.
7. Catalano C, Fraioli F, Laghi A, et al. Infrarenal aortic and lower-extremity arterial disease: Diagnostic performance of multi-detector row CT angiography. Radiology. 2004;231(2):555-63.
8. Schernthaner R, Stadler A, Lomoschitz F, et al. Multidetector CT angiography in the assessment of peripheral arterial occlusive disease: accuracy in detecting the severity, number, and length of stenoses. Eur Radiol. 2008;18(4):665-71.
9. Roditi G, Kusumawidjaja D. Magnetic resonance angiography and computed tomography angiography for peripheral arterial disease. Imaging. 2009;21(2):85-108.
10. Ward EV, Galizia MS, Usman A, et al. Comparison of quiescent inflow single-shot and native space for nonenhanced peripheral MR angiography. J Magn Reson Imaging. 2013;38(6):1531-8.
11. Hodnett PA, Koktzoglou I, Davarpanah AH, et al. Evaluation of peripheral arterial disease with nonenhanced quiescent-interval single-shot MR angiography. Radiology. 2011;260(1):282-93.
12. Amin P, Collins JD, Koktzoglou I, et al. Evaluating peripheral arterial disease with unenhanced quiescent-interval single-shot MR angiography at 3 T. Am J Roentgenol. 2014;202(4):886-93.
13. Foley WD, Stonely T. CT angiography of the lower extremities. Radiol Clin North Am. 2010;48(2):367-96, ix.
14. Crawford ES, DeBakey ME. Popliteal artery arteriosclerotic aneurysm. Circulation. 1965;32(4):515-6.
15. Friesen G, Ivins JC, Janes JM. Popliteal aneurysms. Surgery. 1962;51:90-8.
16. Wright LB, Matchett WJ, Cruz CP, et al. Popliteal Artery Disease: diagnosis and treatment. Radiographics. 2004;24(2):467-79.
17. Diwan A, Sarkar R, Stanley JC, et al. Incidence of femoral and popliteal artery aneurysms in patients with abdominal aortic aneurysms. J Vasc Surg. 2000;31(5):863-9.
18. Jaff MR, White CJ, Hiatt WR, et al. An update on methods for revascularization and expansion of the TASC lesion classification to include below-the-knee arteries: A supplement to the inter-society consensus for the management of peripheral arterial disease (TASC II): The TASC Steering Committee. Catheter Cardiovasc Interv Off J Soc Card Angiogr Interv. 2015;86(4): 611-25.
19. Rholl KS, Durham JD, Sacks D, et al. Peripheral vascular interventions. In: Darcy MD, Vedantham S, Kaufman JA (Eds). Society of Cardiovascular and Interventional Radiology. 2nd edition. SCVIR. 2001.p.391.
20. Block PC, Myler RK, Stertzer S, et al. Morphology after transluminal angioplasty in human beings. N Engl J Med. 1981;305(7):382-5.
21. Bhat R, McBride K, Chakraverty S, et al. Primary cutting balloon angioplasty for treatment of venous stenoses in native hemodialysis fistulas: Long-term results from three centers. Cardiovasc Intervent Radiol. 2007;30(6):1166-1170-2.
22. Vascular and Interventional Radiology: The Requisites. Mosby; 2004.p.744.
23. Bolia A. Percutaneous intentional extraluminal (subintimal) recanalization of crural arteries. Eur J Radiol. 1998;28(3): 199-204.
24. Reekers JA, Bolia A. Percutaneous intentional extraluminal (subintimal) recanalization: How to do it yourself. Eur J Radiol. 1998;28(3):192-8.
25. Pentecost MJ, Criqui MH, Dorros G, et al. Guidelines for peripheral percutaneous transluminal angioplasty of the abdominal aorta and lower extremity vessels. A statement for health professionals from a special writing group of the Councils on Cardiovascular Radiology, Arteriosclerosis, Cardiothoracic and Vascular Surgery, Clinical Cardiology, and Epidemiology and Prevention, the American Heart Association. Circulation. 1994;89(1):511-31.

SECTION

6

Musculoskeletal and Breast Imaging

CHAPTER

152

Current Concepts in Cross-sectional Imaging of Musculoskeletal Diseases

Shivanand Gamanagatti, Ankur Goyal, Raju Sharma

INTRODUCTION

Imaging of musculoskeletal diseases has seen a paradigm shift with increased emphasis on cross-sectional modalities including high-resolution ultrasound (HRUS), computed tomography (CT), and magnetic resonance imaging (MRI). HRUS is fast becoming the modality of choice for evaluation of soft tissue structures while CT serves to accurately assess bone pathology. MRI provides excellent contrast resolution of both marrow disorders as well as soft tissue diseases. This chapter provides an insight into the role of ultrasound (US) and CT and focuses on MRI assessment of musculoskeletal diseases.

Cross-sectional imaging of the musculoskeletal system has made immense progress in the last two decades. The pace of innovation has been maximum in MRI and it has become a versatile and virtually indispensable imaging modality for many musculoskeletal applications. Developments such as high-performance magnetic resonance (MR) systems and optimized coil technology have led to improvements in spatial resolution and signal-to-noise and better cost-effectiveness of MR studies.[1] This in turn has led to improved diagnosis in shorter period of time and better understanding of complex orthopedic disorders. This chapter aims to briefly outline the basic principles of musculoskeletal MRI and highlights the recent advances in this exciting and ever-changing specialty.

ULTRASONOGRAPHY

Musculoskeletal US is currently gaining popularity by leaps and bounds. Not only radiologists, but other specialties are also increasingly using US for both diagnostic and therapeutic purposes. US is a multiplanar cross-sectional imaging modality which provides high-resolution information regarding soft tissue structures. Low cost, dynamic evaluation, and unrestricted field-of-view (FOV) work in its favor along with the opportunity to combine with comprehensive clinical examination. There are no contraindications, radiation exposure or risks involved and US can be repeated any number of times. Portability of the US equipment has enabled its use in the operation theaters as well as in the sports field.

Ultrasound probe frequencies ranging from 5 to 18 MHz are optimal for musculoskeletal imaging. US waves travel through different soft tissues at different speeds based on the propagation speed of that tissue. The propagation speed depends not only on the density of the tissue, but also on the number of internal reflective structures, for example, tendon fibers, which absorb or reflect the sound wave energy. The transducer also acts as a receiver for the reflected sound waves. In brief, less dense structures such as fluid that lack tissue interfaces will appear as dark or hypoechoic, whereas more dense structures with multiple interfaces such as tendon will appear brighter or hyperechoic. The tissue interfaces also produce typical features of a tissue, such as the regular parallel lines of a tendon or ligament, which aid in their identification. US is an operator dependent technique; hence it is important for the radiologist to be well trained for performing musculoskeletal studies.

Ultrasound provides excellent spatial contrast for evaluation of tendons, ligaments, and nerves. The ligaments can be seen as fibrillar structures and any tears can be easily seen **(Fig. 1)**. Stress maneuvers can be applied while doing US so as to diagnose nonretracted tears as well. US is used to evaluate a wide spectrum of tendon diseases such as degenerative/traumatic tears of the rotator cuff, ankle tendons, as well as tenosynovitis, tendinosis, and masses **(Figs. 2 and 3)**. Nerves can be easily scanned throughout their course and comparison with the contralateral side can also be done in equivocal cases **(Figs. 4A and B)**. Panoramic view (extended FOV) function helps to demonstrate longitudinal structures (which are longer than the probe length) by moving the probe along the same. Joint effusions, synovial thickening, and bony erosions are also easily discernible and Doppler signal aids in assessment of active synovitis **(Figs. 5A to D)**. US has become a valuable tool in diagnosis and follow-up of patients with inflammatory arthritis to demonstrate early inflammatory changes such as synovitis, tenosynovitis, enthesitis, and also helps in identification of early bone erosions with added advantage of color Doppler to visualize the vascularity. Tumor and tumor-like masses (including vascular malformations) can also be comprehensively evaluated using US and Doppler. US permits real time imaging, which allows for provocative maneuvers to detect entities which are not well shown on static imaging such as elbow flexion maneuver to elicit ulnar nerve subluxation at cubital tunnel, hip flexion to elicit snapping of iliopsoas tendon, and real-time muscle contraction in diagnosis of myofascial herniation.

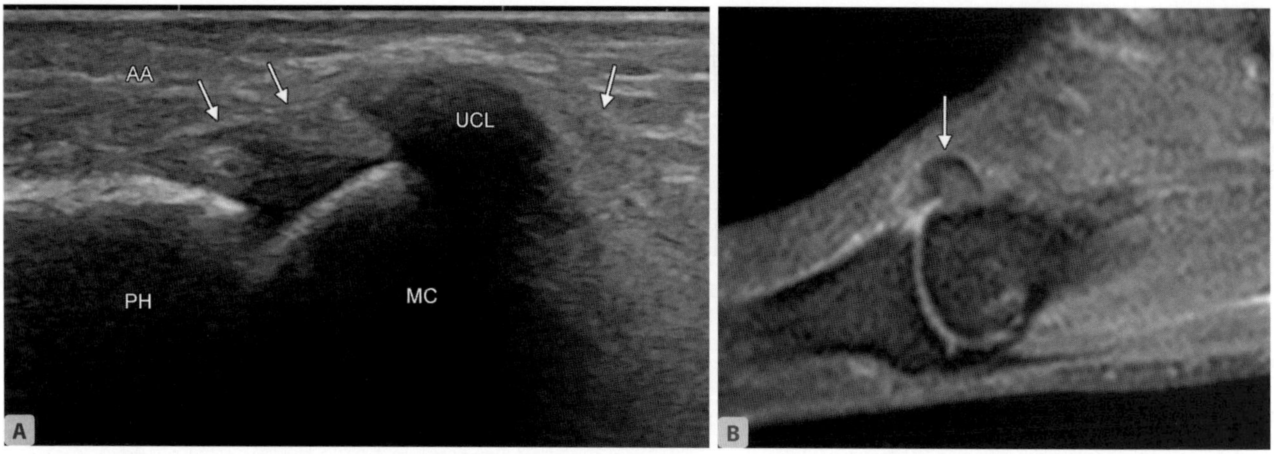

FIGS. 1A AND B: (A) Ultrasound image along the ulnar collateral ligament (UCL) of the thumb shows retracted ligament with adductor aponeurosis (AA) interposed between the ligament and its distal insertion, suggesting Stener lesion; (B) Coronal proton density (PD) fat suppression magnetic resonance image shows the same findings (arrow shows retracted UCL in B). (MC: metacarpal; PH: phalanx).

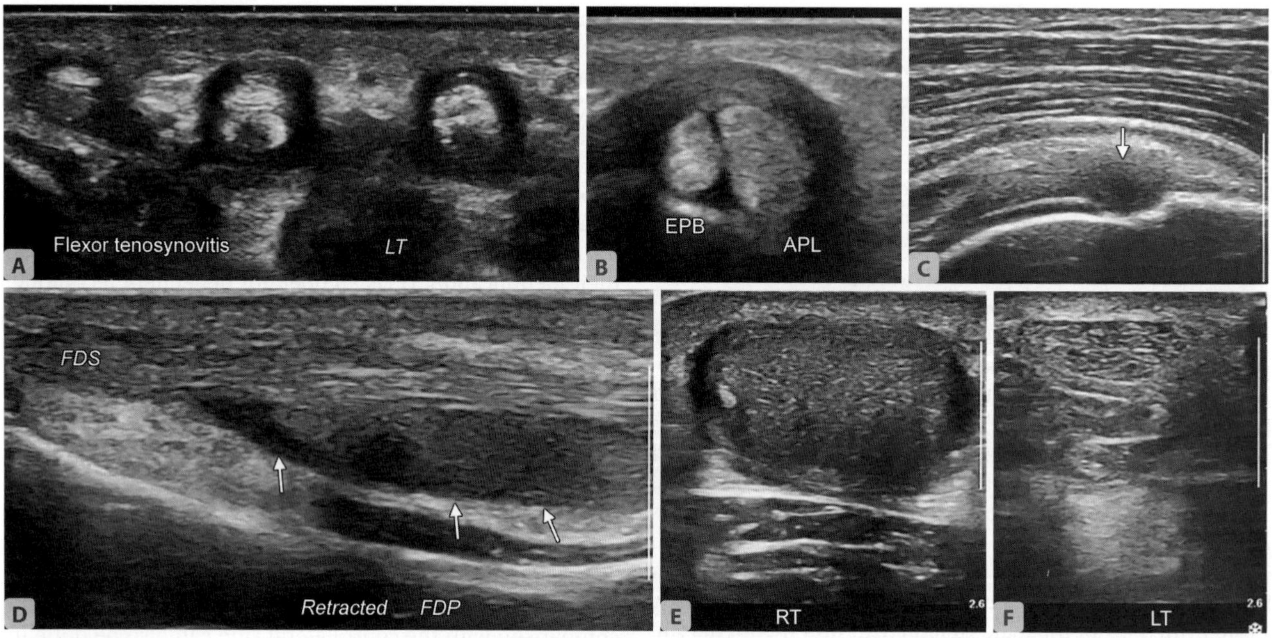

FIGS. 2A TO F: Ultrasound spectrum of tendon disorders. (A) Axial ultrasound image shows presence of hypoechoic tenosynovitis around the flexor tendons of the left hand; (B) Ultrasound image shows de Quervain's tenosynovitis around the first extensor compartment tendons; (C) Ultrasound image in oblique coronal plane along the long axis of supraspinatus shows hypoechogenicity at insertion site (arrow), suggesting tendinosis; (D) Oblique sagittal image shows retracted tendon of flexor digitorum profundus after glass-cut injury of the hand; (E) Axial ultrasound image shows bulky hypoechoic degenerated Achilles tendon in contrast to small echogenic contralateral tendon (F). (APL: abductor pollicis longus; EPB: extensor pollicis brevis; FDP: flexor digitorum profundus; FDS: flexor digitorum superficialis; LT: left; RT: right)

Ultrasound elastography may serve to distinguish benign from malignant soft tissue masses. Also, elastography may detect tendon degeneration before it becomes apparent on gray-scale US. *Contrast-enhanced US (CEUS)* employing gas microbubbles is another addition to US armamentarium, which enables accurate detection of solid viable components in a soft tissue mass. This contrast media is exhaled via lungs and thus can be safely used even in the presence of renal dysfunction. CEUS provides real-time dynamic assessment of perfusion and thus aids in distinguishing high-flow and low-flow lesions. Contrast-enhancement may also serve to assess disease activity in synovial inflammation.

Ultrasound is widely used to guide musculoskeletal interventional procedures such as joint fluid aspiration, drainage of fluid collections, tissue biopsy, injection of tendon sheaths, joints, bursae, and peritendinous soft tissues (e.g., common extensor tendon at lateral epicondyle for tennis elbow) **(Figs. 5A to D)**. Also, US provides a viable imaging method in the presence of metallic prosthesis, to evaluate periprosthetic collections, hematoma, and ligaments, since prosthesis produce artifacts on MRI.

It may be noted however, that US may not be a standalone modality and correlation with radiographs or other cross-sectional modalities may be required to clinch the diagnosis.

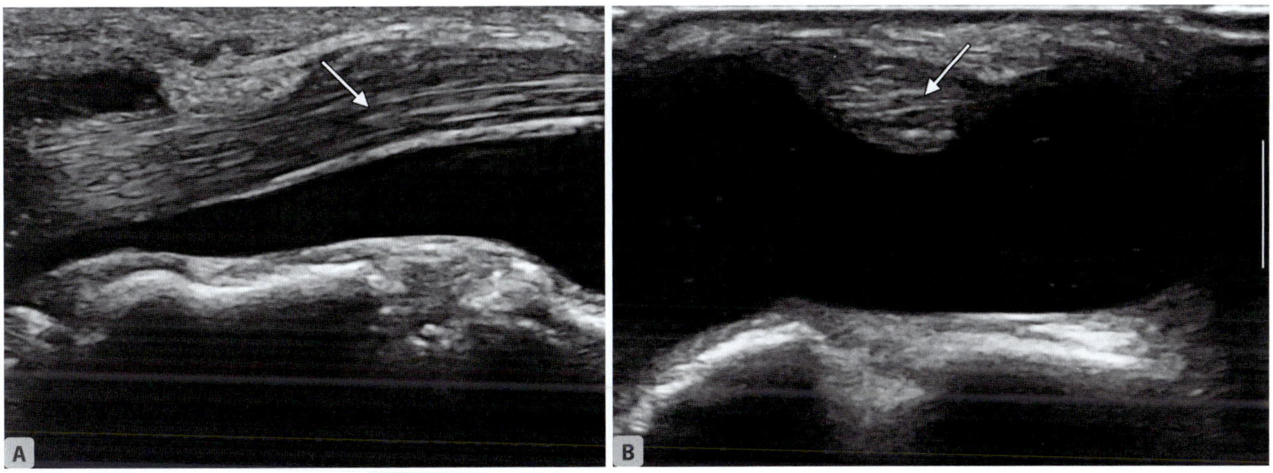

FIGS. 3A AND B: Longitudinal and transverse ultrasound images of ankle showing large fluid collection along the intact tibialis anterior tendon (arrows) suggestive of tenosynovitis.

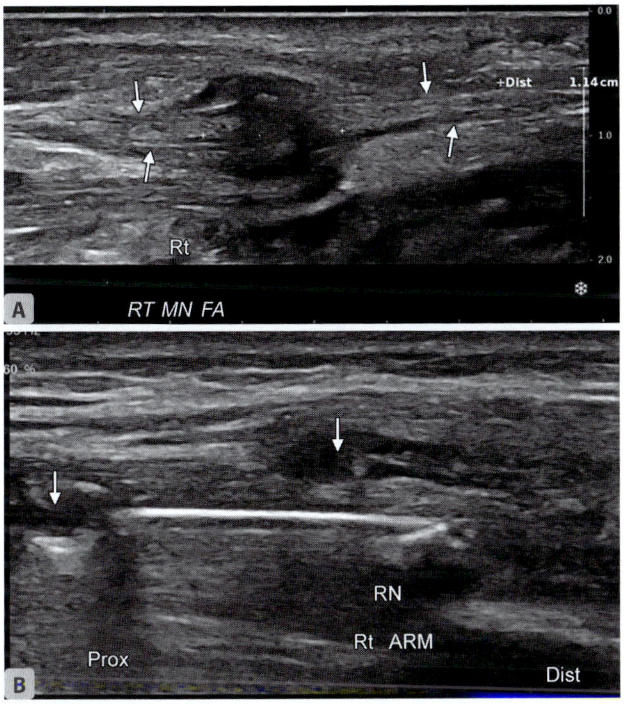

FIGS. 4A AND B: Ultrasound images showing nerve diseases. (A) Long-axis ultrasound image along the median nerve shows complete transection with discontinuity of epineurium and neuroma in continuity; (B) Another patient with radial nerve transection shows separation and retraction of the nerve ends, forming neuromas (arrows).

COMPUTED TOMOGRAPHY

Computed tomography is the investigation of choice for evaluation of bony structures. With the introduction of MRI, role of CT in musculoskeletal imaging has somewhat declined, particularly for soft tissue imaging. Nonetheless, CT has certain inherent advantages that make it a robust tool for some musculoskeletal pathology. CT is most commonly used to evaluate bone trauma, for acute fractures of spine, to detect subtle fractures when the radiograph is normal, fractures of complex anatomical areas such as pelvis, maxillofacial area, and scapula, evaluation of intra-articular fractures, to plan operative reduction of complex fractures, and to diagnose osseous nonunion of fractures. In trauma setting, CT is the workhorse, serving as the gold standard to diagnose complex and multiple fractures. Many classification systems of traumatic fractures are also based on CT and help in deciding the management. CT has obviated the need of taking radiographs at different angulations and projections in sick patients. CT is also used to evaluate various measurements such as after joint replacement, angle of femoral neck anteversion prior to rotation osteotomy, tibial tuberosity-trochlear groove (TT-TG) distance in case of recurrent patellar dislocation, and measurements in evaluation of scoliosis and femoroacetabular impingement. More recently, dual-energy CT has become available and has the capability to provide added information regarding tissue composition, artifact reduction, and image optimization. These advantages of dual-energy CT are used to evaluate crystal deposition disorders like gout, orthopedic implant imaging by reducing metal artifacts (high kV images), trabecular acute bone marrow edema through the use of material decomposition protocol, i.e., virtual noncalcium (VNCa) application **(Figs. 6A to C)**.

Computed tomography is very sensitive for identification of calcium especially to detect matrix mineralization in osseous tumors, chondroid tumors **(Figs. 7A to D)** and to detect calcified nidus in osteoid osteoma **(Figs. 8A to C)**. The other niche indications of CT include suspected partial/stress fractures, bony avulsion fractures, osteoid osteoma, hemangioma, etc. Other applications include, contrast-enhanced CT for evaluation of soft tissue abscess, CT arthrography to evaluate various intra-articular pathology, and CT angiography for vascular encasement **(Figs. 9A and B)** whenever MR is contraindicated or MRI is unavailable or when osteochondral disease is to be evaluated. Low-dose CT is now emerging as a new promising tool to detect early sacroiliitis.

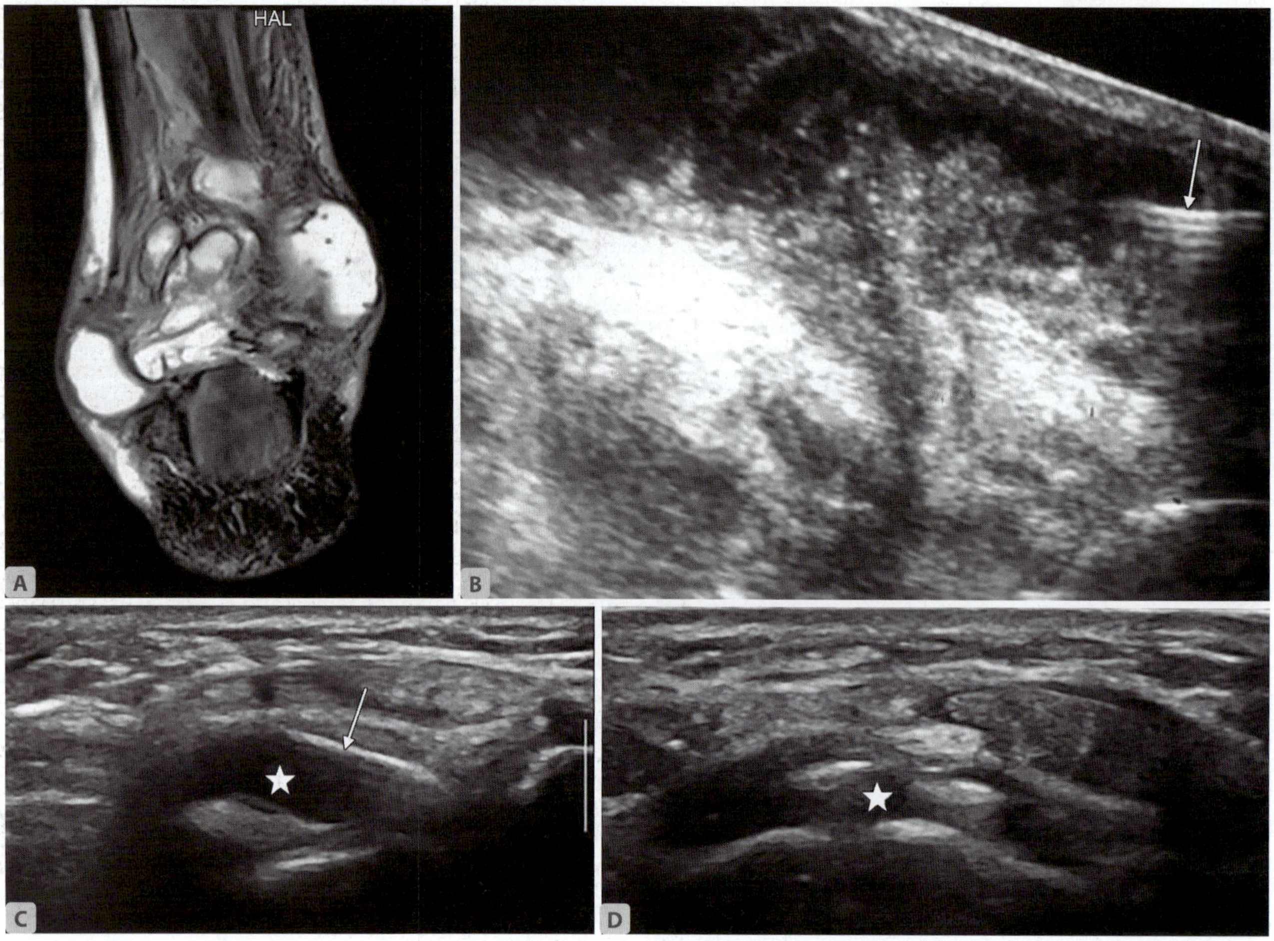

FIGS. 5A TO D: Ultrasound-guided interventions. (A) Coronal short tau inversion recovery (STIR) image shows multiple collections in the ankle joint; (B) Ultrasound image shows severe synovial thickening with effusion with aspiration needle in situ (arrow); (C) Ultrasound image in a different patient of dorsal wrist ganglion (star) shows needle in situ (arrow) for fenestration of the wall; (D) Development of echogenicity within the ganglion cyst (star) after steroid injection.

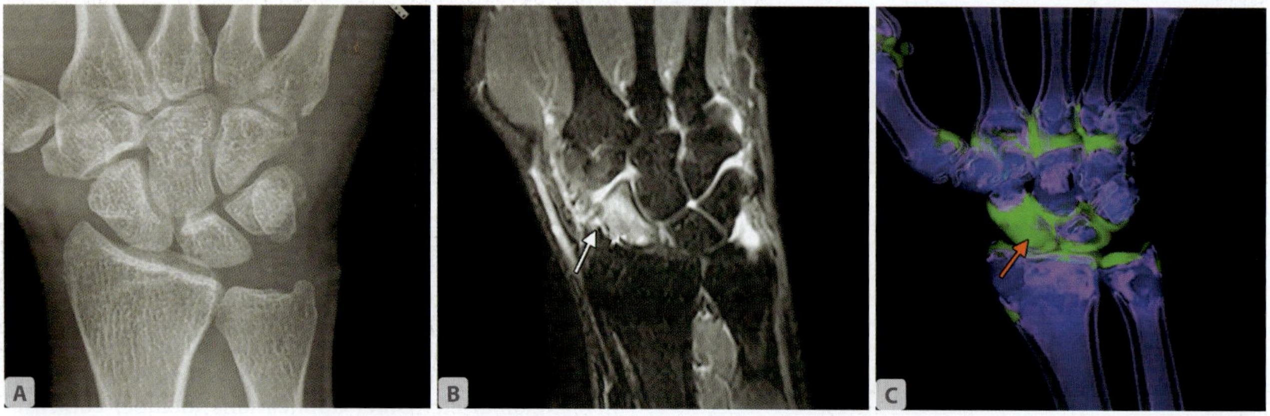

FIGS. 6A TO C: Posteroanterior (PA) radiograph of wrist (A), coronal short tau inversion recovery (STIR) magnetic resonance image (B), and coronal virtual noncalcium (VNCa) image (C) generated from the dual-energy acquisition, show no obvious abnormality on radiograph (A), nonspecific marrow edema involving scaphoid bone (arrow) without any fracture line in magnetic resonance imagining (B) and trabecular acute bone marrow edema (green color) (red arrow) through the use of material decomposition protocol (VNCa).

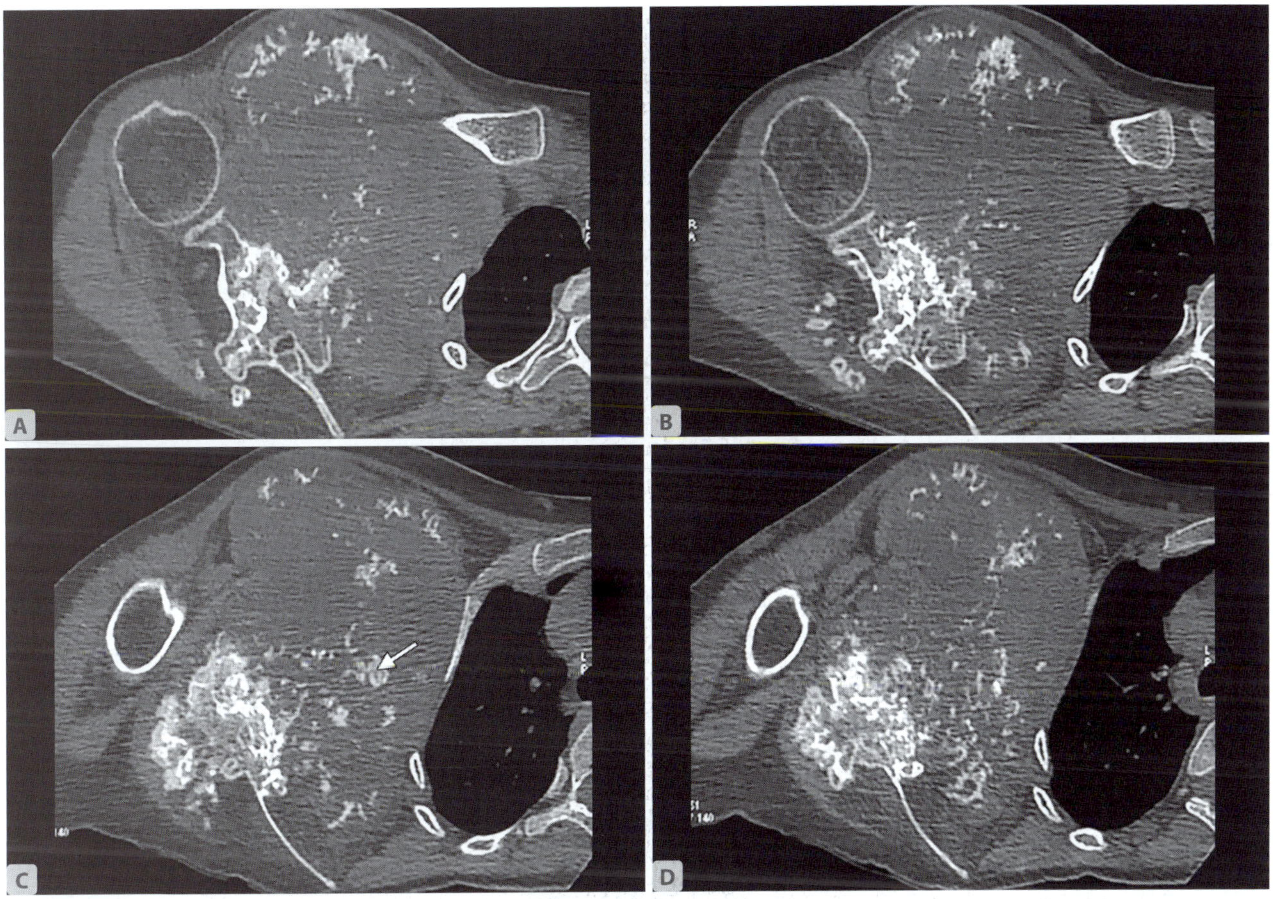

FIGS. 7A TO D: Axial CT images of right shoulder showing large destructive lesion involving body of right scapula associated with large soft tissue component having chondroid type of calcification (arrow) suggestive of chondrosarcoma arising from exostosis.

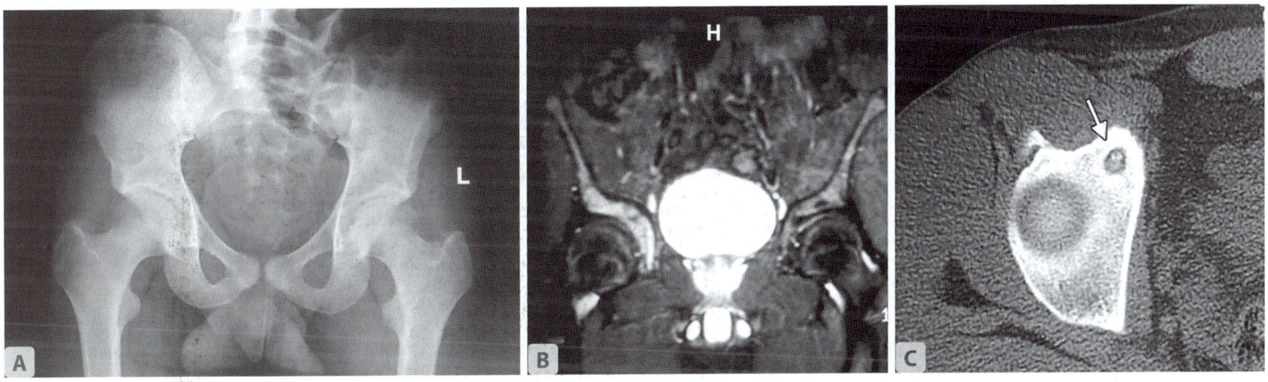

FIGS. 8A TO C: Anteroposterior (AP) radiograph of pelvis (A), coronal short tau inversion recovery (STIR) magnetic resonance image (B) and axial computed tomography section of acetabulum show no obvious abnormality on radiograph (A), nonspecific marrow edema involving acetabulum and right iliac blade (B) and partially calcified nidus within anterior column of acetabulum (arrow) on computed tomography (C).

MAGNETIC RESONANCE IMAGING

Magnetic resonance imaging is currently considered the gold standard imaging investigation for the evaluation of bone marrow and soft tissue structures.

Hardware Issues

The basic prerequisites for optimized MRI of the musculoskeletal system are high spatial and contrast resolution and high sensitivity for the visualization of free water. The high-field systems (3 Tesla) are now widely available and provide very high-quality images of the musculoskeletal system. Faster gradients, improvements in surface coil design, and development of new and faster sequences have all contributed to the fact that MRI has become the modality of choice for evaluation of the musculoskeletal system.[1,2] The use of parallel imaging and motion reduction techniques like periodically rotated overlapping parallel lines with enhanced

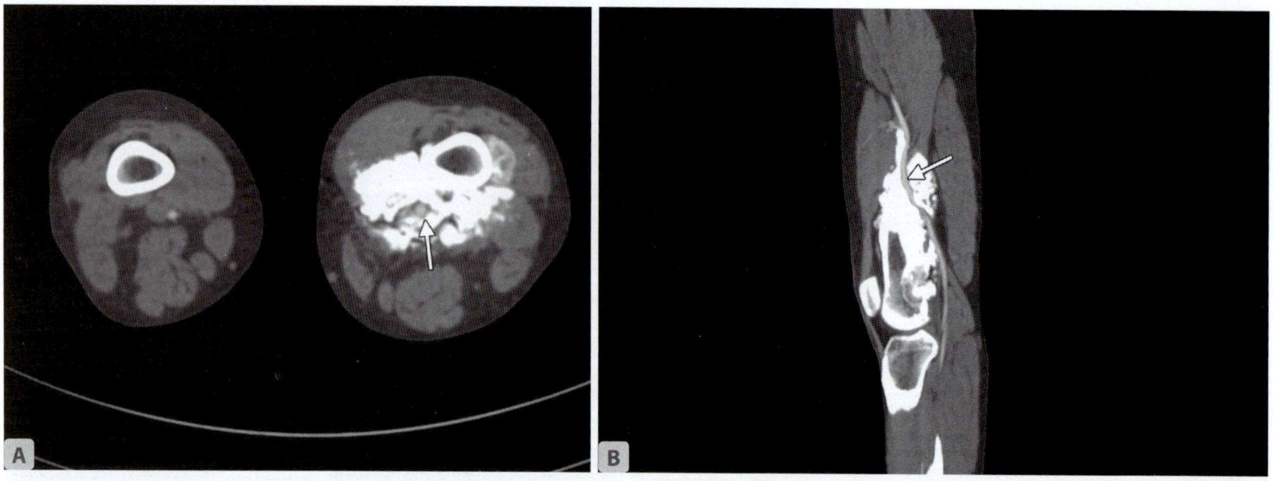

FIGS. 9A AND B: Axial and sagittal CT angiography images showing juxtacortical ossified lesion arising from posterior cortex of left femur which is encasing the superficial femoral artery (arrows).

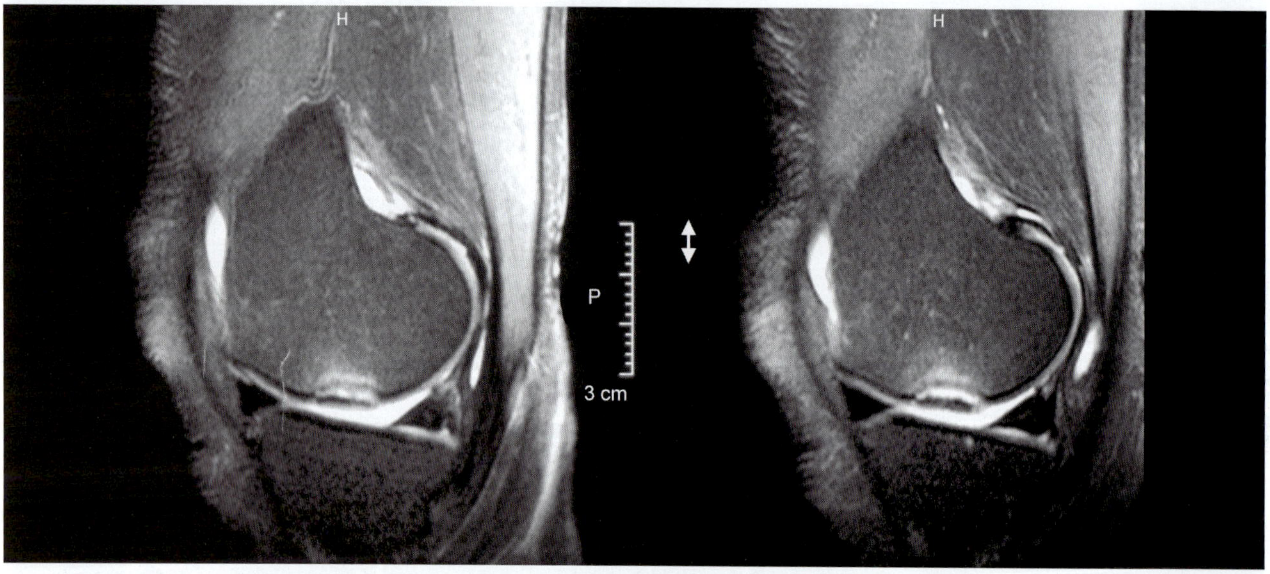

FIG. 10: Sagittal fat suppressed T2-weighted (T2W) image acquired on a 3 Tesla scanner shows a small detached ossific fragment in the articular surface of medial femoral condyle with fluid signal intensity between the fragment and the underlying bone, suggesting osteochondritis dissecans. The image has a high signal-to-noise ratio with excellent delineation of anatomy.

reconstruction (PROPELLER) and BLADE have further enhanced the image quality of MR images.[2] Scanners are now available which allow imaging in the weight bearing, upright position, and also in flexion and extension (kinematic MRI). This allows evaluation of dynamic postural and functional changes in degenerated discs,[3] as well as dynamic evaluation of joints. Upright and kinematic MRI may detect minor neural foraminal compromise related to posture. However, these scanners are open configuration with low magnetic field strength, which may compromise resolution and are therefore suitable for few niche indications.

Choosing the appropriate coil is important to obtain high-quality images. The smallest coil possible, that allows the required anatomical coverage, should be used to get the maximum signal. Surface coils that can be placed on or close to the region of interest should be used. Most new coils are made with a phased array design. These are made of several smaller coils placed in a series and provide the combined advantage of high-resolution images and a wide FOV. 16-channel coils are now available for musculoskeletal applications.

3T Imaging

The 3T imaging has many advantages in the musculoskeletal system. Imaging at higher field strengths gives better signal-to-noise ratio (SNR), resulting in higher resolution images and shorter scan times. The SNR at 3T is about twice that at 1.5T and 3T scanners are being widely used for musculoskeletal imaging **(Fig. 10)**. Research studies are being conducted at 7T systems also. Not only SNR but also spatial resolution and the contrast to noise ratio can be enhanced on 3T scanners.

The collective benefit gives rise to better delineation of the small intrinsic structures of joints. Many studies have documented higher accuracy and greater degree of confidence using 3T imaging, in the diagnosis of meniscal tears, defects in articular cartilage, triangular fibrocartilage pathology, etc. However, 3T imaging is unlikely to replace the need for MR arthrography in lesions like labral tears.[2,4]

The sequences and protocols need to be modified for optimum imaging at 3T. Improved sequence design and widespread use of parallel imaging are likely to improve the image quality at 3T even further.

Sequences

Many different options are available to image the musculoskeletal system. The aim is to get all the diagnostic information necessary in as short a time as possible. This can only be done by adopting a judicious protocol for which it is important to know the merits and demerits of the different types of sequences. It is a good practice to have a standard protocol tailored to a specific clinical indication for a given MR scanner. T1-weighted (T1W) sequence is good for delineation of anatomy and marrow pathology, proton density sequence for meniscal tears, articular cartilage **(Fig. 11)**, and ligament pathology and T2-weighted (T2W) sequence for detecting soft tissue component of tumors **(Figs. 12A and B)**, edema, etc. For most musculoskeletal applications, proton density and T2W sequences are coupled with fat suppression (FS).

Fast Spin-echo Sequences

This group of sequences allows for much more rapid acquisition of images than the conventional spin-echo (SE) method. This is done by acquiring several samples in the time in which one sample is obtained in the conventional SE technique. The time saved is directly proportional to the number of samples also known as the echo train length.[1] This decreases overall imaging time thereby decreasing the motion artifacts and increasing the throughput. Alternatively, the time saved can be used for obtaining additional signal averages and increasing the matrix size to improve the signal and resolution, respectively.

However, the fast spin-echo (FSE) technique has some disadvantages. Firstly the signal intensity of fat remains quite bright on these T2W images. As a result, pathology in subcutaneous fat or marrow may be obscured, due to the similarity in the signal intensity of fat and fluid. This problem can be resolved by combining this technique with fat saturation **(Figs. 12A and B)**, which is now routinely employed.[1,2] Secondly the FSE technique can result in blurring along tissue margins when long echo train lengths

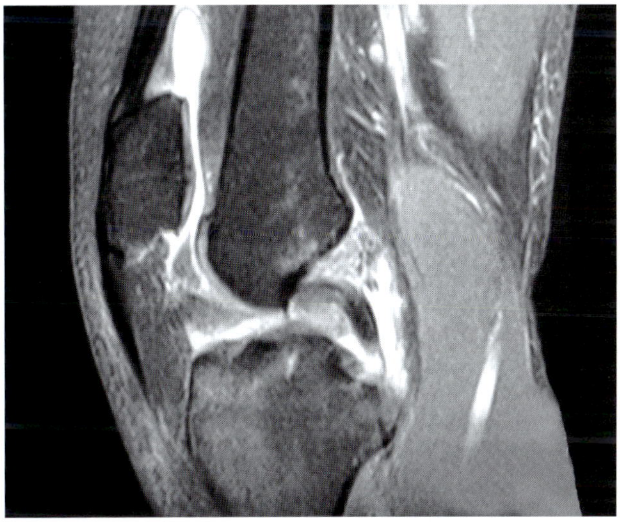

FIG. 11: Sagittal fat suppression proton density (PD) image shows good delineation of hyaline articular cartilage (gray signal intensity along posterior aspect of patella) and cruciate ligaments in the knee. Anterior cruciate ligament is disrupted with no normal fibers identified, and there is buckling of posterior cruciate ligament (PCL), suggesting complete anterior cruciate ligament (ACL) tear.

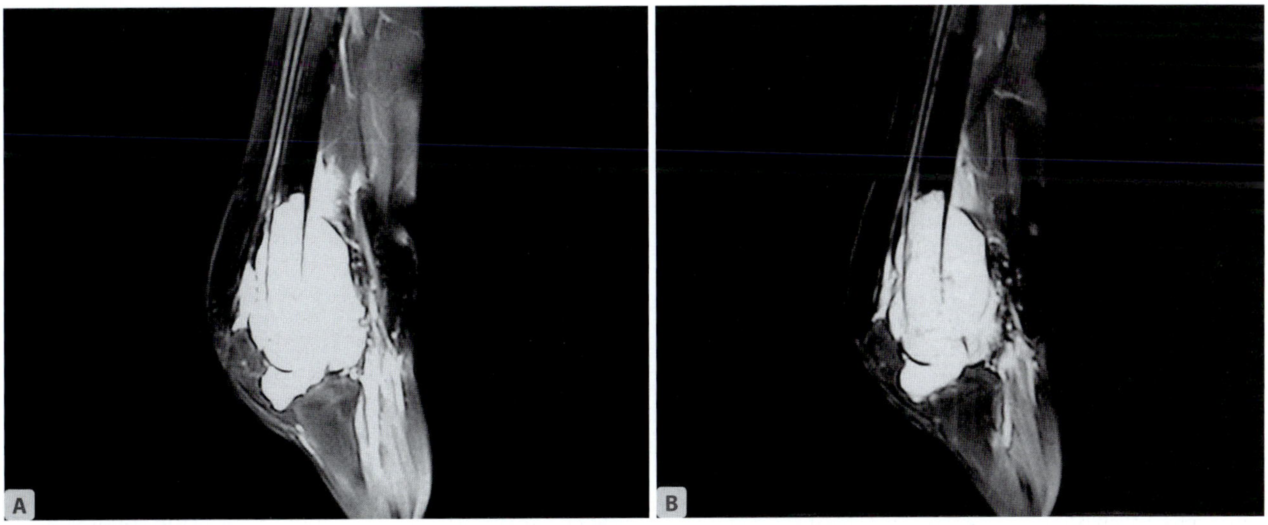

FIGS. 12A AND B: Sagittal fat suppression T2-weighted image of the knee gives excellent depiction of the extraosseous and intraosseous extent of the tumor in a case of osteosarcoma of the distal femoral end. Also note the intra-articular extension of the tumor.

are used. This may result in missing subtle pathology such as meniscal tears in the knee.

Gradient-recalled Echo Sequences

These sequences were originally developed to produce T2W images in less time than was possible with conventional SE techniques. They can be performed either with a two-dimensional (2D) or three-dimensional (3D) volume technique. In 3D imaging, the signal from an entire volume of tissue is obtained at one time and this data can be partitioned into extremely thin slices such that the voxel dimensions are nearly isotropic.[2] This allows for high-resolution imaging and is especially useful when evaluating extremely small structures such as ligaments in the wrist. These 3D sequences also provide the ability to create reformatted images in virtually any plane. Ligaments and articular cartilage are particularly well demonstrated with these sequences. Dual-echo steady state (DESS) is a 3D steady state gradient-recalled echo (GRE) sequence with a good SNR and strong T2 contrast. It is useful for the differentiation of synovial fluid and cartilaginous structures. Multiecho data image combination (MEDIC) is a multiecho GRE sequence that provides good T2W images and has been found useful in joint imaging **(Fig. 13)**.

Gradient-recalled echo sequences are extremely sensitive to susceptibility effects. This is advantageous when searching for subtle areas of hemorrhage, detecting loose bodies and soft tissue gas. Conversely drawbacks of this effect include overestimating the size of osteophytes in spine imaging and gross artifacts when imaging patients with metallic hardware.

Fat Suppressed Sequences

Detection of a pathological process is often hindered by the presence of strong signal from neighboring adipose tissue. In such cases, suppression of the fat signal offers improved conspicuity and sensitivity.[1] FS is commonly employed with FSE T2W sequences on which fat is very bright. It is also frequently coupled with gadolinium enhanced images where the hyperintense signal from enhancing abnormalities may be masked by hyperintense fat. Fat saturated T1W images are also used with gadolinium arthrography. Diffusion-weighted imaging (DWI) also employs FS.

Two main techniques used to accomplish FS are frequency selective (chemical fat saturation) and short tau inversion recovery (STIR) imaging. A problem with the frequency selective fat saturation is the potential for inhomogeneous suppression of fat signal. It relies on adequate separation of fat and water peaks, which occurs only at high-field strength (greater than 1 T), and hence it is not available on low-field scanners.[1] The STIR technique relies on the relaxation properties of fat protons rather than their resonant frequency. It produces more homogeneous FS, because it is not as sensitive to field inhomogeneity as the frequency selective technique **(Fig. 14)**. However, STIR sequence should not be used with intravenous or intra-articular gadolinium because the contrast agent has similar relaxation properties to fat protons and therefore its signal intensity may be saturated along with fat on the STIR images.

A third method of FS is the Dixon technique or fat-water separation technique. This is also based on the difference in the precessional frequency of protons in fat and water. However, unlike chemical fat sat it uses a spectrally nonselective radiofrequency (RF) pulse, with echo times (TEs) that capture the phase difference between fat and water protons. When fat and water are in-phase, the signal is maximal and when they are out-of-phase there is destructive interference between fat and water magnetization vectors. At 1.5 T, the TE for the in-phase image is 4.6 ms or a multiple of 4.6 and the TE for the opposed-phase image is 2.3 ms or a multiple of 2.3. The fat and water in-phase and out-phase images can be added or subtracted to produce water only or fat only images. This two-point Dixon technique is sensitive to

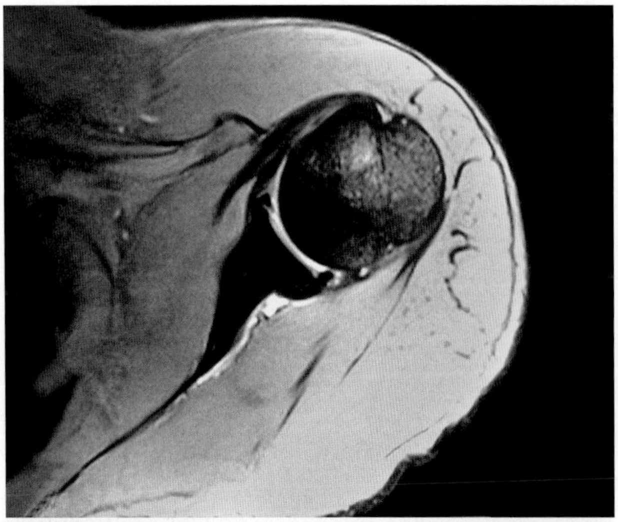

FIG. 13: Axial fat suppression gradient-echo image [multiecho data image combination (MEDIC)] of the shoulder. Anterior and posterior glenoid labrums are well seen as hypointense triangular structures.

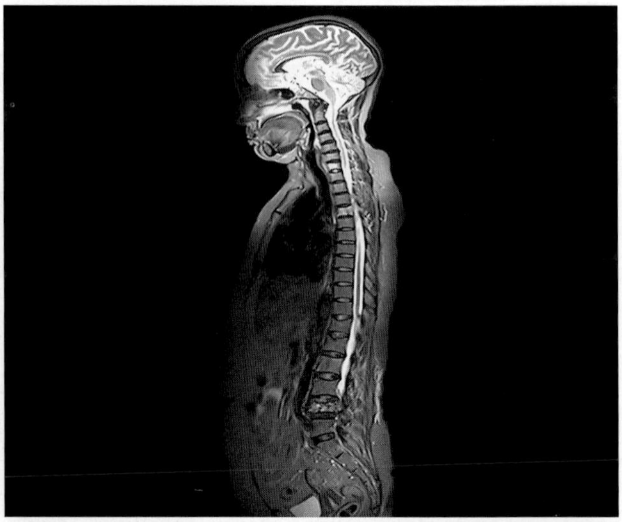

FIG. 14: Sagittal short tau inversion recovery (STIR) image of the whole spine shows hyperintensity and decreased vertebral height involving multiple vertebrae, suggesting multiple metastases in a known case of malignancy. There is homogeneous suppression of fat.

magnetic field inhomogeneity and to overcome this, a three-point Dixon method has been developed where one in-phase and two opposed-phase images (one at 2.3 ms shorter and another sequence with TE 2.3 longer than the nominal TE) are acquired. The three images are analyzed and a phase map is generated from which fat only, water only, and combined images can be created. This technique is called iterative decomposition of fat and water with echo asymmetric and least-square estimation (IDEAL). The Dixon technique can be applied to regions of complex anatomy and can be used with SE, FSE, as well as GRE sequences. Its disadvantages include sensitivity to magnetic field inhomogeneity and potential blurring with FSE sequences.[2]

Role of Contrast

Gadolinium-diethylenetriaminepentaacetic acid (Gd-DTPA) is a paramagnetic compound and is a T1 contrast agent. For musculoskeletal applications it can be administered by the intravenous and intra-articular route. Its major application in musculoskeletal MRI is in the setting of infections **(Fig. 15)**, where it can help to distinguish cellulitis from abscess. It is used in evaluating bone and soft tissue tumors to differentiate cystic from solid lesions for perfusion studies and for directing biopsy to the enhancing viable tumor rather than nonenhancing necrotic component.[1] Time-resolved MR angiography enables rapid acquisition at multiple time points so that scrolling the maximal intensity projection slabs provides images similar to digital subtraction angiography (DSA). This is especially useful in the evaluation of vascular tumors and malformations. Gadolinium is also useful in imaging postoperative spine to differentiate scar tissue from nonenhancing disc material.[2] MR arthrography is useful for the diagnosis of subtle pathology like labral tears.

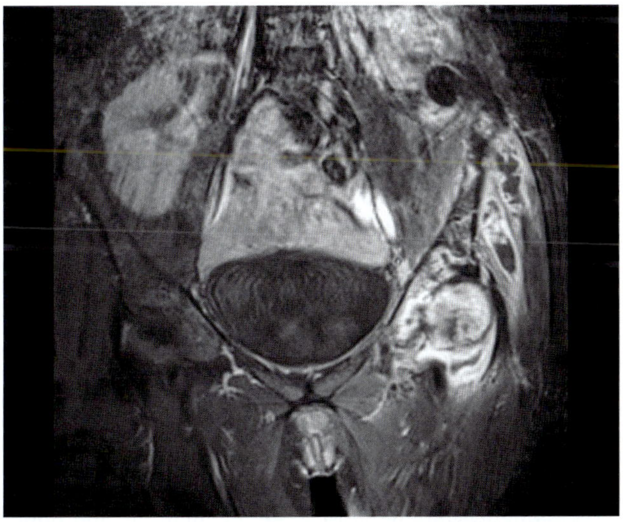

FIG. 15: Utility of contrast administration. Coronal fat suppression postgadolinium T1-weighted image shows abnormal synovial enhancement in a case of tuberculosis (TB) of left hip with multiple rim-enhancing abscesses within the joint cavity and in the surrounding soft tissues.

Reduction of Metallic Artifact from Orthopedic Hardware

Patients with metallic implants and orthopedic hardware frequently need to be imaged. Although they are mostly MR compatible, they can give rise to significant artifact and image distortion. Radiologists should be aware of the steps that can be taken to reduce these artifacts. If there is any doubt of the MR compatibility of the prosthesis, an alternative imaging modality like US should be used.

The degree of metal artifact is related to field strength and imaging at lower field magnets will decrease the metallic artifact. The long axis of the prosthesis should be positioned parallel to the external magnetic field (B0) to minimize artifacts. Other steps that can be taken to reduce in-plane metal artifacts are aligning the frequency encoding direction along the long axis of the implant, increasing the receiver bandwidth, increasing matrix size, and reducing the FOV. FSE sequences with long echo train length are least susceptible to metal artifacts and should be preferred over gradient-echo sequences.[2] STIR and Dixon-based FS work better than chemical-shift in reducing artifacts. Metal artifact reduction sequences (MARS) refer to SE sequences with high bandwidths, increased echo-train length, increased matrix, and decreased echo spacing. MARS may refer to a proprietary sequence but may be better used to refer to an optimized protocol to reduce in-plane distortions. A typical MARS protocol includes STIR coronal, T1 and T2 spin-echo axial and proton-density coronal images. WARP is a proprietary sequence which includes multidirectional view-angle tilting (VAT) to further optimize MARS.

Artifacts due to metal in the adjacent plane (through-plane artifacts) can be reduced by using special multispectral sequences like multiacquisition variable-resonance image combination (MAVRIC) or slice encoding for metal artifact correction (SEMAC). The former uses multiple overlapping acquisitions at different frequencies while the latter uses an additional slice-encoding gradient to FSE. MAVRIC uses multiple frequency-selective excitations, multidirectional VAT, computational postprocessing, and reduces in-plane artifacts as well. Sterile fluid collections are a common complication of metallic prosthesis, especially with metal-on-metal implants **(Figs. 16A to D)**.

Normal Appearance of Musculoskeletal Tissues

It is useful to know the normal appearance of various tissues on different MR sequences and the optimal sequence for each, as this can be applied to any anatomical region. Cortical bone is dark on all sequences whereas the medullary cavity shows a variable signal depending on whether the marrow is hematopoietic or fatty. The distribution of red and yellow marrow changes with age. STIR, fat suppressed FSE T2, and T1W sequences are ideal for imaging marrow pathology, whereas GRE sequences are not useful for bony evaluation. MRI is very sensitive to evaluation of occult osseous trauma **(Figs. 17A and B)** when radiographs are normal and for early diagnosis of marrow infiltrative disorders and for this purpose STIR sequence is the most sensitive.[2]

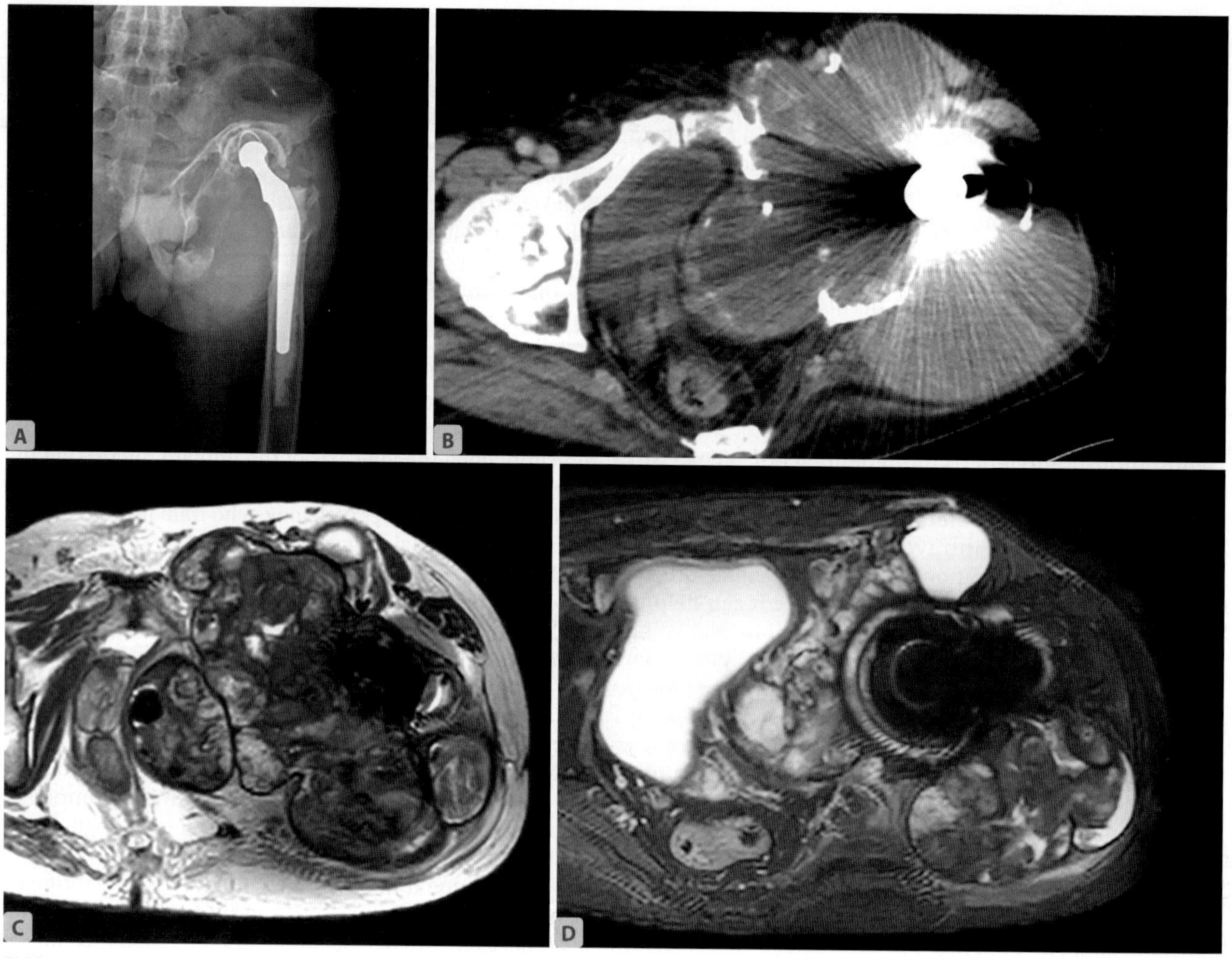

FIGS. 16A TO D: Anteroposterior (AP) radiograph of left hip (A), axial CT section (B), axial T1-weighted (T1W) and T2-weighted (T2W) fat-saturated magnetic resonance images (C and D) of left hip replacement showing lytic destructive lesion involving left ischium, acetabulum, and medial cortex of left femur (A) associated with large soft tissue component (B), which is showing hypointense signal intensity on both T1W and T2W magnetic resonance images suggestive of metallosis.

Articular cartilage is dark gray on STIR and FSE T2W sequences, and is bright on GRE sequences. Fibrocartilage like the menisci and glenoid labrum are dark on all sequences. Meniscal tears are best demonstrated on short TE sequences like T1 and proton density images.

Tendons are generally dark on all pulse sequences. Useful sequences are GRE T2*, T1, and FSE T2. Tendons are usually best imaged in the axial plane. Tears and tendonitis are seen as hyperintense areas but it is important to know some pitfalls for this finding. Tendons may show slightly increased signal intensity close to the site of osseous insertion. This is due to nontendinous fatty material getting interposed between tendon fibers. Another important cause is the magic angle phenomenon, which can give rise to a hyperintense signal in the tendons that are oriented at 55° to the main magnetic field B0. However, this bright signal is seen only on the short TE images (T1W and proton density) and not on T2W images.[1] Common sites where this artifactual hyperintensity may be seen are the posterior tibial tendon in the ankle, rotator cuff in the shoulder, and posterior cruciate ligament in the knee. Changing the position for instance imaging the ankle in 20° plantar flexion can help to overcome this artifact by changing the angle of the tendon with respect to the main magnetic field vector. In addition to hyperintense signal within the tendon, attention should also be paid to any thickening or fluid around the tendon as is seen in tenosynovitis.

Normal synovium is not usually visualized unless it is pathologically thickened. Postgadolinium T1W fat saturated images are useful for delineation of thickened synovium. It may be difficult to distinguish hypertrophied synovium from synovial fluid on T2W and STIR images. Hypertrophied synovium is commonly seen in tubercular and rheumatoid arthritis (RA).

Muscle is of intermediate signal intensity on all sequences. T1W sequences are good to show the anatomy and detect subacute hemorrhage and fatty atrophy. T2W or STIR sequences are sensitive for the diagnosis of muscle strain, myositis, and intramuscular tumors. These sequences are sensitive but unfortunately nonspecific for muscle pathology.

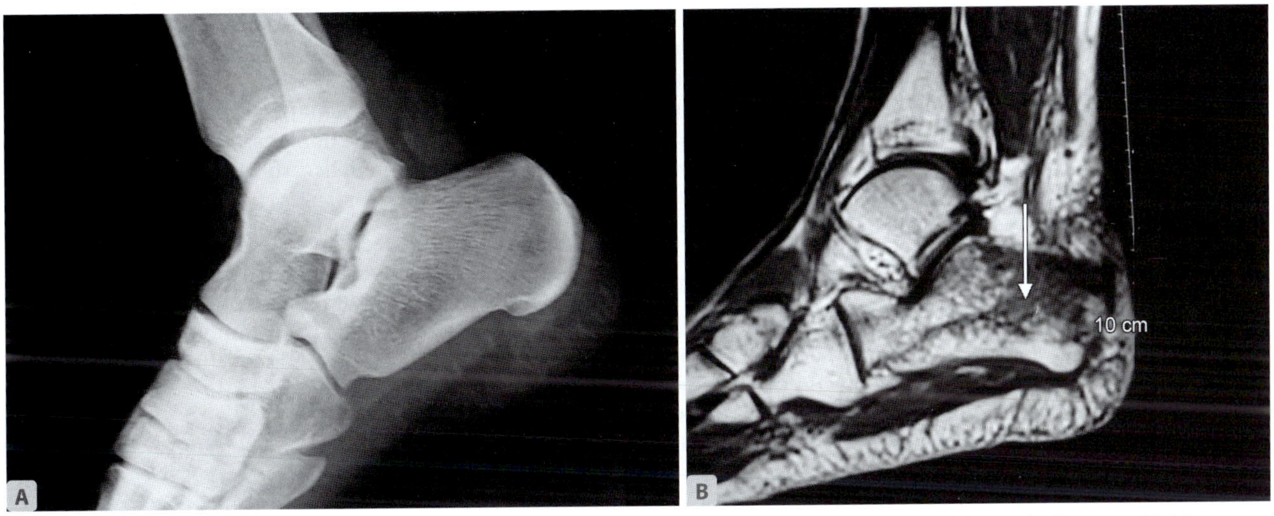

FIGS. 17A AND B: Lateral radiograph (A) and sagittal T1-weighted magnetic resonance image (B) of young adult, who had history of fall from height, showing normal appearing calcaneum without any obvious fracture on radiograph (A) and hypointense fracture line involving calcaneum (B) (arrow) suggesting occult fracture.

Imaging of Articular Cartilage

Articular cartilage imaging has become increasingly important in the setting of aging population where osteoarthritis is a leading cause of chronic disability. Accurate assessment of abnormalities has become essential with advanced surgical and pharmacological treatments proving to be useful in the management of cartilage pathology.

There are two types of cartilage assessment sequences based on their usefulness for morphological or compositional evaluation. To assess the morphology, standard SE and gradient echo sequences, FSE and 3D spin-echo and gradient sequences are available.[5,6] These sequences allow the detection of morphological defects in cartilage and are also used for semiquantitative analysis.

To assess the collagen and proteoglycan content of cartilage matrix, compositional assessment techniques like T2 mapping, delayed gadolinium-enhanced MRI of cartilage (d-GEMRIC), T1ρ (rho) mapping, sodium imaging, and diffusion-weighted techniques are available, but are mostly used at the research level.[2,7]

Morphological Assessment of Cartilage

On SE T1W, proton density **(Fig. 11)** and T2W sequences, articular cartilage is of intermediate signal intensity.[8] With both conventional and advanced MR techniques several investigators have reported a bilaminar, and occasionally, a trilaminar appearance of articular cartilage on MRI. However, the laminar signals may not correspond to the histologic zones. Many MR artifacts like truncation, partial volume, chemical shift, and magic angle can contribute to or obscure the laminated appearance. Routine MR evaluation of a joint includes conventional SE, FSE, and GRE technique.[9] FS methods improve the contrast between the cartilage and fatty marrow. The cartilage appears bright due to an increase in the dynamic range. This technique is easily combined with the routine sequences to provide high contrast images of the cartilage. The use of 3D imaging methods in conjunction with FSE and GRE sequences allows for less than 1 mm slice thickness and greatly improved spatial resolution. 3D spoiled gradient in the steady state (3D SPGR) or 3D fast low-angle shot (FLASH) has been suggested to be one of the most useful techniques for assessment of cartilage lesions. Due to the availability of high-speed gradient MRI systems, interest has recently been renewed in steady-state free precession (SSFP), a rapid GRE imaging technique using a balanced gradient. This is known as balanced turbo field echo (BTFE) or true fast imaging with steady precession (FISP) imaging. SSFP has superior SNR compared with other GRE techniques and has excellent contrast behavior with varying dependence on T1 and T2. Synovial fluid appears bright due to its long T2. The limitation of this sequence is image degradation due to local magnetic field inhomogeneities at a long repetition time (TR). 3D DESS images have been generated by combining images from first and second echoes in a steady state. These images show a high contrast between cartilage and joint fluid.[6,10] Similarly, 3D-water-selective cartilage scan (WATS) (water excitation) shows bright signal in cartilage and fatty bone marrow appears dark, increasing the contrast.

Chondromalacia, osteoarthritic degeneration, osteochondral defects or inflammatory erosions are the common cartilage abnormalities seen on MRI.[8] Cartilage degeneration may be superficial or basal. The MR grading is mainly based on the depth of the abnormality (partial or full-thickness) which is seen as a focal signal alteration. Conventional MR techniques show 52–95% accuracy for lesion detection, which is higher for severe lesions. However, use of FSE 3D SPGR and delayed MR arthrography techniques have increased the sensitivity for early and surface lesions.[10]

Direct (joint injection) or indirect (intravenous injection with delayed imaging) MR arthrography is another cartilage imaging method and is especially useful for detecting superficial lesions. Indirect arthrography with intravenous administration of diluted gadolinium may be performed when direct arthrography is inconvenient or not logistically feasible. It is based on the concept that intravenous contrast over time will diffuse into the joint space, so that semiarthrographic T1W images can be obtained. MR contrast agents do not produce signal themselves but affect the relaxivity of the surrounding structures; consequently a very low concentration can affect numerous surrounding molecules. The advantages are it does not involve a joint injection or fluoroscopic guidance. In addition, vascularized or inflamed tissue will enhance with this method. It works best in joints like the wrist, ankle, and shoulder but not in large joints like the knee.[2]

Compositional Analysis of Cartilage

The macromolecular network of articular cartilage consists of collagen and proteoglycans. The collagen provides the framework for the tissue and is the main source for tensile and shear strength, whereas glycosaminoglycans provide compressive strength.

T2 mapping: T2 of hyaline cartilage is highly sensitive to alterations of cartilage matrix. A multiecho sequence is used to measure T2 values and a quantitative color coded map can be generated representing variations in T2 relaxation time within articular cartilage. Areas of early degeneration are seen as areas of higher T2 as compared to normal cartilage. T2 maps can be used to monitor the effectiveness of cartilage repair.[7,11]

d-GEMRIC: In this technique, the joint is exercised for 10 minutes after the injection of Gd-DTPA and T1 mapping is done 90 minutes after the injection of Gd. The delay is required to allow gadolinium to penetrate the full thickness of the articular cartilage. It is based on the fact that ions in the interstitial fluid of cartilage are distributed on the basis of the concentration of negatively charged glycosaminoglycan molecules. When anionic molecules like Gd-DTPA enter cartilage, they are distributed in areas where the concentration of glycosaminoglycans is low. The concentration of Gd-DTPA can be estimated by measuring T1, T1 mapping of cartilage after administration of Gd-DTPA allows quantitative assessment of glycosamine content. This technique may become the noninvasive method of assessing glycosaminoglycan content in cartilage after various methods of repair.[2,7,11]

T1 rho mapping: This technique assesses both collagen and glycosaminoglycan content and can detect early degenerative changes. However, an additional RF pulse has to be applied after the magnetization has been tipped in the transverse plane. It is a more time-consuming technique and no large trials have been done using this method.[7,11]

Musculoskeletal Tumors

MRI has a vital role in the detection, confirmation, and preoperative evaluation of malignant and aggressive benign musculoskeletal tumors. Though plain radiographs are the initial modality for the diagnosis of bone tumors, MRI is indispensable for elucidation of the intra- and extraosseous extent of the tumor, its categorization as intra- or extracompartmental, assessment of the neurovascular structures and the adjacent joint **(Figs. 18 to 21)**.[1] MRI is also the best technique to detect skip lesions, which are often missed by other imaging means. The plain radiograph is the modality most likely to yield a specific diagnosis **(Fig. 18A)**, whereas MRI is crucial for accurate local staging of a malignant tumor.

In general, musculoskeletal tumors have a nonspecific appearance on MRI and this modality is not reliable in determining the histology of bone tumors in most cases. Occasionally, it may enable a specific diagnosis on account of pathognomonic signal characteristics, for example, vertebral

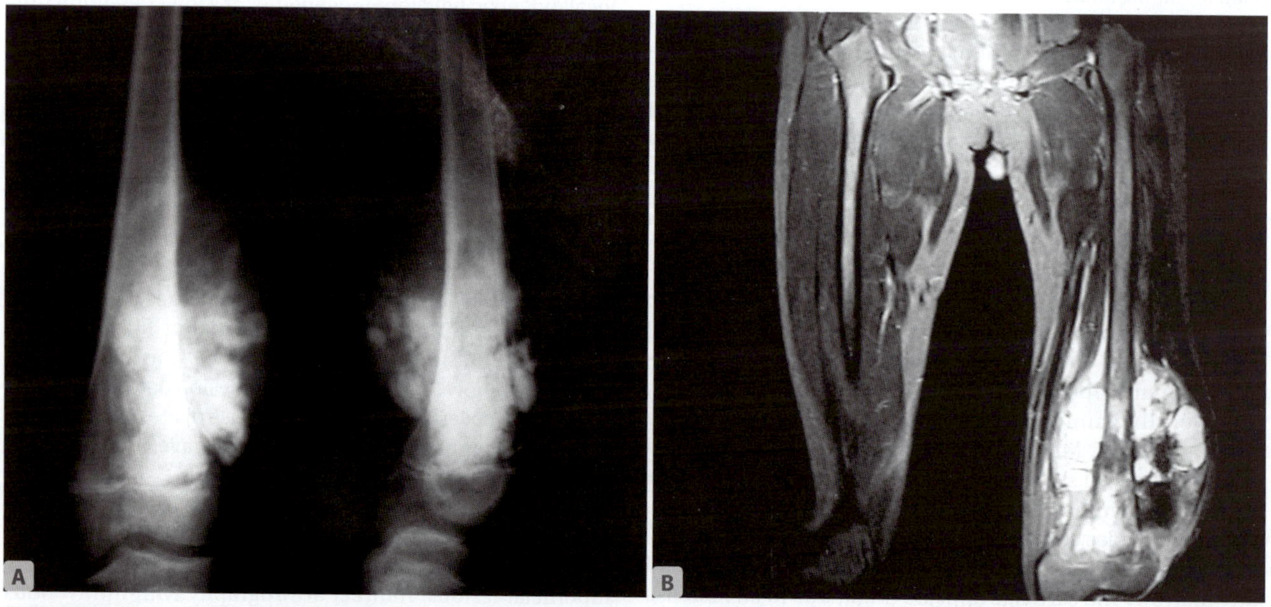

FIGS. 18A AND B: Frontal and lateral radiographs of the knee (A), show osteosarcoma of the distal femoral metaphysis with permeative involvement and osteoid pattern of matrix mineralization extending into the soft tissues. Coronal short tau inversion recovery (STIR) image (B), using body coil shows the complete extent of the tumor, which facilitates optimal surgical management.

hemangioma, soft tissue lipoma **(Figs. 19A and B)**, etc. Therefore, one should be wary of interpreting the MR scan in a suspected tumor without reviewing the radiographs.

Magnetic resonance imaging may detect bone tumors, which are easy to overlook or are not visible on plain radiographs **(Figs. 21A and B)**. This is particularly true in the pelvis and sacrum and in patients with hematological malignancies. In patients with bone pain and a negative plain radiograph, MRI is more sensitive and specific than nuclear scan.[1]

All preoperative imaging of musculoskeletal tumors should be done before a biopsy is performed as it may aid in biopsy planning. Hemorrhage and edema resulting from a biopsy may alter the MR appearance and create difficulty in evaluating the lesion. The tumor should be imaged in at least two planes usually parallel and perpendicular to the long axis of the involved bone. The imaging protocol includes an initial large FOV T1W or STIR study using the body coil **(Fig. 18B)**. This is useful in detection of skip lesions and for planning subsequent sequences. Surface coil images are then obtained in the coronal or sagittal planes to display the extent of the lesion in all three dimensions. The accurate assessment of the craniocaudal extent and exact distance of the proximal and distal margins from a nearby landmark, such as a joint line is crucial for planning a limb-salvage procedure and selection of a suitable prosthesis.[1] Axial images best demonstrate the relationship of the tumor to the neurovascular bundle **(Figs. 19A and B)**. The elucidation of the intraosseous tumor extent as well as the skip lesions needs inclusion of a T1W or STIR sequence **(Figs. 18, 20, and 21)**. However, overestimation of the tumor extent may occur on STIR images due to peritumoral edema. The extraosseous extent is exquisitely demonstrated on a T2W sequence **(Figs. 12A and B)** due to the contrast provided by the low-signal muscles. Adjacent bright fat is best suppressed by a fat saturation technique to further increase the contrast on T2W images. MRI has a high negative predictive value for neurovascular or joint involvement by the tumor, though joint involvement tends to get overdiagnosed based on MRI. A GRE sequence is helpful in clear identification of the neurovascular bundle and contrast administration is not required for extent delineation of bone tumors.[12]

Use of Advanced Magnetic Resonance Techniques

Diffusion-weighted Imaging

Diffusion can be assessed both qualitatively and quantitatively and is a measure of tumor cellularity and cell membrane integrity. It can be used for detection and characterization of bone tumors as well as assess the response to chemotherapy. DWI sequences are done at different b values ranging from 0 to 1,000. Typically, benign lesions lose their signal intensity as b value increases whereas cellular tumors retain their signal intensity. The apparent diffusion coefficient (ADC) can be used for quantitative assessment. Low ADC values are seen in cellular tumors because of restricted diffusion.

Diffusion-weighted imaging can also be used to assess response to chemoradiotherapy. Tumor necrosis caused by these modalities increases the ADC value which can be used as a surrogate marker for response.[13]

Magnetic Resonance Neurography

An MRI of the nerves employs high-resolution thin T1W and T2W SE, 3D isotropic T2 sampling perfection with application optimized contrast (SPACE) or VISTA or CUBE, 3D STIR and volume diffusion-weighted images. 3D diffusion-weighted reverse FISP (3D DW PSIF) has also been advocated especially to evaluate small nerves and differentiate them from vascular signals. Diffusion tensor imaging and color tractography can be done to look for any loss of anisotropy indirectly suggesting the functional status of the nerve fibers.

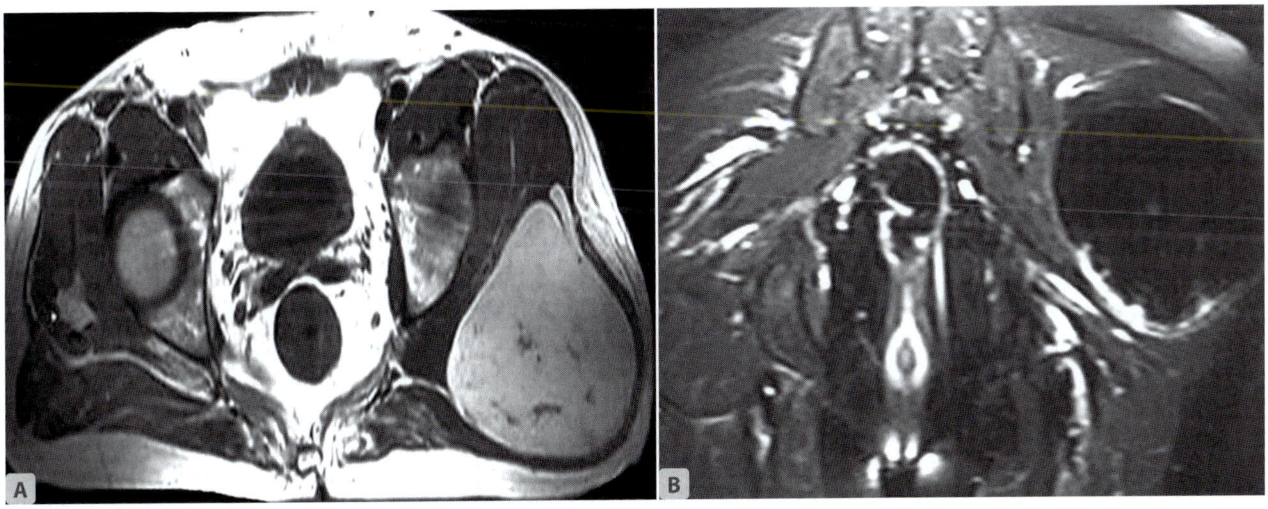

FIGS. 19A AND B: Axial T1-weighted image (A) shows a well-defined hyperintense mass lesion in the left gluteal region which completely loses signal on coronal fat suppressed image; (B) Indicative of fat within, suggesting the diagnosis of soft tissue lipoma. Also note that the signal intensity of the lesion parallels that of subcutaneous fat.

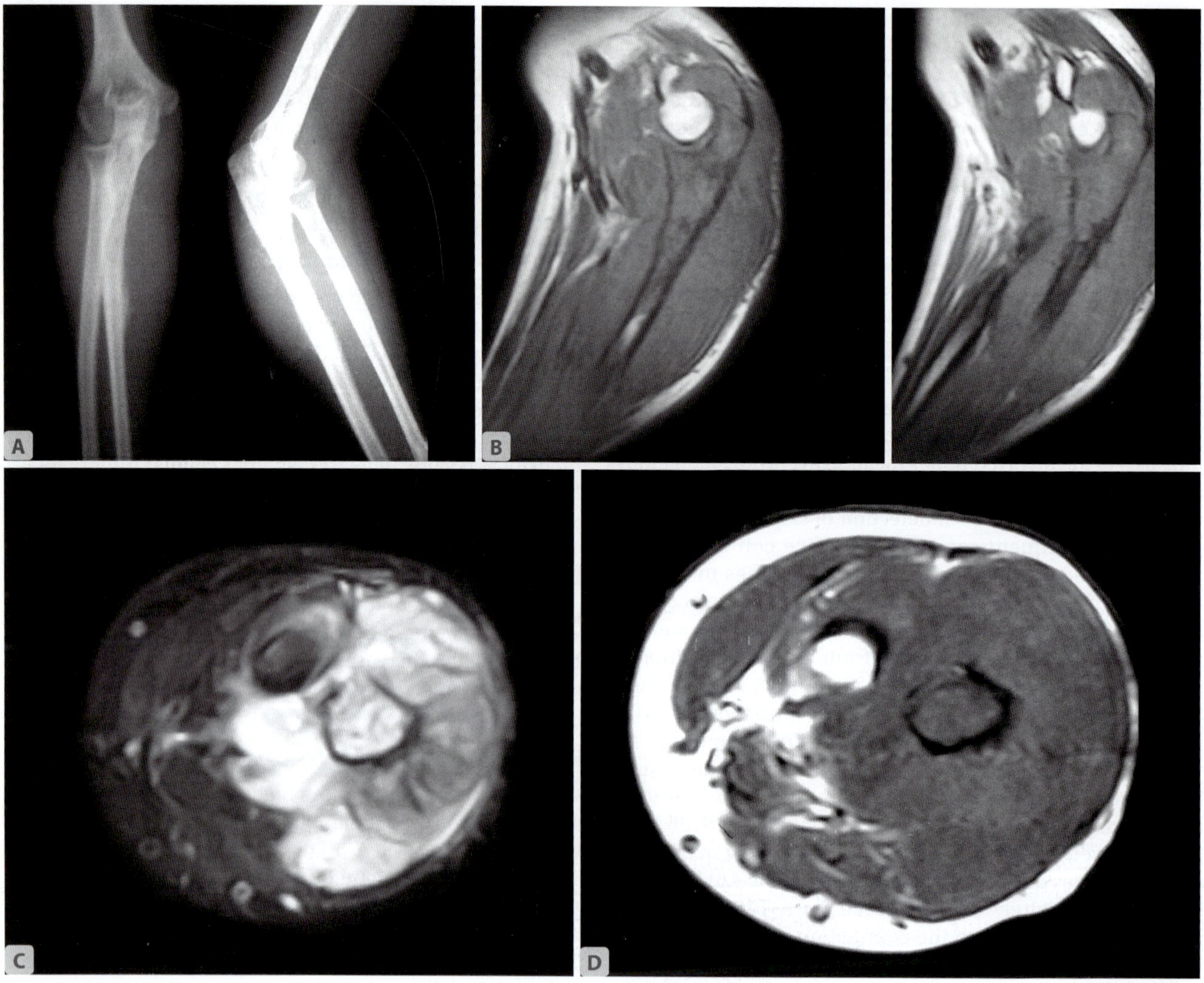

FIGS. 20A TO D: Frontal and lateral radiographs of the elbow (A) show permeative lytic bone destruction with ill-defined margins involving proximal ulna with Codman's triangle, cortical breech, soft tissue extension and osseous mineralization, suggesting osteosarcoma. Sagittal T1-weighted (T1W) image (B), clearly demonstrates the intraosseous extent and extension into surrounding soft tissues. Axial T2-weighted (T2W) (C) and T1W (D) images depict the extent of tumor, cortical disruption, and soft tissue extension with sparing of the neurovascular bundle.

Whole Body Magnetic Resonance Imaging

Whole body MRI (WB-MRI) provides a radiation-free alternative to positron-emission tomography (PET)/CT for evaluation of multifocal and multisystem diseases. Common musculoskeletal indications include detection of lesions, evaluation of tumor load (staging), and follow-up (assessment of treatment response) in case of lymphoma, multiple myeloma, and metastases **(Fig. 22)**.[14] It is also useful in detection of occult primary neoplastic lesion in diseases like oncogenic osteomalacia or identifying the focus of infection in chronic fever of unknown origin. The sequences which are done as part of whole body imaging include STIR, diffusion-weighted imaging with background suppression (DWIBS), and postcontrast T1W imaging. WB-MRI has been found to be more sensitive than bone scan and choline PET/CT for identifying bone metastases from prostatic carcinoma.[14] WB-MRI can aid in evaluating multiple lesions in case of neurofibromatosis and vascular malformations. Quantification techniques have been described for WB-DWI and include calculation of total diffusion volume (TDV) and global ADC. TDV is based on aggregated volume of segmented high signal intensity areas (corresponding to high cellularity tumor) on high b-value DWI image and gives estimate of total disease burden.[15] Corresponding ADC value of the entire volume is known as global ADC and various histogram parameters can be calculated.

Zero Echo Time Magnetic Resonance Imaging

Zero echo time (ZTE) MRI demonstrates increased contrast resolution of the osseous outline and thus may exclude the need to do CT in evaluation of cases like bony Bankart.[16] Ultrashort echo time (UTE) MRI is used in better visualization of tendons, menisci, and calcified zone of hyaline cartilage. ZTE is a further extension of the same concept to evaluate structures with short TE and acquisition is done immediately after the application of RF pulse (TE ~8 ms).[16] ZTE MR allows simultaneous evaluation of marrow edema, bone outline, and subchondral cysts.[15]

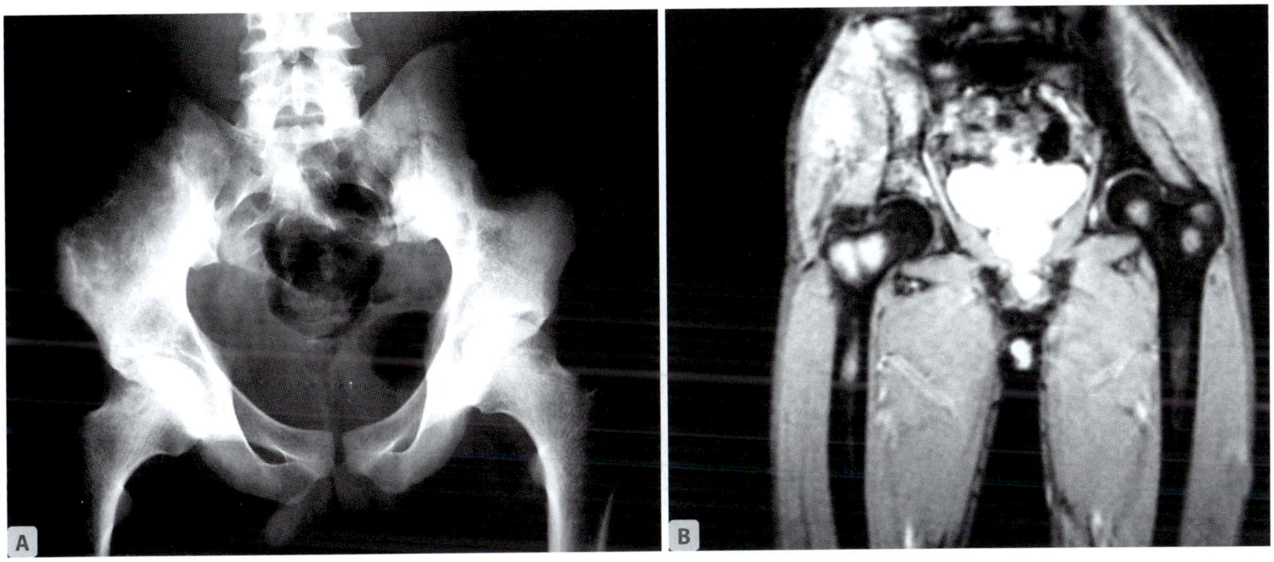

FIGS. 21A AND B: Frontal radiograph of the pelvis (A) shows an ill-defined permeative lytic lesion in the right iliac wing. Short tau inversion recovery (STIR) coronal image (B) clearly shows that there are multiple well-defined hyperintense lesions in bilateral femoral necks also, indicative of bony metastases. These lesions were not apparent on radiographs. The primary tumor was proven to be Ewing's sarcoma.

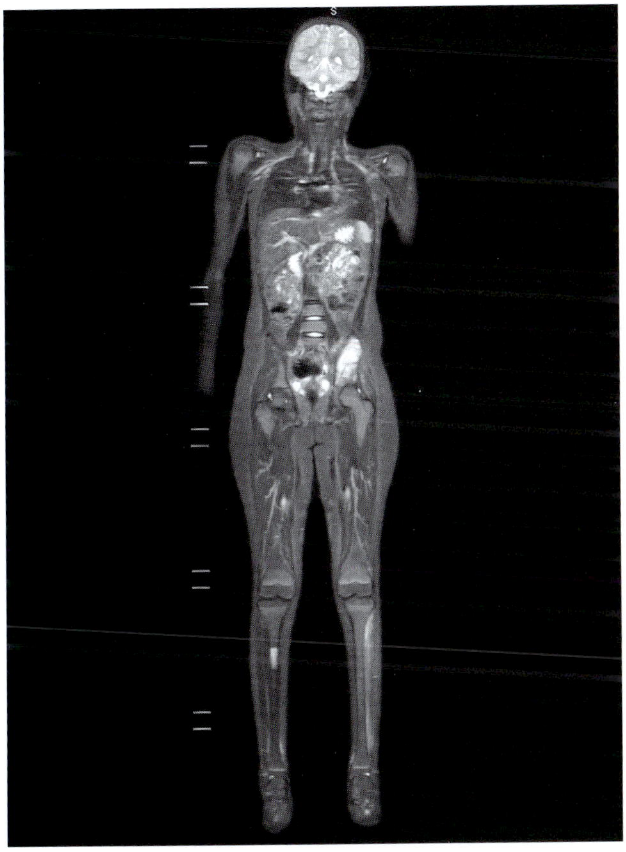

FIG. 22: Whole body short tau inversion recovery (STIR) image shows a large lesion in the left iliac blade and another lesion in the right tibia in a case of multiple metastases.

New Rapid Acquisition Sequences

Compressed sensing serves to accelerate the MR acquisition by acquiring less data via undersampling of the k-space. This is usually combined with parallel imaging to enable high acceleration factors but the role is still investigational in musculoskeletal diseases. Limitations include image blurring and poor visibility of low-contrast structures. Machine-learning reconstructions are also being explored to speed up acquisition. Multislice/multiband imaging employs simultaneous acquisition of information from multiple slices, rather than doing so sequentially [simultaneous multislice (SMS)]. However the problems for musculoskeletal application include altered contrast between the soft tissue structures and loss of image quality.

Conventional MR is unable to provide a specific histologic diagnosis and is unreliable for differentiating benign from malignant neoplasms. Neoadjuvant chemotherapy is used in many bone tumors like osteosarcoma and Ewing's sarcoma. The evaluation of response to chemotherapy on routine MR is based on size reduction, which is unreliable and may take time. These problems can be addressed by using techniques like dynamic contrast-enhanced perfusion imaging, proton spectroscopy, diffusion imaging, intravoxel incoherent motion (IVIM), in-phase/opposed-phase MRI, and texture analysis.[13,17]

Dynamic Perfusion Imaging

T1W gradient echo sequence is repeated rapidly a number of times after an injection of gadolinium bolus (0.1 mmol/kg) followed by a saline chase. Time signal intensity curves are generated in much the same way as is done in breast imaging. In general, malignant tumors show greater enhancement at a faster rate **(Figs. 23A to D)** and a rapid wash out as compared to benign tumors.[17] This technique coupled with conventional MR, spectroscopy and DWI may help in narrowing the list of differential diagnosis, better assess the extent of disease, distinguish responders to chemotherapy from nonresponders, and differentiate residual/recurrent tumor from radiation necrosis. The former enhance early and more rapidly whereas post-therapy changes enhance later and more slowly.[13]

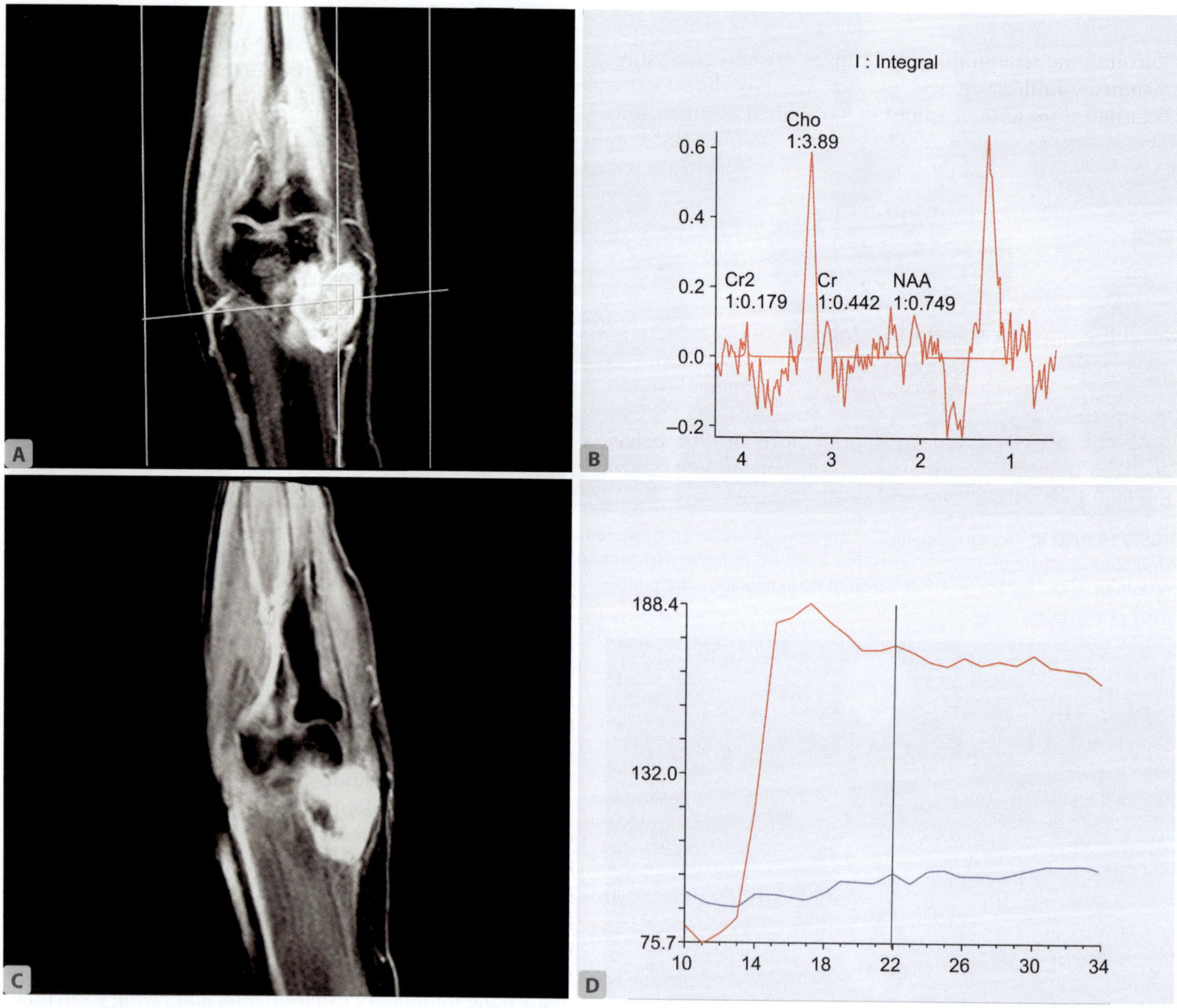

FIGS. 23A TO D: Coronal fat suppression (FS) postgadolinium image (A) of the elbow showing the placement of voxel for single voxel magnetic resonance spectroscopy in enhancing lesion seen in distal humeral metaphysis. There is elevated choline peak (B), suggesting malignant bone tumor. Coronal postgadolinium FS T1-weighted image (C) of the elbow showing the placement of region of interest (ROI) for generation of perfusion map of the lesion to show contrast kinetics. Time signal intensity curve (D) of the same lesion shows rapid uptake and washout of the contrast, indicating malignant neoplasm.

Time-resolved 4D MR angiography is another method of dynamic postcontrast imaging which is useful for characterizing vascular malformations. The principle behind this sequence is that center of the k-space is repeatedly sampled while periphery is sampled only once during acquisition, thus reducing scan time. Commercially this is available as time-resolved angiography with interleaved stochastic trajectories (TWIST) or time-resolved angiography with keyhole method (TRAK) or time-resolved imaging of contrast kinetics (TRICKS). Multiple fast 3D acquisitions of the region of interest are obtained sequentially and almost a real-time effect is perceived.

Proton Spectroscopy

It can be performed using a single voxel technique with a point resolved spectroscopy sequence (PRESS) and TE of 135 ms. The choline peak and choline/creatine ratio has been shown to distinguish benign from malignant bone and soft tissue tumors **(Figs. 23A to D)**. The voxel should be placed on areas showing early and intense enhancement. The caveat is that some metabolically active tumors like giant cell tumor may also show choline peak.[17]

Positron-emission Tomography–Magnetic Resonance Imaging

Hybrid PET-MRI systems offer high-contrast resolution of MRI along with metabolic information from PET. They have been found useful in the T-staging, follow-up, and therapeutic response assessment of musculoskeletal sarcomas.[18] This may also prove useful in multiple myeloma and diffuse metastases. Potential nononcological applications include stress fractures and evaluation of arthritides.

Marrow Imaging

Conventional radiographic techniques are very insensitive to marrow infiltration and tumors. CT may detect gross metastatic disease of the spine but is of limited use in imaging primary and metastatic neoplasms in the rest of the skeleton. Radionuclide bone scanning is insensitive to certain marrow neoplasms such as lymphoma and multiple myeloma. MRI has the major advantage of imaging the bone marrow directly and its excellent contrast resolution allows the differentiation of normal from infiltrated marrow.[1,2]

When diffuse marrow disease is suspected a survey of the entire spine, pelvis, and proximal femora is performed, because this is where the bulk of the hematopoietic marrow exists. For a marrow survey the patient is positioned supine. The phased array coils are used for spine imaging and the body coil is used for the proximal femora and the pelvis. Sagittal images of the spine and coronal images of the pelvis and femora are most useful. WB-MRI can now be routinely performed for metastatic survey and in marrow infiltrative diseases. There is a technique called DWIBS which is ideal for picking up foci of metastatic disease, lymphoma, etc., and may become a competitive modality for PET-CT. T1W and STIR images are most sensitive to marrow pathology.[1]

An MRI can distinguish between hematopoietic or red marrow from yellow marrow. The normal distribution of red and yellow marrow and the conversion of red to yellow marrow occur in a predictable manner based on age.[2] There is a vast array of marrow disorders that can be detected on MRI although the appearance may be nonspecific and only a differential diagnosis may be offered. However, MRI is excellent for establishing the presence of disease and also for directing biopsy to an appropriate site.

Important categories of marrow pathology include marrow proliferative disorders such as leukemia and myeloma and marrow replacement disorders such as metastases and lymphoma.[1] The usual appearance of marrow pathology is low signal intensity (equal to or less than muscle) on T1W scans **(Fig. 24A)** and variable, but usually high-signal intensity on T2W scans.

An MRI is exquisitely sensitive for detection of metastatic disease and surpasses all other imaging techniques in this regard. A common clinical problem is the distinction between metastatic deposits from an acute osteoporotic collapse, especially in a patient with a known primary tumor. Both may show a fractured vertebral body with replacement of normal marrow by low signal intensity on T1W scans. Features that suggest tumor are abnormal signal intensity extending into the pedicles and other posterior elements, involvement of the entire vertebral body by the abnormal signal intensity, associated soft tissue mass, and multiple bone lesions. In osteoporotic fractures, the abnormal signal intensity does not involve the entire vertebral body, but has a horizontal line or band separating the abnormal signal intensity from the normal fatty marrow signal.[1] It has been reported that GRE opposed-phase sequence may be helpful based on the fact that some fat is still present in benign lesions such as osteoporotic fractures. Hence, osteoporotic fractures are supposed to show lower signal intensity than the metastatic lesions. Diffusion-weighted images have also been successfully used for the purpose of this differentiation.[1] The vertebral lesions due to marrow infiltration by tumor become hyperintense on DWI **(Figs. 24B and C)** whereas osteoporotic collapsed vertebra remains hypointense. In- and opposed-phase images have also been used in this context. Collapse due to osteoporosis will retain some normal fatty marrow which will show loss of signal on the opposed-phase image. On the other hand, metastatic and marrow infiltrative disease replaces the fatty marrow completely and hence does not show this signal loss **(Figs. 24D and E)**.

Magnetic resonance can also be used to monitor the response of marrow pathology such as leukemia and metastases to treatment. Serial MRI has been shown to be useful in confirming remission and detecting relapse in patients with leukemia.

Musculoskeletal Infections

Conventional radiographs remain the initial imaging modality of choice for suspected osteomyelitis. However, it is insensitive to the detection of early osteomyelitis. MRI scores over radiography, CT, and scintigraphy in detection of early osteomyelitis. However, the MR appearance is nonspecific and similar to infiltrating neoplasms and stress fractures and the clinical context is important in reaching the correct diagnosis.[19] MR is also superior to other modalities in delineating the soft tissue involvement. The elucidation of the full extent facilitates preoperative planning of the maximal degree of debridement or the level of the amputation. FS techniques combined with gadolinium administration further increase the sensitivity for detection of involved areas. Contrast administration is also helpful in distinguishing abscess **(Fig. 15)** from surrounding cellulitis, increasing the conspicuity of the sinus tracts by causing their walls to enhance and clearly demonstrating the nonenhancing sequestra within enhancing granulation tissue.[20]

In infants and children, involvement of the unossified physis and epiphysis is best shown by MRI.

Inflammatory Arthritis

Radiography has been the imaging modality of choice in RA, primarily because of its reproducibility and feasibility. Currently MRI is being used widely for recruiting patients into clinical trials as well as monitoring disease progression over time, because of its advantage of simultaneous imaging of key structures other than bone (synovium and surrounding soft tissues) that are important in inflammatory arthritis. MRI is also a useful tool in evaluating patients with early RA. It can detect pre-erosive synovitis and can also identify early bone damage before it becomes apparent on radiography. In early RA, wrist and hand involvement is usually bilateral. Some authors perform bilateral MRI of the wrists or hands. However, it is preferred to study the dominant or more painful wrist in order to reduce the study time. The technical recommendations of the OMERACT (Outcome Measures in Rheumatoid Arthritis Clinical Trials) group for MRI studies of RA patients should include at least the following sequences:

- Imaging in two planes (coronal and axial)
- T1-weighted imaging before and after the administration of gadolinium, fat saturated imaging is preferable after administration
- A fat saturated T2W sequence or a STIR sequence.[21]

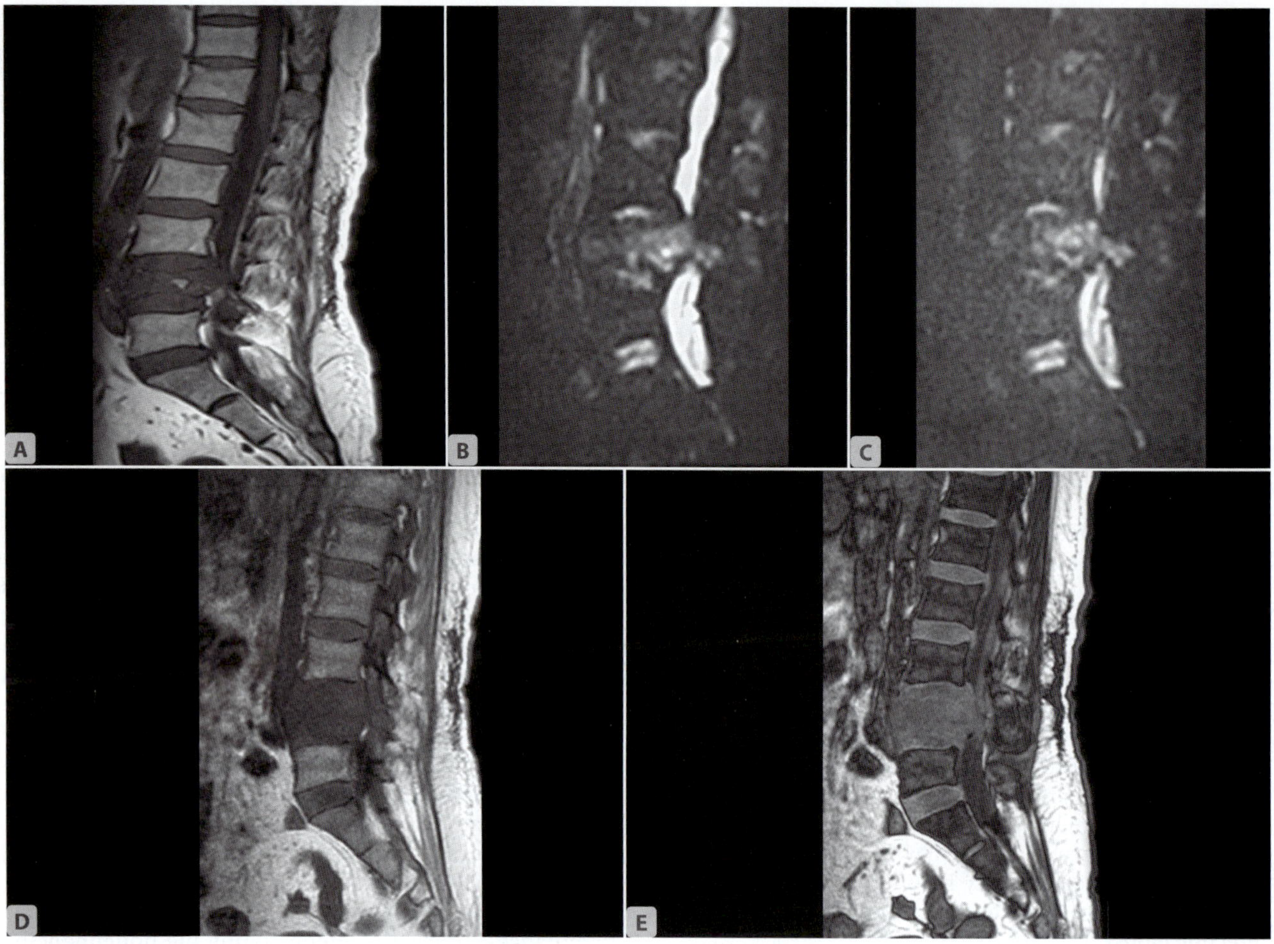

FIGS. 24A TO E: Sagittal T1-weighted (T1W) image (A) of lumbosacral spine shows altered signal intensity with partial collapse of L4 vertebra. Diffusion-weighted images at b 0 s/mm^2 (B) and b 400 s/mm^2 (C) show retention of signal at higher b value, suggesting restricted diffusion. Sagittal T1W in-phase (D) and opposed-phase (E) images show suppression of marrow signal in the normal vertebrae. However, L4 vertebra shows no loss of signal. Diffusion restriction and absence of signal suppression on opposed-phase images are markers of malignant vertebral involvement. This was proven to be metastatic vertebral collapse.

Interventional Magnetic Resonance Imaging

Due to restricted patient access on conventional high and midfield MR machines and unacceptable speed on the older low-field systems, MRI was not considered as a guidance tool for interventional procedures earlier. Since the introduction of open magnet designs offering a nearly free patient access, interest has now focused on interventional MR. In addition, short bore high-field systems presently allow satisfactory patient access combined with high-performance imaging capabilities. A simultaneous creation of an adequate array of MR compatible instruments has made MR interventions viable.[22] Percutaneous biopsies and drainage procedures are currently the easiest procedures to be performed under MR control. These do not require dedicated hard or software modifications and are thus attractive and clinically useful.

Three types of magnets are clinically used for percutaneous biopsies: (1) open low-field magnets (0.2–0.35 T), (2) open midfield system (0.5 T), and (3) closed short bore magnets (1–1.5 T). Improved patient access with open magnet allows interventions in any desired plane and patient position. To begin with, horizontally open magnets were used. Recently, experience with vertically open units has also been reported. Vertically open units permit unrestricted vertical and side access to the patient at the most homogeneous portion of the magnetic field. The other advantage is a horizontally directed main magnetic field along the long axis of the bore, which ensures that the needle trajectory is never parallel to the field.[23] In closed systems, instrument manipulation can only be performed with the patient outside the magnet. However, due to higher field strength, image quality as well as the imaging speed is better.

For instrument visualization, the susceptibility artifact provided by the nonferromagnetic alloys of MR compatible needles is used. The size of the artifact is inversely proportional to the size of the instrument and directly proportional to the field strength and to the angle the instrument makes with the main magnetic field. Typically, biopsy needles are displayed as dark areas surrounded by a brighter rim.[24] Several vendors on the market offer MR compatible needles at present. Fine needles of 20–24G with different tip configurations and cutting needles of 14–18G are commercially available. The overall performance of a MR compatible needle is inferior to a stainless steel needle due to relatively blunt surfaces and softer alloys. For drainage procedures MR compatible sets consisting of MR compatible guidewires, dilators, and drainage catheters are available.

Imaging protocol consists of fast localizers in three planes followed by a fast multislice T2W SE sequence. A postcontrast GRE sequence may be used to select the appropriate biopsy site. In the closed magnet, needle tracking is done by following a procedure similar to that used in CT-guided interventions. After defining the target region, a T1W or T2W compatible grid is fixed to the skin of the patient to aid in selecting needle entry site. The angle and distance from skin to the lesion can be obtained by using standard scanner software. The needle track can be controlled step-by-step during advancement of the needle. In the open magnet, a palpating finger may be used instead of a grid for entry site. The instrument can be tracked by continuous repetition of a fast imaging sequence.[22]

Primary and secondary bone and soft tissue lesions can be accessed by MR-guided interventional procedures. Due to its multiplanar capability, MR allows visualization of the entire planned biopsy pathway including orthogonal and oblique scans. Lack of ionizing radiation is an obvious advantage.[24] The unique advantage of MR interventions is in transcutaneous biopsy of bone marrow lesions of unknown origin, as their display and localization is possible exclusively on MR. However, the available armamentarium to perform MR-guided transcortical bone biopsy is limited, though a MR compatible coaxial bone biopsy system has recently been developed.[22] Although lesion access by MR is good for appendicular skeleton, CT is preferred for biopsy of the axial skeleton due to superior spatial resolution.

CONCLUSION

The scope of musculoskeletal radiology has widened over the last few years and to a large extent this has been possible because of the exquisite detail provided by the versatile technique of MRI. There has been a resurgence of interest in US as a noninvasive simple tool for dynamic evaluation of musculoskeletal pathology. The advent of dual energy CT has led to some new applications like evaluation of gout and marrow imaging based on the VNCa images. High-field MRI, DWI, dynamic contrast-enhanced imaging, MR spectroscopy, and other advances have further enhanced the utility of this modality. However, elegant display of pathology alone does not suffice, as diagnosis based on images alone, especially MR images, is nonspecific. For the optimal use of this technology the radiologist must couple these images with an in depth knowledge of pathophysiology and clinical perspective so that he can guide the referring clinician appropriately. "Seeing better" should be coupled with "knowing more" to make the optimum use of the high tech modality of MRI.[25]

REFERENCES

1. Helms CA, Anderson MW, Major NM, Kaplan P, Dussault R. Musculoskeletal MRI, 2nd edition. Philadelphia: WB Saunders Co; 2009.
2. Stoller DW. Magnetic Resonance Imaging in Orthopaedics and Sports Medicine, 3rd edition. Philadelphia: Lippincott Williams & Wilkins; 2007.
3. Zou J, Yang H, Miyazaki M, Morishita Y, Wei F, McGovern S, et al. Dynamic bulging of intervertebral discs in the degenerative lumbar spine. Spine. 2009;34(23):2545-50.
4. Ramnath RR. 3T MR imaging of the musculoskeletal system (Part II): clinical applications. Magn Reson Imaging Clin N Am. 2006;14(1):41-62.
5. Koff MF, Potter HG. Noncontrast MR techniques and imaging of cartilage. Radiol Clin N Am. 2009;47(3):495-504.
6. Strickland CD, Kijowski R. Morphologic imaging of articular cartilage. Magn Reson Imaging Clin N Am. 2011;19(2):229-48.
7. Choi JA, Gold GE. MR imaging of articular cartilage physiology. Magn Reson Imaging Clin N Am. 2011;19(2):249-82.
8. Suh JS, Lee SH, Jeong EK, Kim DJ. Magnetic resonance imaging of articular cartilage. Eur Radiol. 2001;11(10):2015-25.
9. Sonin AH, Pensy RA, Mulligan ME, Hatem S. Grading articular cartilage of the knee using fast spinecho proton density-weighted MR imaging without fat suppression. Am J Roentgenol. 2002;179(5):1159-66.
10. Reeder SB, Pelc NJ, Alley MT, Gold GE. Rapid MR imaging of articular cartilage with steady-state free precession and multipoint fat-water separation. Am J Roentgenol. 2003;180(2):357-62.
11. Crema MD, Roemer FW, Marra MD, Burstein D, Gold GE, Eckstein F, et al. Articular cartilage in the knee: current MR imaging techniques and applications in clinical practice and research. Radiographics. 2011;31(1):37-61.
12. Peabody TD, Gibbs CP, Simon MA. Current concepts review—evaluation and staging of musculoskeletal neoplasms. J Bone Joint Surg Am. 1998;80(8):1204-18.
13. Garner HW, Kransdorf MJ, Peterson JJ. Posttherapy imaging of musculoskeletal neoplasms. Radiol Clin North Am. 2011;49(6): 1307-23.
14. Petralia G, Padhani AR. Whole-body magnetic resonance imaging in oncology: uses and indications. Magn Reson Imaging Clin N Am. 2018;26(4):495-507.
15. Donners R, Blackledge M, Tunariu N, Messiou C, Merkle EM, Koh DM. Quantitative whole-body diffusion-weighted MR imaging. Magn Reson Imaging Clin N Am. 2018;26(4):479-94.
16. Breighner RE, Endo Y, Konin GP, Gulotta LV, Koff MF, Potter HG. Technical developments: zero echo time imaging of the shoulder: enhanced osseous detail by using MR imaging. Radiology. 2018;286(3):960-6.
17. Costa FM, Canella C, Gasparetto E. Advanced magnetic resonance imaging techniques in the evaluation of musculoskeletal tumors. Radiol Clin North Am. 2011;49(6):1325-58.
18. Kogan F, Broski SM, Yoon D, Gold GE. Applications of PET-MRI in musculoskeletal disease. J Magn Reson Imaging. 2018;48(1): 27-47.
19. Boutin RD, Brossmann J, Sartoris DJ, Reilly D, Resnick D. Update on imaging of orthopedic infections. Orthop Clin North Am. 1998;29(1):41-66.
20. D Towers J. The use of intravenous contrast in MRI of extremity infection. Semin Ultrasound CT MR. 1997;18:269-75.
21. Narváez JA, Narváez J, De Lama E, De Albert M. MR imaging of early rheumatoid arthritis. Radiographics. 2010;30(1): 143-63.
22. Adam G, Bücker A, Nolte-Ernsting C, Tacke J, Günther R. Interventional MR imaging: percutaneous abdominal and skeletal biopsies and drainages of the abdomen. Eur Radiol. 1999;9(8):1471-8.
23. Genant JW, Vandevenne JE, Bergman AG, Beaulieu CF, Kee ST, Norbash AM, et al. Interventional musculoskeletal procedures performed by using MR imaging guidance with a vertically open MR unit: assessment of techniques and applicability. Radiology. 2002;223(1):127-36.
24. Ghelman B. Biopsies of the musculoskeletal system. Radiol Clinics North Am. 1998;36(3):567-80.
25. Feldman F. Musculoskeletal radiology: then and now. Radiology. 2000;216(2):309-16.

CHAPTER

153

Nuclear Medicine Imaging for Musculoskeletal Disorders

Rakesh Kumar, Madhavi Tripathi, Shamim Ahmed Shamim

INTRODUCTION

Musculoskeletal system is a dynamic organ system, which responds to systemic as well as to localized stress and, hence, apart from anatomical visualization, it requires physiological evaluation. Nuclear medicine techniques provide the physician with physiologically detailed images that can give insight, which cannot always be accomplished, from plain radiograph or even with computed tomography (CT) and magnetic resonance imaging (MRI). The major advantage of nuclear medicine imaging stems from the fact that functional changes appear much before anatomical changes. Hence, nuclear medicine imaging allows early detection of diseases affecting musculoskeletal system. The present chapter summarizes the nuclear medicine techniques used for musculoskeletal imaging and their utility in various benign and malignant pathologies involving the musculoskeletal system.

TABLE 1: Radiotracers used for skeletal scintigraphy.

Tracers for skeletal imaging	Nonspecific	Tumor-specific
Planar and SPECT	^{99m}Tc MDP	
	^{99m}Tc HEDP	
PET	18F-Fluoride	*Ga-68 DOTANOC-NET
	*18F FDG	*!Ga-68 PSMA-prostate cancer

*Localizes in bone marrow and bone metastases.

!This tracer localizes to prostate-specific membrane antigen (PSMA) expression on prostate cancer cells and also in neovascularization, thus has been found to localize to bone metastases in breast, anaplastic thyroid cancer, adrenocortical cancer (ACC), etc.

(FDG: fluorodeoxyglucose; HEDP: hydroxyethylidene diphosphonic acid; MDP: methylene diphosphonate; NET: neuroendocrine tumor; PET: positron emission tomography; SPECT: single photon emission computed tomography)

BONE SCINTIGRAPHY

In spite of newer developments in the field of nuclear medicine, bone scintigraphy (BS) remains the most commonly employed method for musculoskeletal imaging. It is performed following the intravenous administration of bone-seeking radiopharmaceuticals. These compounds are usually phosphonates labeled with ^{99m}Technetium (^{99m}Tc). The most widely used is ^{99m}Tc-methylene diphosphonate (MDP) **(Table 1)**. Others are ^{99m}Tc-ethylene hydroxy-diphosphonate (EHDP) and ^{99m}Tc-hydroxymethylene diphosphonate (HDP). The presence of P-C-P bonds makes these compounds resistant to hydrolysis by bone phosphatases, thereby increasing the biological half-life. 3–4 hours after intravenous injection about 25–35% of radiotracer is retained in the normal adult skeleton, the rest is excreted in the urine via the kidney. These phosphorus-containing complexes attach themselves to the hydroxyapatite crystal on the bone surface by chemisorption.[1] Thus, they localize at the site of direct and indirect osteoblastic activation. Autoradiographic studies revealed that the ^{99m}Tc-labeled phosphonates are mainly taken up in the mineral phase of skeletal bone at the site of reactive bone formation. This osteoblastic activation can be seen because of wide array of pathologies, thereby decreasing the specificity. The routine BS employs whole body anterior and posterior sweep images. In addition, dynamic flow and pool images are acquired in selected cases.

SPECT AND SPECT/CT

Given the lack of anatomical information provided by planar BS, especially in the regions of complex anatomy, additional methods are employed. Single photon emission tomography (SPECT) is being routinely used in such a scenario. It gives three-dimensional pictures and is beneficial in patients with normal planar images despite symptoms and in those with equivocal findings.[2] SPECT imaging is most useful for the evaluation of the thoracolumbar spine, skull, and pelvis. These areas have extensive surrounding soft tissue and/or complicated body contours, and thus superior image contrast provided by SPECT improves lesion detection. The decision to perform single field-of-view SPECT studies has been guided by suspicious findings on planar imaging or localized clinical symptoms. However, even with plain SPECT, correlation with anatomical imaging is usually needed. SPECT/CT imaging with hybrid cameras has been introduced to overcome this shortcoming and to provide both anatomical and functional information in a single setting.

PET AND PET/CT

In contrast to routine gamma camera imaging, positron emission tomography (PET) imaging is based on the detection of high energy (511 KeV) annihilation photons emitted by positron-emitting radionuclides. The inherent physics of positron decay allows tomographic imaging without the need for collimators, thereby improving the sensitivity and resolution. The lack of anatomical information on PET alone has been overcome with introduction of hybrid PET/CT. In fact, the availability of hybrid PET/CT systems has made PET alone redundant. Although, PET and PET/CT had greatest impact in the field of cancer imaging, its application for other areas including musculoskeletal disorders is being actively investigated. In clinical practice, most PET studies are performed with 2-[^{18}F] fluoro-2-deoxy-D-glucose (FDG), a glucose analog. It is actively taken up by cells with increased glucose metabolic rate via specific glucose transporters (GLUT-1 and GLUT-4) and is phosphorylated by hexokinases to FDG-6-phosphate, which is retained.[3] Nowadays, FDG-PET is being increasingly used for imaging primary and secondary musculoskeletal tumors as well as infections. Another important tracer in the context of skeletal imaging is ^{18}F-fluoride **(Table 1)**. It can also be used for quantitative studies of skeletal kinetics.[4] Although there are differences between ^{18}F-fluoride and ^{99m}Tc-diphosphonate, it is probable that the mechanism of uptake in bone is the same, i.e., adsorption onto bony surfaces with predilection for sites of active bone formation.[5] The uptake of ^{18}F-fluoride is approximately twofold higher and its blood clearance is significantly faster compared with the ^{99m}Tc-diphosphonates, resulting in an increased bone-to-background ratio. Ga-68 prostate-specific membrane antigen (PSMA) PET-CT is a new addition, is used for prostate cancer staging, particularly for bone metastasis, and shows high sensitivity and specificity for bone metastasis. In addition, PET offers high sensitivity and high resolution, and therefore enables to perform highly accurate whole-body screening for metastases.[6]

MUSCULOSKELETAL TUMOR IMAGING

Metastasis

Skeletal metastasis is the most common bone malignancy. It affects approximately two-thirds of cancer patients, with breast cancer being the leading cause in women, prostate cancer in men, followed by lung cancer in both genders. Accurate assessment of skeletal involvement is essential for optimal management of these patients.[7] Many patients with bone metastases are identified during initial staging, routine follow-up, or on investigation for rising tumor markers. For the past few decades, planar BS has been the most frequently performed imaging study in the evaluation of metastatic bone disease. Although scintigraphic findings alone are often nonspecific for skeletal pathologies, this technique reportedly has an exquisite sensitivity. Radiographs are found to be negative in 30–50% of patients with positive bone scan. The most common pattern of bone metastasis is multiple "hot" spots distributed randomly throughout the skeleton.[8] A lytic metastasis usually presents as a photopenic area with increased activity at the margin of the lesion. False negative results in BS are seen in avascular lesions, in the presence of rapidly growing pure osteolytic metastases with no reactive increased osteoblastic activity, or in lesions with low bone turnover (multiple myeloma and hepatocellular cancer). Specificity of BS is generally lower, due to a known increased blood flow and bone remodeling in response to a variety of disease processes, including trauma, infection, inflammation, and osteoarthritis. Therefore, further assessment with other imaging modalities, mainly CT and MRI, and in some cases, histologic confirmation may be required for precise diagnosis.[9]

Addition of SPECT has been reported to detect 20–50% more lesions in the spine compared with planar scintigraphy.[10] It increases both the sensitivity and specificity of bone scans.[11] The use of SPECT for the assessment of suspicious vertebral lesions on planar BS had a negative predictive value of 98%. The sensitivity and specificity of bone SPECT for diagnosis of bone metastases are 87–92 and 91–93%, respectively.[12] The decision to perform single field-of-view SPECT studies has been guided by suspicious findings on planar imaging or localized clinical symptoms. Newly developed half-time whole body SPECT protocols provide tomographic assessment of the entire skeleton within an acceptable image acquisition time, with subsequent improvement in sensitivity and an increased detection rate of asymptomatic small skeletal metastases.[13] However, even with SPECT correlation with high-quality anatomic images, CT or MRI may still be needed for diagnosis. Hybrid SPECT/CT devices equipped with multislice CT scanners further improve the sensitivity and specificity of BS. It has been shown to be superior to planar BS and SPECT for skeletal metastasis of breast and lung cancers.[14,15] Foci of increased tracer activity on BS, suspicious of representing malignant bone lesions, may not show any morphologic abnormality on CT as functional changes precede anatomical changes, and therefore cannot be confirmed as such. The present consensus is to do SPECT/CT of suspicious planar BS lesions only if the lesion remains equivocal even after SPECT **(Figs. 1A to E)**.

Several studies have shown the superiority of the ^{18}F-fluoride PET over BS for the diagnosis of skeletal metastases; the former demonstrated a higher number of the lesions and a higher contrast between normal and abnormal bone.[16] Although the superb resolution and high abnormal-to-normal bone ratio of ^{18}F-fluoride PET can potentially lower the specificity, hybrid PET-CT imaging should help differentiate benign versus malignant lesions **(Figs. 2A to C)**.[17] ^{18}F-fluoride has shown to be highly sensitive for detecting lytic and sclerotic bone metastasis in breast cancer,[18] prostate cancer,[19] and lung cancer.[20] There has been the suggestion that ^{18}F-fluoride could be more cost effective than the bone scan and that a case can be made for it replacing the bone scan.[21] Increased FDG activity at the sites of skeletal lesions represents active tumor itself, whereas increased ^{99m}Tc-MDP

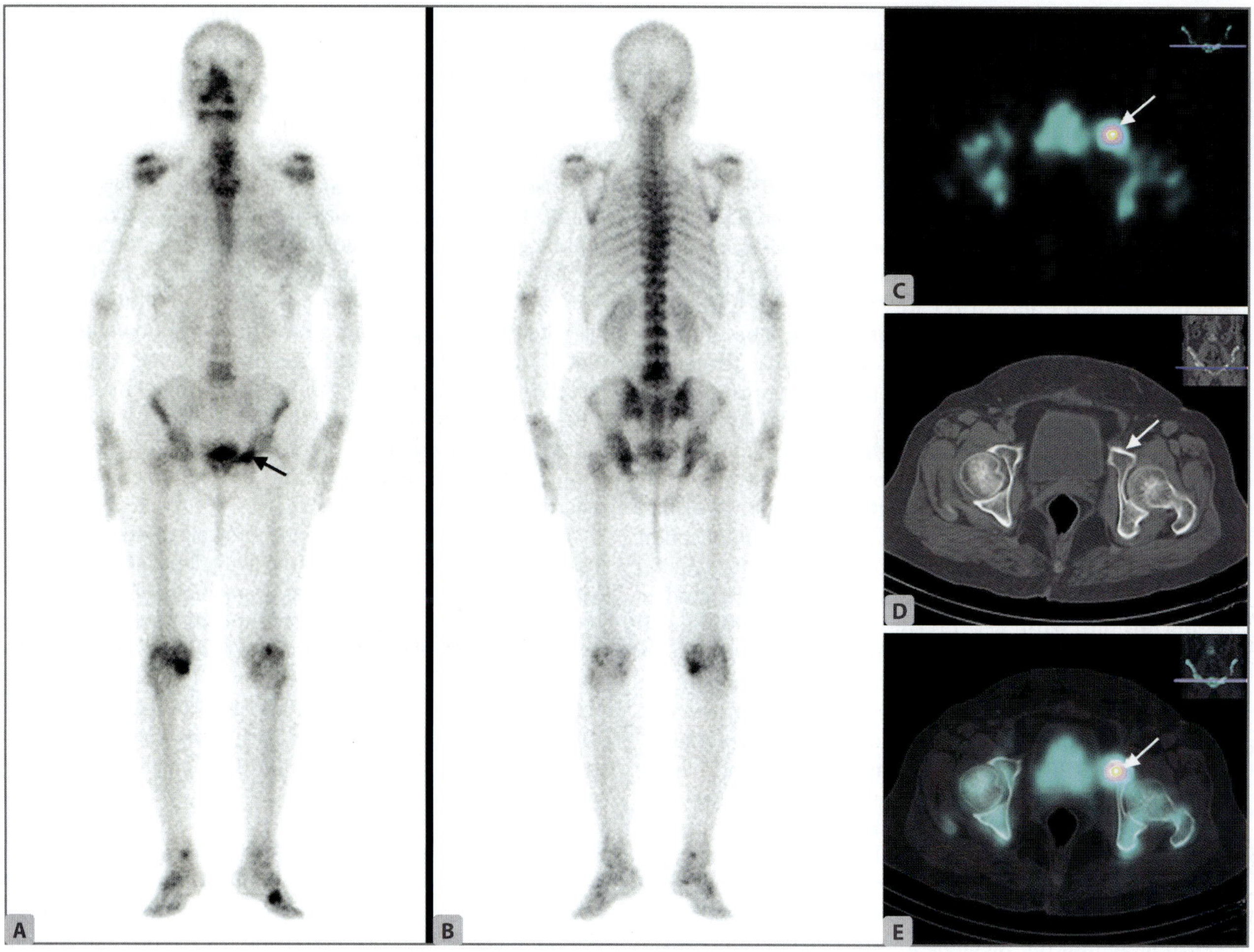

FIGS. 1A TO E: A 37-year-old carcinoma of breast patient for staging. (A and B) Planar bone scintigraphy showed a suspicious focal uptake in left superior pubic rami (arrow). SPECT (C), CT (D), and SPECT (E) images showed lytic lesion with increased tracer uptake (arrows) suggesting metastasis.

or ^{18}F-fluoride activity represents a blastic activity/reparative process in response to tumor and destroyed bone. Compared with BS or ^{18}F-fluoride, FDG-PET is reported to be more sensitive for lytic lesions and bone marrow disease but less sensitive for blastic lesions.[22] It has an additional advantage: the ability to assess extraskeletal metastatic disease, including muscle metastasis.[23] Recent data almost invariably have shown that BS is more sensitive than FDG-PET for detection of blastic/sclerotic lesion, whereas FDG-PET is more sensitive for lytic lesions and bone marrow involvement **(Figs. 3A to D)**.[24] The lower sensitivity of FDG-PET for detecting sclerotic lesions can be complemented by CT, which may obviate the need for BS.[2] For prostatic bone metastasis, Ga-68 PSMA can be used in addition to BS **(Figs. 4A to E)**. It is generally agreed that the overall sensitivity of FDG-PET and BS for all lesions is comparable, but PET has a higher specificity, resulting in an overall higher accuracy. The utility of FDG-PET-CT for bone metastasis has already been shown in breast cancer, lung cancer, lymphoma, multiple myeloma, and neuroblastoma.[25-27] Another very important advantage of FDG-PET-CT is its ability to assess response to therapy in bone metastasis. Although BS has been used to assess the efficacy of treatment and to follow breast cancer patients, the early response to any treatment cannot be assessed by BS. Moreover, BS may show persistent increased activity even in treated lesions for several weeks to months. In most malignancies, FDG-PET has proved an effective modality for early assessment of therapeutic response by showing rapid reduction in FDG uptake by the tumors in responders following chemotherapy.[28] The changes in FDG standard uptake value (SUV) with therapy showed correlation with the overall clinical assessment of response as well as with the change in tumor marker value. Flare phenomenon which is considered to be a marker of response on BS has also been described on FDG-PET but only associated with antiestrogen therapy.[29]

Primary Malignant Tumors

Bone scan has no role in the initial diagnosis or assessment of the extent of primary malignant bone tumors for which MRI is considered the imaging modality of choice. Rather, whole-body BS is generally reserved for evaluation of metastatic bone disease **(Figs. 5A and B)** in these patients. Calcified pulmonary metastases, especially in patients with osteosarcoma, are occasionally identified on BS as focally

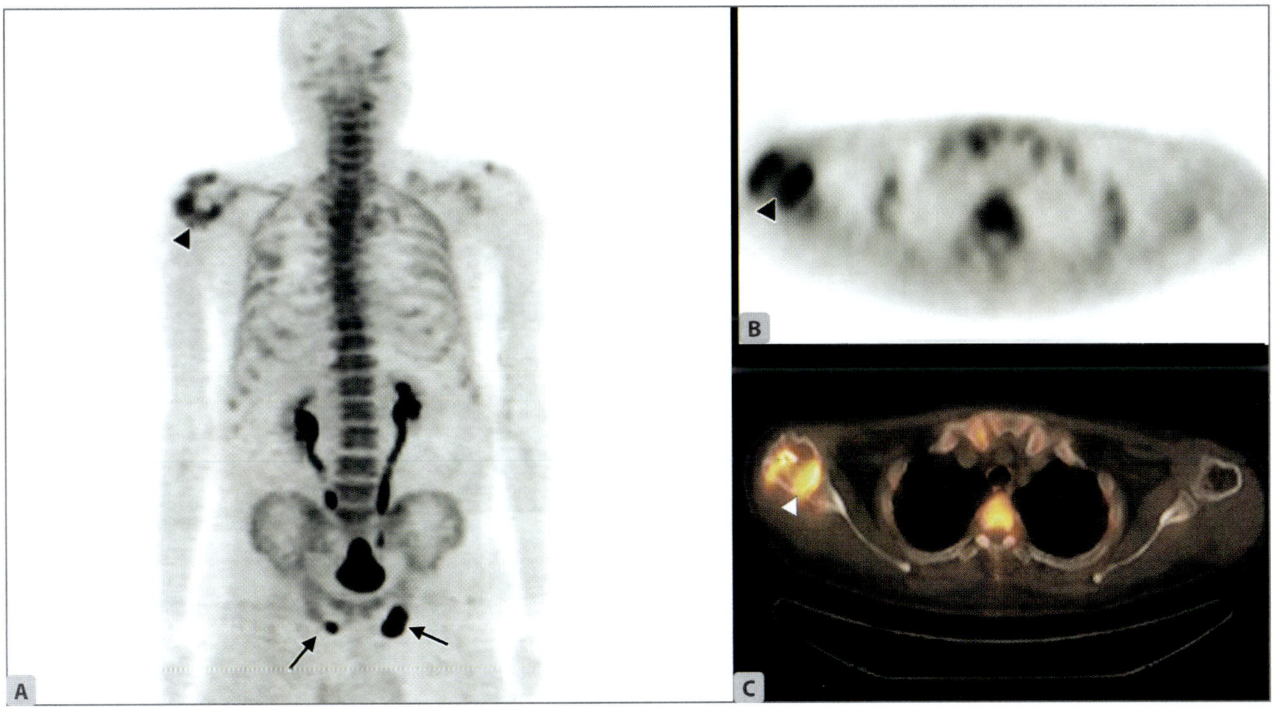

FIGS. 2A TO C: A 60-year-old male with carcinoma of prostate and rising prostate-specific antigen (PSA). (A and B) 18F-fluoride PET maximum intensity projection (MIP) images show focal tracer uptake in bilateral pubic rami (arrows) suggestive of metastasis. Also, noted was tracer uptake in right shoulder (arrowhead); (C) On PET-CT images, this uptake was diagnosed to be degenerative change (arrowhead).

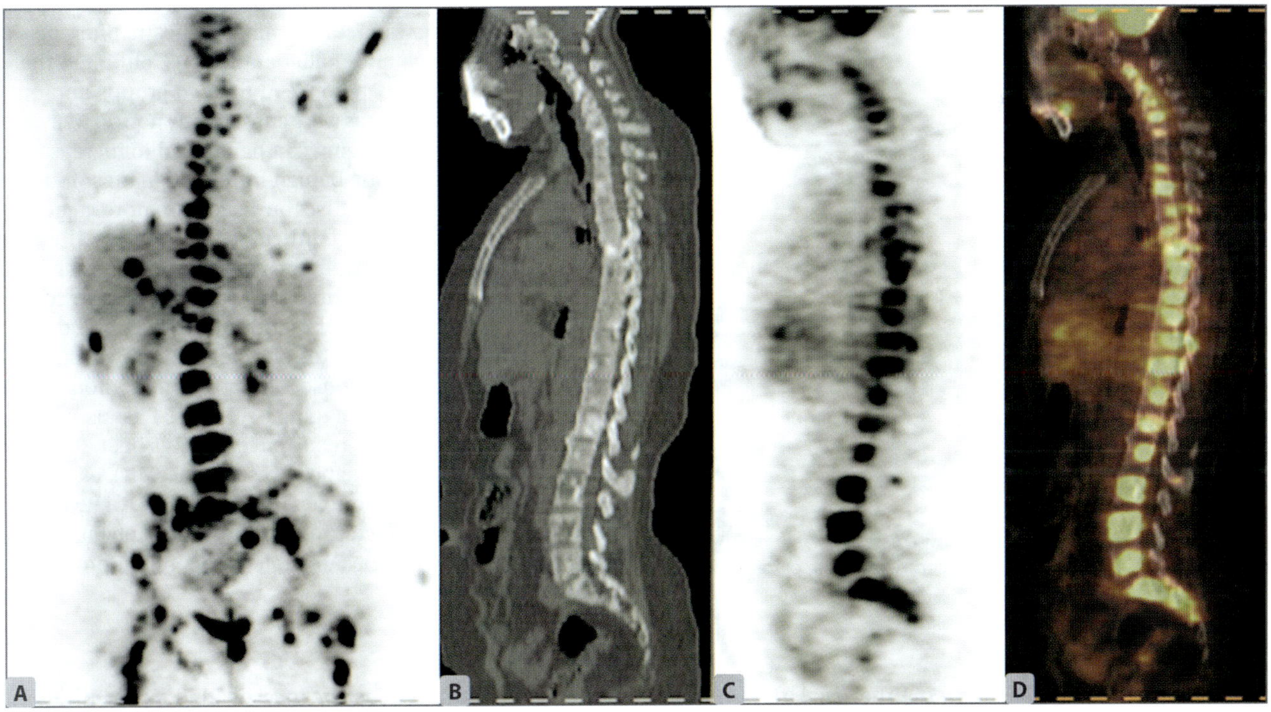

FIGS. 3A TO D: A 35-year-old female with known breast cancer underwent PET-CT scan for staging. 18F-FDG whole body projection image (A) shows focal areas of increased radiotracer uptake suggestive of metastases. Lytic sclerotic bone lesions and FDG uptake in multiple vertebrae in CT, PET, and PET-CT sagittal sections (B to D). There are many lesions showing focal FDG uptake no sclerosis on CT suggestive of marrow metastases.

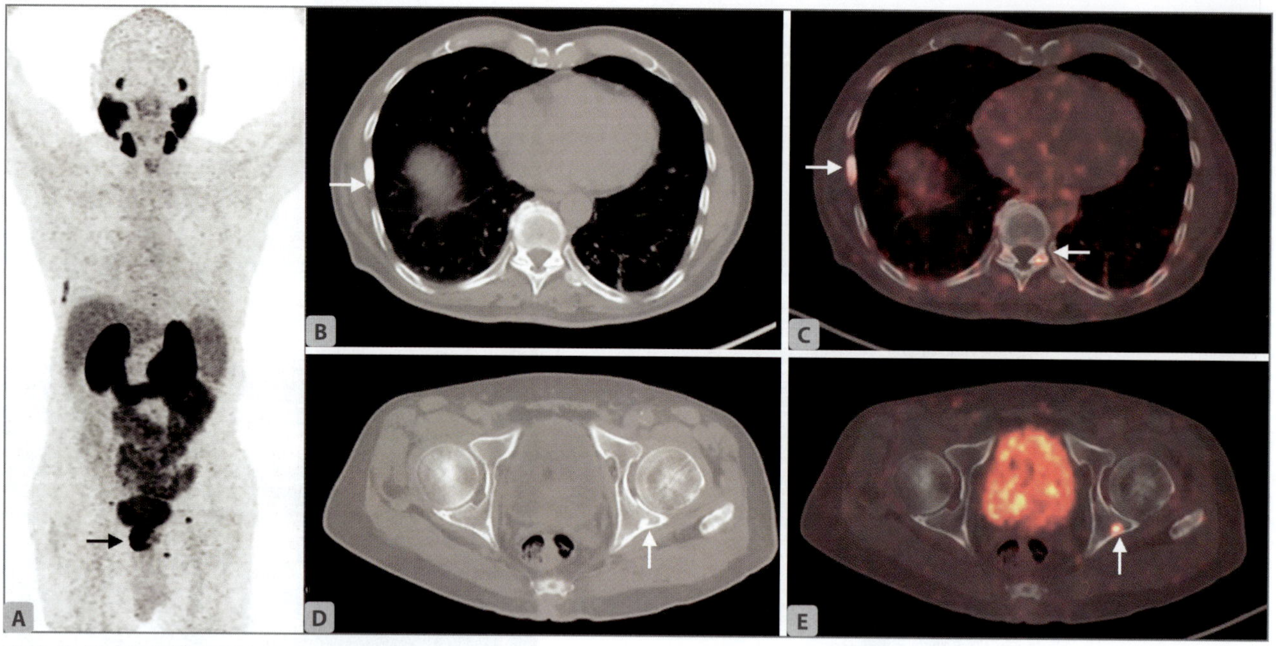

FIGS. 4A TO E: (A) ^{68}Ga-PSMA PET/CT maximum intensity projection image showing heterogeneous increased uptake in prostatic bed with focal uptake in left hip region and physiological uptake in salivary gland, kidney, and bowel loops; (B) Axial CT image showing sclerotic lesion in the rib and left pedicle of vertebra, (C) corresponding fused PET/CT image showing focal uptake (arrows)—consistent with metastases; (D) Axial CT image showing sclerotic lesion in the left acetabulum, corresponding fused PET/CT image (E) showing focal uptake—consistent with metastasis.

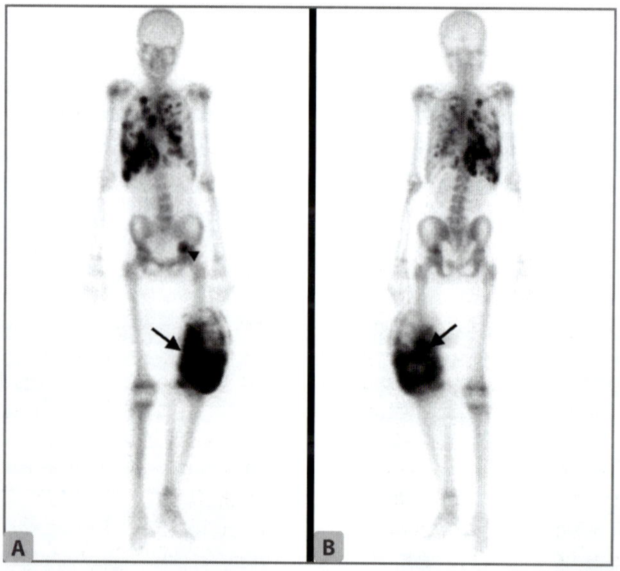

FIGS. 5A AND B: A 16-year-old male with osteosarcoma of left femur. Planar bone scintigraphy (A and B) shows mass in left femoral shaft with heterogeneous tracer uptake (arrows), consistent with primary tumor. In addition, it showed bone metastasis (arrowhead) and osteogenic pulmonary metastasis.

increased tracer uptake **(Fig. 5A)** that can be accurately localized using SPECT/CT. High-resolution CT is the mainstay for the evaluation of pulmonary metastases.

Functional imaging with FDG-PET provides unique information with regard to the metabolic activity of bone and soft tissue tumors **(Figs. 6A to G)**. This may help characterize indeterminate lesions and guide targeted biopsy of the most metabolically active area within larger tumors. This aspect is particularly important in many soft tissue and bone tumors which are of mixed grade and/or cell type. In one study of soft tissue tumors, there was a statistically significant difference in SUV between benign and malignant lesions, although there was considerable overlap between the two groups and only lipomas and hemangiomas were consistently non-FDG avid.[30] Dual-time point PET imaging can be utilized to increase the accuracy of differentiating benign from malignant soft tissue lesions.[31] FDG-PET may also be used for more accurate staging of histologically confirmed tumors, in therapy response assessment to detect progression or response of disease ahead of morphological changes in the tumor and in the early detection of recurrent disease. The degree of FDG uptake by tumors pre- and post-therapy correlates well with histological response, often prior to demonstrable changes on anatomical imaging.[32] FDG-PET is also useful for the detection of tumor recurrence and has been found to be more sensitive than magnetic resonance (MR), especially when MR findings are equivocal.[33] SUV on FDG-PET is an important prognostic factor in most musculoskeletal tumors and has been shown to be a reliable independent prognostic indicator.[34,35]

Benign Tumors

Bone scan is a highly sensitive investigation for the diagnosis of osteoid osteoma. A negative bone scan virtually rules out the diagnosis of osteoid osteoma. A three-phase bone scan shows increased blood flow and blood pool and a "focal" area of intense uptake on delayed images.[36] Some surgeons have used intraoperative scintigraphic probes to localize osteoid osteoma. In addition, BS has been used for detecting

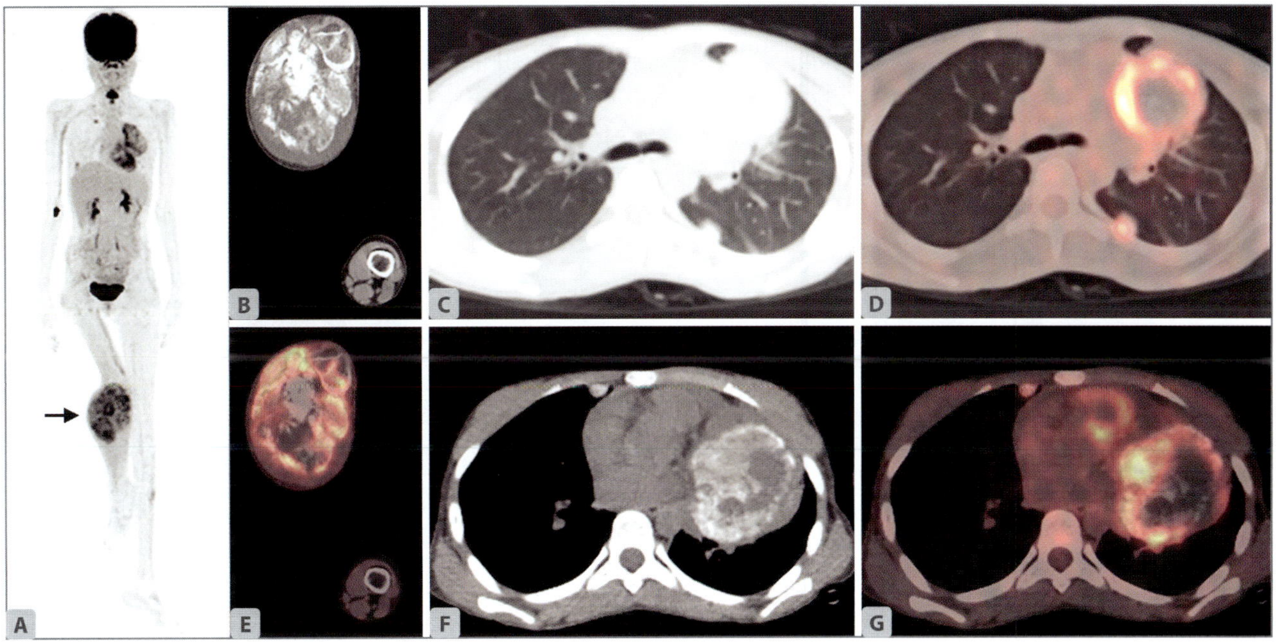

FIGS. 6A TO G: (A) ^{18}F-FDG PET/CT maximum intensity projection images of patient with osteosarcoma of right tibia showing expansile heterogeneous FDG uptake the right knee region (arrow), axial CT and fused PET/CT images at the proximal shaft of right tibia showing FDG avid expansile primary (B and E). Axial CT (C and F) and fused PET/CT (D and G) images at the thoracic level showing multiple calcified masses and nodules (consistent with metastases).

recurrence after radiofrequency ablation of osteoid osteoma. Other benign lesions, which can show increased uptake, are aneurysmal bone cyst, chondroblastoma, enchondroma, etc. However, there is no specific pattern pertaining to these lesions on BS alone. With the availability of hybrid SPECT/CT, these lesions can be characterized with greater certainty by employing their CT characteristics.

INFECTION IMAGING

Acute and Chronic Osteomyelitis

Bone scintigraphy is used as a complementary imaging procedure in the evaluation of infection. The classic findings are increased regional blood flow and blood pool with a corresponding increased uptake on delayed images. This is different from cellulitis where only increase in blood flow and blood pool in the soft tissue with no increased radiotracer uptake on delayed image is seen. ^{99m}Tc MDP has a high sensitivity (82–95%) and accuracy (90%) for detecting acute, uncomplicated osteomyelitis, becoming positive within 28–48 hours after the onset of symptoms. Compared with anatomic modalities, the radionuclide bone scan has the further advantage of detecting multiple foci of disease which can be seen especially in children. However, other conditions (e.g., fractures, neuropathic joints, and arthritis) may mimic osteomyelitis on bone scanning alone, decreasing its specificity.[37] Although adding a fourth phase (24-hour image) is advocated to increase the specificity, with a high accuracy of 85%, the clinical results are not impressive.[38] In addition, in pediatric population, BS can show reduced radiotracer uptake, which is attributed to increased pressure on blood vessels, stripping away of periosteum via the accumulation of pus and interruption of blood supply due to plugging and thrombosis. This can lead to a false negative study. About 30% of patients with acute osteomyelitis will progress to have subacute or chronic osteomyelitis **(Figs. 7A to E)**. Bone scan remains positive for months even after successful treatment of acute osteomyelitis. It is difficult to differentiate healing from chronic active disease.[39]

Other radiotracer, such as ^{67}Ga-citrate and ^{111}In-oxine/^{99m}Tc-hexamethyl-propylene amine oxime (HMPAO)-labeled leukocyte imaging, has been extensively used in musculoskeletal infection, either alone or in combination with BS. ^{67}Ga-citrate localize to the site of infection via several pathway including increased vascular permeability at the site of infection, binding to lactoferrin and direct bacterial uptake.[40] Reported sensitivity for ^{67}Ga-citrate scintigraphy ranges from 25 to 80%, with a specificity of 67%.[41] It has proven to be extremely useful in detecting infection in the immunocompromised population. It is usually done in combination with BS for musculoskeletal infection. However, ^{67}Ga-citrate scintigraphy suffers from poor image quality, long scanning time, and significantly higher patient radiation dose leading to decline in its use with advent of better tracers. Labeled leukocytes can overcome some of the disadvantages of BS. Its uptake is dependent on the chemotaxis of labeled leukocytes at the site of infection. ^{111}In-oxine/^{99m}Tc HMPAO-labeled leukocyte imaging have shown increased specificity—upto 80–90%—compared to BS for detecting infection, particularly when complicating conditions are present. As the majority of leukocytes labeled are neutrophils, the procedure is most useful for identifying neutrophil-mediated inflammatory processes, such as bacterial infections. It is less

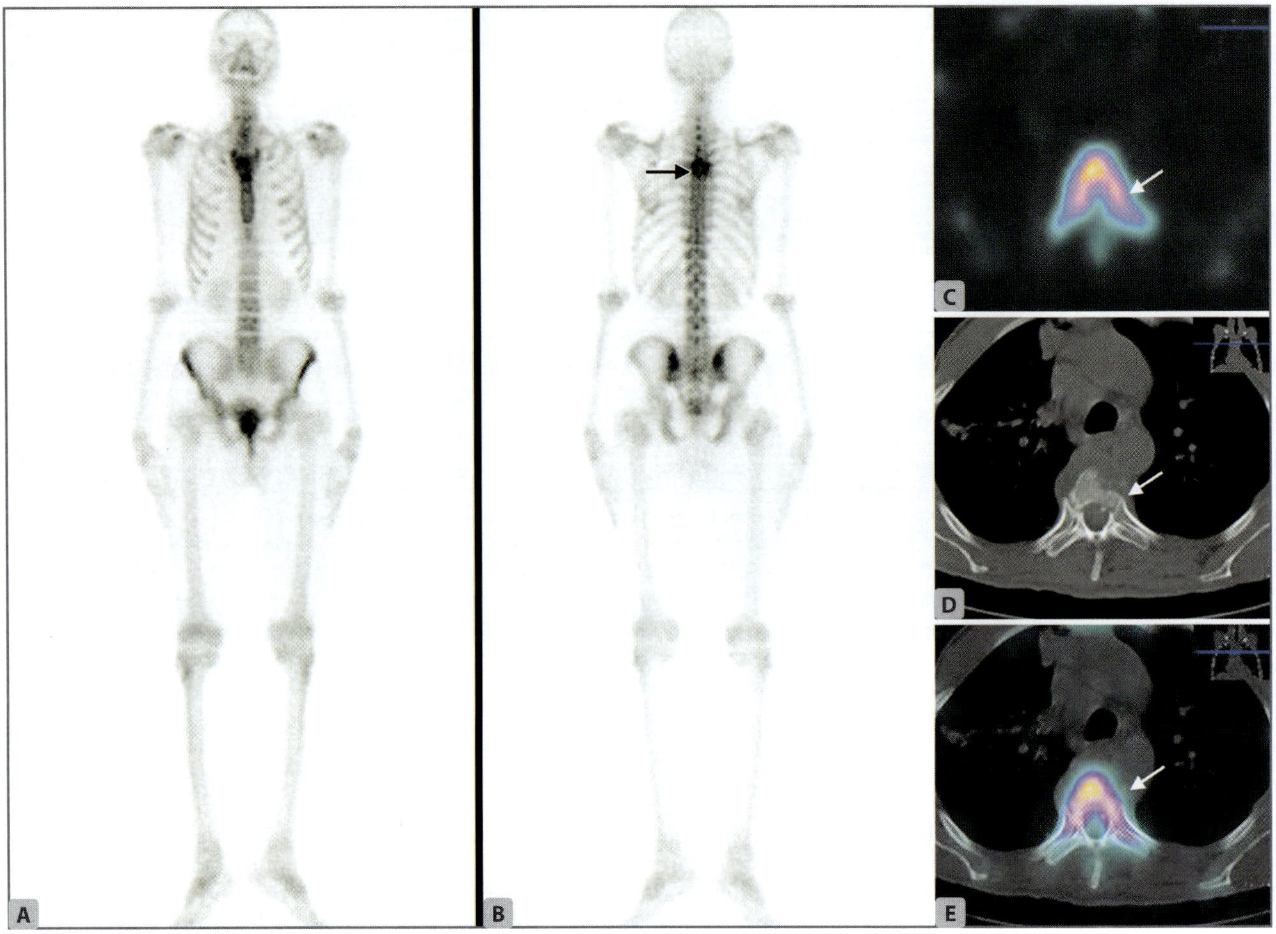

FIGS. 7A TO E: A 35-year-old male with backache. (A and B) Planar bone scintigraphy showed increased irregular tracer uptake in D6 vertebra (arrow). SPECT (C), CT (D), and SPECT-CT (E) images showed destructive changes in D6 vertebra with increased tracer uptake along with paravertebral fluid collection (arrows). The findings were highly suspicious for tuberculosis and confirmed at histopathology.

useful for those illnesses in which the predominant cellular response is other than neutrophilic, such as tuberculosis.[42] Additionally, in contrast to other locations in the skeleton, labeled leukocyte imaging is of limited value for detecting spinal osteomyelitis.[43] Also, their performance requires the withdrawal of a large amount of blood (50 cc); it is also costly, is labor intensive, and has the inherent limitations related to personnel safety, including the risks of infection and cross-contamination from handling blood products. All these factors limit their routine use. Additional use of SPECT/CT with BS, ^{67}Ga-citrate and ^{111}In-oxine/^{99m}Tc HMPAO-labeled leukocyte improves the specificity of these studies for detecting osteomyelitis.[44]

PET-CT-based radiotracers such as ^{18}F-FDG-labeled white blood cell (WBC) and plain ^{18}F-FDG are also being explored for infection imaging. These agents have shown better sensitivity and specificity than SPECT agents and are currently in use for infection imaging **(Figs. 8A to I)**.

Diabetic Foot

Pedal ulcers with or without osteomyelitis is a very common complication in patients with long-standing diabetes. Foot osteomyelitis frequently presents without systemic illness and with no obvious clinical symptoms or signs, besides the ulcer, and imaging studies are often needed to confirm the diagnosis. Although routinely performed, the accuracy of three-phase BS for pedal osteomyelitis is modest with large prospective study demonstrating a sensitivity of 67% and specificity of 43%.[45] With the presence of associated Charcot arthropathy, the diagnosis becomes more difficult. Addition of SPECT-CT in this scenario appears promising.[46] It can show focal bone destruction versus arthropathic changes, thereby clinching the diagnosis **(Figs. 9A to D)**. Labeled leukocyte imaging may be more sensitive for detecting clinically unsuspected pedal osteomyelitis and is useful for monitoring response to medical therapy.[47] But a major drawback is the fact that even neuropathic joints may accumulate labeled leukocyte; hence, it is not useful when both infection and Charcot joint coexist.[48]

Prosthetic Infection

With improving surgical techniques and availability of better prosthetics, the number of patients opting for the same is increasing. Although the clinical results of joint replacement surgery are usually excellent, these implants do fail. Aseptic loosening due to mechanical factors and inflammatory

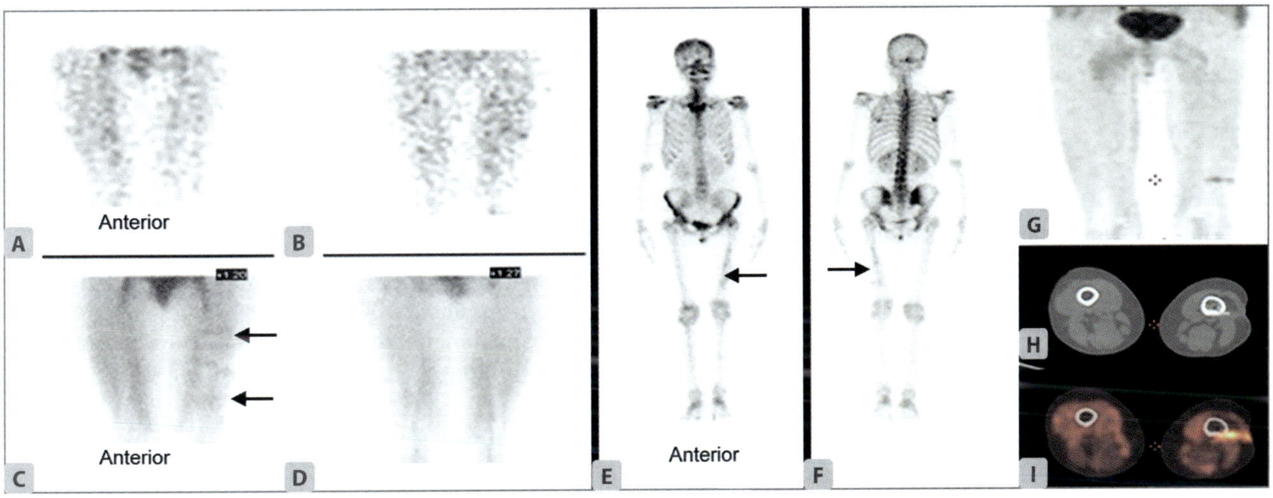

FIGS. 8A TO I: ^{99m}Tc MDP three-phase bone scintigraphy images (Flow A and B, soft tissue/blood pool phase—C and D, delayed phase E and F) and ^{18}F-FDG-PET/CT images (images G to I) of a 37-year-old female with chronic osteomyelitis of left femur. The flow phase images were within normal limits; however, pool showed mild increased radiotracer accumulation in the mid and distal thigh region and delayed phase images showed mild tracer uptake in the mid and distal shaft of femur. FDG-PET/CT was done to rule out infection which showed small area of increased radiotracer uptake in the cortex of distal shaft of femur with calcific changes and increased uptake in the adjacent bone suggestive of residual infection which was confirmed by biopsy culture.

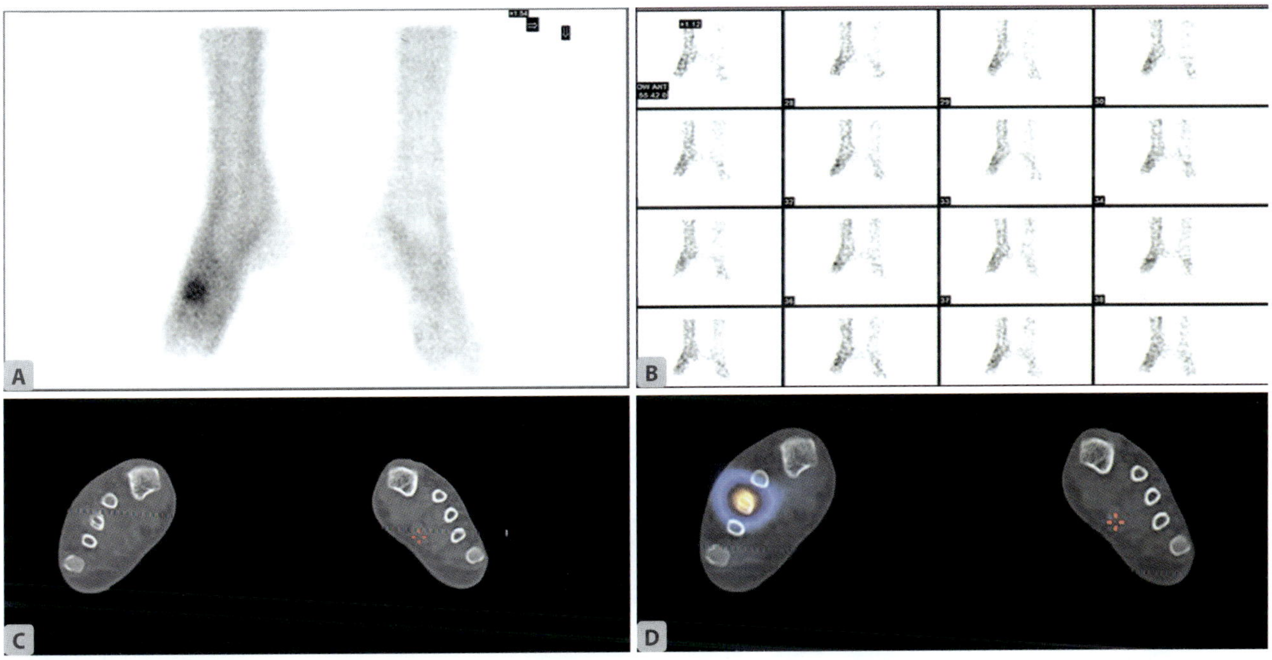

FIGS. 9A TO D: 35-year-old male, known case of diabetic mellitus, having foot ulcer, referred for bone scan to differentiate between cellulitis and osteomyelitis. Blood pool (A) and blood flow (B) images show focal area of increased radiotracer uptake in distal foot region. Axial CT (C) and fused SPECT-CT (D) images showing involvement of right third metatarsal bone—consistent with osteomyelitis.

reaction to prosthetic components is the most common cause for implant failure followed by infection. Infection is perhaps the most serious complication of joint arthroplasty, ranging in frequency from ~1–2% for primary implants to ~3–5% for revision implants.[49] Because their treatments are so different, the importance of distinguishing infection from aseptic loosening of prosthesis cannot be overemphasized. Although BS is sensitive for detecting complications of prosthetic surgery, it cannot reliably distinguish among the causes for failure. Although routinely advocated, periprosthetic uptake patterns are not too useful for differentiating infection from aseptic loosening.[50] Addition of ^{67}Ga-citrate scintigraphy to BS only provides moderate improvement in accuracy.[51] Labeled leukocyte scintigraphy though theoretically presents the advantage of differentiating aseptic loosening from infection, the actual results has been variable.[52,53] Poor sensitivity is ascribed to the chronicity of the process, whereas poor specificity is ascribed to nonspecific inflammation. Addition of BS or marrow scintigraphy might improve the specificity of this test, though there is no general consensus.[54] ^{18}F-FDG-labeled WBC scan and F-18 FDG-PET-CT are also used in these days for distinguishing aseptic and septic loosening **(Figs. 10A to E)**.

FDG-PET-CT for Musculoskeletal Infection

Experimental studies have shown that mononuclear cells and neutrophilic granulocytes have increased FDG uptake when activated during the so-called respiratory burst, which they experience while fighting an infection.[55] This forms the basis for its use in musculoskeletal infections. It provides better resolution and shorter test duration compared to conventional radionuclide procedures, albeit with higher cost and radiation exposure. It should also be remembered that FDG is not specific for infection, and increased FDG uptake also is observed in inflammatory arthritis, osteoarthritis, fractures, normally healing bone, and degenerative changes.[56] For acute and subacute bone and soft tissue infections, sensitivities of 98% and specificities from 75 to 99% have been reported with FDG-PET.[57] It is especially useful in cases of chronic infections where BS has major limitations. It has been shown to be superior to labeled leukocyte imaging for chronic musculoskeletal infections.[58] Its specificity is higher, if recently (<4 months) traumatized or operated bone is excluded. Though initial results were excellent, FDG-PET-CT appears to be less useful for diabetic foot infection.[59] It is inferior to labeled leukocyte imaging for this purpose. Moreover, altered glucose and insulin dynamics in these patients makes FDG technically challenging. Regarding FDG-PET in patients with suspicion of joint prosthesis infection; initial studies showed promising results and reported sensitivities of 90% and specificities of 89% in the diagnosis of infected lower limb prostheses.[60] Accuracy of FDG-PET was 96% for hip prostheses, 81% for knee prostheses, and 100% for other orthopedic devices. However, when associated with loosening, FDG-PET cannot differentiate between septic and aseptic loosening, as both conditions can cause increased FDG uptake.[61] The reason for the increased FDG uptake around the prosthesis in aseptic loosening is likely an inflammatory immune reaction to the prosthetic material. In a large series, the accuracy of FDG-PET for diagnosing infection of the failed prosthetic joint was low, and varied between 47 and 71% depending on different criteria used to evaluate the images.[62] In fact, it was inferior to combined labeled leukocyte/marrow imaging in this series. It should be remembered that image interpretation in patients with prosthetic devices can be affected by attenuation-correction-induced artifacts. Therefore, it is necessary to examine the nonattenuation corrected scans because they show less prominent reconstruction artifacts.[63]

MUSCULOSKELETAL TRAUMA

Stress Fractures

Stress fractures are two types: (1) Fatigue fractures, which are caused by repeated abnormal stress on normal bones, bone scan shows fusiform increased radiotracer uptake involving the posterior tibial cortex and (2) insufficiency fractures resulting from normal stress on abnormal bone. The latter is seen in patients with underlying bone disease such as osteoporosis, osteomalacia, Paget's disease, and fibrous dysplasia. Because clinical assessment usually is not definitive in these injuries, diagnostic imaging is often required. Plain-film radiography is usually the first examination performed when a stress fracture is suspected. Unfortunately, sensitivity of this method for stress fracture may be as low as 15%.[64] BS, however, is extremely sensitive in detecting stress fractures because it assesses bone metabolism rather than bone anatomy **(Figs. 11A to C)**. In fact for stress fracture at certain sites such as metatarsal bones, it is considered to be the reference method. Sacral insufficiency fractures have a classic appearance on BS, highly specific pattern of horizontal uptake in the body of the sacrum and vertical uptake in the alae, resulting in the "Honda" or "H" sign.[36] Addition of SPECT/CT is likely to improve the accuracy of BS, especially by improving the anatomical localization.

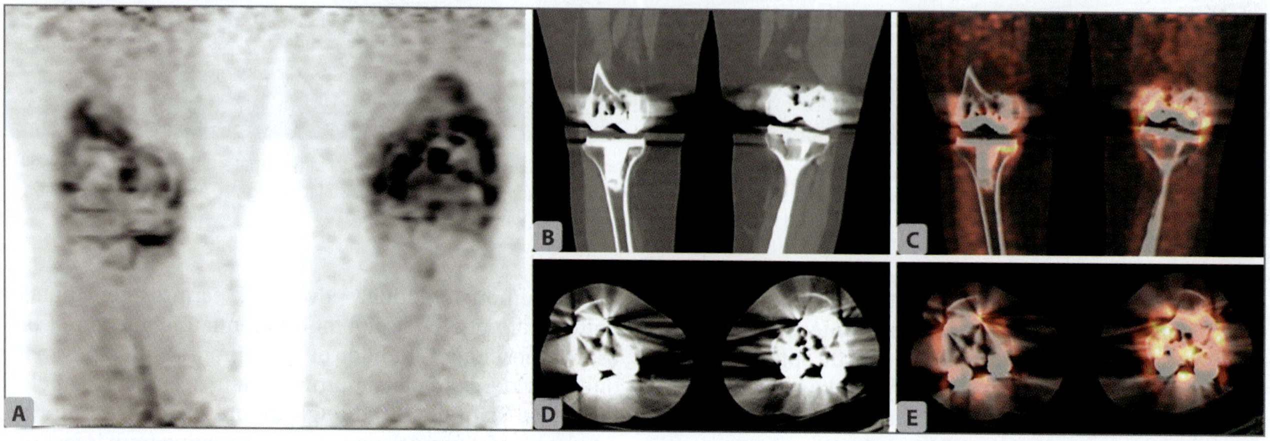

FIGS. 10A TO E: ^{18}F-FDG WBC PET/CT maximum intensity projection image of both knee joint showing increased FDG-labeled WBC accumulation around the prosthesis of left knee joint. Corresponding coronal (A) and axial images of CT (B and D) and fused PET/CT (C and E) show periprosthetic accumulation of labeled WBCs consistent with culture positive prosthetic infection.

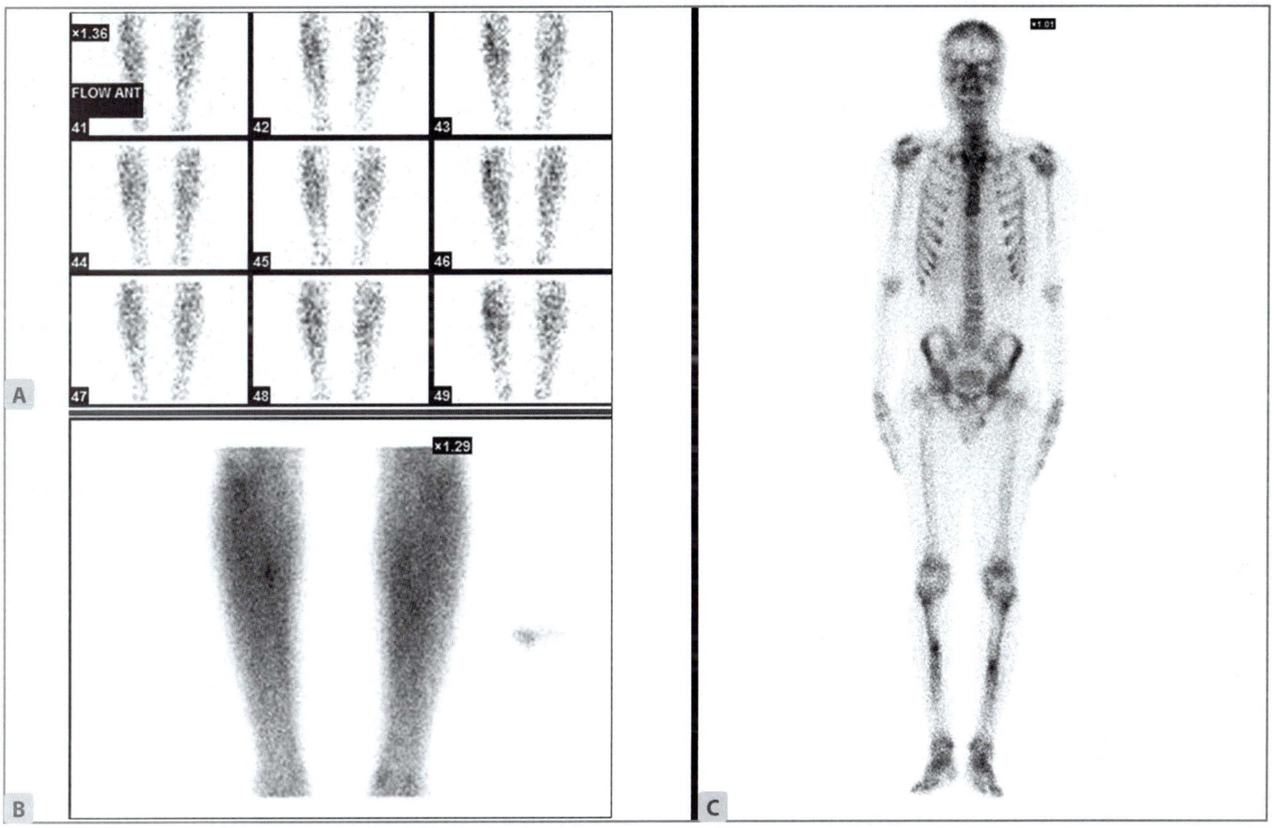

FIGS. 11A TO C: A 25-year-old active male complain of pain in bilateral leg, bone scan showed focal area of increased radiotracer in bilateral tibial region in flow (A), pool (B), and delayed static (C) images suggestive of bilateral stress fractures.

Shin Splints

The clinical entity shin splints is characterized by exercise-induced pain and tenderness on palpation along the posteromedial border of tibia. It results generally from unaccustomed biomechanical stress on the tibia. Shin splints are not fractures and can be distinguished from stress fractures by their linear activity rather than round or fusiform activity.[65] In addition, blood flow and blood pool images are almost always normal. Delayed images of BS demonstrate involvement of the posterior tibial cortex, longitudinally oriented uptake involving one-third of the length of the bone **(Figs. 12A to G)**.

Fractures in Childhood

Very young children may present with failure to move a limb or joint. A history may not be available, especially in preschool children. Bone scans can identify unsuspected sites of fractures in such children. In addition, it can be useful to identify child abuse in children at risk. Radiological skeletal survey and whole-body scintigraphy does offer complementary information that is not available from either study alone.[66] More than 50% of such cases demonstrate diaphyseal injuries.[67] Rarely, fracture of the first rib may be the sole manifestation of abuse. Of course, knowledge of normal BS appearance for the age of child is essential for interpreting such a study.

Sport Injuries

The blood pool phase of BS is very important in detection of soft tissue injuries. Hyperemia is evident in the affected structure with delayed uptake apparent only if there is necrosis/calcification or close apposition of adjacent bony structures, as with tendonitis of the extensor and abductor pollicis tendons and the adjacent radius or tibialis posterior tendonitis and the medial malleolus. SPECT/CT adds by anatomically localizing the site of involvement. It can in addition guide the site of injection, when required.

METABOLIC BONE DISEASE IMAGING

Metabolic bone disorders represent a heterogeneous group of skeletal pathologies that can lead to global or focal changes in bone metabolism. The superior sensitivity of BS can be valuable for diagnosis, detection of complications, and monitoring of treatment response **(Figs. 13A and B)**. The continuous improvement in gamma camera hardware and software with the addition of SPECT, and more recently, hybrid SPECT/CT, has maintained a role for nuclear medicine methods in bone disease despite the improvements seen in morphologic imaging techniques.

Paget's Disease

The initial step in Paget's disease is increased osteoclastic resorption, followed by compensatory osteoblastic activity

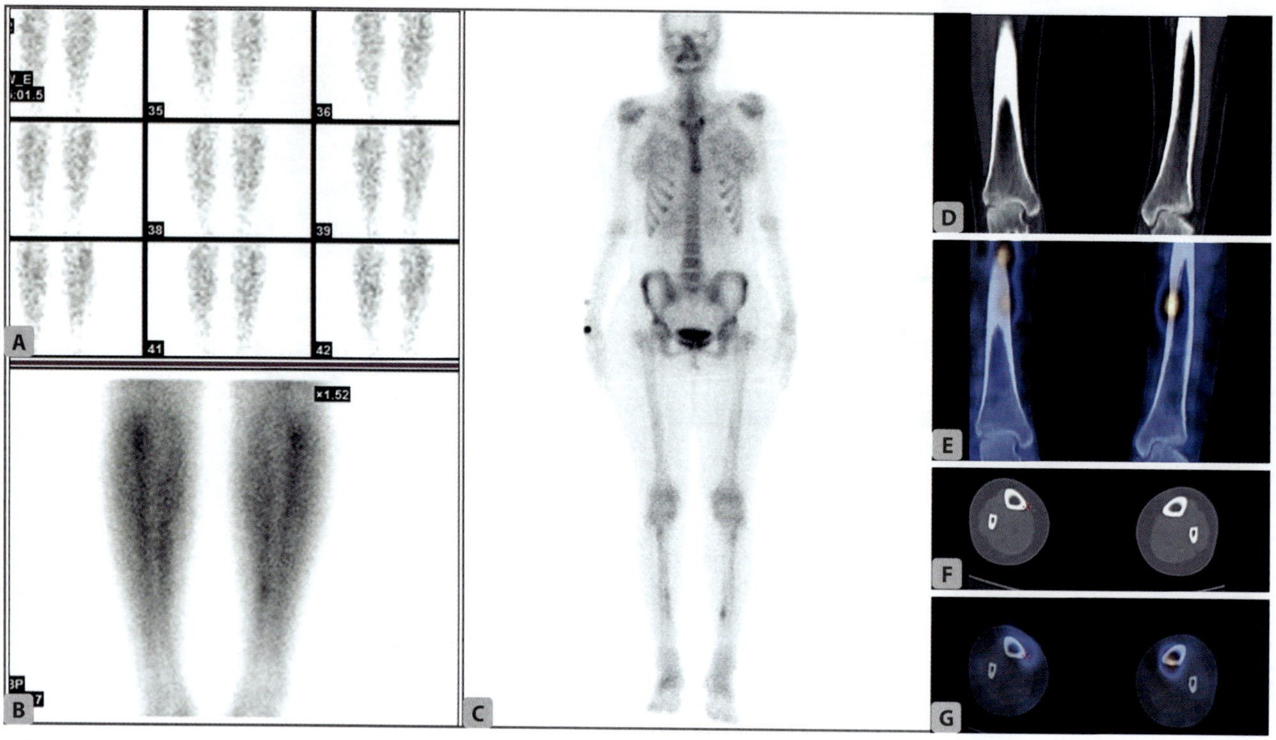

FIGS. 12A TO G: An 18-year-old sports female complains of pain in both legs. Flow (A) and pool (B) images show mild increased radiotracer uptake along the posterolateral border, also noted increased radiotracer along the posterolateral border in delayed static images (C) in addition to focal uptake. CT (D) and fused (E) coronal images, no changes noted on CT images; however, linear uptake noted in the right tibia and focal uptake in mid shaft of the left tibia. Transaxial CT (F) and fused (G) images, on CT, there is no change noted; however, focal uptake noted along the medial boarder of both tibia.

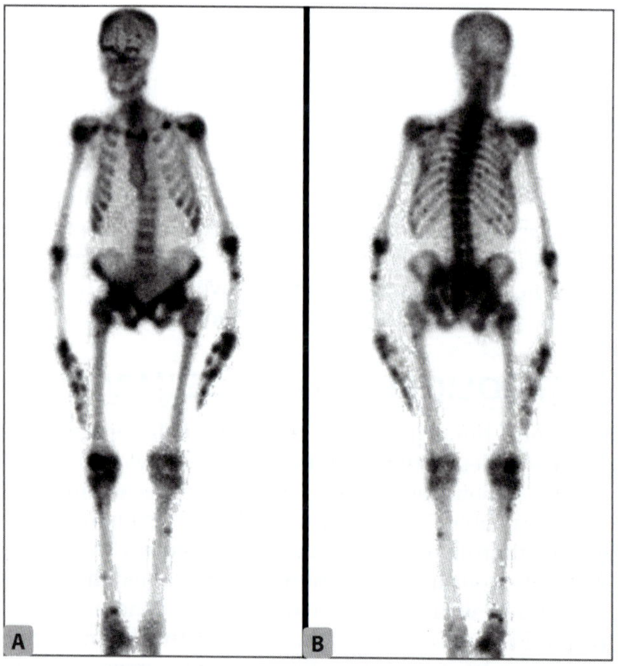

FIGS. 13A AND B: A 29-year-old female presented with multifocal body ache. Biochemical evaluation showed decreased serum calcium. (A and B) Planar bone scintigraphy images showed classical features of metabolic bone disease-increased bone to soft tissue activity, hot calvarium, tie sternum, nonvisualization of kidneys, and multiple pseudofractures classical for osteomalacia.

and increased bone formation. Most patients with Paget's disease have polyostotic disease. Bone scans are a convenient way to evaluate the whole skeleton and has shown a greater sensitivity for detecting affected sites in symptomatic patients in comparison with radiographic skeletal surveys.[68] Characteristically, affected bones show intensely increased activity, extending from the end of a bone and spreading either proximally or distally, often showing a "V"-shaped leading edge **(Figs. 14A to D)**. Many different patterns describing vertebral uptake have been reported as being specific for pagetic involvement, including clover, heart, and Mickey Mouse signs.[69] Apart from localizing the sites of multifocal involvement, another important use of BS is monitoring response to therapy (bisphosphonates). For this purpose, BS is better than measurement of serum alkaline phosphatase alone. The bone scan appearances can be unusual after successful bisphosphonate treatment, resultant heterogeneous uptake sometimes mimicking metastatic disease. As ^{18}F-fluoride PET is better suited to assess bone mineral kinetics, it has also been used to monitor response to bisphosphonate therapy.[70]

Hyperparathyroidism

The diagnosis of hyperparathyroidism is biochemical and BS has no routine role in diagnosis. Bone scans are often used to help differentiate the causes of hypercalcemia, in particular, hyperparathyroidism versus malignancy, so that typical features of metabolic bone disorders may be recognized.

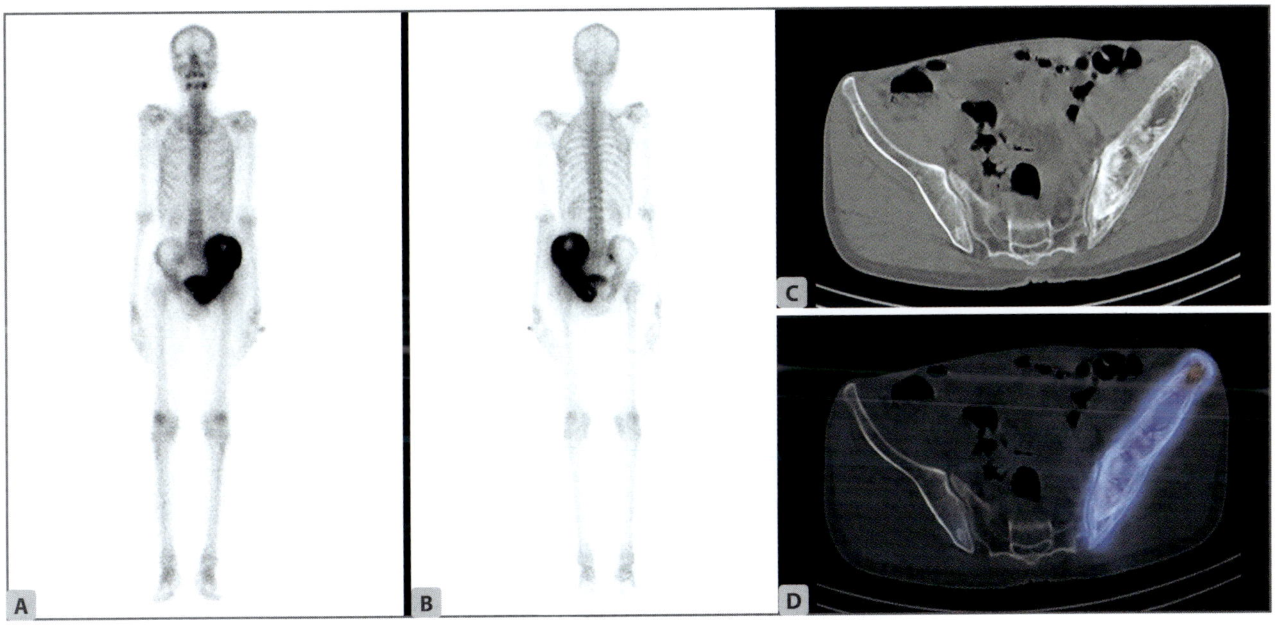

FIGS. 14A TO D: A 57-year-old female complains of pain in the left hip. Anterior (A) and posterior (B) images show intense radiotracer uptake in the left iliac bone in delayed static images. Transaxial CT (C) and fused (D) images, on CT, there is lytic and sclerotic changes in left iliac bone noted. There is no other lesion in the rest of whole body bone scan.

The most common bone scan appearance is similar to a superscan from other metabolic bone disorders, and uptake of diphosphonate in areas of ectopic calcification also may be seen. Multiple focal areas of abnormal radiotracer uptake in bone scan are suggestive of brown tumors in such patients, which can be well characterized on SPECT/CT.[36]

Renal Osteodystrophy

Renal osteodystrophy is due to a combination of bone disorders as a consequence of chronic renal dysfunction, and often demonstrates the most severe cases of metabolic bone disease. It may comprise osteoporosis, osteomalacia, adynamic bone, and secondary hyperparathyroidism in varying degrees. The most common bone scan appearance is similar to a superscan from other metabolic bone disorders. A clue in differentiating this type of scintigraphic pattern from others is that there may be a lack of bladder activity in view of renal failure. Quantitative measurements of bone metabolism in renal osteodystrophy using ^{18}F-fluoride have been compared with bone histomorphometry and have shown a close relationship.[71]

Osteoporosis and Osteomalacia

Bone scans have no routine clinical role in the diagnosis of osteoporosis *per se* but is most often used in established osteoporosis to diagnose fractures, particularly at sites that are difficult to image with plain film radiography (e.g., sacrum and ribs), and may be particularly useful in the diagnosis of vertebral fractures and in distinguishing malignancy-related vertebral fractures from osteoporotic ones. The characteristic appearance of this type of fracture is of intense, linearly increased tracer uptake at the affected vertebral level which in metastatic collapse extends into the posterior elements and is limited to the body only in osteoporotic collapse. In addition, bone scan is extremely helpful in assessing the age of the fracture. Also, other causes of bone pain can be reliably excluded in osteoporotic patients on BS. Osteomalacia on the other hand shows features similar to other metabolic bone disease. This is probably because of increased osteoid formation. The detection of pseudofractures with this technique is more sensitive than that with radiography.[72]

Bone Dysplasias

Fibrous dysplasia is characterized by a slow, progressive, replacement of the medullary cavity by fibrocollagenous tissue. There is usually intense hyperemia and intense uptake with well-delineated margins on BS. Failure of preservation of the bony outline differentiates fibrous dysplasia from Paget's disease. Identification of polyostotic involvement, which is often asymptomatic, is the main indication for BS.[73] In addition, secondary complications in fibrous dysplasia can be demonstrated on BS. In several other uncommon congenital dysplasias, skeletal abnormalities are usually obvious radiologically. BS can occasionally provide images that are of interest but, more importantly, reflect current physiological activity. The BS findings are variable depending on the type and the site of dysplasia. Additionally, BS might be used for monitoring therapy response.

Avascular Necrosis

Avascular necrosis (AVN) is a common condition affecting up to 30% of individuals with underlying medical conditions requiring steroids. Although the hip is most commonly involved, AVN may affect many other bones, such as lunate (Kienböck's disease), navicular (Kohler's disease), scaphoid (post-fracture), and jaw (post-bisphosphonate therapy).

Although MRI is the investigation of choice, a three-phase BS provides useful information to diagnose AVN. A unique advantage of BS is its ability to identify AVN earlier than MRI (72 hours vs. 6 days).[74] Up to 85%, BS may be normal for first 48 hours, the femoral head then shows decreased activity ("cold") for a variable period followed by increased activity due to reparative process. BS is highly sensitive (98%) and specific (95%) for the diagnosis of AVN.[75] SPECT images improve sensitivity to detect AVN. SPECT/CT images are very useful, especially when evaluating small bones.

Complex Regional Pain Syndrome (Reflex Sympathetic Dystrophy)

The complex regional pain syndrome (CRPS) comprises a spectrum of sensory, autonomic, and motor features that predominantly affect the extremities. CRPS I occurs in the absence of definable neurological abnormality. Radiological changes of bone resorption are late findings and hence three-phase BS has been widely utilized in both the diagnosis and the monitoring of treatment. The BS pattern of reflex sympathetic dystrophy (RSD) varies significantly, depending upon the stage of the disease. In early stages, there is increased blood flow and blood pool with increased bone uptake on delayed images **(Figs. 15A to E)**. A characteristic feature is periarticular uptake of radiotracer. In later stages of RSD, bone scan shows normal or even decreased blood flow and blood pool but increased uptake on delayed images on the affected side.[76] In addition, patients with BS abnormalities have higher response rate (90%) to systemic steroid therapy as compared to those without BS findings (36%).[77]

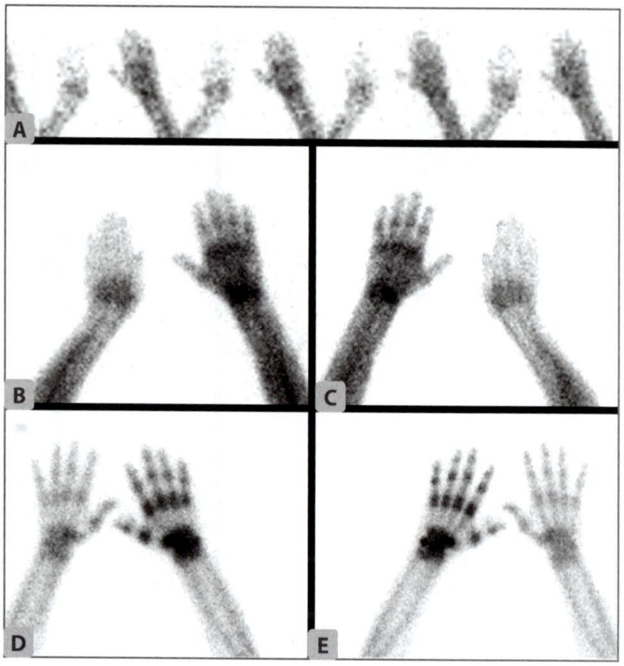

FIGS. 15A TO E: A 42-year-old male presented with swelling and pain in the left hand 3 months after a minor surgery. Three-phase bone scintigraphy showed increased blood flow (A) and pool (B and C) in the left hand along with classical periarticular uptake in small joints (D and E in delayed images, suggestive of CRPS (reflex sympathetic dystrophy).

JOINT IMAGING

The role of BS is usually complementary to anatomical imaging for joint disease. The major role of BS is in the early detection of subclinical synovitis and monitoring its response to treatment. Scintigraphy is sensitive for the early detection of sacroiliitis, although MRI is used routinely. Three-phase bone scans are as sensitive as MRI for identifying early rheumatoid arthritis. Bone scans are very sensitive for the diagnosis of septic arthritis and become abnormal much earlier than radiographs. Multiphase BS shows increased flow and blood pool in soft tissue and joint and diffuses increased uptake in bones around joints on delayed images. This is especially useful in pediatric population.

FUTURE DIRECTION AND THERANOSTICS

Further improvement in imaging technology and development of newer radiopharmaceuticals will keep on strengthening and redefining the role of nuclear medicine imaging. Routine use of SPECT/CT and PET/CT on one hand will improve the accuracy and on the other hand will broaden the range of indications with respect to musculoskeletal imaging. Another exiting development is hybrid PET/MRI, which when clinically available, might revolutionize musculoskeletal imaging providing high quality images (anatomical and functional) with less radiation burden. PET tracers such as ^{18}F-fluoroestradiol, ^{18}F-fluorothymidine, and ^{18}F-fluorocholine will improve the utilization of PET/CT for diagnosis, response monitoring, and prognostication of musculoskeletal tumors. In addition, FDG as well as FDG-labeled leukocyte PET/CT might gain more and more ground for infection imaging.

CONCLUSION

Despite challenges from morphological imaging, nuclear medicine imaging techniques continue to have a major role in a range of neoplastic, infective, inflammatory, metabolic, and traumatic musculoskeletal diseases. In future, with widespread availability of hybrid modalities, its role in musculoskeletal imaging will continue to expand.

REFERENCES

1. Fogelman I. Skeletal uptake of diphosphonates: a review. Eur J Nucl Med. 1980;5(6):473-6.
2. Even-Sapir E. Imaging of malignant bone involvement by morphologic, scintigraphic and hybrid modalities. J Nucl Med. 2005;46(8):1356-67.
3. Kubota R, Yamada S, Kubota K, Ishiwata K, Tamahashi N, Ido T. Intratumoral distribution of uorine-18-uorodeoxyglucose in vivo: high accumulation in macrophages and granulation tissues studied by microautoradiography. J Nucl Med. 1992;33(11):1972-80.
4. Blake GM, Park-Holohan SJ, Cook GJ, Fogelman I. Quantitative studies of bone with the use of 18F-fluoride and ^{99m}Tc-methylene diphosphonate. Semin Nucl Med. 2001;31:28-49.
5. Schirrmeister H, Guhlmann A, Elsner K, Kotzerke J, Glatting G, Rentschler M, et al. Sensitivity in detecting osseous lesions depends on anatomic localization: planar bone scintigraphy versus 18F PET. J Nucl Med. 1999;40(10):1623-9.
6. Schirrmeister H. Detection of bone metastases in breast cancer by positron emission tomography. Radiol Clin North Am. 2007;45(4):669-76.
7. Van der Wall H, Clarke S. The evaluation of malignancy: metastatic bone disease. In: Ell PJ, Gambhir SS, (Eds). Nuclear Medicine in Clinical Diagnosis and Treatment. Edinburgh: Churchill Livingstone; 2004. pp. 641-55.
8. Krasnow AZ, Hellman RS, Timins ME, Collier BD, Anderson T, Isitman AT. Diagnostic bone scanning in oncology. Semin Nucl Med. 1997;27(2):107-41.
9. Tryciecky EW, Gottschalk A, Ludema K. Oncologic imaging: interactions of nuclear medicine with CT and MRI using the one scan as the model. Semin Nucl Med. 1997;27(2):142-51.
10. Gates GF. SPECT bone scanning of the spine. Semin Nucl Med. 1998;28(1):78-94.
11. Savelli G, Mafoli L, Maccauro M, De Deckere E, Bombardieri E. Bone scintigraphy and the added value of SPECT (single photon emission tomography) in detecting skeletal lesions. Q J Nucl Med. 2001;45(1):27-37.
12. Kosuda S, Kaji T, Yokohama H, Yokokawa T, Katayama M, Iriye T, et al. Does bone SPECT actually have lower sensitivity for detecting vertebral metastasis than MRI? J Nucl Med. 1996;37(6):975-8.
13. Even-Sapir E, Flusser G, Lerman H, Lievshitz G, Metser U, et al. SPECT/multislice low-dose CT: a clinically relevant constituent in the imaging algorithm of nononcologic patients referred for bone scintigraphy. J Nucl Med. 2007;48(2):319-24.
14. Sharma P, Singh H, Kumar R, Bal C, Thulkar S, Seenu V, et al. XBone scintigraphy in breast cancer: added value of hybrid SPECT-CT and its impact on patient management. Nucl Med Commun. 2012;33(2):139-47.
15. Sharma P, Kumar R, Singh H, Bal C, Julka PK, Thulkar S, et al. Indeterminate lesions on planar bone scintigraphy in lung cancer patients: SPECT, CT or SPECT-CT? Skeletal Radiol. 2012;41(7):843-50.
16. Petrén-Mallmin M, Andréasson I, Ljunggren O, Ahlström H, Bergh J, Antoni G, et al. Skeletal metastases from breast cancer: uptake of 18F-fluoride measured with positron emission tomography in correlation with CT. Skeletal Radiol. 1998;27(2):72-6.
17. Even-Sapir E, Metser U, Mishani E, Lievshitz G, Lerman H, Leibovitch I. The detection of bone metastases in patients with high-risk prostate cancer: 99mTc-MDP planar bone scintigraphy, single- and multi-field-of-view SPECT, 18F- Fluoride PET, and 18F-Fluoride PET/CT. J Nucl Med. 2006;47(2):287-97.
18. Schirrmeister H, Guhlmann A, Kotzerke J, Santjohanser C, Kühn T, Kreienberg R, et al. Early detection and accurate description of extent of metastatic bone disease in breast cancer with fluoride ion and positron emission tomography. J Clin Oncol. 1999;17(8):2381-9.
19. Langsteger W, Heinisch M, Fogelman I. The role of fluorodeoxyglucose, 18F-dihydroxyphenylalanine, 18F-choline, and 18F-Fluoride in bone imaging with emphasis on prostate and breast. Semin Nucl Med. 2006;36(1):73-92.
20. Schirrmeister H, Glatting G, Hetzel J, Nüssle K, Arslandemir C, Buck AK, et al. Prospective evaluation of clinical value of planar bone scan, SPECT and 18F-labeled NaF PET in newly diagnosed lung cancer. J Nucl Med. 2001;42(12):1800-4.
21. Hetzel M, Arslandemir C, Konig HH, Buck AK, Nüssle K, Glatting G, et al. F-18 NaF PET for detection of bone metastases in lung cancer: accuracy, cost-effectiveness, and impact on patient management. J Bone Miner Res. 2003;18(12):2206-14.
22. Cook GJ, Houston S, Rubens R, Maisey MN, Fogelman I. Detection of bone metastases in breast cancer by 18FDG PET: differing metabolic activity in osteoblastic and osteolytic lesions. J Clin Oncol. 1998;16(10):3375-9.
23. Yilmaz M, Elboga U, Celen Z, Isik F, Tutar E. Multiple muscle metastases from lung cancer detected by FDG PET/CT. Clin Nucl Med. 2011;36(3):245-7.
24. Yang SN, Liang JA, Lin FJ, Kao CH, Lin CC, Lee CC. Comparing whole body (18)F-2-deoxyglucose positron emission tomography and technetium-99m methylene diphosphonate bone scan to detect bone metastases in patients with breast cancer. J Cancer Res Clin Oncol. 2002;128(6):325-8.
25. Cheran SK, Herndon JE 2nd, Patz EF Jr. Comparison of whole-body FDG-PET to bone scan for detection of bone metastases in patients with a new diagnosis of lung cancer. Lung Cancer. 2004;44(3):317-25.
26. Antoch G, Vogt FM, Freudenberg LS, Nazaradeh F, Goehde SC, Barkhausen J, et al. Whole-body dual-modality PET/CT and whole-body MRI for tumor staging in oncology. JAMA. 2003;290(24):3199-206.
27. Kushner BH. Neuroblastoma: a disease requiring a multitude of imaging studies. J Nucl Med. 2004;45(7):1172-88.
28. Stafford SE, Gralow JR, Schubert EK, Rinn KJ, Dunnwald LK, Livingston RB, et al. Use of serial FDG PET to measure the response of bone-dominant breast cancer to therapy. Acad Radiol. 2002;9(8):913-21.
29. Mortimer JE, Dehdashti F, Siegel BA, Trinkaus K, Katzenellenbogen JA, Welch MJ. Metabolic flare: indicator of hormone responsiveness in advanced breast cancer. J Clin Oncol. 2001;19(11):2797-803.
30. Aoki J, Watanabe H, Shinozaki T, Takagishi K, Tokunaga M, Koyama Y, et al. FDG-PET for pre- operative differential diagnosis between benign and malignant soft tissue masses. Skeletal Radiol. 2003;32(3):133-8.
31. Chen YM, Huang G, Sun XG, Liu JJ, Chen T, Shi YP, et al. Optimizing delayed scan time for FDG PET: comparison of the early and late delayed scan. Nucl Med Commun. 2008;29(5):425-30.
32. Evilevitch V, Weber WA, Tap WD, Allen-Auerbach M, Chow K, Nelson SD, et al. Reduction of glucose metabolic activity is more accurate than change in size at predicting histopathologic response to neoadjuvant therapy in high-grade soft-tissue sarcomas. Clin Cancer Res. 2008;14(3):715-20.
33. Dimitrakopoulou-Strauss A, Strauss LG, Schwarzbach MH, Burger C, Heichel T, Willeke F, et al. Dynamic PET 18F-FDG studies in patients with primary and recurrent soft-tissue sarcomas: impact on diagnosis and correlation with grading. J Nucl Med. 2001;42(5):713-20.
34. Adler LP, Blair HF, Makley JT, Williams RP, Joyce MJ, Leisure G, et al. Noninvasive grading of musculoskeletal tumors using PET. J Nucl Med. 1991;32(8):1508-12.

35. Ioannidis JP, Lau J. 18F-FDG PET for the diagnosis and grading of soft tissue sarcoma: a meta-analysis. J Nucl Med. 2003;44(5):717-24.
36. Sartoris DJ. Skeletal System: The Requisites. St Louis: Mosby; 2001. pp. 110-44.
37. Palestro CJ, Torres MA. Radionuclide imaging in orthopedic infections. Semin Nucl Med. 1997;27(4):334-45.
38. Israel O, Gips S, Jerushalmi J, Frenkel A, Front D. Osteomyelitis and soft-tissue infection: differential diagnosis with 24 hour/ 4 hour ratio of Tc-99m MDP uptake. Radiology. 1987;163(3):725-6.
39. Anderson SE, Heini P, Sauvain MJ, Stauffer E, Geiger L, Johnston JO, et al. Imaging of chronic recurrent multifocal osteomyelitis of childhood first presenting with isolated primary spinal involvement. Skeletal Radiol. 2003;32(6):328-36.
40. Palestro CJ. The current role of gallium imaging in infection. Semin Nucl Med. 1994;24(2):128-41.
41. Pineda C, Vargas A, Rodriguez AV. Imaging of osteomyelitis: current concepts. Infect Dis Clin N Am. 2006;20(4): 789-825.
42. Fineman DS, Palestro CJ, Kim CK, Needle LB, Vallabhajosula S, Solomon RW, et al. Detection of abnormalities in febrile AIDS patients with In-111-labeled leukocyte and GA-67 scintigraphy. Radiology. 1989;170(3):677-80.
43. Whalen JL, Brown ML, McLeod R, Fitzgerald RH Jr. Limitations of indium leukocyte imaging for the diagnosis of spine infections. Spine. 1991;16(2):193-7.
44. Linke R, Kuwert T, Uder M, Forst R, Wuest W. Skeletal SPECT/ CT of the peripheral extremities. AJR Am J Roentgenol. 2010;194(4):W329-35.
45. Shults DW, Hunter GC, McIntyre KE, Parent FN, Piotrowski JJ, Bernhard VM. Value of radiographs and bone scans in determining the need for therapy in diabetic patients with foot ulcers. Am J Surg. 1989;158(6):525-30.
46. Heiba SI, Kolker D, Mocherla B, Kapoor K, Jiang M, Son H, et al. The optimized evaluation of diabetic foot infection by dual isotope SPECT/CT imaging protocol. J Foot Ankle Surg. 2010;49(6): 529-36.
47. Newman LG, Waller J, Palestro CJ, Hermann G, Klein MJ, Schwartz M, et al. Leukocyte scanning with 111In is superior to magnetic resonance imaging in the diagnosis of clinically unsuspected osteomyelitis in diabetic foot ulcers. Diabetes Care. 1992;15(11):1527-30.
48. Hayashida K, Ochi T, Fujimoto M, Owaki H, Shimaoka Y, Ono K, et al. Bone marrow changes in adjuvant-induced and collagen-induced arthritis. Interleukin-1 and interleukin-6 activity and abnormal myelopoiesis. Arthritis Rheum. 1992;35(2):241-5.
49. Hanssen AD, Rand JA. Evaluation and treatment of infection at the site of a total hip or knee arthroplasty. Instr Course Lect. 1999;48:111-22.
50. Aliabadi P, Tumeh SS, Weissman BN, McNeil BJ. Cemented total hip prosthesis: radiographic and scintigraphic evaluation. Radiology. 1989;173(1):203-6.
51. Love C, Tronco GG, Yu AK, Marwin S, Nichols K, Palestro C. Diagnosing the infected prosthetic hip: an intraindividual comparison of three- phase bone, bone, gallium, bone/gallium, leukocyte, leukocyte/bone, and leukocyte/marrow imaging. Eur J Nucl Med Mol Imaging. 2007;34(Suppl 2):(P)S384.
52. Pring DJ, Henderson RG, Rivett AG, Krausz T, Coombs RR, Lavender JP. Autologous granulocyte scanning of painful prosthetic joints. J Bone Joint Surg Br. 1986;68(4):647-52.
53. Wukich DK, Abreu SH, Callaghan JJ, Van Nostrand D, Savory CG, Eggli DF, et al. Diagnosis of infection by preoperative scintigraphy with indium labeled white blood cells. J Bone Joint Surg Am. 1987;69(9):1353-60.
54. Love C, Tronco GG, Yu AK, Marwin S, Nichols K, Palestro C, et al. Diagnosing lower extremity prosthetic joint infection: intraindividual comparison of leukocyte/marrow and leukocyte/ bone imaging. J Nucl Med. 2007;48(Suppl):62.
55. Mochizuki T, Tsukamoto E, Kuge Y, Kanegae K, Zhao S, Hikosaka K, et al. FDG uptake and glucose transporter subtype expressions in experimental tumor and inflammation models. J Nucl Med. 2001;42(10):1551-5.
56. Beckers C, Jeukens X, Ribbens C, André B, Marcelis S, Leclercq P, et al. (18)F-FDG PET imaging of rheumatoid knee synovitis correlates with dynamic magnetic resonance and sonographic assessments as well as with the serum level of metalloproteinase-3. Eur J Nucl Med Mol Imaging. 2006;33(3):275-80.
57. Stumpe KD, Dazzi H, Schaffner A, von Schulthess GK. Infection imaging using wholebody FDG-PET. Eur J Nucl Med. 2000;27(7):822-32.
58. de Winter F, van de Wiele C, Vogelaers D, de Smet K, Verdonk R, Dierckx RA. Fluorine-18 fluorodeoxyglucose positron emission tomography: a highly accurate imaging modality for the diagnosis of chronic musculoskeletal infections. J Bone Joint Surg Am. 2001;83(5):651-60.
59. Familiari D, Glaudemans AW, Vitale V, Prosperi D, Bagni O, Lenza A, et al. Can sequential 18F-FDG PET/CT replace WBC imaging in the diabetic foot? J Nucl Med. 2011;52(7):1012-9.
60. Zhuang H, Duarte PS, Pourdehnad M, Maes A, Van Acker F,Shnier D, et al. The promising role of 18F-FDG PET in detecting infected lower limb prosthesis implants. J Nucl Med. 2001;42(1):44-8.
61. Reinartz P, Mumme T, Hermanns B, Cremerius U, Wirtz DC, Schaefer WM, et al. Radionuclide imaging of the painful hip arthroplasty: positronemission tomography versus triple-phase bone scanning. J Bone Joint Surg Br. 2005;87(4):465-70.
62. Love C, Scott EM, Tomas MB, Krauss ES, Tronco GG, Bhargava KK, et al. Diagnosing infection in the failed joint replacement: a comparison of coincidence detection 18F-FDG and 111In-labeled leucocyte/99mTc-sulfur colloid marrow imaging. J Nucl Med. 2004;45(11):1864-71.
63. Goerres GW, Ziegler SI, Burger C, Berthold T, Von Schulthess GK, Buck A. Artifacts at PET and PET/CT caused by metallic hip prosthetic material. Radiology. 2003;226(2): 577-84.
64. Donohoe KJ. Selected topics in orthopedic nuclear medicine. Orthop Clin North Am. 1998;29(1):85-101.
65. Barai S, Kumar R, Dhanpati H, Malhotra R, Dasan JB, Bandopadhyaya GB, et al. Bone scintigraphy in sports injuries. Ortho Today. 2003;5:29-32.
66. Mandelstam SA, Cook D, Fitzgerald M, Ditchfield M, Carty H. Complementary use of radiological skeletal survey and bone scintigraphy in detection of bony injuries in suspected child abuse. Arch Dis Child. 2003;88(5):387-90.
67. Kleinman PK. Shaken babies. Lancet. 1998;352(9130):815-6.
68. Fogelman I, Carr D. A comparison of bone scanning and radiology in the assessment of patients with symptomatic Paget's disease. Eur J Nucl Med. 1980;5(5):417-21.
69. Rotés-Sala D, Monfort J, Solano A, Miralles E, Vila J, Carbonell J. The clover and heart signs in vertebral scintigraphic images are highly specific of Paget's disease of bone. Bone. 2004;34(4):605-8.
70. Installé J, Nzeusseu A, Bol A, Depresseux G, Devogelaer J-P, Lonneux M. 18F-Fluoride PET for monitoring therapeutic response in Paget's disease of bone. J Nucl Med. 2005;46(10):1650-58.
71. Messa C, Goodman WG, Hoh CK, Choi Y, Nissenson AR, Salusky IB, et al. Bone metabolic activity measured with positron emission tomography and 18F-Fluoride ion in renal osteodystrophy: correlation with bone histomorphometry. J Clin Endocrinol Metab. 1993;77(4):949-55.

72. Fogelman I, McKillop JH, Greig WR, Boyle IT. Pseudofractures of the ribs detected by bone scanning. J Nucl Med. 1977;18(12):1236-7.
73. Fukumitsu N, Dohi M, Midda K, Nakada N, Sunagawa Y, Harada J, et al. Bone scintigraphy in polyostotic fibrous dysplasia. Clin Nucl Med. 1999;24(6):446-7.
74. Conway WF, Totty WG, McEnery KW. CT and MRI imaging of the hip. Radiology. 1996;198(2):297-307.
75. Collier BD, Carrera GF, Johnson RP, Isitman AT, Hellman RS, Knobel J, et al. Detection of femoral head avascular necrosis in adults by SPECT. J Nucl Med. 1985;26(9):979-87.
76. Ruffin D. Natural history of reflex sympathetic dystrophy syndrome. J Nucl Med. 1984;25:423-9.
77. Kozin F, Genant HK, Bekerman C, McCarty DJ. The reflex sympathetic dystrophy syndrome. II. Roentgenographic and scintigraphic evidence of bilaterality and of periarticular accentuation. Am J Med. 1976;60(3):332-8.

CHAPTER

154

Angiography and Interventions in Musculoskeletal Lesions

Deep Narayan Srivastava, Madhusudhan KS

INTRODUCTION

With increasing use of computed tomography (CT) and magnetic resonance imaging (MRI) in the diagnosis of bone and soft tissue lesions, angiography is not being used as commonly as before, however, if the procedure is used properly in conjunction with other diagnostic studies, it can play a valuable role in the diagnosis and treatment of bone and soft tissue lesions. The role of angiointerventions and nonvascular musculoskeletal interventions is increasing and will be discussed.

TECHNIQUE

Diagnostic Angiography

The common femoral artery is the commonly used entry site for percutaneous approach because of its accessibility, the ease of compression against the femoral head for hemostasis, and the low rate of complications when punctured. The left or right femoral artery is punctured by Seldinger technique and an arterial sheath is placed. Usually the contralateral femoral artery is used to approach the lesion in lower limb region. Through this, arterial sheath angiographic catheter is advanced into the arteries supplying the lesion. A wide variety of preshaped 4/5 F angiographic catheters are available for selective and superselective catheterization. The catheter is placed selectively in the major vessel supplying the tumor and angiographic runs are taken with contrast medium injection. Various selective injections are taken depending upon the tumor supply.

Visualization of both the arterial and venous circulations is desirable in all cases. The radiographs/frames are obtained initially at two frames/second for 3–4 seconds followed by every 2 seconds for a total of 25–30 seconds. The amount of contrast injection depends on the size and location of the lesion.

Digital subtraction angiograms (DSAs) are superior to conventional angiograms since the superimposed bones, calcifications and also other limb supports in trauma patients can be subtracted resulting in better image quality because of which reliable evaluation of vascular supply of the lesion is possible.

Magnification angiograms are sometimes required for visualization of tiny vessels.

Angioembolization

The term embolization refers to the introduction of an embolic agent into a vessel through a selectively placed catheter to achieve therapeutic vascular occlusion. The advent of catheters with hydrophilic coating, microcatheters, torque control guidewires and various embolic materials has allowed precise and safe delivery of occluding agents to anywhere in the body using the blood vessels as a roadway. In certain situations, these embolizing materials are also injected into the lesion directly under image guidance without angiographic route.

The embolization is usually performed using the access used for diagnostic angiography. After the initial diagnostic angiography, the angiographic catheter is advanced into the artery supplying the tumor before introduction of embolic material. The selective and superselective embolization is a safe interventional procedure for any vascular lesion. Sometimes small caliber catheters like microcatheters (2–3 F) are also used for this. It is also important to weigh the risks of the procedure against those of noninterventional and surgical therapies. The embolization should preferably be performed in angiography suite equipped with C-arm mounted image intensifier with DSA of high-quality resolution. A portable ultrasound scanner is always useful in the assessment of nonpalpable arteries, veins and also for direct percutaneous puncture of lesion.

ANGIOGRAPHY IN BONE TUMORS

The role of angiography in bone tumors is limited because of the following reasons:

- If the definitive angiographic features of malignancy are present, it can be assumed that the lesion is malignant, but a normal arteriogram does not entirely rule out a malignancy.[1]

- It is often not possible to distinguish between various types of bone tumors from the angiographic features alone.

The angiographic features of malignancy include neovascularity, pooling or laking of contrast material, tumor stain or blush, encasement and occlusion of vessels, extension of the tumor vascularity outside the bone, displacement of vessels, arteriovenous shunts, abnormal draining veins, tumor invasion of veins, etc.

Neovascularity and pooling of contrast are important features of malignancy; however, these may also be present in some benign lesions like giant cell tumor, aneurysmal bone cyst, osteoblastoma, Paget's disease, benign nerve sheath tumor and certain hemangiomas **(Figs. 1 to 3)**. These lesions can easily be differentiated by their clinical and plain radiographic features.

The presence of a tumor blush does not indicate malignancy but may suggest the size and extent of the tumor. Angiography, however, does not always define the complete intraosseous extent of the tumor and skip metastases within the bone are not always seen.[2]

The angiographic information about the displacement or encasement of vessel is important if a radical local resection is planned in limb salvage surgeries.

Early arteriovenous shunting is not a reliable sign of malignancy, however, the identification of large abnormal draining veins is important to facilitate early ligation and prevent tumor embolization during surgery.[2]

Some bone tumors in which diagnostic angiography is sometimes indicated are discussed here.

Osteochondroma

These bone tumors because of their size and location may cause vascular complications in the form of thrombosis and pseudoaneurysms[3,4] as well as displacement of vessels. Angiography can show all these complications **(Figs. 4A and B)**. The tumor usually does not show hypervascularity or abnormal vessels.

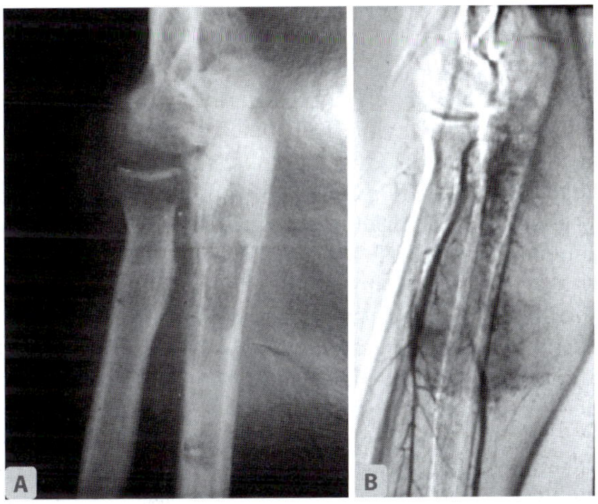

FIGS. 1A AND B: Ewing's tumor. (A) Lytic lesion with periosteal reaction and soft tissue mass of ulna; (B) Pooling of contrast material is seen on digital subtraction angiography (DSA).

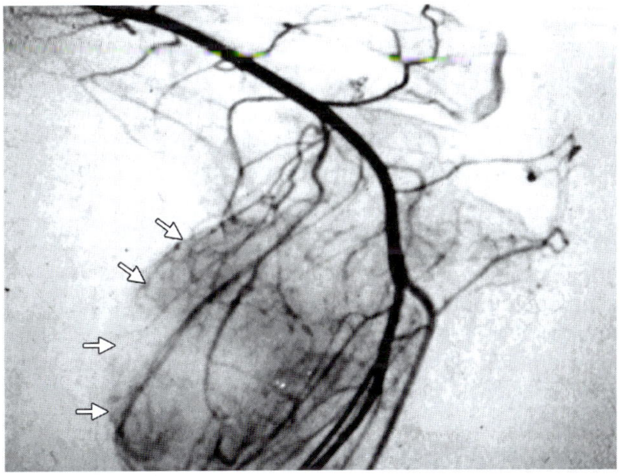

FIG. 2: Benign nerve sheath tumor. The digital subtraction angiography (DSA) showing blush of contrast (arrows).

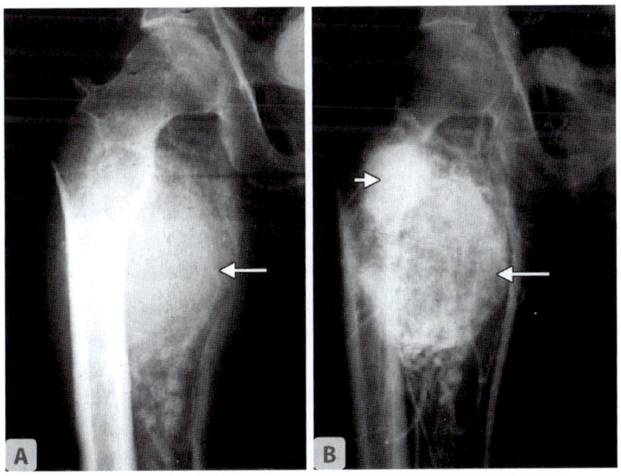

FIGS. 3A AND B: Angiography shows highly vascular mass with pooling of contrast in a case of hemangioma of femur (small arrow) with extraosseous component (large arrows).

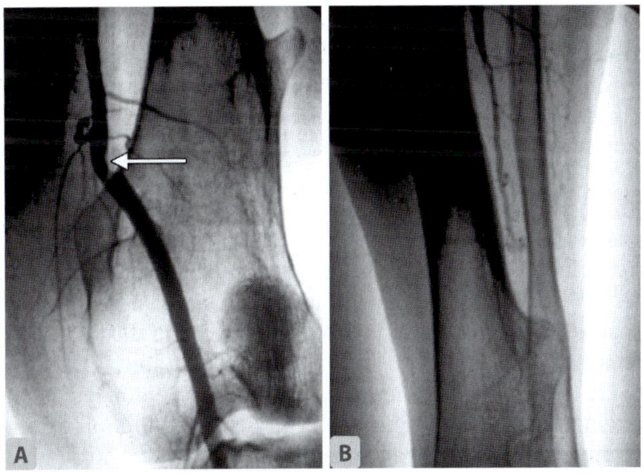

FIGS. 4A AND B: Multiple osteochondroma. (A) Displacement and narrowing (arrow) of femoral artery; (B) Thrombosis of leg vessels.

Osteoid Osteoma

In the absence of classical roentgenographic findings, angiography can be helpful when the diagnosis is in doubt.[5] The angiographic feature is dense, circumscribed blush in the early arterial phase which persists in late venous phase. This feature differentiates it from osteomyelitis, Brodie's abscess and stress fractures that do not have the feature of dense vascular blush.

Osteosarcoma

Angiography can demonstrate that the tumor is malignant, and accurately define the degree of soft tissue extension; however, skip areas within the medullary canal are not always detected.[2] MRI is useful in defining the intraosseous and extraosseous extent of the tumor and its anatomic relationship to nearby structures.

Giant Cell Tumor

Angiography can accurately define the intraosseous as well as extraosseous extent of the tumor because the tumors are usually hypervascular and show neovascularity, intense blush and early venous filling. This is of particular importance in view of the high recurrence rate of the tumor and its ability to become malignant after treatment. The MRI is useful in the limb salvage surgeries in the assessment of extent of tumor and the anatomic relationship to nearby structures and joint.

Aneurysmal Bone Cyst

Angiography can differentiate aneurysmal bone cyst from giant cell tumor. On angiography, it is poorly vascularized tumor, devoid of arteriovenous fistulae and soft tissue invasion.[6] The clinical course and plain radiographic findings are very useful for the diagnosis of this lesion.

ANGIOGRAPHY IN BONE AND SOFT TISSUE LESIONS OF VASCULAR ORIGIN

Hemangioma

Hemangiomas can be grouped into four categories: (1) capillary, (2) cavernous, (3) venous hemangiomas and (4) arteriovenous malformations (AVMs). Hemangiomas usually involve the soft tissues (most commonly skeletal muscles) but can also involve bones.[7] Arteriography can define the extent, degree of vascularity, source of vascular supply, local recurrence in follow-up case and differentiate from AVMs.[8] Angiography may show mild to marked vascularity with coarse, irregular, enlarged arteries and pooling of contrast material **(Figs. 3 and 5)**. Arteriovenous shunting may be seen. The osseous hemangiomas may have dilated vascular spaces **(Figs. 3A and B)**. Venous hemangioma is rarely seen on arteriography but is usually seen on venography[9] **(Figs. 6A to D)**. Sometimes it is difficult to ascertain the entire lesion on angiography.[10] The MRI is useful in depicting the full extent of the lesion and the relationship to surrounding structures **(Figs. 6A to D)**. Angiography sometimes cannot differentiate a benign hemangioma from a malignant vascular tumor.[8]

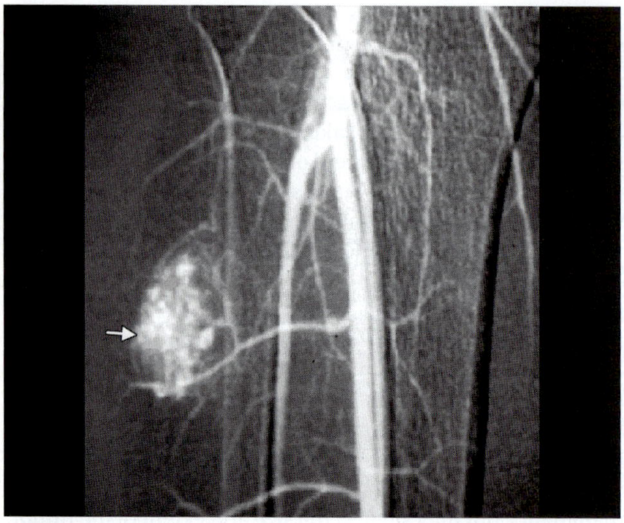

FIG. 5: Soft tissue hemangioma leg. Digital subtraction angiography shows fine vessels with some pooling of contrast (arrow). This painful lesion was successfully treated by percutaneous injection of sclerosing agent.

In cavernous hemangioma, arteriography demonstrates normal sized arteries that may show late venous staining on delayed films. They do not require treatment as they do not change with time and rarely bleed, but a common problem is local pain due to distention of the lesion or superimposed thrombosis. The embolization of regional arterial branches is not always useful, but injection of sclerosing agent by direct puncture technique has shown good results **(Fig. 5)**.

Klippel-Trenaunay syndrome (KTS) is a congenital vascular abnormality consisting of a cutaneous nevus, varicose veins and bone and soft tissue hypertrophy affecting one or more limbs. Venography is very useful in demonstrating the characteristic venous anomaly [Klippel-Trenaunay (KT) vein], which is a large lateral superficial venous channel that often communicates with profunda femoris or iliac veins **(Figs. 7A to C)**. MRI with its multiplanar imaging abilities has the advantage of demonstrating the full extent of venous malformation and the status of muscle and soft tissues.[9]

Arteriovenous malformations tend to grow at the same rate as the individual, unlike the pattern of rapid growth and involution seen in hemangioma. The angiographic findings include enlarged, tortuous feeding arteries, a dense nidus of malformations and early opacification of draining veins. The AVMs are refractory to treatment. Mechanically disturbing a stable lesion (after surgical ligation or proximal embolization of feeding arteries) can result in significant worsening due to development of new collaterals. Transcatheter embolization close to nidus of the lesion has now attained a primary role in the management of AVMs, but proximal occlusion of feeding vessels by an endovascular embolic agent or surgical ligation will provide poor clinical result with recurrence **(Figs. 8A and B)**.[11,12] The angiography can tell about the size, number and location of these lesions **(Figs. 9A and B)**. In lesions of extremities, injection of sclerosing agent or alcohol by direct puncture technique is safe and useful.

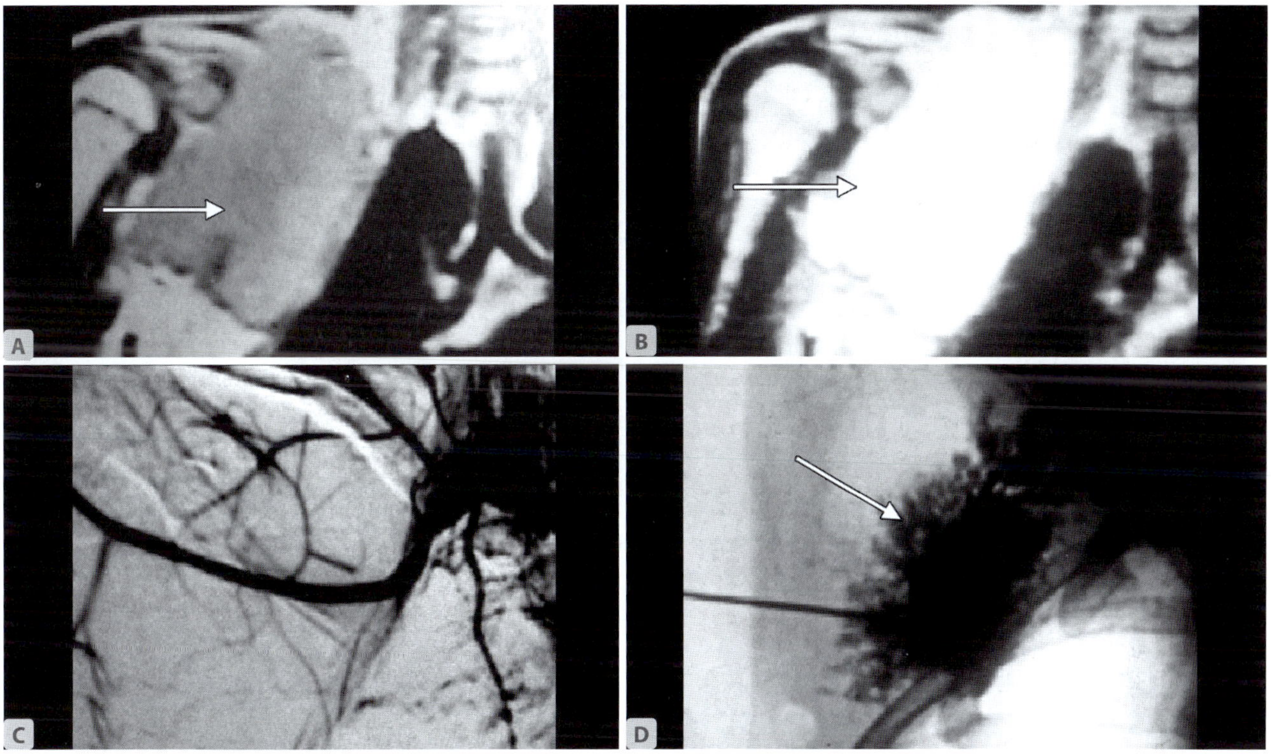

FIGS. 6A TO D: Venous hemangioma (arrows) of axilla with supraclavicular extension. The mass is mildly hyperintense to muscles on T1-weighted image (T1WI) (A) Hyperintense on T2WI; (B) On digital subtraction angiography (DSA), the mass is not vascular with mass effect over axillary artery with splaying of its lateral thoracic and subscapular branches; (C) No early venous filling seen. Percutaneous aspiration and injection of contrast shows multiple dilated vascular spaces; (D) The pain disappeared and the size was reduced after injection of sclerosing agent through the same needle.

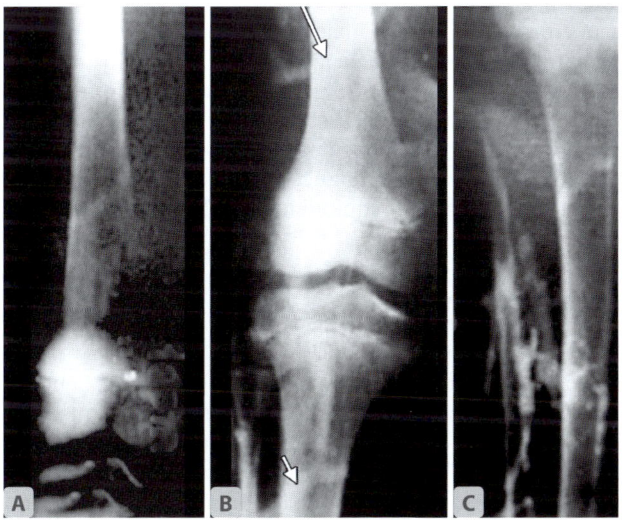

FIGS. 7A TO C: Ascending phlebogram showing two Klippel–Trenaunay veins, one communicating with the popliteal vein (small arrow), and the other with the superficial femoral vein (large arrow).

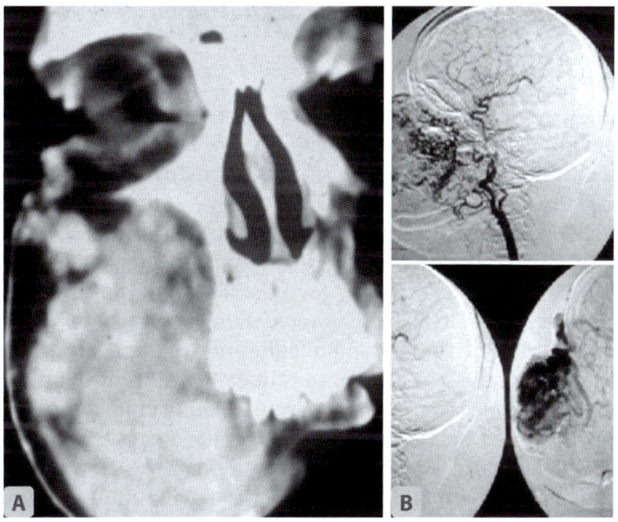

FIGS. 8A AND B: Arteriovenous malformations of cheek. (A) Computed tomography (CT) shows soft tissue vascular mass overlying maxilla, mandible, and inferior orbital margin; (B) On digital subtraction angiography (DSA), the mass is supplied by branches of left external carotid artery with early venous filling.

Hemangiopericytoma

These are hypervascular tumors and are seen as a prolonged dense stain on angiogram.[13] There may be displacement of the major arteries **(Fig. 10)**.

Angiosarcoma

The angiographic features include highly irregular, tortuous arteries with pooling of contrast,[14] arteriovenous shunts and encasement of vessels.

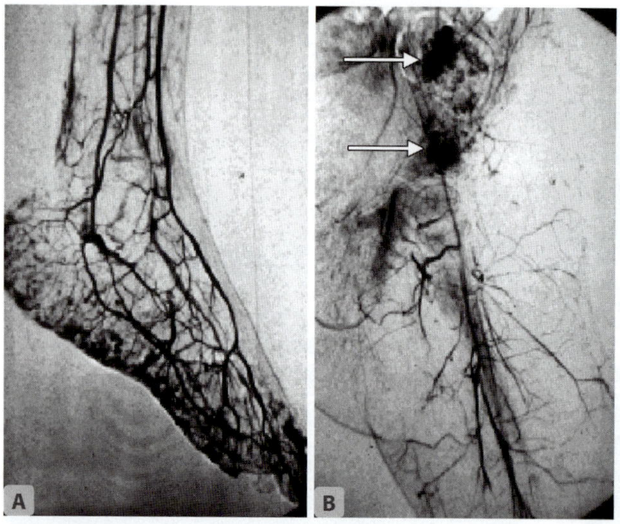

FIGS. 9A AND B: Multiple hemangiomas involving (A) left foot and (B) gluteal muscles (arrows).

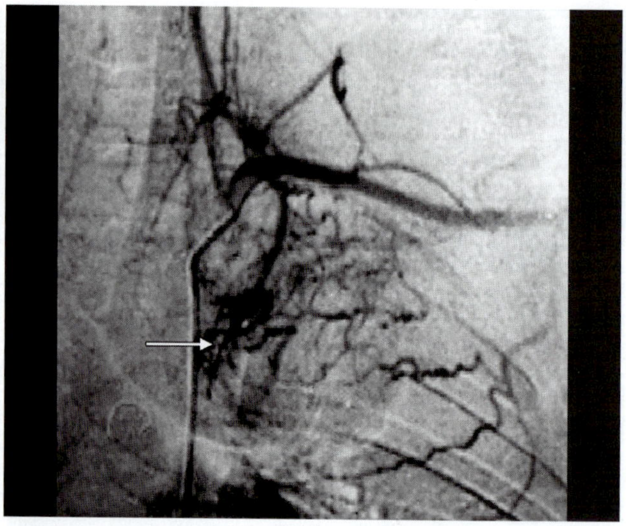

FIG. 10: Hemangiopericytoma. A well-demarcated hypervascular mass (arrow) with homogeneous blush seen on delayed images.

ANGIOGRAPHY IN METASTATIC TUMORS IN BONE AND SOFT TISSUES

Most metastatic lesions have the same vascular characteristics that are exhibited by their primary tumors.[15] Angiography cannot distinguish between different types of metastases. It also cannot distinguish a primary osseous or soft tissue tumor from a secondary growth.

ANGIOGRAPHY IN PERIPHERAL TRAUMA

Angiography has an important role in the management of patients with suspected vascular injury both for diagnosis and treatment. Angiography is both sensitive and specific for the diagnosis of vascular injury (active bleeding, pseudoaneurysms and arteriovenous fistula) **(Figs. 11 and 12)**. Transcatheter embolization is effective, safe and can be a definitive therapy for suitable arterial injuries. In arteriovenous fistula, early intervention is very useful. Early intervention in hemodynamically unstable patients with pelvic fractures is essential to reduce the morbidity of the injury.[16] In pelvic fractures, percutaneous embolization of uncontrolled pelvic hemorrhage is a lifesaving technique **(Figs. 12A and B)**. Small aneurysms can be treated by sonoguided manual compression or coil embolization **(Figs. 13 and 14)**. The intra-arterial thrombolytic therapy can also be used in arterial thrombosis **(Figs. 15A and B)**.

IMAGE-GUIDED INTERVENTIONS IN BONE AND SOFT TISSUE LESIONS

The commonly used image-guided interventions are fine needle aspiration cytology and Trucut biopsies, embolizations, intra-arterial chemotherapies, vertebroplasties, radiofrequency and laser ablation of benign bone lesions.

Aspiration Cytology and Biopsy

The role of aspiration cytology is limited since most lesions require biopsy. Percutaneous biopsy is less invasive, requires smaller dose of anesthetics and analgesics, causes minimal bleeding and biopsy tract contamination, and is a cost-effective method. However, it is less reliable in obtaining an adequate representative specimen for grading and further special studies. For heterogeneous tumors, very myxoid or cystic lesions and bone tumors without soft tissue component, a needle core may not give a high diagnostic yield. The hemangioma and AVMs usually do not require histological confirmation because of characteristic imaging features. For biopsy, various size Trucut needles (11–18G) are used. For bone biopsy, thick needles (11G) with diamond tip are preferred. Ultrasound guidance is always preferred though CT and fluoroscopy is required for vertebral and other bone lesions.

Embolization

Preprocedural Preparations

The patient must be informed about the procedure, benefits, alternative procedures and potential complications. The patient should be well hydrated and standby general anesthesia may be needed for uncooperative patients and children. Severe coagulopathy should be corrected and sometimes antibiotics are also given. The sedation is given during the procedure depending upon the type and duration of the procedure.

Indications

The indications of embolization in bone and soft tissue tumors are as follows:

1. *To control hemorrhage*: If there is internal or external bleeding from the tumor, angioembolization is sometimes done as an emergency procedure.

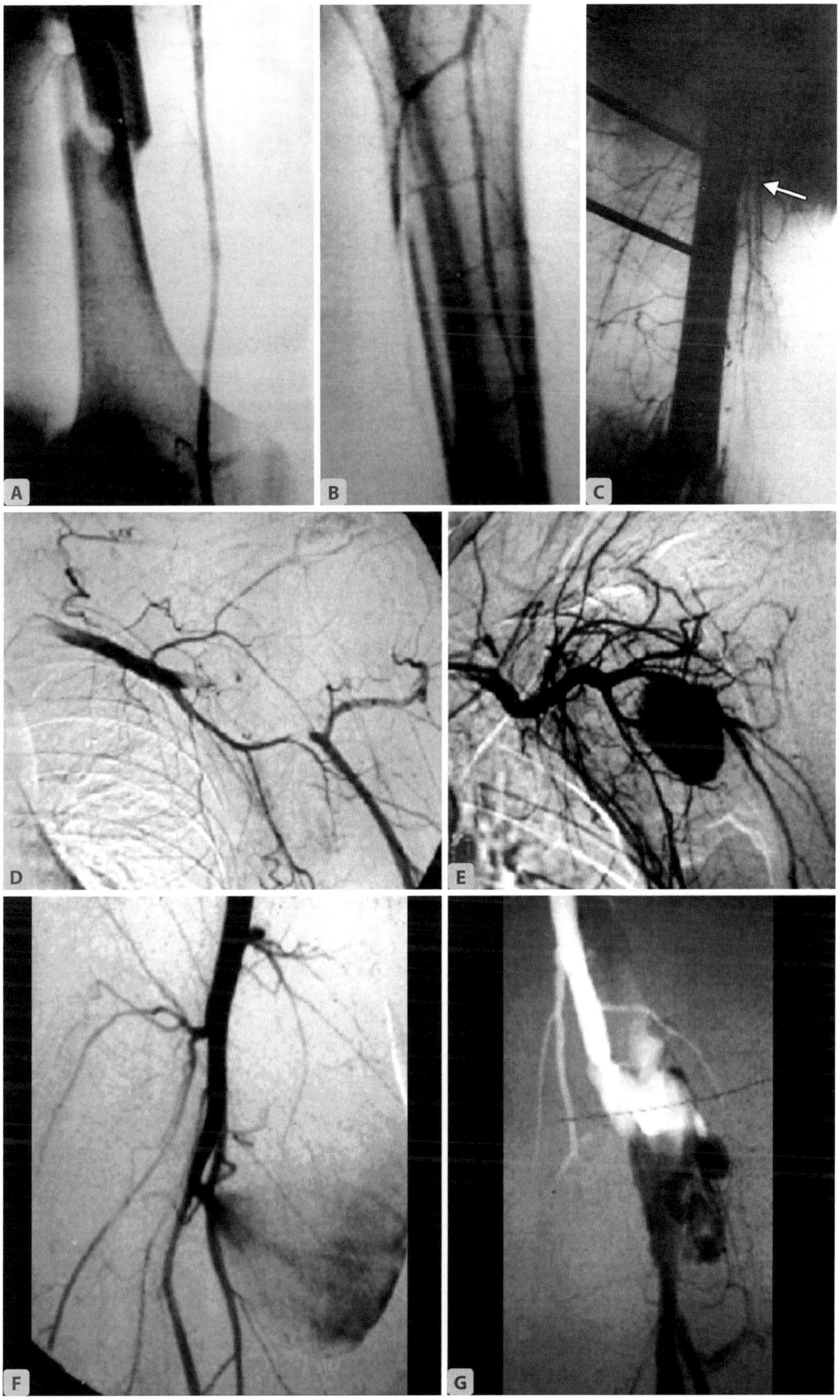

FIGS. 11A TO G: The digital subtraction angiography (DSA) in different patients of trauma. (A and B) Fracture femur and fibula with patent arteries; (C) Fracture femur with thrombosed superficial femoral artery (arrow) with collaterals; (D) Soft tissue injury left shoulder with thrombosed axillary artery-brachial artery is filling from collaterals; (E) Large pseudoaneurysm from axillary artery; (F) Large pseudoaneurysm from right superficial femoral artery; (G) Arteriovenous fistula between popliteal artery and vein.

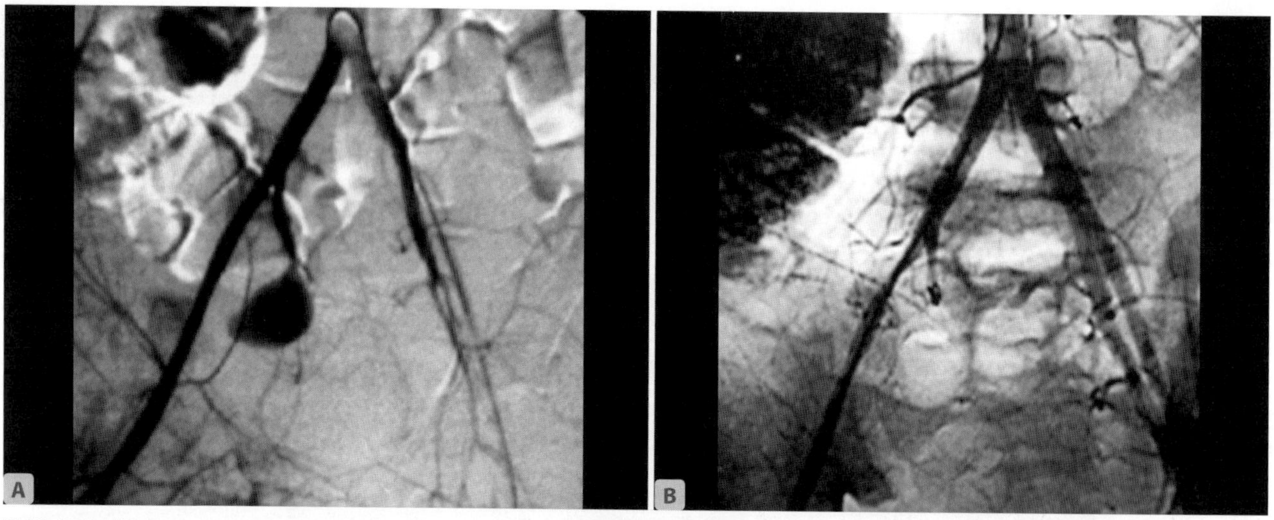

FIGS. 12A AND B: Post-traumatic pelvic bleeding. (A) Digital subtraction angiography (DSA) showing bleeding from right internal iliac artery trunk; (B) Which stopped after steel coil embolization.

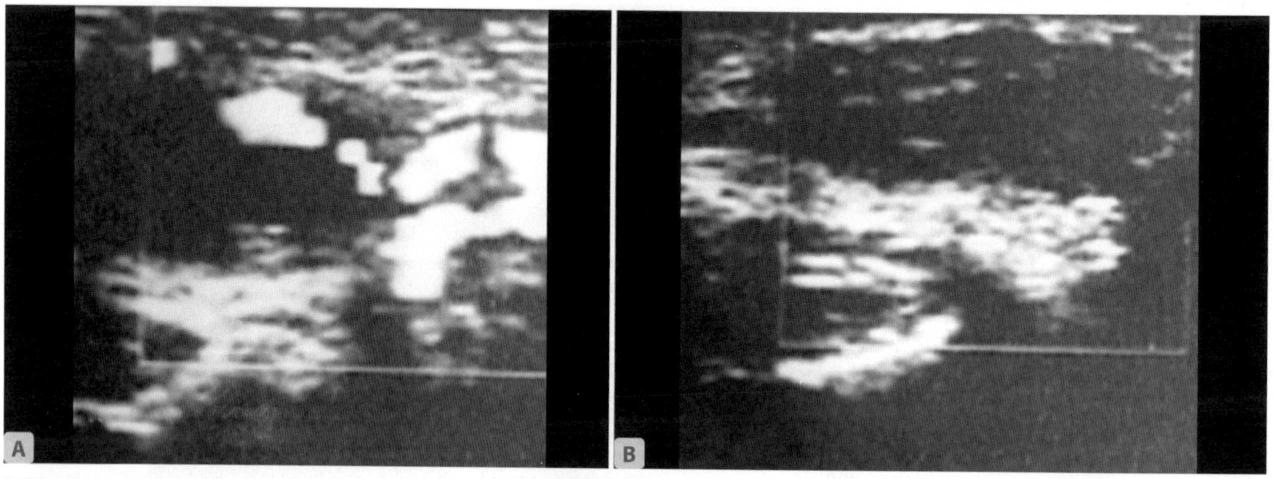

FIGS. 13A AND B: (A) Ultrasound showing pseudoaneurysm of femoral artery; (B) Developed after transfemoral arteriography, treated by manual compression.

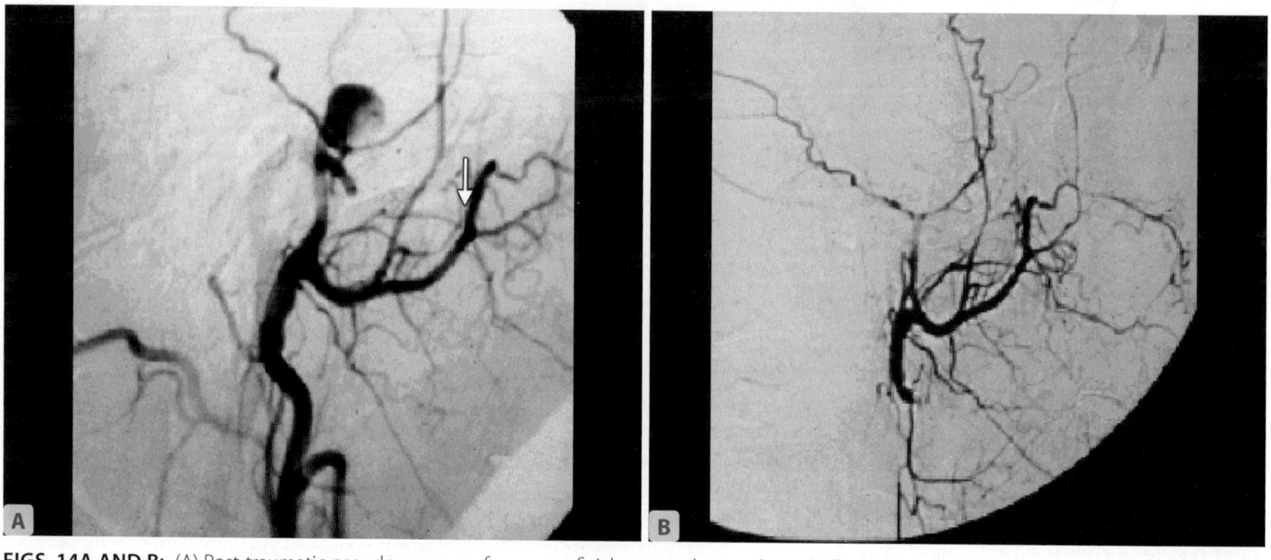

FIGS. 14A AND B: (A) Post-traumatic pseudoaneurysm from superficial temporal artery (arrow). This was treated by ultrasound-guided percutaneous coil embolization; (B) Post-treatment digital subtraction angiography (DSA) is not showing aneurysm.

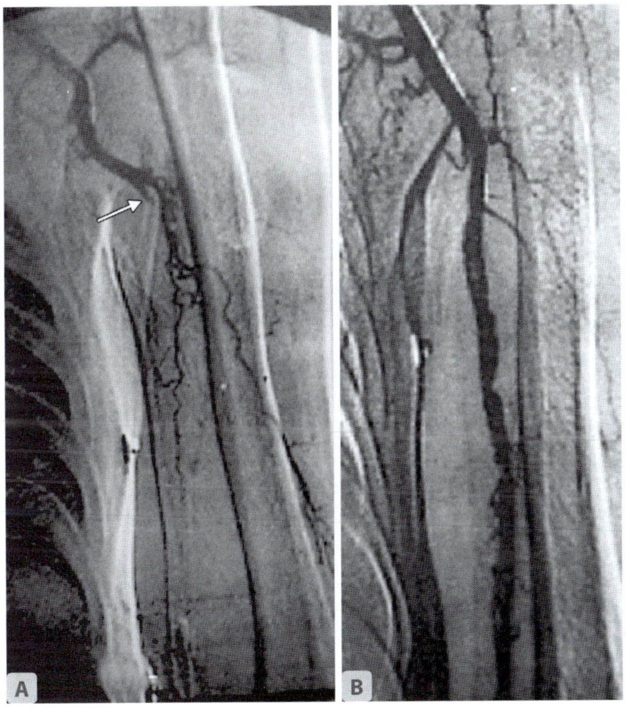

FIGS. 15A AND B: (A) Post traumatic acute thrombosis (arrow) of brachial artery; (B) Recanalized after intra-arterial thrombolytic infusion.

2. *To reduce peroperative bleeding*: It has been used in various soft tissue and bone tumors and hemangiomas to decrease intraoperative blood loss, which improves surgical vision and allows safer and faster surgery.[16,17] Voigt et al. reported the use of Gelfoam embolization in patients with deforming vascular malformations in the craniofacial area.[18] The procedure allows reconstructive surgery to be carried out with decreased blood loss with good cosmetic results **(Figs. 16A and B)**.
3. *As palliative treatment*: In previously treated (surgery and/or embolization) cases of recurrent or residual AVMs if intravascular access is difficult, direct puncture of the symptomatic lesion can be performed[18] by Chiba needle and alcohol or sclerosing agent can be injected directly in tumor bed (nidus) until flow is occluded. The embolization of the soft tissue tumors may result in severe, prolonged muscle pain if acute muscle ischemia takes place. Therefore, for palliation of pain in patients with inoperable tumors, embolization should be cautiously used.
4. *To relieve from chronic pain due to tumors*: It has been reported that therapeutic arterial occlusion in pelvic tumors[19] and in metastatic deposits[16] gives symptomatic relief of pain. The major vessels of supply are embolized with Gelfoam followed by steel coils to occlude the vessels permanently **(Figs. 17A and B)**. Embolization with particles (transcatheter) or percutaneous instillation of sclerosing agent has been used to control pain associated with a peripheral hemangioma **(Fig. 5)**.[20]
5. *As a part of treatment*: In hemangiomas, angio-embolization decreases the chance of recurrence **(Figs. 18A to C)**.[21] A study has shown that this not only decreases the size but also controls a persistent left-to-right shunt.[22]

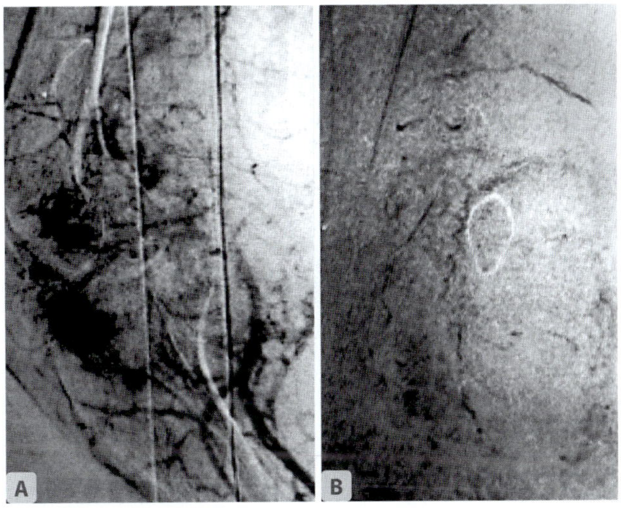

FIGS. 16A AND B: Preoperative embolization of a very large hemangioma around knee for reconstructive surgery. (A) Pre-embolization angiogram; (B) Postembolization angiogram.

Transarterial embolization should be considered in the treatment algorithm of primary or secondary bone tumors. Specific benefit is present where there is a high risk of bleeding at surgery, where there is spinal involvement and neural encroachment, where active bleeding is present or in awkward surgical locations where prolonged surgery is anticipated.[23]

Embolizing Materials

There are various types of embolizing materials available. The selection of the material depends upon the duration, extent and level of occlusion. The materials can be categorized as short, intermediate and long-acting or as particulate or liquid agents depending upon the physical properties. The commonly used embolizing materials have been listed in **Table 1**.

Complications

The common complication is postembolization syndrome in the form of nausea, vomiting, fever and pain due to tissue ischemia. The uncommon complications reported are inadvertent embolization, misplaced or migrated steel coils, abscess formation, spinal cord injury, aneurysm formation or vessel rupture.

Contraindications

The contraindications are patients with hemorrhagic diathesis and puncture site infection.

Intra-arterial Chemotherapy

Patients with sarcomas not amenable to cure by surgical resection alone can benefit from preoperative intra-arterial chemotherapy. Intra-arterial chemotherapy permits limb-sparing resection with less morbidity **(Fig. 19)**.[23,24] In this,

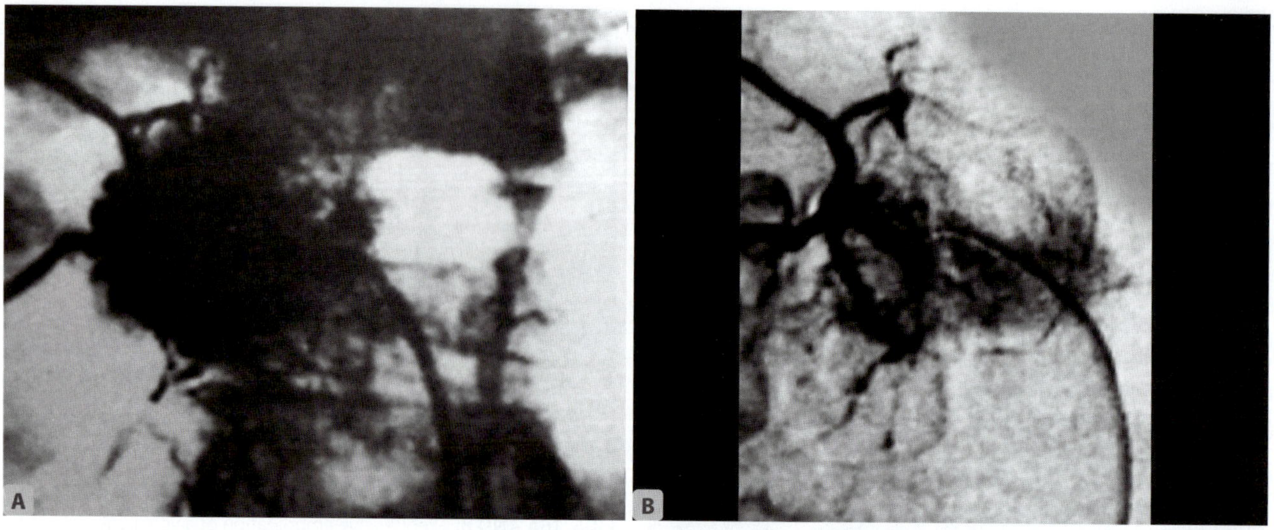

FIGS. 17A AND B: Painful metastatic deposit in the spine treated by therapeutic arterial occlusion. (A) Pre-embolization; (B) Postembolization angiograms.

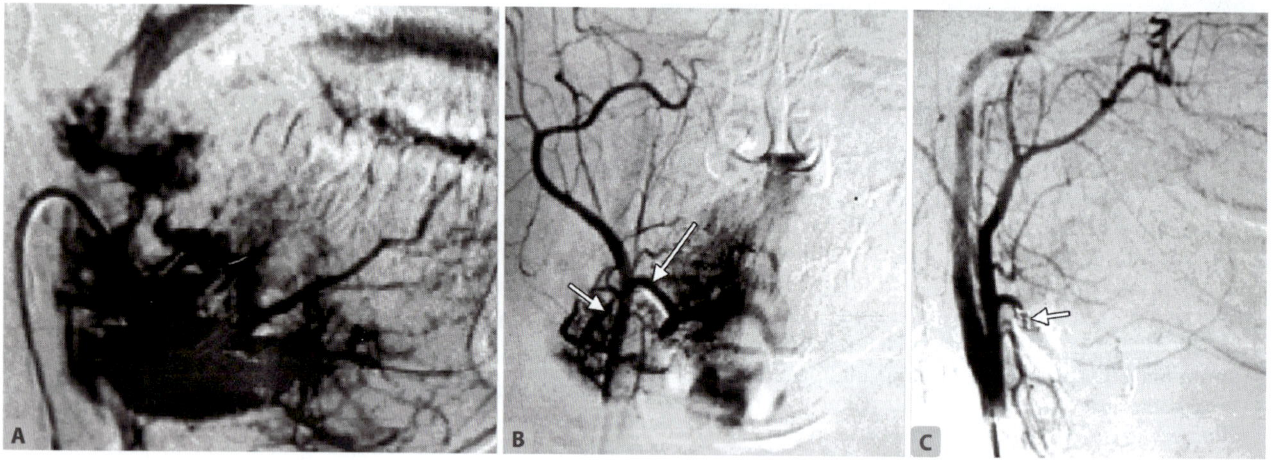

FIGS. 18A TO C: (A) Hemangioma submandibular region; (B) Supplied by right facial and lingual arteries (arrows); (C) The common origin of which embolized by steel coils (arrow).

chemotherapeutic drug is injected in tumor bed with the help of angiographic catheter placed in the artery supplying the tumor.

Neoadjuvant chemotherapy protocols using combined intra-arterial and intravenous agents to treat high-grade osteosarcoma and malignant fibrous histiocytoma of bone in an attempt to improve survival have also been tried with good results.[25]

Percutaneous Vertebral Body Augmentation Procedures

Percutaneous vertebroplasty is a well-accepted interventional procedure for the treatment of painful vertebral lesions. The technique first introduced in 1984[26] for a vertebral hemangioma, has been subsequently used for the treatment of numerous lesions causing back pain associated with vertebral involvement like osteoporotic vertebral collapse,

TABLE 1: Commonly used embolizing materials.

Type of embolizing agent	Examples and duration
Particulate agents	Absorbable (Temporary) • Autologous blood clot • Gelfoam Nonabsorbable (Permanent) • Polyvinyl alcohol particles • Microspheres
Mechanical agents	Nonabsorbable (Permanent) • Steel coils • Detachable balloons
Liquid agents	Nonabsorbable (Permanent) • Isobutyl 2-cyanoacrylate • Ethanol • Sodium tetradecyl sulfate

metastatic disease, multiple myeloma and symptomatic vertebral hemangiomas.

Technique

The procedure consists of instilling acrylic bone cement into the affected vertebra through a bone biopsy needle by a percutaneous approach. The cement consists of polymethyl methacrylate (PMMA) (obtained by mixing liquid monomer to the powdered polymer), which is mixed just before the injection. The cement is injected into the lesion after needle placement, under fluoroscopic control.[27] The cement polymerizes and subsequently sets, affording support to the vertebra **(Figs. 20A to C)**. The steps of the procedure are:

1. Patient is placed in prone position on angiography/ fluoroscopy table.
2. The procedure is performed under sterile conditions. The skin over the center of the pedicle is anesthetized with local anesthesia. A small skin incision is made and bone biopsy needle is positioned with its tip in the center of the midpoint of the pedicle.
3. The needle is advanced under anteroposterior (AP) and lateral fluoroscopy till the junction of the anterior and middle third of the vertebral body. Approximately 6 mL of PMMA cement is injected.
4. Patient is placed in supine position for 3 hours after the procedure and is discharged after 6 hours.

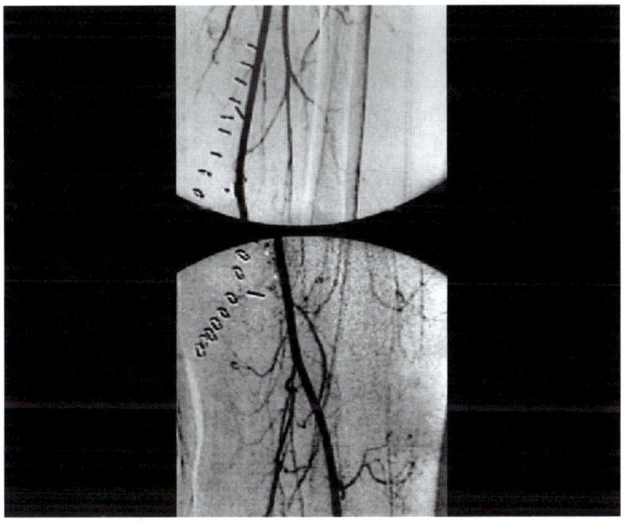

FIG. 19: Soft tissue sarcoma thigh. Postoperative angiogram was done to look for residual mass and intra-arterial chemotherapy.

Results

Vertebroplasty results in relief of pain with decrease in analgesic use. It provides strength so prevents further collapse and pain relief by coagulating the tissue. The relief is obtained irrespective of the cause of pain, and is long-lasting.[27]

Complications

The incidence of complications is less though various complications associated with the procedure are as follows:

- Cement leaks outside the vertebra are mostly inconsequential, but can cause local or radicular pain, neurological damage and pulmonary embolism.
- Inaccurate needle placement can injure nerve root or spinal cord.
- Pain exacerbation may occur due to substantial cement leaks.
- Rarely puncture site infection and bleeding may occur.

Future Directions

Although vertebroplasty can give considerable pain relief, it is not very useful in vertebral body height restoration. A new technique called kyphoplasty[28] involves the inflation of a bone tamp within the vertebral body to restore the height of the vertebra, and subsequently placing bone cement for augmentation of strength.

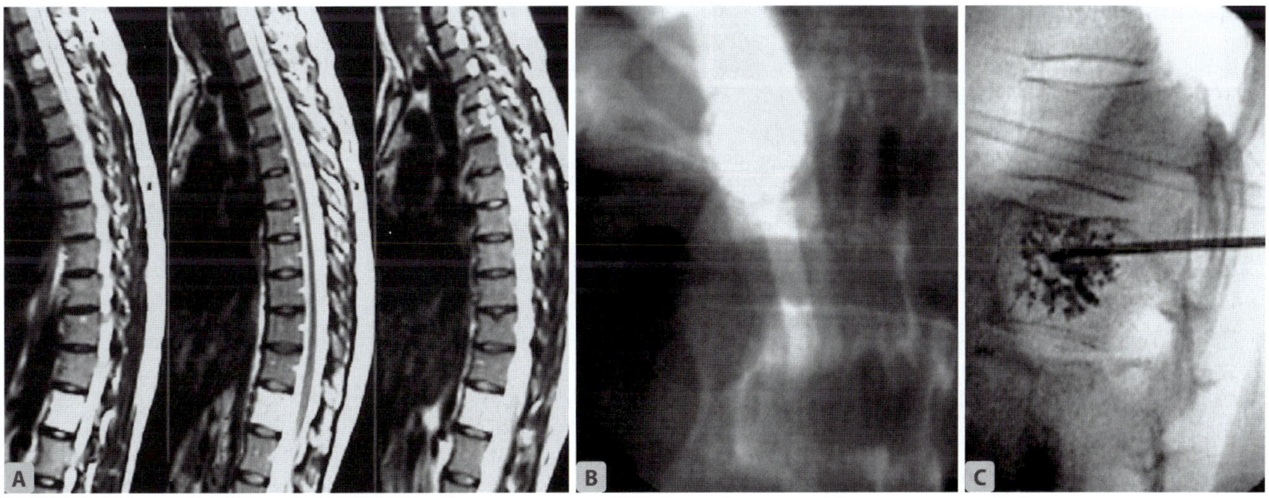

FIGS. 20A TO C: (A) A 30-year-old female with symptomatic D12 vertebral hemangioma, successfully treated with percutaneous vertebroplasty using polymethyl methacrylate bone cement. T2-weighted (T2W) pretreatment magnetic resonance (MR) shows D12 vertebral body hemangioma; (B) The vertebroplasty needle is seen in position with (C) injected bone cement.

Another new technique is vesselplasty, alternative to vertebroplasty and kyphoplasty. It was devised to prevent the leakage of bone cement and restore vertebral body height. In this procedure, cement is injected into a balloon positioned in the vertebral body, thus reducing the incidence of leak. Vesselplasty has shown statistically significant benefits in patients with symptomatic vertebral compression fractures.[29] Recently in the treatment of burst fractures with posterior wall retropulsion and no neurologic deficit, armed kyphoplasty using intravertebral distraction devices, such as vertebral body stents and SpineJack, could be effective in fracture reduction, internal fixation, and indirect central canal decompression. In selected cases, it might represent a suitable minimally invasive treatment option, stand alone or in combination with posterior stabilization.[30]

Vertebroplasty is becoming a well-established modality in the management of the aforementioned conditions, and is relatively safe.[31]

Percutaneous Treatment of Disc Herniation

Low backache is one of the major causes of chronic pain and morbidity. Treatment of herniated disc has evolved from open surgical techniques to minimally invasive or microtherapeutic procedures under local anesthesia. These include percutaneous laser disc decompression (PLDD), percutaneous ozone therapy and percutaneous/endoscopic nucleotomy.

In PLDD, laser energy is delivered into nucleus pulposus by laser fiber, through a needle. The aim of PLDD is to vaporize a small portion of the nucleus pulposus. The ablation of this small volume results in reduction of intradiscal pressure, thus reducing the disc herniation[32] **(Figs. 21A to D)**. This technology has been improved further to deliver proper energy without damaging the nerve.[33]

In percutaneous ozone treatment, mixture of ozone-oxygen gas is administered into nucleus pulposus through the needle. This mixture has a direct effect on the proteoglycans of the nucleus pulposus, resulting in release of water molecules and subsequent degeneration of matrix and reduction of volume[34] **(Figs. 22A to C)**.

Both PLDD and percutaneous ozone therapy are not used for uncontained herniations or sequestered disc. In both the procedures, patient is positioned prone and using either fluoroscopy or CT guidance a lumbar puncture needle (18–21G) is inserted into the center of the disc. After proper position of the needle, for PLDD, an optical fiber is advanced through the needle and proper laser energy is given. For ozone treatment, approximated 4 mL ozone-oxygen mixture is injected with an ozone concentration of 27 μg/mL.[35]

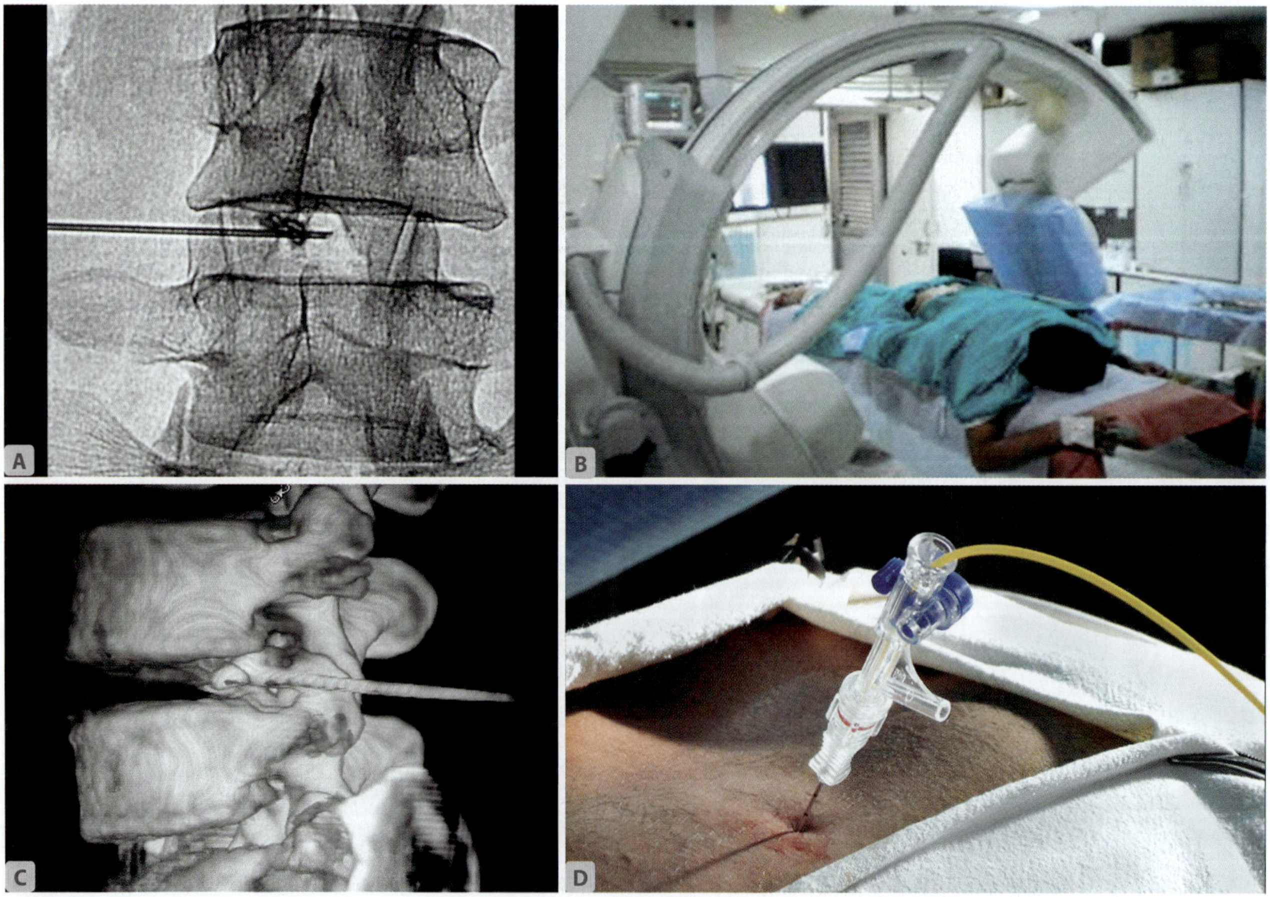

FIGS. 21A TO D: Percutaneous laser treatment of herniated disc. (A) A lumbar puncture needle is placed into the disc under fluoroscopy; (B and C) Needle position can be checked by doing rotation angiogram and three-dimensional (3D) reconstruction image; (D) After proper position of needle, optical fiber is advanced through the needle and laser energy is deposited.

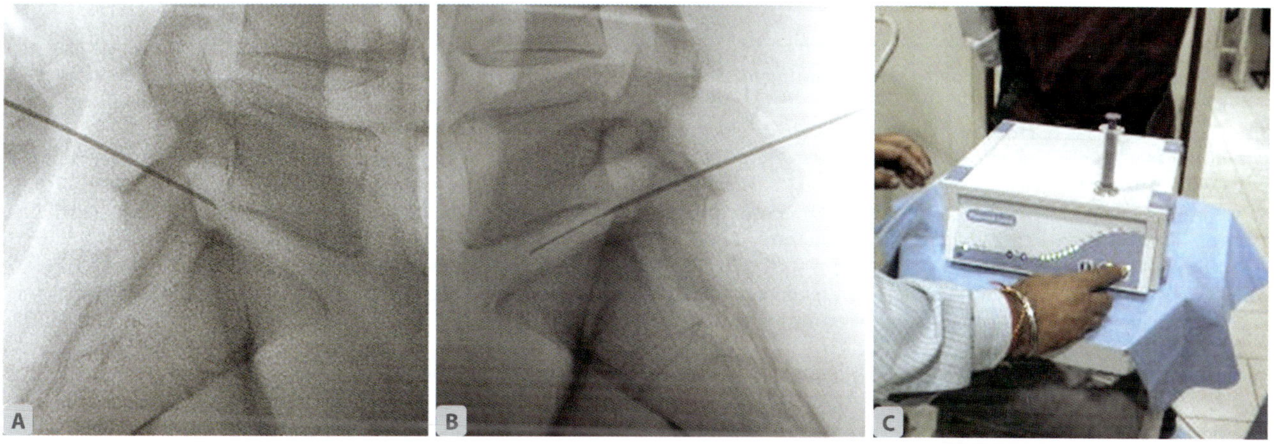

FIGS. 22A TO C: Percutaneous ozone treatment of herniated disc. (A and B) A lumbar puncture needle is placed into the disc under fluoroscopy; (C) Ozone gas is injected after preparing it from ozone generator machine.

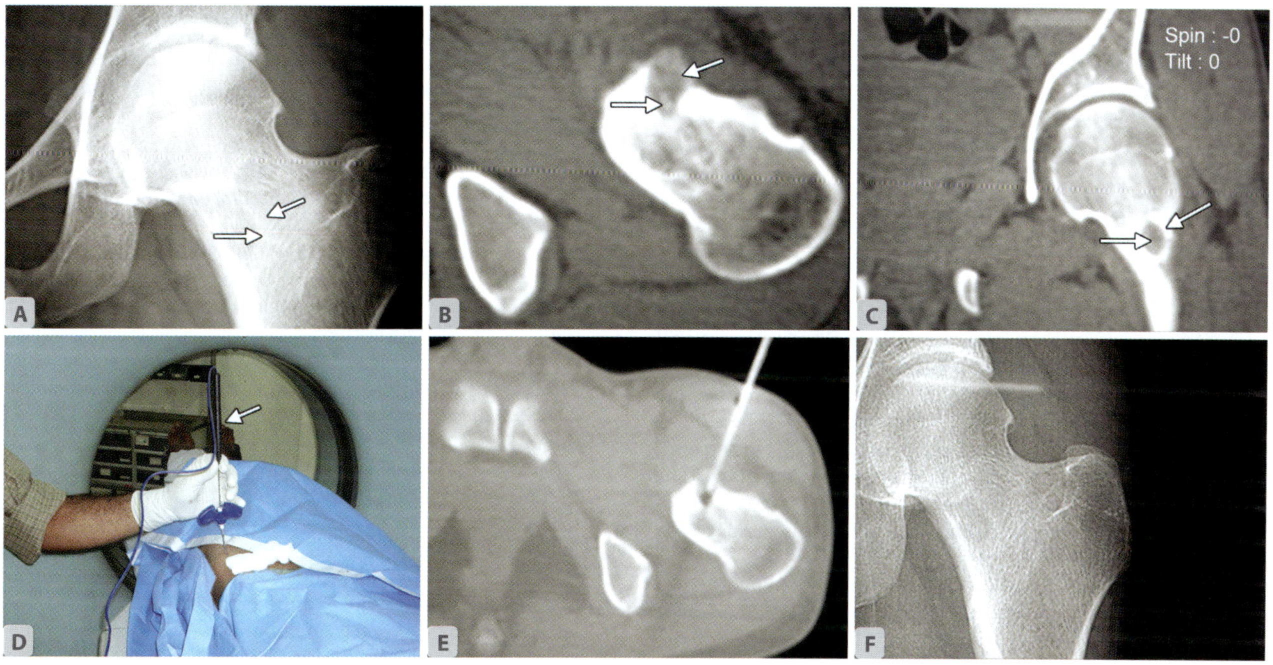

FIGS. 23A TO F: Percutaneous radiofrequency (RF) ablation of osteoid osteoma. Radiograph of left hip anteroposterior (AP) view (A), unenhanced axial (B) and coronal (C) computed tomography (CT) images showing a small calcified nidus (small arrow) with surrounding sclerosis (long arrow). After placement of bone biopsy needle (small arrow) into the lesion under CT guidance, the stylet was withdrawn and the RF probe (long arrow) was introduced (D). Axial CT image at the time of procedure (E) showing tip of the biopsy needle in the lesion. Post-treatment (1 week) AP radiograph (F) does not show nidus and patient is asymptomatic.

PERCUTANEOUS ABLATION OF BONE TUMORS

Percutaneous image-guided tumor ablation with thermal energy source such as radiofrequency, laser or microwave energy is used in the treatment of both benign (osteoid osteoma, osteoblastoma, enchondroma, etc.) and malignant (metastatic) lesions in place of surgery due to potential benefits such as minimal invasiveness, reduced cost and morbidity.[36]

The procedure is performed with CT guidance either under general anesthesia or conscious sedation. A proper bone biopsy needle is placed into the lesion with the help of a hammer or a drill. Radiofrequency probe or laser fiber is introduced through the cannula and proper energy is delivered for ablation **(Figs. 23A to F)**. CT-guided radiofrequency ablation (RFA) is proven to be a safe and effective procedure for the treatment of osteoid osteomas. When compared to surgical excision, it shows a significant reduction in hospitalization cost and duration. With its almost negligible postprocedural complications and a low rate of recurrence, RFA is at the moment is the treatment of choice for these bone tumors.[37]

REFERENCES

1. Voegeli E, Uehlinger E. Arteriography in bone tumors. Skeletal Radiol. 1976;1:3-14.
2. Hudson TM, Haas G, Enneking WF, Hawkins IF Jr. Angiography in the management of musculoskeletal tumors. Surg Gynecol Obstet. 1975;141:11-21.
3. Han SK, Henein MH, Novin N, Giargiana FA. An unusual arterial complication seen with a solitary osteochondroma. Am Surg. 1977;43:471-2.
4. Gomez-Reino JH, Radin A, Gorevic PD. Pseudoaneurysm of the popliteal artery as a complication of an osteochondroma. Skeletal Radiol. 1979;4:26-8.
5. Lateur L, Baert AL. Localisation and diagnosis of osteoid osteoma of the carpal area by angiography. Skeletal Radiol. 1977;2:75-9.
6. deSantos LA, Murray JA. The value of arteriography in the management of aneurysmal bone cyst. Skeletal Radiol. 1978;2:137-41.
7. Bliznak J, Staple TW. Radiology of angiodysplasias of the limb. Radiology. 1974;110:35-44.
8. Levin DC, Grodon DH, McSweeney J. Arteriography of peripheral haemangiomas. Radiology. 1976;121:625.
9. Srivastava DN, Gulati M, Thulkar S, Berry M. Klippel-Trenaunay syndrome: unusual magnetic resonance features. Australas Radiol. 1998;42:88-9.
10. Bartlely O, Wickbom I. Angiography in soft tissue hemangiomas. Acta Radiol. 1959;51:81-94.
11. Bjarnason H. Vascular embolotherapy. In: Ferral H, Bjarnason H, Qian Z (Eds). Synopsis of Castaneda's Interventional Radiology, 1st edition. Philadelphia: Lippincott Williams and Wilkins; 2001. pp. 27-45.
12. Rosen RJ, Riles TS. Arteriovenous malformations. In: Strandness D, van Breda A (Eds). Vascular Diseases: Surgical and Interventional Therapy. New York: Churchill Livingstone; 1994. p. 1126.
13. Yaghmai I. Angiographic manifestations of soft tissue and osseous hemangiopericytomas. Radiology. 1978;126: 653-9.
14. Unni KK, Ivins JC, Beabout JW, Dahlin DC. Hemangioma, hemangiopericytoma, and hemangioendothelioma (angiosarcoma) of bone. Cancer. 1971;27:1403-14.
15. Yaghmai I. Angiography of Bone and Soft Tissue Lesions. New York: Springer; 1979.
16. Hoffer EK, Borsa JJ, Bloch RD, Fontaine AB. Endovascular techniques in the damage control setting. Radiographics. 1999;19:1340-8.
17. Feldman F, Casarella WJ, Dick HM, Hollander BA. Selective intra-arterial embolization of bone tumors: a useful adjunct in the management of selected lesions. Am J Roentgenol Radium Ther Nucl Med. 1975;123:130-9.
18. Voigt K, Schwenzer N, Stoeter P. Angiographic, operative, and histologic findings after embolization of craniofacial angiomas. Neuroradiology. 1978;16:424-7.
19. Doppman JL, Pevsner P. Embolization of arteriovenous malformations by direct percutaneous puncture. AJR Am J Roentgenol. 1983;140:773-8.
20. Wallace S, Granmayeh M, deSantos LA, Murray JA, Romsdahl MM, Bracken RB, et al. Arterial occlusion of pelvic bone tumor. Cancer. 1979;43:322-8.
21. Hemmy DC, McGee DM, Armbrust FH, Larson SJ. Resection of a vertebral hemangioma after preoperative embolization: a case report. J Neurosurg. 1977;47:282-5.
22. Mitty HA, Kleiger B. Partial embolization of large peripheral hemangioma for pain control. Radiology. 1978;127:671-2.
23. Owen RJ. Embolization of musculoskeletal tumors. Radiol Clin North Am. 2008;46(3):535-43.
24. Keus RB, Rutgers EJ, Ho GH, Gortzak E, Albus-Lutter CE, Hart AA. Limb-sparing therapy of extremity sarcomas: treatment outcome and long-term functional results. Eur J Cancer. 1994;30A: 1459-63.
25. Hugate RR, Wilkins RM, Kelly CM, Madsen W, Hinshaw I, Camozzi AB. Intra-arterial chemotherapy for extremity osteosarcoma and MFH in adults. Clin Orthop Relat Res. 2008;466(6):1292-301.
26. Galibert P, Deramond H, Rosat P, Le Gars D. Preliminary note on the treatment of vertebral angioma by percutaneous acrylic vertebroplasty. Neurochirurgie. 1987;33:166-8.
27. Barr JD, Barr MS, Lemley TJ, McCann RM. Percutaneous vertebroplasty for pain relief and spinal stabilization. Spine (Phila Pa 1976). 2000;25:923-8.
28. Ledlie JT, Renfro M. Balloon kyphoplasty: one-year outcomes in vertebral body height restoration, chronic pain, and activity levels. J Neurosurg. 2003;98:36-42.
29. Flors L, Lonjedo E, Leiva-Salinas C, Martí-Bonmatí L, Martínez-Rodrigo JJ, López-Pérez E, et al. Vesselplasty: a new technical approach to treat symptomatic vertebral compression fractures. AJR Am J Roentgenol. 2009;193:218-26.
30. Venier A, Roccatagliata L, Isalberti M, Scarone P, Kuhlen DE, Reinert M, et al. Armed kyphoplasty: an indirect central canal decompression technique in burst fractures. AJNR Am J Neuroradiol. 2019;40(11):1965-72.
31. Gangi A, Guth S, Imbert JP, Marin H, Dietemann JL. Percutaneous vertebroplasty: indications, technique, and results. Radiographics. 2003;23:e10.
32. Gupta AK, Bodhey NK, Jayasree RS, Kapilamoorthy TR, Kesavadas C, Krishnamoorthy T, et al. Percutaneous laser disc decompression: clinical experience at SCTIMST and long-term follow-up. Neurol India. 2006;54:164-7.
33. Meng C, Li Y, Wang S, Yu J, Kou D, Liu C. Application of a modified optical fiber in targeted percutaneous laser disc decompression of lumbar disc herniation: a retrospective study. Exp Ther Med. 2019;18(5):3552-62.
34. Baabor MG, Vazquez PF, Sanchez JA. Automated nucleotomy and nucleolysis with ozone. Acta Neurochir Suppl. 2011;108: 97-101.
35. Andreula CF, Simonetti L, De Santis F, Agati R, Ricci R, Leonardi M. Minimally invasive oxygen-ozone therapy lumber disc herniation. AJNR Am J Neuroradiol. 2003;24:996-1000.
36. Ruiz Santiago F, Garcia MD, Alvarez LG, Montes JL, García MR, Fernández JM. Percutaneous treatment of bone tumors by radiofrequency thermal ablation. Eur J Radiol. 2011;77(1): 156-63.
37. Filippo MD, Russo U, Papapietro VR, Ceccarelli F, Pogliacomi F, Vaienti E, et al. Radiofrequency ablation of osteoid osteoma. Acta Biomed. 2018;89(1):175-85.

CHAPTER

155

Tuberculosis of Bones and Joints

Gaurav Shanker Pradhan, Rashmi Dixit, Jyoti Kumar

INTRODUCTION

Tuberculosis (TB) is endemic throughout the Indian subcontinent.[1] This is of concern, as with the advent of drug-resistant cases and increase in number of immunocompromised patients, the disease prevalence will only increase and management becomes problematic. The causative etiological agent for tubercular affliction of bone is *Mycobacterium tuberculosis*.[2-4]

ETIOPATHOGENESIS

Osteoarticular TB begins in the synovium or in the metaphyseal spongiosa. Synovial infection can occur by contiguous spread or due to hematogenous spread.

Hematogenous spread can occur from lung primary or postprimary focus, or from any other visceral, lymph nodal source of infection. Simultaneous involvement of viscera, lymph nodes, and parts of skeletal system suggest spread of infection through arterial blood supply. The bacillus usually lodges in the spongiosa of the metaphysis. Lesion is usually destructive and accompanied by pus formation. The metaphyseal lesion may infect the joint through subperiosteal space, through capsule or through destruction of the epiphyseal plate. In contrast to pyogenic infections, sequestration and periostitis are not very common. Ischemic necrosis and endarteritis may result in very small sequestrum formation which is usually not radiologically visible. It may become visible as a result of calcification. Marked exudative reaction is, however, a common feature. Granulation tissue spreads onto the free surface of cartilage eroding it in patches, insinuating between cartilage and subchondral bone, advancing from periphery to the center causing loosening and separation of cartilaginous tissue, causing necrosis of cartilage with erosion of exposed bone. Marginal erosions are characteristics of TB in weight-bearing joints such as hip, knee, and ankle. Wedge-shaped necrotic foci may become evident on either side of joint leading to the appearance of "kissing sequestra". Necrosed cartilage, fibrinous material form "rice bodies" in synovial joints, tendon sheaths, and bursae.[5,6] Abscesses that form may track along fascial planes and result in sinus formation. Plaques of irregular bone, if present in walls of chronic abscess or sinus suggest diagnosis of long-standing tubercular infection.

Bacille Calmette-Guérin (BCG) osteitis that can occur following BCG vaccination runs a benign course with localization of the *Bacillus* in epiphysis and metaphysis with extension across growth plate. It resembles chronic osteomyelitis radiologically, but responds to antitubercular therapy (ATT).

Synovial sheath infections are common with nontypical *Mycobacterium* (other than *M. tuberculosis* and *M. bovis*), with history of trauma (puncture wounds), surgery, immunocompromised status, and exposure to contaminated marine life.

Tuberculosis has been seen as a late complication of implant surgery (6–12 months postoperation). This has been attributed to extensive surgery, use of implants, and favorable conditions for circulating mycobacteria such as diabetes mellitus, corticosteroids, and immunocompromised status.[6,7]

CLINICAL FEATURES

Clinical features include insidious onset, low-grade fever, anorexia, weight loss, and night sweats. The patient may present with night pains, painful limitation of movement, muscle wasting, regional lymph node involvement, and neurologic symptoms.

Weight-bearing joints such as hip, knee, and ankle are commonly involved, though any part of the skeleton can get involved by the disease process.[8,9]

RADIOLOGICAL FEATURES

Pathologic affliction of the disease can be categorized as under:

- Inflammatory edema and exudates (predestructive stage)
- Necrosis and cavitation
- Destruction and deformation
- Healing and repair.

Tubercular infection in bones is said to develop 2–3 years after primary focus, so the diagnosis is usually delayed, in contrast to pyogenic infections which are seen 2–3 weeks after clinical presentation. Further changes in bone on plain radiograph, are usually appreciable 2–4 months after onset of disease in the bone. The infection originates in the metaphysis and it can cross the growth plate. There is usually no sclerosis and small sequestra are absorbed. Diaphysial lesions are rare and multiple cystic lucencies are rarer still.

Investigations include anteroposterior and lateral radiographs of the involved region and a radiograph of the chest.

Stage of synovitis: In early synovial disease there is soft tissue swelling and joint widening due to effusion and synovial hypertrophy. The first radiological sign may be juxta-articular osteoporosis. Patchy areas of trabecular or bony destruction may be evident. In the center of osteolytic lesion or cavity, there may be sequestrum or calcification of the caseous tissue, giving appearance of an irregular soft, feathery, coke-like sequestrum **(Fig. 1)**. If there is secondary superadded infection, subperiosteal reaction may result. As a result of localized hyperemia, growth plate may show overgrowth, especially in childhood.

Stage of arthritis: Later in the disease, the articular margin and bony cortices may be hazy (blurring and fuzzy) giving rise to "washed-out appearance". With involvement of articular cartilage there is narrowing and reduction of joint space. Juxta-articular osteopenia, peripherally located osseous lesions, and gradual narrowing of joint space are considered pathognomonic of tubercular osteoarthritis and are referred to as "Phemister triad" **(Fig. 2)**.

Early loss of articular joint space is more typically seen in rheumatoid arthritis and thus helps in differentiating from TB.

Stage of advanced arthritis: In advanced cases, there is collapse of bone, subluxation or dislocation, migration of bone and resultant deformity of joint.[10,11]

With healing, there is remineralization and cortical and articular margins become distinct. Fibrous ankylosis may occur during healing phase. In contrast to pyogenic arthritis, the development of bone ankylosis is uncommon in tuberculous arthritis.

Ultrasonography is helpful in the evaluation of large joints, like hip joint, to demonstrate joint effusion, synovitis, and capsular thickening. Synovial thickening can be seen as hypoechoic intra-articular soft tissue. Fluid in joint space and bursal fluid can be anechoic or hypoechoic (thick exudates). In tenosynovitis, the synovial sheath along tendons is thick and heterogeneous with minimal fluid suggestive of chronic tenosynovitis. It can, in addition, indicate presence of associated soft tissue abscess such as psoas abscess. It can also demonstrate cortical disruption, irregularity of articular margins, and associated soft tissue swelling. Calcification in abscess, if any, can also be seen. Further, evaluation of tendon sheaths and bursal spaces and smaller joints such as wrist, hand, foot, and ankle is also possible. Guided joint fluid aspiration or synovial biopsy is possible under ultrasound guidance.

Computed tomography (CT) is helpful in demonstrating lytic areas and marginal erosions much before plain radiographs.[12]

Swelling in soft tissues, granulation, exudations, abscess, and early calcification can also be demonstrated much earlier. Joint space can also be better evaluated by CT scan.

The predestructive stage can be visualized by magnetic resonance imaging (MRI) and also probably by bone scans. The plain radiographs and CT scan are not likely to detect the stage of inflammatory edema and exudates.

Isotope bone scan or MRI may reveal subclinical active lesion in 40% of patients, in addition to the presenting lesion. Out of technetium-99m, gallium-67, and indium-111 isotopes used in skeletal scintigraphy, technetium-99m is the most sensitive, though not specific. So a positive scan helps in localizing the suspicious region and is also helpful for follow-up.

Fluorine fluorodeoxyglucose positron emission tomography (^{18}F-FDG-PET) has also been found useful in localizing tubercular disease and in differentiating soft tissue infection from osseous infection.[4,5,13]

Synovial hypertrophy is most commonly seen in osteoarticular TB on MRI. Hypointense areas on T2-weighted

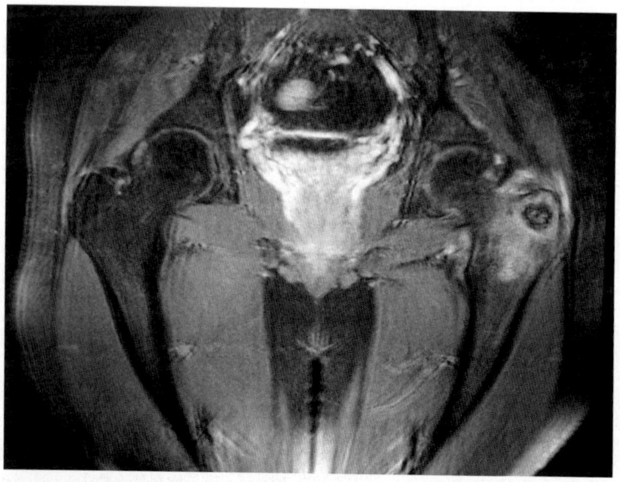

FIG. 1: In the center of osteolytic lesion in left femur, there is a small irregular sequestrum picked up on MRI (image en Grelot).

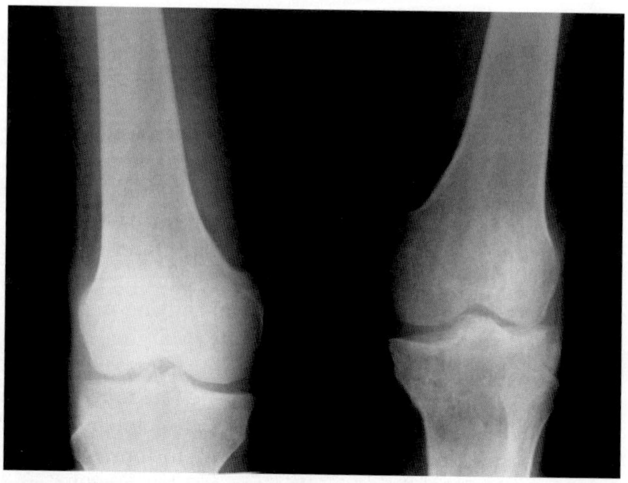

FIG. 2: Diffuse osteopenia with lytic lesion seen at the lateral articular margin of tibia with relative preservation of joint spaces in a case of tuberculosis of left knee.

images (T2WI) suggesting hemosiderin deposition, rim of synovial lesions on pregadolinium T1-weighted images (T1WI) and fluid loculations with enhancing synovial rims and erosions on postgadolinium images may be helpful in characterizing the lesion as tubercular when the radiographs are normal **(Fig. 3)**.

Magnetic resonance imaging can be helpful in diagnostic evaluation:

- *Short-tau inversion recovery (STIR) imaging, inversion recovery [repetition time (TR) >2,000 ms; echo time (TE) >30 ms; inversion-time (TI) = 120–150 ms)]*: Fat-saturation technique that results in markedly decreased signal intensity from fat and strikingly increased signal from fluid and edema. Inversion recovery is an extremely sensitive tool for detecting tissue and marrow pathology. Fast spin echo (FSE)-STIR sequence is used with most of our musculoskeletal protocols.
- T2-weighted sequences are sensitive in picking up high signal of joint fluid and make it a sensitive method to detect joint effusion.

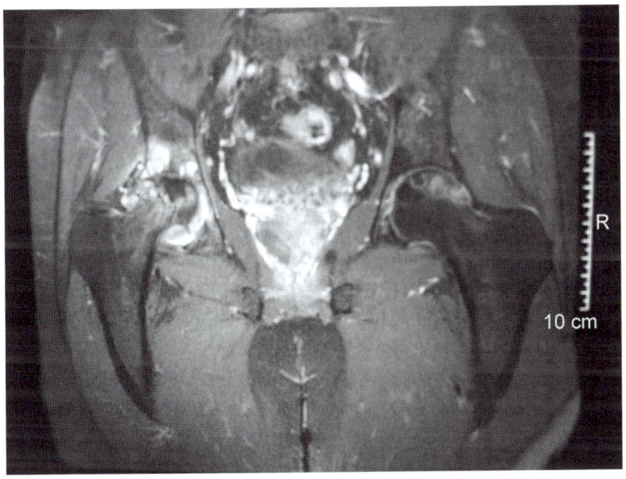

FIG. 3: Fluid loculations with enhancing synovial rims and erosions on postgadolinium images in a case of tuberculosis of right hip.

- T2-weighted images depict synovial proliferation as hypointense, while contrast-enhanced MR shows marked enhancement after gadolinium injection.
- Caseating granulomas with solid centers give a characteristic hypointense signal to the synovium on T2WI.
- Chondral lesions and subchondral bone erosions may be visible at a stage, when the joint space is still well preserved.
- *Penumbra sign* may be present. A thin intermediate signal intensity rim along the periphery of a bone or soft tissue abscess on unenhanced T1WI may be seen, due to layer of granulation tissue along its wall. It is useful in identifying soft tissue abscesses.
- In the pelvis and extremities, routine protocols should include T1, STIR, and postgadolinium T1WI. Section thickness used in the pelvis is 7 mm and in the extremities, 4 mm.
- MRI can be helpful in detecting bone marrow inflammation, intraosseous abscess, sequestrum, cortical destruction, cloaca, and sinus tract formation **(Figs. 4A to C)**.
- Tenosynovitis may be seen in active (hygromatous) and chronic (serofibrinous) phase and bursitis may be seen as distended bursa or multiple small abscesses.[4,9,14]

Skeletal TB involving parts of body other than spine can be classified according to region of involvement:

- *Tuberculosis of joints*: Tubercular arthritis
- *Tuberculosis of long and flat bones*: Tubercular osteomyelitis
- *Tuberculosis of short tubular bones*: Tubular dactylitis.

TUBERCULOSIS OF JOINTS (ARTHRITIS)

Hip Joint

Lesion can arise in acetabulum, synovium, femoral epiphysis or metaphysis (Babcock's triangle) or spread to the hip from foci in the greater trochanter or ischium. If there is tubercular

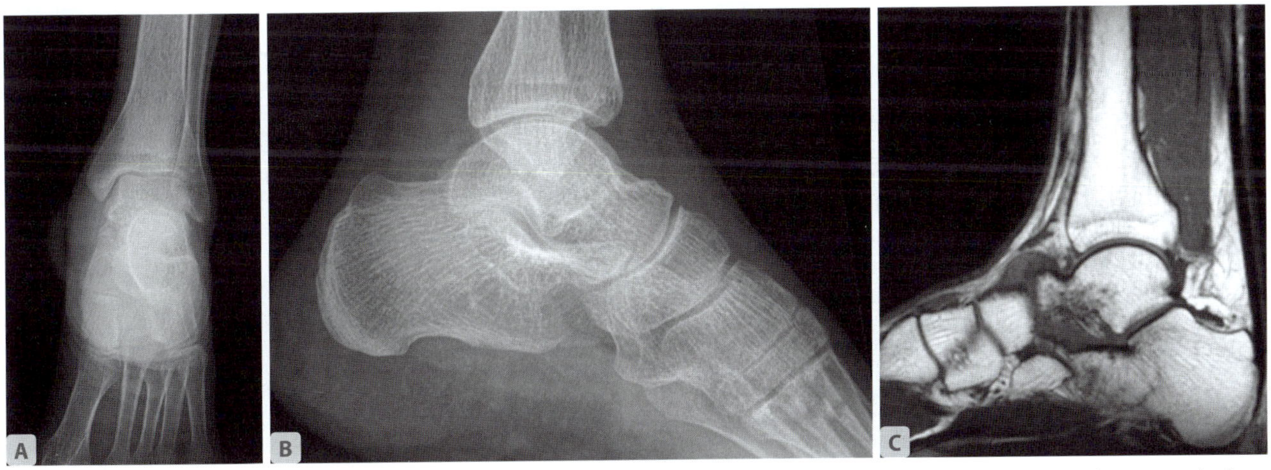

FIGS. 4A TO C: (A and B) Plain X-rays of ankle showing subtle osteolytic lesion in anterior aspect of talus on right side; (C) MRI showing markedly destructive lesion in anterior aspect of talus with associated soft tissue abnormality.

involvement of the upper end of femur (being entirely intracapsular), the joint is involved early in disease and there is destruction of articular margins of femoral head and acetabulum. Hip involvement is seen in about 15% of cases of osteoarticular TB.[15]

Tubercular lesion may start in the greater trochanter or the overlying bursa. There may be surface erosion or lytic lesion may be present in greater trochanter. TB of the greater trochanter may involve the overlying trochanteric bursa without involving the hip joint for a fairly long period of time.

Stage of Synovitis

The patient may present with irritable hip with plain radiograph being normal **(Fig. 5)**. Soft tissue swelling, marked deossification with radiologically significant osteoporosis appearing 12–18 weeks after symptoms may be present. Displacement of fat planes and positive obturator sign occur due to flexion deformity (reduced obturator foramina size).

Ultrasound, CT, and MRI are more sensitive in this stage to detect increased joint space and accumulation of fluid. Investigations may be repeated, at 3–6 weeks' interval, to help in establishing the diagnosis.

Differential diagnosis includes traumatic or nonspecific transient synovitis, Perthes' disease, slipped capital femoral epiphysis, and low-grade pyogenic infections.

Stage of Arthritis

There is deformity of the hip joint. In addition to osteoporosis, localized erosions may be seen in periarticular region **(Fig. 6)**. The destruction of articular cartilage leads to erosion of acetabular margin and femoral head with reduction of joint space. Lesions can usually be picked up on CT, before they are apparent on plain radiographs.[7,9]

Stage of Advanced Arthritis

With progression of disease, there is destruction of articular cartilage, acetabulum, femoral head, capsule, and ligaments. The capsule may also get thickened and contracted **(Figs. 7A to C)**. The upper end of femur may displace upward, dorsally breaking the Shenton's line and leaving the lower part of acetabulum empty (wandering acetabulum; **Fig. 8**). Bone loss can lead to bird-beak appearance with intrapelvic protrusion. If femoral head, neck are grossly destroyed and collapsed in an enlarged acetabulum, this appearance is called "mortar and pestle" appearance **(Fig. 9)**.

Radiological classification for TB of hip (Shanmugasundaram's classification) is useful in assessing relationship between various radiological types and functional outcome in which various radiological types have been described such as traveling acetabulum, dislocated hip, Perthes' type, protrusio acetabuli, atrophic type, and mortar and pestle type **(Figs. 10A to C)**.[16]

Knee Joint

Patients with tubercular involvement of knee can present with pain, limitation of movement or swelling, in addition to general clinical features of TB.

The knee joint has the largest intra-articular space and is involved in about 10% cases of osteoarticular TB. The initial focus may be in synovium or subchondral bone of distal femur, proximal tibia, or patella.[17]

In the synovial stage, there is osteoporosis, soft tissue swelling due to synovial effusion, thickened synovium and capsule. Synovial infection in childhood can lead to effusion, osteoporosis, accelerated growth, and maturation resulting in big bulbous squared epiphysis.[18] Synovitis can also cause widening of the intercondylar notch. Synovial inflammation with cartilage destruction leads to bony involvement in subarticular region and pus formation in joint.

As arthritis sets in, there is loss of definition of articular surfaces, marginal erosions, decreased joint space, and destruction of bones **(Fig. 11)**.

In advanced arthritis, there is bony destruction with joint space reduction and deformity. Translocation of tibia can occur with respect to femur posteriorly, laterally, or superiorly.

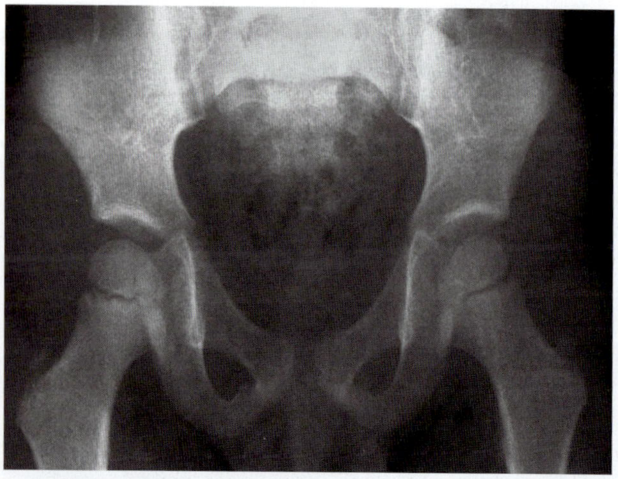

FIG. 5: Plain X-ray of pelvis showing relatively well-maintained hip joint on left side in an early case of tuberculosis of left hip with hip joint effusion on ultrasound.

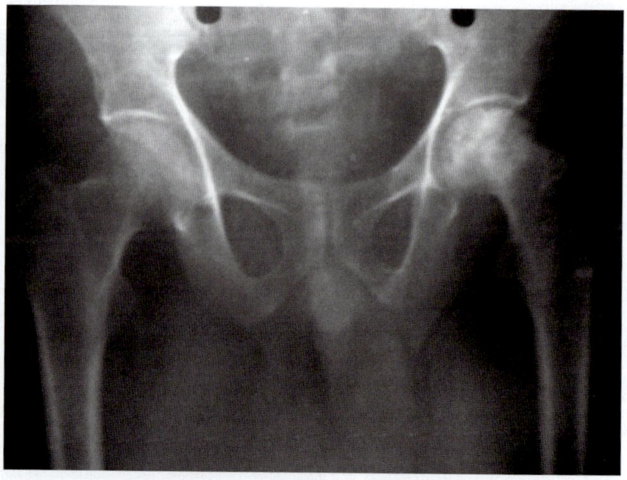

FIG. 6: Tubercular arthritis of left hip showing periarticular osteopenia, indistinct articular surfaces and erosions of femoral head and neck with relative preservation of joint space.

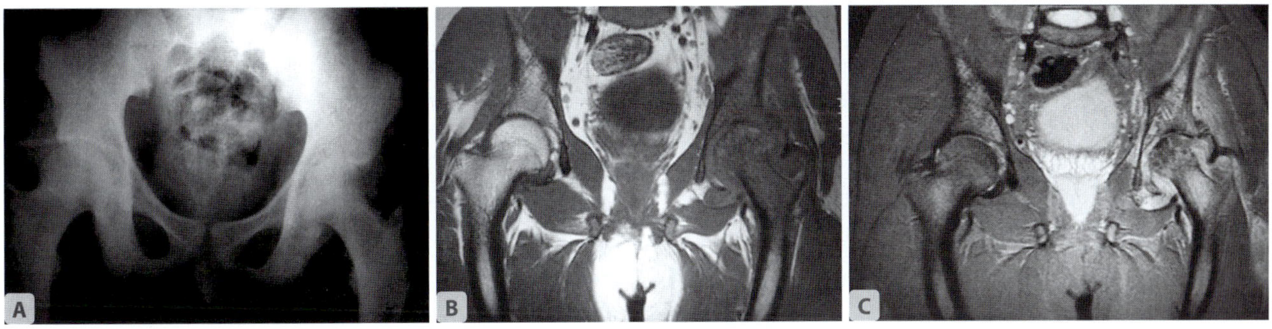

FIGS. 7A TO C: (A) Plain X-ray of pelvis showing erosion of the lateral aspect of femur head and neck with markedly reduced joint space on left side; (B and C) Altered marrow signal intensity in the left femoral head and neck appearing hypointense on T1 and hyperintense on short-tau inversion recovery (STIR) magnetic resonance images.

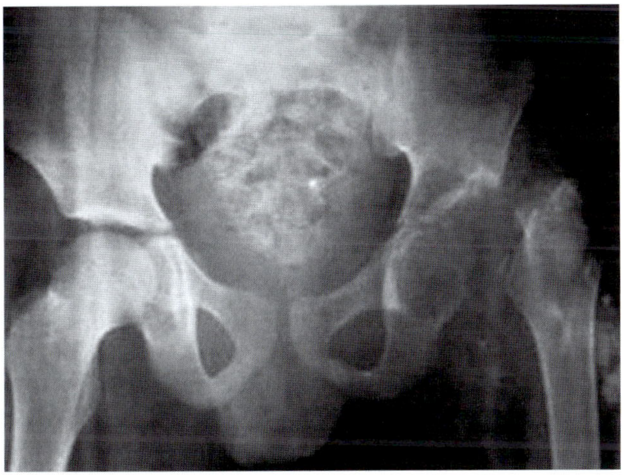

FIG. 8: Plain X-ray of pelvis showing destruction and subluxation of upper end of left femur, being displaced upwards and dorsally resulting in "wandering acetabulum".

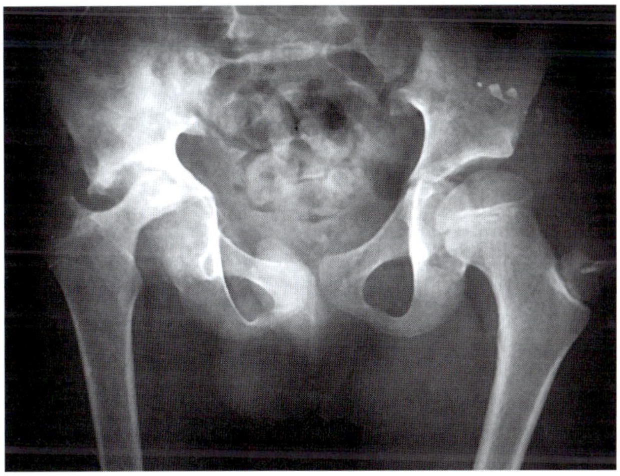

FIG. 9: Plain X-ray of pelvis showing gross destruction of right femoral head and neck with collapse contained within the enlarged acetabulum giving "mortar and pestle appearance".

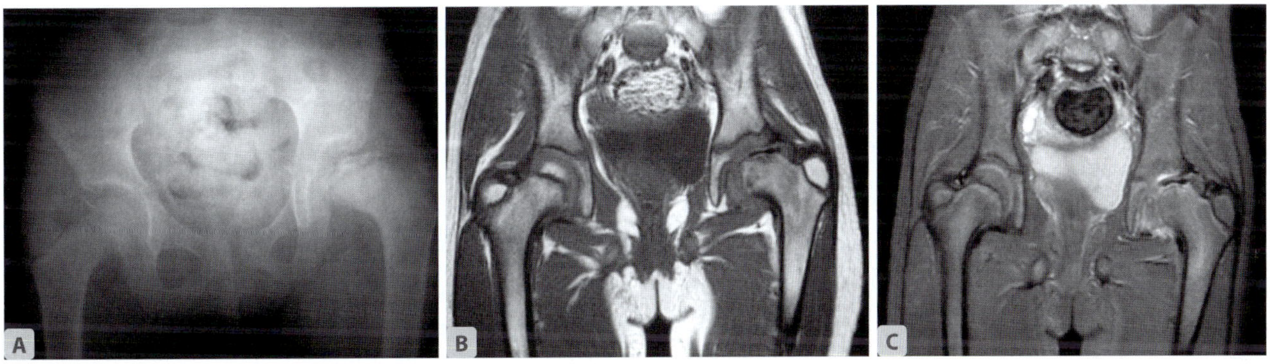

FIGS. 10A TO C: (A) There is evidence of irregularity, partial collapse and sclerosis of epiphysis of left femoral head suggestive of Perthes' type appearance in a case of tuberculosis of left hip joint; (B and C) Flattening of the left femur capital epiphysis in the same case, which appears diffusely hypointense on T1 and short-tau inversion recovery suggestive of sclerosis with marrow signal alteration noted in the left femoral neck.

The differential diagnosis includes juvenile rheumatoid arthritis, villonodular synovitis, osteochondritis dissecans, and hemophilia.

Diagnosis can be aided by clinical sign and symptoms, radiologically by noting regional osteopenia, bony destructive lesions, and joint involvement with pathologic confirmation by fluid analysis or synovial biopsy.

Ankle and Foot

Swelling, limp, and pain may be the early presenting features in TB of ankle joint. The swelling is evident in front of the joint, around the malleoli, and tendoachilles insertion. Marked osteoporosis with or without erosions and osteolytic lesions may be present in active stage of disease. There may

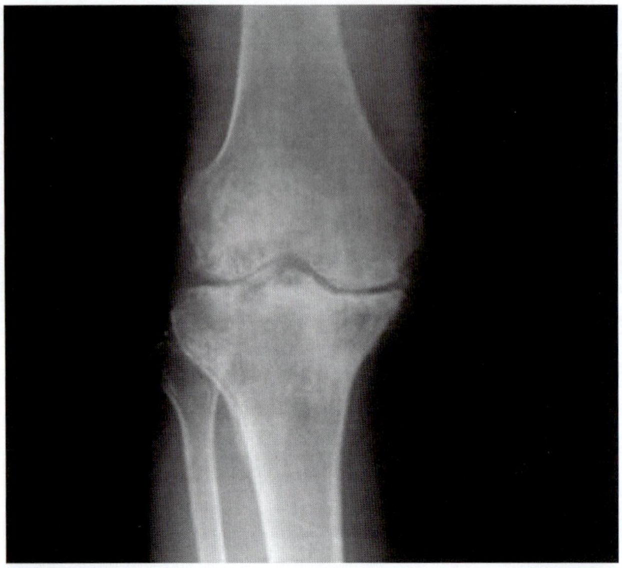

FIG. 11: Plain X-ray of knee joint showing juxta-articular osteopenia with fuzziness of articular margins numerous marginal erosions and loss of joint space.

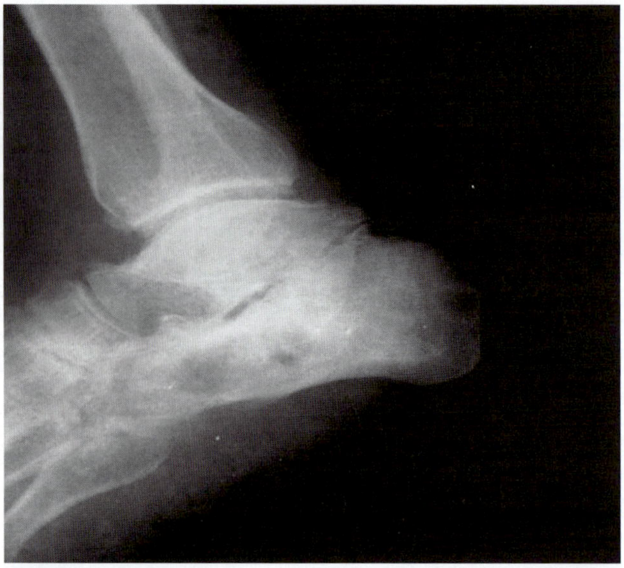

FIG. 12: Plain X-ray of ankle joint showing marginal erosions at subtalar joint with indistinct articular surfaces and loss of joint space.

be unsharpness of articular surfaces along with reduction of joint space **(Fig. 12)**.

In long-standing cases, gross destruction of bones and sinus formation can result. The ankle joint can show pathological anterior dislocation. Rarely, periosteal reaction may occur.

In tubercular affliction of foot, common involvement is seen of calcaneum, subtalar and midtarsal joints, anterior two-thirds of calcaneum being commonly affected.

Talus, metatarsal bones, navicular, cuneiform, cuboid can all get involved.[19] Radiographs can reveal presence of osteolyic lesion with or without coke-like sequestrum. Tubercular infection rapidly spreads across the intercommunicating synovial channels, so multiple bones are commonly involved **(Figs. 13A and B)**.

Differential diagnosis of tubercular affliction includes maduramycosis and neuropathic foot due to various causes, osteochondritis dissecans of talus.

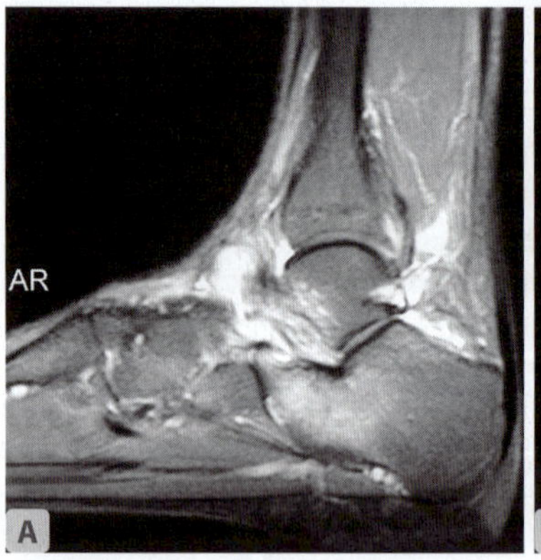

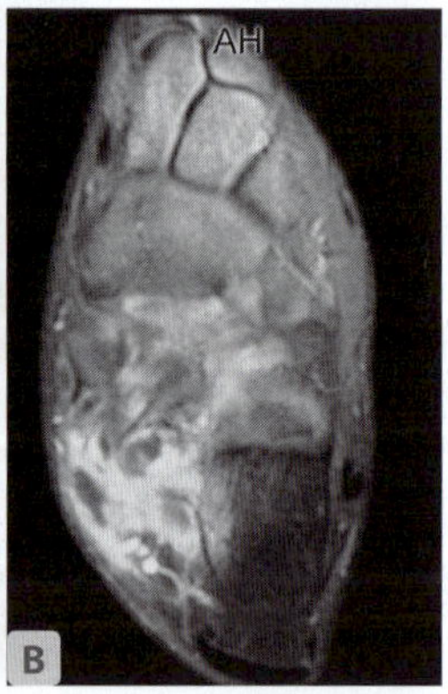

FIGS. 13A AND B: MRI of ankle joint in a case of talocalcaneal tuberculosis showing bony destruction involving talus, multiple collections along with rim enhancement in the subtalar region with cloaca and sinus tract formation.

Shoulder

Tubercular disease involving the shoulder joint is rare. It is more frequent in adults and the incidence of coexisting pulmonary TB is high. The sites of involvement include humeral head, scapula (glenoid, coracoid process, and spine of scapula), and acromioclavicular joint.

In the shoulder joint, the initial tubercular destruction is typically widespread because of the small surface contact area of articular cartilage. There is painful restriction of movement of shoulder in abduction and internal rotation with wasting of associated muscles, as the disease becomes chronic.[20]

Radiologically, there is osteoporosis with erosion of articular margins (fuzzy) with osteolytic lesion involving head of humerus, glenoid or both **(Fig. 14)**. The lesion may mimic giant cell tumor. Sinus formation can also occur. In advanced cases, inferior subluxation of the humeral head and fibrous ankylosis may result **(Fig. 15)**. In atrophic variety of tubercular affliction of shoulder, the disease runs a benign course without pus formation called *caries sicca* and small pitted erosions on the humeral head may be seen. The classical dry type is more common in adults while the fulminating variety with cold abscess or sinus formation is more common in children.[21]

Since the joint space is small, multiple and large osseous destructive lesions are commonly seen. MRI can show synovial lesions as well as the osseous lesions.

Differential diagnosis includes periarthritis, post-traumatic stiff shoulder. Aspiration of joint fluid or biopsy may be required to arrive at the diagnosis.

Elbow

Tubercular involvement is seen in about 2–5% cases.

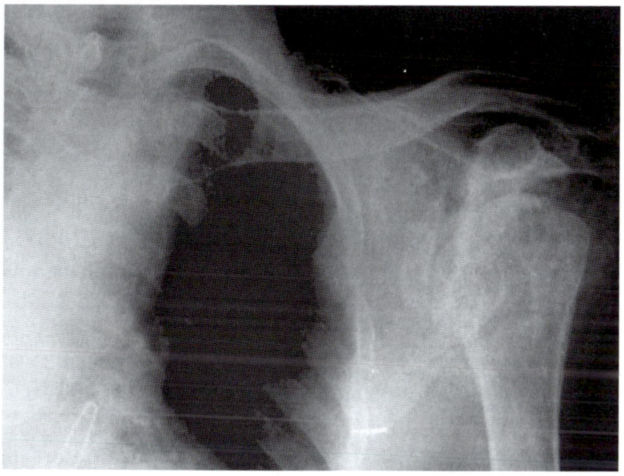

FIG. 14: Plain X-ray of left shoulder joint showing erosions and deformity of humeral head and acetabular margin with osteopenia and periarticular calcification.

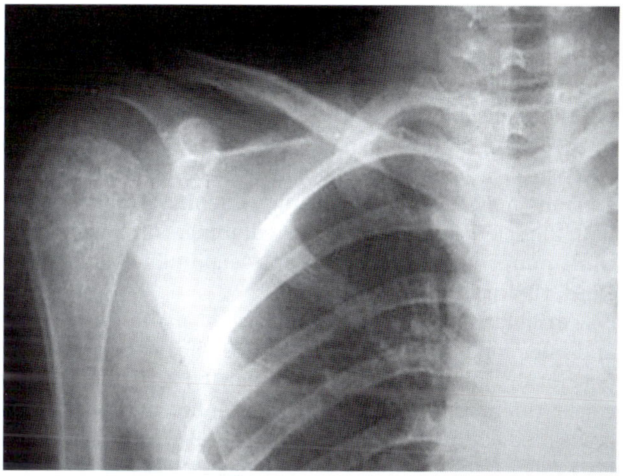

FIG. 15: Plain X-ray of right shoulder joint showing fuzzy articular margins and osteolytic lesions in proximal part of right humerus with pathological subluxation of head of humerus.

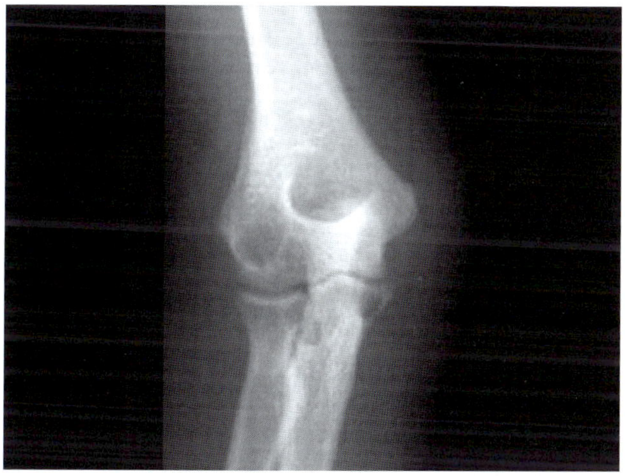

FIG. 16: Plain X-ray of right elbow joint showing multiple osteolytic lesions within the radius, ulna, and capitulum.

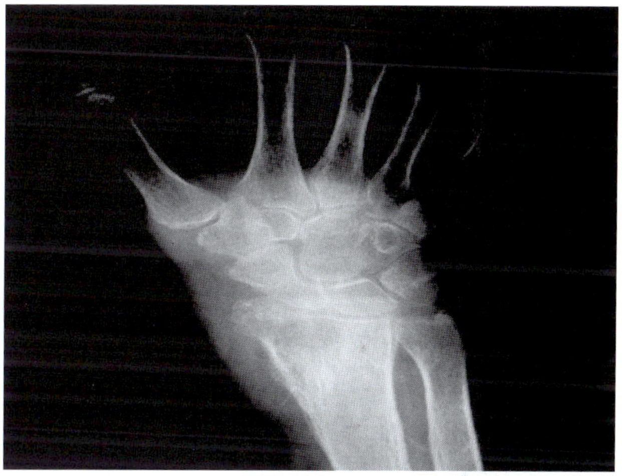

FIG. 17: Plain X-ray of right wrist joint showing irregular area of lytic destruction seen in distal metaphysis of radius with osteoporosis and soft tissue swelling.

Humeral condyles, radial head, and olecranon are frequently involved **(Fig. 16)**. Rarely the disease is synovial in origin.

Radiographic features in articular type include involvement of humerus and ulna, osteoporosis, blurring of articular cortex, and early compromise of joint space, while in extra-articular type ulna is more frequently involved with destructive lesions seen in olecranon or coronoid process.[9,21] Periostitis may also be seen.

Radiographs may depict blurring of articular margins due to synovial involvement. Osteolytic lesions may be seen around the elbow joint. In advanced case, there is decreased joint space and subchondral bone destruction.[20,21] Periostitis commonly affects the ulna.

Osteoid osteoma involving lateral condyle which is intra-articular and osteochondritis dissecans can cause diagnostic dilemma.

Wrist and Carpus

It is a rare site, usually affecting adults. Sites of involvement include distal radius, scaphoid, capitate, and lunate, with or without involvement of adjacent tendon sheaths **(Fig. 17)**.

Radiographic features include intense osteoporosis, soft tissue swelling, erosions of articular margins and cartilage destructions, periosteal reaction, and early appearance of ossification centers.

All carpal bones tend to get involved in adults while more localized lesions are seen in children. This is thought to be due to thicker articular cartilage in children.[22] With cartilage destruction, the carpal bones become crowded and adjacent bones tend to get involved. Intense demineralization is present in carpus, distal radius and ulna, metacarpals being usually spared. This serves as a differentiating feature from rheumatoid arthritis.

Sacroiliac Joints

These are affected more often in young adults than children and the involvement is usually unilateral. Sacroiliac joint infection is usually associated with TB of spine.

Radiographic features include irregularity and fuzziness of articular surfaces starting at the inferior surface. Subarticular erosions may be present causing widening of joint space. Both the sclerosis and erosions predominate on the iliac side while punched out lesions may be seen in ilium or sacrum **(Figs. 18A to D)**.

Articular erosions cause widening of the joint space and infection is associated with abscess formation over the back of the joint which may later calcify. Articular erosion cause widening of the joint space and tubercular infection is associated with abscess formation. This abscess may remain intrapelvic or extend under the glutei muscles.[23]

Magnetic resonance imaging is the ideal means of evaluating the complex anatomy of sacroiliac joints. Coronal imaging of the sacroiliac joints, parallel to the plane of the sacrum allows direct comparison of one sacroiliac joint to the other.[23,24]

BCG OSTEITIS

Bacille Calmette-Guérin is a vaccine of an attenuated bovine tubercular *Bacillus*. Although complications are unusual, generalized BCG infection and bone and joint infection can occur after BCG vaccination. Due to hematogenous spread of BCG infection to the skeleton, it is not usually associated with immunologic disorder and has a favorable prognosis.

Radiologically, BCG osteomyelitis affects children between 6 months and 6 year. It usually affects epiphysis and metaphysis of tubular bone especially around the knee, ribs, the sternum, the small bones of hand and feet. Lesions are more common on same side of the body as the vaccine was injected. Solitary lesions predominate and are seen as well-defined lytic foci.

Foucard and Helmstedt had suggested parameters to establish diagnosis of BCG-induced osteitis as follows:[23]

- BCG vaccination in the neonatal period.
- A period of less than 4 years between vaccination and symptom onset.
- No contact between the child and any adults with TB.

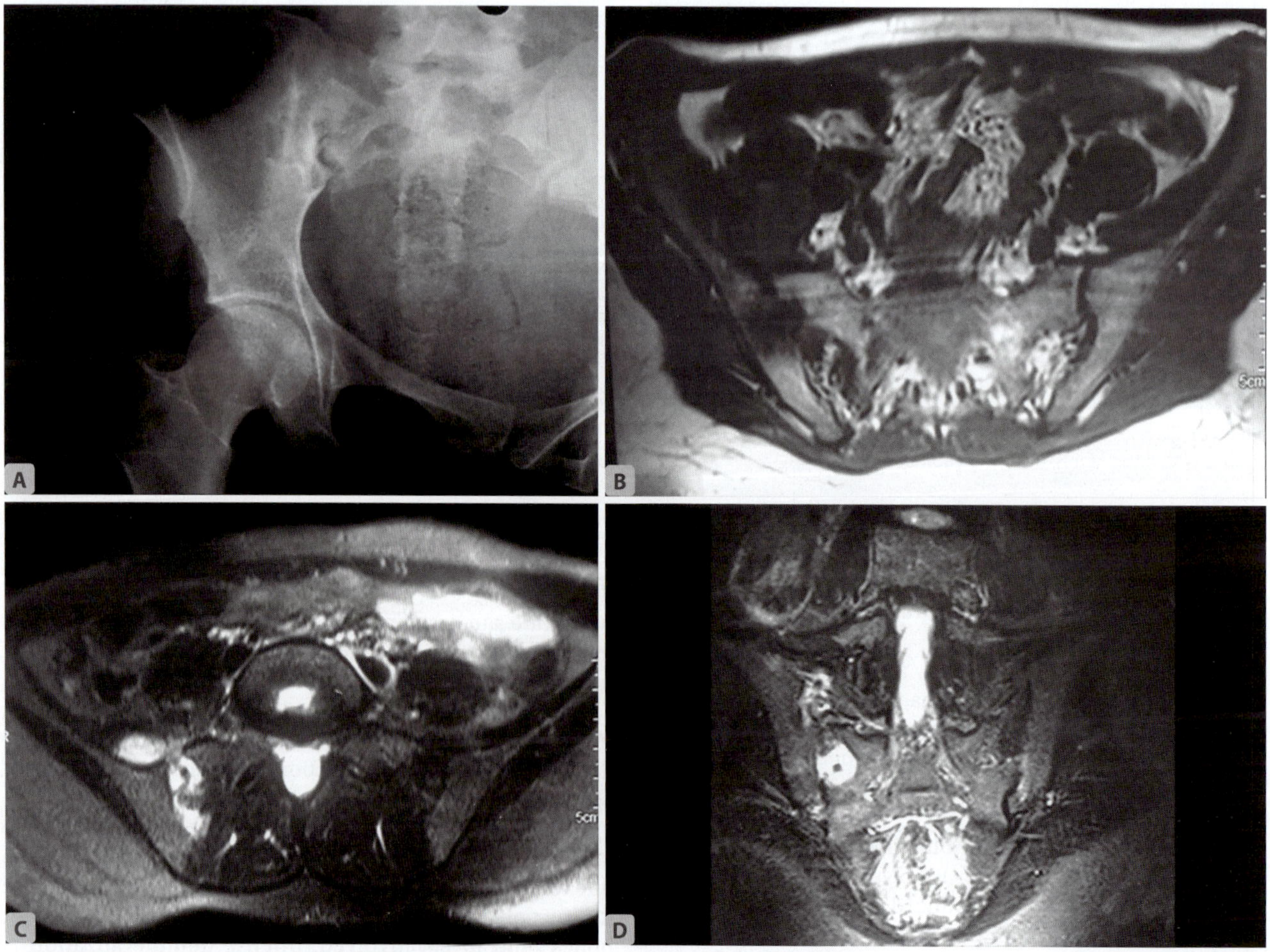

FIGS. 18A TO D: (A) Plain X-ray of pelvis showing large erosions with surrounding sclerosis at right sacroiliac joint; (B and C) Axial T1W and T2W image shows hypointensity along iliac blade with hyperintense signal on T2 likely to be marrow edema with synovial proliferation with altered signal intensity in iliacus muscle; (D) STIR MR image showing hyperintense synovium in right sacroiliac joint.

- A consistent clinical profile
- Histopathology suggestive of TB

TUBERCULOSIS OF LONG AND FLAT BONES

Tubercular osteomyelitis occurs in roughly 3% of patients suffering from bone or joint TB, with multifocal involvement in about 7% cases. Flat bones are commonly involved and include sternum, scapula, ischium, and rarely skull. The lesions tend to be simultaneous in onset and progression and generally affect persons with low immune resistance. Symmetric well round, oval cystic lesions, with little or no periosteal reaction initially, may be present **(Fig. 19)**. In untreated cases, laminated periosteal reaction may be seen **(Figs. 20A to D)**. Sequestra formation is uncommon in adults, though in children large sequestra may be seen as the intraosseous vasculature is more prone to thrombosis. Joint involvement is rare as the lesions are diaphyseal or metphyseal.[24,25] There is no sclerosis, abscess or sinus formation, so it is also called as closed cystic TB.

Differential diagnosis includes polyostotic fibrous dysplasia, eosinophilic granuloma of the bone, and enchondromatosis. Isolated tubercular involvement of bone is rare (2–3% of all cases).

Pathology

Bones are involved as a result of hematogenous spread from a primary focus, usually in the lung or the lymphatic system. Granulomatous lesion develops within the bone at the site of deposition of the *Mycobacterium*, usually metaphysis, which is the site of infection. Earliest lesion appears as eccentric osteolytic lesion in the shaft near the epiphysis or metaphysis. Epiphyseal growth plate offers little resistance resulting in transphyseal spread of infections.

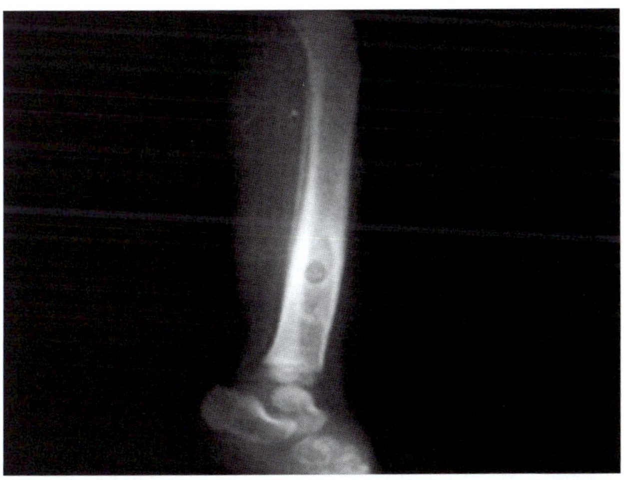

FIG. 19: Plain X-ray of right leg with ankle lateral view showing well- defined round osteolytic area seen in the shaft of tibia, in a case of diaphyseal tuberculosis.

Two types of lesions are described. *Caseous exudative type*, in which there is destruction of bony trabeculae, softening and caseation necrosis followed by formation of tuberculous pus or cold abscess and *granular type caries sicca*, where predominantly granulation tissue is formed with minimal caseation.

Tuberculosis of Long Bones

Two varieties of long bone TB occur:

1. Metaphyseal type, in which oval or round focus in metaphysis ultimately crosses into the epiphysis and further to involve the joint. Femur and tibia being the most commonly affected bones.
2. Cystic (diaphyseal type) generally affecting children and young adults. There is presence of well-defined round or oval lytic areas involving and expanding the diaphysis. Large sequestra may be seen in diaphysis, due to thrombosis of intraosseous vasculature in children. Tibia is the most common bone involved. Joint involvement is infrequent. Solitary involvement is predominant although multifocal involvement can occur. Multiple cystic diaphyseal lesions can occur rarely. The condition is symmetrical in distribution, with simultaneous onset,

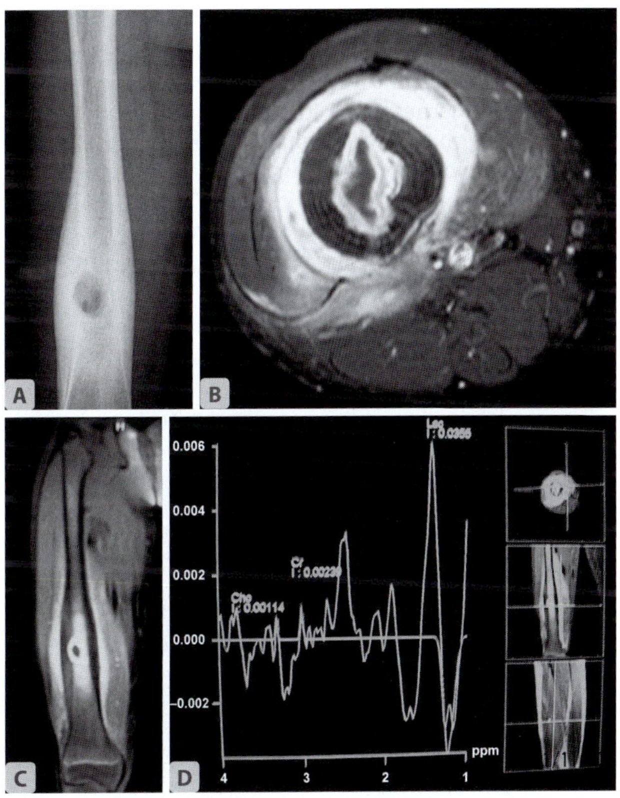

FIGS. 20A TO D: (A) Plain X-ray of right thigh showing well-defined round osteolytic area in the shaft of right femur, along with marked laminated periosteal reaction; (B and C) Magnetic resonance axial and coronal images showing intraosseous abscess in right femur, along with marked laminated periosteal reaction; (D) Magnetic resonance spectroscopic image showing prominent lactate peak in a case of diaphyseal tuberculosis.

progression, and regression. Multifocal tuberculous osteomyelitis also known as *osteitis cystica tuberculosa multiplex.*[25]

Multiple sites of involvement are seen in children, while in adults, involvement is more often confined to a single bone. The earliest lesion appears as an eccentric area of osteolysis in the metaphysis. Little or no surrounding reactive bone and local osteopenia are salient features.

The radiographic appearance may be somewhat different in children as compared to adults. In young patients, the lesions may be symmetrical and favor metaphyseal region. They are usually osteolytic and well-defined, without sclerosis, and may show variable size while in adults, the lesions are smaller, located in the long axis of bone, and may show well-defined sclerotic margins.

On MRI, early focus of altered marrow signal with irregular margins and cortical invasion with ill-defined soft tissue may be seen. Eccentric lesion with cortical breach may show irregular breach or hyperintensity within the cortical black line while small communicating abscesses are better appreciated on postcontrast T1WI as enhancing rings of juxtacortical inflammatory tissue and are a strong predictor of TB.

Flat Bones

Ribs

Rib involvement is seen in about 2% cases of bone TB, adults being generally affected. Nearly one-third of patients will have pulmonary TB or TB at other sites. Patient may present with pain, tenderness, and fluctuant chest wall swelling. There is bony rib expansion with punched out lesions and destruction which may be poorly marginated, posterior half of ribs being most commonly affected **(Fig. 21)**. Associated extrapleural soft tissue abscesses presenting as cold abscesses are commonly seen. The abscess may present as chest wall discharging sinus.[5,7]

Scapula

Scapula is a rare site for tubercular infection. The infective focus may be present in acromion, spine, neck, superior or inferior angle of scapula. The patient can present with pain and swelling around scapula. CT and MRI are helpful in early detection of lesions.[23,24]

Sternum

Sternum is involved in about one and a half percent of cases. An irregular destructive lesion along with presence of retrosternal and presternal soft tissue mass may be seen. There is paucity of sclerosis or periostitis.[24]

Skull

Frontal bone is the most common site to be involved in bones of cranial vault. Ill-defined lytic lesion may be the only radiological feature seen, with overlying cold abscess (Pott's puffy tumor). Button sequestrum can also be sometimes seen **(Fig. 22)**. Facial bones and mandibular involvement is extremely rare.[8,9]

Pelvis

Isolated tubercular lesion may occur in iliac bone, ischial tuberosity, and ischiopubic ramus. Radiologically, lytic lesions without surrounding sclerosis or periosteal reaction may be seen. Infection may extend to involve pubic symphysis **(Fig. 23)**.

Sternoclavicular Joint

Tuberculosis of the sternoclavicular joint is rare. It is usually seen in the region of medial end and presents with a painful swelling. Cold abscess and sinus can result as a complication. MRI can be a useful modality to detect early erosions and associated soft tissue swelling. Biopsy may be necessary in doubtful cases. Differential diagnosis includes rheumatoid arthritis, multiple myeloma, metastasis, and low-grade pyogenic infections.[11,14,24]

Acromioclavicular Joint

Tuberculosis of the acromioclavicular joint is also rare. It is usually seen in the region of lateral end of clavicle and presents with a painful swelling.[24] Clavicle may rarely be involved

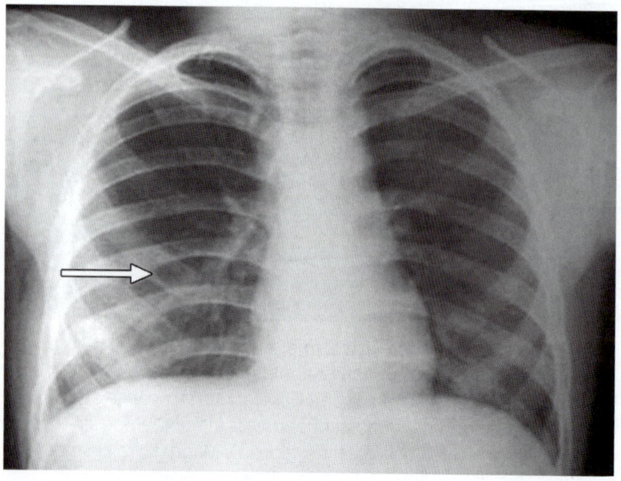

FIG. 21: Plain X-ray of chest showing lytic lesion involving anterior end of right 3rd rib in a case of rib tuberculosis.

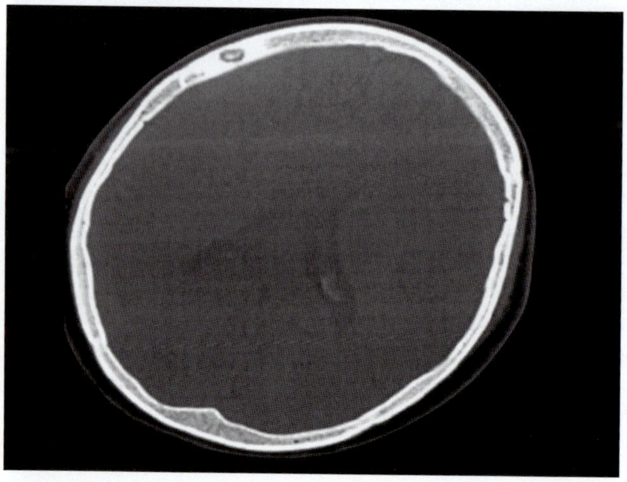

FIG. 22: Plain CT scan of cranium showing button sequestrum in the right parietal bone.

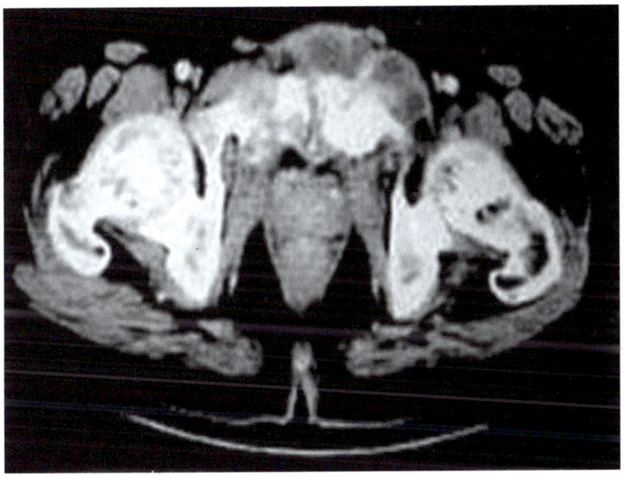

FIG. 23: Axial CT scan showing bilateral pubic bone erosions with subcutaneous small cold abscess.

without involvement of adjoining joints. There may be diffuse thickening and honeycombing, multiple cystic cavities, and sequestra formation such as pyogenic infections. Biopsy may be necessary to confirm the diagnosis.

TUBERCULOSIS OF SHORT BONES

Tuberculosis of short tubular bones is referred to as tubercular dactylitis. It is primarily a disease of childhood. The disease primarily affects short tubular bones of hands and feet.

Hand bones are more commonly affected than bones of feet. Proximal phalanges of 2nd and 3rd fingers and metacarpals of 3rd and 4th fingers are frequently involved in tubercular dactylitis.

Clinical features include soft tissue swelling, which may be followed by pain and numbness. Swelling due to abscess formation may occur. There is usually no fever or other signs of inflammation. Boyer and Nelaton first described tubercular dactylitis. The short tubular bones show cystic expansion as if with air and the condition has been characteristically described as "spina ventosa", spina meaning short bone and ventosa meaning expanded with air.[23]

Initial bony lesion is in the marrow. The disease is characterized by bone destruction and fusiform expansion of the bone, often accompanied by soft tissue swelling. It is more marked in diaphysis of metacarpals and metatarsals in children. Periosteal reaction and sequestra are uncommon. Healing is gradual by sclerosis.[24]

Magnetic resonance imaging may demonstrate intraosseous involvement earlier than with other imaging modalities **(Figs. 24A and B)**.

This condition needs to be differentiated from syphilitic dactylitis, in which there is bilateral and symmetric involvement, more periostitis, less soft tissue swelling and less sequestrations and from pyogenic osteomyelitis in which there is marked periostitis. The differential diagnosis also includes sarcoidosis, hemoglobinopathies, and hyperparathyroidism.[24]

Tuberculosis of Tendon Sheaths and Bursae

While TB can involve any bursa or tendon sheath, the tendon sheaths of hand and wrist and trochanteric bursa are commonly involved.[25]

Primary investigation to confirm the diagnosis of tenosynovitis and to reveal the degree and extent of tendon and tendon sheath involvement is ultrasonography. Sonograms can be quickly obtained along virtually any orientation and very high-frequency transducers provide exquisite spatial and contrast resolution.

In chronic tenosynovitis, tendon and synovial thickening predominate with relatively little synovial sheath effusion, while in acute suppurative tenosynovitis, synovial sheath effusion is the predominant feature.[25]

Magnetic resonance imaging helps in delineating the precise extent of soft tissue involvement and any associated osseous or joint involvement. Three stages of tuberculous tenosynovitis have been described:

1. The *hygromatous stage* is characterized by the presence of fluid inside the tendon sheath without associated sheath thickening.
2. The *serofibrinous stage* is characterized by thickening of the flexor tendons and synovium, with multiple tiny hypointense nodules within the hyperintense synovial fluid on T2WI. These tiny nodules correspond to the *rice* bodies.
3. The *fungoid stage* is characterized by a soft tissue mass involving the tendon and tendon sheath. Among bursal infections, the most commonly affected locations are trochanteric, subacromial, subgluteal, and radioulnar wrist bursa. Plain radiography may demonstrate local osteopenia due to hyperemia in long-standing bursitis or focal osteolytic bone destruction (e.g., greater trochanter or the humeral head) due to local pressure of the enlarged bursa. The wall of the distended bursa may contain calcifications, which may be visible on radiographs.[8,25] On MRI, two patterns of involvement have been reported. A uniform distension of the bursa or multiple small abscesses in the bursa may be seen or low-signal intensity material within the fluid-filled bursa on T2WI may be seen due to the presence of caseous necrosis and fibrotic material.

Atypical Mycobacterial Infection

Infections due to atypical mycobacteria are also seen in specific clinical setting. Skin and pulmonary disease are most frequent, however, skeletal changes may also be noted. The infection may be seen in immunocompromised patients, those with renal transplants or those receiving corticosteroids. Infection can lead to osteomyelitis, septic arthritis, tenosynovitis, and bursitis.[20,23,25]

Radiologically, multiple lesions may be seen, metaphysis and diaphysis of long bones being usually affected. Discrete lesions may be present with sclerotic margins but osteoporosis is not marked. Abscesses and sinus tract can also be seen.

Tubercular Infection of Prosthetic Joint

Prosthetic joint infection may develop, due to reactivation of tubercular arthritis for which the operation had been

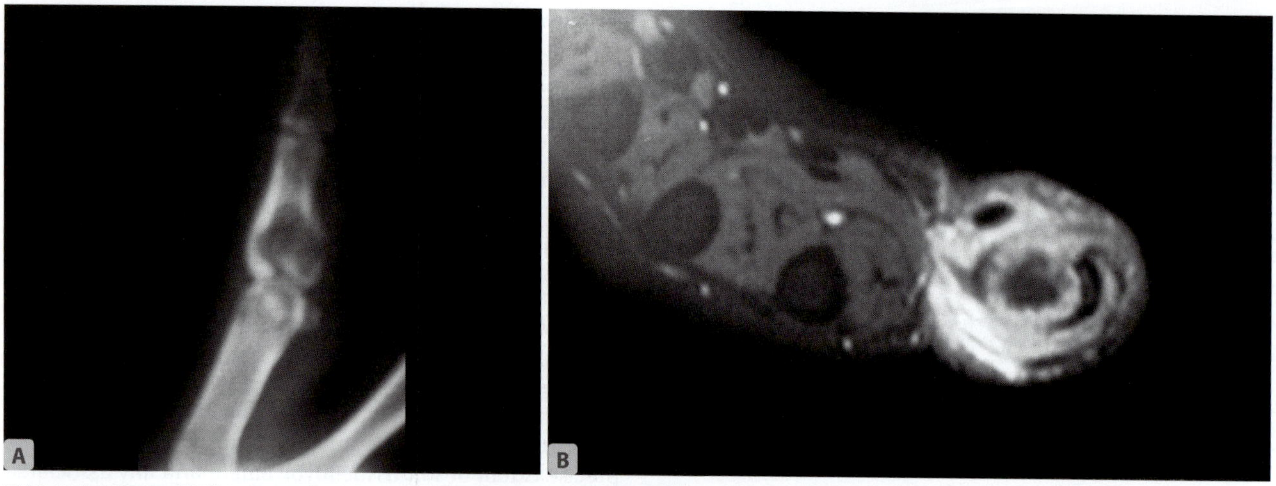

FIGS. 24A AND B: (A) Plain X-ray of right thumb showing cystic expansile lesion of the proximal shaft of proximal phalanx of right thumb with pathological fracture; (B) MRI of the same patient showing bone marrow inflammation along with marked enhancing synovium on postgadolinium images, in a biopsy proven case of tuberculosis.

performed.[26] Arthrocentesis and specimens are required for establishing the diagnosis.

CONCLUSION

It is difficult to diagnose the disease in its earliest stage as the clinical and radiologic findings are nonspecific in initial stages. We should have a high level of clinical suspicion, as the disease is endemic in our country. At this stage, cross-sectional imaging and histological examination can lead to correct diagnosis. In advanced cases, diagnosis is not much of a problem and imaging helps in supplementing and guiding therapeutic procedures.

REFERENCES

1. Yochum TR, Row LJ. Infection: non-suppurative osteomyelitis (tuberculosis). Essentials of Skeletal Radiology, 2nd edition. Philadelphia: Lippincott Williams and Wilkins; 1996.
2. Moore SL, Rafii M. Imaging of musculoskeletal and spinal tuberculosis. Radiol Clin North Am. 2001;39(2):329-42.
3. Bhan S, Nag HL. Skeletal tuberculosis. In: Sharma SK (Ed). Tuberculosis, 2nd edition. New Delhi: Jaypee Brothers Medical Publishers (P) Ltd; 2009. pp. 342-72.
4. Sawlani V, Chandra T, Mishra RN, Aggarwal A, Jain UK, Gujral RB. MRI features of tuberculosis of peripheral joints. Clin Radiol. 2003;58(10):755-62.
5. Grainger and Allison's Diagnostic Radiology: A Textbook of Medical Imaging, 4th edition. UK: Churchill Livingstone; 2005. pp. 2069-70.
6. Greenspan A. Orthopedic Imaging: A Practical Approach, 4th edition. Philadelphia: Lippincott Williams and Wilkins; 2004. pp. 798-9.
7. Tuli SM. Tuberculosis of the Skeletal System. New Delhi: Jaypee Brothers Medical Publishers (P) Ltd; 1997.
8. Sutton D. Textbook of Radiology and Imaging, 7th edition. UK: Churchill Livingstone; 2003. pp. 1166-71.
9. Resnik D, Kransdorf MJ. Bone and Joint Imaging, 3rd edition. Philadelphia: Elsevier Saunders; 2005. pp. 758-65.
10. Riddley N, Shaikh MI, Remedios D, Mitchell R. Radiology of skeletal tuberculosis. Orthopedics. 1998;21(11):1213-20.
11. Ebnezar J. Textbook of Orthopedics, 3rd edition. New Delhi: Jaypee Brothers Medical Publishers (P) Ltd; 2006. pp. 499-519.
12. Morris BS, Varma R, Garg A, Awasthi M, Maheshwari M. Multifocal musculoskeletal tuberculosis in children: appearances on computed tomography. Skeletal Radiol. 2002;31(1):1-8.
13. Yago Y, Yukihiro M, Kuroki H, Katsuragawa Y, Kubota K. Cold tubercular abscess identified by FDG PET. Ann Nucl Med. 2005;19(6):515-8.
14. Griffth JF, Kumta SM, Leung PC, Cheng JC, Chow LT, Metrewell C. Imaging of musculoskeletal tuberculosis: a new look at old disease. Clin Orthop Relat Res. 2002;398:32-9.
15. Babhulkar SS, Pande S. Tuberculosis of the hip. Clin Orthop Relat Res. 2002;398:93-9.
16. Shanmugasundaram TK. A clinicoradiological classification of tuberculosis of hip. Current Concepts in Bone Joint Tuberculosis. Madras: International Bone and Joint Club; 1983.
17. Hoffman EB, Allin J, Campbell JA, Leisegang FM. Tuberculosis of the knee. Clin Orthop Relat Res. 2002;398: 100-6.
18. Lee AS, Campbell JA, Hoffman EB. Tuberculosis of the knee in children. J Bone Joint Surg Br. 1995;77(2):313-8.
19. Dhillon MS, Nagi ON. Tuberculosis of the foot and ankle. Clin Orthop Relat Res. 2002;398:107-13.
20. Singh NV. Fundamental of Orthopedics, 1st edition. New Delhi: New Age International (P) Ltd; 2011. pp. 236-44.
21. Malaviya AN, Kotwal PP. Arthritis associated with tuberculosis. Best Pract Res Clin Rheumatol. 2003;17(2): 319-43.
22. Gardam M, Lim S. Mycobacterial osteomyelitis and arthritis. Infect Dis Clin North Am. 2005;19(4):819-30.
23. Harisinghani GM, McLoud TC, Shepard JO, Ko JP, Shroff MM, Mueller PR. Tuberculosis from head to toe. Radiographics. 2000;20(2):449-70.
24. Babhulkar SS, Pande SK. Unusual manifestations of osteoarticular tuberculosis. Clin Orthop Relat Res. 2002;398:114-20.
25. Boutin RD, Brossmann J, Sartoris DJ, Reilly D, Resnick D. Update on imaging of orthopedic infections. Orthop Clin North Am. 1998;29(1):41-65.
26. Kaya M, Nagoya S, Yamashita, Niiro N, Fujita M. Periprosthetic infection of the hip in a patient with no previous history of tuberculosis. J Bone Joint Surg Br. 2006;88(3):394-5.

CHAPTER

156

Nontubercular Bone and Joint Infections

Anindita Sinha, Manphool Singhal, Kushaljit Singh Sodhi

INTRODUCTION

Osteomyelitis refers to the infection of cortical bone and its marrow space. It is classified into three forms: (1) acute, (2) subacute, and (3) chronic. Subacute osteomyelitis is insidious in presentation as compared to the acute form. Chronic osteomyelitis is a continuous low-grade recurring infection. The pathogens causing osteomyelitis can be bacteria, viruses, mycobacteria or treponemes (syphilis). Pyogenic osteomyelitis is the most common.[1,2] Plain radiographs, scintigraphy, ultrasonography (USG), computed tomography (CT), and magnetic resonance imaging (MRI), all play an important role in the diagnosis of osteomyelitis, but overall diagnostic accuracy does not exceed more than 80–90%.[3] Presence of previous or chronic osteomyelitis, adjoining soft tissue infection, fracture, surgery, and prosthesis are the factors which make the diagnosis difficult.

IMAGING MODALITIES

Plain radiographs are the first imaging study asked for in the workup of osteomyelitis. If cortical irregularity, periosteal reaction, deep soft tissue swelling, and demineralization are detected, additional imaging may not be required to diagnose osteomyelitis.[3] However, only 5% of radiographs are positive in the early course of disease. Less than one-third reveal abnormality by 1 week while 90% are positive only by 3–4 weeks.[4] This delay constrains the utility of plain radiographs in the early diagnosis of osteomyelitis.

Computed tomography offers advantages over conventional radiographs in terms of early detection of bony changes, better visualization of axial skeletal involvement (e.g., spine, pelvis, sternum) and better delineation of overlapping bony abnormalities like thick periosteal reaction or sequestra in chronic osteomyelitis.

Radionuclide scintigraphy is the most sensitive investigation available for diagnosing acute osteomyelitis though the specificity is not as good.[3] 99mTc-labeled methylene diphosphonate (99mTc-MDP), 99mTc-hydroxymethylene diphosphonate (99mTc-HMDP), and gallium-67 (^{67}Ga) citrate are the most commonly used radionuclide agents. The sensitivity and specificity for combined 99mTc ^{67}Ga scanning are 50% and 78%, respectively.[5] Indium-111-labeled white blood cell (leukocyte) scanning (^{111}In WBC) has a higher sensitivity and specificity of 83% and 94%, respectively. Recently introduced Indium-111-labeled polyclonal immunoglobulin (IgG) has the highest sensitivity and specificity of 92% and 95–100%, respectively.[6,7] False negatives occur due to ischemic bone with no isotope uptake.[8] High-resolution USG is being increasingly used for diagnosis of acute osteomyelitis. Positive findings can be detected much earlier than on plain radiographs. Deep soft tissue swelling is the earliest sign which can be detected within 2–3 days of onset. The other changes include periosteal elevation seen as a hyperechoic line and subperiosteal fluid collection **(Fig. 1)**. Cortical breach is seen as a focal defect in the cortex.[9] In a prospective study of 25 patients done to assess the role of ultrasound in acute osteomyelitis, the authors found the presence of deep soft tissue swelling, periosseous fluid **(Fig. 2)**, and periosteal elevation has positive predictive value of 100% in first 3 days after the onset of symptoms.[10]

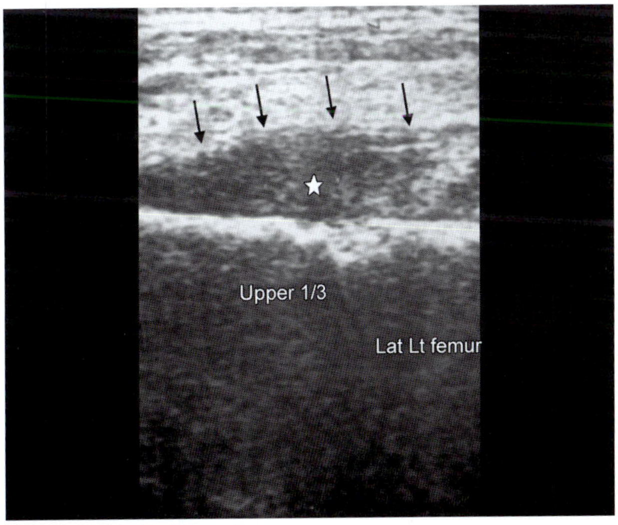

FIG. 1: Acute osteomyelitis. High-resolution ultrasonography (USG) of femur shows periosteal elevation (arrows) (hyperechoic line) with subperiosteal fluid collection (star).

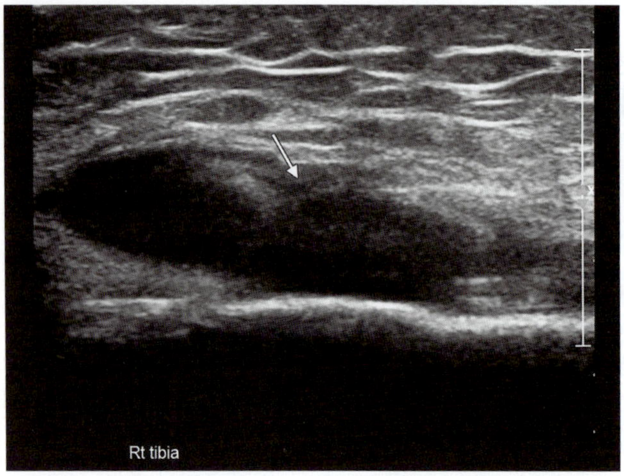

FIG. 2: High-resolution ultrasonography (USG) of tibia shows extraosseous fluid collection in a boy with acute osteomyelitis (arrow).

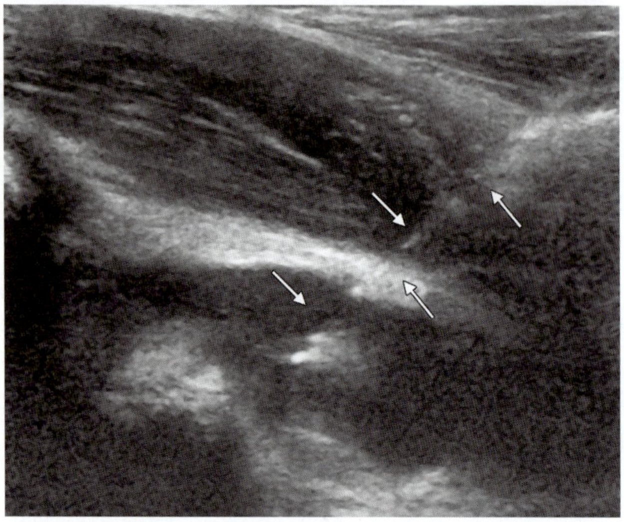

FIG. 3: USG-guided percutaneous aspiration of periosteal fluid. Note the needle in situ (arrows).

Ultrasonography is also an excellent method to detect presence of fluid in the joint which may be an indirect sign to suggest osteomyelitis especially of femur and humerus in an infant. In reactivation of chronic osteomyelitis, USG can demonstrate abscess or sinus tract formation in soft tissues which are characteristic of acute osteomyelitis. USG guidance can also be used for percutaneous aspiration of fluid from the joint or periosteal collection for diagnostic purposes **(Fig. 3)**.

Magnetic resonance imaging due to its multiplanar imaging capability, excellent tissue characterization and high-resolution is now the imaging modality of choice for the early diagnosis of osteomyelitis and overlying soft tissue involvement.[11] It has a sensitivity and specificity of 92–100% and 89–100%, respectively.[12] MRI is better than scintigraphy in evaluation of axial skeletal osteomyelitis because of better anatomical delineation.[13] In addition, MRI can distinguish soft tissue infection with periostitis from osteomyelitis.[14] Moreover, the complications of osteomyelitis like soft tissue and bone abscesses, physeal involvement, and septic arthritis can also be diagnosed which can help in further management such as determining the need for percutaneous or surgical drainage in addition to antibiotic therapy.[15-17]

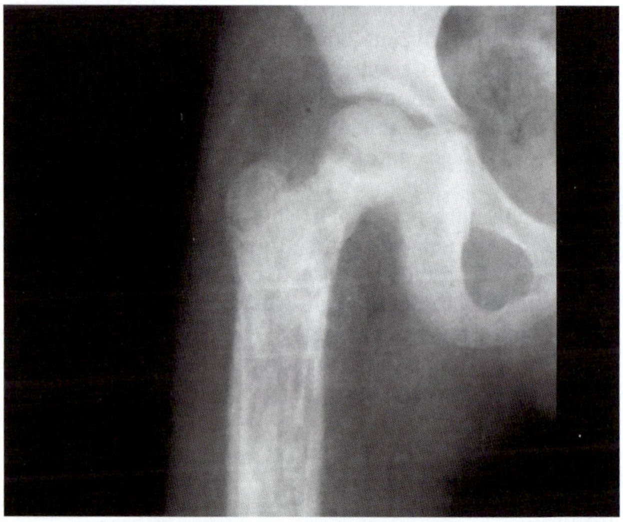

FIG. 4: Chronic osteomyelitis in a child. Radiograph of the right hip showing diffuse ill-defined lytic areas affecting the entire upper shaft of femur with cortical thickening. Note the sparing of epiphysis and the joint.

ACUTE OSTEOMYELITIS

Acute osteomyelitis is usually hematogenous in origin and generally follows skin infection. *Staphylococcus aureus* is the most common offending pathogen. Common age of presentation is 2–16 years with a male preponderance, the latter being attributed to greater exposure to trauma.

Clinical Features

Patients present with local or systemic symptoms with local tenderness, swelling, restriction of motion, fever, irritability, and poor feeding (in infants).

Pathophysiology of osteomyelitis varies in infants, children and adults, being related to the structural and vascular differences of bone at these ages. The blood-borne microbial emboli lodge in the metaphysis because of sluggish blood flow in this region. In children older than 1 year, the epiphyseal plate blocks extension of the infection **(Fig. 4)**, so the infection spreads laterally into the subperiosteal space or to the joint in which synovial reflections extend beyond the epiphysis to metaphysis, such as the shoulder and hip joints. In infants, small capillaries cross the epiphyseal growth plate and thus permit extension of infection to the epiphysis and the joint. In adults, the epiphyseal plate is fused and no longer forms a barrier to the spread of infection from metaphysis to the adjacent joint. Thus, acute pyogenic arthritis is a frequent complication of osteomyelitis in infants and adults **(Fig. 5)**.

The infarcted bone is reabsorbed by formation of granulation tissue and the dead cortex usually forms sequestrum. Reparative new bone formation starts roughly

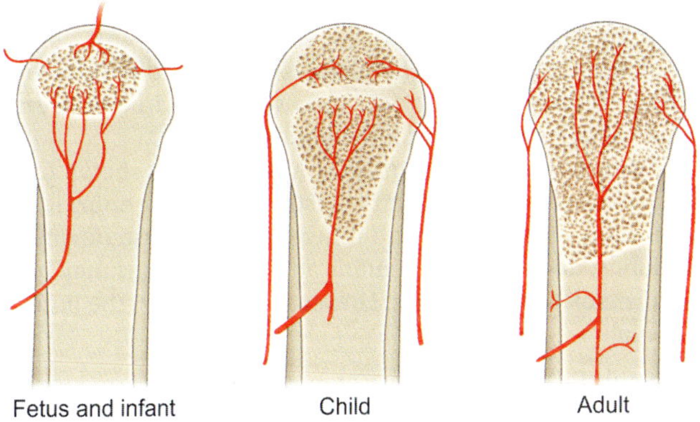

FIG. 5: Schematic diagram of vascular supply of the epimetaphyseal region in the infant, child, and adult.

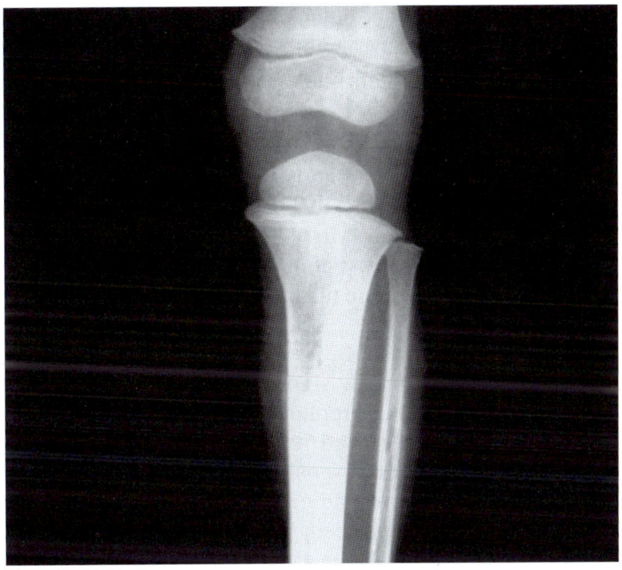

FIG. 6: Acute osteomyelitis of tibia. Radiograph of leg shows small lucencies in the metaphysis along with thin periosteal reaction.

10 days after the onset of infection and new bone is generally laid down along both periosteal and endosteal surfaces resulting in formation of involucrum. Cloacae appear at the site of dead periosteum.

Neonatal osteomyelitis presents with few clinical signs despite multiple sites of involvement, and hence, a complete skeletal survey is warranted in such cases.[18] Premature infants requiring umbilical catheterization are at higher risk for osteomyelitis.[19] Radionuclide bone scintigraphy is advocated in all patients with suspected neonatal osteomyelitis, following initial radiographs.[20]

A soft tissue component, subperiosteal abscess and dense involucrum are more striking in infants than in adults and children. This has been attributed to less rigid bone of infants and easy penetration of periosteum by the abscess.

In adults, direct inoculation from penetrating injury, surgery or adjacent soft tissue infection and periprosthetic infections are common causes of osteomyelitis.[21]

Immunocompromised patients with diabetes mellitus, human immunodeficiency virus/acquired immunodeficiency syndrome (HIV/AIDS), malnutrition, renal or liver failure are prone to developing osteomyelitis. Local factors like lymphedema, vascular stasis, and radiation also predispose to developing osteomyelitis.

Organisms: Bacterial—*Staphylococcus aureus* is the most common organism involved in hematogenous infection or direct inoculation, with methicillin-resistant *S. aureus* being a common pathogen, which is hard to treat. *Pseudomonas*, *Klebsiella* osteomyelitis occur in intravenous (IV) drug users.[22] Fungal osteomyelitis is common in immunocompromised patients.

Radiologic Features

Radiographs

The earliest radiographic changes are seen 7–14 days after onset of infection in the form of soft tissue swelling and small single or multiple osteolytic areas affecting the metaphysis **(Fig. 6)**. Extrusion of infected contents from the medullary cavity due to increased intramedullary pressure, through cortical bone into the subperiosteal space, which is loose in children causes a subperiosteal abscess formation and elevation of the periosteum.[22]

The periosteal reaction is typically lamellar and nodular and layered new bone formation after 3–6 weeks.[2] The dead bone (sequestrum) also forms at 3–8 weeks. It appears dense since it does not participate in normal bone mineral metabolism because of loss of its vascular supply. Osteopenia in the surrounding bone due to hyperemia enhances the density of the sequestrum. Once the acute phase has subsided, remodeling reverts the appearance of bone to normal in infants and children but in adults the sclerosis and cortical irregularity persist.

Patients with sickle cell disease have an unusual propensity for *Salmonella* osteomyelitis. This infection is diaphyseal and difficult to differentiate from a bone infarct. Localized cortical fissuring or tunneling is a characteristic and early feature of this entity.[23]

Despite its low sensitivity in detecting early osteomyelitis, radiographs should be the primary modality of investigation. MRI with or without contrast is the next appropriate investigation. Ultrasound may also be done, especially in cases of foreign body-induced osteomyelitis.[24]

Bone Scintigraphy

The bone scintigraphy shows positive findings much earlier than plain radiographs, usually within 3 days and sometimes within 24 hours of onset of infection. Traditionally, "triple phase" bone scanning is done, using technetium 99mTc agents. The first phase shows the "blood flow", the second phase shows the "blood pool" of the inflamed region and the third phase, which is acquired after 2–4 hours, shows the uptake by bone. Osteomyelitis is "hot" on all phases. However, in patients presenting within 48 hours, the isotope bone scan may reveal a "cold" spot on account of vasospasm. A false-positive result can occur in degenerative disease, healing fracture, inflammatory arthritis, and loose prosthesis. But these conditions do not show increased activity in early (I and II) phases, unlike osteomyelitis. Deep soft tissue infection with periostitis and diabetic osteopathy also cannot be differentiated from osteomyelitis on the basis of bone scanning alone.[3] MRI is considered superior to bone scan in distinguishing these two entities.

Magnetic Resonance Imaging

Magnetic resonance imaging is the modality of choice for early diagnosis of osteomyelitis. Early diagnosis is essential to prevent chronic changes in bone with bone destruction or deformity which are irreversible. MRI shows intramedullary signal change due to bone marrow edema as early as 1 or 2 days after infection.[25]

Magnetic resonance imaging features of acute osteomyelitis include low signal intensity due to pus or edema partially or fully replacing marrow signal on T1-weighted (T1W) image and high-signal intensity on T2-weighted (T2W) and fluid-sensitive images [fat-suppressed T2W and short tau inversion recovery (STIR) sequences] with postcontrast enhancement **(Figs. 7A to C)**. Intraosseous, subperiosteal, and soft tissue abscesses if present appear as well-circumscribed areas of focally decreased signal intensity on T1W images with increased signal intensity equal to that of fluid on fluid-sensitive sequences and rim enhancement on contrast T1W images.[15,26,27]

Rim enhancement of the abscess is useful in differentiating phlegmonous tissue from abscess which needs urgent surgical or image-guided intervention.[28]

Magnetic resonance imaging has also been shown to be more sensitive and specific than isotope bone scanning in the detection, localization, and differentiation of osteomyelitis, cellulitis, and abscess. Cellulitis and osteomyelitis may have similar soft tissue changes. However, in cellulitis, the bone is normal.[29]

Differential diagnosis of osteomyelitis:[22] Tumors such as Ewing's sarcoma, leukemia, Langerhans cell histiocytosis may mimic acute osteomyelitis even on MRI. Presence of intervening interspersed intramedullary fat within the lesion, peripherally enhancing rim of soft tissue (abscess) rather than heterogeneous enhancement of tumor-associated soft tissue go in favor of osteomyelitis. Osteomyelitis also causes more rapid progressive bone destruction.

Stress fractures and osteoid osteoma can also mimic osteomyelitis. Osteoid osteoma enhances rapidly on MRI

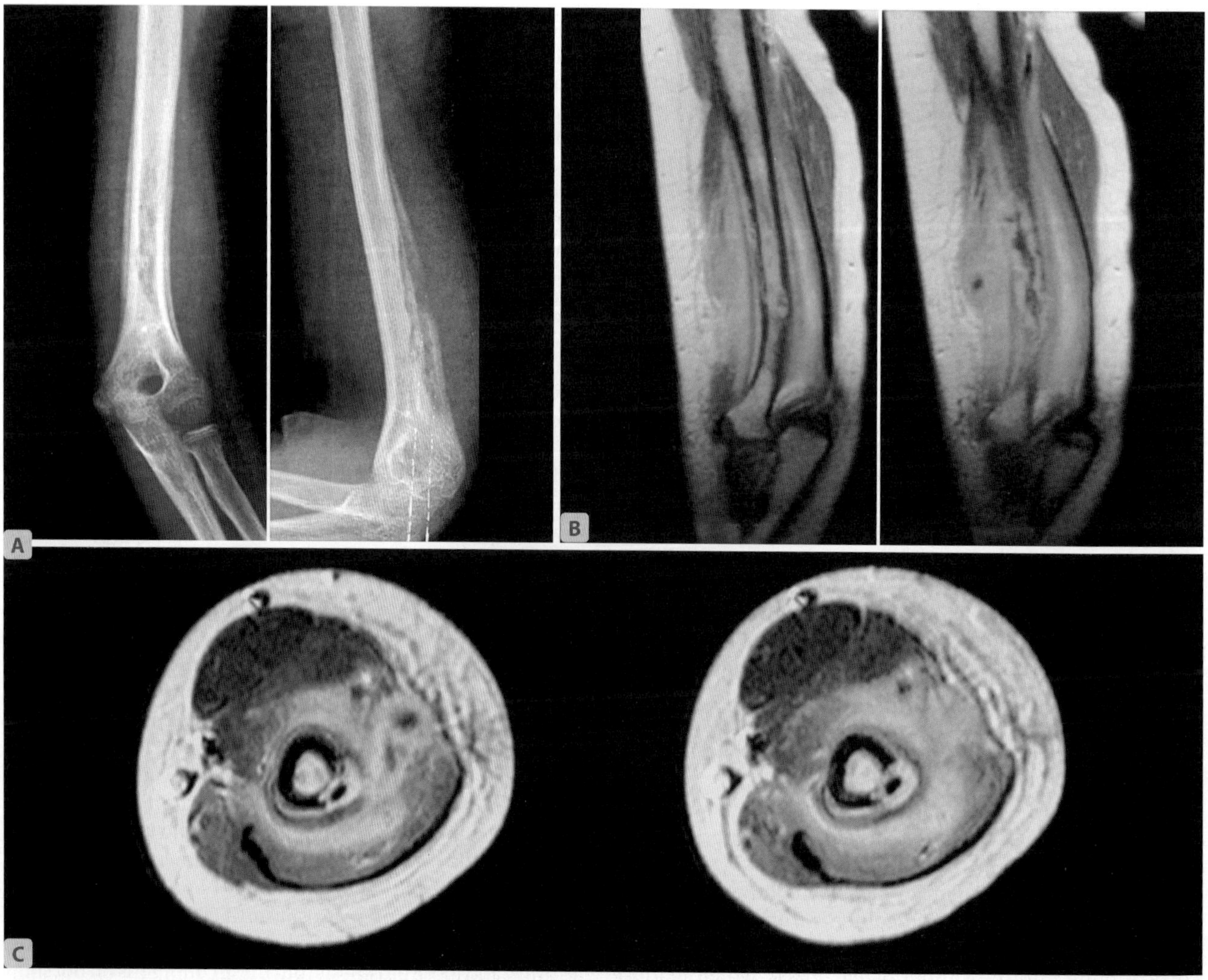

FIGS. 7A TO C: Acute osteomyelitis. (A) Plain X-rays show smooth periosteal reaction with cortical irregularity in the lower third of humerus; Postcontrast sagittal (B) and axial (C) MR images show cortical irregularity with break in the outline and periosseous fluid collection with increased signal in the adjacent soft tissues.

and has a rounded configuration—whereas intraosseous abscesses are irregular or oblong.

LOCALIZED OSTEOMYELITIS (BRODIE'S ABSCESS)

Localized osteomyelitis or Brodie's abscess is a limited osteomyelitis caused either by organisms of low virulence or high resistance in the host. Presentation with insidious pain is most common, which may exacerbate at night and be relieved by nonsteroidal anti-inflammatory drugs (NSAIDs) (like osteoid osteoma). It occurs most frequently at one end of the bone, but it may also occur in the diaphysis. Tibia is most commonly involved bone, followed by femur, although any bone can be affected.[30]

It is seen as a well-circumscribed osteolytic focus surrounded by a sclerotic margin **(Figs. 8A to C)**. Occasionally, a metaphyseal serpiginous channel with sclerotic border marks the tract of infection. This feature is considered characteristic of nontubercular etiology like *Staphylococcus, Streptococcus* or *Haemophilus*.[2] When the lesion is small, it may be difficult to identify on plain radiographs and CT/MRI may be required. The close differential diagnosis of Brodie's abscess is an osteoid osteoma as on imaging both these conditions closely simulate each other (T2 hyperintense nidus, sclerotic rim, and bone edema); however, on T1W MRI scans, a "penumbra sign" has been described as a central intermediate or hypointense zone of pus, a discrete rim of the abscess wall of marginally higher signal intensity than the abscess cavity, sclerosis which is hypointense, and surrounding marrow edema of lower signal intensity than fatty bone marrow, which often enhances after contrast. This has been postulated to be due to the presence of active, vascular, inflammatory granulation tissue around the abscess.[31]

Epiphyseal lesions can be mistaken for aneurysmal bone cyst or chondroblastoma.

CHRONIC OSTEOMYELITIS

Chronic bone infections usually result from inadequately treated acute osteomyelitis or from infection following compound bone fractures. Pain, local swelling, discharge from wound, sinus formation, and systemic signs and symptoms (fever, malaise, nausea, and vomiting) may be present.

Conventional radiographs show cloacae, involucrum or sequestrum **(Figs. 9 and 10)**. There are sclerotic and lucent areas admixed with cortical thickening and deformities. The radiographic impression regarding the activity of infectious process is often equivocal, and one relies heavily on clinical findings such as the presence of a sinus tract.[25] At times, it is imperative to review previous films as it may be difficult to differentiate inactive and active chronic osteomyelitis. In osteomyelitis of the skull, typically no sclerosis is seen **(Figs. 11A and B)**.

Scintigraphy is more useful in determining activity. Routine 99mTc-MDP scanning shows increased uptake, but is often nondiagnostic, since even after 1–2 years following successful treatment, a positive isotope bone scan is not uncommon.[3] ^{67}Ga has been recommended as the optimal agent. Following successful treatment, ^{67}Ga uptake should decrease to a normal level.

Magnetic resonance imaging findings correspond to the pathologic features. On MR images, the involucrum manifests as a well-defined rim of low-signal intensity on all sequences surrounding the infected bone marrow.

Granulation tissue surrounding the infection appears as hypointense on T1W images, hyperintense on T2W and STIR images, and shows enhancement after gadolinium-diethylenetriamine pentaacetic acid (Gd-DTPA).

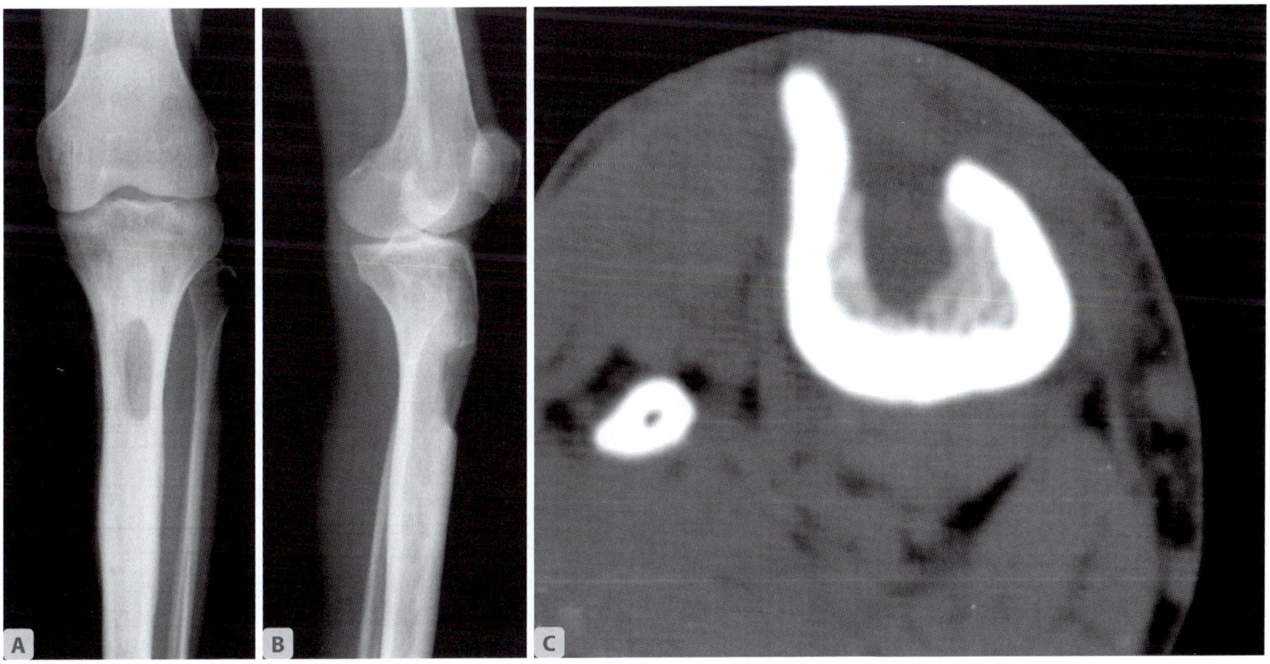

FIGS. 8A TO C: (A and B) Plain X-ray; and (C) Axial CT images showing Brodie's abscess in the upper end of tibia.

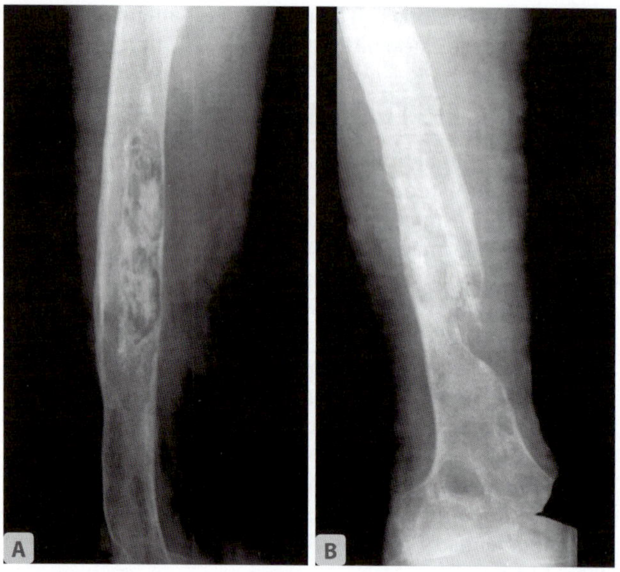

FIGS. 9A AND B: Chronic osteomyelitis of the femoral bone. Diaphyseal lucent areas represent cloacae formation with sequestrum seen as radiodense opacities.

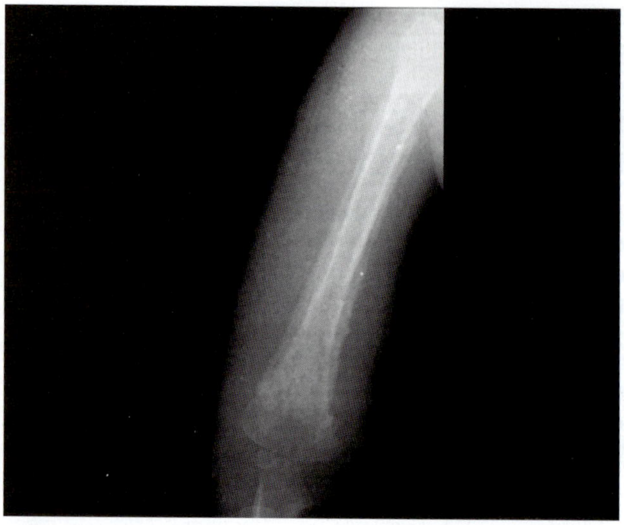

FIG. 10: Chronic osteomyelitis. Radiograph of right arm showing involucrum surrounding distal two-thirds of humerus.

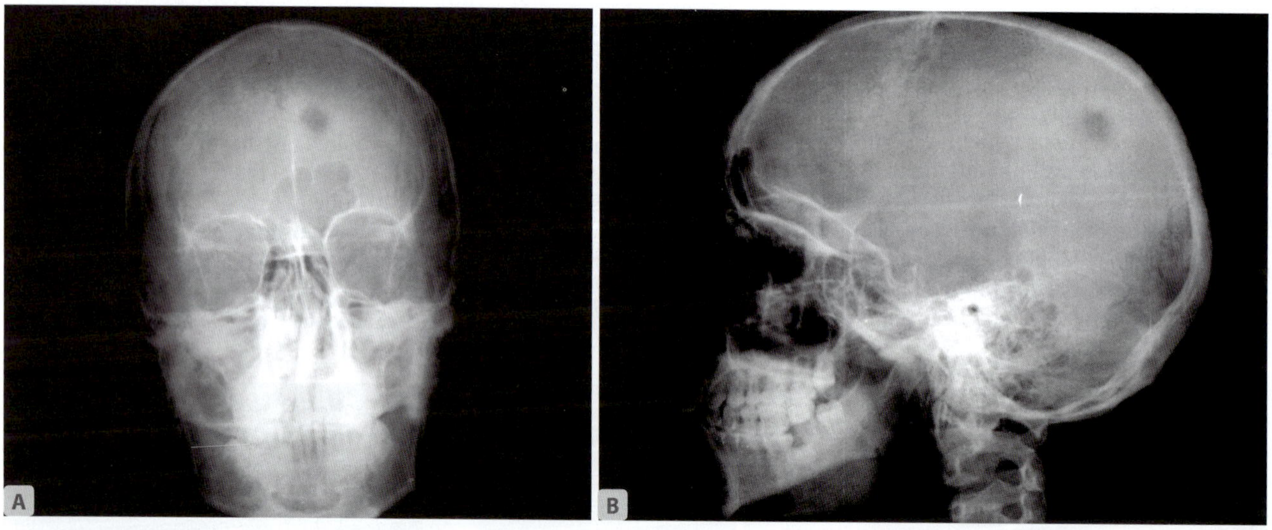

FIGS. 11A AND B: Chronic osteomyelitis of skull vault. Anteroposterior and lateral skull radiographs showing multiple lytic areas with no surrounding sclerosis.

Magnetic resonance imaging has been advocated as the imaging modality to distinguish regions of active infection from uninvolved marrow or fibrotic regions representing scars from previous infection or trauma.[25] Active foci of infection tend to have a low-to-intermediate signal intensity on T1W and high-signal intensity on T2W and fluid-sensitive images which is in marked contrast to the low-signal of thickened, surrounding bone.[32,33]

However, persistent hyperintensity on T2W images may also be seen in postsurgical granulation tissue and does not necessarily imply persistent infection. Comparison with previous imaging is essential as persistent infection leads to progressive increase in intramedullary hyperintensity.[34]

Sequestrum is an isolated fragment of devitalized bone within an area of active infection shows low-signal intensity on all sequences, and does not enhance.

Sinus tract is identified as a linear or curvilinear area of low-signal on T1W and high-signal on T2W and STIR images extending in contiguity from the medullary cavity, with disruption of the cortex, to the skin.

Soft tissue inflammation is seen as bright signal on T2W and STIR images, enhancing after contrast. Sometimes soft tissue abscess may also develop **(Figs. 12A to D)**.[32,33]

SCLEROSING OSTEOMYELITIS OF GARRE

Sclerosing osteomyelitis of Garre is a rare type of chronic osteomyelitis occurring in children and young adults, presenting with insidious onset of local pain. Symptoms recur at intervals for several years and then subside gradually. There is a predilection for involvement of mandible and

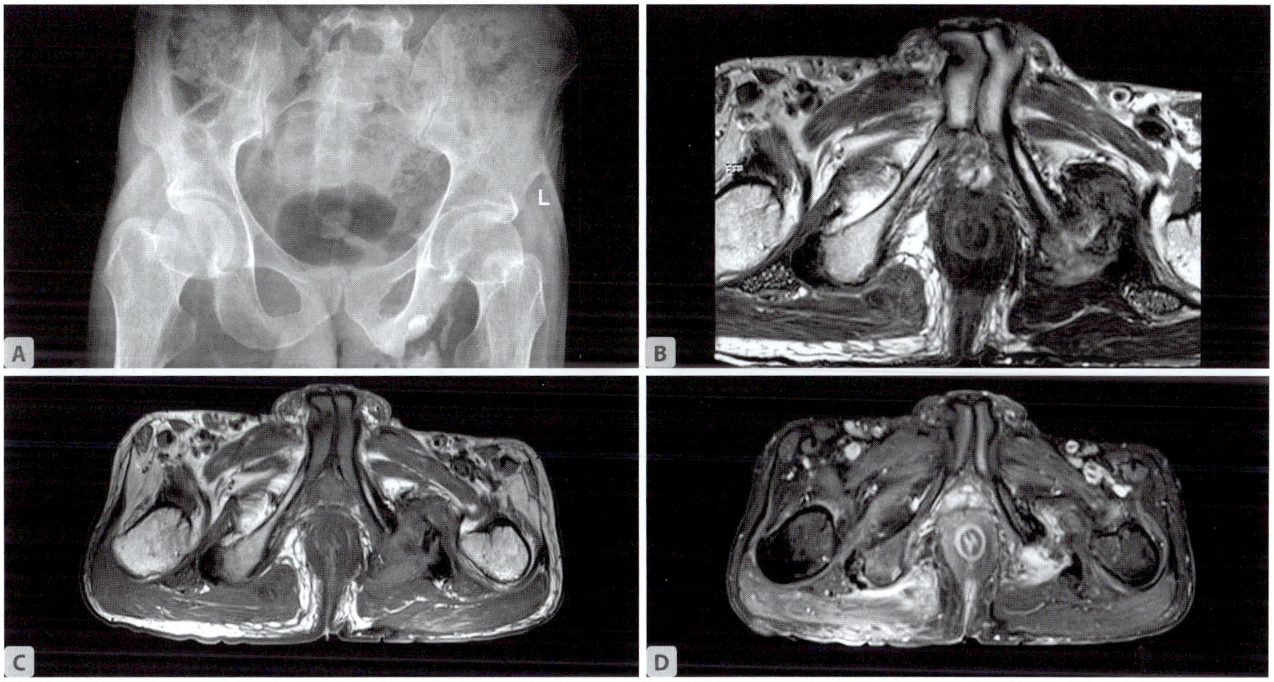

FIGS. 12A TO D: (A) Plain X-ray of hip joints reveals erosions along the inferior border of left ischium with sclerosis; (B) Axial T2-weighted; (C) T1-weighted; and (D) Postcontrast T1 fat-saturated MR images show a large area of lytic destruction involving the left ischium associated with a large inflammatory tissue which is of high signal on T2W and hypointense on T1W images involving the gluteal muscles. The marrow of the left ischium also shows increased signal consistent with marrow edema. Few small peripherally enhancing collections are also seen representing abscesses. The gluteal muscles on the right side also show inflammatory changes.

shafts of long bones. Radiological appearance is of intense sclerosis resulting in thickened bone **(Fig. 13)**. Areas of frank bony destruction are rare. It is distinguished from Ewing's tumor by the absence of lamellations of periosteal reaction and permeative bone destruction.

SYPHILIS OF BONE

Syphilis is caused by *Treponema pallidum* and is of three types:

1. Congenital syphilis, present at birth or in early infancy
2. Late congenital syphilis
3. Acquired syphilis

Congenital (Infantile) Syphilis

Congenital (infantile) syphilis is a systemic disease due to transplacental transmission of the spirochetes. Clinical features include, fever, failure to thrive, saddle nose, Hutchinson's teeth, and pseudoparalysis due to painful bone lesions, etc. Serologic diagnostic tests include the Venereal Disease Research Laboratory (VDRL), fluorescent treponemal antibody absorption (FTA-ABS) tests. Osseous abnormalities include luetic metaphysitis, diaphysitis and periostitis. Radiologically, the earliest change is in the metaphysis, with widening of the zone of provisional calcification. The epiphyseal plate appears wide and dense. The outstanding feature is symmetrical involvement of multiple bones especially at the upper end of tibia and lower end of femur. Symmetrical destruction of medial portion of the proximal tibial metaphysis (Wimberger's sign) is common and pathognomonic of syphilis. It should not be confused with Wimberger's ring sign (around an osteoporotic epiphysis in scurvy) **(Fig. 14)**.

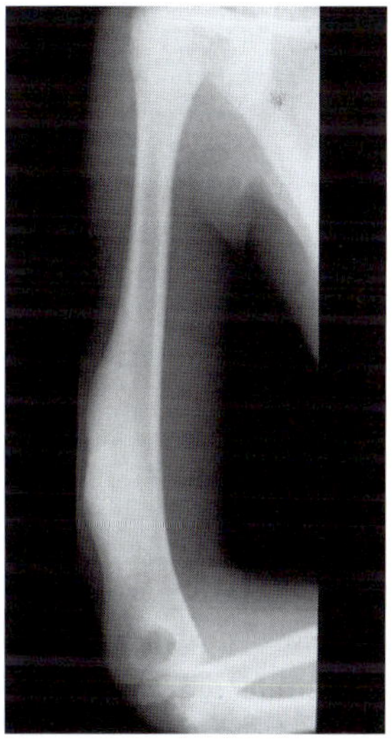

FIG. 13: Chronic sclerosing osteomyelitis of Garre. Long-standing osteomyelitis with endosteal thickening of cortex with obliteration of medullary cavity.

The earliest diaphyseal change is focal cortical destruction. Later there may be extensive destruction of bone. Periosteal reaction can be solid or lamellated. In the skull, irregular, osteolytic lesions are seen.

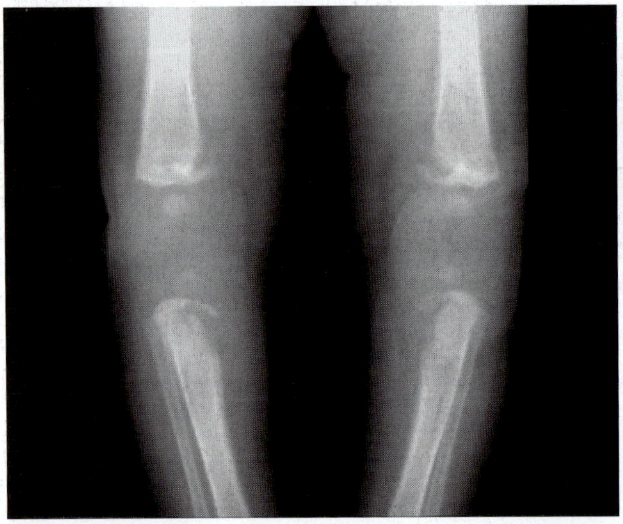

FIG. 14: Congenital syphilis. Radiograph of both knees of an infant showing symmetrical marginal destruction of medial aspect of tibia and femur in juxtaepiphyseal area and metaphyseal bands.

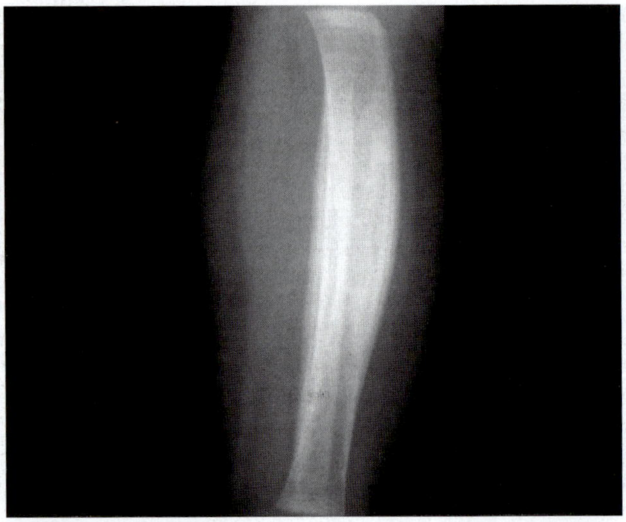

FIG. 15: Saber tibia. Extensive cortical thickening affecting the shaft of tibia which is widened.

Late Congenital Syphilis

In this condition, syphilitic bony lesions do not become evident until childhood or early adult life. The lesions are due to gumma or syphilitic endarteritis. There is minimal bone destruction which is overshadowed by extensive new bone proliferation. This results in diffuse thickening of cortical bone and lamellated periosteal reaction. This lesion causes typical thickening of the upper half of tibial cortex anteriorly and is called "Saber Tibia" **(Fig. 15)**.

Acquired Syphilis

Osseous changes in acquired syphilis manifest as periostitis and osteomyelitis with dense osteosclerosis. Long bones and skull are most frequently involved. The earliest change is periosteal reaction. The affected bone shows thickened cortex with narrowing of medullary canal. Gummas cause osteolytic lesion of variable size and shape. The skull shows predominantly osteolytic lesions, and outer table is more often involved.

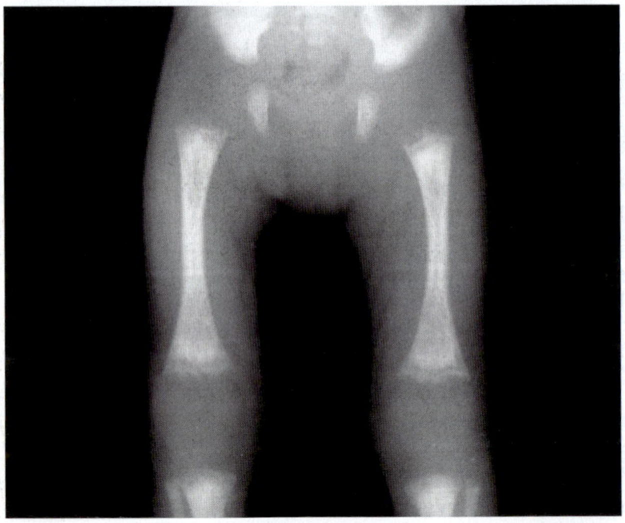

FIG. 16: Rubella. Radiograph of both lower limbs shows the typical metaphyseal bands and trabecular irregularity in metaphysis extending longitudinally. Note absence of periosteal reaction.

RUBELLA OSTEOMYELITIS

Congenital rubella infection occurs following maternal rubella in the early months of pregnancy. The characteristic radiological feature is metaphyseal lucent bands and trabecular irregularity, extending longitudinally from the epiphysis. It is seen in the upper and lower extremities, predominantly in the distal end of femur and proximal end of the tibia (celery stalk appearance) **(Fig. 16)**. Bone changes can be confused with syphilis. Absence of periosteal reaction in congenital rubella helps in differentiating from congenital syphilis.

ACTINOMYCOSIS OF BONE

It is a chronic osteomyelitis caused by gram-positive organism, *Actinomyces israelii*, which grows in colonies and appears as yellow (sulfur) granules in pus. They are common saprophytes in the gastrointestinal tract and infection occurs after a dental procedure or trauma to mouth and jaw. The most common bones involved are vertebrae/mandible, symphysis pubis, tibia, and foot bones. *Actinomyces* is also being isolated increasingly from periprosthetic joint infections.[35]

Radiologically, there is bone destruction without new bone formation. Vertebral osteomyelitis resembles tuberculosis, although discs are usually spared.[2] Ribs respond to actinomycosis by periosteal reaction and thickening, a feature which is most suggestive though, not diagnostic.

MADUROMYCOSIS

Maduromycosis is a form of chronic osteomyelitis due to granulomatous inflammation caused by a wide variety of pathogens including fungi or *Actinomyces*. The infection occurs by entry of organism through minor trauma to skin, usually foot (Madura foot). The disease is painless and presents as swelling, sinus formation and marked deformity **(Figs. 17 and 18)**.

Radiologically, periosteal reaction is the most common lesion and is usually lamellated. The disease arises primarily in soft tissues and secondarily erodes the adjoining cortex and medulla. There is little, if any, osteopenia. The disease is painless, and characteristically, the sequestrum is absent.

LEPROSY OF BONE

Leprosy is a chronic granulomatous infection caused by *Mycobacterium leprae*. In lepromatous leprosy, the disease predominantly affects the skin, mucous membranes, and the viscera. Bone involvement can rarely occur by direct lepromatous granulation tissue or by endarteritis causing bone infarcts. In tuberculoid (neural) type, there is predominant involvement of nerves which become thickened and nodular. The bone changes are secondary to neurotrophic disturbances causing recurrent trauma and infection which go unnoticed.

Radiographically, there is diffuse osteopenia and ill-defined small osteolytic areas with soft tissue swelling are seen. Periosteal reaction is rare. In later stages, erosions or resorption of phalangeal tufts are seen along with soft tissue atrophy **(Figs. 19A and B)**. Nonspecific changes including soft tissue swelling and contractures are also seen. Calcification of nerves, if observed, is classical of leprosy. Nasal septal irregularity, thinning and perforation are not well appreciated on plain radiography, but these abnormalities are very well demonstrated on CT.

DIABETIC FOOT

Infection is the primary problem requiring hospitalization of diabetic patient with foot problems often necessitating amputation. Foot problems account for as much as one-fourth of hospital admissions among diabetic patients.[36] The pathological changes are often a combination of neuropathy, vasculopathy or infection.

Conventional radiographs show osteomyelitis or neuropathic changes in the foot bones (sensitivity and specificity 75% each) **(Fig. 20)**.[37]

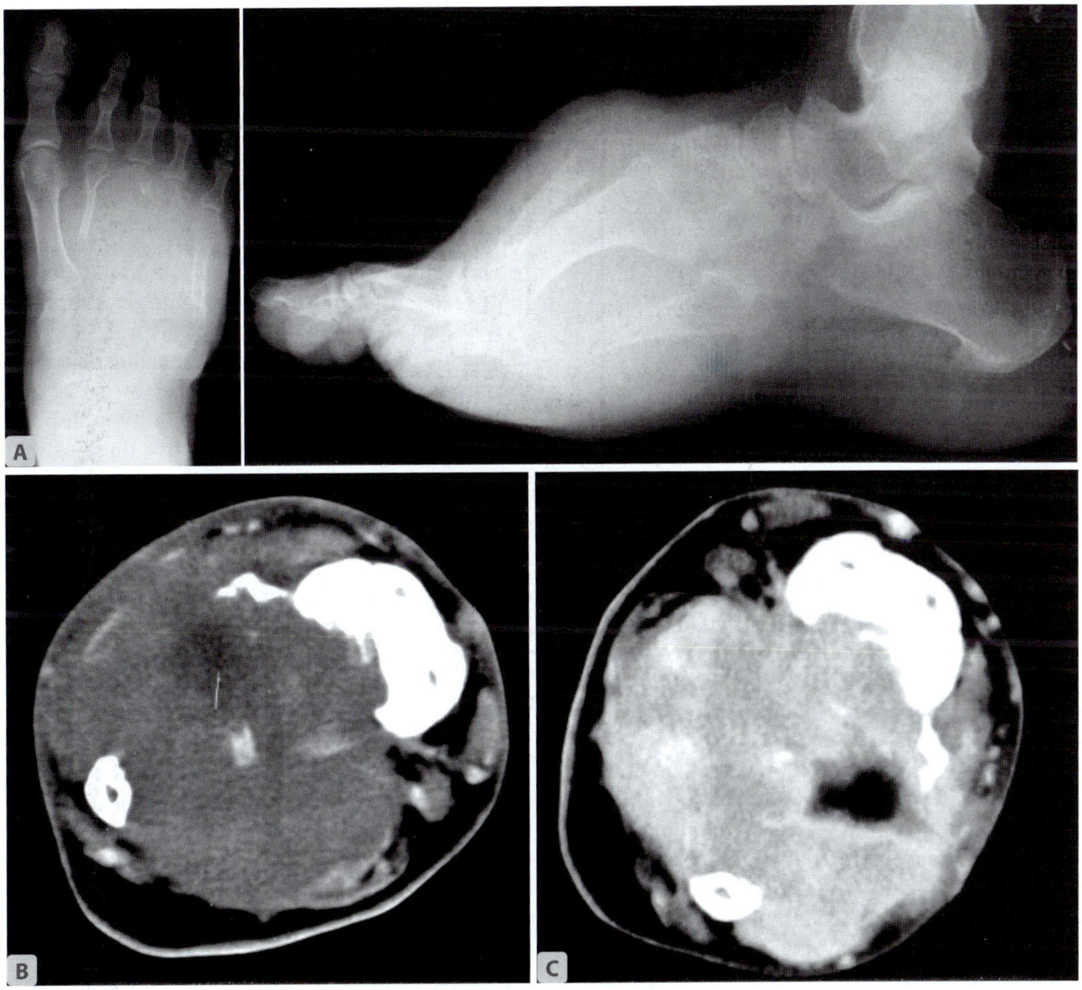

FIGS. 17A TO C: Maduromycosis. (A) Plain X-rays; and (B and C) Axial CT pre- and postcontrast images. There is a large soft tissue swelling in the foot with destruction of 2–4th metatarsals. On CT, an enhancing soft tissue lesion with secondary destruction of metatarsal shafts is seen.

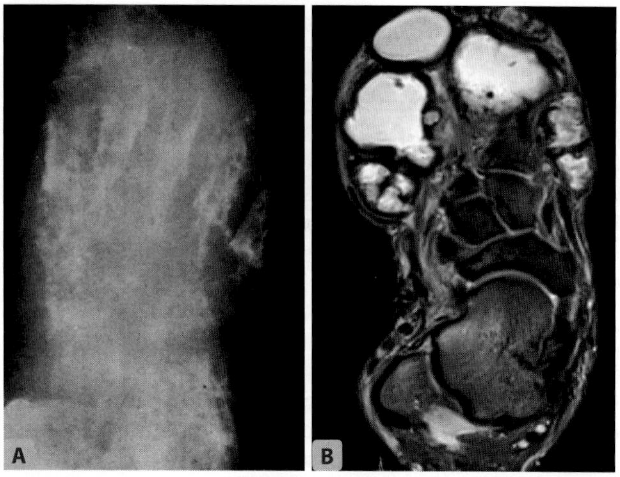

FIGS. 18A AND B: Maduromycosis. (A) Infiltrative destruction of the tarsal and metatarsal bones with large soft tissue component; (B) Axial proton density-weighted fat-saturated image of the foot of another patient with eumycetoma shows multiple hyperintense nodules with hypointense rim in subcutaneous tissue with a central dot-in-circle sign.

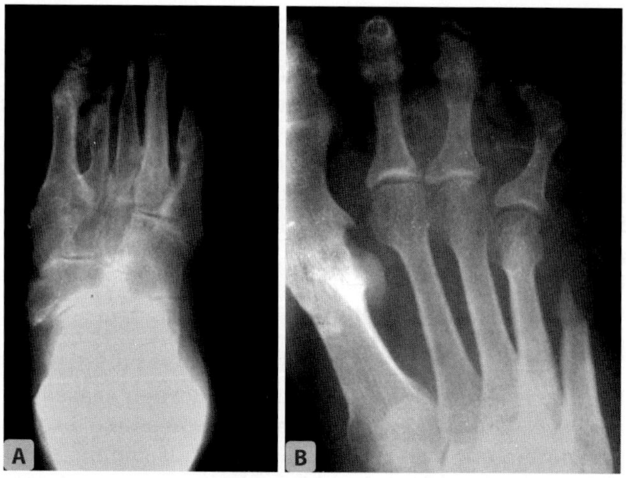

FIGS. 19A AND B: Leprosy. (A and B) Osteopenia with "licked candy appearance" of the metatarsals. Note the absence of the phalanges of the 5th toe (B) due to bony resorption.

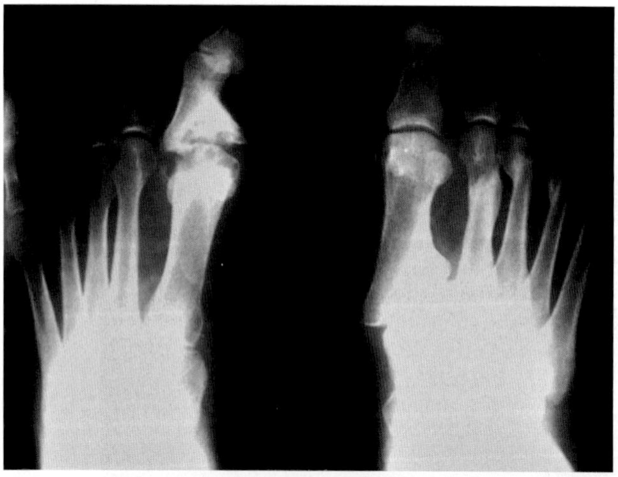

FIG. 20: Diabetic foot. There is narrowing of first metatarsophalangeal joint (right) and tarsometatarsal joint (left) with articular erosion and marked sclerosis of adjacent bone. Lucencies in soft tissues are due to air.

Scintigraphy can identify early osteopathy at a time when the conventional radiograph is normal, but its specificity is very low.[37] ^{111}In WBC scanning is more specific than 99mTc bone scan since it is not affected by increased bone turnover from neuropathy or fracture.[38]

Magnetic resonance imaging can visualize marrow directly and is found to have the lowest false-positive rate compared to both scintigraphy as well as plain radiography.[37]

Early stages of neuroarthropathy may mimic foot osteomyelitis both clinically and on imaging **(Table 1)**. In the early stages where radiography is usually normal, MRI may show soft tissue edema, fluid collections, effusions, and bone marrow abnormalities. Neuropathic changes are primarily periarticular, differentiating it from osteomyelitis which almost occurs secondary to overlying ulcer at predictable sites. Neuroarthropathy usually involves the tarsometatarsal and metatarsophalangeal joints, while calcaneum, cuboid, and malleoli are affected by osteomyelitis. However, both neuropathic changes and osteomyelitis can coexist, making imaging diagnosis difficult.

In neuroarthropathy, MRI typically shows a preserved marrow signal within the marrow on T1W images and subarticular T2 hyperintensity while rest of the bone is normal. Midfoot involvement, periarticular, subchondral or polyarticular involvement favors a neuroarthropathy over osteomyelitis.[39]

This finding is consistently different from early osteomyelitis where a high signal within the nonperiarticular marrow on T2W images is seen with or without changes in T1W images. Abscess, overlying ulcer, and sinus tract are diagnostic of infection; however, imaging goal is to diagnose infections early before these develop.

A trophic ulcer due to neuropathy with bone marrow edema in adjacent bone may cause diagnostic confusion between neuroarthropathy and osteomyelitis. However, 61% of such patients with marrow edema have or eventually developed osteomyelitis in a retrospective study.[40]

Concurrent infection in the adjacent soft tissues, synovium (infectious arthritis), muscles and tendons (tenosynovitis) may reveal increased signal on T2W and STIR images which may enhance on postgadolinium scans, and contrast enhancement is important to differentiate infectious myositis from changes in muscles due to ischemia or neuropathy associated denervation edema since extensive soft tissue and muscle inflammation also occur in acute Charcot neuro-osteoarthropathy (CNO)[41] **(Figs. 21A to F)**.

A sign known as the ghost sign has been described in osteomyelitis where the bones become hypointense and difficult to differentiate from surrounding muscle and inflammation on T1W images, but become prominent after contrast administration due to enhancement.[42]

Contrast should be judiciously administered since many patients have renal dysfunction and is not mandatory for diagnosis. Recent studies on dynamic postcontrast

TABLE 1: Differentiating features between osteomyelitis and neuropathic arthropathy in diabetic foot.

	Osteomyelitis	Neuropathic arthropathy
Distribution	Usually focal involvement	Multiple bones and joints are involved
Location	Peripheral location at weight-bearing areas, e.g., toes, metatarsal heads, calcaneus	Midfoot is predominantly involved
Associated deformity	Usually not seen. Can be ± if associated neuropathic joint	Commonly + along with destruction and debris
Soft tissue changes	Commonly overlying ulcer and draining sinus can be demonstrated	Overlying skin usually intact, edema +
Bone marrow involvement	Hyperintense on T2/STIR, hypointense on T1W image associated with postgadolinium enhancement	Acute stage—mimics osteomyelitis Chronic stage—decreased T1/T2 signal or normal marrow signal
Pattern of bone marrow edema	Usually single bone is affected with diffuse bone marrow edema	Usually periarticular and subchondral in location
Ghost sign	+	–

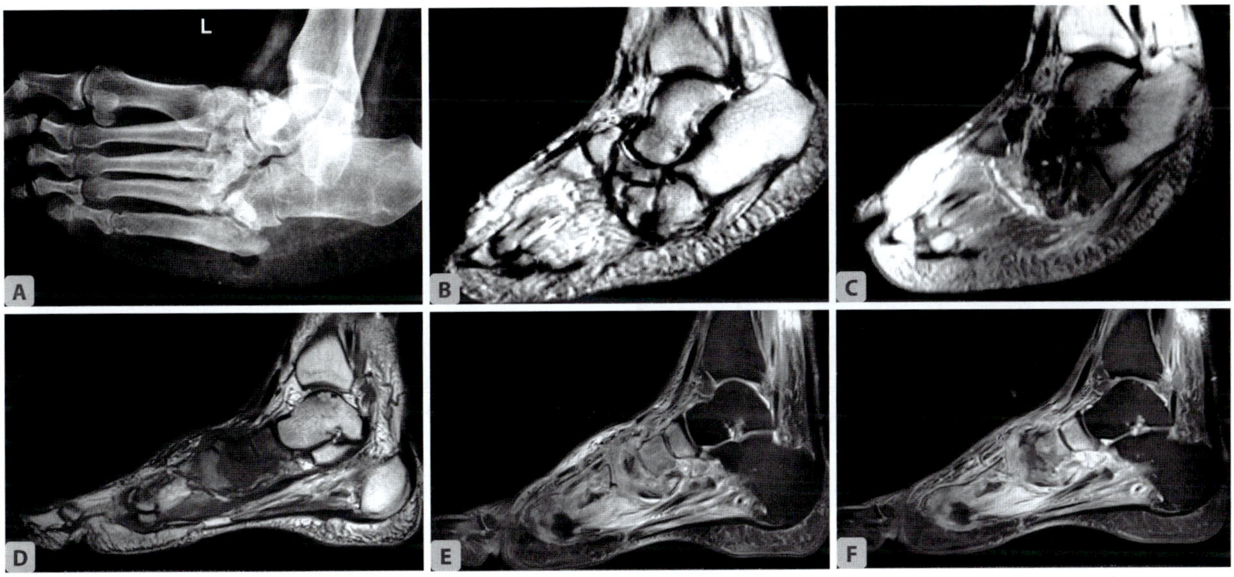

FIGS. 21A TO F: (A to C) Diabetic foot (Charcot's neuroarthropathy). (A) Plain radiograph of foot shows dislocation of joints of midfoot and tarsometatarsal joints and with reduced joint spaces and erosions. The bones show mixed lytic and sclerotic areas; (B) T1-weighted (T1W) MR image shows dislocated-disorganized joints of foot with markedly hypointense areas of bony sclerosis; however, marrow signal is maintained; (C) Postcontrast T1W image shows thickened enhancing synovium at tarsometatarsal joints with enhancing muscles of plantar surface; (D to F) Diabetic foot with osteomyelitis. Sagittal T1W image (D) shows hypointense tarsal bones which show osteitis (E) and intense postcontrast enhancement of bones and adjacent muscles (F).

imaging have demonstrated that it can differentiate between neuroarthropathy and osteomyelitis. Values of K^{trans} (volume transfer constant), K_{ep} (volume of contrast that returns to vascular compartment), and V_e (extracellular volume) are significantly higher in osteomyelitis.[43] Time-intensity curves also may be helpful in differentiating infection from neuropathic changes with rapid wash in and a steep curve in osteomyelitis.[44]

Soft tissue infection of foot occurs especially over pressure points such as metatarsals where organisms enter via superficial ulceration. Gas may be noted in infective tissues, because of gas-producing organisms such as *Escherichia coli*, without implying the presence of gangrene.

HYDATID DISEASE

Bone involvement is rare accounting for 0.5–2% cases. The most commonly involved bones are the spine, pelvis, femur, tibia, ribs, skull, scapula, humerus, and fibula.[45,46] The hydatid disease in the bone and joint begins in childhood and grows at a very slow rate and hence is seldom diagnosed in childhood. The bone offers mechanical resistance; hence cyst cannot assume its typical spherical shape and enlarges along the path of least resistance. Over the time, the trabeculae are absorbed and cortex is breached, resulting in fracture. Then, the disease spreads to surrounding structures and becomes symptomatic.

Hydatid disease should be suspected whenever cystic lesions are seen in the bone especially in the endemic areas.

The bone shows expanded medullary cavity with thinned out cortex with cortical breach or complete fracture. Typically, there is no periosteal reaction or new bone formation. On MRI, the infested bone reveals multiple cysts which exhibit medium-to-low signal on T1W images and high signal on T2W images **(Figs. 22A to D)**.[45,46]

SEPTIC ARTHRITIS

Septic arthritis is usually hematogenous in origin but may follow local trauma, joint aspiration, soft tissue infection or periarticular osteomyelitis. Arthroscopic procedures are complicated by septic arthritis in 0.04–3.4% of patients.[8] *S. aureus* is the most common invader followed by *Neisseria gonorrhoeae*, *Streptococcus*, *Haemophilus*, and anaerobic organisms.[30]

Onset of bacterial arthritis is usually abrupt with high fever, chills, and one or more severely tender swollen joints. Knee joint is most frequently affected (40–50%)

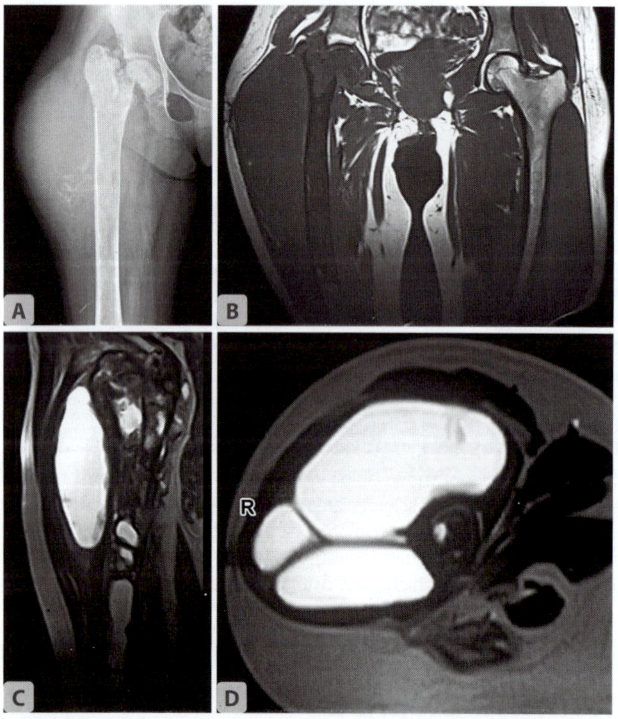

FIGS. 22A TO D: (A) Plain radiograph demonstrates expanded medullary cavity with endosteal scalloping in right femur and thinned out cortex. There is pathological fracture neck of femur with proximal migration of greater trochanter. A large soft tissue shadow is also seen along the lateral aspect with foci of calcifications; (B) Coronal T1W MR image showing altered marrow signal of medullary cavity (hypointense when compared to left femur) with a large hypointense lesion along lateral aspect of upper thigh. Note pathological fracture neck of right femur; (C) Sagittal T2W MR image showing multiple cysts in the medullary cavity of right femur with small cysts in adductor group of muscles and large cysts along lateral aspect of thigh; (D) Axial T2W MR image showing a multiseptated cystic lesion along lateral aspect of femur. Note a small cyst in the medullary cavity.

followed by hip (20–25%), shoulder, wrist, elbow and ankle. Sternoclavicular, sacroiliac, and manubriosternal joints are more often involved in IV drug abusers.

Bone scan is the investigation of choice for early diagnosis of septic arthritis. Although not specific, bone scanning is very sensitive and when negative can rule out the possibility of infected joint.[9] CT demonstrates bone changes much earlier than plain films and is superior in demonstrating the extent of infection. MRI is extremely sensitive in the depiction of joint fluid, cartilage damage, marrow changes, and medullary bone destruction, but cannot differentiate infectious from noninfectious joint effusions.[47]

Radiological patterns are different in adults and infants. Plain radiographs are usually normal in early course of disease. Soft tissue swelling is the first radiographic sign of acute pyogenic arthritis. Hyperemia associated with pyogenic arthritis causes rapid, juxta-articular osteoporosis with disappearance of subchondral white line. Periarticular edema obliterates the adjacent fat planes. At this stage, effusion is identifiable. Earliest bone change occurs 8–10 days after the onset of infection.[48] There is loss of definition of the margins due to osteoporosis with small focal articular erosions followed by progressive destruction of cartilage leading to reduction in joint space. Untreated infection can lead to extensive bone destruction and loss of cortical outline. In later stages, subluxation or even dislocation can occur. With healing, sclerotic bone reaction occurs resulting in irregular articular surface. If the entire cartilage is destroyed, then bony ankylosis follows **(Figs. 23A and B)**.[49]

In infants and children, distention of joint capsule due to fluid can cause joint space widening and even subluxation, especially of the hip and shoulder. In neonates, physiological ossification of femoral head is absent, thus plain radiographs are of limited value. USG in such cases may reveal joint effusion with/without internal echoes **(Fig. 24)**. Thickened synovial membrane is seen as irregular echogenic membrane surrounding the fluid. Joint effusion can also occur as sympathetic response to adjacent focus of osteomyelitis. Arthrocentesis with bacterial cultures is therefore essential in such cases to document joint infection.

In pediatric population, distinguishing transient synovitis from septic arthritis is extremely important and in such cases the USG may not differentiate as both the conditions manifest as synovial thickening, joint effusions, and alteration in surrounding soft tissues. MRI can differentiate these two conditions as in transient synovitis, there are minimal to almost nil marrow changes (high signal changes in T2W and STIR images which show postcontrast enhancement).[50]

Bone changes in gonococcal arthritis are indistinguishable from tuberculosis. Destruction is more rapid and serial films are helpful in distinguishing the two. Similarly, brucellar arthritic changes are also indistinguishable from tubercular joint; however, *Brucella* involves most commonly sacroiliac joints and usually unilaterally.[49] Fungal arthritis is most commonly due to *Candida*, coccidiosis, and blastomycosis. Radiologically, there is soft tissue swelling, periarticular osteopenia, relative joint space preservation and bony erosions but differentiation from tuberculosis is difficult.

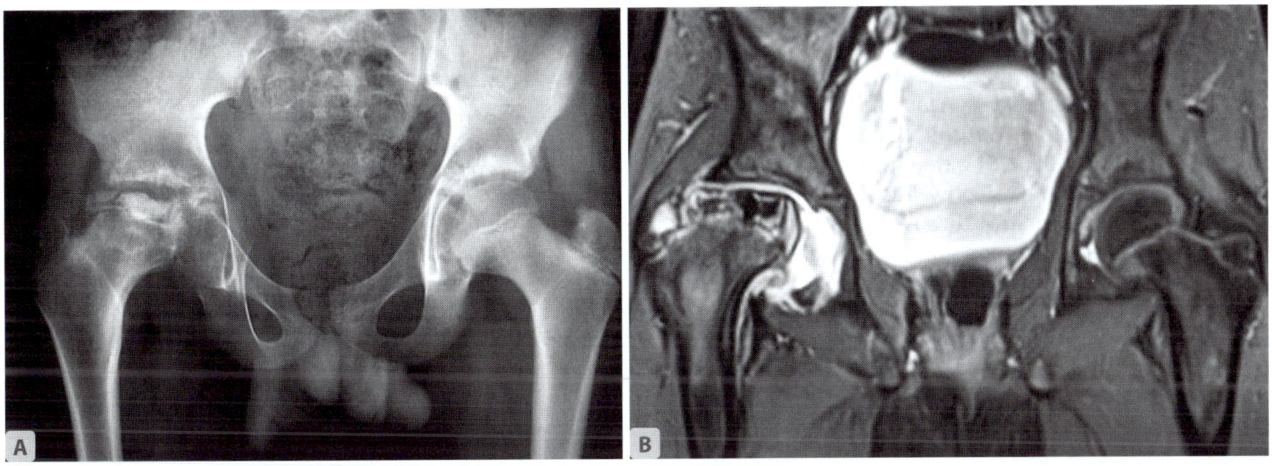

FIGS. 23A AND B: (A) Plain X-ray of hip joints reveals irregular articular margins of right femoral joint with sclerosis. The femoral epiphysis is fragmented, flattened and irregular with superimposed changes of avascular necrosis secondary to infection with increased teardrop distance due to effusion; (B) Postcontrast T1W MR image demonstrates thickened enhancing synovium with intraosseous abscesses in the femoral epiphysis and bone destruction. Also the metadiaphyseal marrow shows enhancement.

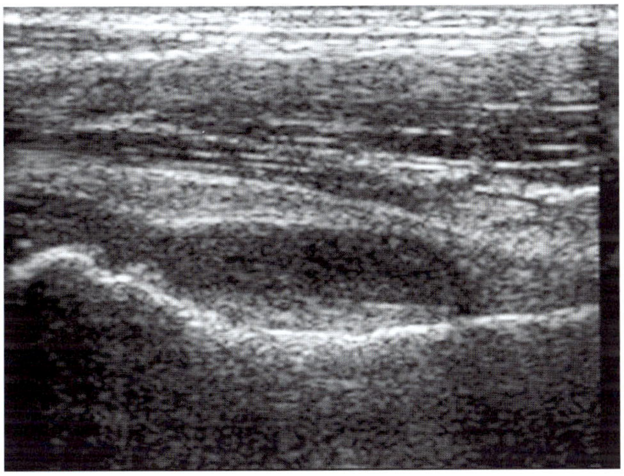

FIG. 24: Ultrasonography image in an infant shows joint effusion in hip joint with dependent debris.

TRANSIENT SYNOVITIS

Transient synovitis is a common self-limiting cause of acute hip pain in children which generally subsides within 2 weeks. Children between 4 and 10 years of age are prone to transient synovitis and the condition is more common in male children.

Clinical Features

Acute hip or groin pain, limp, restriction of motion, refusal to bear weight and systemic symptoms of fever are common. A prior history of upper respiratory tract infection is often present. Erythrocyte sedimentation rate (ESR), C-reactive protein (CRP), and WBC counts may be raised. Although no infectious agent has been isolated, elevated viral titers have been found. Though the disease is self-limiting, recurrence rates range between 0 and 26%.[51] Among the recurrent and persistent cases, a significant proportion progress to Legg-Calvé-Perthes disease.

Common cause of acute hip pain in pediatric age group includes septic arthritis, transient synovitis, and Legg-Calvé-Perthes disease. It is important to differentiate between infectious and noninfectious causes. Dynamic contrast-enhanced MRI shows early decreased enhancement of femoral head epiphysis on time-intensity curves in patients with septic arthritis.[52]

CHRONIC RECURRENT MULTIFOCAL OSTEOMYELITIS

Chronic recurrent multifocal osteomyelitis (CRMO) is an idiopathic autoinflammatory bone disorder of children and adolescents characterized by recurrent episodic osseous pain at one or multiple sites over several years.[53]

It is usually a diagnosis of exclusion once underlying infection and neoplasia has been ruled out. Median age of presentation is of 10 years with a range of 9–14 years, with youngest age at presentation being 6 months.[53] Biopsy of the osseous lesions shows an inflammatory reaction. No organisms are demonstrated.

The combination of synovitis, acne, pustulosis, hyperostosis, and osteitis is designated as SAPHO and is seen as the adult counterpart of CRMO. CRMO is associated with a number of dermatological (psoriasis, palmoplantar pustulosis, etc.), gastrointestinal (Crohn's and ulcerative colitis), genetic (Majeed syndrome), and autoimmune conditions such as Wegener's granulomatosis and Takayasu's arteritis.[53]

The most common sites of disease are the metaphyses or metaphyseal equivalents of the tubular bones, most frequently in the lower limb bones followed by clavicle, spine, ribs, sternum, pelvis, mandible.[53,54] Clavicle involvement is a characteristic finding as this is an uncommon location for hematogenous osteomyelitis. Symmetric involvement is common. In early stages, osteolytic lesion is noted which shows progressive sclerosis during late stages. Lesions can be purely osteolytic, osteolytic with a sclerotic rim, mixed lytic and sclerotic, and purely sclerotic. Characteristically, there is no sequestration.[54] Mild periosteal reaction may be noted. MRI findings include bone marrow edema with heterogeneous contrast enhancement within the affected bone. Abscess formation and soft tissue changes are usually not seen in CRMO **(Fig. 25)** differentiating CRMO from the other types of multifocal osteomyelitis **(Figs. 26A and B)**.

Clinical course of the disease lasts for 7–10 years. Treatment usually includes anti-inflammatory drugs for symptomatic relief.

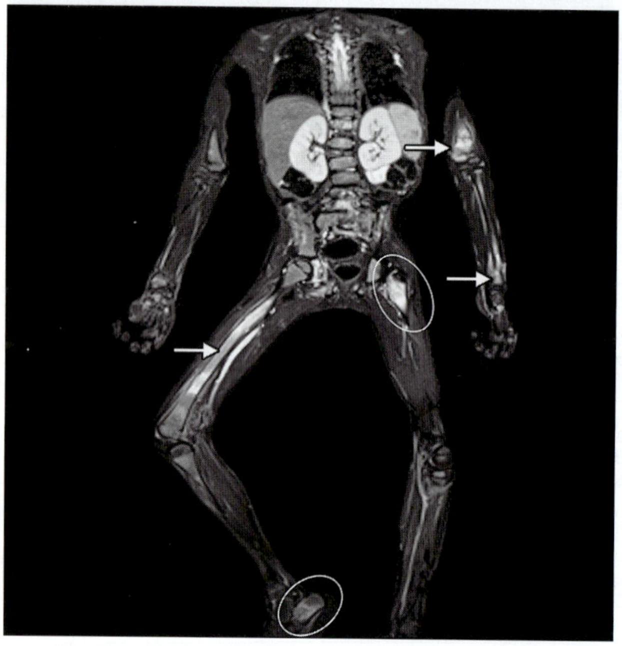

FIG. 25: Whole-body coronal short tau inversion recovery (STIR) sequence in a patient with chronic recurrent multifocal osteomyelitis (CRMO) shows multifocal areas of intramedullary hyperintensity in metaphysis of humerus radii, proximal femur, and calcaneum. Bone marrow edema is seen in diaphysis of right femur.

Major differentials that should be considered are (acute and subacute) osteomyelitis, Langerhans cell osteomyelitis, and Ewing's sarcoma.

FUNGAL OSTEOMYELITIS

The incidence of fungal bone and joint infections has increased in solid organ transplant, chemotherapy, long-term corticosteroid, and HIV-positive individuals. Although pyogenic organisms are the most common type of infection in the immunocompromised patient, but fungal infections have also increased in number in this population. Infection either directly extends from the overlying skin or is hematogenous in origin. In the setting of an indolent infection with associated marked osseous deformity, fungal infection should be considered. Clinical features include pain in the involved region along with signs of systemic illness. No specific imaging features are known till date and it is difficult to differentiate from other infective/inflammatory causes of arthritis.

PERIPROSTHETIC INFECTIONS

Periprosthetic joint infections are a major complication of joint arthroplasties and incidence ranges between 1 and 2.5% in primary arthroplasties to 4% in revision arthroplasties.[55]

Infections can present early within 4 weeks of surgery and are typically caused by highly virulent bacteria (*S. aureus*, streptococci, and enterococci).[55] Clinically, there is evidence of local inflammation, swelling, and pain. Delayed wound healing, wound dehiscence, persistent discharge or a sinus tract can develop.

Delayed infections most commonly occur after the first month but within the first year, though delayed infection can occur at any time, especially in first 3 years. Delayed infections present with insidious clinical symptom of chronic pain, stiffness, and fistula formation.

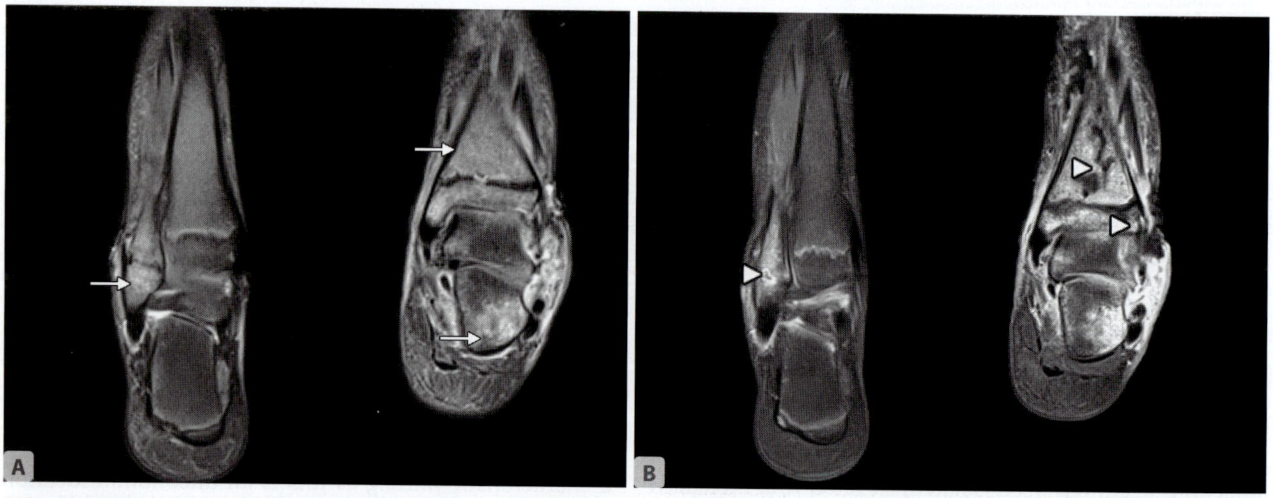

FIGS. 26A AND B: (A) Coronal T2-weighted; and (B) Postcontrast T1-weighted fat-saturated images show multifocal areas of osteitis in right lower fibula, tibia, and calcaneus (arrows in A), with areas of intraosseous and extraosseous abscesses (arrowheads in B) evident after contrast enhancement with surrounding tenosynovitis and soft tissue inflammation.

Imaging

Serial radiographs showing a rapidly developing periprosthetic lucency of >2 mm or a focal osteolysis at the metal-bone or bone-cement interface. Similar findings of lucency can be found in aseptic loosening, which however, does not progress as rapidly as loosening due to infection. Conventional radiographs have a low sensitivity and specificity for periprosthetic infections but should be the first imaging modality. Serial radiographs are essential to evaluate the loosening.

Computed tomography scan evidence of periosteitis and joint distension are indicative of infection.

Magnetic resonance imaging is challenging with metallic artifacts from prosthetic devices and implants. Imaging techniques for metal artifact reduction include increasing bandwidth, decreasing slice thickness, view angle tilting (using a slice selection gradient during read out of the signal) or slice-encoding for metal artifact correction (SEMAC) or multiacquisition variable-resonance image combination (MAVRIC) technique on a 1.5 T MR scanner.[56]

Imaging findings of soft tissue edema, soft tissue mass, fluid around the prosthesis, bone marrow edema, and bone destruction are indicative of infection. Soft tissue mass and bone destruction are indicative of tumor recurrence in patients after tumor resection.[56]

White blood cell labeled with ^{111}In has a high degree of sensitivity, specificity, and accuracy (96–97%) in diagnosing periprosthetic joint infections and is the preferred modality of choice, although fluorodeoxyglucose-positron emission tomography (FDG-PET) also has similar sensitivity and specificity. These modalities remain constrained due to lack of widespread availability.[57,58]

REFERENCES

1. Greenfield GB. Cardinal roentgen features. In: Greenfield GB (Ed). Radiology of Bone Diseases, 5th edition. Philadelphia: JB Lippincott; 1990.
2. Edeiken J. Edeiken's Roentgen Diagnosis of Diseases of Bone, 4th edition. Baltimore: Williams and Wilkins; 1990. pp. 973-1084.
3. Wegener WA, Alavi A. Diagnostic imaging of musculoskeletal infection. Roentgenography; gallium, indium-labeled white blood cell, gammaglobulin, bone scintigraphy. Orthop Clin North Am. 1991;22:401-18.
4. Wheat J. Diagnostic strategies in osteomyelitis. Am J Med. 1985;78:218-24.
5. Markel KD, Brown ML, Dewanjee MK, Fitzgerald RH. Comparison of indium-labeled leukocyte imaging with sequential technetium-gallium scanning in the diagnosis of low grade musculoskeletal sepsis. A prospective study. J Bone Joint Surg Am. 1985;67: 465-76.
6. Rubin RH, Fischman AJ, Callahan RJ, Khaw BA, Keech F, Ahmad M, et al. 111In-labelled nonspecific immunoglobulin scanning in the detection of focal infection. N Eng J Med. 1989;321:935-40.
7. D'Angelo GL, Ogilive-Harris DJ. Septic arthritis following arthroscopy with cost benefit analysis of antibiotic prophylaxis. Arthroscopy. 1988;4:10-4.
8. Mujoomdar M, Russell E, Dionne F, Moulton K, Murray C, McGill S. Appendix 2.5 Diagnosis of acute osteomyelitis. In: Mujoomdar M, Russell E, Dionne F, Moulton K, Murray C, McGill S (Eds). Optimal Use Report: Optimizing Health System Use of Medical Isotopes and Other Imaging Modalities [Internet]. Ottawa (ON): Canadian Agency for Drugs and Technologies in Health; 2012.
9. Esterhai JL Jr, Gelb I. Adult septic arthritis. Orthop Clin North Am. 1991;22:503-14.
10. Desai RV, Khandelwal N, Gupta S, Suri S, Gill SS, Suri S. Role of ultrasound in acute Osteomyelitis. Asian Oceanian J Radiol. 2001;6:159-65.
11. Modic MT, Pflanze W, Feiglin DH, Belhobek G. Magnetic resonance imaging of musculoskeletal infections. Radiol Clin North Am. 1986;24:247-58.
12. Schanwecker DS, Braunstein EM, Wheat LJ. Diagnostic imaging of osteomyelitis. Infect Dis Clin North Am. 1990;4:441-63.
13. Modic MT, Feiglin DH, Piraino DW, Boumphrey F, Weinstein MA, Duchesneau PM, et al. Vertebral osteomyelitis: assessment using MR. Radiology. 1985;157:157-66.
14. Unger E, Moldfsky P, Gatenby R, Hartz W, Broder G. Diagnosis of osteomyelitis by MR imaging. Am J Roentgenol. 1988;150: 605-10.
15. Morrison WB, Schweitzer ME, Batte WG, Radack DP, Russel KM. Osteomyelitis of the foot: relative importance of primary and secondary MR imaging signs. Radiology. 1998;207:625-32.
16. Jaramillo D, Treves ST, Kasser JR, Harper M, Sundel R, Laor T. Osteomyelitis and septic arthritis in children: appropriate use of imaging to guide treatment. Am J Roentgenol. 1995;165: 399-403.
17. Beltran J, Noto AM, McGhee RB, Freedy RM, McCalla MS. Infections of the musculoskeletal system: high-field-strength MR imaging. Radiology. 1987;164:449-54.
18. Brill PW, Winchester P, Krause AN, Symchych P. Osteomyelitis in a neonatal intensive care unit. Radiology. 1979;131:83-8.
19. Mok M, Reilly RJ, Ash JM. Osteomyelitis in the neonate. Radiology. 1982;145:677-82.
20. Bressler EL, Conway JJ, Weiss SC. Neonatal osteomyelitis examined by bone scintigraphy. Radiology. 1984;152:685-8.
21. Cierny G, Mader JT, Pennick JJ. A clinical staging system for adult osteomyelitis. Contemp Orthop. 1985;10:17-37.
22. Lee YJ, Sadigh S, Mankad K, Kapse N, Rajeswaran G. The imaging of osteomyelitis. Quant Imaging Med Surg. 2016;6(2):184-98.
23. Rosen Ra, Morehouse HT, Karp JH, Yu GS. Intracortical fissuring in osteomyelitis. Radiology. 1981;141:17-20.
24. Beaman FD, von Herrmann PF, Kransdorf MJ, Adler RS, Amini B, Appel M, et al. ACR Appropriateness Criteria® suspected osteomyelitis, septic arthritis, or soft tissue infection (excluding spine and diabetic foot). J Am Coll Radiol. 2017;14(5S):S326-37.
25. Jaramillo D. Infection: musculoskeletal. Pediatr Radiol. 2011;41(Suppl 1):S127-34.
26. Connolly SA, Connolly LP, Drubach LA, Zurakowski D, Jaramillo D. MRI for detection of abscess in acute osteomyelitis of the pelvis in children. Am J Roentgenol. 2007;189:867-72.
27. Karchevsky M, Schweitzer ME, Morrison WB, Parellada JA. MRI findings of septic arthritis and associated osteomyelitis in adults. Am J Roentgenol. 2004;182:119-22.
28. Collins MS, Schaar MM, Wenger DE, Mandrekar JN. T1-weighted MRI characteristics of pedal osteomyelitis. Am J Roentgenol. 2005;185:386-93.
29. Cooper C, Cawley MI. Bacterial arthritis in an English Health district. A 10-year-review. Ann Rheum Dis. 1986;45:458-63.
30. Olasinde AA, Oluwadiya KS, Adegbehingbe OO. Treatment of Brodie's abscess: excellent results from curettage, bone grafting and antibiotics. Singapore Med J. 2011;52(6):436-9.
31. Gulati Y, Maheshwari AV. Brodie's abscess of the femoral neck simulating osteoid osteoma. Acta Orthop Belg. 2007;73:648-52.

32. Quinn SF, Murray W, Clerk RA, Cochran C. MR imaging of chronic osteomyelitis. J Comput Assist Tomogr. 1988;12:113-7.
33. Mason MD, Zlatkin MB, Esterhai JL, Dalinka MK, Velchik MG, Kressel HY. Chronic complicated osteomyelitis of the lower extremity evaluation with MR imaging. Radiology. 1989;173:355-9.
34. Pineda C, Espinosa R, Pena A. Radiographic imaging in osteomyelitis: the role of plain radiography, computed tomography, ultrasonography, magnetic resonance imaging, and scintigraphy. Semin Plast Surg. 2009;23:80-9.
35. Könönen E, Wade WG. Actinomyces and related organisms in human infections. Clin Microbiol Rev. 2015;28:419-42.
36. Brodsky JW, Schneidler C. Diabetic foot infections. Orthop Clin North Am. 1991;22:473-89.
37. Yuh WT, Corson JD, Baraniewski HM, Rezai K, Shamma AR, Kathol MH, et al. Osteomyelitis of the foot in diabetic patients: evaluation with plain film, 99mTc-MDP bone scintigraphy and MR imaging. Am J Roentgenol. 1989;152:795-800.
38. Keenam AM, Tindel NL, Alavi A. Diagnosis of pedal osteomyelitis in diabetic patients using current scintigraphy techniques. Arch Intern Med. 1989;149:2262-6.
39. Toledano TR, Fatone EA, Weis A, Cotten A, Beltran J. MRI evaluation of bone marrow changes in the diabetic foot: a practical approach. Semin Musculoskelet Radiol. 2011;15(3):257-68.
40. Duryea D, Bernard S, Flemming D, Walker E, French C. Outcomes in diabetic foot ulcer patients with isolated T2 marrow signal abnormality in the underlying bone: should the diagnosis of "osteitis" be changed to "early osteomyelitis"? Skeletal Radiol. 2017;46(10):1327-33.
41. Leone A, Vitiello C, Gullì C, Sikora AK, MacagninoS, Colosimo C. Bone and soft tissue infections in patients with diabetic foot. Radiol Med. 2020;125(2):177-87.
42. Donovan A, Schweitzer ME. Use of MR imaging in diagnosing diabetes-related pedal osteomyelitis. Radiographics. 2010;30:723-36.
43. Liao D, Xie L, Han Y, Du S, Wang H, Zeng C, et al. Dynamic contrast-enhanced magnetic resonance imaging for differentiating osteomyelitis from acute neuropathic arthropathy in the complicated diabetic foot. Skeletal Radiol. 2018;47(10):1337-47.
44. Noguerol TM, Luna Alcalá A, Beltrán LS, Gómez Cabrera M, Broncano Cabrero J, Vilanova JC. Advanced MR imaging techniques for differentiation of neuropathic arthropathy and osteomyelitis in the diabetic foot. Radiographics. 2017;37(4):1161-80.
45. Pedrosa I, Saiz A, Arrazola J, Ferreirós J, Pedrosa CS. Hydatid cyst: radiologic and pathologic features and complications. Radiographics. 2000;20:795-817.
46. Dhatt S, Singhal M, Tripathy SK, Tahasildar N, Sen R. Primary hydatidosis of femur: a case report and review of the literature. Eur J Orthop Surg Traumatol. 2010;20:401-5.
47. Tang JS, Gold RH, Bessett LW, Seeger LL. Musculoskeletal infection of the extremities: evaluation with MR Imaging. Radiology. 1988;166:205-9.
48. Manaster BJ. Adult chronic hip pain: radiographic evaluation. Radiographics. 2000;20:S3-25.
49. Edeiken J. Edeiken's Roentgen Diagnosis of Diseases of Bone, 4th edition. Baltimore: Williams and Wilkins; 1990. pp. 593-601.
50. Yang WJ, Im SA, Lim GY, Chun HJ, Jung NY, Sung MS, et al. MR imaging of transient synovitis: differentiation from septic arthritis. Pediatr Radiol. 2006;36:1154-8.
51. Asche SS, van Rijn RM, Bessems JH, Krul M, Bierma-Zeinstra SM. What is the clinical course of transient synovitis in children: a systematic review of the literature. Chiropr Man Therap. 2013;21(1):39.
52. Kim EY, Kwack KS, Cho JH, Lee DH, Yoon SH. Usefulness of dynamic contrast-enhanced MRI in differentiating between septic arthritis and transient synovitis in the hip joint. Am J Roentgenol. 2012;198:428-33.
53. Khanna G, Sato TS, Ferguson P. Imaging of chronic recurrent multifocal osteomyelitis. Radiographics. 2009;29(4):1159-77.
54. Iyer RS, Thapa MM, Chew FS. Chronic recurrent multifocal osteomyelitis: review. Am J Roentgenol. 2011;196:S87-91.
55. Izakovicova P, Borens O, Trampuz A. Periprosthetic joint infection: current concepts and outlook. EFORT Open Rev. 2019;4(7): 482-94.
56. Jiang M, He C, Feng JM, Li ZH, Chen Z, Yan FH, et al. Magnetic resonance imaging parameter optimizations for diagnosis of periprosthetic infection and tumor recurrence in artificial joint replacement patients. Sci Rep. 2016;6:36995.
57. Palestro CJ, Kim CK, Swyer AJ, Capozzi JD, Solomon RW, Goldsmith SJ. Total-hip arthroplasty: periprosthetic indium-111-labled leukocyte activity and complementary technetium-99mm-sulfur colloid imaging in suspected infection. J Nucl Med. 1990;31:1950-5.
58. Chryssikos T, Parvizi J, Ghanem E, Newberg A, Zhuang H, Alavi A. FDG-PET imaging can diagnose periprosthetic infection of the hip. Clin Orthop Relat Res. 2008;466:1338-42.

CHAPTER

157

Tuberculosis of the Spine

Rashmi Dixit, Gaurav Shanker Pradhan, Radhika Batra

INTRODUCTION

The spine is the most frequent site of osseous involvement by tuberculosis accounting for about 50% of cases.[1,2] The disease was first described by Sir Percival Pott in 1779, hence, the name Pott's disease.[3] There has been a resurgence of the disease even in developed countries following the human immunodeficiency virus (HIV) pandemic.

Tubercular spondylitis is defined as an infection by *Mycobacterium tuberculosis* of one or more of the extradural components of the spine namely the vertebrae, intervertebral discs, paraspinal soft tissues, and epidural space.[4,5] It is associated with disproportionate amount of morbidity due to its tendency to produce significant deformity and neurologic complications therefore prompt diagnosis and treatment are of utmost importance.

PATHOPHYSIOLOGY

The spread of tuberculosis to the spine is usually by hematogenous route.[2] Hematogenous seeding may arise from a primary focus in the lung or other extraosseous foci such as lymph nodes, gastrointestinal tract (GIT), or any other viscera which may be active or quiescent.[6]

Lower dorsal and lumbar vertebrae are most frequently involved followed by midthoracic and cervical region.[7] The C2-C7 region is reportedly involved in 3–5% of cases[8,9] and the atlantoaxial articulation in less than 1% of cases.[10-12] Usually, two continuous vertebrae are involved but several vertebrae may be affected, skip lesions, and solitary vertebral involvement may also be seen.[7] The so-called skip lesion or a second lesion not contiguous with the more obvious lesion is seen in 4–10% of cases.[4,13]

The infection usually begins in the cancellous, paradiscal area of the vertebral body and less often in the central portion or anterior surface. There is softening of the vertebral body which gets easily compressed to produce either wedging or total collapse. The normal kyphotic curve in the thoracic spine accentuates the pressure on the anterior portion of the vertebral body, producing anterior wedging resulting in kyphus with a gibbus deformity.[6,7]

As infection spreads to the adjacent disc, the disc space narrows. The intervertebral disc is avascular in adults and spread of infection to the disc can occur by extension through the subchondral bone via cartilaginous end plate or beneath the anterior or posterior longitudinal ligament to involve the peripheral disc. Disc space narrowing can also occur due to disc herniation into the weakened vertebral body with subsequent infection of the herniated disc.[6] The intervertebral disc, however, is relatively resistant to infection by *M. tuberculosis*. This is thought to be due to a lack of proteolytic enzymes in the *Mycobacterium* as compared with pyogenic bacteria.[14] The avascularity of the disc may also prevent it from serving as an initial site of infection. Hence it has been suggested that disc involvement occurs only when the disc has lost its nutritional support due to involvement of adjacent vertebral bodies.[2] Disc space narrowing thus occurs later and is less pronounced in tubercular infection than in pyogenic infection.[14-16] Although the vertebral body is involved more often than the posterior elements, these latter structures may be affected initially or predominantly in some persons.[17,18]

A marked exudative lesion due to hypersensitivity reaction to *Mycobacterium* results in formation of thick pus containing serum, leukocytes, caseous material, tubercle bacilli, and bone fragments, which tracks through the pre- and paravertebral soft tissues forming pre- and paravertebral abscesses. The exudate penetrates ligaments and follows the path of least resistance along fascial planes, blood vessels, and nerves to distant sites from the original bony lesion as cold abscess. The abscesses may further extend into the spinal canal producing an epidural abscess and cord compression.[7] Spread of infection can occur beneath the anterior longitudinal ligament, involving adjacent vertebral bodies.

CLINICAL FEATURES

Tuberculous spondylitis can occur in any age group, but, majority of the patients are under 30 years of age at the time of diagnosis. The disease is rare in the first year of life but when it occurs, it tends to be more severe with greater bone destruction and multiple vertebral involvement.[7,8] Symptoms and signs are variable.[4] Some patients may be afebrile and free of systemic symptoms until late stage of the disease, others may present with constitutional symptoms before symptoms related to the spine manifest. The usual presentation is with persistent spinal pain, local tenderness, and limitation of spinal mobility.[4,7]

Paraparesis may be apparent in about 20–30% of all patients with spinal tuberculosis.[4,7] In the cervical region, the incidence is much higher and over 40% cases may be associated with quadriparesis.[4,8] Paraplegia may be *early onset*, which develops during the active phase of the disease or *late onset* which may appear many years after the disease has become quiescent, even without any evidence of reactivation. Early-onset paraplegia is usually due to cord compression by epidural abscess or granulation tissue, pathological subluxation or dislocation, sequestered bone, or disc fragments. Nonmechanical causes include inflammatory cord edema which could be a result of vascular stasis, bacterial toxins, or granulation tissue due extension of tuberculous inflammation through the meninges to the cord. Rarely endarteritis may cause cord infarction. Late-onset paraplegia can occur due to dural fibrosis, severe kyphoscoliotic deformity, spinal canal stenosis, gliosis of cord, or sequestra from vertebral body. Late-onset paraplegia has a less favorable prognosis as compared to early onset paraplegia.[7]

LABORATORY INVESTIGATIONS[19-24]

Blood investigations reveal relative lymphocytosis, low hemoglobin and elevated ESR in active disease. The mantoux test is nondiagnostic in an endemic region and may be negative in immunodeficient individuals. The sensitivity of staining for acid-fast bacilli may vary from 25 to 75%. A long incubation period of 4–6 weeks is required for culture, although BACTEC radiometric culture is faster and takes around 2 weeks. Polymerase chain reaction (PCR) can distinguish between typical and atypical mycobacteria and is an efficient and rapid method of diagnosis. A positive PCR, however, cannot substitute culture and does not indicate disease activity, as it does not distinguish between live and dead microorganisms.

IMAGING MODALITIES

Conventional Radiographs

Radiographs are the usual initial investigation, but they are often negative in early disease **(Figs. 1A to D)**.[25] More than 30–50% of mineral has to be lost before a radiolucent lesion becomes apparent on plain films and 2–5 months are needed for this.[2,7] Plain films are also limited in the evaluation of areas such as craniovertebral junction, cervicodorsal junction, posterior neural arches, and sacrum.

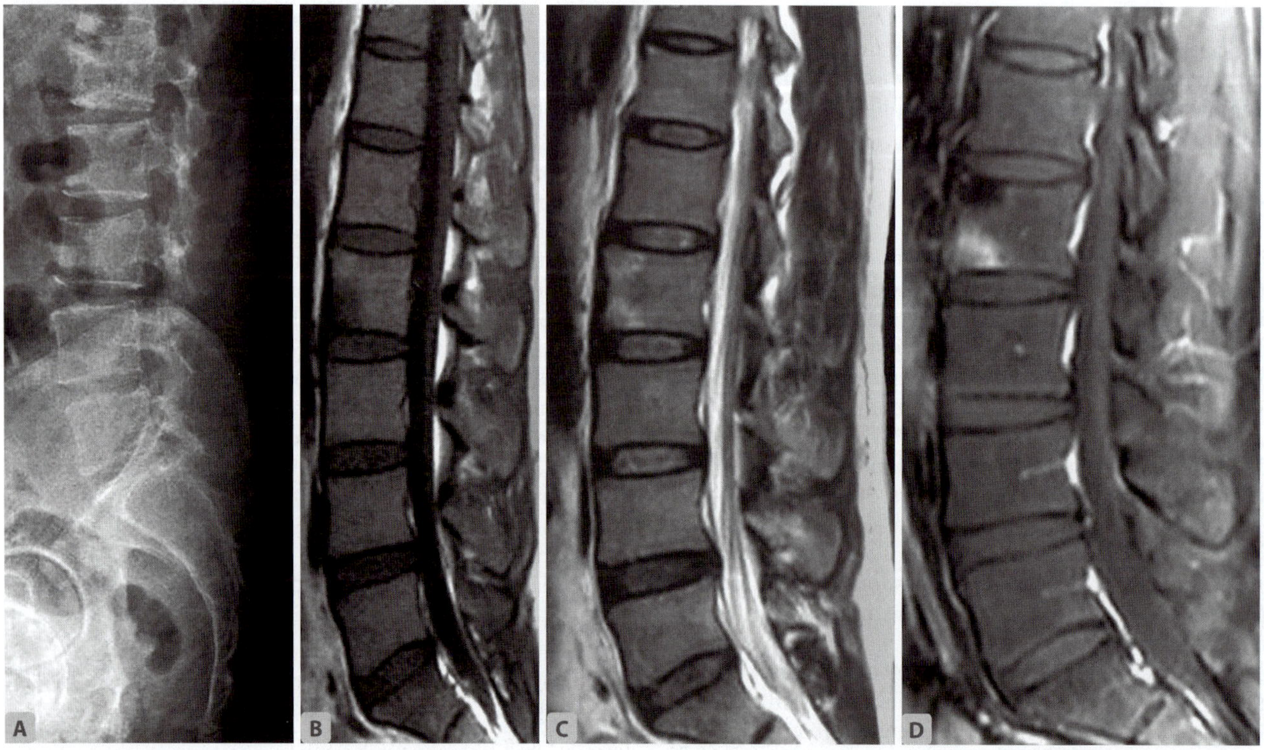

FIGS. 1A TO D: (A) Lateral radiograph L-S spine of a 25-year-old male presenting with low backache and fever reveals normal vertebrae and disc spaces; (B) T1W, (C) T2W, and (D) postcontrast T1W fat suppressed sagittal images of the same patient show an area of signal alteration in the anteroinferior part of L2 vertebral body appearing hypointense on T1W, hyperintense on T2W images and showing patchy enhancement on the postcontrast images.

Computed Tomography

Advantages of computed tomography (CT) evaluation in cases of tubercular spondylitis include early detection of bone and soft tissue changes when plain films are normal, better anatomic localization and characterization of lesions, evaluation of areas difficult to evaluate on plain films such as craniovertebral junction, cervicodorsal junction, and sacrum, and providing guidance for biopsy and surgical approach. It is also an excellent technique for detection of bone fragments, soft tissue calcification, and to demonstrate the exact extent of deformity in chronic cases.[13,26,27] However, a routine CT examination may overlook lesions outside the chosen scan volume.[4] With the use of multirow detector scanners, the entire spine can be covered though with an increased radiation burden **(Figs. 2A and B)**. Furthermore CT is less useful than magnetic resonance for early diagnosis of spondylitis as inflammatory marrow changes in the vertebral body, an early sign of infection, are not well depicted on CT scanning.[28] In addition, soft tissue structures within the bony spinal canal are poorly delineated.[4,28] In the cervicothoracic region, epidural involvement may be missed even on contrast-enhanced CT (CECT), without intrathecal contrast enhancement because of beam hardening artifacts. For this reason, the effect of extradural disease on the thecal sac, spinal cord and neural elements is difficult to evaluate properly.[28]

Magnetic Resonance Imaging

The superiority of magnetic resonance imaging (MRI) in the detection and staging of inflammatory and infective disorders of the spine is generally accepted making MR the imaging modality of choice in these conditions.[15,28,29] MRI is useful to detect disease in areas difficult to evaluate on plain films such as the CV junction. It demonstrates of early bone marrow

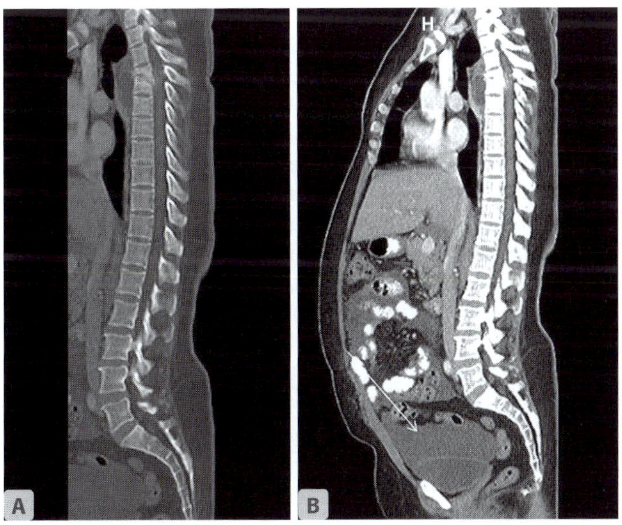

FIGS. 2A AND B: Sagittal reconstructions at bone (A) and soft tissue (B) settings from a multislice CT acquisition for disseminated tuberculosis reveal reduction of disc space between D4 and D5, destruction of endplates and a peripherally enhancing prevertebral abscess due to tubercular involvement. Note the extended coverage and presence of free fluid in the abdomen (arrow).

involvement or edema and allows unparalleled evaluation of the spinal canal and cord. Soft tissue and intraosseous abscesses are also well demonstrated on MRI.[28] It has higher sensitivity for early disease than bone scan and plain films.[2] MRI also scores over CT in the detection of early disease due to its sensitivity to detect bone marrow edema which is best depicted on short tau inversion recovery (STIR) and T1W images.[28] The changes at this stage, however, are nonspecific.

In addition, skip lesions are more easily and more often detected by MRI as compared to CT. Incidence of multilevel noncontiguous vertebral tuberculosis is generally reported to be between 1.1 and 16%, but an incidence as high as 71.4% has been reported when using whole spine MRI **(Figs. 3A to D)**.[30] MR is also superior to CT for detection of epidural, meningeal, and cord involvement.[31,32] Planning the surgical approach can be facilitated by MRI because of the clear display of the extent of the active infection and its complications including involvement of neural arch.

While tuberculosis can be confidently diagnosed when the characteristic imaging features are present, at times it may be difficult to distinguish this from other causes of bone marrow edema in early stages and from other conditions such as metastases and myeloma in atypical cases. Diffusion-weighted (DW)-MRI and apparent diffusion coefficient (ADC) values have been used to help in the differentiation of spinal tuberculosis from other lesions of similar appearance. However, an overlap of ADC values was noted with metastatic disease, hence, these must be interpreted in association with clinical history and routine MR findings.[33,34] MRI does have disadvantages. Calcification, the hallmark of tubercular infection and small bone fragments are not readily detectable by MRI. Small bone fragments in an epidural abscess are important to detect when surgical management is being considered so that they can be accurately removed. Gradient echo (T2*W) images demonstrate calcification better than spin-echo images. The low signal of calcification or bone fragments is more prominent on these images and closely matches calcification seen on CT. Demonstration of bone fragmentation on T2*W images is also considered characteristic of tuberculosis even in the absence of abscess formation.[35] The other disadvantage is that interventional procedures are difficult to perform with MRI.

Nuclear Medicine Scintigraphy[30,32-40]

Bone scintigraphy using technetium diphosphonate is economical but nonspecific for early detection of tuberculous spondylitis. Reported sensitivities vary from 87.5 to 95%. Uptake is usually increased and multiple sites in disseminated disease may be seen which may mimic metastases. However, Lifeso and Weaver reported false-negative bone scan findings in 35% of plain film positive lesions. The authors noted a high incidence of negative Gallium scans as well. This may be explained by a purely lytic and avascular early phase of the disease. False-negative bone scans are seen with disseminated tuberculosis, cervical spine lesions, and isolated neural arch lesions. Posterior neural arch lesions are more readily detectable when cross-sectional nuclear medicine imaging is performed. The pitfalls of limited anatomic resolution, nonspecificity, and false-negative examinations limit the use of scintigraphy in tuberculous spondylodiscitis. These

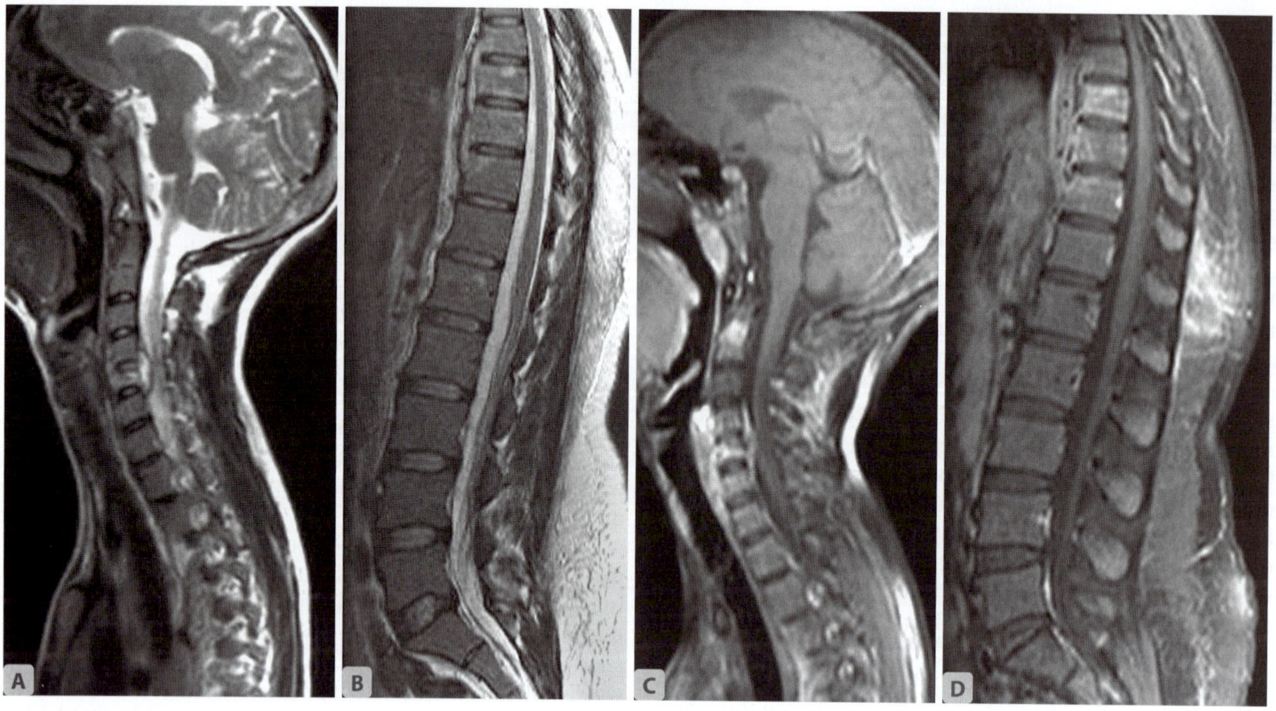

FIGS. 3A TO D: Sagittal T2-weighted images of the cervical (A) and lumbosacral spine (B) in a case of multifocal caries spine reveal hyperintense marrow signal in C5 and D8 to D11 vertebrae. A T2 hyperintense epidural soft tissue is noted at C5 and in the prevertebral region in the lower dorsal spine; (C and D) Postcontrast images reveal abnormal enhancement in the above vertebrae, and soft tissues. Additional foci of enhancement in C2 and posterior to spinous processes in the lumbar region are also seen. Note the relative preservation of the intervertebral discs.

techniques also cannot distinguish between the different causes of infection, but they are useful to identify the area of interest which can then be evaluated further to establish the diagnosis.

Fluorodeoxyglucose-positron emission tomography (FDG-PET) and PET-CT have high sensitivity for detection of chronic osteomyelitis.[41,42] Tubercular lesions are found to have increased FDG uptake in regions of active granulomatous inflammation with cold areas that represent necrosed tissue containing pus. PET-CT can also delineate the sinus tracks without the need for contrast instillation which is an added advantage of PET-CT. If CECT is incorporated along with the PET-CT, the complete extent of osseous, marrow and soft tissue involvement can be delineated. Moreover, it is useful to distinguish active disease from residual fibrotic tissue, detect multiple occult foci, for monitoring response to treatment and providing information on disease spread. It is also a useful tool to guide the site of biopsy or other interventional procedures.

Tuberculosis can be a common cancer mimic on PET/CT, producing uptake patterns that are indistinguishable from that of malignant processes. Though high standardized uptake values (SUVs) >2.5 have been attributed to malignant lesions, high values (up to 21) have been seen in tuberculosis as well. Several groups have attempted to improve the specificity of an ^{18}F-FDG-PET by imaging the abnormal sites at dual time points after its administration including additional delayed imaging at 90–120 minutes.[43,44] At malignant sites, the FDG uptake continues to increase for several hours, which can be demonstrated by the increase in SUVs. On the other hand, in inflammatory lesions, uptake peaks at approximately 60 minutes after administration and the SUVs either stabilize or decline thereafter. Hence, Alavi et al.[35] concluded that imaging at two time points after FDG administration may help distinguish between malignant and inflammatory disorders. However, other authors have found equivocal results with dual point time imaging (45 and 120 minutes post-FDG injection). Another approach to increase the diagnostic accuracy of PET is the combined use of ^{18}F-FDG and C-11 acetate as the latter accumulates in tumors and not in inflammatory lesions.

The exact role of FDG-PET and PET-CT in tuberculosis and other inflammatory diseases is evolving. With the development of newer and more specific radiotracers like positron emitter-labeled antituberculous drug molecules such as isoniazid (INH) and rifampicin in the future, PET/CT may play a significant role in establishing an early diagnosis and effective monitoring of therapeutic response.

IMAGING APPEARANCES

Imaging features in tubercular spondylitis consist of the vertebral, disc space, and the soft tissue changes. Paravertebral abscesses are an important early feature of Pott's spine. Extension of tubercular spondylodiscitis to the adjacent soft tissues is common, incidence varying from 55 to 96%[1,4,45] and rarely may precede any visible vertebral lesion.[6] This extension usually occurs anterolaterally and is less often observed directly posteriorly in the peridural space.[6,45]

Associated changes in the spinal cord and rare variants of disease such as extraosseous extradural granuloma may be detected by modern imaging techniques.

CONVENTIONAL RADIOGRAPHS

The radiographic appearances vary depending on the initial focus of infection within the vertebra. There are mainly four sites of infection in the vertebra, i.e., paradiscal, anterior subperiosteal, central, and appendiceal.

Paradiscal

This is the most common type of lesion, also called marginal, intervertebral, subarticular, or metaphyseal lesion. The disease process most often begins in the anterior vertebral body adjacent to the superior or inferior endplate.[1,15] Two contiguous vertebral bodies are involved in about 50% of cases of tubercular osteomyelitis. Demineralization and loss of definition of the endplates is seen. There is minimal or no periosteal reaction or reactive sclerosis in the remaining part of the vertebra.[1,2,18] Eventually, the adjacent intervertebral disc is narrowed **(Fig. 4)**. Rarely, the disc space may remain intact for a long time. This causes difficulty in diagnosis, as disc space narrowing is an important diagnostic feature It helps to differentiate tuberculosis from traumatic collapse, metastases, solitary myeloma, and porotic collapse where disc space narrowing is absent.[18]

With progressive destruction anterior wedging or collapse occur resulting in varying degrees of kyphosis. The morbidity is greater when three or more vertebral bodies are involved, the angle of kyphosis is more than 25°, and when the vertebrae have lost more than 20% anterior height. Scoliosis may occasionally be seen with asymmetric or unilateral destruction of vertebral bodies and discs and is virtually confined to the lower thoracic and lumbar vertebrae. This is not as frequent as kyphosis.[6]

Central

The central type of lesion starts in the center of the vertebral body. A lytic area with absence of normal trabeculae is seen in the central part of the vertebral body away from the disc margin **(Fig. 5)**.

This gradually enlarges and the vertebral body may expand or balloon out like a tumor. In later stages concentric collapse occurs, almost resembling a vertebra plana. Paravertebral abscesses may be absent or minimal. The disc space is either not affected or only minimally affected.[6,7,18]

Anterior Subperiosteal

This type of infection begins at the anterior vertebral margin underneath the periosteum and spreads beneath the anterior longitudinal ligament producing subtle anterior erosions of multiple vertebrae. The clinical symptoms are out of proportion to the minor radiographic abnormalities **(Figs. 6A and B)**. Disc destruction may be late and anterior erosions may not be apparent on plain radiographs.

Appendiceal or Neural Arch Tuberculosis

The neural arch or vertebral arch includes the spinous process, the laminae, the transverse processes and the pedicle as well as the lateral masses of the atlas, as embryologically, they are equivalent to the neural arch. Overall, the neural arch involvement is reported to range from 2 to 30% of cases usually along with vertebral body involvement.[4,13] Isolated involvement of the neural arch with complete sparing of vertebral bodies and intervertebral discs is rare, constituting less than 2% of all the cases of spinal tuberculosis in nonendemic areas and 5–10% in endemic areas.[4,46] Neural arch tuberculosis (NAT) is being increasingly recognized with the use of cross-sectional imaging **(Figs. 7A to C)**. It is reported NAT usually affects the cervical and upper dorsal

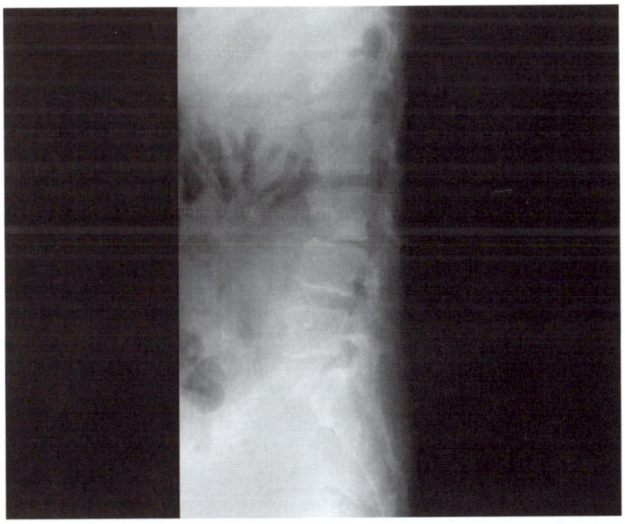

FIG. 4: Lateral radiograph L-S spine showing reduction of L3-L4 disc space with erosion of the anteroinferior aspect of L3 vertebral body—marginal variety of caries.

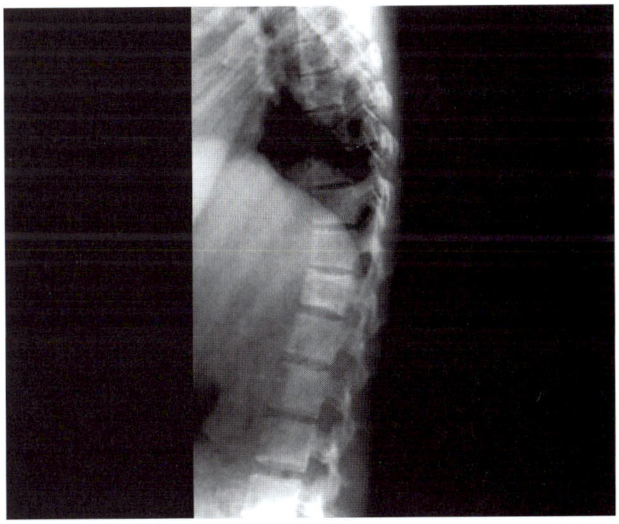

FIG. 5: Lateral radiograph D-L spine showing a lytic area with lack of normal trabeculae in the center of D12 vertebral body. There is mild reduction of vertebral height and minimal sclerosis, adjacent disc spaces are, however, normal—central caries.

spine while the classical variety is the most common at the lumbodorsal region.[47] Radiographic findings in NAT include erosion of pedicles, laminae, the posterior cortex of the vertebra, the adjacent ribs in the dorsal spine with relative sparing of the disc and a large paraspinal mass.[6] Involvement of pedicles (usually unilateral) and laminae is most common in tubercular spondylitis whereas pyogenic spondylitis more often involves the facet joints.[47-49] When there is bilateral involvement of the posterior elements associated with body involvement, gross instability can lead to cord compression and paralysis.

Identification of coexisting posterior and anterior involvement is essential for presurgical planning. Since anterior stabilization depends on posterior stability, anterior, and posterior stabilization must be performed.[2] Simple decompression and debridement with chemotherapy work well for isolated NAT.[50] Paraplegia associated with NAT reportedly has a better prognosis than that with typical spinal tuberculosis.[46]

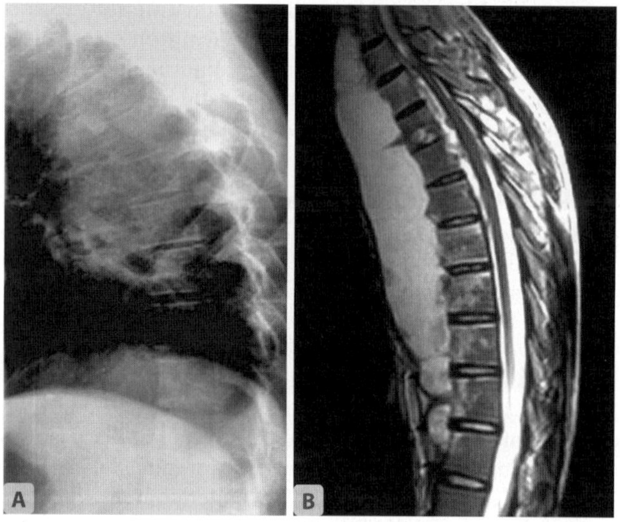

FIGS. 6A AND B: (A) X-ray dorsal spine lateral view in a patient with anterior subperiosteal caries shows indistinct the anterior cortices of multiple dorsal vertebrae; (B) Sagittal T2W MR image of the same reveals the entire extent of pathology with patchy hyperintense signal in multiple dorsal vertebrae, erosions of the anterior cortices and a large prevertebral abscess. A small ventral epidural collection with dorsal displacement of the upper thoracic cord is also noted.

Occasionally, unilateral large bridging osteophytes may occur due to irritation of the bone by inflammatory process with periosteal new bone formation or due to ossification in ligaments. They are more common in the lumbar spine as it bears most of the body weight.

Abscess formation associated with tubercular spondylitis can produce soft tissue opacity on radiographs that appear out of proportion to the bone destruction. The opacity is usually bilateral. It may be globular, which implies pus under tension or fusiform in shape. Involvement of three or more vertebral levels is common paravertebral abscess may be absent or minimal in central caries. A cervical abscess produces widening of the prevertebral soft tissues **(Fig. 8)**. In the thoracic region, the posteromedial pleural line is displaced outward resulting in a characteristic fusiform shape called the "birds nest" appearance.[7] An anterior paravertebral or subligamentous abscess between T4 and T10 vertebrae may produce the so called aneurysmal effect, i.e., erosions or gouge defects on the anterior and lateral surfaces of the vertebral bodies probably due to transmitted aortic pulsations. The intervertebral discs are resistant to pressure atrophy, hence are spared.[6,7,18,51] An abscess at the dorsolumbar junction has a poorly defined lower border and is called a "petering abscess" **(Fig. 9)**. In the lumbar region, tracking of the abscess along the psoas produces bulge of the psoas outline.[6,7,51] Abscesses may calcify which is thought to be characteristic for tuberculosis, since calcification in nontubercular abscesses is uncommon. Psoas abscesses show two patterns of calcification—faint amorphous deposits and tear drop-shaped calcification.[6] Calcification generally becomes more dense as healing occurs, rarely it may decrease or disappear on serial X-rays.[6]

Unusually, sclerotic changes and periosteal reaction mimicking nontubercular infection may be seen. Cystic and

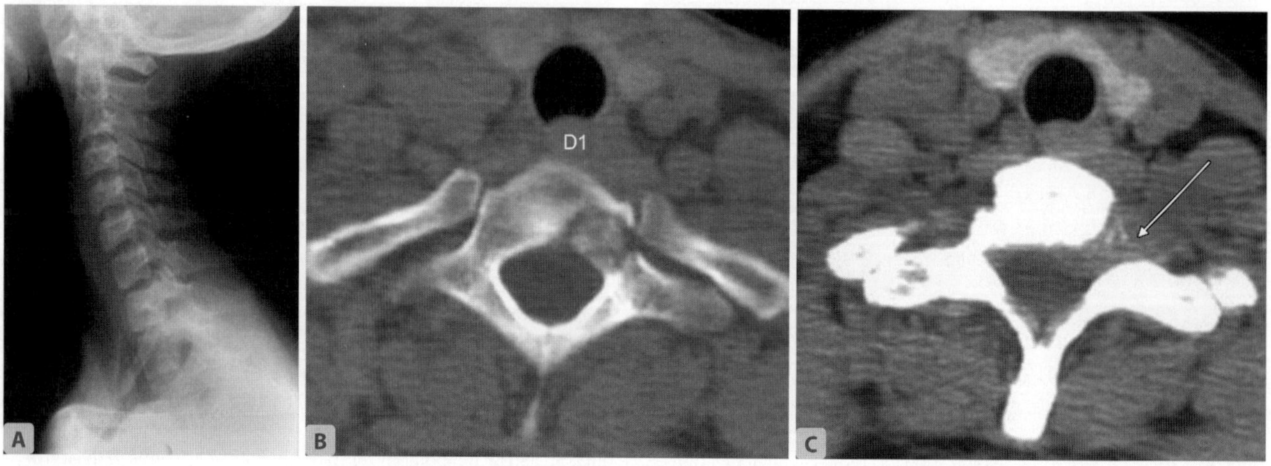

FIGS. 7A TO C: X-ray cervical spine lateral view with the shoulders pulled down reveals no abnormality; (A) Axial CT sections bone (B) and soft tissue (C) windows showing lytic lesions involving the left pedicle and posterior body of D1 vertebra. Associated soft tissue extending into the spinal canal is also seen (arrow)—neural arch tuberculosis.

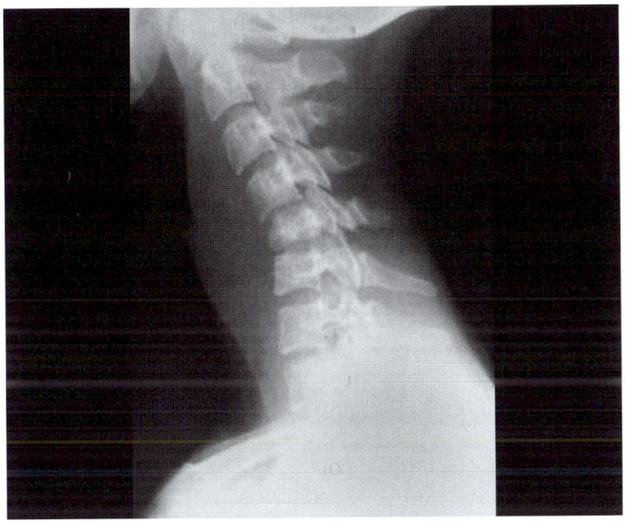

FIG. 8: Lateral radiograph cervical spine in a patient with caries C5 vertebra showing reversal of the cervical lordosis, widening of the prevertebral soft tissues and anterior displacement of the airway due to an associated abscess.

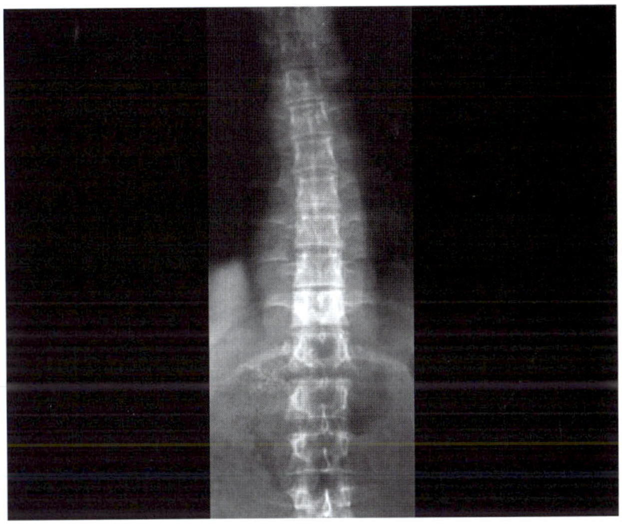

FIG. 9: X-ray D-L spine anteroposterior view of a patient with tuberculosis D10-D11 vertebrae showing a characteristic "petering abscess" with indistinct inferior margins. Subtle amorphous calcification is seen on the right side.

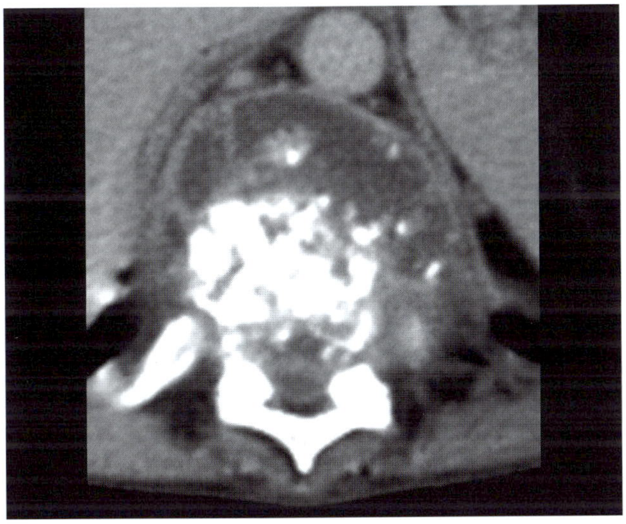

FIG. 10: Postcontrast axial CT scan showing characteristic fragmentary destruction of the vertebral body with an associated multiloculated pre- and paravertebral abscess.

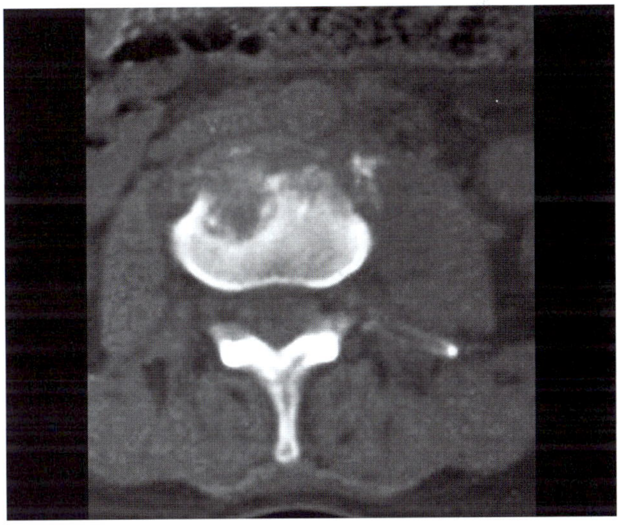

FIG. 11: Axial CT scan showing an osteolytic lesion in the anterior vertebral body in a case of caries spine.

multilocular patterns of involvement may be seen probably due to malnourishment and poor immunological status. However, in general, marked sclerosis, less destruction and collapse, small or no paravertebral abscess more rapid clinical course should suggest a nontubercular etiology on conventional radiographs.[52]

Computed Tomography

Four patterns of bone destruction have been described:[13] on CT, i.e., fragmentary—47% **(Fig. 10)**, osteolytic—33% **(Fig. 11)**, subperiosteal—10% **(Figs. 12A and B)**, and well-defined lytic with sclerotic margins—10%. The fragmentary type is the most common and most typical. In this type numerous residual, small bone fragments are seen embedded in a soft tissue mass. Similar appearance has also been described in involved areas of vertebral appendages.[46] The appearance has been attributed to the absence of proteolytic enzymes required to lyse bone in tuberculosis .[13] Bone fragments may move to the surrounding structures—the spinal canal, paravertebral soft tissues, and psoas muscles. It is especially important to localize such fragments prior to surgical removal which is easily done on CT.[13] Some authors describe that the vertebral bodies appear to have "exploded" with peripheral bony fragments. This is unlike pyogenic spondylitis which shows multiple small erosions like a "pepper pot" and no calcification. Disc space narrowing, multilevel involvement, and kyphosis are also demonstrated and are particularly well seen on multiplanar reconstructions.[4,26]

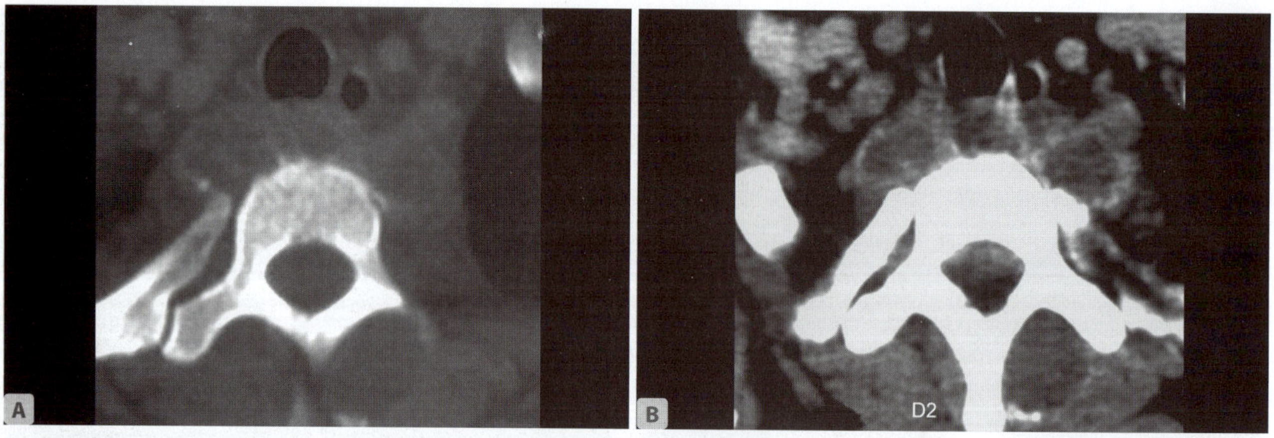

FIGS. 12A AND B: Axial CT scans—bone (A) and soft tissue (B) window settings in a case of subperiosteal caries showing subtle erosions of the anterior cortex of the D2 vertebra. Associated collections are noted in the pre- and paravertebral soft tissues anteriorly. Note another collection in the left posterior paraspinal region.

Computed tomography can also show small amount of calcification not visible on plain radiographs **(Fig. 13)**.[28]

Fat planes around the vertebral body are obliterated early in the course of abscess formation.[4] Soft tissue abscesses are well-demonstrated on axial scans and multiplanar reconstructions.[4,13] These have been characterized by their CT attenuation values with granulation tissue showing high attenuation while abscesses appear as low density lesions with thick a hyperdense rim representing the wall of the inflammatory cavity. Rim enhancement surrounding the low attenuation collection is seen. This is also called the *"rind sign"*.[6] Granulation tissue shows a more homogeneous enhancement **(Figs. 14A and B)**. CT can also demonstrate epidural extension of these soft tissue masses with cord compression but these changes are best delineated on MR.

The combination of a multilocular and calcified paraspinal abscess with thick enhancing rim along with vertebral body fragmentation strongly favors tuberculous rather than pyogenic infection or neoplasm. CT though not always pathognomonic, facilitates CT-guided FNA/biopsy so that histo/cytopathological, or microbiological diagnosis can be established.[4,21,53-55]

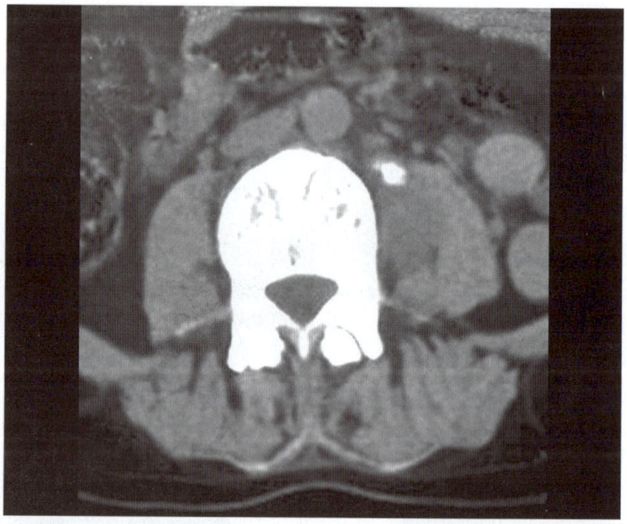

FIG. 13: Axial CT section showing a left psoas abscess with a small speck of calcification.

Magnetic Resonance Imaging

The involved vertebrae show marrow signal alteration appearing hypointense on T1W and relatively hyperintense on T2W images. Loss of cortical definition of the affected vertebrae may also be seen.[4,50] Intervertebral disc is involved in 46–72% of cases though relatively later than pyogenic spondylitis. The internuclear cleft within the disc is a normal finding in patients older than 30 years, and its loss on imaging, in combination with a high-signal intensity, is sign of discitis **(Figs. 15A and B)**.[4,45] In children, the hydrated discs do not form a good barrier to infection and are involved in most patients imaged.[26] Occasionally, the disc space is preserved despite extensive bone destruction, the so-called *floating disc sign*. Involvement of the neural arch is also detected well by MRI **(Fig. 16)**. Enhanced MR studies may demonstrate inhomogeneous enhancement in the region of marrow infiltration.

Paraspinal soft tissue masses are seen in approximately 71% of cases on MRI.[56] On T1W images loss of the uniform psoas muscle signal intensity and enlargement of the affected muscle is seen while on T2W images there is an increase in signal intensity **(Fig. 17)**. Postcontrast studies reveal thick rim enhancement around intraosseous and paraspinal soft tissue abscesses **(Fig. 18)**. More uniform enhancement is seen with granulation tissue or phlegmon.[4,44,56,57] MR is useful in delineating the communication between vertebral and paravertebral components of abscesses with epidural extension being seen 61% of involved vertebrae[45,56] The soft tissue masses displace the thecal sac and the spinal cord is distorted. Postcontrast fat suppressed T1W sequences are the best to demonstrate meningeal and epidural inflammatory soft tissues, with improved definition of cord and nerve root compromise **(Figs. 19A and B)**.[15] Heavily T2W fast spin-echo sequences can also be applied to generate myelographic images showing thecal sac compression.[56]

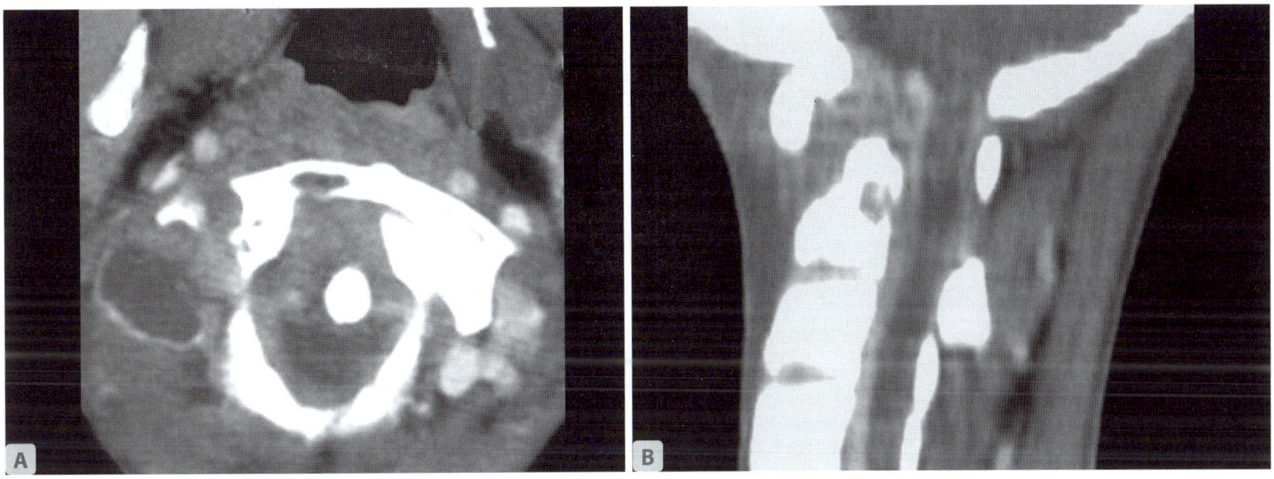

FIGS. 14A AND B: Axial postcontrast CT myelogram (A) with sagittal multiplanar reconstruction (B) in a patient with caries C1-C2 showing atlantoaxial dislocation with erosions of the right lateral mass of C1 and the dens. A peripherally enhancing abscess is noted on the right side while homogeneously enhancing granulation tissue is seen in the predental space.

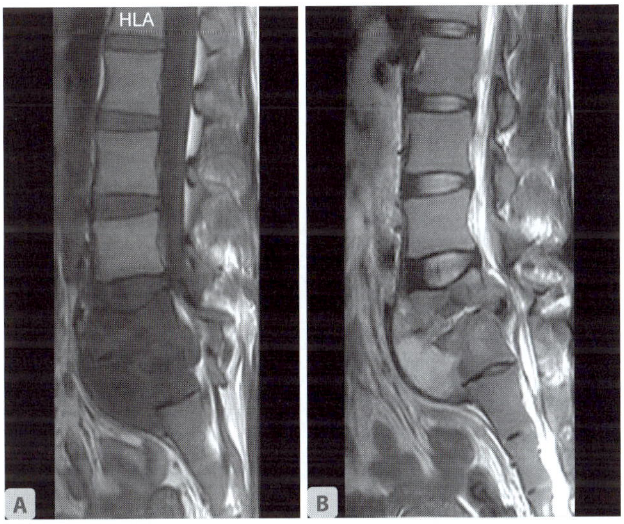

FIGS. 15A AND B: Sagittal T1W (A) and T2W (B) MR scans of a patient with tuberculosis L5-S1 show collapse of L5 vertebral body, hypointense marrow signal of L5-S1 and loss of cortical definition on the T1W image. The intervening disc space is reduced with hyperintense signal on the T2W image suggesting discitis. A prevertebral abscess lifting up the anterior longitudinal ligament and a small ventral epidural collection are also seen.

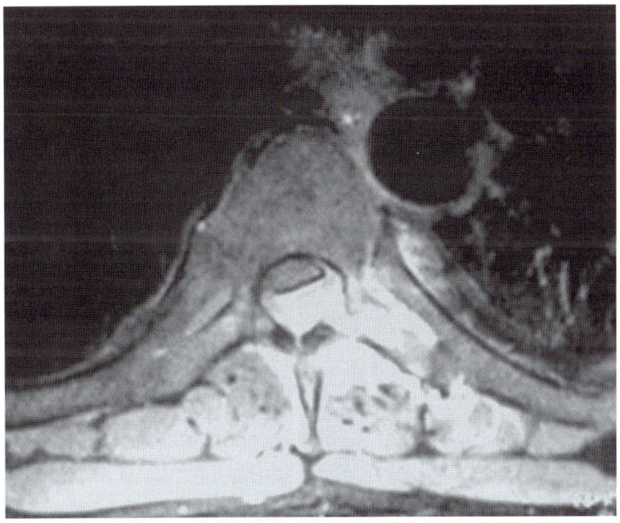

FIG. 16: Postcontrast T1W fat suppressed axial MR section through a thoracic vertebra showing patchy enhancement in the left pedicle, lamina, transverse process, and the adjacent rib. Homogeneously enhancing granulation tissue is noted in the left paraspinal region and dorsal epidural space displacing the cord anteriorly—neural arch tuberculosis.

Disruption of the endplate reportedly has high sensitivity and specificity for diagnosis of spinal tuberculosis,[58] i.e., 100% and 81.4%, respectively. Other features with high sensitivity and specificity include paravertebral soft tissue shadow (96.8% and 85.3%) and a high-signal intensity of the intervertebral disc on the T2W image (80.6% and 82.4%). The overall sensitivity and specificity for diagnosis are 100% and 88.2%, respectively.

Cord Changes

Conventional radiographs provide little information if any, on the status of the cord which is inadequately assessed on CT as well. MRI, on the other hand because of its superior soft tissue contrast is the technique of choice to assess the cord. Cord changes may result in neurological deficit or paraplegia.

Paraplegia in patients with *active disease*—tubercular abscesses, granulation tissue, debris, internal gibbus, or subluxation may cause cord compression due to *mechanical pressure*. The spinal cord may be able with stand some degree of pressure, especially when it develops slowly as in tuberculosis. It is reported that good cord function may be seen even with 40–50% decrease in cord diameter. The midsagittal cord diameter and presence of cerebrospinal fluid (CSF) signal anterior to cord at the apex of the deformity at presentation have been shown to correlate with neurological

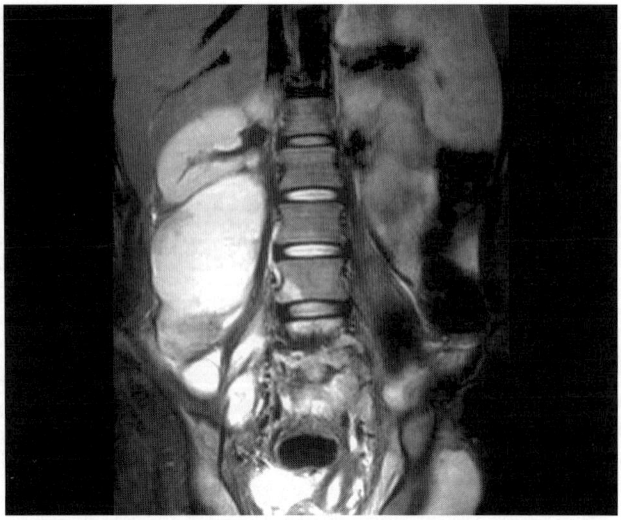

FIG. 17: STIR coronal scan in a patient with lumbosacral caries depicts partial collapse and hyperintense signal involving L4-L5 vertebrae. There is a disproportionately large psoas abscess on the right side lifting up the inferior pole of right kidney.

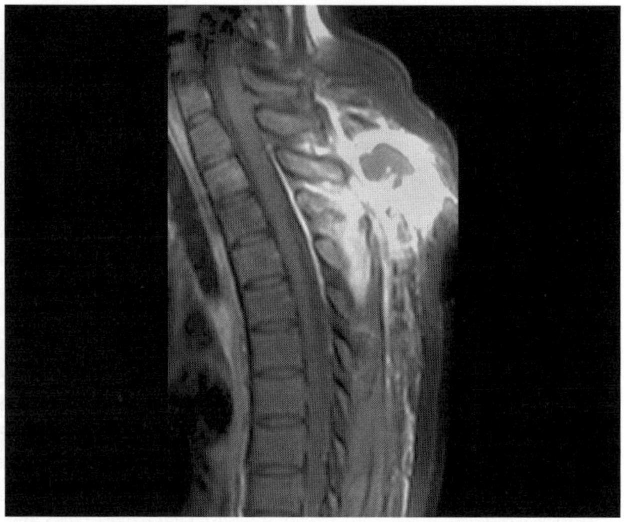

FIG. 18: Postcontrast T1W sagittal MR image of a patient with caries spine showing erosion of the spinous process of D3 vertebra with a large abscess showing thick peripheral rim enhancement.

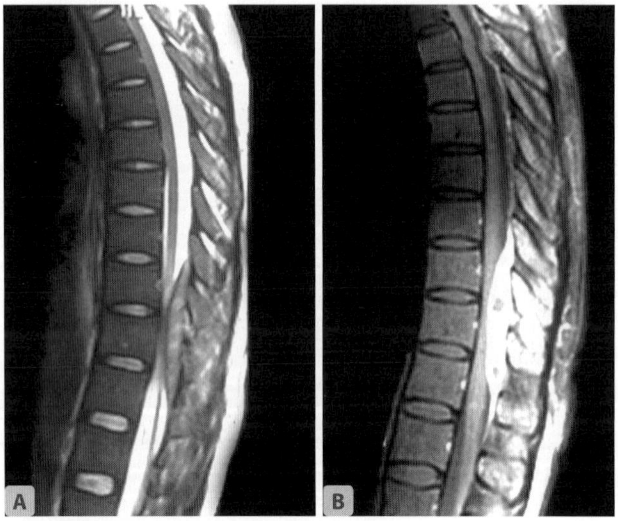

FIGS. 19A AND B: Sagittal T2W (A) and postcontrast fat suppressed T1W (B) MR images in a patient with neural arch tuberculosis D-L spine show nearly homogeneously enhancing dorsal epidural granulation tissue with resultant cord compression. Note the abnormal enhancement in the adjacent spinous processes and interspinous region.

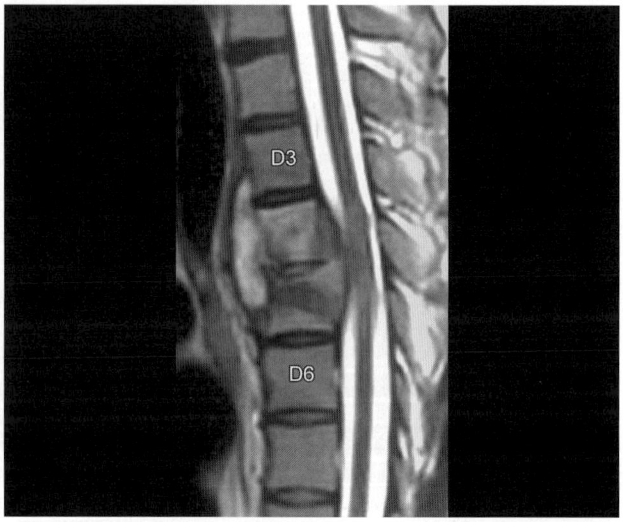

FIG. 20: Sagittal T2W MR image of the cervicodorsal spine in a patient of caries D4-D5 shows reduction in disc space with altered marrow signal in the involved vertebrae and associated prevertebral and ventral epidural collections. The cord is mildly expanded at this level with T2 hyperintense signal due to cord edema.

deficit. Ambulatory patients had greater cord dimensions and CSF signal persisting anterior to cord at the apex of the deformity in this study.[59] Unrelieved compression of the spinal cord results in loss of neurons, gliosis, and demyelination of cord substance in the damaged segment.

Intrinsic changes in the spinal cord may also lead to paraplegia. Spinal cord may show edema, myelomalacia, or syringomyelia **(Fig. 20)**. Edema is seen as hyperintense signal on T2W images but no signal alteration on T1 while myelomalacia shows a T1 hypointense signal (higher than that of CSF) as well and may be associated with thinning of the cord. A syrinx is a tubular, well-defined fluid-filled region within the spinal cord with tapered ends and may be septated. The signal characteristics of a syrinx are typically those of CSF. Edema of the cord is associated with good recovery of neurological function following treatment, while a poor outcome is likely when there is syrinx or myelomalacia. Rarely a small tuberculoma of the cord may be responsible for neurological deficits presenting as spinal tumor syndrome **(Figs. 21A and B)**.[60] Mild atrophy of the cord may persist following treatment even with good neurological outcome.[26,60]

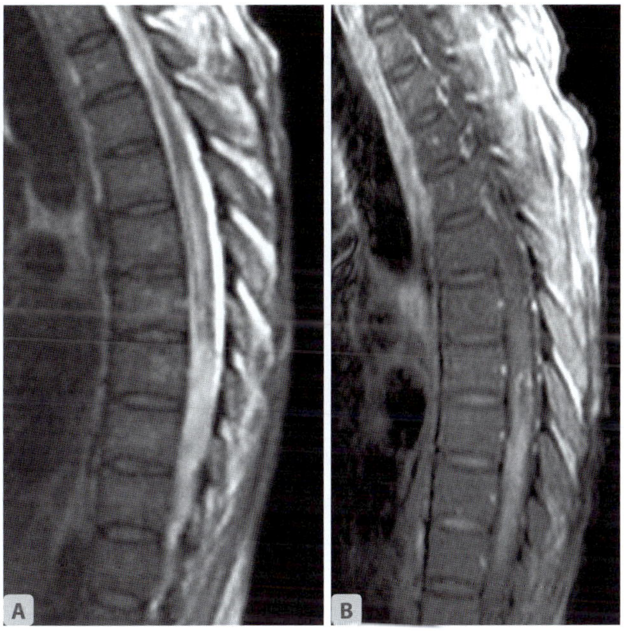

FIGS. 21A AND B: T2W (A) and postcontrast T1W (B) sagittal images of a patient with tubercular myelitis reveal cord swelling and edema appearing hyperintense on the T2W image with patchy enhancement on the postcontrast image.

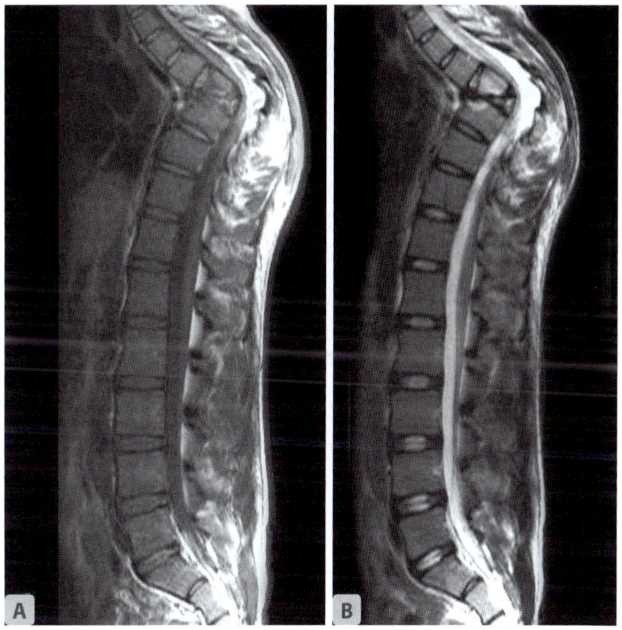

FIGS. 22A AND B: T1W (A) and T2W (B) images of the dorsolumbar spine in an old treated case of tuberculosis spine reveal near complete destruction of D8 vertebra and partial destruction of the adjacent D7 and D9 with fatty marrow signal and gross kyphotic deformity. There is resultant stretching and thinning of the cord but no signal change suggestive of cord atrophy. Note the fibrofatty proliferation along the dorsal epidural space appearing hyperintense on both T1W and T2W images.

According to some authors, MR findings may also be a useful guide to treatment strategy. When MR shows a predominantly fluid collection in the extradural space, compressing the cord with evidence of myelitis or edema only, a good response to conservative treatment is seen. If the extradural compression is due to granulation tissue with little fluid, early surgical decompression may be beneficial.[21] *Paraplegia* with *healed disease*[21] may occur when the initial lesion has healed with a residual severe deformity, even after a gap of 10–20 years. It is produced by stretching of the spinal cord over an internal anterior bony projection, producing gliosis. MRI shows severe atrophy of the cord and/or syringohydromyelia, or constricting scarring of and around the dura **(Figs. 22A and B)**. Symptomatic severe stenosis of the lumbar canal and ossification of the ligamentum flavum adjacent to severe kyphosis may produce an incomplete neurological deficit. Reactivation of the disease is found in 30–40% of old cases on exploration.

ATYPICAL SPINAL TUBERCULOSIS[21]

The classical paradiscal tubercular lesion is easily recognized and treated. Atypical spinal tuberculosis is defined as compressive myelopathy with no visible or palpable spinal deformity and without the radiological appearance of a typical vertebral lesion. Such lesions are not only infrequent, but also difficult to diagnose in the early stages with more chance of neurological complications. Atypical lesions may present as an intraspinal tubercular granuloma, involvement of the neural arch, compressive myelopathy in single vertebral disease, a concertina collapse of a vertebra, or a sclerotic vertebra. Granulomatous lesions of the epidural, intradural, or intramedullary spaces present as a compressive myelopathy, the *spinal tumor syndrome*, without obvious radiological signs. Tubercular granuloma should be considered in the differential diagnosis of spinal tumor syndrome in zones endemic for tuberculosis.

Extraosseous extradural granuloma is a rare variant that leads to an extradural granulomatous lesion in the absence of bone involvement. The route of infection is most likely hematogenous. It is more common in men than women, and usually involves the dorsal epidural space in the thoracic region. Clinically, there are features of compressive radiculomyelopathy. On pathologic examination, a granulomatous membrane is found ensheathing and compressing the spinal cord or cauda equina.[6] MR shows the pathology well. The lesion is T1 isointense and shows mixed signal on T2W images. Uniform enhancement is seen, if the inflammatory tissue is phlegmonous while rim enhancement is seen, if abscess formation or caseation has occurred **(Figs. 23A to C)**.[5] Epidural tuberculous abscess may also be seen in along with arachnoiditis, myelitis, intramedullary tuberculoma, etc.[61]

Post-treatment Follow-up

Conventional Radiographs

While on treatment, sequential radiographs can be repeated to assess the degree of healing. However, radiological evidence of healing is evident late on radiographs. It lags behind by about 3 months.[21] Evidence of bone destruction

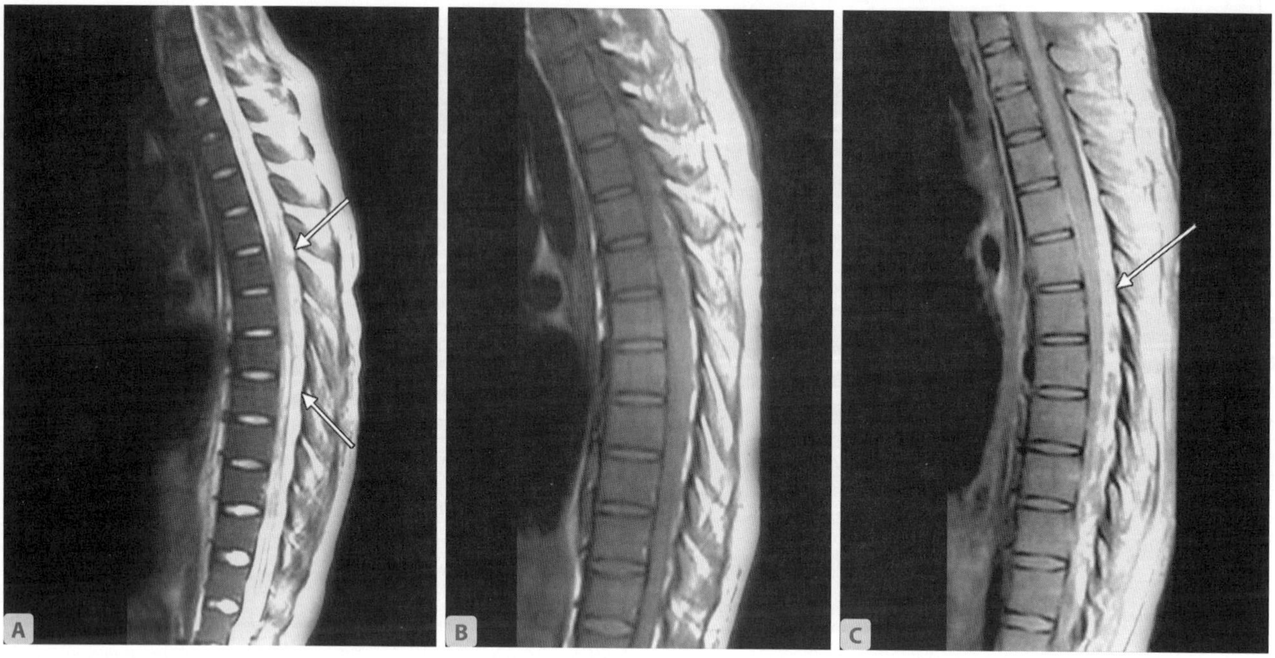

FIGS. 23A TO C: Extraosseous extradural granuloma: Sagittal T2W (A), T1W (B), and postcontrast (C) MR images show normal vertebral and intervertebral disc morphology and signal intensity pattern. A long segment, crescentic dorsal epidural abscess showing heterogeneous signal on T1W and T2W images with irregular peripheral contrast enhancement (arrows) causing anterior displacement of thecal sac is seen.

or loss of vertebral height may progress up to 14 months after treatment initiation and should not necessarily be considered a poor response.[62] Soft tissue paravertebral masses may also progress while on treatment reaching a maximum size within 1.5 months, and may take up to 15 months to resolve. Although MRC trials (multicenter randomized controlled trials of Medical Research Council, UK) have shown persistent changes in plain radiological appearances of the vertebral column up to 3 years after completion of treatment, these changes were attributed to new bone formation and ankylosis.[63] Signs of healing include the lesion remaining static or regressing on serial radiographs, better definition of lesion margin, and sclerosis **(Fig. 24)**. Increased density of the vertebral body with healing can lead to the appearance of an ivory vertebra. The phenomenon is usually seen in the lumbar region **(Fig. 25)**.[6] Calcific debris which progresses to fusion on serial films may be seen in 3 weeks, although it can take up to 27 months for any evidence of fusion to appear.[62] Fusion of contiguous vertebrae is generally regarded as the surest sign of healing tuberculosis although there is no actual proof of this **(Fig. 26)**.[62]

The healed status of disease or end point of treatment is not clearly defined for tuberculosis. Clinical and radiological evidence of healing with no recurrence after 2 years is generally referred to as "healed status."[21] It is, however, well known that reactivation of disease may occur years later.

Computed Tomography

Features of resolution such as increase in vertebral bone density, with reduction in the size of paraspinal soft tissue masses as edema and inflammatory exudate subside are readily apparent on sequential CT examinations.[4]

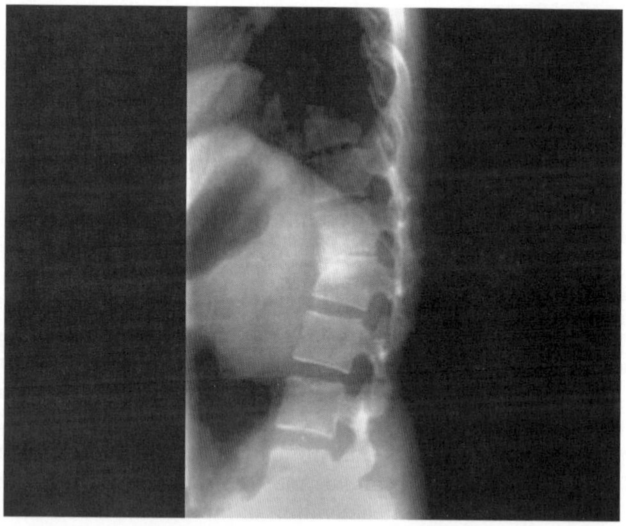

FIG. 24: Lateral radiograph D-L spine in a case of healing tuberculosis shows reduced disc space between D12 and L1 vertebrae with sclerosis adjacent to the vertebral end plates.

The inflammatory reaction in the bone marrow, however, is not well depicted **(Figs. 27A and B)**.[28]

Magnetic Resonance Imaging[40,47,56,64,65]

Post-therapy follow-up can also be done with MR. The earliest sign of healing is a reduction in the amount of soft tissue masses or collections. However, enlargement of the soft tissue mass or bone destruction does not indicate failed treatment. A high-signal intensity rim on the T1W sequences at the edge of the osseous lesion represents healing **(Fig. 28)**.

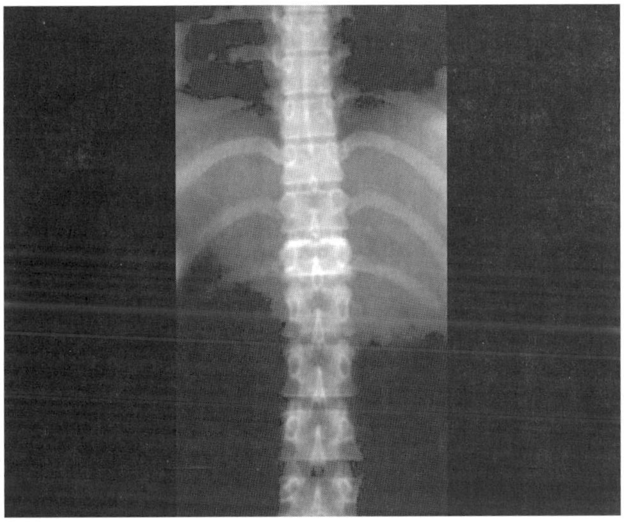

FIG. 25: X-ray D-L spine AP view showing sclerosis of D12 vertebra giving the appearance of ivory vertebra in a patient with healing caries.

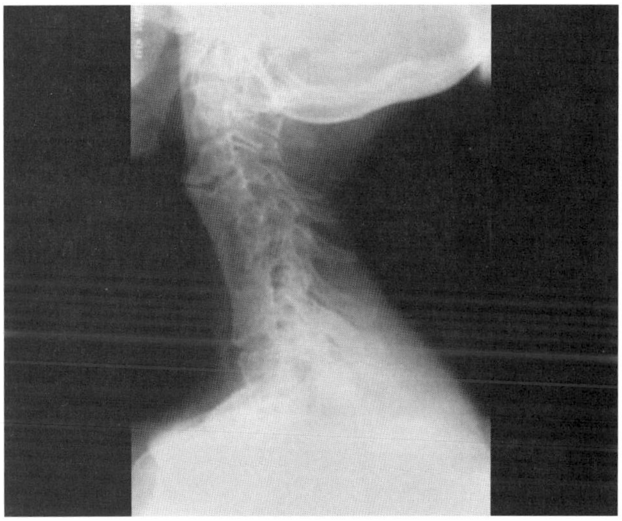

FIG. 26: Lateral radiograph of the cervical spine shows fusion of multiple cervical vertebral forming a large osseous block in a patient with healed tuberculosis of the cervical spine.

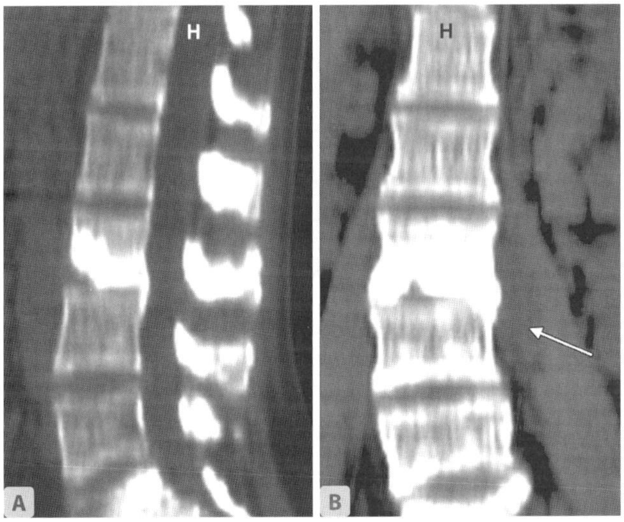

FIGS. 27A AND B: Sagittal and coronal CT reconstructions of the lumbar spine of a patient on anti-tubercular treatment (ATT) showing sclerosis of the inferior body and end plate of L1 vertebra with reduced L1-L2 disc space suggestive of healing disease.

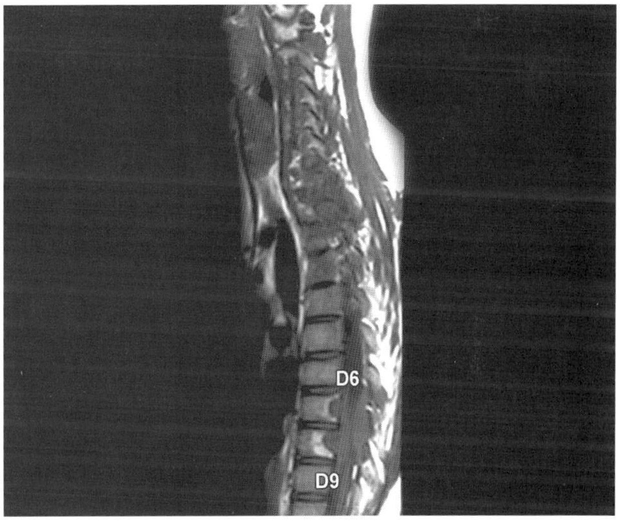

FIG. 28: Sagittal T1W MR image of the cervicodorsal spine of a patient after 3 months of ATT shows erosions of the posterior cortex of D7-D8 vertebrae. These lesions show marginal hyperintense signal signifying healing lesions.

A progressive sequential increase in signal intensity on T1W image is apparent with resolution **(Fig. 29)**. Reduction in gadolinium enhancement and eventual loss of enhancement are useful signs of healing. However, persistent or even increasing enhancement does not necessarily indicate worsening or treatment failure. MRI is also useful in the detection of reactivation of old tubercular spondylitis. The change of signal from low signal in healed tuberculosis to high signal on T2W images suggests active disease. Reactivation may present with an isolated psoas abscess without evidence of bony lesions.

The question whether treatment end point should be determined based on MR findings remains controversial. A significant proportion of patients may have radiological evidence of persistent disease activity in the form of discitis, vertebral body abscess, marrow edema, or multifocal intraosseous abscess with persistent cord compression after 6 months of treatment. Both the British and American Thoracic Societies, based on the evidence of the MRC trials, advocate short course chemotherapy (6 months) for adult uncomplicated fully sensitive spinal tuberculosis. However, the authors felt that in a significant proportion of patients, longer durations of treatment (more than 6 months) may be required as their MR scans were abnormal even though there was apparent disease resolution clinically. Other authors have suggested that the persistence of MRI abnormalities after 12 months of treatment does not require further treatment in patients with good clinical and laboratory outcome.

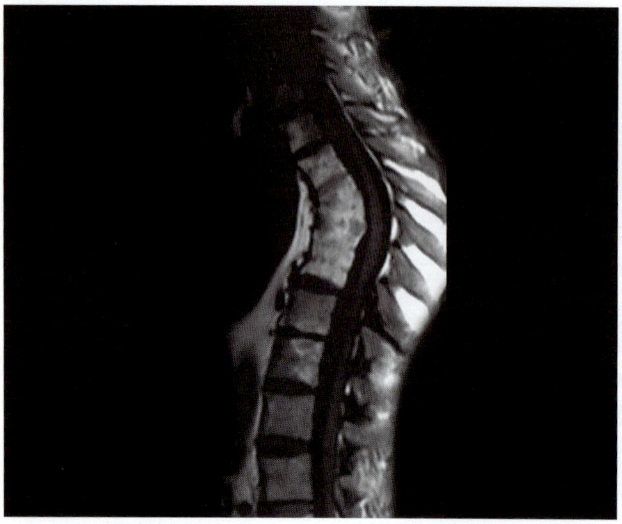

FIG. 29: Sagittal T1W MR image of the dorsal spine in a patient with healed caries spine shows kyphosis with complete absence of disc space between multiple dorsal vertebrae which appear hyperintense on the T1W image due to fatty replacement.

MRI alone should not determine when treatment should be stopped. Repeat MRI is probably not necessary in patients who have a clinical and laboratory improvement during treatment.

Although these studies have evaluated only a limited number of patients they highlight the fact that there are currently no universally accepted guidelines, more studies need to be performed to achieve consensus on the interpretation and use of this powerful modality in the follow-up of spinal tuberculosis patients.

Positron Emission Tomography/ Computed Tomography[66-68]

^{18}F-fluorodeoxyglucose-PET may be useful for discriminating residual and nonresidual spinal infection after treatment healed disease demonstrates absence of uptake. In a recent study, both contrast-enhanced MR and FDG-PET were used for follow-up, with treatment being continued till contrast enhancement or FDG uptake was negative suggestive of healed status. ^{18}F-FDG-PET was considered to be better at demonstrating healed status than MRI.

DIFFERENTIAL DIAGNOSIS

The differential diagnosis of tubercular spondylodiscitis includes pyogenic and fungal infections, degenerative disc disease, brucellosis, neoplasms, etc.

Clinically patients of *degenerative spondylosis* present with radicular pain and no systemic symptoms, but vertebral infection with radicular pain may be misdiagnosed as degenerative disease, if the patient is afebrile. With degenerative disease, the disc space is usually not markedly narrowed, bone density and end plate definition are preserved. On MR disc desiccation produces a low signal on T2W images unlike discitis which is bright. After intravenous contrast infected discs enhance strongly whereas degenerated discs only occasionally minimally.[17]

When infection is considered, a history of chronicity and insidious progression suggests tubercular rather than *pyogenic infection.* In tuberculosis, osteoporosis with absence of sclerosis is seen on plain films. Involvement of multiple contiguous vertebrae, the entire vertebral body, loss of cortical definition, more frequent involvement of posterior elements, disproportionally large paraspinal masses, especially with calcification or a thick rim of enhancement, subligamentous spread to three or more vertebral levels, and presence of skip lesions favor a tubercular etiology. Disc involvement is said to occur later in tuberculosis as compared to pyogenic infections. However, differentiation from pyogenic infection can at times be difficult.[1,17]

Brucellosis is an indolent infection such as tuberculosis. Typically brucellar spondylitis is common in the lower lumbar spine, with minimal paraspinal soft tissue masses, no gibbus deformity, and presence of gas within the disc. On MR images, vertebral body morphology and cortical margins are maintained despite evidence of osteomyelitis.

Sarcoidosis can produce findings identical to those of tuberculosis including multifocal vertebral lesions with paraspinal masses.[1]

When a solitary vertebra is involved, differentiation from *metastatic disease* in adults and from *eosinophilic granuloma* in children may be difficult. Spinal lesions, such as *lymphoma,* that affect consecutive vertebrae or neoplasms, such as *multiple myeloma* and *chordoma,* that involve contiguous vertebrae and discs can add to the diagnostic difficulty.[1,2,4] *Bizarre infections* such as fungal disease and spinal echinococcosis cannot be easily distinguished from tuberculosis or neoplasms.

The morphologic and pathophysiologic changes encountered in spinal tuberculosis are the most severe among infective spondylitides and are also the most varied. Conventional radiographs are the usual initial imaging investigation. However, early in the disease and in atypical cases such as isolated NAT, plain films may be negative and if the clinical suspicion of tubercular infection is strong MRI which is the modality of choice should be considered. The wider availability of CT, high sensitivity and ability to assist in diagnosis by accurately targeting lesions for guided biopsy make it a useful alternative diagnostic tool for early diagnosis when MR is not available.

A delay in diagnosis may lead to irreversible neurologic sequelae and spinal deformity in a high percentage of cases. Hence, a multidisciplinary approach to tubercular spondylitis is essential to ensure prompt assessment of the location, extent and character of spinal pathology to positively affect the clinical management in a timely fashion.

REFERENCES

1. Yao DC, Sartoris ADJ. Musculoskeletal tuberculosis. Radiol Clin N Am. 1995;35(4):679-89.
2. Moore SL, Rafi M. Imaging of musculoskeletal and spinal tuberculosis. Radiol Clin N Am. 2001;39(2):329-42.
3. Pott P. Remarks on that kind of palsy of the lower limbs which is frequently found to accompany a curvature of the spine. London: J Johnson; 1779.
4. Sharif HAS, Morgan JL, al Shahed MS, al Thagafi MY. Role of CT and MR imaging in the management of tuberculous spondylitis. Radiol Clin N Am. 1995;33(4):787-804.
5. Gupta RK. Tuberculosis and other non-tuberculous bacterial granulomatous infections. In: Gupta RK, Lufkin RB (Eds). MR Imaging and Spectroscopy of Central Nervous System Infection. United States: Kluwer Academic/Plenum Publishers; 2001. pp. 95-146.
6. Resnick D. Osteomyelitis, septic arthritis and soft tissue infection: mechanism and situations. In: Resnick D (Ed). Diagnosis of Bone and Joint Disorder, 4th edition. Philadelphia: WB Saunders; 2002. pp. 2377-480.
7. Bhan S, Nag HL. Skeletal tuberculosis. In: Sharma SK, Mohan A (Eds). Tuberculosis. New Delhi: Jaypee Brothers Medical Publishers; 2001. pp. 237-60.
8. Hsu LC, Leong JC. Tuberculosis of the lower cervical spine C2-C7. J Bone Joint Surg Br. 1984;66(1):1-5.
9. Martin NS. Tuberculosis of the spin: A study of results of treatment during the east twenty-five years. J Bone Joint Surg Br. 1970;53:613.
10. Fang D, Leong JCY, Fang HSV. Tuberculosis of the upper cervical spine. J Bone Joint Surg Br. 1983;65(1):47-50.
11. Lal AP, Rajshekar V, Chandy M. Management strategies in tuberculous atlantoaxial dislocation. Br J Neurosurg. 1992;6:529-35.
12. Tuli SM. Tuberculosis of the craniovertebral region. Clin Orthop Res. 1974;104:209-12.
13. Jain R, Sawhney S, Berry M. Computed tomography of vertebral tuberculosis: patterns of bone destruction clinical radiology. 1993;47:196-9.
14. Chapman M, Murray RO, Stoker DT. Tuberculosis of the bones and joints. Semin Roentgenol. 1979;14:266-82.
15. Weaver P, Lifeso RM. The radiological diagnosis of tuberculosis of the adult spine. Skeleltal Radiol. 1984;12:178-88.
16. Kahn DS, Pritzker KPH. Pathophysiology of Bone infection. Clin Orthop. 1973;96:12-9.
17. Sharif HA, Aideyan OA, Clark DC, Madkour MM, Aabed MY, Mattsson TA, et al. Brucellar and tuberculous spondylitis: Comparative imaging features. Radiology. 1989;155:419-25.
18. Golding FC. Tuberculosis of Bone. In: Shanks CS Kerly P (Eds). A Textbook of X-ray Diagnosis by British Authors, 3rd edition; London: H.K.Lewis & Co. Ltd.; 1959. pp. 274-89.
19. Jalleh RD, Kuppuswamy L, Mahayiddin AA, Acob MF, Yusuf NA, Mokhtar A. Spinal tuberculosis—A five year review of cases at the National Tuberculosis Centre. Med J Malaya. 1991;46:269-73.
20. Fam AG, Rubenstein J. Another Look at spinal tuberculosis. J Rheumatol. 1993;20:1731.
21. Jain AK. Afresh look at an old disease. J Bone Joint Surg [Br]. 2010;92-B:905-13.
22. Negi SS, Khan SF, Gupta S, et al. Comparison of the conventional diagnostic modalities, baltec culure and polymerase chain reaction test for diagnosis of tuberculosis. Indian J Med Microbiol. 2005;23:29-33.
23. Jain AK, Jena SK, Singh M, Dhammi IK, Ramachadran VG, Dev G. Evaluation of clinico-radiological, bacteriological, serological, molecular and histological diagnosis of osteoarticular tuberculosis. Indian J Orthop. 2008;42:173-7.
24. Tuli SM. Tuberculosis of the spine: a historical review. Clin Orthop. 2007;460:29-38.
25. Burrill J, Williams CJ, Bain G, Conder G, Hine AL, Misra RR. Tuberculosis: A radiologic review. Radiographics. 2007;27: 1255-73.
26. Pandit HG, Sonsale PD, Shikare SS, Bhojraj SY. Bone scintigraphy in tuberculous spondylodiscitis. Eur Spin J. 1999;8:205-9.
27. Desai S. Early diagnosis of spinal tuberculosis by MRI. J Bone Joint Surg Br. 1994;76:863-9.
28. Nocera RM, Sayle B, Rogers C, Wilkey D. Tc 99m MDP and indium 111 chloride scintigraphy in skeletal tuberculosis. Clin Nucl Med. 1983;8:418-20.
29. Lifeso RM, Weaver P, Harder E. Tuberculous spondylitis in adults. J Bone Joint Surg Am. 1985;67:1405-13.
30. Kaila R, Malhi AM, Mahmood B, Saifuddin A. The incidence of multiple level noncontiguous vertebral tuberculosis detected using whole spine MRI. J Spinal Disord Tech. 2007;20(1):78-81.
31. Stabler A, Reiser MF. Imaging of spinal infection. Radiol Clin N Am. 2001;39(1):115-35.
32. Sharif HA, Clark DC, Aabed MY, Haddad MC, al Deeb SM, Yaqub B, et al. Granulomatous spinal infections MR imaging. Radiology. 1990;177:101-7.
33. Palle L, Reddy MB, Reddy KJ. Role of magnetic resonance diffusion imaging and apparent diffusion coefficient values in the evaluation of spinal tuberculosis in Indian patients. Indian J Radiol Imaging. 2010;20(4):279-83.
34. Pui MH, Mitha A, Rae WI, Corr P. Diffusion-weighted magnetic resonance imaging of spinal infection and malignancy. J Neuroimaging. 2005;15(2):164-7.
35. Gupta RK, Agarwal P, Rastogi H, Kumar S, Phadke RV, Krishnani N. Problems in differentiating spinal tuberculosis from neoplasm on MRI. Neuroradiology. 1996;38:S97-104.
36. Alavi A, Lakhani P, Mavi A, Kung JW, Zhuang H. PET: a revolution in medical imaging. Radiol Clin North Am. 2004;42:983-1001.
37. Andronikou S, Bindapersad M, Govender N, Waner JI, Segwe A, Palliam S, et al. Musculoskeletal tuberculosis-imaging using low-end and advanced modalities for developing and developed countries. Acta Radiol. 2011;52(4):430-41.
38. Buxi TB. Computed tomography in spinal tuberculosis. Ind J Radiol Imag. 1993;3:291-3.
39. Maiuri F, Iaconetta G, Gallicchio B, et al. Spondylodiscitis clinical and magnetic resonance diagnosis. Spine. 1997;22:1741-6.
40. Sharif HA. Role of MR imaging in the management of spinal infections. AJR Am J Roentgenol. 1992;158:1333-45.
41. Harkirat S, Anand SS, Indrajit IK, Dash AK. Pictorial essay: PET/CT in tuberculosis. Indian J Radiol Imaging. 2008;18(2):141.
42. D'Souza MM, Sharma R, Tripathi M, Mondal A. F-18 Fluorodeoxyglucose positron emission tomography/ computed tomography in tuberculosis of the hip: A case report and brief review of literature. Indian J Nucl Med. 2011;26(1):31-3.
43. Hustinx R, Smith RJ, Benard F, Rosenthal DI, Machtay M, Farber LA, et al. Dual time point fluorine-18 fluorodeoxyglucose positron emission tomography: a potential method to differentiate malignancy from inflammation and normal tissue in the head and neck. Eur J Nucl Med. 1999;26(10):1345-8.
44. Zhuang H, Pourdehnad M, Lambright ES, Yamamoto AJ, Lanuti M, Li P, et al. Dual time point 18F-FDG PET imaging for differentiating malignant from inflammatory processes. J Nucl Med. 2001;42:1412-7.
45. Mendonca RA. Spinal infection and inflammatory disorders. In: Atlas SW (Ed). Magnetic Resonance Imaging of the Brain and Spine, 3rd edition. Philadelphia: Lippincot Williams and Wilkins; 2002. pp. 1855-972.

46. Rahman NU, Jamjoom A, Jamjoom ZA, Al-Tahan AM. Neural arch tuberculosis: Radiological features and their correlation with surgical findings. Br J Neurosurg. 1997;11(1):32-8.
47. Loke TK, Ma HT, Chan CS. Magnetic resonance imaging of tuberculous spinal infection. Australas Radiol. 1997;41:7-12.
48. Kumar K. Clinical study and classification of posterior spinal tuberculosis. Int Orthop. 1985;9:147-52.
49. Raglan R, Abdelwahan F, Braffman B, Moss DS. Posterior spinal tuberculosis—a case report. Am J Neuroradiol. 1990;11: 612-3.
50. Abdelwahan IF, Camins MB, Hermann G, Klein MJ. Vertebral arch or posterior spinal tuberculosis. Skeletal Radiol. 1997;26: 737-40.
51. Rodriguez-Takeuchi SY, Renjifo ME, Medina FJ. Extrapulmonary tuberculosis: pathophysiology and imaging findings. Radiographics. 2019;39:2023-37.
52. Jacobs P, Renton P. Periosteal reaction; bone and joint infections; sarcoid. In: Sutton D (Ed). Textbook of Radiology and Medical Imaging, 4th edition. London: Churchill Livingstone; 1987. pp. 71-2.
53. Richards AS. Non-tuberculous pyogenic osteomyelitis of the spine. J Canadian Assoc Radiol. 1960;11:45-9.
54. Kang M, Gupta S, Khandelwal N, Shankar S, Gulati M, Suri S. CT-guided fine-needle aspiration biopsy of spinal lesions. Acta Radiol. 1999;40:474-8.
55. Mondal A, Misra DK. CT-guided needle aspiration cytology (FNAC) of 112 vertebrallesions. Indian J Pathol Microbiol. 1994;37: 255-61.
56. Francis IM, Das DK, Luthra UK, Sheikh Z, Sheikh M, Bashir M. Value of radiologically guided fine needle aspiration cytology (FNAC) in the diagnosis of spinal tuberculosis: a study of 29 cases. Cytopathology. 1999;10:390-401.
57. Gouliamos AD, Kehasgias DT, Lahanis S, Athanassopoulou AA, Moulopoulou ES, Kalovidouris AA, et al. MR imaging of tuberculous vertebral osteomyelitis: Pictoral review Eur. Radiol. 2001;11:575-9.
58. Hong SH, Choi JY, Lee JW, Kim NR, Choi JA, Kang HS. MR imaging assessment of the spine: infection or an imitation? Radiographics. 2009;29:599-612.
59. Danchaivijitr N, Temram S, Thepmongkhol K, Chiewvit P. Diagnostic accuracy of MR imaging in tuberculous spondylitis. J Med Assoc Thai. 2007;90:1581-9.
60. Dunn R, Zondagh I, Candy S. Spinal tuberculosis: magnetic resonance imaging and neurological impairment. Spine (Phila Pa 1976). 2011;36(6):469-73.
61. Kumar R. Spinal tuberculosis: with reference to the children of northern India. Childs Nerv Syst. 2005;21(1):19-26.
62. Trivedi R, Saksena S, Gupta RK. Magnetic resonance imaging in central nervous system tuberculosis. Indian J Radiol Imaging. 2009;19(4):256-65.
63. Boxer DI, Pratt C, Hine AL, McNicol M. Radiological features during and following treatment of spinal tuberculosis. Br J Radiol. 1992;65:476-9.
64. A controlled trial of six-month and nine-month regimens of chemotherapy in patients undergoing radical surgery for tuberculosis of the spine in Hong Kong. Tenth report of the Medical Research Council Working Party on Tuberculosis of the Spine. Tubercle. 1986;67:243-59.
65. Kim SJ, Kim IJ, Suh KT, Kim YK, Lee JS. Prediction of residual disease of spine infection using F-18 FDG PET/CT. Spine. 2009;22(34):2424-30.
66. Cormican L, Hammal R, Messenger J, Milburn HJ. Current difficulties in the diagnosis and management of spinal tuberculosis. Postgrad Med J. 2006;82(963):46-51.
67. Le Page L, Feydy A, Rillardon L, Dufour V, Le Hénanff A, Tubach F, et al. Spinal tuberculosis: a longitudinal study with clinical, laboratory, and imaging outcomes. Semin Arthritis Rheum. 2006;36(2):124-9.
68. Mittal S, Jain AK, Chakraborti KL, Aggarwal AN, Upreti L, Bhayana H. Evaluation of healed status in tuberculosis of spine by fluorodeoxyglucose-positron emission tomography/computed tomography and contrast magnetic resonance imaging. Indian J Orthop. 2019;53(1):160-8.

CHAPTER

158

Nontubercular Infections of the Spine

Sameer Vyas, Manavjit Singh Sandhu, Ujjwal Gorsi

INTRODUCTION

Spinal infections result from several infectious pathologic agents, and have varied and nonspecific clinical presentations.[1-3] Although the spinal infections are rare, there is growing incidence of these due to many factors which make persons more vulnerable to the spinal infections, including immunodeficiency due to human immunodeficiency virus (HIV) infection, chronically debilitated conditions, old age, the extensive use of broad-spectrum antibiotics or corticosteroids and immunosuppressive drugs, parenteral alimentation, and intravenous (IV) drug abuse.[3] The recent developments of medical technologies help in the early detection and appropriate management of spinal infections. Though, these advancements have also increased the occurrence of spinal infections as there are more patients with iatrogenic immunosuppression, increased life expectancy of patients with chronic medical illnesses, and potential infectious complications from the complex spinal procedures. In this chapter, the pathogenesis of spinal infections including the vascular anatomy of the vertebrae, various routes of spread, and anatomic site involved are discussed briefly for better understanding patterns of the spinal infection.

PATHOGENESIS OF SPINAL INFECTIONS

Vascular Anatomy of Vertebrae

The pathogenesis of spinal infections can be explained on the basis of the vascular anatomy of the vertebrae and intervertebral discs.[4] Vertebrae are supplied by the paired segmental arteries which arise from the vertebral arteries, or the aorta, or the iliac arteries depending on the location of the vertebrae. These segmental arteries course along the vertebral body posteriorly, and give rise to multiple small extraosseous anastomotic branches. Each segmental artery gives rise to paired metaphyseal arteries and a single nutrient artery within a vertebral body. These branches are end arteries at the superior and inferior endplates of each vertebral body. The metaphyseal arteries also supply an intermetaphyseal anastomotic arterial network which extends to multiple vertebral body levels. There is significant change in the vasculature of the vertebral bodies and intervertebral discs with age. In children, this arterial network extends to the intervertebral disc and provides vascular supply whereas in adults, these channels involutes and the end arteries end at the superior and inferior endplates of the vertebral bodies. Due to these differences in vascular anatomy in children and adults, intervertebral discs are usually the first site of infection in children followed by involvement of metaphysis, and in adults, the endplates are involved initially followed by disc involvement. Due to multiple extraosseous and intermetaphyseal vascular channels, the spinal infections can extend to multiple vertebrae. The spinal infection can also spread by venous route as there are valveless veins which exit the vertebrae at the dorsal nutrient foramen and communicate with an extradural venous plexus and then drain into the paravertebral venous plexus of Batson. This venous route is responsible for the retrograde spread of infection from abdominal and pelvic organs.

Routes of Spread of the Spinal Infections

The spinal infections can occur principally by three routes of spread: (1) hematogenous route—the arterial route from distant septic foci is more common, though the infections can also spread by venous hematogenous route; (2) contiguous spread from surrounding infected organs such as the pharynx, thoracic or abdominal wall or pleural space of the lung; and (3) direct inoculation (iatrogenically during surgery or interventional procedures).[1,3] The most validated theory for the spinal infection is that it occurs from arterial hematogenous spread from infected microemboli which gets lodged in one of the metaphyseal arteries, causing infarction and resulting in infection. Spondylitis is most common at the endplates because of the more arteries in this region. Anterior subchondral vertebral region is the usual site of infection within the vertebra corresponding to the area rich in arterial supply.[3] The early infectious lesion occurs in the anterosuperior subchondral region of the vertebral body and subsequently extends through the endplate **(Fig. 1)**. Further dissemination may occur via subligamentous spread of infection with resulting anterior vertebral body scalloping

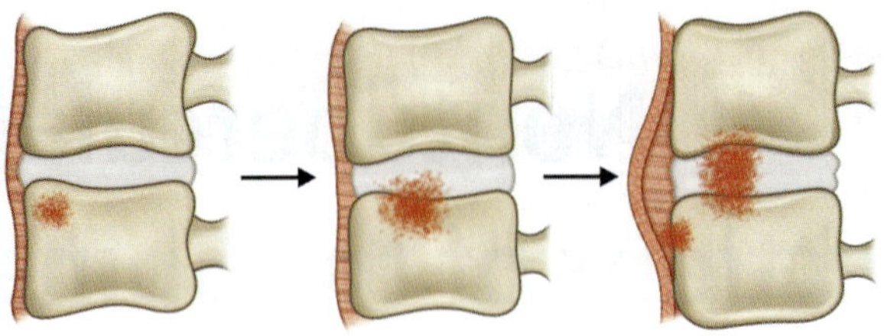

FIG. 1: Pathophysiology of vertebral osteomyelitis: the focus of infection usually begins in the anterosuperior subchondral region and subsequently extends to involve the adjacent disc and vertebral body. Anterior subligamentous spread may also occur.

or rupture of anterior longitudinal ligament. In children, the intervertebral discs receive nutrition by blood vessels that pass through the cartilaginous endplates of adjacent vertebral bodies. Hence, any infection involving the vertebral endplates easily extends to the adjacent disc space, whereas this is not so in the mature adult spine, where the nutrition of the nucleus pulposus occurs primarily by the process of diffusion. Iatrogenic spinal infections are responsible to 2.5% of all the spinal infections. The infection risk of open surgery is reported to be approximately 3–13%.[3] The spinal infections have also been described with radiological procedures such as myelography, discography, chemonucleolysis, vertebroplasty, and kyphoplasty.

Anatomic Sites of the Spinal Infections

Various anatomic sites involved include discs (discitis), vertebrae (spondylitis), discs and vertebral body (spondylodiscitis), facet joints, and epidural and paraspinal spaces (abscesses). Vertebral bodies and intervertebral discs are commonly involved with extension of the infection to epidural space, posterior elements, and paraspinal (paravertebral or psoas muscle and prevertebral space) soft tissues. Occurrence of the spinal infections in various sites is variable. The spondylodiscitis accounts for majority of all spine infections (95%), with nearly one-third of these cases are complicated by secondary epidural and paraspinal abscesses. Primary septic facet joints infections, isolated discitis, spondylitis, and primary epidural abscesses are less common.

IMAGING MODALITIES OF SPINAL INFECTIONS

The various imaging modalities available for evaluation of patients with suspected spinal infection are plain radiography, computed tomography (CT), and magnetic resonance imaging (MRI).[5-8] In these days, the use of myelography is obsolete and CT myelography is not the preferred imaging modality in patients with suspected spinal infection, though it may be very rarely used where MRI is unavailable or contraindicated. Nuclear medicine imaging studies are also useful in spinal infection.[9,10] A wise selection of the modalities is essential for timely patient management, as untreated spinal infections can lead to crippling and even life-threatening situations. Comparison of various imaging modalities in infections is illustrated in **Table 1**.

TABLE 1: Comparison of imaging modalities in spinal infections.

Imaging modality	Advantages	Limitations
Plain radiograph	Readily available and inexpensive	30–50% loss of bone density before becomes abnormal, poor sensitivity
CT	Detects bony changes and surrounding extent	Lacks sensitivity of MRI
MRI	Evaluation of the bone marrow and neural structures	Difficult to distinguish trauma or neoplasm from infection and new from old disease
Nuclear medicine imaging	Scans whole skeleton, sensitive earlier in disease than radiograph and CT	Expensive, long acquisition time, hard to distinguish overlying soft tissue infections

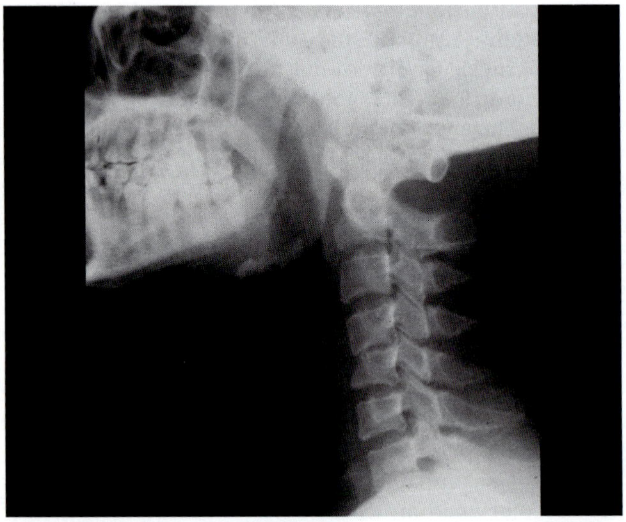

FIG. 2: Bacterial osteomyelitis involving the cervical vertebrae: plain X-ray cervical spine lateral view showing anterior erosion of C5 vertebra, prevertebral soft tissue mass and early loss of disc space height between C4 and 5.

Plain Radiography

Plain radiographs are often done first in patients with suspected spinal pathology. Unfortunately, the changes on plain radiographs appear quite late (2–8 weeks) after the onset of infection. The plain radiographic features of spinal infection **(Figs. 2 to 4)** may include demineralization, loss of definition of endplate margins, narrowing of intervertebral disc space, associated soft tissue swelling (paraspinal or epidural soft tissue masses), and the finally the destruction of the vertebral endplate and the vertebral body (spinal deformity, frank vertebral destruction).[3] Paraspinal extension of the infective process may be appreciated as widened retropharyngeal

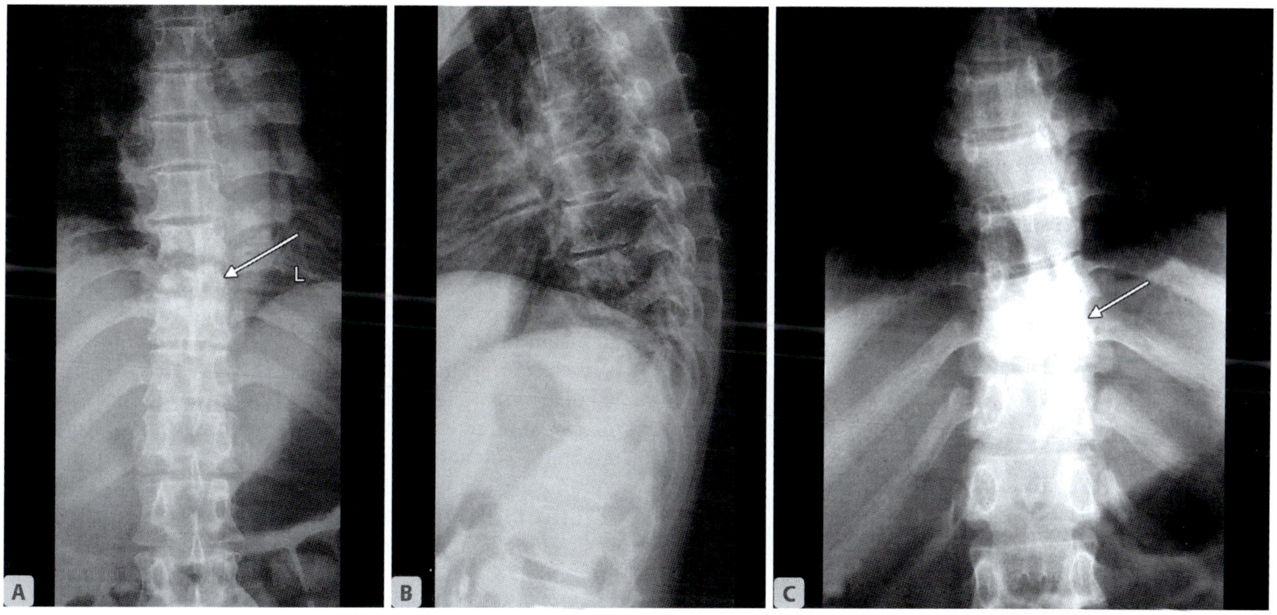

FIGS. 3A TO C: X-ray dorsal spine anteroposterior (A) and lateral view (B) showing contiguous endplate destruction at D8-9 intervertebral disc space and decrease in height of D9 vertebral body (arrow) features suggestive of pyogenic spondylodiscitis. The follow-up X-ray the dorsal spine anteroposterior view (C) demonstrating healing as evidenced by ankylosis of two adjacent vertebrae (arrow).

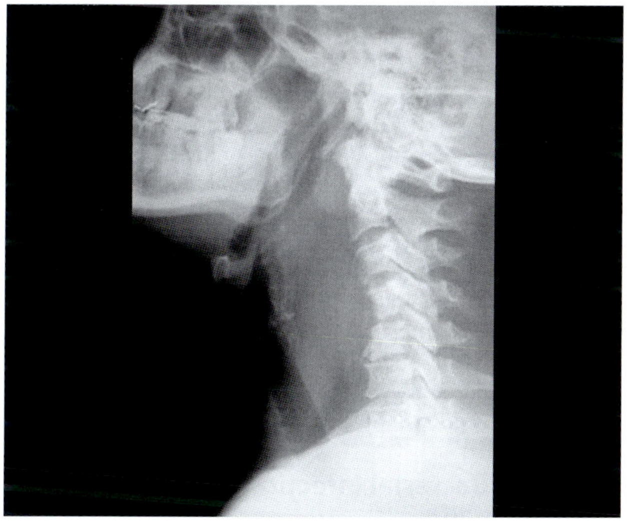

FIG. 4: Case of infective spondylodiscitis in middle-aged female: X-ray cervical spine lateral view showing decreased disc space at C4-C5 level with destruction of anterior vertebral body of C4 vertebra and large prevertebral abscess.

or retrotracheal space in the cervical region, displacement of paraspinal lines in the dorsal region and evidence of unilateral or bilateral paravertebral psoas abscesses in the lumbar region. It is possible to suggest a positive diagnosis if changes are present on plain radiographs, however, there is a significant overlap of findings on radiographs between various infections. Atypical radiographic features at times make it difficult to differentiate infective spinal conditions from other noninfective causes such as spondylodiscitis degenerative changes and neoplastic diseases.

Healed or healing processes may be seen on plain radiographs as areas of sclerosis, reactive new bone formation, spur formation, bony bridging or vertebral fusion. Limitation of plain radiographs is most evident when it comes to differentiate between chronic vertebral osteomyelitis, discogenic degenerative endplate changes, and the presence of superimposed infection in the setting of chronic degenerative disc disease.

Computed Tomography

Computed tomography entails a much better evaluation of the extent of bone destruction **(Figs. 5A and B)**. Involvement of vertebral body and the posterior elements is easily identified by cross-sectional imaging. In addition, CT also demonstrates destruction of disc space and presence of disc space gas. Identification of pre- or paravertebral soft tissue mass and extent of spread into the epidural space with subsequent thecal sac deformity can be well-appreciated on CT. Chronic stages of infection may reveal extensive osseous destruction, sequestrum, and marked heterotropic bone formation. Contrast-enhanced CT (CECT) allows better evaluation of the paravertebral abscesses with psoas involvement. CECT show peripheral enhancement of an epidural abscess causing compression and displacement of the dural sac. The use of multislice CT scans with reformatted images in the various planes depicts better delineation of the lesion extent. In addition to the diagnostic capabilities, CT and fluoroscopy can be used to guide various diagnostic [fine needle aspiration cytology (FNAC) or biopsy in patients of suspected spinal infections] and therapeutic procedures (percutaneous aspiration or catheter drainage of large paraspinal/psoas abscesses).

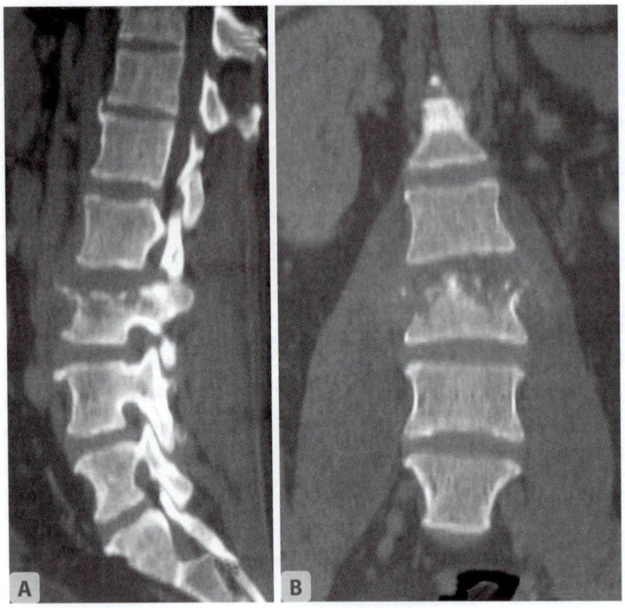

FIGS. 5A AND B: Noncontrast computed tomography (NCCT) lumbar spine sagittal (A) and coronal (B) reformat images showing better depiction of bony changes. There is superior endplate destruction of the L3 vertebra with involvement of the L2-3 intervertebral disc.

Magnetic Resonance Imaging

Magnetic resonance imaging is the imaging modality of choice for evaluating and characterizing the infective lesions of the spine because changes on MRI precede any other radiographic changes, detects marrow inflammation and has superior spatial as well as contrast resolution in imaging the spinal cord and nerve roots.[5-7] MRI has high sensitivity in early stages and with its known multiplanar capabilities and better soft tissue contrast, MRI provides a much better definition of the paravertebral and epidural extension of the disease. Many MRI features have been described for the spinal infection including decreased disc height, altered T1- or T2-signal intensity, enhancement of the disc, effacement of the nuclear cleft, and vertebral endplates erosion on T1-weighted (T1W) MR images.

As in CT, contrast-enhanced MRI allows better definition of the extent of spinal inflammatory lesions. In addition contrast-enhanced images allow better delineation of the paravertebral and intraspinal extension of disease. MRI is also a valuable tool in evaluation of postoperative spinal infections. MRI has a high sensitivity (96%) and a high accuracy (94%) for diagnosing infections.

Though MRI is imaging modality of choice for evaluating the spinal infections, vertebral osteomyelitis may be overlooked in the early course of disease, when there is no exact localization of the disease and when there is sclerosis in or around the lesion.

Nuclear Medicine Imaging Studies

Nuclear medicine imaging studies are important adjunct diagnostic tool to MRI for evaluating the spinal infections. These include radionuclide imaging tests used for detecting inflammatory changes of the spine with technetium-99m (^{99m}Tc) diphosphonate complexes, gallium-67 (^{67}Ga) and indium-111 (^{111}In)-labeled white blood cells (WBC), and ^{18}F-fluorodeoxyglucose (^{18}F-FDG) positron emission tomography (PET) with or without CT.[9,10] The advantages of the radionuclide imaging tests include high sensitivity for early diagnosis of spinal lesions, wide availability, and relatively cheaper. However, main limitation is low specificity as they show increased uptake in cases where there is underlying osseous abnormalities such as trauma, other noninfective inflammatory conditions, and tumors. In addition, the acquisition time for the radionuclide imaging is usually long (hours to days). Gallium-67 scans are mainly used for localization of areas of inflammation, especially for spinal infections. WBC-labeled imaging is not useful for the spinal infections, though it is very useful for diagnosing complicated osteomyelitis.

FDG-PET with or without CT is very useful for imaging of the spinal infections and has evolved as radionuclide modality of choice. Its sensitivity is more than 95% and specificity ranges from 75 to 99% for acute and subacute bone and soft tissue infection. It has a high negative predictive value, and is helpful in differentiating degenerative from infectious vertebral pathologies.

TYPES OF INFECTIONS

Vertebral bodies and intervertebral discs are most frequently involved in the spinal infections. The epidural space, posterior elements, and paraspinal soft tissues are usually involved secondarily due to infection of the vertebrae or discs and, rarely primarily hematogenous route or direct inoculation. In Asia and Africa, majority of the spinal infections are caused by tuberculosis and nontubercular infections are relatively uncommon. These nontubercular infections of the spine can be divided broadly into following subtypes:

- Bacterial [pyogenic and nonpyogenic (e.g., brucellosis, actinomycosis, nocardiosis)].
- Fungal, e.g., coccidioidomycosis, cryptococcosis, blastomycosis, aspergillosis, candidiasis.
- Parasitic, e.g., hydatid disease.

Pyogenic Bacterial Infections

Suppurative infections of the spine comprise only 2–5% of all osteomyelitis.[11,12] A higher incidence is seen in the debilitated, diabetics, and in elderly. *Staphylococcus aureus* is responsible for more than half the cases of infection. Other organisms responsible for infection include *Streptococcus, Pneumococcus*, gram-negative organisms such as *E. coli, Pseudomonas, Salmonella* (in sickle cell disease), and *Klebsiella.*[12] Spine is a common site for infection in IV drug abusers (mainly by *Pseudomonas*) along with sacroiliac and sternoclavicular joints involvement.

Hematogenous spread is common. Infecting organism reach the spine either by arterial antegrade route through the capillary network of the vertebral bodies or by retrograde venous route through the paravertebral Batson venous plexus. There is usually a history of recent primary infection of the skin, urinary tract or the upper respiratory tract, recent surgery or instrumentation. Patients typically present with severe back pain which is constant and aggravated by movement. Other symptoms include fever, malaise, and local tenderness. Development of neurological symptoms usually indicates the spread of infection to the epidural space. Lower lumbar spine involvement may lead to hip pain and contractures. Uncommonly, even radicular pattern of pain may be seen. Examination reveals local tenderness and restriction of movement. Erythrocyte sedimentation rate (ESR) is invariably raised. Diagnosis of spinal infection can be established with blood cultures (positive in less than 25% of cases), image-guided (fluoroscopic or CT guidance) percutaneous FNAC or biopsy sampling of the infected vertebrae or disc (in 68–86% of cases). However, an open surgical biopsy procedure may be performed in cases where percutaneous sampling cannot be performed or fails, or nondiagnostic. Spinal infections are most common in lumbar region (48%), followed by the thoracic spine (35%) and are less common in the cervical spine (6.5%) and sacrum. Infection involves the vertebral body rather than the appendages.

Radiological findings on plain radiographs usually lag behind the symptoms by 2–8 weeks.[11,12] Infection usually starts anteriorly in the subchondral area of the vertebral body, thus, the earliest finding is rarefaction of the endplates. Later frank erosions, scalloping, and destruction of vertebral endplates are noted. Following this, there is a loss of disc space height as the infection spreads to involve the adjacent vertebrae. In most patients, only two vertebrae are involved. Rarely, the infection is confined to one vertebral body. Vertebral destruction occurs and collapse may result with accompanying soft tissue swelling in pre- and paravertebral location. Reparative process can begin as early as 4–6 weeks after the onset of radiologic change and is heralded by increasing sclerosis, reactive new bone going on to spur formation, bony bridging or ankylosis of the adjacent vertebrae. Rarely, ivory vertebrae and soft tissue calcification may be found. Radionuclide scanning may be used to localize the exact site of infection and to search for multifocal lesions.

Computed tomography plays a minor role in cases with bony or soft tissue components. CT findings of vertebral osteomyelitis include: (1) detection of erosion or bone destruction and fragmentation; and (2) presence of adjacent soft tissue swelling with obliteration of fat planes around the vertebral body. CT diagnosis may be problematic if soft tissue lesions are seen in the absence of fragmentation or if fragmentation is seen without associated soft tissue swelling as in the case of previously treated or inactive discitis or hypertrophic degenerative disease. Diagnosis of vertebral osteomyelitis can also be difficult if pathognomonic features of other specific disease entities are present like acute vertebral fractures, metastatic or degenerative disease. Intradiscal or vertebral gas is an extremely uncommon finding in spinal infection and may be detected in clostridial or streptococcal infections. At about 10–12 weeks, an osteoblastic response may occur with sclerotic new bone formation. This is more a feature of pyogenic than tubercular osteomyelitis. Vertebral body ankylosis or fusion may be seen with the process of healing. However, if the therapy is inadequate, collapse with spinal deformity resulting in instability of the vertebral column may occur.

Magnetic resonance imaging is the imaging modality of choice for evaluation of patients with spinal infections. The findings on MR are characteristic and occur early in the disease. A constellation of findings of MR **(Figs. 6 and 7)** indicates pyogenic infection and helps to differentiate it from some of the other disease processes such as TB.[13] These include the following:

- The vertebra usually show homogeneous areas of altered signal intensity (low-signal intensity on T1W images and high-signal intensity on T2W images), but usually at one of the vertebral body metaphyses. These signal alterations mainly represent edema and often precede the destructive changes.
- The intervertebral discs usually show hyperintensity on T2W imaging, with abnormal configuration (absence of the internuclear cleft). The height of the intervertebral disc may be reduced.
- Loss of a margin between disc and vertebral bodies on T2W images.
- Diffuse and homogeneous enhancement is seen in the affected marrow and discs.
- Variable extension of the process into the paraspinal region. The presence of epidural extension and associated meningeal inflammation can be better demonstrated with contrast.
- Osseous and extra-axial abscesses showing restricted diffusion on diffusion-weighted imaging (DWI).

Magnetic resonance imaging may able to differentiate tuberculous spondylitis from pyogenic spondylitis. It is also possible to differentiate between pyogenic infection and other involving the spine, based on clinical and imaging features as described in **Table 2**.[13,14] In tuberculous spondylitis, the paraspinal lesions are more well-defined, abscess wall is thin and smooth, subligamentous spread with multiple vertebral or entire body involvement is seen in contrast to pyogenic spondylitis.

Diffusion-weighted MRI is very useful for the diagnosis of pyogenic spinal infections. It is also helpful for delineating the extent of lesion, treatment planning, and in differentiating the pyogenic spinal infection from nonpyogenic granulomatous infections or malignancy. Pyogenic infection usually shows diffusion restriction due to the pus and the high cellularity. It is important to recognize the MRI artefacts in the spine imaging, like susceptibility artefacts, incomplete fat suppression and volume-averaging artefacts; as these limits the diffusion imaging of the spine.

Pyogenic Disc Space Infections

In adults, since the disc is avascular, hematogenous infection is rare. Most infections occur by contiguous spread from vertebral osteomyelitis or by direct inoculation of bacteria into the disc at the time of surgery or percutaneous procedures such as discography, percutaneous discectomy, and chemonucleosis.[12] *Staphylococcus aureus* is the most common organism implicated and presentation is usually with back pain. ESR is elevated, but this is not a very useful marker especially in postoperative cases where ESR remains elevated even up to 6 months.

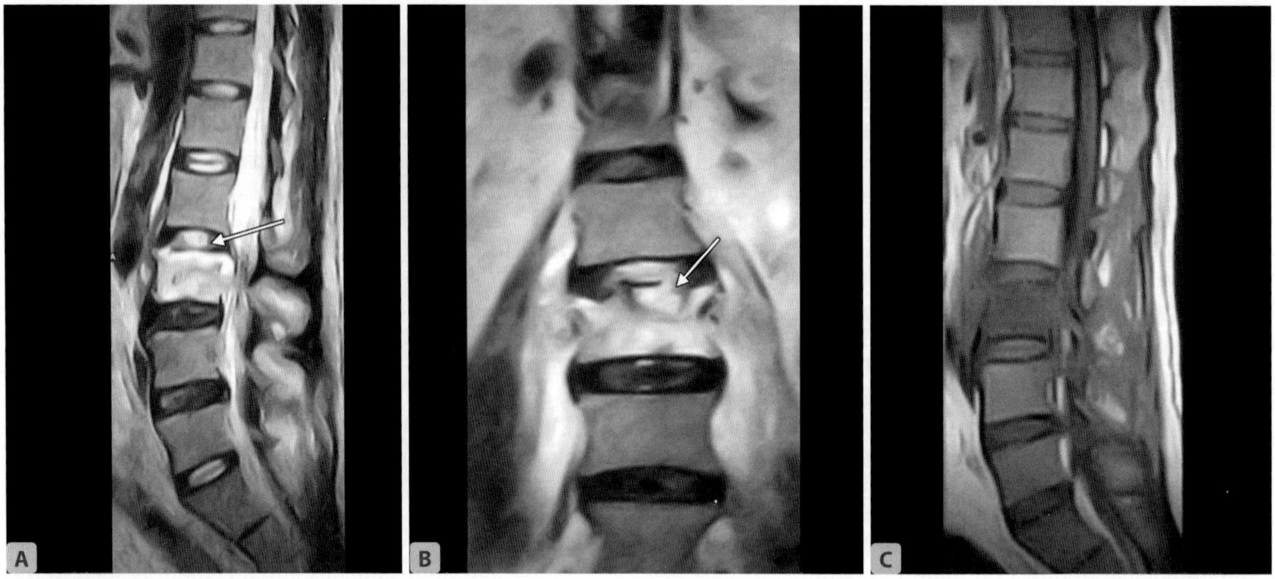

FIGS. 6A TO C: MRI lumbar spine sagittal (A), coronal (B) T2W and T1W (C) images show abnormal signal intensity (arrow) of L3 vertebra, contiguous L2-L3 intervertebral disc and surrounding soft tissue in a case of pyogenic spondylodiscitis. In addition, there is loss of intra-nuclear cleft.

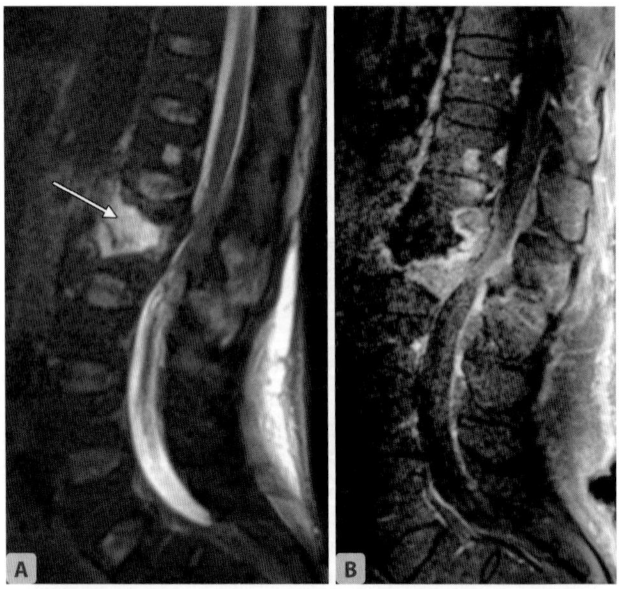

FIGS. 7A AND B: MRI lumbar spine sagittal T2W (A) and T1 fat saturated postcontrast (B) images show destruction of L1-L2 intervertebral disc (arrow) and contiguous vertebral bodies with T2 hyperintense soft tissue that is showing peripheral contrast enhancement and having intraspinal epidural extension in a case of pyogenic spondylodiscitis.

Radiographic features include decreased disc space height and reactive sclerosis of adjacent endplates. Isotope scanning may show increased uptake but it may also be due to recent surgery or percutaneous manipulation. MRI has become the modality of choice for evaluating disc space infection. Septic discitis demonstrates disc space narrowing on MRI. The vertebral endplates are indistinct and show low-signal intensity on T1W images and high-signal intensity on T2W images. The vertebral endplates may be of increased signal intensity but the major finding in the disc space is an abnormal high signal. Paraspinal soft tissue thickening and edematous changes in the paraspinal musculature are also seen. In fact the earliest MR finding in pyogenic septic discitis is obliteration of fat planes between the paraspinal musculature and the outer margin of the disc. Diagnosis is usually confirmed by percutaneous disc aspirates which can be cultured for organisms.

Spinal Infections in Children

Spinal infections in children account for approximately 2–4% of all cases of osteomyelitis.[15,16] The clinical features are nonspecific and include fever, malaise, weight loss, and back pain. These features may be intermittent or constant. Sometimes hip contracture may be seen secondary to psoas muscle irritation. In laboratory findings, ESR is raised, however, leukocyte count may be normal and the blood cultures are positive in less number of cases.

The routes of spread of the spinal infections in children are same as in adults.[15] The most common route of spread is by a hematogenous route, usually by an arterial route or rarely by venous system. In the arterial hematogenous route, there is setting of the initial infection in the subchondral region of the vertebral body, where extensive arterial network leads to the involvement of the disc. The spinal infections in children may be seen with urinary tract and other pelvic infections via the venous hematogenous route, as the direction and extent of blood flow through the valveless Batson's paravertebral venous plexus are affected by changes in intra-abdominal pressure. The spinal infection may also occur due to contiguous spread from a neighboring contaminated source or from direct implantation during punctures of the spinal canal or in postoperative period following laminectomy or other instrumentation such as scoliosis repair.

In contrary to the belief that the spine infections in children begin in the discs as the discs are hypervascular;

TABLE 2: Differentiating features of infectious spondylodiscitis.

Features	Tubercular	Pyogenic	Brucella
Associated with pulmonary site	Yes	No	–
Site of predilection	Dorsolumbar	Lower lumbar	Lower lumbar
Onset of symptoms	Insidious	Acute	Acute
Progression	Slow	Rapid	Rapid
Multifocal involvement	Yes	No	Infrequent
Vertebral body height	Destroyed	Destroyed	Preserved
Posterior elements	May be involved	Spared	Spared
Subligamentous spread	Common	May be seen	No
Disc destruction	Late	Early	Early
Intradiscal gas	Infrequent	May be seen	Frequently
Paraspinal and epidural extension	Common	Common	Uncommon
Paraspinal mass	Large	Small	Small
Enhancement of paraspinal mass	Peripheral	Patchy	Patchy
Calcification in paraspinal mass	Yes	No	No
Spinal deformity	Common	Uncommon	No
Bone sclerosis	May be seen	Yes	Yes

many studies have shown that in children also the spine infection generally starts in the vertebral body adjacent to the endplate with formation of microabscesses.[16] Due to presence of extensive perforating vascular network extending into the endplate and the disc, the infection spread to the disc. Then the infection tends to involve the endplates of the adjoining vertebral bodies. Most common bacteriological agents of the discitis are *Staphylococcus* and *Diplococcus pneumoniae*. With the imaging advancements and early diagnosis, discitis is more than spondylitis. Discitis is more commonly seen in the age group of 1–5 years. Most commonly lumbar region is involved, predominantly the L3-4 and L4-5 intervertebral discs. MRI is the modality of choice for early diagnosis and characterizing the discitis or spondylitis, though there is difficulty in localizing the infection to the osseous and articular structures of the vertebrae. Characteristic radiographic finding is disc space narrowing with destruction of the adjoining surfaces (endplates) of vertebral bodies. It is more sensitive than radiography or CT or nuclear medicine imaging studies. MRI helps in better delineation of the soft tissue extension of the spinal infection in the form of epidural abscess or paravertebral abscess **(Figs. 8A to C)**.

Bacterial Spinal Infections in AIDS

The most common bacterial spinal infection in patients with HIV is *S. aureus*, as in immunocompetent patients. The imaging features are also same as in immunocompetent individuals and show involvement of vertebral body, disc, and epidural space in isolation or combination of these. Features which are suggestive of pyogenic spondylodiscitis are the presence of prevertebral soft tissue involvement, absence of posterior elements involvement, diffuse bone destruction, and absence of marginal sclerosis whereas nonpyogenic infection shows presence of focal lytic bone lesions with marginal sclerosis and paraspinal soft tissue lesions.

Nonpyogenic Bacterial Infections[17,18]

Brucellosis

Brucellosis (undulant fever or Malta fever) is primarily a zoonotic disease, where affected animals (e.g., camels, sheep, goats) are the primary host and humans are the secondary host.[17] It is a granulomatous nontubercular infection which is caused by small, nonmotile gram-negative facultative intracellular *Coccobacilli* of the genus *Brucella*, most common being *Brucella melitensis*. The organisms are usually transmitted by the consumption of uncooked meat or unpasteurized dairy products. The incidence of spinal infection in brucellosis is 2–65%, with males affected more than the females likely due to occupational risks (males mainly work in the stock industry). The spinal involvement in the brucellosis is more commonly seen in the elderly males. Spine is the most common site for skeletal brucellosis. The clinical features of spinal brucellosis are often nonspecific and the onset of the symptom tends to be subacute. The patients present with focal and diffuse forms in the endemic areas and may involve vertebral bodies, intervertebral discs, facet joints, ligaments, paraspinal soft tissues, and epidural space. In the focal form, common site of the spinal infection is anterior aspect of the vertebral endplate (typically superior endplate of L4 vertebra) at the discovertebral junction. In the diffuse form, the vertebral body is involved initially and then the infection extends to involve the adjoining discs and vertebrae.

The lumbar region is more commonly involved, likely due to rich blood supply and higher incidence of endplate degenerative changes. The diagnosis is often difficult because of the significant overlapping radiologic imaging features of the spinal infections which mimics such as brucellosis like

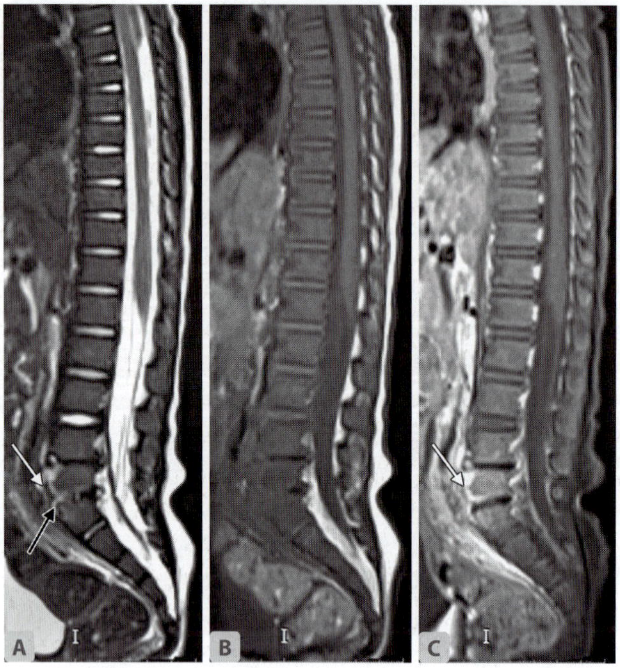

FIGS. 8A TO C: Sagittal T2 (A), T1 (B) and postcontrast fat sat T1(C) MR images of dorsolumbar spine showing altered signal intensity (T2 hyperintensity and T1 hypointensity) involving L5-S1 intervertebral disc (black arrow) and prevertebral soft tissue (white arrow) overlying the L5 vertebra which is showing mild heterogeneous enhancement (arrow) consistent with spondylodiscitis.

tubercular or pyogenic spinal infections and rarely malignancy. The main problem in the diagnosis is its differentiation from other infective processes particularly tuberculosis which is the most common cause of spinal infection in India. In brucellosis, there occur proliferative changes associated with bony repair, which are not seen in tuberculous infection; and in contrast in tuberculosis there occur deformities of the spine, which are rarely seen with brucellosis.

Laboratory tests may show mildly increased sedimentation rates, altered liver function tests, and decreased WBC and platelet counts. Standard tube agglutination test may be helpful for the diagnosis.

Nuclear medicine imaging studies such as bone scan with ^{99m}Tc or PET scan is helpful and sensitive in demonstrating areas of involvement in patients with *Brucella* infection who have musculoskeletal complaints. Plain radiographs mainly show a focal lesion at the superior endplate with maintained vertebral body architecture. Associated sclerosis is frequently seen. Disc space reduction with presence of gas in disc is a hallmark of brucellosis not seen in tuberculosis. Paravertebral soft tissue abscesses are less commonly associated and spinal deformity is rare when compared with tuberculosis.

Computed tomography confirms the presence of focal or diffuse disease in brucellosis. Findings of bone sclerosis, localized endplate destruction simulating Schmorl's nodes, loss of muscle or fat plane, and disc space gas when seen point to a *Brucella* infection, whereas large paraspinal abscesses with enhancing rim, calcification, or bone fragments suggest tubercular nature of infection. CT-guided percutaneous FNAC or biopsy is helpful for making the definitive diagnosis.

On MR, the above findings are further corroborated with evidence of an intact vertebral morphology, normal posterior elements, and a focal lesion which shows decreased signal intensity on T1W images and moderately increased signal intensity or T2W images. Disc destruction is early. There is only a moderate extension into the paraspinal and epidural space by granulation tissue and/or edema and spinal deformity is infrequent.

Actinomycosis

Actinomycosis is a slowly progressive infection caused by gram-positive filamentous bacteria of *Actinomyces* species, most commonly by *Actinomyces israelii.*[19] They are normal commensal of gastrointestinal tract, bronchial, and female genital tracts. Clinical features of the actinomycosis are very nonspecific, and are also referred as the "most misdiagnosed disease". Mandible and spine are most commonly affected. Osseous involvement results from extension of soft tissue infection. Involvement of the spine is rare and usually from the contiguous spread from adjacent sites of infection, especially the lungs and sinuses. Vertebral destruction with deformity is uncommon with *Actinomyces* infection. These infections are usually seen in debilitated persons. Radiological manifestations include lytic lesions with surrounding sclerosis involving several vertebrae and frequently sparing the discs. Posterior elements and ribs are frequently involved, with associated paravertebral abscesses which are not as large as seen in tuberculosis and do not show calcification. Presence of sinus tracts leading to the skin along with above findings suggests the diagnosis.

Nocardiosis

Nocardia are filamentous, branching, gram-positive aerobic bacteria. They are usually associated primarily with pulmonary infection in immunocompromised patients. Spinal involvement is rare with nonspecific radiological findings. There are only about a dozen reported cases of spinal nocardiosis in the literature and occurs both by direct extension of intrathoracic infections and through hematogenous spread.

There are few specific imaging features which have been described for nonpyogenic spondylodiscitis like absence of T2-hyperintensity within the intervertebral discs and the preservation of the intranuclear cleft. However, these finding may also be seen in tubercular spine infections and have been reported in cases of pyogenic spine diseases. In addition, intervertebral discs may also be spared by other nonpyogenic infections caused by *Nocardia, Actinomyces,* and *Coccidioides.* The cause of absence of T2-hyperintensity within the intervertebral disc is unclear and may be multifactorial. The imaging findings may be indicative of absence of invasion of the disc, an altered inflammatory reaction within the involved disc, or an intrinsic characteristic of either the disc before infection (e.g., degenerated disc) or of the invading organisms (e.g., paramagnetic elements in fungi).

Epidural Space Infections

Epidural space is usually involved secondarily to contiguous spread of the infections from surrounding infected spinal structures such as adjacent infected vertebrae, disc space or facet joints (spondylodiscitis or facet joint infection). Primary epidural abscesses due to hematogenous spread of bacteria are relatively less common, and account for less than 2% of all the spine infections. Typically, the epidural abscess presents with intense back pain, usually localized over the infected site of spine. The intense pain is more than the concomitant neurologic deficit. Early diagnosis of the epidural abscess is of paramount importance, as neurological sequelae are severe and may lead to cord compression and paralysis.

Contrast-enhanced MRI with DWI provides the best evaluation of patients with the epidural abscess. Main advantages of MRI include its ability to differentiate the cord from the thecal sac, involvement and extension of the infection to paraspinal soft tissues, or vertebral bone marrow. The epidural abscesses can be clearly seen as soft tissue lesion in the epidural space, usually hypointense on T1W and hyperintense on T2W images which displaces the thecal sac away from the vertebrae with delineation from the dural sac as thin T2-hypointense line. Contrast-enhanced MRI demonstrates two types of enhancement pattern, one with a peripheral enhancement a central hypointense area representing true abscess **(Figs. 9A and B)** and other with a homogeneous enhancement pattern representing the inflammatory changes without purulent contents. Fat-suppressed contract-enhanced MRI helps in better delineation of the extent of the lesion and its differentiation from surrounding structures (interspinous and paraspinal region). DWI plays an important role in the diagnosis of epidural abscesses. It helps in delineation of the extension, and differentiating it from epidural hemorrhage and other neoplastic lesion in the epidural space.

Postoperative Spondylodiscitis

Postoperative spondylodiscitis is an uncommon complication of the spine surgeries or interventional procedures.[3] The patients present with recurrent pain after initial postoperative relief, muscular spasm, and fever. Most likely the cause is intraoperative contamination, though rarely hematogenous spread may occur. The imaging findings are nonspecific initially as it is difficult to differentiate from the postoperative changes and may appear several weeks after the symptoms onset. Characteristic MRI findings of the disc space infection include enhancement of the disc space, annulus, and vertebral body. These imaging findings have to be correlated with laboratory findings like an increased ESR as similar findings may be seen in normal postoperative asymptomatic patients. Thus, main role of imaging is to exclude the diagnosis of postoperative spondylodiscitis by showing no abnormal signal changes and abnormal enhancement in the postoperative site rather than looking for characteristic changes because of the significant overlap of the imaging findings.

Facet Joint Infections

The infection of the facet joints are commonly underdiagnosed and frequently overlooked, though they have distinct clinical and imaging features. The facets joints are diarthrodial joints which consist of opposing cartilage surfaces and

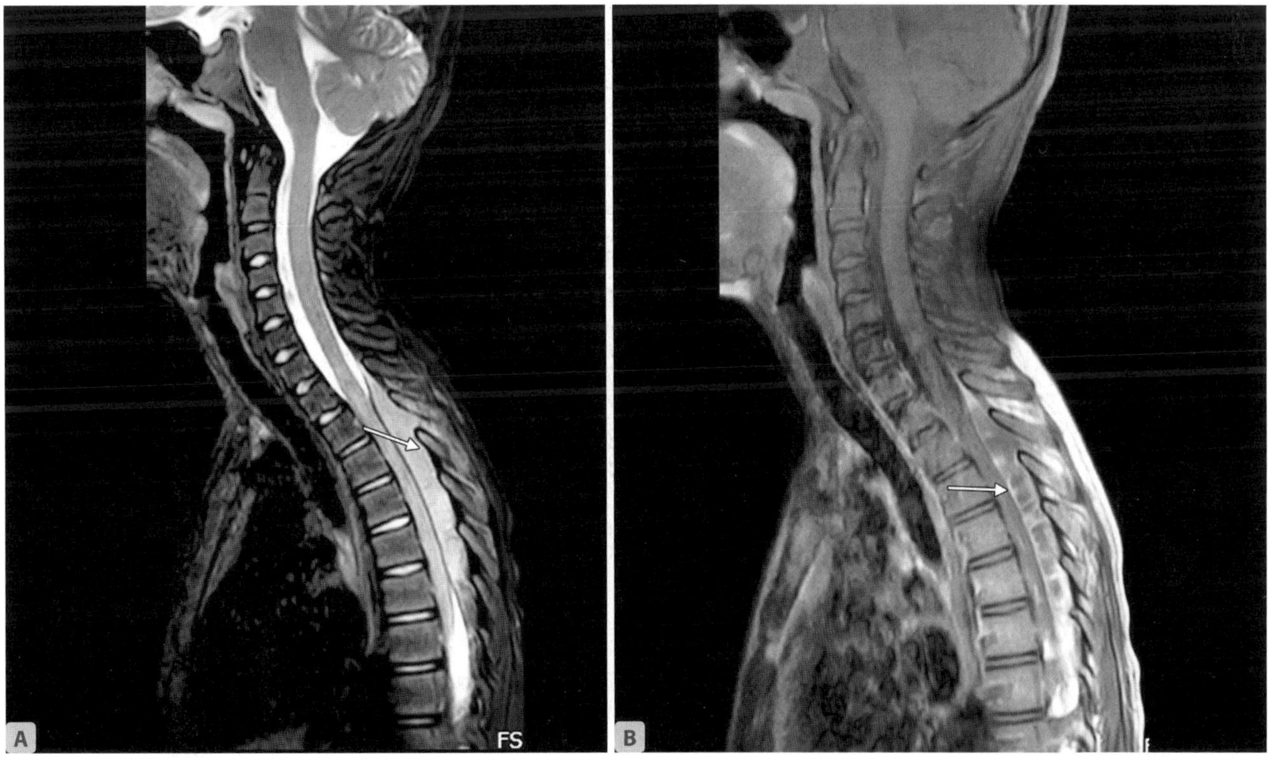

FIGS. 9A AND B: T2 (A) and contrast enhanced T1 (B) sagittal MR images of the child with large epidural abscess (arrows) in the dorsal region showing peripheral enhancement. Upper dorsal cord is compressed and shows cord edema.

interlock adjacent vertebral bodies. The joints are enclosed by a firm ligamentous capsule and contain meniscoids. They transfer load and constrain spine movements along with the intervertebral disc. Route of spread of the infection to the facet joints is commonly by hematogenous route, and rarely iatrogenically by facet injections and instrumentations. Clinical features vary and usually present with acute onset of the symptoms such as unilateral back pain with fever. Plain radiographs are nonspecific and imaging features significantly lag behind, so rarely used. Nuclear imaging studies are useful in indicating the infection. CT may show the erosive changes in affected facets, and soft tissue changes in the epidural space, paraspinal region. However, CT is mainly used for image-guided biopsies if required. MRI is very helpful as it shows changes very early on. It demonstrates the infection of the facet joints as intra-articular fluid, joint space destruction, and abnormal surrounding enhancement.

Fungal Infections[20-22]

Infections of the spine by fungus are uncommon. They are more commonly seen in patients with predisposing conditions such as diabetes, prolonged corticosteroid administration, immunosuppression after organ transplantation, prolonged systemic illness associated with malnutrition and multiple antibiotic use, HIV infection, alcohol or IV drug abuse, and parenteral nutrition. Rarely do they occur due to iatrogenic interventions.

Fungal infections of the spine include aspergillosis, coccidioidomycosis, cryptococcosis, *Candida*, and blastomycosis. Following inhalation of spores, these involve the spine by a hematogenous route. Radiologically, each fungal infection does not have any distinctive features of its own. Most of them resemble tubercular infection, but a few characteristic features have been described for some of the infections.

Aspergillosis

Aspergillus, a ubiquitous species of fungus, is usually pathogenic only in immunocompromised patients. The spinal infections from *Aspergillus* usually extend from contiguous site of infection which is mainly pulmonary, but rarely spread hematogenously. Though rare, *Aspergillus* vertebral infections have been reported in immunocompetent hosts as well.[20] Differentiation must be made from tuberculosis, which can closely mimic aspergillosis of the spine, using serologic testing. There are no characteristic radiographic features and resemble other spinal infection. Imaging may show osseous and disc space destruction, and a paraspinal soft tissue lesion.[19] MRI helps in better delineation of the extent of involvement **(Figs. 10A to C)**.

Coccidioidomycosis

Coccidioidomycosis is caused by *Coccidioides immitis*, a filamentous fungus which infects the lung primarily and disseminates throughout the body in about 0.5% of patients. Osseous involvement is seen in 10–50% of which spine is the most common site.[21] Plain radiographs usually reveal multiple erosive defects involving vertebral bodies and

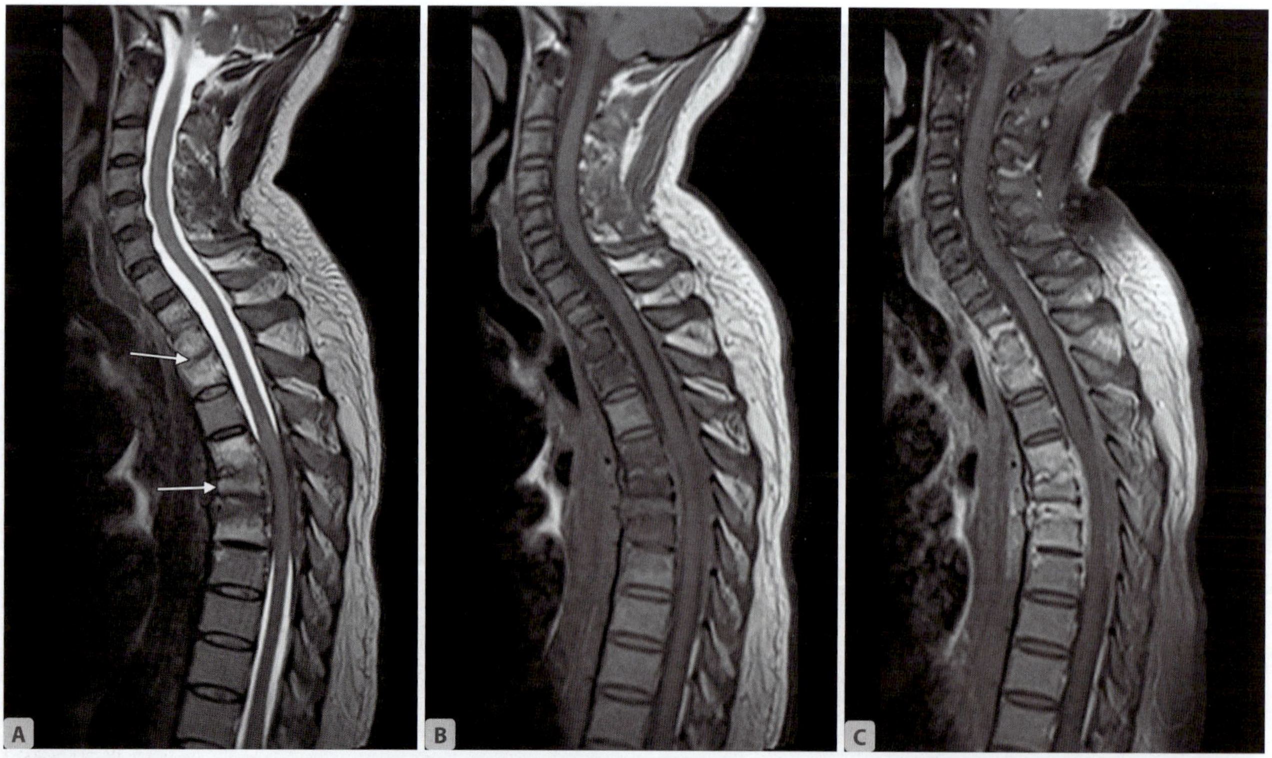

FIGS. 10A TO C: Aspergillus spondylodiscitis in young male. Sagittal T2 (A), T1 (B) and postcontrast T1 (C) weighted MR images of cervico-dorsal region showing diffuse altered marrow signal intensity and contrast enhancement of D1-3 and D5-7 vertebral bodies and intervertebral discs (arrows). There are mild epidural and prevertebral soft tissue signal changes.

appendages. Disc space is usually preserved and spinal deformity is uncommon. Paraspinal masses and adjacent rib involvement is common. Differentiation from tuberculosis can be made by the presence of skull lesions, which although common in coccidioidomycosis, are rare in tuberculosis.[21]

Lumbar spine is commonly affected. MR appearances of the lesion are that of hypo- to hyperintense signal intensity on T1W images and on T2W images, the lesions are almost always hyperintense. Following gadolinium injection, the lesions which are hypo- to isointense on T1W sequence show enhancement.[20] Ring enhancement may be seen in intraosseous abscesses. Presence of paraspinal masses, epidural spread, and subligamentous spread is similar to those seen in tuberculosis.

Cryptococcosis (Torulosis)

Cryptococcosis is caused by *Cryptococcus neoformans*, which has more predilections for the central nervous system. This fungus can be found in soil, pigeon droppings, fruit, and human intestinal tract and skin. The disease is usually acquired by the respiratory route through inhalation of aerosolized spores. This infection tends to occur in immunocompromised patients and is more common in postrenal transplant patients. Disseminated cryptococcal infection may result in osseous involvement in 5–10% of patients and spine is commonly involved. Radiologically, nonspecific well-defined osteolytic areas with sclerotic margins are seen involving the vertebral body and posterior elements **(Figs. 11A to C)**. Again, multifocal involvement and large paraspinal soft tissue abscesses may be present making the picture at times indistinguishable from tuberculosis.

Blastomycosis

This infection caused by *Blastomyces dermatitidis*, which enters the body through skin wound or the respiratory tract. The route of spread to the spine is by hematogenous seeding, or by direct spread from an overlying cutaneous lesion. The vertebra may be involved; however, the radiologic features are not specific. Involvement of the osseous structure is usually secondary, and spine is common site. Common imaging appearance is destructive vertebral lesion with a large paraspinal mass. The lower thoracic and lumbar spine is most often the site of the infection. Features suggestive of blastomycosis of the spine include involvement of the posterior elements of the vertebral body and adjoining ribs, and greater tendency to produce cutaneous fistulae.[20] The definitive diagnosis is typically made by positive cytology or histologic examination of biopsy specimens.

Candidiasis (Moniliasis)

Candidiasis is most commonly caused by *Candida albicans*. Musculoskeletal infections by *Candida* are more common in immunocompromised, especially in IV drug addicts. Osteomyelitis can occur in one or more sites. Spinal involvement is uncommon and seen as involvement of two consecutive vertebral bodies. Usually, the lumbar spine is the region affected and imaging features are nonspecific.[20] The definitive diagnosis as in other spinal fungal infection is typically made by positive cytology or histologic examination.

Parasitic Infections

Echinococcosis or Hydatid

The principal host of echinococcosis is the dog, whereas the intermediate hosts are sheep and humans. The route of transmission is ingestion of ova and then absorption by the bowel. Echinococcosis or hydatid disease of the bones is rare, accounting for approximately 0.5–4% of all patients.[20] Spinal involvement by hydatid disease is seen in about half of these patients. In the spine, sacrum and lower dorsal vertebra are commonly involved. The primary infection from the medullary cavity in the vertebral body spreads to

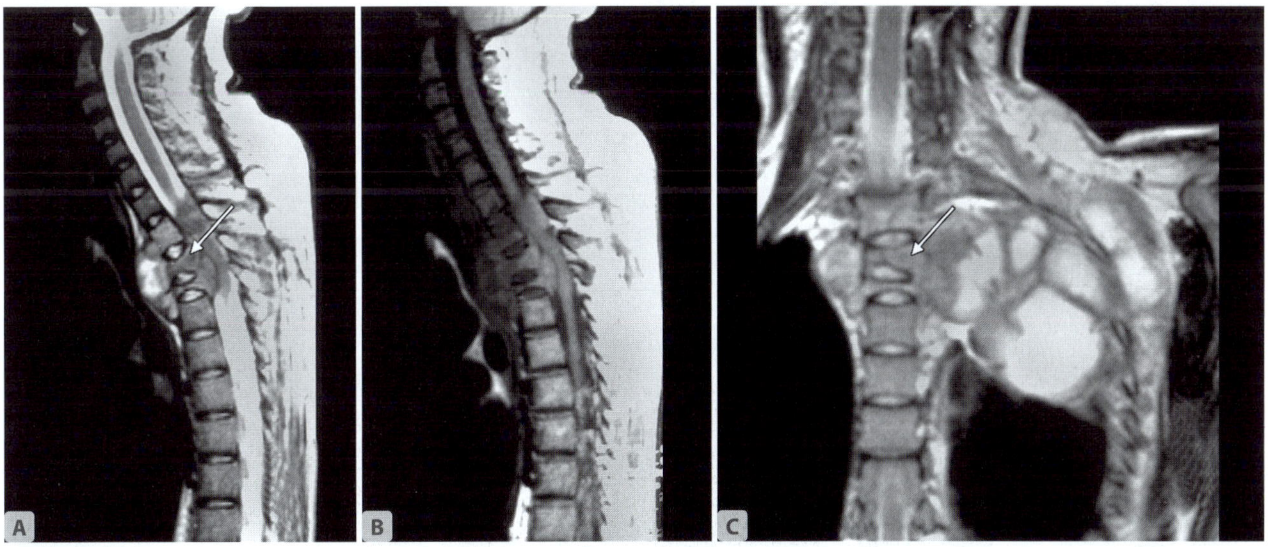

FIGS. 11A TO C: T2 (A), T1 (B) sagittal, and T2 (C) coronal MR imaging in a case of cryptococcosis of the dorsal spine showing multiple contiguous vertebral involvement of the upper dorsal spine (arrows) with vertebral destruction and prevertebral, epidural and posterior paraspinal abscesses with compression of the adjacent cord and relatively preserved disc spaces.

involve the pedicles and laminae. Hydatid disease in the bones differs from disease elsewhere in the soft tissues in that the cysts are always multilocular. Growth occurs along the line of least resistance particularly along the intertrabecular spaces with the formation of diverticulated cysts that may form by exogenous vesiculation. Enlargement of the larvae results in dilatation of the bony spaces of spongiosa and resorption of cancellous bone. Expansion is relatively slow with a smooth well-defined sclerotic margin. Erosion through the periosteum into the adjacent soft tissues proceeds without subperiosteal new bone formation. Extension into extradural space or paraspinal tissues may occur. Contiguous involvement of the rib is a feature.

Spinal hydatid has been classified into: (1) primary cyst in the cord; (2) intradural cyst; (3) extradural cyst; (4) hydatid disease of the vertebrae; and (5) paravertebral hydatid disease. Mid-dorsal and lumbosacral levels are most commonly affected. Plain film findings include a uni- or multiloculated lytic expansile bone lesion with marginal sclerosis involving the vertebral body, posterior elements, and even the adjacent ribs with paraspinal soft tissue mass. Disc space is preserved as the disease propagates beneath the periosteum and ligaments. The findings are at times nonspecific and indistinguishable from other benign cystic bone lesions or metastatic disease.

Computed tomography signs are nonspecific and often reveal bone lysis extending into the posterior elements, adjacent vertebrae, disc space and epidural space, creating a picture of spondylitis. However, costal involvement and lack of enhancement following contrast administration suggest hydatid disease. CT is superior to MR in demonstrating calcified lesions.

On MR, cysts demonstrate inhomogeneous low-signal intensity on T1W images and high signal on T2W images **(Figs. 12A to D)**. T2W images are not helpful in differentiating quiescent from active stage of the cysts. MRI may demonstrate intradural extension to better advantage than CT without the need for subarachnoid contrast.

DIFFERENTIAL DIAGNOSIS OF SPINAL INFECTION[23,24]

Imaging features of the various spinal infections are nonspecific and may mimic other spinal diseases. Imaging features such as signal intensity changes and enhancement patterns seen in various conditions may cause significant overlap with the spinal infection, so it is very important to exclude which mimic like the spinal infections. Important masquerader of the spinal infections include degenerative and inflammatory spinal pathologies such as discogenic vertebral body degeneration in the inflammatory phase (Modic type 1 degeneration), acute cartilaginous node, ankylosing spondylitis, neuropathic spine, dialysis-related spondyloarthropathy, and rarely neoplasm. Modic type 1 disc degeneration is characterized by presence of altered signal intensity in the vertebral endplates (in form of hypointensity on T1 and hyperintensity on T2) with absence of increased T2-signal intensity of the intervertebral disc and absence of soft tissue involvement whereas infectious spondylitis is characterized by endplate destruction, increased disc T2-signal intensity, or a paravertebral or epidural involvement (abscess). In addition, DWI is very useful in differentiating Modic type 1 degenerative changes from infection. Patients with Modic type 1 signal changes show well-marginated, linear region of high signal within the adjacent vertebral bodies at the interface of normal and abnormal marrow, which is referred as "claw sign".

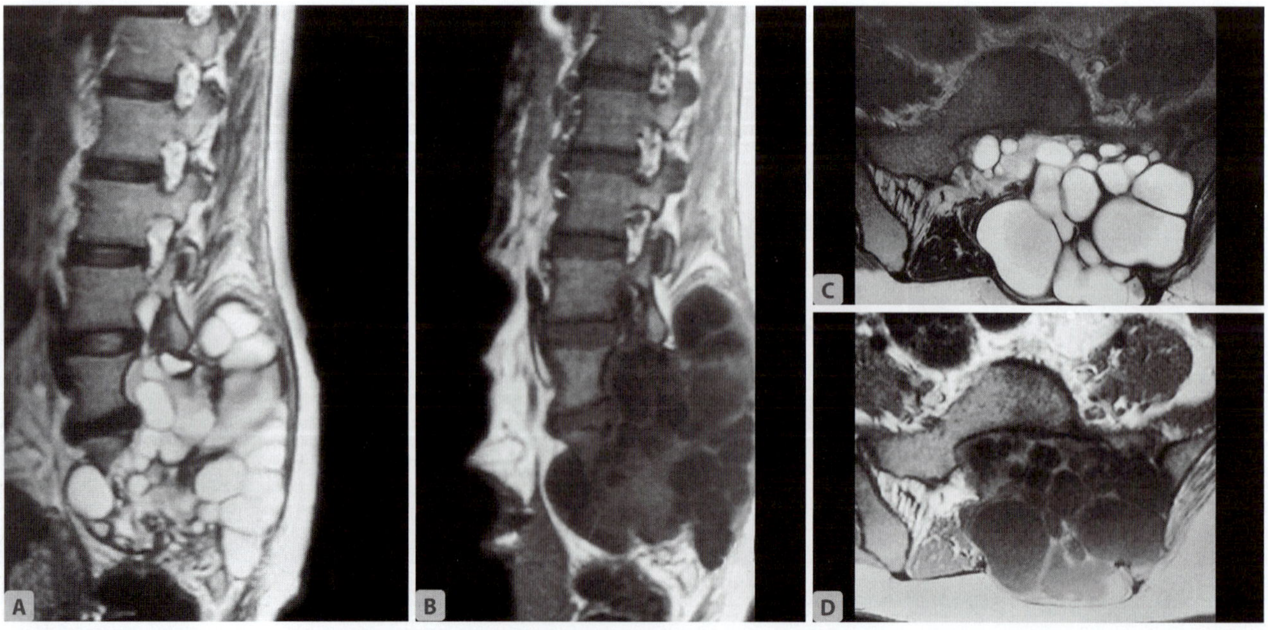

FIGS. 12A TO D: MRI lumbosacral spine parasagittal T2W (A), T1W (B), axial T2W (C), T1W (D) images show large multiloculated, cystic, expansile lesion involving posterior arch elements of L5 and sacrum demonstrating a having both osseous and extraosseous components. The cysts show peripheral T2 hypointense wall and central fluid signal in a case of spinal hydatid.

Acute cartilaginous node may be distinguished by concentric ring of high T2-signal intensity around the node, involvement of only one endplate and no signal intensity changes of the disc. Ankylosing spondylitis can be differentiated by presence of spinal ankylosis and fracture that extends into the posterior column (Andersson lesion). Neuropathic spine is characterized by vacuum phenomenon, facet involvement, lower signal intensity of disc and bone marrow on T2W images whereas in dialysis-related spondyloarthropathy vertebral marrow shows hypointense signal on both T1W and T2W images.

CONCLUSION

Imaging of the spine plays a pivotal role in the early and accurate diagnosis and management of the patient with spinal infection. Imaging helps in delineation of the extent of disease and potential infectious agents; thereby reducing the associated morbidity and mortality. MRI is the imaging modality of choice for the diagnosis and characterization of spinal infection because of the better spatial and contrast resolution. It allows direct evaluation of the bone marrow changes, and simultaneous visualization of the neural structures. However, spinal infections are often indistinguishable on imaging and there is frequent overlap of radiological findings in different types of infections. So it is essential to recognize atypical MRI findings of spinal infection; and imaging features of other noninfectious inflammatory diseases and degenerative disease that may mimic like spinal infections to avoid misdiagnosis and inappropriate treatment.

REFERENCES

1. Babic M, Simpfendorfer CS. Infections of the spine. Infect Dis Clin North Am. 2017;31(2):279-97.
2. Go JL, Rothman S, Prosper A, Silbergleit R, Lerner A. Spine infections. Neuroimaging Clin N Am. 2012;22(4):755-72.
3. DeSanto J, Ross JS. Spine infection/inflammation. Radiol Clin North Am. 2011;49(1):105-27.
4. Esendagli-Yilmaz G, Uluoglu O. Pathologic basis of pyogenic, nonpyogenic, and other spondylitis and discitis. Neuroimaging Clin N Am. 2015;25(2):159-61.
5. Diehn FE. Imaging of spine infection. Radiol Clin North Am. 2012;50(4):777-98.
6. Torres C, Zakhari N. Imaging of spine infection. Semin Roentgenol. 2017;52(1):17-26.
7. Prodi E, Grassi R, Iacobellis F, Cianfoni A. Imaging in spondylodiscitis. Magn Reson Imaging Clin N Am. 2016;24(3):581-600.
8. Moritani T, Kim J, Capizzano AA, Kirby P, Kademian J, Sato Y. Pyogenic and non-pyogenic spinal infections: emphasis on diffusion-weighted imaging for the detection of abscesses and pus collections. Br J Radiol. 2014;87(1041):20140011.
9. Palestro CJ. Radionuclide imaging of musculoskeletal infection: a review. J Nucl Med. 2016;57(9):1406-12.
10. Gemmel F, Dumarey N, Palestro CJ. Radionuclide imaging of spinal infections. Eur J Nucl Med Mol Imaging. 2006;33(10):1226-37.
11. Boody BS, Tarazona DA, Vaccaro AR. Evaluation and management of pyogenic and tubercular spine infections. Curr Rev Musculoskelet Med. 2018;11(4):643-52.
12. Tali ET, Oner AY, Koc AM. Pyogenic spinal infections. Neuroimaging Clin N Am. 2015;25(2):193-208.
13. Harada Y, Tokuda O, Matsunaga N. Magnetic resonance imaging characteristics of tuberculous spondylitis vs pyogenic spondylitis. Clin Imaging. 2008;32(4):303-9.
14. Chang MC, Wu HT, Lee CH, Liu CL, Chen TH. Tuberculous spondylitis and pyogenic spondylitis. Comparative magnetic resonance imaging features. Spine. 2006;31(7):782-8.
15. Tyagi R. Spinal infections in children: a review. J Orthop. 2016;13(4):254-8.
16. Rossi A. Pediatric spinal infection and inflammation. Neuroimaging Clin N Am. 2015;25(2):173-91.
17. Butler JS, Shelly MJ, Timlin M, Powderly WG, O'Byrne JM. Nontuberculous pyogenic spinal infections in adults. A 12 year experience from a tertiary referral center. Spine. 2003;31:2695-700.
18. Tali ET, Koc AM, Oner AY. Spinal brucellosis. Neuroimaging Clin N Am. 2015;25(2):233-45.
19. Young WB. Actinomycosis with involvement of the vertebral column: case report and review of the literature. Clin Radiol. 1960;11:175-82.
20. Chhem RK, Wang SC, Jaovisidha S, Schmit P, Friedman L, Bureau NJ, et al. Imaging of fungal, viral, and parasitic musculoskeletal and spinal diseases. Radiol Clin North Am. 2001;39(2):357-78.
21. Erly WK, Carmody RF, Seeger JF, Lund PJ. Magnetic resonance imaging of coccidioidal spondylitis. Int J of Neuroradiol. 1997;3(5):385-92.
22. Williams RL, Fukui MB, Meltzer CC, Swarnkar A, Johnson DW, Welch W. Fungal spinal osteomyelitis in the immunocompromised patient: MR findings in three cases. Am J Neuroradiol. 1999;20(3):381-5.
23. Hong SH, Choi JY, Lee JW, Kim NR, Choi JA, Kang HS. MR imaging assessment of the spine: infection or an imitation? Radiographics. 2009;29(2):599-612.
24. Ledermann HP, Schweitzer ME, Morrison WB, Carrino JA. MR imaging findings in spinal infections: rules or myths? Radiology. 2003;228(2):506-14.

CHAPTER 159

Imaging in Rheumatological Disorders

Mandeep Kang, Gita Devi, Mahesh Prakash

INTRODUCTION

Rheumatological diseases are the conditions characterized by inflammation affecting connecting or supporting structure of the body, which includes joints, tendons, ligaments, bones, and muscles. Rheumatological disorders are a heterogeneous group which includes inflammatory, autoimmune diseases, degenerative diseases, etc.[1] There is a predilection for the female gender[1] (more common during childbearing age group). Few decades ago, these conditions were grouped under the umbrella term of rheumatism. At present, more than 200 different rheumatic diseases are identified. The common conditions grouped as per etiology are:

- Noninfective inflammatory
  - Rheumatoid arthritis (RA)
  - Juvenile RA
  - Ankylosing spondylitis (AS)
  - Reiter's syndrome (RS)
  - Enteropathic spondyloarthropathy
  - Psoriatic arthropathy (PA)
- Autoimmune
  - Systemic lupus erythematosus (SLE)
  - Systemic sclerosis (scleroderma)
  - Sjögren's syndrome
  - Other connective tissue disorders
- Crystal deposition arthropathy
  - Gout
  - Calcium pyrophosphate dihydrate (CPPD) crystal deposition disease
- Degenerative
  - Degenerative joint disease
  - Diffuse idiopathic skeletal hyperostosis
  - Ossification of the posterior longitudinal ligament
  - Erosive osteoarthritis (OA)
  - Neurotrophic arthropathy
  - Synoviochondrometaplasia
  - Osteoporosis
- Others
  - Idiopathic inflammatory myopathy (IIM)
  - Tendinitis
  - Bursitis
  - Polymyalgia rheumatica (PMR)
  - Behçet's disease
  - Infective arthritis.

Noninfective inflammatory arthritides comprise a group of different, mostly systemic disorders that have one important feature in common; inflammatory granulation tissue eroding and destroying articular cartilage. The noninfective inflammatory arthritides include RA (seropositive) and the seronegative spondyloarthropathies (SSAs), namely—AS, PA, RS and enteropathic arthritis. Although radiologic manifestations of the arthropathies reflect pathologic alterations, joints can react to disease only in limited ways and therefore different pathologic conditions may exhibit similar radiologic features. Many of these are nonspecific, but certain combinations are more likely than others to occur in a particular disease; thus one may consider the "predictive value" of a radiologic feature relative to the clinical condition.[2] A systematic approach with evaluation of various radiological abnormalities helps in arriving at the correct diagnosis. Various features to be evaluated include:

- Distribution of affected joints
- Presence of soft tissue swelling
- Bone density
- Cartilage space narrowing
- Reactive bone formation
- Site and character of erosions
- Subarticular cystic lesions
- Presence of soft tissue calcification
- Joint deformities.[3]

RHEUMATOID ARTHRITIS

Rheumatoid arthritis is the most common inflammatory arthritis, which affects about 0.5–1% of the world's adult population. It is a progressive, chronic, systemic inflammatory disease affecting primarily the synovial joints, which can lead to considerable disability and morbidity. RA may develop at any age, but the peak age of onset is between the 4th and 6th decades. Women are three times more likely to be affected than men.[4] The exact etiology is not known but multiple factors appear to be involved. There is definitely a genetic predisposition with over 70% of the patients expressing HLA-DR4. A role for factors such as smoking and infectious agents has also been suggested in the etiology.[5] Although any synovial joint in the body may be affected, the classical presentation is of a symmetrical polyarthritis affecting the small joints of the hands and feet. However, it may be asymmetrical in 20–25% of cases.[2] Large joints which are commonly involved include the ankle, knee, and shoulder. The axial skeleton is later and less often affected, with the exception of the cervical spine. Characteristically, joints which communicate with one another tend to be affected together, e.g., uniform tricompartmental involvement in the knee joint and simultaneous involvement of the distal radioulnar and radiocarpal joints.[3]

Over the past couple of decades, there has been a fundamental change in the management of RA, which has resulted in significantly improved prognosis. Presently, the management involves two main strategies: first, to initiate treatment as soon as possible which basically translates into early detection and diagnosis of disease and second, to frequently gauge disease activity to monitor response to therapy. New biologic therapies have also emerged such as the antitumor necrosis factor drugs to supplement the conventional disease-modifying antirheumatic agents.[6]

The spectrum of disease manifestations of RA is protean. The diagnostic criteria proposed by the American College of Rheumatology in 1987 were commonly used for the diagnosis of this disease **(Box 1)**.[7] However, these criteria were not fulfilled early in the course of the disease, hence in recent years, the role of imaging like magnetic resonance imaging (MRI) and ultrasound has gained in importance.[8,9]

In 2010, the American College of Rheumatology along with the European League Against Rheumatism (EULAR) revised the diagnostic criteria for RA highlighting features present early in the disease. They included anti-citrullinated protein antibodies (ACPAs) which are a biomarker predicting aggressive disease. Patients with disease of <6 weeks duration are included while patients who already have a bony erosion on radiographs as a sign of structural damage are categorized as RA without applying this scoring system. Four domains are considered, namely (1) the number of joints, (2) serological markers, (3) acute phase reactants and (4) duration of disease **(Table 1)**.[10]

The positive findings in the domains are added according to points appointed and the total is the score assigned. A score of 56 is required to designate RA as the diagnosis.[10] Joint involvement is defined as joint having synovitis on imaging which on clinical examination is swollen and tender.

Pathophysiology

Rheumatoid factors (RFs) are antigammaglobulin antibodies, which are elaborated by the synovium in response to unknown antigens. These antibodies are believed to be the initiating factors, which trigger RA. Deposition of immune complexes in the synovium activates the complement system with influx of inflammatory cells. This leads to synovial proliferation, pannus formation and ultimate cartilage and subchondral bony destruction. In advanced cases, there may be fibrous ankylosis with subsequent bony ankylosis.[11,12]

Box 1: The 1987 diagnostic criteria for the diagnosis of rheumatoid arthritis of the American College of Rheumatology.

- Morning stiffness in and around joints that lasts at least 1 hour before maximal improvement
- Soft tissue swelling of at least three joints that is observed by a physician
- Swelling (arthritis) of the metacarpophalangeal, proximal interphalangeal or wrist joints
- Symmetrical swelling (arthritis)
- Subcutaneous rheumatoid nodules
- A positive test for rheumatoid factor
- Radiographic signs: erosions or periarticular osteopenia in hand or wrist joints

TABLE 1: The American College of Rheumatology (ACR)/European League Against Rheumatism (EULAR) classification criteria for rheumatoid arthritis: domains, categories and point scores.[10]

Domain	Category	Point score
A	*Joint involvement (0–5 points)*	
	1 large joint	0
	2–10 large joints	1
	1–3 small joints (large joints not counted)	2
	4–10 small joints (large joints not counted)	3
	>10 joints including at least 1 small joint	5
B	*Serology (at least one test needed for classification) (0–3 points)*	
	Negative rheumatoid factor (RF) and negative anti-citrullinated protein antibodies (ACPAs)	0
	Low-positive RF or low-positive ACPA	2
	High-positive RF or high-positive ACPA	3
C	*Acute-phase reactants (at least one test needed for classification)*	
	Normal C-reactive protein (CRP) and normal erythrocyte sedimentation rate (ESR)	0
	Abnormal CRP or abnormal ESR	1
D	*Duration of symptoms*	
	<6 weeks	0
	>6 weeks	1

Rheumatoid factors are present in the serum and synovial fluid in 70–80% of patients with a clinical diagnosis of RA. They may be found in the synovial fluid even when the serum is negative. However, they may also be present in the synovial fluid of cases with nonrheumatoid disorders; therefore, only high titers of RF in a joint effusion suggest RA. The RFs may initially be negative and later in the course of disease become positive.[4]

Imaging

The radiologic features of RA may be separated into "early" and "late" changes. The detection of early changes is important because new disease-modifying therapies are more effective when used before severe disability has occurred. Since initial changes are nonosseous in character, sonography and MRI imaging can detect disease earlier than conventional X-rays and computed tomography (CT). Secondly, in the present scenario, RA is treated aggressively with disease-modifying drugs, hence osseous changes are delayed.[5]

Radiographic Features

The earliest changes include joint space widening and soft tissue swelling.

Joint space widening is the earliest but a transient radiographic abnormality, sometimes lasting for only a few weeks. This finding is due to edema and swelling of the synovium and joint effusion. Joint space widening is best detected at the metacarpophalangeal (MCP) joints, especially in the 5th digit.[13] *Soft tissue swelling* results from an amalgam of joint effusion, synovial edema and proliferation, and tenosynovitis which invariably precedes cartilaginous and osseous changes. In the hand, periarticular fusiform swelling may be seen over the proximal interphalangeal (PIP) and 2nd and 5th MCP joints. Soft tissue swelling over the 3rd and 4th MCP joints may be appreciated as a local increased density. Swelling of the soft tissues over the styloid process of the ulna may be better detected on radiographs rather than clinical examination and is due to involvement of the extensor carpi ulnaris sheath. Soft tissue swelling over the styloid process of radius can be seen due to involvement of the radiocarpal joint.[14] In the feet, the soft tissue changes are less evident radiographically but may be seen over the 1st and 5th metatarsal heads. There may be blurring and obliteration of the pre-Achilles fat pad and blurring and thickening of the Achilles tendon.[3]

In the knee, there may be lateral bulging of the fat lines over the distal femur on anteroposterior (AP) radiographs. On lateral views, there is distention of the suprapatellar bursa with blurring of its surrounding fat lines. In the elbow, the anterior and posterior fat lines are displaced away from the joint on the lateral view.[14]

Osteopenia in RA is of two types: (1) local juxta-articular osteopenia is due to synovial inflammation and hyperemia and is a feature of early changes and (2) generalized osteopenia is due to limitation of movement due to pain, muscle wasting or steroid therapy and is therefore seen late in the disease.[3] Osteopenia is seen more often as the disease progresses and 80% of patients demonstrate osteopenia by 2 years after onset of symptoms. It is a precursor of erosive disease and may mask early erosions. Assessment of osteopenia may be difficult and comparison between normal and abnormal joints in the same patient is helpful. However, it is subjective and there may be interobserver as well as intraobserver variability in the assessment. Generalized or solitary terminal phalangeal sclerosis may be seen in up to 35% of patients with RA and other arthropathies and may be seen before any other abnormality.[14]

Joint space narrowing results from damage to the articular cartilage and is virtually always uniform **(Fig. 1)**. It may be more apparent than real in the presence of flexion deformities, and an oblique view may be required to assess the space. Uniform narrowing with an intact subchondral cortex is however not specific for RA as it can also be present in the SSAs or connective tissue diseases. Presence of uniform narrowing on the other hand is an important feature of RA that helps to differentiate it from OA in which the joint space narrowing is characteristically nonuniform or segmental.[2]

Subperiosteal bone apposition is uncommon in adult RA and is almost always subtle. When present, it may be seen at the site of capsular or tendon attachments and probably reflects the effect of tenosynovitis. This relative lack of periosteal reaction, despite advanced and often dramatic joint destruction is a distinctive feature of the disease and is so characteristic that the existence of exuberant periosteal reaction should suggest an alternate diagnosis.[3]

Erosions are the most important diagnostic feature of RA but may not be seen when the patient presents initially. Their incidence rises from <40% at 3 months from symptom onset to 90–95% at 10 years of disease.[14] The detection of erosions indicates irreversible joint damage. The earliest sites of cortical surface erosions are at the bare areas of bone between the margin of the articular cartilage and the attachment of the joint capsule and therefore their distribution is related to the anatomy of the joint.[15]

In the hands, erosions usually involve the wrist, MCP and PIP joints. The distal interphalangeal (DIP) joints are usually

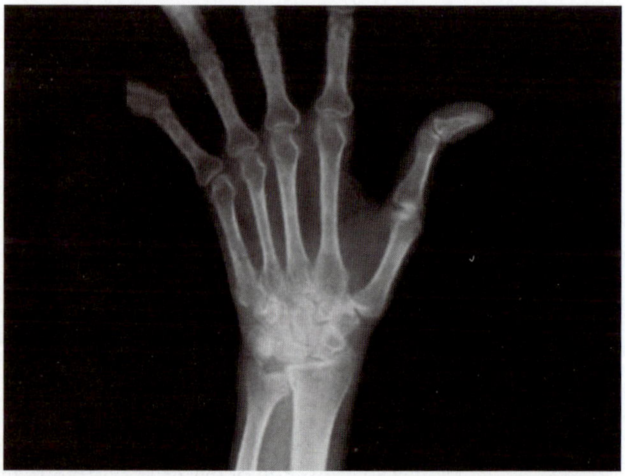

FIG. 1: X-ray of hand reveals the early changes of rheumatoid arthritis with classical juxta-articular osteopenia and uniform narrowing of the distal radioulnar, radiocarpal and intercarpal joints. Subluxations at the 1st metacarpophalangeal (MCP) and interphalangeal (IP) joints cause the classical "Hitchhiker's" deformity.

spared. Erosions involve a wider area on the proximal side of the PIP joints due to the larger bare areas on this side of the joint. At the MCP joints, the metacarpal heads develop the first and most extensive erosions, which are most evident at the radiovolar aspect of the 2nd and 3rd MCP joints. The 5th metacarpal may demonstrate the earliest erosions on its lateral aspect. In the interphalangeal (IP) joint of the thumb, erosions generally develop at the volar aspect on the ulnar side of the base of the distal phalanx. The ulnar styloid is commonly eroded due to inflammation in the prestyloid recess. There may be large erosions of the distal radius at the radioulnar joint. Erosions occur throughout the carpus and may be followed by fusion. However, bony ankylosis is uncommon in other joints in adult RA.[4]

In the feet, erosions appear earlier and are most often seen at the 5th metatarsophalangeal (MTP) joint. The heads of the metatarsals erode before the bases of the proximal phalanges, especially on the medial plantar aspect, although the lateral side of the 5th metatarsal head may be eroded. A characteristic site for erosion in the tarsus is at the posterosuperior aspect of the calcaneum above the insertion of the Achilles tendon. However, tarsal erosions are less often seen in RA as compared to the SSAs.[14] Bone erosions can also appear at extra-articular sites including the upper posterior ribs and ischial margins.[3]

Radiologically, early marginal erosions appear as cortical defects or an indistinctness of the subchondral cortex. This erasure or blurring of the white line of the cortex is first visualized on the radial side of the 4th and 5th metacarpal heads. If seen *en face*, erosions appear entirely within the bone giving a cystic appearance **(Fig. 2)**. Some may be deep or pocketed.

Erosive change is less common in the large joints. There may be a superficial surface irregularity in the presence of diffuse joint narrowing **(Fig. 3)**. In the hip, the medial joint space is characteristically involved with medial migration of the heads of the femora causing protrusio acetabuli. This is distinct from OA, which generally involves the superior compartment of the hip joint.[2]

Rarely, large intraosseous defects or pseudocysts may be seen in patients who have massive proliferation of the synovium. It has been hypothesized that these form due to the high intra-articular pressure, which exceeds the intraosseous pressure resulting in the movement of the synovial fluid into the adjacent subchondral bone. Invariably, there is destruction of the adjacent joint cartilage. Pseudocysts may attain sizes up to 2–3 cm, are usually oval to round, with regular outlines or slightly scalloped margins.[15]

Late Changes

Alignment deformities at joints may result from local synovitis weakening the capsule and tendinitis preventing normal musculotendinous actions causing subluxations and dislocations. Tendons may also rupture in the region of eroded bone. Thus, rotator cuff tears result in upward subluxation of the eroded humeral head. Subluxation at the MCP joints leads to ulnar deviation, which is seen in 50% of patients with chronic disease. There is also increasing palmar flexion due to ulnar deviation of extensor tendons. Other classical deformities in the hands are the "boutonnière" deformity due to flexion at the PIP joint with extension at the DIP joint. The reverse is seen with the "swan-neck" deformity due to PIP joint extension and DIP joint flexion. Flexion at the 1st MCP joint with extension at the IP joint results in the "Hitchhiker's thumb". There may also be dislocation of the carpus causing a bayonet deformity at the wrist.[4]

In the feet, there may be lateral deviation of the toes, especially hallux valgus **(Fig. 4)**. The hallux sesamoids sublux between the 1st and 2nd metatarsal heads and the transverse arch flattens due to ligamentous laxity.[14]

Severe erosive change leads to marked *destruction and narrowing of the joint spaces* with extreme irregularity and destruction of the subchondral bone **(Fig. 5)**. In the hands, the bone ends are often reciprocally eroded and there may be telescoping of the fingers. There is resultant arthritis mutilans, which may also be seen in other conditions such as erosive OA and multicentric reticulohistiocytosis.[3]

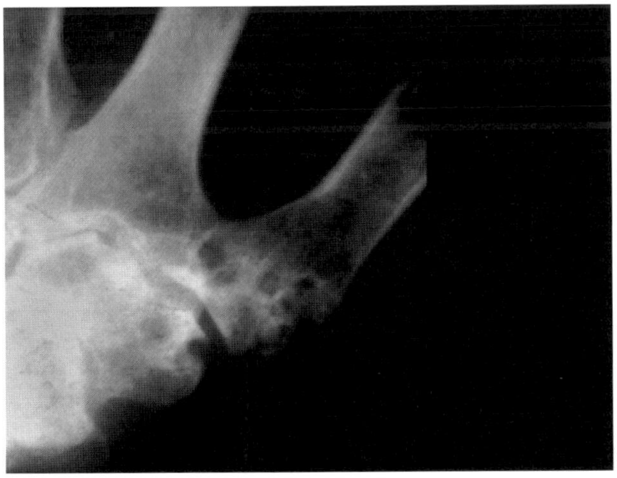

FIG. 2: Rheumatoid arthritis. Magnified view of the carpometacarpal (CMC) joints demonstrates multiple erosions in the bases of the metacarpals and trapezium giving a cystic appearance.

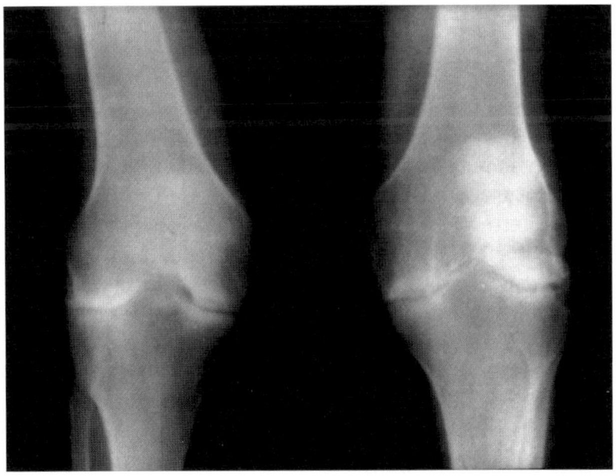

FIG. 3: X-ray of both knee joints in a case of rheumatoid arthritis (RA) reveals diffuse osteopenia with uniform narrowing of the joint spaces. Note the lack of irregularity of the articular margins.

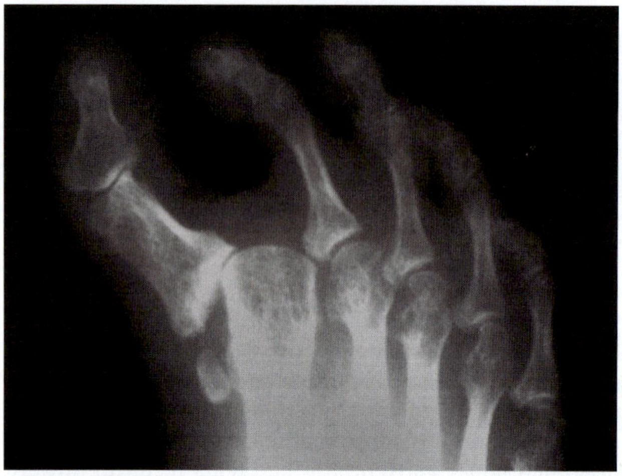

FIG. 4: X-ray of the forefoot shows more advanced changes of rheumatoid arthritis with gross erosions of the metatarsal heads with subluxations at the metatarsophalangeal (MTP) and interphalangeal (IP) joints with hallux valgus.

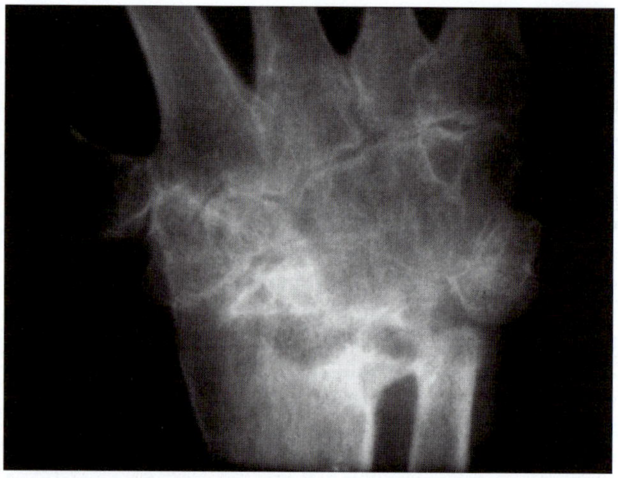

FIG. 5: Magnified view of the wrist joint demonstrating late changes of rheumatoid arthritis with severe osteopenia, gross destruction of the distal ends of the radius and ulna with ankylosis of the carpal bones.

Gross *loss of bone* at the femoral head results in a "bird's beak" appearance. There may be pointing of the adjacent bone ends at the acromioclavicular joints with resorption of the distal clavicles.

Stress fractures may occur due to normal stress on bone with decreased elastic resistance. *Giant synovial* cysts may develop, particularly originating from the knee joint and presenting in the calf. They may also occur around the shoulder, elbow and hip where they may protrude into the pelvis. RA can attack any synovial joint and there may be involvement of the laryngeal joints, sternomanubrial or temporomandibular joints.[3]

Pulmonary involvement may lead to pleural effusions, pulmonary nodules (30%) or interstitial fibrosis (predominantly lower lobe). Pulmonary nodules are usually associated with subcutaneous nodules present at the extensor surfaces of the elbows or other joints. Secondary OA may complicate RA in weight-bearing joints. Reactive sclerosis and new bone formation is not marked in these joints.[14]

Axial Skeleton Involvement

The spondylitis associated with RA is peculiar in that it usually involves the cervical region. Thoracic or lumbar involvement is distinctly uncommon. Osteoporosis, narrowing of the disc along with endplate irregularity are present in the upper cervical vertebrae with minimal reactive new bone formation. This is in sharp contrast to OA which usually involves the lower cervical spine. Erosions at the facet joints can lead to multilevel subluxations in the upper cervical spine giving a step-ladder appearance.[4]

Atlantoaxial (AA) subluxation may be present in up to 20–25% of patients with chronic RA and is primarily due to looseness of the transverse ligament (which is responsible for maintaining the integrity of the AA joint) with/without erosive changes in the odontoid. A gap of >2.5 mm in adults or 4 mm in children between the anterior border of the odontoid and the posterior surface of the anterior arch of the atlas in flexion in children is deemed diagnostic of atlantoaxial dislocation (AAD) **(Figs. 6A and B)**. Although it can be visualized on plain radiographs, three-dimensional (3D) CT and MRI give a better delineation of both the soft tissue and bony involvement **(Figs. 7A to D)**.[15] The eroded odontoid may at times fracture. Resorption of bone at nonarticular surfaces occurs at the spinous processes which become short, sharp and tapered.[3]

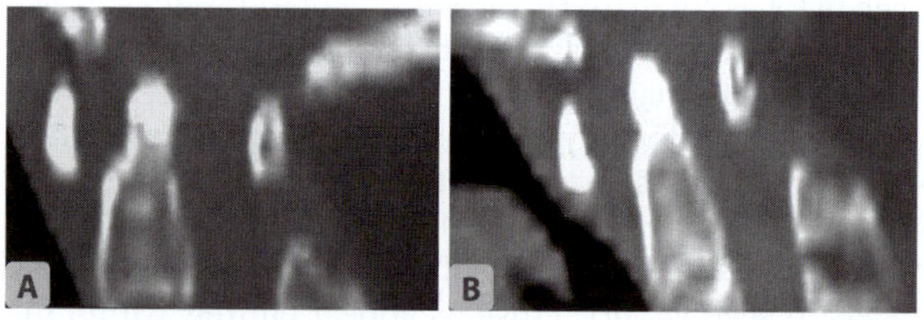

FIGS. 6A AND B: Sagittal reformatted three-dimensional (3D) CT images of the craniovertebral junction in (A) extension and (B) flexion show increase in the atlantoaxial distance on flexion with erosion of the odontoid peg due to rheumatoid arthritis.

Occasionally, the sacroiliac joints exhibit minimal erosions with joint space narrowing; however, reactive sclerosis as seen in AS is typically absent. Rarely, there may be ankylosis of the sacroiliac joints.

Other Imaging Modalities

Ultrasonography

The introduction of high-resolution linear transducers led to the widespread use of ultrasonography (USG) in musculoskeletal imaging. USG may be used for the detection as well as monitoring of the inflammatory changes and osseous damage. A number of studies have demonstrated the ability of USG to identify early synovial inflammation in the form of synovial thickening and joint effusion. Power Doppler has the capacity to discern and measure alterations in the

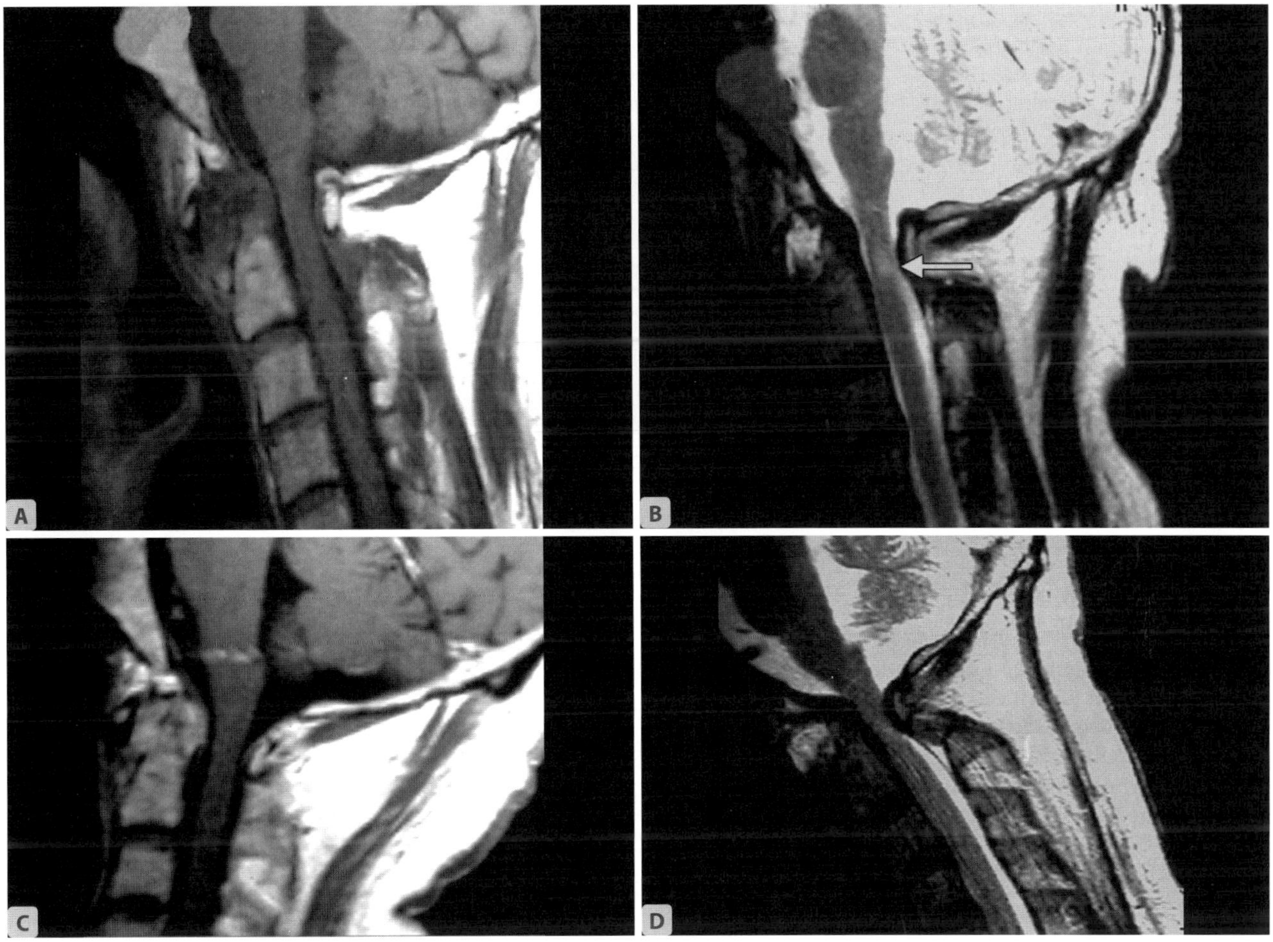

FIGS. 7A TO D: Magnetic resonance (MR) of the craniovertebral junction in a case of rheumatoid arthritis with atlantoaxial dislocation (AAD). (A) T1- and (B) T2-weighted images in neutral position reveal erosion of the odontoid with pannus which appears hypointense on T1 and hyperintense on T2-weighted sequences. Hyperintense signal is seen within the cord at this level due to ischemia/edema; (C) Postgadolinium, there is significant enhancement of the pannus; (D) T2-weighted image in flexion demonstrates compression of the cord due to posterior displacement of the odontoid peg.

vascularity of the synovium due to inflammation **(Figs. 8A and B)**. USG contrast agents have the capability to enhance the sensitivity of power Doppler by increasing the signal from the synovial vessels.

The joint margins can be assessed for the presence of erosions. It has been established that USG has higher sensitivity than conventional radiography for detection of erosion in the small joints.[16] The internal structure of the tendons can be assessed and their integrity or rupture demonstrated by dynamic scanning. Leakage of synovial fluid may also be demonstrated, e.g., a ruptured Baker's cyst which needs to be distinguished from other causes of pain in the calf, such as deep vein thrombosis or muscle tear. USG can also be used to evaluate the response to therapy. Following treatment, USG can detect reduction in the synovial inflammation and vascular flow parameters.[17] Several studies have compared power Doppler with MRI for the detection of early arthritis. A prospective study that included 60 patients demonstrated that USG showed a higher sensitivity than MRI for the detection of synovitis.[18] In another study, sonography was found to be a valuable tool; however, contrast-enhanced magnetic resonance (CEMR) was found to be superior for the evaluation of synovial proliferation as well as erosions.[19] Disadvantages of USG include the user-dependent nature of the modality and the long time required to evaluate multiple joints.

Computed Tomography

Computed tomography is not frequently used routinely in RA as it is inferior to MRI and USG for the detection of early disease along with the disadvantage of using ionizing radiation. It can demonstrate the presence of erosions, particularly in the carpal and tarsal bones. It can also show joint space narrowing or ankylosis. A recent study has reported comparable performance of CT with MRI for the evaluation of synovitis and tenosynovitis using contrast-enhanced CT with digital masking of the bone.[20] However, its main use lies in the diagnosis and management of upper cervical spine abnormalities, particularly for the evaluation of AA subluxation.[15]

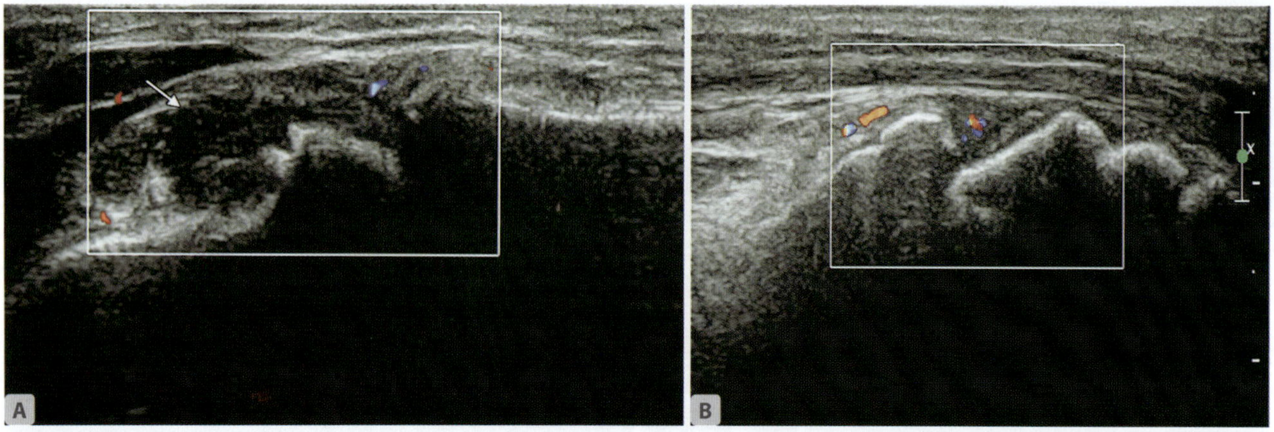

FIGS. 8A AND B: (A) Ultrasound image of the metacarpophalangeal joints shows diffuse synovial thickening (arrow) with convex margin, loss of articular cartilage, fluid and erosions in a case of rheumatoid arthritis; (B) Power Doppler in the same case showing increased vascularity in the synovial thickening.

Radionuclide Scanning

Scanning with ^{99m}Tc-methylene diphosphonate (MDP) is quite sensitive for detection of the inflammatory changes of arthritis but shows poor specificity. In RA, isotopes are at least 70% more sensitive than conventional films and may be used to monitor response to therapy.[11] Findings include increased flow in the synovium in the early or blood pool phase and increased uptake in the delayed 3 hours scans.

Magnetic Resonance Imaging

Over the last two decades, MRI has consolidated its position as the best imaging modality for RA, despite being expensive and time consuming. The Outcome Measures in Rheumatoid Arthritis Clinical Trials (OMERACT) MRI study group was an international, multidisciplinary group which was set up for the purpose of standardizing imaging techniques and definitions of joint pathologies in RA.[6] According to their recommendations, an MRI scan for RA should comprise of the minimum following sequences: (1) imaging in two planes (axial and coronal), (2) T1-weighed sequences before and after gadolinium, and (3) a fat-saturated T2-weighted or a short-tau inversion recovery (STIR) sequence. MRI is also a useful imaging modality for the follow-up of RA to evaluate progression or remission. The typical progression in RA from the stage of synovitis followed by edema of the bone marrow to bony erosion is well demonstrated on MRI.[6]

Synovial Imaging

Magnetic resonance imaging is now believed to be the gold standard for synovial imaging. Inflammatory changes within the soft tissues of the joints which precede the development of erosions and which are not detectable on plain radiographs are well demonstrated on MRI.[21] It has been reported that using the enhancement of MCP and PIP joints as a positive diagnostic criteria, it is possible to diagnose RA with a high sensitivity of 96% and accuracy of 44%.[8] The OMERACT group defines synovitis as an area in the synovial compartment which shows enhancement following contrast administration with thickness which exceeds the width of the normal synovium.[6] MRI depicts irregular thickening of the synovium which is of intermediate signal intensity (SI) compared to darker fluid on T1 and high SI on T2-weighted spin echo sequences. Fat-suppressed T2-weighted sequences more clearly delineate disease extent. Postgadolinium, there can be significant rapid enhancement of the inflamed synovium in contrast to joint effusion which does not show enhancement in the early phase. Images obtained >10 minutes after gadolinium show diffusion of gadolinium into the synovial joint fluid resulting in increased SI.[6] The activity of the synovitis is best assessed on postcontrast fat-suppressed T1-weighted images and there is indirect evidence suggesting that the amount of postcontrast enhancement correlates with the degree of inflammation.[15] Fibrotic pannus and pannus with hemosiderin deposition show low SI on T1- and T2-weighted images and do not enhance on postgadolinium images.

Quantification of synovial volume has been shown to have a significant role to play in the diagnosis as well as follow-up of RA. The baseline synovial volume has been found to correlate significantly with the number of new bone erosions at 1-year follow-up.[6,21]

Bone Marrow Edema

Edema of the bone marrow has been described as a characteristic finding in RA, especially in the early phase. It manifests as ill-defined, high SI on fat-suppressed, T2-weighted and STIR images with enhancement following gadolinium **(Fig. 9)**. It has been reported in up to 39–75% of patients with RA with disease duration of below 1 year.[6] It is commonly found in the subchondral bone and can be seen as an isolated finding or surrounding areas of bone erosions. It is presently considered to be a forerunner of erosions. Some studies have shown the high association of bone marrow edema at baseline with development of erosions later in the course of the illness at 1 and 6 years.[22]

Erosions

On MRI, erosions are seen as focal areas of loss of normal SI from cortical or subchondral bone on T1 with high SI on T2-

weighted or STIR images **(Figs. 10A and B)**. Erosions replace marrow fat and contain inflamed synovium which enhances with gadolinium and are thus easily differentiated from other interosseous fluid-filled cystic lesions.[23]

In early RA, MRI can detect bone erosions in 45–72% of patients with early disease (<6 months duration), in contrast to 8–40% on radiography.[6,9] This is important as MRI can expedite the early diagnosis of RA, allowing treatment to be instituted early in the progression of disease. It is also important to identify those patients in whom progressive disease does not occur as these patients do not require aggressive treatment protocols. In one study, 82% of patients who did not show erosions at the baseline MRI did not develop any radiographic erosions at 2-year follow-up.[6]

Tendons and Ligaments

Rheumatoid arthritis can involve the ligaments or tendons directly which results in predisposition to rupture. Increased signal on T2-weighted spin echo and STIR sequences indicates tendon involvement and may be due to erosion, invasion by pannus or partial tear. Any alterations in the thickness of the tendon are also abnormal.

Tenosynovitis can be diagnosed by the detection of fluid in the tendon sheath, thickening of the tendon sheath or enhancement. The most commonly involved tendon is the extensor carpi ulnaris.[23] Inflammation of the flexor tendons of the wrist results in a greater carpal tunnel volume, which in turn leads to increased mechanical pressure and compression of the median nerve which can also be inflamed resulting in carpal tunnel syndrome. Axial images are most useful for evaluating the anatomy of the carpal tunnel.

Intraosseous cysts show decreased SI on T1 and increased SI on T2- weighted images and may not enhance in the immediate postcontrast phase.[5]

Intra-articular loose bodies are frequently seen due to the destructive inflammatory process and include cartilaginous and osseous fragments. A subset of loose bodies is called "rice bodies" as they resemble polished rice. They are now recognized as a distinctive feature of RA. They may contain various tissues such as collagen, fibrinogen and its products, mononuclear cells, and blood cells along with amorphous material.[5]

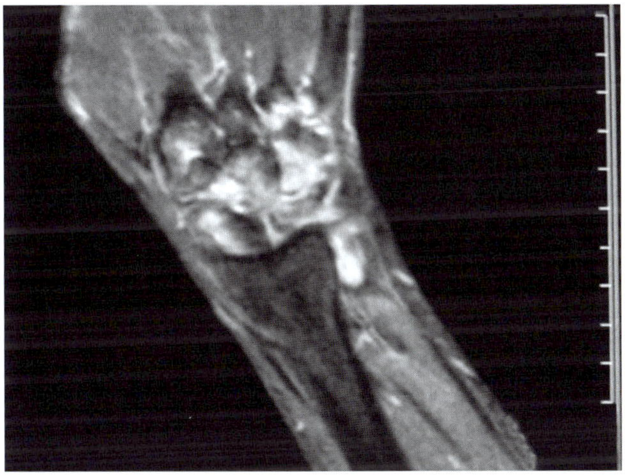

FIG. 9: Coronal short tau inversion recovery (STIR) image shows ill-defined areas of high signal intensity in the carpal bones due to bone marrow edema.

Large Joints

Though involvement of large joints usually occurs after established disease elsewhere, MRI is more sensitive in picking up early change. In the glenohumeral joint, rotator cuff tears, joint effusion, giant synovial cysts and early erosions are best evaluated on MRI. Similarly, involvement of the hip joint with detection of joint effusion, pannus, erosions and articular cartilage destruction is well depicted on MRI **(Figs. 11A and B)**.[22]

Scoring Systems for Rheumatoid Arthritis

Radiographic images establish the degree of structural damage of the joints at a given point in time. Radiographic abnormalities were initially used to develop an index of the damage that was used to assign patients to four stages. However, by the early 1960s, it was realized that assigning

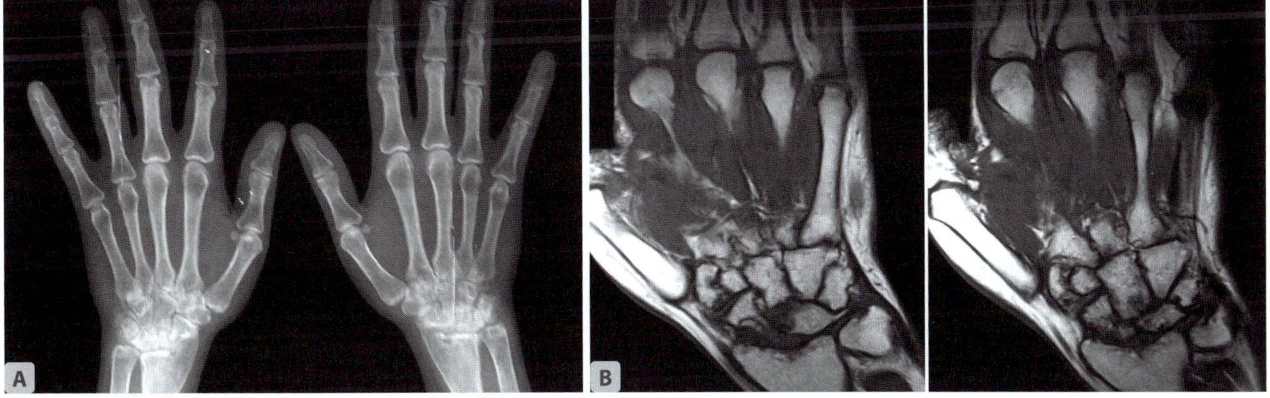

FIGS. 10A AND B: Patient with rheumatoid arthritis. (A) X-ray of both hands posteroanterior (PA) view shows diffuse loss of the joint spaces at the radiocarpal, intercarpal and CMC joints; (B) T1-weighted coronal image demonstrates multiple erosions in the carpal bones, distal ulna and radius.

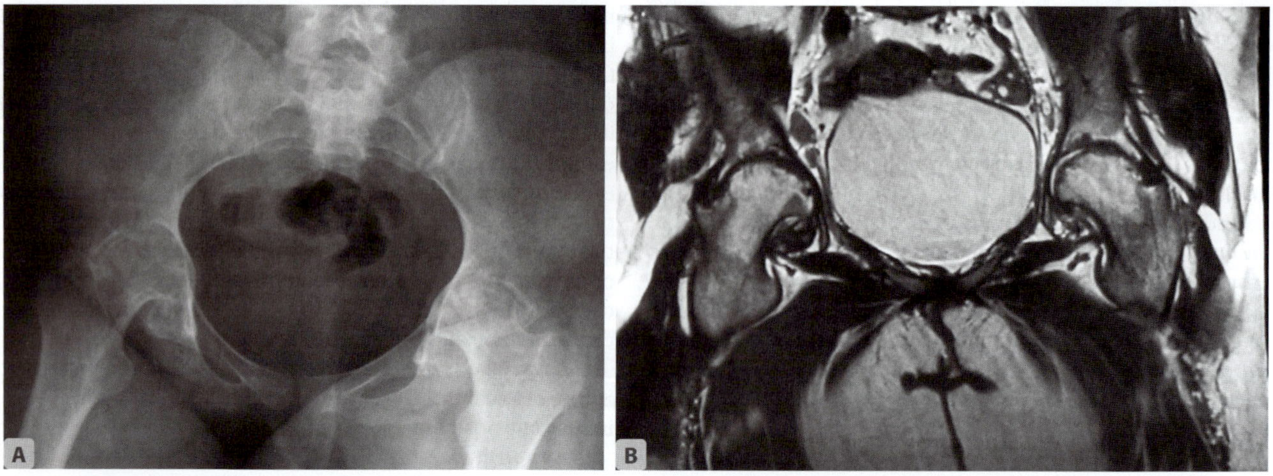

FIGS. 11A AND B: (A) X-ray of pelvis of a patient with rheumatoid arthritis (RA) shows uniform loss of joint space with irregularity of the articular surface in bilateral hip joints. Note the medial migration of the femoral heads; (B) Coronal T2-weighted image better demonstrates the erosions. Note the bone marrow edema manifesting as ill-defined hyperintense signal.

a single score for all radiographic abnormalities lacked sensitivity for detecting disease progression and various scoring systems were developed which rated the severity of bony erosion and degree of joint space narrowing separately. Larsen developed a global scoring system which incorporated the presence of erosions, soft tissue swelling and osteoporosis into a single score. Multiple different modifications and variations of the global or composite methods were extensively used in an attempt to delineate the progression of disease in RA and to effectively assess response to therapy.[24] However, the scoring systems are not exact measurements as they reflect individual readers and so, the error of individual scores can be considerable. Also, the expected progression of bony or soft tissue damage in untreated disease is not possible to ascertain. Development of an accurate, easily reproducible and easily carried out quantitative measurement of bony erosion and cartilage destruction is required.

On MRI at present, the most commonly frequently used method is the Rheumatoid Arthritis Magnetic Resonance Imaging Score (RAMRIS) proposed by OMERACT. In this, the synovitis is rated in three wrist regions: (1) the distal radioulnar joint, (2) the radiocarpal joint, and (3) the intercarpal, carpometacarpal and MCP joints on a scale of 0–3. An assigned score of 0 is normal, while score of 1 (mild), 2 (moderate) or 3 (severe) reflect the increasing volume of enhancing synovium. Similarly, bone marrow edema is scored from 0 to 3 according to the volume: 0 is no edema, 1 is 1–33%, 2 is 34–66%, and 3 is 67–100% of bone that is edematous. Erosions in the bones of the wrist are scored separately. The scores range from 0 to 10 according to the volume of erosions in the assessed bones in increments of 10%. The maximum score in the wrist is 150.[25] However, using the RAMRIS score is difficult, requiring years of dedicated work, is subject to high interobserver variability and is not practical in clinical practice.

Scoring methods have been shown to be effective in determining the benefit from drug treatment and will continue to evaluate the advantages of new drugs in the coming years. Development of a simple, easy to use, accurate and reproducible method would be a powerful tool for both the physician and the clinical investigator.

At present, the aim of the management of RA is to avert disability and damage evident on radiology with early and persistent remission. Treatment efficacy is measured by ACR/EULAR and Disease Activity Score (DAS) which is the first step in disease management.[26]

JUVENILE IDIOPATHIC ARTHRITIDES

A number of separate disorders can lead to chronic arthritis in children; however, there is as yet no uniformly accepted classification for these diseases. The International League of Associations of Rheumatologists (ILAR) Task Force did attempt to establish classification criteria;[27] however, they are not in universal use.

- *Juvenile-onset adult type (seropositive) rheumatoid arthritis*: Seropositive juvenile rheumatoid arthritis (JRA) accounts for 5–15% of juvenile idiopathic arthritis (JIA). The onset is during adolescence and there is a strong female preponderance. It is a peripheral erosive polyarthritis which is nearly identical with adult RA. Large joints like the knee and hips may be affected.
- Seronegative *chronic arthritis*: In this subgroup, systemic or articular symptoms and signs develop in the absence of positive serology for RF.
    - *Classic systemic disease* represents 20% of children with JIA. It affects children below the age of 5 years. Both sexes are equally affected. These children present with an acute febrile onset with anemia, hepatosplenomegaly, lymphadenopathy, anorexia, weight loss, and chronic recurrent arthralgias. Erosive arthritis is uncommon.
    - *Pauciarticular* type is the most common type of JIA responsible for nearly half the cases. Four or less joints are involved, generally the large joints like the knee, elbow and ankle. It typically affects young girls.

- *Polyarticular* type represents approximately 20% of JIA. It may occur at any age and is commoner in females. It is symmetric and involves the large and small joints as well as the cervical spine. Growth retardation is common due to premature fusion of the epiphyses and there may be associated mandibular hypoplasia with antegonial notching.

Generally, the prognosis in JIA is good with fewer than 20% children having progressive destructive disease. The pathophysiology is virtually identical to the adult form with inflammation of the synovium and greater production of joint fluid with effusion. Pannus is less extensive than adult RA but still produces significant cartilage and bony destruction.[4,12,28]

Radiologic Features

The knee is the most common joint to manifest radiographic abnormalities followed by the other large joints, wrist, hand, cervical spine, sacroiliac joints, and sternoclavicular joint.[28] Early changes include soft tissue swelling and osteopenia which may be juxta-articular or diffuse. In early stages, it is probably due to hyperemia, but later, disuse atrophy and steroids contribute to it. Band-like metaphyseal lucent zones (growth arrest lines) may be evident. Pathological fractures may occur.[13] Periostitis appears within weeks following the onset of symptoms and is usually seen along the shafts of the metacarpals, metatarsals, and proximal phalanges.[4]

Later, there is uniform loss of joint space and articular erosions **(Figs. 12A to C)**. Progressive destruction can lead to bony ankylosis. Joining together of the carpometacarpal joint of the middle and index fingers is typical as are multiple, fused cervical vertebrae.[4]

The most distinctive radiographic findings are seen as a result of altered growth patterns. There is accelerated bone maturation with early fusion of epiphyses and bone shortening secondary to hyperemia.[12] This results in large expansile (ballooned) epiphyses while the adjacent metaphysis and diaphysis appear gracile and constricted.[4] Muscle atrophy is generally a prominent feature **(Fig. 13)**.

In the carpus and tarsus, the bones show accelerated maturation, crowding with joint space narrowing and an abnormal angular shape (squashed carpi). The cervical spine is often affected with erosions at the apophyseal joints (usually at C2-3) leading to ankylosis. The associated vertebral bodies fail to develop. AAD is said to occur rarely in children with seronegative disease. The intervertebral discs are narrowed and fusion may occur. There may be ankylosis of the sacroiliac joints. Secondary degenerative changes may occur later.[14]

Radiographs are useful for making the initial diagnosis, and also for staging the disease and for follow-up. They are also useful for excluding other causes of pain like congenital disorders, fractures or tumors. However, they mostly illustrate late changes and indirect signs of synovial disease. USG is a rapid and safe modality which does not utilize ionizing radiation which can directly image the synovium for evidence of proliferation or hypervascularity and joint effusion.[29] USG can also be used as a guidance modality for performing joint aspiration, the sample can be cultured to exclude septic arthritis. In a study on 30 patients, USG demonstrated a higher sensitivity than clinical assessment for the detection of synovial effusion and thickening in cases of JIA.[30] In another

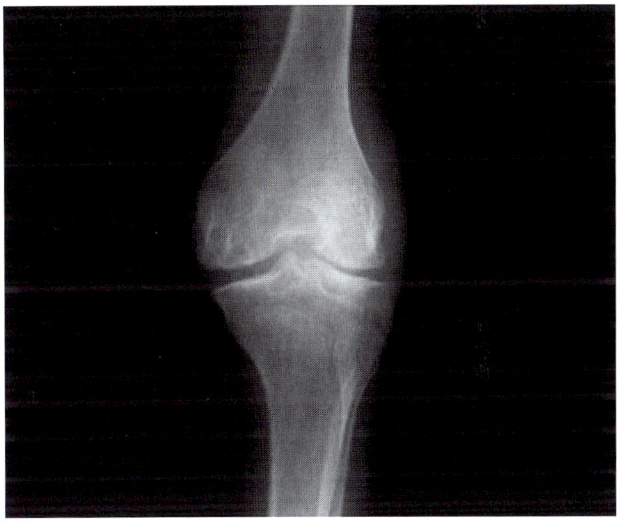

FIG. 13: Juvenile rheumatoid arthritis—X-ray of knee joint antero-posterior (AP) view reveals diffuse osteopenia with large squared femoral condyles, widening with irregularity of the intercondylar notch and subchondral lucencies. Note the reduction in the soft tissue bulk.

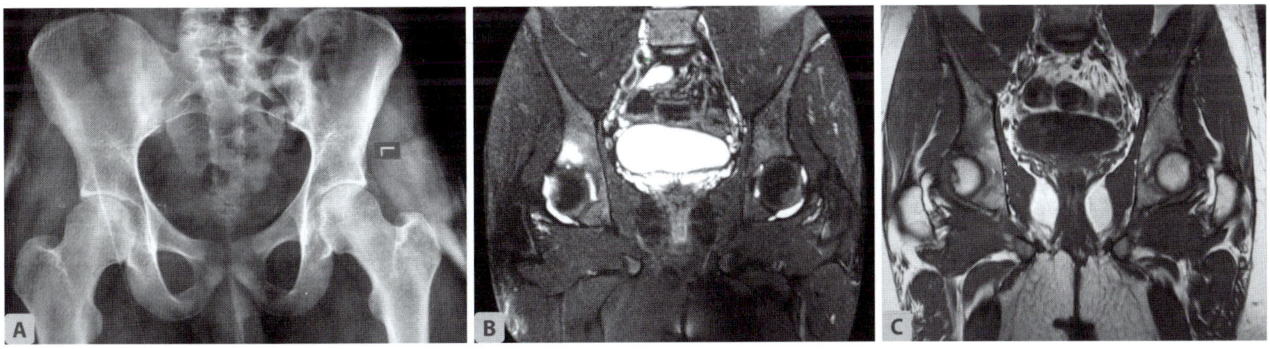

FIGS. 12A TO C: A 12-year-old boy with juvenile idiopathic arthritis (JIA). (A) X-ray of the pelvis shows mild narrowing of the joint spaces in bilateral hips; (B) Coronal T2-weighted image demonstrates the presence of joint effusion and ill-defined hyperintense signal in the acetabulum signifying bone marrow edema; (C) Coronal T1-weighted image shows bone erosions in bilateral hip joints.

study, it was found that power Doppler sonography was highly accurate in monitoring the therapeutic response in cases of JIA.[31]

Magnetic resonance imaging remains the imaging modality of choice for evaluating the early changes of JIA because of its ability to allow direct visualization of nonossified portions of epiphyseal cartilage.[12] It clearly depicts joint effusion, cartilage changes, synovial proliferation, bony erosion or synovial cysts. With long-standing JIA of the knee, chronic inflammation involving the meniscal surfaces can lead to meniscal hypoplasia or even atrophy.[28,32] Radiographic evidence of synovitis may be seen in trauma-induced synovitis or infective arthritis. These disorders are monoarticular in contrast to JIA and history of trauma or acute onset may serve to differentiate them from JIA. If tubercular arthritis involves multiple large joints, it may be indistinguishable from JIA. In hemophilic arthropathy, multiple episodes of bleeding into the joint cavity induce synovial inflammation with hypertrophy resulting in a radiologic picture closely resembling JIA.

SERONEGATIVE SPONDYLOARTHROPATHIES

Seronegative spondyloarthropathies are a category of seronegative arthritic diseases affecting multiple organ systems with clinical and radiological overlap and a significant genetic component. They are characterized by the absence of RF, peripheral arthropathy and sacroiliitis with or without spondylitis. A classification criterion for the entire group of SSA has been developed. These criteria are inflammatory spinal pain or synovitis, in conjunction with minimum one of the following criteria: a positive family history, urethritis, inflammatory bowel disease, psoriasis, acute diarrhea, enthesopathy, alternating buttock pain or radiographically evident sacroiliitis.[33]

ANKYLOSING SPONDYLITIS

Ankylosing spondylitis is a chronic, progressive inflammatory arthritis which chiefly involves the synovial joints of the spine along with the adjacent soft tissues as well as the sacroiliac joints, although peripheral, large joints such as the hips, shoulders and knee can also be involved.[4] There is a strong association with HLA-B27 with >90% of patients with AS having this antigen. It has been shown that AS will develop in 0.6–1.3% of persons who are positive for HLA-B27. Approximately 65% of patients of psoriasis with spondylitis or inflammatory bowel disease with spondylitis also have HLA-B27 and it has been postulated that the antigen is essentially related to spinal changes.[14]

The disease is common in males (4:1) though recently it has been realized that women may be more commonly affected than thought earlier. Women more often have only clinical manifestations without radiographic evidence of disease. The onset of disease is generally between 15 and 35 years.[12]

The archetypal clinical description of AS is of an insidious onset with low back pain which carries on for >3 months. Back stiffness is worse after periods of inactivity and there may be pain over the gluteal and sacroiliac regions. Radiographic evidence of sacroiliitis is mandatory for the definitive diagnosis of AS, but may take several years to appear. Various extra-articular features may be present of which the most common is acute anterior uveitis. Others include aortitis, aortic regurgitation, pulmonary fibrosis, cardiac conduction defects, arachnoiditis, and amyloidosis.[34] Pulmonary involvement can result in cavitation with fibrosis in bilateral lung apices mimicking tuberculosis.[10]

Pathophysiology

Histologically, the synovitis of AS is identical to that of RA. There is a predisposition to develop ankylosis due to metaplasia of the cartilage, endochondral ossification, formation of woven bone and fibrosis. The enthesopathy consists of destruction of ligaments, tendons and local bone with inflammatory infiltrate. This heals by the deposition of new bone at the interface between the tendons and ligaments. This causes bone proliferation at nonarticular sites, syndesmophytes and capsular ossification.[14] It has been suggested that there is a genetic predisposition which permits an antigen or other triggering factor to enter the synovium and evoke an inflammatory response. This inflammatory response causes activation of the lymphocytes which liberate tumor necrosis factor-alpha (TNF-α) and other cytokines leading to destruction of tissue.[34]

Radiologic Features

Sacroiliac Joints

The classic sacroiliitis is bilateral and symmetrical. In about 10% of cases, the sacroiliitis may be unilateral or asymmetrical at presentation but eventually becomes bilaterally symmetrical. Changes occur in both the synovial along with ligamentous (superior and posterior) parts of the sacroiliac joints. The earliest radiographic findings occur in the subchondral cortex which appears blurred or lost. Later, small (rat-bite) erosions appear which are worse along the iliac aspect of the joint. These cause widening of the joint space with hazy margins **(Figs. 14A and B)**. This is followed by larger erosions, subjacent sclerosis and joint space narrowing as irregular new bone bridges the joint space with eventual ankylosis and resolution of the sclerosis.[2,12,14]

The modified New York criteria for grading sacroiliitis established in 1994 are:[35]

- Grade 0: Normal findings
- Grade 1: Suspicious changes
- Grade 2: Minimal abnormality (small localized erosions or sclerosis without alteration in joint width)
- Grade 3: Unequivocal abnormality
- Grade 4: Total ankylosis

Joint changes are assessed using prone views with cephalad angulation or oblique views. However, CT is more sensitive than radiographs in depicting small and early erosions and joint space changes.[34] Recently, it has been suggested that dynamic CEMR shows a higher sensitivity

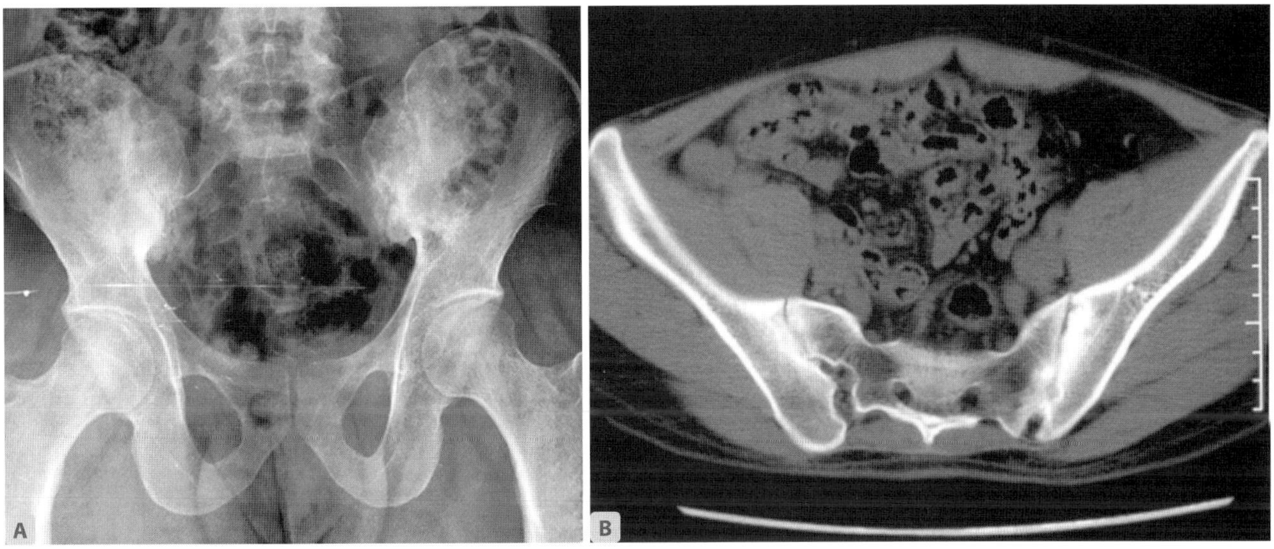

FIGS. 14A AND B: Sacroiliitis in ankylosing spondylitis. (A) X-ray of pelvis anteroposterior (AP) view shows mild irregularity with subarticular sclerosis in both sacroiliac (SI) joints; (B) Axial CT section of the SI joints of the same patient shows irregularity of the articular surfaces with subarticular sclerosis which is more marked in the iliac blades.

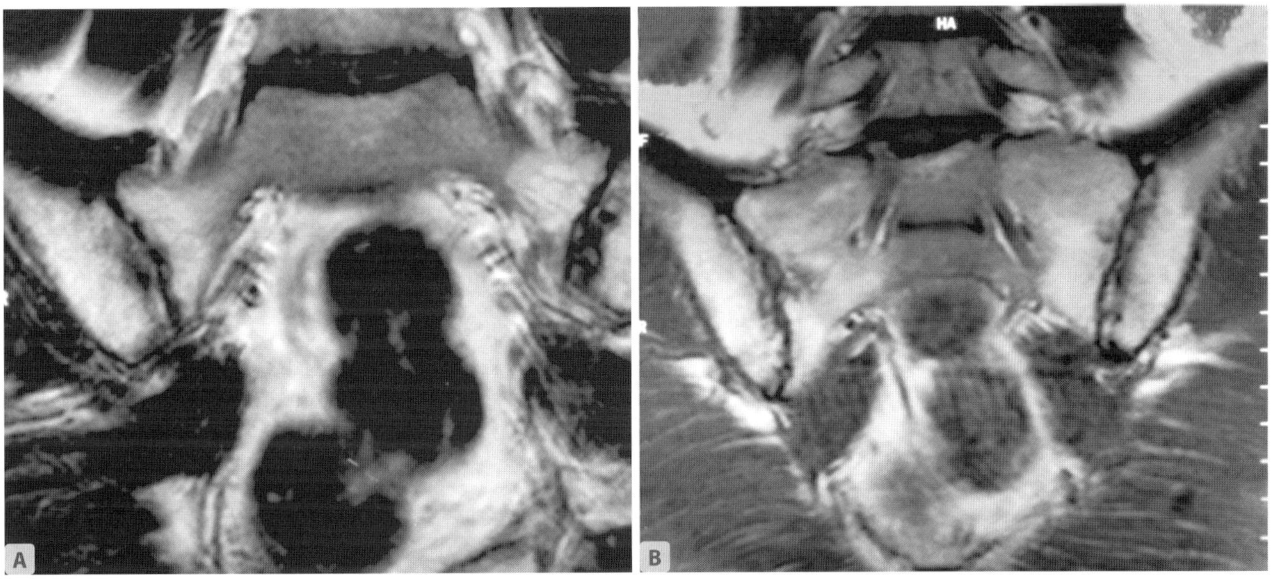

FIGS. 15A AND B: Ankylosing spondylitis. (A) T1- and (B) T2-weighted coronal images show irregularity of the cortex, discrete subchondral erosions, irregular thinning of the articular cartilage and reactive subarticular bone marrow edema and fatty change.

than CT for the detection of sacroiliitis.[36] MRI findings include erosions, subchondral sclerosis, bone marrow edema, intra-articular hyperintensity on T2- and T2*-weighted images with postcontrast enhancement within the joint cavity **(Figs. 15A and B)**. Radionuclide scanning shows nonspecific increased uptake in the presence of active sacroiliitis.

Spine

Spinal involvement classically starts at the dorsolumbar or lumbosacral junction with subsequent progressive involvement of the rest of the spine in an ascending manner. In females, the cervical region may be initially affected. Erosions initially occur at the vertebral margins at the site of attachment of the outer fibers of the annulus fibrosus (Romanus lesions) with adjacent sclerosis (shiny corner sign). In adolescents, these erosions may be quite large mimicking an infectious process (erosive spondylitis). Healing of these erosions or laying down of bone beneath the anterior longitudinal ligament causes "squaring" of the vertebral bodies, best appreciated on lateral radiographs of the lumbar spine. Exuberant new bone formation may even cause anterior convexity of the vertebral body (barrel-shaped vertebrae).[4,14,34] As the disease progresses, there is syndesmophyte formation along the anterior and anterolateral aspects of the body due to ossification in the annulus. Syndesmophytes are paravertebral in location and vertically oriented in contrast to the osteophytes seen in degenerative disease which are horizontally directed. The syndesmophytes seen in AS are classically marginal, symmetrical, fine and delicate. Ankylosis of multiple vertebrae by syndesmophytes gives the bamboo spine appearance. Similar ossifications may be seen in the interspinous ligaments and facet joints causing the dagger and tram-track signs respectively **(Figs. 16A and B)**. Facet joint ankylosis is the major factor causing loss of spinal mobility.[2-4,12]

Studies have demonstrated than MRI can identify active enthesitis in the spine much before Romanus lesions are seen on radiographs. MRI shows an abnormal area of low SI on T1-weighted image which is hyperintense on T2-weighted image and enhances postcontrast.[34]

Spinal fractures are common in the spine through the porotic bone just beneath the endplates. Two categories have been described: (1) the traumatic fractures and (2) stress fractures. Traumatic fractures occur after spinal fusion even with trivial trauma and are of the unstable category with involvement of all three columns. Stress fractures characteristically occur near the cervicothoracic or thoracolumbar junctions, with development of sclerotic pseudoarthrosis with destruction of the disc and vertebral endplates (Andersson lesion) resembling an infective discitis.[14,34]

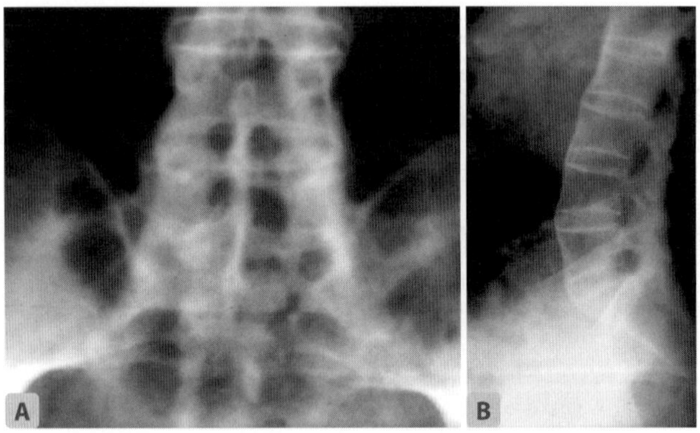

FIGS. 16A AND B: Ankylosing spondylitis: X-rays of lumbosacral spine (A) anteroposterior and (B) lateral views reveal the classical appearance of the bamboo spine on the lateral view and the dagger and tram-track signs on the AP view with bilateral ankylosis of the sacroiliac (SI) joints.

Cauda equina syndrome can result from arachnoiditis with large posterior dural diverticula causing osseous defects in the laminae. Both CT and MRI may delineate peripheral clumping of the nerve roots, laminar erosions, prominent arachnoid diverticula and dural calcifications.[14,34]

Atlantoaxial subluxation can occur but it is much less common than RA. There may be dramatic resorption of bone from the anterior aspects of the lower cervical vertebral bodies.[3]

Peripheral Joints

Ankylosing spondylitis is the only SSA where large joint involvement is not so uncommon. In general, the arthropathy resembles RA with a few differences. Shaggy periostitis and ankylosis are more common, whereas osteoporosis, erosions and joint space narrowing are less prominent.[14]

The hip joints are involved in up to 50% of patients with AS. Radiographic changes include concentric joint space narrowing, axial migration, cuff-like osteophytes on the femoral head and protrusio acetabuli with eventual joint fusion **(Figs. 17A to C)**. The shoulder is the next commonly involved joint and shows narrowing of the acromioclavicular and glenohumeral joint spaces and a hatchet deformity on the humeral head due to enthesitis of the rotator cuff tendon.[34] Small joint involvement is rare and is characterized by an asymmetric distribution, subtle erosions and proliferative bone changes at the involved joints.

Enthesopathies at tendinous and ligamentous insertions can cause erosions with marked sclerosis.[4] These can be frequently seen at the ischial tuberosity (ischial whiskering), iliac crest and the calcaneum.

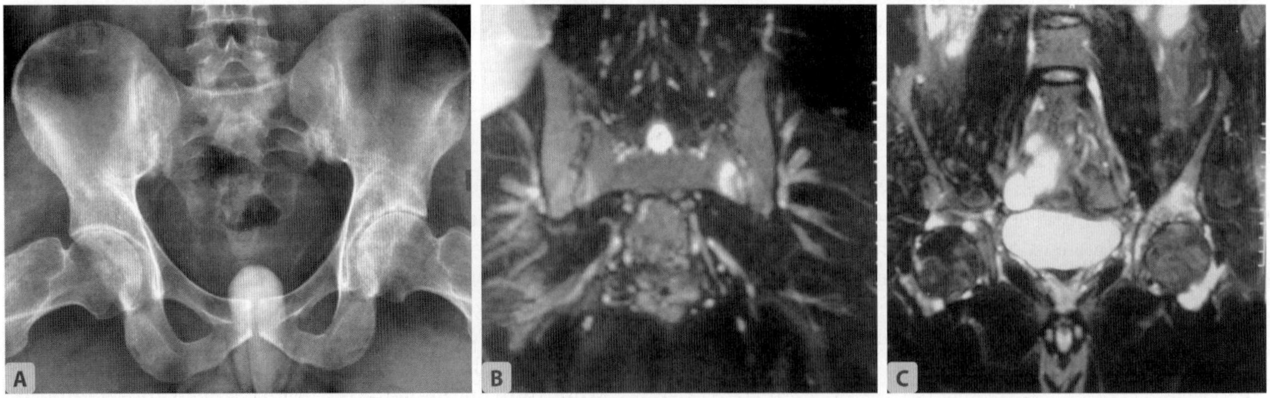

FIGS. 17A TO C: A 32-year-old male with ankylosing spondylitis. (A) X-ray of pelvis shows bilateral sacroiliitis with rat-bite erosions and fuzzy, irregular margins. Note the narrowing of the joint space with erosions in the left hip joint; (B) Coronal short tau inversion recovery (STIR) image shows bilateral sacroiliitis with bone marrow edema; (C) Coronal T2-weighted fat-saturated image demonstrates the narrowing of the left hip joint space, erosions and bone marrow edema.

PSORIATIC ARTHROPATHY

Psoriasis is a chronic inflammatory disease of the skin, which may be associated with a chronic inflammatory arthritis in 5–8% of cases. The incidence is highest between 20 and 39 years in males with females being affected later in the age group of 40–59 years. There is no gender predominance with both sexes being affected. The etiology is unknown. On histopathology, there is a chronic synovitis, which may cause joint destruction with inflammation of the tendon and ligamentous insertion sites.[34]

Skin lesions are usually seen on extensor surfaces, scalp and lumbosacral areas and are well-defined, dry, erythematous plaques with silvery scales. From a clinical standpoint, patients with PA can be broadly classified into three groups:[5,14,34]

1. Mono- or oligoarthritis with enteritis
2. Peripheral polyarthritis resembling RA
3. Predominant axial disease resembling AS with or without peripheral joint disease. This is rare, occurring in only 5% of patients.

The skin lesions precede the arthritis in 70% of patients; however, arthritis may precede skin lesions in 15% of cases. In another 15%, the two appear concomitantly.[14] The joints usually involved are the knee, DIP and PIP joints of the hands and feet, MTP and MCP joints and the ankles. Sacroiliitis may be seen in 35–50% and spondylitis in 30–40% of cases.[37]

Radiologic Features

The radiologic features are quite characteristic and the diagnosis can be strongly suggested on the basis of the presence of bone erosions and prominent bone proliferation which is the most characteristic feature in this condition.

The small joints of the hands and feet are most often involved in PA. A fusiform, soft tissue swelling is seen involving the entire digit (sausage digit). The involvement may be unilateral, if bilateral, it is asymmetric. All the joints of a single row may be affected. The bone density is preserved. Bony erosion classically starts at the joint margins. This may then proceed along either the articular surface (surface erosion) or progress along the joint capsule away from the joint along the metaphysis (enthesitic erosion).[34] This leads to a pencil-like tapering of the ends of the small bones. The joint space may be widened due to fibrous tissue deposition and bone resorption due to severe surface erosions resulting in the "pencil-in-cup" appearance. The enthesitic erosions combined with proliferation of bone may provide an irregular outline to the metaphyses or may widen the end of bone (mouse ears' sign) **(Figs. 18A and B)**.[4] Nail changes may be associated with resorption of the terminal tufts or the distal phalanges may become sclerotic. Calcaneal erosions with fluffy periosteal reaction can be seen at both the posterosuperior and posterior plantar aspects. Periosteal reaction commonly occurs along the diaphysis of the short tubular bones. In the advanced stages, there may be "arthritis mutilans" which is a term used to describe severe destruction of the joints of the hands and feet associated with extensive bone resorption.[14]

The sacroiliac joints may be involved in up to 50% of patients with PA and the involvement is usually bilateral. It may be symmetric or asymmetric and ankylosis is relatively uncommon. Involvement of the spine can happen in the absence of sacroiliitis and is commoner in males than females. This is characterized by coarse, asymmetric paravertebral ossification (nonmarginal syndesmophytes) in the dorsolumbar region in contrast to the symmetric, fine marginal syndesmophytes seen in AS.[2,4] These may be unilateral with skip areas. The anterior surface of the vertebral bodies is spared and squaring of the bodies is distinctly uncommon. There may be diffuse, ill-defined, paravertebral

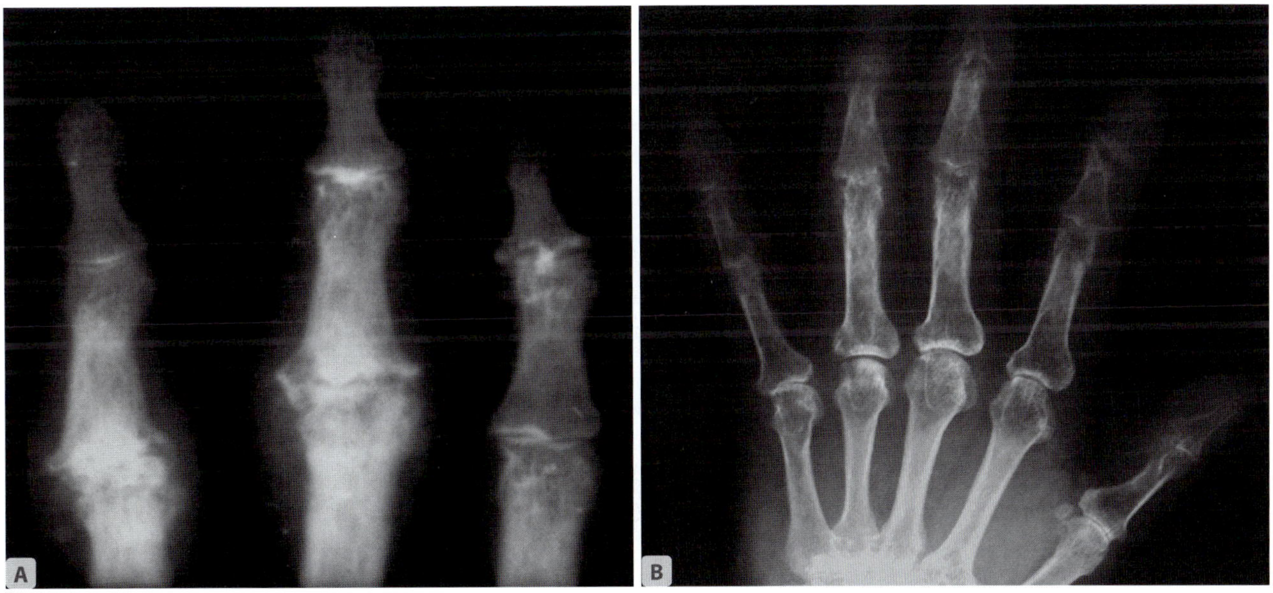

FIGS. 18A AND B: X-rays of the hands—magnified views reveal (A) fusiform soft tissue swelling with gross erosive changes at the distal interphalangeal (DIP) and proximal interphalangeal (PIP) joints. Note the subperiosteal bone apposition causing widening of the bone ends; (B) Erosive changes at the PIP and DIP joints with a "pencil-in-cup" appearance. These features are characteristic of psoriasis.

ossification. Isolated cervical involvement may be seen with apophyseal fusion and AAD.[34]

On MRI, signal changes are often visualized in the soft tissue as well as bone marrow related to the enthesitis reflecting inflammatory changes.[38]

REITER'S SYNDROME

Reiter's syndrome is a sexually transmitted disease commonly affecting young men which is characterized by arthritis, uveitis, and conjunctivitis. In Europe, a similar syndrome occurs in association with bacillary dysentery.[4,14]

Skeletal involvement may eventually occur in up to 80% of cases. There is a peripheral asymmetric arthritis with a predisposition for the joints of the lower limbs especially the feet where erosions occur at the heels, MTP joints and IP joint of the great toe. The DIP joints are rarely involved (in contrast to PA). Periostitis may be fine and lamellar in acute cases or fluffy and irregular in chronic cases. Reactive calcaneal spurs occur in 20% of patients.[3,14]

Sacroiliitis may develop in about 50% of cases and may be unilateral or asymmetrical in contrast to AS where it is classically bilaterally symmetrical **(Figs. 19A to C)**. Ankylosis is also less common. Coarse, asymmetric syndesmophytes similar to those seen in PA may occur, especially in the thoracolumbar region but occur less frequently.[2,4]

A summary of the joints involved, key features and laboratory parameters of RA and the SSAs are given in **Table 2**.[39]

ENTEROPATHIC SPONDYLOARTHROPATHY

This group comprises arthritides associated with inflammatory intestinal diseases such as regional enteritis (Crohn's disease), ulcerative colitis, and Whipple's disease.

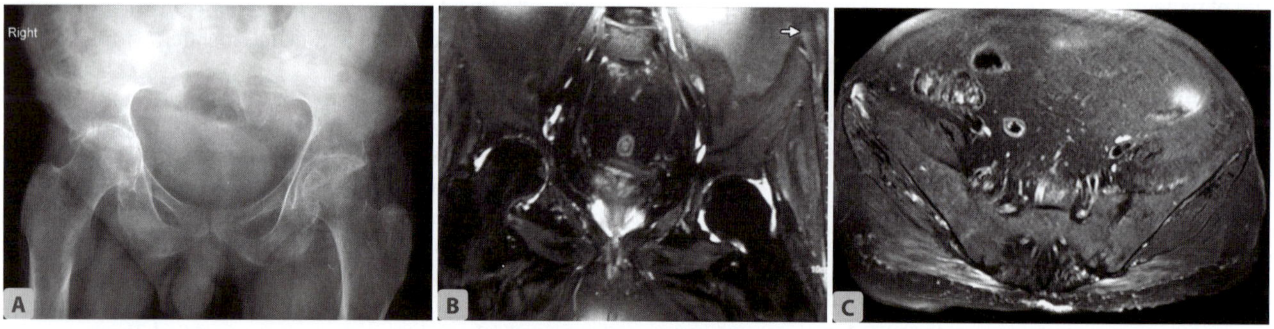

FIGS. 19A TO C: A 32-year-old male with Reiter's arthropathy. (A) X-ray of pelvis shows bilateral sacroiliitis with narrowing and irregularity of the right hip joint; (B) Coronal T2-weighted fat-saturated image shows fluid in bilateral hip joints with erosions and narrowing of the left hip joint; (C) Axial T2-weighted fat-saturated image shows asymmetric ankylosis of the sacroiliac joints.

TABLE 2: Distribution, key signs and laboratory parameters in rheumatoid arthritis and spondyloarthropathy.

Feature	Rheumatoid arthritis	Ankylosing spondylitis	Psoriatic arthritis	Reiter's syndrome
Distribution				
Upper extremity	+++	+	+++	–
(hands)	MCP/wrist	–	DIP/PIP	
Lower extremity	+++	+	+++	+++
Sacroiliac	+	+++	++	++
Bilateral	+	+++	++	++ (asymmetric)
Unilateral	+++	+	++	+++
Spine	++ (cervical)	+++	++	+
Key signs				
Osteoporosis	+++	+++	–	+
Joint space	+++ (narrowing)	++ (narrowing)	++ (widening)	+ (narrowing)
Ankylosis	+	+++	++	–
Periostitis	+ (linear)	+++ (fluffy)	+++ (fluffy)	+++ (fluffy)
Tuft resorption	–	–	+++	–
Soft tissue swelling	+++	+	++	++
Laboratory				
ESR	+++	+++	+	++
RA factor	+++	–	–	–
HLA-B27	6–8% (normal)	90%	30–75%	75%

HLA-B27 is present in most patients with spinal involvement.[4] There are two distinct types of joint involvement:

1. A spondylitis and sacroiliitis, which cannot be differentiated from AS can be seen in 6% of patients with inflammatory bowel disease and may even precede the development of bowel disease. Syndesmophyte formation, squaring of the vertebral bodies and apophyseal ankylosis are seen similar to AS. The sacroiliitis is bilateral and symmetric. These changes do not correlate with the activity of the gut disease and may continue to worsen even if the gut disease becomes quiescent.
2. A peripheral asymmetrical arthropathy with nonspecific features of soft tissue swelling and local periostitis. The activity of the arthropathy approximates the activity of the bowel disease.[14]

CRYSTAL DEPOSITION ARTHROPATHY

Gout

Gout is a metabolic disorder, which typically presents with recurrent attacks of arthritis. This is because of a disturbance in the metabolism of urates resulting in the deposition of monosodium urate (MSU) crystals within the joints along with soft tissues. Primary gout occurs due to inborn defects, either in the metabolism of purine or the secretion of urates by the renal tubules. Secondary gout can be caused by any acquired disorders that result in the increased turnover of nucleic acids (e.g., myeloproliferative disorders), by acquired defects in renal excretion of urates or due to certain drugs like cyclosporine.[40]

Men in the age group of 40–50 years are traditionally affected; however, gout also occurs in postmenopausal women. Four stages are seen clinically:[41]

1. Asymptomatic gout—presence of hyperuricemia.
2. Acute gouty arthritis—episodes of monoarticular peripheral acute arthritis, involving the 1st MTP joint of the great toe in 75% of cases. Later, the arthritis may be polyarticular and chronic and a phase of chronic gouty arthritis results.
3. Intercritical gout—refers to the symptom-free period between acute attacks.
4. Chronic tophaceous gout—this is characterized by the deposition of MSU crystals (tophi) in tendons, ligaments, cartilage, bone and other soft tissues including synovium or in the subcutaneous tissues in a para-articular location.

Definitive diagnosis involves the demonstration of MSU crystals in the synovial fluid. These are needle-shaped and show strong negative birefringence under polarized light microscopy.[4]

Imaging

Gout has several characteristic radiographic features, but these are seldom seen these days as it takes a few years (4–6) for gout to cause radiographically evident disease. By this time, most patients are correctly diagnosed and treated successfully.[2]

The classic findings are the presence of sharply marginated, round to oval erosions, which are oriented in the long axis of the bone, frequently showing sclerotic borders or overhanging edges **(Fig. 20)**. These are initially periarticular in location, but may later extend into the joint. There is a predilection for the 1st MTP joint; however, other joints such as the ankles, knee, elbow and wrist joint may also be affected. Spinal involvement is unusual but the sacroiliac joints may be involved in 5–13% of cases. The bone density is preserved till the late stages of the disease. Punctate, sclerotic foci may be seen in the bones owing to intraosseous deposition of tophi resembling enchondromas.[15] There is uneven articular space narrowing due to cartilage destruction. Para-articular tophi cause asymmetric "lumpy-bumpy" soft tissue swellings, which frequently show fluffy calcification in the presence of renal disease **(Fig. 21)**. These tophi may saucerize the

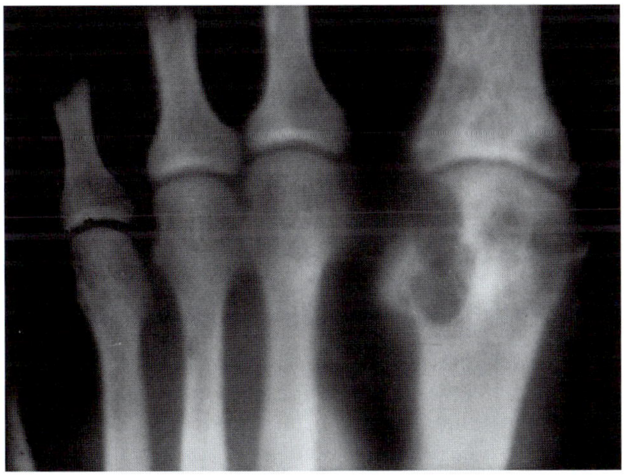

FIG. 20: X-ray of the 1st metatarsophalangeal (MTP) joint shows well-defined periarticular erosions with overhanging edges classical of gout.

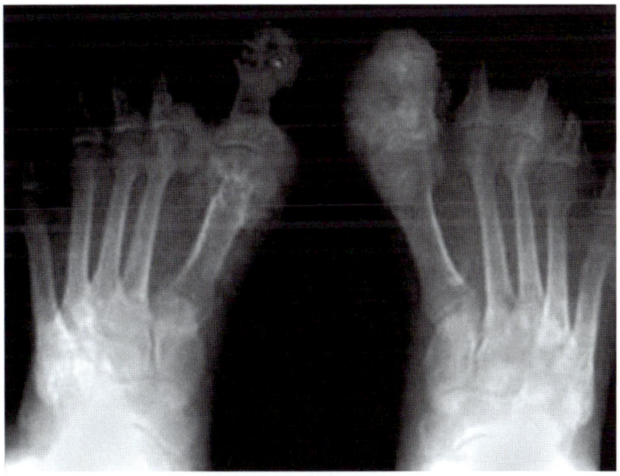

FIG. 21: X-ray of both feet shows advanced changes of gout with multiple soft tissue tophi, some of which are calcified. Gross periarticular erosions are seen in both 1st MTP joints. Note the saucerization of the left 1st proximal phalanx due to overlying soft tissue tophi.

underlying bone. Chondrocalcinosis may be seen because up to 40% of patients with gout have concomitant CPPD deposition disease. Nephrolithiasis may be present in 20% of cases.[2]

On MRI, an inflamed joint will show joint effusion and para-articular edema with enhancement of the para-articular structures postcontrast. Tophaceous deposits show a low to intermediate SI on T1 with high SI on T2-weighted images. If calcified, the tophi demonstrate low signal on T2-weighted images.[40]

Calcium Pyrophosphate Dihydrate Crystal Deposition Disease

Calcium pyrophosphate dihydrate crystal deposition disease occurs due to the deposition of CPPD crystals in hyaline as well as fibrocartilage along with soft tissues. It is characterized by acute, subacute or chronic joint inflammation. The crystals of CPPD are weakly birefringent on polarized light microscopy. The disease may cause intermittent attacks of acute arthritis when it is called pseudogout.[3]

The classic triad consists of pain, cartilage calcification and joint destruction. Chondrocalcinosis can occur in any joint but usually involves the medial and lateral compartments of the knee, the triangular cartilage and lunotriquetral ligament in the wrist and the symphysis pubis **(Fig. 22)**. When CPPD crystals are found in the soft tissues such as the rotator cuff, they cannot be differentiated from calcium hydroxyapatite crystals, which occur in calcific tendinitis.[2]

The arthropathy of CPPD is a degenerative joint disease caused by the crystals eroding the cartilage. However, CPPD has a tendency to involve the shoulder, elbow, wrist and the patellofemoral compartment of the knee, sites which are not usually involved by degenerative joint disease. Occasionally, CPPD arthropathy may accelerate and severe destruction occurs to such an extent that it mimics a neuropathic joint.[2]

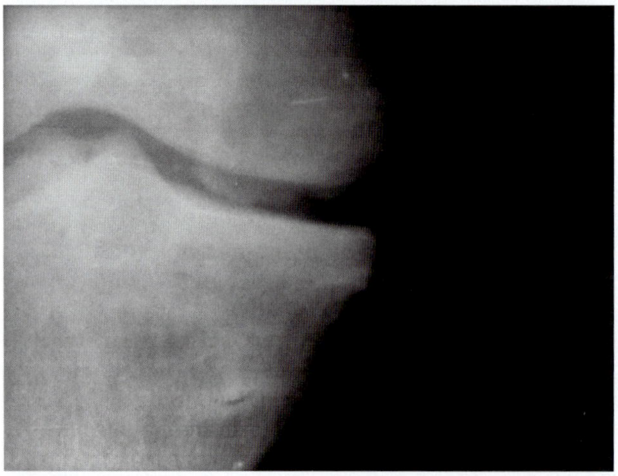

FIG. 22: Magnified view of the knee joint demonstrating chondrocalcinosis.

SYSTEMIC LUPUS ERYTHEMATOSUS

Systemic lupus erythematosus is an autoimmune disease, which can involve multiple organ systems and has a wide age range. Imaging is often done in diagnosed cases to ascertain the extent of the disease and to discover complications. Antiphospholipid antibody syndrome is seen in 27–42% of patients with SLE. Different systems involved in SLE patients would require imaging accordingly like ultrasound or angiography to look for deep venous thrombosis, arterial thrombosis and vasculitis. CT and MRI scans are used to look for strokes, Budd–Chiari syndrome, interstitial lung diseases, arthritis (symmetric and nonerosive), muscle atrophy, insufficiency fractures, etc.[42]

IDIOPATHIC INFLAMMATORY MYOPATHY

Idiopathic inflammatory myopathies are a category of muscle disorders, which are distinguished by proximal muscle weakness as the unique feature. These are rare disorders. Most common of these are dermatomyositis, polymyositis and inclusion body myositis. Biopsy of the muscle should be performed to confirm the diagnosis and exclude other possible causes of proximal myopathy.[43] IIM classification has been improved and according to the recommendation criteria published by EULAR/ACR (2017),[44] the subgroups are: Polymyositis, polymyositis subset includes immune-mediated necrotizing myopathies, inclusion body myositis, amyotrophic dermatomyositis, dermatomyositis, and juvenile dermatomyositis.[44]

Imaging on various modalities shows decrease in the muscle bulk, abnormal attenuation or SI and any destruction of normal muscle morphology, if present. Imaging also helps identifying high-yield biopsy sites to avoid negative biopsies by avoiding fibrotic areas and including inflammation (activity) areas. USG has high sensitivity in detecting myositis, which is comparable with electromyography or serum creatine kinase (CK) activity. Contrast-enhanced USG shows presence of muscle edema and inflammatory hypervascularization, and on follow-up these areas can show normal soft tissue after treatment.[43]

Magnetic resonance imaging shows presence of muscle edema. The most sensitive sequences to differentiate edema from fatty infiltration are the fat-suppressed T2 or STIR sequences. Specific MRI patterns associated with the various subtypes of IIMs have been demonstrated nowadays.[45]

Functional imaging may have a role to play in IIMs but are not yet standardized.[43]

SYSTEMIC SCLEROSIS (SCLERODERMA)

Systemic sclerosis is a chronic autoimmune disease which characteristically causes inflammation of the skin and multiple internal organs.[46] Contractures of the skin are the hallmark of the disease but many patients have joint involvement ranging from mild (arthralgia) to severe (frank arthritis). Joint contractures may occur and tendons can be involved.[47]

Joint involvement may be oligoarticular or polyarticular. Any of the joints can be affected, although there is predominant involvement of the small joints of the hands (in particular the MCP and PIP joints), wrist, and ankle joints.

Fibrinous deposits can occur on the surface of tendon sheaths along with the overlying fascia leading to tendon abnormalities such as a leathery crepitus on palpation of the joints. Bursal involvement may be recurrent. In rare cases, inflammatory proliferative tenosynovitis can result in tendon rupture. RF positivity occurs in up to 30% patients with systemic sclerosis. Presence of anti-citrullinated cyclic peptide (CCP) antibodies helps in the identification of infrequent cases of true systemic sclerosis-RA overlap. On imaging there may be juxta-articular osteoporosis, narrowing of the joint space and even frank erosions involving MCP, PIP and DIP joints (more on the dorsal aspect) and wrist. The 1st carpometacarpal joint may be involved. Pencil-in-cup deformity has also been seen. These articular features occur along with nonarticular features like atrophy of the skin, subcutaneous calcinosis and resorption of the digital tufts on radiography.[48]

FIBROMYALGIA SYNDROME

Fibromyalgia is a syndrome in which patients present with chronic diffuse pain at multiple tendon points along with joint stiffness. Systemic symptoms can occur like mood disorders, cognitive dysfunction, fatigue, and insomnia. Associations with rheumatic pathologies, psychiatric or neurologic disorders, infections and diabetes can be seen.[49]

BURSITIS

Bursae are located where tendons continuously move over bony surfaces or against each other. They are named depending on to their location like subcutaneous, subtendinous, subfascial or submucosal. They are synovial lined sacs that may be communicating or noncommunicating. Bursae near the joints communicate with the joint cavity. Normal bursae cannot be visualized on imaging. They may be seen as cystic, fluid-filled spaces with inflamed walls (thickened and enhancing on imaging) in pathological conditions.[50]

TENDINITIS AND TENOSYNOVITIS

Tendinopathy is a wide term, which is used to describe tendon pain without knowing the specific etiology of the pain. The pain could be due to tears from trauma, inflammatory enthesitis or even chronic degeneration. Tendinitis implies the inflammatory response in arthritis and is associated with decreased function and pain. Tendinosis defines a degenerative state.[51]

Acute tendinitis on imaging presents with increased fluid within the synovial sheath. In chronic tendinitis, there is thickening of the tendon associated with increased fluid in the synovial cavity of the joint. Tenosynovitis is the inflammation of the tendon sheaths caused by various causes like trauma, infections, and RA. Ganglia are the cystic lesions arising from synovial lining of joint or tendon.[52]

BEHÇET'S DISEASE

Behçet's disease is a chronic, systemic disorder distinguished by relapses with recurrent ulcers involving the oral cavity or genitalia, uveitis and involvement of multiple organ systems. Radiologically, its involvement in various body systems shows characteristic features like neuro-Behçet's disease, dural sinus thrombosis, meningitis, vascular occlusions, periaortic pseudoaneurysm, pulmonary thromboembolism, etc.[53]

Arthritis is the most common manifestation of musculoskeletal involvement with the usual pattern being monoarticular involvement. Most commonly, unilateral knee joint involvement is seen. AS without HLA-B5 or HLA-B27 association is seen in around 10% cases.[54]

REFERENCES

1. Østensen M. Drugs in pregnancy: rheumatological disorders. Best Pract Res Clin Obstet Gynaecol. 2001;15: 953-69.
2. Helms CA. Arthritis. In: Helms CA (Ed). Fundamentals of Skeletal Radiology. Philadelphia: WB Saunders; 1989. pp. 135-76.
3. Martel W. Diagnostic radiology in the rheumatic diseases. In: Kelley WN, Harris ED Jr, Ruddy S, Sledge CB (Eds). Textbook of Rheumatology. Philadelphia: WB Saunders; 1982. pp. 580-621.
4. Greenspan A. Inflammatory arthritides. In: Greenspan A (Ed). Orthopedic Radiology: A Practical Approach, 3rd edition. Philadelphia: Lippincott, Williams and Wilkins; 2000. pp. 453-78.
5. Sommer OJ, Kladosek A, Weiler V, Czembirek H, Boeck M, Stiskal M. Rheumatoid arthritis: a practical guide to state-of-the-art imaging, image interpretation, and clinical implications. Radiographics. 2005;25:381-98.
6. Narváez JA, Narváez J, De Lama E, De Albert M. MR imaging of early rheumatoid arthritis. Radiographics. 2010;30:143-65.
7. Arnett FC, Edworthy SM, Bloch DA, McShane DJ, Fries JF, Cooper NS, et al. The American Rheumatism Association 1987 revised criteria for the classification of rheumatoid arthritis. Arthritis Rheum. 1988;31:315-24.
8. Sugimoto H, Takeda A, Hyodo K. Early stage rheumatoid arthritis: prospective study of the effectiveness of MR imaging for diagnosis. Radiology. 2000;216:569-75.
9. Østergaard M, Ejbjerg B, Szkudlarek M. Imaging in early rheumatoid arthritis: roles of magnetic resonance imaging, ultrasonography, conventional radiography and computed tomography. Best Pract Res Clin Rheumatol. 2005;19(1): 91-116.
10. Kay J, Upchurch KS. ACR/EULAR 2010 rheumatoid arthritis classification criteria. Rheumatology (Oxford). 2012;51:vi5-9.
11. Imhof H, Nobauer-Huhmann IM, Gahleitner A, Kainberger F, Krestan C, Sulzbacher I, et al. Pathophysiology and imaging in inflammatory and blastomatous synovial diseases. Skeletal Radiol. 2002;31(6):313-33.
12. Resnick D. Rheumatoid arthritis and the seronegative spondyloarthropathies: radiographic and pathologic concepts. In: Resnick B (Ed). Diagnosis of Bone and Joint Disorders, 4th edition. Philadelphia: WB Saunders; 2002. pp. 837-90.
13. Renner WR, Weinstein AS. Early changes of rheumatoid arthritis in the hand and wrist. Radiol Clin North Am. 1988;26:1185-93.

14. Renton P. Diseases of joints. In: Sutton D (Ed). Textbook of Radiology and Imaging, 7th edition. Churchill Livingstone; 2003. pp. 1201-45.
15. Resnick D. Rheumatoid arthritis. In: Resnick D (Ed). Diagnosis of Bone and Joint Disorders, 4th edition. Philadelphia: WB Saunders; 2002. pp. 891-987.
16. Wakefield RJ, Gibbon WW, Conaghan PG, O'Connor P, McGonagle D, Pease C, et al. The value of sonography in the detection of bone erosions in patients with rheumatoid arthritis: a comparison with conventional radiography. Arthritis Rheum. 2000;43:2762-70.
17. Brown AK, Wakefied RJ, Conaghan PG, Karini Z, O' Connor PJ, Emery P. New approaches to imaging early inflammatory arthritis. Clin Exp Rheumatol. 2004;22(5 Suppl 35):S18-25.
18. Backhaus M, Kamradt T, Sandrock D, Loreck D, Fritz J, Wolf KJ, et al. Arthritis of the finger joints: a comprehensive approach comparing conventional radiography, scintigraphy, ultrasound, and contrast-enhanced magnetic resonance imaging. Arthritis Rheum. 1999;42(6):1232-45.
19. El-Miedany YM, Housny IH, Mansour HM, Mourad HG, Mehanna AM, Megeed MA. Ultrasound versus MRI in the evaluation of juvenile idiopathic arthritis of the knee. Joint Bone Spine. 2001;68(3):222-30.
20. Polster J, Winalski CS, Sundaram M, Lieber ML, Schils J, Ilaslan H, et al. Rheumatoid arthritis: evaluation with contrast-enhanced CT with digital bone masking. Radiology. 2009;252(1):225-31.
21. Tehranzadeh J, Ashikyan O, Dascalos J. Advanced imaging of early rheumatoid arthritis. Radiol Clin North Am. 2004;42:89-107.
22. McQueen FM, Benton N, Perry D, Crabbe J, Robinson E, Yeoman S, et al. Bone edema scored on magnetic resonance imaging scans of the dominant carpus at presentation predicts radiographic joint damage of the hands and feet six years later in patients with rheumatoid arthritis. Arthritis Rheum. 2003;48(7):1814-27.
23. McQueen F, Beckley V, Crabbe J, Robinson E, Yeoman S, Stewart N. Magnetic resonance imaging evidence of tendinopathy in early rheumatoid arthritis predicts tendon rupture at six years. Arthritis Rheum. 2005;52(3):744-51.
24. Larsen A. How to apply Larsen score in evaluating radiographs of rheumatoid arthritis in long-term studies. J Rheumatol. 1995;22:1974-75.
25. Østergaard M, Peterfy C, Conaghan P, McQueen F, Bird P, Ejbjerg B, et al. OMERACT rheumatoid arthritis magnetic resonance imaging studies: core set of MRI acquisitions, joint pathology definitions, and the OMERACT RA-MRI scoring system. J Rheumatol. 2003;30(6):1385-6.
26. Ajeganova S, Huizinga T. Sustained remission in rheumatoid arthritis: latest evidence and clinical considerations. Ther Adv Musculoskelet Dis. 2017;9(10):249-62.
27. Petty RE, Southwood TR, Baum J, Bhettay E, Glass DN, Manners P, et al. Revision of the proposed classification criteria for juvenile idiopathic arthritis: Durban,1997. J Rheumatol. 1998;25:1991-4.
28. Buchmann RF, Jaramillo D. Imaging of articular disorders in children. Radiol Clin North Am. 2004;42:151-68.
29. Doria AS, Kiss MH, Lotito AP, Molnar LJ, de Castro CC, Medeiros CC, et al. Juvenile rheumatoid arthritis of the knee: evaluation with contrast-enhanced color Doppler ultrasound. Pediatr Radiol. 2001;31(7):524-31.
30. Kakati P, Sodhi KS, Sandhu MS, Singh S, Katariya S, Khandelwal N. Clinical and ultrasound assessment of the knee in children with juvenile rheumatoid arthritis. Indian J Pediatr. 2007;74(9): 831-6.
31. Shanmugavel C, Sodhi KS, Sandhu MS, Sidhu R, Singh S, Katariya S, Khandelwal N. Role of power Doppler sonography in evaluation of therapeutic response of the knee in juvenile rheumatoid arthritis. Rheumatol Int. 2008;28(6):573-8.
32. Lamer S, Sebag GH. MRI and ultrasound in children with juvenile chronic arthritis. Eur J Radiol. 2000;33(2):85-93.
33. Dougados M, van der Linden S, Juhlin R, Huitfeldt B, Amor B, Calin A, et al. The European Spondyloarthropathy Study Group preliminary criteria for the classification of spondyloarthropathy. Arthritis Rheum. 1991;34:1218-27.
34. Bennett DL, Ohashi K, El-Khoury GY. Spondyloarthropathies: ankylosing spondylitis and psoriatic arthritis. Radiol Clin North Am. 2004;42:121-32.
35. van der Linden S, Valkenburg HA, Cats A. Evaluation of diagnostic criteria for ankylosing spondylitis: a proposal for modification of the New York Criteria. Arthritis Rheum. 1984;27(4):361-8.
36. Bollow M, Braun J, Hamm B, Eggens U, Schilling A, König H, et al. Early sacroiliitis in patients with spondyloarthropathies: evaluation with dynamic gadolinium-enhanced MR imaging. Radiology. 1995;194(2):529-36.
37. Boumpas DT, Illei GG, Tassiulas IO. Psoriatic arthritis. In: Klippel JH (Ed). Primer on the Rheumatic Diseases, 12th edition. Atlanta: Arthritis Foundation; 2001. pp. 233-8.
38. Weishaupt D, Schweitzer ME, Alam F, Karasick D, Wapner K. MR imaging of inflammatory joint diseases of the foot and ankle. Skeletal Radiol. 1999;28:663-9.
39. Yochum TR, Rowe LJ. Arthritic disorders. In: Yochum TR, Rowe LJ (Eds). Yochum and Rowe's Essentials of Skeletal Radiology. Philadelphia: Lippincott, Williams and Wilkins; 2005. pp. 951-1136.
40. Monu JU, Pope TL. Gout: a clinical and radiological review. Radiol Clin North Am. 2004;42:169-84.
41. Resnick D. Gouty arthritis. In: Resnick D (Ed). Diagnosis of Bone and Joint Disorders, 4th edition. Philadelphia: WB Saunders; 2002. pp. 1519-59.
42. Lalani TA, Kanne JP, Hatfield GA, Chen P. Imaging findings in systemic lupus erythematosus. Radiographics. 2004;24:1069-86.
43. Gazeley DJ, Cronin ME. Diagnosis and treatment of the idiopathic inflammatory myopathies. Ther Adv Musculoskelet Dis. 2011;3(6):315-24.
44. Leclair V, Lundberg IE. New myositis classification criteria: what we have learned since Bohan and Peter. Curr Rheumatol Rep. 2018;20:18.
45. Kubinova K, Dejthevaporn R, Mann H, Machado PM, Vencovsky J. The role of imaging in evaluating patients with idiopathic inflammatory myopathies. Clin Exp Rheumatol. 2018;36:S74-81.
46. Terenzi R, Karalilova R, Lepri G, Bruni C, Bellando-Randone S, Manetti M, et al. Enthesopathy and involvement of synovio-entheseal complex in systemic sclerosis: an ultrasound pilot study. Rheumatology (Oxford). 2020;59:580-5.
47. Sandler RD, Matucci-Cerinic M, Hughes M. Musculoskeletal hand involvement in systemic sclerosis. Semin Arthritis Rheum. 2019;11:1-6.
48. Avouac J, Clements PJ, Khanna D, Furst DE, Allanore Y. Articular involvement in systemic sclerosis. Rheumatology (Oxford). 2012;51:1347-56.
49 Bellato E, Marini E, Castoldi F, Barbasetti N, Mattei L, Bonasia DE, et al. Fibromyalgia syndrome: etiology, pathogenesis, diagnosis, and treatment. Pain Res Treat. 2012;2012:426130.
50. Hirji Z, Hunjun JS, Choudur HN. Imaging of the bursae. J Clin Imaging Sci. 2011;1:22.
51. Charnoff J, Naqvi U. Tendinosis (Tendinitis). In: StatPearls [Internet]. Treasure Island (FL): StatPearls Publishing; 2019.
52. Kharat AT, Singh A, Ranganath P, Kulkarni VM. Tendinitis and tenosynovitis—a pictorial essay. Ind J Radiol Imaging. 2006;16(2): 235-7.
53. Chae EJ, Do KH, Seo JB, Park SH, Kang JW, Jang YM, et al. Radiologic and clinical findings of Behçet disease: comprehensive review of multisystemic involvement. Radiographics. 2008;28(5):e31.
54. Fatemi A, Shahram F, Akhlaghi M, Smiley A, Nadji A, Davatchi F. Prospective study of articular manifestations in Behçet's disease: five-year report. Int J Rheum Dis. 2017;20(1):97-102.

CHAPTER

160

Degenerative Disease of the Spine

Jyoti Kumar, Anju Garg, Anjali Prakash

INTRODUCTION

Degenerative disease of the spine is a ubiquitous collection of conditions that represent some of the most common indications for spine magnetic resonance imaging (MRI). Degenerative changes may arise in the vertebrae, intervertebral discs, facet joints and ligaments. Degeneration at various sites is linked to each other since the main common pathogenetic factor is chronic overload. The intervertebral articulation consists of a three-joint complex consisting of the amphiarthrodial endplate-disc-endplate joint of the anterior column and the two diarthrodial facet joints of the posterior column supported by ligaments and muscle groups. In the cervical spine, uncovertebral joints (joints of Luschka) are the other lateral articulations between the vertebral bodies. The intervertebral disc space consists of the inner nucleus pulposus, outer annulus fibrosus, and hyaline cartilaginous endplates. The ligaments consist of the anterior longitudinal ligament (ALL), posterior longitudinal ligament (PLL), ligamentum flavum (LF), and interspinous ligaments. Since involvement of one site predisposes the other sites to degenerative changes owing to altered biomechanical forces, patients often present with degenerative changes in multiple sites.[1,2]

IMAGING MODALITIES

Back pain requires imaging if it is persistent for >6 weeks or when there is accompanying neurologic deficit, fever, trauma, acute pain in the setting of osteoporosis/cancer/steroid use or history of serious medical condition (e.g., cancer).[3]

Radiographs are often the first imaging modality used to evaluate back pain. However, the role of radiographs is often to exclude other diagnoses than to directly evaluate degenerative disease. The findings that may be seen on radiographs include loss of disc height, irregularity and sclerosis of endplates, osteophytes, Schmorl's nodes (herniation of disc material into the endplate) or intradiscal gas **(Figs. 1A and B)**.

Magnetic resonance imaging is the modality of choice in evaluation of degenerative spine because of its superior soft tissue contrast. It allows direct visualization of intervertebral

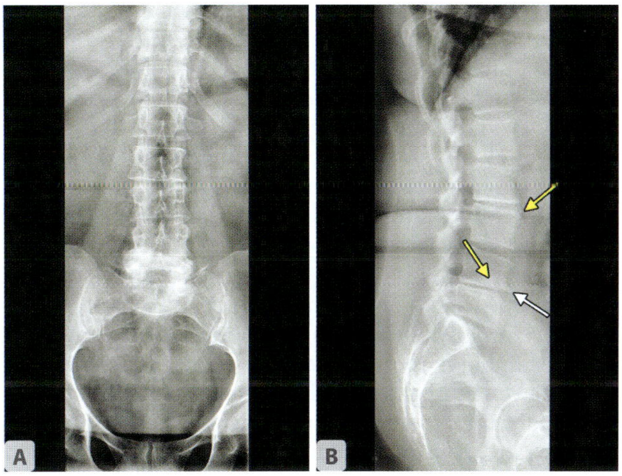

FIGS. 1A AND B: (A) X-rays of lumbar spine anteroposterior and **(B)** lateral views depict reduced disc spaces most marked at L2/L3, L4/L5 and L5/S1 levels with endplate sclerotic changes (yellow arrows) and osteophyte formation (white arrow).

discs and neural elements. Contrast MRI is usually not required and is more used in postoperative examinations to differentiate residual and recurrent herniations from scar tissue. It may also be used sometimes in the preoperative setting to detect annular fissures and inflammatory processes that may accompany acute disc desiccation such as facet joint synovitis and radiculitis. MRI can also pick up other alternative causes of back pain such as inflammation, infection, and tumors.

Computed tomography (CT) is unable to detect early disc desiccation. However, it demonstrates superior spatial resolution and improved conspicuity of osseous and calcified structures and intradiscal gas.[4] It can detect advanced changes like disc space narrowing and sclerotic endplate changes. CT is more sensitive than MRI for detecting the presence of transdiscal gas, predominantly nitrogen. This is known as the vacuum phenomenon and is very specific for disc degeneration and is only rarely encountered in infective discitis.[1] CT is also more accurate in detection of discal calcification and posterior osteophytes which may have therapeutic implications.

On MRI, bright T1 signal may be found with mild to moderate intradiscal calcium deposition.[1,2]

Imaging studies with 6–12 months follow-up have demonstrated that nearly 63% of disc herniations may show spontaneous reduction in size. This may be due to dehydration, fragmentation and phagocytosis of the disc material. This is greatest in extrusions and sequestrations.[2] Radiology is also involved in interventional techniques for therapeutic purpose, e.g., automated discectomy, percutaneous laser disc decompression, intradiscal oxygen-ozone injection. Their success rates range from 70 to 80% with minimal potential complications.[2]

Complementary tests in evaluation of degenerative spine include radiography, discography, conventional myelography, CT myelography, and nuclear scintigraphy. Plain films are inexpensive, widely available and give a panoramic view of the entire spine. Bones can be directly visualized and functional information regarding alignment and stability can be obtained with upright dynamic films in flexion-extension and lateral bending. Myelography is reserved only for patients with contraindications to MRI or in whom subtle instability is suspected but not confirmed by other examinations. Discography is reserved for selected patients before intervention or when the diagnosis of discogenic pain must be confirmed.[2]

Upright MRI is advocated by some groups as axial loading in this position owing to gravity, patient's weight, and spine morphology enables MRI evaluation in natural state of loading. This has also been proven to be useful when there is suspicion of dynamic foraminal stenosis and in patients with positional pain difference. However, there is limited availability of upright MRI with additional problems of poor resolution, increased motion artifacts, and higher false-positive rates. Dynamic flexion extension is also possible in these units.[2] Dynamic plain films, weight-bearing CT or MRI have been used for the study of spinal stenosis. Previously occult abnormalities, including disc herniation, ligamentous infolding, subluxations may all be demonstrated using kinematic MRI. Functional information regarding vertebral stability may also be provided on dynamic examination.

PATHOPHYSIOLOGY

Pathogenetic mechanisms are multiple and chronic overload is the most important factor. The other causes are sequelae to acute trauma, metabolic, toxic, genetic, vascular or infectious causes. The distribution of axial load determines the common sites of spine degeneration. In the cervical spine, it is C5-C6 and C6-C7 levels as these are the sites of lordosis inversion. The dorsal spine is rarely involved as it is less mobile and less involved in dynamic load. In the lumbar spine, L4-L5 and L5-S1 are the sites of highest dynamic and static overload and hence most predisposed to degenerative changes.[2]

In patients with degenerative changes of the spine, there are multiple mechanisms that act in combination to produce pain.[6] These are:

- Biochemical mediators of inflammation resulting from disc degeneration and herniation.
- Mechanical compression of nerves by bone, ligament or disc material.
- Instability or abnormal motion with associated disc degeneration and facet arthropathy.
- Disruption of free nerve endings in the outer annular fibers.

ANATOMY OF INTERVERTEBRAL DISC

The intervertebral disc has an inner nucleus pulposus and an outer annulus fibrosus and is bordered by cartilaginous endplates. The nucleus pulposus is made up of >80% water and consists of hydrated proteoglycans supported by network of elastin and collagen type 2 fibers. Over time, the gelatinous proteoglycans are replaced by fibrocartilage. The nucleus is eccentrically located and more closely related to the posterior surface of the intervertebral disc. The annulus is composed of dense collagen type 1 fibers. The collagen in the inner annulus is less plentiful than in the outer ring. The annular fibers become progressively more compact centrifugally. The outermost fibers are the densest, known as Sharpey's fibers.

The nucleus pulposus converts much of the axial force into radial force and functions to spread the load evenly over the adjacent endplate. Cartilaginous endplates are composed of hyaline cartilage. These are usually not well discernible on imaging. Surrounding the cartilaginous endplate is a ring of dense bone, the ring apophysis that fuses to the vertebra in the 2nd decade of life. Fetal and infantile discs are well vascularized but these branches soon atrophy and the adult disc becomes avascular. It obtains its nutrition by diffusion from vertebral endplates.[4] The intervertebral discs in the lumbar region are thicker than those in the cervical and dorsal region.

MAGNETIC RESONANCE APPEARANCE OF INTERVERTEBRAL DISC

The normal intervertebral discs are of slightly lower signal intensity than bone marrow on T1-weighted images (T1WIs) and with higher T2 signal. The annulus is seen as a peripheral region of low signal intensity on T2-weighted images (T2WIs) and nucleus pulposus is hyperintense, owing to high water content of nucleus pulposus. A horizontal internuclear cleft of fibrous tissue containing collagenous, elastic and reticular fibers may normally be seen on T2WI in over 90% of patients over 30 years of age and is considered a paraphysiologic change.[1,2] On T1WI, the distinction between the nucleus and annular fibers is less discernible **(Figs. 2A to C)**, similar to CT. The endplates are well defined and smooth with intact cortical bone.

DEGENERATIVE CHANGES OF THE SPINE

The intervertebral disc undergoes marked changes with aging. With aging, small concentric and transverse tears may develop in the annulus. The composition of the intervertebral disc may change with decrease in glycosaminoglycans and increase in collagen; and hence a decrease in affinity for water. Therefore, aging can reduce the signal intensity of the disc by a few percent. However, it may be confusing to

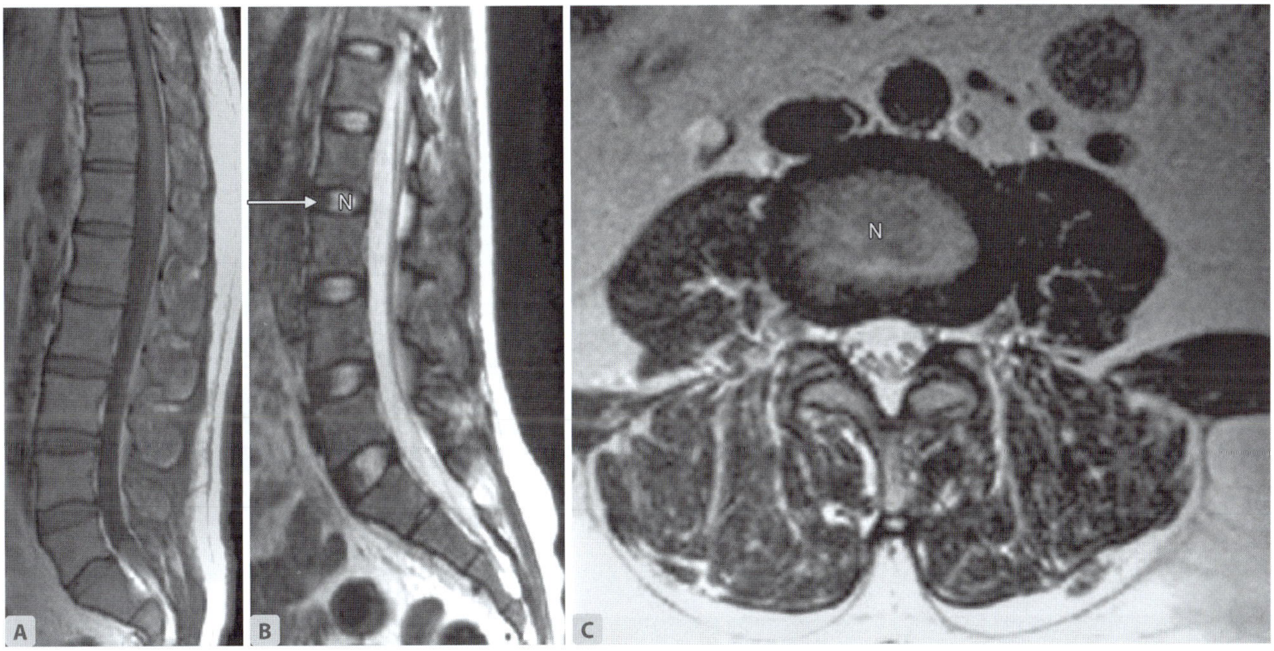

FIGS. 2A TO C: (A) Sagittal T1W, (B) T2W, and (C) axial T2W MR images of lumbosacral spine show normal intervertebral disc that is slightly lower signal intensity than bone marrow on T1W images and with higher T2 signal. The annulus is seen as a peripheral region of low signal intensity on T2W images (arrow) and nucleus pulposus (N) is hyperintense. A horizontal internuclear cleft is seen on T2W sagittal image.

differentiate changes of aging from changes of degeneration. Hence, the term degenerated disc includes the changes of aging as well.[7] Degenerating discs in addition show enhanced inflammatory changes with catabolic metabolism. These undergo desiccation, loss of height, fissures, bulging and herniations. Pfirrmann et al. classified disc degeneration based on the following features—disc structure, distinction between nucleus pulposus and annulus fibrosus, disc signal, and disc height.[8]

Structural Disc Changes

On MR, the earliest appearance of degeneration of the nucleus is desiccation (progressive loss of water), which manifests as low signal intensity on T2WIs instead of high signal of normally hydrated discs **(Fig. 3)**. Although it is usually asymptomatic, it suggests disc overload and is a precursor to further degenerative abnormalities.[1,2] A feature of interest to remember in the cervical spine is that loss of signal intensity of cervical discs may not be helpful in identification of degenerated disc as cervical discs have lower signal intensity compared to lumbar discs.

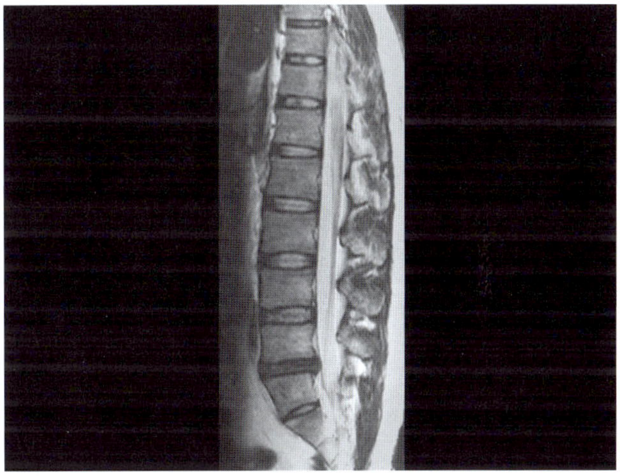

FIG. 3: Sagittal T2W MR image of lumbosacral spine shows decreased T2 signal of L4/L5 disc with loss of differentiation between nucleus and annulus fibrosus suggestive of disc desiccation. Note made of transitional vertebra.

There is progressive loss of disc height. Development of annular fissures results in shrinkage of fibrocartilage in the nucleus pulposus and replacement by dense fibrous tissue and cystic spaces. The disc becomes more and more fibrous and disorganized with no clear distinction between nucleus and annulus.[6] Negative pressure produced by abnormal spaces pulls in gas, predominantly nitrogen resulting in vacuum disc phenomenon **(Figs. 4A and B)**. The disc may show linear or patchy low-signal intensity either due to gas or sometimes, calcification. When occasionally fluid may be pulled instead of nitrogen, there may be paradoxical high signal appearance of the disc on T2WI instead of the low signal intensity of desiccated disc. Associated disc narrowing and endplate changes and osteophytes are pointers that this seemingly hydrated disc is a degenerated disc. With progress of degeneration, disc calcification may occur. This can appear as increased or decreased signal on T1WI. Paradoxical high signal on T1WI may be seen depending on the amount and state of calcium.[6,9]

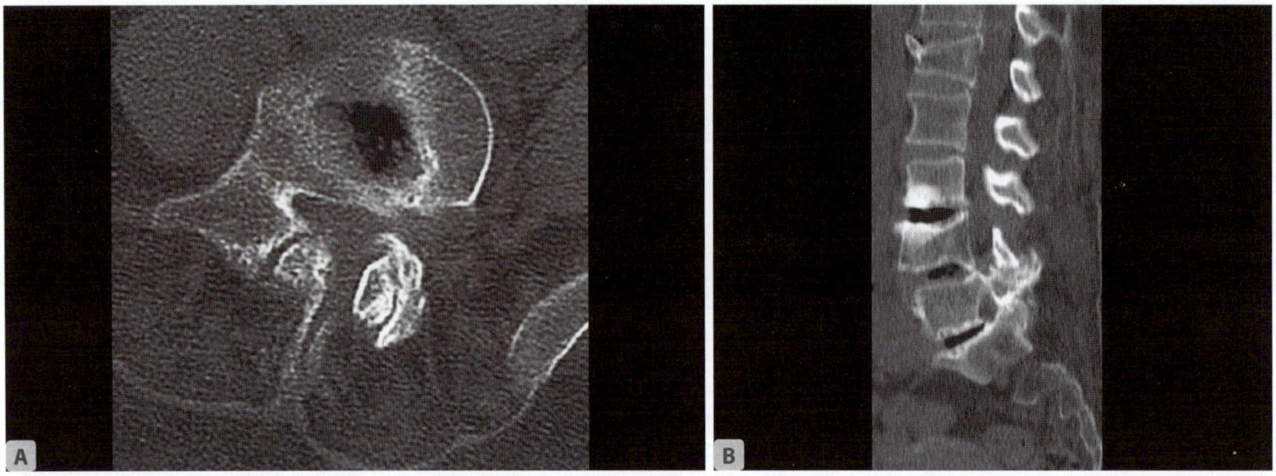

FIGS. 4A AND B: (A) Axial and (B) sagittal multiplanar reformatted CT images show vacuum phenomenon seen as air within multiple intervertebral discs. Note also made of marked hypertrophy of the left facet joint seen on the axial image and wedge compression fracture of L1 vertebra on the sagittal image.

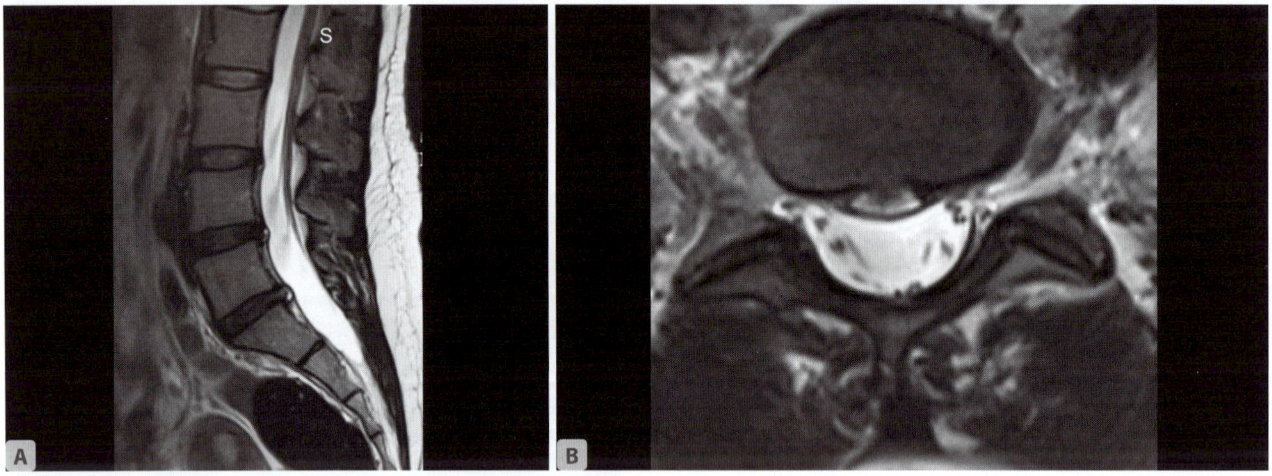

FIGS. 5A AND B: (A) Sagittal; and (B) Axial T2W MR images of lumbosacral spine depict disc desiccation with annular fissure seen as high-intensity zone at L4/5 and L5/S1 level.

Annular Fissures

Annular disruption is a critical factor in degeneration. Annular fiber degeneration may result in fissures:

- Type 1 circumferential or concentric fissures—run longitudinally along the plane of collagen fibers and precede annular bulging. These are seen as focal hyperintense areas in the external aspect of the annulus.
- Type 2 radial fissures—linear rupture of the annulus fibers extending from the nucleus pulposus traversing the entire inner-to-outer dimension of the annulus and correlate with shrinkage and disorganization of the nucleus.
- Type 3 transverse fissures—rupture of Sharpey's fibers adjacent to the ring apophyses and can be seen in normally hydrated disc.

While concentric fissures can be seen in normal discs, transverse and radial fissures are often associated with degenerated discs. As per the Version 2 of lumbar disc nomenclature,[10] annular tear is not the preferred term to be used as the word "tear" may imply a traumatic origin. Although fissures occur in all degenerated discs, not all of these are seen on MR. Magnetic resonance is less sensitive than cryomicrotomy or discography in detecting radial fissures.[7] Even discography cannot demonstrate all the fissures. On MRI, radial fissures appear as hyperintense transverse band into the annulus on MRI **(Figs. 5A and B)**.[1,2] These either represent fluid and/or granulation tissue within the annulus, the latter showing enhancement on gadolinium administration. However, presence of high-intensity zone (HIZ) or even their enhancement is no more thought to be correlated with the acuity of the fissure.

Disc Herniation

Herniation is the term used most commonly to describe the displacement of disc material. It can involve displacement of the nucleus pulposus, endplate cartilage, fragmented apophyseal bone or annular tissue beyond the normal confines of the disc space. Hence, the term "herniated nucleus pulposus" is inaccurate. Also, "rupture", "protrusion", and "prolapse" are considered nonstandard to describe this general diagnosis.

To bring uniformity to reporting of disc degeneration, the North American Spine Society, the American Society of Spine Radiology, and the American Society of Neuroradiology combined their committees, yielding a consensus paper on nomenclature of disc degeneration in 2001 and this has been updated in 2014.[10,11]

Disc Herniation versus Disc Bulge

Disc herniation is localized displacement of the disc material, involving <25% of the circumference of the disc. Disc space is defined by the vertebral endplates on either side and by the edges of the vertebral ring apophysis (excluding osteophytes) as the circumferential borders. It is also important to remember that for disc to be herniated, there needs to be disruption of the annulus or a defect in the vertebral endplate in case of Schmorl's node. Intra-annular displacement not extending beyond the confines of the disc space is not considered herniation. Also, if the annulus is displaced behind one vertebra as an adaptation to subluxation, it should not be considered herniation.

In contrast, disc bulge by definition is not herniation and is the term used when there is a smooth circumferential extension of the disc margin beyond the boundary of the adjacent vertebral endplates for >25% of the disc circumference **(Figs. 6A to C)**. This is usually <3 mm beyond the edges of the vertebral body. The annulus fibrosus is grossly intact, although weakened due to tears in the oblique collagen bridges between the concentric annular fibers. The concentric fibers are intact. On MR, there is uniform circumferential extension of the outer disc margin. There is usually loss of height of the involved disc space and desiccation/dehydration of the nucleus pulposus **(Figs. 7A and B)**.[1,2,12] Apart from degeneration, disc bulge has several etiologies—normal variation, ligamentous laxity, vertebral body remodeling because of osteoporosis or even partial volume averaging.[9]

The use of the either of the terms "bulge" or "herniation" does not suggest any etiology, symptomatology, prognosis, or treatment.

Types of Disc Herniation

Disc herniation can be classified into disc protrusion and disc extrusion **(Figs. 8A to C)**.

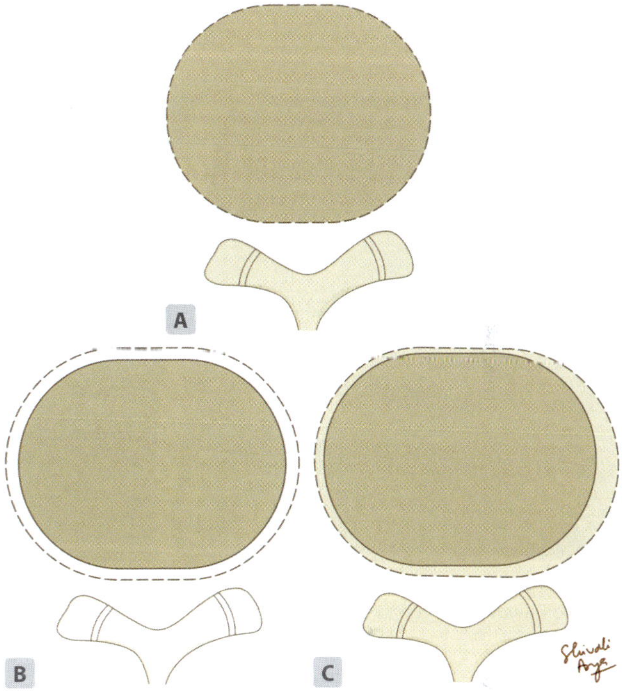

FIGS. 6A TO C: Schematic representation of (A) normal disc, (B) symmetric bulging disc, (C) asymmetric bulging disc. Disc is represented by the broken line.

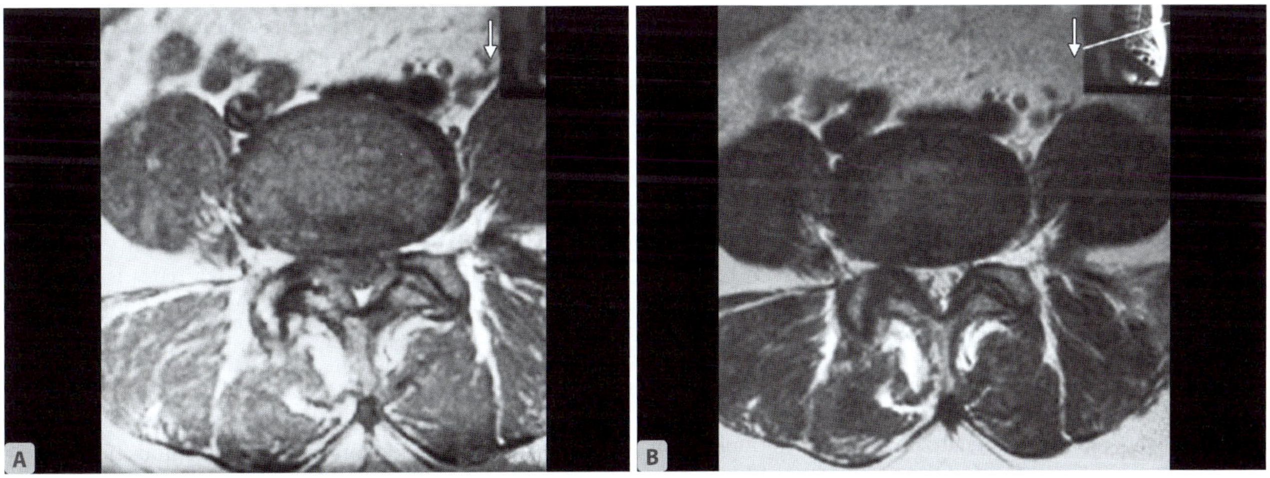

FIGS. 7A AND B: (A) Axial T1W and (B) T2W images at L4-L5 level show diffuse disc bulge with ligamentum flavum (LF) hypertrophy resulting in canal and lateral recess stenosis. Note that LF is better discernible on T1W rather than T2W image.

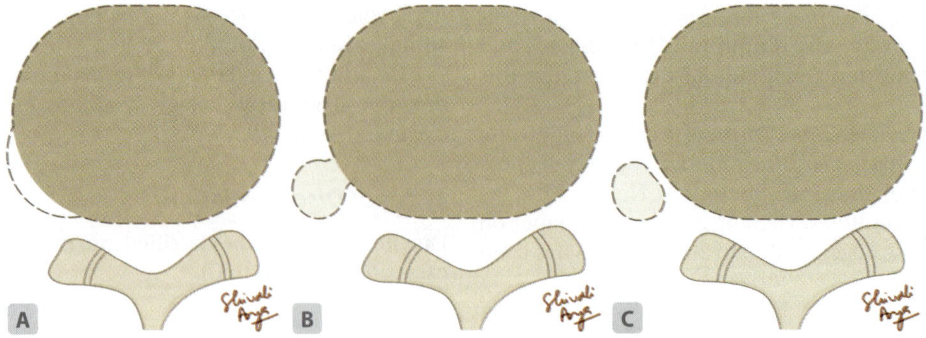

FIGS. 8A TO C: Schematic representation of (A) disc protrusion, (B) disc extrusion, (C) disc sequestration. Disc is represented by the broken line.

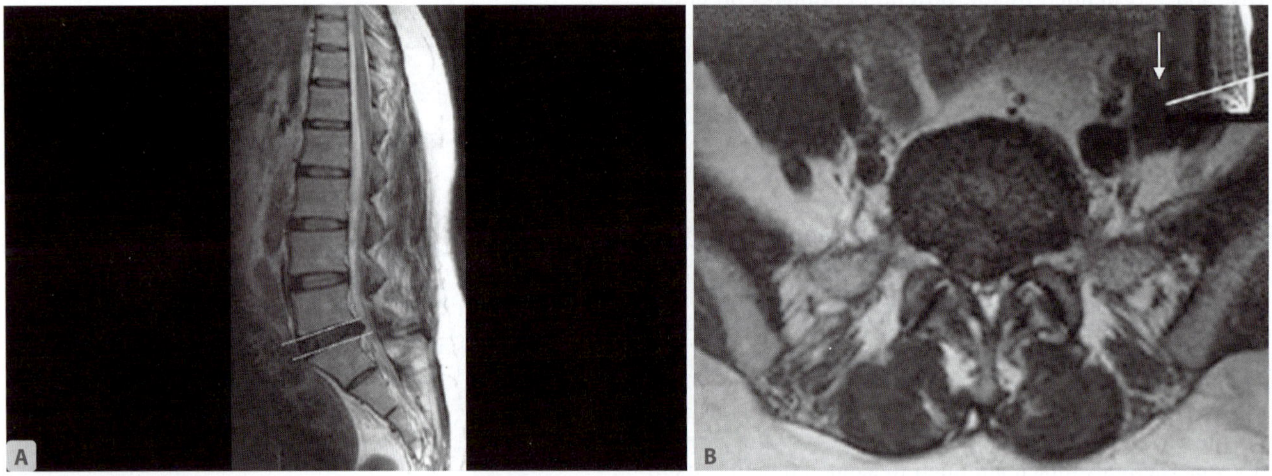

FIGS. 9A AND B: (A) Sagittal and (B) axial T2W MR images depict central disc protrusion at L5/S1 level. On the sagittal image, the herniated disc is seen to lie within the confines of the disc margins.

Disc Protrusion

Disc protrusion is the type of disc herniation which has a broad base (when the maximal length of the herniated disc material beyond the disc space in any plane is less than the distance of the edges at the disc base in the same plane) **(Figs. 9A and B)**. The base of the disc is the width of the disc at its outer margin from where the disc herniates. The disc protrudes through a defect in the inner annulus but the outer annular fibers are intact.

Disc Extrusion

Disc extrusion is the type of disc herniation with narrow base (when the maximal length of the disc is greater than the base of the disc in the same plane) or when there is no continuity of the herniated disc with the parent disc **(Figs. 10A to C)**.

Disc extrusions may be further classified into migrated or sequestrated discs:

- *Disc sequestration*: When the fragment of disc separates from the parent disc. It may be seen anteriorly in the spinal canal and less often in the lateral posterior or even intradural compartment of the spinal canal. This is also known as free fragment.[10,13]
- *Disc migration*: This describes the herniated disc which has migrated away from the site of extrusion, regardless of the continuity with the disc. Continuity with the parent disc may be difficult to establish based on our imaging studies.[10,13]

This is clinically very relevant as a sequestered disc may be a contraindication to minimally invasive therapies such as a microdiscectomies, percutaneous radiofrequency ablations, or the use of intradiscal steroids.[1,2,12]

Contained versus Noncontained Herniation

While protruding discs are contained disc herniations as at least some fibers of the annulus and PLL are intact, extruded discs are uncontained herniations where the annulus and even the overlying PLL is focally disrupted.[10,14]

The differentiation between the two types is often not possible with the current noninvasive imaging techniques (CT and MRI).

The term "subcapsular" is not the preferred term for containment as per the new nomenclature.[10] However, contained herniation may also be referred to as subligamentous and uncontained herniation as transligamentous (when there is extension through the PLL) or transmembranous (when there is extension through the epidural membrane).

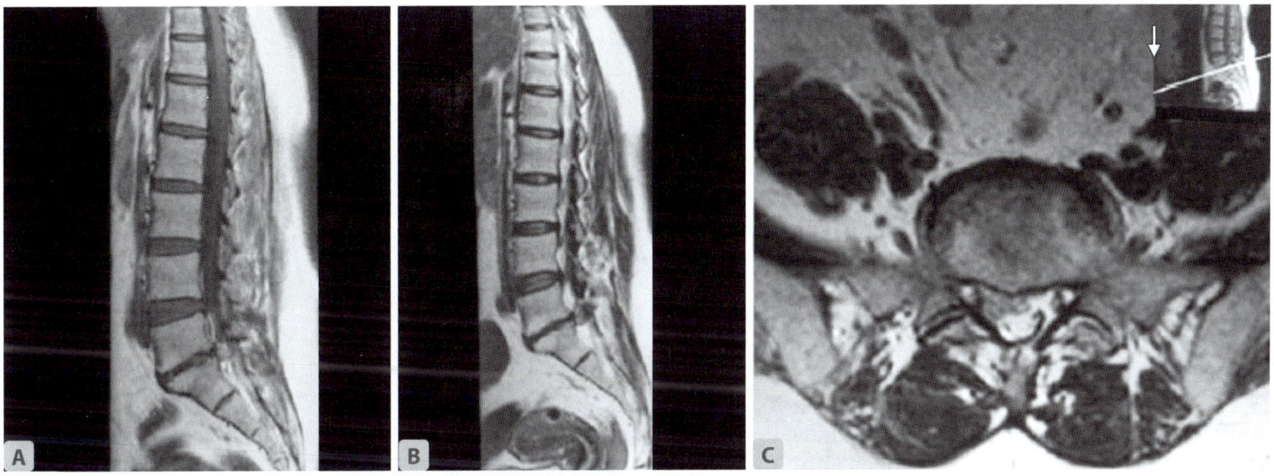

FIGS. 10A TO C: (A) Sagittal T1W, (B) sagittal T2W and (C) axial T2W MR images reveal markedly decreased disc space between L5/S1 with disc extrusion that is seen to extend beyond the confines of the disc space on the sagittal image. On the axial image, the right central extruded disc is seen to impinge on the traversing S1 nerve root on the right side. Note is made of type 2 endplate marrow changes at L5/S1 level seen as hyperintense signal on both T1W and T2W sagittal images.

Classification of Disc Herniation in the Axial Plane

These disc herniations are classified as central, right/left central, subarticular, foraminal, and extraforaminal in the axial plane. The term "paracentral" disc herniation is not preferred. Instead, the discs should be described as right or left central. However, "extraforaminal disc" can be used exchangeably with the term "far lateral disc". The medial edge of the facet articulations and the borders of the pedicles or the neural foramina are used for anatomic landmarks, although they may be difficult to interpret on axial images as they are curved structures.[12]

The axial classification is useful as it describes the herniation relative to the various exiting and traversing nerves. Lumbar disc herniations generally produce symptoms involving the nerve root inferior to the level of herniation as it compresses the transiting inferior root. However, an extraforaminal or foraminal disc herniation may compress the exiting root at the same level. In the cervical spine, disc herniations tend to involve the nerve root at the same level. This information is important to determine whether the patient's symptoms are attributable to MRI findings, for preoperative planning and to avoid surgery at the incorrect spinal level.[1]

Classification of Disc Herniation in the Sagittal Plane

In the sagittal plane, the disc may be classified as suprapedicular, pedicular, infrapedicular, and discal as ascertained by the upper and lower borders of the pedicles.

Endplate Changes

These are a reflection of abnormal stresses—loading or motion stresses. According to Michael Modic, endplate changes can be classified into three categories.[6]

Modic type 1 changes (vascular pattern) correspond to active inflammation, showing decreased signal on T1WI and high signal on T2WI. *Modic type 2 changes* (fatty pattern) reflect fatty infiltration and show bright signal on both T1WI and T2WI **(Figs. 10A and B)**. *Modic type 3 changes* (sclerotic pattern) are seen in advanced chronic stage, and correspond to bone sclerosis. This is seen as decreased signal on both T1WI and T2WI. These changes are also apparent on radiographs and CT **(Fig. 4A)**.[1,2] Sometimes, more than one type of Modic change can be seen at the same level.

The relationship with degenerative disc disease is probably caused by multiple factors—common biomechanical factors, raised mechanical stresses on the endplates induced by disc dehydration and disc metabolism changes. Endplate alterations can also induce disc changes as the disc is an avascular structure supplied by metabolite diffusion from endplate cartilage. The relative lack of blood supply and sparse cell population within the nucleus results in limited ability to recover from metabolic or mechanical injury.[2]

The Modic changes do not necessarily progress in an orderly fashion. Type 1 may progress to type 2 changes or may even revert to normal. Type 1 and type 2 changes may occasionally progress to type 3 changes. Modic type 1 and type 3 changes have been more positively correlated with back pain than Modic type 2 changes.[13] According to Chung et al.,[15] asymptomatic type 1 changes when present are generally focal, involve the anterosuperior endplate and involve midlumbar spine. In contrast, in symptomatic individuals, these are confluent changes superior and inferior to a degenerated disc, and usually seen in the lower lumbar spine.

Mimics

Sometimes type 1 changes may be so extensive that the imaging appearance may simulate infective etiology. However, in an infectious process, there is hyperintensity of the disc on T2WI with enhancement, paraspinal or epidural inflammation and erosion or destruction of endplate. Subchondral enhancement may be seen in both cases.[1,2]

Sclerotic type 3 changes can be rounded and mimic blastic metastatic disease on radiographs and CT. However, the degenerative endplate changes are seen abutting the endplate and there are associated features of disc degeneration like disc narrowing and vacuum phenomenon.[9]

Schmorl's Nodes

Focal herniations of discs through cartilaginous endplates may produce Schmorl's nodes. In most cases, these are remote occurrences of no clinical consequence. However, some of them may be traumatic in etiology and can be related to episodes of sudden pain when MR may show endplate edema representing endplate fracture.[1]

Most Schmorl's nodes occur after axial loading and result in extrusion of nucleus pulposus through the endplate rather than biomechanically stronger annulus fibrosus. Additional predisposing factors are intrinsic abnormalities of the endplate due to vascular channels or notochordal remnant defects. Patients with straight rather than concave endplates are also more predisposed due to less favorable axial loading.[4]

On CT, Schmorl's nodes are seen as focal indentations in the endplate in continuity with the intervertebral disc. There may be surrounding endplate sclerosis. On MR, we can see direct continuity of the disc material into the region of the endplate defect **(Figs. 11A and B)**. In acute/subacute cases, there may be increased T2 signal, typically following the contour of the endplate which may also demonstrate enhancement.[4]

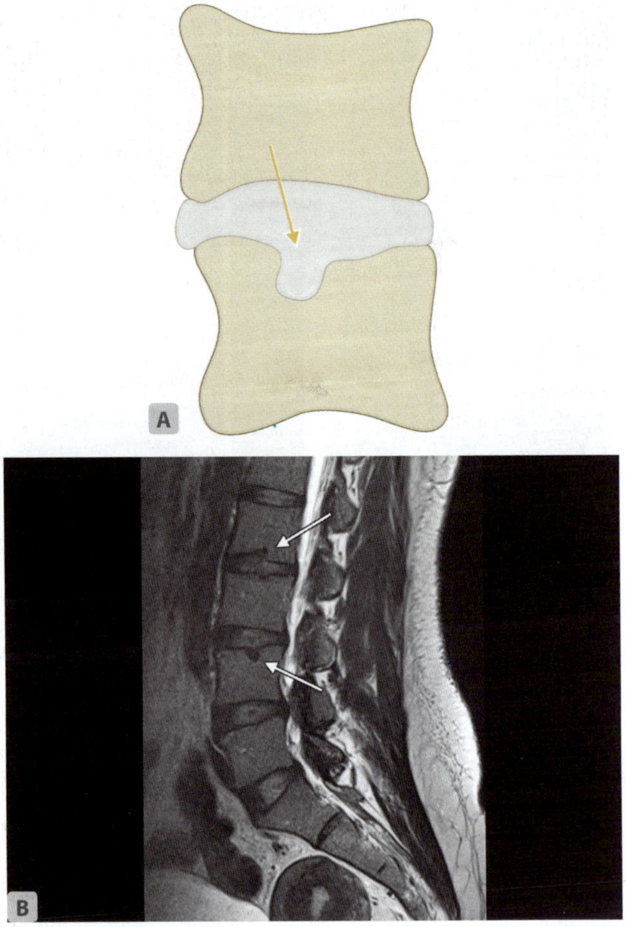

FIGS. 11A AND B: (A) Schematic representation of Schmorl's node; (B) Sagittal T2W MR image of lumbar spine depicts Schmorl's nodes at superior endplate of L4 and inferior endplate of L2 (arrows), which represent herniation of disc material into the endplates.

Facet Osteoarthritis

The facet or zygapophyseal joints are synovium-lined joints. They play an important role in flexion/extension and limiting axial rotation. They are oriented nearly in the sagittal plane in the cervical spine and approximately 40° in the sagittal plane in the lumbar spine. Like other synovial joints, these are predisposed to arthropathy with alterations of articular cartilage.

Facetal joint changes may be primary or secondary to disc degeneration. The latter is believed to be the main inciting factor for facet osteoarthritis. Secondary to disc degeneration, increased loading on facets and increased mobility at a segment can contribute to facet arthropathy. Facet tropism (asymmetry) and more sagittal orientation of facets >45° are other hypothesized causes. It has been postulated that facetal joint degeneration is more likely associated with patient symptoms, especially in the lumbar area, as this is less frequently found in asymptomatic individuals compared to disc degeneration. Patients usually present with axial pain as the capsule, subchondral bone and synovium are highly innervated structures. Involvement of facet joints is rare at the thoracic level owing to restricted mobility.

Facet joint osteoarthritis may trigger radicular pain owing to impingement of the neural foramen or at the site just before the nerve enters the foramen. Facet joint osteoarthritis may also be responsible for instability and spondylolisthesis, with an intact neural arch unlike isthmic spondylolisthesis. In the lumbar spine, facetal degeneration is accompanied by LF hypertrophy and calcification contributing to secondary spinal canal stenosis. This is due to fibrosis and loss of elasticity of the ligament. These ligaments are best assessed on T1WIs as these are difficult to differentiate from cortical bone on T2WI **(Figs. 7 and 12)**. In the lumbar spine, posterior paraspinal muscle atrophy also frequently accompanies facet joint degeneration **(Fig. 13B)**.[1,4]

Computed tomography is more sensitive in detecting early changes than MRI. The imaging findings include joint space narrowing, subchondral sclerosis and cyst formation, osteophyte formation, vacuum phenomenon and hypertrophy of the articular processes **(Figs. 13A and B)**. In addition, MRI can demonstrate congestive edema in the adjacent posterior elements and soft tissues, facet effusion and cysts.[1] MR has the advantage of evaluating the entire spine in a single examination and giving information on the neural and ligamentous components of the spine.

Synovial Cysts

Juxta-articular cysts may also be seen accompanying facet degeneration, most commonly at L4/L5, frequently with degenerative spondylolisthesis. These may represent synovial cysts, ganglion cysts or cysts of the LF. They are much rarer at the cervical spinal level. It is often difficult to differentiate between these entities by radiologic, pathologic or surgical

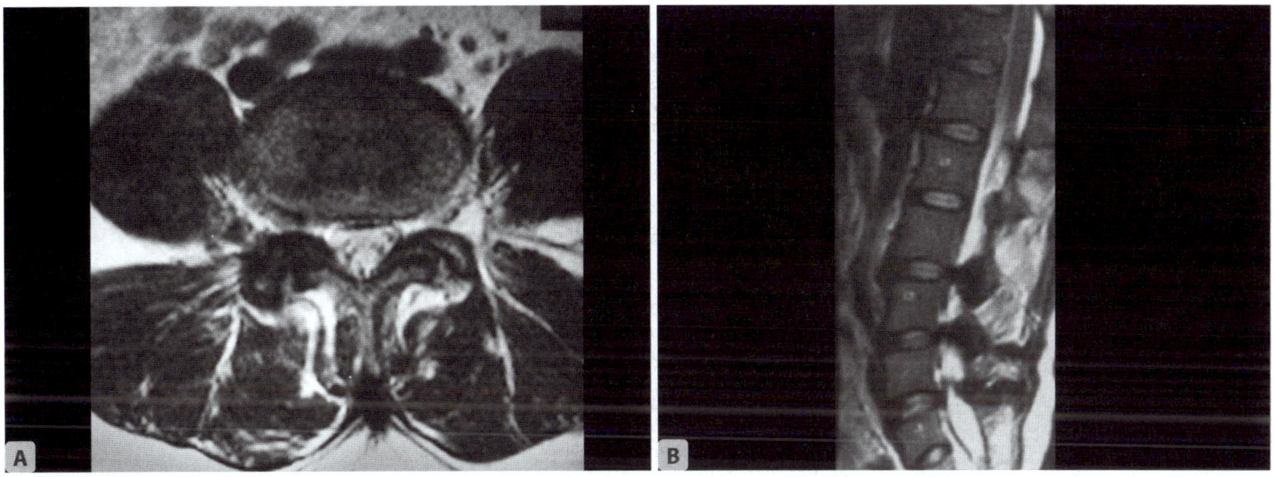

FIGS. 12A AND B: (A) Axial; and (B) Sagittal T2W MR images show degenerative changes involving the right facet joint in the axial image with evidence of ligamentum flavum hypertrophy resulting in narrowing of the spinal canal at L3-L4 and L4-L5 levels.

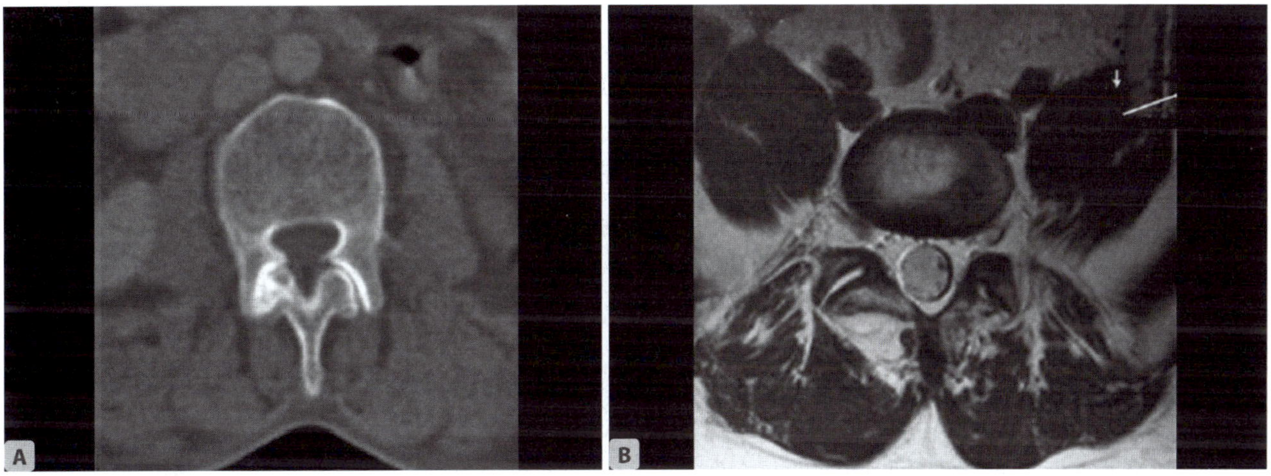

FIGS. 13A AND B: (A) Axial CT image depicts right facet arthrosis seen as erosions, sclerosis and decreased joint space; (B) Axial T2W image of another patient with facet arthritis shows increased fluid within the right facet joint with accompanying paraspinal muscle atrophy.

means. Although posterior cysts are more common, anterior cysts are more likely to be associated with symptoms than posterior cysts as the former project into the spinal canal or neural foramina.[4]

On MRI, these cysts are generally high signal intensity on T2WI. Some portions may be low SI on T2WI due to calcification or gas. These may be treated surgically or percutaneously, while spontaneous regression is also known.[1,4]

Facet Joint Effusion

This may be seen with and without facet degeneration. It may be observed in healthy individuals without any sign of facet degeneration. It is believed by some that if thickness of fluid is >1.5 mm, it could be predictive of degenerative spondylolisthesis at L4/L5 level, even when there is no anterolisthesis evident on supine MRI.[14]

Uncovertebral Joint Degeneration

In the cervical spine, in addition, uncovertebral joints can undergo degeneration **(Figs. 14A to C)**. These develop between the uncinate processes of the lower vertebrae and the lateral margin of the superior vertebrae and are found from C2-C3 level to C6-C7 level. These are variable joints, not present at all levels and not seen in the infants. These joints are lined with cartilage, which is presumably continuous with the adjacent cartilaginous endplate. Degenerative changes may be seen as hypertrophy, subchondral sclerosis and cyst formation, osteophyte formation and narrowing of joint space. These are clinically important as degeneration of these joints plays an important role in foraminal stenosis and nerve root compromise in the cervical spine.[4]

Interspinous Degeneration

Abnormal contact between spinous processes can lead to degeneration of the spinous processes and interspinous ligaments. This may result in interspinous pseudoarthrosis and cyst formation and has been termed Baastrup's disease or "kissing spine". There is localized tenderness that is exacerbated with extension and relieved with flexion, anesthetic injections or surgical excision. Redundant

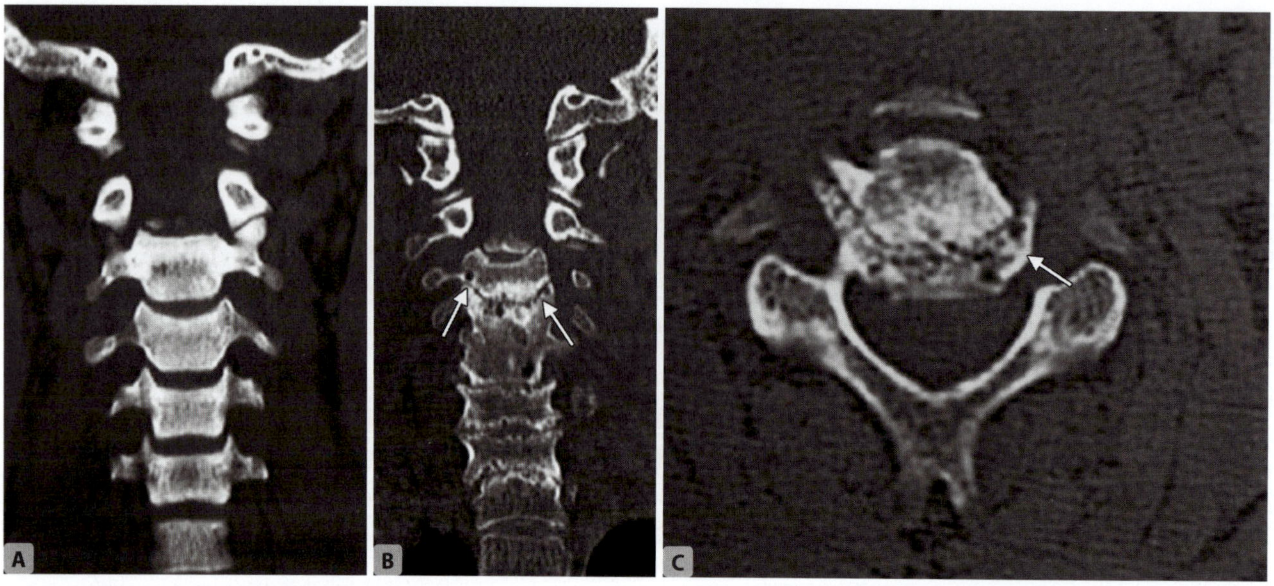

FIGS. 14A TO C: (A) Coronal reformatted CT image shows normal uncovertebral joints in cervical spine; (B) Coronal reformatted CT image in another patient with extensive spinal degenerative changes depicts marked arthrosis involving uncovertebral joints (arrows) as well as endplate changes; (C) Axial CT image of the same patient depicts uncovertebral arthrosis with neural foraminal narrowing.

interspinous ligaments, interspinous bursae, or hypertrophic degeneration may extend anteriorly, contributing to spinal canal stenosis.[4]

The main risk factors in pathophysiology are excessive lumbar lordosis, large spinous processes and degenerative disc disease/fractured vertebra that can lead to decrease in the space within the interspinous joints. The incidence of Baastrup's disease increases as age advances. On CT imaging, there are bone erosions, sclerosis and osteophyte formation with faceted appearance of the spinous processes. On MRI, subchondral edema and bursitis may be seen which are evident as bright signal on T2WIs and enhancement on contrast administration.

Spondylosis Deformans and Intervertebral Osteochondrosis

Degeneration of the disc affects both the nucleus and the annulus simultaneously. The imaging appearance depends on the predominant component.

Spondylosis Deformans

Spondylosis deformans is a degenerative process that essentially affects the annulus fibrosus and adjacent apophyses. The classic sign of spondylosis deformans is osteophytosis where the disc space is essentially preserved or only marginally decreased.[10] Osteophytes are bony spurs that originate from the bone surface and/or ossification of the soft tissue attachment to the bone **(Figs. 15A and B)**. Increased vertebral motility due to weakening and radial degeneration of annular fibers and resultant traction on Sharpey's fibers stimulates osteogenesis. Initially, osteophytes have a triangular horizontal extension (in contrast to syndesmophytes in seronegative arthropathies which are vertically oriented). In more advanced cases, osteophytes become hooked and grow more vertically. These may fuse together on either side of the disc space to form bridging osteophytes. The mucoid matrix of the disc becomes fibrous; however, disc height is normal or only slightly decreased and the disc margins are regular. Posterior osteophytes, although less common, are clinically more relevant because of possible compression of neural structures. They have a triangular shape with marginal location. Large posterior osteophytes may result in spinal stenosis, with compressive myelopathy, especially in the cervical region.[1-4]

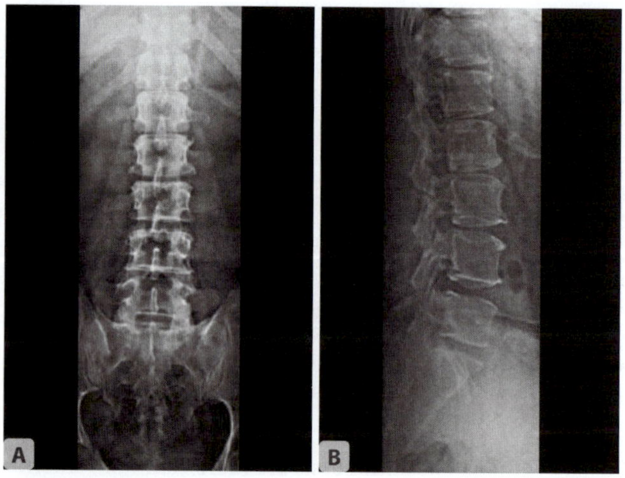

FIGS. 15A AND B: Lumbar spine anteroposterior and lateral radiographs depict marginal osteophytes at L2, L3 and L4 levels with relatively preserved disc spaces.

Intervertebral Osteochondrosis

In contrast to spondylosis, intervertebral osteochondrosis is a degenerative process that involves primarily the nucleus pulposus and vertebral endplates. There is accompanying fissuring of the annulus fibrosus. Early disc changes seen on sagittal fast spin-echo (FSE) T2WI include loss of normal T2 hypointensity within nucleus. Late changes include further decreasing signal within the nucleus pulposus, loss of distinction between nucleus pulposus and annulus fibrosus, disc space narrowing, disc bulges, vacuum phenomenon and endplate changes. Posterior osteophyte formation may also occur at this stage.[2] CT can detect later changes, including disc calcification, gas within disc space and also aid in differentiating osteophytes from degenerated disc.[4]

Complications of Degenerative Spinal Disease

Spinal and Foraminal Stenosis

Congenital and acquired canal stenosis: Lumbar canal stenosis is the most common acquired disorder in elderly population, caused by degenerative changes and primarily manifesting after the sixth decade of life. Congenital stenosis presents earlier in life with multilevel involvement and fewer degenerative changes.[1]

Congenital stenosis is seen in patients with disorders such as achondroplasia and mucopolysaccharidosis or may be idiopathic. It is usually related to short pedicles, short laminae or sagittal orientation of facet joints. Any superimposed pathological process is much more likely to cause symptomatic compression. Acquired stenosis is most commonly due to degenerative changes and usually involves the cervical and lumbar spine. The central canal may be narrowed anteriorly by degenerated disc, posterior bulging of PLL or posterior osteophytes and posteriorly by facet joints and LF.[1,4] This may get aggravated by spondylolisthesis. Other less common causes of acquired spinal canal stenosis include ossification of the PLL (OPLL) and/or LF and epidural lipomatosis.

Cervical spinal stenosis may present with both upper and lower limb motor/sensory deficits and pyramidal symptoms while the typical presentation of lumbar canal stenosis is neurogenic intermittent claudication. The latter may be provoked by prolonged standing/lumbar extension. Cervical canal stenosis is also aggravated by hyperextension when ligamentum flava may further buckle anteriorly.[14]

Imaging Findings

Computed tomography is the gold standard for evaluation of bony abnormalities, and is accurate for identifying posterior osteophytes and calcification of ligaments. It may be more appropriate to evaluate congenital spinal stenosis. MRI depicts the disc pathology and neural structures clearly.[2]

Spinal cord or nerve root compression is a dynamic phenomenon that worsens in erect position or with certain movements. The stenosis can become more evident or sometimes, may only be evident during weight-bearing or dynamic examination.[2,4]

Although absolute measurements may not be clinically relevant in all cases, the diagnosis of spinal canal stenosis should be considered if the anteroposterior diameter of the cervical and lumbar canals is <12 mm and in the thoracic region if it is <10 mm. Stenosis may also be considered if the ratio between canal sagittal diameter and vertebral body sagittal diameter is <0.8. More than objective canal measurements, it is the subjective evaluation of canal morphology and relationship between containing and contained structures that correlates better with patient's symptoms. Epidural fat is reduced or disappears. Multiple anterior and posterior notches can be observed on the dural sac, with disappearance of the subarachnoid space and narrowing of the spinal cord. The stenosis is severe if cerebrospinal fluid (CSF) signal is completely effaced on axial T2WI or CT myelogram images.[1,2]

In severe lumbar canal stenosis, sometimes "redundant nerve root" is seen as enlarged and swollen cauda equina. This may be due to radicular venous congestion, ischemia and edema. The rootlets may not be individually recognizable. In severe stenosis, the epidural fat is not seen posteriorly in addition to unrecognizable roots.[2]

Myelopathy is the most serious complication of canal stenosis. It is thought that continuous pinching of the cord can result in chronic hypoperfusion and result in demyelination and neuronal death. Increased intramedullary signal on T2WI is seen **(Fig. 16)** that indicates the presence of edema, chronic ischemia, myelomalacia or rarely syringomyelic cavitation. Enhancement on T1WI may confirm the abnormality. Low signal on noncontrast T1WI suggests a poor prognosis. However, it must be remembered that absence of abnormal signal does not rule out myelopathy, as clinical and electrophysiological criteria may be more sensitive. Apparent diffusion coefficient (ADC) maps and diffusion tensor imaging may improve the sensitivity in detecting subtle changes, but decrease the specificity.[4]

Facet hypertrophy, PLL thickening or disc herniation can lead to encroachment of lateral recesses. This is best evaluated on axial images and is found most commonly at L4-L5 level **(Figs. 7B and 12B)**. The normal sagittal diameter of the lateral recess is >5 mm; when this space is <4 mm, it is considered stenotic.[2,4]

Foraminal Stenosis

Disc and facet degeneration can also project into the neural foramina, causing their narrowing. Remodeling of the

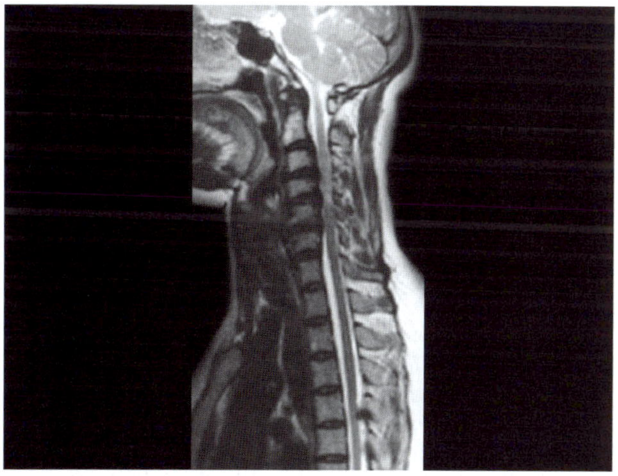

FIG. 16: Sagittal T2W image of the cervical spine shows multiple disc bulges and posterior longitudinal ligament thickening resulting in thecal sac indentation with hyperintense signal within the cord suggesting myelopathy.

endplates secondary to disc degeneration results in wider and shorter vertebral body and this may also cause narrowing of the spinal canal, lateral recesses and neural foramina. Loss of disc height may result in anterosuperior slippage of the facet joint and narrow the craniocaudal diameter of the foramen and hence, contributing to neural foraminal narrowing. In the cervical spine, neural foraminal narrowing is most commonly caused by uncovertebral osteophytes.

Lumbar foraminal herniations are best evaluated on the sagittal plane on T1W images whereas cervical neural foramina are best evaluated on axial MR images.[1,4] On sagittal MRI, foramen is seen as an ovoid structure, filled with CSF and fat. In the lumbar spine, nerve root lies in the superior part of the foramen and the herniated disc may not compress the nerve. When there is clinically significant nerve compression, it is usually due to a multitude of factors that include facetal arthropathy, LF hypertrophy, dorsal spondylophytes in addition to the discal herniation. Mild narrowing is seen as a "keyhole" appearance. Moderate narrowing effaces the inferior portion of the foramen at the level of the disc. Severe narrowing results in effacement of the fat in the foramen. When the fat sleeve around the nerve root is completely lost in this plane, it is consistent with nerve compression.[13] Other signs of nerve compression are contact between the disc and the nerve root with loss of periradicular CSF sleeve, pushed nerve root, increased size of nerve root as well as nerve root enhancement owing to inflammatory changes around the nerve root.[14]

In contrast, the cervical nerve roots lie at the same level or slightly below that of the disc and small herniations can result in nerve compression. At this level, preservation of fat sleeve around the nerve is not considered an accurate sign for ruling out nerve compression. It must be remembered that correlation with symptoms of radiculopathy is essential to diagnose nerve root impingement.[4]

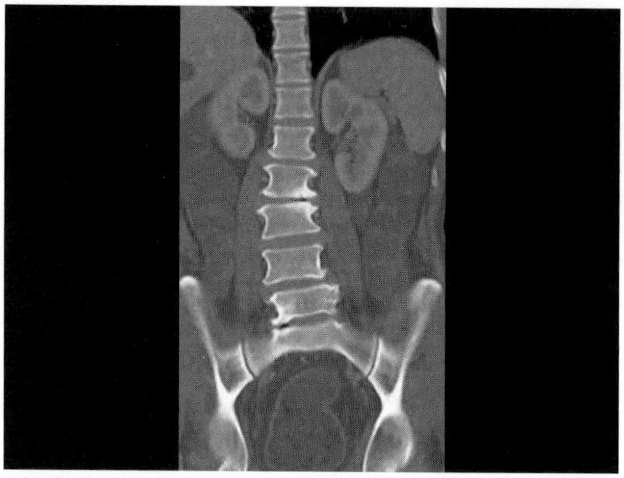

FIG. 17: Coronal reformatted CT image reveals laterally directed osteophytes on the concavity of scoliosis with vacuum phenomenon at multiple levels.

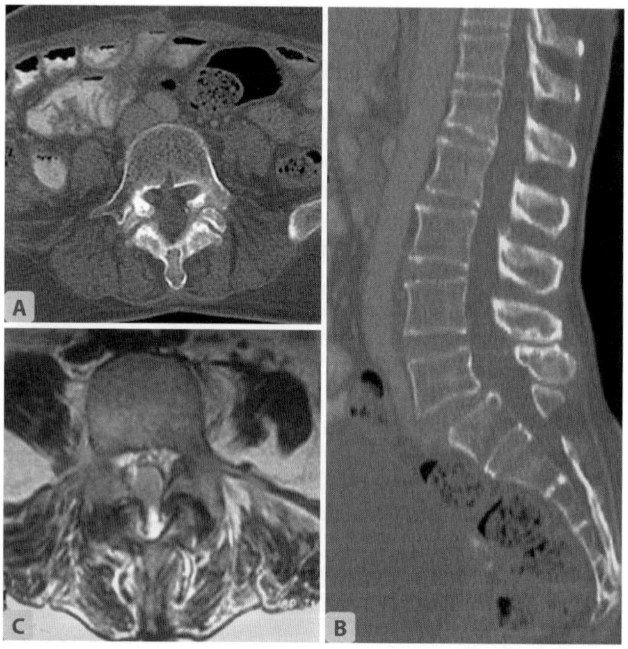

FIGS. 18A TO C: (A) Axial and (B) sagittal reformatted CT images reveal lysis of pars interarticularis of L4 with spondylolisthesis of L4 over L5 resulting in widening of the anteroposterior diameter of the spinal canal; (C) Axial T2W MR image of another patient shows break involving pars interarticularis of L4 with widening of spinal canal.

Scoliosis and Kyphosis

Asymmetric degenerative disc changes can result in degenerative scoliosis **(Fig. 17)**. This tends to produce a positive feedback loop that tends to accelerate the degenerative changes on one side. Compared to idiopathic scoliosis, degenerative scoliosis is usually short segment and most often occurs in the lumbar spine. Also, loss of lumbar lordosis and spinal and foraminal stenosis are more common with degenerative scoliosis. Thoracic kyphosis in adults is frequently secondary to asymmetric degeneration in the anterior portions of the discs.[4]

Segmental Instability

Disc degeneration can lead to narrow disc space and buckling of LF which can further result in an unstable vertebral segment. Resultant malalignment may result in anterolisthesis, retrolisthesis or lateral spondylolisthesis. Degenerative retrolisthesis occurs classically secondary to disc degeneration and results in canal and foraminal stenosis. It may also occur secondary to asymmetric facet degeneration. Anterolisthesis occurs mostly at L4-L5 level, secondary to facet degeneration. In patients with degenerative scoliosis, lateral and retrolisthesis is often encountered.[4] Posterolisthesis, which is associated with facet and disc degeneration, is frequent at more mobile spine segments such as the cervical and upper lumbar spine.[2] The typical sites of degenerative spondylolisthesis are L3-L4 and L4-L5, because of more sagittal orientation of facet joints.

Spondylolisthesis may also result from pars interarticularis defects (spondylolysis) and the most common is the isthmic type of spondylolysis. This is most commonly seen at L5 and L4 vertebrae and is a defect in pars interarticularis which is considered a fatigue fracture. Other less common causes of spondylolisthesis are acute trauma, congenital dysplasias, tumors and iatrogenic causes. Spondylolisthesis due to pars defect may be distinguished from degenerative spondylolisthesis on imaging. The former depicts canal widening at the involved level **(Figs. 18A to C)** whereas the latter demonstrates canal narrowing at the affected level because of slippage of the posterior arch and facet hypertrophy.[1,2]

Secondary to segmental instability, hypertrophy of the ligaments, facet osteoarthritis, and osteophyte formation may develop which have an additive effect on narrowing of the spinal canal and foramina. These osteophytes may aid in stabilizing the spinal segment, which may be shown on kinematic MRI.[4]

Vertebral body movement may be seen on flexion, extension and lateral bending radiographs where instability may be diagnosed as loss of alignment of one or more vertebral lines. Other radiographic signs are vertebral slippage, variations in pedicle length, narrowing of neural foramina, and loss of disc height. Conventional MRI has a limited role. It may show displacement and pseudobulging of disc at the involved level. Axial loaded CT or MRI or upright MRI can provide functional information regarding vertebral stability.[2]

CLINICAL IMPLICATIONS

Natural history of back pain is poorly understood and causes of low backache remain unknown in majority of cases. Nonspecific imaging findings may often be encountered in asymptomatic subjects and findings seen in symptomatic patients do not necessarily correlate with symptoms.[1] The diagnosis should always be based on combined information from clinical findings and imaging studies for determining appropriate patient management strategy.

REFERENCES

1. Rumboldt Z. Degenerative disorders of the spine. Semin Roentgenol. 2006;41(4):327-62.
2. Gallucci M, Limbucci N, Paonessa A, Splendiani A. Degenerative disease of the spine. Neuroimaging Clin N Am. 2007;17(1):87-103.
3. Shah LM, Ross JS. Imaging of degenerative and infectious conditions of the spine. Neurosurgery. 2016;79(3):315-35.
4. Malfair D, Beall DP. Imaging the degenerative diseases of the lumbar spine. Magn Reson Imaging Clin N Am. 2007;15(2):221-38.
5. Bozzao A, Gallucci M, Masciocchi C, Aprile I, Barile A, Passariello R. Lumbar disc herniation: MR imaging assessment of natural history in patients treated without surgery. Radiology. 1992;185(1):135-41.
6. Modic MT, Ross JS. Lumbar degenerative disc disease. Radiology. 2007;245(1):43-61.
7. Kaplan RT, Czervionke LF, Haughton VM. Degenerative disease of the spine. In: Atlas SW (Ed). Magnetic Resonance Imaging of the Brain and Spine (Vol II), 4th edition. Philadelphia: Lippincott Williams and Wilkins; 2009. pp. 1448-507.
8. Pfirrmann CW, Metzdorf A, Zanetti M, Hodler J, Boos N. Magnetic resonance classification of lumbar intervertebral disc degeneration. Spine (Phila Pa 1976). 2001;26:1873-8.
9. Miller TT. Imaging of disc disease and degenerative spondylosis of the lumbar spine. Semin Ultrasound CT MR. 2004;25(6):506-22.
10. Fardon DF, Williams AL, Dohring EJ, Murtagh FR, Gabriel Rothman SL, et al. Lumbar disc nomenclature: version 2.0: recommendations of the combined task forces of the North American Spine Society, the American Society of Spine Radiology and the American Society of Neuroradiology. Spine J. 2014;14(11):2525-45.
11. Fardon DF, Milette PC. Nomenclature and classification of lumbar disc pathology. Recommendations of the combined task forces of the North American Spine Society, American Society of Spine Radiology, and American Society of Neuroradiology. Spine (Phila Pa 1976). 2001;26(5):E93-113.
12. Costello RF, Beall DP. Nomenclature and standard reporting terminology of intervertebral disc herniation. Magn Reson Imaging Clin N Am. 2007;15(2):167-74.
13. Farshad-Amacker NA, Farshad M, Winklehner A, Andreisek G. MR imaging of degenerative disc disease. Eur J Radiol. 2015;84(9):1768-76.
14. Clarençon F, Law-Ye B, Bienvenot P, Cormier É, Chiras J. The degenerative spine. Magn Reson Imaging Clin N Am. 2016;24(3):495-513.
15. Chung CB, Vande Berg BC, Tavernier T, Cotten A, Laredo JD, Vallee C, et al. End plate marrow changes in the asymptomatic lumbosacral spine: frequency, distribution and correlation with age and degenerative changes. Skeletal Radiol. 2004;33(7):399-404.

CHAPTER

161

Skeletal Disorders of Metabolic and Endocrine Origin

Alpana Manchanda, Jyoti Kumar, Swati Gupta

INTRODUCTION

Metabolic bone disease encompasses a diverse group of disorders associated with altered calcium and phosphorus homeostasis.[1,2] Although many of these disorders are quite common, they may be difficult to distinguish on the basis of history, physical examination, and imaging studies.[1,2]

To the clinician, metabolic bone disease is often silent until the patient presents with fracture, the ultimate complication of many metabolic disorders. Other patients may however present with a clinical history of back pain and a nonspecific radiologic finding of generalized osteopenia.[3] At this stage prior to fracture, accurate diagnosis is crucial. Understanding their diverse manifestations on imaging studies may allow early diagnosis, aid in their management, and in taking appropriate preventive measures.

The manifestations of endocrine derangements in the skeletal system depend on the age of the patient at the time of presentation. In general, skeletal manifestations in childhood and infancy consist of disturbances in growth and maturation, and in adulthood, these manifestations consist of disturbances in maintenance and metabolism.

DISORDERS OF METABOLIC ORIGIN

The most common types of metabolic bone diseases are acquired disorders with nutritional deficiencies being an important cause. Nonetheless, rare forms frequently are genetically based and cause intrinsic alterations in the bone cell population.

The various metabolic bone disorders may be grouped according to their underlying defects:

- Defect in osteoid formation: Scurvy
- Defect in mineralization: Rickets/osteomalacia
- Disorder with increased bone resorption: Hyperparathyroidism
- Disorder with no defect in mineralization and osteoid formation but decreased bone mass: Osteoporosis
- Miscellaneous: Fluorosis, heavy metal poisoning, and hypervitaminosis.

Table 1 lists the metabolic profile with reference values.

TABLE 1: Metabolic profile–reference values.

Serum calcium	8.7–10.2 mg/dL
Ionized calcium	4.5–5.3 mg/dL
Serum phosphorus	2.4–4.1 mg/dL
Alkaline phosphatase	223–635 U/L
Vitamin D	>25 ng/mL
Serum parathormone	8–51 pg/mL
Serum ascorbic acid	0.6–1.2 mg/100 mL

The imaging manifestations of metabolic bone disease are varied and the same disease process can have a wide range of skeletal findings.

RICKETS AND OSTEOMALACIA

Rickets in children and osteomalacia in adults are a group of bone disorders in which there is incomplete or inadequate mineralization of normal osteoid tissue. Both conditions usually result from an abnormality in vitamin D metabolism. The biochemical and histological abnormalities are identical in the two conditions while skeletal manifestations differ depending upon the age of the patient at the time of onset of disease. Prior to fusion of the growth plate, features of both rickets and osteomalacia can be seen.

Vitamin D is a steroid hormone which is produced by skin exposure to sunlight and also obtained from the diet.[4] To attain its active form, vitamin D must undergo two hydroxylations—first in the liver and second in the kidneys **(Fig. 1)**. The primary function of vitamin D is to maintain calcium and phosphate homeostasis, thereby ensuring normal mineralization of the skeleton. The target areas for vitamin D action include bone, gastrointestinal tract, kidneys, and parathyroid gland.[1,4,5]

Causes

The term rickets has evolved from the old English word wrick, which means "to twist." This twisting or bending of bones has been found to result from more than one cause.

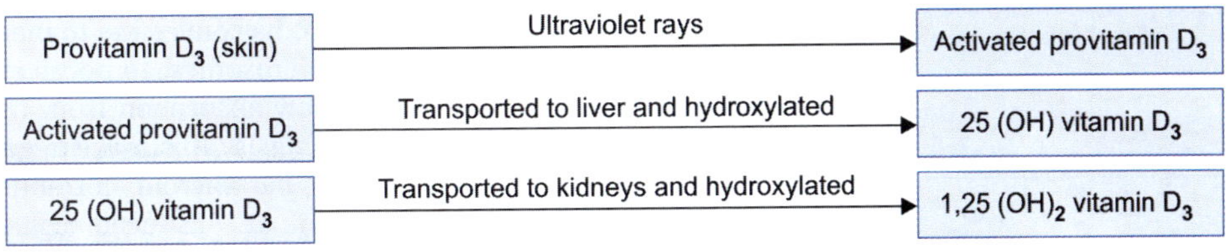

FIG. 1: Pathway for activation of vitamin D_3.

Rickets and osteomalacia occur due to many causes **(Box 1)**, most common being due to dietary deficiency of vitamin D called vitamin D-deficient rickets or nutritional rickets. Many abnormalities in vitamin D metabolism can potentially result in rickets and osteomalacia. These include malabsorption syndromes, hepatobiliary diseases, renal diseases, drugs, and neoplasms.[1,4]

BOX 1: Causes of rickets and osteomalacia.

- Abnormalities of vitamin D metabolism:
  - Deficiency conditions:
    - Dietary deficiency of vitamin D
    - Lack of exposure to ultraviolet light
  - Absorption defects:
    - Gastrointestinal malabsorption
    - Biliary atresia
    - Small bowel bypass surgery
  - Hepatic diseases:
    - Cirrhosis
    - Hepatitis
  - Anticonvulsant therapy
  - Renal insufficiency:
    - Type I VDDR
    - Type II VDDR
- *Rickets and osteomalacia secondary to phosphate loss*:
  - X-linked hypophosphatemia, genetic (Vitamin D-resistant rickets)
  - Primary hypophosphatemic rickets, acquired
  - Renal tubular acidosis (RTA):
    - Type I (distal) RTA
    - Type II (proximal) RTA
  - Tumor-associated phosphate deficiency
  - Chemotherapeutic drug-induced rickets
- *Syndromes with radiographic appearance or osteomalacia but without abnormalities of vitamin D metabolism or renal tubular dysfunction (phosphate loss)*:
  - Metaphyseal chondrodysplasia (Schmid type)
  - Hypophosphatasia
  - Atypical axial osteomalacia

(VDDR: vitamin D-dependent rickets)

Clinical Features

Clinical findings of rickets and osteomalacia are highly variable and depend on the etiology and severity of the disorder as well as the age of patient at the time of presentation.[1,4,5] In the first 6 months of life, rickets can present with tetany or convulsions. In most children with rickets, skeletal growth is stunted and they present with swollen and tender joints. With advanced disease, they may present with irritability, weakness, and bony deformities. The most notable clinical finding is soft-tissue swelling occurring around the growth plates due to hypertrophied cartilage. Clinically, enlargement of wrists and costal cartilage are most suggestive of the disease with a specificity of 81% and 64%, respectively.[6]

In adults, findings of osteomalacia are more subtle. Initial symptoms include fatigue, malaise, or bone pain. With advanced disease, proximal muscle weakness and abnormal gait may be present.[1,5] Typical manifestations of osteomalacia consist of bone pain, especially in the hips and muscle weakness.

Biochemical Findings

On laboratory evaluation, the serum calcium and phosphorus may be normal or slightly reduced while serum alkaline phosphatase levels are increased.

Pathology

There is remarkable similarity in the biochemical and histologic abnormalities in rickets and osteomalacia. The characteristic changes of rickets are identified in the growth plates prior to closure while abnormalities of osteomalacia are seen in the mature areas of trabecular and cortical bone.

In order to understand the changes of rickets, the general structure and organization of growth plate is discussed briefly. The growth plate is a complex structure which is located at the ends of long bones and situated between the epiphysis and metaphysis.[4] Although, it is adjacent to the epiphysis, functionally it is part of the shaft. Histologically, the cellular arrangement of the normal growth plate is characterized by order with progressive increase in the number and size of cartilaginous cells from the epiphysis to metaphysis. The normal epiphysis has four zones. From the epiphyseal ossification center toward the shaft the various zones are—the resting zone, proliferating zone, hypertrophic zone, and zone of primary and secondary spongiosa. The hypertrophic zone is further subdivided into zones of maturation, degeneration, and provisional calcification **(Fig. 2)**.

In rickets, there is disorganization of the growth plate and adjacent metaphysis. The resting and proliferative zones of the cartilaginous growth plate are not significantly altered from the normal pattern. However, the zone of maturation is grossly abnormal with a disorganized increase in the number of cells and a loss of normal columnar pattern. This cell mass results in an increase in length and width of the growth plate. Overall, there is diminished quantity of calcified osteoid and an increase in uncalcified osteoid, which casts increased radiolucency on the radiographs.

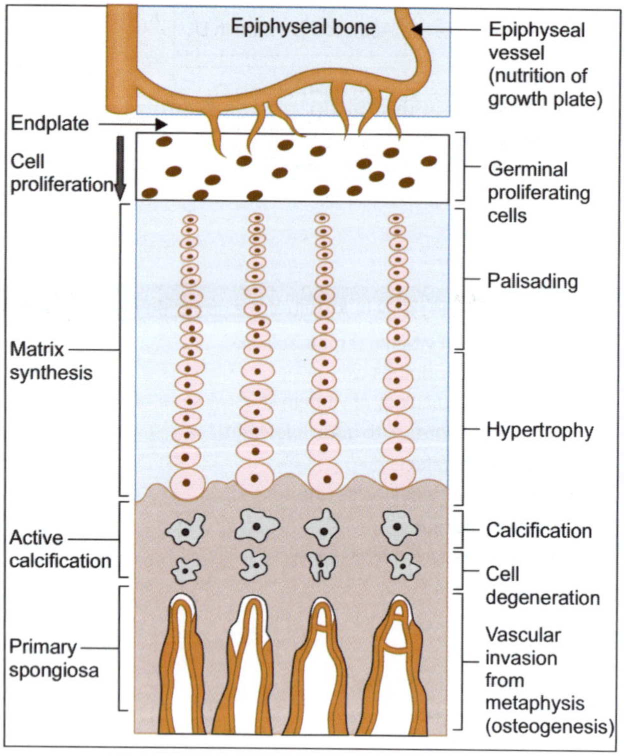

FIG. 2: Structure of the growth plate showing normal cellular organization.

Osteomalacia results from insufficient, delayed, or defective mineralization of cortical and spongy bone. Histologically, it is characterized by abnormal quantities of inadequately mineralized bone matrix called osteoid, coating the surfaces of trabeculae, and lining the haversian canals in the cortex. These layers of osteoid are often referred to as osteoid seams. Osteoid seams are not pathognomonic of osteomalacia and may be found in other active metabolic states associated with high bone turnover. However, there is an increase in both the number and width of the osteoid seams in osteomalacia.

Etiologic Considerations

- *Abnormalities of vitamin D metabolism:*
  - *Deficiency of vitamin D*: It results from a diet which is inadequate in vitamin D or a defect in the synthesis of vitamin D due to poor exposure to sunlight.
  - *Malabsorption of vitamin D*: Defect in absorption of vitamin D may result from small bowel disease, small bowel bypass surgery, rapid intestinal transit, pancreatic insufficiency, or biliary atresia.
  - *Abnormal vitamin D metabolism*: This may occur due to liver diseases such as hepatitis, cirrhosis, or kidney disorders such as chronic renal failure and nephrotic syndrome.
  - *Anticonvulsant therapy*: Epileptic patients require long-term antiepileptic drugs (AED) which are associated with abnormal bone mineral metabolism, osteoporosis, and an increased risk of fracture. A reduction in the active level of vitamin D has been seen which is likely due to induction of liver enzymes by AED leading to its conversion to inactive metabolites in the liver microsomes. Hypocalcemia may also be seen due to low absorption from the gut secondary to hypovitaminosis. This may trigger an increase in circulation of parathyroid hormone and increased bone turnover. AED-induced disturbances of bone integrity are influenced by the type, duration, and dosage of the antiepileptic therapy. The risk of AED-induced bone damage is greater with carbamazepine, phenytoin, and phenobarbital than with other antiepileptic agents.[7]
  - *Renal osteodystrophy*: Renal osteodystrophy is a term which is used to describe the bony changes in patients with chronic renal insufficiency. In children, end-stage renal disease is commonly due to loss of renal parenchyma because of structural abnormalities of the urinary tract. While in adults, chronic glomerulonephritis is the main cause.
    Due to chronic renal disease, there is phosphate retention along with impaired ability to form 1, 25 dihydroxy vitamin D_3. Low levels of vitamin D and an excess of phosphate stimulate an excess parathyroid hormone resulting in secondary hyperparathyroidism. Radiographic changes in renal osteodystrophy, therefore, reflect a combination of different processes including rickets/osteomalacia, secondary hyperparathyroidism, and osteosclerosis. Radiological changes in rickets have already been described. The characteristic radiological changes in secondary hyperparathyroidism consist of bone resorption which may be subperiosteal, intracortical, endosteal, or subligamentous; presence of brown tumors; and soft-tissue and vascular calcification. Increased bone density or osteosclerosis is either focal or diffuse **(Fig. 3A)** and is commonly seen in the spine but also occurs in the pelvis, ribs, skull and tubular bones. The characteristic appearance of the spine is called "rugger jersey spine" because of its resemblance to the striped jersey worn by rugby players and is caused by increased bone deposition in the vertebral endplates **(Fig. 3B)**.
  - *Hereditary Vitamin D-dependent Rickets (VDDR):* Vitamin D-dependent rickets should be considered when rickets presents in early infancy and other usual causes such as inadequate vitamin D intake, intestinal malabsorption, liver disease or kidney disorders have been excluded.
    Two forms have been described which involve problems with the formation or function of $1{,}25(OH)_2\,D_3$.
    - *Type I VDDR:* Type I disorder results from a deficiency (genetic defect) of the renal enzyme 1-alpha-hydroxylase, which converts $25(OH)D_3$ to $1{,}25(OH)_2D_3$. Therefore, the blood levels of $25(OH)D_3$ are normal while those of $1{,}25(OH)_2D_3$ are decreased.
      Clinical presentation is early, often by 3 months of age, with most patients being symptomatic by 1 year of age. The disease is differentiated from X-linked hypophosphatemic rickets by the

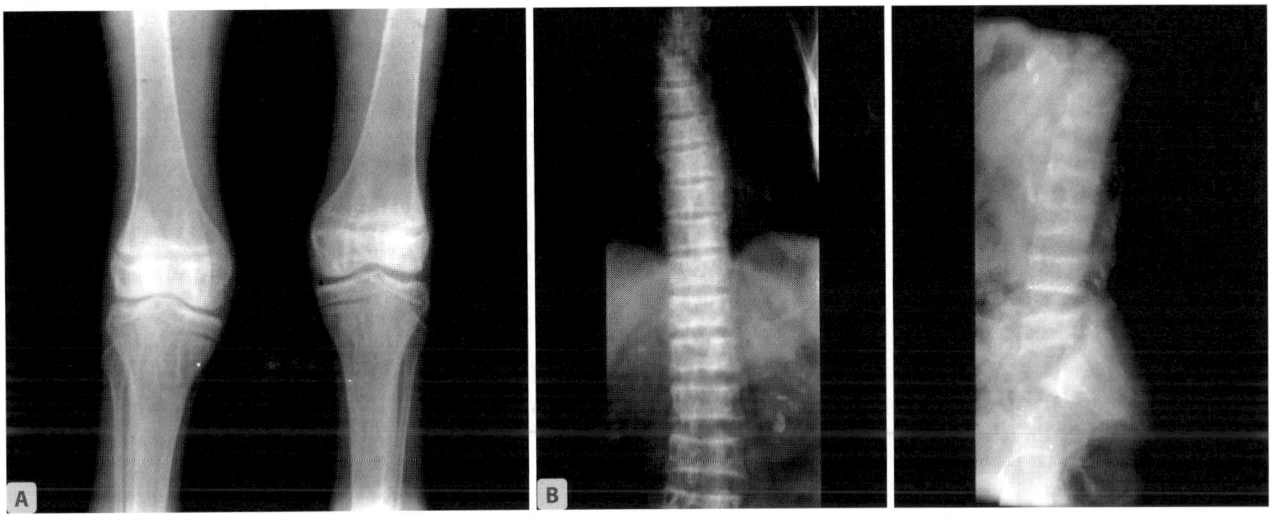

FIGS. 3A AND B: Renal osteodystrophy. (A) X-ray bilateral (B/L) knees showing knock knee deformity and patchy sclerosis at the distal femoral and proximal tibial metaphysis with slight widening of the growth plate; (B) Characteristic "rugger jersey spine" appearance in a patient of chronic renal failure with nephrolithiasis in the left kidney.

presence of convulsions and muscular weakness. Rachitic bone changes may be severe, rapidly progressive, and accompanied by pathologic fractures.[4] Healing occurs with physiologic doses of 1,25 dihydroxy vitamin D_3. This disorder is also known as *pseudovitamin D deficiency rickets* as patients with this condition respond to large doses of vitamin D or physiologic doses of $1,25(OH)_2D$ with resolution of the clinical, biochemical, and radiographic abnormalities.

- *Type II VDDR:* In this type of VDDR serum levels of $1,25(OH)_2D_3$ are elevated, thereby indicating an end-organ resistance to $1,25(OH)_2D_3$. It is also known as *calcitrol-resistant rickets* (CRR) and is a rare autosomal recessive disorder characterized by severe rickets, growth retardation, severe dental changes, and alopecia from early infancy. The diagnosis of type II VDDR should be suspected from the unusual association of severe rickets and alopecia.

- *Rickets and osteomalacia secondary to phosphate loss*: A number of rachitic and osteomalacic syndromes have been identified of both congenital and acquired origin, which share one or several renal tubular abnormalities. Rickets or osteomalacia results from hypophosphatemia secondary to impaired renal tubular resorption of phosphate resulting in phosphate loss. These disorders were described by Albright, Fanconi, and associates who also reported that rickets was resistant to vitamin D therapy in these patients.[4] It includes various conditions with different etiologies, of which increased phosphatonins is a common link. Fibroblast growth factor 23 (FGF23) is the most common studied phosphatonin.
  - *X-linked hypophosphatemia*: It accounts for >80% of familial hypophosphatemic rickets. X-linked hypophosphatemia *(or familial vitamin D-resistant/refractory rickets)* is the most common form of renal tubular rickets and osteomalacia. It is genetically transmitted in an X-linked dominant trait. The syndrome is characterized by lifelong hypophosphatemia. The basic defect lies in impaired reabsorption of phosphate from proximal tubules.[4] In addition, the conversion of $25(OH)D_3$ to $1,25(OH)_2D_3$ is also impaired. Serum calcium levels are in the normal range while the serum inorganic phosphate levels are persistently low. Rickets generally develops between 12 and 18 months of age.
    - *Clinical features*: Clinical features include bowing of legs, limb deformities, short stature, and premature fusion of cranial sutures leading to skull deformities. Dental abnormalities are also seen.
    - *Biochemical findings*: It is characterized by low serum phosphorus, normal serum calcium, normal parathyroid hormone (PTH), and elevated levels of alkaline phosphatase.
    - *Radiological features*: Unlike vitamin D deficiency, craniotabes and rachitic rosary are not seen. Frontal bossing is usually the first finding at 6 months. Radiographically, the rachitic changes may be mild to moderate with bowing of long bones seen, particularly in the lower limbs. As the child starts walking, there are progressive limb deformities leading to disproportionate short stature with short lower limbs.[8] Lower limbs are more affected than upper limbs with coxa vera, genu varum, and valgus. Coarsening of trabecular pattern is seen with increasing age. In adults, generalized increase in bone density, especially of the axial skeleton, is characteristic. The spine and pelvis may show changes in the form of calcification and ossification in the paravertebral

ligaments, ligamentum flavum, and iliolumbar and sacroiliac ligaments. The spinal changes may resemble to those of ankylosing spondylitis or diffuse idiopathic skeletal hyperostosis (DISH). However, the sacroiliac joints in X-linked hypophosphatemia show no bone erosions in contrast to that seen in ankylosing spondylitis. The appendicular skeleton also shows multiple sites of new bone formation at various muscle and ligament attachments. Osteoarthritis is common, particularly in the ankle, knees, wrists, and sacroiliac joints.

The above radiographic findings in the axial and appendicular skeleton are distinctive and the diagnosis may be suggested prior to the clinical recognition of the disorder.

- *Primary hypophosphatemic rickets*: It is a form of rickets characterized by low serum phosphate levels and resistance to treatment with UV radiation or vitamin D therapy.
- *Renal tubular acidosis*: Renal tubular acidosis (RTA) comprises a group of tubular transport defects characterized by inability to appropriately acidify the urine with resultant metabolic acidosis. The underlying abnormalities consist of an impairment of bicarbonate resorption or excretion of hydrogen ions or a combination of both. Detailed biochemical tests are essential for reaching at a correct diagnosis in RTA.[9]
  - *Type I (distal) RTA*: It is characterized by persistent severe metabolic acidosis with continuous bicarbonaturia and is an important cause of severe rachitic abnormalities.[9] In untreated cases, nephrocalcinosis/renal calculi are formed.
  - *Type II (proximal) RTA*: This type of RTA may occur in children in an isolated form or as part of global proximal tubular dysfunction called *Fanconi's syndrome.* In this condition, phosphaturia of tubular origin is associated with glycosuria and various aminoacidurias in addition to bicarbonaturia. Unlike type I RTA, children with type II RTA do not progressively accumulate acid.[9] Rachitic deformities and nephrocalcinosis are uncommon in isolated proximal RTA but are common in Fanconi's syndrome.
- *Tumor-associated rickets and osteomalacia*: Tumor-associated rickets and osteomalacia (also termed *oncogenic osteomalacia*) is a syndrome characterized by hyperphosphaturia, with resultant hypophosphatemia, decreased levels of 1,25$(OH)_2D_3$ (refractory to vitamin D_3 administration), and various neoplasms.

  The syndrome is more common in adults than children. The tumors are benign, of connective tissue origin, located either in soft tissues or bones. They are typically vascular and often show foci of new bone formation.

  Patients with this syndrome frequently have long-standing generalized muscle weakness and proximal myopathy. Radiographic changes of rickets and osteomalacia may be advanced at the time of initial presentation.

  The cause of rickets in association with these tumors has been attributed to the secretion of a humoral agent termed "phosphatonin" which directly inhibits the absorption of phosphates in the proximal tubule.[10] The tumors are usually small, benign, and of vascular origin (hemangiopericytoma), but there is now known to be a wide spectrum of tumors, some of which may be malignant.[11]

  Biochemically, serum calcium is normal with marked decrease in serum phosphate. These patients are resistant or refractory to vitamin D. However, resection of the tumor results in the reversal of metabolic, clinical, and osseous abnormalities.
- *Chemotherapeutic drug-induced rickets:* High doses of a chemotherapeutic agent, *"ifosfamide"* used in the treatment of solid tumors, especially in children have been known to result in Fanconi syndrome with hypophosphatemic rickets. This complication is seen as a result of nephrotoxic metabolites of the drug and may be irreversible.[10] Renal toxicity is predominantly tubular, although glomerular abnormalities may also occur. Any part of the nephron may be damaged by ifosfamide. The major cause of rickets and osteomalacia is hyperphosphaturia with resultant hypophosphatemia.

- *Syndromes with the radiographic appearance of rickets or osteomalacia but without abnormalities of vitamin D metabolism or renal tubular dysfunction (phosphate loss)*:
  - *Metaphyseal chondrodysplasia (Schmid type)*: It is a disorder in which there is generalized symmetric disturbance of endochondral bone formation, primarily at the metaphysis.[4] It is manifested in childhood as short stature and bowing of the long bones, having a benign course. The radiographs show widening of the growth plate. Multiple, small, and bony projections extend from the metaphysis into the growth plate. In contrast to the usual rickets, the metaphysis is well mineralized and may show increased density.[4] There is absence of Looser's zones. The serum calcium, phosphorus, and alkaline phosphatase levels are normal. Spontaneous improvement occurs and patients do not respond to vitamin D therapy.
  - *Hypophosphatasia*: Hypophosphatasia is a rare disorder that is genetically transmitted that may resemble rickets both clinically and radiologically. However, the serum calcium and phosphorus levels are normal. The characteristic diagnostic features are:
    - Defective skeletal mineralization, resembling rickets radiologically
    - Low serum alkaline phosphatase level (in contrast to rickets in which it is increased)
    - Increased amounts of phosphoethanolamine, an amino acid, in the blood and urine.

  A wide spectrum of clinical severity is noted with most patients being diagnosed in infancy and childhood. The most severely affected neonates usually die soon after birth. *Radiologically,* there is reduced mineralization. Fractures with deformity and shortening may suggest a dwarfing syndrome. Radiographic changes at the growth plate may be seen soon after birth, and are similar to those of rickets but show characteristic multiple radiolucent extensions into the metaphysis that represent uncalcified bone matrix.[4] Coarse trabecular pattern, bowing deformities with or without healing fractures may be present. Wormian bones and craniosynostosis may be present.

- *Atypical axial osteomalacia*: It is a rare condition in which the radiographic abnormalities are confined to the axial skeleton, with sparing of appendicular sites. A dense, coarse trabecular pattern is most marked in the cervical region. The lumbar spine, pelvis, and ribs are also involved. Looser's zones have not been identified in this condition.[10] The biochemical findings are normal with no response to vitamin D therapy.

Radiological Features

Although there is a significant overlap between rickets and osteomalacia, their radiologic findings are quite different and hence, they will be discussed separately.

Rickets

Rickets occurs when the orderly development and mineralization of the growth plate is interrupted. In the earliest stage, rachitic changes are not detectable radiologically. Biochemical and histologic changes develop several weeks prior to the appearance of the conclusive changes in the radiographs.[12]

The most common and nonspecific radiologic finding in patients of rickets is osteopenia.[1,4,5] Characteristic changes occur at the open growth plate.[5] The findings are seen on the metaphyseal side of the growth plate as the unmineralized osteoid is concentrated there. These changes are best seen in those areas showing most active growth. The distal ends of radius and ulna are the optimal sites for the demonstration of the earliest lesion.[11] Significant changes are often seen in the ulna when the radius appears to be normal as the distal ulnar growth plate grows more rapidly than the distal radius. Therefore, the ulna is a more sensitive indicator of rickets at the wrist.

Radiographic abnormalities reflect the disordered proliferation of cartilaginous cells in the zone of hypertrophy along with the deficient mineralization in the zone of provisional calcification.[4,5] The zone of provisional calcification is a band of calcification which marks the end of the radiolucent growth plate and beginning of the radiographically calcified metaphysis.

As the rachitic changes are more advanced at the fastest growing growth plates, radiographs of the most active sites should be undertaken. In order of decreasing activity, the most active growth plates are costochondral junction of the middle ribs, the distal femur, the proximal humerus, both ends of tibia, and the distal ulna and radius.

The characteristic radiologic features of rickets seen at the end of long bones in order of occurrence the radiologic findings are:

- *Widening of the growth plate* is the *earliest specific radiologic change* which occurs as a result of increase in cartilaginous cell mass.[4]
- *Irregular metaphyseal margins* (paint brush metaphyses) occurs due to fraying and disorganization of the spongy bone in the metaphyseal region.
- Further progression of the disease leads to *widening and cupping* of the *metaphysis* **(Figs. 4A and B)**. This can be explained by the protrusion of the bulky mass of cartilaginous cells in the zone of hypertrophy into the poorly mineralized metaphysis. Cupping of the distal end of the ulna in younger infants is not necessarily abnormal as it has been observed in some nonrachitic infants during the first months of life.[12] Cupping is common in both ends of the fibula and the distal ends of the ulna and tibia. Metaphyseal cupping is however never found in the bones of the elbow.[13]
- Similar process occurs on the epiphyseal side of the growth plate. The defective maturation and mineralization result in an *epiphysis* that is *osteopenic* and has irregular, indistinct borders and shows *delayed appearance of ossification centers.*
- The shafts of long bones may appear normal when changes are first detected in the metaphysis. *Rarefaction* of the *shaft* becomes evident a few weeks later due to loss of mineral content. The cortex becomes thin with a coarse texture.
- *Skeletal deformities* are the most common complication detected radiologically, the appearance and location of which depend on age and the part in which disease develops.[4]
    - *Skull*: It is particularly affected in the early months of life as it has to accommodate the rapidly growing brain. There is excess osteoid deposition in frontal and parietal regions and posterior flattening due to supine posture of the infant. This results in squared configuration of the skull known as "craniotabes" **(Fig. 5A)**.
    - *Long bones*: In early childhood, more rapid growth occurs in the long bones and bowing deformities of arms and legs are common which can be related to the sitting position assumed by infants and children. Bowing also is a result of displacement of the growth centers owing to the asymmetrical musculotendinous pulls on the weakened growth plate[14] **(Fig. 5B)**. Bulbous enlargement of the costochondral junctions, particularly those of the middle ribs can be seen (rachitic rosary **Fig. 5C**), which can indent the pleural surface or even the thymic shadow.[6]
    - *Spine*: Scoliosis and vertebral end plate deformities may develop in older children as the effects of weight bearing become more important. Scoliosis coupled with bending deformities of long bones results in an overall decrease in height of the child.
    - *Pelvis*: The protrusion of the hip and spine into the soft pelvis produces a triradiate configuration of the pelvis. Such a pelvic deformity may cause considerable difficulty during parturition.
    - *Fractures*: In long-standing cases of rickets, trivial trauma may result in fracture of the weakened undermineralized bone **(Figs. 6A and B)**.

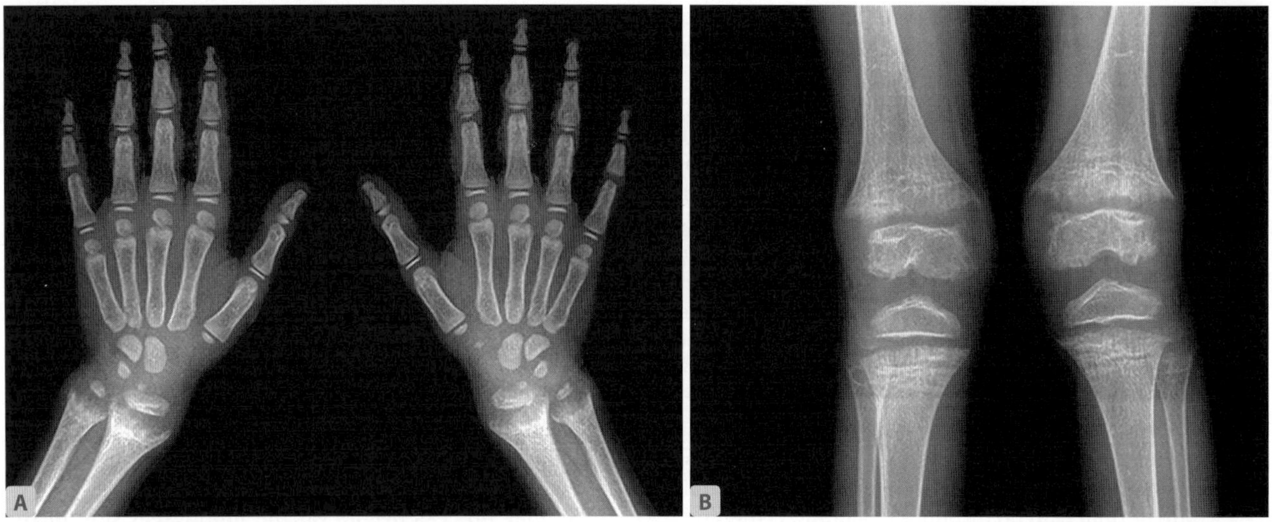

FIGS. 4A AND B: Rickets: X-ray bilateral wrists (A) and knees (B). Anteroposterior (AP) view: Typical changes of active rickets consisting of fraying, irregularity of distal radius and ulnar metaphysis and distal femoral and proximal tibial metaphysis with widening of the growth plates at the wrists and knees. The adjacent epiphysis and diaphysis are osteopenic.

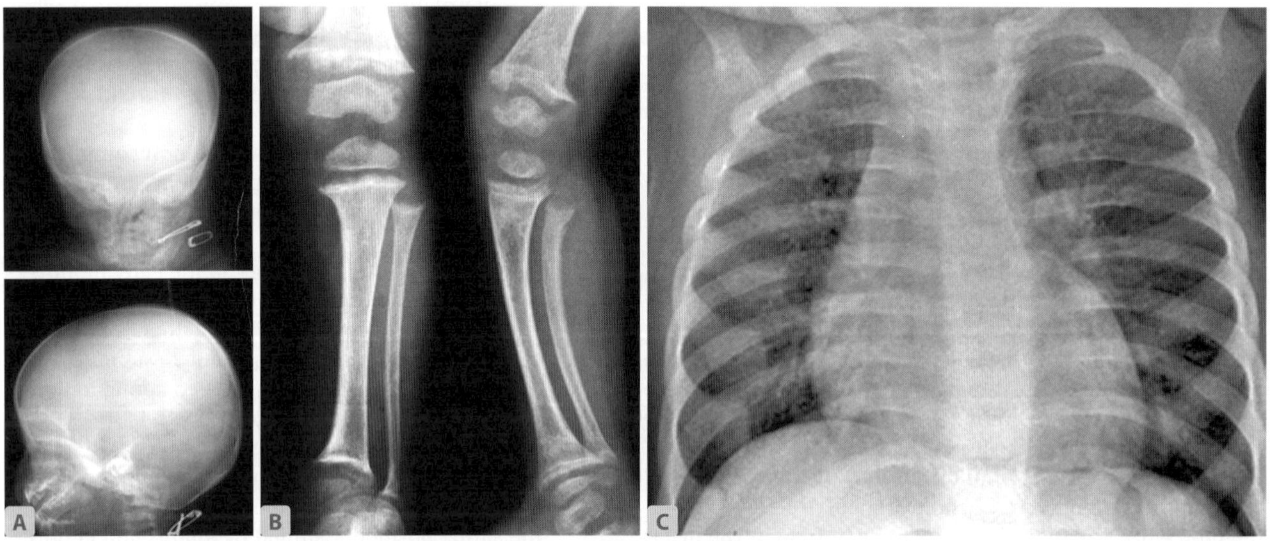

FIGS. 5A TO C: Skeletal deformities in rickets. (A) Squared configuration of the skull in the neonatal period: "Craniotabes"; (B) Marked anterior bowing of the tibia and fibula with rachitic changes. The visualized bones are osteopenic; (C) "Rachitic rosary": Widened anterior ends of ribs due to hypertrophy of costochondral junction.

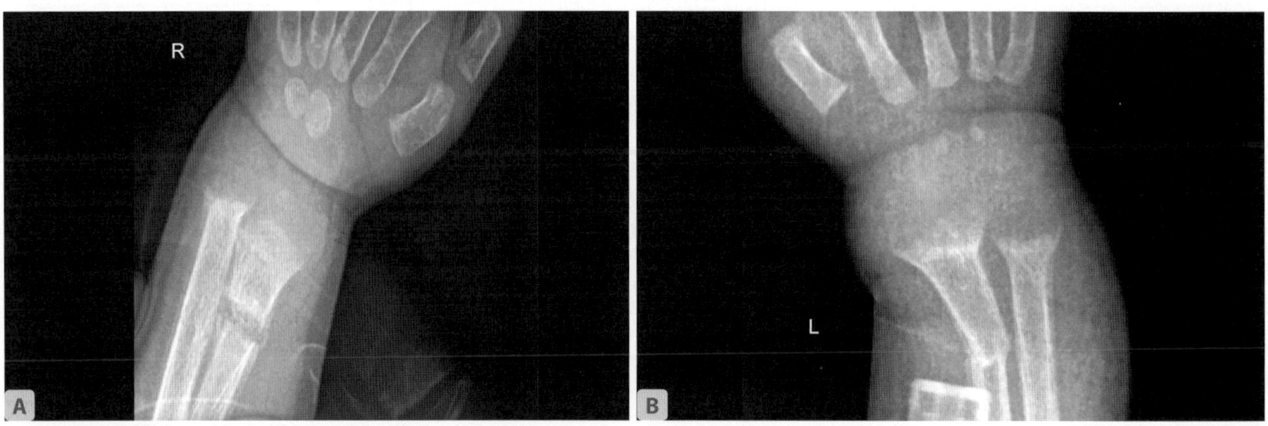

FIGS. 6A AND B: X-ray of wrists of two infants with rickets. The bones are markedly osteopenic with fracture of distal ends of radius in both.

In severe malnutrition, rickets may be associated with scurvy and protein deficiency.

Signs of Healing

Radiological evidence of healing is seen within 2–3 weeks of adequate therapy and total recalcification is usually complete in 2 months.[15] The signs of healing rickets are:

- Reappearance of the dense zone of provisional calcification: This is the first evidence of healing and is seen radiologically as a transverse line of increased density, which appears beyond the visible end of shaft with a metaphysis interposed between the two radiolucent areas **(Fig. 7)**. Further mineralization of the osteoid unites this with the metaphysis.
- Increase in cupping of the healing metaphysis is seen as compared to the cupping seen in the active stage of rickets.
- Recalcification of the subperiosteal osteoid may produce a thick envelope of cortex that surrounds the shaft. This thick, opaque envelope along the shaft may be of uniform density or lamellated.
- Epiphyseal ossification center which were ill-defined and osteopenic in the active stage of rickets become sharply defined in the healing stage. In severe cases, the ossification centers may become invisible during the active stage of rickets and reappear when they are recalcified during healing, erroneously suggesting a rapid advance in skeletal maturation.

When the patient is on intermittent or inadequate treatment, the process of calcification and repair is irregular. Radiologically, patchy sclerosis of the metaphysis is seen, sometimes with alternating sclerotic and lucent bands.

Sequelae

Complete healing and restoration of normal structures is the rule in rickets even when severe changes are present during the active stage.[12]

Central rarefaction of ossification centers and cortical thickening of tubular bones may remain for a long time. Bowing and angulation deformities are not uncommon due to weakened bones.

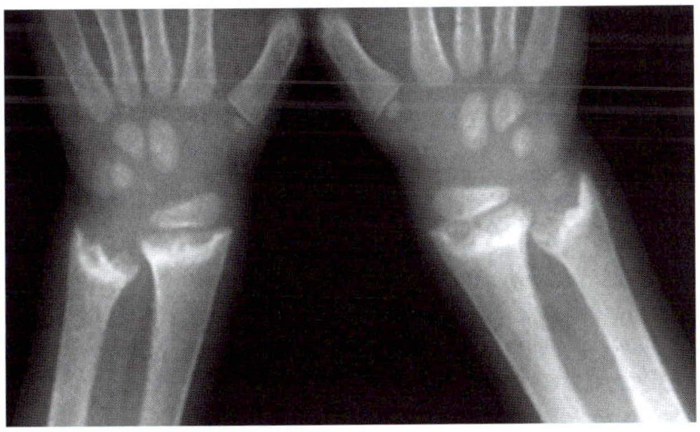

FIG. 7: Healing rickets: X-ray bilateral (B/L) wrists showing reappearance of the dense zone of provisional calcification at the metaphysis.

Osteomalacia

The term osteomalacia literally means *"soft bones."*

Radiological Changes

The radiological findings of osteomalacia are often nonspecific.[4] Correlation with appropriate laboratory and clinical data are often required for reaching a correct diagnosis. The major skeletal changes observed are:

- *Osteopenia:* It is the most common radiologic sign due to decreased bone mineral content.[4] It is usually uniform involving all the bones.
- *Coarse indistinct trabecular pattern:* It is in combination with generalized osteopenia and suggests osteomalacia.[4] An overall decrease in number of bony trabeculae within all the bones enhances the contrast of the remaining trabeculae giving a coarse, mottled appearance **(Figs. 8A and B)**.
- *Cortical involvement:* The cortices of long bones become thin, with indistinct definition, especially on the endosteal surface.
- *Pseudofractures or Looser's zones:* These are a more specific but less common manifestation of osteomalacia.[16] Looser's zones are linear radiolucent bands of undermineralized osteoid that occur in a bilateral and symmetric distribution[16,17] **(Figs. 9A and B)**. They are oriented at right angles to the cortex, i.e., perpendicular to the long axis of the bone.[15] The characteristic sites include:
    - Axillary margins of scapula
    - Superior and inferior pubic rami
    - Medial femoral necks
    - Posterior margins of the proximal ulna
    - Ribs.[4,17]

Looser's zones are considered to be either insufficiency type stress fracture or due to vascular pulsations acting on the softened bone.[6,14] However, in contrast to fatigue type stress fractures, pseudofractures do not necessarily involve weight-bearing bones and may remain unaltered over long

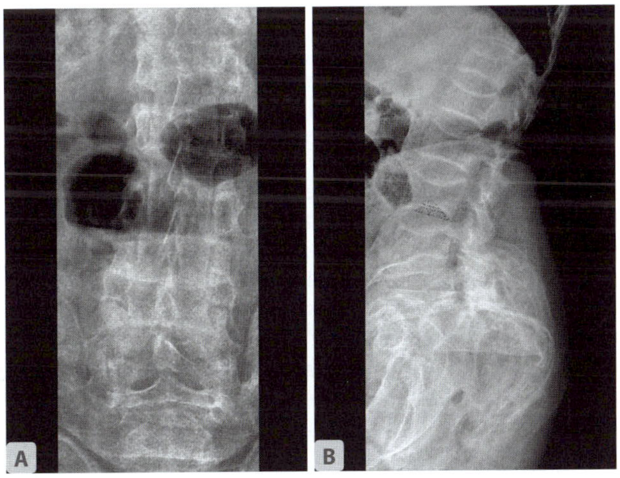

FIGS. 8A AND B: X-ray lumbosacral spine anteroposterior (AP) and lateral views reveal marked diffuse osteopenia with reduced vertebral height with biconcave appearance giving cod fish appearance. The sacral spine is acutely kyphotic: Osteomalacia.

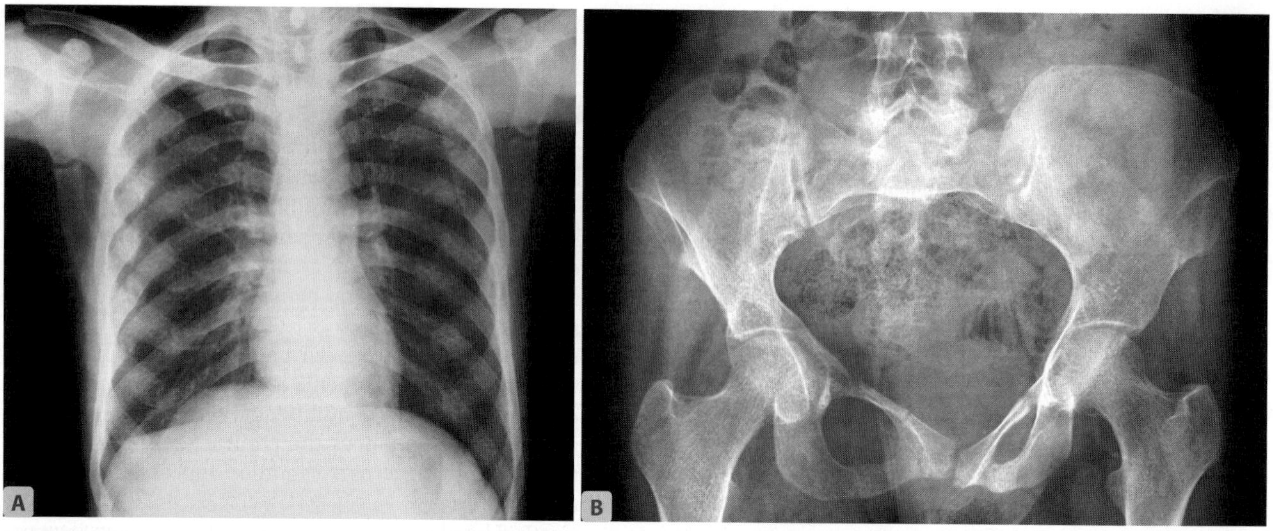

FIGS. 9A AND B: (A) Chest radiograph showing typical appearance of Looser's zone in bilateral lateral and medial borders of scapulae and ribs; (B) X-ray of pelvis [anteroposterior (AP)] showing characteristic appearance of Looser's zones in bilateral superior pubic rami and mild right protrusio acetabuli with resultant asymmetric shape of the pelvic cavity.

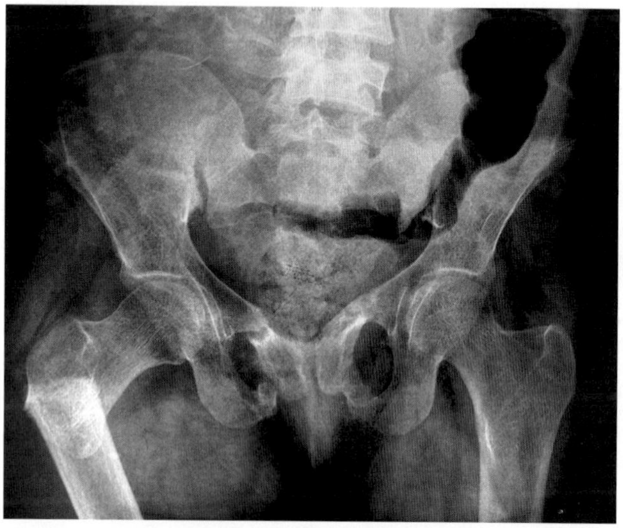

FIG. 10: X-ray of pelvis [anteroposterior (AP)] in a 28 years' female with sudden-onset pain over right thigh following trivial trauma reveals fracture of upper end of the right femur. The visualized bones are osteopenic with coarse trabecular pattern. Looser's zones are seen in bilateral superior and inferior rami: Osteomalacia.

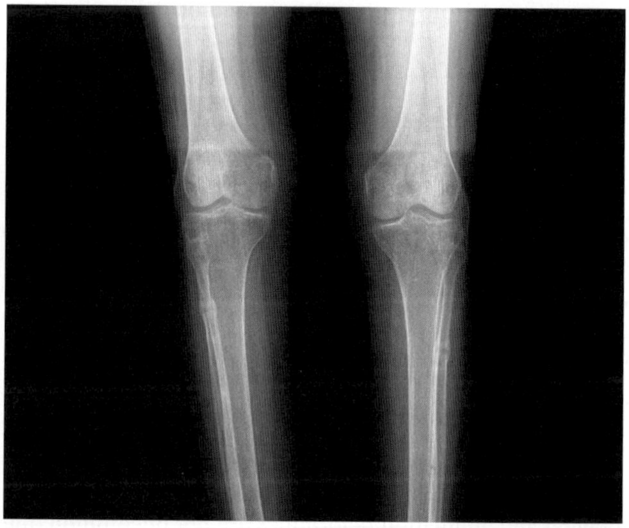

FIG. 11: Radiograph bilateral legs [anteroposterior (AP)] showing Looser's zone in upper one-third bilateral fibula with surrounding sclerosis. There is osteoporosis with cortical thinning of the bones.

periods of time. True fractures may develop later at these sites because they represent areas of weakened bone[14] **(Fig. 10)**. In addition, Looser's zones show mild-to-moderate sclerosis with an absence of callus. Radiolucent areas similar to pseudofractures may be seen in bones affected by Paget's disease and fibrous dysplasia.[14,16]

The terms *Milkman's fracture, increment fracture and umbauzonen* have also been used to describe osteomalacic pseudofractures.[4,6] Pseudofractures occur at sites of increased stress and therefore, accelerated bone turnover. They are classically seen at the concave (compressive) side of a bony deformity.[31] The osteoid which is laid down in the replacement process is inadequately mineralized, which accounts for its radiolucent appearance **(Fig. 11)**.[4,14]

Pseudofractures may be identified by radionuclide bone scan or MR imaging before being evident on radiographs.[14]

Bone scintigraphy has been found to be more sensitive than blood biochemistry and radiographic findings in the detection of osteomalacia. The typical features of osteomalacia seen on whole-body scintigraphy are widening of mandible, rachitic rosary sign, the tie sign of the sternum, pseudofracture sign, and prominent epiphysis of the knees.[18]

- *Bony deformities:* These occur mainly in weight-bearing joints. In the pelvis, there is medial acetabular migration (protrusio acetabulae) and inferior displacement of

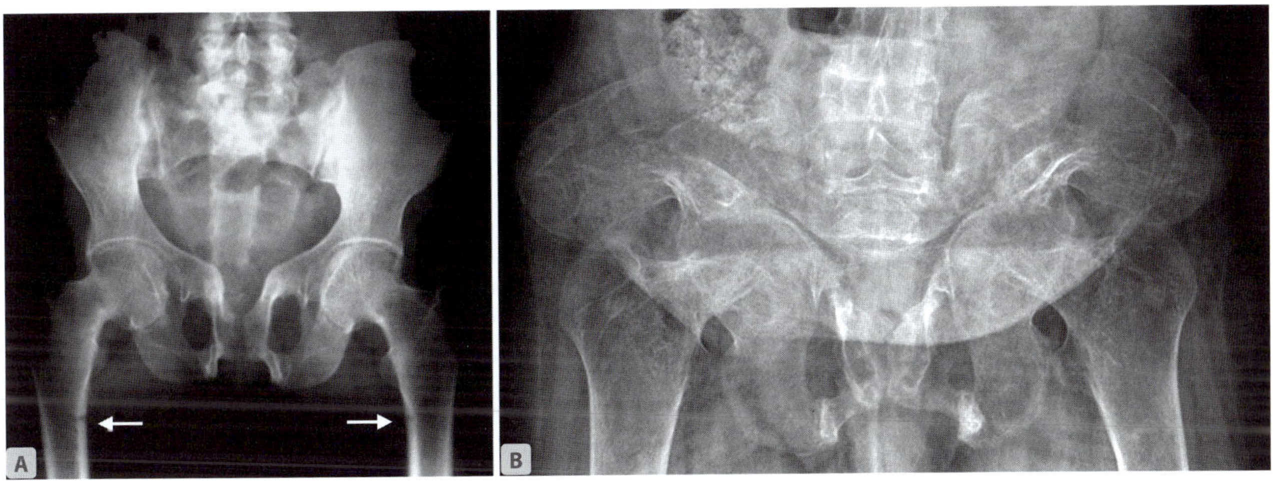

FIGS. 12A AND B: Pelvis [anteroposterior (AP)] in two different patients of osteomalacia. (A) Looser's zones in bilateral symmetric distribution in inner margins of proximal femora and superior and inferior pubic rami; (B) Severe osteomalacic changes with triradiate pelvis due to bilateral (B/L) protrusio acetabuli and inferior displacement of sacrum. The visualized bones are markedly osteoporotic. Old healed Looser's zones are seen in B/L superior and inferior pubic rami.

sacrum thereby producing a triradiate shape of the pelvis[9] (**Figs. 12A and B**). Both the femur and tibia show bowing deformity, vertebral bodies may develop a biconcave shape ("codfish" vertebrae), and kyphoscoliosis is not an uncommon finding. Basilar invagination of the skull may occur.[9]

Radiographs of the spine in osteoporosis (characterized by decrease in bone mass but there is no defect in mineralization) and osteomalacia may appear to be similar but they can be differentiated on the basis of coarse and indistinct trabeculae in osteomalacia while the trabeculae are thin and sharp in osteoporosis. Also, the spinal deformity in osteomalacia is uniform unlike osteoporosis wherein it is nonuniform.[4]

HYPERPARATHYROIDISM

Hyperparathyroidism (HPT) is a pathological state characterized by excessive production of parathyroid hormone (PTH). In the normal state, parathyroid hormone promotes release of calcium into the blood from the bone. It also stimulates extensive bone remodeling. Alterations of parathyroid function cause a breakdown in calcium homeostasis leading to increased renal absorption of calcium, phosphaturia, increased synthesis of 1,25-dihydroxy vitamin D_3, which increases intestinal calcium resorption, and increased bone turnover, thereby resulting in characteristic pathologic and radiologic abnormalities.[19] Hyperparathyroidism is divided into primary, secondary, and tertiary types.

Primary Hyperparathyroidism

Primary HPT refers to inappropriate or unregulated overproduction of PTH occurring as a result of abnormality in one or more of the parathyroid glands. The cause in most cases is a single parathyroid adenoma (90% of cases); less common causes include double adenomas (4%), hyperplasia of multiple glands (6%), and parathyroid carcinoma (<1%).[20] Hyperplasia of the parathyroid glands can occur as an isolated finding or as part of multiple endocrine neoplasia (MEN) syndromes.

Secondary Hyperparathyroidism

Secondary HPT is more common than primary HPT. It is associated with abnormalities in function of the parathyroid glands induced by a sustained hypocalcemic stimulus. The most common cause is chronic renal failure in which chronically elevated serum phosphate levels depress the serum calcium level leading to compensatory hypertrophy of the chief cells of the parathyroid gland. Occasionally, malabsorption states and dietary abnormalities leading to hypocalcemia may be responsible.[21]

Tertiary Hyperparathyroidism

Tertiary HPT occurs in patients with long-standing secondary HPT who develop autonomous parathyroid function and hypercalcemia.

Pathophysiology

The clinical, pathological, and radiological manifestation of HPT can be understood by understanding the interrelated roles of parathyroid hormone (PTH) and vitamin D in the regulation of calcium metabolism.

Parathyroid hormone influences many tissues in the human body and is essential for the proper transport of calcium and other ions in bone, intestine, and kidney. The synthesis and secretion of PTH is regulated by the ionized serum calcium level. The normal serum calcium levels are maintained within a normal physiologic range by the intestines and kidneys which balance intake and excretion. Ninety-nine percent of the elemental calcium is bound to the skeleton and PTH works to increase the serum calcium by increasing the resorption with liberation of calcium and phosphorus.

In the kidneys, PTH inhibits resorption of phosphate in the proximal and distal tubules. This causes a decrease in the plasma phosphate concentration which in turn helps to maintain the serum calcium level. PTH also increases the renal tubular reabsorption of calcium.

Parathyroid hormone has no documented direct effect upon intestinal calcium absorption. PTH along with a decreased serum calcium and phosphate stimulates synthesis of 1,25 dihydroxy vitamin D the primary mediator of intestinal calcium and phosphorus absorption, and also acts on bone to produce resorption. Thus, functioning renal tissue is critical to the metabolism of both PTH and vitamin D and is a major target organ for the action of these hormones **(Fig. 13)**.

Therefore, there exists a negative feedback loop between serum calcium and PTH. An abrupt fall in calcium will actively stimulate PTH secretion **(Fig. 14)**.

Clinical Features

The clinical features of primary HPT relates to hypercalcemia which results from:

- Increased intestinal absorption of calcium
- Increased bone turnover
- Increased tubular resorption of calcium.

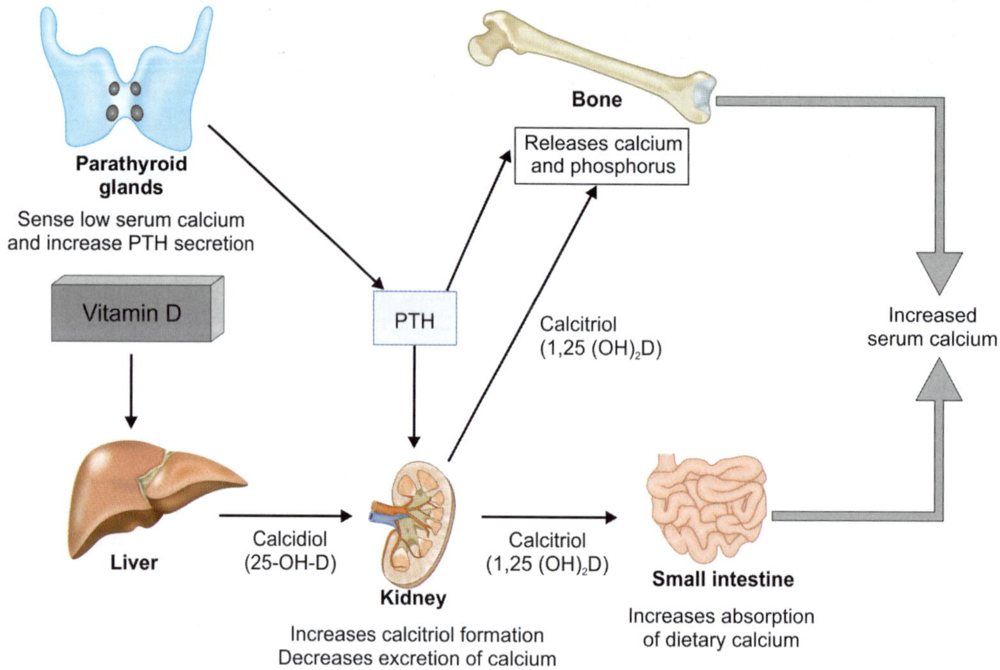

FIG. 13: Overview of vitamin D metabolism. (PTH: parathyroid).

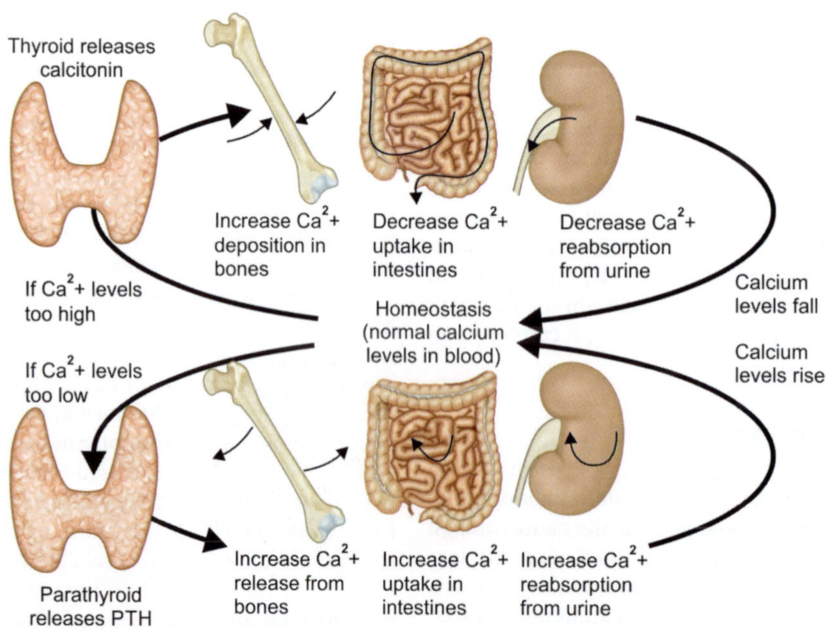

FIG. 14: Role of parathyroid (PTH) and calcitonin in the regulation of calcium metabolism.

Patients may present with tiredness, lethargy, polyuria, anorexia or nausea, or to bone or renal complication.

The true incidence of primary HPT is not known but biochemical screening identifies the condition in unsuspected persons. It is found at all ages from birth to old age, with the highest incidence between 20 and 60 years, with women being affected two to four times more often than men.[15]

There appears to be a relationship between the severity of the disease and the type of symptoms that predominate. Patients with renal calculi are younger, have a chronic course, and are associated with hyperplasia of the parathyroid gland. Those with bone changes have a subacute progressive course characterized by a marked elevation in serum calcium levels, and these patients generally have adenomas.[21]

Nephrolithiasis is the most common clinical manifestation, followed by hypertension, peptic ulcers, pancreatitis, psychiatric disorders, and bone pain.[22]

Biochemical Findings

In most cases, the diagnosis of hyperparathyroidism can be made on the basis of clinical symptomatology and laboratory tests. Sustained elevation of serum calcium and serum parathormone levels are the most accepted means for the establishment of diagnosis of primary HPT.[19] Multiple measurements of serum calcium are often recommended due to the variations in the amount of circulating parathyroid hormone at any given time. Also, hypercalcemia is a feature of other disease states such as malignancy, endocrinological disorders, secondary to drugs, granulomatous disorders, etc. **(Box 2)**. About 10–20% of patients with malignancy have elevated serum calcium levels (normal reference range = 9–11 mg%) with majority of these patients having direct involvement of the skeleton by a malignant lesion.[23]

The term pseudohyperparathyroidism is referred to the syndrome consisting of hypercalcemia of malignancy in the absence of demonstrable skeletal metastasis or primary hyperparathyroidism.

Elevated urinary cyclicAMP and elevated alkaline phosphatase levels signify increase in bone turnover and skeletal involvement.

In secondary HPT, the plasma calcium levels are normal or low and the serum inorganic phosphate levels are high (chronic renal failure) or low (intestinal malabsorption).

Radiological Approach

The value of radiological studies in primary and secondary HPT lies not in the initial diagnosis, but in assessing the severity of the condition, and in noninvasive localization of the parathyroid glands prior to surgery as well as in the follow-up of the patient.[21]

Radiological Findings

The skeletal changes in HPT are characteristic and reflect the histologic changes of increased resorption of cortical and cancellous bone with substitutive fibrosis. Conventional radiography can assess the extent of bone involvement and the presence of bone changes is an accepted indication for parathyroid surgery in primary HPT.[21] The bone changes of primary and secondary HPT are identical, except for the associated changes of renal osteodystrophy in secondary HPT.

In the past, for earlier diagnosis of subtle osseous abnormalities, magnification radiography was done. But now, with advances in digital radiography routine hand radiographs are considered the most effective method.

Bone Resorption

The incidence of bone lesions varies from 30 to 40%.[21] The initial bone changes may not be seen on radiographic or gross pathologic examination, although, microscopic evaluation shows osteoclastic activity.[19] Bone resorption is a hallmark of HPT and is one of the effects of increased PTH production. The bone resorption is due to increased osteoclastic activity and can be detected on the subperiosteal, intracortical, endosteal, subchondral, and trabecular surfaces. Overall cortical bone is affected more severely than cancellous bone. These changes are reflected radiologically by poor definition of cortical surfaces, increased cortical striations ("tunneling"), cortical thinning, and distortion and blurring of trabecular bone.[21]

BOX 2: Differential diagnosis of hypercalcemia.

- *Malignancy*:
  - Solid tumors (primarily breast cancer)
  - Hematologic disorders
  - Myeloma
  - Lymphoma
  - Leukemia
- *Enocrinological disorders*:
  - Primary hyperparathyroidism
  - Multiple endocrine neoplasias (types I and II)
  - Ectopic hyperparathyroidism (malignancy predominantly lung cancer)
  - Secondary hyperparathyroidism (renal failure)
  - Hyperthyroidism
  - Hypoadrenalism
- *Drugs*:
  - Vitamin A intoxication
  - Vitamin D intoxication
  - Thiazides
  - Calcium
  - Milk alkali syndrome
  - Dialysis
- *Granulomatous disorders*:
  - Sarcoidosis
  - Tuberculosis
  - Histoplasmosis
  - Berylliosis
  - Rheumatoid arthritis
- *Pediatric disorders*:
  - Infantile hypercalcemia
  - Hypophosphatasia
- *Miscellaneous*:
  - Immobilization
  - Paget's disease

Subperiosteal Resorption

Subperiosteal resorption of cortical bone is considered pathognomonic of HPT.[19,21] Although it may be seen at various skeletal sites, the earliest and best recognized changes are seen in the hands.[24] The earliest site of subperiosteal resorption is the radial aspect of middle phalanges of middle and index fingers **(Figs. 15A and B)**. Some authors have cited the earliest radiographic evidence of subperiosteal resorption to occur in the terminal tufts of the fingers.[21,24] Loss of fine cortical outline around the tufts results in a lace-like irregular appearance of external surface of bone with significant erosion of tufts being more obvious in advanced cases. A distinctive pattern of band-like appearance of acroosteolysis may be seen in the terminal phalanges of the hands (less commonly the feet), consisting of band-like radiolucent areas that may separate the tuft and the base of the phalanx separately.

Other sites of subperiosteal resorption include the medial aspect of the proximal end of tibia, humerus and femur, superior and inferior margins of the ribs, and lamina dura surrounding the teeth[24] **(Fig. 16)**. Loss of lamina dura once considered pathognomonic of HPT is now considered as nonspecific as it may accompany dental sepsis, fibrous dysplasia, Paget's disease, osteomalacia, and other endocrine disorders.[19,24] Subperiosteal resorption may also occur in the marginal areas of joints, particularly in the hands and feet, and may mimic erosive changes of rheumatoid arthritis or other inflammatory arthropathies. A feature to differentiate the erosions in HPT from that of rheumatoid arthritis is that they are located slightly away from the joint margin and are almost always associated with typical subperiosteal resorption of the adjacent phalangeal tufts.

Intracortical Bone Resorption

Intracortical bone resorption or cortical tunneling is one of the hallmarks of rapid bone turnover wherein groups of osteoclasts tunnel through the Volkman's and haversian canals.[21] This finding is also not specific for HPT and may be seen in hyperthyroidism, acromegaly, and disorders causing rapid osteoporosis. They are radiographically seen as subtle linear striations or scalloping within the cortex parallel to the long axis of the bone, best seen in the tubular bones of the hand and feet, especially in the cortex of the second metacarpal. Intracortical resorption of bone is almost always associated with subperiosteal resorption **(Fig. 17)**.

Richardson et al. quantified the degree of intracortical tunneling in the metacarpal shafts and found it to be a sensitive indicator of the extent of bone disease in HPT.[21,24,25] This method known as the "cortical striation index" requires detailed magnification radiographs.[21,24] A grading system is used to determine the degree of cortical striation present in the first and second metacarpals of each hand.

- Grade 0 Solid cortex with up to one striation
- Grade 1 Mild increase in striations
- Grade 2 Increased striations, but with involvement of <50% of the cortex
- Grade 3 Extensive striations throughout the cortex

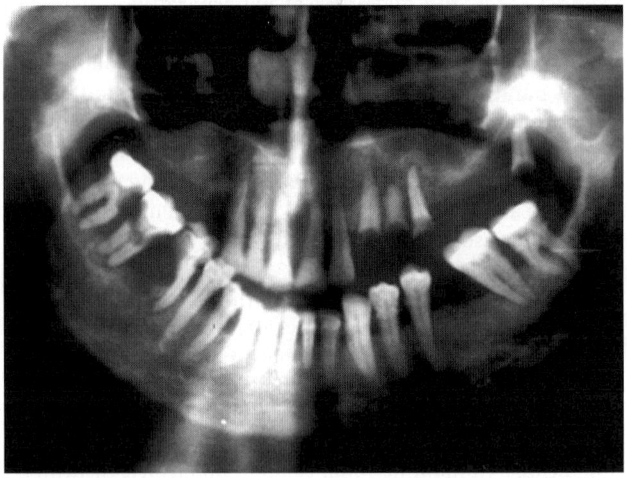

FIG. 16: Pantomogram showing extensive subperiosteal resorption with loss of lamina dura in a patient with parathyroid adenoma.

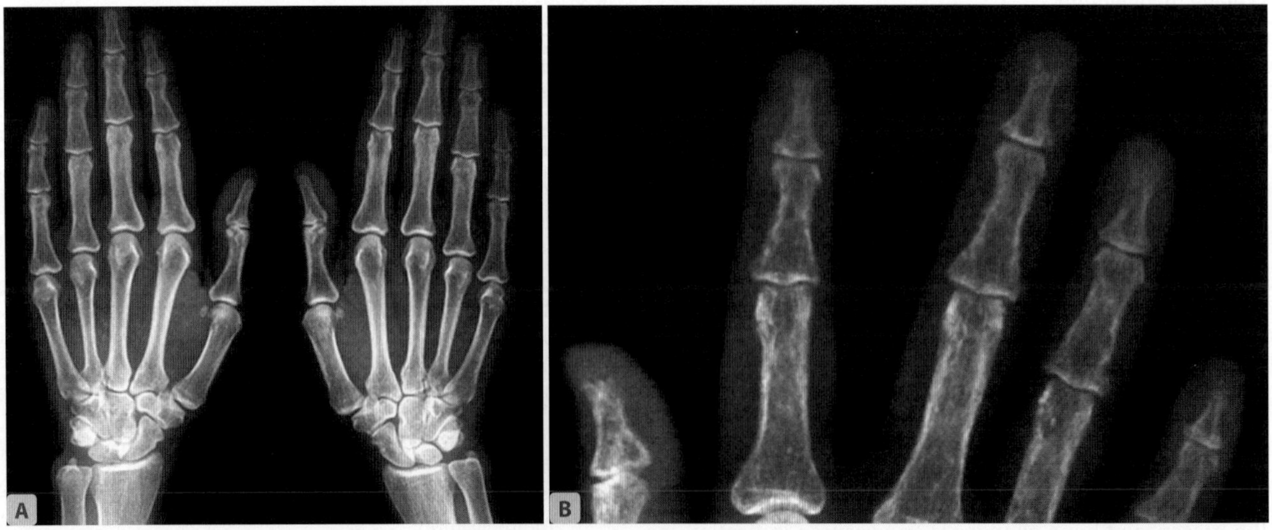

FIGS. 15A AND B: Hyperparathyroidism. (A) Hands showing resorption of the subperiosteal bone on the radial aspect of the middle phalanges of the index and middle fingers with magnified view; (B) Resorption of the tufts of terminal phalanges as well.

The second and third metacarpals of each hand are graded separately. In normal individuals, the "mean cortical index" is 1 or <1. Increased striations are seen in patients with primary HPT, renal osteodystrophy, and osteomalacia. The importance of cortical striation measurement in patients with HPT is in monitoring the response to treatment.[21]

Endosteal Bone Resorption

It leads to cortical thinning, scalloping, and irregularity of the endosteal surface and may obscure the corticomedullary junction, especially in the bones of the hand. Endosteal bone resorption may occur more commonly in conjunction with subperiosteal and intracortical resorption rather than an isolated finding.

Subchondral Bone Resorption

Subchondral bone resorption is a common manifestation of hyperparathyroidism, particularly in the joints of the axial skeleton, such as the sacroiliac, sternoclavicular, acromioclavicular joints, pubic symphysis, and discovertebral junctions causing surface irregularity and increase in joint space.[21,24] The changes are most severe in the distal clavicles. The peripheral joints may also show subchondral bone resorption, and these changes may mimic infective arthritis.

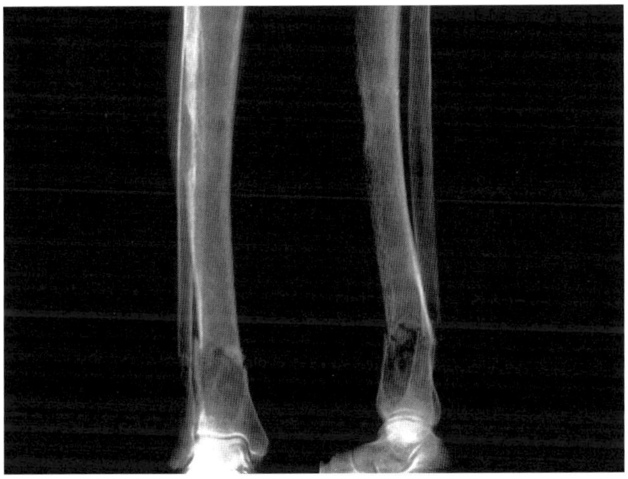

FIG. 17: Anteroposterior and lateral radiograph of leg shows resorption of anterior tibial cortex, intracortical striations, and brown tumor with pathological fractures: Hyperparathyroidism (HPT).

Subphyseal Bone Resorption

In children with primary or secondary HPT, irregular radiolucent areas may appear in the metaphysis adjacent to the growth plate. This finding is reminiscent of the abnormalities accompanying rickets.[23]

Subligamentous and Subtendinous Bone Resorption

Resorption of bone occurs at sites of tendon and ligament attachment to bone. The frequently involved sites are greater and lesser trochanter, ischial, and humeral tuberosities, elbow, inferior surface of calcaneus, and inferior aspect of distal end of clavicle.

Trabecular Bone Resorption

Trabecular resorption occurs throughout the skeleton in HPT, especially in the advanced stages of the disease, though changes in the skull vault are characteristic.[19,21] Osteoclasts on the surface of bone dissect through the center of trabecula, with loss of sharp trabecular pattern giving a stippled, mottled, and granular appearance termed radiologically as *"salt and pepper skull"*[19,21] **(Figs. 18A and B)**. The definition of outer and inner table is lost. Focal areas of osseous thickening in the cranial vault may be observed on radiographs as well-defined or poorly defined radiopaque areas.

Brown Tumors

They are also known as *osteitis fibrosa cystica or osteoclastomas*. Brown tumors are cyst-like well-circumscribed lytic lesions within bone and are an end result of extensive bone resorption.[19] They have initially been described characteristic of primary hyperparathyroidism, but seen with

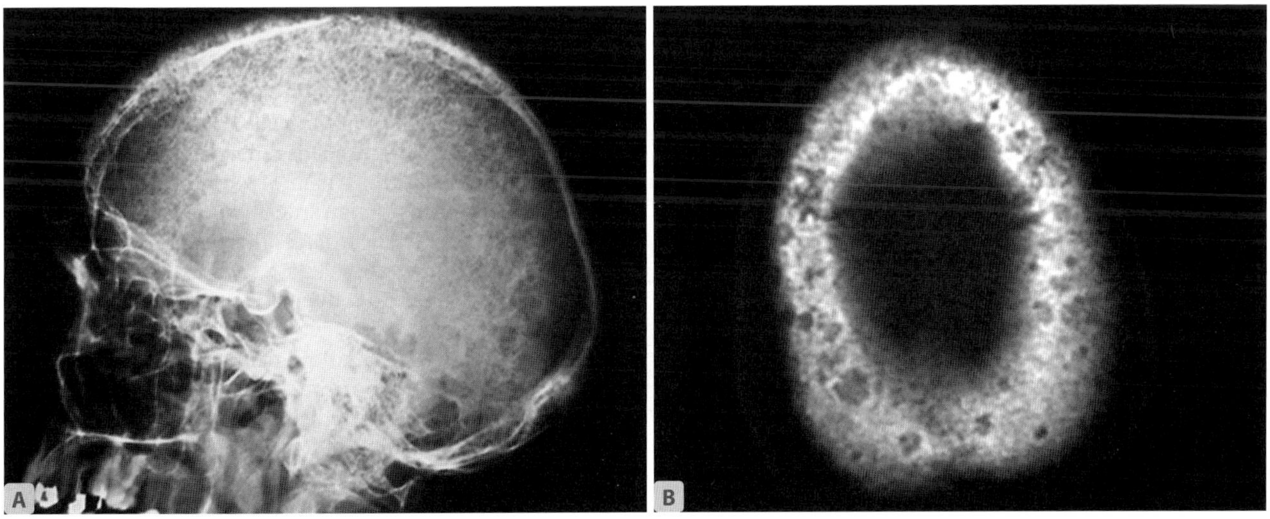

FIGS. 18A AND B: (A) Osteoporosis with loss of definition of inner and outer tables of the skull causing a classical mottled appearance of the skull vault: "salt and pepper skull"; (B) Computed tomography (CT) bone window reveals multiple variable-sized lytic lesions scattered throughout the calvarium with loss of differentiation of outer and inner tables.

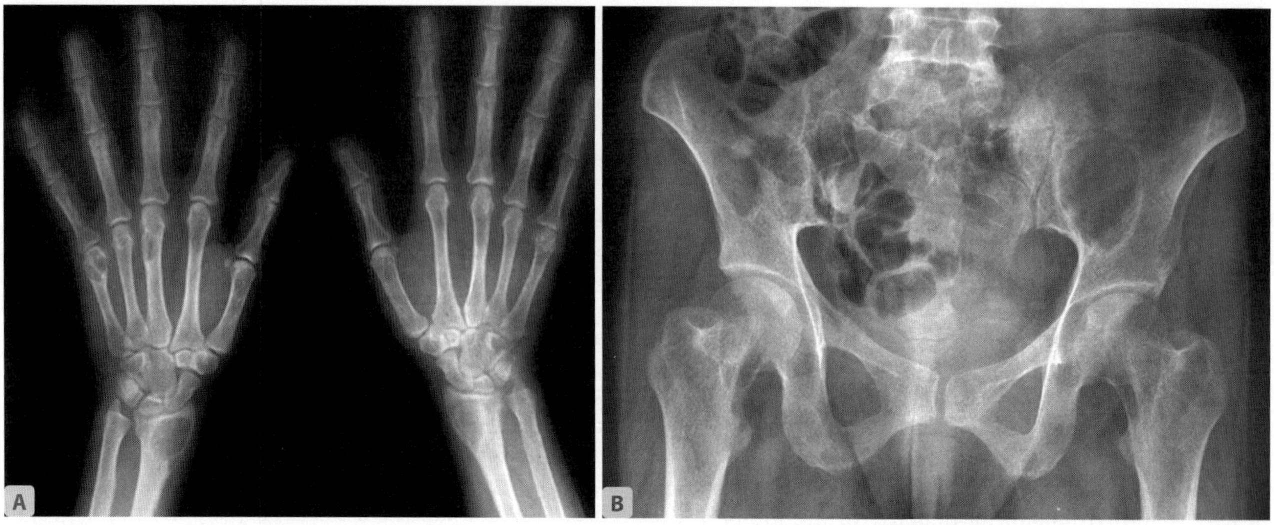

FIGS. 19A AND B: (A) X-ray bilateral hands in primary hyperparathyroidism (HPT) showing multiple, well-defined, expansile lytic lesions in lower end of radius, head, and distal ends of third and fifth metacarpals of right hand; (B) A large well-defined, oval lytic lesion with sclerotic rim in left iliac bone with multiple smaller ill-defined lesions in bilateral ischium: Brown tumors.

increasing frequency in secondary hyperparathyroidism as well.[24] They represent hemorrhage and deposition of breakdown products of hemoglobin. Brown tumors may cause swelling, pathological fracture, and bone pain in the skeletal system. Histologically, the cavities are filled with fibrous tissue and osteoclasts with necrosis and hemorrhagic liquefaction. *Radiographically,* brown tumors are seen as lytic, expansile, and cystic lesions which are solitary but are often multiple. They appear as well-defined lesions of the axial or appendicular skeleton, and are frequently eccentric or cortical in location, can be central **(Figs. 19A and B)**. The common sites of involvement are the mandible, clavicle, ribs, pelvis, and tubular bones.[19,21,25] Other manifestations of HPT are generally present, although occasionally a brown tumor may be the only finding radiologically. With removal of the parathyroid adenoma, brown tumors may demonstrate healing with sclerosis.[21,25]

The presence of multiple osteolytic lesions in an elderly patient with complaints of bone pain is suggestive of a mitotic/metastatic etiology. However, other etiologies such as multiple myeloma or brown tumor should be considered and serum phosphate, calcium, and PTH levels and serum protein electrophoresis should also be checked.

Brown tumors with hemorrhagic or cystic component in weight-bearing bones are associated with a higher risk of pathological fracture. MR imaging can aid in determining hemorrhage and cystic component and indirectly in estimation of fracture risk.[26]

It has been seen that there is a risk of pathological fracture when the brown tumor involves more than two-thirds of the cortex of the long bone, especially in the weight-bearing area. Preventive internal fixation is indicated if the tumor involves more than two thirds of the cortex of the weight-bearing long bone.[27]

In the past, advanced cases of hyperparathyroidism presenting with severe bone resorption was not an uncommon finding. However, use of more sophisticated diagnostic techniques along with an increased awareness of this condition, have led to an earlier diagnosis, when the degree of bone resorption is somewhat limited.[17] Fine detail and magnification skeletal radiography in primary HPT will not only detect mild disease but will also reveal intracortical, endosteal, and trabecular resorption.[19]

The combined effect of all the patterns of bone resorption is generalized osteopenia in a majority of patients.[19,24] On radiographs, osteopenia is frequently a subjective finding that is difficult to interpret and is identifiable only after 30–50% of mineral content is lost. This difficulty can be overcome by using quantitative bone mineral analysis which will indicate not only the degree and rate of bone loss in the disease but also partial recovery of the loss that is seen after successful parathyroidectomy.[19]

Joint Disorders

Erosive arthropathy of the hands, wrists, and shoulders may occur in patients with HPT, simulating rheumatoid arthritis. These changes are almost always associated with typical subperiosteal resorption of the phalanges and occur on the ulnar aspect of metacarpal heads unlike rheumatoid arthritis.

Another feature that is more common in primary hyperparathyroidism is chondrocalcinosis or calcification in hyaline cartilage or fibrocartilage. This occurs due to calcium pyrophosphate dihydrate (CPPD), calcium hydroxy apatite, or calcium oxalate crystal deposition. It may also occur in chronic renal disease, although its frequency is much lower than in primary HPT. Radiologically, chondrocalcinosis is seen in 18–40% patients with primary HPT.[19,24] Chondrocalcinosis may be seen in hyaline cartilage and fibrocartilage of the knee, symphysis pubis, and triangular cartilage of the wrist.[22] The deposition of crystals may lead to episodes of pseudogout. In contrast, soft-tissue and vascular calcification is more common in secondary HPT than in primary HPT.

Osteosclerosis

Increased bone density or osteosclerosis may be seen due to stimulation of osteoblastic activity by PTH in addition to its osteoclastic activity. The bone sclerosis can be either focal or diffuse.[24] Even though the bone shows increased density, it is structurally weak and prone to stress fractures.[30] In patients with secondary HPT, a diffuse increase in bone density is seen while in patients of primary HPT bone sclerosis is localized or patchy. Focal bone sclerosis is apparent in the metaphyseal regions of the long bones, the skull or the vertebral endplates. In the evaluation of hyperparathyroidism, one must keep in mind that osteosclerotic changes may also occur as a manifestation of healing, either spontaneous or as a result of treatment.[28]

Renal Osteodystrophy

Renal osteodystrophy is a term applied to the bone changes present in patients with chronic renal failure. In chronic renal failure, secondary HPT often coexists with rickets, osteomalacia, osteosclerosis, and osteoporosis as part of spectrum of findings called renal osteodystrophy. The skeletal changes of primary and secondary HPT are identical, except for associated changes of renal osteodystrophy seen in secondary HPT. **Table 2** highlights the features differentiating primary from secondary HPT.

TABLE 2: Primary versus secondary HPT.

Primary HPT	Secondary HPT
• Consists of skeletal features of HPT only	• Skeletal features of HPT with features of renal osteodystrophy (rickets/osteomalacia and osteosclerosis)
• Skeletal changes are less florid	• More florid
• Sclerosis rarely seen	• Commonly seen
• Brown tumors are more common	• Less common
• Chondrocalcinosis more common	• Less common
• Soft-tissue and vascular calcification are less common	• More common

The most common cause is chronic glomerulo-nephritis.[29] It can also result from bilateral chronic pyelonephritis, often associated with vesicoureteric reflux. In both conditions, small contracted kidneys are an evidence of the end-stage renal disease. The findings in renal osteodystrophy in children and adults are distinctive.

The most common finding in secondary HPT of renal osteodystrophy is subperiosteal resorption although other manifestations may be seen. The osseous resorption has shown to increase from 10% in the early stage of disease to 50–70% after 3–9 years of dialysis.[29] Conversely, following parathyroidectomy, bone resorption has shown to regress. Calcification of arteries, articular cartilage, and periarticular tissues also occur in renal osteodystrophy.

Osteosclerosis may occasionally be the only manifestation of renal osteodystrophy. It has a predilection for the axial skeleton **(Figs. 20A and B)**, with deposition of bone in the subchondral areas of the vertebral bodies.[30] This results in the appearance of radiodense bands across the superior and inferior vertebral margins known as "rugger jersey" spine appearance similar to stripes on an English rugby shirt. Other sites of osteosclerosis include the pelvis, ribs, and clavicles **(Fig. 21)**. It also involves the metaphysis of long bones and the skull. Post renal transplantation, the osteosclerosis may regress.[31]

Osteopenia has been reported in up to 85% of patients in renal osteodystrophy and is the end result of effect of osteomalacia, bone resorption, and a decrease in bone quantity (osteoporosis).[29]

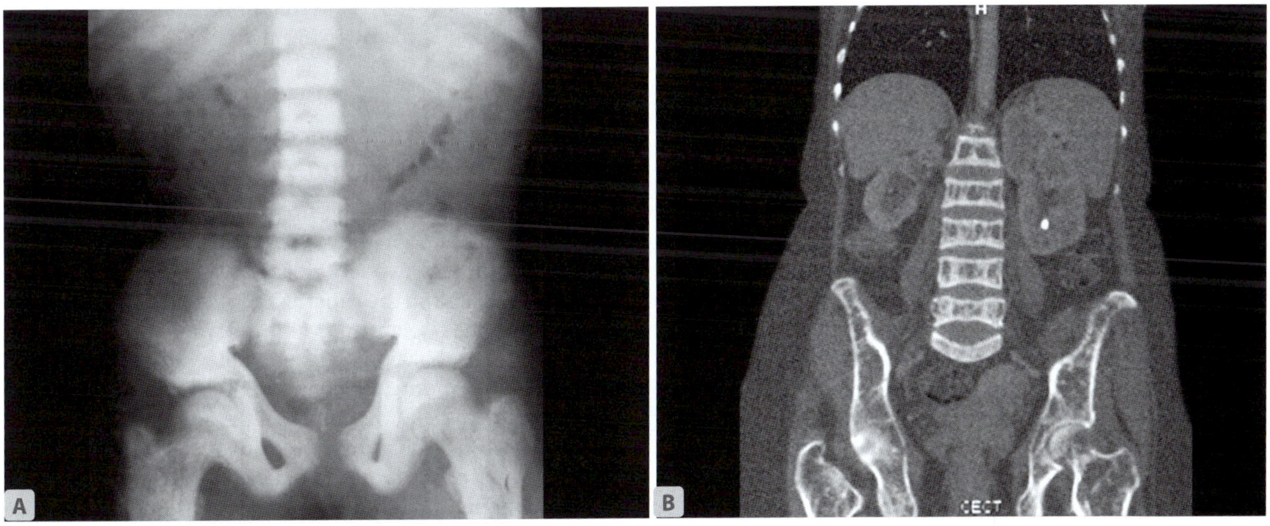

FIGS. 20A AND B: Renal osteodystrophy. (A) Diffuse increase in bone density of the pelvis and lumbar vertebrae with coarsened trabecular pattern; (B) Computed tomography (CT) abdomen bone window in another patient of secondary hyperparathyroidism (HPT) reveals diffuse osteopenia with coarsened trabecular pattern, loss of height of multiple lumbar vertebrae with mild sclerosis of superior and inferior end plates, patchy areas of sclerosis in the right ilium. Renal calculus noted in lower pole of the left kidney.

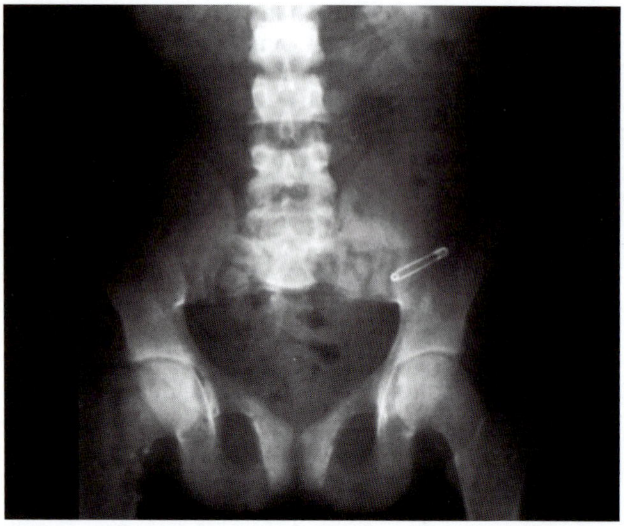

FIG. 21: Typical features of renal osteodystrophy in form of osteosclerosis of the axial skeleton with osteomalacic changes in the pelvis.

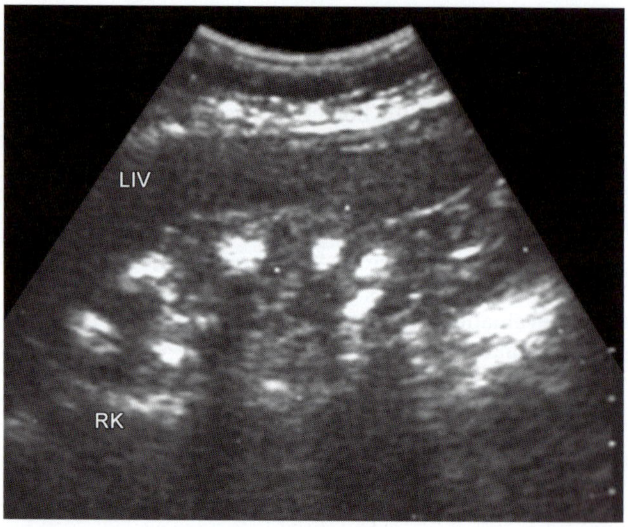

FIG. 22: Ultrasound of the right kidney (RK) shows medullary nephrocalcinosis in a patient of secondary hyperparathyroidism (HPT).

In children, metaphyseal changes resembling rickets are seen. This together with cortical erosions can give rise to the "rotting fencepost" appearance, particularly in the femoral neck. Slipped capital epiphysis may also be seen as a complication, most commonly involving the proximal femur.

Renal Lesions

Renal tubular dysfunction results from the direct effect of parathyroid hormone on the kidney and is corrected by parathyroidectomy. Renal calculi have been reported in 50% patients. These calculi are often small and the patient often presents with a renal colic.

Nephrocalcinosis

This is less common than renal calculi. Deposition of calcium is generally in the region of the renal pyramids **(Fig. 22)**, but forms no diagnostic pattern. Uremia is a major cause of death in untreated HPT.

Parathyroid Localization

The standard treatment for primary hyperparathyroidism is surgical removal of the abnormal parathyroid gland or glands.[21,32] This is because untreated HPT leads to bone loss, renal calculi, and nephrocalcinosis. The presence of bone changes is an accepted indication of parathyroid surgery in primary HPT.[21]

Following parathyroidectomy, the subperiosteal resorption resolves, bone turnover decreases, and bone density improves. Patients with nephrolithiasis develop fewer newer stones and renal function improves. Patients with peptic ulcer disease improve and symptoms of depression, weakness, and fatigue often disappear.[21]

Preoperative localization of abnormal parathyroid is not routinely advocated by all surgeons due to a high success rate of 90–95% in localizing the lesion in previously unoperated patients.[32] However, imaging can assist the surgeon in preoperatively identifying a persistent or ectopic parathyroid adenoma or parathyroid hyperplasia, thereby increasing surgical success from 60–90%.[32]

Preoperative Localization Techniques

The noninvasive tests for parathyroid localization are:
- High-resolution ultrasound
- High-resolution computed tomography (HRCT)
- Magnetic resonance imaging (MRI)
- Dual isotope thallium-201 chloride-^{99m}Technetium subtraction scanning
- ^{99m}Technetium sestamibi scintigraphy
- Single-photon emission computed tomography (SPECT)
- Parathyroid digital subtraction angiography
- Selective venous sampling.

The success of all these techniques, except venous sampling depends to a varying degree on the size of the abnormal gland.

Anatomical and Pathological Considerations Important for Localization

Embryology and Anatomy

In the majority of population (84%), the parathyroid glands are four in number—two superior and two inferior. The glands are symmetrical, with the superior parathyroid glands usually lying behind the superior third of the two thyroid lobes and the inferior parathyroid glands just below the inferior poles of the thyroid. About 3–5% population has five glands, and 1–3% have three glands. Supernumerary glands are seen approximately 3–5% of time.[33]

The superior parathyroid glands are derived from the fourth branchial pouch along with the lateral lobes of the thyroid. The inferior glands arise from the third branchial pouch along with thymus gland. These embryologic relationships help to explain the normal and variable anatomic location of the superior and inferior parathyroid glands. The superior parathyroid glands being closely related to the thyroid gland undergo minimal descent and their position are relatively constant.[20] More than 90% glands are located deep in relation to the mid portion of the superior pole of the thyroid near the cricothyroid junction.[33]

The incidence of ectopic parathyroid glands is 20%. Ectopic superior parathyroids may be found within the thyroid gland (1–2%), in retrotracheal or retroesophageal location (1% cases), within the carotid sheath (1% of cases) or may descend into the posterosuperior mediastinum (5% of cases). The inferior parathyroid glands along with the thymus descend a greater distance and therefore are more variable in location but most commonly are located inferior, posterior, or lateral to the lower thyroid pole (69%). Ectopic inferior parathyroid glands are more common and can lie anywhere from the angle of the mandible to the pericardium, i.e., along the path of migration of the thymus.[34] They can be found more inferiorly in the neck, in the thyrothymic ligament, in the thymic tongue, or in the cervical portion of the thymus gland (29%). Persistent hypercalcemia after parathyroid surgery can be due to mediastinal parathyroid glands in as many as one third of cases.

Surgical Treatment

Definitive treatment of primary hyperparathyroidism involves the surgical excision of hyperfunctioning parathyroid glands. In the past, this was achieved with bilateral neck exploration and removal of the enlarged gland or glands. Improved presurgical imaging localization, intraoperative PTH assays, and hand-held gamma detectors have made the selective excision of hyperfunctioning parathyroid glands possible.[20]

Over the past decade, the development of minimally invasive techniques to parathyroid surgery has made accurate preoperative localization of parathyroid disease absolutely critical for effective surgical treatment.

Currently practiced minimally invasive techniques include unilateral open parathyroidectomy, video-assisted parathyroidectomy, and videoscopic parathyroidectomy. All of these techniques involve a more focused approach wherein the procedure is limited to the abnormal parathyroid gland, thereby reducing the operating time substantially.[33] The extent of minimally invasive parathyroidectomy is often guided by rapid intraoperative PTH testing. A greater than 50% drop in the serum PTH to normal or near-normal levels 10 minutes after parathyroid resection is suggestive of a single parathyroid adenoma as the cause of primary HPT.[20] Thus, the primary benefit of preoperative imaging studies is the accurate determination of uniglandular disease to help select patients most appropriate for unilateral and minimally invasive approaches.

The Guidelines for the Management of Asymptomatic Primary Hyperparathyroidism from the Fourth International Workshop were formulated in 2014. As per the committee, the following are the recommendations for surgery in asymptomatic patients with primary HPT:[35]

- Serum calcium >1 mg/dL
- Peri- or postmenopausal women and men >50 years with T score ≤–2.5 on bone mineral density (BMD)
- Premenopausal women and men <50 years with Z score ≤–2.5
- Creatinine clearance <60 mL/min
- If renal stones or nephrocalcinosis is present
- 24-hour urinary calcium >400 mg/dL.

Parathyroid Imaging

High-resolution sonography and ^{99m}Tc sestamibi scintigraphy are the main imaging techniques for preoperative location of parathyroid adenomas with similar sensitivities and specificities for solitary adenoma detection by these techniques.

Localization accuracy improves when both sonography and scintigraphy are obtained preoperatively. Contrast-enhanced CT and MRI can also effectively locate parathyroid adenomas but are less commonly used for preoperative location and are more commonly used in the setting of failed parathyroidectomy for the detection of suspected ectopic (mediastinal) glands.[33]

Sonographic Evaluation

Ultrasonography is the modality of choice for preoperative localization of the pathological gland in all patients of proven HPT. Transducers of 12–15 MHz are used for imaging giving a tissue resolution of 1–2 mm. Solid lesions can be differentiated from blood vessels. High-resolution sonography is an established procedure with a sensitivity of 80% and specificity of 90% in detecting cervical parathyroid adenomas.[21]

Normal parathyroid glands are 2–7 mm in length, 2–4 mm in width, and 0.5–2 mm in thickness and weigh 35–55 mg.[34] They are normally not visible on ultrasound, CT, or MRI.

Most cases of primary hyperparathyroidism are caused by a single parathyroid adenoma (90%). Hyperplasia of all four glands (6%), double adenomas (4%), and rarely parathyroid carcinoma are the other causes. Parathyroid adenomas are benign neoplasms, composed of chief cells, oncocytic cells or transitional oncocytic cells, with frequently a mixture of cell types being seen. Adenomas are considerably larger, having a mean mass of greater than 10 times the normal parathyroid gland and are thus often identified at cross-sectional imaging.[29]

At sonography, *parathyroid adenomas* are typically seen as homogeneously hypoechoic solid masses. This is due to the compact cellularity of the gland that is characteristic of adenomas at sectioning.[33] They may sometimes have a hyperechoic capsule. The echogenicity of vast majority of parathyroid adenomas is substantially less than that of thyroid tissue; normal thyroid parenchyma having a characteristic sonographic appearance of homogeneous medium to high level echoes. Around 90% of adenomas are found at the poles of the thyroid gland and are easily discernable sonographically **(Figs. 23A and B)**. Imaging of the lower poles can be enhanced by asking the patient to swallow, which momentarily raises the thyroid gland in the neck. They are usually oval or bean shaped, but larger adenomas can be multilobulated.

Parathyroid carcinomas are usually larger than adenomas, on an average measuring >2 cm as compared to 1 cm for adenomas. Carcinomas generally have a lobulated contour, heterogeneous echotexture, and cystic components. However, they may be indistinguishable from parathyroid

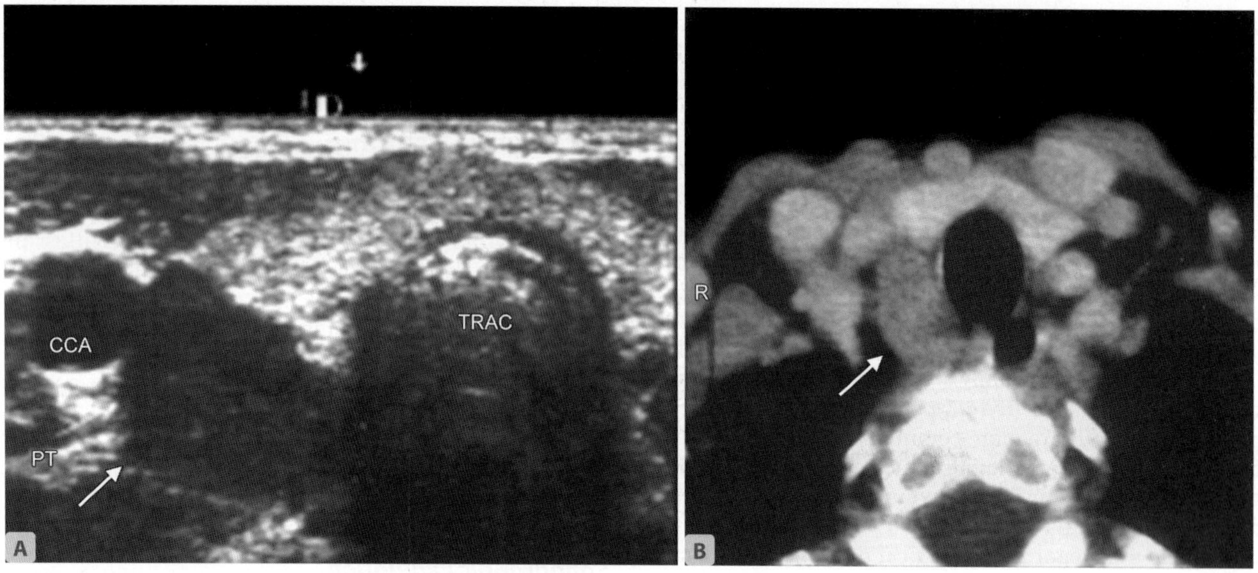

FIGS. 23A AND B: (A) Transverse ultrasound scan reveals a hypodense mass posteroinferior to the right lobe of thyroid (arrow) in a patient with parathyroid adenoma; (B) Contrast-enhanced computed tomography (CECT) also shows a hypodense solid mass in the same location (arrow).

adenomas in all imaging studies except when local invasion of neighboring structures is present.[21]

When parathyroid gland enlargement is not found in the region of the thyroid, the entire neck from mandible to suprasternal notch should be examined sonographically, including the retrotracheal region via a lateral approach.[32] However, ectopic parathyroid glands in the neck may be missed on ultrasonographic evaluation. Ultrasonography cannot be used to identify mediastinal parathyroid adenomas. Rarely, parathyroid adenomas may be intrathyroid in location. These are completely surrounded by thyroid tissue and are oriented with their greatest dimension in the cephalocaudal direction. Sonographically, they are well visualized because they are hypoechoic in contrast to the echogenic thyroid parenchyma. However, percutaneous biopsy may often be required to reliably differentiate an intrathyroid adenoma from a thyroid nodule.

Gray-scale imaging should be supplemented by color and power Doppler imaging to look for feeding vessels and vascularity of suspected adenomas seen at initial gray-scale imaging. As per literature, color and power Doppler imaging commonly show a characteristic extrathyroidal feeding vessel (typically a branch of the inferior thyroidal artery), which enters the parathyroid gland at one of the poles. Internal vascularity is also commonly seen in a peripheral distribution. The artery feeding the adenoma tends to branch around the periphery of the gland before penetrating deeper, resulting in a characteristic arc or rim of vascularity. In addition, color Doppler sonography of the overlying thyroid gland may show an area of asymmetric hypervascularity that may help to locate an underlying adenoma. When gray-scale and Doppler imaging fail to show an abnormal parathyroid gland, graded compression of subcutaneous tissues and strap muscles may show a relatively incompressible gland which may help differentiate an adenoma from surrounding soft tissue. This technique is often helpful in detection of ectopic glands in the lower neck.[33]

Hyperplasia is also a more difficult diagnosis to make sonographically because the single gland size is generally much smaller than an adenoma. However, similar to adenomas, compact cellularity may render hyperplastic glands hypoechoic relative to the overlying thyroid.

Pitfalls in Interpretation

Normal cervical structures such as perithyroid veins, esophagus, and Longus colli muscles of the neck can simulate parathyroid adenomas, producing false-positive results during neck sonography. Performing real-time sonography in multiple planes, color Doppler flow imaging, and use of certain maneuvers by the patient help to differentiate the above normal structures from a suspected parathyroid adenoma. Pathologic structures that are potential causes of false-positive results include thyroid nodules and cervical lymph nodes.

Several features may help in distinguishing lymph nodes from adenomas. An echogenic fatty hilum usually indicates a benign lymph node. At color Doppler examination, lymph nodes are supplied by small hilar vessels, whereas a polar, peripheral distribution of color flow is commonly seen with parathyroid adenomas.

Concomitant thyroid disease also contributes to imaging pitfalls. Enlarged multinodular thyroid gland can limit the sonographic evaluation of parathyroid adenomas. Anatomy is distorted and posterior nodules may mimic parathyroid disease. Posterior thyroid nodules can have a similar sonographic appearance to intracapsular parathyroid glands, although the typical vascular pattern of a parathyroid adenoma is uncommonly seen in thyroid nodules.[33]

Thyroid nodules more often show a heterogeneous echotexture with calcification and or cystic changes;[32] while parathyroid adenomas are of a homogeneous, hypoechoic echogenicity. A hyperechoic capsule favors a parathyroid adenoma. However, these sonographic features are inconsistent and it may not be always possible to differentiate abnormal parathyroid glands from lymphadenopathy and thyroid masses.

Percutaneous Aspiration/Biopsy

Fine-needle aspiration cytology (FNAC) of the parathyroid masses has increased the specificity of sonography by reliably differentiating parathyroid pathology from thyroid nodule and cervical lymph nodes. In addition to the cytologic or histologic analysis of the specimen, the aspiration can be diluted with 1 mL of saline and analyzed for parathyroid hormone (PTH) by radioimmunoassay.[21]

Although PTH aspiration is rarely necessary for routine cases, this procedure can be particularly helpful in cases in which prior thyroid or parathyroid surgery has distorted neck anatomy or when preoperative confirmation of unusual-appearing or ectopic glands is needed. A theoretic complication of the procedure is seeding of abnormal parathyroid tissue along the biopsy track resulting in an entity known as parathyromatosis. This has been described in cases of recurrent hyperparathyroidism after parathyroidectomy in which the capsule of the parathyroid gland was disrupted during the procedure.

Although it is primarily used as a therapy to treat tertiary hyperparathyroidism (most often in the setting of renal failure), sonographically guided parathyroid ablation with ethanol is a potential treatment option for patients with primary hyperparathyroidism. The procedure involves placement of the needle in the parathyroid gland and slowly injecting a volume of ethanol equal to approximately 50% of the volume of the gland until the absence of blood flow to the gland is confirmed on color Doppler sonography.[33]

Contrast-enhanced Computed Tomography

Contrast-enhanced computed tomography (CECT) has a sensitivity of up to 87% in detecting parathyroid adenoma. It is superior to sonography in patients with failed parathyroidectomy, in cases of altered anatomy and in delineating ectopic mediastinal parathyroid masses, thereby aiding in operative planning. Computed tomography has the advantage of larger field of view and ability to image all areas of neck and mediastinum. Spiral CT has enabled excellent visualization of neck vasculature and their separation from other neck structures[21] **(Figs. 24A and B)**.

Four-dimensional Computed Tomography

Four-dimensional computed tomography (4D CT) of the parathyroid is a technique for preoperative localization of parathyroid adenomas which was introduced as an alternative to conventional CT by Rodgers et al. in 2006. The technique consists of CT performed in multiple phases and reformatted images in three planes, i.e., axial acquisition with coronal and sagittal reformations combined. The "fourth dimension" of 4D CT consists of change in contrast enhancement over time.[36] Thus, it provides both functional and anatomic information enabling localization of eutopic and ectopic parathyroid adenomas and can also depict multiglandular disease which may be missed on other imaging modalities.[37]

The protocol for 4D CT involves a noncontrast multiple detector computed tomography (MDCT) of the neck followed by two or more contrast-enhanced phases. The multiple phases are performed to determine the pattern of enhancement as this is one of the main features which enables identification of a parathyroid adenoma and its differentiation from thyroid nodules and lymph nodes which it can mimic.[38]

The first phase is a nonenhanced scan acquired with a smaller z-axis that only covers the thyroid glands so as to reduce the radiation exposure. Two contrast-enhanced phases are then acquired from the angle of mandible to the carina after intravenous administration of 75 mL of nonionic

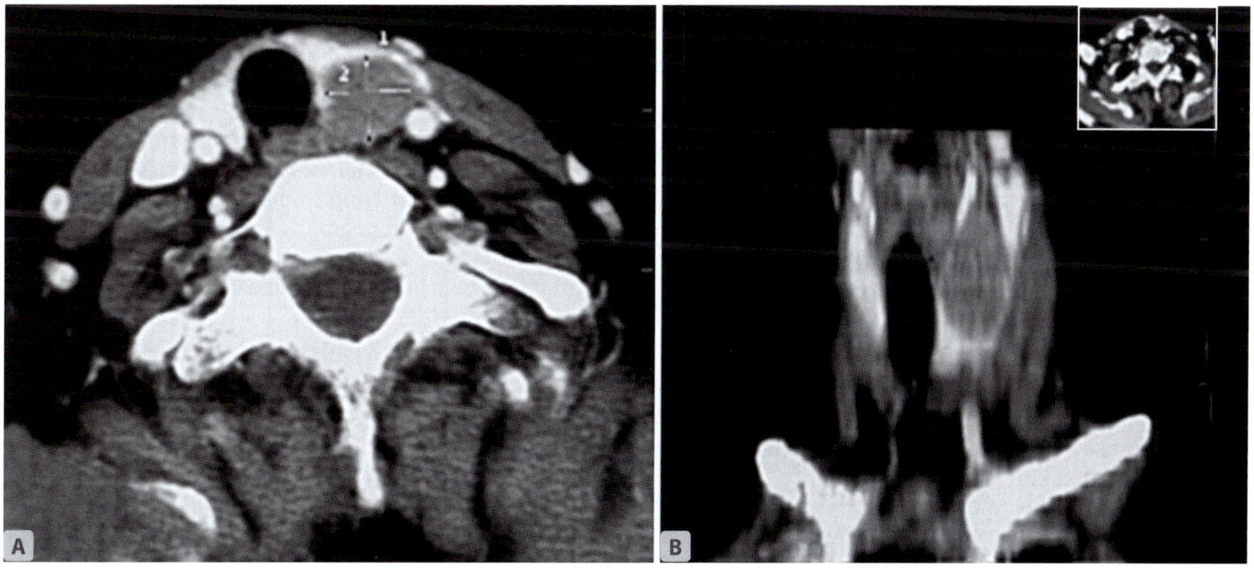

FIGS. 24A AND B: Axial computed tomography (CT) section (A) and coronal reconstruction (B) showing a solid mass posterior to the left lobe of thyroid extending to the inferior part of neck in a patient of multiple parathyroid adenomas.

TABLE 3: Phases of 4D CT protocol.

Number of phases	Phase of CT	Region scanned	Scan timing after start of contrast injection
First phase	NCCT	From hyoid bone to clavicular head (to cover thyroid gland)	-
Second phase	Arterial phase	From angle of mandible to carina (so that ectopic parathyroid is not missed)	25 seconds
Third phase	Delayed (venous phase)		80 seconds

(NCCT: noncontrast computed tomography)

contrast (300 mg of iodine per mL) followed by a 25 mL-saline chase.

Table 3 depicts the various phases of 4D CT protocol described by Hoang et al.

On the noncontrast phase, a parathyroid adenoma appears as a lesion with lower attenuation than the thyroid gland. On arterial phase, the characteristic enhancement pattern is avid enhancement with peak enhancement greater than that of the thyroid and a washout of contrast in the delayed phase.

The peak enhancement has been described between 25 and 60 seconds after contrast injection, ranging from 138 to 180 HU, while lymph nodes show a peak enhancement at 90 seconds corresponding to the delayed phase.

The morphologic features of a parathyroid adenoma should also be evaluated on CT. It appears as an oval or rounded soft-tissue lesion with smooth or slightly lobulated margins in the typical locations around the thyroid gland. When large, an adenoma can have a low attenuation component due to either cystic degeneration, fibrosis, or hemorrhage.

The vascular imaging features on 4D CT have been described as the "polar vessel sign" depicted on the arterial phase. It consists of a feeding artery which is usually a branch of the inferior thyroid artery and typically enters the parathyroid gland at the upper or lower pole. On a 4D CT scan, the "polar vessel sign" may be seen in around 63% of adenomas.

The 4D CT has shown to be useful in many clinical situations such as:

- In patients with previous neck surgery
- Mild hyperparathyroidism
- Multigland disease
- Patients in whom sestamibi and USG examinations are negative.

Studies have compared 4D CT with sestamibi and ultrasound in recent years and have found 4D CT to be superior to both in accurately lateralizing the parathyroid adenoma, thereby allowing the surgeon to perform minimally invasive parathyroidectomy. Such a directed surgical approach has been adopted since the last two decades because of improved preoperative imaging and use of intraoperative parathyroid hormone assay.[39]

An intraoperative parathyroid hormone (IOPTH) measurement is used to confirm the complete resections of abnormally secreting parathyroid tissue. When IOPTH decreases >50% within 10 minutes of resection, it confirms the removal of hyperfunctioning parathyroid tissue.[40]

There is considerable radiation exposure to the patient due to the multiple phases of 4D CT. Reported effective doses for 4D CT is 10.4 mSv compared to 7.8 mSv for nuclear scintigraphy. However, the radiation organ dose to the thyroid has been found to be >50 times higher with 4D CT. Hence, 4D CT should be used with caution, especially in young patients and the benefit of detecting an adenoma and curing the patient following resection as well as the advantage of minimally invasive surgery over bilateral neck exploration along with radiation risk should be considered.[36]

Magnetic Resonance Imaging

Magnetic resonance imaging is less commonly used for preoperative localization than sonography and scintigraphy though it has similar sensitivity to other techniques in the detection of abnormal parathyroid tissue. MRI is the accepted modality for localizing parathyroid lesion in persistent or recurrent hyperparathyroidism, despite previous parathyroidectomies with a sensitivity of 88%.[34] MRI has an equally high sensitivity when the gland is in the mediastinum.[34]

On MR scans, parathyroid adenomas are soft-tissue masses that are of low-to-medium signal intensity on T1-weighted images, are medium-to-high signal intensity on T2-weighted images, and show moderate enhancement on gadolinium-enhanced images. Approximately 10–35% of enlarged glands do not have high-signal intensity on T2-weighted images. This may be due to fat content, hemorrhage, or fibrosis. The size of the gland is the most important factor affecting detection on MRI.[34]

The typical signal intensities of abnormal parathyroid gland on T1-weighted and T2-weighted images may not be distinguishable from lymph nodes. This differentiation is more often based on topography and shape of the structures. A location medial to the carotid sheath is mostly due to parathyroid while nodes are located laterally.[21]

Parathyroid Scintigraphy

Nuclear medicine computer subtraction images of thallium and technetium can aid in the localization of the abnormal parathyroid gland. This technique relies on the differential uptake of the two isotopes by the thyroid and parathyroid glands. Thallium-201 chloride accumulates in tissues with high blood flow which includes both thyroid and parathyroid glands as well as in thyroid nodules and parathyroid adenomas. ^{99m}Technetium accumulates only in the thyroid. Digital images are produced with each isotope. The technetium scan is then subtracted from the thallium leaving an image of only the parathyroid concentration of thallium.

The primary disadvantage of nuclear medicine techniques is limited spatial resolution. The maximum resolution of thallium-technetium scanning is 7–8 mm and it is very difficult to detect glands weighing <500 mg with this technique.[32]

The *radiopharmaceutical of choice* for imaging parathyroid enlargement is *^{99m}Tc sestamibi.* ^{99m}Tc sestamibi has replaced ^{201}Tl for parathyroid scintigraphy because of superior image quality, more favorable dosimetry, and improved detection sensitivity with its use. Three general techniques of radionuclide scintigraphy are commonly used for the detection and visualization of hyperfunctioning parathyroid glands: Single-phase dual isotope subtraction imaging, dual-phase single-isotope imaging, and a combination of the two. In *dual-isotope subtraction imaging technique*, one radiopharmaceutical (^{99m}Tc sestamibi) is used for visualization of the hyperfunctioning parathyroid gland and the thyroid gland, and a second (^{123}I or ^{99m}Tc pertechnetate) is used for visualization of the thyroid gland only. The second set of images is then digitally subtracted from the first set. Evidence of residual radioactivity on the subtraction image represents a hyperfunctioning parathyroid gland **(Fig. 25)**. Disadvantages of this subtraction method include the necessity of two radionuclide injections and of a cooperative and immobile patient, identically positioned for the two studies. In addition, there is an increased likelihood of artifacts on images obtained with digital subtraction. Dual agent studies with ^{99m}Tc sestamibi and iodine 123 or ^{99m}Tc pertechnetate subtraction have produced a sensitivity of 95 percent for adenomas and 64–80% for hyperplastic glands.[32] The *single-isotope dual-phase imaging technique* was proposed on the basis of the frequently observed difference between the rate of ^{99m}Tc sestamibi washout from the thyroid gland and the rate of washout from hyperfunctioning parathyroid glands, which is typically slower. This technique requires a single injection of ^{99m}Tc sestamibi, followed by imaging at approximately 10–15 minutes and 1.5–3 hours after the injection. Increased mitochondrial content in parathyroid adenomas is believed to be responsible for the observed sestamibi concentration. Due to the high sensitivity of sestamibi scintigraphy (82–100%), it is generally considered the standard initial imaging modality to detect a parathyroid adenoma.

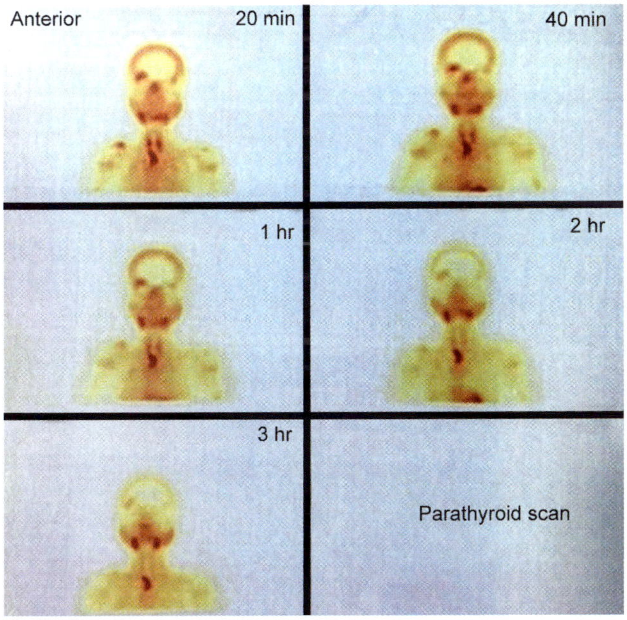

FIG. 25: Sestamibi scan: There is evidence of increased uptake of 99-Tc-Sestamibi in the region of right parathyroid gland which persists on delayed phase image (3 hours). Increased uptake is also seen in the region of right orbit due to a brown tumor.

Single-photon Emission Computed Tomography

Single-photon emission computed tomography is a technique whereby images of diseased glands which have absorbed a radioactive marker can be obtained. It increases the sensitivity and specificity by 2–3% over routine sestamibi scanning. SPECT can be performed anytime within the first several hours after a patient is injected with sestamibi. SPECT is used with increasing frequency as it provides three-dimensional information (lateral, superoinferior and anteroposterior). The major reason for the superiority of SPECT is the improved contrast resolution (target to background). The fusion of CT images with SPECT images, either by using software or by performing the studies sequentially on hybrid SPECT/CT imaging systems, has the advantage of combining the physiologic three-dimensional information from SPECT and anatomic information from CT. The most important use for SPECT scanning is when ordinary sestamibi scans are inconclusive or when a more detailed anatomic localization is required such as when patients are being reoperated.[21]

HYPOPARATHYROIDISM

The most common cause of hypoparathyroidism is excision or trauma to the parathyroid glands during thyroid surgery.[19] It can also occur as idiopathic hypoparathyroidism in which the parathyroid glands are absent or atrophied.

It usually occurs in childhood with girls being affected more commonly than boys. The disorder may be characterized by the presence of circulating antibodies to the parathyroid, adrenal, and thyroid glands supporting the concept that idiopathic hypoparathyroidism may be part of a generalized autoimmune disease.

Rare forms of hypoparathyroidism are seen after radiation damage to the gland and as a response of an infant to hyperparathyroidism in the mother owing to transplacental transport of calcium with suppression of fetal parathyroid activity.

Clinical Presentation

Patients with hypoparathyroidism usually present with neuromuscular dysfunction precipitated by hypocalcemia.[16] Premature closure of the growth plate may lead to short stature. Dental abnormalities may occur in the form of delay or failure of tooth eruption.

Biochemical Findings

Laboratory findings in hypoparathyroidism consist of decreased serum levels of parathyroid hormone (PTH) and calcium with elevated phosphate levels.

Radiological Findings

- The most common finding in hypoparathyroidism is bony sclerosis, which may be focal or generalized.[16,19] Localized osteosclerosis is more common, reported in 23% of patients while generalized osteosclerosis is seen in 9%.[23] Bones involved more commonly are pelvis, proximal femur, and vertebral bodies.
- Other findings include calvarial thickening and hypoplastic dentition.
- Band-like areas of increased radiodensity in the metaphysis of long bones may also be seen in hypoparathyroidism.
- The abnormalities in the spine resemble those of diffuse idiopathic skeletal hyperostosis (DISH) including calcification and ossification of the anterior longitudinal ligament and spinal osteophytes. The sacroiliac joints are generally spared. This feature along with lack of erosive arthropathy differentiates it from ankylosing spondylitis.
- Subcutaneous calcification may be seen around the hip and shoulder joints.
- Calcium deposition in the basal ganglia is a characteristic finding and occasionally also seen in the cerebrum and cerebellum. It is also a feature of pseudohypoparathyroidism. It is also seen in infectious disorders such as toxoplasmosis and cytomegalic inclusion disease, in Fahr's syndrome (ferrocalcinosis), after radiation therapy and exposure to toxic substances such as carbon monoxide.[23]

PSEUDOHYPOPARATHYROIDISM

Pseudohypoparathyroidism (PHP) is an inherited disorder that manifests as end-organ resistance to parathyroid hormone rather than from deficient secretion of the hormone. This may be due to a defect in the adenyl-cyclase-cyclic AMP system in the renal tubules and bones. It is transmitted as an autosomal dominant trait and shares many features with hypoparathyroidism.

Clinical Findings

The patients are usually short, obese, mentally retarded, and may have brachydactyly.[16,19]

Pseudohypoparathyroidism is more frequent in women than men and is usually diagnosed in the second decade of life.

Biochemical Findings

Hypocalcemia and hyperphosphatemia are seen similar to that in hypoparathyroidism. However, the levels of serum parathyroid hormone (PTH) are elevated.

Radiological Findings

- The best known sign of PHP is *shortening of the fourth metacarpal*. Although not specific for PHP as it is also seen in pseudopseudohypoparathyroidism (PPHP), this is a characteristic finding **(Fig. 26)**.
    - The metacarpal sign has been used to determine whether this shortening is present. To use the sign, a line is drawn tangential to the heads of the fourth and fifth metacarpals. Normally the line does not intersect the third metacarpal bone or just contacts its distal aspect. The sign is considered positive if the line intersects the third metacarpal, indicating disproportionate shortening of the fourth and fifth metacarpal bone. Other congenital conditions with positive metacarpal sign are basal cell nevus syndrome, multiple epiphyseal dysplasia, Beckwith-Wiedemann syndrome as well as acquired conditions such as juvenile chronic arthritis, sickle cell anemia with infarction, trauma, and neonatal hyperthyroidism. This sign may be unreliable in diagnosing PHP and PPHP as the third metacarpal may also be short in these conditions.[23]
    - Other radiological findings in PHP are similar to those of hypoparathyroidism and consist of bony sclerosis, soft-tissue calcification, dense metaphyseal bands, calvarial thickening, and basal ganglia calcification. Basal ganglia calcification is more common than in idiopathic hypoparathyroidism **(Fig. 27)**.[29]
- *Soft-tissue calcification and ossification.* This occurs in approximately 55% of patients with PHP and is seen commonly in the hands and feet. The calcifications may be present at birth and are superficial in location and usually periarticular in distribution.
- Radiographic findings of secondary hyperparathyroidism may be seen in some patients with PHP.
- In addition to short metacarpals, metatarsals; phalanges may be short and exostoses and cone shaped epiphysis may be seen. The exostoses are frequently located centrally and project at right angles to the bone and differ from the appearance of multiple hereditary exostoses in which the outgrowths are usually directed away from joints.

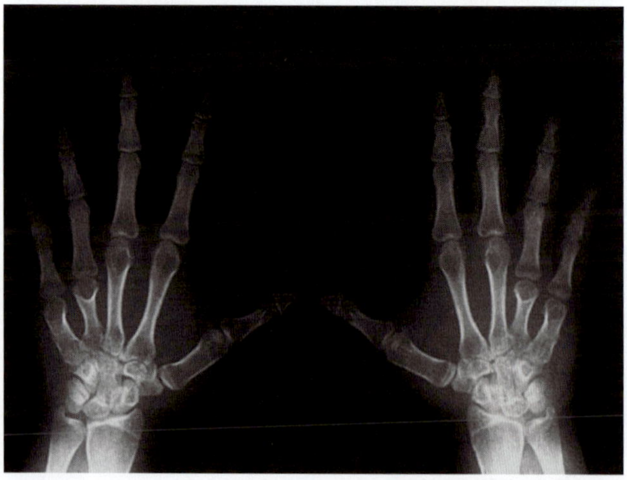

FIG. 26: Shortening of fourth and fifth metacarpal bones seen in both hands in a patient of pseudohypoparathyroidism (PHP) along with shortening of the middle phalanges of the fifth fingers.

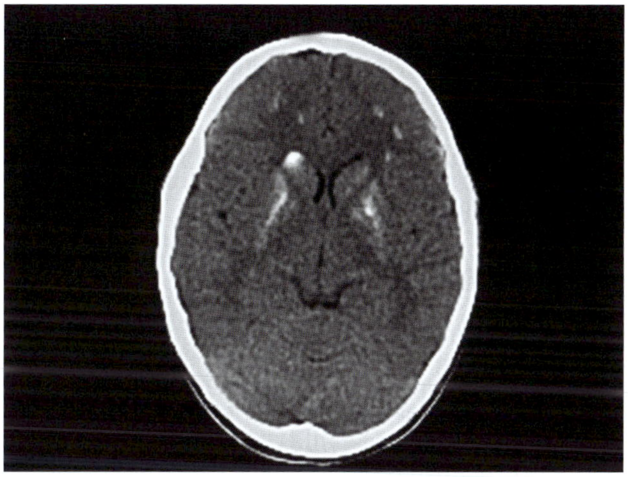

FIG. 27: Pseudohypoparathyroidism (PHP): Axial computed tomography (CT) section of the cranium reveals calcification in bilateral basal ganglia and frontal lobes in a 13-year-old child.

- Growth deformities in the form of bowing of long bones may be seen.

PSEUDOPSEUDOHYPOPARATHYROIDISM

This is the result of incomplete genetic manifestation of PHP and like PHP is caused by an end-organ resistance to parathyroid hormone. PHP and PPHP share most of their clinical and radiological features. The main difference between the two is that patients with PPHP are normocalcemic.

Radiographic abnormalities of the hand in PHP and PPHP are almost identical, except for a relatively higher rate of occurrence of short distal phalanges in PHP and relatively shorter metacarpals in PPHP.[19]

The differential diagnosis of short fourth metacarpal includes Turner's syndrome and physeal trauma. Other radiologic features of PHP may resemble fibrodysplasia ossificans progressiva or multiple hereditary exostoses syndrome.

DISORDERS OF ENDOCRINE ORIGIN

Normal skeletal maturation requires the presence of certain hormones in addition to vitamin D and other metabolites. The principal endocrine glands that influence this process are pituitary, thyroid, adrenals and gonads. Deficient production of hormones from any of these glands may disturb normal skeletal maturation and ossification (**Table 4** lists the normal reference values).

The various skeletal disorders of endocrine origin may be grouped as:
- *Disorders due to excessive corticosteroids*:
  - Hypercortisolism
- *Growth hormone disorders*:
  - Acromegaly
  - Gigantism
- *Thyroid disorders*:
  - Hypothyroidism
  - Hyperthyroidism

TABLE 4: Endocrine profile–reference value.

• Serum cortisol	Fasting: 8 am–12 noon: 5–25 g/dL; 12 noon–8 pm: 5–15 g/dL; 8 pm–8 am: 0–10 g/dL
• Serum ACTH	6–76 pg/mL
• Serum TSH	0.34–4.25 μIU/mL
• Free T3	2.4–4.2 pg/mL
• Total T4	5.4–11.7 μg/dL
• Serum growth hormone	0.5–17 ng/mL
• Serum LH: - Follicular phase - Ovulatory phase - Luteal phase	 2–15 IU/L 22–105 IU/L 0.6–19 IU/L
• Serum FSH: - Follicular phase - Ovulatory phase - Luteal phase	 3–20 IU/L 9–26 IU/L 1–12 IU/L
• Serum free testosterone: - Male - Female	 47–244 pg/mL 0.6–6.8 pg/ml
• Serum calcitonin (male/female)	3–26 pg/mL; 2–17 pg/mL

(ACTH: adrenocorticotropic hormone; FSH: follicle-stimulating hormone; TSH: thyroid-stimulating hormone; T3: triiodothyronine; T4: thyroxine)

- *Gonadal disorders*:
  - Hypogonadism
  - Hypergonadism.

HYPERCORTISOLISM

Hypercortisolism or *Cushing's syndrome* is the clinical manifestation of exposure to excessive amounts of cortisol-like corticosteroids (glucocorticoid). It is caused by a tumor of the adrenal glands (adenoma and carcinoma), ectopic ACTH production by a tumor (bronchial carcinoma), or iatrogenically by treatment with glucocorticoids. Cushing's disease caused by a basophil pituitary adenoma is an uncommon cause of hypercortisolism. Hypercortisolism is most frequently the result of excessive administration of exogenous corticosteroids.[41]

The effects of glucocorticoids on the skeleton are numerous and complex and consist of inhibition of bone formation, stimulation of bone resorption by osteoclast, decrease in intestinal absorption and increase in renal excretion of calcium, and decrease in synthesis of collagen. The net result of hypercortisolism on the musculoskeletal system is osteoporosis, osteonecrosis, and muscle wasting.[41]

Radiological Findings

- Generalized loss of bone density (osteoporosis) occurs which is more prominent in the spine, pelvis, ribs, and cranial vault as trabecular bone is affected more severely than cortical bone.

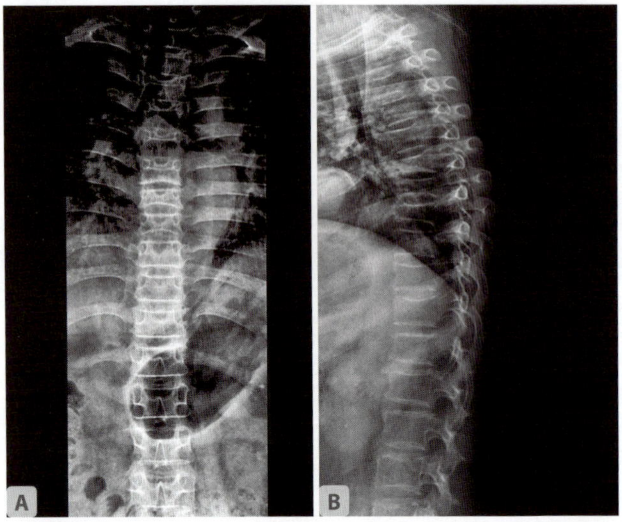

FIGS. 28A AND B: Cushing's syndrome due to increased adrenocorticotropic (ACTH) production in a 16-year-old. X-ray dorsolumbar spine [anteroposterior (AP)] and (lateral) views reveal reduced height of vertebral bodies with endplate sclerosis and osteoporosis.

- There is accentuation of primary trabeculae, with central endplate depressions in the vertebral bodies giving them a biconcave fish-like appearance.
- Increased radiodensity of the superior and inferior margins of compressed or collapsed vertebral bodies is a characteristic feature due to exuberant callus formation called marginal condensation, resulting, from combination of insufficiency compressive microfractures and subsequent healing **(Figs. 28A and B)**. Exuberant callus may also be seen at fracture sites in long bones and ribs. Although the vertebral end-plate sclerosis with osteoporosis is typical of hypercortisolism, in most cases it may be indistinguishable from generalized osteoporosis resulting from other causes such as hyperthyroidism, hyperparathyroidism, acromegaly, and hypogonadism.
- Local regions of osteonecrosis may be seen especially after treatment with exogenous corticosteroid. The typical sites of avascular necrosis are femoral and humeral heads which may be involved months or years after the corticosteroid treatment has begun or end.
- Hypercortisolism during skeletal immaturity suppresses growth, resulting in a short child with osteoporosis, truncal obesity, and delayed bone age. Osteonecrosis at growing epiphyses may lead to abnormal development at the ends of bone and eventually result in early development of degenerative osteoarthropathy.

HYPOPITUITARISM

This is due to deficiency of anterior pituitary hormones, particularly growth hormone resulting from damage to the pituitary gland by neoplasms, infections, vascular insults or post-therapeutic ablations. If the deficiency in growth hormone occurs in combination with deficiencies in other pituitary hormones, it is called panhypopituitarism.[41]

Radiological Findings

- There is delay in skeletal maturation manifested radiologically by a delay in appearance and closure of epiphysis.
- Skeletal growth is retarded.
- There is overall loss of bone density due to decreased bone formation.

HYPOTHYROIDISM

Deficiency of thyroid hormones (T3 and T4) produces a spectrum of musculoskeletal abnormalities termed "cretinism" in infants, "juvenile myxedema" in children, and "myxedema" or "hypothyroidism" in adults.[22] The deficiency may result from disorders that affect the thyroid gland (primary hypothyroidism) or from a deficiency of thyroid stimulating hormone (secondary hypothyroidism). Primary hypothyroidism occurs as a result of thyroiditis, neoplastic disorders, thyroid ablation, or disturbances in iodine metabolism.

Clinical Findings

Clinical manifestations of hypothyroidism vary according to the age of the patient at the time of presentation.[16] In infants, there is mental retardation and developmental abnormalities as thyroid hormone is essential for postnatal growth. In children, mental retardation, obesity, developmental delay, growth retardation, lethargy, and constipation may be seen. The clinical presentation in adults includes fatigue, lethargy, paresthesias, dry coarse skin and hair, constipation, and bradycardia.

Radiological Findings

The radiologic findings also depend on the patient's age at presentation.

Congenital hypothyroidism is characterized by delayed skeletal maturation with bone age lagging behind the chronological age. This is evident by short stature and the late appearance of epiphyseal ossification centers. Bone age can be assessed by getting a plain radiograph of the knee.[41] Normally, the distal femoral epiphysis is usually ossified at 36 weeks' gestational age and the proximal tibial epiphysis at 38 weeks' gestational age. Decreased size or absence of distal femoral or proximal tibial epiphyses is a marker for intrauterine hypothyroidism. When they appear, the ossification centers are deformed and irregularly shaped (*epiphyseal dysgenesis*). These changes are bilateral and symmetrical. Such changes in the hip must be differentiated from bilateral Perthes disease and multiple epiphyseal dysplasia. There is also delayed closure of the epiphyseal plates in hypothyroidism.

In the *skull,* the sutures may remain open and show the formation of intrasutural (Wormian) bones. The sella is either small and bowl shaped in young children or large, rounded in older children. The paranasal sinus are underdeveloped.

In the *spine,* anteriorly wedged bullet-shaped vertebral bodies are seen, especially at the thoracolumbar junction, where kyphosis may develop.

In the *pelvis*, the incidence of slipped capital femoral epiphysis is increased. The pelvis is often narrow with coxa vara deformities.

In adult or acquired hypothyroidism, skeletal manifestations are usually mild compared to severe skeletal abnormalities in congenital hypothyroidism. Generalized osteoporosis is the most common finding.

HYPERTHYROIDISM

Hyperfunction of the thyroid gland usually occurs as a result of Graves' disease (toxic diffuse goiter) or toxic multinodular goiter.[22] Excessive production of thyroid hormones, both triiodothyronine (T3) and thyroxine (T4) by the overactive gland cause a hypermetabolic state. This results in increase in both formation and resorption, with bone resorption being dominant.[16] Catabolism of protein and loss of connective tissue manifests as muscle wasting.

Hyperthyroidism in children causes accelerated skeletal maturation and advanced bone age. In adults, it causes generalized osteoporosis leading to vertebral fractures and kyphosis.

Clinical Findings

Patients may present with weakness, fatigue, nervousness, weight loss, tachycardia, palpitations, diarrhea, or intolerance to heat.[16] Myopathy is a common clinical feature of hyperthyroidism whose symptoms may mimic that of arthritis. Muscle wasting is also known to occur, especially in the proximal muscle groups.[41]

Biochemical Findings

Biochemical findings show elevated levels of calcium, phosphorus and alkaline phosphatase and elevated urinary calcium.

Radiological Findings

Skeletal finding in hyperthyroidism are more common in men and patients with radiologic abnormalities have had the disease for at least 5 years.

- *Osteoporosis* is the most common radiological finding particularly in the spine, pelvis, skull, hands, and feet. Older patients show rapidly progressive generalized osteoporosis. It has been seen that the progression of thyrotoxic osteoporosis is much more rapid than postmenopausal osteoporosis,[41] even though the two are radiologically indistinguishable. An overall decrease in bone density is seen as a result of bone resorption. Changes in the spine are more common in the dorsal and lumbar vertebrae and consist of biconcave vertebral bodies, wedge deformities, and resultant kyphosis. Fractures may also occur, especially in femoral neck.
- The predominant radiographic pattern of increased osteoblastic and osteoclastic activity consists of *cortical tunneling or striations.* This is more evident in the tubular bones of the hand and feet occurring in up to 50% of patients.[22]
- *Thyroid acropachy* is a rare complication that occurs in 0.5–1%of patients after treatment for hyperthyroidism by surgery or antithyroid medication.[16,41] It may appear years after the initial presentation of hyperthyroidism and the patients are often euthyroid but may be hypo or hyperthyroid. The cause is unknown with no apparent age or gender predilection. Patients may present with exophthalmos, soft-tissue swelling of the fingers and toes, pretibial myxedema, or clubbing.[16,41]

The radiologic findings of thyroid acropachy are virtually diagnostic and consist of dense, solid, and periosteal new bone formation with feathery margins. The periostitis is commonly seen in an asymmetric distribution and is most prominent along the radial margin of metacarpals and phalanges in the diaphyseal region. Uncommonly, long bones may be involved. The bony changes are not progressive.[41]

Thyroid acropachy must be distinguished from hypertrophic osteoarthropathy, a very painful condition wherein the long bones are considerably more likely to be involved than are hands and feet, and the feathery contour is absent. Another differential of thyroid acropachy is pachydermo-periostitis where the periostitis affects the long bones more than the hands with extension of the periosteal new bone to the metaphysis and epiphysis. There is associated soft-tissue prominence of the hands with bilateral symmetrical periosteal bone formation in tibia, fibula, radius, and ulna.[42] The radiological appearance of venous stasis, leukemia, and osteomyelitis may mimic thyroid acropachy but differentiation is usually possible on the basis of characteristic clinical presentation of these disorders.[16] Fluorosis is associated with more extensive abnormality of the axial skeleton and long bones, while leukemic acropachy is particularly prominent in the terminal phalanges.[42]

HYPERGONADISM

Hypergonadism may be caused by overproduction of sex hormones by the testes or ovaries or by the overproduction by the adrenal cortex. In congenital adrenal hyperplasia, a deficiency in the synthesis of cortisol leads to high levels of ACTH. A secondary effect of high ACTH leads to excessive levels of adrenal sex steroids. A central nervous system lesion may also lead to gonadotropin excess and hypergonadism.

The skeletal manifestation of hypergonadism in the child is precocious growth and maturation. The epiphyseal ossification centers appear early. The long bones grow rapidly and the growth plates close early. Although there is initial precocious growth spurt, the early closure of the growth plate results in short stature, with a tall child becoming a short adult.[41] The morphology of the skeleton is otherwise normal.

HYPOGONADISM

Hypogonadism may be secondary to low production of gonadotropins (luteinizing hormone and follicle-stimulating hormone) from the pituitary, or deficient production of hormones by the gonads themselves.[22] The latter is termed "primary gonadal deficiency" and, when present in growing boys is referred to as *eunuchoidism. Turner's syndrome* is a female sex-linked disorder in which there is ovarian dysgenesis due to an XO genotype. In older women, primary gonadal deficiency occurs with menopause.

Radiological Findings

The radiographic features of hypogonadism in males consist of:

- Generalized decrease in bone density.
- Delay in skeletal maturation which manifests in the form of delayed closure of epiphysis. This results in long extremities with relatively short trunks.

Turner's Syndrome

- More than 50% of the patients do not have any radiographic abnormalities. In the remaining patients, skeletal maturation is usually normal until 15 years of age, following which delayed epiphyseal closure becomes evident, particularly in the apophysis of the iliac crests[22] and unusually long and slender tubular bones in the extremities.
- There may be depression or slanting of the medial tibial plateau with concomitant overgrowth of the medial condoyle of the femur.
- The fourth and fifth metacarpals are often short producing a positive metacarpal sign. The heads of the third and fourth metacarpals may appear flattened and cubitus valgus may be seen. This is seen in 50% of patients.
- Other findings include narrow ribs, small sella turcica, hypertelorism, and android pelvis.

GROWTH HORMONE DISORDERS

Growth hormone disorders occur as a result of excess or deficient production of growth hormone.

Acromegaly

Acromegaly results from excessive production of growth hormone (somatotropin) in a skeletally mature individual. It is usually caused by a pituitary adenoma that produces growth hormone autonomously. Elevated serum growth hormone reactivates endochondral bone formation, stimulates periosteal bone formation along with connective tissue proliferation leading to characteristic clinical and radiological features.

The overgrowth of bone in association with enlargement of soft tissue is particularly prominent in the acral parts (hands, feet, and lower jaw) of the skeleton leading to the term acromegaly for this condition.[43]

Clinical Findings

Acromegaly is typically seen in the third or fourth decade of life with an equal incidence in men and women.

The clinical features are distinctive and include coarse facial features, thick skin, poor dental occlusion, thick calvarium, deepening of voice, lantern jaw, prominent tongue, broad hand and feet, and organomegaly.[16] Rheumatologic complaints like backache and arthropathy are common.

Definitive Diagnosis

The definitive diagnosis of acromegaly is made by measurement of 24-hour serum growth hormone levels and demonstration that growth hormone secretion is not suppressed by an oral glucose challenge. Measurement of serum levels of insulin-like growth factor 1 (IGF-1 or somatomedin C) is a sensitive screening test.[41]

Radiological Findings

The radiographic findings of bony and soft-tissue overgrowth are quite characteristic in patients of acromegaly.

- Collagen tissue demonstrates a marked response to excessive amounts of growth hormone which manifests in the form of thickening of the skin. *Soft-tissue thickening* is classically seen in the heel pads and digits. The measurement is obtained by calculating the shortest distance between the calcaneus and plantar surface of the skin **(Fig. 29)**. According to Kho and associates, the thickness of the heel pad in acromegaly is related to the severity and chronicity of disease and is correlated with serum levels of growth hormone (GH).[43] Values >23 mm in men and 21.5 mm in women are suggestive of acromegaly and values >25 mm in men and 23 mm in women are diagnostic, if local causes of skin thickening are excluded.[43]
- In the *skull, changes* include:
  - Thickening of the cranial vault
  - Prominence of the supraorbital ridges and zygomatic arches
  - Prominence of the external occipital protuberance
  - Enlargement of the sella turcica with distinctive changes
  - Prominence and enlargement of the frontal and maxillary sinuses
  - Excessive pneumatization of the mastoid

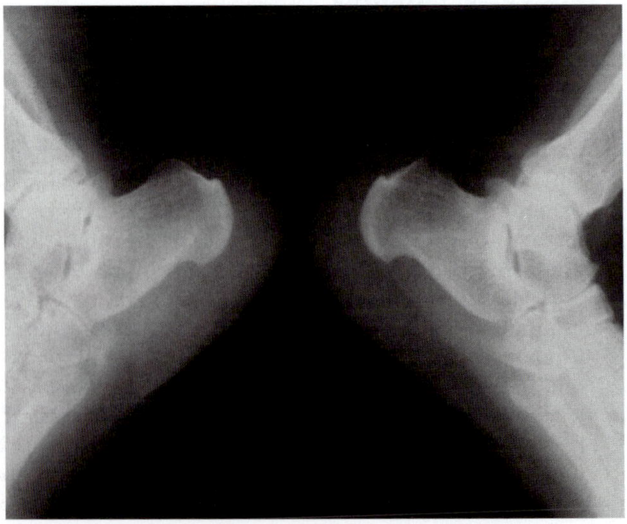

FIG. 29: Acromegaly with increase in soft-tissue thickness of the heel pad.

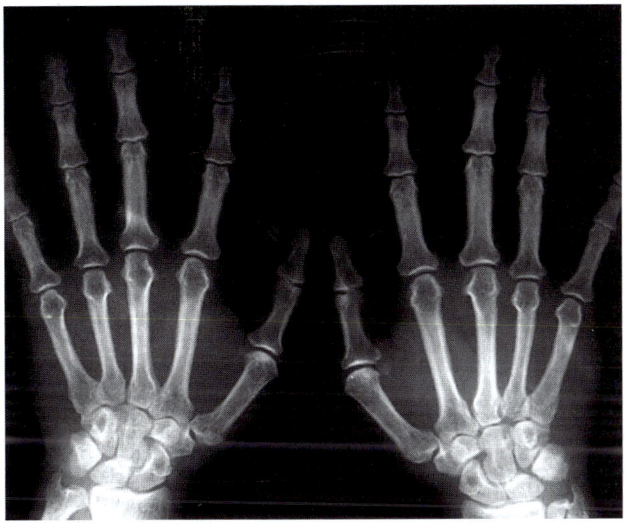

FIG. 30: Acromegaly. There is enlargement of the soft tissues with thickening of fingers and prominent joint spaces due to cartilage hypertrophy. The distal phalanges show the characteristic arrow-head appearance, more marked in the first finger.

- Enlargement and elongation of the mandible with widening of the mandibular angle.
- *Abnormalities in the hands and wrists* include soft tissue thickening of fingers, thickening, and squaring of the phalanges and metacarpals, tubulation, or overconstriction of the shafts of the phalanges, abnormally wide articular spaces, bony excrescences at sites of tendon and ligament attachment to bone and prominence of the ungual tufts which may assume a spade-like appearance.[43] An increase in soft tissue **(Fig. 30)** and bony measurements at certain specific sites has been described. One such measurement in the *Sesamoid index* which is the greatest product of the medial first metacarpophalangeal sesamoid and its maximum perpendicular diameter. This index >40 mm in men and 32 mm in women is suggestive of acromegaly. No single measurement is specific for acromegaly and the concomitant findings which are suggestive of acromegaly include:
  - Increased phalangeal soft tissue thickness ≥27 mm (men) (at proximal mid phalanges) ≥26 mm (women)
  - Widening of second metacarpophalangeal joint >2.5 mm in men and women
  - Bone excrescences and marginal spurs
  - Increased width of phalanges
  - Large sesamoid index >40 mm (men) >32 mm (women)
  - Increased interstyloid distance.
- The abnormalities in the *vertebral column* in acromegaly consist of:
  - Elongation and widening of vertebral bodies
  - Anterior and lateral osteophytes
  - Increased height of intervertebral disc
  - Scalloping of the posterior margins of vertebral bodies
  - Increased thoracic kyphosis
  - Exaggerated lumbar lordosis.
- *Thoracic cage abnormalities* consist of an enlarged thorax due to elongation of ribs and prominence of costochondral junction.
- In *pelvis*, in addition to articular alteration in sacroiliac joints and hip, enlargement and beaking of symphysis pubis is seen.
- In the *feet*, the radiographic changes resemble those in hands with:
  - Soft-tissue enlargement
  - Prominence of tufts and base of terminal phalanges
  - Bone proliferation at sites of tendon and ligament attachment like under surface of calcaneum.
- *Articular abnormalities* are most frequently seen in the knees, hip, and glenohumeral joints. Proliferation of chondrocytes in the articular cartilage result in widening of articular space seen at metacarpophalangeal, metatarsophalangeal, and interphalangeal joints.

In the later stages of the disease, cartilaginous and osseous degeneration occurs leading to secondary degenerative changes. Superficially, the appearance of acromegalic arthropathy is similar to osteoarthritis, but the joint spaces tend to be widened rather than narrowed. The distribution of involvement usually includes the large joints and the lumbosacral spine which are normally spared by osteoarthritis.

Gigantism

Excess of growth hormone during skeletal development results in gigantism, which is a rare condition. The direct hormonal stimulation of activity at the growth plates and other sites of bone formation by growth hormone leads to progressive enlargement of length and width of the bones. The most striking feature of patients with gigantism is extreme height with normal body proportions.[41] An autonomously functioning pituitary adenoma is the most common cause of gigantism. Unless treated, the growth hormone excess continues after growth plate closure with patients of gigantism developing progressively more striking features of acromegaly.[41]

SCURVY

Scurvy, also known as Barlow's disease, is the result of long-term deficiency of vitamin C. Infantile scurvy is found in infants fed on pasteurized or boiled milk formula since the pasteurization and boiling processes destroy the vitamin C content.[12,22] Children with developmental or psychological disorder, who have a vitamin C-poor diet, are at a risk of developing scurvy. Scurvy is rare before 6 months of age as for scurvy to manifest itself the deficiency must be present for at least 4–6 months.[22] It is seen much less frequently than rickets.[44]

Clinical Findings

Scurvy usually occurs in the age group of 6 months to 2 years. Child presents with progressive irritability, with tender, edematous limbs, and weakness of lower limbs resulting in pseudoparalysis. Musculocutaneous manifestations are seen in 80% of patients with scurvy, such as arthralgia, myalgia, hemarthrosis, and muscular and subperiosteal hemorrhage. Lower extremities are more commonly involved than the upper extremities with knee being more commonly involved. Subcutaneous and mucous membrane hemorrhages occur and a secondary anemia may develop. Scurvy is rare in adults, being seen in patients suffering from chronic severe malnutrition.

Biochemical Findings

Serum ascorbic acid: 0.6–1.2 mg/100 mL (normal range).

Pathophysiology

The pathological changes seen in scurvy are the result of depression of normal cellular activity.[22] There is suppression of osteoblastic activity resulting in cessation of normal bone formation. However, bone resorption continues leading to the development of osteoporosis.

At the growth plate, although cartilage proliferation is decreased, mineralization is unimpaired, resulting in the zone of provisional calcification becoming wide and dense. Similar changes occur around epiphyseal ossification centers, resulting in a thin ring of *increased* density surrounding the *epiphysis*. Vascular invasion of the zone of provisional calcification is arrested and with suppressed osteoblastic activity there is decreased formation of bony matrix. Thus, the trabecular bone mass is decreased in the zone of primary and secondary spongiosa. This is seen radiographically as a *transverse band* of *radiolucency* adjacent to the zone of provisional calcification. This zone, called Trümmerfeld zone represents an area of weakened bone and shows a tendency to fracture. The zone of provisional calcification extends beyond the margins of the metaphysis, resulting in periosteal elevation and marginal spur formation. Large subperiosteal hemorrhages resulting in soft tissue edema occur in late stages of the disease.

The optimal sites for detection of scurvy in the skeleton are bones of the lower extremities. Diagnostic changes may be demonstrable at the knees when minimal changes are present at the wrists.[12]

Radiological Findings

Radiographically, characteristic signs are seen which reflect the pathological changes occurring as a result of lack of vitamin C.

- Osteoporosis.
- *White line of Frankel* is the dense, white line in the zone of provisional calcification at the growing metaphysis.
- Beneath the Frankel's line, there is a radiolucent zone in the metaphysis called *Trümmerfeld zone or Scorbutic zone*, due to lack of mineralization of osteoid **(Fig. 31)**.
- The epiphysis is small, sharply marginated by a sclerotic rim while the central portion is more radiolucent, called *Wimberger's sign*.
- Finally, as the metaphysis is weakened, it is prone to fractures, which manifest themselves at the cortical margin, giving rise to *Pelkan spur*, that project perpendicular to the long axis of the shaft.
- In addition, due to capillary permeability, *subperiosteal hemorrhages* occur which may give rise to periosteal elevation and subsequent new bone formation, particularly following treatment. The hemorrhages appear as soft-tissue density adjacent to the cortical bones such as femur, tibia, and humerus. Upon healing, the subperiosteal hemorrhages calcify, and cast shadows of increased density in the soft tissues surrounding the bone **(Fig. 32)**.

The above findings constitute the classic signs of infantile scurvy. These changes are less apparent as the patient ages. On healing, all changes are reversible on vitamin C

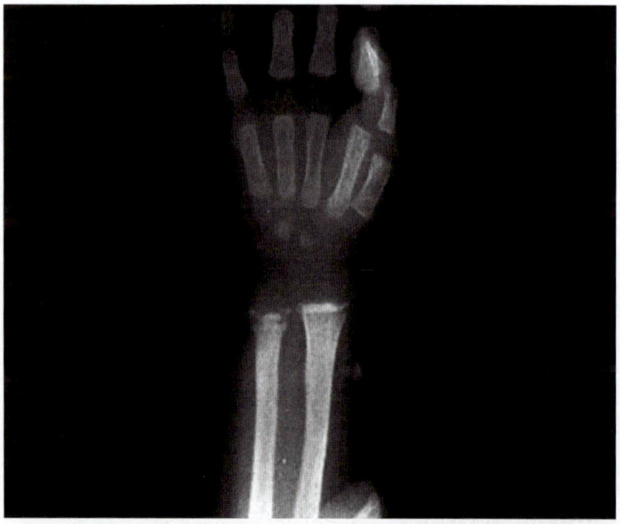

FIG. 31: Scurvy. X-ray wrist anteroposterior (AP) view reveals increased density of the zone of provisional calcification (Frankel's line) with a lucent zone beneath it (Trümmerfeld zone) in the distal radial and ulnar metaphysis.

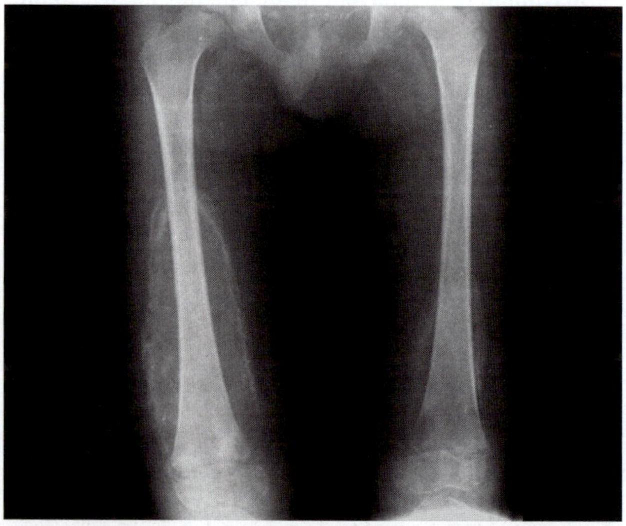

FIG. 32: Calcified subperiosteal hemorrhages seen along bilateral femoral shafts, more extensive on the right side: Healing scurvy.

therapy though a single growth arrest line may remain in the metaphysis as a residual of Frankel's line, an indicator of prior vitamin C therapy.

Diagnosis

The diagnosis of scurvy is by clinical and radiographic findings and may be supported by additional findings of low level of vitamin C in the serum or Buffy coat of leukocytes.

Ultrasound Evaluation

Though the clinical and radiological changes described in scurvy are the best diagnostic tool, effective use of ultrasonography in pediatric patients has been described, both in diagnosis and follow-up as it does not involve any ionizing radiation. High-resolution ultrasonography of the affected limb very well depicts the recurrent and multiple subperiosteal hemorrhage as heterogeneous hypoechoic lesions beneath the periosteum with absence of vascularity on color Doppler, thereby ruling out the likelihood of a malignant process[45] **(Figs. 33A to C)**.

Magnetic Resonance Imaging

Magnetic resonance imaging findings of scurvy have also been described in the literature. It consists of heterogeneous signal of the marrow on T1- and T2-weighted sequences, subperiosteal hemorrhage and surrounding edema **(Figs. 34A to D)**. These findings can also be seen in osteomyelitis, subperiosteal abscess, or leukemia which need to be excluded. However, an increase in the subperiosteal hemorrhage on follow-up scans due to recurrent hematoma is a pointer toward the diagnosis of scurvy.[46]

Treatment

Since scurvy is rare with nonspecific symptomatology, the best evidence in diagnosis is the improvement in symptoms that usually start within few days of start of vitamin C therapy.

Oral vitamin C supplementation with a dose of 100–300 mg in children should be given until the serum level improves. Spontaneous hemorrhages stop in 24 hours while muscle and body aches disappear in a few days with complete relief from symptoms observed within 3 weeks.[45]

FLUOROSIS

It is a chronic metabolic bone disease caused by chronic ingestion of excessive amounts of fluoride.

The alterations in bone metabolism in fluorosis are not clearly understood but seem to be multifactorial. A generalized increase in bone density is seen which is due to osteoclastic response to the fluorine rather than fluorine deposition *per se*.[15] The synthesis of normal collagen is also disturbed.

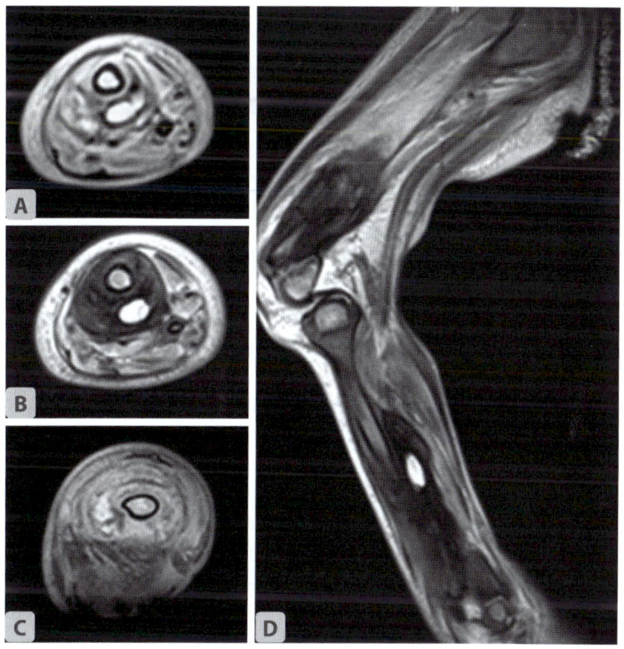

FIGS. 34A TO D: Magnetic resonance imaging of the lower limb of the same child was done. T2 sagittal, T1 and T2W axial images and post contrast TW FS images show elevation of distal femoral periosteum with altered signal in the subperiosteal space extending from epiphysis to midshaft appearing isointense on T1W images (A) and iso- to hypointense on T2W/STIR images; (B) showing no enhancement on postcontrast images; (C) suggestive of hematoma of varying stage; (D) Similar findings are seen along the tibial diaphysis. Overlying muscles appear atrophic with heterogeneous signal intensity suggestive of fatty infiltration; features suggestive of nutritional deficiency likely scurvy.

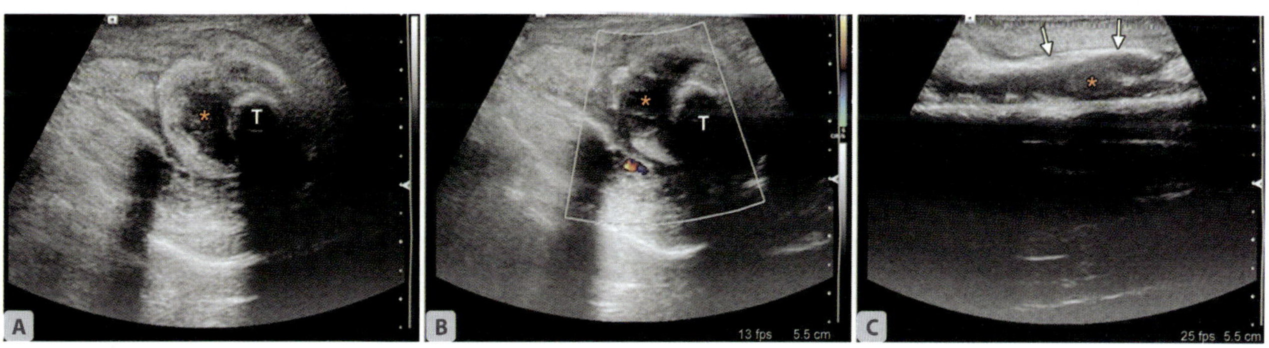

FIGS. 33A TO C: (A) Ultrasound left leg in a 5-year-old child with mixed cerebral palsy with cellulitis reveals heterogeneous hypoechoic areas (*) beneath the periosteum of left tibial (T) shaft, with no vascularity within on color Doppler (B) suggestive of subperiosteal hemorrhage due to scurvy. Arrows in the longitudinal image (C) depicts the elevated periosteum.

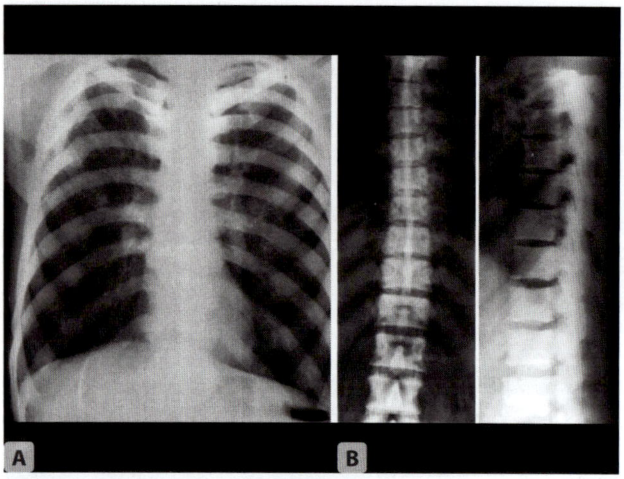

FIGS. 35A AND B: Fluorosis. (A) Frontal chest X-ray reveals diffuse osteosclerosis; (B) Osteosclerosis and osteophytosis of the dorsal vertebral bodies with posterior longitudinal ligament ossification.

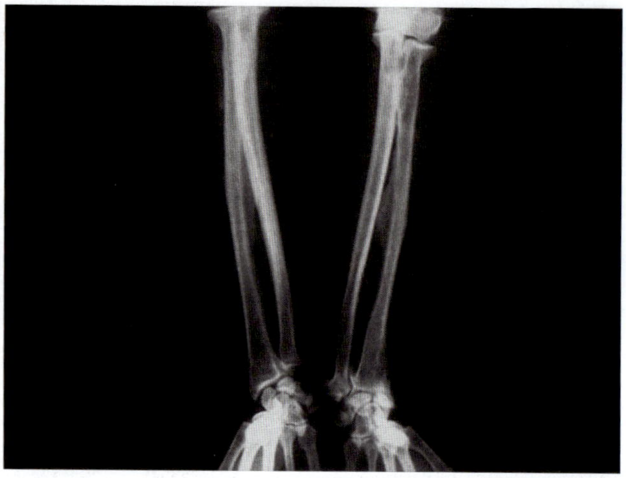

FIG. 36: Interosseous membrane ossification—diagnostic of fluorosis.

Clinical Findings

Clinically, there is marked variation in presentation. The most pronounced feature is mottled dental enamel. Bone changes produce few symptoms. However, exceptionally high levels of fluorine may be associated with crippling stiffness and pain.[15] Criteria for diagnosing fluorosis clinically consist of:[47]

- Residing in endemic area for >10 years
- Mottled tooth enamel
- Urine fluoride levels >10 mg/L (normal level <1.5 mg/L)
- Typical symptoms and findings on clinical examination
- No evidence of any other metabolic bone disease on clinical evaluation.

Radiographical Findings

Radiological evaluation is considered the best method for diagnosing fluorosis, especially when the patient is asymptomatic.

Radiographically, the changes are diffuse increase in bone density (osteosclerosis), osteophytosis, and calcification/ossification of the attachments of tendons, muscles, and ligaments.

- *Osteosclerosis* is a common finding in fluorosis and involves all bones, but is most marked in the spine, pelvis, and ribs **(Figs. 35A and B)**. Initially, there is a thickening of the bony trabecular pattern which then progresses to a dense, uniform, symmetrical sclerosis that obliterates the bony architectural landmarks. The skull and tubular bones of the appendicular skeleton are relatively spared in the sclerotic process. The only change in the calvarium may be a sclerosis of the base of the skull and posterior clinoids.[44] One needs to remember that osteosclerosis alone is a nonspecific finding seen in many conditions such as metastasis, myelofibrosis, Paget's disease, renal osteodystrophy, etc.
- Thickening of the cortex of the affected bones occurs at the expense of the medullary cavity.
- The inferior margins of the ribs may show characteristic irregularity/fringed appearance called "rose-thorn appearance."
- *Ligamentous calcification* and *ossification*, particularly of sacrospinous and sacrotuberous ligaments, is another characteristic radiographic feature.
- *Ossification* in the *interosseous membranes* of paired bones is *diagnostic* **(Fig. 36)**.
- *Osteophytosis* of the vertebrae can be severe and at times encroach on the spinal canal and intervertebral foramina. Paraspinal and intraspinal ligament ossification is known to occur and may cause compressive myelopathy **(Fig. 37)**.

Magnetic resonance imaging is a useful imaging modality in the early diagnosis of fluorosis and in planning surgical intervention in a symptomatic patient as the extent of soft tissue, spinal cord changes and associated abnormalities are well visualized. Typical MRI findings in fluorosis of spine consist of diffusely sclerotic bones, ossification of posterior longitudinal ligament and ligamentam flavum, and spinal canal and neural foramina narrowing. Osteosclerosis is typically seen as low-signal intensity on both T1- and T2-weighted images. In endemic regions, MRI may show diffuse low signal on all pulse sequences and help in early detection of fluorosis and save the patients from serious manifestations such as fluorotic myelopathy which may require surgical decompression.

Diagnosis is based on characteristic ligament calcification, history of long-term heavy exposure to fluoride, and high urinary fluoride levels.

CONCLUSION

To conclude, plain radiographs are the primary imaging tools for the evaluation of suspected skeletal disorders of metabolic and endocrine origin. By and large, these disorders involve the skeleton as a whole. The radiographic changes are therefore predominantly diffuse or at least multifocal involving many areas of the skeleton. An understating of the diverse manifestations of these disorders including their findings on imaging helps in reaching an early diagnosis. Imaging also plays a role in evaluation of severity of disease, assessment of disease activity, and in monitoring the effect of treatment.

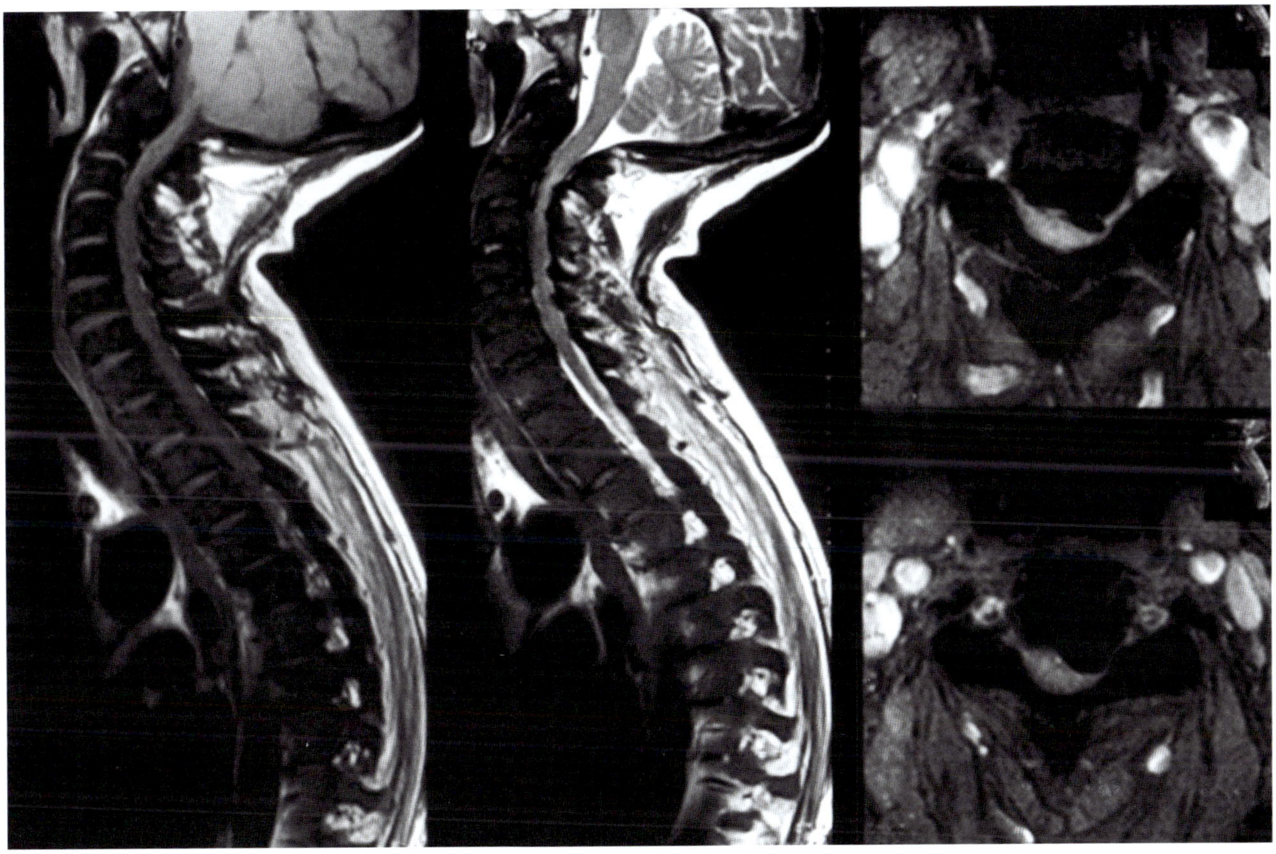

FIG. 37: Fluorosis: T1W and T2W sagittal MR scans of cervicodorsal spine reveals diffuse decrease in marrow signal intensity of vertebral bodies, appearing more hypointense than intervening intervertebral discs consistent with sclerosis. The vertebral bodies show osteophytic changes. Axial images depict ossification of posterior longitudinal ligament with resultant spinal canal stenosis.

REFERENCES

1. Mankin HJ. Metabolic bone disease. J Bone Joint Surg Am. 1994;76:760.
2. Reynolds WA, Karo JJ. Radiologic diagnosis of metabolic bone disease. Orthop Clin North Am. 1972;3(3):521-43.
3. Pitt M. Osteopenic bone disease. Orthop Clin North Am. 1983;14(1): 65-80.
4. Pitt MJ. Rickets and osteomalacia are still around. Radiol Clin North Am. 1991;29(1):97-118.
5. Mankin HJ. Rickets, osteomalacia and renal osteodystrophy: Part I. J Bone Joint Surg Am. 1974;56.101.
6. Rowe LJ, Yochum TR. Nutritional metabolic and endocrine disorders: In: Yochum, Rowes (Eds). Essentials of Skeletal Radiology, 3rd edition. Philadelphia: Lippincott Williams and Wilkins; 2005. pp. 1497-545.
7. Chaudhari JR, Mridula KR, Rathnakishor C, Balaraju B, Bandaru VS. Association of 25-Hydroxy vitamin D deficiency in pediatric epileptic patients. IJCN. 2017;11(2): 46-56.
8. Jagtal VS. Hypophosphatemic rickets. IJEM. 2012;16(2): 177-82.
9. Gupta AK. Rickets and osteomalacia. In: Berry M, Chowdhury V, Suri S, Mukhopadhyay S (Eds). Diagnostic Radiology-Musculoskeletal and Breast Imaging, 1st edition. Delhi: Jaypee Brothers Medical publishers (P) Ltd.; 1998. pp. 162-75.
10. Pitt MJ. Rickets and osteomalacia. In: Resnick D (Ed). Diagnosis of Bone and Joint Disorders, 4th edition. USA: WB Saunders Company; 2002. pp. 1901-45.
11. Judith EA. Metabolic and endocrine skeletal disease. In: Adams A, Dixon AK (Eds). Grainger and Allison's Diagnostic Radiology: A Textbook of Medical Imaging, 5th edition. London: Churchill Livingstone Elsevier; 2008. pp. 1083-113.
12. Silverman FN. Dysostoses, miscellaneous syndromes and metabolic abnormalities. In: Silverman FN, Kuhn JP (Eds). Caffey's Pediatric X-ray Diagnosis, 9th edition. USA: Mosby. 1993. pp. 1746-81.
13. Kottamasu SR. Metabolic bone diseases. In: Silverman FN, Kuhn JP (Eds). Caffey's Pediatric X-ray Diagnosis, 10th edition. USA: Mosby; 2003. pp. 2242-68.
14. Pitt MJ. Rickets and osteomalacia. In: Resmick D, Krausdorf MJ (Eds). Bone and Joint Imaging, 3rd edition. USA: Elsevier Saunders; 2005. pp. 563-75.
15. Murray RO, Stoker DJ. Skeletal disorders of metaboloic and endocrines origin. In: Sutton D (Ed). Textbook of Radiology and Imaging, 4th edition. London: Churchill Living Stone. 1987;1: 229-63.
16. Lenchik L, Sartoris DJ. Orthopaedic aspects of metabolic bone disease. Orthop Clin North Am. 1998;29(1):103-34.

17. Steinbach HL, Noetzli M. Roentgen appearance of the skeleton in osteomalacia and rickets. AJR. 1964;91:955.
18. Chuang TL, Kuo JL, Chang XY, Chiu JS, Wang YF, et al. Scintigraphic evidence of osteomalacia: Usefulness and typical signs. Ann Nucl Med Sci. 2007;20:115-20.
19. Resnick D. Parathyroid disorders and renal osteodystrophy. In: Resnick D (Ed). Diagnosis of Bone and Joint Disorders, 4th edition. Philadelphia: WB Saunders Company. 2002;2:2043-111.
20. Eslamy HK, Ziessman HA. Parathyroid Scintigraphy in patients with primary Hyperparathyroidism: ^{99m}Tc sestamibi SPECT and SPECT /CT. Radiographics. 2008;28:1461-76.
21. Chowdhury V. Hyperparathyroidism. In: Berry M, Chowdhury V, Suri S, Mukhopadhyay S (Eds). Diagnostic Radiology: Musculoskeletal and Breast Imaging, 1st edition. Delhi: Jaypee Brothers Medical Publishers (P) Ltd; 1998. pp. 186-200.
22. Volger JB, Kim JH. Metabolic and endocrine disease of the skeleton. In: Grainger RG, Allison DJ, Adam A, Dixon AK (Eds). Diagnostic Radiology. A Textbook of Medical Imaging, 4th edition. London: Churchill Livingstone; 2001. pp. 1925-66.
23. Resmick D. Parathyroid disorders and renal osteodystrophy. In: Resmick D, Krausdorf MJ (Eds). Bone and Joint Imaging, 3rd edition. USA: Elsevier Saunders. 2005;2:603-22.
24. Hayes CW, Conway WF. Hyperparathyroidism. Radiol Clin North Am. 1991;29(1):85-96.
25. Richardson ML, Pozz-Mucelli RS, Kanter AS. Bone mineral changes in primary hyperparathyroidism. Skeletal Radiology. 1986;15:85-95.
26. Sahan MH, Guner S, Guner SI. Radiological findings in the primary hyperparathyroid case with multiple brown tumors: a case report. Eastern Journal of Medicine. 2008;13:30-4.
27. Su AW, Chen CF, Huang CK, Chen PC, Chen WM, Chen TH.. Primary hyperparathyroidism with brown tumor mimicking metastatic bone malignancy. J Chin Med Assoc. 2010;73(3): 177-80.
28. Greenspan A. Hyperparathyroidism. In: Greenspan A (Ed). Orthopaedic imaging: A practical approach, 4th edition. USA: Lippincott Williams and Wilkins; 2004. pp. 837-42.
29. Young WR. Metabolic and Endocrine disorders affecting bone. In: Sutton D (Ed). Textbook of Radiology and Imaging, 7th edition. London: Churchill Livingstone. 2003;1:1351-69.
30. Chang CY, Rosenthal DI, Mitchell DM, Handa A, Kattapuram SV, Huang AJ. Imaging findings of metabolic bone disease. Radiographics. 2016;36:1871-87.
31. Patel AA, Ramanathan R, Kuban J, Willis MH. Imaging findings and evaluation of metabolic bone disease. Hindawi; 2015.
32. Larson TC, Smith MM, Chong WK, Martin WH. Imaging of the thyroid and parathyroid glands. In: Hagga JR, Lanzieri CF, Gilkeson RC (Eds). CT and MR Imaging of the Whole Body, 4th edition. USA: Mosby. 2003;1:663-90.
33. Johnson NA, Tublin ME, Ogilvie JB. Parathyroid imaging: Technique and role in the preoperative evaluation of primary hyperparathyroidism. AJR. 2007;188(6):1706-15.
34. Mc Dermott VG, Spritzer CE. Parathyroid and thyroid glands. In: Stark DD, Bradley WG Jr (Eds). Magnetic Resonance Imaging, 3rd edition, volume III. USA: Mosby, Inc; 1999. pp. 1807-20.
35. Bilezikian JP, Brandi ML, Eastall R, Silverberg SJ, Udelsman R, Marcocci C, et al. Guidelines for the management of asymptomatic hyperthyroidism: Summary statement from the 4th International workshop. J Clin Endocrinol Metab. 2014;99(10): 3561-9.
36. Hoang JK, Sung W, Bahl M, Philips CD. How to perform parathyroid 4D CT: Tips and traps for technique and interpretation. Radiology. 2014;270(1):15-24.
37. Bann DV, Zacharia T, Goldenberg D, Goyal N. Parathyroid localization using 4D-computed tomography. Ear Nose Throat J. 2015;94(4-5):E55-7.
38. Bahl M, Sepahdari AR, Sosa JA, Hoang JK. Parathyroid adenomas and hyperplasia on four-dimensional CT scans: three patterns of enhancement relative to the thyroid gland justify a three-phase protocol. Radiology. 2015;277(2): 454-62.
39. Yeh R, Tay YD, Tabacco G Dercle L, Kuo JH, Bandeira L. Diagnostic performance of 4D CT and Sestamibi SPECT/CT in localizing parathyroid adenomas in primary hyperparathyroidism. Radiology. 2019;291(2):469-76.
40. Lundstroem AK, Trolle W, Soerenses CH, Myschatzky. Preoperative localization of hyperfunctioning parathyroid glands with 4D-CT. Eur Arch Otorhinolaryngol. 2016;273: 1253-9.
41. Chew FS. Radiologic manifestations in the musculoskeletal system of miscellaneous endocrine disorders. Radiol Clin North Am. 1991;29(1):135-47.
42. Resnick D. Pituitary disorders. In: Resnick D (Ed). Diagnosis of Bone and Joint Disorders, 4th edition. USA: WB Saunders Company; 2002. pp. 2003-25.
43. Resnick D. Pituitary disorders. In: Resnick D (Ed). Diagnosis of Bone and Joint Disorders, 5th edition. USA: WB Saunders Company; 2005. pp. 589-96.
44. Greenfield GB. Epiphyseal region. In: Greenfield (Ed). Radiology of Bone Diseases, 5th edition. Philadelphia: JB Lippincott Company; 1990. p. 235.
45. Polat AV, Bekci T, Say F, Bolukbas E, Selcuk MB. Osteoskeletal manifestations of scurvy: MRI and ultrasound findings. Skeletal Radiology. 2015;44(8):1161-4.
46. Choi SW, Park S, Kwon YS, Oh IS, Lim MK, Kim WH, et al. MR imaging in a child with scurvy: a case report. Korean J Radiol. 2007;8(5):443-7.
47. Nair N, Gupta N. Radiology of skeletal fluorosis: A review. Annals of Orthop Rheumatol. 2016;4(2):1069-71.

CHAPTER

162

Osteoporosis

Chirag Kamal Ahuja, Mukesh Kumar Yadav, Vikas Bhatia, Ajay Kumar

INTRODUCTION

Osteoporosis, one of the common metabolic bone disorders, is a manifestation of compromised bone strength. It is defined by the World Health Organization (WHO) as "a skeletal disease, characterized by low bone mass and microarchitectural deterioration of bone tissue, with a consequent increase in bone fragility and susceptibility to fracture."[1] The strength of the bone is a constituent of two features, namely, its quality and density (mass/volume). Bone quality is a composite of bone architecture, turnover, mineralization, and damage incurred. The bone mineral density (BMD) can be subject to measurement and has been used in the quantitative WHO definition of osteoporosis, with bone density <2.5 standard deviations (SD) qualifying for the diagnosis of osteoporosis.[2] Histologically, there occurs a decrease in cortical thickness along with reduction in the size and number of the trabeculae of cancellous bone. There may be fractures of the trabecular as well as compromise of the trabecular connectivity. The structure of organic matrix (osteoid) is preserved with no obvious defect in mineralization. Thus, osteoporosis is histologically distinguishable from osteomalacia, in which mineralization of osteoid matrix is impaired with an increase in the ratio of organic matrix to mineral.

PATHOGENESIS

Bone remodeling (its production and resorption) is a continuous process, which is regulated by systemic and locally produced agents. A number of metabolic, nutritional, and mechanical factors are also involved in the procedure. A fine balance in bone formation and resorption maintains the skeletal mass. Tipping of the balance toward resorption results in reduced bone mass resulting in osteoporosis.[2]

Aging also leads to reduced bone mass. Although skeletal growth ceases by the end of adolescence and there occurs closure of the endochondral growth plate, bone mass continues to increase by radial growth until peak is achieved at about the age of 35 years. Thereafter, a balance is achieved for a few years when there is an equivalence of new bone formation and bone resorption. After a few years of growth, in around fourth to fifth decade, bone resorption starts to increase more than bone formation and skeletal mass decreases. Different areas of the skeleton show different bone loss. There is progressive reduced rate of loss of cortical bone of about 0.3–0.5% per year subsequently in both genders. The rate of bone loss in women may be accelerated around the time of menopause, which is attributable to estrogen deficiency. The cumulative loss of bone mass ranges from 20 to 30% in men and 40 to 50% in women over the last four to five decades of life.[2,3]

ETIOLOGY

Table 1 highlights the various causes, which may contribute to osteoporosis. The various types and causes are briefly discussed in the following text.

Primary Osteoporosis

Type I (Postmenopausal) Osteoporosis

It occurs in women between 51 and 75 years of age in which there is disproportionate accelerated loss of trabecular bone.[4] Fractures of vertebral bodies and distal forearm are common. Biochemically, both circulating parathormone and 1,25$(OH)_2$ vitamin D are reduced.

Type II (Senile) Osteoporosis

It occurs in both sexes over 70 years of age. There is proportionate loss of both cortical and trabecular bone, and the fracture sites are also those which contain both types of bone, i.e., femoral neck, proximal humerus, proximal tibia, and pelvis. Biochemically, circulating parathormone is increased but 1,25$(OH)_2$ vitamin D is reduced.

Juvenile Osteoporosis

Juvenile osteoporosis is a rare disease, which occurs in children between 8 and 15 years of age. Clinical features include bone pain, fractures with minimal trauma (mostly metaphyseal fractures of distal tibia and vertebral crush fractures), reduced bone density at areas of new bone growth, and loss of height. Spontaneous recovery occurs within 4–5 years, but deformities may persist. Biochemical investigations are normal and most forms of treatment are ineffective.

TABLE 1: Various causes of osteoporosis.

Cause unknown	Causes known	Miscellaneous causes
• Primary osteoporosis (senile, postmenopausal) • Juvenile osteoporosis	Endocrine disorders: • Acromegaly • Adrenal atrophy in Addison's disease • Cushing's syndrome • Eating disorders • Endometriosis • Gonadal insufficiency (primary or secondary) • Hyperparathyroidism • Hyperprolactinemia • Hyperthyroidism • Hypogonadism • Type 1 diabetes mellitus • Nutritional disorders • Tumor secretion of parathyroid hormone-related peptide Gastrointestinal disease: • Alcohol-related liver diseases • Celiac disease • Chronic active hepatitis • Chronic cholestatic diseases • Gastrectomy • Inflammatory bowel disease • Jejunoileal bypass • Malabsorption syndromes • Pancreatic insufficiency • Parenteral nutrition • Primary biliary cirrhosis • Severe liver disease Marrow-related disorders: • Amyloidosis • Hemochromatosis • Hemophilia • Leukemia • Lymphoma • Mastocytosis • Multiple myeloma • Pernicious anemia • Sarcoidosis • Sickle cell anemia • Thalassemia Organ transplantation: • Bone marrow • Heart • Kidney • Liver • Lung	• Ankylosing spondylitis • Chronic obstructive pulmonary disease • Congenital porphyria • Epidermolysis bullosa • Hemophilia • Idiopathic hypercalciuria • Idiopathic scoliosis • Multiple sclerosis • Rheumatoid arthritis • Immobilization Genetic disorders: • Hypophosphatasia • Osteogenesis imperfect • Homocystinuria • Ehlers–Danlos syndrome • Marfan syndrome Drugs associated with bone loss: • Aluminum • Anticoagulants • Anticonvulsants • Cigarette smoking • Cytotoxic drugs • Excessive alcohol • Excessive vitamin A • Glucocorticoids and adrenocorticotropin • Gonadotropin-releasing hormone agonists • Heparin • Lithium • Tamoxifen (in the premenopausal patient) • Beta carotene • Bile-acid binding resins

Endocrine Causes

Glucocorticoid Excess

Cushing's syndrome or glucocorticoid excess from exogenous or endogenous sources results in osteoporosis. There are a number of mechanisms responsible for this, and it has been shown by various studies that both dose and duration of steroid treatment correlate with bone loss. Glucocorticoid-induced bone loss predominantly affects the trabecular bone. Once osteoporosis develops in adults with Cushing's syndrome, the abnormality may persist indefinitely even after the cause is removed.

Hypogonadism

Whether due to primary gonadal failure or secondary to gonadotropin deficiency, hypogonadism is associated with osteoporosis, particularly of trabecular bone. It is a well-known fact that estrogen is important in preventing bone loss in normal premenopausal women, and estrogen deficiency due to any cause can lead to osteoporosis.[5] Similarly, testosterone deficiency appears to be the major factor responsible for reduced bone mass in men.

Thyrotoxicosis

Significant bone loss is rare in thyrotoxicosis due to its early diagnosis and treatment. Both bone formation and resorption are increased in this disorder, but the formation is unable to match the resorption which leads to reduced bone mass.

Hyperprolactinemia

In women with hyperprolactinemia, reduced estrogen secretion is the key factor for osteoporosis. Even in men with hyperprolactinemia, there is reduced bone density due to associated hypogonadism.

Diabetes Mellitus

In insulin-dependent (type 1) diabetes mellitus, there is reduction in the bone mass. The mechanism is not clear. Though the calcium levels are high, there is reduced tubular reabsorption of phosphate that may be a contributing factor for osteoporosis. A primary decrease in bone formation due to reduced insulin action has also been postulated.

Hyperparathyroidism

Generalized loss of bone density is a prominent feature in primary or secondary hyperparathyroidism, which is followed by endosteal resorption. Osteoporosis may be seen in patients with primary hyperparathyroidism who may not have subperiosteal resorption or brown tumor or elevated serum alkaline phosphatase. Increased osteoclastic activity is responsible for osteoporosis.[5]

Malignant Diseases

Several malignant tumors may cause diffuse osteopenia. Multiple myeloma is the most common. Other tumors include lymphoma, leukemia, systemic mastocytosis, etc. The neoplastic plasma cells secrete osteoclast-activating factor which may be involved in mediating bone loss. Heparin or possibly other agents released by mast cells or lymphoma cells may be the effector molecule for osteoporosis.

Immobilization

Increased bone resorption resulting from decreased weight bearing is the cause of bone loss.

Drugs

Long-term heparin administration potentiates parathyroid hormone (PTH)-mediated bone resorption and activation of collagenase, which leads to bone loss. Ethanol may also cause or contribute to bone loss. There is a long list of medications associated with bone loss.

Genetic Abnormalities in Bone Collagen Synthesis

Osteogenesis imperfecta (brittle bone syndrome) is described under four types. *Type I* osteogenesis imperfecta is an autosomal dominant form characterized by mild-to-moderate bone fragility, blue sclerae, and premature deafness. *Type II* is a lethal perinatal disorder. *Type III* is characterized by severe bone fragility, progressive bone deformity, and white sclerae. *Type IV* shows features of type I with white sclerae. Defective gene encoding leading to decreased collagen formation of type I leads to osteoporosis. It is postulated that what is now diagnosed as idiopathic or postmenopausal osteoporosis is due to defect in these genes (*COLIA1* and *COLIA2*) in absence of other features of osteogenesis imperfecta.

Osteoporosis also occurs in patients with homocystinuria due to cystathionine synthetase deficiency, an autosomal recessive trait associated with ectopia lentis, various deformities of the extremities, mental retardation, decreased pigmentation of hair and skin, and thromboembolism. The osteoporosis may be due to the effect of homocysteine or other metabolites in interfering with cross linking of collagen.

In Marfan syndrome, an autosomal dominant disease, osteoporosis is due to defective collagen formation. It is characterized by arachnodactyly, posterior scalloping of vertebral bodies, high arched palate, lenticular subluxation, and dissecting aneurysm.

Gastrointestinal Diseases

In diffuse liver diseases, malabsorption or defective metabolism of vitamin D can cause osteopenia. Primary biliary cirrhosis is a well-known example. In addition, many other gastrointestinal diseases are associated with osteoporosis.[5]

Organ Transplantation

Organ transplantation as the effective therapy for end-stage diseases of kidney, lung, liver, and cardiac patients has shown improved outcomes leading to increase in the number of transplant patients. These patients require lifelong medications such as steroids, immunosuppressant drugs, and anticoagulation. Varying mechanisms are responsible for osteoporosis in these patients.[5]

CLINICAL FEATURES

Osteoporosis becomes clinically significant when bone mass is reduced to the extent that the skeleton is insufficient to perform its normal function. Generalized skeletal pain is uncommon, and between fractures most patients are free of symptoms. Pain usually results from collapse of vertebra, especially in the dorsal and lumbar regions, typically acute in nature, and may radiate along the distribution of the respective intercostal nerve and into the abdomen.[6] These may occur even with trivial trauma. The collapse fractures usually cause anterior wedging of the vertebrae and result in loss of height with kyphosis (dowager's or widow's hump). Scoliosis is also common. There may be recurrent episodes of vertebral collapse at different levels resulting in increasing spine deformity with loss of height.

INVESTIGATIONS

Bone Mineral Analysis

With the advent of bone mass measurement, the fracture risk in osteoporosis can be quantified before the fracture occurs. This is the major advancement in the field of osteoporosis.

The advances in radiological sciences have set in motion the development of various noninvasive, accurate, and sensitive techniques for measuring the mineral content of bone.[7] The various modalities which may be utilized are listed in **Box 1**.

Standard Radiography

Qualitative assessment of bone mineral content from standard radiographs of skeleton is usually based on subjective criteria. The assessment is commonly done on metacarpal, calcaneum, talus, femoral neck, vertebral bodies, etc. The findings are:

- Generalized osteopenia, most prominent in the axial skeleton, especially the vertebral column **(Fig. 1A)**
- Reduces thickness and accentuation of cortex
- Accentuation of primary trabeculae with thinning of secondary trabeculae
- Changes in vertebral body shape—wedge shape, biconcave, and compression **(Fig. 1B)**
- Insufficiency fractures as a result of weakened bone resulting from normal stress. Sacrum, supra-acetabular regions, os pubis, etc., are common sites. The fracture may be occult radiographically and detected on computed tomography (CT) or scintigraphy.
- Fractures at other sites (especially wrist and hip)

The major disadvantage is that it is subjective and gets affected by body habitus, radiographic exposure factors, presence of overlying soft tissue, and patient positioning. Approximately, >30% bone loss must be there to be appreciated on plain radiographs.[3,7]

Magnification radiography by either optical or direct geometric means has a small but significant role in the assessment of osteoporosis. Subperiosteal and intracortical bone absorption, even subtle, may be appreciated on magnification radiography.

BOX 1: Various modalities for the detection of osteoporosis.

- Standard radiography
- Radiogrammetry
- Photodensitometry
- Compton scattering
- Neutron activation analysis
- Single and dual photon absorptiometry
- Dual energy X-ray absorptiometry
- Quantitative computed tomography
- Quantitative ultrasound
- Magnetic resonance imaging
- Multidetector computed tomography

Radiogrammetry

Radiogrammetry is one of the simplest methods of quantitative bone mineral assessment. Conventional anteroposterior (AP) radiograph of a tubular bone (like metacarpal) is taken. The cortical thickness on either side of the medullary space is measured with a measuring device, and their sum is expressed as the combined cortical thickness (CCT). This technique is most commonly used at the midshaft of second metacarpal. Cortical bone volume (BV) is calculated from the CCT.[8] This technique is imprecise and insensitive.

Photodensitometry

In this technique, images of bone of interest and of reference aluminum wedge of known density are exposed on the same film. The optical density of the bone is then compared with that of the wedge with a photodensitometer. The information

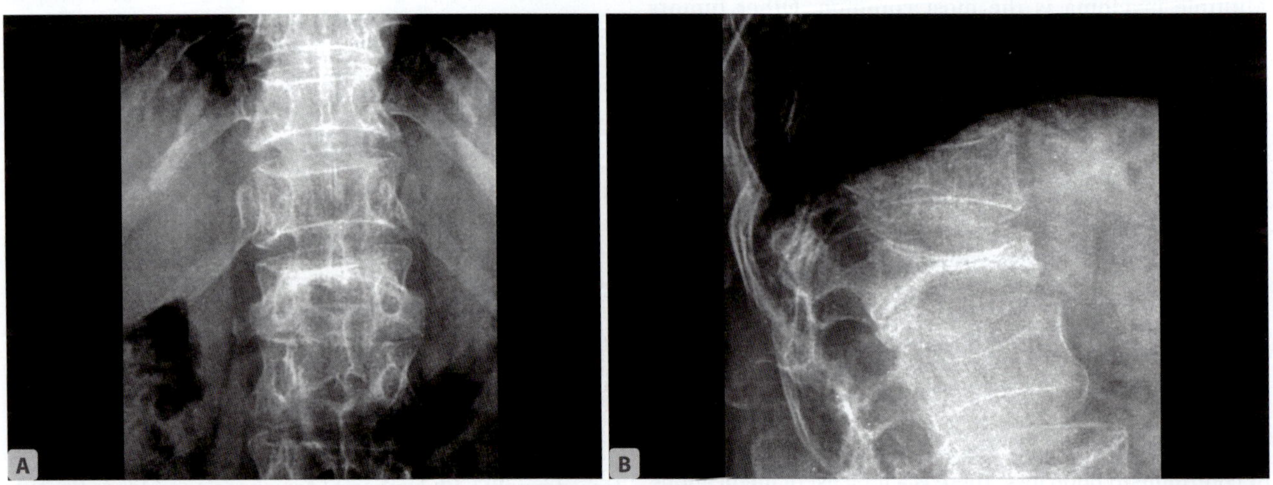

FIGS. 1A AND B: Radiographs of dorsolumbar spine anteroposterior (A) and lateral (B) views demonstrating decreased bone density with thinning of vertebral endplates, which appear as fine dense lines in contrast to the center of the vertebral body and the presence of multiple biconcave vertebrae.

obtained is comparable to that of single-photon absorptiometry but with slightly lower precision, sensitivity, and accuracy.

Neutron Activation Analysis

In this method, neutrons from an accelerator or a reactor bombard a small fraction of the total ^{48}Ca in the body, changing it to ^{49}Ca which is a radioactive isotope. By counting its activity, the total calcium content of the body is estimated. The precision and accuracy are in the order of 2–5%. However, it does not clearly reflect the state of trabecular bone and does not correlate well with spinal mineral measurements. Another disadvantage is a relatively large radiation dose (200–300 mrem).

Compton Scattering

This technique measures the absolute density of a volume of tissue based on its electron density and is the only method other than CT that can measure purely trabecular bone. It is based on the measurement of scattered radiation from a source of 100–700 keV gamma rays and is used for calcaneum, spine, and radius. The precision of this method is about 3–5% and the radiation dose varies from 200 to 2000 mrem. At present, it is largely a research tool.

Single-energy Photon Absorptiometry

Single-energy photon absorptiometry (SPA) technique requires a gamma ray source (^{125}I), a detector, and intervening electronics that measure the beam attenuation through bone and express the result in bone mineral per cm^2 scanned. Usually, the radius is measured at two sites, the mid-diaphysis, which consists of nearly 100% cortical bone, and the distal radial metaphysis, which contains about 75% cortical bone and 25% trabecular bone.

This technique is useful in population studies. The precision of coefficient of variance (CV) of this technique is about 2% and the accuracy about 6% along with low-radiation exposure (<10 mrem). However, because of dosimetric and statistical considerations, the low-energy ^{125}I source cannot be used for body parts thicker than the forearm. A major clinical limitation of this technique, therefore, is that it reflects the status of peripheral long bone and measures primarily the cortex.

Dual-energy Photon Absorptiometry

Dual-energy photon absorptiometry (DPA) technique utilizes a radioisotope that emits photons at two different energy levels. The chief advantage is that the gamma-ray energy of the source is higher (^{153}Gd with photons of 42 and 100 keV) and it has a uniform path length. The lumbar spine from L1 to L4 is usually scanned. This technique yields integral of all minerals within the scan path including the vertebral bodies, endplates, and posterior elements. The major disadvantage is that vertebral compression fractures (VCFs) with callus formation, kyphoscoliosis, articular facet hypertrophy, discogenic sclerosis, marginal osteophytosis, and extraosseous calcification (aorta) are also included in the integral measurement and may result in inaccurate and poorly reproducible vertebral measurements. In healthy subjects, the precision is in the order of 2–3% with accuracy of 4–10% of CV. The usual radiation dose is about 15–20 mrem. It is also used to determine the total body mineral content.

Dual-energy X-ray Absorptiometry

Dual-energy X-ray absorption (DXA) was first described in 1987 and has stood the test of time, representing the most commonly used method of diagnosing osteoporosis in clinical practice. The WHO chose this modality in 1994 for diagnosing osteopenia and osteoporosis. Consequentially, DXA measurements became the standard of reference for the clinical diagnosis of osteoporosis with bone densitometry.[9,10] DXA employs an X-ray beam formed by two different photon energies for generating BMD. Once the high-energy and low-energy photons are transmitted through bones and soft tissue, they are analyzed separately. This is followed by subtraction of the attenuation values of soft tissues with the remainder being the attenuation values of bone. Development in technology has led to significant changes in the DXA equipment. Fan-beam is a wider beam, which has replaced the previously used pencil-thin beam. This, along with a bank of detectors, allows more rapid scanning (approximately 3–5 minutes per site) resulting in better image quality and a high spatial resolution (0.5–0.7 mm).

The variably attenuated X-ray beams received on the detectors are further analyzed and quantified to generate measurements, namely bone mineral content (in grams) at the projected area of the measured site (calculated in square centimeters). BMD is calculated by dividing bone mineral content by the area (expressed in grams/cm^2). BMD is expressed in terms of SD as a T-score and a Z-score.[11] The T-score compares the BMD of the interrogated subject/patient with the mean BMD of a standard young adult individual (between 20 and 30 years of age). The Z-score reflects the difference between the examined BMD of the patient and the mean BMD of age and gender-matched controls. The WHO classifies BMD on the basis of the T-score: with the categories being normal (≥–1.0), osteopenia (<–1.0 but >–2.5), osteoporosis (≤–2.5), and severe osteoporosis (≤–2.5 with a fragility fracture).[12] It should be noted that this definition is applied to DXA measurements made **(Table 2)** in the lumbar spine **(Fig. 2)**, proximal femur **(Fig. 3)**, and forearm. Similar values obtained with other techniques (e.g., quantitative CT) or values similar to DXA measurements made at other anatomic sites (e.g. calcaneus) are not considered in the definition.

Bone mineral density examination serves three principal purposes, namely the diagnosis of osteoporosis, the assessment of patients' risk of fracture, and monitoring response to treatment. BMD is a reasonably strong predictor of fracture risk, reflecting approximately 75–85% of bone strength. It has been found that there is an approximately 1.5 times increase in the fracture risk for each SD decrease of BMD from age-adjusted value.[13,14] Bone density examination is useful for evaluating a host of clinical indications contributing to increased bone resorption/faulty bone formation, which has been published by the International Society for Clinical Densitometry (ISCD) and is summarized in **Box 2.**[12]

There are many advantages of central DXA as summarized in **Box 3**.

Dual-energy X-ray absorptiometry is currently the only procedure, which can be used with the fracture risk assessment tool or FRAX, for identifying patients who are at higher risk for fracture.[13] *FRAX* is a useful tool, based on DXA, which provides an estimate of the fracture risk of the individual. The calculation is based on the BMD of the femoral neck;[14] the patient's gender, age, weight, and height; and seven clinical risk factors (history of previous fracture, hip fracture in parent, current smoking, glucocorticoid use, rheumatoid arthritis, secondary osteoporosis, and ingestion of three or more units of alcohol daily). Once this information is fed into the automated software along with the name of the manufacturer of the DXA scanner used, the algorithm estimates the 10-year probability of a major osteoporotic fracture in various regions of the body (hip, spine, distal forearm, etc.). As is evident from the variables used for FRAX generation, FRAX values are different for different ethnicity of population. To cater to our population, Indian data is used to establish age-specified BMD reference range for Indian females and males using DXA.[15] Few studies have shown a lower BMD for Indian population in comparison with age-matched US females, which extends across all age groups.

TABLE 2: The World Health Organization (WHO) definitions of osteoporosis and osteopenia.

Terminology	T-score definition
Normal	$T \geq -1.0$
Osteopenia	$-2.5 < T < -1.0$
Osteoporosis	$T \leq -2.5$
Severe osteoporosis	$T \leq -2.5$ in the presence of one or more fragility fractures

Apart from axial skeleton (lumbar spine and proximal femur), DXA scan can also be done at peripheral sites such as distal radius and calcaneus. The calcaneus is particularly useful for monitoring changes in BMD secondary to treatment as it contains high percentage (95%) of metabolically active trabecular bone.

Though peripheral DXA (pDXA) is a much easier examination to perform requiring less compact scanners, its fracture predictive ability for vertebral and global fragility fracture risk in postmenopausal women is weaker than central DXA, according to ISCD guidelines. However, pDXA

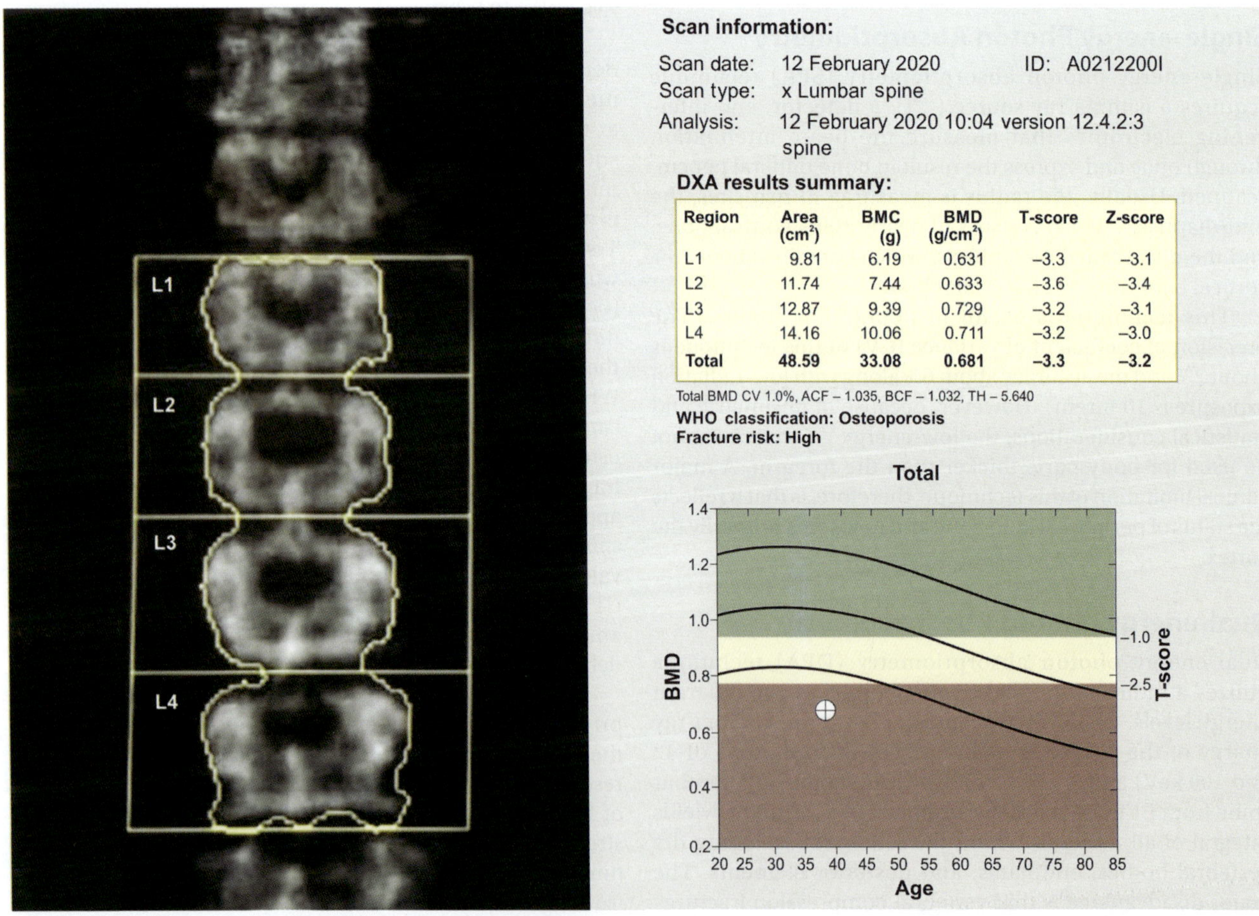

FIG. 2: Axial dual-energy X-ray absorptiometry (DXA) report of a patient demonstrating the L1-L4 vertebrae being interrogated with results generated in the form of T- and Z scores as well as absolute bone mineral density (BMD) measurements. Graphical display of the BMD serves well for patient understanding. Note that the WHO classification (osteoporosis) and fracture risk (high) have also been interpreted and mentioned based on BMD scores.

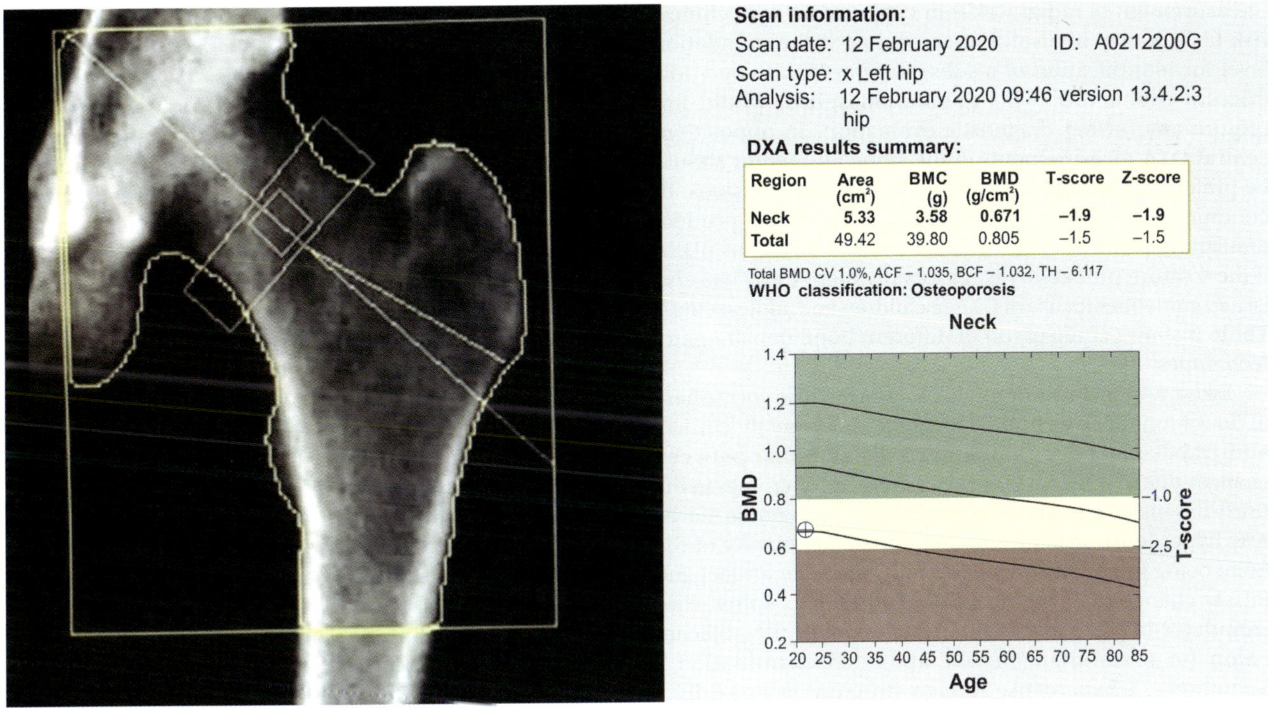

FIG. 3: Femoral dual-energy X-ray absorptiometry (DXA) report of a patient demonstrating the femoral bone being interrogated with generation of T- and Z-scores along with absolute bone mineral density (BMD) measurements. The BMD falls into the category of osteopenia.

BOX 2: Indications for bone mineral density (BMD) testing.[12]

- Women aged 65 years and older
- *For postmenopausal women younger than age 65 years, a bone density test is indicated if they have a risk factor for low bone mass such as:*
  - *Low body weight*
  - *Prior fracture*
  - *High-risk medication use*
  - *Disease or condition associated with bone loss*
- Women during the menopausal transition with clinical risk factors for fracture, such as low body weight, prior fracture, or high-risk medication use
- Men aged 70 years and older.
- *For men <70 years of age, a bone density test is indicated if they have a risk factor for low bone mass such as:*
  - Low body weight
  - Prior fracture
  - High-risk medication use
  - Disease or condition associated with bone loss
- Adults with a fragility fracture
- Adults with a disease or condition associated with low bone mass or bone loss
- Adults taking medications associated with low bone mass or bone loss
- Anyone being considered for pharmacologic therapy
- Anyone being treated, to monitor treatment effect
- Anyone not receiving therapy in whom evidence of bone loss would lead to treatment

Women discontinuing estrogen should be considered for bone density testing according to the indications listed above.

BOX 3: Clinical advantages of hip and spine DXA.

- Proven ability to predict fracture risk
- Consensus that BMD results can be interpreted using WHO T-scores
- Proven for effective targeting of antifracture treatments
- Effective for monitoring response to treatment
- Basis of new WHO algorithm for predicting fracture risk
- Short scan times
- Easy patient setup
- Low radiation dose
- Good precision
- Acceptable accuracy
- Availability of reliable reference ranges
- Stable calibration
- Effective instrument quality control procedures

(BMD: bone mineral density; DXA: dual-energy X-ray absorptiometry; WHO: World Health Organization) (measurement of radial BMD) in conjunction with clinical risk factors may be useful in screening at the population level for identification of a subset among it with very low fracture probability. This population subset would not require any further diagnostic evaluation. In opposition, central DXA measurements at the spine and femur should be preferentially used for making therapeutic decisions. In conditions where central DXA is not feasible, it is prudent to institute pharmacologic treatment based on radius pDXA if the fracture probability is reasonably high. ISCD has also issued guidelines for use of DXA in children and adolescents.[12] **Table 3** shows comparison of different bone densitometry techniques.

Like any other imaging modality, DXA has also got its share of limitations such as limited ability to differentiate cortical and trabecular bone, inability to discriminate between changes due to different bone geometry (e.g., increases in the third dimension), and bone density along with some artifacts. Any hyperdense structure in the immediate vicinity of the bone being interrogated by DXA may induce an artifact and falsely change the generated DXA values, e.g., spinal cord stimulator implant and iodinated contrast in the adjacent colon for a simultaneous CT abdomen examination.[16] Sometimes, a hyperdense foreign structure in immediate contact with the vertebral body may cause it to be mistakenly included in the region of interest (ROI) during estimation of BMD leading to falsely elevated values, e.g., staple and gastric band. A study by Bolotin pointed out inherent fallacies in DXA being contaminated by sizable, unavoidable, inextricable independent soft-tissue contributions leading to erroneous BMD measurements as concerns to the adoption of DXA as a sole medium to describe bone density.[17] Nevertheless, it seems to be the most easily understandable, simple, reproducible imaging modality for BMD estimation currently available.

Quantitative Computed Tomography

Quantitative computed tomography (QCT) is an addition to the field of bone mineral analysis. Quantitative CT differs from DXA in that it has the capability to generate estimates of trabecular and cortical bone BMD as a true volumetric mineral density in mg/cm^3.[3,18] This method uses a mineral calibration phantom that is placed in the CT scanner with the patient and provides corrections for machine drifts. A lateral computed radiograph (scout view) is first obtained for localization and then single axial scans are obtained through the midplane of two to four lumbar vertebral bodies **(Figs. 4 and 5)**. Quantitative readings are obtained from a ROI over trabecular bone comprising 3–4 cm^3 of each vertebral body and from four different reference solutions in the phantom. These readings are averaged and used to calculate the mineral density of trabecular bone in mineral equivalents of K_2HPO_4 (mg/cm^3), which subsequently is used for generating T- and Z-scores **(Figs. 6 and 7)**. In addition to estimating the BMD, QCT now can also determine the future risk of osteoporotic fractures.[19]

The precision of this method is 1–3% for single-energy (80 kVp) and 3–5% for dual-energy (80/140 kVp) techniques with an accuracy of 5–10%. The radiation dose is approximately 2 Sv.

The theoretical advantages of QCT[20] over other modalities include: (1) transaxial display of data permitting identification of the anatomy and separate measurement of cortical, cancellous, or integral bone mineral; (2) capability of determining the linear absorption coefficient for a readily defined volume of bone and thereby providing a measure of density, and (3) in the dual-energy mode, the ability to determine mineral content with high accuracy in the presence of variable fat and soft-tissue content.

Quantitative CT serves pretty well for prediction of vertebral fractures in postmenopausal women and for serially measuring bone loss. Its sensitivity is generally considered better than DXA because the trabecular bone located in the center of the vertebral body, which represents the metabolically active bone, is selectively analyzed, unlike in DXA where the entire bone is evaluated. This property of selective assessment of trabecular bone also makes quantitative CT sensitive to detecting BMD changes over short follow-up times. Quantitative CT scores are better than DXA in having the:

- Ability to exclude from the measurement of structures that do not contribute to spine mechanical resistance (which falsely change the DXA values as these cannot be excluded in DXA measurements)

TABLE 3: Comparison of different bone densitometry techniques.

	Central DXA	Peripheral DXA	QCT	QUS
Compatible with WHO T-scores	✓	×	×	×
Proven to predict fracture risk	✓	✓	✓	✓
Compatible with new WHO fracture risk algorithm	✓	×	×	×
Proven for effective targeting of treatment	✓	?	?	?
Suitable for patient follow-up	✓	×	✓	×
Stable calibration	✓	✓	✓	×
Good precision	✓	✓	✓	×
Reliable reference ranges available	✓	?	?	?

(✓) Indicates where an alternative technique is known to perform in a comparable manner to central DXA.
(?) Indicates where our knowledge is limited by an absence of suitable studies.
(×) Indicates that alternative types of measurement are definitely unsuitable in these roles.
(DXA: dual energy X-ray absorptiometry; QCT: quantitative computed tomography; QUS: quantitative ultrasound; WHO: World Health Organization)

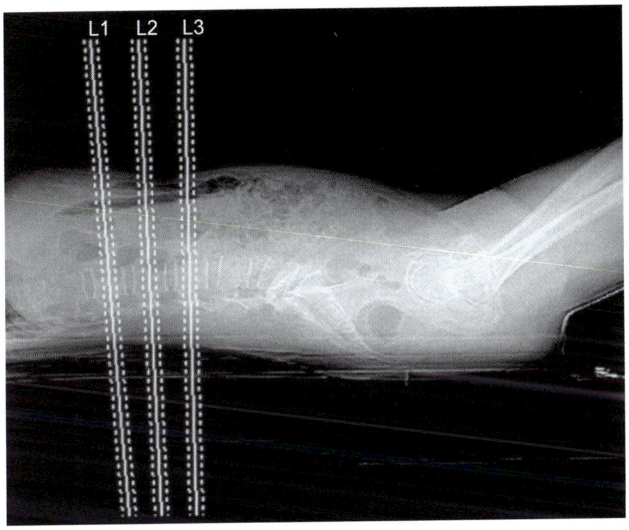

FIG. 4: Lateral topogram (scout view) showing automatic determination of midvertebral slices of L1, L2, and L3.

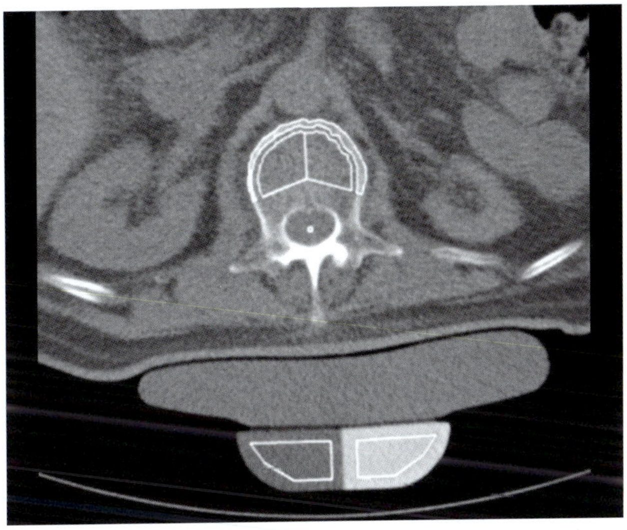

FIG. 5: Midvertebral slice on quantitative computed tomography showing automatic contour determination separating cortical (outer semicircle) and trabecular bone (inner semicircle). Note the phantom and calculation marker.

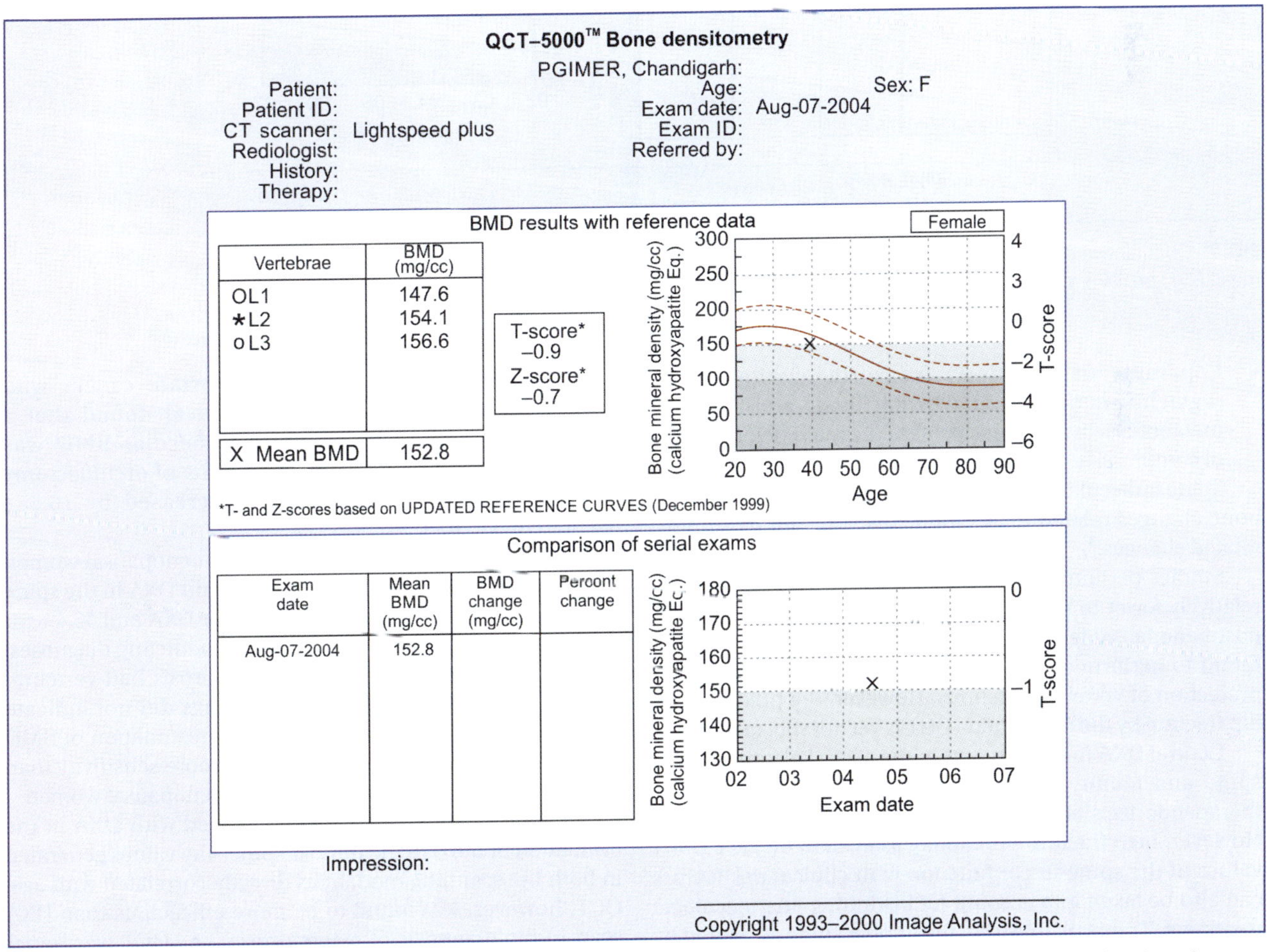

QCT–5000™ Bone densitometry

PGIMER, Chandigarh:

Patient:
Patient ID:
CT scanner: Lightspeed plus
Rediologist:
History:
Therapy:

Age: Sex: F
Exam date: Aug-07-2004
Exam ID:
Referred by:

BMD results with reference data

Vertebrae	BMD (mg/cc)
OL1	147.6
∗L2	154.1
oL3	156.6
X Mean BMD	152.8

T-score* –0.9
Z-score* –0.7

*T- and Z-scores based on UPDATED REFERENCE CURVES (December 1999)

Comparison of serial exams

Exam date	Mean BMD (mg/cc)	BMD change (mg/cc)	Peroont change
Aug-07-2004	152.8		

Impression:

Copyright 1993–2000 Image Analysis, Inc.

FIG. 6: Quantitative computed tomography (QCT) determination of bone mineral density (BMD) of a normal 36-year-old female with a mean BMD of 152.8 mg/cc with T-score of –0.9 and Z-score of –0.7.

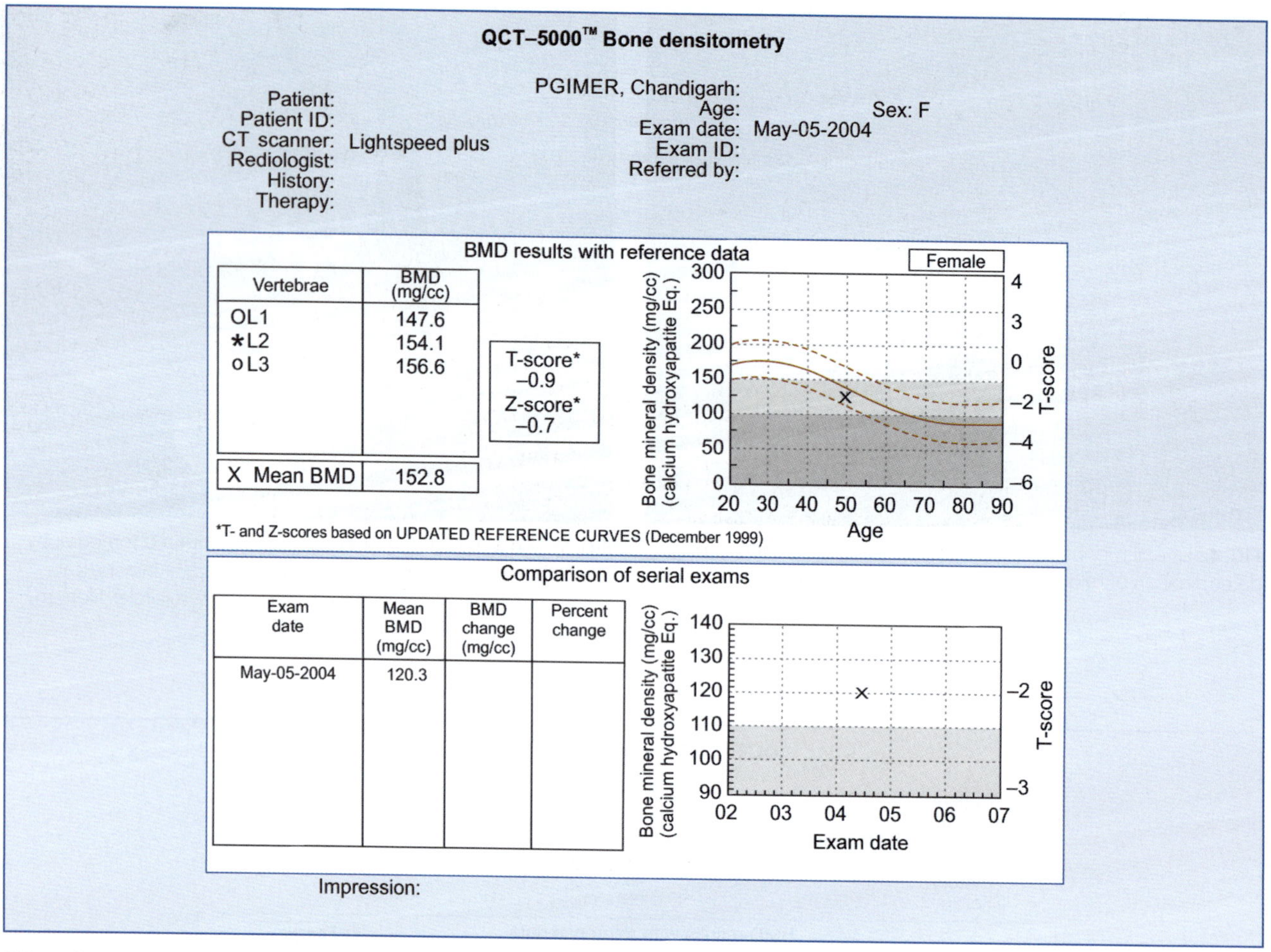

FIG. 7: Quantitative computed tomography (QCT) determination of bone mineral density (BMD) of an osteopenic 50-year-old female with mean BMD of 120.3 mg/cc with T-score of –2.0 and Z-score of –0.7.

- Capability of selectively measuring various bony segments, namely the trabecular tissue and the most metabolic active tissue which are the main determinants of compressive strength in the vertebrae.[21]

Spine trabecular BMD by QCT can also be used to monitor bone changes related to age, bone disease, and treatment-related changes.[22]

Studies pertaining to fracture prediction using QCT are relatively fewer in number than the ones related to DXA. In postmenopausal females though, QCT of the spine has been found to perform as well as, if not better than, DXA in the prediction of vertebral fractures. However, the prediction of hip fracture by the use of spine QCT is yet not substantiated.[22]

Central DXA measurements in the axial skeleton, namely spine and femur, are the preferred method for making therapeutic decisions and should be used wherever possible.[23] However, high fracture probability as evident on QCT BMD values of the spine in conjunction with clinical risk factors can also be taken into account for instituting pharmacologic treatment. Trabecular BMD of the lumbar spine measured by QCT can be also be used to monitor disease and treatment-related BMD changes and even for assessing the age. The disadvantage of QCT is that the accuracy of BMD decreases to 20–25% in elderly osteoporosis populations.

In a study of 55 patients of prostate cancer who underwent orchidectomy, Agarwal et al. found that a statistical reduction in vertebral trabecular BMD was observed in all patients within 6 months of orchidectomy **(Figs. 8A to C)**.[24] Average BMD decreased by 16.5 ± 8.6 mg/cm^3 (13.8%).

Li et al.[25] evaluated BMD in 140 postmenopausal women for detection of osteoporosis with QCT and DXA in the spine and hip. The detection rate was 17.1% for DXA and 46.4% for QCT ($p < 0.01$). Of the 41 patients with conflicting diagnoses, 7 whose diagnosis by QCT was osteoporosis had vertebral fractures even though their DXA findings did not indicate osteoporosis. QCT thus avoided the overestimation of BMD by DXA. It was thus concluded to have more sensitivity than DXA for detecting osteoporosis in postmenopausal women.

In another study, QCT was compared with DXA in the evaluation of BMD in the lumbar spine. The values generated in both the scanning modalities directly correlated with age. QCT, however, was found to be more efficacious than DXA scan in the diagnosis of osteoporosis, i.e., QCT was better discriminated between normal and osteoporotic subjects than DXA.[26]

Although spinal QCT has many advantages over the DXA technique, it is also fraught with several limitations,

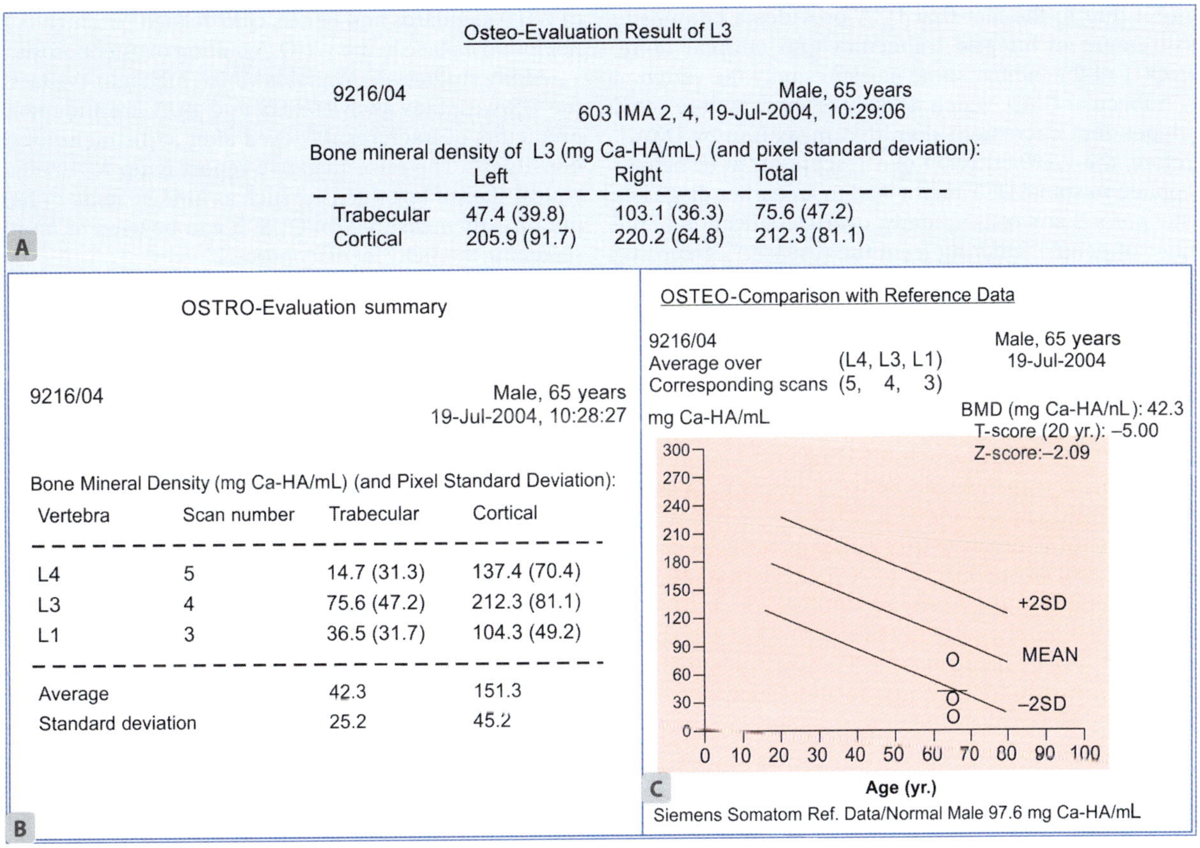

FIGS. 8A TO C: Quantitative computed tomography determination of bone mineral density of a 65-year-old postorchidectomy male patient at an (A) individual vertebra and (B and C) average of three lumbar vertebrae.

TABLE 4: Radiation exposure of QCT protocols and other procedures involving ionizing radiation for comparison.

Techniques	Voltage (kV)	Time current product (mAs)	Approximate effective dose (mSv)
Single-slice QCT spine L1–L3 10 mm slice thickness	80	120	<0.2
	120	200	Approximately 1.0
3D QCT spine L1 and L2 (10 cm scan length)	120	100	Approximately 1.5
3D QCT proximal femur (15 cm scan length)	120	200	Approximately 2.5–3
pQCT forearm clinical CT scanner (10 cm scan length)	120	100	<0.01
pQCT forearm/tibia on dedicated single-slice pQCT scanners per slice	<70	<1	<0.003
High-resolution pQCT forearm (XtremeCT) (15 cm scan length)	60	1	<0.005
Annual naturally occurring background radiation (UK)			2.7
Return transatlantic flight			0.08
Chest radiograph			0.02
Lumbar spine radiograph			0.7
CT imaging, e.g., abdomen/pelvis			2.5–4
Radionuclide bone scan			3

(pQCT: peripheral quantitative computed tomography; QCT: quantitative computed tomography)

the most notable ones being high radiation dose (**Table 4**), poor precision limiting its applicability to longitudinal assessments, higher scanner costs involved, a high degree of operator dependence, and the need for a considerable amount of space. Moreover, it is difficult to assess volumetric BMD of the hip due to its complex shape and inability to generate appropriate phantoms. The WHO definition of osteoporosis of a T-score "at or below" 2.5 applies to DXA of the lumbar spine, femoral neck, total hip, and distal 33% radius. Other sites and modalities are not currently within its ambit due to the fact that DXA provides a composite measurement of integral trabecular and cortical bone, while QCT of the lumbar spine measures only the vertebral body trabecular BMD, which is likely to show a more rapid age-dependent decrement than that measured by DXA.[27] Therefore, the WHO criterion of a T-score of "at or below" 2.5 applied to spinal QCT might lead to an earlier diagnosis of osteoporosis and consequently, over-classification of the number of people suffering from the disease.[28] According to one study, individuals with an absolute BMD <80 mg hydroxyapatite (HA)/cm^3 could be classified as osteoporotic whereas the ones having BMD between 80 and 120 mg/cm^3 may be labeled as having osteopenia.[29]

Over the last decade, technical developments in the CT technique have resulted in development of dedicated peripheral CT scanners, which are smaller, more mobile, and less expensive than whole-body CT scanners to assess peripheral skeletal sites.

A number of bones were assessed previously as part of detection of BMD by peripheral QCT (pQCT). In its current form, it is applied to the nondominant forearm. In view of its lesser radiation-related side effects, pQCT is preferable to central QCT in pediatric patients for assessment of bone development in children.[30,31] Age-related changes can be monitored by pQCT measurement of trabecular and total BMD of the ultradistal radius.

Quantitative Ultrasound

Ultrasound (US) has been successfully used for several years for testing of nonpenetrative materials. Many characteristics, notable ones being scattering capability and US velocity changes, have been used to understand the mechanical competence of various types of material. US variables are speed of sound (SUS) and broadband ultrasound attenuation (BUA). These quantitative ultrasound (QUS) parameters are indirect markers of the material properties of trabecular bone and the degree of fragility of the bones being tested. QUS of bone is performed at substantially lower frequencies, i.e., between 200 and 1.5 MHz, and signals are acquired in the transmission mode. In addition to assessing bone density, these variables reflect parameters such as elasticity and microarchitecture, which are important in assessing fracture risk in osteoporotic subjects. US is currently being performed at peripheral sites such as patella, fingers, tibia, and calcaneum. The calcaneum is the most favored site as it is a weight-bearing bone and composed almost entirely of trabecular bone. The US wave is generated by piezoelectric crystals located in the US probe used for scanning, emitted as a sinusoid impulse, and detected once it has passed through the medium. The emitting and receiving probes are placed on either side of the skeletal segment that is being interrogated for bone density.

Quantitative US results can be expressed as absolute values or as T-scores and Z-scores, similar to other forms of modalities for bone evaluation. This has been made possible due to availability of well-established and validated normative reference curves, allowing bone loss to be followed up over time.[32] However, discrepancy has been found in using these parameters for defining bone density according to WHO standards and hence, QUS-related parameters have not found a place in the WHO definition of osteoporosis.

Many studies are available which highlight the fact that the US variables such as SUS and BUA are independent predictors of fractures risk even after adjustment for bone density.[33,34] The false-negative report is up to 10% as the typical sites of bone density such as lumbar spine or hip are not directly measured on QUS. It can be used as an initial screening modality for osteoporosis.[33]

The main advantage of US is lack of ionizing radiation.[35] It is less bulky and portable as well as cheaper than CT or DXA machines. Therefore, QUS has a potential for wider applicability, including preventive screening for osteoporosis. However, the major disadvantage is that there is no standardized method of calibration and expression of measurement results since QUS devices employ diverse technology and different methods of calibration.

Presently, US assessment serves as a screening tool in many centers, with DXA being subsequently done for confirmation of diagnosis in all suspected cases identified. Many studies have demonstrated the utility of quantitative US in predicting osteoporotic fractures of the calcaneus, especially in elderly women aged 65–70 years or older.[36] According to the latest ISCD guidelines for QUS, calcaneus may be used to predict fragility fracture in postmenopausal women (vertebral, hip, and global fracture risk) and men over the age of 65 years (hip and all nonvertebral fractures), independently of central DXA BMD. As highlighted in the recommendations, the combination of heel QUS and clinical risk factors may be used to identify a population at very low fracture probability, which does not warrant any further diagnostic evaluation. In case central DXA is not available as an indicator of BMD, fracture probability information on heel QUS in conjunction with clinical risk factors may be used for instituting pharmacologic treatment. QUS, however, should not be used to monitor the effects of drugs or other forms of therapy on the bony changes in osteoporosis.

High-resolution Bone Imaging

The usefulness of assessing the microarchitectural make-up of bony trabeculae (bone quality) along with mineral density (bone quantity) in the context of osteoporosis cannot be over-emphasized as has been highlighted in a number of publications. Currently, magnetic resonance imaging (MRI) and high-resolution peripheral quantitative imaging (HR-pQCT) are the best modalities available to study the bony make-up. MRI outscores HR-pQCT in that the latter is limited to evaluation of peripheral bony areas, namely the wrist and ankle, while the former can also image other sites, e.g., proximal femur, though with compromised spatial resolution.

Magnetic Resonance Imaging

Magnetic resonance imaging has revolutionized the field of medical imaging with the unique capability of analyzing cortical and trabecular bone in vivo by means of high-resolution images. It is a radiation-free imaging modality and is well-suited for assessing bone structure in a clinical setting. In MRI, bone is usually seen with a negative contrast relative to the high-background signal from bone marrow. Once the images are obtained, segmenting information pertaining to various aspects such as topology, structure, and orientation of the trabecular bone network as well as cortical thickness and area can be done by application of digital postprocessing techniques. The analytical parameters of trabecular and cortical bone are discussed in the following text.

Trabecular Bone Assessment

Signal-to-noise ratio (SNR) and spatial resolution: Excellent soft-tissue spatial resolution is the hallmark of MRI. Increase in resolution, however, occurs at the expense of SNR, which may compromise the image quality. A balance has to be struck between the two parameters such that the optimal quality of resolution and SNR can be achieved. Li et al. investigated the influence noise and limited spatial resolution on structural parameters.[37] They noted systematic changes in the derived structural parameters with decreasing SNR below a certain threshold. Nevertheless, it became evident that at smaller SNR levels, these errors were correctable by using simple methods such as simple linear transformations. Imaging the peripheral bones has inherent advantages with researchers making considerable efforts to develop trabecular bone imaging of peripheral sites such as the radius, femur, calcaneus, and tibia.[38]

Bone imaging may be performed by using two main types of pulse sequences, namely gradient-echo (GE)-based and spin-echo (SE)-based pulse sequences. Choosing an appropriate sequence depends on the following considerations:

- Higher SNR is provided by a three-dimensional (3D) excitation sequence than a 2D sequence.
- The acquisition of GE should be immediate after the excitation pulse as it would avoid signal loss due to T2 relaxation.
- The acquisition time should be in a clinically feasible range.

The simplest sequence that fulfills the above-mentioned requirements is the basic GE sequence. Further improvements in SNR efficiency are also possible by fully balancing all magnetic gradients during one repetition. The so-called balanced steady-state gradient-echo free precision (bSSFP) pulse sequence optimizes and maximizes SNR efficiency but has a flip side of being susceptible to magnetic field in homogeneities. Krug et al., however, proposed that it may be used to one's advantage.[39] This proved to be a boon for the enhanced visualization of smaller trabeculae, which normally vanish due to partial volume effects. The reason was increased signal cancelation when using bSSFP compared to an SE approach.[40] In the current scheme of things, SSFP has become the sequence of choice among GE-based pulse sequences for trabecular bone imaging due to its high SNR efficiency.[41,42] With the availability of accelerated image acquisition techniques (parallel imaging methods), the imaging time can be remarkably decreased.

Image analysis: The various postprocessing steps involved in image analysis of trabecular bone images in MRI are the correction of the coil sensitivity, outlining of the trabecular bone ROI, and bone/marrow segmentation followed by structural calculations.

Image Postprocessing

There are many methods described for extracting structural information from 3D images of the trabecular bone. The final parameter that needs to be determined is bone volume fraction (BVF), which is a ratio of BV to total volume (TV).

Trabecular Bone Analysis

The various structural parameters required for trabecular bone analysis are topology, scale, and orientation.[43,44] Investigating the plate or rod-like structure of the trabecular network, as is reflective by its name, can assess topology. Scale refers to the volume of bone in a circumscribed ROI with respect to the spacing between the trabeculae or the actual thickness of the trabeculae. The orientation is a marker of the degree of anisotropy of the structure.

The three parameters of scale, topology, and anisotropy can be analyzed by the novel technique of geodesic topological analysis (GTA) described by Carballido-Gamio et al.[45] GTA, which is a measure of bone quality combined with BMD, a bone quantification method, allows for better discrimination than BMD alone [area under the curve (AUC) = 0.95; $p < 0.001$]. It can also be used for treatment monitoring. It should, however, be ensured that the same trabecular sections should be analyzed at baseline and follow-up for detecting microlevel changes in the fine trabecular structure.

Cortical Bone Assessment Using MRI

Cortical bone thickness is an important determinant of the strength of bone as demonstrated by Hyun et al.[46] They have demonstrated significant differences in the cortical thickness of postmenopausal osteopenic versus osteoporotic women, which underscores the importance of geometric measurements of the cortical bone. A study showed that there is an increase in bone water content in the postmenopausal group compared to the premenopausal group.[47] The differential water content may be due to the presence or absence of marrow in the cortical pores. For efficiently imaging the intracortical microstructure, ultra-short echo times (UTE) have to be employed.

Pulse Sequences

The 3D fast gradient recalled echo (FGRE) pulse sequence was employed by Hyun et al. for evaluating cortical bone of the distal radius at 1.5 Tesla. They used a slice thickness of 2 mm.[46] Goldenstein et al. used a balanced steady-state free precession (bSSFP) pulse sequence using a dedicated quadrature wrist coil on a 3T MR scanner.[48] The image acquisition resulted in an image resolution of 156 μm × 156 μm × 500 μm. Hyun et al. formulated a semiautomatic segmentation algorithm to measure cortical thickness.[46]

Clinical Applications

Magnetic resonance imaging has found a distinct place in the analysis of almost all regions of the body due to significant technological developments that have taken place in this field in the last couple of decades. Its noninvasive radiation-free nature has added to this effect. Quantitative bone evaluation has proven to be one of its key uses currently and with the ability to provide structural information, it can contribute to fracture discrimination in unison with BMD estimation. Wehrli et al. demonstrated that MRI-based topological bone parameters had better capability to discriminate fracture group from nonfracture group than BMD alone.[49] Many researchers are of the opinion that MRI-based in vivo analysis of trabecular bone can be used as a potential tool for monitoring osteoporosis treatment. However till now, no recommendations are there from ISCD to use it in diagnosis of osteoporosis, prediction of fracture risk, or monitoring of treatment.

High-resolution Peripheral Quantitative Computed Tomography

There has been ongoing work on dedicated peripheral body scanners, being less bulky and possibly more cost-effective in specific scenarios. A dedicated extremity imaging scanner has been designed for trabecular-scale imaging. It is seen to generate higher SNR and spatial resolution compared to multidetector CT (MDCT) and MRI. The radiation is limited to the interrogated body part, namely the extremity not involving critical, radiosensitive organs, and is considerably lower compared to whole-body CT. However, its major limitation is evaluation of only peripheral skeletal sites. Moreover, presently only a limited number of devices are installed.

Image Acquisition Scan Setup

Due to its limited presence in a clinical setup, a fixed manufacturer-recommended scan protocol needs to be run for generation of optimal results.[50] The protocols have, however, been modified to suit the differences in patient sizes and to avoid radiation exposure to epiphyseal growth plate in evaluating children. Smaller field of view (FOV) (approximately 12–13 cm) is used for optimum imaging. The dataset acquired is reconstructed using a modified Feldkamp algorithm, yielding submillimeter isotropic voxels.[51] The total scan time is around 3 minutes with a significantly attenuated radiation dose (approximately 4.2 μSv), which is remarkably less than a body CT scan and is comparable to DXA.

Image Analysis and Postprocessing

The dataset obtained is analyzed using a standard manufacturer-provided protocol, which includes segmentation and approximate contour delineation. The cortical bone is segmented using a 3D Gaussian smoothing filter. This component is subtracted digitally from the periosteal contour to generate the trabecular compartment. Using beam-hardening correction and phantom calibration procedures, the linear attenuation values of the tomographic images are converted to HA mineral densities, which are used for designating bone details of that region.

Morphometric Analysis

The high isotropic resolution of HR-pQCT (82 μm) permits direct, 3D assessment of important measurements such as intertrabecular distances, trabecular number, average trabecular thickness, and bone volume fraction (BV/TV) which is in contradistinction to CT and MRI, which base the measurements on large-slice thickness relative to the in-plane resolution.

According to ISCD, pQCT of the forearm at the ultradistal radius is a useful predictor of fragility fractures of the hip in postmenopausal females. This value, however, does not hold true for spinal fractures.

Multidetector Computed Tomography

Spiral CT generates densitometric data, which is used to assess mass lesions. Efforts are being made to use this data to assess BMD in the lumbar spine. A recent study calculated BMD from spiral CT data by using equation BMD = 0.77 × mean BMD MDCT, where mean BMD on MDCT is the average of densities of L1 to L3 vertebrae as calculated on spiral CT and 0.77 is the conversion factor. They found significant correlation between BMD data obtained from spiral CT and QCT.[52] Few studies have in fact demonstrated that MDCT depicted trabecular microarchitecture of the dorsal spine outscored BMD obtained by DXA in identifying patients with vertebral fractures from those who did not.[53]

In addition, the advent of MDCT enabled trabecular analysis of the hip (which is a clinically important site of fracture). However, a high radiation dose remains a matter of concern.

MACHINE-BASED ARTIFICIAL INTELLIGENCE IN PREDICTING BONE MINERAL DENSITY

Artificial intelligence has had a significant role to play in the field of medical sciences in the recent past. With the stupendous increase in the performance of machine-learning algorithms, the scope of technology in the diagnosis, prediction, and even management of various disorders in medicine has shown a phenomenal rise. On similar lines, there has been a surge in the models for prediction of BMD using basic imaging modalities such as US and CT by using deep learning methods.[54-56] The bone fragility can be analyzed based upon vertebral bone attenuation on CT done for other indications.[57]

Several newer methods have been described for prediction of fracture risk in osteoporosis along with models to help with the identification and segmentation of bone images from a host of imaging modalities, namely acoustics, MRI, CT, and radiographs.[58]

Radiomics is playing a leading role in developing predictive models to classify osteoporosis, osteopenia, and normal patients in susceptible population. Panoramic dental radiographs,[59] spine radiographs, and CT (lumbar, femoral trochanteric, intertrochanteric, and neck)[60] images have been used as substrates for application of feature selection and classification methods to generate models of osteoporosis classification based on bone mineral densitometry image features.

INTERVENTIONAL MANAGEMENT OF OSTEOPOROTIC COMPRESSION FRACTURES—PERCUTANEOUS VERTEBROPLASTY

Treatment of acute osteoporotic fractures has been largely conservative, with medical therapy emphasizing pain control using various analgesics and anti-inflammatory medications in combination with immobilization.[61] Vertebroplasty aims to alleviate pain and improve mobility, with the secondary goal of stabilizing the vertebral body. Klazen et al. have shown that vertebroplasty outperformed conservative management with significantly greater pain relief.[62] Another large study concluded that percutaneous vertebroplasty was considerably effective in relieving pain associated with osteoporosis-induced VCFs, and the analgesic effect of the procedure was long lasting.[63] The outcome of single-level vertebroplasty is not dependent on the age of the vertebral fracture, with good outcomes noted among acute, subacute, and chronic stages.[64]

Indications

Percutaneous vertebroplasty can be offered for the following indications:

- Painful VCF refractory to medical therapy
- Painful VCF associated with osteonecrosis (Kümmell's disease)
- Unstable VCF that demonstrates mobility at the wedge deformity
- Conditions which warrant reinforcement of the vertebral body or pedicle, before a posterior surgical stabilization procedure or interbody fusion, in patients with osteoporosis
- Although routine prophylactic treatment is not advocated, unaffected vertebra in patients with multiple compressions in whom further collapse may lead to pulmonary compromise as a result of kyphosis may rarely be considered for vertebroplasty

Conservative medical therapy still forms the frontline management of osteoporotic VCFs with intractable pain, in spite of optimum medical management, forming the prime clinical criteria for performing vertebroplasty. Some operators avoid treating patients who have >20–30% spinal canal compromise from retropulsed fracture fragments.[61] Vertebroplasty in such cases may aggravate spinal stenosis and may even lead to compressive myeloradiculopathy.

Procedure

The procedure is done under conscious sedation under fluoroscopy/CT/CT-fluoroscopy guidance. The patient is placed prone on the fluoroscopic/CT table. A vertebroplasty needle (11/13G needle with biopsy set) is introduced under fluoroscopic guidance through the pedicle into the involved vertebral body up to the junction of anterior third and posterior two-thirds and bone cement, an acrylic polymer—PMMA (polymethylmethacrylate), is injected with the aim of almost completely filling the osteoporotic collapsed vertebral body, care being taken not to have any spillage beyond the posterior margin of the vertebral body **(Figs. 9A to F)**.

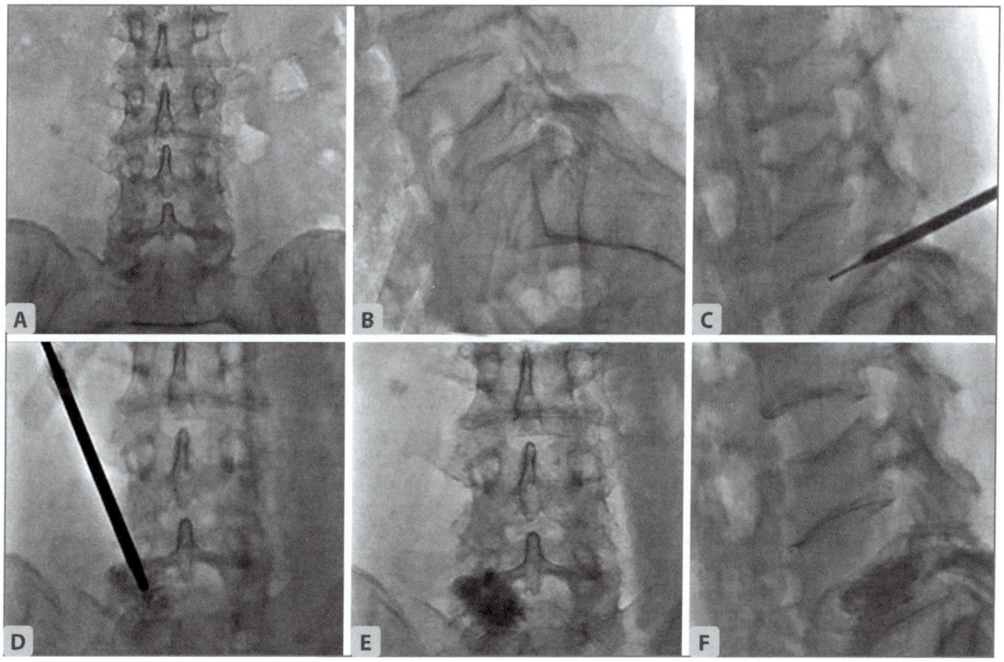

FIGS. 9A TO F: Vertebroplasty. (A) Anteroposterior; and (B) Lateral lumbar spine radiographs showing L5 vertebral body collapse; (C and D) Percutaneous transpedicular insertion of the cannula with injection of polymethylmethacrylate cement; (E) Anteroposterior; and (F) Lateral radiographs demonstrating the bone cement.

Postprocedure Care

Nowadays, the procedure is routinely being done on an outpatient basis, with a 2-hour observation period after vertebroplasty. Focal pain at the puncture sites may last 2 for days, which usually responds to analgesics.

Complications

The complication rate of vertebroplasty procedure ranges from 1 to 10% with higher rates being reported in the treatment of neoplastic collapse than the osteoporotic collapse.

- Extravasation of PMMA into the adjoining structures due to vertebral cortical destruction/fracture, causing nerve root/spinal cord compression
- Injection into vertebral venous plexus leading to pulmonary embolism
- Rib fracture
- Fracture of the pedicle or transverse process
- Paravertebral hemorrhage
- Epidural infection (abscess formation)
- Sedation-related adverse effects, namely seizure/respiratory arrest
- Swallowing difficulties from esophageal compression in a cervical vertebroplasty
- Death from massive PMMA pulmonary embolization

There were initial concerns that there may be a potential for increased risk of fractures at an adjacent level following vertebroplasty. However, many studies have proved otherwise.[65] Many workers postulate that these new fractures are more likely to be the result of natural history of osteoporosis rather than the imbalance created secondary to vertebroplasty.

Bone health is an important component of the overall health of the human body. With the better understanding of the bone morphology and various means to identify reduced bone density, there has been an impetus toward improvement in bone health of the population to prevent the morbidity associated with various fractures.

REFERENCES

1. Assessment of fracture risk and its application to screening for postmenopausal osteoporosis. Report of a WHO Study Group. Geneva, World Health Organization, 1994 (WHO Technical Report Series, No. 843).
2. Kanis JA. Diagnosis of osteoporosis and assessment of fracture risk. Lancet. 2002;359(9321):1929-36.
3. Lane JM, Riley EH, Wirganowicz PZ. Osteoporosis: diagnosis and treatment. JBJS. 1996;78-A:618-31.
4. NIH Consensus Development Panel on Osteoporosis Prevention, Diagnosis, and Therapy. Osteoporosis prevention, diagnosis, and therapy. JAMA. 2001;285(6): 785-95.
5. Fitzpatrick LA. Secondary causes of osteoporosis. Mayo Clin Proc. 2002;77:453-68.
6. Jergas M, Gluer CC. Assessment of fracture risk by bone density measurements. Semin Nuclear Med. 1997;27(3):261-75.
7. Sartoris DJ, Resuik D. Current and innovative methods for noninvasive bone densitometry. RCNA. 1990;28(2): 257-78.
8. Bach-Mortensen P, Hyldstrup L, Appleyard M, Hindsø K, Gebuhr P, Sonne-Holm S. Digital X-ray radiogrammetry identifies women at risk of osteoporotic fracture: results from a prospective study. Calcif Tissue Int. 2006;79(1):1-6.
9. Kanis JA, on behalf of the World Health Organization Scientific Group. Assessment of osteoporosis at the primary healthcare level: technical report. University of Sheffield, UK: World Health Organization Collaborating Centre for Metabolic Bone Diseases; 2008.
10. Kanis JA. An update on the diagnosis of osteoporosis. Curr Rheumatol Rep. 2000;2(1):62-6.
11. Blake GM, Fogelman I. The clinical role of dual energy X-ray absorptiometry. Eur J Radiol. 2009;71:406-14.
12. International Society of Clinical Densitometry (ISCD) (2013). Official positions of the International Society for Clinical Densitometry. [online] Available from https://www.iscd.org/official-positions/2013-iscd-official-positions-adult/ [Last accessed March, 2020].
13. World Health Organization. FRAX WHO fracture risk assessment tool. [online] Available from https://www.sheffield.ac.uk/FRAX/index.aspx.
14. Kanis JA, McCloskey EV, Johansson H, Oden A, Ström O, Borgström F. Development and use of FRAX in osteoporosis. Osteoporos Int. 2010;21(Suppl 2):S407-13.
15. Marwaha RK, Tandon N, Kaur P, Sastry A, Bhadra K, Narang A, et al. Establishment of age-specified bone mineral density reference range for Indian females using dual-energy X-ray absorptiometry. J Clin Densitom. 2012;15(2):241-9.
16. Spiro AJ, Hoang TD, Shakir MK. Artifacts affecting dual-energy X-ray absorptiometry measurements. AACE Clin Case Rep. 2019;5(4):e263-6.
17. Bolotin HH. DXA in vivo BMD methodology: An erroneous and misleading research and clinical gauge of bone mineral status, bone fragility, and bone remodelling. Bone. 2007;41(1):138-54.
18. Cann CE. Quantitative CT for determination of bone mineral density—a review. Radiology. 1988;166:509-22.
19. Ryan PJ. Overview of role of BMD measurements in managing osteoporosis. Semin Nuclear Med. 1997;27(3):197-209.
20. Sartoris DJ. Clinical value of bone densitometry. AJR. 1994;163:133-5.
21. Engelke K, Adams JE, Armbrecht G, Augat P, Bogado CE, Bouxsein ML, et al. Clinical use of quantitative computed tomography and peripheral quantitative computed tomography in the management of osteoporosis in adults: the 2007 ISCD Official Positions. J Clin Densitom. 2008;11(1):123-62.
22. Ito M, Hayashi K, Ishida Y, Uetani M, Yamada M, Ohki M, et al. Discrimination of spinal fracture with various bone mineral measurements. Calcif Tissue Int. 1997;60(1):11-5.
23. Grampp S, Jergas M, Wang P, et al. Quantitative CT assessment of the lumbar spine and radius in patients with osteoporosis. AJR. 1996;167:133-40.
24. Agarwal MM, Mandal AK, Khandelwal N, Singh SK. Need for measurement of bone mineral density in patients of prostate cancer before and after orchidectomy: role of quantitative computer tomography. J Assoc Physicians India. 2007;55:486-90.
25. Li N, Li XM, Xu L, Sun WJ, Cheng XG, Tian W. Comparison of QCT and DXA: Osteoporosis Detection Rates in Postmenopausal Women. Int J Endocrinol. 2013;2013:895474.
26. Bansal SC, Khandelwal N, Rai DV, Sen R. Comparison between the QCT and the DEXA scanners in the evaluation of BMD in the lumbar spine. J Clin Diagn Res. 2011;5(4):694-9.
27. Miller P. Controversies in bone mineral density diagnostic classification. Calcif Tiss Int. 2000;66:317-9.
28. Faulkner R, von Stetten E, Miller P. Discordance in patient classification using T-scores. J Clin Densitom. 1999;2:343-50.

29. Felsenberg D, Gowin W. Bone densitometry by dual energy methods. Radiology. 1999;39(3):186-93.
30. Zemel B, Bass S, Binkley T, Ducher G, MacDonald H, MacKay H, et al. Peripheral quantitative computed tomography in children and adolescents. J Clin Densitom. 2008;11(1):59-74.
31. Brennan BM, Mughal Z, Roberts SA, Ward K, Shalet SM, Eden TO, et al. Bone mineral density in childhood survivors of acute lymphoblastic leukemia treated without cranial irradiation. J Clin Endocrinol Metab. 2005;90:689-94.
32. Ekman A, Michaëlsson K, Petrén-Mallmin M, Ljunghall S, Mallmin H. Dual X-ray absorptiometry of hip, heel ultrasound, and densitometry of fingers can discriminate male patients with hip fracture from control subjects: A comparison of four different methods. J Clin Densitom. 2002;5(1):79-85.
33. Langton CM, Langton DK. Comparison of bone mineral density and quantitative ultrasound of the calcaneus: Site matched correlation and discrimination of axial BMD status. BJR. 2000;73:31-5.
34. Cepollaro C, Gonnelli S, Pondrelli C, Martini S, Montagnani A, Rossi S, et al. The combined use of ultrasound and densitometry on the prediction of vertebral fractures. BJR. 1997;70:691-6.
35. Huda W, Morin RL. Patients doses in bone mineral densitometry. BJR. 1996;69:422-5.
36. Khaw KT, Reeve J, Luben R, Bingham S, Welch A, Wareham N, et al. Prediction of total and hip fracture risk in men and women by quantitative ultrasound of the calcaneus: EPIC-Norfolk prospective population study. Lancet. 2004;363(9404):197-202.
37. Li CQ, Magland JF, Rajapakse CS, Guo XE, Zhang XH, Vasilic B, et al. Implications of resolution and noise for in vivo micro-MRI of trabecular bone. Med Phys. 2008;35:5584-94.
38. Krug R, Banerjee S, Han ET, Newitt DC, Link TM, Majumdar S. Feasibility of in vivo structural analysis of high-resolution magnetic resonance images of the proximal femur. Osteoporos Int. 2005;16:1307-14.
39. Krug R, Han ET, Banerjee S, Majumdar S. Fully balanced steady-state 3D-spin-echo (bSSSE) imaging at 3 Tesla. Magn Reson Med. 2006;56:1033-40.
40. Krug R, Carballido-Gamio J, Burghardt AJ, Kazakia G, Hyun BH, Jobke B, et al. Assessment of trabecular bone structure comparing magnetic resonance imaging at 3 Tesla with high-resolution peripheral quantitative computed tomography ex vivo and in vivo. Osteoporos Int. 2008;19:653-61.
41. Krug R, Stehling C, Kelley DA, Majumdar S, Link TM. Imaging of the musculoskeletal system in vivo using ultra-high field magnetic resonance at 7 T. Invest Radiol. 2009;44:613-8.
42. Kazakia GJ, Hyun B, Burghardt AJ, Krug R, Newitt DC, de Papp AE, et al. In vivo determination of bone structure in postmenopausal women: a comparison of HR-pQCT and high-field MR imaging. J Bone Miner Res. 2008;23:463-74.
43. Wehrli FW, Song HK, Saha PK, Wright AC. Quantitative MRI for the assessment of bone structure and function. NMR Biomed. 2006;19:731-64.
44. Wehrli FW. Structural and functional assessment of trabecular and cortical bone by micro magnetic resonance imaging. J Magn Reson Imaging. 2007;25:390-409.
45. Carballido-Gamio J, Krug R, Huber MB, Hyun B, Eckstein F, Majumdar S, et al. Geodesic topological analysis of trabecular bone microarchitecture from high-spatial resolution magnetic resonance images. Magn Reson Med. 2009;61:448-56.
46. Hyun B, Newitt DC, Majumdar S. Assessment of Cortical Bone Structure Using High-Resolution Magnetic Resonance Imaging. Proceedings 13th Scientific Meeting, International Society for Magnetic Resonance in Medicine; Miami; 2005.
47. Techawiboonwong A, Song HK, Leonard MB, Wehrli FW. Cortical bone water: in vivo quantification with ultrashort echo- time MR imaging. Radiology. 2008;248:824-33.
48. Goldenstein J, Kazakia G, Majumdar S. In vivo evaluation of the presence of bone marrow in cortical porosity in postmenopausal osteopenic women. Ann Biomed Eng. 2010;38(2):235-46.
49. Wehrli FW, Gomberg BR, Saha PK, Song HK, Hwang SN, Snyder PJ. Digital topological analysis of in vivo magnetic resonance microimages of trabecular bone reveals structural implications of osteoporosis. J Bone Miner Res. 2001;16:1520-31.
50. Laib A, Hauselmann HJ, Ruegsegger P. In vivo high resolution 3D-QCT of the human forearm. Technol Health Care. 1998;6: 329-37.
51. Feldkamp LA, Davis LC, Kress JW. Practical cone-beam algorithm. J Opt Soc Am A. 1984;1:612-9.
52. Thomas ML, Boris BK, Thomas L, Bauer J, Lu Y, Rummeny EJ. *In vitro* and *in vivo* spiral CT to determine bone mineral density: initial experience in patients at risk for osteoporosis. Radiology. 2004;231:805-11.
53. Ito M, Ikeda K, Nishiguchi M, Shindo H, Uetani M, Hosoi T, Orimo H, et al. Multidetector row CT imaging of vertebral microstructure for evaluation of fracture risk. J Bone Miner Res. 2005;20(10):1828-36.
54. Nakamoto T, Hatsuta S, Yagi S, Verdonschot RG, Taguchi A, Kakimoto N. Computer-aided diagnosis system for osteoporosis based on quantitative evaluation of mandibular lower border porosity using panoramic radiographs. Dentomaxillofac Radiol. 2020;20190481.
55. Pahr DH, Zysset PK. Finite element-based mechanical assessment of bone quality on the basis of in vivo images. Curr Osteoporos Rep. 2016;14(6):374-85.
56. Yasaka K, Akai H, Kunimatsu A, Kiryu S, Abe O. Prediction of bone mineral density from computed tomography: application of deep learning with a convolutional neural network. Eur Radiol. 2020;10.1007/s00330-020-06677-0.
57. Kim YW, Kim JH, Yoon SH, Lee JH, Lee CH, Shin CS, et al. Vertebral bone attenuation on low-dose chest CT: quantitative volumetric analysis for bone fragility assessment. Osteoporos Int. 2017;28(1):329-38.
58. Ferizi U, Honig S, Chang G. Artificial intelligence, osteoporosis and fragility fractures. Curr Opin Rheumatol. 2019;31(4): 368-75.
59. Lee KS, Jung SK, Ryu JJ, Shin SW, Choi J. Evaluation of transfer learning with deep convolutional neural networks for screening osteoporosis in dental panoramic radiographs. J Clin Med. 2020;9(2):E392.
60. Rastegar S, Vaziri M, Qasempour Y, Akhash MR, Abdalvand N, Shiri I, et al. Radiomics for classification of bone mineral loss: a machine learning study [published online ahead of print, 2020 Feb 4]. Diagn Interv Imaging. 2020;pii: S2211-5684(20) 30025-5.
61. Jensen ME, Dion JE. Percutaneous vertebroplasty in the treatment of osteoporotic compression fractures. Neuroimag Clin North Am. 2000;10(3):547-68.
62. Klazen CA, Lohle PN, de Vries J, Jansen FH, Tielbeek AV, Blonk MC, et al. Vertebroplasty versus conservative treatment in acute osteoporotic vertebral compression fractures (Vertos II): an open-label randomised trial. Lancet. 2010;376(9746):1085-92.
63. Tanigawa N, Kariya S, Komemushi A, Nakatani M, Yagi R, Kohzai M, et al. Percutaneous vertebroplasty for osteoporotic compression fractures: long-term evaluation of the technical and clinical outcomes. AJR. 2011;196:1415-8.
64. Rad AE, Kallmes DF. Correlation between preoperative pain duration and percutaneous vertebroplasty outcome. Am J Neuroradiol. 2011;32:1842-5.
65. Yang W, Yang J, Liang M. Percutaneous Vertebroplasty Does Not Increase the Incidence of New Fractures in Adjacent and Nonadjacent Vertebral Bodies. Clin Spine Surg. 2019;32(2): E99-106.

CHAPTER

163

Diagnostic Approach to Focal Bone Lesions

Shivanand Gamanagatti, Raju Sharma

INTRODUCTION

Plain radiography remains the first-line choice of imaging modality for the initial evaluation of a bone lesion following clinical examination. Radiographs can be obtained quickly, easily, and at low cost. At least two views of the affected bone including anteroposterior and lateral views are usually adequate for the assessment of an osseous abnormality. Computed tomography (CT) and magnetic resonance imaging (MRI) provide complimentary information that is extremely useful in the work-up of focal bone lesion. CT scan is particularly useful in evaluating the cortex and matrix. MRI is useful in determining the intramedullary extent and soft tissue extent of focal bone lesion, and also plays a vital role in detecting skip lesions.[1]

A methodical approach is essential for the evaluation of bone tumors, with particular consideration to the location, multiplicity, margins, zone of transition, type of periosteal reaction, matrix mineralization, cortical integrity, and presence of a soft-tissue component. However, it becomes difficult to define the exact origin of a skeletal lesion in small bones of hand and foot, because whole width of the bone may get involved. It becomes challenging to establish whether the lesion is arising from medullary cavity, cortex, or is juxtacortical.

GENERAL PRINCIPLES OF FOCAL BONE LESION EVALUATION

- Prior to the analysis of the radiographic features of focal bone lesion, certain clinical information is essential to narrow down the differential diagnosis, such as age of the patient, the location of the lesion, and is it single or multiple?
- Within long bones, plane of the lesion must be determined with reference to long axis (epiphysis, metaphysis, and diaphysis) and horizontal axis (medullary, cortical, and juxtacortical). Juxtacortical lesions may be parosteal or periosteal.
- Radiograph is essential for lesion detection and characterization. Radiograph should be systematically assessed for:
    - Type of bone destruction
    - Margins/transition zone
    - Cortical status
    - Type of matrix mineralization
    - Type of periosteal reaction
    - Presence or absence of soft tissue component
    - Lesion number (single or multiple)
- The bone lesion can be classified as nonaggressive or aggressive from its radiographic appearance.
- Nonaggressive versus aggressive pattern on radiograph is not always equivalent to benign versus malignant, e.g., osteomyelitis can have an aggressive pattern on radiograph.
- Do not "overdiagnose" a benign bone tumor and do not "underdiagnose" a malignant bone tumor.
- Do not misdirect the biopsy approach to the lesion so as to convert more conservative operation (compartment resection or limb salvage procedure) into more radical operation (amputation).
- Any skeletal lesion detected on a well-penetrated radiograph rule out infection, eosinophilic granuloma, subchondral degenerative cyst, lesion related to metabolic bone disease such as Brown tumor, post-traumatic changes such as stress fracture or is it normal variant.
- If the lesion is unchanged from old films (at least 2 years old), then consider for a clinical/radiographic follow-up of the patient.
- If there are multiple lesions, rule out metastases, especially in adults or other causes of multiple skeletal lesions such as multiple enchondromas, multiple osteochondromas, fibrous dysplasia, fibrous cortical defects/nonossifying fibromas, and sarcoidosis.
- If there is solitary lesion, characterize the lesion further based on age, location, pattern of destruction, margins, cortical response, matrix, and periosteal reaction.

AGE OF THE PATIENT

Most bone tumors have a predilection for a specific age group; therefore, patient's age is an important clinical information while assessing a bone tumor. Typical peak ages of different lesions are listed in **Table 1**. For example, simple bone cysts (SBCs) and chondroblastomas occur in skeletally immature people, while giant cell tumors (GCTs) occur in

TABLE 1: Bone tumors predilection for specific age groups.

	0–10	10–20	20–30	30–40	40–50	>50
Metastatic neuroblastoma	<2years					
Simple bone cyst	▨	■				
Fibrous cortical defect	■	■				
Aneurysmal bone cyst	▨	■				
Ewing's sarcoma		■				
Osteosarcoma		■				
Giant cell tumor			■	■		
Chondrosarcoma				■	■	■
Multiple myeloma						■
Metastasis						■

skeletally mature people. Ewing's sarcoma typically occurs in 10–20 year-old patients, while conventional osteosarcoma has two age peaks, one, arising de novo, in teenagers and the second, arising in background of Paget's disease or previously irradiated bone, in adults older than 50 years. A malignant bone lesion in an adult over 40 years old is much more likely to be metastatic carcinoma, myeloma, or metastatic non-Hodgkin lymphoma rather than a primary bone sarcoma.[2]

LOCATION OF LESION (FIG. 1)

Most bone tumors, regardless of whether they are benign or malignant, often occur in a characteristic location in the skeleton (i.e., axial vs. appendicular skeleton or long vs. flat bone). Thus, some tumors (e.g., osteosarcoma) have a predilection for sites of rapid bone growth, usually the metaphyseal region, while other tumors (e.g., Ewing's sarcoma) tend to follow the distribution of red marrow. Furthermore, lesions such as enchondroma in a long bone are usually located centrally within the medullary cavity, while an aneurysmal bone cyst is located eccentrically in the medullary cavity **(Fig. 1)**. However, in short or thin tubular bones, such as the metacarpals, metatarsals, phalanges, and fibula, the entire diameter of the bone can be involved, sometimes making it difficult to determine in which part of the bone the lesion originated. An apophysis (a growth center that does not contribute to the length of a bone) is the equivalent of an epiphysis (a growth center at the end of a bone that does contribute to length); thus, one should use the "end-of-bone" differential list for a lesion in such sites as the greater trochanter of the femur and the tibial tubercle **(Fig. 1)**. Similarly, other growth centers such as the patella; the small bones of the wrist, hindfoot, and midfoot; and the subarticular portions of flat bones, such as those around the sacroiliac joints and acetabuli in the pelvis, and the glenoid of the scapula are also end-of-bone equivalents.

The differential diagnosis can then be further narrowed by knowing the age of the patient. For example, a lytic lesion in the epiphysis of a long bone of an adolescent is likely to be a chondroblastoma, whereas a lytic lesion at the end of a long bone in a young adult is likely to be a GCT. Ewing's sarcoma and Langerhans cell histiocytosis have a predilection for the diaphysis of long bones in people younger than 20 years and a predilection for flat bones, such as the pelvis and skull, in people older than 20 years, reflecting the normal change in the distribution of red marrow as a person ages.

Some lesions have a predilection for a particular bone and location, such as an adamantinoma and osteofibrous dysplasia for the anterior cortex of the tibia, periosteal desmoids for the posterior distal aspect of the femur, and hemangioma for vertebral bodies.[2]

PATTERNS OF BONE DESTRUCTION

Three patterns of bone destruction have been described as follows **(Figs. 2A to C)**:[3]

1. Type I—geographic bone destruction
2. Type II—moth-eaten bone destruction
3. Type III—permeative bone destruction

Geographic Bone Destruction

This type of bone destruction is the least aggressive form and suggests a slow growing lesion. It is seen as a well-circumscribed lytic lesion with a narrow zone of transition. The slow growth rate results in sharp demarcation between the destructive lesion and adjacent normal bone. The margin of the lesion represents the true histological margin of destruction; however, malignant lesions such as metastasis or myeloma may also demonstrate a similar pattern.

This pattern is further divided into three subtypes:

1. Type IA—geographic lesion with sclerotic margin
2. Type IB—geographic lesion with no marginal sclerosis
3. Type IC—geographic lesion with ill-defined margins

Geographic Lesion with Sclerotic Margin

The slow growth of the lesion permits the development of a reactive bone around the lesion so as to accommodate the transmission of forces. The sclerotic margin may vary

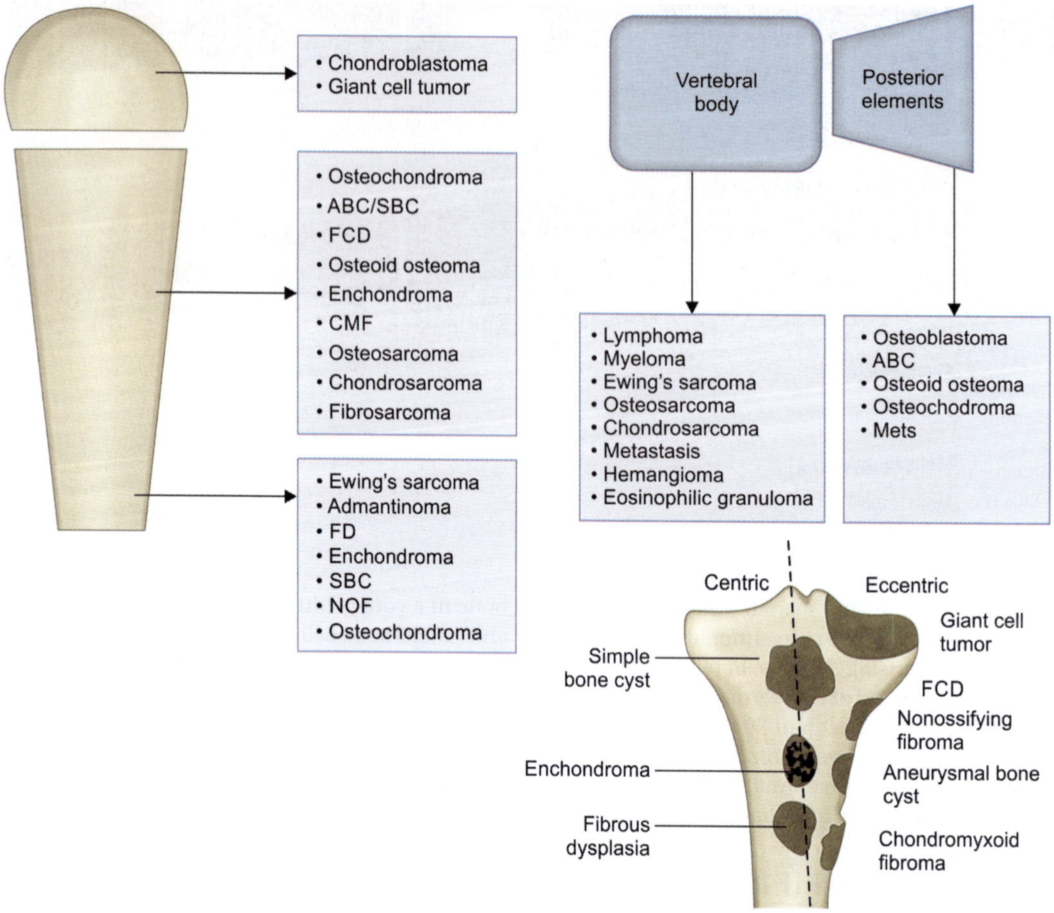

FIG. 1: Diagrammatic representation of the locations of various focal bone lesions. (ABC: aneurysmal bone cyst; CMF: chondromyxoid fibroma; FCD: fibrous cortical dysplasia; FD: fibrous dysplasia; NOF: nonossifying fibroma; SBC: simple bone cyst).

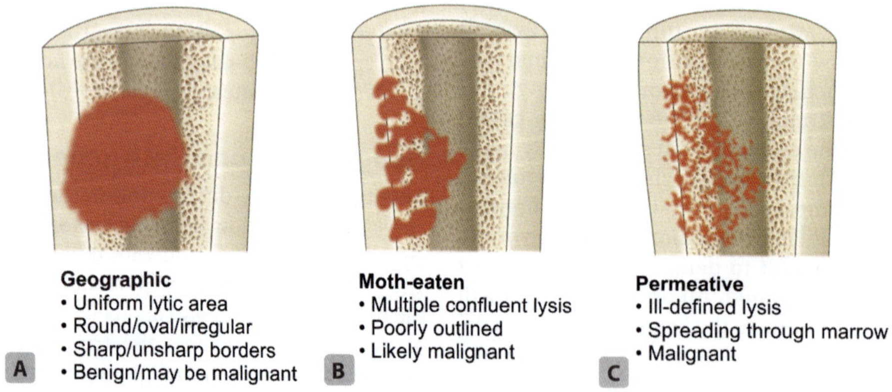

FIGS. 2A TO C: Patterns of bone destruction.

in thickness and is especially thick in lesions occurring in weight-bearing bones such as femur and tibia. This type of lesion is commonly seen in SBC **(Fig. 3A)**, enchondroma, chondromyxoid fibroma, Brodie's abscess, and fibroxanthoma. Fibrous dysplasia often displays a peripheral thick sclerotic rim resembling a "rind" of orange **(Fig. 3B)**. In some lesions such as Brodie's abscess **(Fig. 3C)** and eosinophilic granuloma, the sclerotic rim is rather fuzzy and appears to be fading gradually into adjacent cancellous bone. The sclerotic rim is a mechanical adaptation designed to accommodate forces transmitted around the space-occupying mass.

Geographic Lesion with No Marginal Sclerosis

This type of lesion shows sharp margins with narrow zone of transition, referred to as a punched-out lesion with no

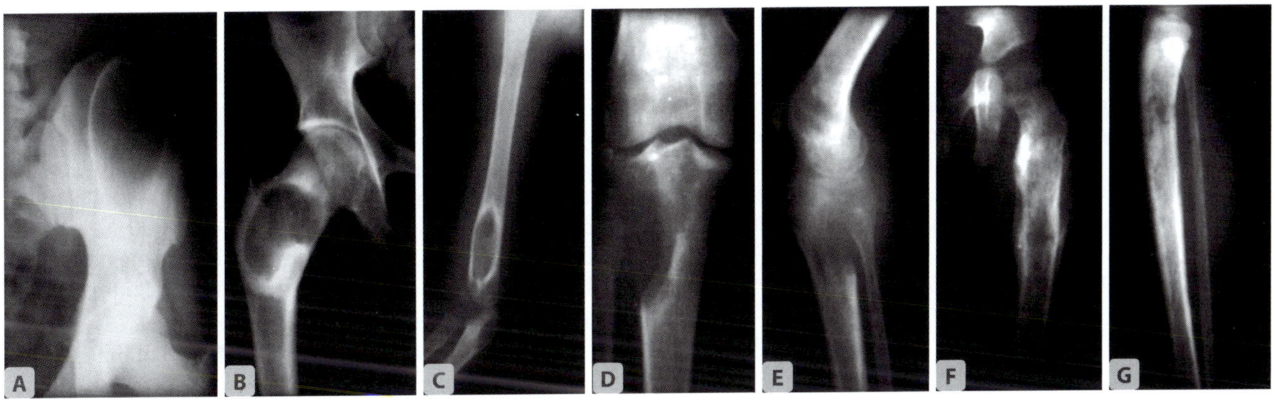

FIGS. 3A TO G: Patterns of bone destruction. (A) Type IA—geographic destruction with sclerotic margins in a simple bone cyst seen in the left iliac bone; (B) Type IA—geographic destruction with thick sclerotic margins, "rind sign," seen in fibrous dysplasia involving neck of right femur; (C) Type IA—geographic destruction with sclerotic margin which is fuzzy and facing peripherally, in Brodie's abscess involving lower end of humerus; (D) Type IB—geographic destruction with punched-out lesion seen in giant cell tumor involving upper tibia—note its typical eccentric subarticular position; (E) Type IC—geographic destruction with ill-defined margins seen in another patient of giant cell tumor involving upper tibia; (F) Type II—moth-eaten destruction seen in osteomyelitis involving left upper femur in a child—also note associated single lamellar periosteal reaction; and (G) Type III—permeative bone destruction involving upper tibia with osteomyelitis, note the tunneling in the anterior cortex.

sclerosis **(Fig. 3D)**. The margins seen on radiograph reflects the true histological edge of the lesion. GCT typically displays this pattern. Many lesions associated with type IA pattern may also show this pattern, e.g., bone cyst, enchondroma, and chondroblastoma.

Geographic Lesion with Ill-defined Margins

This type indicates locally infiltrative process. The margins are poorly defined suggesting more aggressive pattern than type IB lesions **(Fig. 3E)**. The destructive process extends in the marrow between the trabeculae beyond the radiographic destructive edge. This type of lesion is seen characteristically in GCT, osteosarcoma, chondrosarcoma, fibrosarcoma, aneurysmal bone cyst, eosinophilic granuloma, and osteomyelitis.

Moth-eaten Bone Destruction

This type of lesion is relatively more aggressive, suggesting more rapidly growing lesion. It is characterized by multiple small varying sized lytic lesions that coalesce and involve both cancellous and cortical bone **(Fig. 3F)**. In cancellous bone, normal trabeculae may be seen in between the lytic lesions while in cortical bone, the lytic lesion starts from endosteal surface and extends outward. This may progress to complete cortical destruction with extension into adjacent soft tissues. The lesion has less well-defined margins with wide zone of transition and is more extensive on histopathology than suggested on a radiograph. This pattern is usually seen in malignant neoplasms such as lymphoma, osteosarcoma, chondrosarcoma, fibrosarcoma, round cell tumor (including Ewing's sarcoma), and also osteomyelitis.

Permeative Bone Destruction

This pattern represents the most aggressive form and suggests a rapidly destructive bone lesion. This type is characterized by multiple, tiny oval lucent lesions or lucent streaks, mostly involving cortical bone **(Fig. 3G)**. Progressive cortical destruction occurs with exuberant cortical tunneling by osteoclasts, and the lesions are ill-defined. The highly aggressive nature does not allow bone to react and stop its further progress. These lesions are much more widespread than they appear on a radiograph. This type of lesion is seen in Ewing's sarcoma, lymphoma, high-grade chondrosarcoma, fibrosarcoma, angiosarcoma, leukemia, and metastasis.

Combination and Changing Pattern

This is characterized by combination of type IA, IB, and IC; type II; or type III patterns in a single lytic lesion and suggests more aggressive local growth. This pattern is usually seen in some benign lesions, when they become active, undergo malignant change or fracture. Pressure from tumor growth or active hyperemia are some of the factors that contribute to this pattern. A changing pattern is discernible when a change in the nature of margin is observed radiographically over time.

MARGIN OF THE LESION AND RATE OF GROWTH

The margin of the lesion relates to the radiographic appearance of the interface between the lesion and adjacent normal bone. This is determined by reaction of the host bone to the lesion and rate of growth of the lesion. Well-marginated lesions have a narrow zone of transition **(Fig. 3A)**, while poorly-defined lesions have a wide zone of transition **(Fig. 3G)**. The aggressiveness and rate of growth of the lesion can be assessed from its margin. Sharply- defined margin or a sclerotic margin suggests slow growth rate, while ill-defined margins indicate aggressive lesion and rapid growth rate. Some benign lesions may, however, show a rapid growth rate, and some malignant lesions may be slow growing and have well-defined margins. Therefore, assessment of radiographic margin does not always indicate benign or malignant nature of a lesion.[4,5] Aneurysmal bone cyst, eosinophilic granuloma, majority of GCTs, and chondromyxoid fibroma may display aggressive appearance on radiographs and yet be benign. On the other hand, malignant lesions such as plasmacytoma and juxtacortical osteosarcoma are slow growing and may appear nonaggressive on plain radiograph. Treatment can also alter the appearance of malignant bone tumors; following radiation or chemotherapy, they may exhibit significant sclerosis as well as a narrow zone of transition.[3]

Inflammatory lesions usually produce marked reactive bone formation compared with neoplasms. Typically, these lesions show a sclerotic margin with sharp inner border and hazy outer border. However, osteoid osteoma also shows extensive osteosclerosis around the margin of similar nature. Benign tumors or tumor-like conditions and slow growing malignant tumors usually show sclerotic rim with sharp outer and inner margins **(Fig. 3B)**, while inflammatory lesions show a sclerotic margin with sharp inner border and a hazy outer border **(Fig. 3C)**.

Sometimes, a lesion may demonstrate a scalloped margin. This occurs in lesions of cartilage, fibrous tissue, fat, and vascular tissue, where the cells grow in clumps or lobules at different growth rates. The scalloped margin is seen typically in nonossifying fibroma. The assessment of growth rate on radiographs correlates well with virulence of organisms, host response, degree of spread of infection in inflammatory lesions, and with aggressiveness of the tumors. However, the radiographic rate of growth is not synonymous with actual biological behavior and growth rate of the lesion as seen in acute osteomyelitis and Ewing's sarcoma. Both these lesions may show similar radiographic appearance of aggressive pattern of bone destruction. However, such an appearance develops in a relatively short period of time in acute osteomyelitis in contrast to Ewing's sarcoma, which may take a longer period. Nonetheless, assessment of growth rate may help in narrowing the differential diagnosis.

CORTICAL RESPONSE

Presence of an intact cortex usually suggests nonaggressive nature of the lesion. Cortex responds in different ways (thinning, scalloping, expansion, or complete destruction) to underlying focal lesion. Cortical thinning (trabeculation) implies a slow-growing nature of lesion, usually benign lesion such as SBC and GCT **(Fig. 4A)**. Endosteal scalloping suggests the lobular growth pattern of the underlying tumor seen in chondral **(Fig. 4B)** or fibrous lesion, but does not help to differentiate benign from malignant lesion. Cortical expansion is a misnomer but implies that endosteal bone removal due to tumor growth is occurring at a similar speed to periosteal bone production, again suggesting slow growth. Sometimes, the outer cortical layer may be too thin to be seen on plain radiographs but evident on CT **(Figs. 4C and D)**. Highly aggressive lesions show complete destruction of the cortex with soft tissue component, sometimes saucerization of the cortex may be seen due to pressure erosion by the soft tissue without obvious cortical destruction **(Fig. 4E)**. Destruction of the cortex suggests rapid growth of the lesion. These two features (penetration of an apparently intact cortex and cortical saucerization) are most frequently seen with malignant round cell tumors, particularly Ewing's sarcoma.

MATRIX MINERALIZATION

Matrix refers to the acellular intercellular substance produced by the mesenchymal cells, namely osteoblasts, cartilage cells, and fibroblasts, and this includes osteoid, chondroid, myxoid, and collagen tissue. Matrix becomes visible on the radiograph only when it is mineralized sufficiently with calcium salts.[6]

Evaluation of matrix is valuable for two reasons:

1. Identification of particular configuration of matrix helps in suggesting specific diagnosis.
2. It is an indirect indicator of biological activity, e.g., transition from mineralized to nonmineralized matrix on follow-up radiographs indicates increased biologic activity and suggests this as an optimal site for biopsy.

The plain radiographs remain the best modality for assessing the pattern of matrix mineralization; however, the presence of subtle matrix mineralization can be seen only on CT.

Osseous Matrix

Osseous matrix is produced either by normal or tumor osteoblasts. The presence of bony trabeculae, appearing as thin interlacing radiodense struts within a lesion, is pathognomonic of a bone matrix. This occurs in myositis ossificans produced by normal osteoblasts, and in low-grade parosteal osteosarcoma produced by tumor osteoblasts. The osseous matrix may appear fluffy, amorphous, hazy **(Fig. 5A)**, cloud-like or ivory pattern **(Fig. 5B)** on radiograph, when ossified sufficiently and is seen in high-grade osteosarcoma, parosteal osteosarcoma, and osteoblastoma.

Osseous matrix is also produced by the modulation of fibroblasts into osteoblasts and occurs in fibrous dysplasia and appears diffuse, hazy, or poorly defined but not as radiodense as seen in tumor new bone. Necrosis of fat tissue may result in the development of bone matrix which appears as clumps of radiodensity.

Cartilage Matrix

The cartilage matrix, when sufficiently calcified, is seen as flecks, punctate **(Fig. 5C)**, or flocculated **(Fig. 5E)** in appearance (enchondroma and osteochondroma). When the cartilage matrix is sufficiently ossified, it shows appearance of arcs **(Fig. 5D)** or rings **(Fig. 5D)** hazy, cloud-like or ivory-pattern. The punctate calcification of cartilage occurs in disrupted zone of provisional calcification while ring or arc appearance originates from disrupted enchondral bone formation. Both these patterns may exist alone or in combination. The ossified rings in cartilage tumor suggest low-grade nature of the tumor.

PERIOSTEAL REACTION

Periosteum is like an envelope that separates the bone from surrounding soft tissues. This consists of two layers, the outer fibrous and inner cellular. It is firmly adherent to the

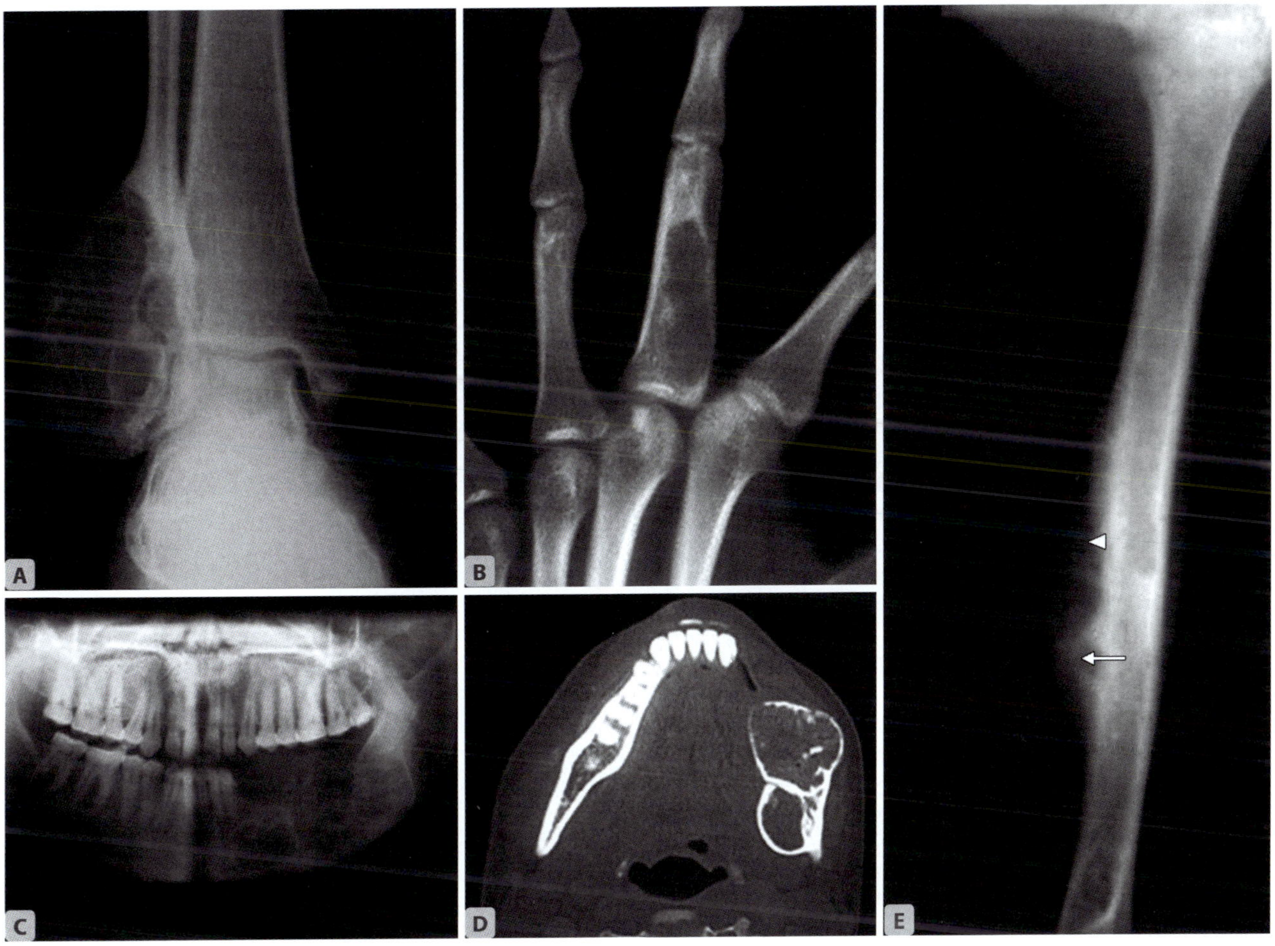

FIGS. 4A TO E: Cortical response. (A) Giant cell tumor showing expansile lytic lesion with intact cortex in lower end of fibula reaching up to subarticular location suggestive of cortical trabeculation indicating slow growth; (B) Enchondroma showing mildly expansile intramedullary lytic lesion in proximal phalanx causing endosteal scalloping indicating lobular growth; (C and D) Aneurysmal bone cyst showing expansile lytic lesion in body of mandible, cortical integrity is not well seen on plain radiograph, CT section of same patient showing the intact cortex around the expansile lytic lesion; and (E) "Saucerization" (arrowhead) of the medial humeral diaphysis in Ewing's sarcoma caused by the pressure erosion of the soft mass.

underlying bone in adults but less so in children. Normally, periosteum is not visible and even when it is elevated, it cannot be appreciated on radiographs till mineralization occurs. The periosteal reaction can be stimulated by hyperemia, inflammation, or spread of tumor. Its presence is an indicator of biologic activity and reflects the duration and intensity of underlying process.[4]

The type of periosteal reaction can be considered under three subgroups **(Fig. 6A)**:

1. Continuous
2. Discontinuous or interrupted
3. Complex

Continuous Periosteal Reaction

Continuous periosteal reaction may occur either with intact or destroyed underlying cortex. It may be solid, single lamellar, multilamellar, or parallel spiculated. An underlying inflammatory or neoplastic process incites hyperemia that activates fibroblasts to osteoblasts that produce osteoid and mineralized layers of new bone. It takes 10–21 days, from the initial insult, for the periosteum to become radiographically visible.

Single lamellar periosteal reaction **(Fig. 6B)** is seen as a thin 1–2 mm faint radiopaque line from the cortical surface and usually occurs in osteomyelitis, histiocytosis, some benign tumors, and healing fractures.

In multilamellated periosteal reaction **(Fig. 6H)**, there are multiple layers of concentric periosteal reaction resembling an onion skin. Repeated insults from underlying disease process with alternating periods of rapid and slow growth first result in ossified layer of periosteum to be elevated, and later subsequent layers of periosteum are formed as the lesion waxes and wanes during its progression. This type of periosteal reaction occurs in osteomyelitis, histiocytosis, aneurysmal bone cyst, Ewing's sarcoma, and osteosarcoma. Interruptions in the lamellated periosteal reaction indicates more aggressive behavior of the lesion.

Solid periosteal reaction **(Fig. 6C)** indicates a slow process and is almost always associated with benign pathology. This occurs as a result of ossified matrix filling the spaces between lamellations and cortex. This is seen as

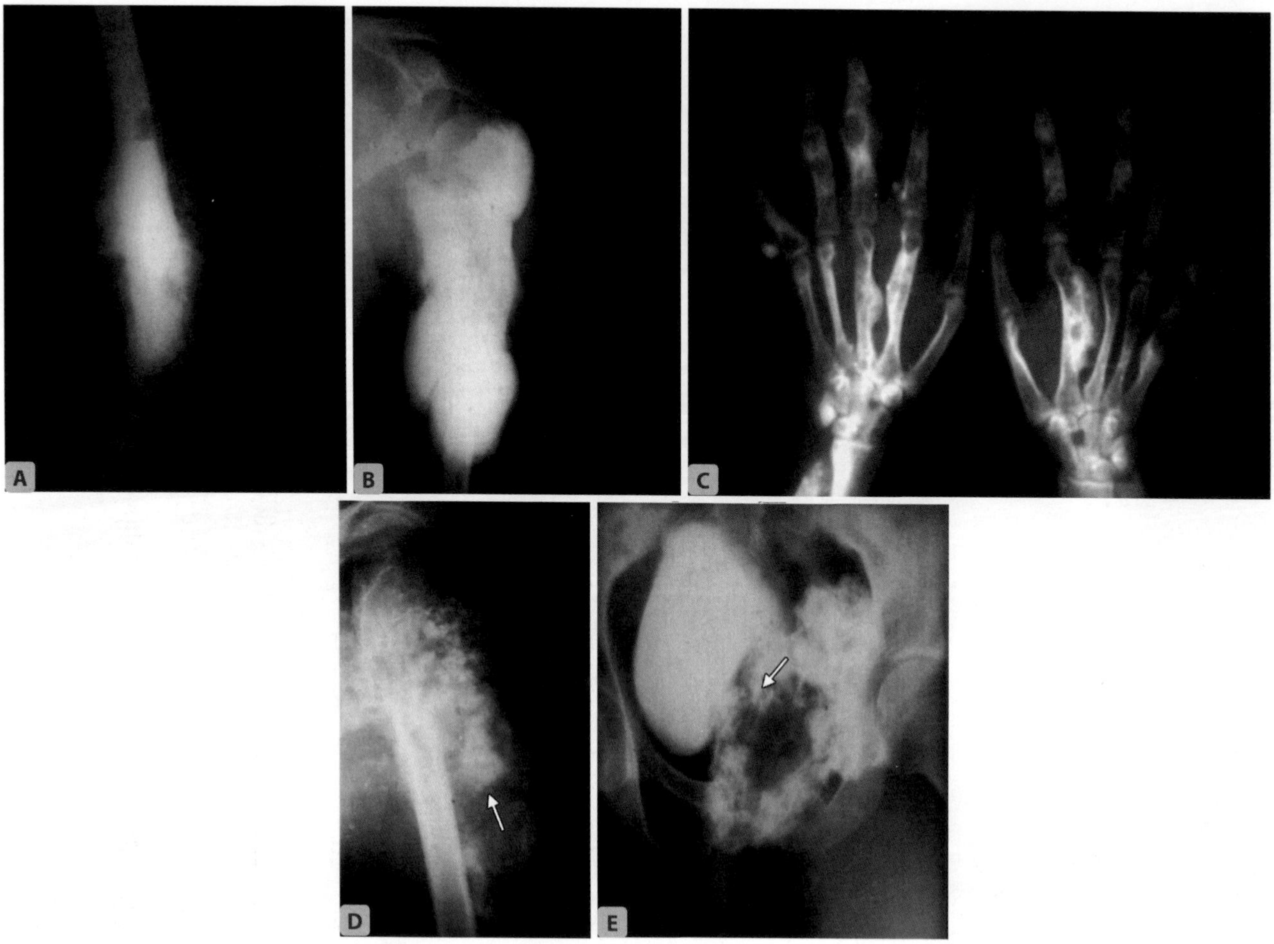

FIGS. 5A TO E: Patterns of matrix mineralization. (A) Cloud-like pattern of osteoid matrix in mid-diaphysis and ivory-like pattern in metaphyseal region of femur in osteosarcoma—note the single lamellar periosteal reaction along the anterior cortex; (B) Ivory-like pattern of osteoid matrix in a case of parosteal osteosarcoma involving proximal humerus—note that underlying humeral shaft can be seen through the tumor new bone in the lower part; (C) Punctate pattern of chondroid matrix in enchondromas involving multiple bones of hands in Maffucci syndrome—note multiple phleboliths with soft tissue swellings suggestive of cavernous hemangiomas; (D) Flocculent and arc-like (arrow) pattern of chondroid matrix involving upper third of femur with sarcomatous change in diaphyseal aclasis; and (E) Extensive flocculent and ring-like (arrow) chondroid matrix in chondrosarcoma involving left pubic bone, showing mass effect on urinary bladder.

marked thickening of the periosteal surface of the cortex on plain radiographs. It may be smooth or irregular. Lesions that show solid periosteal reaction include osteoid osteoma and eosinophilic granuloma.

Undulating periosteal reaction **(Fig. 6D)** is a variant of solid periosteal reaction, seen in low-grade osteomyelitis, long-standing varicosities, pulmonary osteoarthropathy, and chronic osteitis, but rarely in neoplasms.

Parallel spiculated continuous periosteal reaction represents an underlying malignant pathology. Bony spicules may appear perpendicular to the cortex—"hair-on-end" **(Figs. 6E and F)**, fan out in focal divergent manner—"sunburst pattern" **(Fig. 6G)**, appear to slope in a focal manner ("velvet pattern"), or show an unorganized pattern. The direction of the spicules is determined by the direction in which the tumor grows. This type of periosteal reaction suggests a more rapid process than lamellated or solid reaction. The spicules may show uniform, fine velvet-like pattern to long linear shadows with a gradual reduction in height in each direction along the shaft from the mid-zone of the reaction. *Hair-on-end* periosteal reaction commonly occurs in Ewing's sarcoma, osteosarcoma, metastasis, and thalassemia. These spicules are composed of normal reactive bone. Loose areolar tissue between the spicules may be replaced by tumor tissue in Ewing's sarcoma, osteosarcoma, and metastasis, while these may be replaced by hyperplastic red marrow in thalassemia **(Fig. 6F)** and sickle cell anemia. *Sunburst appearance* is more often seen in osteosarcoma, osteoblastic metastasis, and hemangioma **(Fig. 6G)**. In osteosarcoma, the divergent spicules are composed mainly of tumor bone but may also be composed of reactive bone or a combination of both. In *velvet pattern* of periosteal reaction, the spicules are short and sloped. This is seen rarely in chondrosarcoma. In unorganized form of periosteal reaction, the spicules are seen in various directions and indicate marked aggressive nature of the lesion, seen in Ewing's sarcoma as it extends into soft tissues.

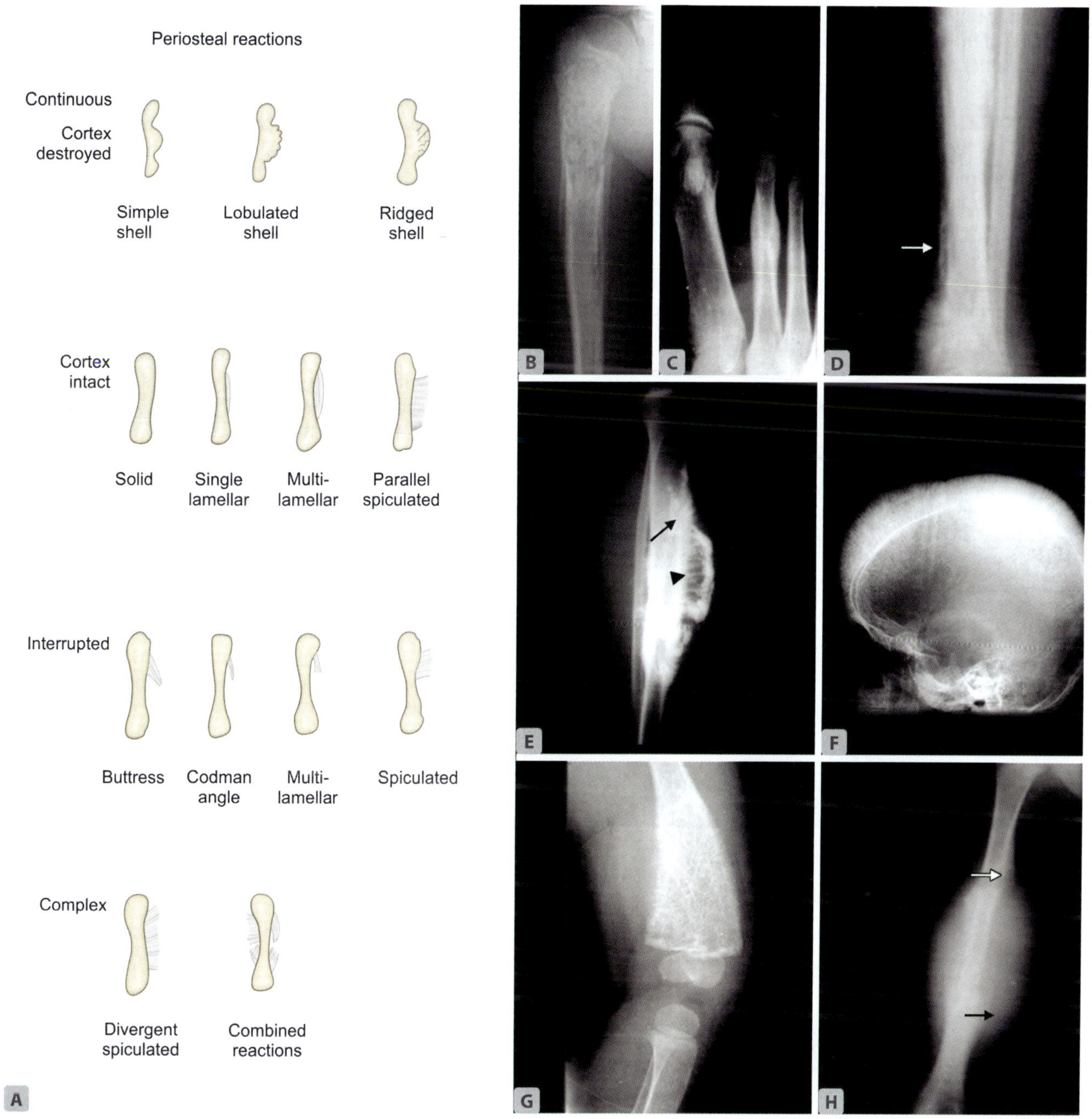

FIGS. 6A TO H: Various types of periosteal reaction: (A) Schematic diagram showing various types of periosteal reactions; (B) Single lamellar periosteal reaction in osteomyelitis involving upper-half of tibia—note type III—permeative bone destruction; (C) Solid periosteal reaction in stress fracture involving second metatarsal; (D) Undulating periosteal reaction (arrow) in chronic osteomyelitis of tibia; (E) Parallel (hair-on-end) (arrow) and divergent (sunburst) (arrowhead) spiculated periosteal reaction in diaphyseal osteosarcoma of tibia—note ivory pattern of osteoid tumor matrix; (F) Hair-on-end periosteal reaction involving the skull vault in thalassemia with marked thickening of outer table in frontoparietal region; (G) Sunburst periosteal reaction with coarse and striated trabecular pattern seen in hemangioma involving distal femoral metaphysis in a child; and (H) Complex periosteal reaction in Ewing's sarcoma of humeral diaphysis—note interrupted multilamellar (onion skin) reaction, buttress formation (white arrow) in the upper part, and Codman's angles (black arrow) in the lower part of the tumor both on medial and lateral aspects of bone.

Interrupted Periosteal Reaction

In this type, continuous mineralization of the periosteal reaction does not occur, resulting in the formation of Codman angles, buttresses, or truncated lamellae.

Codman Angles

The periosteal reaction forms an angular configuration with underlying cortex, resembling two sides of an angle **(Fig. 6G)** and indicates an aggressive pathology. This is formed by elevation of the periosteum by tumor, blood, edema, or pus. The angle of the triangle may or may not contain tumor. This is nonspecific, seen in both benign and malignant lesions.

Buttresses

In this type, solid reactive bone is formed at the lateral extraosseous margins of slowly growing bone lesions, the cortex beneath the buttress is frequently intact **(Figs. 6H and 7)**.

Truncated Lamellae

In aggressive neoplasms and virulent infections, the lamellations are sometimes interrupted or truncated **(Fig. 6H)**, because they are resorbed faster than they can be formed.

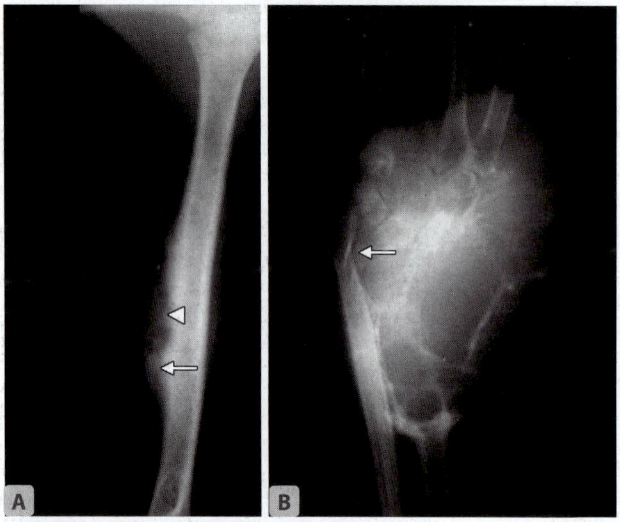

FIGS. 7A AND B: Saucerization. (A) "Saucerization" (arrowhead) of the medial humeral diaphysis in Ewing's sarcoma—note the buttress type (arrow) of periosteal reaction in the distal part; (B) Expansile, lytic, and multiseptate lesion in a patient with giant cell tumor of lower end of radius—note saucerization (arrow) of lateral ulnar cortex due to soft tissue component of tumor and ridged shell periosteal reaction.

Complex Periosteal Reaction

Complex periosteal reaction includes combinations of lamellated, divergent spiculated periosteal reaction, buttresses, and Codman angles **(Fig. 6H)**. The more extensive and complex the periosteal reaction, the greater is the biologic activity of the underlying pathology.

SOFT TISSUE EXTENSION

Normally, the soft tissue shadow of muscle bundles when visualized on a radiograph is sharp with no displacement. It appears obscured when there is infiltration of intermuscular fat planes by inflammation, hemorrhage, or tumor. It may show displacement by organized hemorrhage or abscess. Presence of fat density in a soft tissue mass suggests a lipoma **(Fig. 8A)**. The presence of phleboliths indicates low flow vascular malformation or angiomatous lesion **(Fig. 5C)**. In myositis ossificans, focal rounded or streak-like areas of amorphous radiodensity are seen with areas of bone formation in the peripheral part as the lesion matures. Parosteal osteosarcoma also appears as an amorphous mass of increased density, but it matures earliest centrally in contrast to myositis ossificans. Both these lesions may or may not demonstrate a cleavage plane between the mass and underlying bone. Synovial sarcoma shows punctate clumps of calcific density and is usually present around a joint or along a tendon sheath **(Fig. 8B)**.[5]

Soft tissue mass is often associated with primary bone tumor, but less commonly with a secondary deposit. It may displace adjacent intermuscular fat planes **(Fig. 8C)** and may or may not erode the contiguous bony cortex.

MULTIPLICITY

Multiplicity of malignant lesions usually indicates metastatic disease **(Fig. 9A)**, multiple myeloma, or lymphoma. Very rarely, primary malignant bone lesions, such as Ewing's sarcoma or osteosarcoma, present as multifocal disease. Benign lesions, which tend to involve multiple sites, are

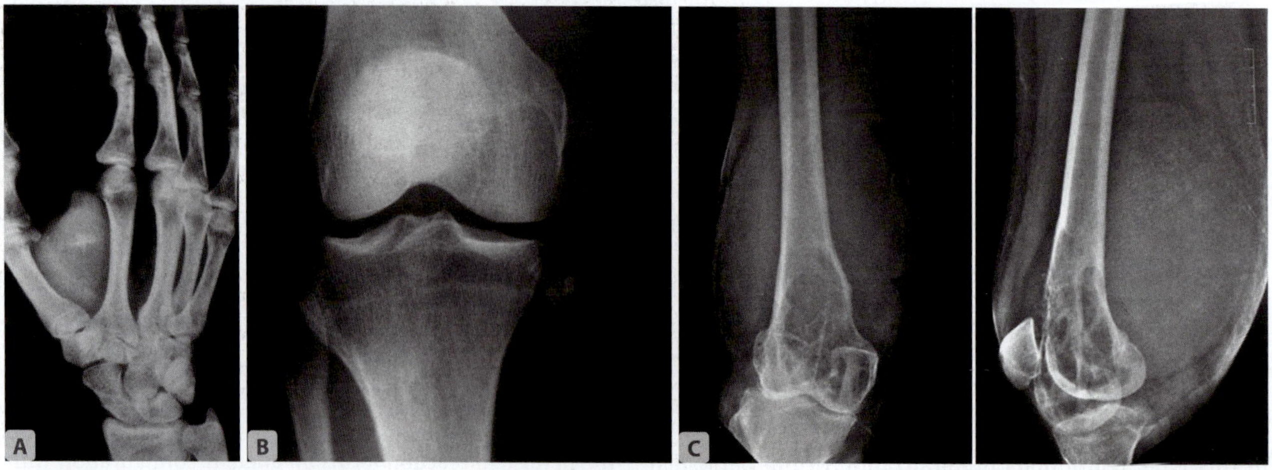

FIGS. 8A TO C: Soft tissue components. (A) Radiograph of hand showing low-density lesion in first web space (due to presence of fat density) suggests a lipoma; (B) Radiograph of knee joint showing punctate clumps of calcific density around the joint due to synovial sarcoma; (C) Radiograph of thigh including the knee joint showing lytic destructive lesion in the lower end of femur associated with large soft tissue component displacing the adjacent intermuscular fat planes.

polyostotic fibrous dysplasia, multiple osteochondromas, enchondromatosis **(Fig. 9B)**, Langerhans cell histiocytosis **(Fig. 9C)**, hemangiomatosis, hemophilia pseudotumors **(Fig. 9D)**, and fibromatosis.[7]

MISCELLANEOUS

Septations (Table 2)

Lytic expansile lesions often show septations which represent residual normal bone that has not been resorbed or destroyed. These include aneurysmal bone cyst, GCT, nonossifying fibroma, etc. These septations are left behind by the lobules of growing lesion that advance asymmetrically at a more rapid rate. The septae are thin in GCT **(Fig. 10A)**, while they are thick in nonossifying fibroma and chondromyxoid fibroma **(Fig. 10B)**.[8]

Saucerization

Some tumors invade the cortex of a tubular bone in such a way that the area of bone destruction resembles a saucer when the long bone radiograph is viewed in profile. Ewing's sarcoma and metastasis may show typical saucerization configuration. In Ewing's sarcoma, the tumor breaks through the cortex, extends subperiosteally and erodes from its paracortical location to produce saucerization **(Fig. 7A)**. Metastasis also invades subperiosteal region in the same way as Ewing's sarcoma or may invade cortex directly. Large soft tissue masses may erode bone in a similar manner **(Fig. 7B)**.[8]

Floating Fragment Sign

A fractured fragment may be seen within a radiolucent lesion. This fragment changes its location with change in extremity position, a characteristic feature seen in unicameral bone cyst. This sign is also known as "fallen fragment sign" **(Fig. 11)**. When the fractured fragment remains attached at the fracture site, it is seen in the form of a trapped door due to hydrostatic pressure of the fluid contained within the cyst. This is called "trap door sign". Both these signs are typical of unicameral bone cyst.

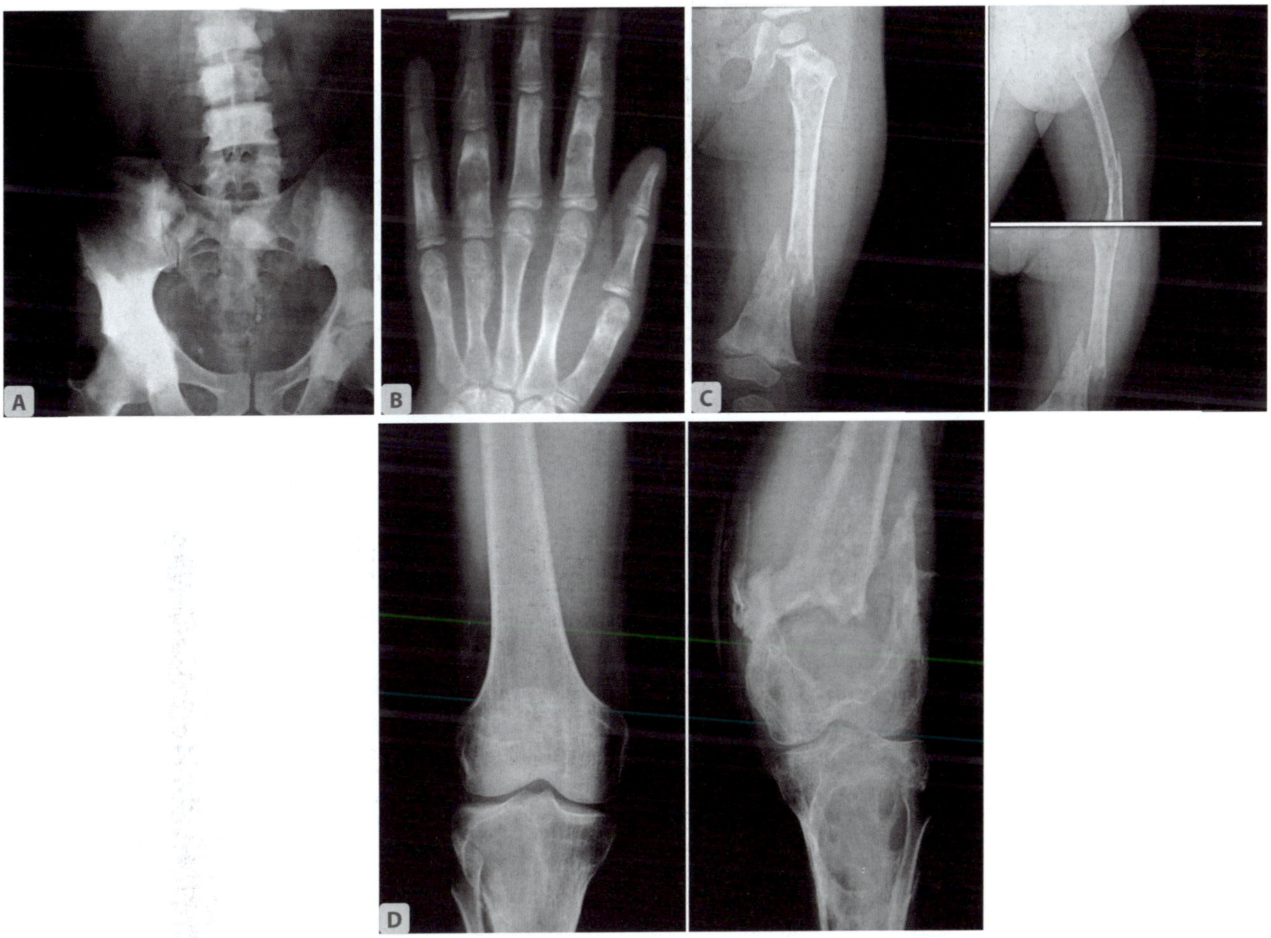

FIGS. 9A TO D: Multiplicity of lesions. (A) Multiple sclerotic lesions involving pelvis and lumbar spine in elderly patient suggestive of metastases; (B) Multiple intramedullary lytic lesions with chondroid type of calcification in short bones of hand suggestive of multiple enchondromatosis; (C) Multiple lytic lesions involving long bone both metaphysis and diaphysis with pathological fracture in a child suggestive of Langerhans cell histiocytosis; (D) Multiple lytic lesions involving tibia and femur in patient with history of bleeding diathesis suggestive of hemophilic pseudotumors.

TABLE 2: Examples of septated lesions.

Septations	Lesions
Coarse and thick	Chondromyxoid fibroma
Delicate and thin	Giant cell tumor
Delicate and horizontally oriented	Aneurysmal bone cysts
Lobulated	Nonossifying fibroma
Striated and radiating	Hemangioma

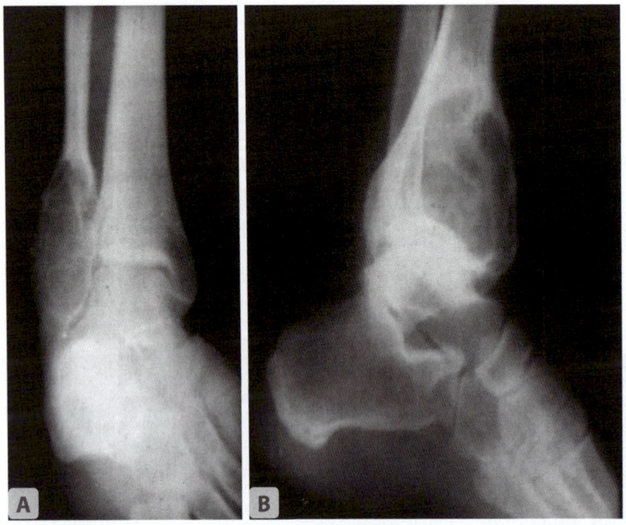

FIGS. 10A AND B: Septations. (A) Expansile, lytic, and multiseptate lesion in a patient with giant cell tumor of lower end of radius—note saucerization of lateral ulnar cortex due to soft tissue component of tumor and ridged shell periosteal reaction; (B) Eccentric expansile lytic lesion showing thick septa and ridged shell reaction in chondromyxoid fibroma involving the lower end of tibia.

BENIGN VERSUS MALIGNANT

Although it is sometimes very difficult to distinguish benign from malignant bone lesions on the basis of plain radiographs alone; however, certain key characteristic features may favor one over the other. Benign tumors usually present with well-defined, sclerotic borders, a geographic type of bone destruction, an uninterrupted solid periosteal reaction, and no soft tissue extension. Malignant lesions, on the other hand, tend to demonstrate poorly-defined borders with a wide zone of transition, a moth-eaten or permeative pattern of bone destruction, an interrupted periosteal reaction of the sunburst or onion-skin type, and an adjacent soft-tissue mass. As noted earlier, it should be kept in mind that some benign tumors can also exhibit aggressive features **(Table 3)**.[9]

When all the clinical and radiographic information concerning a patient with a bone lesion has been analyzed, the most important diagnostic decision is whether the lesion is definitely benign and not to be biopsied, but rather monitored or completely ignored (a "do not touch lesion") **(Table 4)**, or whether it has an ambiguous and an aggressive appearance and should be further investigated via percutaneous or open biopsy. The results of the histopathologic examination would then determine whether further management in a given case would be surgical, chemotherapeutic, radiotherapeutic, or a combination of these.

TABLE 3: Benign lesions with aggressive features.

Lesion	Radiographic presentation
Osteoblastoma	Bone destruction and soft (aggressive) tissue extension similar to osteosarcoma
Desmoplastic fibroma	Expansive destructive lesion, frequently trabeculated
Periosteal desmoid	Irregular cortical outline, mimics osteosarcoma or Ewing's sarcoma
Giant cell tumor	Occasionally aggressive features—osteolytic bone destruction, cortical penetration, and soft tissue extension
Aneurysmal bone cyst	Soft tissue extension, occasionally mimicking malignant tumor
Osteomyelitis	Bone destruction and aggressive periosteal reaction, occasionally, features resembling Ewing's sarcoma
Pseudotumor of hemophilia	Bone destruction and periosteal reaction, occasionally mimics malignant tumor
Myositis ossificans	Features of parosteal or periosteal osteosarcoma
Brown tumor of hyperparathyroidism	Lytic bone lesion and resembling malignant tumor

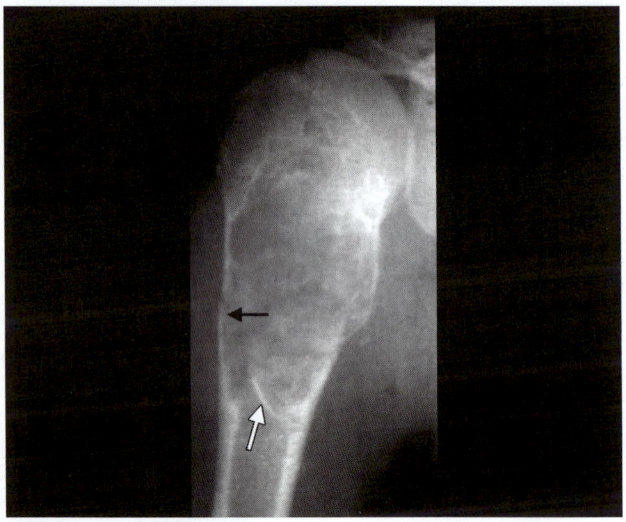

FIG. 11: Simple bone cyst involving humerus showing "fallen fragment" (white arrow) and "trap-door" (black arrow) signs.

ULTRASONOGRAPHY

It is of limited utility in the evaluation of primary osseous lesions. In particular, ultrasonography can be used for the initial evaluation of soft-tissue masses in patients with contraindications to MRI. Sonography can confirm the presence of the mass, characterizing it as solid or cystic, and assessing its dynamic features such as compressibility and vascularity. Perhaps one of the most widely used applications

TABLE 4: Lesions that should not be biopsied.

Tumors and tumor-like lesions	Non-neoplastic conditions
Fibrous cortical defect	Avulsion fracture (healing phase)
Nonossifying fibroma	Bone infarct
Periosteal (cortical) desmoid	Bone island (enostosis)
Small and solitary focus of fibrous dysplasia	Pseudotumor of hemophilia
Myositis ossificans	Degenerative and post-traumatic cysts
Intraosseous ganglion	Brown tumor of hyperparathyroidism
Enchondroma in a short, tubular bone	Discogenic vertebral sclerosis

of ultrasonography is image-guided intervention. Ultrasonography can be used to guide a minimally invasive technique to guide the placement of the needle during biopsy into an area of solid tissue. Ultrasound also plays an important role in detecting soft issue recurrence in postoperative cases, in patients with metallic implants.

COMPUTED TOMOGRAPHY ANALYSIS OF BONE LESIONS

Computed tomography gives better morphological assessment of the lesion as well as the surrounding area, thereby helping in the evaluation of lesion margin with great advantage. Hence, a lesion with well-defined border and localized within the cortex implies slow growth, while features of cortical destruction suggest aggressive nature of the lesion.

Like radiographic evaluation, CT also has a grading system for evaluating bone lesions:

- *Grade I*: Lesions within the bone or causing thinning of cortex and contained by thick periosteal new bone suggest slow growth process.
- *Grade II*: Lesions with localized destruction of cortex associated with periosteal reaction suggest aggressive nature.
- *Grade III:* Lesions completely penetrate through the cortex but show no localized bone destruction associated with soft tissue, suggest highly aggressive nature.

In the evaluation of focal bone lesion, CT is usually used to get "radiographic" evidence, in areas with complex anatomy, particularly for lesions in vertebrae and flat bones such as ilium, sacrum, and scapula[5] **(Figs. 12A and B)**. CT is better than radiography in showing the exact site of the lesion within the bone (medullary, cortical, periosteal, and parosteal). This is very useful for making the diagnosis of certain entities such as nonossifying fibroma and juxtacortical chondroma.

Computed tomography helps not only in defining the margins of the lesion but also helps in detecting subtle cortical alterations and sclerotic reactions. It has the superior ability to show subtle periosteal reactions that may not be visible on radiographs due to superimposition or inadequate contrast resolution. Additionally, CT plays a valuable role in detecting subtle matrix mineralization, making it a very useful modality in confirming the diagnosis of osteoid or chondroid forming lesions.[10]

Computed Tomography Grading System of Bone Lesions

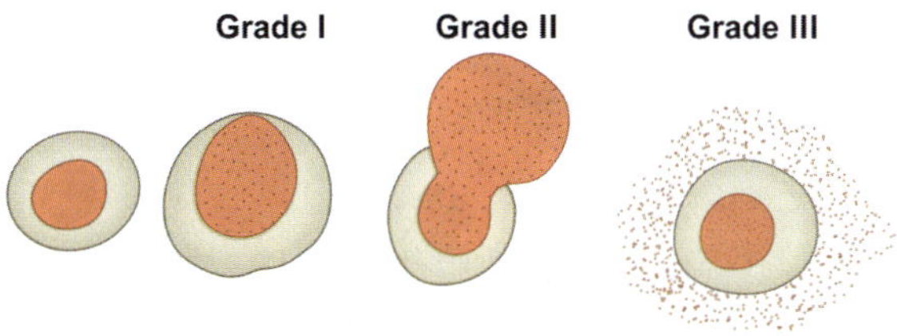

MAGNETIC RESONANCE IMAGING OF BONE LESIONS[11,12]

Magnetic resonance imaging is exquisitely sensitive to lesions that replace marrow and destroy bone. It shows the full extent of lesions and extension into soft tissues. MRI is of minor value in the estimation of the malignant potential of an osseous lesion. Although many bone tumors and tumor-like lesions present similar morphology at MRI, some entities can be diagnosed with good reliability. These include chondrogenic tumors **(Fig. 13A)**, solitary **(Fig. 13B)**, and aneurysmal bone cysts **(Fig. 13C)**; GCTs; lesions containing fatty tissue; and, to a certain extent, osteoid osteomas and osteoblastomas.

The differential diagnosis for benign bone lesions surrounded by extensive marrow edema includes osteoid osteoma/osteoblastoma, chondroblastoma, Langerhans cell histiocytosis, and osteomyelitis. As a general (but not absolute) guideline, the greater the extent of surrounding marrow edema, the more likely the bone lesion is benign. Marrow edema may be present around malignant bone tumors, as well, in which case it constitutes the reactive zone of the tumor.

However, its main role is for preoperative staging of tumor extent (precise compartmental localization), involvement of critical structures such as joints and neurovascular bundles and also plays a vital role in detection of skip lesions **(Fig. 13D)**.

Magnetic resonance imaging is particularly useful to evaluate aggressive lesions such as malignant tumors and infective lesions **(Fig. 13E)**. It depicts transcortical infiltration which is a sign of highly aggressive lesions **(Fig. 13F)**. It also depicts intratrabecular infiltration, a sign of infiltrative growth in case of malignant bone tumor. It also shows active tumor growth in periosteal and endosteal extension at tumor margins. Unless it is contraindicated, contrast should be administered when evaluating soft-tissue component of bone tumor. Contrast enhancement delineates areas of necrosis within the lesion.

CONCLUSION

- The guidelines mentioned in this chapter usually permit us to make a correct diagnosis or offer a narrow differential diagnosis **(Flowchart 1)**.
- The pattern of bone destruction, margins, cortical response, location, and site of lesion on radiographs helps in the differential diagnosis of bone tumor and tumor-like lesions.

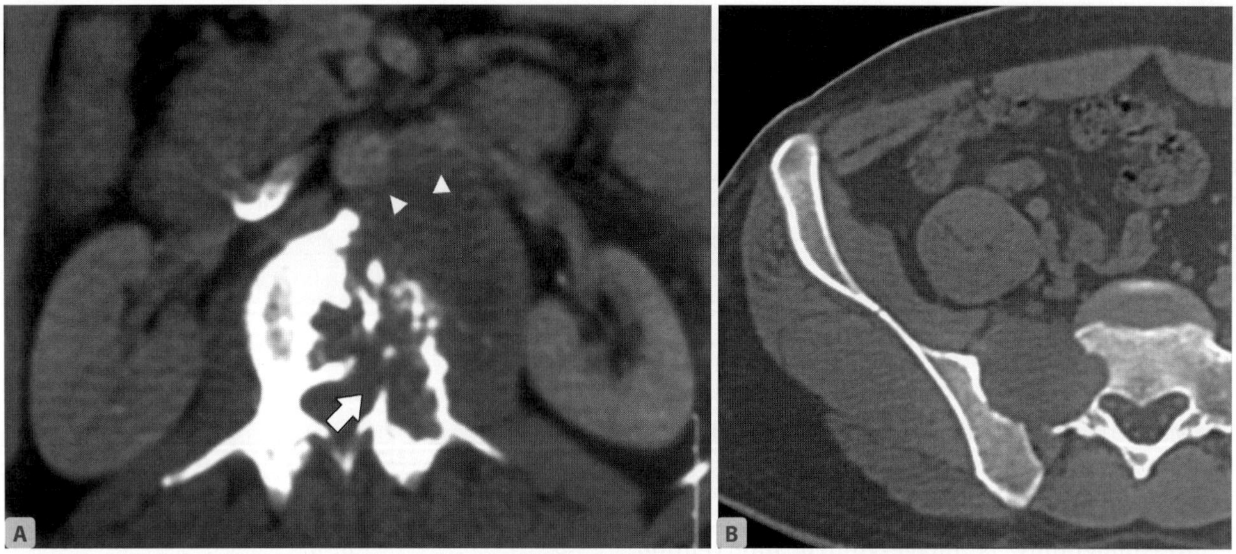

FIGS. 12A AND B: Role of CT scan in assessment of focal bone lesion: (A) Axial CT of the lumbar vertebra at the level of the renal hilum shows marked tumoral destruction of the left half of the vertebral body and the left pedicle by a proven chondrosarcoma. Matrix mineralization and residual trabeculae are seen inside. The tumor is extending into the left psoas muscle and is lifting the aorta and the left renal vain anteriorly (arrowheads). The fat plane with the aorta is obliterated. Posteromedially, the mass is extending into the spinal canal and causing an impression on the theca (arrow); (B) Axial CT section of sacrum showing expansile lytic lesion in right sacral ala a case of giant cell tumor.

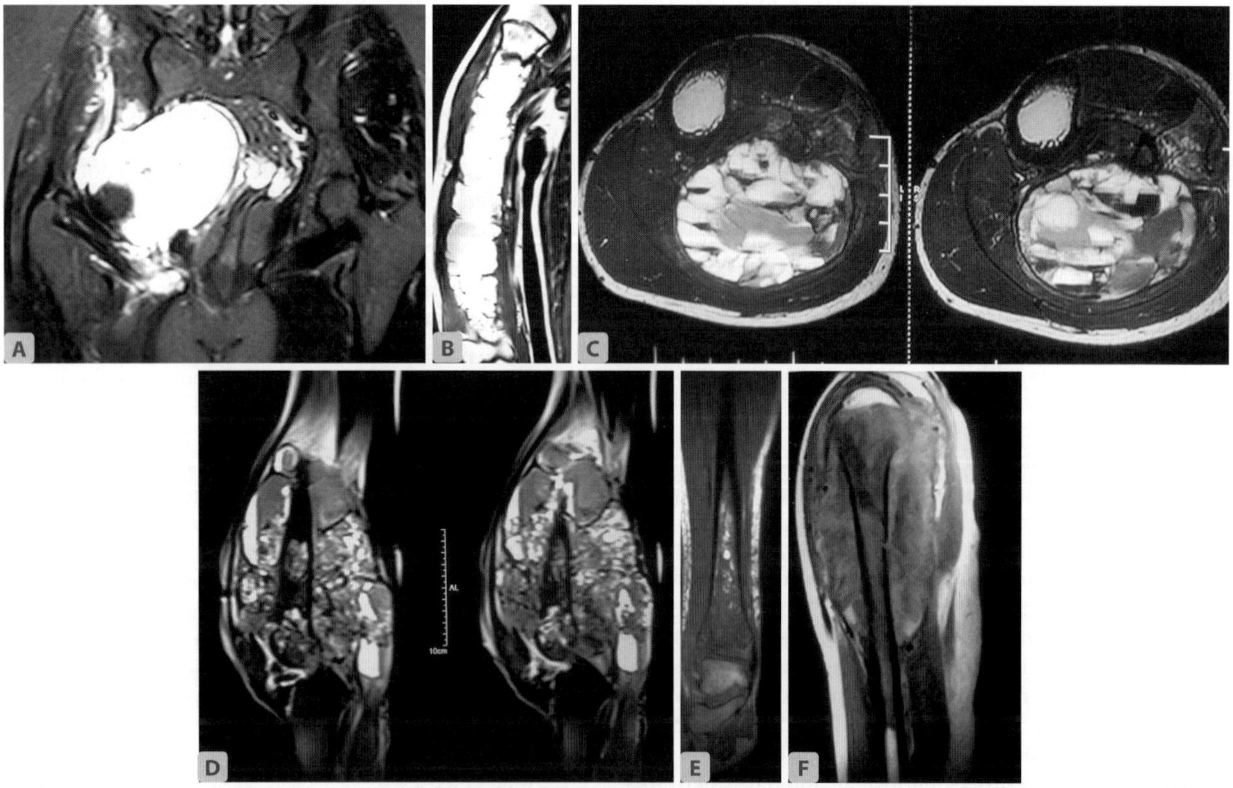

FIGS. 13A TO F: Role of magnetic resonance imaging (MRI) in assessment of focal bone lesion. (A) Coronal T2-weighted (T2W) MR image showing brightly hyperintense lobulated mass lesion arising from the right acetabulum in elderly patient suggestive of chondrosarcoma; (B) Coronal short tau inversion recovery (STIR) MR image showing elongated hyperintense lesion involving the shaft of humerus in a child suggestive of simple bone cyst; (C) Axial T2W MR image showing expansile lesion with multiple blood fluid levels suggestive of aneurysmal bone cyst; (D) Sagittal T2W MR image of a patient with biopsy-proven case of osteosarcoma showing altered signal intensity involving the metaepiphysis of lower end of femur associated with large soft tissue component which is extending into knee joint; (E) Coronal T1-weighted (T1W) image of a child with osteomyelitis showing heterogenous signal intensity involving the diaphysis, metaphysis, and epiphysis of lower end of tibia suggestive of aggressive lesion; (F) Sagittal T1W MR image of arm in patient with known case of osteosarcoma showing altered signal intensity involving upper end of humerus associated with large surrounding soft tissue component without obvious cortical destruction suggestive of transcortical infiltration.

FLOWCHART 1: Assessing focal bone lesion.

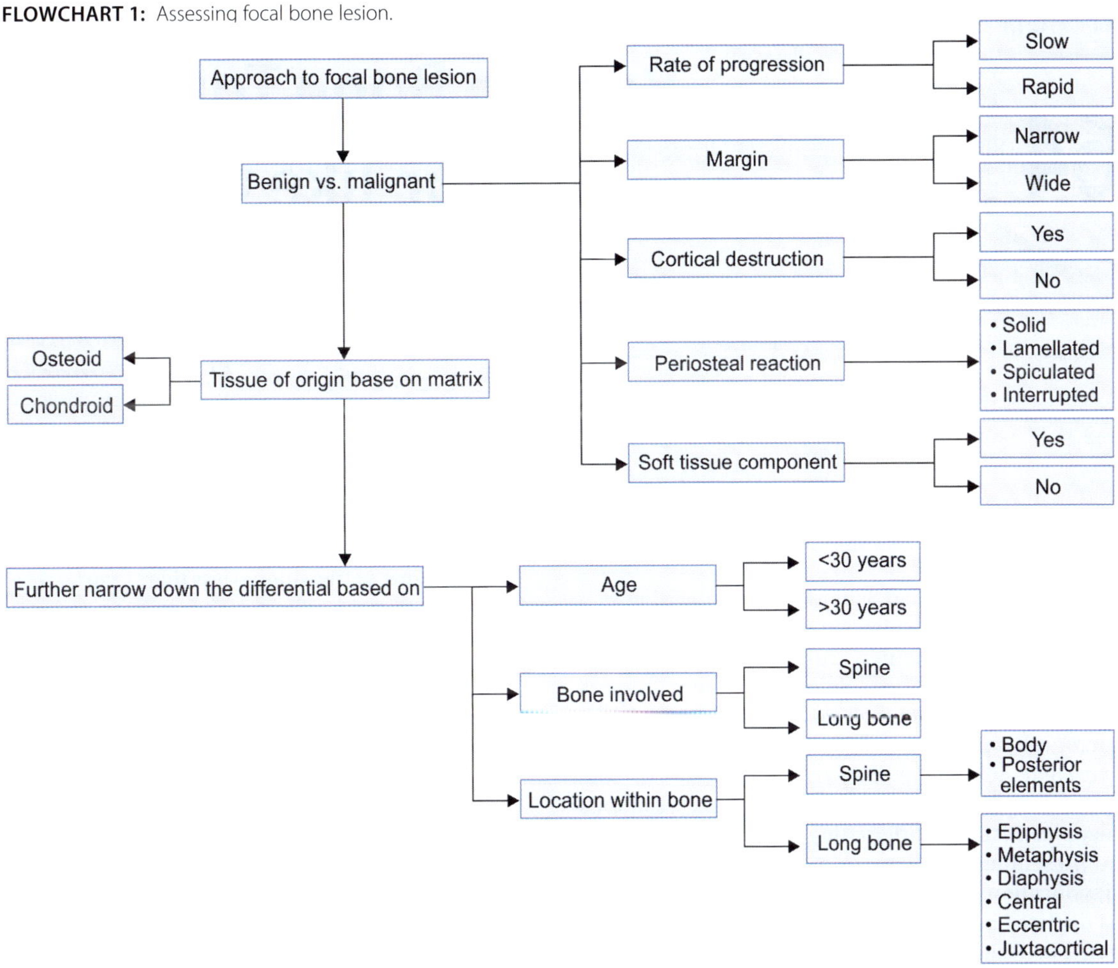

- Because of high specificity in detecting lesion features, radiography is integrated with clinical findings that allows the differential diagnosis between neoplastic and non-neoplastic lesions including trauma (healing or stress fractures, myositis ossificans), infection (acute osteomyelitis, Brodie's abscess), eosinophilic granuloma, such as Brown tumors of hyperthyroidism.
- Radiography is not sufficient to evaluate the lesions in complex anatomical sites such as spine, pelvis, and scapula nor does it define the intra- and extraosseous extent of the tumor. In such cases, cross-sectional imaging such as CT and MRI helps to define the extent of lesions.
- The radiologist should never interpret the CT or MRI of a suspected bone tumor without first reviewing the plain radiographs. The orthopedic surgeon, radiologist, and pathologist must collaborate as a multidisciplinary team to make the diagnosis more accurately and improve patient care.

REFERENCES

1. O'Donnel P. Evaluation of focal bone lesions: basic principles and clinical scenarios. Imaging. 2003;15(4):298-323.
2. Miller TT. Bone tumors and tumorlike conditions: analysis with conventional radiography. Radiology. 2008;246(3):662-74.
3. Madewell JE, Ragsdale BD, Sweet DE. Radiologic and pathologic analysis of solitary bone lesions. I. Internal margins. Radiol Clin North Am. 1981;19(4):715-48.
4. Ragsdale BD, Madewell JE, Sweet DE. Radiologic and pathologic analysis of solitary bone lesions. II. Periosteal reactions. Radiol Clin North Am. 1981;19(4):749-83.
5. Brown KT, Kattapuram SV, Rosenthal DI. Computed tomography analysis of bone tumors: patters of cortical destruction and soft tissue extension. Skeletal Radiol. 1986;15(6): 448-51.
6. Sweet DE, Madewell JE, Ragsdale BD. Radiologic and pathologic analysis of solitary bone lesions. III. Matrix patterns. Radiol Clin North Am. 1981;19(4):785-814.
7. Priolo F, Cerase A. The current role of radiography in the assessment of skeletal tumors and tumor-like lesions. Eur J Radiol. 1998; 27(Suppl 1):S77-85.
8. Moser RP, Madewell JE. An approach to primary bone tumors. Radiol Clin North Am. 1987;25(6):1049-93.
9. Ma LD, Frassica FJ, Scott WW, Fishman EK, Zerhouni EA. Differentiation of benign and malignant musculoskeletal tumors: potential pitfalls with MR imaging. Radiographics. 1995;15(2):349-66.
10. Woertler K. Benign bone tumors and tumor-like lesions value of cross-sectional imaging. Eur Radiol. 2003;13(8):1820-35.
11. Pettersson H, Gillespy T 3rd, Hamlin DJ, Enneking WF, Springfield DS, Andrew ER, et al. Primary musculoskeletal tumors: examination with MR imaging compared with conventional modalities. Radiology. 1987;164(1):237-41.
12. Zimmer WD, Berquist TH, McLeod RA, Sim FH, Pritchard DJ, Shives TC, et al. Bone tumors: magnetic resonance imaging versus computed tomography. Radiology. 1985;155(3):709-18.

CHAPTER

164

Benign Bone Tumors and Tumor-like Conditions

Mahesh Prakash, Anindita Sinha, Akshay Kumar Saxena

INTRODUCTION

Bone tumors may be defined as a new growth arising in a bone or derived from cells which are components of skeletal tissue.[1] The majority of benign true tumors of bone are detected in children and young adults. Benign bone tumors can be classified according to their matrix production and/or predominant cell type into cartilage forming, bone forming, fibrous, vascular, and other connective tissue lesions.[2,3] The term "tumor-like lesions of bone" denotes various conditions of non-neoplastic nature originating from or affecting the bone and presenting as solitary or multiple bone lesions. A broad classification of benign bone tumor and tumor-like lesions is depicted in **Table 1**. For diagnosis of bone tumors and tumor-like lesion, there is need for close cooperation of radiologist, orthopedician, and pathologists; however, the role of radiologist is most important. The primary aim of imaging should be to make specific diagnosis (if possible) or narrowing of the differential diagnosis which can be a guide for further intervention and management.

IMAGING MODALITIES

Before radiological evaluation, consideration of patient's data (age, gender) and clinical information of concerned patient are very useful for diagnosis as many lesions of bone show predilection for particular age group and gender.[2,3]

Radiography

Despite availability of a host of imaging modalities, plain radiographs continue to play a major role in the diagnostic evaluation of bone neoplasms. Plain radiographs demonstrate location of the tumor in the body; segment involved—whether epiphysis, metaphysis, or diaphysis; growth characters of the lesion such as margin—well-defined/ill-defined; presence or absence of periosteal reaction and the appearance of tumor matrix—whether calcified or not, which are all important parameters to arrive at a proper diagnosis.

The pointers to the benign nature of a bone tumor include the following:

- Area of geographic bone destruction which is well-circumscribed and is characterized by a sharp transition between the destroyed area and the normal bone (i.e., narrow zone of transition—less than 1 cm).
- Sclerotic margin indicates slow growth and is generally seen in benign lesions located at the metaphysis. Certain tumors stimulate surrounding sclerosis which may obscure the central lytic area such as osteoid osteoma.
- *Periosteal reaction*: In general, periosteal reaction is not a feature of benign bone tumors unless a fracture has occurred except in a very few lesions such as osteoblastoma, osteoid osteoma, and chondromyxoid fibroma. Periosteal reaction is radiographically described as solid or interrupted. Solid periosteal reaction is defined

TABLE 1: Benign bone tumors and tumor-like lesions.[4]

Benign bone tumors	Tumor-like lesions
Bone-forming tumors • Enostosis • Osteoma • Osteoid osteoma • Osteoblastoma	Fibro-osseous lesions • Nonossifying fibroma • Fibrous dysplasia • Osteofibrous dysplasia • Periosteal desmoid
Cartilage forming tumors • Enchondroma • Osteochondroma • Periosteal chondroma • Chondroblastoma • Chondromyxoid fibroma	Cystic lesions • Simple bone cyst • Aneurysmal bone cyst • Intraosseous ganglion • Epidermoid cyst • Subchondral cyst
Connective tissue tumors • Desmoplastic fibroma • Benign fibrous histiocytoma • Ossifying fibroma • Myxoma • Lipoma	Giant cell containing lesions • Giant cell reparative granuloma • Brown tumor • Pigmented villonodular synovitis
Vascular tumors • Hemangioma • Lymphangioma • Glomous tumor	Others • Eosinophilic granuloma • Pseudotumors
Others/semimalignant • Giant cell tumor • Ameloblastoma	

as a single layer of new bone >1 mm in thickness which is usually of uniform density. When seen, solid periosteal reaction indicates benign pathology.[1,3] It is seen in osteoid osteoma and osteoblastoma.

- *Tumor matrix*: Presence of calcification in the form of rings, flocculant patches, or stippled flecks point to the cartilaginous origin of the tumor. A ground-glass haze indicates fibrous lesions. Osteoid matrix is seen in bone-forming tumors.

Computed Tomography

Computed tomography (CT) can be used for radiographic information where conventional radiography has limited information such as in the region of complex anatomy and superimposition of bony elements (pelvis, spine, and scapula). CT is superior to radiography in determination of the epicenter of a bone lesion, whether it is in cortex, medulla, or periosteal in location.[3,5,6]

Other advantages of CT over radiography are to detect cortical alteration (breech, scalloping, expansion) and detection of periosteal reaction. CT is most valuable imaging modality in detection of subtle matrix calcifications and therefore it is very useful for diagnosis of a bone- or cartilage-forming benign bone tumor.[3-6]

Magnetic Resonance Imaging

Magnetic resonance imaging (MRI) is the most accurate method for demonstrating extent of tumors especially intramedullary component.[7] MRI has also demonstrated significant potential for tumor characterization. On T1-weighted (T1W) images, most bone tumors show decrease in signal intensity because of marked contrast with hyperintense fat of the marrow. On T2-weighted (T2W) images most of the tumors are of high-intensity making it difficult to separate tumor from fat but easy to differentiate tumor from surrounding muscles. Presence of atypical signal patterns help in predicting a dominant tissue component, e.g., high-signal intensity on T1W images may be due to fat, as seen in lipoma, hemangioma, medullary bone infarct or hemorrhage as seen in aneurysmal bone cyst.[8]

Magnetic resonance is the best technique for demarcating the soft tissue component of bone tumors and its relationship to adjacent joint and neurovascular structures.[7,8]

Generally, only few bone tumors have a classical radiological picture. Similarly, biopsy of the lesion is not always the ultimate answer. On the other hand, some tumors are difficult to diagnose histologically but have a typical radiographic appearance, e.g., osteoid osteoma. Others with unusual radiographic features exhibit a characteristic histological appearance, e.g., aneurysmal bone cysts. Thus, close correlation of clinical history, histology, and radiology are always essential to achieve highest diagnostic accuracy.

BONE-FORMING TUMORS

Enostosis

These lesions are commonly known as "bony islands" are usually asymptomatic. Histologically, bony islands consist of dense intramedullary lamellar bone with normal haversian canals. Enostosis is commonly found in spine, ribs, and pelvis.[9] It is usually seen as oval, densely sclerotic intramedullary lesions. Usually a bone island is aligned in the long axis of trabeculae **(Figs. 1A and B)**. Its only significance lies in the fact that it may be confused with osteoblastic metastases. Scintigraphy and MRI are helpful in the differentiation, as bony islands usually do not exhibit an increase tracer uptake on bone scans. On MRI, enostosis shows hypointense signal on both T1W and T2W sequences **(Figs. 2A and B)** while sclerotic metastasis shows halo of surrounding marrow edema on fluid sensitive sequences.[10]

Osteoma

Histologically, an osteoma is composed of both dense and woven bone and arises from the cortex. Common sites include

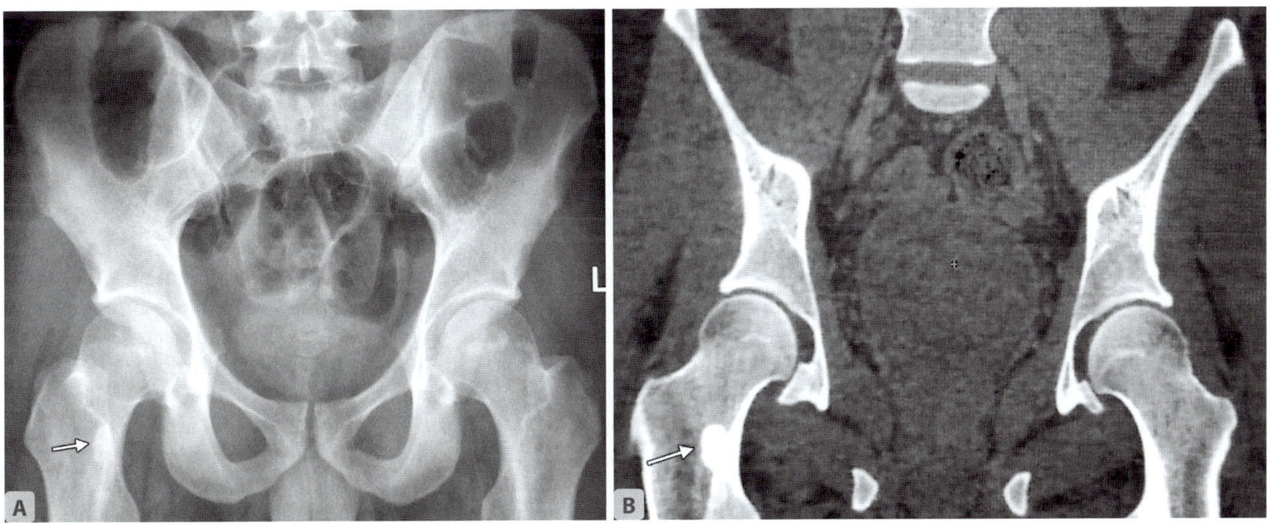

FIGS. 1A AND B: Enostosis. Radiograph (A) and CT coronal reconstruction (B) of pelvis show well-defined oval sclerotic lesion (arrow) in intertrochanteric region of right femur.

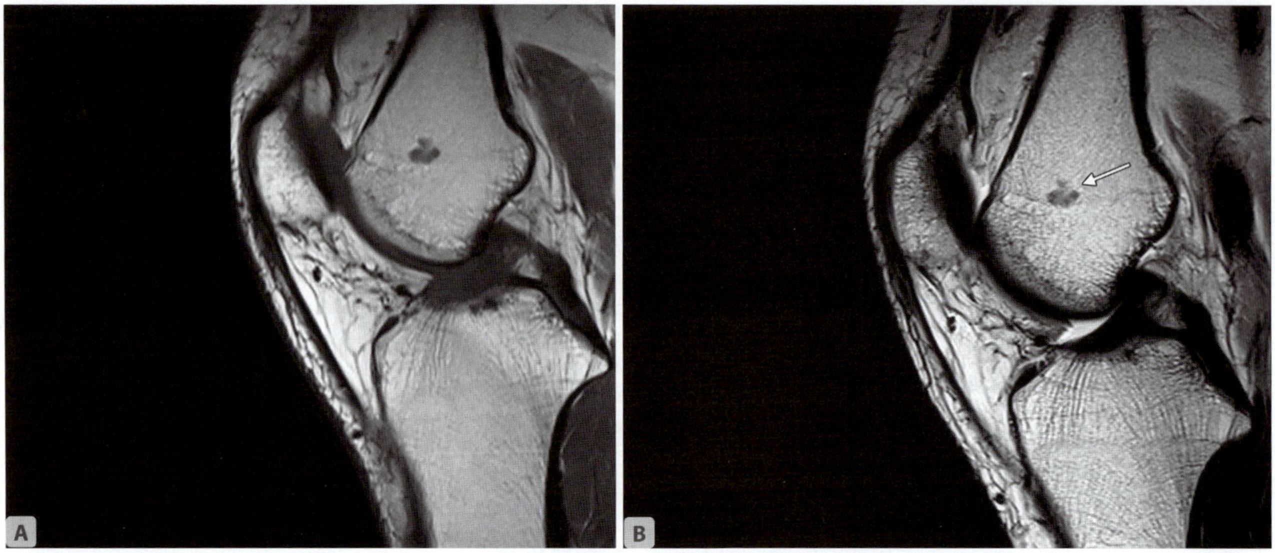

FIGS. 2A AND B: Enostosis. T1W (A) and T2W (B) sagittal MR images show well-defined lobulated lesion in lower end of femur which shows hypointense signal on both sequences (arrow).

outer table of skull, paranasal sinuses (frontal/ethmoid), and mandible. They are generally asymptomatic, but may cause sinus obstruction, proptosis, etc. Radiologically, osteoma is seen as a well-circumscribed lesion arises from the cortex, which protrudes from the surface of the affected bone. It demonstrates same density as cortex on X-ray and CT scan **(Fig. 3)**. On MRI, osteoma shows hypointense signal on both T1W and T2W images.[11] Multiple osteomas occur as a part of Gardner's syndrome.

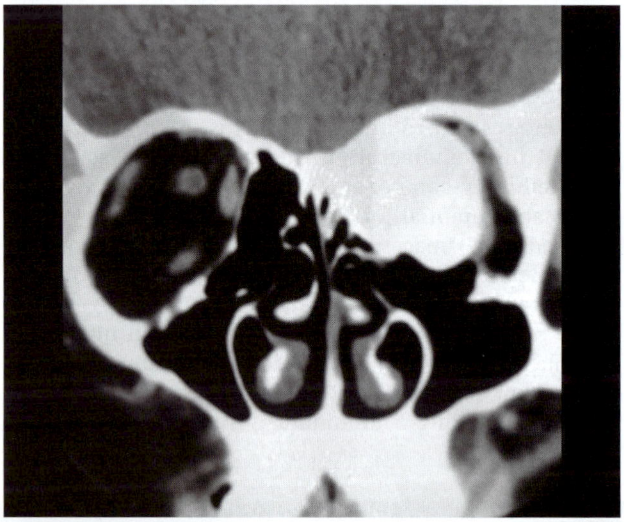

FIG. 3: Large osteoma. CT scan (coronal section) of paranasal sinus shows large well-defined bony lesion arising from ethmoid sinus causing compression of left orbital structures.

Osteoid Osteoma

Osteoid osteoma is a fairly common tumor, accounting for approximately 10–12% of all benign tumors.[12] These tumors usually affects patients between 5 and 25 years of age. Clinically most patients presents with pain that is especially severe at night and relieved by aspirin or other nonsteroidal anti-inflammatory agents.

More than half of tumors are located in proximal femur and tibia. They occur less frequently in the upper extremities than in the lower extremities. Osteoid osteoma also frequently affects the tubular bones of the hands and feet. They are however, less common in the spine, where they affect the posterior arches of the vertebrae. Histologically, the lesion consists of a nidus which is usually less than 1 cm in diameter and surrounded by variable degree of sclerotic bone depending upon location. The nidus contains interlacing trabeculae at various stages of ossification within a stroma of loose, vascular connective tissue. Osteoid osteoma can be cortical (the most common type), cancellous or medullary, and subperiosteal.[11] The latter two types produce less sclerotic bone than those in the cortex do, making radiologic diagnosis difficult.

Radiographically, the lesion appears as well-defined lytic lesion, surrounded by reactive sclerosis **(Figs. 4A and B)**. Nidus may be purely radiolucent or contain a dense center. Intraarticular osteoid osteomas may be either cancellous or periosteal and have little reactive bone or periosteal new bone formation.[11]

Computed tomography is very useful in showing the nidus, which can vary in its degree of ossification. CT appears to display the nidus better than MRI. Intense bone marrow edema adjacent to nidus is very useful to detect and localized the lesion on MRI **(Fig. 5)**; however, nidus may not readily visible if it is very small.[13] The tumor nidus typically shows hypo- to intermediate signal on T1W images and low to high signal on T2W images. The nidus shows enhancement with gadolinium. Intra-articular osteoid osteomas produce joint effusions and synovial proliferation. Radionuclide bone scans have been used for many years to help diagnosis of osteoid osteomas. Bone scintigraphy, which is a highly sensitive

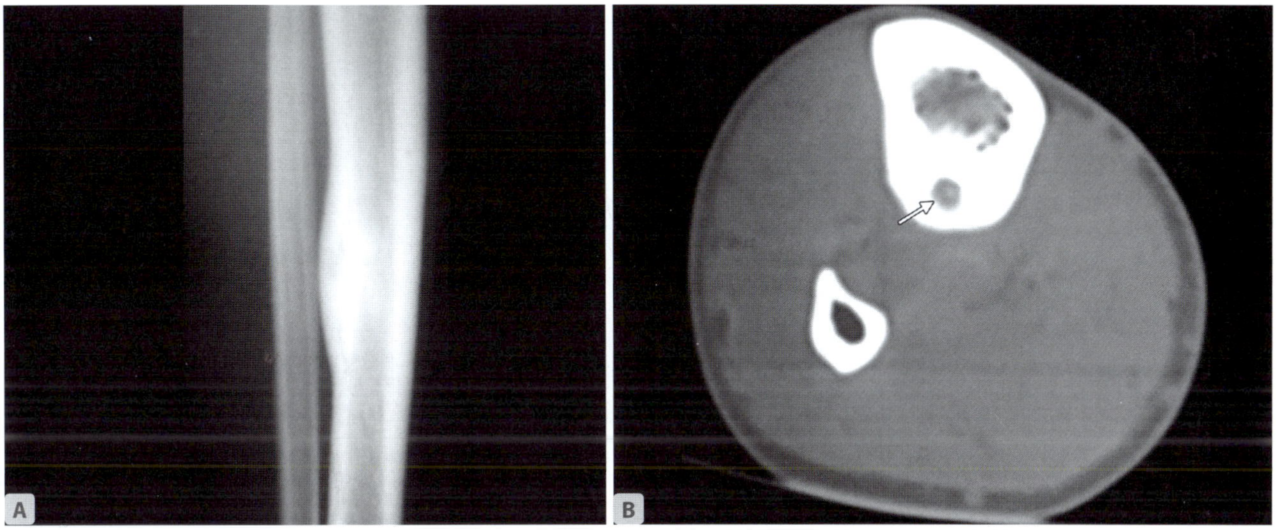

FIGS. 4A AND B: Osteoid osteoma. (A) Radiograph of leg shows dense sclerosis and solid periosteal reaction in the diaphysis of tibia; (B) CT scan (axial section) reveals well-defined lytic lesion with calcified nidus (arrow) associated with gross adjacent sclerosis.

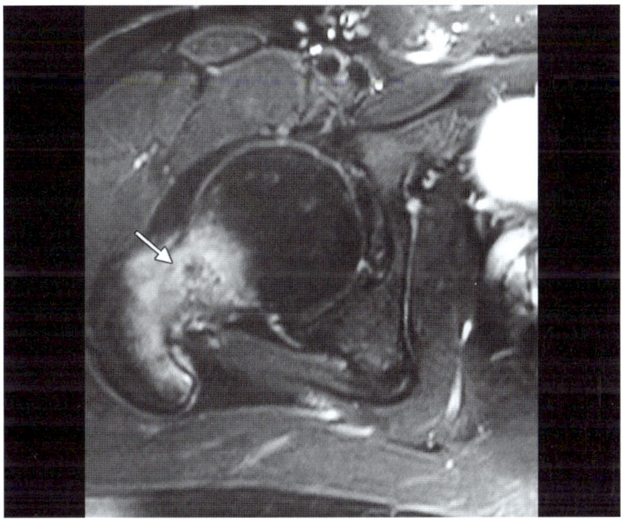

FIG. 5: Osteoid osteoma. T2W fat suppressed MRI (axial section) shows small nidus in neck of femur associated with extensive surrounding edema.

method of detecting osteoid osteoma, typically shows increased flow to the lesion on immediate images and a focus of increased activity on skeletal equilibrium images with double density sign.[14] Many times, osteomyelitis can mimick osteoid osteoma clinically as well radiographically, however, presence of soft tissue extension favors the diagnosis of osteomyelitis.

Osteoblastoma

Osteoblastomas are rare bone-forming tumors and most commonly occurs in patients in the second and third decade of life. This tumor is more common in males than in females. Histologically, the osteoblastoma is closely related to osteoid osteomas except that bony trabeculae are broader and longer with absence of surrounding sclerotic halo. Size is an important consideration in distinguishing between these two types of tumors. If the size of lesion is less than 2 cm in diameter than it is likely of be osteoid osteomas, whereas tumors larger than 2 cm are usually osteoblastoma.[15]

The most common location of osteoblastoma is spine where it classically affects posterior elements **(Figs. 6A to C)**. The other common locations are proximal femur and talus. On plain X-ray, spinal osteoblastoma is osteolytic lesion with destruction of overlying cortex and may extend to in the spinal canal. In the long bones, osteoblastoma appears radiologically as round or oval lucent tumors in the medulla. Periosteal reaction is common. CT demonstrates extent of lesion in complex bony structures such as spine and pelvis better than radiography. MRI features may be nonspecific but helps to determine extension of vertebral lesion into spinal canal and spinal foramina.[16]

CARTILAGE-FORMING TUMORS

Osteochondroma

Osteochondromas are common lesions of the growing skeleton. It is the most common benign neoplasm and constitutes 20–50% of all benign tumors.[17] They arise from bony metaphysis with cartilage cap covering. These tumors are either pedunculated or sessile **(Fig. 7)**. Multiple osteochondroma occur as a manifestation of diaphyseal aclasia, an inherited disorder with autosomal dominance **(Fig. 8)**. The long axis of the osteochondroma pedicle or stalk is almost always directed away from the adjacent joint. The direct communication between the osteochondroma and the cortex and marrow cavity of the bone from which it arises is a distinctive feature, that is particularly well demonstrated on CT and MRI. T2W proton density (PD) MR images are useful to demonstrate a cartilaginous cap **(Figs. 9A and B)**. The cap can be quite thick in early childhood like the normal physis,

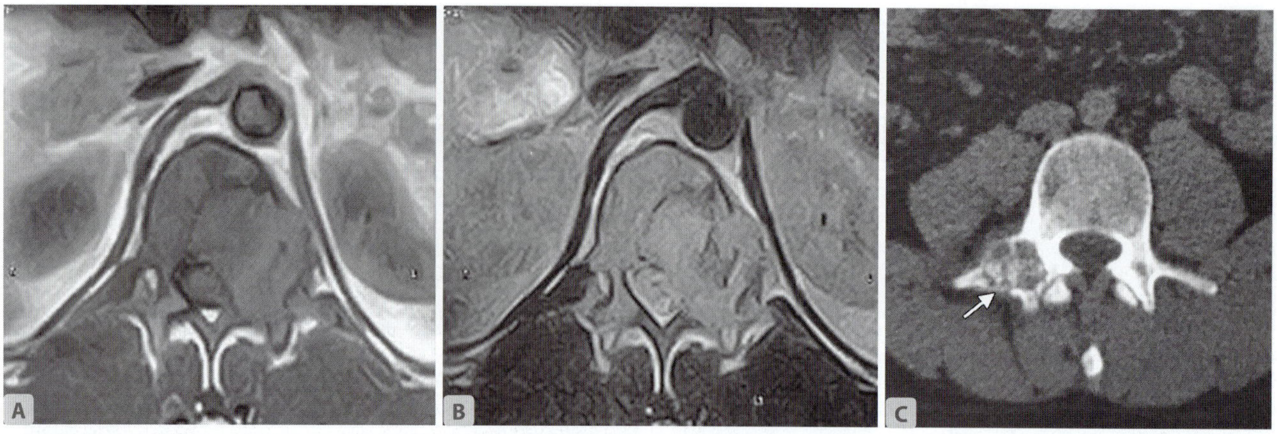

FIGS. 6A TO C: Osteoblastoma. (A and B) T1W and T2W MR (axial section) images reveal heterogeneous signal mass lesion, predominantly involving posterior elements of vertebra extending into spinal canal; (C) CT scan of spine of another patient shows expansile lytic lesion in right posterior elements with internal matrix mineralization suggestive of osteoblastoma.

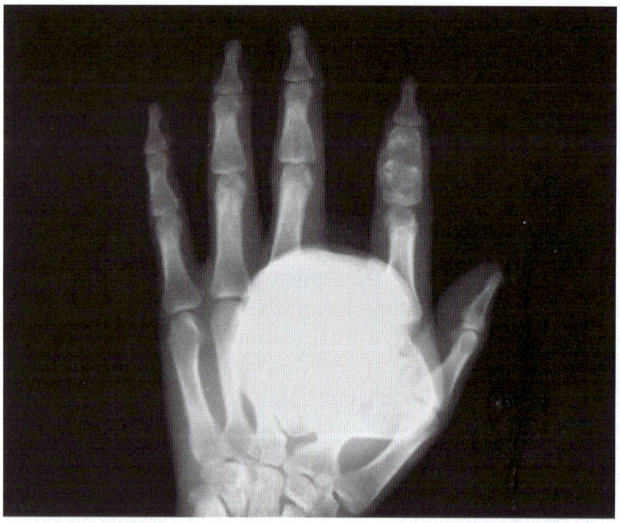

FIG. 7: Sessile osteochondroma. Radiograph of the left hand shows a large well-defined calcified lesion having a broad-based attachment to second metacarpal. An enchondroma showing typical central spotty calcification is also present in the middle phalanx of the index finger.

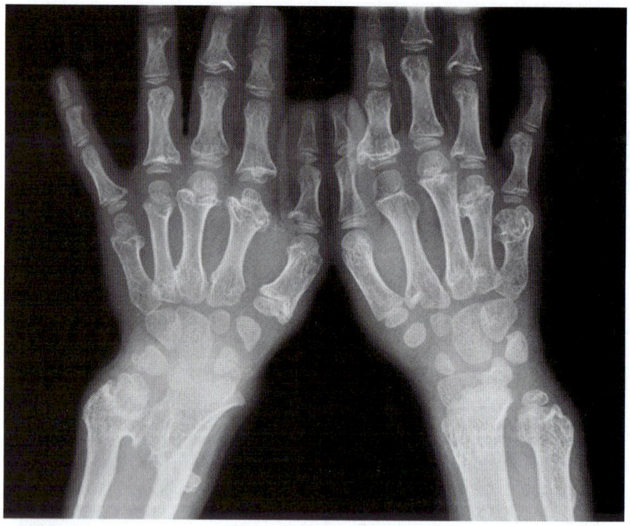

FIG. 8: Diaphyseal aclasia. Radiograph of bilateral hands (PA view) shows multiple osteochondromas and deformities involving multiple bones of hands and forearm.

becomes thinner with age. After epiphyseal closure, growth of the osteochondroma ceases. Because most osteochondromas are asymptomatic, they are usually discovered incidentally. However, mechanical irritation of adjacent soft tissues or nerves, vascular injuries, fracture of the stalk, or malignant transformation can produce symptoms.

Malignant transformation into low-grade chondrosarcoma occurs in 1% of osteochondromas; however, the risk is 10–30% in cases of multiple osteochondromatosis.[17] Malignant transformation should be considered when the osteochondroma grows after epiphyseal closure. Malignancy occurs in the cartilaginous cap, which becomes thickened. After skeletal maturity, the cartilage cap should not be thicker than 2 cm. Pain and cartilage cap growth are the signs of malignant transformation.[10]

Enchondroma

Enchondromas accounts for 12% of benign bone tumors.[18] These are most frequently located in the large and small tubular bones of the hands and feet **(Fig. 10)**. Like other cartilaginous tumors, enchondromas exhibit a lobulated growth pattern that results in asymmetric expansion of the medullary cavity and endosteal scalloping. Tumor matrix may be radiolucent or show calcification. Characteristic cartilaginous ring and arc pattern of calcifications is seen on radiographs and CT images. On MRI, the tumor is isointense to muscle on T1W and exhibits a heterogeneous, predominantly high T2W signal.[19] Contrast-enhanced MRI may demonstrate a pattern of thin arcs and rings.

Ollier's disease is a nonheritable disorder of cartilage proliferation in which enchondromas involve multiple

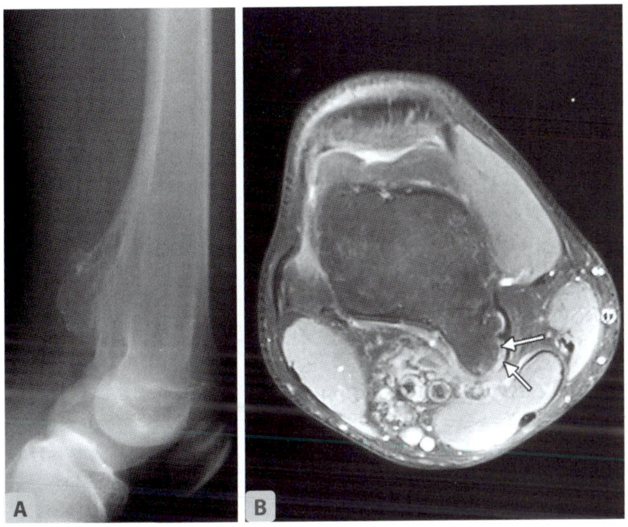

FIGS. 9A AND B: Pedunculated osteochondroma. (A) Radiograph of lower end of femur (lateral view) shows large well-defined bony outgrowth, with broad-based attachment to femur; (B) MRI (Proton density fat saturation, axial section) of the same patient shows clear demonstration of continuity of marrow and cortex of host bone into osteochondroma with covering cartilage cap (arrows).

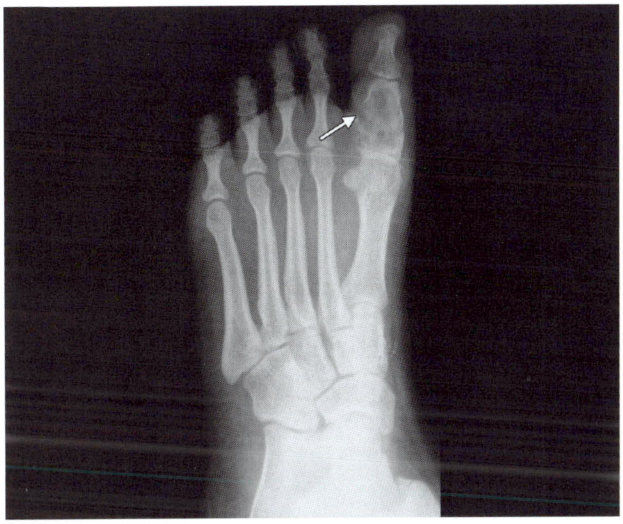

FIG. 10: Enchondroma. Radiograph of foot shows sharply demarcated expansile lesion in proximal phalanx of great toe having endosteal scalloping and cortical breech (arrow).

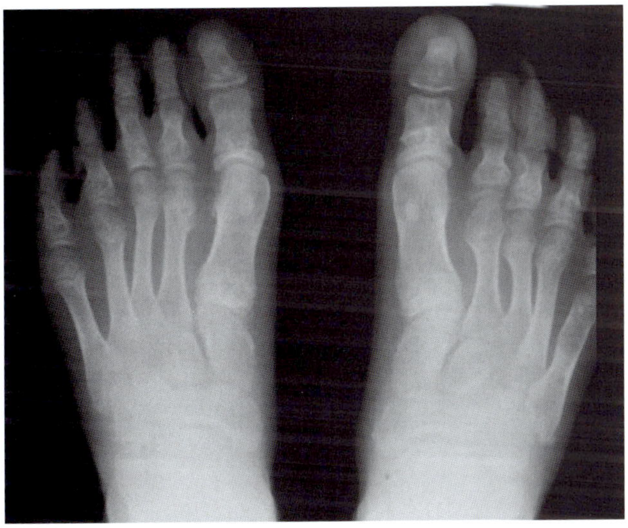

FIG. 11: Ollier's disease. Radiograph of feet shows relatively well-defined expansile lytic lesions involving most of the phalanges, with varying amounts of calcification within them.

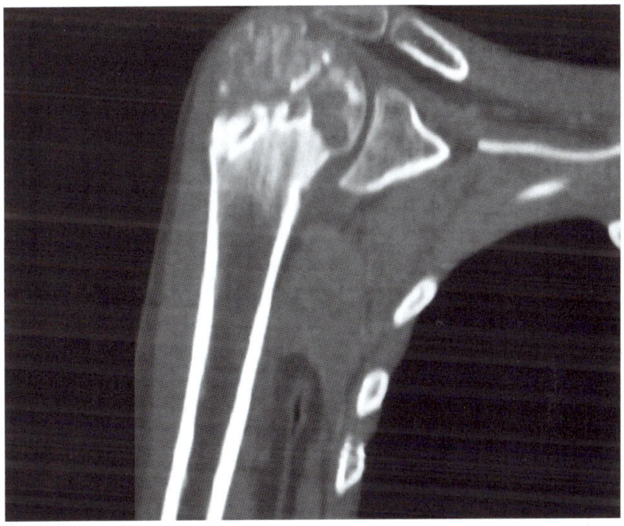

FIG. 12: Chondroblastoma. CT scan (coronal reformation) shows expansile lytic lesion in epiphysis (characteristic location) of upper humerus with matrix calcification.

bones, especially those of the hands and may result in skeletal deformity **(Fig. 11)**. Enchondromatosis accompanied by multiple hemangiomas is known as Maffucci syndrome. Calcified phleboliths may be demonstrated radiographically in the hemangiomatous soft tissue masses. Lesions associated with both Ollier disease and Maffucci syndrome carry a significant risk of malignant degeneration.[20]

Chondroblastoma

It is less common than enchondroma. Chondroblastoma is composed of primitive cartilage cells, usually occurs in the age group of 10–25 years. It is typically located in epiphysis and apophysis of bone, most often the proximal humerus, distal femur, and proximal tibia.[17] On plain X-ray, chondroblastoma is an eccentric, lucent, well-defined lesion with sclerotic borders. Periosteal reaction, far from the lesion is another common feature suggesting an accompanying inflammatory process. Approximately, one-third of chondroblastoma have a calcified matrix which can be better seen on CT scan **(Fig. 12)**.

The tumor shows signal intensity similar to that of muscle on MRI; however, the rim of the tumor has lower signal intensity. On T2W images, the signal intensity of the tumor is low to intermediate. This tumor also shows extensive surrounding inflammation which may be confused with more aggressive lesion. Malignant transformation of chondroblastoma is extremely uncommon.[21] The differential diagnosis of epiphyseal lesions includes giant cell tumor (GCT), osteomyelitis, subchondral cyst, and Langerhans cell histiocytosis.

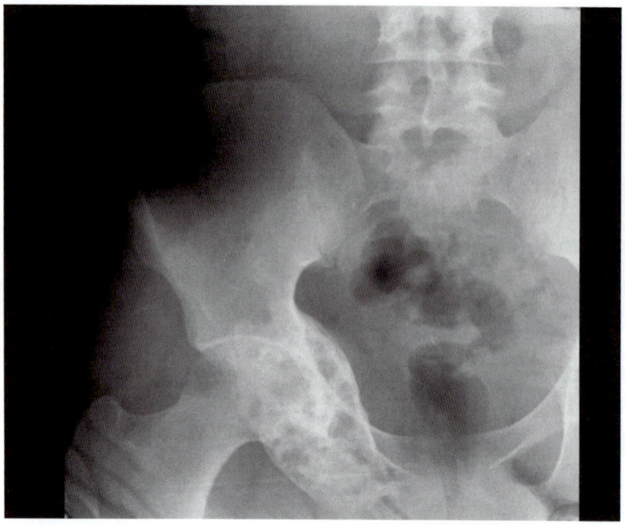

FIG. 13: Chondromyxoid fibroma. Radiograph of right hip shows large expansile lesion with sclerotic border and trabeculations involving right acetabulum.

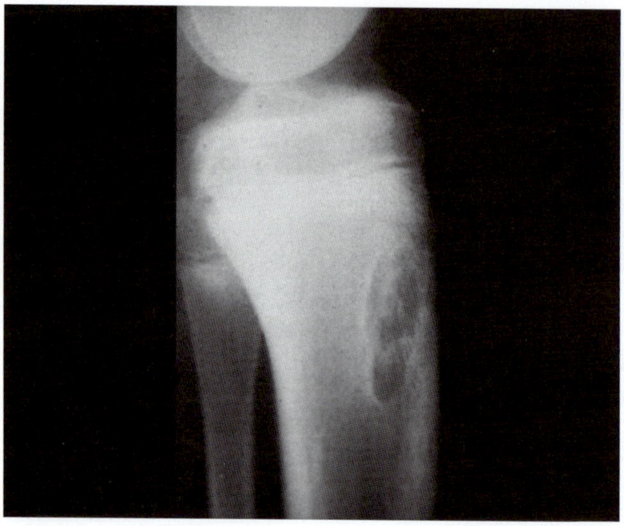

FIG. 14: Nonossifying fibroma. Lateral radiograph of leg shows an eccentric geographic lytic lesion in the medulla of proximal tibial metaphysis.

Chondromyxoid Fibroma

Chondromyxoid fibroma is rare and commonly affects males and patients younger than 35 years.[18] Histologically, it is composed of chondroid, myxoid, and fibrous tissue in varying amounts. The common locations of tumor are ilium, tibia, and bones of foot. These tumors are located characteristically in metadiaphyseal location unlike chondroblastoma and do not cross an open growth plate. On plain radiograph, it appears as a well-marginated central or eccentric lucent lesion, with sclerotic margins and cortical thinning **(Fig. 13)**. Half of the lesions may show parallel orientation to the long axis of the involved bone. Matrix calcification and periosteal new bone formation usually do not occur.

FIBROUS TUMORS/LESIONS

Fibrous Cortical Defects and Nonossifying Fibroma

Fibrous cortical defect and nonossifying fibroma are basically similar benign fibrous lesions located slightly differently, nonossifying fibroma being located eccentrically in the medullary cavity **(Fig. 14)**, and fibrous cortical defect seen superficially affecting the cortex **(Fig. 15)**. Pathologically, these lesions are composed of fibrous tissue, xanthoma cells, and giant cells. The common location of lesion is in the bones around the knee joints. These lesions are usually asymptomatic and do not require specific treatment. On plain radiography, the lesion appears as well-marginated eccentric lytic lesion with scalloped margin. Its inner border is often sclerotic and may appear multilocular due to corrugations. Differential diagnosis includes unicameral bone cyst, aneurysmal bone cyst, fibrous dysplasia, and chondromyxoid fibroma. The signal intensity of nonossifying fibroma is equal to or less than muscle on T1W MR images and hypointense on T2W images.[22] Postcontrast images usually show heterogeneous enhancement.

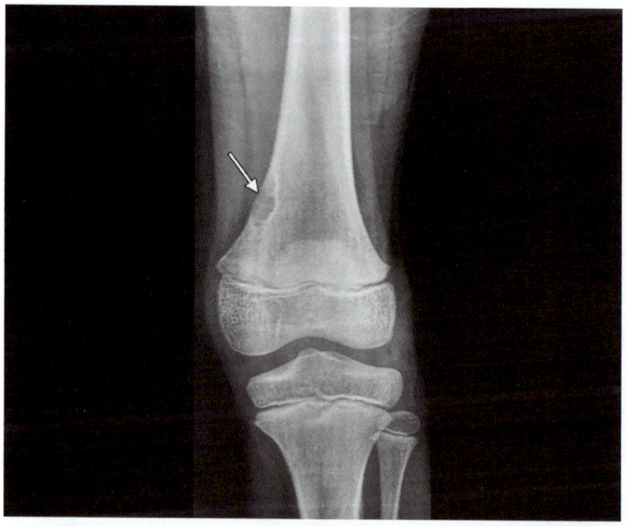

FIG. 15: Fibrous cortical defect. Radiograph of knee (AP view) shows eccentric well-defined lytic lesion in lower end of femur which is limited to cortex (arrow).

Fibrous Dysplasia

Fibrous dysplasia is a disorder where bone is replaced by abnormal fibrous tissue. Fibrous dysplasia can be monostotic, polyostotic, monomelic, or polymelic. It is more common in young females. It is occasionally seen in the first decade of life. In a small percentage of cases (2–3%), fibrous dysplasia is associated with endocrine disorders, especially precocious puberty in girls (McCune-Albright syndrome).[23,24] Although it is not a true neoplasm, fibrous dysplasia involving a long bone may mimic a bone tumor or cyst. This type of fibrous dysplasia causes expansion of the medullary cavity of tubular bones, endosteal scalloping, and trabeculation. The margin is sclerotic **(Fig. 16)**. The lesion may appear as ground glass or radiolucent, and this depends upon amount of fibrous tissue within the lesion. Bowing of the affected

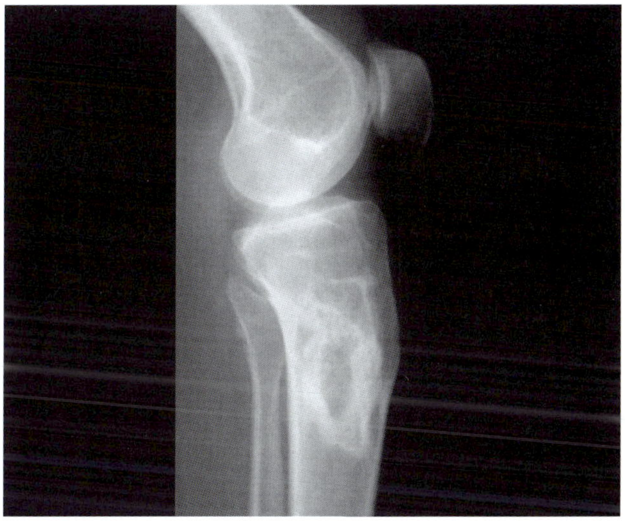

FIG. 16: Fibrous dysplasia. Lateral radiograph of knee joint shows a well-defined lytic lesion in proximal tibial metaphysis with surrounding sclerotic rind which is characteristic of fibrous dysplasia.

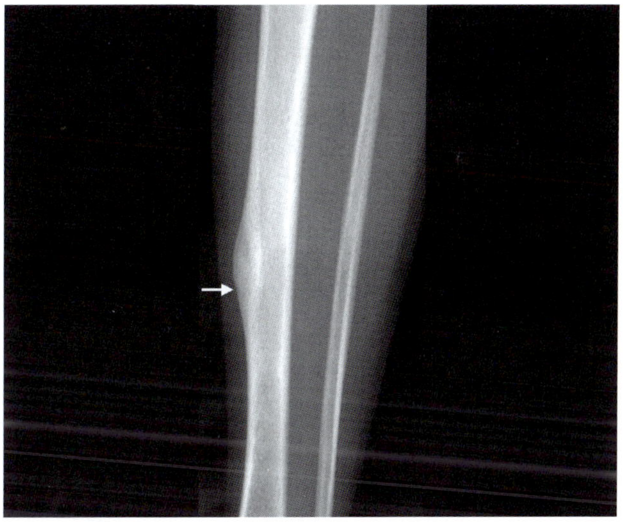

FIG. 18: Radiograph of leg shows well-defined lytic lesion in anterior cortex of tibia characteristic of osteofibrous dysplasia (arrow).

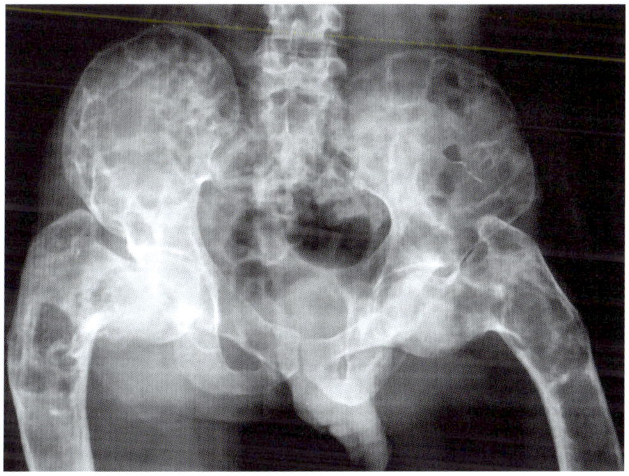

FIG. 17: Polyostotic fibrous dysplasia. Radiograph of pelvis shows multiple lytic lesions involving pelvic bones and bilateral femora with characteristic shepherd's crook deformity.

long bone may occur, when the affected bone is femur, the resulting deformity is called a "shepherd's crook" **(Fig. 17)**. Thinning and destruction of the bony cortex may be seen on CT or MR images. Soft tissue extension of the lesion is unusual. On T1W MR images, the signal intensity of fibrous dysplasia is similar to that of skeletal muscle. Although the signal of pure fibrous tissue is hypointense on T2W images, the signal of fibrous dysplasia is variable.

Osteofibrous Dysplasia

It is a rare lesion that is usually confined to the tibia but can also involve the fibula. Most cases occur during the first decade of life. On plain X-ray, the lesion appears as an eccentric, lucent, solitary, or multiloculated, lesion involving the anterior aspect of tibia **(Fig. 18)**. CT is very helpful in determining its intracortical location, an important feature in distinguishing osteofibrous dysplasia from fibrous dysplasia.[25]

Desmoplastic Fibroma

Desmoplastic fibroma is rare accounting for only 0.1% of benign bone tumors. This lesion is usually seen in the second and third decade of life. Histologically, there is infiltration of abnormal fibrous tissue in the bone and at times it is confused with low-grade fibrosarcoma of bone. They are mostly located in the metadiaphysis of long bones but may invade the epiphysis. Femur, tibia, and humerus are most commonly affected.[26] On radiography, the lesion has aggressive appearance and present as lytic expansile lesion with internal trabeculation and sclerotic margin. CT may demonstrate cortical breech and adjacent soft tissue if any. MRI typically shows intermediate to low signal on fluid sensitive sequences.[27]

VASCULAR AND CONNECTIVE TISSUE TUMORS

Hemangioma

Hemangioma is slowly growing lesions of bone composed of newly formed vascular spaces. About 50% of hemangiomas of bone occur in vertebrae and are most commonly located in lower thoracic and upper lumbar regions.[28] About 20% of hemangiomas occur in skull. Small bones of the hand and feet may also be affected.

Hemangioma of the vertebra has a typical radiographic picture in the form of coarse vertical striations on the plain radiographs and polka dot appearance on CT[29] **(Figs. 19A and B)**. It shows high intensity on both T1W and T2W images. In the skull, hemangioma generally affects the calvarium and is seen as an expansile lytic lesion which has a sunburst appearance with striations radiating from the center. In the short and long bones, the lesion lacks characteristic features and may be difficult to differentiate from other expansile central lesions such as aneurysmal bone cyst, chondromyxoid fibroma, or enchondroma.

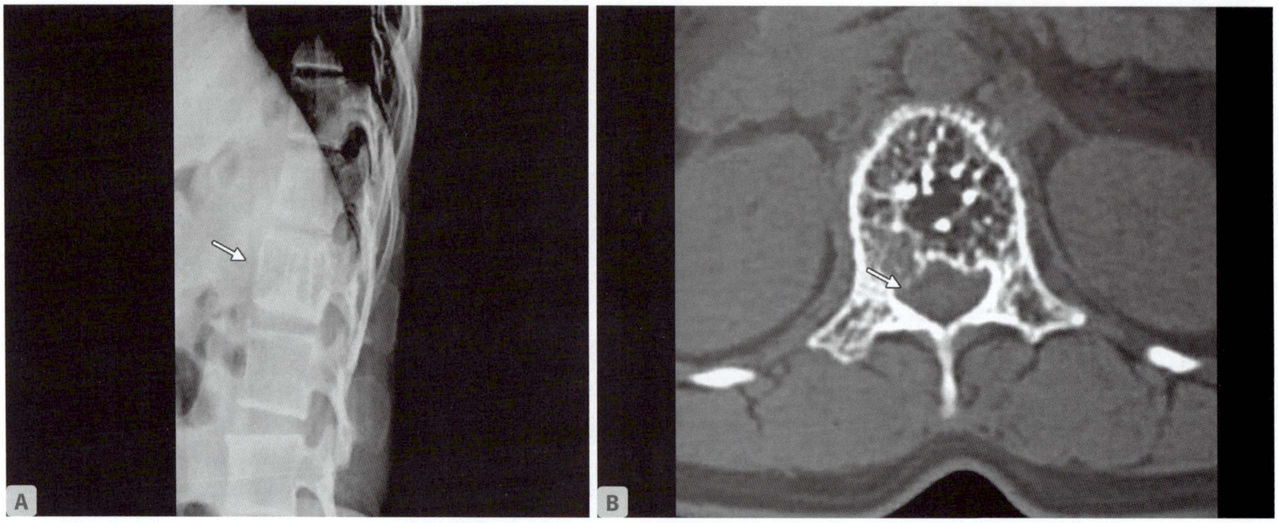

FIGS. 19A AND B: Hemangioma of vertebra. (A) Lateral radiograph of dorsolumbar spine shows mild expansion of L1 vertebral body with coarse vertical striations (arrow); (B) Axial CT scan of the same patient shows "polka dot" appearance due to vertical trabeculae cut in cross-section. In addition, there is focal disruption of the posterior cortex of vertebral body (arrow).

Lipoma

Intraosseous lipoma is a rare benign neoplasm that occurs between 5 and 70 years of age. The proximal femur, tibia, and calcaneum are the most common sites of involvement. On plain radiographs lipoma appears as a well-defined osteolytic lesion with a thin sclerotic rim. Bone expansion and trabeculations may be seen within the lesion. Cortical erosion and periosteal reaction are characteristically absent. In the calcaneum, the lesion usually occurs along the plantar margin where a "triangle" is formed by major trabecular groups and there may be a calcified nidus. CT scan shows typical "fat" density (-60 to -120 HU) and lack of contrast enhancement **(Fig. 20)**. On MRI, lipoma typically shows high signal intensity on T1W image and iso to hyperintense signal on T2W image.[30]

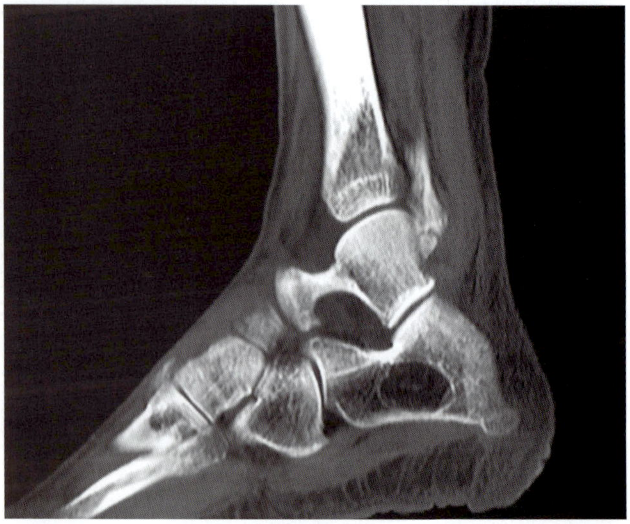

FIG. 20: Sagittal CT (MIP) image of ankle and foot shows well-defined lucent (fatty) lesions in calcaneum suggestive of lipoma.

OTHER TUMORS

Giant Cell Tumor

Giant cell tumor constitutes about 5% of all bone tumors and slightly less than 20% of all benign tumors.[31] The tumor originates from undifferentiated cells of the supporting tissues of bone marrow. As opposed to other benign tumors, GCT has a female predilection and mostly occurs after the closure of epiphysis, with a peak in the third decade.

Giant cell tumors arise eccentrically in the metaphysis with tendency to approach the adjacent subarticular cortex as they enlarge **(Fig. 21)**. About 40–50% of lesions occur around the knee.[31] Involvement of distal radius is seen in 10–12% which otherwise is an uncommon site for bone tumors. Other sites are sacrum, short tubular bones, and vertebral bodies. Classical radiographic picture is that of a well-defined eccentric lytic lesion which expands the bone and is usually not surrounded by a sclerotic rim **(Fig. 22)**. Cortical penetration with or without an associated soft tissue mass is seen in 33–50% of cases. The solid portion of a GCT is usually low to intermediate signal intensity at T1W and T2W images. This has been attributed to its high collagen content, high cellularity, or presence of hemosiderin.[32] GCT is the most common lesion associated with secondary aneurysmal bone cyst. Following contrast administration, there is diffuse enhancement of the solid component and peripheral or septal enhancement of cystic areas **(Figs. 23A and B)**. GCTs are aggressive benign neoplasms with a high rate of recurrence.

TUMOR-LIKE LESIONS

Simple Bone Cyst

A bone cyst is a fluid-filled lesion with fibrous lining. It occurs in metaphysis of long bones and adjacent to physis in children

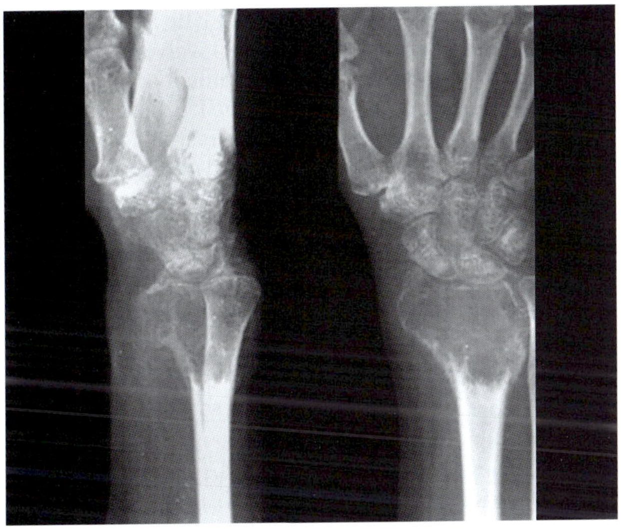

FIG. 21: Giant cell tumor. Radiograph of the left wrist shows an expansile subarticular lytic lesion in the distal end of radius. Cortex appears intact.

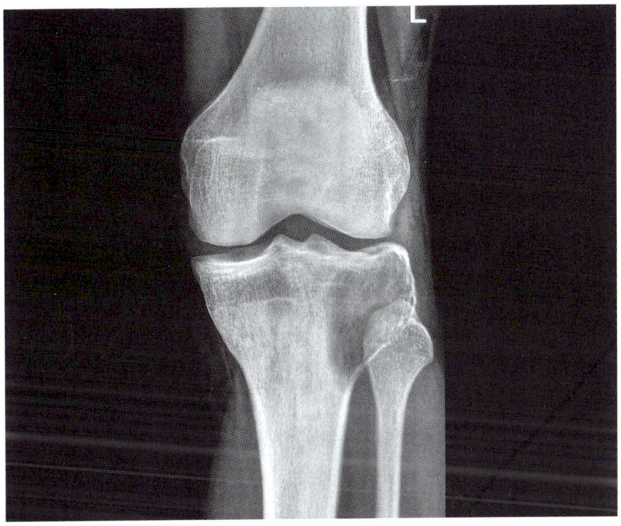

FIG. 22: Giant cell tumor. Radiograph of the knee shows an eccentric expansile subarticular lytic lesion in proximal end of tibia without sclerotic margin.

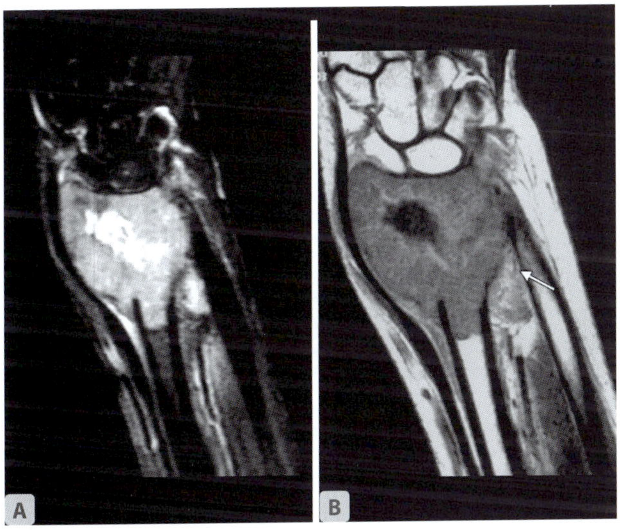

FIGS. 23A AND B: Giant cell tumor. (A) Coronal MR images of left forearm of the patient (Fig. 19) showing expansile subarticular epiphyseal lesion of radius which is hyperintense on T2W image with central cystic area; (B) Postcontrast image shows homogeneous enhancement of solid component and no enhancement of cystic area. The cortical line on the lateral side is intact but shows disruption with extension of the tumor into the soft tissues on the medial aspect (arrow).

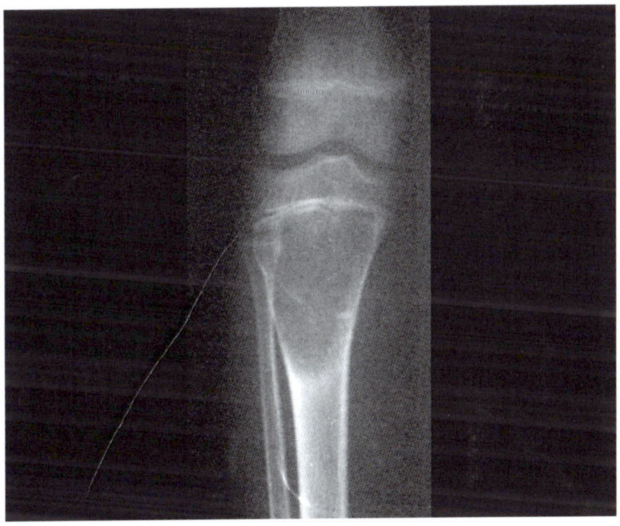

FIG. 24: Bone cyst. Radiograph of knee joint shows mildly expansile lytic lesion in metaphysis of tibia with thinning of cortex and septation.

and young adults. Common locations are proximal humerus and femur.[28] Calcaneum and ileum are less common sites. On plain radiograph, the lesion appears as moderately expansile, well marginated with or without sclerosis **(Fig. 24)**. The cortex may be thinned out and may lead to pathological fracture. "Fallen fragment" sign has been described as pathognomonic features of bone cyst when fragment of bone settles at the base of lesion due to simple nature of fluid. "Rising bubbles" sign is also based on similar principles.[33] CT and MRI can confirm the cystic nature of the lesion. The fluid contents are usually of low intensity on T1W images and hypertense on T2W images.[34] However, hemorrhage into the cyst can alter the signal characteristics of the lesion.

Aneurysmal Bone Cyst

Aneurysmal bone cyst is solitary, expansile radiolucent lesion and generally located in metaphysis of long bones. Other sites are dorsolumbar spine, small bones of hand, feet, and pelvis. Pathologically, the lesion contains multiples cystic spaces containing various stages of blood. Radiologically the lesion appears as expansile, lytic sharply circumscribed with thin cortex. The characteristic features are its ballooned out appearance and trabeculated appearance **(Fig. 25)**. CT may demonstrate fluid-fluid level and thin rim of bone overlying the lesion. MRI shows the various stages of blood products which appear as layers of different signal intensity on both T1W and T2W images[28] **(Figs. 26A and B)**. The differential diagnosis includes GCT, osteoblastoma, chondroblastoma, osteosarcoma, and simple bone cyst.

Eosinophilic Granuloma

Eosinophilic granuloma is the most benign form of histiocytosis X, which is a disease of unknown etiology characterized by proliferation of histiocytes. Eosinophilic granuloma constitutes 60–80% of Langerhans cell histiocytosis. Bone lesion may be solitary (85%) or multiple (20%) with peak incidence between 5 and 10 years.[35] The preferred sites being skull, mandible, spine, and long bones. The skull lesion on radiographs is seen as a punched out lytic lesion having a bevelled appearance due to unequal involvement of outer and inner table, with a variably sclerotic margin **(Fig. 27)**. The center of the lesion has a sclerotic focus which is often termed as a button sequestrum. In the mandible, lytic lesion may cause floating teeth. In the spine, typically the vertebral body is affected, and there may be complete lysis resulting in a solitary collapsed vertebra with a preserved disc space. In the long bones, the lesions are generally diaphyseal or metaphyseal in location and cause endosteal scalloping. Benign type of periosteal reaction is considered typical.

Pseudotumor of Hemophilia

Hemophilia is a bleeding disorder that occurs in males. Repetitive hemorrhage within the bone may result expansile geographic lesion which can simulate neoplasm **(Fig. 28)**. The common locations are femur, pelvis, tibia, and hand. CT scan

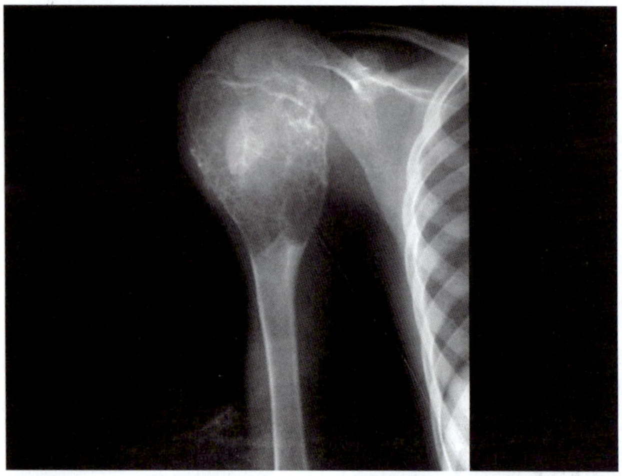

FIG. 25: Aneurysmal bone cyst. Radiograph of shoulder joint shows multiloculated very expansile lytic lesion, involving upper end of humerus.

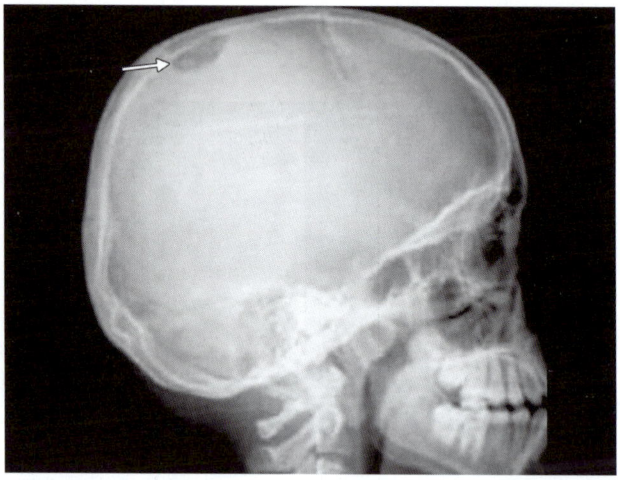

FIG. 27: Eosinophilic granuloma. Lateral radiograph of skull shows a well-defined lytic lesion with bevelled edges in the parietal bone (arrow).

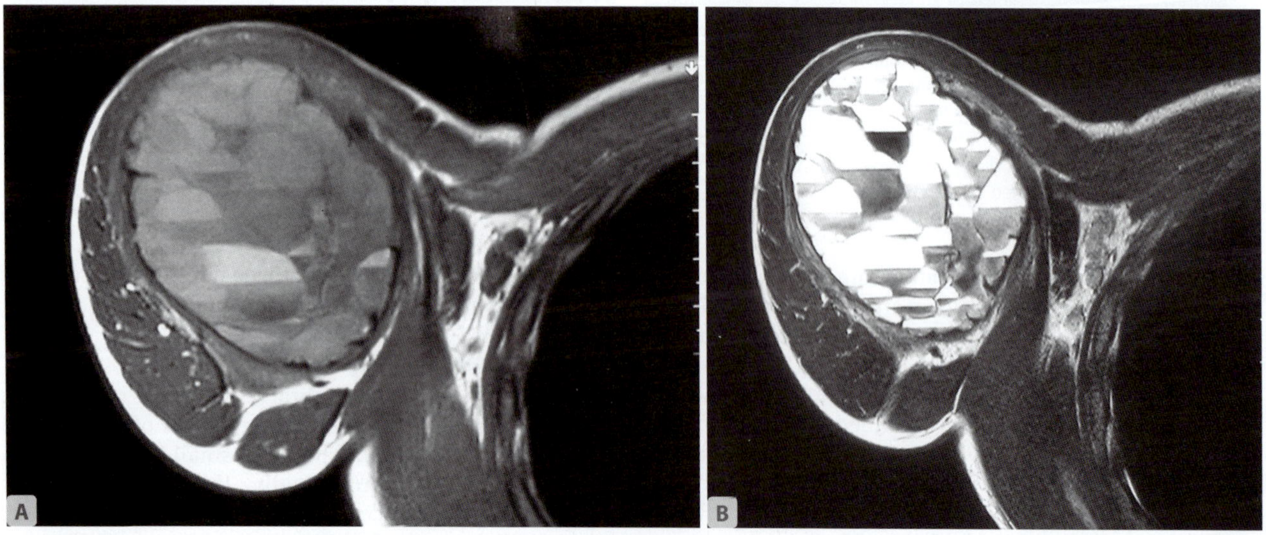

FIGS. 26A AND B: Aneurysmal bone cyst. MRI of the same patient, axial T1W (A) and T2W (B) images show well-defined multiloculated expansile lesion with extensive fluid–fluid/hemorrhage levels.

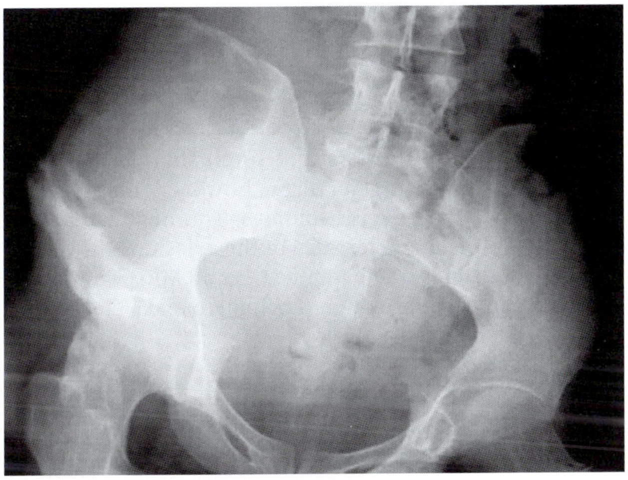

FIG. 28: Hemophilic pseudotumor. Radiograph (anteroposterior view) of pelvis reveals a large well-defined lytic lesion in the right iliac bone with an associated soft tissue mass.

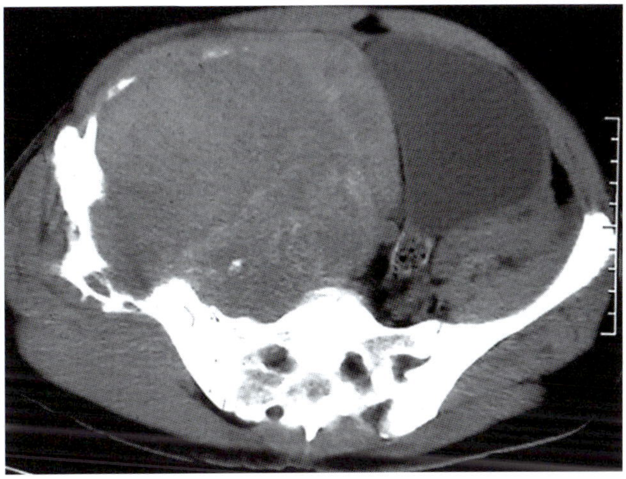

FIG. 29: Axial noncontrast computed tomography (NCCT) scan of the same patient shows erosion of the right ilium with a large soft tissue mass that has a variegated appearance with hyperdense areas within it suggestive of hemorrhage.

better demonstrates the bony erosion/destruction with adjacent hematoma **(Fig. 29)**. MRI shows variable heterogeneous signals, in form of various stages of blood products.[36]

Brown Tumor of Hyperparathyroidism

Brown tumors represent focal, bone replacing lesions, encountered both in primary or secondary hyperparathyroidism. They represents hemorrhage and breakdown product of hemoglobin. The lesions most often occur in metaphyses and diaphyses and the common bones involved are mandible, pelvis, ribs, and femur.[37]

On plain radiographs, the lesions are seen as slightly trabeculated, solitary, or multiple expansile lytic lesions with well-defined margins **(Fig. 30)**. Differentiation from a simple bone cyst is difficult when the lesion is solitary. Associated skeletal osteoporosis and biochemical changes, sclerotic appearance of brown tumor after removal of parathyroid adenoma, and the marked activity with scintigraphy are helpful in the diagnosis.[37,38]

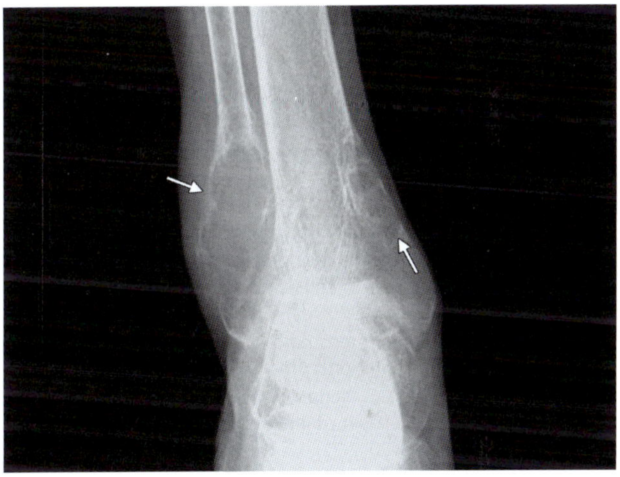

FIG. 30: Brown tumors. Radiograph of left ankle of young man with hyperparathyroidism shows multiple well-defined expansile multiloculated lytic lesions in lower end of tibia and fibula.

ROLE OF ADVANCE MAGNETIC RESONANCE IMAGING

Apart from conventional T1W/T2W MR sequences, there has been advancement in MRI in last two decades with sequences such as diffusion-weighted imaging (DWI), perfusion-weighted imaging, and spectroscopy. Most of them being used in diagnosis and management in malignant bone tumors, however, some authors have tried these sequences in benign bone tumors also.

Diffusion-weighted Imaging

DWI is a method of functional imaging.[39] This method measures the Brownian motion of water at a microscopic level. Corresponding ADC (apparent diffusion coefficient) maps provide quantitative assessment of the diffusivity of the lesion. ADC is marker of cellularity and tumor density. High cellularity tumor has low ADC, and low-density tumor shows more ADC. Various authors have tried to differentiate benign and malignant bone tumors by using DWI and reported with good results with some overlap features.[40,41]

Perfusion-weighted MRI

Perfusion sequences provide insight of vascularity of tumor. The most common method of perfusion is dynamic contrast-enhanced MRI (DCMR). This is done by using GRE sequence for particular volume of tumor after injecting intravenous contrast and creating time intensity curve (TIC) and using semiquantitative measurements. Authors have used DCMR to differentiate malignant from benign bone lesions with good sensitivity and specificity.[42] Sometime osteoid osteoma can mimic chronic osteomyelitis on radiographs. Although CT is best to show nidus in osteoid osteoma; however, MRI can help by showing typical TIC curve by using DCMR. Most osteoid osteoma shows arterial enhancement with rapid washout.[43]

MR Spectroscopy

Proton MR spectroscopy is noninvasive method form molecular characterization of tumor. Some of the authors have shown choline peaks and different choline ratio for differentiating benign and malignant musculoskeletal tumors.[44,45] The method is technically challenging and may have overlapping features as choline may not be feature of tumor aggressiveness and malignancy.[46]

These advance methods are although promising but should be additional to conventional MRI sequence and should not read in isolation without plain radiographs to avoid misdiagnosis.

CONCLUSION

Some of the bony tumors and tumor-like lesions have characteristic imaging features; however, many others may have overlap imaging findings. Thorough knowledge of radiographic characteristics of these lesions on various imaging modalities (radiography, CT, and MRI) with patient data and clinical information is helpful to make diagnosis or to reach differential diagnosis.

REFERENCES

1. Greenfield BG. The solitary lesion. Radiology of Bone Disease, 5th edition. Philadelphia: JB Lippincott; 1990. pp. 580-732.
2. Forest M, Coindre JM, Diebold J. Pathology of tumors. In: Forest M, Tomeno B, Vanel D (Eds). Orthopedic Surgical Pathology: Diagnosis of Tumors and Pseudotumoral Lesions of Bone and Joints. Epindburgh: Churchill Livingstone; 1997. pp. 71-516.
3. Resnick D. Tumors and tumor-like lesions of bone: Radiographic principles. In: Resnick D (Ed). Diagnosis of Bone and Joint Disorders. Philadelphia: Saunders; 1995. pp. 3613-27.
4. Woertler K. Benign bone tumor and tumor-like lesions: value of cross sectional imaging. Eur Radiol. 2003;13:1820-35.
5. Resnick D, Kyriakos M, Greenway GD. Tumors and tumor- like lesions of bone: imaging and pathology of specific of bone lesions. In: Resnick D (Ed). Diagnosis of Bone and Joint Disorders. Philadelphia: Saunders; 1995. pp. 3628-938.
6. Magid D. Two-dimensional and three-dimensional computed tomographic imaging in musculoskeletal tumors. Radiol Clin North Am. 1993;31:425-47.
7. Berquist TH. Magnetic resonance imaging of primary skeletal neoplasms. Radiol Clin North Am. 1993;31:411-24.
8. Moulton JS, Bvaley SE, Biedel JS. Bone and soft tissue tumors. Clinical Magnetic Resonance Imaging, 2nd edition. Philadelphia: Saunders; 1996. pp. 2042-77.
9. Greenspan A. Bone island (enostotsis): current concept—a review. Skeletal Radiol. 1995;24:111-5.
10. Schweitzer ME, Levine C, Mitchell DG, Gannon FH, Gomella LG. Bull's eyes and halos: useful discriminators of osseous metastases. Radiology. 1993;188:249-52.
11. Cerase A, Priolo F. Skeletal benign bone forming lesions. Eur J Radiol. 1998;27:91-7.
12. Bloem JL, Kroon HM. Osseous lesions. Radiol Clin North Am. 1993;31:261-5.
13. Davies M, Cassar-Pullicino VN, Davies MA, McCall IW, Tyrrell PN. The diagnostic accuracy of MR imaging in osteoid osteoma. Skeletal Radiol. 2002;31:559-69.
14. Brown LM. Bone scintigraphy in benign and malignant tumors. Radiol Clin North Am. 1993;31:731-8.
15. Motamedi K, Seeger LL. Benign bone tumors. Radiol Clin N Am. 2011;49:1115-34.
16. Motamedi K, Ilaslan H, Seeger LL. Imaging of lumbar spine neoplasms. Semin Ultrasound CT MR. 2004;25:474-89.
17. Giudici MA, Moser RP, Kransdorf MJ. Cartilaginous bone tumors. Radiol Clin North Am. 1993;31:237-59.
18. Robbin MR, Murphey MD. Benign chondroid neoplasms of the bone. Semin Musculoskeletal Radiol. 2000;4:45-58.
19. Steven S, Srinivas K, Javicr B. MR imaging of tumors and tumor like lesions of the upper extremity. Magn Reson Imaging Clin N Am. 2004;12:349-59.
20. Holtz P, Sundaram M. Enchondroma. Orthopaedics. 1995;18:509-10.
21. Mermelstein LE, Friedlaender GE, Katz LD. Chondroblastoma. Orthopaedics. 1997;20:67-71.
22. Jee Wh, Choe BY, Kang HS, Suh KJ, Suh JS, Ryu KN, et al. Nonossifying fibroma: Characteristics at MR imaging with pathologic correlation. Radiology. 1998;209:197-202.
23. Hudson TM, Stiles RG, Monson DK. Fibrous lesions of bone. Radiol Clin North Am. 1993;31:279-97.
24. Lucas E, Sundaram M, Boccini T. Polyostotic fibrous dysplasia. Orthopaedics. 1995;18:311-3.
25. Zeanah WR, Hudson TM, Springfield DS. Computed tomography of ossifying fibroma of the tibia. J Comput Assist Tomogr. 1983;7:688-91.
26. Robbin MR, Murphey MD, Temple HD, Kransdorf MJ, Choi JJ. Imaging of musculoskeletal fibromatosis. Radiographics. 2001;21:585-600.
27. Frick MA, Sundaram M, Unni KK, Inwards CY, Fabbri N, Trentani F, et al. Imaging findings in desmoplastic fibroma of bone: Distinctitive T2 characterstics. Am J Roentgenol. 2005;184:1762-7.
28. Conway WF, Hayes CW. Miscellaneous lesions of bone. Radiol Clin North Am. 1993;31(2):339-58.
29. Persaud T. The polka dot sign. Radiology. 2008;246:980-1.
30. Propeck T, Bullard MA, Lin J, Doi K, Martel W. Radiologic pathologic correlation of intraosseous lipomas. Am J Roentgenology. 2000;175:673-8.
31. Manaster BJ, Doyle AJ. Giant cell tumors of bone. Radiol Clin North Am. 1993;31(2):299-323.
32. George N, Murphey M, Kransdof MJ. Primary bone tumors of the lower extremities. Radiol Clin North Am. 2002;40:971-90.
33. Jordanov MI. The "rising bubble" sign: a new aid in the diagnosis of unicarmeral bone cyst. Skeletal Radiol. 2009;38:597-600.
34. Parman LM, Murphey MD. Alphabet soup: cystic lesions of bone. Semin Musculoskelet Radiol. 2000;4:89-101.
35. Marin C, Warrier RP. Langerhans cell histiocytosis. Orthop Clin North Am. 1996;27(3):615-23.
36. Wilson DA, Prince JR. MR imaging of hemophilic pseudotumors. Am J Roentgenol. 1988;150:349.
37. Richardson ML, Pozz-mucelli RS, Kanter AS. Bone mineral changes in primary hyperparathyroidism. Skeletal Radiol. 1986;15: 85-95.
38. Hayes CW, Conway WF. Hyperparathyroidism. Radiol Clin North Am. 1991;29:85-96.

39. Einarsdóttir H, Karlsson M, Wejde J, Bauer HC. Diffusion-weighted MRI of soft tissue tumours. Eur Radiol. 2004;14(6):959-63.
40. Pekcevik Y, Kahya MO, Kaya A. Diffusion-weighted magnetic resonance imaging in the diagnosis of bone tumors: Preliminary results. J Clin Imag Sci. 2013;3:63.
41. Rao A, Sharma C, Parampalli R. Role of diffusion-weighted MRI in differentiating benign from malignant bone tumors. BJR Open. 2019;1:20180048.
42. Cao J, Xiao L, He B, Zhang G, Dong J, Wu Y, et al. Diagnostic value of combined diffusion-weighted imaging with dynamic contrast enhancement MRI in differentiating malignant from benign bone lesions. Clin Radiol. 2017;72(9):793.e1-793.e9.
43. Chai JW, Hong SH, Choi JY, Koh YH, Lee JW, Choi JA, et al. Radiologic diagnosis of osteoid osteoma: from simple to challenging findings. Radiographics. 2010;30(3):737-49.
44. Fayad LM, Barker PB, Jacobs MA, Eng J, Weber KL, Kulesza P, et al. Characterization of musculoskeletal lesionson 3-T proton MR spectroscopy. Am J Roentgenol. 2007;188(6):1513-20.
45. Fayad LM, Wang X, Salibis N, Barker PB, Jacobs MA, Machado AJ, et al. A feasibility study of quantitative molecular characterization of musculoskeletal lesions by proton MR spectroscopy at 3 T. Am J Roentgenol. 2010;195(1):W69-75.
46. Ratnaparkhi CR, Tayade KA, Mitra KR. Magnetic resonance spectroscopy of giant cell tumor of bone. J Clin Diagn Res. 2018;12(11):TC07-TC10.

CHAPTER

165

Malignant Bone Tumors

Anju Garg, Radhika Batra, Sapna Singh

Primary malignant bone tumors are rare and they account for only 0.2% of all primary malignancies and 5.0% of all pediatric malignancies.[1,2] Metastatic tumors, benign tumors, and tumor mimics (e.g., bone cysts, nonossifying fibroma, inflammatory lesions, fibrous dysplasia, and Paget's disease) are more commonly seen than primary bone malignancies. There is a peak at the age of 10–20 years, with a second peak seen after the age of 40 years, although primary bone malignancies may occur at any age.[1,3]

The determination of the nature and the extent of the tumor is critical for appropriate decision making regarding the utility of limb salvage procedures, chemotherapy, radiation therapy, or combined therapy in managing skeletal neoplasms. The correct diagnosis and an accurate staging therefore become more than just an academic exercise, as they determine the appropriate therapy and prognosis. Conventional radiography along with cross-sectional imaging modalities, particularly magnetic resonance imaging (MRI), plays a very important role in detecting, establishing the nature, assessing the extent, and in follow-up in all suspected cases of bone tumors.

CLASSIFICATION OF PRIMARY MALIGNANT BONE TUMORS

The bone tumors have been classified according to their cell of origin or histogenesis (e.g., osteogenic, chondrogenic, fibrogenic, fibrohistiocytic, notochondral, and vascular tumors). They have been further broadly divided into benign, intermediate—locally aggressive and rarely metastasizing, and malignant categories. An updated classification of soft-tissue and bone tumors has been published by the World Health Organization (WHO) in 2013. The updates have been established on the identification of new genetic findings in different tumors. This revision has led to reproducible and reliable classification of the tumors enabling more effective treatment stratification. Hemangiopericytoma and malignant fibrous histiocytoma (MFH) have been removed from the 2013 WHO classification with the recognition that these groups include tumors which can be classified as specific sarcoma types.[4,5] **Table 1** gives a modified version of malignant tumors of the WHO classification.

Hematopoietic neoplasms include plasma cell myelomas, solitary plasmacytoma of bone, and primary non-Hodgkin lymphoma of bone which have been discussed elsewhere in the book.

GENERAL PRINCIPLES OF DIAGNOSIS

A reasonable differential diagnosis can be achieved for most bone tumors using the patient's age, location of the lesion and its imaging appearance. However, the final diagnosis is histological, often requiring an imaging-guided biopsy.

The *age* of the patient plays an important role in establishing the diagnosis and may lead to the correct histological diagnosis even when the tumor is radiographically atypical. The preferential time of origin of the various tumors is summarized in **Table 2**. In very young patients, malignant bone tumors are likely to be metastases from neuroblastoma or leukemia. In the first decade, the most likely primary bone tumors are Ewing sarcoma and, later, osteosarcoma. In adolescence and adult life, various primary tumors are probable. In older age groups, most bone tumors are metastatic carcinomas. Multiple myeloma also occurs in this age group.

The *site of origin or location* of a lesion is also of diagnostic significance with respect to which bone is involved and which portion of the bone, i.e., epiphysis, metaphysis, or diaphysis, is the tumor situated in. **Table 3** summarizes the preferential sites of origin of various malignant bone tumors. Many primary osseous neoplasms develop in the areas of rapid bone growth, especially the distal femur, proximal tibia, and proximal humerus. As the tumors of a given cell type typically arise in a location where the homologous normal cells are most active, the predilection of many bone tumors for the metaphysis and physeal regions of an enlarging tubular bone is not unexpected.[6] Furthermore, the vascular anatomy peculiar to this region, consisting of looped vessels and sinusoidal channels, promotes sluggish blood flow and, with it, metastatic seeding of tumor (and infection).

TABLE 1: WHO classification of malignant bone tumors.

Osteogenic tumors	• Low-grade central osteosarcoma • Conventional osteosarcoma • Chondroblastic osteosarcoma • Fibroblastic osteosarcoma • Osteoblastic osteosarcoma • Telangiectatic osteosarcoma • Small cell osteosarcoma • Secondary osteosarcoma • Parosteal osteosarcoma • Periosteal osteosarcoma • High-grade surface osteosarcoma
Chondrogenic tumors	• *Chondrosarcoma*: Grade II and III • Dedifferentiated chondrosarcoma • Mesenchymal chondrosarcoma • Clear cell chondrosarcoma
Fibrogenic tumors	Spindle cell sarcoma (fibrosarcoma)
Fibrohistiocytic tumors	Malignant fibrous histiocytoma of bone was removed from the current classification and renamed undifferentiated high-grade pleomorphic sarcoma of bone
Ewing sarcoma	
Osteoclastic giant cell rich tumors	Malignancy in giant cell tumor of bone
Hematopoietic tumors	• Plasma cell myeloma • Solitary plasmacytoma • Primary non-Hodgkin lymphoma of bone
Notochordal tumors	Chordoma
Vascular tumors	• Epithelioid hemangioendothelioma • Angiosarcoma
Myogenic, lipogenic, and epithelial tumors	• Leiomyosarcoma • Liposarcoma • Adamantinoma
Undifferentiated high-grade pleomorphic sarcoma	

TABLE 2: Age and malignant tumors.

Age (years)	Tumors
<1	Neuroblastoma
1–10	Ewing sarcoma—tubular bones
10–30	Osteosarcoma and Ewing sarcoma—flat bones
30–40	Spindle cell sarcoma (fibrosarcoma), undifferentiated pleomorphic sarcoma, parosteal sarcoma, malignant giant cell tumor, and lymphomas
>40	Metastatic carcinoma, multiple myeloma, and chondrosarcoma

TABLE 3: Preferential site of origin of various malignant tumors of bone.

Epiphysis	Giant cell tumor (after fusion of growth plate)
Metaphysis	• Osteosarcoma • Parosteal sarcoma • Chondrosarcoma • Spindle cell sarcoma (fibrosarcoma) • Giant cell tumor (before fusion of growth plate)
Diaphysis	• Ewing tumor • Myeloma • Reticulum cell sarcoma • Adamantinoma • Undifferentiated pleomorphic sarcoma

Certain tumors, because of their derivation, predominate in one or more particular areas of the skeleton, e.g., chordomas, developing from the remnant of the primitive notochord, are typically seen at the cranial and caudal limits of the vertebral column, whereas a variety of neoplasms related to dentition are virtually confined to the mandible or maxilla.

The *morphological features* of the bone tumors generally reflect their tissue of origin. The pattern of bone destruction, the growth rate of the lesion, the presence and the nature of the visible tumor matrix, internal trabeculation, cortical erosion, penetration, expansion, and the periosteal response are some of the features which need to be analyzed.

Predisposing conditions: Certain benign lesions can transform into bone malignancies. Radiation to healthy bone and radiation of preexisting lesions can lead to malignancy. Osteosarcoma can be seen in 10–29% of children <5 years of age who receive 1,500–5,000 cGy of radiation with a latent period of 3–18 years. Osteosarcoma or spindle cell sarcoma can also occur after radiation exposure. The tumors develop in the periphery of the radiation field where cell mutation occurs without cell death.

Malignant transformation can be seen with Paget's disease, more commonly seen in men in the sixth to seventh decades of life. The most common sarcoma to develop is osteosarcoma followed by spindle cell sarcoma and chondrosarcoma. These tumors occur most commonly in the femur, pelvis, and humerus. Lymphoma and leukemia can also arise in the bone in Paget's disease.

Bone infarction is also a predisposing factor for the development of sarcomas. Malignancy can arise sporadically in patients with fibrous dysplasia, most common being osteosarcoma followed by fibrosarcoma. Most cases of malignancy from fibrous dysplasia are secondary to radiation.

Other predisposing factors include chronic osteomyelitis, orthopedic implants, aneurysmal bone cysts (ABCs), giant cell tumors (GCTs), and neurofibromatosis 1.

Determining the *histological type* of the tumor, by fine-needle aspiration cytology or by biopsy, should be the last step in the patient's pretreatment evaluation as the reaction of tissue to the biopsy alters the imaging appearance of tumor obscuring its true anatomic extent and local aggressiveness. Also, if the biopsy is done at the final stage of evaluation, the definitive surgical procedure can be done at the same operation setting with the diagnosis made on the frozen section. Imaging studies can be of value in identifying the specific area of a tumor that should be biopsied and in planning how to get there without undue tissue contamination.

STAGING OF BONE TUMORS

Enneking system for staging malignant musculoskeletal tumors and the American Joint Committee on Cancer (AJCC) system for staging bone sarcomas are the commonly used staging systems for malignant bone tumors.[7] The universal TNM staging system used for most carcinomas is not commonly used for bone sarcomas because of the rarity with which these sarcomas metastasize to lymph nodes.

Enneking and coauthors described a staging system that gained acceptance in which malignant bone tumors are staged by the assessment of the histological grade (G), the local extent (T), and the presence or absence of regional or distant metastases **(Table 4)**.

Grade

The grade of a tumor is a measure of its potential to metastasize. It is based primarily on histological features and therefore requires a preoperative biopsy. A sarcoma is classified as either low-grade or high-grade. Low-grade lesions are well differentiated, have less mitoses, display only moderate cellular atypia, and have low risk of metastases (<25%). They require a relatively conservative surgical procedure. High-grade lesions are poorly differentiated and show high mitotic rate and high cell-to-matrix ratio. Conversely, a high-grade lesion usually necessitates a more radical procedure, because of its more aggressive nature.

Local Extent

The anatomic extent is either intracompartmental (A) or extracompartmental (B). A "compartment" is defined as an anatomic structure or space bounded by natural barriers to tumor extension. Tumors confined to the compartment of origin usually are less aggressive and require less radical surgery than those extending into the adjacent compartment. Small nodules of tumor may be found separate from the main body of the tumor, but usually remain within the same anatomic compartment. Extracompartmental spread may occur via direct tumor invasion of an adjacent compartment or by contamination resulting from fracture, hemorrhage, or an operative procedure, such as an unplanned resection or poorly planned biopsy.

Metastases

The third component of the staging system is the presence or absence of nodal or distant metastases. Regional lymph node involvement is much less common with musculoskeletal sarcomas than are pulmonary metastases, but both are equally poor prognostic factors.

The AJCC system for bone sarcomas is based on tumor grade, size, presence, and location of metastases **(Table 5)**. Stage I includes low-grade tumors and stage II includes high-grade tumors, which are subdivided based

TABLE 4: Enneking surgical staging of musculoskeletal sarcoma.

Stage (M)	Grade	Site (T)	Metastasis
IA	Low (G1)	Intracompartmental (T1)	No (Mo)
IB	Low (G1)	Extracompartmental (T2)	No (Mo)
IIA	High (G2)	Intracompartmental (T1)	No (Mo)
IIB	High (G2)	Extracompartmental (T2)	No (Mo)
III	Any (G)	Any (T)	Yes (M1)
			Regional/distant

TABLE 5: American Joint Committee on Cancer system for staging bone sarcomas.

Stage	Grade	Size	Metastasis
IA	Low	<8 cm	None
IB	Low	>8 cm	None
IIA	High	<8 cm	None
IIB	High	>8 cm	None
III	Any	Any	Skip metastasis
IVA	Any	Any	Pulmonary metastases
IVB	Any	Any	Nonpulmonary metastases

on tumor size; stages IA and IIA are 8 cm or less in their maximum linear dimension and stages IB and IIB are more than 8 cm. Stage III tumors show skip metastases, which are defined as discontinuous lesions within the same bone or within the immediately adjacent bone. Stage IVA has pulmonary metastases and stage IVB has nonpulmonary metastases. There is subdivision in stage IV as patients with nonpulmonary metastases have worse prognosis than patients with only pulmonary metastases.

IMAGING MODALITIES

Conventional radiographic techniques still remain the mainstay in initial diagnosis and work-up of a patient suspected to have any bony pathology. Cross-sectional studies are required following conventional radiography, in cases of suspected malignant bone tumors for (1) staging of tumor, (2) determining the site and route of biopsy, (3) providing measurements needed for an anticipated surgical procedure, and (4) evaluation of residual and/or recurrent disease after therapy.

Conventional Radiography

Plain radiographs can demonstrate the location of the lesion, the pattern of bone destruction, size and shape of the lesion, presence and nature of the visible tumor matrix, trabeculation, periosteal response, and the presence and characteristics of the adjacent soft-tissue mass. This information combined with the site of the lesion and the age of the patient allows formulation of a reasonable diagnosis in most cases. Malignant lesions are generally poorly defined lesions with a wide zone of transition, a moth-eaten or permeative pattern of bone destruction, an interrupted periosteal reaction of the sunburst or onion-skin type, and an adjacent soft-tissue mass. However, some aggressive benign lesions may also show the same pattern on plain radiographs.

Chest radiographs should be obtained in all cases of malignant skeletal tumors to evaluate for pulmonary metastases, particularly in patients with osteosarcoma.

Magnetic Resonance Imaging

Due to its excellent contrast resolution and multiplanar capabilities, MRI has now virtually replaced computed tomography (CT) as the imaging modality for assessing the local extent, local staging, and follow-up of malignant bone tumors. MRI is the best imaging modality (1) in assessing intra- and extracompartmental extent of bone tumors, (2) in assessing neurovascular and juxta-articular involvement, and (3) in detecting skip lesions, leading to a more accurate staging.[8] Evaluation for intra-articular extension needs careful interpretation. When the lesion is far from the joint or obviously within the joint, the diagnosis is easy, but when the tumor abuts the joint, involvement of the joint is often overevaluated. Involvement is suggested when the hyaline cartilage is penetrated or more commonly when the tumor extends through the capsule. Joint effusion does not necessarily mean involvement.[9]

The MRI protocol for bone tumor evaluation should include an initial large field of view T1 or inversion recovery sequence to detect any skip lesions and for planning subsequent sequences. T1 and T2 or inversion recovery sequences of the involved area should then be acquired in axial, coronal, and/or sagittal planes, using the surface coil, to show the complete extent of the tumor in all three dimensions, along with its relation to the adjacent joint and neurovascular bundle.

Magnetic resonance imaging features are usually nonspecific in differentiating benign from malignant tumors. Both benign and malignant tumors are generally seen as low signal on T1-weighted (T1W) and high signal on T2-weighted (T2W) images. Thus, intraosseous extent and skip lesions are well evaluated on T1W images due to the contrast between the high signal marrow and the low signal tumor, whereas the extraosseous extent is better assessed on T2W images due to the contrast provided by the low signal muscles to the high signal tumor. Fat-suppression techniques can suppress the adjacent bright fat to further increase the contrast on T2W images **(Figs. 1A to C)**. Contrast enhancement delineates the exact extent of the tumor, defines viable tumor and necrotic areas, and helps in differentiating edema from tumor tissue and identifying residual/recurrent tumor from scar or fibrotic tissue in treated cases.

Dynamic contrast-enhanced (DCE) perfusion MRI provides physiologic information that cannot be determined from conventional anatomic MRI, including information regarding tissue vascularization and perfusion, capillary permeability, and the volume of the interstitial space. DCE perfusion MRI has been frequently used in the evaluation of musculoskeletal tumors as it helps in tissue characterization, staging of local extent, identification of areas of viable tumor to guide biopsy, monitoring of preoperative chemotherapy,

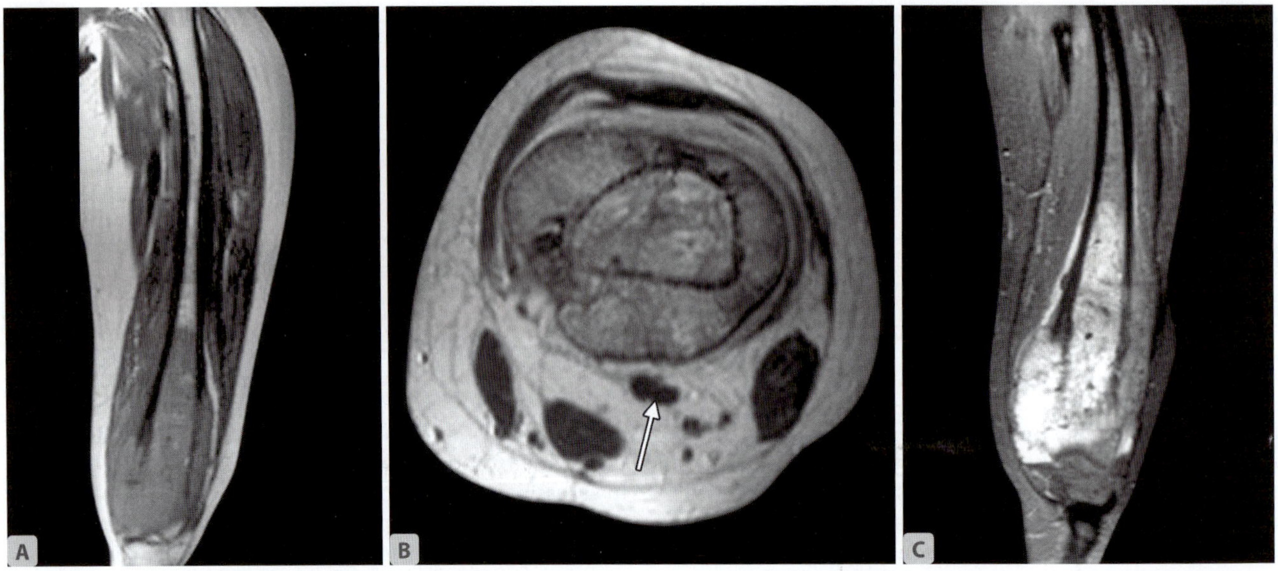

FIGS. 1A TO C: MRI (magnetic resonance imaging) showing local staging of distal femoral osteosarcoma. Coronal T1-weighted (T1W) sequence (A) demonstrates the intraosseous extent and axial T2-weighted (T2W) sequence (B) demonstrates the extraosseous extent. The periosteum is intact and the neurovascular bundle (arrow) is well separated from the tumor. Coronal short tau inversion recovery (STIR) image (C) shows the soft tissue extension well; however, the intramedullary extension is not well appreciated.

detection of residual or recurrent tumor, and differentiating tumor from fibrosis. Time-intensity curves can be obtained, type IV curve may be seen in malignant tumors (e.g., synovial sarcoma and leiomyosarcoma) and type V curve can be found in tumors after radiation or chemotherapy treatment or in tumors with a large interstitial space such as myxoid tumors.[10]

Dynamic contrast-enhanced MRI can be used to obtain pharmacokinetic parameters, such as the volume transfer constant (Ktrans), the volume rate constant (Kep, which represents the transfer of the contrast agent from the extravascular extracellular space to the blood plasma), and the extravascular extracellular volume fraction (Ve). In a study done by Oh et al., Ktrans and Kep showed significant differences between benign and malignant bone tumors; however, a significant difference could not be found for Ve. This is the first report using a composite parameter derived from DCE-MRI and diffusion-weighted imaging (DWI) to evaluate musculoskeletal tumors. The Ktrans, Kep, and Ktrans/apparent diffusion coefficient (ADC) were significantly higher and the ADC value was significantly lower in the malignant bone lesions than in the benign bone lesions. These findings suggest that the multiparametric approach with a hybrid parameter derived from DCE MRI and DWI could be potentially useful.[11]

Diffusion-weighted MRI: Densely cellular areas with restricted diffusion have lower ADCs as compared to less cellular areas with higher ADCs. ADC values are significantly higher in benign than in malignant tumors.

Diffusion-weighted MRI has also been found useful in assessing tumor response to therapy. Effective therapy in bone tumors leads to breakdown of tumor cell membranes resulting in increased diffusion of water in the tumor on diffusion-weighted images. Even though the tumor bulk may not reduce significantly, increase in the ADC value indicates a response to treatment.[12]

^{1}H magnetic resonance spectroscopic imaging (MRSI) can be used as a noninvasive approach to the evaluation of musculoskeletal tumors, providing a means of molecular characterization of bone and soft-tissue malignancies. This method can characterize lesions based on their metabolic constituents, such as choline, a phospholipid constituent of cell membranes. Diagnostically, ^{1}H MRSI is used to detect increased levels of choline compounds, which are markers of increased cell membrane turnover, a feature of malignancy.

Multivoxel ^{1}H MRSI has been shown to be feasible for characterizing musculoskeletal tumors. The choline peak is used to differentiate benign and malignant tumors. The presence of a choline peak (identified visually at 3.2 ppm in a spectrum obtained with TE = 135 ms) is supportive of malignancy, although some metabolically active benign tumors and abscesses may also show a choline peak.[10]

Computed Tomography

With the easier availability of MRI, the role of CT in the evaluation of malignant bone tumors has reduced considerably. However, CT still remains superior to MRI in detection and characterization of matrix mineralization (osteoid or chondroid), in picking up subtle calcification, and in the assessment of cortical involvement, bone trabeculation, and periosteal reaction. CT can be used to demonstrate the morphological features of the tumor in areas which are not well evaluated by plain radiography, e.g., pelvis, shoulder, and vertebrae and where MRI is contraindicated. CT is also the investigation of choice for detecting pulmonary metastases.

It helps to evaluate treatment response as bone tumors ossify as they heal. CT-guided procedures allow accurate placement of biopsy needles. It also guides probes for tumoral ablation with ultrasound radiofrequency, microwave, chemical, or cryoablation.[13]

Fluoroscopy

Fluoroscopy is used for localization of bone tumors at the time of surgery and for angiography used in chemoembolization treatments and preoperative embolization of vascular tumors.[13]

Nuclear Medicine

Radionuclide scanning using both traditional technetium-labeled phosphonate compounds and newer positron emitters is an important adjunctive modality.

^{99m}Technetium methylene diphosphonate (^{99m}Tc MDP) bone scan has traditionally been used as the first additional investigation in most instances to detect whether the lesion is monostotic or accompanied by other skeletal lesions. The major limitation of bone scanning is its lack of specificity as a number of bone disorders may have similar scintigraphic appearances. These lesions need to be characterized further by other imaging modalities. The role of ^{99m}Tc MDP bone scan for monitoring response to treatment is limited because it is not always possible to distinguish active disease from healing.

Assessment of tumor response to therapy can be affected by flare phenomenon. An increased uptake of the radioactive substance can be detected up to 6 months after the treatment of metastases and distinguishing this phenomenon from disease progression is difficult and requires additional evaluation with other imaging modalities such as MRI.

Fluorodeoxyglucose positron emission tomography (FDG-PET) is assuming an increasingly important role in the evaluation of skeletal metastatic disease. FDG accumulation in skeletal lesions reflects direct uptake by tumor, in contrast to ^{99m}Tc MDP activity on conventional bone scans, which reflects increased new bone formation in response to destruction of bone by tumor. The role of FDG-PET in the imaging algorithm of primary musculoskeletal tumors is not well defined. Its role in the initial diagnosis is limited. It cannot replace biopsy because it cannot consistently differentiate benign from malignant bone tumors. In the patient with a documented bone tumor, it can (1) guide a biopsy to the most active tissue, (2) predict overall survival, (3) distinguish recurrent tumor from post-therapeutic changes, (4) monitor response to neoadjuvant chemotherapy, and (5) may also identify poorly responding patients earlier in therapy.[14]

Recently, another positron emitter fluorine-18 sodium fluoride (NaF) has been used as a PET bone imaging agent. The bone uptake of this agent is twofold higher and blood clearance is much faster than ^{99m}Tc MDP which makes it much more sensitive and selective than conventional bone scan for diagnosis and detection of bone metastases.[15] It has higher spatial image resolution as compared to ^{99m}Tc MDP bone scan. It is potentially useful in staging and follow-up of bone forming malignancies such as osteosarcoma and osteoblastic osseous metastases.[13]

The use of low-dose CT or MRI in conjunction with PET improves the sensitivity and specificity of the PET imaging techniques.

Angiography

Angiography has limited specificity in differentiating between benign and malignant tumors as there are no characteristic angiographic features of malignancy. However, two signs, i.e., encasement of normal vessels and presence of tumor vessels, occur with greater frequency in malignant tumors.

Currently, conventional angiography has been largely replaced by noninvasive CT and magnetic resonance (MR) angiography techniques. Conventional angiography still remains useful for pretherapy planning in selected cases and in therapeutic interventions. In planning limb salvage procedures, it can be used to map the vascular supply of a potential vascularized bone graft. Preoperative selective arterial embolization can substantially lower the risk of hemorrhage from hypervascular bone tumors, such as GCT and metastatic renal cancer. Conventional angiography also has been used to deliver intra-arterial infusion chemotherapy to some malignant bone tumors.

Ultrasonography

With the advent of CT and MRI, ultrasonography (USG) has been relegated to the role of an adjunct imaging modality in the evaluation of musculoskeletal tumors. USG plays no useful role in diagnosis or staging but has proven to be of value in guiding needle biopsy of those lesions with a large extraosseous component.[14] It can also help detect the solid/cystic nature of the soft-tissue component.[13] Color Doppler flow imaging with duplex analysis has a role in monitoring tumor response to chemotherapy in patients with high-grade sarcomas, provided there is a soft-tissue component. Response is predicted on the basis of changes in intratumoral blood flow and changes in resistive indices in the limb arteries. Postsurgery USG can be of value in detecting sarcoma recurrence, particularly when orthopedic hardware is present.[16]

TREATMENT FOR PRIMARY MALIGNANT BONE TUMORS

- *Surgery*: Surgery remains the primary treatment for most of symptomatic or malignant bone tumors.
  - *Wide excision*: This involves removal of the entire lesion along with reactive tissue surrounded by intact cuff of normal tissue.
  - *Radical excision*: The lesion along with the entire muscle, bone, or other involved tissues in the compartment is removed.

Limb Salvage Considerations

Limb salvage should be considered only if functional result is likely which involves restoration of the musculoskeletal and neurovascular structures. Growing children present a special difficulty in that limb salvage may not be sensibly attempted if the growth plate cannot be maintained. Preoperative imaging should provide specific information including:

- Proximal, distal, and transverse extent of osseous and soft-tissue involvement
- Location of either of the proximal or distal end of the lesion relative to a palpable anatomic landmark
- Specific muscles and compartments involved by tumor must be identified
- Major neurovascular involvement
- Joint involvement
- Tumor extension relative to epiphyseal plate; mostly approximately 2 cm of tumor free bone adjacent to metaphyseal side of growth plate for adequate limb salvage surgery seeking to retain the physis.
- *Chemotherapy*: It is the first-line treatment for Ewing sarcoma and lymphoma and serves as an adjuvant therapy for most other malignant bone tumors. Lesions such as low-grade chondrosarcoma, periosteal osteosarcoma, and parosteal osteosarcoma are not responsive to chemotherapy. Chemotherapy can be used for conventional osteosarcoma and other high grade osteosarcomas, prior to definitive surgical treatment which helps in shrinking the soft-tissue mass and allows easier tumor resection, especially surrounding the neurovascular bundles. Chemotherapy may also help in controlling systemic micrometastases. Evaluation of tumor response to chemotherapy helps in directing further postoperative treatment.
- *Radiotherapy*: Radiotherapy with chemotherapy is considered first-line therapy for Ewing sarcoma and primary bone lymphoma. It helps in decreasing and controlling the tumor mass in high-grade lesions. Postoperatively, it can be used for lesions with marginal resection. Radiotherapy can also be used in the treatment of local recurrence. Low-grade chondrosarcomas and low-grade osteosarcomas are not responsive to radiation.
- Radiofrequency ablation may be used for painful bony metastases which are not responding to other treatment.

Image Fusion for Computer-assisted Bone Tumor Surgery

Adequate tumor resection without excessive removal of normal tissue is required for a successful limb salvage surgery. Imaging modalities such as CT, MRI, and PET scans have been adapted for use with computer navigation to provide more accurate intraoperative assessment and resection. The fusion of images obtained with CT and MRI is a software-dependent processing technique that allows integration and analysis of preoperative images for planning complex musculoskeletal tumor resections. Integration of various imaging modalities into one imaging data set facilitates preoperative image analysis and planning of navigation computer-assisted bone tumor resection and reconstruction. CT and MRI are essential for preoperative assessment for complex bone tumor surgery. Fusion of CT and MRI yields hybrid images that combine the key characteristics of each technique, allowing better interpretation and accurate localization of the lesion.[17]

It yields an excellent picture of anatomic tumor location and extent of infiltration into surrounding tissues. Image fusion might not be restricted to plain CT or MRI data sets, CT angiography, and MRI fusion can provide information regarding regional vascular anatomy. Functional imaging such as F-18 FDG-PET scans can also be incorporated into the navigation software. PET images have low spatial resolution; therefore, they should be combined with anatomic CT or MRI data sets for interpretation. Metabolic information regarding the tumor is particularly useful in patients with previous surgery and radiotherapy as it helps in distinguishing tumor from scar tissue or postradiotherapy changes on anatomic imaging data sets. The fusion images are excellent for surgical planning as they provide better intraosseous and extraosseous extent of the tumors. Merging of postoperative with preoperative images and precise fitting of custom tumor prostheses might allow validation of the accuracy of a resection as planned.[17,18]

OSTEOGENIC ORIGIN

Osteosarcoma

Osteosarcoma is the most common primary osseous malignancy excluding malignant neoplasms arising from the marrow (myeloma, lymphoma, and leukemia); it accounts for approximately 20% of bone cancers. It mostly affects patients younger than 20 years of age.[7] It is characterized by the production of osteoid or bone by the tumor cells. The malignant cells also retain the potential to form fibrous tissue or cartilage. Thus, the constituents of the tumor matrix are highly variable and can include osteoid tissue, calcification, fibrous tissue, cartilaginous tissue, or a combination of these tissues. Demonstration of osteoid formation by malignant cells on histopathology is essential for diagnosing osteosarcoma. Defects in RB and p53 genes play an important role in the development of osteosarcoma. Abnormalities in INK4a, which encodes p16 (a cell cycle regulator) and p14 (which aids and abets p53 function), are also seen.[7] They can be classified according to their main tissue component and their site of origin **(Box 1)**.

Osteosarcomas can be associated with various syndromes such as McCune-Albright syndrome, Mazabraud syndrome, familial Paget's disease, retinoblastoma, Li-Fraumeni syndrome, and Bloom syndrome.[19]

Conventional Osteosarcoma

Conventional intramedullary osteosarcoma is the most common subtype of osteosarcoma and accounts for approximately 75–85% of all cases.

Clinical Presentation

Age

It is commonly seen in the second and third decades of life with peak incidence seen between 10 and 15 years. Conventional osteosarcoma is rare in patients <6 years or >60 years.[19] The median age of patients with osteosarcoma arising

BOX 1: Classification of osteosarcoma.

- *Primary osteosarcomas*:
  - Conventional intramedullary/central high grade (osteoblastic, chondroblastic, and fibroblastic)
  - Telangiectatic
  - Small cell
  - Low-grade central
- *Surface osteosarcoma*:
  - Juxtacortical/parosteal
  - Periosteal
  - High-grade surface
- Secondary osteosarcomas can occur in Paget's disease and after radiation exposure
- Unusual forms of osteosarcoma given below are viewed as subtypes of conventional osteosarcoma as their biological behavior is similar
- Osteoblastic osteosarcoma—sclerosing type
- Osteosarcoma resembling osteoblastoma
- Chondromyxoid fibroma such as osteosarcoma
- Chondroblastoma such as osteosarcoma
- Clear cell osteosarcoma
- Malignant fibrous histiocytoma such as osteosarcoma
- Giant cell rich osteosarcoma
- Epithelioid osteosarcoma

in tubular bones is 17 years. Flat bones are affected at median age of 25 years.

Sex

The male:female ratio is 2:1.

Clinical Picture

Most patients present with pain and a palpable mass. Symptoms are usually present for several months, the swelling having been attributed to trauma or infection in the first place. Systemic symptoms and pathological fractures are common. Serum alkaline phosphatase may be elevated with larger tumors.

Site

The typical lesion affects the metaphyseal region of the growing end of a long bone. About 50–75% are found in the distal femur or the proximal tibia. Other common sites include proximal humerus and femur. Rarer sites include the ilium, ribs, vertebrae, and jaw bones. Extension of the tumor into the diaphysis and/or epiphysis is common. About 10% of the tumors arise in the diaphysis. Skip metastases may be seen in approximately 5% of patients.[19] Distant spread is mainly via the bloodstream with early metastases to the lungs.

Imaging Features

On plain radiographs, the tumor may be predominantly osteosclerotic (25%) or osteolytic (25%), but more frequently, it is of the mixed osteosclerotic/osteolytic type (50%). The classical appearance is that of a focal lesion in the metaphyseal end of a long bone showing a moth-eaten or permeative pattern of destruction with a wide zone of transition. The tumor breaks through the cortex early in the course of the disease leading to a soft-tissue mass. This mass is first unmineralized but later shows ill-defined tumor bone within it. Mineralization of the tumor osteoid leads to a cloud-like density in the region known as the *cumulus cloud* appearance. The medullary lesion is predominantly lytic but mineralization leads to a characteristic-associated medullary sclerosis. A Codman triangle may form at the margin of the lesion due to subperiosteal extension of the tumor lifting the periosteum **(Figs. 2A and B)**. Bone spicules can be seen perpendicularly or radially in a "sunburst" or "sunray" pattern following the line of extended Sharpey's fibers **(Figs. 3A and B)**. A lamellated (onion skin) pattern of periosteal reaction resembling that of Ewing sarcoma may sometimes be seen. In contrast to cortical bone, the articular cartilage is more resistant to tumor invasion and is not violated until late in the course of the disease.[20,21]

Magnetic resonance imaging is the investigation of choice following conventional radiographs. The entire bone should be scanned to look for skip metastases. An obvious heterogeneous tumor can be seen within the bone, often associated with a soft-tissue mass, with low-signal intensity on T1W images and high-signal intensity on short tau inversion recovery (STIR) or T2W images **(Figs. 4A to D)**. Areas with increased sclerosis may show lower signal intensity on both T1W and T2W images. Peritumoral edema in the marrow tends to be of an intermediate signal intensity on STIR and T1W images and does not disrupt the normal architecture.[22] Both intramedullary and extraosseous extensions are accurately demonstrated as is the involvement of the neurovascular bundle and extension into the adjacent joint **(Figs. 5A to D)**. Intramedullary "skip" lesions may also be identified.

The classical osteosarcoma has been described above, but a variety of appearances may be observed. The tumor bone may be entirely sclerotic **(Figs. 6A and B)** or the tumor may be entirely lytic when it is difficult to differentiate from Ewing sarcoma. A chondroblastic variety of osteosarcoma may occur when a large part of the tumor is composed of cartilage.

Telangiectatic Osteosarcoma

The rare *telangiectatic osteosarcoma*[23] is characterized by the formation of large septated blood-filled cavities with a rim containing high-grade osteosarcomatous cells. It accounts for 2.5–12% of osteosarcomas and presents usually as a lytic lesion resembling an aggressive ABC.[19] The femur, tibia, and humerus are most commonly involved. It arises frequently in the diaphysis and extends into the metaphysis. It lacks visible bone production. A predominant expansile, lytic lesion with remodelling, cortical destruction, and periosteal reaction is seen on plain radiographs **(Fig. 7A)**. Subtle matrix mineralization may be demonstrated by CT. Extensive hemorrhage and blood-fluid levels can be seen on both CT and MRI **(Fig. 7B)**, mimicking ABC. However, the presence of thick peripheral, septal, and nodular enhancement of solid viable tissue on postcontrast studies **(Fig. 7C)** helps to distinguish telangiectatic osteosarcoma from ABC. Although the prognosis for this type of osteosarcoma is poor as compared

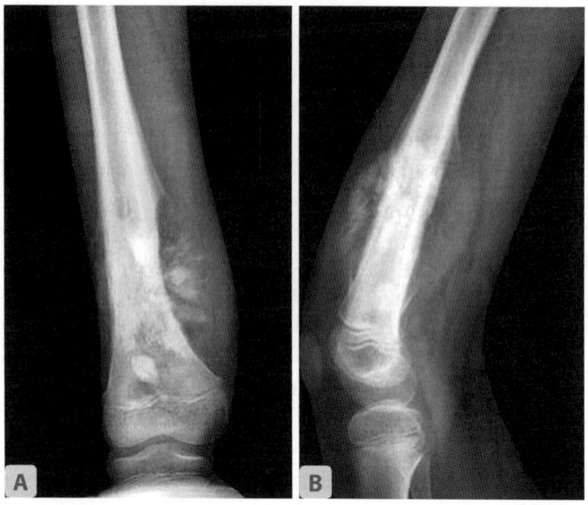

FIGS. 2A AND B: Conventional central osteosarcoma. Anteroposterior (AP) (A) and lateral (B) radiographs of the distal femur in a 14-year-old boy showing a classical osteosarcoma with mixed lytic and sclerotic areas, extraosseous mass with tumor bone formation, and Codman triangles at the upper and lower margins of the lesion.

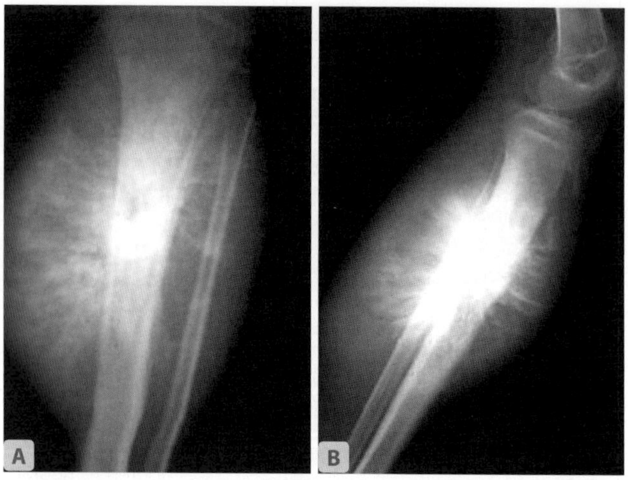

FIGS. 3A AND B: Osteosarcoma of the tibia. Anteroposterior (AP) (A) and lateral (B) radiographs of the leg show a mixed lesion in metadiaphyseal region of tibia with a large soft tissue component and the characteristic "sunburst" or spiculated periosteal reaction.

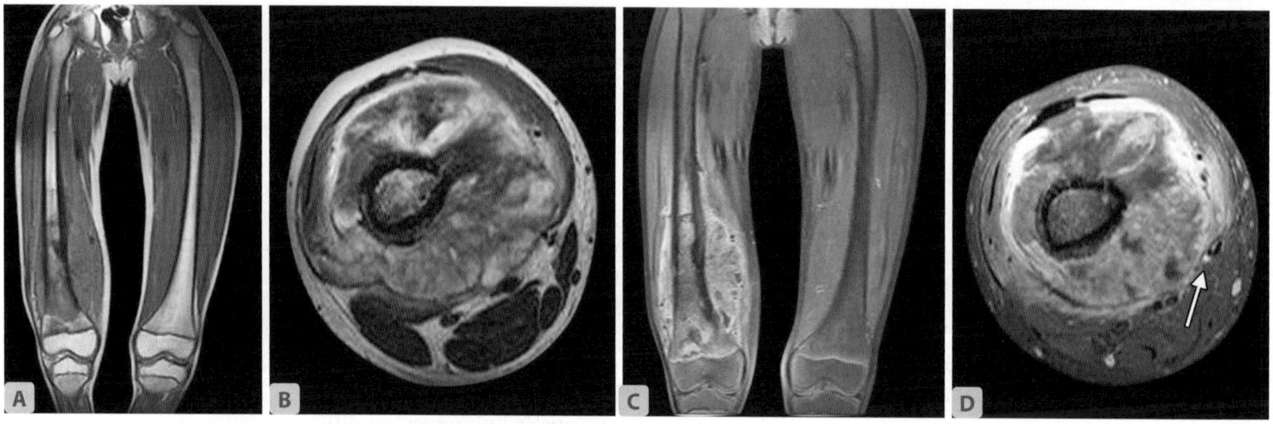

FIGS. 4A TO D: MRI of the osteosarcoma (same case as in Fig. 2). Coronal T1-weighted (T1W) magnetic resonance (MR) image (A) shows the large tumor as a predominantly hypointense mass with evidence of cortical destruction and axial T2-weighted (T2W) image (B) shows the cortical disruption with soft tissue extension of the tumor mass with loss of fat planes with the neurovascular bundle. Contrast-enhanced coronal (C) and axial (D) MR images show heterogeneous enhancement of the tumor mass.

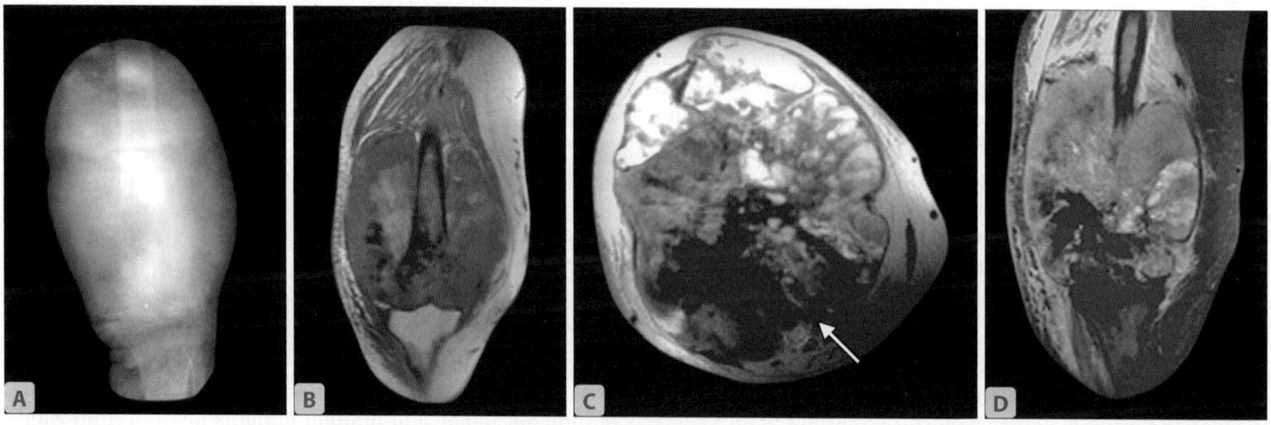

FIGS. 5A TO D: Osteosarcoma of distal femur. Anteroposterior (AP) radiograph (A) showing a destructive lesion in the distal femur with extensive cloud-like mineralization in the intra- and extraosseous component. Coronal T1-weighted (T1W) magnetic resonance (MR) image (B) shows the large tumor as a predominantly hypointense mass with evidence of cortical destruction. An axial T2-weighted (T2W) image (C) shows a heterogeneous mass which is completely encasing the neurovascular bundle (arrow). T2W (fat-suppressed) coronal image (D) shows the intra-articular extension of the tumor into the knee joint.

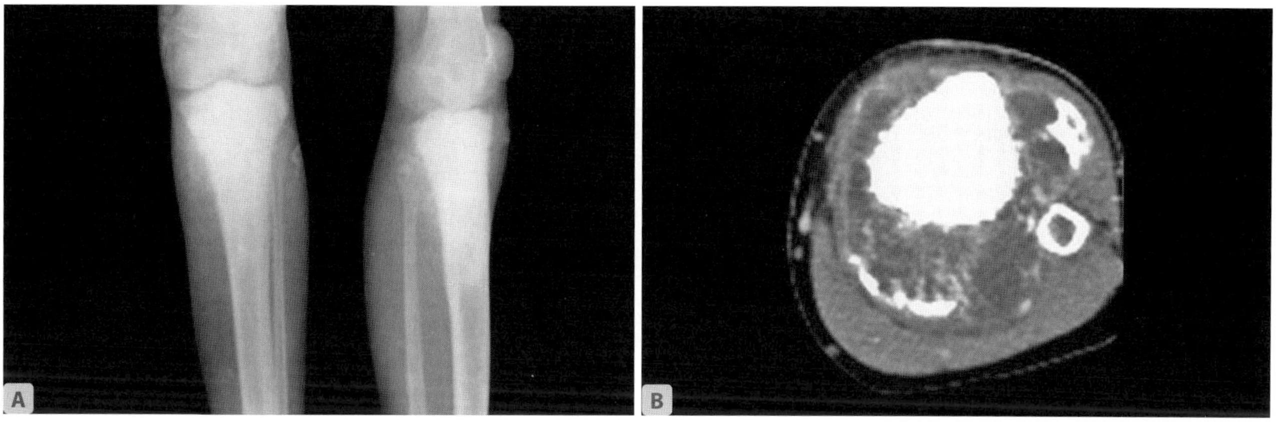

FIGS. 6A AND B: Osteosarcoma—osteoblastic variety. Anteroposterior (AP) and lateral (A) radiographs show a purely osteosclerotic lesion of the proximal metaphysis of the tibia. Computed tomography (CT) (B) shows mineralization of tumor matrix within the soft tissue component and a spiculated periosteal reaction.

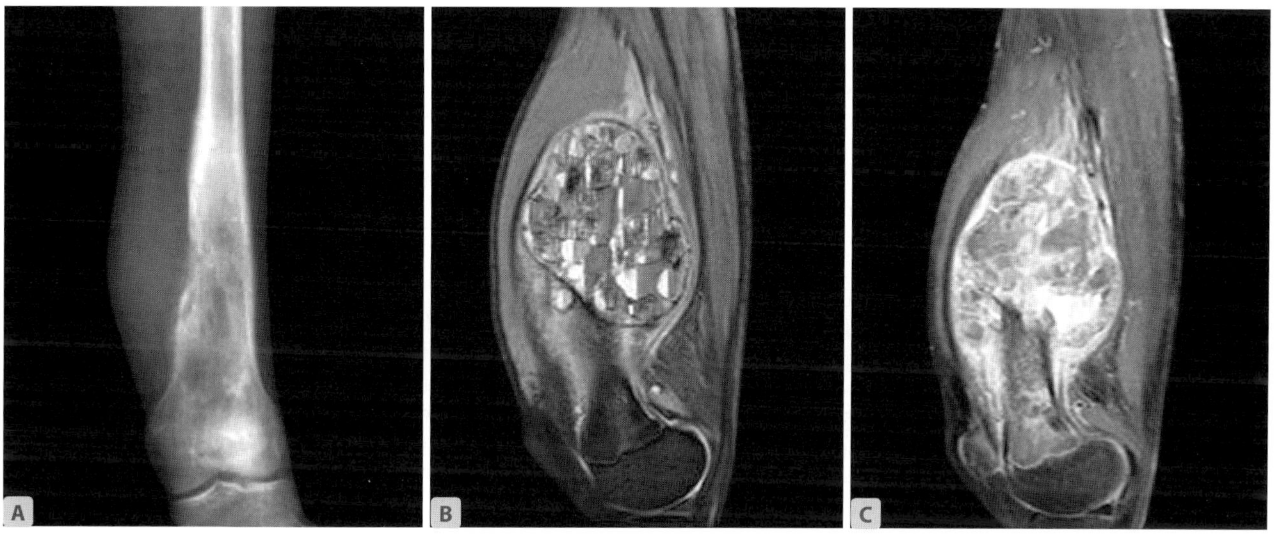

FIGS. 7A TO C: Telangiectatic osteosarcoma. Anteroposterior (AP) radiograph (A) of the distal femur shows a predominantly lytic lesion in the distal femur with irregular cortical destruction and a large soft tissue component and sagittal T2W fat-suppressed magnetic resonance (MR) image (B) shows the characteristic blood–fluid levels within the tumor. On contrast-enhanced image (C), marked peripheral and septal enhancement is seen.

to conventional osteosarcoma, effective chemotherapy has improved survival.

Small cell osteosarcoma[24] (approximately 1–4%) is a rare subtype and is similar to conventional osteosarcomas in its clinical presentation and radiographic appearance. Equal number of men and women are affected; lesions are seen in the metaphysis most commonly and may extend into the diaphysis occasionally. Isolated diaphyseal lesions can be seen in 15%.[19] They are seen as intramedullary, permeative lesions with ill-defined margins associated with cortical destruction, periosteal reaction, and soft-tissue mass. Histologically, it contains solid areas of small round cells or spindle-shaped cells resembling those seen in Ewing sarcoma. The significance of this entity is its extremely poor prognosis.

Low-grade osteosarcoma,[25] also referred to as intraosseous well-differentiated osteosarcoma, is a rare type of osteosarcoma (around 1–2%), which presents in an older age group (median age 30 years) with a long-standing history. The radiographic features vary from predominantly osteolytic or ground glass to predominantly sclerotic. The tumor may show geographic destruction and is frequently expansile with regular cortical destruction and solid periosteal reaction. It has a good prognosis. Due to its relatively benign appearance, the tumor may be mistaken for fibrous dysplasia, osteoblastoma, or a low-grade chondroid tumor. However, CT and MRI will show extraosseous extension, which should aid in the diagnosis.

The main *differential diagnoses* of osteosarcoma in its early stages are osteomyelitis and trauma. A long history may

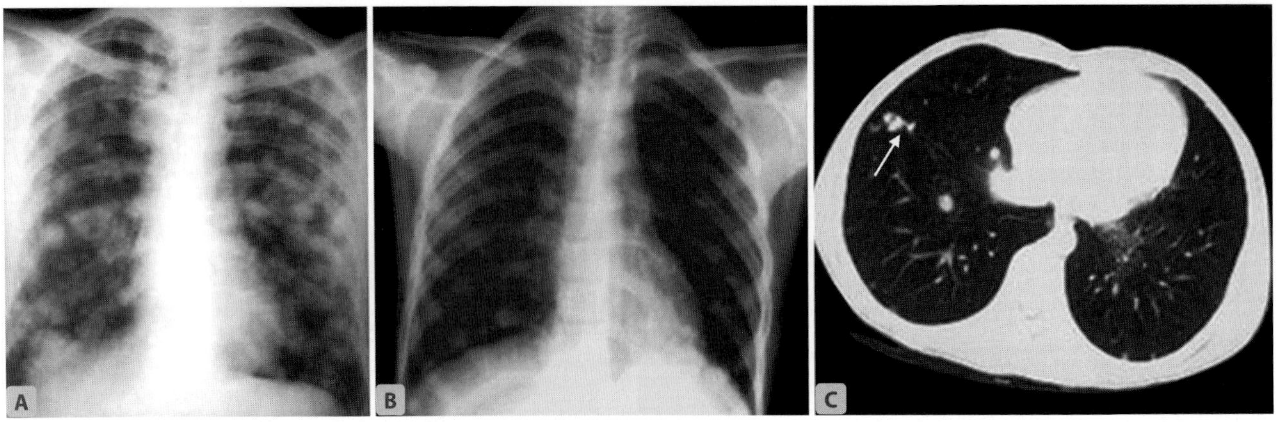

FIGS. 8A TO C: Pulmonary metastases from osteosarcoma. (A) Multiple dense rounded opacities are seen scattered through both the lung fields suggestive of osteoblastic metastases; (B) In another case, plain radiograph of the chest shows a few ill-defined opacities suspicious of metastases; and (C) Axial computed tomography (CT) scan shows multiple nodular metastatic lesions scattered in both lung fields. Ossification can be seen in some (arrow).

indicate that infection is unlikely. Once the plain radiograph reveals a medullary lesion, the diagnosis usually lies between osteosarcomas and other malignancies, including metastasis. Of the benign lesions, osteoblastoma, GCT, osteoid osteoma, and osteomyelitis, particularly the sclerosing variety of Garré, have to be considered.

Osteosarcoma spreads via the bloodstream leading to pulmonary metastases. These contain osteoid, take- up bone-seeking isotopes, and ultimately ossify. The metastases are often subpleural in location and commonly associated with a pneumothorax. It is essential to exclude the presence of lung metastases with CT for purposes of staging before starting therapy **(Figs. 8A to C)**.

The prognosis of osteosarcoma has improved greatly with the use of chemotherapy and limb-preserving surgery. Presently, the treatment requires multiple cycles of chemotherapy before surgical resection. DCE MRI has been used with considerable success in some centers to predict the degree of chemotherapy response and to identify active tumor remnants in recurrences.[26] Biochemical markers such as alkaline phosphatase and lactate dehydrogenase can be used to assess prognosis and treatment response.

Surface Osteosarcomas

Surface osteosarcomas arise from the surface of the bone and account for 4–10% of osteosarcomas. They include the periosteal, parosteal, high-grade surface, and intracortical osteosarcomas.

Periosteal Osteosarcoma

Periosteal osteosarcoma is an intermediate-grade chondroblastic osteosarcoma that originates from deep periosteal layer. It accounts for 25% of surface osteosarcomas. It is seen in the second and third decades with a slight male preponderance. This entity is characteristically diaphyseal in location with the involvement of 50% of osseous circumference and the center of the tumor is located on the surface of the bone with a saucer-like shallow area of adjacent cortical bone destruction.[19] The crater contains striated, radiating mineralization. It is found in the tibia and femur followed by ulna and humerus. Tumor mineralization is best shown by CT. Absence of marrow involvement is easily seen on CT/MRI. MRI classically shows hyperintensity on T2W images due to the chondroblastic nature of the lesion. Reactive marrow changes may be seen in >50% cases, appearing hypointense on TIW images and hyperintense on T2W images adjacent to but not contiguous with the lesion.

Juxtacortical/Parosteal Osteosarcoma

Parosteal osteosarcomas account for around 65% of all surface osteosarcomas. They arise from the outer layer of the periosteum and are attached to the surface of the affected bone and have a tendency to encircle it. They occur in the third and fourth decades and are more common in women. This tumor is almost exclusively found in long bones, with 70% occurring around the knee, especially the posterior aspect of the femur.[19]

The characteristic feature is a dense ossific mass abutting or enveloping the distal femoral metaphysis **(Fig. 9A)**. A broad-based soft-tissue mass with perpendicular periosteal reaction is seen on the surface of the bone with cortical thickening and cortical scalloping. Codman triangle can be seen at upper or lower margins. In its early growth, a well-defined radiolucent line separates the tumor from the normal cortex. Cortical thickening without aggressive periosteal reaction may be seen. Medullary involvement needs to be evaluated on CT or MRI **(Figs. 9B to D)**. MRI shows a low signal equivalent to normal cortex in the poorly cellular ossified element with a variable increase in the signal intensity from the peripheral more active element of the tumor.[27] Eventually, both cortex and medulla become involved by the tumor. Most parosteal osteosarcomas are low grade; however, high-grade foci can be seen in 22–64% of cases and appear as nonmineralized soft-tissue components >1 cm^3 on CT and MRI. The differential diagnosis includes a heavily mineralized osteochondroma and juxtacortical myositis ossificans, which is differentiated by its peripheral mineralization pattern and lack of attachment to the cortex.

Parosteal osteosarcoma is associated with an excellent prognosis with a 10-year survival rate of 80%.[19]

High-grade Surface Osteosarcoma

This is a very rare lesion arising from the surface of the bone but having the same histological features as conventional central osteosarcomas. It, therefore, has a very much poorer prognosis than other osteosarcomas. High-grade surface osteosarcoma is more common in second and third decades with male preponderance. It involves diaphysis of long bones (femur, humerus, and fibula). The radiological features are similar to those of periosteal osteosarcoma but more aggressive in that the tumor is usually larger and there is a greater degree of cortical erosion.[28] It involves entire circumference of bone with invasion of medullary cavity.

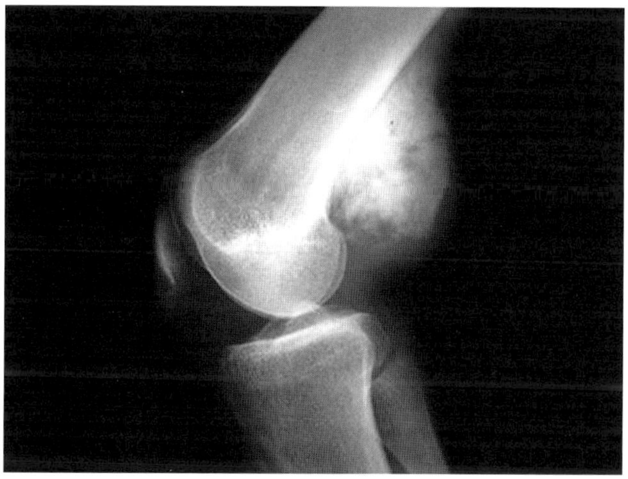

FIG. 9A: Parosteal osteosarcoma. Lateral radiograph of the knee shows a dense, lobulated mass arising from the posterior distal femur. This is the classical location for parosteal osteosarcoma.

Intracortical Osteosarcomas

Intracortical osteosarcomas are the rarest form of osteosarcoma, accounting for <1% of cases. They are usually seen in the second decade and in men.[19] All reported cases had arisen in the cortex of femur or tibia. The tumor appears as a small lytic lesion surrounded by thickened cortex, resembling an osteoid osteoma or osteoblastoma. These tumors have a better prognosis than the conventional intramedullary osteosarcoma. Medullary invasion is rare.

Extraosseous Osteosarcoma

Occasionally, osteosarcomas may arise in an extraosseous site. The most common site is the soft tissue of the thigh, but they can also be found in the pleura, dura of brain, heart valves, retroperitoneum, axilla, breast, etc. These rare tumors present the same histological pattern as other osteosarcomas. They usually present as large soft-tissue masses, which may not be close to bone. The radiological appearance is nonspecific. Mineralization of the matrix can suggest the diagnosis, but differentiation from other soft-tissue sarcomas which calcify (e.g., chondrosarcoma, fibrosarcoma, and synovial sarcoma) is difficult.[29]

Multifocal Osteosarcoma

This condition is characterized by multiple intraosseous osteosarcomas that was earlier thought to represent multicentric osteosarcomas, but it is now believed to represent rapidly progressive multicentric metastatic disease. It accounts for approximately 3–4% of all osteosarcomas. It is bilaterally symmetrical in skeletally immature patients but asymmetrical in skeletally mature older patients. The dominant lesion is large and has osteoid, or it may be purely lytic with metastatic foci which are smaller, sclerotic, well-defined with absent periosteal reaction, and cortical destruction **(Fig. 10)**. It is associated with poor prognosis with mean survival being only around 12 months.[19]

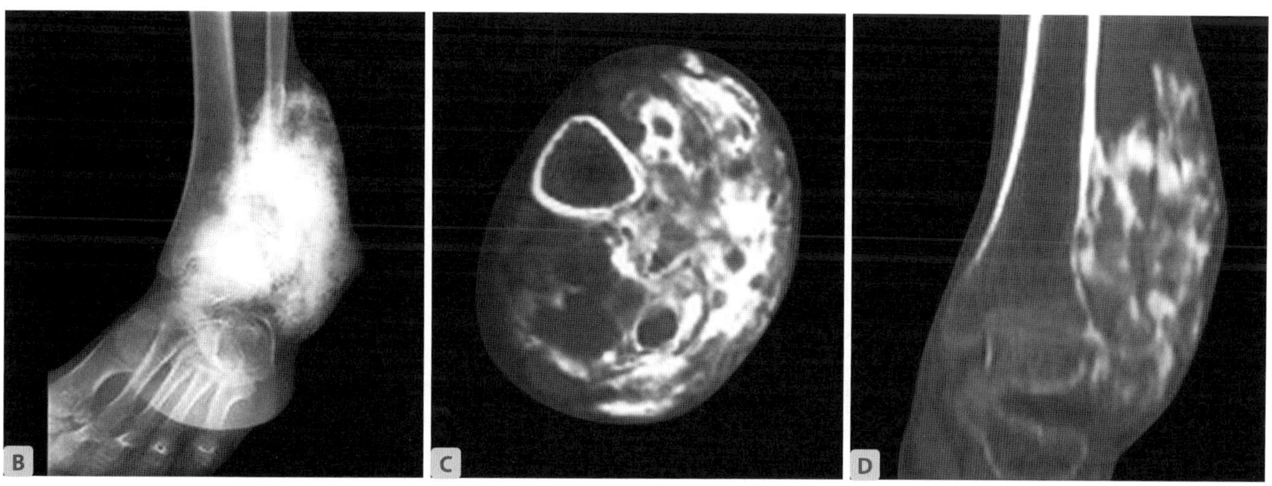

FIGS. 9B TO D: Parosteal osteosarcoma. In another case, anteroposterior (AP) radiograph of the ankle shows a dense homogeneous mass of bone overlying the distal fibula and tibia (B); Axial and coronal reformatted computed tomography (CT) sections show the cleavage plane separating the lesion from the underlying bone (C and D).

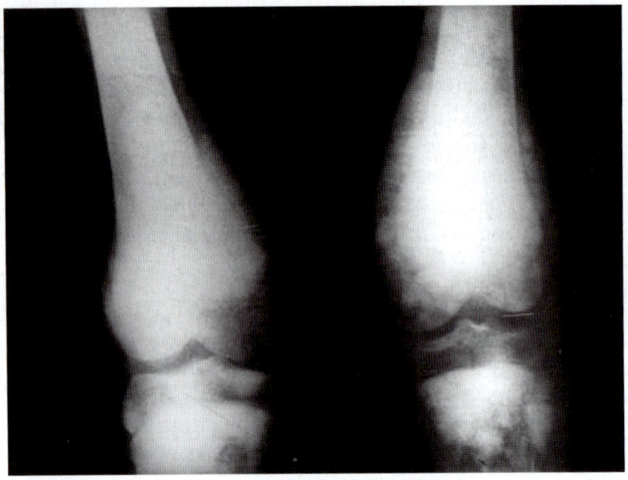

FIG. 10: Multifocal osteosarcoma. Anteroposterior (AP) radiograph of bilateral knees of a 16-year-old boy shows dense osteoblastic lesions involving the metaphyses of both femora and tibia.

Secondary Osteosarcoma

Secondary osteosarcomas occur following malignant degeneration of benign disorders, most commonly seen after radiotherapy and in Paget's disease. Rarely, osteosarcoma develops in the association with osteonecrosis, fibrous dysplasia, osteogenesis imperfecta, metal prosthesis, and chronic osteomyelitis.[29]

Radiation therapy may lead to the development of osteosarcoma. The criteria for diagnosing a *postradiation sarcoma (PRS)* include: (1) a history of radiation therapy, (2) development of a neoplasm in the radiation field, (3) a latent period of several years, and (4) histological proof of a sarcoma, which differs significantly from that initially treated.

Precise threshold dosage is unknown, but it is considered that a minimal dose of 30 Gy is required to induce a PRS and it is also suggested that concurrent chemotherapy increases the risk of sarcoma development. The treated tumors, which most commonly result in the development of PRS, are breast carcinoma, lymphoma, head and neck cancers, and gynecological malignancies. The most common sites are pelvic and shoulder girdle and the most common PRS is an osteosarcoma followed by undifferentiated pleomorphic sarcoma (UPS). Radiologically, there is an evidence of bone destruction, soft-tissue mass, matrix mineralization, and periosteal reaction. There may also be associated features of radiation changes in the underlying bone in the form of radiation osteitis and marrow infarction. The prognosis is usually poor.[30]

Malignant change has also been reported to occur in about 5% patients with Paget's disease. Most common malignancy is osteosarcoma (73–84%), fibrosarcoma (9–16%), chondrosarcoma (14%), or UPS (5%).[19] Radiologically, the most common sites for Paget's disease, the pelvis, and the femur are common locations for malignant change. CT and MRI show an area of bone destruction with a wide zone of transition and a large soft-tissue mass.[29]

CHONDROGENIC ORIGIN

Chondrosarcoma

Chondrosarcoma is a malignant tumor of chondrogenic origin that remains essentially cartilaginous throughout its evolution. It arises from chondroblasts and collagenoblasts, thus producing only cartilage and collagen. It is the third most common primary malignant tumor of bone after multiple myeloma and osteosarcoma, accounting for about 25% of all primary bone tumors.[19] It usually develops later in life than osteosarcoma and carries a much better prognosis because metastases often occur late. A high-grade chondrosarcoma, however, behaves in a fashion very similar to an osteosarcoma.

Chondrosarcoma can be divided into two broad categories: primary and secondary. A primary chondrosarcoma is believed to be malignant from the outset while a secondary chondrosarcoma arises in a preexisting bony lesion, usually an enchondroma or an osteochondroma and rarely in chondromyxoid fibroma or chondroblastoma. A chondrosarcoma may also be classified according to its histological grade as low grade (grade 1: 45–50% of cases), myxoid (grade 2: 30–40% of cases), high grade (grade 3: 8–25% of cases) or dedifferentiated, which refers to the development of an adjacent high-grade nonchondroid neoplasm, typically osteosarcoma or UPS. Chondrosarcoma grade I (now officially termed atypical cartilaginous tumor) is reclassified as an intermediate (locally aggressive) tumor better reflecting its clinical behavior.[5] Other varieties include mesenchymal, clear cell, and dedifferentiated chondrosarcoma on the basis of histology. According to its epicenter, chondrosarcoma can be classified into two types: central, when it is intramedullary, and peripheral, when it arises from the surface of the bone. Rarely, chondrosarcomas may arise in an extraosseous site.

Chondrosarcomas may be associated with osteochondromatosis and Maffucci syndrome.

Central Chondrosarcoma

It is the most common type of chondrosarcoma (approximately 90%).

Clinical Presentation

Age

It is most commonly seen in the sixth decade.[19] It is rare in children and should be differentiated from the chondroblastic variety of osteosarcoma.

Sex

Male:female incidence is 1.5–2:1.

Site

The common sites are the pelvis, the ribs, and the proximal ends of the femur and the humerus. It is relatively rare distal to the knee and elbow joints. In the long bones, chondrosarcoma is located in the metaphysis or metadiaphysis.

Imaging Features

Radiologically, the *central tumors* are seen as large, osteolytic, expansile, round, or oval lesions which are well marginated with endosteal thickening or thinning **(Figs. 11A and B)**. There is evidence of cartilaginous matrix mineralization which may be stippled, nodular, or conglomerate (popcorn), sometimes showing rings or arcs. CT may show calcification of the matrix when it is not visible on plain radiographs **(Figs. 12A and B)**. As chondrosarcomas are slow-growing tumors, reactive changes occur in the normal bone, so that as endosteal resorption takes place, periosteal new bone is laid down and bone expansion occurs. Deep endosteal cortical scalloping (greater than two-thirds) is suggestive of chondrosarcoma as opposed to chondroma. Periosteal reaction is common and is seen in almost 50% of cases.[31,32]

As the tumor grows, tumor margination may be lost and the tumor tissue may invade the overlying cortex to extend into the adjacent soft tissues. A soft-tissue mass out of proportion to the size of the intraosseous lesion may be present **(Figs. 13A to F)**. In the pelvic tumors, this mass is not easily demonstrated on conventional radiography. CT and MRI can demonstrate the soft-tissue extension with much greater accuracy. On MRI, cartilage shows characteristic increased signal intensity on T2W images and a multilobulated and septated appearance. The lesion is slightly hypointense to muscle on T1W images **(Figs. 14A to C)**.

Most chondrosarcomas are poorly vascularized and therefore show minimal enhancement after intravenous contrast on CT and MRI, typically showing a peripheral or septal enhancement pattern **(Fig. 14D)**. The presence of clear cut enhancement, especially if it is only in a part of the tumor, is a feature which favors dedifferentiation into a more malignant tumor, usually a UPS, with a more adverse prognosis.

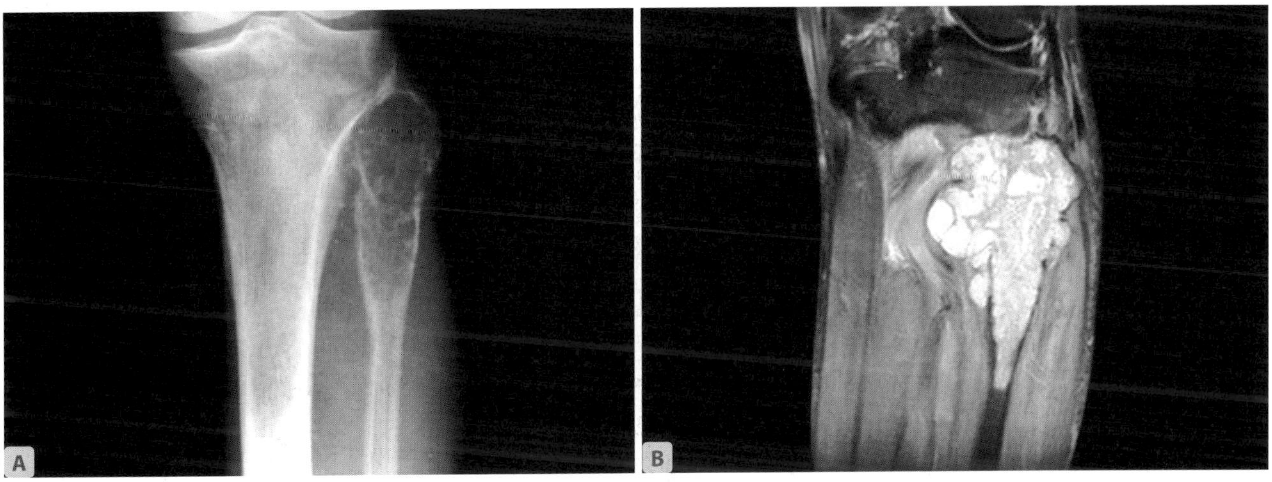

FIGS. 11A AND B: Conventional chondrosarcoma. Plain radiograph (A) shows an osteolytic, expansile lesion in the upper end of the fibula with faint calcification seen within. Coronal T2-weighted (T2W) fat-suppressed magnetic resonance (MR) image (B) shows the characteristic hyperintense, lobulated lesion with internal septations.

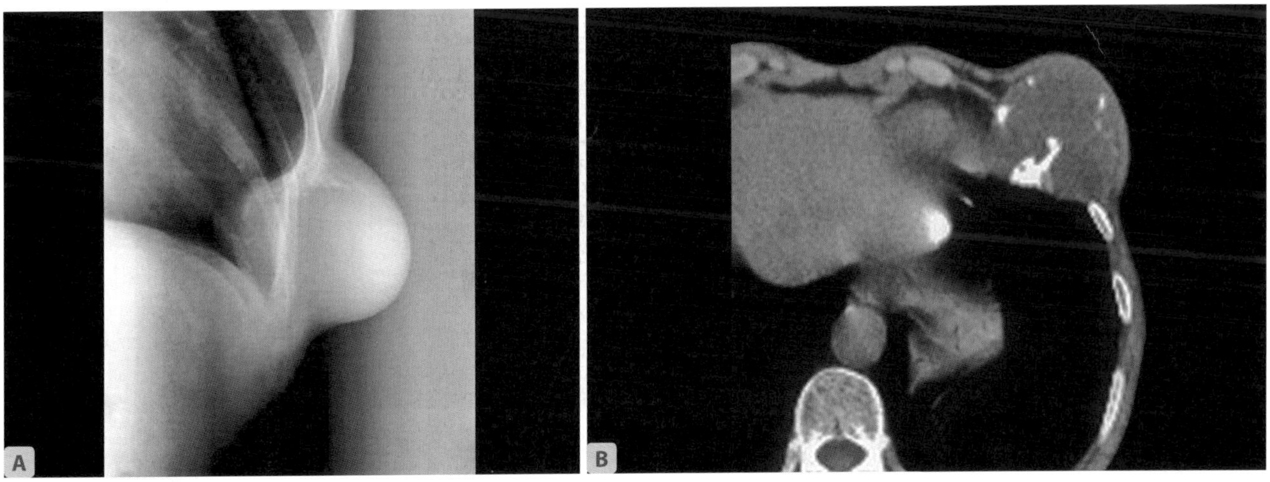

FIGS. 12A AND B: Chondrosarcoma. (A) A large expansile lesion is noted in the anterior end of the left 7th rib; (B) Computed tomography (CT) shows specks of calcification within the lesion.

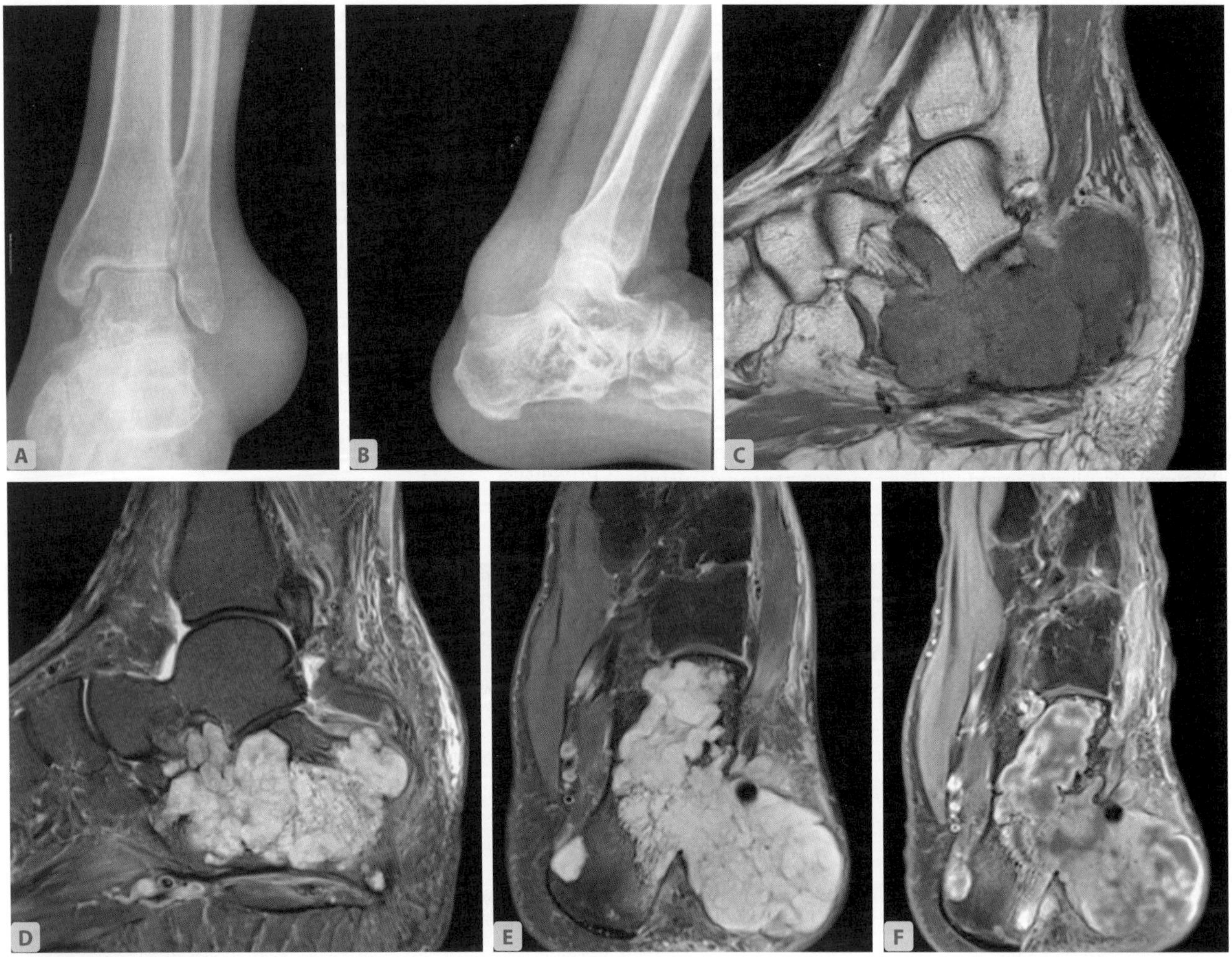

FIGS. 13A TO F: Chondrosarcoma calcaneum. Anteroposterior (AP) (A) and lateral (B) radiographs of the ankle show an ill-defined lytic sclerotic lesion involving the calcaneum with a large soft tissue swelling along the posterolateral aspect of the ankle joint. T1-weighted (T1W) sagittal (C), short tau inversion recovery (STIR) sagittal (D), and proton density (PD) fat-saturated (FS) axial (E) magnetic resonance (MR) images show a lobulated lesion in the calcaneum with a large extraosseous soft tissue component extending laterally, the lesion appears hypointense on T1W image and hyperintense on STIR and PD FS images with heterogeneous enhancement on postgadolinium image (F). Another smaller similar lesion is seen in the medial aspect of the calcaneum.

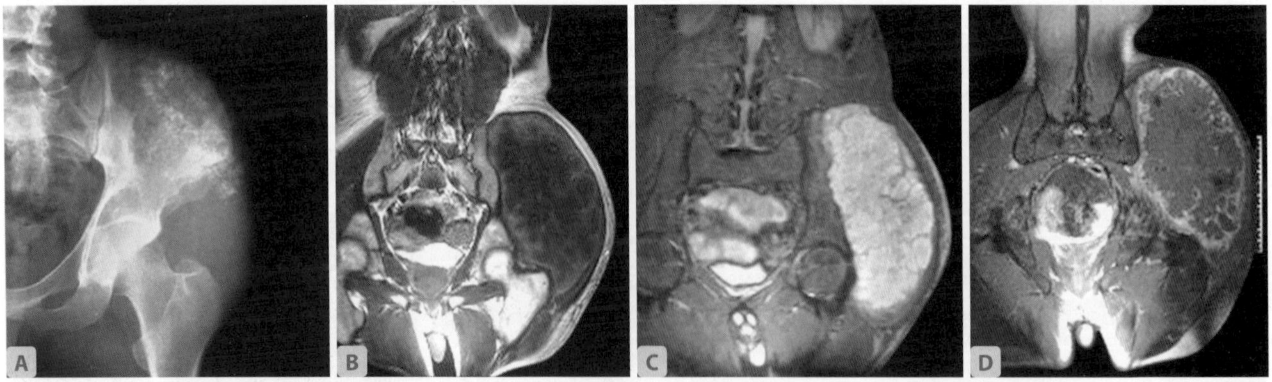

FIGS. 14A TO D: Conventional chondrosarcoma. Radiograph of the hemipelvis (A) shows a mass extending from the left iliac blade with the characteristic "popcorn" calcification of a cartilaginous matrix. T1-weighted (T1W) magnetic resonance (MR) image (B) shows the large soft tissue component of the chondrosarcoma as a low signal intensity lobulated mass. On coronal T2-weighted (T2W) MR image (C), the tumor is seen as lobulated mass of high signal intensity with septations of low signal intensity. After intravenous administration of gadolinium, a coronal T1W MR image (D) shows irregular peripheral and septal enhancement.

Peripheral Chondrosarcoma

Most of the *peripheral chondrosarcomas* probably arise from benign osteochondromas. Risk of conversion is more in the presence of multiple lesions such as osteochondromatosis (5–25%), enchondromatosis (10–25%), or Maffucci syndrome. It is more common in men and has a younger age distribution as compared to conventional chondrosacrcoma.[19] The distinction between active osteochondroma and low-grade chondrosarcoma can be extremely difficult. Clinical features such as recent onset of pain or presence of an enlarging mass may suggest a malignant transformation. Radiologically, there may be destruction of part of a well-formed calcified cap or ossified stem of such a structure. The thickness of the cartilage cap cannot be assessed radiographically unless it abuts some other structure, e.g., a vessel or viscus filled with contrast medium. It can be readily identified by USG, CT, or MRI, and the thicker the cap, the more likely it is that malignant degeneration has supervened. Most osteochondromas have cartilage caps <5 mm thick, and a cap in excess of 20 mm is likely to be malignant. Unfortunately, the wide separation between these figures makes this observation of limited value.[33]

The prognosis of chondrosarcoma is good when complete resection is achieved before metastatic spread. When metastatic spread occurs, it is generally owing to invasion by the tumor of regional venous channels. Parenchymal metastases to the lungs are therefore not uncommon. Metastases elsewhere, particularly to the skeleton, are rare; similarly, regional lymph nodes are also only rarely involved. The prognosis is better for peripheral tumors in the limbs than with central tumors, e.g., in the pelvis. Failure to remove the complete tumor leads to local recurrence and often breakdown of the overlying skin. The tumor shows a poor response to radiotherapy and cytotoxic drugs.

Other Varieties of Chondrosarcoma

Mesenchymal Chondrosarcoma

Mesenchymal chondrosarcoma is an uncommon entity. It occurs typically in the spine, ilium, or the nonpelvic flat bones (craniofacial bones and ribs) and at a younger age as compared to the conventional chondrosarcomas. Histologically, it has a much more cellular malignant matrix than the conventional chondrosarcoma. Radiologically, it is indistinguishable from a conventional chondrosarcoma. About 75% show chondrogenic calcification. Local recurrence and disseminated metastases occur earlier and more frequently.[19,34]

Clear Cell Chondrosarcoma

Clear cell chondrosarcomas are low-grade, slow-growing variant of chondrosarcomas with a long history. They are seen in third and fourth decades being more common in men and almost always involve the ends of long bones (femur or humerus) after closure of the epiphyseal plate. Less commonly, they may be seen in ribs, skull, spine, hands, and feet. Radiographically, they are usually lytic and may show a loculated or a "soap-bubble" appearance. Lesions may show well-defined margins with thin sclerotic rim or may appear expansive with cortical thinning. One-third may show chondrogenic calcification; periosteal reaction is rare. They may be indistinguishable from chondroblastoma or even chondromyxoid fibroma. The presence of a painful lesion and a soft-tissue mass suggests the provisional diagnosis of chondrosarcoma and makes a biopsy obligatory.[19,35]

Dedifferentiated Chondrosarcoma

Dedifferentiated chondrosarcoma (around 10% of chondrosarcomas) shows a bimorphic pattern of well-differentiated chondrosarcoma and high-grade noncartilaginous lesion. It is seen in fifth to ninth decades with a male preponderance. Dedifferentiated chondrosarcoma is seen in pelvis, femur, and humerus. On imaging, an intramedullary lesion is seen with a bimorphic appearance with a cartilaginous component showing calcification and an aggressive osteolytic component with ill-defined margins and soft-tissue mass.[19]

Juxtacortical Chondrosarcoma

Juxtacortical chondrosarcoma is rare and originates on the surface of long bones. Age of patients varies from 17 to 65 years and it is more common in women. It most commonly occurs in the distal posterior femoral metaphysis. Juxtacortical osteosarcoma is seen as a surface mass causing scalloping of the cortex; it may show matrix calcification. MRI may show reactive marrow involvement and a thick radial periosteal reaction.[19]

FIBROGENIC TUMORS

Spindle Cell Sarcoma (Fibrosarcoma)

Spindle cell sarcomas, originally called fibrosarcomas of bone, are rare malignant tumors that contain spindle-shaped cells that produce no osteoid in either the primary lesion or in any metastatic deposits. They may be primary or can occur secondarily in Paget's disease, chondrosarcoma, bone infarction, following irradiation, and even in the sinus tracts of osteomyelitis.

Clinical Presentation

Age

Most of the tumors occur between 20 and 50 years.

Sex

Equal in both sexes.

Clinical Picture

Pain, swelling, and pathological fractures are the common presenting features.

Site

The tubular bones are more frequently involved in younger patients, the flat bones in older patients. Almost 50% of these tumors arise in the lower limbs, particularly around the knee. The femur, tibia, and humerus account for approximately two-thirds of the tumors and the classical locations within these bones are the condyles of the femur and the epicondyles of the humerus. Other frequent sites include the innominate bones, skull, and facial bones. Lesions are mostly seen in the metaphysis but may extend into the epiphysis. The majority develop primarily in bone and may be either medullary or periosteal in location, while a few arise primarily in soft tissue and cause secondary bone changes. Metastases occur to the lungs, central skeleton, and viscera in a large percentage of cases.

Imaging Features

The tumor is essentially osteolytic with moth-eaten pattern of bone destruction and wide zone of transition; it provokes little new bone formation and usually lacks calcification or ossification **(Figs. 15A and B)**. The medullary variety is characterized by an irregular area of radiolucency. With very low-grade tumors, a minimal degree of sclerosis may surround the radiolucency. Slowly growing tumors may thin and expand the cortex, but with a diffuse infiltrative pattern, it is more usual for cortical destruction to occur. The subsequent soft-tissue extensions are without calcification or ossification, and periosteal new bone formation is unremarkable. This feature may differentiate it from osteosarcoma or chondrosarcoma.[36]

Periosteal tumors, however, frequently exhibit shaggy ill-defined periosteal new bone formation. Destruction of the outer side of the cortex frequently takes place, but the erosion is usually clearly defined, almost as though a piece of bone has been removed surgically. In this respect, considerable variance is shown from the poor definition of the edge of most malignant tumors. Secondary involvement of bone may result also from a spindle cell sarcoma arising in the soft tissue.

The major differential diagnoses are lytic osteosarcoma, dedifferentiated chondrosarcoma, and metastases. The more aggressive ill-defined varieties may be indistinguishable from malignant round cell tumors.

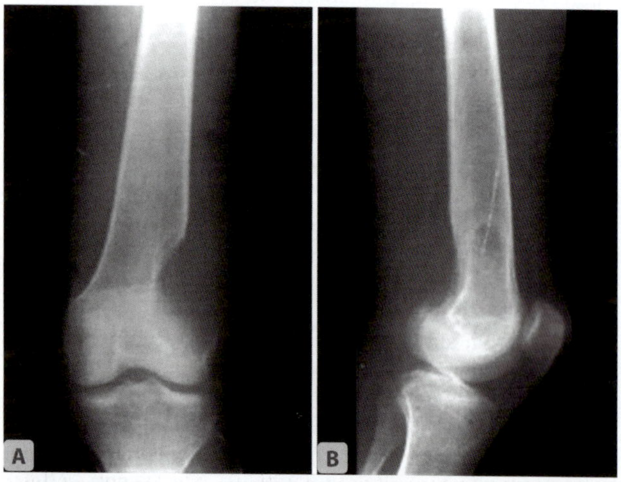

FIGS. 15A AND B: Spindle cell sarcoma. Anteroposterior (AP) (A) and lateral (B) radiographs of the knee show an osteolytic lesion with a short zone of transition in the distal femur. Note the absence of a periosteal reaction and tumor matrix mineralization.

SMALL ROUND BLUE CELL TUMORS

Small round blue cell tumors (SRBCTs) are comprised of a group of undifferentiated embryonal tumors that show aggressive behavior and include neuroblastoma, rhabdomyosarcoma, non-Hodgkin lymphoma, and the family of Ewing sarcomas. These tumors display similar histologic features and immunohistochemistry, and other molecular techniques are required for their diagnosis.[10]

EWING SARCOMA FAMILY OF TUMORS

The Ewing sarcoma family of tumors includes osseous Ewing sarcoma, extraskeletal Ewing sarcoma, primitive neuroectodermal tumor of bone (PNET), and Askin tumor which share a karyotype abnormality with translocation involving chromosomes 11 and 22. These lesions show sheets of small round blue cells on histopathology.[37]

Ewing Sarcoma

Ewing first identified this tumor in the early 1920s. Ewing sarcoma is the second most common primary malignant bone tumor in children and adolescents after osteosarcoma. It is also the fourth most common malignant bone tumor after multiple myeloma, osteosarcoma, and chondrosarcoma.

Clinical Presentation

Age

It is most frequently seen in the first three decades of life with 95% of cases occurring between 4 and 25 years of age.[37]

Sex

Slight male preponderance is seen (male-to-female ratio of 1.5:1).

Clinical Picture

The patient presents with pain and mass or swelling and symptoms are mostly present for >6 months before diagnosis. The presence of fever and raised erythrocyte sedimentation rate (ESR) can simulate an infectious cause. Pathological fractures at presentation are uncommon.

Site

Most commonly affected sites include femur, ilium, tibia, humerus, fibula, ribs, and sacrum. Less frequently involved sites include mobile portion of spine, scapula, hand, foot, radius, ulna, mandible, maxilla, clavicle, calvaria, facial bones, and sternum. Long tubular bone involvement is more common proximally than distally, the lesion is seen in the diaphysis but the involvement can often be metadiaphyseal.

Usually, a single bone is involved, but multiple lesions occur at presentation in 10% of cases and more commonly later in the disease as Ewing sarcoma spreads by direct infiltration and hematogenous route to other bones and the lungs **(Figs. 16A to C)**. About 60% have bone metastases at autopsy.[38]

Imaging Features

On radiography, Ewing sarcoma appears as an aggressive lesion with bone destruction showing a moth-eaten or

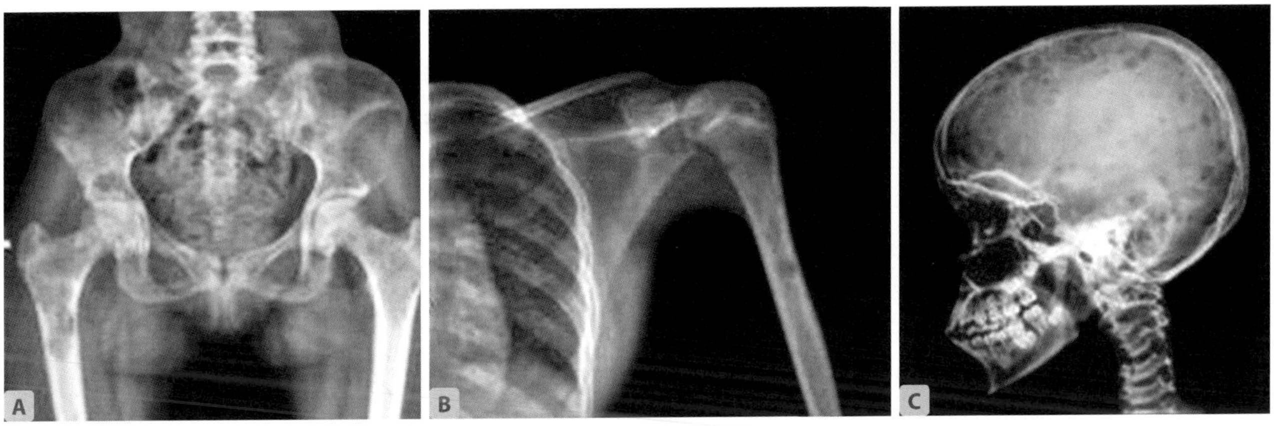

FIGS. 16A TO C: Ewing sarcoma with skeletal metastases. Pelvic radiograph (A) shows the primary tumor as a large predominantly lytic lesion in the left iliac bone with multiple lytic bony metastases in the right iliac blade and both the femora, humeral shaft (B), and skull (C).

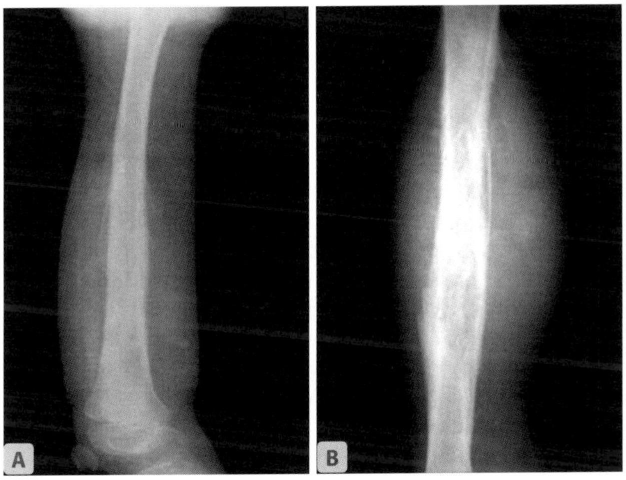

FIGS. 17A AND B: (A) Ewing sarcoma of the femur shows an ill-marginated, lytic-sclerotic lesion with cortical irregularity, laminar periosteal reaction, with a large soft tissue mass in the metadiaphyseal region; (B) In another case involving the femoral diaphysis, "saucerization" is well seen, with peripheral Codman triangles and a large soft tissue mass.

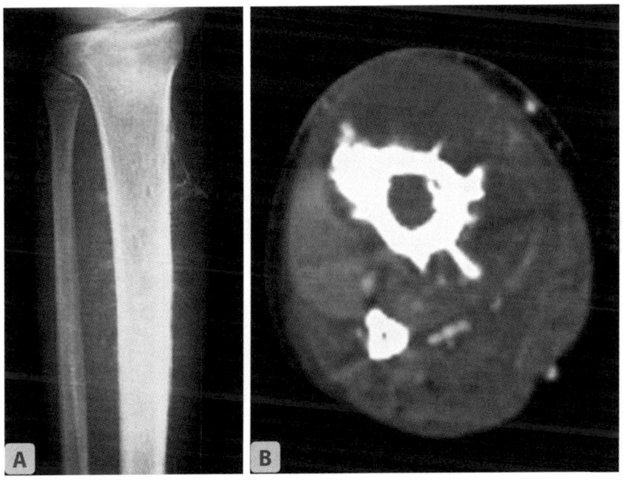

FIGS. 18A AND B: Ewing sarcoma. (A) Conventional radiograph shows a permeative lesion in the tibial diaphysis with a soft tissue component with spiculated periosteal reaction better appreciated on the axial computed tomography (CT) scan (B).

permeative pattern. The lesion shows a wide zone of transition. Cortical destruction associated with a soft-tissue mass is also commonly seen **(Figs. 17A and B)**. Periosteal reaction is also frequently seen and can be lamellated (onion skin), spiculated (sunburst or hair on end) **(Figs. 18A and B)**, or marginal (Codman triangle).

Sclerotic components can be seen that are often noted in the intraosseous component of lesions, in flat bones and spine; it appears dense, cloud-like, and represents reactive bone formation. Less common imaging features include cortical thickening, pathological fracture, expansile bone remodeling, soft-tissue calcification, saucerization, vertebra plana, or a well-marginated lesion. A soft-tissue mass may be the predominant abnormality with the osseous destruction being subtle at radiography. Saucerization of the outer bone cortex is often seen in cases extending from medullary canal.

Computed tomography demonstrates aggressive bony destruction with soft-tissue mass **(Figs. 19A and B)**, areas of focal cortical destruction with continuity between intraosseous and soft-tissue component can be seen. Hypodense linear channels extending through the high attenuation cortex representing tumor extension along neurovascular channels and haversian canals are also common and indicate subtle cortical involvement.[37]

Magnetic resonance imaging shows marrow replacement, cortical destruction, and soft-tissue mass which is circumferential but asymmetric around the osseous involvement **(Figs. 20A to D)**. It shows homogeneous and intermediate signal on T1W images with homogeneous, low-to-intermediate signal on T2W images. Heterogeneity and high T2W signal intensity can also be seen which are more common in larger lesions due to hemorrhage or necrosis **(Figs. 21A to I)**. Large areas of cortical destruction

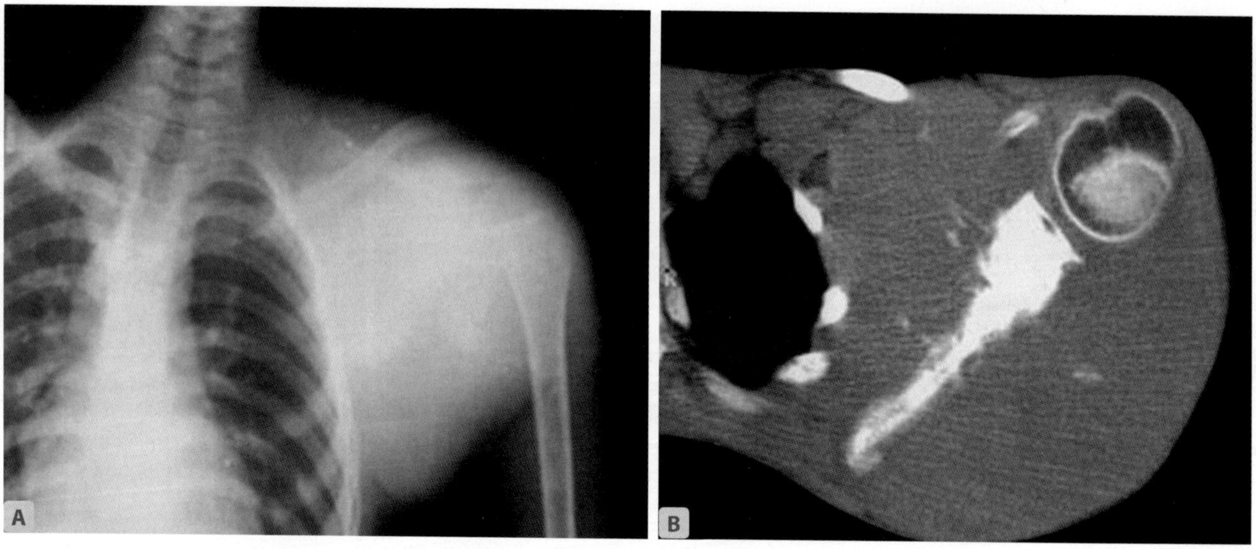

FIGS. 19A AND B: Ewing sarcoma. (A) Plain radiograph; (B) Axial computed tomography (CT) section of left shoulder shows a dense sclerotic involvement of the scapula with a large soft tissue mass.

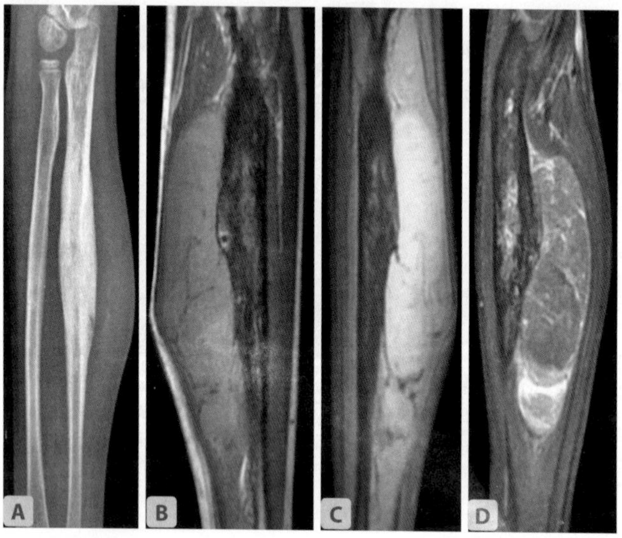

FIGS. 20A TO D: Ewing sarcoma of ulna. Anteroposterior (AP) radiograph of forearm (A) in a young girl presenting with pain and swelling reveals an aggressive lesion with a wide zone of transition involving the diaphysis of the ulna with cortical thickening and periosteal reaction. T1-weighted (T1W) (B), T2-weighted (T2W) (C), and T1-weighted (T1W) fat-saturated postcontrast (D) images show marrow replacement in the diaphysis of the ulna with a large associated soft tissue component appearing hypointense on T1W and hyperintense on T2W images showing heterogeneous postcontrast enhancement.

with continuity between medullary cavity and soft-tissue component are common at MRI **(Figs. 22A to D)**. Subtle cortical involvement as seen on CT is also evident on MRI with intermediate signal intensity channels extending through low signal intensity cortex; this imaging feature strongly suggests an SRBCT such as Ewing sarcoma, lymphoma, or leukemia. Contrast enhancement can be peripheral and nodular or diffuse.[37]

Ewing sarcoma is one of the more aggressive tumors with a tendency toward recurrence and metastases. It is the most common primary malignant tumor to metastasize to bone. Skip lesions are common. Secondary spread to the lungs also occurs frequently involving the lung parenchyma and pleura. FDG-PET is more sensitive than bone scan in the detection of bone metastases, with accuracy similar to whole body MRI.

Differential diagnosis in the early stages is with osteomyelitis or occasionally trauma. Each of these may produce a periosteal reaction with little bone destruction. In Ewing sarcoma, a well-defined soft-tissue mass is seen, while in infection, the soft-tissue component is ill-defined. In later stages, Ewing sarcoma may be indistinguishable from a lytic osteosarcoma. Primary lymphoma is differential in patients over the age of 30 years. Langerhans cell histiocytosis may occasionally mimic Ewing sarcoma, especially when presenting at an early destructive stage and involving the pelvis.[29]

Ewing sarcoma is usually treated with multiple cycles of multidrug chemotherapy for local and metastatic disease and radiation therapy or limb salvage for local control of tumor. Resectable lesions in the extremities have a better prognosis than those found in the pelvis or other bones of the axial skeleton.[39] Pretreatment DCE MRI has a potential role for determining the outcome and may be used in the decision to intensify treatment.[40] With treatment, the soft-tissue mass decreases in size and the intraosseous portion becomes necrotic with a higher signal on T2W imaging. MRI is also more accurate than standard radiography, CT, or scintigraphy in the diagnosis of recurrent Ewing sarcoma.

Rarely, extraskeletal Ewing sarcoma (EES) may develop in the soft tissues at any location. The most common sites of occurrence of EES are the trunk, extremities, and retroperitoneum. Although it is a soft-tissue primary tumor, it can cause changes in the cortex of the adjacent bone. EES is more common in adults and is associated with a high incidence of local recurrence and distant metastases.[41]

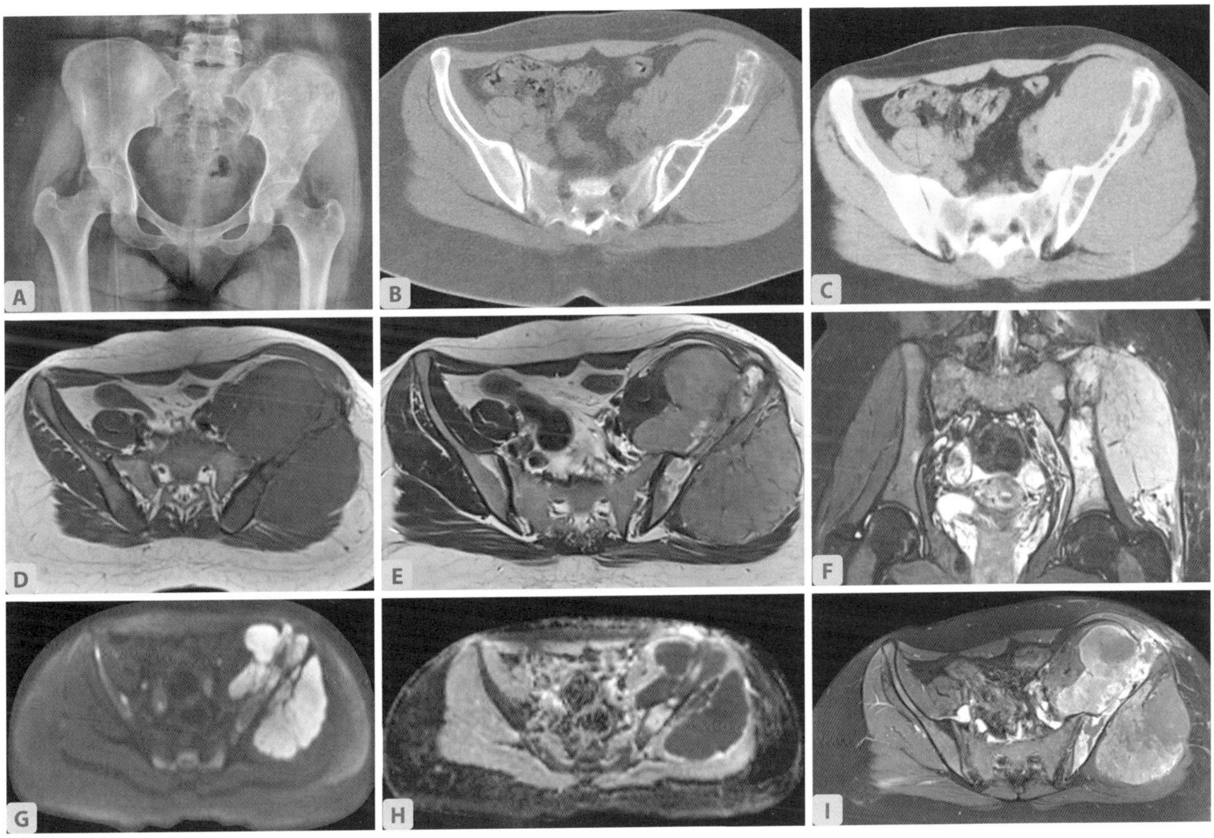

FIGS. 21A TO I: Ewing sarcoma of left iliac blade. Anteroposterior (AP) radiograph of the pelvis (A) in a young female with complaints of pain and swelling in gluteal region shows a large lytic lesion with permeative pattern of bony destruction involving the left iliac blade. Axial computed tomography (CT) images in the bone (B) and soft tissue (C) windows show the large, ill-defined lytic lesion in the left iliac blade associated with a large soft tissue component. Axial T1-weighted (T1W) (D), axial T2-weighted (T2W) (E), and short tau inversion recovery (STIR) coronal (F) images of the same patient show diffusely altered marrow signal intensity within the left iliac blade with a large soft tissue component seen along both sides of the bone, appearing hypointense to isointense to the surrounding muscle on T1W image and heterogeneously hyperintense on T2W and STIR images. Two small hyperintense focal lesions are seen in the left sacral ala and right iliac bone on STIR images suggestive of metastases. The lesion shows restricted diffusion on diffusion-weighted image (G) and appears hypointense on the corresponding apparent diffusion coefficient (ADC) map (H); heterogeneous enhancement with few nonenhancing necrotic areas are seen within the soft tissue component on postgadolinium scan (I).

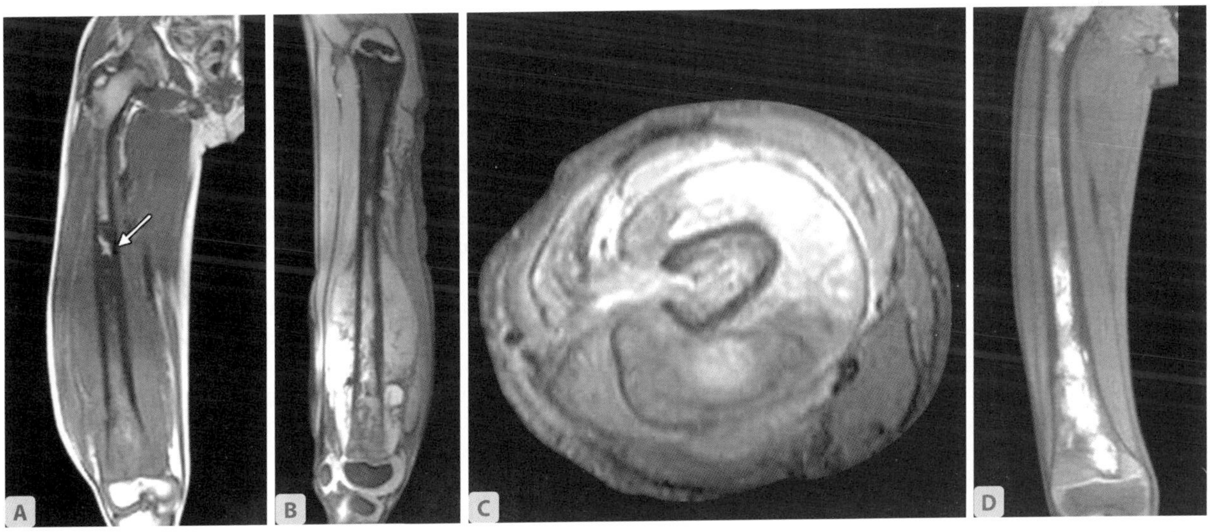

FIGS. 22A TO D: Ewing sarcoma. A T1-weighted (T1W) coronal scan (A) shows the intramedullary extent of the tumor as low signal intensity of the marrow with a small "skip" lesion proximally (arrow). The extraosseous component is better appreciated on the short tau inversion recovery (STIR) coronal image (B). The axial T2-weighted (T2W) image (C) shows the tumor within the femur as high signal intensity with cortical discontinuity. Soft tissue component can be seen surrounding the femoral diaphysis, displacing the neurovascular bundle posteromedially (D). After radiotherapy, there is marked reduction in the soft tissue mass with well-defined high signal intensity mass within the bone suggesting necrotic change.

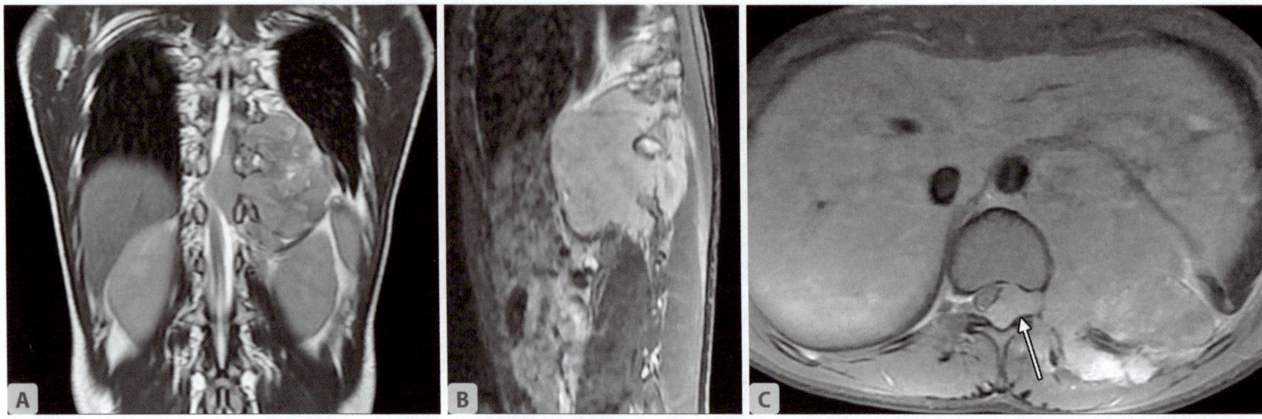

FIGS. 23A TO C: Askin tumor of chest wall in a young male presenting with lower back pain and difficulty in walking, T2-weighted (T2W) coronal (A) and short tau inversion recovery (STIR) sagittal images (B) show a relatively well-marginated paraspinal mass of high signal intensity in the left dorsolumbar region. Postcontrast axial (C) image shows the enhancing lesion with associated rib destruction, intradural extension, and mass effect on spinal cord (arrow in C).

Primitive Neuroectodermal Tumor of Bone

These rare tumors of bone resemble Ewing tumors clinically except that they are more common in the female sex. They arise in the metaphyses and diaphyses of the lower limbs, humerus, pelvis, and scapula. Radiologically, they resemble Ewing sarcoma in being destructive ill-defined neoplasms which readily spread into the soft tissues. *Askin tumor* is a rare PNET of the thoracopulmonary region occurring in children and young adults. Radiologically, in 70% of patients, it presents as a pleural disorder **(Figs. 23A to C)**. A soft-tissue mass involving the chest wall is seen in about half of the patients and a subpleural pulmonary mass with pleural involvement in about one quarter.[29]

NOTOCHORDAL ORIGIN

Chordoma

Chordoma is a rare, low-to-intermediate grade malignant tumor which arises from ectopic cellular remnants of the notochord which have persisted within the nucleus pulposus of the intervertebral disc or from aberrant cell rests of notochord tissue within the vertebral bodies. This tumor has a predilection for the sacrococcygeal and spheno-occipital regions.[19,42]

Clinical Presentation

Age

It is most common in the fifth and sixth decades.

Sex

Incidence is more common in males with male:female ratio varying from 2:1 to 3:1.

Clinical Picture

Patients present with pain. Other symptoms relate to pressure on local structures—rectal/vesical dysfunction in the sacral region and cranial nerve palsies in the spheno-occipital region.

Site

It usually occurs as a solitary lesion and is exclusively seen in the axial skeleton, in midline of sacrococcygeal region, more commonly below S3 level (50%), spheno-occipital region (40%), or vertebrae (5%). Spheno-occipital tumors are seen in younger patients and are smaller in size as compared to sacrococcygeal lesions. Vertebral chordomas can occur equally in both men and women, it can affect children and is more common in cervical region. Distant metastases are rare, mainly involving lymph nodes, liver, and lungs.

Imaging Features

Clinical presentation is delayed due to the slow-growing nature of these tumors and radiologically, these lesions appear advanced. Radiographs reveal a destructive lytic lesion associated with a soft-tissue mass that may show nonspecific, amorphous calcification **(Fig. 24A)**. A sclerotic margin and narrow zone of transition may be present as a result of slow growth, especially in spinal lesions. In the spheno-occipital region, the dorsal aspect of the sella and clivus may be destroyed, with a soft-tissue mass indenting the nasopharyngeal airway.

Computed tomography scans show a destructive expansive lesion and a large lobulated soft-tissue mass containing calcification **(Fig. 24B)**. Due to the gelatinous matrix, the soft-tissue mass shows low attenuation on CT and intermediate-to-low signal intensity on T1W images and high signal intensity on T2W images on MRI **(Figs. 25A to C)**. Hemorrhage, when present, appears as a high T1 signal. Variable contrast enhancement is seen, appearing minimal in myxoid-containing lobules and moderate in vascular septa, which produces a crisscross pattern. Sacral nerve root involvement is best seen on coronal MR images. Assessment should include extension to sacroiliac joints, spinal nerves, and plexus. The differential diagnosis for this condition includes chondrosarcoma, plasmacytoma, metastasis, and lymphoma.

Vertebral chordoma lesions begin in the center of the body and extend to involve the posterior elements, with

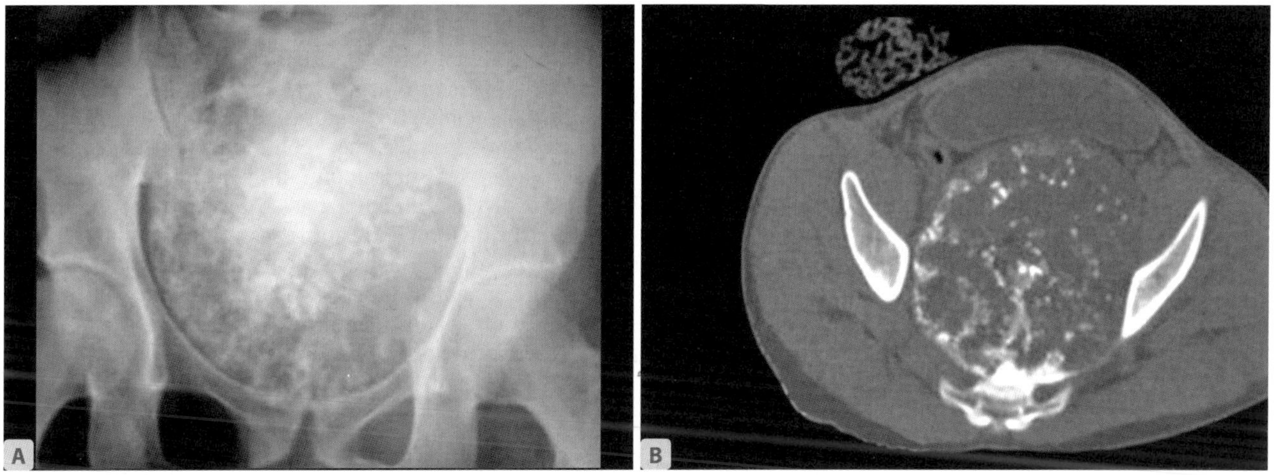

FIGS. 24A AND B: Chordoma of the sacrum. Plain radiograph (A) and computed tomography (CT) (B) showing a large pelvic mass with calcification.

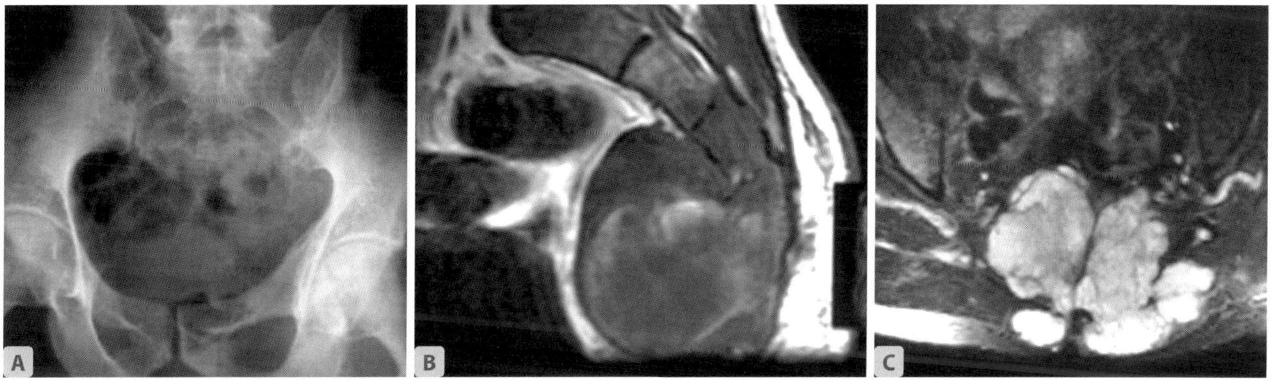

FIGS. 25A TO C: Chordoma of the sacrum. (A) Plain radiograph shows a lytic lesion destroying the distal half of the sacrum (B) and (C) T1-weighted (T1W) sagittal and T2-weighted (T2W) axial magnetic resonance (MR) images show the large tumor with inhomogeneous signal intensity arising from the distal sacrum.

soft-tissue masses seen anterior, posterior, and lateral to the bodies. With involvement of the epidural space, the soft-tissue mass may extend to involve multiple craniocaudal contiguous levels. Discal involvement is seen very late in the disease and as chordoma and discs show the same signal on MRI, disc involvement is not diagnosed based on MRI signal, but on the loss of end-plate integrity. The differential diagnosis for vertebral chordoma includes tuberculosis, chondrosarcoma, and metastasis from renal adenocarcinoma.

Treatment for chordoma includes wide resection and surgical debulking; rectal involvement necessitates a colostomy. Radiotherapy may be done in operable cases, where wide resection is not possible. Younger patients and those with lesions that are small or sacrococcygeal have a better prognosis. Metastasis occurs late in the disease in 10% of the patients with sacrococcygeal lesions and in 30–40% of patients with spinal lesions. Although metastasis is relatively uncommon, it is locally aggressive, often resulting in severe neurologic symptoms. High rate of local recurrence (around 40%) is noted, especially in the surgical bed, which is treated with radiation.

The chondroid variant of chordoma (approximately 15% of chordomas) contains cartilaginous areas with most present in the skull base. Imaging features for this variant are similar to those of chondrosarcoma. CT and MRI reveal a lobulated tumor, with low attenuation areas and calcification and with low T1 and high T2 signal. Contrast enhancement is not lobular, but there is only mild septal enhancement compared with the lobular, nodular, or diffuse enhancement of chondrosarcomas. Occasionally, a rings-and-arcs pattern of enhancement may be seen.

Chordomas (chondroid and nonchondroid) stain for cytokeratins, epithelial membrane antigen (EMA), and carcinoembryonic antigen (CEA), but these antigens are not expressed by chondrosarcomas.

Dedifferentiated chordomas (around 6–9% of chordomas) can occur in either primary or recurrent chordoma. It is more common in the sacrococcygeal region, particularly after radiation. Extra-axial chordomas have also been reported; patients with these lesions tend to have a better prognosis because the tumors are not near vital structures in the midline. CT and MRI show destructive lesions with internal hemorrhage and cyst formation.[1]

VASCULAR TUMORS OF THE BONE

Malignant vascular lesions of the bone are rare and usually present with nonspecific clinical and radiological features. Tumors in this group include hemangioendothelioma, epithelioid hemangioendothelioma, and angiosarcoma. Vascular tumors of the bone should be considered in the presence of multifocal bony lesions, especially distal to elbow or knee joints in young or middle-aged patients.

Angiosarcoma

Angiosarcoma is a rare, high-grade malignant vascular tumor of bone, affecting all ages, although peak incidence is seen in third and fourth decades. Male:female ratio is 2:1. Any bone can be affected, but the vertebrae and the femur are most commonly involved. Multiple lesions occur in one-third of the cases.[19,43]

Radiologically, a multilocular or "soap bubble" appearance may be seen. The lesion often involves a considerable length of bone. It may be seen as a lytic lesion with ill-defined margins, mixed lytic and sclerotic lesions have also been described. Purely sclerotic lesions are rare. Endosteal erosion, cortical destruction, and extraosseous extension can be seen; however, periosteal reaction and pathological fractures are rare. CT and MRI appearances are nonspecific. This is a highly malignant tumor usually treated by surgery including amputation, limb salvage, radical local resection, and radiotherapy with a 5-year survival rate of under 10%. Differential diagnosis includes primary sarcomas and metastases.

Hemangioendothelioma

Hemangioendothelioma is a rare low-grade endothelial neoplasm that can occur between the ages of 10 and 60 years and is more commonly seen in males. Sites of involvement include lower limb (femur and tibia) followed by vertebrae, upper limb, and flat bones. It is common in diaphysis but may also be seen in metaphysis or metaepiphysis. Twenty-five percent of patients may have multicentric disease.[19] Multiple lesions in one bone or extremity or multifocal lesions in various bones may suggest this diagnosis. Usually, the lesion is lytic, although mixed lytic sclerotic and purely sclerotic lesions may be seen. Osseous expansion, cortical thinning, and endosteal erosions can be present; periosteal reaction, cortical destruction, and soft-tissue masses are uncommon.

In children, differential diagnosis for a multifocal lesion includes Langerhans cell histiocytosis, fibrous dysplasia, brown tumor, and metastasis; and in adults, the differential diagnosis includes metastasis, multiple myeloma, lymphoma, brown tumors, and fibrous dysplasia. A solitary lesion may be confused with fibrous dysplasia, fibrous cortical defect, solitary bone cyst, osteosarcoma, spindle cell sarcoma (fibrosarcoma), or Ewing sarcoma. These patients have variable prognosis which depends on the histologic grade, level of differentiation, and unifocal or multifocal nature of the tumor. Treatment includes surgery and adjuvant therapy for unifocal lesions and radiation for multifocal lesions.

Epithelioid Hemangioendothelioma

Epithelioid hemangioendothelioma is a rare malignant vascular neoplasm that involves multiple skeletal sites; it has nonspecific imaging features. This condition can occur across a wide age range, most commonly in the second and third decades. It is more commonly seen in men. Typical sites of involvement include calvarium, spine, femur, tibia, and feet. In the long bones, it is seen in the metaphysis or epiphysis. Radiographs reveal lytic lesions, 40% of which are multifocal and usually involve a single anatomic site or extremity. Cortical destruction and expansion are commonly seen, whereas periosteal reaction and matrix mineralization are rare. A soft-tissue mass is seen in 40% of cases.[19]

MYOGENIC, LIPOGENIC, AND EPITHELIAL TUMORS

Liposarcoma

Primary intraosseous liposarcoma is extremely rare despite the extensive fatty content of the bone marrow. It is four times as common in males as in females, and is seen between 24 and 45 years of age.[19]

Most tumors affect the long bones of the lower limbs, the femur and the tibia. The lesion can be seen in the epiphysis, metaphysis, or diaphysis. Radiologically, appearance varies from local geographic bone destruction to a permeative pattern. Fluid–fluid levels may be seen. CT and MRI provide characteristic diagnostic information due to the nonhomogeneous fatty content of the tumor. Although fat-containing lesions are usually considered benign, biopsy is essential in the presence of cortical destruction and soft-tissue mass which can indicate malignancy.

Adamantinoma of Long Bones

This is a rare low-grade epithelioid malignant lesion which is characterized by squamous, alveolar, and vascular tissues of unknown origin. It most commonly involves the midshaft of the tibia. Although it has some histological resemblance to maxillofacial adamantinoma, the two conditions are not related.

Clinical Presentation

Age

It is commonly seen in the second and third decades.

Sex

It is more common in men.

Clinical Picture

Local pain and tenderness of several months to several years' duration is the most common presenting complaint.

Site

Most commonly seen in tibia (83%) followed by fibula, humerus, and femur. It is classically located in the anterior tibial diaphysis in its mid or proximal portions. Tumors with multiple foci in the same long bone may sometimes occur.

Imaging Features

Adamantinomas can be situated in the cortex or the medullary space. Radiographs reveal an eccentric, intracortical, expansile mixed lytic lesion that can extend longitudinally in the cortex or it can destroy the cortex and extend into the medulla. Soap bubble appearance can be seen with multilocularity and thin walls. A multiloculated appearance and satellite lesions are useful diagnostic features. Periosteal reaction is uncommon. MRI is invaluable in the local staging of adamantinoma for features such as extension into the marrow cavity, extraosseous extension, and multifocal lesions. A lobulated growth pattern is typical, but there are no specific signal characteristics. Intense, uniform enhancement is seen following contrast-enhanced studies.[44]

Differential diagnosis includes metastatic carcinoma, plasmacytoma, ABC, fibrous dysplasia, and osteofibrous dysplasia. However, fibrous dysplasia is seen at a younger age and shows ground-glass opacity with anterior tibial bowing without periosteal reaction or moth-eaten destruction. Unlike adamantinoma, osteofibrous dysplasia occurs in patients younger than 10 years and is typically intracortical with no medullary extension. Age is a helpful differentiating factor when imaging findings overlap.

Adamantinomas grow at a slow rate but are characterized by local recurrences and eventual metastases to the lung. Metastases to the bones and lymph nodes can also occur. Extensive local resection is the usual form of treatment.

Differentiated adamantinoma (osteofibrous dysplasia-like adamantinoma) is a variant of adamantinoma, a diagnosis that is based on histology. It has a prolonged course similar to osteofibrous dysplasia and is treated less aggressively.

UNDIFFERENTIATED PLEOMORPHIC SARCOMA (MALIGNANT FIBROUS HISTIOCYTOMA)

Malignant fibrous histiocytomas were replaced by the term undifferentiated pleomorphic sarcoma (UPS) which denotes the anonymity of the entity but confirms its mesenchymal origin and malignant nature.[45]

Most of these lesions arise de novo; about 22–43% of the lesions arise secondary to preexisting osseous lesions that are caused by previous irradiation, bone infarcts, Paget's disease, chronic osteomyelitis, fibrous dysplasia, ABC, GCT, neurofibromatosis 1, or orthopedic implants.[19]

Clinical Presentation

Age

Most commonly seen in fifth to seventh decades with peak incidence in the fifth decade.

Sex

Males are more commonly affected, with male-to-female ratio of 3:2.

Clinical Picture

The patient presents with localized pain and swelling of insidious onset. Pathological fracture is common.

Site

Lesions involve the ends of long bones commonly, especially the distal diametaphysis of the femur and proximal metaphysis of the tibia. Other bones involved are the humerus, the ribs, the craniofacial bones, and the spine.

Imaging Features

An aggressive lytic lesion with permeative type of bony destruction is seen on radiographs with involvement of soft tissue being a common feature. Periosteal reaction is rare. Occasionally punctate, soft-tissue calcification is present. Most cases present with multiple skeletal lesions and the initial impression is of skeletal metastases rather than of a primary or multifocal bone tumor. The main differential diagnosis is a malignant round cell tumor.

The lesions show variable appearance on MRI, ranging from isointense to slightly hyperintense relative to muscle on T1W images and intermediate to slightly hyperintense relative to muscle on STIR and T2W images, with nodular and inhomogeneous enhancement pattern. This appearance makes it one of the few lytic malignant lesions without a very high T2 signal, similar to lymphoma and leiomyosarcoma, because of the histologic fibrous tissue matrix and variable cellularity in these lesions. Predominantly, hypointense T1 and hyperintense T2 signals in the lesion have also been reported. In secondary cases, the underlying bone lesion is seen along with UPS. Extraosseous disease is seen in almost all patients with UPS. UPS is associated with a high rate of local recurrence and metastasis, particularly to lungs, bones, brain, kidneys, and heart.

MALIGNANT GIANT CELL TUMOR

Malignant GCTs are a heterogeneous group of tumors, which contain giant cells that have aggressive local behavior and systemic metastasis. The malignant GCT classification can be divided into categories of malignancy in GCT, giant cell-containing sarcoma, secondary malignant GCT, and benign metastasizing GCT. Malignancy in GCT and secondary malignant GCT account for about 6% of all GCTs. Malignancy in GCT have sarcomatous areas juxtaposed with typical benign GCT in patients with no history of radiation, resection, or curettage.

When a sarcoma develops in patients with a history of radiation, resection, or curettage of conventional GCT, the lesion is labeled secondary malignant GCT (87%). A history of radiation is present in 76% of these secondary GCT cases, with a latent period of 10 years or longer. Secondary malignant GCT in the absence of radiation is extremely rare. Malignancy in GCT is said to occur in an older population than conventional GCTs. Giant cell-containing sarcoma is an anaplastic variant of the typical benign GCT, but without the evidence of tumor osteoid, bone, or cartilage. It is often associated with Paget's disease and should be differentiated pathologically from giant cell-rich sarcoma variants, such as osteosarcoma and fibrosarcoma.

Benign metastasizing GCT is a term used for skeletal GCT with pulmonary metastasis that is histologically identical to GCT. It is seen in 1.8–5% of GCTs. Local recurrence is seen in 48% of these patients. The prognosis for these patients is good. Metastasectomy is recommended when feasible.[19]

METASTATIC BONE DISEASE

Skeletal metastases are defined as tumors involving bone, which originate from another distal site. Metastases are the most common malignant tumors of the skeletal system. Approximately 70% of all malignant tumors are metastatic in origin, with only 30% being primary in nature.[46] Postmortem studies show that their incidence is much higher than may be detected in vivo. Bony metastases are present in approximately 25% of all deaths from malignant diseases.[47] Most of the osseous metastases are from a primary extraskeletal focus; the majority are epithelial in origin. The most common primary sites are in the breast, lung, prostate, kidney, thyroid, and bowel. With the exception of tumors of the central nervous system and basal cell carcinoma of the skin, almost every malignant tumor can metastasize to bone.

Bone involvement in metastases occurs by means of three main mechanisms: (1) direct extension, (2) retrograde venous flow, and (3) seeding with tumor emboli via the blood circulation which is the most common route of spread. Venous tumor emboli get arrested at a distant capillary bed. As the tumor emboli have to pass through the pulmonary bed, metastatic cancer to bone is a relatively late occurrence and generally occurs after pulmonary metastases have appeared.[48] Retrograde venous embolism is probably the major mechanism when spread from intra-abdominal cancer involves the vertebrae. Increased intra-abdominal pressure causes blood to be diverted from the systemic caval system to the valveless vertebral venous plexus of Batson; this diversion allows the caudal and cranial flow of blood.

Clinical Presentation

Age

Most patients are older than 40 years. In children <5 years, skeletal metastases usually occur from neuroblastoma. Metastases between the age group of 10 and 25 years commonly occur from Ewing sarcoma and osteosarcoma, and between 20 and 35 years, they occur from Hodgkin lymphoma.

Sex

In females, the carcinoma of the breast is responsible for majority of all bone metastases followed by the carcinomas of thyroid, kidney, and uterus. In males, carcinoma prostate is the most common primary focus, followed by the carcinoma of the lung.

Site

They are most often found in the axial skeleton and other sites of residual red marrow. Thus, the common sites for metastases are vertebrae, pelvis, proximal femora and humeri, skull, sternum, and ribs. Metastases to bones of hand and feet are rare and almost 50% of these are due to the carcinoma of the lung.

Clinical Picture

The lesions may be entirely asymptomatic or present with vague bone pains. Occasionally, a pathological fracture through the metastatic lesion may bring it to notice. Weight loss, cachexia, anemia, and even fever may be seen in the later stages.

Imaging Features

Plain Radiographs

Bone metastases may be lytic, sclerotic, or mixed lytic and sclerotic. As a metastatic lesion grows in the medullary cavity, the surrounding bone is remodeled by means of either osteoclastic or osteoblastic processes. The relative degree of resultant bone resorption or deposition is highly variable and depends on the type and the location of the tumor. The relationship between the osteoclastic and osteoblastic remodeling processes determines whether a predominant lytic, sclerotic, or mixed pattern is seen on radiographs. The majority (75%) of metastases is osteolytic. Lesions usually appear in the medullary cavity, spread to destroy the medullary bone, and then involve the cortex, usually without the development of much periosteal reaction. Soft-tissue extension is relatively uncommon. At least 30–50% bone destruction is necessary before the lytic lesions can be detected on plain radiographs.

Some metastases (15%) are predominantly osteoblastic, e.g., from prostate, stomach, and carcinoid. The increased density of the blastic metastases is due to the laying down of new bone, which is non-neoplastic in nature, but is a reactive response of the local osteoid tissue to the presence of the tumor. Mixed osteolytic and osteosclerotic metastasis (10%) occur from carcinoma of the breast and occasionally, lung.

Breast in females and prostate in males are the most common primary tumors metastasizing to bone. Breast metastases are commonly lytic **(Figs. 26A and B)**, but 10% may be osteoblastic and in another 10% can be mixed. Diffuse infiltration of the whole marrow may occur and may only become evident radiologically when sclerosis occurs after therapy. Skeletal metastases from prostate are predominantly blastic or mixed **(Figs. 27A and B)**. Purely lytic lesions are rare. Individual lesions may sometimes show a florid "sunburst' appearance, simulating osteosarcoma **(Fig. 28)**. Metastases from the lung occur most commonly to the axial skeleton **(Figs. 29A to D)**; however, metastases to hand and foot are most commonly from bronchogenic carcinoma **(Fig. 30)**. The squamous cell and oat cell carcinomas of lung produce lytic metastases, while adenocarcinomas and bronchial carcinoid which metastasize to bone in about 10% of cases, produce focal, or diffuse densely blastic lesions.

Hypernephroma and thyroid carcinoma generally show lytic, expansile metastases, also called "blow-out metastases" **(Fig. 31)**. The incidence of skeletal metastases from the gastrointestinal tract is under 7%, but as these malignancies are more common than kidney and thyroid, they are encountered commonly. They are usually lytic, but sclerotic metastases may occur. Calcification is also a feature. Cervical carcinoma usually involves bone by contiguous spread to the bony pelvis. Blood-borne metastases are uncommon

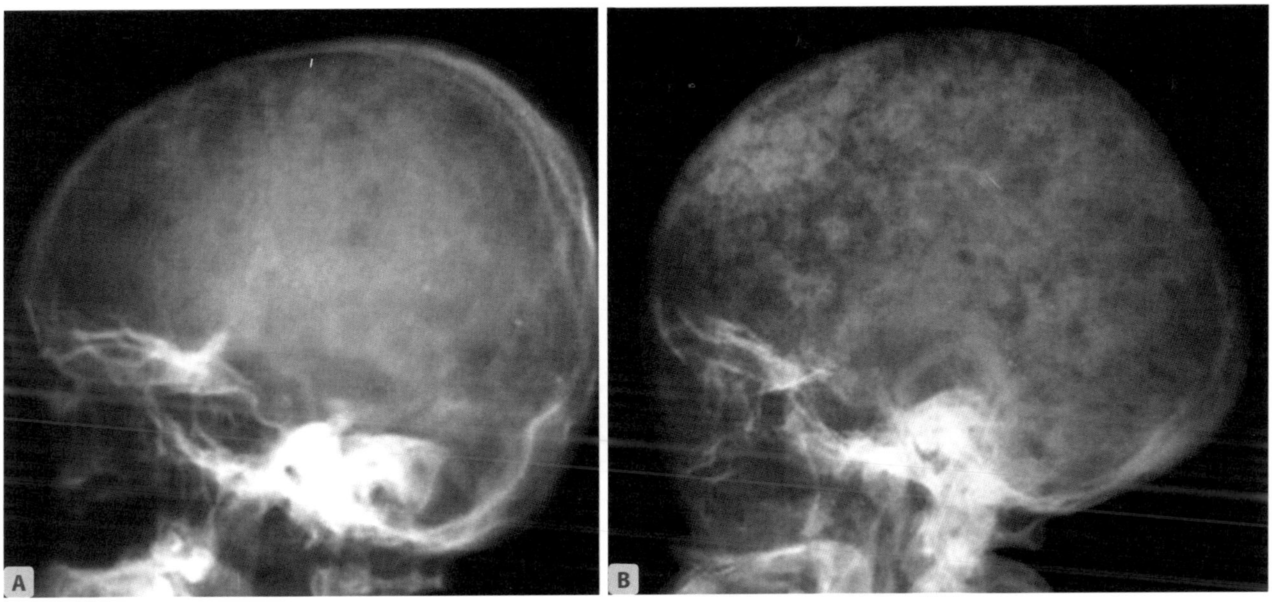

FIGS. 26A AND B: Skeletal metastases. Lateral radiographs (A and B) of the skull of two different patients show multiple ill-defined lytic lesions of varying sizes in the calvarium.

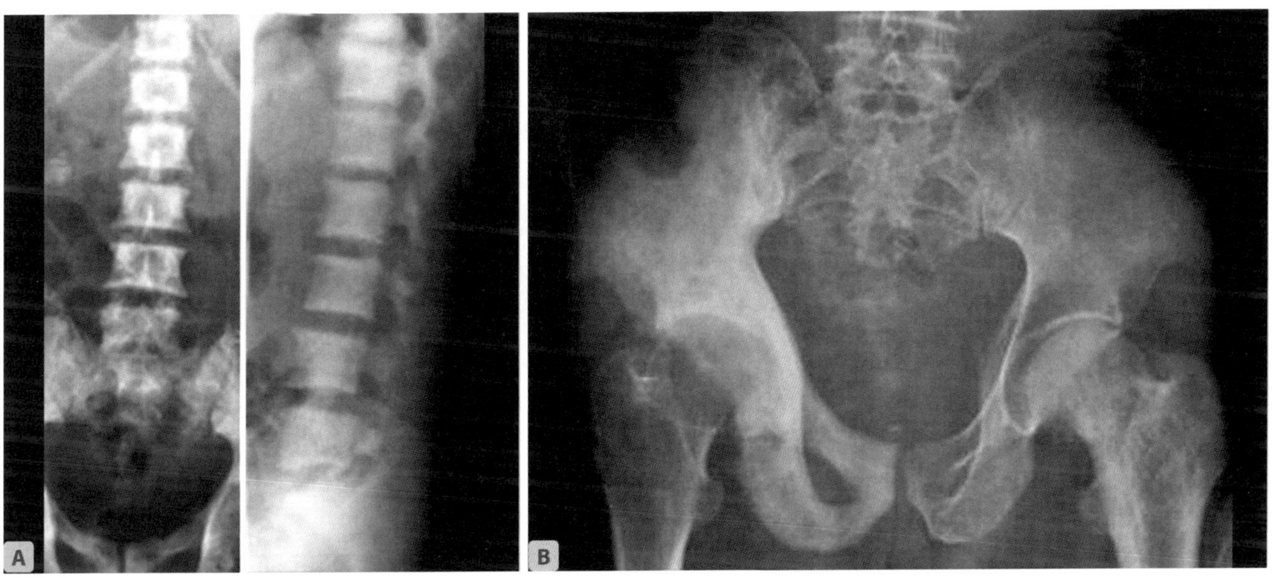

FIGS. 27A AND B: Metastases from carcinoma prostate. (A) Anteroposterior (AP) and lateral radiographs of the lumbar spine show characteristic osteoblastic metastases; (B) Radiograph of pelvis shows diffuse sclerosis in the right iliac bone and left femoral head.

and usually lytic, but may rarely be osteoblastic or mixed. Carcinoma of the uterine body is an adenocarcinoma and, like that of the ovary, may produce osteoblastic metastases, particularly of the vertebrae.

Nuclear Medicine

The value of establishing the presence of multiple skeletal lesions cannot be overemphasized, as individual metastatic lesions may mimic primary malignant tumors of bone. For this purpose, bone scintigraphy remains the most cost-effective method.[49] Several patterns of scintigraphic abnormality may be seen. The most common is one of multiple sites of increased skeletal activity typically in the axial skeleton **(Fig. 32)**. The abnormal uptake on scintigraphy depends upon intact local blood flow and increased osteoblastic activity. Lesions which outgrow their blood supply or stimulate no osteoblastic response may appear as photopenic or "cold spots." Occasionally, a combination of both "hot" and "cold" lesions may be seen. A super scan appearance, i.e., generalized increase in skeletal activity with reduced or absent renal activity is typically seen in diffuse osteoblastic metastatic disease from breast or prostate **(Fig. 33)**.

The specificity of bone scintigraphy is generally lower, due to a known increased blood flow and bone remodeling in response to a variety of disease processes, including trauma, infection, inflammation, and osteoarthritis. Therefore, further assessment with other imaging modalities, mainly CT and MRI, and in some cases, histologic confirmation may be required for precise diagnosis.

Single photon emission computed tomography (SPECT) imaging of the skeleton uses ^{99m}Tc-MDP, the same radionuclide used in conventional skeletal scintigraphy; however, images are acquired in a cross-sectional rather than a planar fashion. Whereas planar imaging is limited by superimposition of structures, SPECT can show axial slices through the body, providing better localization of abnormal radionuclide uptake. Addition of SPECT has been reported to detect 20–50% more lesions in the spine compared with planar scintigraphy. It increases both the sensitivity and the specificity of bone scans.

FDG-PET is more sensitive and specific than bone scan for detecting bone metastases. It detects all types of bone metastases; however, it is more sensitive for detecting lytic metastases than sclerotic metastases **(Figs. 34A to E)**.

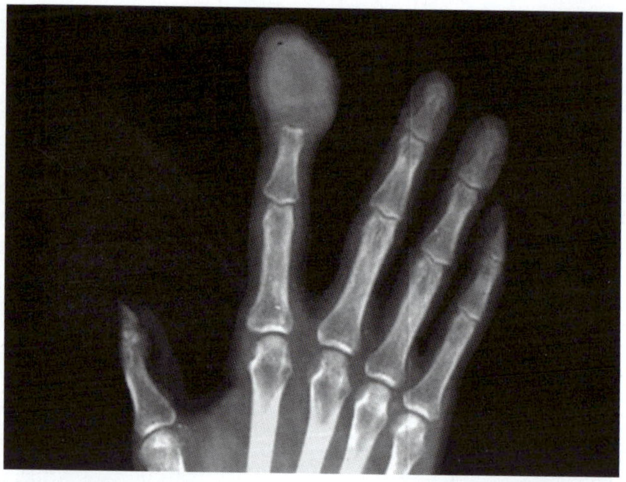

FIG. 30: Metastasis from carcinoma lung. A lytic lesion involves the terminal phalanx of the index finger.

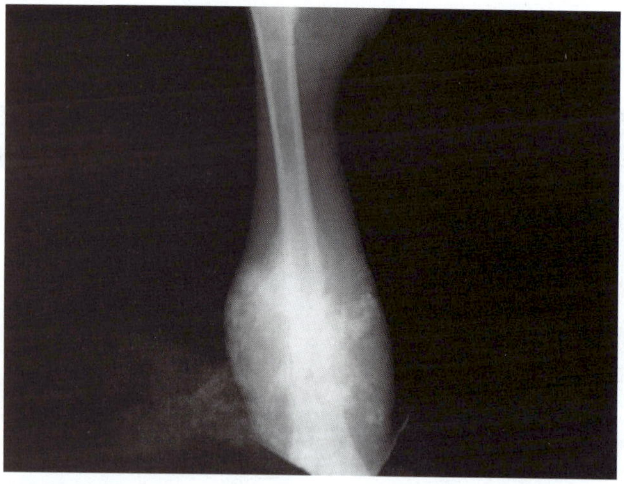

FIG. 28: Metastasis from carcinoma prostate. Anteroposterior (AP) radiograph of the femur shows osteoblastic metastasis with extensive "sunburst" periosteal reaction resembling osteosarcoma.

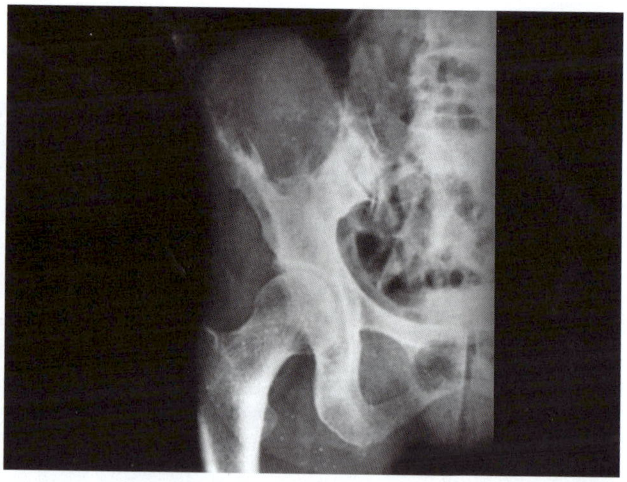

FIG. 31: Metastasis from a hypernephroma. A large lytic lesion is seen in the left iliac blade.

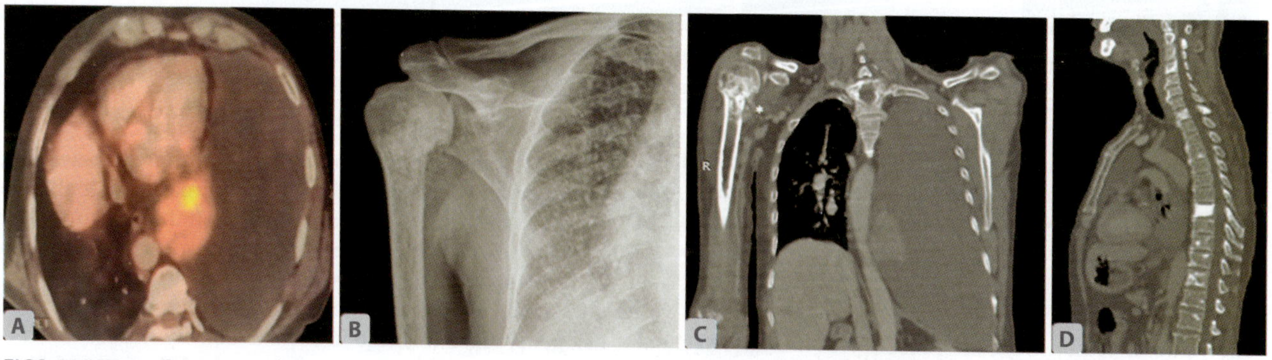

FIGS. 29A TO D: Carcinoma of the left lung with metastases to right humerus and vertebrae in an adult male patient. Positron emission tomography computed tomography (PET-CT) (A) reveals a malignant lesion showing increased uptake in the collapsed left lung with massive left pleural effusion. Anteroposterior (AP) radiograph of right shoulder (B) shows a sclerotic lesion in the humeral head and proximal shaft with associated irregularity along the medial aspect of the humeral head and neck. Coronal (C) and sagittal (D) CT images in bone window shows the sclerotic lesion in head and shaft of right humerus with associated soft tissue in axilla and multiple sclerotic lesions involving vertebrae at various levels.

The increased avidity of lytic lesions for FDG is because of the high glycolytic rate and relative hypoxemia that are characteristic of these lesions in contrast to sclerotic lesions, which are relatively acellular, less aggressive, and not prone to hypoxia.[14] FDG-PET has the additional advantage of detecting extraskeletal metastatic disease as well. FDG-PET has also proved to be an effective modality for the assessment of therapeutic response by showing rapid reduction in FDG uptake by the tumors in responders following chemotherapy. The changes in standard uptake value (SUV) with therapy showed good correlation with the overall clinical assessment of response as well as with the change in tumor marker value.

Sodium fluoride PET is very sensitive for detecting both osteolytic and osteoblastic lesions and is superior to bone

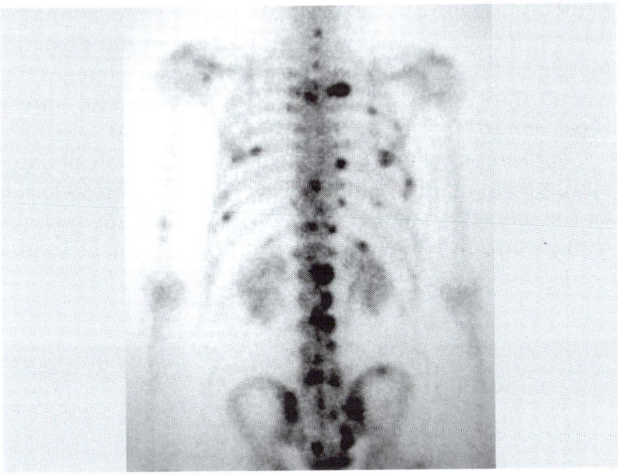

FIG. 32: Skeletal scintigraphy in metastatic disease of the skeleton shows multiple randomly distributed focal lesions scattered throughout the skeleton, particularly the spine, ribs, and pelvis.

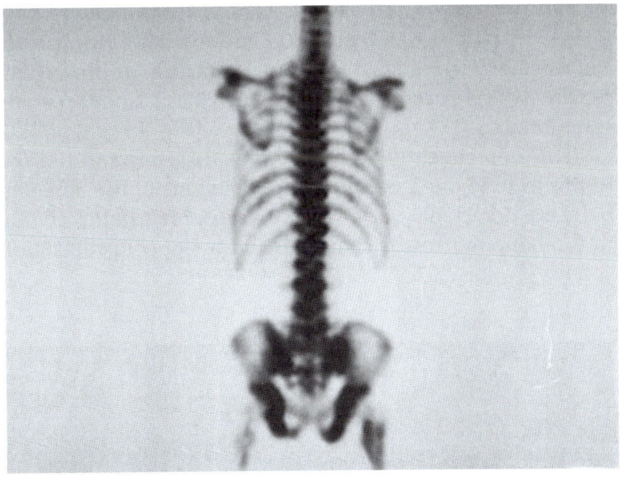

FIG. 33: Technetium-99m bone scintiscan in a case of prostatic carcinoma. This image shows diffuse and intense uptake in most of the bones. Patchy rib lesions are also seen, but renal uptake is absent.

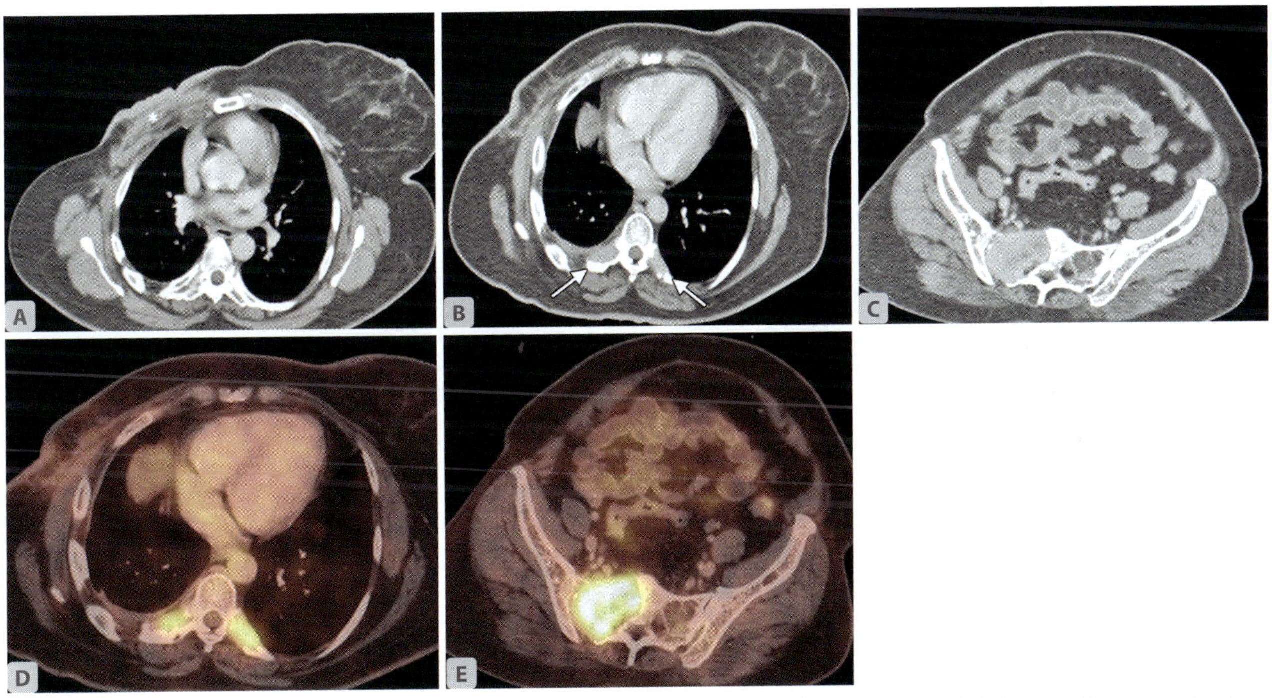

FIGS. 34A TO E: Bone metastases in a postoperative postradiotherapy case of invasive ductal carcinoma right breast with neuroendocrine differentiation. Axial contrast-enhanced computed tomography (CECT) images of the chest (A and B) show right mastectomy with postradiotherapy changes involving chest wall on the right side, lytic lesions with associated soft tissue noted at the vertebral ends of bilateral ribs (arrows). Axial CECT image at the level of sacrum (C) shows an expansile soft tissue density lesion in the right sacral ala. Axial positron emission tomography computed tomography (PET-CT) images (D and E) show avid fluorodeoxyglucose (FDG) uptake in the lesions involving the ribs and sacrum.

scintigraphy for diagnosing skeletal metastases. Evan-Sapir et al. compared bone scintigraphy, NaF-PET, and NaF-PET/CT in patients with high-risk prostate cancer and found that NaF-PET/CT was the most accurate modality for detecting bone metastases.[50] Increased FDG activity at the sites of skeletal lesions represents active tumor itself, whereas increased ^{99m}Tc-MDP or 18F-fluoride activity represents a blastic activity/reparative process in response to tumor and destroyed bone.

Gallium-68 prostate-specific membrane antigen (Ga-68 PSMA) PET-CT is a new addition and is useful for prostate cancer staging, particularly for bone metastasis. It shows high sensitivity and specificity for bone metastasis from prostatic carcinoma.

MRI depicts early hematogenous dissemination of the tumor to the bone marrow before reactions in the adjacent bone are detectable on ^{99m}Tc scintiscans. Metastatic seeding in the bone marrow is characterized by long T1 relaxation times, whereas T2 relaxation times are variable, depending on tumor morphology. Lesions are seen as focal or diffuse areas of hypointensity on T1W images and as areas of intermediate or high signal intensity on T2W images. Tumor deposits typically appear hyperintense against a dark background of suppressed signal intensity within fat on STIR images. Osteoblastic metastases may appear hypointense on all pulse sequences. The identification of a "halo" of high signal intensity around a lesion is a highly specific feature of metastasis on T2W sequences.[51] In vertebrae, additional criteria for malignancy include bulging of the posterior margin of the vertebral body, signal intensity changes that extend into the pedicle, and paraosseous tumor spread **(Figs. 35A to D)**.

Diffusion-weighted MRI is highly sensitive to cellularity and the mobility of free water molecules, which are responsible for the differences between benign and malignant fractures. Using a single-shot echo-planar DWI pulse sequence with a

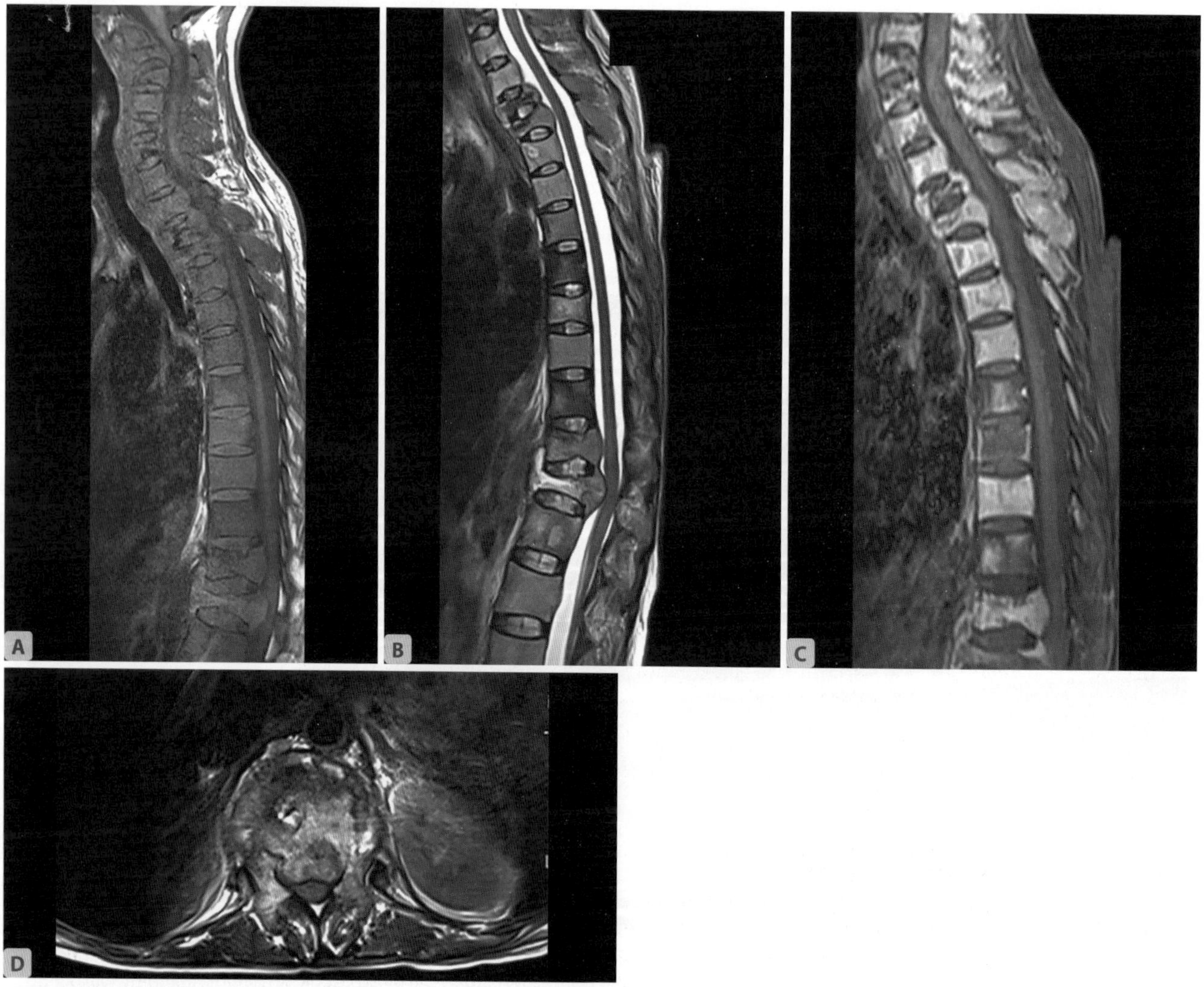

FIGS. 35A TO D: Skeletal metastases from carcinoma breast. T1-weighted (T1W) sagittal (A), T2-weighted (T2W) sagittal (B), and postcontrast sagittal (C) magnetic resonance (MR) images of the dorsolumbar spine show multiple lesions with collapse of the vertebrae appearing hypointense on T1W and hyperintense on T2W sequences with heterogeneous postcontrast enhancement. The disc spaces are spared and the collapsed vertebral bodies show posterior convexity. Axial T2W MR image (D) shows the presence of paraspinal soft tissue.

high B factor, Chan et al. showed that ADC values are useful in differentiating benign osteoporotic fractures from malignant vertebral body compression fractures.[52]

Whole-body MRI, using fast pulse sequences over multiple anatomic stations to acquire a survey of the entire body, has resulted in the ability to use unenhanced T1W spin echo and STIR sequences to screen the whole body for marrow abnormalities with a sensitivity and specificity superior to skeletal scintigraphy.[53] One limitation of MRI is that cortical bone, due to its very short T2 relaxation time, is not well seen, and therefore, bones with a low marrow volume such as the ribs are better evaluated with CT. Whole body MRI with diffusion weighting allows qualitative and quantitative evaluation of the focal lesions through signal intensity evaluation on DWI images and the reconstruction of the ADC map.

Differential Diagnosis

A solitary metastasis may resemble a primary malignant bone tumor, a primary benign tumor of aggressive nature, e.g., a GCT, infection, and miscellaneous disorders such as Paget's disease. The most important factor in the differential diagnosis is the patient's age. The second important factor is the presence of multiple bone deposits. Other features are the diaphyseal location, involvement of vertebral bodies and then pedicles, the lack of bone expansion, absence of florid periosteal reaction, and tumor bone or soft-tissue mass. No one investigation, apart from biopsy, can provide a specific diagnosis of a metastasis or its site of origin.

CONCLUSION

Conventional radiographic techniques remain of fundamental importance in the diagnosis and analysis of bone tumors and tumor-like lesions. Radiographic information combined with data concerning the clinical presentation, the site of the lesion, and the age of the patient allows the formulation of a reasonable diagnosis in most cases. CT and MRI are useful in determining the intraosseous and extraosseous spread of the lesions. MRI has virtually replaced CT in its ability to detect the presence of a lesion and demonstrate its extent with respect to compartmental anatomy, i.e., in the staging of the tumor. MRI also plays an important role in prognosticating and follow-up after therapy to look for recurrence or residual disease.

REFERENCES

1. Dorfman HD, Czerniak B. Bone cancers. Cancer. 1995;75(Suppl 1):203-10.
2. Unni KK, Inwards CY, Bridge JA, Kindblom LG, Wold LE. Tumors of the bones and joints. In: AFIP Atlas of Tumor Pathology, Series 4. Washington, DC: American Registry of Pathology; 2005.
3. Kindblom LG. Bone tumors: epidemiology, classification, pathology. In: Davies AM, Sundaram M, James SJ (Eds). Imaging of Bone Tumors and Tumor-like Lesions. Berlin: Springer; 2009. pp. 1-15.
4. Fletcher C DM, Bridge JA, Hogendoorn P, Mertens F. WHO Classification of Tumours of Soft Tissue and Bone, Fourth edition. WHO 2013; IARC WHO Classification of Tumours, No. 5.
5. Doyle LA. Sarcoma classification: An update based on the 2013 World Health Organization Classification of Tumors of Soft Tissue and Bone. Cancer. 2014;120(12):1763-74.
6. Johnson LC. A general theory of bone tumors. Bull N Y Acad Med. 1953;29(2):164-71.
7. Kundu ZS. Classification, imaging, biopsy and staging of osteosarcoma. Indian J Orthop. 2014;48(3):238-46.
8. Nomikos GC, Murphey MD, Kransdorf MD, Bancroft LW, Peterson JJ. Primary bone tumors of lower extremities. Radiol Clin North Am. 2002;40(5):971-90.
9. Stoller DW. Bone and Soft Tissue Tumors in Magnetic Resonance Imaging in Orthopaedics and Sports Medicine, 3rd edition. Philadelphia: Lippincott Williams and Wilkins; 2007.
10. Costa FM, Canella C, Gasparetto E. Advanced Magnetic Resonance Imaging Techniques in the Evaluation of Musculoskeletal Tumors. Radiol Clin N Am. 2011;49(6):1325-58.
11. Oh E, Yoon YC, Kim JH, Kim K. Multiparametric approach with diffusion-weighted imaging and dynamic contrast-enhanced MRI: a comparison study for differentiating between benign and malignant bone lesions in adults. Clinical Radiology. 2017;72(7):552-9.
12. Hayashida Y, Yakushiji T, Awai K, Katahira K, Nakayama Y, Shimomura O, et al. Monitoring therapeutic response of primary bone tumors by diffusion-weighted image: initial results. Eur Radiol. 2006;16(12):2637-43.
13. Mintz DN, Hwang S. Bone tumor imaging, then and now: review article. HSS J. 2014;10(3):230-9.
14. Hwang S, Panicek DN. The evolution of musculoskeletal tumor imaging. Radiol Clin North Am. 2009;47(3):435-53.
15. Evan-Sapir E. PET/CT in malignant bone disease. Sem Musculoskeletal Radiol. 2007;11(4):312-21.
16. Van der Woude HJ, Vandershueren G. Ultrasound in musculoskeletal tumours with emphasis on its role in tumour follow up. Radiol Clin North Am. 1999;37(4):753-66.
17. Wong KC, Kumta SM, Antonio GE, Tse LF. Image fusion for computer-assisted bone tumor surgery. Clin Orthop Relat Res. 2008;466(10):2533-41.
18. Wong KC, Kumta SM. Use of computer navigation in orthopedic oncology. Curr Surg Rep. 2014;2(4):47.
19. Rajiah P, Ilaslan H, Sundaram M. Imaging of primary malignant bone tumors (Nonhematological). Radiol Clin North Am. 2011;49(6):1135-61.
20. Ellis JH, Siegel CL, Martel W, Weatherbee L, Dorfman H . Radiologic features of well-differentiated osteosarcoma. AJR Am J Roentgenol. 1988;151(4):739-42.
21. Kumar R, David R, Madewell JE, Lindell MM Jr. Radiographic spectrum of osteogenic sarcoma. Am J Roentgenol. 1987;148:767-72.
22. Miller SL, Hoffer FA. Malignant and Benign bone tumours. Radiol Clin North Am. 2001;39(4):673-99.
23. Murphey MD, wan Jaovisidha S, Temple HT, Gannon FH, Jelinek JS, Malawer MM. Telangiectatic osteosarcoma: radiologic-pathologic comparison. Radiology. 2003;229(2):545-53.
24. Edeiken J, Raymond AK, Ayala AG, Benjamin RS, Murray JA, Carrasco HC. Small-cell osteosarcoma. Skeletal Radiol. 1987;16(8):621-8.
25. Choong PF, Pritchard DJ, Rock MG, Sim FH, McLeod RA, Unni KK. Low grade central osteogenic sarcoma. A long-term follow-up of 20 patients. Clin Orthop Relat Res. 1996;322:198-206.
26. Van der Woude HJ, Bloom JL, Hogendoorn PC. Preoperative evaluation and monitoring chemotherapy in patients with high grade osteogenic and Ewing sarcomas: A review of current imaging modalities. Skeletal Radiol. 1998;27(2):57-71.

27. Jelinek JS, Murphey MD, Kransdorf MJ, Shmookler BM, Malawer MM, Hur RC. Parosteal sarcoma: Value of MR imaging and CT in the prediction of histologic grade. Radiology. 1996;201(3):837-42.
28. Okada K, Kubota H, Ebina T, Kobayashi T, Abe E, Sato K. High grade surface osteosarcoma of the humerus. Skeletal Radiol. 1995;24(7):531-4.
29. Stoker DJ, Saifuddin A. Bone tumours (2): Malignant lesions. Grainger and Allison's Diagnostic Radiology. London: Churchill Livingstone; 2007. pp. 1059-81.
30. Sheppard DG, Libshitz H. Post-radiation sarcomas: a review of the clinical and imaging features in 63 cases. Clin Radiol. 2001;56(1):22-9.
31. Murphey MD, Walker EA, Wilson AJ, Kransdorf MJ, Temple HT, Gannon FH. From the Archives of the AFIP: Imaging of primary chondrosarcoma: radiologic-pathologic correlation. Radiographics. 2003;23(5):1245-78.
32. Brien EW, Mirra JM, Luck JV Jr. Benign and malignant cartilage tumors of bone and joint: Their anatomic and theoretical basis with an emphasis on radiology, pathology and clinical biology. II. Juxta cortical cartilage tumors. Skeletal Radiol. 1999;28(1):1-20.
33. Lee YK, Yao L Wirth CR. MR imaging of solitary osteochondromas: Report of eight cases. AJR Am J Roentgenol. 1987;149(3):557-60.
34. Nakashuma Y, Unni KK, Shives TC, Swee RG, Dahlin DC. Mesenchymal chondrosarcoma of bone and soft tissue. A review of 111 cases. Cancer. 1986;57(12):2444-53.
35. Collins NS, Koyama T, Swee RG, Inwards CY. Clear cell chondrosarcoma: radiographic, computed tomographic and magnetic resonance findings in 34 patients with pathologic correlation. Skeletal Radiol. 2003;32(12):687-94.
36. Taconis WK, Mulder JD. Fibrosarcoma and malignant fibrous histiocytoma of long bone: Radiographic features and grading. Skeletal Radiol. 1984;11(4):237-45.
37. Murphey MD, Senchak LT, Mambalam PK, Logie CI, Klassen-Fischer MK, Kransdorf MJ. From the radiologic pathology archives: Ewing sarcoma family of tumors: radiologic-pathologic correlation. Radiographics. 2013;33(3):803-31.
38. Eggli KD, Quiogue T, Moser RP Jr. Ewing's sarcoma. Radiol Clin North Am. 1993;31(2):325-37.
39. Sailer SL, Harmon DC, Nakin HJ, et al. Ewing sarcoma: Surgical resection as a prognostic factor. Int J Radiat Oncol Biol Phys. 1988;15(1):43-52.
40. Miller SL, Hoffer FA, Reddick WE, Wu S, Glass JO, Gronemeyer SA, et al. Tumor volume or dynamic contrast enhanced MRI for prediction of clinical outcome of Ewing sarcoma family of tumors. Pediatric Radiol. 2001;31(7): 518-23.
41. Weshi AS, Allam A, Ajarim D, Al Dayel F, Pant R, Bazarbashi S, et al. Extraskeletal Ewing sarcoma family of tumors in adults: Analysis of 57 patients from a single institution. Clin Oncol. 2010;22(5):374-81.
42. Papagelopoulos PJ, Mavrogenis AF, Galanis EC, Savvidou OD, Boscainos PJ, Katonis PG, et al. Chordoma of the spine: clinicopathological features, diagnosis and treatment. Orthopaedics. 2004;27(12):1256-63.
43. Lomasney LM, Martinez S, Demos TC, Harrelson JM. Multifocal vascular lesions of bone: Imaging characteristics. Skeletal Radiol. 1996;25(3):255-61.
44. Van der Woude HJ, Hazelbag HM, Bloem JL, Taminiau AH, Hogendoorn PC. MRI of adamantinoma of long bones in correlation with histopathology. AJR. 2004;183(6):1737-44.
45. Sarode SC, Sarode GS, Ingale Y, Ingale M, Raj AT, Patil S. Malignant fibrous histiocytoma of the mandible—A case report and review of published case reports. J Oral Biol Craniofac Res. 2019;9(2):221-5.
46. Yochum TR, Rowe LJ. Tumors and tumor-like processes. In: Yochum TR, Rowe LJ (Eds). Essentials of Skeletal Radiology, 3rd edition. Philadelphia: Lippincott Williams and Wilkins; 2005. pp. 1137-372.
47. Abrams HL, Sprio R, Goldstein N. Metastasis in carcinoma; analysis of 1000 autopsied cases. Cancer. 1950;3(1):74-85.
48. Galasko CSB. The anatomy and pathways of skeletal metastases. In: Weiss L, Gilbert HA (Eds). Bone Metastasis. Boston: GK Hall Publishers; 1981. pp. 49-63.
49. Rosenthal DI. Radiological diagnosis of bone metastases. Cancer. 1997;80(S8):1595-607.
50. Evan-Sapir E, Mester U, Mishani G, Lievshitz G, Lerman H, Leibovitch I. The detection of bone metastases inpatients with high risk prostate cancer: ^{99m}Tc-MDP planar bone scintigraphy, single and multi-field-of-view SPECT, ^{18}Fluoride PET, and ^{18}Fluoride PET/CT. J Nucl Med. 2006;47(2): 287-97.
51. Schweitzer ME, Levine C, Mitchell DG, Gannon FH, Gomella LG. Bull's eyes and halos: Useful MR discriminators of osseous metastases. Radiology. 1993;188(1):249-52.
52. Chan JH, Peh WC, Tsui EY, Chau LF, Cheung KK, Chan KB, et al. Acute vertebral body compression fractures: discrimination between benign and malignant causes using apparent diffusion coefficients. Br J Radiol. 2002;75(891):207-14.
53. Choi J, Raghavan M. Diagnostic imaging and image-guided therapy of skeletal metastases. Cancer Control. 2012;19(2): 102-12.

CHAPTER

166

Imaging in Marrow Disorders: Benign and Malignant

Swati Gupta, Sapna Singh, Alpana Manchanda

INTRODUCTION

The bone marrow lies within the skeleton and it provides red blood cells, platelets and white blood cells to meet the requirements for oxygenation, coagulation and immunity. It is composed of a combination of red marrow and yellow marrow, and its composition changes throughout life in response to normal maturation (red marrow to yellow marrow conversion) and stress (yellow marrow to red marrow reconversion).

Normal bone marrow has following three primary components:

1. The osseous component consisting of primary and secondary trabeculae of cancellous bone, which provide the structural framework for myeloid and fat cells.
2. The red marrow is hematopoietically active and supplies red blood cells, white blood cells, and platelets.
3. The yellow marrow contains fat, which is hematopoietically inactive.

The chemical composition and vascular supply of these various components of bone marrow are different from each other.[1-4] Although red marrow and yellow marrow are described as discrete elements for convenience, they are actually intermixed within the medullary space. Their proportions determine the overall distribution of fat and water.[5] **Table 1** describes the composition of marrow.

A variety of imaging techniques can be used in bone marrow assessment which is mentioned here.

TABLE 1: Cellular and chemical components of bone marrow in adults.[6]

Component of bone marrow	Cellular composition	Chemical composition
Yellow marrow	95% fat cells 5% nonfat cells	80% fat 15% water 5% protein
Red marrow	40% fat cells 60% hematopoietic cells	40% fat 40% water 20% protein

Conventional radiographic techniques are insensitive to marrow infiltration and are not helpful in accurate bone marrow characterization. Indirect evidence of pathology may be seen in the form of trabecular destruction or sclerosis.

Radionuclide imaging uses various different tracers to evaluate specific components of bone such as reticuloendothelial system, erythroid precursors, myeloid components or active bone production. This may allow different bone marrow disorders to be distinguished. In addition, positron emission tomography (PET) tracers are useful to assess the metabolic and proliferative activity in the bone marrow.

Hybrid techniques such as PET-CT (positron emission tomography-computed tomography) and PET-MR (positron emission tomography-magnetic resonance), which fuse the functional and morphological data, are playing an increasing role in the evaluation of marrow disorders. PET and magnetic resonance imaging (MRI) are combined either by retrospective spatial registration of data from PET and MRI obtained on separate PET and MR machines or sequential data acquisition on combined PET-MR scanners. PET-MRI is superior to PET-CT because of the improved intrinsic soft-tissue contrast and direct bone marrow depiction using MRI. The SUV_{max} of normal bone marrow is approximately 1.[7] An SUV_{max} ≥4 has been shown to allow distinction between benign and malignant bone marrow lesions.[8]

Computed tomography has a low sensitivity and specificity for detection of marrow disorders. Trabecular destruction can be visualized on CT, and obvious asymmetry in marrow attenuation on visual or quantitative inspection may warrant further evaluation. Characterization of marrow changes is however not feasible on CT.

Magnetic resonance imaging is a useful technique for noninvasive evaluation of pathologic bone marrow conditions.[1,2] MRI with its excellent spatial and contrast resolution, allows direct visualization of the bone marrow. The signal intensity, morphology, and location of pathological findings on MRI can be used to provide more accurate diagnosis, to guide treatment and to follow therapy-related changes. Various MRI techniques are utilized to accentuate chemical and cellular composition of normal marrow and marrow diseases. MRI is more sensitive than specific in marrow disorders but an integration of clinical and radiologic data helps in suggesting an accurate diagnosis.

MAGNETIC RESONANCE APPEARANCE OF NORMAL MARROW

The differences in signal intensities of yellow and red marrow result primarily from differences in their proportional amounts of water and fat. The normal MR appearance of red and yellow marrow includes the following features **(Figs. 1 and 2)**:

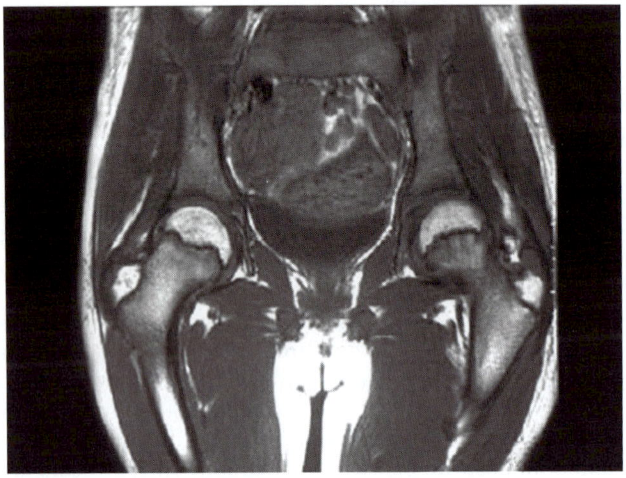

FIG. 1: Normal marrow pattern in childhood (1–10 years). T1-weighted (T1W) coronal magnetic resonance (MR) image of the pelvis showing high-signal yellow marrow (signal identical to subcutaneous fat) in the femoral epiphysis, apophysis, and the femoral diaphysis. Red marrow has intermediate signal intensity (higher than adjacent muscle), is seen present in the proximal femoral metaphysis and in the pelvic bones. Marked symmetry of distribution seen bilaterally.

- Red marrow demonstrates low-signal intensity on T1-weighted (T1W) images, reflecting its increased water content, and intermediate-signal intensity with progressive T2 weighting. Normal red marrow demonstrates T1 signal that is equal to or higher than adjacent muscle or intervertebral discs.
- With suppression of the signal from fat on short tau inversion recovery (STIR) images, areas of red marrow demonstrate higher signal intensity than areas of yellow marrow.
- On T1W and conventional T2-weighted (T2W) images, yellow marrow demonstrates the bright signal intensity of fat.
- Yellow marrow demonstrates low signal intensity on STIR images, in which signal from fat is nulled. The signal intensity is also reduced on fat-suppressed T2W spin-echo (SE) and fat-suppressed T2W fast SE sequences, and it appears darker when using fat-suppression techniques with sequences having longer repetition times (TR) and echo times (TE).[9]
- Red and yellow marrow contrast differences become less distinct on heavily T2W protocols with TR >2,500 ms.

NORMAL DISTRIBUTION OF MARROW

Hematopoiesis begins in utero, at approximately 19 gestational days, within the yolk sac. By week 16 of gestation, the main sites of fetal hematopoiesis are the liver and the spleen. After week 24 of gestation, marrow becomes the main organ of hematopoiesis. At birth, active hematopoiesis (i.e. red marrow) is present throughout the entire skeleton, including the epiphyses. Early in the normal ossification process, yellow marrow replaces the hyaline cartilage template in the epiphysis and the apophysis. Conversion of red to yellow marrow commences in the terminal phalanges of hand and feet. Bone marrow conversion occurs from appendicular to axial skeleton.

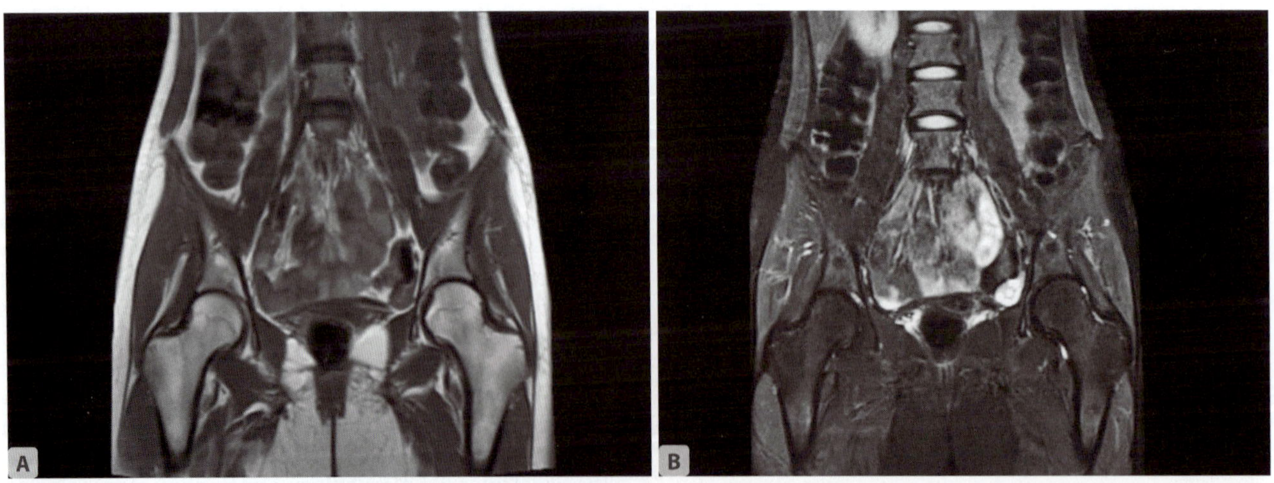

FIGS. 2A AND B: Normal red and yellow marrow. T1-weighted (T1W) coronal image (A) of the pelvis and the femora. Yellow marrow has signal identical to that of the high signal subcutaneous fat. It is present in the apophyses, the epiphyses, the femoral diaphyses, and the focal regions in the pelvis. Red marrow is intermediate signal and located in the pelvis and the proximal femoral metaphyses. Note the striking symmetry of the distribution of red and yellow marrow bilaterally. Short tau inversion recovery (STIR) coronal image (B) of the pelvis and the femora. Fatty marrow becomes black from fat suppression in this sequence. Red marrow is intermediate signal, similar in appearance to the muscle; this is best seen in the pelvis.

Within the long bone, marrow conversion first starts in the diaphysis and progresses bidirectionally toward the metaphyses, faster distally than proximally as described in **Table 2**.

In the femoral diaphysis, on T1W images, high-signal intensity yellow marrow is observed as early as when the subject is 3 months old, with marrow heterogeneity at 12 months, and homogeneous high-signal intensity after the age of 5 years.

In <10 years of age, yellow marrow is seen in most of the diaphysis of long bones of arms and legs.

From the age of 10–20 years, yellow marrow is seen predominantly in the limbs with residual red marrow in the femoral and humeral metaphysis.

Conversion happens continuously from peripheral to central with respect to the skeleton and is complete by the age of 25 years, when the adult pattern is established, characterized by the distribution of red marrow limited to the axial skeleton (skull, vertebrae, ribs, sternum, and pelvis) and proximal aspects of the appendicular skeleton (femora and humeri) **(Figs. 3A to C)**.

At 60 years of age, the percentage of fat in red marrow can be as high as 70% **(Figs. 4A and B)**. These changes are also described in **Table 3 (Fig. 5)**.

TABLE 2: Progression of conversion from red to yellow marrow.[10]

Skeletal segment (extremities to axial skeleton)	Individual long bones (peripheral to central)
Hands/feet	Epiphyses/apophyses
↓	↓
Forearms/lower legs	Diaphysis
↓	↓
Humeri/femora	Distal metaphysis
↓	↓
Pelvis/spine	Proximal metaphysis

This conversion is not entirely symmetric. These changes vary and are dependent on factors such as diseases, athletic activities, and therapies.[11-13] Regional differences between the two sexes have been demonstrated. Small differences in the amount and distribution of red marrow from side to side are normal, but marked asymmetry is indicative of a marrow-infiltrating disease process.

The appearance of vertebral marrow has been explained by Sebag et al.[14] He explains that vertebral marrow remains hypointense before the age of 1 year and hyperintense after the age of 5 years due to progressive red to yellow marrow conversion on T1W images **(Figs. 6A and B)**. Marrow around the basivertebral venous plexus is first to get converted, followed by subchondral marrow adjacent to end plates **(Figs. 7A and B)**. Focal islands of yellow marrow are common in the spine around the central venous channels in the vertebral bodies.

Heterogeneous pattern of marrow distribution is a normal variant. Chronic stresses and biomechanical stimuli cause a decrease in the vascularity to specific sites in marrow and stimulate conversion of red to yellow marrow, which probably accounts for many focal areas of conversion to fat. A classic example of this phenomenon occurs in the marrow adjacent to vertebral end plates that border on a degenerated disc. A band-like focal alteration in marrow signal occurs as a result of the ischemia associated with the disc disease **(Figs. 8A to C)**. Islands of red marrow may also occur in predominantly yellow marrow **(Figs. 9A and B)**. Presence of yellow marrow within the islands of red marrow, known as the "Bull's eye appearance," indicates benign appearance. Other helpful features in distinguishing heterogeneous red marrow from a pathologic process include higher signal intensity relative to skeletal muscle on T1W images, feathery margins representing red marrow elements interdigitating with the adjacent yellow marrow, relative bilaterality, and the absence of mass effect in red marrow.

Red marrow may extend in the epiphyses and is considered a normal variant as described by Mirowitz.[15]

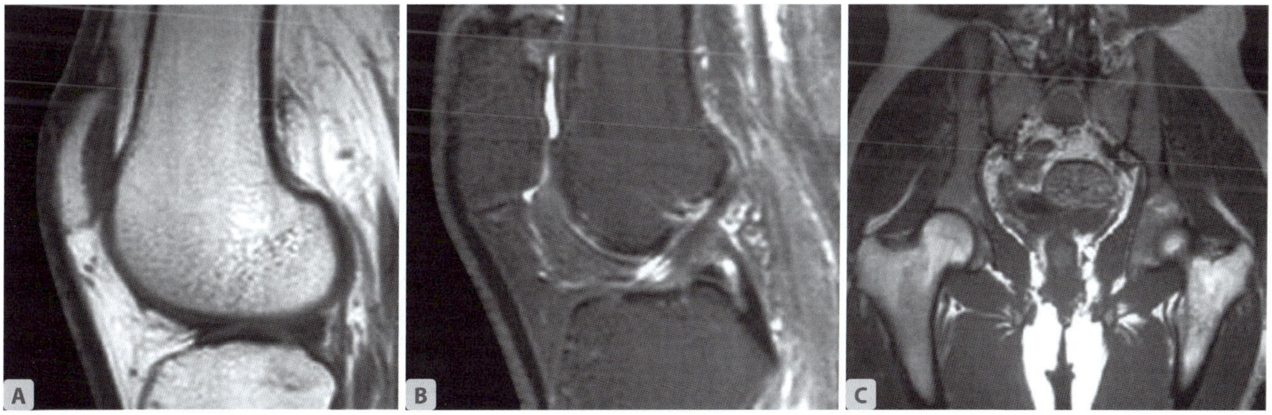

FIGS. 3A TO C: Normal marrow pattern in an adult >25 years of age. T1-weighted (T1W) sagittal (A), short tau inversion recovery (STIR) sagittal (B) magnetic resonance (MR) images of the knee showing normal yellow marrow in the diaphysis and the distal metaphysis of the femur. T1W coronal image of the pelvis (C) showing intermediate signal intensity red marrow in the proximal femoral metaphysis and the pelvic bones.

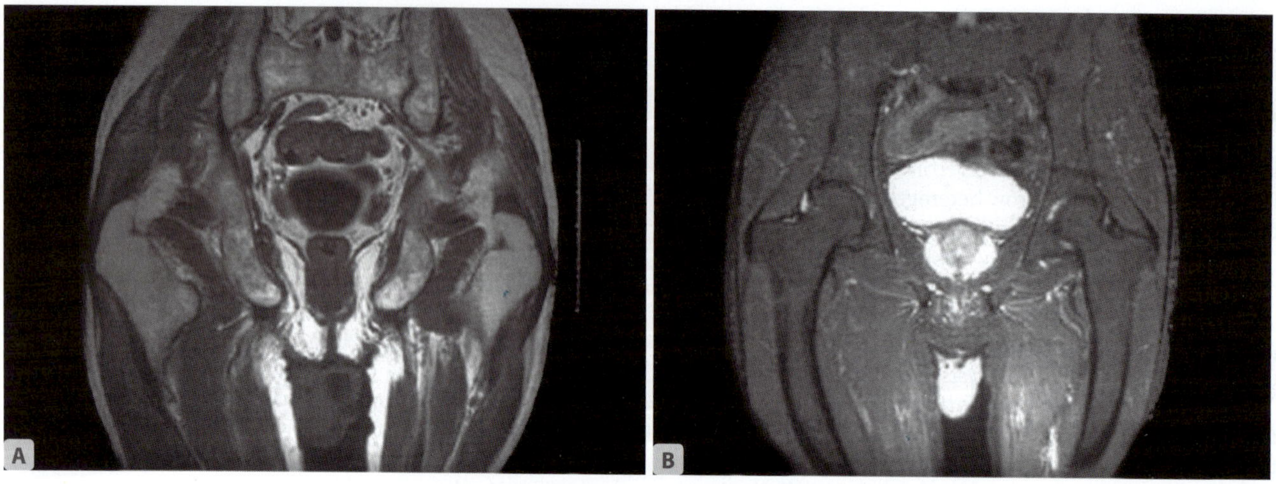

FIGS. 4A AND B: T1-weighted (T1W) coronal image of the pelvis (A) in a 70-year-old showing high-signal yellow marrow in the proximal femoral metaphyses and foci of yellow marrow in the pelvic bones. Short tau inversion recovery (STIR) coronal image of the pelvis (B) shows complete suppression of the signal indicating fatty marrow. Normal marrow pattern for >60 years of age.

TABLE 3: Age-related conversion from red to yellow marrow.[10]

Age group	Marrow findings
Infants (<1 year)	Diffuse red marrow except for ossified epiphyses and apophysis
Children (1–10 years)	Yellow marrow below knees and elbows, and in diaphysis of femora and humeri
Adolescents (10–20 years)	Progressive yellow marrow in distal and proximal metaphyses of proximal long bones
Adults (>25 years)	Yellow marrow except in axial skeleton and proximal metaphyses of proximal long bones

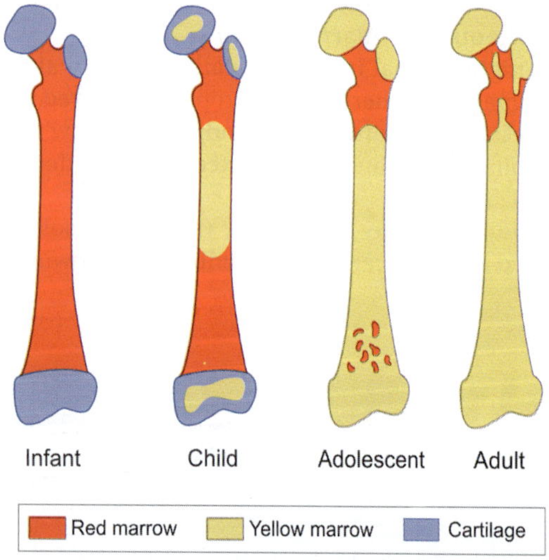

FIG. 5: Diagram of marrow maturation in the long bones from left to right and pattern of reconversion from right to left.

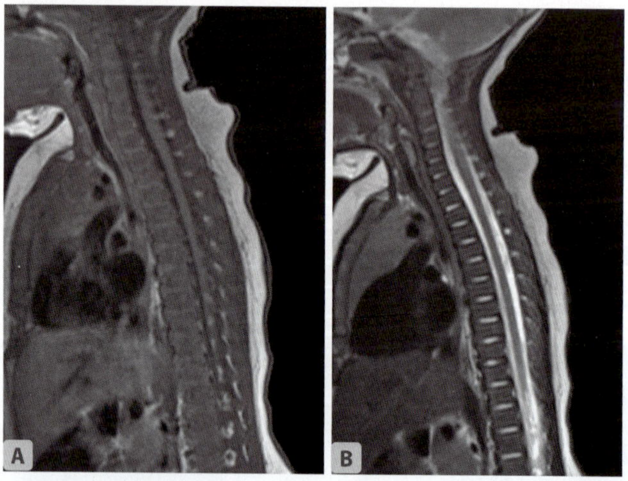

FIGS. 6A AND B: Marrow signal in a 1-month-old child. T1-weighted (T1W) sagittal (A) and T2-weighted (T2W) sagittal magnetic resonance (MR) images (B) of cervical and dorsal spine showing vertebral marrow that is hypointense to intervertebral disc on both T1- and T2-weighted images.

MAGNETIC RESONANCE IMAGING TECHNIQUES

The MRI protocol includes T1W SE sequences, fat-suppression sequence (STIR-sequences), chemical shift imaging (in-phase image/opposed-phase image), diffusion-weighted imaging (DWI), and T1 SE with fat presaturation (FS) before and after contrast (Gadolinium-Gd) injection with subtraction manipulation, if possible.

T1-weighted Sequence

T1-weighted sequence is the most fundamental sequence in marrow imaging. There is high tissue contrast between

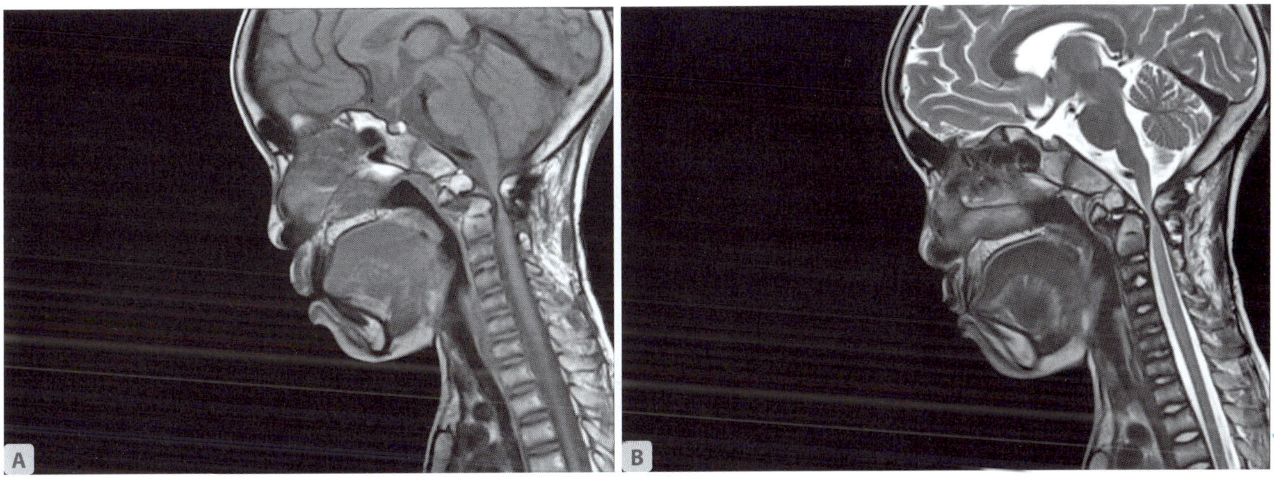

FIGS. 7A AND B: Marrow signal in a 10-year-old child. T1-weighted (T1W) sagittal (A) and T2-weighted (T2W) sagittal magnetic resonance (MR) images (B) of cervical spine in a patient with craniovertebral junction anomaly showing vertebral marrow that is hyperintense to intervertebral disc on T1W image. The conversion begins around basivertebral venous plexus.

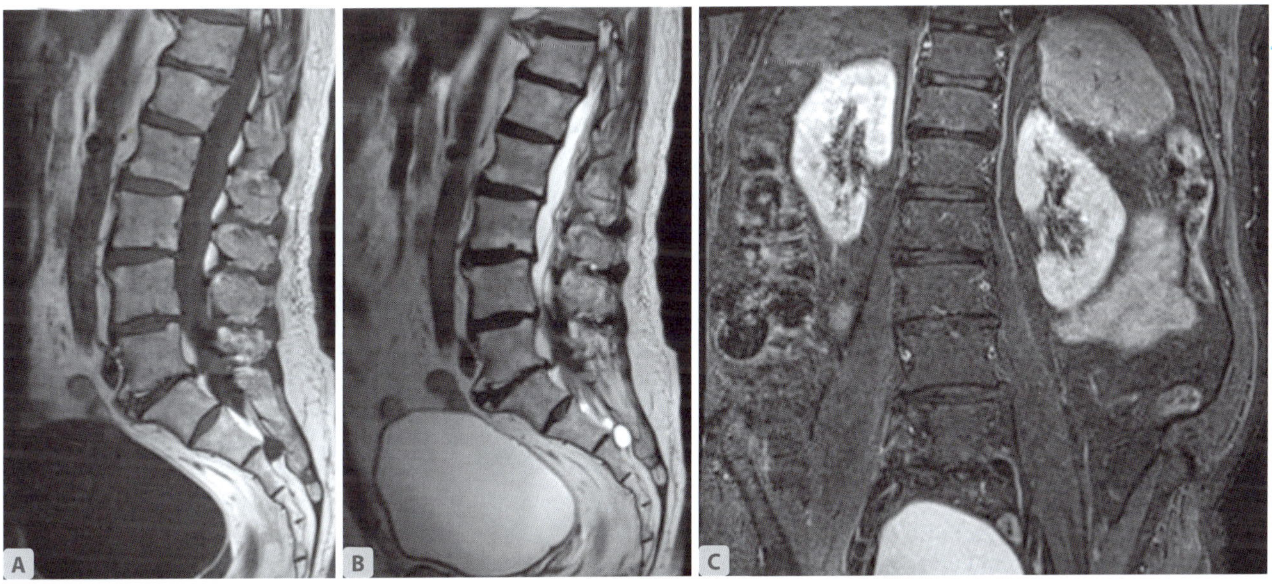

FIGS. 8A TO C: Degenerative disc disease. T1-weighted (T1W) sagittal (A), T2-weighted (T2W) sagittal (B) and short tau inversion recovery (STIR) coronal (C) magnetic resonance (MR) images showing a band-like focal alteration in marrow signal adjacent to end plates, more prominent at L3 and L4 level which shows suppression on STIR image suggestive of fatty replacement, associated with the disc disease.

yellow and red marrow as well as between yellow marrow and disease on this sequence. Fat has a bright signal on T1W images and pathologic lesions have a low signal; hence, the lesions are easily detected on T1W images as the contrast is maximized on T1W images. There is little contrast between red marrow and pathologic lesions as both have a low-signal intensity. The differentiating feature is that the signal intensity of pathological lesions is usually less than that of the intervertebral discs in the spine and less than that of the muscle in the extremities.

T2-weighted Sequence

On fluid-sensitive images, the signal intensity difference between red and yellow marrow is less apparent. Also, the difference between the pathologic marrow and yellow marrow is minimal as both show a high signal on the sequence. Fat-suppressed sequences are useful to increase the contrast. The two widely used fat suppression techniques are the STIR sequence and the fat-saturated SE sequence.[3,16]

STIR Sequence

The STIR sequence is of great value for pathological lesions associated with prolonged T1 and T2 values. The STIR sequence has a high sensitivity but a low specificity. Pathological lesions have a high-signal intensity due to increased cells, fluid, and edema. Normal yellow marrow is seen as signal void, red marrow as low-signal intensity, and pathological lesions are seen as high-signal intensity.

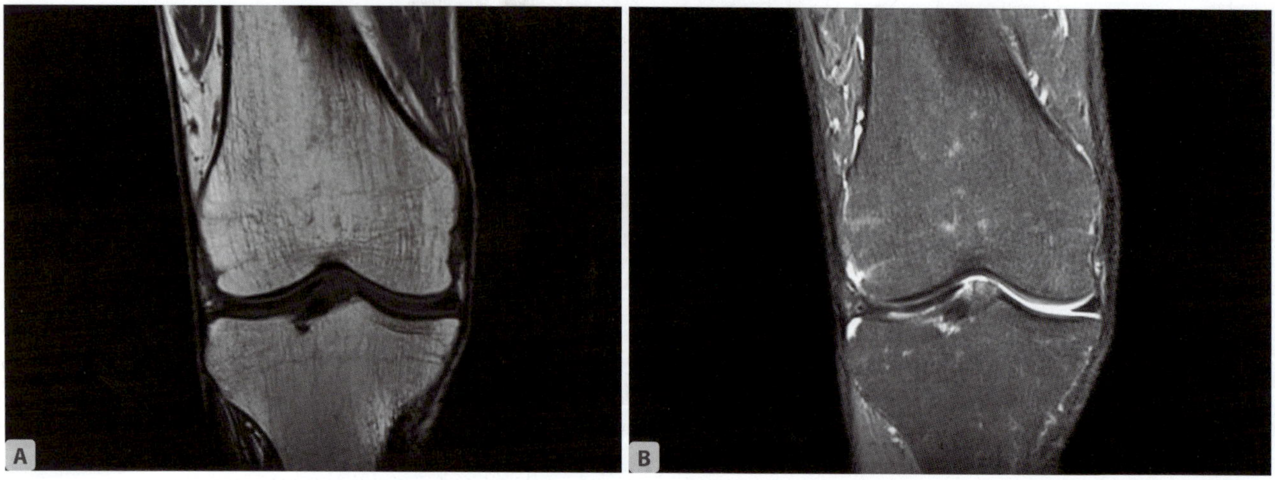

FIGS. 9A AND B: Heterogeneous marrow in an adult (normal variant). T1-weighted (T1W) coronal (A) and short tau inversion recovery (STIR) coronal (B) magnetic resonance (MR) images of knee show foci of red marrow that are hypointense on T1 and of intermediate intensity on STIR image in distal femur metaphysis on a background of yellow marrow.

Fibrous tissue, calcification, and hemosiderin deposits are low in signal intensity, whereas fluid, edema, and recent hemorrhage are bright. Muscle remains intermediate in signal intensity.

The main drawback of the STIR sequence is that it cancels every signal identical to fat, e.g., blood in hematoma or contrast-enhanced tissue. Further, a very homogeneous magnetic field is required for this sequence; therefore, it is not efficient on every MR unit. The other disadvantages include a relatively long imaging time and a low signal-to-noise ratio. The combination of T1W SE sequence with an STIR or fat-suppressed fast SE T2W sequence forms the basis of most bone marrow imaging protocols.[16]

Chemical Shift Imaging

Chemical shift imaging uses the difference in resonance frequency between fat and water photons to cancel their signal on out-of-phase images. Since fat is present in both red and yellow marrow but not in neoplastic lesions, neoplastic lesions do not demonstrate the normal loss of signal on out-of-phase images. It has been suggested that a decrease in signal intensity >20% on out-of-phase images compared with in-phase images should be used as a cut-off threshold for normalcy **(Figs. 10A and B)**. Any lesion, which is not composed of fat on T1W images, and which decreases <20% of its signal intensity on out-of-phase images compared to in-phase images, should be considered suspicious for malignancy.[17] A further refinement of this technique is the development of quantitative chemical shift imaging where the quantitative assessment of fat fraction can be done.[3,18,19] Two main families of techniques have been emerging for proton-dependent fat fraction quantification: single-voxel proton magnetic resonance spectroscopy (MRS) and chemical shift encoding-based water–fat imaging.[20]

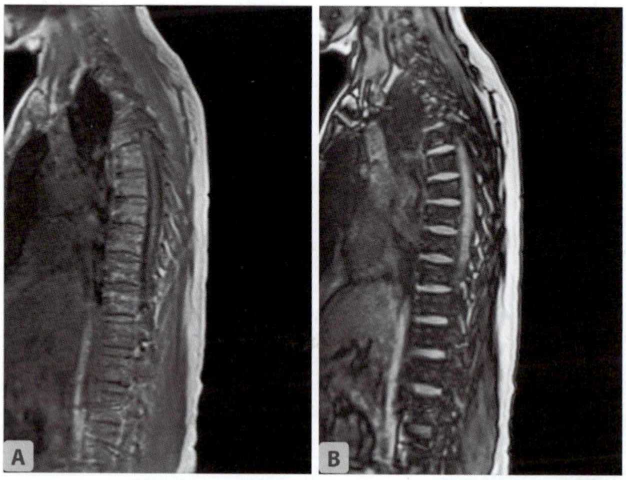

FIGS. 10A AND B: Normal appearance of marrow on chemical shift imaging. Magnetic resonance (MR) images of the dorsolumbar spine in-phase (A) and opposed phase (B) showing drop of signal on the opposed phase images as compared to the in-phase images due to the presence of fat.

Diffusion-weighted Imaging

Red marrow has higher apparent diffusion coefficient (ADC) values and signal intensity on high-*b*-value images due to higher cellularity and water content; yellow marrow, on the other hand, has lower cellularity mainly represented by large adipose cells, poorer water content, and lower perfusion.

Diffusion-weighted imaging (DWI) has proven to be a useful method in identification of marrow pathology. As red marrow restricts diffusion, DWI must be used with caution in infants and children.[21] ADC values lower than 1.1–1.2 $\times 10^{-3}$ mm^2/s are usually seen in cases of high cellularity or malignancy.

Diffusion-weighted MRI is useful in differentiating benign fracture edema and tumor infiltration of the vertebral body **(Figs. 11A and B)**.[3,18,19] DWI is also useful in distinguishing progressive changes in bone marrow among treatment sequelae, fracture, or tumor, which can be difficult on conventional MRI. In addition to the tumor evaluation, DWI may be useful in differentiation of degenerative and infectious

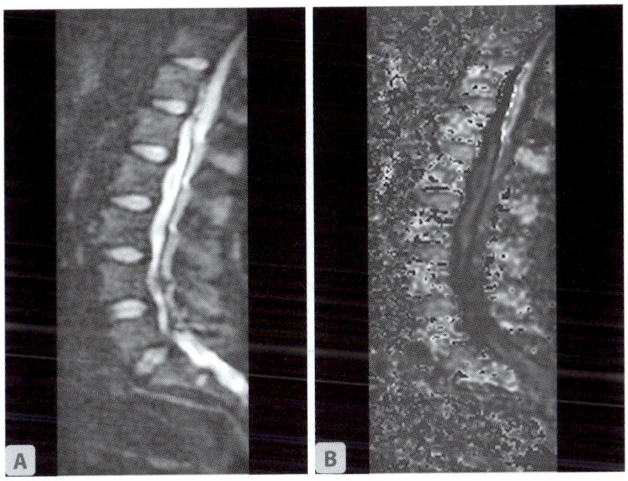

FIGS. 11A AND B: Normal appearance of marrow on diffusion-weighted imaging. Diffusion-weighted magnetic resonance (MR) images of the spine showing the normal vertebral bodies as hypointense with the normal apparent diffusion coefficient (ADC) map.

endplate abnormalities. DWI showed hyperintensity in patients with infection, and no hyperintensity in degenerative end plates; ADC values of infectious end plates were significantly lower than normal and degenerative end plates. In a study on spine metastasis, decreased DWI signal of the spine was seen after 2 months of therapy in patients with clinical improvement, whereas persistent abnormal hyperintense signal was found when there was no clinical improvement.[22]

Proton Magnetic Resonance Spectroscopy

There is paucity of literature on the use of MRS in the evaluation of marrow due to signal dropout from cortical bone and spectral peak contamination from adipose tissue. In this technique, the global MR signal from bone is divided into the two major segments of water and lipid separated by 3.1 ppm. The spectra of proton MRS have a water peak, originating mostly from red marrow, and a lipid peak, arising from yellow marrow. Signal peaks can vary among subjects, and are influenced not only by the water-lipid proton quantity and the tissue environment but also by the surface coil and the distance between the voxel and surface coil. Because of these variables, instead of measuring the absolute signal peak for signal quantification, a lipid-water ratio is often measured. The fat fraction value determined from MRS has been adopted as a predictor of bone marrow fat content in most studies. It has been shown that a decrease in cancellous bone is accompanied by a corresponding increase in fat cells and decrease in arterial capillaries and sinuses in bone marrow. Data also suggests that an elevated choline signal may be used to discriminate malignant from benign lesions.[23,24]

Contrast Enhancement

The enhancement of the normal marrow in adults is usually <35% from baseline on intravenous gadolinium administration.[25] The uptake is best seen on T1W fat presaturated sequences.[3,4,26] Contrast enhancement is less useful as both normal red marrow and various diseases (infection, inflammation, and tumor) can enhance. It has been stated that in case of normal STIR images no relevant additional information is found with contrast-enhanced T1W images, while in the case of abnormal STIR images, additional information is obtained on administration of gadopentetate dimeglumine.[27]

Dynamic Contrast-enhanced Magnetic Resonance Studies

Dynamic gadolinium-enhanced MR scans show increased enhancement of the neoplastic infiltration compared to normal marrow. They can be used to generate estimates of the volume of normal or pathological marrow before and after treatment. The enhancement is significantly higher in marked marrow infiltration and in lesions with higher vessel density as compared to those with mild or no infiltration. Bone marrow perfusion assessed by dynamic contrast-enhanced MR has also been studied in patients with osteoporosis. Studies have shown that decreasing marrow perfusion and increasing marrow fat content accompany a reduction in bone density.[28]

MAGNETIC RESONANCE PROTOCOL FOR SURVEY OF MARROW

Magnetic resonance imaging of suspected bone marrow abnormalities should be directed to the site of clinical symptoms or where abnormalities or confusing findings are present on other imaging studies. When diffuse marrow disease is suspected, a marrow survey of the entire body or, more commonly, of the entire spine, pelvis, and proximal femora is performed. These areas are surveyed because the bulk of red marrow (and marrow pathology) exists there.

The protocol for an MR survey examination includes:

- T1W coronal images of the pelvis and proximal femori, which are adult sites of red marrow concentration. These images are acquired with large (40 cm) fields of view to include assessment of lumbosacral spine marrow.
- Coronal STIR images are obtained to null fat signal and identify abnormal T1 or T2 prolongation.
- Sagittal T1W and STIR images are routinely acquired to evaluate suspected spinal malignancies.

In addition, components of survey include:

- Axial T1W, STIR images may be obtained at specific sites of suspected pathologic processes and are important in determining cross-sectional marrow involvement. T1W images are particularly valuable in evaluating blastic processes, which are low in signal on STIR images.
- Gadolinium-enhanced axial images, especially in cases with soft-tissue or cord involvement.
- Additional techniques on case-to-case basis.

WHOLE BODY MAGNETIC RESONANCE IMAGING

Whole body magnetic resonance imaging (WBMRI) has demonstrated huge potential for evaluation of malignant marrow disorders because of advantages such as absence of ionizing radiation, superior diagnostic performance, one-step staging, and ability to assess therapeutic response.[29] WBMRI is also useful in targeting marrow biopsy due to the favorable contrast between tumors and normal tissue on the STIR sequences.

Magnetic resonance imaging pulse sequences can be divided into anatomic (or morphologic), i.e., the classic T1W, T2W, and STIR pulse sequences that provide tissue delineation and basic physicochemical information about tissue content; and functional (or metabolic), i.e., DWI and perfusion sequences that provide information on tissue cellularity and/or vascularity.

Whole body T1, STIR is performed in coronal or axial planes. The coronal plane is preferred because of increased coverage. DWI sequences using high-diffusion sensitizing gradients (b values) are usually performed in the axial plane at consecutive anatomic stations. Sagittal study of the spine is recommended for detecting small lesions, lesions at risk or responsible for neurologic complications, and vertebral compression fractures. Gadolinium-based contrast scan is performed if liver and brain scanning is planned.

For scanning, it is preferable to use multiple surface coils. Depending upon the indication, WBMR can be limited from "eyes to thighs" or can cover the entire body.

Whole-body magnetic resonance imaging has been shown to be comparable to PET/CT, and better than bone scintigraphy, in detection of neoplastic marrow with sensitivities of 98, 90, and 30%, respectively.[30] WBMRI is useful in lymphomas with poor fluorodeoxyglucose (FDG) avidity and it also detects extramedullary lesions such as lymph nodes in non-Hodgkin lymphoma (NHL).[31,32] In multiple myeloma, consensus statement by the International Myeloma Working Group presents WBMRI as the imaging reference standard for the detection of bone marrow involvement and recommends systematic WBMRI in patients with smoldering myeloma and asymptomatic patients. Interpretation of WBMR is however challenging because of huge amount of information. It is also associated with a high false-positive rate and low sensitivity in early stage of a disease.

BONE MARROW PATHOLOGY

Abnormalities of bone marrow sometimes have a diagnostic appearance, but they are often nonspecific in their features. Five broad categories of marrow diseases can be used to facilitate an approach to evaluate the images and form an appropriate differential diagnosis. These categories are elaborated in **Table 4**. The categories are as follows:

- Marrow proliferative disorders
- Marrow replacement disorders
- Marrow depletion
- Vascular abnormalities
- Miscellaneous marrow diseases.

MARROW PROLIFERATIVE DISORDERS

Marrow proliferative disorders are diseases that arise from proliferation of cells that normally exist in the marrow. MRI of marrow proliferative disorders can have several appearances. Normal appearance of marrow on MRI does not eliminate the possibility of a significant marrow disease. Proliferation of abnormal cells may be indistinguishable from normal red marrow early in the disease, when the tumor burden is low. This is the situation in about 10–20% of patients with multiple myeloma and leukemia, and it is important to understand this weakness of the imaging technique.

The major abnormalities we look for on an MRI to indicate a marrow proliferative disease are as follows:

- Abnormal signal intensity
- Abnormal distribution of what appears to be normal signal intensity red marrow
- Both abnormal marrow distribution and signal intensity.

Reconversion of Yellow Marrow to Red Marrow

Reconversion of yellow marrow to red marrow takes place when demand of the body exceeds the capacity of the existing red marrow store. It occurs in people with obesity, chronic infection, chronic cardiac decompensation, hyperparathyroidism, endurance athletes, and heavy smokers.[2,33] It also occurs in hematologic disorders such as severe chronic anemia, thalassemia **(Figs. 12A to F)**, sickle cell disease, and hereditary spherocytosis. This happens because of the erythrocytes produced in the bone marrow being either less efficient at transporting oxygen or having a shorter life than normal or due to a combination of both these factors.[1,2,34]

The pattern of reconversion is opposite of that of physiological marrow conversion. Reconversion begins in the axial skeleton in the vertebrae and flat bones of the pelvis and progresses peripherally to the long bones of the extremities, the proximal bones before the distal long bones. Epiphyses are usually spared and reconversion occurs only in the severely affected patients.[1,2,35]

Imaging

On radiography, changes related to expansion of medulla, thinning of cortical bone, and reduction in bone density may be seen in patients with extensive reconversion such as thalassemia. In the skull, widening of diploic space occurs with hair-on-end appearance. Hypopneumatization of sinuses, premature fusion of epiphyses, and coarsened trabeculae may also be seen. Extramedullary hematopoietic soft-tissue masses are common.

Hyperplastic hematopoietic cells lead to a reduction in signal intensity on T1W images although the signal intensity is still equal to or greater than that of muscle. On T2W images, the signal intensity may be equal or hypointense to that of yellow marrow. The reconversion tends to be symmetrical **(Figs. 13A and B)**. It is however difficult to differentiate foci of reconverted bone marrow in an atypical location, e.g., diaphysis of long bones from a malignant process and metastases.

Differentiating criteria between reconversion and malignancy are tabulated in **Table 5**.[1,2,34,36]

TABLE 4: Categories of bone marrow pathology.[10]

Category	Comment	Distribution	Causes
Marrow proliferative disorder	Arises from existing marrow elements	Mostly diffuse except plasmacytoma	• Reconversion • Myelofibrosis • Polycythemia vera • Mastocytosis • Myelodysplastic syndrome • Leukemia • Multiple myeloma • Amyloidosis • Waldenström macroglobulinemia • Langerhans cell histiocytosis
Marrow replacement disorder	Implantation of cells in marrow that do not normally exist there	Mostly focal	• Primary bone tumors • Osteomyelitis • Metastases • Lymphoma
Marrow depletion	Ablation of red marrow elements	Diffuse or regional distribution	• Aplastic anemia • Chemotherapy • Radiation therapy
Vascular abnormalities: Hyperemia	Hyperemia causes bone marrow edema	Focal lesions, often involving epiphyses	• Trauma • Transient osteoporosis of hip • Regional migratory osteoporosis • Complex regional pain syndrome • Infection • Tumors • Joint abnormalities • Early osteonecrosis
Vascular abnormalities: Ischemia	Ischemia causes osteonecrosis in poorly vascularized fatty marrow	Focal lesions in epiphyses or diaphyses	• Trauma • Steroids • Sickle cell anemia • Dysbaric causes • Systemic lupus erythematosus • Gaucher's disease • Alcoholism • Pancreatitis • Idiopathic
Miscellaneous marrow diseases	These abnormalities do not fit neatly into the other categories of marrow disease		• Gaucher's disease • Paget's disease • Osteopetrosis • Hemosiderosis • Serous atrophy (gelatinous transformation) of marrow

Red marrow, being more vascular and active, is more commonly involved by malignancy. Normal red marrow is mildly hyperintense to muscle and intervertebral disc on T1W images. Hypointensity to muscle has 81% accuracy and hypointensity to vertebral disc has 78% accuracy for identification of an infiltrative process.[36]

Myelofibrosis

Myelofibrosis refers to a spectrum of bone marrow disorders that result in replacement of red marrow with fibrotic tissue. It occurs due to neoplastic process leading to abnormal proliferation of fibroblasts and collagen deposition.

Primary myelofibrosis (PMF) is believed to arise from a somatic mutation of a pluripotent hematopoietic progenitor cell and has an incidence of approximately 0.4–1.4 per 100,000 individuals. Janus kinase 2 *(JAK2)* mutation is believed to play a role in PMF.

Secondary myelofibrosis can be a complication of variety of benign and malignant disorders like acute leukemia, polycythemia vera, essential thrombocythemia, myelodysplasia, and renal osteodystrophy.

The most common signs and symptoms include easy bruising, weight loss, anemia, extramedullary hematopoiesis, and hepatosplenomegaly. Replacement of bone marrow can lead to deficiency of all blood cell lineages and related clinical manifestations. Hemorrhage and infection can be severe and are often the presenting clinical complaint. Primary acute myelofibrosis is a rapidly progressing disease with a high mortality rate. Leukemic conversion can be seen in up to 20% of affected individuals.

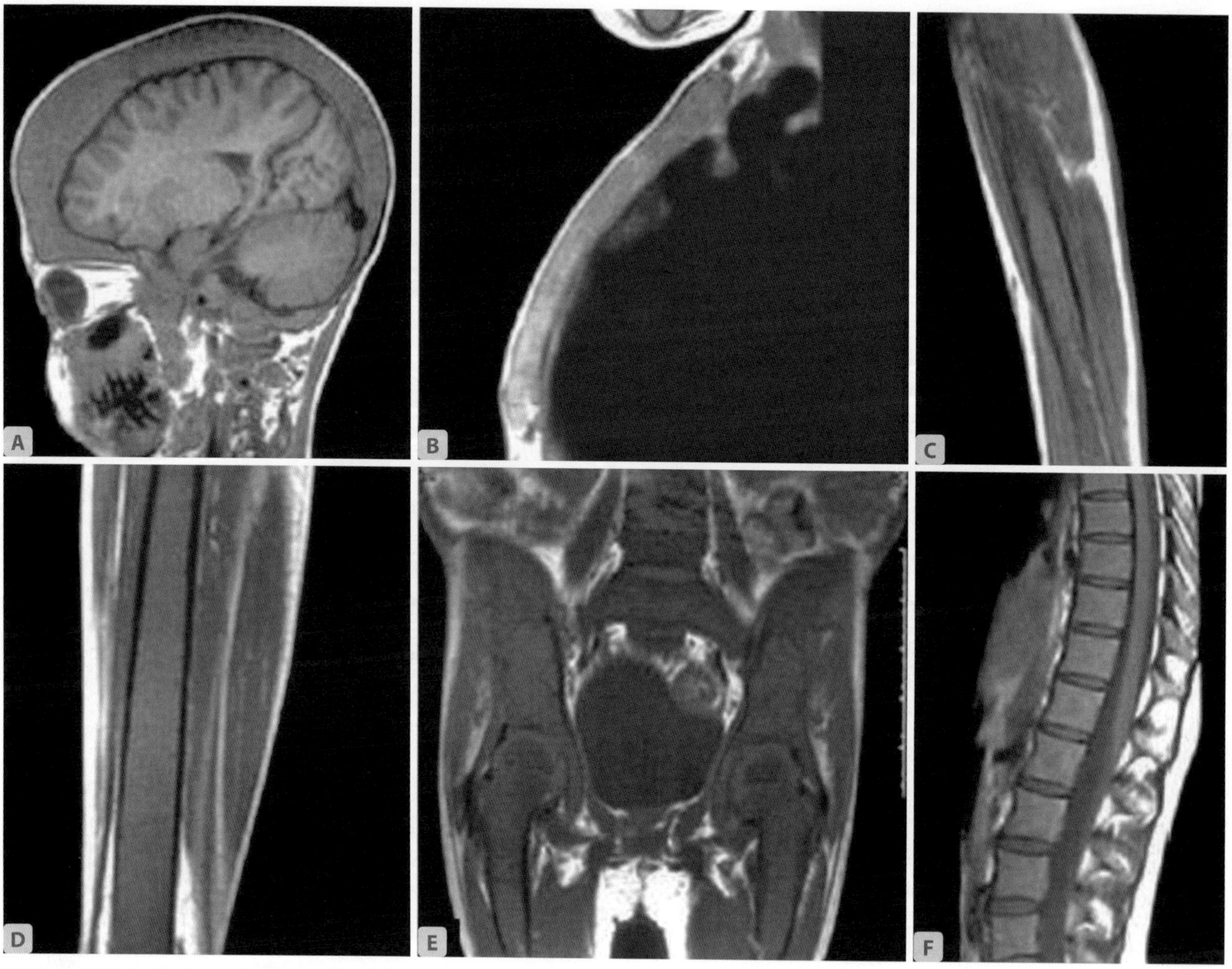

FIGS. 12A TO F: Thalassemia. T1-weighted (T1W) magnetic resonance (MR) images of skull (A), sternum (B), humerus (C), femur (D), pelvis (E), and dorsolumbar spine (F) showing medullary expansion and red marrow reconversion. The hematopoietic marrow is seen as decreased signal intensity on these T1W images throughout the axial and appendicular skeleton.

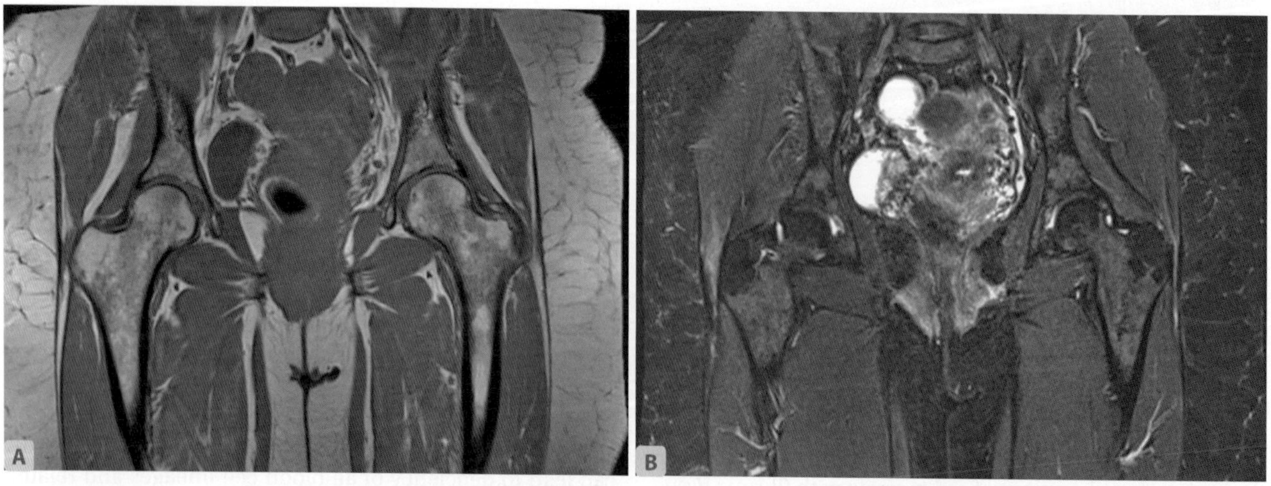

FIGS. 13A AND B: Reconverted marrow in a 70-year-old female. T1-weighted (T1W) coronal (A) and short tau inversion recovery (STIR) coronal (B) magnetic resonance (MR) images of the pelvis with red marrow in proximal metaphyses, diaphyses of bilateral femori, and pelvis due to chronic anemia. Yellow marrow is hyperintense on T1W image with suppression of signal on STIR image. Red marrow is hypointense on T1W image and intermediate signal intensity on STIR image.

TABLE 5: Differences between reconverted and malignant infiltration of marrow.

Reconversion marrow	Malignancy
Follows the normal pattern of marrow distribution and is bilaterally symmetrical	Asymmetric and geographic in distribution
Signal intensity equal to muscle on STIR and fat-saturated T2W images	Signal intensity more than muscle on STIR and fat-saturated T2W images
No cortical break or soft tissue mass	Cortical break with mass may be seen
Significant contrast enhancement not present; changes do not extend beyond the growth plate line, sparing the articular ends	Contrast enhancement present; changes can extend beyond growth plate line and involve articular ends
On chemical shift imaging, signal drop on out-of-phase image is >20% when compared to in-phase image	Malignancy does not show signal drop on out-of-phase image

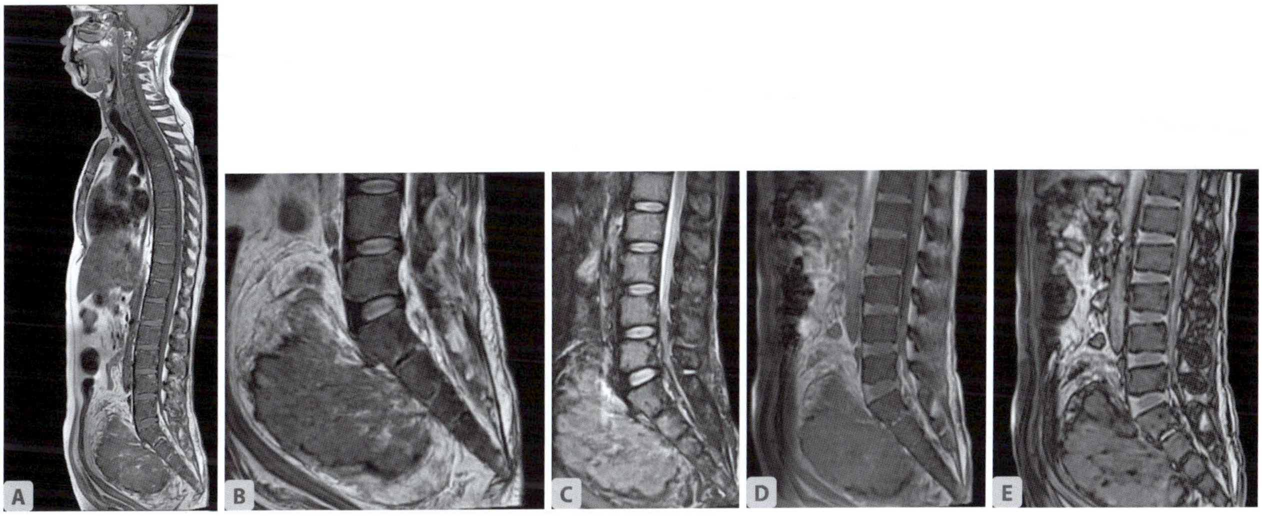

FIGS. 14A TO E: Myelofibrosis. T1-weighted (T1W) sagittal (A), T2-weighted (T2W) sagittal (B) magnetic resonance (MR) images showing a diffuse low signal in all the vertebral bodies. Presacral lobulated soft tissue with similar signal intensity suggestive of extramedullary hematopoietic mass. Short tau inversion recovery (STIR) sagittal (C) image showing diffuse increase in signal intensity and no drop of signal on opposed phase image (E) as compared to in-phase image (D).

Imaging

The predominant radiographic feature of myelofibrosis is osteosclerosis, typically seen in axial skeleton, ribs, proximal femur, and humerus; a finding that occurs in approximately 30–70% of patients. Other features may include hepatosplenomegaly and extramedullary hematopoietic soft-tissue masses.

Bone scan may give superscan appearance.

Magnetic resonance imaging findings include low T1 and T2 signal of bone marrow without associated enlargement of the affected bones. On STIR images, the signal intensity is greater than muscle. Opposed-phase imaging does not show a drop in signal as typically noted in normal red marrow; however, drop may be seen in areas of reconverted marrow. Extramedullary hematopoiesis is a common associated finding in the paraspinal soft tissue **(Figs. 14A to E)**.

Other causes of low marrow signal are listed in **Table 6**.

In Gaucher's disease (GD), associated bone infarcts may be present; while in hemosiderosis, excessive iron deposition can cause almost a complete signal loss resulting in a "black marrow."[37]

Bone marrow and stem cell transplantation appear to improve prognosis of the disease, with some patients demonstrating long-term remission. Mild cases can be monitored and blood counts managed with medication or transfusions. JAK2 inhibitors appear to be a promising developing treatment option.[38]

TABLE 6: Differential diagnosis for low T1 and T2 signal marrow.[10]

	Distribution	
	Focal	**Diffuse**
Conditions	• Bone islands **(Figs. 15A to C)** • Sclerotic metastases • Intraosseous vacuum phenomenon	• Myelofibrosis • Mastocytosis • Hemosiderosis • Osteopetrosis • Gaucher's disease

Leukemia

Leukemia is a malignant condition arising due to excess production of immature or abnormal leukocytes, which eventually suppresses the production of normal blood cells in marrow. Malignant transformation usually occurs

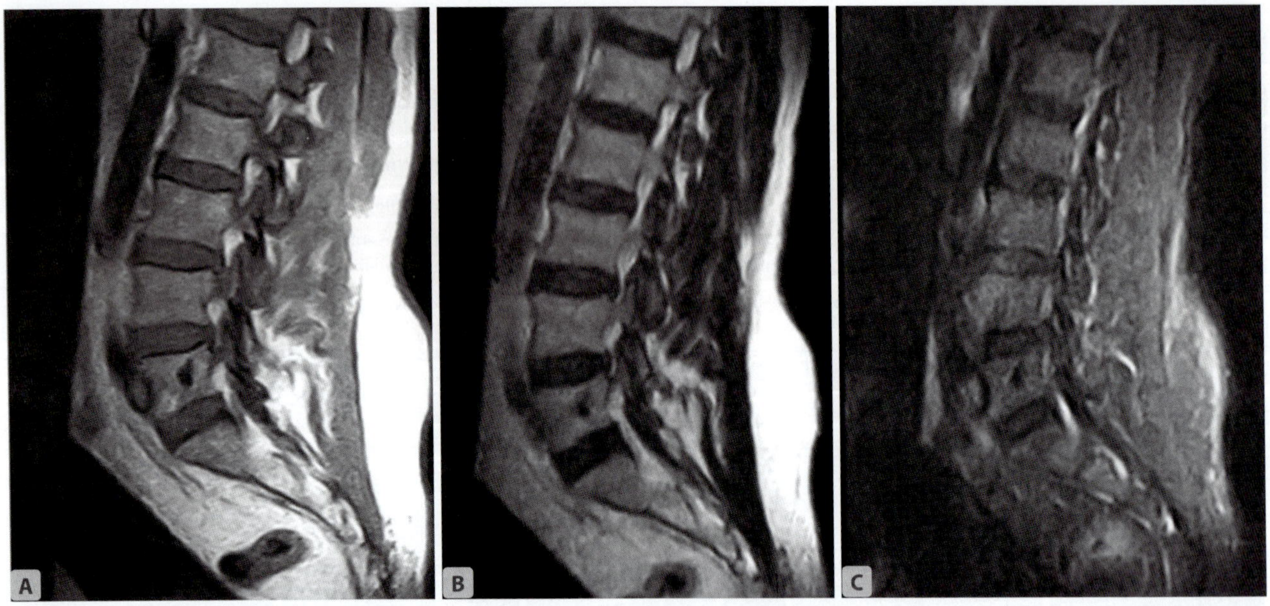

FIGS. 15A TO C: Bone island. T1-weighted (T1W) sagittal (A), T2-weighted (T2W) sagittal (B) and short tau inversion recovery (STIR) sagittal (C) magnetic resonance (MR) images showing hypointense focus in L5 vertebral body suggestive of bone island.

at the pluripotent stem cell level, although it sometimes involves a committed stem cell with limited capacity for self-renewal. Abnormal proliferation, clonal expansion, aberrant differentiation, and diminished apoptosis (programmed cell death) lead to replacement of normal blood elements with malignant cells.

Classification of Leukemia

The current approach to classifying leukemia is based on the 2016 World Health Organization (WHO) system. The WHO classification is based on a combination of clinical, morphologic, immunophenotypic, and genetic features. Leukemias are commonly also categorized as:

- *Acute or chronic*: Based on the percentage of blasts or leukemia cells in bone marrow or blood.
- *Myeloid or lymphoid*: Based on the predominant lineage of the malignant cells.

The four most common leukemias are:

1. Acute myeloid leukemia (AML)
2. Acute lymphoblastic leukemia (ALL)
3. Chronic myeloid leukemia (CML)
4. Chronic lymphocytic leukemia (CLL).

Leukemia comprises one-third of all malignancies in childhood and ALL is the most common. In adults, CLL and AML are the common subtypes.

Risk factors for leukemia include exposure to radiation, chromosomal abnormalities such as Down syndrome, oncoviruses such as human T-cell leukemia virus type 1 (HTLV-1), cigarette smoking (AML), obesity, family history (CLL), and chemical exposures (AML).

Common signs and symptoms of chronic or acute leukemia include pain in the bones or joints, lymphadenopathy, fever, fatigue, bleeding and bruising, frequent infections, hepatosplenomegaly, weight loss, etc.

The red marrow is preferentially infiltrated by leukemic cells ultimately leading to anemia, neutropenia, and thrombocytopenia. The calvaria, spine, flat bones, proximal end of the long bones and subsequently the appendicular skeleton are involved. Extramedullary sites of involvement include lymph nodes, thymus, central nervous system (chronic meningitis), infiltration of salivary glands, skin, lungs, liver, spleen, pleura, pericardium, and testis.

Imaging

The diagnosis of leukemia may be missed on radiographs as the findings are subtle and do not appear till advanced stage of disease. Osteopenia with coarse trabeculation may be seen.[39-42] Other findings include periosteal reaction, radiolucent metaphyseal bands (classically in pediatric cases) **(Figs. 16A to D)**.[42] Leukemic bone marrow infiltration may also cause collapse of vertebral body (vertebra plana).[43]

The pattern of involvement of marrow may be diffuse or multifocal. On MRI, infiltration by leukemic cells is seen as decreased signal intensity on T1W images and increased signal intensity on STIR images[44] **(Figs. 17 to 19)** with increased enhancement of involved areas. The signal intensity is increased or unchanged on T2W images because of the high water content of leukemic cells. Leukemic marrow shows restriction of diffusion and DWI has been shown to be predictive of leukemia even before bone marrow biopsy.[45-47] Although marrow aspiration or biopsy is required for definitive diagnosis, MRI has been shown to demonstrate leukemic infiltration of the bones even with a negative bone marrow biopsy in pediatric cases.[41]

Bone marrow necrosis (BMN) is an unusual entity that has been reported to occur in close association with malignancy, particularly acute lymphocytic leukemia. BMN is characterized by a loss of myeloid tissue and marrow fat

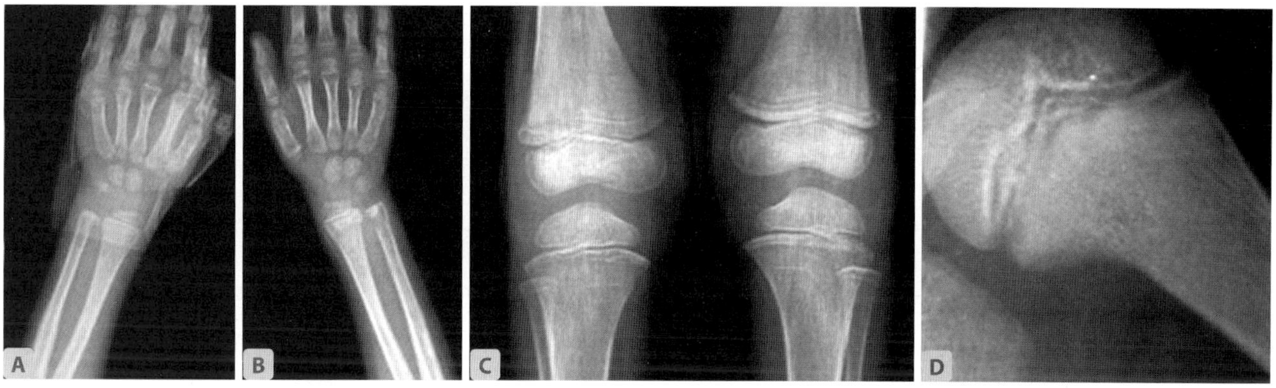

FIGS. 16A TO D: Leukemia: Radiographs bilateral wrist anteroposterior (AP) view (A and B), bilateral knees AP view (C), and left shoulder AP view (D) reveal diffuse osteopenia with radiolucent metaphyseal bands. Area of osteolysis is seen in the radial aspect of bilateral distal ulnar metaphyses.

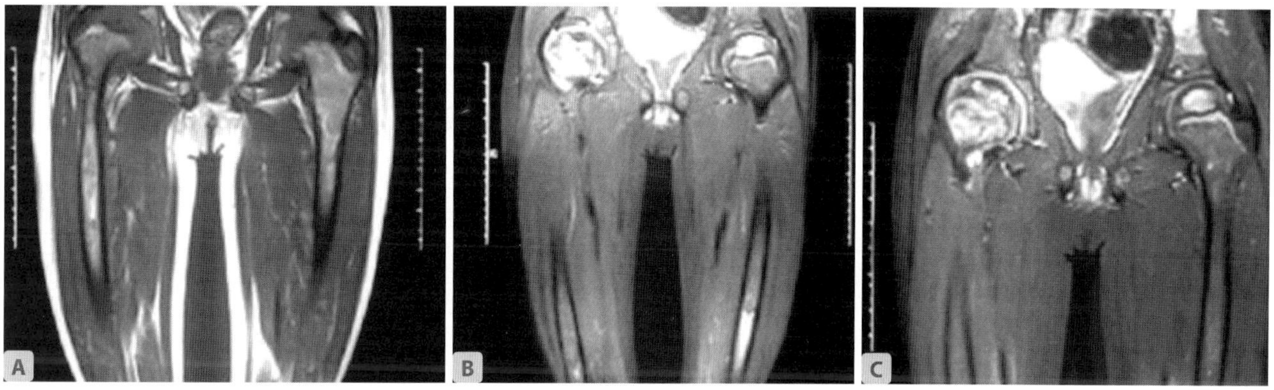

FIGS. 17A TO C: Leukemic infiltration of marrow. T1-weighted (T1W) coronal magnetic resonance (MR) image of the pelvis (A) in a 5-year-old child showing abnormal low-signal in the femoral head instead of the high-signal fat normally seen at this age. Few foci of abnormal signal are also seen in the femoral diaphysis. Short tau inversion recovery (STIR) coronal images of the pelvis (B and C) show these foci in the femoral head, diaphysis, and iliac blades to be high-signal (higher than muscle) which is abnormal.

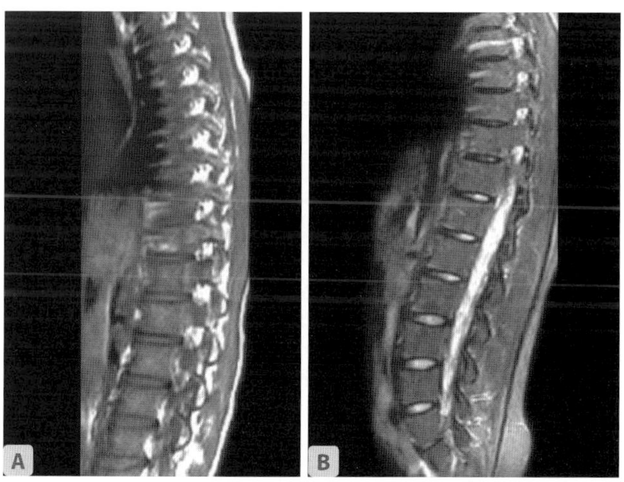

FIGS. 18A AND B: Leukemic infiltration of marrow. T1-weighted (T1W) sagittal magnetic resonance (MR) image of the dorsolumbar spine (A) showing diffuse abnormal signal in the vertebrae, the signal being lower than the adjacent intervertebral discs. T2-weighted (T2W) sagittal image (B) showing no increase in signal.

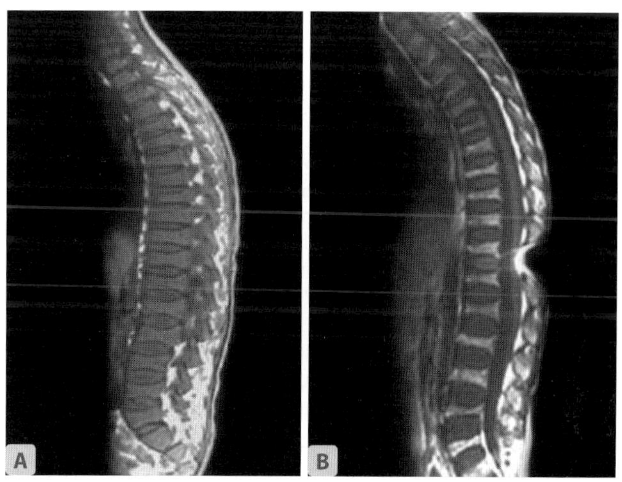

FIGS. 19A AND B: Acute lymphocytic leukemia (ALL). T1-weighted (T1W) magnetic resonance (MR) images of the spine in a case of ALL showing a diffuse low signal of the vertebral bodies in the active stage. The vertebrae also show reduced height (A). In the stage of remission (B), the vertebral bodies show a replacement of the marrow with fat.

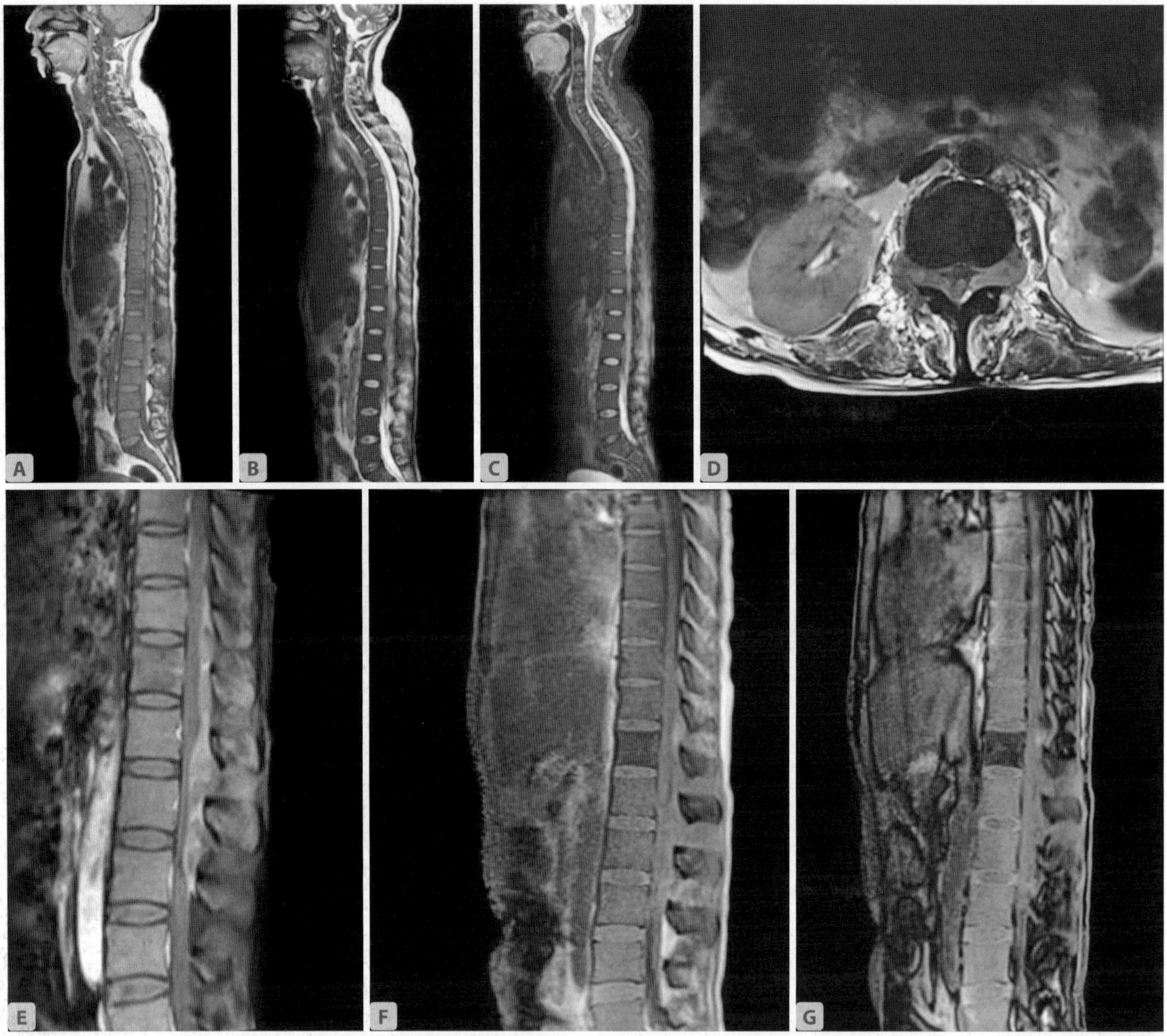

FIGS. 20A TO G: Chronic myeloid leukemia with granulocytic sarcoma. T1-weighted (T1W) (A), T2-weighted (T2W) (B), short tau inversion recovery (STIR) (C) sagittal magnetic resonance (MR) images show diffuse infiltration of marrow that is hypointense on T1W with hypointense signal on T2W and STIR images. T2W axial (D) and contrast-enhanced sagittal (E) image reveals heterogeneously enhancing soft tissue within the posterior and lateral epidural space causing narrowing of the spinal canal and compressive myelopathy suggestive of granulocytic sarcoma. In-phase (F) and opposed phase (G) images show no drop in the signal of the vertebral marrow except one vertebral body which shows some preserved fatty marrow.

without trabecular destruction which is unlike avascular necrosis (AVN). About 91% of patients with BMN have malignancy, with acute lymphocytic leukemia representing 18% of cases.[48] MR findings of BMN are similar to those of AVN but are more diffuse and involve the axial skeleton without vertebral collapse.

Chloroma (also known as granulocytic sarcoma) is a rare manifestation of AML, but it may also occur with other myeloproliferative and myelodysplastic disorders. It is a solid tumor composed of mass-like *extramedullary* proliferation of primitive cells of myeloid lineage. Most common sites of chloroma are the bone and periosteum, which is explained by the direct spread from the adjoining infiltrated marrow. Other frequently involved sites are skin (leukemia cutis), lymph nodes, and orbit, although any site may be potentially affected. On MRI, it is iso-/hypointense on T1 and mildly hyperintense on T2W images **(Figs. 20A to G)**.

On FDG-PET/CT and FDG-PET/MRI, increase in uptake is seen in involved marrow. Further research needs to be performed before it can be accepted as a staging tool.[49,50]

Treatment options for leukemia include chemotherapy regimens, bone marrow or peripheral blood stem cell transplant, and antibody-mediated medications such as ibrutinib or idelalisib for CLL and imatinib for CML.[51] Although acute leukemia is more aggressive than chronic leukemia, the former responds better to treatment than the latter.

Multiple Myeloma

Multiple myeloma refers to a spectrum of disorders arising due to malignant clonal proliferation of plasma cells of B-cell origin. There is production of an abnormal paraprotein leading to a wide M-band on plasma electrophoresis. Multiple myeloma is the third most common blood cancer in adults.[51] This is a disease of the elderly. About 75% of those affected are over the age of 50 years with a peak over 80 years. A male predominance of up to 2:1 is seen. Risk factors for multiple myeloma include male sex, increasing age, African-American ethnicity, monoclonal gammopathy of undetermined significance (MGUS), and radiation exposure. MGUS often precedes frank multiple myeloma.

TABLE 7: Definitions of multiple myeloma and related conditions.[52]

	Definition
Multiple myeloma	Monoclonal proliferation of plasma cells with myeloma-defining CRAB* findings
MGUS	Monoclonal proliferation of plasma cells without myeloma-defining CRAB* findings
Solitary plasmacytoma	Monoclonal plasma cells manifesting as a single tumor
Smoldering myeloma	Monoclonal proliferation of plasma cells in bone marrow and/or serum/urine with abnormal levels of monoclonal protein

*CRAB = calcium level elevation, renal failure, anemia, or bone lesions. (MGUS: monoclonal gammopathy of undetermined significance)

Production of light-chain immunoglobulins results in Bence Jones proteinuria in over half the patients. Multiple systemic effects, including hypercalcemia, renal failure and/or hematologic dyscrasias may also occur. Diseases in the multiple myeloma spectrum have been described in **Table 7**.

Persistent bone pain is the most common symptom which is worse during the day, is relieved by rest, and aggravated by weight bearing. Pathological fracture is a common complication. Associated weight loss, anemia and, cachexia occur. Bacterial infections occur in 10% of cases, most of which are respiratory in nature.

Laboratory findings reveal a normochromic, normocytic anemia, thrombocytopenia, hypercalcemia, hyperglobulinemia with a reversed A:G ratio, hyperuricemia, and Bence Jones proteinuria. Erythrocyte sedimentation rate (ESR) is often raised to over 100 mm/h. Bone marrow biopsy confirms the plasma cell dyscrasia. The spine, pelvis, skull, ribs, and scapula are the most frequently involved bones.

Imaging

On radiography, multiple myeloma may be seen as diffuse or focal osteolysis. The involved bones show well-defined, small, punched-out lytic lesions, most characteristic in the skull **(Figs. 21A to C)**. These lesions can also be seen in the pelvic bones, clavicles, ribs, and long bones. Osteolytic lesions involving long bones tend to show signs of cortical erosion from the medullary side, i.e., endosteal cortical scalloping. These lesions may be differentiated from lytic metastatic lesions by the more uniform size of the lesions in multiple

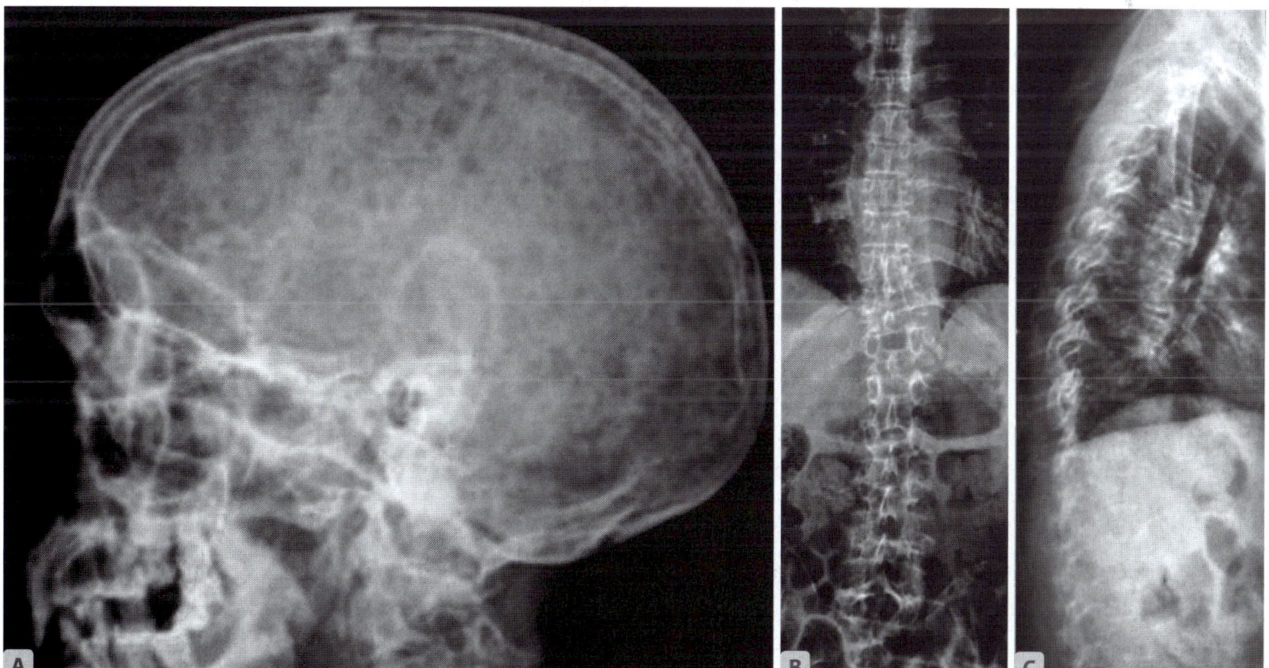

FIGS. 21A TO C: Multiple myeloma. X-ray of skull lateral view (A), dorsolumbar spine anteroposterior (AP) (B) and lateral view (C) reveal diffuse osteopenia with multiple well-defined punched out lesions in the skull.

myeloma. Generalized osteopenia is another important form of presentation. A pathological fracture affects about half of the patients at some time or the other. Examples of purely sclerotic myeloma have been occasionally reported. They may take the form of diffuse osteosclerosis, patchy sclerotic areas throughout the skeleton and, very rarely, small numbers of focal sclerotic lesions.

Involvement of the spine is usually in the lower thoracic and upper lumbar regions, and is seen as diffuse osteopenia. Pedicular involvement, although rare, can occur in multiple myeloma patients; and so the usefulness of this feature to differentiate multiple myeloma from metastatic disease appears doubtful.

On CT, well-circumscribed, lytic "soap bubble" osseous lesions, with a narrow zone of transition, are seen. The attenuation of lesions is 40–80 HU of attenuation, similar to soft tissue **(Figs. 22A and B)**.

Multiple myeloma generally has no osteoblastic activity and is thus typically negative on ^{99m}Tc bone scans. FDG-PET/CT has high specificity and sensitivity for multiple myeloma lesions and is especially good at demonstrating extramedullary disease.[53] FDG-PET/CT can be used to monitor treatment response because the ^{18}F-FDG uptake of osseous lesions will decrease with successful treatment.

On MRI, bone marrow in multiple myeloma shows elevated signal intensity on T2W images and decreased signal intensity on T1W images **(Figs. 23 and 24)**. MRI correlates with the clinical severity. Stabler et al. have found five infiltration patterns of multiple myeloma on MRI. These are as follows:

1. Normal appearing marrow with low-grade interstitial infiltration
2. Focal pattern
3. Diffuse
4. Mixed focal and diffuse
5. Salt and pepper appearance.

The infiltration patterns correlated with the clinical staging in their study. They concluded that MR is of prognostic value and can be a supporting pillar in the staging and planning treatment of patients with multiple myeloma.[54]

Vertebral body compression fractures occur frequently in patients with multiple myeloma. The differentiation between osteoporotic vertebral collapse and that due to myeloma may be difficult even on MRI. DWI and opposed-phase (in-phase–out-of-phase) imaging have been advocated to help differentiate insufficiency fractures from pathologic compression fractures.

The most important differential diagnosis in this age group is metastases. Features, which help in distinguishing the two, are summarized in **Table 8**.

Early- or low-grade infiltration of myeloma in the bone marrow may demonstrate normal bone marrow signal intensity at MRI, underlining the importance of correlation with the laboratory tests and bone marrow biopsy. Greater than 40% increase in signal intensity compared with the baseline after contrast administration correlates with diffuse tumor infiltration of marrow.[55]

Despite the widespread use of the radiographic skeletal survey, MRI has been shown to be useful in the assessment of multiple myeloma patients; and considering the increased sensitivity of FDG-PET/CT and MRI in identifying bone marrow infiltration, the staging system has been revised. The Durie-Salmon PLUS system replaces the radiographic skeletal survey with MRI and FDG-PET/CT.[53] The Durie-Salmon PLUS system divides patients with multiple myeloma into three groups (each of which has two subgroups) on the basis of the number of focal lesions or the severity of diffuse bone infiltration noted on imaging.

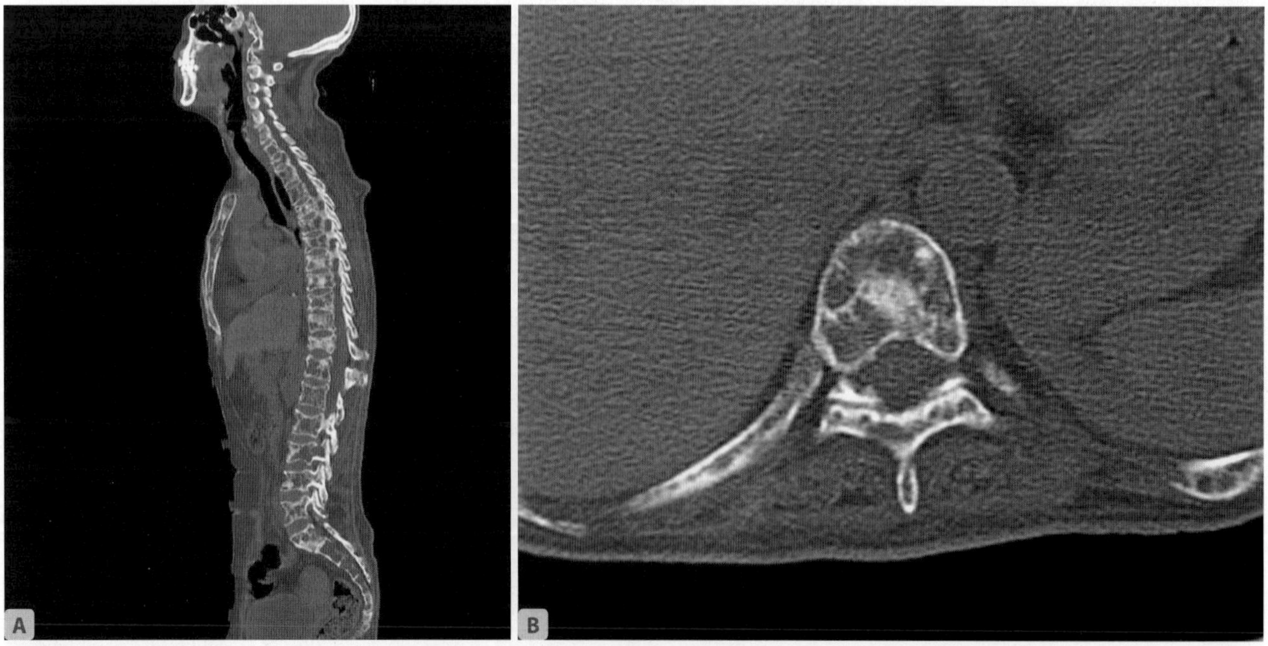

FIGS. 22A AND B: Multiple myeloma. Computed tomography (CT) bone window sagittal (A) and axial (B) images show multiple well-defined lytic lesions in visualized bones.

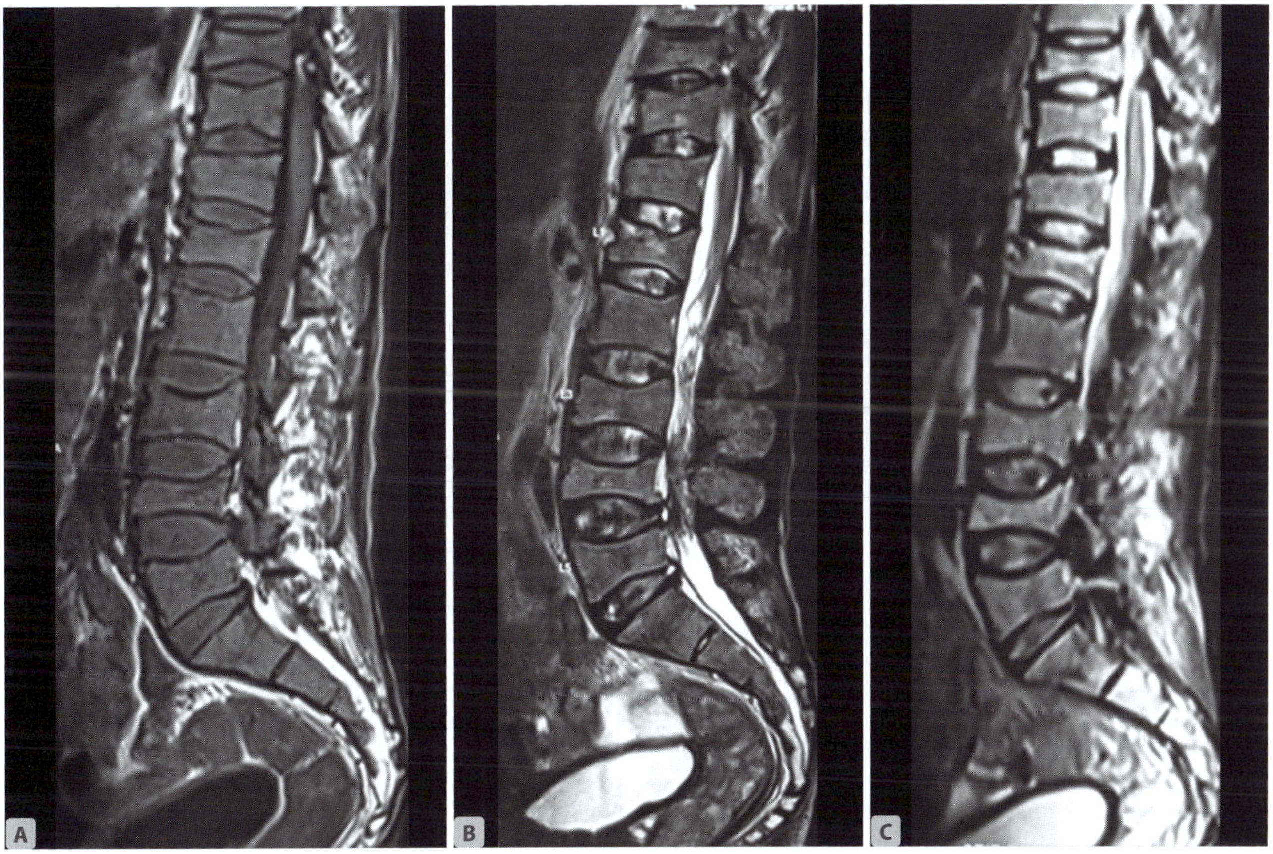

FIGS. 23A TO C: Multiple myeloma. T1-weighted (T1W) sagittal (A), T2-weighted (T2W) sagittal (B), and short tau inversion recovery (STIR) sagittal (C) magnetic resonance (MR) images of the lumbar spine showing diffuse alteration of marrow signal appearing hypointense on T1W and mildly hyperintense on T2W and STIR images.

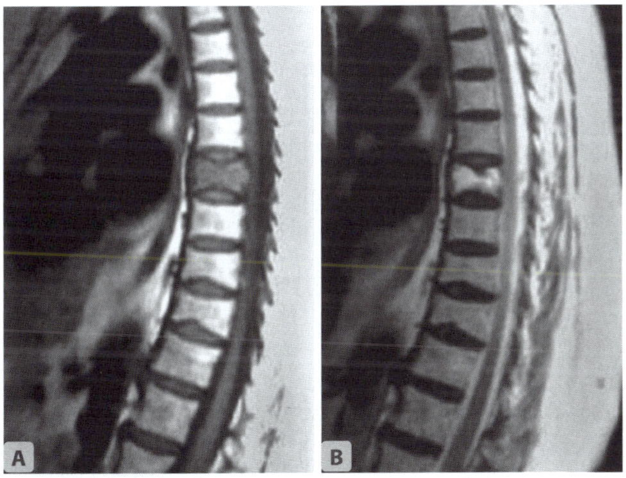

FIGS. 24A AND B: Multiple myeloma. T1-weighted (T1W) (A) and T2-weighted (T2W) (B) sagittal magnetic resonance (MR) images of the dorsal spine show complete alteration of the marrow signal in the seventh thoracic vertebra, hypointense on T1W and hyperintense on T2W images, with evidence of collapse. A posterior convexity of the involved vertebra suggests a malignant etiology.

TABLE 8: Distinguishing features between multiple myeloma and metastases.

Multiple myeloma	Metastases
Vertebral pedicles and posterior elements less commonly involved; destruction of intervertebral disc may occur	Destruction of vertebral pedicles
Soft-tissue mass associated with a bony lesion	Soft tissue extension is relatively uncommon
Mandible involved commonly	Mandible involved rarely
Radionuclide studies may give false negative results	Radionuclide studies are very sensitive
Serum alkaline phosphatase may be normal	Serum alkaline phosphatase is always raised in disseminated disease

Durie-Salmon PLUS staging system—MRI findings, FDG-PET/CT findings, or both.

MGUS: All negative.

Stage IA, smoldering or indolent: Can have single plasmacytoma or limited disease at imaging.

Stage IB: <5 focal lesions, mild diffuse disease.

Stage IIA or IIB: 5–20 focal lesions, moderate diffuse disease.

Stage IIIA or IIIB: >20 focal lesions, severe diffuse disease.

The criteria for subgroup A classification is a serum creatinine level <2.0 mg/dL and no extramedullary disease, whereas the criteria for subgroup B classification is serum creatinine level >2.0 mg/dL or the presence of extramedullary disease.

Magnetic resonance may also help guide the biopsy and also to confirm the response to therapy. Complete response to chemotherapy includes the following postcontrast enhancement patterns:

- Complete resolution of abnormality
- Persistent abnormality with no enhancement
- Peripheral rim enhancement only.[56]

A partial response to chemotherapy can show conversion of diffuse pattern to a focal or variegated pattern with persistent contrast enhancement. Reconstituted fatty tissue is seen as multifocal, diffuse increase in signal intensity on T1W images with less contrast enhancement[3] **(Figs. 25A to C)**

Treatment options for multiple myeloma include chemotherapy, steroid therapy, stem cell transplant, radiation therapy, biologic therapy, and watchful waiting.

Plasmacytoma

A plasmacytoma represents a localized form of plasma cell proliferation, which is apparently solitary at presentation and may remain localized for many years, but is potentially capable of transition to generalized myelomatosis.

Although few cases present below the age of 40 years, the overall age of presentation tends to be earlier, and the age range wider, than in generalized myelomatosis.

Presentation may be with local pain as a result of fracture, but uncomplicated plasmacytoma may cause no symptoms. The lesion predominantly affects sites containing persistent red marrow. The mandible, ilium, vertebrae, ribs, and proximal femur are the commonly involved bones. Peripheral lesions are rare.

Imaging

A plasmacytoma arises in the medulla and the bone changes usually resemble a benign lesion. The characteristic appearance is that of a geographic, radiolucent lesion which is highly expansile with apparent trabeculation or a "soap bubble" appearance.

Involvement of the vertebral body is common, sometimes leading to early collapse. Sometimes a whole vertebral body is lost, with geographical destruction of the margins of the adjoining vertebral bodies, usually posteriorly. Coarse trabecular strands of increased density may give a network appearance in the area of destruction. Exceptionally, the lesion may be entirely sclerotic. Scintigraphy and CT/MRI do not give any specific information; however, the finding

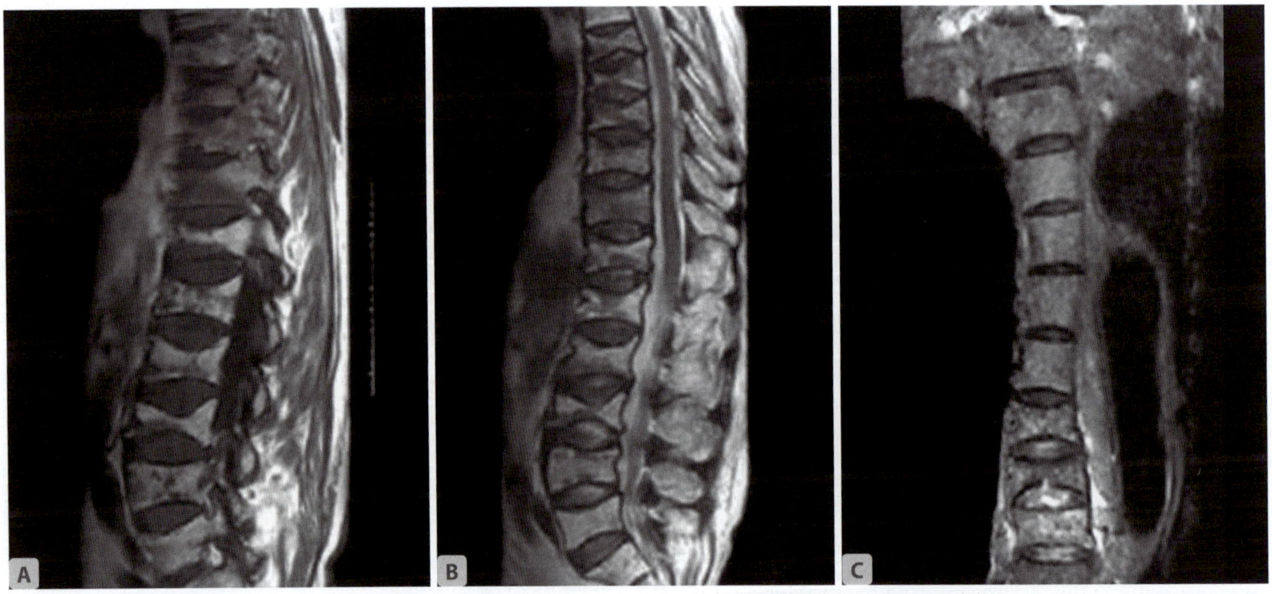

FIGS. 25A TO C: Multiple myeloma on treatment. T1-weighted (T1W) sagittal (A), T2-weighted (T2W) sagittal (B) and short tau inversion recovery (STIR) coronal (C) magnetic resonance (MR) images showing collapse of multiple vertebrae with heterogeneous marrow signal of vertebral bodies predominantly hyperintense on both T1W and T2W images s/o fatty marrow replacement. Areas of active marrow infiltration/edema are noted involving D11 and few other lower dorsal and lumbar vertebrae seen as hypointense on T1, hyperintense on T2, and STIR images with associated (L) paravertebral mass. Proven case of multiple myeloma on treatment showing fatty marrow replacement with residual active marrow infiltration in few vertebrae.

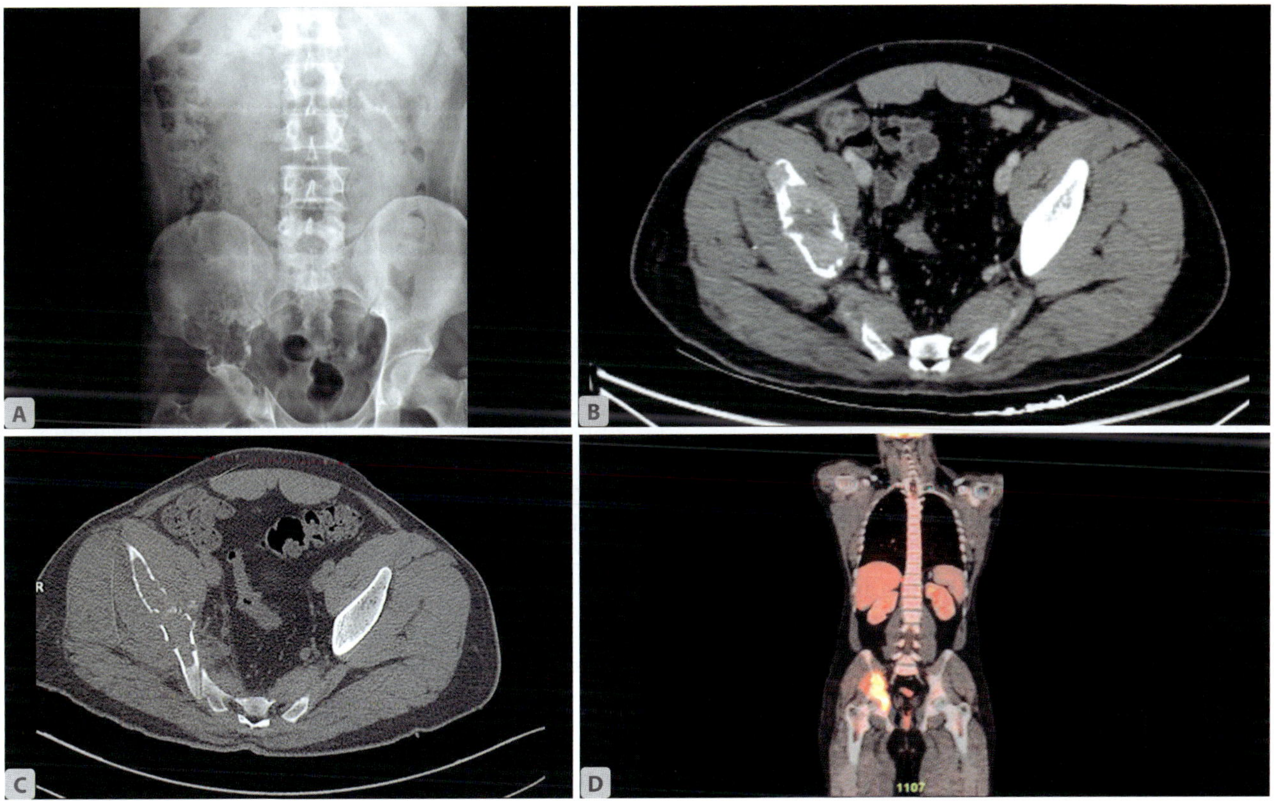

FIGS. 26A TO D: Plasmacytoma. A 30-year-old male patient presented with pain in right gluteal region. Plain anteroposterior (AP) radiograph (A) of the pelvis shows a lytic expansile lesion in the supra-acetabular region of right iliac bone causing erosion and thinning of overlying cortex. The computed tomography (CT) axial soft tissue (B) and bone window (C) of the pelvis of the same patient show a soft tissue lesion in the right iliac bone causing bony erosion. Coronal positron emission tomography (PET)-CT image (D) shows increased fluorodeoxyglucose (FDG) uptake in the lesion.

of apparently solitary plasmacytoma in the spine should be investigated with whole spine MRI to identify further radiographically occult lesions **(Figs. 26A to D)**.

The most important differential diagnosis is an osteolytic metastasis. In the vertebrae, such metastases are likely to involve the pedicles. Chordoma, brown tumors of hyperparathyroidism, hemophilic pseudotumor, hydatid cyst, fibrous dysplasia, and giant cell tumor can also be considered in the differential diagnosis.

A study of patients initially diagnosed with solitary plasmacytoma found that there was evidence of additional sites of intramedullary involvement in one-third of cases at MRI screening of the thoracic and lumbosacral spine.[57] This is significant, as these cases were initially thought to have only a single focus of disease.

The International Myeloma Working Group has recommended that low-dose whole-body CT, FDG-PET/CT or whole-body, and/or spine MRI be performed in all patients with a clinical presentation of smoldering multiple myeloma and solitary plasmacytoma; equivocal or small lesions should be reassessed with prompt (3–6-month) follow-up MRI.[53]

POEMS Syndrome, also known as Takatsuki Disease or Crow–Fukase Syndrome

An uncommon condition with the acronym POEMS is characterized by a chronic, progressive polyneuropathy, organomegaly (hepatosplenomegaly), endocrinopathy (commonly diabetes mellitus), M-proteins (plasma cell dyscrasia), and skin changes (hirsutism, pigmentation, and edema). In POEMS syndrome, there is also a monoclonal proliferation of plasma cells, but at a lower level than in multiple myeloma.[53] It is usually seen in young men. Imaging findings of POEMS syndrome include organomegaly and sclerotic osseous lesions that can have the same ^{18}F-FDG avidity as a normal bone. Findings include multiple sclerotic lesions, most commonly in the spine and pelvis. The lesions may be uniformly sclerotic or appear target-like, with a peripheral margin of bone sclerosis. Ivory vertebrae and areas resembling bone islands may be seen. Bone proliferation is seen at sites of tendon and ligament attachments. Irregular bony excrescences involving the posterior elements of the spine are characteristically seen. Digital clubbing and periostitis in tubular bones simulate the findings of hypertrophic osteoarthropathy.[58]

Langerhans Cell Histiocytosis

Langerhans cell histiocytosis (LCH) is a rare multisystem disease with a wide and heterogeneous clinical spectrum and variable extent of involvement. There is abnormal proliferation of cells derived from myeloid dendritic cells that exhibit the same antigens (CD1a, S100, and CD207) and the same unique intracytoplasmic organelles as in Langerhans cells. The intracytoplasmic organelles appear racquet-shaped on electron microscopy, and are known as Birbeck granules.

Langerhans cell histiocytosis is divided into three groups, on the basis of the number of lesions and systems involved.

1. *The unifocal (localized) form*: Patients usually present between 5 and 15 years of age and involvement is limited to a single bone or a few bones. This form is seen in approximately 70% of LCH cases. Patients may be asymptomatic or may present with focal pain and swelling and are at risk for pathologic fractures. It may involve the lungs. Patients with mandibular involvement may present with gingival bleeding and facial swelling.
2. *The multifocal unisystem (chronic recurring) form*: Patients with this form of disease present between 1 and 5 years of age. The disease involves multiple bones as well as the reticuloendothelial system (i.e., the spleen, liver, lymph nodes, and skin). It comprises approximately 20% of LCH cases and is accompanied by diabetes insipidus when the pituitary gland is involved.
3. *The multifocal multisystem (fulminant) form*: It is typically diagnosed in the first 2 years of life and is characterized by disseminated involvement of the reticuloendothelial system, thrombocytopenia, and anemia.[59] It constitutes approximately 10% of LCH cases and is often fatal.

Eosinophilic granuloma, Hand-Schüller-Christian disease, and Letterer-Siwe disease respectively are older names for the three groups.

Imaging

The most common radiographic manifestation of LCH are bone lesions and occurs in approximately 80% of patients. Any bone can be affected by LCH, but the involvement of flat bones is more common.[60] The skull is the most common flat bone involved. The lesions in skull are well-defined lytic "punched-out" and show beveled margins. This appearance is caused by asymmetric destruction of the inner and outer cortices **(Figs. 27A and B)**.[60] When the skull lesions grow in size, they may coalesce, creating a map-like appearance referred to as a *geographic skull*. The differential diagnosis for calvarial lesions includes lymphoma, multiple myeloma, leukemia, and metastases for multiple lesions and dermoid and epidermoid cysts for single lesions. Osteomyelitis must also be considered in the list of differential diagnoses.

Severe mandibular lesions may destroy the alveolar ridge, resulting in a radiographic appearance of "floating teeth".

The vertebral body is the most commonly affected part of the spine in LCH. Early lesions appear lytic at radiography and computed tomography (CT). As the disease progresses, the early lytic lesions can result in symmetric uniform collapse of the vertebral body with preservation of the intervertebral disc spaces.[60] The flattened vertebral body has been termed *vertebra plana* and may result in substantial neurologic defects and pain. Although vertebra plana can have additional causes in children, such as leukemia, aneurysmal bone cyst, metastatic neuroblastoma, or Ewing sarcoma, the most common cause in children is LCH.

Long bone involvement is more common in children than in adults. Lesions typically occur in the metaphysis or diaphysis, with femur, humerus, and tibia being the most commonly involved long bones. Early lesions often appear expansile, lytic, and aggressive. Less aggressive lesions have been associated with imaging findings of smooth periosteal reaction and cortical thickening. As lesions become chronic, they may resolve or appear sclerotic from periosteal new bone formation.

Bone scintigraphy typically shows increased radiotracer uptake. However, bone scan should be evaluated in conjunction with radiographic findings, as false-negative bone scan findings are common, particularly in patients with older lesions.[60]

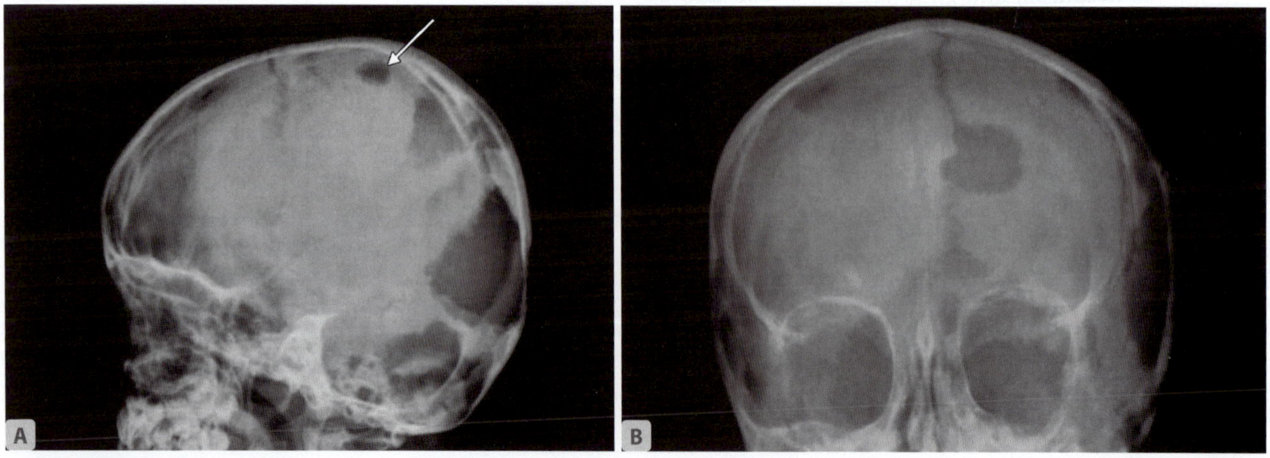

FIGS. 27A AND B: Langerhans cell histiocytosis. X-ray of skull—lateral (A) and anteroposterior (AP) (B) view showing multiple well-defined lytic areas in skull bones. On lateral view, one of the lesions in parietal bone shows characteristic beveled margin (arrow).

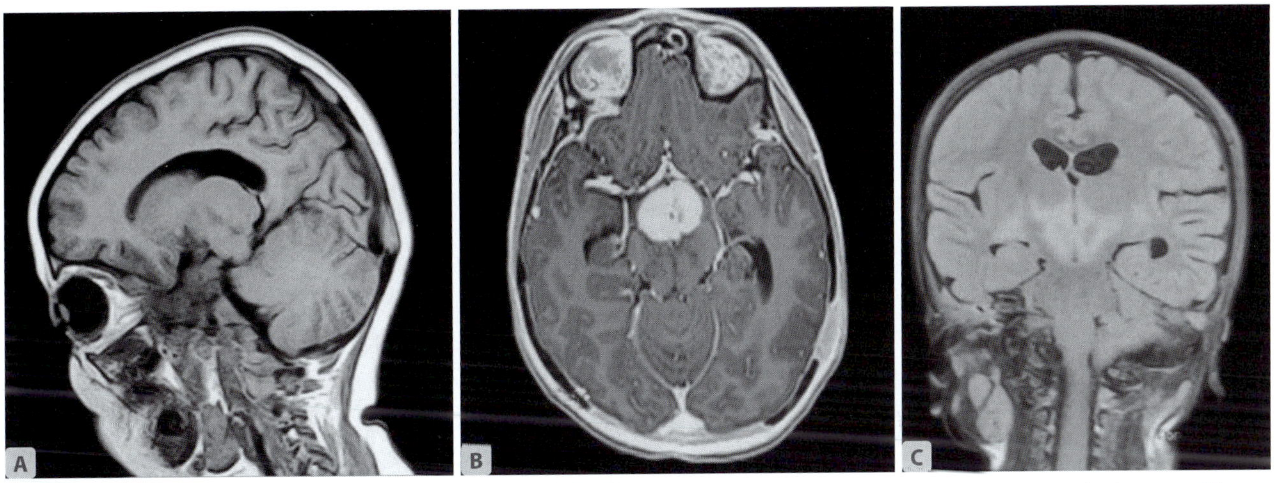

FIGS. 28A TO C: Magnetic resonance (MR) of same patient as Figure 27 with T1 sagittal image (A) and postcontrast axial MR images (B) showing enhancing T1 hypointense lesion in hypothalamus with multiple enhancing lesions in parietal bones. Coronal fluid-attenuated inversion-recovery (FLAIR) (C) image shows the presence of cervical lymphadenopathy.

Magnetic resonance imaging shows intramedullary lesions with extramedullary soft-tissue components. The soft-tissue component is isointense on T1W images and hyperintense on T2W images, with enhancement after gadolinium-based contrast agent administration **(Figs. 28A to C)**.[60]

Diagnosis of LCH is made by corroborating clinical features, immunohistochemistry, histopathology, and radiologic findings. Treatment of single lesion includes radiation therapy, curettage, or curettage with intralesional steroid injection. Oral systemic steroids and chemotherapy may be used to treat multiple lesions or to prevent central nervous system (CNS) extension in cases of a skull lesion. Radiation therapy is the treatment of choice for vertebral lesions that are at risk for collapse.

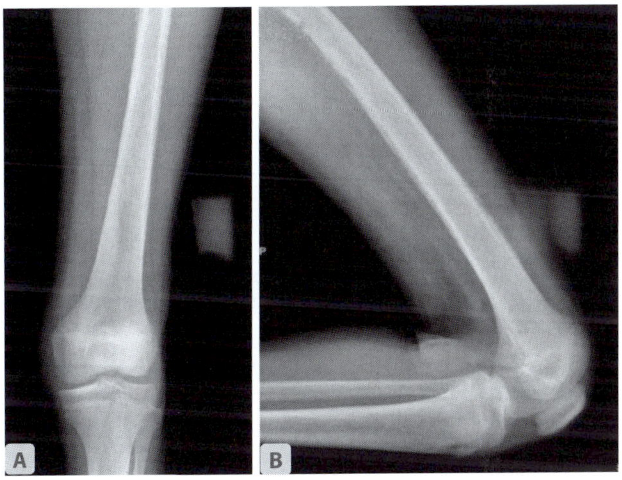

FIGS. 29A AND B: Acute osteomyelitis. X-ray of the left femur anteroposterior (AP) (A) and lateral view (B) in a 13-year-old girl showing subtle changes of acute osteomyelitis as evidenced by periosteal reaction, areas of osteolysis in the diaphysis, and blurred fat planes.

MARROW REPLACEMENT DISORDERS

In contrast to marrow proliferative diseases, which are usually diffuse and arise from cells that originate in the bone marrow, the most common marrow replacement diseases are usually focal abnormalities that arise from cells other than those inherent in the bone marrow.

Benign Marrow Replacement Disorder

Osteomyelitis

Osteomyelitis is an infection of medullary bone caused by bacteria and the most common infecting organisms are *Staphylococcus aureus*, *Streptococcus*, and *Pneumococcus*. Less common organisms are *Haemophilus influenzae*, *Escherichia coli*, and *Pseudomonas*. Occasionally fungi, viruses, and parasites are the causative agents.[2,3]

There are three major routes of pathogenesis which are as follows:

1. Hematogenous, beginning in the metaphysis of long bones, juxtachondral portion of flat bones, or spiral end plates. This is commonly seen in infancy and childhood. In neonates, the intact vascular communication between metaphysis and epiphysis leads to epiphyseal involvement in up to 70% cases. Between 1 year and skeletal maturity, the cartilage provides a barrier to joint involvement, except in the hip where the femoral head is intra-articular.
2. Direct inoculation due to trauma/surgery.
3. Via contiguous spread from an adjacent infection.[1-3]

Imaging

Radiographs are insensitive in the first 2 weeks. Routine radiographs are fairly specific in the late stages **(Figs. 29A and B)**. Early changes include soft-tissue swelling and loss of fat planes. Other changes include osteopenia with periosteal thickening and lytic areas.

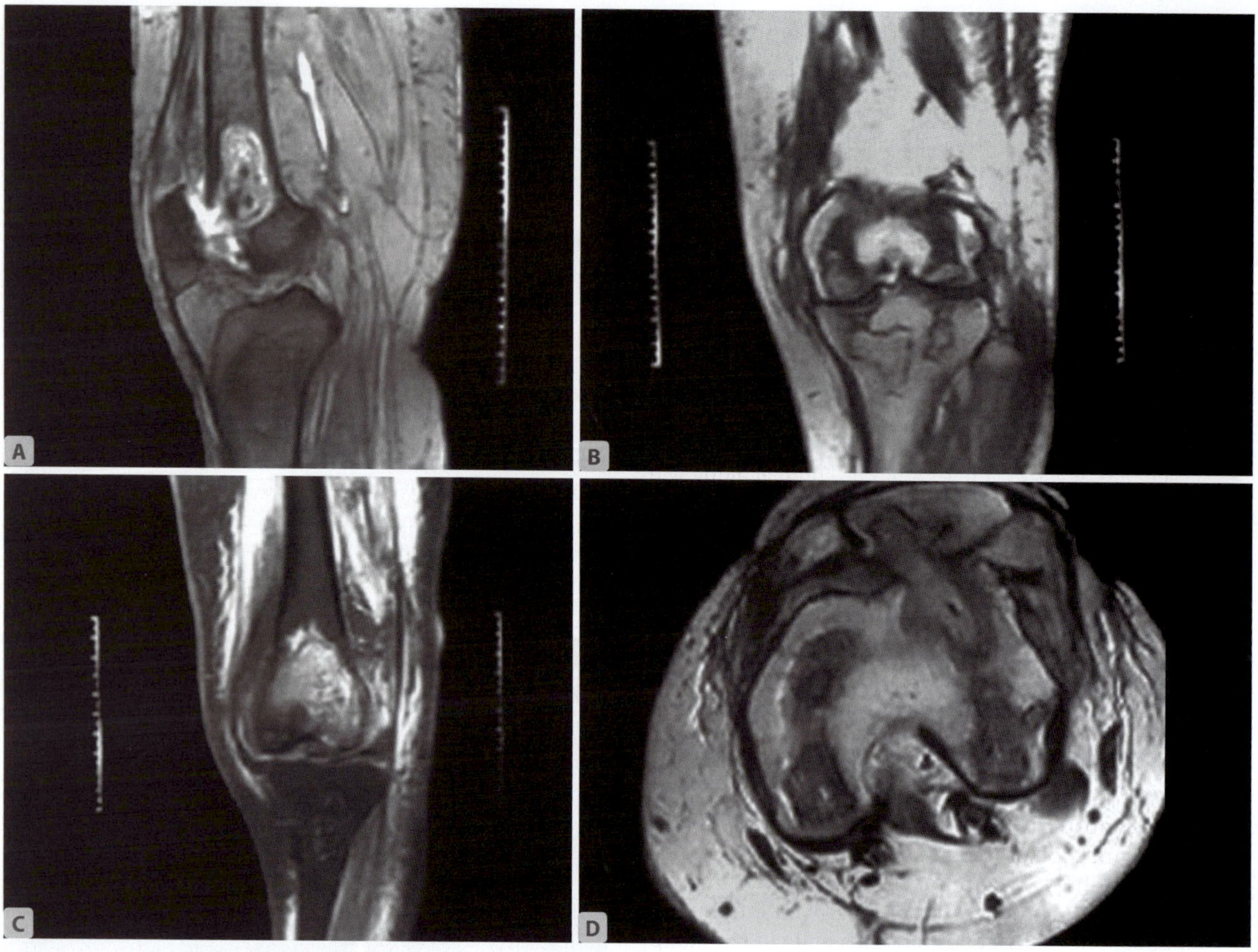

FIGS. 30A TO D: Chronic osteomyelitis of the femur with intramedullary abscess and associated infective arthritis. Fat-suppressed sagittal (A), T1 coronal (B), short tau inversion recovery (STIR) coronal (C) and T2 axial (D) magnetic resonance (MR) images of the knee showing an area of marrow signal alteration in the metadiaphyseal region of lower femur. Signal alteration is also seen in the patella and the upper end tibia. Cortical destruction with cloacae formation seen in anterior aspect of the femur, posterior aspect of the patella, and joint effusion with edema seen in the muscles.

Osteomyelitis causes marrow replacement with inflammatory cells resulting in increased extracellular water or fluid, which causes a decreased signal intensity on T1W images and increased signal intensity on T2W fat-saturated, STIR images as well as contrast-enhanced images. Fat-suppressed images increase the specificity and conspicuity of bony changes. Edema on STIR images and enhancement on contrast administration are the two most common findings in osteomyelitis **(Figs. 30A to D)**.

Acute osteomyelitis causes marrow replacement due to infiltration by inflammatory cells, hemorrhage, fibrin, debris, and edema. The margins are typically ill-defined against the surrounding marrow. Secondary signs of infection such as cellulitis, cortical disruption, sinus tracts, soft tissue abscesses, and periosteal reaction help establish the diagnosis of osteomyelitis.[2,3,61]

Healed osteomyelitis appears as localized fat replacement within red marrow.

Chronic osteomyelitis is defined as persistent infection after 1 month of treatment. On radiograph, it is seen as thickening and irregularity of cortex with mixed sclerotic and lucent areas. Involucrum and cloacae are also seen. It exhibits the same signal pattern as acute osteomyelitis, but the foci are surrounded by a sclerotic rim seen as a signal void, which clearly delineates the extent of the lesion. Sequestrated bone appears as a signal void, while infarct is seen as "double line" with associated muscle infarction.[61,62]

Malignant Marrow Replacement Disorder

Metastasis

Metastatic infiltration of the marrow occurs by hematogenous spread. The red marrow is predominantly affected because of its rich vascular supply. The most common metastasis in children are from neuroblastoma, rhabdomyosarcoma, and Ewing's sarcoma; while in adults, they are from the prostate, breast, lung, and kidney **(Figs. 31A to D)**. They are discussed in detail elsewhere in this book.

Lymphoma

Lymphomas are a heterogeneous group of tumors of the lymphoid tissue which can arise anywhere in the body.

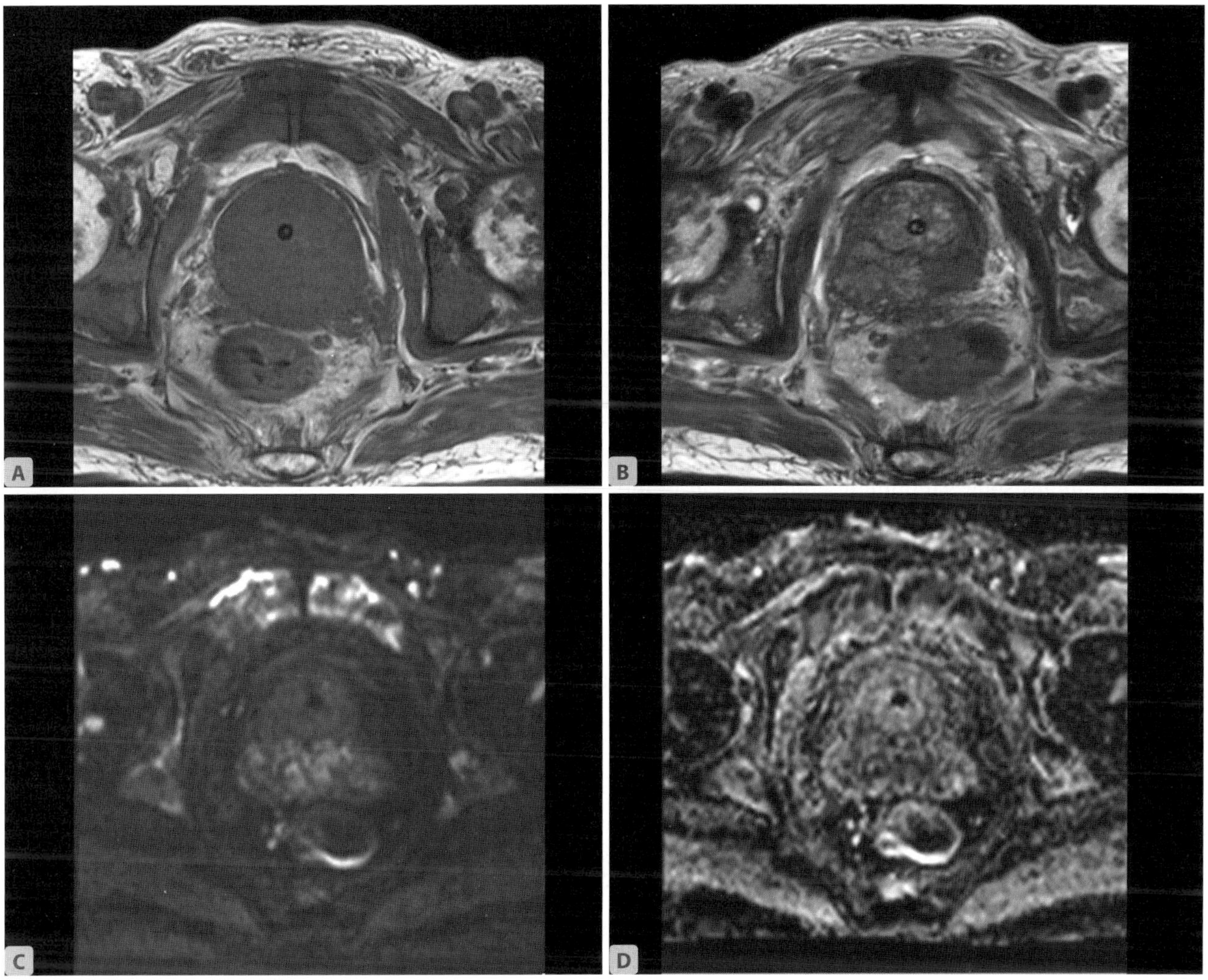

FIGS. 31A TO D: Metastases. T1 axial (A) and T2 axial magnetic resonance (MR) images (B) show hypointense marrow in the pelvic bones with the presence of restriction of diffusion (C and D) in a patient with skeletal metastases from carcinoma prostate.

They arise more commonly from B lymphocytes than T lymphocytes.

Infiltration of bone marrow is found in 20–40% of patients with NHL and 5–15% of patients with Hodgkin lymphoma (HL).[63]

Risk factors for lymphoma include Epstein Barr virus, immunosuppressant medications, severe autoimmune conditions, obesity, family history [human leukocyte antigen (HLA) subtype] and chronic *Helicobacter pylori* infection in the case of gastric mucosa-associated lymphoid tissue (MALT) lymphoma.[51] HL tends to affect young adults and adolescents, while the median age of diagnosis for NHL is 66 years.

Lymphoma is characterized as *primary osseous lymphoma* when bone is the only known site of disease for 6 months.[64] It accounts for <5% of all bone malignancies.[65] Synonyms for primary osseous lymphoma include reticulum cell malignant lymphoma of bone, sarcoma, and osteolymphoma.[66] Primary osseous lymphoma typically affects the metadiaphysis or diaphysis of long bones in the appendicular skeleton or the flat bones of the axial skeleton.

Secondary osseus lymphoma occurs due to metastatic spread from another primary site. Secondary or metastatic osseous lymphoma tends to favor the axial skeleton.[65]

Imaging

The findings on radiography can be subtle, nonspecific, or even inapparent. Osseus lymphoma is seen as the area of permeative osteolysis or mixed lytic sclerotic pattern with broad zone of transition. Periosteal reaction, when present, is usually aggressive and lamellar.[66] In the more common lytic destructive pattern, channels of bone loss can be seen parallel to long axis of bone with focal devascularization and sequestrum formation.[53] However, a bony sequestrum can also be seen in other conditions, such as radiation necrosis, osteomyelitis, osseous tuberculosis, and in tumors such as fibrosarcoma or eosinophilic granuloma. The mixed lytic-sclerotic pattern may be seen after therapeutic intervention and is more common in secondary osseous lymphoma.[66] Lymphoma should also be considered in the differential diagnosis for an ivory vertebrae or sclerotic vertebral lesion. A soft-tissue mass may be seen around an apparent intact or minimally involved cortical bone. This occurs due to spread through the Volkmann and haversian canals of bone cortex and may also be found in small cell malignancies.

At FDG-PET/CT, patterns of multifocal or focal uptake of ^{18}F-FDG on a background of diffuse uptake in bone marrow should be considered positive for bone marrow involvement. HL most commonly shows a multifocal pattern. Higher SUV has been correlated with more aggressive disease.[53] FDG-PET/CT is sensitive in detecting bone marrow involvement; with a pooled meta-analysis sensitivity of 88.7%.[67,68] The concordance rate for bone marrow biopsy and FDG-PET/CT is higher for more aggressive subtypes of lymphoma as compared to more indolent varieties.[69]

On the MR, patterns of bone marrow involvement in lymphoma can be diffuse or focal. These appear as areas of decreased signal intensity of T1W images and increased signal intensity on STIR images **(Figs. 32A to J)**. Contrast-enhanced studies show gadolinium enhancement of the lesions.[66,70] The nodular nature of lymphomatous marrow deposits allows MR mapping to select the site of biopsy because blind bone marrow biopsy may give false negative results.[7,8] In HL, marrow involvement is detected more often with MR than with marrow biopsy. In low-grade NHL, the involvement is diffuse, and biopsy is superior. In high-grade lymphomas, the involvement is more focal, and MRI is more efficient.[65]

The diagnosis of bone marrow involvement by lymphoma can be made by ^{18}F-FDG or with percutaneous biopsy, usually of the posterior iliac bone.[53] Currently, FDG-PET/CT is more widely used due to greater availability, although more research may prove ^{18}F-FDG-PET/MR and WBMRI to be useful, especially in patients who need protection from excess radiation, such as children and young women.[71]

There are many treatment regimens for NHL, including radiation therapy, chemotherapy, targeted drug therapy (e.g., rituximab), and peripheral blood stem cell or bone marrow transplant. Yttrium 90 (^{90}Y)-tagged ibritumomab tiuxetan is a beta-emitting radiopharmaceutical agent that is effective as an adjunct to chemotherapy and autologous stem cell transplant in treating certain cases of refractory NHL. ^{90}Y-tagged ibritumomab tiuxetan binds to the CD20 surface antigen, present in mature B lymphocytes, but not in precursor cells, and causes selective beta radiation-induced cell death.[72] Treatment of HL usually involves a combination of radiation therapy and chemotherapy, directed by the histologic grade and stage of the disease.[69]

MARROW DEPLETION

Myeloid depletion refers to the loss of hematopoietic tissue. Diffuse or regional absence of normal red marrow may occur as a consequence of aplastic anemia, chemotherapy, and/or radiation therapy.

Aplastic Anemia

Aplastic anemia is a pan myelopathy thought to result from suppression of the multipotent myeloid cells. The myeloid depletion manifests as cytopenia of the erythrocytes, leukocytes, and thrombocytes. There is a resultant decrease in the cellularity due to decrease in the hematopoietic marrow, which is replaced by fatty marrow.

Causes of aplastic anemia have not been identified yet but its provoking factors are viral infections, drugs, toxic substances, hepatitis, and unknown causes.[3,73]

Imaging

Two MRI patterns have been seen with aplastic anemia. One pattern is that of diffuse yellow marrow throughout the skeleton in areas where red marrow is expected to exist (**Figs. 33A and B**). This pattern may be difficult to recognize as abnormal in older individuals, in whom large proportions of fatty marrow are normal. The second pattern is seen in patients who have been treated for aplastic anemia and develop focal islands of red marrow regeneration scattered throughout the yellow marrow. These islands of red marrow can be very focal in appearance and may simulate other diseases. The hematopoietically active cell nests return mainly in the marrow space of the vertebral body.[3,73]

Treatment-related Changes

Chemotherapy, radiation, granulocyte colony-stimulating factor, and bone marrow transplant are routinely used in the treatment of neoplasms and can result in temporary or permanent changes in marrow composition. It is crucial to understand the expected post-treatment changes for identifying recurrent or residual neoplastic marrow involvement.

Chemotherapy changes are diffuse and influenced by time duration since the last cycle. In the first week, increased dilatation and permeability of the sinusoids in marrow leads to edema. In the following weeks, the cytotoxic effect leads to fatty marrow transformation and reduction of myeloid precursors. Within 3–4 weeks, numerous small foci of red marrow may be seen due to regeneration.[74] There may be no changes in the MRI study of some patients receiving chemotherapy.

Granulocyte colony-stimulating factor is administered in conjunction with chemotherapy to stimulate myeloid cell production. Stimulation of red marrow proliferation typically occurs in a diffuse or patchy pattern and can mimic disease. The effect occurs rapidly, maximizes at 2 weeks, and normalizes 6 weeks after discontinuation of the growth factor.

Radiation therapy causes changes restricted to the region covered by the radiation port. Altered marrow signal intensity can occur in adjacent structures due to a combination of indirect effects and/or scattered radiation.[75,76] In the first 2 weeks, hemorrhage and edema is seen leading to a variable imaging appearance. After 3–6 weeks, there is preferential disappearance of the red marrow. After 6 weeks, the fatty marrow transformation becomes more homogeneous **(Fig. 34)**. Recovery of normal marrow signal intensity is largely dependent on the patient's age and the radiation dose. Younger patients and patients receiving <30–40 Gy are more likely to recover with full marrow regeneration. At doses >40–50 Gy, little or no regeneration occurs due to sinusoidal destruction.[77] Complications after radiation therapy include growth disturbance in the skeletally immature,

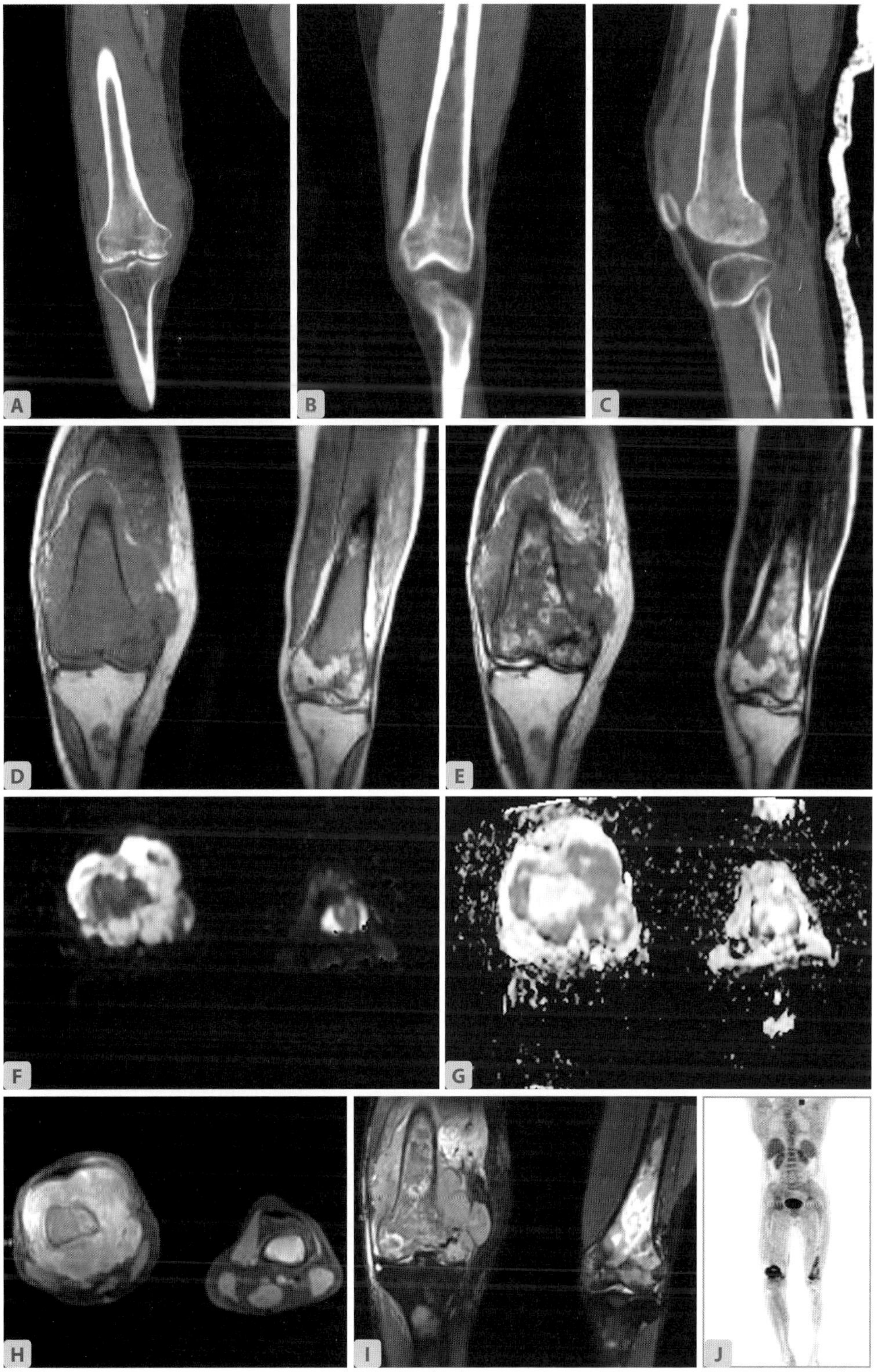

FIGS. 32A TO J: Lymphoma. Coronal (A and B) and sagittal (C) computed tomography (CT) images of right knee (bone window) show e/o an ill-defined permeative type of bony lesion involving femoral condyles and supracondylar region causing marrow expansion and erosion of the articular margin with heterogeneous soft tissue around the femoral shaft. Coronal T1-weighted (T1W) (D) and T2-weighted (T2W) (E) magnetic resonance (MR) images, respectively, showing the above described lesion appearing isointense on T1W image and hypointense on T2W image. Similar lesion is also noted in the distal left femur. There is associated soft tissue mass involving the muscles of various compartments with edema. The lesion is showing restricted diffusion (F and G). T1 fat saturation postgadolinium axial (H) and coronal (I) MR images show heterogeneous avid postcontrast enhancement in the lesion. Left femoral shaft also shows similar lesion. Coronal positron emission tomography (PET)-CT (J) image shows fluorodeoxyglucose (FDG) avid lesion in the bilateral femori.

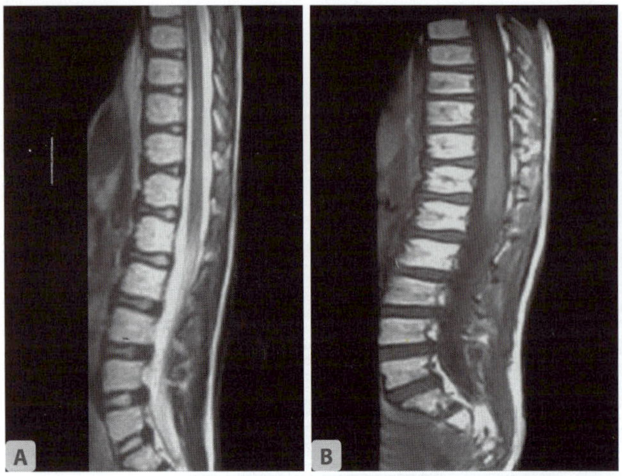

FIGS. 33A AND B: Aplastic anemia. Sagittal T2-weighted (T2W) (A) and sagittal T1-weighted (T1W) (B) magnetic resonance (MR) images of the dorsolumbar spine showing high-signal of the vertebral marrow on both T1W and T2W images s/o fatty marrow.

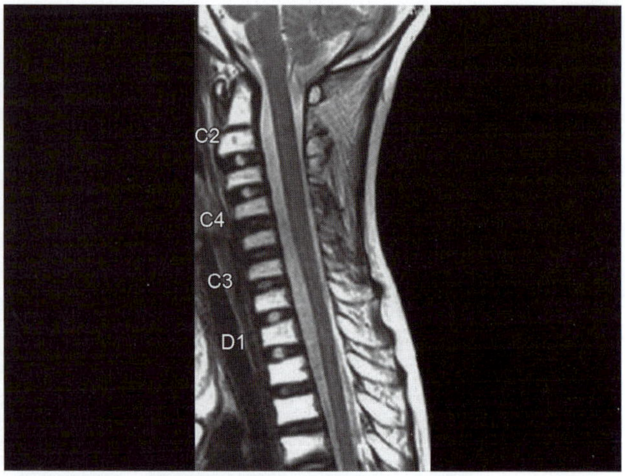

FIG. 34: T2-weighted (T2W) sagittal magnetic resonance (MR) image of the cervical spine in a case of carcinoma breast (postradiation) revealing increased signal in the vertebral marrow s/o fatty replacement.

osteonecrosis, insufficiency fractures, and secondary radiation-induced benign and malignant neoplasms, most commonly osteochondroma and osteosarcoma. *Bone marrow transplant* involves ablation of the patient's native marrow and infusion of either autologous or allogenic stem cells to reconstitute a new marrow free of neoplastic cells. 2–4 weeks after stem cell infusion, a peripheral band-like pattern of mildly increased T1W signal intensity relative to muscle appears, which reflects regenerating hematopoietic cells repopulating along the subendosteal sinusoids. In other areas, a multifocal pattern with numerous small foci of red marrow can be present. Post-transplant changes typically stabilize by 3 months. In patients with successfully reconstituted marrow, T1W signal intensity often remains increased compared with that of age-matched controls.[74]

Angiogenesis-inhibiting drugs, such as thalidomide, depend on neovascularization to be useful for treating hematologic malignancy; these agents were added to some treatment regimens for patients with advanced myeloma. The antiangiogenesis is intended to stop cancer progression by suppressing tumor recruitment of new blood supply. One sign of a response to this treatment is a rather delayed, less steep, and smaller bone marrow enhancement after intravenous administration of small molecular Gd-chelates, compared to pretreatment studies.

Treatment effects of various chemotherapeutic regimen on the bone marrow in patients with leukemia and lymphoma can be detected with ^{31}PMR spectroscopy. The treatment-induced change in tumor pH with an alkaline shift is related temporally to increases in the phosphodiester/beta-adenosine triphosphate ratio and occurs before alterations in tumor size are documented. The changes in the ^{31}PMR spectral profile can also be detected by investigations of serum of the patients.[74]

VASCULAR ABNORMALITIES (HYPEREMIA AND ISCHEMIA)

The underlying cause of extracellular bone marrow edema is usually hyperemia. Different clinical abnormalities may lead to localized bone marrow edema, including trauma, transient osteoporosis of the hip, regional migratory osteoporosis, complex regional pain syndrome, osteonecrosis (early), infection, tumors, and joint abnormalities.

The MRI appearance of marrow edema is that of intermediate-signal intensity on T1W images, and very high-signal intensity on T2W images. The signal characteristics are the result of yellow marrow cells intermixed with the edema fluid. It has a heterogeneous appearance without a discrete pattern. Tumor and infection generally have edema at the periphery of the underlying lesion.

Trauma

Bone Contusion

Direct or indirect trauma can involve the bone marrow, and mild marrow changes have been termed as bone bruises. These can be caused by edema, hemorrhage, and hyperemia. Conventional radiographs are generally normal. On MR, these are seen as geographic areas of decreased signal intensity on T1W and increased signal intensity on T2W images **(Figs. 35A and B)**. Bone bruises are most often seen in the juxta-articular and subchondral areas of the distal femur and proximal tibia in association with ligamentous and meniscal injuries. Bone bruises resolve within 6–9 weeks.

Occult Fractures

These are trabecular bone microfractures which may be diagnosed on MR in the absence of conventional

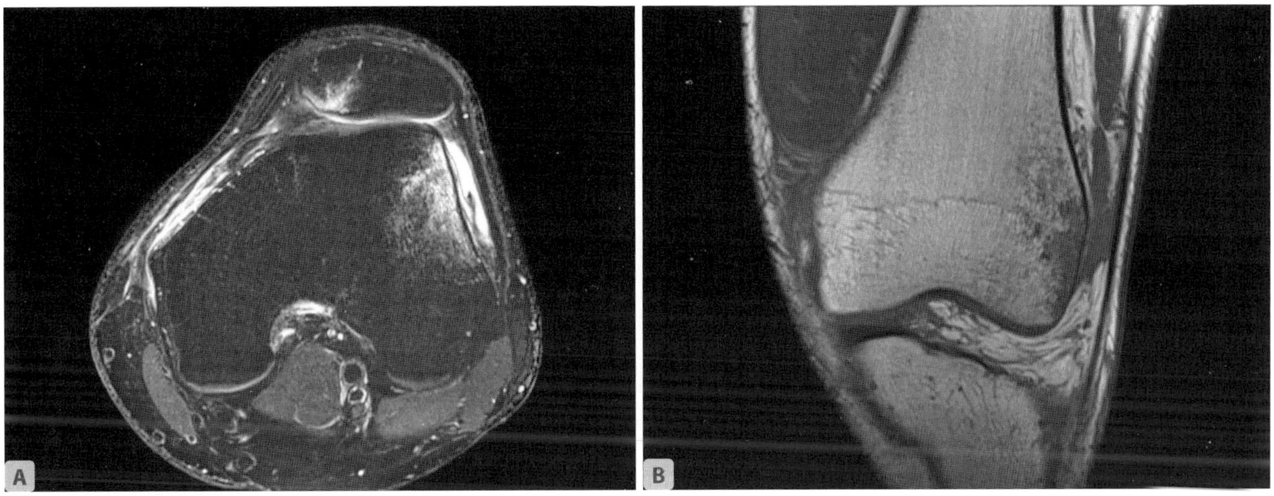

FIGS. 35A AND B: Contusion. Short tau inversion recovery (STIR) axial (A) magnetic resonance (MR) image showing focal areas of increased signal intensity in lateral femoral condyle and medial aspect of patella due to kissing contusion caused by transient patellar subluxation. T1 coronal image (B) showing area of hypointensity in that area in lateral femoral condyle.

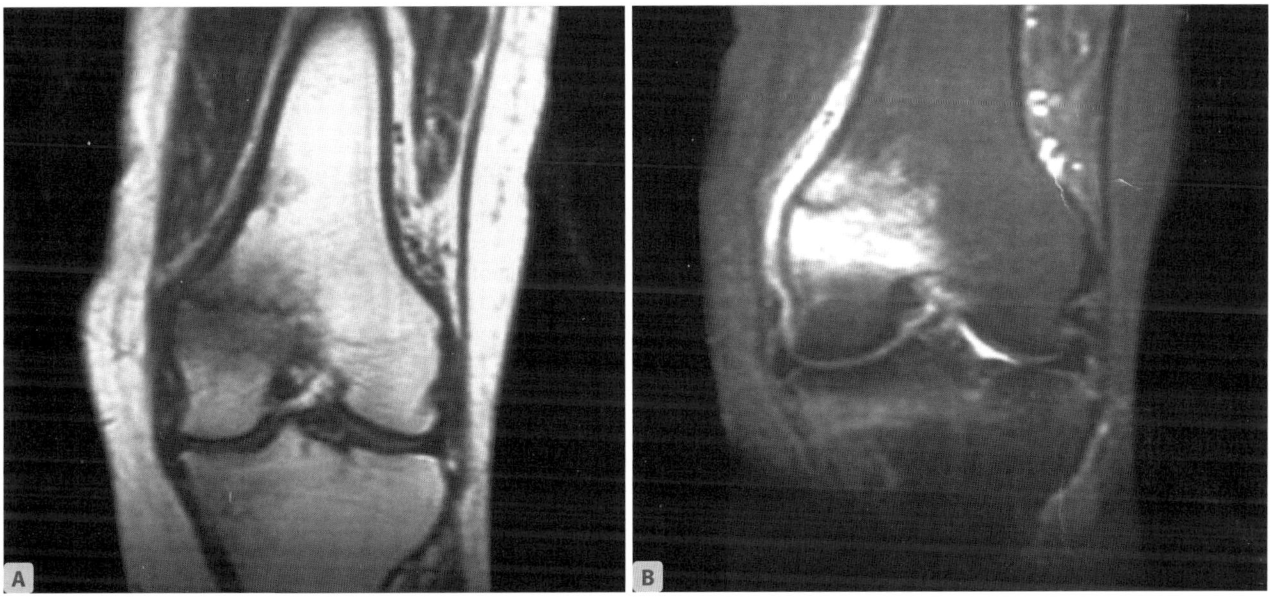

FIGS. 36A AND B: Occult fracture knee. T1-weighted (T1W) coronal (A) and short tau inversion recovery (STIR) coronal (B) magnetic resonance (MR) images of the knee showing a linear fracture line in the medial femoral condyle with surrounding bone marrow edema in a case where X-ray of knee appeared normal.

radiographic signs. The use of STIR or a fat-suppressed T2W sequence is helpful for screening for an occult fracture. These subchondral occult fractures are well seen as a linear signal void on all sequences surrounded by an ill-defined band of decreased signal intensity on T1W, and increased signal intensity on T2W images[78] **(Figs. 36A and B)**.

Stress Fractures

Stress fractures are caused by an imbalance between the strength of the bone and the stress applied. These may be seen after marching, jogging, chronic cough, etc.[79]

Conventional radiographs show a juxtacortical transverse or oblique sclerotic band with a thin radiolucent line within this band. MRI can visualize the pathophysiologic changes accompanying a stress fracture. This consists of a band-like signal void surrounded by marrow edema. The signal void band represents trabecular microfractures and intratrabecular callus formation.

Differentiation of stress fractures from occult intraosseous fractures is difficult. Stress fractures are almost always metaphyseal or diaphyseal, while occult fractures are typically subchondral or epiphyseal and have a precipitating cause.

Transient Osteoporosis

Mainly young and middle-aged men are affected by transient osteoporosis of the hip/painful bone marrow edema

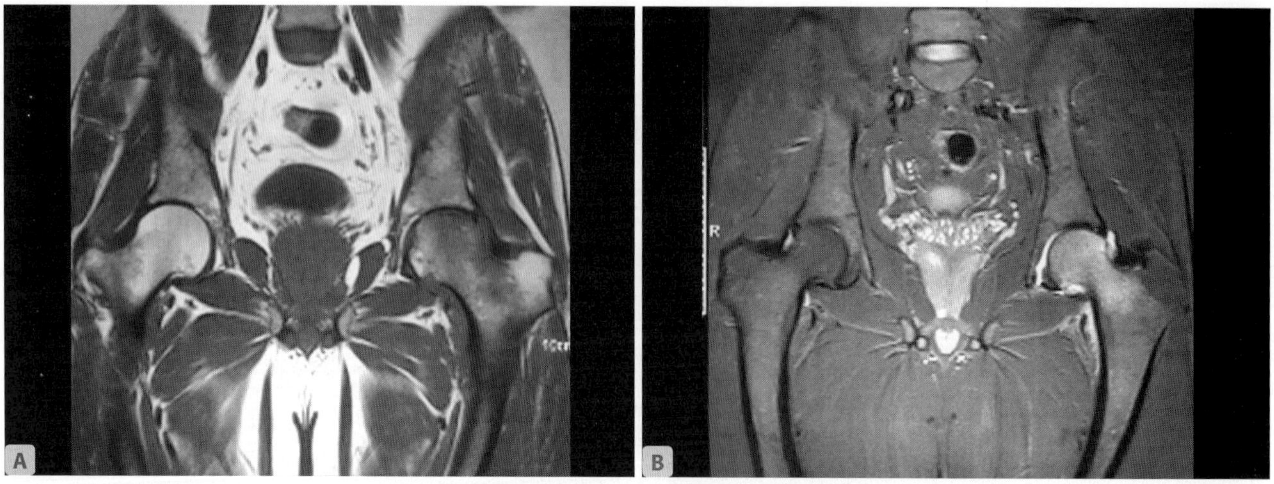

FIGS. 37A AND B: Transient osteoporosis. T1 coronal (A) and short tau inversion recovery (STIR) coronal (B) magnetic resonance (MR) images showing the area of reduced intensity on T1 and increased intensity on STIR image in proximal metaphysis and epiphyses of left femur.

syndrome. Women with transient osteoporosis of the hip are often affected in the last trimester of pregnancy, with a predilection for the left hip. Osteoporosis may also be severe enough to cause fracture.

Imaging

The joint space remains normal, but joint effusions are common. Bone marrow edema usually affects the femoral head and neck, down to the intertrochanteric region. Follow-up studies show resolution of edema and osteoporosis as the clinical symptoms subside in 3–12 months **(Figs. 37A and B)**.[80-82]

Regional Migratory Osteoporosis

Regional migratory osteoporosis has the same MRI and clinical features as transient osteoporosis of the hip. The major difference is that abnormalities are not confined to the hip and are migratory in nature. The subchondral regions of the knee, ankle, and hip, each may be affected in turn, and both extremities may be involved over several years. Spontaneous recovery also occurs in this entity.

The pathogenesis of transient osteoporosis of the hip and regional migratory osteoporosis is unknown, but clinical similarities to reflex sympathetic dystrophy syndrome are striking. The MRI findings for all of these entities are compatible with ischemic changes of the small vessels that supply proximal nerve roots, with a majorly distal loss of control of the normal vascular supply, leading to localized hyperemia.

The relationship between transient osteoporosis of the hip and regional migratory osteoporosis to osteonecrosis is unclear. Biopsy of these lesions shows areas of bone necrosis. There have been reports of typical changes of transient osteoporosis of the hip that, rather than undergoing spontaneous resolution, went on to develop typical MRI and biopsy changes of osteonecrosis in the femoral heads. It is unclear why this should occur and in which patients.

Imaging

MR findings include patchy areas of intermediate-signal intensity (isointense or higher than muscle or disc) on T1W images that become bright on T2W images.

Complex Regional Pain Syndrome

Complex regional pain syndrome affects children aged 5–17 years, and is more common amongst adolescent girls.[44] Inciting events include fracture (in up to 40% of cases), blunt trauma, and surgery. It occurs due to sensitization of nociceptive receptors and subsequent hyperalgesia consequent to an increased inflammatory or immune response. Abnormal sudomotor and vasomotor function in the form of skin discoloration, temperature changes, hyperhidrosis, and edema occurs due to sympathetic dysfunction. Muscle contractures and loss of function may occur in the late stages.

Imaging

Within 2–8 weeks, patchy subchondral and subperiosteal osteopenia can be seen, which progresses to diffuse severe periarticular osteopenia. In adults, upper extremity involvement is more common, whereas in children, the lower extremity is five times more likely to be affected.

Magnetic resonance imaging demonstrates extensive subcortical and patchy marrow edema with occasional articular erosions in the acute stage. Extraosseous manifestations include skin thickening, muscle atrophy, joint effusion, and periarticular soft-tissue edema. In some cases, the abnormal findings may be limited only to the soft tissues.

In the chronic stages, there is periarticular soft-tissue atrophy. The imaging appearance is nonspecific and often overlaps with those of altered and disuse biomechanics. A complex treatment may result in favorable outcome in 1–43% of patients.[38]

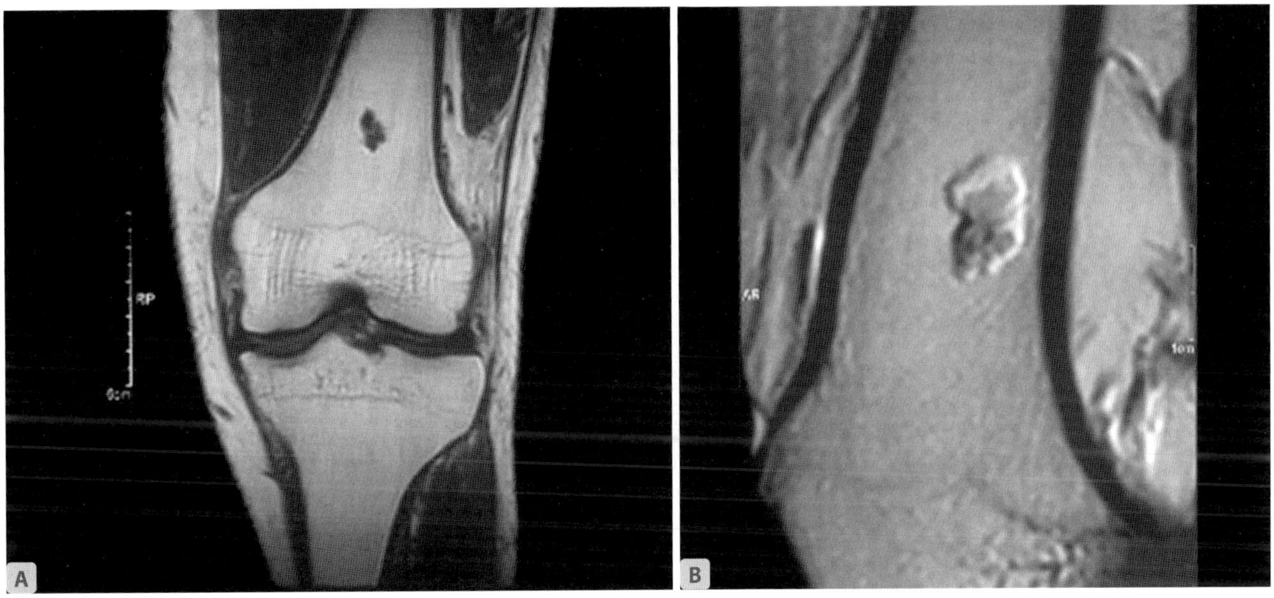

FIGS. 38A AND B: Osteonecrosis. T1-weighted (T1W) coronal magnetic resonance (MR) image (A) showing a geographic hypointense lesion in distal femoral metaphysis. T2-weighted (T2W) coronal MR (B) image showing hyperintense line inside the low-signal intensity line suggestive of "double line" sign.

Ischemia

The causes of ischemia of bone marrow are numerous and include traumatic disruption of the blood supply, steroids, sickle cell anemia, hyperglobulinemia, GD, alcoholism, pancreatitis, dysbaric causes, systemic lupus erythematosus, and others. Many clinicians refer to ischemic changes in the epiphyses as AVN and to changes in the shafts of bone as bone infarction. The MRI findings are similar, regardless of location of the lesions. Osteonecrosis most commonly affects areas where yellow marrow (with its poor vascular supply) predominates the epiphyses and diaphyses of long bones. Hematopoietic cells die within the first 6 hours of anoxia, while osteocytes, osteoblasts, and osteoclasts survive for up to 48 hours. Fat cells become vulnerable in 2–5 days following the insult. An adequate circulation allows repair to begin with a fibrous demarcation of necrotic area.

Imaging

On radiography, there is initial minor osteopenia. Gradually, microfractures of the subchondral bone accumulate in the dead bone, which is unable to repair leading to collapse of the articular surface. Eventually, the cortex collapses and fragments, with superimposed secondary degenerative change.

The MRI appearance of osteonecrosis varies based on the age and stage of the lesion. The earliest manifestation seen with MRI is a nonspecific focal area of what looks like marrow edema-intermediate-signal intensity on T1W images and high-signal intensity on T2W images, in the typical anatomic locations for infarction, i.e., in the epiphyses and diametaphyses. This pattern rapidly progresses to a distinctive, well-defined pattern that allows a specific diagnosis to be made.

A characteristic, low-signal intensity serpentine rim develops in >90% of cases on T1W and T2W images. This serpentine line represents the interface at the junction between the living and the dead bone. This is the site of active bone repair, where a new bone and an advancing front of granulation tissue is seen histologically. In approximately 80% of cases of osteonecrosis, a high-signal intensity line is present on T2W images, just inside the low-signal intensity serpentine line, producing the *double-line sign* **(Figs. 38A and B)**. This line probably occurs as a result of chemical shift misregistration or perhaps reflects the pathologic changes at the reactive bone interface. A "double line" sign consisting of two parallel stripes of low- and high-signal indicates irreversibility.[2,83]

The area of bone within the infarcted segment usually has signal intensity identical to fat. Occasionally, the infarcted bone has signal that is low intensity on T1W images and high signal on T2W images (edema), or low-signal intensity on T1W and T2W images (fibrosis, sclerosis, and trabecular collapse). Due to partial blood supply to the peripheral marrow cavity, the infarct exhibits a peripheral line, with a subcortical double contour giving the "bone-in-bone" appearance. Symptoms tend to be least severe in lesions that are isointense with fat and most severe in lesions with low-signal intensity on all pulse sequences. Joint effusions are usually present in cases of painful osteonecrosis that involve the epiphysis of a bone that makes up the joint.

Magnetic resonance imaging can be used to determine the volume and location of bone involved with osteonecrosis. MRI also can show if there is a collapse of the bone or if degenerative changes are present. Infarcts may become infected leading to osteomyelitis.[83]

MISCELLANEOUS MARROW DISEASES

There is an important group of abnormalities that affect bone marrow, but these abnormalities do not fit neatly into the other categories of marrow disease. This group includes Gaucher's disease (GD), Paget's disease, osteopetrosis, hemosiderosis, and serous atrophy (gelatinous transformation) of marrow.

Gaucher's Disease

Gaucher's disease is the most common lysosomal storage disorder which is caused by a genetic deficiency of glucocerebrosidase, leading to an increase in the deposition of glucosylceramide in macrophages in the brain, spleen, liver, and bone marrow. Consequently, these macrophages get enlarged with a build-up of glycolipids, and are called Gaucher cells. About 80% of patients with GD have skeletal abnormalities.

Imaging

On radiography, an array of bone findings is seen in GD, including growth retardation in children, osteopenia, lytic lesions, pathologic fractures, osteonecrosis, cortical and medullary infarcts. Marrow replacement with Gaucher cells can lead to the expansion of the medullary cavity with thinning of the cortex, endosteal scalloping, and Erlenmeyer flask deformity in distal femori. Nonskeletal manifestations include hepatomegaly and splenomegaly. Focal splenic masses are common and may represent clusters of Gaucher cells or extramedullary hematopoiesis. They may be detected with sonography, CT or MRI.

Magnetic resonance imaging can be used in the early diagnosis of GD and for demonstrating improvement after enzyme therapy. Accumulation of Gaucher cells leads to osteoporosis, localized destruction, and ischemic necrosis. Infiltration of the marrow increases the T1 relaxation time and shortens the T2 relaxation time causing a low-signal intensity of the affected marrow on both T1W and T2W images. These appearances are similar to those in other infiltrative processes but the low-signal intensity on T2W images allows differentiation from tumor processes. This low-signal intensity is due to fibrosis.[1,2,84] Bone marrow infiltration starts proximally and increasingly affects more peripheral areas of the appendicular skeleton. Bone marrow infarction is also a typical finding related to GD and is characterized by a serpiginous pattern with a bright signal in fat-saturated T2W or STIR sequences. Erlenmeyer flask deformities of the distal femora are obvious on MRI.

Other causes of bone marrow changes with osteonecrosis include sickle cell anemia, Waldenström macroglobulinemia, and marrow disorders treated with steroid.

Treatment of GD may consist of administration of an enzyme to break down the glucocerebroside. MRI is often used for monitoring the changes in the liver, spleen, and marrow in these patients. Decreased amounts of marrow infiltration are evident on serial images in patients who respond to the therapy.

Iron Overload (Hemosiderosis)

This disorder occurs due to hemosiderin (iron) deposition in macrophages located in the bone marrow and other organs. Causes include chronic breakdown of red blood cells (sickle cell anemia and thalassemia), chronic blood transfusions, metabolic abnormalities in chronic inflammatory disorders, and acquired immunodeficiency syndrome (AIDS).

Imaging

The iron deposition can be patchy or uniform in distribution involving the pelvis, spine, and metaphysis or diaphysis of long bones. On MRI, the marrow appears hypointense on T2W and gradient recalled echo (GRE) images. In severe hemosiderosis, the signal also decreases on T1W images. Excessive iron deposition can cause nearly a complete signal loss resulting in a "black marrow" **(Figs. 39A to C)**.[26,36] Sickle cell disease can be further complicated by bone infarction. The liver and spleen have the same low-signal intensity as bone marrow, which helps to distinguish this process from similar appearing diseases on MRI.

Paget's Disease

Paget's disease of bone (PDB), also known as osteitis deformans, was originally described by Sir James Paget in 1877. It is a chronic disorder characterized by excessive and abnormal remodeling of bone, often leading to osseous deformities. PDB has osteolytic and osteoblastic phases, with the lytic phase predominating early on in the course of the disease process. It primarily affects the pelvis, spine, skull, and femur. PDB is polyostotic in 66% cases. The etiology is unclear but likely multifactorial. There is epidemiologic data to support an autosomal dominant trait and a possible causative role of paramyxoviral infection.

Paget's disease affects the aging population, with affected individuals usually older than 55 years at diagnosis. Patients younger than 40 years are rarely affected. The prevalence of PDB varies greatly between different countries.

Imaging

On radiography, the classically described radiological appearance is an expanded bone with a coarsened trabecular pattern. Plain radiographic features will depend upon the phase of the disease. The early phase features osteolytic (lucent) regions which are later followed by coarsened trabeculae and bony enlargement. Sclerotic changes occur much later in the disease process. Additional destructive features may become apparent if malignant transformation occurs.

Characteristic vertebral body findings have been described as "picture frame" appearance secondary to central osteopenia and a peripheral coarse and thickened trabecular pattern. Findings may also include increased size and diffuse sclerosis of the vertebral body, referred to as "ivory" vertebra. Vertebral enlargement could lead to neural foraminal and/or central canal stenosis with associated neurologic symptoms.

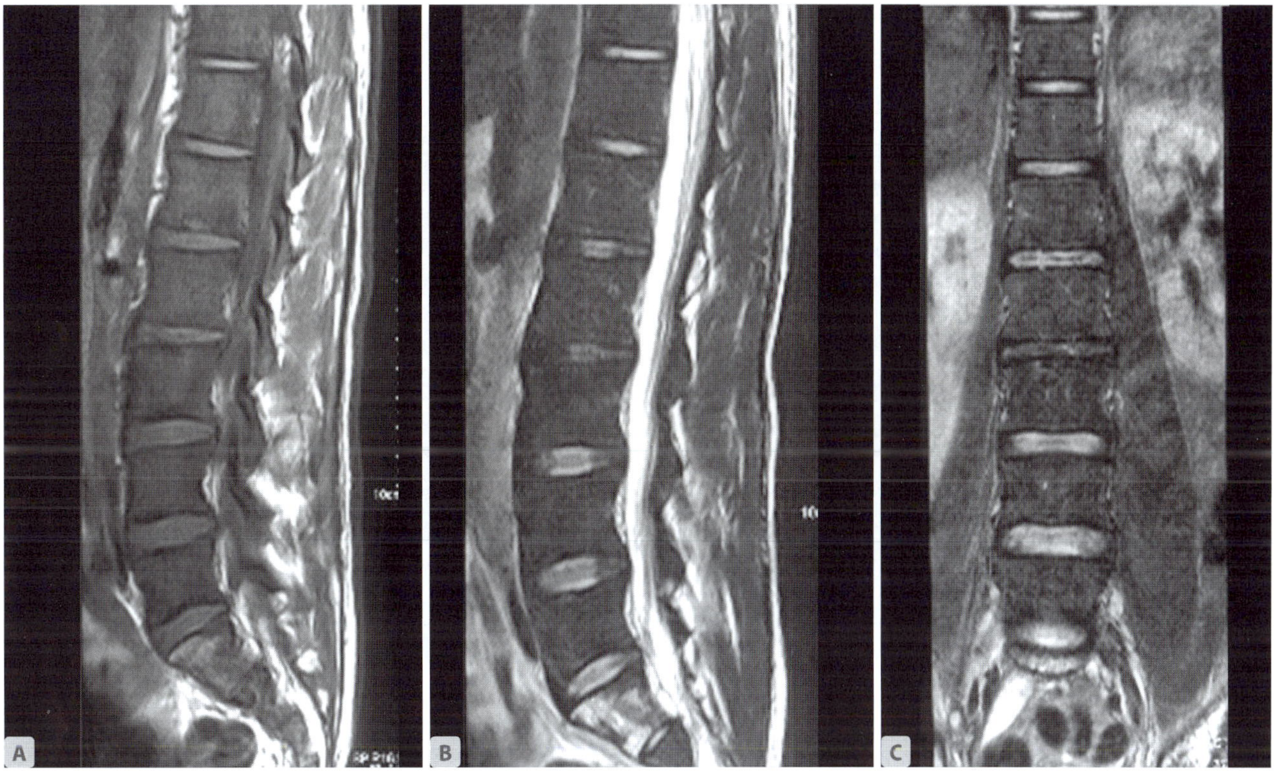

FIGS. 39A TO C: Hemosiderosis. T1-weighted (T1W) sagittal (A), T2-weighted (T2W) sagittal (B) and short tau inversion recovery (STIR) coronal (C) magnetic resonance (MR) images showing diffuse reduction in signal intensity of marrow.

Bone scan is highly sensitive but not specific and may aid with polyostotic disease. There is marked increased uptake in all phases of the disease, although in the burnt-out sclerotic quiescent phase uptake may be normal.

Common MRI findings in pagetic bone include areas of normal high-signal intensity from fat and areas of intermediate- or low-signal intensity on T1W images due to fibrovascular connective tissue, dilated vascular channels, or uncalcified osteoid. Thick bone trabeculae and cortical bone can be seen but not as easily as on conventional radiographs or CT. Areas of active lysis demonstrate increased T2 signal intensity. Contrast-enhanced CT or MRI may demonstrate significant marrow enhancement in the active or lytic phase. There is preservation of the normal marrow in unaffected areas.

Secondary complications of Paget's disease include basilar invagination, kyphoscoliosis, fractures due to bone softening, extramedullary hematopoiesis, and congestive heart failure. If there is interval change in imaging characteristics, soft tissue component, or increasing pain, further cross-sectional contrast-enhanced imaging should be performed to evaluate for rare sarcoma formation. Osteosarcoma is the most common type of sarcoma associated with Paget's disease, representing approximately 50% of cases.[85] Sarcomatous transformation is highly fatal, with a 3-year mortality rate >90%.[86]

Differential diagnosis for Paget's disease involving the spine includes metastatic disease and vertebral hemangioma. Although PDB has a distribution similar to metastatic disease, greater involvement of the ribs has been described with the former. There is also typically no enlargement of the affected osseous structures with metastatic disease. However, sometimes the distinction is difficult and biopsy is necessary. Vertebral hemangiomas have a delicate trabecular pattern, in contrast to the coarse and enlarged trabecular pattern seen in pagetoid bone. Additionally, typical vertebral hemangiomas demonstrate high T1- and T2-signal intensity on MRI.

Alkaline phosphatase, which reflects the level of new bone formation, is used as an adjunct in the diagnosis and also plays a role in evaluating treatment response. However, it is nonspecific and values are normal in up to 15% of symptomatic patients with monostotic disease. Disease activity and response to therapy can be followed with measurements of alkaline phosphatase and other serum markers.

Treatment of PDB is mostly targeted at symptomatic relief with analgesic medication. Medications that inhibit osteoclastic activity (e.g., bisphosphonate) also play a role. Surgical intervention is sometimes needed.

MAGNETIC RESONANCE APPROACH TO MARROW DISEASE

An attempt at systematic approach toward categorization of the bone marrow lesions has been made in the past. One of the articles by Del Grande et al.[87] divides the bone

TABLE 9: MRI characteristics of various categories of bone marrow lesions.

MR technique	MR sequences	Category 1	Category 2	Category 3
Conventional	T1W SE	Signal intensity > muscle	Signal intensity < muscle/disc	Heterogeneous signal intensity
	PD-W/T2W TSE	Signal intensity approaching or similar to fat	Signal intensity approaching or similar to fat	Heterogeneous
	STIR/T2 fat sat	Increased signal intensity—generally no focal lesions	Increased signal intensity, focal lesions	Heterogeneous with or without focal lesions
	Postcontrast T1W	Minimal enhancement	Intense enhancement	Minimal or no enhancement
Problem-solving techniques	CSI	>20% signal loss on out-of-phase imaging	Neoplasm <20% signal loss on out of phase imaging. Infection: signal loss on out-of-phase imaging	>20% signal loss on out-of-phase imaging
	DWI	Usually no diffusion restriction	Neoplasm/pus-diffusion restriction	Usually no diffusion restriction
	MRS	No choline peak	Neoplasm–choline peak	No choline peak

(CSI: chemical shift imaging; DWI: diffusion-weighted imaging; MR: magnetic resonance; MRS: magnetic resonance spectroscopy; PD: proton density; SE: spin echo; STIR: short tau inversion recovery; T1W: T1-weighted; T2W: T2-weighted)

marrow lesions into three categories based on the imaging appearances as described in **Table 9**. Category I includes bone marrow lesions related to trauma, insufficiency injury, aseptic necrosis, biomechanical, disuse, CRPS, transient osteoporosis of hip, or degenerative/inflammatory etiologies. Category II includes aggressive processes, such as infections or neoplastic conditions. Category III includes pathologies with complex/mixed phenomena, such as metabolic, hematopoietic, treated infiltrative malignancies, human immunodeficiency virus (HIV) treatment-associated lipodystrophy, serous marrow lesions, and Paget's disease.

CONCLUSION

Imaging characteristics of normal bone marrow change throughout life and familiarity with these changes is important to correctly approach bone marrow pathology. Neoplastic disease of the bone marrow is a frequent pathology and has different morphologic patterns. For standard imaging of bone marrow, T1W and STIR sequences are the fundamental sequences. The addition of newer imaging techniques and advances in MRI has enabled a better characterization of the various pathologies and helped in narrowing the differential diagnosis.

REFERENCES

1. Moore SG, Bisset GS III, Siegal MJ, Donaldson JS. Pediatric musculoskeletal MR imaging. Radiology. 1991;179(2):345-60.
2. Siegel MJ, Luker GD. Bone marrow imaging in children. Magn Reson Imaging Clin N Am. 1996;4(4):771-96.
3. Vogler JB III, Murphy WA. Bone marrow imaging. Radiology. 1988;168(3):679-93.
4. Waitches SG, Zanvin JK, Poznanski AK. Sequences and rate of bone marrow conversion in the femora of children as seen on MR imaging: Are accepted standards accurate? Am J Roentgenol. 1994;162(6):1399-406.
5. Cohen MD, Klatte EC, Baehner R, Smith JA, Martin-Simmerman P, Carr BE, et al. Magnetic resonance imaging of bone marrow disease in children. Radiology. 1984;151(3):715-8.
6. Małkiewicz A, Dziedzic M. Bone marrow reconversion - imaging of physiological changes in bone marrow. Pol J Radiol. 2012;77(4):45-50.
7. Mettler FA, Guiberteau MJ. Essentials of Nuclear Medicine Imaging, 5th edition. Philadelphia: Saunders/Elsevier; 2006.
8. Tian R, Su M, Tian Y, Li F, Li L, Kuang A, et al. Dual–time point PET/CT with F-18 FDG for the differentiation of malignant and benign bone lesions. Skeletal Radiol. 2009;38(5):451-8.
9. Mirowitz SA, Apicella P, Reinus WR, Hammerman AM. MR imaging of bone marrow lesions: Relative conspicuousness on T1-weighted, fat-suppressed T2-weighted, and STIR images. Am J Roentgenol 1994;162(1):215-21.
10. Helms CA, Major NM, Andersson MW, Kaplan PA, Dussault R. Musculoskeletal MRI, 2nd edition. Philadelphia: Saunders Elsevier; 2009. pp. 20-49.
11. Moore DG, Dawson KL. Red and yellow marrow in the femur: Age-related changes in the appearance at MR imaging. Radiology.1990;175(1):219-23.
12. Dooms GC, Fischer MR, Hricak H, Richardson M, Crooks LE, Genant HK. Bone marrow imaging: Magnetic resonance studies related to age and sex. Radiology.1985;155(2):429-32.
13. Taccone A, Oddone M, Dell Acqua AD, Occhi M, Ciccone MA. MRI "road map' of normal age-related bone marrow: Thorax, pelvis and extremities. Pediatric Radiology.1995;25(8):596-606.
14. Sebag GH, Dubois J, Tabet M, Bonato A, Lallemand D. Pediatric spinal bone marrow: Assessment of normal age- related changes in the MRI appearance. Pediatr Radiol 1993;23(7):515-8.
15. Mirowitz SA. Hematopoietic bone marrow within the proximal humeral epiphysis in normal adults: Investigation with MR imaging. Radiology 1993;188(3):689-93.
16. Jones KM, Unger EC, Granstrom P, et al. Bone marrow imaging using STIR at 0.5 and 1-5T. Magn Reson Imaging.1992;10(2):169-76.
17. Zajick DC, Morrison WB, Schweitzer ME, Parellada JA, Carrino JA. Benign and malignant processes: Normal values and differentiation with chemical shift MR imaging in vertebral marrow. Radiology. 2005;237(2):590-6.

18. Glover GH. Multipoint Dixon technique for water and fat proton and susceptibility imaging. J Magn Reson Imaging. 1991;1(5):521-30.
19. Subhawong TK, Jacobs MA, Fayad LM. Diffusion-weighted MR imaging for characterizing musculoskeletal lesions. RadioGraphics. 2014;34(5):1163-77.
20. Karampinos DC, Melkus G, Baum T, Bauer JS, Rummeny EJ, Krug R. Bone marrow fat quantification in the presence of trabecular bone:initial comparison between water–fat imaging and single-voxel MRS, Magn Reson Med. 2014;71(3):1158-65.
21. Herrmann J, Krstin N, Schoennagel BP, Sornsakrin M, Derlin T, Busch JD, et al. Age-related distribution of vertebral bone-marrow diffusivity. Eur J Radiol 2012;81(12):4046-9.
22. Byun WM, Shin SO, Chany Y, Lee SJ, Finsterbusch J, Frahm J. Diffusion weighted MR imaging of metastatic disease of the spine: assessment of response to therapy. AJNR. 2002;23:906-12.
23. Zhang J, Cheng K, Ding Y, Liang W, Ding Y, Vanel D, et al. Study of single voxel 1H MR spectroscopy of bone tumors: Differentiation of benign from malignant tumors. Eur J Radiol. 2013;82(12):2124-8.
24. Fayad LM, Bluemke DA, McCarthy EF, Weber KL, Barker PB, Jacobs MA. Musculoskeletal tumors: Use of proton MR spectroscopic imaging for characterization. J Magn Reson Imaging. 2006;23(1):23-8.
25. Vande Berg BC, Lecouvet FE, Galant C, Simoni P, Malghem J. Normal variants of the bone marrow at MR imaging of the spine. Semin Musculoskelet Radiol. 2009;13(2):87-96.
26. Enlcmann R, Vassollo B, Bongartz G, Müller-Miny H, Rummeny E, Stöber U, et al. Musculoskeletal neoplasms with fast low angle shot MR imaging with and without Gd-DTPA. Radiology. 1990;176(2):489-95.
27. Mahnken AH, Wildberger JE, Adam G, Stanzel S, Schmitz-Rode T, Günther RW, et al. Is there a need for contrast enhanced T1 weighted MRI of the spine after inconspicuous short T inversion recovery imaging? Eur Radiol. 2005;15(7):1387-92.
28. Griffith JF, Yeung DKW, Antonio GE, Lee FKH, Hong AWL, Wong SYS, et al. Vertebral bone mineral density, marrow perfusion and fat content in healthy men and men with osteoporosis: Dynamic contrast enhanced MR imaging and MR spectroscopy. Radiology. 2005;236(3):945-51.
29. Ghanem N, Altehoefer C, Kelly T, Lohrmann C, Winterer J, Schäfer O, et al. Whole body MRI in comparison to skeletal scintigraphy in detection of skeletal metastases in patients with solid tumours. In Vivo. 2006;20(1):173-82.
30. Kumar J, Seith A, Kumar A, Sharma R, Bakhshi S, Kumar R, et al. Whole-body MR imaging with the use of parallel imaging for detection of skeletal metastases in pediatric patients with small-cell neoplasms: Comparison with skeletal scintigraphy and FDG PET/CT. Pediatr Radiol 2008;38(9):953-62.
31. Goo HW. Regional and whole-body imaging in pediatric oncology. Pediatr Radiol. 2011;41(Suppl 1):S186-94.
32. Padhani AR, Koh DM, Collins DJ. Whole-body diffusion-weighted MR imaging in cancer: Current status and research directions. Radiology. 2011;261(3):700-18.
33. Shellock FG, Morris E, Deutsch AL, Mink JH, Kerr R, Boden SD. Hematopoietic bone marrow hyperplasia, high prevalence on MR images of the knee in asymptomatic marathon runners. Am J Roentgenol. 1992;158(2):335-8.
34. Levin TL, Sheth SS, Ruzal-Shapiro C, Abramson S, Piomelli S, Berdon WE. MRI marrow observations in thalassemia: The effects of primary disease, transfusional therapy and chelation. Pediatr Radiol. 1995;25(8):605-13.
35. Emery JL, Follet GF. Regression of bone marrow haematopoiesis from the terminal digits in the foetus and infants. Br J Haematol. 1964;10:485-99.
36. Chan BY, Gill KG, Rebsamen SL, Nguyen JC. MR imaging of pediatric bone marrow. RadioGraphics. 2016;36(6):1911-30.
37. Kaplan KR, Mitchell DG, Steiner RM, Murphy S, Vinitski S, Rao VM, et al. Polycythemia vera and myelofibrosis: Correlation of MR imaging, clinical and lab findings. Radiology. 1992;183(2):329-34.
38. Mesa RA, Tefferi A. Emerging drugs for the therapy of primary and post essential thrombocythemia, post polycythemia vera myelofibrosis. Expert Opin Emerg Drugs 2009;14(3):471-9.
39. Bancroft LW. Hematopoietic tumors. In: Davies AM, Sundaram M, James SLJ (Eds). Imaging of Bone Tumors and Tumor-like Lesions: Techniques and Applications. Berlin: Springer-Verlag; 2009. pp. 351-63.
40. Kim SH, Smith SE, Mulligan ME. Hematopoietic tumors and metastases involving bone. Radiol Clin North Am. 2011;49(6):1163-83.
41. Kato M, Koh K, Kikuchi A, Toyama D, Mochizuki S, Uchisaka N, et al. Case series of pediatric acute leukemia without a peripheral blood abnormality, detected by magnetic resonance imaging. Int J Hematol. 2011;93(6):787-90.
42. Tafaghodi F, Aghighi Y, Rokni Yazdi H, Shakiba M, Adibi A. Predictive plain X-ray findings in distinguishing early stage acute lymphoblastic leukemia from juvenile idiopathic arthritis. Clin Rheumatol. 2009;28(11):1253-8.
43. Desmond R, McDerra J, Kelly K, Smith O. Multiple vertebral collapse as a presentation of childhood acute lymphoblastic leukaemia. Br J Haematol. 2009;144(5):627.
44. Silva JR Jr, Hayashi D, Yonenaga T, Fukuda K, Genant HK, Lin C, et al. MRI of bone marrow abnormalities in hematological malignancies. Diagn Interv Radiol. 2013;19(5):393-9.
45. Nishii T, Kono AK, Akasaka Y, Mori T, Hayakawa A, Iijima K, et al. Bone marrow magnetic resonance imaging of the clivus in pediatric leukemia patients and normal controls. Jpn J Radiol. 2015;33(3):146-52.
46. Wang J, Zhang X, Niu J. Clinical significance of magnetic resonance imaging of bone marrow in patients with leukemia. J Tongji Med Univ. 2001;21(3):242-5.
47. Nöbauer I, Uffmann M. Differential diagnosis of focal and diffuse neoplastic diseases of bone marrow in MRI. Eur J Radiol. 2005;55(1):2-32.
48. Janssens AM, Offner FC, Van Hove WZ. Bone marrow necrosis. Lancet. 2000;88(8):1769-80.
49. Hutchings M, Specht L. PET/CT in the management of haematological malignancies. Eur J Haematol 2008;80(5):369-80.
50. Mauro FR, Chauvie S, Paoloni F, Biggi A, Cimino G, Rago A, et al. Diagnostic and prognostic role of PET/CT in patients with chronic lymphocytic leukemia and progressive disease. Leukemia. 2015;29(6):1360-5.
51. American Cancer Society. Cancer facts and figures 2015. Atlanta: American Cancer Society; 2015.
52. Rajkumar SV, Dimopoulos MA, Palumbo A, Blade J, Merlini G, Mateos MV, et al. International Myeloma Working Group updated criteria for the diagnosis of multiple myeloma. Lancet Oncol. 2014;15(12):e538-48.
53. Navarro SM, Matcuk GR, Patel DB, Skalski M, White EA, Tomasian A, et al. Musculoskeletal imaging findings of hematologic malignancies. RadioGraphics. 2017;37(3):881-900.
54. Stäbler A, Baur A, Bartl R, Munker R, Lamerz R, Reiser MF. Contrast enhancement and quantitative signal analysis in MR imaging of multiple myeloma: Assessment of focal and diffuse growth patterns in marrow correlated with biopsies and survival rates. Am J Roentgenol. 1996;167(4): 1029-36.
55. Hwang S, Panicek DM. Magnetic resonance imaging of bone marrow in oncology part 2. Skeletal Radiol. 2007;36(11):1017-27.

56. Moulopoulos LA, Dimopoulos MA, Alexanian R, Leeds NE, Libshitz HI. Multiple myeloma: MR patterns of response to treatment. Radiology. 1994;193(2):441-6.
57. Moulopoulos LA, Dimopoulos MA, Weber D, Fuller L, Libshitz HI, Alexanian R. Magnetic resonance imaging in the staging of solitary plasmacytoma of bone. J Clin Oncol. 1993;11(7):1311-5.
58. Moulopoulos LA, Dimopoulos MA, Varma DG, Manning JT, Johnston DA, Leeds NE, et al. Waldenström macroglobulinemia. MR imaging of the spine and CT of the abdomen and pelvis. Radiology. 1993;188(3):669-73.
59. Zaveri J, La Q, Yarmish G, Neuman J. More than just Langerhans cell histiocytosis: A radiologic review of histiocytic disorders. RadioGraphics. 2014;34(7):2008-24.
60. Stull MA, Kransdorf MJ, Devaney KO. Langerhans cell histiocytosis of bone. RadioGraphics. 1992;12(4):801-23.
61. Cohen MD, Cary DA, Kleiman M, Smith JA, Broderick NJ. Magnetic resonance differentiation of acute and chronic osteomyelitis in children. Clinical Radiology. 1990;41(1):53-6.
62. Erdman WA, Tamburno F, Jayson HT, Weatherall PT, Ferry KB, Peshock RM. Osteomyelitis: Characteristics and pitfalls of diagnosis with MR imaging. Radiology. 1991;180(2):533-9.
63. Cortés-Romera M, Sabaté-Llobera A, Mercadal-Vilchez S, Climent-Esteller F, Serrano-Maestro A, Gámez-Cenzano C, et al. Bone marrow evaluation in initial staging of lymphoma: 18F-FDG PET/CT versus bone marrow biopsy. Clin Nucl Med. 2014;39(1): e46-52.
64. Coley BL, Higinbotham NL, Groesbeck HP. Primary reticulum-cell sarcoma of bone: Summary of 37 cases. Radiology. 1950;55(5):641-58.
65. Ruzek KA, Wenger DE. The multiple faces of lymphoma of the musculoskeletal system. Skeletal Radiol. 2004; 33(1):1-8.
66. Krishnan A, Shirkhoda A, Tehranzadeh J, Armin AR, Irwin R, Les K. Primary bone lymphoma: Radiographic–MR imaging correlation. RadioGraphics. 2003;23(6):1371-83.
67. Chen-Liang TH, Martin-Santos T, Jerez A, Senent L, Orero MT, Remigia MJ, et al. The role of bone marrow biopsy and FDG-PET/CT in identifying bone marrow infiltration in the initial diagnosis of high grade non-Hodgkin B-cell lymphoma and Hodgkin lymphoma: Accuracy in a multicenter series of 372 patients. Am J Hematol 2015;90(8):686-90.
68. Adams HJ, Kwee TC, de Keizer B, Fijnheer R, de Klerk JM, Nievelstein RA. FDG PET/CT for the detection of bone marrow involvement in diffuse large B-cell lymphoma: Systematic review and meta-analysis. Eur J Nucl Med Mol Imaging. 2014;41(3): 565-74.
69. Adams HJ, Kwee TC, Fijnheer R, Dubois SV, Nievelstein RA, de Klerk JM. Bone marrow 18F-fluoro-2-deoxy-D-glucose positron emission tomography/computed tomography cannot replace bone marrow biopsy in diffuse large B-cell lymphoma. Am J Hematol. 2014;89(7):726-31.
70. Vande Berg BC, Lecouvet FE, Michaux L, Ferrant A, Maldague B, Malghem J. Magnetic resonance imaging of the bone marrow in hematological malignancies. Eur Radiol. 1998;8(8):1335-44.
71. Heacock L, Weissbrot J, Raad R, Campbell N, Friedman KP, Ponzo F, et al. PET/MRI for the evaluation of patients with lymphoma: Initial observations. Am J Roentgenol 2015;204(4):842-8.
72. Auger-Quittet S, Duny Y, Daures JP, Quittet P. Outcomes after (90) yttrium-ibritumomab tiuxetan-BEAM in diffuse large B-cell lymphoma: A meta-analysis. Cancer Med. 2014;3(4):927-38.
73. Kaplan PA, Asleson RJ, Klanen LW, Duggan MJ. Bone marrow patterns in aplastic anaemia: Observations with 1.5T MR imaging. Radiology. 1987;164(2):441-4.
74. Daldrup-Link HE, Henning T, Link TM. MR imaging of therapy-induced changes of bone marrow. Eur Radiol. 2007;17(3):743-61.
75. Otake S, Mayr NA, Ueda T, Magnotta VA, Yuh WT. Radiation-induced changes in MR signal intensity and contrast enhancement of lumbosacral vertebrae: Do changes occur only inside the radiation therapy field? Radiology. 2002;222(1):179-83.
76. Blomlie V, Rofstad EK, Skjønsberg A, Tverå K, Lien HH. Female pelvic bone marrow: Serial MR imaging before, during, and after radiation therapy. Radiology. 1995;194(2):537-43.
77. Sacks EL, Goris ML, Glatstein E, Gilbert E, Kaplan HS. Bone marrow regeneration following large field radiation: Influence of volume, age, dose, and time. Cancer. 1978;42(3):1057-65.
78. Lee JK, Yao L. Stress fractures: MR imaging. Radiology. 1988;169(1):217-20.
79. Staffard SA, Rosenthal DI, Gebhardt MC, Brady TJ, Sott JA. MRI in stress fractures. Am J Roentgenol. 1986; 147:553-6.
80. Wilson AJ, Murphy WA, Hardy DC, Totty WG. Transient osteoporosis—transient bone marrow oedema. Radiology. 1988;167(3):757-60.
81. Pory NT, Singer WS, Bartel E. Hip pain in three children accompanied by transient abnormal findings on MR images. Radiology.1989;171(1):147-9.
82. Bloem JL. Transient osteoporosis of the hip: MR imaging. Radiology.1988;167(3):753-5.
83. Imhof H, Breitenseher M, Trattnig S, Kramer J, Hofmann S, Plenk H, et al. Imaging of avascular necrosis of bone. Eur Radiol. 1997;7(2):180-6.
84. Rosenthal DI, Scott JA, Barianger J, Mankin HJ, Saini S, Brady TJ, et al. Evaluation of Gaucher's disease using magnetic resonance imaging. J Bone Joint Surg Am. 1986;68(6):802-8.
85. Hadjipavlou A, Lander P, Srolovitz H, Enker IP. Malignant transformation in Paget disease of bone. Cancer. 1992;70(12):2802-8.
86. Smith SE, Murphey MD, Motamedi K, Mulligan ME, Resnik CS, Gannon FH. From the archives of the AFIP. Radiologic spectrum of Paget disease of bone and its complications with pathologic correlation. RadioGraphics. 2002;22(5):1191-216.
87. Del Grande F, Farahani SJ, Carrino JA, Chhabra A. Bone marrow lesions: A systematic diagnostic approach. Indian J Radiol Imaging. 2014;24(3):279-87.

CHAPTER

167

Magnetic Resonance Imaging of Shoulder and Temporomandibular Joints

Mahesh Prakash, Paramjeet Singh

SHOULDER JOINT

INTRODUCTION

Various imaging modalities have been used to assess the shoulder joint, like radiography, computed tomography (CT), ultrasonography (USG), and magnetic resonance imaging (MRI). Although each modality has its own advantages and disadvantages, MRI provides the comprehensive and accurate assessment of shoulder.[1] Clinical examination is important and usually help in providing the proper choice of subsequent investigative modality. Radiographs and CT are useful to demonstrate osseous structures of shoulder girdle; however, they provide poor or limited evaluation of soft tissue anatomy. USG has also been used to visualize pathology of rotator cuff and bursae of the joint with variable success.[2-4] This technique however is operator dependent and needs high end equipment.[5] The MRI, because of its excellent soft tissue contrast and imaging capability in any desired plane and nonionizing noninvasive nature, is an ideal modality for evaluation of shoulder joint.[6]

MAGNETIC RESONANCE IMAGING PROTOCOLS

Improved coil designs have helped to improve the signal-to-noise ratio and provide adequate spatial resolution in MRI of shoulder. Proper immobilization and comfort of the patient, off axis small FOV imaging capability, high matrix size, and elimination of phase wrap are desirable requisites for imaging the shoulder.

During MRI of shoulder, patient is placed in supine position with their arm on the side of body in partial external rotation. After localizer images, joint should be imaged in axial, coronal-oblique, and sagittal-oblique planes.[7] Coronal-oblique plane is selected parallel to the course of supraspinatus tendon (SST). The sagittal-oblique images are done parallel to glenoid surface. The imaging sequences may vary in different institution and depends on available hardware and other factors and have seen changing over the years. Previously we had used proton/T2 turbospin-echo (TSE) and gradient-echo sequences in axial planes, T1 SE and proton/T2 TSE sections oblique coronal planes, and oblique sagittal sections using T1 SE and T2 TSE sequences. An STIR, turbo inversion recovery or fat suppressed T2 TSE sequence, was additionally used in one of the planes. The basic sequences presently done in our institution on 3 Tesla MR machine are listed in **Table 1**.

MAGNETIC RESONANCE ARTHROGRAPHY

Magnetic resonance arthrography with intra-articular contrast is performed by injecting 12–15 cc mixture of gadolinium dimeglumine (2 mmol/L), normal saline, lidocaine, and iodinated contrast media into joint cavity with a 20G spinal needle through either anterior or posterior approach under fluoroscopic guidance.[8,9] The gadolinium concentration of 2 mmol/L is achieved by mixing 0.5 mL of contrast in 50 mL of saline. T1 fat suppressed sections are

TABLE 1: Standard pulse sequences for MRI examination of the shoulder at 3 Tesla.

Pulse sequence	FOV (cm)	Slice thickness (mm)	Matrix	TR/TE
Axial PD with fat saturation	14	3	256 × 256	3,000/43
Sagittal oblique PD with fat saturation	14	3	256 × 256	3,000/43
Coronal oblique T1	14	3	256 × 256	650/24
Coronal oblique T2 with fat saturation	14	3	256 × 256	3,000/89
Sagittal oblique T1	14	3	256 × 256	650/24

taken in axial, oblique coronal, and sagittal planes. Additional imaging in an abducted externally rotated (ABER) arm may also be done to assess capsule-labral pathology. Some people are comfortable using USG guidance for injecting contrast in the joint cavity.

NORMAL ANATOMY

Shoulder joint is a ball and socket joint formed by articulation between head of humerus and glenoid of scapula. Structurally, it is a weak joint because of disparity of articulating surface area between small and shallow glenoid cavity in comparison to the humeral head. However, this arrangement provides the glenohumeral joint with the greatest range of motion of any articulation in human body. Stability to this unstable joint is provided by following structures.

- Coracoacromial arch (CCA) consisting of acromian, coracoacromial ligament (CAL), coracoid process, and the acromioclavicular joint (AC joint).
- Musculotendinous cuff of shoulder.
- Glenoid labrum along with capsule and glenohumeral ligaments (GHL).
- The muscles attaching the humerus to pectoral girdle, i.e., long head of biceps and triceps, coracobrachialis, teres major, etc.

Osseous Structures

The osseous structures of shoulder joint include proximal humerus, scapula, and clavicle. The proximal humerus consists of head, neck, and greater and lesser tuberosities. The humeral head is typically round with slight flattening of posteroinferior surface. This flattening should not be confused with Hill-Sachs lesion which is seen at or above the level of coracoid process.[10] The anatomic neck forms the oblique circumference and separates head from tuberosities. The acromian and glenoid of scapula makes articulation with humeral head and clavicle to become components of shoulder joint. The acromian is posterior landmark and articulates with clavicle. The coracoid process is anterior landmark of shoulder with variable morphology.[11] The glenoid is important structure, which articulates with humeral head to form shoulder joint. The glenoid is pear or oval shaped in coronal plane.[12] The lateral end of clavicle articulates with acromian to form AC joint.

Ligaments

The joint capsule is loose and permits free movements. It is least supported inferiorly where dislocations are common. Medially the capsule is attached to the scapula beyond the supraglenoid tubercle and margins of the labrum and laterally to the anatomical neck of humerus. The capsule is reinforced anteriorly and inferiorly by several thickenings, namely the anterior and posterior bands of inferior glenohumeral ligament (IGHL) with an inferior axillary recess, the more variable middle GHL (MGHL) and the smallest superior GHL (SGHL). They all extend to the anatomical neck of humerus and stabilize the joint variably. The coracohumeral ligament (CHL) extends from lateral aspect of coracoid process to the neck of humerus and is a key structure in impingement and instability syndromes. Transverse humeral ligament bridges the bicipital groove and holds tendon of long head of biceps brachii. The glenoid labrum is a fibrocartilaginous ovoid rim attached to the margins of the glenoid cavity. It is often deficient anterosuperiorly. It functions to deepen the glenoid cup and is a site of capsuloligamentous attachment. It is more mobile superiorly and functions with biceps tendon as a mobile "biceps labral complex" that slides over the superior glenoid.

MUSCULOTENDINOUS ANATOMY

From anterior to posterior, subscapularis muscle (SCM), biceps, supraspinatus muscle (SSM), infraspinatus muscle (ISM), and teres minor (TM) muscles together with their tendons form the rotator cuff. All originate from the scapula and insert on the humerus. Of these tendons, the SST, infraspinatus tendon (IST), and teres minor insert on their respective notches on the greater tuberosity while subscapularis tendon (SCT) attaches to the lesser tuberosity. The SST and IST fibers may partially fuse posteriorly to form a conjoint tendon (an area sometimes referred to as posterior rotator interval). The gap between SCT and SST, named anterior rotator cuff interval (RCI), is filled with fibrofatty tissue. The CHL, SGHL, and biceps tendon (BT) lie beneath it in that order. The long head of BT originates from the supraglenoid tubercle, crosses the joint obliquely through RCI, attaches to superior labrum, and exits the joint into bicipital groove. The bicipital groove is hooded by transverse humeral ligament.

Bursae

Numerous bursae are related to shoulder joint, which can be communicating or noncommunicating with the joint. The subscapularis, subcoracoid, infraspinatus, and peribicipital bursae are communicating bursae. Bursa superior to AC joint and those related to coracobrachialis, teres major, long head of triceps, and lattisimus dorsi do not communicate with the joint. The subacromial-subdeltoid bursa (SASDB), the largest bursa in the body, is lined with areolar tissue and synovium, which allow free sliding motion of adjacent structures. They are fused and considered as one and do not communicate with the joint.

NORMAL MAGNETIC RESONANCE APPEARANCE

(*Refer to Abbreviations in Table 2*)

Axial Sections (Figs. 1 and 4)

The cuff muscles appear as intermediate signal intensity structures on T1W. Highest sections show SSM, followed posteriorly by ISM and TM and their tendons. The tendons appear darker than muscles and can be traced to greater tuberosity. Biceps tendon is seen anterosuperiorly and SCT anterior to the scapula at midsuperior head level. Bicipital groove is best seen on these sections lateral to lesser tuberosity. Anterior and posterior labra are particularly

TABLE 2: Abbreviations used for Figures 1 to 4.

1. AC	Acromian process	13. IST	Infraspinatus tendon
2. BT	Biceps tendon	14. MGHL	Middle glenohumeral ligament
3. CAL	Coracoacromial ligament	15. QS	Quadrilateral space
4. CCL	Coracoclavicular ligament	16. RCI	Rotator cuff interval
5. CHL	Coracohumeral ligament	17. SASD	Subacrominal subdeltoid bursa
6. CL	Clavicle	18. SCT (m)	Subscapularis tendon/muscle
7. CP	Coracoid process	19. SGHL	Superior glenohumeral ligament
8. D	Deltoid muscle	20. SST(m)	Supraspinatus tendon/muscle
9. GL	Glenoid	21. TM	Teres minor
10. HH	Humeral head	22. TMj	Teres major
11. IGHL	Inferior glenohumeral ligament	23. TR	Trapezius
AB—	anterior band, PB—posterior band	24. PL	Post labrum
12. ISM	Infraspinatus muscle		

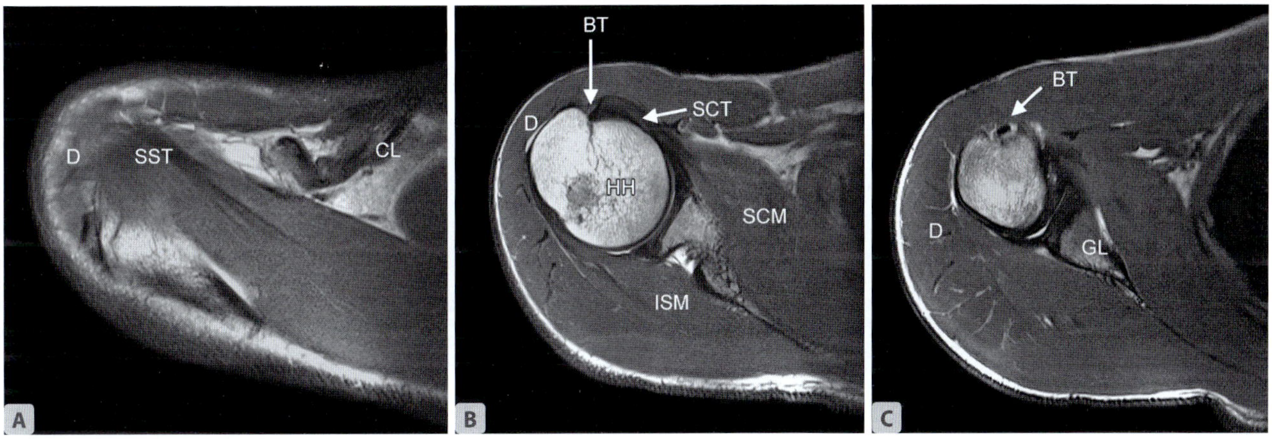

FIGS. 1A TO C: Axial T1-weighted sections of shoulder (normal anatomy).

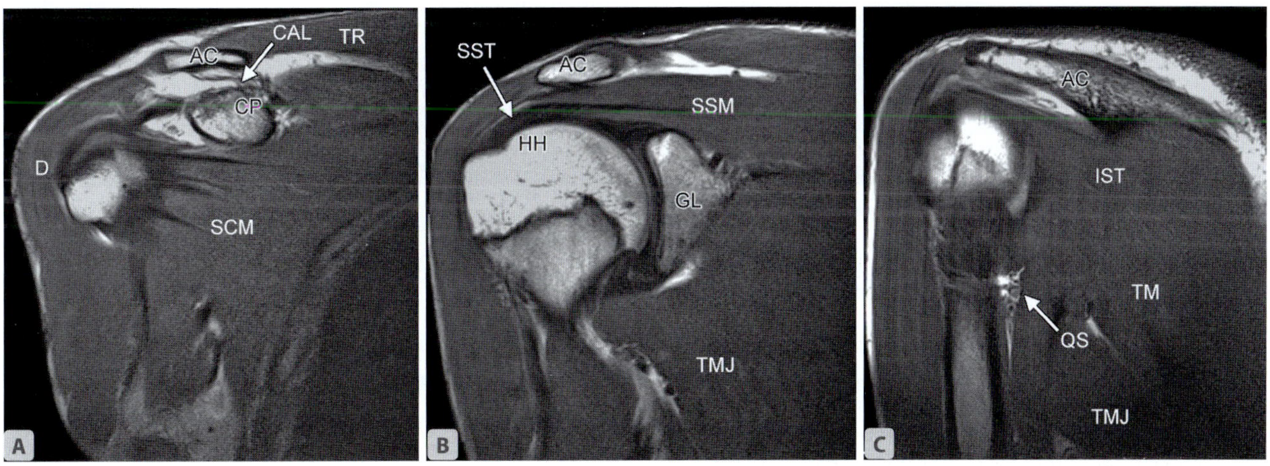

FIGS. 2A TO C: (A to C—anterior to posterior) Oblique coronal T1-weighted sections (normal anatomy).

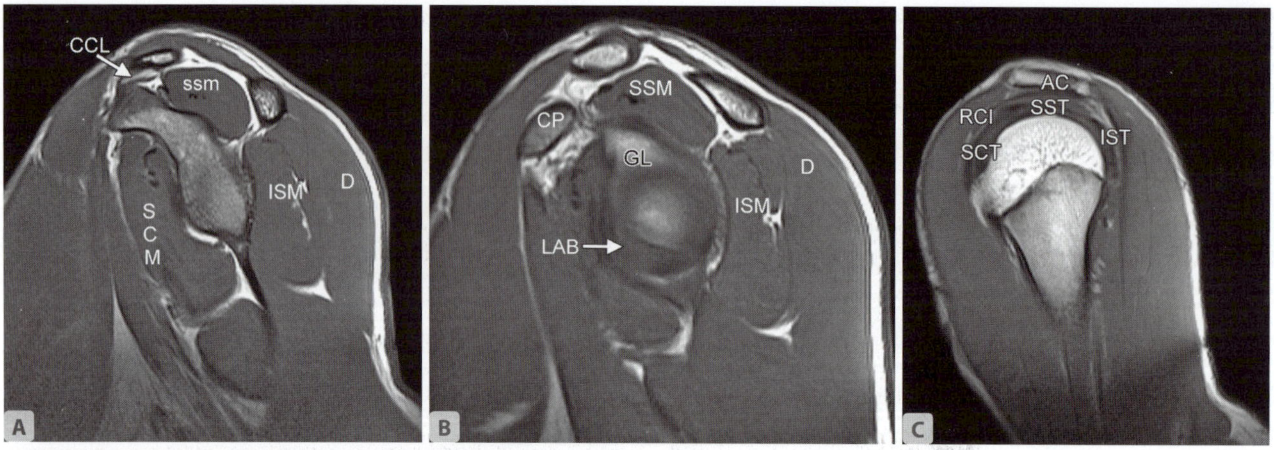

FIGS. 3A TO C: Oblique sagittal T1-weighted sections (normal anatomy).

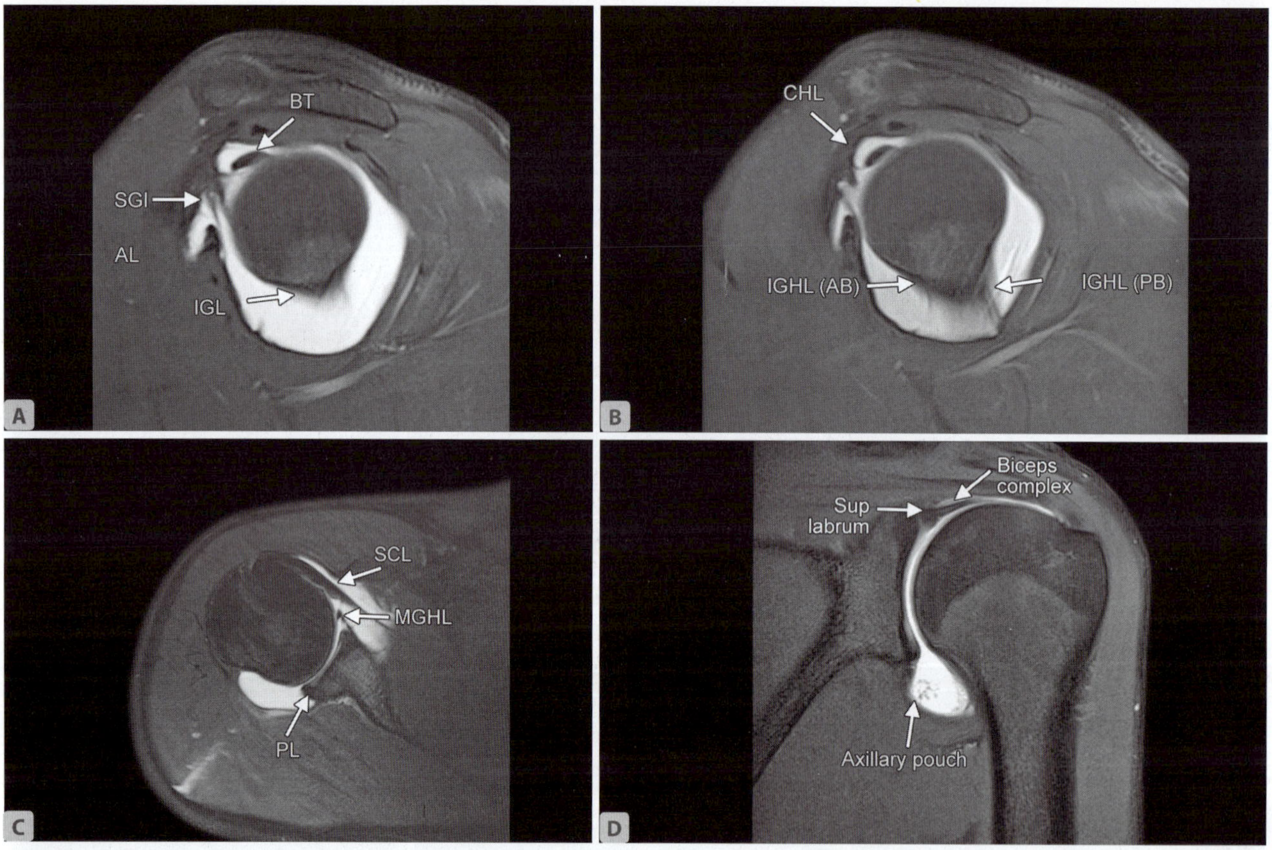

FIGS. 4A TO D: (A and B) Sagittal; (C) Axial; and (D) Coronal T1-weighted fat saturated arthrogram images show ligamentous anatomy. The superior glenohumeral ligament (SGHL) is seen coursing down from its coracoid attachment. Inferior glenohumeral ligament (IGHL) is seen with thick anterior and posterior bands outlining a distended axillary recess. The middle glenohumeral ligament (MGHL) is seen as a thin hypointense band beneath subscapularis tendon (SCT). The biceps-labral complex is firmly attached to the glenoid rim.

well seen on axial sections. The GHLs are low-intensity structures and better seen in presence of fluid in the joint or on MR arthrogram. The SGHL lies superiorly and follows the concavity of coracoid on its lateral aspect. The MGHL closely follows posterior margin of SCT and IGHL lies at lower head level. The articular cartilage appears bright on T2 and gradient images and best evaluated in axial sections.

Coronal Sections (Figs. 2 and 4)

The rotator cuff tendon structures are best evaluated on oblique coronal sections. The mid to anterior sections show the SST (along with AC joint). The sections posterior to this show conjoint tendons of SST and IST and TM. The tendons can be traced to greater tuberosity. The SASDB appears as a thin bright line beneath the deltoid muscle on T2W.

The anterior sections also show SST and biceps tendon passing beneath it as well as coracohumeral, coracoacromial, and coracoclavicular ligaments. The superior labrum is best evaluated in the coronal plane. Axillary pouch is seen medial and inferior to humeral head.

Sagittal Sections (Figs. 3 and 4)

These sections provide a cross-sectional view of all the muscles of shoulder. Mid and lateral sagittal images show the SST/IST conjoint tendon as a low signal structure between humeral head and acromion. The morphological abnormalities of acromion (i.e., anterior sloping) are best shown on these images. The long head of biceps can be seen passing anteroinferiorly between SST and SCT through the rotator cuff interval. More medially coracoacromial ligament can be seen arching over the rotator cuff interval along with AC joint in profile. The SGHL can be seen lying beneath the long head of biceps, the MGHL anterior to medial humeral head, and IGHL along with a thick inferior labrum along the inferior aspect of the glenoid cavity.

SHOULDER IMPINGEMENT SYNDROME

Impingement syndrome is a clinical diagnosis in which pain is felt in shoulder due to encroachment of the rotator cuff and associated soft tissues between the humeral head and overlying CCA. The CCL is a triangular strong structure limiting the space available to rotator cuff during abduction. Abnormalities involving one or more of the components of CCA results in narrowing of the acromiohumeral distance.

Rotator cuff impingement can be classified as:
- Primary extrinsic impingement
- Secondary extrinsic impingement
- Intrinsic impingement.

Primary Extrinsic Impingement

This is due to the abnormalities of the CCA and can be subacromial or subcoracoid types.

Possible etiologies of subacromial impingement are:
- Subacromial spur
- Hypertrophic changes in AC joint
- Unstable os acromial (failure to fuse by 25 years)
- Subacromial subdeltoid bursitis
- Thickening of the coracoacromial ligament
- Laterally downsloping acromian process (type 3).

As seen on oblique sagittal plane (outlet view on plain radiographs) the anterior acromion is straight in type I, curved in type II, and anteriorly hooked in type III morphology **(Figs. 5A to C)**.[13] Type II configuration is most common and type III is most commonly associated with rotator cuff pathology. Anterior part of SST is most commonly affected in subacromial type impingement alone or along with other tendons in 95% cases. The cuff along with subacromial bursa is entrapped along the undersurface of CCA.

The subcoracoid impingement can be due to reduced distance between coracoid process and the medial aspect of humeral head leading to compression of SCT and biceps long head.

Secondary Extrinsic Impingement

Here the abnormality lies in the stability of the glenohumeral joint in the setting of a normal CCA. It usually occurs in young athletes involved in sports demanding overhead arm movements. Possible underlying defect of static stabilizers (glenohumeral ligaments) leads to overload on secondary stabilizers (cuff structures) and a reduced acromiohumeral gap.

Internal Impingement

It is due to contact between undersurface of rotator cuff and glenoid rim due to throwing with arm in abduction and maximal external rotation. Supraspinatus hypertrophy or an abnormality of the greater tuberosity may also be contributory factors.

ROTATOR CUFF TENDINOPATHY AND TEARS

Rotator cuff disease is one of the most common causes of shoulder pain and indication for MRI evaluation of shoulder. Multiple etiologies have been implicated in the

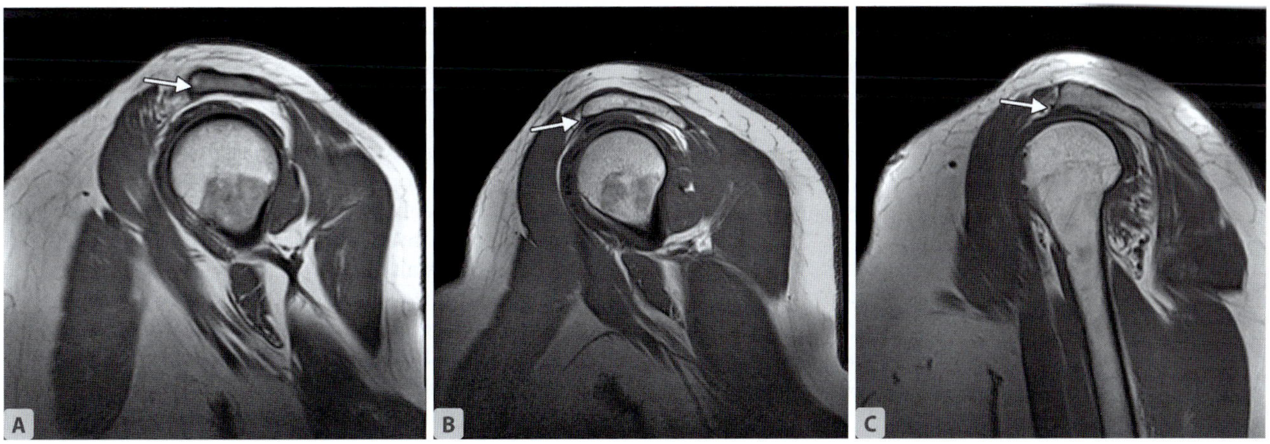

FIGS. 5A TO C: (A) Type I; (B) Type II; and (C) Type III acromion morphologies.

development of degenerative changes (tendinopathy) in the rotator cuff tendons near greater tuberosity. Aforementioned rotator cuff impingement between CCA and humeral head is most often implicated. Acute and chronic trauma, sports, overuse, aging, collagen vascular, and metabolic diseases are also associated with rotator cuff tendinopathy and tears. Vascular insufficiency leading to degeneration in critical zone may also plays a role in rotator cuff tears (RCTs). Critical zone, approximately 1 cm from the insertion of the SST at the greater tuberosity, is the most susceptible area for tears.

Neer described three clinicopathologic stages of impingement.[14]

Stage I

There is reversible edema and hemorrhage within the distal SST usually in young patient (<25 years) and is managed conservatively.

Stage II

There is tendinitis and thickening with fibrosis. Bursal pathology aggravates the condition by compromising subacromial space. Patient are usually between 25 and 40 years of age. No radiographic changes are seen in stage I and II.

Stage III

These are characterized by partial or a full thickness tears of rotator cuff or biceps tendon usually seen in patients older than 40 years of age. Osseous changes in the form of degenerative changes at greater tuberosity and acromial osteophyte formation are seen on radiographs.

Impingement is a process of progressive wear and tear. MR interpretation in early stages is often equivocal. The injured tendon may appear thickened due to mucoid degeneration; however, histology of tendons of asymptomatic people also shows similar changes. The term "tendinosis or tendinopathy" is preferred over tendinitis as no inflammatory changes are seen within these tendons. In contrast to these intrasubstance changes of tendinosis, "tendon surface degeneration" is seen as irregularity of surface and may be indistinguishable from or coexist with "partial tears." There may also be associated features of bursal and peribursal inflammation.

Magnetic Resonance Appearance

Seeger[15] has classified impingement on coronal MR images into three types:

Type 1

Normal low-signal intensity on T1 and T2WI and normal morphology of the SST. Areas of increased signal intensity are noted on proton and GRE images.

Type 2

High-signal intensity of SST on T1WI. If T2WI also reveal high signal intensity, which is not involving the entire thickness, it may represent partial tear (bursal or articular surface or intra substance).

Type 3

High-signal intensity is found on T1 and T2WI traversing full thickness suggestive of complete RCT, with or without tendon retraction.

Carrino et al.[16] described more extensive MR grading for RCTs.

Grade 0 (Normal)

Uniform low-signal intensity of the tendons.

Grade I

Increased signal intensity in tendon, more obvious on T1WI and proton images but not seen or less obvious on T2WI **(Figs. 6A and B)**.

Grade II (Tendinosis/Tendinitis)

Increased signal intensity on T2WI that does not involve articular or superior surface. The tendon may be thin, thick, or irregular, similar to Neer stage II **(Figs. 7A and B)**.

Grade III (Degeneration)

Increased signal intensity on T2WI in one or multiple areas but signal changes do not meet criteria for partial or complete tear.

Grade IV (Partial Tear)

Increased signal intensity on T2WI that involve the inferior (articular) or superior (bursal) surface of the tendons **(Fig. 8)**.

Grade V

Full thickness tear with few spared fibers.

Grade VI

Full thickness tear without tendon retraction **(Fig. 9)**.

Grade VII

Full thickness tear with tendon retraction **(Fig. 10)**.

An increase in T2 signal intensity along with abnormality in tendon morphology increases the confidence level of diagnosing a tear. Partial tears are better shown on T2WI (with fat suppression), particularly in presence of joint effusion as a discontinuity or fraying of the tendon **(Fig. 8)**. Partial tears are classified as grade I, II, or III depending on involvement of less than 25%, 25–30%, or more than 50% of the tendon thickness.

Complete RCTs occur at sites of previous tendinopathy and can be diagnosed with greater confidence on MRI than the debatable early tendon pathology and partial tears. Full thickness tears can be classified as small (<1 cm or involvement of one tendon only) **(Fig. 11)**, medium (1–3 cm or involvement of two tendons), and massive (>3–5 cm or involvement of three or more tendons). Massive tears of the rotator cuff may also involve the subscapularis and biceps with or without dislocation **(Fig. 12)**. Both anteroposterior and mediolateral measurements of tears as well as quality of torn margins should be noted as these are important information from surgical point of view. Undersurface tears of posterior SST and IST, humeral head chondromalacia, and

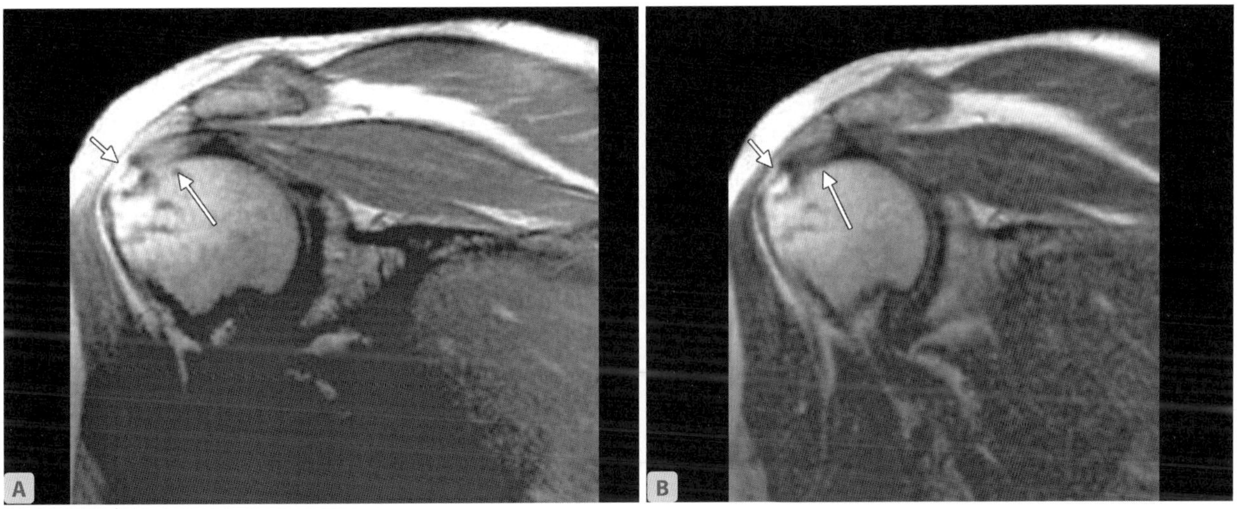

FIGS. 6A AND B: (A) Proton; and (B) T2 turbospin-echo (T2 TSE) coronal sections show increased signal within the supraspinatus tendon (SST) (A, long arrow); however, T2WI (B) shows less pronounced signal changes in the tendon suggesting tendinopathy. Partial retraction at the insertion site with cyst formation is also noted (short arrow).

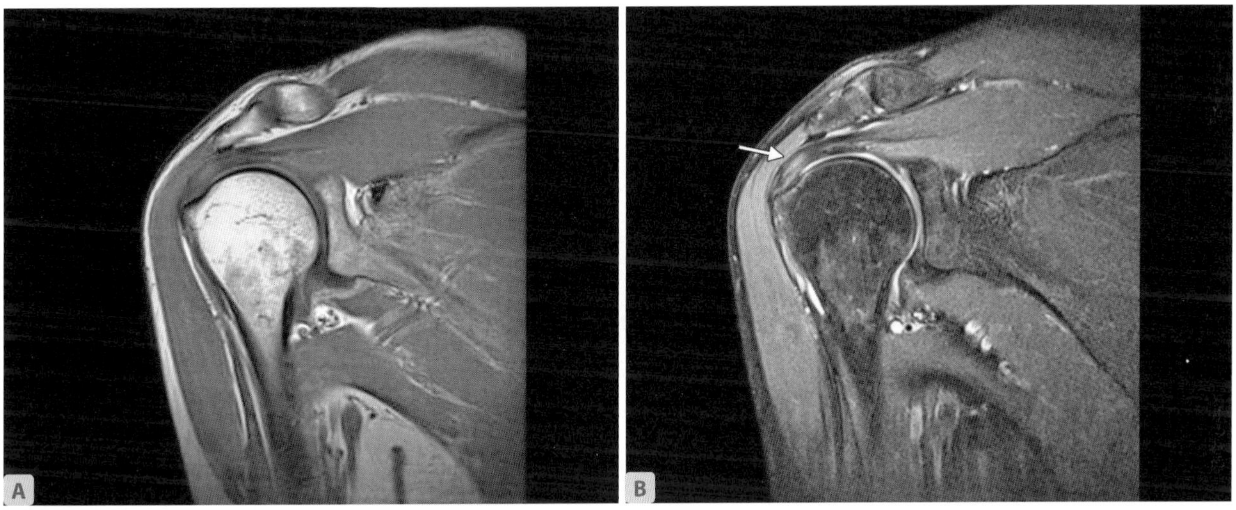

FIGS. 7A AND B: (A) T1; and (B) T2 fat saturated coronal sections show intrasubstance increased signal (tendinosis) in the supraspinatus tendon on both the images (arrow).

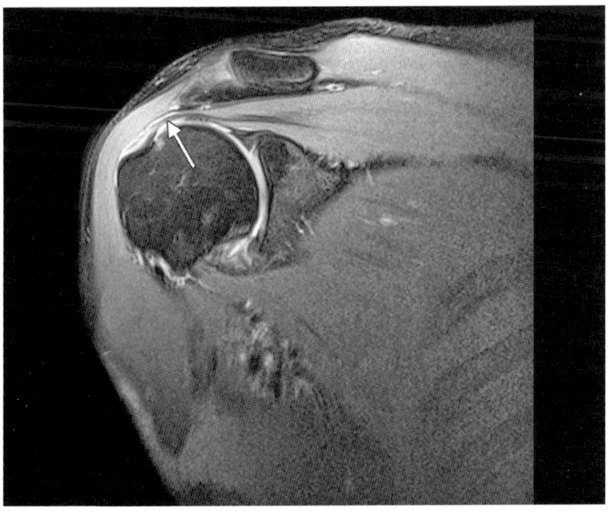

FIG. 8: Proton density (fat saturated) coronal section shows articular surface tear as a focus of bright signal area along the undersurface of the supraspinatus tendon (SST) (arrow).

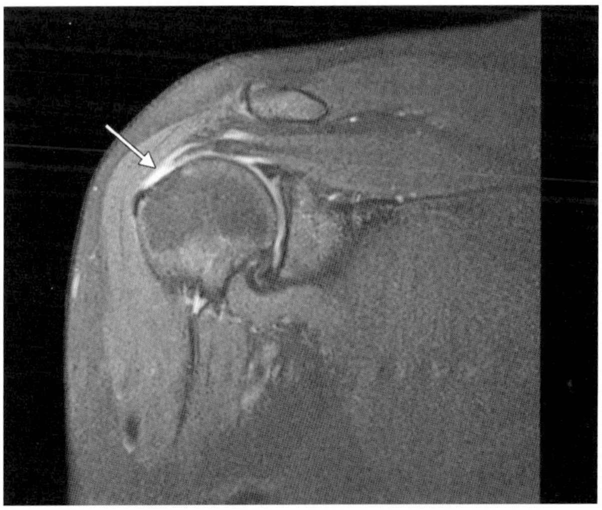

FIG. 9: Proton density (fat saturated) coronal section shows full thickness tear of supraspinatus tendon (SST) without retraction (arrow).

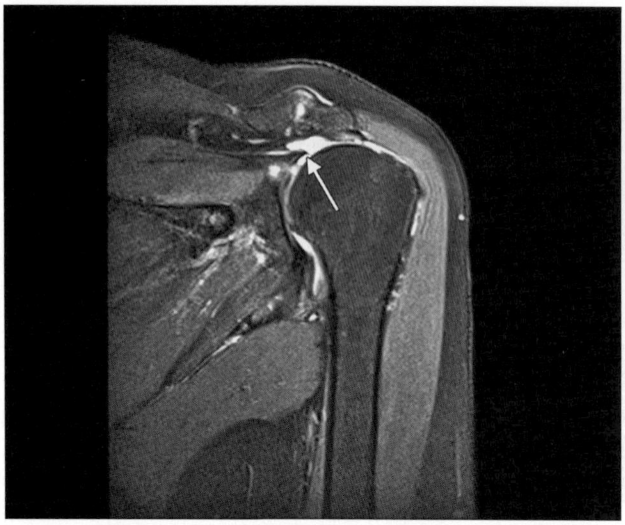

FIG. 10: Proton density (fat saturated) coronal section shows full thickness tear of supraspinatus tendon (SST) with retraction of fibers (arrow). Acromian osteophyte is also noted.

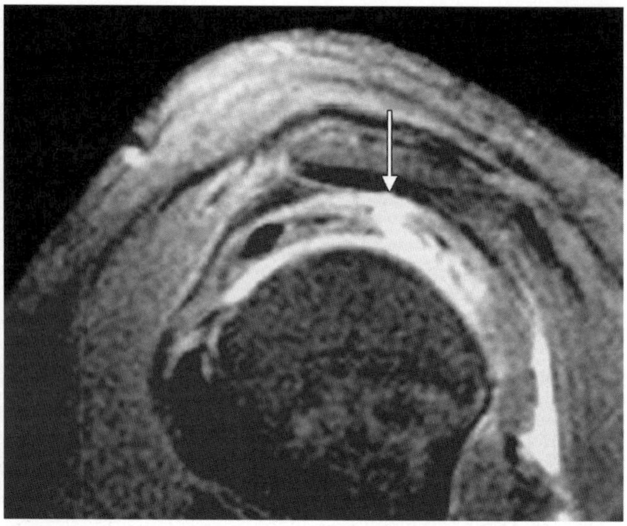

FIG. 11: Sagittal fat-suppressed T1 MR arthrographic image is showing tear of posterior supraspinatus tendon (SST) and possibly infraspinatus tendon (IST) (conjoint tendon) with a full thickness defect outlined by the contrast in posterior rotator interval (arrow).

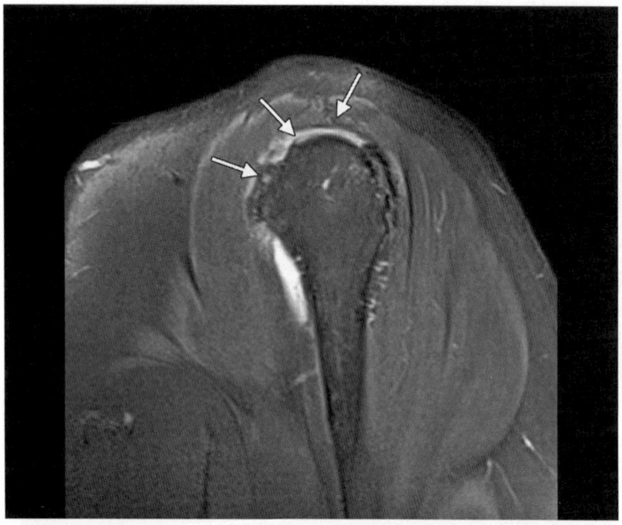

FIG. 12: Oblique sagittal proton density (fat saturated) section through the rotator cuff shows a massive tear involving subscapularis tendon (SCT), supraspinatus tendon (SST) as well as the infraspinatus tendon (IST) (from anterior to posterior-arrows) are seen as increased signal replacing normal low signal of the tendons.

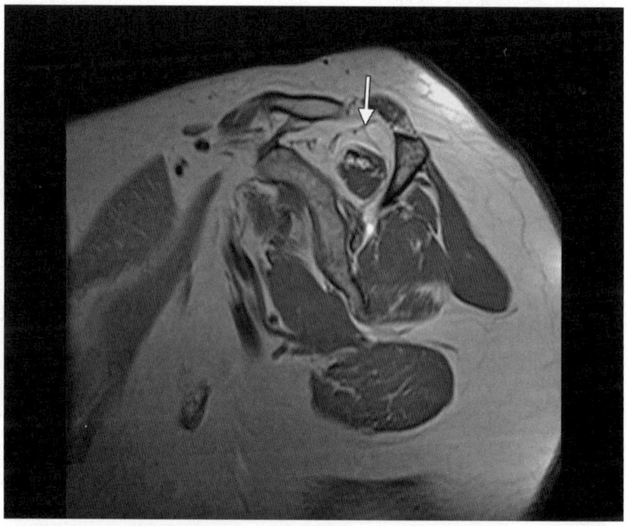

FIG. 13: T1 oblique sagittal section shows atrophy of the rotator cuff muscles and fatty changes are seen as T1 hyperintensity (arrow).

fraying of posterosuperior labrum are hallmarks of internal impingement syndrome seen in overhead throwers **(Fig. 11)**.

Sometimes tears may not show T2 hyperintensity due to granulation or fibrosis and appear to be normal. Although less specific, knowledge of secondary signs of RCT is useful in such difficult cases. MR may show fatty atrophy of muscle belly in complete tears as T1 hyperintensity and loss of volume **(Fig. 13)**. Humeral head may be apposed to the acromion in such chronic cases. Tendons may be completely nonvisualized due to musculotendinous retraction in complete tears. Tendon retraction, loss of peribursal/subdeltoid fat plane, and fluid in the subdeltoid subacromial bursa can be seen in 92% patients with complete RCT **(Figs. 14A and B)**.[17] However, bursal fluid can also be found in impingement (43%), labral abnormality (29%), bursitis (19%), tendinitis (14%), and even in asymptomatic people **(Fig. 15)**.[18] Joint effusion can be seen in both partial and complete tears. Marrow signal changes and cyst formation in the greater tuberosity on fat suppressed T2 WI and osseous changes like AC joint osteophytosis and subacromial spurs are secondary signs of cuff tendinopathy and indicate advanced disease **(Fig. 10)**. Artifactually increased signal may be noted within the tendons on proton images due to "magic angle effect" in areas where the tendon courses at 55° angle in relation to

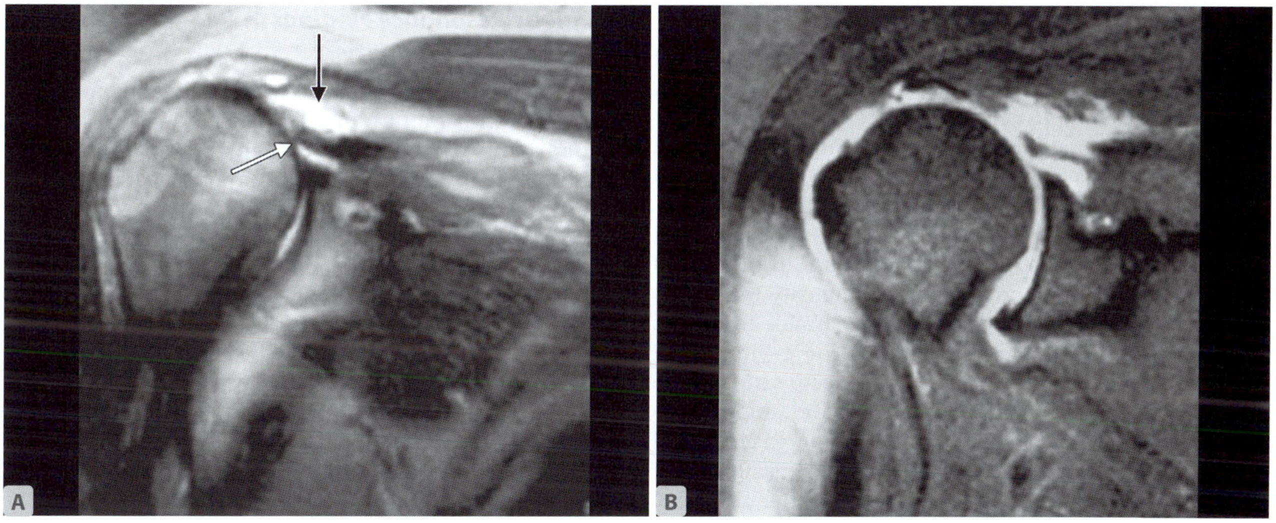

FIGS. 14A AND B: T2 turbospin-echo (T2 TSE) and arthrographic coronal sections show complete tear of SST (white arrow) with tendon retraction and fluid in the subacromial-subdeltoid bursa (SASDB) (black arrow) (A). There is free spillage of intraarticular contrast into the SASDB (B).

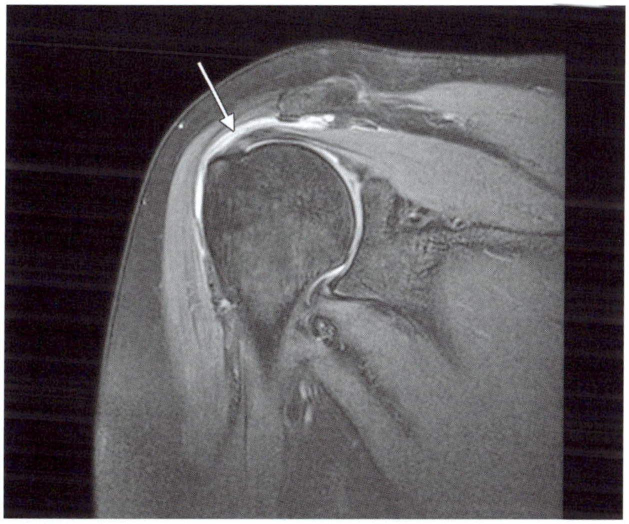

FIG. 15: Proton density (fat saturated) coronal section: The subacromial-subdeltoid bursa (SASDB) shows fluid (arrow) in absence of any visible rotator cuff tear.

the magnetic field. Normal signal on T2WI differentiates this from actual tendinopathy.

According to Zlatkin and colleagues,[19] sensitivity and specificity of MR for imaging partial and full thickness tears are 91% and 88%, respectively, with 89% accuracy. MR arthrography though not used routinely is useful in difficult cases and is gaining in popularity **(Fig. 14B)**.[20] It is superior to conventional T2WI for evaluating partial tears particularly on the articular side and differentiating small complete tears (with fibrosis) from partial tears. It is also helpful for diagnosing associated instability and capsulolabral disorders.

Instability

Shoulder joint is one of the most mobile joints in the body. But this mobility comes at the expense of stability as the joint architecture, which allows maximum mobility, also predisposes it to dislocation.

Glenohumeral joint is relatively shallow with a large humeral head in comparison to glenoid fossa. The structures responsible for maintaining joint stability are dynamic stabilizers (rotator cuff) and static stabilizers (glenoid labrum, joint capsule, GHL and periarticular soft tissue) **(Fig. 4)**. Pathology of any of these structures can predispose to instability.

Anterior and posterior bands are thickenings of anterior and posterior margins of IGHL, which prevent anterior and posterior dislocation respectively. Most important static stabilizer of shoulder is anterior band of inferior GHL, which prevents anterior dislocation.[21]

For practical purpose, shoulder instability can be broadly classified into two types: (1) unidirectional traumatic instability and (2) multidirectional nontraumatic instability, former being more common.[22] As the name implies unidirectional traumatic instability follows trauma, is unidirectional, usually anterior and is unilateral. Anterior instability is often associated with anteroinferior labral tear with or without glenoid rim fracture (Bankart lesion). This condition usually requires surgery and has been given a name traumatic, unidirectional, Bankart, surgery (TUBS).[22] MRI aids in planning surgical management in these patients as it can show associated capsulolabral-ligamentous defects, rotator cuff injury as well as osseous lesions.

Multidirectional nontraumatic instability is seen in young without history of trauma. It is often bilateral and invariably has an inferior component. These patients can voluntarily dislocate their shoulders. Basic pathology here seems to be capsular laxity which is difficult to assess by MRI. Treatment is usually conservative. These lesions are also named as AMBRI (atraumatic, multidirectional, bilateral, rehabilitation, inferior capsular shift).[22] As MR plays little role in evaluation of multidirectional instability, subsequent discussion will mainly focus on unidirectional instability (labral tears).

Imaging Techniques for Labral Tears

The shape of labrum varies from individual to individual (triangular, rounded, blunted, crescent shaped, etc). Most commonly, it is triangular anteriorly and rounded or triangular posteriorly **(Fig. 16)**. Few horizontal notches and vertical clefts along anterior aspect of labrum are considered normal. When seen posteriorly, these are considered tears.

Labral tear is seen as either complete absence of a portion of labrum, displacement of labrum from glenoid rim or linear area of increased signal intensity within the labrum on T2WI. Abnormal labral appearance in MRI is classified into four types as follows: Type 1—increased signal within the labrum not extending to the surface consistent with degeneration. Type 2—frayed appearance of labrum with normal signal. Type 3—increased signal within labrum extending to the surface consistent with tear and Type 4—combined features of Type 2 and Type 3. Type 2 to 4 labra are considered pathological. MR arthrography is the technique of choice for diagnosing labral pathology **(Fig. 17)**. Injected contrast distends the joint cavity and better delineates morphology of labrum and GHL. Contrast entering the labrum or tracking beneath the labrum to the external surface of joint also suggests tear **(Fig. 18)**. Positioning the arm is abduction and external rotation (ABER) has been shown to increase the sensitivity of MR arthrography.[23] This position puts tension on and improves evaluation of anterior band of IGHL and anterior inferior labrum.

Magnetic resonance arthrography has sensitivity of 91% and specificity of 93% for labral tears.[24] Conventional MRI, CT arthrography, and radiographic arthrography are alternative techniques for evaluation of labrum. Conventional MRI has shown variable accuracy with sensitivity ranging from 78 to 93% and specificity from 68 to 87%.[25,26] Relatively few studies have compared the accuracy of various techniques. However, one study by Chandnani et al.[27] compared CT arthrography, MR, and MR arthrography and showed MR arthrography to be the most sensitive modality among these (96%).

Magnetic Resonance Findings in Patients with Instability

Findings in anterior instability typically include anteroinferior labral tear with rupture of scapular periosteum (Bankart lesion), Bankart fracture (bony Bankart), and Hill Sach's lesion **(Figs. 17 and 19)**. When humeral head dislocates anteriorly, it can cause fracture of anterior glenoid rim (Bankart fracture) and can produce impaction fracture in superior posterolateral aspect of humeral head (Hill-Sach's lesion). On axial images, this is identified as a compression defect in the normally round posterolateral humeral head superior to the coracoid process (as opposed to normal defect of head below it)[28] **(Figs. 19 and 20)**. There may be associated marrow edema in recent injuries. Identification of these lesions is important as they predispose to recurrent dislocation with minimal trauma and may affect surgical planning.[29]

Some terms are used to describe Bankart variants. Glenolabral articular disruption (GLAD) lesions are described as tears of anteroinferior glenoid labrum with injury to glenoid articular cartilage. Scapular periosteum remains intact and holds labrum in place in GLAD. Loose bodies can occur in joint from detached avulsed articular cartilage fragment.[30] In ALPSA (anterior labroligamentous periosteal sleeve avulsion) lesion, there is tear of anterior labrum with periosteal stripping and displacement of labrum medially. Healing occurs typically with synovial fibrosis.[31] HAGL (humeral avulsion of GHL) lesions include detachment of capsule and IGHL from their anterior humeral attachment site. These lesions are uncommon cause of instability.[32] Perthe's lesion is described as an anterior labral tear having a scapular attachment with an intact periosteal sleeve[31] **(Fig. 21)**.

Three variations in anterior capsule insertion have been described.[33] Type I capsule inserts near the labrum, in type II, it inserts just medial to the labrum, and in type III, capsule is attached greater than 1 cm from the labral margin.

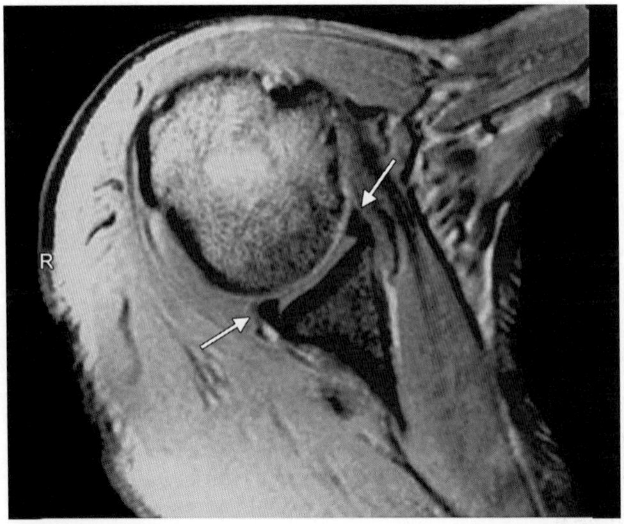

FIG. 16: Gradient-echo axial section shows normal anterior and posterior triangular labra undercut by a bright appearing articular cartilage (arrows).

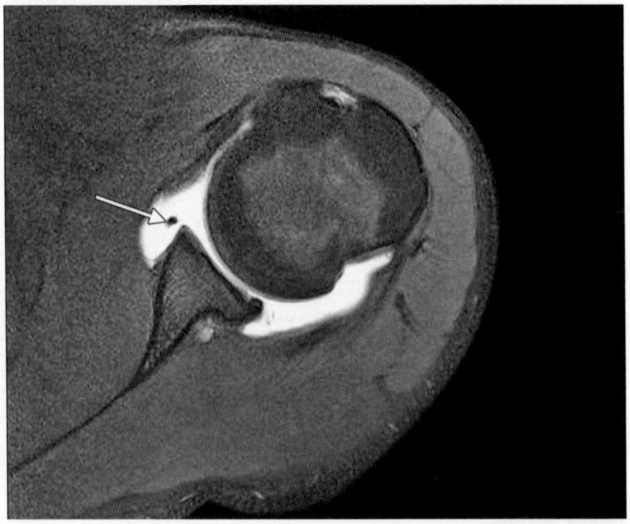

FIG. 17: T1 fat saturated arthrogram (axial section) at the inferior head level: Bankart lesion is seen as a separated anterior inferior labrum (arrow).

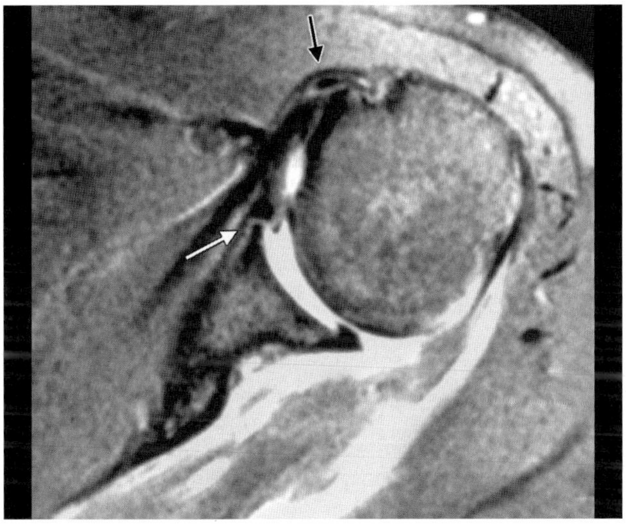

FIG.18: MR arthrogram shows a detached labrum with contrast outlining its base (white arrow). Partially sectioned middle glenohumeral ligament (MGHL) may at times mimic a labral fragment. Also note the medially dislocated biceps tendon from its groove and lying anterior to the subscapularis tendon (SCT) (black arrow).

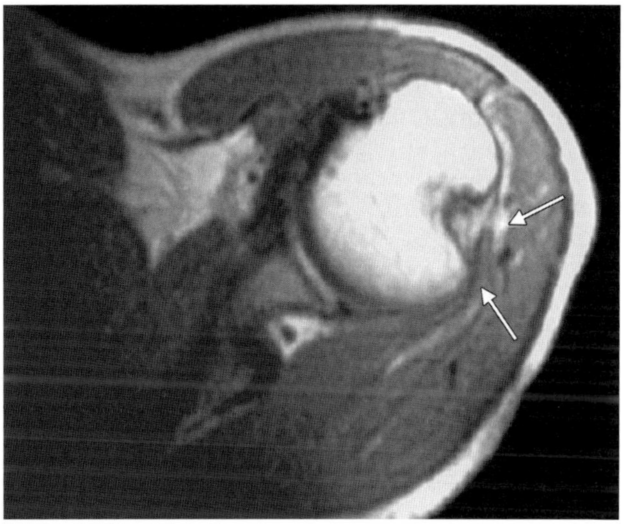

FIG. 19: T1 spin-echo axial section: There is a wedge-shaped defect at the posterosuperior aspect of the humeral head representing Hill-Sach's lesion (arrows) due to anterior dislocation of shoulder.

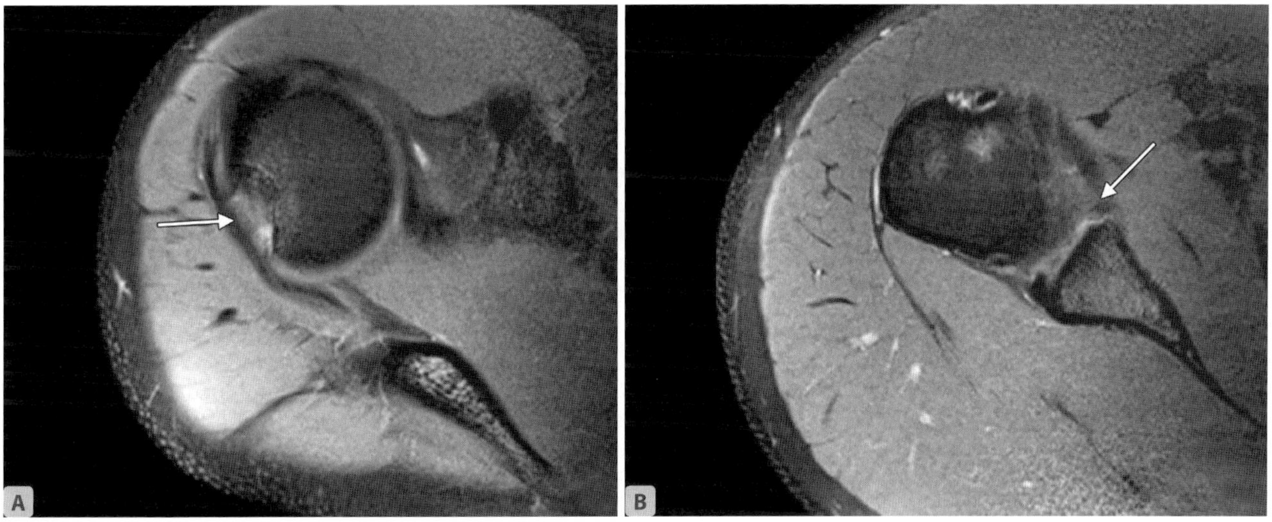

FIGS. 20A AND B: Proton density fat saturated axial sections (A and B) in another patient show typical Hill-Sach's defect in humeral head with anteroinferior glenoid injury (arrows).

Whether type III capsule predisposes to or is the result of anterior instability is not clear and debatable. However, a large capacious anterior pouch/subscapularis bursa is a frequent secondary finding in patients with recurrent anterior subluxation.

A close scrutiny of rotator cuff interval should also be done in all patients of clinical instability with RCT as capsule is weak in this area. The tear of the capsule may be isolated or associated with SST/SCT tears as well as biceps tendon dislocation.[34]

Superior labrum anterior to posterior (SLAP) lesions are important cause of traumatic instability. These lesions are typically seen in young people involved in sports activity requiring overhead movement of humeral head, like bowlers. They are believed to be caused by repetitive contact of humeral head with posterosuperior labrum. Consequently labrum becomes weak and tears away **(Fig. 22)**. Gradually tear progresses from posterior to anterior direction. The SLAP lesions were originally classified into four types by Snyder,[35] depending on the nature of labral injury and whether there is associated biceps tendon damage.

Type I

Fraying of glenoid labrum, but biceps tendon and labrum are not torn from glenoid (managed conservatively).

Type II

Stripping of labrum along with biceps tendon from glenoid (repaired surgically).

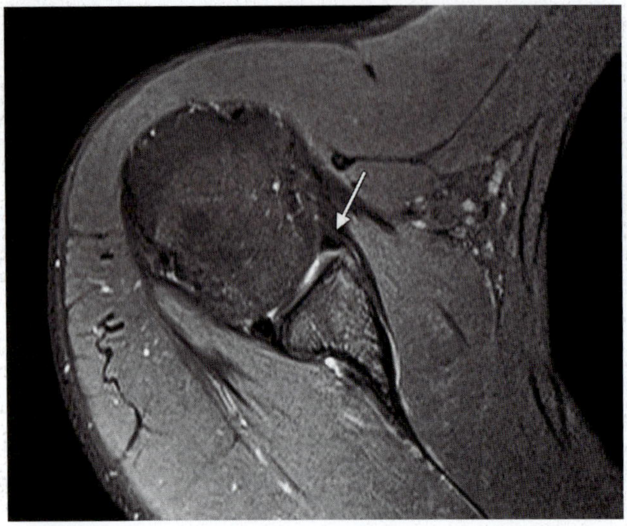

FIG. 21: Proton density fat saturated axial section showing avulsed labrum with a sleeve attached to the periosteum consistent with Perthe's variation of Bankart lesion (arrow).

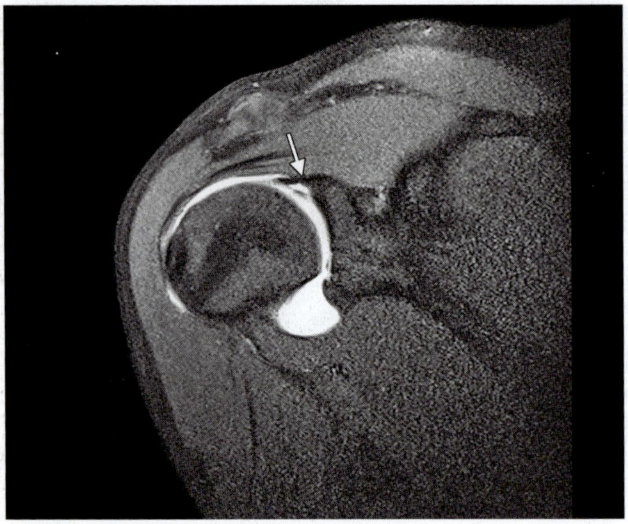

FIG. 22: T1 fat saturated arthrogram (coronal section) shows irregular shape tear with contrast filling in superior labrum suggestive of superior labrum anterior to posterior (SLAP) tear (arrow).

Type III

Bucket handle tear of labrum leaving biceps attachment to glenoid intact.

Type IV

Extension of bucket handle tear into biceps tendon.

This original classification was later expanded on the basis of arthroscopic findings however their clinical implication is questionable.

Type V

Bankart tear extending posterosuperiorly to biceps labral complex.

Type VI

Unstable flap or radial tear with separation of biceps from its anchor.

Type VII

Superior labral tear extending anteriorly beneath the middle GHL.

Type IX

Circumferential labral tear.

The SLAP lesions are associated with anterior instability and cuff tears. They are difficult to diagnose but important to identify as they respond well to arthroscopic repair.

Labral tears can be associated with labral cysts or ganglia which can cause compression neuropathy **(Fig. 23)**. These form because of one way valve mechanism leading to accumulation of joint fluid within them.

Anterior instability may also result from subscapularis injury. Subscapularis tears are seen after anterior dislocation over 40 years of age and after posterior dislocation at any age. Plain films and MRI may show lesser tuberosity fracture **(Fig. 24)**. Pfirrman et al.[36] graded subscapularis injury into four grades. Grade 0 tear is normal morphology. Grade I tear involves less than one-fourth and grade II tears involve greater than one fourth of subscapularis width. Grade III is complete detachment.

Posterior instability is much less common than anterior (2–4%). It is usually a result of anterior direct blow on shoulder or seizures. Imaging findings in addition to subscapularis tears include teres minor injury, posterior labral and capsular tear and anteromedially located reverse Hill-Sach's lesion **(Figs. 25A and B)**.[37]

Pitfalls

Some anatomic variants that can mimic labral tear should be kept in mind while interpreting shoulder MR. The most significant normal variation is a deficient attachment of labrum in the anterosuperior quadrant of glenoid (sublabral foramen or recess). At superior portion of the labrum three types of attachments are seen.

Type I

Labrum firmly attached to glenoid rim.

Type II

A small recess is present between labrum and the cartilage.

Type III

A large sublabral recess is present.

Sublabral recess is seen in 30% of patients[38] and should be differentiated from an SLAP tear on MR arthrography by observing location and configuration of contrast. The SLAP tears are usually seen at or posterior to biceps tendon attachment while the recess is seen anterior to it. Contrast in sublabral recess is seen as a thin line with smooth margins that runs along the glenoid. Contrast in a tear has irregular

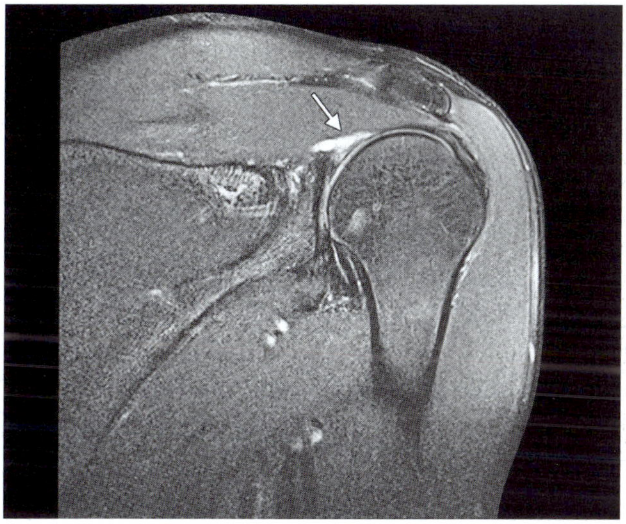

FIG. 23: Proton density fat sat coronal section shows superior labral tear with ganglion (arrow).

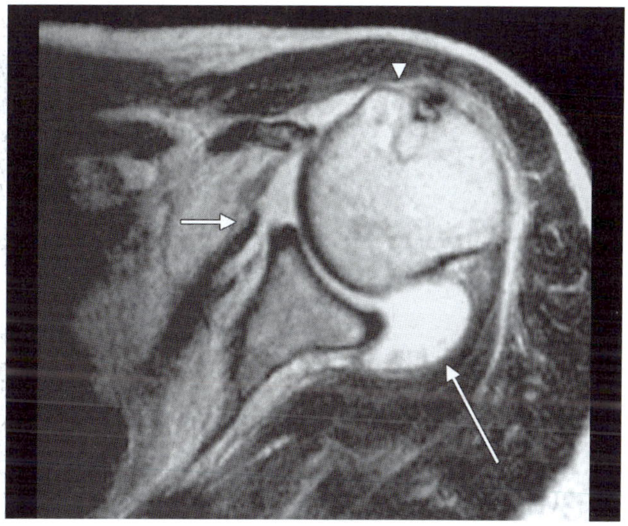

FIG. 24: T2 turbo spin-echo (T2 TSE) axial section shows a subscapularis tendon (SCT) tendon tear in a case of massive rotator cuff tear (RCT). The retracted tendon fibers (short arrow) and marrow edema at the lesser tuberosity (arrowhead) can be seen. A redundant posterior capsule indicates shoulder instability (long arrow).

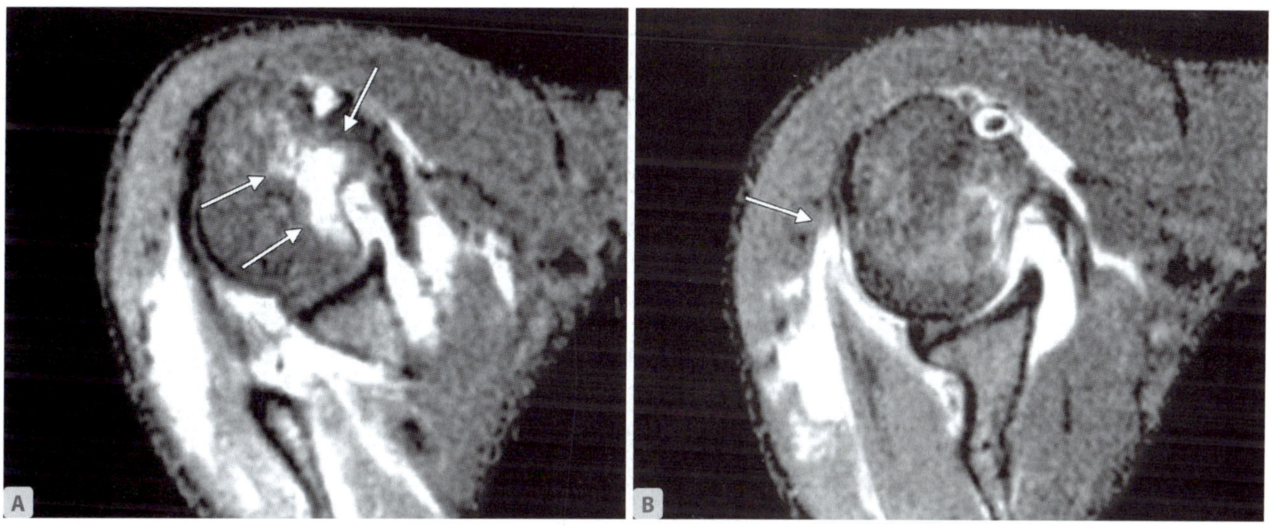

FIGS. 25A AND B: Turbo inversion recovery axial sections show classical anteromedial bony defect of reverse Hill-Sach's lesion due to posterior dislocation (A, arrows) and associated teres minor tendon tear (B, arrow). The posterior labrum is infolded and heterogeneous in signal.

margins, globular shape, and is seen to enter into labral substance.[39] Occasionally, contrast may be seen filling both sublabral recess and tear. This has been likened to a double chocolate or cream-filled cookie (Oreo sign).

A sublabral hole is seen in 17% normal people and is present at 2 O'clock position in pear-shaped glenoid cavities. Association of thick MGHL and an absent anterosuperior labrum has been termed as "Buford complex" and is also a normal variant.

The bright signal of hyaline cartilage between glenoid rim and labrum and the gap between MGHL and anterior glenoid can mimic tears of labrum. Following GHL on consecutive images can solve this problem.

ABNORMALITIES OF BICEPS TENDON

Bicipital Tendinopathy/Rupture

This usually occurs in middle aged or older patients with rotator cuff disease due to impingement of biceps tendon during flexion at shoulder joint beneath coracoacrominal ligament and anterior acromian.

This impingement may cause tendinopathy (or tenosynovitis) with flattening and thinning of tendon that may lead to complete rupture of the tendon **(Figs. 26A and B)**. Bicipital tendinopathy may also occur in patients with glenohumeral instability and attrition at the groove. Early bicipital tendinopathy often goes undetected on MR studies.

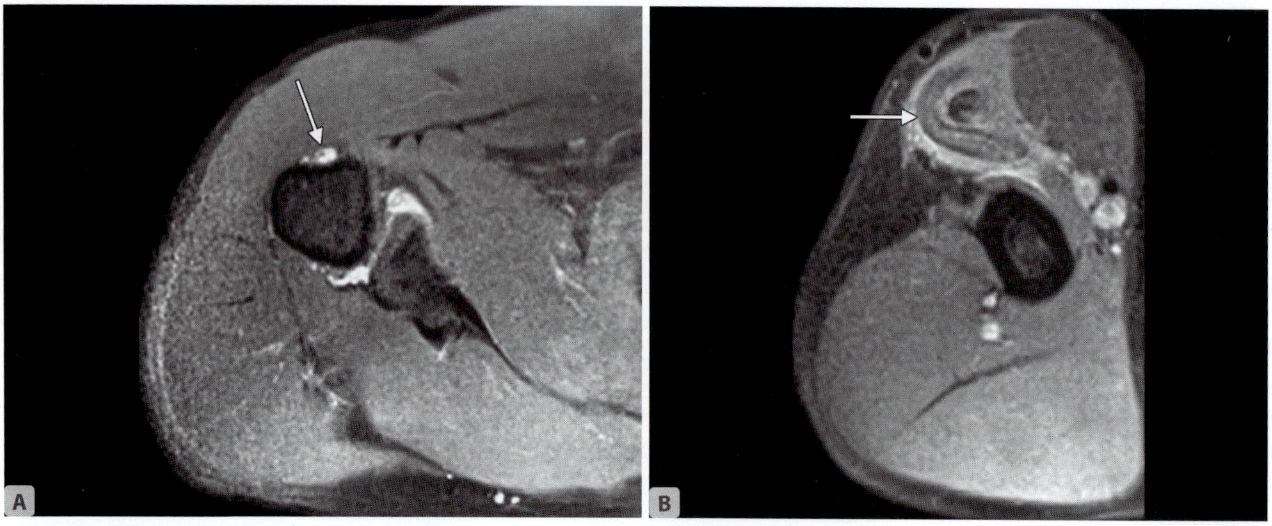

FIGS. 26A AND B: Proton density fat saturated axial section at the level of glenoid (A) shows empty bicipital groove suggestive of complete rupture of biceps tendon. Retracted biceps tendon (arrow) is seen in upper arm (B).

MRI reveals increased signal intensity within the abnormal tendon.[40] "Magic angle effect" can also lead to fallacious increased signal intensity within the tendon.

Morphologic abnormalities such as fraying, flattening, and absence of tendon may sometime be identified. Disproportionate amount of fluid in bicipital tendon sheath as compared to the joint fluid may suggest bicipital abnormality, i.e., tenosynovitis.

Bicipital Tendon Dislocations

Bicipital tendon dislocation usually occurs with the chronic RCTs that have extended to involve the subscapularis tendons. The symptoms are usually masked by those of RCTs.

Some fibers of subscapularis along with deep fibers of coracohumeral and the superior GHL complex forms the pulley for biceps tendon and the bicipital groove is hooded by transverse humeral ligament. When all the three structures are disrupted, tendons of long head of biceps dislocates medially posterior to subscapularis tendon into the joint, where it may be mistaken for a detached anterior labrum. Rarely when subscapularis tendon remains intact, with the disruption of other two ligaments, biceps tendon displaces extra-articularly, anterior to SCM.[41] On axial MR images, bicipital groove is empty with medially dislocated tendon in cases of biceps dislocations **(Fig. 27)**.

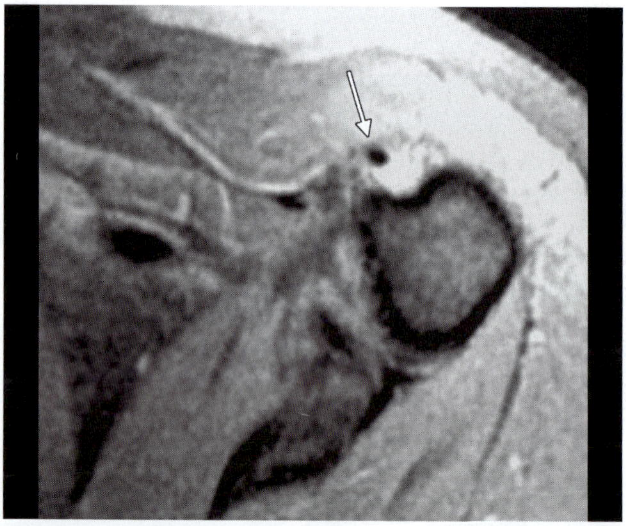

FIG. 27: Fat-suppressed T2 turbo spin-echo (T2 TSE) axial section: Biceps tendon is seen dislocated medially (arrow) with an empty bicipital groove.

NERVE ENTRAPMENT SYNDROMES

The following two nerve entrapment syndromes are uncommon but important causes of shoulder pain.

Quadrilateral Space Compression Syndrome

Quadrilateral space is bounded by teres minor superiorly, teres major inferiorly, shaft of humerus laterally, and long head of biceps medially. Axillary nerve and posterior humeral circumflex artery and vein pass through it. Patients present with pain and paresthesia in axillary nerve distribution and muscle atrophy of teres minor and major muscles. MRI does not show actual entrapment but excludes other causes of shoulder pain and only shows atrophy of teres minor with major muscle.[42] MR angiography or DSA (digital subtraction angiography) may be helpful by showing occlusion of posterior circumflex humeral artery.

Suprascapular Nerve Entrapment

Suprascapular nerve passes through supraspinatus notch to enter supraspinatus fossa beneath supraspinatus muscles. Further posteriorly it passes through spinoglenoid notch to enter into the intraspinatus fossa. It supplies both supraspinatus as well as infraspinatus muscle. Compression of nerve at the level of suprascapular notch results in atrophy of both muscles **(Fig. 28)** and compression at the level of spinoglenoid notch results in atrophy of infraspinatus muscle only. Compression may be because of neoplasm, hematoma, or most commonly ganglion cyst. MR shows fatty replacement of involved muscle and soft tissue lesion responsible for compression.[43]

Ganglion cysts are either associated with labral tears or typically arise from a posterior capsular defect and present at spinoglenoid notch. They appear isointense to muscle on T1WI and hyperintense on T2WI. They are often septate and may show rim enhancement on gadolinium administration.

Adhesive Capsulitis

Adhesive capsulitis (frozen shoulder) is a clinical syndrome of pain and restricted joint movement secondary to thickening and contraction of the synovial sheath and joint capsule. It is most commonly seen in 40–60 years old females. It may be associated with trauma, osteoarthritis, or rheumatic disorders.

On MRI, abnormal soft tissue may be seen in the rotator cuff interval encasing SGHL or CHL and may extend to undersurface of the biceps anchor.

Joint capsule and synovial thickening of more than 4 mm at the level of axillary recess is a useful MR criterion to diagnose this condition[44] **(Figs. 29A and B)**. Postgadolinium enhancement of the rotator cuff interval or axillary recess may be present, increasing the diagnostic accuracy.

Magnetic resonance arthrography, though not preferred for diagnosis, reveals decreased joint volume (<10 cc), decreased fluid volume in biceps tendon sheath and axillary recess, corrugations of capsule with thickening, and rotator interval abnormality.

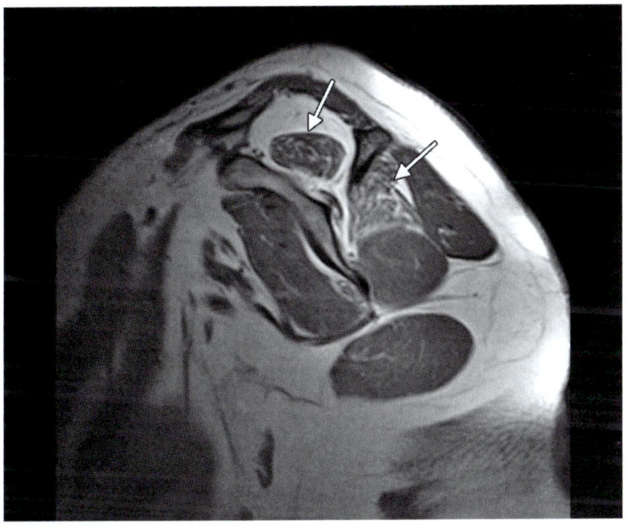

FIG. 28: T1 oblique sagittal section shows atrophy and fatty changes in supraspinatus and infraspinatus (arrows) secondary to impingement of suprascapular nerve.

Calcific Tendinitis

Formation of calcific deposits in the tendon is a degenerative process. Calcification of rotator cuff most commonly occurs in supraspinatous tendon but can occur in other tendons.[45] The size of deposition may vary from few millimeter to several centimeter. MR examination shows linear or globular area of decreased signal in all pulse sequences; however, T2* GRE has more sensitivity and specificity to demonstrate hypointensity in the tendon **(Figs. 30A and B)**.

ARTHRITIS

The shoulder joint is frequently involved in osteoarthritis and other infective/inflammatory arthropathies. MRI can demonstrate early inflammatory soft tissue and osseous changes and can be used as a sensitive monitoring tool.

Osteoarthritis

Osteoarthritis of shoulder is characterized by chondral erosions, osteophyte formation, subchondral cyst, sclerosis, and synovitis.[46] Humeral head sclerosis and cartilage loss are usually central or superior in location. MRI is very good to

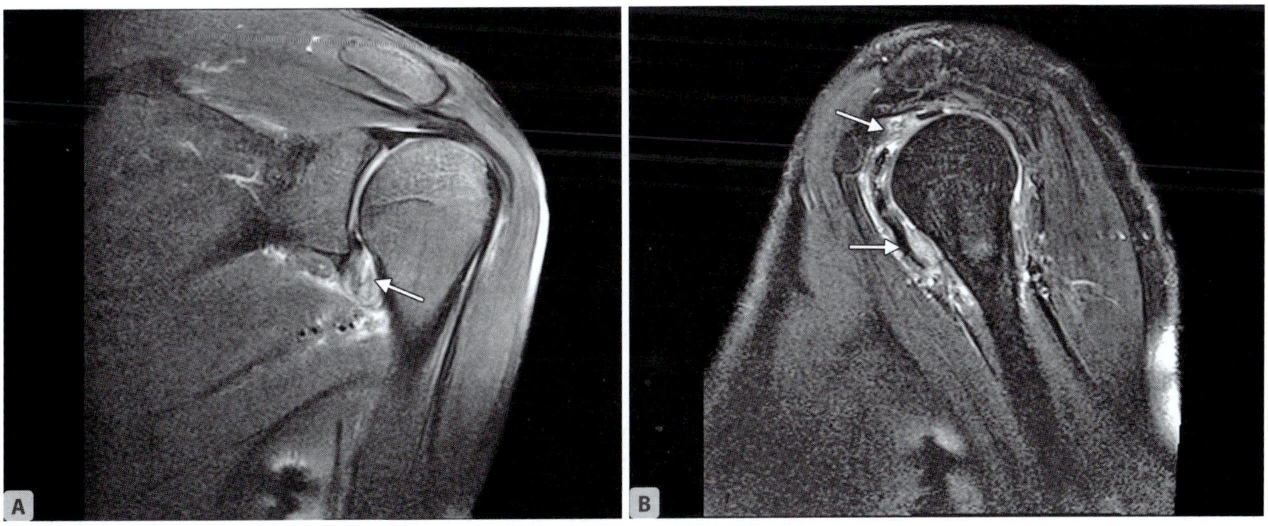

FIGS. 29A AND B: Proton density fat coronal section (A) and sagittal oblique (B): Thickened axillary pouch (arrows) with capsular edema and soft issue in rotator interval are indicative of adhesive capsulitis in a patient with frozen shoulder.

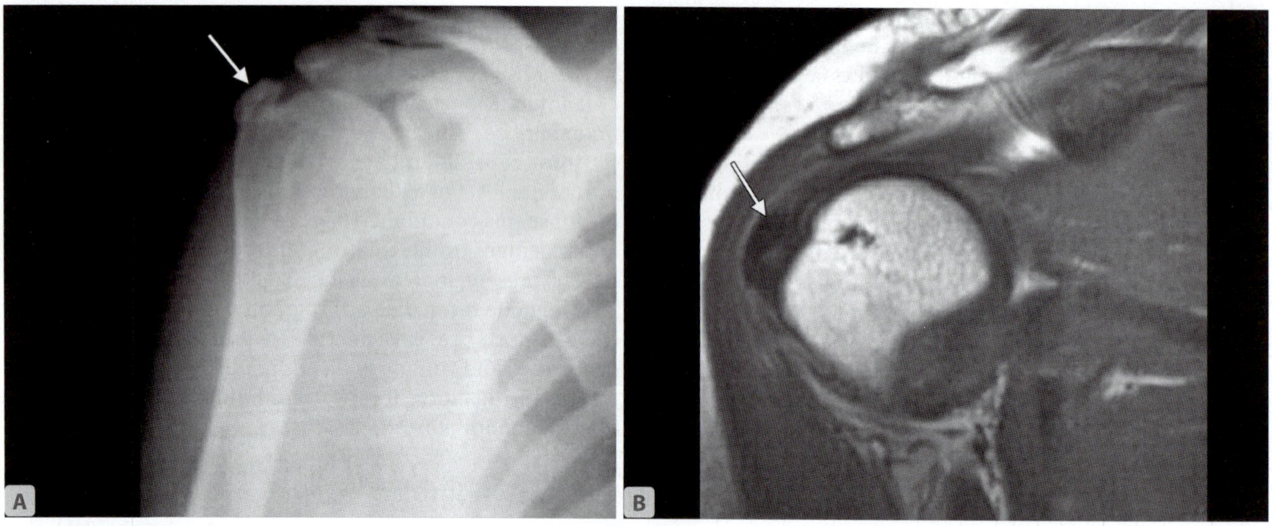

FIGS. 30A AND B: (A) Radiograph of shoulder shows globular calcification near greater tuberosity; (B) T1W coronal section shows globular area of hypointense signal (arrow) in the supraspinatus tendon suggestive of calcific tendinitis.

identify cartilage thinning and loss. Subchondral cysts are seen in both humeral head and glenoid **(Fig. 31)**. Inferior capsule may be enlarged with contraction of anterior capsule. Loose bodies occur in glenohumeral joint and subacromial bursa which appear isointense to bone or hypointense on T2W images.

Infective Arthritis

Septic arthritis is a clinical diagnosis relying on physical and laboratory parameters and microbiologic assessment of joint aspirate. Usually it affects older age group (average 65 years). The source of infection is either hematogenous or local. Immunocompromised status and pre-existing degenerative joint disease increases risk of septic arthritis. However, typical systemic and local symptoms may be absent in indolent infections like tuberculosis. Conventional radiographs may show associated osteoarthritis, osteomyelitis, or serve as a baseline study to monitor disease progression or response to treatment, but are insensitive to pick up early marrow or soft tissue changes. MR demonstrates these well along with bone changes; however, its specificity is low.[47]

Inflammation of synovial lining and joint effusion, the earliest pathologic changes, and associated bone marrow edema are seen well on fat-saturated T2WI and postcontrast T1WI **(Figs. 32A and B)**. Further progression of disease leads to cartilage destruction manifesting as joint space narrowing and marginal erosion of bare area. Subchondral bone changes in form of edema, subchondral cyst formation, and bone destruction follow when disease becomes subacute. Osteomyelitis, bone destruction, and joint ankylosis are features of chronic septic arthritis. RCTs can also be seen in subacute and chronic disease. MR cannot distinguish septic from nonseptic arthritis. Combination of bone erosions with marrow edema favors infectious etiology. Tuberculosis of shoulder joint is infrequent and has indolent clinical presentation. Patients usually presents with pain and restriction of movement for long duration. MRI is very useful to demonstrate synovial thickening, erosions, bone edema, and periarticular collections **(Figs. 33A and B)**.

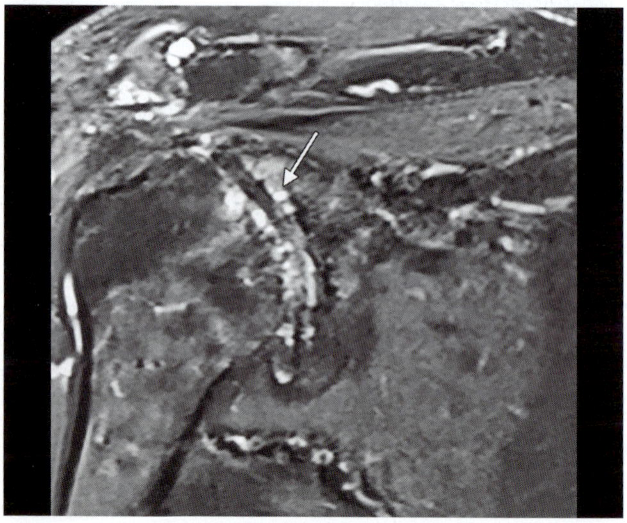

FIG. 31: T2 fat suppressed coronal section shows osteophytes, cartilage loss, and subchondral cysts which are typical findings of osteoarthritis.

Rheumatoid Arthritis

Rheumatoid arthritis (RA) is a chronic inflammatory joint disease, which involves synovial lining of joints. With disease progression there is involvement of articular cartilage, bone at joint margins, and periarticular soft tissue. Shoulder joint becomes involved later in the disease process. Proliferative synovitis involves glenohumeral joint, AC joint, and bursae around shoulder. Rotator cuff also becomes involved as disease progresses.

Magnetic resonance imaging is useful for detecting early changes of RA including synovitis, joint effusion, and marginal erosions. Marginal erosions are seen as low-signal areas on T1WI and variable signal intensity on T2WI. MRI may

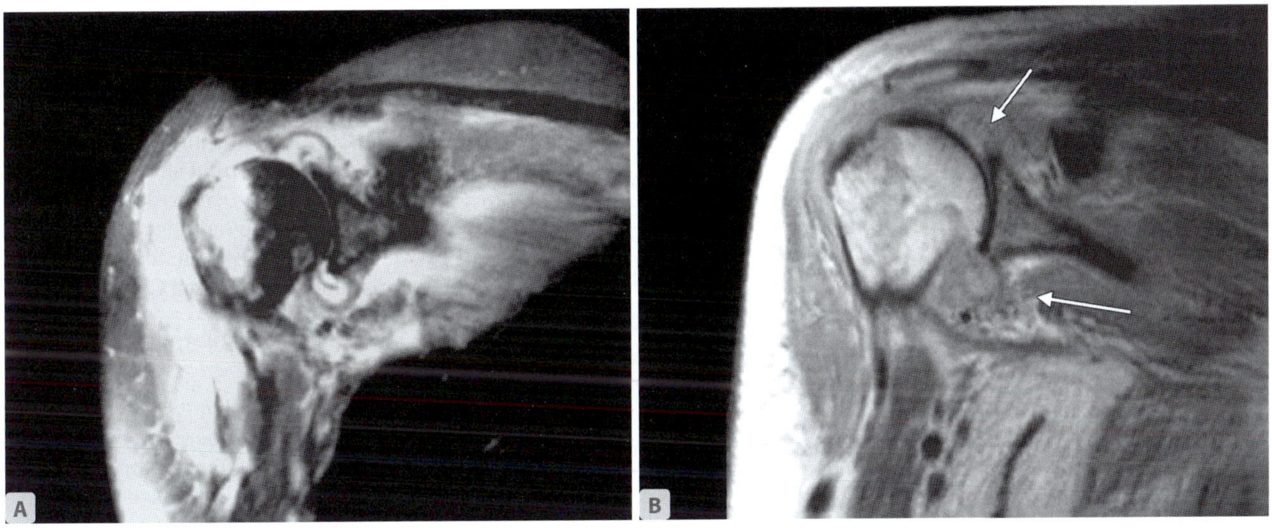

FIGS. 32A AND B: T2 turbo spin-echo (T2 TSE) fat-suppressed coronal section (A) reveals marked bone marrow and periarticular soft tissue edema and synovial thickening in a case of septic arthritis. T1 SE postcontrast (B) shows enhancement of the synovium and the periarticular tissue (arrows).

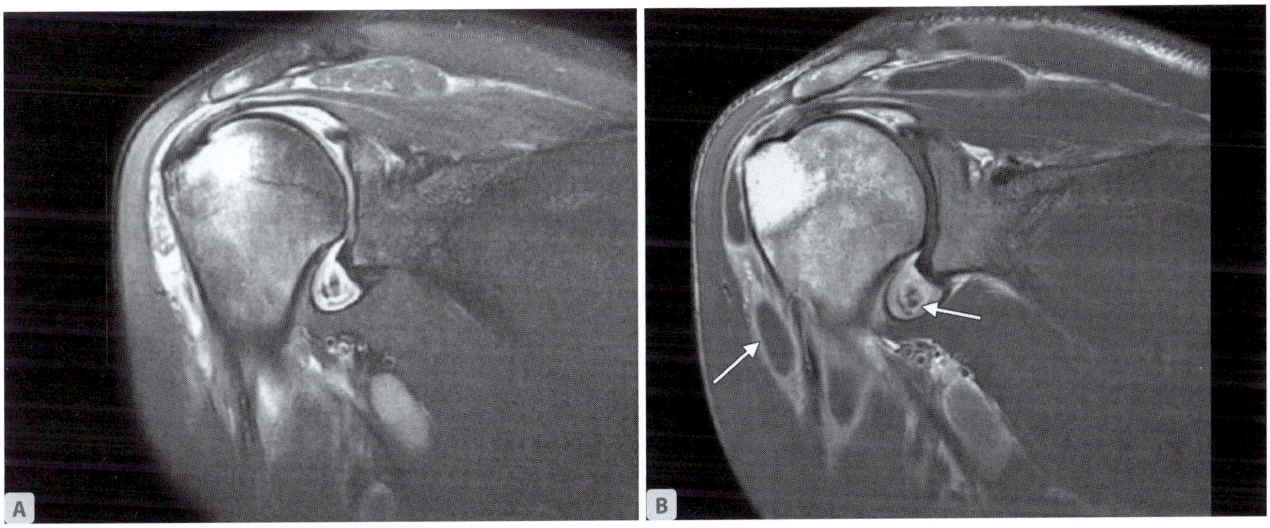

FIGS. 33A AND B: Tubercular arthritis: T2W fat saturated (A) and T1 fat saturated postcontrast coronal section (B) show joint effusion, synovial thickening, erosions, and periarticular collections.

be superior to ultrasound, CT, or conventional radiographs for detecting marginal erosions.[48]

Cartilage destruction is difficult to evaluate with routine shoulder protocol including MR arthrography, as it is very thin. RCTs are commonly seen in RA due to destructive synovitis near greater tuberosity.

Presence, size, and extent of synovial cysts, clinically evident soft tissue swellings of subacromial, and subdeltoid bursitis and simultaneous arthritic involvement of AC joint, all well-known manifestations of RA can be well shown by MR.

AVASCULAR NECROSIS

It is associated with trauma, steroid use, sickle cell anemia, and alcoholism. It can be differentiated from osteoarthritis by signal abnormality confined to the humeral head and sparing of glenoid. The Neer classification for shoulder AVN is similar to Ficat classification for hip osteonecrosis.[49] MR may show focal subarticular dark signal, a dark line encircling normal marrow, or a double line sign early on and fragmentation and collapse of head later **(Fig. 34)**. Metadiaphyseal lesions may show classical serpiginous low-intensity line surrounding high-intensity center (in chronic infarcts) and high-intensity rim in more acute infarcts.

NEOPLASMS

Magnetic resonance imaging is the imaging modality of choice for characterizing and staging both primary and secondary musculoskeletal neoplasms and tumor like lesions. MR shows joint involvement, soft tissue, and osseous components, involvement of neurovascular structures as well as helps in tissue characterization. T1WI (for marrow involvement), T2WI (for soft tissue extension), STIR, and postgadolinium fat-suppressed T1WI diagnose and stage tumors well. Metastatic disease is by far the most common malignant tumor around shoulder followed by myeloma, osteosarcoma, chondrosarcoma, and Ewing's sarcoma **(Figs. 35A and B)**. Frequent benign lesions comprise osteochondroma, chondroma, chondroblastoma, and giant cell tumor. Common soft tissue lesions around the shoulder are hemangioma **(Figs. 36A and B)**, lipoma **(Figs. 37A and B)**, and extra-abdominal desmoid.[50]

ADVANCE MAGNETIC RESONANCE TECHNIQUES IN SHOULDER JOINT

The routine protocols used for MR examinations of shoulder are quite good to detect shoulder injuries and related pathologies; however, there has been advancement in MR techniques to answer some particular clinical queries.[51]

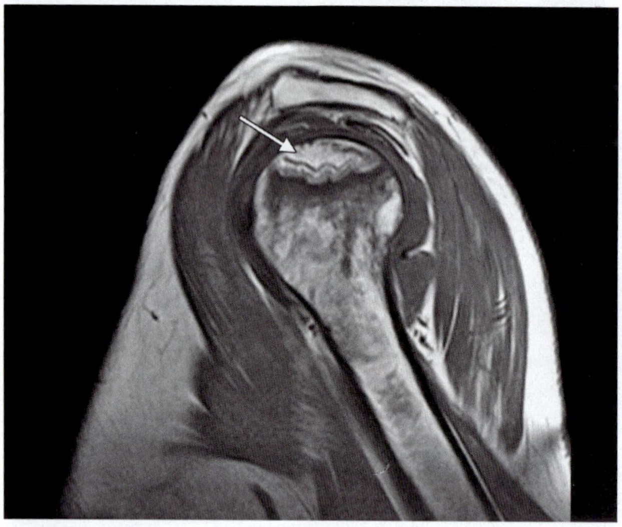

FIG. 34: T1 oblique sagittal section shows well-defined serpiginous area in humeral head suggestive of AVN (arrow).

Axial 3D Dual Echo-time T1-weighted FLASH Sequence

Assessment of bony injuries involving humeral head and glenoid are important for management of shoulder injuries. CT scan with 3D reconstructions provides details of bony injuries; however, it is associated with radiation exposure. 3D dual echo-time T1-weighted FLASH sequence can provide 3D reconstruction comparable to traditional CT.[52-53]

Oblique Sagittal 3D Volume-interpolated Breathhold Examination (VIBE)

Rotator cuff tear may be associated with fatty degeneration of cuff muscle. The assement of fatty degeneration is important at it is important factor for outcome after rotator cuff repair. Goutallier classification system is established qualitative assessment method however recent studies have focused on the quantitative assessment of fat fractions to see relationship between muscular atrophy and fatty infiltration of the rotator cuff by using a 3D oblique sagittal volume-interpolated breathhold examination (VIBE) sequence with the 2-point Dixon method.[54-56]

Three-dimensional MRI Reconstruction of the Rotator Cuff

3D imaging can depict the exact shape of cuff tear which is useful for preoperative planning of these patients. Tendon tears can be classified as either longitudinal or crescent shaped. Longitudinal tears are those with length greater than its width. Crescent-shaped tears has more width then length. Longitudinal tear may be subdivided in U- or L-shaped tears.[57-58]

Radial MRI of the Shoulder

There can be partial averaging of insertional fibers of rotator cuff with concealment of smaller tear. Radial MRI can improve the detection of small tear. Radial imaging has

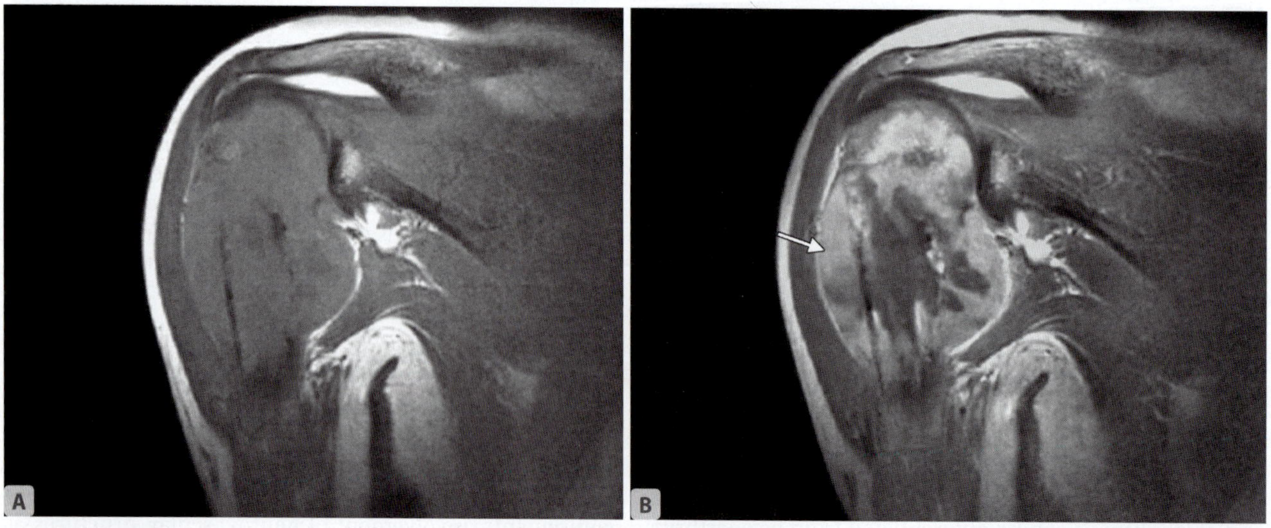

FIGS. 35A AND B: Ewing's sarcoma: T1W coronal (A) and postcontrast T1W, coronal section (B) shows malignant mass arising from metadiaphysis of right humerus associated with cortical destruction and adjacent soft tissue.

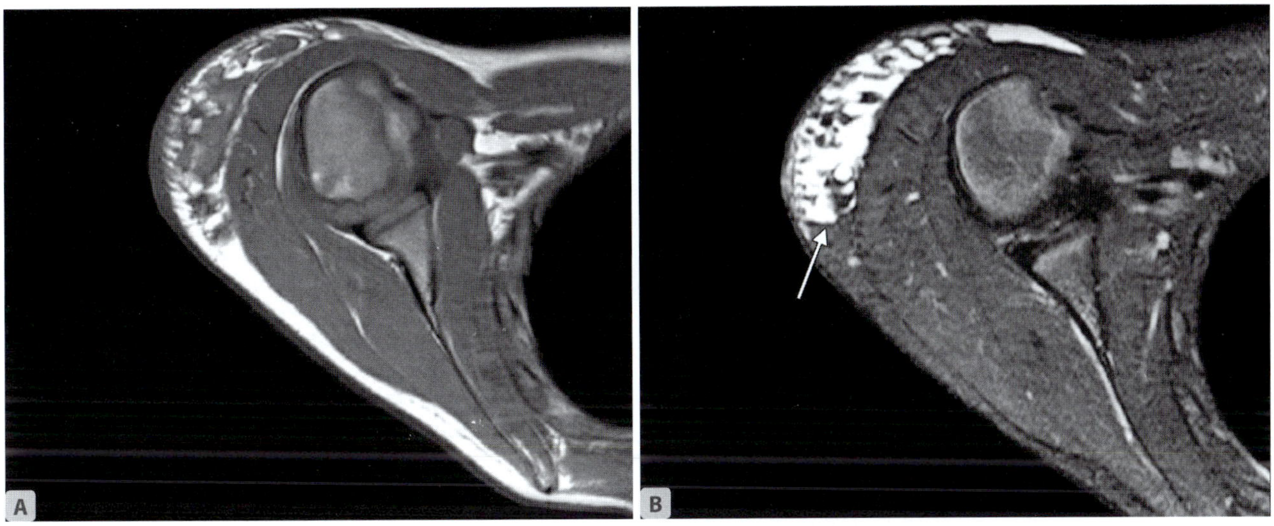

FIGS. 36A AND B: Soft tissue hemangioma: T1W axial (A) and T2W fat saturated axial section (B) of shoulder show altered signal soft tissue lesion superficial to deltoid muscle limited to subcutaneous tissue.

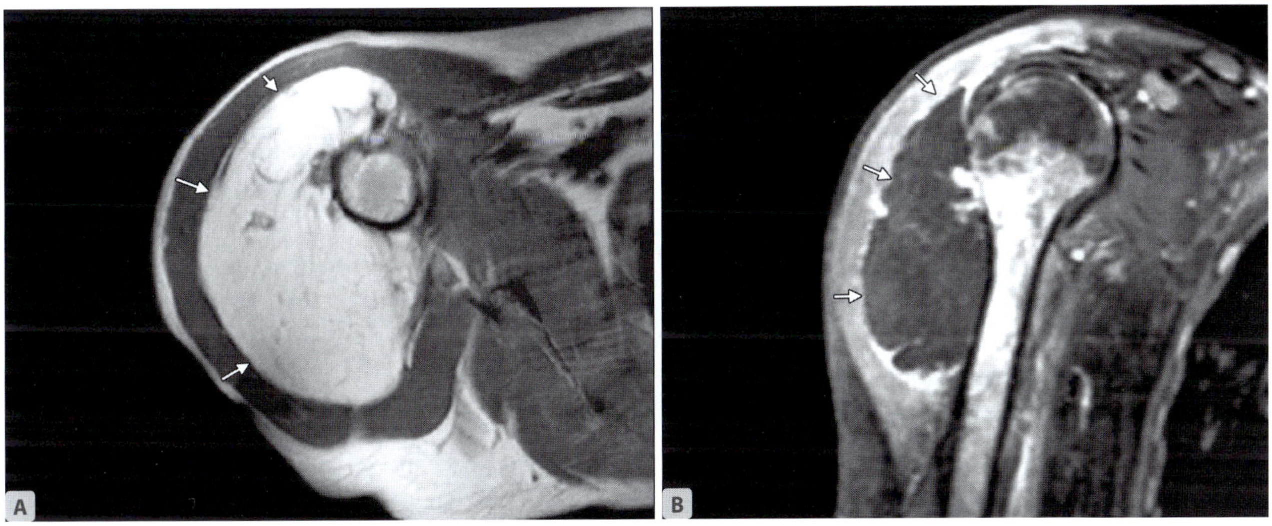

FIGS. 37A AND B: T1 axial section: A lipoma (arrows) in relation to the subacromial-subdeltoid bursa (SASDB) showing high-signal of fat (A). The inversion recovery image shows dark signal due to fat saturation (B).

shown excellent promise in the evaluation of subtle RCTs, especially those involving the subscapularis tendon.[59]

Diffusion Tensor Imaging (DTI)

It is an advanced method for quantify direction-dependent water diffusion. Rotator muscle fibers tracts are visualized by advanced postprocessing. As a functional MR technique, DTI may show muscle abnormalities before they become evident at conventional morphologic MR sequences.[60]

TEMPOROMANDIBULAR JOINT

INTRODUCTION

Temporomandibular joint (TMJ) dysfunction is a common condition that may affect up to 28% of the population.[61]

The most common cause of TMJ dysfunction is internal derangement, which is defined as an abdominal relationship of the disc to the condyle. The TMJ dysfunction is best evaluated with MRI due to excellent demonstration of disc morphologic changes, disc displacement, and various other abnormalities of TMJ.[62]

MAGNETIC RESONANCE IMAGING TECHNIQUE

Magnetic resonance imaging of TMJ is performed by using the body coil as transmitter and dual surface coils as receiver (simultaneous examination of both sides is preferred as TMJ disorders often involve both sides). Axial plane is used for localization of condyle and planning of sagittal and coronal images. Sagittal images are obtained in both closed and open mouth positions, in a plane perpendicular to the horizontal

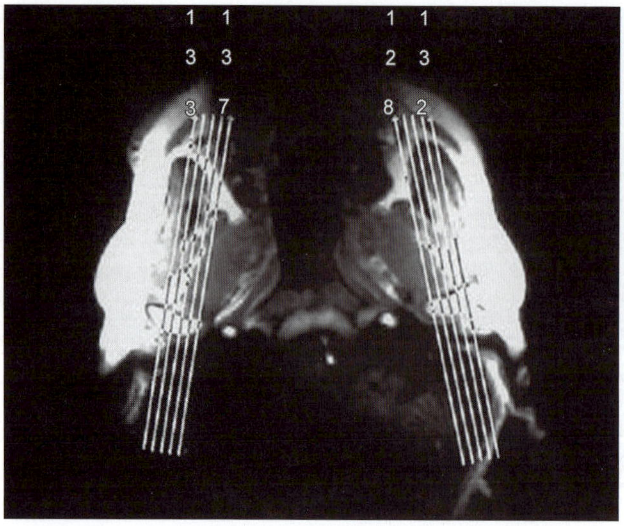

FIG. 38: For temporomandibular joint imaging, sagittal images are planned perpendicular to the horizontal axes of mandibular condyles on axial scout images as shown. The coronal images are planned perpendicular to the above prescribed sagittal plane.

long axes of mandibular condyles **(Fig. 38)**. Coronal images are acquired along the horizontal long axes of condyles in closed mouth position. Out of these sagittal plane is standard plane of imaging. The preferred sequences are T1 spin echo (shows fat as bright), T2 turbo spin echo (fluid sensitive), and proton density images. Functional joint dynamics at incremental mouth opening can be shown with small flip angle gradient echo imaging.

NORMAL ANATOMY AND MAGNETIC RESONANCE APPEARANCE (FIGS. 39 TO 42)

Temporomandibular joint is a diarthrodial synovial joint. Its articular surfaces are formed by articular eminence and anterior part of mandibular (glenoid) fossa superiorly and head of mandibular condyle inferiorly **(Figs. 39A and B)**. Articular surfaces are covered by a fibrocartilage. Mandibular condyles are elliptical in shape with their long axes converging posteriorly at around 15° **(Fig. 40C)**.[63] An intra-articular disc divides the joint into upper and lower compartments **(Figs. 39 and 40)**. The disc is composed of avascular fibrous connective tissue which merges with peripheral capsule. It is oval in shape, measuring approximately 18 mm in anteroposterior dimension and 20 mm in mediolateral extension. It is biconcave in sagittal plane and crescent shaped in coronal plane. Two localized thickenings are present in the disc, called anterior and posterior bands. Posterior band is thicker than the anterior band. Consequently, the disc is 2 mm thick in its anterior part, 1 mm centrally, and 3 mm in its posterior part.[64] Normally, in a closed mouth position, posterior band is located directly above the condyle, central thin zone between articular eminence and condyle and anterior band below articular eminence. Disc is attached posteriorly to temporal bone and posterior subcondylar area through a fibrofatty vascular connective tissue called posterior attachment, retrodiscal tissue, or bilaminar zone through its superior and inferior lamina. This structure restrains its anterior movement. Joint is covered by a loose connective tissue capsule, attached superiorly to articular eminence and circumference of mandibular fossa and inferiorly to neck of condyle. The superior head of lateral pterygoid inserts on anterior capsule and adjacent condylar neck with its tendinous fibers directly attaching to the anterior band of the disc and helps in mouth opening. Medial pterygoid and temporalis muscles with their mandibular insertions also assist mandibular movements. Temporomandibular and sphenomandibular/stylomandibular ligaments reinforce the lateral and medioposterior capsule, respectively.

Normal Magnetic Resonance Appearance

The cortices of condyle and temporal component of the TMJ have smooth outline and low-signal intensity **(Fig. 40A)**. The articular covering and synovium show high-signal. Intra-articular disc shows low-signal intensity as it is composed of fibrous tissue; however, the posterior disc attachment has relatively high-signal intensity because of fatty tissue. The attachment of superior belly of lateral pterygoid to anteromedial disc and adjacent condyle can also be demonstrated as low-intensity structure. The medial pterygoid muscle lies inferiorly. The low-signal maxillary vessels can be seen between pterygoid muscles and mandibular condyle. The low-signal temporomandibular ligament can be seen as laterally supporting structures on coronal images **(Fig. 40B)**.

MOVEMENTS

The TMJ movements take place at both compartments. Translation occurs predominantly in the upper compartment and both rotation and translation in the lower compartment. During jaw opening, initially the condyles rotate in lower compartment followed by translatory movement in upper and subsequently in the lower joint compartment. During translation there is sliding movement of intraarticular disc along with condyle in relation to mandibular fossa. During all movements the central disc remains located between the condyle and the articular tubercle with anterior and posterior bands acting as functional guides. In contrast to the 12 O'clock location of posterior band in closed mouth position, in open mouth position the apex of the condyle lies opposite the articular eminence with interposed central thin zone between the two and there is marked expansion of the tissue in the region of posterior attachment **(Figs. 39 to 41)**. The disc does not move in the mediolateral direction unless these attachments are torn.

DISEASES OF TEMPOROMANDIBULAR JOINT

Temporomandibular joint disorders are more prevalent in young and middle age females. Patients with TMJ disorders present with complaints of myofacial pain syndrome (pain

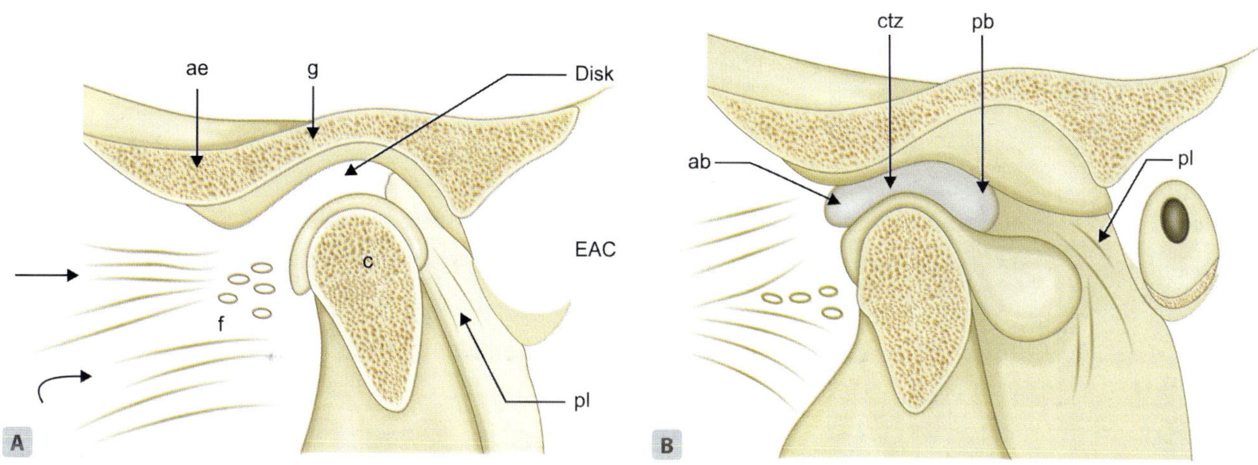

FIGS. 39A AND B: Diagrammatic representation of temporomandibular joint (TMJ) anatomy. (A) Close mouth position—oval disc lies between the condyle (c) and glenoid fossa (g). More anteriorly the articular eminence is seen (ae). The retrodiscal tissue (pl) acts as the posterior attachment. Bright lateral pterygoid fat plane (f), external auditory canal (EAC), superior (straight arrow) and inferior (curved arrow) bellies of lateral pterygoid muscles are also labeled; (B) Open mouth position—the condyle and the disc move anteriorly together to a position below the articular eminence with central thin zone interposed between the two. (ab: anterior band; ctz: central thin zone; pb: posterior band).

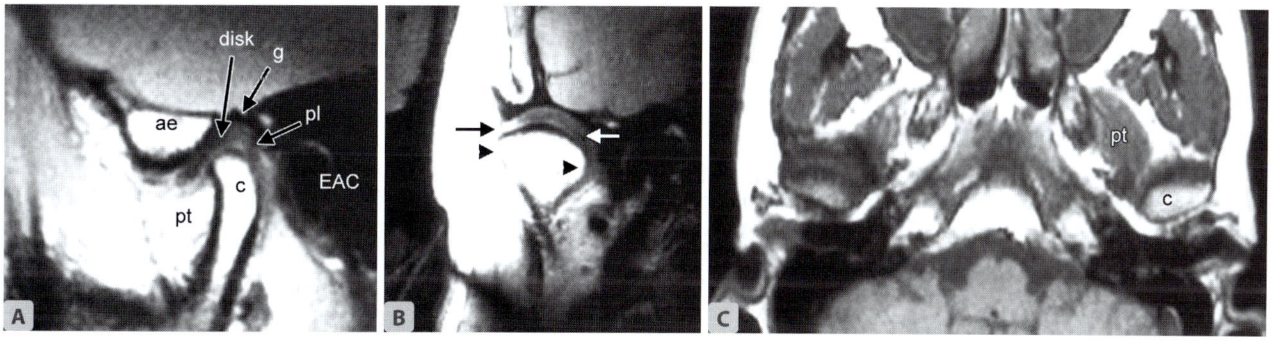

FIGS. 40A TO C: (A) Sagittal proton WI showing normal anatomy (compare with Fig. 2). The marrow in the condyle and articular eminence appears bright in signal. The articular margins of temporal bone are dark and well-defined. The disc shows intermediate signal; (B) Coronal proton WI: The crescent-shaped disc (white arrow), and lateral attachment of disc (black arrow) are seen. The lateral and medial poles of the condyle (arrow heads) can be seen with disc attaching just beneath them; (C) Axial anatomy T1WI: Elliptical condyles with posteriorly converging horizontal axes in relation to skull base. (c: condyle; pt: inferior belly of lateral pterygoid muscle).

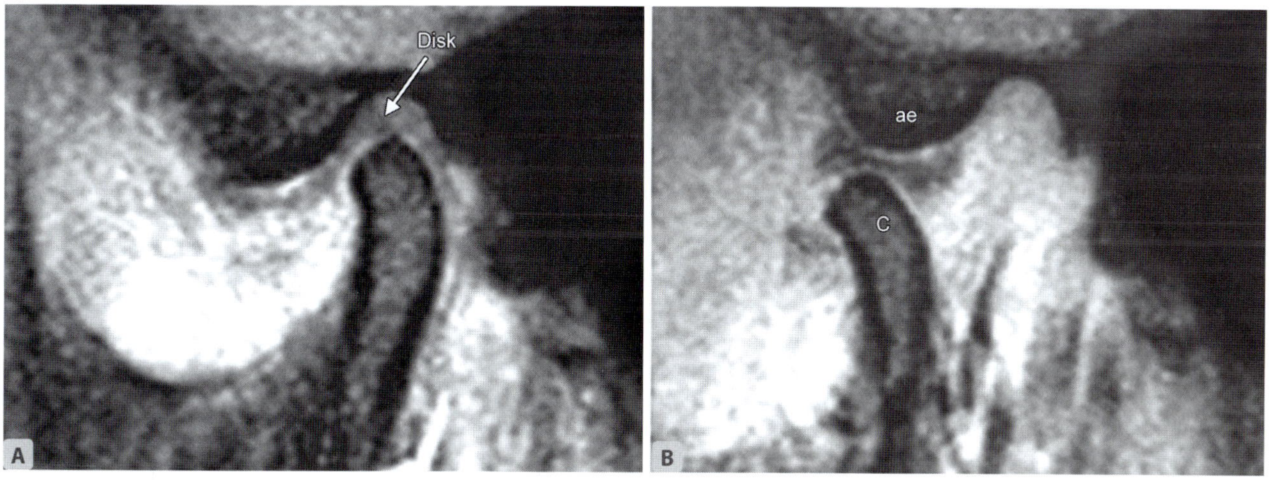

FIGS. 41A AND B: (A) Close mouth; and (B) Open mouth positions showing location of disc (arrow) in relation to the condyle. The posterior band lies just superior to condyle in (A) and the condyle lies opposite the articular eminence with interposed thin zone between them in open mouth position (B).

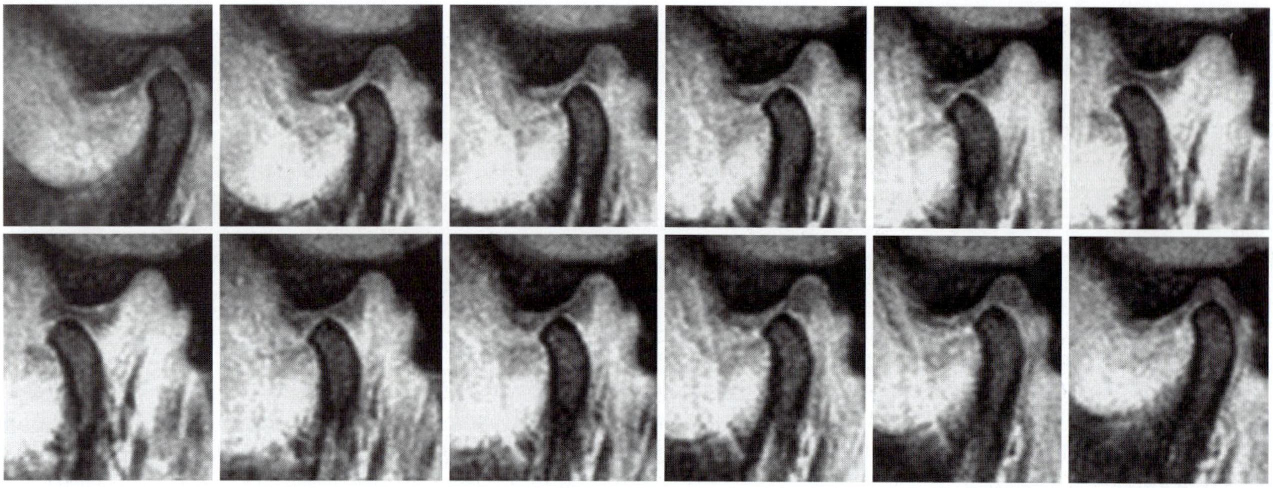

FIG. 42: Fast gradient echo serial sagittal sections showing condylar translation in the glenoid fossa and its constant relationship with the disc. (upper row—mouth opening and lower row—mouth closing). The posterior band at 12 O'clock position in the closed mouth position (first frame upper row). The head opposed to articular eminence with thin zone of disc interposed between the two (last frame upper row). Note expansion of the posterior soft tissues as mouth opens.

and muscle tenderness around the joint) and biomechanical dysfunction (clicking, crepitus, and limitation of jaw movements).

Internal Derangement

Internal derangement is defined as altered morphological and functional relationship between articular surface of the temporal bone, disc, and mandibular condyle.

Disc Displacements

This is the most common TMJ disorder.[65] Normally the posterior band is at 12 O'clock position in relation to mandibular condyle. Displacement is said to have occurred when this relationship is altered. Disc can displace in anterior, posterior, anteromedial, anterolateral, and sometimes purely in lateral and medial directions.[66] Anterior and posterior displacements are seen best in sagittal images. Lateral and medial displacements are best seen in coronal images.

Disc displacement is further categorized into "displacement without reduction" and "displacement with reduction." When an anteriorly displaced disc fails to return to normal position on jaw opening it is called displacement without reduction **(Figs. 43A and B)**. These patients can not open their mouths fully (closed lock jaw).[67] In displacement with reduction, displaced disc returns to normal position relative to condyle during jaw opening leading to reciprocal clicking[68] **(Figs. 44A and B)**.

Most common disc displacement is anterior however often it also has an anteromedial or anterolateral component **(Figs. 45A and B)**. Such displacements are also called rotational displacements. Further the disc displacement may be complete or partial when only the medial or lateral part of the disc is displaced. In pure medial and lateral disc displacements sagittal images will show no disc between condyle and mandibular fossa. Instead pulled up lateral or medial capsular tissue, respectively, will be seen, giving it an empty appearance (empty fossa sign).

Disc Deformity and Osteoarthritis

Internal derangements of TMJ are progressive disorders. The reducing disc leads to nonreducing disc in due course of time and a chronically displaced disc slowly gets deformed and later leads to osteoarthritis of the joint.[69] The above stages of displaced disc are also graded as acute (reducing disc with normal morphology), subacute (nonreducing disc with deformity), and chronic (adhesions, fibrosis, perforation, and degenerative joint disease).[70] Disc deformity is important to identify as it is treated with discectomy while disc repositioning is done for disc displacements.

Earliest MR findings of disc deformity is thickening of posterior band. As the disease progresses disc assumes rounded, biconvex, or sigmoid shaped instead of normal biconcave configuration. It may also show fissuring and surface irregularity. In some of the cases, the disc may show severely diminished volume.

Another tissue alteration seen in association with chronic disc displacement is formation of "pseudodisc." This appearance is because of fibrosis and anterior displacement of posterior attachment which comes to occupy the normal position of disc between condyle and mandibular fossa and simulates disc because of its low-signal intensity. Perforations are seen in 5–15% patients with disc displacement, more frequently at posterior disc attachment.[71] Secondary changes because of disc deformity include synovitis and joint effusion. It is best seen on T2 WI as increased signal intensity in upper, lower, or both compartments.

Marrow abnormality in form of marrow edema, osteonecrosis, or sclerosis in the condyle can be secondary to disc deformity **(Fig. 46)**. Normal marrow in condyle shows high signal intensity on both T1 and T2 WI. Marrow edema is seen as low-signal intensity on T1WI and high-signal intensity on T2WI. Osteonecrosis and sclerosis show low-signal

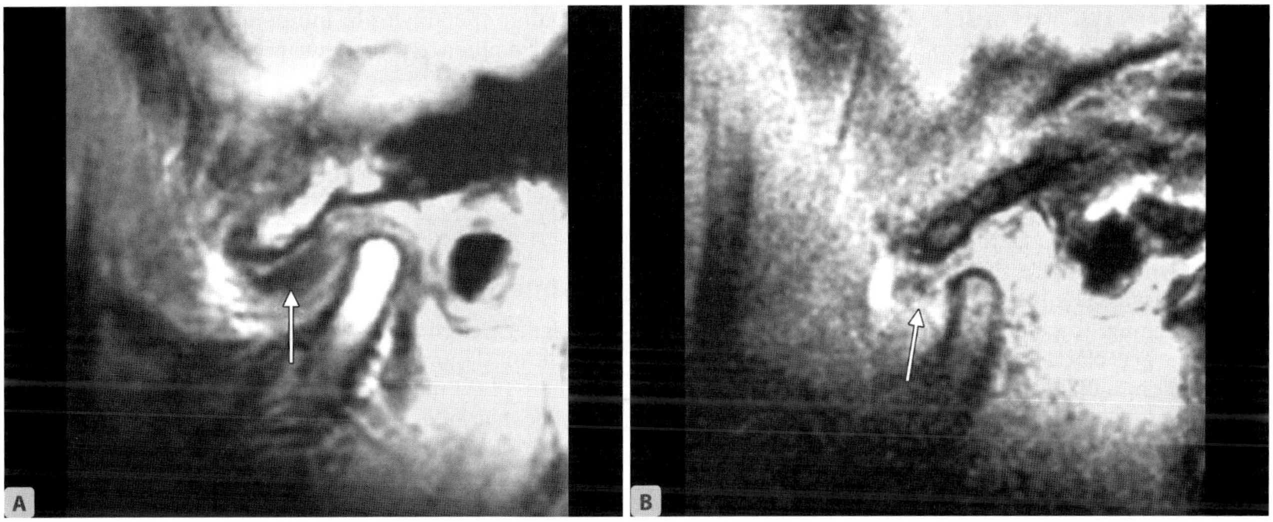

FIGS. 43A AND B: Nonreducing disc. Sagittal section (A) closed mouth and (B) open mouth. The nonreducing anteriorly displaced disc is shown (arrows).

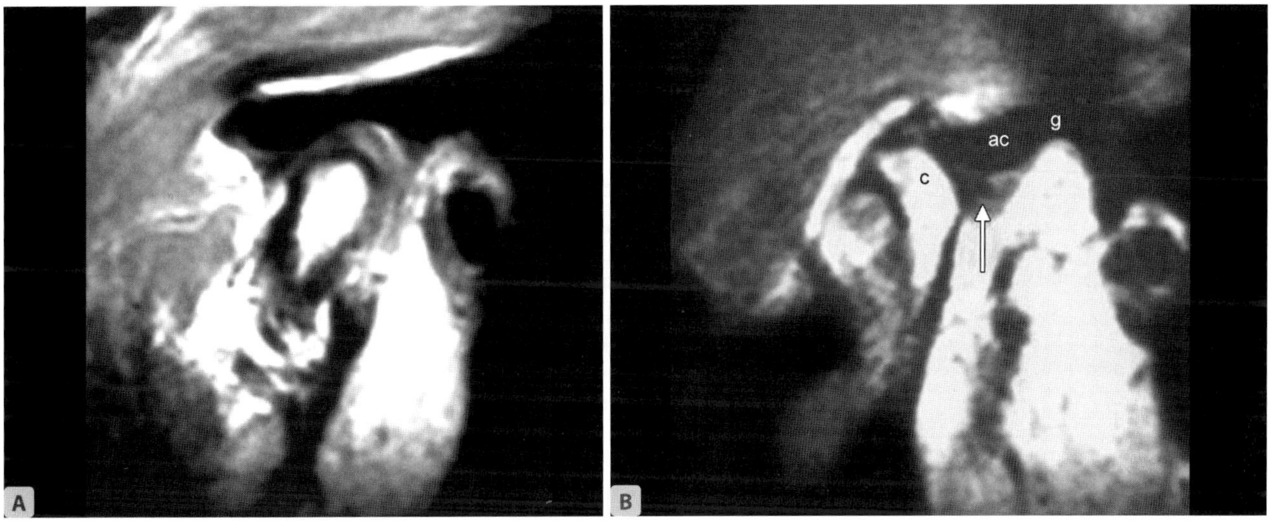

FIGS. 44A AND B: Reducing disc. Sagittal section (A) closed mouth and (B) open mouth. (A) There is mild anterior displacement of the disc; (B) Dislocation of condyle into infratemporal fossa anterior to the articular eminence. The eminence and the reduced disc (arrow) prevents condyle from returning to the glenoid fossa.

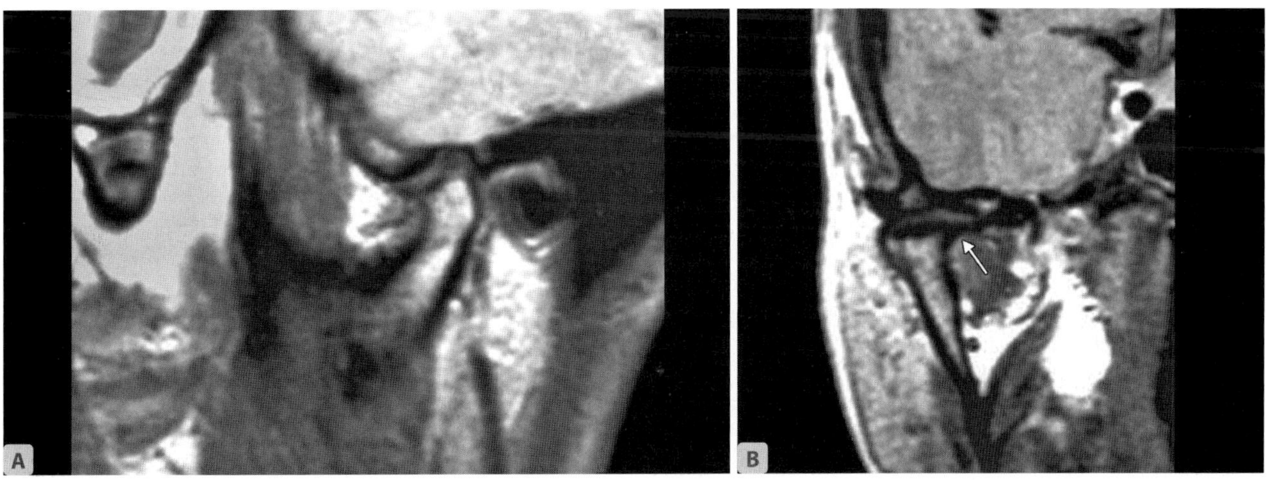

FIGS. 45A AND B: (A) Proton weighted sagittal section: The disc is not well seen in the glenoid fossa; (B) Coronal section: The disc is anteromedially displaced (arrow).

intensity on T1WI and variable signal intensity on T2WI. Long-standing disc displacement without reduction can lead to osteoarthritis in TMJs. It is characterized by osteophyte formation with flattening and irregularity of articular surfaces **(Figs. 47A and B)**.

Stuck Disc

Upper compartment permits translational movements only, in which the disc slides or translates relative to the mandibular fossa. This movement is important in later part of jaw opening. In pathology of upper compartment, this movement gets blocked, consequently the patients is not able to open his mouth fully. This can cause pain and discomfort.

Open Lock Jaw

In contrast to "closed lock state" described above, in "open lock jaw," after wide opening of the mouth patient is not able to close mouth temporarily or permanently due to the dislocation of condyles in infratemporal fossa anterior to articular eminence. The latter prevents the condyle from returning back into glenoid fossa. On the other hand, a reducing disc may do the same **(Figs. 44A and B)**.

Further indications of imaging of TMJ are demonstration of loose bodies, postoperative evaluation, mandibular asymmetry, trauma, infective/noninfective arthritis, and neoplasia.

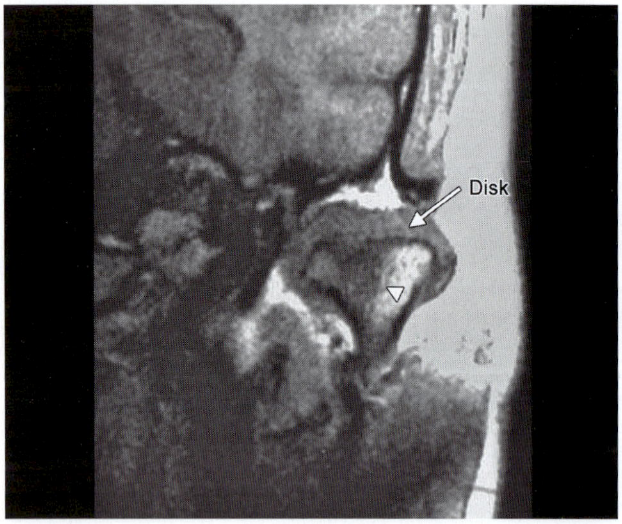

FIG. 46: Coronal T1WI: Low-intensity area in the medial part of the condyle (arrowhead) in case of displaced disc (arrow) likely representing a focus of avascular necrosis.

Osteonecrosis and Osteochondritis Dissecans

Low-signal areas on T1WI within the marrow of mandibular condyle may represent above two conditions. Increased signal on T2 WI may indicate presence of edema and may be a precursor of osteonecrosis. The probable precipitating factors are local trauma and disc displacement[72] **(Fig. 46)**. Loose bodies may be seen within the joint in osteochondritis dissecans as hypointense structures.

POSTOPERATIVE IMAGING

Magnetic resonance is valuable in demonstrating joint mobility and postoperative adhesions/fibrosis after disc repositioning surgery and discectomy and also for evaluation of alloplastic implants. Contrast administration may be useful in postoperative evaluations of the joint.

EVALUATION OF MANDIBULAR ASYMMETRY

This is multifactorial and could be due to trauma or internal derangement. Unilateral condylar hyperplasia on long side may be seen in these patients.[73] In children with facial asymmetry, decreased condylar growth, or degenerative joint changes on short side may be demonstrated in response to displaced disc[74] **(Figs. 48A to C)**.

INFECTIONS AND ARTHRITIDES

Infections of TMJ are rare and seen postoperatively or through spread from adjacent structures, i.e., ear cavity.[75]

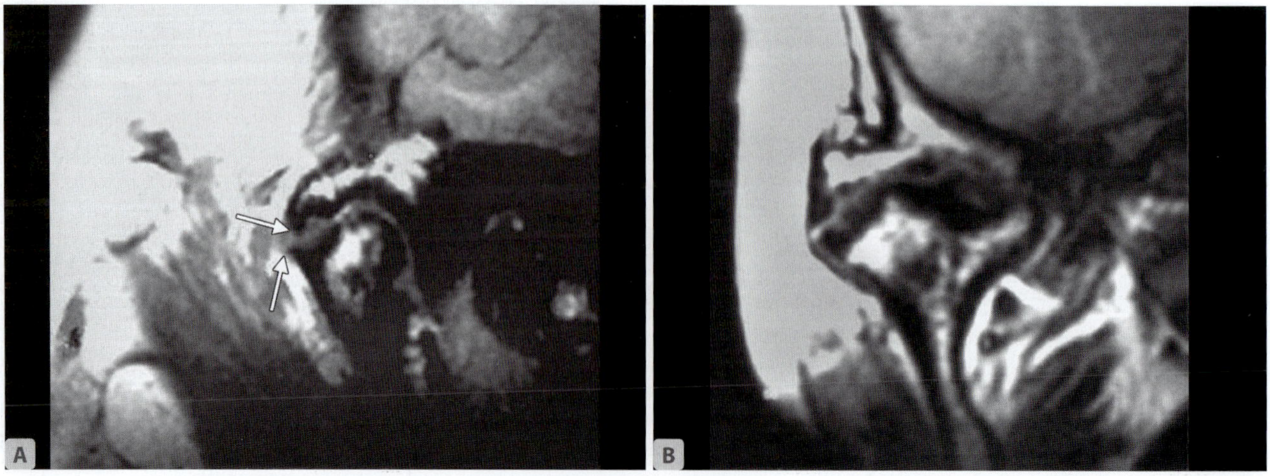

FIGS. 47A AND B: Sagittal (A) and coronal (B) T1-weighted sections: Articular surface irregularity, subchondral sclerosis, and osteophytes (arrows) along anterior glenoid rim and condyle in a case with osteoarthritis of TMJ.

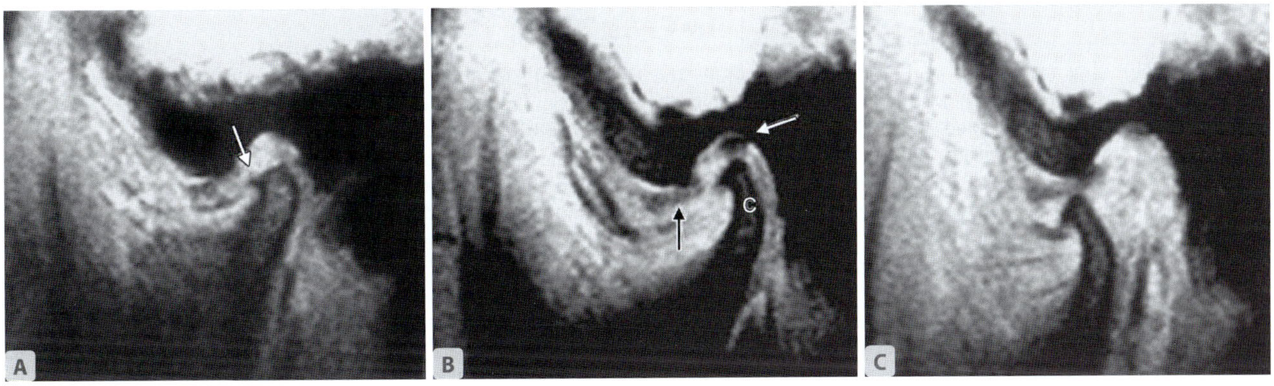

FIGS. 48A TO C: Mandibular asymmetry due to disc dislocation. (A) Right side—closed mouth; (B) Left side—closed mouth; (C) Left side—open mouth. The left condyle is hypoplastic (B). There is anterior dislocation of the disc on this side (black arrow) with fibrosis of posterior attachment (white arrow). The disc is nonreducing (C). The right-sided disc also shows features of degeneration (arrow—A).

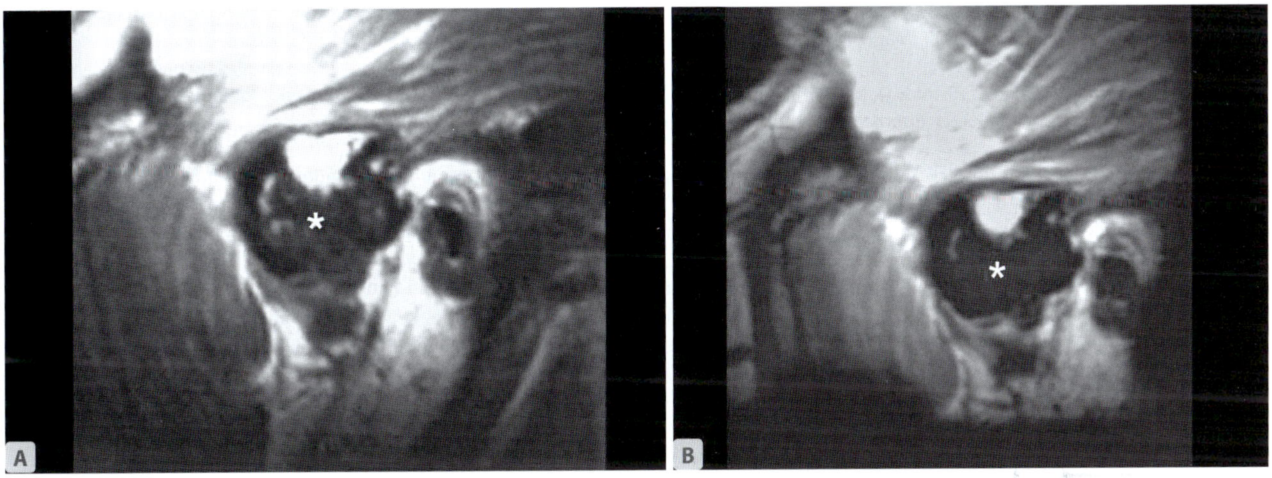

FIGS. 49A AND B: T1WI (A) and T2WI (B) show a densely sclerotic lesion in the articular eminence (asterisk) suggestive of osteoma.

Fluid sensitive sequences (T2 TSE) and postcontrast imaging provide valuable information in infections. TMJ is involved in 50% of patients with RA, ankylosing spondylitis, psoriatic arthritis, and pseudogout. MRI shows soft tissue involvement, erosions, and synovial proliferation.[76]

TUMORS AND TUMOR-LIKE CONDITIONS

Tumors of TMJ region are uncommon and more than two-thirds are benign.[77] Synovial chondromatosis has been reported in TMJ,[78,79] and MR may show joint expansion, synovial thickening with low-intensity foci within it. Osteochondroma is also a common tumor of the mandibular condyle and needs to be differentiated from osteoma and hypertrophic condylar changes **(Figs. 49A and B)**. Pigmented villonodular synovitis is uncommon but reported in TMJ. MR features include synovial thickening/mass with hypointensities on both TI and T2W images **(Fig. 50)**.[80] Metastatic diseases from a remote site (mostly adenocarcinoma from breast) can present around the TMJ in less than 1% cases. Synovial cysts, aneurysmal bone cyst, eosinophilic granuloma, chondrosarcoma, and lymphoma are reported in TMJ or mandibular condyle.[81-82]

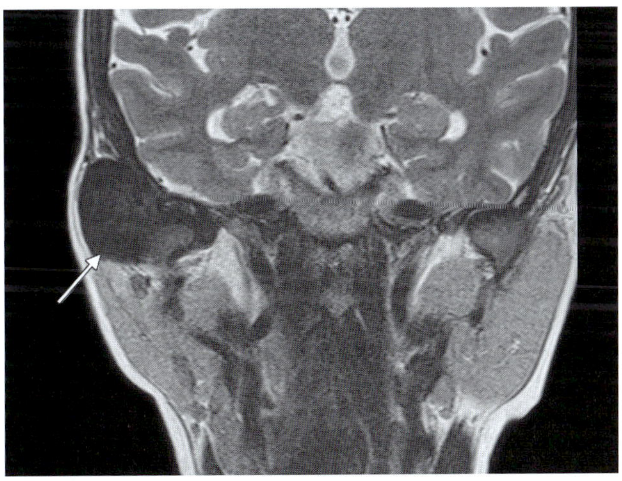

FIG. 50: T2W coronal section shows lobulated hypointense mass in right temporomandibular joint with widened joint space (arrow) suggestive of pigmented villonodular synovitis (PVNS).

REFERENCES

1. Stoller DW, wolf EM, LI AE, Nottage WM, Tirman FJP. The shoulder. In: Stoller DW (Eds). Magnetic Resonance Imaging in Orthopaedics and Sports Medicine, 3rd edition. Philadelphia: Lippincott, Williams and Wilkins; 2007. p. 1131.
2. Mack LA, Matsen FA III, Kilcoyne RF, Davies PK, Sickler ME. US evaluation of rotator cuff. Radiology. 1985;157:205-9.
3. Middleton WD, Edelstein G, Reinus WR, Melson GL, Totty WG, Murphy WA. Sonographic detection of rotator cuff tears. Am J Roentgenol. 1985;144:349-53.
4. Van Holsbeeck M, Strouse PJ. Sonography of the shoulder: Evaluation of the subacromial subdeltoid bursa. AJR Am J Roentgenol. 1993;160:561-4.
5. Martinoli C, Bianchi S, Prato N, Pugliese F, Zamorani MP, Valle M, et al. US of the shoulder: Nonrotator cuff disorders. Radiographics. 2003;23:381-401.
6. Berquist TH. MRI of the Musculoskeletal System, 3rd edition. New York: Raven Press; 1990. pp. 517-607.
7. Cook TS, Stein JM, Simonson S, Kim W. Normal and variant anatomy of the shoulder on MRI. Magn Reson Imaging Clin N Am. 2011;19:595-608.
8. Chung CB, Dwek JR, Feng S, Resnick D. MR arthrography of the glenohumeral joint: A tailored approach. Am J Roentgenol. 2001;177:217-19.
9. Chung CB, Corrente L, Resnick D. MR arthrography of the shoulder joint. MRI Clinics North Am. 2004;12:217-9.
10. Rudez J, Zanetti M. Normal anatomy, variants and pitfalls on shoulder MRI. Eur J Radiol. 2008;68:25-35.
11. Gumina S, Postacchini F, Orsina L, Cinotti G. The morphometry of the coracoid process - its aetiologic role in subcoracoid impingement syndrome. Int Orthop. 1999;23:198-201.
12. Prescher A, Klompen T. The glenoid notch and its relation to the shape of glenoid cavity of the scapula. J Anat. 1997;190:457-60.
13. Bigliani LU, Morrison DS, April EW. Morphology of acromion and its relationship to rotator cuff tears. Orthop Trans. 1986;10:228.
14. Neer CS. Anterior acromioplasty for the chronic impingement syndrome: A preliminary report. J Bone Joint Surg (Am). 1972;54:41-50.
15. Seeger LL, Gold RH, Bassett LW, Ellman H. Shoulder impingement syndrome: MR findings in 53 shoulders. AJR Am J Roentgenol. 1988;150:343-7.
16. Carrino JA, McCauley TR, Katz LD, Smith RC, Lange RC. Rotator cuff: Evaluation with fast spin echo versus conventional spin echo imaging. Radiology. 1997;202:533-9.
17. Zlatkin MB, Reicher MA, Kellerhouse ME, McDade W, Vetter L, Resnick D. The painful shoulder: MR imaging of the glenohumeral joint. J Comput Assist Tomogr. 1988;12:995-1001.
18. Mirowitz SA. Normal rotator cuff: MR imaging with conventional and fat suppression techniques. Radiology. 1991;180:735-40.
19. Zlatkin MB, Iannotti JP, Roberts MC, Esterhai JL, Dalinka MK, Kressel HY, et al. Rotator cuff tears: Diagnostic performance of MR imaging: Comparison with arthrography and correlation with surgery. Radiology. 1989;172:223-9.
20. Hoddler J, Kursunoglu-Brahme S, Syndler SJ, Cervilla V, Karzel RP, Schweitzer ME, et al. Rotator cuff disease: Assessment with MR arthrography versus standard MR imaging in 36 patients with arthroscopic confirmation. Radiology. 1992;182:431-3.
21. Turkel SJ, Panio MW, Marshal JL, Girgis FG. Stabilizing mechanisms preventing anterior dislocation of the glenohumeral joint. J Bone Joint Surg Am. 1981;63:1208-17.
22. Cleeman E, Flatow EL. Shoulder dislocations in the young patient. Orthop Clin North Am. 2000;3:217-29.
23. Kwak SM, Brown RR, Trudell D, Resnick D. Glenohumeral joint: Comparison of shoulder positions at MR arthrography. Radiology. 1998;208:375-80.
24. Palmer WE, Caslowitz PL. Anterior shoulder instability: Diagnostic criteria determined from prospective analysis of 121 MR arthrograms. Radiology. 1995;197:819-25.
25. Garneau RA, Renfrew DL, Moore TE, el-Khoury GY, Nepola JV, Lemke JH. Glenoid labrum: Evaluation with MR imaging. Radiology. 1991;179:519-22.
26. Legan JM, Burkhard TK, Goff WB II, Balsara ZN, Martinez AJ, Burks DD, et al. Tears of the glenoid labrum: MR imaging of 88 arthroscopically confirmed cases. Radiology. 1991;179:241-6.
27. Chandnani VP, Yeager TD, De Berardino T, Christensen K, Gagliardi JA, Heitz DR, et al. Glenoid labral tears: Prospective evaluation with MR imaging, MR arthrography and CT arthrography. Am J Roentgenol. 1993;161:1229-53.
28. Richards RD, Sartoris DJ, Pathria MN, Resnick D. Hill Sach's lesion and normal humeral groove: MR imaging features allowing their differentiation. Radiology. 1994;190:665-8.
29. Sugaya H, Moriishi J, Dohi M, Kon Y, Tsuchiya A. Glenoid rim morphology in recurrent anterior glenohumeral instability. J Bone Joint Surg Am. 2003;85:878-84.
30. Sanders TG, Tirman PF, Linares R, Feller JF, Richardson R. The glenolabral articular disruption lesion: MR arthrography with arthroscopic correlation. Am J Roentgenol. 1999;172:171-5.
31. Levine WN, Flatow EL. The pathophysiology of shoulder instability. Am J Sports Med. 2000;28:910-7.
32. Bui-Mansfield LT, Taylor DC, Uhorchak JM, Tenuta JJ. Humeral avulsions of the glenohumeral ligament: Imaging features and a review of the literature. AJR Am J Roentgenol. 2002;179:649-55.
33. Mosley HF, Overgaard B. The anterior capsular mechanism in recurrent anterior dislocation of the shoulder morphological and clinical studies with special reference to glenoid labrum and the glenohumeral ligaments. J Bone Joint Surg. 1962;44:913-27.
34. Bigoni JB, Christine B, Chung MD. MR imaging of the rotator cuff interval. Magn Reson Imaging Clin North Am. 2004;12:61-73.
35. Snyder Sj, Karzel RP, Del Pizzo, Ferkel RD, Friedman MJ. SLAP lesions of the shoulder. Arthroscopy. 1990;6:274-9.
36. Pfirrman CWA, Zannette M, Weishaupt D, Gerber C, Hodler J. Subscapularis tendon tears: Detection and grading at MR arthrography. Radiology. 1999;213:709-14.
37. Tung GA, Hou DD. MR arthrography of the posterior labrocapsular complex: Relationship with glenohumeral joint alignment and clinical posterior instability. Am J Roentgenol. 2003;180:369-75.
38. Stoller W. MR arthrography of the glenohumeral joint. Radiolol Clin North Am. 1997;35:97-116.
39. Jee WH, McCauley TR, Kalz LD, Matheny JM, Ruwe PA, Daigneault JP. Superior labral anterior posterior (SLAP) lesions of the glenoid labrum: Reliability and accuracy of MR arthrography for diagnosis. Radiology. 2001;218:127-32.
40. Erickson SJ, Fitzgerald SW, Quinn SF, Carrera GF, Black KP, Lawson TL. Long bicipital tendon of the shoulder: Normal anatomy and pathologic findings on MR imaging. Am J Roentgenol. 1992;158:1091-6.
41. Bennet WF. Visualisation of the anatomy of the rotator interval and bicipital sheath. Arthroscopy. 2001;17:107-11.
42. Linker CS, Helms CA, Fritz RC. Quadrilateral space syndrome: Findings at MR imaging. Radiology. 1993;188:675-6.
43. Fritz RC, Helms CA, Steinback LS, Genant HK. Suprascapular nerve entrapment: Evaluation with MR imaging. Radiology. 1992;183:437.

44. Emig EW, Schweitzer ME, Karasick D, Lubowitz J. Adhesive capsulitis of the shoulder: MR diagnosis. Am J Roentgenol. 1995;164:1457-9.
45. Rockwood C, Uhthoff HK, Dervin G, et al. Calcifying tendinitis. In: Rockwood C, Matsen III F, Wirth M, Lippt S (Eds). The Shoulder, 3rd edition. Philadelphia: Saunders; 2004. p. 1033.
46. Lee E, Flatow, E. The shoulder and arm. In: Weinstein S, Buckwalter J (Eds). Turek' Orthopedics, 6th edition. Philadelphia: Lippinkot Williams and Wilkins; 2005. p. 345.
47. Learch TJ, Farooki S. Magnetic resonance imaging of septic arthritis. Clin Imaging. 2000;24:336-42.
48. Alasaarela E, Suramo I, Tervonen O, Lähde S, Takalo R, Hakala M. Evaluation of humeral head erosions in rheumatoid arthritis: A comparison of ultrasonography, magnetic resonance imaging, computed tomography and plain radiography. Br J Rheumatol. 1998;37:1152-6.
49. Neer CS. Shoulder Reconstruction. Philadelphia: WB Saunders; 1990. p. 194.
50. Enzinger FM, Weiss SW. Soft Tissue Tumors. St. Louis, MO: CV Mosby; 1983.
51. Gottsegen CJ, Merkle AN, Bencardino JT, Gyftopoulos S. Advanced MRI techniques of the shoulder joint: Current applications in clinical practice. Am J Roentgenol. 2017;209(3):544-51.
52. Gyftopoulos S, Yemin A, Mulholland T, Bloom M, Storey P, Geppert C, et al. 3DMR osseous reconstruction of the shoulder using a gradient-echo based two-point Dixon reconstruction: A feasibility study. Skeletal Radiol. 2013;42:347-52
53. Gyftopoulos S1, Beltran LS, Yemin A, Strauss E, Meislin R, Jazrawi L, et al. Use of 3D MR reconstructions in the evaluation of glenoid bone loss: A clinical study. Skeletal Radiol. 2014;43:213-8.
54. Schiefer M, Mendonca R, Maganini MM, Fontenelle C, Pires Carvalho AC, Almeida M, et al. Intraobserver and interobserver agreement of Goutallier classification applied to magnetic resonance images. J Shoulder Elbow Surg. 2015;24:1314-21.
55. Lee YH, Kim S, Lim D, Song H, Suh J. MR quantification of the fatty fraction from T2*-corrected Dixon fat/water separation volume-interpolated breathhold examination (VIBE) in the assessment of muscle atrophy in rotator cuff tears. Acad Radiol. 2015;22:909-91.
56. Nozaki T, Tasaki A, Horiuchi S, Osakabe C, Ohde S, Saida Y, et al. Quantification of fatty degeneration within the supraspinatus muscle by using a 2-point Dixon method on 3-TMRI. Am J Roentgenol. 2015;205:116-22.
57. Burkhart SS, Danaceau SM, Pearce CE. Arthroscopic rotator cuff repair: Analysis of results by tear size and by repair technique—margin convergence versus direct tendon to bone repair. Arthroscopy. 2001;17:905-12.
58. Davidson JF, Burkhart SS, Richards DP, Campbell SE. Use of pre-operative magnetic resonance imaging to predict rotator cuff tear pattern and method of repair. Arthroscopy. 2005;21:1428.
59. Furukawa R, Morihara T, Arai Y, Ito H2, Kida Y1, Sukenari T, et al. Diagnostic accuracy of magnetic resonance imaging for subscapularis tendon tears using radial-slice magnetic resonance images. J Shoulder Elbow Surg. 2014;23:e283-90.
60. Budzik JF, Balbi V, Verclytte S, Pansini V, Le Thuc V, Cotten A. Diffusion tensor imaging in musculoskeletal disorders. Radiographics. 2014;34:E56-72.
61. Guralnick W, Kaban LB, Merrill RG. Temporomandibular joints afflictions. N Engl J Med. 1978;299:123-9.
62. Tomas X, Pomes J, Berenguer J, Quinto L, Nicolau C, Mercader JM, et al. MR imaging of temporomandibular joint dysfunction: A pictorial review. Radiographics. 2006;26:765-81.
63. Yale SH. Radiographic evaluation of the temporomandibular joint. J Am Dent Assoc. 1969;79:102-7.
64. Hansson T, Nordström B. Thickness of soft tissue layers and articular disc in the temporomandibular joint. Acta Odontol Scand. 1977;35:77-83.
65. Paesani D, Westesson PL, Hatala M, Tallents RH, Kurita K. Prevalence of internal derangement in patients with craniomandibular disorders. Am J Orthod Dentofacial Orthop. 1992;101: 41-7.
66. Katzberg RW, Westesson PL, Tallents RH, Anderson R, Kurita K, Manzione JV Jr, et al. Temporomandibular joint: MR assessment of rotational and sideways disc displacements. Radiology. 1988;169:741-8.
67. Wikes CH. Arthrography of the temporomandibular joint in patients with temporomandibular joint pain dysfunction syndrome. Minn Med. 1978;39:319-23.
68. Farrar WB. Characteristics of the condylar path in internal derangement of the TMJ. J Prosthet Dent. 1978;39:319-23.
69. Wikes CH. Internal derangement of the temporomandibular joint: Pathological variations. Arch Otolaryng Head Neck Surg. 1989;115:469-77.
70. Hasso AN, Christiansen EL, Alder ME. The temporomandibular joint. Radiol Clin North Am. 1989;27:301.
71. Westesson PL, Bronstein SL, Leidberg JL. Internal derangement of the temporomandibular joint: Morphological description with correlation to joint function. Oral Surg Oral Med Oral Path. 1985;59:323-31.
72. Schellhas KP, Wikes CH, Fritts HM, Omlie MR, Lagrotteria LB. MR of osteochondritis dissecans and avascular necrosis of the mandibular condyle. AJNR. 1989;10:3-12.
73. Jonck LM. Facial asymmetry and condylar hyperplasia. Oral Surg Oral Med Oral Pathol. 1975;40:567-73.
74. Katzberg RW, Tallents RH, Hayakawa K, Miller TL, Goske MJ, Wood BP. Internal derangements of the temporomandibular joint: Findings in paediatric age group. Radiology. 1985;154: 125-7.
75. Thomson HG. Septic arthritis of the temporomandibular joint complicating otitis externa. J Otolaryngol Otol. 1989;103: 319-21.
76. Smith HJ, Larheim TA, Aspestrand F. Rheumatic and non-rheumatic disease in the temporomandibular joint: Gadolinium enhanced MR imaging. Radiology. 1992;185:229-34.
77. Poveda-Roda R, Bagán JV, Sanchis JM, Margaix M. Pseudotumors and tumors of the temporomandibular joint: A review. Med Oral Patol Oral Cir Bucal. 2013;18:e392-402.
78. Heffez LB. Imaging of internal derangements and synovial chondromatosis of the temporomandibular joint. Radiol Clin North Am. 1993;31:149-62.
79. Benslama L, Schouman T, Toure S, Chardain J, Goudot P. Synovial chondromatosis of the temporomandibular joint: Report and analysis of 12 cases. J Stomatol Oral Maxillofac Surg. 2019;120(5):476-9.
80. Bravo SM, Winalski CS, Weissman BN. Pigmented villonodular synovitis. Radiol Clin North Am. 1996;34: 311-26.
81. Rai KK, Dharmendrashinh R, Shiva Kumar HR. Aneurysmal bone cyst: A lesion of the mandibular condyle. J Maxillofac OralSurg. 2012;11:238-42.
82. Giorgione C, Passali FM, Varakliotis T, Sibilia M, Ottaviani F. Temporo-mandibular joint chondrosarcoma: Case report and review of the literature. Acta Otorhinolaryngol Ital. 2015;35(3):208-11.

CHAPTER

168

Magnetic Resonance Imaging of Wrist

Anindita Sinha, Harish Bhujade, Mahesh Prakash

INTRODUCTION

Wrist is composed of complex joint formed by small bones, ligaments, tendons, and cartilage. Magnetic resonance imaging (MRI) is an important diagnostic tool in evaluation of common wrist disorders and ligamentous injuries. For accurate diagnosis of various pathologies of wrist, it is important to know detailed anatomy of wrist.

BONES AND JOINTS

Wrist is formed by distal radius and ulna, eight carpal bones and bases of metacarpals. The proximal row is formed by scaphoid, lunate, triquetrum, and pisiform; the distal row is formed by trapezium, trapezoid, capitate, and hamate (from lateral to medial). The distal ends of radius and ulna form the distal radioulnar joint (DRUJ). The radius has a triangular articular surface for the scaphoid and a quadrilateral articular surface for the lunate at its distal end to form the radiocarpal joint.

The two rows of carpal bones form *Gilula's arc*, which comprised of Arc I along the proximal surfaces of proximal carpal bones (scaphoid, lunate, and triquetral), Arc II along the distal surfaces of these proximal carpal bones, and Arc III along the proximal surfaces of capitate and hamate **(Fig. 1)**.[1]

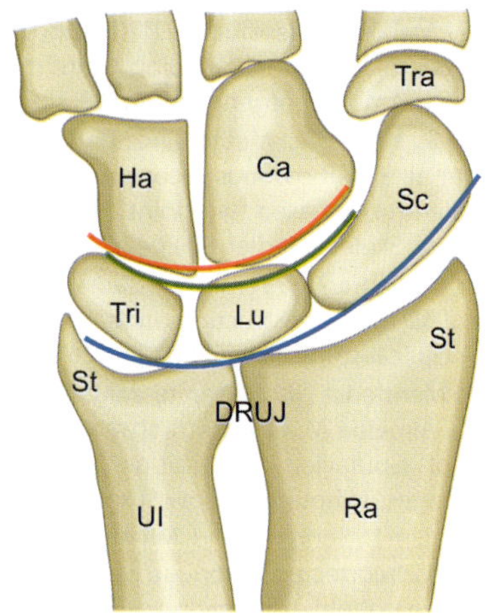

FIG. 1: Bones of the wrist with carpal bones forming the three arcs of Gilula. Proximal row (blue) is formed by the proximal articulating surfaces of scaphoid (Sc), lunate (Lu), and triquetral (Tri). The II arc (green) is formed by the distal articulating surfaces of the proximal carpal bones. The III arc (red) is formed by the proximal articulating surface of capitate (Ca) and hamate (Ha). The radius (Ra), ulna (Ul), and the styloid processes (St) and the distal radioulnar joint (DRUJ) are shown. Note the neutral ulnar variance.

Ulnar Variance or Hulten Variance

It is the difference in lengths of articular surfaces of distal ends of radius and ulna.[2] This can be neutral when both articular surfaces are at the same level, negative (ulnar articular surface >2 mm proximal to the radial articular surface), and positive (ulnar articular surface >2 mm distal to radial articular surface) **(Figs. 2A to C)**.

Ligaments of Wrist

For convenience, the wrist ligaments are grouped into intrinsic ligaments, extrinsic ligaments, and ligaments of thumb.

Intrinsic ligaments attach only to carpal bones and include scapholunate ligament, lunotriquetral ligament, and triangular fibrocartilage complex (TFCC) **(Fig. 3)**.

Extrinsic ligaments attach to other structures besides carpal bones. These are further divided into volar extrinsic and dorsal extrinsic ligaments.

- *Volar extrinsic ligaments* consist of volar radioscaphocapitate, volar radiotriquetral, volar ulnolunate, volar ulnotriquetral, and volar radioulnar ligaments.
- *Dorsal extrinsic ligaments* consist of dorsal intercarpal, dorsal radiotriquetral, and dorsal radioulnar ligaments.

Scapholunate Ligament (Fig. 3)

Scapholunate ligament is a U-shaped ligament and has three components—Volar, dorsal, and interosseous.[3] The volar component, which courses obliquely, is thinner (1 mm in thickness) and weaker. The dorsal component is the thickest component (3 mm). The volar and dorsal components are best seen on axial images, appearing as

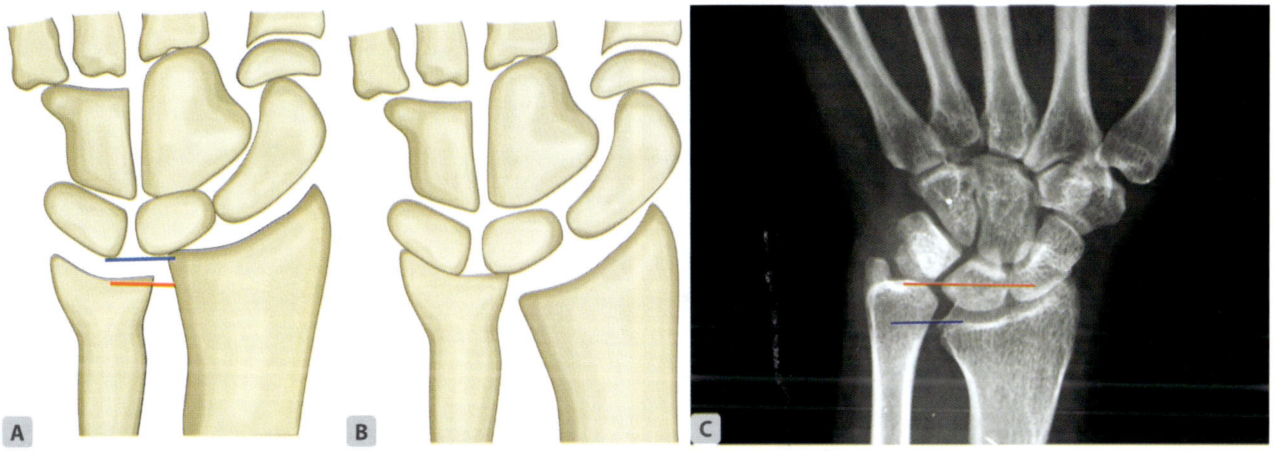

FIGS. 2A TO C: Ulnar variance. Ulnar variance is measured as the distance between two lines, one drawn tangential to the lunate fossa of radius (blue line) and another drawn tangential to the ulnar articular surface of ulna. (A) Negative ulnar variance with a short ulna; (B) Positive ulnar variance with ulna longer than the distal radius; (C) Radiograph of the wrist showing positive ulnar variance.

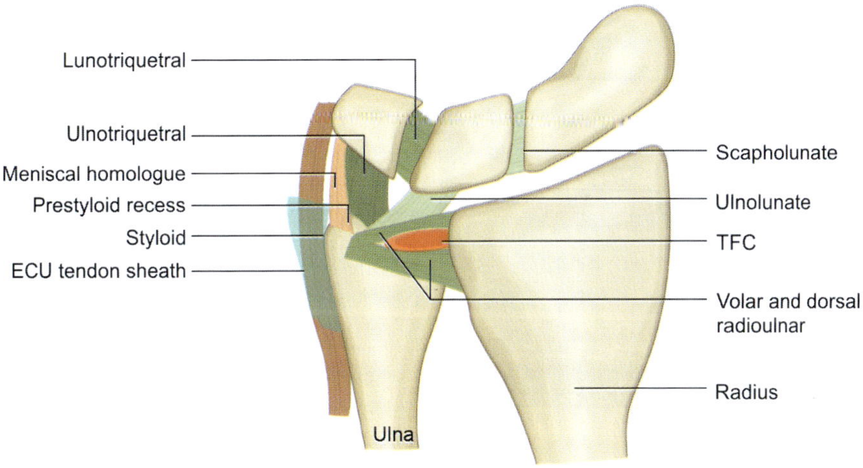

FIG. 3: Components of triangular fibrocartilage complex. The triangular articular disc (TFC disc proper), the volar, and dorsal radioulnar ligaments, the ulnolunate ligament, the ulnotriquetral ligament, the ulnar collateral ligament, the meniscus homologue, and part of the sheath of the extensor carpi ulnaris tendon. The scapholunate and lunotriquetral ligaments are also shown. (ECU: extensor carpi ulnaris; TFC: triangular fibrocartilage).

band-like structures, the dorsal showing homogeneous-signal intensity and the volar showing heterogeneous-signal intensity. The interosseous component is best viewed on coronal sections. It appears band-like at its dorsal aspect, triangular at its central aspect, and trapezoidal at its volar aspect.

Lunotriquetral Ligament (Fig. 3)

Lunotriquetral ligament appears V-shaped and has volar, dorsal, and proximal components. The dorsal component is important for carpal stability and resistance to rotation.[3] The volar and dorsal components appear band-like on axial images.

Triangular Fibrocartilage Complex (Fig. 3)

Triangular fibrocartilage complex lies between the distal end of ulna and proximal carpal bones (lunate and triquetral). It consists of a triangular articular disc [triangular fibrocartilage (TFC) disc proper], dorsal radioulnar ligament, volar radioulnar ligament, ulnolunate ligament, ulnotriquetral ligament, ulnar collateral ligament, meniscus homologue, and part of the sheath of the extensor carpi ulnaris (ECU) tendon. The appearance of TFCC varies with ulnar variance. It is thicker and short with negative ulnar variance and thin and stretched with positive ulnar variance.

Triangular fibrocartilage disc appears as an asymmetric bowtie structure, which is best seen on coronal sections as a low-signal intensity structure on all pulse sequences. The triangular ligament has two bands, which attach the disc proper to the tip and fovea of the styloid process of ulna **(Figs. 4A to C)**. The vascularized tissue between the two bands is called the ligamentum subcruentum. TFC is supplied by the palmar and dorsal branches of the anterior interosseous artery and branch of the ulnar artery. The central and radial part of TFC is avascular while the periphery is vascularized. The tears of the vascularized part of TFC get healed while those of the central and radial part do not heal.[3]

The meniscal homologue appears as a triangular fat intensity structure between the ulnar styloid and triquetrum.

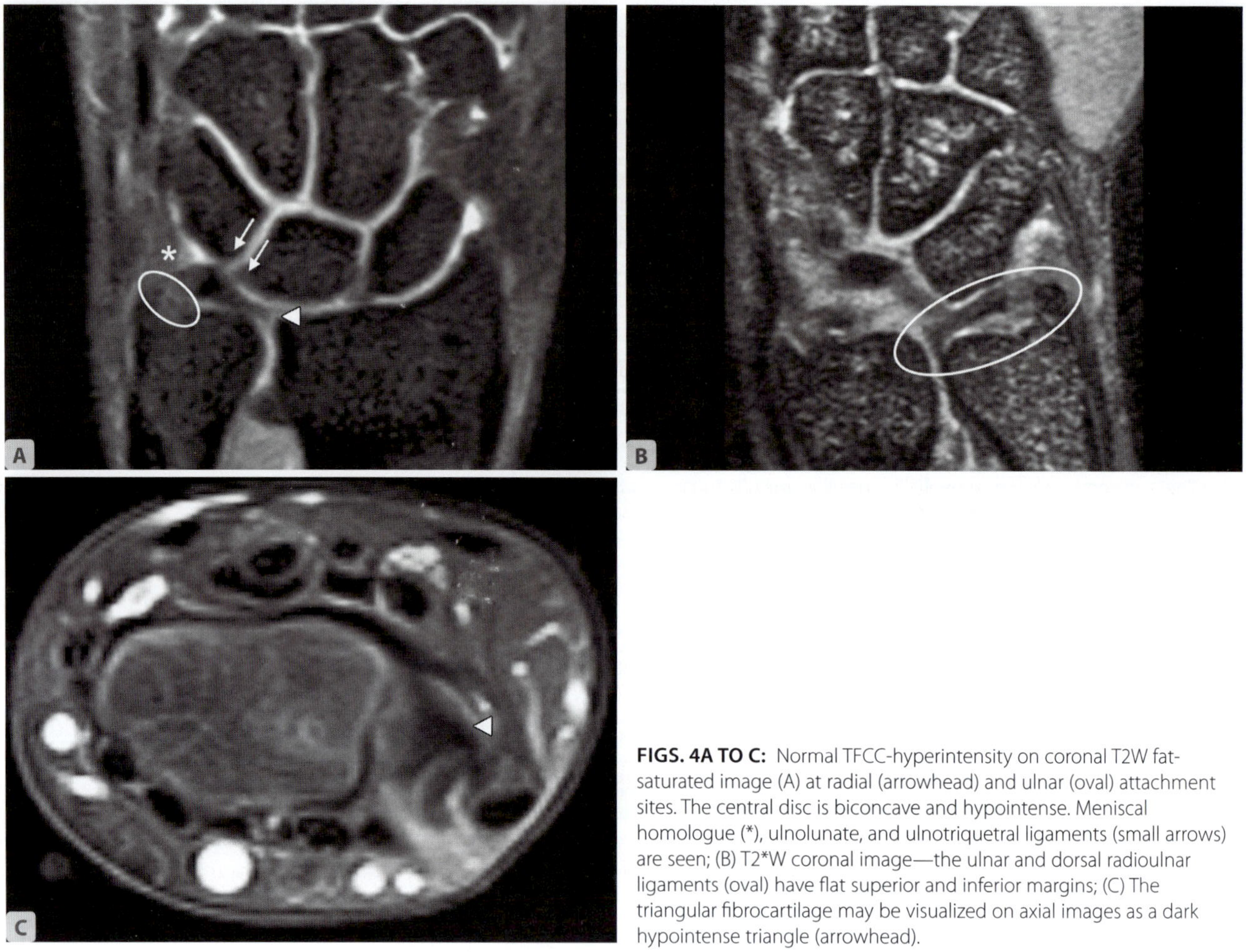

FIGS. 4A TO C: Normal TFCC-hyperintensity on coronal T2W fat-saturated image (A) at radial (arrowhead) and ulnar (oval) attachment sites. The central disc is biconcave and hypointense. Meniscal homologue (*), ulnolunate, and ulnotriquetral ligaments (small arrows) are seen; (B) T2*W coronal image—the ulnar and dorsal radioulnar ligaments (oval) have flat superior and inferior margins; (C) The triangular fibrocartilage may be visualized on axial images as a dark hypointense triangle (arrowhead).

It joins the ECU tendon sheath and joint capsule to form a ligamentous stabilizer.[4]

The radioulnar ligaments (dorsal and volar) are the main stabilizers of the wrist and DRUJ. It has superficial and deep fibers, both arising from the ulnar side of the distal radius at the sigmoid notch. The deep fibers insert on the fovea of the styloid process of ulna and are most important for joint stability, and the superficial fibers attach to the tip of the ulnar styloid.[5]

The volar ulnolunate ligament arises from the volar radioulnar ligament. It attaches distally to the lunate, parallel to the long axis of the wrist and forearm. Some of its fibers also attaches to the lunotriquetral ligament. The volar ulnotriquetral ligament also arises at the volar radioulnar ligament, medial to the volar ulnolunate ligament. This ligament then broadens and attaches on the triquetrum. Both these volar ligaments can be best seen on coronal images. The volar radioscaphocapitate ligament arises from the radial styloid and courses distally and medially to the capitate. Few of its fibers attach to the waist of scaphoid.

The volar radiolunate ligament also arises from the radial styloid, adjacent to the radioscaphocapitate ligament origin. The volar radiolunate ligament extends obliquely to attach on the lunate.

The dorsal radiotriquetral ligament arises from the dorsal styloid process of radius and attaches to the dorsal tubercle of the triquetrum. It courses in an oblique fashion, attaching and crossing the medial aspect of the lunate. The dorsal intercarpal ligament spans from the dorsal tubercle of the triquetrum to the dorsal groove of the scaphoid. The dorsal radiotriquetral and dorsal intercarpal ligaments are best evaluated on coronal images.[3]

Extensor Compartment (Fig. 5)

The extensor retinaculum stretches between the ulnar styloid process, the medial margin of pisiform and triquetrum, and the lateral radius margin. From the radial to the ulnar side, the extensor tendons are arranged under the extensor retinaculum into six extensor compartments. The extensor tendons are best evaluated on axial images.

1. *Compartment I:* The abductor pollicis longus (APL) and extensor pollicis brevis (EPB) tendons
2. *Compartment II:* The extensor carpi radialis longus and brevis tendons
3. *Compartment III:* The extensor pollicis longus (EPL) tendon
4. *Compartment IV:* The extensor digitorum and indices tendons

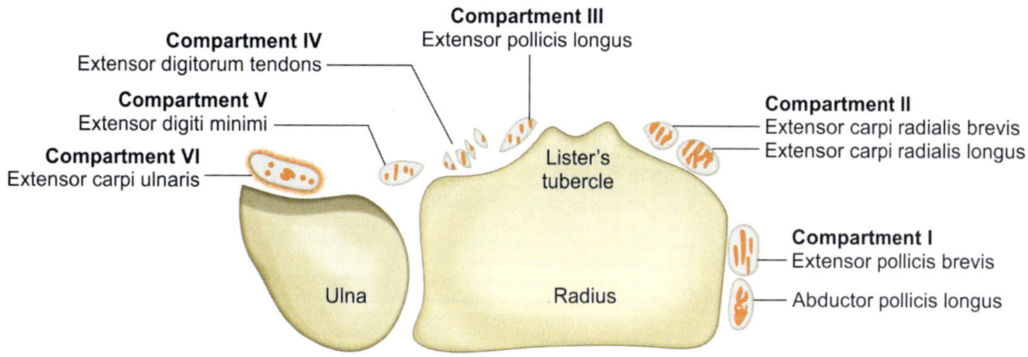

FIG. 5: From the radial to the ulnar side, the extensor tendons are arranged under the extensor retinaculum into six extensor compartments. Lister's tubercle is a landmark dividing compartments II and III.

5. *Compartment V:* The extensor digiti minimi tendon
6. *Compartment VI:* The ECU tendon.

Flexor Compartment (Figs. 6A to C)

A total of nine tendons traverse the carpal tunnel passing under the flexor retinaculum, which includes the four deep flexor digitorum profundus (FDP) tendons, the four superficial flexor digitorum superficialis (FDS) tendons, and the single flexor pollicis longus (FPL) tendon.

- *Guyon's canal* is a small anatomic space containing the ulnar nerve.
- *The medial border:* Pisiform bone and the hook of the hamate
- *The roof:* The palmar carpal ligament, palmar fascia, and palmaris brevis muscle
- *The floor:* FDP tendons, transverse carpal ligament (flexor retinaculum), pisohamate and pisometacarpal ligaments, and opponens digiti minimi muscle
- *Contents:* Ulnar nerve and vessels.

Carpal Tunnel (Figs. 6A to C)

Carpal tunnel is formed on the volar aspect of the wrist joint by the flexor retinaculum (transverse carpal ligament) forming the fibrous roof. The floor is formed by the carpal bones. The flexor retinaculum attaches to the scaphoid proximally on the radial side and tubercle of trapezium distally. The retinaculum attaches to the pisiform proximally and hook of hamate distally on the ulnar side.

The carpal tunnel contains the median nerve, the flexor tendons (four each of FDS and FDP surrounded by a single synovial sheath), and the FPL in a separate synovial sheath.

IMAGING TECHNIQUE OF WRIST

Magnetic Resonance Imaging

The wrist can be imaged at 1.5 Tesla. The 3 Tesla scanner is preferable for high-resolution imaging of the small intrinsic ligamentous structures of the wrist.[6]

Positioning

Patients can be placed in prone position with arms outstretched above the level of head (Superman position).

Patients unable to stay in this position can stay in supine position with hand beside the body. In this position, a single hand and wrist can be imaged by a phased array coil; however, image quality including fat suppression may be suboptimal due to distance of wrist and hand from the isocenter of the magnet. Additional manual shimming and use of fat suppression techniques such as IDEAL (iterative decomposition of water and fat with echo asymmetry and least-squares estimation) can overcome these problems.[6]

Coil

A dedicated 8–16-channel wrist (surface) coil is ideal for wrist. Small flex or loop coils can be used for cases where only a small field of view is needed for imaging of a dedicated structure. These coils can be closely wrapped around the anatomical part to be imaged.

The suggested protocol is given in **Table 1**.

Sequences are given in **Table 2**.

The three-dimensional fast spin-echo (3D FSE) isotropic sequences are better than GRE for cartilage, ligament, and osseous evaluation. These techniques can be quickened by parallel imaging, driven equilibrium techniques, compressed SENSE, or variable flip angles of the radiofrequency (RF) refocusing pulse [e.g., SPACE (Sampling Perfection with Application optimized Contrasts using different flip angle Evolution), CUBE, VISTA (volume isotropic turbo spin-echo acquisition) are techniques in various scanners].[7]

Cartilage Imaging

Cartilage imaging has the potential of early detection of degenerative changes and tears of TFCC and articular cartilage of carpal bones. Preliminary studies have suggested changes in T1rho (T1ρ) and T2 relaxation times in torn ligaments and in degenerative and inflammatory conditions, as well as changes in response to different medications in inflammatory arthritis.[8,9]

Magnetic Resonance Arthrography of Wrist

Magnetic resonance arthrography of wrist can be single-compartmental (most commonly radiocarpal), two-compartmental, or rarely three-compartmental (radiocarpal, DRUJ, and midcarpal) arthrography. The fluoroscopic guidance is used for injections into the joint. The dorsal

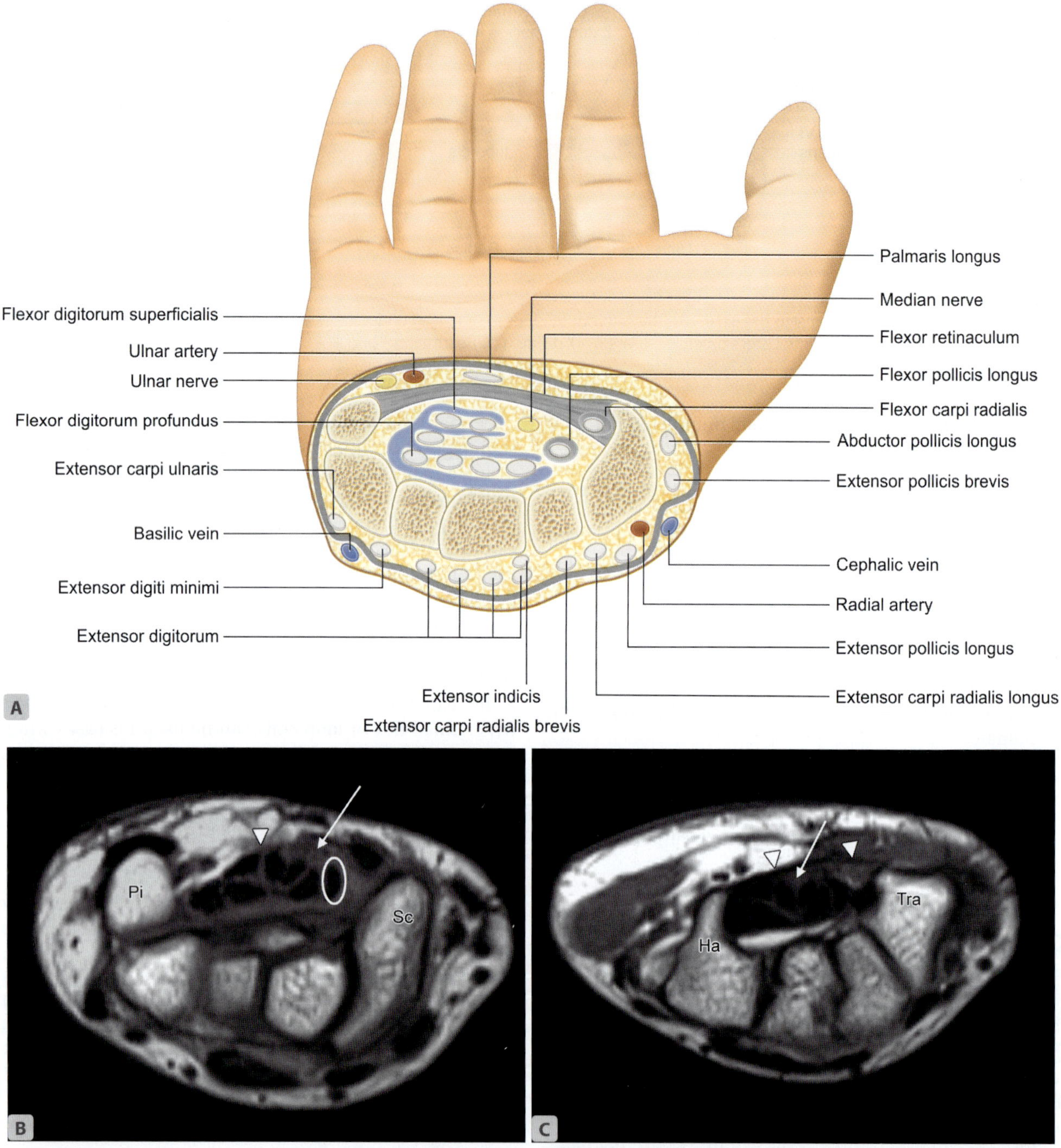

FIGS. 6A TO C: (A) Carpal tunnel and Guyon's canal. Normal magnetic resonance (MR) anatomy of the carpal tunnel; Axial T1W MR images at the level of pisiform (B) and at the level of hook of hamate (C) show the fibro-osseous carpal tunnel bounded by the carpal bones posteriorly, by the pisiform and hook of hamate on the ulnar side, and the scaphoid and tubercle of trapezium on the radial side. Superiorly, the hypointense linear flat flexor retinaculum (arrowheads) forms the roof of the carpal tunnel. The hypointense flexor digitorum superficialis and profundus tendons and the fasciculated speckled median nerve (arrow) are seen traversing the tunnel. The tendon of flexor pollicis longus (oval) is deep to the median nerve.

approach is commonly used for radiocarpal injections. The lateral approach can be used for radiocarpal injections.[10] The radiocarpal joint is visualized, and skin surface is marked at the level of the midscaphoid. Local anesthesia is given with a 22–26 gauge, hypodermic needle on the dorsum of the wrist. 3-5 mL of 1:1 contrast media (diluted iodinated contrast and gadolinium) is injected till the resistance is felt under fluoroscopic/cine guidance after advancing the needle into radiocarpal joint.

The dorsal approach can also be used for midcarpal and DRUJ injections. For midcarpal injections, the needle is advanced into the central part of the junction of the hamate, lunate, capitate, and triquetrum. For DRUJ injection, the needle extends to the radial aspect of the ulnar head.[11]

TABLE 1: MRI protocol planning routine imaging of the wrist.

FOV	8–10 cm
Matrix	416 × 192, 224 × 224 (for 3D sequences)
Slice thickness	2–2.5 mm with no interslice gap
Imaging plane	Axial scout-to-plan coronal (coronal should be the first sequence)
Coronal	Coronal-parallel to ulnar and radial styloid process [coverage from bases of metacarpals to distal radioulnar joint (DRUJ)]
Axial	Coronal scout-to-plan axial
	Axial images should include carpometacarpal joints and DRUJ
Sagittal	Use axial images to plan
	Sagittal images should be perpendicular to volar tips of the scaphoid tubercle and pisiform

(FOV: field of view)

TABLE 2: MRI sequences.

Coronal	• T2 FS • T1 • PD FS* (keep TE at 40, not less for PD sequences)
Axial	• T2 FS • T1
Sagittal	PD FS
Coronal 3D isotropic sequence[7]	T2 *GRE, 3D volumetric FSE PD FS turbo spin echo with <1 mm slice thickness

*Keep TE at 40, not less for PD sequences.
(FS: fat-saturated; FSE: fast spin-echo; GRE: gradient recalled-echo; PD: proton density; TE: echo time)

Indications for MR arthrography include peripheral TFC tears, undersurface TFCC tears as well as for evaluation of the postoperative TFCC where the injection site should be DRUJ. MR arthrography also increases diagnostic confidence in detecting tears of scapholunate and lunotriquetral ligaments.[12]

The contraindications for wrist injections include local skin infections. Pain and swelling may be seen after the injections, which is likely due to overdistension of joints.

Magnetic resonance arthrography is performed after the injections on 1.5 T or higher tesla machine. The position of patient is like conventional MR wrist (superman position). Fat-suppressed (FS) T1 fast spin-echo sequences in axial, coronal, and sagittal planes are acquired with 2 mm slice thickness. Additional sequences, T2 fat-saturated coronal and T1 coronal can be taken.[13]

Scaphoid Fracture

Scaphoid is the most common carpal bone to fracture; 70% of the fractures around the carpal bones are scaphoid fractures.

The mechanism of injury is a fall on the outstretched hand with pain in the anatomical snuffbox.

Fractures through the waist of scaphoid are most common.

Fractures through tubercle of scaphoid and incomplete scaphoid waist fractures are stable. Fractures through proximal pole, fracture dislocations, distal pole oblique fractures, and complete fractures through waist are unstable fractures (Herbert classification) **(Figs. 7A to C)**.

The Russe classification divides the fractures according to the orientation of the fracture line—horizontal oblique, vertical oblique, and transverse. The vertical oblique orientation has the most propensity to displace.[14]

However, none of the classifications can predict nonunion.

Clinical Symptoms

May be minimal with very little restriction of movement, leading to delay in diagnosis as fractures may be radiologically occult.

Radiographs should be obtained in posterior-anterior and lateral views, hand in 45° ulnar deviation and pronation and an oblique view in 45–60° pronation.

Radiologically occult fractures may be evident on computed tomography (CT) or MRI. About 80% of scaphoid is covered by articular cartilage, and the space left for blood supply from the recurrent radial artery branch is minimal. The neglected fractures are at a risk of nonunion due to tenuous blood supply of the scaphoid from the dorsal branch of the radial artery, which enters distal to the waist.[15]

Stable scaphoid fractures are treated conservatively by casts. Delayed union can occur even in stable fractures, which is evident as a persistently visible fracture line 16 weeks after fracture.[16]

Magnetic Resonance Imaging of Scaphoid Injuries

Chronic scaphoid delayed union or nonunion results in sclerosis in radiographs or CT. However, sclerosis does not imply avascular necrosis.

Presence of sclerosis and fluid in the cleft of the fracture fragment are signs of nonunion on MRI **(Figs. 8A to C)**. MRI is superior to CT or bone scintigraphy in detecting possible avascular necrosis due to its superior resolution.

The proximal pole is prone to avascular necrosis in scaphoid waist fractures due to blood supply from the distal pole traversing through the waist to reach the proximal pole.

Magnetic resonance appearance of hypointensity of >50% of the proximal pole on both T1-weighted (T1W) and T2-weighted (T2W) images suggests avascular necrosis.[17]

However, sensitivity and specificity of noncontrast-enhanced MRI is low in detecting avascular necrosis due to a common finding of a heterogeneous signal on T2W images, and hypointensity on both T1W and T2W images also found in ischemic bone (**Figs. 9A to C**).

Hyperintensity on T2W images may also be present in avascular necrosis and hypointensity is seen in only 50% of the cases.[18]

Contrast-enhanced MRI is necessary to distinguish between ischemic and necrotic bone. Complete lack of enhancement on postcontrast fat-saturated T1W images suggests severe ischemia or avascular necrosis.[19]

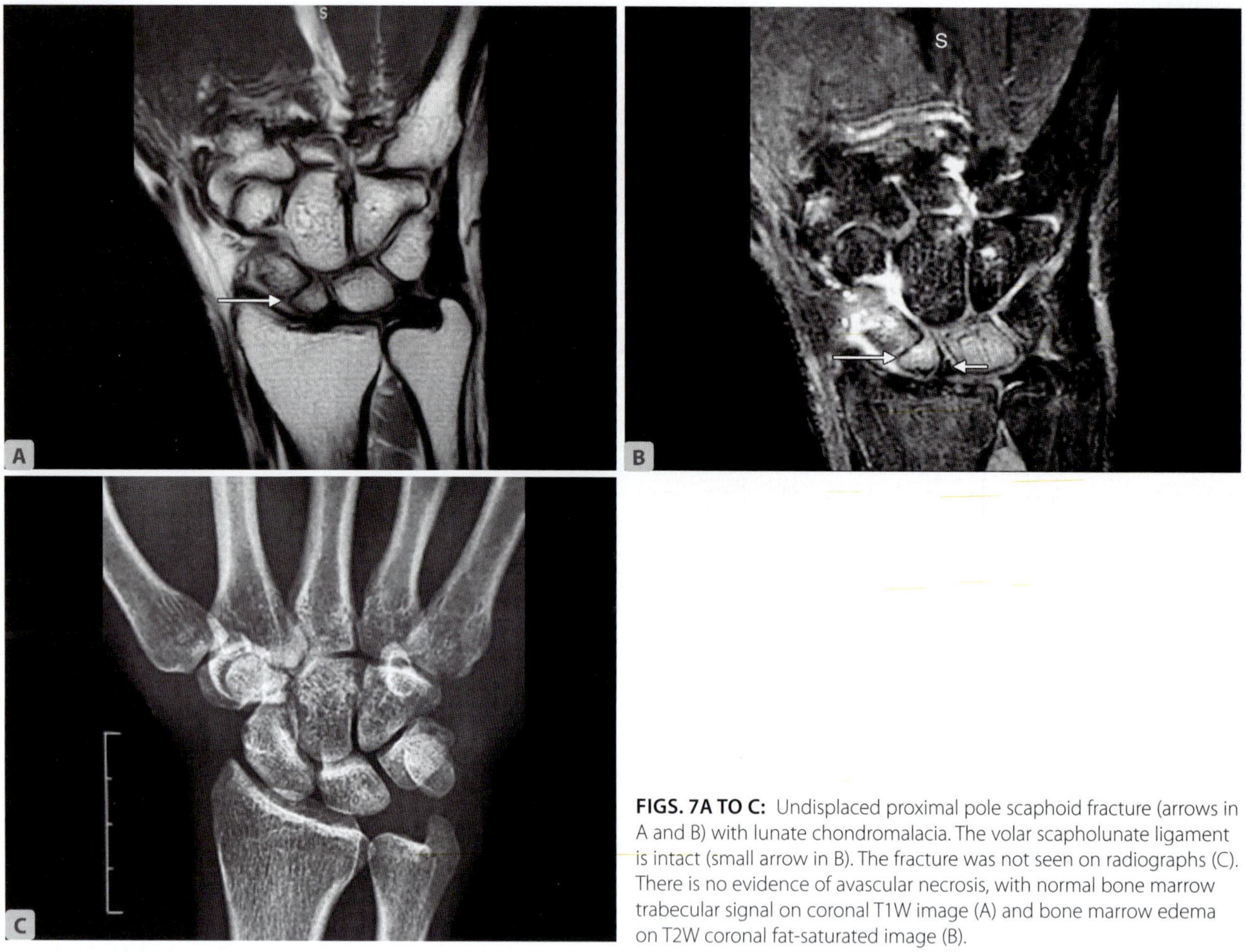

FIGS. 7A TO C: Undisplaced proximal pole scaphoid fracture (arrows in A and B) with lunate chondromalacia. The volar scapholunate ligament is intact (small arrow in B). The fracture was not seen on radiographs (C). There is no evidence of avascular necrosis, with normal bone marrow trabecular signal on coronal T1W image (A) and bone marrow edema on T2W coronal fat-saturated image (B).

However, some patients have increased enhancement of the proximal pole on postcontrast images, possibly due to ingrowth of fibrovascular tissue or diffusion of contrast into necrotic bone from the surrounding tissue.[20]

Diagnostic Algorithm

Recent recommendations in imaging of scaphoid fractures suggest that CT be acquired/reformatted in sagittal-oblique and coronal-oblique planes in cases of normal or equivocal radiographs. CT is better in demonstrating a fracture pattern including fracture orientation and dislocation or fragmentation. However, CT is inferior to MRI in detecting microtrabecular fracture and nondisplaced fractures. MRI is useful in detecting all scaphoid fractures, and additional sequences should be acquired in sagittal-oblique and coronal-oblique planes along long axes of scaphoid. However, diagnostic confusion may persist in cases of bone marrow edema (bone contusion) and nondisplaced fracture.[21]

Fractures of Other Carpal Bones

Fractures of other bones are uncommon. Hook of hamate fractures also occurs due to a fall on the outstretched hand and can occur due to avulsion at the flexor retinaculum attachment site.[15] Hook of hamate fractures can be easily missed on radiographs, where absence of visibility of hook of hamate can be the only sign on routine posteroanterior (PA) views. Ulnar styloid fractures can lead to DRUJ instability, when associated with the base of styloid fractures which disrupt the TFCC. Pisiform is also prone to fractures due to its superficial location and can be detected on routine radiographic views or carpal tunnel view; undiagnosed pisiform fractures lead to pisotriquetral chondromalacia, intra-articular loose bodies, and ulnar nerve impingement.[22]

Kienböck's Disease

Kienböck's disease is referred to avascular necrosis of the lunate bone. It was first described by the Austrian radiologist Robert Kienböck's in 1910.[23]

The etiology of Kienböck's disease is multifactorial. Predisposing factors include trauma, disruption of venous outflow and local vascular anatomy, ulnar variance, metabolic factors, and repetitive mechanical load. A negative ulnar variance has been found in 78% of cases.[24] Type II lunate with an articulating facet with the hamate also shows higher risk of Kienböck's disease **(Figs. 10A and B)**.[25]

The terminal arterial branches without sufficient collateral vessels and cases with a single palmar vessel are more prone to Kienböck's disease **(Table 3)**.

The onset of disease is seen between the ages of 20 and 40 years with a 2:1 ratio of men to women. It commonly affects

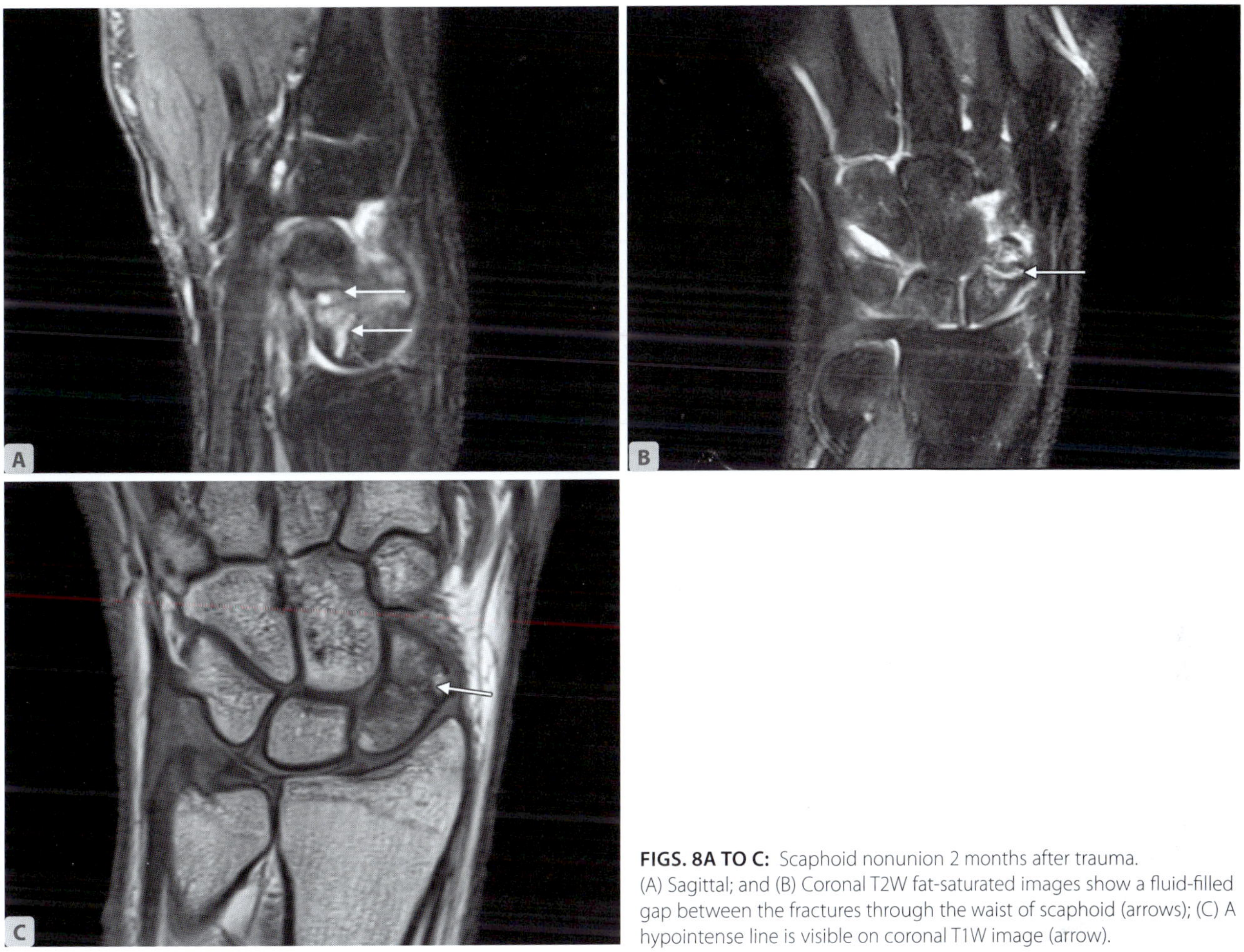

FIGS. 8A TO C: Scaphoid nonunion 2 months after trauma. (A) Sagittal; and (B) Coronal T2W fat-saturated images show a fluid-filled gap between the fractures through the waist of scaphoid (arrows); (C) A hypointense line is visible on coronal T1W image (arrow).

the dominant wrist, but bilateral disease can be seen. The clinical onset can be abrupt or insidious and patients can also remain asymptomatic in the precollapse stage.[26]

Patients present with dorsally located central wrist pain with dorsal tenderness around the lunate, swelling, reduced wrist motion, and grip after acute or repetitive trauma.[27]

Contrast-enhanced MRI helps in differentiation between bone marrow edema and partial or complete necrosis. Enhancement is homogeneous in non-necrotic edematous bone. Partial necrosis shows a heterogeneous enhancement pattern and complete necrosis shows absence of enhancement.[28]

The Lichtman classification may help in treatment decision-making. Options include nonoperative management in early stage disease (stages I to IIIA) to vascularized grafting, proximal row carpectomy, or arthrodesis in late stages (stages IIIB to IV). However, treatment remains controversial and may not alter the natural history of the disease.[29]

Triangular Fibrocartilage Complex Lesions

Triangular fibrocartilage is a hypointense, biconcave, or bow-tie shaped on coronal sections, discoid or biconcave on sagittal, and triangular on axial sections[30] **(Figs. 11A to C)**. The volar and dorsal radioulnar ligaments of the TFCC have parallel upper and lower margins **(Figs. 12A and B)**.

At the radial attachment, minimal hyperintensity due to hyaline cartilage may be seen and may be mistaken for a tear.[30]

At the ulnar attachment, there are two laminae, one from the styloid process of ulna and one from fovea which are striated but hypointense. Intervening ligamentum subcruentum may appear hyperintense normally.

Triangular fibrocartilage complex lesions can occur due to trauma or repetitive overuse. The Palmer classification divides TFCC injuries into two classes—traumatic (Class I) and degenerative (Class II) **(Table 4)**.[22]

However, the Palmer classification does not classify tears of volar or dorsal radioulnar ligaments or subclassify type IB ulnar avulsions further into distal (styloid) avulsions or proximal (foveal) avulsions, which have prognostic and therapeutic significance, since the foveal attachment damage is more disabling and styloid avulsion fractures associated with distal lamina tears can cause instability. Combinations of different tears and partial tears are also common and have not been classified.[31]

Type IA tears are central perforations of the TFC, often found in asymptomatic individuals and do not result in any dysfunction of the DRUJ. Central perforations are seen as fluid-signal intensity or contour irregularity within the central or paracentral portion of the triangular fibrocartilage proper and may be partial-thickness tear of either the proximal or

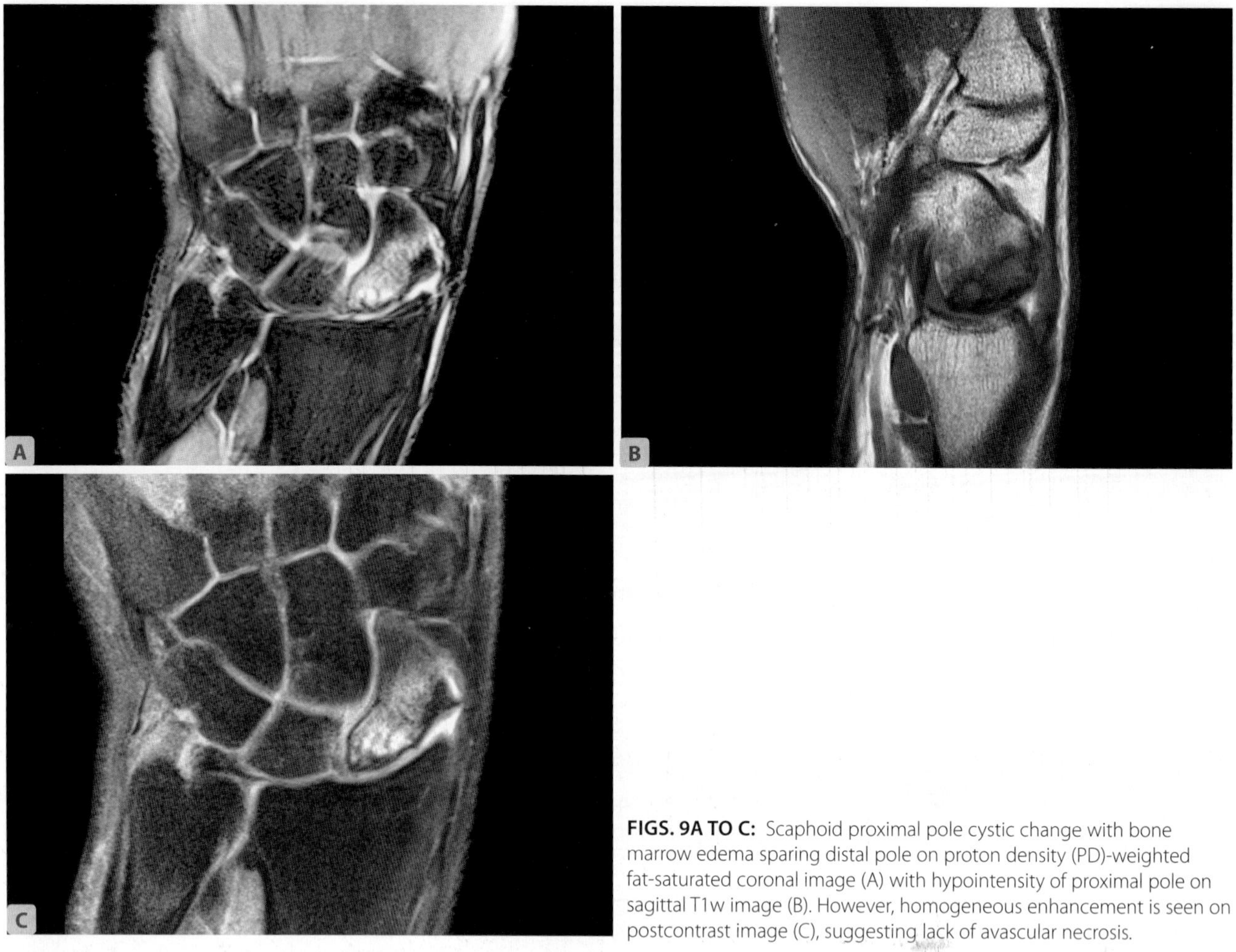

FIGS. 9A TO C: Scaphoid proximal pole cystic change with bone marrow edema sparing distal pole on proton density (PD)-weighted fat-saturated coronal image (A) with hypointensity of proximal pole on sagittal T1w image (B). However, homogeneous enhancement is seen on postcontrast image (C), suggesting lack of avascular necrosis.

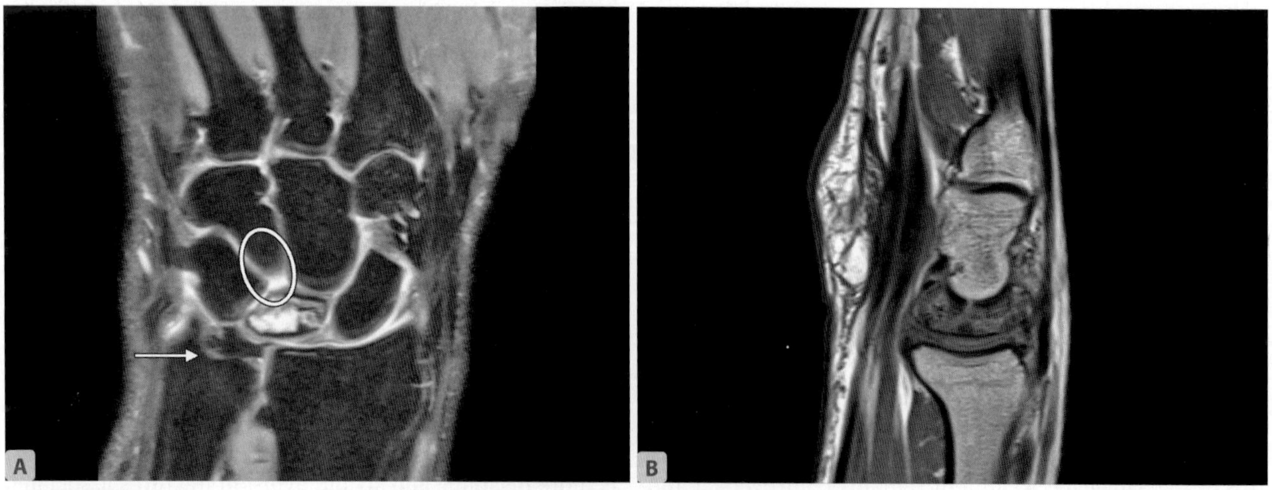

FIGS. 10A AND B: Kienböck's disease with negative ulnar variance with flattened type II lunate. Proton density fat-saturated coronal image (A) shows flattened lunate bone with hyperintensity on fat-saturated images involving the entire lunate (A) and hypointensity of the lunate on the T1w image (B). The lunate has a facet for articulation with hamate (oval in A). The articular surface of distal ulna is proximal to that of the radius (negative ulnar variance) (arrow in A), another predisposing factor for Kienböck's disease.

TABLE 3: Lichtman staging of Kienböck's disease.[28]

Stages	Radiographic and CT findings	MRI findings
I	Normal morphologic findings	• Morphologic preservation • Edema pattern in bone marrow
II	• Normal morphologic findings • Sclerosis in bone marrow	• Morphologic preservation • Signal intensity low on T1W images, variable on T2W images
IIIA	• Collapse of lunate bone • Radioscaphoid angle <60°	• Morphologic collapse of lunate bone • Signal intensity low on T1W images, variable on T2W images
IIIB	• Collapse of lunate bone • Radioscaphoid angle >60°	• Morphologic collapse of lunate bone • Signal intensity low on T1W images, variable on T2W images
IIIC	• Collapse of lunate bone • Coronal lunate fracture (chronic)	• Morphologic collapse of lunate bone • Signal intensity low on T1W images, variable on T2W images Coronal lunate fracture (chronic)
IV	Radiocarpal or midcarpal degenerative arthritis	• Radiocarpal or midcarpal degenerative arthritis • Signal intensity low on T1W images, variable on T2W images

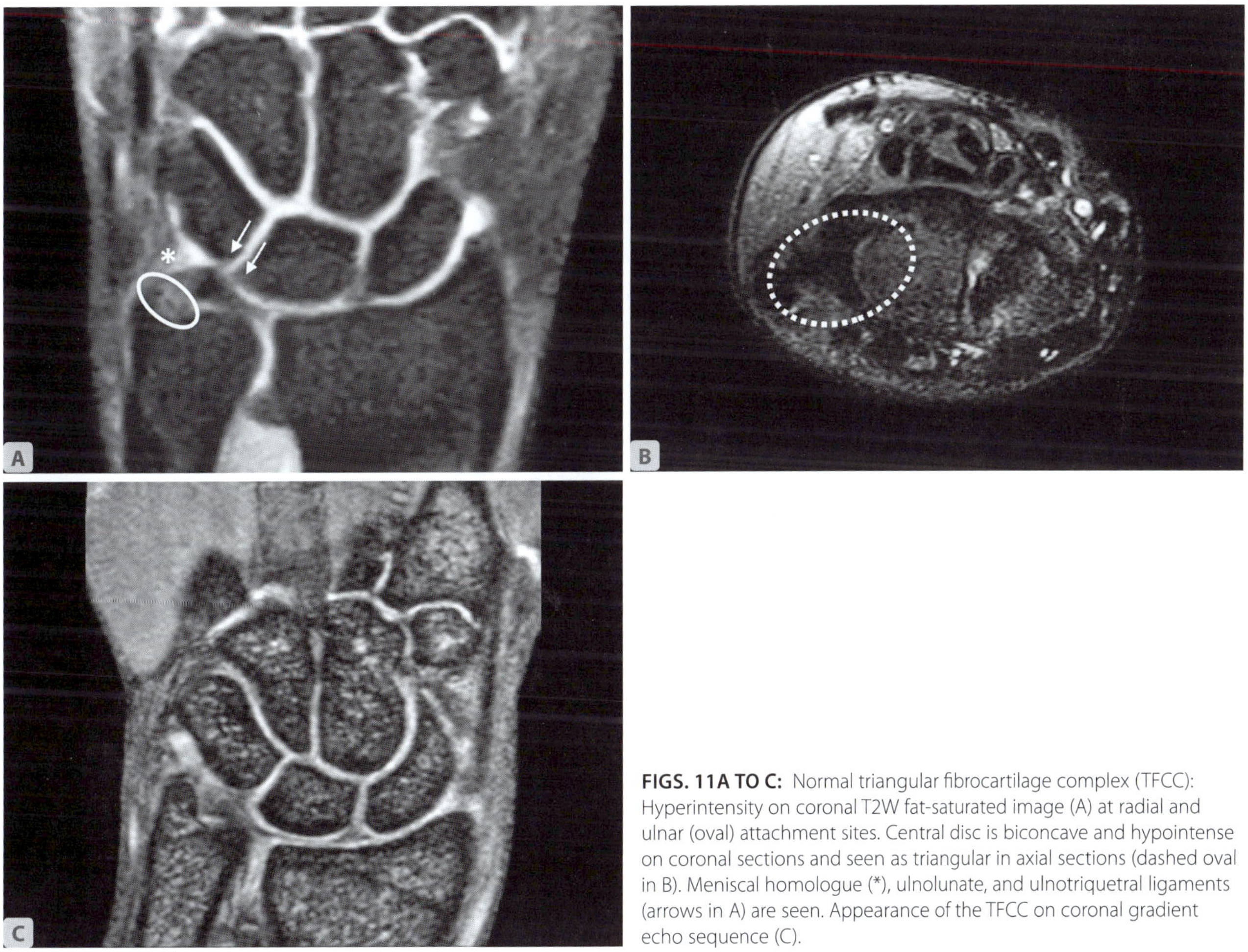

FIGS. 11A TO C: Normal triangular fibrocartilage complex (TFCC): Hyperintensity on coronal T2W fat-saturated image (A) at radial and ulnar (oval) attachment sites. Central disc is biconcave and hypointense on coronal sections and seen as triangular in axial sections (dashed oval in B). Meniscal homologue (*), ulnolunate, and ulnotriquetral ligaments (arrows in A) are seen. Appearance of the TFCC on coronal gradient echo sequence (C).

the distal (less common) articular surface. Type IA tears are in the avascular zone and cannot be surgically repaired **(Figs. 13A and B)**.

Type IB tears near the ulnar attachment are difficult to diagnose on MRI; features of ulnar-sided synovitis and focal fluid on the ulnar side are clues to diagnosis. Ulnar-sided tears and type IC tears are vascular and respond well to interventions.[31] MR arthrography with DRUJ injections have better sensitivity in detecting type IA and IB lesions **(Figs. 14A and B)**.

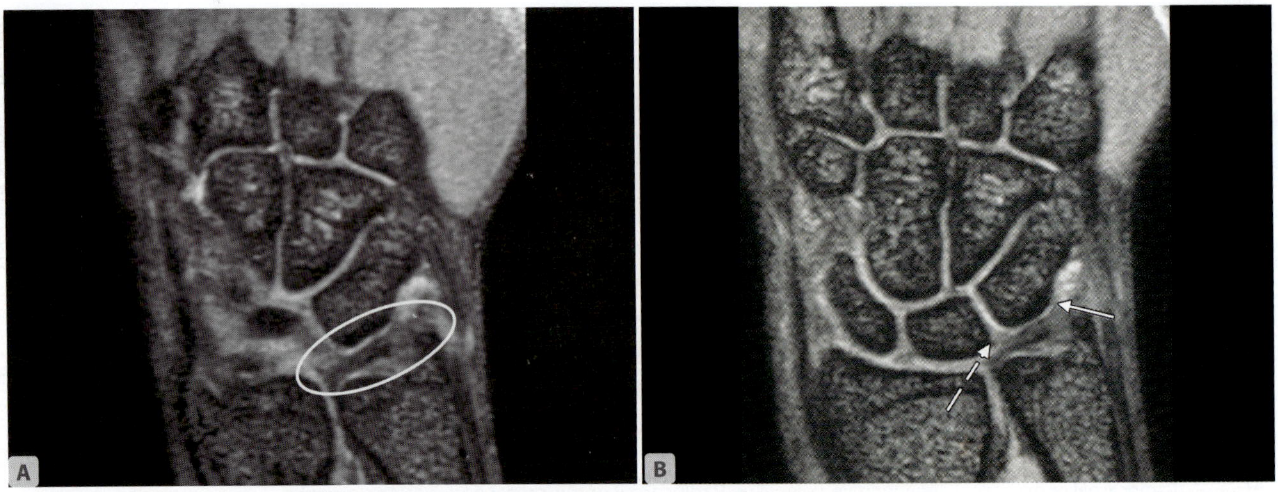

FIGS. 12A AND B: (A) Dorsal radioulnar ligament (oval) which has horizontal superior and inferior margins unlike the biconcave triangular fibrocartilage articular disc proper; (B) Ulnolunate (dashed arrow) and ulnotriquetral ligaments (arrow).

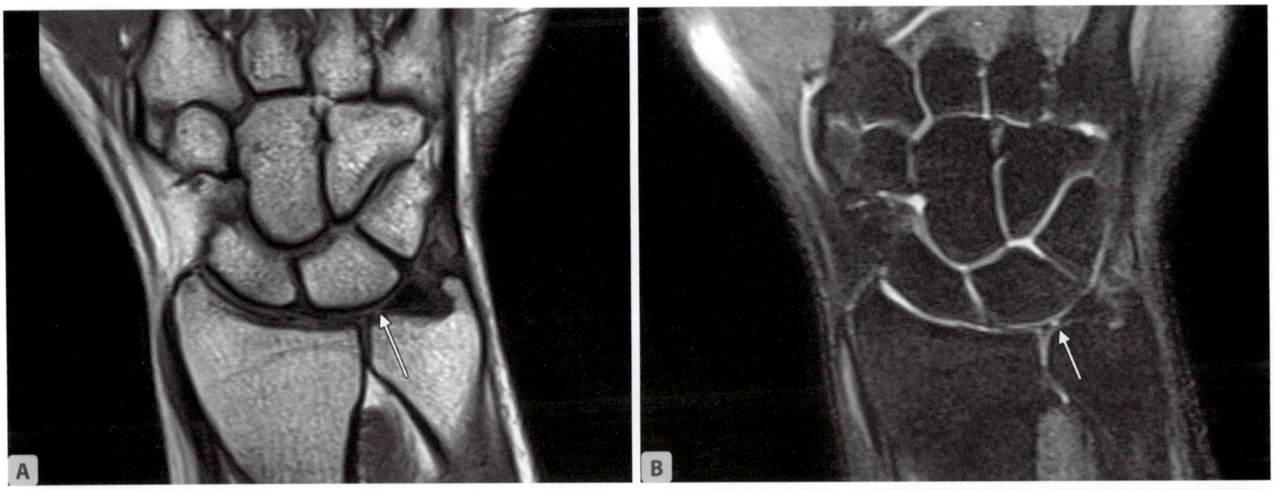

FIGS. 13A AND B: Central triangular fibrocartilage complex (TFCC) tear. Coronal PD weighted (A) and T2W fat saturated (B) images show a central perforation of the TFCC (arrow), with fluid signal within the central portion of the disc. These tears are often asymptomatic.

TABLE 4: Classification of triangular fibrocartilage complex (TFCC) tears.

Class I tears (traumatic)	
IA	Central perforations
IB	Ulnar avulsion with or without distal ulnar fracture
IC	Distal avulsion at carpal attachment
ID	Radial avulsion with or without sigmoid notch fracture
Class II tears (degenerative)	
IIA	TFCC wear
IIB	TFCC wear with lunate and/or ulnar chondromalacia
IIC	TFCC perforation with lunate and/or ulnar chondromalacia
IID	C and lunotriquetral ligament perforation
IIE	D and ulnocarpal arthritis

Type IC tears appear as thickening with edema within the ligament on long TE sequences.[31] Type ID tears near the radial attachment can be associated with radial avulsion fractures of sigmoid notch.

Degenerative Tears

Triangular fibrocartilage complex degeneration manifests as intrasubstance hyperintensity not communicating with the articular surface. The disc may appear diffusely thinned in degenerative tears. Degenerative tears are common with aging and rarely seen before 30 years and are associated with positive ulnar variance and ulnar impaction with chondromalacia of lunate or degenerative subchondral cysts.[31]

Three-dimensional Imaging

Three-dimensional isotropic imaging is specifically useful for evaluating the TFCC since in the imaging position, the TFCC is

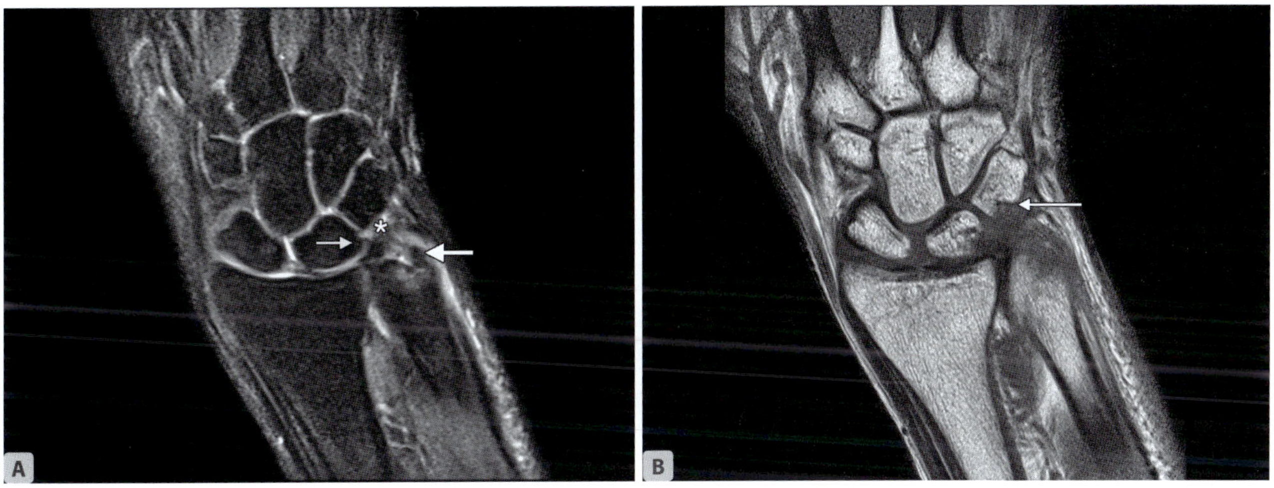

FIGS. 14A AND B: (A) PD-weighted fat-saturated coronal MRI reveals fracture of base of ulnar styloid (thick arrow) with thickened and hyperintense proximal and distal lamina of TFC (thick arrow). The ulnolunate ligament is hypointense (thin arrow). Hyperintensity and thickening of ulnotriquetral ligament is seen (*); (B) Coronal T1W image shows osteochondral impaction injury at the proximal radial side of triquetrum (arrow) at the ulnolunate ligament attachment site.

not orthogonal to the coronal plane but oblique to it, resulting in false-positive diagnosis of tears as the entire ligament may not be visualized in one section due to its obliquity. 3D sequences with a section thickness of 1 mm or less with no interslice gap can be reconstructed with multiplanar reconstructions for better evaluation of the TFCC. Punctate hypointensity on 3D gradient echo sequences is an early sign of degeneration.[32]

Radioulnar Ligament Lesions

Injuries of dorsal and volar radioulnar ligaments result in DRUJ dysfunction with ulnar-sided wrist pain.

The dorsal and volar radioulnar ligaments have flat superior and inferior margins unlike the biconcave margins of the TFC and are hypointense on all pulse sequences, but mildly more hyperintense than the TFC proper.

Disruptions of the radioulnar ligaments should be carefully evaluated on the peripheral MRI sections. The ulna commonly subluxates dorsally relative to the sigmoid notch due to tear of the dorsal radioulnar ligament with loss of concentric relation between sigmoid notch of radius and ulnar head **(Figs. 15A to C)**.[30]

Ulnar Impaction Syndrome (Ulnocarpal Abutment)

This is a common cause of ulnar-sided wrist pain and is occasionally associated with positive ulnar variance causing excessive load on the ulnar side of the wrist with ulnar impaction on the TFCC and ulnar-sided carpal bones. The condition can also be seen in neutral or negative ulnar variance.[22]

Radiography with forearm in pronation with hand gripped may show the actual increase in positive ulnar variance and impaction. Foreshortened radius may also be found postsurgically, post-traumatically in malunited foreshortened radius, due to premature physeal fusion of the distal radius (congenitally or in post-traumatic cases in skeletally immature patients).[2,22]

Magnetic resonance imaging is useful in detecting early changes since radiographic findings may be subtle or normal even in advanced disease. MRI shows the ulnar-sided degenerative changes involving ulnar-sided carpal bones (ulnar side of lunate, triquetrum) and ulnar head. Cartilage thinning, subchondral cysts, marrow edema, and sclerosis along the ulnar aspect of the lunate and/or triquetrum may be seen **(Figs. 16A and B)**.[22] Degenerative changes in the thinned-out TFCC are also seen. Advanced cases lead to ulnocarpal joint arthritis.

Ulnar Styloid Impaction Syndrome

This causes ulnar-sided wrist pain due to impaction between a long styloid process of ulna (>6 mm) and a nonunited styloid process fracture fragment and the triquetral bone.

Magnetic resonance imaging findings: Degenerative changes are noted in a long or curved ulnar styloid process and in triquetrum with bone marrow edema, cartilage changes, subchondral cysts, and sclerosis along the styloid process and triquetrum **(Fig. 17)**.[22]

Ulnar Impingement Syndrome

In this condition, a shortened ulna, which lies proximal to the sigmoid notch, impinges against the radius. MRI shows a foreshortened ulna with bone marrow edema at the level of impingement on the radius proximal to sigmoid notch. Later stages show sclerosis, scalloping along the ulnar margin of distal radius, and degenerative changes with osteophytes.[22]

Hamatolunate Impingement

Hamatolunate impingement occurs due to a type II lunate where there is an additional facet on the distal articular surface of the lunate where the hamate and lunate articulate.

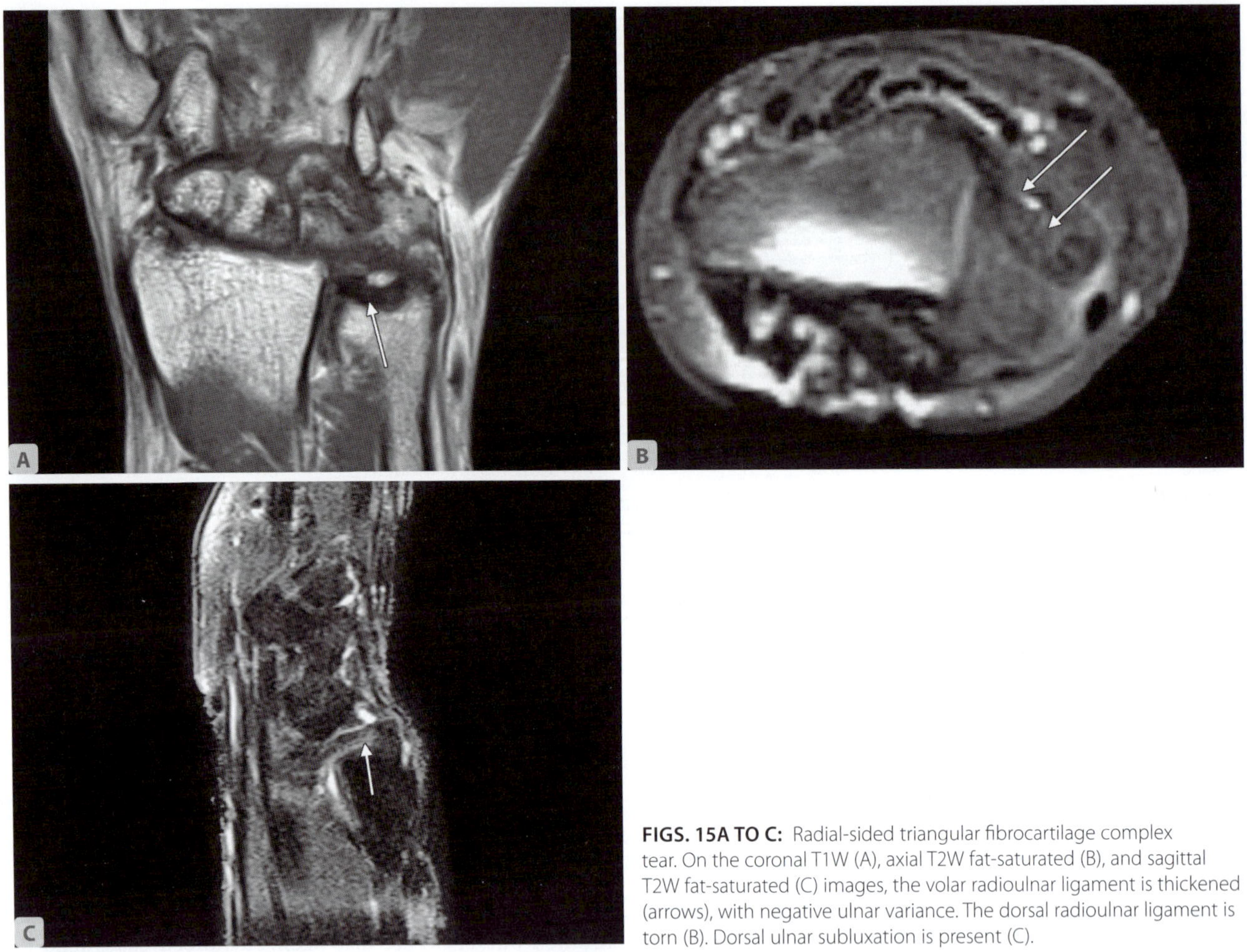

FIGS. 15A TO C: Radial-sided triangular fibrocartilage complex tear. On the coronal T1W (A), axial T2W fat-saturated (B), and sagittal T2W fat-saturated (C) images, the volar radioulnar ligament is thickened (arrows), with negative ulnar variance. The dorsal radioulnar ligament is torn (B). Dorsal ulnar subluxation is present (C).

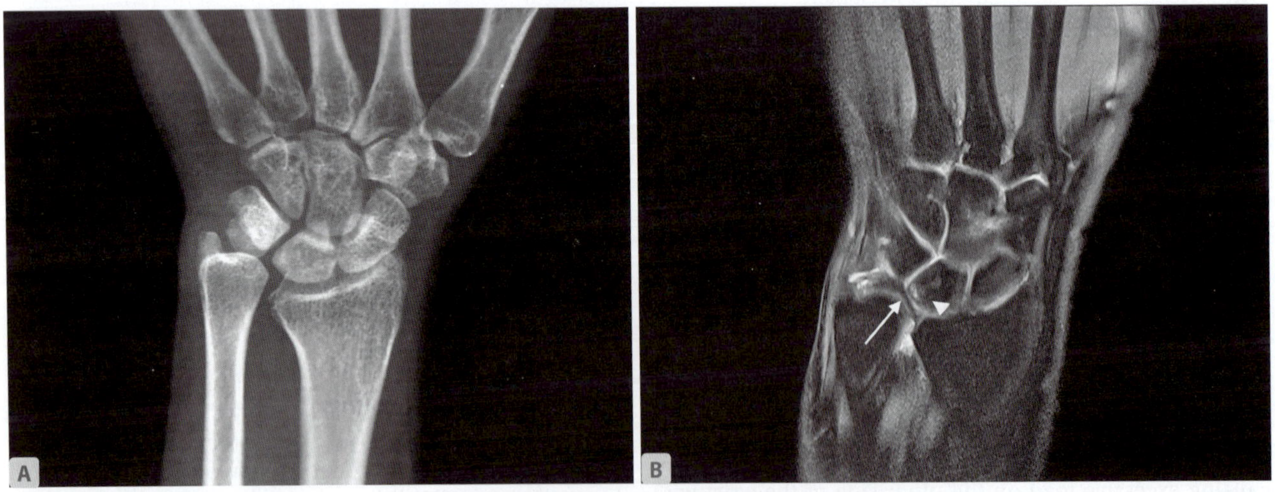

FIGS. 16A AND B: Ulnocarpal abutment. (A) Radiograph; and (B) Coronal T2W fat-saturated image. Positive ulnar variance with thinned-out TFC and chondromalacia along the ulnar aspect of the lunate (arrowhead).

Impingement at this articulation can cause chondromalacia and pain.[33]

Carpal Instability

Carpal instability is defined as the inability to bear physiological load.

Carpal instabilities are most commonly caused by injuries to the intrinsic ligaments of the wrist, though inflammatory and congenital conditions can also lead to instability. Based on the type of injury, carpal instability is classified into four types according to the Mayo classification **(Table 5)**.

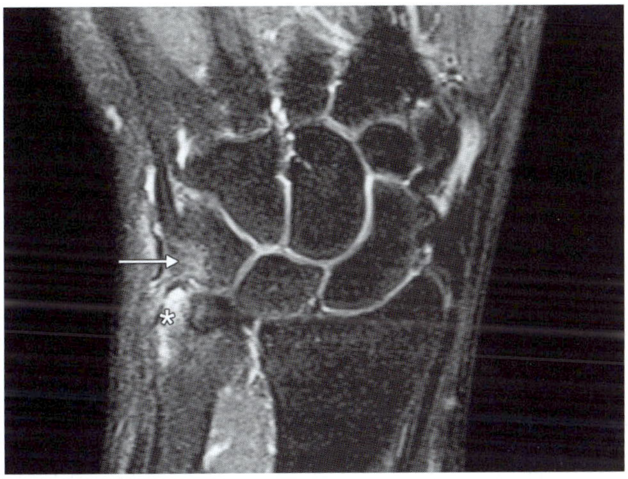

FIG. 17: Coronal T2w fat-saturated image shows ulnar styloid impaction with edema of the ulnar styloid process (*) and ulnar aspect of triquetrum (arrow).

Carpal Instability Dissociative

Scapholunate instabilities are the most common carpal instabilities, and the scapholunate and lunotriquetral ligament injuries are the most common causes of dissociative carpal instability. Scaphoid fractures, Kienböck's disease, and rheumatoid arthritis (RA) also cause scapholunate instability.[34]

Scapholunate Ligament Injury

Scapholunate ligament injuries are associated with radial-sided wrist pain and popping or clicking on physiological loading of the wrist joint. Scapholunate ligament injury can result in scapholunate dissociation, scapholunate advanced collapse (SLAC), and scaphoid nonunion advanced collapse (SNAC).[35]

The scapholunate ligament has three components—dorsal, interosseous, and volar. The dorsal component is most important for maintaining stability. The dorsal intercarpal ligaments also act as secondary stabilizers.[36]

Scapholunate dissociation causes widening of the scapholunate interval to >3 mm on radiographs. This is known as Terry Thomas sign. However, routine radiographs may be normal even in complete scapholunate ligament tears and stress radiographs may be required with clenched fist views or wrist in ulnar and radial deviation. MRI or MR arthrography can demonstrate the ligament tear.

Scapholunate ligament injuries cause a pattern of injury known as dorsal intercalated segment instability (DISI) with a dorsal tilt of the concave distal articular surface of the lunate and volar tilt of the scaphoid with an increase in the scapholunate angle (>60°). These injuries occur due to damage to scapholunate ligament along with secondary stabilizers such as radioscaphocapitate and scaphocapitate ligaments.[34,35]

Further progression leads to degenerative changes in the radioscaphoid articulation and ultimately carpal collapse **(Figs. 18A to C)**. Nontraumatic scapholunate dissociation and SLAC are seen in patients with calcium pyrophosphate deposition disease.

TABLE 5: Classification of carpal instability.	
Nomenclature	**Area of abnormality**
Carpal instability dissociative (CID)	Between the proximal row (most common) and distal row of carpal bones in the same row
Carpal instability nondissociative (CIND)	Between radiocarpal and midcarpal rows
Carpal instability complex	Combination of the above two
Adaptive carpus	Due to abnormality proximal or distal to carpal rows

On MRI, partial tears may appear as an elongated or a focally thin ligament or a focal area of high-signal intensity. Complete tears appear as a complete discontinuity.[12] Double-compartment MR arthrography can demonstrate tears with greater sensitivity and specificity.[12,37]

Lunotriquetral Ligament Injury

The lunotriquetral ligament, like the scapholunate ligament, has three components (dorsal, interosseous, and volar) and plays an important role in maintaining stability of the proximal carpal row. The volar component of the lunotriquetral ligament is the strongest. Lunotriquetral ligament injuries present with ulnar-sided wrist pain.

Lunotriquetral ligament injury along with injury of the secondary stabilizers (dorsal radiotriquetral and dorsal scaphotriquetral ligaments) leads to volar intercalated segment instability (VISI). The lunate rotates in a volar direction.[38]

The lunotriquetral ligament is triangular or linear. The tears of this ligament are not easily detected on MRI, and MR arthrography has greater sensitivity in detecting tears. Widening of the lunotriquetral interval is rarely seen, unlike scapholunate ligament tears.[12]

Distal Radioulnar Joint

The distal radius, ulna, TFCC, and joint capsule form the DRUJ. The head of ulna forms a pivot joint after it articulates with the sigmoid notch on the ulnar aspect of the distal radius. Forearm movement of pronation and supination occur at the DRUJ, which also plays an important role in stabilization of the forearm. The foveal attachment of the radioulnar ligaments of the TFCC and the ulnotriquetral ligament also have a role in maintaining stability. Distal radial fractures are also associated with DRUJ injuries, which often go unrecognized.[39]

The clinical features of DRUJ instability include pain or audible clicking on pronation/supination or restricted movement. The empty groove of extensor carpi ulnaris can be palpated. The ulna which subluxates dorsally can also be palpated.[39]

Associated osseous injuries—Colles', Smith's (reverse Colles, fracture), Essex-Lopresti, Galeazzi, Chauffeur's, and Barton's fractures—can be associated with DRUJ instability. DRUJ instability causes ulnar-sided pain and early onset of degenerative arthritis in patients with distal radial fractures.[13,39]

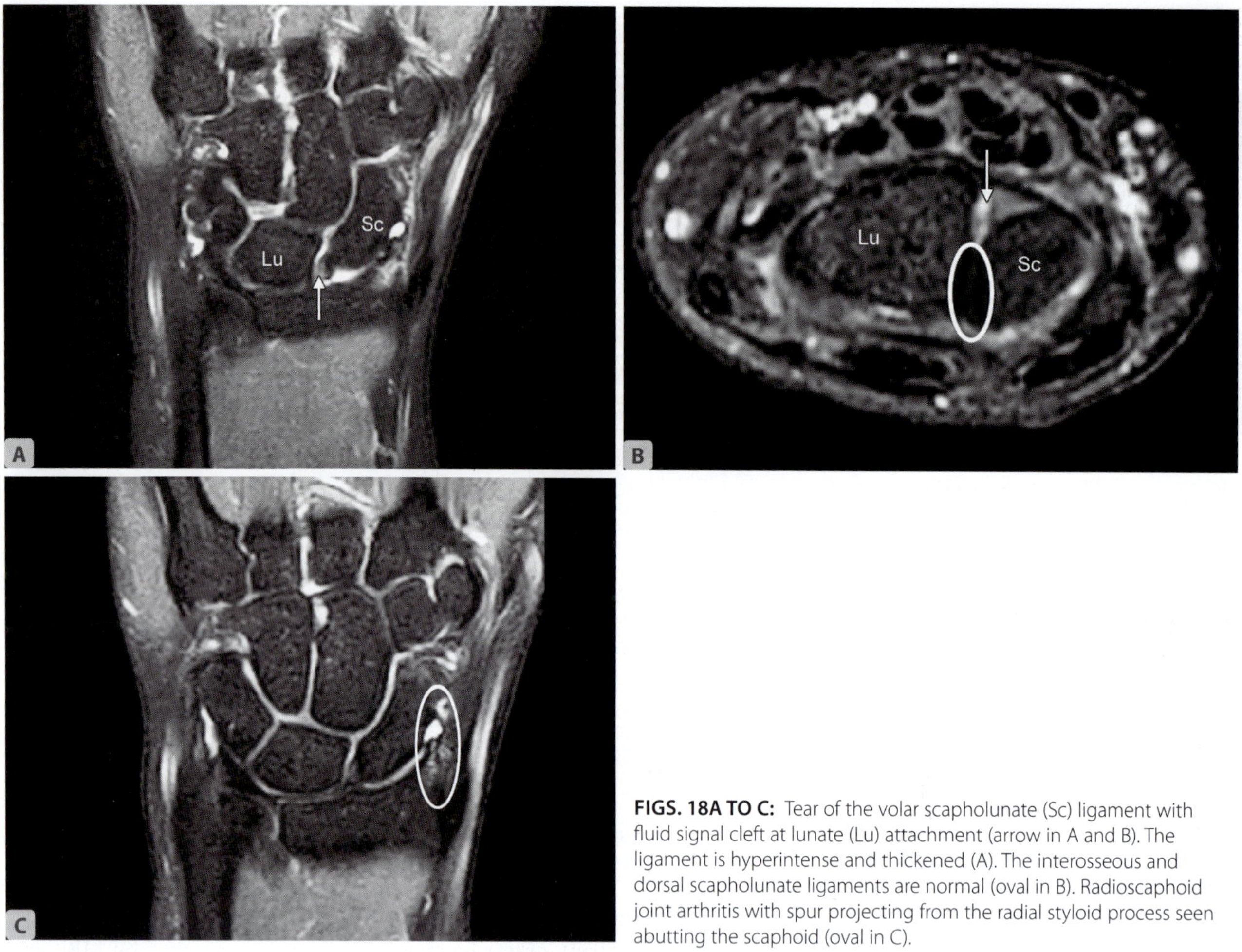

FIGS. 18A TO C: Tear of the volar scapholunate (Sc) ligament with fluid signal cleft at lunate (Lu) attachment (arrow in A and B). The ligament is hyperintense and thickened (A). The interosseous and dorsal scapholunate ligaments are normal (oval in B). Radioscaphoid joint arthritis with spur projecting from the radial styloid process seen abutting the scaphoid (oval in C).

Radiography is the primary investigation of choice and in a well-positioned lateral radiograph, the ulnar anterior and posterior margins overlap with the radius. However, positioning may be difficult and subtle subluxations may be missed.

The CT and MRI are useful for detecting the congruence of the DRUJ on axial images. In addition to ligamentous and osseous injuries, entrapment of ECU may also be detected, which may result in failure of closed reduction in certain osseous injuries such as Barton's fracture.[40]

Post-traumatic fractures of ulnar styloid, especially base of ulnar styloid, are also associated with DRUJ instability due to concomitant injury to foveal attachment of TFCC. Chronic unstable styloid fractures or malunited ulnar styloid fractures also results in repetitive trauma and dislocation or tears of ECU. Post-traumatic distal radial fractures and physeal fusion can lead to positive ulnar variance and DRUJ instability due to TFCC tears.[39]

Tendon Disorders

Tendons have low-signal intensity on all pulse sequences due to a parallel arrangement of fibers with low water content. APL can have a normally striated appearance due to multiple tendon slips with interspersed fat. Magic angle artifact can cause artifactual intermediate-signal intensity, especially in the FPL and ECU.[41]

De Quervain's Tenosynovitis

De Quervain's tenosynovitis affects the first extensor compartment containing the APL and EPB. This is commonly seen in middle-aged females and can be bilateral in 30%.[41] It is also common in the peripartum period.[33] Positive Finkelstein's test with pain on ulnar deviation of the thumb is diagnostic.

The MRI findings include tendon thickening, fluid around the tendon sheath, and surrounding edema. A septum may be found between the tendon sheaths **(Figs. 19A and B)**. Ultrasound is an alternative tool to MRI to look for septum between the two tendons.

Intersection Syndrome

The first compartment tendons of APL and brevis cross from ulnar to radial side over the second compartment extensor tendons of extensor carpi radialis longus and brevis. Overuse or repeated friction at this intersection 3–4 cm proximal to Lister's tubercle of the radius causes tenosynovitis of the second compartment with pain in the distal forearm.

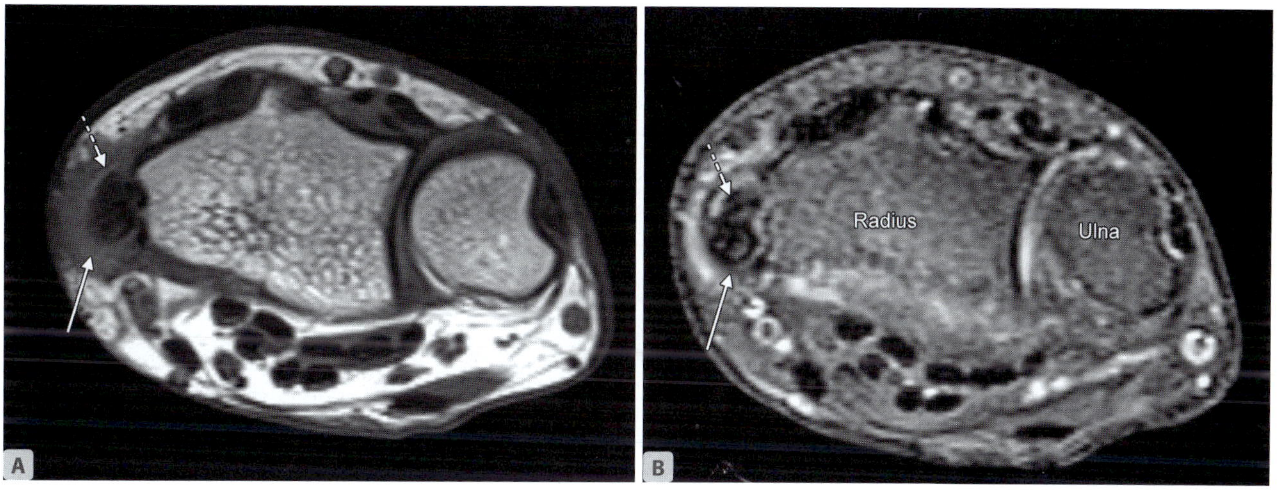

FIGS. 19A AND B: De Quervain's tenosynovitis. (A) Axial T1W and (B) T2W fat-saturated images show thickening and intratendinous intermediate signal of abductor pollicis longus (arrow) and extensor pollicis brevis (dashed arrow). Fluid seen surrounding the tendons and mild surrounding soft tissue edema are also present.

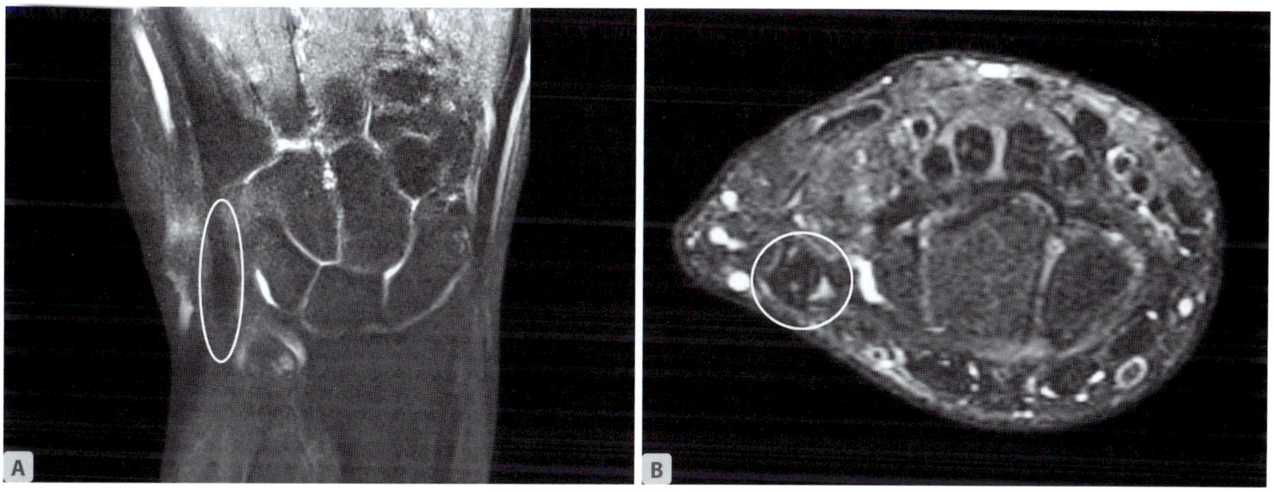

FIGS. 20A AND B: Flexor carpi ulnaris tendinopathy in a patient with ulnar wrist pain. Coronal PD-weighted fat-saturated images show a focal thickening of flexor carpi ulnaris with mild fluid (ovals in A and B). Fluid is also seen in the adjacent distal radioulnar joint.

The site of pain is proximal to the site of pain in de Quervain's tenosynovitis, at the site of intersection. Overhead racket players and weight-lifters are prone to this overuse injury.

Distal Intersection Syndrome

This is a rare cause of pain on the dorsal side of the wrist over Lister's tubercle at the point of crossing of the third compartment tendon of extensor pollicis longus (EPL) over the second compartment tendons of extensor carpi radialis brevis and longus.

Extensor Carpi Ulnaris Tenosynovitis

Extensor carpi ulnaris tenosynovitis is common and seen most commonly in patients with RA and in patients with subluxation of the ECU due to DRUJ instability, which may be postinflammatory or post-traumatic **(Figs. 20A and B)**.

Flexor Tenosynovitis

Flexor tenosynovitis occurs commonly in patients with RA or tubercular arthritis, both of which can lead to synovial thickening and intrasynovial rice bodies. Distension of the common flexor tendon sheath can present as carpal tunnel syndrome (CTS) **(Figs. 21A and B)**.

Carpal Tunnel Syndrome

Carpal tunnel syndrome accounts for approximately 90% of all entrapment neuropathies and is caused by compression of the median nerve at the carpal tunnel in the volar aspect of the wrist. Patients present with complaints of pain, numbness, or tingling feeling in the hands in the median nerve distribution.[42] Nerve conduction studies remain the gold standard for diagnosing and grading CTS, but provide limited information about the exact location, extent, and possible cause of nerve entrapment and is also uncomfortable

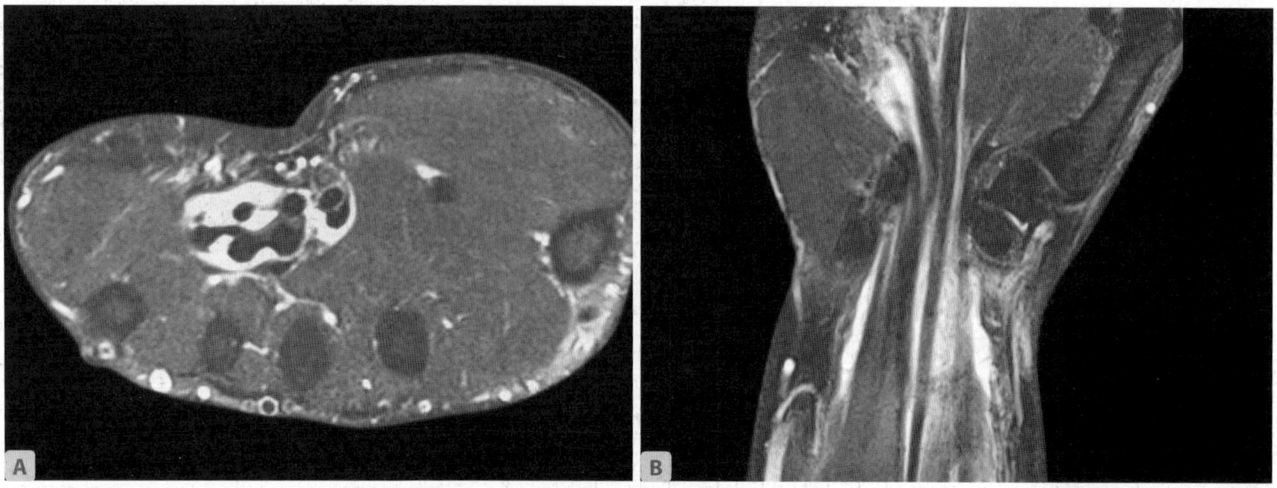

FIGS. 21A AND B: Flexor tenosynovitis. Fluid is seen around the flexor tendons in the axial (A) and coronal (B) T2W fat-saturated sequences.

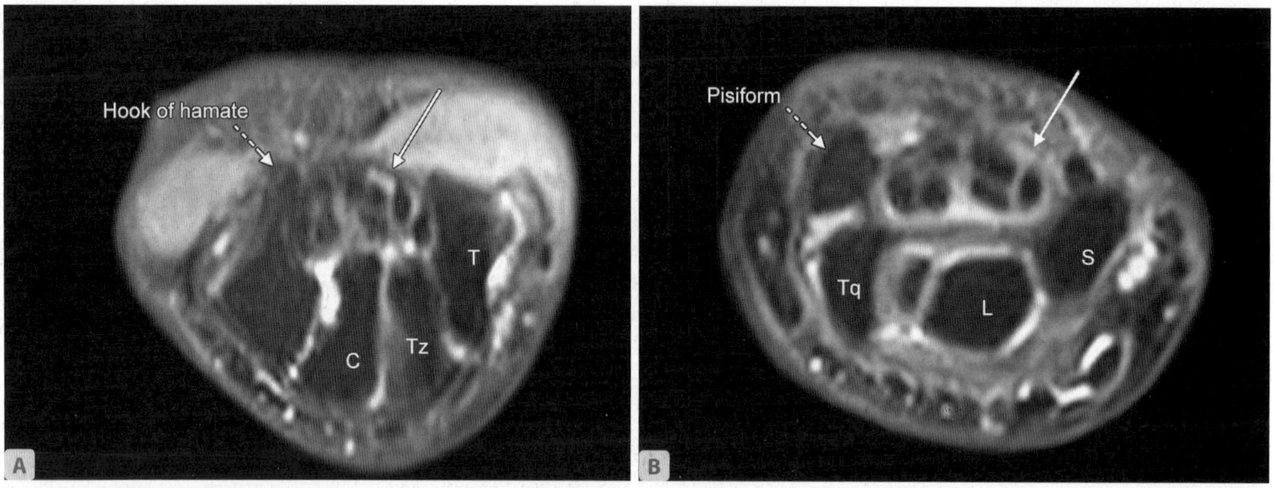

FIGS. 22A AND B: Normal median nerve on MRI. Axial T2 SPAIR images at the (A) hamate hook level (dashed arrow in A), (B) level of pisiform bone (dashed arrow in B) depicting normal size and signal intensity of the median nerve (arrow) at the CT in the right wrist of a patient in the control group. (C: capitate, L: lunate; R: radius; S: scaphoid; T: trapezium; Tq: triquetrum; Tz: trapezoid; U: ulna; SPAIR: spectral adiabatic inversion recovery).

for the patient.[43] Magnetic resonance neurography (MRN) is a specific MR technique to enhance the peripheral nerve visualization with the help of high-resolution and high-contrast pulse sequences. MRI has the advantage of excellent soft-tissue resolution, the capacity to delineate the site of nerve injury, and to demonstrate the secondary causes of CTS.[44]

Magnetic resonance neurography sequences recommended include axial T1W pulse sequence, axial FS pulse sequence, preferably T2-spectral adiabatic inversion recovery (SPAIR) sequence, coronal proton density sequence, and 3D nerve imaging.[45] The advantage of the 3D isotropic technique lies in the ability to allow thinner slices and multiplanar reconstructions derived from isotropic voxels for clear display of nerves along the long axis. A diffusion-based 3D reversed fast imaging with steady-state free precession (3D PSIF) is another sequence which can be used to cause vascular signal suppression in peripheral nerves creating nerve specific images.[44,45] Diffusion tensor imaging can also be performed as a problem-solving tool for quantification of the fractional anisotropy (FA). Axial T2 SPAIR sequence is adequate for assessing the median nerve; T2 fat-suppressed 3D PSIF sequence is useful to delineate the margins and course of the median nerve.[46]

Cross-sectional area (CA) of the median nerve is the most well-studied parameter, with measurement just proximal to the tunnel or at the site of the most marked swelling of the nerve being the most useful.[47-50] A cutoff value of CA of >0.165 cm^2, 1 cm proximal to the pisiform, had the highest sensitivity of 91.1% and specificity of 87.5% **(Figs. 22A and B)**.[46] Koh et al. found a value of 0.143 cm^2 at the same level to give a sensitivity of 76.2% and specificity of 73.8%.[47] Klauser et al. found a cutoff value of 0.575 for FA to have sensitivity and specificity of 73.9% and 80%, respectively, and a maximum CA value of 0.17 cm^2 to have a sensitivity of 93.3% and specificity of 93.3%.[51]

Median nerve signal intensity on MRI relative to the hypothenar muscle is significantly different between patient and control group **(Figs. 23A and B)**.[47,52] Retinacular bowing of >0.122 cm has a sensitivity and specificity of 60.0% and

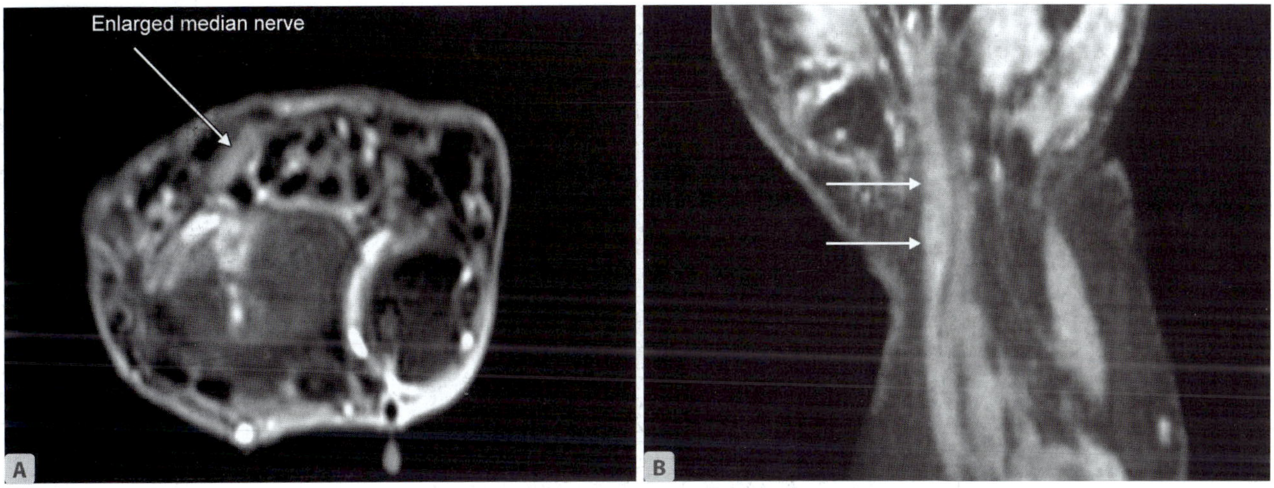

FIGS. 23A AND B: (A) T2 SPAIR axial image showing enlarged median nerve; (B) 3D PSIF curved reformatted image showing focal thickening of the median nerve just proximal and at the carpal tunnel in a patient with severe carpal tunnel syndrome (CTS) on nerve conduction studies.

65.6%, respectively.[46] Associated findings of extraosseous ganglion cysts and flexor tenosynovitis may be found.

Guyon's Canal Syndrome

Guyon's canal syndrome is a rare ulnar neuropathy. The ulnar nerve while traversing through the narrow Guyon's canal in the wrist can be compressed by ganglion cysts. Repetitive trauma can cause ulnar artery thrombosis or aneurysm, a condition known as hypothenar hammer syndrome.[53]

Wartenberg's Syndrome

Wartenberg's syndrome is pain or paresthesia along the radial aspect of dorsal forearm and over dorsal thumb and index finger due to injury or compression of the superficial radial nerve, which emerges and courses between the brachioradialis and extensor carpi radialis longus tendon.

Inflammatory Arthritis

Rheumatoid Arthritis

Changes of RA can be detected early before radiographic evidence of the disease by both ultrasound and MRI, as early as 4 months from clinical onset. Synovitis, erosions, and tenosynovitis can be detected by both modalities. However, MRI can also reveal bone marrow edema, which is a precursor of erosions[54] **(Figs. 24A to C)**.

Contrast-enhanced MRI can differentiate between synovitis, which enhances, and effusion, which is nonenhancing. However, in late acquisitions, gadolinium can diffuse into the synovial fluid and this occurs more rapidly in small joint.[55] Dynamic gadolinium-enhanced MRI can quantify the degree of synovial enhancement. The extent of erosions and bone marrow edema on MRI can also be used for longitudinal follow-up and assessment of response.

Synovitis, erosions, and bone marrow edema can be graded with scores of 0–3 according to the Outcome Measures in Rheumatology Clinical Trials (OMERACT) and European League Against Rheumatism (EULAR) Rheumatoid Arthritis Magnetic Resonance Imaging Score (RAMRIS) system.[56]

Seronegative Spondyloarthropathies

Magnetic resonance imaging is sensitive in diagnosing erosions, edema, and synovitis but not specific. Similar findings can be detected in other causes of inflammatory arthritis including seronegative spondyloarthropathies such as psoriatic arthritis and Reiter's disease. Involvement of the axial skeleton and enthesitis helps in differentiating between RA and seronegative arthropathies.[54]

Infections

Infectious Tenosynovitis

Acute suppurative tenosynovitis is bacterial and commonly spreads from the adjacent soft-tissue infections after a penetrating injury. Fluid or pus within the tendon sheath along with heterogeneous tendon thickening may be found. In chronic tenosynovitis due to tubercular infections, intrasynovial hypointense rice bodies may be found **(Fig. 25)**.[57]

Palmar Space Infections

There are many potential spaces in the wrist joint and hand—thenar space, midpalmar space, hypothenar space, and space of Parona (between the pronator quadratus and the FDP tendon). The radial bursa, which is a sheath covering FPL, and ulnar bursa, which is a continuation of the flexor tendon sheath of the little finger, communicate with the space of Parona.[58] Infections in these spaces can occur after penetrating injury or rupture of the radial or ulnar bursa into space of Parona.

Chronic Infectious Arthritis

Tubercular arthritis can present with heterogeneous synovial thickening, erosions, and tenosynovitis. Sinus tracks and

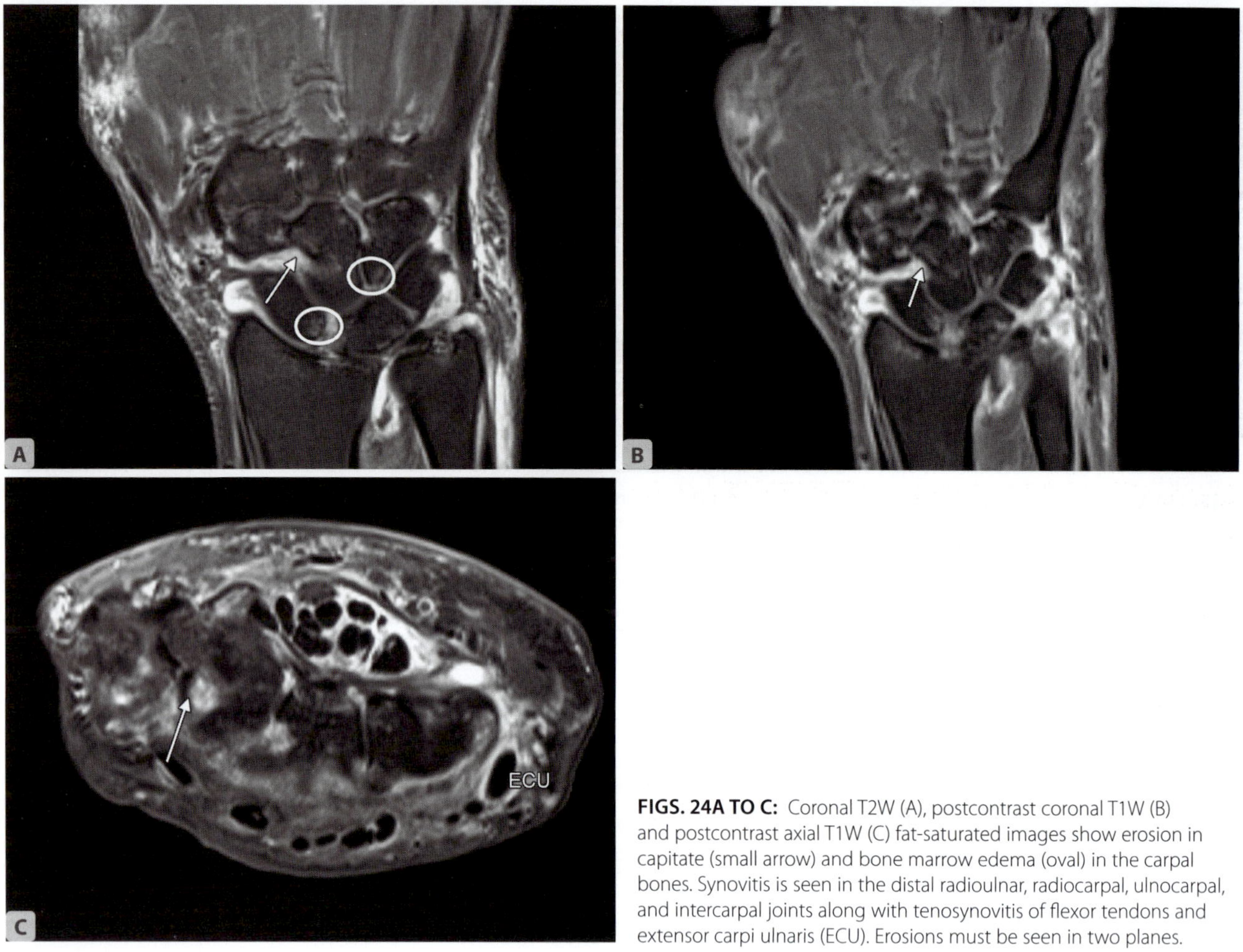

FIGS. 24A TO C: Coronal T2W (A), postcontrast coronal T1W (B) and postcontrast axial T1W (C) fat-saturated images show erosion in capitate (small arrow) and bone marrow edema (oval) in the carpal bones. Synovitis is seen in the distal radioulnar, radiocarpal, ulnocarpal, and intercarpal joints along with tenosynovitis of flexor tendons and extensor carpi ulnaris (ECU). Erosions must be seen in two planes.

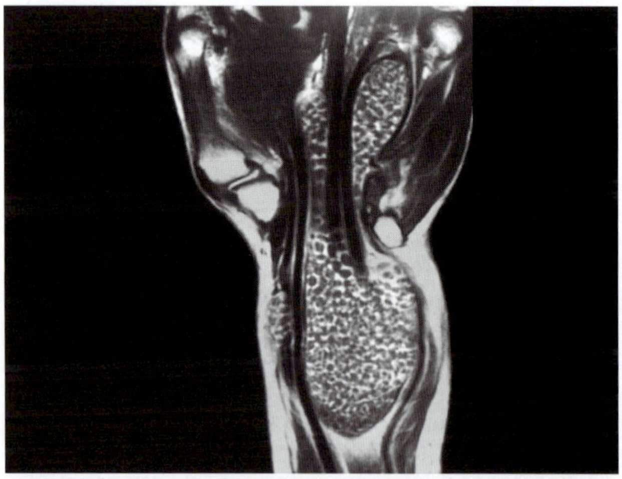

FIG. 25: Intrasynovial hypointense rice bodies in the common flexor tendon sheath on a coronal T2W image. Rice bodies can also be seen in inflammatory arthritis like rheumatoid arthritis.

ulcers or abscesses or periarticular soft-tissue nodules or masses may also be seen and should raise the suspicion of atypical bacterial or fungal infections.[58]

Degenerative Arthritis

Wrist osteoarthritis (OA) occurs most commonly as post-traumatic sequelae after SLAC or scaphoid nonunion advanced collapse which progresses from radiocarpal arthritis to midcarpal arthritis, involving scaphocapitate and capitolunate joints. Patients with inflammatory arthritis and pyrophosphate deposition disease also develop OA. Idiopathic OA may also develop and in some studies, idiopathic OA is more common than post-traumatic arthritis of the wrist.

Radiographs show osteophytes, subchondral sclerosis and cysts, joint space narrowing, and marginal erosions (in erosive OA). Although scoring systems for hand and wrist OA on radiographs exist (Kellgren-Lawrence Scale), there is poor correlation between clinical severity and radiographic findings.[59]

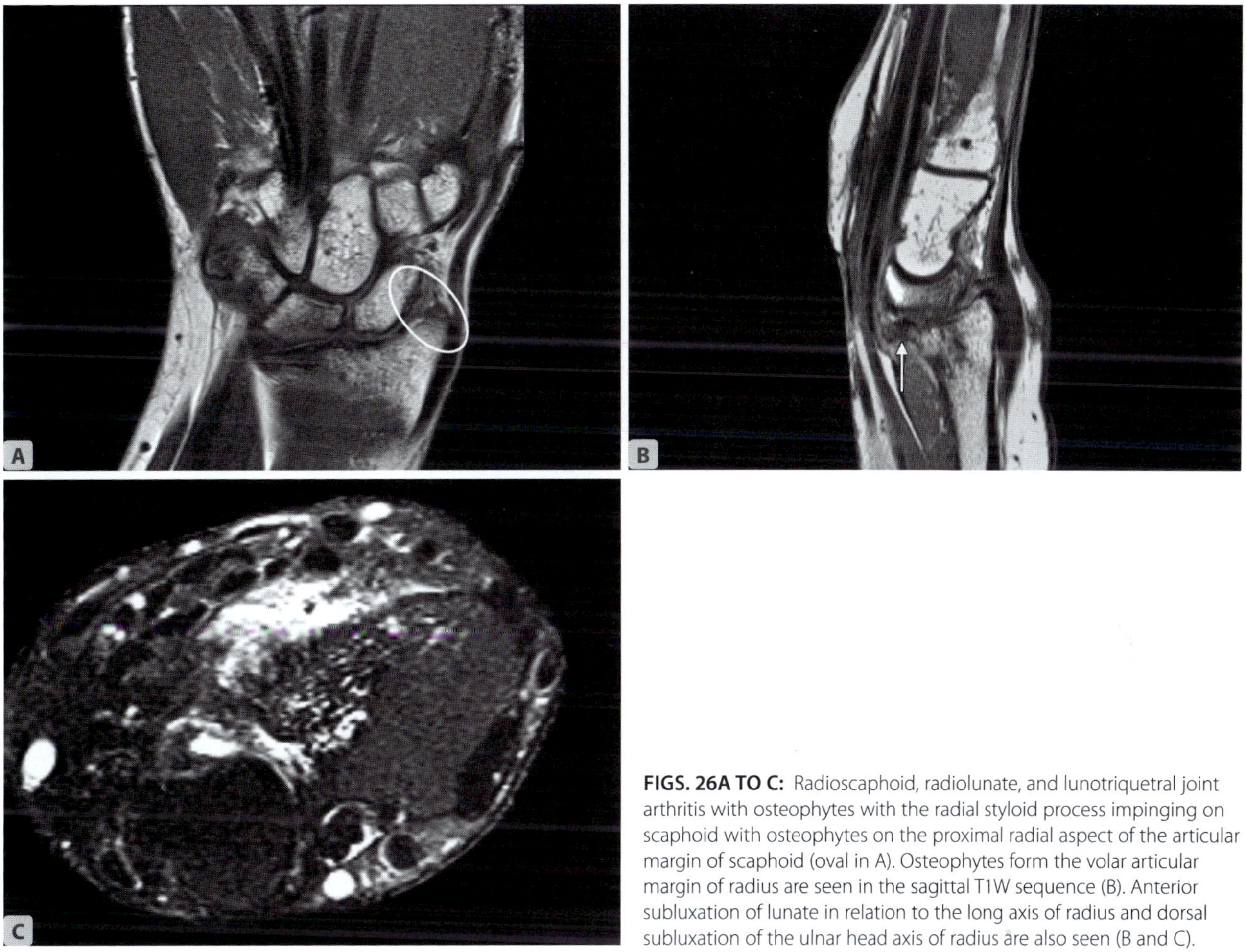

FIGS. 26A TO C: Radioscaphoid, radiolunate, and lunotriquetral joint arthritis with osteophytes with the radial styloid process impinging on scaphoid with osteophytes on the proximal radial aspect of the articular margin of scaphoid (oval in A). Osteophytes form the volar articular margin of radius are seen in the sagittal T1W sequence (B). Anterior subluxation of lunate in relation to the long axis of radius and dorsal subluxation of the ulnar head axis of radius are also seen (B and C).

The MRI is more reliable and sensitive in detecting radiocarpal arthritis, especially radiolunate arthritis, which has implications in deciding the arthrodesis procedure **(Figs. 26A to C)**.[60]

Tumors

Tumors include ganglion, intraosseous synovial cyst/ganglion/soft-tissue giant cell tumor (GCT) of the tendon sheath (GCTTS) and tumors like neurofibromas and schwannomas.

Soft Tissue Tumors

The common soft tissue tumors in the wrist joint are cystic, and ganglion cyst is the most common soft tissue tumor commonly seen. Ganglion cysts or synovial cysts are associated with ligamentous injury or degenerative conditions where increased intra-articular pressure causes extrusion of joint fluid, or there is mucoid degeneration of the collagenous tissue. On imaging, a small communication may be visible with the joint space, most commonly on the dorsal radial aspect of the wrist. An uncomplicated cyst appears isointense on T1W image and hyperintense on T2W image **(Figs. 27A and B)**. However, a hemorrhagic or ruptured cyst may have internal debris and content and mimic a neoplasm. On contrast enhancement, peripheral enhancement can be noted in a ganglion cyst and is helpful in differentiating it from a solid neoplasm.[61,62]

Benign soft tissue tumors are more common than malignant tumors. Soft tissue tumors commonly seen in the wrist joint are lipomas, vascular malformations **(Figs. 28A to C)**, GCTTS, neurogenic tumors, and lipofibromatous hamartoma of the median nerve **(Figs. 29A and B)**.

Giant cell tumor of the tendon sheath, also known as pigmented villonodular synovitis, presents as a firm multinodular nontender mass. It is the second most common tumor after ganglion cysts. Long-standing tumors can cause pressure erosion over bone. They appear as hypointense on both T1W and T2W imaging, and can also be located along the carpal bones.[63] GCTTS can be classified as type I with a single round or multilobulated tumor and type II where there are two or more distinct tumors which are not joined.[64] These tumors have a high recurrence rate if they are not completely excised or in type II tumors[63] **(Figs. 30A to C)**.

Among the malignant tumors, epithelioid sarcoma, synovial sarcomas, and malignant peripheral nerve sheath tumors are common in adults and rhabdomyosarcomas in pediatric population.

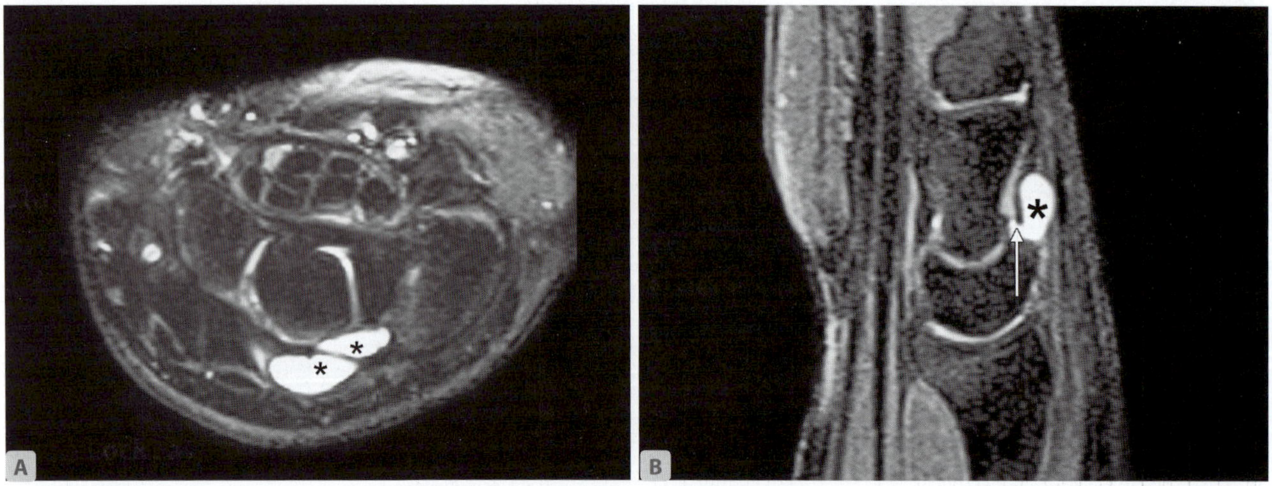

FIGS. 27A AND B: Ganglion. A lobulated hyperintense lesion (*) seen in the dorsal wrist with a small beak-like extension (arrow in B) from the capitolunate joint.

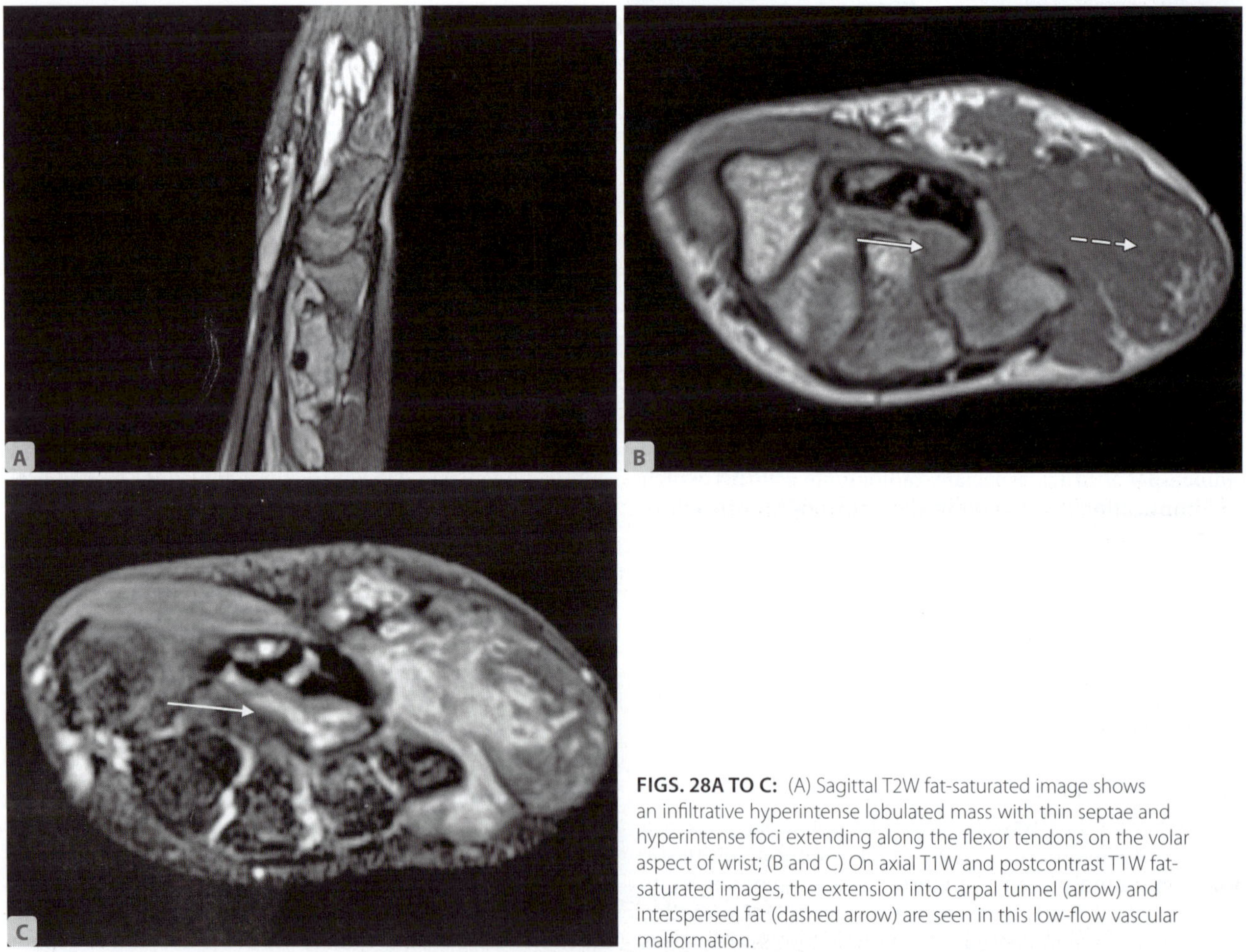

FIGS. 28A TO C: (A) Sagittal T2W fat-saturated image shows an infiltrative hyperintense lobulated mass with thin septae and hyperintense foci extending along the flexor tendons on the volar aspect of wrist; (B and C) On axial T1W and postcontrast T1W fat-saturated images, the extension into carpal tunnel (arrow) and interspersed fat (dashed arrow) are seen in this low-flow vascular malformation.

Osseous Lesions

Intraosseous ganglion is a very common cystic lesion of the hand and wrist, in a carpal bone.[62]

Benign bone tumors are far more common than malignant lesions. Enchondromas, GCTs, giant cell reparative granulomas, osteoid osteomas, and aneurysmal bone cysts are found in the metacarpals and phalanges and rarely in the carpal bones. Lymphomas, eosinophilic granulomas, chondrosarcomas, and osteosarcomas and rarely Ewing's sarcoma can affect the hand and wrist.

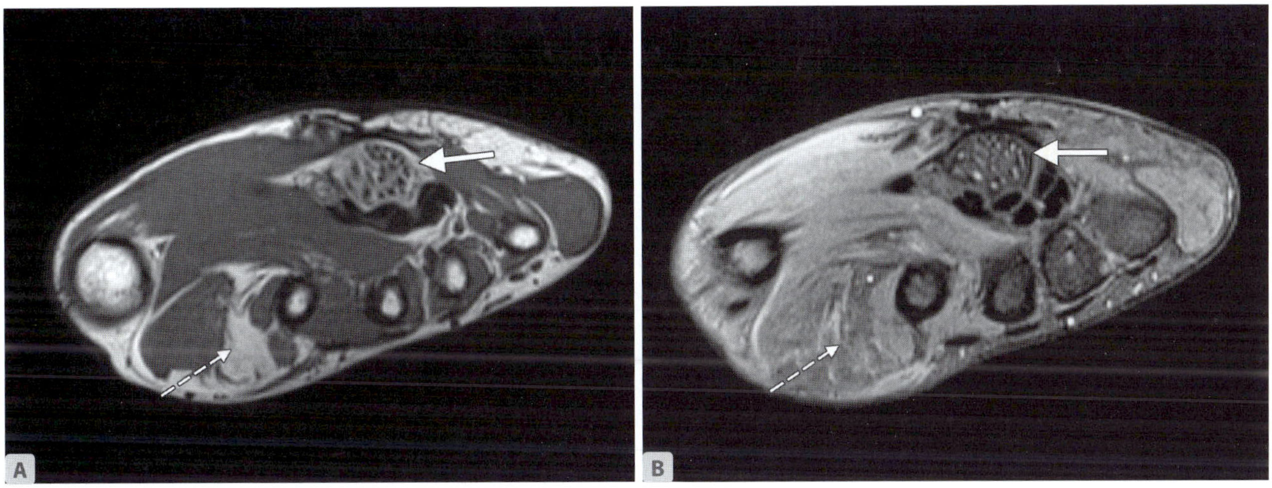

FIGS. 29A AND B: Fibrolipomatous hamartoma of the median nerve. The median nerve is thickened with a stippled appearance (arrow) with separation of the enlarged fascicles by fat, which is suppressed on the PD-weighted fat-saturated images. The digital branch of the median nerve is also involved (dashed arrow).

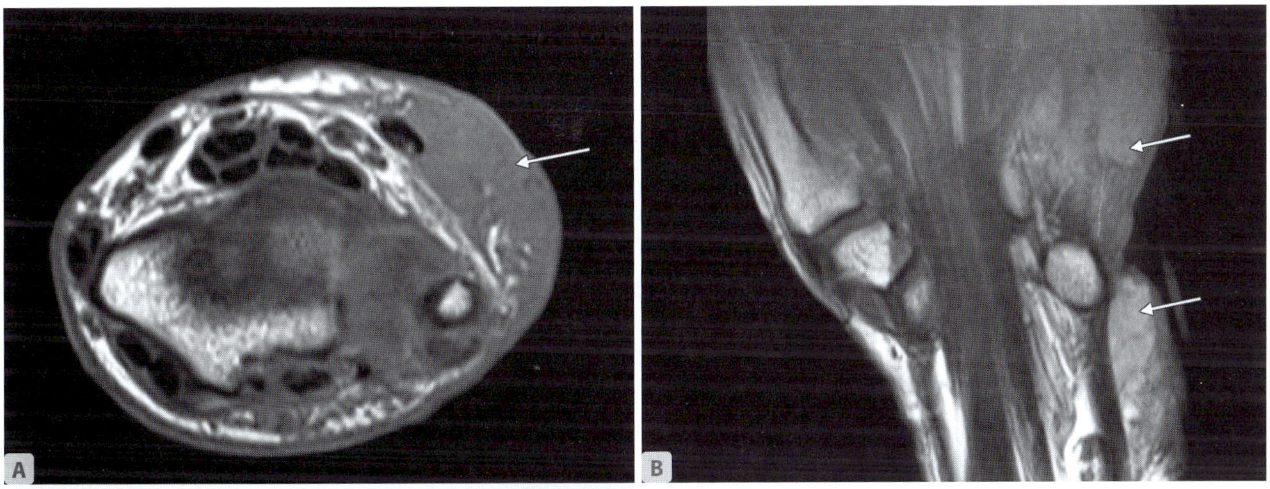

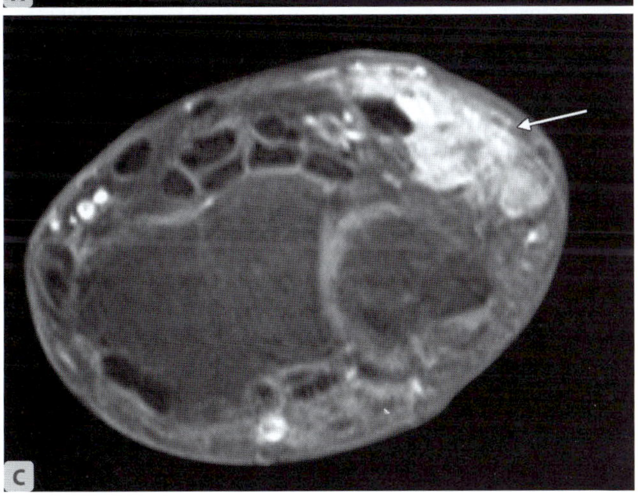

FIGS. 30A TO C: Giant cell tumor of the tendon sheath. Multilobulated mass around the flexor carpi ulnaris, isointense on T1W axial image (arrow in A), intermediate to hyperintense on T2W coronal image (B) and showing contrast enhancement (C).

Ulnar-sided Wrist Pain

The causes of ulnar-sided wrist pain are given in **Table 6**.

Radial-sided Wrist Pain

The causes of ulnar-sided wrist pain are given in **Table 7**.

TABLE 6: Causes of ulnar-sided wrist pain.[2,22]

Ligamentous injuries	• Triangular fibrocartilage complex (TFCC) lesions
Impaction syndromes	• Ulnar impaction syndrome • Ulnar impingement syndrome • Ulnar styloid impaction syndrome • Hamatolunate impingement syndrome
Osseous injuries	• Kienböck's disease • Ulnar styloid fracture • Hamate fracture • Pisiform fracture • Base of fifth metacarpal fracture
Joint disorders	• Carpal instability • Distal radioulnar joint disorders
Tendon disorders	• Extensor carpi ulnaris disorder • Flexor carpi ulnaris tendinitis
Nerve impingement	• Guyon's canal syndrome

TABLE 7: Causes of radial-sided wrist pain.

Ligamentous injuries	• Scapholunate ligament injury
Osseous injuries	• Scaphoid fracture and avascular necrosis (AVN) of scaphoid
Joint disorders	• Scapholunate advanced collapse and scaphoid nonunion advanced collapse • Trapeziometacarpal joint arthritis
Tendon disorders	• De Quervain's tenosynovitis • Intersection syndromes (between I and II compartments proximal and II and III compartments distal to Lister's tubercle) • Flexor carpi radialis tenosynovitis
Nerve impingement	• Wartenberg's syndrome

REFERENCES

1. Mann FA, Gilula LA. Post-traumatic wrist pain and instability: a radiographic approach to diagnosis. In: Lichtman DM, Alexander AH (Eds). The Wrist and Its Disorders, 2nd edition. Philadelphia PA: Saunders; 1997. pp. 91-108.
2. Cerezal L, Del piñal F, Abascal F, García-Valtuille R, Pereda T, Canga A. Imaging findings in ulnar-sided wrist impaction syndromes. Radiographics. 2002;22(1):105-21.
3. Bateni CP, Bartolotta RJ, Richardson ML, Mulcahy H, Allan CH. Imaging key wrist ligaments: what the surgeon needs the radiologist to know. Am J Roentgenol. 2013;200(5):1089-95.
4. Buck FM, Gheno R, Nico MA, Haghighi P, Trudell DJ, Resnick D. Ulnomeniscal homologue of the wrist: correlation of anatomic and MR imaging findings. Radiology. 2009;253(3):771-9.
5. Haugstvedt JR, Berger RA, Nakamura T, Neale P, Berglund L, An KN. Relative contributions of the ulnar attachments of the triangular fibrocartilage complex to the dynamic stability of the distal radioulnar joint. J Hand Surg Am. 2006;31(3):445-51.
6. Johnson D, Stevens KJ, Riley G, Shapiro L, Yoshioka H, Gold GE. Approach to MR imaging of the elbow and wrist: technical aspects and innovation. Magn Reson Imaging Clin N Am. 2015;23(3):355-66.
7. Chang AL, Yu HJ, von Borstel D, Nozaki T, Horiuchi S, Terada Y, et al. Advanced imaging techniques of the Wrist. Am J Roentgenol. 2017;209(3):497-510.
8. Akella SV, Regatte RR, Borthakur A, Kneeland JB, Leigh JS, Reddy R. T1rho MR imaging of the human wrist in vivo. Acad Radiol. 2003;10(6):614-9.
9. Ku E, Pedoia V, Tanaka M, Heilmeier U, Imboden J, Graf J, et al. Evaluating radiocarpal cartilage matrix changes 3-months after anti-TNF treatment for rheumatoid arthritis using MR T1ρ imaging. J Magn Reson Imaging. 2017;45(5):1514-22.
10. Medverd JR, Pugsley JM, Harley JD, Bhargava P. Lateral approach for radiocarpal wrist arthrography. Am J Roentgenol. 2011;196(1):W58-60.
11. Limarzi GM, O'Dell MC, Scherer K, Pettis C, Wasyliw CW, Bancroft LW. Magnetic resonance arthrography of the wrist and elbow. Magn Reson Imaging Clin N Am. 2015;23(03):441-55.
12. Cerezal L, Abascal F, Garcia-Valtuille R, del Pinal F. Wrist MR arthrography: how, why, when? Radiol Clin N Am. 2005;43(4):709-31.
13. Squires JH, England E, Mehta K, Wissman RD. The role of imaging in diagnosing diseases of the distal radioulnar joint, triangular fibrocartilage complex, and distal ulna. Am J Roentgenol. 2014;203(1):146-53.
14. Ten Berg PW, Drijkoningen T, Strackee SD, Buijze GA. Classifications of acute scaphoid fractures: a systematic literature review. J Wrist Surg. 2016;5(2):152-9.
15. Cockenpot E, Lefebvre G, Demondion X, Chantelot C, Cotten A. Imaging of sports-related hand and wrist injuries: sports imaging series. Radiology. 2016;279(3):674-92.
16. Amadio PC, Berquist TH, Smith DK, Ilstrup DM, Cooney WP 3rd, Linscheid RL. Scaphoid malunion. J Hand Surg [Am]. 1989;14(4):679-87.
17. Trumble TE, Irving J. Histologic and magnetic resonance imaging correlations in Kienböck's disease. J Hand Surg Am. 1990;15(6): 879-84.
18. Desser TS, McCarthy S, Trumble T. Scaphoid fractures and Kienböck's disease of the lunate: MR imaging with histopathologic correlation. Magn Reson Imaging. 1990;8(4):357-61.
19. Cerezal L, Abascal F, Canga A, García-Valtuille R, Bustamante M, del Piñal F. Usefulness of gadolinium-enhanced MR imaging in the evaluation of the vascularity of scaphoid nonunions. Am J Roentgenol. 2000;174(1):141-9.
20. Anderson SE, Steinbach LS, Tschering-Vogel D, Martin M, Nagy L. MR imaging of avascular scaphoid nonunion before and after vascularized bone grafting. Skeletal Radiol. 2005;34(6):314-20.
21. Schmitt R, Rosenthal H. Imaging of scaphoid fractures according to the New S3 guidelines. Fortschr Röntgenstr. 2016;188(5): 459-69.
22. Watanabe A, Souza F, Vezeridis PS, Blazar P, Yoshioka H. Ulnar-sided wrist pain. II. Clinical imaging and treatment. Skeletal Radiol. 2010;39(9):837-57.
23. Kienböck R. Über traumatische malazie des mondbeins und ihre folgezustände: entartungsformen und kompressionsfrakturen. Fortschr Geb Roentgenstrahlen. 1910;16:77-103.
24. Hulten O. Über anatomische variationen der hand-gelenkknochen. Acta Radiol. 1928;9:155-68.
25. Antuña Zapico JM. Malacia del semilunar. Vall-adolid, Spain: University of Valladolid; 1966.

26. van Leeuwen WF, Janssen SJ, ter Meulen DP, Ring D. What is the radiographic prevalence of incidental Kienböck disease? Clin Orthop Relat Res. 2016;474(3):808-13.
27. Stoller DW. Magnetic Resonance Imaging in Orthopaedics and Sports Medicine, 3rd edition. Baltimore, MD: Lippincott Williams & Wilkins; 2007
28. Arnaiz J, Piedra T, Cerezal L, Ward J, Thompson A, Vidal JA, et al. Imaging of Kienböck disease. Am J Roentgenol. 2014;203(1):131-9.
29. Kennedy C, Abrams R. Lichtman classification for Kienbock disease. Clin Orthop Relat Res. 2019;477(6):1516-20.
30. Helms C, Major N, Anderson M, Kaplan PE, Dussault R (Eds). Musculoskeletal MRI, 2nd edition. Philadelphia: Saunders; 2009. pp. 252-9.
31. Ng AW, Griffith JF, Fung CS, Lee RK, Tong CS, Wong CW. MR imaging of the traumatic triangular fibrocartilaginous complex tear. Quant Imaging Med Surg. 2017;7(4):443-60.
32. Bae WC, Ruangchaijatuporn T, Chang EY, Biswas R, Du J, Statum S, et al. MR morphology of triangular fibrocartilage complex: correlation with quantitative MR and biomechanical properties. Skeletal Radiol. 2016;45(4):447-54.
33. Moser TP, Martinez AP, Andoulsi S, Jeantroux J, Cardinal E. Radiographic/MR imaging correlation of the wrist. Magn Reson Imaging Clin N Am. 2019;27:601-23.
34. Kani KK, Mulcahy H, Chew FS. Understanding carpal instability: a radiographic perspective. Skeletal Radiol. 2016;45(8):1031-43.
35. Treiman ML, Strle NA, Matthews CR, von Borstel D. Carpal instability: clarification of the most common etiologies and imaging findings. J Am Osteopath Coll Radiol. 2019;8(4):5-10.
36. Shahabpour M, Staelens B, Van Overstraeten L, De Maeseneer M, Boulet C, De Mey J, et al. Advanced imaging of the scapholunate ligamentous complex. Skeletal Radiol. 2015;44(12):1709-25.
37. Schmitt R, Christopoulos G, Meier R, Coblenz G, Fröhner S, Lanz U, et al. Direct MR arthrography of the wrist in comparison with arthroscopy: a prospective study on 125 patients. Rofo Fortschr Geb Rontgenstr Neuen Bildgeb Verfahr. 2003;175(7):911-9.
38. Lee DJ, Elfar JC. Carpal ligament injuries, pathomechanics, and classification. Hand Clin. 2015;31(3):389-98.
39. Mespreuve M, Vanhoenacke F, Verstraete K. Imaging findings of the distal radio-ulnar joint in trauma. J Belgian Soc Radiol. 2015;99(1):1-20.
40. Amrami KK, Moran SL, Berger RA, Ehman EC, Felmlee JP. Imaging the distal radioulnar joint. Hand Clin. 2010;26(4):467-75.
41. Bencardino JT. MR imaging of tendon lesions of the hand and wrist. Magn Reson Imaging Clin N Am. 2004;12(2):333-47.
42. Ghasemi-Rad M, Nosair E, Vegh A, Mohammadi A, Akkad A, Lesha E, et al. A handy review of carpal tunnel syndrome: from anatomy to diagnosis and treatment. World J Radiol. 2014;6(6):284-300.
43. Filler AG, Kliot M, Howe FA, Hayes CE, Saunders DE, Goodkin R, et al. Application of magnetic resonance neurography in the evaluation of patients with peripheral nerve pathology. J Neurosurg. 1996;85(2):299-309.
44. Chhabra A, Lee PP, Bizzell C, Soldatos T. 3 Tesla MR neurography—technique, interpretation, and pitfalls. Skeletal Radiol. 2011;40(10):1249-60.
45. Chhabra A, Flammang A, Padua A Jr. Carrino JA, Andreisek G. Magnetic resonance neurography: technical considerations. Neuroimaging Clin N Am. 2014;24(1):67-78.
46. Bagga B, Sinha A, Khandelwal N, Modi M, Ahuja CK, Sharma R. Comparison of magnetic resonance imaging and ultrasonography in diagnosing and grading carpal tunnel syndrome: a prospective study. Curr Prob Diagn Radiol. 2020;49(2):102-15.
47. Koh SH, Kwon BC, Park C, Hwang SY, Lee JW, Kim SS. A comparison of the performance of anatomical MRI and DTI in diagnosing carpal tunnel syndrome. Eur J Radiol. 2014;83(11):2065-73.
48. Uchiyama S, Itsubo T, Yasutomi T, Nakagawa H, Kamimura M, Kato H. Quantitative MRI of the wrist and nerve conduction studies in patients with idiopathic carpal tunnel syndrome. J Neurol Neurosurg Psychiatry. 2005;76(8):1103-8.
49. Britz GW, Haynor DR, Kuntz C, Goodkin R, Gitter A, Kliot M. Carpal tunnel syndrome: correlation of magnetic resonance imaging, clinical, electrodiagnostic, and intraoperative findings. Neurosurgery. 1995;37(6):1097-103.
50. Monagle K, Dai G, Chu A, Burnham RS, Snyder RE. Quantitative MR imaging of carpal tunnel syndrome. Am J Roentgenol. 1999;172(6):1581-6.
51. Klauser AS, Abd Ellah M, Kremser C, Taljanovic M, Schmidle G, Gabl M, et al. Carpal tunnel syndrome assessment with diffusion tensor imaging: value of fractional anisotropy and apparent diffusion coefficient. Eur Radiol. 2018;28(3):1111-7.
52. Radack DM, Schweitzer ME, Taras J. Carpal tunnel syndrome: are the MR findings a result of population selection bias? Am J Roentgenol. 1997;169(6):1649-53.
53. Hui-Chou HG, McClinton MA. Current options for treatment of hypothenar hammer syndrome. Hand Clin. 2015;31(1):53-62.
54. Jbara, M, Patnana M, Kazmi F, Beltran J. MR imaging: arthropathies and infectious conditions of the elbow, wrist, and hand. Magn Reson Imaging Clin N Am. 2004;12:361-79.
55. McQueen FM. Magnetic resonance imaging in early inflammatory arthritis: what is its role? Rheumatology. 2000;39(7):700-6.
56. Ejbjerg B, McQueen F, Lassere ME, Haavardsholm P, Conaghan P, O'Connor P, et al. The EULAR–OMERACT rheumatoid arthritis MRI reference image atlas: the wrist joint. Ann Rheum Dis. 2005;64:i23-i47.
57. Plotkin B, Srihari SC, Srinath SC, Motamedi K. MR imaging and US of the WRIST Tendons. Radiographics. 2016;36(6):1688-700.
58. Patel DB, Emmanuel NB, Stevanovic MV, Matsuk GR, Gottsegen CJ, Forrester DM, et al. Hand infections: anatomy, types and spread of infection, imaging findings, and treatment options. Radiographics. 2014;34(7): 1968-86.
59. Haugen IK, Bøyesen P. Imaging modalities in hand osteoarthritis—status and perspectives of conventional radiography, magnetic resonance imaging, and ultrasonography. Arthritis Res Ther. 2011;13:248.
60. Li AE, Lee SK, Rancy SK, Burge AJ, Potter HG, Wolfe SW. Comparison of magnetic resonance imaging and radiographs for evaluation of carpal osteoarthritis. J Wrist Surg. 2017;6(2):120-5.
61. Vanhoenacker FM, Eyselbergs M, Van Hul E, Van Dyck P, De Schepper AM. Pseudotumoural soft tissue lesions of the hand and wrist: a pictorial review. Insights Imag. 2011;2(3):319-33.
62. Plate AM, Lee SJ, Steiner G, Posner MA. Tumor-like lesions and benign tumors of the hand and wrist. J Am Acad Orthop Surg. 2003;11(2):129-41.
63. Di Grazia S, Succi G, Fragetta F, Perrotta RE. Giant cell tumor of tendon sheath: study of 64 cases and review of literature. G Chir. 2013;3(5-6):149-52.
64. Al-Qattan M. Giant cell tumors of tendon sheath: classification and recurrence rate. J Hand Surg Br. 2001;26(1):72-5.

CHAPTER

169

Magnetic Resonance Imaging of the Hip and Pelvis

Anjali Prakash, Alpana Manchanda, Rashmi Dixit

INTRODUCTION

The hip joint is a primary weight-bearing joint. The pelvis transmits the weight of the body to both the feet and at the same time allows extensive movement of the hip. Pain in the hip is one of the most common orthopedic complaints which has a broad differential diagnosis and includes both intra and extra-articular causes.

Conventional radiography is used as a first-line tool in trauma, arthritis, and suspected tumors; however, it is insensitive to early osseous changes and may depict only advanced stage of the disease where treatment options are limited to hip replacement. It is also unable to detect soft tissue injury, cartilage, and labral pathology. Magnetic resonance imaging (MRI) has become the imaging study of choice for diagnosing most hip disorders.

NORMAL ANATOMY

The pelvis is a complex structure composed of an osseous ring formed by the innominate bones and the sacrum with numerous muscles attached for support and ambulation. The sacroiliac joints allow little movement and the articulating surfaces serve to transmit weight. These surfaces are covered by hyaline cartilage and bound together by strong ligaments—the interosseous anteriorly and by the sacroiliac ligaments posteriorly.

The hip is a ball and socket joint formed by the articulation of the spherical femoral head with the acetabulum. The acetabulum covers 40% of the femoral head and is formed by the ilium, ischium, and the pubis. In infants, the acetabulum is united by a Y-shaped cartilage. The acetabulum is tilted anteriorly, making hip flexion easier than extension. The concave shape of the acetabulum adds to stability of the joint. The semilunar surface of the acetabulum is covered by hyaline cartilage shaped like an inverted horseshoe. It contains nonarticulating central depression, the acetabular fossa. The depth of the acetabulum is increased by the fibrocartilaginous labrum that surrounds it.

The femoral head is almost completely covered by hyaline cartilage sparing only the depression of the acetabular fovea where the ligamentum teres attaches. The ligamentum teres carries an artery which supplies blood to the femoral head in children and involutes with age.

The trochanters are apophysis which add to the width of the bone. There are four distinct facets in the greater trochanter of the hip three of which have corresponding tendon attachment sites. The tendons of the gluteus medius and minimus, the obturator internus and externus, and piriformis muscle attach to the greater trochanter. The facets of the greater trochanter have bursae that are intimately associated with them. These include the subgluteus minimus and medius bursae, these bursae lay beneath the gluteus minimus and medius tendon osseous attachment sites, respectively. In addition, there is a subgluteus maximus bursa, the largest of the three. The iliopsoas tendon inserts at the lesser trochanter **(Figs. 1 and 2)**.

Similarly, the attachment sites of the proximal hamstring tendons correspond to changes in osseous contour. The proximal hamstring attachment complex is composed of the semimembranosus, semitendinosus, and biceps femoris tendons. All three, except for the short head of the biceps femoris, arise from the posterolateral ischial tuberosity, lateral and inferomedial facets. The semimembranosus tendon originates from the superolateral facet while the semitendinosus and long head of the biceps femoris form a conjoint tendon that attaches to the inferomedial facet. Rarely, the conjoint tendon is absent and the two tendons arise separately. The coronal plane on MR imaging is superior in visualization of the proximal hamstring attachment to these facets. In the transverse plane, the semimembranosus tendon can be found anterolaterally to the conjoint tendon. More distally, the tendon runs more medial and anterior to the other two hamstring tendons.

The trabecular pattern within the femoral head and neck is reinforced by two regions of increased trabeculation corresponding to areas of relative increase in stress. The largest of these areas runs from the apex of the femoral head inferolaterally crossing the physeal plate to the medial femoral neck. This region is referred to as primary weight-bearing trabecula. Primary weight-bearing trabeculae produce a fan-shaped area of lower signal within the femoral head and neck, produced by increased concentration of calcium relative to fat. A second area of trabecular prominence runs from the

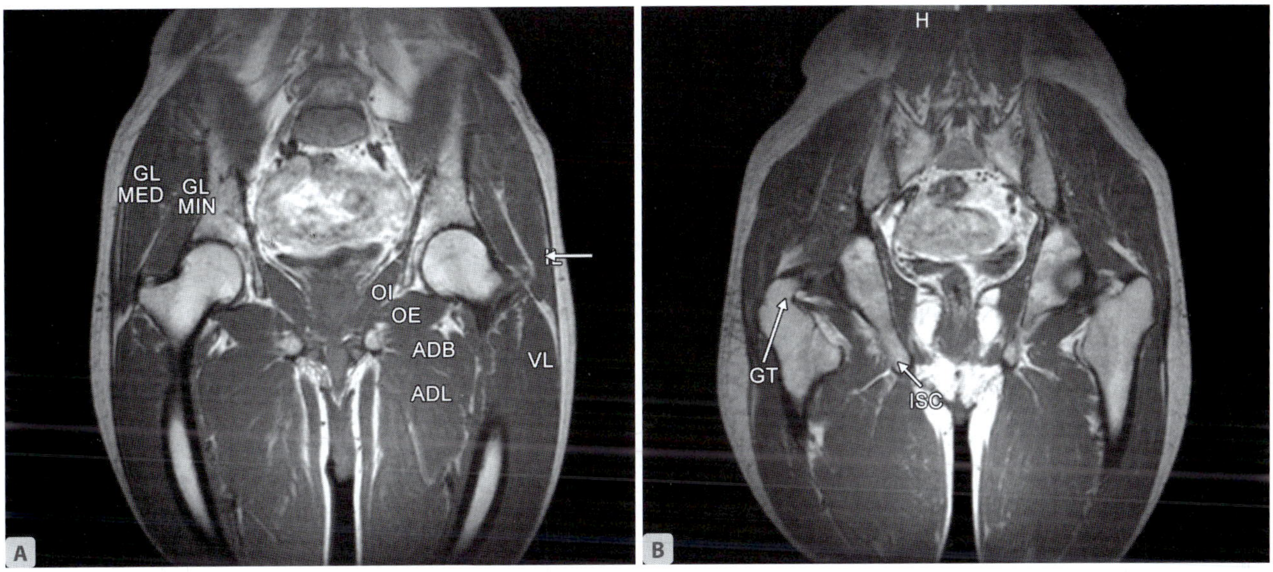

FIGS. 1A AND B: T1-weighted coronal image of both hips anterior (A) to posterior (B) depicting normal anatomy. (ADB: adductor brevis; ADL: adductor longus; GL MED: gluteus medius; GL MIN: gluteus minimus; GT: greater trochanter; IL: iliofemoral ligament; ISC: ischium; OE: obturator externus; OI: obturator internus; VL: vastus lateralis).

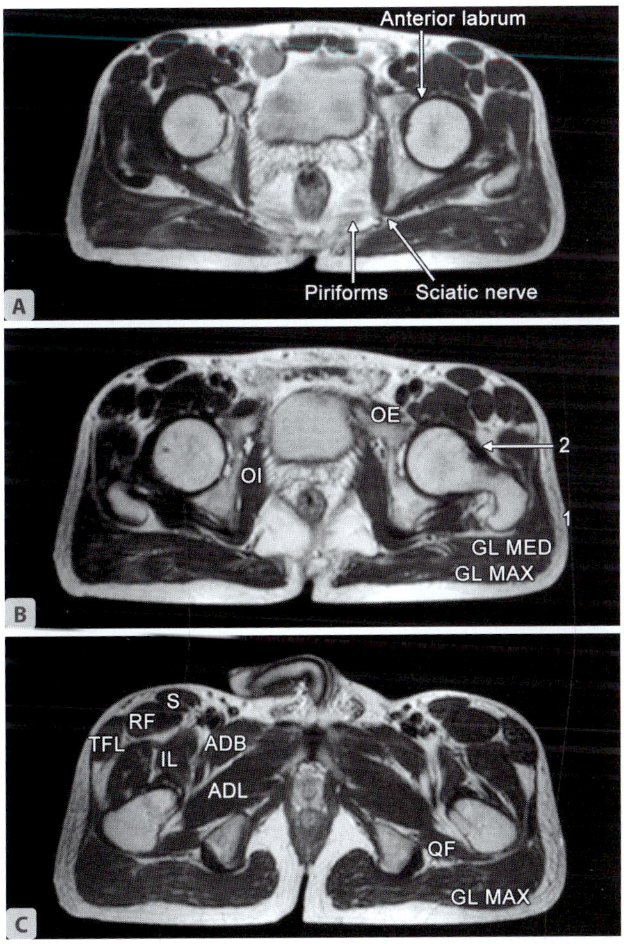

FIGS. 2A TO C: T1-weighted axial image of both hips depicting normal anatomy superior to inferior. Arrow marked 2-iliofemoral ligament (anterior fold of the hip capsule). (ADB: adductor brevis; ADL: adductor lingus; GL MAX: gluteus maximus; GL MED: gluteus medius; IL: iliopsoas muscle; OE: obturator externus; OI: obturator internus; QF: quadratus femoris; RF: rectus femoris; S: sartorius; TFL: tensor fascia lata).

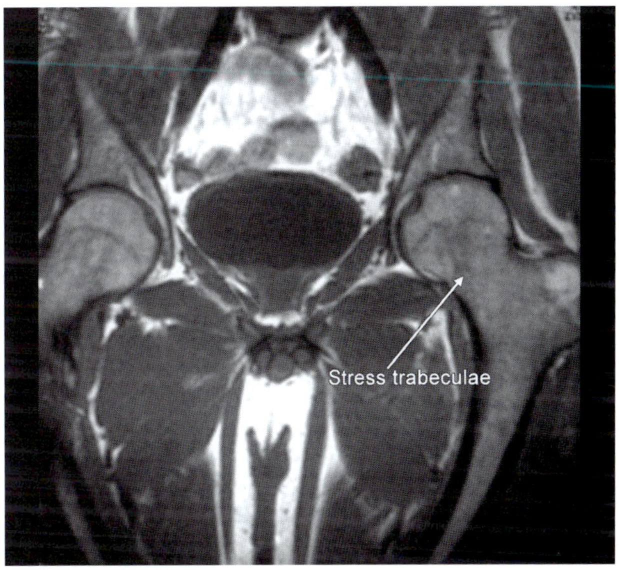

FIG. 3: T1-weighted coronal image of both hips—stress trabeculae seen as fan-shaped region of hypointensity in the femoral neck.

inferomedial femoral head laterally and across the neck toward the greater trochanter **(Fig. 3)**.

MAGNETIC RESONANCE IMAGING TECHNIQUE

Conventional Magnetic Resonance Imaging

The technique for performing MRI of the hip is designed to image the entire pelvis and both hips. Hip MRI is best performed on a 1.5 or 3 Tesla magnet. The patient is placed in a supine position as straight as possible with the toes taped together to maintain slight internal rotation of the hip and to immobilize. A multichannel body coil with a large field of view is used to get an overview of the entire pelvis.[1]

Magnetic resonance examination of the hip begins with a triplane localization which is a low resolution gradient recalled echo imaging technique. This allows accurate positioning. Imaging is done in three standard planes **(Figs. 4A to C)**. Coronal images should cover the insertion of the adductor tendons and the iliopsoas. An axial whole pelvis sequence should extend from the level of sacroiliac joints to the level of insertion of iliopsoas at the lesser trochanter. Sagittal images must include from the medial acetabular wall to the greater trochanter. Images in axial oblique plane to look for abnormal femoral head-neck offset are also obtained. The axial oblique plane is obtained by using a coronal localizer and angling the slices parallel to the femoral neck **(Figs. 5A and B)**.

Standard hip MR protocol **(Table 1)** consists of anatomical sequences such as nonfat saturated T1W TSE. Fluid sensitive sequences such as T2W FSE with fat saturation and short tau inversion recovery (STIR in coronal plane) are also obtained. Postcontrast fat saturated T1W images are obtained as a routine in suspected cases of tumor and infection.

This is followed by a tailored high-resolution protocol for the area of interest. There is no true hip coil and hip imaging is best performed with a shoulder coil or a small field of view surface coil. The hip is centered in the magnetic field. Specific protocols for deep gluteal syndrome, adductor tendinitis, gluteal tendons, rectus femoris, and athletic pubalgia can be used based on patient symptomatology and clinical findings.

Radial Imaging

The nearly spherical femoral head, anteverted orientation, and anatomically abducted hip joint make imaging of the hip in conventional planes a challenge due to volume averaging. The regions most affected are the anterior and posterosuperior regions of the hip joint in the axial plane and the superior part in the sagittal plane. Labral and cartilage pathology in these regions may be masked.

Radial imaging plane is perpendicular to the curved surfaces of the joint with the imaging plane going through the center of the joint or along the radius of the sphere. This provides a cross section of the cartilage and labrum. Radial sections are obtained in the plane of the acetabular opening and are planned on the enface view of the acetabulum **(Fig. 6)**. Acquisition of the enface view requires the use of

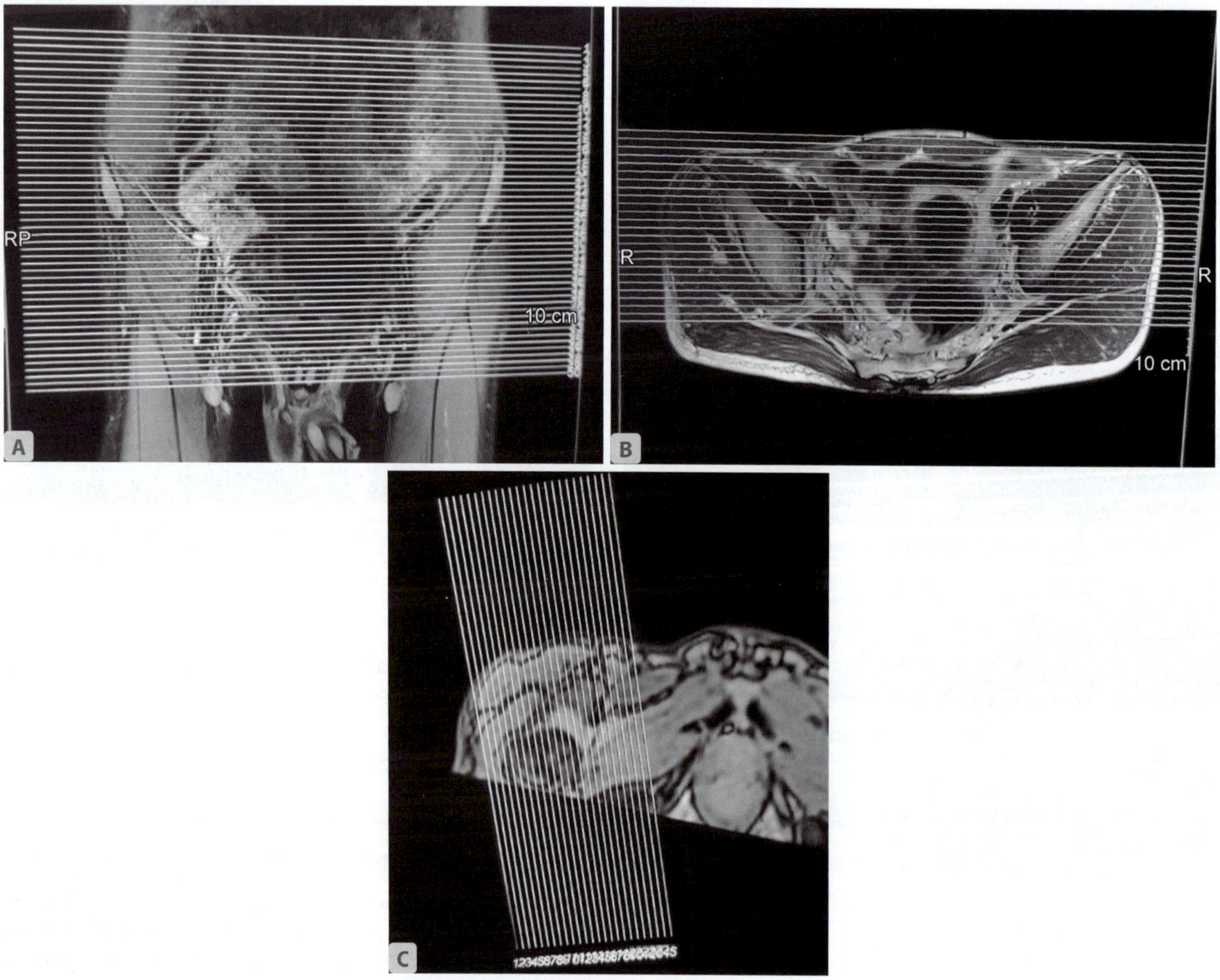

FIGS. 4A TO C: Triplane localizer on which planning is done for MR pelvis and hip.

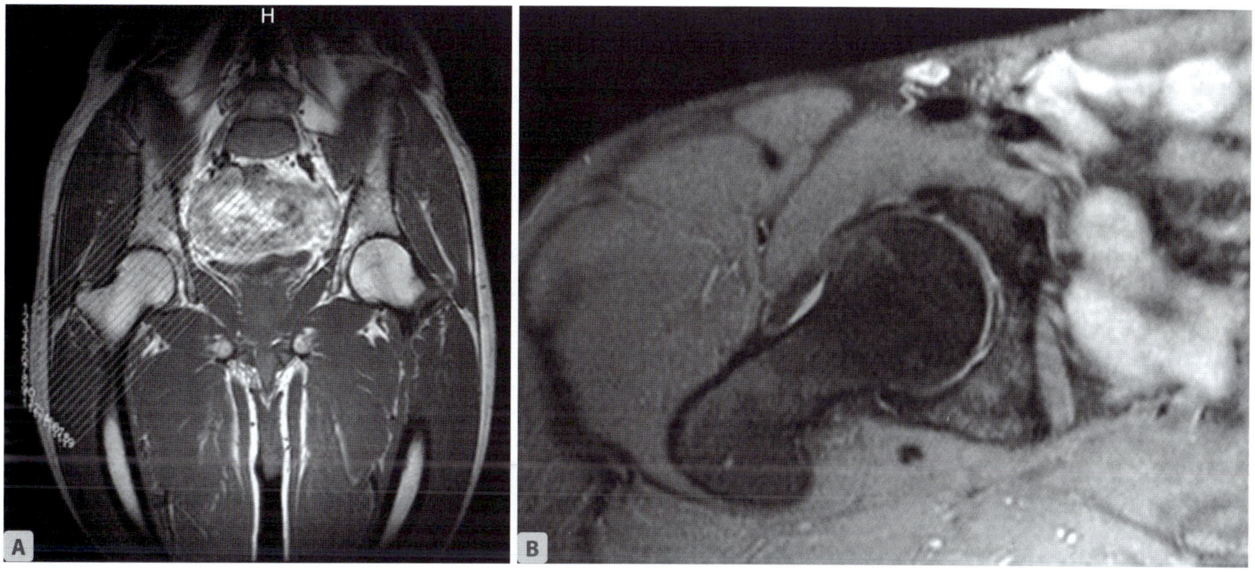

FIGS. 5A AND B: (A) T1-weighted coronal image, used as localizer to obtain axial-oblique proton density-weighted image (PDWI) (B).

TABLE 1: Magnetic resonance protocol for routine examination of hip.

Sequence	FOV (mm)	Matrix	TR (ms)	TE (ms)	TI (ms)	Bandwidth (kHz)	Echo train length
Coronal STIR (pelvis)	360	320 × 192	4,060	48	200	200	7
Axial PD FSE	200	256 × 256	2,730	9	-	300	5
Coronal T1 FSE	200	384 × 307	650	15	-	303	5
Coronal T2 FSE FS	200	256 × 256	3,070	60	-	250	11
Sagittal PD FSE	200	384 × 307	3,500	43	-	303	7
Oblique axial PD FSE FS	160	384 × 257	3,640	48	-	303	5
Axial T2 FSE FS	200	256 × 154	4,000	69	-	250	11

(FS: fat saturation; FSE: fast spin echo; PD: proton density image; STIR: short tau inversion recovery)

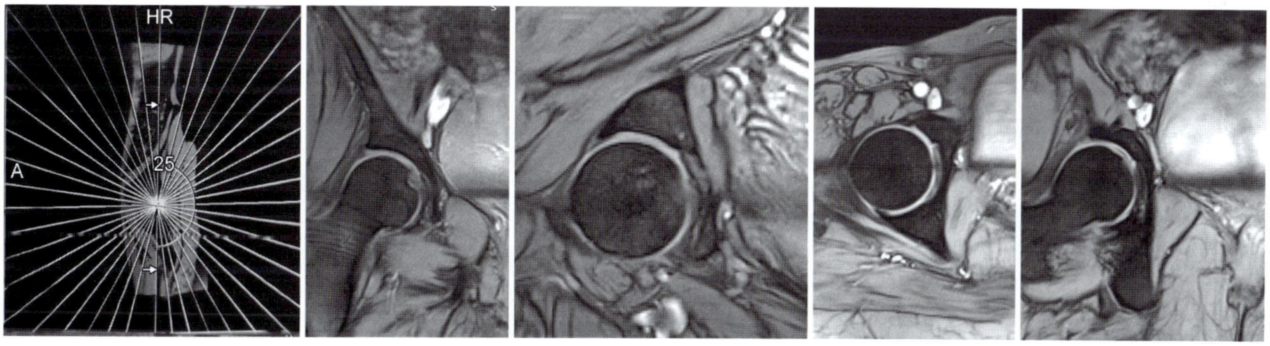

FIG. 6: Radial sections obtained around the enface view of acetabulum.

a double oblique orientation. Two localizers are obtained—first is axial oblique, second is the coronal localizer. Plane of section is adjusted to go through the edge of the acetabular rim on both localizer images. Sections are obtained with a spectral presaturation attenuated inversion recovery with proton density weighting. Each section provides information about diametrically opposite positions in the joint.[2,3]

Magnetic Resonance Arthrography

Direct magnetic resonance arthrography (MRA) is the mainstay in hip imaging to detect labral and chondral pathology. It is the current gold standard for detection of intra-articular lesions.[4] Injection of gadolinium into the joint distends it and increases the intra-articular pressure forcing contrast into cartilage and labral tears and detachments. Recent studies

TABLE 2: Magnetic resonance arthrogram protocol.

Routine hip MR arthrogram protocol						
Sequence	**FOV (mm)**	**Matrix**	**TR (ms)**	**TE (ms)**	**Bandwidth (kHz)**	**Echo train length**
Coronal T1 FSE	160	448 × 269	610	15	302	3
Coronal T1 FSE FS	160	384 × 230	570	15	237	3
Oblique axial T1 FSE	160	384 × 230	650	14	237	3
Axial T2 FSE FS	160	384 × 230	3,500	82	237	11
Coronal T2 FSE FS	160	384 × 230	3,960	82	210	11
Sagittal T1 FSE FS	160	448 × 318	640	13	211	3

(FS: fat saturation; FSE: fast spin echo; STIR: short tau inversion recovery)

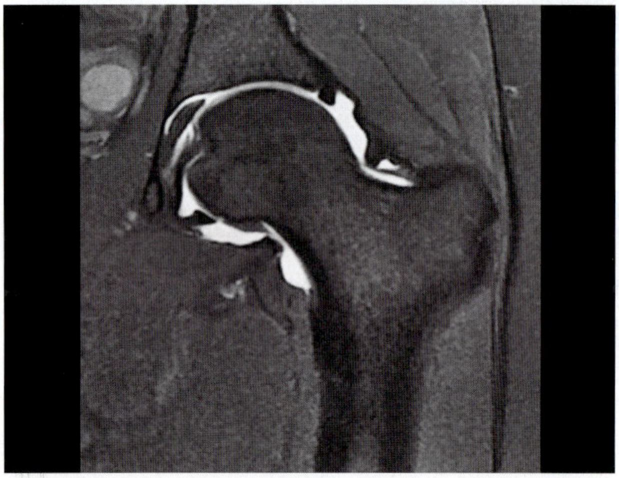

FIG. 7: MR arthrogram-contrast injected directly into the joint. Labrum appreciated as low signal triangular structure.

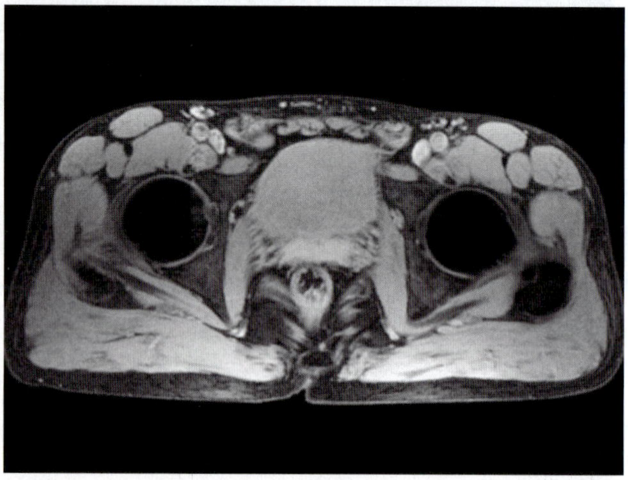

FIG. 8: Indirect MR arthrogram—diffuse enhancement seen within the joint.

have suggested that due to a higher signal-noise ratio (SNR), noncontrast MRI imaging at 3T MRI could replace direct MR arthrography at 1.5T MRI.[5]

Direct MR arthrography of the hip consists of two steps. Initially, the joint injection is performed in the fluoroscopic suite. After instillation of iodinated contrast material to document the intra-articular position of the needle, 10 mL of 1:200 dilution of gadolinium contrast is injected into the joint. The second step is the actual MR imaging in the MR suite. MR arthrogram protocol is given in **Table 2**. Concurrent injection of local anesthetic into the joint and performing provocative maneuvers can help correlate symptoms to pathology **(Fig. 7)**.

Indirect MRA is an alternate technique that is performed after intravenous injection of gadolinium. The contrast eventually enters the joint by diffusion and bulk flow from the synovium producing an arthrogram-like effect. Imaging is done 30 minutes after the injection. Exercise after injection helps to promote contrast accumulation into the joint **(Fig. 8)**. This technique can be helpful in certain select patients. High sensitivity and specificity for this technique performed at 3T MRI has been found for labral pathology with lower accuracy for acetabular and femoral head cartilage lesions.

Indirect MRA suffers from several drawbacks, as there is no increase in intra-articular pressure, some labral tears may not be detected. Presence of contrast in multiple compartments in the joint does not imply abnormal communication as it would in direct MRA.[6,7]

MAGNETIC RESONANCE APPEARANCES OF NORMAL HIP

The appearance of the hip on MRI varies depending on the type of sequence and the skeletal maturity of the patient. Cortical bone produces a thin sharply defined black line. Thicker cortex is noted in the femoral diaphysis. Higher signal is always present within the medullary cavity of both the femoral head and acetabulum. In the adult, the epiphysis is filled completely with fatty marrow that is high in signal on all sequences, except STIR and fat saturation techniques, in which the epiphysis becomes dark. The nonossified epiphyseal cartilage of the child is homogeneous and moderately high in signal. Maturation replaces the cartilage with larger amounts of fatty marrow within the bony epiphysis **(Figs. 9 and 10)**.

The immature metaphysis contains hematopoietic marrow and is intermediate in signal on all sequences.

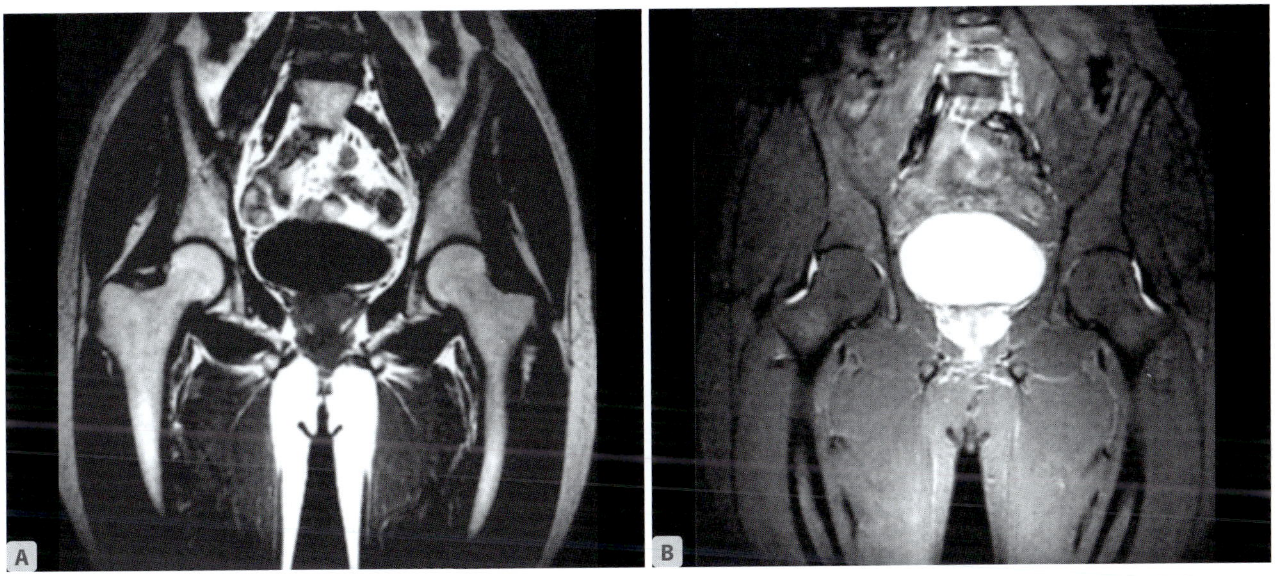

FIGS. 9A AND B: (A) T1-weighted coronal image of bilateral hips and pelvis; and (B) Short tau inversion recovery (STIR) coronal image showing fatty marrow of the femoral head, which is suppressed on STIR. Cortical outline is sharply defined and black on both sequences—normal appearance.

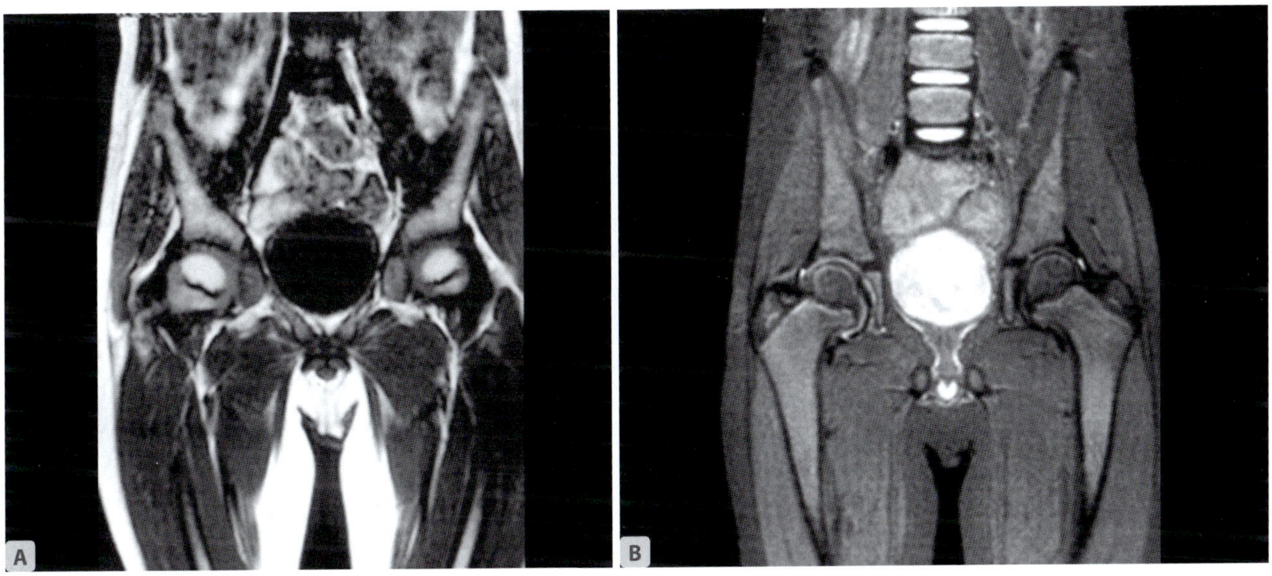

FIGS. 10A AND B: (A) T1-weighted coronal image; and (B) Short tau inversion recovery (STIR) coronal image shows moderately high signal in the epiphyseal cartilage with ossifying femoral head exhibiting fatty marrow in a child.

The adult metaphysis contains a mix of fatty and hematopoietic marrow that is lower in signal than the epiphysis and is often heterogenous. Hematopoietic marrow dominates in younger patients and fatty marrow in older patients. This may be due to decreased blood supply of the marrow with age and a change from the sinusoidal blood flow of hematopoietic marrow to the more sparse capillary flow in fatty marrow. The physeal scar separating the epiphysis from the metaphysis is seen on all MR examinations of the hip **(Fig. 11)**. The inability to identify some part of the physeal scar indicates an examination of inadequate quality. The physeal scar, best seen on T1W images is seen as a thin black line on all sequences.

Labrum is seen as a triangular structure, hypointense on all sequences. The articular cartilage of the femoral head and acetabulum produces a thin, smooth uniform intermediate signal, the signal being higher on STIR, gradient, and fat saturation sequences **(Fig. 12)**.

The structures to be evaluated on a hip MRI are given in **Box 1**.

Pathological Conditions of the Hip

Avascular Necrosis

Osteonecrosis (ON) **(Box 2)** refers to bone death secondary to interruption of the blood supply. The term avascular

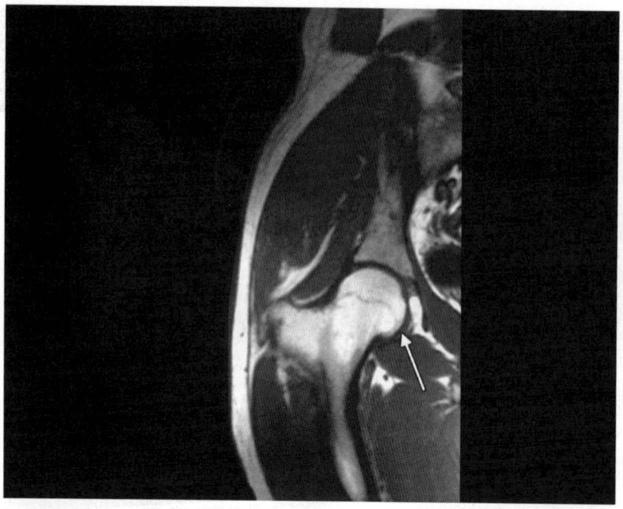

FIG. 11: T1-weighted coronal image of the right hip showing normal physeal scar seen as a thin hypointense line separating epiphysis from metaphysis.

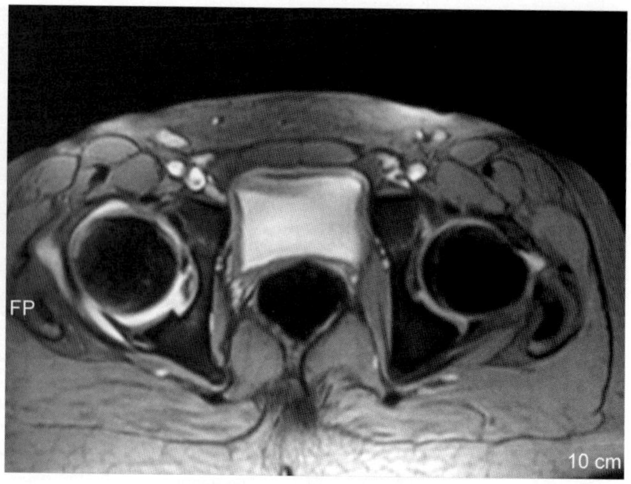

FIG. 12: T2-weighted fat-saturated fast spin-echo (FSE)—axial scan depicts normal hypointense labrum and intermediate signal articular cartilage.

necrosis (AVN) describes the occurrence of ON in the epiphysis or subarticular bone and the term bone infarction to ischemia occurring at metadiaphyseal sites.

Etiopathogenesis

Avascular necrosis has a varied etiology, the most common causes being idiopathic, trauma, use of corticosteroids and alcoholism.[8,9]

In the hip, AVN occurs as a complication of displaced femoral neck fracture or hip dislocation. The risk of AVN is related to the degree of fracture displacement and a delay in reduction. Blood supply to the femoral head is derived primarily from the medial circumflex artery. The medial and lateral circumflex artery sends branches with the capsular reflections (retinacula) of the hip joint to the femoral head. These branches are oriented along the long axis of the femoral head. Consequently, a subcapital fracture or a fracture of the femoral neck traverses these branches, which renders the head susceptible to ischemic necrosis. In some individuals, blood supply to the femoral head reaches via the foveal artery, which runs in the ligamentum teres. This artery may also be disrupted in the setting of trauma. Traumatic AVN is typically unilateral.

The pathogenesis of corticosteroid-induced ON is due to fatty embolization with osteoporosis-induced microfractures and increased blood viscosity. Long duration of steroid therapy, high and divided doses increases the likelihood of ON.

The first phase is interruption of blood supply. This leads to cell death and loss of cellular metabolic activity. Bone marrow is composed of three separate cell types—hematopoietic cells, osteocytes, and marrow fat cells. When these cells are exposed to an ischemic insult, they die at a different rate. Hematopoietic cells tend to die within 6–12 hours after insult, whereas osteocytes live up to 12–48 hours after blood flow is interrupted while fat cells live up to 5 days after the ischemic insult.

BOX 1: Structures to evaluate in different planes

- Coronal:
  - *Osseous structures:*
    - Acetabulum
    - Femoral head, neck
    - Greater, lesser trochanter
    - Sacrum
    - Ilium
    - Sacroiliac joints
  - Muscles:
    - Gluteal muscles
    - Adductors
    - Abductors
    - Hamstrings
    - Quadriceps
  - Labrum
  - Pulvinar
- *Axial:*
  - Osseous structures:
    - Femoral head, neck
    - Greater, lesser trochanter
    - Sacrum
    - Sacroiliac joints
    - Acetabulum
  - Muscles:
    - Gluteus maximus, medius, and minimus
    - Sartorius, rectus femoris
    - Gracilis, pectineus, adductor longus, brevis, and magnus
    - Tensor fascia lata
    - Piriformis
    - Obturator internus, externus
    - Gemelli superior and inferior
    - Quadratus femoris
  - Labrum
  - Pulvinar
- *Sagittal*
  - Osseous structures
    - Femoral head
- *Labrum*

BOX 2: Causes of osteonecrosis.

- Trauma
- Corticosteroids (exogenous and endogenous)
- Idiopathic
- Sickle cell anemia
- Collagen vascular disease
- Alcoholism
- Pancreatitis
- Renal transplantation
- Drug therapy [immunosuppressive, cytotoxic therapy bisphosphonates (jaw)]
- Pregnancy
- Radiation therapy
- Occlusive vascular disease (thromboembolic disease and arteriosclerosis)
- Infection (including immunodeficiency virus)
- Leukemia/lymphoma
- Vasculitis
- Diabetes
- Dysbaric conditions (caisson disease)
- Hemophilia
- Gout
- Thermal injury (burn, frostbite)
- Gaucher disease
- Langerhans cell histiocytosis
- Neuropathic arthropathy
- Polycythemia vera
- Multiple epiphyseal dysplasia

The second pathological phase of AVN is characterized by a rim of hyperemia surrounding the infarcted marrow. This marks an attempt to wall off and repair the ON area. Centripetal neovascularization of the necrotic zone characterizes the third pathological phase. This reactive interface is an attempt to repair the necrotic area and is called the *creeping zone of substitution*. The dead bone is resorbed and trabecular structure gets weakened. This initiates early fracture of the overlying cartilage with cleavage of the subchondral fracture plane and has a crescentic appearance in the femoral head. During this time, the weakened articular surface collapses with consequent joint space narrowing and degenerative arthritis.

Clinical Features

The condition is seen mainly in young men in the third to fourth decade and is bilateral in up to 72% of cases. There are no specific symptoms. Patients may present with intermittent groin pain of gradual onset that is present at rest, exacerbated by weight bearing and it may radiate to the knee or buttocks. Movement of hip is associated with pain particularly on internal rotation. AVN does not always produce pain. Hips with stage I, II disease may be completely asymptomatic. Initially the pain is due to increased intramedullary pressure due to marrow edema.

Imaging

Plain radiographs are used in the initial workup of clinically suspected AVN; an anteroposterior (AP) and frog leg lateral projection should be obtained (this increases the likelihood of detecting a subchondral fracture.

Early changes of AVN may take several months to appear on radiographs; hence, they are insensitive for early disease detection. In late stages, the appearances are characteristic, if the radiographs are positive for advanced disease, further imaging is unnecessary except in the determination of clinically occult contralateral disease in patients at risk for AVN. A negative radiographic examination requires additional imaging. At the initial stages, plain radiograph may show nonspecific patchy areas of sclerosis and lucency. The earliest manifestation of advanced disease seen on radiographs is the *crescent* like subchondral fracture which will eventually lead to articular collapse followed by osteoarthritis.[10]

Radionuclide imaging for AVN is performed with a bone-seeking agent ^{99m}Tc-methylene diphosphonate (^{99m}Tc MDP) or marrow-seeking agent such as ^{99m}Tc sulfur colloid. Early in the course of disease, a cold photopenic zone may be observed in the anterosuperior part of the femoral head, which is virtually pathognomic for AVN. Later the reactive hyperemia and reparative response may result in a doughnut sign. Between the two phases is a window where bone scan may be normal.[11,12]

Computed tomography is not indicated for early detection, as it is less sensitive to MR and scintigraphy. Alteration of the normal asterisk of the femoral head (condensation of compressive and tensile trabeculae) is seen in early stages. Later changes include serpentine sclerotic margins. Multidetector row computed tomography (MDCT) is useful in providing information on the location of articular collapse and extent of the epiphyseal ON. CT is required in surgical planning for rotational arthroplasty.[10]

Magnetic resonance imaging is the most sensitive and specific modality for the identification of ON with reported 97–100% accuracy.[9,10] MR imaging findings were reported to appear within a week of vascular insult in animal models.[13]

The most common MR appearance of AVN is that of a circumscribed subchondral geographic area of yellow marrow surrounded by a low signal intensity rim on all pulse sequences in the anterosuperior portion of the femoral head. This site represents the most peripheral site in the intraosseous circulation of the proximal femur and correlates histologically with the reactive interface between viable and nonviable bone **(Figs. 13A and B)**. The yellow marrow signal intensity is maintained because viable and nonviable fat have similar MR appearance. The rim of sclerosis is cresenteric/band like/rings like or wedge shaped.[14]

Another sign, seen on T2W images, in patients who have AVN is the "double line" sign.[11] This consists of an outer low intensity rim and an inner high intensity band on T2W images **(Fig. 14)** and has been described in up to 80% of cases. The high intensity component of this sign is believed to represent a zone of hyperemia and granulation tissue at the reactive interface between viable and nonviable bone. This sign was introduced by Mitchell and was considered as pathognomonic for AVN. It has been noted that transposition of the frequency and phase encoding axis results in the reversal of the positions of the bright and dark rims, suggesting the possibility of a chemical shift artifact as the etiology behind this sign. The artifactual nature of the double line sign does not reduce its diagnostic value for the diagnosis of AVN when

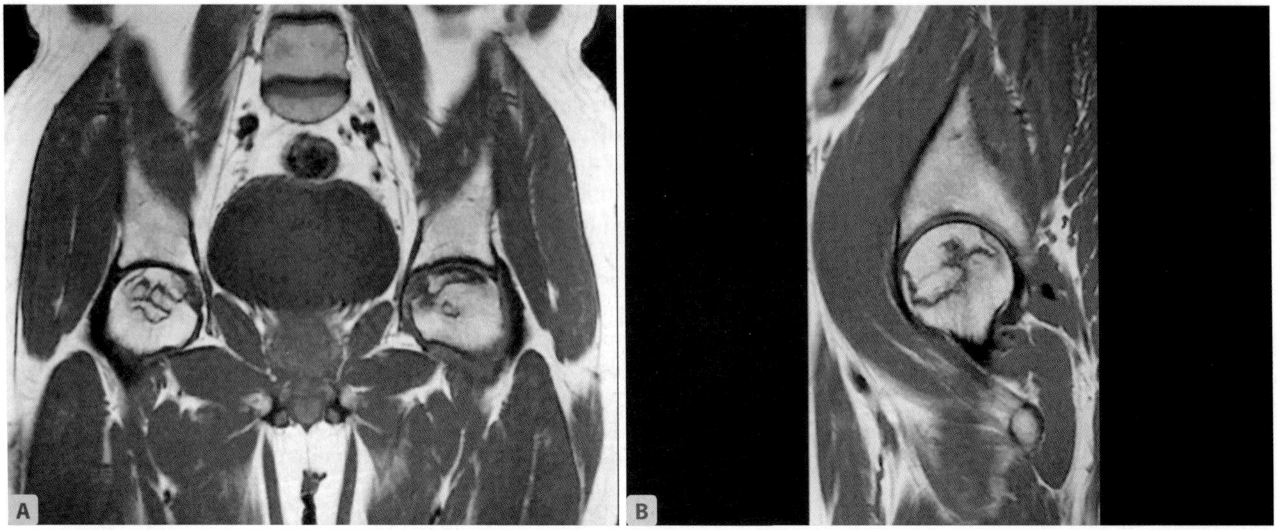

FIGS. 13A AND B: (A) T1-weighted (T1W) axial image of both hips; (B) T1W sagittal image of right hip showing characteristic serpiginous area of altered signal intensity of the anterosuperior part of the femoral head—avascular necrosis.

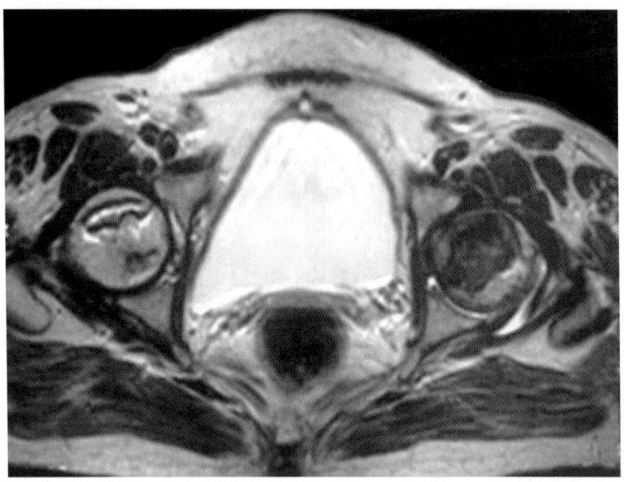

FIG. 14: T2-weighted axial image of both hips showing the "Double line" sign—outer hypointense and inner hyperintense rim—avascular necrosis.

conventional T2W SE or nonfat suppressed turbo spin echo sequences are applied. The newer high field scanners do not show this sign as spectral presaturation is applied with T2WFSE/TSE sequences.[15,16]

The MR signal intensity in the area of ON may show signal other than fat. Mitchell proposed a classification system based on the appearance of the center region signal, bounded by a low signal rim on T1 and T2W images.[11] Class A lesions have fat-like signal, class B has signal similar to subacute blood, Class C has fluid signal while low signal corresponding to fibrosis is seen in Class D lesions. This classification is not widely used as it does not correlate with radiographic staging and prognosis.

Subchondral fractures may occur in AVN. These are seen as low signal intensity lines on T1-weighted MR images and can be differentiated from subchondral insufficiency fractures based on the shape of the lesion. In AVN, the low signal band is smooth, concave to the articular surface and circumscribes the entire necrotic segment, whereas in insufficiency fractures, the low signal intensity band is irregular, discontinuous, and convex to the articular surface **(Figs. 15A and B)**. Unlike in most cases of AVN, the subchondral fragment and distal bone are edematous because both fragments are viable.[17,18]

Joint effusion is seen in 58–72% of patients and is due to associated synovitis **(Fig. 16)**.[19] This is often associated with bone marrow edema (BME) and is considered to be a cause of pain. BME may be seen in up to 30–59% of patients with AVN **(Figs. 17A and B)**. It is located within the femoral head, neck, and intertrochanteric region, as a reaction to subchondral fracture and blockage of venous drainage. BME is never found in the early stages of AVN as earlier thought. It develops after the onset of pain, typically in advanced disease, correlates with necrotic volume and articular collapse. Presence of BME is a poor prognostic indicator associated with failure of core decompression, failure of vascularized bone grafting.[19]

The use of contrast-enhanced MR is not necessary for the diagnosis or assessment in most cases. Lack of enhancement of the necrotic part with a peripheral rim of enhancement is seen **(Figs. 18A and B)**. Dynamic contrast-enhanced MR shows increased peak enhancement and delayed time to peak enhancement. Use of contrast-enhanced MR to predict risk of development of AVN post femoral neck fractures has also been studied.[20,21]

Use of advanced MR techniques such as diffusion-weighted imaging,[22] perfusion weighted imaging, T2 mapping, and magnetic resonance spectroscopy are being researched to increase the accuracy of MRI in AVN. The ADC values in hip AVN are significantly higher than normal marrow but diffusion weighted MRI fails to distinguish between different stages of AVN **(Box 3)**. Preliminary studies have shown that proton MR spectroscopy can detect changes

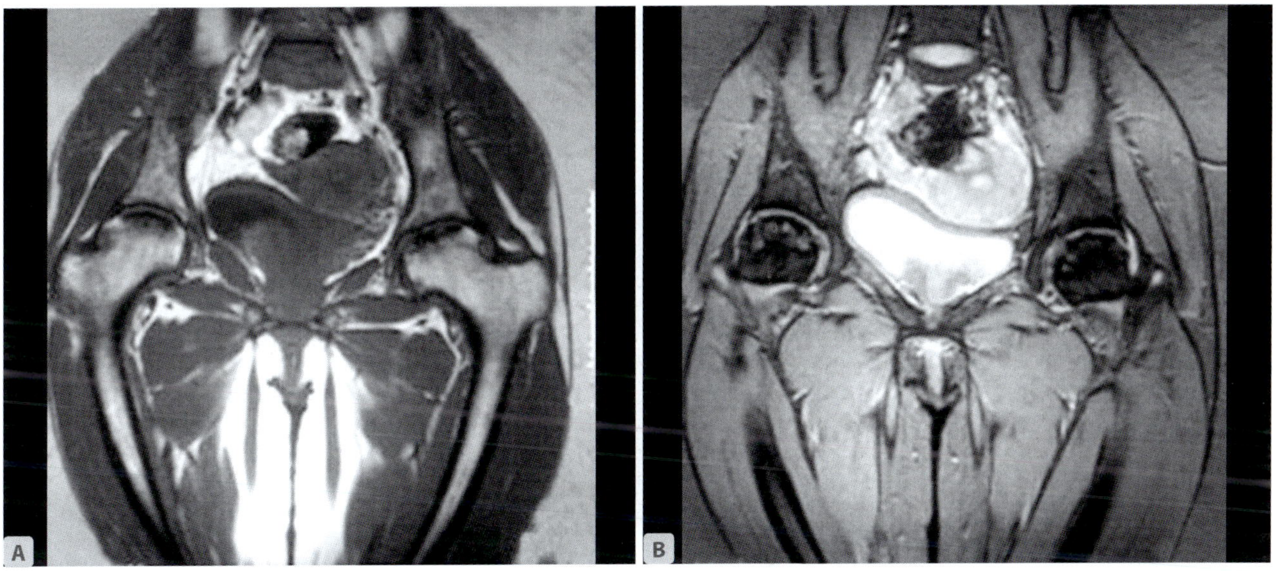

FIGS. 15A AND B: (A) T1-weighted coronal; and (B) Short tau inversion recovery (STIR) coronal depict insufficiency fracture of osteoporosis as irregular, discontinuous low signal intensity lines.

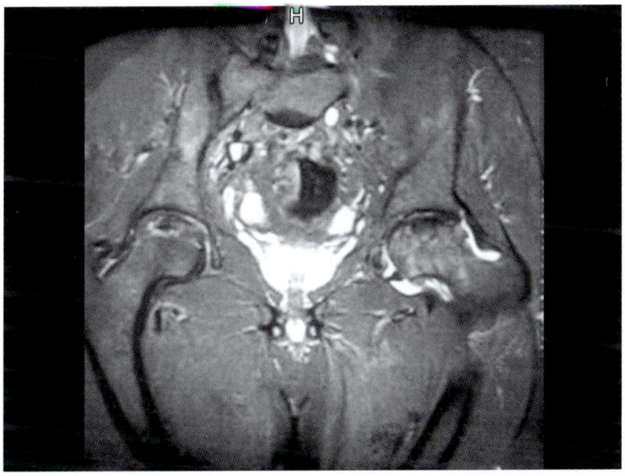

FIG. 16: Short tau inversion recovery (STIR) coronal image of both hips showing joint effusion on the left side with bilateral avascular necrosis.

in the lipid/water spectra of patients with AVN before any morphological changes are evident.[23]

Staging

Various staging systems have been developed for the assessment of femoral head ON. These are the Ficat and Arlet, Steinberg **(Table 3)** and the association research circulation osseous (ARCO). All systems progress from radiologically occult disease to imaging findings consistent with femoral head collapse and degenerative arthritis.

Ficat and Arlet devised a staging system for hip AVN, based on clinical and plain radiographic findings.[24]

- *Stage 0*: Represents biopsy proven AVN in asymptomatic patients with normal radiographs and bone scan.
- *Stage 1*: Patients may have normal radiographs, abnormal bone scans and is associated with hip pain and decreased range of motion.
- *Stage 2*: Femoral head osteoporosis with areas of cystic lucency and sclerosis.
- *Stage 3*: There is subchondral collapse (crescent sign) of the femoral head with preservation of joint space.
- *Stage 4*: There is frank cortical collapse of the femoral head.
- *Stage 5*: Superimposed degenerative joint disease.

Magnetic resonance is an integral part of several staging systems. The most critical part in all systems is the loss of spherical contour of the femoral head; MRI is to be used in precollapse stages of AVN.

The Toulouse, France-based Association *Internationale de Recherche sur la Circulation Osseuse (the association research circulation osseous)*[26] has proposed a more comprehensive staging system (*ARCO Classification,* **Table 4).**

MAGNETIC RESONANCE IMAGING AND PROGNOSTIC INDICATORS

A normal MR image is a good predictor of disease absence and is rare in case of biopsy proven disease. The natural history of AVN is typically of progression, though the rate of progression is unpredictable. The lesions themselves do not increase in size and small lesions remain stable. The larger the area involved, the more likely it is to collapse. As the lateral weight-bearing portion gets involved, the likelihood of collapse increases. In case of chronic renal failure, MRI positive asymptomatic, radiographically occult lesions have been seen to disappear without therapy.

When AVN is present, the percentage of weight bearing surface that is involved by the AVN lesion is the most reliable

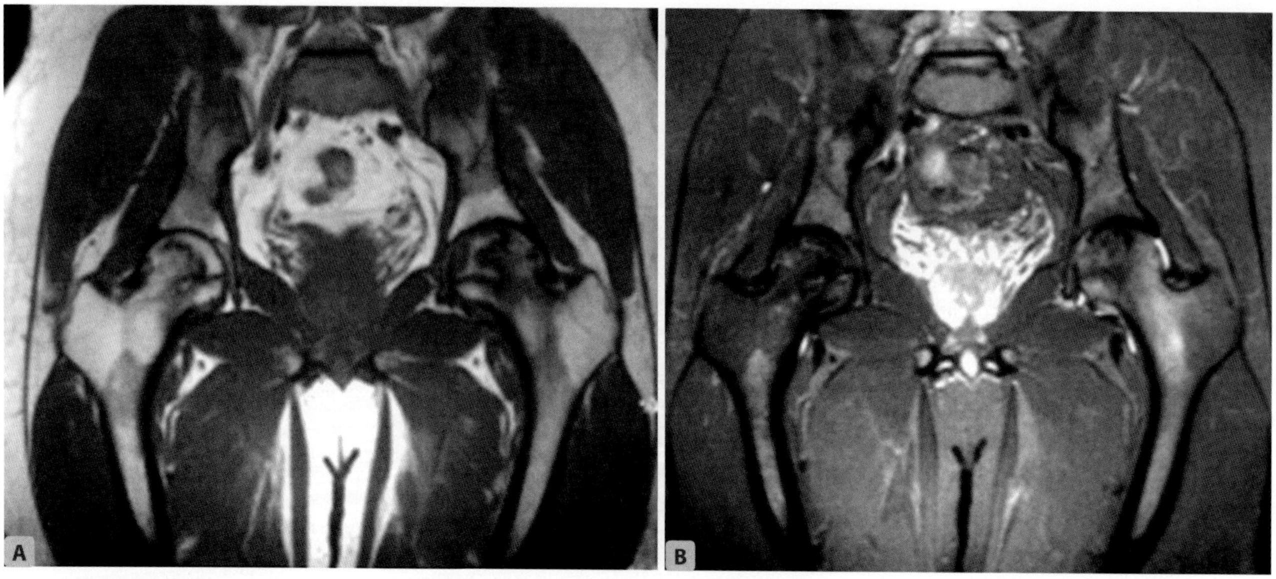

FIGS. 17A AND B: (A) T1-weighted coronal; and (B) Short tau inversion recovery (STIR) coronal images of both hips, showing increase in intertrochanteric fatty marrow on the right side with marrow edema on the left side with bilateral avascular necrosis.

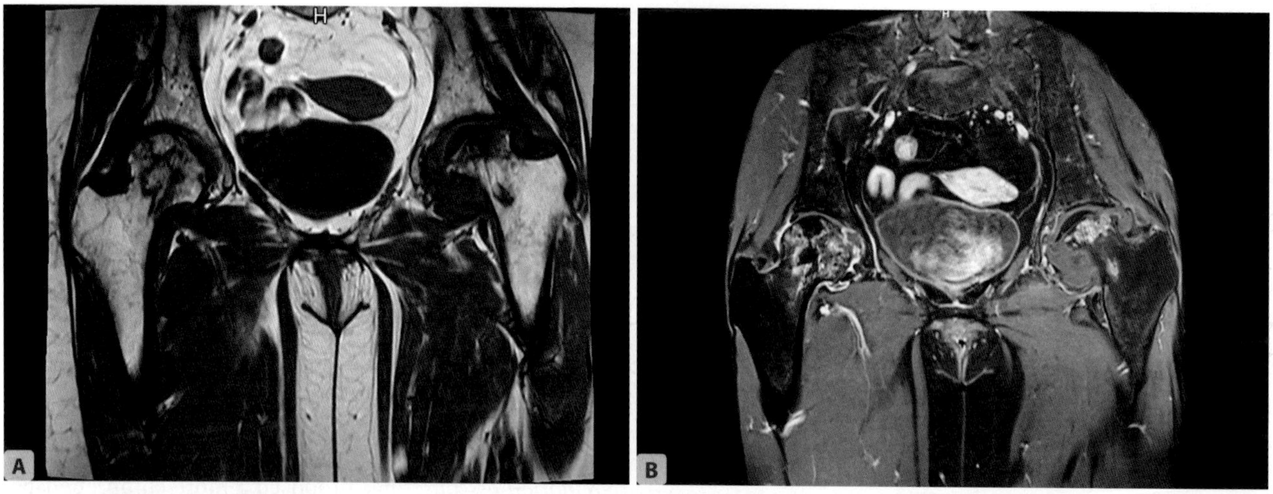

FIGS. 18A AND B: Bilateral avascular necrosis. (A) T1-weighted coronal; and (B) T1-weighted coronal fat suppressed, postgadolinium image of both hips showing necrotic nonenhancing areas with enhancing viable interface.

BOX 3: Avascular necrosis: Magnetic resonance imaging.

- Anterior femoral head affected first
- 10 O'clock–2 O'clock position on coronal images
- Diffuse bone marrow edema
- Focal serpiginous low signal line
- Double line sign
- Focal subchondral low signal lesion on T1 with variable signal on T2

factor in predicting outcome. The size of the necrosis is important in predicting whether a fracture and further joint destruction will occur. Methods of quantification vary from the simple to the sophisticated, requiring advanced software. The extent of femoral head involvement has been estimated with MR imaging as percentage of the weight-bearing area, index of necrotic extent, and absolute necrotic volume. The extent and location of the necrotic fragment can be assessed using coronal MR images. The femoral head is viewed as a circle. If the necrotic fragment involves less than 25% of the diameter of the circle, there is less likelihood of lesion progressing to collapse. The location of the lesion is also important to determine future deterioration. The weight-bearing surface of the femoral head is defined as a segment extending from the medial aspect of the acetabulum to the lateral aspect of the acetabular roof. If more than 2/3rd of the weight-bearing surface is involved, there is 74% chance of collapse of the femoral head. Sagittal MR imaging can also be used to assess the extent and location of the necrotic fragment. If the reactive interface crosses the zenith (12 O'clock position), there is an 82% chance of collapse **(Figs. 19A and B)**.[27-29]

TABLE 3: Steinberg classification of avascular necrosis (AVN).[25]

Stage	Clinical features	Radiologic findings	Histologic findings
0	No symptoms	Normal radiographs and MR images	ON present
I	Presence or absence of symptoms	Normal radiographs Abnormal MR images	ON present
II	Symptoms present	Radiographs with trabecular bone changes without subchondral bone changes and preserved joint spaces Diagnostic MR images	ON present
III	Symptoms present	Variable trabecular bone changes with subchondral bone fracture (crescent sign and/or subchondral bone collapse) Preserved femoral head shape and hip joint space	ON present
IV	Symptoms present	Altered shape of femoral head with variable joint space	ON present

TABLE 4: ARCO staging system for avascular necrosis (AVN).

Stage	Clinical features	Radiologic findings	Histologic findings
0	No symptoms	Normal radiographs and MR images	ON present
I	Presence or absence of symptoms	• Normal radiographs • Abnormal MR images	ON present
II	Symptoms present	• Radiographs with trabecular bone changes without subchondral bone changes and preserved joint spaces • Diagnostic MR images	ON present
III	Symptoms present	• Variable trabecular bone changes with subchondral bone fracture (crescent sign and/or subchondral bone collapse) • Preserved femoral head shape and hip joint space	ON present
IV	Symptoms present	Altered shape of femoral head with variable joint space	ON present

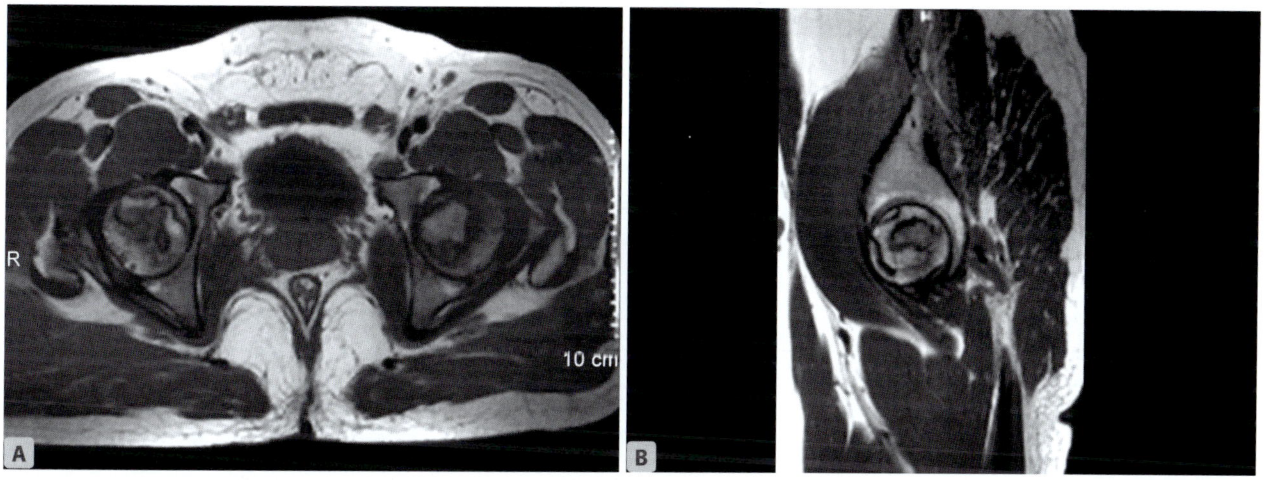

FIGS. 19A AND B: (A) T1-weighted axial image (T1W) of bilateral hips; and (B) T1W sagittal image of right hip shows bilateral avascular necrosis with >30% involvement of femoral head; the lesion is seen to cross the 12 O'clock position with an increased likelihood of collapse on the right side.

Two high-risk markers of disease may be observed in patients who have clinically suspected AVN. These are an early conversion from hematopoietic to fatty marrow and a dense intact physeal scar. The presence of either of these findings and the absence of definite disease warrants a follow-up in patients with risk factors for AVN and hip pain.[30,31]

Treatment

Patients, whose disease is discovered prior to articular collapse, are candidates for a host of operative and nonoperative interventions aimed at preserving the femoral head. These include administration of bisphosphonates, core decompression, nonvascularized and vascularized bone grafting, porus tantalum implant, mesenchymal stem cells, rotational osteotomy, etc. Hip arthroplasty is performed in cases of femoral head collapse and intractable pain. The results of hip replacement in patients with AVN are poorer than those of age-related controls.

Monitoring of Treatment

The MR features indicating normal incorporation of the graft includes enhancement surrounding the graft, revascularization of the previously necrotic area, reduction in BME, and an increase in signal of the necrotic bone. Dynamic CEMRI shows vascular ingrowth at 1–7 months postsurgery.

Pitfalls in Diagnosis[1]

- Occasionally normal red marrow can be present in the femoral head, leading to a misinterpretation.
- Synovial herniation pit, which represents a tiny defect in the bone that allows joint fluid to fill this space, can be erroneously identified as an area of AVN **(Fig. 20)**.
- Subchondral bone cysts resulting from degenerative joint disease of the hip may appear similar to AVN but the low signal margins of the cyst are smooth and regular, rather than serpiginous as with AVN **(Figs. 21A and B)**.
- Fovea centralis, a normal anatomic finding, can be diagnosed as a site of AVN **(Fig. 22)**.

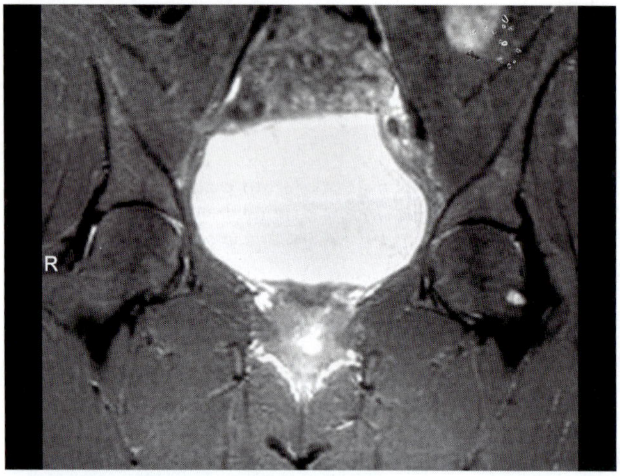

FIG. 20: T2-weighted fat suppressed coronal image of both hips shows herniation pit in the characteristic location on the left side.

Minimal Avascular Necrosis

This entity is seen as a small and eccentrically located focal lesion at the femoral head, believed to be as a result of single episode of infarction rather than recurrent ischemia. This does not lead to articular collapse. Differential diagnosis includes bone tumors and synovial herniation pits.[32]

ACUTE BONE MARROW EDEMA SYNDROME

The term "acute BME syndrome" refers to two clinical entities—transient osteoporosis of the hip and regional migratory osteoporosis. Both conditions present with pain of acute onset in middle-aged men and women in the peripartum period. The symptoms gradually resolve with conservative treatment. BME is noted on MR in both conditions.[33,34]

The pathophysiology of the BME remains unknown. Links with ischemia, fractures, neurogenic compression, intraosseous thrombosis, and reflex sympathetic dystrophy syndrome have been suggested. The appearance of BME is nonspecific and probably results from different causes.

Transient osteoporosis of the hip (TOH) **(*Box 4*)** was first described by Curtiss and Kincaid in pregnant women during third trimester since then most cases have been observed in middle-aged men.[35] TOH has a predilection for hip, though similar changes may be seen in knee, ankle, and foot.

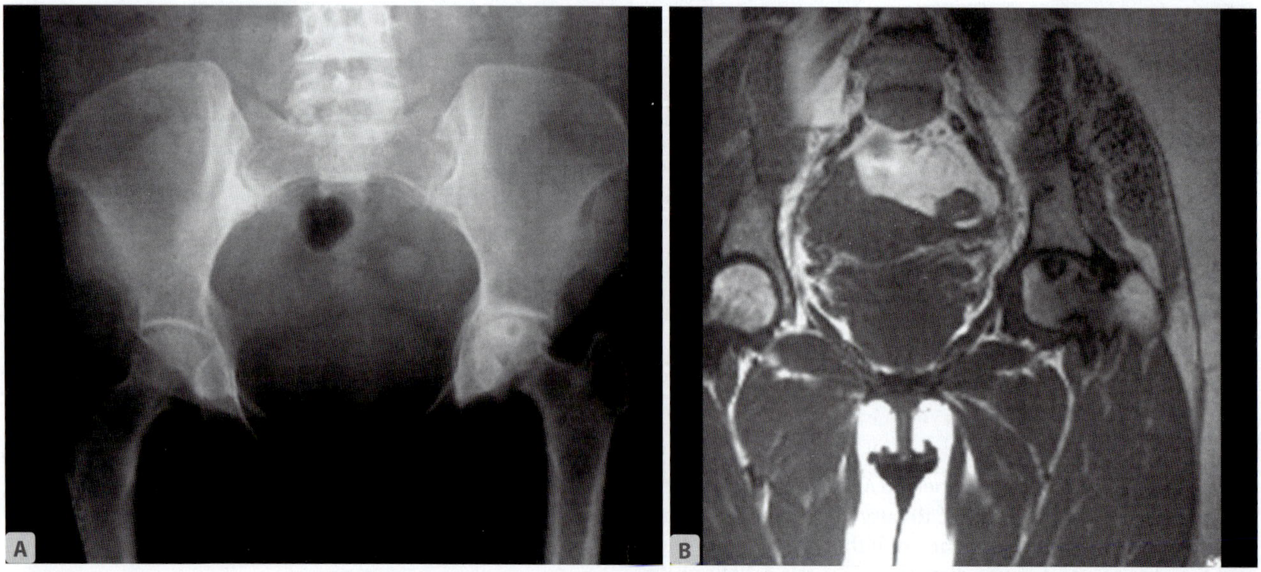

FIGS. 21A AND B: X-ray pelvis and both hips—(A) AP view shows decreased joint space on the left with subchondral cystic changes and osteophytes; (B) T1-weighted coronal image of both hips depicting subchondral cyst with osteophytes—degenerative changes.

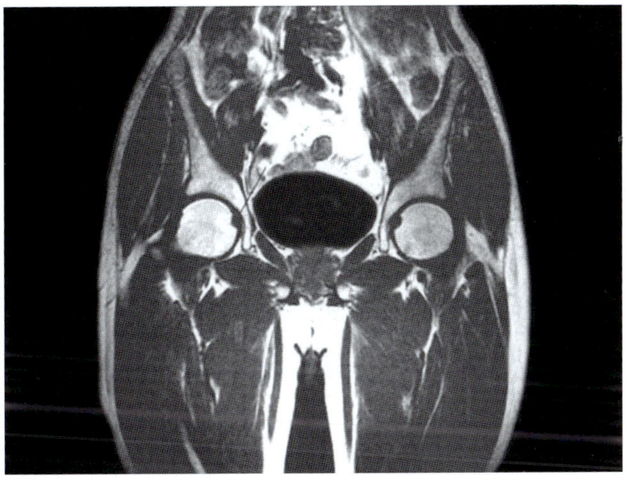

FIG. 22: T1-weighted coronal image of both hips—normal fovea central is seen on both sides.

Generally, only one hip is involved. Unilateral hip pain begins spontaneously without history of trauma, may be rapid or gradual in onset, and is aggravated by weight bearing. After a plateau phase, pain progressively decreases until complete regression by 6–12 months after the onset without residual sequelae.

Regional migratory osteoporosis presents as migratory arthralgia of the weight-bearing joints of the appendicular skeleton. Migration follows a predicted pattern of proximal to peripheral location and time of symptom occurrence from 4 to 12 months.[36]

Imaging

Initial radiographs are normal but marked osteoporosis of the femoral head with preserved joint space is seen on radiographs obtained several weeks (at least 5 weeks) after the onset of symptoms. The bone resorption can be so intense that the subchondral bone plate becomes indistinguishable on conventional radiographs. Follow-up radiographs demonstrate a return to a normal appearance. Radionuclide studies with bone-seeking agents reveal abnormal accumulation. The severity of osteopenia does not correlate with the extent of marrow edema

Magnetic resonance imaging shows extensive BME of the proximal femur within 48 hours of the onset of symptoms. It appears moderately hypointense on T1-weighted images and intermediate to high on T2-weighted images. Edema may spare the inferomedial part of the femoral head and the greater trochanter called the "sparing sign." This is noted in a majority of patients, however, the specificity of this sign is not yet known. Edema may extend into the femoral neck. The lesion lacks definite margins and the transition zone between the lesion and the adjacent marrow is large. The lesion is homogeneous in signal, without obvious focal round or lobulated changes and without residual intralesional fatty areas **(Figs. 23A to C)**. After intravenous contrast injection, homogeneous and moderate to marked enhancement is seen. Moderate joint effusion is usually present and surrounding soft tissue edema.[37,38]

BOX 4: Transient osteoporosis of the hip.

- Middle-aged men
- Pregnant women
- Male:female 3:1
- No history of trauma
- Low T1, high T2 signal femoral head to intertrochanteric line
- Spontaneous resolution (6–8 months)
- Differential diagnosis—AVN, osteoid osteoma, septic hip

Small subchondral areas of low signal intensity (on T2W or T1W postcontrast) are seen in 30% of patients with BME syndrome. Subchondral low signal lesions that were <4 mm thick or 12.5 mm long returned to normal as opposed to those that were larger and continued on to collapse, representing progression to AVN. In transient osteoporosis, diffuse homogenous enhancement is seen in contradistinction to AVN where enhancement is heterogeneous with avascular foci of low signal. Dynamic contrast-enhanced MR shows distinct patterns, with transient bone marrow edema showing a subchondral spot of marked hyperfusion while ON showing high flow surrounding a subchondral area without detectable flow.

Bone marrow edema is a frequent MR imaging finding that is seen in a spectrum of hip conditions with wide variability in terms of prognosis and treatment options. Knowledge of various patterns of BME along with laboratory and clinical data is helpful in narrowing the differential **(Table 5)**.[39]

Analysis of the T1-weighted SE images is mandatory to differentiate a true "bone marrow edema syndrome" from other lesions in which marrow edema can also be a predominant feature like tumors, infection, cysts and systemic ON. After confirmation of the BME on T1-weighted SE images, high-resolution T2-weighted SE sequences are useful to assess (1) the articular cartilage, (2) the subchondral bone plate, and (3) the subchondral marrow.

If the articular cartilage is abnormal, the lesion is clinically irreversible (osteoarthritis or ON); if the subchondral bone plate is interrupted and the epiphysis lacks sphericity, the lesion is irreversible; if a fluid-like signal intensity plane is visible underneath the epiphyseal contour (cleft fracture), the lesion is irreversible.

After exclusion of a cartilage lesion and obvious fracture of the subchondral bone plate, detection and quantitative assessment of possible focal subchondral changes (low signal intensity subchondral area on T2- or enhanced T1-weighted SE images) are done. The lack of any additional focal changes in the subchondral edematous marrow area indicates a favorable prognosis, i.e., spontaneous resolution of the lesions and symptoms. The presence of a crescent-shaped low signal intensity area in the subchondral region with a thickness equal or superior to 4 mm on T2-weighted images suggests an irreversible lesion. In some situations, the prognosis remains uncertain and follow-up MR studies obtained 3 months later represent a valid alternative to further evaluate the femoral head lesion.

Labrum

The labrum is present in approximately three-fourths of the circumference of the acetabulum and absent along its

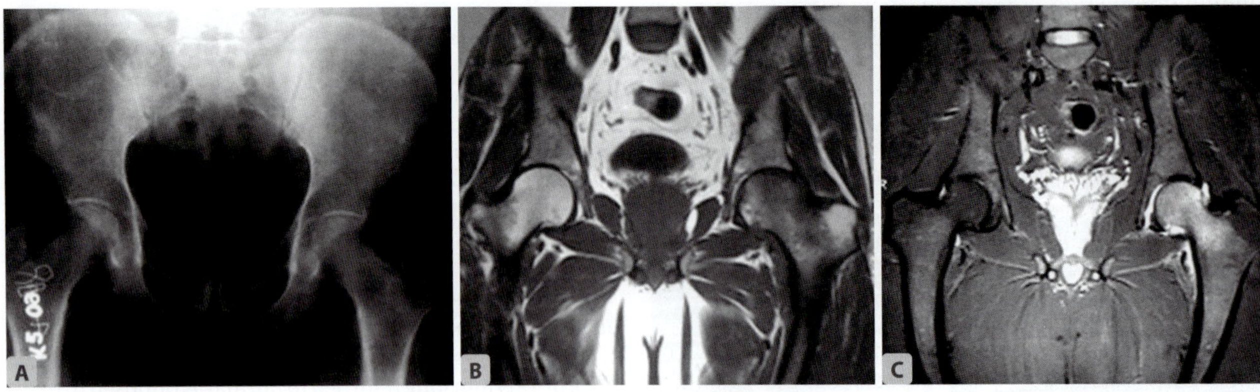

FIGS. 23A TO C: (A) X-ray of pelvis and both hips of a patient with hip pain shows no abnormality; (B) T1-weighted coronal image; (C) Short tau inversion recovery (STIR) coronal image of the same patient show homogeneous area of altered signal intensity seen as hypointense on T1-weighted and bright on STIR images involving the left femoral head, extending to intertrochanteric region—bone marrow edema.

TABLE 5: Various causes of bone marrow edema and their differentiation.

	Avascular necrosis	Transient osteoporosis of hip	Regional migratory osteoporosis
Patients age	3rd–4th decade	4th–6th decade	4th–6th decade
Patients sex predominance	Males	Males Females (3rd trimester of pregnancy/postpartum)	Males
Onset of symptoms	Subacute	Acute	Acute
Most common location	Hip	Hip	Weight-bearing joints of appendicular skeleton
Migration	-	-	Yes; typically within 4–12 months from initial involvement
Plain radiographs	Normal in early stage lucency and surrounding sclerosis Subchondral fracture (crescent sign) Articular collapse osteoarthritis	osteopenia	osteopenia
MR imaging	Band-like lesion Double-line sign Crescent sign (subchondral fracture) BME (late stages following articular collapse)	BME (initial stages) With or without subchondral fracture, Not progressing to collapse	BME (initial stages) With or without subchondral fracture not progressing to collapse
Main associations	Corticosteroids Alcohol consumptions Idiopathic Trauma Hematologic diseases Irradiations	Osteopenia Osteoporosis Pregnancy	Osteopenia Osteoporosis Pregnancy
Treatment	Medical Surgical (core decompression Vascularized grafting, total arthroplasty)	Weight-bearing restriction Analgesics	Weight-bearing restriction Analgesics

inferior aspect. It is innervated by nerves that play a role in proprioception and pain production. The normal labrum has low signal on all imaging sequences and appears as a triangular structure attached to the acetabulum on all imaging planes **(Box 5)**.

Labral tears occur due to acute injury, impingement or developmental dysplasia. Patient has pain, clicking and restricted motion. MR arthrography is the recommended imaging technique for the labrum.

The shape of the acetabular labrum shows a tendency to become rounded and irregular with age. When degeneration is present, the labrum shows globular foci of increased signal intensity on the T2 and proton density weighted images frequently associated with a volume increase of the labrum.

BOX 5: Labrum.

- *Normal*
  - Triangular, low signal on all sequences
  - Best seen with use of surface coil and MR arthrography
- *Abnormal*
  - Complaints of clicking, pain ± decreased range of motion
  - High signal in or through labrum
  - Deformed contour
  - Detached from acetabulum

A labral tear is established when contrast material can be seen traversing or undercutting the labrum. Displacement of the labrum or the presence of a para-labral cyst can increase diagnostic confidence. Since most labral tears occur in the anterior/superior labrum, oblique coronal, oblique axial, and sagittal planes are most useful in detection. In Asian population, the labral tear is most commonly posterior in location.

An absent labral segment at MR arthrography should always been considered abnormal in patients with symptoms suggesting a pathologic labral condition. A normal cleft along the anteroinferior and posteroinferior labrum near its junction, with the transverse ligament, which spans the inferior aspect of the acetabulum along the acetabular notch, is seen. The presence of gadolinium in this cleft should not be misinterpreted as a labral tear. In addition, there is a normal recess superficial to the superior labrum and as gadolinium enters this recess, the appearance can mimic a labral tear. The iliopsoas tendon crosses anterior to the labrum and is potential mimic of a tear.[40]

FEMOROACETABULAR IMPINGEMENT

Femoroacetabular impingement (FAI) is a recently recognized cause of hip pain in all age groups and a proposed mechanism in the development of early osteoarthritis. FAI occurs due to an abnormal relationship between the femur, typically the junction between the anterior/superior femoral head and neck, and the acetabular rim. Repetitive contacts between the two may instigate chondral lesions and labral tears leading to early degenerative disease. A number of predisposing conditions have been described with deformities of the femur and/or the acetabulum which result in abnormal contact between these two structures, such as Legg-Calve-Perthes, slipped capital femoral epiphysis, coxa magna, hip dysplasia, and fractures of the femoral neck are known to predispose to FAI. However, a subset of patients who have no history of developmental or acquired disease of the hip joint may also be predisposed to FAI. Clinically, FAI is characterized by anterior inguinal pain and decreased range of motion with flexion, adduction, and internal rotation.[41-44]

Classically, two types of FAI have been described. The first has been labeled cam impingement and is most often seen in young athletic males. The second is pincer impingement and is more common in middle-aged and older females.

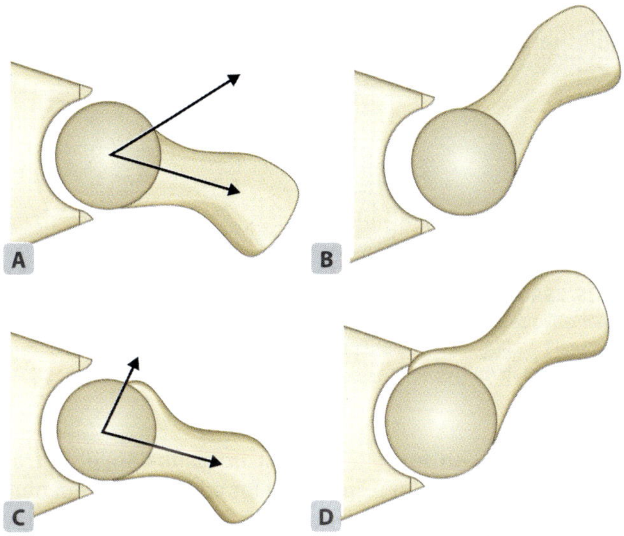

FIGS. 24A TO D: Schematic diagram through the femoral neck in the axial-oblique plane (A) alpha angle is measured, the normal angle = 42°; (B) A normal femoral head/neck junction allows clearance of the acetabular labrum during flexion of the hip; (C) Abnormal head/neck offset with an alpha angle greater than 55°; and (D) This creates an abnormal contact on the acetabular labrum during hip flexion cam impingement.

Cam Impingement

In cam type impingement of the hip, the predominant abnormality is in the contour of the anterior/superior femoral head-neck junction with a normal morphology of the acetabulum. Normally, the anterior/superior femoral head-neck junction has a concave configuration. However, this junction is either flattened or convex in cam type impingement. In addition, the femoral head may become somewhat aspherical due to this morphologic abnormality. During forceful motion, especially flexion, the nonspherical portion of the femoral head is squeezed under the acetabular rim. This abnormal contact results in damage predominately to the acetabular cartilage in a rather constant location along the anterosuperior acetabular rim. Chondral abrasion or avulsion in turn leads to a tear or detachment of the acetabular labrum **(Figs. 24A to D)**. Repetitive osseous impingement can then result in osteophyte formation on the anterior femoral neck, further exacerbating the problem.[45,46]

Pincer Impingement

In pincer type impingement, the predominant abnormality is with the morphology of the acetabulum with a relatively normal contour of the proximal femur. Abnormalities in acetabular morphology include acetabular retroversion, anterior and/or lateral over-coverage, and protrusio acetabulae. All these conditions increase either the relative depth of the acetabulum or the circumferential overcoverage of the femoral head. Continued impact of the relatively normal femoral neck against the acetabular rim leads to pincer abutment and lesions in the acetabular rim **(Figs. 25A and B)**. The first lesion to appear is degeneration of

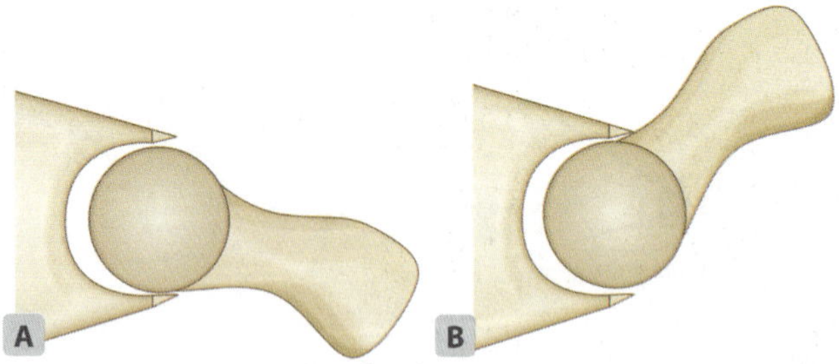

FIGS. 25A AND B: Schematic diagram through the femoral neck in the axial-oblique plane. Redundant acetabulum with over coverage of the femoral head (A), which causes abnormal linear contact with the labrum during flexion (B) Pincer impingement.

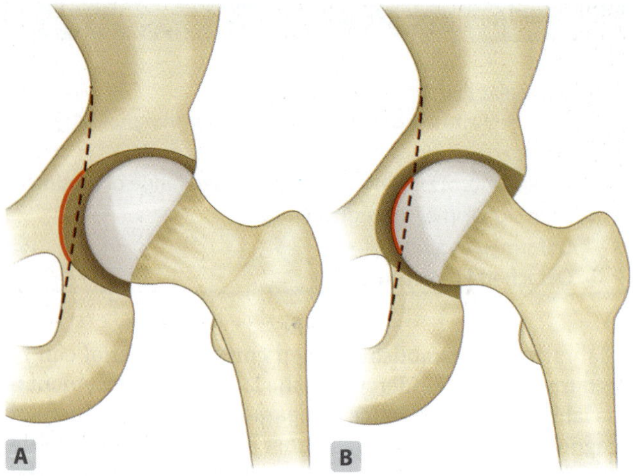

FIGS. 26A AND B: Schematic diagram depicting (A) Coxa profunda—the medial border of the acetabular fossa contacts or is medial to the ilioischial line; and (B) Coxa protrusio—the medial border of the femoral head contacts or is medial to the ilioischial line.

the labrum with formation of an intrasubstance cyst or ossification of the rim responsible for additional deepening of the acetabulum and worsening of the overcoverage. The repetitive abutments occur more often anteriorly and can result in chondral injury in the conter-coup region of the posteroinferior acetabulum. Acetabular cartilage lesions are typically limited to a small region on the acetabular rim. In contrast, cam impingement is characterized by deeper cartilage lesions (some of which are very large flaps) and more extensive labral tears.

Imaging

Femoroacetabular impingement is assessed with radiography and MR arthrography. Radiography depicts osseous abnormalities while MR imaging allows multiplanar visualization of the same and stages soft tissue.

Radiography in Femoroacetabular Impingement

High quality radiography in AP projection without rotation or tilt is mandatory for assessment of FAI. Centering of the radiograph has to be the patient's midline and not the hip. The patient position should be upright for the AP projection. A lateral view—frog leg lateral is also required. Suboptimal radiographs may overestimate, underestimate or falsely diagnose FAI. Comprehensive radiographic assessment is done following a suggested checklist.[47,48]

Radiographs in patients with impingement may initially appear normal because the abnormalities can be subtle.

Cam—on an AP view of the hip, the normal concavity along the lateral aspect of the femoral head-neck junction becomes flattened or slightly convex. This abnormal waisting at femoral head-neck junction has been referred to as the pistol-grip deformity or an abnormal epiphyseal extension. Loss of the normal concavity along the anterior femoral head-neck junction can also be appreciated on a true lateral view. Qualitative assessment is performed by approximating the femoral head with a circle; no bone should extend beyond this circle in normal morphology. Femoral head neck offset (FHNO) is assessed on lateral view with FHNO <10 mm indicating Cam morphology **(Box 6)**.

Pincer impingement—assessment of pincer morphology begins with qualitative assessment of global acetabular depth.

BOX 6: Cam morphology.

- Asphericity of the femoral head
- Abnormal waisting at the FHNJ
- Femoral head-neck offset <10 mm
- Femoral head-neck offset to femoral head diameter ratio <0.17
- Alpha angle >55°

(FHNJ: femoral head neck junction)

Coxa profunda occurs when the medial border of the acetabular fossa contacts or is medial to the ilioischial line **(Fig. 26A)**.

Coxa protrusio occurs when the medial border of the femoral head contacts or is medial to the ilioischial line **(Fig. 26B)**.

Various signs for retroversion of the acetabulum have been described **(Figs. 27A to C)**.

- *Crossover sign*: The anterior rim of the acetabular fossa normally is medial to the posterior rim. If the anterior rim extends lateral to the posterior rim in the superior part, a crossover sign is present.
- *Posterior wall sign*: The posterior rim should cross at or near the femoral head center. If posterior rim is lateral then posterior wall over coverage is said to be present. A deficient posterior wall is present if the posterior rim is medial.
- *Ischial spine sign*: The ischial spine is normally largely obscured by the medial acetabulum. Visualization of prominent ischial spine is seen in acetabular retroversion.

Care must be taken as slight craniocaudal or transverse angulation can either mimic or obscure true retroversion of the acetabulum.[49]

Global acetabular overcoverage can also be assessed by measuring the center edge angle (normal = 25 acetabular overcoverage = 39°) and acetabular index (normal-2-10°).

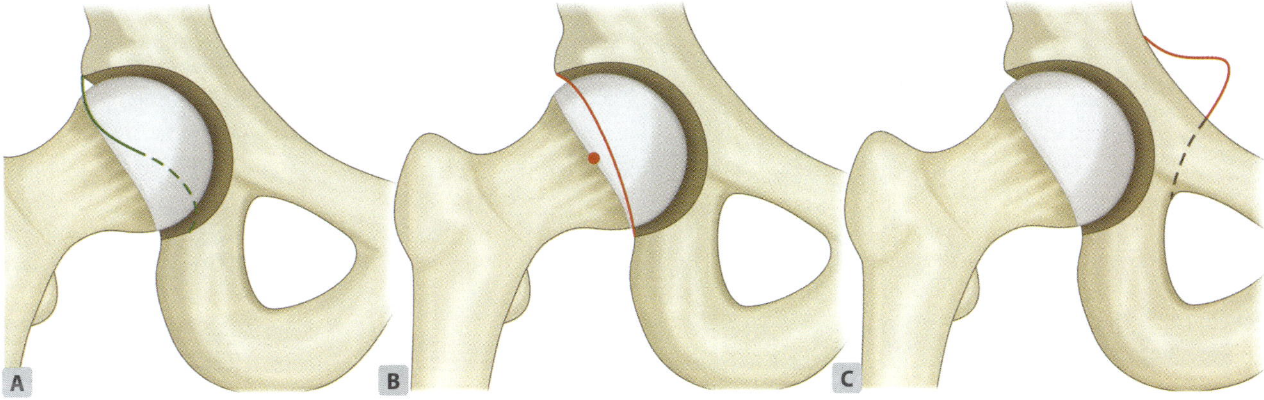

FIGS. 27A TO C: Schematic diagram of signs of acetabular retroversion—(A) Crossover sign; (B) Posterior wall sign; (C) Ischial spine sign.

TABLE 6: Magnetic resonance imaging (MRI) sequences for suspected femoroacetabular impingement.

Axial oblique (Swiss axial)	Obtained parallel to the femoral neck Allows better visualizations of the anterior and posterior labrum with decreased geometric distortions
Radial imaging	Images are perpendicular to a double oblique en face view of the acetabulum. Minimizes geometric distortion and partial volume average effects inherent when imaging spherical structures using routine anatomic planes
3D GRE	Obtained with 1.5 mm isotropic voxels Allows multiplanar assessment of osseous morphology
SS-FSE of knee and hip	To assess for femoral torsion

An association between an os acetabuli and hip impingement has also been suggested. Some believe that this heterotopic bone formation on the acetabular rim is due to abnormal contact with the femur. The mineralization may be seen in the soft tissues or in the labrum. There is a high prevalence of herniation pits in patients with FAI.

Magnetic Resonance Imaging

Apart from routine imaging of the hip to be assessed and a survey of the entire pelvis, sequences **(Table 6)** to look specifically for FAI are obtained. MR arthrography is usually done and can be done using leg traction to break the seal effect of labrum with potential improvement in visualization of cartilage injury.

The same morphologic osseous abnormalities as seen on radiography are seen at MR imaging. Epiphyseal extension is best seen on coronal sequences as they most closely approximate the AP view of the hip. The abnormal femoral head-neck offset on the anterior/superior head-neck junction is often best seen on oblique (oblique axial or oblique sagittal) images that parallel the femoral neck to measure the sphericity of the femoral head as well as the abnormal offset at the femoral head-neck junction.

Quantitative measurement is done by measuring the alpha angle. The alpha angle is measured on an oblique image through the center of the femoral neck. A line is drawn along the long axis of the femoral neck bisecting a circle which outlines the femoral head. A second line is then drawn from the center of the circle to the point at which the femoral head or neck protrudes beyond the confines of the circle anteriorly. The angle formed by these two lines comprises the alpha angle. An alpha angle >50° is abnormal although using a threshold of 55° may be more specific to impingement. The alpha angle will be greater in many causes of impingement due to an abnormality of the shape of the femoral head-neck junction such as a wide femoral neck, osteophytes or posterior displacement of the femoral head **(Figs. 28A to C)**.[50]

Magnetic resonance arthrography helps visualize the cartilage and labral lesions that are often associated with FAI **(Fig. 29 and Box 7)**.

A triad of MR arthrographic findings has been described in patients with cam type FAI. The triad consists of an abnormally increased alpha angle, an anterior/superior acetabular cartilage lesion, and an anterior/superior acetabular labral tear.[51-54]

Femoroacetabular impingement is often bilateral but one hip may be asymptomatic, therefore both hips must be assessed. A large number of patients with cam FAI have an associated acetabular deformity (Pincer) **(Table 7)**.

Role of preventive treatment in asymptomatic patients with FAI morphology is unclear. Symptomatic patients, however, benefit from early noninvasive and surgical interventions.

Herniation Pits

Conversion defects (herniation pits) result from an abrasive effect of the anterior hip capsule in an area of the anterosuperior subcapital region of the femoral neck. This phenomenon is common, affecting 4–5% of adults and occurs in an area where there are normal cortical defects. The medullary canal is exposed to erosion from the overlying soft tissue and synovium, which create a subcortical pit. Previously considered an incidental finding, these are now considered as potential imaging indicators for FAI.

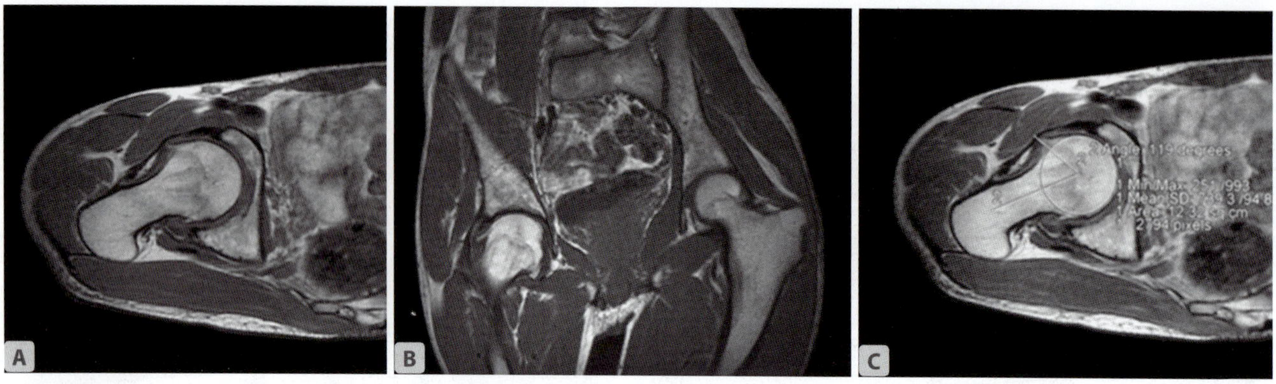

FIGS. 28A TO C: Abnormal head/neck offset in the right hip of a young adult, appreciated on the axial oblique image (A), with degenerative changes seen on T1-weighted coronal image (B), alpha angle measures 119° (C).

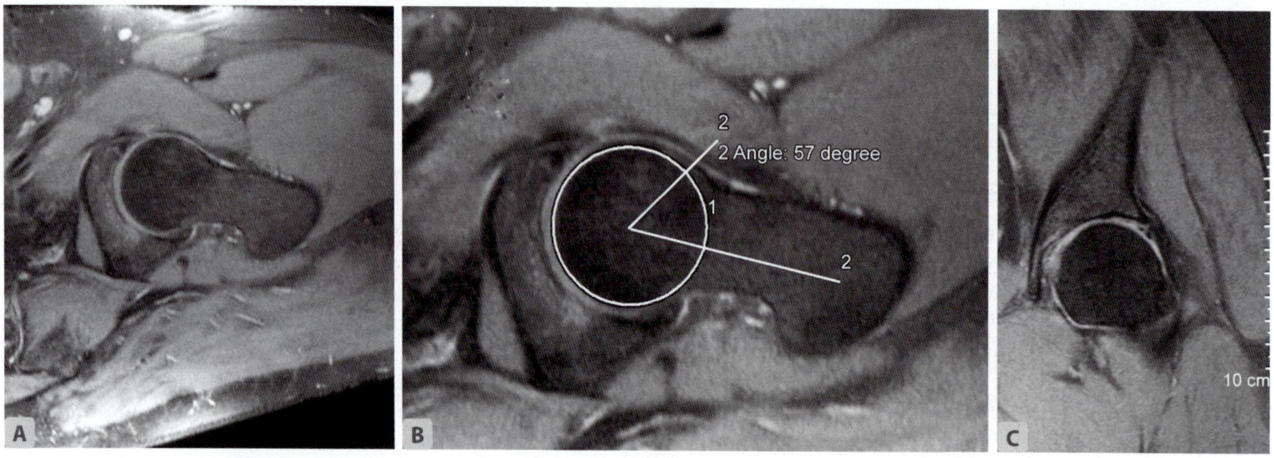

FIGS. 29A TO C: Indirect MR arthrogram shows abnormal femoral head neck offset in axial oblique image (A), increased alpha angle (B) and an anterior labral tear seen on coronal image (C).

BOX 7: Magnetic resonance (MR)/magnetic resonance arthrography (MRA) checklist in the assessment of femoroacetabular impingement.

- Presence and character of acetabular over-coverage of the femoral head
- Femoral head asphericity or morphologic alterations of the femoral head neck junction
- Articular cartilage injury
- Acetabular labral injury
- Additional injuries to the soft tissues about the hip
- Presence of osteoarthritis
- Bone marrow abnormalities

On MR images, herniation pits show marrow replacement in the subcapital region with a rim of low signal on all pulse sequences corresponding to an area of sclerosis. Internally, the lesions are composed primarily of fibrocartilaginous tissue and fluid components. Lesions show a low to intermediate signal intensity on T1 and are of variable signal intensity on T2WI; those with fibrous component being low and those with fluid being hyperintense on T2WI **(Figs. 30A and B)**.[55]

TABLE 7: Pincer morphology.

Global acetabular over-coverage	Acetabular retroversion
• Negative acetabular depth (femoral head center medial to line connecting anterior and posterior acetabular rims) • Center-edge angle >39°	Negative cranial or equatorial acetabular version

HIP TRAUMA

Hip fractures are seen with increasing frequency in older population due to falls and in younger population with high impact motor vehicle accidents. Fractures of the pelvis, hip, and proximal femur are usually identified at radiography. CT adds substantially in further evaluation of complex pelvic fractures. MR imaging adds another dimension to the study of hip trauma as immediate changes in the appearance of marrow are identified on MR **(Figs. 31A and B)**. Thus, it is useful in nondisplaced fractures, stress fractures, insufficiency fractures, and fractures in axial plane that cannot be identified on CT.

Magnetic resonance imaging is the method of choice in detecting 2–10% occult fractures of the hip.[56] Additional

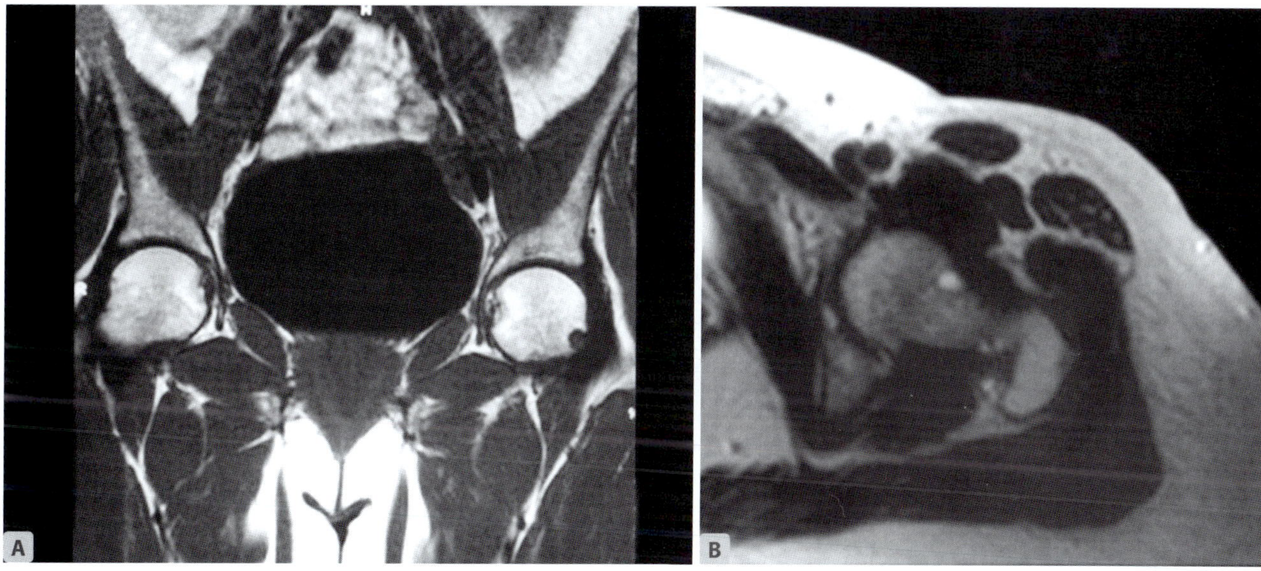

FIGS. 30A AND B: Herniation pit seen as a smooth well-marginated lesion in anterosuperior aspect of left femoral head with fluid characteristics on (A) T1-weighted coronal image; and (B) T2-weighted axial image of both hips.

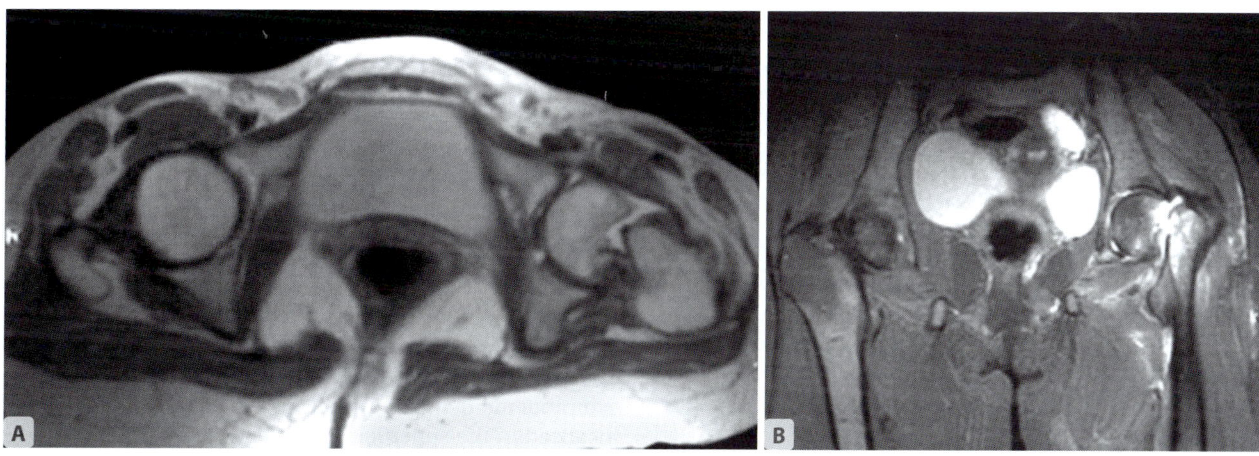

FIGS. 31A AND B: Fracture neck left femur. (A) T2-weighted axial; and (B) Short tau inversion recovery (STIR) coronal images of both hips show marrow edema and fluid at the fracture site.

information about soft tissue pathology is provided by MRI specifically in fractures of the greater trochanters. All avulsion fractures of the greater or lesser fractures of the adults without history of significant trauma necessitate investigation for potential metastatic disease.

A low signal intensity linear or curvilinear line with surrounding BME on T1W images is seen in fractures. It is best appreciated in coronal plane. This single sequence is considered sufficient for the diagnosis of occult fracture of the hip. Contrast-enhanced MR perfusion of the femoral head may be useful to assess femoral head perfusion after femoral neck fracture to aid the clinician in deciding between joint preserving surgery and hip arthroplasty.[57,58]

Stress Fractures

Stress fractures can be further divided into fatigue and insufficiency fractures.

Fatigue fractures occur commonly in pelvis and hips. Fatigue fractures result from increased or abnormal stress applied to normal bone. MRI is sensitive and specific because it shows the fracture line as a linear low signal band/line on both T1W andT2W images with surrounding marrow edema. Increased signal may be seen within the fracture site on fluid sensitive sequences because of hemorrhage within the fracture site. The signal alterations related with stress injury resolve by 6–12 weeks. Stress reactions occur along the medial aspect of the femoral neck (compressive surface) or superior surface (tensile surface). Additional locations include pubic rami and sacrum **(Figs. 32A to C)**.[59]

In the pelvis, fatigue fractures are seen in the sacrum. These are frequently bilateral in the supra-acetabular region of ilium.

Insufficiency fractures occur from normal strain on a bone weakened by osteoporosis, osteomalacia, steroids,

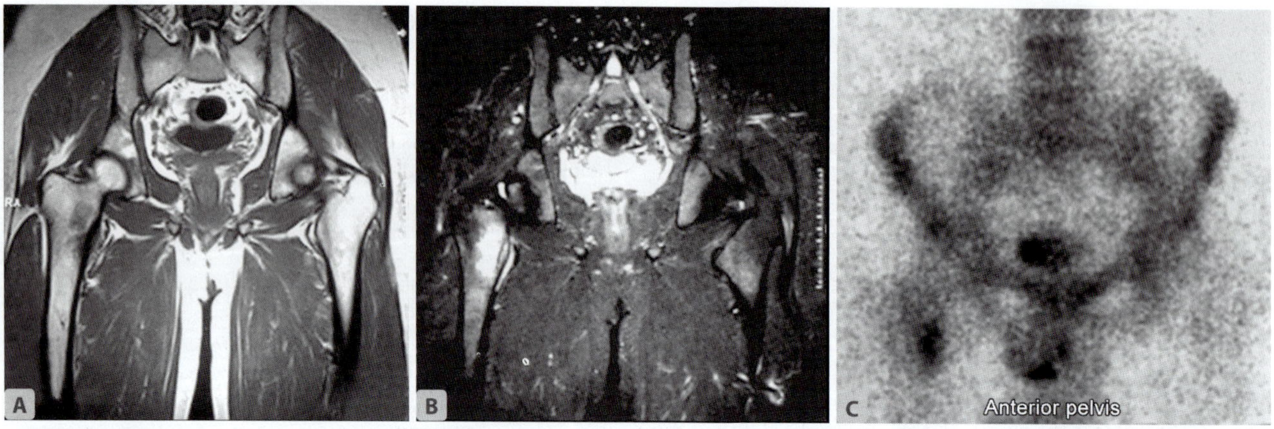

FIGS. 32A TO C: T1-weighted (T1W) coronal image of both hips (A) and short tau inversion recovery (STIR) coronal image of both hips (B), showing an area of edema on the compressive medial surface of the right femur (hypo on T1W image and hyper on STIR) with associated soft tissue swelling and corresponding hot spot on the bone scan; (C) Stress reaction.

rheumatoid arthritis (RA), etc. In a clinical setting of osteoporosis and a painful hip, even in absence of trauma an occult fracture may be present. A limited MRI examination consisting of coronal and axial images of the entire pelvis using T1 and fat suppressed T2W sequences can be used. MR demonstrates low signal fracture line surrounded by marrow edema. Multiple fractures coexist. The most common locations for insufficiency fractures of hip and pelvis are subcapital, intertrochanteric, sacral, supra-acetabular, pubic bones, and pubic rami.

Salter Fracture

Traumatic epiphyseal slip can occur in skeletally immature individuals in setting of infant abuse or birth trauma. A fast spin echo T2W sequence with fat suppression and STIR imaging shows edema and the hemorrhage through the physis and is diagnostic of shear injury.

Traumatic Musculotendinous Injury

Musculotendinous injuries are among the most common form of sport-related injury to the pelvis and hip. The pelvic ring and proximal femur are the sites of origin or insertion for several major muscle groups including the abdominal, gluteal, adductors, hamstrings, and iliopsoas muscles. The injuries occur as a result of blunt direct trauma or secondary to indirect trauma from excessive tension or forceful contraction. The injuries can be categorized based on the mechanism of trauma and the site of involvement. These include tendinous avulsion injury, muscle contusion, and myotendinous strain.[60-62]

Avulsion Injury

Acute avulsion injury at the tendinous insertion site results from forceful eccentric muscle contraction or passive lengthening. It is manifested on MR as a hematoma and periosteal stripping at the tendinous attachment site. Waviness and retraction of the torn end of the tendon along with a fragment of bone or cartilage may be present. Avulsion injuries about the hip joint occur primarily at six sites.

- Ischial tuberosity
- Anterosuperior iliac spine
- Anteroinferior iliac spine
- Lesser trochanter
- Greater trochanter
- Pubic bone.

Nondisplaced bony avulsions appear on T1W images as curved sharply marginated bone fragment adjacent to the apophysis from which it has originated. Increased distance between a displaced fragment and the parent bone is a poor prognostic indicator and may lead to fibrous union and disability.

Muscle Contusions

These are secondary to direct trauma usually by a blunt object. They often occur deep in the muscle belly and tend to be less symptomatic than strains because the latter are commonly localized in the superficial muscle layers. Common sites of muscle contusion about the hip joint include the gluteal region and proximal thigh. Muscle contusions are seen in MR examinations of clinically suspected hip fractures and negative radiographs.

The MR imaging appearance varies according to the severity of the lesion. Diffuse edematous changes of the muscle are manifested by a feathery MR imaging appearance on STIR and T2W images along with an increased muscle girth. Intramuscular hemorrhages may develop with more severe trauma.

Muscle Strain—Myotendinous Strain

Strain injuries affect the myotendinous junction, the weakest point of the musculotendinous unit. The most common strained muscles about the hip joint are the rectus femoris and the hamstrings. In the first-degree strains implying minor degrees of fiber disruption, there is interstitial edema and hemorrhage at the myotendinous junction extending into the fascicles producing a feathery pattern. Partial tears without retraction characterize the second-degree tears. Hematoma and perifascial fluid collections may also be seen. Third-degree tears refer to complete rupture of the myotendinous unit. MRI is used for preoperative assessment of the extent of retraction.

Gluteus Medius Tendon Tear—Greater Trochanteric Pain Syndrome

The rotator cuff lesions of the hip involve tears of the abductor musculature, namely the gluteus medius and minimus. Proposed causes include friction of the iliotibial band with the underlying tendons, abnormal gait leading to altered biomechanics, repetitive stress in runners, and trauma. It more commonly affects middle-aged to elderly women who complain of chronic pain around hip or groin region, mimicking intra-articular hip pathology. It is also seen in recreational runners and participants of step aerobics. The most common symptom is lateral hip pain which has a broad differential diagnosis including entities such as bursitis, tendonitis, muscle insufficiency fractures, nerve entrapment, muscle strain, and bursitis **(Figs. 33A and B)**. Small focal tears are more common than diffuse avulsions. Various MR findings such as increased T2 signal superior to the greater trochanter and atrophy of the gluteal muscles may be seen.[63]

Morel-Lavallée Lesion

It is a post-traumatic encapsulated fluid collection between the superficial and deep layers of the fascia in the lateral thigh, in the trochanteric region adjacent to fascia lata. It is distinct from trochanteric bursitis. Vessels perforating the facial layers get damaged due to compression in closed space or due to shear forces and leak into this space. It does not resolve spontaneously and requires surgical drainage. If chronic, it may mimic a soft tissue sarcoma.

Snapping Hip Syndrome

A cause of hip pain in athletes in high energy sports like soccer; this is due to sudden movements of the iliopsoas tendon over the iliopectineal eminence, the femoral head or a paralabral cyst. It can be associated with iliopsoas tendinopathy and iliopsoas bursitis. Thickened iliopsoas tendon with increased signal on fluid sensitive sequences is seen. Iliopsoas tendon tears at its tendinous part while the muscular insertion into the iliacus remains intact.[64]

ATHLETIC PUBALGIA

Athletic pubalgia was formerly called as "sports hernia." It is seen as groin injury in professional soccer players. Pubalgia is caused by injuries to the rectus abdominis insertion, origin of the hip adductors tendons, and the pubic symphysis. Tears of the aponeurosis connecting the rectus abdominis muscle and the adductor longus muscle can be detected as fluid-like areas underneath the aponeurosis. Sagittal and oblique coronal planes that are perpendicular to the aponeurosis and a small field of view are recommended for imaging. Separation of the aponeurotic plate from the underlying pubic bone causes a fluid filled cleft. Tendon avulsion from the parent bone may be seen. Signal changes are seen in the involved muscles **(Fig. 34)**. Osteitis pubis may be noted in chronic changes.[65,66]

ARTHRITIS

Arthropathies commonly affect the following joints of the pelvis: The sacroiliac joint, the hips, and to a lesser extent of the symphysis pubis. Primary and secondary arthritis are common, RA can affect the hip in a small percentage, often bilaterally symmetrically with axial joint space narrowing. Hip involvement in ankylosing spondylitis is seen in 24–36% of patients. Calcium pyrophosphate dihydrate deposition (CPPD) disease and occasionally gout also involve the hip. The hip is a preferred site for several unusual articular diseases including pigmented villonodular synovitis (PVNS) and primary synovial chondromatosis.

Radiography remains the primary modality by which arthropathy of the hip is evaluated. With the advent of

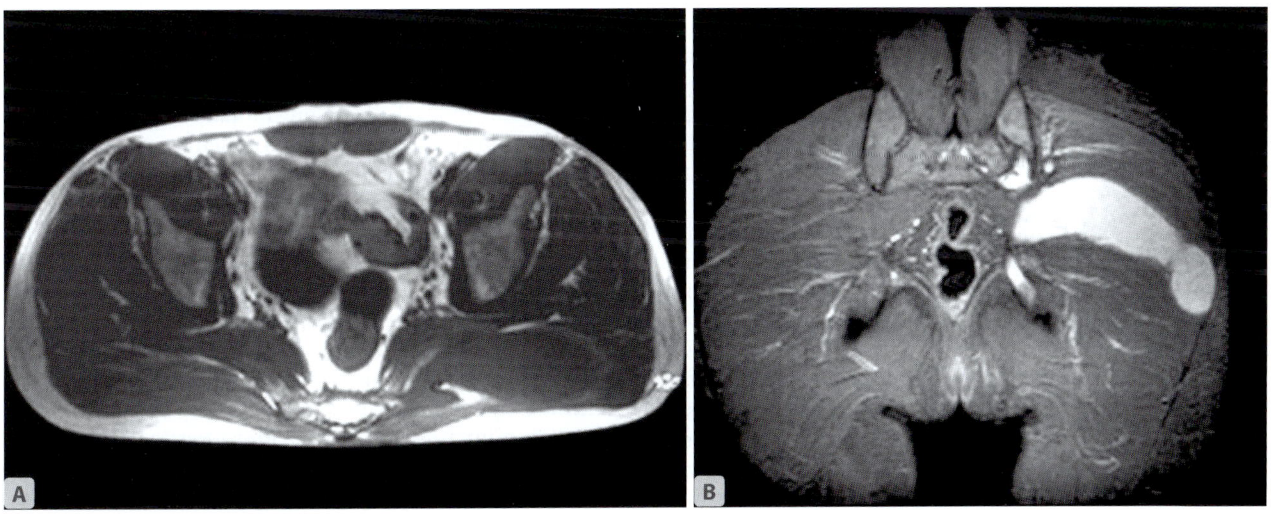

FIGS. 33A AND B: (A) T1-weighted axial image; and (B) Short tau inversion recovery (STIR) coronal image of the pelvis shows well-marginated area of altered signal in the gluteus maximus suggestive of a tear.

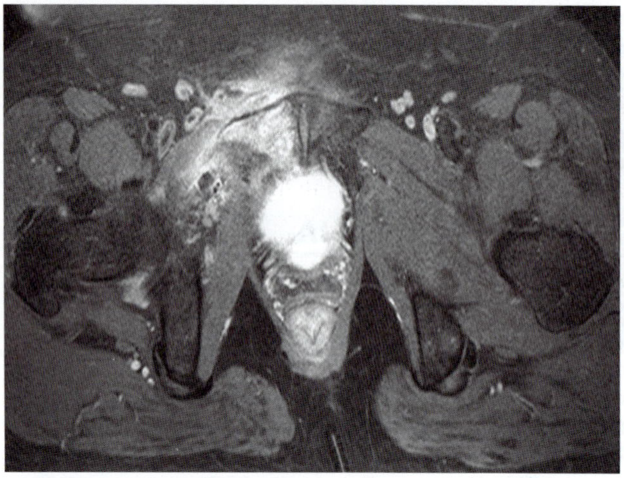

FIG. 34: T2-weighted fat-saturated fast spin-echo (FSE)—marrow edema right pubic bone with soft tissue edema in a case of pubalgia.

aggressive and advanced treatment options, MRI can demonstrate extent of synovial hypertrophy (pannus) that is common to all inflammatory arthritis but not evident on radiographs. Pannus shows low signal on T1 and high signal intensity on T2 images. It may be difficult to differentiate from synovial fluid. Pannus shows slightly higher signal intensity on short TR images and has more heterogenous and mildly lower signal intensity on long TR images. Pannus and synovitis enhance more dramatically and diffusely compared to synovial fluid which enhances only peripherally. Fibrotic component of pannus may be of low SI on T2W images. These are often more prominent in seronegative spondyloarthropathy and reflect inactive disease or therapeutic effect.

Magnetic resonance imaging also depicts the degree of bone erosion and cartilage thinning. MRI can be used to monitor therapy by quantitating the volume of pannus.

Rheumatoid Arthritis

BME is seen as an early marker in patients with RA. It correlates with the presence of acute phase reactants in the blood. Seen in subchondral regions or with bone erosions, BME is a marker of synovitis and subsequent erosive damage which may occur after a lag of almost a year. Intense contrast enhancement, effusions, and erosions (seen as sharply marginated juxta-articular enhancing lesions) are other features on MRI.[67,68]

Pigmented villonodular synovitis (PVNS) is an uncommon disorder characterized by synovial proliferation with hemosiderin deposition in the involved synovial tissue. Pressure erosions of bone by the synovial masses may occur. Pigmented villonodular synovitis occurs most commonly in 2nd and 5th decade and is usually monoarticular. The knee is the most often involved joint but it can also occur in the hip.

Magnetic resonance imaging: Hemosiderin deposition is pathognomic of the condition and is seen as large globular areas of low signal intensity on all imaging sequences with blooming on gradient echo imaging. Pigmented villonodular synovitis is characterized by low signal intensity on T1W and T2W images distinguishing it from almost all tumors and inflammatory conditions, which have high signal on T2W images.[69]

Primary Synovial Chondromatosis

This results from metaplastic proliferation of synovium with formation of multiple cartilaginous or osseous loose bodies. It is not associated with degenerative change until later in the course of disease. On conventional radiography, it is not possible to differentiate it from PVNS.

Magnetic Resonance Imaging

MRI makes the differentiation possible as synovial chondromatosis follows the signal characteristics of cartilage. Cartilaginous loose bodies are low in signal on T1 and higher in signal on T2 images. Ossified loose bodies may be diffusely dense and sclerotic (low signal on all pulse sequences) or may have low signal cortical margin with a fatty center (chewy nougat).[70]

Amyloid arthropathy is a rare entity and typically presents in patients of renal failure with clinical features similar to RA. There may be erosions within acetabulum and femoral head and neck that show low signal on T1 and low to intermediate signal on T2 images. History and absence of hemosiderin, allows it to be differentiated from PVNS.

SACROILIITIS

This is a nonspecific term suggesting an inflammatory process involving the sacroiliac joints. A variety of disease process affect this joint including HLA-B27 spondyloarthropathies such as ankylosing spondylitis, psoriasis, and Reiter's syndrome. Other common conditions that affect these joints include osteoarthritis, gout, RA, and infection including tuberculosis.

In contrast to the hip, conventional radiography of the sacroiliac joints is often difficult even with specialized projections. The complex shape of the sacrum and iliac bones, curved nature of SI joints, and the overlapping bowel gases make the assessment suboptimal with early changes being difficult to interpret.

Magnetic resonance imaging is an accurate method for assessing early sacroiliac joint disease. The advantages of MR evaluation are direct visualization of cartilage, imaging in the oblique coronal plane for evaluation of synovial compartment, and lack of ionizing radiation as most patients of sacroiliitis are young and of reproductive age group. It is more sensitive than CT in detecting cartilage loss, edema, and small erosions.

The normal sacroiliac joint is well depicted with MR imaging. It clearly distinguishes the synovial and ligamentous compartments of the sacroiliac joint. The ligamentous part of the joint is posterior and obliquely oriented and contains adipose tissue with focal areas of low signal intensity representing loose connective tissue and the interosseous sacroiliac ligaments. The synovial compartment of the sacroiliac joint is anterior and more vertically oriented corresponding to the inferior one-half to two-thirds on plain radiographs MR imaging allows identification of the hyaline cartilage in the synovial compartment as a thin zone of intermediate signal, the maximum thickness of the cartilage is 5 mm. The iliac and sacral cortices are seen as areas of low signal intensity on either side of the cartilage **(Fig. 35)**. The most characteristic finding of sacroiliitis at MR imaging is loss of the normal thin band of intermediate signal intensity representing cartilage on T1W images. Altered signal intensity in the sacral and iliac cortices with adjacent marginal irregularity and deeper defects in the juxtaposed marrow are seen on T1W images. Erosions are more prominent anteroinferiorly and on the iliac side of the synovial compartment where cartilage is thinned and subchondral bone is not well protected. Area of increased signal is seen on T2 images in the synovial compartment.

The use of dynamic gadolinium-enhanced MR imaging has shown to be more sensitive than conventional MR imaging. Rapid (>90%) increase in signal intensity of articular and periarticular region represents active sacroiliitis.

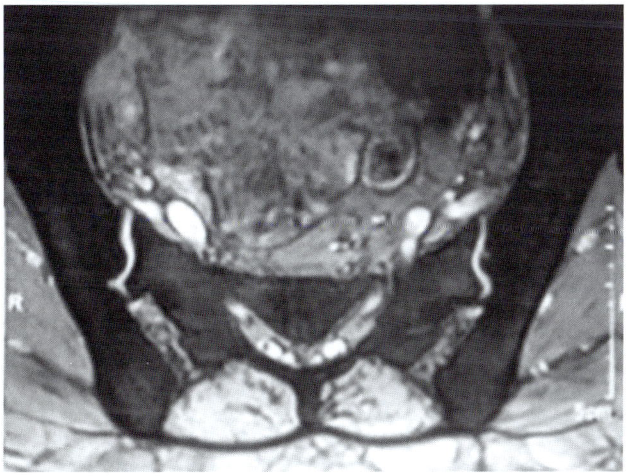

FIG. 35: Gradient T2-weighted axial image shows vertical anterior synovial part of the joint and posterior obliquely oriented ligamentous part—normal sacroiliac joint.

Intra-articular enhancement is noted in patients with active sacroiliitis. The fluid within the joint space does not enhance whereas the inflammatory reaction (phlegmon) may enhance **(Figs. 36 and 37)**.[71,72]

The cause of sacroiliitis cannot be distinguished with MR imaging. The asymmetry of appearance aids the differential diagnosis, as ankylosing spondylitis is generally bilateral and symmetric. Unilateral disease with prominent edema in the soft tissue and marrow adjacent to the joint suggests infection.

INFECTION

The MRI protocol for diagnosis of soft tissue infections and osteomyelitis differs from the routine protocol. Additional imaging sequences using fat suppressed T1 FSE sequences pre- and post-IV gadolinium are performed to enable the diagnosis of sinus tracts and abscesses. The presence of BME and enhancement on MR images is very sensitive for osteomyelitis and the absence of these findings excludes the presence of acute osteomyelitis. The distinction between para-articular cellulitis and osteomyelitis can be made with MR imaging, which is also useful in defining the extent of osteomyelitis before surgery.[73]

Soft tissue infection about the hips can involve the joint or surrounding muscles. Hip joint infection is common in infancy and childhood. MRI shows early cartilage destruction. Any case of monoarticular arthritis should be considered infectious unless proved otherwise.

Tubercular Arthritis

Articular manifestations of musculoskeletal TB are second to spinal disease in frequency of presentation. The most commonly involved are the hip and knee followed by the sacroiliac joint, shoulder, elbow, and ankle. Magnetic resonance demonstrates synovitis and joint effusion. Indolent infections such as tuberculosis result in prominent

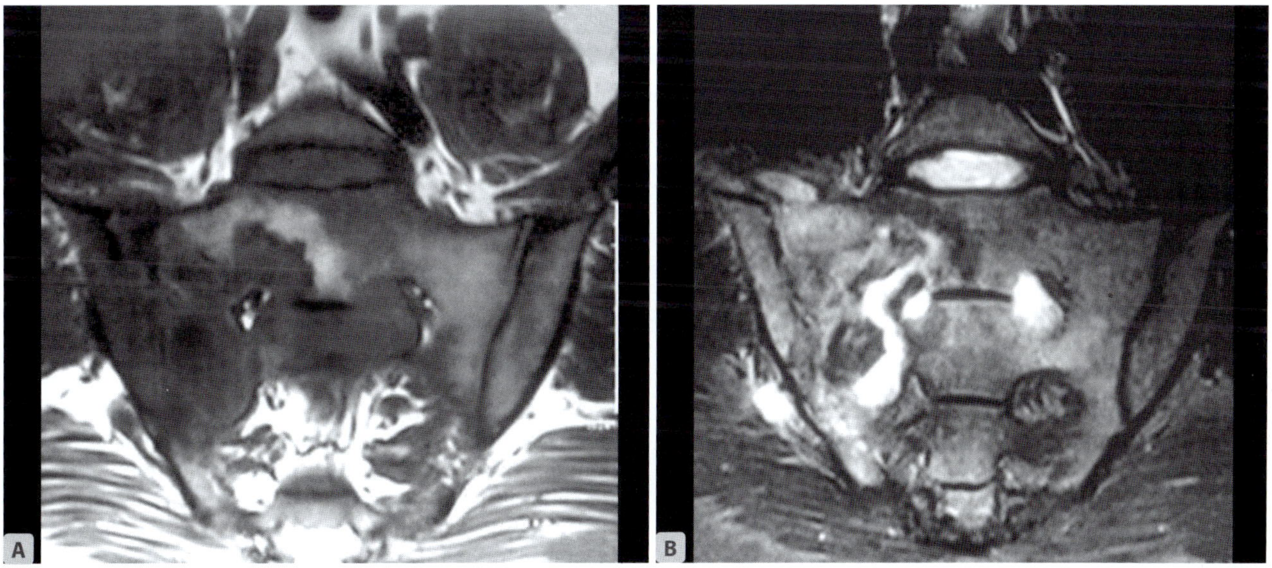

FIGS. 36A AND B: (A) T1-weighted coronal image of both sacroiliac joints; and (B) T2-weighted coronal image show altered signal in the right sacral ala and iliac blade, with articular erosion and decreased joint space—right sacroiliitis.

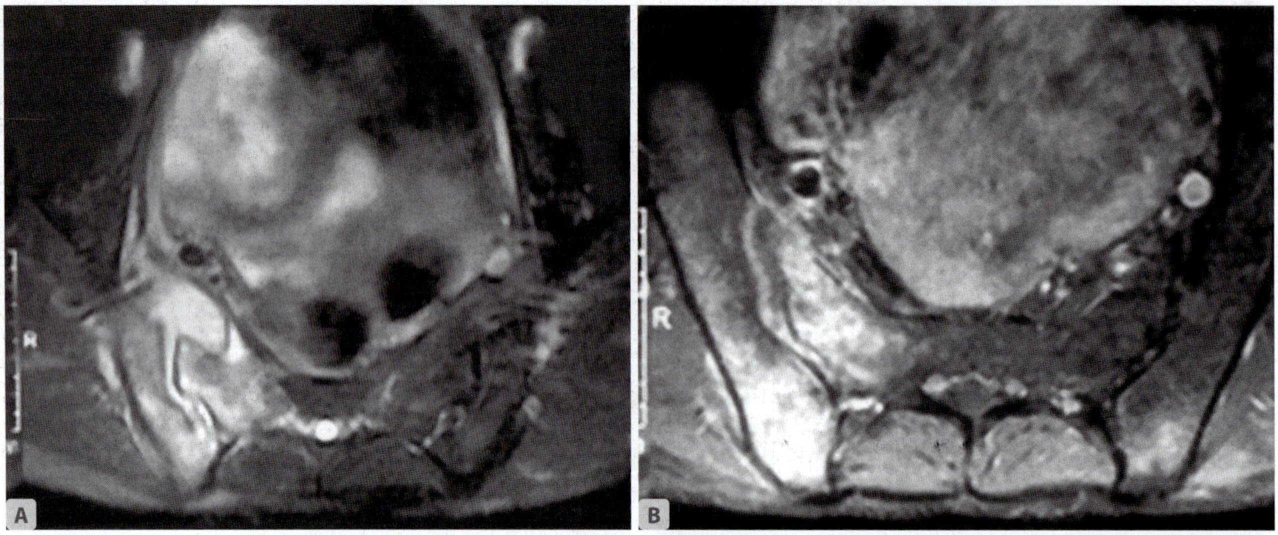

FIGS. 37A AND B: (A) T2-weighted axial; and (B) Short tau inversion recovery (STIR) axial image of both sacroiliac joints showing altered signal in right sacroiliac joint with widened joint space and periarticular collection—tubercular sacroiliitis.

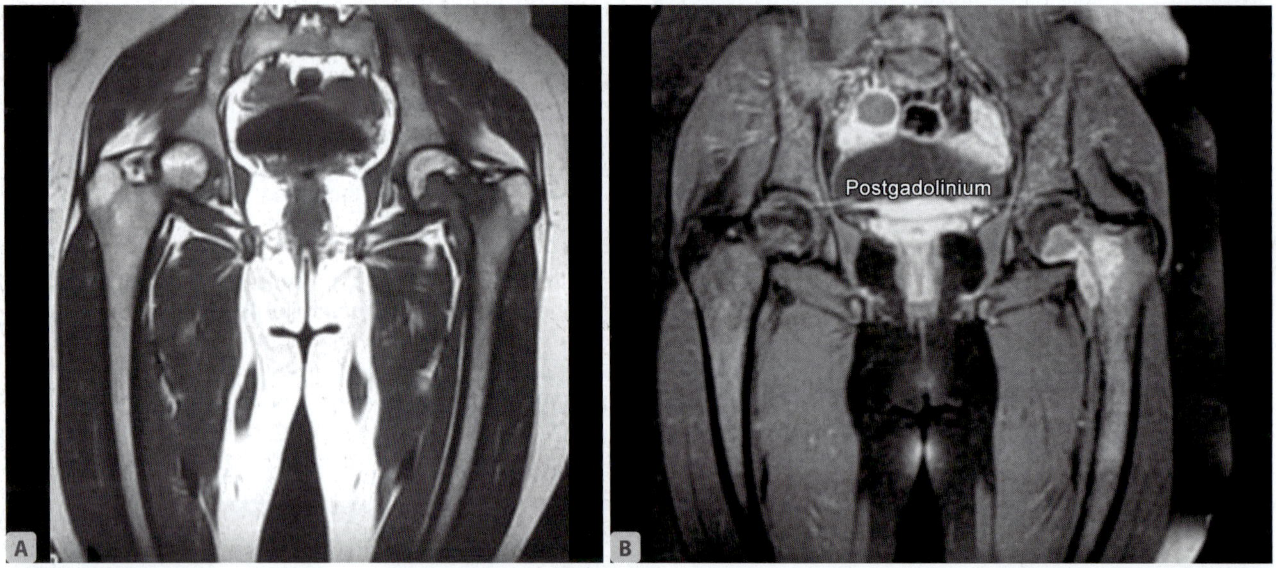

FIGS. 38A AND B: (A) T1-weighted (T1W) coronal image of the pelvis; and (B) T1W coronal postgadolinium image show an area of cortical erosion in the femoral neck with associated marrow edema—tubercular arthritis.

synovitis and MRI can then simulate a noninfectious inflammatory arthritis. MRI may demonstrate intraosseous involvement earlier than with other modalities **(Figs. 38A and B)**. Tuberculosis of the joints is discussed in detail elsewhere in the book.

BURSAE

There are several bursae in the hip region, which can get inflamed. *The iliopsoas bursa* is the largest bursa in the body and communicates with the hip joint in 15% of population. The iliopsoas bursa is located anterior to the hip joint and adjacent to femoral vessels. It lies between the psoas muscle and the anteromedial surface of the hip joint. The bursa measures 3–7 cm in length and is 2–4 cm in width. It gets distended in inflammatory, infective or degenerative disease. Patient may have groin pain and a palpable mass. It is not seen unless distended with fluid. Postcontrast scanning delineates the bursa better as the lining of the bursa enhances and the fluid does not. Asymptomatic bursal fluid may occur in the presence of joint effusion due to communication with the joint.

Greater trochanteric bursitis is another cause of hip pain, with patient localizing the pain to lateral aspect of the hip; this results from repetitive hip flexion. The findings on MR consist of no perceptible abnormality on T1W images. On T2 images, there is increased signal paralleling the greater trochanter. Instead of a well-defined fluid collection, a focus of interdigitating high signal may be seen around the tendons of the greater trochanter. Clinically, it may not

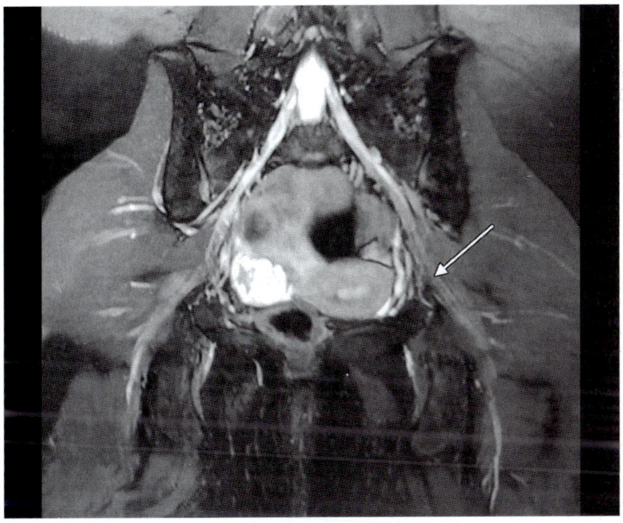

FIG. 39: MR neurography—maximum intensity projection (MIP) image depicting the sciatic nerve on both sides (marked with arrow on the left).

be possible to differentiate bursitis from gluteus medius/minimus tears.

NERVES

The largest nerve adjacent to the hip joint is the sciatic nerve. It is located immediately posterior to the posterior column of the acetabulum and lateral to the L4-S3 nerve roots. The nerve exits the infrapiriformis portion of the greater sciatic foramen and courses between the ischial tuberosity and greater trochanter surrounded by fat. It is located between quadratus femoris muscle anteriorly and gluteus maximus posteriorly. On MRI, the sciatic nerve is identified as intermediate signal intensity stippled structure surrounded by fat just lateral to the ischial tuberosity on axial images. MR neurography depicts the sciatic nerve in detail **(Fig. 39)**.[74]

The sciatic nerve can be compressed by a nearby mass or may be traumatized by a direct blow resulting in swelling of the nerve with an increased signal on T2W images.

Magnetic resonance imaging of acetabular fractures can be used to detect subclinical injury to the sciatic nerve. The injured nerve shows perineural or intraneural enhancement. Preoperative detection of such abnormalities warrants intraoperative monitoring as these patients would be at risk for further (iatrogenic) nerve injury. Compared with neurological examinations and somatosensory-evoked potential (SEP) monitoring, MR may be a more sensitive indicator of sciatic nerve trauma.[75]

Fibrolipomatous hamartoma may be seen in relation to the sciatic nerve in which fascicles of the nerve are surrounded by fat.

PIRIFORMIS SYNDROME

The sciatic nerve exits the pelvis at the greater sciatic notch and is located immediately anterior to the piriformis muscle. The sciatic nerve can split through piriformis and a portion of the nerve can be superficial to the piriformis muscle. Due to this variation in location of the sciatic nerve, compression, hypertrophy or injury to the piriformis muscle can cause irritation to the sciatic nerve, mimicking radicular symptoms of disc disease.

Magnetic resonance imaging may show asymmetry in size of one piriformis compared to opposite side. In case of trauma, high signal may be noted.

MAGNETIC RESONANCE IMAGING IN POSTARTHROPLASTY HIP

Complications of hip replacement procedures can be hardware failure, periprosthetic fractures, implant loosening, infections, and adverse tissue reactions. Tendinopathy, heterotopic ossification, neuropathy, and component-induced synovitis are other complications. MR plays an important role in the diagnosis and grading of adverse tissue reactions because of poor sensitivity of radiography and CT.

Imaging of the hip after total hip arthroplasty was a challenge due to susceptibility artifacts. With pulse modifications designed to reduce artifacts, better hardware, MRI is now being used to detect postoperative complications. MRI protocols to image implants include use of sequences with high spatial resolution, smaller fields of view, and higher imaging matrices. A lower strength magnet (1.5T instead of 3T),with stronger gradients, use of Spin echo instead of gradient echo sequences, increasing receiver bandwidth, and use of STIR (instead of frequency selective fat suppression) for a more uniform fat saturation are other steps to reduce susceptibility. Newer techniques such as slice encoding for metal artifact correction (SEMAC), multiacquistion variable resonance image combination (MAVRIC), and view angle tilting are now available which have improved imaging around prosthesis.[76,77]

Initially metal on metal (MOM) arthroplasties were done which were replaced by metal on polymer (MOP) implants due to high incidence of aseptic loosening in the former. MOP arthroplasties have metallic femoral head prosthesis and a polyethylene liner within the prosthetic acetabular cup. Aseptic loosening and shedding of polyethylene fragments from this led to periprosthetic loosening and aseptic loosening (particle disease) of second-generation MOM implants constructed from chromium cobalt and molybdenum alloy were introduced in the late 1990s. These are now known to have complications like adverse reaction to metal debris (ARMD) due to reaction to shed metallic microparticles. Granulomatous inflammation and aseptic lymphocytic vacuities associated lesions (ALVAL) have also been documented. Clinical long-term follow-up and monitoring of cobalt and chromium levels are used to detect ARMD.[78]

Direct visualization by MRI is the least invasive technique to determine the occurrence of ARMD. Periprosthetic collections are seen in both types of implant. They may have signal like simple fluid, others have more ill-defined solid debris with thicker, irregular pseudocapsule, appreciated on fluid sensitive sequences. MRI plays a significant role in the assessment of soft tissues adjacent to the prosthesis and can detect insertional tears of gluteal tendons, muscle edema/atrophy, and periprosthetic marrow edema. Metallosis is noted as a low signal intensity halo around the prosthesis on all sequences.

Trochanteric bursitis, avulsion of the gluteus tendons, and short external rotators can be identified on MRI.

HIP AND PELVIS-BONE TUMORS

Any bone tumor or tumors-like lesion can occur in and round the hip and pelvis, but there are certain tumors that are preferentially seen in this region **(Box 8)**.

BOX 8: Common bone tumors of the hip and pelvis.

- *Benign*
  - Osteochondroma
  - Enchondroma
  - Chondroblastoma
  - Giant cell tumor
  - Osteoid osteoma
  - Geode
- *Malignant*
  - Metastasis
  - Chondrosarcoma
  - Ewings sarcoma
  - Plasmacytoma

The pelvis and proximal femur contain hematopoietic red bone marrow that persists throughout life and a mix of red and yellow marrow is seen in adults. Both the apophysis and epiphysis should have yellow marrow. Fat marrow can convert to red marrow in times of increased physiological demands. Variations in the red marrow pattern are a source of diagnostic errors. Normal red marrow has serpiginous margins which do not disrupt normal anatomical barriers and appear iso to hyperintense to skeletal muscles on T1W images after neonatal period.

Most bone tumors in the pelvis are malignant and most tumors in proximal femur are benign in the adults. Metastasis and multiple myeloma are very common in the pelvis in patients >40 years of age and must be excluded in patients presenting with a lytic/blastic lesion in the pelvis. The most common primary malignant bone tumors of the pelvis are chondrosarcoma **(Figs. 40A to C)**, followed by Ewing's sarcoma and the osteosarcoma.[79] Same are also seen in proximal femur (chondrosarcoma being the most common followed by osteosarcoma and Ewing's sarcoma). The most common primary benign tumors in pelvis are osteochondroma, giant cell tumors, and Langerhans cell histiocytosis, and in the proximal femur are fibrous dysplasia, solitary bone cyst, and osteoid osteoma.

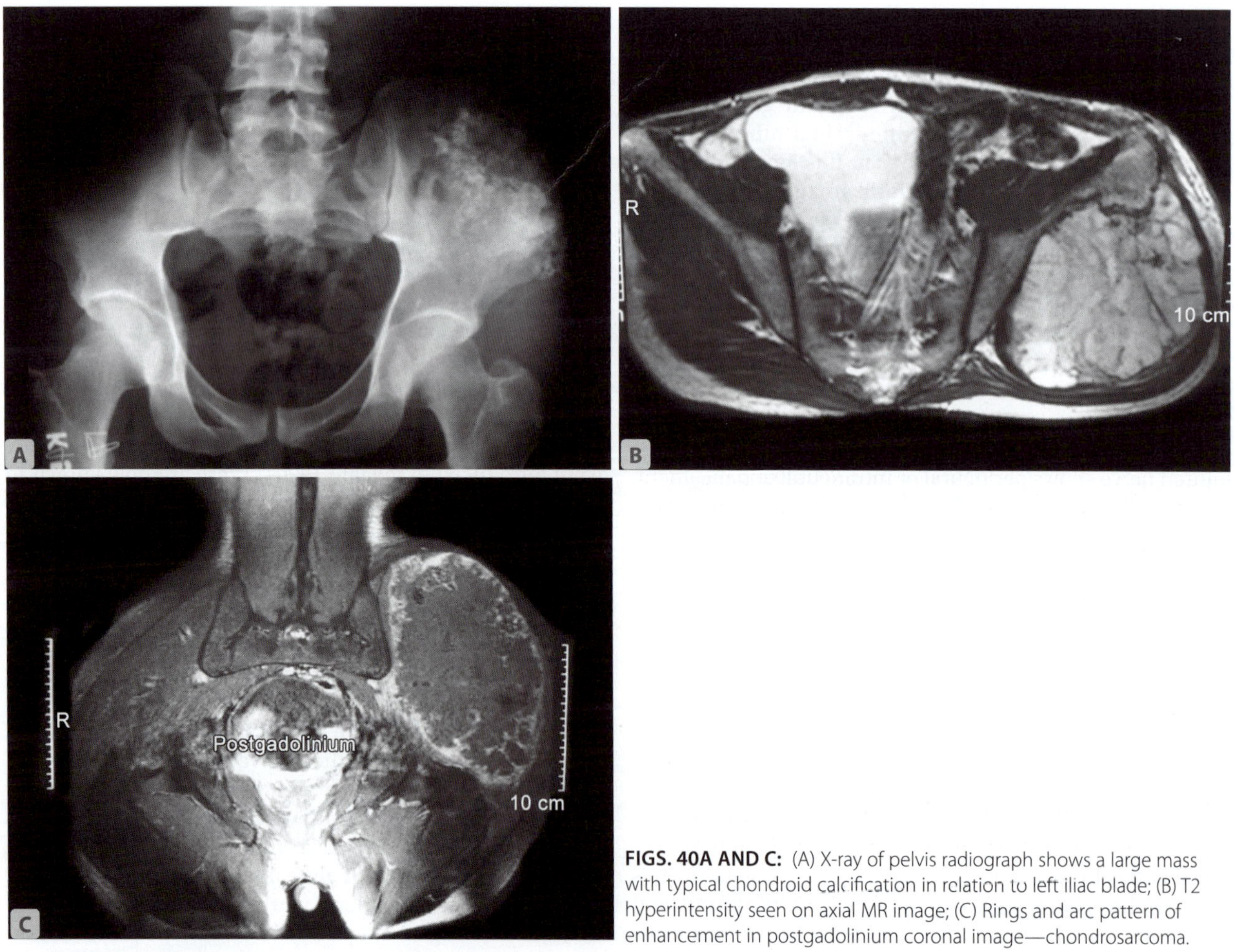

FIGS. 40A AND C: (A) X-ray of pelvis radiograph shows a large mass with typical chondroid calcification in relation to left iliac blade; (B) T2 hyperintensity seen on axial MR image; (C) Rings and arc pattern of enhancement in postgadolinium coronal image—chondrosarcoma.

Transarticular spread across joints—sacroiliac, symphysis pubis, and a hip via ligamentum teres is mostly seen with aggressive lesions such as chondrosarcoma, osteosarcoma, metastasis, and giant cell tumor.

Bone islands (enostosis) are common incidental and asymptomatic findings with pelvis and sacrum being common sites. Suspicion of metastasis may be raised in patients with a known malignancy. Clinical correlation, metabolic profile, and review with previous imaging are required to reach a diagnosis.

CONCLUSION

Magnetic resonance imaging is the diagnostic modality of choice for most disorders of the hip and pelvis in evaluating cases with radiographic findings that are inconclusive or do not explain the patient's complaints. In the evaluation of hip and pelvis, MRI is often the problem solving technique bypassing bone scintigraphy and CT. With MRI, one can stage the pathology of the hip and pelvis to prognosticate and influence therapeutic decisions.

REFERENCES

1. Hips and pelvis. In: Helms C, Major N, Anderson MW, Kaplan P, Dussault R (Eds). Musculoskeletal MRI, 2nd edition. Philadelphia: WB Saunders; 2009. pp. 324-51.
2. Sutter R, Zanetti M, Pfirrmann CWA. New developments in hip imaging. Radiology. 2012;264(03):651-67.
3. Petchprapa CN, Dunham KS, Lattanzi R, et al. Demystifying radial imaging of the hip. Radiographics. 2013;33:E97–112.
4. Llopis E, Fernandez E, Cerezal L. MR and CT arthrography of the hip. Semin Musculoskelet Radiol. 2012;16(01):42-56.
5. Crespo-Rodríguez AM, De Lucas-Villarrubia JC, Pastrana-Ledesma M. The diagnostic performance of non-contrast 3-Tesla magnetic resonance imaging (3-T MRI) versus 1.5-Tesla magnetic resonance arthrography (1.5-T MRA) in femoro-acetabular impingement. Eur J Radiol. 2017;88:109-16.
6. Morrison WB. Indirect MR arthrography: concepts and controversies. Semin Musculoskelet Radiol. 2005;9:125-34.
7. Zlatkin MB, Pevsner D, Sanders TG, Hancock CR, Ceballos CE, Herrera MF. Acetabular labral tears and cartilage lesions of the hip: indirect MR arthrographic correlation with arthroscopy–a preliminary study. Am J Roentgenol. 2010;194:709-14.
8. Hungerford DS, Zizic TM. Pathogenesis of ischemic necrosis of the femoral head. Hip; 1983. pp. 249-62.
9. Malizos KN, Karantanas AH, Varitimidis SE, Dailiana ZH, Bargiotas K, Maris T. Osteonecrosis of the femoral head: Etiology, imaging and treatment. Eur J Radiol. 2009;63:16-28.
10. Murphey MD, Foreman KL, Klassen-Fischer MK, Fox MG, Chung EM, Kransdorf MJ. From the radiologic pathology archives imaging of osteonecrosis: Radiologic-pathologic correlation. Radiographics. 2014;34(04):1003-28.
11. Mitchell DG, Rao VM, Dalinka MK, Spritzer CE, Alavi A, Steinberg ME, et al. Femoral head avascular necrosis: Correlation of MR imaging, radiographic staging, radionuclide imaging and clinical findings. Radiology. 1987;162(3):709-15.
12. Beltran J, Herman LJ, Burk JM, Zuelzer WA, Clark RN, Lucas JG, et al. Femoral head avascular necrosis: MR imaging with clinical pathological and radionuclide correlation. Radiology. 1988;166:215.
13. Nadel DN, Debatin JT, Richardson LW. Detection of acute avascular necrosis of the femoral head in dogs: Dynamic contrast enhanced MR imaging vs spin echo and STIR sequences. Am J Roentgenol. 1992;159:1255.
14. Karantanas AH, Drakonaki EE. The role of MR imaging in vascular necrosis of the femoral head. Semin Musculoskelet Radiol. 2011;15:281-300.
15. Duda SH, Laniado M, Schick F, Claussen CD. The Double line sign of osteonecrosis: Evaluation on chemical shift MR images. Eur J Radiol. 1993;16(3):233-8.
16. Omar I, Blount J. Magnetic Resonance Imaging of the hip. Top Magn Reson Imaging. 2015;24:165-87.
17. Ikemura S, Yamamota T, Motomura G, Nakashima Y, Mawatari T, Iwamoto Y. MRI evaluation of collapsed femoral head in patients 60 years old or older: Differentiation of subchondral insufficiency fracture from osteonecrosis of the femoral head. Am J Roentgenol. 2010;195(1):W63-8.
18. Yeh LR, Chen CK, Huang YL, Pan HB, Yang CF. Diagnostic Performance of MR imaging in the assessment of subchondral fractures in avascular necrosis of the femoral head. Skeletal Radiol. 2009;38(06):559-64.
19. Huang GH, Chan WP, Chang YC, Chang CY, Chen CY, Yu JS. MR imaging of bone marrow edema and joint effusion in patients with osteonecrosis of the femoral head: relationship to pain. Am J Roentgenol. 2003;181:545-9.
20. Vande Berg B, Malghem J, Labaisse MA, Noel H, Maldague B. Avascular necrosis of the hip. Comparison of contrast enhanced and nonenhanced MR imaging with histological correlation. Radiology. 1992;182:445-50.
21. Chan WP, Liu YJ, Huang GS, Lin MF, Huang S, Chang YC, et al. Relationship of the idiopathic osteonecrosis of the femoral head to perfusion changes in the proximal femur by dynamic contrast enhanced MRI. Am J Roentgenol. 2011;196:637-43.
22. Oner AY, Aggunlu L, Akpek S, Celik A, Le Roux P, Tali T, et al. Staging of hip avascular necrosis: Is there a need for DWI? Acta Radiol. 2001;52:111-4.
23. Hou CH, Shih TT, Liu CY, Li YD, Enright T. Proton MR spectroscopy of the femoral head-evaluation of patients at risk for vascular necrosis. J Magn Reson Imaging. 2006;24(2):409-17.
24. Arlet J, Ficat RP. [Diagnosis of primary femur head osteonecrosis at stage 1 (preradiologic stage)]. Rev Chir Orthop Reparatrice Appar Mot. 1968;54(7):637-48.
25. Steinberg ME, Hayken GD, Steinberg DR. A quantitative system for staging avascular necrosis. J Bone Joint Surg Br. 1995;77(1): 34-41.
26. Association for Research on Osseous Circulation. Committee on Terminology and Classification. ARCO News. 1992;4:41-6.
27. Shimizu K, Moriya H, Akita T, et al. Prediction of collapse with magnetic resonance imaging of avascular necrosis of the femoral head. J Bone Joint Surg. 1994;76A:215-21
28. Bradway JK, Morrey BF. The natural history of the silent hip in bilateral atraumatic osteonecrosis. J Arthroplasty. 1993;8(4): 383-7.
29. Hu LB, Huang ZG, Wei HY, Wang W, Ren A, Xu YY. Osteonecrosis of the femoral head: Using CT, MRI and gross specimen to characterize the location, shape and size of the lesion. Br J Radiol. 2015;88(1046):20140508
30. Mitchell DG, Rao UM, Dalinka MK, Spritzer CE, Axel L, Gefter W, et al. Hematopoietic and fatty bone marrow distribution in the normal and ischemic hip: New observations with 1.5T MR imaging. Radiology. 1986;161(1):199-202.

31. Jiang CC, Shih TT. Epiphyseal scar of the femoral head: Risk factor of osteonecrosis. Ra diology. 1994;191(2):409-12.
32. Coleman BG, Kressel HY, Dalinka MK, Scheibler ML, Burk DL, Cohen EK. Radiographically negative avascular necrosis detection with MR imaging. Radiology. 1988;168:525-8.
33. Vande Berg BC, Lecovet FE, Koutaissoff S. Bone marrow edema of the femoral head and transient osteoporosis of the hip. Eur J Radiol. 2008;67:68-77.
34. Kaplan SS, Stegman CJ. Transient osteoporosis of the hip. J Bone Joint Surg Am. 1985;67A:490-2.
35. Curtiss PH, Kincaid WE. Transitory demineralisation of the hip in pregnancy. J Bone Surg Am. 41A:1237-1333.
36. Uzun M, Ayhan E, Beksac B, Karaman O. Regional migratory osteoporosis and transient osteoporosis of the hip: Are they all the same? Clin Rheumatol. 2013;32(6):919-23.
37. Vande Berg BE, Malghem JJ, Labaisse MA, Noel HM, Maldague BE. MR imaging of avascular necrosis and transient marrow edema of the femoral head. Radiographics. 1993;13(3):501-20.
38. Klontzas ME, Vassalou EE, Zibis AH, Bintoudi AS, Karantanas AH. MR imaging of transient osteoporosis of the hip: an update on 155 hip joints. Eur J Radiol. 2015;84(3):431-43.
39. Klontzas ME, Zibis AH, Vassalou EE, Karantanas AH. MRI of the hip: current concepts on bone marrow oedema. Hip Int. 2017;27(4):329-35.
40. Naraghi A, White LM. MRI of labral and chondral lesions of the hip. Am J Roentgenol. 2015;205:479-90.
41. Kassarjian A, Brisson M, Palmer WE. Femoroacetabular impingement. Eur J Radiol. 2007;63:29-35.
42. Anderson SE, Siebenrock KA, Tannast M. Femoroacetabular impingement: evidence of an established hip abnormality. Radiology. 2010;257(1):8-13.
43. Ganz R, Parvizi J, Beck M, Leuing M, Notzli H, Siebenrock KA. Femoroacetabular impingement: A cause of osteoarthritis of the hip. Clin Orthop Relat Res. 2003;417:112-20.
44. Amanatullah DF, Antkowiak T, Pillay K, Patel J, Refaat M, Toupadakis CA, et al. Femoroacetabular impingement: Current concepts in diagnosis and treatment. Orthopedics. 2015;38:185-99.
45. Siebenrock KA, Wahab KH, Werlen S, Kalhor M, Leunig M, Ganz R. Abnormal extension of the femoral head epiphysis as a cause of cam impingement. Clin Orthop Relat Res. 2004;418:54-60.
46. Notzli HP, Wyss TF, Stoecklin CH, Schmid MR, Treiber K, Hodler J. The contour of the femoral head-neck junction as a predictor for the risk of anterior impingement. J Bone Joint Surg Br. 2002;84:556-60.
47. Ghaffari A, Davis I, Storey T, Moser M. Current concepts of femoroacetabular impingement. Radiol Clin North Am. 2018;56(6):965-82.
48. Sutter R, Pfirrmann CWA. Update on femoroacetabular impingement: What is new, and how should we assess it? Semin Musculoskelet Radiol. 2017;21(5):518-28.
49. Siebenrock KA, Kalbermatten DF, Ganz R. Effect of pelvic tilt on acetabular retroversion: A study of pelvis from cadavers. Clin Orthop Relat Res. 2003;407:241-8.
50. Ito K, Minka A, Leunig M, Werlen S, Ganz R. Femoroacetabular impingement and the cam effect: An MRI based quantitative anatomical study of the femoral head-neck offset. J Bone Joint Surg Br. 2001;83:171-6.
51. Schmaranzer F, Lerch TD, Strasser U, Vavron P, Schmaranzer E, Tannast M. Usefulness of MR arthrography of the hip with and without leg traction in detection of intra-articular bodies. Acad Radiol. 2019;26(9):e252-9.
52. Pfirrmann CWA, Mengiardi B, Dora C, Kalberer F, Zanetti M, Hodler J. Cam and pincer femoroacetabular impingement: Characteristic MR arthrographic findings in 50 patients. Radiology. 2006;240(3):778-85.
53. Li AE, Jawetz ST, Greditzer HG 4th, Burge AJ, Nawabi DH, Potter HG. MRI for the preoperative evaluation of femoroacetabular impingement. Insights Imaging. 2016;7(2):187-98.
54. Kassarjian A, Yoon LS, Belzile E, Connolly SA, Millis MB, Palmer WE. Triad of arthrographic findings in patients with cam type femoroacetabular impingement. Radiology. 2005;236:588-92.
55. Nokis SR, Vogler JB, Spritzer CE, Martinez S, Herfkens RJ. Herniation pits of the femoral neck: Appearance at MR imaging. Radiology. 1989;172(1):231-4.
56. Rehman H, Clement RG, Perks F, White TO. Imaging of occult hip fractures: CT or MRI? Injury. 2016;47(6):1297-1301.
57. Nachtrab O, Cassar-Pullicino VN, Lalam R, Tins B, Tyrrell PN, Singh J. Role of MRI in hip fractures, including stress fractures, occult fractures, avulsion fractures. Eur J Radiol. 2012;81(12):3813-23.
58. Lang P, Mauz M, Schörner W, Schwetlick G, Henkes H, Berthezene Y, et al. Acute fracture of the femoral neck: Assessment of femoral head perfusion with gadopentetate Dimeglumine—Enhanced MR imaging. Am J Roentgenol. 1993;160(2):335-41.
59. Steele CE, Cochran G, Renninger C, Deafenbaugh B, Kuhn KM. Femoral neck stress fractures: MRI risk factors for progression. J Bone Joint Surg Am. 2018;100(17):1496-502.
60. Kassarjian A, Rodrigo RM, Santisteban JM. Current concepts in MRI of rectus femoris musculotendinous (myotendinous) and myofascial injuries in elite athletes. Eur J Radiol. 2012;81(12):3763-71.
61. Bencardino JT, Palmer WE. Imaging of hip disorders in athletes. Radiol Clin North Am. 2002;40(2):267-87.
62. Boutin RD, Newman JS. MR imaging of sports-related hip disorders. Magn Reson Imaging Clin N Am. 2003; 11(2):255-81.
63. Kingzett-Taylor A, Tirman PF, Feller J, McGann W, Prieto V, Wischer T, et al. Tendinosis and tears of gluteus medius and maximus muscles as a cause of hip pain: MR imaging findings. Am J Roentgenol. 1999;173(4):1123-6.
64. Lee KS, Rosas HG, Phancao JP. Snapping hip: Imaging and treatment. Semin Musculoskelet Radiol. 2013;17(3):286-94.
65. Mullens FE, Zoga AC, Morrison WB, Meyers WC. Review of MRI technique and imaging findings in athletic pubalgia and the "sports hernia.". Eur J Radiol. 2012;81(12):3780-92.
66. Agten CA, Sutter R, Buck FM, Pfirrmann CWA. Hip imaging in athletes: Sports imaging series. Radiology. 2016;280(2):351-69.
67. Narváez JA, Narváez J, De Lama E, De Albert M. MR imaging of early rheumatoid arthritis. Radiographics. 2010;30(1):143-63; discussion 163-5.
68. Hetland ML, Ejbjerg B, Hørslev-Petersen K, Jacobsen S, Vestergaard A, Jurik AG, et al. MRI bone oedema is the strongest predictor of subsequent radiographic progression in early rheumatoid arthritis. Results from a 2-year randomised controlled trial (CIMESTRA). Ann Rheum Dis. 2009;68:384-90.
69. Flandry F, Hughston J, McCann S, Kurtz DM. Diagnostic features of diffuse pigmented villonodular synovitis of the knee. Clin Orthop. 1994;298:212-20.
70. Hermann G, Abdelwahab IF, Klein M, Kenan S, Lewis M. Synovial chondromatosis. Skeletal Radiol. 1995;24:298-300.
71. Murphey MD, Wetzel LH, Bramble JM, Levine E, Simpson KM, Lindsley HB. Sacroiliitis: MR imaging findings. Radiology. 1991;180:239-44.
72. Bollow M, Braun J, Hamm B, Eggens U, Schilling A, König H, et al. Early sacroiliitis in patients with spondyloarthropathy: Evaluation with dynamic gadolinium enhanced MR imaging. Radiology. 1995;194:529-36.
73. Maj L, Gombar Y III, Morrison WB. MR imaging of hip infection and inflammation. Magn Reson Imaging Clin N Am. 2013;21(01): 127-39.
74. Chhabra A, Chalian M, Soldatos T, Andreisek G, Faridian-Aragh N, Williams E, et al. 3-T high-resolution MR neurography of sciatic neuropathy. AJR Am J Roentgenol 2012;198(4):W357-64.

75. Potter HG, Montgomery KD, Heise CW, Helfet DL. MR imaging of acetabular fractures: Value in detecting femoral head injury, intra-articular fragments and sciatic nerve injury. Am J Roentgenol. 1994;163(4):881-6.
76. Berkowitz JL, Potter HG. Advanced MRI techniques for the hip joint: focus on the postoperative hip. Am J Roentgenol. 2017;209(3):534-43.
77. Fritz J, Lurie B, Miller TT, Potter HG. MR imaging of hip arthroplasty implants. Radiographics. 2014;34(4):E106-32.
78. Müller GM, Lundin B, von Schewelov T, Müller MF, Ekberg O, Månsson S. Evaluation of metal artifacts in clinical MR images of patients with total hip arthroplasty using different metal artifact-reducing sequences. Skeletal Radiol. 2015;44(3): 353-9.
79. Afonso PD, Weber MA, Issac A, Bloem JL. Hip and pelvis bone tumours: Can you make it simple. Semin Musculoskelet Radiol. 2019;23:e37-57.

CHAPTER

170

Magnetic Resonance Imaging of the Knee

Sapna Singh, Anjali Prakash, Gaurav Shanker Pradhan

INTRODUCTION

The knee is one of the important weight bearing (WB) joints capable of performing complex and extensive movements. It is therefore most frequently affected by traumatic and degenerative conditions.

Since its inception, magnetic resonance imaging (MRI) has been found to be a very informative imaging method widely accepted by the orthopedic community for evaluating the knee joint. MRI has reduced the number of diagnostic arthroscopies and has enabled selection of patients for therapy-oriented arthroscopy.[1,2] Soft tissue discrimination with MRI is excellent and differentiation can be made between cortex, marrow, ligaments, tendons, muscles, synovium, vascular, and cartilage elements.[3] This differentiation is not possible with conventional radiographic techniques. Additional advantages of MRI are its multiplanar and thin section capabilities and the ability to evaluate subchondral bone and marrow. MR is the recommended imaging modality over CT for the evaluation of bone contusions and occult knee fractures including the tibial plateau fractures. It has supplanted nuclear scintigraphy in the characterization of osteonecrosis and can be used to assess the integrity of overlying articular cartilage surfaces. Kinematic and dynamic MR techniques provide an improved perspective for assessing the biomechanics of the patellofemoral joint and the normal functions of the ligamentous structures of the knee.

3 Tesla (3T) MRI has revolutionized musculoskeletal imaging. The gain in the signal-to-noise ratio (SNR) improves image quality with increased signal and higher spatial resolution leading to an improved diagnostic accuracy. The ligamentous and cartilaginous structures are elucidated in better details on a 3T MR scanner. The smaller structures such as the posterolateral corner (PLC) are also assessed better.

IMAGING PROTOCOLS/TECHNICAL FACTORS

An ideal MR technique should yield images of the osseous and soft tissue structures of the knee with good contrast and spatial resolution in a reasonable time to maximize patient acceptability. The use of a dedicated knee coil is mandatory for a quality study because it improves the SNR. Using a small field of view (FOV) in the range of 10–14 cm greatly improves spatial resolution and facilitates optimal assessment of the small anatomical structures of the knee. A matrix of 256 × 256 is usually standard.

Patient Positioning

The patient is placed supine, feet first with the leg in full extension. The knee is placed in 10–15° of external rotation to realign the anterior cruciate ligament (ACL) parallel with the sagittal imaging plane. This is typically the position of the knee in the relaxed state and no effort at externally rotating the knee needs to be made in the majority of patients. The knee is placed in a dedicated knee coil to produce a uniform signal intensity across the image and foam pads are used to immobilize the knee within the center of the coil. Only one knee can be imaged at a time.

Slice Thickness

Four millimeter sections are used for axial, coronal, and sagittal images of the knee.[4] When needed, submillimeter resolution can be obtained with three-dimensional Fourier transformation (3D FT) volume protocols. In children, 3 mm slices allow optimal medial to lateral joint coverage in the sagittal plane and anterior to posterior coverage in the coronal plane.

Imaging Planes and Pulse Sequences

Acquisition of images in three orthogonal planes is helpful in defining and characterizing abnormalities.[4,5] An axial acquisition through the patellofemoral joint is used as the initial localizer for subsequent sagittal and coronal plane images. Menisci and cruciate ligaments are best evaluated on sagittal images with coronal views for secondary visualization and confirmation of pathology. The medial and lateral collateral ligaments are best displayed on coronal images. The articular cartilage surfaces of medial and lateral compartments are assessed in both coronal and sagittal planes. The patellofemoral joint including patellar facet and trochlear groove is best seen on axial images.

Standard MR Pulse Sequences

Short echo time (TE) conventional spin echo (CSE) images generally provide the best contrast for anatomical evaluation. The more rapidly acquired, fast spin echo (FSE) pulse sequences with short echo train length provide high SNR, excellent soft tissue contrast, high in-plane spatial resolution, and shorter scan times compared to CSE sequences. Short tau inversion recovery (STIR) and fat-saturated FSE pulse sequences are best for the evaluation of bone contusions and other marrow abnormalities. A knee protocol that works well includes FSE proton density (PD) and T2-weighted (T2W) sequence in the sagittal plane, a STIR sequence in the coronal plane, T1-weighted (T1W) coronal images, T2W axial images, and a sequence for articular cartilage.

Isotropic 3D Fast Spin Echo Acquisition

Many 3D techniques with gradient echo (GRE) based and fat suppressed (FSE) based sequences are available which have been discussed in detail in the section on articular cartilage. These sequences provide thinner sections and reduce partial volume averaging excellent for the depiction of subtle cartilaginous defects.

Metallic Artifact Reduction Sequences (MARS)

The metallic susceptibility artifacts cause both through plane and in plane distortions which can be corrected by view angle tilting (VAT), slice-encoding for metal artifact correction (SEMAC), and multiple-acquisition with variable resonance image combination (MAVRIC) sequences.[6]

Intravenous gadolinium is useful in assessment of inflammatory arthritides as it causes enhancement of the pannus. The biomechanics of patellar tracking can be assessed with kinematic technique with a cine loop display of acquired images.

MR EVALUATION OF THE KNEE

The structures that are studied can be broadly categorized as:

- Menisci
- Central structures of the knee [ACL, posterior cruciate ligament (PCL)]
- Medial structure of the knee [medial collateral ligament (MCL)]
- Corner based anatomy [PLC, posteromedial corner (PMC), anterolateral corner (ALC), anteromedial corner (AMC) or the extensor mechanism of the knee]
- Patellofemoral joint and MR kinematics
- Articular cartilage
- Synovium
- Bone marrow
- Subchondral bone

MENISCI

Magnetic resonance imaging is the modality of choice for evaluating a patient with suspected meniscal pathology. By displaying the morphology of meniscal tear, MR provides valuable information for determining the need for operative intervention and predicting the feasibility of meniscal repair.

Microanatomy of the Menisci

The menisci are predominantly made up of type I collagen arranged into bundles. Most of the bundles course circumferentially parallel to the long axis of the meniscus. A smaller number of fibers are oriented in a radial fashion functioning as stabilizing tie fibers. With axial loading of the joint, the circumferential orientation of most of the collagen bundles allows for meniscal deformation, the development of "hoop stresses", and a relatively even distribution of the load across the joint surfaces. Up to one-third of the peripheral meniscus is vascularized and innervated (the "red zone") whereas the remaining inner two-thirds or more is strictly fibrocartilaginous (the "white zone").[7,8]

Macroanatomy and MRI Appearance

The menisci are C-shaped structures that are conventionally described as having three segments **(Figs. 1A to C)**:

1. Anterior horn
2. Body
3. Posterior horn

Each meniscus measures approximately 5 mm in height along its periphery and tapers to a thin inner edge and hence shows a triangular shape when cut in cross section **(Fig. 2)**. The upper margin is called the superior articular surface whereas the lower margin is called the inferior articular surface. The superior articular surface is completely visible to the arthroscopist, the inferior to some extent, while the outer nonarticular capsular surface is not seen.

The menisci demonstrate diffusely low signal on all MRI pulse sequences because of their fibrocartilaginous nature. Meniscal pathology is best demonstrated on sequences that use a short TE (<20 ms), i.e., T1W, PD, and gradient echo images. If a FSE technique is used, the echo train length should be kept below 4–5 and the interecho space minimized to reduce the blurring effect inherent to this technique that can obscure a meniscal tear.[9,10] The menisci can also be evaluated by 3D volumetric acquisitions and radial imaging. Radial imaging in which multiple planes are rotated from the center of each meniscus or center of tibia can section portions of both the medial and lateral meniscus in views similar to conventional arthrogram.

Medial Meniscus

The semicircular medial meniscus has a wide posterior horn, narrows anteriorly, and has a more open C-shaped configuration than the more circular lateral meniscus. The anterior horn is roughly one-third to one-half as large as the posterior horn on sagittal images. The body of the meniscus is seen as a bow tie-shaped structure on the two most peripheral sagittal slices through the meniscus when 3- or 4-mm thick slices are obtained.[11]

The medial meniscus is attached to the joint capsule along its entire peripheral circumference. It is attached to medial femoral condyle and tibial plateau by the coronary ligament [deep fibers of medial collateral ligament (MCL)].

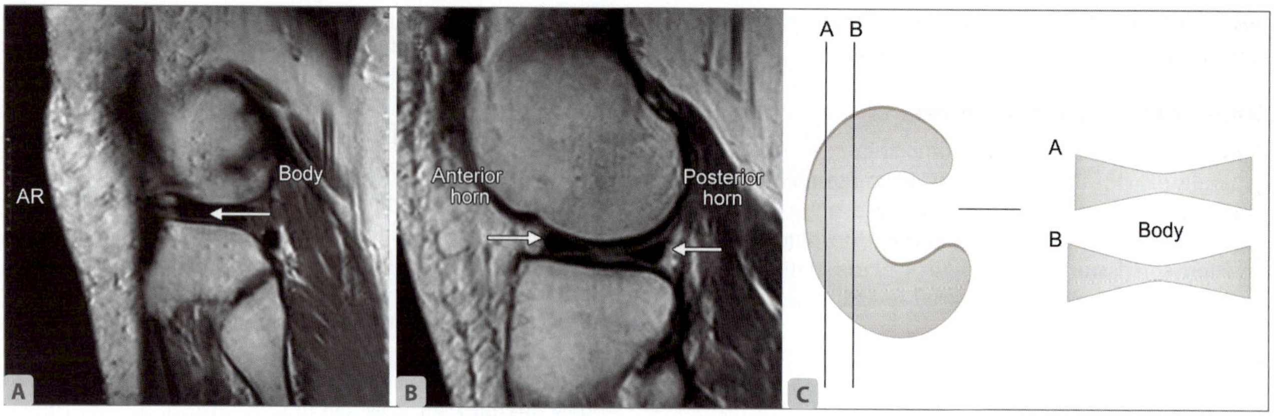

FIGS. 1A TO C: Sagittal T2W MR images of the knee showing a bow-tie configuration of the body of the lateral meniscus (A) and the symmetric equal size anterior and posterior horns (B). (C) Schematic diagram of the body of the meniscus seen as a bow-tie. Normal diffuse low-signal intensity of the meniscus is seen throughout—normal lateral meniscus.

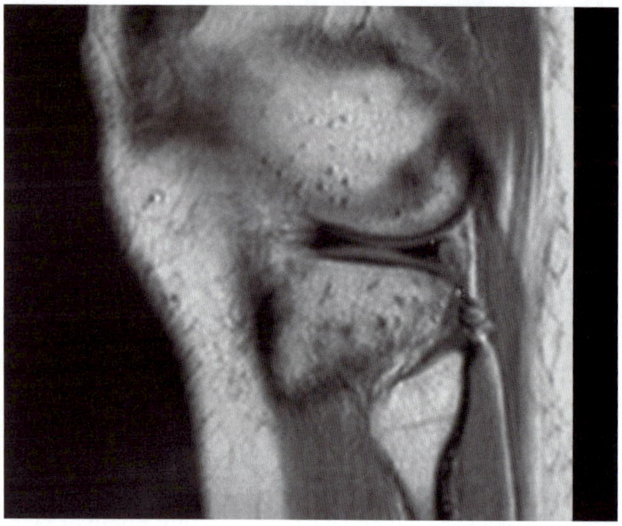

FIG. 2: Sagittal proton density MR image through the lateral meniscus showing the normal triangular shape of the meniscus thick peripherally and tapering to a thin inner edge. The normal meniscus measures 3–5 mm in height along its periphery.

The less mobile medial meniscus attachment to the deep layer of the MCL and the capsule makes the medial meniscus more susceptible to injury.

Lateral Meniscus

The lateral meniscus forms a tight C-shape (more circular than the medial meniscus) and is symmetric in width from anterior to posterior. The lateral meniscus is relatively mobile, it is more loosely attached to the joint capsule especially along its posterolateral aspect where the popliteus tendon courses through its intra-articular tunnel. There is no direct attachment of the lateral meniscus to the fibular collateral ligament or lateral collateral ligament. The meniscofemoral ligaments course from the posterior horn of the lateral meniscus, along either side of PCL, to attach to the inner margin of the medial femoral condyle. The ligament of Humphry courses anterior to PCL whereas the ligament of Wrisberg passes posterior to it. One of these two limbs is present in approximately 70% of the knees, both are present in only 6%.[6]

Anatomic Variants

Discoid Meniscus

A discoid meniscus is a dysplastic meniscus in which the meniscus is disc-shaped rather than C-shaped. The lateral meniscus is most commonly affected with a reported incidence of around 3%. Often a discoid meniscus is enlarged and affects the anterior or posterior horns of the meniscus asymmetrically. On sagittal images using 4–5 mm slice thickness, a discoid meniscus exhibits a continuous or bow tie appearance on three or more consecutive images **(Figs. 3A to C)**. Central tapering seen in normal menisci is lost in discoid fibrocartilage. Coronal images show the extension of the discoid meniscus apex toward or into the intercondylar notch and can be diagnosed when the body of the meniscus is more than 15 mm on a midline coronal image. Although often encountered incidentally, discoid menisci are more prone to undergo cystic degeneration with subsequent tears and multiple tears within the same meniscus are not uncommon.[12]

Meniscus Flounce (Buckled Meniscus)

Occasionally, the medial meniscus demonstrates an undulating or buckled appearance on sagittal MR images. This redundancy is a normal variant that is related, at least in part, to knee position. Close inspection of the meniscus is needed however because a meniscal tear may occasionally result in a similar appearance.[13]

Meniscal Ossicle

This is an embryologic variant or sequelae of prior trauma. It is a small focus of ossification within the meniscus and usually involves the posterior horn of the medial meniscus.[14] Although mostly asymptomatic, a meniscal ossicle may cause mechanical symptoms or pain and can be mistaken for a loose body on radiographs or MRI.

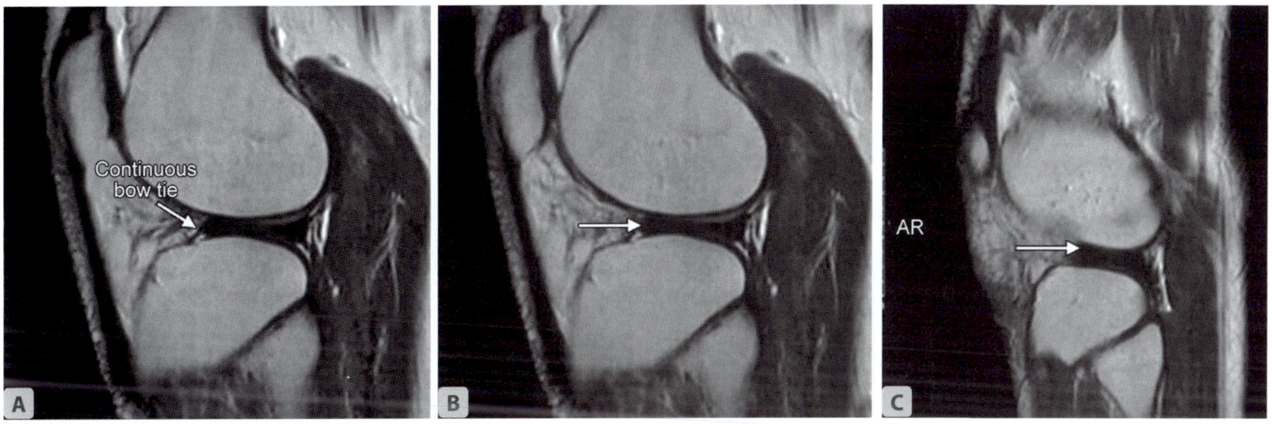

FIGS. 3A TO C: Consecutive 4 mm T2W sagittal MR images through the lateral meniscus showing a continuous bow-tie appearance on three sections—discoid meniscus.

Abnormal Meniscus

Meniscal Degenerations and Tears

The rotation of femur against a fixed tibia during flexion and extension places the menisci at risk for injury. Degeneration and tears of the meniscus demonstrate increased signal attributed to the imbibed synovial fluid.

MR Grading of Meniscal Tears

The MRI diagnosis of a meniscal tear is based on the alteration of intrameniscal signal characteristics. An MRI grading system divides increased intrameniscal signal into three grades according to their configuration and relation to articular surface.[15]

Grade I

In grade I, a nonarticular focal or globular intrasubstance increased signal is seen **(Fig. 4)**. Histologically, grade I signal intensity correlates with foci of early mucinous degeneration and chondrocyte deficient or hypocellular regions. Grade I signal intensity may be observed in asymptomatic athletes and normal volunteers and is not clinically significant.[16]

Grade II

In grade II, a linear intrasubstance horizontal increased signal extends from the capsular periphery of the meniscus. However, it does not involve an articular meniscal surface **(Figs. 5A and B)**. Areas and bands of mucinous degeneration are more extensive in grade II than in grade I.

Grade III

The increased signal intensity of the meniscus extends to at least one of the two articular surfaces **(Figs. 6A and B)**.

Abnormal Morphology

In addition to abnormal signal intensity, the morphology, i.e., size and shape of the meniscus should be assessed when evaluating meniscal lesions. The normal meniscus measures 3–5 mm in height. The medial meniscus varies in width from 6 mm at the anterior horn to 12 mm at the posterior horn. The lateral meniscus is approximately 10 mm in width throughout its length. Irregularity of the meniscal margin, a focal defect in one of its articular surfaces or an abnormally small meniscal segment, may be indicative of a tear **(Figs. 7A and B)**. Focal step such as contour deformities and wedge defects in the contour of the articular surface "Notch sign" may be the only sign present in some tears.[17] If a smaller than normal meniscal segment is observed, a thorough search should be performed to identify a displaced fragment.

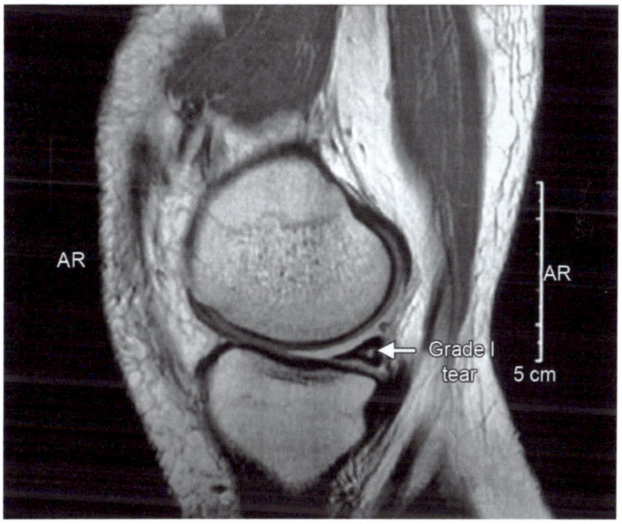

FIG. 4: Proton density sagittal MR image showing intrasubstance focal/globular increased signal within the posterior horn of the medial meniscus—Grade I meniscal signal.

"Two-slice-touch" Rule

Meniscal distortion in the absence of prior surgery and intrasubstance signal intensity extending to the articular surface, if seen on two or more consecutive images, is called the two-slice-touch rule. The positive predictive value of this sign is 94% in the medial meniscus and 96% in the lateral meniscus and should be reported as a meniscal tear.[18]

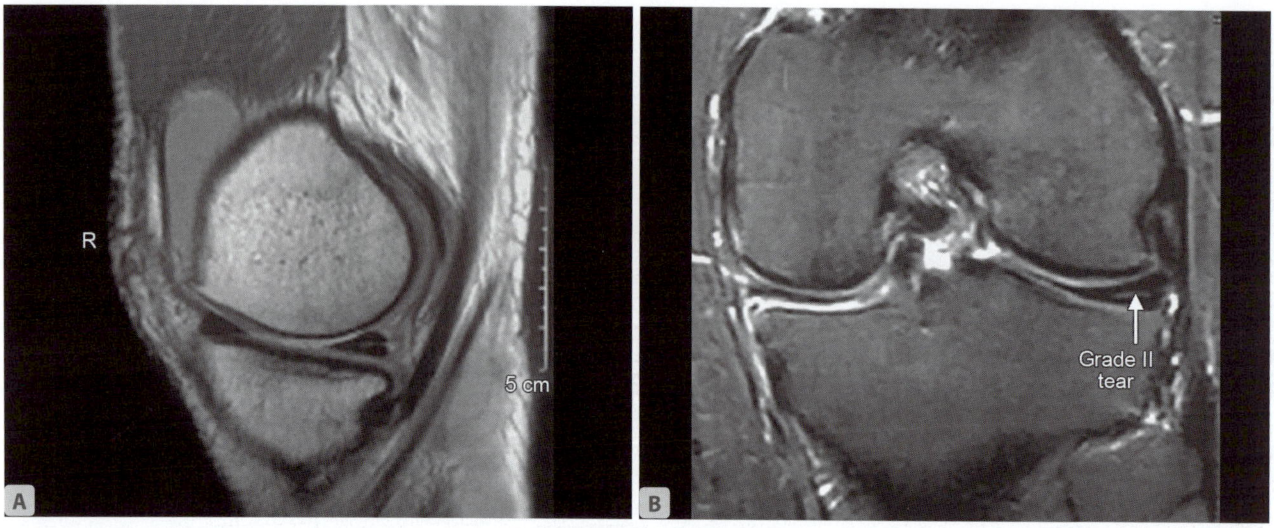

FIGS. 5A AND B: (A) T2W sagittal MR; and (B) STIR coronal images showing a horizontal, linear intrasubstance increased signal extending from the capsular periphery of the meniscus but not involving an articular meniscal surface—Grade II meniscal signal.

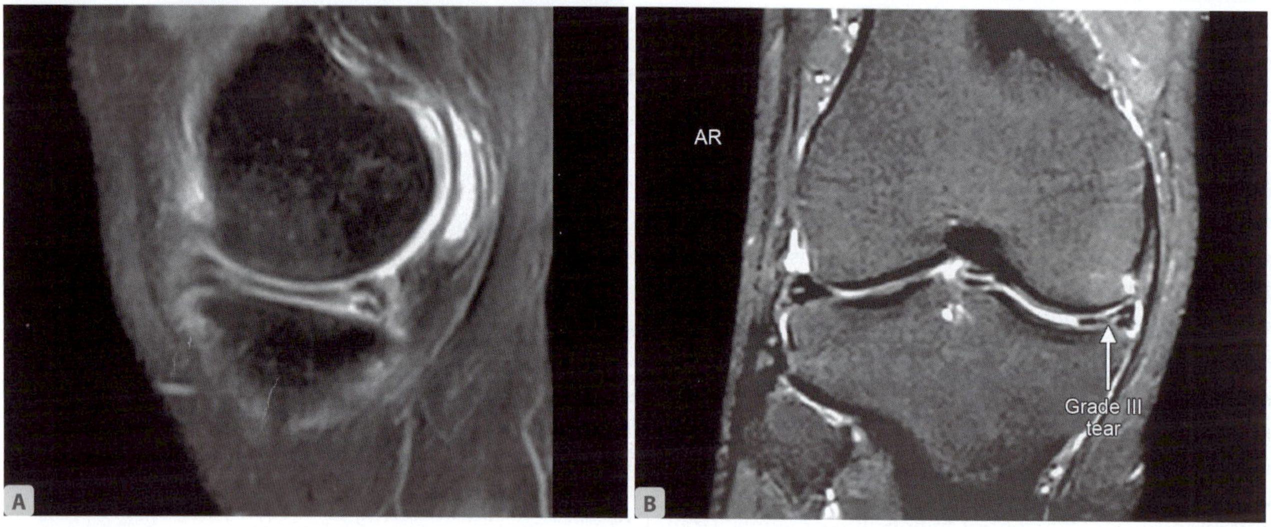

FIGS. 6A AND B: T2W fat suppressed sagittal (A) and (B) STIR coronal MR images showing increased signal intensity within the meniscus communicating or extending to the inferior articular surface—Grade III meniscal signal.

Classification of Meniscal Tears

Meniscal tears are divided into two basic types—vertical and horizontal. Vertical tears are often of a traumatic origin whereas horizontal tears are usually secondary to meniscal degeneration.

Vertical Tears

Vertical tears are further subdivided into radial (perpendicular to the long axis of the meniscus) and longitudinal (parallel to the long axis) varieties **(Fig. 8)**.

Horizontal Tears

A horizontal or oblique tear extends through the meniscus along a plane parallel to the tibial plateau, separating the meniscus into superior and inferior fragments **(Fig. 9)**. Also called a horizontal cleavage tear, this is the most common type of tear to be associated with a meniscal cyst.[19] The cyst occurs as a result of fluid extending through the tear by a ball valve effect and collecting either within the meniscus (intrameniscal cyst) **(Figs. 10A and B)** or at the meniscocapsular junction (parameniscal cyst) **(Figs. 11A and B)**. If a cyst is seen along the meniscocapsular junction, an underlying meniscal tear should be excluded because the cysts tend to recur after resection if the underlying tear is not repaired. There are three criteria for the diagnosis of a meniscal cyst:

1. A tear which is horizontal in morphology
2. Accumulation of fluid seen as high-signal intensity on T2W images
3. Flat lining against the outer margin of the meniscus.

A meniscal cyst does not communicate with the joint space and is hence not opacified by contrast on MR arthrography.

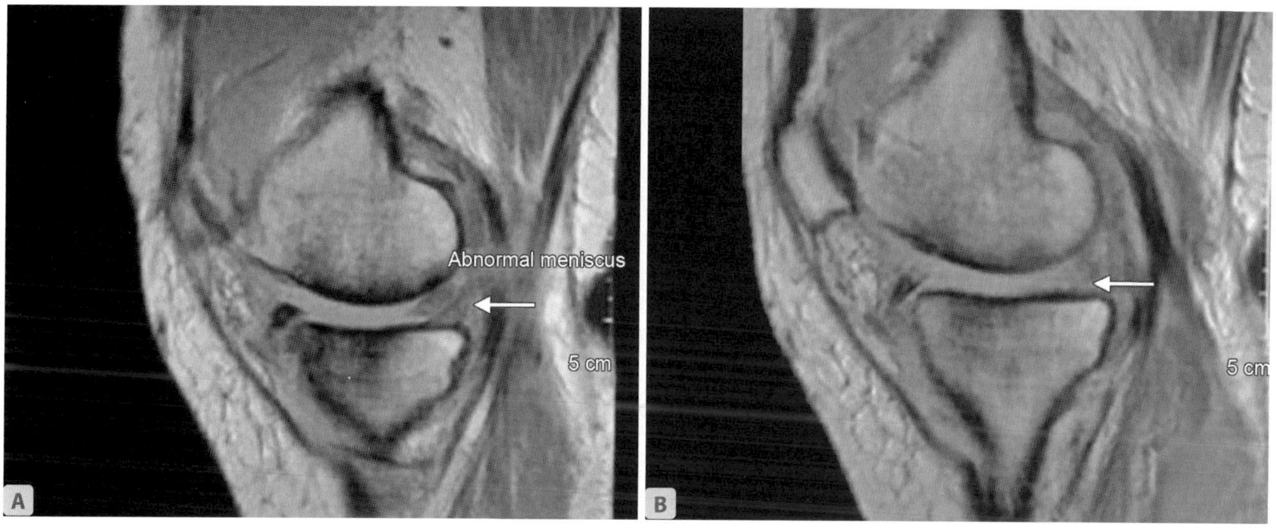

FIGS. 7A AND B: Consecutive proton density sagittal MR images of the knee showing irregularity and abnormally small posterior horn of the medial meniscus suggestive of a tear.

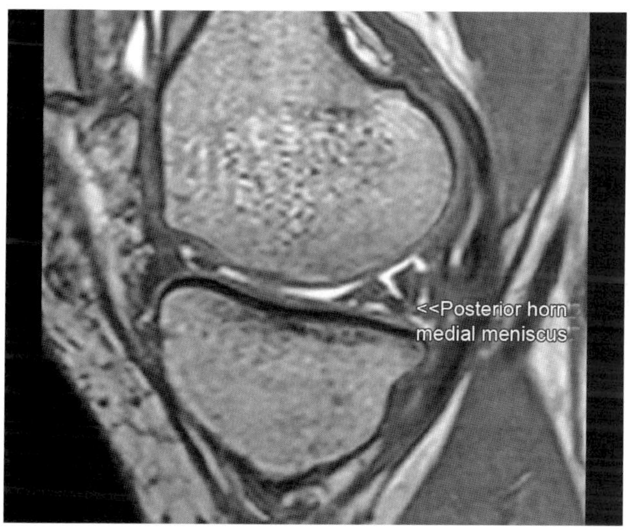

FIG. 8: Double echo steady state (DESS) sequence sagittal MR image showing a vertical longitudinal tear of the posterior horn of the medial meniscus seen as a vertically oriented linear focus of abnormal signal intensity within the substance of the meniscus along its long axis.

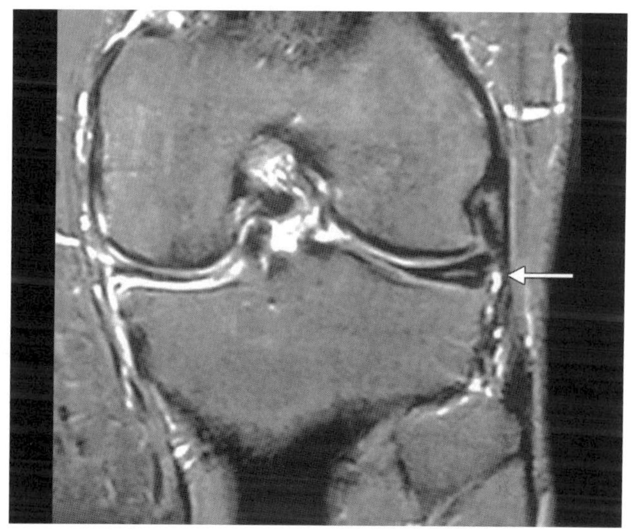

FIG. 9: STIR coronal MR image showing a horizontal tear in the body of the lateral meniscus.

Radial/Free Edge Tears

Radial tears extend perpendicular to the long axis of the meniscus. These range from a small injury along its free edge to a large tear extending through its entire circumference. MR images obtained perpendicular to the orientation of a radial tear demonstrate the tear as a small gap or cleft in the meniscus *(cleft sign)* which can sometimes be observed to move across the meniscus on successive images *(marching cleft sign)*.[20] If the orientation of the imaging plane is in the same direction as a full-thickness radial tear, a section through the same plane of the tear will demonstrate an absent meniscus or high-signal intensity resulting in the so called *ghost sign*. A partial-thickness radial tear will demonstrate blunting or abrupt truncation of the apex of the meniscus *(truncated triangle sign)*. A full-thickness radial tear severely compromises meniscal function by disrupting the critical circumferential collagen bundles such that the meniscus can no longer develop the "hoop stresses" necessary to disperse an axial load.[21] The middle third of the lateral meniscus is a common location for radial tears, probably because of its more circular shape and decreased radius of curvature, its increased mobility, and excessive loading during valgus stress.

Root Tears

Root tears are full-thickness radial tears at the central tibial attachments of the menisci. Root tears should be suspected in cases of peripheral subluxation of the involved meniscus.[22] On posterior coronal MR images, abrupt loss or blunting of the normal meniscotibial attachment and foreshortening of the meniscus toward the posterior aspect of the intercondylar notch are seen.

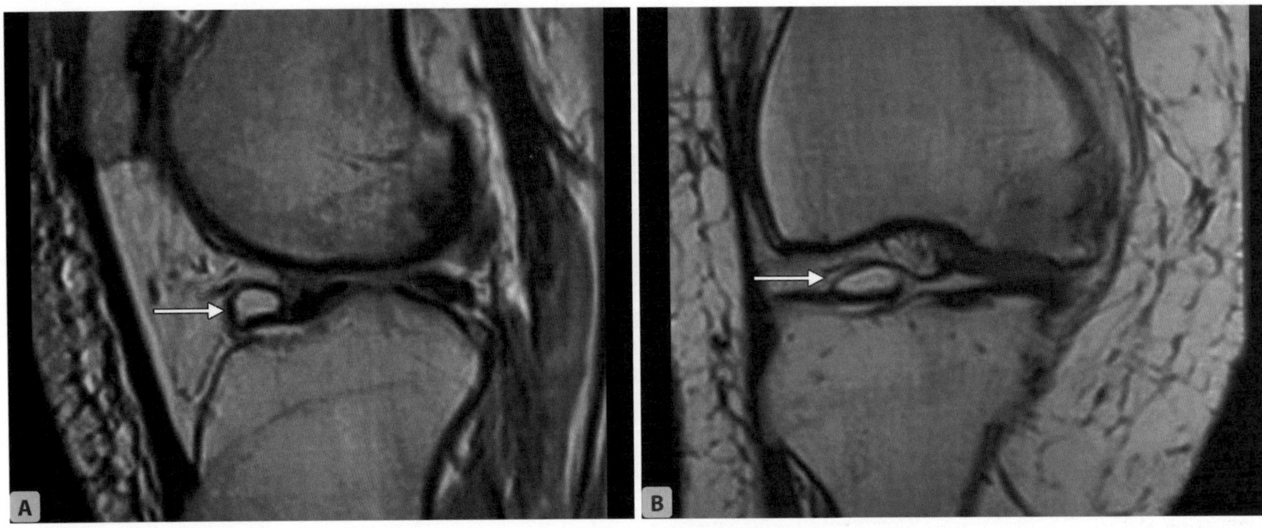

FIGS. 10A AND B: Sagittal and coronal MR images showing a meniscal cyst giving a slightly swollen appearance to the meniscus.

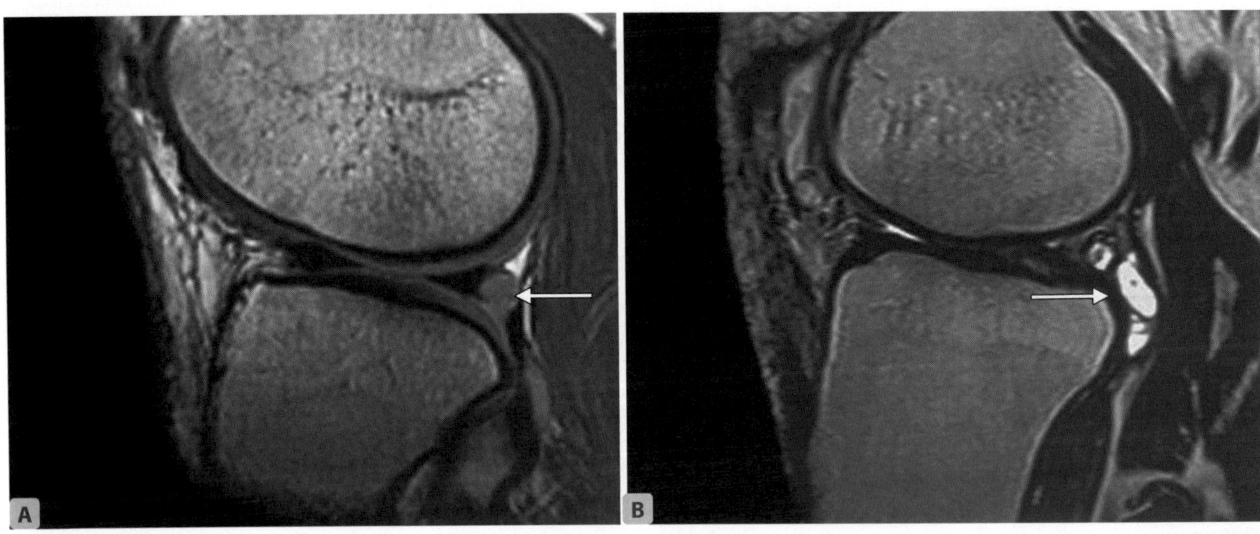

FIGS. 11A AND B: (A) Sagittal proton density; and (B) T2W MR images showing a fluid signal intensity structure at the meniscocapsular junction—parameniscal cyst.

Longitudinal Tears

Vertical longitudinal tears make up the common bucket handle tear that occurs in about 10% of meniscal tears. The normal meniscus has a body width of about 9 mm which is seen on sagittal images as a single slab of meniscal tissue that has a shape similar to a bow tie. When the inner edge of the meniscus displaces, a bucket handle tear is easily diagnosed by noting only one instead of the normal two body segments present on the outermost sagittal images through the meniscus. This is called the "absent bow tie sign"[10] and may be the only indication of a bucket handle tear. The anterior and posterior cruciate ligaments are the only two structures seen in the intercondylar fossa in a normal knee. A structure, in addition to these two, in the intercondylar fossa, is abnormal and is most likely to be a displaced meniscal fragment. A displaced meniscal fragment, usually, but not always, can be found especially in the intercondylar notch and a careful inspection for a fragment should always be made when only one body segment is seen on the sagittal images **(Fig. 12)**.[23,24] The displaced meniscal fragment can lie in front of the PCL which is called a "double PCL sign" **(Figs. 13A to C)**. The displaced fragment may also flip over the anterior horn of the affected meniscus which is called an "anterior flipped meniscus sign". On coronal images, a truncated appearance of the meniscus may be seen **(Figs. 14A to C)**. A new sign has been described recently for the diagnosis of bucket handle tears called the "V sign". The V sign is seen on the axial images and is seen at the junction of the displaced fragment and the meniscus, which is in place. The acute angle created accounts for the appearance as an inverted V. The V sign, when seen on axial images, is highly suggestive of a bucket handle tear.[25]

Peripheral Tear

If a tear is confined to the outer one-third of the meniscus, it is described as a peripheral tear because this changes the therapeutic plan for the patient. Except for the peripheral 10–25% of the meniscus which is supplied by the perimeniscal capillary plexus, the meniscus in adults is relatively avascular. Because of the rich vascularity in peripheral portion of the meniscus (red zone), this type of tear is more likely to heal with conservative therapy or operative repair, whereas tears confined to the inner white zone of the meniscus (avascular) have to be debrided or resected.[26]

Complex Tear

A combination of horizontal, longitudinal, and radial components constitutes a complex tear. The tear extends in more than one plane and the meniscus appears fragmented.[27]

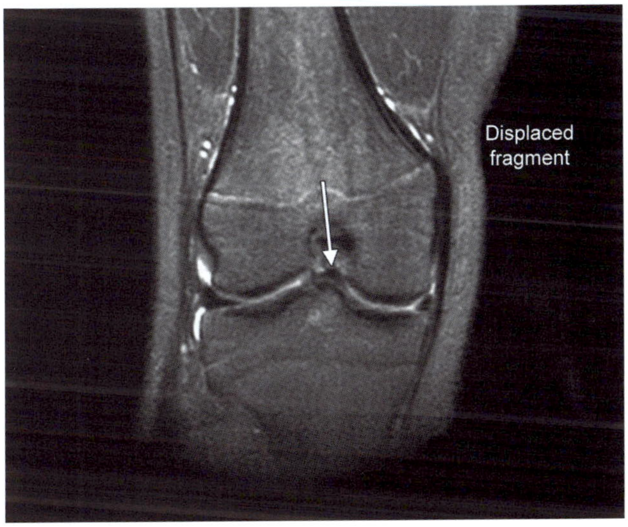

FIG. 12: STIR coronal MR image showing the displaced fragment lying within the intercondylar notch—bucket handle tear of the medial meniscus.

Meniscocapsular Separation

A meniscocapsular separation refers to an injury in which the meniscus separates from the adjacent capsule. This can lead to meniscal instability if unrecognized and is most commonly seen along the medial meniscus, which is more tightly adherent to the joint capsule. It can also occur along the PLC of the joint where the lateral meniscus is attached by the popliteal meniscal fascicles. This injury is diagnosed when true fluid signal intensity is seen interposed between the meniscus and adjacent capsule or when the popliteal meniscal fascicles are disrupted.

Indirect Signs of the Meniscal Tear

There are some indirect signs that suggest a meniscal tear.[27]

Parameniscal Cysts

A parameniscal cyst when present suggests a horizontal tear of the meniscus. These represent the peripheral escape of joint fluid through a meniscal tear. Parameniscal cysts are differentiated from bursae and ganglion cysts owing to their intimate contact with a meniscus either directly or via a fluid track.

Meniscal Extrusion

It is said to be present when the peripheral margin of the meniscus extends 3 mm or more beyond the tibial plateau edge. There is a close association between meniscal extrusion and root tears.

Subchondral Marrow Edema

Linear subchondral bone marrow edema adjacent to the meniscal attachment site less than 5 mm deep and paralleling the articular surface can be seen with 90% of lateral meniscus tears and 60% of medial meniscus tears.[28] Contusions/bone bruises in the posterior medial tibial

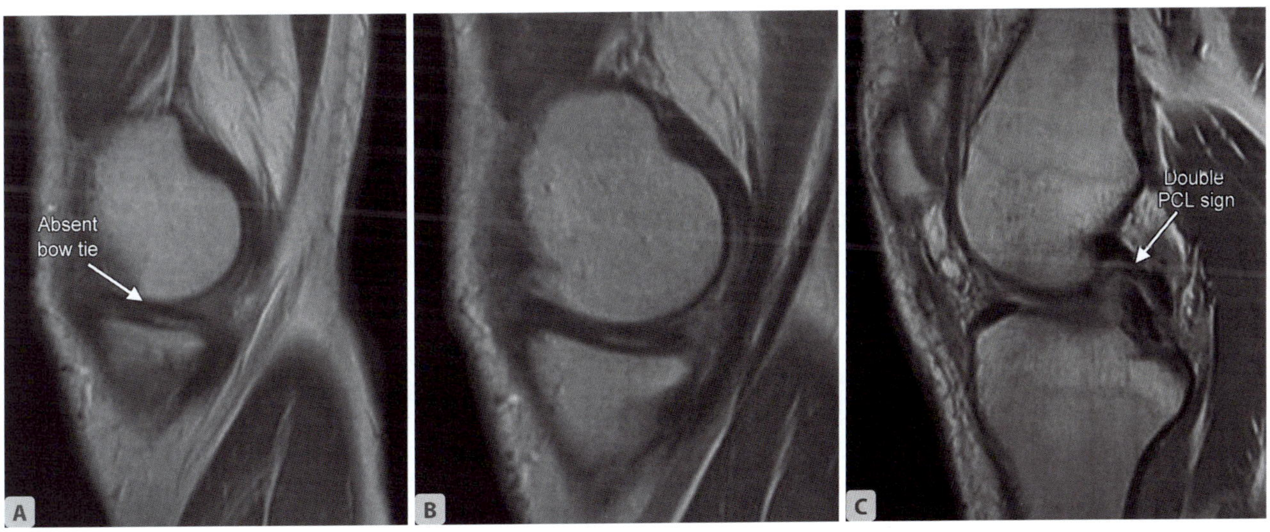

FIGS. 13A TO C: T2W sagittal MR images showing absent bow tie sign (A and B) and a displaced meniscal fragment beneath the posterior cruciate ligament (PCL) designated as a double PCL sign (C)—bucket handle tear of the medial meniscus.

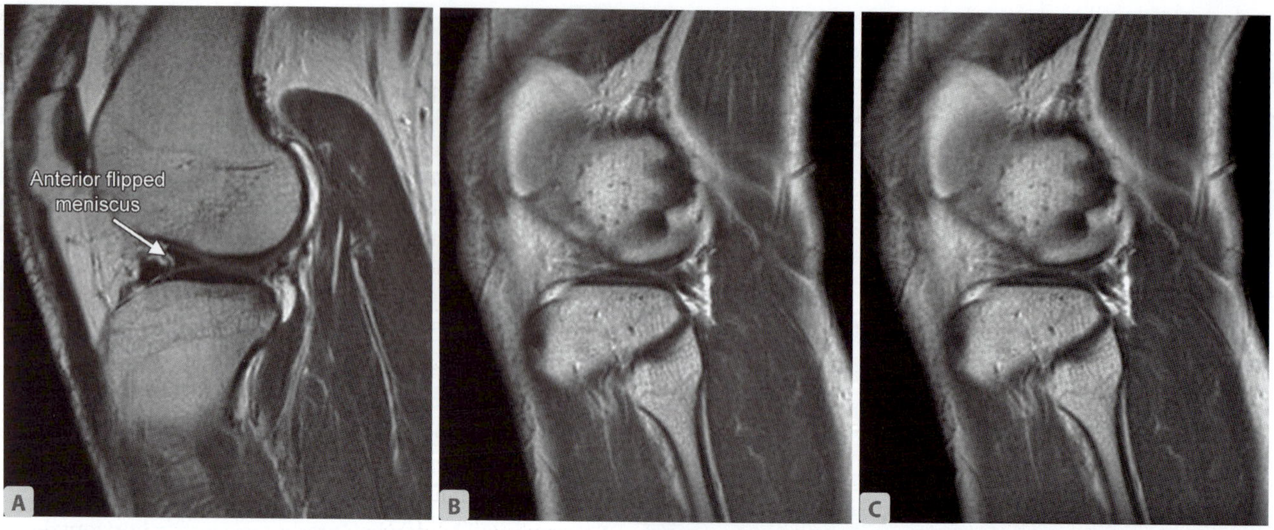

FIGS. 14A TO C: T2W sagittal MR images showing the displaced fragment flip over the anterior horn of the lateral meniscus (A) with an absent bow-tie sign (B and C)—bucket handle tear of the lateral meniscus.

plateau have an associated tear of the posterior horn of the medial meniscus.

Imaging Challenges

Although MRI is extremely accurate in diagnosing meniscal pathology, there are numerous imaging pitfalls and artifacts that may simulate a tear and lead to an erroneous diagnosis. These are especially common in the posterior horn of the lateral meniscus.

Potential Pitfalls

Transverse Intrameniscal Ligament

On sagittal scans, the attachment of the transverse ligament to the anterior horn of the medial or lateral meniscus may be mistaken for a tear. This pitfall is avoided by following the meniscal fragment on successive sagittal scans, recognizing that it is contiguous with the normal ligament coursing across the infrapatellar fat.

Meniscofemoral Ligaments

Similarly, the attachment of the meniscofemoral ligaments of Humphry or Wrisberg to the posterior horn of the lateral meniscus may be mistaken for a tear on sagittal scans. Again, examination of sequential sagittal or appropriate coronal scans should allow for accurate diagnosis.[29]

Popliteus Tendon

There is usually at least a small amount of fluid within the popliteus tendon sheath that can be mistaken for a tear at the junction of the posterior horn and body of the lateral meniscus on sagittal or coronal scans.[30]

Magic Angle Effect

The posterior horn of the lateral meniscus courses slightly upward as it extends into the posterior intercondylar notch. As a result, artifactually increased signal may be seen within the meniscus on short TE sequences because of the magic angle artifact. This is due to the magic angle phenomenon caused by 55° orientation of this meniscus with respect to the static magnetic field. The signal, however, is often of a rather diffuse nature and disappears on long TE images (>40 ms).[31]

Pulsation Artifact from the Popliteal Artery

Phase artifacts propagating from the popliteal artery may mimic a tear in the posterior horn of the lateral meniscus on sagittal scans. Misdiagnosis can be avoided by recognizing the alternating lines of increased and decreased signal propagating across the entire image at that level.

Surgical Considerations in Meniscal Tear

When faced with a meniscal tear, the surgeon has three options—(1) leave the tear alone, (2) attempt a primary meniscal repair, and (3) perform a partial or complete meniscectomy. The paramount goal is to preserve as much meniscal tissue as possible to lessen the probability of developing osteoarthritis (OA).[32] Several features have been shown to be correlated with a higher probability of a successful meniscal repair and these features should be included in the MRI report by the radiologist.

Tear Location

The most important factor in predicting the success of a meniscal repair is where the tear is located in the meniscus, e.g., a tear in the periphery of the meniscus (within 3 mm of its capsular surface) has the highest probability for healing because of the excellent vascularity in that region.[26]

Blind spots for the arthroscopist include the anterior horn of each meniscus, the extreme inner portion of the posterior horn of the medial meniscus, and the undersurface of both menisci. It is also important to describe any meniscal tissue that has become displaced into a para-articular "gutter" so that the arthroscopist is able to probe for and resect the fragment, which might otherwise be missed.

Tear Morphology and Length

Vertical longitudinal tears have the best prognosis for healing because they do not disrupt the circumferential collagen bundles that are important for maintaining normal meniscal function.

Small partial tears (involving less than half the height of the meniscus) and radial tears measuring less than 5 mm in length also have a higher rate of healing than do larger tears.[26,33] A radial tear extending through the meniscus to the capsule is essentially unrepairable because of the complete disruption of the circumferential collagen bundles. Most horizontal tears are also not amenable to repair and the surgeon typically resects either the superior or inferior flap, leaving the other *in situ*.

Accuracy of MR in the Diagnosis of the Meniscal Tears

The accuracy of MR imaging of meniscal tears is greater than 90% in most series and the negative predictive value approaches 100%.[34,35] An additional advantage of MRI is the ability to evaluate extra-articular cause of knee pain masquerading as meniscal disease.

CENTRAL STRUCTURES OF THE KNEE

Anterior Cruciate Ligament

Anatomy

The ACL provides central support of the knee joint, contributing the most significant stabilizing mechanism against excessive anterior translation of the tibia. The ACL is a fan-shaped structure, with a tightly bound femoral attachment that expands broadly at the tibial attachment. The ACL is 11 mm wide and 31–38 mm long. The individual fascicles of the ACL are divided into two longitudinal fiber bundles, the longer and stronger anteromedial bundle (AMB) and the shorter posterolateral bundle (PLB).[36]

MR Appearance

T2W sagittal 3–4 mm thickness images are recommended for evaluating the ACL. It is also well-visualized on the axial and coronal images. The normal ACL has straight, taut fibers that run parallel to the roof of the intercondylar notch **(Figs. 15A and B)**. It typically has a striated appearance with some high signal within it especially at its insertion on the tibia.

ACL Tears

The most common mechanism of ACL tear is external rotation of femur on a fixed tibia combined with valgus force (i.e., twisting injury).

On MRI, an ACL tear is diagnosed by alterations in signal intensity, morphology, and the course of the ligament. An increased signal intensity within the ACL on PD and T2W images indicates an acute or subacute injury. A cloud-like amorphous mass of increased signal intensity may be evident within the ligament reflecting edema or hemorrhage **(Figs. 16A and B)**.

A complete ACL tear can be diagnosed when the ligament is either absent ("empty notch sign" in coronal images) **(Figs. 17A and B)** or discontinuous. An irregular or wavy contour and disruption of fibers also suggests a complete tear.[37]

Indirect signs of ACL tear include:

- Buckling (abnormal high arc) of the PCL giving rise to a "question mark" configuration **(Fig. 18)**.
- Undulation and redundancy of the patellar tendon.
- *Uncovered lateral meniscus sign*: This sign is positive if a vertical line drawn tangentially to the most posterior margin of the lateral tibial plateau intersects any part of the posterior horn of the lateral meniscus. A positive uncovered lateral meniscus sign indicates that the lateral

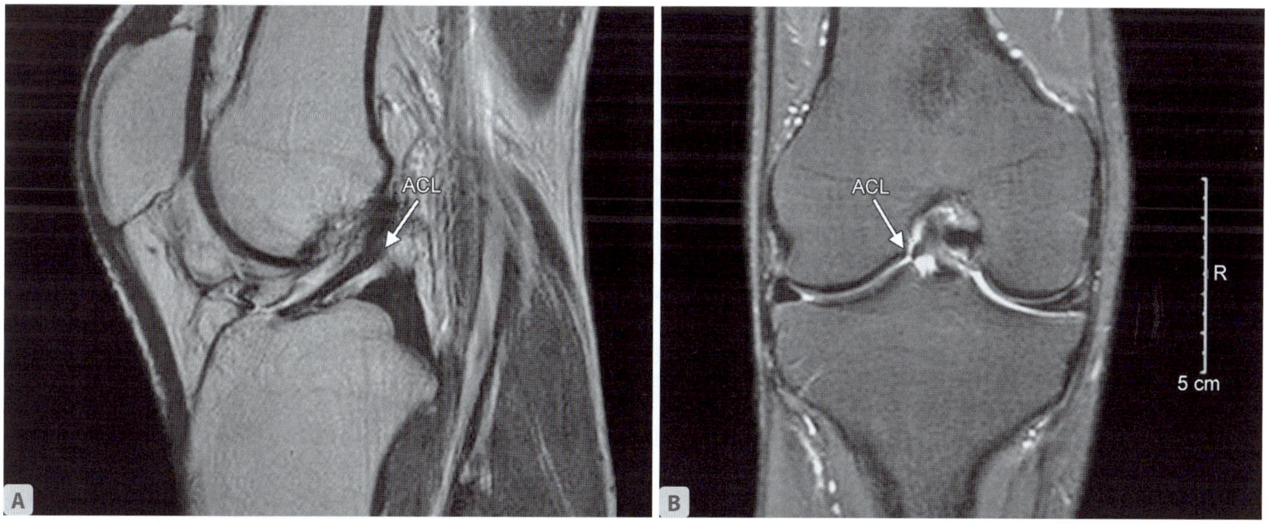

FIGS. 15A AND B: (A) T2W sagittal MR image of the knee depicting the normal anterior cruciate ligament (ACL) with straight, taut fibers that run parallel to the roof of the intercondylar notch; (B) STIR coronal MR image showing the ACL as a triangular structure within the notch.

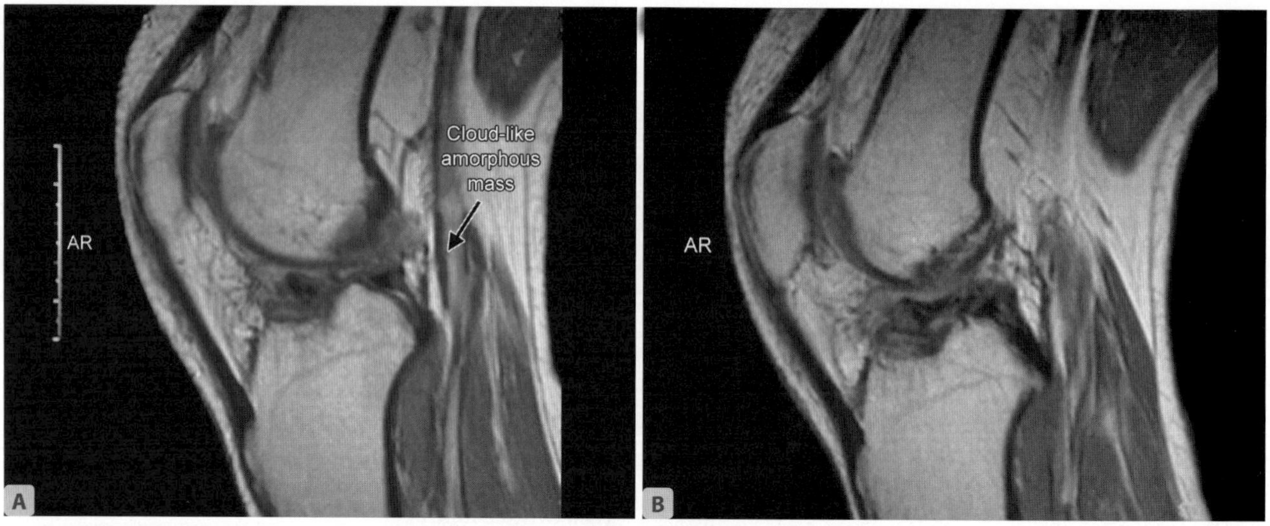

FIGS. 16A AND B: T2W sagittal MR images of the knee showing complete disruption of anterior cruciate ligament (ACL) fibers with a cloud-like amorphous mass of increased signal intensity in the region of ACL reflecting edema and hemorrhage—complete ACL tear.

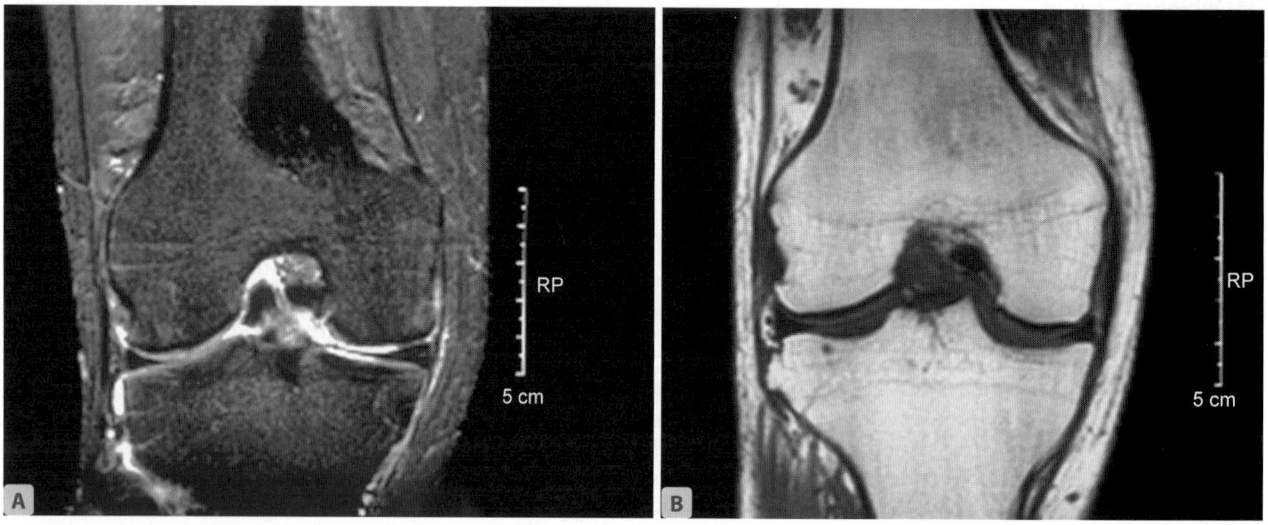

FIGS. 17A AND B: (A) STIR coronal image of the knee showing normal anterior cruciate ligament (ACL) and posterior cruciate ligament (PCL) in the intercondylar notch; (B) T1W coronal image shows the ACL to be absent (empty notch sign) in a case of ACL tear.

meniscus does not subluxate anteriorly with the tibia in an ACL injury.

- Anterior tibial subluxation larger than 5 mm with respect to femur is a very sensitive and specific sign of complete ACL tear. If the distance between two parallel lines drawn tangential to the posterior lateral femoral condyle and posterior lateral tibial plateau is more than 5 mm, it is a sensitive ancillary sign of complete ACL tear **(Figs. 19A and B)**. This sign offers improved discrimination of complete from partial tears which is clinically important since the presence of partial tear is not considered an indication for surgical reconstruction.[38]
- Lateral notch sign in which the deep lateral femoral notch exceeds 2 mm in depth.
- Bone bruises/contusions in the midportion of the lateral femoral condyle and posterior portion of the lateral tibial plateau.[39,40] These so-called kissing contusions are representative of edema and hemorrhage caused by impaction trabecular microfractures that occur when the ACL ruptures **(Figs. 20A to C)**.
- Avulsion fracture of the lateral tibial rim (Segond fracture) is also suggestive of ACL tear.
- Joint effusion/hemarthrosis is a common finding associated with ACL injuries **(Fig. 20C)**.[41]
- A tibial spine avulsion is an uncommon but specific finding for ACL injury. Chronic tears of ACL may present with slumping of the distal fragment over the tibial indicating increased laxity of the ligament which may also be attenuated. In chronic tears, edema and synovitis are usually not present. MR also has an important role in defining partial tears of the ACL because these injuries are difficult to differentiate from complete ACL tears clinically. The detection of a discrete area or focus of increased signal intensity within the substance of the ACL is consistent with a diagnosis of partial tear **(Figs. 21A and B)**. In partial tear, although the bulk of the ligament

appears to be intact with a relatively normal axis, there may be localized angulation of the ligament at the site of fiber disruption. False-negative diagnosis may result from the formation of scar tissue with adherence of ACL to the postcruciate ligament simulating a normal course and signal of the ACL. A partial volume averaging with the lateral femoral condyle and periligamentous or intraligamentous fat should be differentiated from partial ACL tears to avoid false positive diagnosis. A false positive diagnosis may also be seen in mucoid degeneration and ganglion cyst of the ACL. However, the ligament in these cases has a striated appearance on T2W images with interspersed intact ligamentous fibers resembling a "celery stalk".[42] Often an intraosseous ganglion cyst is seen at the tibial insertion of the ACL. Typically, there is no previous history of trauma.

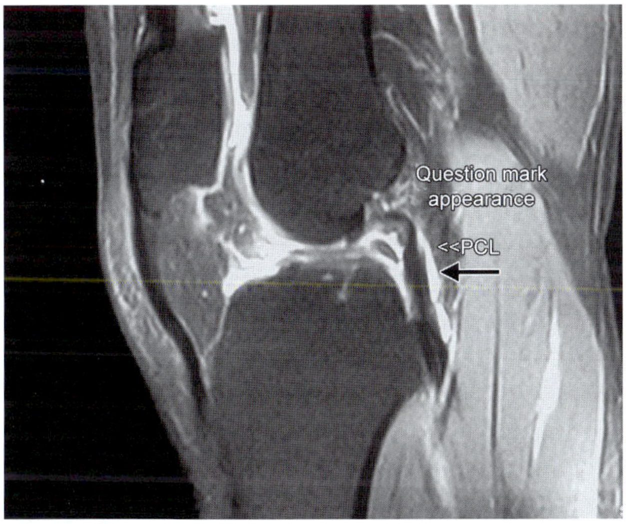

FIG. 18: T2W fat suppressed sagittal image of knee showing abnormal high arc (buckling) of the posterior cruciate ligament (PCL) giving rise to a "question mark" configuration—indirect sign of anterior cruciate ligament tear.

O'Donoghue Triad

A triad of ACL injury associated with MCL disruption and medial meniscus tear is known as O'Donoghue triad **(Figs. 22A to C)**.

Accuracy of MR in ACL Tears

Accuracy of MRI for tears of the ACL is extremely high approaching 95–100% in almost all reported series.[4]

Posterior Cruciate Ligament

Anatomy

The PCL originates in the lateral aspect of the medial femoral condyle, crosses the ACL, and attaches to the posterior intercondylar fossa of tibia.[43] It averages 38 mm in length and 13 mm in width at its midportion. The PCL provides central support to the knee joint and protects against excessive posterior translation of tibia, stabilizes the joint against excessive varus and valgus stress, and restricts external rotation of tibia.

MR Appearance

On MRI, the PCL is normally depicted as a band-like structure of low signal intensity. In sagittal images, it has an arcuate shape with the knee in neutral position **(Figs. 23A and B)**.

PCL Injury

MR findings of PCL injury are anatomic disruption, increased signal intensity in the ligament, and redundancy of an avulsed ligament.[44]

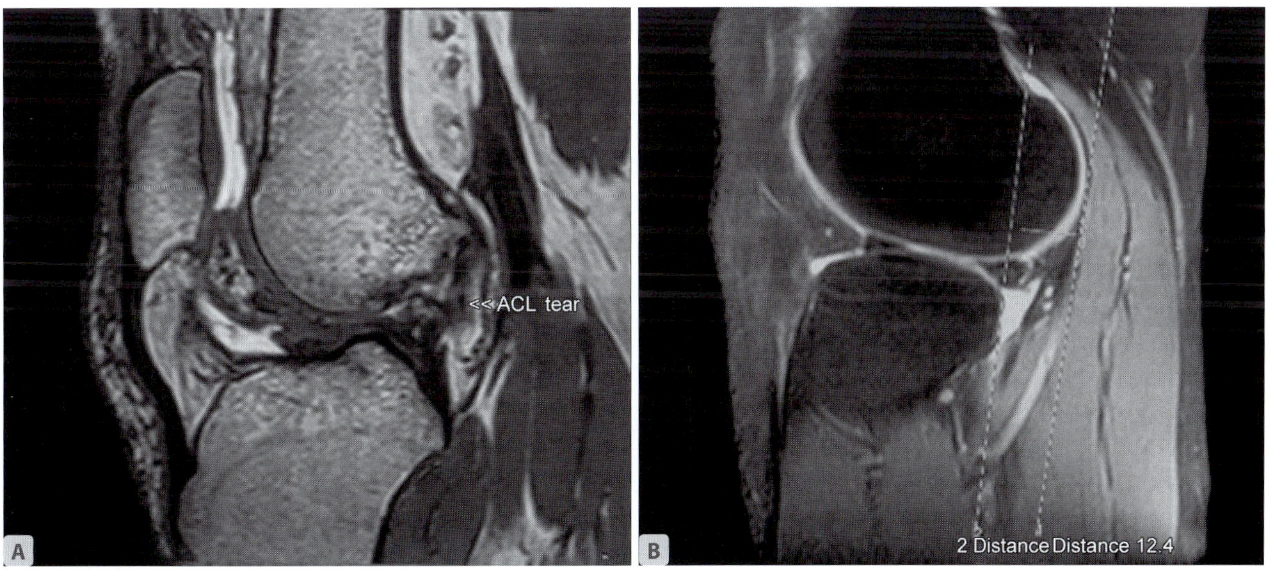

FIGS. 19A AND B: (A) Double echo steady state sagittal; and (B) T2W fat suppressed sagittal MR images of the knee showing cloud-like amorphous mass of increased signal in the region of anterior cruciate ligament (ACL) with anterior tibial translation larger than 5 mm with respect to femur—indirect sign of complete ACL tear.

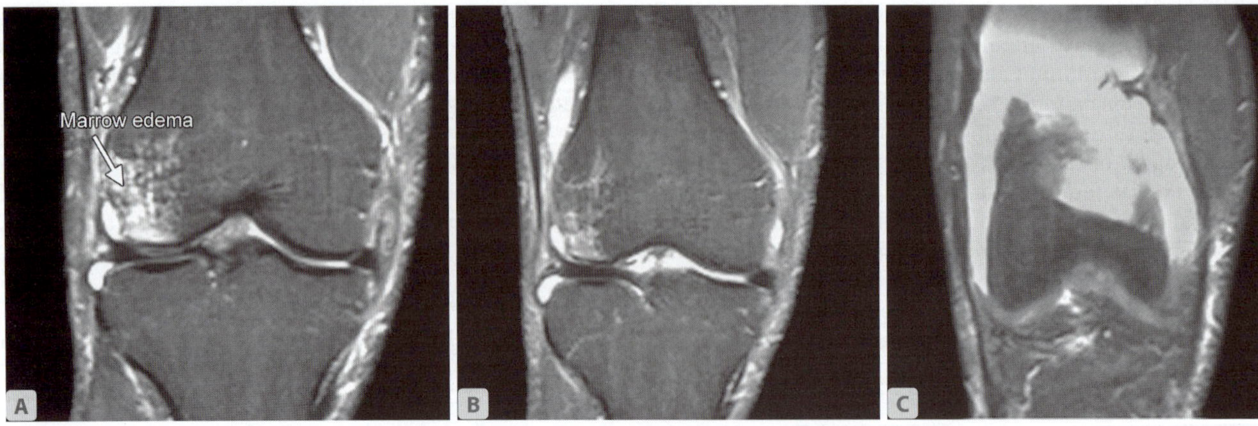

FIGS. 20A TO C: STIR coronal MR images of the knee showing marrow edema in the lateral femoral condyle and suprapatellar joint effusion—indirect signs of anterior cruciate ligament tear.

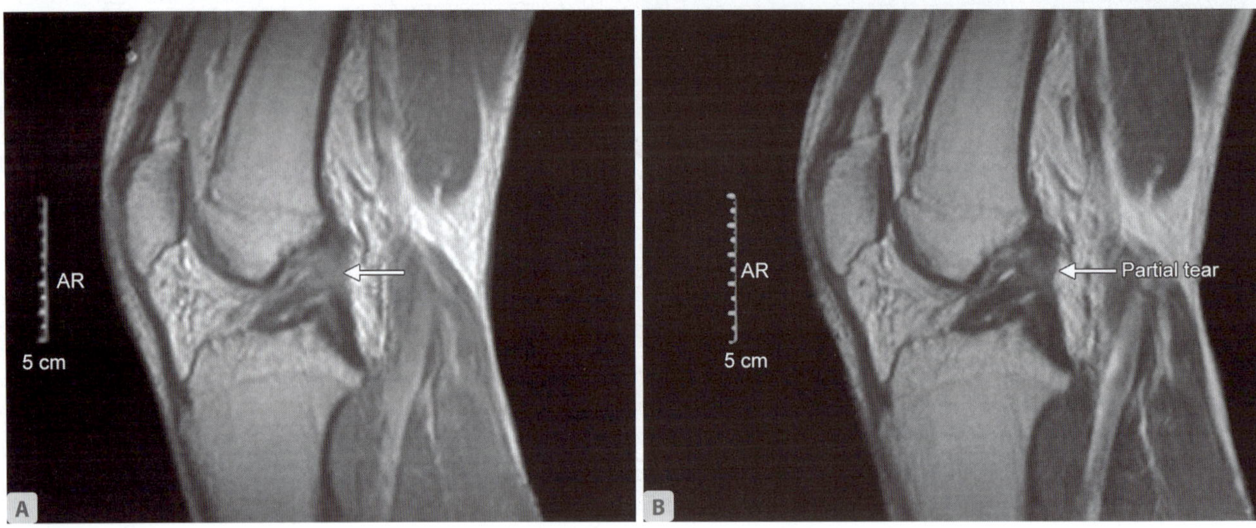

FIGS. 21A AND B: (A) Proton density; and (B) T2W sagittal MR images showing a discrete area of increased signal intensity within the substance of the anterior cruciate ligament (ACL), the ligament appearing intact—partial tear of ACL.

Injuries to the PCL are classified as **(Figs. 24A to C)**:

- *Grade I* is consistent with intraligamentous edema and hemorrhage and appears as foci of increased signal in a ligament with otherwise intact borders.
- *Grade II* injuries represent partial tears.
- *Grade III* abnormalities represent complete tears.

Aggressive surgical treatment of PCL tears is recently becoming more common since chronic knee instability with early degenerative arthritis has become better appreciated with chronic injuries of the PCL.

MEDIAL STRUCTURES OF THE KNEE

Anatomy

Medially, the supporting structures of the knee are arranged in three layers. The invested deep fascia of the sartorius muscle, which overlies the gastrocnemius muscle, forms the most superficial layer.[45] The tibial collateral ligament and the superficial component of the MCL forms the middle layer. The deepest layer is comprised of the meniscofemoral and meniscotibial ligaments, which constitute the deep components of the MCL. The MCL stabilizes the knee against excessive valgus force and hyperextension. The tibial collateral ligament, the primary support structure, extends from the medial epicondylar region of the femur to the medial surface of the proximal tibia and spans about 8–9 cm in length.[46]

Magnetic Resonance Imaging

On MRI, the MCL is best displayed on coronal images and appears as a smooth structure of low signal intensity that extends from the medial femoral epicondyle to the proximal tibial metaphysis **(Fig. 25)**. At the level of the joint line, the superficial and deep portions of the ligament are separated by a bursa and surrounding fat which should not be mistaken for a localized meniscocapsular separation.

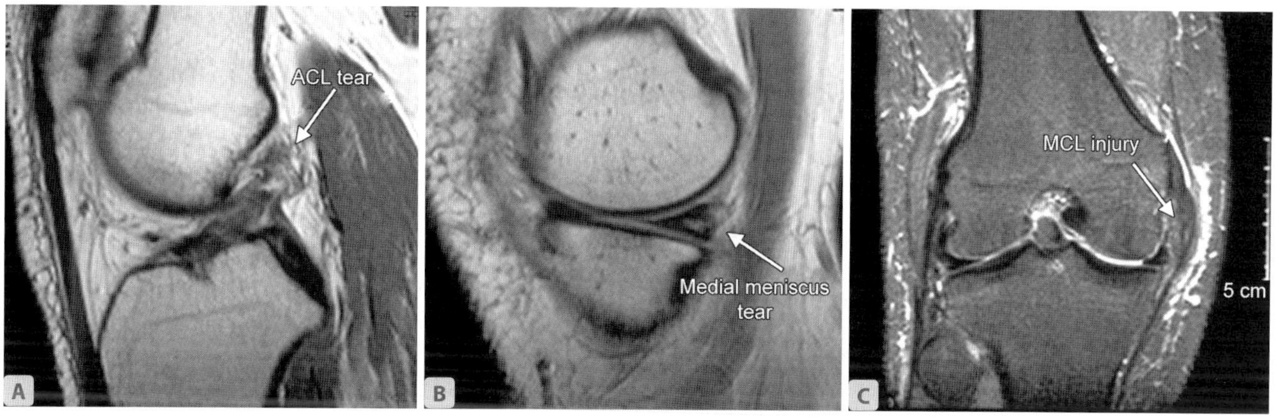

FIGS. 22A TO C: (A and B) T2W sagittal; and (C) STIR coronal MR images showing anterior cruciate ligament tear, medial meniscus tear, and injury of the medial collateral ligament—O'Donoghue triad.

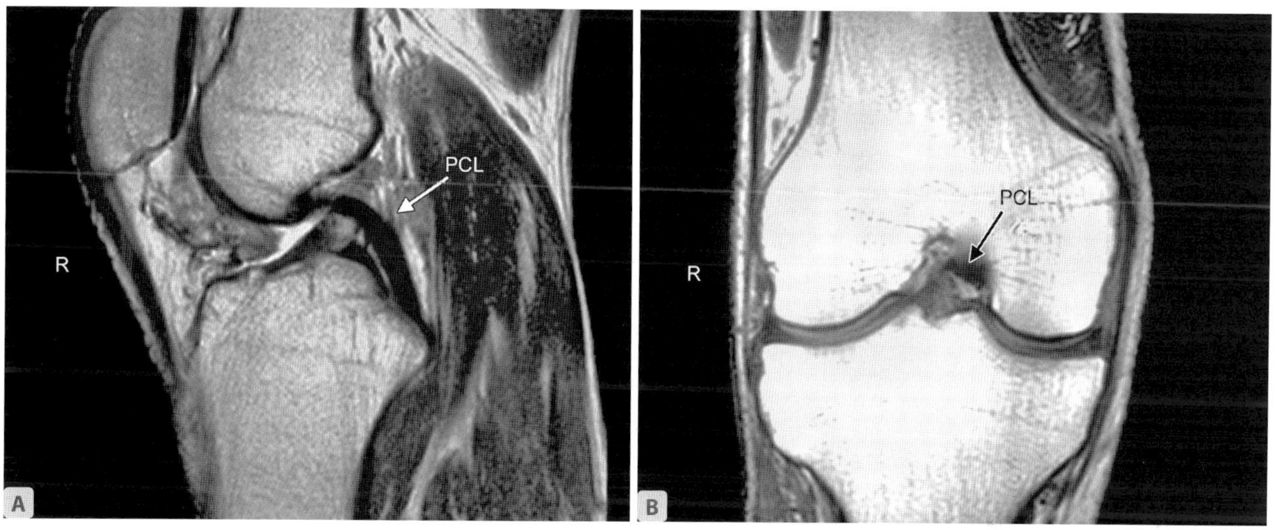

FIGS. 23A AND B: (A) T2W sagittal MR image of knee showing normal posterior cruciate ligament (PCL) as a band-like structure of low-signal intensity having an arcuate shape; (B) T1W coronal MR image showing the normal PCL as a triangular structure within the intercondylar notch.

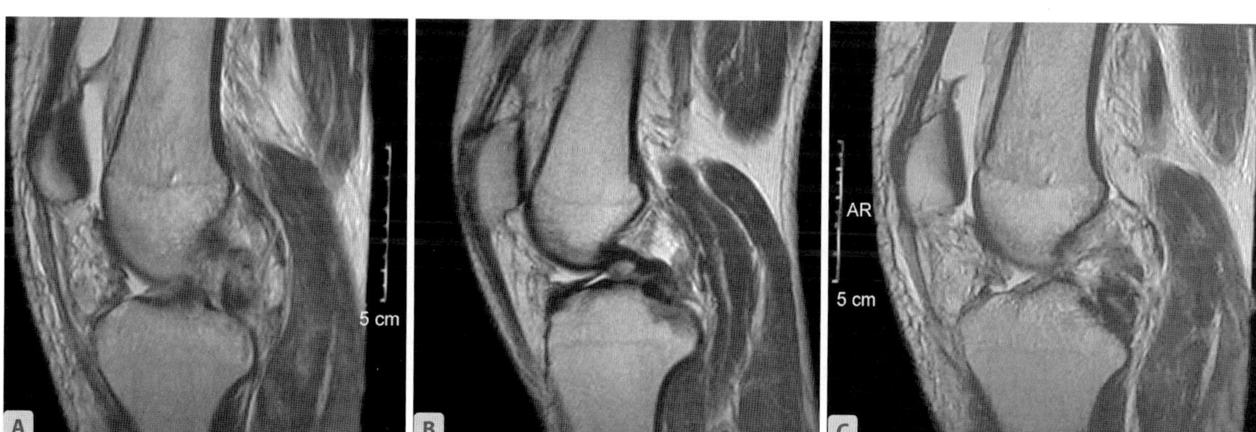

FIGS. 24A TO C: T2W sagittal MR images showing (A) grade I tear of the posterior cruciate ligament seen as intraligamentous edema and hemorrhage; (B) Grade II tear seen as partial tear of the tibial attachment; and (C) Grade III tear seen as a complete disruption of the ligament.

MCL Injury

Twisting injuries cause a large number of MCL injuries.

- In grade I injury, a slight contour irregularity or thickening of the ligament may be seen but there is no discontinuity of its fibers. Edema and hemorrhage are identified in the soft tissue and subcutaneous fat paralleling the MCL **(Figs. 26A and B)**.
- In grade II, discontinuity of some fibers may be evident.
- In grade III, frank discontinuity of all its fibers is seen **(Figs. 27A and B)**. Two findings that may be encountered on conventional radiography are predictive of underlying MCL injury. Pellegrini–Stieda disease or calcification around the medial femoral condyle represents chronic partial or complete tears of the MCL.[47] The reverse Segond fracture is an avulsion fracture of medial tibial plateau at the attachment of the deep fibers of the MCL. This finding is associated with PCL disruption and peripheral medial meniscal tear.

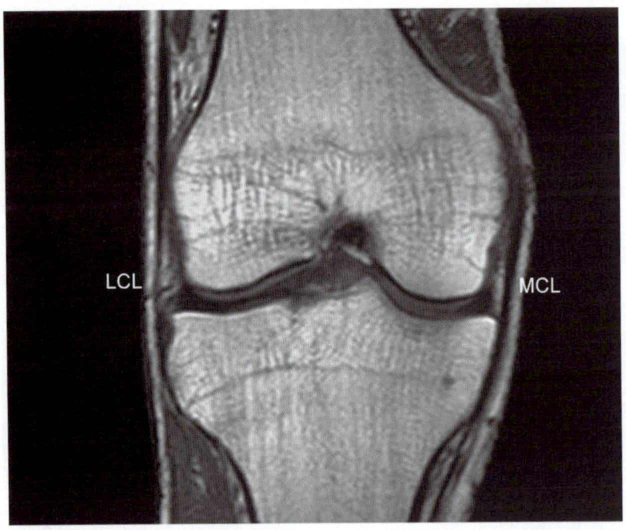

FIG. 25: T1W coronal MR image of the knee showing the normal medial collateral ligament (MCL) as a low-signal intensity structure that extends from the medial femoral epicondyle to the proximal tibial metaphysis.

CORNER-BASED ANATOMY OF THE KNEE

The secondary stabilizers of the knee can be thought of in terms of "corner"-based anatomy. The corners of the knee include PLC, PMC, ALC, and AMC or the extensor mechanism of the knee.

Posterolateral Corner of the Knee

Of all the corners about the knee, the PLC has received the greatest attention. Once regarded as the "dark side of the knee", the fine anatomic details of the region have now been elucidated owing to the advances in imaging.[48] Timely diagnosis and interventions of the PLC injuries are imperative to prevent chronic knee instability, cartilage damage, and failed ligament reconstruction.

Anatomy

The PLC of the knee is composed of ligaments, muscles, and tendons that are static and dynamic restraints to posterior translation, varus angulations, and external rotation of the knee. Also called the arcuate ligament complex, they include the fibular ligament or lateral collateral ligament (LCL), popliteus muscle and tendon, popliteofibular ligament, biceps femoris tendon, fabellofibular ligament, and the arcuate ligament. The components are summarized in **Box 1**.

The fibular collateral ligament or LCL is 5–7 cm long, arising from a tubercle on the lateral femoral condyle directly above the groove of the popliteus tendon origin. It inserts on the lateral surface of the head of the fibula, joining the biceps femoris tendon to form the conjoined tendon **(Figs. 28A and B)**.

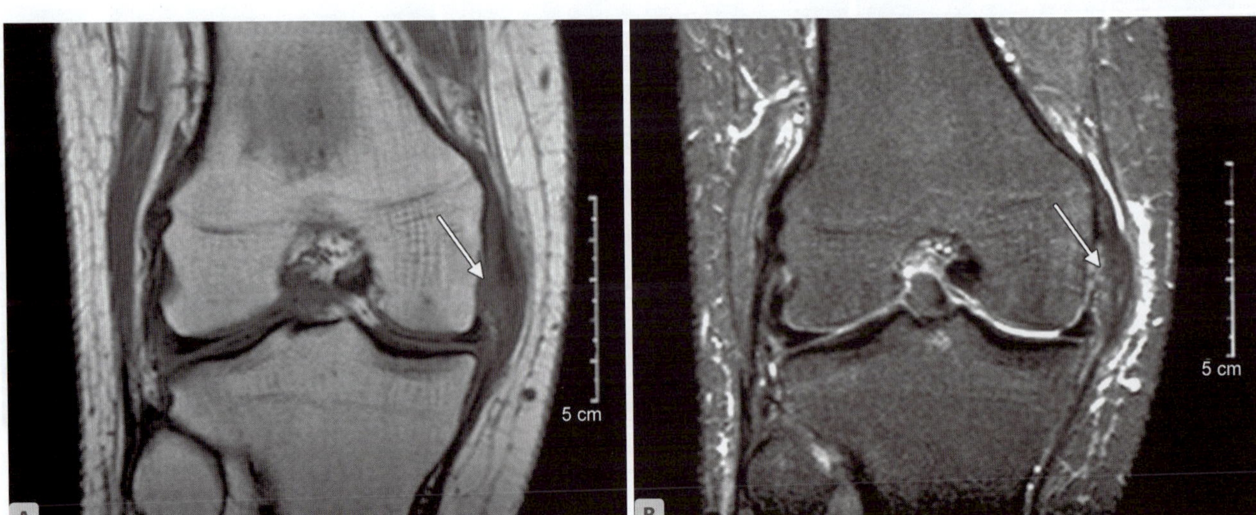

FIGS. 26A AND B: (A) T1W coronal MR; and (B) STIR coronal images showing grade I medial collateral ligament (MCL) injury as edema and hemorrhage in the soft tissue and subcutaneous fat paralleling the MCL with slight contour irregularity of the ligament.

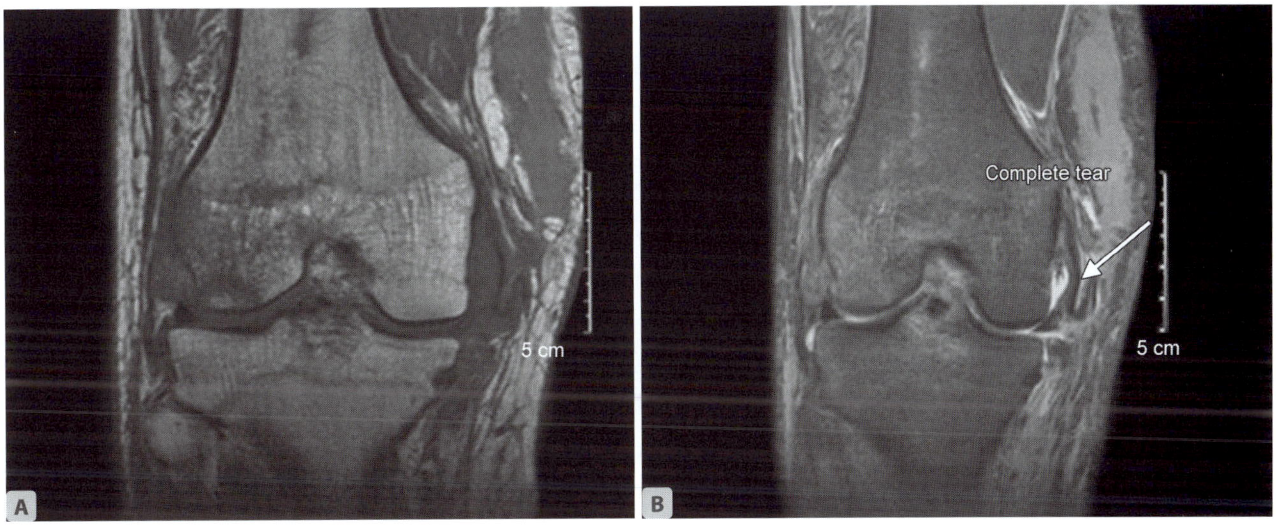

FIGS. 27A AND B: (A) TIW; and (B) STIR coronal MR images showing a complete disruption of the medial collateral ligament (MCL) with extensive edema and hemorrhage in the adjacent soft tissues and subcutaneous fat. Extensive bone marrow contusions are also noted—complete MCL tear.

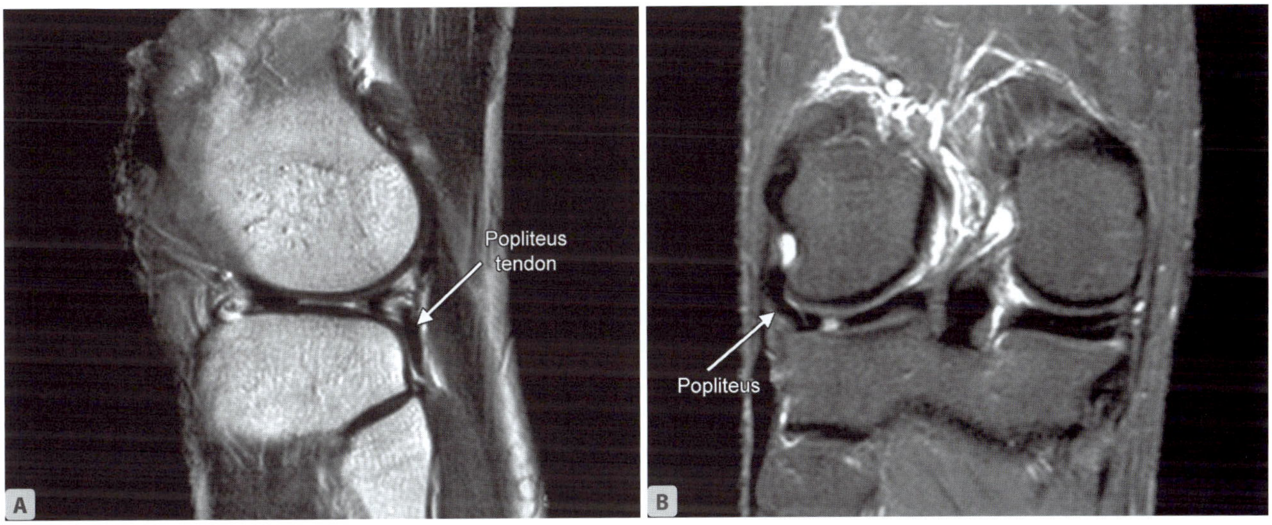

FIGS. 28A AND B: (A) Proton density sagittal; and (B) STIR coronal MR images of the knee showing the popliteal muscle that arises as a tendon from the lateral femoral condyle just anterior and inferior to the lateral collateral ligament, courses in a posteromedial direction to insert at the medial aspect of tibia, attaches to the lateral meniscus forming the popliteomeniscal ligament, and has a third attachment site on the styloid process of the fibula.

BOX 1: Components of the posterolateral corner.[48,49]

- Fibular collateral ligament
- Popliteus tendon and muscle complex
- Arcuate ligament
- Fabellofibular ligament
- Posterolateral joint capsule
- Popliteofibular ligament

The main function of the LCL is to stabilize the knee against varus forces.[50]

The fabellofibular ligament courses from the fibular styloid process to the fabella, a normal sesamoid bone within the lateral gastrocnemius tendon. The arcuate ligament is a Y-shaped structure that represents thickening of the posterolateral joint capsule.[49]

Magnetic Resonance Imaging

The LCL is most vulnerable when a varus force is applied to the knee when it is in flexion or internal rotation. The LCL is best visualized in entirety in the coronal plane. It is seen as low-signal intensity structures on all pulse sequences and nearly uniform in thickness. Soft tissue edema characterizes the MRI findings associated with acute LCL injuries. Contour changes, such as thickening and irregularity, are more typical of subacute or old injuries. Complete tears with discontinuity and retraction of the fibers may produce a ribbon-like deformity of the LCL **(Figs. 29A to C)**. Most complete ruptures involve the conjoined tendon and may produce a

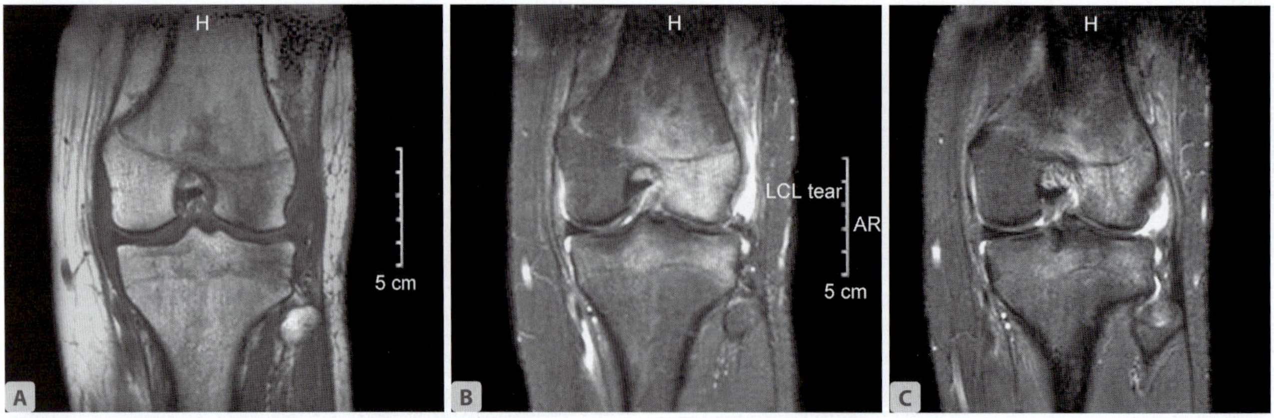

FIGS. 29A TO C: (A) T1W; and (B and C) STIR coronal MR images showing complete discontinuity and retraction of the fibers of the lateral collateral ligament (LCL) producing a ribbon-like deformity. Extensive contusions are seen in the lateral femoral condyle and lateral aspect of the tibial plateau—complete LCL tear.

small avulsion of the styloid process of the fibular head. When this occurs, marrow edema in the proximal fibula is usually evident on T2W and STIR images.

Most injuries involving the posterolateral structures are optimally depicted using a coronal oblique plane that is oriented parallel to the popliteus tendon.[51] Acute injuries of the popliteus muscle most commonly involve the myotendinous junction, whereas avulsion injuries of fibular insertion are less common. When the popliteal tendon tears, hemorrhage and edema in the muscle and tendon produce focal and high signal on T2W sequences. Edema of the adjacent soft tissue structures can also be observed. Complete tears of the popliteal tendon cause enlargement of the muscle belly and the retracted tendon terminates abruptly. Isolated popliteal injuries are rare because most are associated with concomitant injuries of the arcuate ligament complex. PLC injuries are very often associated with cruciate ligament injuries, more commonly with the PCL **(Figs. 30A to F)**.

Posteromedial Corner of the Knee

Anatomy

The tendon of the semimembranosus muscle and the posterior oblique ligament are the main support structures in the posteromedial aspect of the knee.[52] The posterior oblique ligament is formed by the union of the posterior fibers of the MCL and the medial capsular ligament. The semimembranosus muscle originates from the posterolateral portion of the ischial tuberosity, and inserts on the posteromedial surface of the medial tibial condyle. The components of PMC are enumerated in **Box 2**.

Magnetic Resonance Imaging

Posteromedial corner injuries usually result from a valgus stress combined with rotational forces. The semimembranosus tendon is the largest tendon in the popliteal fossa. It has a fusiform configuration and appears uniformly hypointense on all imaging sequences. A strain of the semimembranosus tendon is manifested by loss of continuity at the insertion and high signal on T2W and STIR sequences owing to edema and hemorrhage. Accompanying fluid within the tendon sheath is a common finding. A focus of marrow edema may be present when the posterior oblique ligament avulses.

Anterolateral Corner of the Knee

Normal Anatomy

Anterolateral corner of the knee includes the anterolateral ligament (ALL), the iliotibial band (ITB), the anterior oblique band (AOB) of the LCL, and the capsular ligament **(Box 3)**.

Together, these structures contribute to anterior and posterolateral stability. The ALL arises from the femur and courses anteroinferiorly to attach at anterolateral aspect of proximal tibia. The ITB is an extension of the tensor fasciae latae with distal attachments to the lateral femoral condyle, the lateral patella, and the tubercle of Gerdy at the anterolateral aspect of the tibia.

Iliotibial Band Injury

Iliotibial band injury is the most common injury to the ALC. Tearing most often involves the posterior fibers that interdigitate with the AOB. These are usually well demonstrated on coronal MR images.

Segond Fracture

The Segond fracture, or avulsion of the anterolateral aspect of the lateral tibial plateau, is a radiographic entity that signifies underlying trauma to the ALC structures of the knee. These lesions such as all anterolateral corner injuries, are highly suggestive of the presence of an underlying ACL tear (75–100%), meniscal tear (66–75%) or PLC injury.

Iliotibial Band Friction Syndrome

Iliotibial band friction syndrome (ITBFS) refers to lateral knee pain arising from the friction that occurs as the ITB passes over the lateral femoral epicondyle during repetitive flexion and extension of the knee. This injury is seen most often in individuals who participate in long-distance running and cycling. On MR images, ill-defined signal abnormality

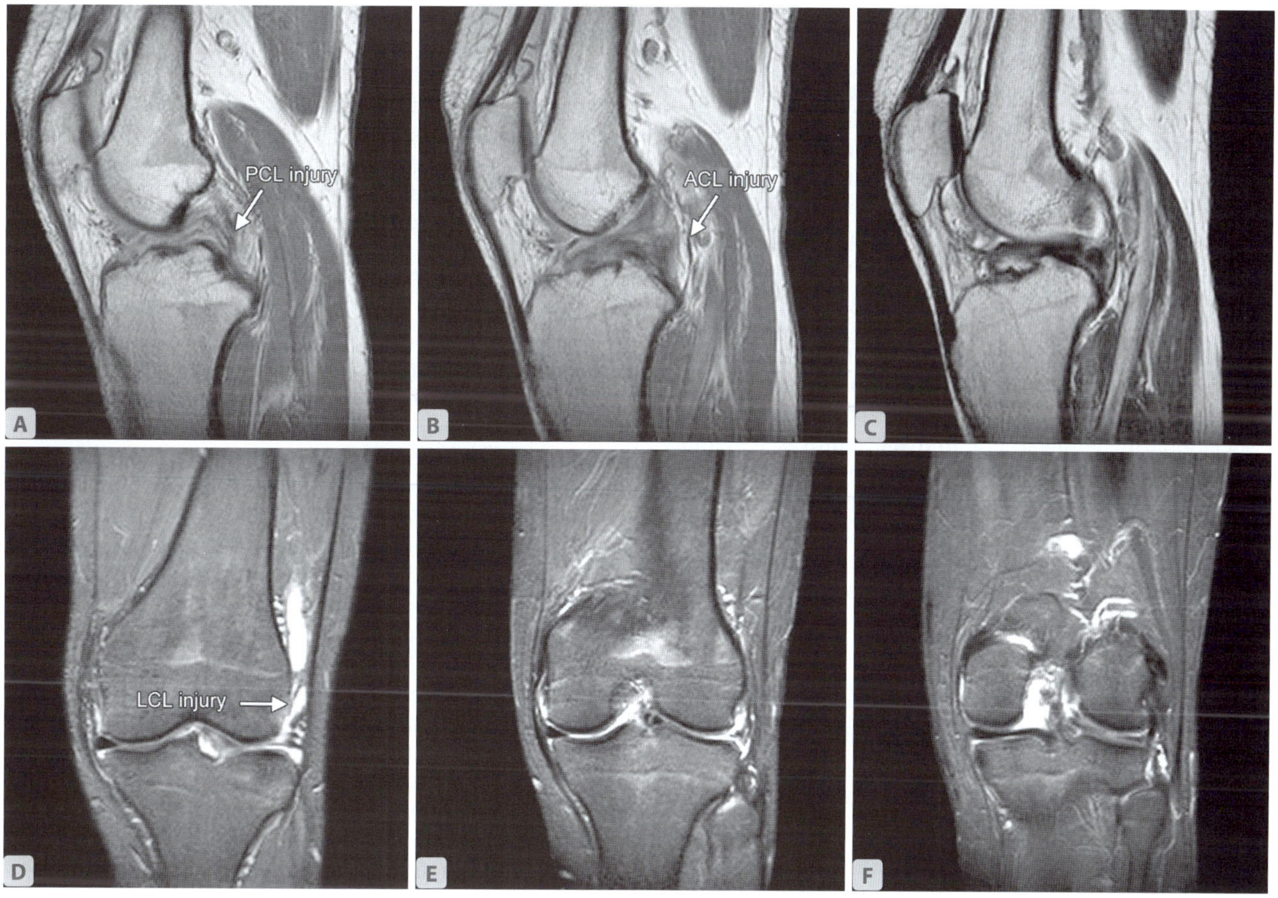

FIGS. 30A TO F: (A to C) T2W sagittal; and (D to F) STIR coronal MR images showing a tear of the posterior cruciate ligament (PCL), anterior cruciate ligament (ACL), and lateral collateral ligament (LCL)—multiligament injury of the knee.

signifying soft tissue edema is present within the fat deep to the ITB.

POSTERIOR STRUCTURES OF THE KNEE

Anatomy

The gastrocnemius, soleus, and plantaris muscles form the superficial muscles of the calf. The gastrocnemius muscle arises as two heads from the posterior surface of the medial and lateral femoral condyles. The tendons of the gastrocnemius muscles along with the soleus tendon form the Achilles tendon, which inserts on the posterior tubercle of the calcaneus. The primary action of the gastrocnemius muscle is plantar flexion of the foot but also serves as a passive supportive structure of the posterior joint capsule.

Magnetic Resonance Imaging

Gastrocnemius injuries are most commonly caused by hyperextension of the knee or when the tibia posteriorly dislocates during knee flexion.[54] Acute injuries of the proximal gastrocnemius include interstitial edema of the myotendinous junction and surrounding soft tissues.[55] Occasionally, an intramuscular hematoma forms a space-occupying mass in the muscle. MRI can assess the chronicity of the hematoma by the general appearance of the products of hemoglobin degradation. A complete rupture of the gastrocnemius head is associated with retraction of the muscle belly.

BOX 2: Components of the posteromedial corner.[53]

- Semimembranosus tendon and aponeurotic expansions
- Posterior oblique ligament
- Posteromedial capsule
- Oblique popliteal ligament
- Posterior horn medial meniscus
- Deep components of medial collateral ligament complex (meniscofemoral and meniscotibial)

KNEE DISLOCATIONS

A dislocation of the knee is a severe injury that is caused by high-energy trauma, such as motor vehicle and motorcycle accidents, falls, and industrial accidents. Knee dislocations are important because they produce extensive disruption of the ligaments that stabilize the knee and the surrounding soft tissue structures, including the popliteal artery.[56]

Magnetic Resonance Imaging

A knee dislocation is classified according to the position of the tibia relative to the femur. There are five different types of dislocations—(1) anterior, (2) posterior, (3) lateral, (4) medial, and (5) posterolateral. Posterior and posterolateral dislocations have a high association with complete tears of the popliteus and conjoined tendons, manifested by retraction, hemorrhage, and muscle edema. In general, both cruciate ligaments are likely to be torn. Complete disruption of one or both of the collateral ligaments is expected with this severe injury. Concomitant meniscal injury is also common. Frequently, the pattern of bone contusions allows definition of the type of knee dislocation. This is an important observation because posterior and posterolateral dislocations have a high association with peroneal nerve injury.[56] Neurovascular injury is the most dreaded complication of knee dislocation. It can result in irreversible neurologic deficits with consequent limb loss. Being relatively fixed in the popliteal fossa, the popliteal artery is at an increased risk in up to 40% of dislocations. Amputation rate is as high as 85% if revascularization is not done within 8 hours.

ANTERIOR STRUCTURES OF THE KNEE OR THE EXTENSOR MECHANISM OF THE KNEE

Anatomy

The main soft tissue structures in the anterior aspect of the knee are the components of the extensor mechanism and include the quadriceps tendon, patellar tendon, and the medial and lateral patellar retinacula.[57] The four muscle groups that form the quadriceps tendon include the rectus femoris, vastus lateralis, vastus medialis, and the vastus intermedius. The quadriceps tendon inserts on the superior pole of the patella and causes extension of the knee joint **(Fig. 31A)**. The medial and lateral patellar retinacula are extensions of the vastus medialis and lateralis, respectively and contribute to passive stabilization of the patella **(Fig. 31B)**.

The layers of the quadriceps tendon can be visualized best in sagittal plane on MRI as uniform low-signal intensity bands with intervening higher signal intensity fat separating each layer. The layered configuration of the quadriceps tendon enables discrimination between partial and full tears. Discontinuity of any of the tendinous layers is consistent with partial tears often involving the rectus femoris component. Transection of all the layers is diagnostic of a complete rupture and may be associated with a mass of edematous tissue and hemorrhage seen as high signal on T2W images.[58] A patella baja (low-riding patella) and undulating appearance of the patellar tendon is associated.

The patellar tendon also has homogeneous low-signal intensity appearance except for small occasional triangular areas of intermediate signal intensity directly below the patella and adjacent to the tibial tuberosity. The normal thickness of the tendon does not exceed 7 mm in its proximal part. A large collection of adipose tissue, the infrapatellar fat pad of Hoffa, rests just posterior to the patellar tendon. The patellar tendon ruptures less frequently than the quadriceps tendon.

BOX 3: Components of the anterolateral corner.

- Anterolateral ligament
- Iliotibial band
- Anterior oblique band
- Capsular ligament

Patellar Tendonitis (Jumper's Knee)

Most patellar ligament injuries are the result of repetitive forced extension of the knee as seen in the context of basketball, volleyball, soccer, tennis, and track events—hence the name jumper's knee. This form of injury manifests as thickening and partial tearing of the proximal patellar tendon

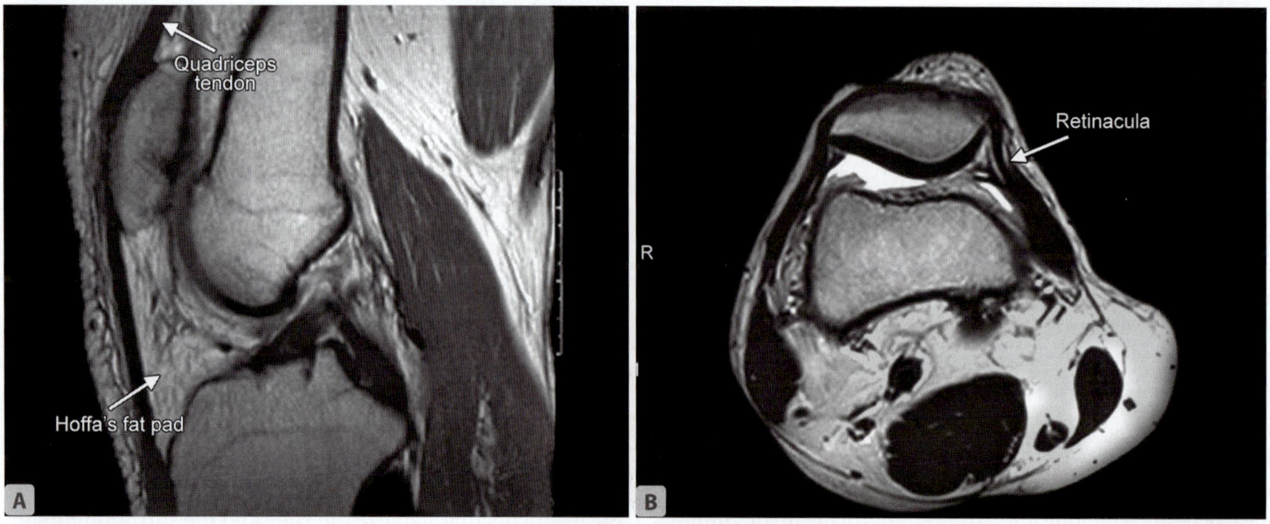

FIGS. 31A AND B: (A) T2W sagittal MR image showing the normal quadriceps tendon inserting on the superior pole of the patella, the patellar tendon, and the infrapatellar Hoffa's fat pad; (B) T2W axial MR image showing the medial and lateral patellar retinacula.

and is well seen on sagittal MR images as increased tendon thickness greater than 7 mm or as intrasubstance high-signal intensity. Similar changes can be seen in both symptomatic and asymptomatic individuals. In symptomatic patients, the findings may be accompanied by patellar tracking disorders in as many as 45% of patients.

Acute Patellar Tendon Disruption

A minority of patellar ligament injuries are complete tendon disruption resulting from acute macrotrauma in the setting of sports-related activity. This most commonly occurs near the patellar attachment and is best seen on sagittal MR images as discontinuity of the patellar ligament with buckling of the tendon, retraction of the patella, and fluid signal in the intervening gap.

Patellar Tendon-lateral Femoral Condyle Friction Syndrome

Patellar tendon-lateral femoral condyle friction syndrome refers to the constellation of MRI findings that correspond to the clinical entity known as fat pad impingement syndrome. Affected patients are both athletes and nonathletes who experience chronic anterior knee pain that localizes to the inferior patellar pole on physical examination. The etiology is unknown, but it is likely related to friction onto the fat interposed between the patellar ligament and the lateral femoral condyle due to abnormal patellar tracking or alignment. MRI findings include abnormal obliteration of the fat planes, abnormal signal, and enhancement within the lateral soft tissues of the inferior patellofemoral joint. Most patients demonstrate patellar alignment abnormality, such as patella alta or lateral subluxation. Patients typically respond well to conservative treatment, which usually entails taping the superior pole of the patella.

Retinacular tears are characterized by areas of high signal on T2W and STIR sequences secondary to edema and hemorrhage.[59] The medial retinaculum is thinner than the lateral and frequently tears. The avulsed free end of the retinaculum is often frayed and thickened and fluid may dissect around a muscular slip of the vastus medialis muscle.

PATELLOFEMORAL JOINT AND KINEMATIC MRI

Patellofemoral Joint Anatomy

The shape of the patella and femoral trochlear groove is important for the function of the patellofemoral joint.

Patellar Shape

Wiberg has proposed a three-part classification to encompass the majority of patellar facet configurations. In type I configuration, both facets are gently concave, symmetrical, and nearly equal in size. In type II, which is the most common, the medial facet is smaller than the lateral. In type III configuration, the medial facet is distinctly markedly smaller with marked lateral predominance.[60] Dysplastic patellar shapes have a variety of unusual configurations and are commonly observed with chondromalacia, recurrent dislocation, and patellofemoral instability.

The medial stabilizers prevent lateral subluxation of patella and include the medial patellar retinaculum and the medial patellofemoral ligament. The lateral stabilizers include the lateral patellar retinaculum and the lateral patellofemoral ligament.

MRI of Patellar Instability

The predisposing factors for patellar instability include trochlear dysplasia, excessive lateral distance between the tibial tubercle and the trochlear groove (lateralization of tibial tuberosity), and patella alta. For a safe tracking of the patella throughout the range of patellofemoral flexion, the femoral sulcus must be deep enough and the lateral trochlea high enough. Patellar dislocation is characterized by a complete loss of contact between the patellofemoral joint surfaces with the patella dislocating laterally in almost all cases.

Trochlear Dysplasia

This refers to a flattening of the joint surface. It can be evaluated on MR imaging by measuring the lateral trochlear inclination, trochlear facet asymmetry or trochlear depth.[61]

Lateral Trochlear Inclination

The most superior section showing trochlear cartilage is selected from axial section. A line is drawn along the subchondral bone of the lateral trochlear facet and another along the posterior aspect of the femoral condyles. The angle between the two lines is then measured. An inclination angle of less than 11° suggests trochlear dysplasia **(Figs. 32A and B)**.[61]

Trochlear Facet Asymmetry

This is calculated as the ratio of the length of the medial trochlear facet to the length of lateral trochlear facet. A trochlear facet ratio of less than 40% indicates trochlear dysplasia **(Figs. 33A and B)**.

Trochlear Depth

If the depth of the trochlear groove is less than 3 mm, it is indicative of trochlear dysplasia.[61]

Sulcus Angle

The femoral trochlear groove provides a mechanical restraint that helps stabilize and serve as a guide for the patella as it articulates with the groove during joint function. In the axial plane, the posterior apex of a normal patella is centered directly above the intercondylar femoral sulcus. The sulcus angle is formed by the highest points of the medial and lateral femoral condyles and the lowest point of the intercondylar sulcus and measures 138° ± 6° **(Figs. 34A and B)**. Shallow sulcus angles (larger sulcus angle measurements) predispose to patellar instability.

Distance from Tibial Tubercle to Trochlear Groove[61]

A distance between tibial tubercle and trochlear groove less than 15 mm is normal, distances between 15 and

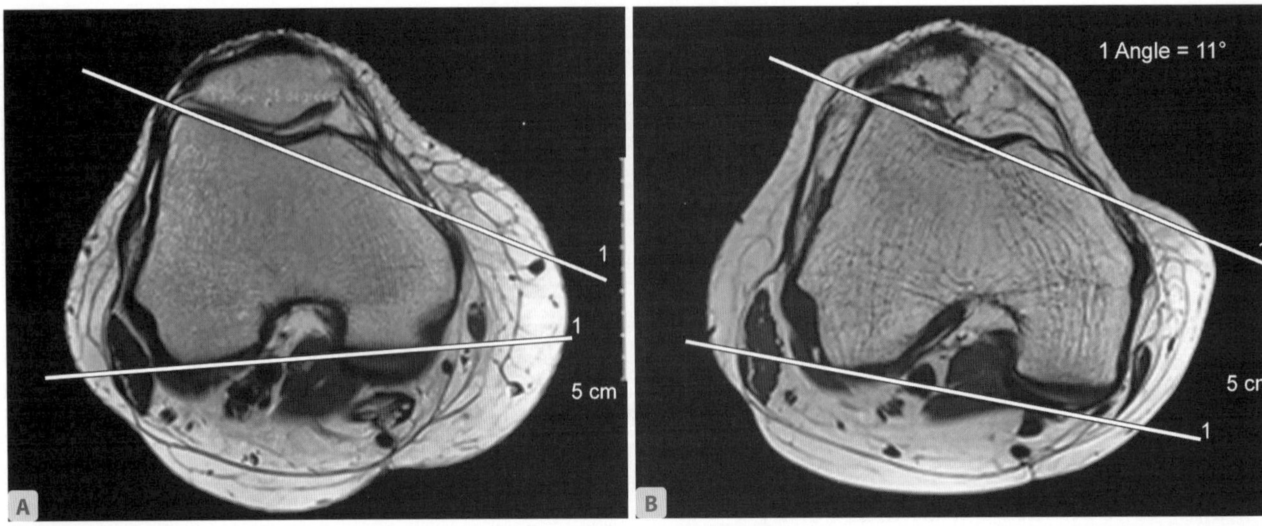

FIGS. 32A AND B: MR images showing the normal trochlear inclination (A) and abnormal (<11°) in a case (B).

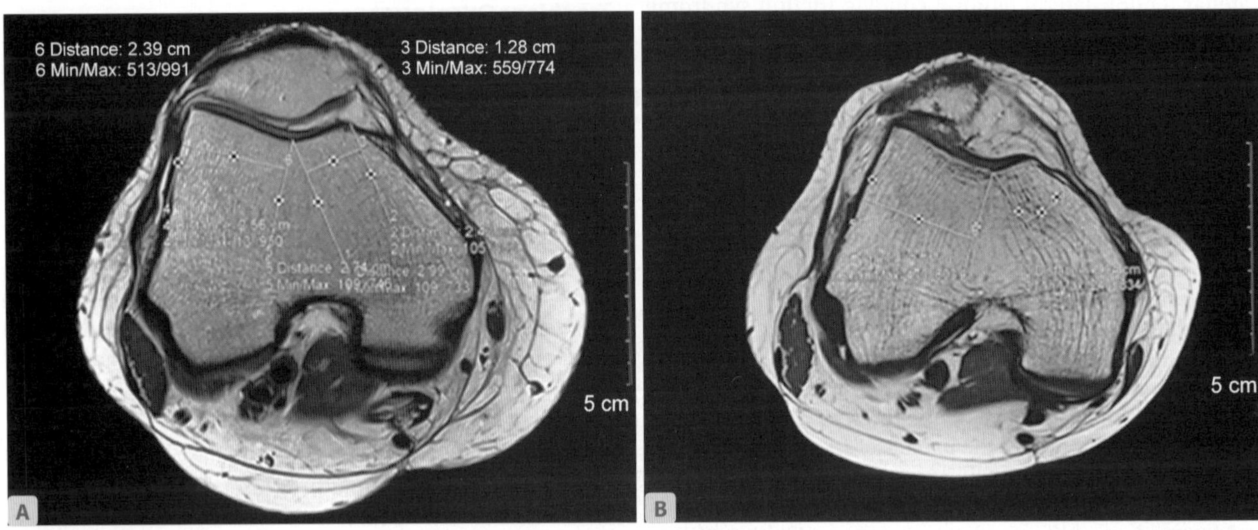

FIGS. 33A AND B: MR images showing the normal trochlear facet ratio (>40%) in a case (A); (B) Abnormal facet ratio (<40%) seen in another.

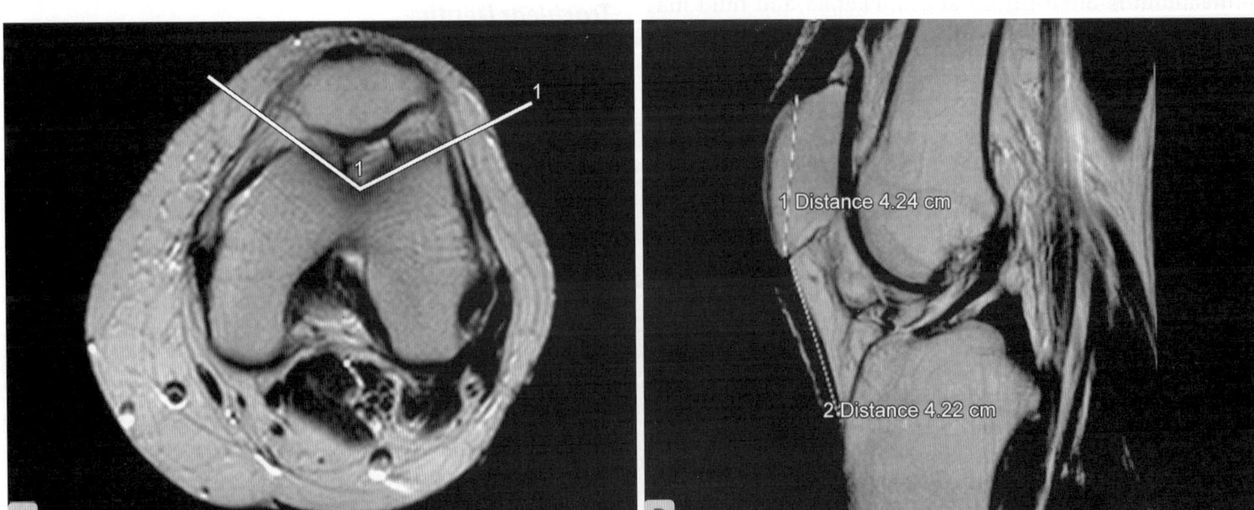

FIGS. 34A AND B: (A) T1W axial image showing the normal sulcus angle formed by the highest points of the medial and lateral femoral condyles and the lowest point of the intercondylar sulcus; (B) T2W sagittal MR image showing the normal position of the patella (the greatest diagonal length of the patella equals the patellar tendon length).

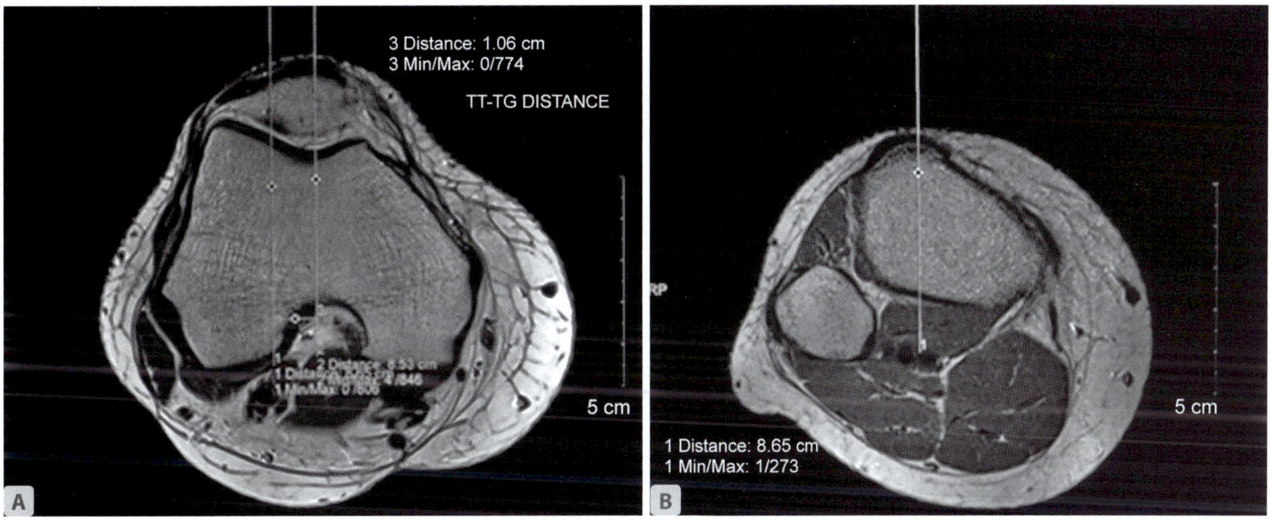

FIGS. 35A AND B: MR images showing the normal tibial tubercle to trochlear groove distance <15 mm.

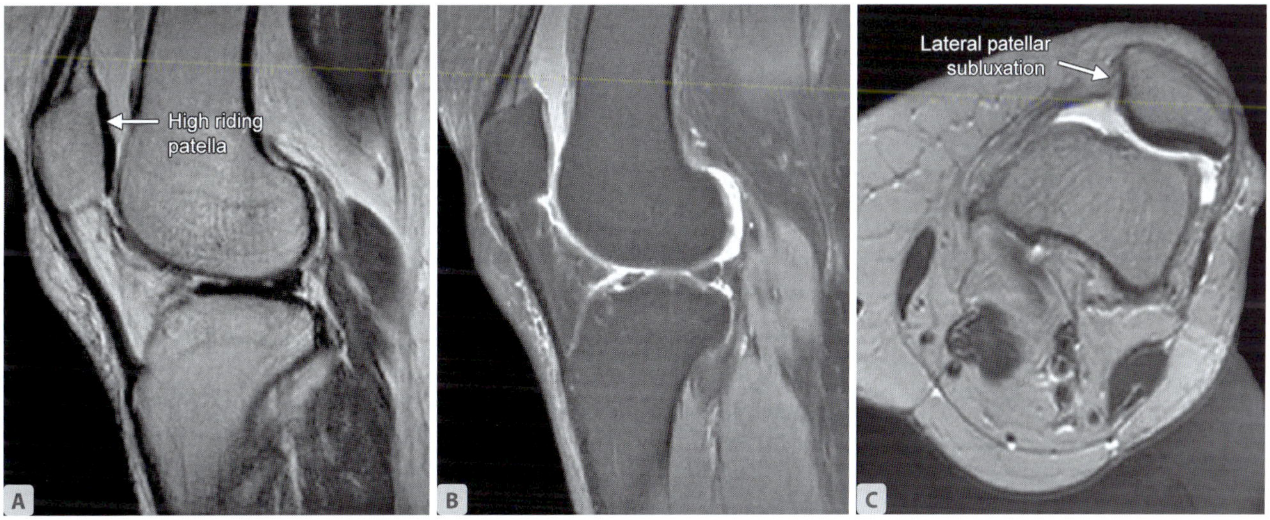

FIGS. 36A TO C: (A) Proton density; and (B) T2W fat suppressed sagittal MR images showing a high-riding patella with (C) Axial T2W MR image revealing a lateral patellar subluxation—patella alta.

20 mm are borderline and distances of more than 20 mm are indicative of lateralization of tibial tuberosity **(Figs. 35A and B)**. This causes the patella to be pushed laterally during flexion predisposing to lateral dislocation.

Patella Alta and Patella Baja

In the sagittal plane, the patella is in normal position when in semiflexion of the knee the greatest diagonal length of the patella approximately equals the distance between the inferior pole of the patella and the tibial tuberosity (patellar tendon length). A truly high-riding patella (patella alta) most commonly results from a patellar tendon tear but is also associated with lateral patellar subluxations, recurrent dislocations, and spastic neuromuscular disorders[61] **(Figs. 36A to C)**. A low-riding patella (patella baja or profunda) occurs in quadriceps tendon rupture but is also found with paralytic neuromuscular disorders, achondroplasia, and juvenile rheumatoid arthritis (JRA).

Kinematic MRI

Kinematics is a term to describe movement of a body without reference to force or mass. Although conventional computed tomography (CT) and cine CT have also been used to perform kinematic studies of the patellofemoral joint, kinematic MRI has the advantage of showing the various soft tissue components (i.e., medial and lateral retinacula, patellar tendon, quadriceps muscles) that are involved in the stability and function of the joint.

Techniques

Incremental, Passive Positioning Technique

The technique involves obtaining multiple axial images at different section locations and both the patellofemoral joints are passively flexed into incremental positions using a nonferromagnetic positioning device. The use of a special positioning device is crucial because direct anterior or lateral pressure may occur with the patient placed in prone position that is sufficient to displace the patella and give an erroneous appearance of patellar subluxation.

The MR images are obtained using a T1W spin echo, or spoiled gradient echo pulse sequences at several different slice locations while the joint is progressively flexed at 5° increments from 5° to 30°. This procedure should be repeated at three different section locations so that the entire excursion of the patella can be evaluated as it articulates with the femoral trochlear groove.[60]

Active Movement or Dynamic Technique

Faster MRI techniques, e.g., ultrafast spoiled gradient recalled acquisition in the steady state (GRASS), turbo fast low-angle shot (FLASH) have been developed recently that provide significant improvements in temporal resolution and allow images to be obtained during active or dynamic movement of the patellofemoral joint. MR images typically are obtained at a temporal resolution of one image per second or faster using these fast scan techniques. The primary advantage of using active movement kinematic MRI technique is that the patellofemoral joint may be examined in terms of influence of the activated muscles and other related soft tissue structures on patellar alignment and tracking. Compared with the incremental, passive positioning technique, a more physiological examination is obtained and in certain instances, abnormal patellar tracking is more apparent during active movement. Dynamic MRI has the potential to characterize and quantify mechanics of internal structures in vivo.

Motion Triggered Cine Technique

In this technique, a special nonferromagnetic device incorporates a trigger system that senses the motion of the patella. The patient is placed supine on the positioning device and a single patellofemoral joint is flexed and extended repeatedly while gradient echo images are obtained using a circular surface coil.

Active Movement, Loaded Technique

In this, active movement against an externally applied load or resistance is applied.[62] With the patient in prone position, the movement against this resistance primarily requires activation of the extensor mechanism of the knee. This method enables identification of abnormalities that may not be observed during unloaded examination.

Abnormalities that may be seen on kinematic MR include lateral or medial subluxation of patella and lateral patellar tilt or excessive lateral pressure syndrome.

Kinematic MR study can be combined with routine MR study of the knee since both the procedures can be completed within an acceptable time and can provide a more thorough examination of the knee especially in cases of suspected patellofemoral incongruency.

Weight-bearing MRI of the Knee

Imaging in nonrecumbent position under physiological stress allows detection of load-induced physiological and pathological variations. WB-MRI is dedicated open MR unit in which the patient is positioned standing upright or sitting.[63] Such systems allow flexion and extension views to be obtained (multipositional MRI). This instrument enables detection of unstable meniscal lesions as there occurs a modification of the meniscal morphology resulting in a posterior subluxation of the posterior horn of the medial meniscus in unstable lesions during passage from supine to upright position. Upright MRI also allows one to understand patellofemoral kinematics. This helps in understanding the etiology of patellofemoral pain, differentiates non-maltrackers from maltrackers, and helps improve treatment for patellofemoral instability by pinpointing the exact cause.[63]

MRI OF THE ARTICULAR CARTILAGE

The articular surfaces of the knee are covered by hyaline cartilage. By deforming under pressure, the articular cartilage greatly increases the effective contact area between femoral condyles and tibial plateaus, significantly decreasing the pressure transmitted across these joints. The menisci are also helpful in distributing forces across the knee joint. The cartilaginous matrix of articular cartilage allows the knee to withstand large local pressures up to 5 times the normal pressures.

Initial evaluation of the articular cartilage used primarily T1W images. Because of its hydropic composition, normal hyaline cartilage demonstrates intermediate signal intensity on T1W images compared with the low signal intensity of the cortex and fibrocartilaginous menisci. On conventional T2W images also, hyaline cartilage displays an intermediate signal intensity. In the presence of joint effusion, T2W images create an arthrogram like effect with hyperintense synovial fluid improving the delineation of thinner cartilage surfaces (e.g., medial and lateral compartments). There is poor contrast, however, between articular cartilage and subchondral bone on conventional T2W images and in the absence of joint effusion, surface or contour irregularities may not be resolved.

STIR and gradient echo images can also depict morphological changes of the articular cartilage. With STIR image contrast, it is possible to differentiate the brighter signal intensity of fluid from intermediate-to-high signal intensity of articular cartilage. This sequence is also useful in demonstrating early changes of subchondral bone in areas of overlying articular cartilage damage. Areas of fluid within articular cartilage fissures and fragmentation can also be visualized on STIR images. Gradient echo imaging is useful with respect to imaging geometry, speed, and contrast. 3D imaging significantly improves SNR at high spatial resolution. With gradient echo techniques, articular cartilage demonstrates high signal intensity. However, articular cartilage and articular fluid show similar high-signal intensity, and significant cartilaginous injuries may be missed using gradient echo techniques if joint fluid and articular cartilage are isointense.

The demand for improved preoperative detection and characterization of articular cartilage damage has resulted in recent improvements in the accuracy of MRI of articular cartilage with use of sequences optimized for articular cartilage evaluation. Fat suppressed T2W FSE techniques are useful in separating the cartilage-fluid interface and identifying early changes of articular cartilage degeneration **(Fig. 37A)**.[64] A fat suppressed three-dimensional spoiled gradient echo technique (3D SPGR) is also used.[65-67] The sequence, dual echo steady state (DESS), combines the principles of heavily T2W steady state sequence and gradient echo imaging **(Fig. 37B)**. 3D MR pulse sequences commonly used for articular cartilage have different vendor specific abbreviations as given in the **Table 1**.[68]

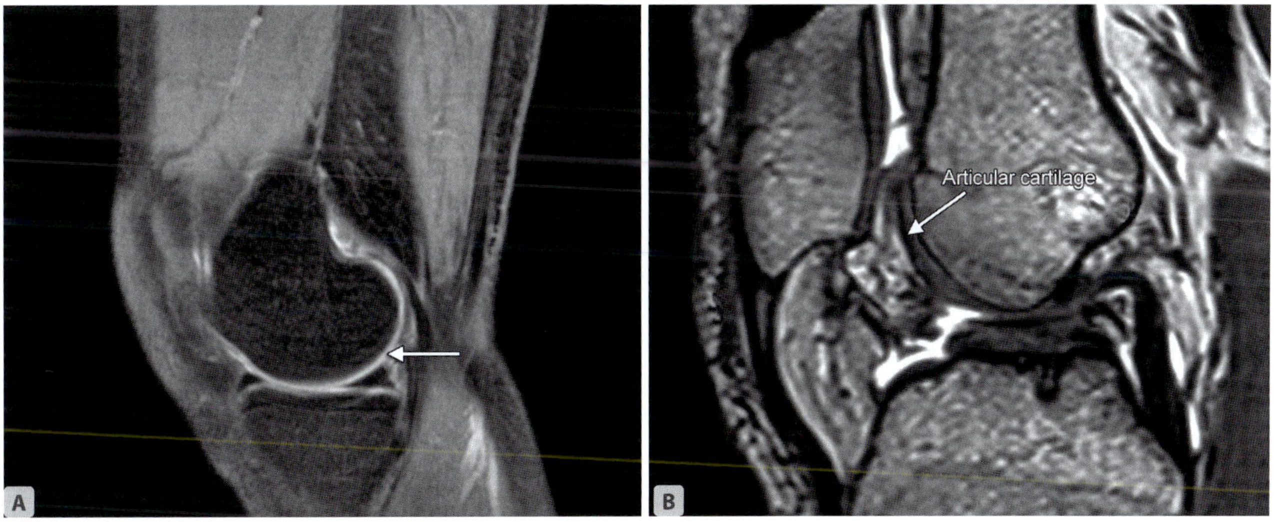

FIGS. 37A AND B: (A) Sagittal fat suppressed T2W MR image showing the articular cartilage as high-signal intensity; (B) DESS sequence for articular cartilage showing the intermediate gray signal articular cartilage. The thickness of the cartilage varies with the thickest cartilage seen at the patella and thinnest seen at the tibial plateau.

TABLE 1: Three-dimensional MRI pulse sequences commonly used in musculoskeletal imaging.

Sequences	Fluid signal intensity	Vendor abbreviation		
		GE	Siemens	Philips
GRE-based sequences				
Spoiled GRE	Dark	SPGR (Spoiled gradient-recalled echo)	FLASH (Fast low-angle shot)	T1 FFE (Fast field echo)
Steady-state sequences				
Postexcitation refocused (Coherent gradient echo)	Bright	GRASS (Gradient-recalled acquisition in steady state), Fast MPGR (Multiplanar gradient-recalled)	FISP (True fast imaging with steady-state free precession)	FFE (Fast field echo)
Fully refocused (bSSFP)	Bright	FIESTA (Fast imaging using steady-state free acquisition)	True FISP (true fast imaging with steady-state free precession)	Balance FFE (Fast field echo)
Pre-excitation refocused (Steady-state free precession)	Bright	SSFP (Steady-state free precession)	PSIF (reversed FISP) (reverse fast imaging with steady-state free precession)	T2 FFE (Fast field echo)
Derivative bSSFP	Bright	VIPR-SSFP (Vastly undersampled isotropic projection steady-state free precession)		
Dual/multiecho steady-state balanced imaging	Bright	MENSA (Multiecho in steady-state acquisition)	DESS (Dual-echo in steady state)	
Spin-echo-based sequences				
Fast spin-echo	Variable	CUBE, XETA (Extended echo train acquisition)	SPACE (Sampling perfection with application optimized contrast with different flip-angle evolutions)	VISTA (Volume isotropic turbo spin-echo acquisition)

Source: Adapted from Naraghi A, White LM. Three-dimensional MRI of the musculoskeletal system. Am J Roentgenol. 2012;199(3):W283-93.68

The new 3D FSE sequences such as SPACE from Siemens, VISTA from Philips, and 3D MVOX (multivoxel) from Hitachi provide contrast that equals the 2D FSE sequences in contrast, offer submillimeter isotropic resolution, can be reconstructed in any imaging plane, and have a scan time which is shorter than the scan time needed to acquire three 2D sequences.[68]

All three imaging planes are useful, however, the sagittal plane is the best single plane for evaluation of articular cartilage because it provides near orthogonal images of most of the articular cartilage surfaces in the knee. Intra-articular contrast or MR arthrography is useful for detection of loose bodies or for evaluation of osteochondral defects for assessment of integrity of overlying articular cartilage.

MRI Assessment of Articular Cartilage Injury

Arthroscopic grading system for correlation with MR findings is:

- Minimal articular cartilage change with localized softening and minimal or no break in the articular surface.
- Areas of fibrillation or fissuring with an irregular roughened surface.
- Definite fibrillation with fissuring extending to the subchondral region and a classic "crab meat" appearance.
- Absence of articular cartilage with possibly eburnated subchondral bone.

MR can thus be used for grading and determining the extent of cartilage damage.[69,70] MR also has a role in the follow-up of cartilaginous injuries. Arthroscopy is too invasive for follow-up of these lesions.[60]

Chondromalacia Patellae

The term chondromalacia patellae meaning softening of the patellar cartilage is widely used to designate a clinical syndrome of retropatellar pain, patellofemoral crepitus, and quadriceps wasting which is associated with softening or fibrillation of the articular cartilage of patella.[71] The clinical observations that symptoms are self-limiting, may settle spontaneously, and that chondromalacia patellae does not progress to fully-developed OA in later life, suggest that the two diseases are different entities. Patients with chondromalacia patellae have cartilaginous thinning, focal signal or focal contour defects in the patellar cartilage on T2W MR images.

Osteoarthritis

Osteoarthritis affects the knee more frequently than any other joint. The MR findings in degenerative arthrosis/osteoarthritis vary from osteophytic spurring to compartment collapse, denuded articular cartilage, torn and degenerative meniscal fibrocartilage, and diminished marrow signal intensity in areas of subchondral sclerosis **(Figs. 38A to C)**. The various alterations in the subchondral bone microstructure associated with the different stages of OA include:[72]

- *Bone marrow edema-like lesions*: Bone marrow edema-like lesions (BMELs) are defined on MRI as monocystic subchondral areas of ill-defined hyperintensity on STIR and T2W sequences and areas of hypointensity on T1W sequences. BMELs may increase or decrease over time and larger BMELs are seen more frequently in subjects who have pain.[73]
- *Subchondral cyst-like lesions*: These lesions have a characteristic appearance on MRI and are seen as well-defined round areas of fluid like signal intensity on nonenhanced imaging. They are a consequence of traumatic bone necrosis following impact of two opposing articular surfaces.
- *Synovitis*: Synovitis occurs not only as a secondary phenomenon related to cartilage degeneration but also plays a role in the progression of cartilage loss. Synovial inflammation is believed to contribute to pain in patients who have knee OA.
- *Joint effusion*: Joint effusion is commonly detected in patients who have moderate-to-advanced OA and reflects synovial activation secondary to ligament injury, loose bodies, hyaline cartilage deterioration, and meniscal damage. Only contrast-enhanced images can differentiate between synovium and joint effusion.
- *Subchondral bone attrition*: Subchondral bone attrition is defined as a depression or flattening of the subchondral bony surface unrelated to gross fracture. It is considered to be a predictor of knee pain in cases of OA.

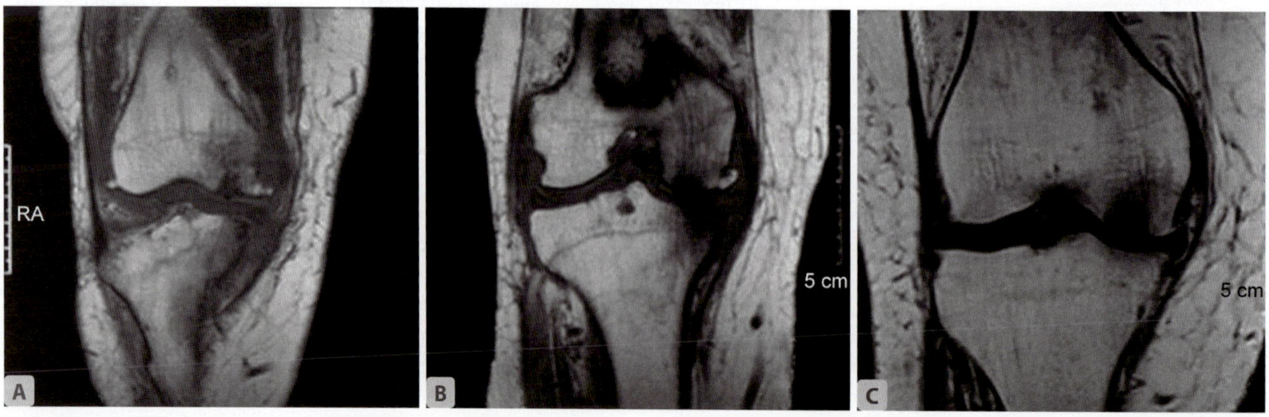

FIGS. 38A TO C: T1W coronal MR images of the knee showing osteophytic spurring, denuded articular cartilage, mild medial compartment collapse, and subchondral sclerosis—osteoarthritis.

- *Periarticular cysts*: A wide spectrum of periarticular cystic lesions may be encountered in knee OA like parameniscal cysts and ganglion cysts may be seen. Ganglion cysts are viscous synovium filled masses with mucopolysaccharide rich contents. Septations are common within ganglia. There is usually a connection or stalk traceable to the joint.
- *Loose bodies*: Chondral fragments (intermediate-signal intensity) and loose bodies (high-signal intensity of marrow fat) may be associated with more advanced degenerative disease. A T1W image in at least one plane should be included in the study to improve the identification of loose bodies that contain marrow fat. The exclusive use of fat suppressed sequences may lead to the loose bodies being missed. In addition to the patellofemoral, medial, and lateral compartments of the knee, changes in the tibiofibular joint which may also be affected by degenerative arthrosis are well seen by MRI **(Figs. 39A to D)**.

The ability of MRI to accurately assess hyaline cartilage surfaces may give MR an advantage over plain film radiography in preoperative planning for joint replacement procedures, especially in unicondylar arthroplasties for OA.[74] Therapeutic techniques such as chondrocyte transplantation requires high resolution and volumetric MRI studies for accurate identification of focal articular cartilage defects and generalized cartilage loss. Creation of cartilage models by 3D MR image rendering may be helpful for preoperative planning of orthopedic surgical procedures in advanced cases of OA. Also, tailored MRI producing high spatial and contrast resolution images is proving to be an important tool in the early detection and surveillance of progression of OA.[75]

NOVEL SEQUENCES AND TECHNIQUES FOR DETECTION OF EARLY OSTEOARTHRITIS

Biochemical MR Imaging of Knee Articular Cartilage/Compositional MRI[76]

The various routine MRI sequences allow for an evaluation of the morphology of articular cartilage but do not provide much information about its biochemical properties **(Figs. 40A and B)**. The main constituents of the articular cartilage are an extracellular matrix composed of 80% water, proteoglycan molecules, and type II collagen fibers. The biochemical changes of early OA include a decrease in the proteoglycan content, an increase in the free water content, and a disorganization of the collagen fibers.[76] The MR

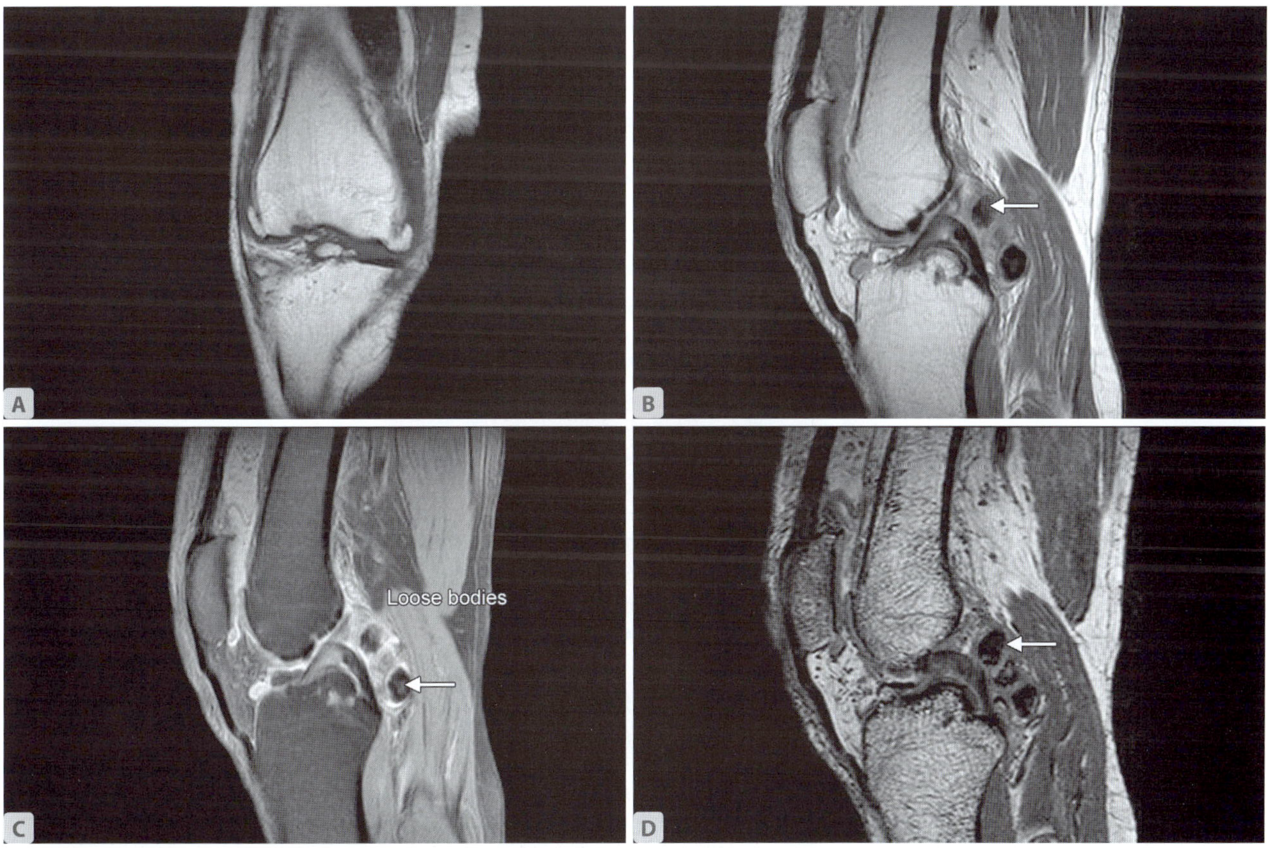

FIGS. 39A TO D: (A) T1W coronal; (B) T2W sagittal; (C) Fat suppressed T2W sagittal; and (D) Double echo steady state sequence showing osteophytic spurring at femur, patella, and multiple loose bodies. The loose bodies show high-signal marrow fat on T1W image (A) with signal suppression on fat suppressed image (B).

techniques which allow a study of these early biochemical changes include T1 rho and T2 mapping **(Figs. 40C to E)**.

T1 Rho

In T1 rho mapping, a low power RF pulse follows the critical RF pulse for a user defined time period called the spin lock time (TSL). As a result, the protons relax with a different time constant called T1 rho rather than the time constant T2 of conventional MR imaging.[77] T1 rho value of a given tissue is always higher than the corresponding T2 value of the tissue for a given RF pulse strength. In cases of early OA, there is depletion of proteoglycan resulting in fewer water molecules bound to proteoglycans resulting in increased T1 rho values. The acquired T1 rho values for a region of cartilage can be displayed in the form of a color-coded map. High T1 rho values are represented by warm colors (red tones) and low T1 rho values are represented by cool colors (blue tones) **(Figs. 40F to H)**.

T2 Mapping

In normal healthy articular cartilage, water protons are bound by well-organized collagen fibers allowing for a rapid dephasing and hence low T2 values. T2 values are reflective of the collagen disorganization and

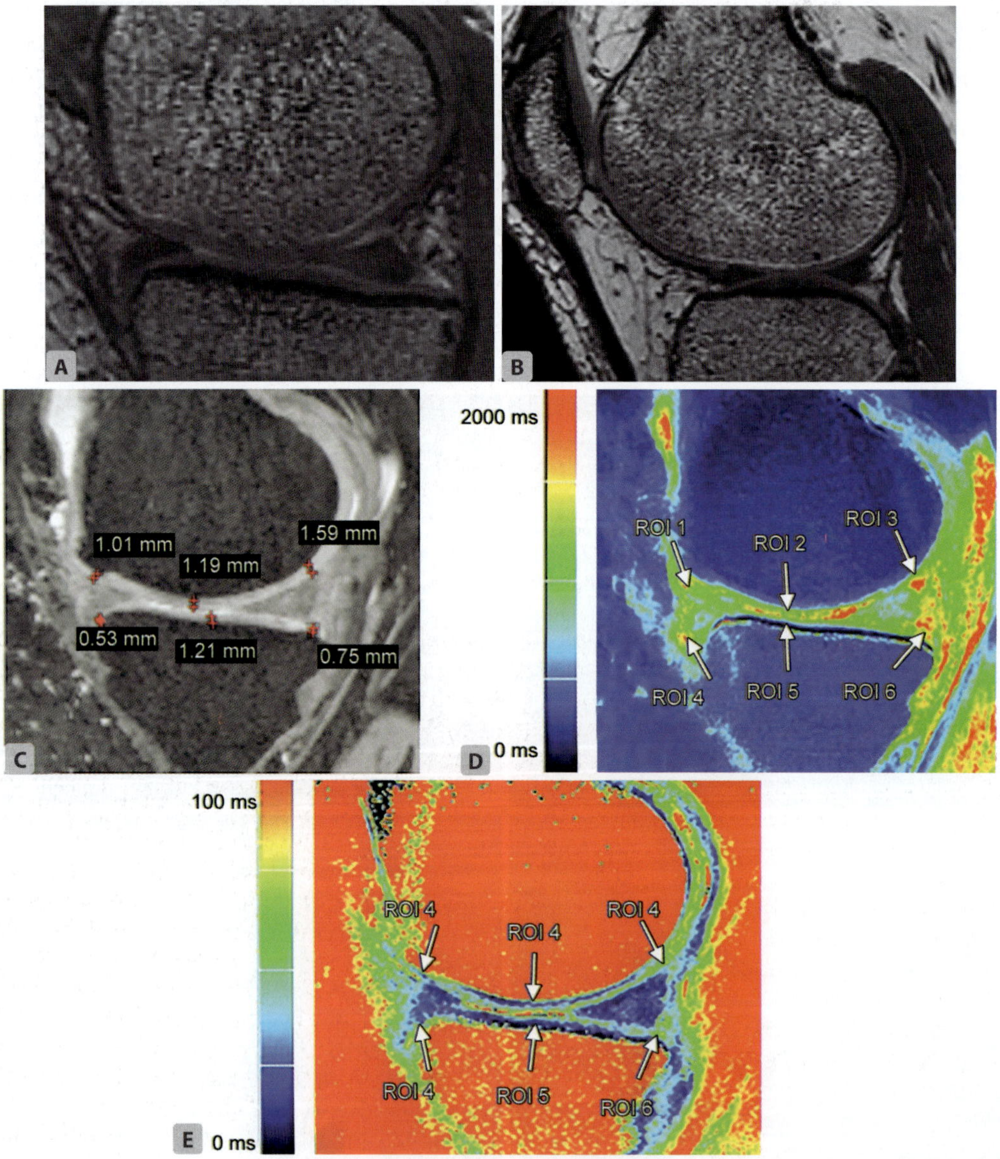

FIGS. 40A TO E: (A) T1W sagittal SPGR image shows thinning of medial femoral and tibial articular cartilage; (B) T1W sagittal SPGR image shows thinning of lateral femoral and tibial articular cartilage; (C) T2W sagittal double echo steady state Image showing medial femorotibial compartment (average thickness of articular cartilage in MFC ~1.28 mm and MTC ~0.83 mm); (D) Corresponding color coded sagittal T1 map of medial femor-tibial compartment [average T1 relaxation time of articular cartilage (in ROI 1, 2, and 3) for MFC ~1068.54 ms and (in ROI 4, 5, and 6) MTC ~957.8 ms]; (E) Color-coded sagittal T2 map of medial femorotibial compartment [average T2 relaxation time of articular cartilage (in ROI 1, 2, and 3) for MFC ~63.25 ms and (in ROI 4, 5, and 6) for MTC ~59.14 ms].

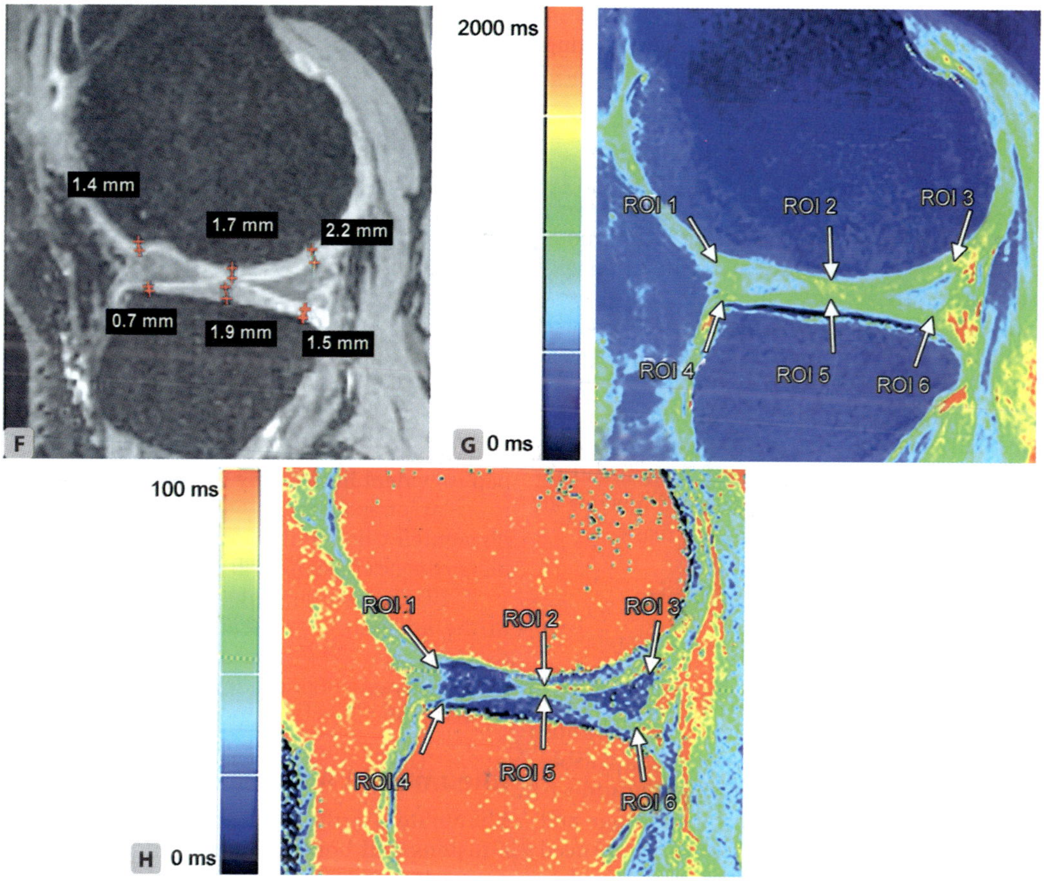

FIGS. 40F TO H: (F) T2W sagittal double echo steady state image showing lateral femorotibial compartment (average thickness of articular cartilage in LFC ~1.76 mm and LTC ~1.36 mm); (G) Corresponding color-coded sagittal T1 map of lateral femorotibial compartment [average T1 relaxation time of articular cartilage (in ROI 1, 2, and 3) for LFC ~1098.39 ms and (in ROI 4, 5, and 6) for LTC ~1098.89 ms]; (H) Color-coded sagittal T2 map of lateral femorotibial compartment [average T2 relaxation time of articular cartilage (in ROI 1, 2, and 3) for LTC ~60.6 ms and (in ROI 4, 5 and 6) for LTC ~65.54 ms].

increased water content that begins with OA in addition to the proteoglycan depletion.[77] T2 mapping can also be represented in the form of a color coded map, similar to the T1 rho maps with the red tones standing for high T2 values and blue tones standing for low T2 values. T2 mapping also permits differentiation among the three zones of articular cartilage. The superficial zone shows a higher signal compared to the deep layers owing to the more organized radial orientation of collagen fibers in the deep layers. This zonal differentiation is important as the osteoarthritic changes affect the more superficial layers much before the deeper layers. T1 rho and T2 mapping can also be used to study the degeneration of fibrocartilaginous structures like menisci in addition to the articular cartilage and both provide complementary information **(Figs. 40I to N)**.

Cartigram

T2 maps can be automatically generated by MR scanner when a special sequence is applied, e.g., Cartigram on General Electric MR scanners. T1 rho and T2 maps can also be generated using postprocessing methods like voxel-based relaxometry.

Quantitative Cartilage Imaging—Delayed Gadolinium-enhanced MRI of Cartilage

The normal cartilage is rich in glycosaminoglycans (GAG) which have negatively charged carboxyl and sulfate groups. Negatively charged contrast agents such as Gd-DTPA are injected intravenously or (intra-articularly) and these get distributed in the cartilage by diffusion. Because both GAG and gadolinium are negatively charged, gadolinium diffuses to articular cartilage in inverse proportion to local GAG concentration. Gd-based contrast agents thus show only a minimal enhancement in the normal healthy cartilage, owing to the high GAG concentration and accumulate in areas of cartilage loss with low GAG content.[78] The protocol consists of intravenous administration of Gd-DTPA (0.2 mmol/kg), 10 minutes of cycling or exercise to enhance its distribution and image acquisition 90 minutes (1–2 hours) using a 3D inversion recovery spoiled gradient echo sequence. Since there is a delay between contrast administration and image acquisition, the technique is called delayed gadolinium-enhanced MRI of cartilage (dGEMRIC). The concentration of Gd-DTPA in cartilage can be quantified and these quantitative findings have a particularly important role in evaluating early OA where changes are still reversible. dGEMRIC uses a T1 mapping technique after intravenous application of Gd-DTPA. dGEMRIC has been found helpful in monitoring therapy and interventions such as cartilage repair and oral medications.[79]

Sodium Imaging

Owing to the GAG content of the cartilage being negatively charged, cations such as Na^+ are attracted in the cartilaginous interstitial matrix. Thus the GAG content can be estimated using the sodium content. This, however, requires a dedicated sodium MRI which suffers from low SNR because of very low sodium concentration (~260–400 times lower than proton concentration in healthy cartilage). Sodium MRI, thus, has a limited clinical applicability as it requires dedicated coils, has low SNR, limited resolution, and long acquisition time (15–30 minutes). Further improvements in hardware and software combined with high field imaging at 7 T are required to make sodium MRI clinically feasible.[79,80]

Glycosaminoglycan Chemical Exchange Saturation Transfer Imaging

This is the newest compositional cartilage imaging technique. In chemical exchange saturation transfer (CEST) experiments, exogenous or endogenous compounds containing either exchangeable protons or exchangeable molecules are selectively saturated.[80] The saturation is then transferred to bulk water by chemical exchange and detected indirectly through the water signal with enhanced sensitivity. In cartilage, CEST exploits the exchangeable protons including NH, OH, and NH_2 proton groups on the GAG side chains of proteoglycans. The technique is still in the experimental stages and requires higher magnetic field strengths like 7 T.

Ultrashort Echo Time Imaging of Articular Cartilage

Tissues with a very short transverse relaxation time (T2) include bone, ligaments, tendons, menisci, and calcified cartilage. When conventional MR sequences are used, the signal from the tissues with a short T2 decays very rapidly. The result of the rapid decay is that signal from these tissues is zero or close to zero by the time the receive mode of a clinical MR system is enabled. The tissues thus appear hypointense in conventional MRI. Ultrashort echo time (UTE) sequences use TEs of <100 ms. These pulse sequences enable materials with short T2 to be assessed. UTE imaging in the knee enables detection of subtle matrix alterations and holds promise in the diagnosis of early degenerative changes.

In Vivo Diffusion MRI

Water mobility is restricted in the intact collagen network. In early degenerative disease of articular cartilage, an increased mobility of water is found leading to increased apparent diffusion coefficient values. Diffusion tensor imaging can measure the diffusion anisotropy of cartilage and provide information on the mechanical function of articular cartilage. It is a promising technique but requires sophisticated and high field imaging making it less suitable for routine clinical application.

Hybrid MRI

A combination of PET and MRI (PET/MRI) allows a combination of structural and molecular (metabolic) imaging techniques for the detection of early OA.[79]

EVALUATION OF THE SYNOVIUM

Synovial reaction and proliferation are characterized on MR images by changes in the contour of synovial reflections. Although the synovium cannot be imaged directly, a corrugated surface along Hoffa's infrapatellar fat pad is evident in the early stages of synovial irritation. This irregular infrapatellar fat pad sign is seen in patients with RA, pigmented villonodular synovitis (PVNS), hemophilia, and hemorrhagic effusions with reactive synovium.

Gd-DTPA contrast-enhanced T1W MR images are useful in the accurate identification of pannus tissue. Pannus tissue is seen as an area of increased signal intensity on these contrast-enhanced images adjacent to the low-signal intensity joint fluid.[81]

Rheumatoid Arthritis

Rheumatoid arthritis (RA) typically presents with joint effusions and bony and cartilaginous erosions. Marginal and subchondral erosions with diffuse loss of hyaline articular cartilage are evident on both medial and lateral femoral articular surfaces. An irregular fat pad may be seen in the more active stages of the disease. Hypertrophied synovial masses remain relatively low in signal intensity on T1W and T2W images. The Gd-DTPA contrast-enhanced images are useful in identifying the pannus or granulation tissue that grows on the surfaces of articular cartilage in RA **(Figs. 41A to D)**.[81]

The ability to map out pannus is useful in examining patients with inflammatory arthritis when synovectomy is considered. MRI determined synovial membrane and effusion volumes are sensitive markers and predictors of disease activity and treatment outcome in RA. Osteonecrosis and infarcts in rheumatoid arthritis can also be identified on MR scans before radiographic changes are evident.

Tuberculosis of the Knee

Magnetic resonance imaging is excellent for detecting early changes of tuberculosis. Synovial proliferation seen in TB is typically hypointense on T2W images. On administration of IV contrast, the hypertrophied synovium is intensely enhancing. Marrow edema, osteomyelitis, cortical erosions, myositis, cellulitis, abscesses, and skin ulceration/sinus formation can be seen in the bone and adjacent soft tissues **(Figs. 42A to C)**.

Juvenile Rheumatoid Arthritis

In JRA or Still's disease, MRI studies demonstrate synovitis with irregularity of Hoffa's infrapatellar fat pad in the early

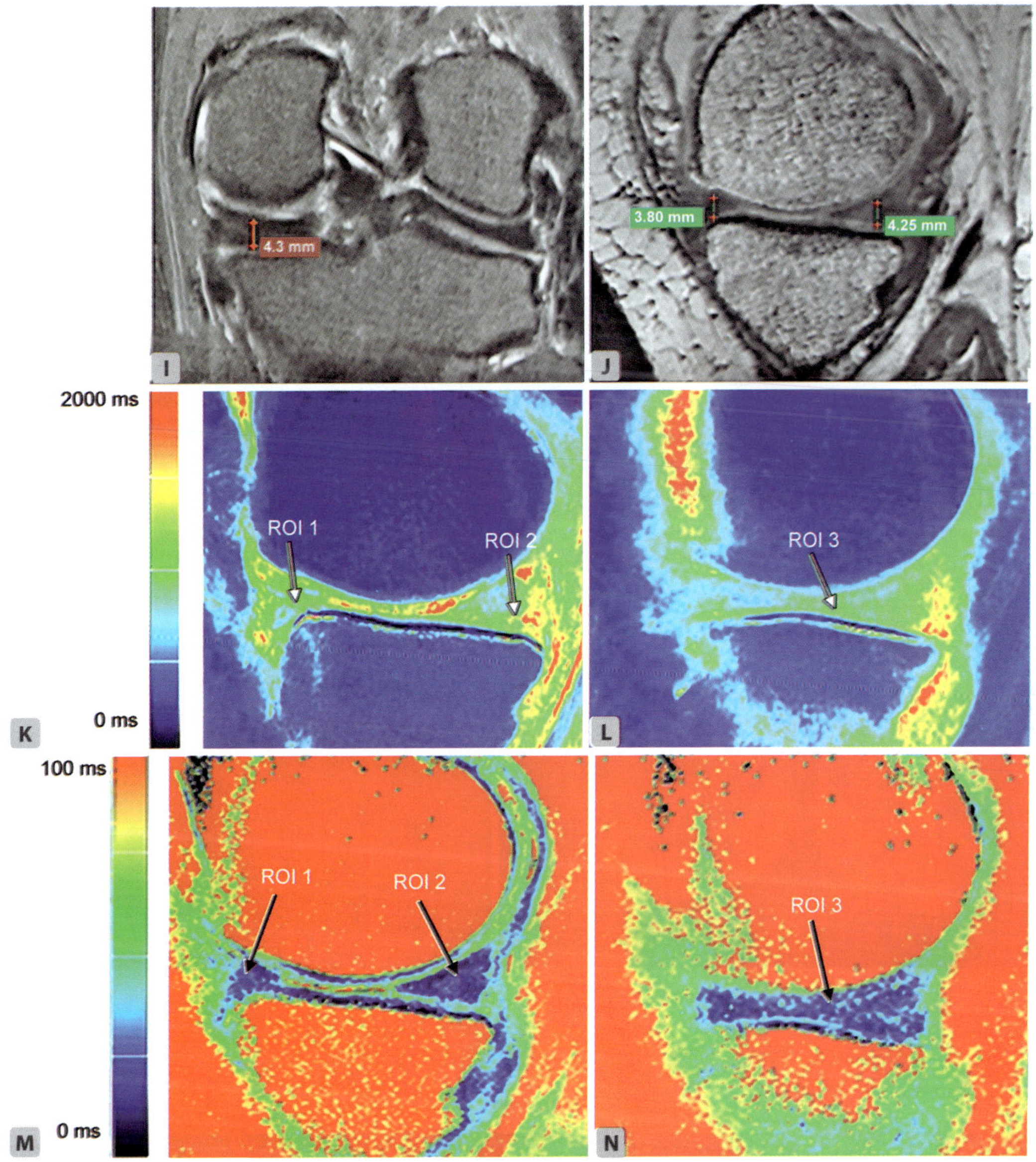

FIGS. 40I TO N: (I) T1W coronal STIR image shows average thickness of body of medial meniscus; (J) T1W sagittal SPGR image shows average thickness of anterior and posterior horn of medial meniscus; (K and L) Color-coded sagittal T1 maps show average T1 relaxation time (in ROI 1, 2, and 3) of medial meniscus ~924.79 ms; (M and N) Color-coded sagittal T2 maps show average T2 relaxation time (in ROI 1, 2, and 3) of medial meniscus ~25.54 ms.

stage. Articular cartilage erosions and synovial hypertrophy can also be identified. Hypoplastic menisci, with small anterior and posterior horns and body, have also been described in patients with JRA on MR studies. An enlarged epiphysis, widening of the intercondylar notch, and squaring of the inferior margin of the patella are radiographic findings also detected on MR. MR evaluation of signs of disease progression such as pannus tissue changes may be a cost-effective way of monitoring the effectiveness of therapy. MR studies may also be used for serial follow-up of functional status in patients with JRA.

Pigmented Villonodular Synovitis

Pigmented villonodular synovitis may also affect the knee. PVNS may present as a focal mass but more frequently is monoarticular. Histologically, the lesions present with fibrous synovial proliferation, infiltration by histiocytes, multinucleated giant cells and hemosiderin laden macrophages, and hemosiderin staining of the synovium presumably from recurrent hemorrhage. These lesions present on MRI as characteristic proliferative synovial focal masses containing hypointense signal on all pulse sequences **(Figs. 43A to D)**. The signal loss results from

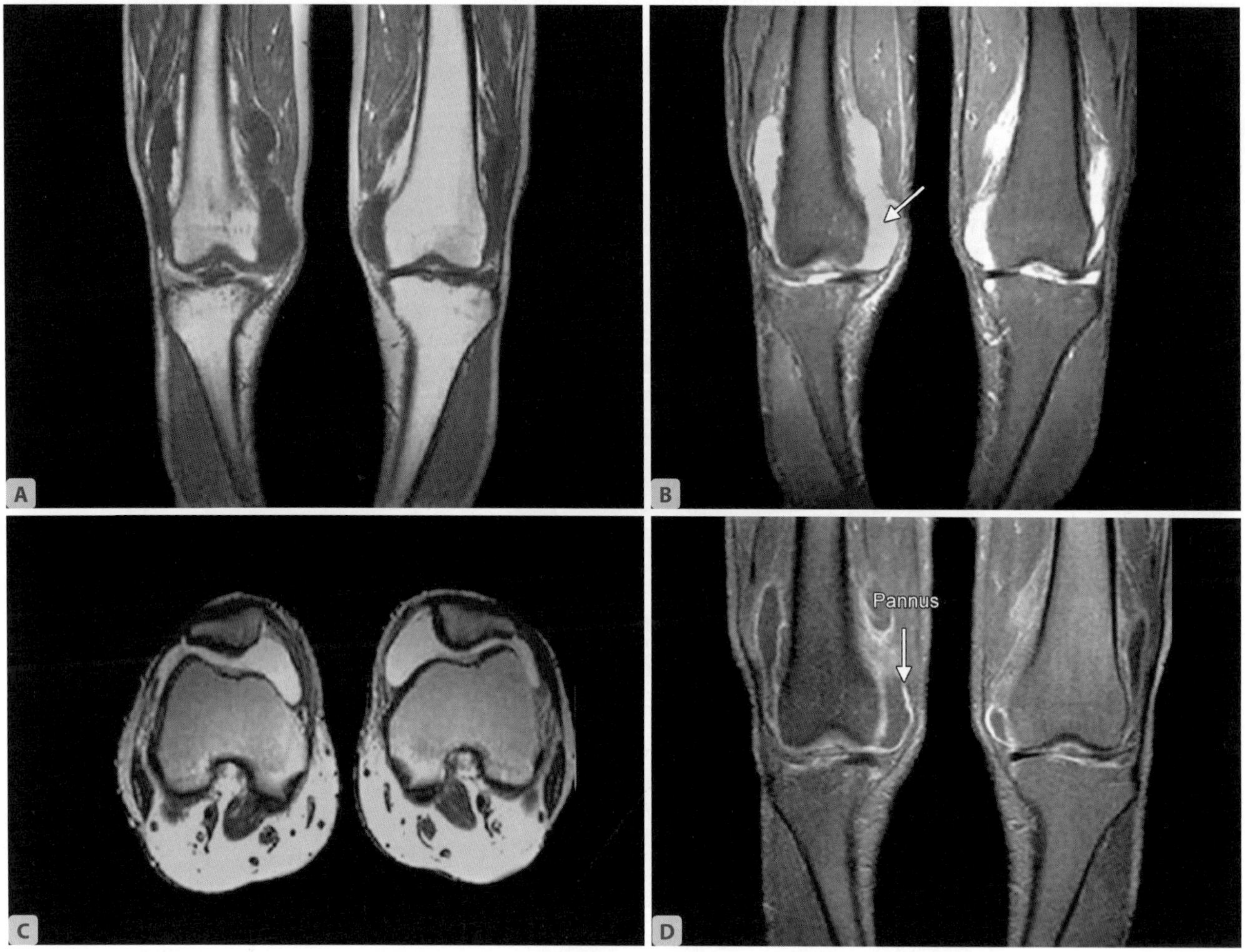

FIGS. 41A TO D: (A) T1W coronal; (B) STIR coronal; (C) Axial T2W; and (D) Postcontrast T1W coronal images showing joint effusion with enhancing pannus growing on the surface of the articular cartilage in both the knees—rheumatoid arthritis.

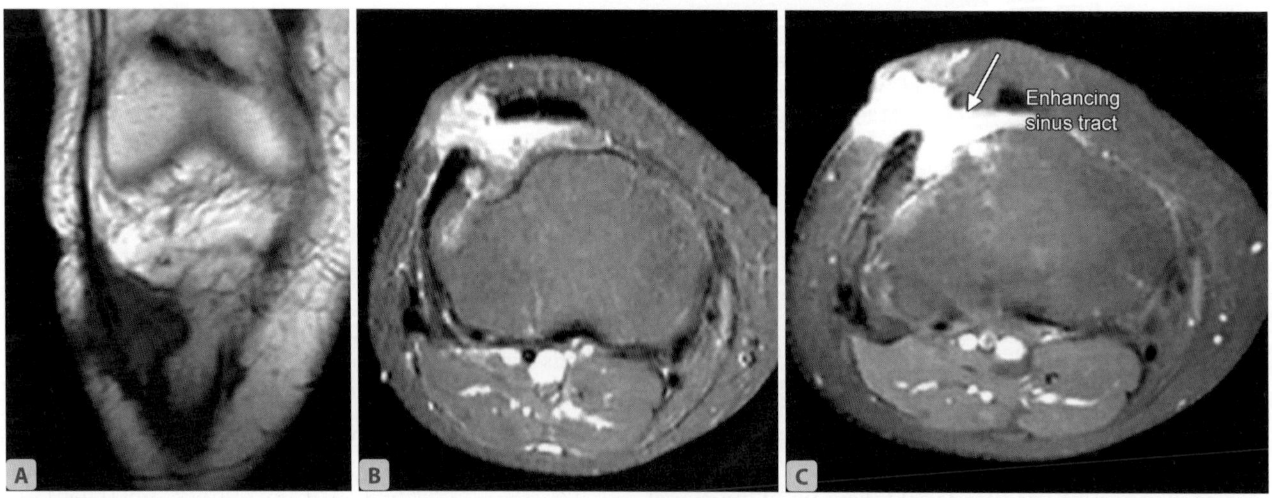

FIGS. 42A TO C: T1W coronal (A) and postcontrast T1W axial (B and C) MR images showing irregularity of the lateral tibial plateau with enhancing synovium and an enhancing sinus tract from the bone to the skin surface—tuberculosis.

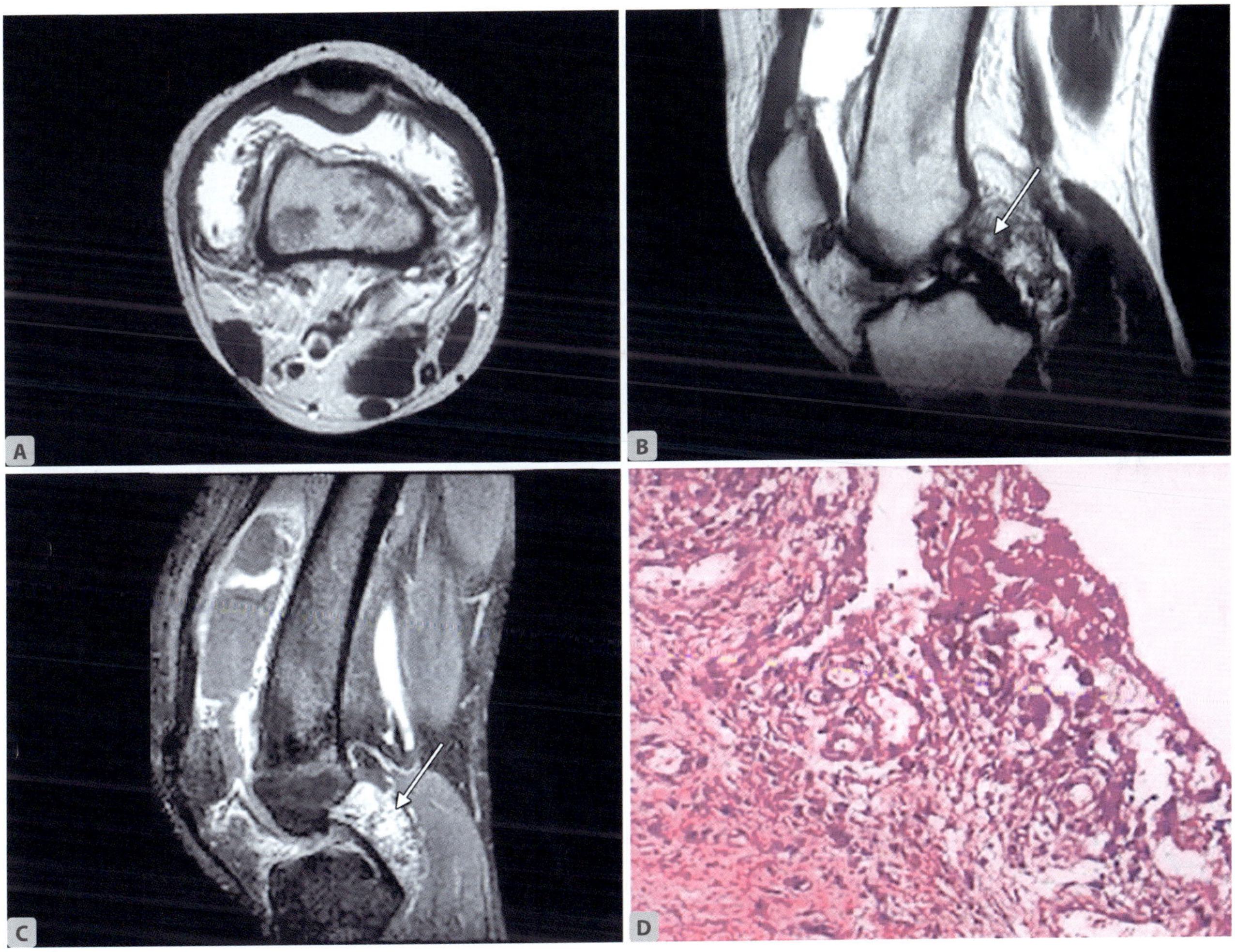

FIGS. 43A TO D: (A) Axial T2W; and (B) Sagittal images showing synovial thickening and associated effusion with scattered low signal areas of hemosiderin within. Low signal mass seen posterior to posterior cruciate ligament (PCL); (C) Postcontrast image showing enhancement of the thickened synovium and the focal mass posterior to PCL; (D) Biopsy showing histiocytes with hemosiderin pigment—pigmented villonodular synovitis.

proton dephasing from local magnetic field inhomogeneity caused by magnetic susceptibility effects of the iron containing byproducts of hemoglobin. Bony erosions are better visualized on MR than on plain films.[5,60]

Hemophilia

Subchondral and intraosseous cysts or hemorrhage can be identified on coronal and sagittal MR images. Hemosiderin and fibrous tissue formed from repeated episodes of joint hemorrhage demonstrate low-signal intensity on T1W and T2W images **(Figs. 44A to C)**. Signal loss in these conditions is usually more uniform in its involvement of the joint synovium and focal masses characteristic of PVNS are not usually seen in chronic hemorrhagic conditions.

Synovial Chondromatosis of the Knee

It is a process associated with metaplastic changes within the synovium that produce multiple cartilaginous islands in the synovium. These cartilaginous islands may become dislodged producing both calcified and noncalcified loose bodies. Lesions contain enough calcium to be detected on plain films. They are low in signal intensity on all MR pulse sequences.

Deferiprone-induced Arthropathy

Deferiprone (DFP) is widely used as an iron chelator in thalassemia patients. The arthropathy consists of musculoskeletal stiffness, joint pain, and joint effusion. Arthroscopy reveals excess iron in the synovium and cartilage. MRI in these cases reveals irregular thickening of the cartilage with subchondral erosions and cartilage intrusions in the subchondral defects. Synovial thickening and enhancement, synovial bands, and effusions have been described. The symptoms decrease with dose reduction or temporary discontinuation of drug **(Figs. 45A to C)**.

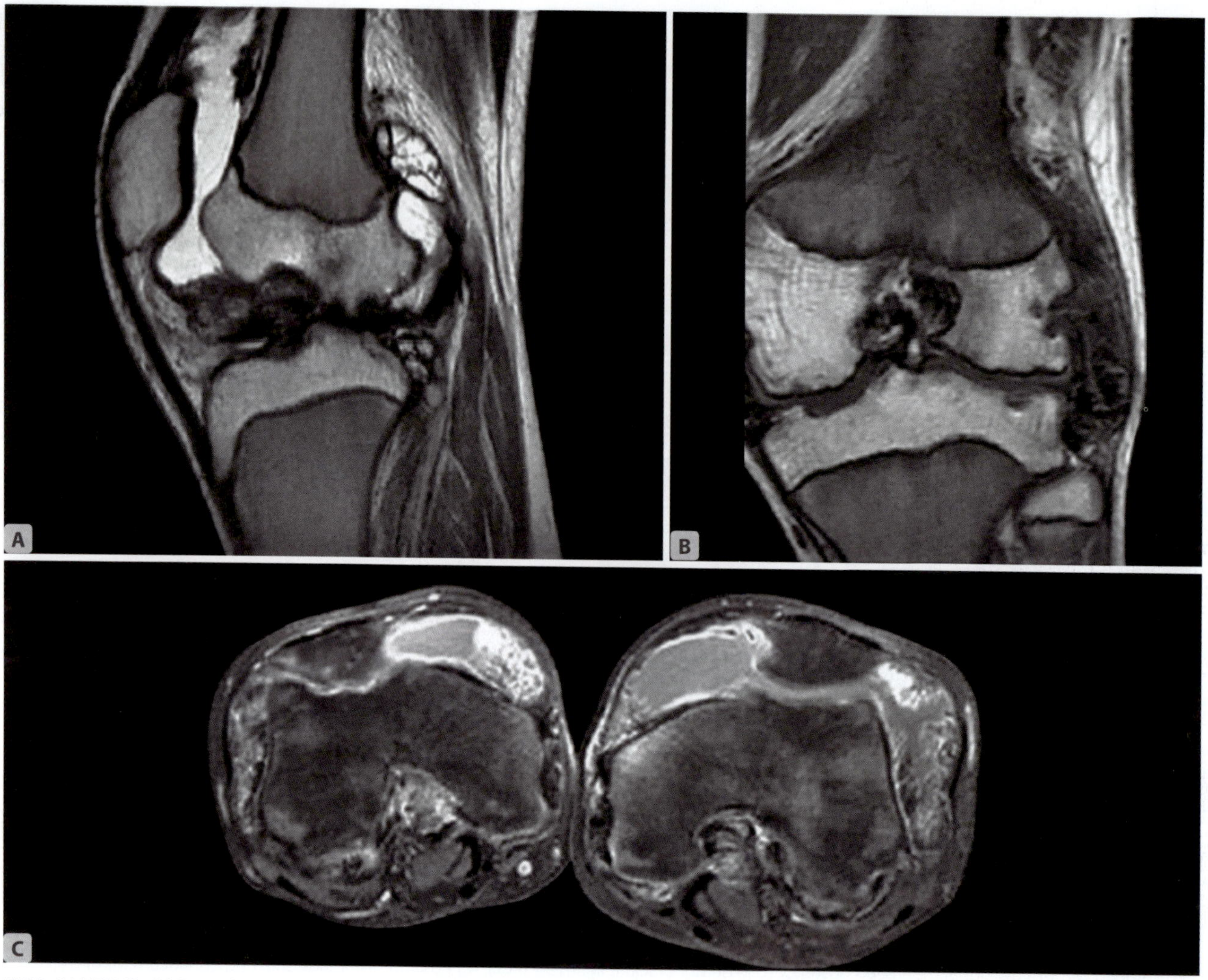

FIGS. 44A TO C: (A) Sagittal T2W; (B) Coronal T1W; and (C) Postcontrast T1W axial MR images showing thickening of the joint synovium with low signal areas within due to hemosiderin and fibrous tissue. There is fuzziness and irregularity of the articular margins. Changes are seen in both the knees—hemophilic arthropathy.

TRAUMATIC BONE MARROW ABNORMALITIES OF THE KNEE

The ability of MRI to detect clinically significant bony injuries that are undetected on radiographic studies has probably been MRI's most important attribute in clinical practice. MRI may be very helpful in evaluating patients with acute knee pain. Occult bony injuries are an important component of the cause of symptoms. Lynch has classified bony injuries as:[60]

Lynch Type I

An acute impaction force on a bone results in marrow hemorrhage and edema, disruption of trabeculae, and interstitial fluid leakage within the marrow space. On MRI, these type I bony injuries known as bone bruises/contusions are identified by the vague, geographic, edema-like pattern hypointense on T1 and hyperintense on T2 and STIR images **(Fig. 46)**. Majority of the bone bruises show signal resolution at 3 months. A minority <5% fail to resolve by 3 months probably secondary to repetitively applied trauma. A method of grading severity of marrow edema, particularly trauma-induced marrow edema, is based on diffusion imaging. Diffusion imaging represents a precise method of evaluating water movement. Trabecular disruption leads to increased multidirectional movement of water, hence a recorded change in marrow diffusion is an objective marker of the severity of marrow injury. A high recorded diffusion coefficient can be used as an early indicator of severe marrow injury and can be optimally managed by a nonweight bearing regimen.[82] Five classic contusion patterns have been described in the knee include:

1. The *pivot shift injury* occurs in skiers and American football players as a result of rapid deceleration with simultaneous change in direction. The tibia undergoes external rotation with the knee in flexion. On MRI, bone bruises are seen in the posterolateral tibial plateau and midportion of the lateral femoral condyle. This pattern is highly suggestive of an ACL injury.[83]

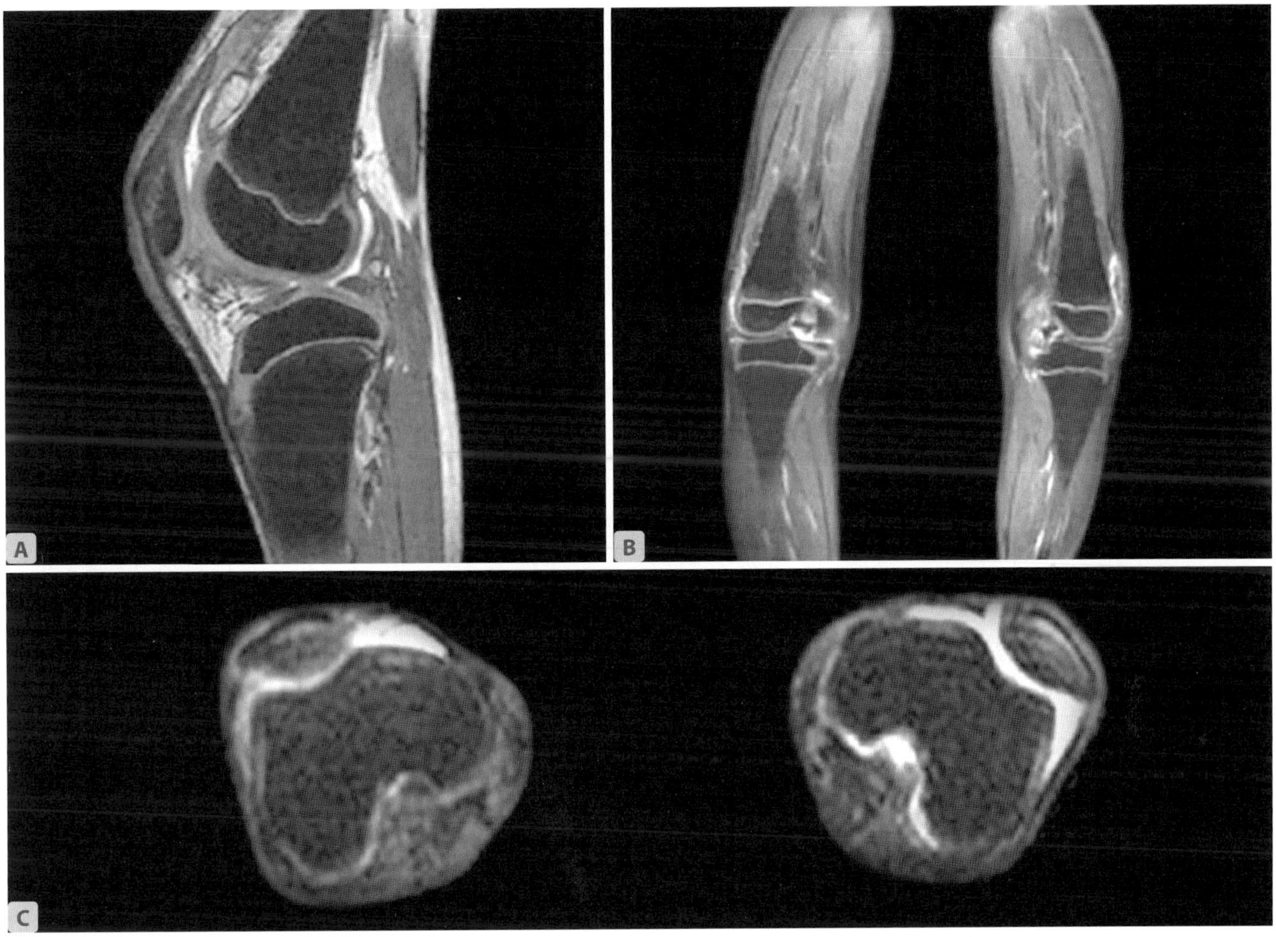

FIGS. 45A TO C: Sagittal (A) and coronal (B) GE images showing black out in the metaphyseal marrow, irregular thickening of the articular cartilage of femoral condyles, and patella with synovial thickening; (C) Postcontrast image showing synovial thickening and enhancement—deferiprone-induced arthropathy.

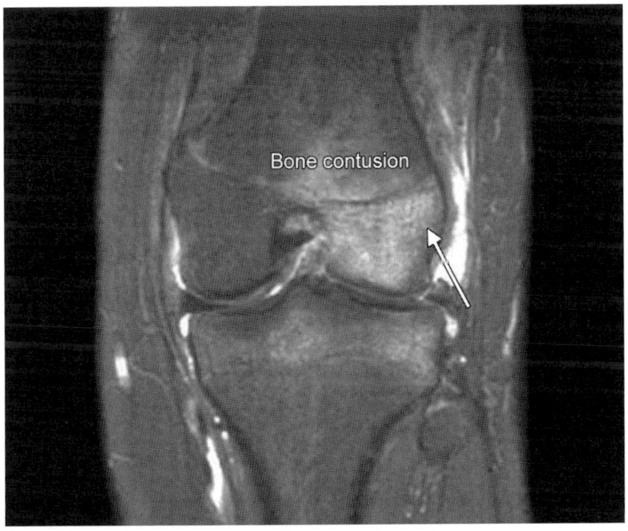

FIG. 46: STIR coronal MR image in a case of trauma showing areas of geographic bone marrow edema seen as hyperintense signal in the lateral femoral condyle and the posterolateral tibial plateau—type I bony injury.

2. The *dashboard injury* occurs in passengers in automobiles who undergo traumatic impact of the anterior proximal tibia with the dashboard while their knee is in flexion. An identical injury pattern can result from a fall onto bent knee. This injury will manifest on MRI as a bone contusion at the site of impact. A significant association has been demonstrated with injury to the PCL.
3. *Hyperextension injury* of the knee occurs with a direct blow to the anterior tibia on to the planted foot, results in "kissing contusions" of the anterior aspect of the proximal tibia and the distal femur. This finding on MRI is suggestive of additional trauma to the PCL, ACL, or menisci.
4. The *clip injury* results from pure valgus stress onto the partially flexed knee joint. Classically, this injury is seen in American football players who experience a blow to the lateral knee with the foot planted. It may also occur in a pedestrian struck by a car. The direct impact to the lateral knee will result in bone contusion at the lateral femoral condyle and lateral tibial plateau. The distractive forces at the medial joint compartment may result in coexisting MCL and medial meniscal tears (O'Donoghue triad).

A smaller contusion in the medial femoral condyle at the MCL attachment may also be present as a result of the avulsive stress. Small contusion at the posterior lip of the medial tibial plateau has been described and attributed to contrecoup impaction as the knee relocates following the ACL tear.

5. *Lateral patellar dislocation* occurs in the setting of internal rotation of the femur with the knee in flexion. The resultant contraction of the quadriceps tendon in this configuration causes the patella to dislocate laterally. Bone contusions occur at the inferomedial patella and the anterior aspect of the lateral femoral condyle from the contact that occurs on relocation.

Lynch Type II

These lesions reveal an interruption in the cortical bone on T1W scans **(Fig. 47A)**. These are seen as regions of increased signal intensity on T2W images and those lesions usually represent acute traumatic injuries with medullary hemorrhage and edema.

Lynch Type III

Lesions present as regions of profound signal loss immediately adjacent to the cortical bone on both T1W and T2W scan. Type III lesions most likely represent degenerative type subchondral sclerosis.[74]

Acute and Chronic Avulsive Injuries

Distraction injuries result in a small avulsion fracture related to a tendinous, ligamentous or capsular attachment on the bone. The associated marrow edema is much less extensive than the marrow edema seen with an impaction injury because cortical rather than medullary bone is involved.[84] The avulsed fragment is difficult to detect on MRI as the disproportionate edema and hemorrhage in the adjacent soft tissues masks the small osseous fragment. An example is Segond fracture. A Segond fracture represents an avulsion of the lateral tibial rim at the attachment site of the lateral capsular ligament **(Fig. 47B)**. Although the fracture fragment is typically small, cortical and obscured by soft tissue edema, this injury is important to identify because it indicates substantial meniscoligamentous injury and anterolateral instability of the knee which may cause long-term disability if not recognized.

Thigh and shin splints cause traction periostitis.[85] In addition to the expected periosteal edema or fluid, MRI reveals marrow edema and even cortical signal abnormalities that indicate osseous stress injuries of varying degrees.

Fatigue and Insufficiency Fractures

Fatigue fractures occur when abnormal stress is applied to normally mineralized bone whereas insufficiency fractures result from normal activities applied to the weakened bone. MRI reveals a spectrum of findings from periosteal edema alone to progressively severe marrow edema **(Figs. 48A and B)** to a hypointense fracture line in cancellous or cortical bone. MR has been advocated as a problem-solving modality in suspected stress fracture in a patient[86] with negative plain radiographs and equivocal bone scan. MR may secure the diagnosis if the fracture line is identified.

Stress Fractures

Stress fractures can result from either normal stress placed on deficient bone, as would occur in the osteoporotic elderly individual or, excessive stress placed on normal bone, as would occur in the running, jumping, or hurdling athlete.

Radiography is unreliable for detecting these lesions, particularly in the early stages. MRI, with a reported sensitivity and specificity as high as 88% and 100%, respectively, is the modality of choice. On MRI, stress fractures appear as as linear low-signal intensity bands, away from the joint on T1W and T2W images. Increased signal intensity may be seen around the impacted fracture site on T2W images, reflecting the associated edema.

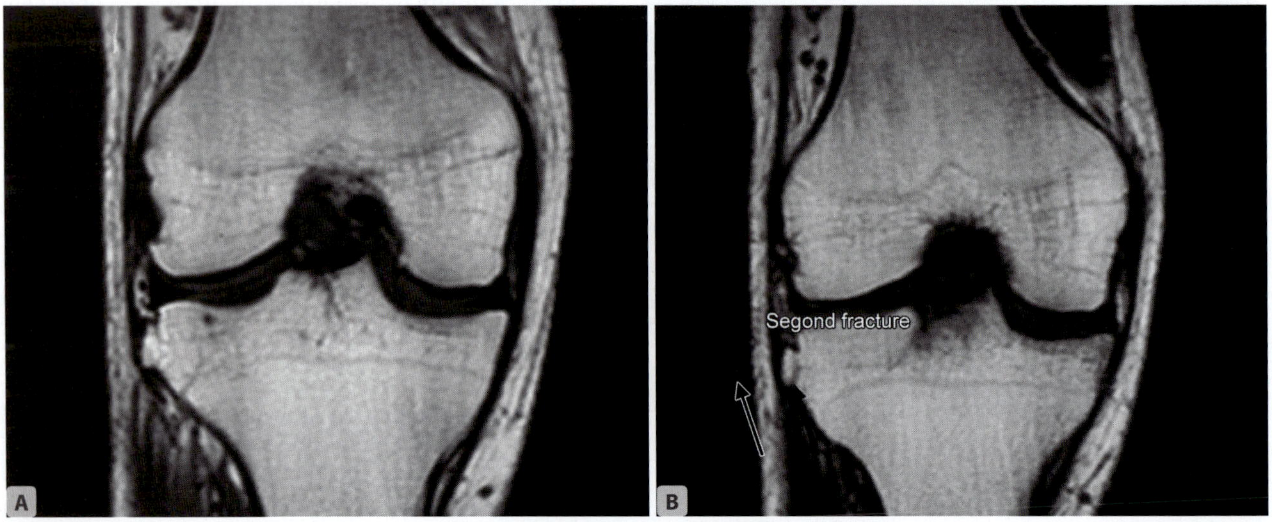

FIGS. 47A AND B: T1W coronal images showing an interruption in the cortical bone seen as linear low signal in the tibial spine—Grade II bony injury. Also seen is avulsion of the lateral tibial rim slightly below the level of the joint—Segond fracture.

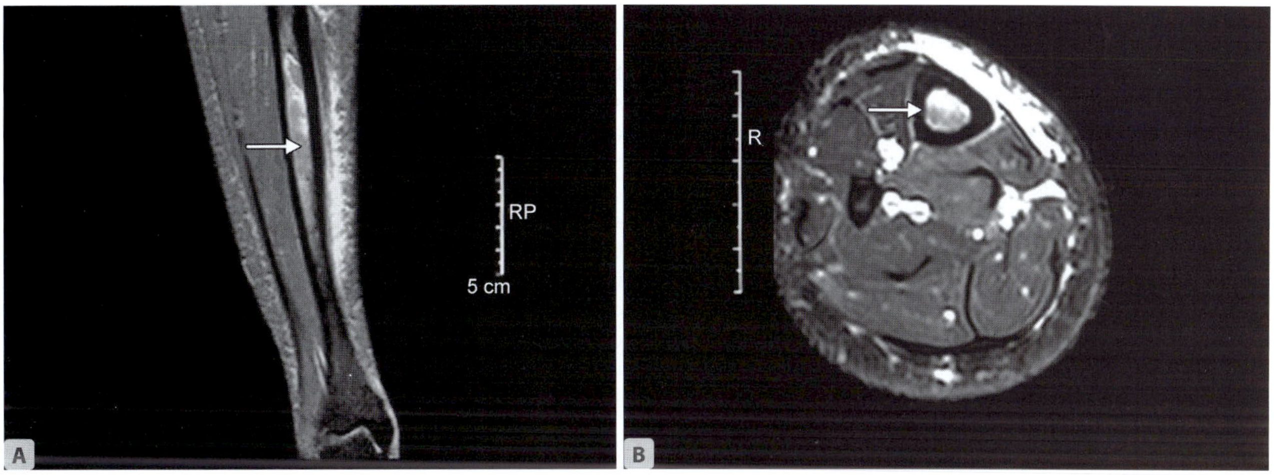

FIGS. 48A AND B: (A) STIR coronal, and (B) STIR axial images showing edema in the subcutaneous tissues, extensive bone marrow edema seen as hyperintense signal with no evidence of cortical irregularity or periosteal reaction—stress fracture in tibia.

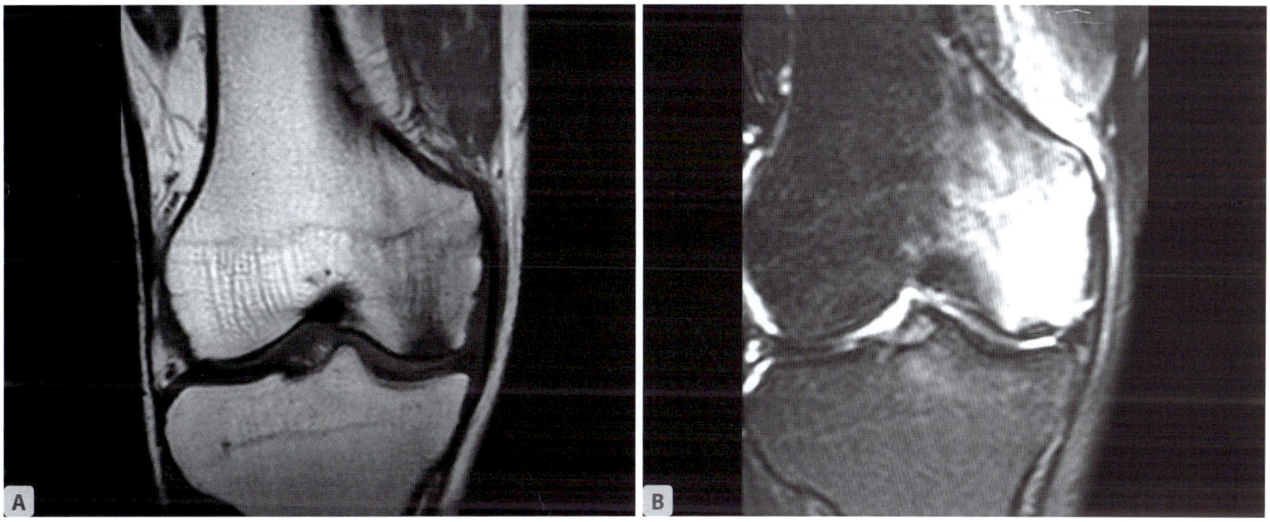

FIGS. 49A AND B: (A) T1W coronal; and (B) STIR coronal MR images showing extensive marrow edema in the medial femoral condyle along with a crescentic subchondral focus of low-signal intensity—spontaneous osteonecrosis of the knee.

OSTEOCHONDRAL LESIONS OF THE KNEE

The term "osteochondral lesion" refers to a localized abnormality of the articular cartilage and subchondral bone. This may be seen as a scalloped defect along the articular surface of the bone.

Spontaneous Osteonecrosis

As the name implies, spontaneous osteonecrosis of the knee (SPONK/SONK) is a condition that affects the knee and results in an area of subchondral necrosis. Although long thought to represent a form of primary osteonecrosis, recent studies have concluded that this lesion is actually a subchondral insufficiency fracture (SIF) that results in a devitalized segment of bone between the fracture line and overlying articular cartilage.[87] The primary event is thus a SIF followed by secondary necrosis limited to the area between the fracture line and the subchondral bone. SONK is basically a SIF that progresses into collapse. Hence, the term spontaneous osteonecrosis is a misnomer and is a condition completely different from primary osteonecrosis of the knee.

Spontaneous osteonecrosis is a distinct clinicopathological entity characterized by an older age of onset (most commonly an elderly woman), an abrupt onset of symptoms, acute onset of pain, a predilection for the weight bearing surface of medial femoral condyle, and a unique MRI appearance. The patients who develop osteonecrosis are elderly and osteoporotic. The osteoporotic bone is susceptible to microfracture leading to accumulation of fluid within the subchondral bone seen as extensive edema on the MR images. Initial radiographs are often normal in spontaneous osteonecrosis even though the pain is severe, and the patient is unable to ambulate. On MRI, extensive edema-like signal is seen in the medial femoral condyle along with a linear subchondral focus of low-signal intensity that represents the insufficiency fracture[88] **(Figs. 49A and B)**. A length of 14 mm and a thickness of

4 mm for these subchondral low-signal intensity areas are indicative of evolution to collapsed osteonecrosis. Deeply located low signal lines with respect to subchondral bone also indicate irreversible osteonecrosis. Medial meniscal tears have also been reported in association with spontaneous osteonecrosis.

This entity needs to be differentiated from osteochondritis dissecans (OCD) and from transient bone marrow edema syndrome. The lesion in OCD is typically in a different location on the lateral aspect of medial femoral condyle.[89] Histologically, the osteochondritic lesion is composed of hyaline articular cartilage covering a metabolically active ossific nucleus. The lesion in osteonecrosis consists of dead bone. Loose bodies are a frequent result of osteochondritis—in fact they may be the presenting symptom in OCD but they are unusual in osteonecrosis.[90]

Juvenile and Adult Osteochondritis Dissecans[91]

Osteochondritis dissecans is an idiopathic focal alteration of subchondral bone that carries the risk for instability and disruption of adjacent articular cartilage. OCD may result in premature OA. While acute traumatic osteochondral lesions first affect the articular cartilage and the bone later ("outside in" mechanism), OCD lesions involve the cartilage later (inside out mechanism). The condition manifests itself either in childhood (juvenile OCD) or middle age (adult OCD), but the most frequent age of onset is preadolescence. Several theories have been postulated for its etiology. It has been suggested by some to result from repetitive trauma that causes shear forces across the cartilage. The alternative theory, more popular recently, is that OCD is an avascular lesion attributed to an insufficient end arterial blood supply to the subarticular trabeculae and poor anastomoses with the neighboring systems resulting in the infarctions of small wedge-shaped pieces of bone immediately beneath the articular cartilage. Whatever be the etiology, the insult causes a disturbance of a small area of epiphyseal growth plate which results in localized delay or cessation of normal ossification. The affected epiphyseal segment remains cartilaginous while the rest of the epiphysis continues to ossify and expand in a centrifugal fashion. This creates an appearance of a radiolucent crater which basically represents hindered cartilage ossification and is called a "progeny" segment. The progeny segment may later develop laminar calcifications in the deep areas or may ossify partially or completely.[91] When the OCD lesion cannot withstand forces applied to the joint, it separates from the "parent" bone. The sequence of events is as follows 5 cleft/rim at the interface between the fragment and adjacent bone -> fragment instability -> disruption of the bone and overlying articular cartilage -> fragment separation. The fragment may separate completely to form a loose body or it may remain in its crater in the femoral condyle.

The typical location of an OCD lesion is the lateral aspect of the medial femoral condyle. Radiographic findings include a geographic subchondral lucency along the nonweight bearing surface of the medial femoral condyle. MRI plays an important role in detecting the lesion if plain films are normal. It usually shows a crescentic or ovoid focus of subchondral signal abnormality. MRI can also allow characterization of various tissue components of the progeny fragment. Gradient recalled echo sequences show nonmineralized portions of the fragment. The primary concern when evaluating a focus of OCD is whether the fragment of subchondral bone is unstable or stable. The four signs of instability described on MRI include **(Figs. 50A to C)**:

1. T2W MR images reveal a high-signal intensity rim at the interface between the fragment and adjacent bone.
2. Fluid-filled cysts beneath the lesion.
3. A high-signal intensity line extending through the articular cartilage overlying the lesion.
4. A focal osteochondral defect filled with joint fluid.

All four criteria when present indicate a 100% sensitivity and 100% specificity for instability in adult OCD. However, these criteria are not specific for juvenile OCD. These criteria have been revised for juvenile OCD with the addition of three secondary signs:[91]

1. A high-signal intensity rim surrounding a juvenile OCD lesion indicates instability only if it has the same signal intensity as that of joint fluid.
2. A second outer rim of T2W low-signal intensity.

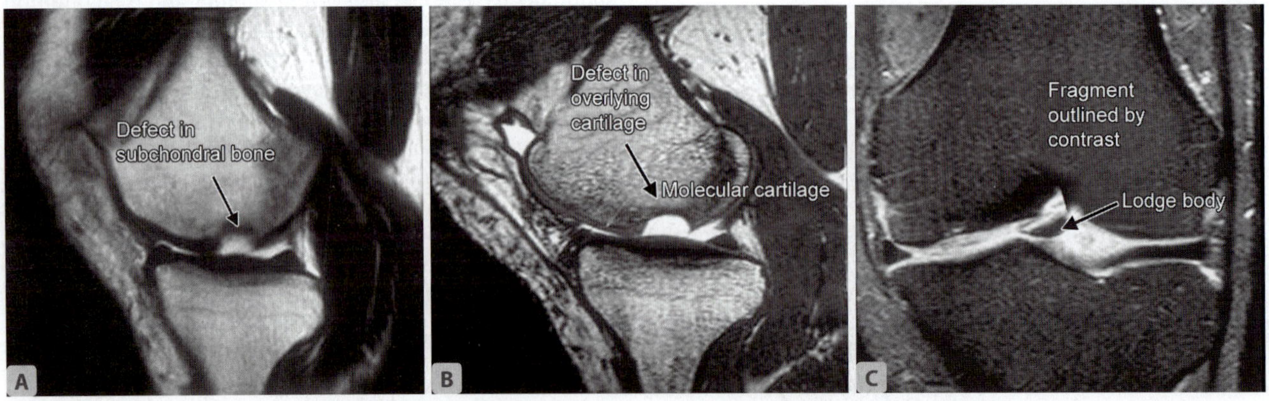

FIGS. 50A TO C: (A) Sagittal T2W; (B) DESS sagittal plane images showing a defect in the subchondral bone and overlying cartilage; and (C) Indirect MR arthrography showing the displaced fragment outlined by contrast—osteochondritis dissecans.

3. Multiple breaks in the subchondral bone plate on the T2W MR images.

The rim of fluid-filled signal intensity surrounding an OCD lesion represents a cleft filled with fluid between the parent bone and progeny. The outer rim of low-signal intensity represents fibrous tissue and subchondral cysts should be multiple and larger than 5 mm for the lesion to be unstable.

MRI of the knee is an excellent diagnostic tool that provides information about the composition, integrity, and stability of the OCD segment.

These osteochondral lesions may predispose to OA. An assessment of the overlying articular cartilage is important to guide appropriate treatment. Once OA occurs, it may be impossible to determine the original cause and treatment options may be limited to joint replacement.

Transient Bone Marrow Edema Syndrome (Transient Osteoporosis)

Transient bone marrow edema syndrome (also known as transient osteoporosis) was first described in the hip. In the knee, the lateral femoral condyle is usually involved, although involvement of the medial femoral condyle and tibial plateau has also been described. Affected patients present with an acute onset of pain usually not associated with trauma. Resolution of pain and edema usually takes place within 6 to 12 months. Long-term sequelae do not occur. MRI findings include diffuse edema (low signal on T1W images and high signal on T2W or STIR sequences) without a focal area of signal abnormality typical of osteonecrosis.[92]

There is a considerable difference in clinical prognosis and treatment of transient osteoporosis as compared to spontaneous osteonecrosis. Hence, it is important to differentiate between these two entities. The differentiating features include:

- Absence of low-signal intensity in subchondral areas on T2W MR images is indicative of complete reversibility.
- Absence of focal deformity of the epiphyseal contour is indicative of complete reversibility.
- Spontaneous osteonecrosis of the knee typically involves medial femoral condyle while transient osteoporosis is more commonly seen in the lateral femoral condyle.

MISCELLANEOUS LESIONS

Bursae[1]

Several bursae may be seen around the knee joint. At times, these can mimic intra-articular pathology and need to be differentiated.

Popliteal (Baker's Cysts)[4]

Popliteal (Baker's cysts) of the gastrocnemius semimembranosus bursae arise between medial head of the gastrocnemius muscle and the more medial semimembranosus tendon. A narrow neck connecting the cyst to the joint may be seen on axial images **(Figs. 51A and B)**. Popliteal cysts may arise from any condition that causes an increase in synovial fluid within the joint and are frequently seen in association with tears of the posterior horn of the medial meniscus.[60] Popliteal cysts at times can become very large and cause compartment syndrome. The rupture in the adjacent musculature can cause intense inflammation, mimic deep vein thrombosis, and be very symptomatic.

Prepatellar Bursa

Also called the housemaid's knee, prepatellar bursitis is a common cause of anterior knee pain. It is seen as a fluid collection anterior to the patella.

Pes Anserinus Bursa

Also called the "goose's foot" (webbed foot appearance), it refers to the configuration of the insertion of the pes tendons on to the tibia. Gracilis, sartorius, and semitendinosus constitute the pes anserinus tendons. The bursa lies beneath the tendons and on being inflamed may be seen to extend

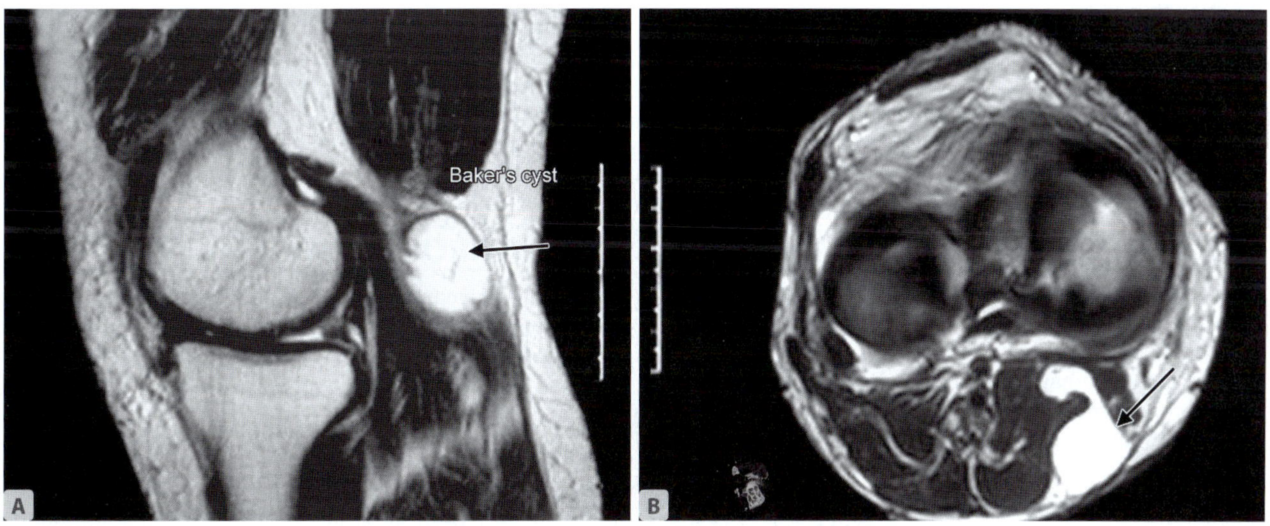

FIGS. 51A AND B: (A) T2W sagittal; and (B) T2W axial MR images of the knee showing fluid intensity cystic structure between the medial head of gastrocnemius and the more medial semimembranosus tendon—popliteal/Baker's cyst.

proximally toward the joint. Pes Anserinus bursitis is seen just below the joint line on the anteromedial tibia.[4]

Semimembranosus-tibial Collateral Ligament Bursa

This bursa occurs on the joint line and drapes like a horseshoe over the semimembranosus tendon. It may mimic a meniscal cyst but no connection to a meniscus is, however found.

Tibial Collateral Ligament Bursa

This lies deep to the MCL and extends vertically above and below the joint line. The finding of the fluid being well contained and cyst like rather than being diffusely distributed separates it from meniscocapsular separation.

Medullary Infarction

Several factors, e.g., steroids, trauma, vasculitis are known to predispose to the development of focal areas of medullary infarction. Medullary infarcts result in geographic areas of ischemic and devitalized marrow that produce a characteristic MRI appearance; a geographic focus of typically heterogeneous signal within the marrow that is surrounded by characteristic low-signal intensity, serpentine border on T1W images. This border often demonstrates a classic double-line sign on T2W images. This is one of the few medullary lesions that usually contain some central fat. The presence of central fat is characteristic of this lesion.

Reflex Sympathetic Dystrophy

The exact cause of reflex sympathetic dystrophy (RSD) is unclear but it is believed to represent sequelae from hyperactivity of the sympathetic nervous system. In many cases, it occurs after a recent episode of trauma. It results in circulatory changes and may progress to muscle atrophy, contractures, pale skin, and loss of hair on the extremity. MRI reveals diffuse, patchy bone marrow edema, which does not progress to the subchondral collapse seen in osteonecrosis. MRI findings which suggest the diagnosis of RSD include skin thickening, contrast enhancement, muscular atrophy, soft tissue edema, and joint effusions.[93]

BONE INFECTIONS

Capsular distension and joint effusions can be seen in MR scans of infected joints but are nonspecific findings.[94] A septic joint may be further characterized by intra-articular debris and synovitis from hematogenous seeding. In cases of osteomyelitis, the metaphysis, an active site of bone formation in children may show signal abnormalities (low signal on T1, bright signal on T2 or STIR images) restricted to this region. Marrow infiltration and soft tissue extension of osteomyelitis can be demonstrated using STIR and fat suppressed T2W image **(Figs. 52A to D)**. Supportive findings include overlying cortical destruction and an abscess or fistula extending to bone. A low-signal intensity rim sign has been described in chronic infection resulting from trauma. This rim of fibrous tissue or reactive bone displays low signal on all pulse sequences and surrounds the area of active bone disease.

Magnetic resonance is also used to evaluate subacute osteomyelitis including Brodie's abscess. In Brodie's abscess, the focus of involvement of osteomyelitis is hyperintense on STIR and fat suppressed T2W images. The sclerotic margin displays low signal on all pulse sequences and there may be fluid in communication with the central infected focus.[5]

BONE NEOPLASMS

Magnetic resonance imaging has become an important component in the evaluation of primary bone neoplasms because of its ability to detect and accurately determine the local extent of disease. MRI and MR spectroscopy may also be helpful in following a patient's response to therapy. Osteogenic sarcoma is one of the most common primary bone tumors emanating from the distal femur. The extent of intramedullary disease is best defined with T1W spin echo or STIR images while T2W images may provide information about full extent disease and edema into the soft tissues. Encasement of major vessels and nerves as well as involvement of multiple muscular compartment may all be evaluated by MR and may decrease the efficacy of limb salvage surgery **(Figs. 53A to D)**.[95]

Infiltrative neoplasms such as leukemia and lymphoma may present with knee pain indistinguishable from that caused by internal derangements of knee. These lesions need to be distinguished from signal inhomogeneity of normal marrow bone in metaphyses caused by variations in extent of hematopoietic marrow. Most types of marrow pathology result in signal intensity that is lower than that of skeletal muscle or intervertebral disc on T1W images whereas hematopoietic marrow demonstrates signal intensity that is slightly higher than that of skeletal muscle or disc on T1W images (owing to the relatively high amount of fat present even in red marrow). Other features of red marrow include signal intensity that parallels the signal intensity of other areas of known hematopoietic marrow, bilateral symmetry, scattered foci of fatty signal within the region of concern, and an abrupt margination at the level of a closed physis. Also, in contrast to the normal hematopoietic marrow, infiltrative disorders usually present a homogeneous low signal intensity mass on T1W images and show well-defined margin.

Magnetic resonance imaging is also helpful in evaluating benign bony neoplasms. MRI characterizes the components of an osteochondroma better than other imaging techniques such as CT. The cartilaginous cap is well-visualized by MRI and should be less than 1 cm in the non-neoplastic disease.[51]

MR ARTHROGRAPHY

Intra-articular contrast material enhances the diagnostic capabilities of MRI especially in the depiction of small structure and subtle disease.

Technique

The direct MR arthrographic technique does not differ from conventional arthrography. The knee is placed in a slightly bent, recumbent position for the usually used anterolateral access. The patella is pulled laterally and the puncture is

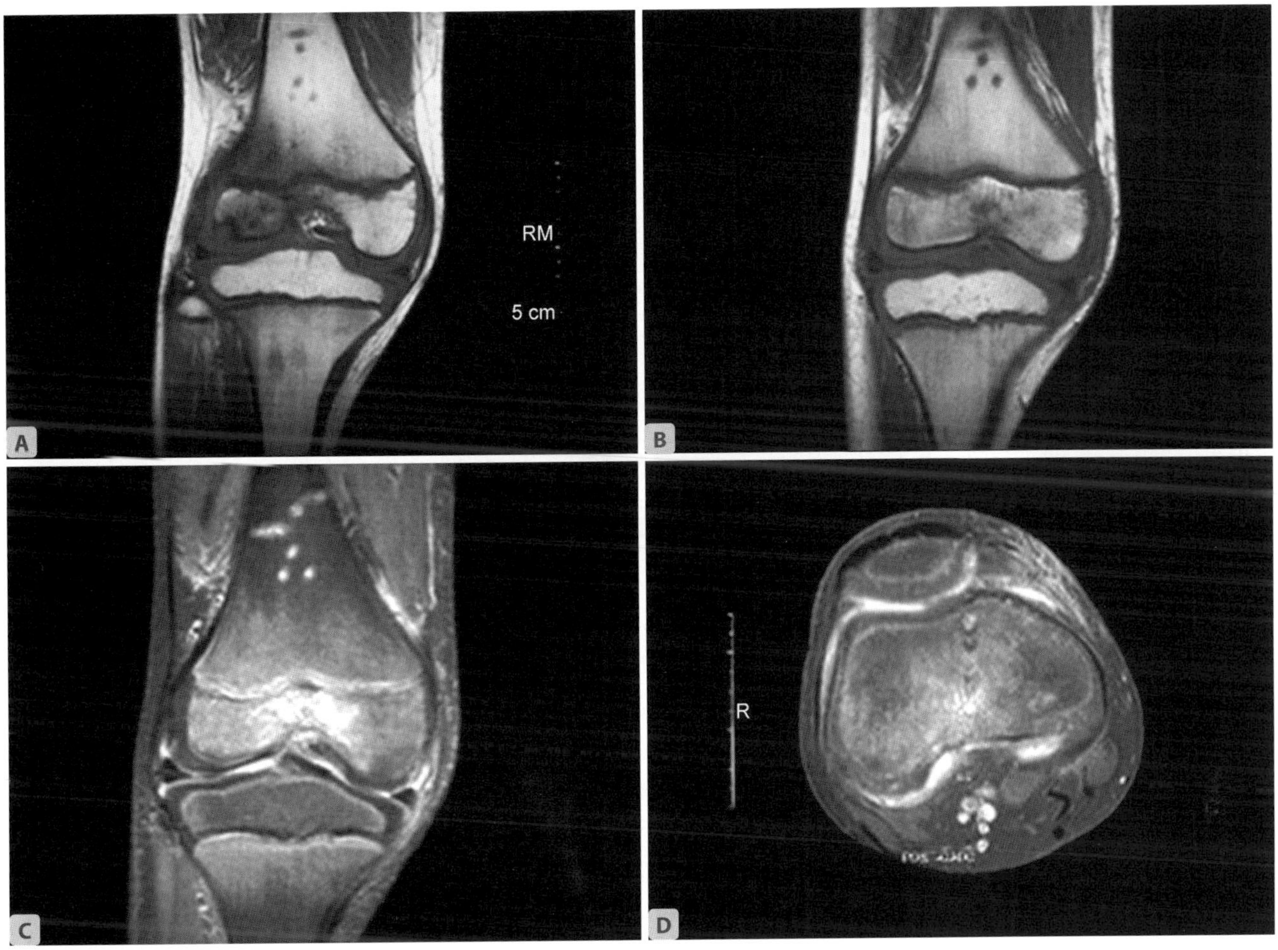

FIGS. 52A TO D: T1 coronal (A) and (B) postgadolinium coronal (C) postgadolinium T1 axial (D) images showing erosion of the articular margin of femur, fuzziness of the articular margins, marrow signal alteration, joint effusion, and thick enhancing synovium—septic arthritis.

made mid-patella or above with the needle entering the joint beneath the surface of the patella. To be able to fill the knee joint with a small volume of dissolved contrast medium, compression is applied to the soft tissues 15–20 cm above the joint cavity with an elastic bandage to prevent entry of the contrast medium into the suprapatellar recess. The injection is carried out under sterile conditions. The total amount of the dilute contrast mixture (Gd-DTPA) injected should be 30–40 mL. After the injection, active and passive movements of the knee joint are carried out several times to achieve uniform distribution in the joint. An arthrographic effect or indirect MR arthrography can also be achieved with joint fluid enhancement following intravenous injection of Gd-DTPA. This method is referred to as indirect MR arthrography since no articular injection is required. The role of MR arthrography is in the following lesions:

- *Meniscal lesions*: MR arthrography has been shown to have a greater accuracy than conventional MRI for the detection of meniscal retears.[96] Because gadolinium-based contrast material has a lower viscosity than synovial fluid, it is more likely to be imbibed into a small cleft and thereby highlight the presence of a tear.
- *Cartilage lesions*: Administration of intra-articular contrast agent allows excellent delineation of the cartilage surface and provides good discrimination of cartilaginous lesions which have been graded from I to IV.[97] MR arthrography allows detection of grade II to IV lesions, however, grade I lesions still remain difficult to detect by arthrography since grade I lesions have no surface abnormality that is detected by intra-articular Gd-DTPA solution. On delayed sequences, however, an enhancement effect in cartilaginous areas with altered intrachondral structures can be observed. This is caused by diffusion of contrast material into the hyaline cartilage, although the thickness and surface of the cartilage may still appear normal in grade I lesions.
- *Osteochondritis dissecans*: OCD is a lesion that characteristically affects the articular cartilage and subchondral bone with the potential of fragmentation and separation. Early detection of osteochondral lesion is desirable because the onset of degenerative arthritis in patients with OCD is estimated to occur 10 years earlier than in normal individuals. Management and prognosis of these osteochondral lesions depend on the stability of the fragment within its bony crater and the status of the overlying articular cartilage. MR arthrography is more accurate than MR in staging these osteochondral lesions of the knee.[98]

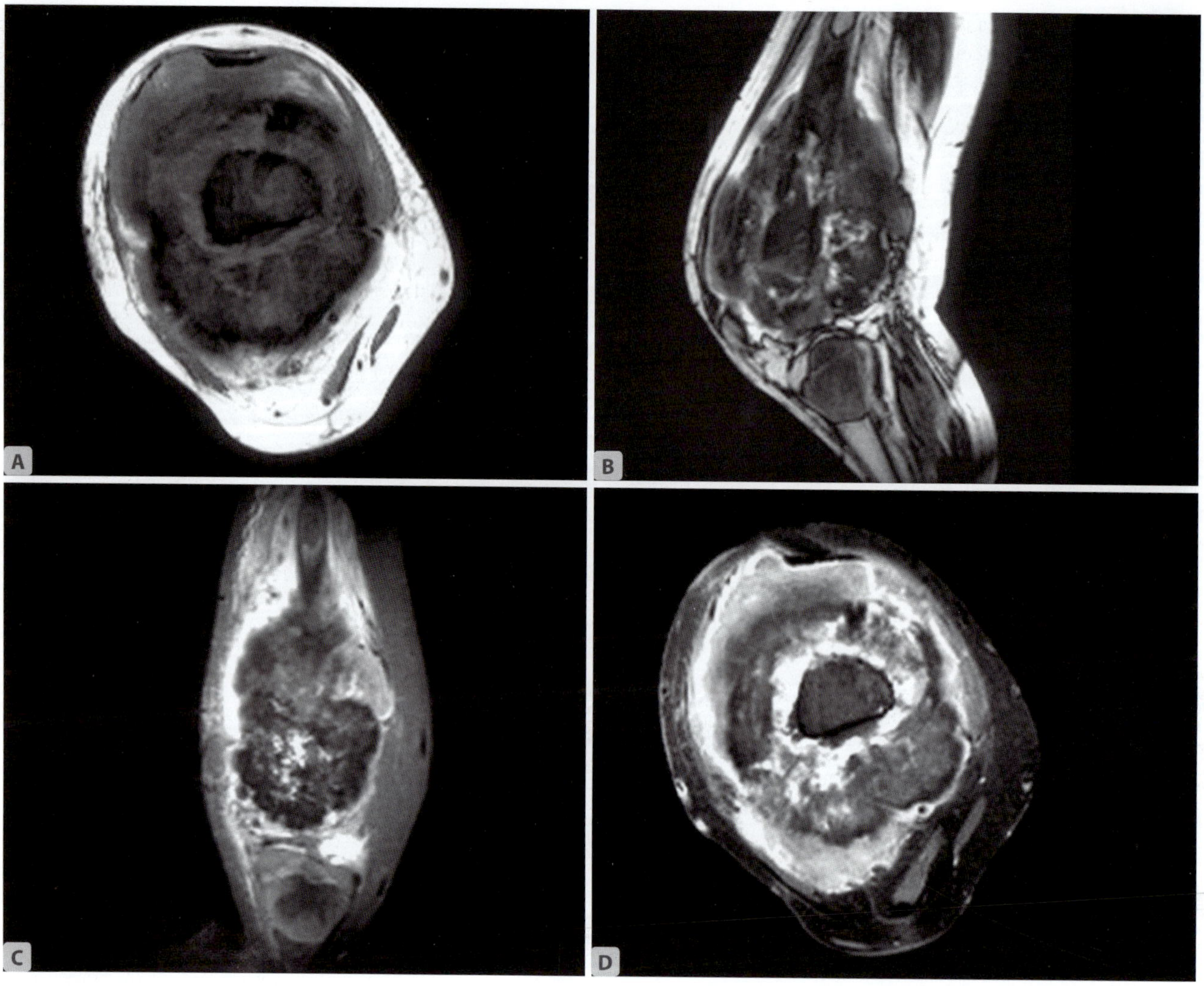

FIGS. 53A TO D: (A) T1 axial; (B) T2 sagittal; (C) T1 postcontrast coronal; and (D) Axial MR images showing an irregular circumferential heterogeneous mass arising from the lower metadiaphyseal region of femur with cortical destruction, spiculated periosteal reaction, new bone formation, infiltration of medulla and multicompartment muscle involvement. Skip/metastatic focus also seen in upper tibia—osteogenic sarcoma lower end femur.

- *Intra-articular bodies*: The knee is affected most commonly by intra-articular bodies. These may consist of bone, cartilage or both bone and cartilage. Imaging is necessary to confirm the clinical diagnosis and to localize these bodies before surgery, because intra-articular bodies may be missed during arthroscopy. Radiography and conventional tomography are useful only when radiopaque intra-articular bodies are present. MR arthrography has the greatest sensitivity (86%) which is significantly more sensitive than conventional MRI.[99]
- *Plica synovialis*: The three plicae of the knee (suprapatellar plica, medial patellar plica, and infrapatellar plica) are remnants of the embryologic synovium that separate the joint into different compartments during gestation. Partial plical remnants are often identified at arthroscopy but are incidental findings without clinical significance. Some plicae may persist into adult life and cause anterior knee pain, clicking, catching or locking of the knee when these plicae become inflamed and thickened by trauma or overuse.

The mediopatellar plica which extends from underneath the quadriceps and slides over the medial femoral condyle with knee movement is of great pathologic importance. The plica is usually attached closely to the femoral condyle and is not visualized when there is insufficient synovial fluid to outline. Differentiation between knee injuries and mediopatellar plica is important to avoid unnecessary arthroscopy. MR arthrography enables assessment of thickened plicae and should be considered as an alternative to diagnostic arthroscopy in patients with mediopatellar plica.[100]

POSTOPERATIVE EVALUATION OF THE KNEE

New developments and improvements in the ligamentous and meniscal surgery and cartilage repair procedures have led to an increased incidence of these procedures being performed. Subsequently there is an increase in the postoperative imaging studies and it is imperative for the radiologist to know the normal imaging appearance and complication of these procedures.

Imaging of the ACL Graft

The most commonly injured ligament in the knee is the ACL. ACL-deficient knees can result in changes in mechanics causing secondary meniscal and cartilage injury. Hence, reconstruction of ACLs is being undertaken more commonly. FSE is preferred over conventional spin echo because of the decreased metallic artifact seen with FSE.[101] An addition, an oblique sagittal scan, is often performed in the plane of the graft to allow better visualization of the ACL graft on one slice. Use of thinner 3 mm sections reduces volume averaging artifacts and provides better delineation of the neoalignment. An ACL neoalignment is considered intact if a smooth well-defined low-signal intensity band is seen along its entire course on both T1W and T2W images. The MR criteria used to assess disruption are contour irregularity, increased signal intensity within the ligament on T2W images, and discontinuity of the ligament.

Graft Rupture

Spontaneous graft rupture is rare and is frequently secondary to trauma. The same criteria used to diagnose a torn native ACL are used to diagnose a ruptured ACL graft and include discontinuity of normal fibers **(Figs. 54A and B)** and abnormal signal intensity within the substance of the graft which is usually fluid signal intensity interrupting the graft.

Graft Impingement

Graft impingement occurs when the graft abnormally contacts either the wall or the roof of the intercondylar notch. Impingement can lead to stretching, erosion, remodeling, and tearing of the graft.

In impingement, MRI shows the tibial tunnel to project anterior to a line drawn along the intercondylar roof and extended to the tibial plateau (Blumensaat's line). The distal two-thirds of the graft show increased signal intensity on T2W images,[102] however, this is never fluid signal intensity unlike in graft rupture.

Arthrofibrosis

Following ACL reconstruction loss of terminal extension (extension lag) is one of the major causes of morbidity. One of the major etiologies causing extension lag is localized anterior arthrofibrosis. In this condition, a focal fibrous nodule develops anterior to the distal portion of the ACL within the intercondylar notch. The nodule physically impairs terminal extension of the knee. The bluish discoloration of this rounded lesion resembles an eyeball on arthroscopy and has been named the cyclops lesion.[103] Cyclops lesion can be identified on MRI. On T1W and PD-weighted images, nodular intermediate-signal intensity mass is seen at the anterior distal aspect of the graft in the intercondylar notch. On T2W images, the nodule has a heterogeneous but predominantly low-signal intensity.

Postoperative Meniscus

The criteria for diagnosing meniscal tears in the virgin meniscus do not apply to the post-meniscectomy knee because there can be residual abnormal signal intensity and morphology. This is especially important when greater than 25% of the meniscus is removed in which the remaining meniscus can appear foreshortened with an irregular margin. In addition, abnormal signal can also be seen in stable meniscal remnants. The specificity of these findings for meniscal retear is lower than that for tears in nonoperative menisci. Several studies have reported an accuracy of 66–80% in the postoperative meniscus.[96]

Signal changes within the meniscus at a site distant from the original tear, *fluid signal intensity* in the meniscus

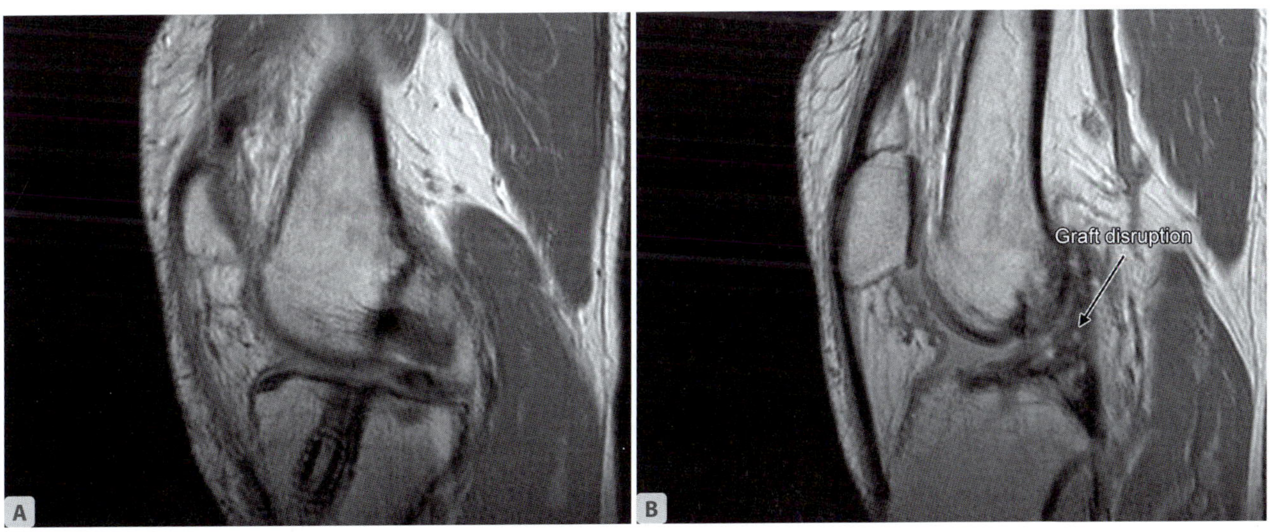

FIGS. 54A AND B: T2W sagittal MR images in a postoperative knee with anterior cruciate ligament graft showing discontinuity of the graft fibers with high-signal intensity within—graft disruption.

remnant and a displaced fragment are specific signs of a meniscal retear but are not very sensitive. Direct MR arthrography increases the accuracy of diagnosing retears of the postoperative meniscus.

Postoperative Articular Cartilage

The development of new cartilage repair procedures that transplant or potentially reform hyaline-like articular cartilage has led to an accurate noninvasive evaluation of the cartilage lesions following repair procedures.

Magnetic resonance imaging has been used to assess incorporation of grafts, assess vascularity of grafts, evaluate the congruency between the graft and the native cartilage and bone, and assess the donor site. One complication associated with this procedure is incongruence of the graft. Other complications include loose bodies, avascular necrosis of the donor site, and condylar fracture which are all detected by MRI.

Autologous chondrocyte implantation involves harvesting chondrocytes from the relative nonweight bearing surfaces such as intercondylar notch. The chondrocytes are grown *ex vivo* and replaced into the periosteal covered site of the cartilage defect. Chondrocytes progress through several stages. Initially in the proliferative stage there is formation of a jelly-like substance. The second stage (7–12 weeks), known as the transition stage, involves formation of a type II collagen framework. From 13 weeks to 3 years, the maturation stage involves remodeling of the collagen framework resulting in firm hyaline tissue. MRI can assess the rate of and characteristics of growth cartilage and its incorporation within the native cartilage. The state of the underlying subchondral bone can also be assessed by MRI.

Magnetic resonance imaging and arthroscopy are complementary examinations for follow-up of autologous chondrocyte implants in knee. Arthroscopy is better used for assessing the cartilage surface and MR is better used for assessing lesions deep within the cartilage and underlying bone.[104,105]

ARTIFICIAL INTELLIGENCE IN THE EVALUATION OF KNEE PATHOLOGY[106]

The integration of artificial intelligence (AI) algorithms into the workflow of MSK radiology has the potential to improve diagnostic accuracy, reduce reader fatigue, expedite cases with urgent findings, and provide decision support. The CNNs or convolutional neural networks can detect pathology (tear of ligaments/meniscus, cartilage lesion), help in classification (grading OA on knee radiographs, meniscal tears), and provide cartilage and meniscus segmentation. AI thus holds the potential for lesion detection, characterization, and disease monitoring but a lot of work is needed to achieve this.[106]

CONCLUSION

Magnetic resonance imaging is clearly the imaging modality of choice for detecting and exploring joint, osseous, and soft tissue injuries in the knee. MRI plays a pivotal role in making a precise diagnosis and then guiding treatment decisions. It is also extremely helpful in imaging the postoperative knee and in determining the response to therapy. It should be the goal of any radiologist who interprets MRI examinations of the knee to be able to recognize not only the normal anatomy and accurately diagnose pathology but also to develop a better grasp of the surgical implications of the imaging findings. By thinking like an arthroscopist, one can provide a more clinically relevant report and by doing so, add value to the workup of a patient with any knee pathology.

REFERENCES

1. Reicher MA, Bassett LW, Gold RH. High resolution MRI of the knee joint. Pathologic correlations. AJR. 1985;145(5):903-9.
2. Reicher MA, Hartzman S, Duckwiler GR, Bassett LW, Anderson LJ, Gold RH. Meniscal injuries. Detection using MR imaging. Radiology. 1986;159(3):753-7.
3. Hartzman S, Reicher MA, Bassett LW, Duckwiler GR, Mandelbaum B, Gold RH. MR imaging of the knee. Chronic disorder. Radiology. 1987;162:553-7.
4. Kaplan PA. Knee. In: Kaplan PA, Helms CA, Dussault R, Anderson MW, Major NM (Eds). Musculoskeletal MRI, 1st edition. US: WB Saunders; 2001.
5. Stoller DW, Cannon WD, Anderson LJ. The knee. In: Stoller DW (Ed). Magnetic Resonance Imaging in Orthopaedics and Sports Medicine, 2nd edition. Philadelphia: Lippincott Raven; 1997.
6. Ariyachaipanich A, Bae WC, Statum S, Chung CB. Update on MRI pulse sequences for the knee: Imaging of cartilage, meniscus, tendon and hardware. Semin Musculoskeletal Radiol. 2017;21(2):45-62.
7. Bassett GC. The meniscus. Orthopaedics. 1992;15:35-42.
8. Koski JA, Ibarra C, Rodeo SA, Warren RF. Meniscal injury and repair. Clinical status. Orthop Clin North Am. 2000;31:419-35.
9. Escobedo EM, Hunter JC, Zink-Brody GC, Wilson AJ, Harrison SD, Fisher DJ. Usefulness of turbo spin-echo MR imaging in the evaluation of meniscal tears. Comparison with a conventional spin echo sequence. Am J Roentgenol. 1996;167(5):1223-7.
10. Kowalchuk RM, Kneeland JB, Dalinka MK, Siegelman ES, Dockery WD. MRI of the knee. Value of short echo time fast spin echo using high performance gradients versus conventional spin echo imaging for the detection of meniscal tears. Skeletal Radiol. 2000;29(9):520-4.
11. Helms CA, Laorr A, Cannon WD. The absent bow-tie sign in Bucket handle tears of the menisci in knee. Am J Roentgenol. 1998;170(1):57-61.
12. Ryu KN, Kim IS, Kim EJ, Ahn JW, Bae DK, Sartoris DJ, et al. MR imaging of tears of discoid lateral menisci. Am J Roentgenol. 1998;171(4):963-7.
13. Yu JS, Cosgarea AJ, Kaeding CC, Wilson D. Meniscal flounce MR imaging. Radiology. 1997;203(2):513-5.
14. Schnarkowski P, Tirman PF, Fuchigami KD, Crues JV, Butler MG, Genant HK. Meniscal ossicle: radiographic and MR imaging findings. Radiology. 1995;196(1):47-50.
15. Hajek PC, Gylys Morin VM, Baker LL, Sartoris DJ, Haghighi P, Resnick D. The high signal intensity meniscus of the knee magnetic resonance evaluation and *in vivo* correlation. Invest Radiol. 1987;22(11):883-90.

16. Kaplan PA, Nelson NL, Garvin KL, Brown DE. MR of the knee. The significance of high signal in the meniscus that does not clearly extend to the surface. Am J Roentgenol. 1991;156(2):333-6.
17. Davis SJ, Teresi LM. The "Notch" sign: meniscal contour deformities as indicators of tear in MR imaging of the knee. J Comput Assist Tomography. 1990;14:975-80.
18. Seung JY, Seunghun L, Song Y. Two slice touch rule in meniscal tear. Radiology. 2016;280(2):649-50.
19. Campbell SE, Sanders TG, Morrison WB. MR imaging of meniscal cysts: incidence, location and clinical significance. Am J Roentgenol. 2001;177(2):409-13.
20. Harper KW, Helms CA, Lambert HS III, Higgins LD. Radial Meniscal tears: significance incidence and MR appearance. AM J Roentgenol. 2005;185(6):1429-34.
21. Tuckman GA, Miller WJ, Remo JW, Fritts HM, Rozansky MI. Radial tears of the menisci: MR findings. Am J Roentgenol. 1994;163(2):395-400.
22. Ozkor G, Circi E Gone U, Irgit K, Pourbagher A, Tandogan RN. Radial tears in the root of the posterior horn of the medial meniscus. Knee Surg Sports Traumatol Arthrosc. 2008;16(9):849-54.
23. Wright DH, De Smet AA, Norris M. Bucket handle tears of the medial and lateral menisci of the knee: value of MR imaging in detecting displaced fragments. Am J Roentgenol. 1995;165(3):621-5.
24. Singson R, Feldman F, Staron R, Kiernan H. MR imaging of displaced meniscal bucket handle tear of the medial meniscus. Am J Roentgenol. 1991;156(1):121-4.
25. Rao N, Patel Y, Opsha O, Chen Q, Owen J, Elsemon E, et al. Use of the V-sign in the diagnosis of bucket handle meniscal tear of the knee. Skeletal Radiol. 2012;41(3):293-7.
26. Belzer JP, Cannon WD. Meniscus tears: treatment in the stable and unstable knee. J Am Acad Orthop Surg. 1993;1(1):41-7.
27. Nguyen JC, Smet A, Graf BK, Rosas HG. MR imaging based diagnosis and classification of meniscal tears. Radiographics. 2014;34(4):981-99.
28. Bergin D, Hochberg H, Zoga AC, Qazi N, Parker L, Morrison WB. Indirect soft tissue and osseous signs on knee MRI of surgically proven meniscal tears. Am J Roentgenol. 2008;191(1):86-92.
29. Vahey TN, Bennett HT, Arrington LE, Shelbourne KD, Ng J. MR imaging of the knee: pseudotear of the lateral meniscus caused by the meniscofemoral ligament. Am J Roentgenol. 1990;154(6):1237-9.
30. Watanabe AT, Carter BC, Teitelbaum GP, Seeger LL, Bradley WG Jr. Normal variations in MR imaging of the knee: appearance and frequency. Am J Roentgenol. 1989;153(2):341-4.
31. Peterfy CG, Janzen DL, Tirman PF, van Dijke CF, Pollack M, Genant HK. Magic-angle phenomenon: a cause of increased signal in the normal lateral meniscus on short TE MR images of the knee. Am J Roentgenol. 1994;163(1):149-54.
32. Henning CE, Lynch MA. Current concepts of meniscal function and pathology. Clin Sports Med. 1985;4(2):259-64.
33. Matava MJ, Eck K, Totty W, Wright RW, Shively RA. Magnetic resonance imaging as a tool to predict meniscal reparability. Am J Sports Med. 1999;27(4):436-43.
34. Reicher MA, Hartzman S, Bassett LW, Mandelbaum B, Duckwiler G, Gold RH. MR imaging of the knee traumatic disorders. Radiology. 1987;162(2):547-51.
35. Crues JV, Mink J, Levy TL, Lotysch M, Stoller DW. Meniscal tears of the knee: accuracy of MR imaging. Radiology. 1987;164(2):445-8.
36. Bencardino JT, Rosenber ZS, Brown RR, Hassankhani A, Lustrin ES, Beltran J. Traumatic musculotendinous injuries of the knee: diagnosis with MR imaging. Radiographics. 2000;20:103-20.
37. Lee JK, Yao L, Phelps CT, Wirth CR, Czajka J, Lozman J. Anterior cruciate ligament tears. MR imaging compared with arthroscopy and clinical tests. Radiology. 1988;166(3):861-4.
38. Chan WP, Peterfy C, Fritz RC, Genant HK. MR diagnosis of complete tears of the anterior cruciate ligament of the knee: importance of anterior subluxation of tibia. Am J Roentgenol. 1994;162(2):355-60.
39. Kaplan PA, Gehl RH, Dussault RG, Anderson MW, Diduch DR. Bone contusions of the posterior lip of the medial tibial plateau (countercoup injury) and associated internal derangements of the knee at MR imaging. Radiology. 1999;211(3):747-53.
40. Graf BK, Cook DA, De Smat AA, Keene JS. Bone bruises on magnetic resonance imaging evaluation of anterior cruciate ligament injuries. Am J Sports Med. 1993;21(2):220-3.
41. Tung GA, Davis LM, Wiggins ME, Fadale PD. Tears of the anterior cruciate ligament: primary and secondary signs at MR imaging. Radiology. 1993;188(3):661-7.
42. Vanhoenacker F, Vos ND, Dyck PV. Common mistakes and pitfalls in magnetic resonance imaging of the knee. Journal of the Belgian Society of Radiology. 2016;100(1):1-17.
43. Covey DC, Sapega AA. Anatomy and function of the posterior cruciate ligament. Clin Sports Med. 1994;13(3):509-18.
44. Hansford BG, Yablon CM. Multiligamentous injury of the knee: MRI diagnosis and injury pattern. Semin Musculoskeletal Radiol. 2017;21(2):63-74.
45. D Maesaneer M, Von Roy F, Lenchik L, Barbaix E, De Ridder F, Osteaux M. Three layers of the medial capsular and supporting structures of the knee: MR imaging-anatomic correlation. Radiographics. 2000;20:83-9.
46. Schweitzer MS, Tran D, Deely DM, Hume EL. Medial collateral ligament injuries: evaluation of multiple signs, prevalence and location of associated bone bruises and assessment with MR imaging. Radiology. 1995;194(3):825-9.
47. Mendes LF, Preeterklieber ML, Cho JH, Garcia GM, Resnick DL, Chung CB. Pellegrini Stieda disease: A heterogeneous disorder not synonymous with ossification/calcification of the tibial collateral ligament—anatomic and imaging investigation. Skeletal Radiol. 2006;35(12):916-22.
48. Rosas HG. Unraveling the posterolateral corner of the knee. Radiographics. 2016;36(6):1776-91.
49. Jadhav S, Mone S, Riascos R, Lemos DF, Swischuk LE. Comprehensive review of the anatomy, function and imaging of the popliteus and associated pathologic conditions. Radiographics. 2014;34(2):496-513.
50. Recondo JA, Salvador E, Villanua JA, Barrera MC, Gervás C, Alústiza JM. Lateral stabilising structures of the knee: functional anatomy and injuries assessed with MR imaging. Radiographics. 2000;20:91-102.
51. Yu JS, Salonen DC, Hodler J, Haghighi P, Trudell D, Resnick D. Posterolateral aspect of the knee: improved MR imaging with a coronal oblique technique. Radiology. 1996;198(1): 199-204.
52. Loredo R, Hodler J, Pedowitz R, Yeh LR, Trudell D, Resnick D. Posteromedial corner of the knee: MR Imaging with gross anatomic correlation. Skeletal Radiol. 1999;28(6):305-11.
53. Lundqnist RB, Matcuk GR, Schein AJ, Skalski MR, White EA, Forrester DM, et al. Posteromedial corner of the knee: the neglected corner. Radiographics 2015,35(4):1123-37.
54. Hayes CW, Brigido MK, Jamadar DA, Propeck T. Mechanism based pattern approach to classification of complex injuries of the knee depicted at MR imaging. Radiographics. 2000;20:121-34.
55. Menz MJ, Lucas GL. Magnetic resonance imaging of a rupture of the medial head of the gastrocnemius muscle. J Bone Joint Surg Am. 1991;73(8):1260-1.
56. Yu JS, Goodiwn D, Salonen D, Pathria MN, Resnick D, Dardani M, et al. Complete dislocation of the knee: Spectrum of associated soft tissue injuries depicted by MR imaging. Am J Roentgenol. 1995;164(1):135-9.

57. Yu JS, Petersilge C, Sartoris DJ, Pathria MN, Resnick D. MR imaging of injuries of the extensor mechanism of the knee. Radiographics. 1994;14(3):541-51.
58. Nance EP, Kaye JJ. Injuries of the quadriceps mechanism. Radiology. 1982;142(2):301-7.
59. Quinn SF, Brown TR, Demlow TA. MR imaging of patellar retinacular ligament injuries. J Magn Reson Imaging. 1993;3(6):843-7.
60. Crues JV, Manji SA, Shellock FG. Knee. In: Stark D, Bradley WG (Eds): Magnetic Resonance Imaging, 3rd edition. US: Mosby; 1999.
61. Diederichs G, Issever AS, Scheffler S. MR Imaging of patellar instability. Radiographics. 2010;30(4):961-81.
62. Shellock FG, Mink JH, Deutsch AL, Foo TK, Sullenberger P. Patellofemoral joint: identification of abnormalities with active movement 'unloaded' versus 'loaded' kinematic MR imaging techniques. Radiology. 1993;188(2):575-8.
63. Bruno F, Barile A, Arrigoni F, Laporta A, Russo A, Carotti M, et al. Weight bearing MRI of the knee: a review of advantages and limits. Acta Biomed. 2018;89:78-88.
64. Bradella MA, Tirman PFJ, Peterfy CG, Zarlingo M, Feller JF, Bost FW, et al. Accuracy of T2 weighted fast spin-echo MR imaging with fat saturation in detecting cartilage defects in the knee: comparison with arthroscopy in 130 patients. AJR. 1999;172(4):1073-80.
65. Hardy PA, Recht MP, Piraino DW. Fat suppressed MRI of articular cartilage with spatial-spectral excitation pulse. J Magn Reson Imaging. 1998;8(6):1279-87.
66. Disler DG, McCauley TR, Kelman CG, Fuchs MD, Ratner LM, Wirth CR, et al. Fat suppressed three-dimensional spoiled gradient-echo MR imaging of hyaline cartilage defects in the knee: comparison with standard MR imaging and arthroscopy. Am J Roentgenol. 1996;167(1):127-32.
67. Erickson SJ, Waldochmidt JG, Czervionke LF, Prost RW. Hyaline cartilage truncation artifact as a cause of trilaminar appearance with fat suppressed three dimensional spoiled gradient recalled sequences. Radiology. 1996;201(1):260-4.
68. Naraghi A, White LM. Three-dimensional MRI of the musculoskeletal system. Am J Roentgenol. 2012; 199(3):W283-93.
69. Kijowski R, Blankenpaker DG, Davis KW, Shinki K, Kaplan LD, De Smet AA. Comparison of 1.5 and 3.0 T MR imaging for evaluating the articular cartilage of the knee joint. Radiology. 2009;250(3):839-48.
70. Wong S, Steinbach L, Zhao J, Stehling C, Ma CB, Link TM. Comparative study of imaging at 3.0 T versus 1.5 T of the knee. Skeletal Radiol. 2009;38(8):761-9.
71. McCauley TR, Kier R, Lynch KJ, Jokl P. Chondromalacia patellae: diagnosis with MR imaging. Am J Roentgenol. 1992;158(1):101-5.
72. Crema MD, Roemer FW, Marra MD, Guermazi A. MR Imaging of intra and periarticular soft tissues and subchondral bone in knee osteoarthritis. Radiol Cl N Am. 2009;47(4):687-701.
73. Kijowski R, Stanton P, Fine J, Smet AD. Subchondral bone marrow edema in patients with degeneration of the articular cartilage of the knee joint. Radiology. 2006;238(3):943-9.
74. Waldochmidt JG, Braunstein EM, Buckwalter KA. Magnetic resonance imaging of osteoarthritis. Rheum Dis Clin North Am. 1999;25:451-65.
75. Buckwalter JA, Mankin HJ. Articular cartilage repair and transplantation. Arthritis Rheum. 1998;41:1331-42.
76. Le J, Peng Q, Sperling K. Biochemical magnetic resonance imaging of knee articular cartilage: T1 rho and T2 mapping as cartilage degeneration biomarkers. Ann NY Acad Sci. 2016;1383(1):34-42.
77. Sophia Fox, Bedi AJA, Rodeo SA. The basic science of articular cartilage: structure, composition and function. Sports Health. 2009;1(6):461-8.
78. Link TM, Stahl R, Woertler K. Cartilage imaging, motivation, techniques, current and future significance. Eur Radiol. 2007;17(5):1135-46.
79. Hayashi D, Roemer FW, Guermazi A. Recent advances in research imaging of osteoarthritis with focus on MRI, ultrasound and hybrid imaging. Clin Exp Rheumatol. 2018;36:S43-52.
80. Schmitt B, Zbyn S, Stelzeneder D, Jellus V, Paul D, Lauer L, et al. Cartilage quality assessment by using glycosaminoglycan chemical exchange saturation transfer and 23Na MR Imaging at 7 T. Radiology. 2011;260(1):257-64.
81. McGonagle D, Gibbon W, O'Connor P, Green M, Pease C, Emery P. Characteristics magnetic resonance imaging entheseal changes of knee synovitis in spondyloarthropathy. Arthritis Rheum. 1998;41(4):694-700.
82. Sanders TG, Medynski MA, Feller JF, Lawhorn KW. Bone contusion patterns of the knee at MR imaging: footprint of the mechanism of injury. Radiographics. 2000;20:135-51.
83. Baltazar R, Ma C, Shankman S, Beltran J. Knee. In: Haaga JR, Dogra VS, Forsting M, Gilkeson RC, Kwon HA H, Sundaram M (Eds). CT and MRI of the Whole Body, 5th edition. US: Mosby; 2009.
84. Palmer WE, Levine SM, Dupuy DE. Knee and shoulder fractures: Association of fracture detection and marrow oedema on MR images with mechanism of injury. Radiology. 1997;204(2): 395-401.
85. Anderson MW, Ugalde U, Batt M, Gacayan J. Shin splints: MR appearance in a preliminary study. Radiology. 1997;204(1): 177-80.
86. Anderson MW, Greenspan A. Stress fractures. Radiology. 1996;199(1):1-12.
87. Yamamoto T, Bullough PG. Subchondral insufficiency fracture of the femoral head and medial femoral condyle. Skeletal Radiol. 2000;29(1):40-4.
88. Frosberg PK, Braunstein EM, Buckwalter KA. Osteonecrosis, transient osteoporosis and transient bone marrow edema. Radiol Clin North Am. 1996;34(2):273-91.
89. Hughston JC, Hergenroeder PT, Courtenay BG. Osteochondritis dissecans of the femoral condyles. J Bone Joint Surg. 1984;66(9):1340-8.
90. DeSmet A, Fisher DR, Graf BK, Lange. Osteochondritis dissecans of the knee: value of MR imaging in determining lesion stability and the presence of articular cartilage defects. Am J Roentgenol. 1990;155(3):549-53.
91. Gorbachova T, Melenevsky Y, Cohen M, Cerniglia BW. Osteochondral lesions of the knee: differentiating the most common entities at MRI. Radiographics. 2018;38(5):1478-95.
92. Wambeek N, Munk PL, Lee MJ, Meek RN. Intra-articular regional migratory osteoporosis of the knee. Skeletal Radiol. 2000;29(2):97-100.
93. Schweitzer ME, Mandel S, Schwartzman RJ, Knobler RL, Tahmoush AJ. Reflex sympathetic dystrophy revisted: MR imaging findings before and after infusion of contrast material. Radiology. 1995;195(1):211-4.
94. Graif M, Schweitzer ME, Deely D, Matteucci T. The septic versus nonspecific inflamed joint: MRI characteristics. Skeletal Radiol. 1999;28(11):616-20.
95. Sundaram M, McGuire MH, Herbold DR. Magnetic resonance imaging in planning limb salvage surgery for primary malignant tumours of bone. J Bone Joint Surg. 1986;68:809-19.
96. Applegate GR, Flannigan BD, Tolin BS, Fox JM, Del Pizzo W. MR diagnosis of recurrent tears in the knee: Value of intra-articular contrast material. Am J Roentgenol. 1993;161(4):821-5.
97. Kramer J, Recht MP, Imhof H, Stiglbaüer R, Engel A. Postcontrast MR arthrography in assessment of cartilage lesions. J Comput Assist Tomography. 1994;18(2):218-24.
98. Kramer J, Stiglbauer R, Engel A, Prayer L, Imhof H. MR contrast arthrography in osteochondrosis dissecans. J Comput Assist Tomography. 1992;16(2):254-60.

99. Brossmann J, Priedler KW, Daenen B, Pedowitz RA, Andresen R, Clopton P, et al. Imaging of osseous and cartilaginous intra-articular bodies in the knee: Comparison of MR imaging and MR arthrography with CT and CT arthrography in cadavers. Radiology. 1996;200(2):509-17.
100. Kobayashi Y, Murkami R, Tajima H, Yamamoto K, Ichikawa T, Mase Y, et al. Direct MR arthrography of plica synovialis mediopatellaris. Acta Radiol. 2001;42(3):286-90.
101. Schatz JA, Potter HG, Rodeo SA. MR imaging of anterior cruciate ligament reconstruction. Am J Roentgenol. 1997;169:223-8.
102. Howell SM, Berns GS, Farley TE. Unimpinged and impinged anterior cruciate ligament grafts: MR signal intensity measurements. Radiology. 1991;179(3):639-43.
103. Recht MP, Piraino DW, Cohen MA, Parker RD, Bergfeld JA. Localised anterior arthrofibrosis (cyclopos lesion) after reconstruction of the anterior cruciate ligament: MR imaging findings. Am J Roentgenol. 1995;165(2):383-5.
104. Ho YY, Stanley AJ, Hui JH, Wang SC. Postoperative evaluation of the knee after autologous chondrocyte implantation: what Radiologists Need to Know. Radiographics. 2007;27(1):207-20.
105. Gnannt R, Chhabra A, Theodoropoubs JS, Hodler J, Andreisek G. MR imaging of postoperative knee. Journal of Magnetic Resonance Imaging. 2011;34(5):1007-21.
106. Garwood ER, Tai R, Joshi G, Watts V GJ. The use of Artificial Intelligence in the evaluation of knee pathology. Semin Musculoskeletal Radiol. 2020;24(1):21-9.

CHAPTER

171

Magnetic Resonance Imaging of Ankle

Anindita Sinha, Mahesh Prakash

INTRODUCTION

Ankle joint is formed by the lower end of tibia, fibula, and talus and is a hinge joint allowing plantar flexion and dorsiflexion. The ankle mortise is formed by the medial and lateral malleoli and tibial plafond articulating with the talar dome or trochlea of talus, which is broader anteriorly, making the foot more stable in dorsiflexion. The lower ankle joint is formed by the talus articulating with the calcaneus forming the subtalar joint and the navicular **(Fig. 1)**. The subtalar joint allows inversion and eversion of the foot **(Figs. 2A and B)**. The ankle joint is stabilized by ligaments on the lateral [anterior and posterior talofibular and calcaneofibular ligaments (CFL)], medial (deltoid), and plantar aspects. Ankle injuries are the most common indication for imaging the ankle joint, and inversion injuries are most common with tear of the lateral ligaments; most commonly anterior talofibular ligament. Chronic

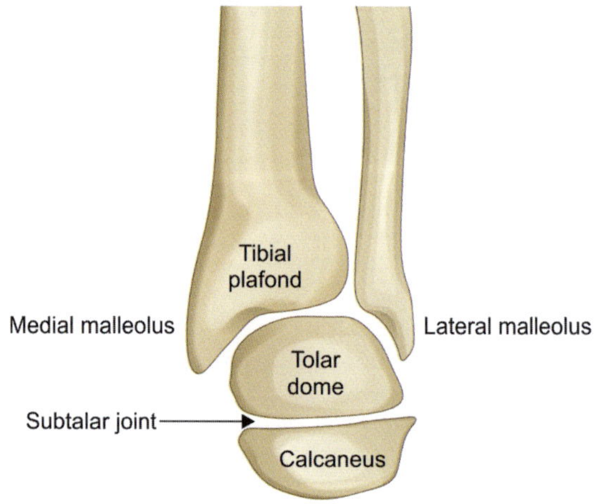

FIG. 1: Ankle joint.

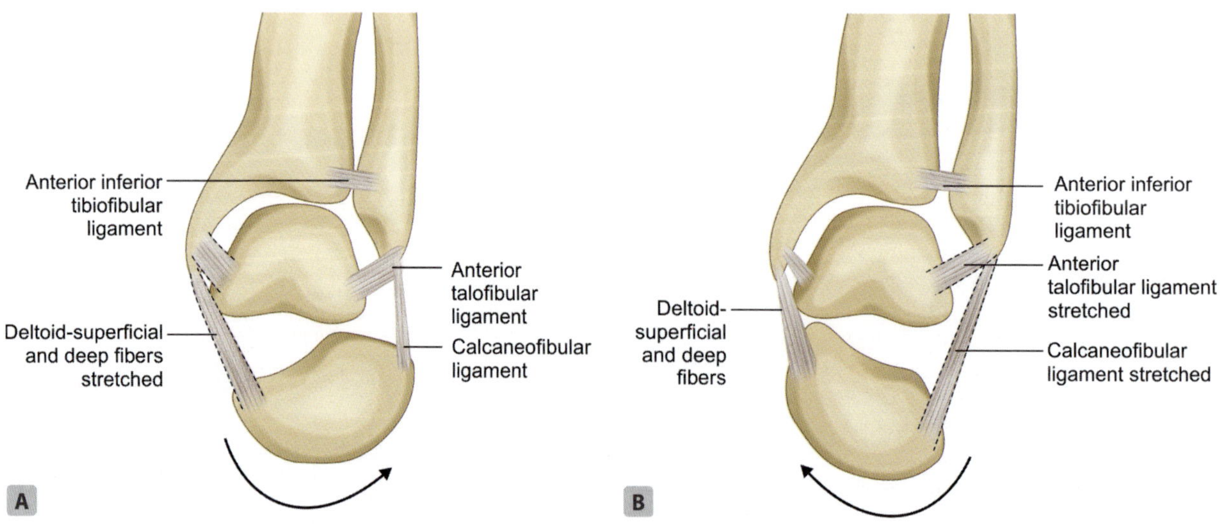

FIGS. 2A AND B: Eversion (A) and inversion (B) injuries of the foot. Inversion injuries (B) are much more common than eversion injuries.

pain as a result of previous injury leading to instability and impingement and congenital or acquired causes of flat foot are among the other common indications. Differentiating between infection and neuropathic joint in diabetic foot is also a major diagnostic concern. Detailed knowledge of osseous, ligamentous and tendon, and neurovascular anatomy in the various compartments (anterior, medial, lateral, and posterior) is a prerequisite for proper diagnosis.

IMAGING PROTOCOLS/TECHNICAL FACTORS

An ideal magnetic resonance (MR) technique should yield images with good contrast and spatial resolution of the osseous and soft tissue structures of the ankle.

Patient Positioning and Coils

1.5 or 3.0 T scanners are the most common MR units for musculoskeletal (MSK) imaging. Conventional closed bore, open bore, and extremity units are used for ankle imaging. Closed-coupled coil should be used to achieve optimal signal-to-noise ratios and spatial resolution. Standard extremity coil is routinely used.

The patient is placed supine with foot in the neutral position. The foot should be at right angle to the lower leg or 20° plantar flexion. The foot should be supported and immobilized with padding or straps to maintain the alignment and prevent movement.

With surface coils, it is recommended to use FOV (field of view) of 8–16 cm and 256 × 256 or 256 × 192 matrix. Foot and ankle are not scanned simultaneously and hence an ankle MRI should not include the toes, and a forefoot examination should not include the ankle.

Slice Thickness

A 2–4 mm slice thickness with 0.2–0.5 mm interslice gaps is best for defining complex foot and ankle anatomy.

Imaging Planes and Pulse Sequences

Coronal, axial, and sagittal image planes are commonly used for foot and ankle examination.

An ankle protocol includes T1-weighted axial and sagittal images, proton density (PD) and T2-weighted images in the sagittal plane, STIR sequence in the axial and sagittal plane.

The scan planning is initially done on axial or sagittal localizer with sagittal plane preferred.[1]

Axial images are first obtained (most valuable), parallel to the axis of the calcaneus, covering from distal tibial metadiaphyseal junction to the distal most part. Base of the metatarsals should be included in the axial images.

Coronal images are acquired next perpendicular to the axials. The coronal images should cover the base of the metatarsals. Next on the axial scout images, sagittal images are planned covering from lateral to medial malleolus.[1]

Sagittal images are best used to evaluate Achilles tendon, sinus tarsi, and plantar fascia. Axials of ankle are best for evaluation of tibiofibular ligaments, anterior and posterior talofibular ligaments (PTFLs), spring ligament complex, and the osseous structures.

Coronal images of ankle are best for detailed review of the deltoid ligaments, deep and superficial CFL, and the tarsal tunnel.

MAGNETIC RESONANCE ANATOMY

- *Anterior*: From medial to lateral the structures are **(Figs. 3A and B)**—
    - Tendons of tibialis anterior (TA), extensor hallucis longus (EHL), extensor digitorum longus (EDL)
    - Anterior tibial artery located between EHL and EDL
    - Deep peroneal nerve crosses the artery from medial to lateral.
- *Lateral* **(Figs. 3 to 6)**:
    - Ligaments:
        - Anterior talofibular ligament—attaches on anterior margin of fibular malleolus and on the talus it attaches just anterior to lateral articular surface—anterior talofibular ligament (ATFL) is the weakest and most frequently torn ligament in ankle sprains.
        - Posterior talofibular ligament—thick and striated and infrequently torn.
        - Calcaneofibular ligament—descends vertically deep to the peroneal tendons to attach to the trochlear tubercle on the lateral surface of calcaneum.
    - Tendons—peroneus longus and peroneus brevis:
        - Peroneus longus—attaches to plantar surface of the base of medial cuneiform and first metatarsal and is located behind the peroneus brevis tendon and on axial sections is rounded in shape.

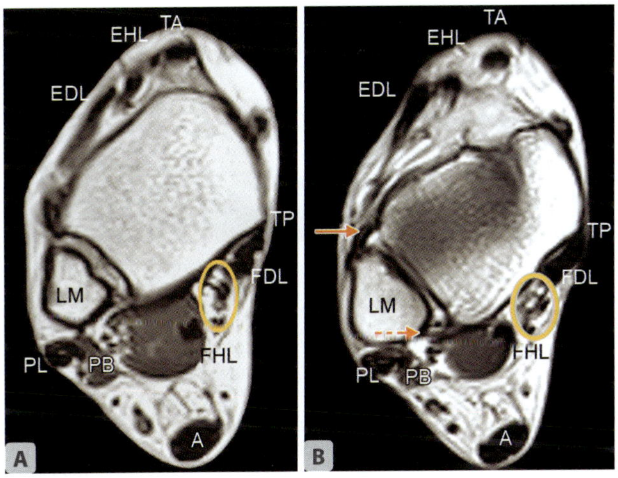

FIGS. 3A AND B: Anterior tendons from medial to lateral-tibialis anterior (TA), extensor hallucis longus (EHL), and extensor digitorum longus (EDL). Peroneus longus (PL) and peroneus brevis (PB) seen posterior to lateral malleolus (LM); peroneus brevis tendon is smaller and flat. Medial group of tendons are tibialis posterior (TP), flexor digitorum longus (FDL), and flexor hallucis longus (FHL) most posteromedially. Lower section of inferior tibiofibular joint shows the anterior inferior tibio-fibular ligament (AITFL) (arrow) and posterior inferior tibiofibular ligament (PITFL) (dashed arrow). The neurovascular bundle is between FDL and FHL (oval). Achilles tendon (A) shows mild focal anterior convexity which may be a normal finding.

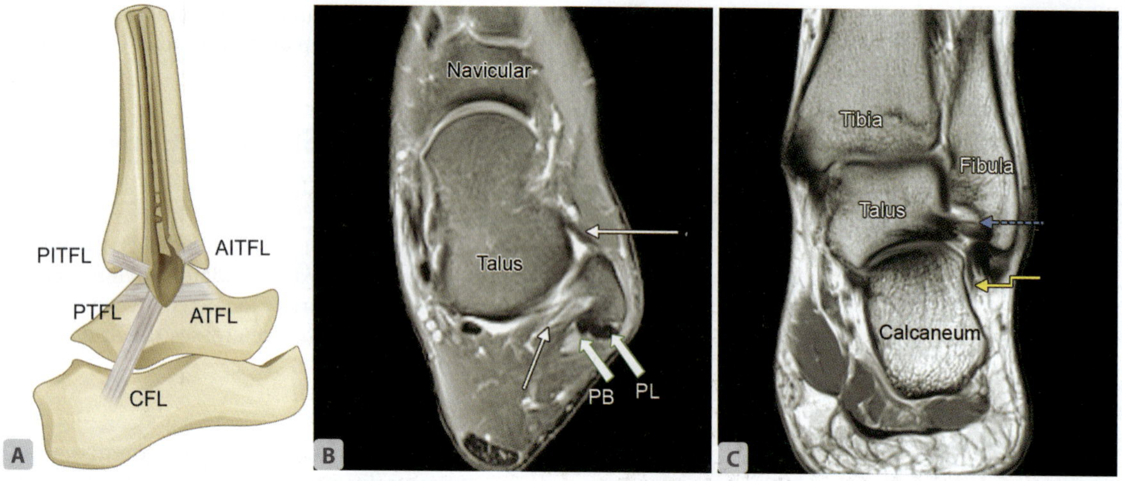

FIGS. 4A TO C: (A) Ligaments on the lateral aspect of the ankle. Anterior and posterior inferior tibiofibular ligaments (AITFL and PITFL) or syndesmotic ligaments, anterior and posterior talofibular ligaments (ATFL and PTFL), and calcaneofibular ligament (CFL); (B) Axial PD-weighted fat-saturated image shows the thin hypointense ATFL (arrow), and the striated appearance of PTFL (small arrow); (C) Coronal PD-weighted image shows the PTFL (dashed arrow) and the CFL (step arrow) abutting the lateral margin of the calcaneus deep to the peroneal tendons. The peroneal tendons are seen behind the fibular retromalleolar groove, which here is flat and not concave. The peroneus brevis (PB) is anteromedial and peroneus longus (PL) is larger.

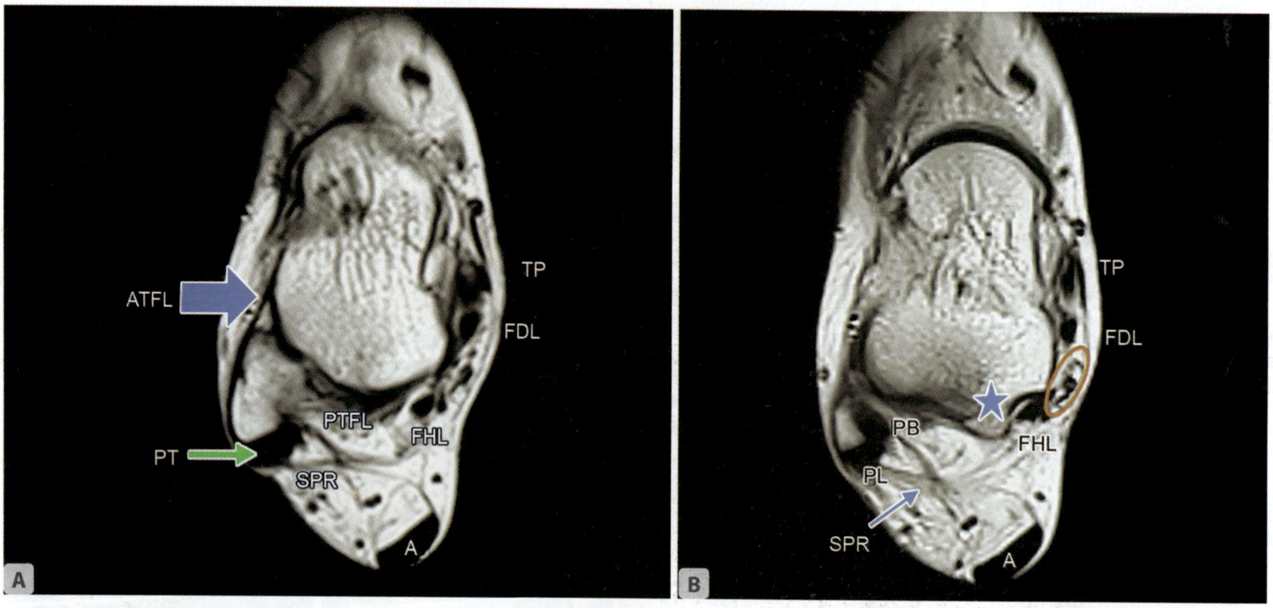

FIGS. 5A AND B: Axial proton density-weighted images at the level of lateral malleolar fossa demonstrates the uniform thickness hypointense band of anterior talofibular ligament (ATFL-arrow) from the anterior ridge of lateral malleolus to the lateral surface of talus. Note that tibia is not seen at the level of ATFL. The striated and thicker posterior tibiofibular ligament (PTFL) is seen posteriorly. PTFL is rarely torn in isolation. The peroneal tendons are seen behind the lateral malleolus which has a flat retromalleolar groove in this case. The peroneal tendons (PT in A) are enclosed within a thin triangular hypointense fascial layer known as superior peroneal retinaculum (SPR-arrow in B). Posteriorly the hypointense Achilles tendon with a concave anterior margin is seen. Medially from anterior to posterior the tibialis posterior tendon (TP), flexor digitorum longus (FDL) is visualized. The posterior tendon of flexor hallucis longus (FHL) lies behind the neurovascular bundles of posterior tibial artery and nerve (oval) and lodges between posterior tubercles of talus (*).

- Peroneus brevis—attaches to base of the fifth metatarsal. Located just posterior to fibular retromalleolar groove, and is adjacent to bone. Peroneus brevis tendon is smaller and flatter on axial views.
- Both tendons are enclosed in a thin sheath known as superior peroneal retinaculum (SPR) superiorly at malleolar level, which extends from the posterior fibular ridge laterally to the calcaneus or Achilles tendon posteriorly.
- Due to their curved course, both tendons can show magic angle effect with artefactual high signal mimicking a tear or tendinopathy on short TE images.

○ *Superior peroneal retinaculum:* It encases and stabilizes the peroneal tendons at the level of the

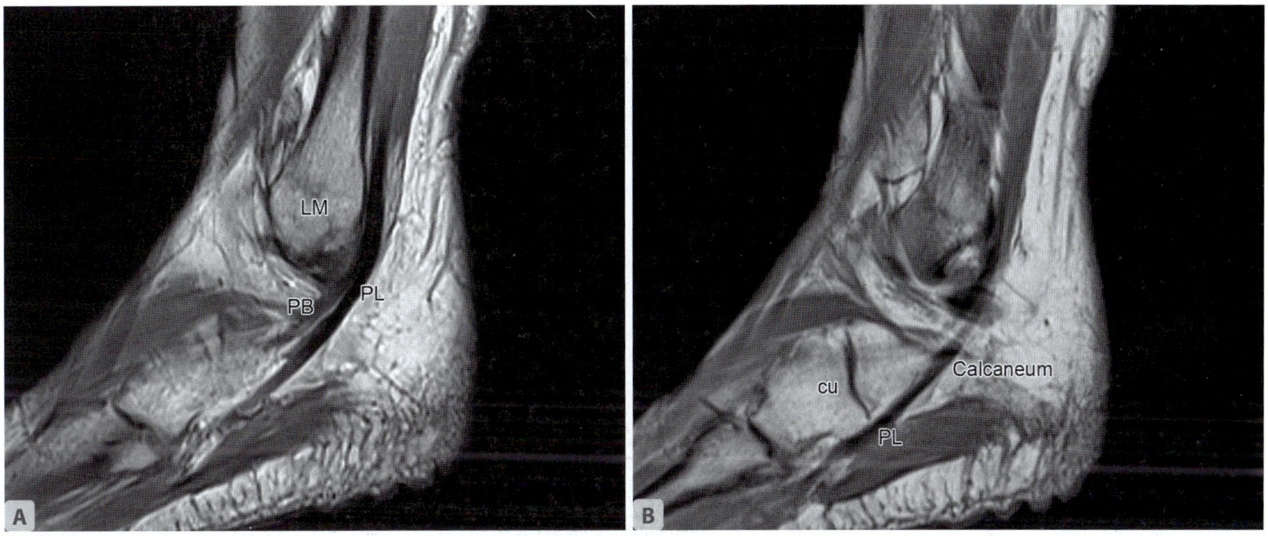

FIGS. 6A AND B: Sagittal proton density-weighted images show peroneus longus tendon (PL) coursing behind lateral malleolus (LM). Peroneus brevis is seen anteriorly (PB). A more medial sagittal section shows the peroneus longus curving around groove in cuboid (cu); the tendon in this area is intermediate in signal intensity due to magic angle artefact.

retromalleolar groove. SPR is visible on MRI as a thin hypointense band extending from the lateral malleolus to the lateral calcaneus.

- *Medial* **(Figs. 3A and B)**:
  - Tendons of **T**ibialis posterior, flexor **D**igitorum longus, flexor **H**allucis longus (FHL)
  - Posterior tibial **A**rtery
  - Tibial **N**erve
  - Arrangement is **T**om **D**ick **An**d **H**arry from anterior to posterior
  - Deltoid ligament—a triangular/fan-shaped ligament from medial malleolus—is divided into **(Figs. 7 and 8)**:
    - *Superficial layer*:
      - Extends from medial malleolus to navicular, spring ligament, calcaneus
      - Tibiocalcaneal, tibiospring, tibionavicular
    - *Deep layer*:
      - Extends from medial malleolus to talus
      - Anterior tibiotalar and posterior tibiotalar (thickest)
      - Stronger than superficial layer
  - Spring ligament **(Figs. 9A to D)**:
    - One of the important stabilizers of medial longitudinal arch of foot and stabilizes talar head
    - Has three components:
      - Superomedial calcaneonavicular—from sustentaculum tali to medial portion of navicular bone—most important ligament
      - Two other components are the inferoplantar longitudinal calcaneonavicular ligament and medioplantar oblique calcaneonavicular ligament
- *Posterior* **(Figs. 3 and 10)**:
  - *Achilles tendon* is formed by soleus, medial, and lateral head of gastrocnemius.
  - It inserts into calcaneal tuberosity.

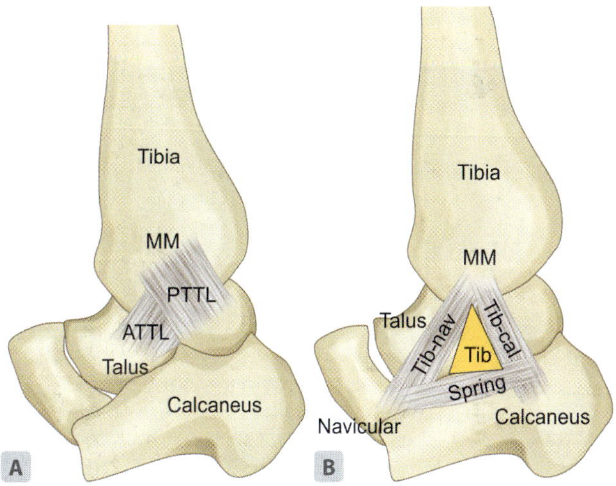

FIGS. 7A AND B: Diagrammatic representation of the deltoid ligament. (A) The deep deltoid ligament attaching the tibia to the talus—the anterior (ATTL) and posterior tibiotalar ligament (PTTL); (B) Components of the deep deltoid ligaments—from anterior to posterior-tibionavicular (Tib-nav), tibiospring (Tib), and tibiocalcaneal ligaments (Tib-cal). (MM: medial malleolus).

  - The tendon does not have a lining synovial sheath, but is surrounded by fibrous connective tissue known as paratendon.
  - The myotendinous junction is formed in mid-calf and tendon length is around 15 cm.
  - MRI appearance is hypointense on all sequences.
  - Best seen in axial and sagittal views
  - Axial—anterior margin is concave. Sagittal—tendon margins are parallel.
  - Bursa around Achilles tendon:
    - Retro-Achilles bursa—behind Achilles tendon

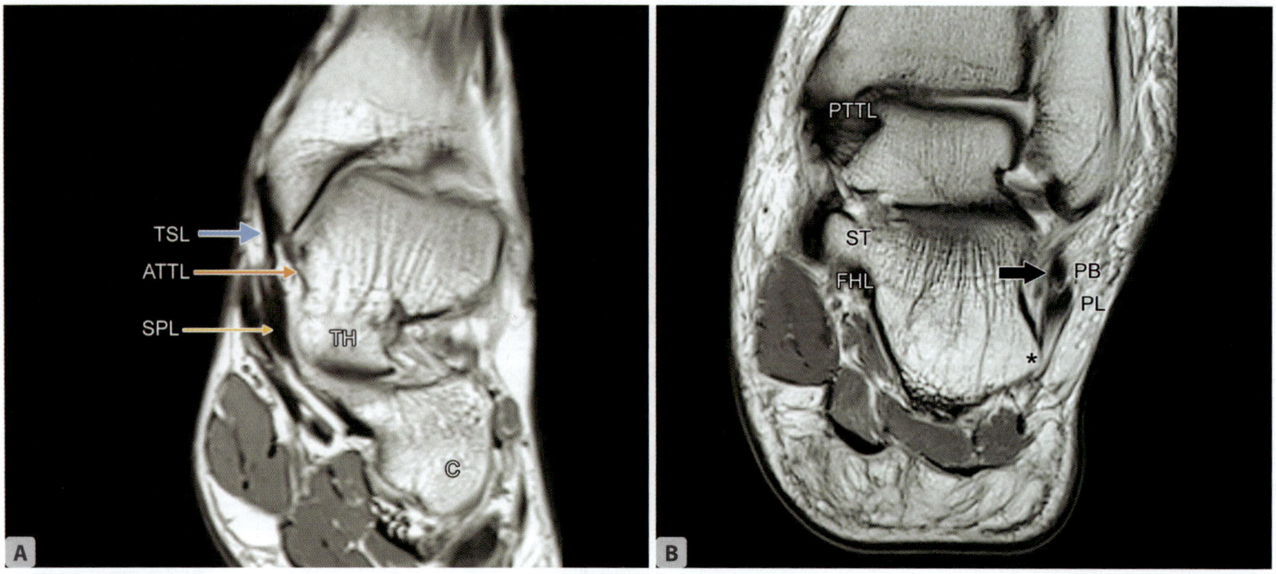

FIGS. 8A AND B: Coronal T1-weighted image (A) shows thin strand of anterior tibiotalar ligament (ATTL)—a deep portion of the deltoid ligament, which is very thin and variably seen. The tibiospring ligament (TSL), part of the superficial deltoid, attaches to the spring ligament (SPL) near the talar head (TH); (B) On a more posterior section, the striated posterior tibiotalar ligament (PTTL) is seen. On the lateral aspect, the calcaneofibular ligament (CFL) (arrow) can be seen in its entirety attaching to the calcaneal tuberosity (*) deep to the peroneal tendons [peroneus brevis and peroneus longus (PB and PL)].

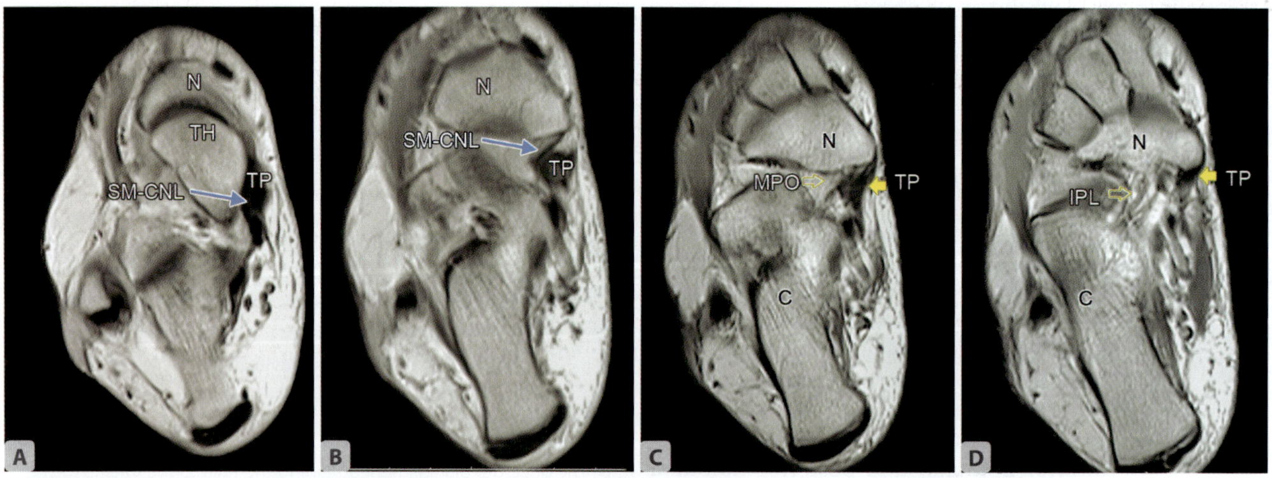

FIGS. 9A TO D: Spring ligament. (A and B) Axial proton density-weighted consecutive images show the hypointense band of superomedial calcaneonavicular ligament (SM-CNL) deep to the tibialis posterior (TP) tendon, adjoining the medial aspect of the talonavicular joint. Talar head (TH) and navicular bone is marked N; (C and D) Hypointense band of medioplantar oblique calcaneonavicular (MPO) and inferoplantar longitudinal (IPL) calcaneonavicular portions of the spring ligament. Navicular bone is marked by (N) and calcaneum by (C). The tibialis posterior has attached to the tuberosity of navicular (TP). Posteriorly the Achilles tendon attachment is seen at the calcaneal tuberosity.

- Retrocalcaneal bursa—in front of the anterior margin of distal Achilles tendon between tendon and posterior calcaneus.

○ Plantaris tendon—may be present medial to Achilles tendon and inserts within or anteromedial to Achilles tendon insertion on calcaneus. An intact plantaris can simulate a partial tear of a completely torn Achilles tendon.

○ Kager's fat pad is a triangular area seen anterior to Achilles tendon.

Joints (Figs. 1 and 10)

The ankle joint is formed by three joints:

1. Tibiotalar joint (talocrural or ankle joint mortise)—formed by tibial plafond, dome of talus, and medial and lateral malleolus
2. Subtalar joint formed between the talus and calcaneum (there are three articulations—anterior, middle, and posterior)
3. Inferior tibiofibular joint (joined by syndesmotic ligaments—anterior and posterior inferior tibiofibular ligament) **(Fig. 1B)**.

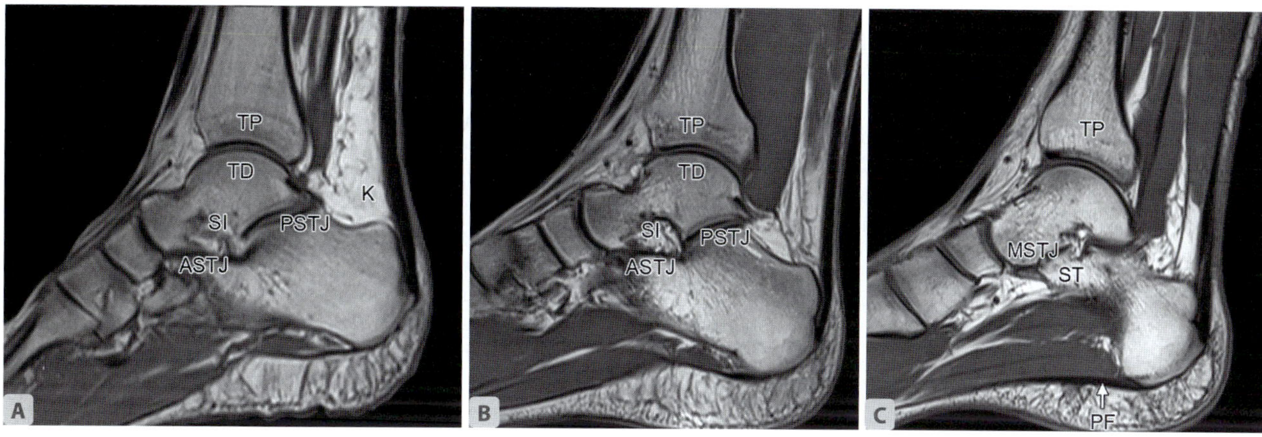

FIGS. 10A TO C: Sagittal proton density-weighted images show Achilles tendon-straight and hypointense and attaching to calcaneal tuberosity. The Kager's fat pad (K) is seen anterior to Achilles tendon. The anterior, middle, and posterior subtalar joints (talocalcaneal joints) are marked ASTJ, MSTJ, and PSTJ. The middle subtalar joint is formed by the articular facet of sustentaculum tali (ST). In these medial sections the hypointense plantar fascia (PF) is seen at calcaneal attachment. The fat and interosseous ligaments of a portion of the sinus tarsi (SI) are also seen. The tibial plafond (TP) and talar dome (TD) form the tibiotalar joint.

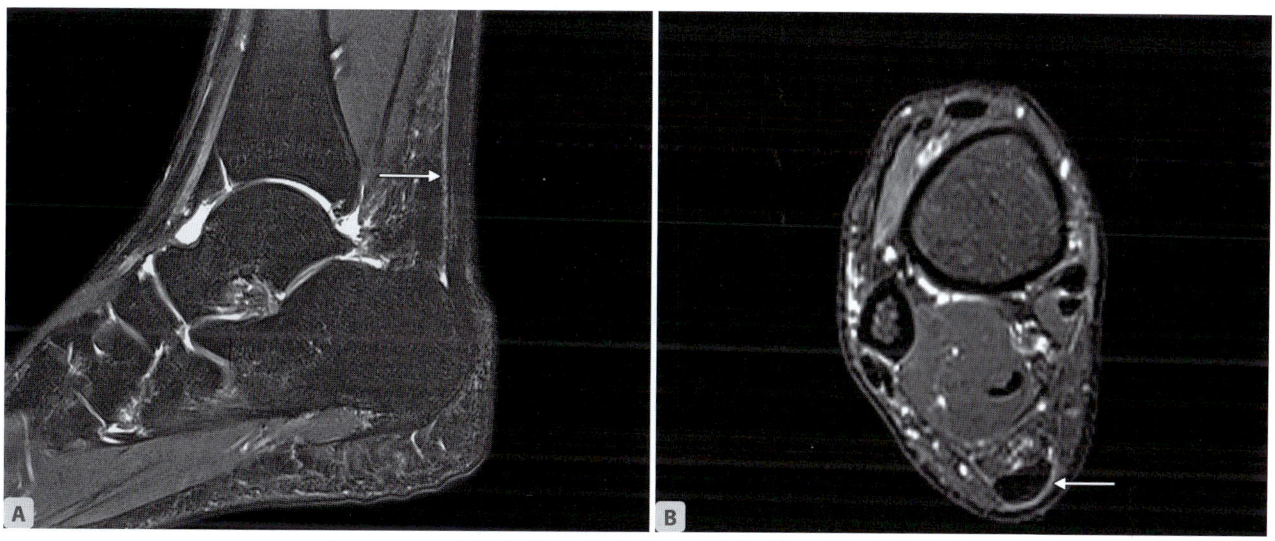

FIGS. 11A AND B: Achilles paratendinosis: Sagittal and axial T2-weighted images show a thin sliver of fluid (arrow) surrounding the Achilles tendon, which remains hypointense and maintains its anterior concave margin on axial sections.

Achilles Tendon Pathologies

Achilles tendon is the strongest and largest tendon in the body. Achilles tendon injuries are common and can be due to acute trauma or due to chronic overuse in athletes.

Acute Injuries

Acute tendon injuries are most commonly seen due to sudden forced ankle movement in elderly otherwise fit individuals. Spontaneous acute rupture is seen in individuals with connective tissue disorders or diabetes.

Chronic Injuries

Tennis leg rupture of the myotendinous junction of the medial head of gastrocnemius or a myofascial injury is more common than a plantaris rupture. Fluid signal is seen between medial head of gastrocnemius and soleus.

Tendinopathy/Tendinosis

- Achilles tendinopathy can appear as focal or diffuse thickening with loss of normal anterior concavity in axial plane. Signal may remain hypointense or become hyperintense in mucoid degeneration.[2,3]
- Achilles paratendinopathy—diffuse thin fluid is seen around the Achilles tendon, since the tendon itself does not have a true synovium-lined tendon sheath but is surrounded by fibrous connective tissue to allow for its gliding action **(Figs. 11A and B)**.

Tendon Ruptures

- Partial or complete ruptures of the Achilles tendon are caused by acute sudden dorsiflexion.
- Site prone to tear is a relatively avascular zone 2–6 cm proximal to insertion.

- Patients with pre-existing connective tissue disorders or diabetes are prone to tendon rupture following minor trauma.
- MRI appearance—a fluid-filled gap is seen between the torn ends. Hemorrhage with heterogeneous signal may be present. Tendon itself may be thickened in cases of pre-existing tendon degeneration **(Figs. 12A to C)**.
- Partial tears can be longitudinal split tears.
- Chronic tears with intervening fibrotic tissue may make diagnosis difficult.[2,4,5]

Haglund's Syndrome (Fig. 13)

- Haglund's syndrome causes posterior ankle pain and is caused by ill-fitting shoes pressing the retro-Achilles bursa against the posterior calcaneal tuberosity.
- Chronic irritation causes edema or enlargement of the calcaneal tuberosity (Haglund's deformity).
- Fluid-filled retrocalcaneal and retro-Achilles bursa can be seen.
- Achilles tendinosis can be associated with Haglund's syndrome.

Achilles Tendon Xanthomas

- Achilles tendon xanthomas present as painless soft tissue masses, may often be present bilaterally.
- Histopathologically, they are lipid-laden macrophages due to cholesterol deposits in tissues—may be associated with familial hypercholesterolemia and cerebrotendinous xanthomatosis.[6]
- MRI appearance:
  - Diffuse or focal tendon enlargement with speckled appearance is seen on MRI.
  - The lesions are hyperintense on T1- and T2-weighted images.[6]
- Differential diagnosis includes tendinopathy and gout.

Peroneal Tendon Pathologies

- Peroneal tears or tendinopathies are seen in athletic young individuals as well as in elderly and are often associated with other injuries.
- Common presentations are lateral hind foot pain, popping or snapping in patients with peroneal subluxations or dislocations.
- Peroneus brevis tendon tears/tendinopathies.
- Overuse and friction against an abnormally-shaped retromalleolar groove is a common cause.
- *Shape of retromalleolar groove:* Retromalleolar groove is generally concave. Flat or convexity or irregular protuberance posteriorly causes chronic injury especially in the peroneus brevis located adjacent to fibular malleolus.[7]

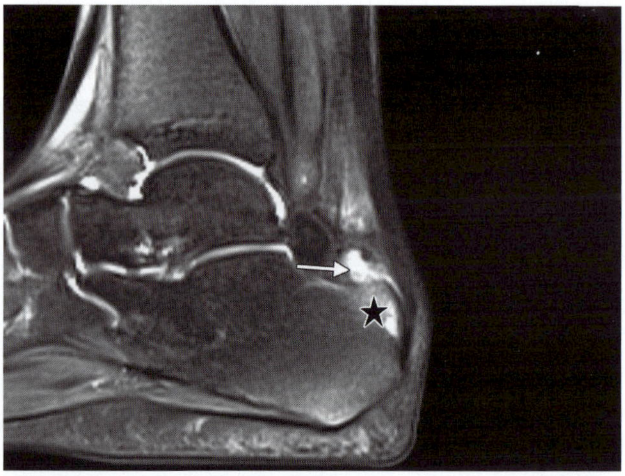

FIG. 13: Haglund's syndrome. Edema and prominence of the calcaneal tuberosity (*) with retrocalcaneal bursitis (arrow).

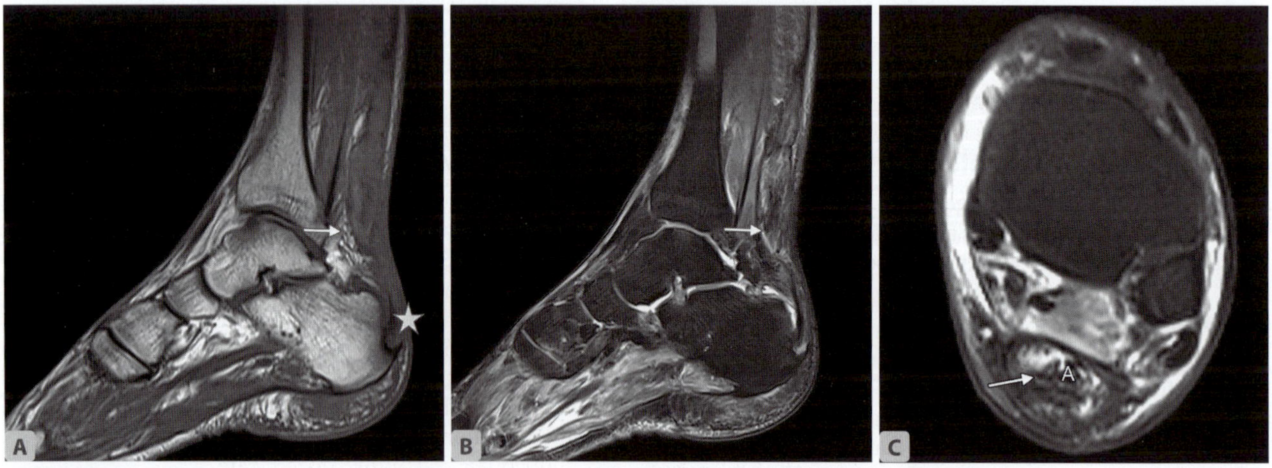

FIGS. 12A TO C: Complete tear of Achilles tendon (A) with hemorrhage-sagittal T1-weighted and T2-weighted images shows heterogeneous T1 hyperintense area (arrow) 4 cm from insertion of the Achilles tendon (*). This is heterogeneously hypointense on T2-weighted image (arrow in B), due to hemorrhage. The tendon insertion is also hypointense and shows erosion and sclerosis of the calcaneal tuberosity, suggesting a pre-existing tendinopathy with enthesitis. A gap is seen between the proximal and distal ends of the torn tendon (arrow in B). Intratendinous thickening and heterogeneity is seen on axial images (C).

Tendinopathy (Figs. 14A and B)

- Common sites of friction are:
  - Peroneal tubercle of the calcaneus—a bony prominence on the lateral surface of the calcaneum that separates the peroneus brevis from the peroneus longus—enlargement >5 mm is associated with chronic tears or tendinopathies.
  - Cuboid notch—where the peroneus longus turns toward the plantar aspect of the foot toward its ultimate insertion to the plantar aspect of base of medial cuneiform and first metatarsal.
- Patients with rheumatoid arthritis, psoriatic arthritis, and diabetes are prone to tendinopathies.
- *MR appearance:* Tendon is thickened with increased intrasubstance signal abnormality.[8]

Tenosynovitis

- Peroneal tenosynovitis can be postinfective or post-traumatic (acute trauma associated with CFL injury causes false-positive appearance of tenosynovitis due to accumulation of joint fluid within the tendon sheath)
- Chronic inflammatory arthritis is a risk factor for tenosynovitis.
- Patients present with pain, tenderness, and swelling along the lateral ankle
- *MRI appearance:* Fluid distension of the tendon sheath (a sliver of fluid is normal; >3 mm thickness of fluid is a sign of tenosynovitis)
- The fluid signal may be heterogeneous; low-signal intensity bands may be seen in stenosing tenosynovitis
- Peroneal tendons may be thickened
- Synovial enhancement is commonly seen on postcontrast images.[8]

Peroneal Tendon Injuries

- Tendon injuries are often associated with ankle sprains and can be easily overlooked

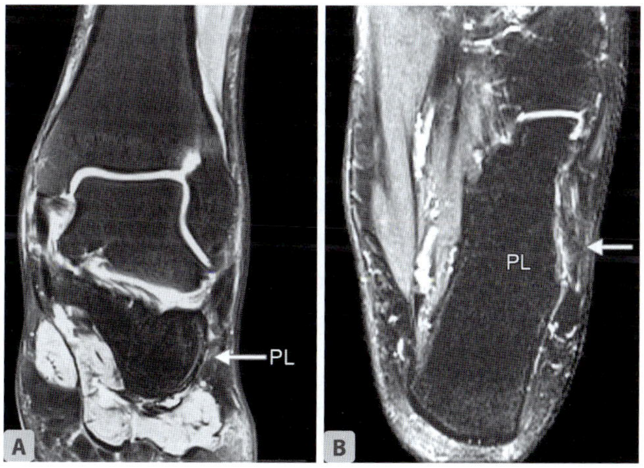

FIGS. 14A AND B: Peroneal tendinopathy. Coronal (A) and axial (B) T2-weighted fat-saturated images show tendinopathy of peroneus longus (PL) just beyond the peroneal tubercle. The tendon appears intermediate in signal intensity (arrow) and has a thin sliver of fluid surrounding it.

- Preexisting tendinopathy and microtrauma are other predisposing factors for tendon tears
- Partial tears can be associated with tendon thinning or thickening—a thickened tendon makes it difficult to differentiate between a thickened partially torn tendon and a tendinopathy
- Complete tears show discontinuity.

Peroneus Brevis Tears (Figs. 15A to D)

- Peroneus brevis is prone to tears due to friction between retromalleolar groove and anteriorly peroneus longus posteriorly.
- This anterior position against the retromalleolar groove makes the peroneus brevis more prone to tendinopathies and tears than the peroneus longus.[7]
- Predisposing factors include associated tears of ATFL, flat, convex or irregular retromalleolar groove, accessory muscle, low lying muscle belly of peroneus brevis and injuries and tears of superior peroneal retinaculum.
- *MRI appearance*:
  - *Boomerang or "C" shape:* A boomerang or "C" shaped peroneus brevis tendon engulfs the peroneus longus.
  - *Split tear:* Tears may progress to a longitudinal split with two separate tendon components of peroneus brevis and tendon of peroneus longus subluxating anteriorly between the torn tendon components (intrasheath subluxation).[8,9]

Peroneus Longus Tears

- Peroneus longus tears can also be partial or complete split tears at ankle or mid foot.
- Peroneus longus tears are less common than peroneus brevis tears and are often associated with peroneus brevis tears.
- Partial tears are more common in retromalleolar region and complete tear in midfoot at the point of the tendon curving around the cuboid on toward its plantar course.[8]
- Osseous abnormalities accompanying peroneus longus tears on MRI are:[7-9]
  - Hypertrophied peroneal tubercle
  - Edema of cuboid
  - Avulsion fracture of os peroneum (with separation of the avulsed fragments by >2 mm)
  - The entire os peroneum may be edematous and dislocated posteriorly from its normal position near the lateral calcaneocuboid joint.

Subluxation/Dislocation/SPR Injuries (Figs. 16A and B)

- Peroneal tendon subluxation and dislocations result from injury to the superior peroneal retinaculum.
- SPR injuries result from acute trauma in athletic individuals and mimic ankle sprain.
- SPR injuries can occur at the fibular attachment, with a complete tear or stripping off of the periosteum. A bony avulsion from lateral malleolus can also be present. Anterolateral subluxation or dislocation of the peroneal tendons may occur into the pouch formed by the stripped off periosteum.

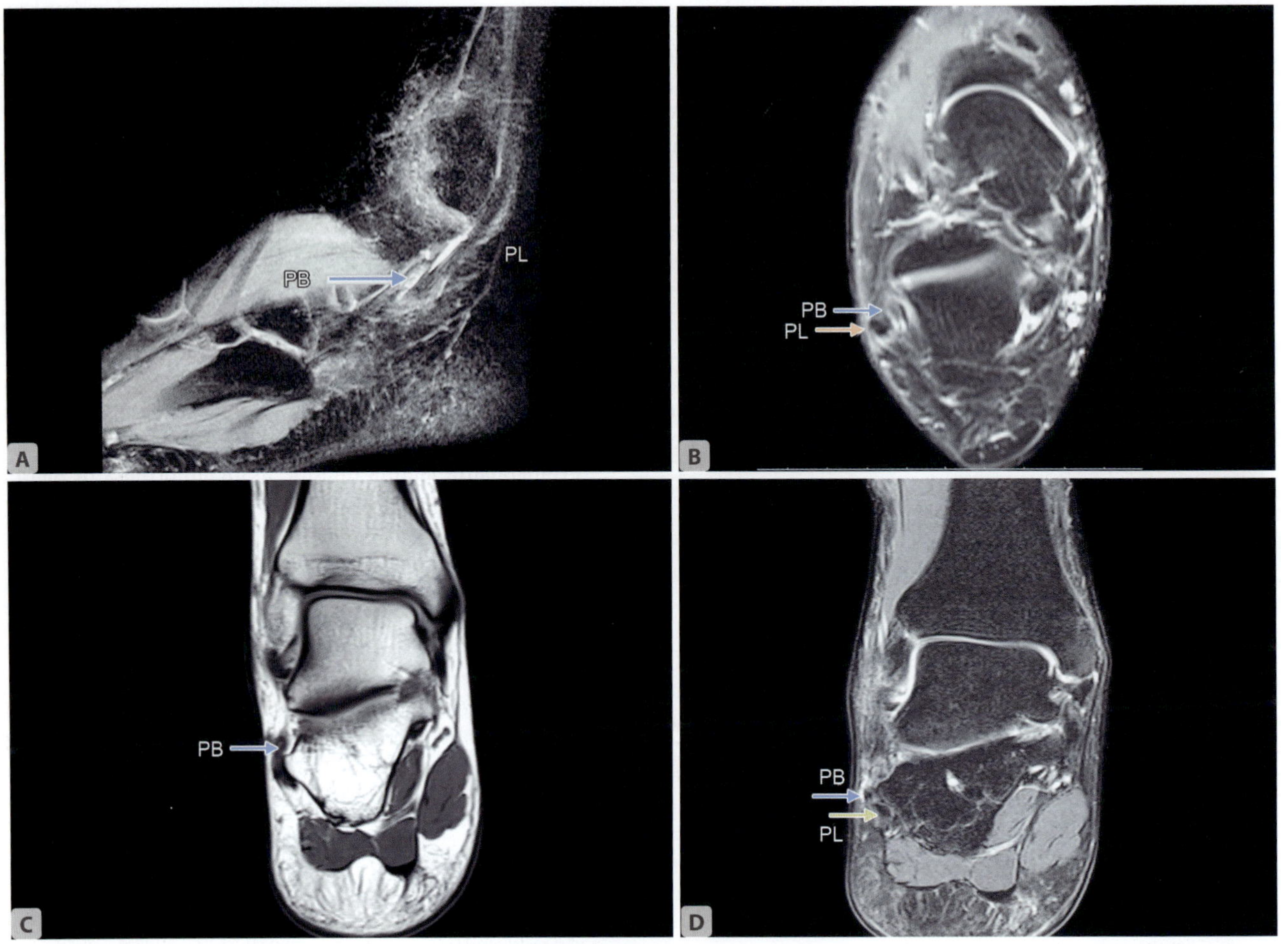

FIGS. 15A TO D: Partial tear of peroneus brevis (PB) tendon. On sagittal T2-weighted fat-saturated images there is partial fluid-filled discontinuity within the peroneus brevis, which may appear sometimes due to volume averaging on the sagittal images (A). However, tendon is thinned and shows a linear intermediate signal due to partial tear on axial T2-weighted fat-saturated image (B) and also on coronal proton density-weighted and T2-weighted fat-saturated images (C and D). (PL: peroneus longus).

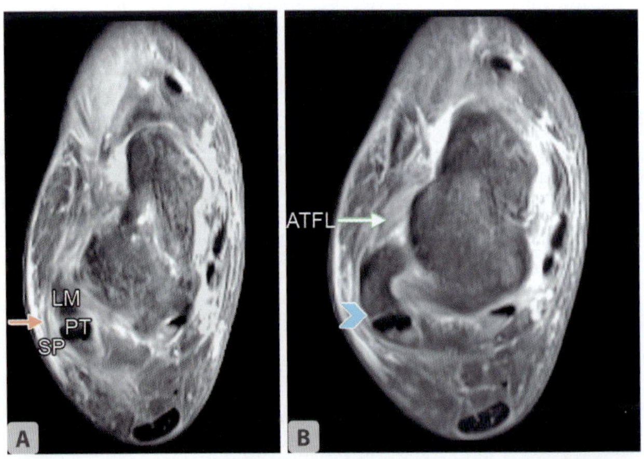

FIGS. 16A AND B: Acute SPR injury and ATFL injury. (A) The superior peroneal retinaculum is hyperintense and stripped off from the lateral malleolus (LM) (small arrow); peroneal tendons (PT) are not subluxated and remain behind lateral malleolus. A superior axial proton-density-weighted image (B) reveals a thickened, hyperintense, and torn anterior talofibular ligament at fibular attachment. The retromalleolar fossa is flat (arrowhead in B). Extensive edema seen along medial aspect of joint. (ATFL: anterior talofibular ligament; SPR: superior peroneal retinaculum).

- Transient peroneal subluxations can be difficult to identify on MRI, and dynamic ultrasound is essential to demonstrate the subluxation.
- Secondary evidence with hyperintensity along the retinaculum and nonvisualized or partially visualized retinaculum, edema along the adjacent lateral malleolus suggest retinacular injuries.[9]

Medial Compartment Tendon Abnormalities (Figs. 17A to C)

- *Tibialis posterior:* Tibialis posterior tenosynovitis, tendinopathies, and tears cause adult-acquired flat foot (planovalgus).
- Tendon dysfunction is common in elderly females. Patients present with chronic pain in the medial side of the arch of foot.
- Tibialis posterior tendon sheath normally contains a sliver of fluid, however, circumferential fluid >2 mm in thickness suggests tenosynovitis.
- Tenosynovitis progresses to tendinopathy and tears.

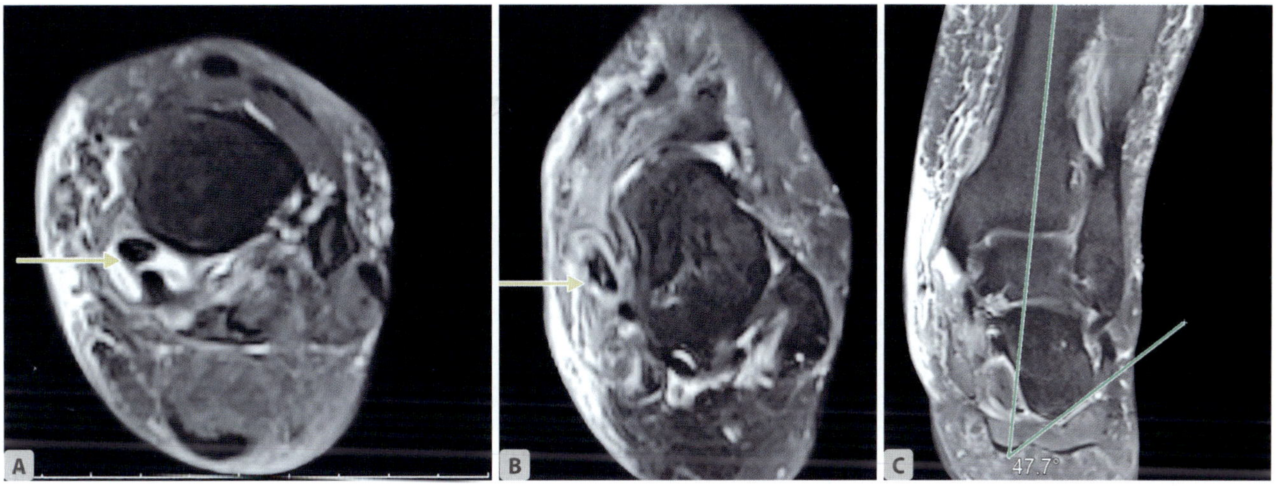

FIGS. 17A TO C: Tibialis posterior tenosynovitis with partial split tear and valgus deformity. Fluid seen surrounding the proximal tibialis posterior (arrow in A) in the axial T2-weighted fat-saturated image. Distal axial section shows intratendinous increased signal due to an interstitial tear (arrow in B). The patient presented with progressive flat foot due to posterior tibial dysfunction and had calcaneal valgus (C).

- Tendinopathy is characterized by fusiform enlargement of tendons and mild-to-moderate increased signal on T2-weighted images.[10,11]
- Complete tears of tibialis posterior are uncommon; partial or interstitial tears are more common and present as thinning and intrasubstance hyperintensity.
- Normal tibialis posterior is double the size of FHL and thinner than TA or combined diameters of peroneal tendons.
- Healed partial tears can present with hypertrophic thickening due to fibrotic scarring.
- A mixed hypertrophic-atrophic pattern of chronic tears can also be seen with hypertrophic proximal tendon.[11,12]

Ligament Injuries—Lateral

- *Mechanism of injury*: Plantar flexion with inversion causes the typical "ankle sprain."
- *Indications for imaging*: Most acute ankle sprains are not imaged. Indications for imaging are in professional athletes and to rule out syndesmotic injury, prolonged pain or ankle instability.
- *Ligaments most commonly torn*—ATFL and CFL. PTFL is the strongest and is rarely torn except in severe trauma associated with dislocations.

Anterior Talofibular Ligament and Posterior Talofibular Ligament

- ATFL is the weakest and the commonly injured ligament.
- *MRI appearance*: Normal ATFL has a hypointense band-like appearance on all pulse sequences and attaches to anterolateral aspect of lateral malleolar tip and lateral surface of talar neck. A striated appearance due to interposed fat may be seen.
- Normal PTFL is the thickest and has a striated appearance.
- PTFL attaches to malleolar fossa of fibula and posterolateral tubercle on posterior surface of talus.
- Low-grade ATFL injuries result in interstitial tear with intermediate intraligamentous signal intensity and intra- and periligamentous edema on proton density and fat saturated T2-weighted images.
- Injured ligament is seen as thickened, irregular, lax and wavy, or discontinuous ligament with intraligamentous or periligamentous edema.[13]
- Partial tear is seen as a focal discontinuity within the ligament.
- Full thickness tears can cause thinned out appearance or complete discontinuity at attachment or midsubstance of the ligament **(Figs. 17 and 18)**.
- Bright rim sign of tiny hyperintense foci at the torn site of attachment of ATFL has been reported by Lee et al.[14]
- Healing of ATFL tear takes 6–12 months and imaging appearances vary from ill-defined intermediate edematous signal with thickening of the ligament in initial stages to a more hypointense well-defined ligament with decrease in thickening as the scar tissue matures.[13]
- MRI has a 76–84% accuracy and 83–92% sensitivity in the diagnosis of chronic ATFL tears. Redundant or discontinuous ligament is more likely to be associated with instability.[13]
- *PTFL injuries*: PTFL is normally striated and hyperintense. This normal appearance should not be mistaken for a tear.

Calcaneofibular Ligament

- CFL is the second common ligament to be torn in inversion injuries after ATFL.
- CFL connects the lower tip of the lateral malleolus with the trochlear eminence on the lateral calcaneal surface.
- It has a vertical oblique course, best seen deep to the peroneal tendons.
- *MRI appearance*: It is best seen as a 6–8 mm hypointense structure deep to peroneal tendons and parallel to and adjacent to calcaneal lateral wall on axial and coronal images.

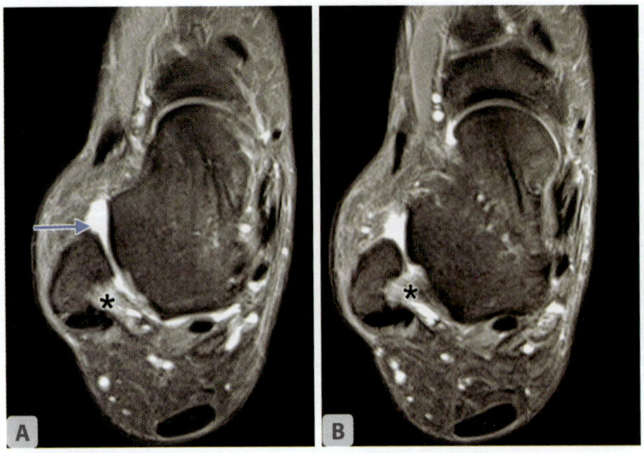

FIGS. 18A AND B: ATFL complete tear-nonvisualized ATFL (arrow in A) in a case of chronic tear. PTFL (*) is normal and striated in appearance (B). Another patient with thickened and heterogeneous wavy PTFL with loss of striation due to acute partial tear. No discontinuity seen either at attachment sites or within the ligament. Complete ATFL tear was also seen in this patient. (ATFL: anterior talofibular ligament; PTFL: posterior talofibular ligament).

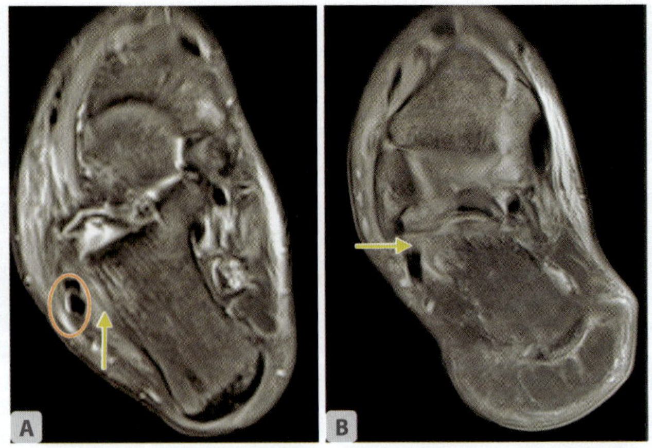

FIGS. 19A AND B: Calcaneofibular ligament tear. Axial and coronal proton density-weighted fat-saturated images show intermediate signal of the CFL medial to the peroneal tendons with periligamentous edema. The acutely kinked course on coronal images suggests a mid-substance tear. Adjacent osseous edema at the calcaneal attachment is seen. Peroneal tendons (oval) are intact. (CFL: calcaneofibular ligament).

- Tears can cause thickening and intermediate- or high-signal intensity with indistinct ligament, irregular wavy margins medial to peroneal tendons as well as fluid within the peroneal tendons **(Figs. 19A and B)**.
- In complete tears, the peroneal tendons about the lateral surface of the lateral malleolus.
- *Anatomical classification of ankle sprains*:[15]
  - First degree sprain—a partial or complete tear of the ATFL
  - Second degree sprain—partial or complete tearing of the both the ATFL and CFL
  - Third degree sprain—injury to all of the lateral ligaments, including the PTFL.

Syndesmotic Ligaments[16]

- *Injury of distal tibiofibular syndesmotic ligaments:* Anterior inferior tibiofibular ligament, posterior inferior tibiofibular ligament, and interosseous ligament injury result in high ankle sprain.
  - *Anterior-inferior tibiofibular ligament (AITFL)* inserts between anterior aspect of lateral malleolus and fibular tubercle on the anterolateral aspect of inferior tibia **(Fig. 3B)**
  - Posterior-inferior tibiofibular ligament (PITFL) attaches at the posterior tubercle of tibia and posterior lateral malleolus **(Fig. 3B)**.
  - *Interosseous ligament* is the thickened inferior portion of the interosseous membrane.[16]
- *Mechanism of injury* is hyperdorsiflexion and external rotation, commonly seen in footballers.
- *Radiography* is essential and may show avulsion fractures of lateral process or posterolateral talar process, talar dome, base of 5th metatarsal, and ankle fractures. Fibular fractures are commonly associated with syndesmotic injury so radiographs of both ankle and proximal tibiofibular joint are needed to detect Maisonneuve fractures.[13]
- AITFL is the most frequently injured syndesmotic ligament. Normal ligament is band like.
- *MRI appearance*:[16,17] Normal AITFL is hypointense on all pulse sequences.
- Adjacent osseous edema or osteochondral injury may be present.
- Fluid tracking up the tibiofibular recess above the level of the talar dome for a height of >1 cm is also indicative of syndesmotic ligament injury.
- Ankle arthrography may help in demonstrating intra-articular gadolinium extending high up into the recess.

Ligament Injuries—Medial (Figs. 20A to C)

- Deltoid ligament injuries comprise 15% of ligament injuries of ankle.[18]
- Common mode of injury is eversion.
- Lateral malleolar fracture and lateral talar dislocation are commonly associated.
- Avulsion fractures of medial malleolus at the site of superficial ligamentous attachment may be found.
- Lateral ligament complex injuries and syndesmotic injuries are also frequently found along with deltoid ligament injury.

Anatomy

- *Deep component:*
  - *Anterior tibiotalar ligament*—the thinnest and variably present in 50% of the population.
  - It attaches to the anterior tip of the anterior colliculus of medial malleolus and to fovea of the talus just distal to anterior part of medial articular surface.
  - *Posterior tibiotalar ligament*:[18] This is the thickest medial ligament; it originates from posterior surface of anterior colliculus of medial malleolus, intercollicular groove and posterior colliculus. It inserts into medial surface of talus under the medial articular

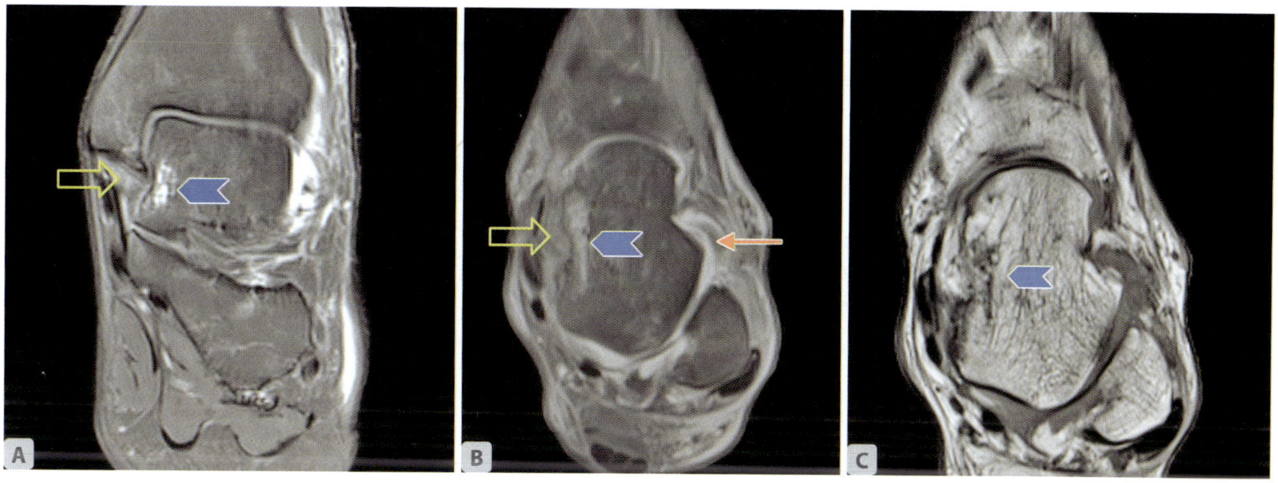

FIGS. 20A TO C: Deep deltoid injury with complete ATFL tear. Coronal and axial proton-density weighted fat saturated image (A) shows hyperintensity within the posterior tibiotalar ligament (arrow) with bone bruise (arrowhead) along medial margin of talus. The linear hypointense microtrabecular fractures are better appreciated on T1-weighted images (arrowhead in C). A completely torn ATFL is seen (small arrow). (ATFL: anterior talofibular ligament).

facet, posteriorly extending up to the posteromedial tubercle of talus.

- *MRI of tear:*[18] Focal tears are more common than full thickness tears.
- Hematoma, complete absence of ligament, and soft tissue edema are seen in full thickness tears.
- The most common site of tear of the superficial component is at medial malleolus and that of the deep posterior tibiotalar component is at the talar attachment.[19]

Deltoid ligament injuries are also found in chronic lateral ankle instability, which causes recurrent ankle sprain after a single episode of lateral sprain.[20]

Ankle Impingement

- Ankle impingements can occur due to post-traumatic synovitis, malunion, recurrent sprain, scarring, and osseous abnormalities.[21]
- *Anatomical locations of impingement:* Impingements can be anterior, anteromedial, anterolateral, posterior, and posteromedial.
- Clinically patients present with painful and restricted range of motion.

Anterior Impingement

- Patients present with restricted dorsiflexion.
- Anterior impingement occurs at the anterior recess between talar dome and anterior tibial plafond **(Fig. 21)**.
- Commonly seen in football players due to repeated dorsiflexion.
- Radiographs show osteophytes from anterior inferior margin of tibial plafond and from talar neck (forming a talar beak); however, these traction spurs may also be asymptomatic.[22]
- MRI is useful for diagnosing soft tissue abnormalities like anterior capsular and synovial thickening and fibrous bands in addition to anterior osteophytes.[23,24]

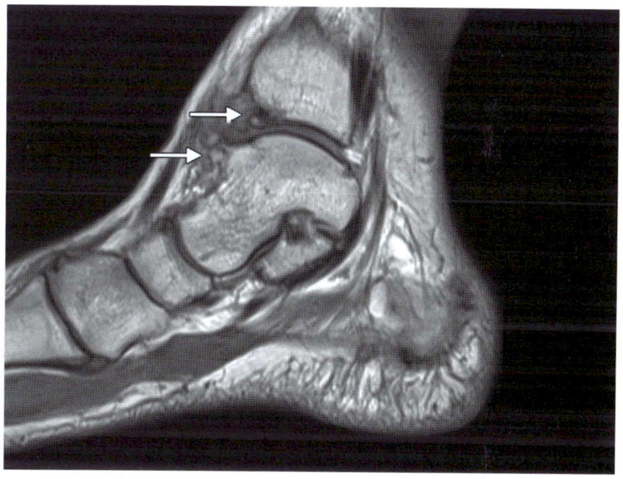

FIG. 21: Anterior impingement. Sagittal T1-weighted image shows osteophytes from anterior tibial plafond and from adjacent dome of talus.

Anterolateral Impingement

- Uncommon and is a diagnosis of exclusion in patients presenting with chronic anterolateral ankle pain exacerbated on dorsiflexion accompanied by swelling
- Usually caused by prior inversion injuries of the ankle
- Pain is caused by pathology in anterolateral recess
- Anatomical boundaries of anterolateral recess—anteriorly—ATFL
- Superiorly—anterior inferior tibiofibular ligament, medially-tibia, laterally fibula
- Normal content is minimal fluid
- Impingement can occur due to chronic synovial proliferation or torn or thickened ATFL or fibrotic tissue
- The fibrotic tissue can appear like triangular meniscus—known as meniscoid lesion
- Osteophytes in anterolateral tibial plafond can also cause impingement.[24]

Differential diagnosis of lateral ankle pain—peroneal tendon pathologies (tendinopathy, tears or subluxations), sinus tarsi syndrome, osteoarthritis, and ganglia.[21]

Anteromedial Impingement

- Uncommon cause of anteromedial ankle pain
- Caused by injury to anterior tibiotalar ligament (component of deep deltoid ligament), leading to thickening, soft tissue (meniscoid lesion), osteophytes or spurs along talar dome or anteromedial tibial plafond or medial malleolus

Posterior Impingement (Figs. 22A and B)

- Posterior impingement is clinically characterized by posterior ankle pain on plantar flexion.
- Commonly seen due to chronic repetitive injury in football players due to repeated plantar flexion causing impingement soft tissues between posterior calcaneal process and posterior tibia.
- Osseous abnormalities associated with posterior impingement include elongated lateral posterior process of talus (Stieda process) or os trigonum (formed by failure of fusion of the secondary ossification center of the lateral process).
- Edema of the posterior process or os trigonum can be seen.
- Soft tissue abnormalities include posterior capsular thickening, injuries of posterior talofibular, and tibiofibular ligament.[25]

Tarsal Coalitions (Figs. 23A to C)

- Patients with tarsal coalitions may be asymptomatic or present with hind-foot pain or flat foot.
- Calcaneonavicular and talo-calcaneal coalitions are most common; calcaneocuboid or talonavicular coalitions or multiple tarsal coalitions are rare.
- X-ray—45° internal oblique view can easily diagnose calcaneonavicular coalitions, with typical elongation of anterior process of calcaneus forming the "ant-eater sign." Reverse ant-eater sign is used to describe a hyperplastic navicular and a "drunken waiter" sign or C sign to describe a dysplastic sustentaculum tali.[26]
- Coalitions can be fibrous (hypointense on T2-weighted images), cartilaginous [hyperintense on T2-weighted images or osseous (bone marrow signal)]. Joint space is reduced or irregular and hypointense in fibrous coalitions, and obliterated in cases of osseous coalitions.[27]
- Bone marrow edema adjacent to the involved joint may be found and may lead to diagnosis of unsuspected coalition.[27]
- Sagittal MR images best depict the calcaneonavicular coalition.
- Coronal sections are best to visualize talocalcaneal coalitions, which generally involves the middle facet of talocalcaneal joint.
- CT and X-ray may be normal in patients with fibrous or cartilaginous coalitions, whereas MRI can directly show the area of abnormality.[27,28]

Adult-acquired Flat Foot[10]

- Acquired flat foot deformity in adults occurs due to lesions in the stabilizers of the medial side of the ankle-deltoid ligament complex, spring ligament or posterior tibial tendon.[10]
- Spring ligament consists of superomedial calcaneo-navicular ligament, medioplantar oblique calcaneo-navicular ligament, and inferoplantar longitudinal calcaneonavicular ligament.
- Superomedial calcaneonavicular ligament is the most frequently injured important component.
- MRI shows thickening and heterogeneity of the ligament (>6 mm) or thinned out or discontinuity within the ligament.[10]

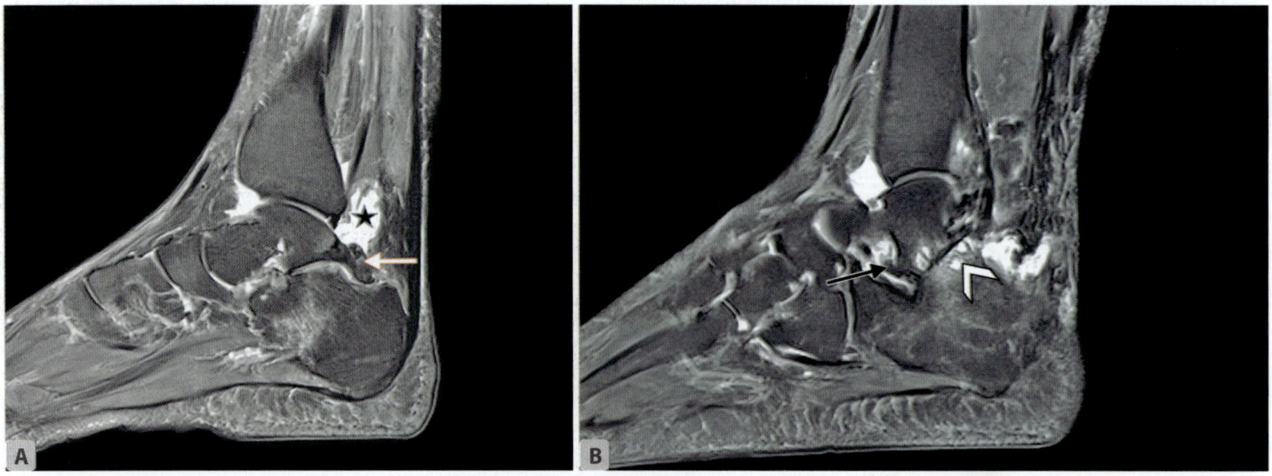

FIGS. 22A AND B: Posterior impingement due to elongated Stieda process (arrow in A) with osteophytes with subtalar arthritis (arrowhead). Complete replacement of sinus tarsi fat is also seen with edema and osteophytes (black arrow in B). Adventitious bursitis is seen superior and posterior to the Stieda process (* in A).

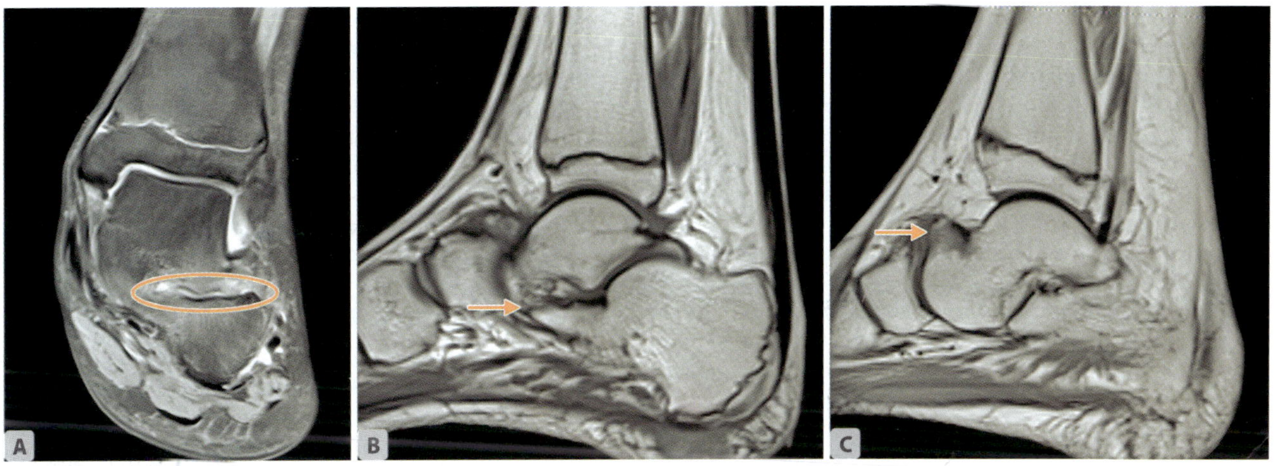

FIGS. 23A TO C: Coalition of anterior facet of talocalcaneal joint (oval in A) with absence of normal cartilage signal and irregular decreased joint space. (B) An elongated anterior process of calcaneus is seen (arrow). A talar beak is also seen (arrow in C).

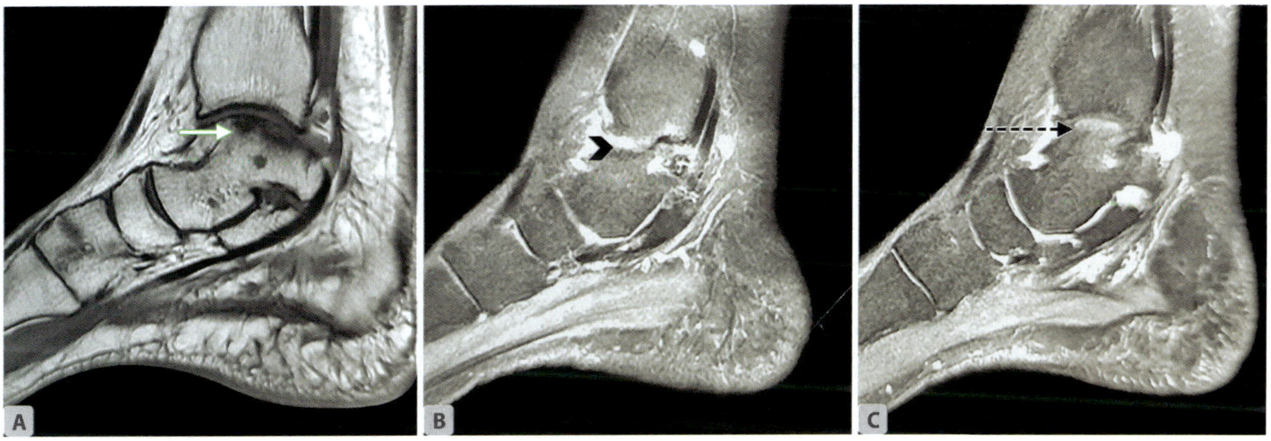

FIGS. 24A TO C: AVN of talus. (A) Sagittal T1-weighted image shows a subchondral area of hypointensity in the talar dome (arrow). On PD-weighted fat-saturated images (B and C), subchondral hyperintensity is seen in the talar dome (dashed arrow) along with subchondral collapse (arrowheads) and articular cartilage loss. (AVN: avascular necrosis).

- Adult-acquired flat foot is often associated with posterior tibial tendinopathy or tears.

Bones

Avascular Necrosis of Talus (Figs. 24A to C)

- *Anatomical considerations* predisposing to avascular necrosis (AVN)—talus is predominantly covered by cartilage (60%) with a tenuous arterial supply through the bare areas of the bone, predisposing it to ischemia in cases of traumatic disruption of blood supply.[29]
- *Atraumatic AVN*—predisposing factors include corticosteroid intake, alcoholism, SLE, renal transplant, and hyperlipidemia.
- *Traumatic AVN*—occurs most commonly as a sequelae of displaced talar neck fracture with subtalar dislocation. Associated ankle joint dislocation or talonavicular dislocation increases risk of AVN to 100%. Talar body fractures also have a high risk of AVN and a worse prognosis.[29]
- *"Hawkins sign"*—a linear radiolucent area parallel to talar dome is a well-described sign on radiographs; post-traumatic "Hawkins sign" implies an area of revascularization with reduced chances of AVN.
- However, radiographs are insensitive in early AVN, where ischemic or necrotic bone and healthy bone cannot be differentiated.
- *MRI* is sensitive in detecting bone marrow edema in early AVN.[29]
- T1-weighted images show the typical serpiginous low-signal intensity line in the talar dome.
- On T2-weighted images, a hyperintense line demarcating avascular bone is seen.
- Advanced AVN presents with articular cartilage damage and subchondral collapse **(Figs. 24A to C)**.[29]
- Other bones of foot prone to AVN are navicular and heads of metatarsals (Freiberg disease).

Osteochondral Lesions of Talus

- Osteochondral lesions of the talus have a predilection for the medial talar dome, (due to greater frequency of inversion injuries) and are areas of articular cartilage and subchondral bone changes.

- Osteochondral lesions denote a wide spectrum of changes including bone marrow edema to osteochondral fragment to osteoarthritic changes.[30]
- Clinical symptoms vary and patient can remain asymptomatic and this lesion can be incidentally detected.
- Patients can also present with persistent pain and instability.
- Lesions can be associated with acute as well as chronic injuries.[31]
- Routine radiographs may miss subtle lesions and weight bearing views and mortise views are recommended
- MRI demonstrates both articular cartilage changes as well as the condition of the subchondral bone.
- Articular cartilage in ankle is thinner and more difficult to assess but has the same trilaminar appearance with intermediate signal (higher on fat-saturated sequences).
- The innermost of basal layer of cartilage is relatively hypointense and adjacent subchondral bone is linear and hypointense.[31]
- Chondral damage can be limited to fissuring (which is difficult to detect without high resolution imaging) and fragmentation.
- Frank delamination of the basal layer of chondral cartilage leads to a flap which can remain in situ without any displacement.[31]
- Hyperintense fluid signal cleft may be found with minimal displacement. Since the fluid which insinuates may be minimal and intermediate in signal, these changes are difficult to appreciate.
- Underlying bone may be normal or show edema or an osteochondral fracture in acute injury.
- Chronic changes may be in the form of subchondral bone cysts or subchondral sclerosis **(Fig. 25)**.[31]

Degenerative

- Osteoarthritis (OA) of ankle joint is rare as compared to osteoarthritis of knee and most cases are idiopathic and occur in younger individuals.
- Post-traumatic osteoarthritis can also occur, after osteochondral injury with cartilage damage and ligamentous injuries **(Figs. 26A to C)**.
- *MRI findings* include bone marrow edema around tibiotalar and talofibular joint. Subtalar joint arthritis may cause periarticular bone marrow edema around talus and calcaneum.
- Bone marrow changes may be absent in early osteoarthritis even with radiographic evidence of OA.[32]

Nerve Entrapment-Tarsal Tunnel Syndrome

- *Anatomical boundaries*—tarsal tunnel is a fibro-osseous tunnel located on medial side of ankle.[1]
- It is bounded laterally by talus and sustentaculum tali of calcaneus, medially by flexor retinaculum and abductor hallucis muscle.
- *Contents*—tibialis posterior, FHL, flexor digitorum longus, posterior tibial artery, and tibial nerve

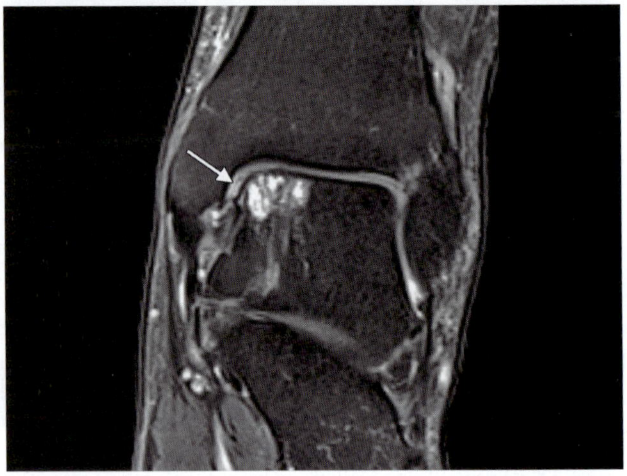

FIG. 25: Osteochondral lesion talus: Subchondral bone cysts in the medial talar dome with overlying cartilage showing loss of the trilaminar appearance and an area of hyperintensity (arrow). No definite osteochondral flap is seen.

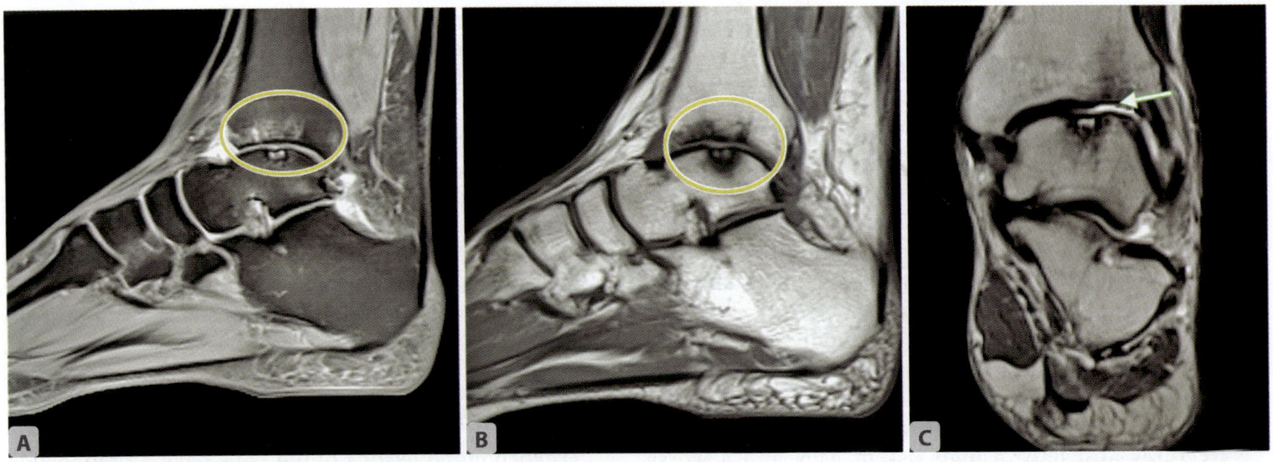

FIGS. 26A TO C: Degenerative arthritis with osteochondral lesion of talus. Subchondral cysts and edema seen in tibial plafond and talar dome (oval in A) with subchondral sclerosis (oval in B). There is an osteochondral lesion in mid-talar dome with subchondral cyst and mild flattening of talar dome. Cartilage denudation seen on coronal T2-weighted image (arrow in C).

- *Clinical presentation* of tarsal tunnel syndrome—burning and pain in sole and toes.
- *Common causes* are compression of posterior tibial nerve by ganglion cyst, tenosynovitis, neurogenic tumors, pannus, fibrosis, and varicosities **(Fig. 27)**. Post-traumatic scarring and hind foot valgus can also cause tarsal tunnel syndrome. Many cases are idiopathic.[33]
- *MRI findings* depend on the cause. Ganglion cysts are common.

Sinus Tarsi Syndrome

- *Anatomical boundaries*—sinus tarsi is a cone-shaped space located between talus and calcaneus, open laterally.
- *Contents*—fat, neurovascular structures, cervical ligament, interosseous ligament, and joint capsule insinuation from posterior subtalar joint.
- *Clinical presentation*—sinus tarsi syndrome is characterized by lateral ankle pain and instability.
- *Cause*—chronic inversion injuries with disruption of the cervical and interosseous ligaments along with injuries to lateral ligaments; inflammatory arthritis.
- *MRI findings*—complete obliteration of fat in the sinus tarsi replaced by high-signal intensity due to fluid or low signal in fibrosis (partial obliteration of fat is nonspecific)
- In the setting of acute ankle sprain, fluid or hemorrhage may accumulate in sinus tarsi, and should not be diagnosed as sinus tarsi syndrome.[1]

Infections

Untreated infectious arthritis causes rapid destruction of articular cartilage.[34] MRI is sensitive in detecting osteomyelitis as early as 1–2 days after infection. Osteitis with hypointense signal on T1-weighted images is the earliest finding.

In patients with diabetic neuropathy, a common indication for imaging is differentiating between neuropathic joint (Charcot's neuropathic osteoarthropathy) and osteomyelitis or osteomyelitis complicating neuropathic joint. MRI is sensitive and more specific than bone scintigraphy. Negative MRI rules out Charcot's neuroarthropathy.[35]

Early stages can present with subchondral bone marrow edema with or without microfractures on MRI, and early diagnosis is important for early offloading of the ankle joint to prevent chronic damage. The pattern of involvement can be tarsometatarsal, tarsal or subtalar, and ankle joints. Early stages progress to marked muscle and soft tissue edema **(Figs. 28A and B)**.[36] Untreated patients progress to chronic stage with subluxation, dislocation, and fractures with joint distension with debris and fluid. In later stages, MRI can be useful for diagnosing complications like infections with intraosseous or soft tissue abscesses, sinus tracts or causes of internal derangement due to ligament or tendon tears or tendinopathy due to impingements caused by subluxations or dislocations.[36]

Atypical infections like actinomycosis (actinomyces is a filamentous bacteria) or eumycetomas (true fungi) are chronic granulomatous suppurative infections of the foot with typical clinical presentation of blackish or yellowish granular discharge through draining sinuses depending upon the causative agent. A dot-in-circle sign has been described in mycetomas, which are a hypointense speck within a hyperintense lesion.[37]

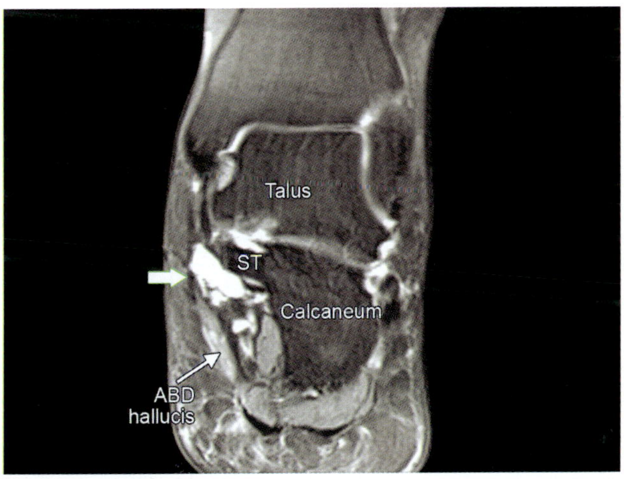

FIG. 27: Tarsal tunnel syndrome. Lobulated ganglion cyst (large arrow) causing mass effect on the tarsal tunnel. (ABD hallucis: abductor hallucis; ST: sustentaculum tali).

Inflammatory Arthritis

The ankle is affected by rheumatoid arthritis, seronegative arthropathies, reactive arthritis as well as gout. Erosions and synovitis and bone marrow edema along with effusions are seen earlier with MRI than on radiographs. Seronegative arthropathy and reactive arthritis presents with enthesitis with edema at insertion of Achilles tendon with or without tendinopathy along with plantar fasciitis **(Figs. 29A and B)**. MRI appearance of gouty arthritis with gouty tophi is nonspecific with hypointensity or intermediate signal on T1-weighted sequences and heterogeneous signal on T2-weighted images.[38] Erosions and synovitis are also seen.

Plantar Fasciitis (Figs. 30A and B)

- The plantar fascia originates from the plantar aspect of calcaneal tuberosity.
- It has three components—a central portion which originates from medial aspect of calcaneal tuberosity and medial and lateral expansions.[1]
- Normal thickness should not exceed 4 mm near the calcaneal attachment.[1]
- Clinical symptoms—pain or tenderness on the plantar aspect of ankle near plantar fascia attachment. Middle-aged women and patients with seronegative arthropathy are prone to develop this condition.[1]
- MRI appearance of plantar fasciitis—thickening of the plantar fascia near calcaneal attachment with high signal on T2-weighted sequences.
- Adjacent calcaneum may show edema or erosions.

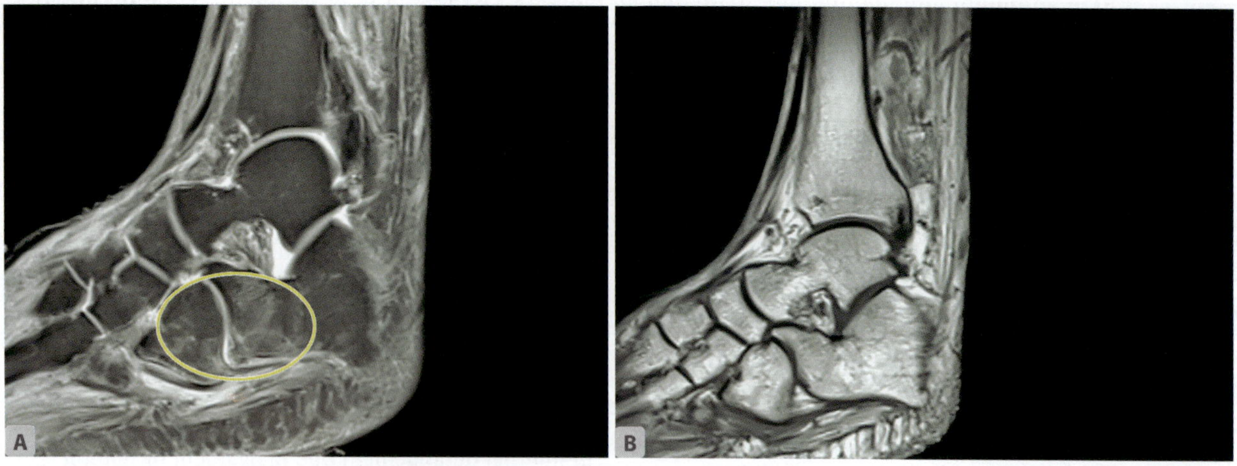

FIGS. 28A AND B: Early Charcot's neuroarthropathy with subarticular bone marrow edema at calcaneocuboid joint (oval in A) which is showing patchy hyperintensity in sagittal PD-weighted fat-saturated sequence (A). No hypointensity seen on sagittal T1-weighted image (B) suggesting absence of infection. Extensive muscle and soft tissue edema is seen.

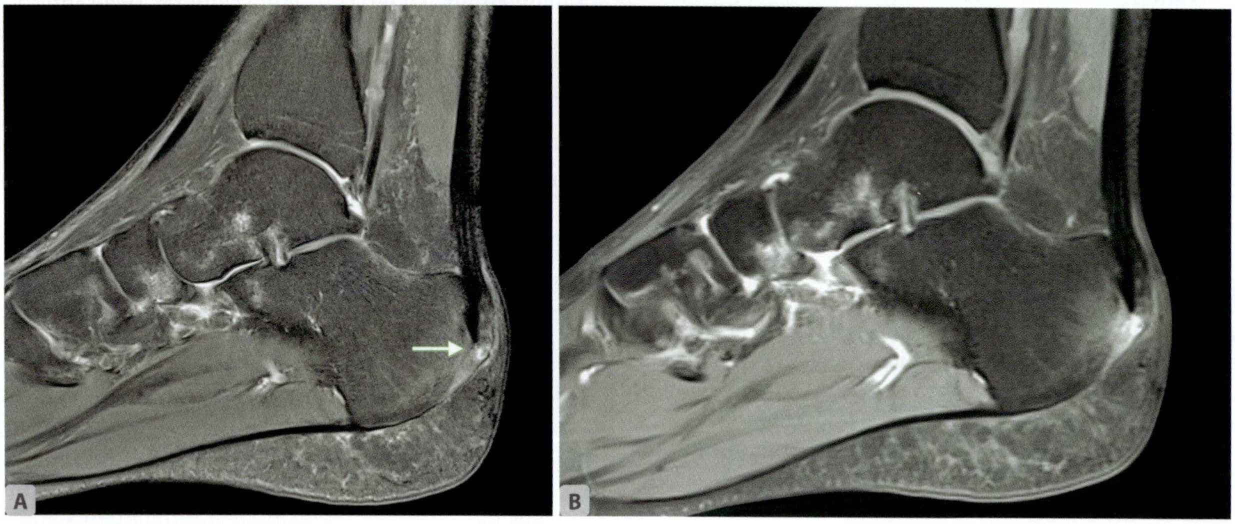

FIGS. 29A AND B: Seronegative arthropathy with enthesitis at Achilles tendon insertion (arrow in A) on sagittal PD-weighted fat-saturated image, with subarticular bone marrow edema in subtalar joint and navicular, which shows enhancement on postcontrast T1-weighted fat-saturated images (B).

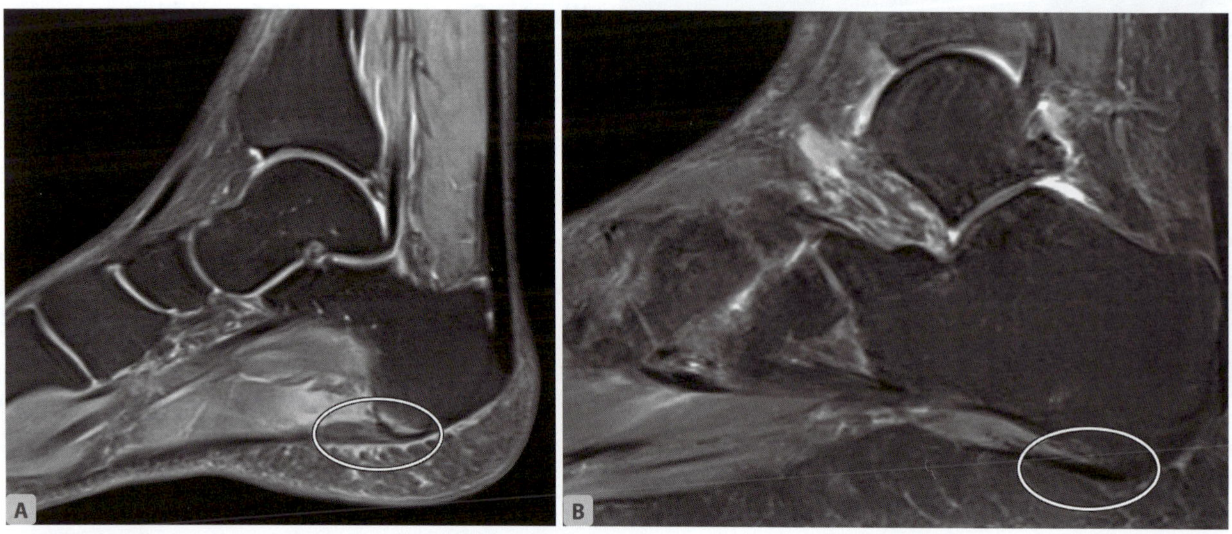

FIGS. 30A AND B: (A) Plantar fasciitis. The plantar fascia (oval) is thickened and hyperintense on the PD fat-saturated sagittal sequence. Adjacent bone marrow edema is seen in the calcaneum; (B) Normal hypointense thin plantar fascia.

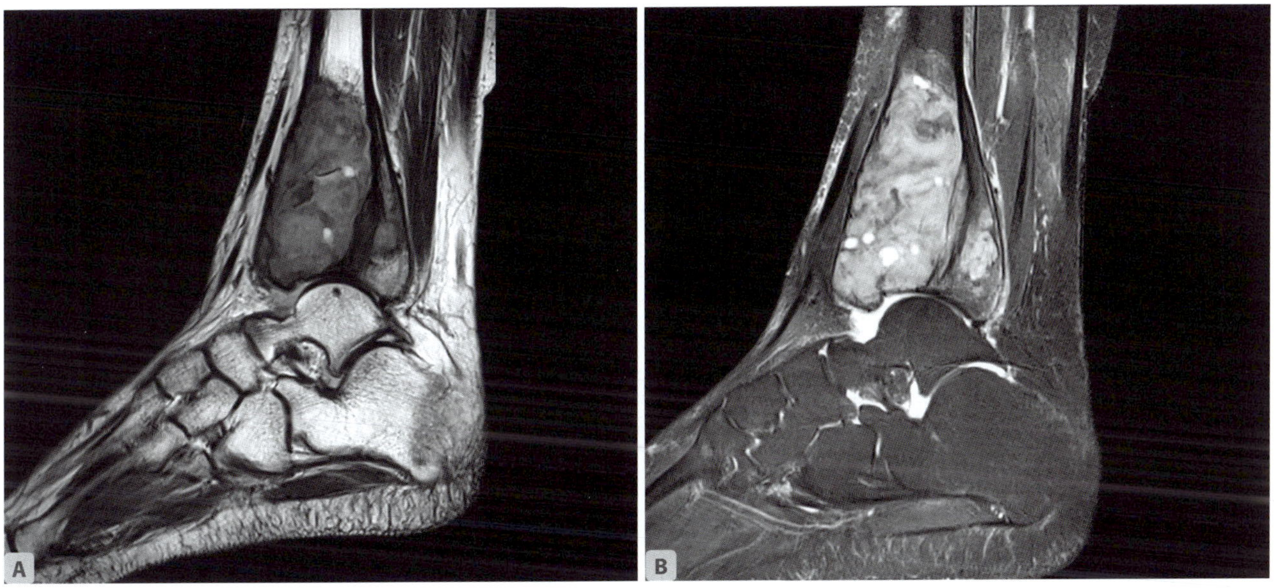

FIGS. 31A AND B: Giant cell tumor of the lower end of tibia. (A) A subarticular mildly expansile lesion with hypointense margins and predominantly hypointense internal contents with few hyperintense areas on sagittal T1-weighted image; (B) The lesion is hyperintense on sagittal T2-weighted fat-saturated image. No cortical breech or soft tissue is noted.

Tumors

Tumors of the ankle and foot are rare.

Osseous Tumors

Tumors of distal tibia and fibula most commonly seen are nonossifying fibromas, giant cell tumors **(Figs. 31A and B)**, aneurysmal bone cysts, enchondromas, and osteochondromas.[39]

Intraosseous lipoma and simple bone cyst are typically found anteriorly in midportion of calcaneus, whereas giant cell tumors and aneurysmal bone cysts are located posteriorly. Ewing's sarcoma and osteosarcoma rarely can involve the ankle and foot.[1] In the older adult, chondrosarcoma is common.[40]

Soft Tissue Tumors

Benign—plantar fibromatosis, vascular malformations, ganglion cysts, giant cell tumors of the tendon sheath, pigmented villonodular synovitis, and neurogenic tumors are common benign soft tissue tumors of the ankle and foot.

Malignant tumors—synovial sarcomas, epithelioid sarcomas, and pleomorphic sarcomas the common soft tissue are common soft tissue sarcomas in the ankle and foot.[40]

REFERENCES

1. Helms C, Major N, Anderson M, Kaplan PE, Dussault R, (Eds). Musculoskeletal MRI, 2nd edition. USA: Saunders; 2009. p. 435.
2. Schweitzer ME, Karasick D. MR imaging of disorders of the Achilles tendon. Am J Roentgenol. 2000;175(3):613-25.
3. Tam KF, Lui TH. MR imaging of the Achilles tendon after surgical repair. Open Orthop J. 2017;31(11):697-703.
4. Pierre-Jerome C, Moncayo V, Terk MR. MRI of the Achilles tendon: A comprehensive review of the anatomy, biomechanics, and imaging of overuse tendinopathies. Acta Radiol. 2010;51(4): 438-54.
5. Lawrence DA, Rolen MF, Abi Morshed K, Moukaddam H, Moukaddam H. MRI of heel pain. Am J Roentgenol. 2013;200(4):845-55.
6. Griffith JF, Hu M, Yeung DKW, Guo P, Lam SL, Xiao F, et al. Achilles tendon xanthomas: Fat-water separation at baseline and after treatment. Radiology. 2017;285(3):876-84.
7. Schubert R. MRI of peroneal tendinopathies resulting from trauma or overuse. Br J Radiol. 2013;86(1021):20110750.
8. Taljanovic MS, Alcala JN, Gimber LH, Rieke JD, Chilvers MM, Latt DL. High-resolution US and MR imaging of peroneal tendon injuries. Radiographics. 2015;35 (1):179-99.
9. Wang XT, Rosenberg ZS, Mechlin MB, Schweitzer ME. Normal variants and diseases of the peroneal tendons and superior peroneal retinaculum: MR imaging features. Radiographics. 2005;25(3):587-602.
10. Mengiardi B, Pinto C, Zanetti M. Spring ligament complex and posterior tibial tendon: MR anatomy and findings in acquired adult flatfoot deformity. Semin Musculoskelet Radiol. 2016;20(1):104-15.
11. Schweitzer ME, Karasick D. MR imaging of disorders of the posterior tibialis tendon. Am J Roentgenol. 2000;175(3):627-35.
12. Schweitzer ME. Magnetic resonance imaging of the foot and ankle. Magn Reson Q. 1993;9(4):214-34.
13. Linklater JM, Hayter CL, Vu D. Imaging of acute capsuloligamentous sports injuries in the ankle and foot: Sports imaging series. Radiology. 2017;283(3):642-65.

14. Lee MH, Cha JG, Lee YK, Choi GC, Paik SH, Lee HK, et al. The bright rim sign on MRI for anterior talofibular ligament injury with arthroscopic correlation. Am J Roentgenol. 2012;198(4):885-90.
15. Rosenberg ZS, Beltran J, Bencardino JT. From the RSNA refresher courses. Radiological Society of North America. MR imaging of the ankle and foot. Radiographics. 2000;20:S153-79.
16. Evans JM, Schucany G. Radiological evaluation of a high ankle sprain. Proc (Bayl Univ Med Cent). 2006;19:402-5.
17. Brown KW, Morrison WB, Schweitzer ME, Parellada JA, Nothnagel H. MRI findings associated with distal tibiofibular syndesmosis injury. Am J Roentgenol. 2004;182(1):131-6.
18. Mengiardi B, Pinto C, Zanetti M. Medial collateral ligament complex of the ankle: MR imaging anatomy and findings in medial instability. Semin Musculoskeletal Radiol. 2016;20(1):91-103.
19. Jeong MS, Choi YS, Kim YJ, Kim JS, Young KW, Jung YY. Deltoid ligament in acute ankle injury: MR imaging analysis. Skeletal Radiol. 2014;43(5):655-63.
20. Chun KY, Choi YS, Lee SH, Kim JS, Young KW, Jeong MS, et al. Deltoid ligament and tibiofibular syndesmosis injury in chronic lateral ankle instability: Magnetic resonance imaging evaluation at 3T and comparison with arthroscopy. Korean J Radiol. 2015;16(5):1096-103.
21. Berman Z, Tafur M, Ahmed SS, Huang BK, Chang EY. Ankle impingement syndromes: An imaging review. Br J Radiol. 2017;90(1070):20160735.
22. Stoller SM, Hekmat F, Kleiger B. A comparative study of the frequency of anterior impingement exostoses of the ankle in dancers and nondancers. Foot Ankle. 1984;4(4):201-3.
23. Haller J, Bernt R, Seeger T, Weissenback A, Tuchler H, Resnick D. MR-imaging of anterior tibiotalar impingement syndrome: agreement, sensitivity and specificity of MR imaging and indirect MR-arthrography. Eur J Radiol. 2006;58(3):450-60.
24. Cerezal L, Abascal F, Canga A, Pereda T, García-Valtuille R, Pérez-Carro L, et al. MR imaging of ankle impingement syndromes. Am J Roentgenol. 2003;181(2):551-9.
25. Robinson P, White LM. Soft-tissue and osseous impingement syndromes of the ankle: Role of imaging in diagnosis and management. Radiographics. 2002;22(6):1457-71.
26. Nalaboff KM, Schweitzer ME. MRI of tarsal coalition: Frequency, distribution, and innovative signs. Bull NYU Hosp Jt Dis. 2008;66(1):14-21.
27. Guignand D, Journeau P, Mainard-Simard L, Popkov D, Haumont T, Lascombes P. Child calcaneonavicular coalitions: MRI diagnostic value in a 19-case series. Orthop Traumatol Surg Res. 2011;97(1):67-72.
28. Newman JS, Newberg AH. Congenital tarsal coalition: Multimodality evaluation with emphasis on CT and MR imaging. Radiographics. 2000;20(2):321-32.
29. Pearce DH, Mongiardi CN, Fornasier VL, Daniels TR. Avascular necrosis of the talus: A pictorial essay. Radiographics. 2005;25(2):399-410.
30. Posadzy M, Desimpel J, Vanhoenacker FM. Staging of osteochondral lesions of the talus: MRI and cone beam CT. J Belg Soc Radiol. 2017;101(S2):1.
31. Linklater JM. Imaging of talar dome chondral and osteochondral lesions. Top Magn Reson Imaging. 2010;21(1):3-13.
32. Nakamura Y, Uchiyama S, Kamimura M, Komatsu M, Ikegami S, Kato H. Bone alterations are associated with ankle osteoarthritis joint pain. Sci Rep. 2016;6:18717.
33. Erickson SJ, Quinn SF, Kneeland JB, Smith JW, Johnson JE, Carrera GF, et al. MR imaging of the tarsal tunnel and related spaces: normal and abnormal findings with anatomic correlation. Am J Roentgenol. 1990;155(2):323-8.
34. Pioro MH, Mandell BF. Septic arthritis. Rheum Dis Clin North Am. 1997;23(2):239-58.
35. Rogers LC, Frykberg RG, Armstrong DG, Boulton AJ, Edmonds M, Van GH, et al. The Charcot foot in diabetes. J Am Podiatr Med Assoc. 2011;101(5):437-46.
36. Mautone M, Naidoo P. What the radiologist needs to know about Charcot foot. J Med Imaging Radiat Oncol. 2015;59(4):395-402.
37. Sarris I, Berendt AR, Athanasous N, Ostlere SJ. MRI of mycetoma of the foot: Two cases demonstrating the dot-in-circle sign. Skeletal Radiol. 2003;32(3):179-83.
38. Gandikota G, Glazebrook KN, Jacobson JA. Advanced imaging in gout. Am J Roentgenol. 2013;201(3):515-25.
39. Toepfer A, Harrasser N, Recker M, Lenze U, Pohlig F, Gerdesmeyer L, et al. Distribution patterns of foot and ankle tumors: A university tumor institute experience. BMC Cancer. 2018; 18:735.
40. Mascard E, Gaspar N, Brugières L, Glorion C, Pannier S, Gomez-Brouchet A. Malignant tumours of the foot and ankle. EFORT Open Rev. 2017;2(5):261-71.

CHAPTER

172

Radiological Evaluation of Appendicular Trauma

Atin Kumar, Devasenathipathy Kandasamy, Arun Kumar Gupta

INTRODUCTION

Skeletal trauma is one of the most common forms of injuries suffered by people in everyday life. The extremities are the most often affected. The emergency radiologist plays a key role in the workup of such patients as the initial evaluation requires radiographic examination. The radiograph has to be well-performed and accurately interpreted. It provides diagnostic evidence of the presence of fracture or dislocation along with the severity and extent of the trauma. The radiographs are also essential to check for accuracy of fracture reduction and to monitor bone healing.

CLINICAL EVALUATION

The features pointing toward underlying fracture include deformity, swelling, ecchymosis, marked local tenderness, abnormal mobility and crepitus on palpation, and impairment of function. It is important to assess the state of the circulation and neural integrity in the limb distal to the fracture, both at the time of initial presentation and after any intervention.

The radiologist should also be aware of the mechanism of the injury as well as the time interval from the injury to the radiographic examination. This helps the radiologist to know what and where to look for in the radiograph. The radiologist can also look for specific injuries that are known to be associated with the mechanism of the injury.

RADIOLOGICAL EVALUATION

Definitions and Classification

A *fracture* is a disruption in the continuity of the bone. A *dislocation* is a complete disruption of a joint with loss of congruity between the articular surfaces. *Subluxation* is a minor disruption of the joint where some part of the articular surfaces remain in contact.

The fractures are clinically classified into open or closed fractures. The open fractures are those which penetrate the overlying skin and the fracture site is exposed to the external environment whereas closed fractures are those with intact overlying skin and hence no exposure to the environment. This makes the open fractures amenable to the risk of infection because of contamination by microorganisms.

The radiographic evaluation of fracture should work on the basic principle of obtaining at least two views of the involved bone, ideally perpendicular to each other, with each view including two joints adjacent to the involved bone. This helps the radiologist eliminate the risk of missing an associated dislocation or subluxation at a site remote from the apparent primary injury. Additional views should be obtained if there is any doubt or in specific situations like an oblique view for scaphoid fracture. It is estimated that about 5% of fractures are seen only on one view and about 5% of fractures require additional views to be detected **(Figs. 1A and B)**. In children, especially if there is involvement of the ossification centers which are not fused, it may be necessary to obtain a radiograph of the normal, unaffected side for comparison.

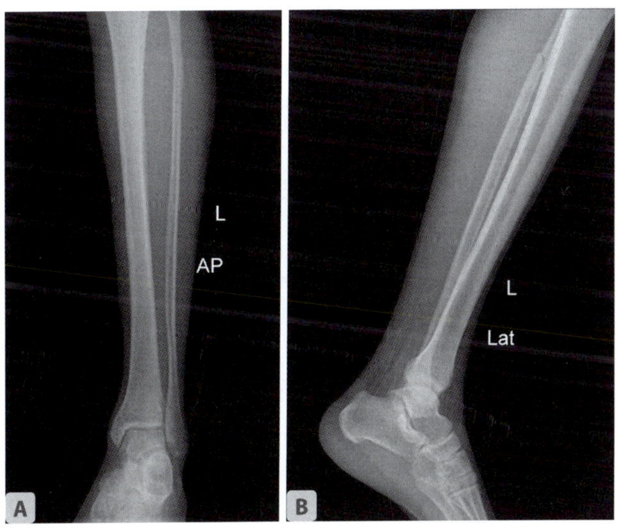

FIGS. 1A AND B: Anteroposterior (AP) and lateral (Lat) radiographs of the leg show a fracture of the upper shaft of fibula which is visualized only on the lateral view and is almost not seen on the AP view.

The complete radiographic evaluation of a trauma patient should consist of:
- Osseous evaluation
- Soft tissue evaluation

Osseous Evaluation

Presence or Absence of Bony Injury

A careful examination of all the bones included in the radiograph must be done for detection or ruling out a fracture. A fracture can appear as any of the following—an obvious disruption in continuity of bone, abnormal line of radiolucency, cortical irregularity or increase in bone density (due to impacted or compression fractures). Sometimes the fracture may be "occult" which are clinically suspected but are not visualized on the initial radiograph. They may be detected subsequently on a follow-up radiography or scintigraphy. Scaphoid fractures are an example.

Anatomic Location and Extent of the Fracture

When describing a fracture it is important to specify the location within the long bone. In case of a fracture involving shaft of a long bone it should be described whether it is located in proximal, middle or distal thirds of bone, or at junction of any two parts. It can also be described in terms of involvement of anatomic point of reference, e.g., supracondylar fracture of humerus. For fractures located near bone ends, mention should be made of any intra-articular extension as this will alter the subsequent management of the patient.

Types of Fracture

Complete or incomplete: The fracture is classified as complete if it involves the entire width of the bone to involve both the cortices and incomplete if only some of the bony trabeculae are completely severed while others are bent or remain intact.[1] Incomplete fractures are more likely to be seen in children. Angular deformities are common without any displacement in incomplete fractures **(Table 1)**.

The complete fractures are further classified as:
- *Simple*: One fracture line separating the bone into two fragments.
- *Comminuted*: Two or more fracture lines with three or more fragments. A "butterfly" fragment can be seen if a small triangular fragment gets isolated on the concave side of the injury.

The incomplete fractures can be of following types:
- *Greenstick (Hickory stick) fractures* ***(Figs. 2A and B)***: Fractures occurring due to angulation forces primarily in infants and young children below 10 years of age because of the relatively greater component of pliable woven bone. The fracture affects the tension or the convex side of the bone. The bone bends with the convex side showing a horizontal break in the continuity of the cortex whereas the other concave side remains intact.[1] The greenstick fractures heal without any complications in most instances.
- *Torus (buckling) fractures*: Fractures occurring due to longitudinal compressive forces over a soft bone of young child. The fracture affects the compressive (concave) side of the bone. The cortex bulges outward due to compressive forces at the site of injury. They occur mostly in the metaphysis and are very painful.[1]
- *Plastic bowing fractures* ***(Figs. 3A and B)***: No true fracture is seen. It occurs when the force on the bone is not sufficient enough to cause a cortical disruption but instead leads to bowing of the bone.

TABLE 1: Fracture types.

Complete fracture	Incomplete fracture
• Simple—one fracture line, two bony fragments • Comminuted—two or more fracture lines with three or more fragments	• Greenstick—cortical break in convex side, intact concave side • Torus—compression fracture in concave side • Plastic bowing—no fracture, just bowing seen

Direction of the Fracture Line

This is described with respect to the longitudinal axis of the bone.[2] Based on this, the fractures can be classified into:
- *Transverse fracture* ***(Figs. 4A and B)***: The fracture line is perpendicular to the long axis of the bone. In long bones it occurs as a result of angulation force. This type of fracture is usually stable and unlikely to be displaced after reduction.
- *Oblique fracture*: The fracture line runs oblique to the long axis of the bone and the angle is <90°.
- *Spiral fracture* ***(Fig. 5)***: The fracture line turns and twists around the shaft and encircles it at least once. It occurs as a result of twisting force to the limb. This type of fracture is prone to be displaced after reduction.[2]

Spatial Relationship of the Fragments

This is described in terms of apposition/displacement, alignment/angulation, rotation and distraction/over-riding.

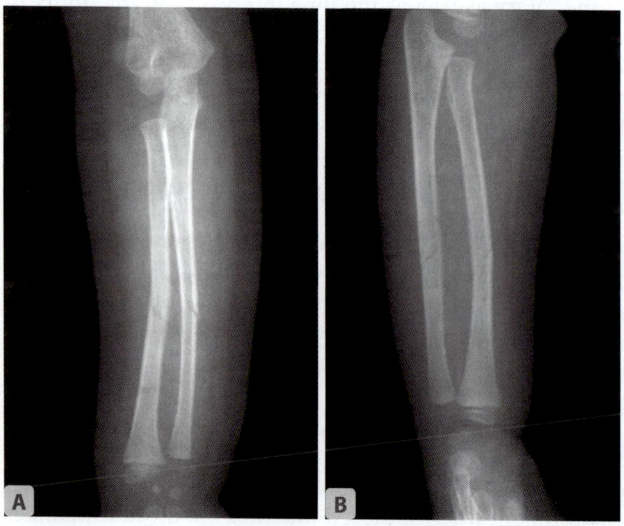

FIGS. 2A AND B: Anteroposterior and lateral radiographs of the forearm show greenstick fractures of the shaft of radius and ulna.

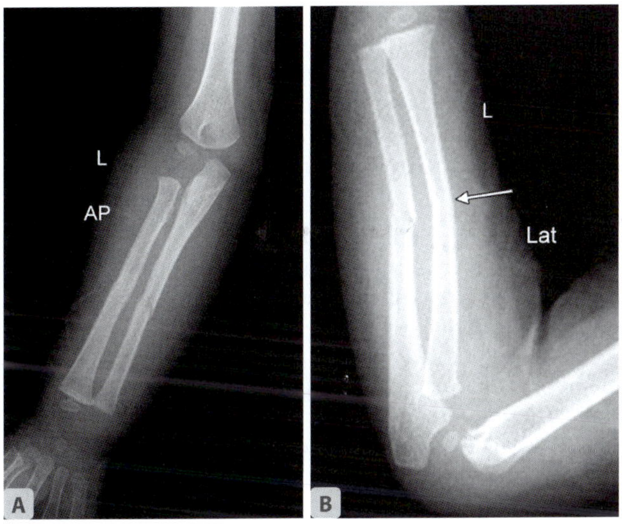

FIGS. 3A AND B: Anteroposterior and lateral radiographs of the forearm show plastic bowing fracture without an obvious cortical break in the midshaft of radius (arrow). A complete fracture of the adjacent ulna is associated.

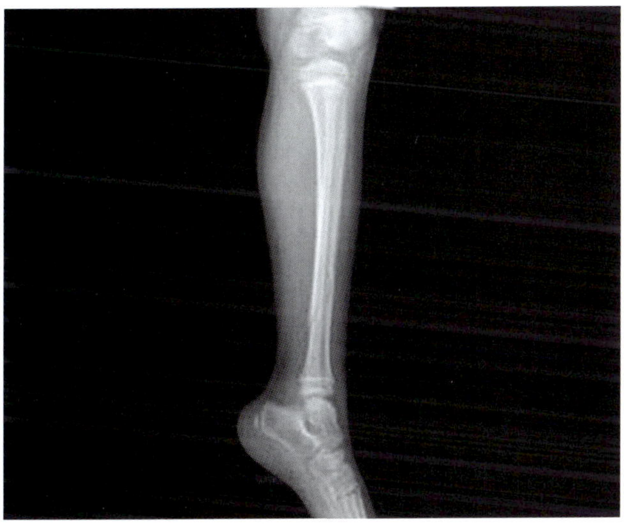

FIG. 5: Lateral radiograph of the leg showing a spiral fracture through the lower shaft of tibia.

- *Apposition*: It refers to the state of bony contact at the fracture site and the resultant shift of the fragments relative to each other. This classifies fractures into undisplaced and displaced. The displacement is described with reference to the direction of shift of the distal fragment. An undisplaced fracture with a fine fracture line is termed as "hairline" fracture.
- *Alignment*: It refers to the position of the distal fragment with respect to the proximal fragment. It can be lateral/medial displacement or tilt/angulation. The angulation of the distal fragment medially is termed "varus" and laterally is termed "valgus"
- *Rotation*: It refers to the rotation of the distal fragment over the longitudinal axis. It can be internal or external

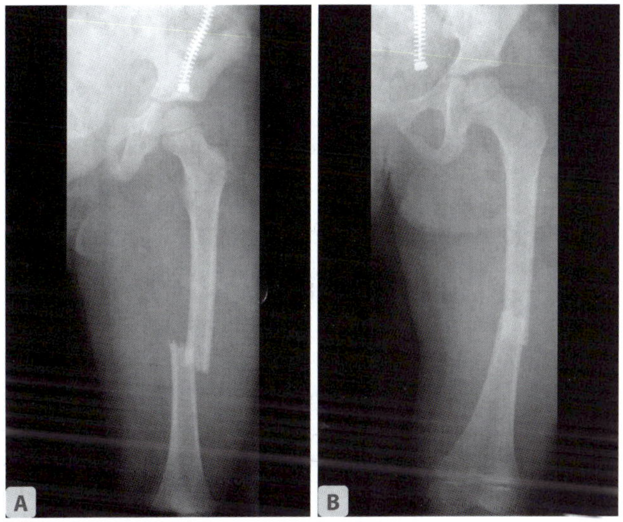

FIGS. 4A AND B: Anteroposterior and oblique radiographs of the left thigh show a transverse fracture of the shaft of ulna with overriding of the bone fragments.

rotation. To comment on rotation, the proximal and distal joints must be included in the radiograph.
- *Overriding/distraction*: A longitudinal separation of the bony fragments in the long axis of the bone with resultant increased distance between the two fragments is termed distraction. If the bony fragments overlap on each other, it is termed overriding and leads to foreshortening of the limb **(Figs. 4A and B)**.

Presence of Special Features

The special features that need to be commented upon in a radiograph include:

- *Impaction*: When the two fragments are driven into each other. This occurs due to compressive forces. The classical radiolucent fracture line is not seen but instead a subtle radiopaque line is seen at the site which may be the only marker of the fracture. It is important to obtain additional views in this situation in case of a doubt.
- *Depression*: It represents an inward bulging of the outer bony surface. It is a type of impaction fracture. This gives rise to a "double cortical line". It is seen most commonly at tibial plateau and radial head in extremities and in frontal bone in the skull.
- *Compression*: It represents an impaction fracture involving the spinal vertebral body due to hyperflexion forces.
- *Avulsion*: It involves tearing away of a portion of the bone usually at insertion of a muscle or ligament due to forceful pulling. The frequent sites are tuberosities of tubular bones, elbow, lateral metatarsal and lower cervical spinous processes. A small cortical avulsion is termed a "flake" fracture. "Chip" or "corner" fracture represents avulsion of a small fragment of bone from the corner of a phalanx or other short or long tubular bone. Corner chip fractures at metaphyseal ends in children should raise the suspicion of battered baby syndrome.

Presence of Associated Abnormalities of the Adjacent Joints

It may be commonly associated with certain types of mechanisms of injuries and some specific fractures. Examples include a femoral shaft fracture associated with hip joint dislocation, a lower end tibial fracture associated with upper end fibula fracture, etc. The joints may be dislocated or subluxated. When dislocation is associated with a fracture, it is termed as fracture dislocation. A fracture through a joint surface may involve the cartilage only (chondral fracture) or cartilage and underlying bone (osteochondral fracture).

Presence of Special Types of the Fractures

The fractures may be due to excessive stress or due to underlying bone weakening disorder. A normal classical fracture occurs due to excessive trauma to a normal bone without underlying abnormality. The ends of the fracture are sharply marginated and the adjacent bone appears healthy in acute settings. However, if the underlying bone is weakened by a localized (tumor) or systemic disease process (osteopenia due to any cause, metastases, multiple myeloma), then even a normal trauma (which is otherwise insufficient to cause fracture) can lead to a fracture. Such fractures are termed "pathological fractures." These fractures are usually transverse with smooth margins. A "stress (fatigue)" fracture is caused by repetitive stress on normal bone. The stress itself is insufficient to cause fracture but over a period of time it leads to the development of fracture. These are commonly seen in runners, dancers, and gymnasts. The metatarsals, tibia, and fibula are commonly affected bones. These fractures become radiologically evident about 2–4 weeks after trauma as a faint transverse radiolucent line often surrounded by a callus **(Figs. 6A and B)**. "Insufficiency fractures" are special type of fractures which occur as a result of chronic repetitive normal stress on a pathological (often osteoporotic) bone. They can occur even with normal walking in a person with underlying osteopenia. They occur commonly in patients of osteomalacia, Paget's disease, and rickets. Radiographically they are seen as linear lucencies on the convex surface of the bone that are oriented perpendicular to the long axis of the bone. They are often multiple and bilateral.

Involvement of Growth Plate/Physis: Seen in Children

These fractures result in growth arrest and deformity. The *Salter-Harris* classification is used most commonly for such fractures.[3] This classifies the physeal injuries into the five types **(Table 2)**.

Radiographs may not detect the epiphyseal injuries or their displacement especially if only one side alone is radiographed. Hence, it is important to radiograph the opposite limb for comparative evaluation.

Soft-tissue Evaluation

- *Soft-tissue swelling*: Almost always present adjacent to the site of acute fracture.
- *Obliteration or displacement of fat stripes*: Also gives a clue to underlying soft tissue swelling associated with a fracture. Commonly seen in fractures around the wrist joint.
- *Joint capsular swelling*: May be seen due to joint effusion/hemarthrosis secondary to an intra-articular fracture. The capsular distension is also evident by bulging of fat planes around it. It is a good sign to detect fractures near elbow joint. If there is leak of bone marrow fat from within the medullary cavity into the joint along with blood (lipohemarthrosis), then a fat-fluid level may be visualized. It is better evident on computed tomography (CT) or magnetic resonance imaging (MRI).

FRACTURE HEALING

The pathological process of healing of fractures occurs in following phases which last for about 10 days each.[4]

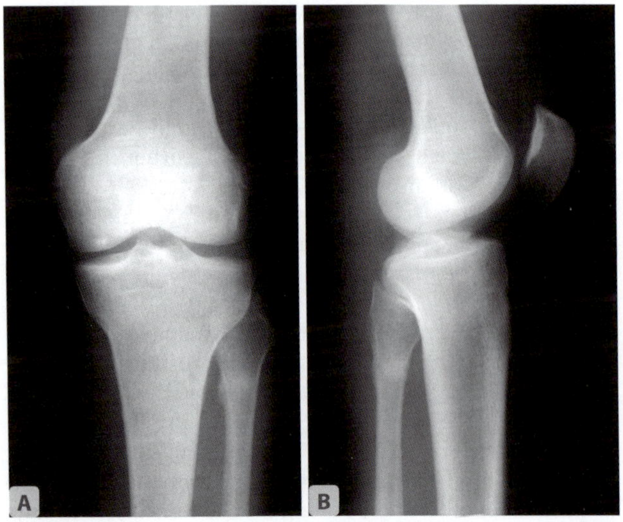

FIGS. 6A AND B: Anteroposterior and lateral radiographs of the knee joint show a stress fracture of the proximal shaft of fibula.

TABLE 2: Salter-Harris classification of physeal injuries.

Types	Imaging features
Type 1	Fracture through the growth plate. The radiograph appears normal
Type 2	Fracture through the displaced growth plate with involvement of the metaphysis. The metaphyseal fragment is known as the "Thurston Holland" sign. This type is the most common seen in about 75% of cases
Type 3	Fracture through the growth plate with involvement of the epiphysis. The resultant intra-articular fracture often requires open reduction treatment
Type 4	Obliquely oriented vertical fracture passing though the metaphysis, growth plate, and epiphysis
Type 5	Crush fracture leading to compressive deformity of the growth plate. The initial radiographs are normal. Subsequently due to growth arrest there occurs progressive angulation deformity. Hence, it is advisable to follow-up these children for at least 2 years following injury

- Circulatory or inflammatory phase—it comprises:
  - Stage of hematoma
  - Stage of subperiosteal and endosteal cellular proliferation
  - Stage of callus formation
- Consolidation or reparative phase
- Remodeling or mechanical phase.

Radiologically, the fracture line shows increase in its width in the first few days due to resorption of its margins. In the next 2–4 weeks the healing occurs by formation of callus. In cases of simple undisplaced fractures the healing occurs by primary union wherein the predominant callus formation is endosteal (internal) which obliterates the fracture line. In cases of complex displaced fractures the healing occurs by secondary union wherein the predominant callus formation is periosteal (external). The callus is initially radiolucent when it contains fibrous tissue and cartilage. At this stage the fracture may be clinically united. Gradually the callus gets remodeled and also gets ossified to give the radiodense white line appearance consistent with radiographic union. In a young adult the total process takes around 4–6 weeks while it may take up to 12 weeks in elderly.[5]

COMPLICATIONS OF FRACTURE

The various complications occur at multiple time intervals postinjury. They are divided into immediate, intermediate, and delayed complications **(Table 3)**.

Immediate Complications

- *Vascular injury*: Most commonly with penetrating trauma, sharp bony fragments in open or comminuted fractures or even due to operative manipulation. The popliteal artery, distal superficial femoral artery, and the brachial artery are involved most frequently.
- *Nerve and soft tissue injury*: The adjacent nerves, muscles, ligaments, and tendons may show varying severity of injury.
- *Compartment syndrome*: Results from increased pressure within a muscular compartment secondary to hemorrhage and edema. It leads to muscle necrosis and may be limb or life threatening. Anterior compartment of leg and anterior compartment of forearm are common sites.
- *Fat embolism*: Associated with fracture of a major bone most commonly femur. Usually, it is not of any clinical significance as it occurs in minor degree. It leads to emboli of fat globules from the bone marrow into the vessels and get lodged in small vessels of lung and brain. There is a classical symptom free period of about 2 days between the injury and symptoms of fat embolism. It is clinically evident by cerebral disturbance, drowsiness, coma, tachypnea, dyspnea, and petechial rash over the body.[6,7] Chest radiograph may reveal bilateral diffuse air space consolidation in peripheral distribution with normal sized heart. Brain changes are best evident on MRI in the form of bilateral small T2-hyperintense lesions in deep white matter and corpus callosum which may show restricted diffusion.[8]
- *Gas gangrene*: Occurs in open wounds which get infected by *Clostridium perfringens*.

TABLE 3: Complications of fractures.

Immediate complications	Intermediate complications	Delayed complications
• Vascular injury • Nerve and soft tissue injury • Compartment syndrome • Fat embolism • Gas gangrene	• Infection • Post-traumatic ossification • Sudeck's post-traumatic osteodystrophy • Post-traumatic osteolysis • Synostosis	• Abnormal healing process • Avascular necrosis • Disuse osteoporosis • Post-traumatic arthritis

Intermediate Complications

- *Infection*: It occurs in the form of osteomyelitis and is seen in open fractures and those which have undergone operative intervention. Most commonly by *Staphylococcus aureus*. Tibia and femur are the frequently involved bones.
- *Post-traumatic ossification* ***(Fig. 7)***: It is also known as myositis ossificans which is a misnomer as there is no infective lesion of the muscle. It is heterotopic bone formation occurring deep to the muscles. The common sites are elbow and thigh. The new bone formation occurs in the hematoma beneath the stripped periosteum and the joint capsule. The children are more prone as the periosteum is loosely attached and gets stripped following trauma. On radiograph the classical hallmark is the clearly recognizable pattern of its evolution over a period of 2 months. At the end of 2 months when the lesion is fully formed, the characteristic zonal appearance may be seen. The central part is radiolucent representing immature bone formation. It is surrounded by a dense peripheral zone of ossification. The outermost part of this ossification zone shows definite well-organized cortical bone. A thin lucent zone may separate this cortical layer from the ossific mass. If the ossification reaches up to the bone surface it mimics parosteal osteosarcoma. CT and MRI may help to confirm the diagnosis. Biopsy is conformatory.[9]
- *Sudeck's post-traumatic osteodystrophy*: Also known as reflex sympathetic dystrophy syndrome or post-traumatic painful osteoporosis. The hands or feet are commonly involved. The patient presents about 2 months after injury with extremely painful and tender swollen extremity which hyperemic and glossy with marked stiffness of the small joints. Colles' fracture is the most common cause in upper limb. The radiograph shows diffuse soft-tissue swelling with gradually progressive patchy osteoporosis which is more than that expected by disuse osteoporosis. The bone scan may show diffuse area of increased uptake.
- *Post-traumatic osteolysis*: It refers to dissolution of bone following trauma. Most commonly involves distal end of clavicle and pubic bones.
- *Synostosis*: It may occur between bones which are closely opposed such as radius-ulna and tibia-fibula.

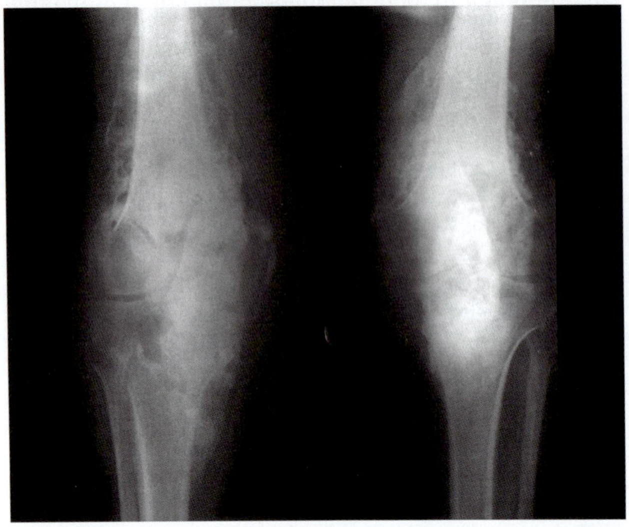

FIG. 7: Anteroposterior radiograph of the bilateral knee joints shows extensive soft tissue ossification around bilateral knee joints suggestive of myositis ossificans.

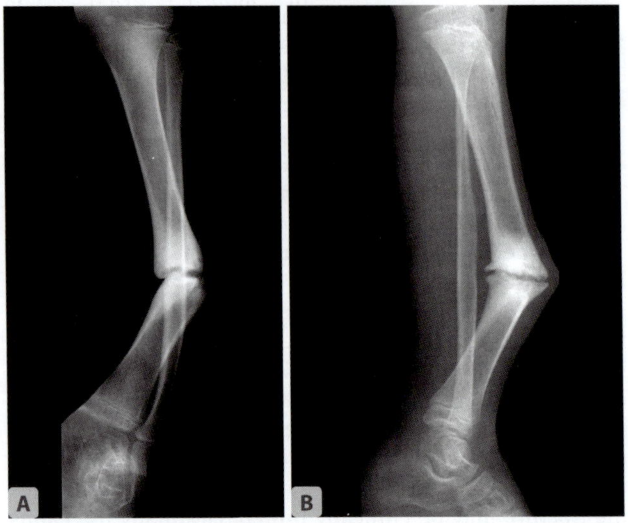

FIGS. 8A AND B: Anteroposterior and lateral radiographs of the leg. 6 months after trauma shows an old nonunited fracture of the shaft of tibia with rounding of fracture edges, marginal sclerosis, gap between the fracture ends and formation of pseudoarthrosis.

Delayed Complications

- *Abnormal healing process*: These occur secondary to multiple factors including inadequate blood supply, distraction, inadequate immobilization, interposition of soft tissues, infection, and pathological weakness of bone. The term delayed union is used to describe a fracture which does not unite within a reasonable period of time (16–18 weeks) depending on patient's age and the fracture site. Nonunion is diagnosed if the fracture fails to unite. The most common sites are midclavicle, ulna, and tibia. The radiograph shows characteristic features after few months which include rounding of fracture edges, smoothening of margins with sclerosis, gap between the two fragments, demonstration of mobility (on serial stress radiographs or on fluoroscopy), lack of callus formation, and pseudoarthrosis **(Figs. 8A and B)**. Pseudoarthrosis refers to formation of false joint-like cavity with synovial-like capsule between the ends of the two fragments. If formed, a pseudoarthrosis requires refracture and removal for the process of healing. Malunion refers to a union of fracture fragments in an imperfect anatomical position which results in unacceptable deformity. It usually requires surgical correction.
- *Avascular necrosis* ***(Fig. 9)***: It is also known as osteonecrosis. It occurs due to loss of blood supply secondary to fracture. The process may take months to years. The most commonly affected bones are femoral head, scaphoid, humeral head and talus. On radiograph it appears as a sharply defined dense bone in contrast to the surrounding disuse osteoporosis. This progresses to loss of height of the involved part with shrunken, crumpled appearance. Bone scan with ^{99m}Technetium may be helpful. MRI shows the features earliest.
- *Disuse osteoporosis*: Mild-to-moderate degree osteoporosis secondary to pain and immobilization.

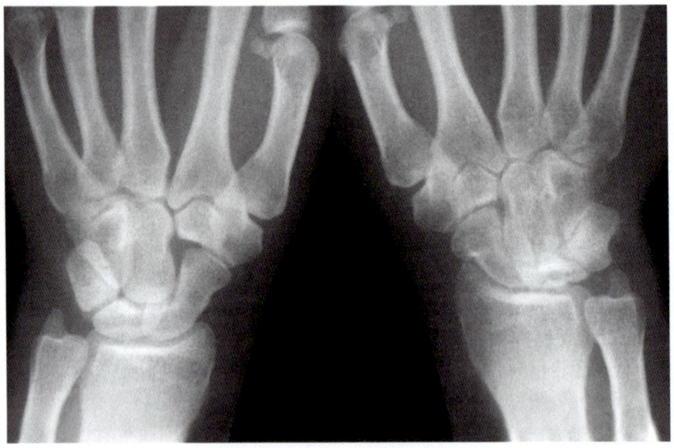

FIG. 9: Posteroanterior radiograph of the bilateral wrist joints. The left lunate is showing an old fracture with marked sclerosis of the bone consistent with avascular necrosis (Kienböck's disease).

- *Post-traumatic arthritis*: Degenerative changes in the joint. The predisposing factors include intra-articular fracture, malaligned fracture and avascular necrosis. Seen most commonly in weight bearing joints such as knee, hip and ankle.

IMAGING MODALITIES

Plain radiograph: It is the first-line investigation for any skeletal trauma of the extremities. A minimum of two radiographic projections ideally perpendicular to each other should be acquired to conclusively rule out fracture. Additional views are taken if necessary. The detailed radiographic evaluation has been discussed earlier.

Ultrasonography: It has been shown to have an increasing role in the detection of fractures in the acute setting of trauma as well as monitoring of fracture healing. It is also helpful in joint pathologies for detection of effusion (hemarthrosis), ligaments, and tendinous injuries.

Radioisotope scanning: With ^{99m}Technetium diphosphonate is useful in detection of occult fractures. The scan may take become positive after 24 hours in acute setting. It is also helpful in detection of stress fractures.

Computed tomography: It is markedly superior to radiograph for detection of bony injuries. It is reserved for areas of complex bony anatomy or where the radiographs are equivocal. Multiplanar reformats in all three planes gives a complete overview of the presence and extent of the bony injury along with its relation to surrounding structures. In addition, the soft tissues can also be well evaluated which gives it an added advantage over radiographs. It is commonly used to assess fractures of tibial plateau, ankle, and epiphyseal injuries. In addition it can assess complications such as vascular injury by CT angiography.

Magnetic resonance imaging: It has become the investigation of choice for detailed evaluation of injuries of joints and soft tissues. It has advantages of excellent depiction of soft tissue injuries including those of ligaments, tendons, menisci, and cartilage besides detection of bony injuries by marrow edema. It can detect subtle bone injuries such as occult fractures and bone contusions which may sometimes not be evident on both radiographs and CT. It is also the best modality to detect complications such as avascular necrosis. Use of contrast MR arthrography also enables better depiction of articular and periarticular injuries such as those related to labrum, cartilage, and menisci.

UPPER LIMB TRAUMA

Dislocation of the Shoulder

Glenohumeral joint is the most common joint of the body to dislocate. It is seen usually in adults and elderly. It is classified into subtypes depending upon the direction of displacement of the humeral head into anterior, posterior, superior and inferior direction.

Anterior Dislocation

It is the most frequent (95% cases). The humeral head can dislocate anteriorly to lie in subglenoid, subcoracoid, or subclavicular position. The subglenoid dislocation is accompanied by fracture of greater tuberosity whereas subcoracoid dislocation can occur without bony injury and is prone to recurrence **(Fig. 10)**. The Hill-Sachs defect (impaction of the humeral head) and avulsion of the inferior glenoid rim (Bankart's lesion) are often seen especially with recurrent dislocations. Magnetic resonance imaging with MR arthrography is more sensitive in detecting these lesions.[10]

Posterior Dislocation

It occurs as a result of violent muscle contraction as in epileptic convulsion or following electric shock.

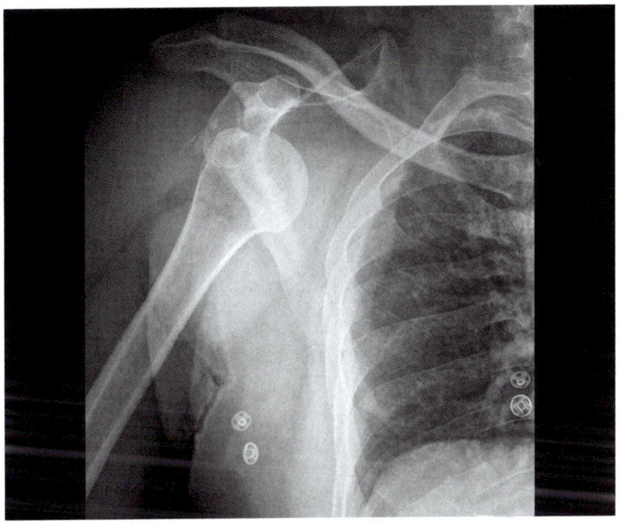

FIG. 10: Anteroposterior radiograph of the right shoulder shows anteroinferior dislocation of the right humerus.

Inferior Dislocation

It is also known as *luxatio erecta*. It occurs secondary to severe hyperabduction trauma with humeral head locked in abduction under the subglenoid position.

Superior Dislocation

It is rare. It occurs secondary to considerable force and most commonly occurs secondary to rotator cuff tear.

The radiological evaluation of shoulder dislocation should consist of a true anteroposterior and a trans-scapular view since it may be missed in the anteroposterior views with internal and external rotation which are routinely done for any shoulder pathology.[11] The AP view can diagnose a shoulder dislocation but the anterior and posterior varieties cannot be differentiated on it. Fracture of the glenoid rim or the greater tuberosity may be seen in this view. Recurrent anterior dislocations would show the Hill-Sachs deformity. In posterior dislocations, on AP radiograph the normal parallelism between the humeral head and the anterior rim of glenoid is absent. The "light bulb" or the "tennis racquet" appearance on the AP view along with widening of the joint space more than 6 mm are clue to diagnosis of posterior dislocation of shoulder. Since the head is fixed in internal rotation, there occurs no change in the appearance of the head on external rotation view.[12]

Fracture of the Neck of Humerus

The frontal AP views of the shoulder with humerus in internal and external rotation are usually sufficient to detect majority of humeral fractures. The fractures of the neck are described by Neer classification[13] which includes four different areas of involvement—the anatomic neck, surgical neck, greater tuberosity, and lesser tuberosity. The total number of fractures and their angulations are taken into account to classify the fractures into four parts—1, 2, 3, and 4. The fragments are considered displaced if there is at least 1 cm of separation or 45° angulation. Most common (80%) are one part fractures. The surgical neck which lies immediately distal to the tuberosities is the most commonly fractured region **(Fig. 11)**. The axillary nerve may be involved by these fractures. It is important to note that an impacted fracture can be easily overlooked in this region. Undisplaced fractures in this region may be managed conservatively. However, significant displacement of the greater or lesser tuberosity is an indication for surgical repair.

Fracture of the Shaft of Humerus

These can involve the proximal, middle, or distal shaft of the humerus. The fracture orientation can be transverse, oblique, or spiral. There can be marked angulation, overlap, or displacement of the fragments. Transverse fracture of the middle shaft is the most common fracture in this region. A fracture in the proximal shaft should be carefully evaluated to look for underlying pathology as metastatic deposits are common in this part of the bone.

Fracture of the Distal Humerus

The fractures of this region are classified according to their relationship with humeral condyles and the shape of the fracture line.

- *Supracondylar fractures*: The fracture line runs superior to the level of condyles. This is seen most commonly in children after fall on outstretched hand. The distal fragment is displaced and angulated posteriorly. The lateral view shows the displacement and the fracture best. Elevation of anterior and posterior fat pads is also indirect signs of underlying fracture. The fracture may be associated with development of Volkmann's ischemic contracture. The brachial artery may also be injured.
- *Intercondylar fractures*: The fracture line runs between the medial and lateral condyles and extends into the supracondylar region to form a "T" or "Y" configuration. This is more commonly seen in adults. If the fracture involves both condyles it is termed transcondylar fracture.
- *Condylar fractures*: Fracture running through either of the lateral or medial humeral condyle. Fracture of the lateral condyle is the second most common fracture of this region in children and can often result in nonunion. The ulnar nerve may be injured in lateral condyle fractures. If a small fragment gets detached it can lead to loose body within the joint.
- *Epicondylar fractures*: They are avulsion injuries of the epicondyles due to strong pull of the flexor or extensor tendons. The medial epicondyle fractures are seen in sportspersons with throwing action. In children, due to the apophysis being unossified, the fracture may not be radiologically evident.

Dislocation of the Elbow

It is the most common joint to be dislocated in children and third most common in adults (after shoulder and interphalangeal joints).[14] The most common type is posterior or posterolateral dislocation which describes the position of the radius and ulna relative to the humerus **(Figs. 12A and B)**. It is often associated with fractures of the radial head, coronoid process, capitulum, or the medial epicondyle. Post-traumatic ossification can also be seen following posterior dislocations.

The other form of dislocation of the elbow is "pulled elbow." It occurs in young children less than 5 years of age due to traction to the elbow as in lifting the child from the floor by holding the hand. It leads to slippage of the humeral head out of the annular ligament. It leads to immediate crying of the child with forearm held in midpronation. It is not evident radiographically. The treatment involves just simple supination of the forearm.

Fracture of the Head and Neck of Radius

It is the most common injury of the elbow region in young adults and occurs due to fall on outstretched hand. It usually is a hairline fracture oriented vertically involving the

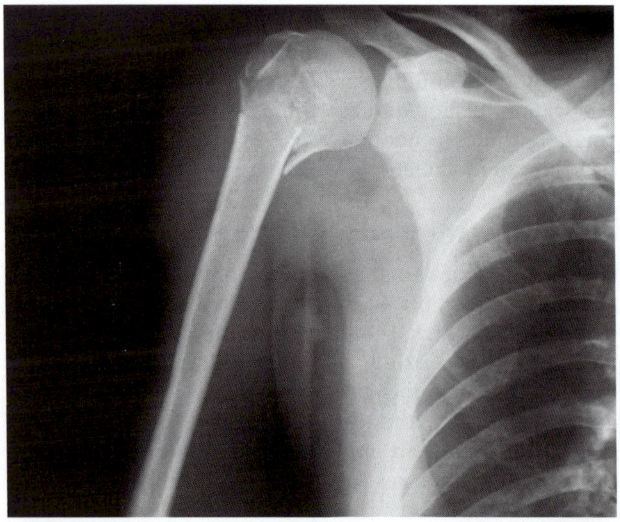

FIG. 11: Anteroposterior radiograph of the right arm shows fracture at the surgical neck of the humerus.

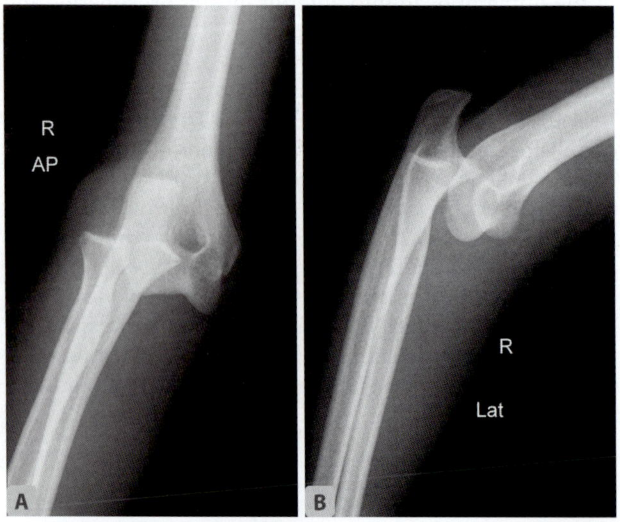

FIGS. 12A AND B: Anteroposterior and lateral radiographs of the elbow show posterolateral dislocation of the elbow.

articular surface. Since the fracture is often nondisplaced, it is sometimes difficult to visualize on routine AP and lateral views of the elbow. Displacement of anterior and posterior fat pads on the lateral view may aid in the diagnosis. The presence of posterior fat pad is a more reliable and consistent indicator of underlying fracture of the radial head. The radial neck fracture is usually an impacted fracture at its junction with the head. Comminuted fractures of the radial head are often dealt with complete excision of the radial head surgically.

Fracture of the Upper End of Ulna

Olecranon fractures are the second most common fractures of this region in adults. They occur after fall on the point of elbow. The fracture line is best visualized on lateral view. The coronoid process may rarely be fractured in association with posterior dislocation of the elbow or by avulsion by brachialis muscle.

Fractures of the Shaft of Radius and Ulna

The radius and ulna can be fractured in isolation but are both fractured in association in a large number of patients when it is called both bones ("B-B") fracture. The fractures of this region are prone to displacement with angulation and rotation and hence often require surgical correction. There are increased chances of compartment syndrome after fractures of this region.

A fracture of the proximal ulnar shaft with dislocation of the radial head is known as *Monteggia fracture-dislocation* **(Figs. 13A and B)**.

An isolated fracture of distal ulnar shaft is termed as *Nightstick* or *Parry fracture.*

A fracture of the distal shaft of radius at the junction of middle and distal third with dislocation of the distal radio-ulnar joint is termed as *Galeazzi* or *"reversed" Monteggia fracture.*

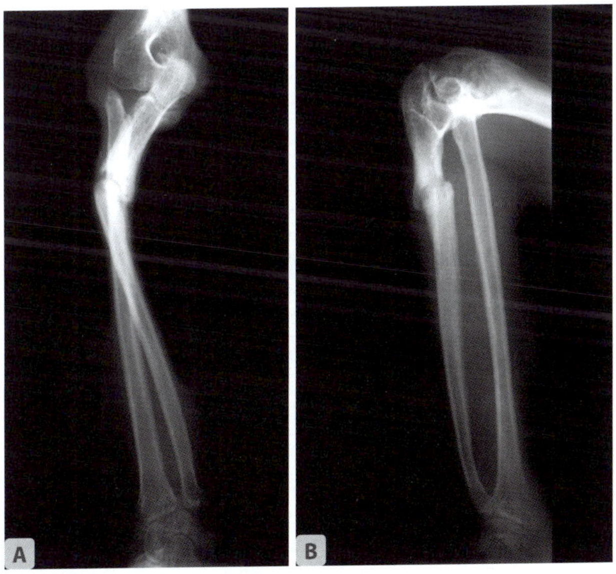

FIGS. 13A AND B: Anteroposterior and lateral radiographs of the forearm show an old nonunited fracture of the upper shaft of ulna with dislocation of the radial head consistent with *Monteggia fracture-dislocation.*

Fractures of the Distal End of Radius

Fractures of the distal part of radius are common injuries of adulthood especially in females.[15]

A fracture of the distal end of radius with posterior angulation of the distal fragment is termed as *Colles' fracture* **(Figs. 14A and B)**. The fracture line is seen around 2–3 cm proximal to the articular surface of the radius. The distal fragment is tilted dorsally so that on lateral view it gives rise to classical "dinner-fork" deformity. A fracture of ulnar styloid process is associated in 60% of cases. Complications include malunion and Sudeck's post-traumatic osteodystrophy.

A fracture of the distal radius with anterior angulation of the distal fragment is termed as *Smith's fracture* or *Reversed Colles' fracture.*

A fracture of the posterior rim of the distal radial articular surface with associated proximal dislocation of the carpus is termed *Barton's fracture.* The involvement of volar radial rim is termed *Reverse Barton's fracture.*

Fracture of the radial styloid process is termed *Chauffeur's fracture.*

A fracture through the distal radial epiphysis is common in children. The epiphysis gets slipped posteriorly and is usually associated with a small metaphyseal fracture making it a Type 2 Salter Harris injury. This is equivalent to a *Colles' fracture* of adult.

Fractures of the Carpal Bones

Scaphoid is the most common carpal bone to be fractured. It is usually seen in adults with fall on outstretched hand. Clinically, there is tenderness in the anatomical snuffbox. The standard views to detect a scaphoid fracture include PA, lateral, external oblique, and a PA view with ulnar deviation.[16] About 70% of fractures involve the waist of scaphoid followed by proximal and distal poles **(Figs. 15A and B)**. Nondisplaced fractures are difficult to identify. If there is high clinical suspicion but no fracture line is visible on initial radiograph, then precautionary immobilization is done and the radiograph is repeated after 2 weeks. The fracture line may be better evident by this time. A bone scan may detect the fracture earlier. Fractures through the waist or proximal to it make the proximal part of scaphoid prone to avascular

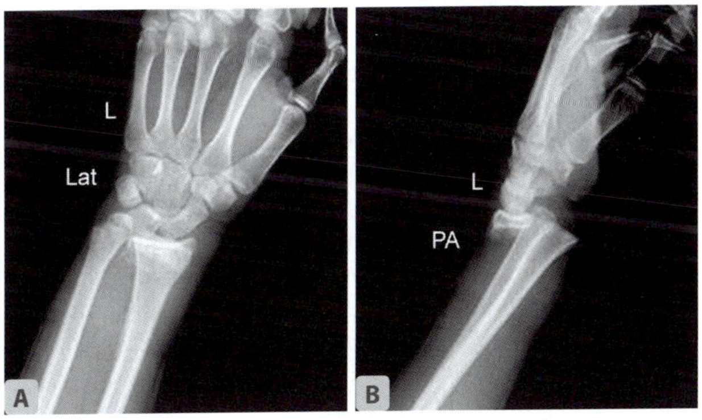

FIGS. 14A AND B: Posteroanterior and lateral radiographs of the hand show *Colles' fracture* of the radius.

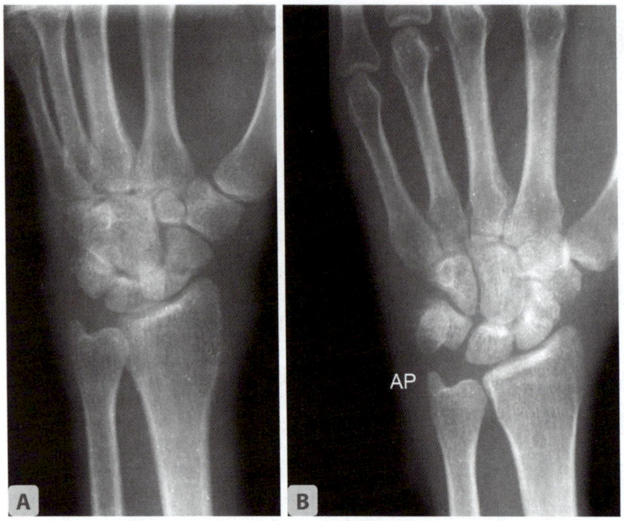

FIGS. 15A AND B: Posteroanterior and oblique radiographs of the wrist joint show a fracture through the waist of scaphoid bone.

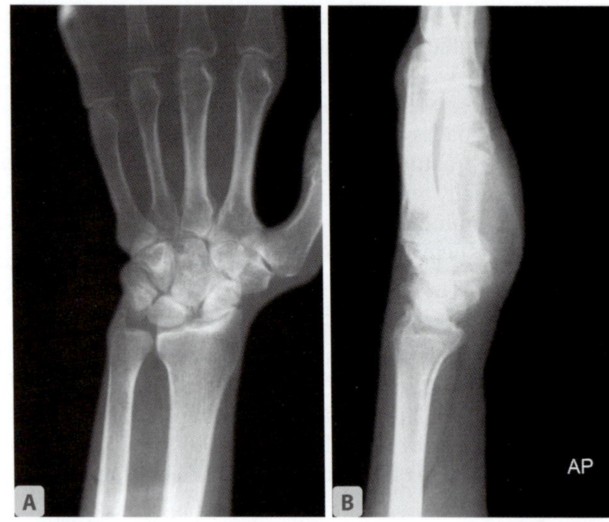

FIGS. 16A AND B: Posteroanterior and lateral radiographs of the wrist show scapholunate dislocation with increased distance between the scaphoid and lunate (*Terry Thomas sign*) and signet ring appearance of the scaphoid.

necrosis as the nutrient artery enters the bone through the distal part of the waist. The chances of avascular necrosis increase with more proximal fracture line. The avascular part is seen as more dense compared to the rest of the bone and the other surrounding bones. The scaphoid fractures are also more prone to nonunion.

Triquetrum is the second most common carpal bone to be fractured. An avulsion fracture at the site of attachment of the radiocarpal ligament is termed *Fischer's fracture.* It is identified on lateral radiograph of the wrist.

Lunate fractures are uncommon. *Kienböck's disease* is avascular necrosis of the lunate which may be secondary to a fracture **(Fig. 9)**.

Dislocation of the Wrist

Dislocations affecting the wrist are mainly of two types:

1. Single carpal dislocations
2. Multiple carpal dislocations.[17]

Single Carpal Dislocations

Lunate dislocation is the most common of all carpal bones. The lunate displaces anteriorly with forward tilt so that the concave lower articular surface faces anteriorly. This is best seen on the lateral view.

The scaphoid is the second most common bone to subluxate. It usually undergoes rotatory subluxation so that it rotates anteriorly and moves laterally to cause scapholunate dissociation. The distance between the scaphoid and lunate on AP view is increased to more than 4 mm (known as *Terry Thomas sign).* In addition the scaphoid appears small and circular in shape (*signet ring sign)* **(Figs. 16A and B)**.

Multiple Carpal Dislocations

The most common in perilunate dislocation where the lunate bone maintains its spatial relationship with the radius but rest of all the carpal bones get dislocated dorsally. It is best visualized on lateral view. This type of dislocation may be associated with fracture of the scaphoid.

Fractures and Dislocations of the Hand

Posteroanterior, lateral, and oblique projections are the most commonly used views to image injuries of this region. Collimated views may be required if a single digit is to be evaluated.

Among the metacarpals, the first metacarpal base is most commonly injured. An oblique intra-articular fracture through the base of first metacarpal with dorsal and radial displacement of the shaft is known as *Bennet's fracture.* A comminuted Bennet's fracture is termed *Ronaldo's fracture.* A transverse fracture of the neck of the fifth metacarpal with volar angulation of the distal fragment is termed *Boxer's fracture.*

Fractures of the phalanges are more common than metacarpal fractures. An avulsion chip fracture at the base of distal phalanx at the insertion of extensor tendon leads to *Mallet finger* with the finger fixed in moderate flexion and cannot be extended.

LOWER LIMB TRAUMA

Dislocations of the Hip

The dislocations of the hip are classified as posterior and anteriors dislocations.[18]

Posterior Dislocation

It is the most common type accounting for approximately 80% of hip dislocations. It occurs when there is a blow to the knee with hip in flexed position. The femoral head displaces posteriorly to lie outside the acetabulum on its lateral and superior aspect. This often produces a fracture of the posterior acetabular rim with rarely a small fracture of the anterior femoral head. These fractures are best seen on CT scan. The sciatic nerve may also be injured. Clinically, there is medial rotation of the leg with limb shortening.

Anterior Dislocation

It accounts for about 15% of hip dislocations and is caused by forced abduction and extension of the femur. Clinically the limb is seen to lie in abduction. The head may be dislocated anteriorly and superiorly (subspinous or iliac type) with the femur extended and abducted or the head may get dislocated anteriorly and inferiorly (obturator type) with the femur abducted and externally rotated. The acetabulum usually does not show any fracture.[19]

Fractures of the Proximal Femur

Fracture of the neck of femur is a common injury seen in elderly especially in females with underlying osteoporosis.[20] Complications include avascular necrosis, osteoarthritis, and nonunion. AP view of pelvis, coned AP view of ipsilateral hip, and horizontal beam lateral view are the usual radiographs for detection. The fractures of this region are classified into intracapsular and extracapsular types depending upon the relationship of the fracture line to the joint capsule.

Intracapsular Fractures

The intracapsular fractures include all fractures above the level of trochanters. They account for about 60% of all proximal femoral fractures. The intracapsular fractures are more prone to undergo nonunion and avascular necrosis.

Subcapital fracture occurs at the junction of head with neck and is the most common type of intracapsular fracture. These fractures may be impacted without displacement or may show variable degrees of displacement.

Midcervical fracture at the middle part of the neck and basicervical fractures just above the level of trochanters are the other types of intracapsular fractures. These regions may be more commonly fractured with underlying pathological lesion.

Extracapsular Fractures

These include all fractures at or below the level of the trochanters.

The intertrochanteric fractures constitute of a fracture line running obliquely to involve both the trochanters **(Fig. 17)**. These fractures are generally comminuted. These fractures unite easily without significant complications.

The trochanteric fractures involve avulsion injuries of the greater or the lesser trochanter.

Subtrochanteric fractures occur below the level of the trochanters or may be seen as an extension of intertrochanteric fractures. It is usually seen in younger patients with significant trauma or superimposed over pathological bone in elderly.

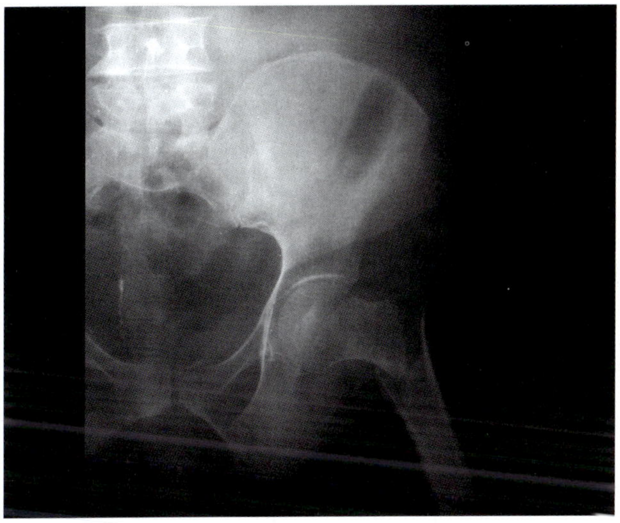

FIG. 17: Anteroposterior radiograph of the left hip joint shows an intertrochanteric fracture of the left femur.

Fractures of the Shaft of Femur

These occur at all ages and are a result of severe violence. The fracture orientation may be spiral, oblique, or transverse. The fractures may be associated with significant soft tissue hemorrhage. The femoral artery may commonly get injured most commonly at the level of the adductor canal. Radiograph should always include both the proximal hip and the distal knee joint because of high incidence of ipsilateral associated injuries.

The supracondylar fracture of the femur produces posterior angulation and displacement of the distal fragment due to the pull of the gastrocnemius muscle.

The condylar fractures often involve the articular surface and need to be corrected to prevent delayed osteoarthritis. The condyles may be injured in isolation or there may be extension of a supracondylar fracture into the intercondylar area with a "T" or "Y" configuration. Injury of the popliteal artery must be looked for with these fractures.

Fractures of the Patella

The patella gets fractured either by direct trauma or by indirect mechanism of strong quadriceps contraction. Direct trauma often leads to a comminuted fracture while the quadriceps mechanism usually results in a transverse or oblique fracture **(Figs. 18A and B)**. The transverse fracture line is at the mid part. These fractures at best visualized on AP and lateral view except a rare vertical fracture which may be seen only on the sunrise or the skyline view. A superolateral accessory ossification center in a bipartite patella may simulate an acute fracture but can be differentiated by its typical location, well-defined sclerotic margins, and being bilateral.

Dislocation of the Patella

The patella most commonly dislocates laterally. It may occur secondary to a sudden change in direction while dancing or running or may occur following direct trauma. The dislocation is usually transient and gets reduced easily. The patella may rarely get dislocated in vertical direction with locking in the intercondylar notch or in horizontal direction with inversion and locking of superior pole of patella in the knee joint.

The dislocations may be associated with an osteochondral fragment on the medial facet of the patella or the lateral

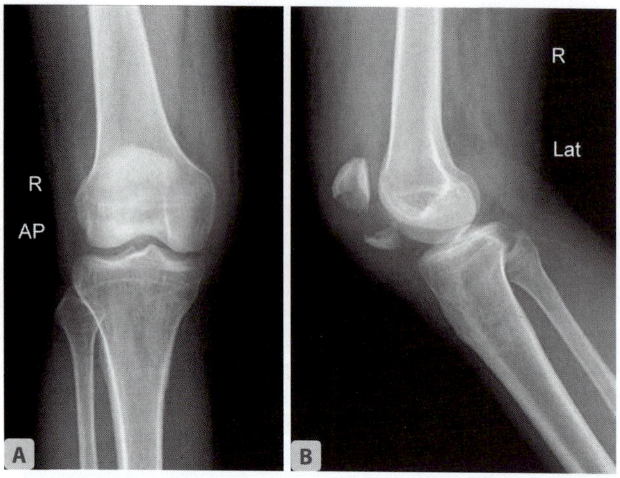

FIGS. 18A AND B: Anteroposterior and lateral radiographs of the knee joint show a fracture through the mid part of patella with separation of the fracture fragments due to associated muscle pull.

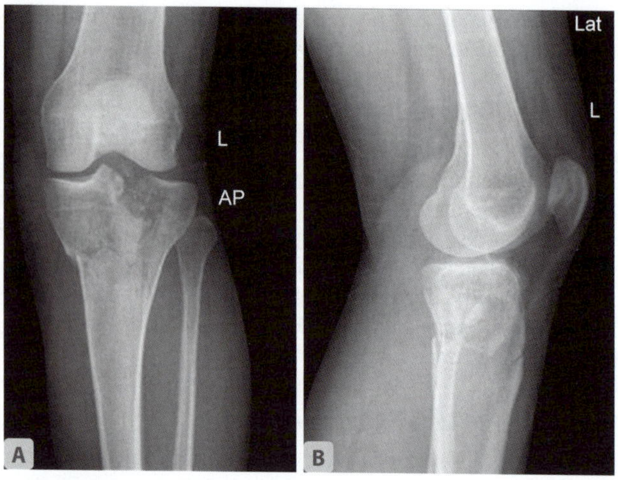

FIGS. 19A AND B: Anteroposterior and lateral radiographs of the knee joint show fracture of the lateral tibial plateau extending into the proximal metaphysis.

femoral condyle. CT scan may be required for the diagnosis as the fragment needs to be removed to prevent future occurrence of osteoarthritis.

Fractures of the Proximal Tibia

Fracture of the lateral tibial plateau is much more common than that of the medial tibial plateau **(Figs. 19A and B)**. It is also known as bumper fracture as is commonly seen in car accidents but this mechanism constitutes only 25% of etiology.[21] It may be more commonly seen in various other injury mechanisms including vertical compression and twisting. The common classification followed is the Hohl classification:[22] Type 1 is a vertical split of the joint margin, Type 2 is a compression of lateral plateau by impaction of lateral femoral condyle, Type 3 is a split peripheral vertical fracture with compression of the medial articular surface of the lateral tibial plateau, Type 4 is fracture of medial tibial plateau, and Type 5 is bicondylar fracture with "Y" or "T" configuration.

These fractures may be associated with ligament injuries. Hence, on radiograph it is important to look for avulsion fractures at the site of ligamentous attachments. Lipohemarthrosis may be seen in tibial plateau fractures and is identified on horizontal beam lateral radiograph. CT scan and MRI are often indicated to look for the exact extent of the fracture and the associated ligamentous injuries.

An avulsion fracture of the lateral tibial plateau at the site of attachment of the iliotibial tract is termed as *Segond fracture*. It is commonly associated with injuries of the anterior cruciate ligament and meniscal injuries.

Fractures of the anterior and posterior tibial spine (intercondylar eminence) usually result from avulsion injuries at the origin of anterior and posterior cruciate ligaments.

Fractures of the Shaft of Tibia and Fibula

Fractures of shaft of the tibia are often associated with fractures of fibula **(Figs. 20A and B)**. The fibular fracture is commonly at upper- and middle-third region whereas the tibial fractures are usually at middle and lower-third region. Hence, it is important to image the complete length of both bones in the radiograph so as to avoid missing associated fracture. The fractures of this region are prone to development of compartment syndrome.

An undisplaced spiral fracture in a child around 2 years of age is called as toddler's fracture.

Midshaft of the tibia along with proximal tibial metaphysis, fibular shaft, and femoral neck are the common sites for stress fractures. They are seen in athletic individuals or those involved in strenuous running. Clinically, it presents with pain during activity with relief on rest.

Fractures of the Distal Tibia and Fibula

Fractures of the medial and lateral malleoli occur due to adduction and abduction injuries. The medial malleolus fractures are generally transverse or oblique whereas those of the lateral malleolus are usually spiral **(Figs. 21A and B)**. There may also be avulsion injuries at the malleoli. The distal tibiofibular joint may also show diastasis associated with the malleolar fractures.

Fractures of the Talus

Fractures of the talus are second only to the calcaneus as a site of injury in the ankle region. Most common injuries are the avulsion fractures. It occurs at the anterosuperior part of the talar neck at the site of attachment of the joint capsule. The other common type of fracture is the vertical fracture of the talar neck occurring in an automobile accident. Such fractures are often complicated by avascular necrosis of the proximal part of talus. The likelihood of developing avascular necrosis increases with more anterior neck fracture. The talar dome is also a common site for development of osteochondral fractures.[23] These occur in typical location of middle third of lateral margin or posterior third of the medial margin of talar dome. If there is doubt in detection of osteochondral fractures on plain radiograph, CT scan can be done which clearly shows the fracture line.

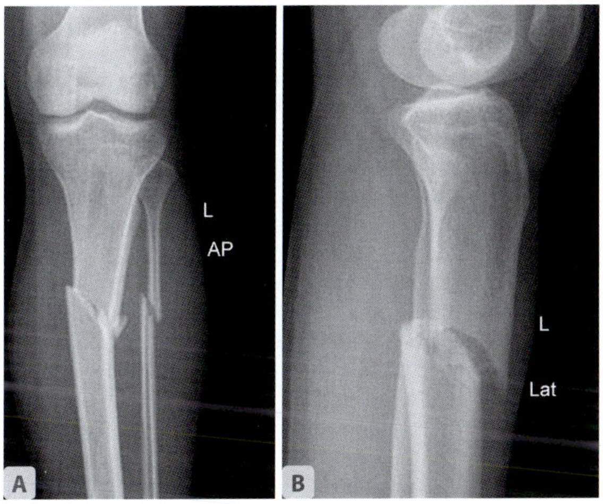

FIGS. 20A AND B: Anteroposterior and lateral radiographs of the proximal leg show fractures of upper shafts of both tibia and fibula.

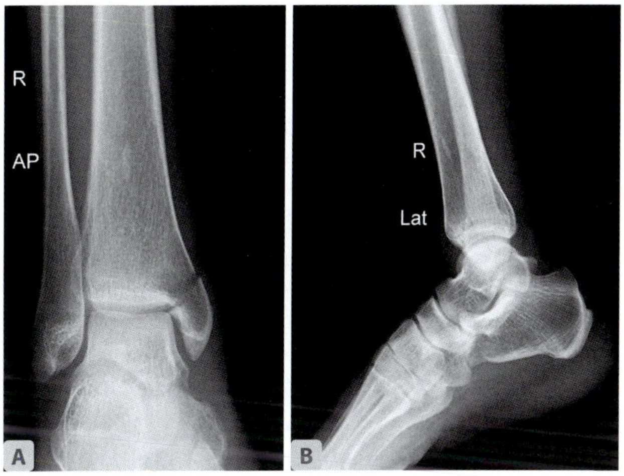

FIGS. 21A AND B: Anteroposterior and lateral radiographs of the ankle joint show a transverse fracture of the medial malleolus.

Fractures of the Calcaneum

The calcaneus is the most frequent tarsal bone to get injured. About 75% of the fractures are intra-articular with involvement of the subtalar joint and the rest 25% are extra-articular.[24,25] The intra-articular fractures are most commonly caused by fall from height and are compression fractures. They are often bilateral (10%) and/or associated with fractures of the thoracolumbar spine. These fractures usually have associated depression of the posterior facet of the subtalar joint. The subtle compression fractures of the calcaneum can be best detected on lateral radiograph of ankle by measuring the Böhler's angle. It is the angle between a line joining the superior most part of anterior process of calcaneum to the superior point of posterior facet and a line joining the superior point of posterior facet to posterosuperior margin of calcaneum tuberosity. Normally the angle between these two lines ranges from 28° to 40°. A Böhler's angle of less than 28° represents a depression of the calcaneus and hence a fracture. The extra-articular fractures are mainly avulsion injuries and may involve the anterior process (most common), superior aspect of tuberosity, plantar aspect of tuberosity, or the sustentaculum tali. The extra-articular fractures are usually managed conservatively whereas significant involvement of articular surface of subtalar joint is an indication for operative repair.[26,27]

Dislocations of the Foot

The talus is the most common foot bone to dislocate. The dislocation may involve the talotibial, talocalcaneal (subtalar), and the talonavicular joints.

Lisfranc's dislocation is a dislocation at tarsometatarsal junction. The second, third, and fourth metatarsals dislocate laterally, with or without associated fractures. Fracture of the base of second metatarsal is characteristic. The first metatarsal may dislocate laterally with other metatarsals (homolateral type) or may deviate medially (divergent type).

Chopart's dislocation is medial dislocation of the talonavicular and calcaneocuboid joints of the foot.

CONCLUSION

For an accurate interpretation of a radiograph of skeletal trauma, it is important for the radiologist to be aware of the clinical details including the time interval from injury and mechanism of injury. The traumatized region should always be imaged in at least two different planes with inclusion of both the proximal and distal joints to the injured bone. A knowledge of the common injuries, their radiographic manifestations, the special radiographic views for that region if any, the pitfalls in diagnosis and the associated injuries is paramount for the radiologist. It is important not to miss an injury not only because of the treatment implications but also because many of these are medicolegal cases in which the radiograph forms part of concrete irrefutable radiological evidence. Comparative evaluation with the contralateral normal limb may be required especially in children. The use of other imaging modalities including ultrasound, CT, MRI, and scintigraphy may be indicated in specific situations as and when indicated. The radiologist also has a role in the detection of post-traumatic early and delayed complications during the follow-up of the patient.

REFERENCES

1. Felson B. Roentgenology of Fractures and Dislocations. New York: Grune and Stratton; 1978.
2. Rogers LF. Radiology of Skeletal Trauma, Vols 1 and 2, 3rd edition. Philadelphia PA: Churchill Livingstone; 2002.
3. Dalinka MK. Imaging of skeletal trauma. In: Hodler J, Zollikofer CL, Von Schulthess GK (Eds). Musculoskeletal Diseases 2009–2012. Milano: Springer; 2009.
4. Salter RB, Harris WR. Injuries involving the epiphyseal plate. J Bone Joint Surg. 1963;45:587.
5. Cruess RL, Dumont J. Current concepts, fracture healing. Can J Surg. 1975;18:403.
6. Hulth A. Current concepts in fracture healing. Clin Orthopaed. 1989;249:265.
7. Bulger EM, Smith DG, Maier RV, Jurkovich GJ. Fat embolism syndrome: a 10-year review. Arch Surg. 1997;132:435-9.
8. Shaikh N, Parchani A, Bhat V, Kattren MA. Fat embolism syndrome: clinical and imaging considerations: Case report and review of literature. Indian J Crit Care Med. 2008;12:32-6.
9. Gupta B, Kaur M, D'souza N, Dey CK, Shende S, Kumar A, et al. Cerebral fat embolism: a diagnostic challenge. Saudi J Anaesth. 2011;5(3):348-52.
10. Bashir WA, Aziz A, Jidaal I. Imaging of skeletal extremity trauma: a review. Trauma. 2014;16(4):300-17.
11. Nuovo MA, Norman A, Chumas J, Ackerman LV. Myositis ossificans with atypical clinical, radiographic, or pathologic findings: a review of 23 cases. Skeletal Radiol. 1992;21:87-101.
12. Workman TL, Burkhard TK, Resnick D, Goff WB 2nd, Balsara ZN, Davis DJ, et al. Hill Sach lesion: comparison of detection with MR imaging, radiography and arthroscopy. Radiology. 1992;185:847.
13. Pavlov H, Freiberger RH. Fractures and dislocations about the shoulder. Semin Roentgenol. 1978;13:85-91.
14. Kerr R. Diagnostic imaging of upper extremity trauma. Radiol Clin North Am. 1989;27(5):891-908.
15. Neer CS II. Displaced proximal humeral fractures. Part 1-classification and evaluation. J Bone Joint Surg (Am). 1970;52:1077.
16. Linscheid RL, Wheeler DK. Elbow dislocations. JAMA. 1965;194:1171.
17. Goldfarb CA, Yin Y, Gilula LA, Fisher AJ, Boyer MI. Wrist fractures: What the clinician wants to know. Radiology. 2001;219:11-28.
18. Munk PL, Lee MJ, Logan PM, Connell DG, Janzen DL, Poon PY, et al. Scaphoid bone waist fractures, acute and chronic: Imaging with different techniques. Am J Roentgenol. 1997;168:779-86.
19. Fisher MR, Rogers LF, Hendrix RW. A systematic approach to the diagnosis of carpometacarpal dislocations. Radiographics. 1982;2:612-27.
20. Newberg AH, Greenstein R. Radiographic evaluation of tibial plateau fracture. Radiology. 1978;126:319.
21. Epstein HC. Traumatic dislocations of the hip. Clin Orthop. 1973;92:116.
22. Erb RE, Steele JR, Nance EP Jr, Edwards JR. Traumatic anterior dislocation of the hip: spectrum of plain film and CT findings. Am J Roentgenol. 1995;165:1215-9.
23. Hohl M. Tibial condylar fractures. J Bone Joint Surg (Am). 1967;49:1455.
24. David S. Textbook of Radiology and Imaging, 7th edition. London: Churchill Livingstone; 2003. pp. 1371-416.
25. Canale ST, Belding RH. Osteochondral lesions of the talus. J Bone Joint Surg (Am). 1980;62A:97-102.
26. Greenspan A. Imaging of the foot and ankle. Curr Opin Orthop. 1996;7:61-8.
27. Karasick D. Fractures and dislocations of the foot. Semin Roentgen. 1994;24:152.

CHAPTER

173

Imaging of Soft Tissue Tumors

Ashu Seith Bhalla, Ankur Goyal, Priyanka Naranje

INTRODUCTION

Soft tissue tumors (STTs) encompass a wide spectrum of entities. Patients often present with nonspecific clinical findings, such as an ill-defined soft tissue swelling or a discrete palpable mass, with or without accompanying tenderness or pain. With equivocal clinical findings, imaging can confirm the presence of a soft tissue mass or identify a suspected "mass" as normal tissue. The objectives of initial imaging evaluation are detecting the suspected lesion, establishing a diagnosis or formulating a differential diagnosis and radiological staging (if the lesion is neoplastic). The evaluation of STTs has undergone dramatic evolution with advances in magnetic resonance imaging (MRI). Soft tissue sarcoma (STS) is a broad term used for tumors of mesenchymal origin and encompasses the various subtypes described in the classification below. While these constitute <1% of malignancies encountered in the adults, the incidence is more in children which is approximately 12%.[1]

CLASSIFICATION

The classification currently followed for STTs is the 4th edition of the WHO classification (2013).[2] This system is based not only on the histopathological features but also clinical behavior and molecular and genetic features.[3] The broad categories of STT according to WHO classification are illustrated in **Flowcharts 1 and 2**. Further two of these groups also include tumors of uncertain differentiation and undifferentiated sarcomas (or unclassified).

The WHO classification is based on the tissue that the tumor morphology is similar to (e.g., smooth muscle/skeletal muscle) and not necessarily the one that it arises from. Apart from histopathology, immune histochemistry (IHC) and molecular techniques (for genetics) govern the diagnosis.

Immune Histochemistry

Some important IHC markers are summarized in **Table 1**.

FLOWCHART 1: Groups of soft tissue tumors (STTs) according to the WHO classification.

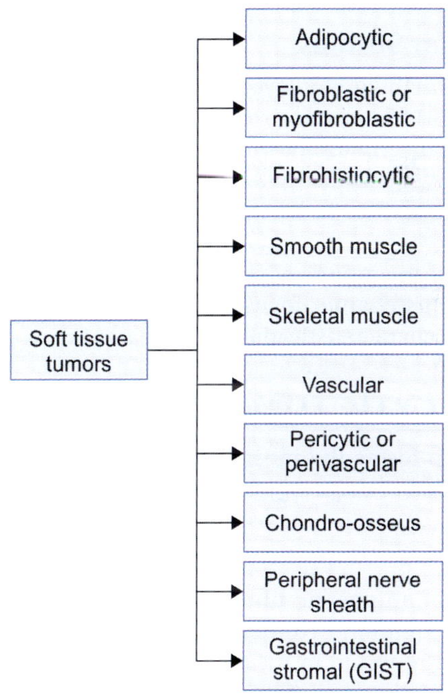

FLOWCHART 2: The WHO classification based on biological behavior (applies to each category).

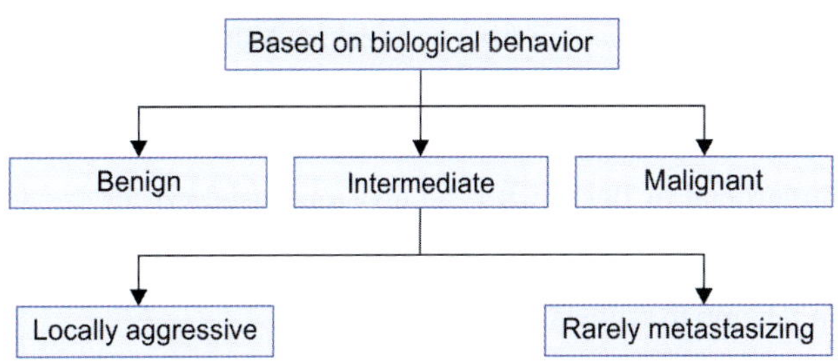

TABLE 1: Important immune histochemistry markers.

Desmin	S-100	Cytokeratin
Myogenic differentiation • Rhabdomyosarcoma • Leiomyosarcoma	• Nerve sheath tumors • Ossifying fibromyxoid tumor	*Rare* • Synovial sarcoma • Epitheloid sarcoma • Absent in fibrosarcoma

TABLE 2: Classification of adipocytic tumors.

Benign	Intermediate (locally aggressive)	Malignant
• Lipoma • Lipomatosis • Lipoblastoma • Angiolipoma	• Atypical lipomatous tumor • Well-differentiated liposarcoma	Liposarcoma • Dedifferentiated • Myxoid • Pleomorphic • NOS

(NOS: not otherwise specified).

Molecular Studies

Common methods employed for detecting genetic mutations include FISH (fluorescence in situ hybridization) and RT-PCR (reverse transcriptase polymerase chain reaction). Affected chromosomes include EWSR1 with various translocations of the gene described in Ewing's sarcoma, clear cell sarcoma, among others.[4]

Each of the groups of classification includes numerous entities. This chapter focuses on common lesions and/or those with characteristic imaging appearances.

ADIPOCYTIC TUMORS

This group forms the most frequently encountered STTs. Classification of these tumors is shown in **Table 2**.

Lipoma

Majority of adipocytic tumors are benign and lipoma is the most common.[5] Numerous chromosomal aberrations have been reported in these tumors with HMGA2 protein truncation being one of the effects.[6] Typical patient profile is that of an overweight, middle aged person; though these are encountered at any age including children. Most of these tumors do not cause pain unless they compress nerves. The classical lipoma on imaging displays an appearance of homogeneous fatty lesion similar to subcutaneous fat **(Figs. 1A to F)**. Fine septae may be present. Many categories of lipomas are often discussed.[7]

Based on Location

Superficial or deep, with the division based on the fascia covering the muscles. In the deep lipomas, parosteal or intramuscular forms are known. Lipoma arborescens occurs in relation to synovial lining of a joint.

Based on Capsule

Lipomas may have a capsule (encapsulated). Those without capsule can appear infiltrative with infiltrative intramuscular lipoma being one form. These can be challenging to differentiate from liposarcomas (LPSs).

Based on Content

Lipomas may have a mixed histology with other components such as bone or cartilage.

Lipoblastoma

Lipoblastoma is a rare tumor encountered typically in infants or early childhood (less than 3 years). It is mostly painless; however, nerve compression can result in pain or even Horner's syndrome (in cervicothoracic tumors) or even thoracic cage compression in case of large tumors. Appendicular location is commoner than trunk or head and neck.

Unlike lipoma, the tumor is composed of immature fatty tissue, which on MRI shows less hyperintensity (on T1WI) compared to mature fat. Also, there may be components of myxoid or fibrous tissues found within, further giving it a heterogeneous appearance. The tumor is known to regress spontaneously or mature into a lipoma, as the child grows. Hence, this should be kept in mind when a decision regarding surgery or conservative approach is taken. On imaging and even histology, the lesion resembles an LPS **(Figs. 2A to C)**; however, the typical age of presentation aids in the distinction. A diffuse, infiltrative form of the neoplasm is referred to as "lipoblastomastosis."[8]

Other Benign Tumors

Other benign adipocytic tumors mostly include entities, which have elements of other tissues and include:

- *Angiolipoma*: Mature fatty tissue with small vessels. Small subcutaneous lesions, often multiple **(Figs. 1A to F)**.
- *Myolipoma*: Mature fat plus mature smooth muscles. Deep location is more frequent.
- *Chondroid lipoma*: Chondroid or myxoid matrix with mature fat.
- *Spindle cell lipoma (SCL)*: Synonym pleomorphic lipoma, more frequent in men.

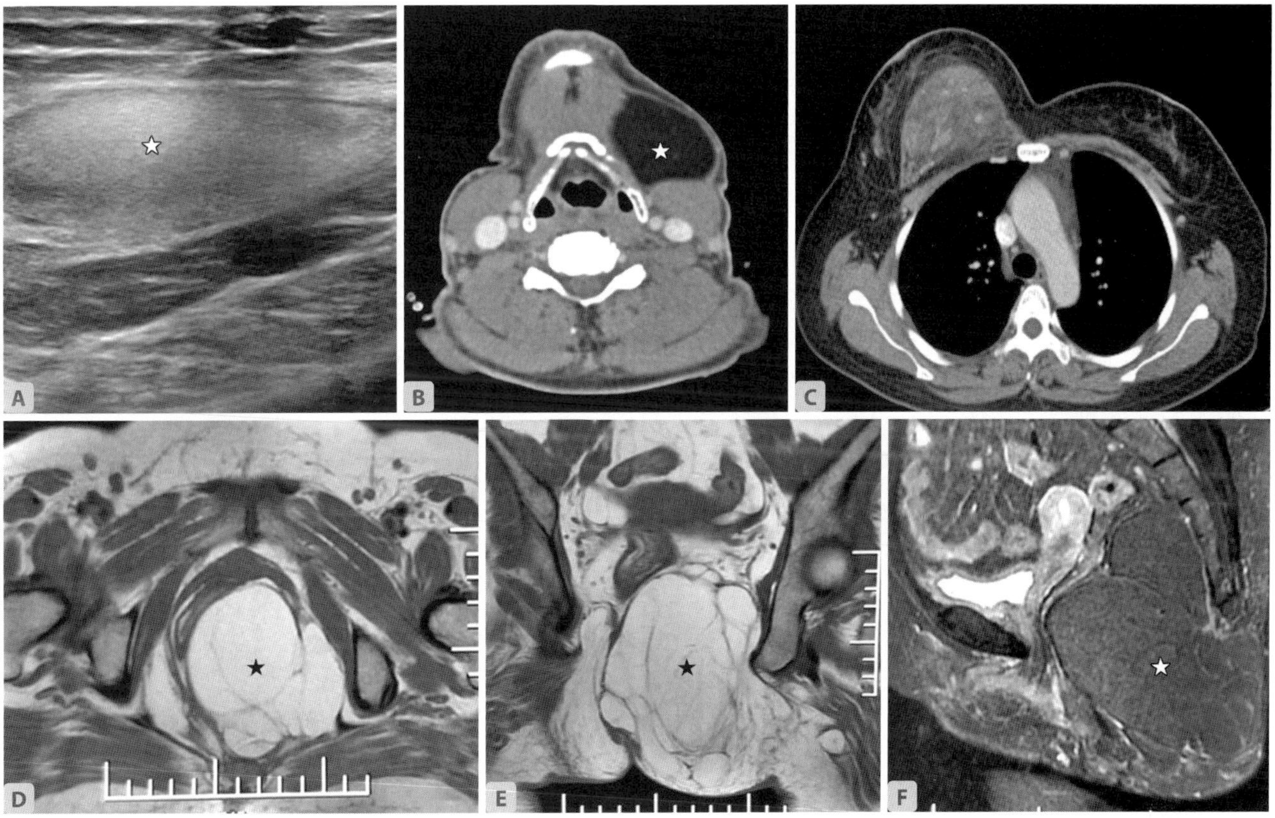

FIGS. 1A TO F: Lipomas. (A) Ultrasound image shows homogeneously echogenic lesion (asterisk) in the gluteal subcutaneous location, suggestive of lipoma; (B) Axial computed tomography (CT) image shows homogeneous fat-attenuation lesion (asterisk) anterior to left sternocleidomastoid; (C) Axial CT image shows heterogeneous lesion in RT chest wall (retromammary location) with mixed soft tissue and fat attenuation with prominent vessels. Histology revealed angiolipoma; (D) Axial; and (E) Coronal T1-weighted (T1W) magnetic resonance (MR) images show fat signal intensity hyperintense lesion (asterisks) in left ischiorectal fossa with thin septations, suggestive of lipoma; (F) There is complete suppression of lesion signal on fat-suppressed image.

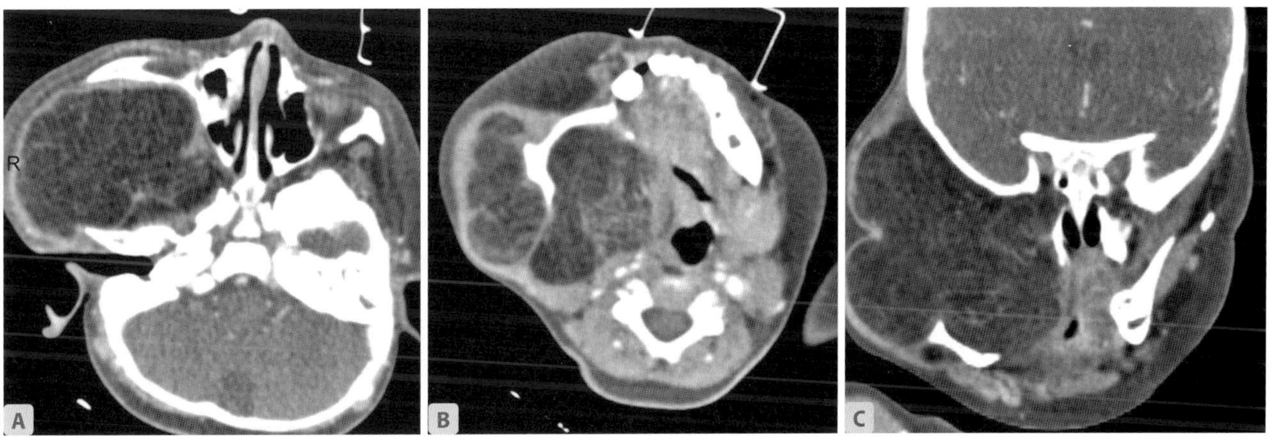

FIGS. 2A TO C: Lipoblastoma. (A and B) Axial; and (C) Coronal contrast-enhanced computed tomography (CECT) images in an infant show fat attenuation infiltrative lesion in RT face and infratemporal fossa with septations within, suggesting the diagnosis of lipoblastoma.

- *Lipomatosis of nerve (LN)*: Synonym fibrolipomatous hamartoma. The most common location of this lesion is the wrist, occurring in relation to median nerve/branches.
- *Lipomatosis*: These lesions involve proliferation of mature adipose tissue in various locations (often deep) in an infiltrative manner **(Figs. 3A to D)**. These can be part of spectrum of "overgrowth syndromes" when involving an extremity.
- *Hibernoma*: Neoplasm of brown fat which is seen in neck or back and can resemble LPS on imaging.

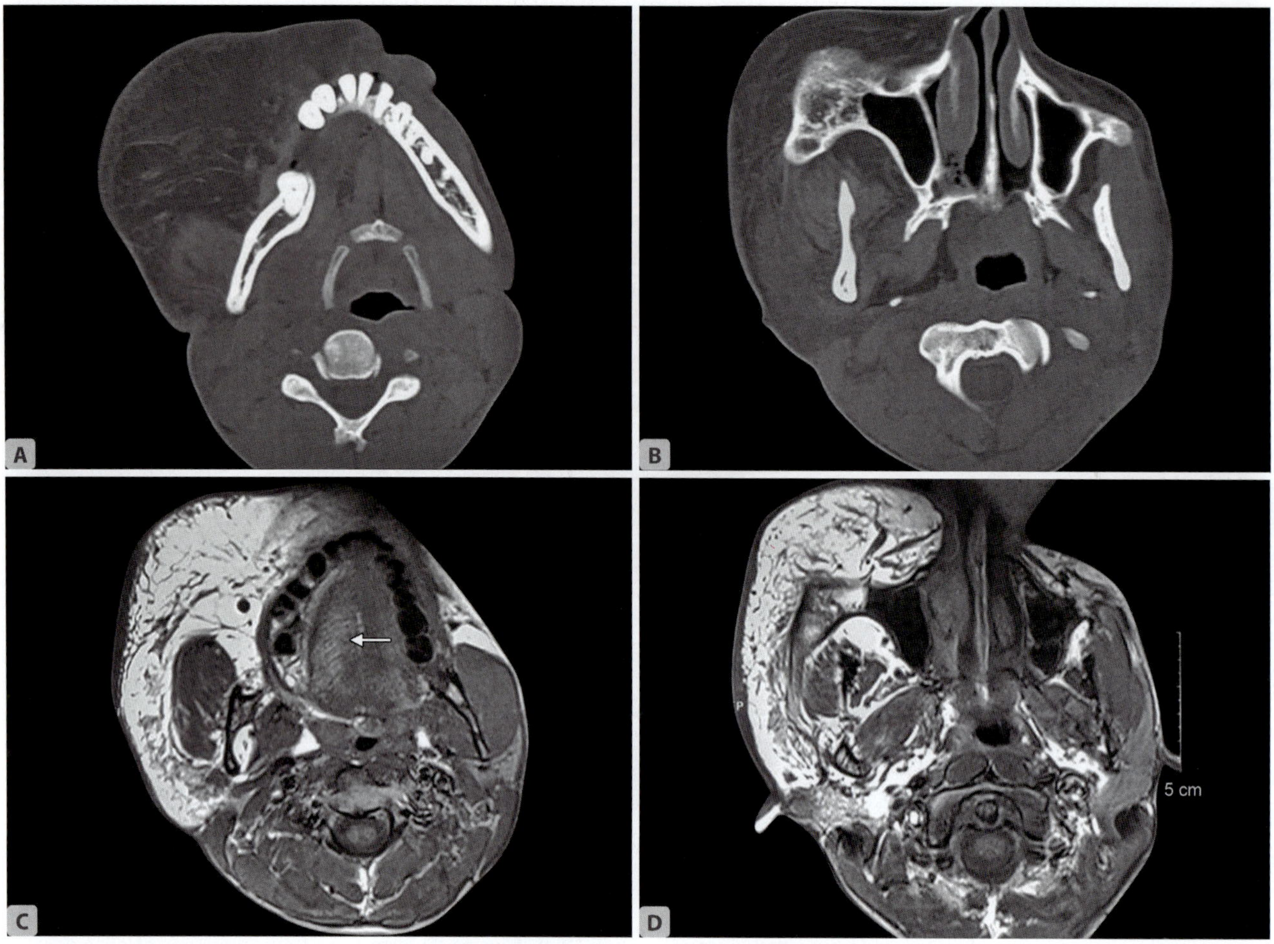

FIGS. 3A TO D: Lipomatosis. (A and B) Axial computed tomography (CT) images show diffuse fatty hypertrophy involving the right side of face, predominantly in subcutaneous region but also involving mastication muscles and parotid. There is bony overgrowth of the maxilla as well; (C and D) T1-weighted (T1W) magnetic resonance (MR) images better show hyperintense fat signal intensity. The right part of tongue also shows lipomatosis (arrow).

FLOWCHART 3: Classification of liposarcoma.

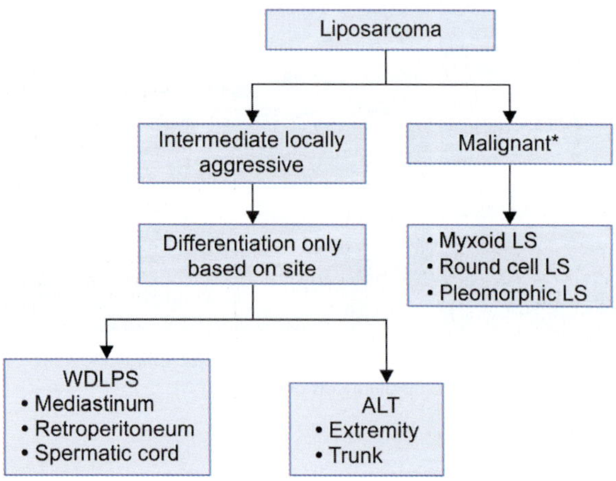

*Among these, pure myxoid LPSs are low-grade sarcomas, others are high grade.

(WDLPS: well-differentiated liposarcomas; ALT: atypical lipomatous tumor; LS: liposarcoma)

Liposarcoma

The classification of LPS group of tumors is shown in **Flowchart 3**.

Intermediate Well-differentiated Liposarcoma/Atypical Lipomatous Tumor

The tumors of this grade can be locally aggressive, have a higher recurrence rate but do not metastasize, unless they evolve into a high-grade sarcoma which is seen up to 17% of those in the retroperitoneum (RP).[9]

On imaging, while the predominant component of the mass remains fatty (as in lipomas), there is presence of thick septations (>2 mm) which may be nodular, with or without nonfatty components appearing as soft tissue attenuation (<2 cm) **(Figs. 4 and 5)**. Calcifications can be seen in up to one-third of the masses on CT. Further most fatty lesions in RP or mediastinum are well-differentiated liposarcoma (WDLPS) rather than a benign lipoma. Management is surgical, i.e., wide local excision (WLE).

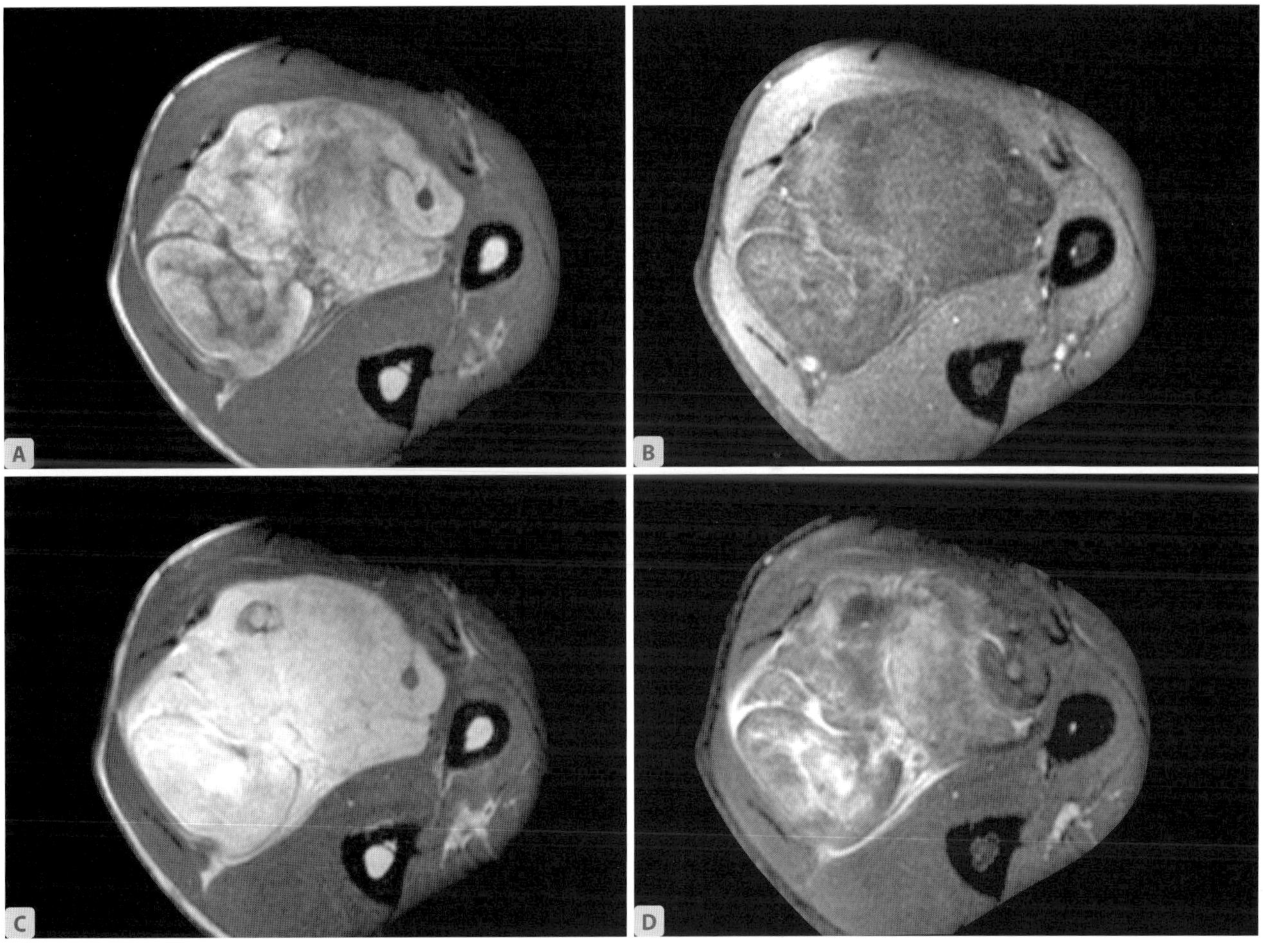

FIGS. 4A TO D: Atypical lipomatous tumor. (A) Axial T1-weighted (T1W); (B) T1W fat-suppressed; (C) T2-weighted (T2W); and (D) T2W fat-suppressed images depict large intramuscular heterogeneous lesion showing fat signal intensity areas which are suppressed on fat-saturated (FS) images. There are intermingled areas of soft-tissue signal intensity as well which appear hyperintense on T2W FS image (D). Histology revealed atypical lipomatous tumor.

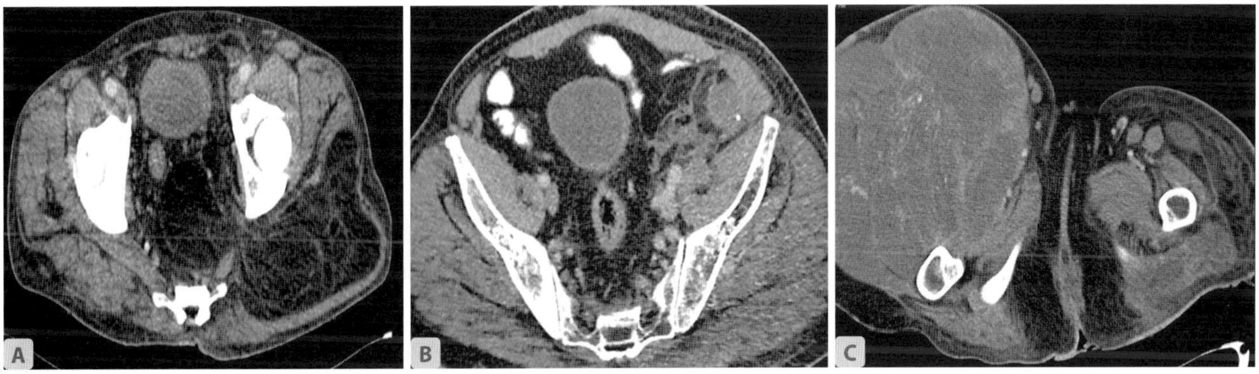

FIGS. 5A TO C: Liposarcomas. (A) Axial contrast-enhanced computed tomography (CECT) image shows fat-attenuation lesion in the left hemipelvis herniating into gluteal region with thin soft-tissue strands within in a case of well-differentiated liposarcoma; (B) Ill-defined lesion in left side of pelvis with relatively demarcated areas of fat and soft-tissue attenuation, (latter >2 cm and nodular) along with a speck of calcification. Histology revealed dedifferentiated liposarcoma; (C) Myxoid liposarcoma shows a large hypodense enhancing mass in the right thigh without any evident fat on imaging.

Well-differentiated liposarcoma and atypical lipomatous tumor (ALT) are similar on histology and molecular markers (positive for MDM 2, HMGA2, CDK4); the only differentiation being based on site. ALT refers to tumors in extremity and trunk which are easier to resect **(Figs. 4A to D)**; WDPLS are lesions in mediastinum/RP wherein complete resection is challenging due to involvement of vital structures, and hence has higher recurrence rate and poor prognosis.

Malignant Liposarcoma

Dedifferentiated liposarcoma: The most common site of dedifferentiated liposarcoma (DDLPS) is RP, occurring in elderly patients. The tumor can arise de novo or result from dedifferentiation of WDPLS. Essentially the nonfatty component is malignant and of variable histology, e.g., rhabdomyosarcoma (RMS) or osteosarcoma. Four morphological types of appearance are described.[10]

- *Category I*: Mainly fatty, nonfatty part is small.
- *Category II*: Mainly nonfatty, fatty part is small.
- *Category III*: Both the components are well delineated, lying adjacent to each other **(Figs. 5A to C)**.
- *Category IV*: Similar to III but both components are mainly nonfatty.

Treatment of choice is WLE; however, likelihood of incomplete resection is high.

Myxoid Liposarcoma/Round Cell Liposarcoma

Pure myxoid LPS is a low-grade sarcoma that typically occurs in the extremities, in the deep location (typically thigh), and in younger patients. It has a characteristic MR appearance with T1 hypointensity and striking high T2 signal, resembling a myoma or even a cyst. The lesion however shows contrast enhancement **(Figs. 5A to C)**. These lesions can have a round cell component, with myxoid and round cell LPS being considered two ends of same spectrum. Those tumors with more than 5% component being round cell are considered as high grade.[8] Such tumors have a more heterogeneous MR signal and poor prognosis. Myxoid LS shows a high propensity for extrapulmonary metastasis (bone/soft tissues).

Pleomorphic Liposarcoma

This variant of LPS is a high-grade sarcoma encountered in extremities off middle aged patients and less commonly in the RP/mediastinum.[11] Among the three variants of malignant LPS, this form has the lowest incidence. On imaging, it is mostly a soft tissue nonfatty mass measuring more than 10 cm, with areas of necrosis and hemorrhages. Fatty component is the small, and differentiation from other STS is often not possible. It is an aggressive lesion with high incidence of pulmonary metastases.

The imaging differences between lipoma, WDLPS, and malignant LPS are summarized in **Table 3**.

FIBROBLASTIC OR MYOFIBROBLASTIC TUMORS

This group of tumors is more common in children than adults.[12] **Table 4** enumerates the entities constituting fibroblastic or myofibroblastic tumors. The more common entities are discussed in **Figures 6 to 8**.

Myositis Ossificans

This is the most commonly encountered lesion in this group, and is reparative process in majority of the patients.

TABLE 3: Differentiating imaging features of lipoma, well-differentiated liposarcoma (WDLPS), and malignant liposarcoma (LPS).

	Lipoma	WDLPS	Malignant LPS
Attenuation	• Homogeneous • Fat • Thin septae • <2 mm	• Soft tissue, nonfatty components (<2 cm) • Thick septae (nodular/interrupted) • >2 mm	• Soft tissue component • >2 cm • Large size • Myxoid LPS: Typical T2 hyperintensity • *High-grade sarcomas*: Large size (>10 cm) • Necrosis, hemorrhage, size of fatty component small
Location	Rare in mediastinum/RP	Mediastinum/RP	*DDLPS*: RP/mediastinum *Myxoid/Pleomorphic*: Extremities

TABLE 4: Classification of fibroblastic or myofibroblastic tumors.

Benign	Intermediate (locally aggressive)	Intermediate (rarely metastasizing)	Malignant
• Fasciitis – Nodular – Proliferative • Myositis ossificans • Fibrous hamartoma of infancy • Calcifying fibrous tumor	• Fibromatosis – Palmar/plantar – Desmoid type – Lipofibromatosis	• Dermatofibrosarcoma • Protuberans – Solitary fibrous tumor – Inflammatory myofibroblastic tumor – Infantile fibrosarcoma	• Adult fibrosarcoma • Myxoid fibrosarcoma

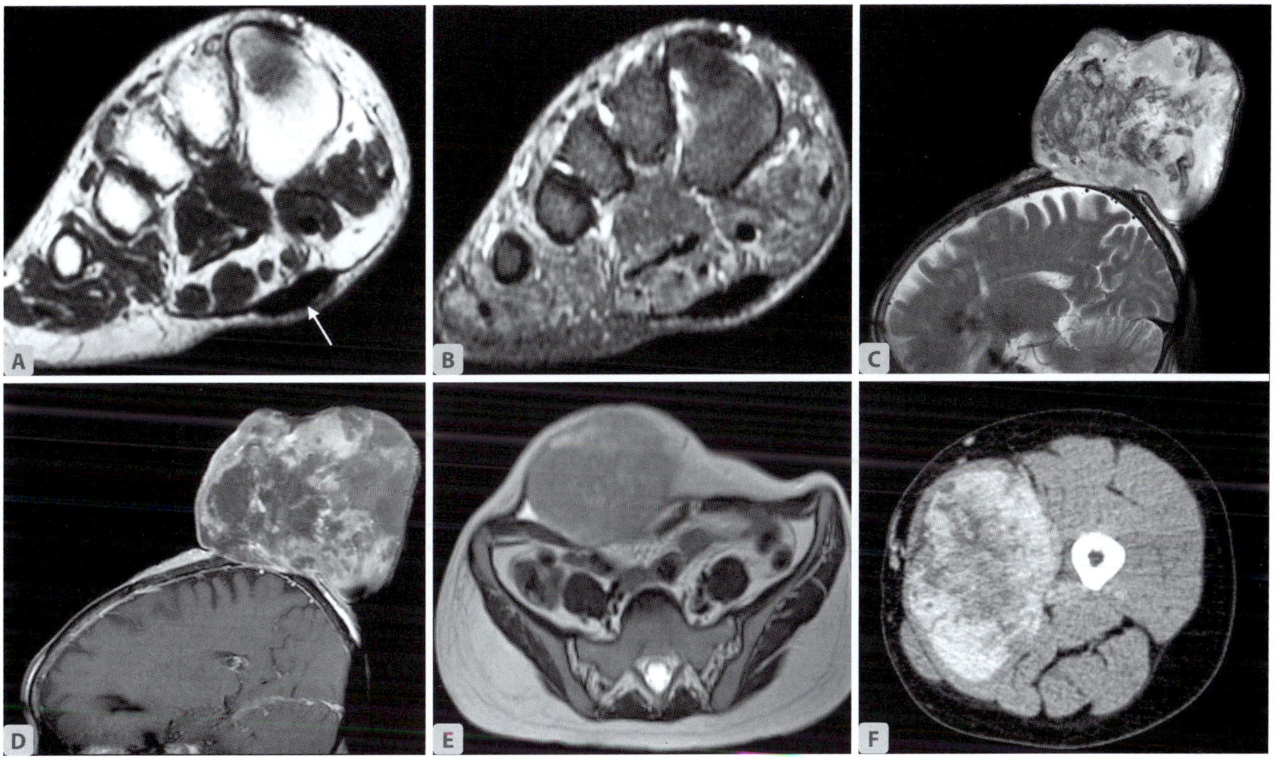

FIGS. 6A TO F: Myofibroblastic tumors. (A) T2-weighted (T2W); and (B) T2W fat-saturated (FS) images show hypointense nodular thickening of plantar fascia (arrows) in a case of plantar fasciitis; (C) Sagittal T2W; and (D) Postcontrast images show heterogeneous appearing large tumor in case of dermatofibrosarcoma protuberans; (E) Axial T2W image shows intermediate signal intensity mass arising from abdominal wall in case of fibromatosis; (F) Axial contrast-enhanced computed tomography (CECT) image in a case of solitary fibrous tumor shows intensely enhancing thigh mass.

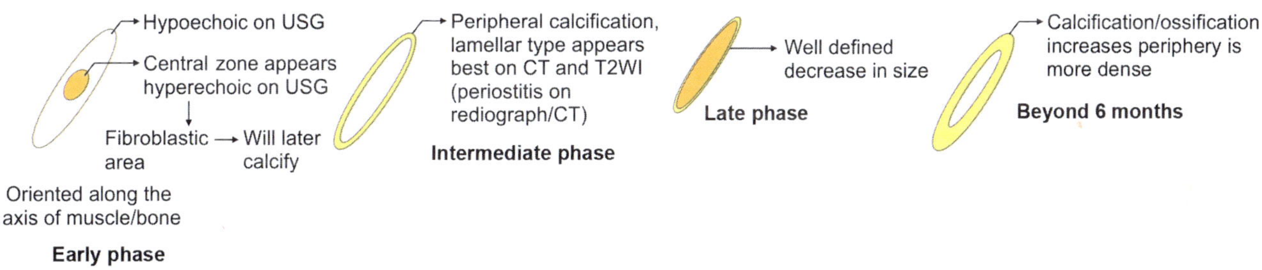

FIG. 7: Schematic diagram showing phases of post-traumatic myositis ossificans. (CT: computed tomography; T2WI: T2-weighted image; USG: ultrasonography).

The frequent sites being skeletal muscles, tendons, and fat, wherein there is formation of metaplastic bone. There are three subtypes of myositis ossificans (MO).

1. Post-traumatic (most common, three-fourths of the patients)[13]
2. Nontraumatic
3. Myositis ossificans progressive.

Post-traumatic Myositis Ossificans

The stages observed on imaging reflect the progressive ossification on histology. The time period stated is in the relationship to the time of trauma **(Table 5; Figs. 7 and 8)**.

In the early phase, clinically and radiologically, it is difficult to differentiate the lesions from other tumors including sarcomas. Patients present with swelling, pain, erythema, and even fever.

Features that aid in distinction from STSs on MRI in early phase include:

- Surrounding edema
- Long axis of lesion
- Periostitis
- Peripheral rim enhancement, however can be diffuse
- Intact bone cortex.

As the lesion matures, the peripheral calcification and subsequent increasing ossification is best seen on T2-

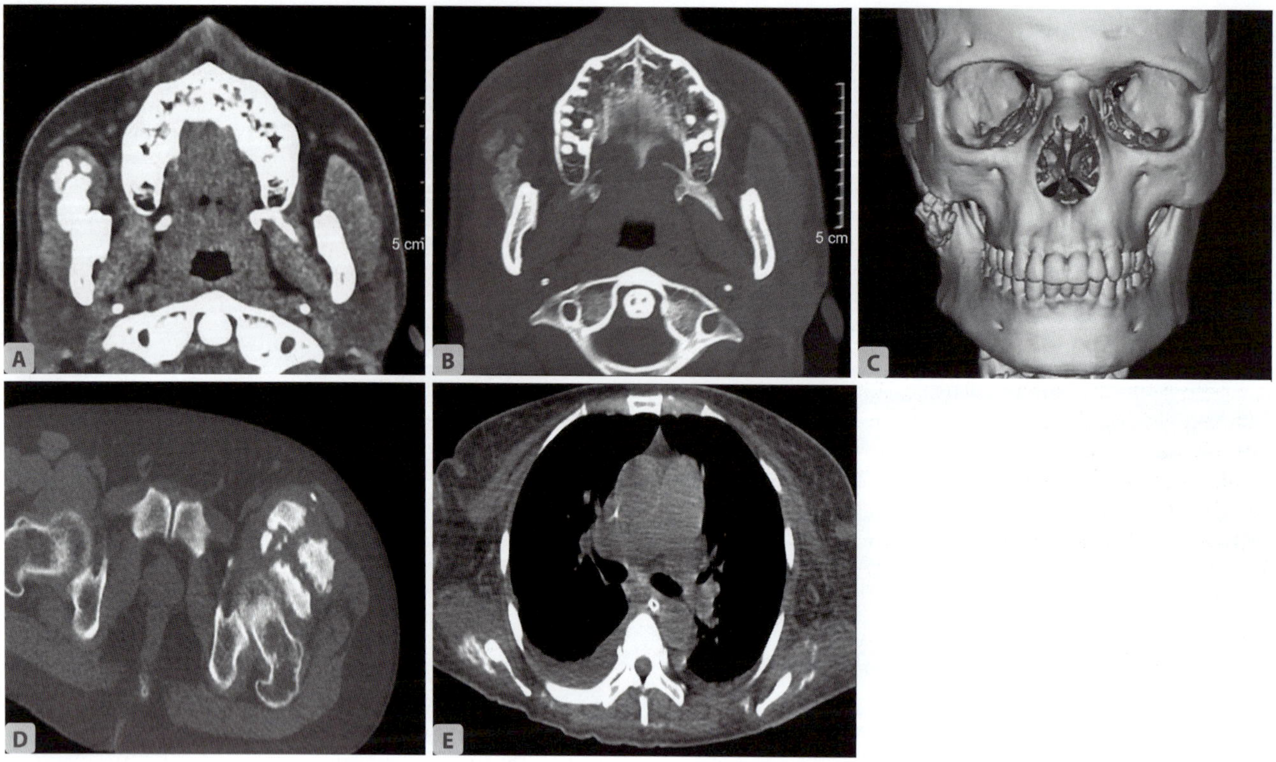

FIGS. 8A TO E: Myositis ossificans. (A) Axial soft tissue; and (B) Bone window computed tomography (CT) images show chunky calcification in the right masseter in a case of myositis ossificans. Periphery is denser than the center; (C) Volume-rendered image depicts the calcified lesion; (D) Myositis ossificans in muscles of the anterior thigh, separate from the underlying bone; (E) Another case of myositis ossificans with calcified lesions in both shoulder girdles.

TABLE 5: Imaging appearance of myositis ossificans according to various phases.

Phases	Time frame	Imaging appearance
Early proliferative phase	Less than 3 weeks	• Nonspecific soft tissue • Along the long axis of muscle/bone
Intermediate phase (calcification plus ossification)	3–7 weeks	Peripheral calcification
Mature ossification phase	More than 7 weeks	• Progressive fall in calcification, increase in ossification • Clear margins • Size reduction (beyond 6 months)

weighted images. Also edema and periostitis resolve with time and the size of lesion decreases.

Nontraumatic Myositis Ossificans

Synonym: Pseudomalignant myositis ossificans

This form of MO occurs in patients with burns or long-standing paralysis (beyond 2 months). It is more frequent in adults and typically occurs below the level of paralysis, also connective tissues are involved more than skeletal muscle.

Myositis Ossificans Progressiva

Synonym: Fibrodysplasia ossificans progressiva

This is an autosomal dominant inherited disorder of the connective tissues resulting from mutation of *ACVR1* gene.[14] In early childhood, patients present with recurrent episodes of soft tissue swellings. These are associated with pain and followed by a trivia trauma. These eventually develop heterotropic ossification. Some characteristic features are:

- Multiple compartment involvement.
- Skeletal muscles, fascia, and ligaments/tendons can be involved.
- *Progression*: Axial to appendicular; cranial to caudal.

The condition is not treatable and patients have severe limitation of mobility, and eventually difficulty in breathing, resulting in mortality. The disease begins in early childhood, and worsens significantly by second or third decade of life.

Desmoid Fibromatosis

Desmoid fibromatosis (DF) is a locally aggressive tumor encountered in children and young adults (it has a bimodal peak—one in first decade and then in third decade). It is common in extremities, truncal region, and less frequent in head and neck. If the lesion develops in a pre-existing fibroma, it has a more aggressive behavior. Association with familial adenomatous polyposis/Gardner syndrome is described.[15] Also, intra-abdominal lesions are more aggressive.

On imaging, the masses can be well-delineated or infiltrative. The stroma of the tumors may predominantly have a stroma that is composed of collagen, or one that is predominantly mucous. The imaging appearance will vary accordingly. Collagen-rich tumors are hypoechoic on USG and show posterior acoustic shadowing, have similar attenuation to muscles on CT, T1 hypointense with variable T2 signal (collagen rich—hypointense, cellular—hyperintense). Mucus-rich tumors are also T1 hyperintense. Tumor may cause scalloping/pressure erosion of adjoining bone. Another sign described on imaging is the "fascial tail sign"—these results from extension of the neoplasm along the fascia.[12] Significant, heterogeneous contrast enhancement is seen on MR.

Management Strategy

- *Conservative*: Clinicoradiological follow-up
- *Chemotherapy*: Rapidly growing tumor or those in critical location
- *Surgical resection*: Only if surgery is possible without undue morbidity
- Recurrence rates are high and particularly higher in those with neurovascular bundle involvement.

Inflammatory Myofibroblastic Tumor

Inflammatory myofibroblastic tumor (IMT), earlier called inflammatory pseudotumor, is an intermediate grade tumor (rarely metastasizing type). Up to one-fourth of the tumors recur post resection, but metastases is rare.[13] It is encountered most commonly in first to third decades of life with common sites being chest, head and neck, and abdomen. The tumor secretes interleukins which are inflammatory mediators and can hence be associated with systemic symptoms.

The tumor is composed of fibroblasts and myofibroblasts in combination with lymphocytes, plasma cells as well as eosinophils. It is this variable combination of fibrotic and cellular elements which will govern the imaging appearance, particularly the T2 signal. These tumors can be large and are characterized by moderate enhancement, which is characteristically persistent. Calcification is frequent **(Figs. 9A to D)**.[16]

In the chest, peripheral tumors are more common than central ones, though IMT may occur in both locations **(Figs. 9A to D)**. In the abdomen, infiltration of soft tissues around the porta (in case of liver IMT) and bowel involvement (in mesenteric/omental location) is described.[17] Surgery is the treatment of choice, though recurrence is frequent. Chemotherapy is only employed in case of unresectable neoplasms.

FIBROHISTIOCYTIC TUMORS

The term used for these tumors by WHO classification is "so-called fibrohistiocytic tumors." The term "so-called" has been attached to the tumors, as HPE IHC and genetic analysis show that these tumors do not arise from histiocytes but only resemble them.[18] The term MFH or malignant fibrous histiocytoma is now eliminated from this category, and only four neoplasms are included. Entities under this group are enumerated in **Table 6.**

Tenosynovial Giant Cell Tumor

Tenosynovial giant cell tumor (TSGCT) basically arise from the synovium lining joints, tendon sheaths, or even bursae, hence, can be extra-articular or intra-articular. These are further divided into localized or diffuse forms[19] **(Table 7 and Fig. 9)**.

SMOOTH MUSCLE TUMORS

This group includes two entities: (1) leiomyoma (benign) and (2) leiomyosarcoma (malignant). Leiomyomas are most frequent in the uterus and the GI tract, with other sites including soft tissues being rare. These have a nonspecific MR appearance, and calcification may be seen in leiomyomas but is rare in the leiomyosarcomas. Leiomyosarcomas are larger and more heterogeneous with necrosis. Both the tumors tend to remodel bone (rather than cause permeative destruction).

PERICYTIC (PERIVASCULAR) TUMORS

These tumors resemble pericytes, which are contractile smooth muscle cells located around vessels and include glomus tumors, myopericytoma, and angioleiomyoma. Glomus tumors in this category are not the same as paragangliomas (also called "glomus"). Glomus tumors of this form occur in the extremities, with less frequent site being paranasal sinuses. These tumors are rare and occur in middle age/elderly, are intensely enhancing, unencapsulated, and locally aggressive lesions **(Figs. 9A to D)**. The tumors are iso/hypointense on T2WI.[20]

Angioleiomyoma is typically encountered in middle-aged females and displays flow voids and avid enhancement due to its mixed composition.

SKELETAL MUSCLE TUMORS

The benign tumor in this group is rhabdomyoma and the malignant neoplasm is RMS.

Rhabdomyosarcoma

Rhabdomyosarcoma is frequent in the pediatric age group, particularly in children less than 10 years of age, among whom it constitutes about half of the STSs.[21] It is a high-grade, small round cell neoplasm, with the more differentiated components resembling skeletal muscle. On IHC, tumors are positive for desmin and myogenin. The types of RMS are illustrated in **Flowchart 4**. The main differences between the major types are enlisted here.[22]

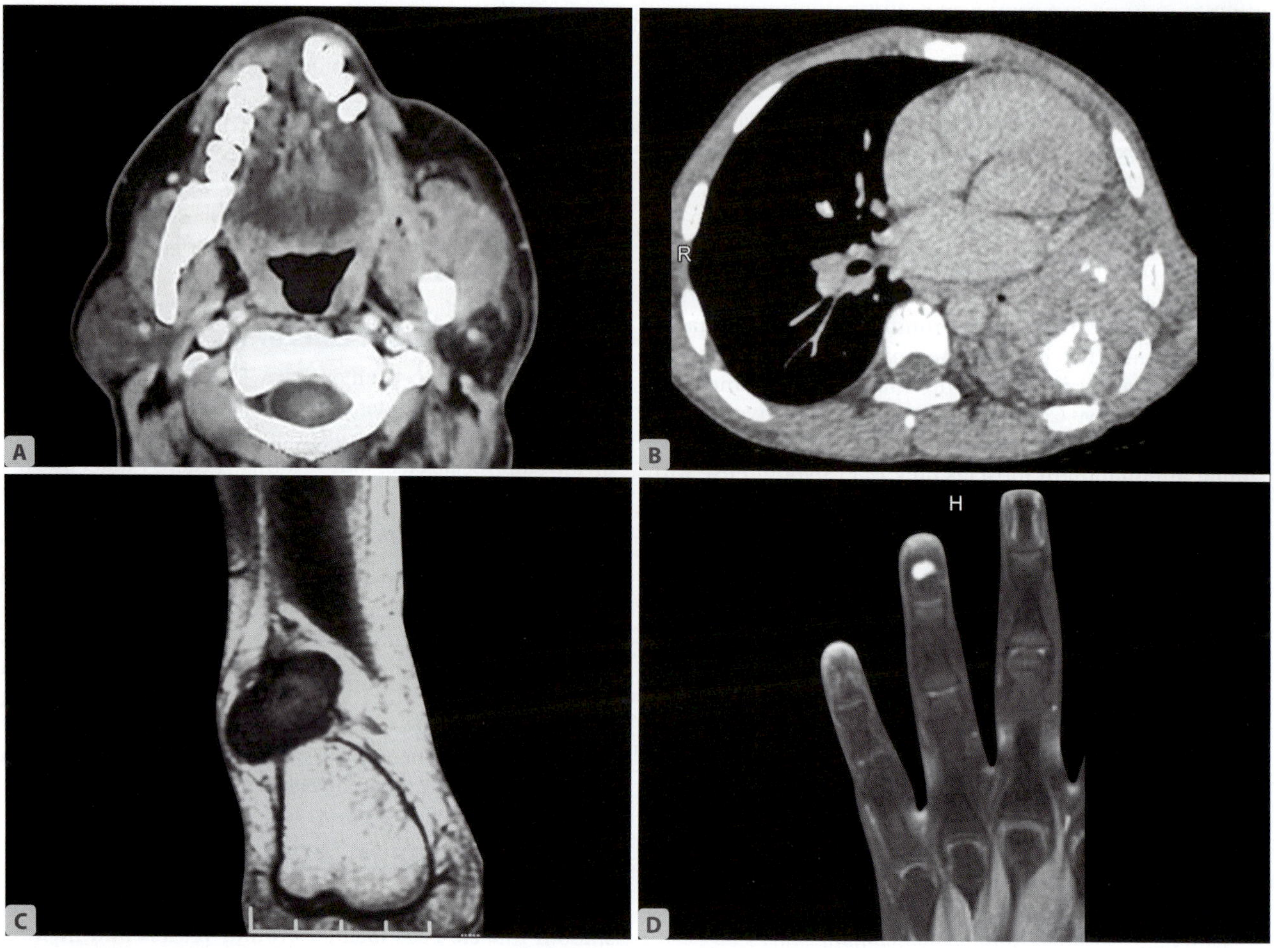

FIGS. 9A TO D: Inflammatory pseudotumor, giant cell tumor, and glomus tumor. (A) Axial contrast-enhanced computed tomography (CECT) image shows bulky left masseter with fatty replacement of ipsilateral parotid. Biopsy revealed inflammatory myofibroblastic tumor (IMFT); (B) Another patient with chest IMFT shows large mass filling in the left thoracic cavity with chunky calcification; (C) Coronal T2-weighted (T2W) image shows round hypointense lesion posterior to the ankle joint, suggestive of localized giant cell tumor; (D) Postcontrast coronal image shows intensely enhancing subcentimetric lesion in soft tissues of the finger tip, suggesting glomus tumor.

TABLE 6: So-called fibrohistiocytic tumors.

Benign	Intermediate (rarely metastasizing)	Malignant
Tenosynovial giant cell tumor	Plexiform fibrohistiocytic tumor	No entity
Deep benign fibrous histiocytoma	Giant cell tumor of soft tissue	

Embryonal RMS

- More common (more than two-thirds)
- Younger age group
- Better prognosis.

Alveolar RMS

- Less than one-third cases
- Older group
- Worse prognosis.

Head and neck is the most common site (over one-third cases), followed by genitourinary or extremities **(Figs. 10A to D)**. In the head and neck, masses may be orbital, parameningeal (involving skull base), or nonparameningeal. Common genitourinary sites include bladder, prostate, or vagina. Other sites include biliary, trunk, thorax, or extremities. RMS is an aggressive neoplasm and is frequently metastatic with common sites being pulmonary, osseous, or lymph nodal. These can be associated with Li-Fraumeni syndrome or DICER1 syndrome among other predisposing factors.

The imaging appearance of RMS is nonspecific. It is the presence of a soft tissue mass in described locations that is aggressive with no fatty component in a young patient that raises the suspicion. Embryonal forms can cause bowing of adjoining bones, while bone destruction is seen in up to one-fifth of the patients. Calcification is uncommon. Necrosis is seen in alveolar and pleomorphic forms, while the embryonal type is mostly homogeneous. MR signal is also nonspecific. The lesion may show flow voids. Contrast enhancement is moderate **(Figs. 10A to D)** and the pleomorphic form may show "ring like" enhancement. Staging is similar to other STS, as is addressed later in the chapter.

TABLE 7: Clinical and imaging features of localized and diffuse forms of tenosynovial giant cell tumor (TSGCT).

	Localized TSGCT	**Diffuse TSGCT**
Synonym	• GCT of tendon sheath • Nodular tenosynovitis	• Diffuse type GCT • Pigmented villo-nodular synovitis/tenosynovitis
Behavior	Benign	Locally aggressive (nonmetastasizing)
Age	• 30–50 years • F>M	<40 years
Location	Hand	• Large joints • Knee, hip, elbow, shoulder
Presentation	• Slow growth • Painless	Painful, tender
Radiograph/CT	• Soft tissue mass, well defined • Pressure erosion of adjoining bone	• Ill-defined soft tissue mass • No calcification • Bone erosion • Joint effusion • Joint space preserved • Bone density normal
USG	• Solid • Well defined • Hypoechoic • Homogeneous/heterogeneous • Adjoining a tendon/joint • Internal vascularity+	• Ill defined • Joint effusion+
MRI (modality of choice)	• *T1WI*: Low intermediate • *T2WI*: Variable • Hypointense foci (hemosiderin deposits) • *Gradient echo*: Blooming • *CEMR*: Diffuse enhancement	• Similar features • *Synovial thickening:* Diffuse or plaque like or nodular • Subchondral cysts/erosions • Effusion with septae
Recurrence rates	Less	More
Treatment of choice	Excision	Wide excision

FLOWCHART 4: Histological subtypes of rhabdomyosarcoma (RMS).

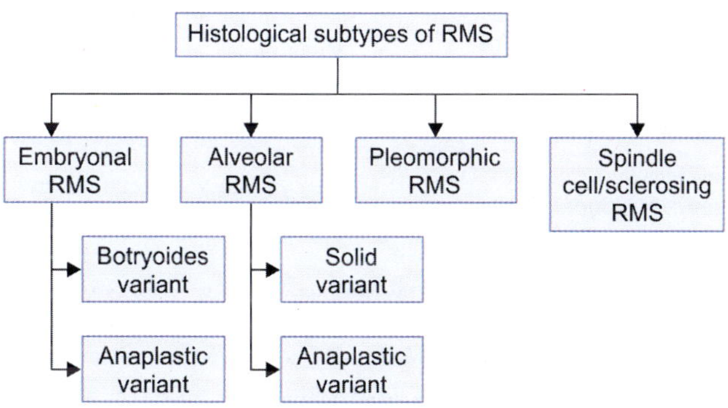

VASCULAR TUMORS

The discussion on this group of tumors encompasses concepts both from the WHO classification as well as the ISSVA (International Society for Study of Vascular Anomalies) classification, primarily the ISSVA concepts[23] **(Table 8).**

Infantile Hemangioma

Superficial infantile hemangioma is associated with skin discoloration (strawberry mark) while in deep lesions overlying skin/mucosa maybe normal. It is encountered during infancy or neonatal period, increases during the next few months, and then regresses. It is characterized by the following phases **(Table 9)**. Beta-blockers have shown to be effective in proliferating phase.[24] These tumors are often GLUT-1 positive.[25]

Congenital Hemangioma

It includes two forms: (1) rapidly involuting congenital hemangioma (RICH) and (2) noninvoluting CH (NICH). The main difference between IH, RICH, or NICH is the age of presentation/regression. CH tumors peak at birth or in some instances have already begun to involute by that time. The rapidly involuting form completely regresses by about 1 year of age. NICH on the other hand does not regress.[26] CH tumors are usually GLUT-1 negative.

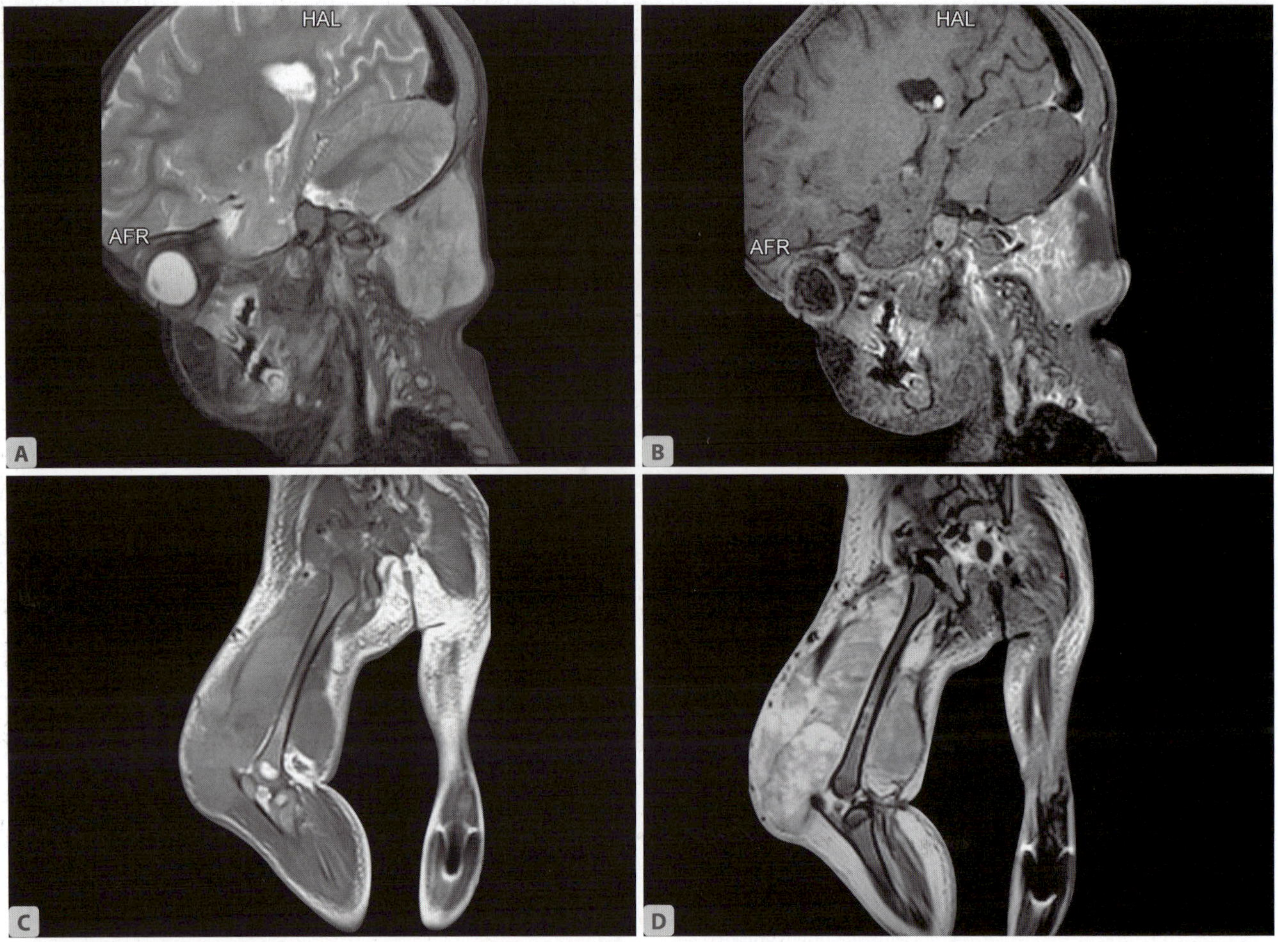

FIGS. 10A TO D: Rhabdomyosarcoma. (A) Sagittal T2-weighted (T2W); and (B) Postcontrast magnetic resonance (MR) images show mildly hyperintense mass in the soft tissues of the neck, showing heterogenous contrast enhancement; (C) Sagittal T1-weighted (T1W); and (D) T2W MR images in another child show large heterogeneous thigh mass in a case of alveolar rhabdomyosarcoma.

TABLE 8: Vascular tumors.

Benign	Intermediate (locally aggressive)	Intermediate (rarely metastasizing)	Malignant
Hemangioma	Kaposiform hemangioendothelioma	Hemangioendothelioma • Retiform • Composite • Pseudomyxogenic	Epitheloid hemangioendothelioma Angiosarcoma

TABLE 9: Imaging appearance of infantile hemangioma according to phases.

Phases	Period	USG	MRI
Proliferative phase	• Neonatal/early infancy • Up to about one and a half years of age	• Well defined mass with variable echogenicity (low or high) • Lobulated • Doppler–arterial flow	• Well defined • Lobulated – *T1WI*: hypo/isointense – *T2WI*: Hyperintense • Flow voids • Early, persistent enhancement
Involuting phase	• After 1 year • Continues for years • Slow regression	Decrease in size and vascularity	• Decrease in size • T2 hyperintensity and enhancement reduce • Fatty replacement

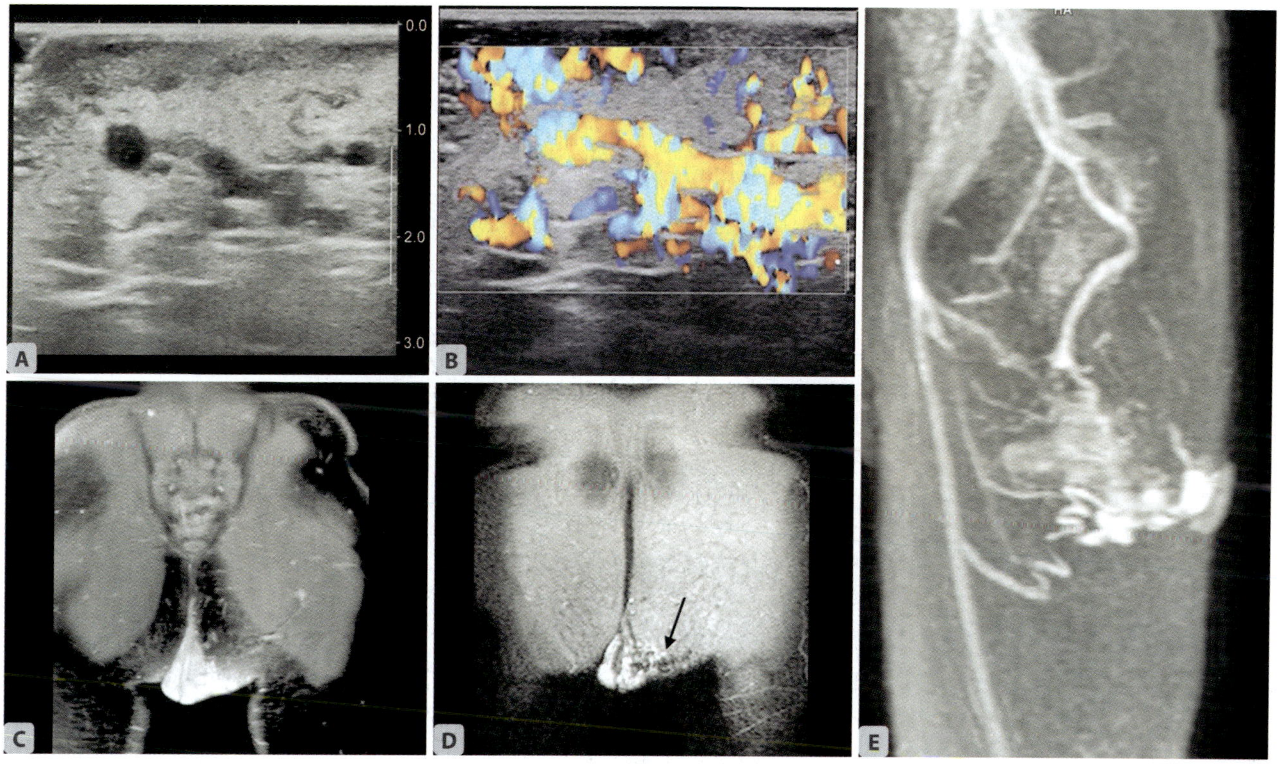

FIGS. 11A TO E: Lobular capillary hemangioma in a young female patient. (A) Gray-scale ultrasound image shows echogenic mass with anechoic vascular channels, showing intense color flow on Doppler image (B); (C and D) Coronal short tau inversion recovery (STIR) images show hyperintense mass involving skin, subcutaneous tissues in perineal region with flow voids (arrow); (E) Time-resolved magnetic resonance (MR) angiography depicts early intense enhancement with arteriovenous shunting.

While imaging features of CH and IH are broadly similar, CH displays some differences:

- More heterogeneity
- Ill-defined margins
- Aggressive features on angiography-aneurysms or arteriovenous shunts **(Figs. 11A to E)**
- Calcification may be present.

Kaposiform Hemangioendothelioma

Kaposiform hemangioendothelioma (KHE) is so-called due to its resemblance to Kaposi's sarcoma on pathology. It is a locally aggressive neoplasm which occurs in infants or children. KHE has an association with Kasabach-Merritt syndrome (a consumption coagulopathy with thrombocytopenia). On imaging, the tumors are similar to hemangiomas but has ill-defined infiltrative margins and may show osseous invasion.[27] The tumor does not metastasize.

Angiosarcoma

Angiosarcoma is a locally aggressive tumor, which occurs most frequently in skin, followed by soft tissues or bone. It is more common in the elderly. Tumor has both vascular/lymphatic components. The tumor displays early and widespread metastases, with lung being the most common site. On imaging, it shows similar features as the other vascular tumors. However, it displays a restriction on diffusion due to high cellularity.[28] A variant described is the "Stewart-Treves syndrome," wherein the neoplasm arises in post-treatment breast carcinoma patients with lymphedema of long duration.

TABLE 10: Chondro-osseous tumors.

Benign	Malignant
Soft tissue chondroma	• Mesenchymal chondrosarcoma • Extraskeletal osteosarcoma

CHONDRO-OSSEOUS TUMORS

The presence of characteristic chondroid/osteoid matrix in extra-osseous masses alerts to the possibility of these tumors. Soft tissue chondro-osseous neoplasms are uncommon/rare tumors encountered in the extremities or head and neck **(Table 10)**.

GASTROINTESTINAL STROMAL TUMORS

The discussion of this tumor is beyond the scope of this chapter.

PERIPHERAL NERVE SHEATH TUMORS

The subtypes of peripheral nerve sheath tumors (PNSTs) are given in **Table 11**.

Benign Peripheral Nerve Sheath Tumors

Of the PNSTs, benign tumors constitutes almost a tenth of all STT. Both schwannomas and neurofibromas share a similar imaging appearance; however, many differential features are also described. Both the tumors are well circumscribed, longitudinally oriented in the direction of nerve and may be homogeneous/heterogeneous **(Figs. 12 and 13)**. The key differences among them are:

- Nerve is eccentric in schwannomas, hence separable; but located within the tumor in neurofibromas.
- Heterogeneity, necrosis, and cystic degeneration are more frequent in schwannomas **(Figs. 13A to D)**.
- Schwannomas are encapsulated tumors, neurofibromas are not. Pseudocapsule can be present.
- "Split-fat sign" can be seen in both, much more often in schwannoma. It refers to the presence of fat around the tumor.[29]
- On MRI, both are iso/hypointense (to muscle) on T1-weighted images, and mildly hyperintense on T2-weighted images with moderate enhancement.
- "Target sign" on MR may be seen in neurofibromas, which refers to low-signal intensity in the center

TABLE 11: Benign and malignant peripheral nerve sheath tumors (PNSTs).

Benign	Malignant
• Schwannoma • Neurofibroma - Plexiform neurofibroma • Granular cell tumor	• Malignant PNST • Malignant triton tumor

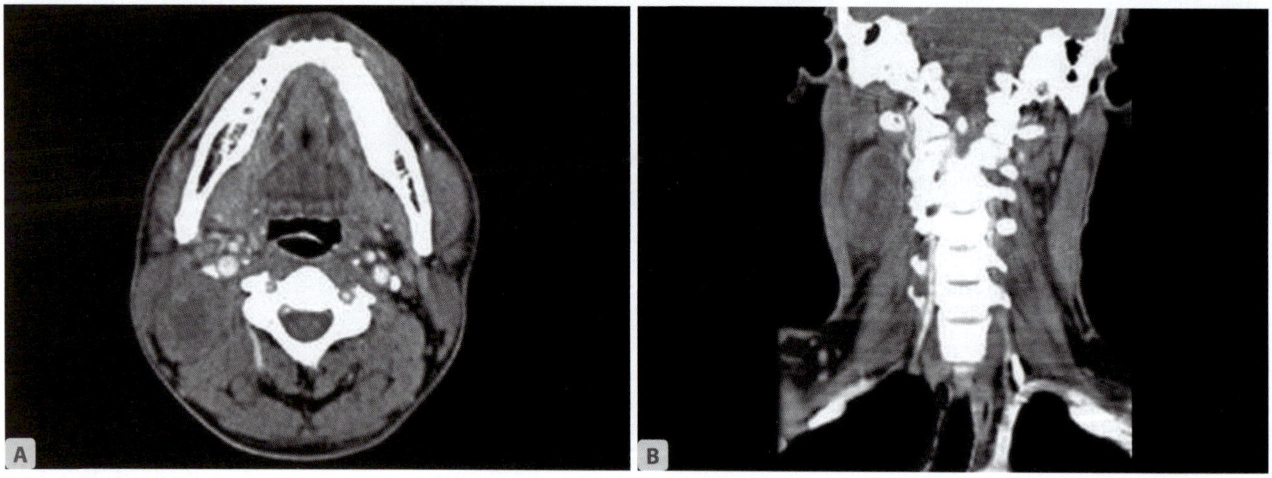

FIGS. 12A AND B: Neurogenic tumor. Contrast-enhanced computed tomography (CECT) images show a longitudinally ovoid, heterogeneous right carotid space mass lesion displacing the vessels anteriorly, suggestive of vagal neurogenic tumor.

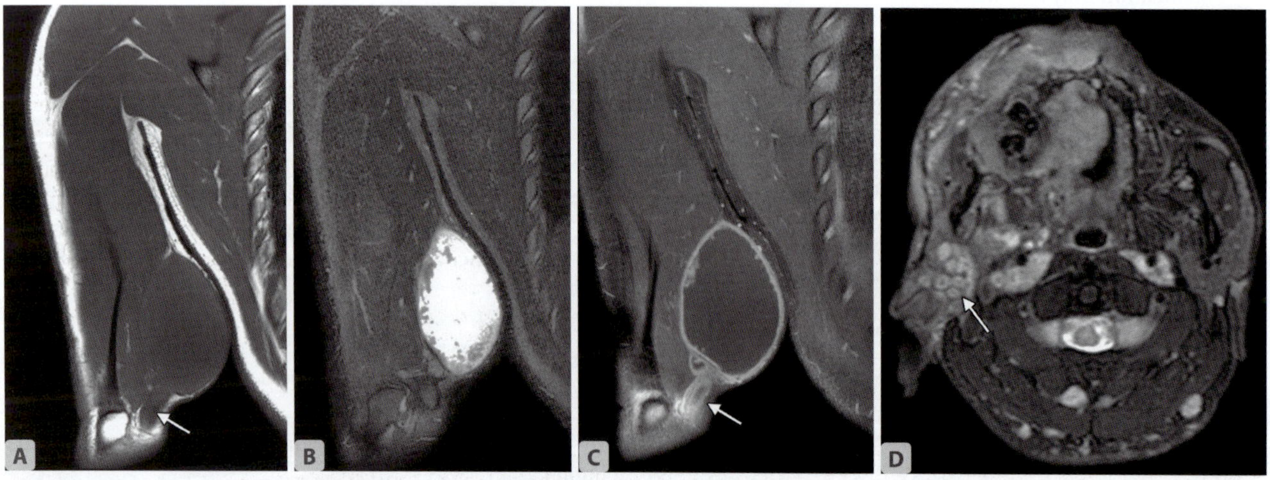

FIGS. 13A TO D: Schwannoma and plexiform neurofibroma. (A) Coronal T1-weighted (T1W); (B) T2-weighted (T2W); and (C) Postcontrast images show longitudinal ovoid lesion, in continuity with the ulnar nerve (arrow), brightly hyperintense on T2W image and showing peripheral contrast enhancement in case of ulnar nerve schwannoma; (D) Another patient with plexiform neurofibroma of the right side of face shows central hypointensity of target sign (arrow).

(fibrocollagenous tissue), with hyperintense periphery (myxoid areas) on T2-weighted image **(Figs. 13A to D)**.

Malignant Peripheral Nerve Sheath Tumors

Malignant PNSTs (MPNSTs) can be challenging to differentiate from benign PNSTs on imaging. The features that suggest malignancy are:

- Large size
- Loss of definition of margins (even if partial or focal) should is the suspicion of MPNST
- Rapidly increasing size
- Heterogeneity and necrosis.

Malignant PNSTs are more frequent in patients with neurofibromatosis (NF-1) and can often developed in preexisting benign PNST. Multiple PNSTs are encountered in NF-1 both in soft tissues and deeper locations (chest and abdomen).

TUMORS OF UNCERTAIN DIFFERENTIATION

These include uncommon/rare entities such as acral fibromyxoma, hemosiderotic fibrolipomatous tumors, and synovial sarcoma. Among these, the malignant counterpart synovial sarcoma is the most frequently encountered.

Synovial Sarcoma

Synovial sarcoma (SS) is an intermediate to high-grade, slow-growing STT, which occurs most frequently in young adults, particularly seen around the joints, especially in popliteal fossa. It does not arise in intra-articular location or synovial structures, but tends to occur near the joints. Pathologically, the cells resemble the normal synovium but stain for epithelial markers and have monophasic, biphasic, or poorly differentiated subtypes. Over 90% of cases demonstrate t(X;18) translocation which is highly specific for SS.[30]

Imaging features are nonspecific, but a juxta-articular soft tissue mass with calcification (which is seen in 30% of cases) in a young patient is very suggestive of SS. On CT or MRI, the tumor shows lobulated margins and heterogeneity with presence of hemorrhage, septations, calcification, or fluid levels **(Figs. 14A to C)**. Such marked heterogeneity gives rise to the "triple sign" which represents the cystic degeneration; and high-signal on T2WI along with presence of hypointense internal fibrotic bands and calcifications. "Bowl of grapes" sign arise due to presence of multiple fluid–fluid levels secondary to recurrent bleeds. Bone involvement can occur in the form of extrinsic erosion or periosteal reaction.

The tumor has high metastatic potential and cannon ball pulmonary metastasis is well known.[31] SS most commonly affects the lower extremities, and is less commonly seen in head and neck region, and is rare in chest wall and viscera. Management constitutes surgery along with pre- and postoperative radiotherapy/chemotherapy. SS has a tendency to locally recur (30–50% local recurrence rates).[30]

UNDIFFERENTIATED/UNCLASSIFIED SARCOMAS

This category contains only malignant lesions not included in the other categories. The types of undifferentiated sarcomas include spindle cell, pleomorphic, round cell, epitheloid, and NOS (not otherwise specified). Prior to 2013, these were labeled as "malignant fibrous histiocytoma."

Staging of Soft Tissue Sarcomas

American Joint Committee on Cancer (AJCC), 8th edition, staging system is recommended for staging of STS.[32] Similar to bone tumors, STS staging also accounts grade based on histopathology (G); in addition to primary tumor (T), lymph nodes (N), and metastases (M). STS are considered under four categories, based on location:

1. Trunk and extremity

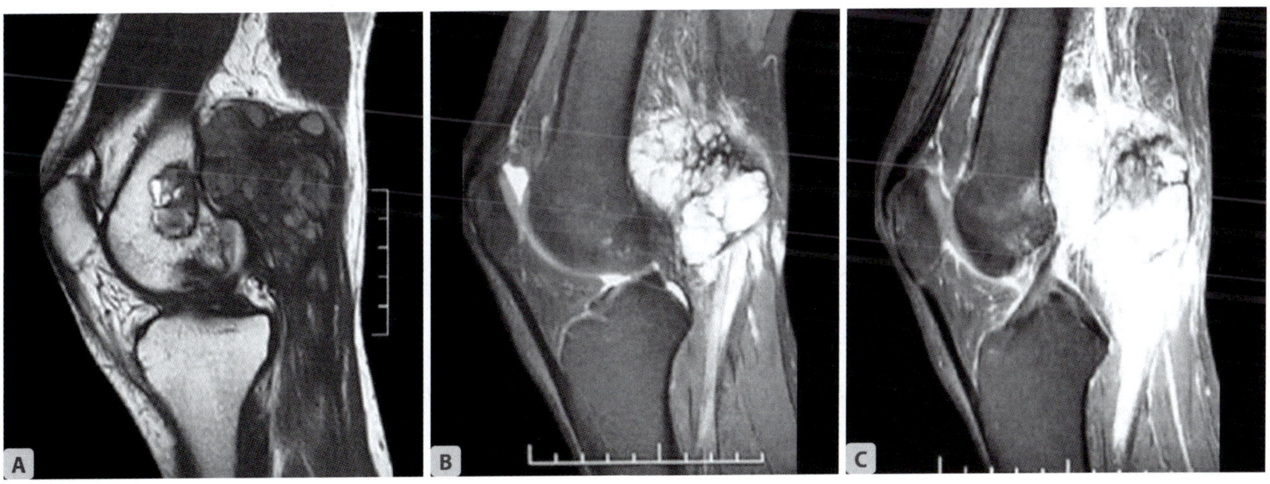

FIGS. 14A TO C: Synovial sarcoma. (A) Sagittal T1-weighted (T1W); (B) T2-weighted (T2W); and (C) Postcontrast magnetic resonance (MR) images of a young male show a heterogeneous, solid, lobulated extra-articular mass located just behind the knee joint. The lesion is brightly hyperintense on T2W image and shows intense enhancement. Intraosseous extension is seen into the adjoining femur.

2. Head and neck
3. Retroperitoneum
4. Visceral.

Tumor Grades

The AJCC staging system includes three tumor grades, based on the French Federation of Cancer Centers Sarcoma Group (FNCLCC) system: high grade (poorly differentiated) is the highest grade 3, followed by intermediate grade (moderate differentiated 2), and low- or well-differentiated which is labeled as grade 1.

Steps of Staging (Flowchart 5)

T Stage

T stage definition differs according to the site of the tumor. Tx category is common to all sites, i.e., that the tumor is not assessable. **Table 12** shows the T descriptors according to site.

Size refers to largest tumor dimension.

The staging of STS is applicable to most histological subtypes; however, some unusual tumors/sites have been excluded from the common staging system. The discussion of these entities and of gastrointestinal stromal tumor is beyond the scope of this chapter.

FLOWCHART 5: Steps of staging.

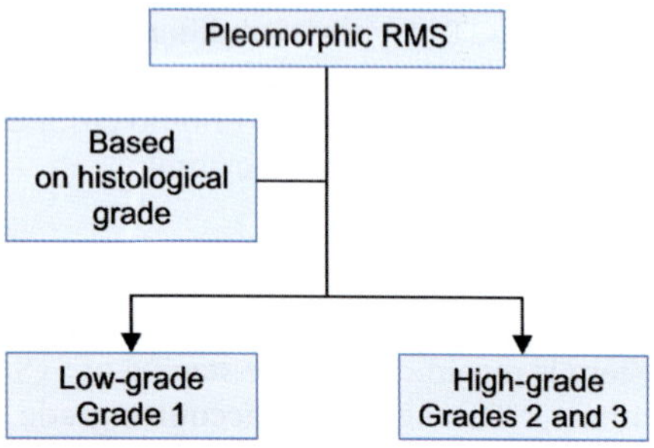

The stage groupings are essentially dependent on the stage and histological grade (G), as presence of positive nodes or metastases places the tumor in stage III or IV depending on site **(Table 13)**. There are some differences in the staging systems advocated by AJCC and UICC (Union for International Cancer Control). In this chapter, the AJCC system is followed for discussion. The 8th edition introduced two new sites: (1) "Head and neck" and (2) "Abdomen and thoracic visceral organs." While separate T descriptors for these sites have been detailed **(Table 12)**, separate stage groupings have not been given. The only difference in stage groupings of trunk, extremity vs. RP is that in the latter N1 is placed in III B group.

In the head and neck region, T4 category has been further divided based on which surrounding organs are infiltrated.

- *T4a*: Orbit, skull base or dura, viscera, facial bones, pterygoid muscles.
- *T4b*: Invasion of cerebral parenchyma, carotid artery, prevertebral muscle, perineural spread (to CNS).

On the other hand, the subdivision of T4 category in abdomen and thoracic is based on number sites involved: 2 sites being T4a, 3–5 sites being T4b, and more than 5 sites being T4c.

IMAGING MODALITIES AND APPROACH

Ultrasonography

Ultrasonography (USG), due to its obvious advantages, is advocated as the first level screening modality for evaluation

TABLE 12: T descriptor according to various sites.

T descriptor	Trunk/extremity/RP	Head and neck	Abdominal and thoracic visceral organs
T0	No primary tumor	No primary tumor	No primary tumor
T1	Size ≤5 cm	Size ≤2 cm	Limited to the organ
T2	Size >5 cm, ≤10 cm	Size >2 cm, ≤4 cm	Spread beyond the organ
T3	Size >10 cm, ≤15 cm	Size >4 cm	Infiltration of a different organ
T4	Size >15 cm	When there is surrounding infiltration/invasion	Multifocal

TABLE 13: Staging groups.

Applicable to trunk and extremities					
Stage I		**Stage II**	**Stage III**		**Stage IV**
A	B		A	B	
T1	T2–T4	T1	T2	T3	N1 or M1 with any T
Gx or G1	Gx or G1	G2 or G3	G2 or G3	G2 or G3	
Applicable to retroperitoneum					
Similar	Similar	Similar	Similar + any T, any G N1 included		M1 (any T any G)

of soft tissue masses **(Box 1)**.[33] Although, it suffers from limitations, particularly in evaluation of deep seated lesions, it can categorize several lesions definitely avoiding biopsy or further evaluation **(Table 14)**. Addition of tissue harmonic imaging, compound imaging, and Doppler is advocated depending on nature of lesion. USG is also useful for image-guided interventions. Elastography is an adjunct tool to high-resolution USG in the evaluation of soft tissue lesions. Assessment of stiffness of masses using elastography helps in their characterization.[34] Contrast-enhanced US (CEUS) has been shown to have some role in characterization of STTs into benign and malignant forms. One of the studies have shown an inhomogeneous pattern of contrast uptake, and

BOX 1: Lesions that can be labeled as clearly benign on USG.

- Cystic lesions
  - Simple cyst
  - Ganglion cyst
  - Bursae
- *Lipoma*: If superficial, well defined, stable in size
- Vascular malformations
- Superficial fibromatosis
- Superficial nerve sheath tumors in known patients of neurofibromatosis
- Motor neuroma
- Aneurysms

TABLE 14: Magnetic resonance (MR) acquisition protocol.

System	**1.5 T or 3 T (minimum 1 T)**
FOV (field of view)	Not only include complete lesion but also adjoining edema plus normal surrounding tissues Skin markers can be used
Matrix	≥256
Slice thickness	3 mm or 4 mm depending on tumor size
Sequences	
Precontrast T1W	Axial
Fat-sat fluid sensitive sequences (e.g., STIR)	Parallel to tumor long axis
T2W: Fat saturated (FS) or PD-FS	Axial
Intravenous gadolinium-based contrast	Preferable to use unless contraindicated *Dose*: 0.1 mm/kg
Postcontrast T1W FS	In long axis and in one additional plane Subtraction images should be generated
Dynamic contrast enhanced MR	Optional
Diffusion weighted imaging	b-values 400–1000

FLOWCHART 6: Choice of imaging modalities for evaluation of suspected soft tissue tumors (STT).

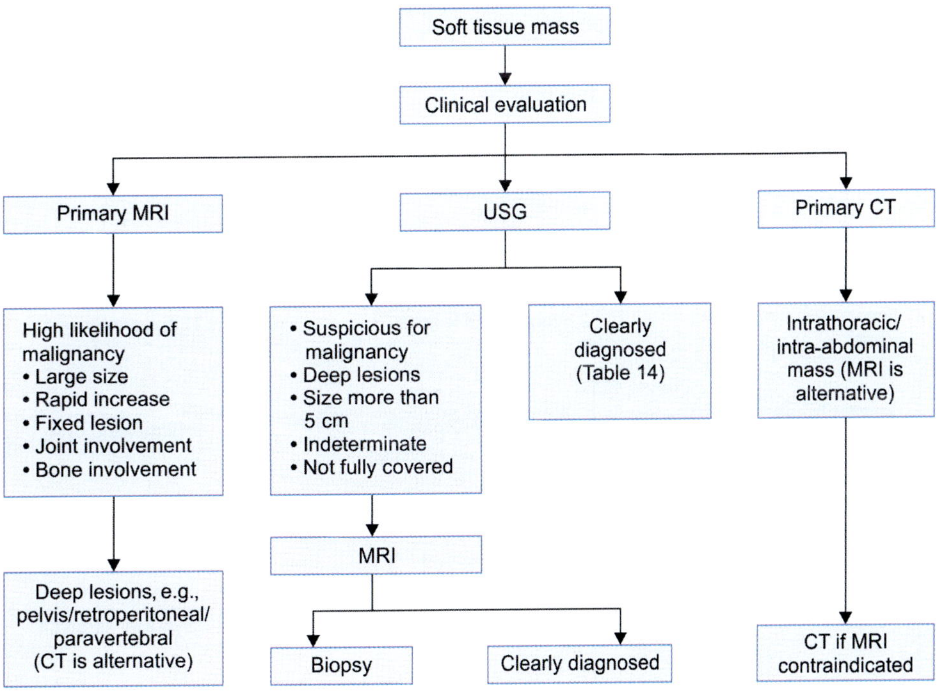

arterial phase enhancement is associated with high risk of malignancy.[35]

Algorithmic approach to choice of imaging modalities for evaluation of suspected STT is outlined in **Flowchart 6.**[36]

MRI

Magnetic resonance imaging is the work-horse of imaging of STTs. It may be performed upfront if clinical suspicion of malignancy is high (primary MRI), or subsequent to another imaging modality.[37] MRI aids in both characterization and tumor mapping **(Table 14).**

Some lesions which can be clearly diagnosed on MRI. These include the list given under USG. Additional lesions which can be diagnosed on MR include:
- Hamartoma
- Myositis ossificans
- PVNS
- Muscle tears.

Further, the MR signal also guides further diagnosis **(Flowchart 7)**.

CT Scan

Computed tomography has been largely replaced in the evaluation of soft tissue masses, except when MRI is contraindicated or unavailable. It can be performed upfront (primary CT) for abdominal/pelvic/retroperitoneal or thoracic masses; or subsequent to USG. In intrathoracic lesions it is often the preferred primary modality. It may be required even subsequent to MRI even, for better assessment of calcification/ossification/bone involvement in abdominal or chest masses.

Radiographs

Plain radiography may be performed initially if the distinction from an osseous origin mass is unclear clinically. It is mostly used as a "complimentary modality" to USG/MRI to better visualize calcification/ossification in the soft tissue mass; or underlying osseous involvement. It is mostly used for appendicular lesions for this purpose; with CT being the preferred modality for truncal lesions.

Biopsy

Biopsy is indicated in all masses suspicious for malignancy and in indeterminate masses. In suspected malignant masses recommended gauge of the biopsy needle is a minimum of 14 G. Also, at least 3–4 cores should be obtained. FNAC is not adequate for diagnosis. Also, biopsy should be performed where facility for appropriate molecular/genetic evaluation is available besides histopathology. If not, patient may require a rebiopsy at a specialist center. Currently, image-guided biopsies are preferred over excision biopsy, unless the lesion is small (<2 cm).

STRUCTURED REPORTING FORMAT

Ultrasound and MRI would suffice for evaluation of most soft tissue lesions, while plain radiographs and CT are useful adjuncts to demonstrate associated osseous changes or matrix mineralization/ossification. MRI is the method of choice for their assessment and staging but MRI does not provide histologic diagnosis. Soft tissue involvement is often underestimated by CT. Indeterminate lesions will require biopsy and careful follow-up. Once histology has confirmed that a lesion is malignant, CT scanning of thorax is required to determine the presence or absence of intrapulmonary metastases. Use of a structured reporting format enhances the quality of the report. The structured reporting format of USG/MRI of soft tissue lesions is shown in **Table 15.**

In addition, morphological features as detailed under USG should also be mentioned in the MRI report.

FLOWCHART 7: Approach based on magnetic resonance (MR) signal.

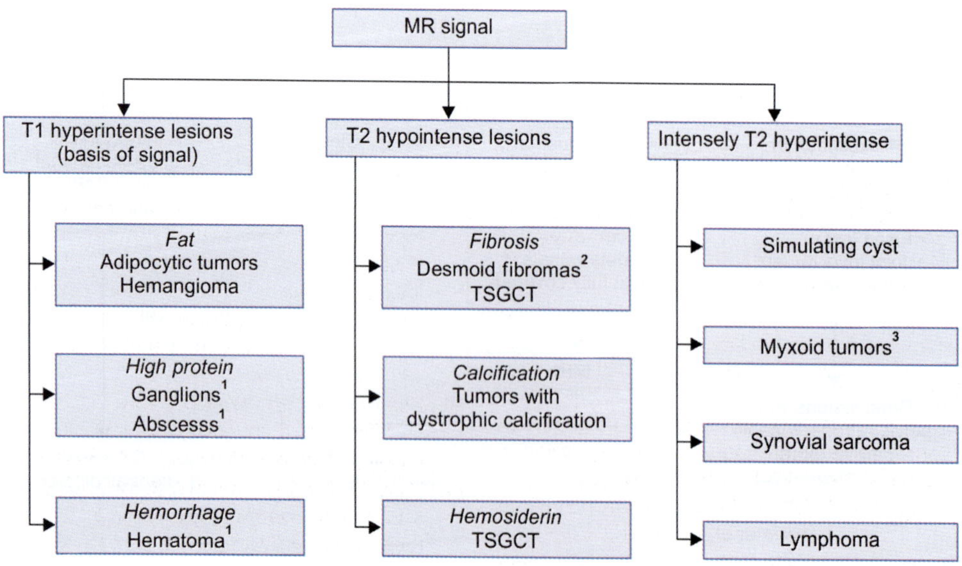

[1]Not neoplasms.

[2]*Fibromas:* Plantar fibroma, elastofibroma, fibrosarcoma.

[3]*Myxoid tumors:* Myxoid LPS, intramuscular myxoma.

TABLE 15: Systematic reporting of USG and MRI of soft tissue masses.

USG	
Morphology: Echogenicity of lesion	• Cystic • Solid • Mixed solid cystic
Margins	Well-defined/ill-defined/infiltrative
For solid masses	• Homogeneous • Heterogeneous with necrosis
For cystic lesion	• Internal echoes • Septae • Walls
Vascularity	
Calcification	Posterior acoustic shadowing (present/absent)
Size	In all three dimensions
Location or relationship to/infiltration of adjoining structures	• Fascia (superficial and deep) • Compartment • Adjoining bone/joints • Vessels and nerves
Elastography strain ratio	
MRI	
T1WI signal	Hypointense, intermediate, hyperintense
T2WI signal	Hypointense, intermediate, hyperintense
DWI	Restricted/facilitated (ADC value)
Postgadolinium enhancement pattern	Homogeneous/heterogeneous/rim
Capsule/pseudocapsule	±
Peritumoral edema/surrounding infiltration	±
Satellite lesion/multiple lesions	±
Nodes	± with size and location
Any specific sign if present	e.g., split-fat sign, target sign
T stage	In case of STS
N stage	In case of STS

REFERENCES

1. Siegel RL, Miller KD, Jemal A. Cancer statistics, 2020. CA Cancer J Clin. 2020;70(1):7-30.
2. Fletcher C, Bridge J, Hogendoorn P, Mertens F. World Health Organization Classification of Tumours of Soft Tissue and Bone, 4th edition. Lyon: IARC Press; 2013.
3. Vilanova JC. WHO classification of soft tissue tumors. In Vanhoenacker FM, Parizel PM, Gielen JL (Eds). Imaging of Soft Tissue Tumors. Chcam: Springer; 2017. pp.187-96.
4. Wei S, Henderson-Jackson E, Qian X, Bui MM. Soft tissue tumor immunohistochemistry update: Illustrative examples of diagnostic pearls to avoid pitfalls. Arch Pathol Lab Med. 2017;141(8):1072-91.
5. Bancroft LW, Kransdorf MJ, Peterson JJ, O'Connor MI. Benign fatty tumors: Classification, clinical course, imaging appearance, and treatment. Skeletal Radiol. 2006;35(10):719-33.
6. Dreux N, Marty M, Chibon F, Vélasco V, Hostein I, Ranchère-Vince D, et al. Value and limitation of immunohistochemical expression of HMGA2 in mesenchymal tumors: About a series of 1052 cases. Mod Pathol. 2010;23(12):1657-66.
7. Burt AM, Huang BK. Imaging review of lipomatous musculoskeletal lesions. SICOT J. 2017;3:34.
8. Gupta P, Potti TA, Wuertzer SD, Lenchik L, Pacholke DA. Spectrum of fat-containing soft-tissue masses at MR imaging: The common, the uncommon, the characteristic, and the sometimes confusing. Radiographics. 2016;36(3): 753-66.
9. Weiss SW, Rao VK. Well-differentiated liposarcoma (atypical lipoma) of deep soft tissue of the extremities, retroperitoneum, and miscellaneous sites. A follow-up study of 92 cases with analysis of the incidence of "dedifferentiation". Am J Surg Pathol. 1992;16(11):1051-8.
10. Hong SH, Kim KA, Woo OH, Park CM, Kim CH, Kim MJ, et al. Dedifferentiated liposarcoma of retroperitoneum: Spectrum of imaging findings in 15 patients. Clin Imaging. 2010;34(3):203-10.
11. El Ouni F, Jemni H, Trabelsi A, Ben Maitig M, Arifa N, Ben Rhouma K, et al. Liposarcoma of the extremities: MR imaging features and their correlation with pathologic data. Orthop Traumatol Surg Res. 2010;96(8):876-83.

12. Sargar KM, Sheybani EF, Shenoy A, Aranake-Chrisinger J, Khanna G. Pediatric fibroblastic and myofibroblastic tumors: a pictorial review. Radiographics. 2016;36(4):1195-214.
13. Coffin CM, Alaggio R. Fibroblastic and myofibroblastic tumors in children and adolescents. Pediatr Dev Pathol. 2012;15(1 Suppl):127-80.
14. Giacopelli F, Cappato S, Tonachini L, Mura M, Di Lascio S, Fornasari D, et al. Identification and characterization of regulatory elements in the promoter of ACVR1, the gene mutated in Fibrodysplasia Ossificans Progressiva. Orphanet J Rare Dis. 2013;8:145.
15. Ferrari A, Alaggio R, Meazza C, Chiaravalli S, Vajna de Pava M, Casanova M, et al. Fibroblastic tumors of intermediate malignancy in childhood. Expert Rev Anticancer Ther. 2013;13(2):225-36.
16. Patnana M, Sevrukov AB, Elsayes KM, Viswanathan C, Lubner M, Menias CO. Inflammatory pseudotumor: The great mimicker. AJR Am J Roentgenol. 2012;198(3): W217-27.
17. Kim SJ, Kim WS, Cheon JE, Shin SM, Youn BJ, Kim IO, et al. Inflammatory myofibroblastic tumors of the abdomen as mimickers of malignancy: Imaging features in nine children. AJR Am J Roentgenol. 2009;193(5):1419-24.
18. Kang HS. So-Called Fibrohistiocytic Tumors, 1st edition. Singapore: Springer; 2017.
19. Gouin F, Noailles T. Localized and diffuse forms of tenosynovial giant cell tumor (formerly giant cell tumor of the tendon sheath and pigmented villonodular synovitis). Orthop Traumatol Surg Res. 2017;103(1S):S91-7.
20. Razek AA, Huang BY. Soft tissue tumors of the head and neck: imaging-based review of the WHO classification. Radiographics. 2011;31(7):1923-54.
21. Jawad N, McHugh K. The clinical and radiologic features of paediatric rhabdomyosarcoma. Pediatr Radiol. 2019;49(11): 1516-23.
22. Leiner J, Le Loarer F. The current landscape of rhabdomyosarcomas: An update. Virchows Arch. 2020;476(1): 97-108.
23. Nozaki T, Matsusako M, Mimura H, Osuga K, Matsui M, Eto H, et al. Imaging of vascular tumors with an emphasis on ISSVA classification. Jpn J Radiol. 2013;31(12):775-85.
24. Léauté-Labrèze C, Dumas de la Roque E, Hubiche T, Boralevi F, Thambo JB, Taïeb A. Propranolol for severe hemangiomas of infancy. N Engl J Med. 2008;358(24): 2649-51.
25. Restrepo R, Palani R, Cervantes LF, Duarte AM, Amjad I, Altman NR. Hemangiomas revisited: The useful, the unusual and the new. Part 1: overview and clinical and imaging characteristics. Pediatr Radiol. 2011;41(7):895-904.
26. Restrepo R, Palani R, Cervantes LF, Duarte AM, Amjad I, Altman NR. Hemangiomas revisited: The useful, the unusual and the new. Part 2: endangering hemangiomas and treatment. Pediatr Radiol. 2011;41(7):905-15.
27. Gruman A, Liang MG, Mulliken JB, Fishman SJ, Burrows PE, Kozakewich HP, et al. Kaposiform hemangioendothelioma without Kasabach-Merritt phenomenon. J Am Acad Dermatol. 2005;52(4):616-22.
28. Walker EA, Salesky JS, Fenton ME, Murphey MD. Magnetic resonance imaging of malignant soft tissue neoplasms in the adult. Radiol Clin North Am. 2011;49(6):1219-34, vi.
29. Kakkar C, Shetty CM, Koteshwara P, Bajpai S. Telltale signs of peripheral neurogenic tumors on magnetic resonance imaging. Indian J Radiol Imaging. 2015;25(4):453-8.
30. Murphey MD, Gibson MS, Jennings BT, Crespo-Rodríguez AM, Fanburg-Smith J, Gajewski DA. From the archives of the AFIP: Imaging of synovial sarcoma with radiologic-pathologic correlation. Radiographics. 2006;26(5):1543-65.
31. Bakri A, Shinagare AB, Krajewski KM, Howard SA, Jagannathan JP, Hornick JL, et al. Synovial sarcoma: Imaging features of common and uncommon primary sites, metastatic patterns, and treatment response. AJR Am J Roentgenol. 2012;199(2):W208-15.
32. Tanaka K, Ozaki T. New TNM classification (AJCC eighth edition) of bone and soft tissue sarcomas: JCOG Bone and Soft Tissue Tumor Study Group. Jpn J Clin Oncol. 2019;49(2):103-7.
33. Catalano O, Varelli C, Sbordone C, Corvino A, De Rosa D, Vallone G, et al. A bump: What to do next? Ultrasound imaging of superficial soft-tissue palpable lesions. J Ultrasound; 2019.
34. Li S, Liu L, Lv G. Diagnostic value of strain elastography for differentiating benign and malignant soft tissue masses. Oncol Lett. 2017;14(2):2041-4.
35. De Marchi A, Prever EBD, Cavallo F, Pozza S, Linari A, Lombardo P, et al. Perfusion pattern and time of vascularisation with CEUS increase accuracy in differentiating between benign and malignant tumours in 216 musculoskeletal soft tissue masses. Eur J Radiol. 2015;84(1):142-50.
36. Wu JS, Hochman MG. Soft-tissue tumors and tumorlike lesions: A systematic imaging approach. Radiology. 2009;253(2):297-316.
37. Manaster BJ. Soft-tissue masses: Optimal imaging protocol and reporting. Am J Roentgenol. 2013;201(3):505-14.

CHAPTER

174 Imaging of Peripheral Nerves

Mahesh Prakash, Harish Bhujade, Anindita Sinha

INTRODUCTION

The peripheral nervous system (PNS) consists of nerves, ganglions, receptors which carry signal from central nervous system to the peripheral organs and vice-versa. There are many acquired, traumatic, or rarely congenital conditions which are seen in PNS. Traditionally, clinical examination and electrophysiological studies are the mainstay to make diagnosis of disorders of PNS. However, due to the patchy distribution of conduction block and slow conduction, accurate diagnosis is challenging in certain cases on electrophysiological studies.[1] The accuracy of electrophysiological studies may be affected by a many other factors such as age, gender, built, temperature, and body mass index.[2] Accurate diagnosis of peripheral nerve disorders is very important to guide correct patient management.[3] Many neuropathies are often remain undiagnosed on clinical examination or nerve conduction studies. Imaging of PNS is not only useful in direct demonstration of nerves but also helpful in assessing surrounding tissue.[3] Recent advances in high resolution ultrasound (US) and magnetic resonance imaging (MRI) permit precise evaluation and diagnosis of various diseases of peripheral nerves.[4] Improvements in technology (developments in transducer materials, enhanced software, higher fields MR scanner and availability of MR selective sequences) permit accurate diagnosis of various disorders of PNS. Especially the MR neurography, which is a noninvasive technique, allows assessment of the underlying cause of injury and differentiate between surgically curable and noncurable etiologies.[5]

ANATOMY OF PERIPHERAL NERVOUS SYSTEM

The nerve consists of multiple axons, which is covered by a tissue layer known as endoneurium. Many axons are grouped together to form the fascicles. Every fascicle is surrounded by tissue layer known as perineurium. These bundles of fascicles are covered by a tissue layer known as epineurium which is outermost layer of nerve **(Fig. 1)**. The PNS consists of spinal nerves and cranial nerves. The dorsal and ventral roots of spinal nerves composed of sensory and motor axons,

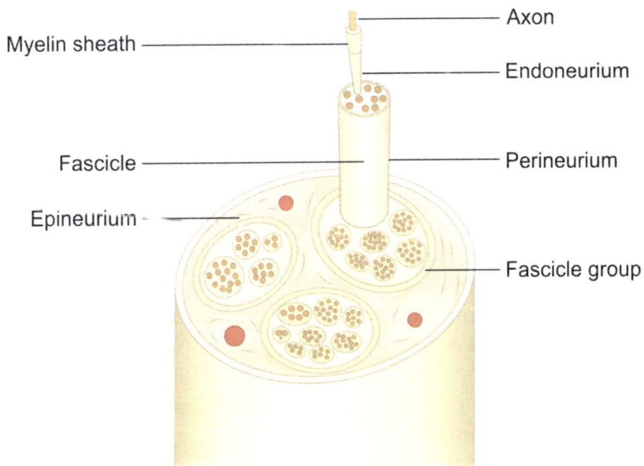

FIG. 1: Anatomy of nerve.

respectively. The spinal nerves divided into anterior (ventral) and posterior (dorsal) rami innervating muscles and the skin. These rami are hybrids containing sensory and motor fibers.

CURRENT IMAGING IN PERIPHERAL NERVOUS SYSTEM

Radiological imaging of PNS is very good in assessing the size, appearance, course, and continuity of nerves and also in evaluating surrounding soft tissue and bones. The indications of imaging of PNS include localization of the pathology, visualization of anatomical definition of a nerve, traumatic grading of the nerve injury, response to therapy, evaluation of radiation injury to a nerve or plexus, and evaluation of cases of chronic pain. Preprocedural imaging is also helpful for planning of image-guided intervention. Evaluation of PNS mainly depends on US and MRI.

Conventional Radiography

Conventional radiography has very limited role, may be useful to look for bony abnormalities.[6] It is initial screening technique to rule out any osseous or joint pathology.

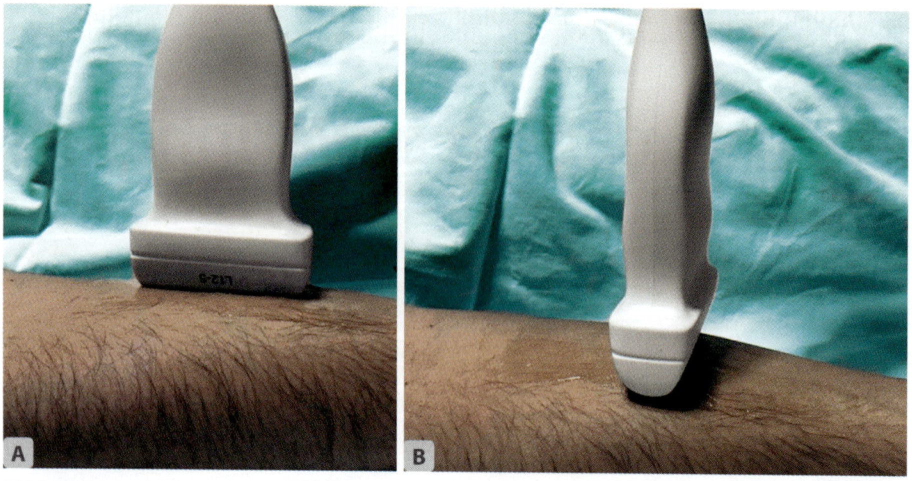

FIGS. 2A AND B: Ultrasound (US) technique is showing position of transducer in long (A) and short axis (B).

Computed Tomography

The role of computed tomography (CT) in imaging of PNS is often limited to assessment of bony structures. It is useful in diagnosis of nerve compression by osseous pathology[6] CT angiography can be sometimes useful in cases of nerve compression by vascular causes or aberrant vessel. The peripheral nerve tumors can be visible on CT imaging, however, it is inferior to MRI in characterization and origin of peripheral nerve masses.[7] The larger peripheral nerve such as sciatic nerve may be seen on CT, however, morphology of nerve and various pathologies cannot be assessed due to poor contrast resolution.[8]

Ultrasound

A recent advancement in high-resolution US has made increase use of US for initial assessment of peripheral nerve. Newer high end on US machine and higher frequency linear transducer enables better visualization of peripheral nerves.[9] The special resolution of US is comparable to MRI and scores over MRI due to ability of US to perform dynamic study, cost effective, and easy availability and less time consuming. However, there is long learning curve in accurate assessment of PNS to make accurate diagnosis.

Technique

High frequency linear transducer with 12–18 MHz is generally used to assess the peripheral nerves. The nerves are assessed by placing the transducer on skin surface in transverse and longitudinal sections **(Figs. 2A and B)**. Proper depth and focus are of utmost importance for optimal visualization of nerves. An extended field of view and panoramic view **(Fig. 3)** are helpful for entire nerve length visualization. Color Doppler study is useful for assessing the vascularity of nerve pathology. Normal nerve shows no or minimal vascularity on Doppler. Dynamic scanning is the most useful to identify the neuropathy due to instability. The advantages and limitation of US are mentioned in **Table 1**.

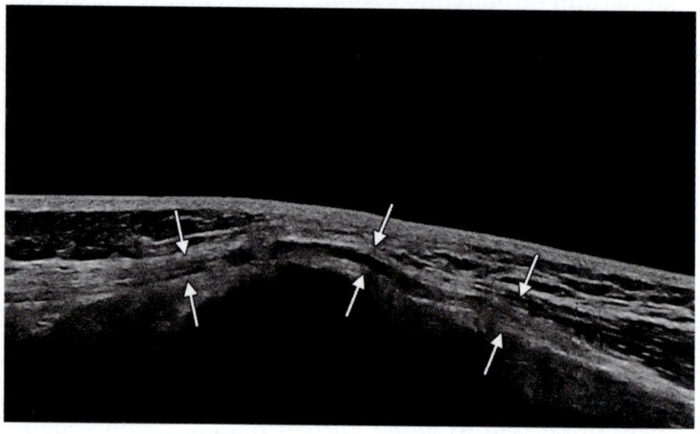

FIG. 3: Ultrasound (US) panoramic view shows extended length of ulnar nerve (arrows) in arm and forearm.

US Appearance

In transverse plane, nerve appears as round to oval with hypoechoic areas corresponding to fascicles separated by hyperechoic interfascicular perineum (honey-combing appearance). In longitudinal plane, it appears as bundles of hypoechoic linear areas with hyperechoic lines in between, corresponding to perineurium giving fibrillary appearance.[10] The epineurium is seen as thin hyperechoic layer surrounding in nerve **(Figs. 4A and B)**. On US, nerves show minimal anisotropy compared to tendons. US assessment of peripheral nerve includes size of nerve, echotexture, fascicular morphology, course and continuity of nerve, vascularity of nerve, and status of adjacent structures. Abnormal nerve may show diffuse or focal nerve enlargement, enlarged fascicles, loss of fascicular pattern, or increased vascularity on Doppler study **(Figs. 5A and B)**. Perineural soft tissue changes can also be assessed on US. In addition, US can identify changes in muscle such as muscle atrophy in denervation when compared to contralateral side.[11]

TABLE 1: Advantages and limitations of ultrasound (US) and magnetic resonance imaging (MRI).

Imaging	Advantages	Limitations
US	• Very good spatial resolution • Dynamic assessment • Low cost • Easily available • Nonionizing • US-guided procedures or biopsy • Quick	• Operator dependent • Long learning curve • Deeper structures cannot be evaluated • Poor resolution in obese patients • Bony lesion may not be seen
MRI	• Excellent contrast and spatial resolution • Three dimensional • Deeper structures can be evaluated • Less operator dependent • Evaluation of muscles • Bony lesions/marrow edema can be seen • Research potential	• Higher cost • Contraindications to MR (Pace maker, claustrophobia, MR incompatible implants) • Long duration time • Static examination

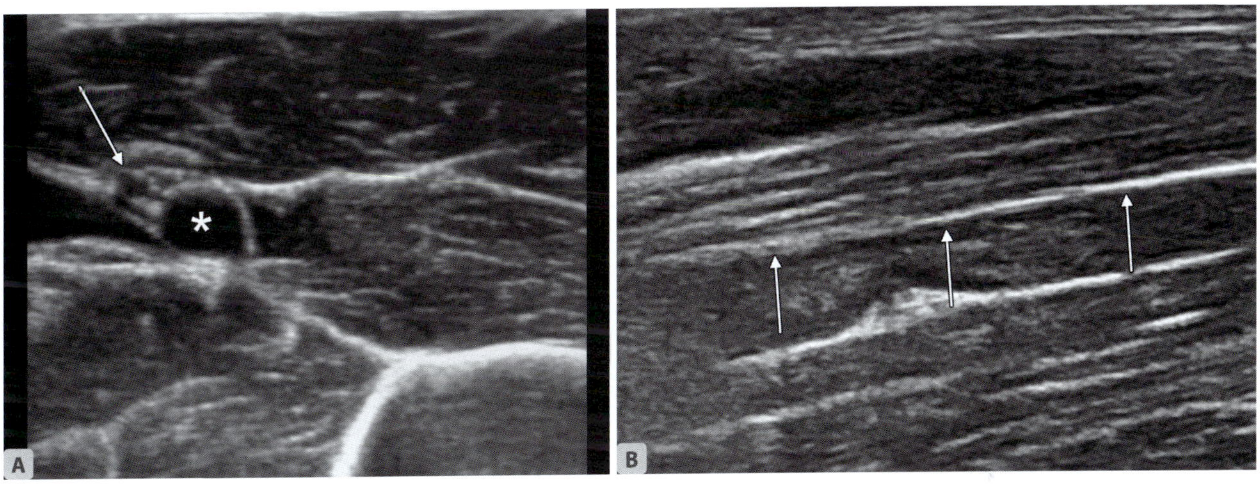

FIGS. 4A AND B: Ultrasound (US) appearance of normal nerve. (A) Short axis image showing honeycomb appearance of median nerve (arrow); (B) Long-axis image showing fascicular pattern of median nerve (arrows). Star (*) depicts brachial artery.

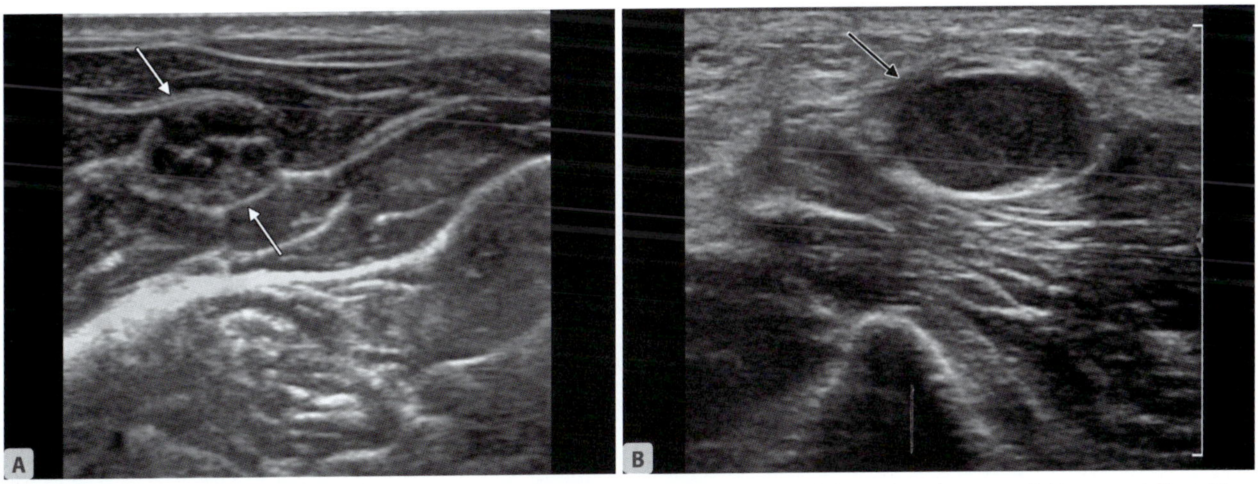

FIGS. 5A AND B: Abnormal US appearance of nerve. (A and B) The images show thickening with fascicular enlargement (white arrows) (A) and loss of fascicular pattern (black arrow) (B).

Magnetic Resonance Imaging

Magnetic resonance imaging is a noninvasive, radiation-free technique and useful in direct visualization of peripheral nerve trunk. Due to high special resolution of MRI, the fascicular patter can be identified. Perineural soft tissue and deeper structures can be easily evaluated on MRI. It is less operator dependent as compared to US. The advantages and limitation of MRI are mentioned in **Table 1**. The MR protocols for nerve imaging may be different at various institutes or organizations. The routine sequences for MR neurography at our institute are given here.

- T1W nonfat suppressed axial
- T2W fat-suppressed axial
- T2 W fat-suppressed coronal or sagittal (optional)
- T2 space (sampling perfection with application optimized contrast)
- 3D PSIF (reversed FISP, fast imaging with steady-state free precession)
- Diffusion-weighted imaging (DWI)/diffusion tensor imaging (DTI)
- Postcontrast T1W fat-saturated axial and coronal (on case basis in infection/inflammatory conditions or tumors).

The MR neurography is often done by using heavily T2-weighted acquisition with long echo times (>90 ms) and saturation bands to decrease signal from surrounding vascular structure.[12] The 3D diffusion-weighted PSIF (reversed FISP) sequence is also obtained using heavily T2-weighted MR technique with suppression of adjacent the vessel signal. Additionally, 3D sequences enable formation of multiplanar reconstruction (MPR) and maximum intensity projection (MIP) images **(Figs. 6A and B)**.

"Magic angle phenomenon," similar to tendons, can be seen in nerves, when their orientation is at around 55° angle to magnetic field in T2-weighted sequences with long TE.[13] The magic angle signal changes should be considered while reading MR images, especially when only abnormal nerve signal present and there are no associated changes.

Intravenous gadolinium can be useful to see enhancement when there is breach in blood brain barrier. It is especially helpful in infectious or inflammatory and neoplastic conditions of nerve. Normally, the nerve shows little or no contrast enhancement.[14]

Diffusion tensor imaging uses tissue anisotropy to produce images. The measurements caused by water molecules motion in anisotropic media is used to give information about architecture and orientation of tissues. The DWI can be useful in the evaluation of larger peripheral nerves compared to smaller nerves.[15,16] Tractography is the mathematical rendered technique derived from DTI used to obtain 3D images of fiber tracts and evaluation of the course and direction of nerve fibers **(Fig. 7)**.[17,18] It consists of mean apparent diffusion coefficient (ADC) and mean fractional anisotropy (FA). Fiber tracking acquisition uses a spin-echo single-shot diffusion-weighted EPI sequence with fat suppression. Color coding is given to the direction of anisotropic structures. Any disease or injury to the nerve fibers will change nerve architecture which can be depicted by this technique.[19,20] The tractography is currently useful for evaluation of large nerve bundles.

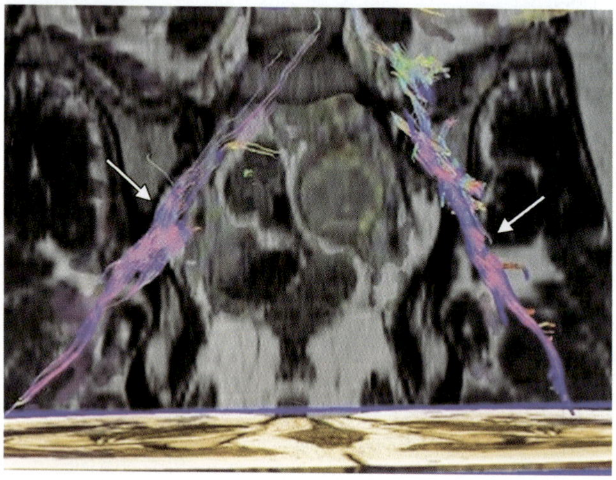

FIG. 7: Diffusion tensor imaging with tractography of bilateral sciatic nerves (arrows).

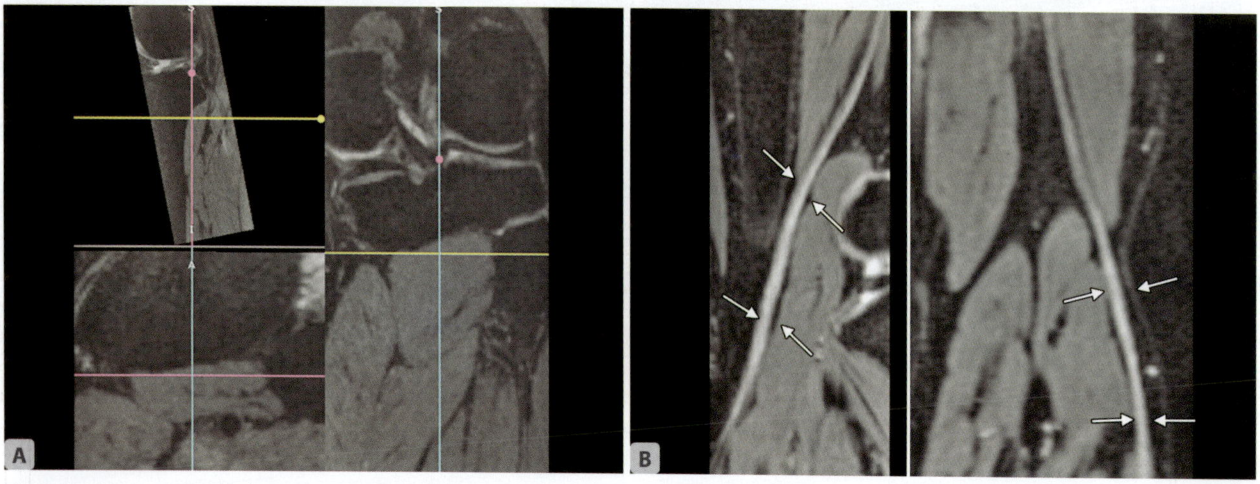

FIGS. 6A AND B: (A) Multiplanar reconstruction (MPR) technique; (B) Curved MPR images show better visualization of course of nerve (arrows).

The MR evaluation of peripheral nerves includes assessment of signal intensity of nerves, size of nerve, morphology or fascicular pattern, course and continuity of nerves, perineural fat and surrounding soft tissue, status of muscles, and tendons.[21] The appearance of nerve on magnetic resonance neurography is depicted in **Table 2.**[22]

Signal Intensity

On T1WI, normally nerves have intermediate signal intensity compared to muscles **(Fig. 8A)**. Nonfat-saturated T1 images are best to evaluate the nerve anatomy and course. On T2WI normal nerves show isointense signal intensity to that of muscle.[11] On fluid sensitive fat-suppressed sequences such as SPAIR, T2WIFS or STIR sequences peripheral nerves show as isointense or minimally hyperintense to that of muscle **(Fig. 8B)**. PSIF sequence suppressed the signal from adjacent vascular structures and nerve appears minimally hyperintense with clear demarcation **(Fig. 8C)**. Increased signal intensity on fluid-sensitive sequences which is similar to adjacent vessels suggests nerve pathology. Most of the nerve tumors appears hyperintense on fluid-sensitive sequences and hypo- to isointense T1 images.

Size and Fascicular Pattern of Peripheral Nerve

The neural injury/neuropathy is suggested by presence of enlargement or thinning of nerve, enlarged single or multiple fascicles, loss of the normal fascicular appearance, or ill-defined perifascicular fat. The anatomic changes can be easily picked up on MR in large nerve such as sciatic, median, or ulnar nerve. Fascicular pattern of larger nerve are often visible on axial nonfat-saturated T1- and T2-weighted images.

Course and Continuity

Normal peripheral nerves have regular course without any lump or bumps. Branches of peripheral nerve normally directed to supplying muscles. The peripheral nerves have well-defined margins surrounding by perineural fat which can easily identified on nonfat saturated T1- and T2-weighted images. Normal variant in course of peripheral nerve sometime can be seen in form of bifid nerve.[23] The abnormal nerve may have deviated course or discontinuous which can be seen on MR neurography. However, one should be careful for interpreting MR artifacts such as metallic artifacts as nerve pathology.

Perineural Fat

There is layer of fat surrounding the nerve trunk, which can be easily seen in T1- or T2-weighted images. At times it may be difficult to recognize perineural fat in poorly build individuals. Increased signal intensity of perineural fat is often seen on fluid-sensitive sequences like STIR images in cases of inflammatory pathologies.

Muscles

In acute setting, muscle denervation is best depicted by the STIR or T2 fat-suppressed sequences which occur due to muscle edema.[24] There are minimal changes in T1-weighted images in acute setting. The early stages there is increase in extracellular fluid within the muscles which show increase signal intensity. However, muscle bulk is not affected in early stages. Nerve injury leads to denervation of the muscles supplied by the nerve. Identification of denervated muscles helps to recognize the peripheral nerve involved and also helps to differentiate between other muscle pathologies such as myositis, muscle infections, or infarcts.

In chronic denervation, there is muscle atrophy and fatty replacement of muscles. This leads to increased T1-signal intensity on nonfat-saturated images. There is also increased signal intensity on T2-weighted images and STIR images. Reduced muscle bulk can be identified easily if comparison is made to contralateral side.

Specific Peripheral Nerve Pathologies

Nerve Injury

Peripheral nerve injury occurs due to trauma, various mechanisms of traction, shear stress and ischemia, in isolation or combination.[19] The various imaging features

TABLE 2: Normal and abnormal appearance of nerve on magnetic resonance neurography.[22]

Features	Normal nerve	Abnormal nerve
Size of nerve	Similar to adjacent arteries, gradually decreases distally	Focal or diffuse enlargement, larger than adjacent arteries
Signal intensity	Isointense to skeletal muscle on T1- and T2-weighted imaging; isointense to minimally hyperintense on STIR and fat-suppressed T2-weighted imaging	Hyperintense on T2-weighted imaging similar to adjacent veins
Fascicular morphology	Seen on T1- and T2-weighted imaging	Enlargement or disruption of single or multiple fascicles
Course	Smooth without focal deviations, outlined by perineural fat	Focal or diffuse deviations, discontinuity
Continuity	Maintained	Discontinuous or complete transaction
Postcontrast	Absent except in areas of deficient blood-nerve barrier, such as dorsal nerve root ganglion	Present in tumors and infections because of disruption of blood-nerve barrier
Perineural fat	Preserved best seen on T1 non-FS	Effaced

(FS: fat saturated)

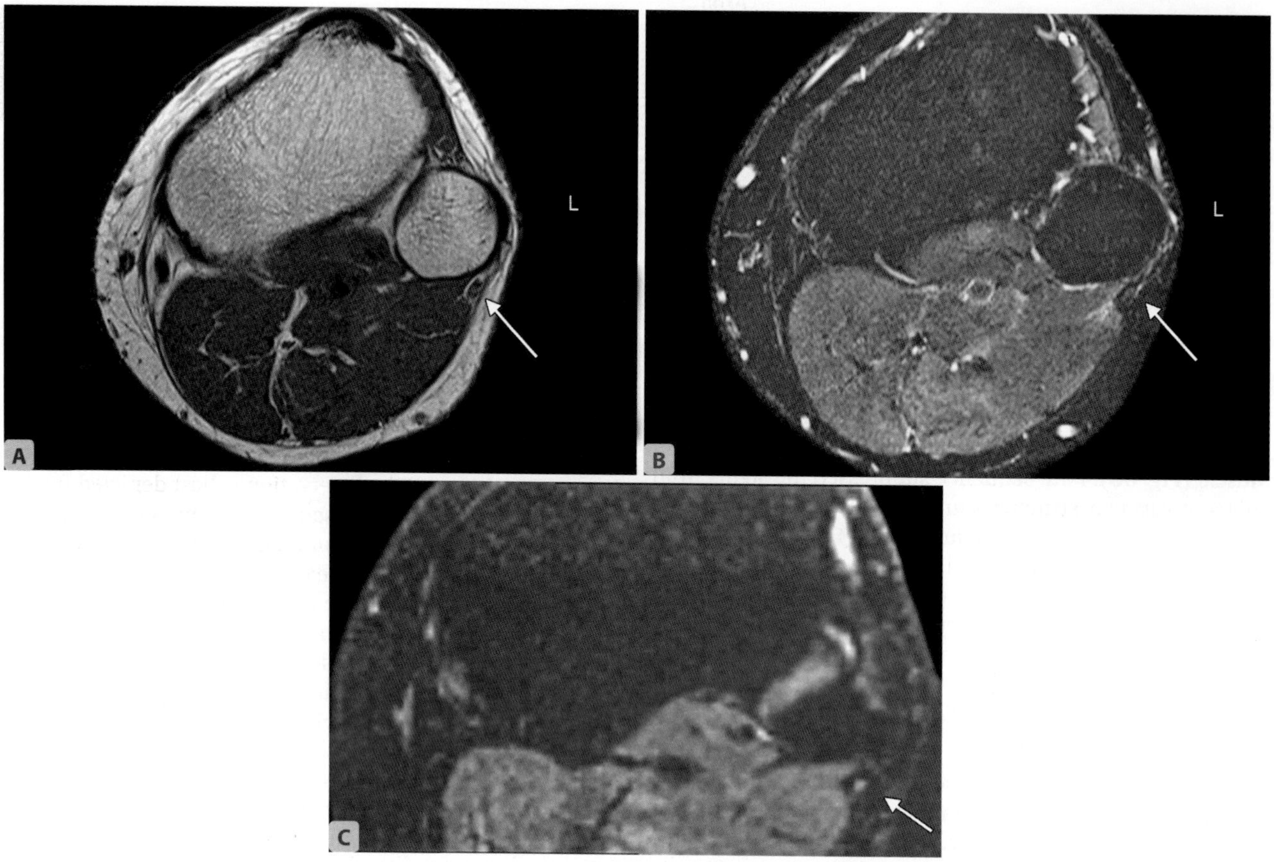

FIGS. 8A TO C: Normal MR appearance of nerve. (A and B) Nonfat-suppressed T1 weighted image and fat-suppressed T2-weighted image showing common peroneal nerve (arrows) at the level of fibular neck. Note the hyperintense perineural fat on T1WI; (C) PSIF sequence shows minimally hyperintense normal nerve with clear demarcation (arrow).

depend on congestion of nerve, edema, fibrosis, and axonal damage.

Wallerian degeneration is response to nerve injury distal to site of nerve injury by the axon, Schwann cell, and macrophages. It starts immediately within few minutes after the nerve injury. Initially there is degeneration of axon with increase in immune and inflammatory response distal to site of injury followed by the regrowth of axon stump toward distal stump. If regeneration of nerve may take months to years, if regeneration does not happen, the injury segment is replaced by fibrous tissue. There is focal swelling of axon stump known as neuroma.[25] The classification of nerve injury was given by Seddon, who categorized nerve injuries into three grades, from least to most severe, as neurapraxia, axonotmesis, and neurotmesis **(Fig. 9, Table 3)**.[19,26,27] The neuropraxia refers to the transient nerve conduction block causing transient sensory and motor loss followed by full rapid and complete recovery. Axonotmesis referred to damage to axon but intact epineurium. In neurotmesis there is complete transaction or discontinuity of nerve. The Sunderland classification **(Table 3)** is currently used by most of the surgeons. It has five grades and these grades are similar to Seddon classification of increasing severity of nerve injury. Dellon and MacKinnon described the sixth grade that includes incomplete or mixed nerve damages.[28] In incomplete damage, a part of the nerve fibers (circumference) is damaged while the rest of the fibers are intact. In mixed nerve damages, all tissues of the nerve are involved. The recovery of nerve injury depends on type of damage and severity of every nerve fiber.

In neurapraxic injury, the nerve may appear as swollen with hypoechoic appearance on US **(Fig. 10)** and hyperintense on T2 fat-suppressed and PSIF sequences **(Figs. 11A and B)**. In axotomies, the nerve appears swollen and hypoechoic with enlarged fascicles on US and MR with more marked findings than neuropraxic injury. Neuroma-in-continuity is seen as fusiform hypoechoic thickened nerve with decreased nerve echotexture on US **(Fig. 12)** and fusiform thickened hyperintense nerve on MRI **(Figs. 13A and B)**.[26] The complete disruption of nerve fibers can be identified on US in cases of transaction injury due to glass and sharp objects, etc. A neuroma formation can be seen at both ends of transacted nerve which appear as hypoechoic thickening or a bulbous mass at nerve ends **(Figs. 14 and 15)**. High resolution US or MR neurography, both can depict the nerve injury. The various features of imaging are given in **Table 3**.

Nerve Compression

Nerve compression can occur due to kinetic and static causes. Kinetic compression often arises during motion or mobility of

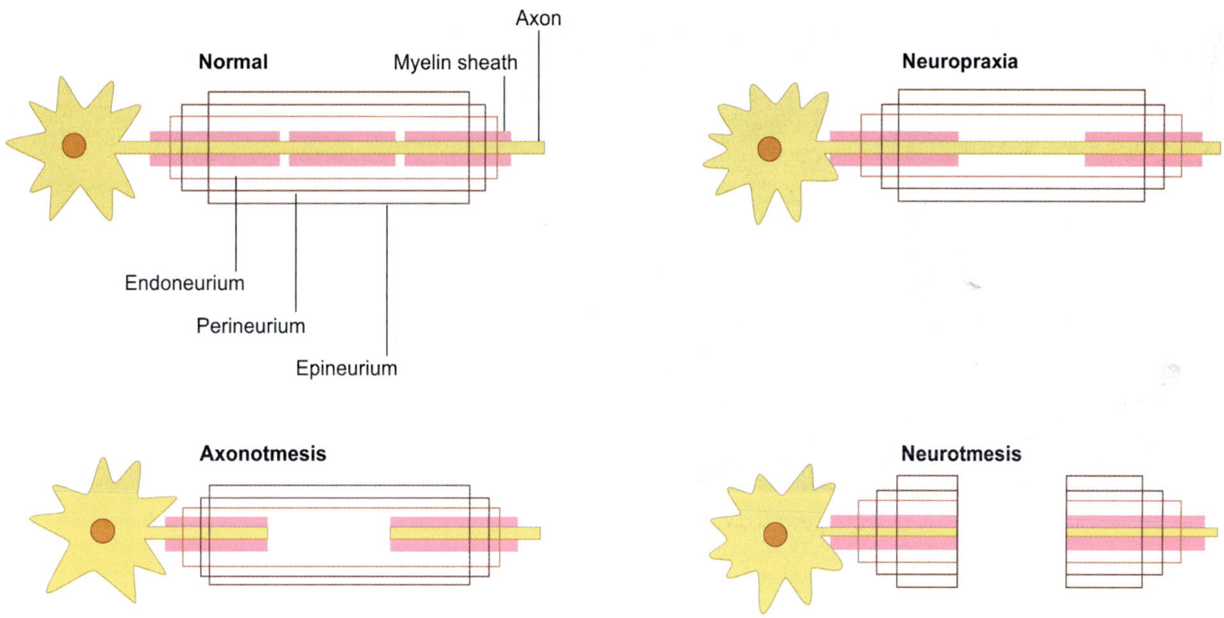

FIG. 9: Grading of nerve injury.

TABLE 3: Seddon and Sunderland classifications of peripheral nerve injury with the magnetic resonance (MR) and ultrasound (US) features.[26,27]

Sunderland (grade)	Seddon	Nerve injury	MR features	US features
I	Neuropraxia	Focal demyelination	Nerve: Hyperintense ± increased caliber	Nerve: Hypoechoic ± increased caliber
II	Axonotmesis	Axon	Nerve: Hyperintense ± increased caliber. Expanded fascicles Denervation changes in muscles	Nerve: Hypoechoic ± increased caliber Expanded fascicles
III	Axonotmesis	Axon endoneurium	Nerve: Hyperintense ± increased caliber. Expanded fascicles (More marked than grade II) Denervation changes in muscles	Nerve: Focal hypoechogenicity with increase in caliber with muscle: Altered echogenicity of the denervated muscles
IV	Axonotmesis	Axon endoneurium perineurium	Nerve: Neuroma at ends with discontinuous fascicles Denervation changes in muscles	Nerve: Hypoechoic neuroma in continuity with the nerve with loss of fascicular pattern Muscle: Altered echogenicity of the denervated muscles
V	Neurotmesis	Complete nerve transection	Nerve: End bulb neuroma with separation Denervation changes in muscles	Nerve : Hypoechoic neuroma at end with surrounding heterogenicity Muscle: Altered echogenicity of the denervated muscles
VI	Neurotmesis	Mixed level of injury	Combination of above findings Fibrosis with sudden signal changes of the nerves.	Nerve: Hypoechoic enlarged with mixed findings of fibrosis, discontinuity or neuroma formation

joints. Static causes include compression of nerve by adjacent tissue, which may be pathological such as infections, tumor, bony fragment, or aberrant/anomalous in nature.[4] Commonly, the compression occur at specific locations where the nerves passes through the anatomic space or tunnels such as cubital and carpal tunnels **(Figs. 16 to 18)**, or in an unspecified location where a space occupying lesion can cause compression of the nerve **(Figs. 19 and 20)**. Mostly, the sensory component is arranged in periphery compared to the motor component in the mixed nerves. Therefore, nerve compression is more likely to have early sensory signs. Presently, the peripheral nerve compression is commonly graded based on symptoms, clinical examination results, and electrodiagnostic findings. The various tunnels and known

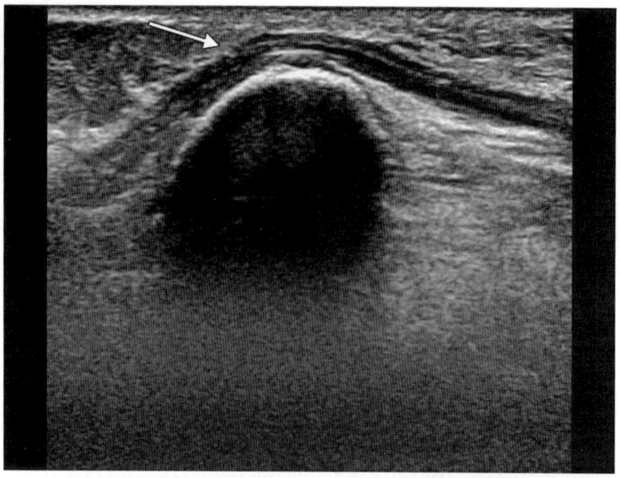

FIG. 10: High-resolution ultrasound (US) of ulnar nerve shows hypoechoic appearance of nerve (arrow) in stretch injury (neuropraxia).

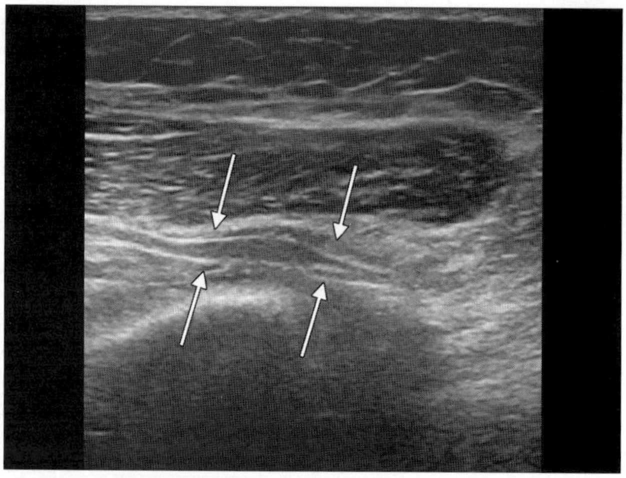

FIG. 12: High-resolution ultrasound (US) in post-traumatic case shows ulnar nerve injury with neuroma in continuity of nerve (arrows).

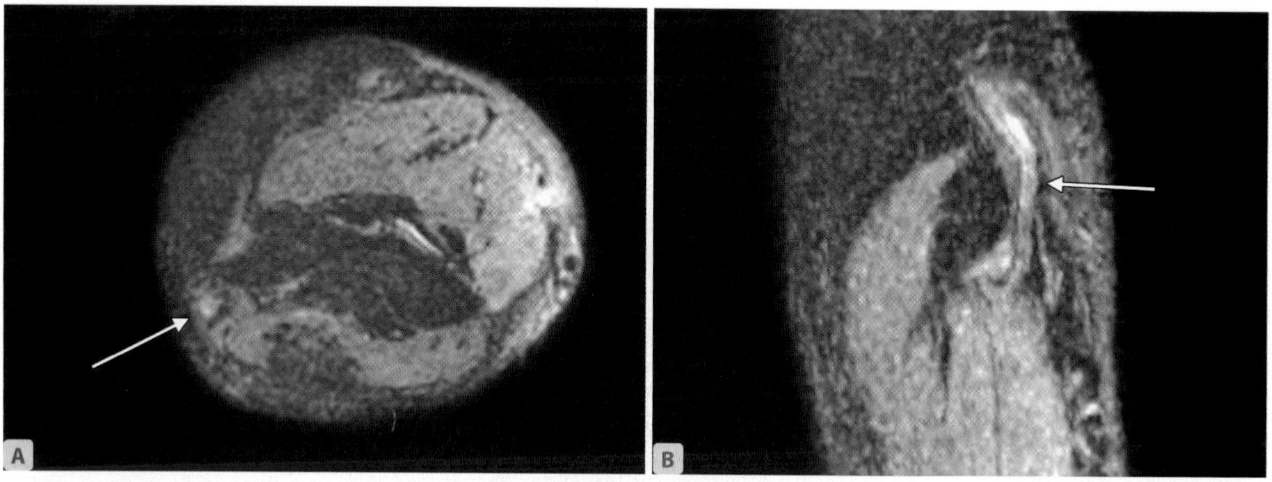

FIGS. 11A AND B: Neuropraxia of ulnar nerve. 3D PSIF axial (A) and sagittal (B) reconstruction shows patchy hyperintensities in ulnar nerve without disruption (arrows).

entrapment sites along the course of the commonly imaged peripheral nerves are described in **Table 4**.[29]

The compression of nerve can be detected on careful examination with high resolution US. Various US features of compression include thinning of nerve or reduction in diameter or cross sectional area, enlargement of nerve proximal or distal to compression site.[9] The nerve cross-sectional area can be calculated on US. In larger-sized nerves such as sciatic, median, ulnar nerves or common peroneal nerve, loss of fascicular morphology can be seen. For smaller nerve, careful examinations with higher frequency transducer (17–24 MHz) are very useful in assessment of morphology of nerve.

Nerve Infections

Mycobacterium leprae is the causative organism of a chronic disease "leprosy," which is common cause of curable peripheral neuropathy. The ulnar nerve is often involved in leprosy. Other nerves such as median, posterior auricular, fibular, and posterior tibial nerves are also involved. The disease process causes enlargement of nerve which can be detected on imaging US or MRI.[30] Subacute phase may show calcifications of nerve in leprosy. On US, the abnormal nerve appears as hypoechoic enlarged nerve with enlarged fascicles **(Figs. 21A and B)**, loss of fascicular pattern, or asymmetry of fascicles **(Figs. 22 and 23)**.[31,32] Color Doppler can be helpful which may show increased vascularity in lepromatous nerve **(Figs. 22A and B)**. Sometimes, infection of nerve results in abscess formation which appears as homogeneous fusiform collection hyperintense T2 and hypointense on T1 images. DWIs may show central diffusion restriction **(Figs. 24A to C)**. US shows hypoechoic collection along the course of nerve in cases of nerve abscess. Pyogenic infections of nerve are often direct extension of infection from adjacent tissue **(Fig. 25)**.

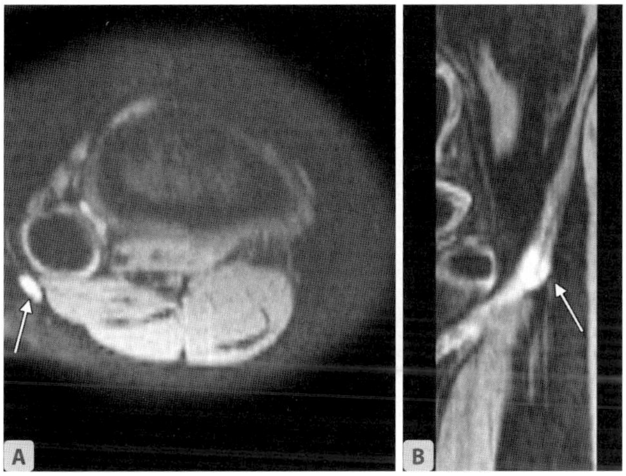

FIGS. 13A AND B: Neuroma in continuity. 3D PISF axial (A) and coronal reformatted (B) MR neurography images show focal fusiform thickening (arrows) of common peroneal nerve near fibular head with continuation of nerve fibers.

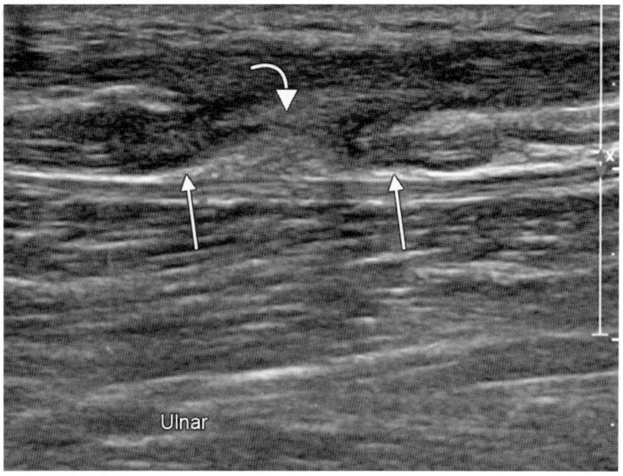

FIG. 14: High-resolution ultrasound (US) in post-traumatic case show complete transaction of ulnar nerve (curved arrow) in forearm with end nerve neuroma formation at both ends (white straight arrows).

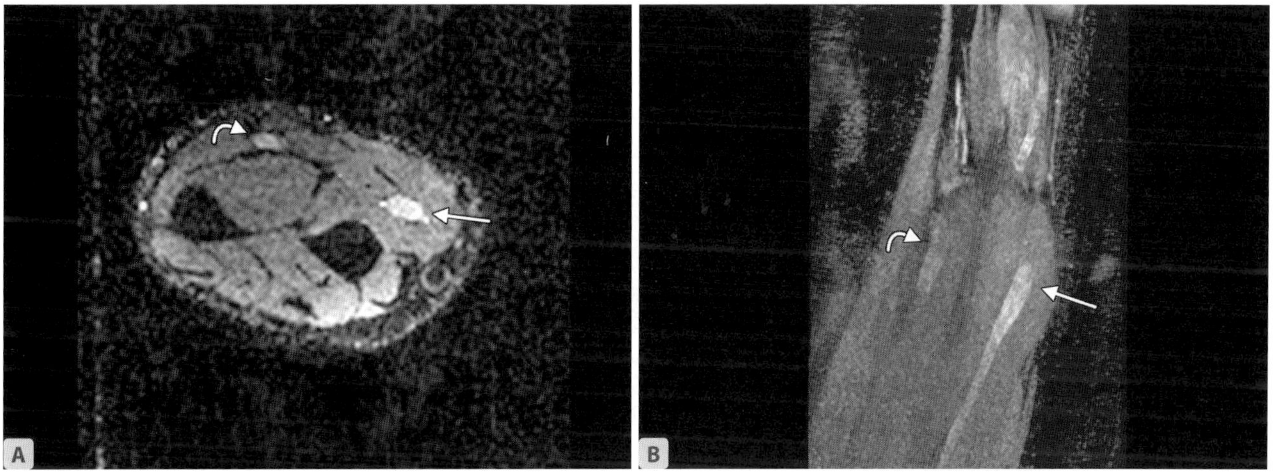

FIGS. 15A AND B: Cut injury at the level of forearm. 3D PSIF axial (A) and coronal reconstructed neurography images (B) show complete transaction of median (straight arrows) and ulnar nerve (curved arrows) with end neuroma formation.

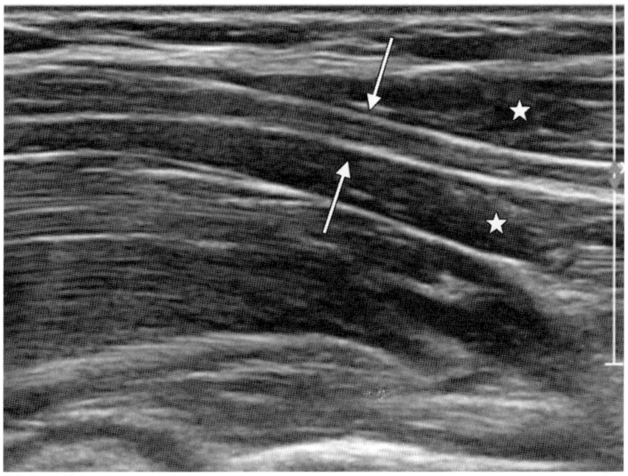

FIG. 16: High-resolution ultrasound (US) (long axis) showing compression of median nerve (white arrows) between two heads of pronator teres (stars).

Nerve Tumors and Tumor-like Conditions

Peripheral nerve sheath tumor (PNST) is the most commonly seen tumor of peripheral nerve. If regional muscle denervation changes are seen in the adjacent or distal to the tumor, one should look for the PNST. Also the large mass tends to impinge the nerve may lead to muscle denervation changes. The nerve tumor is suggested by the "tail sign" (where the mass tapers at one end) or "fusiform-shaped" tumor (where the mass tapers at both ends), "fascicular sign" (enlarged nerve fibers seen in cross-section as multiple small ring-like shapes), target sign (central low signal due to collagenous tissue with peripheral myxoid change on a fluid-sensitive sequence), and "split-fat sign" (fat separating the tumor from adjacent muscles, best seen at tapering margins of the tumor showing its slow growth consequently leading to displacement of the perineural fat planes) **(Figs. 26A to C)**.[25] These lesions show diffuse homogeneous enhancement.[33] Different features of common PNSTs are depicted in **Table 5**.[34]

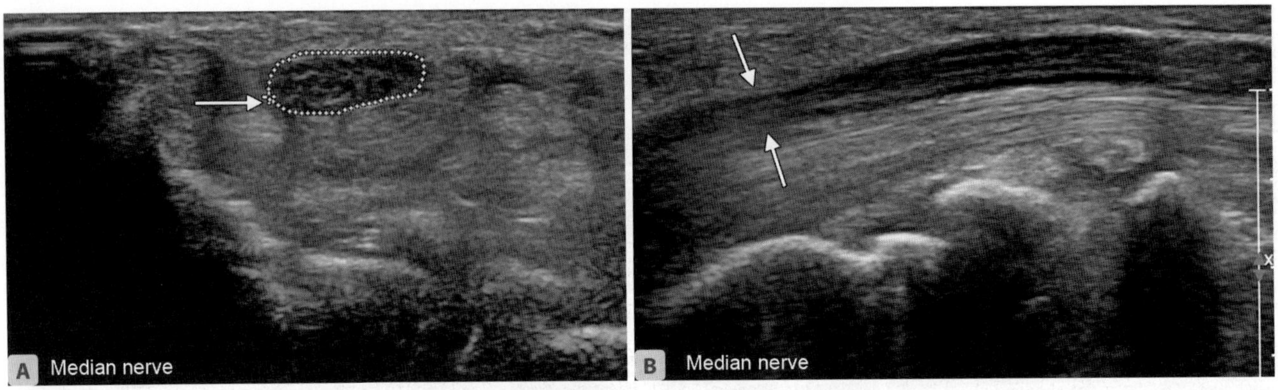

FIGS. 17A AND B: Carpal tunnel syndrome. High-resolution ultrasound (US), short axis (A) and long axis (B) shows increased cross sectional area of median nerve (arrow in A) with typical compression at flexor retinaculum (arrows in B).

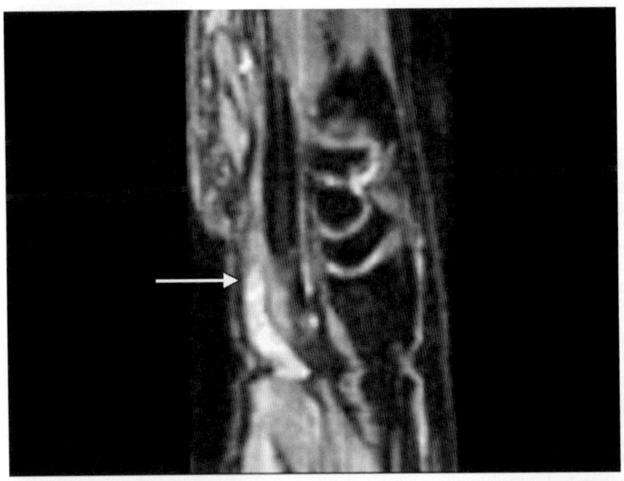

FIG. 18: Sagittal reformatted 3D PSIF images of wrist show focal enlargement and hyperintensity of median nerve (arrow) in carpal tunnel syndrome.

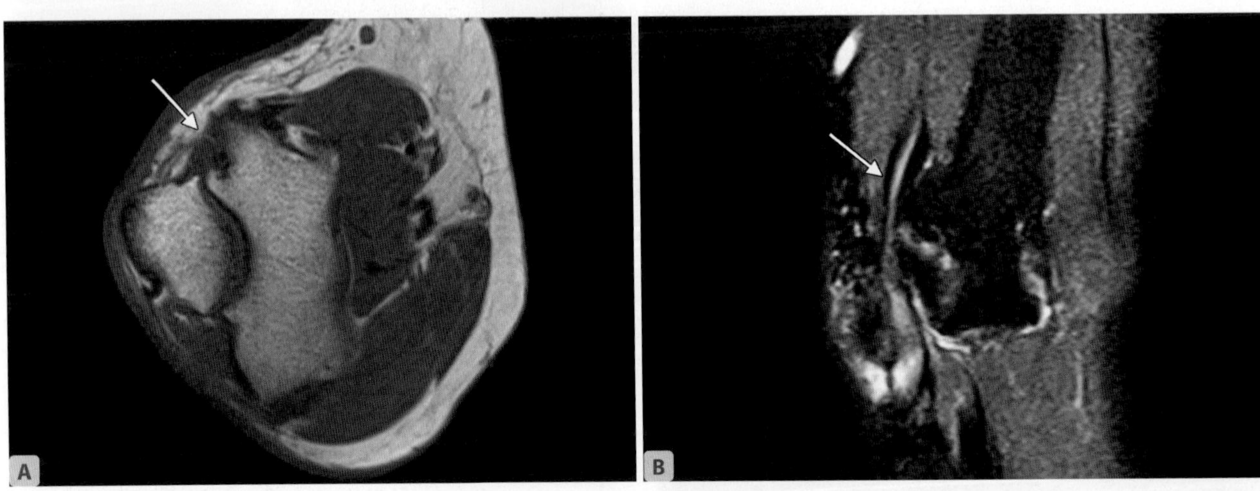

FIGS. 19A AND B: Compression of ulnar nerve at cubital fossa. Axial nonfat-suppressed T1-weighted image (A) and oblique fat-suppressed T2-weighted image (B) showing compression of ulnar nerve (arrows) by osteophytes and fibrotic tissue due to old injury of elbow.

The ultrasound appearance of peripheral nerve masses are seen as hypoechoic fusiform soft tissue lesion along the course of nerve. The entry or exit of nerve may be seen on careful US examination. The most of the tumors of PNS are generally benign. Heterogeneous appearance of tumor on US may be due to internal hemorrhages or cystic changes.

Schwannoma is more prevalent than neurofibroma, and often shows cystic changes, calcification, and internal hemorrhage **(Figs. 27 and 28)**. Slow growth, stability on follow-up, or underlying history and genetics are useful indicators of benign diagnosis.

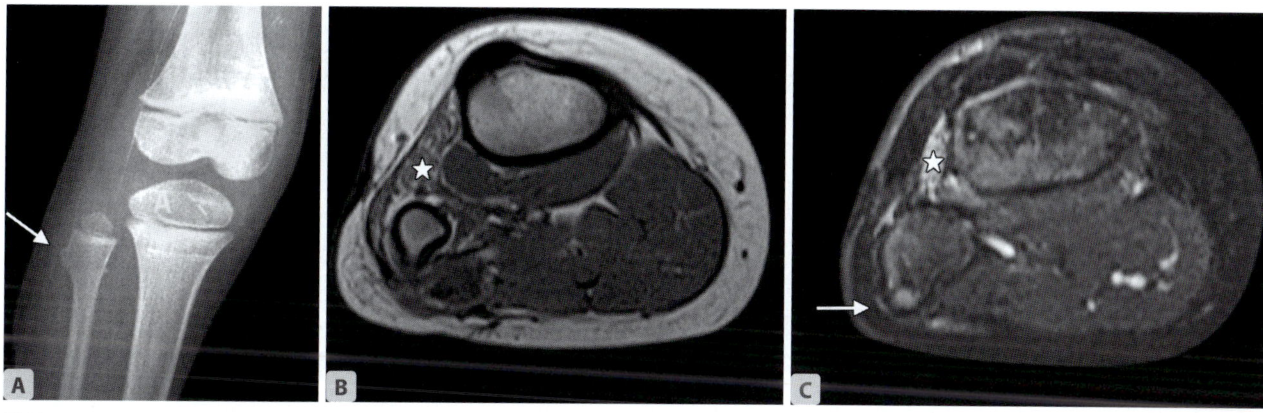

FIGS. 20A TO C: Nerve compression due to osteochondroma. AP radiograph of knee (A), axial T1 nonfat-suppressed image (B) and axial T2 fat-suppressed image (C) showing compression of common peroneal nerve (white arrow) by fibular osteochondroma (black arrow) with denervation changes (atrophy, increased T1 signal and fatty infiltration) in extensors muscles (stars).

TABLE 4: Various sites of compression of peripheral nerves.[29]

Nerve	Sites	Remarks
Ulnar nerve	• The arcade of Struthers • Medial epicondyle at the entry the cubital fossa • Within the cubital fossa • Proximal forearm at pronator teres • Guyon canal	The arcade of Struthers, a fibrous space posteriorly made up of intermuscular septum, the internal brachial ligament, deep fascia
Median nerve	• Distal arm by Struthers ligament • At elbow by biceps aponeurosis • At Elbow between two heads of the pronator teres. • Proximal forearm by flexor digitorum superficialis muscle • Carpal tunnel by retinaculum	Struthers ligament is a fibrous residue, between anteromedial distal humerus to medial epicondyle in 2.7 % individuals The most common nerve entrapment is carpal tunnel syndrome
Radial nerve	• At radial head between the brachioradialis and joint capsule • At radial neck by the leash of Henry, branches of the radial recurrent artery • Margin of the extensor carpi radialis brevis muscle • The arcade of Frohse • At wrist (Wartenberg syndrome)	The arcade of Frohse is a thick tendinous proximal margin of the superficial head of the supinator Wartenberg syndrome or cheiralgia paresthetica, is entrapment of the superficial branch of the radial nerve in the distal forearm or wrist
Femoral nerve	At the level of the inguinal ligament • The iliacus compartment • At Groin in hernia repair, femoral puncture, gynecological and hip surgeries	Iliacus compartment, a space between the ilio-psoas and iliacus fascia
Sciatic nerve	• Greater sciatic notch (piriformis muscle syndrome) • At the level of the ischial tuberosity by the biceps femoris	The sciatic nerve at greater sciatic notch may compressed by the pyriformis muscle or its pathology, known as piriformis syndrome
Common peroneal nerve	• Fibular neck. • Proximal attachment of peroneus longus	Extrinsic compression, stretching or trauma can cause nerve injury at these sites
Posterior tibial nerve	Tarsal tunnel (Tarsal tunnel syndrome)	Tarsal tunnel syndrome caused by trauma (fracture, surgery, and scarring), adjacent tissue pathologies (tumor, ganglia, varicosities), anomalous muscles and foot deformities
Interdigital nerve	Intermetatarsal space (Morton neuroma)	The entrapment of the nerve against the transverse metatarsal ligament or nerve ischemia causes formation of neuroma

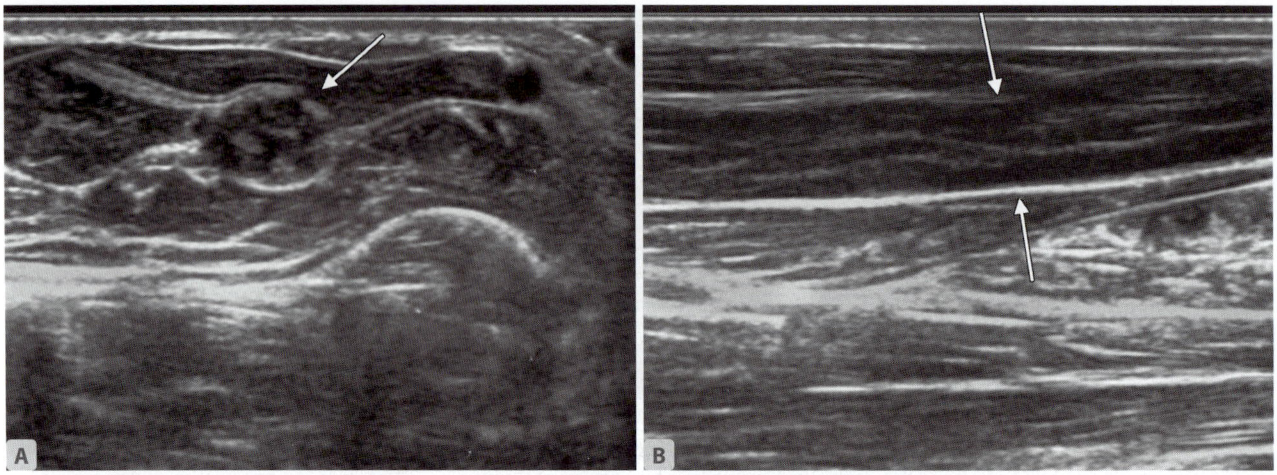

FIGS. 21A AND B: Leprotic neuropathy of ulnar nerve. High-resolution ultrasound (US) short axis (A) and long axis (B) shows diffuse enlarged ulnar nerve with symmetric enlargement of fascicles (white arrows).

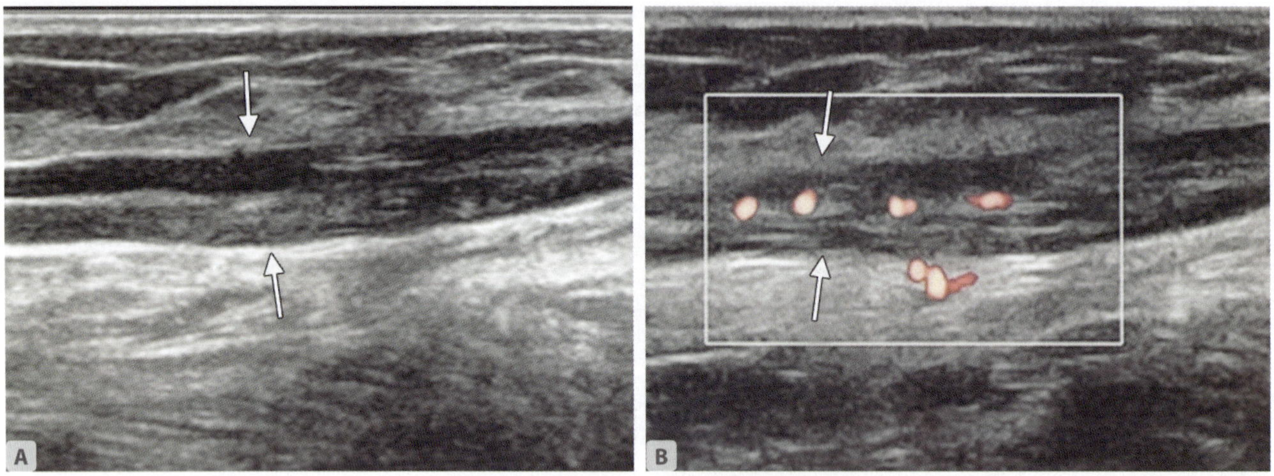

FIGS. 22A AND B: Asymmetric fascicular pattern. High-resolution ultrasound (US) long axis, gray scale (A) and color Doppler (B) images showing enlarged thickened ulnar nerve with asymmetric fascicles (arrows in A) with increased color flow (arrows in B) in leprotic neuropathy.

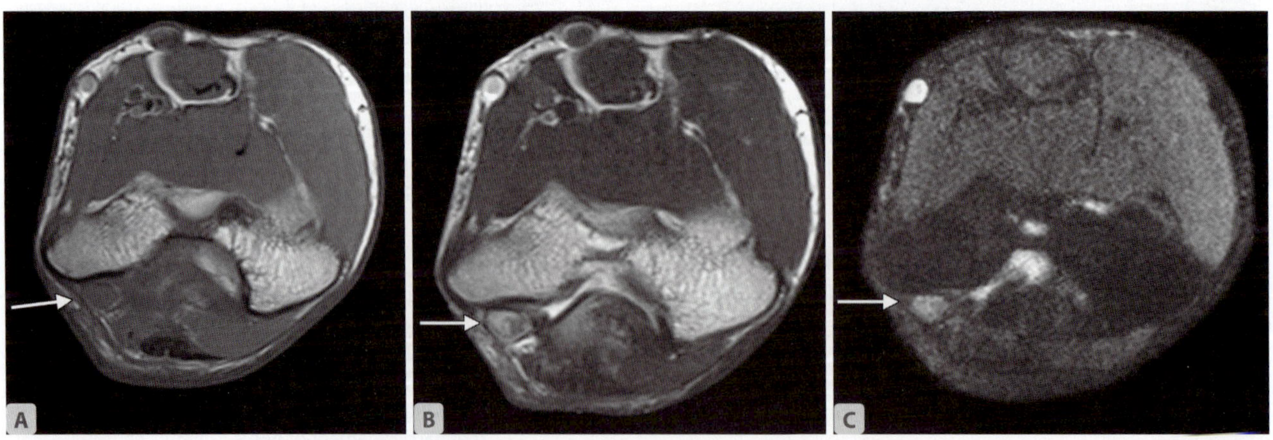

FIGS. 23A TO C: MRI of leprotic nerve. Axial T1 nonfat suppressed (A), T2 nonfat-suppressed (B) and T2 fat-suppressed (C) images showing enlarged and thickened ulnar nerve with asymmetric fascicles (arrows) in leprotic neuropathy.

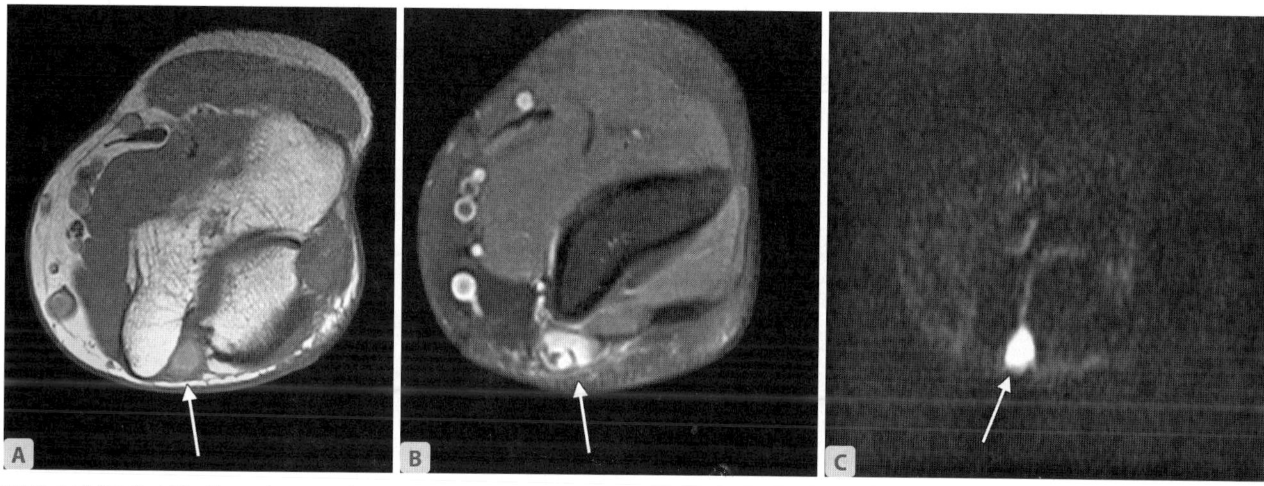

FIGS. 24A TO C: MRI of leprotic nerve abscess. (A and B) Axial T1 nonfat-suppressed and PD fat-suppressed images at elbow level showing T1 hypointense and PD hyperintense lesion in ulnar nerve (arrows); (C) DWI shows diffusion restriction within the abscess (arrow).

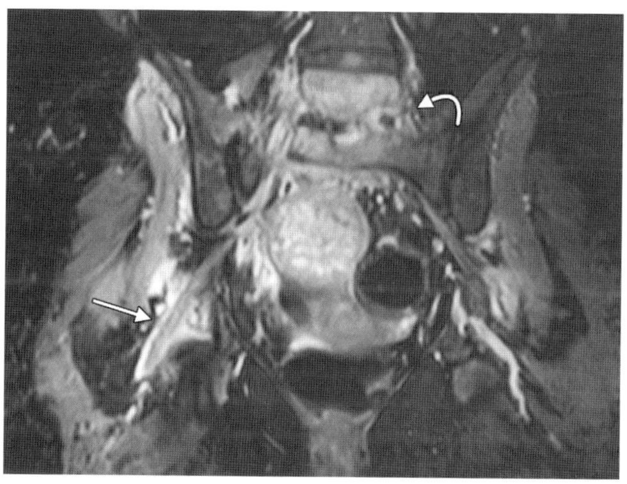

FIG. 25: Pyogenic infective neuritis: T2 fat-suppressed coronal MR image shows hyperintensity of sciatic nerve (straight arrow) with surrounding inflammation in case of pyogenic discitis (curved arrow) and pyogenic collections. Sciatic nerve was secondarily involved.

Plexiform neurofibroma shows diffuse infiltrative mass lesion and/or associated skin thickening. Plexiform neurofibroma or schwannoma may additionally show "bag of worms" appearance.[35] Schwannomatosis is characterized by numerous schwannomas without bilateral acoustic neuromas. It is a distinct entity from NF type II which shows acoustic neuromas and exhibits different genetic aberrations.

Malignant PNST can occur in a sporadic fashion (older age and less aggressive) or as part of NF type I (earlier age, increased incidence, and more aggressive). The imaging features which suggest malignant lesion includes large size (>5 cm), heterogeneous appearance, internal hemorrhage and/or necrosis, local tissue invasion or extracompartmental extension, surrounding edema, heterogeneous enhancement **(Fig. 29)**, and low ADC values on DTI (<1.1 mm^2/s) with disrupted and disorganized tracts on tractography.[36]

In lymphoma, there is diffuse infiltration of nerve with nodularity **(Fig. 30)**. The postcontrast MR shows homogeneous contrast enhancement. Diagnosis is often made on nerve biopsy.

Fibrolipomatous hamartomas of nerves is a rare tumor-like condition, characterized by fatty deposition within nerve sheaths. The median nerve is the most commonly affected. Macrodactyly is seen into 30–35% of the cases with involvement of median nerve. On MR neurography, there is prominent serpentiform fascicles bounded by fibrous and fatty tissue within the expanded nerve sheath **(Figs. 31A and B)**.[37,38]

Interdigital neuroma or Morton's neuroma may present with chronic foot pain due to vascular compromised or entrapment of the digital nerve in web spaces of foot against the transverse intermetatarsal ligament (commonly 3rd web space).[39] On US, it appears as hypoechoic ill-defined soft tissue lesion in web space. It may show internal vascularity on Doppler. On MR neurography, it shows hypointense to intermediate signal on T1-weighted images and hypointense on T2-weighted images **(Figs. 32A and B)**. T2 hypointensity can be used to differentiate Morton's neuroma from other lesions of web spaces like bursitis or Schwannoma. On postcontrast MR images, it often shows variable contrast enhancement.[40]

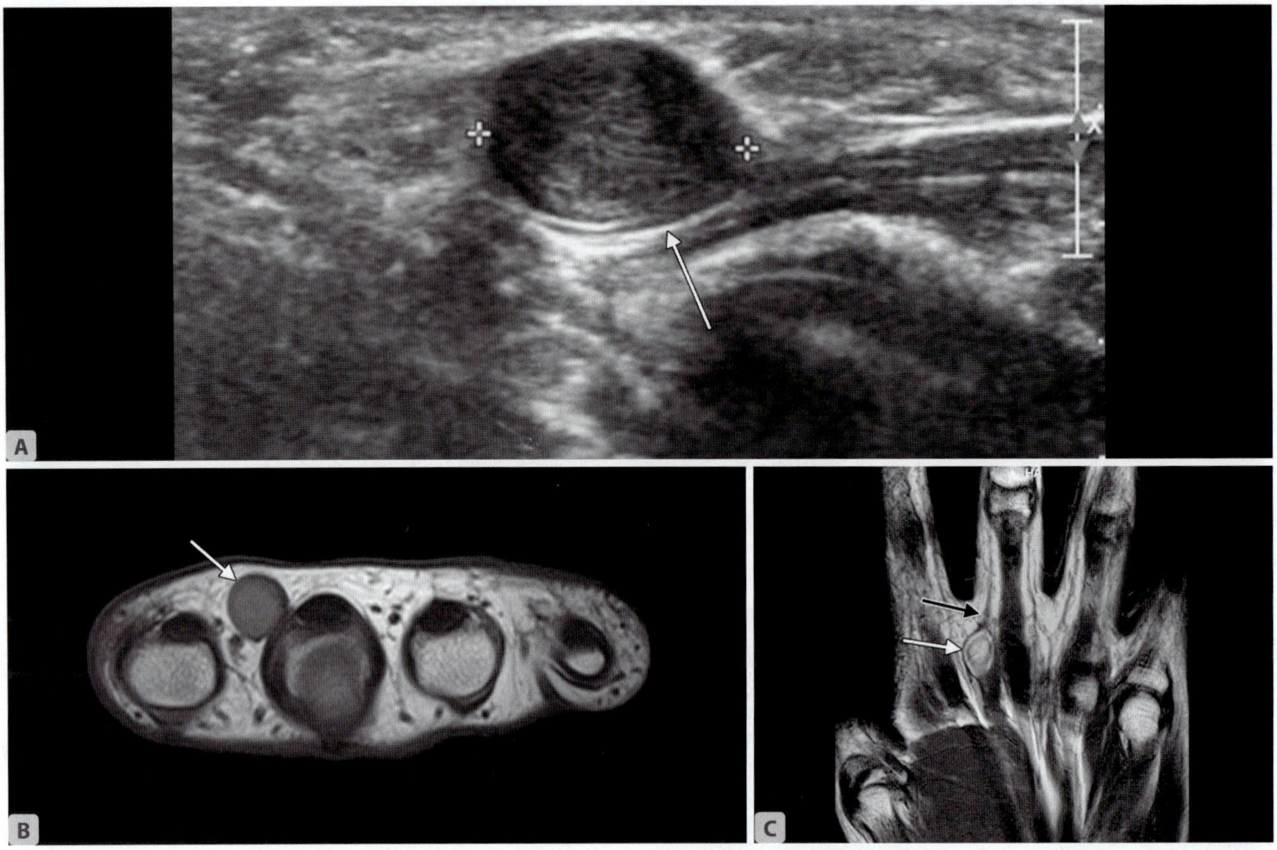

FIGS. 26A TO C: Schwannoma of digital nerve. High-resolution US in long axis (A) show well-defined fusiform hypoechoic lesion along the course of digital nerve. MRI of same patient: Axial T1 nonfat-suppressed (B) and coronal T2 nonfat-saturated section (C) showing well-defined T1 hypointense and T2 hyperintense "fusiform" lesion with "target sign" (white arrow) and "tail sign" (black arrow) along the course of digital nerve of hand.

TABLE 5: Imaging characteristics of common nerve tumors.[34]

Imaging features	Neurofibroma	Schwannoma	MPNST
Location	Central	Eccentric	Central
Target sign	+++	+	-
Fascicular sign	+++	+++	+/-
Split fat sign	+++	+++	-
T2 hyperintense thin rim	+	++	-
Cystic degeneration	+/-	++	+/-
Surrounding fat strandings	-	-/+	++
Hemorrhage	-	++	+++
Enhancement	Central and homogeneous	Peripheral, may be heterogeneous	Heterogeneous, with areas of necrosis
Adjacent tissue invasion	-	-	++

(MPNST: malignant peripheral nerve sheath tumor)

Systemic Etiologies of Neuropathy

Multiple systemic disease can cause neuropathy such as Guillain-Barré syndrome (GBS), chronic inflammatory demyelinating neuropathy (CIDP), multifocal motor neuropathy (MMN), Hirayama disease, drug-induced neuropathy, metal toxicity, hereditary neuropathy (Charcot-Marie-Tooth disease), vasculitis, diabetes mellitus, thyroid disease, deposition disease (amyloidosis), neurocutaneous syndromes, hyperlipidemia, etc. Clinical examinations with electrophysiologic studies are helpful for the diagnosis of these disorders.[41] Imaging is useful for exclusion or confirmation of neuropathy. Imaging plays

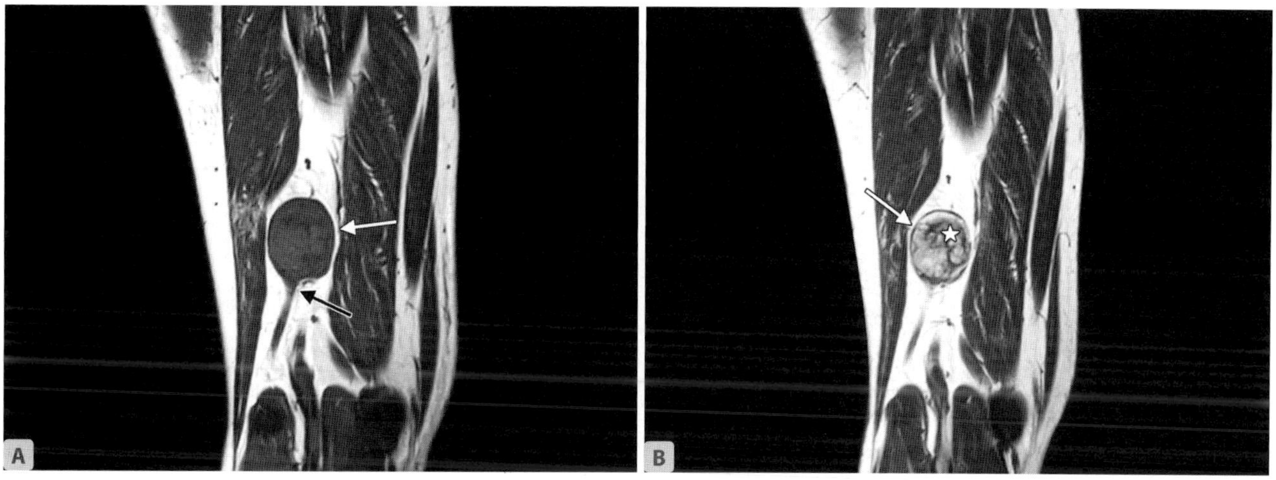

FIGS. 27A AND B: Coronal nonfat-suppressed T1 (A) and T2 (B) images of thigh showing eccentric well-defined T1-hypointense and T2-hyperintense lesion (white arrows) suggestive of Schwannoma. Note is made of tail sign (black arrow) and few hemorrhagic areas are also seen within the lesion (star).

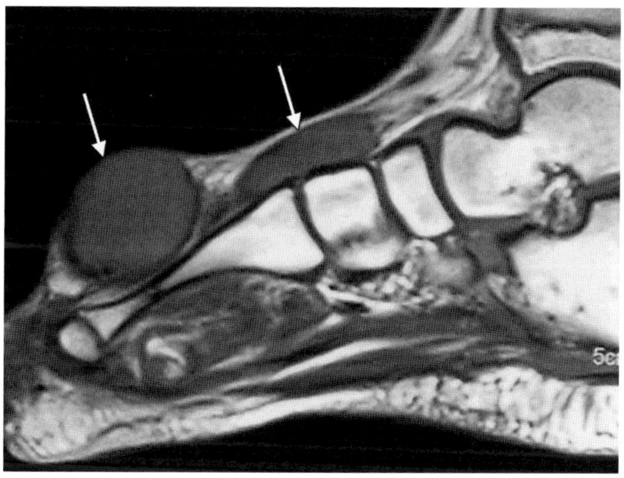

FIG. 28: Neurofibromas. Sagittal T1 nonfat-suppressed section of foot in known case of neurofibromatosis showing T1 hypointense well-defined variable sized and shaped lesions on dorsum of foot.

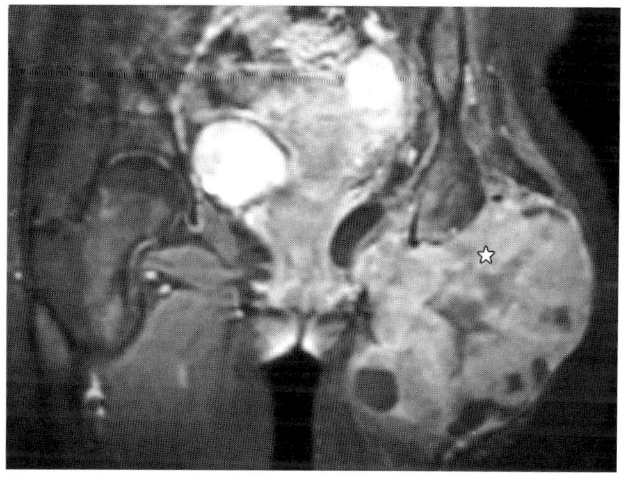

FIG. 29: Malignant peripheral nerve sheath tumor. Postcontrast T1FS coronal section showing heterogeneously enhancing lobulated mass lesion (star) in hip region extending along sciatic notch with local infiltrations of adjacent muscles and bones.

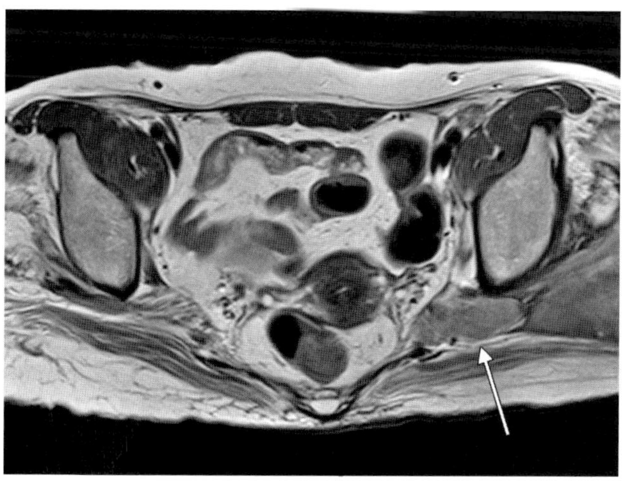

FIG. 30: Lymphomatous involvement of nerve. Axial T2 nonfat-suppressed image showing minimally hyperintense signal intensity with diffuse nodular enlargement of sciatic nerve in known case of lymphoma.

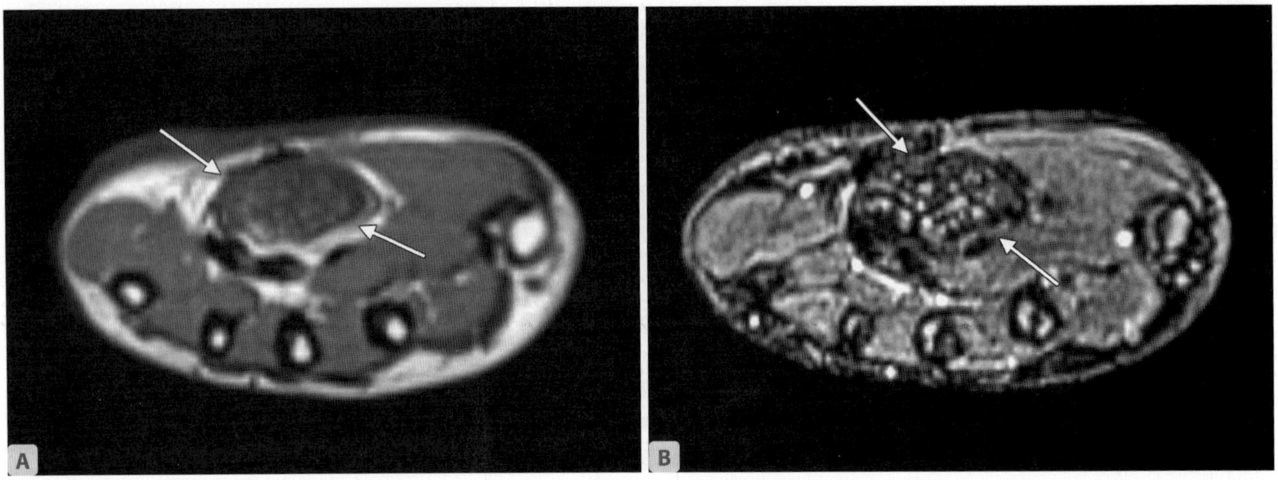

FIGS. 31A AND B: Fibrolipomatous hamartoma of median nerve. Axial T1 nonfat-suppressed (A) and T2 fat-suppressed (B) images of hand showing grossly enlarged median nerve (arrows) with fatty deposition giving cable-like appearance.

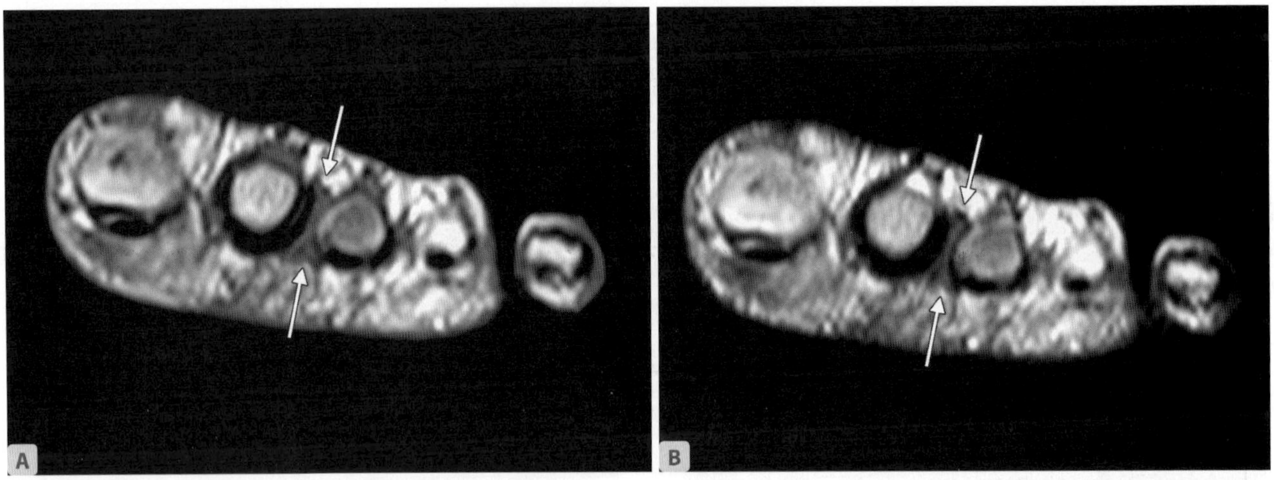

FIGS. 32A AND B: Morton's neuroma: Coronal nonfat-suppressed T1 (A) and T2 (B) images of forefoot showing hypointense lesion in 2nd intermetatarsal web space (arrows).

important role to detect superimposed complications, such as secondary lymphoma (nodular lesions in the nerve). Multiple nerve abnormalities or multifocal nerve disease, diffuse disease, abnormality at unexpected sites of nerve, nodularity or focal/multifocal nerve thickening points to the diagnosis of lymphoma, amyloid deposition, or neurocutaneous syndrome.[41]

There are useful clinical and biochemical tests in the diagnosis of systemic etiologies. These includes history, nature and course of weakness, blood work up, autoimmune work up, cerebrospinal fluid (CSF) analysis, and history of drug intake, etc.

In GBS, apart from specific clinical features, MR shows diffuse nerve thickening and increased signal intensity of affected nerves on T2/STIR sequences, such as in cauda equina nerve roots.[42] In CIDP, on imaging there is diffuse or patchy nerve thickening **(Figs. 33A and B)**.[43] In CMT type 1A, pseudo masses may be seen mimicking neurofibromatosis.[44]

Vasculitis or chemotherapy-induced neuropathy causes bilateral patchy nerve involvement, often seen in sciatic nerve. In diabetes mellitus, there is diffuse nerve thickening, increase signal intensity, and intraepineurial fat deposition. Amyloidosis is usually presenting with bilateral sciatic nerve thickening with or without nodularity and patchy enhancement. Neurocutaneous syndromes show diffuse nerve thickening and multifocal nodularity.[41]

Radiation Neuropathy

Postradiation neuritis or neuropathy may be seen in patient who underwent radiation therapy for other diseases. Radiation neuropathy may be seen after some period (weeks to years) postradiation therapy. It is generally diagnosis of exclusion. The severity of radiation neuropathy depends on dose of radiation exposure.[45] The affected nerve shows nonspecific features on imaging such as enlargement of nerve **(Figs. 34A to C)**.

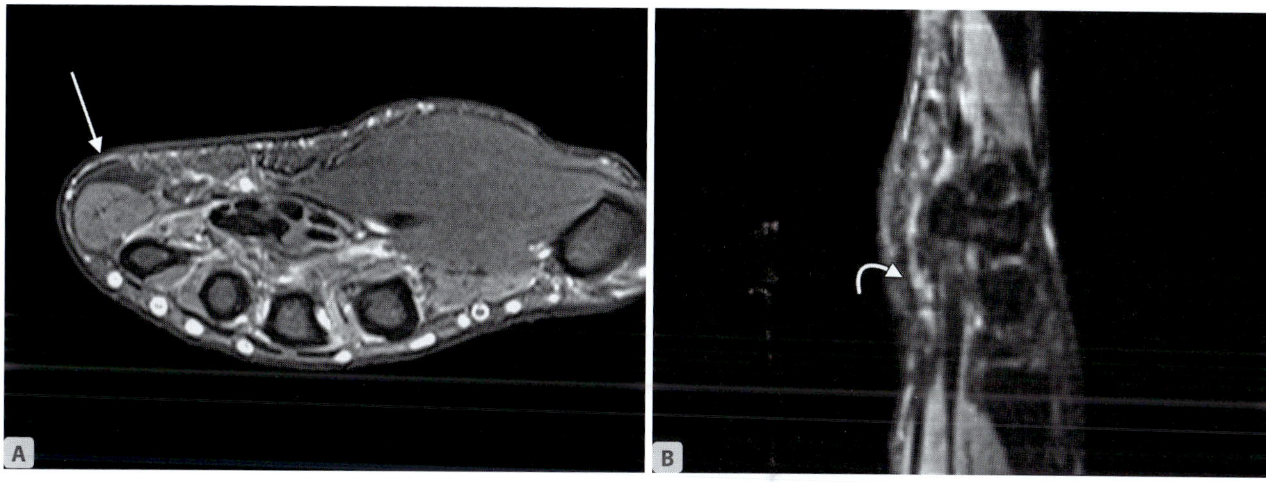

FIGS. 33A AND B: Chronic inflammatory demyelinating neuropathy (CIDP) involving ulnar nerve. Axial T2 fat-suppressed (A) and 3D PSIF sagittal reformatted (B) images showing atrophy and denervation edema of hypothenar muscles (straight arrow) and nodular hyperintense ulnar nerve (curved arrow).

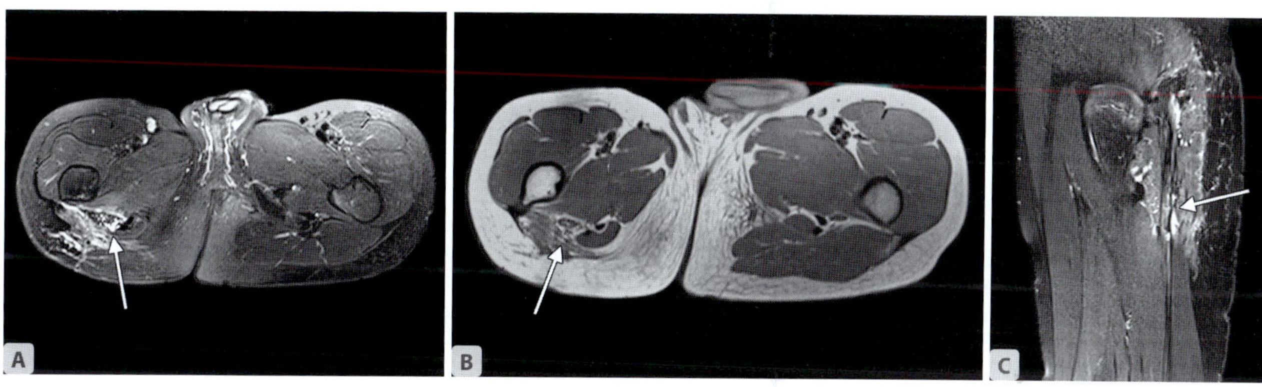

FIGS. 34A TO C: Radiation neuropathy of right sciatic nerve. Axial T2 fat-suppressed (A) and axial T1 nonfat-suppressed (B) and sagittal T2 fat-suppressed (C) images shows mildly thickened right sciatic nerve with heterogeneous signal. This patient received radiotherapy for malignant tumor thigh and hip region.

RECENT ADVANCES IN PERIPHERAL NERVE IMAGING

Microneurography

In microneurography, very high magnetic fields (>9 T) with powerful gradients (400 mT/m) and coils are used which provides very high special resolution. This is similar to use of higher frequency US, which increases the spatial resolution.[46]

Dedicated Contrast Media

The contrast agents can be helpful in MR assessment of peripheral nerve:

- Superparamagnetic MR contrast agents (SPIO: Endorem or Resovist) and ultrasmall superparamagnetic contrast agents (USPIO: Sinerem), having iron oxide particles and have their affinity for the macrophage which gives hypointense signal on gradient-echo sequences through a paramagnetic effect.[25,47]
- Gadofluorine have affinity to demyelinating area of injured nerve, which gives low T1 signal until remyelination is over. It has high sensitivity and specificity in detecting focal demyelinating areas. This can be useful in post-therapy follow-up of demyelinating diseases.[25,48]

Contrast-enhanced Ultrasound

The contrast-enhanced US may be useful in peripheral nerve imaging, providing quantitative measures of PNS perfusion. The applications have been suggested, particularly in trauma cases to monitor grafted nerve injuries[49]

Elastography

Ultrasound elastography is a measure of the elasticity of tissues. It is a noninvasive technique in which both qualitative and quantitative evaluation of nerve tissue constitution can be done.[50] Many studies found that in peripheral neuropathy, the nerve rigidity increases due to loss of less rigid myelin and restoration with connective tissue. The qualitative

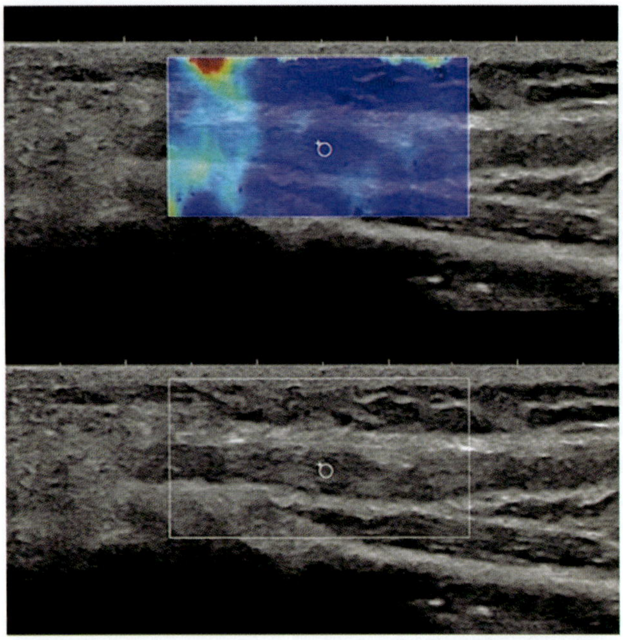

FIG. 35: Elastography of ulnar nerve. Shear-wave elastographic images with color mapping in case of leprotic neuropathy.

evaluation is represented by the color coded mapping. The quantitative shear modulus maps can be measured by shear-wave velocities in meters per second or tissue elasticity in kilopascals **(Fig. 35)**.

Spinal Ganglion Morphometry

In a study by West et al., they showed quantification of spinal ganglion volume corresponded to with histological quantification, which corresponded to the number of nerve cell bodies.[51] The loss of neurons corresponds to decrease in spinal ganglion volume which may be useful in objective and early method of measuring sensory neuronal injury. In chronic inflammatory demyelinating polyneuropathy, inherited neuropathies or lymphomatous infiltration of nerve, there is increase in volume of spinal ganglion.[25]

MR Spectroscopy

The contrast resolution (~7–10 mm) of MRS is not promising in imaging of PNS at present. The muscle metabolism was studied by Baldassarri[52] in nerve regeneration using 31P MRS to specify high-energy metabolites and calculate muscle pH. The study showed that muscle tissue pH was alkaline in the denervation phase and returned to normal after reinnervation.

REFERENCES

1. Franssen H, Wieneke GH, Wokke JH. The influence of temperature on conduction block. Muscle Nerve. 1999;22:166-73.
2. Grant GA, Goodkin R, Maravilla KR, Kliot M. MR neurography: diagnostic utility in the surgical treatment of peripheral nerve disorders. Neuroimaging Clin N Am. 2004;14(1):115-33.
3. Goedee HS, van der Pol WL, Hendrikse J, van den Berg LH.. Nerve ultrasound and magnetic resonance imaging in the diagnosis of neuropathy. Curr Opin Neurol. 2018;31:526-33.
4. Möller I, Miguel M, Bong DA, Zaottini F, Martinoli C. The peripheral nerves: Update on ultrasound and magnetic resonance imaging. Clin Exp Rheumatol. 2018;114(5):145-58.
5. Petchprapa CN, Rosenberg ZS, Sconfienza LM, Cavalcanti CF, Vieira RL, Zember JS. MR imaging of entrapment neuropathies of the lower extremity part 1. The pelvis and hip. Radiographics. 2010;30:983-1000.
6. Hochman MG, Zilberfarb JL. Nerves in a pinch: Imaging of nerve compression syndromes. Radiol Clin North Am. 2004;42(1): 221-45.
7. Pilavaki M, Chourmouzi D, Kiziridou A, Skordalaki A, Zarampoukas T, Drevelengas A. Imaging of peripheral nerve sheath tumors with pathologic correlation: Pictorial review. Eur J Radiol. 2004;52(3):229-39.
8. Floch H, Naux E, Pham Dang C, Dupas B, Pinaud M. Computed tomography scanning of the sciatic nerve posterior to the femur: Practical implications for the lateral mid-femoral block. Reg Anesth Pain Med. 2003;28(5):445-9.
9. Ellis JRC, McNally EG, Scott PM. Ultrasound of peripheral nerves. Imaging. 2002;14(3):217-22.
10. Martinoli C, Bianchi S, Derchi LE. Ultrasonography of peripheral nerves. Semin Ultrasound CT MR. 2000;21:205-13.
11. Kim S, Choi JY, Huh YM, Song HT, Lee SA, Kim SM, et al. Role of magnetic resonance imaging in entrapment and compressive neuropathy-what, where, and how to see the peripheral nerves on the musculoskeletal magnetic resonance image: Part 2. Upper extremity. Eur Radiol. 2007;17(2):509-22.
12. Maravilla KR, Bowen BC. Imaging of the peripheral nervous system: Evaluation of peripheral neuropathy and plexopathy. Am J Neuroradiol. 1998;19(6):1011-23.
13. Chappell KE, Robson MD, Stonebridge-Foster A, Glover A, Allsop JM, Williams AD, et al. Magic angle effects in MR neurography. Am J Neuroradiol. 2004;25:431-40.
14. Martinoli C, Derchi LE, Bertolotto M, Gandolfo N, Bianchi S, Fiallo P, et al. US and MR imaging of peripheral nerves in leprosy. Skeletal Radiol. 2000;29:142-50.
15. Takahara T, Hendrikse J, Yamashita T, Mali WP, Kwee TC, Imai Y, et al. Diffusion-weighted MR neurography of the brachial plexus: Feasibility study. Radiology. 2008;249(2):653-60.
16. Zhang ZW, Song LJ, Meng QF, Li ZP, Luo BN, Yang YH, et al. High-resolution diffusion-weighted MR imaging of the human lumbosacral plexus and its branches based on a steady-state free precession imaging technique at 3T. Am J Neuroradiol. 2008;29(6):1092-4.
17. Hiltunen J, Suortti T, Arvela S, Seppä M, Joensuu R, Hari R. Diffusion tensor imaging and tractography of distal peripheral nerves at 3T. Clin Neurophysiol. 2005;116:2315-23.
18. Skorpil M, Karlsson M, Nordell A, Peripheral nerve diffusion tensor imaging. Magn Reson Imaging. 2004;22:743-5.
19. Chhabra A, Madhuranthakam AJ, Andreisek G. Magnetic resonance neurography: Current perspectives and literature review. Eur Radiol. 2018;28:698-707.
20. Kabakci N, Gürses B, Firat Z, Bayram A, Uluğ AM, Kovanlikaya A, et al. Diffusion tensor imaging and tractography of median nerve: Normative diffusion values. Am J Roentgenol. 2007;189:923-27.
21. Hormann M, Traxler H, Ba-Ssalamah A, Mlynarik V, Shodaj-Baghini M, Kubiena H, et al. Correlative high-resolution MR-anatomic study of sciatic, ulnar, and proper palmar digital nerve. Magn Reson Imaging. 2003;21(8):879-85.
22. Chhabra A, Andreisek G, Soldatos T, Wang KC, Flammang AJ, Belzberg AJ, et al. MR neurography: Past, present, and future. Am J Roentgenol. 2011;197:583-91.

23. Kraus E, Tenforde AS, Beaulieu CF, Ratliff J, Fredericson M. Piriformis syndrome with variant sciatic nerve anatomy: A case report. PMR. 2016;8(2):176-9.
24. Kamath S, Venkatanarasimha N, Walsh MA, Hughes PM. MRI appearance of muscle denervation. Skeletal Radiol. 2008;37: 397-404.
25. Ohana M, Moser T, Moussaoui A, Kremer S, Carlier RY, Liverneaux P, et al. Current and future imaging of the peripheral nervous system. Diagnos Intervent Imag. 2014;95:17-26
26. Chhabra A, Ahlawat S, Belzberg A, Andreseik G. Peripheral nerve injury grading simplified on MR neurography: as referenced to Seddon and Sunderland classifications. Indian J Radiol Imaging [Serial Online]. 2014;24:217-24.
27. Agarwal A, Chandra A, Jaipal U, Bagarhatta M, Mendiratta K, Goyal A, et al. Can imaging be the new yardstick for diagnosing peripheral neuropathy?—a comparison between high resolution ultrasound and MR neurography with an approach to diagnosis. Insights Imaging. 2019;10:104.
28. Mackinnon S, Dellon AL. Diagnosis of nerve injury. Surgery of the peripheral nerve. New York: Thieme Publications; 1988. pp. 74-8.
29. Miller TT, Reinus WR. Nerve entrapment syndromes of the elbow, forearm, and wrist. Am J Roentgenol. 2010;195:585-94.
30. Benedetti PF, Anderson MW, Maselli R, Rogero GW. Hypertrophic peripheral neuropathy due to leprosy: MR features. J Comput Assist Tomogr 1994,18:995-6.
31. Zaidman CM, Al-Lozi M, Pestronk A. Peripheral nerve size in normals and patients with polyneuropathy: An ultrasound study. Muscle Nerve. 2009;40(6):960-6.
32. Martinoli C, Schenone A, Bianchi S, Mandich P, Caponetto C, Abbruzzese M, et al. Sonography of the median nerve in Charcot-Marie-Tooth disease. Am J Roentgenol. 2002;178(6):1553-6.
33. Bhargava R, Parham DM, Lasater OE, Chari RS, Chen G, Fletcher BD. MR imaging differentiation of benign and malignant peripheral nerve sheath tumors: Use of the target sign. Pediatr Radiol. 1997;27:124-9.
34. Kakkar C, Shetty CM, Koteshwara P, Bajpai S. Telltale signs of peripheral neurogenic tumors on magnetic resonance imaging. Indian J Radiol Imaging. 2015;25:453-8.
35. Wilkinson LM, Manson D, Smith CR. Best cases from the AFIP: Plexiform neurofibroma of the bladder. Radiographics 2004; 24:S237–S242.
36. Li CS, Huang GS, Wu HD, Chen WT, Shih LS, Lii JM, et al. Differentiation of soft tissue benign and malignant peripheral nerve sheath tumors with magnetic resonance imaging. Clin Imaging. 2008;32:121-7.
37. Walker CW, Adams, BD, Barnes CL, Roloson GJ, Fitzrandolph RL. Case report 667. Fibrolipomatous hamartoma of the median nerve. Skeletal Radiol. 1991;20:237-9.
38. Choi W, Jung JY, Song IS, Lee JS, Lee TJ, Jung YY, et al. Fibrolipomatous hamartoma of digital branch of the median nerve without macrodystrophy: Two case reports with magnetic resonance imaging findings. J Korean Soc Radiol. 2012;67(6): 483-7.
39. Bencardino J, Rosenberg ZS, Beltran J, Liu X, Marty-Delfaut E. Morton's neuroma: Is it always symptomatic? AJR Am J Roentgenol. 2000;175(3):649-53.
40. Espinoza N, Schmitt JW, Saupe N, Maquieira GJ, Bode B, Vienne P, et al. Morton neuroma: MR imaging after resection-postoperative MRI and histologic findings in asymptomatic and symptomatic metatarsal spaces. Radiology. 2010;255:850-6.
41. Chhabra A. Peripheral MR neurography. Neuroimaging Clin North Am. 2014;24(1):79-89.
42. Sureka J, Cherian RA, Alexander M, Thomas BP. MRI of brachial plexopathies. Clin Radiol. 2009;64:208-18.
43. Bradley LJ, Wilhelm T, King RH, Ginsberg L, Orrell RW. Brachial plexus hypertrophy in chronic inflammatory demyelinating polyradiculoneuropathy. Neuromuscul Disord. 2006;16:126-31.
44. Cartwright MS, Brown ME, Eulitt P, Walker FO, Lawson VH, Caress JB. Diagnostic nerve ultrasound in Charcot-Marie Tooth disease type 1B. Muscle Nerve. 2009;40(1):98-102.
45. Mondrup K, Olsen NK, Pfeiffer P, Rose C. Clinical and electrodiagnostic findings in breast cancer patients with radiation-induced brachial plexus neuropathy. Acta Neurol Scand. 1990;81:153-8.
46. Bilgen M, Heddings A, Al-Hafez B, Hasan W, McIff T, Toby B, et al. Microneurography of human median nerve. J Magn Reson Imaging. 2005;21(6):826-30.
47. Bendszus M, Stoll G. Caught in the act: In vivo mapping of macrophage infiltration in nerve injury by magnetic resonance imaging. J Neurosci. 2003;23(34):10892-6.
48. Wessig C, Jestaedt L, Sereda MW, Bendszus M, Stoll G. Gadofluorine M-enhanced magnetic resonance nerve imaging: Comparison between acute inflammatory and chronic degenerative demyelination in rats. Exp Neurol. 2008;210(1):137-43.
49. Wang Y, Tang P, Zhang L, Guo Y, Wan W. Quantitative evaluation of the peripheral nerve blood perfusion with high frequency contrast-enhanced ultrasound. Acad Radiol. 2010;17(12):1492-7.
50. Zakrzewski J, Zakrzewska K, Pluta K, Nowak O, Miłoszewska-Paluch A. Ultrasound elastography in the evaluation of peripheral neuropathies: A systematic review of the literature. Pol J Radiol. 2019;84:e581-e591
51. West CA, Davies KA, Hart AM, Wiberg M, Williams SR, Terenghi G. Volumetric magnetic resonance imaging of dorsal root ganglia for the objective quantitative assessment of neuron death after peripheral nerve injury. Exp Neurol. 2007;203(1):22-33.
52. Baldassarri AM, Zetti G, Masson S, Gatti S, Albani AP, Ferla G, et al. Magnetic resonance (MR) imaging and MR spectroscopy of nerve regeneration and target muscle energy metabolism in a model of prosthesis-guided reinnervation in rats. Acad Radiol. 1995;2(2):128-34.

CHAPTER

175

Imaging in Prosthetic Joints

Ankur Goyal, Shivanand Gamanagatti

INTRODUCTION

Most commonly performed orthopedic procedures include fracture fixations and joint arthroplasties.[1] Thus, there is a need for the radiologist to know about the imaging interpretation of commonly performed arthroplasties. The common indications of arthroplasty include severe pain due to advanced osteoarthritis, postinflammatory or infective arthritis, complex fractures, and avascular necrosis.[1] Neuropathic joint, morbid obesity, and active infection are the usual contraindications.

This chapter focuses on basic concepts of arthroplasty and imaging evaluation of three most commonly performed prosthetic joints, namely hip, knee, and the shoulder. First and foremost, we should be able to recognize the proper positioning of the implant and secondly any associated complications.

BASIC CONCEPTS

The purpose of arthroplasty is to alleviate the joint pain while preserving function, stability, and mobility.

Primary fixation of an implant is based on tight press-fit with the stem being inserted more than the bony crevice. This compression generates hoop stress, providing stability. *Secondary or definitive fixation* is due to bony ingrowth, providing anchorage for longevity of the implant.

Osseointegration refers to formation of lamellar bone around the implant, which enables tight fit. If the degree of motion at the implant-bone interface is <20 mm, then there is predominantly bone formation at the interface, stabilizing the implant. Motion >150 mm leads to formation of fibrous tissue and 40–150 mm leads to both bone and fibrous tissue formation. The center of the prosthesis needs to be placed in anatomical position without any offset. Any deviation leads to increased wear and loosening of the implant.

Wearing in refers to loss of material of the articulating prosthesis surfaces when they slide against each other under load. This is the most common cause of implant failure. Wear in produces particulate debris, inciting foreign body reaction, osteolysis, and asymmetric joint space narrowing.

Prosthesis leads to diminution of normal stress from the periprosthetic bone leading to osteopenia (Wolff's law) and is known as *stress shielding*. This bone loss leads to failure of osseointegration and it is the most common cause of implant loosening. It is more pronounced with large or long implants or those with extensive porous-coated stems.

Resistance of the implant to a particular degree of motion is referred to as *constraint*. Accordingly, implants may be fully constrained (restricted motion in a particular axis), semiconstrained or nonconstrained (allow full movement in a particular axis). For example, in knee, nonconstrained prostheses retain the cruciate ligaments; semiconstrained ones include large anterior tibial spine and corresponding rectangular space to prevent posterior tibial subluxation; and constrained prostheses are hinged ones used in tumors and revision arthroplasties.

Conformity refers to the degree of the geometric articulation fit between the prosthetic components. Greater conformity means more contact area, resulting in reduced stress and wear but more deformation of polyethylene and early loosening.

Modularity refers to the option of adding stems, augmentations, and wedges to the implant components so as to customize the prosthesis intraoperatively.

Custom prosthesis refers to preoperatively designed implant which is different from the standard one to cater to the specific needs of the patient. One example is long-stem implant in limb salvage procedures in case of tumors **(Fig. 1A)**.

Fixation of the prosthesis to the underlying bone may be done with bone cement [polymethylmethacrylate (PMMA)] or without (cementless/uncemented implants; **Fig. 1B**). In latter, implants are specially textured and porous coated (hydroxyapatite or titanium) to promote bony fixation. Cemented implants are used when the bone is fragile (osteopenia/postinflammatory arthritis) and enable early weight-bearing. However, they are prone to loosening.

PROSTHETIC MATERIALS

Commonly used prosthetic materials include metal, ceramics, polyethylene, and bone cement. Metals used in making the

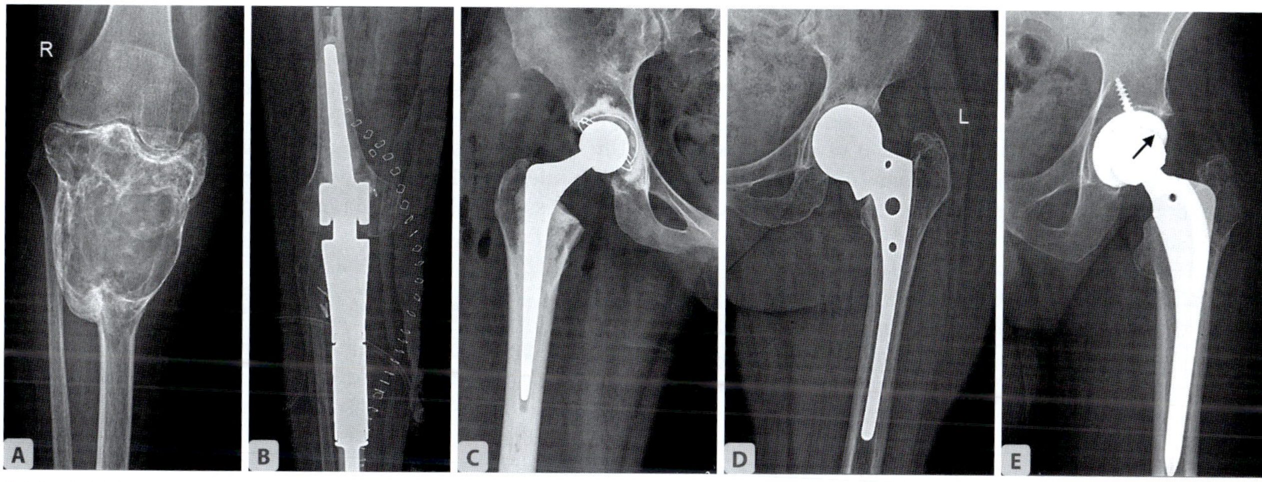

FIGS. 1A TO E: (A) Radiograph depicts expansile lytic soap-bubble lesion in proximal tibia in a case of giant cell tumor; (B) Radiograph shows custom hinged prosthesis with long-stem implant; (C) Radiograph following total hip arthroplasty shows cemented fixation of both femoral (metal) and acetabular components (polyethylene) in total hip replacement (THR); (D) Radiograph shows noncemented fixation of femoral stem which articulates with native acetabulum in unipolar hemiarthroplasty; (E) Radiograph depicts bipolar hemiarthroplasty, where acetabular component is fixed using a screw. Arrow denotes radiolucent polyethylene cup at the articulation of the prosthetic femoral head and the acetabulum.

implants include stainless steel, titanium, and alloys based on titanium and cobalt. Smaller crystal size provides better strength and resistance. However, there may be long-term harmful effects of metal ions and loosening due to allergic response.

Ultra-high-molecular-weight polyethylene (UHMWPE) plastic has high strength, chemically inert, biocompatible with good fatigue resistance.

Ceramics (aluminum or zirconium oxide) are harder than metals and resistant to oxidative wear, but more susceptible to breakage. Ceramics have the lowest wear rate.[2]

Bearing (contact) surfaces can be made of polyethylene, metal or ceramic and accordingly the implant combinations (nomenclature) can be of the following types:

- Hard-on-soft (metal on polyethylene or ceramic on polyethylene)
- Hard-on-hard (metal-on-metal, ceramic-on-ceramic and metal-on-ceramic).

Most commonly used combination is metal-on-polyethylene **(Fig. 1C)**. For example, in hip prosthesis, femoral stem is metallic, head can be metallic or ceramic, cup is metallic or of polyethylene, and cup liner is usually ceramic or polyethylene.

The particulate polyethylene debris due to wear-in can however result in aseptic loosening of the implant. To decrease the particulate debris from abrasive wear, hard-on-hard combinations were developed to improve the life of implant.

Fixation materials include PMMA cement, calcium phosphate ceramic-coating or porous metal surfaces and promote osseointegration **(Figs. 1D and E)**. Bone cement is used less as an adhesive and more to fill the space between the implant and the bone.[2] Porous metal surface, fiber mesh, and sintered microsphere beads allow bony ingrowth whereas textured surface allows bony ongrowth. Surfaces can be textured by grit blasting with aluminum oxide or plasma spraying.[2] Bioactive coatings (hydroxyapatite) also promote bone growth.

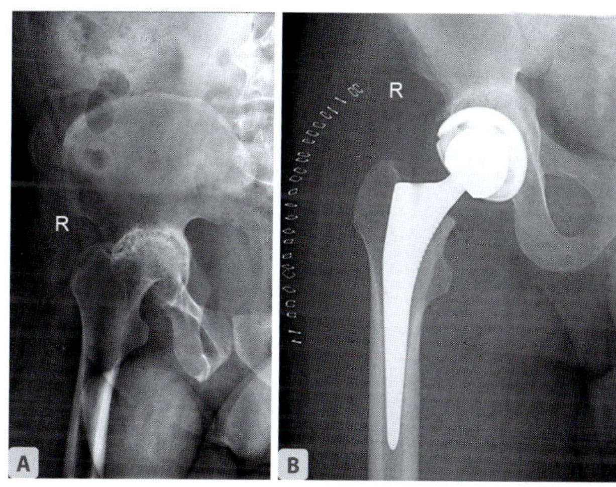

FIGS. 2A AND B: (A) Frontal radiograph shows severe osteoarthritis on right hip; (B) Immediate postoperative radiograph after bipolar hemiarthroplasty (metal-on-polyethylene bearing surfaces).

IMAGING MODALITIES

Radiographs

Radiographs are very useful for initial assessment as well as postoperatively to look for type of prosthesis, alignment of components and to look for complications such as osteolysis, loosening, and implant failure and fractures **(Figs. 2A and B)**. Serial radiographs are very useful to identify stress shielding, implant wear in and loosening. Various measurements can be done on radiographs for early detection of implant offset.

Computed Tomography

Computed tomography (CT) provides comprehensive multiplanar evaluation with high spatial resolution. This is helpful for assessment of acetabular and femoral neck version, measuring rotational alignment of knee prosthesis **(Fig. 3A)**, assessing periprosthetic bone **(Fig. 3A)**, evaluation of collections and masses, and taking treatment decisions for revision surgery.

However, the beam hardening artifacts are a major problem and hamper with the image interpretation **(Fig. 3B)**. **Table 1** depicts the factors affecting metal- related artifacts. Thus, the methods to reduce them include: Increasing tube voltage (kVp) and tube current and exposure time product (mAs), using narrow detector collimation and low pitch, using lower frequency or iterative deblurring reconstruction algorithms, increasing section thickness while scrolling and using extended CT scale technique for multiplanar reformation (MPR) and wide window settings to accentuate border of osseous structures.[3] It may be kept in mind that most of these remedies also increase the radiation dose to the patient.

Ultrasound

Sonography is an excellent modality for evaluation of periprosthetic soft tissues. Any adjacent collections or effusions can be assessed and aspirated **(Figs. 4A and B)**. Ultrasound is also useful in distinguishing aseptic loosening from infection. It is also useful in evaluation of any nerve compression or hematoma in the immediate postoperative period **(Fig. 4C)**.

Magnetic Resonance Imaging

The indications of magnetic resonance imaging (MRI) in prosthetic joint imaging include:

- Evaluation of adjacent soft tissues
- Metallosis or particle disease **(Fig. 5)**
- Infection
- To assess tendon or muscle injuries
- Characterize collections and masses.

Most of the metallic implants used nowadays are MR compatible. However, metallic components cause artifacts by inducing magnetic field heterogeneity **(Fig. 5)**. This leads to

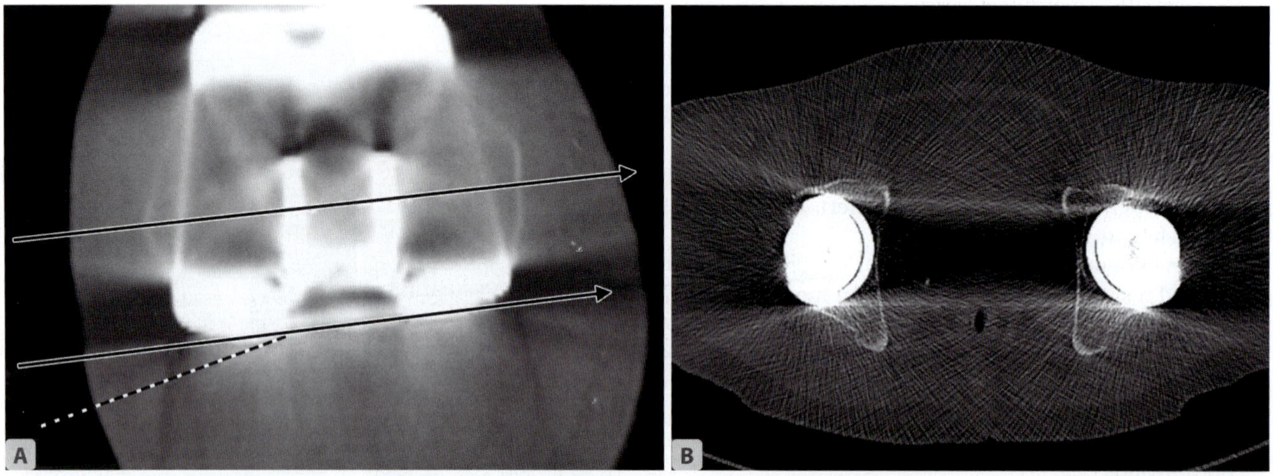

FIGS. 3A AND B: (A) Axial thick multiplanar reconstruction (MPR) image shows the transepicondylar line and femoral component posterior condylar line drawn to measure femoral component rotation post-knee arthroplasty; (B) Axial computed tomography (CT) image postbilateral total hip replacement (THR) shows beam hardening artifacts.

TABLE 1: Factors which affect metal-related artifacts on computed tomography (CT).

Factor	Effect
Metal composition	Titanium < Stainless steel < Cobalt-chrome (more dense metal produces more artifacts)
Prosthesis shape	More artifacts with complex shape
Orientation	More artifact along the long axis in axial plane
Collimation	Less artifact with narrow collimation
Pitch	Less artifact with low pitch (most important parameter affecting image quality in prosthesis cases)
Tube voltage (kVp)	Less artifact with high kVp
Tube current and exposure time product (mAs)	Less artifact with high mAs
Reconstruction algorithm	Less artifact with lower spatial frequency algorithm ("smooth" images)
Reconstruction section thickness	Less artifacts with thicker sections

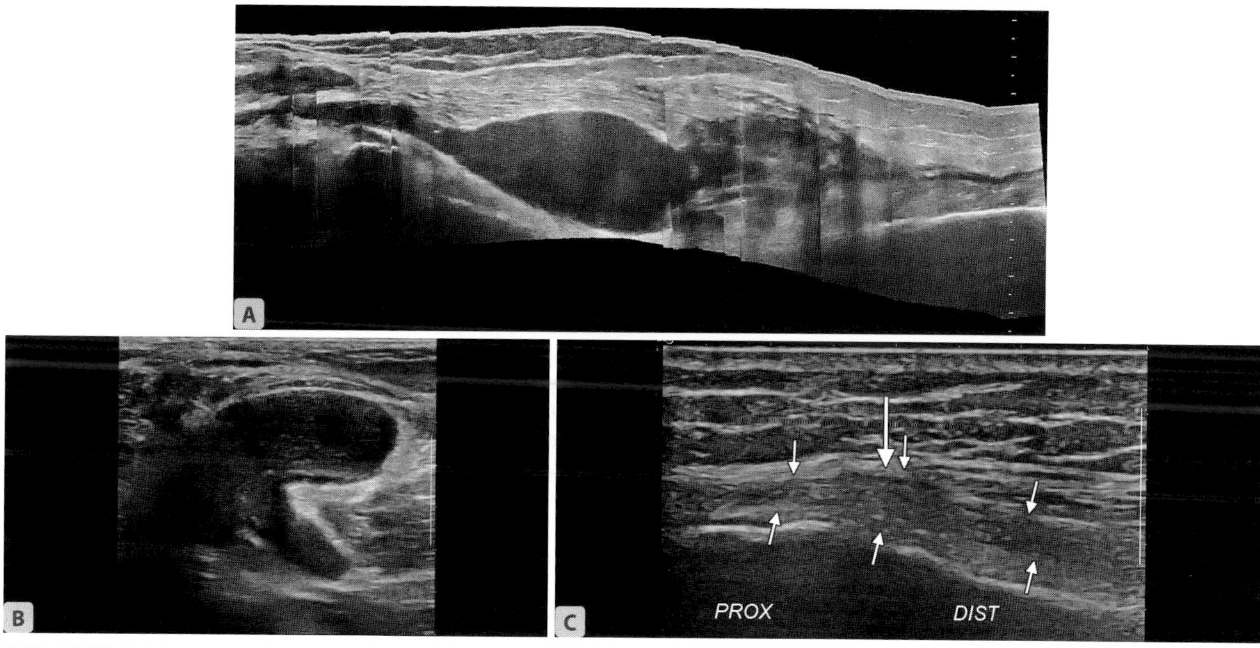

FIGS. 4A TO C: (A) Extended field-of-view panoramic ultrasound image shows large fluid collection in a patient who underwent total hip replacement (THR) 1 month ago. Aspiration revealed purulent material; (B) Another patient with Baker's cyst post-THR showing echogenic debris within; (C) Ultrasound of common peroneal nerve in another patient who developed foot drop post-THR. There is focal bulkiness of the nerve (long arrow) with preserved fibrillar architecture and continuity suggesting neuropraxia.

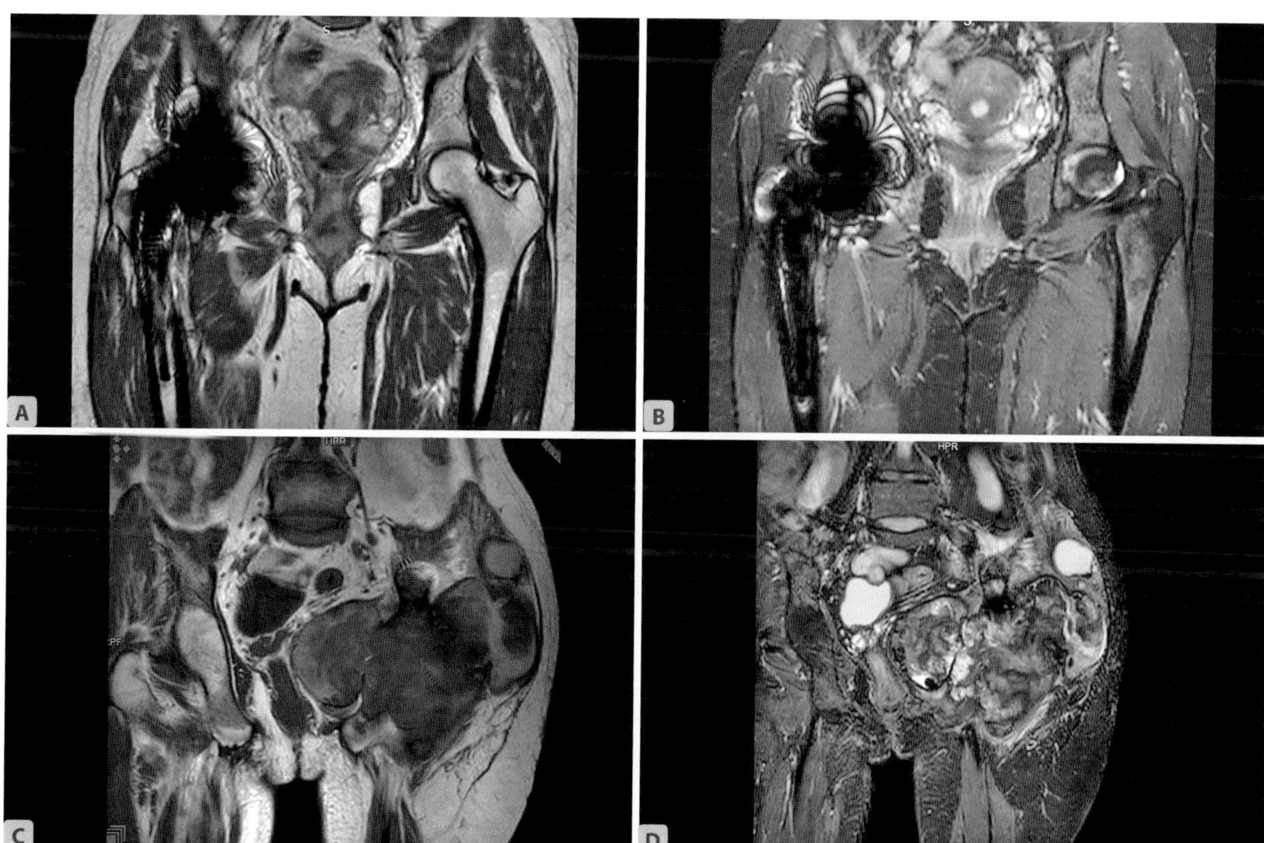

FIGS. 5A TO D: (A) Coronal T2-weighted (T2W) and (B) Fat-suppressed T2W images show susceptibility artifacts due to metal component, exaggerated in (B); (C and D) Coronal T1W and short-tau inversion recovery (STIR) images show large hypointense mass around the hip prosthesis due to metallosis.

in-plane distortion (pileup artifacts and signal loss, latter due to T2* dephasing), poor fat suppression, geometric distortion through section distortion. These artifacts are more on 3T compared with 1.5T and also depend on the type of prosthesis (size, shape, and configuration) and metal (titanium < cobalt-chromium < stainless steel).

Methods to Reduce Metal Artifacts in MRI

- Long axis of the prosthesis to be positioned parallel to the magnetic field and frequency encoding direction along the long axis of the implant.
- Fast spin echo with long echo-train length and short echo time (TE).
- Increasing the receiver bandwidth (reduces geometric distortion) and image matrix size.
- Reducing the field-of-view (FOV).
- Reducing slice thickness (reduces through section distortions).
- Fast spin-echo sequences with long echo-train length are least susceptible to metal artifacts and should be preferred over gradient-echo sequences.
- Short-tau inversion recovery (STIR) and Dixon-based fat suppression produce lesser artifacts than spectral fat suppression.

Based on these methods, the first integrated approach to reduce in-plane MR artifacts was described by Olsen et al. and termed metal artifact reduction sequences (MARS).[4] The typical MARS protocol includes STIR coronal, T1 and T2 spin-echo axial and proton-density coronal images. WARP includes multidirectional view-angle tilting (VAT) to further optimize MARS, however it results in image blurring.

Artifacts due to metal in the adjacent plane (through-plane artifacts) can be reduced by using special multispectral sequences such as multiacquisition variable-resonance image combination (MAVRIC) or slice-encoding for metal artifact correction (SEMAC). The former uses multiple overlapping acquisitions at different frequencies while the latter uses an additional slice-encoding gradient to fast spin echo. MAVRIC uses multiple frequency-selective excitations, multidirectional VAT, computational postprocessing, and reduces in-plane artifacts as well. SEMAC is a two-dimensional (2D) fast spin-echo sequence where there is phase encoding in the third dimension (Z-axis) for each slice so that exact delineation of the distortion due to magnetic susceptibility is there.[4]

Nuclear Medicine Scans

Various scintigraphy techniques are available for evaluation of postimplant complications. A standard three-phase bone scan is sensitive to detect failed joint replacement. Combining gallium scintigraphy enables differentiation between infection and aseptic loosening of the implant with moderate accuracy **(Figs. 6 and 7)**. Radiolabeled leukocyte scintigraphy is however the investigation of choice to identify neutrophil-mediated processes **(Figs. 6 and 7)**. Combined in vitro labeled leukocyte or bone marrow scintigraphy is the gold standard imaging modality to diagnose infection with higher accuracy than even ^{18}F-fluorodeoxyglucose-positron-emission tomography (FDG-PET) and single photon emission computed tomography (SPECT).

COMMON ARTHROPLASTIES: INDICATIONS, TERMINOLOGY, AND MEASUREMENT

The common indications of any arthroplasty include severe pain due to osteoarthritis, ankylosis secondary to prior infection/inflammatory arthritis/trauma, complex fractures, avascular necrosis, and tumors around the joint.

Hip Arthroplasty

Hip arthroplasty is of two types. *Total hip replacement or arthroplasty (THR/THA)* means replacing both the femoral and acetabular articulating surfaces and is usually done when both native surfaces are abnormal and is the most common type of hip arthroplasty. There are two components in THR implants: an acetabular part and a stemmed femoral part with

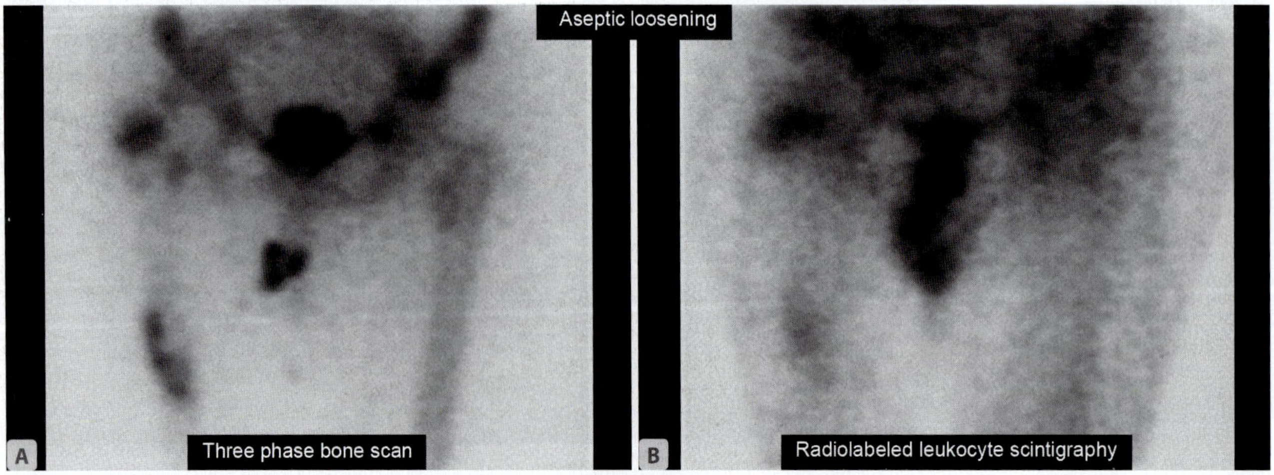

FIGS. 6A AND B: (A) Bone scan shows increased periprosthetic uptake on right side but no significant uptake is seen on leukocyte scintigraphy (B). This was a case of aseptic loosening of total hip replacement (THR).

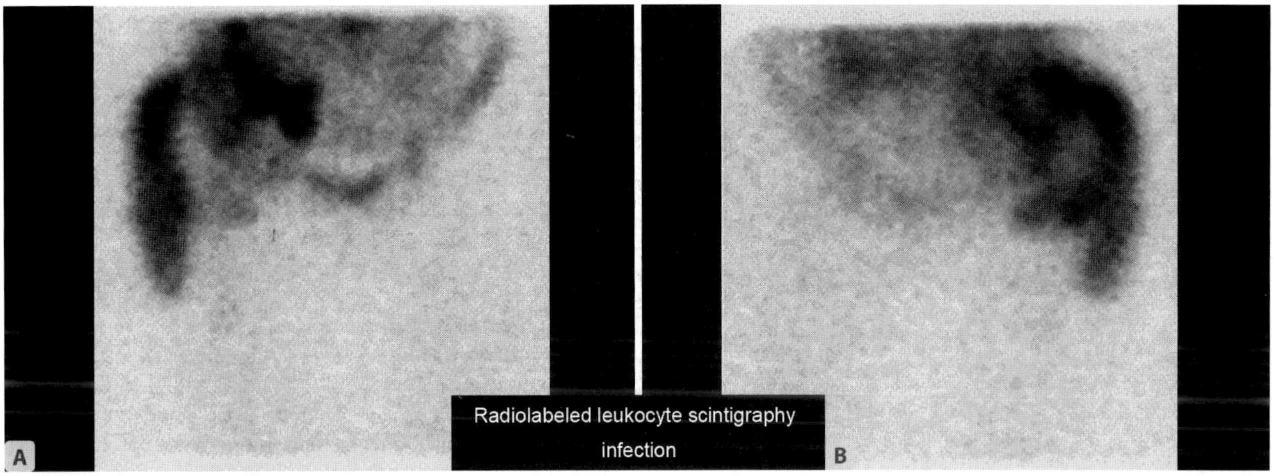

FIGS. 7A AND B: Leukocyte scintigraphy in periprosthetic infection shows increased uptake on right side (A is anterior projection and B is posterior projection).

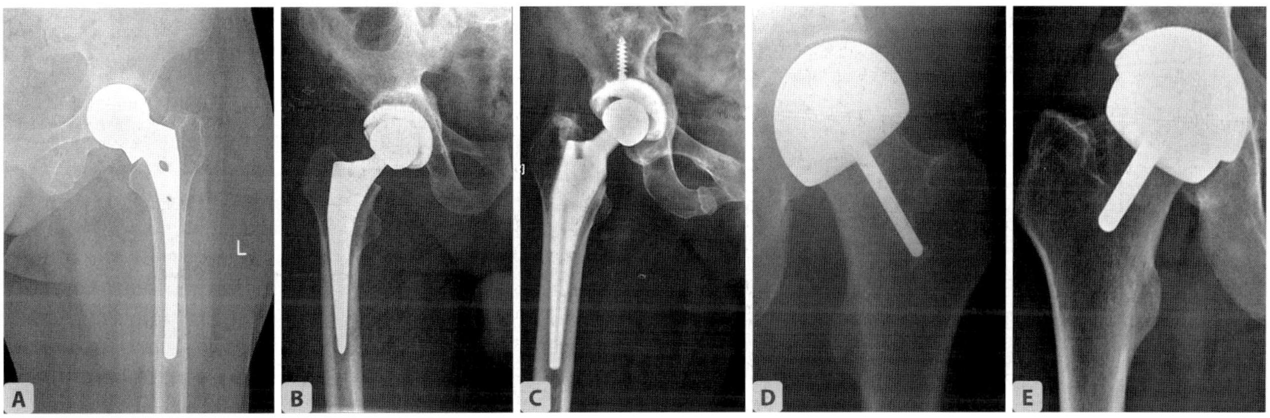

FIGS. 8A TO E: Different types of hip arthroplasty: (A) Unipolar noncemented hemiarthroplasty; (B) Bipolar hemiarthroplasty. Native sclerotic acetabulum is preserved with acetabular articular cartilage evident as thin lucency between acetabulum and the acetabular cup; (C) Total hip replacement (THR; acetabular component is attached to reamed acetabulum); (D) Resurfacing hemiarthroplasty; (E) Resurfacing total hip arthroplasty.

head **(Fig. 8)**. Former is fixed after removing the acetabular articular cartilage and the underlying sclerotic bone. Latter is fixed after removing the femoral head and neck and reaming the intramedullary cavity.[2] Hybrid THR comprises cemented femoral part and uncemented acetabular part whereas reverse hybrid THR employs reverse fixation.[2]

Hemiarthroplasty or partial hip replacement refers to replacing the femoral head which articulates with native acetabular cartilage (done in case of severe subcapital femoral neck fractures). Hemiarthroplasty may employ unipolar prosthesis (no movement within the implant) or bipolar prosthesis (movement occurs between the implant components; **Figs. 8A and B**). Bipolar hip implant has two parts: a femoral stem with head and a polyethylene-lined acetabular cap **(Fig. 8B)**. Thus, motion can occur between the head and acetabular cap as well as between the cap and the native acetabulum. Bipolar implants have better longevity (due to less wear of the acetabular articular cartilage), less prone to dislocation and can be more easily converted to THR later in life. Thus, unipolar hemiarthroplasty of hip is commonly done only in elderly patients (with limited life expectancy) for intracapsular hip fractures.[1]

In *resurfacing arthroplasty*, only the articular surface is replaced and the underlying bone is retained to reduce complications but the pain relief is suboptimal. Resurfacing arthroplasty can be done for both the articular surfaces (resurfacing THA) or only the femoral head (resurfacing hemiarthroplasty) and is usually employed in young active patients **(Figs. 8D and E)**.

In the initial postoperative evaluation of hip arthroplasty patient, following measurements are commonly done: Femoral stem alignment, acetabular version, and femoral anteversion.

Femoral Stem Alignment

On anteroposterior (AP) radiograph, femoral stem should be along the axis of femoral shaft (neutral alignment) with tip in center of the femoral shaft **(Fig. 9A)**. Varus malpositioning leads to implant failure. In resurfacing arthroplasty, femoral implant is placed in mild valgus position (5–10°) relative to femoral neck.[5]

Acetabular Version

The angulation of the acetabular axis from the coronal plane on a lateral radiograph is termed acetabular anteversion. Normal values are 5–25° to allow adequate flexion. Excessive anteversion predisposes to anterior dislocation while retroversion makes the prosthesis prone to posterior dislocation. On CT, one line is drawn between the lateral anterior and posterior margins of the acetabular component and another line (sagittal plane) is drawn perpendicular to the line connecting two identical points on either side of pelvis (interischial line) and the corresponding angle is measured **(Figs. 9B and C)**.[6] Normal range is same as in radiographs.

Femoral Version

Femoral component version is calculated on CT as the angle between femoral head-neck line (between center of head and neck of femoral prosthesis) and posterior intercondylar line (between posterior aspect of medial and lateral femoral condyles; **Fig. 10**). Normal range of femoral neck anteversion is 10–20°. It is also termed femoral antetorsion or femoral neck version.

Knee Arthroplasty

Knee arthroplasty is resurfacing arthroplasty in which articular surfaces are resurfaced using metal and polyethylene. Unlike hip, knee arthroplasty always involves replacement of both the opposing joint surfaces. There are three compartments in the knee joint: medial, lateral, and patellofemoral. *Unicompartmental arthroplasty (partial knee replacement or hemiarthroplasty)* is mostly done for isolated medial compartment arthritis (medial compartment arthroplasty; **Fig. 11**).[1] Patellofemoral arthroplasty is reserved for trochlear dysplasia or malalignment of the patellofemoral joint; however, has not shown encouraging results.[1]

Total knee replacement (TKR) includes replacing femoral, tibial, and patellar articular surfaces (tricompartmental replacement; **Fig. 11**). Multiradius metal component replaces the surface of both the femoral condyles as well as the trochlear notch, tibial component is high-density

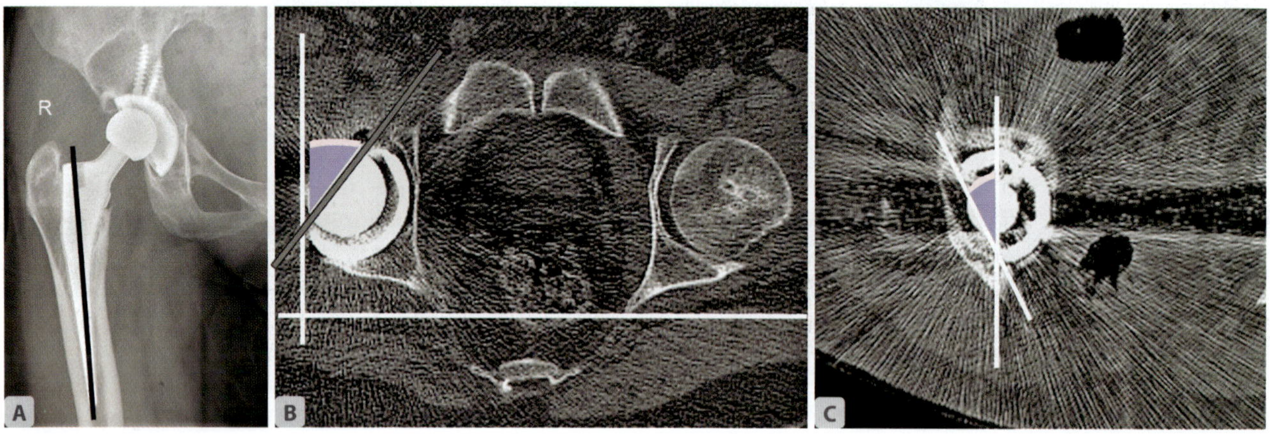

FIGS. 9A TO C: Measurements in hip arthroplasty: (A) Anteroposterior (AP) radiograph shows normal alignment of femoral stem along the shaft; (B) Acetabular anteversion angle measurement on CT; (C) Acetabular retroversion.

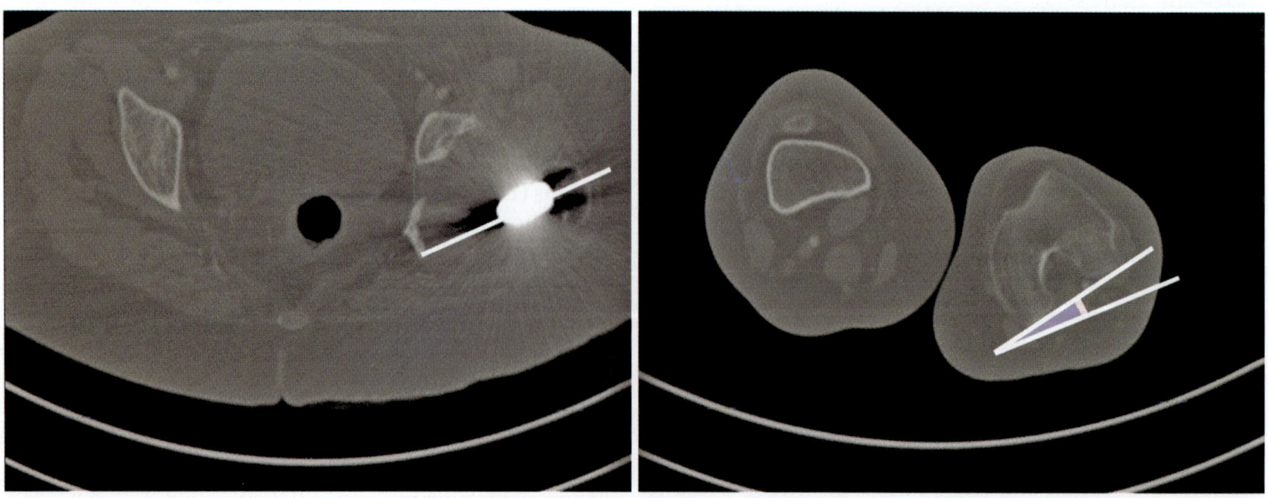

FIG. 10: Measurement of femoral anteversion (angle between the femoral neck line and posterior condylar line).

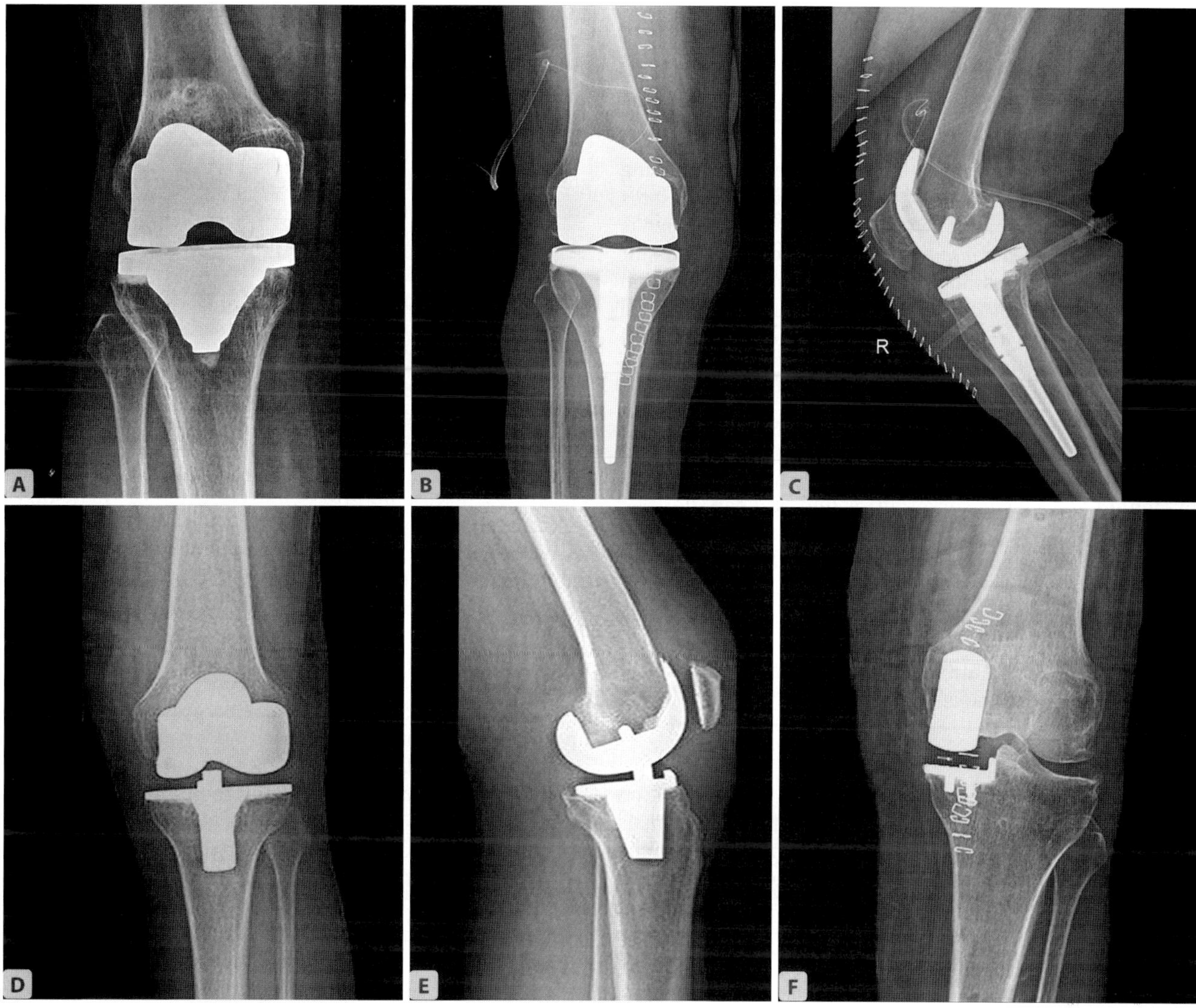

FIGS. 11A TO F: Different types of knee arthroplasty: (A) Cemented total knee replacement (TKR) with cruciate retaining arthroplasty; (B and C) Cemented long-stem tibial implant in TKR (cruciate retaining arthroplasty); (D and E) Cruciate substituting arthroplasty; (F) Medial joint hemiarthroplasty.

polyethylene commonly with metal backing and patellar surface is replaced by polyethylene (with or without metal backing).

Multiple designs of TKR implants are available. *Cruciate-retaining implants* are most commonly used; they preserve the posterior cruciate ligament (PCL), are nonconstrained and done in patients with healthy surrounding muscles and ligaments.

Cruciate-substituting arthroplasty employs semi-constrained implants and done when there is ligament injury or deformed knee joint. PCL is resected and posterior stability is provided by including a post or spine in the tibial polyethylene which articulates with a box-like defect in the center of femoral component. Mobile-bearing designs allow additional motion between the tibial polyethylene and tibial metal component in the region of tibial spacer.

Constrained (hinged) prostheses are used in case of tumors and revision surgeries **(Figs. 1A and B)**. The stem of these implants can be cemented, noncemented or anchored with screws.

Computed tomography enables accurate measurement of rotational alignment of tibial and femoral components. *Rotational alignment of femoral component* is determined by measuring angle between transepicondylar line (connecting lateral epicondyle with base of medial sulcus adjacent to medial epicondyle) and femoral prosthesis posterior condylar line **(Fig. 3A)**. Normal is mild internal rotation. Abnormal femoral rotation leads to increased tibiofemoral wear and dislocations.

Tibial component rotation refers to angle subtended between the tibial component line and tibial tubercle line, measured at the geometric center of proximal tibia.[7] A perpendicular line is drawn to the posterior surface of tibial component and is termed tibial component line. In the next caudal section, the geometric center of proximal tibia is established. The next caudal section through tibial tubercle is superimposed on the geometric center image and then a line is drawn from the apex of tibial tubercle to the geometric center. Following this, the tibial component image is also superimposed and angle between the tibial tubercle line and tibial component line is measured to assess the rotational position of tibial component.

Shoulder Arthroplasty

Similar to hip, hemiarthroplasty consists of only humeral component (metallic stem with modular head) articulating with native glenoid and in total arthroplasty it articulates with glenoid component **(Figs. 12A and B)**.[1] Former is done in case of proximal humeral fractures or severe rotator cuff tears where glenoid is normal. Resurfacing humeral head implants are also available. Glenoid component is of two types: polyethylene with wire loop (keeled) or metal (pegged). Former is cemented while latter is secured by screws. The functionality of shoulder implant depends on the competency of the rotator cuff and these prostheses are less constrained than those of the hip. Another type is reverse total shoulder arthroplasty, in which metal sphere is fixed on glenoid and plastic socket forms humeral cap, done in patients who requires shoulder arthroplasty but their rotator cuff muscles are either atrophic or damaged **(Fig. 12C)**.

COMPLICATIONS

Complications occur due to failure of fixation, failure of implant material or wear and tear **(Figs. 13A to D)**.

Polyethylene Wear

Abnormal loading stress on the implant leads to wear of the polyethylene on the superolateral aspect of the hip. This is the most common cause of arthroplasty failure. The normally expected molding is in superomedial aspect and leads to slight polyethylene thinning in the area of weight-bearing (known as creep). While creep is normal postoperative phenomenon, wear is pathological. Wear results in loss of particulate debris from the prosthetic surface due to abrasion, adhesion, or fatigue. Scratching over of one surface by another is termed abrasion. Transient bonding of the bearing surfaces due to poor lubrication is known as adhesion. Fatigue refers to excessive stress on the implant material, more than the mechanical limits. Loss of the particle debris leads to asymmetric joint space narrowing and eventual metal-on-metal contact. Also, the debris incites foreign body granulomatous reaction, manifested in the form of synovitis and osteolysis **(Flowchart 1)**.

Classification of wear is as follows:
- *Type 1*: Normal.
- *Type 2*: One articulating surface is worn (thinning of polyethylene liner so that metal backing is exposed and articulates with prosthetic head).
- *Type 3*: Third-body (fragment) interposition and abrasion between normal articulating surfaces.
- *Type 4*: Articulation or motion between two nonbearing surfaces.

Particle disease on MRI manifests as intermediate high-signal intensity collections on T2-weighted (T2W) images with synovial thickening (represented by peripheral T2-hypointense foci; **Fig. 13**) and areas of bone lysis (cortical thinning or disruption).

Osteolysis

It refers to bony resorption around the prosthesis and is an important cause of aseptic loosening, eventually requiring revision surgery. Osteolysis results because of poor initial fixation, mechanical stress leading to poor fixation or due to granulomatous reaction to particulate debris from the prosthesis and is common in THR than TKR due to larger particles in former. In the knee, tibial component failure is more common.

Loosening can occur at the implant-bone interface, implant-cement or cement-bone interface. Patients present with chronic persistent pain and there may be mild increase in serum inflammatory markers.

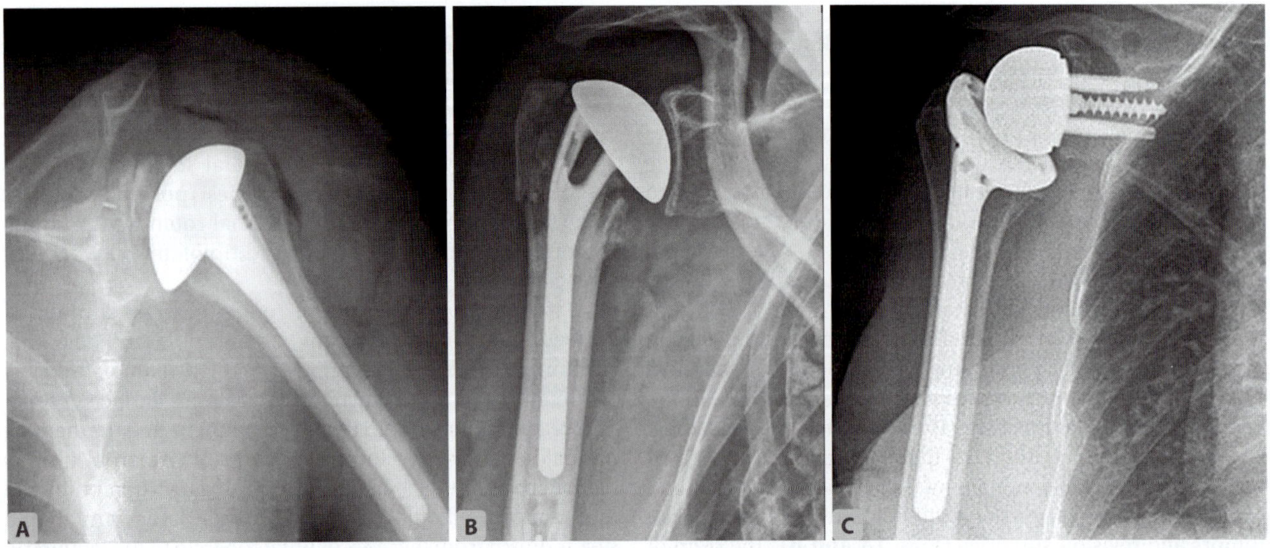

FIGS. 12A TO C: Types of shoulder arthroplasty: (A) Total shoulder arthroplasty; (B) Hemiarthroplasty for proximal humeral fractures; (C) Reverse shoulder arthroplasty.

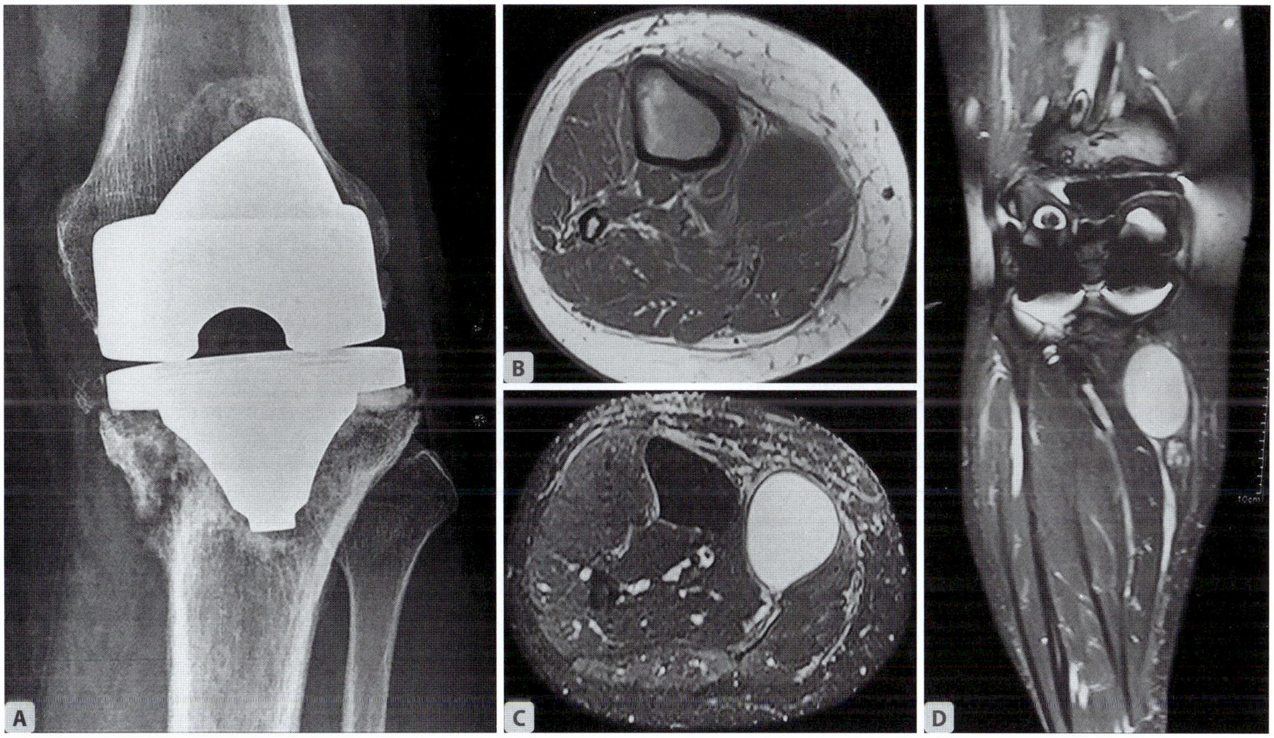

FIGS. 13A TO D: Complications of joint prosthesis: (A) Aseptic loosening of tibial component with periprosthetic fracture and implant malalignment; (B) Axial T1-weighted (T1W); (C) T2W; and (D) Short-tau inversion recovery (STIR) coronal images showing periprosthetic fluid collection.

FLOWCHART 1: An algorithmic approach to show how polyethylene wear leads to failure of implant.

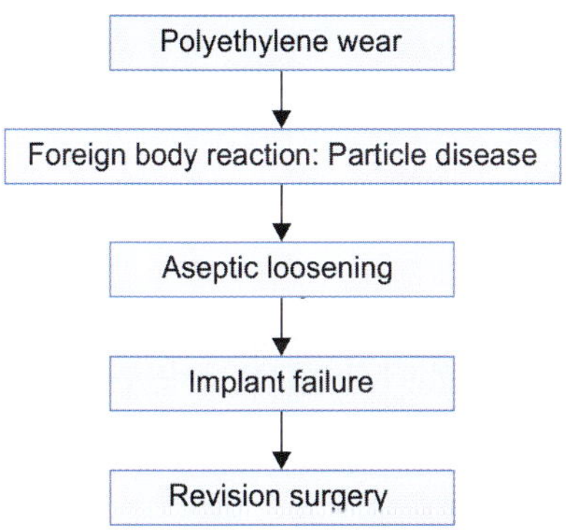

Imaging shows periprosthetic lucency >2 mm or progressive increase in lucency on serial radiographs, especially at the margins of the implant **(Figs. 13 and 14)**. There may be fracture of the cement mantle, bead shedding (punctate metal pieces around the bony ingrowth) and pedestal formation (sclerosis in medullary cavity distal to the tip of implant) as well. Progressive increase in periprosthetic radiolucency and component motion, fracture, change in position or migration is highly suggestive of aseptic loosening. However, this entity has to be differentiated from infection. Prior researchers have suggested standard zones to describe the location of periprosthetic lucencies on radiographs (three zones from lateral to medial for acetabular component on AP view, 7 zones each on AP and lateral views for the femoral component, 7 zones for tibial component; **Figs. 15A to C**).[8,9]

Infection

Infection is a mimicker of aseptic loosening and may be difficult to differentiate. Infection also leads to osteolysis and loosening of the implant with resultant change in position or migration. Diagnosis may be aided by increased erythrocyte sedimentation rate (ESR), C-reactive protein (CRP), leukocyte counts or joint aspiration may be needed. Demonstration of sinus tract on CT or MRI communicating with the implant clinches the diagnosis **(Figs. 16A to D)**. Presence of bone erosions, periosteal reaction, or collection in the soft tissues is suggestive of infection but not commonly seen. Ultrasound or MRI may show collections and joint effusions which may be aspirated under ultrasound guidance. Associated marrow and soft tissue edema is often present and serves to differentiate from sterile collections.[4] Radionuclide imaging is helpful and leukocyte bone marrow scintigraphy is the imaging gold standard to diagnose infection.

Instability

The causes of prosthetic instability include implant failure either due to aseptic loosening or infection, pre-existing deformity, component malalignment or tears of the ligaments and tendons.[10] In knee, mediolateral instability is the most common. Plain radiographs play important role in identifying instability. Ultrasound helps to identify ligament and tendon injuries especially quadriceps and patellar tendon ruptures.

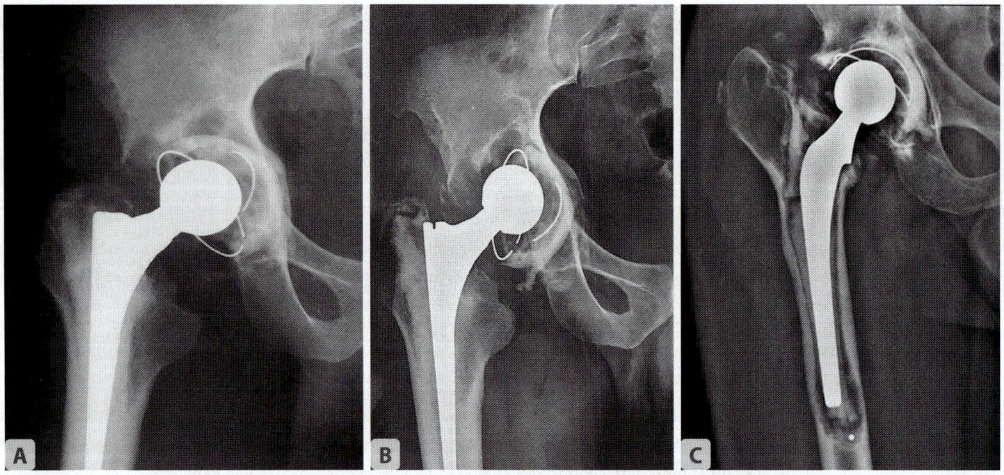

FIGS. 14A TO C: Complications of joint prosthesis: (A and B) Serial radiographs show development of lucency around acetabular implant (due to particle disease) causing osteolysis, protrusio, and implant failure; (C) Another patient with aseptic osteolysis and development of periprosthetic radiolucency.

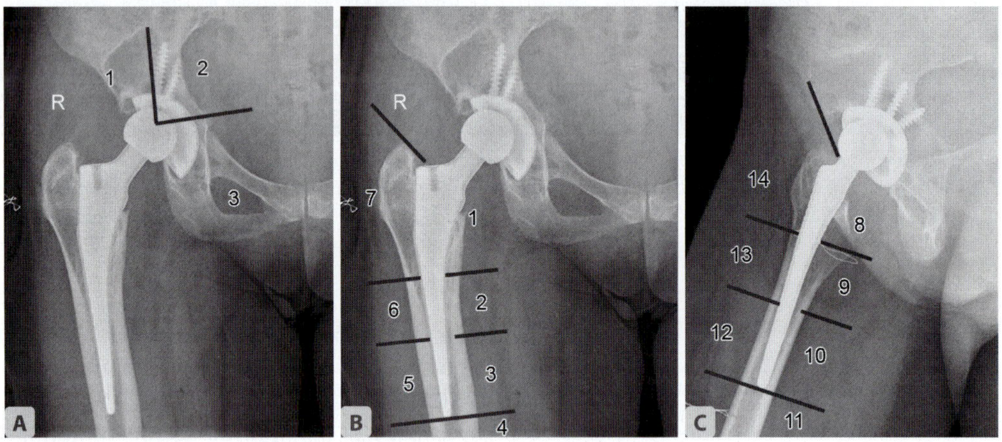

FIGS. 15A TO C: (A and B) Anterioposterior (AP); and (C) Lateral radiographs showing three zones to describe acetabular lucency, seven zones for femoral lucency on frontal and seven zones on lateral projection.

Fracture/Dislocation

Fractures can occur intraoperatively or after surgery secondary to trauma. In the hip, femoral component is more prone to fracture while in TKR, patella has the maximum propensity to fracture followed by femur and tibia. The propensity of implant fractures has reduced because of the use of high strength metal alloys. Fracture of the femur may occur in THR during the placement of the stem of the femoral implant. Causes of fracture include osteolysis, osteoporosis, falls in elderly patients or prosthetic malalignment **(Figs. 17A and B)**. Dislocation is rare after primary arthroplasty; however, is common in revision THR.[11]

Metallosis/Pseudotumors

Toxicity of metal ions can incite lymphocyte predominant immunological response (similar to type 4 hypersensitivity reaction). This is known as adverse reaction to metal debris or metallosis and histologically it is known as aseptic lymphocyte-dominated vasculitis-associated lesion (ALVAL).[4] These present as mass-forming collections, known as pseudotumors, which are neither neoplastic nor infective. Metal-on-metal THRs are the usual culprits with elevated serum chromium and cobalt levels (>17 µg/L and >19 µg/L respectively) in corresponding prosthesis associated with metallosis. Radiographs may show soft tissue density mass around the implant, which can cause erosions or bony destruction, and may mimic like aggressive bone tumor **(Figs. 18A to C)**. Ultrasound demonstrates these lesions as collections which may be anechoic or filled with echogenic debris and associated synovial thickening. On MRI, these lesions usually have a well-defined T2-hypointense wall. The contents are usually hypointense on T2W and hyperintense on T1W images **(Figs. 5 and 18)**.

Heterotopic Ossification

Another complication of joint prosthesis (especially hip) is heterotopic ossification and risk factors include elderly (>65 years) age, male gender, seronegative spondyloarthropathy, and diffuse idiopathic skeletal hyperostosis.

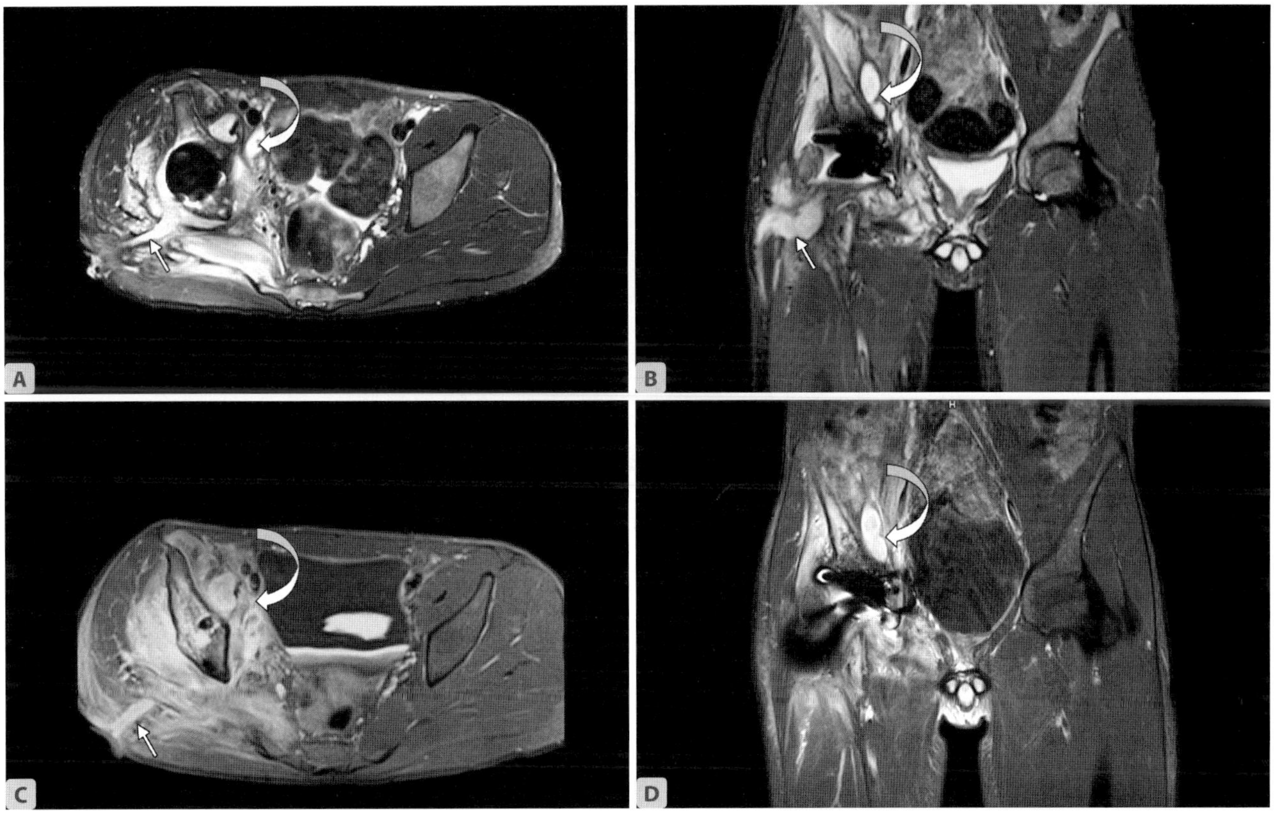

FIGS. 16A TO D: (A) Axial short-tau inversion recovery (STIR); (B) Coronal STIR; (C) Axial; and (D) Coronal postcontrast magnetic resonance (MR) images show presence of right hip synovitis and soft tissue edema. Note made of multiple fluid collections and lymphadenopathy (curved arrows) in addition to sinus tract reaching the skin (arrow), suggesting active infection.

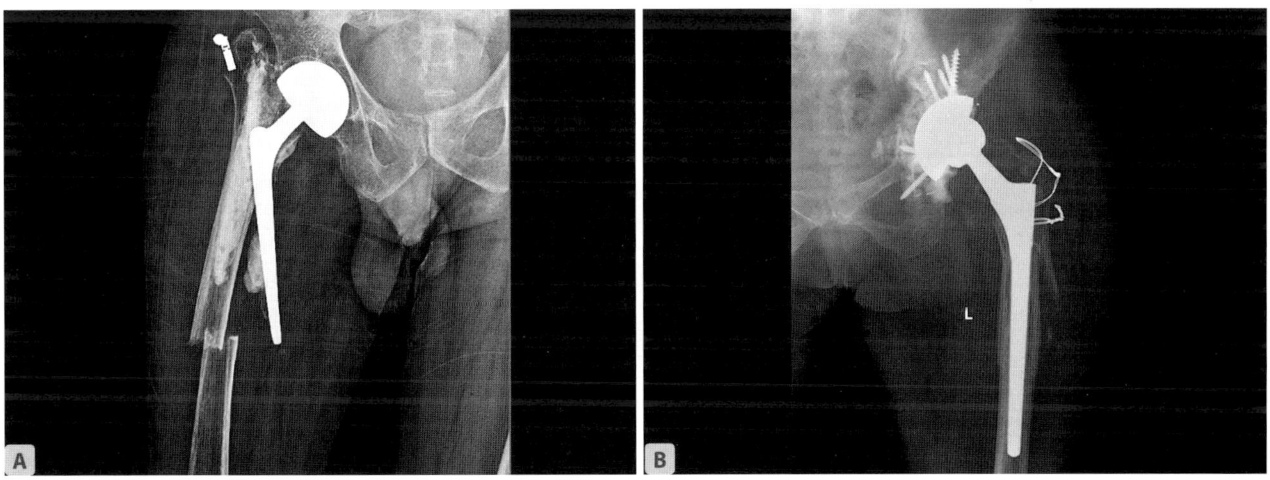

FIGS. 17A AND B: Postimplant periprosthetic fractures: (A) Radiograph shows fracture femoral shaft; (B) Osteolysis in femoral neck with fracture proximal shaft.

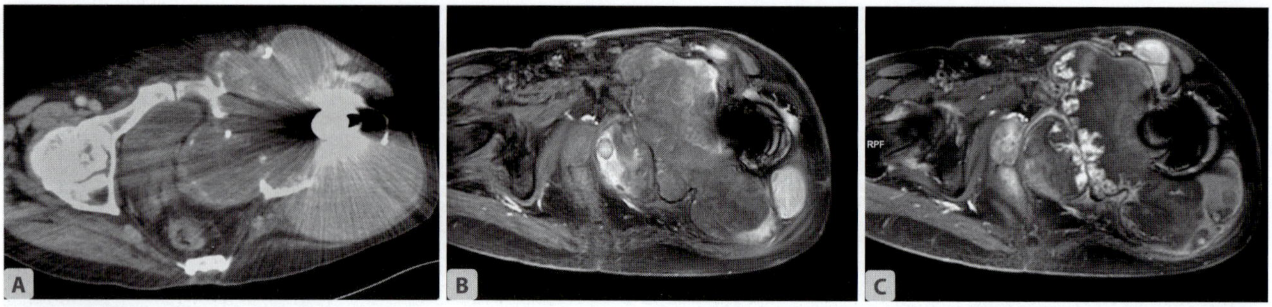

FIGS. 18A TO C: (A) Axial computed tomography (CT) image shows large destructive mass post left total hip replacement (THR) causing expansion and bone lysis; (B) Axial T1-wighted fat-suppressed image shows heterogeneous signal mass with peripheral hyperintensity; (C) Axial postcontrast image shows heterogeneous enhancement of soft tissue mass. Aspiration revealed sterile viscous dark colored fluid, consistent with the diagnosis of pseudotumor.

It is graded as per Brooker classification, which depends of the extent of involvement of the space between the femur and pelvis.

Soft Tissue Injury

There may be injury to the tendon and muscles leading on to tears and tendinosis, especially at the myotendinous junctions. Predisposed structures include abductor tendons of the hip, the iliopsoas, quadriceps, and patellar tendon and the rotator cuff tendons of the shoulder.[4]

CONCLUSION

With increasing number of joint replacements performed these days, it is imperative for the radiologists to be aware of the normal expected postoperative findings and interpret any abnormality diligently for early detection of complications. Radiographs are the most commonly used imaging modality and serial follow-up is important. Ultrasound, CT, and metal-suppression MRI are used for further evaluation and leukocyte scintigraphy is helpful to diagnose infection.

REFERENCES

1. Taljanovic MS, Jones MD, Hunter TB, Benjamin JB, Ruth JT, Brown AW, et al. Joint arthroplasties and prostheses. Radiographics. 2003;23(5):1295-314.
2. Mulcahy H, Chew FS. Current concepts of hip arthroplasty for radiologists: part 1, features and radiographic assessment. AJR Am J Roentgenol. 2012;199(3):559-69.
3. Roth TD, Maertz NA, Parr JA, Buckwalter KA, Choplin RH. CT of the hip prosthesis: appearance of components, fixation, and complications. Radiographics. 2012;32(4):1089-107.
4. Talbot BS, Weinberg EP. MR imaging with metal-suppression sequences for evaluation of total joint arthroplasty. Radiographics. 2015;36(1):209-25.
5. Vanrusselt J, Vansevenant M, Vanderschueren G, Vanhoenacker F. Postoperative radiograph of the hip arthroplasty: what the radiologist should know. Insights Imaging. 2015;6(6):591-600.
6. Fujishiro T, Hayashi S, Kanzaki N, Hashimoto S, Kurosaka M, Kanno T, et al. Computed tomographic measurement of acetabular and femoral component version in total hip arthroplasty. Int Orthop. 2014;38(5):941-6.
7. De Valk EJ, Noorduyn JCA, Mutsaerts EL. How to assess femoral and tibial component rotation after total knee arthroplasty with computed tomography: a systematic review. Knee Surg Sports Traumatol Arthrosc. 2016;24(11):3517-28.
8. DeLee JG, Charnley J. Radiological demarcation of cemented sockets in total hip replacement. Clin Orthop Relat Res. 1976;121:20-32.
9. Johnston RC, Fitzgerald RH, Harris WH, Poss R, Müller ME, Sledge CB. Clinical and radiographic evaluation of total hip replacement. A standard system of terminology for reporting results. J Bone Joint Surg Am. 1990;72(2):161-8.
10. Fritz J, Lurie B, Potter HG. MR imaging of knee arthroplasty implants. Radiographics. 2015;35(5):1483-501.
11. Manaster BJ. From the RSNA refresher courses. Total hip arthroplasty: radiographic evaluation. Radiographics. 1996;16(3):645-60.

CHAPTER

176

A Systematic Approach to Imaging of Breast Lesions

Smita Manchanda, Smriti Hari, Manisha Jana, Arun Kumar Gupta

INTRODUCTION

Imaging plays a crucial role in the early detection and accurate diagnosis of breast cancer, the first-line investigations being mammography and ultrasound (US). Magnetic resonance imaging (MRI) has a high sensitivity for breast pathology and is a valuable second-line investigation. Mammographic early detection of breast cancer has proven reduction in mortality.[1] In the screening setup, the sensitivity of mammography in detection of breast malignancy is in the range of 83–95%.[2] But in radiographically dense breasts, this sensitivity decreases to as low as 30–48%.[3]

IMAGING TECHNIQUES

MAMMOGRAPHY

Mammography is technically challenging as it requires excellent soft tissue contrast, high spatial resolution, and wide image latitude especially in denser breasts combined with a low radiation dose. The mammography equipment and technique has to account for the wide variation in breast size and also the relative amounts of fat, glandular and stromal tissue. Also, there is a low inherent contrast between normal and abnormal breast tissue.

Mammography Equipment

Dedicated mammography X-ray equipment **(Fig. 1)** with following features is necessary for producing high-quality images:

- *Tube current:* As high as possible to keep exposure time short.
- *Target-filter combination:* Molybdenum target with 0.03 mm molybdenum filter.
  - *Special X-ray tubes with molybdenum or rhodium anodes:* Low energy X-rays required necessary to achieve high tissue contrast.
  - *Adding filters at the source of the X-ray beam:* This removes the very low energy photons which are likely to be absorbed in the breast (do not contribute in the image formation).

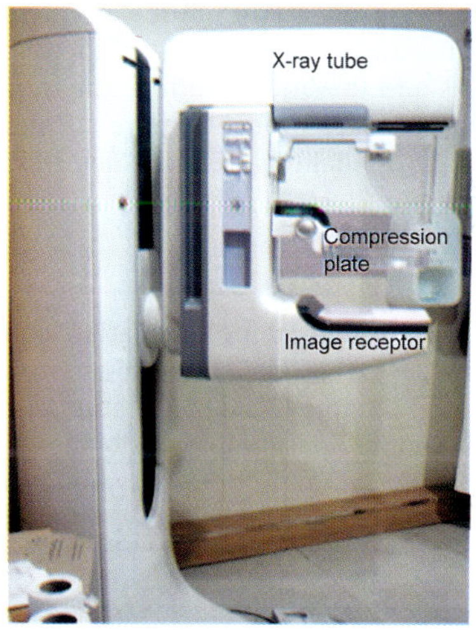

FIG. 1: Mammography equipment. Modern mammography machines automatically select target/filter combination, peak kilovoltage (kVp) and tube current according to breast density and the thickness of the compressed breast.

- *Peak kilovoltage (kVp):* Range 26–30 kV.
- High spatial resolution is essential to identify microcalcifications measuring in the order of 100 μm.
  - Small focal spot of the X-ray tube (0.3 mm for routine mammography and 0.1 mm for magnification mammography).
  - High-resolution film-screen combinations.
- Grids are used to reduce scattered radiation and to increase contrast, especially in the dense or thick breast.
- *Automated exposure control:* Modern equipment automatically selects target/filter combination, kVp and tube current according to breast density and the thickness of the compressed breast, e.g., higher energy X-ray spectrum for large breasts for sufficient penetration. These devices also control the exposure duration so that the optimum optical density of the mammograms is maintained over a wide range of breast densities and sizes. The automatic exposure control device (phototimer or ionization chamber) is normally positioned 3 cm

posterior to the nipple, where the most dense glandular tissue is likely to be seen.
- *Single side emulsion film with a single intensifying screen:* For optimum resolution. Specially designed cassettes ensure good film-screen contact.
- *Breast compression:* Good breast compression with radiolucent compression paddle is essential for mammography. This results in uniform thickness and hence uniform exposure and density in most parts of the breast. Separation of the overlapping tissues improves their visualization. Firm compression of the breast closer to film/image receptor also helps to reduce the geometric blur and magnification. As the breast is stabilized, the movement blur is also reduced. Mammography cannot be performed if breast compression is not possible (example in uncooperative women, tender breasts, presence of wound or recent surgery).
- *Quality control:* Good quality control is essential and includes periodic maintenance of the equipment, positioning and exposure, film processing, viewing conditions and the interpretation. The requirements of mammography are probably more stringent than any other imaging modality for accurate detection and disease characterization.

Mammography Projections

The standard mammographic evaluation consists of two orthogonal images for basic imaging evaluation of each breast: (1) mediolateral oblique (MLO) view and (2) craniocaudal (CC) view. The entire breast cannot be included in any single mammographic view. More breast tissue is shown on the MLO projection than on any other view.

Mediolateral Oblique View

It is obtained with the tube angled at 45° to the horizontal, with compression applied obliquely across the chest wall, perpendicular to the long axis of the pectoralis major muscle **(Fig. 2A)**.

Craniocaudal View of Breast

It is obtained with a vertical X-ray beam. The breast is pulled up and forward, away from the chest wall and compression is applied from above **(Fig. 2B)**. It demonstrates the subareolar, medial and lateral portions of the breast; however, tissue in the posterolateral aspect of the breast may not be documented completely. The criteria for well-positioned MLO and CC views are given in **Box 1**.

Supplementary Views

These can be taken to solve specific diagnostic problems.

Rolled View

These separate normal fibroglandular elements into their individual components. The breast tissue is "rolled" and compressed in the same projection in which the finding was first noted. On the rolled view, true masses will retain their shape and persist; whereas if it is separated into its normal fibroglandular components, it represents a summation shadow.

Magnification View (Figs. 4A and B)

Magnification is required for analysis of microcalcifications and the margins of small mass lesions. This can be done by increasing the film-object distance, producing an "air gap", and using a fine focal spot to increase resolution.

Spot Compression View

This is obtained by using a small compression paddle with or without magnification. Compression displaces the breast tissue overlying a small lesion and there is better delineation of morphologic features. Spot compression view also helps to differentiate the cause of asymmetrical soft tissue shadows as normal glandular tissue or underlying mass lesion.

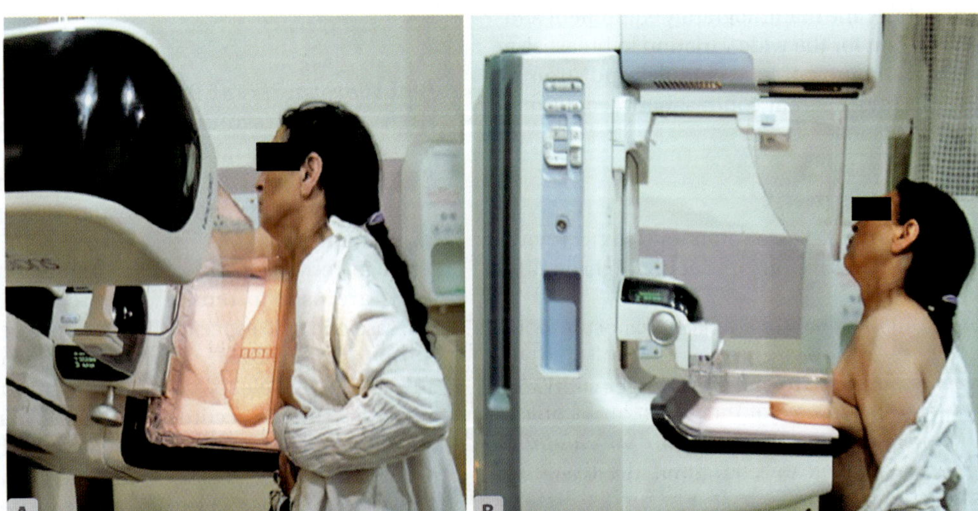

FIGS. 2A AND B: Positioning for mediolateral oblique (MLO) and craniocaudal (CC) views. (A) MLO view. The MLO view is obtained with the tube angled at 45° to the horizontal, with compression applied obliquely across the chest wall, perpendicular to the long axis of the pectoralis major muscle; (B) CC view. Positioning is achieved by pulling the breast up and forward, away from the chest wall, with compression applied from above.

Box 1: Criteria for well-positioned mediolateral oblique (MLO) and craniocaudal (CC) views.

Criteria for a well-positioned MLO view ***(Fig. 3A)***:

- Nipple to be seen in profile
- Pectoralis muscle should extend inferior to the posterior nipple line (PNL)

  (PNL is an imaginary line drawn from the nipple to the pectoralis muscle or film edge and is perpendicular to pectoralis muscle)
- Visible open inframammary fold
- No superimposition of skin folds on the breast

Criteria for a well-positioned CC view ***(Fig. 3B)***:

- Nipple to be demonstrated in profile
- The PNL on the CC view is drawn from the nipple to the pectoralis muscle or film edge. Length of PNL on the CC view should be within 1 cm of its length on the MLO view

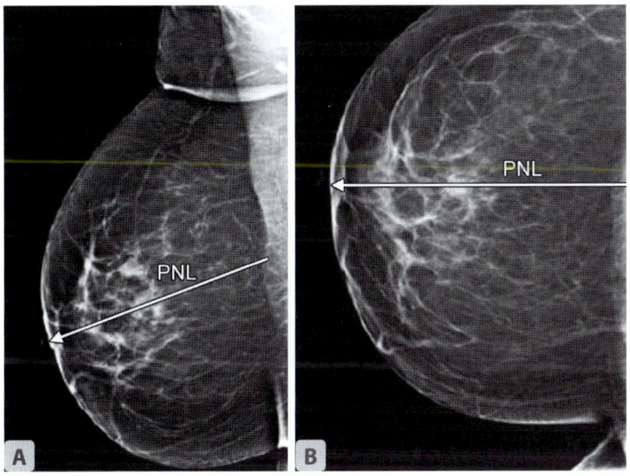

FIGS. 3A AND B: Well-positioned mediolateral oblique (MLO) and craniocaudal (CC) views. (A) A well-positioned MLO view should include breast tissue from high in the axilla to just below the inframammary fold. The pectoralis muscle should extend inferior to the posterior nipple line (PNL) an imaginary line drawn from the nipple to the pectoralis muscle or film edge and perpendicular to the pectoralis muscle; (B) An adequately positioned CC view should demonstrate the subareolar, medial and lateral portions of the breast. The PNL on the CC view is drawn from the nipple to the pectoralis muscle or film edge. The length of the PNL on the CC view should be within 1 cm of its length on the MLO projection.

Extended Craniocaudal View

This view is performed by rotating the patient's body to display the lateral or medial breast tissue better than possible with a standard CC view. When the patient is rotated medially, the lateral part of the breast and axillary tail is brought over the film and the medial portion of the breast is excluded. This well demonstrates the tissue in most posterolateral part of the breast. For medial breast lesions, the patient is rotated laterally to bring the medial part of the breast over the film and the outer breast tissue is excluded.

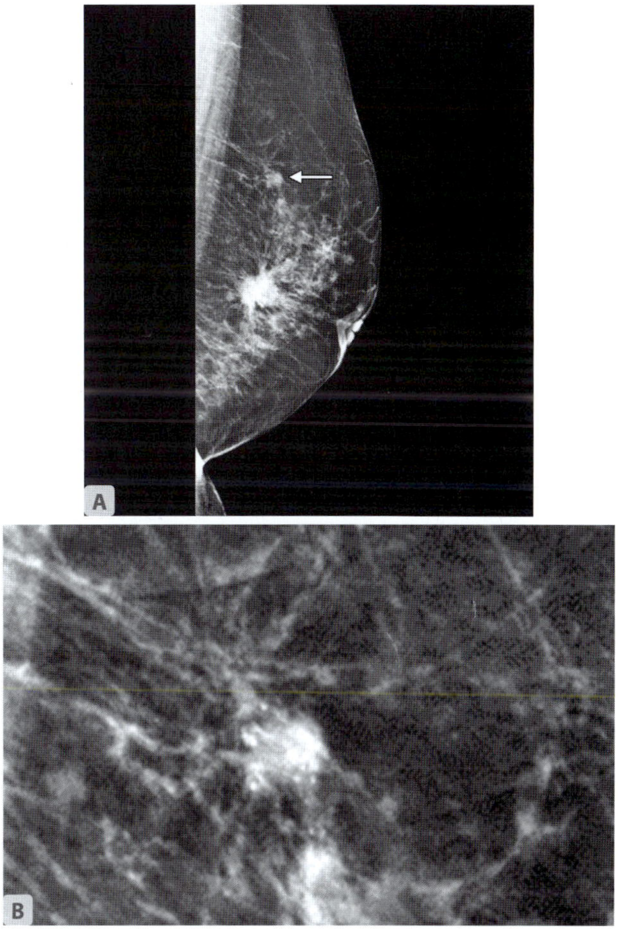

FIGS. 4A AND B: Left mediolateral oblique (MLO) (A) and magnification mammography (B). Margins of the mass in upper outer quadrant of left breast (arrow in A) are better seen on magnification mammography.

Indications for Mammography

Mammography is not usually done in pregnant or lactating women and is generally avoided in women below 30 years of age. The major indications for mammography are listed in **Box 2**.

Normal Mammographic Anatomy

There are 15–20 lobes in the breast. A single lactiferous duct drains each lobe and repeatedly branches within breast. Terminal ducts are the distal most branches and they have extralobular and intralobular portions **(Fig. 5)**. Lobule is formed by the intralobular portion and the acini. The lobule and extralobular duct form the terminal ductal lobular unit (TDLU). This TDLU is the site of beginning of most malignant and benign disease of the breast.

Mammographic Appearance

It depends on the relative amounts of fat and glandular tissue.

- *Young woman's breast:* Large amount of glandular tissue (soft tissue density)

- *Older women:* Involution of glandular tissue has occurred and mostly fatty density.

Normal lymph node: An oval or lobulated dense mass with a radiolucent fatty hilum.

- *Intramammary lymph nodes:* Within the breast in the upper outer quadrant
- Normal lymph nodes often seen in the axilla.

Nipple:
- Usually everted
- Should be seen in profile on at least one mammographic view (retroareolar region can be visualized without superimposition of nipple)
- It can be inverted since birth as a normal variant
- Recent nipple inversion is of concern for a retroareolar mass.

Box 2: Indications for mammography.

- Screening asymptomatic women age ≥50 years
- Screening asymptomatic women aged ≥35 years with high risk of developing breast malignancy
  - Women with have one or more first-degree relatives diagnosed with premenopausal breast malignancy
  - Women with histologic risk factors at previous surgery, e.g., atypical ductal hyperplasia
- Symptomatic women aged 35 years with breast lump or any other clinical evidence of breast tumor
- For occult primary tumor, search in patients presenting with metastases
- Postoperative surveillance of breast following local excision of breast cancer
- Breast lump in a male

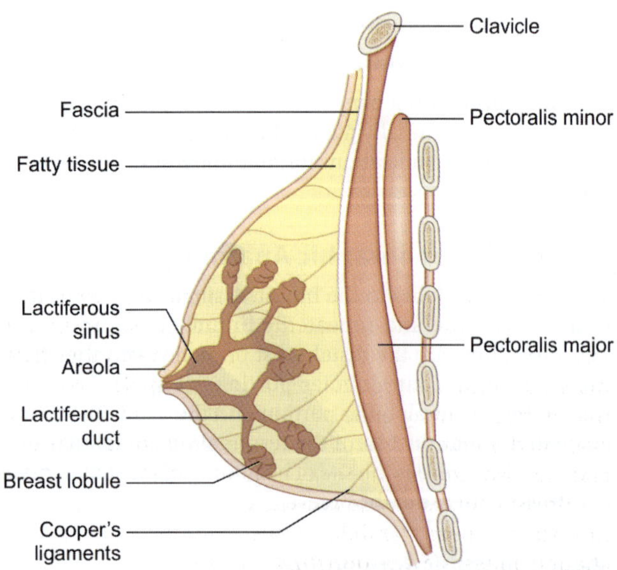

FIG. 5: Schematic representation of the breast anatomy.

Interpretation and Reporting of Mammograms

Viewing:
- Ideally on console [two-dimensional (2D) and tomosynthesis images]

Films:
- In optimum lighting conditions and exclude light from around the films and inessential light in the viewing room
- Check for correct labeling and for radiographic quality
- Standard MLO and CC views studied with right and left breast films "back to back"
- Essential to examine the symmetry of breast tissue.

Breast Imaging—Reporting and Data System

The American College of Radiology (ACR) has devised the Breast Imaging-Reporting and Data System (BI-RADS) for mammogram, US, and MRI. This is a standardized method to describe the morphology of breast lesions and categorize these findings in a definite report. For this lesion description and assessment, there is a lexicon of descriptive terms and the main intention is to provide a common language and ensure consistency in reports. Currently the 5th edition, which was released in 2013, is in use.[4]

Breast Density

The breast density/composition is an evaluation of the relative amounts of fat and fibroglandular tissue in the breast and should be evaluated first while interpreting a mammogram. It is important to remember that the diagnostic accuracy of mammogram falls with increased density of breast. In the 4th edition of ACR lexicon, percentage values of fibroglandular tissue were assessed and reported in increments of 25%. The current ACR BI-RADS divides breast composition into four major categories (from least dense to most dense) based on visual assessment of the mammographic density **(Box 3)**.

The abnormal mammographic finding is then categorized as a mass, calcification, architectural distortion or asymmetry. Other findings include intramammary lymph node, skin lesion, and solitary dilated duct.

Mass

A breast mass is defined as a three-dimensional (3D) space-occupying lesion, seen in two mammographic views (ACR BI-RADS lexicon). Mass evaluation is optimally done in a spot compression magnification view in which the mass is superimposed over the surrounding fat.

Box 3: ACR BI-RADS categories of breast density (Figs. 6A to D).

- Breast tissue almost entirely fatty
- Scattered fibroglandular tissue
- Heterogeneously dense breasts
- Extremely dense breast (lowers the sensitivity of mammograhy)

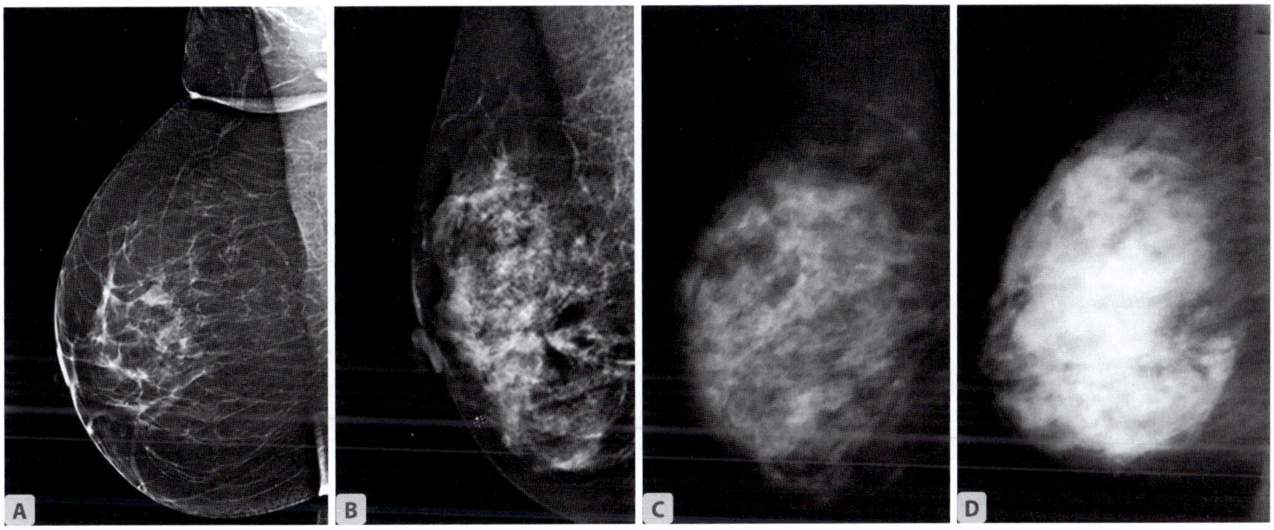

FIGS. 6A TO D: The American College of Radiology (ACR) categories of breast parenchymal density. (A) Category A: breast tissue almost entirely fatty; (B) Category B: scattered fibroglandular tissue; (C) Category C: heterogeneously dense breasts; (D) Category D: extremely dense breast.

TABLE 1: ACR BI-RADS mass descriptors in mammography.

Characteristic	Term	Description
Shape	Round	Spherical
	Oval	Elliptical
	Irregular	Neither round nor oval
Margin	Circumscribed	Margins form a sharp, abrupt transition with the surrounding tissue
	Obscured	Normal surrounding tissue hides the true edge of the lesion
	Microlobulated	Short undulations at the surface of the lesion
	Indistinct	Demarcation between the mass and surrounding tissue is not clearly defined
	Spiculated	Sharp lines radiating from the margins of the mass
Density	High	High density relative to glandular parenchyma
	Equal	Similar density relative to glandular parenchyma
	Low	Less dense relative to glandular parenchyma
	Fat containing	Internal lucent area suggestive of fat

Mass should be described under the following headings:
- Size, morphology (shape, margin), density, associated calcifications, associated features, and location **(Table 1)**.

Size and Location: This should be clearly mentioned in the report in terms of quadrant and approximate clock of position.

Morphology

Shape

The shape of a mass may be round, oval or irregular **(Figs. 7A to C)** and as the shape becomes more irregular, the probability of malignancy increases. It is important to note that lobular shape descriptor is no longer used according to the ACR 5th edition.[5,6] Hence, a mass with two or three lobulations will be oval and further morphological description would be in terms of margins.

Margins

The margins can be circumscribed (sharply defined), obscured, microlobulated, indistinct or spiculated **(Figs. 8A to E)**. In general, this margin categorization is from least suspicious to most suspicious for malignancy. Benign masses have *well-circumscribed* borders as these do not invade tissue margins. Term *obscured margin* is used when all or part of the margin abuts glandular parenchyma and cannot be evaluated precisely. *Microlobulations* are small undulations and are suspicious for malignancy.

Breast cancers invade basement membrane and extend into surrounding glandular tissue resulting in irregularly shaped masses with indistinct or spiculated margins. *Spiculated margin* is highly suspicious for malignancy and is characterized by thin lines radiating from the central portion of the mass. Intense fibrotic reaction to tumor or growth of the cancer into surrounding glandular tissue can result in spiculations.

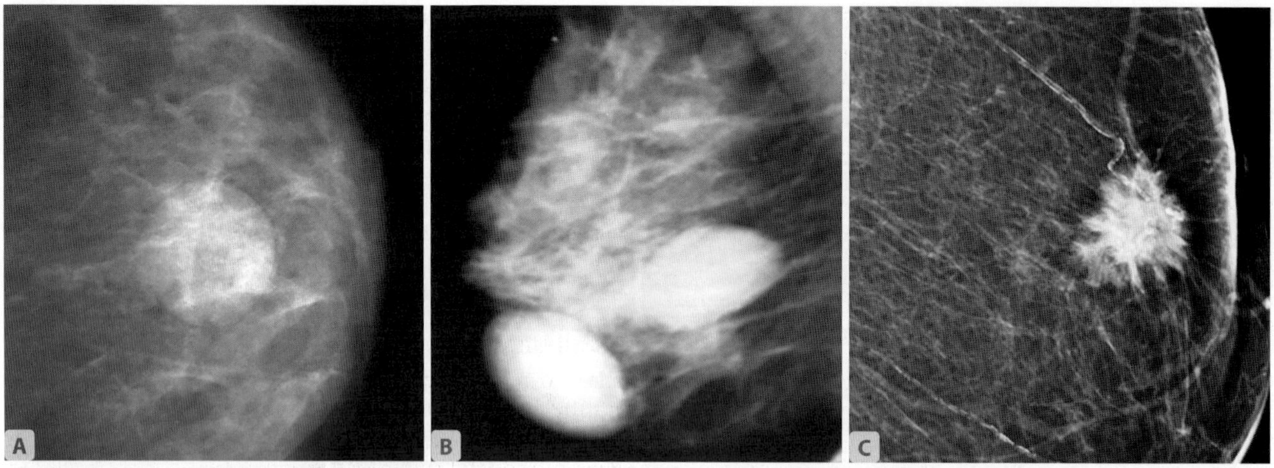

FIGS. 7A TO C: The American College of Radiology Breast Imaging-Reporting and Data System (ACR BI-RADS) descriptors for mass shape on mammography. (A) Round; (B) Oval; (C) Irregular.

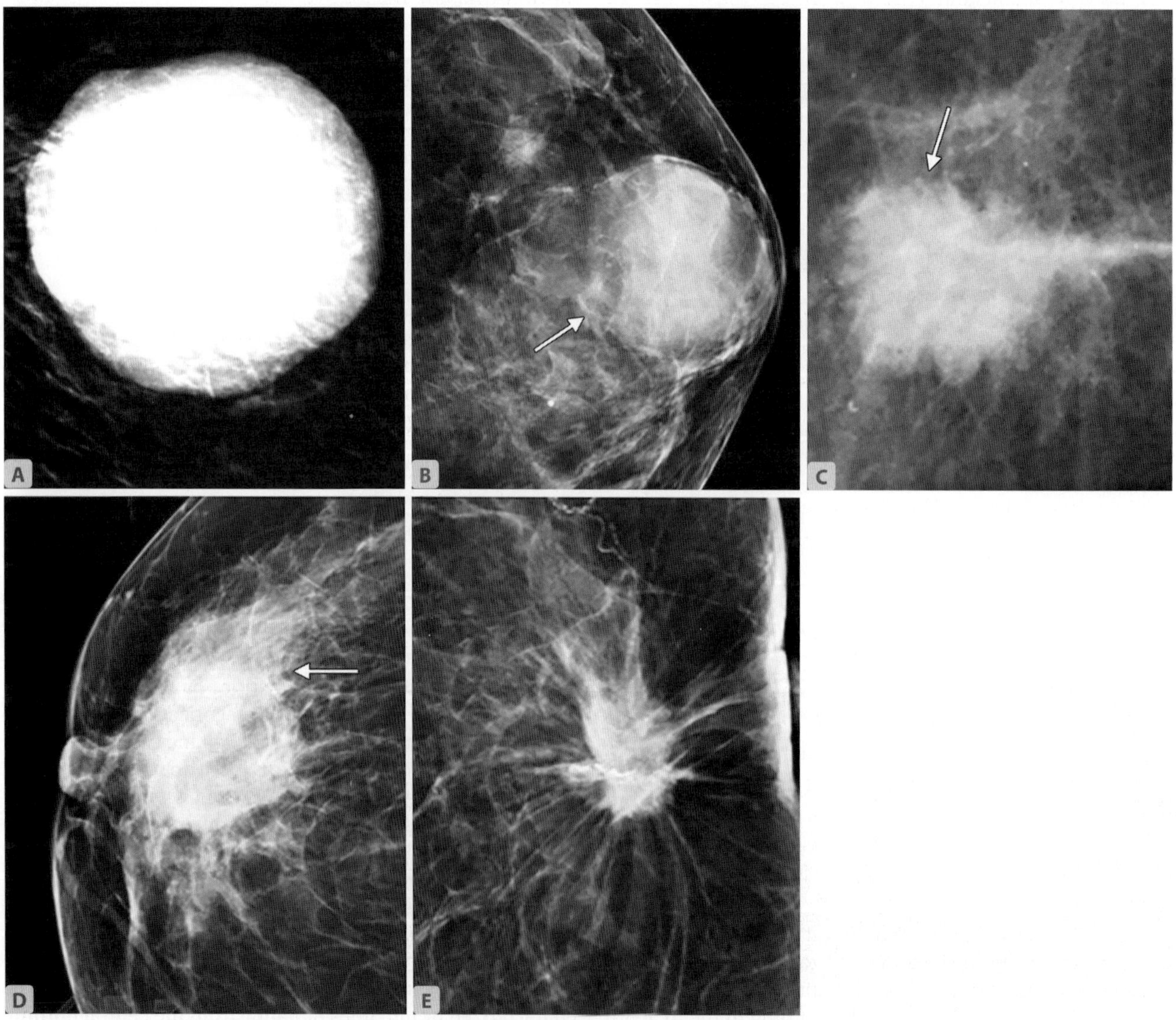

FIGS. 8A TO E: ACR BI-RADS descriptors for mass margins on mammography. (A) Circumscribed (sharply defined); (B) Obscured (arrow); (C) Microlobulated (arrow); (D) Indistinct (arrow); (E) Spiculated.

Density

Density is termed as high, equal or low relative to glandular breast parenchyma **(Figs. 9A to C)**. Density of the mass is not effective in characterization of the masses. Exception is fat-containing masses which are always benign and are described as such. The term "radiolucent" has been omitted in the current lexicon.

Calcification

Calcifications are commonly encountered on mammograms but majority of these are the result of benign processes. For description of calcifications, the following descriptors are used: morphology, distribution, associated features, and location.[6,7]

Morphology

Calcifications are broadly classified into typically benign calcifications and those of suspicious morphology **(Table 2)**.

Benign Calcifications (Figs. 10A to F)

Most benign calcifications are >0.5 mm. Typically benign calcifications include lucent-centered calcifications (skin calcifications or fat necrosis), vascular calcifications, popcorn calcifications of involuted fibroadenoma, eggshell or rim calcifications, long rod-like ductal calcifications and coarse dystrophic calcifications. The new lexicon includes eggshell and lucent-centered calcifications under the term "rim". The term "round" includes round and punctate calcifications.

Suspicious Morphology Category (Figs. 11A to D)

Amorphous: Tiny, roundish "flake-like" particles too small and vague to characterize further, 27% probability of malignancy. Edges not as sharply defined as in the pleomorphic category. These are often difficult to detect as their density is only slightly higher than surrounding glandular tissue.[5]

Coarse Heterogeneous

Irregular, conspicuous and >0.5 mm, 13% probability of malignancy.

Fine pleomorphic: Varying in shape and density, irregular, <0.5 mm (microcalcifications), 50% probability of malignancy.

Fine Linear or Fine-linear Branching (Casting) Calcifications

These form an irregular cast of the duct and appear as little broken needles with sharp ends or "dot-dash" appearance with both linear and round shapes, 78% probability of malignancy. Ductal carcinoma in situ (DCIS) develops in breast duct epithelium, remains within the duct basement membrane, and grows along the duct. Individual calcifications form within the DCIS tumor because of cell death and necrosis in the comedo form of DCIS.

Distribution

The distribution of calcifications **(Table 2 and Figs. 12A to D)** within the breast often may allow benign and malignant categorization. The TDLU is the anatomic site of origin of most intraductal carcinomas. Thus, calcifications oriented in a "linear" or multiple linear ("segmental") orientation are more suspicious. For example, linear or segmental arrangements of coarse heterogeneous calcifications are more worrisome than a regional distribution of the same calcifications.[5,7]

Grouped microcalcifications occupy <1 cm^3 of tissue and are composed of at least five elements. The new lexicon also includes "a larger number of calcifications within 2 cm of each other" under this category of grouped calcifications.

Architectural Distortion

Architectural distortion implies focal distortion/tethering of trabeculae, focal spiculations and retraction of parenchyma.

Imaging

Architectural distortion is characterized by multiple thin, straight lines or spiculations radiating from an area with no obvious features of an underlying mass or focal asymmetry **(Fig. 13)**. It is important to remember that these radiating spicules can also be seen from the edge of a mass or focal asymmetry where it is a margin descriptor. At times, it is difficult to differentiate spiculated mass from architectural distortion; however, the presence of these radially oriented lines is highly suspicious for malignancy.

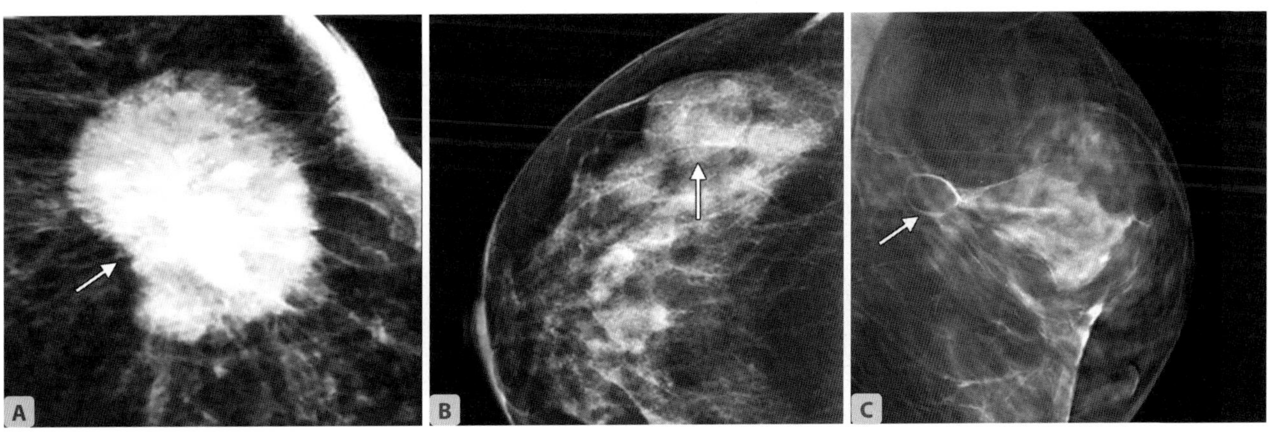

FIGS. 9A TO C: ACR BI-RADS descriptors for mass density (as compared to the fibroglandular parenchyma) on mammography. (A) High-density mass (arrow); (B) Isodense mass (arrow); (C) Fat attenuation (arrow).

TABLE 2: Specific ACR BI-RADS terms for description of calcifications.

Characteristic	Term	Description
Distribution	Segmental	Five or more calcifications in a cubic centimeter of tissue constitutes a cluster
	Linear	Fine-linear branching pattern produced by calcification of necrotic cancer cells within a duct
	Grouped	Calcifications within a single duct network of a lobe
	Regional	Randomly distributed calcifications not conforming to a duct and usually occupying a quadrant or more
	Diffuse	Randomly distributed calcifications throughout the entire breast
Morphology (typically benign)	Skin	Sharply defined with lucent center
	Vascular	Parallel tram-track calcification
	Coarse or "popcorn-like"	Characteristic of involuting fibroadenoma
	Large rod-like	Secretory calcifications—calcified debris in the duct lumen (solid rods), calcified inflammatory reaction around a duct (lucent-centered rods)
	Round	Concretions formed in the acini of microcystically dilated lobules
	Rim	Very thin, benign calcifications that appear as calcium deposited on the surface of a sphere
	Dystrophic	Large (>0.5 mm), irregular (post-trauma or radiotherapy)
	Milk of calcium	
	Suture	Typically linear or tubular in appearance, and knots are frequently visible
Suspicious morphology	Amorphous	Round or flake-shaped deposits those are too small or hazy to characterize
	Coarse heterogeneous	Irregular, dense calcifications >0.5 mm in size
	Fine pleomorphic	Irregular, vary in size and shape, and are <0.5 mm
	Fine linear or fine-linear branching	Thin, discontinuous, irregular particles that form in a linear pattern and are < 1 mm in width (calcifications of necrotic tumor in the lumen of a duct that is irregularly involved by breast cancer)

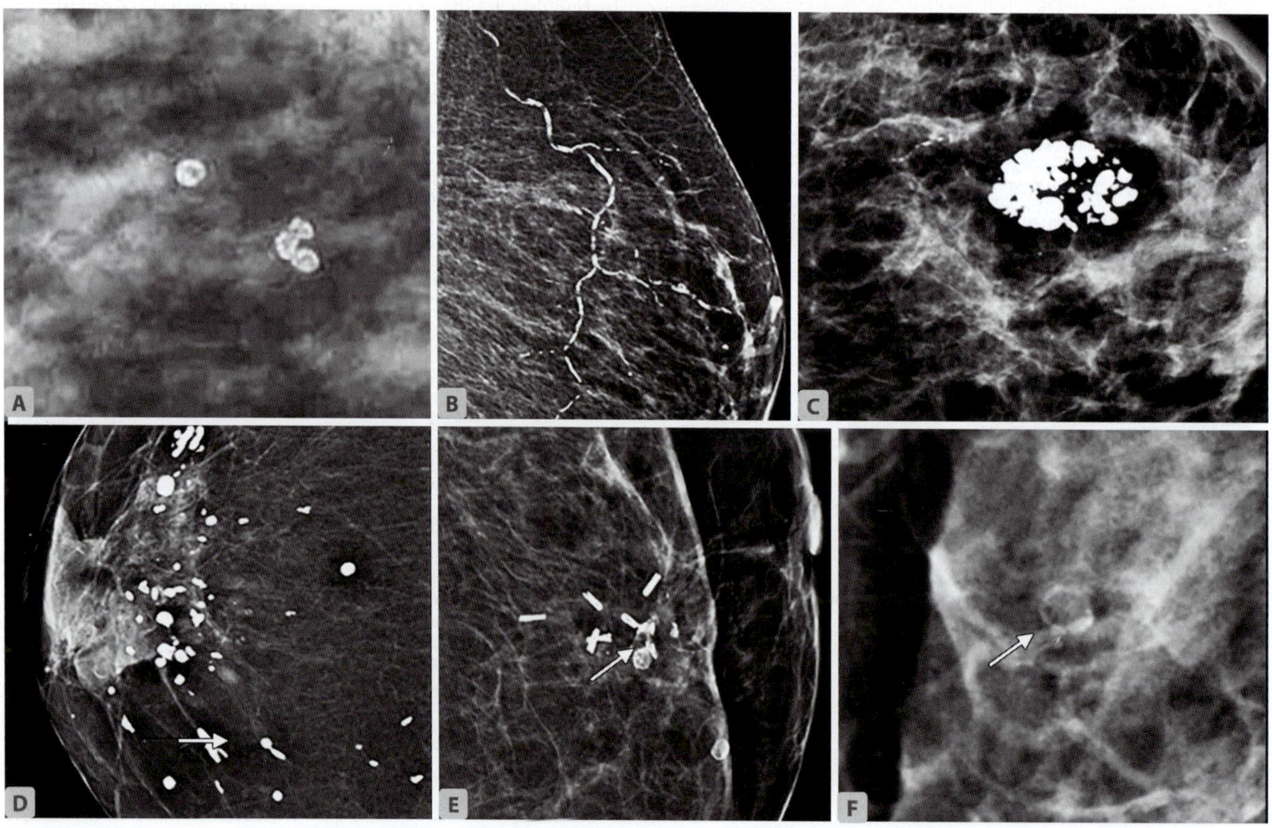

FIGS. 10A TO F: Typically benign calcifications. (A) Lucent-centered calcifications consistent with skin calcifications; (B) Vascular calcification; (C) Popcorn calcifications within involuted fibroadenoma; (D) Large rod-like (arrow) and round calcifications; (E) Coarse dystrophic calcifications (arrow) and sutures seen in a postoperative breast; (F) Milk of calcium (secretory) (arrow).

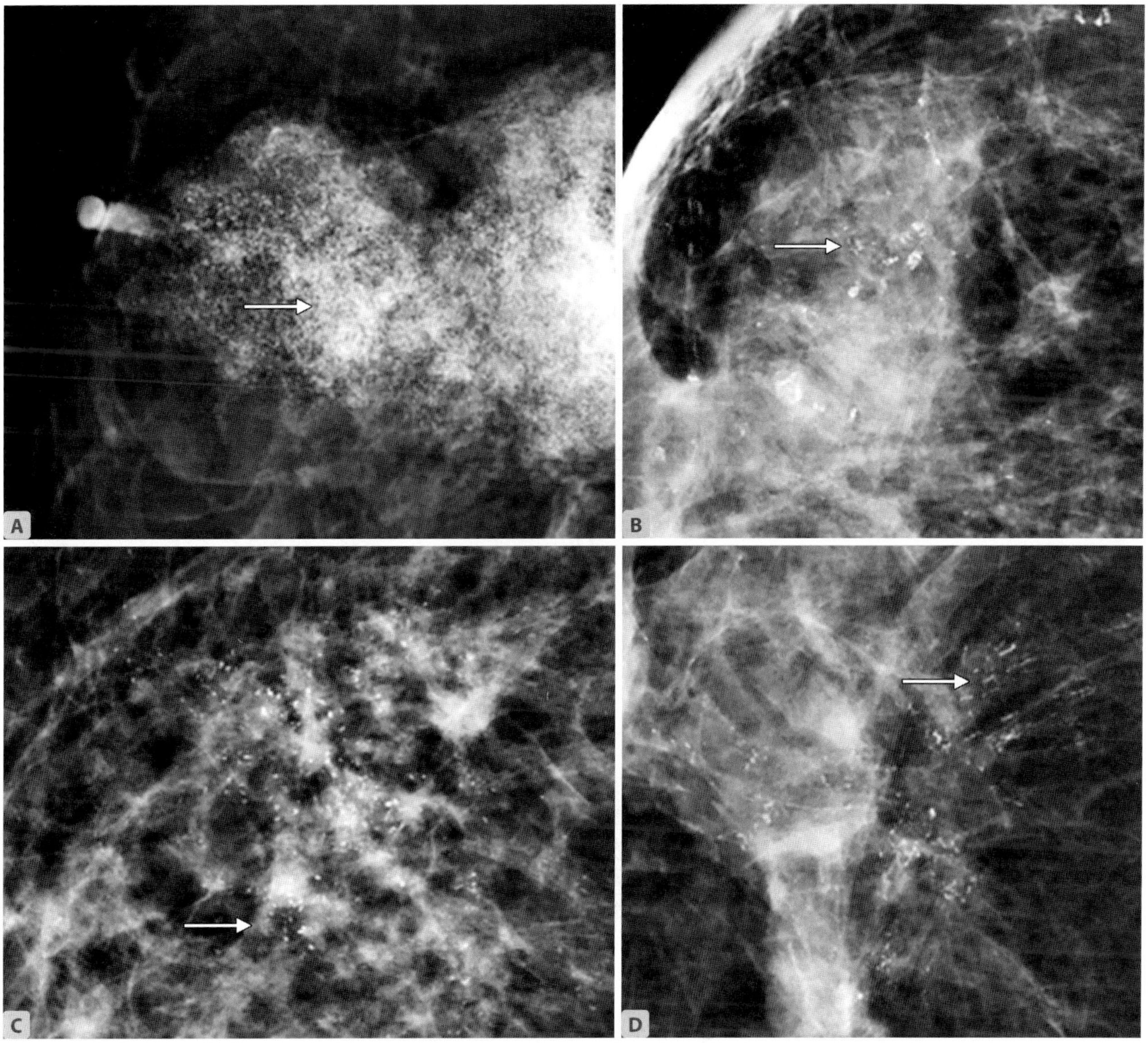

FIGS. 11A TO D: Calcifications of suspicious morphology. (A) Amorphous (arrow); (B) Coarse heterogeneous (arrow); (C) Fine pleomorphic (arrow); (D) Fine linear or fine-linear branching (arrow).

Differential Diagnosis[5,6]

This includes radial scar/complex sclerosing lesion, malignancy and postoperative scarring. In absence of surgical history, this finding requires a histological diagnosis.

Asymmetries

It is important to differentiate an asymmetry versus a focal asymmetry versus a mass.[6]

Asymmetry

Soft tissue finding identified only on one view, without matching tissue in a similar location in the contralateral breast.

Focal Asymmetry and Mass

These are seen on two views at a comparable depth with similar density and shape.

Mass: Consistent convex margins

Focal asymmetry: It lacks convex outward borders on both views **(Figs. 14A and B)** and usually confined to a small area of the breast.[6]

Global Asymmetry

In a larger portion of the breast (>1 quadrant). It can be a normal variation or secondary to the effects of hormone replacement therapy (HRT).

Developing Asymmetry

This is a new term introduced in the ACR 5th edition and is defined as "a focal asymmetry which is new or becomes more conspicuous over time". Developing asymmetry is of concern because if seen at screening mammography, there is 12.8% risk for malignancy and persistence at diagnostic mammography carries a 26.7% risk for malignancy.[8]

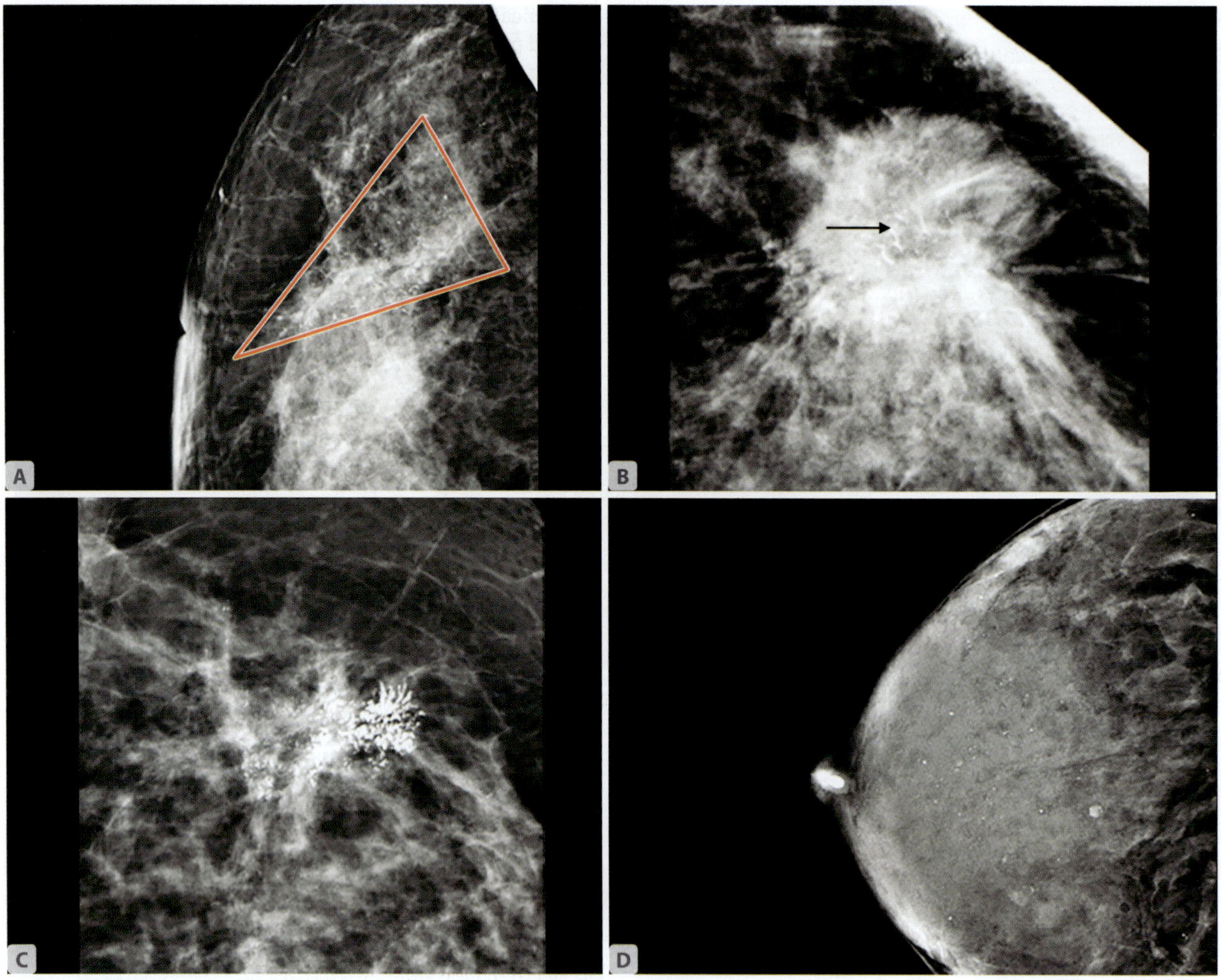

FIGS. 12A TO D: ACR BI-RADS descriptors for distribution of calcifications. (A) Segmental; (B) Linear (arrow); (C) Grouped; (D) Diffuse.

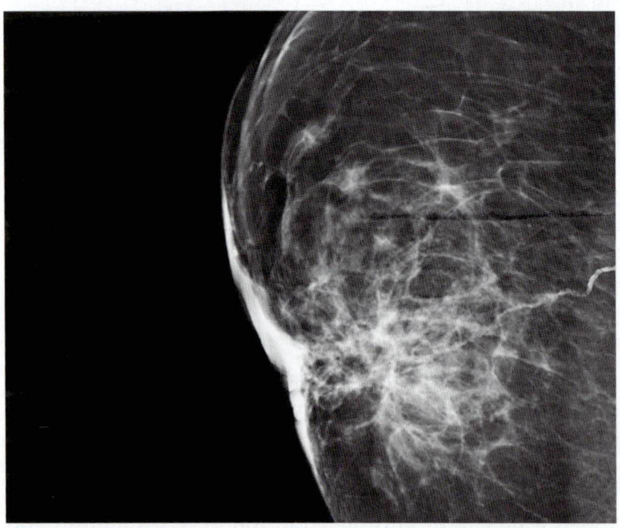

FIG. 13: Architectural distortion (postoperative breast). Mammogram showing multiple thin, straight lines radiating from a central area that does not have features of a mass. There is associated focal skin thickening and retraction.

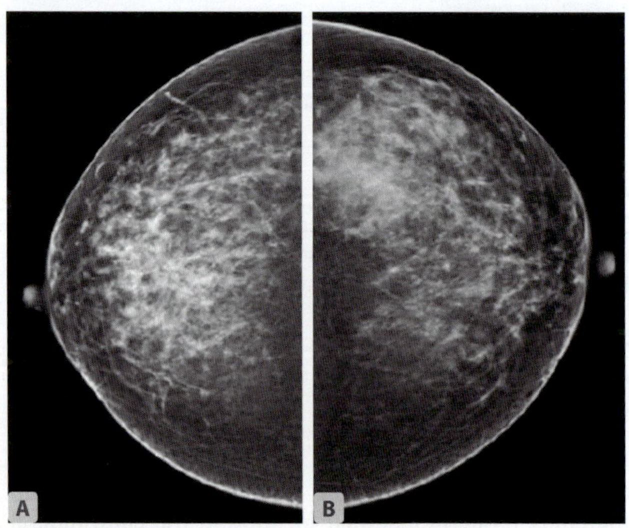

FIGS. 14A AND B: (A and B) Focal asymmetry. Bilateral craniocaudal (CC) views showing focal asymmetry in the left breast outer quadrant which was also seen on the mediolateral oblique (MLO) view. Ultrasound showed a suspicious mass. Invasive ductal carcinoma on histopathology.

Associated Features

Certain associated features have been described in the 5th edition for further characterization of mass, calcification and asymmetry. These include nipple retraction, skin retraction, trabecular thickening, skin thickening, axillary lymphadenopathy, architectural distortion, and calcifications.

Location of Lesion

This should include laterality, the depth of lesion, distance from nipple and quadrant and clock face.[4]

Special Cases

The terms intramammary lymph node, solitary dilated duct and skin lesion are the same as in BI-RADS fourth edition. Asymmetric tubular structure is no longer used now.[5,6] Breast edema and axillary lymph nodes are detailed here.

Breast Edema

Breast edema is recognized on mammograms as diffusely increased density and coarse trabecular pattern in an enlarged breast with thickened skin. The causes of an edematous breast are:

- Primary breast cancer. Lymphatic spread from an advanced primary tumor or inflammatory carcinoma can lead to breast edema.
- Axillary lymph node metastasis.
- Breast abscess.
- Radiotherapy (RT). Postradiotherapy treatment there is gradual progression of breast edema which reaches a maximum at 6 months. There is resolution approximately 18 months after RT treatment.
- Cardiac or renal failure: unilateral or bilateral breast edema.

Abnormal Axillary Lymph Nodes

Normal lymph nodes:

- Commonly seen on mammograms
- Typically, well-defined with central lucency (fatty hilum) and peripheral soft tissue attenuation
- Intramammary lymph nodes: Commonly in the upper outer quadrant with similar features.

Pathological lymph nodes:

- Enlarged and show loss of central fatty lucency
- Benign conditions like infection, sarcoidosis
- Malignant conditions like lymphoma, leukemia or metastasis.

Calcification in lymph nodes:

- Metastatic lymph nodes from breast cancer: Microcalcification
- Tubercular nodes: Coarse calcification.

ACR BI-RADS Assessment Categories

The mammographic findings are categorized from BI-RADS 0 to BI-RADS 6, which are primarily aimed for communication of significance of the mammographic findings to the referring physician and to recommend the most appropriate management **(Table 3)**.[4-6]

Mammographic Assessment is Incomplete

Category 0—Incomplete Evaluation

This category needs additional evaluation by imaging and/or comparison with previous mammograms.

Mammographic Assessment is Complete—Final Categories

Category 1—Negative

In this category, there is nothing specific to mention. Both the breasts are symmetric and there is no evidence of any mass, suspicious calcification or architectural distortion.

Category 2—Benign Finding

This category is also a normal assessment; however, lesions with characteristically benign findings are described here.

TABLE 3: ACR BI-RADS mammographic assessment categories.

Category	Description	Likelihood of malignancy	Examples	Next step in evaluation
0	Incomplete; need additional imaging evaluation, or comparison with previous examinations	Unknown	Asymmetry, mass, calcifications on screening mammography	Special mammographic views, US, MRI; obtain previous examinations
1	Negative	No mammographic evidence of malignancy	Normal mammography	Routine screening
2	Benign finding	No mammographic evidence of malignancy	Intramammary lymph node, oil cyst, vascular calcifications, calcifying fibroadenoma	Routine screening
3	Probably benign finding	<2%	Benign-appearing solid mass or clustered calcifications	Follow-up imaging (mammography or US) at 6 and 12 months
4	Suspicious abnormality	5–95%	Complex or solid mass, indeterminate clustered calcifications	Biopsy
5	Highly suggestive of malignancy	>95%	Spiculated mass	Biopsy
6	Known malignancy	100%	Biopsy-proven	Definitive treatment

This includes multiple secretory calcifications and involuting or calcified fibroadenomas. The fat-containing lesions (oil cysts, galactoceles, lipomas, hamartomas) also have characteristic appearances.

Other findings like intramammary lymph nodes, implants, vascular calcifications, or postoperative changes (architectural distortion/sutures) can also be mentioned in this category clearly stating that there is no mammographic evidence of malignancy.

Category 3—Probably Benign Finding

A finding in this category would have >0% chance of malignancy but <2%. This includes a nonpalpable well-circumscribed mass on mammogram, or cluster of punctate calcifications or a focal asymmetry. It is essential to document lesion stability on an initial short-term interval follow-up at 6 months; followed by additional examinations till long-term 2- or 3-year stability is documented.[7]

Category 4—Suspicious Abnormality

In this category, the probability of malignancy is large from 5 to 95% and it is further subdivided into 4A, 4B, and 4C.

BI-RADS 4A category: Lesions with a very low probability for malignancy. They are sampled but a malignant histopathology report is not expected. In these cases, a 6-month follow-up after a benign biopsy is suitable. Examples: palpable, partially circumscribed solid mass with sonography features suggestive of a fibroadenoma, a breast abscess or a palpable complicated cyst.

BI-RADS 4B category: Lesions with an intermediate probability of malignancy. Biopsy is recommended and close radiopathological correlation is warranted. If there is a benign biopsy report, follow-up depends on the concordance between imaging and pathological features.

For example, a partially circumscribed mass with ill-defined margins with a fibroadenoma result is satisfactory, but in case of a diagnosis of papillary lesion, surgery should be advised.

BI-RADS 4C category: These findings are of moderate concern, but not classical for malignancy and a malignant biopsy result is expected in this category. In case of a benign result, 6-month follow-up is essential to rule out a false-negative report.

Examples of findings placed in this category are recent cluster of fine pleomorphic calcifications solid, irregular masses with ill-defined margins.

Category 5—Highly Suggestive of Malignancy

Findings typical for classic breast cancers, with a >95% likelihood of malignancy.

Examples of findings suggestive of this category are: segmental or linear arrangement of fine-linear calcifications; spiculated, irregular high-density mass or irregular spiculated mass **(Figs. 15A and B)** with associated pleomorphic calcifications.

Category 6—Known Biopsy-proven Malignancy

In this category, lesions are identified on the imaging study of patients with biopsy diagnosis of malignancy.

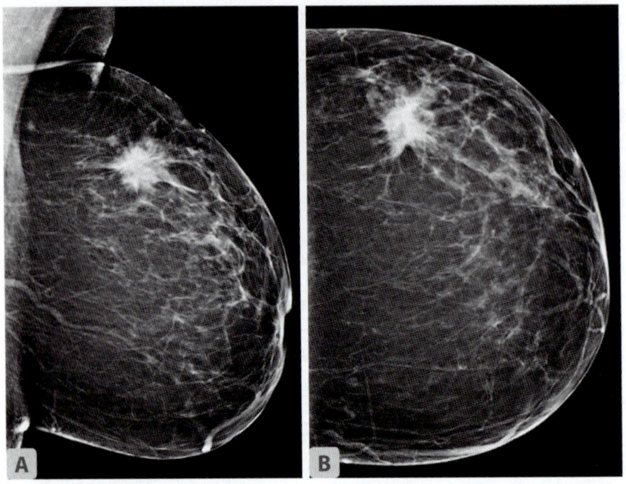

FIGS. 15A AND B: Illustrative example for ACR BI-RADS mammographic assessment categories. (A) Craniocaudal (CC) view; (B) Mediolateral oblique (MLO) view. High density, irregular shaped mass with spiculated margins in upper outer quadrant of left breast. Highly suggestive of malignancy lesion—BI-RADS 5.

Digital Mammography

Full-field digital mammography (FFDM) is now gradually replacing screen-film (conventional) mammography. The diagnostic yield is increased by newer applications of digital mammography like digital breast tomosynthesis (DBT) and contrast-enhanced mammography.

Full-field Digital Imaging

Digital systems may be direct radiography (DR) units, which have a built-in digital detector, thus completely replacing screen-film mammography (SFM) or computed radiography (CR) units, which consist of add-on digital conversion detectors that only replace the screen-film cassette system in a screen-film unit.

Computed Radiography Systems

These use photostimulable phosphor imaging plates that can be loaded into a conventional bucky assembly. Image acquisition in CR is a two-stage process and requires transfer of the CR plate to the readout device. The CR mammography screen and cassettes are different from CR radiography and have higher detective quantum efficiency (DQE) and reduced noise. The CR image can be displayed on a high-resolution monitor or printed on film.

Digital Radiography Systems

The digital detector converts the X-rays into digital signals and replaces the film and are of two types.

1. *Indirect digital detectors*: These convert X-rays into light and then into a digital signal. These detectors use photostimulable phosphors, amorphous silicon or charge-coupled devices (CCDs).
2. *Direct digital detectors*: Also known as flat panel detectors, they use a photoconductive material that is able to directly convert X-ray photons into a digital image. Examples

include amorphous selenium detectors and crystal silicon detectors.[9]

The overall design of the mammography unit (including X-ray tube, gantry, compression paddles), technique of doing the mammography and amount of radiation involved remains similar to those of the film-screen mammography.

Radiation Dose

The mean glandular dose in FFDM is comparable to or less than SFM. The average single view mean glandular dose for FFDM is 1.86 mGy, which is 22% lower than the average film-screen mammography mean glandular dose of 2.37 mGy.[10]

Advantages and Applications of the Digital Mammography

Digital mammography images are available for immediate viewing and dark room, which is frequently a major source of image degradation and artifacts, is eliminated. The advantages of digital mammography over SFM are:

- Better contrast characteristics and dynamic range. There is no loss of contrast in over or underexposed portions of the digital image and similar contrast is seen over the entire dynamic range of the detector.
- Postprocessing such as manipulations of the brightness, contrast, zoom-pan and edge enhancement and adjustment of image display.
- Better archival, storage and communication, i.e. picture archiving and communication system (PACS) and telemammography.

When compared with the SFM, major limitations of digital mammography are the cost and lower spatial resolution. FFDM systems have spatial resolutions from 5 to 10 lp/mm, whereas the SFM combinations have a linepair resolution of 18–20 lp/mm. This lower spatial resolution of FFDM is compensated by an increase in contrast resolution. The digital system has wider dynamic range and hence it can record and differentiate minor variations in contrast better than SFM.

Newer applications of the digital mammography are exciting. These include computer-aided detection (CAD) and diagnosis, DBT and dual-energy contrast-enhanced mammography.

Computer-aided Detection

Computer-aided detection is a computer software system that is designed to aid the film reader by highlighting the areas of concern (calcifications and masses). The software highlights the suspicious areas for careful evaluation by the radiologist. The CAD thus decreases the chances of overlooking these abnormalities. It may help inexperienced radiologists, and also acts as a second opinion to the experienced radiologists. Use of CAD in screening setups increases the cancer detection rates.[11] There is lower specificity with high false-positive rates.

Digital Breast Tomosynthesis

The dense glandular tissue may hide an underlying mass, or it may simulate a mass when none exists. DBT is a digital imaging technique, which helps to distinguish glandular breast tissue from true lesions, especially in dense breasts. It is more helpful in characterization of asymmetries, architectural distortion and masses than in the assessment of calcifications.[12]

Multiple projections are acquired at different depths by a digital detector from a mammographic X-ray source that moves gradually in a small arc over the compressed breast. These projection image datasets are reconstructed using specific algorithms in the form of sections similar to the CT. Each individual slice presents a planar mammogram in either the CC or MLO view. As each reconstructed slice may be as thin as 0.5 mm, masses and mass margins that may otherwise be superimposed with out-of-plane structures are more visible in the reconstructed slice **(Figs. 16A to D)**.

As the technique involves number of exposures compared to single exposure per view for nontomosynthesis FFDM, the radiation dose is slightly increased. However, all FFDM systems produce DBT images with dose below the Food and Drug Administration (FDA) limit of 300 millirad (mrad) per exposure.

The potential benefits of DBT include an increase in screening sensitivity, improvement in lesion size at detection, better characterization, and decrease in recall rates.[13] It is useful in both screening and diagnostic evaluation of the breast. The primary benefit of DBT is for evaluation of noncalcified mammographic findings such as masses, distortion and asymmetries.

BREAST ULTRASOUND

Ultrasound is the most valuable adjunct to mammography for the diagnosis of breast diseases. The additional advantages include lack of ionizing radiation, easy availability and low cost. US can be used as a primary imaging modality; and a secondary adjunct modality for targeted evaluation of any lesion detected on mammography/MRI.

Technique

Breast US should be performed with linear high-frequency transducers. The center frequency should be 10 MHz, with frequency ranging as high as 17 MHz in the near field and as low as 5 MHz deeper in the image field, thus enabling greater penetration of the posterior breast tissue and pectoralis muscle. The patient is examined in the supine oblique position. The side being examined is raised and the arm is placed above the head to ensure that the breast is evenly distributed over the chest wall. If the US is being done as a targeted examination, proper area to scan must be determined from the mammogram or clinical examination. The direction of scanning is in the transverse and longitudinal directions. A systematic approach should be followed (e.g., center to periphery). Scanning in the radial (parallel to the ducts) and antiradial (perpendicular to ducts) planes is of value in demonstrating ductal abnormalities. If lesion is identified, its presence should be confirmed with 90° rotation of the transducer. The morphology of the lesion should be carefully assessed. For the purpose of accurate follow-up, it is crucial to consistently and completely document the lesion size and location. The specific location, including laterality (right or left breast), the clock-face location, and

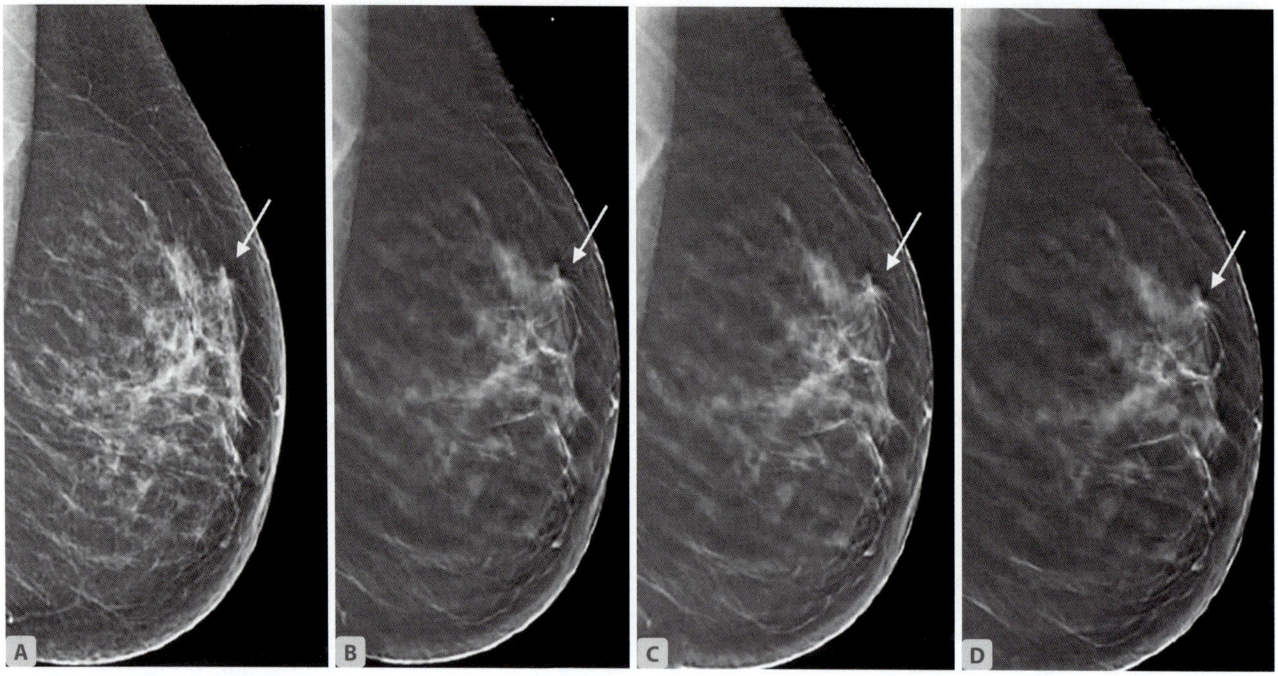

FIGS. 16A TO D: Digital breast tomosynthesis. (A) Conventional mediolateral oblique (MLO) view shows a subtle area of architectural distortion (arrow) in the upper part of right breast; (B to D) 1-mm thin contiguous tomographic slices convincingly show the irregular spiculations radiating from this area (arrows), thus increasing the diagnostic confidence.

the distance from the nipple, should be accurately annotated on the images and documented in the reports. The length of the transducer face (footprint), usually between 3.5 and 5 cm, can be used to estimate the distance from the nipple. Extended field of view (FOV) imaging is a helpful tool to image large lesions that extend beyond the width of the transducer footprint or to better depict relationships among multiple lesions. Evaluation of the nipple and retroareolar region requires should be done carefully. It is often helpful to place the transducer slightly off center to the nipple and then use angulation to image the retroareolar tissues. "Rolled nipple" technique is another maneuver of visualization of retroareolar area. Whenever in doubt; a comparison with the contralateral side should be done to exclude any artifacts or normal variation.

Investigations into the use of Doppler US of breast lesions have produced mixed results. Because Doppler technique relies on increased vascularity (which can be seen in both benign and malignant lesions), significant overlap of positive findings is not unexpected. As color Doppler equipment has become more and more sensitive, vascular signals can been found in normal, benign, and malignant tissue. Penetrating vessels are more likely to be present in malignant tumors.[14] There are several potential causes of false-positive Doppler results (inflammatory lesions, recent fine-needle aspiration, and some vascular fibroadenomas) and false-negative results (poorly vascularized tumors, insensitive Doppler parameters, and incidental cancers) on color Doppler US.

Indications for Breast Ultrasound

In current clinical practice, the indications for breast US can be in two broad categories: (1) screening and (2) diagnostic. The European Society of breast imaging has divided the indication into three categories: (1) definite, (2) possible, and (3) inappropriate[14] **(Table 4)**. US is indicated in young (30–35 years) high-risk women who cannot undergo MRI screening for various reasons. In older high-risk women, US can be used as an adjunct to mammographic screening.[15] BRCA mutation carriers are more prone to develop radiation-induced cancers; hence, US is a suitable modality in screening them, especially at a young age.[16]

In the absence of a suspicious clinical lesion, a negative US and mammography has a very high negative predictive value for malignant disease. Main disadvantage of US is that its performance is operator-dependent and can be time consuming. Whereas mammogram is superior to US in lesion detection in older women with fatty breast composition; US is superior in lesion detection in dense breasts. It should be kept in mind that US is not always an alternative to mammography; rather they play a complementary role.

Normal Anatomy

The skin, which is normally 1–3 mm thick, appears as two parallel echogenic lines. The subcutaneous fat layer is demonstrated superficially as hypoechoic tissue compared to the glandular tissue from which it is separated by a well-defined scalloped margin. Normal ducts are often visible in the subareolar region, as anechoic tubular structures. The US appearance of the glandular tissue depends on how much involution of the glandular tissue has taken place. The young glandular breast contains a well-defined layer of glandular tissue, within which round or oval well-defined, hypoechoic fat lobules may be present. As involution takes place, more of the breast is composed of fat. In the

TABLE 4: Indications for breast ultrasound (US).[14]

Definite	Possible	Inappropriate
• Screening in high-risk population (where MRI could not be performed) • First investigation in any young patient (<40 years) with clinical breast abnormality • Pregnancy and lactation with clinical breast abnormality • Suspicious abnormality in MRI or mammography • Locoregional staging in diagnosed breast cancer (when MRI is not done) • Breast cancer patients receiving neoadjuvant treatment, for monitoring (when MRI could not be done) • Surgical scar abnormality after mastectomy or conservation surgery • Symptomatic patients with breast implants • Patients with suspicious nipple discharge, recent onset nipple inversion/skin thickening/inflammatory changes • Percutaneous breast intervention guidance	• 40–74 years age group women with dense breast; as an adjunct to mammography • Patients who previously have had a mammographically occult tumor • Normal clinical examination; in the setting of complaint of lump palpable by the patient • New onset noncyclical breast pain • Intraoperative ultrasonography (USG)	• Screening average risk young patients (<40 years) • As a sole investigation for screening in average risk patients >40 years; replacing mammography • As a sole investigation in follow-up in previous breast cancer patients, without mammography • Asymptomatic breast implants • Diffuse premenstrual breast pain

completely involuted breast, US shows hypoechoic fat lobules separated by fine curvilinear septa of increased echogenicity. Fat lobules can be distinguished by their unique spindle shape, which merges with the rest of the parenchyma at different angles and planes of imaging. By contrast, masses remain discrete with distinctive borders in all planes of imaging. Deep to the glandular tissue, a retromammary fat layer is seen and behind this pectoral muscle can be seen sharply demarcated by its echogenic fascia. Costochondral cartilages appear as hypoechoic oval masses deep to the muscle and calcified ribs show prominent shadowing. Beneath the thoracic wall, a linear echogenic interface can be seen that includes chest wall, pleura, and lung border. Anatomic structures that can be seen in axilla include blood vessels, lymph nodes, and the proximal portions of the pectoral muscles.

ACR BI-RADS Ultrasound Lexicon Descriptors

The 5th edition of ACR BI-RADS lexicon has been in use since its release in 2014[4] **(Table 5)**. US BI-RADS category was first introduced in the 4th edition of BI-RADS lexicon in 2003.

On US, a mass is evaluated by its shape, orientation, margin, echo pattern and posterior features. A mass can be oval, round or irregular **(Figs. 17A to C)**. By definition, orientation refers to the relationship the mass has to the skin **(Figs. 18A and B)**. In general, benign solid masses are parallel to the skin. When a mass is taller than it is wide, it is a suspicious sonographic finding. When describing mass margins, the most important distinction is between circumscribed and noncircumscribed margins **(Figs. 19A to E)**. Circumscribed margins are well defined or sharp, with an abrupt transition between the lesion and the surrounding tissue. Noncircumscribed margins encompass the remaining margin descriptors, including microlobulated, indistinct, angular, and spiculated. Microlobulated margins demonstrate a scalloped appearance. Indistinct margins are not clearly demarcated from the surrounding tissue. Angular margins demonstrate sharp corners, often with acute angles, in distinction from spiculated margins, which appear more as lines projecting from a mass. The BI-RADS US descriptors shown to have a high predictive value for benignity include a circumscribed margin (90%), parallel orientation (78%), and an oval shape (78%).[17] The features most predictive of malignancy are an irregular shape (62%), spiculated margins (86%), and nonparallel orientation (69%). The internal echogenicity of the mass may be anechoic, hyperechoic, complex cystic and solid, hypoechoic, isoechoic or heterogeneous **(Figs. 20A to D)**. The patient's fat should serve as the internal control to which the echogenicity of all lesions should be compared. Generally, lesions that are hyperechoic to the subcutaneous fat are benign. Because a majority of both malignant and benign solid breast masses are hypoechoic, other features, such as margin characteristics, establish the level of suspicion.

Posterior features **(Figs. 21A and B)** may or may not be seen when imaging solid masses. Posterior acoustic shadowing is a suspicious finding and may be seen in cases of invasive carcinoma, postoperative scar, complex sclerosing lesion, or macrocalcifications. Posterior enhancement is an indeterminate US finding that can be associated with a variety of entities, including simple cysts, complicated cysts, fibroadenoma, papilloma, complex cystic mass, invasive ductal carcinoma, and lymphoma.

In the 5th edition of ACR BI-RADS Atlas, there are a few changes which are highlighted in **Table 6.**[5,6]

After complete US evaluation, the appropriate ACR BI-RADS category should be assigned to guide further management **(Table 7)**.

TABLE 5: ACR BI-RADS ultrasound lexicon descriptors for breast lesions.

Characteristic	Term	Description
Shape	Oval	Elliptical (may include 2–3 undulations)
	Round	Spherical
	Irregular	Neither round nor oval in shape
Orientation	Parallel	Wider than tall
	Not parallel	Taller than wide
Margin	Circumscribed	Well-defined or sharp margin with an abrupt transition between the lesion and the surrounding tissue
	Angular	Some or all of the margin has sharp corners, often forming acute angles
	Indistinct	No clear demarcation between a mass and its surrounding tissue
	Microlobulated	Short cycle undulations impart a scalloped appearance to the margin of the mass
	Spiculated	Margin characterized by sharp lines projecting from the mass
Echo pattern	Anechoic	Without internal echoes
	Hyperechoic	Increased echogenicity relative to fat
	Complex cystic and solid	Mass contains both anechoic and echogenic components
	Isoechoic	Same echogenicity as fat
	Hypoechoic	Decreased echogenicity relative to fat
	Heterogeneous	Heterogeneous hypo- and hyperechoic appearance
Posterior features	No posterior acoustic features	No posterior shadowing or enhancement
	Enhancement	Increased posterior echoes
	Shadowing	Decreased posterior echoes; edge shadows are excluded
	Combined pattern	
Associated features	Duct changes	Abnormal caliber
	Edema	Increased echogenicity of surrounding tissue
	Architectural distortion	Disruption of normal anatomic planes
	Skin thickening/retraction	Normal skin is 2 mm or less in thickness except in the periareolar area and lower breast
	Vascularity (absent/internal vascularity/vessels in rim)	Doppler US signal in a mass
	Elasticity assessment (soft/ intermediate/hard)	Elasticity value measurement of the mass in comparison with the adjacent breast tissue
Calcifications	Calcification within a mass	Echogenic foci within a mass
	Calcifications outside a mass	Echogenic calcific foci outside the mass
	Intraductal calcifications	Echogenic foci within the ducts
Special cases	Clustered microcysts	A cluster of tiny anechoic foci 2–3 mm in diameter with thin intervening septations and no discrete solid components
	Simple cyst	Completely anechoic cyst
	Complicated cysts	Cysts having homogeneous, low-level echoes. May also have fluid-fluid, or fluid debris levels
	Mass in or on skin	These masses are clinically apparent and may include sebaceous or epidermal inclusion cysts, keloids, moles and neurofibromas
	Lymph nodes	Bean-shaped, well-defined with an echogenic hilum
	Foreign body including implants	
	Vascular abnormalities	Arteriovenous malformations or Mondor's disease
	Postsurgical fluid collection	Anechoic fluid collection (seroma) or collection with variable degree of internal echoes (hematoma)
	Fat necrosis	Well-circumscribed echogenic lesion/anechoic cystic lesion (oil cyst) with rim calcification

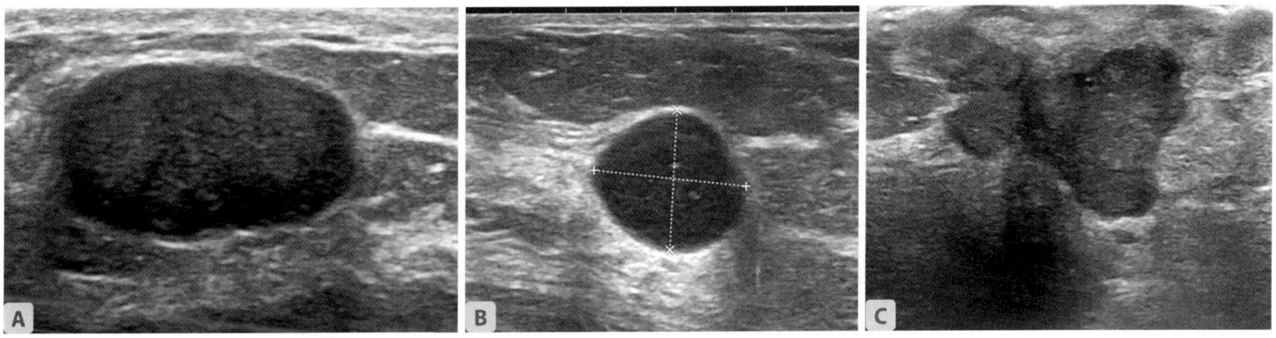

FIGS. 17A TO C: ACR BI-RADS descriptors for mass shape on ultrasound. (A) Oval; (B) Round; (C) Irregular.

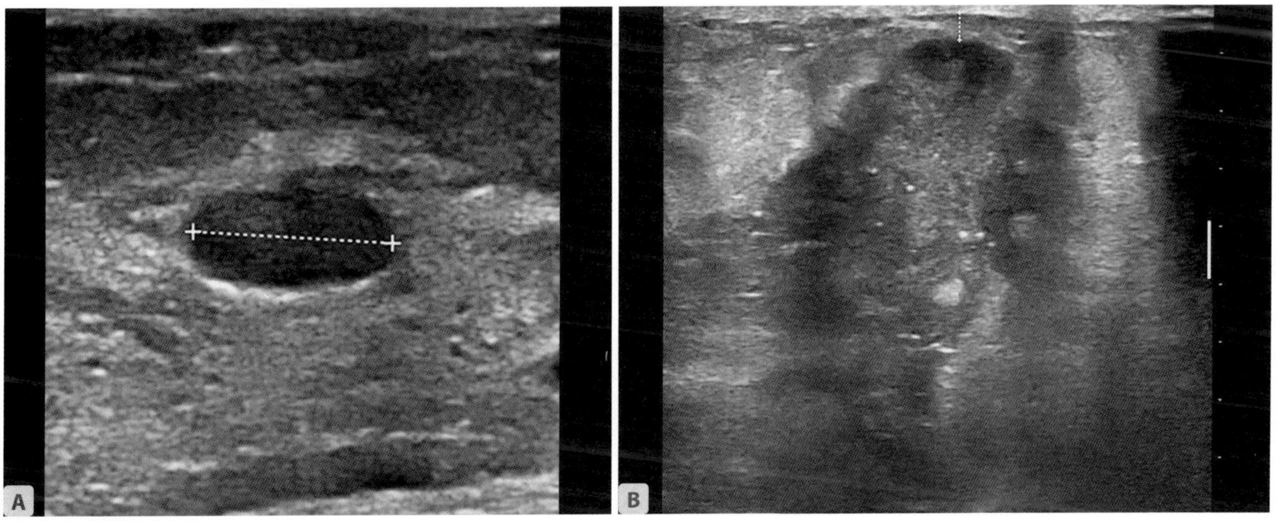

FIGS. 18A AND B: Orientation of a mass to skin on ultrasound. (A) Parallel orientation (wider than taller); (B) Antiparallel orientation (taller than wider).

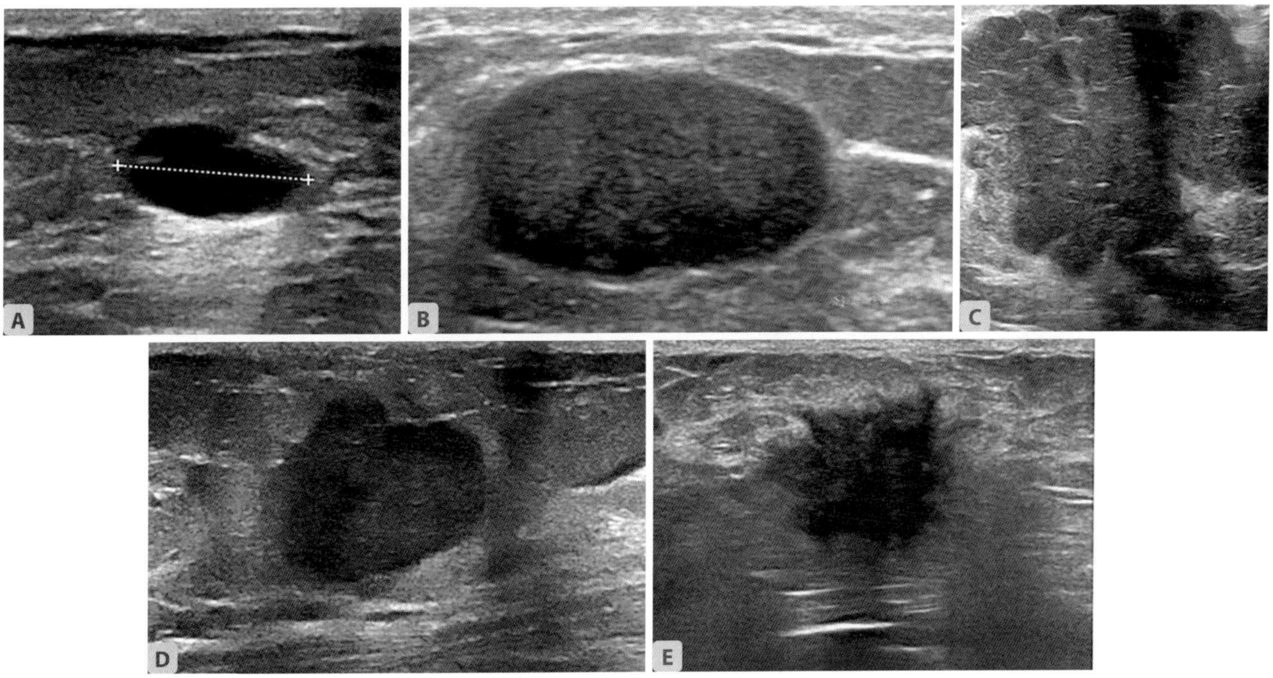

FIGS. 19A TO E: ACR BI-RADS descriptors for mass margins on ultrasound. (A) Circumscribed; (B) Microlobulated; (C) Indistinct; (D) Angular; (E) Spiculated.

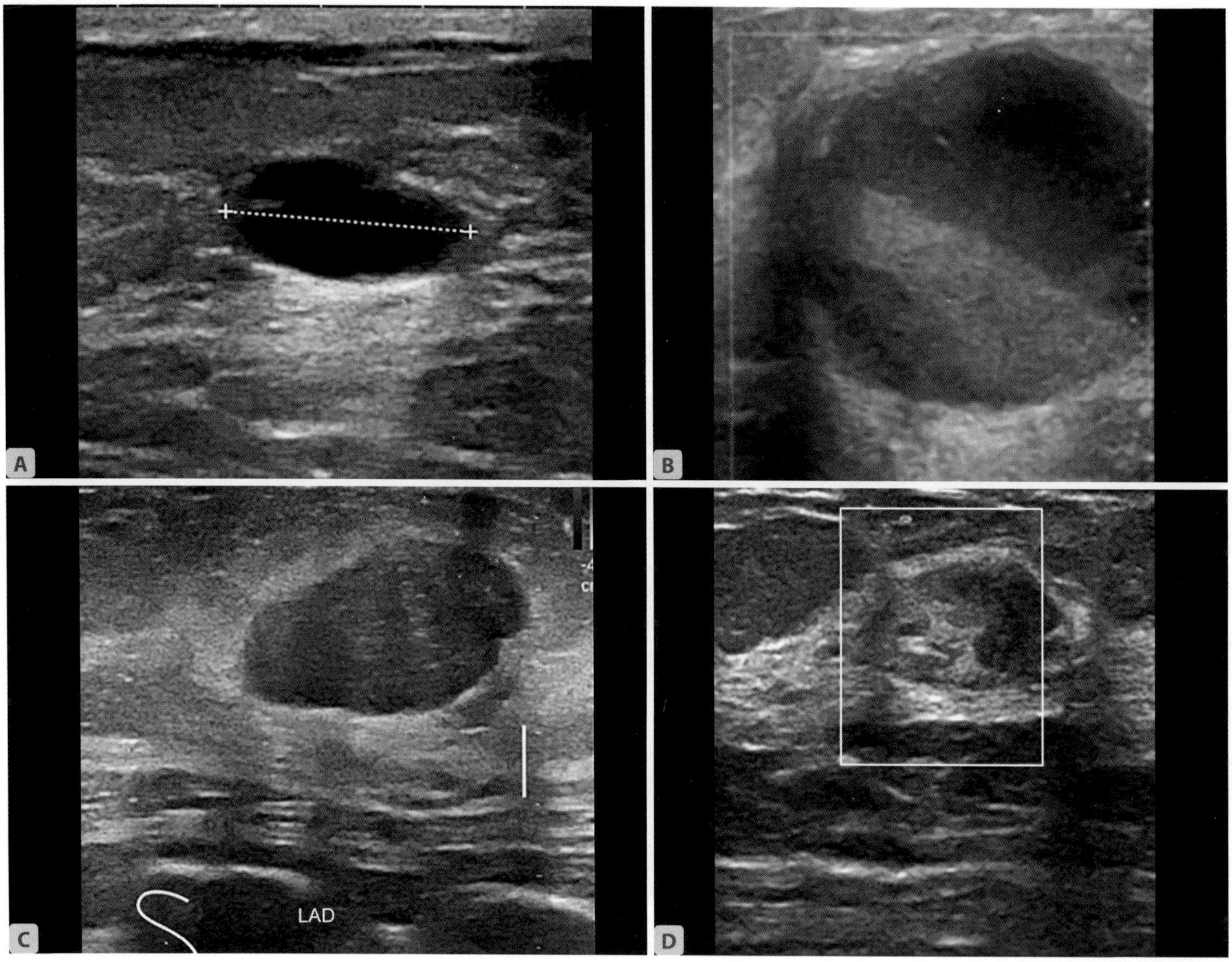

FIGS. 20A TO D: ACR BI-RADS descriptors of mass echogenicity. (A) Anechoic; (B) Complex solid cystic; (C) Hypoechoic; (D) Hyperechoic. (LAD: left anterior descending).

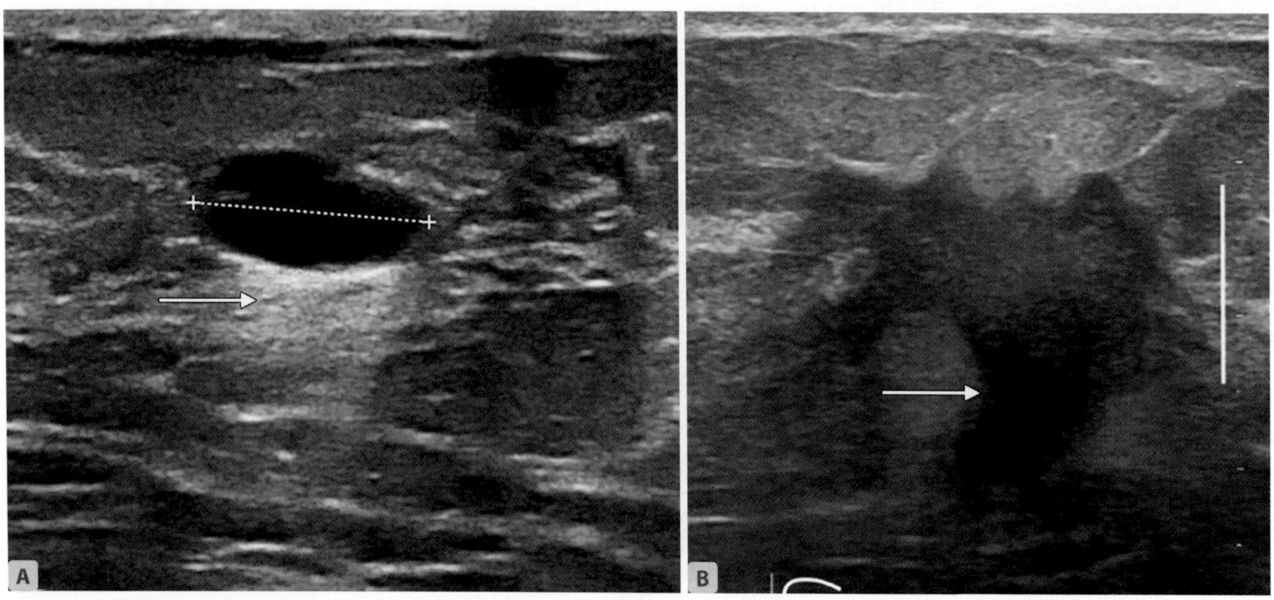

FIGS. 21A AND B: Posterior features of a mass on ultrasound. (A) Posterior enhancement (arrow); (B) Posterior shadowing (arrow).

TABLE 6: Modifications in ACR BI-RADS 5th edition ultrasound lexicon.

Section	4th edition	5th edition	Change
Background echotexture	Background echotexture • Homogeneous background echotexture-fat • Homogeneous background echotexture-fibroglandular • Heterogeneous	Tissue composition • Homogeneous background echotexture-fat • Homogeneous background echotexture-fibroglandular • Heterogeneous	Renamed as "tissue composition"
Masses	Lesion boundary		Omitted
	Echo pattern • Anechoic • Hyperechoic • Complex • Hypoechoic • Isoechoic	Echo pattern • Anechoic • Hyperechoic • Complex cystic and solid • Hypoechoic • Isoechoic • Heterogeneous	"Complex" renamed as "complex cystic and solid" Addition: "Heterogeneous"
	Surrounding tissues • Ducts • Changes in Cooper's ligaments • Edema • Architectural distortion • Skin thickening • Skin retraction/irregularity	Associated features • Architectural distortion • Duct changes • Skin changes • Edema • Vascularity • Elasticity assessment	Moved to another category "Associated features" after a few changes
Calcifications	• Macrocalcifications • Microcalcifications – In a mass – Outside a mass	• Calcification in a mass • Calcification outside a mass • Intraductal calcification	Micro/macrocalcification differentiation omitted "Intraductal" category added
Special cases	• Clustered microcysts • Complicated cyst • Mass in or on skin • Foreign body • Lymph nodes	• Simple cyst • Clustered microcysts • Complicated cyst • Mass in or on skin • Foreign body • Lymph nodes • Vascular abnormality • Postsurgical fluid collection • Fat necrosis	New conditions added

Challenges in Assigning Final Assessment Categories and the Influence of Clinical Factors

For a lesion with benign characteristics, although data support follow-up of probably benign lesions, an important clinical factor that influences BI-RADS final assessment categorization is the age of the patient. For an older patient, the threshold for biopsy should be lowered, and biopsy may be warranted even in the setting of probably benign imaging features.

Despite benign imaging features at US or mammography, palpable solid lesions are frequently subjected to biopsy, which leads to a large number of benign results of biopsies and incurs both financial and psychologic costs. Recent data support the fact that a solid mass need not be subjected to biopsy simply because it is palpable.[18] For palpable masses with benign imaging characteristics, the range of reported negative predictive values is 97–100%.[19] Therefore, such lesions should be managed with short-interval follow-up rather than with biopsy.

There are situations in which clinical factors are more important than the imaging appearance of a lesion. An abscess often demonstrates a complex internal echo pattern and can be indistinguishable from an invasive carcinoma. However, in the correct clinical setting (a young lactating patient with clinical signs of infection and a mass that is tender to palpation), the likelihood of malignancy is low and it should be categorized as a BI-RADS 3 lesion with recommendation of follow-up.

Contrast-enhanced Ultrasound

During the last few years, US contrast agents have been developed that increase blood echogenicity and improve US image quality by detection of slow and low-volume blood flow

TABLE 7: ACR BI-RADS ultrasound assessment categories.

Category	Description	Likelihood of malignancy	Examples	Next step in evaluation
0	Incomplete; need additional imaging evaluation, or comparison with previous examinations	Unknown	Postoperative scar/recurrence	MRI; obtain previous examinations
1	Negative	No ultrasound evidence of malignancy	Normal ultrasound	Negative findings at US do not exclude breast cancer in the setting of a suspicious mammographic finding. If the patient is being evaluated for a palpable abnormality and the findings with both US and mammography are negative, the report should stress the importance of clinical assessment and further management should be based on the clinical level of concern
2	Benign finding	No ultrasound evidence of malignancy	Simple cysts, breast implants, stable postsurgical changes, and probable fibroadenomas noted to be unchanged at successive US studies	Routine screening
3	Probably benign finding	<2%	A solid mass with circumscribed margins, an oval shape, and parallel orientation	Follow-up imaging (mammography or ultrasound) at 6 and 12 months
4	Suspicious abnormality	3–95%	Solid masses with benign features (e.g., fibroadenomas) if the lesion is clinically palpable. Complicated cysts and some complex cystic and solid masses (e.g., clinically apparent abscesses)	Fine-needle aspiration, percutaneous or surgical biopsy
5	Highly suggestive of malignancy	>95%	Spiculated mass	Percutaneous or surgical biopsy
6	Known malignancy	100%	Biopsy-proven	Definitive treatment

in small tumor vessels (<5 mm) within the focal lesions in the breast. Commonly used US contrast agents include Sonovue (sulfur hexafluoride microbubbles coated with phospholipids) and Levovist (galactose microparticles coated with palmitic acid). Various studies involving contrast-enhanced US (CEUS) in breast masses have shown differences in the vascularity pattern in benign and malignant lesions. Malignant lesions tend to have greater number of vessels, irregular vessels running to the center of the mass and greater enhancement **(Figs. 22A and B)**. In spite of being in clinical use for quite a long duration,[20,21] it is still listed as "upcoming applications"; and not recommended in the current EFSUMB guidelines.[22]

Ultrasound Elastography

Elasticity assessment has been introduced in the present ACR BI-RADS lexicon 5th edition.

Ultrasound elastography explores the simple principle of tissue response to a given amount of external pressure; a harder tissue (breast malignancies tend to be scirrhous and therefore harder) resists deformation by external pressure and hence retains its original shape while benign lesions are softer and get easily deformed by external pressure.

Elastography can be broadly divided into two categories: (1) static US elastography and (2) shear wave elastography (SWE). Static US elastography requires external application of pressure by the operator and provides a color-coded map of elasticity that is superimposed on the real-time grayscale image. SWE is a new quantitative technique of obtaining elastography images where an acoustic radiation force impulse (ARFI) is induced in the tissues by a focused US beam and an ultrafast imaging sequence captures in real-time the propagation of the resulting shear waves. The production of ARFI impulse by the probe rather than the operator (as in static US elastography) means SWE is more reproducible than static elastography.

The parameters measured in a quantitative SWE **(Fig. 23)** are listed in **Table 8**. The region of interest (ROI) placement in 2D SWE should be done with caution, as it affects the measurement parameters. Invasive breast cancers have been shown to be stiffer than benign or normal tissues. Various studies[23-25] have provided wide cutoff elasticity values for differentiation of benign from malignant masses [33.3–80 kPa (median, 59.35 kPa) for E_{mean}; 46.7–93.8 kPa (median, 79.25 kPa) for E_{max}]. Addition of SWE to grayscale US can improve the sensitivity and specificity in reclassifying BI-RADS category 3 and 4a lesions.[26]

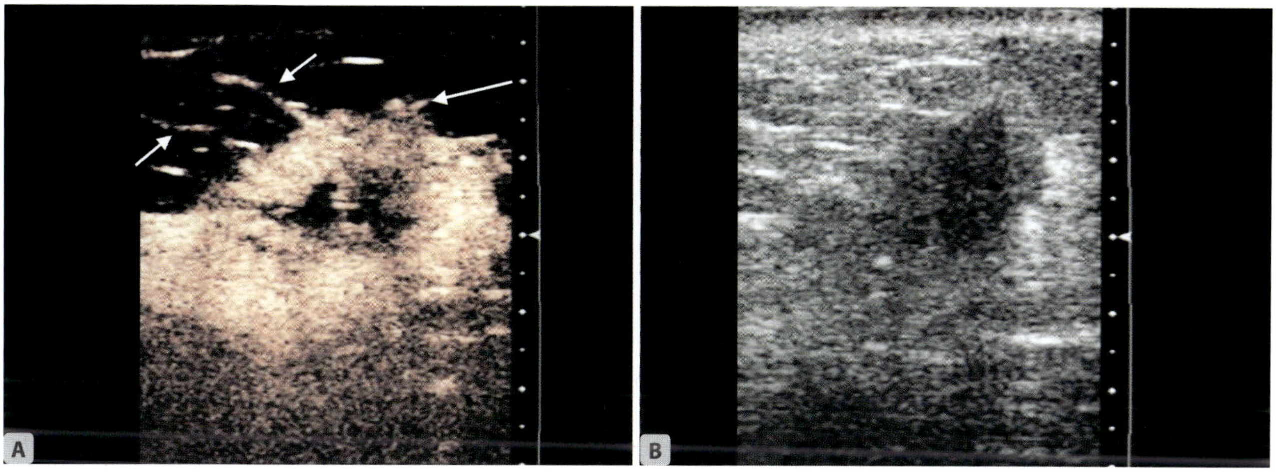

FIGS. 22A AND B: Contrast-enhanced ultrasound in a 43-year-old lady with invasive ductal carcinoma. Ultrasound image obtained 30 seconds after contrast injection shows intense early enhancement of the irregular mass lesion with ductal extension (arrows).

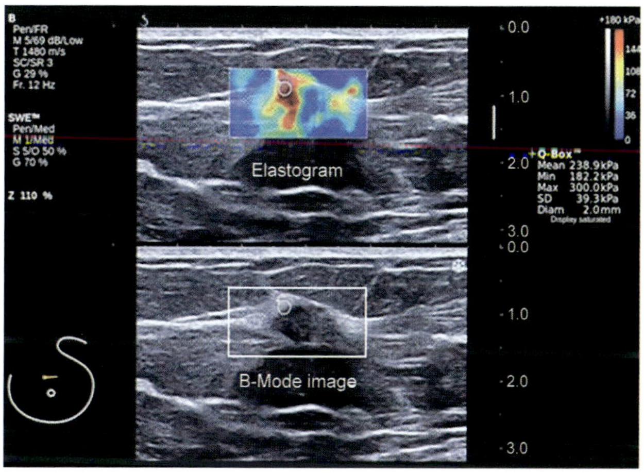

FIG. 23: Shear wave elastography. B-mode ultrasound image shows a subtle, 7 mm size, irregular solid mass. The real-time elastography image shows peritumoral stiffness (red areas) with high mean elasticity value of 238.9 kPa in the operator marked region of interest (ROI). Ultrasound-guided core biopsy confirmed invasive ductal carcinoma.

TABLE 8: Measurement parameters in shear wave elastography (SWE).

Parameter	Meaning	Effect of region of interest (ROI) size
E_{mean}	Sum of all elasticity values of each pixel within the ROI divided by the number of pixels	Decreases with an increase in ROI size
E_{max}	Maximum elasticity value (elasticity value of the stiffest pixels)	Not affected
E_{SD}	Average difference in elasticity value within the ROI to E_{mean}	Increases with size of ROI

Three-dimensional SWE is a new technique in which volumetric color-coded tissue stiffness maps are generated upon a single acquisition. Studies have demonstrated that 3D SWE can demonstrate the stiffest part of the tumor much easily than a 2D SWE.[27,28]

Other promising applications of elastography as an adjunct to gray scale US include prediction of breast cancer prognosis and prediction of response to neoadjuvant therapy.

Recent advances in breast US (including automated breast volume US) will be discussed in a separate chapter.

BREAST MAGNETIC RESONANCE IMAGING

Since the early development of breast MRI, numerous technical developments, variations, and innovations have been described. This section describes the indications, techniques, ACR BI-RADS lexicon for MRI breast.

Indications of Breast Magnetic Resonance Imaging

The indications of breast MRI are listed in **Table 9**. Broadly, they can be divided into three categories: (1) screening, (2) diagnostic, and (3) as a problem solving tool. While there are conflicting reports regarding the utility of breast MRI in each of these scenarios; few of them have been unanimously proven to be of use.[29-33]

Technique

Coils and Patient Positioning

For breast MRI, the patient is placed in the prone position with the breasts in the "cups" of the coil, with judicious padding to minimize patient motion and transmitted vibration. Immobilization should be achieved by gently fixating the breast in the section-encoding direction (CC direction for transverse protocols).

TABLE 9: Indications for breast magnetic resonance imaging.[29-33]

Clinical scenario	Suitable candidate/present status
Screening	High-risk women (lifetime cancer risk 20% or higher); as a supplemental imaging technique to mammography • Several genetic mutations (e.g., BRCA1, BRCA2, PALPB2, TP53, PTEN, CHECK2, CDH1, ATM, and STK11) • Women who received chest radiation treatment before the age of 30 years Contralateral breast screening in known cancers
Preoperative staging in known breast cancer	• Young age at diagnosis • Interval cancer • Dense breasts • Hormone receptor-negative cancers • Breast conservation surgery (BCS) without radiation therapy contemplated • Invasive lobular carcinoma
Known cancers on treatment	• Presurgical treatment before BCS, and after neoadjuvant chemotherapy • Tumor response assessment on chemotherapy
Problem solving tool	• Discrepancy in mammography, US and clinical examination findings • Mammographic asymmetric density

Prone patient positioning minimizes the effects of respiratory motion on images and helps to move the breasts away from the chest wall and the resulting artifacts from cardiac and respiratory movement. Patient comfort is vital, as the breast MRI examination can last 30 minutes or longer, and any patient discomfort is likely to manifest as movement during or between scans.

MRI Field Strength

The current recommendations require that breast MRI be performed at 1.5 tesla (T) or higher. The higher field strength enables the acquisition of high-resolution imaging with adequate signal-to-noise ratio (SNR) and enables the use of fat suppression. Imaging at 3.0 T provides an opportunity for even greater improvement in SNR, increased image resolution, and faster imaging.

Imaging Protocols

Dynamic contrast-enhanced MRI is the key sequence of a breast MRI. It relies on the principle of neoangiogenesis in a cancer; the new vessels being "leaky" capillaries. Hence, the cancers tend to show a very early enhancement.

Multiparametric Breast MRI

The most widely used multiparametric MRI consists of the following sequences: T1-weighted spin-echo (T1W-SE), T2-weighted turbo spin-echo (T2W-TSE), diffusion-weighted imaging (DWI), and postcontrast sequences. T2W imaging can depict nonenhancing structures that correlate to mammographic or palpable findings, including simple or complex cysts, and dilated retroareolar ducts. T2W imaging can also help characterize certain benign lesions such as simple cysts, myxoid fibroadenoma or lymph nodes as these have very high signal intensity on T2W scans, whereas most cancers are dark. The contrast sequences can be acquired as an ultrafast dynamic contrast-enhanced series (for the first 1 minute); or the routine dynamic contrast-enhanced sequences. It is to be kept in mind that while imaging for the detection of post-neoadjuvant chemotherapy (NACT) residual disease; a delayed phase is more useful. To the contrary, the early dynamic imaging is useful for assessing tumor chemotherapy response.[29] Ultrafast dynamic contrast-enhanced MRI follows the same principle as the routine dynamic scans. The malignant lesions tend to show more early contrast wash-in, whereas benign lesions show enhancement at a later phase (>15 seconds).[29]

Implementation of the routine dynamic enhanced imaging requires careful monitoring by the radiologist. Precontrast T1W imaging should be checked carefully to ensure adequate breast coverage and lack of severe artifacts. A 0.1 mmol/kg gadolinium diethylenetriamine penta-acetic acid (Gd-DTPA) should be injected via an intravenous catheter placed in an antecubital vein before the patient is positioned in the coil. The patient must not be moved in and out of the magnet for the injection, to prevent motion and unnecessary time loss in the early postcontrast phase. The contrast agent is injected with a power injector at a rate of 3 mL/s, followed by a 20 mL saline flush. The first postcontrast acquisition is started after the volume of contrast material has been injected (i.e., during the application of the saline flush). Hand injections can also be used. T1-weighted scans are obtained at every 1 minute for at least 5–7 minutes after contrast injection. It is important to use the same T1 sequence and scan technique which was used for precontrast scan.

Bilateral imaging helps to avoid diagnostic errors (e.g., in patients with nonmass-like enhancement or enhancing foci). To categorize these areas or foci, it is very helpful to be able to assess symmetry by comparing with the contralateral breast.

Abbreviated Breast MRI

This refers to a short MRI protocol consisting of only one pre- and one postcontrast T1W sequence. After its introduction in 2014;[34] it has been extensively evaluated worldwide for its accuracy in cancer detection. The results are promising, claiming a diagnostic accuracy similar to a full protocol.[35]

Plane of Imaging

Sagittal or axial planes of acquisition are preferred, as these planes allow for better depiction of the ductal organization of the breast glandular tissue than the coronal plane. Sagittal imaging provides the opportunity for much higher in-plane resolution because of the small imaging FOV obtainable. However, simultaneous bilateral sagittal imaging requires longer imaging time, and can lead to inadvertent exclusion of breast tissue in the axillary region. Axial imaging is therefore often used for bilateral breast MRI.

Fat Suppression

The ACR guidelines encourage the use of fat suppression techniques because, after contrast injection, enhancing lesions may become isointense to adjacent fatty tissue. Active fat suppression means that the signal from fatty tissue is specifically eliminated by additional radiofrequency pulses or by choosing selective water excitation. Both types add to the acquisition time and require a very homogeneous magnetic field across the entire FOV, which is difficult to achieve with bilateral imaging.

Subtraction does not require extra acquisition time and is not influenced by magnetic field inhomogeneities, which is why it is the preferred type of fat suppression for dynamic bilateral imaging. The main disadvantage of subtraction is that it may suffer from patient motion: Subtraction errors occur if the precontrast mask and the postcontrast image are not entirely congruent due to even subtle patient motion.

Kinetic Analysis

Kinetic data can be evaluated by visually assessing the lesion enhancement pattern, by placing an ROI to obtain kinetic curves, and by using a CAD system. The ROIs should be placed with wide window settings into the area that exhibits strongest enhancement on the first postcontrast image. Softwares which demonstrate color-coded areas of high enhancement with respect to predetermined threshold have now been developed and should be used if available, to place the ROI accurately. The ROI should include not >3–4 pixels, and care should be taken to ensure that the ROI is within the lesion throughout the entire dynamic series. If there is unrecognized patient movement during dynamic scans, the lesion moves out of the prescribed ROI after the first postcontrast image leading to false washout pattern. To quantify enhancement, the increase in signal intensity relative to baseline precontrast signal intensity is measured and is plotted over time.

Normal Magnetic Resonance Imaging Appearances

Normal glandular tissue has intermediate signal intensity on T1W and T2W sequences, whereas fat is of high signal. The fibrous trabeculae are seen as fine low signal intensity structures traversing the subcutaneous fat. Low axillary and intramammary lymph nodes can be recognized through their characteristic bean shape and central fatty hilum. The skin is of intermediate signal and uniformly thin except in the areolar region where it may be and few millimeters in thickness. After intravenous gadolinium, the nipple, blood vessels and lymph nodes normally enhance. Normal glandular parenchyma can also enhance gradually, especially in the second half of the menstrual cycle, reflecting hormonal-induced glandular proliferation. This enhancement, referred to as background enhancement, is often diffuse, patchy and progressive. Rarely, it may be intense or focal and difficult to interpret. Hence, if possible, breast MRI should be performed after menstruation in second week of the cycle.

Interpretation of Breast Magnetic Resonance Imaging

For differential diagnosis of enhancing lesions in breast MRI, morphologic information (type of enhancement, mass shape and margins, distribution of nonmass-like enhancement, internal architecture), kinetic information (initial enhancement increase and delayed phase enhancement), and information related to lesion signal intensity on T2W and T1W precontrast nonfat-suppressed images are analyzed systematically.

When interpreting breast MRI studies, the first step is to categorize any abnormal enhancement according to the 5th edition of ACR BI-RADS-MRI lexicon, published as a part of the American College of Radiology's Breast Imaging Reporting and Data System Atlas: a mass, an area of nonmass-like enhancement or a focus.

Focus

In the 4th edition of ACR BI-RADS Atlas, lesions smaller than 5 mm were termed as "foci". In the 5th edition, the size criteria are no more valid; rather the differentiation between mass/foci is largely based on morphology. A focus is a small isolated enhancing dot, too small for applying morphologic descriptors.[5,6]

Mass

A mass is a 3D space occupying lesion within the breast. Usually, it has a visible correlate on precontrast T1- or T2-weighted images. Masses are described in terms of shape, margin, and internal enhancement characteristics **(Table 10)**.

- *Shape*: A mass can be round, oval, or irregular **(Figs. 24A to C)**. "Lobulated" shape has been included in the "oval" category in the 5th edition. Irregular masses have an uneven shape that cannot be characterized as round or oval.
- *Margin*: Margins can be described as circumscribed (earlier designated "smooth") or noncircumscribed (includes irregular and spiculated) **(Figs. 25A to C)**. Spiculated margins frequently are a feature of malignant breast lesions and radial scars.
- *Internal enhancement characteristics*: Enhancement patterns of masses **(Figs. 26A to C)** have been divided into the following four types:
  1. Homogeneous enhancement is uniform and confluent enhancement throughout the mass.
  2. Heterogeneous enhancement is nonuniform enhancement that shows variations within the mass.
  3. Rim enhancement is enhancement mainly concentrated at the periphery of the mass. This type

TABLE 10: ACR BI-RADS mass descriptors in magnetic resonance imaging.

Characteristic	Term	Description
Shape	Round	Spherical
	Oval	Elliptical
	Irregular	Uneven shape
Margin	Circumscribed	Smooth
	Noncircumscribed • Irregular • Spiculated	 Sharp lines projecting from the mass
Internal enhancement	Homogeneous	Uniform enhancement
	Heterogeneous	Nonuniform enhancement
	Rim enhancing	Enhancement concentrated at the periphery
	Internal nonenhancing septations	Dark septations within an enhanced lesion

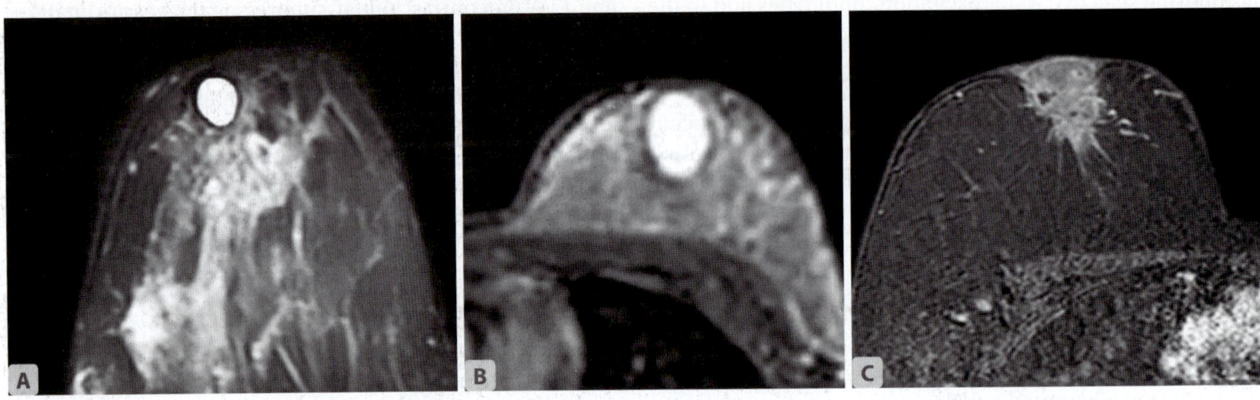

FIGS. 24A TO C: ACR BI-RADS descriptors for mass shape on magnetic resonance imaging (MRI). (A) Round; (B) Oval; (C) Irregular.

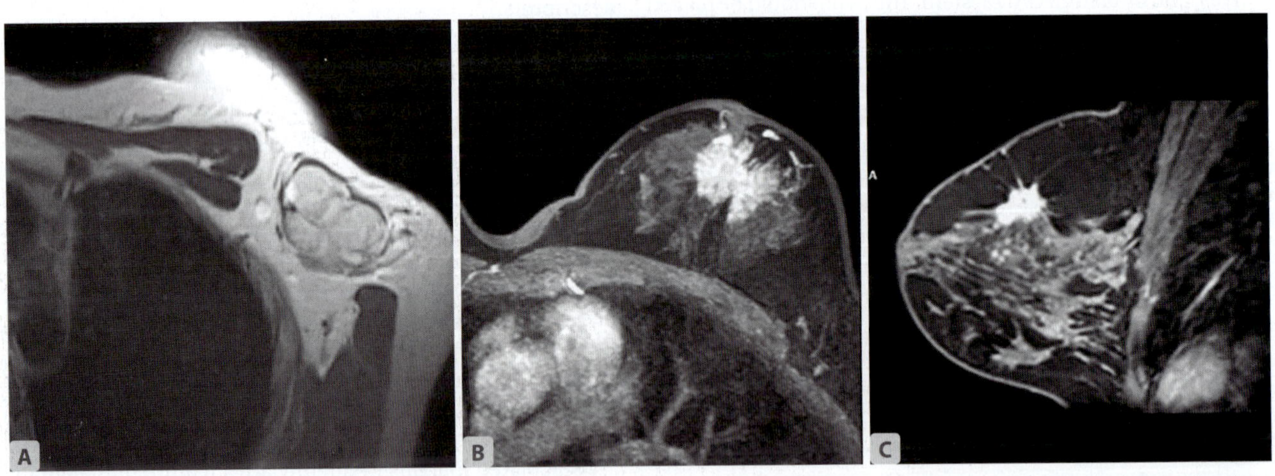

FIGS. 25A TO C: ACR BI-RADS descriptors for mass margin on magnetic resonance imaging (MRI): (A) Circumscribed; (B) Irregular; (C) Spiculated.

of enhancement is most frequently a feature of high-grade invasive ductal cancer, fat necrosis, and cysts with inflammation.

4. Dark internal nonenhancing septations within an enhanced lesion are typical of fibroadenomas, especially when the lesion has smooth or lobulated borders.

Two types (enhancing internal septations and central enhancement) have been omitted in the 5th edition.

Nonmass-like Enhancement

Nonmass-like enhancement means that enhancement occurs in an area of the fibroglandular tissue that otherwise appears

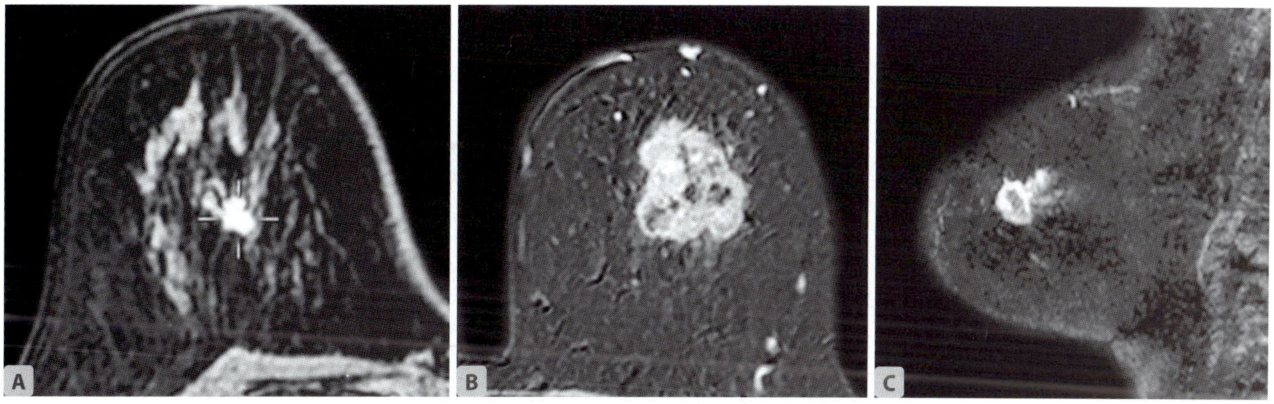

FIGS. 26A TO C: ACR BI-RADS descriptors for mass internal enhancement on magnetic resonance imaging (MRI): (A) Homogeneous; (B) Heterogeneous; (C) Rim enhancement.

normal on precontrast images. There is no space-occupying effect **(Fig. 27)**. The enhancing area usually has no correlate on fat-suppressed or nonfat-suppressed T2-weighted images. The distinction between mass and nonmass-like enhancement is important for further differential diagnosis. In a mass, the differential diagnostic consideration is either invasive breast cancer or a benign solid tumor (e.g., fibroadenoma). In nonmass-like enhancement, the main differential diagnosis is between intraductal or diffuse (e.g., lobular) cancer and mastopathic changes (focal adenosis), hormonal stimulation, or inflammatory changes. Features of nonmass-like enhancement[36] such as internal enhancement pattern, symmetry, and the distribution are assessed **(Table 11)**.

Distribution (Figs. 28A to C)

- A focal area is enhancement occupying <25% of the volume of a breast quadrant that has fat or normal glandular tissue between abnormally enhanced components. This type of enhancement usually manifests as clumped, irregular contrast enhancement.
- Linear enhancement is a sheet of enhancement that does not conform to the shape of a ductal system.
- Segmental enhancement is conical and probably represents one or more ductal systems. Segmental distribution of enhancement may be associated with in situ ductal cancer or invasive ductal cancer, atypical ductal hyperplasia, papillary neoplasms, or sclerosing adenosis.
- Regional enhancement is geographic enhancement involving one or more segments of the breast. A specific ductal or segmental configuration cannot be discerned.
- Multiple regions of enhancement are distributed in several areas of the breast.
- Diffuse enhancement is uniform enhancement of the entire parenchyma of the breast, usually associated with benign processes or normal fibroglandular tissue.

In the 5th edition, "ductal" enhancement has been omitted.

Internal Enhancement Pattern

The internal enhancement patterns are homogeneous, heterogeneous, clumped, and clustered ring. In the clustered ring pattern, the normal fat glandular tissue interface is lost. This finding is usually associated with inflammatory breast cancer or lymphatic involvement.

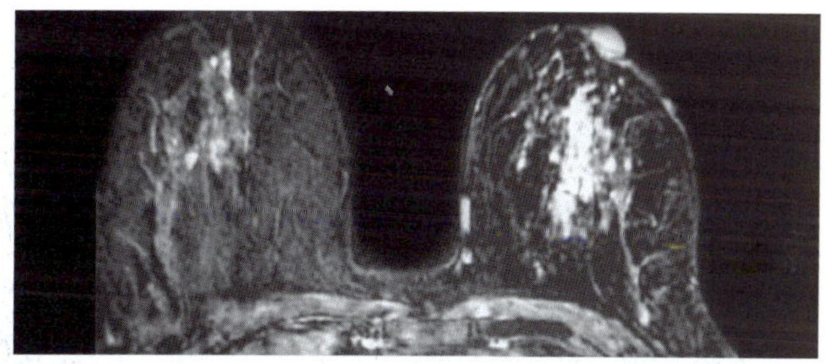

FIG. 27: Nonmass-like enhancement. Enhancement occurs in an area of the fibroglandular tissue that otherwise appears normal on precontrast images and there is no space-occupying effect.

Symmetry is helpful in further characterization of nonmass-like enhancement. Bilateral symmetric nonmass-like enhancement in any distribution is more often caused by benign changes than by malignant lesions.

A new enhancement pattern "clustered ring" has been added in the 5th edition. Stippled/punctate calcification has been omitted.

Associated Findings

Associated findings have been expanded in the 5th edition; and divided into six categories.

1. Intramammary lymph node
2. Skin lesions
3. Nonenhancing findings (include cyst, seroma, nonenhancing mass, foreign body/surgical clip, architectural distortion, etc.)
4. Associated findings (nipple retraction, nipple invasion, skin retraction, skin thickening, skin invasion, axillary adenopathy, chest wall/pectoralis muscle invasion, etc.)
5. Fat-containing lesions
6. Implants (a detailed evaluation of implants is newly added in the 5th edition).

Kinetic Curve Assessment

The analysis of enhancement kinetics is achieved by measuring the signal intensity in a small area of a lesion and

TABLE 11: ACR BI-RADS descriptors of nonmass-like enhancement in magnetic resonance imaging.

Characteristic	Descriptor	Illustration
Distribution	Focal	
	Linear	Enhancement in a line that may not conform to a duct
	Segmental	Triangular area of enhancement, apex pointing to nipple, suggesting a duct and its branches
	Regional	Enhancement in a large volume of tissue not conforming to a ductal distribution
	Multiple	Enhancement in at least two large volumes of tissues not conforming to a ductal distribution, multiple geographic areas, patchy areas of enhancement
	Diffuse	Enhancement distributed uniformly throughout the breast
Internal enhancement pattern	Homogeneous	Confluent uniform enhancement
	Heterogeneous	Nonuniform enhancement in a random pattern
	Clumped	Punctuate dot-like, enhancing foci
	Clustered ring	Enhancement with finger-like projections extending toward nipple (earlier included in reticular/dendritic pattern)

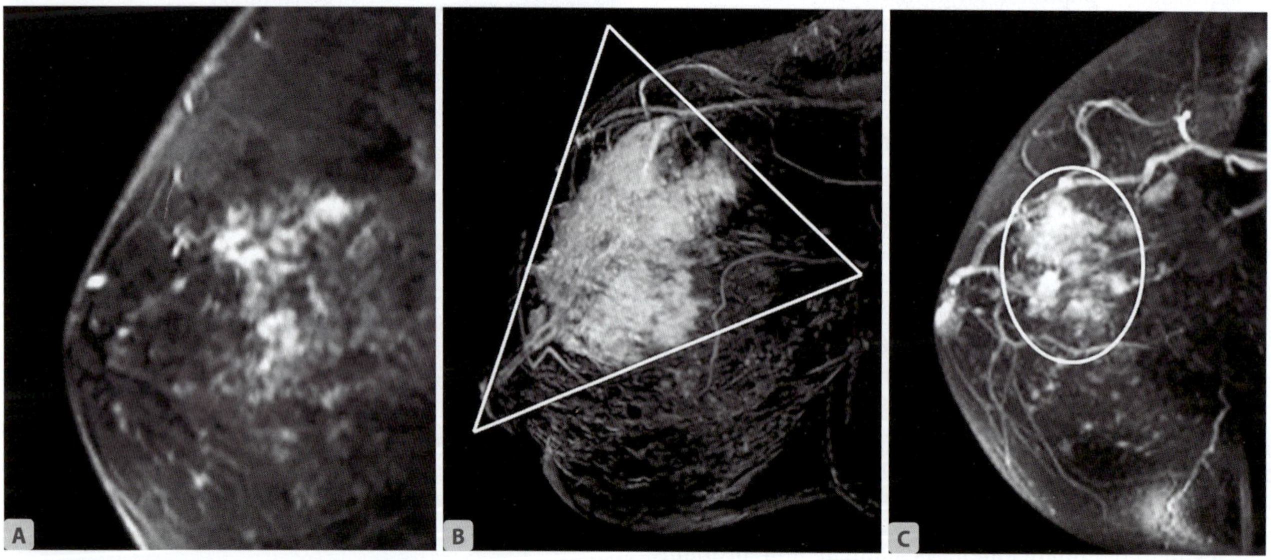

FIGS. 28A TO C: ACR BI-RADS descriptors of distribution of nonmass-like enhancement in magnetic resonance imaging (MRI). (A) Linear; (B) Segmental; (C) Regional.

tracking its course over the dynamic series to yield the kinetic curve (also referred to as time-signal intensity curve).

The most suspicious curve pattern derived from the fastest-enhancing part of a lesion is chosen to describe the enhancement curve. *Early phase enhancement*, i.e., enhancement within the first 2 minutes after contrast injection or until the curve starts to change, indicates the velocity and degree with which enhancement occurs and may be slow, medium, or fast.

Delayed phase enhancement refers to signal intensity changes that occur immediately after the early signal intensity increase, as early as 3 minutes after injection. Immediately after the early initial increase, the signal intensity may decline again, yielding a so-called washout curve (**type 3**) (**Fig. 29**); (1) exhibit a sharp bend and plateau (**type 2**); or (2) continue to rise after the early phase, yielding persistent enhancement until the delayed postcontrast phase (**type 1**). The main difference is that in types 2 (plateau) and type 3 (washout) curves, peak enhancement is reached early, usually within the first 2 minutes. This is the time course observed in most invasive breast cancers. Lesions with rapid early enhancement followed by a delayed phase plateau or washout have a positive predictive value of 77% for malignancy.[37] In persistent kinetics, the enhancement continues until the delayed postcontrast phase. This is the time course observed in most benign changes.

While enhancement kinetics is useful for the differential diagnosis of morphologically equivocal masses, it may be misleading and should, therefore, not be used for classification of nonmass-like enhancement. The reason is that in nonmass-like enhancement, the differential diagnosis includes DCIS and lobular cancers—two disease states known to exhibit inconsistent angiogenic activity.

Diffusion-weighted Imaging

Invasive breast cancers demonstrate restricted diffusion (lower apparent diffusion coefficient) relative to normal breast tissue or benign breast lesions.[38] This restricted diffusion of water in invasive cancers renders these lesions bright on diffusion-weighted images **(Figs. 30A and B)** and can potentially help identify malignant lesions when dynamic contrast-enhanced imaging is equivocal. Benign lesions with high intrinsic T2 signal intensity can also appear bright on DWI because of the phenomenon of "T2 shine-through". An apparent diffusion coefficient (ADC) pixel map should be generated from the component diffusion-weighted images produced from two or more DWI sets as hypointensity on these images confirms the restriction of diffusion. Thus, use of ADC quantification rather than DWI inspection alone is recommended for breast lesion characterization. The use of optimized ADC cutoff improves breast lesion characterization without decreasing sensitivity[39] with a potential reduction in the number of negative biopsies.

The changes in MRI section in BI-RADS 5th edition are highlighted in **Table 12**.

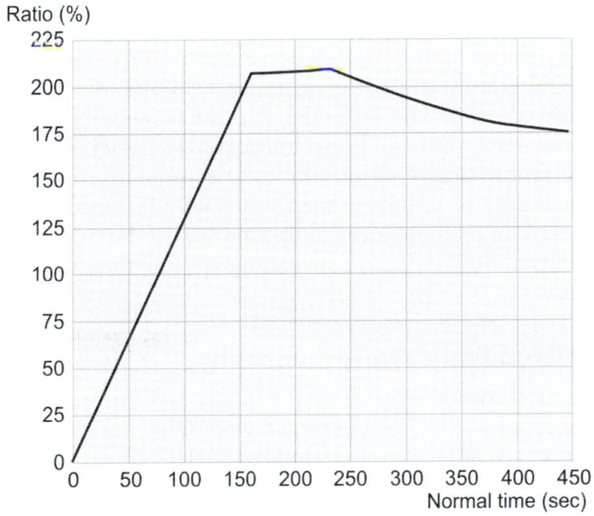

FIG. 29: Kinetic analysis of enhancing mass lesions on dynamic contrast-enhanced magnetic resonance imaging (DCE-MRI) showing type 3 curve. Immediately after the early initial increase, the signal intensity declines rapidly yielding a type 3 or washout curve.

Sensitivity and Specificity of Magnetic Resonance Imaging

Detection of invasive breast carcinoma is extremely reliable on MRI as the sensitivity approaches 100%.[36] The sensitivity of breast MRI is not impaired by the density of the fibroglandular tissue or by scar tissue (e.g., after lumpectomy), radiation therapy, or prosthetic breast implants. It can, therefore, detect cancers which are occult on mammography and US. Normal breast MRI excludes the presence of gross focus of invasive cancer with high reliability. However, breast MRI has lower specificity and this is one of its biggest limitations. The detection of cancer relies on contrast enhancement but this can also be seen in many benign conditions like fibroadenoma, papilloma, fibrocystic disease, and lymph nodes. This results in significant false-positive examinations and hence unnecessary biopsies. False-negative breast MRI examinations can also occur but these are rare. Nonenhancing invasive breast cancers are exceedingly rare. More often, the reason for failure to diagnose invasive cancer with breast MRI is early and strong enhancement in the surrounding normal fibroglandular tissue that may mask the enhancing cancer. Invasive lobular carcinoma, well-differentiated invasive ductal carcinoma and few DCIS may be missed on breast MRI. A recent meta-analysis of 44 studies has estimated the sensitivity and specificity of MRI for the diagnosis of breast cancer as 90% and 72% respectively.[37] Because of the potential issue of a false-negative examination, a negative MRI examination should not deter biopsy of a suspicious lesion (BI-RADS 4 or 5) on mammography or US. Breast MRI is best used as an

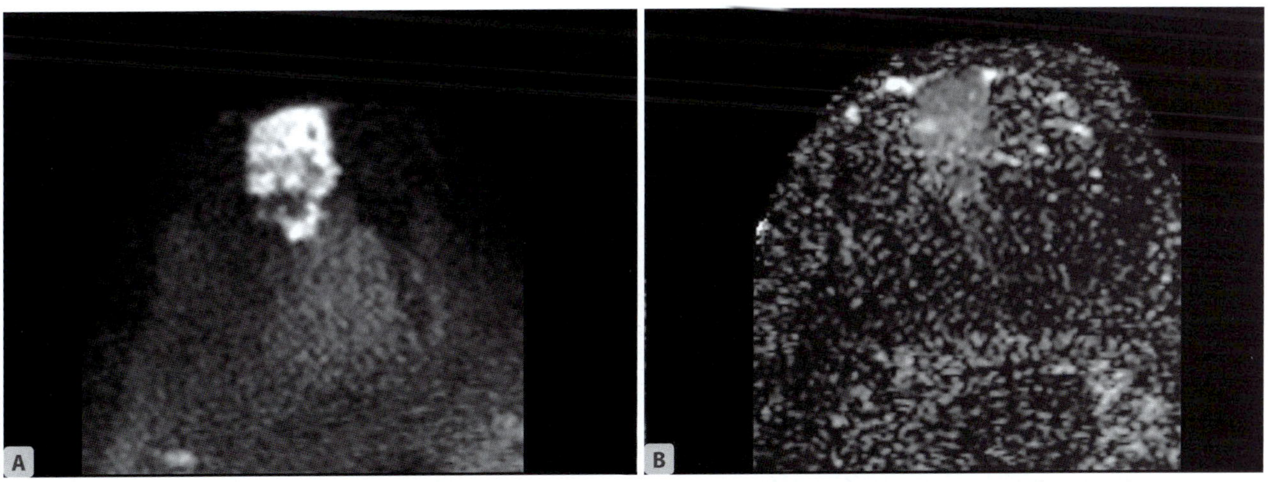

FIGS. 30A AND B: Diffusion-weighted magnetic resonance (MR) imaging. (A) Diffusion-weighted image; and (B) Apparent diffusion coefficient (ADC) pixel map in a malignant lesion showing marked restriction of diffusion.

TABLE 12: Changes in 5th edition ACR BI-RADS MRI section.[5]

Section	Changes in 5th edition
Amount of fibroglandular tissue	Newly added section (divided in four categories)
Background parenchymal enhancement	Newly added section (two categories with several subcategories included)
Focus	Definition changed (vide supra)
Mass descriptors: shape	Omitted "lobulated"
Mass descriptors: internal enhancement	Omitted two categories: enhancing internal septations and central enhancement
Nonmass-like enhancement: distribution	Omission of ductal distribution
Nonmass-like enhancement: internal enhancement patterns	Omission of stippled/punctate pattern Addition of "clustered ring" pattern
Associated findings	Expanded and divided in six categories (vide supra)

Box 4: Challenges in MRI interpretation.

False-positive
- Fibrocystic change
- Hormone-related enhancement
- Focal fibrosis, scar, fat necrosis
- Intraductal papilloma
- Fibroadenomas
- Intramammary lymph node

False-negative
- Strong background enhancement
- Nonenhancing ductal carcinoma *in situ* (DCIS)
- Nonenhancing invasive lobular carcinoma
- Recent radiotherapy

adjunct to conventional imaging, complementing but never replacing basic mammography and US.

Challenges in MRI interpretation have been shown in **Box 4**.

NUCLEAR MEDICINE IN BREAST IMAGING

Nuclear medicine techniques require intravenous administration of a radiotracer [technetium-99m-methoxyisobutyl isonitrile (MIBI)] and a camera that detects radiotracer activity. 99mTc-sestamibi preferentially accumulates in malignant tissue and this differential uptake is imaged. Its uptake and retention in the lesion depends on the regional blood flow, angiogenesis, and metabolic activity. The use of traditional gamma camera and radiotracer to image the breast is termed scintimammography,[40,41] where patients lie prone with breast dependent and imaging is performed in the lateral and anteroposterior positions. Malignant lesions are seen as focal increased uptake.

Breast-specific Gamma Imaging

Breast-specific gamma imaging (BSGI)[42] addresses the limited tumor visibility (minimum size, 15–20 mm) of large FOV sestamibi imaging. It provides optimal spatial resolution and sensitivity and is targeted at 95% detection rate of lesions 5 mm in diameter. For BSGI, the breast is positioned and compressed in a manner similar to a mammogram examination after intravenous injection of 20 mCi of technetium sestamibi. Routine CC and MLO views are obtained, with additional images as necessary resulting in an approximate 45-minute total examination time. If a focal area of uptake is seen, especially if there was no concern on mammogram, a directed US can be performed to determine if there is a suspicious finding that warrants biopsy.

Positron Emission Tomography

The ^{18}F-fluorodeoxyglucose (^{18}F-FDG) positron emission tomography (PET) has emerged as another imaging tool for many malignancies, including breast cancer. Rapidly dividing neoplastic cells have higher glucose metabolism compared with nonmalignant cells and hence, show preferential uptake of ^{18}F-FDG. The ^{18}F-FDG-PET, however, has poor anatomic resolution like other nuclear medicine techniques. Introduction of the hybrid FDG-PET/CT scanner, in which the FDG-PET scanner is equipped with a high-resolution multidetector CT for simultaneous acquisition of the FDG-PET and CT data, has greatly enhanced the spatial resolution of this technique. The FDG-PET/CT has proved to be useful in:

- Detection of breast cancers in mammographically dense breast, those with implants and those presenting with occult primary when other imaging modalities are indeterminate. A positive FDG-PET scan of the breast is highly suspicious for cancer with a high positive predictive value of 96%.
- *Locoregional staging of breast cancer*: Whole body FDG-PET can correctly estimate the true local and distant extent of the disease. PET can detect metastases to axillary lymph nodes as well as nodes at unsuspected areas such as internal mammary or supraclavicular lymph nodes owing to its large FOV.
- *Detection of unsuspected distant metastases*: 99mTc-methylene diphosphonate (MDP) bone scan has better sensitivity for sclerotic bone metastases and PET is more

sensitive for lytic bone metastases. PET is unsatisfactory for detection of brain and small pulmonary metastases.

- Detection of recurrences in soft issues.
- *Early prediction of tumor response in patients with locally advanced breast cancer undergoing NACT.* Decreased uptake with chemotherapy suggests that pathologic remission may be achieved. Persistent high uptake with treatment predicts poor response.[43]
- Differentiation of scar tissue from cancer recurrence.

Limitations

Diagnostic accuracy of FDG-PET is dependent on tumor size and histology. The sensitivity of FDG-PET is 92% for lesions larger than 2 cm but is only 53% for primary lesions <5 mm.[44] PET also has poor sensitivity for detection of DICS and slow growing cancers such as invasive lobular carcinoma. PET is not suitable for screening even for high-risk patients, as negative study has limited value.

Positron Emission Mammography

Positron emission mammography (PEM) is a high spatial resolution (2 mm), dedicated breast PET device that can provide functional and anatomical information.[45] Dual moving head detectors are mounted opposite each other on compression paddles attached to a portable compact scanner to obtain tomographic images of the breast in the CC and MLO positions. It is primarily used for patients unable to undergo MRI.

CONCLUSION

The BI-RADS is a standardized system of reporting breast pathology on mammogram, ultrasonography (USG) and MRI and the standardized lexicon should be followed to ensure consistency between reports. The reporting structure should be such that there is clear communication to the clinician regarding diagnosis and management recommendations.

REFERENCES

1. Tabár L, Vitak B, Chen TH, Yen AM, Cohen A, Tot T, et al. Swedish two-county trial: impact of mammographic screening on breast cancer mortality during 3 decades. Radiology. 2011;260(3):658-63.
2. Mushlin AI, Kouides RW, Shapiro DE. Estimating the accuracy of screening mammography: a meta-analysis. Am J Prev Med. 1998;14:143-53.
3. Boyd NF, Guo H, Martin LJ, Sun L, Stone J, Fishell E, et al. Mammographic density and the risk and detection of breast cancer. N Engl J Med. 2007;356:227-36.
4. D'Orsi C, Sickles EA, Mendelson EB, Morris EA. ACR BI-RADS Atlas: Breast Imaging Reporting and Data System, 5th edition. Reston, VA: American College of Radiology; 2013.
5. Rao AA, Feneis J, Lalonde C, Ojeda-Fournier H. A pictorial review of changes in the BI-RADS fifth edition. Radiographics. 2016;36: 623-39.
6. Spak DA, Plaxco JS, Santiago L, Dryden MJ, Dogan BE. BI-RADS® fifth edition: a summary of changes. Diagn Interv Imaging. 2017;98: 179-90.
7. Rominger M, Wisgickl C, Timmesfeld N. Breast microcalcifications as type descriptors to stratify risk of malignancy: a systematic review and meta-analysis of 10,665 cases with special focus on round/punctate microcalcifications. Rofo. 2012;184(12):1144-52.
8. Price ER, Joe BN, Sickles EA. The developing asymmetry: revisiting a perceptual and diagnostic challenge. Radiology. 2015;274(3): 642-51.
9. D'Orsi CJ, Newell MS. Digital mammography: clinical implementation and clinical trials. Semin Roentgenol. 2007;42(4):236-42.
10. Hendrick RE, Pisano ED, Averbukh A, Moran C, Berns EA, Yaffe MJ, et al. Comparison of acquisition parameters and breast dose in digital mammography and screen-film mammography in the American College of Radiology Imaging Network Digital Mammographic Imaging Screening Trial. AJR Am J Roentgenol. 2010;194(2):362-9.
11. Noble M, Bruening W, Uhl S, Schoelles K. Computer-aided detection mammography for breast cancer screening: systematic review and meta-analysis. Arch Gynecol Obstet. 2009;279(6):881-90.
12. Poplack SA, Tosteson TD, Kogel CA, Nagy HM. Digital breast tomosynthesis: initial experience in 98 women with abnormal digital screening mammography. AJR Am J Roentgenol. 2007;189:616-23.
13. Gur D, Abrams GS, Chough DM, Ganott MA, Hakim CM, Perrin RL, et al. Digital breast tomosynthesis: observer performance study. AJR Am J Roentgenol. 2009;193:586-91.
14. Evans A, Trimboli RM, Athanasiou A, Balleyguier C, Baltzer PA, Bick U, et al. Breast ultrasound: recommendations for information to women and referring physicians by the European Society of Breast Imaging. Insights Imaging. 2018;9(4):449-61
15. Berg WA, Blume JD, Cormack JB, Mendelson EB, Lehrer D, Böhm-Vélez M, et al. Combined screening with ultrasound and mammography vs mammography alone in women at elevated risk of breast cancer. JAMA. 2008;299:2151-63.
16. Colin C, Foray N, Di Leo G, Sardanelli F. Radiation induced breast cancer risk in BRCA mutation carriers from low-dose radiological exposures: a systematic review. Radioprotection. 2017;52(4):231-40.
17. Stavros AT, Thickman D, Rapp CL, Dennis MA, Parker SH, Sisney GA. Solid breast nodules: use of sonography to distinguish between benign and malignant lesions. Radiology. 1995;196(1):123-34.
18. Graf O, Helbich TH, Fuchsjaeger MH, Hopf G, Morgun M, Graf C, et al. Follow-up of palpable circumscribed noncalcified solid breast masses at mammography and US: can biopsy be averted? Radiology. 2004;233(3):850-6.
19. Raza S, Goldkamp AL, Chikarmane SA, Birdwell RL. US of breast masses categorized as BI-RADS 3, 4, and 5: pictorial review of factors influencing clinical management. Radiographics. 2010;30(5): 1199-213.
20. Sorelli PG, Cosgrove DO, Svensson WE, Zaman N, Satchithananda K, Barrett NK, et al. Can contrast-enhanced sonography distinguish benign from malignant breast masses. J Clin Ultrasound. 2010;38:177-81.
21. Jia WR, Chai WM, Tang L, Wang Y, Fei XC, Han BS, et al. Three-dimensional contrast-enhanced ultrasound score and dynamic contrast-enhanced magnetic resonance imaging score in evaluating breast tumor angiogenesis: correlation with biological factors. Eur J Radiol. 2014;83:1098-105.
22. Sidhu SP, Cantisani V, Dietrich CF, Gilja OH, Saftoiu A, Bartels E, et al. The EFSUMB guidelines and recommendations for the clinical practice of contrast-enhanced ultrasound (CEUS) in non-hepatic applications: update 2017 (Long Version). Ultraschall Med. 2018;39:e2-44.

23. Youk JH, Son EJ, Gweon HM, Kim H, Park YJ, Kim JA. Comparison of strain and shear wave elastography for the differentiation of benign from malignant breast lesions, combined with B-mode ultrasonography: qualitative and quantitative assessments. Ultrasound Med Biol. 2014;40:2336-44.
24. Chang JM, Moon WK, Cho N, Yi A, Koo HR, Han W, et al. Clinical application of shear wave elastography (SWE) in the diagnosis of benign and malignant breast diseases. Breast Cancer Res Treat. 2011;129:89-97.
25. Au FW, Ghai S, Moshonov H, Kahn H, Brennan C, Dua H, et al. Diagnostic performance of quantitative shear wave elastography in the evaluation of solid breast masses: determination of the most discriminatory parameter. AJR Am J Roentgenol. 2014;203: W328-36.
26. Berg WA, Cosgrove DO, Dore CJ, Schafer FK, Svensson WE, Hooley RJ, et al. Shear-wave elastography improves the specificity of breast US: the BE1 multinational study of 939 masses. Radiology. 2012;262:435-49.
27. Youk JH, Gweon HM, Son EJ, Chung J, Kim JA, Kim EK. Three-dimensional shear-wave elastography for differentiating benign and malignant breast lesions: comparison with two-dimensional shear wave elastography. Eur Radiol. 2013;23:1519-27.
28. Lee SH, Chang JM, Kim WH, Bae MS, Cho N, Yi A, et al. Differentiation of benign from malignant solid breast masses: comparison of two-dimensional and three-dimensional shear-wave elastography. Eur Radiol. 2013;23:1015-26.
29. Mann RM, Cho N, Moy L. Breast MRI: state of the art. Radiology. 2019;292:520-36.
30. National Comprehensive Cancer Network. (2018). Breast cancer screening and diagnosis. [online] Available from: https://www.nccn.org/professionals/physician_gls/pdf/breast-screening. pdf [Last accessed March, 2018].
31. National Institute for Health and Care Excellence. (2018). Early and locally advanced breast cancer: diagnosis and management. NICE guideline (NG101). [online] Available from: https://www.nice.org.uk/guidance/ng101 [Last accessed March, 2018].
32. Houssami N, Abraham LA, Kerlikowske K, Buist DS, Irwig L, Lee J, et al. Risk factors for second screen-detected or interval breast cancers in women with a personal history of breast cancer participating in mammography screening. Cancer Epidemiol Biomarkers Prev. 2013;22(5):946-61.
33. Lee JM, Abraham L, Lam DL, Buist DS, Kerlikowske K, Miglioretti DL, et al. Cumulative risk distribution for interval invasive second breast cancers after negative surveillance mammography. J Clin Oncol. 2018;36(20):2070-7.
34. Kuhl CK, Schrading S, Strobel K, Schild HH, Hilgers RD, Bieling HB. Abbreviated breast magnetic resonance imaging (MRI): first postcontrast subtracted images and maximum-intensity projection: a novel approach to breast cancer screening with MRI. J Clin Oncol. 2014;32(22):2304-10.
35. Leithner D, Moy L, Morris EA, Marino MA, Helbich TH, Pinker K. Abbreviated MRI of the breast: does it provide value? J Magn Reson Imaging. 2019;49:e85-100.
36. Saslow D, Boetes C, Burke W, Harms S, Leach MO, Lehman CD, et al. American Cancer Society guidelines for breast screening with MRI as an adjunct to mammography. CA Cancer J Clin. 2007;57(2):75-89.
37. Peters NH, Borel Rinkes IH, Zuithoff NP, Mali WP, Moons KG, Peeters PH. Meta-analysis of MR imaging in the diagnosis of breast lesions. Radiology. 2008;246:116-24.
38. Kuroki Y, Nasu K, Kuroki S, Murakami K, Hayashi T, Sekiguchi R, et al. Diffusion-weighted imaging of breast cancer with the sensitivity encoding technique: analysis of the apparent diffusion coefficient value. Magn Reson Med Sci. 2004;3(2):79-85.
39. Partridge SC, DeMartini WB, Kurland BF, Eby PR, White SW, Lehman CD. Quantitative diffusion-weighted imaging as an adjunct to conventional breast MRI for improved positive predictive value. AJR Am J Roentgenol. 2009; 193(6):1716-22.
40. Liberman M, Sampalis F, Mulder DS, Sampalis JS. Breast cancer diagnosis by scintimammography: a meta-analysis and review of the literature. Breast Cancer Res Treat. 2003;80(1):115-26.
41. Khalkhali I, Villanueva-Meyer J, Edell SL, Connolly JL, Schnitt SJ, Baum JK, et al. Diagnostic accuracy of 99mTc-sestamibi breast imaging: multicenter trial results. J Nucl Med. 2000;41(12):1973-9.
42. Brem RF, Floerke AC, Rapelyea JA, Teal C, Kelly T, Mathur V. Breast-specific gamma imaging as an adjunct imaging modality for the diagnosis of breast cancer. Radiology. 2008;247(3):651-7.
43. Smith IC, Welch AE, Hutcheon AW, Miller ID, Payne S, Chilcott F, et al. Positron emission tomography using [(18)F]-fluorodeoxy-D-glucose to predict the pathologic response of breast cancer to primary chemotherapy. J Clin Oncol. 2000;18:1676-88.
44. Kumar R, Das CJ. Hybrid PET-dynamic CECT in the management of breast cancer. Eur J Nucl Med Mol Imaging. 2009;36(3):413-5.
45. Berg WA, Madsen KS, Schilling K, Tartar M, Pisano ED, Larsen LH, et al. Breast cancer: comparative effectiveness of positron emission mammography and MR imaging in presurgical planning for the ipsilateral breast. Radiology. 2011;258(1):59-72.

CHAPTER

177

Benign and Malignant Lesions of the Breast

Smriti Hari, Smita Manchanda, Ekta Dhamija

INTRODUCTION

The primary role of breast imaging is to detect and characterize abnormalities that could represent malignancy. A large number of benign conditions of the breast are diagnosed and managed clinically. Imaging of benign conditions is required to detect underlying suspicious abnormalities, if any, and to evaluate patients of symptomatic breast diseases with equivocal clinical findings. Mammography is the primary breast imaging modality; ultrasound and magnetic resonance imaging (MRI) have an important complimentary role. Imaging findings are generally suggestive but not specific for most breast lesions.

PROLIFERATIVE BENIGN LESIONS OF THE BREAST

Benign proliferative breast disease is a pathological term used to describe breast conditions wherein there is more glandular and/or fibrotic tissue than expected for the patient's age and parity. It involves the lobules or ducts or both. The tissue is also morphologically abnormal. These conditions include fibrocystic disease, adenosis, fibroadenoma, cyst, ductal hyperplasia, and papilloma. These may coexist.

Fibrocystic Disease

This is the most common benign diagnosis in symptomatic women. It is a nonspecific term, which includes variations in the breast that histologically range from normal physiological changes to premalignant proliferative conditions. The breast is an end organ for cyclic hormonal changes during normal menstruation. The breast parenchyma is hyperemic and edematous in luteal phase of the menstruation. The response of the breast parenchyma to these hormonal changes varies considerably, from minimal to severe, time to time, and woman to woman. This heterogeneous response of breast leads to variable symptoms such as cyclical pain and lumpiness with clinical findings of nonspecific nodularity and tenderness. In addition, there is a long-term age-related actual involution resulting in replacement of glandular tissue with fat. The range of breast changes is often included under the broad heading of aberrations in normal development and involution (ANDI) of the breast.

Imaging findings are also variable. These include increased mammographic density or heterogeneous echotexture of the breast. Diffuse imaging findings do not correlate with histological changes and there is overlap in the normal and pathological conditions. Hence, imaging diagnosis of fibrocystic disease is discouraged.[1] Indication of imaging in symptomatic patient is to detect the underlying focal lesion, if any. If detected, further characterization and management such as biopsy or follow-up should be recommended.

Adenosis

Adenosis represents enlargement of the lobule secondary to a benign proliferation of the blunt ending intralobular ductules (acini). This proliferation is primarily an elongation and multiplication of the acini accompanied by overgrowth of epithelial and connective tissue elements in the lobule. If connective tissue proliferation is a predominant finding, then the term "sclerosing adenosis" is used. Adenosis is a relatively common benign condition of the breast, which is included under benign proliferative conditions.

Mammographically, adenosis rarely forms a visible mass. On occasion, it may be the cause of isolated cluster of uniform microcalcifications. These are extremely small deposits that precipitate in the acini of the lobule and their cystic dilated ends. These calcifications may be diffuse and scattered bilaterally. Adenosis may also cause nonspecific patchy or homogeneous areas of increased density. Adenosis is not visible by ultrasound.

Fibroadenoma

Fibroadenoma is the most common benign tumor of the breast in women of childbearing age. Fibroadenoma develops from overgrowth of the stromal connective tissue within the lobule. This idiopathic proliferation of collagen expands the lobule while simultaneously surrounding and compressing the acini and terminal ducts. Histologically, the proportion of stromal elements found in a fibroadenoma may vary, producing very cellular adenomas or preponderantly fibrotic lesions.

Clinical breast examination (CBE) reveals a firm, mobile, nontender mass. Fibroadenoma may be single or multiple, unilateral, or bilateral, vary in size from few millimeters to a very large size, though most are <3 cm in diameter. Fibroadenomas in women older than 35 years or those which are rapidly growing are excised. Fibroadenomas are hormone-dependent lesions. They regress with age and necrosis within the tumor results in coarse calcification. Fibroadenomas are not premalignant lesions. As there is epithelium within fibroadenoma, cancer can develop just as it can in normal ductal epithelium. Hence, ill-defined margins, microcalcifications, and increase in size on follow-up should raise concern.

On mammography, fibroadenoma is seen as a well-defined, round or oval mass with smooth margins **(Figs. 1A and B)**. Fibroadenomas may have somewhat flattened contours which if present help to distinguish them from cysts. Because, fibroadenomas follow the structure of the lobule, their margins are often lobulated. Occasionally, they have microlobulated margins. In the presence of microlobulations, however, cancer should be suspected. Fibroadenoma may partly or completely be surrounded by a radiolucent halo. Many fibroadenomas calcify as they undergo myxoid degeneration with age. There may be heavy, central, amorphous calcification or coarse, sharp, intermittent popcorn calcification. In postmenopausal age, there may be complete resolution of the soft tissue component of the fibroadenoma resulting in no residual soft tissue density on mammogram, but calcification remains unchanged.

On ultrasound, fibroadenomas are typically solid, round, or oval, well-circumscribed, homogeneously hypoechoic masses that are wider than taller. Like any round or oval masses, fibroadenomas may exhibit lateral wall refractive shadowing, the side lobe artifact. Posterior acoustic enhancement is frequently seen. Fibroadenomas can, however, produce varying sonographic and elastography appearances including ill-defined margins and posterior acoustic shadowing in more fibrotic adenomas.[2,3]

Magnetic resonance imaging is not recommended for a mammographically well-defined mass that is suspected to be a fibroadenoma. If MRI is performed, predominantly fibrous fibroadenomas are hypointense on all sequences and show no enhancement. Fibroadenomas, which are cellular and contain adenomatous or myxoid tissue, show an intermediate- to high-signal intensity on T2-weighted images and most have circumscribed margins with low-intensity internal septae. The enhancement is significant and homogeneous, usually delayed (type 1). Visualization of nonenhancing septae is diagnostic of fibroadenoma.[4]

A fibroadenoma with a diameter of >6 cm is defined as a giant fibroadenoma. It may fill a large part of the breast. It is a benign lesion and most commonly seen in adolescent females. Phyllode tumor is a close differential diagnosis; however, it is generally seen in later decades of life. Lactating fibroadenoma occurs in young females and is associated with pregnancy or lactation. The lactating fibroadenoma may attain enormous size. Juvenile fibroadenoma is another variant which may be seen in teenage females. It often grows rapidly and becomes very large.

Cysts

Breast cysts develop when lumina of ducts or acini become dilated and are lined by atrophic epithelium. Simple cysts are common lesions and vary in size from microscopic to large palpable masses. These are frequently bilateral and multiple but all may not be identified clinically or by imaging. Cysts are common in perimenopausal age but may be seen in women of all ages. Cysts are benign lesions. Cysts may remain stable for many years or spontaneously resolve.

On mammography, a cyst is typically seen as well-defined, round or oval mass. The cyst may be of variable size, solitary or may occur in clumps. A tense cyst is round, but a lax cyst may vary in shape depending upon the degree of compression applied. Calcification is infrequent and it may be seen as a thin peripheral rim or flecks of calcium near the periphery. Rarely, microcysts may contain milk of calcium fluid which on erect lateral mammography layers on the cyst floor forming so-called "tea-cup" calcification. Cysts cannot be accurately diagnosed by mammography, because they

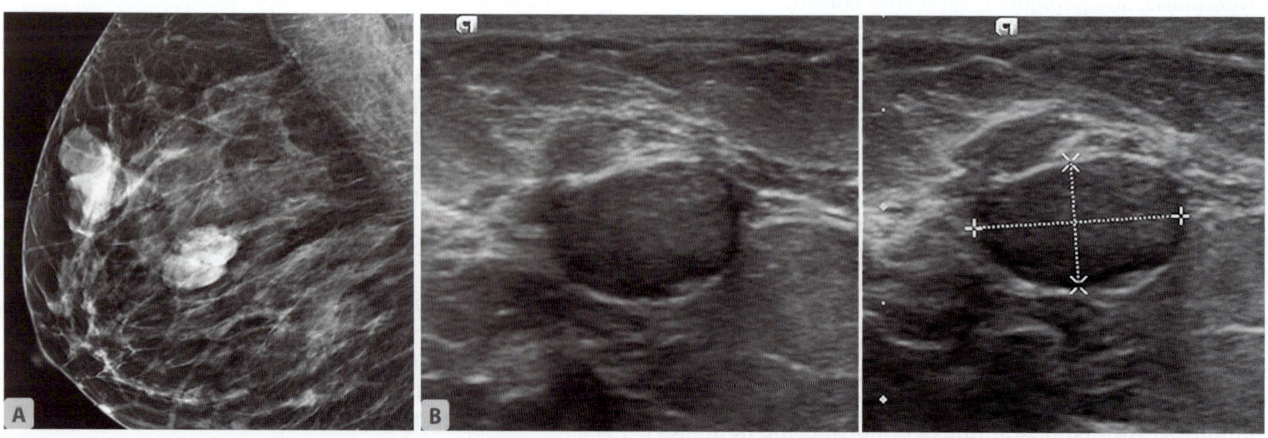

FIGS. 1A AND B: Fibroadenoma. (A) Mammogram shows two well-defined circumscribed masses with lobulations in upper outer quadrant of right breast. No internal calcification or surrounding architectural distortion is noted; (B) Corroborative ultrasound shows these lesions to have circumscribed margins and homogeneously hypoechoic echopattern.

cannot be distinguished from other circumscribed masses, unless they display characteristic pattern of calcification. However, bilateral multiple benign morphology masses on mammography most commonly represent cysts.[1] Ultrasound has an important role in the diagnosis of breast cysts. Typical simple breast cyst is sharply marginated, anechoic with posterior acoustic enhancement **(Fig. 2)**. It may have angular margins, few thin septations, or echogenic debris in the dependent part. These features do not necessarily make it suspicious for malignancy and can be ignored.[4] Posterior enhancement may not be seen if the cyst is small or close to the chest wall. Sometimes, multiple cysts may be seen forming a cluster. Ultrasound diagnosis of simple breast cyst is important as it obviates the need of any fine needle aspiration cytology (FNAC), treatment, or follow-up. Cysts with debris, wall thickening, and septations are referred to a complicated cysts. Chances of malignancy in a complicated cyst are < 0.5% and hence, most complicated cysts are appropriately assigned BIRADS 3 (Breast Imaging Reporting and Data System 3) category.[5] Intracystic tumors are rare. If present, these are commonly intracystic papillomas; intracystic cancer is extremely rare. Indications for aspiration of complicated cysts include suspicion of cyst being an abscess, significant enlargement on follow-up, solid mass in the cyst, or suspicious mammographic findings. Symptomatic cysts may also require ultrasound-guided aspiration; however, half of these recur over 2 years.

On MRI, most cysts are hypointense on T1-weighted images and brightly hyperintense on T2-weighted images. The presence of proteinaceous contents or blood products can modify the signal intensity pattern.

Intraductal Papilloma

Papilloma results from proliferation of the ductal epithelium. They project into the lumen of the duct and connected by a fibrovascular stalk to the epithelial lining. The duct around them can dilate forming a cystic structure giving the appearance of an intracystic papilloma. Benign papilloma is the most common cause of unilateral nipple discharge.[6] Most are located within few centimeters from the nipple in the major subareolar ducts and are usually single.

On mammography, most papillomas are not seen. Larger papillomas are seen as round or oval mass with benign morphology **(Fig. 3A)**. Sometimes, they grow over along length of the duct filling, but not enlarging it. Occasionally, mulberry-like calcification may be seen in the subareolar region. Ultrasound is the preferred modality for the evaluation of nipple discharge. On ultrasound, a typical finding of papilloma is a dilated duct with solid round or oval intraluminal mass **(Fig. 3B)**. Ductography shows dilated duct with intraluminal filling defect or complete obstruction of a duct with a meniscus **(Fig. 3C)**. On MRI, large papillomas behave similar to fibroadenomas.[7] Multiple papillomas arise more distally and are associated with increased risk of cancer.[8]

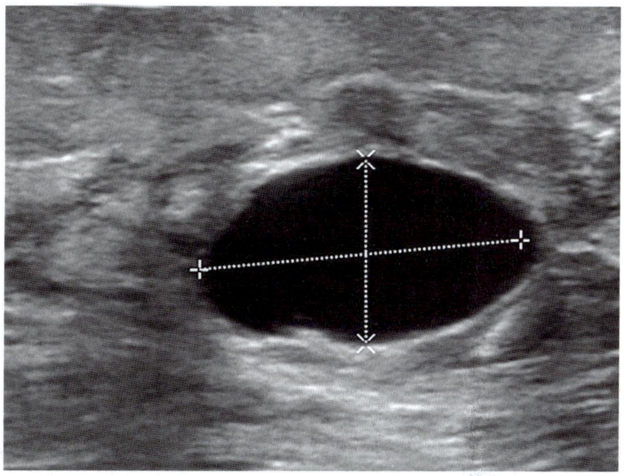

FIG. 2: Breast cyst. Ultrasound shows circumscribed anechoic lesion with smooth walls and posterior acoustic enhancement consistent with simple cyst. No internal septations or solid mural nodule is seen.

Duct Ectasia

Duct ectasia primarily affects the major ducts in the subareolar region. There is nonspecific dilatation of one or more ducts. It is generally associated with periductal inflammation. The distended ducts are filled with secretions and cellular debris.

On mammography, dilated ducts may or may not be appreciated. Ectatic ducts with thickened walls or periductal fibrosis are more visible. Intraluminal debris may calcify and produce calcifications called secretory deposits, resembling broken sticks. Ultrasound shows one or more dilated ducts without intraluminal mass. Depending on the composition of the contents, the duct may be anechoic, show debris or may be hyperechoic. Ductography is usually unnecessary and it shows a dilated duct with attenuated peripheral branches.

Ductal Epithelial Hyperplasia

Ducts are lined with a single layer of epithelial cells. In ductal hyperplasia, there is the benign multilayered cellular proliferation of the epithelium. If atypical cells are found in these, it is called atypical ductal hyperplasia (ADH). It is a high-risk condition as some of these progress into ductal carcinoma in situ (DCIS). Ductal hyperplasia is incidentally diagnosed on biopsy and does not have specific clinical or imaging features. Sometimes, suspicious masses or calcifications may be seen on mammography.

MISCELLANEOUS BENIGN BREAST CONDITIONS

Lipoma

As fat is frequently the preponderant tissue in the breast, it is difficult to differentiate a true lipoma from normal fat. Most lipomas are superficial and form a palpable mass. These are freely movable and generally soft. On mammography, they are lucent, have thin capsule and mass effect with displacement of surrounding structures **(Fig. 4)**. They are hypoechoic on ultrasound, just like the normal breast fat.

Fat Necrosis

Fat necrosis is an inflammatory process of breast related to prior trauma or surgery. Patients are mostly asymptomatic

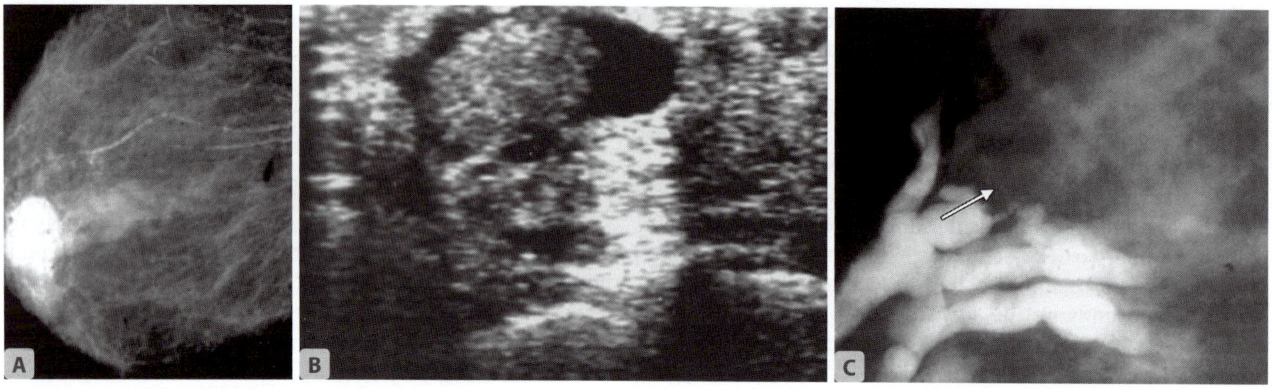

FIGS. 3A TO C: Duct papilloma. (A) Mammogram shows a small well-defined mass in subareolar location along with dilated duct; (B) Ultrasound shows a papilloma within a dilated duct; (C) Ductogram shows an abrupt cut-off of a duct with meniscus formation (arrow).

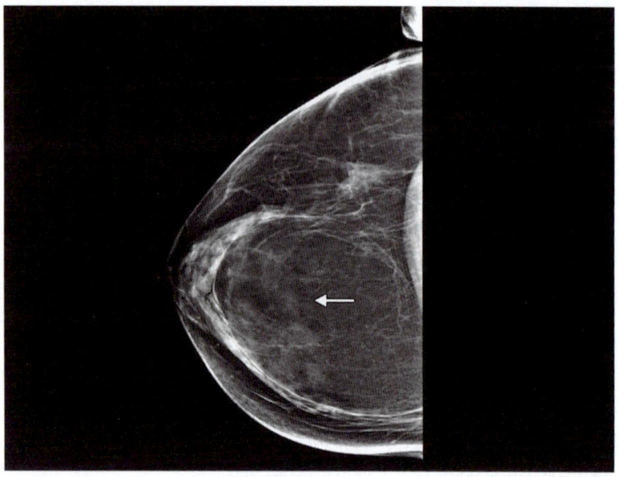

FIG. 4: Lipoma. Mammogram shows a well-defined fat density mass with a capsule (arrow).

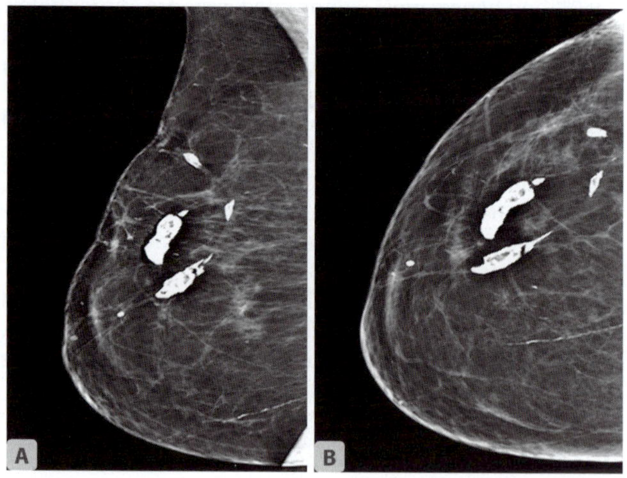

FIGS. 5A AND B: Fat necrosis. Mammogram shows multiple round and oval-calcified nodules suggestive of oil cyst formation at the operative site.

and history of definite trauma is not always present. Some patients have a palpable painful mass with skin thickening or retraction. Occasionally, necrosed fat may form a gelatinous oil cyst with fibrous wall. Fat necrosis is an important lesion because it comes in the differential diagnosis of carcinoma and abscess on mammography.

On mammography, there is a wide spectrum of appearances. Most lesions are superficial in location. Surgical bed is also a common site. Fat necrosis may appear as a spiculated or irregular mass. Calcification is common in fat necrosis and may produce several patterns. Oil cyst shows a round smooth lucent mass, sometimes with calcified thin rim with egg shell appearance **(Figs. 5A and B)**. Cluster of microcalcifications or coarse calcification may also be seen. Post-traumatic oil cysts show varying echogenicity on ultrasound. MRI features of fat necrosis are variable and cannot be distinguished from malignancy. If a fat density is demonstrated within the center of the lesion on nonfat suppressed unenhanced T1-weighted images, fat necrosis can be confirmed.

Galactocele

Galactocele is a cyst filled with inspissated milk. It occurs during pregnancy or lactation and may persist long after cessation of lactation. It may be unilateral or bilateral or may present with multiple palpable masses.

Mammographic features vary with the fat content of the cyst. It may be a well-defined dense lesion like a cyst or a radiolucent mass surrounded by dense lactating breast parenchyma. The usual site is the retroareolar central breast area. Ultrasound shows features of a simple or complicated cyst or a solid mass with posterior enhancement **(Figs. 6A and B)**.

Radial Scar

Radial scar, also known as sclerosing duct hyperplasia, is a lesion of unknown etiology, possibly related to chronic inflammatory process or obliterative changes in blood vessels. There is no palpable mass and no history of trauma. Most are found incidentally on histopathology and some are detected on mammography. Radial scars cannot be accurately diagnosed on core biopsy and require an excisional biopsy. Radial scar is not a premalignant condition but it may rarely contain ADH and DCIS.

Mammographically, it is a spiculated lesion that cannot be differentiated from a cancer **(Figs. 7A and B)**. Central dense mass may or may not be seen. If central mass is absent, it appears like a spiculated architectural distortion only, which is well seen in one view but difficult to appreciate in the other.[9] Microcalcifications are rare. With the advent of digital breast tomosynthesis (DBT), the incidence of detection of radial scars have increased as it demonstrates architectural distortion better than standard two-dimensional (2D) digital mammography.[10] However, its association or upgradation to malignancy is less when seen only on DBT.[11] Ultrasound appearance is also similar to cancer and it shows an irregular, ill-defined, hypoechoic mass. On MRI, an irregular mass with variable contrast enhancement is seen.

Hamartoma

Hamartoma or fibroadenolipoma is an uncommon lesion, which results from fibrous and adenomatous proliferation. The mammographic appearance is characteristic and is seen as sharply defined mass containing admixture of both fatty- and soft-tissue density. Ultrasound appearance is also similar and shows hypoechoic and hyperechoic areas within a well-defined mass.

Desmoid Tumor

Desmoid tumor, also known as fibromatosis, is a locally invasive, benign spindle cell tumor. It usually occurs in abdominal wall but may rarely be seen in the breast. It tends to develop deep in the breast, along the pectoralis fascia. Most patients have history of trauma or surgery. On mammography, it is seen as round or irregular mass with ill-defined or spiculated margins.[4]

Diabetic Mastopathy

It is a rare fibrous tumor that is found in young women with type 1 diabetes. It probably represents an autoimmune inflammatory process. They present with a hard palpable breast mass. Usual mammographic appearance is that of an asymmetric density. Ultrasound shows an ill-defined hypoechoic mass with posterior shadowing.[12]

Superficial Thrombophlebitis (Mondor's Disease)

It is a thrombophlebitis of superficial veins of the breast. It is clinically diagnosed and characterized by thickened and painful cord like veins. History of trauma, surgery, or breast biopsy may be present in some patients. It is a self-limiting process. It is difficult to demonstrate on mammography. The thrombosed vein may be seen as an elongated and beaded cord-like opacity on mammography **(Fig. 8A)**. A thrombosed

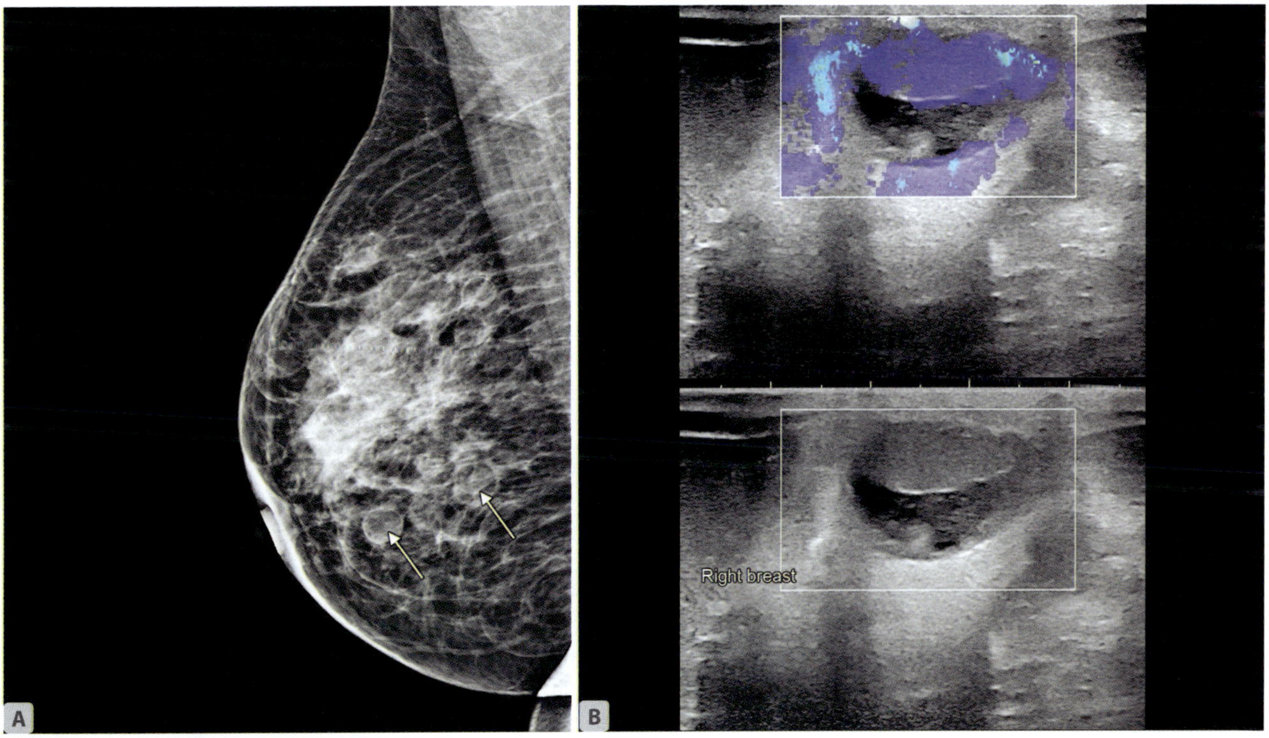

FIGS. 6A AND B: Galactocele. (A) Mammogram shows architectural distortion in upper quadrant with presence of multiple well-defined low-density circumscribed lesion; (B) Corroborative ultrasound shows cysts with debris in vicinity of a prominent duct. The apparent hypodense material in the cyst shows no vascularity and low elasticity on elastography.

subcutaneous vein can also be demonstrated on ultrasound **(Fig. 8B)**.

Breast Infections

Breast infections may be in the form of acute mastitis associated with lactation or a breast abscess. Acute mastitis may progress to form an abscess. Patient presents with painful, localized, or diffuse enlargement of the breast, with erythematous and edematous overlying skin. Breast infections are usually diagnosed and managed clinically.

Mammography is not required in acute mastitis. Breast abscess is painful and mammography is also difficult to perform. If performed, abscess formation is easily missed through the dense, edematous breast. In others, it is usually seen as a well- or ill-defined mass. Overlying skin thickening is often present. Ultrasound is preferred in evaluation of painful and tender breast as it does not require breast compression. It is useful to localize the abscess, to exclude underlying inflammatory breast cancer (IBC), and for diagnostic or therapeutic aspiration.[13] On ultrasound, an abscess is seen as a complex irregular mass with solid/cystic components **(Figs. 9A and B)**. Gross subcutaneous edema is usually associated, which is seen as multiple thin, fluid-filled clefts beneath the skin. MRI is not required for evaluation of breast infections. If performed, it shows intense enhancement and secondary changes such as skin thickening, retraction, or architectural distortion. The enhancement tends to be delayed and diffuse but it cannot be differentiated from inflammatory carcinoma.

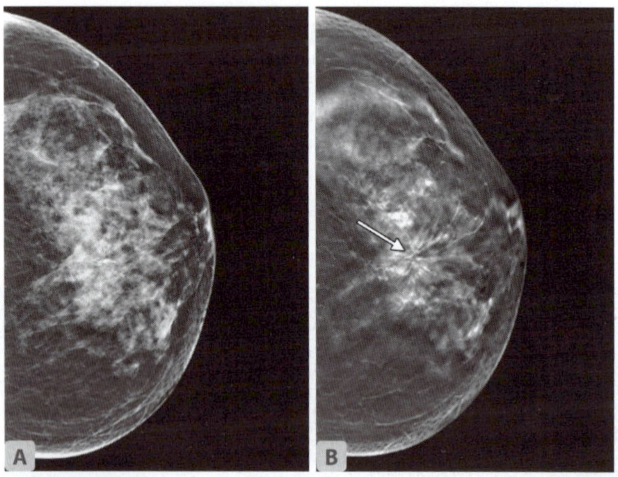

FIGS. 7A AND B: Radial Scar. Digital breast tomosynthesis shows area of architectural distortion in central inner quadrant (arrow in B) which was not appreciable on 2D mammogram (A).

Granulomatous Mastitis

Granulomatous mastitis is a chronic inflammatory condition of breast for which underlying cause is uncertain. In developed countries, autoimmune etiology has been postulated whereas infection is thought to be the etiology in developing countries. Patients usually present with vague lumps. Clinical evaluation may mimic cancer. Mammography shows nonspecific features such as asymmetric increased density or an ill-defined mass with architectural distortion/trabecular thickening. Ultrasound may show an irregular mass, abscess, fluid-filled tracking channels, edema, or sinus tracts **(Figs. 10A and B)**.[14] Diagnosis is established on biopsy only.

Since tuberculosis is endemic in our country, it is thought to be the most common cause of any unresolving breast infection/mastitis. It has variable mammographic appearances. There are three types of lesions seen on mammography.[15] Nodular form is seen as a dense mass with irregular or spiculated margin, with or without calcification. It is the most common mammographic feature of breast tuberculosis and may mimic carcinoma.[16] Diffuse involvement produces multiple caseating confluent foci of tuberculosis. These also result in skin thickening, ulceration, and sinus formation. Mammography shows dense breast, or skin thickening with or without lymphadenopathy. These findings may mimic inflammatory carcinoma. Sclerosing form of breast tuberculosis is a slow-growing process with excessive fibrosis rather than caseation. Entire breast is hard with nipple retraction. Mammography is not contributory

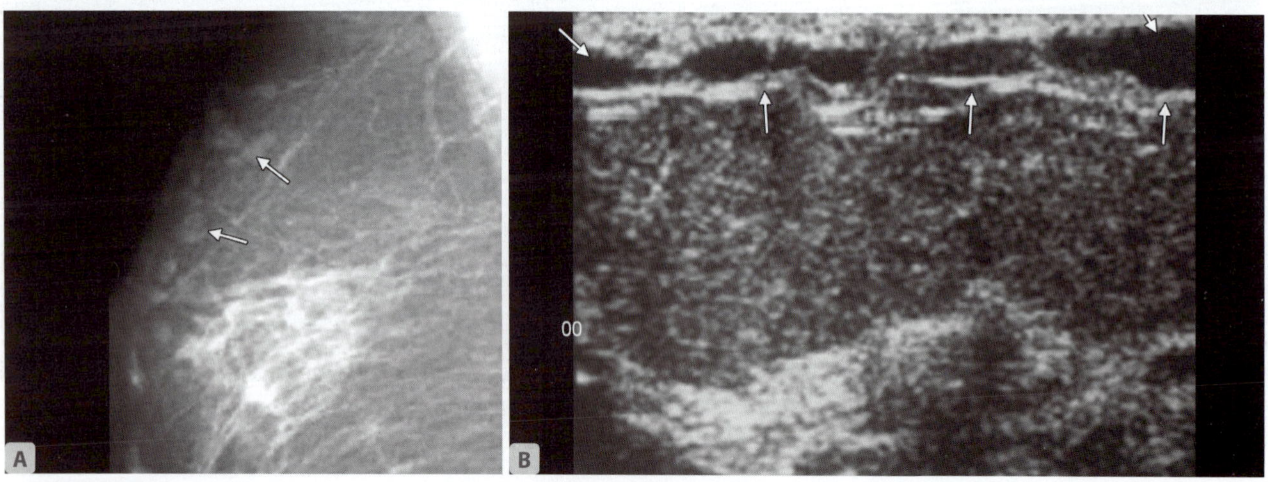

FIGS. 8A AND B: Mondor's disease. (A) Mammogram shows superficial tortuous linear opacities (arrows) representing a thrombosed vein; (B) Thrombosed subcutaneous vein (arrows) can be seen on ultrasound also.

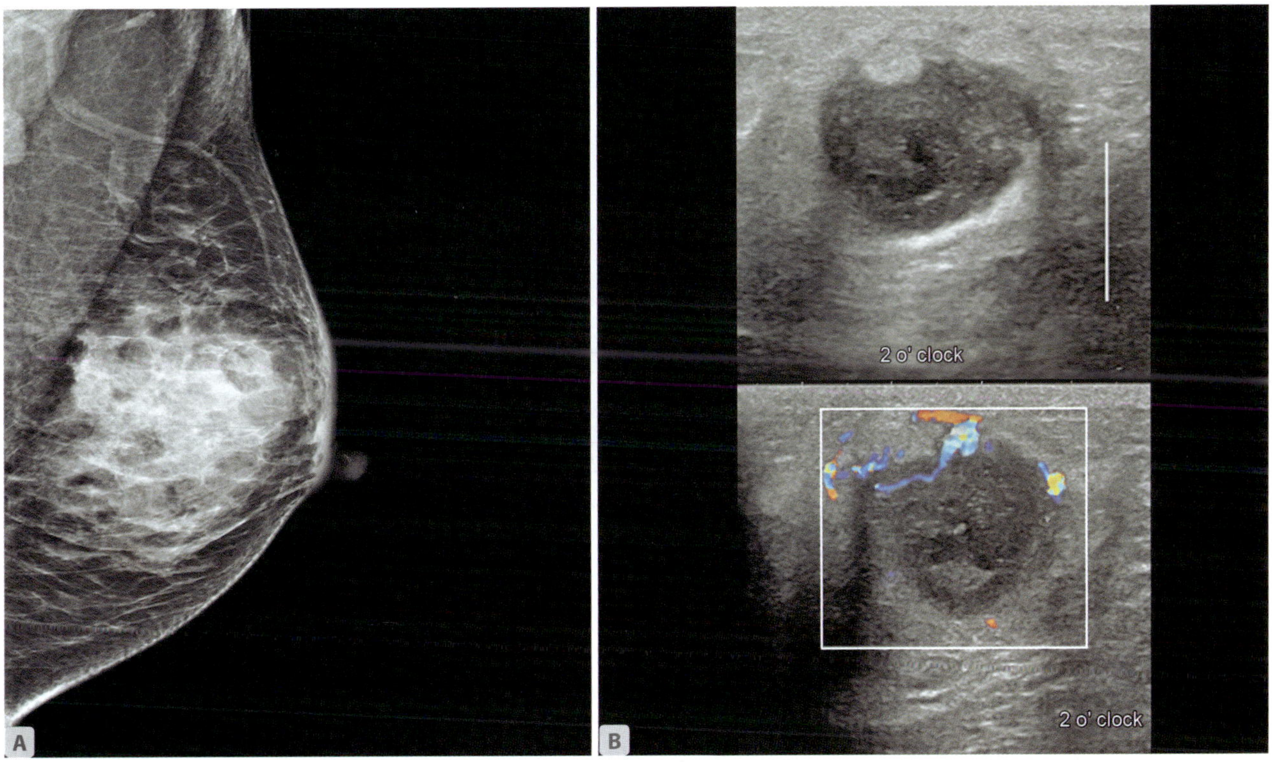

FIGS. 9A AND B: Breast abscess. (A) Left breast MLO view demonstrating irregular mass with obscured margins in central quadrant with overlying skin thickening in periareolar location; (B) Correlative ultrasound shows irregular complex solid cystic mass with surrounding inflammatory changes and vascularity in the periphery only. (MLO: mediolateral oblique).

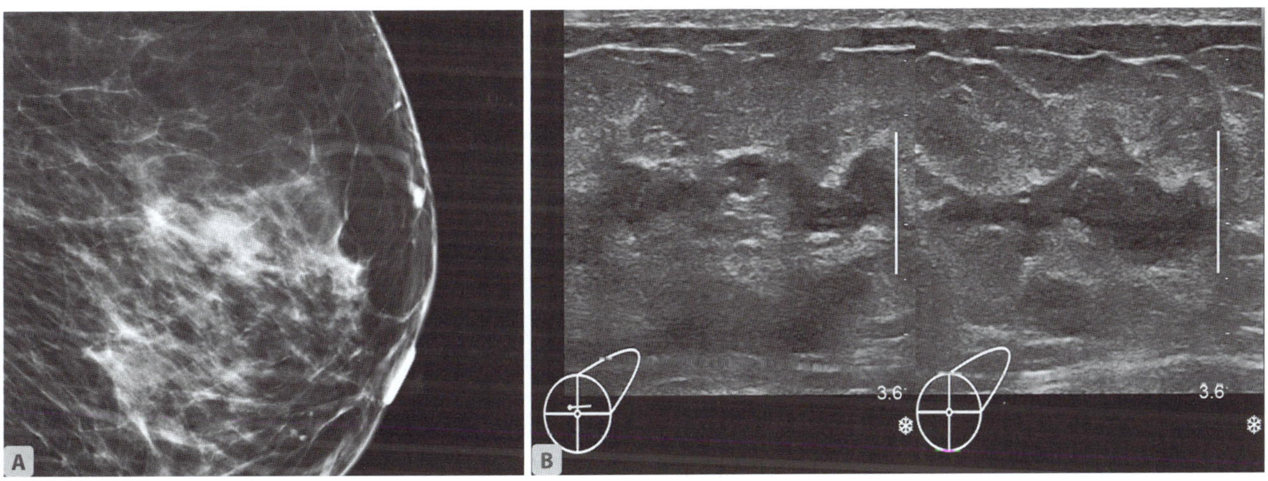

FIGS. 10A AND B: Granulomatous mastitis. (A) Mammogram shows an area of architectural distortion and trabecular thickening in central quadrant of left breast which is seen as fluid-tracking channels on ultrasound (B).

as it shows uniformly increased density of one breast. Ultrasound features of breast tuberculosis are nonspecific and these include a hypoechoic mass or abscess, skin thickening, sinuses, and duct ectasia. Computed tomography (CT) is useful in demonstrating the underlying chest wall involvement.

Breast Implants

Implants are used for cosmetic augmentation of the breast or for breast reconstruction after mastectomy. These are silicone rubber bags filled with silicone gel or saline. These are usually placed behind the breast tissue and anterior to pectoralis muscle. A fibrous capsule normally forms around the implant because of foreign body reaction. Implants appear semiovoid and opaque on mammography and these are anechoic on ultrasound **(Figs. 11A and B)**. During mammography, only the breast tissue anterior to implant can be pulled forward and compressed. Hence, complete visualization of breast parenchyma is not possible on mammography and this interferes with cancer detection. Ultrasound and MRI are

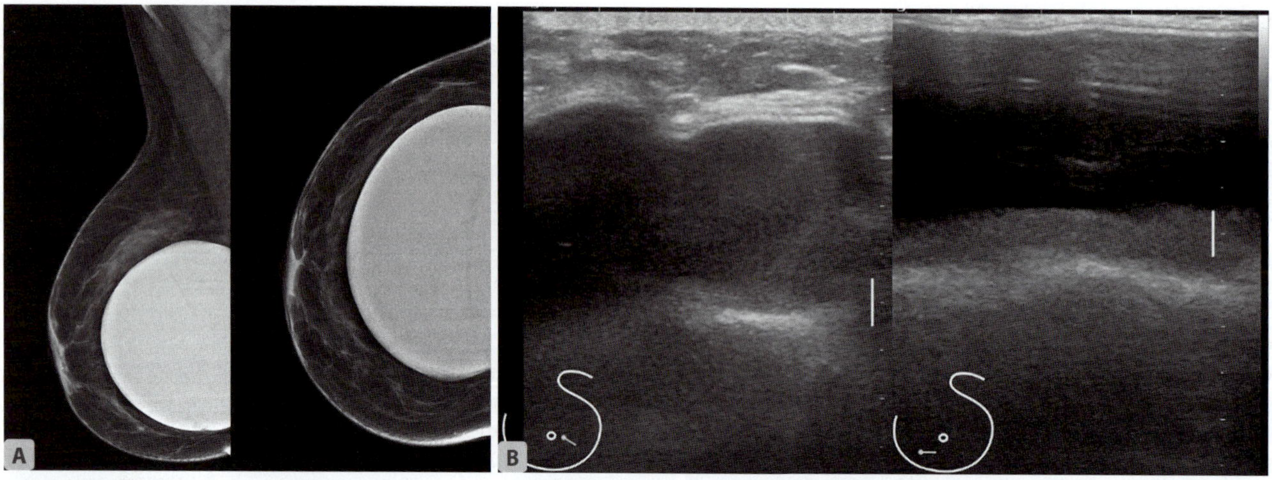

FIGS. 11A AND B: Breast implant. (A) Mammogram shows the implant as a large, semiovoid well-defined opacity; (B) Implant shows anechoic fluid content on ultrasound.

useful for evaluation of implants. MRI is the modality of choice. Plain MRI is sufficient. Water- and fat-suppressed (silicone only) T2-weighted magnetic resonance (MR) sequences are particularly useful. Silicone is hypointense on T1-weighted images and hyperintense on T2-weighted images.

Common complications of implants are capsular contractions causing pain and deformity of the breast and implant rupture. Rupture may occur spontaneously due to capsular contracture or during the closed capsulotomy, a procedure in which a surgeon manually compress the capsule to break it and relieve the pain. Rupture can be intracapsular in which the extravasated gel remain inside fibrous capsule or it may be extracapsular leading to spread of the gel in breast parenchyma. The sequelae of noncontained silicone include granuloma formation, fibrosis, and migration. Migration of silicone into the axilla can involve the brachial plexus, resulting in neuropathy.

On ultrasound, intracapsular rupture is seen as folded membranes representing collapsed envelope in step-ladder pattern within the anechoic gel. On MRI, collapsed envelope is seen as low-intensity membranes floating in hyperintense gel on T2-weighted sequences.[17] With extracapsular rupture, ultrasound shows multiple hyperechoic foci in the breast. Extravasated gel in the parenchyma is very echogenic and produces shadowing.[18] On MRI, the extravasated gel appears as foci of low-signal intensity on T1-weighted sequences and high-signal intensity on T2-weighted sequences.[19]

MALIGNANT LESIONS OF THE BREAST

Breast cancer is the most common cancer in female population worldwide with over 2 million new cases detected in 2018 itself.[20] According to GLOBACON 2012, it constitutes approximately 25.1% of all cancers and is more common in developed countries but has more mortality in developing nations.[21] In India, breast cancer is number one cancer among females with age adjusted rate of 25.8 per 100,000 women and mortality of 12.7 per 100,000 women.[22]

Risk Factors for Breast Cancer

Female gender and increasing age are the most important risk factors for development of breast cancer. Other risk factors include early menarche, late menopause, nulliparity or late first pregnancy, and decreased breast feeding. All of these factors increase the overall duration of endogenous estrogen exposure, a hormone known to play a major role in the development of breast cancer. Exogenous estrogen exposure in hormonal replacement therapy (HRT) also increases the risk of breast cancer. Family history of breast cancer in a first-degree relative is also a risk factor, especially if they had breast cancer at an early age. The familial inheritance of the risk may be associated with or without genetic mutations. Women with Li-Fraumeni and Cowden syndromes have a high risk. History of benign breast disease, especially atypical hyperplasia also increases the risk of breast cancer. Mammographic breast density has also been identified as a risk factor. Women with >75% glandular density on mammogram are at fourfold greater risk for breast cancer development.[23]

BRCA1 and *BRCA2* genes mutations are major risk factors and these account for 5–10% of all breast cancers. The chances of breast cancer in the carriers of these mutations are variable in different races and range from 45 to 85%.[24] They also have an increase a risk for ovarian cancer, especially with *BRCA1* mutation. Breast cancer arising in these women is frequently aggressive and triple negative; negative for estrogen receptor (ER), progesterone receptor (PR), and human epidermal growth factor receptor (HER2). Management options in BRCA mutation carriers include close surveillance, chemoprevention, and prophylactic bilateral mastectomy with or without salpingo-oophorectomy.

Diagnosis of the Breast Cancer

Breast cancer may be detected in preclinical stage on screening mammography. Others are detected by self-breast examination (SBE) or CBE. Symptomatic breast cancers present with a palpable mass, focal tenderness, nipple discharge, skin retraction or ulceration, or sometimes as a metastatic disease with occult primary site. Mammography is the primary modality for detection of breast cancer; tomosynthesis, ultrasound, and MRI complement mammography in detection of breast cancer. Approach to the breast imaging and role of various imaging modalities in detection of breast cancer has been covered in the preceding chapter. However, there are no characteristic features of breast cancer on imaging. It is interesting to note that mammographic interpretation has a category of definitely benign lesions (BIRADS 2) but there is no category of definitely malignant lesions. Mammography only detects lesions which are either suspicious (BIRADS 4) or highly suspicious (BIRADS 5) for malignancy. Hence, all such lesions need to be subjected to biopsy for the definitive diagnosis of breast cancer. Image-guided breast biopsy is an important tool for the diagnosis of breast cancer, and it is described in detail in the following chapter. Pathological analysis routinely consists of assessment of invasion, histopathological characterization, and immunohistochemical analysis for ER, PR, and HER2 receptor status.[25] Classification of breast cancer into luminal and basal type, based on genetic expressions and molecular biology may also be performed.

BREAST CANCER SCREENING

Cancer screening is aimed at detection of a cancer when it is small, asymptomatic, and early stage. Chances of cure are highest with such cancers. Primary purpose of any screening program that targets healthy population is to reduce deaths from the disease and not just its early diagnosis. Mammography screening achieves this goal.

Mammography Screening

Mammography screening is the most widely used cancer screening modality in the world. It has been studied extensively and no other imaging modality has been subjected to as large scale and extensive research as mammography. There is level 1 evidence to suggest that mammography screening reduces the breast cancer mortality significantly in the screened population and it is cost effective. This evidence has primarily come from eight large randomized screening trials [randomized controlled trials (RCTs)] started in 1970s and early 80s in which half of women were invited to screening and the other half were not. These trials along with early benefits from these are given in **Table 1**.[26] Many of these trials are continuously analyzed. Health Insurance Plan (HIP) of New York was the first trial and it also included CBE along with mammography. Twin county trial consisted of two simultaneous trials conducted at Swedish counties of Ostergotland and Kopparberg. It is the largest screening trial for which longest follow-up is available. National Breast Screening Studies (NBSS) of Canada performed two separate screenings for women of age groups 40–49 and 50–75 years, respectively. These were similar to HIP. The data and long-term follow-up of these trials have been analyzed and debated several times to determine the exact quantum of benefits from mammography screening. Overall, mammography screening effectively reduces the overall breast cancer mortality by 28–45%.[27] Most recent meta-analysis for US Preventive Services Task Force (USPSTF) also confirmed that mammography screening significantly reduces breast cancer mortality in women aged 39–69 years.[28] A three decade follow-up of the twin county trial has shown that cost-effectiveness and number of deaths prevented by screening improve over time.[29] Analysis of community screening programs, outside the RCTs, in developed countries of Europe, America, and Australia have also shown that the implementation of screening mammography reduces breast cancer deaths by as high as 35–50%.[28-31] Reviews and data analysis from the RCTs have been performed several times and using variable methods.[32] Some concluded that there is no benefit with screening mammography.[33] However, such reviews are few and their analysis is considered flawed by most experts.[34] Early detection is beneficial for diagnosis and treatment of any cancer and breast cancer is certainly not an exception to this logic.[35]

There are some variations in the recommendations for mammography screening. American College of Radiology and American Cancer Society recommend mammography every year from 40 to 74 years of age. However, USPSTF recommends 2 yearly mammography in the 50–75 years age group.[36] In some European countries, mammography is offered every 2 years from 50 to 70 years or 74 years.[37-39] After the age of 75 years, mammography is not cost-effective in term of number of lives saved as there are other competing causes of death.

TABLE 1: Randomized controlled trials (RCTs) of mammography screening.

RCT	Years of start	Number of women	Age group (years)	Mammography interval (months)	Early mortality reduction
HIP, New York, USA	1963	62,000	40–64	12	29%
Two county, Sweden	1978	162,981	40–74	24	37%
Malmo, Sweden	1976	42,000	45–69	18	18%
Stockholm, Sweden	1981	59,176	40–64	24	20%
Gothenburg, Sweden	1982	52,000	39–59	18	14%
Edinburg, UK	1978	45,130	45–64	12	16%
NBSS 1, Canada	1980	50,430	40–49	12	Nil
NBSS 2, Canada	1980	39,476	50–59	12	30%

(HIP: Health Insurance Plan; NBSS: National Breast Screening Studies)

Mammography screening must be organized and optimized for it to be successful. Mammography is the most regulated and legislated imaging modality in Europe and America. Licensing and accreditation of the facilities, regular QA programs, tests and training programs of radiographers and radiologists, reporting standards are regularly monitored, and audit of the outcome performed.

Screening mammography is a high-cost venture. At least 414 women must be screened for 7 years to prevent one breast cancer death.[27] It has several other drawbacks as well, which frequently generates controversies. Most important among these are false-positive mammograms and overdiagnosis. After a regular screening round, some women are recalled at the facility for additional imaging and/or biopsy. Although majority of them will not have a cancer, it causes anxiety in all of them and also increases the cost of screening. About half of women screened for 10 years have at least one recall and may be a biopsy. Screening mammography has also led to many fold increase in the DCIS detection rates.[40] This leads to biopsy and surgery, including mastectomies, in women with mammographic lesions. This may be unnecessary in some women since all DCIS do not grow into invasive carcinoma and cancer would have never been diagnosed in their lifetime, had screening not been done. Overdiagnosis and overtreatment of such indolent breast cancers is considered a major disadvantage of mammographic screening and often criticized. However, since there is no way to predict which DCIS will progress into invasive ductal carcinoma (IDC), this limitation of mammographic screening should be accepted for overall benefits. Screening mammography also does not detect all breast cancers. Some aggressive cancers may get diagnosed in between two sequential rounds of the screening. These are called interval cancers and their incidence may range from 10 to 43% in different age groups.[41]

True benefits from screening mammography have also been debated. In recent years, improved breast cancer treatment with better chemo/hormonal therapy and targeted therapy have improved the survival and it is difficult to determine the absolute contribution of screening mammography in reducing overall breast cancer mortality.[42] It is estimated that mammography has contributed by two-thirds and adjuvant treatment by one-third in present day breast cancer mortality reduction in developed countries.[30]

Magnetic Resonance Imaging Screening

Familial breast cancers account for 10–15% of all breast cancers and about half of these patients are *BRCA1* and *BRCA2* mutations carriers. Cancer occurs in these women at younger age and hence, screening must be started much earlier. Mammographic breast density is high in young women and as expected, the performance of mammography is poor in detection of breast cancer in these women. MRI does not depend on breast density and it is the most sensitive tool for breast cancer detection in these women.[43,44] Breast MRI is recommended for screening of high-risk women, if risk quantification is >25%.[44,45] Generally, annual breast MRI and mammograms are performed with 6-month gap between these two tests, resulting in imaging surveillance at every 6th month. Screening should be started at younger age of 25–30 years. Higher sensitivity of breast MRI comes with high false-positive rates. This leads to higher number of benign breast biopsies, when compared with mammographic screening.

Ultrasound Screening

Ultrasound, as a sole modality, has never been used for breast cancer screening. However, it is routinely used to evaluate mammographically dense breasts. It can show mammographically occult breast cancers in asymptomatic women with negative mammograms. However, the detection rate is <1%.[46,47] A blinded screening trial [ACRIN (American College of Radiology Imaging Network) 6666] comparing ultrasound and mammography for cancer detection in high-risk women found mammographic detection rate of 7.6 cancers per 1,000 women screened. It increased to 11.8 cancers with combined mammography and ultrasound use.[48] Additional cancers detected on ultrasound were invasive and node negative and hence, these women actually benefited from ultrasound screening. However, ultrasound is not likely to be used for population screening because of its inability to visualize microcalcifications, operator dependency, time consuming nature, and high false-positive rates, mostly from complicated cysts.

Breast Cancer Screening in Developing Countries

Population-based screening mammography is expensive and resource intensive. Hence, it is not an immediate option in countries with limited resources. SBE and CBE are widely encouraged for early diagnosis, or more precisely, to decrease the proportion of advanced breast cancers at presentation. However, the only RCT on SBE for breast cancer screening has shown no benefits.[49] Breast Health Global Initiative (BHGI), a nonprofit organization working in this area, has recommended the use of traditional "triple test" assessment comprising CBE, imaging (diagnostic mammography or ultrasound), and FNAC or biopsy for early diagnosis of breast cancer in low-resource countries.[50]

IMAGING FEATURES OF BREAST CANCER

Breast cancer is a group of malignant breast lesions. All breast cancers are believed to arise from the terminal duct lobular unit (TDLU). It is the distal most part of the ductal branching system which opens into the lobule of the gland and is the site of most active cellular proliferation. Breast cancers are classified into various pathological subtypes according to the World Health Organization (WHO) system. These cannot be determined on imaging. There are no imaging features which are specific to any pathological subtype of the breast cancer. Actually, imaging features are not even specific for cancer. However, some imaging characteristics are somewhat more commonly associated with particular type of cancer than others.

Preinvasive Breast Lesions

Preinvasive breast lesions include DCIS and lobular carcinoma in situ (LCIS). DCIS is the precursor of invasive breast cancer. On the other hand, most LCIS do not become invasive and this entity is hence, regarded as a high-risk condition rather than a true cancer.

Ductal Carcinoma In Situ

Ductal carcinoma in situ lies along a spectrum of preinvasive lesions of the breast tissue, with histologic progression from ADH to DCIS and then to the IDC. The pathological classification of DCIS is based on the nuclear grade of the tumor cells (low, intermediate, or high), the architectural pattern of tumor growth (solid, papillary, micropapillary, or cribriform), and the presence or absence of comedo necrosis.

Ductal carcinoma in situ is usually small but can grow to large size and become symptomatic. Presentations of DCIS include mammographically detected mass or calcification, palpable mass, Paget's disease, or an incidental finding on breast biopsy. DCIS is a precursor of IDC; however, only some of DCIS develop into invasive cancer, while other remains indolent forever. True incidence of IDC in patients with DCIS is unknown. On mammography, DCIS is characterized by microcalcifications, usually of linear branching type **(Fig. 12)**. Less commonly, DCIS can produce a mass with ill-defined or lobulated borders, with or without calcification. Ultrasound is unsuitable to detect microcalcifications. Associated soft tissue component and architectural distortion may be appreciated as a hypoechoic mass on ultrasound. It may be suspected if there is an area of altered echotexture with parenchymal echogenicity, ductal changes, or few nonspecific cysts on ultrasound. Atypical ductal and parenchymal changes in comparison to normal rest of the breast parenchyma should be evaluated carefully to rule out possibility of DCIS. Calcifications are not seen on MRI; however, overall sensitivity of MRI is higher than mammography in detection of DCIS.[51] Both can detect DCIS not detected by the other modality. On MRI, about half of DCIS are seen as enhancing masses. Others show nonmass-like enhancement or no enhancement.[52] All three patterns of enhancement curves can be seen with DCIS. DCIS is treated with mastectomy or breast conservation treatment [lumpectomy followed by radiotherapy (RT)]. Since, it is not an invasive cancer, axillary dissection is not required.

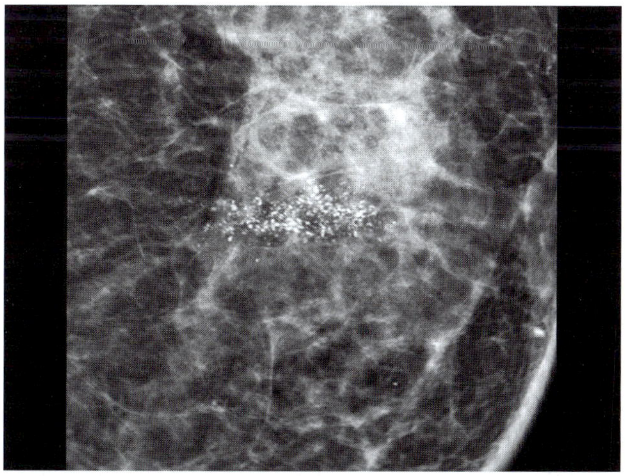

FIG. 12: DCIS. Mammogram shows pleomorphic, linear branching microcalcifications in the ductal orientation. (DCIS: ductal carcinoma in situ).

Lobular Carcinoma In Situ

Atypical lobular hyperplasia (ALH) and LCIS are not true cancers but are high-risk or premalignant conditions. These are asymptomatic and incidentally detected on breast biopsy. Pathologically, these represent spectrum of atypical proliferation of loosely cohesive cells in the TDLU. LCIS is often multifocal and bilateral. It does not cause any clinical or imaging abnormalities. About one-third of the women with LCIS ultimately develop invasive lobular carcinoma (ILC) in the same or contralateral breast.[1] Management options include close surveillance or prophylactic mastectomy.

Invasive Breast Cancer

Invasive or infiltrating ductal carcinoma (IDC) is the most common histologic subtype of breast cancer. It is designated not otherwise specified (NOS) as it is not categorized into specific types such as medullary, lobular, mucinous, etc. In SEER data of National Cancer Institute, IDC (NOS) constituted 83.9% of all invasive breast cancers.[53] Others include invasive lobular (7.4%), medullary (3.1%), mucinous (2.3%), and Paget's disease (1%). Other subtypes accounted for <1% each. Depending on the nuclear pleomorphism and mitotic activity, all breast cancers are also graded histologically into grade 1 (well differentiated), grade 2 (moderately differentiated), and grade 3 (poorly differentiated). This tumor grading has prognostic significance.

Invasive Ductal Carcinoma

Invasive ductal carcinoma (NOS) is undifferentiated and has no specific histologic pattern. Desmoplastic reaction is common in IDC which accounts for its most common presentation of hard mass on palpation and spiculated mass on mammography **(Figs. 13A to C)**. It may also be seen as malignant calcifications, architectural distortion, or any combination of these. Ultrasound and MRI show a mass having one or more malignant features described in Chapter 25 **(Figs. 13A to C)**. Irregular mass with rim enhancement or heterogeneous internal enhancement is the most common MR appearance of IDC.

Invasive Lobular Carcinoma

Invasive lobular carcinoma is the second most common invasive breast cancer and a large number of these are multicentric or bilateral. Histologically, these show diffuse tumor foci invading the stroma. They spread in the form of a single file (line) of noncohesive malignant cells through intervening normal parenchyma, instead of a well-formed mass. They do not evoke desmoplastic response. Because of these features, ILC are difficult to detect on clinical examination, mammography, and even on MRI. Clinical presentation may be of an ill-defined mass, nonspecific

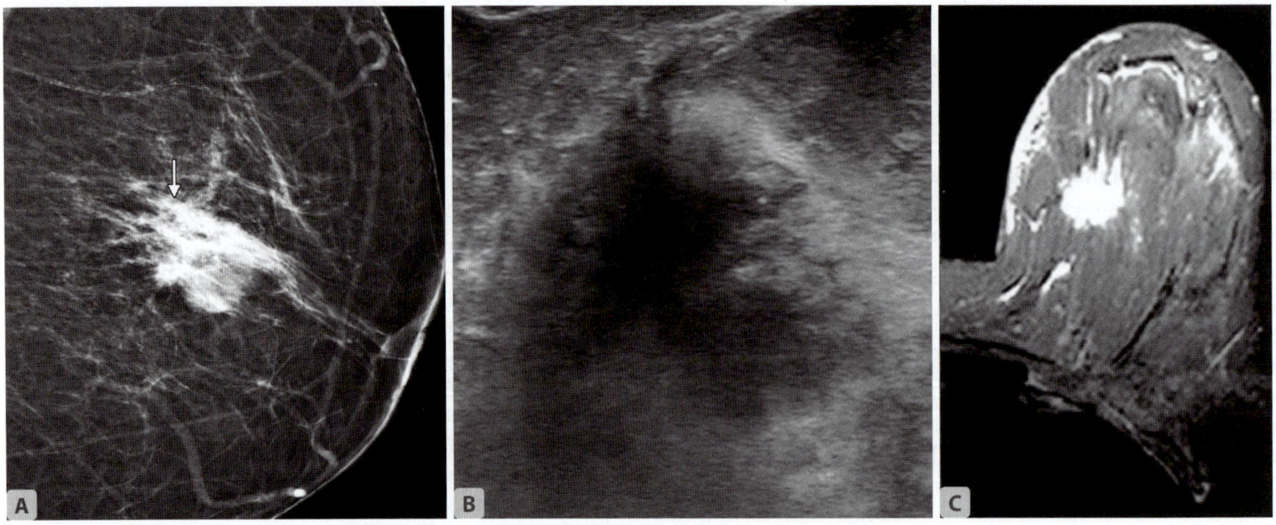

FIGS. 13A TO C: IDC. (A) Mammogram shows a high-density, irregular, spiculated mass (arrow); (B) Ultrasound shows a hypoechoic, irregular, spiculated mass with distal acoustic shadowing; (C) Contrast-enhanced T1-weighted MRI scan of another woman shows a spiculated, intensely enhancing mass. (IDC: invasive ductal carcinoma; MRI: magnetic resonance imaging).

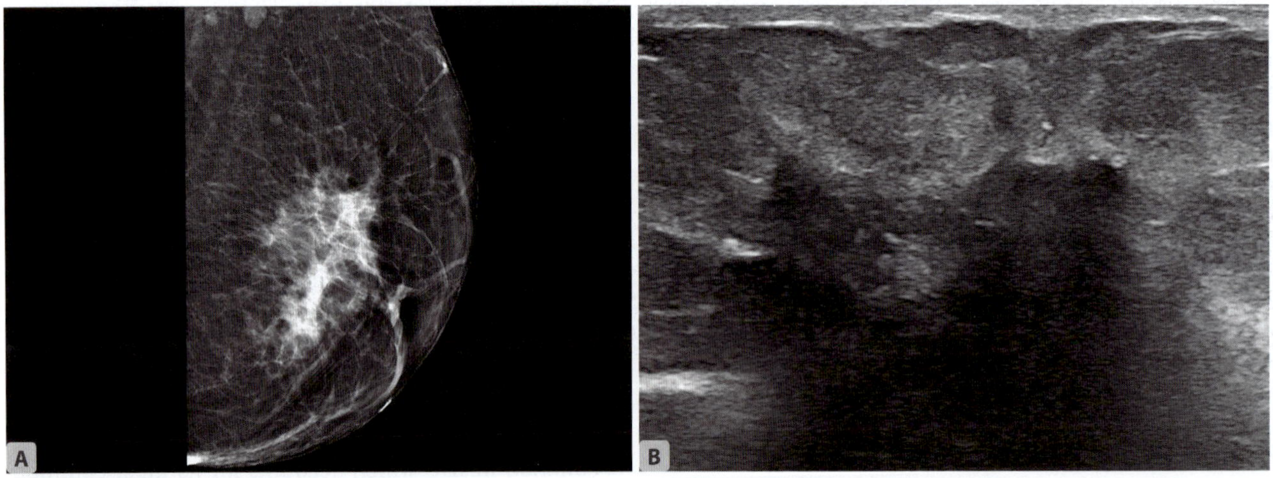

FIGS. 14A AND B: Invasive lobular carcinoma. (A) Left MLO view shows architectural distortion causing nipple retraction in the breast; (B) Ultrasound shows ill-defined hypoechoic mass with radiating spiculated margins. (MLO: mediolateral oblique).

induration, or tenderness. Other patients may present with symptoms from distant metastases. Mammographically, asymmetric breast density is the most common finding. Other mammographic findings include spiculated or ill-defined mass, or a normal mammogram.[1] Calcifications are distinctly rare. Ultrasound is useful to detect underlying mass in an asymmetric density seen on mammography **(Figs. 14A and B)**. MRI does not detect all ILC; however, it is more accurate than mammography for detection of ILC.[54] On MRI, ILC are most commonly seen as enhancing mass with variable contrast enhancement patterns. Others may be seen as diffuse area of enhancement that is difficult to differentiate from normal parenchyma.[55] MRI detects additional foci of cancer in >50% of patients diagnosed with ILC.[56]

Medullary Carcinoma

Medullary carcinoma is usually seen in younger age. It is a rapidly growing tumor and often large in size when detected.[1] Histologically, they are high-grade tumors with abundant infiltration by inflammatory cells. Desmoplastic process is uncommon. The prognosis is poor as most have early lymphovascular invasion, lymph node, and distant metastases. On mammography, a well-defined or ill-defined mass, without spiculations or calcification is seen **(Fig. 15)**. On ultrasound, they are hypoechoic, well-circumscribed, or lobulated. Distal acoustic enhancement may be seen. These ultrasound features often simulate benign masses.

Mucinous Carcinoma

Mucinous (or colloid) carcinoma is a well-differentiated, slow growing tumor. It is generally seen in older women and has a better prognosis. It is characterized by abundant mucin production. Usual mammographic finding is of a low-density mass with ill-defined or microlobulated margins **(Figs. 16A and B)**. Calcification or desmoplastic reaction is uncommon. Ultrasound shows a well-defined, iso- or hypoechoic mass with microlobulated margins and posterior acoustic enhancement insome.[57] Rarely, it is seen as a complex cystic-solid mass on ultrasound. MR features are similar to mammography; however, the contrast enhancement pattern is frequently of benign type. Unlike most other breast cancers, mucinous cancer can demonstrate high-signal intensity on T2-weighted images.

Tubular Carcinoma

Tubular carcinoma is a rare well-differentiated invasive carcinoma which demonstrates poorly formed ductal structures. About one-third of these are multicentric and bilateral. They are slow growing and have better prognosis. On mammography, a small spiculated or ill-defined mass is usually seen.[1] Uncommonly, calcifications may be seen. There are no specific MR features.

Papillary Carcinoma

Papillary carcinoma is seen with advanced age. There is villous epithelial proliferation that eventually fills the ductal lumen. Papillary carcinoma can develop as an intracystic lesion, although it is likely that the cyst represents a secondarily dilated duct.[1] These are slow growing and do not have desmoplastic reaction. On mammography, papillary carcinomas are seen as well-circumscribed masses because of their cystic nature. This is the only breast cancer which is commonly cystic on ultrasound; usual sonographic appearance is a complex solid-cystic mass or intracystic tumor with multiple fronds projecting into the lumen of the cyst **(Fig. 17)**.

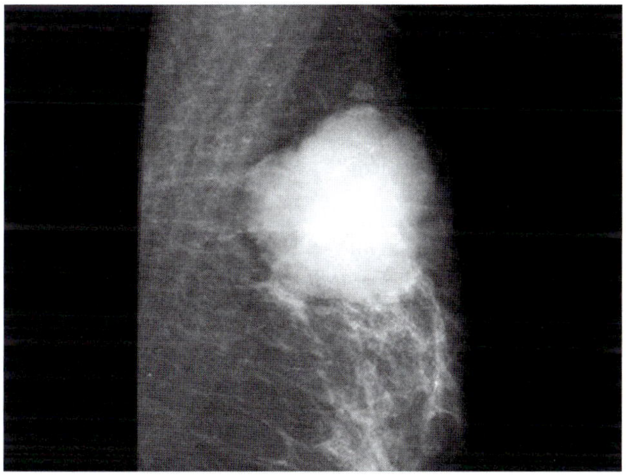

FIG. 15: Medullary carcinoma. Mammogram shows a round mass with lobulated, partially indistinct margin.

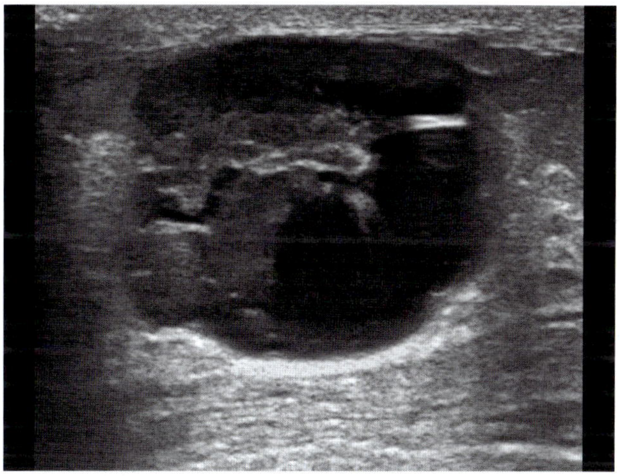

FIG. 17: Intracystic papillary carcinoma: ultrasound shows a complex cyst with irregular solid component projecting intraluminally from the lateral wall.

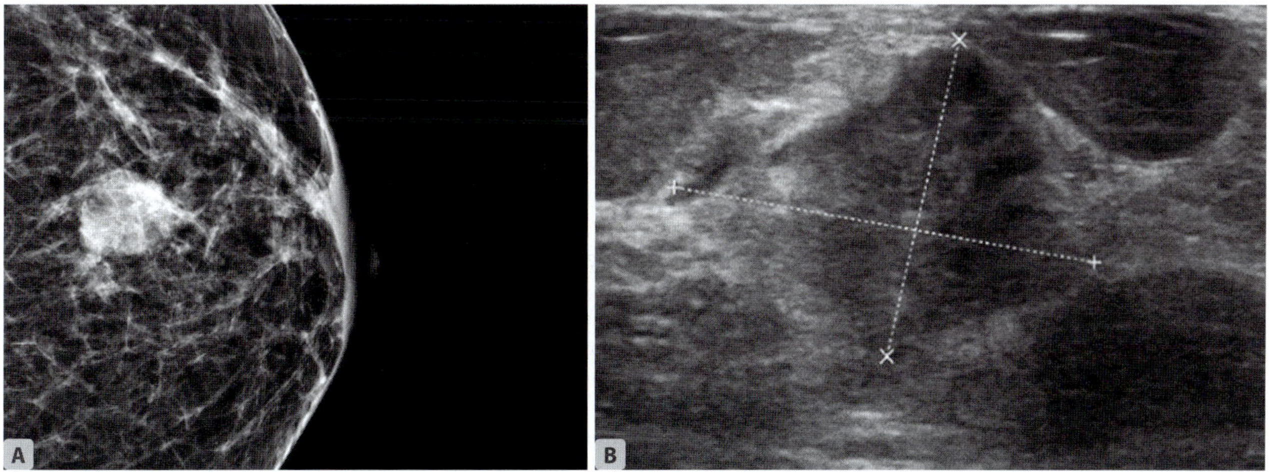

FIGS. 16A AND B: Mucinous carcinoma. (A) Mammogram shows an irregular high-density mass in central quadrant with partially obscured margins; (B) Ultrasound shows irregular, isoechoic mass with focal angular margins.

Triple Negative Breast Cancer

Triple negative breast cancer (TNBC) is the term used for invasive breast cancers of any histologic type, which are negative for ER, PR, and HER2 receptors on immunohistochemistry. These are now separately classified because of their distinct clinical, radiological, and prognostic features. TNBC are characterized by occurrence at younger age, aggressive behavior, early metastases, and are refractory to treatment. TNBC are also difficult to diagnose on mammography. These are usually seen as well-defined or ill-defined masses. Spiculations and calcifications are rare. Hence, these may be difficult to differentiate from benign masses.[58] On ultrasound also, these have benign features of circumscribed masses with frequent posterior acoustic enhancement. MRI is most useful for their diagnosis. These are seen as mass- or nonmass-like lesions with intense type 3 enhancement curve. These are frequently multicentric and are well-demonstrated on MRI.[59]

STAGING AND TREATMENT OF BREAST CANCER

Breast cancer is staged according to the TNM (Tumor size, Lymph Nodes affected, Metastases) staging system of AJCC (American Joint Committee on Cancer). An overview of the staging system is given in **Table 2**. After the diagnosis of breast cancer, clinical staging is performed based on both clinical as well as imaging findings. The clinical stage is denoted as cTNM. For metastatic workup, chest X-ray, ultrasound of the abdomen, and bone scan is sufficient in stage I and II tumors. CT or positron-emission tomography (PET) is recommended for stage III cancers. Surgery is the primary treatment of breast cancer in resectable patients and this includes breast conservation therapy (BCT) or mastectomy. After surgery, a final or pathological stage is assigned and it is denoted as pTNM. Final stage of the disease and other risk factors are considered to decide for adjuvant (postoperative) treatment with RT, chemotherapy, and hormone therapy.[60]

TABLE 2: Overview of staging of breast cancer.

Tis	**Carcinoma in situ**	**T-stage**	
T1	<2 cm		T1a: Up to 5 mm T1b: Up to 1 cm T1c: Up to 2 cm
T2	2–5 cm		
T3	>5 cm		
T4	Chest wall/skin involvement		T4a: Chest wall invasion T4b: Skin invasion T4c: Both chest wall and skin invasion T4d: Inflammatory breast cancer
N-stage			
N0	No lymphadenopathy		
N1	Mobile level I, II axillary LN		
N2	Fixed level I, II axillary LN or internal mammary LN		N2a: Fixed or matted level I/II axillary LN N2b: Internal mammary LN without axillary LN
N3	Level III axillary, internal mammary, supraclavicular LN		N3a: Level III axillary LN N3b: Both axillary and internal mammary LN N3c: Supraclavicular LN
M-stage			
M0	No distant metastases		
M1	Distant metastases		

Stage groups					
	N0	N1	N2	N3	M1
T1	IA	IIA	IIIA	IIIC	IV
T2	IIA	IIB	IIIA	IIIC	IV
T3	IIB	IIIA	IIIA	IIIC	IV
T4	IIIB	IIIB	IIIB	IIIC	IV

(LN: lymph node)

Preoperative Breast Imaging

Surgery, either mastectomy or breast conservation surgery (BCS), is the mainstay of breast cancer treatment. Preoperative mammography, sometimes complimented with MRI, is important in patient selection for breast conservation. If mastectomy is planned, the role of mammography is limited to evaluation of the contralateral breast.

Main purpose of mammographic evaluation prior to BCS is to assess the extent and size of the tumor and to exclude multiple cancers. Breast cancers that are >5 cm are generally not treated with BCT. Mammography detects additional cancer in about 10% patients. Multifocal (located in same quadrant or within 4 cm) tumor can be considered for BCT **(Fig. 18)**. However, the extent of surgical resection will be wide and may not achieve the desired cosmesis. Also, women with multiple cancers have propensity to develop more cancers after the surgery resulting in treatment failure.[61] Multicentric (located in different quadrant) cancer is an absolute contraindication for BCT. Presence of suspicious calcification in and around the tumor should be carefully assessed. Clustered calcifications away from the tumor may indicate skip tumor areas. Invasive carcinoma frequently has associated component of DCIS which might extend along the ducts over a large area away from the tumor. This is known as extensive intraductal component (EIC). It is a frequent cause of positive margins in the surgically resected specimen.[62] Presence of linear branching calcifications extending from the primary tumor is a strong indicator of presence of EIC. Indeed, tumor may be more extensive than suspected on mammography. Many DCIS, especially the noncomedo type, are not always calcified and hence, not appreciated on mammography.[63,64] Contralateral breast must also be carefully evaluated on mammography to detect additional cancer, if any.

Preoperative mammographic evaluation is unsatisfactory in women with dense glandular breasts. Breast MRI is superior to mammography for preoperative evaluation of both breasts.[65] Routine preoperative MRI in women already diagnosed with breast cancer detects mammographically occult ipsilateral multicentric cancer in 20% women and contralateral synchronous cancer in 3–5% women **(Fig. 19)**.[66,67] Extent of surgical resection may be increased if multifocal cancer is detected. Similarly, BCS is converted into mastectomy if multicentric cancer is detected on MRI. Women in whom contralateral breast cancer is detected by MRI are also benefited as both cancers can be treated at the same time. Overall, preoperative breast MRI changes surgical management in 13% women; however, it may be due to false-positive MRI finding in half of these.[67] False-positive MRI, which results in unnecessarily more extensive breast surgery or mastectomy, is an important area of concern.[60] MRI is also useful for assessment of pectoralis muscle in patients with deep-seated tumors, as this cannot be evaluated on mammography.[68] Abnormal enhancement of the muscle is a specific indicator of muscle invasion; loss of fat plane is unreliable to diagnose muscle invasion. Breast MRI is the most preferred modality for preoperative breast evaluation, but not yet considered mandatory. Mammography remains the basic requirement of preoperative evaluation of the breasts before BCT.

Breast Conservation Therapy

Breast conservation therapy consists of wide local excision of the tumor with negative margins (BCS), followed by RT of the breast. It retains the affected breast and hence, has a cosmetic, and psychological advantage over mastectomy. BCT has low recurrence rates and its overall survival rates are comparable with those of mastectomy.[69,70] BCT is the preferred treatment modality for breast cancer in carefully selected patients. It is generally offered for the tumors up to 5 cm in size (T2). Ratio of tumor size and breast size is also considered. Patients with small breasts and large tumor size may be unsuitable, although some use neoadjuvant chemotherapy (NACT) for reduction of tumor size and to make it suitable for BCT.

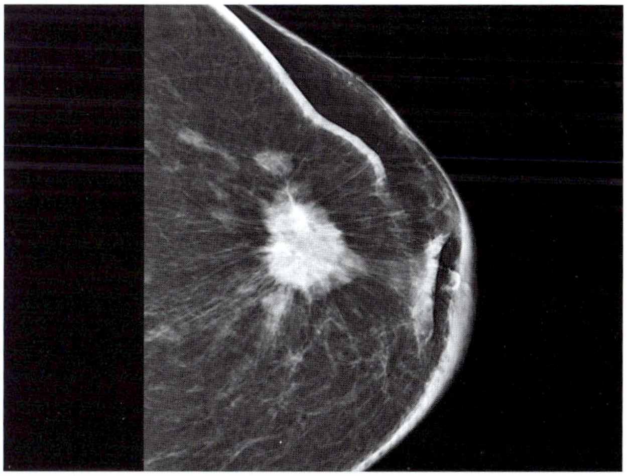

FIG. 18: Multifocal breast cancer. Mammogram shows multiple small ill-defined masses adjacent to an already diagnosed spiculated index tumor.

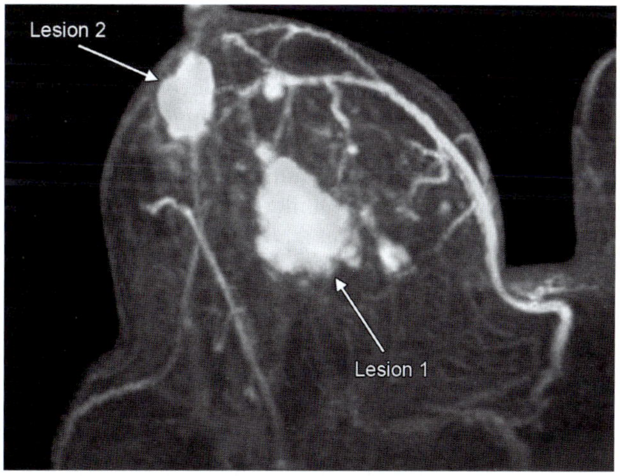

FIG. 19: Multicentric breast cancer. MIP image of a contrast-enhanced MRI shows a subareolar cancer in addition to an already diagnosed index tumor (MIP: maximum-intensity projection; MRI: magnetic resonance imaging).

Large or multicentric tumors, pregnancy, and collagen vascular diseases are contraindications for BCT. Finally, patient's preference is also taken into account while selecting BCT or mastectomy.

Mastectomy

Mastectomy is the traditional surgery for breast cancer. It is performed in patients with contraindications for BCS or in those who opt for it. Total mastectomy removes skin, nipple-areola, and fascia anterior to pectoralis major along with the entire breast parenchyma. When combined with simultaneous axillary dissection, it is termed as modified radical mastectomy (MRM). Reconstruction of the breast for cosmetic purpose is also possible after skin sparing mastectomy. It is done in same sitting using myocutaneous flaps with intact vascular pedicle, such as transverse rectus abdominis muscle (TRAM) flap or latissimus dorsi (LD) flap to create a breast mound. Silicone or saline implants are also used for breast reconstruction.

Management of Axilla

Axillary lymph node involvement is the most important prognostic indicator for breast cancer survival. Axillary lymph node dissection is a standard part of surgery, whether BCS or mastectomy, in patients with invasive breast cancer. It is performed in same sitting. It is both therapeutic as well as a staging procedure used to determine pathological N-stage. Axillary lymph nodes are divided into three groups: level, II, and III which are located lateral, posterior, and medial to pectoralis minor muscle, respectively. Level III axillary nodes are also called as infraclavicular nodes. Axillary lymph node dissection, however, is a morbid procedure. It causes disruption of major lymphatic channels and fibrosis, which may be further complicated by axillary irradiation. This leads to various problems such as lymphedema of the arm, sensory loss, and restricted shoulder movements. This may be reported by up to one-third of the patients after axillary dissection and it is difficult to treat.

Sentinel lymph node mapping and biopsy is a technique, which helps to avoid axillary dissection in some of the patients who do not have axillary lymph nodes on clinical examination. In this, a radiotracer (^{99m}Tc labeled sulfur colloid) along with a blue dye is injected in or around the tumor. The lymphatics draining the tumor take up this dye with the radiotracer and course toward axilla. Intraoperatively, the first lymph node (sentinel node) draining the tumor is identified using a hand-held gamma camera sensor. This lymph node is removed and analyzed with frozen sections. If it is free of tumor, it is presumed that axillary nodes are also uninvolved and axillary dissection is avoided. If the sentinel node is involved, axillary dissection is performed to pathologically stage the axilla. False-negative rates of sentinel lymph node biopsy are low and its ability to correctly stage the axilla is comparable with direct axillary dissection.[71]

However, sentinel lymph node biopsy is a time-consuming and expensive procedure. The sentinel lymph node may not be localized in some patients and axillary dissection has to be performed. Allergic reactions to dye may also occur. Preoperative ultrasound evaluation of the axilla in patients selected for sentinel lymph node biopsy is fast gaining acceptance. It helps to avoid sentinel lymph node biopsy in some patients. A detailed description of ultrasound and ultrasound-guided FNAC of axillary lymph nodes is given in Chapter 27.

Perioperative Breast Imaging

If the tumor is nonpalpable, preoperative mammography or ultrasound-guided Hookwire localization is required before the BCS. These procedures are described in detail in Chapter 27. Although uncommonly utilized, intraoperative ultrasound is useful to assess gross tumor margins more accurately. Use of intraoperative ultrasound results in better margins of resection and lowers the chances of residual tumor.[72] Immediate postoperative mammograms may sometimes be requested but these are difficult to perform and interpret. The breast is tender and adequate compression cannot be given to the recently operated breast. The postoperative hematoma and edema also makes the mammographic interpretation difficult and residual mass, if any, cannot be reliably excluded on mammogram. Diagnosis of residual breast cancer after surgery and the decision to re-excise is primarily based on detection of positive tumor margins on postoperative histopathology and not on imaging. However, postoperative MRI after positive margins is desirable, if it was not performed preoperatively. It can identify gross residual tumor or unsuspected multifocal cancer and aid in planning of the extent of re-excision or to consider mastectomy.[73]

Adjuvant Treatment

Adjuvant (postoperative) treatment is given to treat microscopic disease. RT is used for local adjuvant treatment and is aimed at eradicating microscopic residual disease if any, so that chances of local recurrence are reduced. Systemic adjuvant treatment consists of chemotherapy or hormonal therapy, or more commonly, both. It is aimed at eradicating circulating micrometastases, if any, so that chances of distant metastatic recurrence are reduced.[74]

Radiotherapy is given to all patients after BCS. Generally, a total of 45–50 Gy of whole breast RT is given, which may be followed by 10–16 Gy of boost RT to the tumor bed. After mastectomy, RT is given to patients with adverse factors only, such as those with large tumors, close margins, lymphovascular invasion, and axillary lymph node involvement.[57]

Chemotherapy and hormonal therapy is the mainstay of systemic adjuvant treatment of breast cancer. All tumors of >1 cm require adjuvant chemotherapy. Standard anthracycline-based chemotherapy includes combination of 5 fluorouracil (5 FU) and cyclophosphamide along with doxorubicin or epirubicin [5-fluorouracil, adriamycin, cyclophosphamide (FAC)]. Newer regimes also incorporate taxanes.[57] Hormonal therapy with tamoxifen, an estrogen analog, is given for 5 years to all patients with ER-positive breast cancers. It significantly improves the disease-free survival and overall survival in these patients.[74] HER2 overexpression by the breast cancer is associated with high risk of early recurrence and resistance to standard chemotherapy and hormonal therapy. Trastuzumab (Herceptin) is a monoclonal antibody against HER2 protein.

It improves survival in HER2 positive patients when given for 1 year, along with or after adjuvant chemotherapy.[60]

ADVANCED BREAST CANCER

Locally Advanced Breast Cancer

This term is used for breast cancers which are inoperable at presentation but without distant metastases **(Fig. 20)**. It includes all T4 tumors (invasion of chest wall, skin, or both), those with fixed axillary lymph nodes, and IBC. Some breast surgeons also include large (>5 cm) but operable tumors in locally advanced breast cancer (LABC). The pretreatment workup includes core biopsy for the diagnosis and receptors status, as well as metastatic workup to exclude distant metastases. These patients are treated with NACT with the intention of downstaging the tumor and making it operable.

Inflammatory Breast Cancer

Inflammatory breast cancer is an aggressive form of invasive duct carcinoma and accounts for 2.5% of all breast cancers.[75] Histopathologically, there is diffuse infiltration and obstruction of dermal lymphatics. It is characterized by younger age, rapid progression, early metastases, and high mortality. Patients present with enlarged painful breast with diffuse erythema, edema, sloughing, and ulceration of the skin over the breast. Clinical presentation mimics acute mastitis and the tumor though sizable, is difficult to palpate.

The diagnosis is usually clinical. Mammography is difficult to perform in a painful breast. Usual mammographic finding is of a dense edematous breast with skin and trabecular thickening **(Figs. 21A and B)**. Hence, primary tumor is uncommonly identified on mammography. Ultrasound is useful and it locates the primary tumor in more than half of patients.[73] It is seen as irregular or lobulated mass on ultrasound, usually large in size. Multicentric and diffusely infiltrating IBC is not localized on ultrasound. MRI and PET-CT are most accurate for evaluation of primary tumor as well as distant metastases.[76] MRI detects primary tumor in nearly all patients with IBC. The primary tumor is most often seen as single or multiple confluent masses with type three enhancement curve and skin involvement in majority of lesions.[77]

Neoadjuvant Chemotherapy

Locally advanced breast cancer is the most common indication for NACT. Patients with large but operable tumors who desire for BCT instead of mastectomy are also offered NACT. Traditional anthracycline-based chemotherapy is used. Majority of tumors respond well to chemotherapy and become operable. Mastectomy or BCT is offered after successful NACT, depending on the residual tumor size. About 15–25% patients achieve pathological complete response with NACT.[78]

Response to NACT is assessed with clinical examination and imaging. Mammography, ultrasound, MRI, and PET have been used for response assessment. Prediction of response after initial one or two cycles is important. Good responders can be continued with NACT, while it can be stopped in nonresponders. For this purpose, combination of mammography and ultrasound is more useful than clinical assessment alone.[78] PET-CT is also useful but MRI is most accurate.[79] Response to NACT is depicted by decrease in size and degree of contrast enhancement on MRI and decrease in standard uptake value (SUV) on PET.[80,81] Diffusion-weighted MRI evaluation is also useful to predict the response to NACT. Low-pretreatment apparent diffusion coefficient (ADC) values and high post one cycle ADC values predict good response.[82,83] After completion of NACT, residual tumor size is an important consideration for surgical planning. Both MRI and PET are highly sensitive to identify patients with pathological complete response, however, with moderate specificity.[84] Hence, all patients need to be operated, even if complete resolution of tumor is seen on post-NACT scans. It is prudent to insert a metallic marker clip in these tumors before starting NACT. If the tumor disappears on mammography,

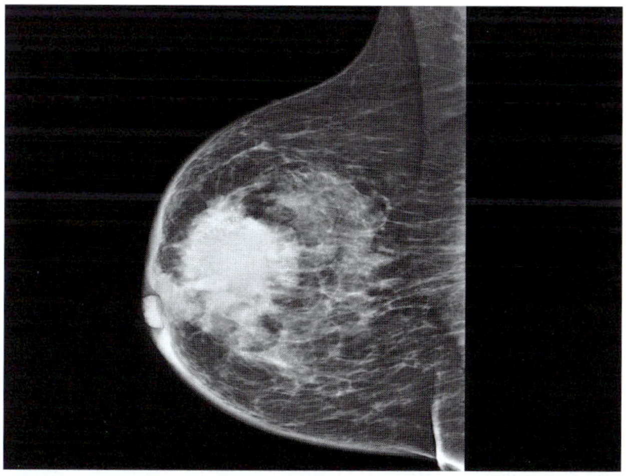

FIG. 20: Locally advanced breast cancer. Mammogram shows a large, infiltrating, spiculated mass with thickening of overlying skin.

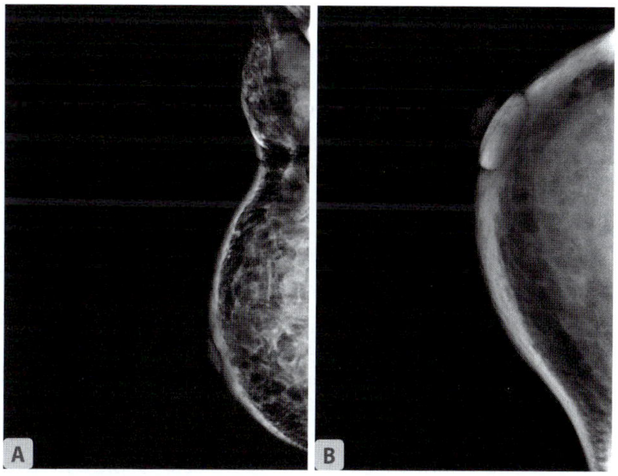

FIGS. 21A AND B: Inflammatory breast cancer. Mammogram shows diffuse increase in breast density along with thickening of trabeculi and skin. No definite mass is seen.

the marker clip is used to perform preoperative hook wire localization and surgery.[85]

Metastatic Breast Cancer

Metastatic breast cancer (MBC) is stage IV breast cancer that has spread beyond the breast, regional lymph nodes, and chest wall. Common sites of breast cancer metastases are liver, bone, lung, distant lymph nodes, and brain; however, any organ in the body can be involved. ER/PR positive cancers tend to spread to bones while receptor-negative cancers are more likely to involve the liver. Lobular carcinoma has propensity for serosal deposits involving pleura and peritoneum. Most women with MBC have already diagnosed breast cancer but small proportion of women present with symptoms of metastatic disease and breast cancer is subsequently diagnosed during workup for the occult primary cancer. Symptoms of MBC are nonspecific and include cough or dyspnea, bone pain, lymphadenopathy, or fatigue. Radionuclide bone scan, ultrasound, CT scan, and PET-CT are usually employed for diagnosis and response assessment of breast cancer metastases.

Bone is the most common site of distant metastases from breast cancer.[86] These preferentially involve spine and pelvis but any bone can be involved. Radionuclide bone scan is the primary imaging modality for detection of bone metastases.[87] It is sensitive, however, specificity is moderate. False-positive bone scan results are mainly from degenerative and inflammatory lesions. X-ray or CT-evaluation is required if metastases cannot be differentiated reliably from these on bone scan. On radiographs, bone metastases of breast cancer may be osteolytic, sclerotic, or mixed **(Fig. 22)**. PET is equally sensitive as bone scan but more specific. MRI is the most accurate modality for diagnosis of bone metastases from breast cancer.[88] However, it is not used as a routine investigation. PET-CT and MRI are also useful to monitor treatment response of the bone metastases. Liver metastases are hypovascular and hence, are identified on venous phase of the CT **(Fig. 23)**. Some liver metastases may be small and diffuse giving rise to the appearance of pseudocirrhosis.[89] Ascites and shrinkage of liver outline may also be present with these. Focal fatty infiltration is common in patients on chemotherapy or hormonal therapy. This may also be misinterpreted as metastases on CT. Lack of mass effect and preserved liver architecture is helpful to differentiate these from metastases. MRI is required in equivocal cases. Lung metastases from breast cancer are usually seen as single or multiple nodules. Breast cancer is a common cause of unusual manifestation of lung metastases such as lymphangitis carcinomatosis, airspace consolidation, and endobronchial metastases.[90] Breast cancer is the most common cause of ovarian metastases and its clinicoradiological features are usually similar to that of primary ovarian cancer. Breast cancer metastases to small bowel produce long segment strictures and those to stomach may produce antral narrowing similar to linitis plastica.

Clinical and imaging diagnosis of metastases is usually unequivocal in majority. In others, biopsy may be required. If not already known, ER, PR, and HER2 status must be determined on biopsy, either from the breast lesion or the metastatic site.

Treatment of MBC is aimed at palliation and prolonging survival. Patients with less extensive metastases, fewer symptoms, and late development of metastases perform better. Chemotherapy is the mainstay of treatment in all MBC. Patients with ER/PR positive MBC are initially treated with hormonal therapy. HER2 positive patients benefit from trastuzumab. Other treatment options include bisphosphonates (pamidronate or zoledronic acid) to patients with bone metastases and RT to brain metastases and painful bone metastases.[60]

Occult Primary Breast Cancer

Mammography is standard part of workup in women presenting with metastatic adenocarcinoma anywhere from an occult primary site. Women presenting with axillary lymphadenopathy only are also evaluated with mammography. If clinical examination and mammography are negative but axillary lymph node biopsy is suspicious

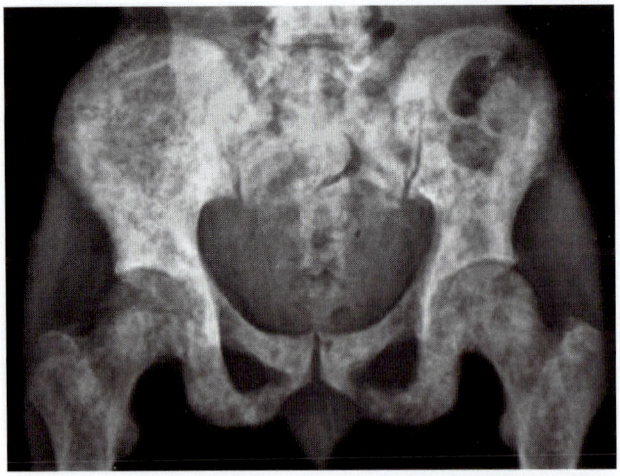

FIG. 22: Bone metastases. Pelvic radiograph shows multiple diffuse lytic and sclerotic metastases in all pelvic bones and both proximal femoral bones.

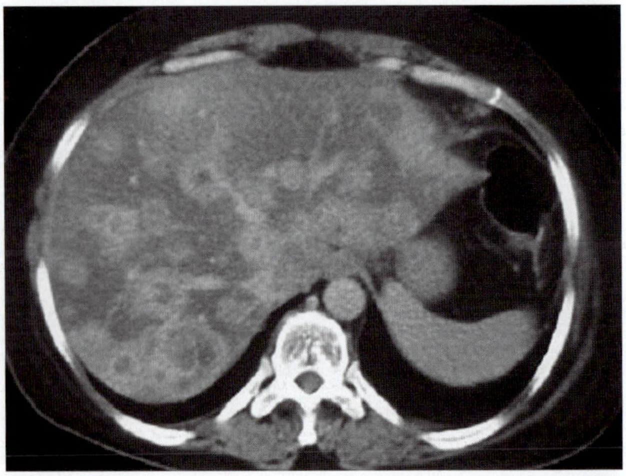

FIG. 23: Liver metastases. Multiple liver metastases are seen. In spite of being hypovascular, they appear hyperdense in the background of fatty infiltration of the liver.

of primary breast carcinoma, MRI is recommended. MRI identifies mammographically occult breast cancer in majority of these patients.[91] If primary is not identified, the patients are treated with mastectomy or RT.

POST-TREATMENT BREAST IMAGING AND FOLLOW-UP

Patients treated with BCT need regular bilateral mammographic follow-up. It is primarily required to detect recurrence of cancer in treated or contralateral breast. A baseline mammogram of the treated breast should be obtained at 3–6 months after completion of the RT. This mammogram is compared with future serial mammograms. Patients treated with mastectomy are also followed with annual screening mammograms of the contralateral breast, as they are at high risk for development of second breast cancer. Breast cancer survivors have threefold increased risk of developing contralateral breast cancer. They are also at some risk for endometrial cancer, lung cancer, angiosarcoma, and acute leukemia.[58]

Several postsurgery and RT changes are apparent on follow-up mammogram after the BCT. A *fibrous scar* develops at the operative site, which is seen as an ill-defined density with adjacent architectural distortion **(Figs. 24A and B)**. Metallic surgical clips, intended to mark the tumor bed for boost radiation, may also be seen at the operative site. Sometimes, the fibrous scar has spiculated appearance and appears suspicious **(Figs. 25A and B)**. However, it does not have high-central density as in the case of a true mass. Exact site of the lumpectomy site must be known and review of preoperative mammograms is useful to determine this. Careful evaluation of scar in both craniocaudal (CC) and mediolateral oblique (MLO) views is also helpful. Unlike solid mass, the scar is a 2D structure formed by approximation and fibrosis of the lumpectomy cavity. Hence, size and density of the scar varies considerably in two views. *Seroma* is a fluid collection that is frequently seen at the operative site. It is usually seen as a round or oval mass which may persist for up to 2 years **(Figs. 26A to C)**.[92] It can be reliably characterized on ultrasound. Debris or septations are commonly seen in seroma and this should not lead to ultrasound-guided aspiration.

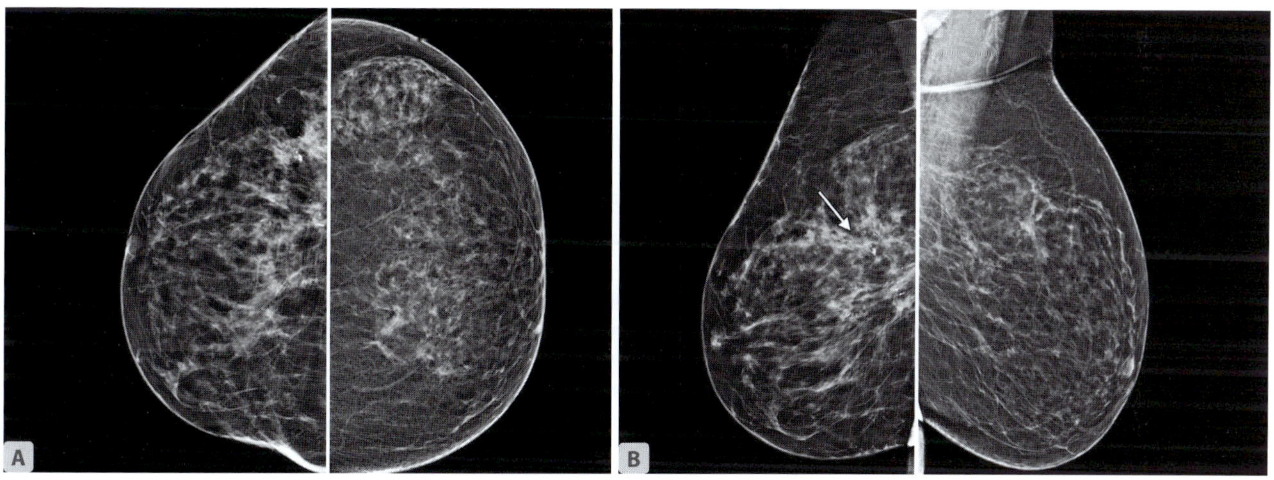

FIGS. 24A AND B: Post-treatment bilateral mammogram: Right breast shows fibrous scar at the operative site (arrow) with foci of dystrophic calcifications. There is diffuse trabecular thickening and increased density of the left breast, secondary to radiotherapy, as compared to the left breast.

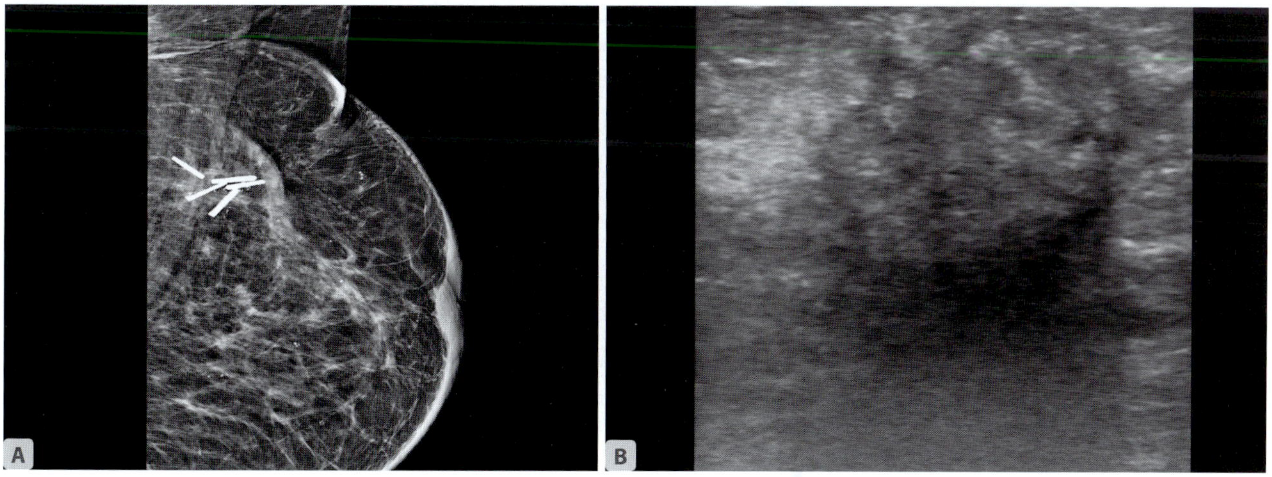

FIGS. 25A AND B: Postoperative scar. Mammogram shows architectural distortion and ultrasound shows spiculated scar at the operative site. This is an expected finding and does not suggest recurrence.

Radiation changes are seen in the form of diffuse thickening of trabeculi and skin, along with an overall increase in breast density. The changes are similar to breast edema due to any other cause. The severity of these changes varies in different patients; however, these remain stable or decrease on follow-up mammograms. Some distortion of the breast outline is also apparent after BCT and the degree of this depends on the extent of the excision. In addition to above changes, there may be development of benign calcifications in post-treatment mammograms. The causes include fat necrosis, sutural calcifications, and radiation-induced dystrophic calcifications.

Local recurrence at operative site occurs rarely and is seen in 2–7% of women followed for 10 years.[57] Younger age at diagnosis, high grade, and ER/PR negative breast tumors are more prone for local recurrence. Mammography is the primary modality of follow-up and detection of recurrences. However, its accuracy is lowered because of distortion of breast parenchyma by the post-treatment changes. Majority of local recurrences are detected by mammography or by patients themselves on self-breast examination, while few are diagnosed on CBE.[93] The recurrences are most often seen as increased density and/or size of the scar, new mass, or suspicious calcifications on mammography. Their morphology is usually similar to that of the primary breast cancers in these patients and hence, review of the preoperative mammogram is useful for the detection of a recurrence.[94] MRI and percutaneous biopsy should be promptly obtained in case of suspicion of recurrence on mammogram.[95]

MISCELLANEOUS MALIGNANT LESIONS OF THE BREAST

Paget's Disease

In this condition, a centrally located ductal carcinoma grows along the ducts into the nipple with eczematous changes at the summit of the nipple (pagetoid changes). Nipple changes range from mild itching to extensive scaling, erosions, and ulceration in the nipple. Erosion extends to the areola and may cover a larger area of the skin. Fifty percent patients have a palpable mass. This disease is usually unilateral.

On mammography and ultrasound, underlying malignant mass or calcification is seen in most patients **(Figs. 27A and B)**. Nipple and areolar thickening is also present.[96] Malignant type of calcifications may be seen extending from deeper carcinoma to the nipple. MRI is recommended if mammogram is equivocal or normal.

Phyllodes Tumor

Phyllodes tumor (or phylloid tumor) is a stromal tumor composed of the epithelial elements of connective tissue stroma, similar to fibroadenoma. Its malignant potential is variable from completely benign lesion to fully malignant sarcoma. Most are benign. Clinically, they present as round multinodular palpable tumors like fibroadenomas. On mammography and ultrasound, they are well-defined and indistinguishable from fibroadenomas **(Figs. 28A and B)**. Occasionally, cystic component may be seen on ultrasound.[2] Phyllodes tumors are treated with wide local excision. Approximately 20% of these recur, if margins of excision are inadequate.[57] As malignant phyllodes tumor is a sarcoma, axillary lymphadenopathy is less common and lung metastases are more common.

Sarcoma

Sarcomas are rare tumors of breast. These include phyllodes tumor, angiosarcoma, fibrosarcoma, liposarcoma, malignant fibrous histiocytoma, and osteosarcoma. Their imaging features are nonspecific. Angiosarcoma is an aggressive, rapidly growing vascular tumor of young age. Presentation is similar to IBC. MRI shows a strongly enhancing, ill-defined, infiltrative mass with skin invasion. It metastasizes early and is rapidly fatal.

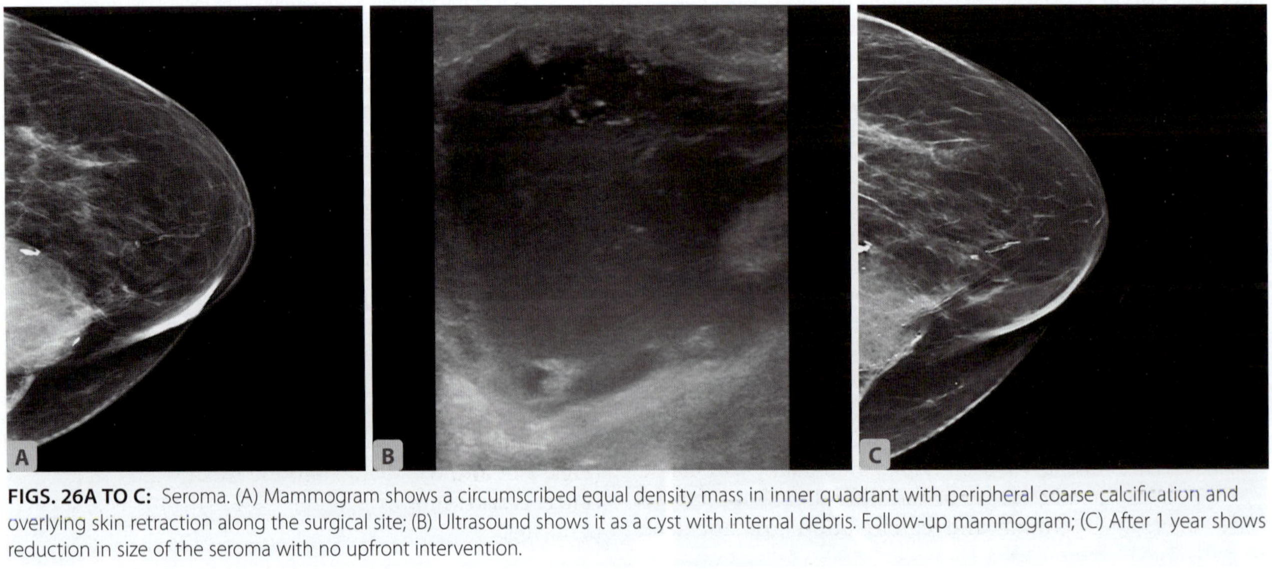

FIGS. 26A TO C: Seroma. (A) Mammogram shows a circumscribed equal density mass in inner quadrant with peripheral coarse calcification and overlying skin retraction along the surgical site; (B) Ultrasound shows it as a cyst with internal debris. Follow-up mammogram; (C) After 1 year shows reduction in size of the seroma with no upfront intervention.

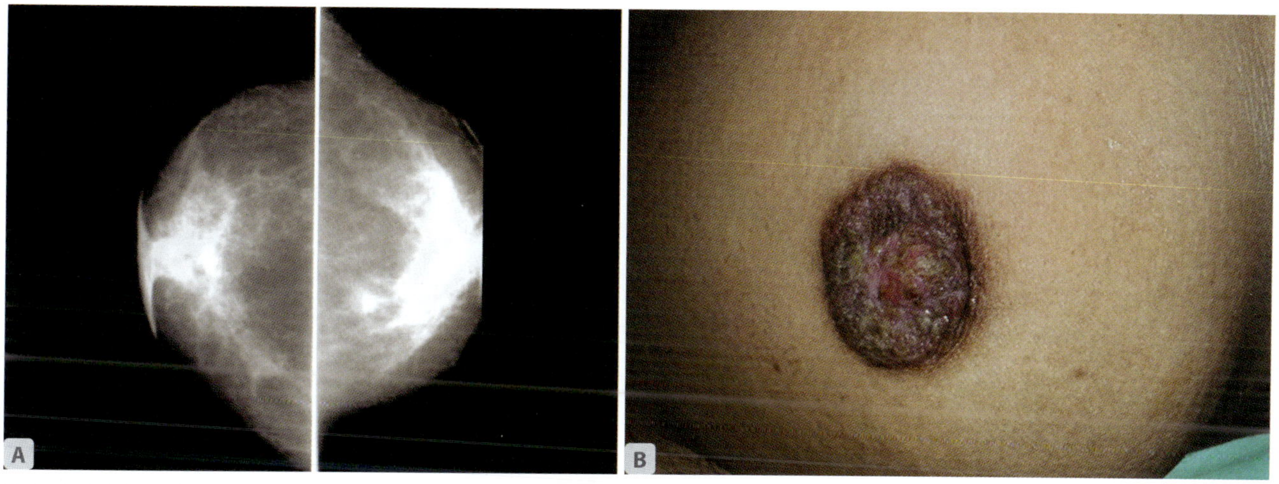

FIGS. 27A AND B: Paget's disease. Mammography shows nipple and areolar thickening in right breast with a subareolar mass. The NAC thickening corroborates with clinical picture of the patient. (NAC: nipple-areolar complex).

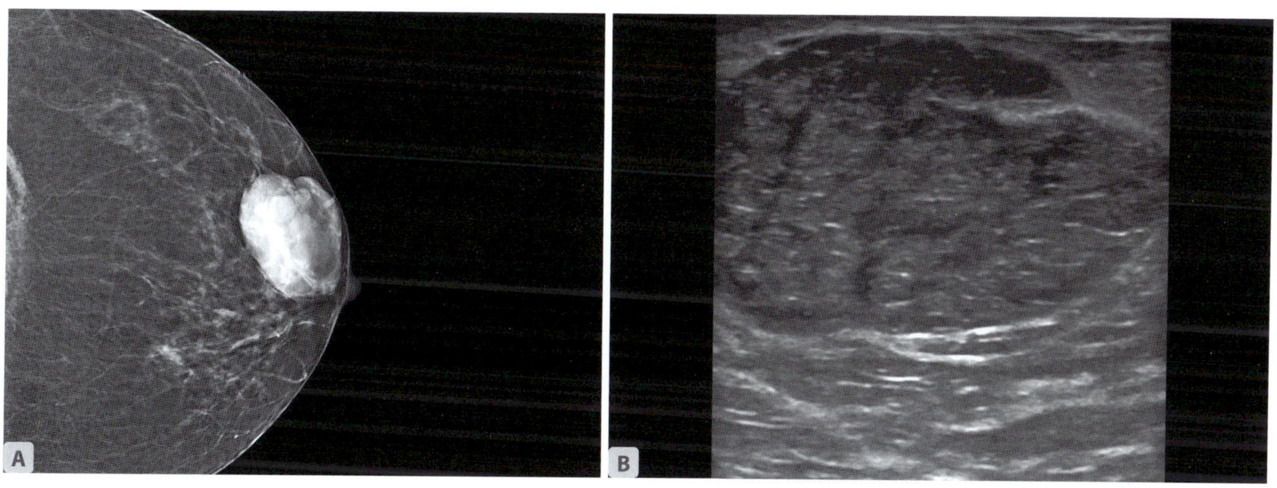

FIGS. 28A AND B: Phyllodes tumor. (A) Mammogram shows a dense breast with an irregular large mass in the anterior third of the breast; (B) Ultrasound shows a large hypoechoic mass with fluid clefts within.

Metastases to Breast

Metastases to breast from other sites are rare. Usual primary sites of cancer are melanoma, lung, stomach, cervix, and ovary. Clinically, there are multiple palpable masses. In one-third of these patients, this may be the first manifestation of an occult primary cancer.[57] Another form of metastasis to breast is cross-lymphatic spread from the contralateral advanced breast cancer causing localized thickening of the skin.

On mammography, metastases to breast are usually multiple and bilateral **(Figs. 29A and B)**. These are seen as well-defined or ill-defined masses. Spiculations and calcifications are not commonly seen.

Although rare, *lymphoma* can secondarily involve the breasts. Large axillary lymph nodes are usually associated. Mammographically, single or multiple ill-defined masses are seen. Spiculations and calcification are not seen. Lymphomatous lesion may also be seen as increased asymmetric density in the breast. Ultrasound shows single or multiple nonspecific solid masses.[97]

Male Breast Cancer

Male breast cancer accounts for about 1% of all breast cancers. Breast cancer in male patients occurs at an older age group than in female patients. Risk factors include Klinefelter's syndrome, BRCA mutation carriers, undescended testis, chronic liver disease, and alcoholism.[57] Gynecomastia is not a risk factor. Clinically, there is a painless hard mass. Nipple discharge or ulceration is seen in 25% cases. Mammographic features of male breast cancer are similar to those in females **(Figs. 30A and B)**.[98] Pathology and treatment of male breast cancer is also same. Due to small size of the breast, BCT is not performed.

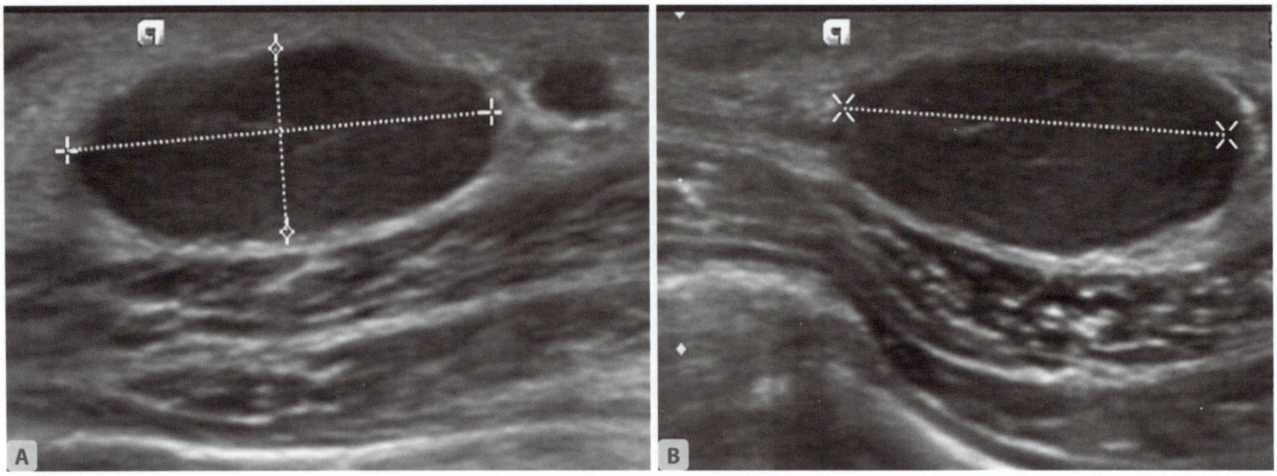

FIGS. 29A AND B: Metastases. Mammogram shows multiple variable-sized metastatic masses in the breast from Ewing's sarcoma (FNAC proven mets). (FNAC: fine needle aspiration cytology).

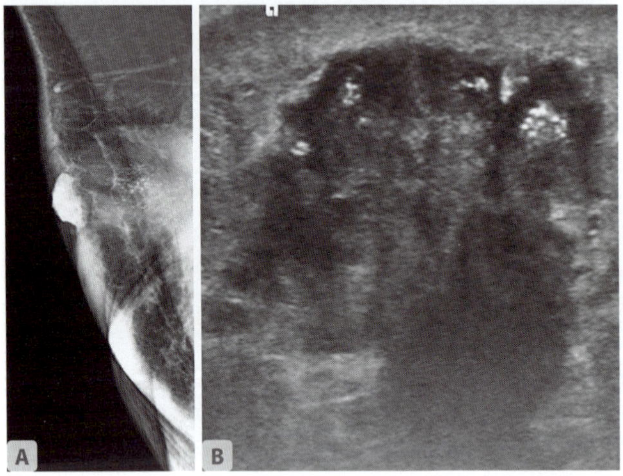

FIGS. 30A AND B: Male breast cancer. (A) Mammogram shows irregular retroareolar mass with pleomorphic calcification within; (B) Ultrasound confirms presence of an irregular hypoechoic mass with angular margins and internal microcalcifications.

REFERENCES

1. Kopans DB. Histologic, pathologic and imaging correlation. In: Kopans DB (Ed). Breast Imaging, 3rd edition. Philadelphia: Lippincott, Williams and Wilkins; 2007. pp. 783-888.
2. Goel NB, Knight TE, Pandey S, Riddick-Young M, de Paredes ES, Trivedi A. Fibrous lesions of the breast: imaging-pathologic correlation. Radiographics. 2005;25:1547-59.
3. Elseedawy M, Whelehan P, Vinnicombe S, Thomson K, Evans A. Factors influencing the stiffness of fibroadenomas at shear wave elastography. Clin Radiol. 2016;71(1):92-5.
4. Liberman L, Morris E, Lee MJ, Kaplan JB, LaTrenta LR, Menell JH, et al. Breast lesions detected on MR imaging: Features positive predictive value. AJR. 2002;179:171-8.
5. Venta LA, Kim JP, Pelloski CE, Morrow M. Management of complex breast cysts. AJR. 1999;173:1331-6.
6. Berg WA, Sechtin AG, Marques H, Zhang Z. Cystic breast masses and ACRIN 6666 experience. Radiol Clin N Am. 2010;48: 931-87.
7. Lau S, Kuchenmeister I, Stachs A, Gerber B, Krause A, Reimer T. Pathologic nipple discharge: Surgery is imperative in post menopausal women. Ann Surg Oncol. 2005;12:546-51.
8. Orel SG, Dougherty CS, Reynolds C, Czerniecki BJ, Siegelman ES, Schnall MD. MR imaging in patients with nipple discharge: Initial experience. Radiology. 2000;216:248-54.
9. Neal L, Tortorelli CL, Nasser A. Clinicians guide to imaging and pathologic findings in benign breast disease. Mayo Clin Proc. 2010;85:274-9.
10. Phantana-Angkool A, Forster MR, Warren YE, Livasy CA, Sobel AH, Beasley LM, et al. Rate of radial scars by core biopsy and upgrading to malignancy or high-risk lesions before and after introduction of digital breast tomosynthesis. Breast Cancer Res Treat. 2019;173(1):23-9.
11. Alshafeiy TI, Nguyen JV, Rochman CM, Nicholson BT, Patrie JT, Harvey JA. Outcome of architectural distortion detected only at breast tomosynthesis versus 2D mammography. Radiology. 2018;288(1):38-46.
12. Wong KT, Tse GM, YangWT. Ultrasound and MR imaging of diabetic mastopathy. Clin Radiol. 2002;57:730-5.
13. Hook GW, Ikeda DM. Treatment of breast abscess with US guided percutaneous needle drainage without indwelling catheter placement. Radiology. 1999;213:579-82.

14. Memis A, Bilgen I, Ustun EE, Ozdemir N, Erhan Y, Kapkac M. Granulomatous mastitis: Imaging features with histopatholgical correlation. Clin Radiol. 2001;57:1001-6.
15. Sabate JM, Clotet M, Gomez A, Heras PD. Radiologic evaluation of uncommon and reactive breast disorders. Radiographics. 2005;24:411-24.
16. Sakr AA, Fawzy RK, Fadaly G, Baky MA. Mammographic and sonographic features of tuberculous mastitis. Eur J Radiol. 2004;51:54-60.
17. Herborn CU, Marincek B, Erfmann D, Meuli-Simmen C, Wedler V, Bode-Lesniewska B, et al. Breast augmentation and reconstructive surgery: MR imaging of implant rupture and malignancy. Eur Radiol. 2002;12:2198-206.
18. Debruhl ND, Gorczyca DP, Ahn CY, Shaw WW, Bassett P. Silicone breast implants: US evaluation. Radiology. 1993;189:95-8.
19. Caskey CI, Berg WA, Hamper UM, Sheth S, Chang BW, Anderson ND. Imaging spectrum of extracapsular silicone: Correlation of US, MR imaging, mammographic and histopathologic findings. Radiographics. 1999;19:S39-51.
20. Breast cancer statistics. (2018). World Cancer Research Fund. [online] Available from https://www.wcrf.org/dietandcancer/cancer-trends/breast-cancer-statistic [Last accessed March 2020].
21. Ghoncheh M, Pournamdar Z, Salehiniya H. Incidence and mortality and epidemiology of breast cancer in the world. Asian Pac J Cancer Prev. 2016;17(S3):43-6.
22. Malvia S, Bagadi SA, Dubey US, Saxena S. Epidemiology of breast cancer in Indian women. Asia Pac J Clin Oncol. 2017;13(4):289-95.
23. Boyd NF, Guo H, Martin LJ, Sun L, Stone J, Fishell E, et al. Mammographic density and the risk and detection of breast cancer. N Engl J Med. 2007;356:227.
24. Brose MS, Rebbeck TR, Catzone KA, Stopfer JE, Nathanson KL, Weber BL. Cancer risk estimates for BRCA1 mutation carriers identified in a risk evaluation program. J Natl Cancer Inst. 2002;94:1365.
25. Perou CM, Sorlie T, Eisen MB, van de Rijn M, Jeffrey SS, Rees CA, et al. Molecular portraits of human breast tumours. Nature. 2000;406:747-52.
26. Kopans DB. Screening mammography. In: Kopans DB (Ed). Breast Imaging, 3rd edition. Philadelphia, PA: Lippincott, Williams and Wilkins; 2007. pp. 121-90.
27. Tabar I, Vitak B, Chen HH, Yen MF, Duffy SW, Smith RA. Beyond randomized controlled trials: Organized mammographic screening substantially reduces breast cancer mortality. Cancer. 2001;91:1724-31.
28. Nelson HD, Tyne K, Naik A, Bougatsos C, Chan BK, Humphrey L. Screening for breast cancer: An update for the US Preventive Services Task Force. Ann Intern Med. 2009;151:727-42.
29. Tabar L, Vitak B, Chen THH, Yen AM, Cohen A, Tot T, et al. Swedish two county trial: Impact of mammographic screening on breast cancer mortality during 3 decades. Radiology. 2010;260:658-63.
30. Paci E, Duffy SW, Giorgi D, Crocetti E, Vezossi V, Bianchi S, et al. Quantification of the effect of mammographic screening on fatal breast cancers: The Florence programme 1990-96. Br J Cancer. 2002;87:65-9.
31. Elmore JG, Armstrong K, Lehman CD, Fletcher SW. Screening for breast cancer. JAMA. 2005;293:1245-56.
32. Elmore JG, Barton MB, Moceri VM, Polk S, Arena PJ, Fletcher SW. Ten year risk of false positive screening mammograms and clinical breast examinations. N Engl J Med. 1998;338:1089.
33. Schopper D, de Wolf C. How effective are breast cancer screening programs by mammography? Review of current evidence. Eur J Cancer. 2009;45:1916-23.
34. Gotzsche PC, Olsen O. Is screening for breast cancer with mammography justifiable? Lancet. 2000;355:129-34.
35. Bock K, Borisch B, Cawson J, Damtjernhaug B, de Wolf C, Dean P, et al. Effect of population based screening on breast cancer mortality. Lancet. 2011;378:1775-6.
36. US Preventive Services Task Force. Screening for breast cancer: US preventive services task force recommendation statement. Ann Intern Med. 2009;151:716-26.
37. ACOG. Breast cancer risk assessment and screening in average-risk women. [online] Available from https://www.acog.org/Clinical-Guidance-and-Publications/Practice-Bulletins/Committee-on-Practice-Bulletins-Gynecology/Breast-Cancer-Risk-Assessment-and-Screening-in-Average-Risk-Women?IsMobileSet=false [Last accessed March 2020].
38. Seely JM, Alhassan T. Screening for breast cancer in 2018—what should we be doing today? Curr Oncol. 2018; 25(Suppl 1):S115-24.
39. Breast Cancer Screening Guidelines for Women. [online] Available from https://www.cdc.gov/cancer/breast/pdf/breastcancerscreeningguidelines.pdf [Last accessed March 2020].
40. Ernster VL, Ballard BR, Barlow WE, Zheng Y, Weaver DL, Cutter G, et al. Detection of ductal carcinoma in situ in women undergoing screening mammography. J Natl Cancer Inst. 2002;94:1546-54.
41. Bordas P, Jonsson H, Nystom L, Lenner P. Interval cancer incidence and episode sensitivity in Norrbotten mammography screening programme. Sweden J Med Screen. 2009;16:39.
42. Kalager M, Zelen M, Langmark F, Zheng Y, Weaver DL, Cutter G, et al. Effect of screening mammography on breast cancer mortality in Norway. N Engl J Med. 2010;163:1203-10.
43. Warner E, Plewes DB, Hill KA, Causer PA, Zubovits JT, Jong RA, et al. Surveillance of BRCA1and BRCA2 mutation carriers with magnetic resonance imaging, ultrasound, mammography and clinical breast examination. JAMA. 2004;292:1317-25.
44. Gilbert FJ, Warren RM, Kwan-Lin G, Thompson DJ, Eeles RA, Evans DG, et al. Cancers in BRCA1 and BRCA2 carriers and in women with high risk for breast cancer: MR imaging and mammographic features. Radiology. 2009;254:358-68.
45. Saslow D, Boetes C, Burke W, Harms S, Leach MO, Lehman CD, et al. American Cancer Society guidelines for breast screening with MRI as an adjunct to mammography. CA Cancer J Clin. 2007;57:75-89.
46. Corsetti V, Houssami N, Ferrari A, Ghirardi M, Bellarosa S, Angelini O, et al. Breast screening with ultrasound in women with mammography negative dense breasts: Evidence on incremental cancer detection, false positives and associated cost. Eur J Cancer. 2004;4:539-44.
47. Nothaker M, Duda V, Hahn M, Warm M, Degenhardt F, Madjar H, et al. Early detection of breast cancer: Benefits and risks of supplemental breast ultrasound in asymptomatic women with mammographically dense breasts. A systematic review. BMC Cancer. 2009;9:335.
48. Berg WA, Blume JD, Cormac JB, Mendelson EB, Lehrer D, Böhm-Vélez M, et al. Combined screening with ultrasound and mammography vs mammography only in women at elevated risk of breast cancer. JAMA. 2008;299:2151-63.
49. Thomas DB, Gao DL, Ray RM, Wang WW, Allison CJ, Chen FL, et al. Randomized trial of breast self examination in Shanghai: Final results. J Natl Cancer Inst. 2002;94:1445-57.
50. Anderson BO, Shyyan R, Eniu A, Smith RA, Yip CH, Bese NS, et al. Breast cancer in limited resources countries: An overview of the Breast Health Global Initiative 2005 guidelines. Breast J. 2006;12:S3-15.
51. Kuhl CK, Shrading S, Bieling HB, Wardelmann E, Leutner CC, Koenig R, et al. MRI for diagnosis of pure ductal carcinoma *in situ*: A prospective observational study. Lancet. 2007;370:485-92.
52. Morris EA. Breast cancer imaging with MRI. RCNA. 2002;40: 443-86.

53. Stalsberg H, Thomas DB. Age distribution of histologic types of breast cancer. Int J Cancer. 1993;54:1-7.
54. Weinstein SP, Orel SG, Heller R, Reynolds C, Czerniecki B, Solin LJ, et al. MR imaging of the breast in patients with invasive lobular carcinoma. AJR. 2001;176:399-406.
55. Yeh ED, Slanetz PJ, Edmister WB, Talele A, Monticciolo D, Kopans DB. Invasive lobular carcinoma: Spectrum of enhancement and morphology on magnetic resonance imaging. Breast J. 2003;9:13-8.
56. Liberman L, Morris EA, Dershaw DD, Abramson AF, Tan LK. MR imaging of ipsilateral breast in women with percutaneously proved breast cancer. AJR. 2003;180:901-10.
57. Lam WW, Chu WC, Tse GM, Ma TK. Sonographic appearance of mucinous carcinoma of the breast. AJR. 2004;182:1069-74.
58. Yang WT, Dryden M, Broglio K, Gilcrease M, Dawood S, Dempsey PJ, et al. Mammographic features of triple negative primary breast cancers in young premenopausal women. Breast Cancer Res Treat. 2008;111:405-10.
59. Dogan BE, Gonzalez-Angulo AM, Gilcreae M, Dryden MJ, Yang WT. Multimodality imaging of triple negative breast tumours with mammography, ultrasound and MRI. AJR. 2010;194: 1160-6.
60. Burstein HJ, Harris JR, Morrow M. Malignant tumours of the breast. In: DeVita VT, Lawrence TS, Rosenberg SA (Eds). Cancer: Principles and Practice of Oncology, 9th edition. Philadelphia: Wolter Kluwer, Lippincott, Williams and Wilkins; 2011. pp. 1401-46.
61. Kutz JM, Jacquemier J, Amalric R, Brandone H, Ayme Y, Hans D, et al. Breast conserving therapy for macroscopically multiple cancers. Ann Surg. 1991;212:38-44.
62. Kurniawan ED, Wong MH, Windle I, Rose A, Mou A, Buchanan M, et al. Predictors of surgical margin status in breast conserving surgery within a breast screening program. Ann Surg Oncol. 2008;15(9):2542-9.
63. Holland R, Hendricks J, Verbee K, Mravunac M, Schuurmans Stekhoven JH. Extent, distribution and mammographic/ histologic correlations of breast ductal carcinoma *in situ*. Lancet.1990;335:519-22.
64. Umetsu T, Yuen S, Kasami M, Uchida Y. Comparison of magnetic resonance imaging, multidetector row computed tomography, ultrasonography and mammography for tumour extension of breast cancer. Breast Cancer Res Treat. 2008;112:461-74.
65. Berg WA, Gutlerrez L, NessAlver MS, Carter WB, Bhargavan M, Lewis RS, et al. Diagnostic accuracy of mammography, clinical examination, US, and MR imaging in preoperative assessment of breast cancer. Radiology. 2004;233:830-49.
66. Lehman CD, Gatsonis C, Kuhl CK, Hendrick RE, Pisano ED, Hanna L, et al. MRI evaluation of contralateral breast in women with recently diagnosed breast cancer. N Engl J Med. 2007;356:1295-303.
67. Plana MN, Carreira C, Muriel A, Chiva M, Abraira V, Emparanza JI, et al. Magnetic resonance imaging in preoperative assessment of patients with primary breast cancer: Systematic review of diagnostic accuracy and meta-analysis. Eur Radiol. 2012;22: 26-38.
68. Morris EA, Schwartz LH, Drotman MB, Kim SJ, Tan LK, Liberman L, et al. Evaluation of pectoralis major muscle in patients with posterior breast tumours on breast MR images: Early experience. Radiology. 2000;214:67-72.
69. Veronesi U, Cascinelli N, Mariani L, Greco M, Saccozzi R, Luini A, et al. Twenty year follow up of a randomized study comparing breast conserving surgery with radical mastectomy for early breast cancer. N Engl J Med. 2002;347:1227-32.
70. Fisher B, Anderson S, Bryant J, Margolese RG, Deutsch M, Fisher ER, et al. Twenty year follow up of a randomized trial comparing total mastectomy, lumpectomy, and lumpectomy plus irradiation for the treatment of invasive breast cancer. N Engl J Med. 2002;347:1233-7.
71. Mansel RE, Fellowfield L, Kissin M, Goyal A, Newcombe RG, Dixon JM, et al. Randomized multicenter trial of sentinel node biopsy versus standard axillary treatment in operable breast cancer: The ALMANC trial. J Natl Cancer Inst. 2006;98:599.
72. Moore MM, Whitney LA, Cerilli I, Imbrie JZ, Bunch M, Simpson VB, et al. Intraoperative ultrasound is associated with clear lumpectomy margins for palpable infiltrating ductal breast cancer. Ann Surg. 2001;233:761-8.
73. Lee JM, Orel SG, Czerniecki BJ, Solin LJ, Schnall MD. MRI before re-excision surgery in patients with breast cancer. AJR. 2004;182:473-80.
74. Early Breast Cancer Trialist Group. Effects of chemotherapy and hormonal therapy for early breast cancer on recurrence and 15-year survival: An overview of the randomized trials. Lancet. 2005;365:1687.
75. Le-Petraus H, Uppendahl L, Stafford J. Sonographic features of inflammatory breast cancer. Semin Roentgenol. 2011;46:275-9.
76. Le-Petross H, Cristofanilli M, Carkaci S, Krishnamurthy S, Jackson EF, Harrell RK, et al. MRI features of inflammatory breast cancer. AJR. 2011;197:W769-6.
77. Robertson FM, Bondy M, Yang W, Yamauchi H, Wiggins S, Kamrudin S, et al. Inflammatory breast cancer: The disease, the biology, the treatment. CA Cancer J Clin. 2010;60:351-75.
78. Peintinger F, Kuerer HM, Anderson K, Boughey JC, Meric-Bernstam F, Singletary SE, et al. Combination of mammography and sonography is useful in predicting tumor response in breast cancer patients after neoadjuvant chemotherapy. Ann Surg Oncol. 2006;13:1443-9.
79. Choi JH, Lim HI, Lee SK, Kim WW, Kim SM, Cho E, et al. The role of PET CT to evaluate the response to neoadjuvant chemotherapy in advanced breast cancer: Comparison with ultrasonography and magnetic resonance imaging. J Surg Oncol. 2009;4:1-6.
80. Yeh E, Slanetz P, Kopans DB, Rafferty E, Georgian-Smith D, Moy L, et al. Prospective comparison of mammography, sonography and MRI in patients undergoing neoadjuvant chemotherapy for palpable breast cancer. AJR. 2006;184:868-77.
81. Wang Y, Zhang C, Liu J, Huang G. Is ^{18}F-FDG PET accurate to predict neoadjuvant therapy response in breast cancer? A meta-analysis. Breast Cancer Res Treat. 2012;131:357-69.
82. Park SH, Moon WK, Cho N, Song IC, Chang JM, Park IA, et al. Diffusion weighted MRI imaging: Pretreatment prediction of response to neoadjuvant chemotherapy in patients with breast cancer. Radiology. 2010;257:56-63.
83. Fangberget A, Nilsen LB, Hole KH, Holmen MM, Engebraaten O, Naume B, et al. Neoadjuvant chemotherapy in breast cancer response evaluation and prediction of response to treatment using dynamic contrast enhanced and diffusion weighted MRI imaging. Eur Radiol. 2011;21:1188-99.
84. Park SH, Moon WK, Cho N, Chang JM, Im SA, Park IA, et al. Comparison of diffusion weighted MR imaging and FDG PET/CT to predict pathological complete response to neoadjuvant chemotherapy in patients with breast cancer. Eur Radiol. 2012;22:18-25.
85. Nadeem R, Chagla LS, Harris O, Desmond S, Thind R, Flavin A, et al. Tumour localization with a metal coil before administration of neoadjuvant chemotherapy. Breast. 2005;14:403-7.
86. Hamaoka T, Madewell JE, Podoloff DA, Hortobagyi GN, Ueno NT. Bone imaging in metastatic breast cancer. J Clin Oncol. 2004;22:2942-53.
87. Costelloe CM, Rohren EM, Madewell JE, Hamaoka T, Theriault RL, Yu TK, et al. Imaging bone metastases in breast cancer: Techniques and recommendations for diagnosis. Lancet Oncol. 2009;10:606-14.
88. Liu T, Cheng T, Xu W, Yan WL, Liu J, Yang HL. A meta-analysis of ^{18}FDG-PET, MRI and bone scintigraphy for diagnosis of bone metastases in patients with breast cancer. Skeletal Radiol. 2011;40:523-32.

89. Brookes M, MacVicar D, Husband J. Metastatic carcinoma of the breast: The appearances of metastatic spread to abdomen and pelvis as demonstrated by CT. Br J Radiol. 2007;80: 284-92.
90. Jung JM, Kim HH, Park SH, Song SW, Chung MH, Kim HS, et al. Thoracic manifestations of breast cancer and its therapy. Radiographics. 2004;24:1269-85.
91. Olson JA Jr, Morris EA, Van Zee KA, Linehan DC, Borgen PI. Magnetic resonance imaging facilitates breast conservation for occult breast cancer. Ann Surg Oncol. 2000;7:411-5.
92. Brenner RJ, Pfaff JM. Mammographic features after conservation therapy for malignant breast disease: Serial findings standardized by regression analysis. AJR. 1996;167:171-8.
93. Montgomery DA, Krupa K, Cooke TG. Follow-up in breast cancer: Does routine clinical examination improve outcome? A systematic review of literature. Br J Cancer. 2007;97:1632-41.
94. Gunhan-Bilgen I, Oktay A. Mammographic features of local recurrence after conserving surgery and radiation therapy: Comparison with that of the primary tumour. Acta Radiologica. 2007;48:390-7.
95. Dao TH, Rahmount A, Campana F, Laurent M, Asselain B, Fourquet A. Tumour recurrence versus fibrosis in the irradiated breast: Differentiation with dynamic gadolinium contrast enhanced MR imaging. Radiology. 1993;187:751-5.
96. Gunhan-Bilgen I, Oktay A. Paget's disease of breast. Clinical, mammographic, sonographic and pathologic findings in 52 cases. Eur J Radiol. 2006;60:256-63.
97. Yang WT, Lane DL, Le-Petross HT, Abruzzo LV, Macapinlac HA. Breast lymphoma: Imaging findings in 32 tumours. Radiology. 2007;245:692-702.
98. Dershaw DD, Borgen PI, Deutch BM, Liberman L. Mammographic findings in men with breast cancer. AJR. 1993;160:267-70.

CHAPTER

178

Breast Interventions

Surabhi Vyas, Smriti Hari, Smita Manchanda

INTRODUCTION

Breast interventions primarily comprise of biopsy of suspicious breast lesions to obtain accurate pathological diagnosis. Breast biopsy is the mainstay of definitive and timely diagnosis of breast cancer and its treatment. Preoperative wire localization has both diagnostic and therapeutic applications. Ablative procedures for breast cancer treatment are still considered investigational.

BREAST BIOPSY

Mammography and other breast imaging modalities can detect nonpalpable breast abnormalities which may represent breast cancer and hence imaging-guided procedure for their sampling is mandatory for timely diagnosis of the breast cancer. The techniques and instrumentation of these procedures have evolved over years with improvement in accuracy of the diagnosis. Although palpable lesions can be sampled without image guidance, the sampling accuracy improves when the procedure is conducted under image guidance. For non-palpable lesions, imaging guidance is mandatory.[1] Special skills beyond those acquired in general radiology are required for radiologist who performs these procedures. As several of these techniques involve special equipment, assistance of an experienced technologist is desirable. The radiologist must have the basic knowledge of diagnostic breast imaging, limitations of imaging, cancer risks and treatment options for breast cancer so as to select appropriate lesion and the biopsy technique. This knowledge is also required for meaningful discussion with the patient, referring clinician and the pathologist. After the biopsy, follow-up of patient to diagnose and treat any complications is mandatory. Pathology results of the biopsy must also be correlated with baseline imaging findings to ensure that these are concordant with imaging.

BREAST BIOPSY TECHNIQUES

Surgical Biopsy

Surgical excision biopsy is the most accurate technique for the diagnosis of breast cancer as it completely removes the abnormality and hence there is no chance of sampling error. For nonpalpable lesions, this is performed after preoperative hookwire localization, so as to guide the surgeon to the exact location of the lesion. Surgical excision biopsy is the gold standard of breast cancer diagnosis and it is still routinely performed at few centers. However, the procedure is invasive and disfiguring. This disadvantage is especially important considering the fact that majority of breast biopsy results are benign and resultant scar and disfigurement of breast may be unacceptable to these patients. Even in patients with malignant diagnosis, this leads to two surgical procedures, one diagnostic and then another for treatment, leading to increased patient anxiety and cost of the treatment.

Percutaneous needle biopsy expedites the breast cancer diagnosis and is cost-effective. With modern biopsy techniques and instrumentations, the diagnostic accuracy is also nearly comparable to that of surgical excision biopsy. Percutaneous biopsy can be a fine needle aspiration cytology (FNAC) or core biopsy.

Fine Needle Aspiration Cytology

Fine needle aspiration cytology is a simple, less expensive and less traumatic technique. Generally, a 20-gauge (20G) to 22G needle is used to make multiple excursions in the lesion and fluid-containing dislodged cells is aspirated to make smears for cytological diagnosis. Results of FNAC are immediately available. However, FNAC has several limitations. It requires the availability of an experienced breast cytologist who can establish the adequacy of aspirated sample on site and also interpret it accurately. It has high insufficiency and false-negative rates. A negative FNAC cannot reliably exclude the presence of breast cancer. FNAC is especially unsuitable for nonpalpable breast lesions as up to 34% of FNAC samples may be insufficient for diagnosis.[2] Insufficiency rate is much higher for calcifications than for masses. FNAC gives cytological diagnosis only, i.e., it cannot differentiate in situ from invasive cancer. Modern treatment protocols often require immunohistochemical analysis for hormonal receptor status and this is difficult to obtain on FNAC. Benign FNAC results are often nonspecific and definitive diagnosis of a benign condition is rarely made. This affects the radiologic-pathologic correlation and may be a limitation in deciding further management. Diagnosis of papillary lesions is inaccurate on FNAC and it cannot differentiate fibroadenoma from phyllodes tumor.[3] FNAC results are frequently interpreted as atypical or suspicious only, which leads to a second more invasive biopsy. This leads to increased cost and delay in the diagnosis of breast cancer.[4] Although extremely rare, false-positive results on FNAC leading to an unnecessary surgery are also known. Because of these disadvantages, breast FNAC is less commonly employed at present and most breast care centers do not rely on breast FNAC to make the management decisions.

Core Needle Biopsy

Several of the disadvantages of FNAC have been addressed by percutaneous core needle biopsy (CNB) of the breast and this has become the standard of care for biopsy of breast lesions; whether palpable or not. Accuracy of CNB is better than FNAC and it allows cellular and architectural evaluation. With this, specific diagnosis of benign and malignant conditions can be made. The cores are also suitable for immunohistochemical and genetic analysis. However, CNB of breast is more traumatic, more expensive and requires higher skills to perform when compared with FNAC. Results of CNB are not immediately available and take few days at least.

Breast CNB is commonly performed using spring-loaded automated core biopsy needles, commonly known as biopsy guns. Earlier smaller gauge (16G or 18G) biopsy needles were used, but these suffered from lower sample sufficiency rates. Introduction of 14G core needles significantly improved the accuracy of breast CNB[5] **(Figs. 1A and B)**. False-negative rates of 14G CNB range from 0 to 9%.[6] Long throw (2 cm), 14G caliber is the standard size of biopsy guns used for breast CNB and smaller gauge biopsy guns which are routinely used in other body parts are not recommended for breast CNB. Typically, a minimum of 4–5 cores are obtained during a breast CNB.

Vacuum-assisted Biopsy

Directional vacuum-assisted biopsy (VAB) of breast is a modified and improved technique of large core breast biopsy. It was introduced in late 1990s.[7] It can be used under ultrasound, stereotactic or magnetic resonance (MR) guidance. The VAB device consists of a main unit housing the vacuum generator and the operating console and disposable biopsy probe (needle) attached to it **(Fig. 2)**. The probe consists of an outer cannula with a sample notch and an inner cutting cannula. When activated, a vacuum is applied which sucks and holds the tissue at the sample notch. Next, the inner cannula advances with high speed rotation to cut and enclose the tissue core within. Without removing the probe from the breast, the cut sample is then transported outside to the sample chamber using activation of another vacuum. Vacuum is also used to aspirate the oozed blood preventing hematoma formation. Saline irrigation or instillation of local anesthetic at the biopsy site through the probe is also possible during the procedure. All the steps of VAB are automated and contiguous multiple cores of tissue can be harvested without removing the probe from the breast. Some of the currently available VAB devices include Mammotome® (previously Johnson and Johnson; now Devicor, Cincinnati, USA), Eviva® and Atec® (previously Suros; now Hologic, Bedford, USA) and Encore® (previously Senorx; now Bard, Tempe, USA). Thick caliber (11G–7G) probes are typically used in VAB.

Advantages of Vacuum-assisted Biopsy

Major advantage of the VAB is that it allows fast acquisition of multiple, large and contiguous tissue cores with single needle insertion into the breast. When compared with CNB using biopsy guns, a 10-fold greater tissue volume is obtained per core.[8] The probe can be rotated 360° within the lesion facilitating removal of tissue around the probe. Small lesions can be completely removed thereby eliminating the chances

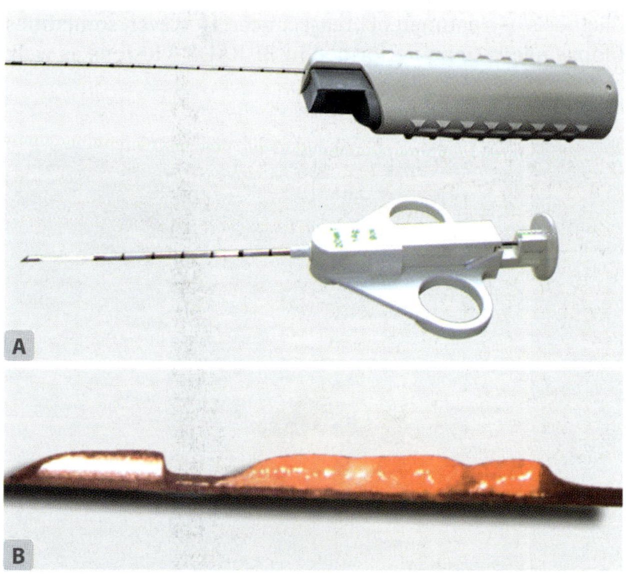

FIGS. 1A AND B: Core needle biopsy of breast: (A) 14G biopsy guns; (B) Open sample notch of the biopsy gun showing harvested tissue specimen.

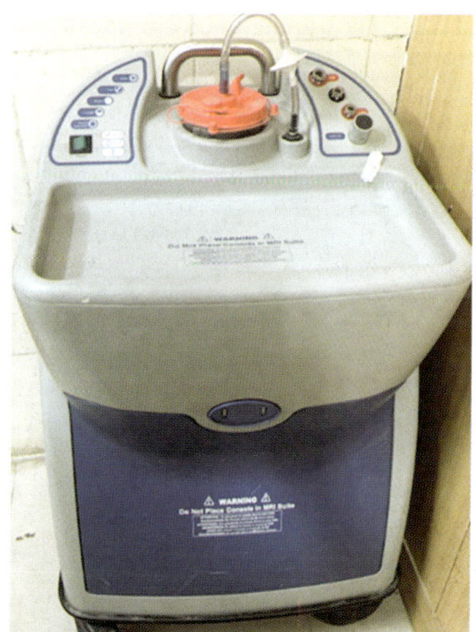

FIG. 2: Vacuum-assisted biopsy (VAB) device. Suros unit for vacuum-assisted breast biopsy.

of sampling errors. Unlike biopsy guns, very accurate needle placement is not mandatory for VAB. The sample notch can be directed to the lesion and it can pull the lesion into the notch. This feature is particularly valuable when a small cluster of calcification is targeted. In VAB, the probe is placed close to or within the lesion before actually taking the biopsy and hence chance of cutting needle sliding by the side of the lesion, rather than penetrating it, is also eliminated. After the first few cores obtained during CNB, subsequent cores tend to contain tissue as well as clots. This does not happen in VAB as the oozing blood is continuously removed and all the harvested cores are of good quality.

Larger tissue removal with VAB increases the accuracy of breast biopsy. False-negative rates of VAB range from 0.6 to 5.2%.[6] The results of VAB are almost as good as surgical biopsy and negative predictive value as high as 99.9% can be achieved with VAB.[9,10] VAB is also more accurate than CNB in terms of frequency of histological underestimation, false negatives, and need for rebiopsy.[11,12]

Marker Clip Placement with Vacuum-assisted Biopsy

Vacuum-assisted biopsy probes also allow placement of radiopaque marker clips at the biopsy site before the removal of the probe from the breast **(Figs. 3A and B)**. If the small lesion is completely removed during the biopsy and histopathology result is positive for cancer, this clip can be used to direct preoperative hookwire placement to guide breast conservation surgery. If the result is benign, the small marker clip is left as such in the breast. Some marker clips have both metal and a gel which expands into the tissue. This type of clip can be visualized both on mammography and ultrasound for hookwire localization. Placement of marker clip is also important for breast mass of any size that is being considered for neoadjuvant chemotherapy.[13,14] After chemotherapy, some breast cancers may completely disappear on imaging and in this situation, tumor site can be identified with marker clip only and the surgery can be performed after performing hookwire localization of the marker clip.

Disadvantages of Vacuum-assisted Biopsy

Vacuum-assisted biopsy is more expensive than CNB using biopsy guns. The main unit with operating console as well as disposable biopsy probes is expensive. VAB probes are up to 10 times more expensive than the biopsy guns. One of the approaches toward better cost-effectiveness is that it could be selectively used as an alternative to open surgical biopsy for patients with nondiagnostic initial biopsy.[15] This approach is currently followed at author's institute. VAB also lacks the convenience of CNB. The probe is heavier and an experienced assistant is required during the procedure. However, advantages of VAB far outweigh the disadvantages and it has become the standard of breast biopsy in most breast care centers.

Complete Lesion Removal with Vacuum-assisted Biopsy

It is important to note that VAB instrument is intended for tissue sampling only and not for therapeutic removal of the lesion. Even if complete imaging evidence of the malignant lesion is removed with VAB, cancer is still found on surgery in majority of the patients.[16,17] Surgery for breast cancer requires en bloc removal of the tumor with adequate margins of normal parenchyma around it and not just the gross tumor removal. However, this is not an issue with the benign lesions. Although uncommonly performed, VAB has been used as a minimally invasive technique to remove small benign breast masses with high patient satisfaction rates.[18,19] VAB leaves a very small, 3–4 mm, scar on the breast and results in excellent cosmetic outcome when compared with surgical removal of a benign mass.

Lesion Selection for Breast Biopsy

Breast biopsy is indicated in all lesions classified as BI-RADS 4 (suspicious) or BI-RADS 5 (highly suspicious). BI-RADS 3 lesions have <2% chance of malignancy and these are best managed with imaging follow-up without significant delay in diagnosis or treatment of breast cancer. However, sometimes biopsy needs to be performed in BI-RADS 3 lesions as well.

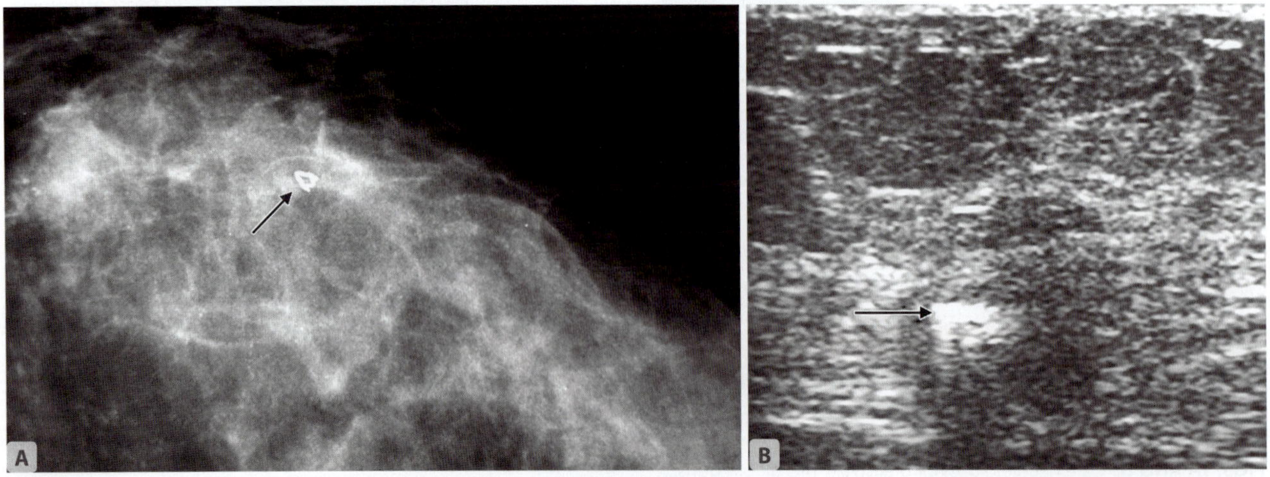

FIGS. 3A AND B: Marker clips. (A) Metallic marker clip Mammomark® deployed at the biopsy site (arrow) after VAB is seen on postbiopsy mammogram; (B) Gel-coated marker clip (arrow) can also be visualized on ultrasound.

Such situations include inability to follow-up, anxious patient who refuses for follow-up, planned pregnancy, and presence of another breast lesion which is already diagnosed as breast cancer.

Selection of Guiding Modality

Image-guided breast biopsy can be performed under ultrasound, mammographic (stereotactic) or MR guidance. Ultrasound is the most commonly used modality, if the breast lesion is unequivocally demonstrated on ultrasound. No special ultrasound equipment is required and the modality as well as expertise is widely available. The procedure is real time and fast. The lying position is also comfortable to the patient. Ultrasound-guided procedures also allow greater flexibility of the approach and the puncture site. The needle can be inserted oblique or near parallel to the chest wall. Lesions located close to the chest wall, in the axillary tail or in the subareolar location may be difficult to position under stereotactic biopsy but these can be readily targeted with ultrasound guidance.

Microcalcifications only or masses which are seen on mammography only are indications for stereotactic breast biopsy. Personal preference and experience with biopsy techniques also govern the selection of guiding modality. At some centers, stereotactic biopsy is the preferred modality for all types of lesions, including masses that can be seen on ultrasound. MR-guided biopsy is cumbersome, expensive and time consuming. However, with increasing use of breast magnetic resonance imaging (MRI) and its higher sensitivity, MR-guided biopsy is required for lesions which are visible on MRI only. It is worthwhile to perform a careful "second look" targeted breast ultrasound in an attempt to localize the MRI-detected lesion. Many of the MR positive breast lesions can be demonstrated like this and ultrasound-guided biopsy can be performed.[20,21]

Suspicious areas of focal asymmetry or architectural distortion are generally not subjected to percutaneous biopsy. Excision biopsy is preferred in these situations. A suspicious dilated duct is also excised surgically unless there is an associated mass or calcification which can be used as a target for image-guided percutaneous biopsy.

Prebiopsy Assessment

Imaging on basis of which the breast biopsy has been recommended must be carefully evaluated. It should be ensured that a clearly visible abnormality is present which can be targeted accurately. Appropriate biopsy technique and guiding modality is then selected. If the imaging is inadequate or presence of the lesion is doubtful, additional imaging must be done before scheduling the biopsy. A brief history should be obtained from the patient and at the same time biopsy procedure, its risks and postbiopsy instructions may also be conveyed to the patient. History of allergy to Betadine or lignocaine, if any, should also be asked. No claims about outcome of the biopsy or future management should be made. The patient should be aware that a rebiopsy or excision may be required if the biopsy specimen is considered inadequate for definite pathological opinion. Informed consent must be obtained before the biopsy. Preprocedural coagulation profile is not required, unless patient has a bleeding tendency or is taking anticoagulants. Patients on aspirin or nonsteroidal anti-inflammatory drugs (NSAIDs) should stop it 3–5 days before the biopsy. Prophylactic antibiotics are not routinely required; however, these can be considered based on individual clinical judgment in patients with diabetes, rheumatic heart disease, artificial heart valves or joint replacement.

Ultrasound-guided Breast Biopsy

Wide availability, low cost, and ease of convenience to both the radiologist and the patient makes ultrasound the preferred modality for breast biopsy. Linear, 7.5 MHz (or more) transducer should be used. CNB must be performed with 14G long throw (2 cm or more) biopsy guns, even for a small subcentimeter lesion. Preprocedure test fire of the biopsy gun should be avoided. Correct patient positioning is important for ultrasound-guided breast biopsy. Ipsilateral arm of the patient should be raised above the head. Supine patient position is good for medial quadrant lesions. For lateral quadrant lesions, ipsilateral anterior supine oblique position should be made, preferably with a pillow under the patient's shoulder. This helps to spread and thin out the breast parenchyma over the lesion. Ultrasound unit should be aligned in such a way that a right-handed radiologist can conveniently scan with left hand and hold the needle in right hand, without twisting his or her body to see the image on the monitor.

Technique

After preliminary scanning, skin puncture site should be carefully chosen. Free hand technique with needle visualization in longitudinal plane of the scan field is used for ultrasound-guided breast biopsy. Instead of choosing shortest skin to lesion distance, puncture site should be at least 1 cm or more away from the edge of the transducer. This increases the distance which the needle has to travel in the breast, but it makes the needle path parallel to chest wall, thereby reducing the chances of injury or penetration of the chest wall. The needle remains parallel to the transducer improving the needle visibility **(Fig. 4)**.

The skin should be cleaned with Betadine and the draped with sterile sheets. Transducer surface is also cleaned or covered with sterile cover, as per the local practice. Local anesthesia should be given using 5–10 cc of 1% lignocaine and 22G or 23G needle. Local anesthetic should be injected under ultrasound guidance, first close to the lesion, then along the needle tract and finally, in the subcutaneous tissue at the puncture site. Raising a skin wheal with local anesthetic at the puncture site greatly reduces the pain during biopsy. A small skin incision is given at the puncture site using number 11 scalpel blade. Needle is then carefully inserted and turned horizontally. Some resistance may be felt initially as the needle penetrates through the fascia and ligaments attached to the skin, the needle advancement should be carefully controlled so as to avoid sudden give-in and deep penetration. In hard breast, counter pressure from opposite direction may be required to facilitate needle penetration. The needle should always be kept parallel to the chest wall and in the plane of the long axis of the transducer, i.e., the scan plane. Otherwise, the needle tip may not be seen. To achieve this transducer-needle alignment, sometimes the transducer needs to be rotated or repositioned during advancement of the needle. The needle tip should just pierce the lesion, if it is large enough, and has been stabilized with the transducer pressure **(Fig. 5A)**. Patient should be warned that a "thud" sound will be heard and she should not get scared or make sudden jerky moves. If an assistant is helping in taking the samples, phrases like "fire now" should be avoided as it may upset or scare the patient. The gun is then fired under real-time guidance. Before removing the needle, scanning in longitudinal and transverse planes should be done so as to ensure that the sample notch part of the gun is truly within the lesion **(Figs. 5B and C)**. It does not matter if the needle tip has crossed beyond the lesion. The needle is withdrawn; sample is retrieved and transferred to the sample bottle containing 10% formalin. The needle should not be dipped in formalin; instead, a scalpel blade should be used to remove the tissue from the sample notch. In this way multiple, at least four to five samples are collected and sample bottle is labeled. After the biopsy, light compression is applied at the biopsy site for about 10 minutes.

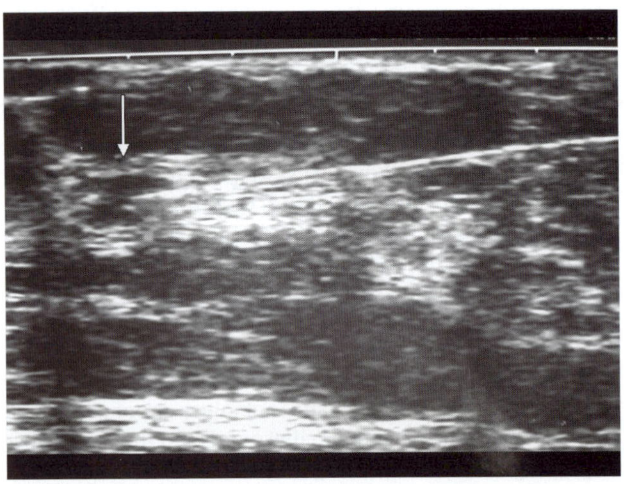

FIG. 4: Ultrasound-guided core needle biopsy (CNB). Horizontal needle approach improves the needle visualization, especially for targeting of small mass (arrow).

Technique of ultrasound-guided VAB is similar to that of ultrasound-guided CNB using biopsy gun **(Fig. 6A)**. The skin incision should be little wider so as to accommodate the large caliber VAB probes. The probe (needle) of VAB is not fired inside the lesion. Instead of hitting the lesion from the side, the probe tip is positioned below the lesion, in such a way that the sample notch remains just beneath the lesion **(Fig. 6B)**. This helps to obtain contiguous core of the lesion, beginning from the deeper part of the lesion and then probe gradually moves superficially through the lesion for each subsequent core. The probe of the VAB is thick and not removed from the breast until the end of the biopsy procedure. If it is placed in the superficial part, most part of the lesion will be obscured beneath the acoustic shadowing of the probe after obtaining initial cores. If a small lesion is completely removed during VAB, a marker clip must be deployed at the biopsy site through the probe before taking it out from the breast.

Stereotactic Breast Biopsy

The principle of stereotactic biopsy is based on the trigonometric determination of depth of the target lesion in the breast. The breast is positioned and compressed in the stereotactic unit and pair of mammographic spot exposures (stereo images) is obtained with +15° and –15° tube angulations. Relative position of the target will change in both views because of the parallax shift due to different tube angulations. Lesion situated close to the detector moves less and lesion situated away from the detector moves more in these two images. This movement is compared with the movements of a marker with known depth (reference marker at the base) to determine the depth (z-coordinate) of the target lesion in the breast. Actual process involves complex trigonometric calculations, which are fortunately performed by the system computer. The x- and y-coordinates are same in both views.

Equipment

Stereotactic biopsy equipment are of two types: (1) dedicated prone table and (2) add-on erect stereotactic device. Both of these were film-based in past but now digital systems are used as they make the procedure simpler and faster. In dedicated prone table unit, the patient lies prone on the table and the breast hangs down through an opening in the table **(Figs. 7A and B)**. The patient is comfortable and breast remains

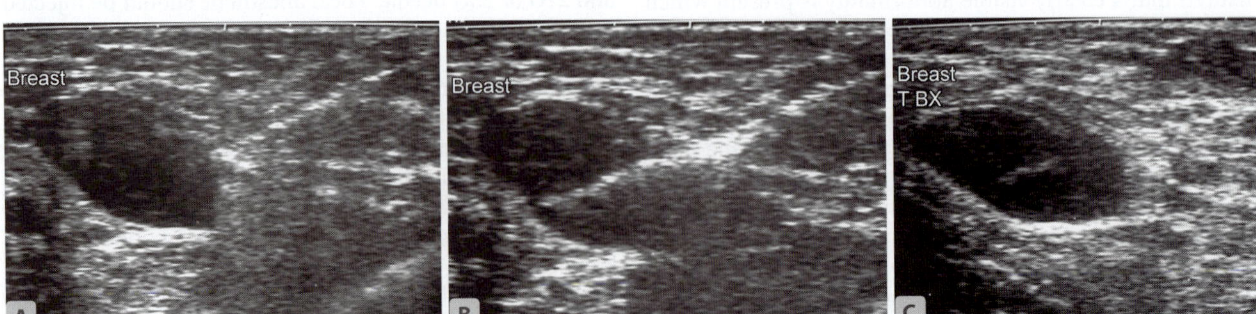

FIGS. 5A TO C: Ultrasound-guided core needle biopsy (CNB). (A) The tip of the biopsy needle is positioned at the periphery of the mass; (B) The mass and the needle are stabilized and the needle is fired. Area of sample notch is seen within the center of the mass indicating accurate positioning and sampling; (C) After withdrawal of the needle, small echogenic area of hemorrhage is seen within the mass at the site of biopsy.

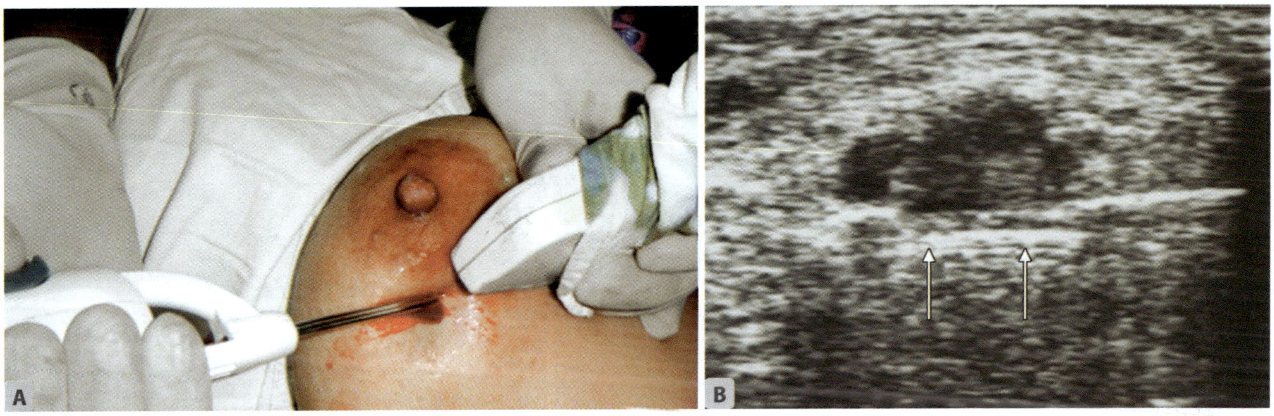

FIGS. 6A AND B: Ultrasound-guided vacuum-assisted biopsy (VAB). (A) Biopsy procedure is being performed with Mammotome® probe and transducer aligned in the same plane; (B) The open sample notch (arrows) is positioned just beneath the mass.

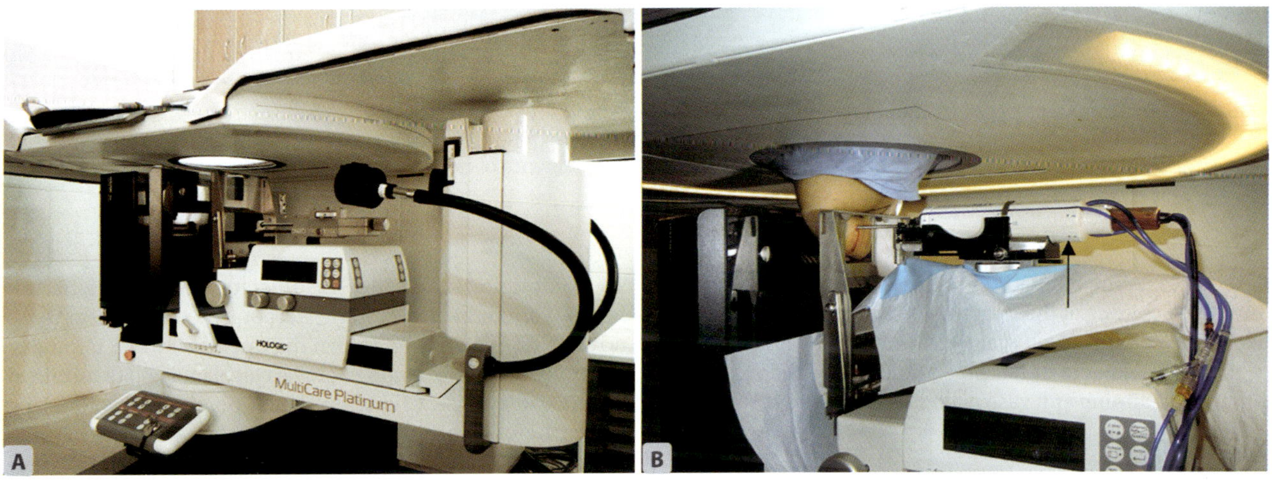

FIGS. 7A AND B: Dedicated prone table stereotactic biopsy. (A) Equipment (Mutlicare®, Hologic); (B) Stereotactic biopsy being performed using Atec® VAB device.

stable during the procedure which is performed below the table. As the patient does not see the procedure, her anxiety is reduced. There is also more working space for the radiologist. The lesion can be approached from any side (360°) around the breast. Dedicated prone table stereotactic biopsy units are more expensive, require large space and cannot be used for diagnostic mammography. Hence, these are cost-effective only if stereotactic biopsy is being routinely performed in the department. As thickness of the table will always remain between the chest wall and the breast, lesions situated too close to the chest wall may be difficult to access.

Add-on stereotactic biopsy device is actually an accessory device which can be attached to a standard diagnostic mammography unit to perform stereotactic biopsy **(Figs. 8A and B)**. It is cheaper and cost-effective. However, the biopsy can be performed in erect (sitting) patient position only. It is inconvenient to both the patient and the radiologist as working space is limited. The needle must be inserted from cranial aspect only, even if the lesion is located in caudal part

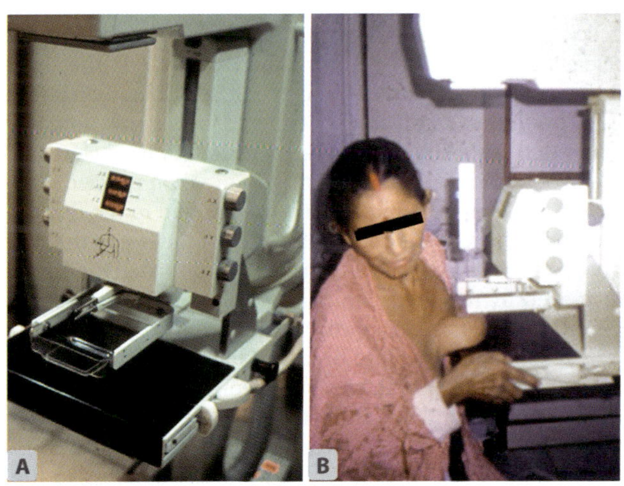

FIGS. 8A AND B: Add-on erect stereotactic biopsy equipment. (A) Biopsy unit (Opdima®, Siemens); (B) Stereotactic biopsy is being performed with biopsy gun in a sitting position.

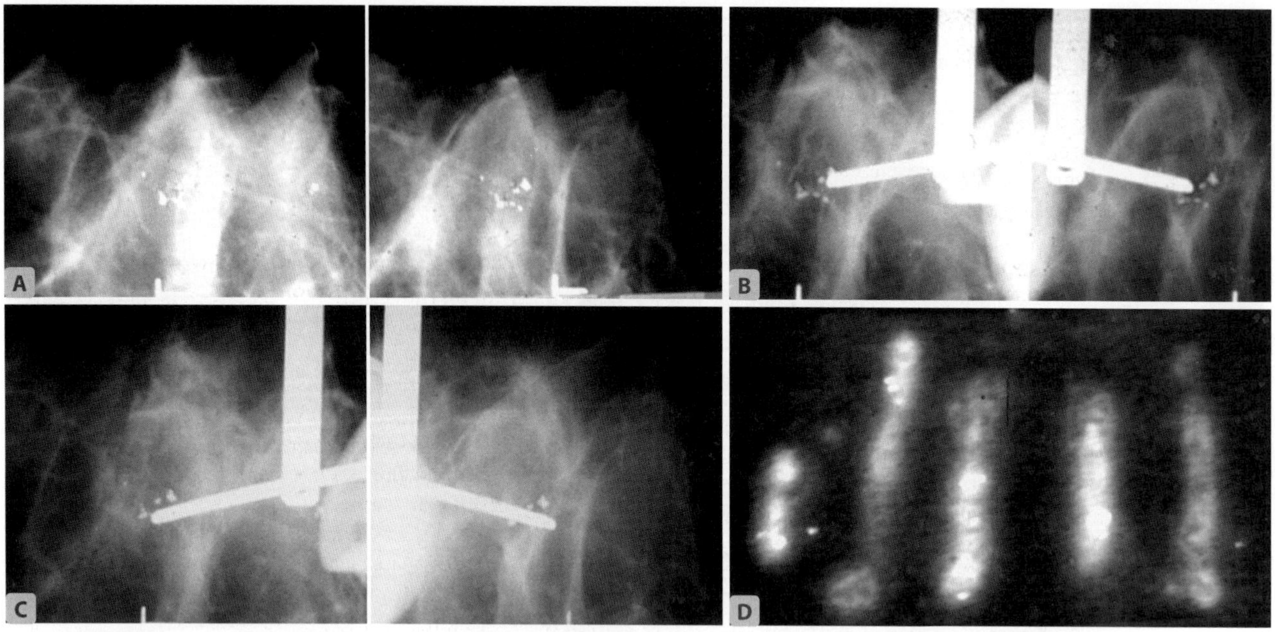

FIGS. 9A TO D: Stereotactic biopsy. (A) Pair of stereo images obtained at +10° and –10°. Targets are marked in both images on the lesion, i.e., cluster of calcifications in this case; (B) Prefire pair of images show needle tip close to the lesion in both images; (C) Postfire images show that needle has traversed the lesion; (D) Specimen radiography of the samples shows presence of calcifications in multiple cores, confirming accurate targeting and sampling.

of the breast. The chances of breast movement resulting in unnoticed shifting of the target lesion during biopsy are more likely. The patient closely watches the approach and insertion of the biopsy needle in her breast and hence there are high chances of fainting and vasovagal reactions.

Technique

The technique of stereotactic biopsy is same for both types of units. The breast is positioned and compressed with a compression plate having an open window. An initial spot image is obtained without tube angulation to ensure that the lesion is seen in the center of the window. Once this is confirmed, a pair of stereo images is obtained without releasing the breast compression **(Fig. 9A)**. At the user interface of the computer, total needle length and distance from tip of the needle to the center of the sample notch is entered. Needle length must be measured in fired status of the needle. Single or multiple targets are then marked with mouse clicks in both images and transmitted to the device. Care must be taken to mark same part of the lesion in both images. The x-, y- and z-coordinates are calculated and displayed by the unit. The needle holder position is then moved and adjusted to appropriate position.

Presence of adequate breast tissues (thickness), both proximal and deep to the lesion, in compressed position of the breast is essential in stereotactic breast biopsy. The core biopsy sample is obtained from the sample notch and not from the tip of the needle. If the lesion is too close to the skin, the gun will have to be fired while the sample notch is partially outside the breast. This is not recommended. Similarly, if the lesion is too close to the table (bucky), the needle tip will puncture the skin and hit the table. These situations are called insufficient stroke margins and biopsy cannot be done. Some stereotactic units detect these errors automatically and warn the operator, while in others, safety of the stroke margin has to be calculated and determined by the radiologist. Changing breast position or rolling the breast before compression is sometimes useful in such situations. Prone table biopsy units are better in these situations as they allow greater flexibility in choosing the direction of needle entry.

Site preparation and biopsy procedure is same as that for ultrasound-guided breast biopsy. Needle is inserted through the needle holder in its selected final position. A prefire pair of stereo images is obtained with needle fully inserted **(Fig. 9B)**. In both of these images, the needle tip should be seen just before and at the same distance from the target. After that, the gun is fired and another set of postfire stereo images is obtained **(Fig. 9C)**. The needle tip should have symmetrically crossed the lesion in both of these images. The biopsy gun is then removed and sample retrieved. Subsequently, each target is selected, transmitted and fresh needle insertions are made to obtain multiple cores. It is not necessary to obtain pre- and postfire images for each subsequent core if these images are satisfactory during first sample. However, if the lesion has moved or if there is asymmetry of needle tip—lesion relationship in pre- or postfire images, a fresh pair of stereo images without needle should be obtained and biopsy continued with fresh target setting. When biopsy is being performed with vacuum-assisted probe, the probe is rotated in the same position to obtain multiple cores from all directions around the probe. At the end, the needle is withdrawn from the breast and compression is released.

Tomosynthesis-guided Core Biopsy

Digital breast tomosynthesis is a technique which improves detection and characterization of a breast lesion, by reconstructing the data into thin sections. It is especially helpful in dense breasts where the margin of a lesion may be obscured by overlapping fibroglandular parenchyma.[22] Tomosynthesis-guided core biopsy is a recent advance that allows histopathological diagnosis without resorting to more invasive surgical intervention.

Benefits

Tomoguided biopsy allows easier sampling of focal asymmetry, architectural distortion, calcifications and noncalcified masses by automatically providing a depth estimation without having to calculate the z-coordinate. It allows a sitting/upright biopsy and thus do away with the discomfort associated with prone biopsy. Posteriorly located lesions are also easily sampled compared to prone biopsy. However as some patients may experience vasovagal reaction, prone tomoguided setups are also now available. Studies have shown it to be a faster technique compared to the stereotactic biopsy as there is no intervening step of stereo-pair images.[23]

Technique

The steps of acquiring a tomoguided biopsy are similar to a stereotactic biopsy with few exceptions. After assessing the lesion on prior imaging and clinical examination, the approach for biopsy is planned as either craniocaudal/caudocranial or mediolateral/lateromedial, depending on the location of lesion and its nearest skin distance. After appropriate positioning, tomosynthesis data is acquired instead of the scout and stereo pairs. The suspicious area can then be targeted based on which tomo slice shows the lesion to best advantage. The depth calculation is not required. Further steps of biopsy, check view, clip placement and specimen radiography are similar to the stereotactic biopsy.

Disadvantages

Visualization of subtle and faint calcifications may sometimes be limited on tomosynthesis and may require two-dimensional (2D) imaging and 2D stereotactic biopsy.

Specimen Radiography

If the target lesion has calcifications, specimen radiography of the harvested cores is essential to document retrieval of calcifications in the specimen **(Fig. 9D)**. This is recommended both after ultrasound-guided and stereotactic core biopsy. The cores may be placed on a wet slide or film so that they do not stick to it and specimen radiography is performed on standard mammography unit using lowest exposure factors. Demonstration of calcifications in cores eliminates the risk of sampling error and improves the chances of specific diagnosis. If the calcifications are not demonstrated, pathological diagnosis can still be made; however, the accuracy of the diagnosis is lower than when calcifications are demonstrated.[24,25] Specimen mammography of cores is not required when the target is a mass lesion without calcification.

Postbiopsy Care

After ultrasound-guided or stereotactic core biopsy of the breast, a continuous light pressure is maintained over the biopsy site (and not at the skin puncture site) at least for 10 minutes to achieve good hemostasis. Sometimes, a longer compression is needed. After that the skin is cleaned with alcohol and the incision is closed using sterile adhesive tape. Procedure and instructions must be written in postbiopsy notes and explained to the patient. The patient should be advised to keep the biopsy site dry and watch for obvious bleeding or sudden breast enlargement; the latter would indicate internal bleed and hematoma formation. Although this is rare, the patient can apply light pressure herself and contact the radiologist immediately should this happen. A telephone number of the radiologist should be provided to her for this purpose. Patient should be asked to avoid strenuous ipsilateral arm movements, such as lifting heavy weights, pushing something exercise or cooking activities. The tape on the wound can be removed after 48 hours.

Mild pain and some heaviness of the breast may be experienced by the patient immediately after the biopsy. Ice fomentation using ice cubes in a plastic bag is useful to relieve postbiopsy pain and also to reduce chances of bleeding. Routine analgesics are not required and should be avoided as far as possible. Patients should also be told that small bruising or discoloration of the skin due to ecchymosed blood can occur and this clears subsequently. Local skin inflammation or small serous ooze from incision site may rarely be seen which is also self-limiting. The wound should be kept clean and dry and no ointment, etc., should be applied. Prolonged bloody or purulent discharge from the wound however, should be evaluated clinically as well radiologically to determine if any treatment is required.

COMPLICATIONS OF BREAST BIOPSY

Percutaneous core biopsy breast is a safe procedure and complications are rare. Vasovagal reaction, hematoma formation, and infection are main complications. Excessive bleeding or pain during biopsy necessitating termination of the procedure is extremely rare. Minor complication rate is 1.4%.[9] Significant hematoma formation or infection, defined as those requiring medical or surgical treatment, occurs only in 0.1% cases. Small hematoma formation at the biopsy site is an expected finding and it can be seen on ultrasound for a week in majority of patients.[26] Complication rates of biopsy with biopsy gun and VAB are similar.[27]

Vasovagal reaction is a potential but unpredictable risk of breast biopsy. It is caused by anxiety, fear, and pain. It is characterized by complaints of lightheadedness or fainting and signs of sweating, skin flushing and bradycardia. Distracting light conversation with patient during the biopsy procedure is helpful to avoid it. The patient should not be left alone during the biopsy. If vasovagal reaction occurs, she should be immediately placed in a supine position with feet raised and pulse and blood pressure monitored. This is usually adequate and active treatment with atropine is not generally required. Strict aseptic precautions during the biopsy are essential to minimize the chances of infection. A good compression after the biopsy and patient compliance of the postbiopsy instructions are important to reduce the chances of major hematoma formation.

Although complications of breast biopsy are uncommon, psychological impact of breast biopsy is important. The patient is worried and disturbed ever since she is told that there is a suspicious lesion in her breast that could be a cancer. Anxiety about the biopsy procedure itself is an additional cause of fear. These factors must also be considered while interacting with the patient.

Percutaneous breast biopsy does not cause seeding of tumor cells along the biopsy tract so as to cause spread or recurrence of the tumor in the breast or skin.[28] Although displaced tumor cells can be rarely found along the needle tract on histological examination of excised specimen, these cells probably do not sustain long enough to produce tumor seeding.[29,30] Needle tract cell displacement is more common with automated gun biopsies than with VAB, as unlike with biopsy guns, only single-time needle insertion is required with VAB.

Percutaneous breast biopsy generally does not produce any long-term changes, scarring or architectural distortion on follow-up mammograms. In <2% cases, a tiny round opacity may develop, which is seen in only one view of the mammogram.[31]

Magnetic Resonance Imaging-guided Breast Biopsy

Magnetic resonance imaging of breast is generally used as a problem-solving modality. It is also being used for high-risk screening and preoperative staging of breast cancer. Contrast-enhanced breast MRI is the most sensitive modality for breast cancer detection, which means that some breast lesions are seen only on MRI and not on conventional imaging. These are the lesions which require biopsy using MR guidance.

Magnetic resonance imaging-guided breast biopsy is performed with special breast coils and needle guide known as aiming device. It allows access on lateral aspect of breast only and hence, medially located lesions require deep needle insertion. Two types of localization devices are available. Most commonly used is a grid type device, a plate with multiple holes. The patient is positioned prone with breast in the coil. Mild compression is given with grid plate itself and contrast-enhanced MRI is performed. A fiducial (marker), usually a vitamin E capsule, is also placed in one of the holes. The lesion is localized in axial and sagittal planes. Its location and distance with respect to fiducial is determined. The needle holder is fixed in the grid hole which is in line with the lesion. Depth is determined by counting the sagittal slices between needle holder and the lesion. A coaxial needle is first introduced up to the lesion, through which biopsy is taken using MR compatible biopsy gun or VAB probe.[32] The other type of aiming device has a bar and column, which can be moved in horizontal and vertical directions respectively, instead of a grid. The lesion and fiducial are localized and bar and columns moved to align the needle holder with the lesion for performance of biopsy.

Magnetic resonance imaging-guided breast biopsy is difficult, time-consuming and expensive. It requires special hardware in the form of a special imaging coil with window for biopsy and localization device and MR compatible needles, usually made of titanium of nickel alloys. The biopsy must be done with contrast-enhanced MRI, which means that the procedure must be completed within 30–40 minutes when the lesion is enhancing and hence visible. The patient needs to be moved in and out of the gantry several times during the biopsy, making it cumbersome and time-consuming. As the lesion is seen only because of contrast enhancement in vivo, specimen imaging cannot be done.

Histopathological Correlation

Core biopsy is a reliable method of diagnosis of breast abnormalities. When malignancy is found, definitive surgery is undertaken. However, some cancers can be missed on core biopsy. False-negative rates of core breast biopsy can be as high as 9% for gun biopsy and 5% for VAB.[6] Core biopsy is a sampling procedure and sampling error cannot be eliminated altogether. However, steps should be taken to achieve best possible accuracy of the procedure. Accurate target setting and relationship of the needle with the lesion should be verified on imaging during breast biopsy. Whenever applicable, specimen radiography must be done to verify presence of calcifications in the harvested samples. After biopsy, the results of the biopsy should always be correlated with imaging findings. A rebiopsy is essential if the sample is considered inadequate for definitive pathological diagnosis. Rebiopsy, preferably a surgical excision biopsy, should also be performed when there is imaging-histologic discordance or if a high-risk lesion like atypical ductal hyperplasia (ADH) is reported on core biopsy. Imaging-histologic discordance is a situation when imaging findings are not consistent with the pathology report. Benign core biopsy diagnosis for a spiculated mass lesion or pleomorphic microcalcifications is not expected. Imaging-histologic discordance occurs in 3–7% of core biopsies and malignancy is found in about one-fourth of these cases on surgical excision.[33,34] Even if benign diagnosis of core biopsy is acceptable, such as for BI-RADS 4 lesions, it should be closely followed up with 6 monthly mammograms to rule out any sampling error.[35,36] Any suspicious development on follow-up mammogram is an indication for rebiopsy.

Histological underestimation is another limitation of core biopsy. When core biopsy result are correlated with final histopathology of the surgical specimen, a lesion diagnosed as atypical ductal hyperplasia or ductal carcinoma in situ (DCIS) on core biopsy may turn out to be DCIS or invasive carcinoma respectively. Biopsy may turn out to be DCIS or DCIS on core biopsy may turn out to be an invasive cancer. Histological underestimation occurs when core biopsy samples do not represent the pathologically most aggressive part of the lesion and this can occur in up to 40% of gun biopsies and 16% of VABs.[37] Hence, high-risk lesions like ADH should be subjected to rebiopsy with excision.

Close audit of the biopsy results at an individual center should be regularly performed to maintain the standard and accuracy of breast biopsy. Overall, malignant results are expected in 20–40% of all breast biopsies performed. This is known as positivity rate or positive predictive value (PPV) of the breast biopsy. If higher PPV is encountered, it indicates low index of suspicion on breast imaging. This means that some lesions which could have been cancers are not being recommended for biopsy and therefore, missed. On the other hand, if the PPV is low, the index of suspicion is very high and some lesions best suited for follow-up only are being referred for unnecessary biopsies.

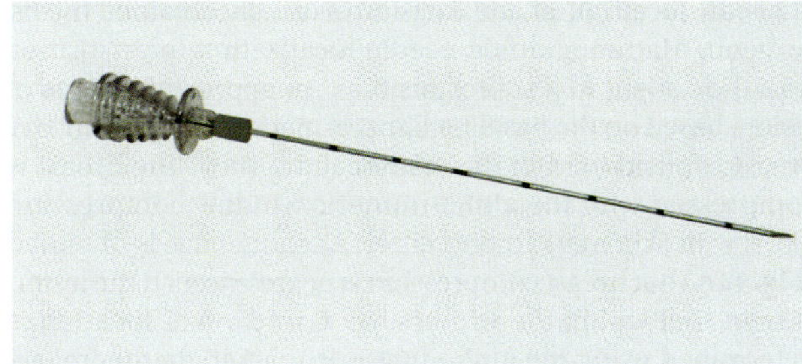

FIG. 10: Kopans needle-hookwire assembly. It consists of a 20G needle and a hookwire.

PREOPERATIVE HOOKWIRE LOCALIZATION

Needle-hookwire localization followed by surgical excision was the standard procedure for obtaining pathological diagnosis of nonpalpable but suspicious breast lesions seen on the mammograms. With development of accurate percutaneous core biopsy techniques, hookwire localization is now rarely performed for initial diagnosis. At present, it is mainly used as a preoperative localization procedure for therapeutic excision (breast conservation surgery) of already diagnosed but nonpalpable breast cancer. Hookwire localization prior to breast conservation surgery helps to precisely resect the cancer with clear margins. Indications of hookwire localization for diagnostic surgical excision biopsy include nonavailability of stereotactic biopsy facility or rebiopsy after inconclusive or discordant percutaneous core breast biopsy. It is also recommended for biopsy of vaguely defined breast abnormalities lesions; such as suspicious focal asymmetry or architectural distortion without associated mass. Needle localization for excision biopsy helps to achieve accurate lesion retrieval with minimal removal of breast parenchyma.

Early preoperative localization procedures were performed using various types of dyes, such as methylene blue or Evans blue, mixed with iodinated contrast. The dye was injected in the lesion through a needle introduced under mammographic guidance. The dye could be seen on postlocalization films and also intraoperatively. However, spread of the dye and amount of tissue stained was unpredictable, leading to missed lesions or excision of much larger breast tissue than actually required. Charcoal powder was also used instead of aqueous dyes, so as to restrict the spread over large area, but this was also not very accurate.

Accuracy and reliability of preoperative needle localization greatly improved after the development of various needle-hookwire combinations. Kopans needle-hookwire assembly is most widely used. It consists of a 20G needle and a thin flexible wire which can be introduced through it. The distal end of the wire is folded back forming a sharp angle and overbent so that it has a spring action **(Fig. 10)**. The needle is introduced under mammographic guidance. After correct needle placement, the hookwire is introduced and needle withdrawn over it. This exposes the hook of the wire which then anchors itself in the lesion. Then it can only be removed surgically. A modification of this hookwire has a thick stiffened segment just proximal to the hook. This rigid segment of wire is useful to the surgeon as it allows manual palpation of the target lesion intraoperatively. Some versions of hookwire have double-folded hook forming a barb, which prevent their displacement with in or out of the breast. Another type of needle-hookwire assembly has a retractable curved J-tip instead of the angled hook. In this design, after positioning of the needle, the wire is advanced. The end of the wire which comes out of the needle forms a J-shaped curve and gets anchored. If final hookwire position is unsatisfactory, the curved part of the wire can be retracted back into the needle and repositioning can be performed. The needle stays in the breast after deployment and it provides a stiff guide to the surgeon.

Equipment

Needle localization is usually performed under mammographic guidance. However, it may also be performed under ultrasound guidance if the lesion is clearly defined on ultrasound. MR compatible needle-hookwire assemblies are also available to localize the lesions seen only on MRI. Needle localization can be performed on all standard mammography machines. Only requirement is a special compression plate for needle localization. There are two types of compression plates. Alpha-numeric plate is the most widely used. It has a rectangular open window under which the lesion is positioned. There are radiopaque alpha-numeric centimeter markers on the margins of the window. The fenestrated compression plate has rows of multiple small round holes, like a sieve, instead of a single open window. These are also marked. The needle is introduced through the hole overlying the lesion. This type of compression is not preferred by many, as lesion frequently gets positioned under the solid part of the plate, rather than under the hole. Both digital and film-based mammography machines are suitable for needle localization. However, digital systems are preferred as images at each step are immediately available and procedure is therefore much faster.

Technique

Films on the basis of which needle localization has been recommended are reviewed and appropriate guiding modality and approach is selected. The procedure is scheduled just before the surgery. Informed consent inclusive of needle localization and excision is usually obtained by the surgeon. Mammographic needle localization is performed with the patient in a sitting position. An approximate area of lesion, based on the baseline films, is marked on the skin and breast is positioned in the craniocaudal view. The breast is compressed with the alpha-numeric window compression plate, with skin mark in the center. A scout image is obtained **(Fig. 11A)** but breast compression is not released. If the lesion is seen well within the window, its x- and y-axis location is determined using the alpha-numeric markers in the image. The point is marked on the skin at the crossing of same coordinates, as visible on the compression plate. Availability of movable cross-hair shadow marker in the light beam of mammography unit is greatly useful to mark the exact point on the skin.

After the skin entry point is marked, skin is prepared and local anesthetic is injected. If the target lesion is a mass or architectural distortion, care should be taken not to inject too much local anesthetic as it can obscure lesion. The localization needle without hookwire is then inserted vertically into the

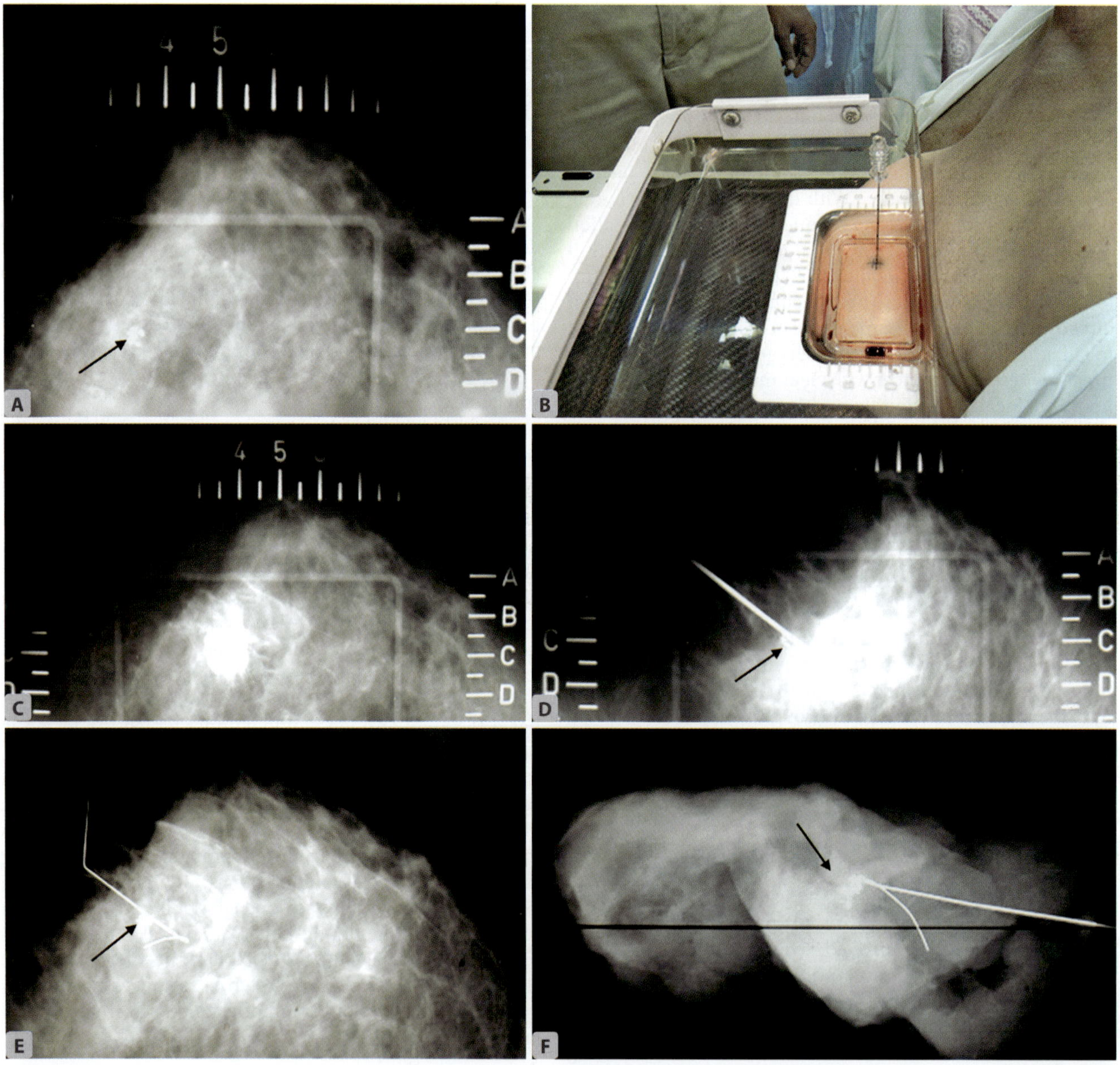

FIGS. 11A TO F: Preoperative hookwire localization. (A) Craniocaudal scout view shows cluster of calcification (arrow) in the center of the window of the compression plate. Its coordinates are determined in this film and skin entry point is marked; (B) Needle is inserted vertically. Note that the needle entry point is in the center of the shadow of the hub; thereby ensuring correct needle alignment in the direction of X-ray beam; (C) Another film is obtained. Needle is seen end on with its hub overlapping the lesion in this view; (D) Mediolateral view obtained thereafter shows that the needle tip has just crossed the lesion (arrow). Then the hookwire is inserted and the needle is withdrawn; (E) Posthookwire localization mammogram shows hookwire anchored correctly within the lesion (arrow); (F) Specimen radiograph of the excised tissue confirms accurate removal of the lesion (arrow).

breast. To improve the accuracy of needle hitting the target, the light beam of the mammography unit is turned on during insertion. It should be ensured that the shadow of the needle hub on the breast surrounds the needle entry point **(Fig. 11B)**. This maintains the needle in the direction of the X-ray beam and the needle remains perfectly perpendicular to the lesion. The needle is inserted to maximum depth and another image is obtained. With perfect positioning, the needle is seen enface in the form of a dot superimposed on the lesion **(Fig. 11C)**. Needle positioning is inaccurate if some length of the shaft is seen or if the needle is >5 mm away from the target. If this occurs, the needle should be withdrawn and reinserted. After satisfactory positioning, the compression released gradually. While the compression is being released, the breast bounces back and this may cause needle tip to come out from the lesion. To prevent this, the needle should be firmly supported and mild pressure is maintained to keep the needle tip deep in the breast during compression release. If the needle is not held, the needle hub may get entangled at the border of the compression plate window and come out with it. The breast is then repositioned in orthogonal (mediolateral) view using same compression plate. Then the exposure is made and the image obtained **(Fig. 11D)**. The needle should be seen crossing the lesion with tip about 1 cm beyond the lesion in this image. If this is not the case, then needle should be withdrawn accordingly while the breast is still compressed. Exact length to be withdrawn can be determined with the help of centimeter markings seen in the image. Presence of centimeter marks on the needle is useful in this depth adjustment.

After needle tip adjustment, the hookwire is inserted into the needle with the hook closed. The wire is inserted till a black mark on the wire reaches the hub. The tip of the hook is just at the needle tip at this position. A slight resistance to further advancement of wire is also be felt. The outside wire is then firmly held in position and needle withdrawn over it, releasing the hook in the breast. Wire should not be pushed during the withdrawal of the needle, as the hook may move further beyond the lesion, especially in fatty breasts.

After hookwire deployment, a mediolateral film is obtained for the surgeon **(Fig. 11E)**, craniocaudal view is not necessary. Procedure is considered successful if the hookwire is in the lesion or within 1 cm of it. If the wire is further away, procedure should be repeated with additional hookwire placement. The wire entry site is lightly covered with a gauze piece taking care that the wire is free to move in and out of the breast with changes in breast shape in supine and erect position of the patient. The wire should not be plastered to the breast at the skin entry site; otherwise the hook end of the wire inside the breast may get dislodged as the patient moves. The patient is then sent to the operation theater (OT) along with postlocalization film, with lesion marked on it, and a written note about the procedure and final hookwire-lesion relationship.

Other Localization Techniques

Hookwire localization is the most commonly performed and standard localization technique for nonplapable breast cancers. It requires a coordinated effort by breast intervention radiologist and breast surgeon, so that both are performed on the same day; however, there is a possibility of displacement or migration of the wire during patient transport from radiology to the operating theater.[38] The protruding wire has a bearing on route of dissection and may prove bothersome to the patient. There are recent advances in the localization techniques namely radioactive seed localization, magnetic seed for localization (Magseed) and infrared light/microimpulse radar reflector (SAVI scout).

1. *Radioactive seeds*: It was the first alternative to the wire localization systems and uses radioactive Iodine-125 seeds contained in a titanium shell. The placement of the seed can be performed under mammography or ultrasound guidance using 18G needle or by a preloaded assembly. The seed is localized at the time of surgery by a gamma probe, and confirmation is obtained by obtaining a specimen radiograph which shows the metallic seed within the resected specimen. Studies have shown it to be an effective alternate to wire localization with improved efficiency and convenience for the patient, intervention radiologist and the operating surgeon. The seed can be placed up to 5 days prior to the surgery. Disadvantages include exposure to radioactive material and the associated precautions required by the nuclear regulatory authorities, proper retrieval and safe disposal of the seed once it is used for localization.
2. *SAVI scout*: It is the first nonradioactive, nonwire localization method approved for use in humans. The localizer includes a reflector with antennae and is inserted in the breast lesion by a preloaded 16G introducer assembly. The reflector can be inserted as early as 30 days prior to surgery and remains inactive till it is activated by an extrinsic handpiece at the time of surgery.[39] It then reflects the RADAR signal and the location of the localizer can be deduced, which helps in guiding the surgery. The disadvantage of the system is that the reflector can be disabled by the electrocautery used during surgery. Also the antenna may be damaged during surgical dissection, causing failure of localization.
3. *Magseed*: Magseed is a paramagnetic seed made of steel and iron oxide of size 1 × 5 mm that may be used to localize a nonpalpable breast lesion up to 30 days prior to surgery under ultrasound or mammography guidance. It is also available in a preloaded 18G needle. Its location is detected with a probe that generates magnetic field and thus detects the magnetic influx generated by the seed. A potential disadvantage is the interference created in its localization by other ferromagnetic instruments and equipment including electrocautery used in surgery, thereby necessitating use of special nonferromagnetic instruments. Moreover, the seed has to be placed after any MRI procedure.[38]

Specimen Radiography

The surgeon dissects the breast using hookwire in situ. The approach is usually along the wire. Rarely, a separate incision is made guided by the palpation of the thickened part of the wire and lesion approached. The breast tissue around the hook and the thickened wire segment is resected and sent to the mammography room for specimen radiography. The specimen radiography is done on mammography unit with minimal exposure factors **(Fig. 11F)**. Mild compression may be required, if the specimen is large. The specimen mammogram should confirm that the target lesion, along with good margins, has been removed within the resected specimen. The specimen mammogram must be correlated carefully with baseline mammogram for this purpose. This is especially important if the lesion has calcifications; all foci of suspicious calcifications should be within the specimen. Successful lesion removal should be communicated to the surgeon, who is waiting in the OT, so that the breast can be closed and sutured. If the lesion is incompletely seen or seen extending up to the margins, this should also be communicated in details, so that additional resection at the appropriate site is attempted.[40]

Complications

Preoperative hookwire localization is a well-established safe procedure. Complications are rare. These mainly include vasovagal reaction, bleeding, and pain. Unusual complications include hooking of pectoralis muscle and pneumothorax due to entry of the needle into the chest.

Migration of the hookwire after successful placement is an uncommon but serious problem. Risk factors for this include entirely fatty breast, excessive arm movements after the wire placement, and delay in surgery. Hookwire migration can also occur intraoperatively. Surgeon may hold and pull the wire during dissection and wire may come out. The wire may also get cut during dissection. The deeper segment of the wire then gets retracted and lost in the breast. If the surgeon is not familiar with this procedure, he should be cautioned about these complications.

Special Techniques of Localization

Placement of two or more hookwires in the same breast may be required for multiple lesions or to mark the extent of a large lesion (hookwire bracketing) before breast conservation surgery.[41] Stereotactic guidance is generally not preferred for needle localization procedures but this may be required for lesions seen in one view only. Needle localization can be accurately and quickly performed under ultrasound guidance and this modality should be preferred if the lesion is visible on ultrasound. Another advantage of ultrasound-guided needle localization is that it can be performed with anterior approach. Most surgeons prefer anterior approach for dissection. As with mammographic needle localization, postlocalization mammogram and specimen radiography should also be performed after ultrasound-guided localization. MRI-guided hookwire localization is also possible with MR compatible needle-hookwire devices. It is required for the lesions seen on MRI only.

Hematoma-guided localization has also been found useful for breast conservation surgery of nonpalpable breast cancers.[42,43] After a core biopsy, a small hematoma is always formed at the biopsy site. If the biopsy result is malignant and surgery is planned within 4–5 weeks, the small hematoma can be identified with intraoperative ultrasound. This can be used as a guide for dissection, without the need for any preoperative localization procedure. Radioguided occult lesion localization (ROLL) is another technique in which a radioisotope-containing colloid (also used for sentinel lymph node mapping) is injected into the tumor. Tumor is then localized intraoperatively using handheld gamma probe.[44]

Ultrasound-guided Intraoperative Excision

The use of intraoperative ultrasound is a relatively newer use of sonography in breast surgery. Palpable lesions are easy to identify and localize during surgery; however, nonpalpable, deep set, or smaller lesions may require use of ultrasound to objectively guide excision. Ultrasound-guided intraoperative excision helps in achieving tumor-free resection margins with sparing of surrounding healthy parenchyma and thus obtaining an optimum resection volume. It has been found that there is a difference in the adequacy of resection margins by ultrasound and wire localization with the former achieving 89% negative resection margins compared to around 50% in later.[45]

Various studies have shown that the use of ultrasound allows nearly 100% detection of nonpalpable lesions; however, smaller lesions of <5 mm may be missed, especially in obese patients.[46] In patients planned to undergo breast conservation surgery, ultrasound reduces the margin positivity rates and also reduces the reduction of breast volume thus achieving optimum cosmetic outcome.[47] There is also a consequent reduction in the re-excision rates.[48]

Technique

There are three basic techniques employed for ultrasound in intraoperative settings. The *first* involves a continuous use of ultrasound during resection to measure the distance of the resected margin from the ultrasound visualized mass. However, this technique offers some challenges due to fluid and air insinuating in the tissue planes during surgery which may preclude the proper visualization of the mass. Also, when the probe is inserted into the surgical bed, there is compression or displacement of the surrounding structures. The *second* technique involves marking the tumor margins on the skin prior to the resection in the OT. However, in this technique there may be mismatch of the surface markings and the actual tumor location, especially when there is mobilization of the breast during surgery. Moreover, depth measured prior to the surgery may not stay true after the mass is partially resected. The *third* technique involves a use of ultrasound-guided markers in the form of ultrasound contrast agents, visible dye, needle or wires to localize the mass with ultrasound so as to guide the surgeon during the procedure. All techniques include the ex vivo sonography of the resected specimen to ensure optimum margin to tumor distance.

MISCELLANEOUS BREAST INTERVENTIONS

Ductography

Ductography (or galactography) was a commonly performed procedure for evaluation of patients with nipple discharge, as ductal anatomy is not well seen on mammogram. With the advent of high-resolution ultrasound and contrast-enhanced MRI of the breast, ductal evaluation is now possible with reasonable accuracy with these modalities and hence ductography is rarely performed at present.

Indications of ductography include spontaneous solitary duct discharge that is serosanguineous, or bloody. Causes of such duct discharge are papilloma, fibrocystic disease, duct ectasia, and carcinoma.[49] Bilateral nipple discharge or discharge elicited by squeezing only is physiological not requiring ductography.

Ductography should be performed during active discharge. A 27G or 30G ductography cannula is used which is connected to a syringe containing 3–5 mL of nonionic contrast. All air from the cannula, tube and syringe must be removed. The duct is identified with a gentle squeeze and cannulated with gentle probing. The contrast is slowly injected till the patient feels some fullness. Usually, <1 cc of contrast is required. The cannula is then securely taped on the breast and mediolateral and craniocaudal mammographic views are obtained. Additional contrast can be injected if ductal opacification is incomplete.

Ductography demonstrates ductal anatomy of the drainage territory of the cannulated duct **(Fig. 12A)**. The size of the ductal territory is highly variable; this may be a small segment of the breast or it may cover a large area of the breast. Normal ducts show uniform and orderly branching of the ducts with smooth tapering from nipple to periphery. Single or multiple filling defects in the duct are most commonly produced by papillomas **(Fig. 12B)**, sometime by fibrocystic disease, blood clots, air bubbles or rarely by carcinoma. Abrupt cutoff may be produced by papilloma or a carcinoma. Ductal dilatation with abrupt tapering of distal ducts is a characteristic feature of duct ectasia **(Fig. 12C)**. Beaded appearance of the duct with multiple opacified cysts is seen in fibrocystic disease.[50]

Cyst Aspiration

Percutaneous cyst aspiration may be required for analysis of the contents of complex breast cysts. These usually represent inflammatory pathology, and extremely rarely, malignancy. Breast cyst aspiration may also be performed for symptomatic relief of large simple breast cysts. Breast cyst aspiration is best performed under ultrasound guidance using 18G needle **(Fig. 13)**. Complete evacuation of the cyst should be attempted. If the fluid is clear or serous, cytological evaluation is not required.[51] If the fluid is bloody or purulent, it should be sent for cytological examination. Residual solid lesion after cyst aspiration is an indication for biopsy.

Ultrasound-guided Axillary Lymph Node FNAC

All patients with breast cancer require axillary lymph node dissection for sampling and pathological staging of the nodes, irrespective of their clinical nodal status. However, this procedure is morbid and many of the patients develop shoulder stiffness and lymphedema of the arm subsequently. Sentinel lymph node staging helps to avoid axillary lymph dissection in some of the patients who do not have axillary lymphadenopathy on clinical examination. In this procedure, a dye and radionuclide (99mTc-labeled sulfur colloid) is injected around the tumor. The first node draining the tumor area is localized with scintigraphy probe and excised.

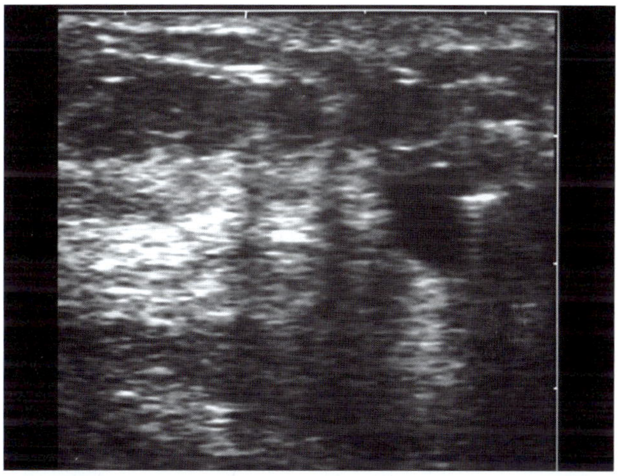

FIG. 13: Ultrasound-guided cyst aspiration. Needle tip is seen within the cyst with accompanied reverberations characteristically seen during cyst aspiration.

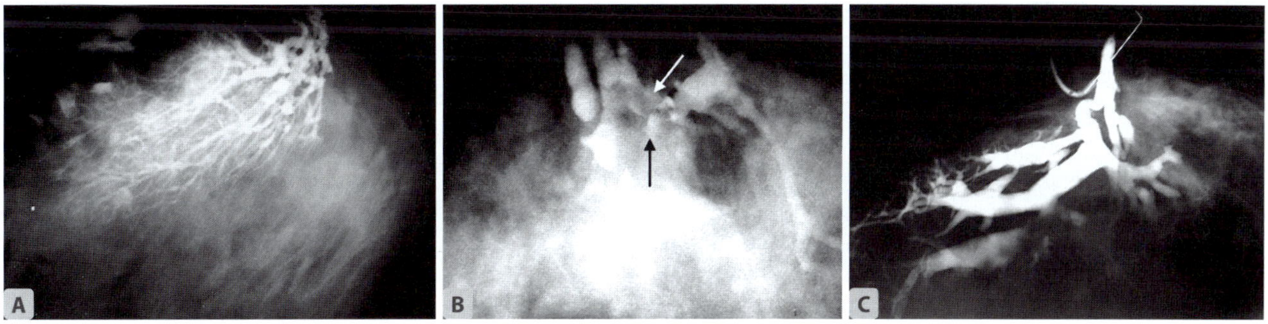

FIGS. 12A TO C: Ductogram. (A) Normal ductogram shows uniform branching pattern of the nondilated ducts opacified in segment of the breast; (B) Subareolar papilloma is seen as a filling defect (arrows) within a mildly dilated duct; (C) Duct ectasia is seen as moderately dilated ducts with pruning of side branches.

If this node is not pathologically involved, distal axillary lymph nodes are considered to be disease free and axillary dissection is avoided. However, the technique of sentinel lymph node staging is cumbersome, time-consuming and expensive.

Ultrasound of axilla in clinically node-negative patients, with ultrasound-guided FNAC of abnormal lymph nodes so detected, is fast gaining acceptance. Patients with confirmed axillary lymph node involvement can then be spared of sentinel lymph node staging and directly taken for axillary lymph node dissection. On ultrasound, size criteria or Doppler evaluation are not useful for identification of abnormal axillary lymph nodes. Lymph nodes of any size with focal or diffuse cortical thickening (>3 mm) or presence of hypoechoic deposits are considered suspicious[52] **(Figs. 14A and B)**. Absence of fatty hilum is also a reliable feature.[53] Abnormal lymph nodes are subjected to ultrasound-guided FNAC. Core biopsy is also done at some centers but FNAC is generally sufficient, as aim is to confirm the presence of malignancy and histological analysis is not essential. Overall, ultrasound-guided FNAC of axillary lymph nodes has high sensitivity and specificity of 80% and 98% respectively for axillary lymph node staging.[54]

ABLATIVE PROCEDURES FOR BREAST CANCER

There are various image-guided ablative procedures increasingly used in both benign and malignant diseases. There is increasing data regarding potential of using radiofrequency ablation (RFA), cryoablation, high-intensity focused ultrasound (HIFU), laser ablation and electroporation in breast cancers and focal benign diseases like fibroadenoma. These methods are less invasive and give better cosmetic results due to small incision, if any, with reduced time and expenditure of hospitalization. Their role is proving useful especially in small early stage cancers and in poor surgical risk patients. Several studies have reported good pathological tumor ablation in most patients in both benign and malignant breast pathologies.[55,56] RFA seems the most promising modality as complete ablation of tumor and adjacent margin of breast parenchyma can be achieved with it[57-59] **(Figs. 15A and B)**.

Radiofrequency Ablation

Similar to tumors throughout body, RFA has been used for breast cancers as well. It involves insertion of a needle electrode in the center of the tumor through which alternating current passes which cause heating and tumor necrosis. Ultrasound is the preferred modality for guidance as RFA may cause artifacts with MRI. Skin burns and injury to the underlying pectoralis muscle may complicate the procedure, especially when the tumor is abutting or invading these structures. Instillation of saline may be performed in such cases to increase the distance between skin/pectoralis and the tumor.

Cryoablation

Cryoablation is the only ablative method available which involves freezing for achieving tumor death instead of heating. It involves insertion of the cryoprobe through the skin under ultrasound/MRI or computed tomography (CT) guidance after a small skin incision. The procedure involves two phases of freezing and intervening thawing and formation of ice ball. The tumor cells are destroyed by means of intracellular ice formation, osmotic dehydration

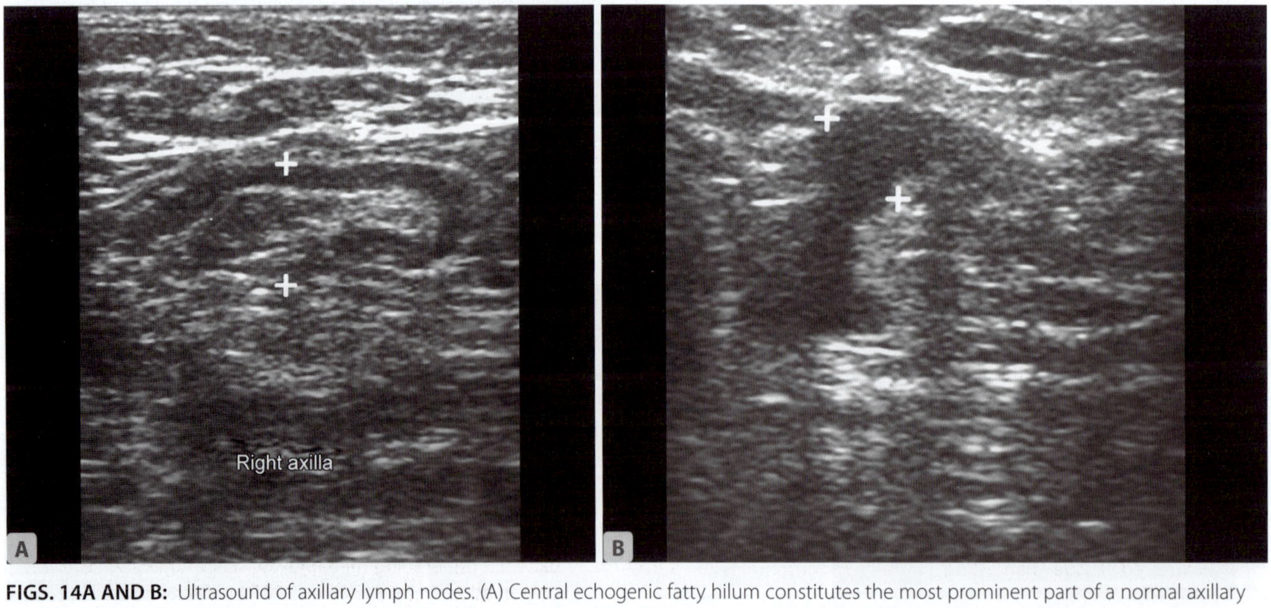

FIGS. 14A AND B: Ultrasound of axillary lymph nodes. (A) Central echogenic fatty hilum constitutes the most prominent part of a normal axillary lymph node. Peripheral cortex is seen as a thin hypoechoic rim of uniform thickness around the hilum; (B) A metastatic axillary lymph node showing irregular cortical thickening with normal fatty hilum.

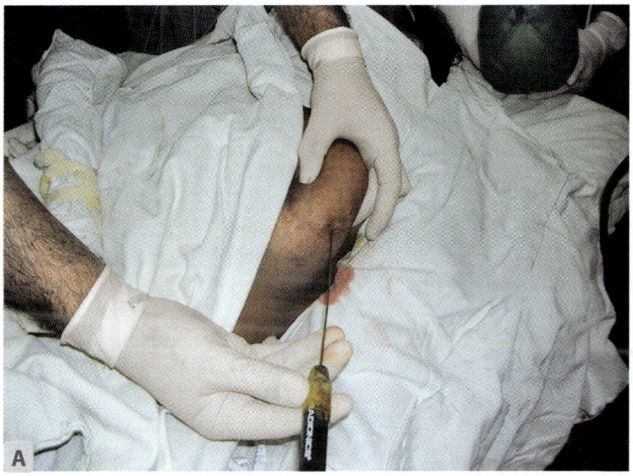

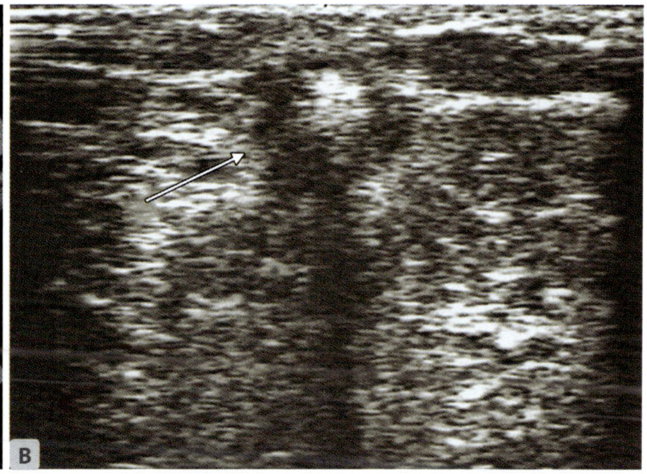

FIGS. 15A AND B: Breast cancer radiofrequency ablation (RFA). (A) RFA probe is percutaneously inserted into the breast mass using same technique as that for biopsy; (B) An echogenic area forms within the tumor (arrow) as energy is deposited during RFA procedure.

and ischemia followed by an enhanced immunological response by means of release of cytokines and stimulation of cytotoxic lymphocytes. Advantage of the technique is the added anesthetic effect due to freezing; however, the risk of skin injury remains.

Laser Ablation

Laser ablation uses a laser light energy delivered to the target tissue by a thin optical wire introduced into the tumor under either ultrasonography (USG), CT or MRI guidance. Skin burn and pneumothorax are potential complications.

Microwave Ablation

It uses electromagnetic waves which causes heating of the water molecules, and localized tissue destruction in breast cancer. An advantage of microwave ablation is that the tissue with lower water content like fat and glandular parenchyma of the breast remains unaffected. Complications include skin flap necrosis and skin blistering.

REFERENCES

1. Liberman L, Ernberg LA, Heerdt A, Zakowski MF, Morris EA, LaTrenta LR, et al. Palpable breast masses: is there a role of percutaneous imaging-guided core biopsy? AJR Am J Roentgenol. 2000;175:774-87.
2. Pisano ED, Fajardo LL, Tsimikas J, Sneige N, Frable WJ, Gatsonis CA, et al. Rate of insufficient samples from fine-needle aspiration for nonpalpable breast lesions in an multicenter clinical trial: the Radiologic Diagnostic Oncology Group 5 study. The RDOG5 investigators. Cancer. 1998;82:679-88.
3. Tse MG, Tan PH. Diagnosing breast lesions by fine needle aspiration cytology or core biopsy: which is better? Breast Cancer Res Treat. 2010;123:1-8.
4. Hukinen K, Kiwisaari L, Heikkelis PS, Von Simitten K, Leidenius M. Unsuccessful preoperative fine needle aspiration cytology or core biopsy, lead to increased cost of the diagnostic work-up in breast cancer. Acta Oncol. 2008;47:1037-45.
5. Parker SH, Jobe WE, Dennis MA, Stavros AT, Johnson KK, Yakes WF, et al. US-guided automated large-core breast biopsy. Radiology. 1993;187:507-11.
6. O'Flynn EA, Wilson AR, Michell MJ. Image-guided breast biopsy: state-of-the-art. Clin Radiol. 2010;65:259-70.
7. Burbank F, Parker SH, Fogarty TJ. Stereotactic breast biopsy: improved tissue harvesting with mammotome. Am Surg. 1996;62:738-44.
8. Berg WA, Krebs TL, Campassi C, Magder LS, Sun CC. Evaluation of 14- and 11-gauge directional vacuum-assisted biopsy probes and 14-gauge biopsy guns in a breast parenchymal model. Radiology. 1997;205:203-8.
9. Kettritz U, Rotter K, Schreer I, Murauer M, Schulz-Wendtland R, Peter D, et al. Stereotactic vacuum-assisted breast biopsy in 2,874 patients: a multicenter study. Cancer. 2004;100:245-51.
10. Jackman RJ, Marzoni FA Jr, Rosenberg J. False-negative diagnosis at stereotactic vacuum-assisted needle breast biopsy: long-term follow-up of 1,280 lesions and review of literature. AJR Am J Roentgenol. 2009;192:341-51.
11. Shah VI, Raju U, Chitale D, Deshpande V, Gregory N, Strand V. False-negative core needle biopsies of the breast: an analysis of clinical, radiologic, and pathologic findings in 27 consecutive cases of missed breast cancer. Cancer. 2003;97: 1824-31.
12. Cho N, Moon WK, Cha JH, Kim SM, Kim SJ, Lee SH, et al. Sonographically guided core biopsy of the breast: comparison of 14-gauge automated gun and 11-gauge directional vacuum-assisted biopsy methods. Korean J Radiol. 2005;6: 102-9.
13. Nadeem R, Chagla LS, Harris O, Desmond S, Thind R, Flavin A, et al. Tumour localisation with a metal coil before administration of neo-adjuvant chemotherapy. Breast. 2005;14:403-7.
14. Oh JL, Nguyen G, Whitman GJ, Hunt KK, Yu TK, Woodward WA, et al. Placement of radiopaque clips for tumor localization in patients undergoing neoadjuvant chemotherapy and breast conservation therapy. Cancer. 2007;110:2420-7.
15. Carpentier E, Maruani A, Michenet P, Bonneau C, Degand P, Lebas P. Can US-guided vacuum-assisted biopsies be an alternative to diagnostic surgery in cases of non-diagnostic core needle biopsy? J Radiol. 2005;86:475-80.

16. Liberman L, Dershaw DD, Rosen PP, Morris EA, Abramson AF, Borgen PI. Percutaneous removal of malignant mammographic lesions at stereotactic vacuum-assisted biopsy. Radiology. 1998;206:711-5.
17. March DE, Coughlin BF, Barham RB, Goulart RA, Klein SV, Bur ME. Breast masses: removal of all US evidence during biopsy by using a handheld vacuum-assisted device—initial experience. Radiology. 2003;227:549-55.
18. Fine RE, Whitworth PW, Kim JA, Harness JK, Boyd BA, Burak WE Jr. Low-risk palpable breast masses removal using a vacuum-assisted hand-held device. Am J Surg. 2003;186:362-7.
19. Thurley P, Evans A, Hamilton L, James J, Wilson R. Patient satisfaction and efficacy of vacuum-assisted excision biopsy of fibroadenomas. Clin Radiol. 2009;64:381-5.
20. LaTrenta LR, Menell JH, Morris EA, Abramson AF, Dershaw DD, Liberman L. Breast lesions detected with MR imaging: utility and histopathologic importance of identification with US. Radiology. 2003;227:856-61.
21. Meissnitzer M, Dershaw DD, Lee CH, Morris EA. Targeted ultrasound of the breast in women with abnormal MRI findings for whom biopsy has been recommended. AJR Am J Roentgenol. 2009;193:1025-9.
22. Hari S, Surabhi V, Chandrashekhara SH. Digital mammography. In: Gupta AK, Garg A, Sandhu S (Eds). Diagnostic Radiology: Recent Advances and Applied Physics in Imaging, 3rd edition. New Delhi, India: Jaypee Brothers Medical Publishers (P) Ltd.; 2019. pp. 279-86.
23. Shin K, Teichgraeber D, Martaindale S, Whitman GJ. Tomosynthesis-guided core biopsy of the breast: why and how to use it. J Clin Imaging Sci. 2018;8:28.
24. Liberman L, Smolkin JH, Dershaw D, Morris EA, Abramson AF, Rosen PP. Calcification retrieval at stereotactic 11-gauge directional vacuum-assisted breast biopsy. Radiology. 1998;208:251-60.
25. Margolin FR, Kaufman L, Jacobs RP, Denny SR, Schrumpf JD. Stereotactic core biopsy of malignant calcifications: diagnostic yield of cores with and without microcalcifications on specimen radiographs. Radiology. 2004;233:251-4.
26. Huber S, Wagner M, Medl M, Czembirek H. Benign breast lesions minimally invasive vacuum-assisted biopsy with 11-gauge needles: patient acceptance and effect on follow-up imaging. Radiology. 2003;226:783-90.
27. Philpotts LE, Hooley RJ, Lee CH. Comparison of automated versus vacuum-assisted biopsy methods for sonographically guided core biopsy of the breast. AJR Am J Roentgenol. 2003;180: 347-51.
28. Parker SH, Burbank F, Jackman RJ, Aucreman CJ, Cardenosa G, Cink TM, et al. Percutaneous large-core breast biopsy: a multi-institutional study. Radiology. 1994;193:359-64.
29. Diaz LK, Wiley EL, Venta LA. Are malignant cells displaced by large-gauge needle core biopsy of the breast? AJR Am J Roentgenol. 1999;173:1303-13.
30. Hoorntje LE, Schipper ME, Kaya A, Verkooijen HM, Klinkenbijl JG, Borel Rinkes IH. Tumour cell displacement after 14G breast biopsy. Eur J Surg Oncol. 2004;30:520-5.
31. Lamm RL, Jackman RJ. Mammographic abnormalities caused by percutaneous stereotactic biopsy of histologically benign lesions evident on follow-up mammograms. AJR Am J Roentgenol. 2000;174:753-6.
32. Heywang-Köbrunner SH, Sinnatamby R, Lebeau A, Lebrecht A, Britton PD, Schreer I, et al. Interdisciplinary consensus on the uses and technique of MR-guided vacuum-assisted breast biopsy (VAB): results of a European consensus meeting. Eur J Radiol. 2009;72:289-94.
33. Liberman L, Drotman M, Morris EA, LaTrenta LR, Abramson AF, Zakowski MF, et al. Imaging-histologic discordance at percutaneous breast biopsy. Cancer. 2000;89:2538-46.
34. Ciatto S, Houssami N, Ambrogetti D, Bianchi S, Bonardi R, Brancato B, et al. Accuracy and underestimation of malignancy of breast core needle biopsy: the Florence experience of over 4,000 consecutive biopsies. Breast Cancer Res Treat. 2007;101:291-7.
35. Jackman RJ, Nowels KW, Roderiguez-Soto J, Marzoni FA Jr, Finkelstein SI, Shepard MJ. Stereotactic, automated, large-core needle biopsy of nonpalpable breast lesions: false-negative and histologic underestimation rates after long-term follow-up. Radiology. 1999;210:799-805.
36. Youk JH, Kim EK, Kim MJ, Oh KK. Sonographically guided 14-gauge core needle biopsy of breast masses: a review of 2,420 cases with long-term follow-up. AJR Am J Roentgenol. 2008;190:202-7.
37. Hoorntie LE, Peeters PH, Mali WP, Rinkes IH. Vacuum-assisted breast biopsy: a critical review. Eur J Cancer. 2003;39:1676-83.
38. Jeffries DO, Dossett LA, Jorns JM. Localization for breast surgery: the next generation. Arch Pathol Lab Med. 2017;141(10): 1324-9.
39. Mango V, Ha R, Gomberawalla A, Wynn R, Feldman S. Evaluation of the SAVI scout surgical guidance system for localization and excision of nonpalpable breast lesions: a feasibility study. AJR Am J Roentgenol. 2016;207:W69-72.
40. Schaefer FK, Eden I, Schaefer PJ, Peter D, Jonat W, Heller M, et al. Factors associated with one step surgery in case of non-palpable breast cancer. Eur J Radiol. 2007;64(3):426-31.
41. Kirstein LJ, Rafferty E, Specht MC, Moore RH, Taghian AG, Hughes KS, et al. Outcome of multiple wire localization for larger breast cancers: when can mastectomy be avoided? J Am Coll Surg. 2008;207:342-6.
42. Thompson M, Tillman RH, Margulies A, Thostenson J, Bryant-Smith G, Fincher R, et al. Hematoma-directed ultrasound guided (HUG) breast lumpectomy. Ann Surg Oncol. 2007;14:148-56.
43. Arentz C, Baxter K, Boneti C, Henry-Tillman R, Westbrook K, Korourian S, et al. Ten-year experience with hematoma-directed ultrasound-guided breast lumpectomy. Ann Surg Oncol. 2010;17:378-83.
44. Nadeem R, Chagla LS, Harris O, Desmond S, Thind R, Titterrell C, et al. Occult breast lesions: a comparison between radioguided occult lesion localisation (ROLL) vs. wire-guided lumpectomy (WGL). Breast. 2005;14:283-9.
45. Rahusen FD, Bremers AJ, Fabry HF, van Amerongen AH, Boom RP, Meijer S. Ultrasound-guided lumpectomy of nonpalpable breast cancer versus wire-guided resection: a randomized clinical trial. Ann Surg Oncol. 2002;9:994-8.
46. Ngô C, Pollet AG, Laperrelle J, Ackerman G, Gomme S, Thibault F, et al. Intraoperative ultrasound localization of nonpalpable breast cancers. Ann Surg Oncol. 2007;14:2485-9.
47. Fisher CS, Mushawah FA, Cyr AE, Gao F, Margenthaler JA. Ultrasound-guided lumpectomy for palpable breast cancers. Ann Surg Oncol. 2011;18:3198-203.
48. Davis KM, Hsu CH, Bouton ME, Wilhelmson KL, Komenaka IK. Intraoperative ultrasound can decrease the re-excision lumpectomy rate in patients with palpable breast cancers. Am Surg. 2011;77:720-5.
49. Tabar L, Dean PB, Pentek Z. Galactography: the diagnostic procedure of choice for nipple discharge. Radiology. 1983;149:31-8.
50. Bassett LW, Kim CH. Ductography. In: Dershaw DD (Ed). Imaging-Guided Interventional Breast Techniques. New York: Springer-Verlag; 2003. pp. 1-30.
51. Ciatto S, Cariaggi P, Bularisis P. The value of routine cytologic examination of breast cyst fluid. Acta Cytol. 1987;31:301-4.

52. Choi YJ, Ko EY, Han BK, Shin JH, Kang SS, Hahn SY. High-resolution ultrasonographic features of axillary lymph node metastasis in patients with breast cancer. Breast. 2009;18:119-22.
53. Cho N, Moon WK, Han W, Park IA, Cho J, Noh DY. Preoperative sonographic classification of axillary lymph nodes in patients with breast cancer: node-to-node correlation with surgical histology and sentinel node biopsy results. AJR Am J Roentgenol. 2009;193:1731-7.
54. Houssami N, Ciatto S, Turner RM, Cody HS 3rd, Macaskill P. Preoperative ultrasound-guided needle biopsy of axillary nodes in invasive breast cancer: meta-analysis of its accuracy and utility in staging the axilla. Ann Surg. 2011;254:243-51.
55. Manenti G, Bolacchi F, Perretta T, Cossu E, Pistolese CA, Buonomo OC, et al. Small breast cancers: in vivo percutaneous US-guided radiofrequency ablation with dedicated cool-tip radiofrequency system. Radiology. 2009;251:339-46.
56. Zhao Z, Wu F. Minimally invasive thermal ablation of early-stage breast cancer: a systematic review. Eur J Surg Oncol. 2010;36:1149-55.
57. Grotenhuis BA, Vrijland WW, Klem TM. Radiofrequency ablation for early-stage breast cancer: treatment outcomes, and practical considerations. Eur J Surg Oncol. 2013;39(12): 1317-24.
58. Mauri G, Sconfienza LM, Pescatori LC, Fedeli MP, Ali M, Di Leo G, et al. Technical success, technique efficacy and complications of minimally-invasive imaging-guided percutaneous ablation procedures of breast cancer: a systematic review and meta-analysis. Eur Radiol. 2017;27(8):3199-210.
59. Zhang W, Zhan-Qiang J, Baikpour M, Li JM, Zhang H, Liang T, et al. Clinical application of ultrasound-guided percutaneous microwave ablation for benign breast lesions: a prospective study. BMC Cancer. 2019;19:345.

CHAPTER

179

Advances in Breast Imaging

Tulika Singh, Veenu Singla, Uma Debi

INTRODUCTION

Among the cancers affecting women in the modern era, breast cancer has been at the forefront. In fact, it accounts for a major chunk of cancer-related mortality among women. Breast imaging plays an important role in screening as well as in diagnosis of breast cancer. In the last decade, many technological advancements have happened in the field of breast imaging. In this chapter, we have reviewed them with their clinical applications.

DIGITAL BREAST TOMOSYNTHESIS

Screen-film mammography (SFM) is being used for diagnostic and screening mammography for >30 years. For the last 10–15 years, it has been replaced by full-field digital mammography (DM) at most of the places.[1] It shows slightly higher sensitivity than SFM, but low density in women with dense breasts remain the limitation of conventional mammography.[2,3] The sensitivity of mammography ranges from about 30 to 48% in women with dense breasts, thus increasing the risk of interval cancer.[4,5] It is attributed mainly to overlapping of tissues which can obscure the breast cancer with similar attenuation as the breast tissue resulting in false-negative cases. In addition, overlapping of normal breast tissue can produce a pseudolesion, i.e., summation artifact resulting into false-positive cases. Digital breast tomosynthesis (DBT) is an emerging modality which can resolve this limitation to some extent. It acquires a series of low-dose projection images and then thin sections are reconstructed from the volumetric data on the workstation.[6] This has shown better sensitivity in various studies.[7,8]

Digital Breast Tomosynthesis Technology

Digital breast tomosynthesis is a mammography-based technology which uses X-rays but forms the image slices of the tissue volume. It has got US Food and Drug Administration (FDA) approval in 2012. These slices can be seen as thin as 1 mm in sharp focus with the tissue above and below out of focus.[9] Acquisition is similar to two-dimensional (2D) mammography and involves compression of the breasts between the compression paddle and the detector. A series of low-dose images is obtained by an X-ray tube head rotating in the arc across the breast from 15 to 50°, each from a different angle **(Fig. 1)**.[10] The time of acquisition varies between 5 and 25 seconds depending on the vendors. The total radiation exposure depends on breast density and thickness, but overall DBT radiation exposure is equivalent to that of SFM or DM. It usually acquires standard mammographic views which are craniocaudal (CC), mediolateral oblique (MLO), and mediolateral. Images can also be acquired with spot compression and implant displacement views. However, magnification view cannot be done with DBT.

The overall number of reconstructed images obtained depends on the thickness of the compressed breast. Images can be reviewed on the special workstation for tomosynthesis which allows the radiologist to scroll through the images. We can also adjust the slice thickness according to the lesion. DBT images are usually acquired in a combination mode which is FDA approved.[11] In a combination mode, DBT and 2D full-field DM are obtained in single breast compression. It acquires DBT first followed by 2D mammography; then 2D and 3D database can be coregistered and the radiologist

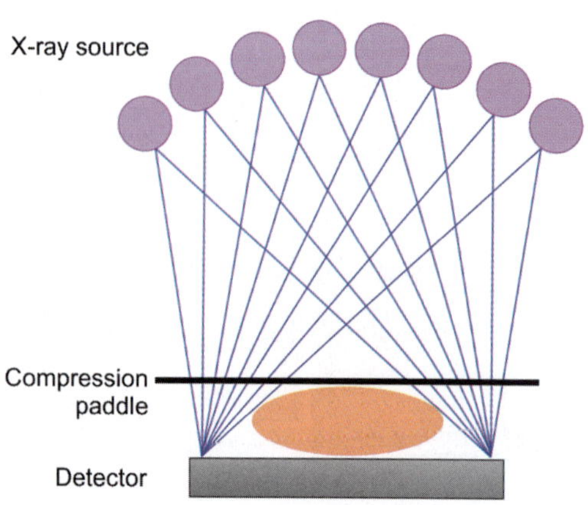

FIG. 1: Pictorial diagram of digital breast tomosynthesis image acquisition showing the X-ray tube movement in an arc, executing multiple sequential low-dose exposures of the compressed breast tissue with a sweep.

can shuffle between 2D and 3D database. A synthesized 2D image reconstruction algorithm has been recently developed (C-View Hologic) to create a reconstructed 2D image from the volume of the DBT database.[12] It can reduce the patient radiation dose by acquiring only DBT and create a synthesized 2D view without acquiring any additional 2D view. Its performance is comparable to a conventional 2D mammogram in many studies.[13] DBT has demonstrated improved visibility of small invasive breast cancer which is subtle or occult on conventional mammography leading to interval cancer.[14] Mammographic visualization varies for different types of breast cancer. In invasive lobular carcinoma, the tumor growth is nonmass-like and sometimes it is difficult to detect on 2D and is better seen with DBT.[15] Several studies have concluded that DBT can also replace the need of additional compression view which is routinely done in diagnostic mammography. It also reduces the need of second-look ultrasound for better characterization of the lesion. Use of DBT can reduce the number of BI-RADS 3 (Breast Imaging Reporting and Data System 3) in a diagnostic setting by better characterization of breast lesions and changing these lesions into BIRADS 2 or 4.[16]

Digital Breast Tomosynthesis in a Screening Setting

Many studies done on screening with DBT show a decreased recall rate with increased cancer detection. These studies have been done by performing both conventional 2D mammography and DBT which resulted in increase in radiation dose as compared to mammography alone, but it was below the permissible limit.[7] The need of additional 2D mammography along with DBT screening is due to its better visualization of microcalcification which is an important sign of ductal carcinoma in situ (DCIS), for the comparison of previous mammography.

Use of Digital Breast Tomosynthesis in Diagnostic Workup

In clinical practice, DBT is generally used for the assessment of noncalcified lesions. Evaluation of calcification on DBT is limited; it may depict only a limited number of calcification with poor characterization.

Architectural Distortion

Architectural distortion is a subtle finding better seen on DBT which is difficult to visualize on conventional imaging. It is a common manifestation of cancer. Architectural distortion on DBT shows a higher percentage of invasive lobular carcinoma (20%).[14] DBT also gives better visualization of radial scar; which are seen as a radiating lines converging to a point **(Figs. 2A and B)**. DBT is especially helpful in detection of suspected distortion at the fat–glandular interface and apex of the breast where summation shadows are frequent.

Focal Asymmetry

Focal asymmetry is called when a small abnormal area of the fibroglandular density is seen in a similar shape in both views of a mammogram. The recent BI-RADS lexicon uses the term "asymmetry" when the finding is seen only in one view and is unilateral. DBT can be used to differentiate true asymmetry from the superimposed fibroglandular tissue or it can reclassify into a mass **(Figs. 3A and B)**. It has shown higher sensitivity (93%) in better characterization of focal asymmetry than the spot compression imaging (50%).[17]

Masses

Masses are described in terms of shape, margin, and density. These features are better visualized on DBT and a radiologist can give a better and accurate degree of suspicion of masses **(Figs. 4A and B)**. Use of an irregular shape descriptor is reduced with DBT, and the shape of masses is usually

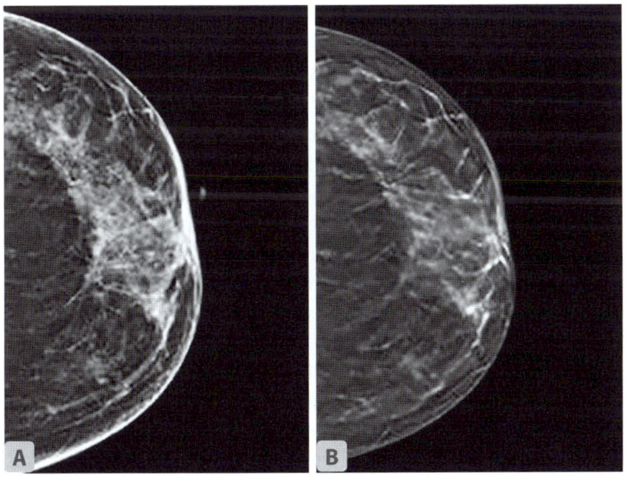

FIGS. 2A AND B: Better visualization of architectural distortion on digital breast tomosynthesis (DBT) (B) as compared to a 2D craniocaudal view (A). DBT image shows a multiple line radiating from a point in the lateral breast which is a suspicious finding. On stereotactic biopsy, it came out to be radial scar without atypia.

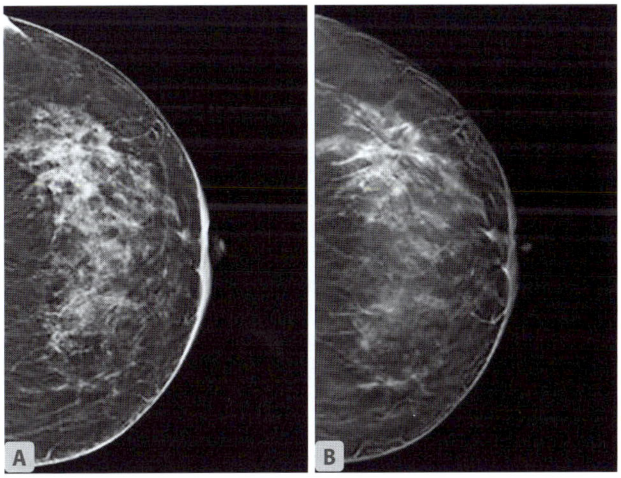

FIGS. 3A AND B: Better evaluation of focal asymmetry. 2D craniocaudal view (A) showing a focal asymmetry which on digital breast tomosynthesis image (B) shows well-defined mass with spiculated margins. Biopsy showed invasive ductal carcinoma.

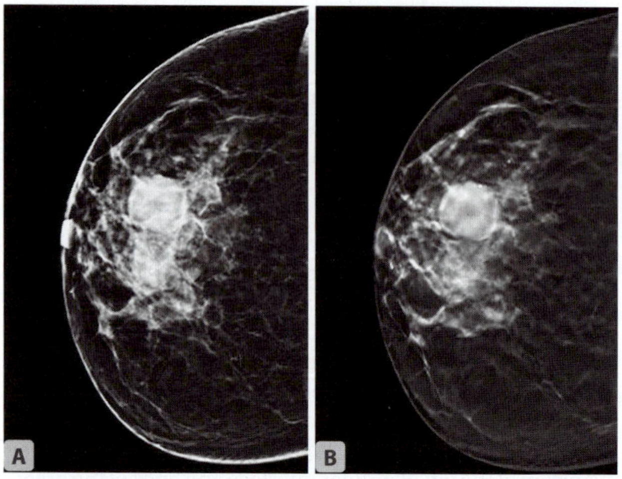

FIGS. 4A AND B: Improved visualization of mass shape and margins. (A) Right craniocaudal 2D image shows equal-density mass with obscured margins in the central breast; (B) Digital breast tomosynthesis image shows well-defined, round, equal-density mass with well-circumscribed margins. Biopsy showed fibroadenoma.

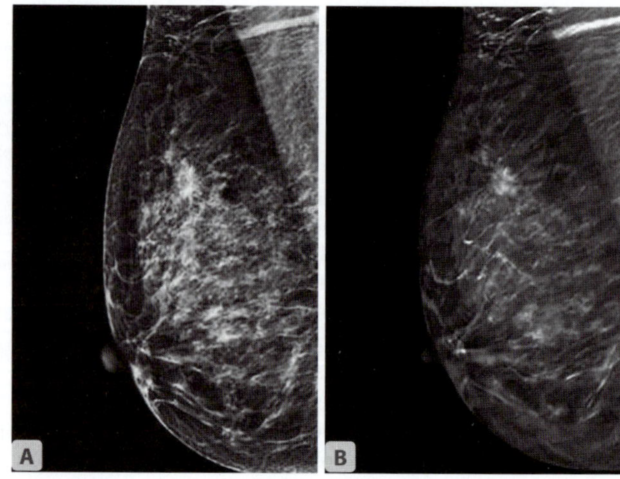

FIGS. 5A AND B: Improved visualization of mass margins. (A) Right mediolateral oblique 2D image shows high-density mass with indistinct margins in the upper breast; (B) Digital breast tomosynthesis image shows irregular mass with spiculated margins. Biopsy demonstrated invasive ductal carcinoma.

recategorized as round or oval, specially in benign masses.[18] Margins of malignant masses are also better seen on DBT with improved details **(Figs. 5A and B)**. DBT is also useful in differentiation of spiculated and indistinct margins, which is difficult with 2D mammography. Associated architectural distortion is also better seen on DBT. Overall improved details result in an increase in degree of suspicion of malignant masses. Although the shape and margin of masses are better seen with DBT, the density of the mass is better appreciated on 2D mammography. Masses which are of high density on 2D mammography usually show lower density on 1-mm thin sections of DBT.

The overall need of spot compression decreases with DBT. It gives more patient satisfaction and is time-saving without any loss of diagnostic details for noncalcified lesions. Visualization of microcalcification is variable on DBT[19] and it needs dedicated magnification views for characterization which is currently recommended for microcalcification. However, if we adjust the slab thickness, we can evaluate the distribution of calcification better.

The drawbacks of DBT include radiation dose, cost, and workflow. The radiation dose is twice that of conventional DM, if we combine 2D mammography and DBT. Although it is less than the permitted limit, for screening population it may be of little concern. With the development of synthesized reconstructed 2D images which are made from a DBT volume dataset, we can eliminate the 2D mammography and reduce the radiation dose. The other limitation of DBT is the longer interpretation time for mammography plus DBT images as DBT can have 200 or more images. But it is compensated by decreasing the recall rate and additional views.[16] The cost of the DBT system is also higher than the cost of the 2D mammography system and with DBT there is additional expense of large storage space for large file size of DBT.

CONTRAST-ENHANCED MAMMOGRAPHY

Contrast-enhanced mammography (CEM) is an emerging imaging modality which combines intravenous (IV) contrast administration and DM. It utilizes the principle of dual-energy X-ray, also called contrast-enhanced dual-energy mammography (CEDM). CEM got FDA approval in 2011 as an adjunct to mammography. With the advanced full-field DM units, it can perform low-energy tomosynthesis in the same compression. Breast cancer is diagnosed on CEM by density, morphology, and neovascularity associated with malignancy.[20,21]

Contrast-enhanced Mammography Acquisition and Image Analysis

Contrast-enhanced mammography is done by using a standard DM system which is upgraded with a copper filter and special software to perform dual-energy scan.

For CEM, a nonionic iodinated contrast agent is first injected intravenously at 1.5 mL/kg at a rate of 3 mL/s. After 2 minutes of contrast injection, standard two-view mammography is performed. MLO and CC views using dual energy technique. In dual energy, low-energy imaging is done at kilovoltage which is below the K-edge of iodine (33.2 keV). In this image, no iodine is visualized and it appears similar to conventional digital 2D mammography with the same diagnostic performance.[22,23] High-energy imaging is acquired at above the K-edge of iodine, and it shows contrast agent uptake with other diagnostic information. The total duration of examination is around 5–6 minutes. Dual-energy images can be acquired up to 10 minutes after the contrast injection, if any extra view is required **(Fig. 6)**. These dual-energy images are subsequently postprocessed and the

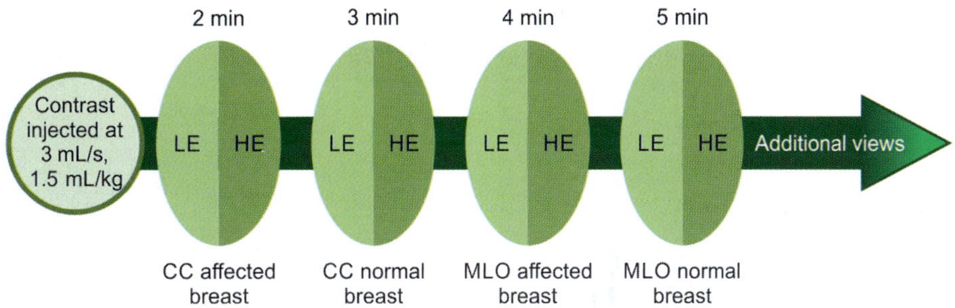

FIG. 6: Standard protocol of performing contrast-enhanced mammography. Low-energy (LE) images followed by high-energy (HE) images are taken for each view. (CC: craniocaudal; MLO: mediolateral oblique).

reconstructed image is formed which shows highlighted areas of contrast enhancement with suppression of background breast tissue densities. Both recombined and low-energy images are used for diagnostic evaluation. Additional spot compression and magnification views can be done after CEM, if needed. These can be done without the dual-energy technique.[24] Any abnormality found on a recombined image should be correlated with a low-energy image; if no correlate is identified on the low-energy image, additional ultrasound or magnetic resonance imaging (MRI) should be performed.

At present, there is no CEM-specific BI-RADS lexicon for image interpretation. Currently, mammography BI-RADS descriptors are used for low-energy images and MRI BI-RADS descriptors are used for evaluation of recombined images.[25,26]

Contrast-enhanced Mammography in Screening

The utility of CEM for breast cancer screening is being studied, but only limited data is available. Mammography is the first and best imaging modality for breast cancer screening, although its sensitivity is low in women with dense breast.[27] In these women, ultrasound is commonly used for additional screening. Women with a high risk of breast cancer were screened with supplemental MRI.[28] Doing MRI for these women is a challenge as MRI is expensive with long examination time and its lack of availability to all patients. Few studies have been done to evaluate the performance of CEM as an alternative to MRI in these patients. A study by Jochelson et al., which included 307 high-risk women for comparison of CEM and MRI, found that CEM and MRI are comparable with specificity of 94.1% and 94.7%, respectively.[29] These studies are preliminary, and more studies are needed to validate.

Diagnostic Performance of Contrast-enhanced Mammography

Breast Mass

CEM can be used for diagnostic workup of a palpable lump or a lesion found on imaging is diagnostic mammography. A retrospective study by Lalji et al., evaluated patients with breast lump in screening recall with mammography and CEM and found sensitivity of 97% and specificity of 70%.[22]

There are few studies that have compared the CEM with mammography and ultrasound in the setting of newly diagnosed cancer. CEM does not provide additional information in characterization of masses except the enhancement. However, it helps in identifying any additional lesion in breast **(Figs. 7A and B)**.[30]

Architectural Distortion

Architectural distortion is difficult to distinguish in mammography. It can be due to a benign or malignant cause and biopsy is the standard care as its chances of being malignant are as high as 50–70%.[31] In a study done with MRI, absence of enhancement with architectural distortion is more reliable on benign etiology.[32] Both CEM and MRI help differentiate the benign from the malignant cause of architectural distortion. Patel et al., conducted CEM in patients with architectural distortion and subsequent biopsy was performed in these patients, and 97% of patients who showed enhancement on CEM had malignancy.[33] CEM has high sensitivity and negative predictive values (NPV). It is useful to evaluate subtle architectural distortions detected on screening mammography which are not reproducible. If these do not show enhancement on CEM, then biopsy can be avoided.

Microcalcification

The most common cause of recall in screening mammography is microcalcification. Risk assessment of microcalcification is done by BI-RADS descriptors. Morphology of microcalcification can be well evaluated with the low-energy images in CEM and the recombined images can show any associated enhancement. Many studies have been done to evaluate the role of CEM in a setting of microcalcification but they have shown mixed results. The overall results from these studies suggest that the presence of enhancement can suggest malignancy, but lack of enhancement cannot rule out malignancy. Suspicious calcification has to be biopsied. So, the role of CEM in the microcalcification is debatable and more studies are needed to evaluate this application.

Contrast-enhanced Mammography as an Alternative to Magnetic Resonance Imaging

With its comparable performance to show tumor enhancement, CEM can be used as an alternative to MRI evaluate the disease extent for the local staging. It can show a satellite lesion in ipsilateral or contralateral breast **(Figs. 8A and B)**. Many studies showed comparable performance

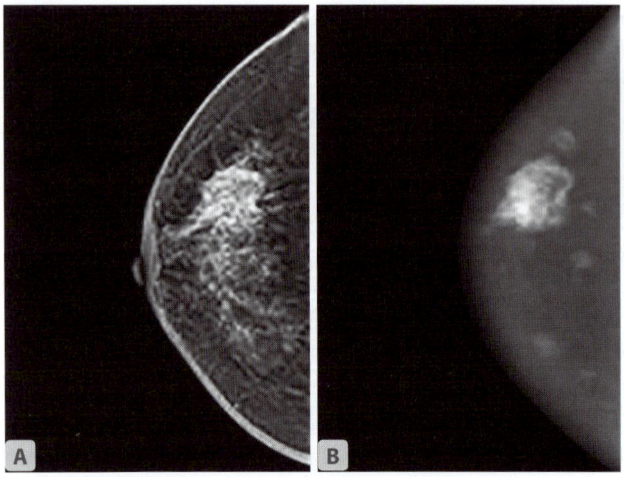

FIGS. 7A AND B: (A) Conventional craniocaudal view of right breast showing heterogeneously dense breast tissue suspicious of breast mass; (B) Contrast-enhanced subtracted image: Intensely enhancing right upper outer quadrant mass with multiple additional enhancing small masses in the same and other quadrants—s/o multicentric carcinoma right breast.

Source: Dr Rashmi Sudhir. Senior Consultant Radiologist, Indo American Cancer Hospital and Research Centre.

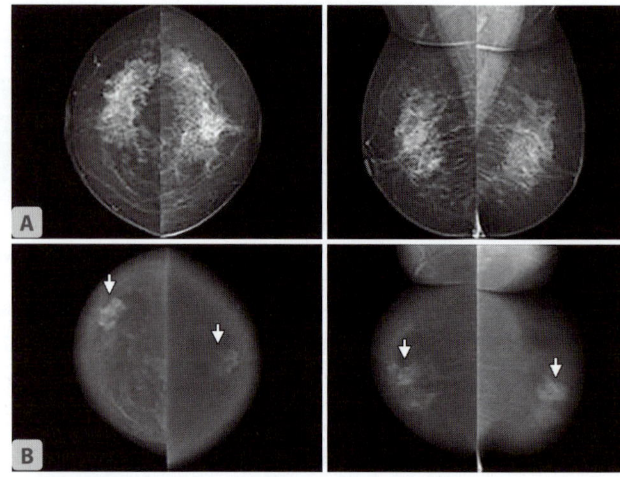

FIGS. 8A AND B: (A) Conventional mammogram shows heterogeneous dense breast tissue [American College of Radiology (ACR) category C] with asymmetric density and architectural distortion in retroareolar and upper outer quadrant of right breast. No definite mass lesion is seen in the left breast; (B) Contrast-enhanced subtracted mammogram shows enhancing mass lesions in bilateral breast (arrows).

Source: Dr Rashmi Sudhir. Senior Consultant Radiologist, Indo American Cancer Hospital and Research Centre.

and sensitivity for evaluating the disease extent in newly diagnosed breast cancer with satisfactory size correlation.[34,35] It can also be used as an alternative to MRI to evaluate the response assessment after neoadjuvant chemotherapy which is current practice for evaluating response. Multiple studies have been done to evaluate comparison of these two modalities in response assessment. Iotti et al., evaluated CEM and MRI before, during, and after neoadjuvant chemotherapy in patients of breast cancer.[36] CEM shows pathological complete response to treatment better than MRI.

Contrast-enhanced mammography may be used as an alternative to MRI to evaluate the disease extent and the chemotherapy response. It is especially useful in those places where MRI is not easily available. It is easy to upgrade the standard mammography machine with CEM and it costs less than MRI.

AUTOMATED BREAST VOLUME SCAN

Automated breast volume scan (ABVS) has recently developed for breast imaging and got FDA approval in 2012. These scanners are mainly developed to overcome few limitations of doing conventional handheld ultrasound for adjunct screening for women with dense breast on mammography. Although handheld ultrasound is the gold standard for breast ultrasound, the major limitation is that it is user dependent. In ABVS, continuous acquisition of B-mode pictures is done from which data is extrapolated and subsequent three-dimensional (3D) reconstruction of breast volume is done. Another advantage is that this data can be shared and analyzed separately by a specialist.[37]

Automated breast volume scan devices utilize wide linear-array transducers and making 3D imaging of whole breast volume possible.

A literature review comparing handheld ultrasound vis-a-vis ABVS has shown that although both these techniques allow detection of early breast cancer which are not detected on mammography, they tend to increase the false-positive recall rates. Screening programs utilizing mammography have mainly been successful due to their ability to detect breast cancer at an early stage albeit their sensitivity falls to as low as 61% in women with dense breasts, thus leading to an increase in the number of interval cancers in women with dense breasts. Small cancers are notorious in that they are silhouetted by normal glandular tissue reducing their rate of detection. Prospective trials in recent times have highlighted the ability of handheld ultrasound in the detection of early stage invasive breast cancer in apparently normal women with dense breasts which are not picked up on mammography.[38]

Optimum visualization using the ABVS system requires acquisition of minimum two, on an average three, consecutive B-mode ultrasound volumes per breast using high-frequency linear array transducers. The transducer utilizes a mechanical arm that automatically acquires in excess of 300 sections with the minimum thickness of 0.5 mm/volume. The technician is thus given the luxury of imaging the area of the breast between the midsternal line and the midaxillary line as a consequence of obtaining overlapping volumes.

Anteroposterior acquisition involves placement of nipple at the center of the ABVS image. Although lateral acquisition has some similarities with the anteroposterior acquisition, it involves placing the transducer in such a way that the lateral boundary of the transducer is kept in line with the midaxillary line so that the lateral part of breast sections can be imaged.

Water-based media need to be applied to the whole breast in order to prevent the air contact artifact. The patient should be instructed to breathe superficially and not to talk during ABVS acquisitions.

Automated breast volume scan acquisitions require a good workstation which can reconstruct the transverse images obtained to coronal and sagittal ones. These are subsequently displayed and interpreted using a multiplanar hanging protocol under appropriate conditions. Reporting of ABVS examinations generally requires 3–5 minutes for a normal case. The diagnostic accuracy and interpretation of ABVS are similar to those of handheld ultrasound.

Supplemental ABVS screening shows increased detection of small early stage invasive cancer specially in dense breast as compared to mammography alone. Detection of DCIS with ABVS is difficult, and this is the main cause for false-negative results in screening with ABVS. False-positive results on ABVS are mainly due to artifacts by Cooper's ligament and presence of a large number of benign lesions in healthy women.

The diagnostic performance of ABVS is comparable with handheld ultrasound. The commonly seen benign lesions on ABVS are cysts and fibroadenomas **(Fig. 9)**. It also beautifully depicts the intraductal papillary lesion **(Fig. 10)**. The other benign lesion is a complex sclerosing lesion which may raise suspicion of malignancy as it shows a retraction pattern on coronal ABVS images making it difficult to differentiate from malignancy.

The characteristics of a malignant lesion are the same as in handheld ultrasound. But a specific descriptor of the malignant mass on ABVS is the retraction phenomenon **(Fig. 11)**, commonly seen in breast cancer as stellate pattern around the mass likely a result of desmoplastic reaction in the surrounding tissue.[39] It is more common in low-profile indolent cancer and is usually not seen with fast-growing cancer like high-grade triple negative cancer.[40] ABVS is a novel technique that allows the whole breast ultrasound to be done by a technician in a standard way. The radiologist can read the images on the workstation and they are reproducible. It is useful as a supplemental screening tool for breast cancer in women with dense breast, and its diagnostic performance is comparable with conventional handheld ultrasound. There is a learning curve for the technologist as well as the radiologist for both acquisition and interpretation of ABVS images.

BREAST ELASTOGRAPHY

Elastography derives the information about the stiffness of the lesion under evaluation. It is a known fact that the malignant breast masses are harder than the adjoining normal breast parenchyma or any benign lesions, due to their desmoplastic reaction. The evaluation of breast masses to differentiate a benign lesion from a malignant one is one

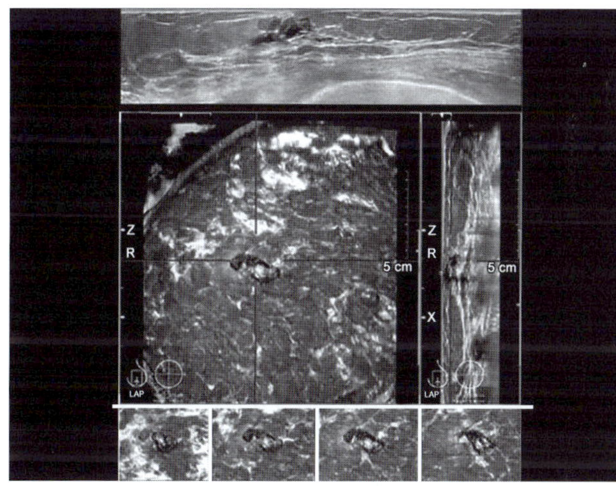

FIG. 10: Automated breast volume scan (ABVS) image showing a dilated duct at 10 o'clock position in the periareolar region reaching up to the nipple with an intraluminal polypoidal lesion. The course of the duct is better visualized in the coronal plane images of ABVS. (Biopsy showed intraductal papilloma).

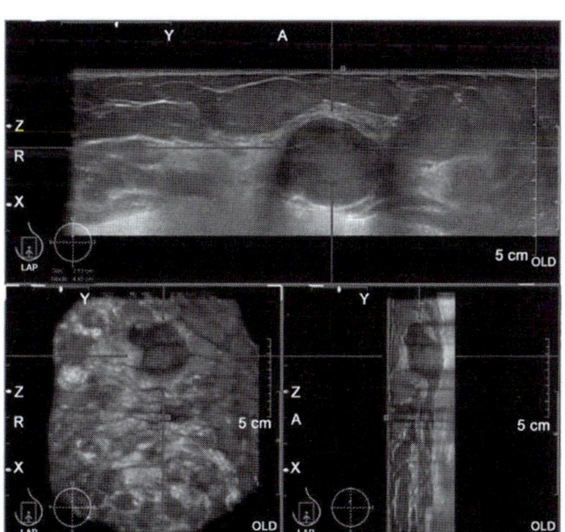

FIG. 9: Well-circumscribed iso- to hypoechoic mass with smooth margin at 12 o'clock position of left breast showing posterior acoustic enhancement by automated breast volume scan in three orthogonal planes. Biopsy showed fibroadenoma.

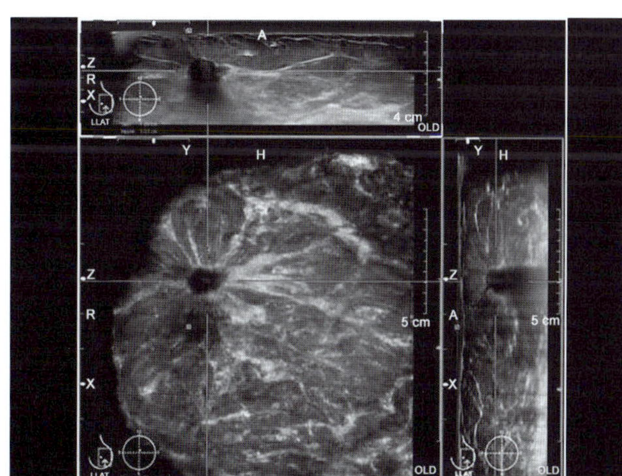

FIG. 11: Retraction phenomenon seen as converging bands of hyper- and hypoechogenicity in the coronal plane images of automated breast volume scan in a case of infiltrating ductal carcinoma.

of the initial applications of the ultrasound elastography.[41] The evaluation of the stiffness has the same principle of that of conventional clinical examination just like palpation of any breast lump. Early works done in this area in 1997 showed that cancer generally appeared stiffer (darker) than a benign lesion and surrounding normal breast tissue on elastography.[42]

After that, many studies supported that when elastography is used as an adjunct to gray-scale ultrasonography, it can help a radiologist to give a more appropriate category of BI-RADS classification. Recently, elasticity of the breast masses was included as an associated feature in the 5th edition of BI-RADS ultrasound lexicon. Two most commonly used elastography techniques in breast are strain elastography and shear-wave elastography. This classification of elastography is based on the type of excitation for a region of interest (ROI) and measurement of induced disturbance. When this disturbance is measured as displacement in the field of view, it is called strain elastography. When it is measured as the velocity of an induced shear wave, it is called shear-wave elastography.[43,44]

Strain Elastography

Strain elastography utilizes different parameters to differentiate benign and malignant breast masses. The commonly used parameter is elasticity score (Tsukuba score).[45] It is a proposed scoring system for the lesions on color maps which is based upon the elastographic properties of the tissue (For details refer to Ultrasound Elastography chapter in Recent Advances and Applied Physics book).

When the elastography score cutoff point was taken between 3 and 4 for the malignant masses, it showed 86.5% sensitivity, 89.8% specificity, and 88.3% accuracy in the initial study.[45] This gives information about the strain at a given location in tissues, although the mechanical properties of the surrounding influence it. Another disadvantage is that it is not quantitative.[46] Therefore, other semiquantitative methods have been developed; one of them is the distance ratio in which the size of the lesion measured on elastogram is divided by the lesion size on gray-scale ultrasonography. It is noted that malignant masses almost invariably appeared larger on elastography due to stromal response to breast cancer. Distance ratio cutoffs >1 as malignant and <1 as benign show sensitivity and specificity (100% and 95%) in differentiating malignant from benign breast masses.[47] Other methods of semiquantitative assessment are the strain ratio of the nodule to the adjoining normal breast tissue for the differentiation of the benign verses malignant masses **(Fig. 12)**.[48]

Shear-wave Elastography

Shear-wave elastography gives information linked to the local elastic properties of the tissue, with a quantitative approach to elasticity values.[49] The interpretation and measurement of elasticity is done in terms of Young's modulus (in kilopascals, kPa). It is evaluated either as a single value in a small ROI or can be taken for each point in box (FOV) displayed as a color map **(Fig. 13)**.[50] On a color map, the scale ranges from 0 kPa (dark blue-soft) to 180 kPa (red-hard) for breast masses.[51] It is reported that mean elasticity values are significantly higher in malignant masses (153.3 ± 58.1 kPa) than in benign masses (46.1 ± 42.9 kPa).

With these methods, elastography can help in upgrading a mass of low suspicion, BI-RADS 3 which would be sent for biopsy otherwise or in downstaging a mass which is classified as BI-RADS 4A, when used as an adjunct to gray-scale ultrasound.[52]

Recently, elastography is also being used for the assessment of neoadjuvant chemotherapy response. Breast cancers stiff on strain elastography were less likely to have a pathological complete response after neoadjuvant chemotherapy than cancers which were soft on elastography **(Figs. 14A to C)**.[53]

Few studies show correlation between histological types of breast cancer with elastography features, but it is still an area of research and needs more studies for validation.

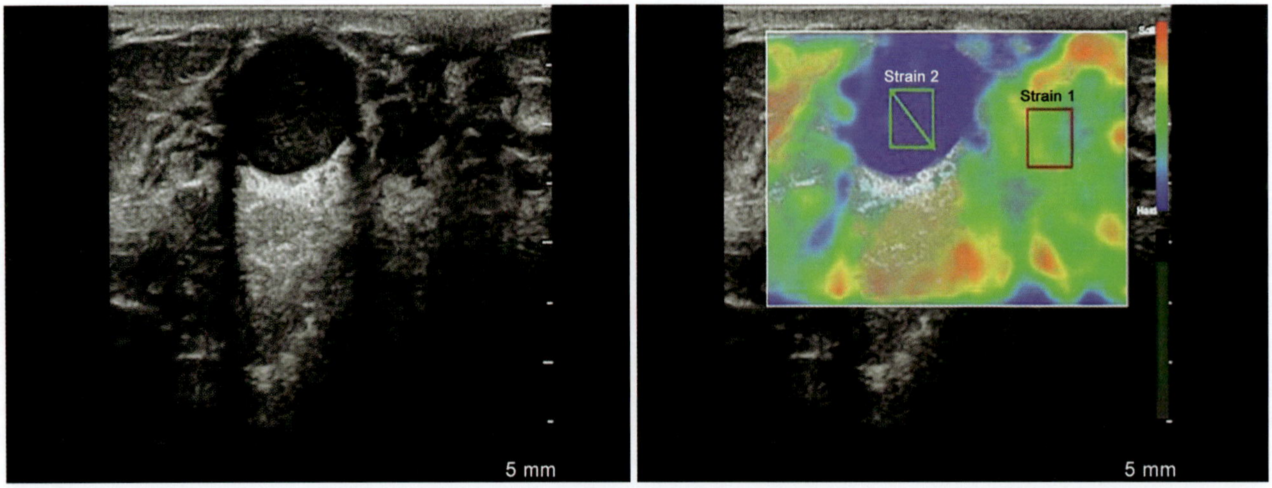

FIG. 12: Strain elastography image showing blue color in the lesion as well as in the surrounding parenchyma suggestive of malignancy. It is also showing a strain ratio of 4.5 between the lesion and the normal breast parenchyma which is highly suggestive of malignancy. Biopsy showed infiltrating ductal carcinoma.

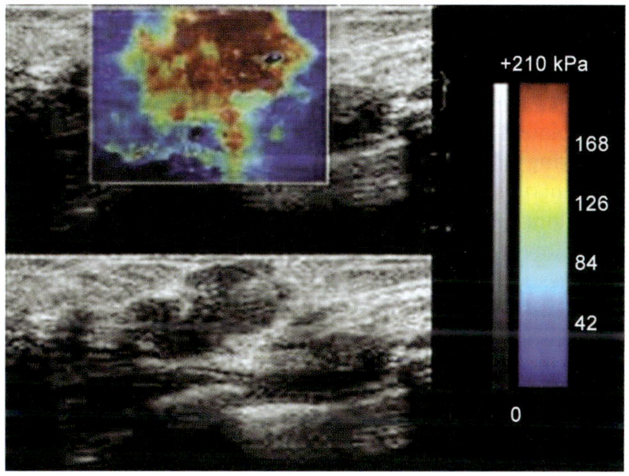

FIG. 13: On shear-wave elastography, image breast mass is showing red color suggestive of hard mass, with mean elasticity 210 kPa suggestive of malignancy. Biopsy showed invasive ductal carcinoma.

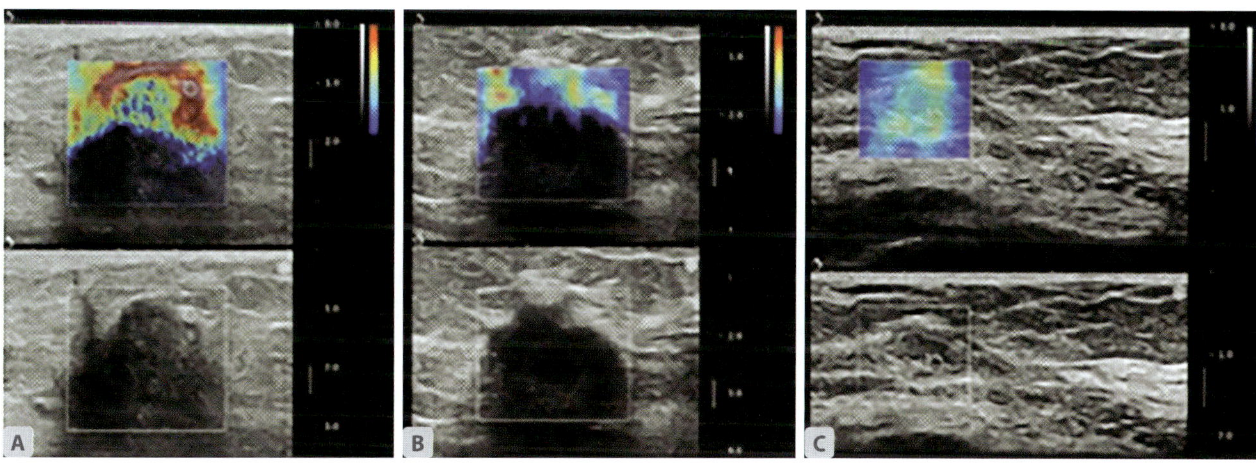

FIGS. 14A TO C: Change in mean elasticity after two cycles of neoadjuvant chemotherapy in a responder patient. (A and B) Elasticity measurements prechemotherapy and after two cycles, respectively. On completion of chemotherapy (C) the mass is faintly visible with marked reduction in elasticity.

There are few limitations for the elastography of the breast masses. It is difficult to characterize complex masses with mixed solid and cystic components. Some benign masses such as hyalinized fibroadenoma and fat necrosis with fibrosis can also be stiff and some mucinous carcinoma can be soft. Posterior breast masses are difficult to assess with strain elastography.[54]

CONTRAST-ENHANCED ULTRASOUND

The role of contrast-enhanced ultrasound (CEUS) has been studied in the imaging of focal hepatic tumor, renal tumor, and gallbladder masses. Angiogenesis is the basic physiologic change which is growth of new microvessels, and it is essential for tumor growth and its prognostication. Color Doppler is commonly used for evaluation of vascularity on ultrasound in soft-tissue masses, but its role in detecting low flow and small vessels is limited. This limitation can be overcome by adding microbubble contrast agents along with specialized software. It enhances the signal of blood flow with suppression of intrinsic tissue signals making it as effective as MRI for the evaluation of soft-tissue masses.[55] CEUS was first utilized for the evaluation of the breast masses in the early 1990s. Early studies were focused on the enhancement pattern for the differential diagnosis of the breast lesions. Over the last decade, CEUS with quantitative and qualitative analysis studies has been developed for the breast masses for differentiating benign and malignant lesions.

Ultrasound Contrast Agent and Basic Principles

Ultrasound contrast agents are gas-filled microbubbles with phospholipid covering. The size of the microbubbles is <7 m to pass through capillaries. There are two generations of an ultrasound contrast agent depending on the type of gas in microbubbles. The first generation has air covered by a galactose shell. These agents undergo early destruction.

The second-generation agents contain sulfur hexafluoride gas with a phospholipid shell on outside. These agents stay longer and can be used for continuous imaging. It is injected intravenously and it acts like a blood-pool contrast agent and improves the detection of blood flow. It causes an acoustic impedance difference causing ultrasound signal backscattering and vascular enhancement on the ultrasound images. It increases echoes from blood 500–1,000 times. Previous CEUS studies used Doppler flow signals to visualize the microbubbles but they were associated with many artifacts. Now with contrast-specific nonlinear harmonic imaging, pulse sequences are used to actually separate nonlinear microbubble signals at the second harmonic and suppress the linear tissue signals from the surrounding stationary tissues.[56] Ultrasound contrast agents are excreted via breathing and through liver. No renal excretion makes it valuable in patients with kidney disease.[55]

Contrast-enhanced Ultrasound Acquisition and Evaluation

For contrast-enhanced imaging, 2–4 mL of an ultrasound contrast agent is injected in a peripheral vein in a bolus followed by 5–10 mL of saline flush. Continuous imaging is done just after the injection for 2–3 minutes and video clips are stored. Acquired clips can be analyzed on a qualitative or quantitative basis. Qualitative analysis of breast masses includes the following features:

- Lesion enhancement as compared to the surrounding parenchyma. There can be hyperenhancement, isoenhancement, or hypoenhancement.
- *Internal homogeneity*: It can be homogeneous enhancement or heterogeneous enhancement.
- *Enhancement direction*: It can be centripetal or centrifugal.
- *Perfusion defect*: It can be present or absent.
- Presence or absence of radially penetrating vessels.[57]

Benign masses usually show slow wash-in with homogeneous and centrifugal enhancement with clear margins and the size will be equal to or less than the size on the 2D gray-scale images **(Figs. 15A to C)**. No perfusion defect will be seen. Malignant masses will show hyperenhancement with centripetal perfusion, irregular shape, and perfusion defects **(Figs. 16 and 17)**. The size will appear larger than the size on a 2D gray-scale image. Penetrating vessels can be seen **(Fig. 18)**. This is because malignant masses show abnormally arranged clusters of cells with increased desmoplastic stroma. There is increased vascularity in tumors with abnormally arranged vessels. As the tumor size increases, blood vessel formation increases in periphery which is more tortuous and dilated. Rapid growth of tumors leads to difference in demand and supply of oxygen causing hypoxia and necrosis. These are the factors responsible for irregular heterogeneous enhancement of contrast radially penetrating vessels and central perfusion defect seen on CEUS.

Quantitative Analysis

It is derived from the time–intensity curve and the following parameters can be analyzed:

- *Peak intensity (PEAK)*: It is the maximum intensity value of the time-intensity curve, calculated by the formula

$$\frac{\text{Postcontrast intensity} - \text{Precontrast intensity}}{\text{Precontrast intensity}} \times 100\%$$

- *Time to peak (TTP)*: It is the time taken between the point when the contrast medium reaches first in the lesion and the time of maximum intensity of contrast enhancement.
- *Mean transit time (MTT)*: It is the total duration of contrast enhancement.[57]

For *qualitative analysis*, malignant masses show significantly higher and faster enhancement than the benign masses and their TTP is usually shorter. They also show larger wash-in area under the curve (AUC) and shorter MTT.[58]

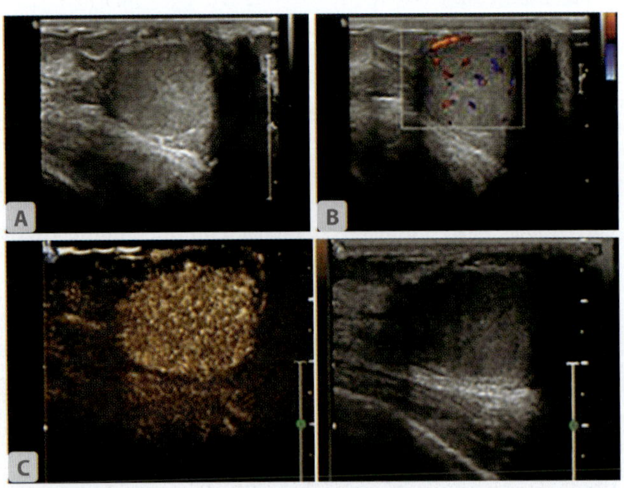

FIGS. 15A TO C: (A) Gray-scale ultrasound shows oval circumscribed isoechoic mass in parallel orientation; (B) Color Doppler shows significant internal vascularity; (C) Contrast-enhanced ultrasound shows well-defined hyperenhancing mass with uniform postcontrast appearance with a regular shape and no enlargement of diameter. Biopsy showed fibroadenoma.

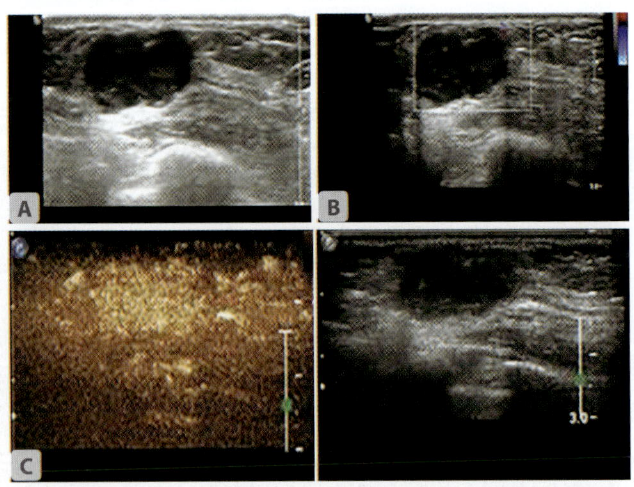

FIGS. 16A TO C: (A) Gray-scale ultrasound shows hypoechoic mass with a microlobulated outline in parallel orientation; (B) Color Doppler shows mild internal vascularity; (C) Contrast-enhanced ultrasound shows poorly defined hyperenhancing mass with irregular margins. Biopsy demonstrated invasive ductal carcinoma.

Lymphosonography is another area in which CEUS has a promising role in breast imaging. Identification and localization of the first line of lymph nodes in the tumor pathway that is called the sentinel node are important for staging. Conventionally, lymphography is done with the dermal injection of lymphatic dye and visualizing tracking the lymphatic channels directly into surgical bed[59] and it also performed with the radiotracer dye and the node with gamma probe.[60]

Lymphosonography is also done with the same method of periareolar dermal injection and visualization of the nodes after 5 minutes of ultrasound contrast injection. Initial studies of lymphosonography have shown the sentinel node in breast cancer patients.[61]

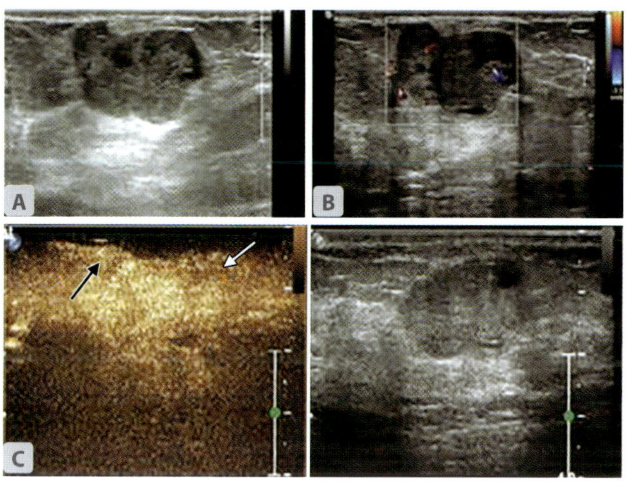

FIGS. 17A TO C: (A) Gray-scale ultrasound shows heterogeneously hypoechoic mass with a microlobulated outline in parallel orientation; (B) Color Doppler shows internal vascularity and surrounding vessel; (C) Contrast-enhanced ultrasound shows poorly defined heterogeneously hyperenhancing mass areas of perfusion defect within (white arrow) and surrounding vessel (black arrow). Biopsy showed intraductal carcinoma.

Use of CEUS combined with gray-scale ultrasound for breast imaging is a promising technique with significant clinical application. More research is being done to develop newer techniques in this field for better visualization and quantifying breast masses vascularity.

THERMAL IMAGING

Thermography, or thermal imaging, is a noninvasive and radiation-free modality of breast imaging. This was extensively evaluated in the 1970s and 1980s and was approved by US FDA as an adjunct tool for diagnosis of breast cancer.

A special type of camera is used to measure the temperature of the skin on the breast's surface based on infrared radiation which the human body normally emits. It gives a pictorial representation. The physiological principle behind this imaging modality is that as the cancer cells grow and multiply very fast as compared to normal tissue, the blood flow and metabolism are higher in that area. So, the skin temperature in that area also becomes higher than the surrounding skin which can be detected in thermal imaging.

The infrared cameras used in thermal imaging are ultrasensitive. Sophisticated computers are used to detect the small temperature variations. The data is then analyzed to produce high-resolution images of the skin temperature.

Thermal imaging has been in use for many decades, but till now no concrete evidence exists to prove that it can be used as a good screening tool for early detection of breast cancer. The US FDA has given a safety communication that thermal imaging is not to be used as a substitute for mammography.

ARTIFICIAL INTELLIGENCE IN BREAST IMAGING

Various attempts have been made previously in order to augment human perception, such as computer-aided detection (CAD) used in breast imaging. Artificial intelligence (AI) has become an umbrella term and includes various

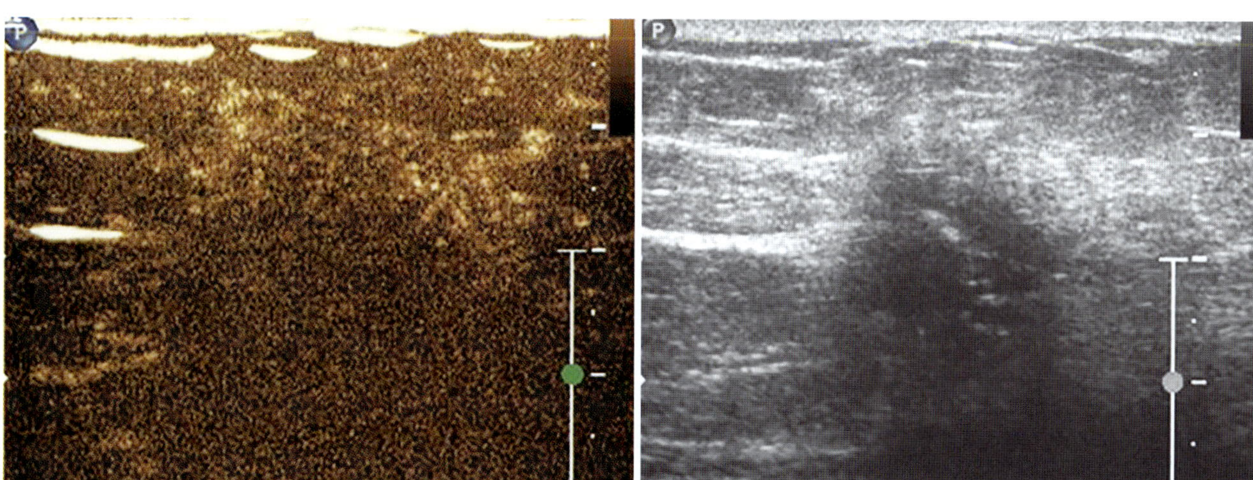

FIG. 18: Contrast-enhanced ultrasound shows poorly defined heterogeneously enhancing mass (predominantly peripheral) with enlargement of transverse diameter and surrounding vessel. Biopsy showed invasive ductal carcinoma.

training techniques, such as machine learning (ML), artificial neural networks (ANNs), and deep learning (DL).[62]

Artificial intelligence has been used in various other fields such as military, communications, finance, corporate, and entertainment sectors. Recently, there is a growing focus on health care, especially radiology. The techniques used in AI are well suited for radiology because images themselves, whose pixel values can be quantitated, are primary source data that can inform and train some AI algorithms.

Recent breast imaging studies have focused on ways to improve multimodality detection and diagnosis, workflow, and clinical decision-making. Beginning in the 1990s, articles about CAD appeared in the radiology literature as aids to radiologists in marking calcifications and masses on mammograms, findings that might have gone undetected or misclassified.[62] Many false-positives reduced the benefit-to-harm ratio before sensitivity and specificity thresholds were calibrated better to attain the desired location on a receiver operating characteristic curve (ROC).

A 2011 study undertaken to determine whether an ANN could predict breast cancer from analysis of patient age and mammographic and ultrasound BI-RADS features of masses in 800 patients with biopsy established breast cancer yielded disease prediction of 90.5%, thus validating the process.[62] AI research based on voxel analysis in 3D CT and MRI is not as far as is image analysis based on pixel quantification.

Reading mammograms in a screening setting is one of the most difficult tasks in radiology. A system that supports radiologists with the decision to refer a woman for further examination appears to be more effective than a classical CAD system. AI systems are now available for mammography analysis with accuracy that is on par with that of average but dedicated, breast radiologists on heterogeneous datasets of mammograms. Deep learning will contribute significantly to increase the application areas of MRI and make it an economically viable breast cancer screening method. AI will open more ways to detect breast cancer earlier and reduce mortality, decrease the variance in performance between radiologists, and improve the screening program as a whole by supporting less-experienced radiologists with their decisions. High-quantity and quality data are needed to train such algorithms. Various algorithmic errors are possible in AI and still there is no solid evidence supporting it. AI should not be relied on solely for a clinician's decisions that may affect survival.

CONCLUSION

Breast imaging has an important place in the field of radiology. Mammography is the first and best method of breast cancer screening. DBT has been developed to overcome few limitations of conventional mammography with an improved cancer detection rate. CEM has a promising role as it has comparable results as MRI in detecting enhancing masses in breast. ABVS has shown significant benefit over conventional mammography in women with dense breast. Other emerging ultrasound techniques such as breast elastography and contrast-enhanced breast ultrasound are expected to continue to expand their role in breast imaging.

REFERENCES

1. Lee CI, Lehman CD. Digital breast tomosynthesis and the challenges of implementing an emerging breast cancer screening technology into clinical practice. J Am Coll Radiol. 2013;10(12):913-7.
2. Pisano ED, Gatsonis C, Hendrick E, Yaffe M, Baum JK, Acharyya S, et al. Diagnostic performance of digital versus film mammography for breast-cancer screening. N Engl J Med. 2005;353(17):1773-83.
3. Bick U, Diekmann F. Digital mammography: what do we and what don't we know? Eur Radiol. 2007;17(8):1931-42.
4. Mandelson MT, Oestreicher N, Porter PL, White D, Finder CA, Taplin SH, et al. Breast density as a predictor of mammographic detection: comparison of interval- and screen-detected cancers. J Natl Cancer Inst. 2000;92(13):1081-7.
5. Kolb TM, Lichy J, Newhouse JH. Comparison of the performance of screening mammography, physical examination, and breast US and evaluation of factors that influence them: an analysis of 27,825 patient evaluations. Radiology. 2002;225(1):165-75.
6. Lei J, Yang P, Zhang L, Wang Y, Yang K. Diagnostic accuracy of digital breast tomosynthesis versus digital mammography for benign and malignant lesions in breasts: a meta-analysis. Eur Radiol. 2014;24(3):595-602.
7. Skaane P, Bandos AI, Gullien R, Eben EB, Ekseth U, Haakenaasen U, et al. Comparison of digital mammography alone and digital mammography plus tomosynthesis in a population-based screening program. Radiology. 2013;267(1):47-56.
8. Skaane P, Bandos AI, Gullien R, Eben EB, Ekseth U, Haakenaasen U, et al. Prospective trial comparing full-field digital mammography (FFDM) versus combined FFDM and tomosynthesis in a population-based screening programme using independent double reading with arbitration. Eur Radiol. 2013;23(8):2061-71.
9. Caumo F, Bernardi D, Ciatto S, Macaskill P, Pellegrini M,Brunelli S, et al. Incremental effect from integrating 3D-mammography (tomosynthesis) with 2D-mammography: increased breast cancer detection evident for screening centres in a population-based trial. Breast. 2014;23(1):76-80.
10. Andersson I, Ikeda DM, Zackrisson S, Ruschin M, Svahn T, Timberg P, et al. Breast tomosynthesis and digital mammography: a comparison of breast cancer visibility and BIRADS classification in a population of cancers with subtle mammographic findings. Eur Radiol. 2008;18(12):2817-25.
11. Gur D, Zuley ML, Anello MI, et al. Dose reduction in digital breast tomosynthesis (DBT) screening using synthetically reconstructed projection images: an observer performance study. Acad Radiol. 2012;19(2):166-71.
12. Zuley ML, Guo B, Catullo VJ, Chough DM, Kelly AE, Lu AH, et al. Comparison of two-dimensional synthesized mammograms versus original digital mammograms alone and in combination with tomosynthesis images. Radiology. 2014;271(3):664-71.
13. Skaane P, Bandos AI, Eben EB, Jebsen IN, Krager M, Haakenaasen U, et al. Two-view digital breast tomosynthesis screening with synthetically reconstructed projection images: comparison with digital breast tomosynthesis with full-field digital mammographic images. Radiology. 2014;271(3):655-63.
14. Dang PA, Humphrey KL, Freer PE, Halpern EF, Saksena MA, Rafferty EA. Comparison of lesion detection and characterization in invasive cancers using breast tomosynthesis versus conventional mammography [abstr]. In: Radiological Society of North America Scientific Assembly and Annual Meeting Program. Oak Brook, Ill: Radiological Society of North America, 2013;156.

15. Hilleren DJ, Andersson IT, Lindholm K, Linnell FS. Invasive lobular carcinoma: mammographic findings in a 10-year experience. Radiology. 1991;178(1):149-54.
16. Raghu M, Hooley RJ, Philpotts LE, et al. Digital breast tomosynthesis in diagnostic mammography: can tomo affect the final assessment categories? [abstr]. In: Radiological Society of North America Scientific Assembly and Annual Meeting Program. Oak Brook, Ill: Radiological Society of North America, 2013;156.
17. Nicholson BT, Raymond S, Rochman CM, Peppard HR, Harvey JA. Comparison of tomosynthesis in the diagnostic setting to 2D mammography for the evaluation of focal asymmetry recalled from screening. Presented at the annual meeting of the American Roentgen Ray Society, San Diego, California, May 4-9, 2014.
18. Zuley ML, Bandos AI, Ganott MA, Sumkin JH, Kelly AE, Catullo VJ, et al. Digital breast tomosynthesis versus supplemental diagnostic mammographic views for evaluation of noncalcified breast lesions. Radiology. 2013;266(1):89-95.
19. Destounis SV, Arieno AL, Morgan RC. Preliminary clinical experience with digital breast tomosynthesis in the visualization of breast microcalcifications. J Clin Imaging Sci. 2013;3:65.
20. Dromain C, Thibault F, Muller S, Rimareix F, Delaloge S, Tardivon A, et al. Dual-energy contrast-enhanced digital mammography: initial clinical results. Eur Radiol. 2011;21(3):565-74.
21. Lewin JM, Isaacs PK, Vance V, Larke FJ. Dual-energy contrast-enhanced digital subtraction mammography: feasibility. Radiology. 2003;229(1):261-8.
22. Lalji UC, Jeukens CR, Houben I, Nelemans PJ, van Engen RE, van Wylick E, et al. Evaluation of low-energy contrast-enhanced spectral mammography images by comparing them to full-field digital mammography using EUREF image quality criteria. Eur Radiol. 2015;25(10):2813-20.
23. Francescone MA, Jochelson MS, Dershaw DD, Sung JS, Hughes MC, Zheng J, et al. Low energy mammogram obtained in contrast-enhanced digital mammography (CEDM) is comparable to routine full-field digital mammography (FFDM). Eur J Radiol. 2014;83(8):1350-5.
24. Dromain C, Balleyguier C, Adler G, Garbay JR, Delaloge S. Contrast-enhanced digital mammography. Eur J Radiol. 2009;69(1):34-42.
25. Knogler T, Homolka P, Hoernig M, Leithner R, Langs G, Waitzbauer M, et al. Application of BI-RADS descriptors in contrast-enhanced dual-energy mammography: comparison with MRI. Breast Care (Basel). 2017;12(4):212-6.
26. Kamal RM, Helal MH, Mansour SM, Haggag MA, Nada OM, Farahat IG, et al. Can we apply the MRI BI-RADS lexicon morphology descriptors on contrast-enhanced spectral mammography? Br J Radiol. 2016;89(1064):20160157.
27. Patel BK, Davis J, Ferraro C, Kosiorek H, Hasselbach K, Ocal T, et al. Value Added of Preoperative Contrast-Enhanced Digital Mammography in Patients With Invasive Lobular Carcinoma of the Breast. Clin Breast Cancer. 2018;18(6):e1339-45.
28. Mainiero MB, Moy L, Baron P, Didwania AD, diFlorio-Alexander RM, Green ED, et al. (2017). ACR Appropriateness Criteria: Breast Cancer Screening. American College of Radiology. [online] Available from https://acsearch.acr.org/docs/70910/Narrative/. [Last accessed March 2019].
29. Jochelson MS, Pinker K, Dershaw DD, Hughes M, Gibbons GF, Rahbar K, et al. Comparison of screening CEDM and MRI for women at increased risk for breast cancer: A pilot study. Eur J Radiol. 2017;97:37-43.
30. Patel BK, Garza SA, Eversman S, Lopez-Alvarez Y, Kosiorek H, Pockaj BA. Assessing tumor extent on contrast-enhanced spectral mammography versus full-field digital mammography and ultrasound. Clin Imaging. 2017;46:78-84.
31. Luczyńska E, Heinze S, Adamczyk A, Ryś J, Mituś JW, Hendrick E. Comparison of the mammography, contrast-enhanced spectral mammography and ultrasonography in a group of 116 patients. Anticancer Res. 2016;36(8):4359-66.
32. Si L, Zhai R, Liu X, Yang K, Wang L, Jiang T. MRI in the differential diagnosis of primary architectural distortion detected by mammography. Diagn Interv Radiol. 2016;22(2):141-50.
33. Patel BK, Naylor ME, Kosiorek HE, Lopez-Alvarez YM, Miller AM, Pizzitola VJ, et al. Clinical utility of contrast-enhanced spectral mammography as an adjunct for tomosynthesis-detected architectural distortion. Clin Imaging. 2017;46:44-52.
34. Fallenberg EM, Dromain C, Diekmann F, Engelken F, Krohn M, Singh JM, et al. Contrast-enhanced spectral mammography versus MRI: Initial results in the detection of breast cancer and assessment of tumour size. Eur Radiol. 2014;24(1):256-64.
35. Lee-Felker SA, Tekchandani L, Thomas M, Gupta E, Andrews-Tang D, Roth A, et al. Newly diagnosed breast cancer: Comparison of contrast-enhanced spectral mammography and breast MR imaging in the evaluation of extent of disease. Radiology. 2017;285(2):389-400.
36. Iotti V, Ravaioli S, Vacondio R, Coriani C, Caffarri S, Sghedoni R, et al. Contrast-enhanced spectral mammography in neoadjuvant chemotherapy monitoring: a comparison with breast magnetic resonance imaging. Breast Cancer Res. 2017;19(1):106.
37. Wojcinski S, Farrokh A, Hille U, Wisklrchen J, Gyapong S, Soliman AA, et al. The automated breast volume scanner (ABVS): initial experiences in lesion detection compared with conventional handheld B-mode ultrasound: a pilot study of 50 cases. Int J Womens Health. 2011;3:337-46.
38. Van Zelst JCM, Mann RM. Automated three-dimensional breast us for screening: technique, artifacts, and lesion characterization. Radiographics. 2018;38(3):663-83.
39. Chen L, Chen Y, Diao XH, Fang L, Pang Y, Cheng AQ, et al. Comparative study of automated breast 3-D ultrasound and handheld B-mode ultrasound for differentiation of benign and malignant breast masses. Ultrasound Med Biol. 2013;39(10):1735-42.
40. Zheng FY, Lu Q, Huang BJ, Xia HS, Yan LX, Wang X, et al. Imaging features of automated breast volume scanner: correlation with molecular subtypes of breast cancer. Eur J Radiol. 2017;86:267-75.
41. Cespedes I, Ophir J, Ponnekanti H, Maklad N. Elastography: elasticity imaging using ultrasound with application to muscle and breast in vivo. Ultrasonic imaging. 1993;15(2):73-88.
42. Garra BS, Cespedes EI, Ophir J, Spratt SR, Zuurbier RA, Magnant CM, et al. Elastography of breast lesions: initial clinical results. Radiology. 1997;202(1):79-86.
43. Barr RG, Sonographic breast elastography. J Ultrasound Med. 2012;31(5):773-83.
44. Barr RG. Elastography in clinical practice. Radiol Clin North Am. 2014;52(6):1145-62.
45. Itoh A, Ueno E, Tohno E, Kamma H, Takahashi H, Shiina T, et al. Breast Disease: Clinical Application of US Elastography for Diagnosis. Radiology. 2006;239(2):341-50.
46. Burnside ES, Hall TJ, Sommer AM, Hesley GK, Sisney GA, Svensson WE, et al. Differentiating benign from malignant solid breast masses with US strain imaging. Radiology. 2007;245(2):401-10.
47. Barr RG. Real-time ultrasound elasticity of the breast: initial clinical results. Ultrasound Q. 2010;26(2):61-6.
48. Zhi H, Xiao Y, Yang HY, Wen Y, Ou B, Luo B-M, et al. Semi-quantitating stiffness of breast solid lesions in ultrasonic elastography. Acad Radiol. 2008;15(11):1347-53.
49. Tanter M, Bercoff J, Athanasiou A, Deffieux T, Gennisson JL, Montaldo G, et al. Quantitative assessment of breast lesion viscoelasticity: initial clinical results using supersonic shear imaging. Ultrasound Med Biol. 2008;34(9):1373-86.

50. Cosgrove D, Piscaglia F, Bamber J, Bojunga J, Correas JM, Gilja O, et al. EFSUMB guidelines and recommendations on the clinical use of ultrasound elastography. Part 2: Clinical applications. Ultraschall Med. 2013;34(3):238-53.
51. Lee SH, Chang JM, Cho N, Koo HR, Yi A, Kim SJ, et al. Practice guideline for the performance of breast ultrasound elastography. Ultrasonography. 2014;33(1):3-10.
52. Shiina T, Nightingale KR, Palmeri ML, Hall TJ, Bamber JC, Barr RG, et al. WFUMB guidelines and recommendations for clinical use of ultrasound elastography: Part 1: basic principles and terminology. Ultrasound Med Biol. 2015;41(5):1126-47.
53. Hayashi M, Yamamoto Y, Ibusuki M, Fujiwara S, Yamamoto S, Tomita S, et al. Evaluation of tumor stiffness by elastography is predictive for pathologic complete response to neoadjuvant chemotherapy in patients with breast cancer. Ann Surg Oncol. 2012;19(9):3042-9.
54. Faruk T, Islam MK, Arefin S, Haq MZ. The Journey of elastography: background, current status and future possibilities in breast cancer diagnosis. Clin Breast Cancer. 2015;15(5):313-24.
55. Cosgrove D. Ultrasound contrast agents: An overview. Eur J Radiol. 2006;60(3):324-30.
56. Wan C, Du J, Fang H, Li F, Wang L. Evaluation of breast lesions by contrast enhanced ultrasound: qualitative and quantitative analysis. Eur J Radiol. 2012;81(4):e444-50.
57. Vraka I, Panourgias E, Sifakis E, Andreas K, Galanis P, Dellaportas D, et al. A correlation between contrast-enhanced ultrasound characteristics (qualitative and quantitative) and pathological prognostic factors in breast cancer. In Vivo. 2018;32(4): 945-54.
58. Ji CL, Li XL, He YP, Li DD, Gu XG, Xu HX. Quantitative parameters of contrast-enhanced ultrasound in breast invasive ductal carcinoma: The correlation with pathological prognostic factors. Clin Hemorheol Microcirc. 2017;66(4):333-45.
59. Goldberg BB, Merton DA, Liu JB, Forsberg F, Zhang K, Thakur M, et al. Contrast-enhanced ultrasound imaging of sentinel lymph nodes after peritumoral administration of Sonazoid in a melanoma tumor animal model. J Ultrasound Med. 2011;30(4):441-53.
60. Rautiainen S, Sudah M, Joukainen S, Sironen R, Vanninen R, Sutela A. Contrast-enhanced ultrasound-guided axillary lymph node core biopsy: diagnostic accuracy in preoperative staging of invasive breast cancer. Eur J Radiol. 2015;84(11):2130-6.
61. Omoto K, Matsunaga H, Take N, Hozumi Y, Takehara M, Omoto Y, et al. Sentinel node detection method using contrast-enhanced ultrasonography with sonazoid in breast cancer: preliminary clinical study. Ultrasound Med Biol. 2009;35(8):1249-56.
62. Mendelson EB. Artificial intelligence in breast imaging: potentials and limitations. Am J Roentgenol. 2019;212(2):293-9.

CHAPTER

180

Male Breast Imaging

Veenu Singla, Tulika Singh, Nidhi Prabhakar

INTRODUCTION

The male breast is structurally identical to that of the female breast at birth. However, the testosterone surge during puberty causes atrophy and involution of the ductal units, making it nonfunctional and rudimentary. The male breast is susceptible to similar pathologies as that of the female breast. The incidence of breast-related complaints in males is on the rise, though the pathologies affecting the male breast are predominantly benign. The incidence of breast cancer in males is approximately 1%. More than half of men over 44 years show palpable stroma.[1]

IMAGING METHODS

Imaging of the male breast has been a challenge as there are no set protocols for its evaluation and because of the lesser breast volume, breast malignancies tend to involve the chest wall much earlier. The use of mammography and ultrasound for radiological evaluation of the male breast varies among different radiologists. Mammography is a reliable imaging investigation to differentiate between gynecomastia and breast cancer as it allows accurate assessment of relationship of mass with nipple, and eccentric location of mass favors malignancy. In daily practice, all masses which are suspicious clinically in patients >25 years of age should undergo mammography as the first imaging investigation. Bilateral mammograms should always be obtained as they allow comparison, and as risk factors predisposing to carcinoma on one breast are also applicable to the other breast. Despite the lesser breast volume in males, mammography is easy to acquire and standard craniocaudal (CC) and mediolateral oblique (MLO) views should be routinely done. Magnification and spot compression views should be done as per case-based requirement. Ultrasonography is performed if mammography findings are questionable or not typical of gynecomastia. Ultrasonography is easy to perform because of the small breast size and can also guide tissue sampling. Magnetic resonance imaging (MRI) is technically difficult to perform in males and is recommended when lesion identification is difficult because of associated gynecomastia, for evaluating chest wall or skin invasion, and for demonstrating primary breast mass in cases of axillary metastasis when both ultrasound and mammography are negative.

ANATOMY

Knowing the anatomy of male breast is crucial to identify and differentiate various benign and malignant processes on imaging. The male breast extends from the 2nd to 6th anterior ribs craniocaudally, and from the sternum in the midline to the midaxillary line mediolaterally. It comprises skin, subcutaneous tissue, fibroglandular stroma and involuted ducts. However, the fatty component of the breast predominates in the male breast, unlike fibroglandular stromal predominance in females. The suspensory ligaments of Cooper are not seen in male breasts. As the lobular development is dependent on estrogen and progesterone, pathologies that involve the lobular units viz., fibroadenoma, phyllodes tumor, lobular carcinoma in situ, and invasive lobular carcinoma are rare, with the gamut of diseases affecting the ductal and stromal units predominating in males.[2] The male breast receives its blood supply from the branches of the axillary artery, internal mammary artery and intercostal arteries, with the venous drainage into the intercostal veins. Lymphatics of the breast drain into the axillary, internal mammary, and the supraclavicular nodes.[3]

NORMAL IMAGING APPEARANCE

On mammography, due to the predominant fatty component, male breast appears homogeneously radiolucent, with minimal retroareolar ductal tissue and a prominent pectoralis muscle **(Fig. 1)**. On ultrasonography, the nipple appears as an echogenic nodule with posterior acoustic shadowing. The skin is hyperechoic. The subcutaneous tissue is hypoechoic with echogenic fibrous septa **(Fig. 2)**. The rudimentary fibroglandular tissue appears hypoechoic.[3]

Though gynecomastia and breast cancer are considered mainly in a male patient with a palpable breast mass, masses arising from skin and subcutaneous tissue like lipomas and epidermal inclusion cysts are also common.

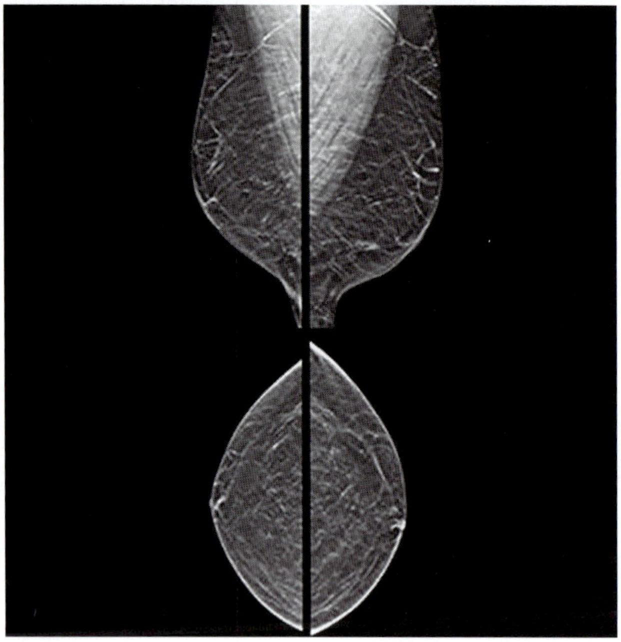

FIG. 1: Mammographic appearance of a normal male breast showing predominantly fatty tissue and minimal fibroglandular component.

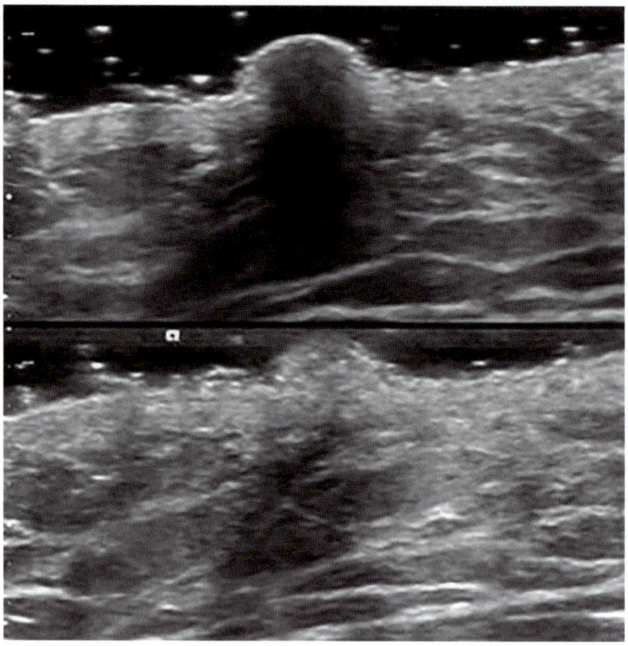

FIG. 2: Ultrasonographic appearance of the normal male breast. The nipple appears as a small heteroechoic nodule with mild posterior attenuation. The small volume of glandular tissue appears hypoechoic. The overlying skin is hyperechoic, and the subcutaneous tissue is hypoechoic with hyperechoic streaks that represent fibrous striae.

Gynecomastia

It is the most common breast abnormality in males and is due to benign proliferation of the stromal and ductal elements. Gynecomastia presents with clinical manifestations and imaging signs which may be unilateral or bilateral. Gynecomastia can be physiological during infancy, puberty and senescence, when there is increased estrogen and reduced testosterone. It can also be seen with the use of drugs (such as marijuana, steroids, leuprolide, thiazides, etc.), in patients with cirrhosis, syndromic hypogonadism, hyperthyroidism, chronic kidney disease and neoplasms such as germ cell tumors, Sertoli and Leydig cell tumors, adrenocortical tumors, and pituitary tumors.[2]

Men commonly present with a palpable, tender lump, or burning sensation. Clinically, gynecomastia is seen as a concentric subareolar mass contrary to other pathologies, which show eccentric growth in relation to the nipple-areola complex. This should also be differentiated from pseudogynecomastia, which occurs due to fat proliferation with no significant proliferation of the stroma.

On mammography, three characteristic patterns of gynecomastia are seen, namely—(1) nodular, (2) dendritic and (3) diffuse glandular.[2,4] The *nodular pattern* is seen as a *fan-shaped* density which radiates from the nipple. It is usually more prominent in the upper outer quadrant. This correlates with the pathological class of early phase of gynecomastia known as "florid gynecomastia", where there is hyperplastic ductal epithelium, with loose stroma and edema surrounding it. Clinically, it correlates with the phase of a painful lump. On mammography, a fan-shaped or triangular density is seen behind the nipple. On ultrasonography, it is seen as a focal hypoechoic nodular discoid structure or triangular hypoechoic area in the retroareolar location, with long axis parallel to the skin. It is reversible if the precipitant stimulus is removed. The *dendritic pattern* of gynecomastia is seen as a *flame-shaped* soft tissue density in the retroareolar location. This form correlates with the pathological class of long-standing, quiescent, or "fibrous gynecomastia", which shows dense fibrotic stroma. On mammography, it is seen as a dendritic density in the subareolar location with finger-like projections extending into deeper fatty tissue. On ultrasonography, irregular subareolar hypoechoic is seen with linear projections extending into surrounding adipose tissue. As fibrosis has set in, the process becomes irreversible from this phase **(Figs. 3A and B)**.[5] The *diffuse glandular pattern* resembles that of a heterogeneously dense breast seen in females and is seen in patients on high-dose estrogen therapy.[2] On mammography, there is generalized increase in breast density; and on ultrasonography, there is increase in volume and echogenicity of breast tissue resembling sonologically dense female breast. Gynecomastia may be confused with malignancy, although malignancies rarely involve the subareolar location. However, careful history with special attention to patient's medical history, and clinical examination can help in differentiating gynecomastia from malignancy.

As breast malignancy is uncommon in younger males, nearly all men <30 years of age having breast symptoms have gynecomastia. Imaging features that favor gynecomastia over malignancy are central/subareolar location of mass, lack of spiculations and absence of secondary signs of malignancy like skin changes. Occasionally, it becomes

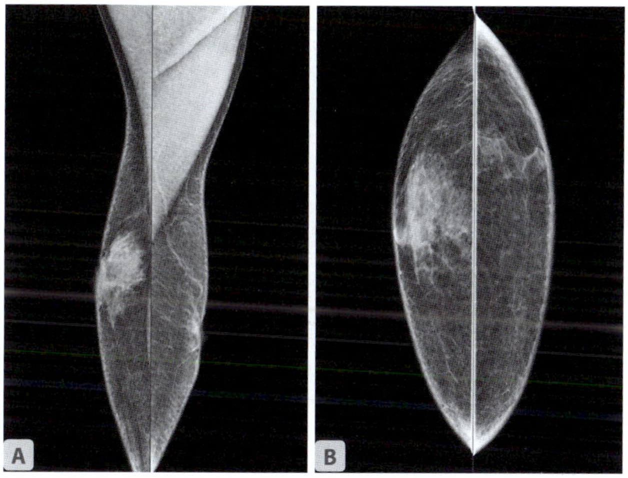

FIGS. 3A AND B: Mammography of a male patient showing dendritic subareolar density interdigitating into underlying fatty tissue. Features suggestive of gynecomastia—dendritic type.

difficult to differentiate gynecomastia from malignancy on imaging,[6] and biopsy is required for confirmation of the diagnosis.[2]

Gynecomastia is self-regressing and may resolve when the precipitating factors are eliminated. However, in later stages, when the disease is refractory to medical management, reduction mammoplasty can be undertaken.

BENIGN NEOPLASMS OF THE MALE BREAST

Angiolipoma

It is a common fatty tumor in rest of the body; however, its occurrence in the breast is rare. On mammography, it appears as a mixed density mass having fatty as well as soft tissue components. On ultrasonography, it is seen as a homogeneously hyperechoic mass. The patient is usually kept on imaging follow-up. The tumor is rarely treated by excision.

Schwannoma

They are extremely rare neoplasms in the male breast; however, when associated with neurofibromatosis type 2, they have increased malignant potential. They present as soft, smooth, and often painless mass. On mammography, they are seen as nonspecific, round or oval, well-defined masses. On ultrasonography, they are seen as well-demarcated, solid hypoechoic masses with variable degrees of posterior acoustic enhancement. Occasionally, these tumors may show central cystic regions.

Intraductal Papilloma

It is characterized by proliferation of the ductal epithelium, supported by a core of fibrovascular stroma and myoepithelial cells. Men usually present with a palpable lump in the subareolar location or with discharge from the nipple. Ultrasonography has shown increased sensitivity in the detection of these lesions, which are seen as an intraluminal masses within a dilated duct. On color Doppler, the fibrovascular stalk shows internal vascularity. When the duct is not dilated at the time of the ultrasound examination, the intraluminal mass may be become inconspicuous and may lead to false-negative results.[2] Surgical excision is the preferred diagnostic as well as therapeutic modality as core biopsy may underestimate the lesion histologically.[2]

Lipomas

They are the second most common benign lesion of the male breast after gynecomastia; and are characterized by benign proliferation of mature adipocytes. They present as nonpainful, soft palpable masses. On mammography, they are seen as a well-defined, encapsulated lesion showing fat density; and on ultrasonography as mildly echogenic, avascular masses. However, they may also appear isoechoic or hypoechoic to the surrounding fat. They do not warrant surgery unless they are cosmetically disturbing.

Benign Spindle Cell Neoplasms

These are rare mesenchymal lesions, which include myofibroblastoma, spindle cell lipoma, leiomyoma, solitary fibrous tumor, and fibrous histiocytoma. The imaging features are nonspecific, and often, histopathology is needed for validation of diagnosis. Mammography and ultrasonography may show well-defined masses with coarse calcifications. Myofibroblastomas have been reported to occur in cases of previous malignancies of pancreas, kidney, and prostate.

BENIGN NON-NEOPLASTIC LESIONS OF MALE BREAST

Pseudogynecomastia

This is a bilateral or less commonly unilateral condition, which is seen commonly in obese adolescent males, overweight persons, or in neurofibromatosis. It occurs due to excessive fat deposition. On clinical examination, it is non-nodular, diffuse, and symmetrical. On mammography, there is excessive fatty tissue in the breast without any fibroglandular tissue. On ultrasonography, homogeneously hypoechoic lobules of adipose tissue are seen to be separated from one another by thin hyperechoic bands representing fibrous tissue.

Intramammary Lymph Nodes

They are common lesions, usually seen in the upper outer quadrant, however, can be located anywhere within the breast. On mammography, they appear oval with radiodense peripheral cortex and radiolucent central fatty hilum. On ultrasonography, normal lymph nodes appear homogeneous with a cortical thickness of <2–3 mm, with hyperechoic fatty hilum and echogenic cortex. Lymph nodes which measure >10 mm in short axis diameter, rounded nodes, irregular nodes, or nodes with cortical thickening >3 mm are taken as abnormal.

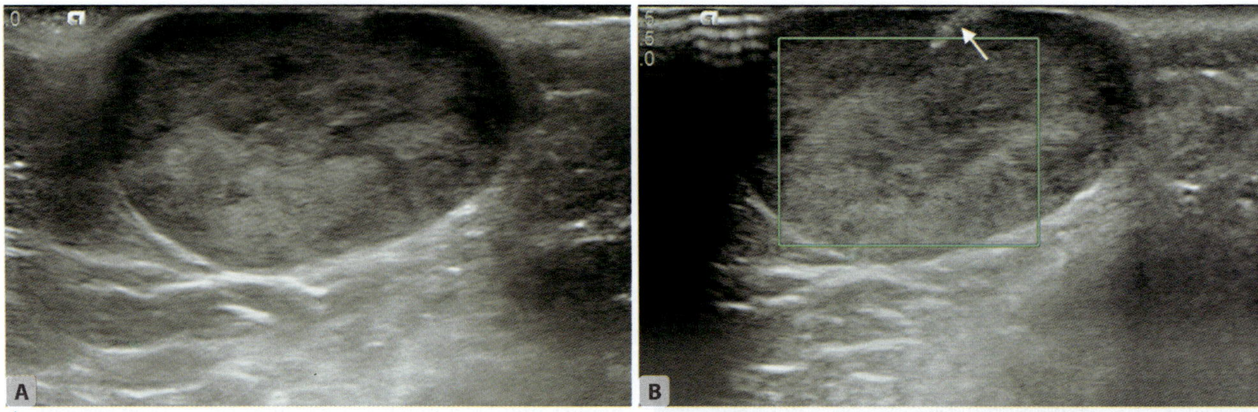

FIGS. 4A AND B: Epidermal inclusion cyst. Ultrasonography of the breast showing presence of a superficial, well-defined heteroechoic lesion lying parallel to the chest wall and showing positive "claw sign" with the surrounding subcutaneous tissue and an echogenic tract (arrow) reaching up to the skin surface. Color Doppler shows no vascularity within the lesion.

Epidermal Inclusion Cyst

They are benign intradermal lesions, which occur secondary to obstruction of hair follicles and contain lamellated keratin within a wall of epidermis. They are the third most common benign lesion in male breast. On imaging, they are indistinguishable from sebaceous cysts, which occur due to obstruction of hair follicles. On mammography, both are seen as a well-defined high density, superficial lesion, which is continuous with the skin. On ultrasonography, they are seen as oval, well-demarcated, hypoechoic, subcutaneous lesions adjacent to the skin surface with no internal vascularity **(Figs. 4A and B)**. However, infected cysts may show peripheral hyperemia. Due to the lamellated keratin, they may give onion skin appearance on sonography, with alternate hypoechoic and hyperechoic concentric rings. Such lesions are seldom sampled for diagnosis as their rupture may lead to inflammatory response and subsequent formation of breast abscess, hence these are considered "no biopsy" lesions and diagnosis should be clinched on imaging.

Duct Ectasia

Duct ectasia is rare in men. It may present with signs of chronic inflammation and nipple discharge. Imaging reveals dilated subareolar ducts with inspissated secretions. These secretions may occasionally calcify. As benign duct dilatation is present centrally; if located peripherally, malignancy needs to be ruled out.

Diabetic Mastopathy

It is a rare fibroinflammatory disease seen in patients with a long-standing history of type 1 diabetes mellitus. On mammography, it may appear as a discrete, nonspecific mass, or focal asymmetry. On ultrasonography, appearance may be as solitary or multiple hypoechoic masses which show minimal or no internal vascularity, and may show posterior acoustic attenuation. Imaging appearance may be similar to that of malignancy; hence biopsy is often required for diagnosis. On histopathology, it shows sclerosis of the stroma with dense infiltration by lymphocytes. Diagnosed cases do not necessitate surgery as these lesions have no increased malignant potential.

Post-traumatic Hematoma/Fat Necrosis

It is usually seen following breast trauma or surgery, however, may follow a trivial trauma in patients with coagulopathy or patients on anticoagulant medications. In acute phases, hematoma as well as fat necrosis may appear as an atypical mass, which shows associated thickening of skin and accentuation of the trabeculae. On mammography, hematomas are radiopaque, circumscribed or irregular, having appearance that may be similar to that of an abscess or malignancy. With time, hematomas progress to discrete masses showing fluid-fluid levels due to conversion of acute blood into serum; and fat necrosis may evolve to masses showing fat-fluid levels due to necrosis/liquefaction of fat. Acute hematomas are hyperechoic on sonography. However, on ultrasonography, both hematoma and fat necrosis may appear similar as well-defined masses showing fluid-debris level and internal septations with no internal vascularity. Ultrasound examination in the decubitus views is crucial to look for the mobility of debris and exclude underlying soft tissue. Internal vascularity suggests an underlying neoplastic etiology. Chronic hematomas and fat necrosis may appear as persistent masses, architectural distortion, and dystrophic calcifications on imaging **(Fig. 5)**.

Mastitis

It is a diffuse inflammation of the breast which may present with or without abscess formation within ectatic ducts. It is usually caused by staphylococci or less commonly streptococci. These bacteria enter the nipple due to trauma or nipple piercing. On mammography, they appear as diffuse enlargement of the breast with thickened trabeculae **(Figs. 6 and 7)**. In the presence of an abscess, ill-defined masses are seen which may or may not show calcifications. They may be confused with gynecomastia; however, presence of skin thickening helps in differentiating between them. Treatment is by percutaneous drainage and antibiotics with or without excision of ectatic ducts.

Subareolar Abscess

It is due to a localized infection, which occurs secondary to ductal ectasia, chronic ductal obstruction, and inflammation. Men present with nipple swelling, discharge and pain. On mammography, they are seen as an ill-defined mass with trabecular thickening. On ultrasonography, they are seen as an ill-circumscribed mass showing complex fluid within and showing peripheral hyperemia and no internal vascularity (**Figs. 8A and B**). Treatment is by surgical excision of the abscess and the regional ducts to avoid recurrence of the disease.

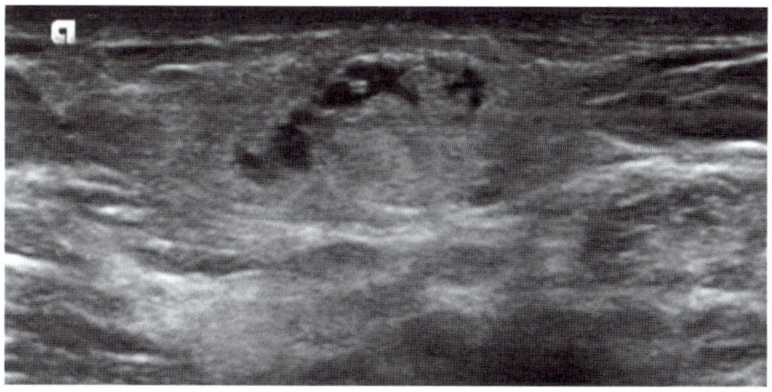

FIG. 5: Ultrasonography of breast in a male with history of chest trauma showing a superficial, ill-defined, predominantly echogenic lesion with few hypoechoic areas within which show internal debris. Features suggestive of traumatic fat necrosis.

Tuberculosis of the Breast

Primary tuberculosis of the male breast is rare, as its incidence increases in females during pregnancy and lactation due to increased vascularity as well as dilated ducts. HIV infection is also a major risk factor. Commonly it presents with lump with surrounding inflammatory signs with or without axillary lymphadenopathy. They can be of three types, namely—(1) nodular tuberculosis (characterized by a malignant looking mass with or without sinus formation), (2) diffuse or disseminated mastitis (characterized by multiple foci which may lead to the formation of draining sinuses) and (3) sclerosing type (characterized by hard, painless lump with nipple retraction due to extensive fibrosis).

Pseudoangiomatous Stromal Hyperplasia

Pseudoangiomatous stromal hyperplasia (PASH) is a benign proliferation of the stroma which is commonly seen incidentally on biopsy specimens, which were done for other indications. However, it may also present with a palpable lump. On mammography and ultrasonography, it may show well defined or partially defined margins. Symptomatic or fast

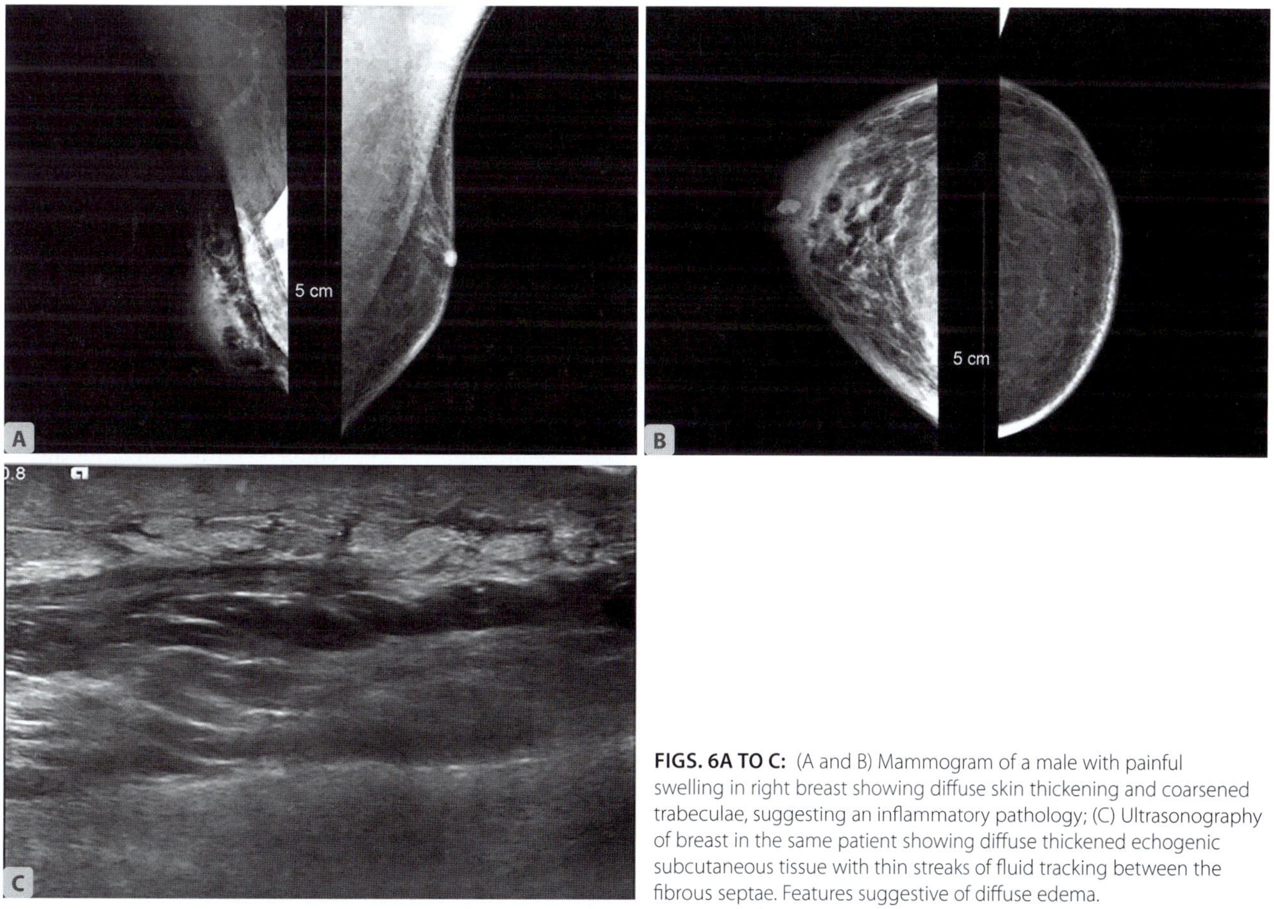

FIGS. 6A TO C: (A and B) Mammogram of a male with painful swelling in right breast showing diffuse skin thickening and coarsened trabeculae, suggesting an inflammatory pathology; (C) Ultrasonography of breast in the same patient showing diffuse thickened echogenic subcutaneous tissue with thin streaks of fluid tracking between the fibrous septae. Features suggestive of diffuse edema.

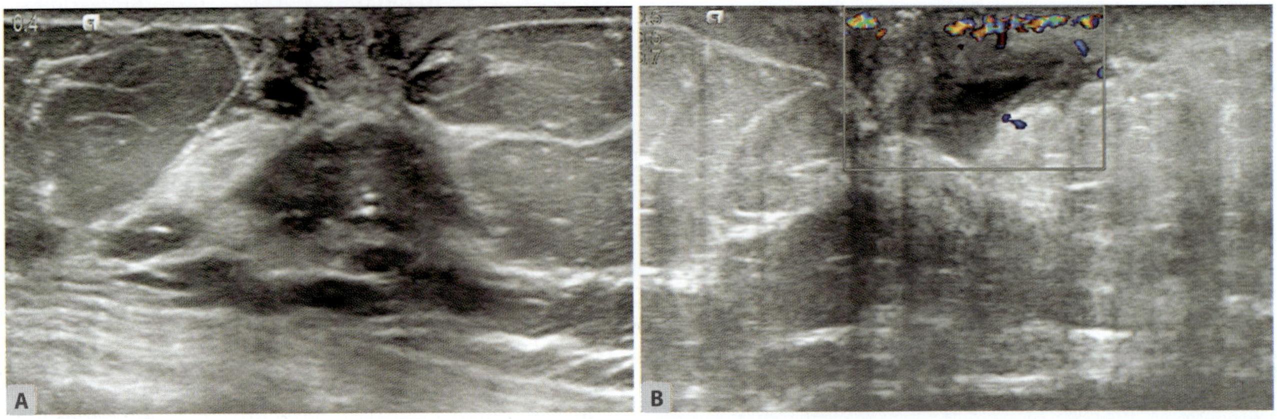

FIGS. 7A AND B: Ultrasonography of breast in a male presenting with painful lump showing presence of focal heteroechoic area in the subareolar location with increased peripheral vascularity. Features suggestive of mastitis.

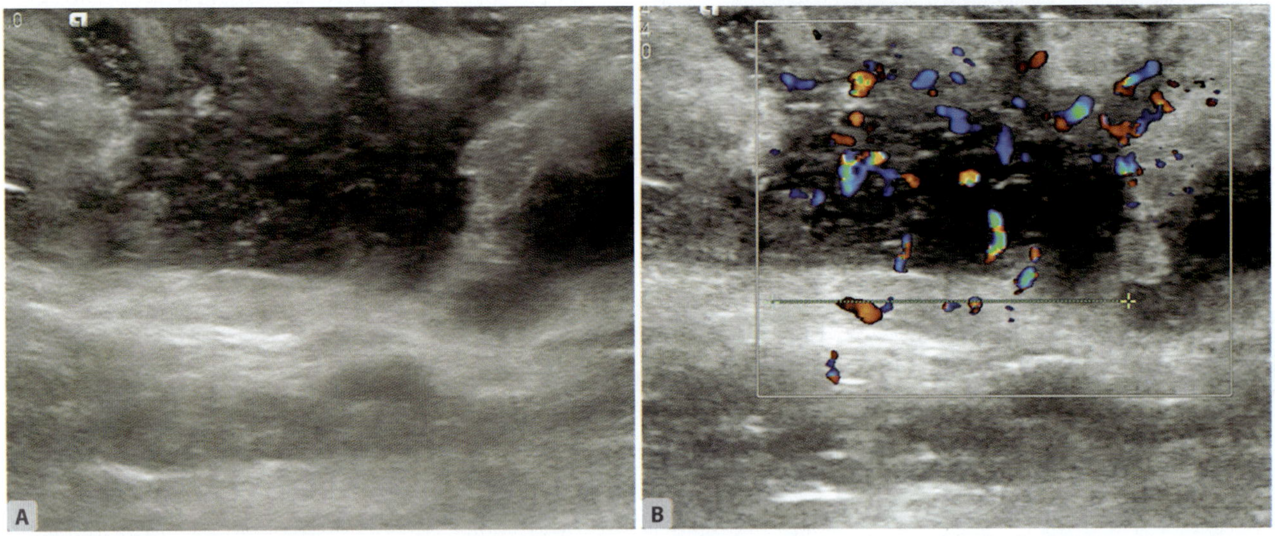

FIGS. 8A AND B: Ultrasonography of breast in a male presenting with painful breast lump showing presence of a heteroechoic lesion in the subcutaneous tissue showing shaggy walls and dense internal echoes within. Color Doppler showing hypervascularity. Features suggestive of evolving breast abscess.

growing lesions can be treated by wide local excision taking 1–2 cm surgical margins, as they carry high rates of recurrence.[1]

Hamartomas

They are uncommon lesions containing fibroglandular and fatty elements of the breast. These lesions rarely can harbor foci of ductal carcinoma within them. On mammography, these lesions are well defined with stromal as well as fat density areas within. On ultrasonography, they have varied appearances and can appear hyperechoic, heteroechoic, or isoechoic well-defined lesions.

Augmented Male Breasts

Hormonal therapy is used as a nonsurgical option in transsexual patients for breast augmentation. This is done by the administration of exogenous estrogen and suppression of androgen secretion. This results in dense breasts similar to that of female breasts. In addition, injected high viscous fluids (like petroleum jelly, paraffin, automobile transmission fluid, etc.) may show extensive calcifications, which in some cases may cause extensive surrounding inflammation leading to a condition called sclerosing lipogranulomatosis. Sclerosing lipogranulomatosis may require treatment by radical debridement and even mastectomy.

Venous Malformation

It is the most common vascular malformation of the male breast, which is characterized by slow flow and absence of arteriovenous shunting. It usually presents as unilateral painless, gradual breast enlargement. On mammography, they are seen as multiple serpiginous densities. On ultrasonography, they show multiple tubular, anechoic cystic spaces showing internal color flow, which differentiate them from a lymphatic malformation. They may show associated features such as phleboliths or thrombosis.

Secondary Syphilis

It can be transmitted during vaginal delivery in cases of congenital syphilis or sexually transmitted in cases of acquired syphilis. Secondary syphilis manifests several months after the primary chancre and shows periareolar mucous excrescences, nipple retraction, and skin thickening. On mammography, they are seen as diffuse skin thickening and diffuse asymmetry of fibroglandular pattern. Similar mammographic appearances can be seen in cases of Paget's disease of the breast, subareolar abscesses, and inflammatory carcinomas.

Nodular Fasciitis

It is a benign, reactive fibroblastic proliferation, usually affecting forearms and rarely affecting the breast presenting as a firm mass. On mammography, they are seen as ill-defined irregular densities. On ultrasonography, they are seen as solid hypoechoic masses which may mimic malignancy, and hence biopsy is often needed for confirmation of diagnosis.

MALE BREAST CANCER

Male breast cancer constitutes <1% of all breast cancers. Hence, the screening for male breast cancer is not justified, and imaging of the male breast is usually for diagnostic purposes. It is associated with multiple risk factors such as advanced age, Klinefelter's syndrome, mutations of *BRCA1* or *BRCA2*, history of breast cancer in a first-degree male or female relative, hyperestrogenic states, cryptorchidism, testicular injury, liver dysfunction, and prior irradiation to the chest. There is two- to four times increased risk of breast cancer in patients with a positive family history. These cancers are more commonly unilateral, with the incidence of bilateral cancers being <1% of all male breast cancers. The mean age of diagnosis of male breast cancers is about 5–10 years later than that of female breast cancers; with more than half the men (>50%) presenting with axillary nodal metastasis at presentation. Majority of the cancers are infiltrating ductal carcinoma of "not otherwise specified" subtype (up to 80%) or ductal carcinoma in situ (DCIS); with the rarer subtypes being infiltrating mammary carcinoma and invasive papillary carcinoma.[7] However, papillary carcinomas are seen to be more commoner in men than in women.[8]

Men usually present with a palpable painless breast lump which may be associated with skin thickening, nipple retraction, nipple discharge or axillary lymphadenopathy. The mass can be immobile and fixed to the skin or the subcutaneous tissue. These lesions most commonly occur at the subareolar location, eccentric to the nipple or less commonly in the peripheral breast. The predominance in subareolar location can be explained by the fact that in females breast tissue is mainly present in upper outer quadrant, while in males, breast tissue is confined mainly to subareolar location. Nipple discharge may be the only presenting symptom in carcinoma *in situ*.[9] Mammography remains the initial imaging modality, and a supplementary ultrasonographic examination is done whenever necessary. On mammography, bilateral CC and MLO views should be acquired. These lesions can have a wide spectrum of mammographic appearances, ranging from having well-defined, ill-defined, to spiculated margins; and round, oval to irregular shapes **(Figs. 9 and 10)**. In contrary to the female breast cancers, calcifications are fewer, more coarser and scattered and seldom rod-shaped. In other words, the benign patterns of calcifications in female breast lesions need not necessarily be benign in male breast lesions, i.e., calcifications which are accepted as benign in female breast (e.g., punctate), may indicate malignancy in male breast . On ultrasonography, these lesions may appear as taller than wider hypoechoic masses with angulated or microlobulated or spiculated margins with or without calcifications. Lesions may also show variable degrees of posterior acoustic attenuation or enhancement or both. Rarely these lesions can also appear as complex cystic masses as in cases of papillary carcinomas. On color Doppler, they may show variable degrees of internal vascularity.[10] Ultrasonography provides added advantage of assessment of chest wall or nipple invasion and axillary nodal assessment. Any suspicious lesion on any of the modalities should be sampled for diagnosis.

Imaging of cancer in men with concomitant gynecomastia is challenging and has similar pitfalls of imaging a female breast cancer with background breast dysplasia. The increase in mammographic density in gynecomastia can mask the presence of an underlying malignancy. Also, a mass appearing benign on imaging can turn out to be malignant on histology and vice versa. The differentiating features of male breast carcinoma from gynecomastia are summarized in **Table 1**.

Although no standard guidelines are available for the screening of high-risk patients for cancer, it is recommended that screening should be done in patients with a strong family history of breast cancer, genetic predispositions for breast cancers, and men with previous history of breast cancer. Screening should be done in the form of:

- Self-examination of the breast every month
- 6 monthly clinical examination, after the age of 35
- Baseline mammography, at 40 years of age and annually thereafter if the breast density is increased on baseline imaging [National Comprehensive Cancer Network (NCCN) clinical practice guidelines in oncology].[11]

OTHER MALIGNANT NEOPLASMS OF THE MALE BREAST

Primary Lymphoma

Primary lymphoma affecting the breast is extremely rare and shares a similar frequency of occurrence as that of the female breast. Majority of the patients show lesions as a part of disseminated disease. Mammographic findings of the disease are nonspecific and show a wide spectrum of features, of which the most typical pattern is the presence of a well-defined lesion with a thin radiolucent halo. On ultrasonography, the lesions commonly appear hypoechoic and parallel to the chest wall; however, findings are nonspecific. These masses are usually hypervascular **(Figs. 11A and B)**. Axillary lymphadenopathy may be seen as a part of disseminated disease.

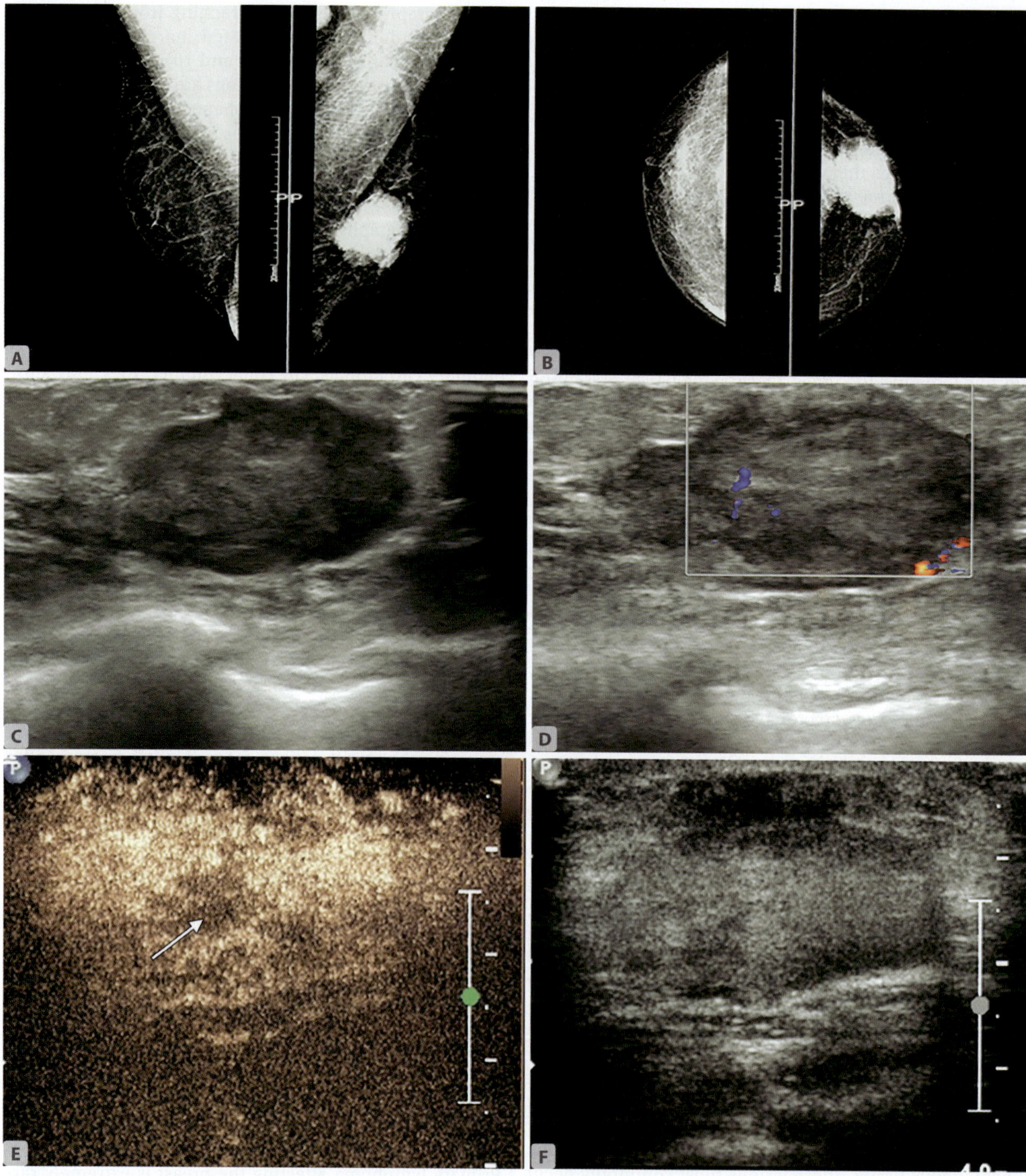

FIGS. 9A TO F: (A and B) Mediolateral oblique and craniocaudal views of mammogram of a male presenting with painless breast lump showing presence of an oval, high-density lesion with microlobulated margins in the outer central aspect of left breast showing surrounding architectural distortion and associated axillary lymphadenopathy. Note the eccentric location of the lesion; (C and D) Ultrasonography of breast shows presence of an oval heteroechoic mass with lobulated margins with mild architectural distortion. Color Doppler shows peripheral as well as internal vascularity; (E and F) Contrast-enhanced ultrasound showed florid enhancement with central perfusion defect (arrow). Biopsy from the lesion revealed infiltrating ductal carcinoma.

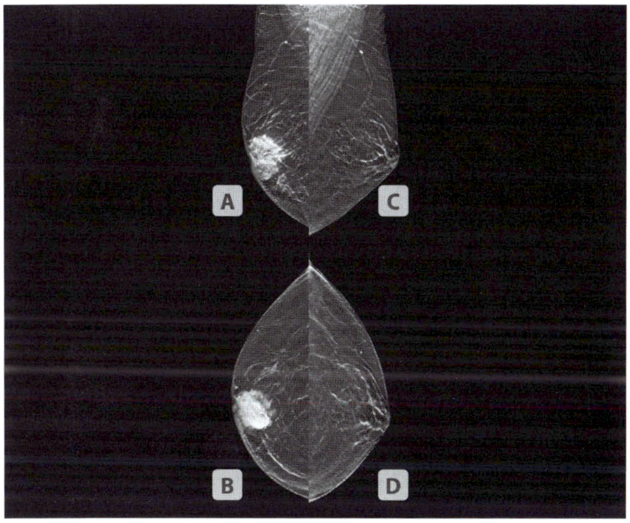

FIGS. 10A TO D: Mammogram of another male patient. (A and B) Mediolateral oblique (MLO) and craniocaudal (CC) views of right breast showing an irregular high-density mass with spiculated margins present in retroareolar location. There is associated skin thickening and nipple retraction. This mass was proven to be breast carcinoma on biopsy; (C and D) MLO and CC views of left breast of the same patient showing normal mammogram.

TABLE 1: Differentiating features of male breast carcinoma from gynecomastia.

S. No.	Gynecomastia	Carcinoma
1.	Age: infancy, puberty, senescence	Age >60 years
2.	Soft	Hard
3.	Mobile	Immobile
4.	Tender in acute phase	Painless
5.	Subareolar (central) in location	Eccentric in location
6.	Unilateral or bilateral	Usually unilateral
7.	No skin thickening or nipple retraction	Skin thickening or nipple retraction may be present

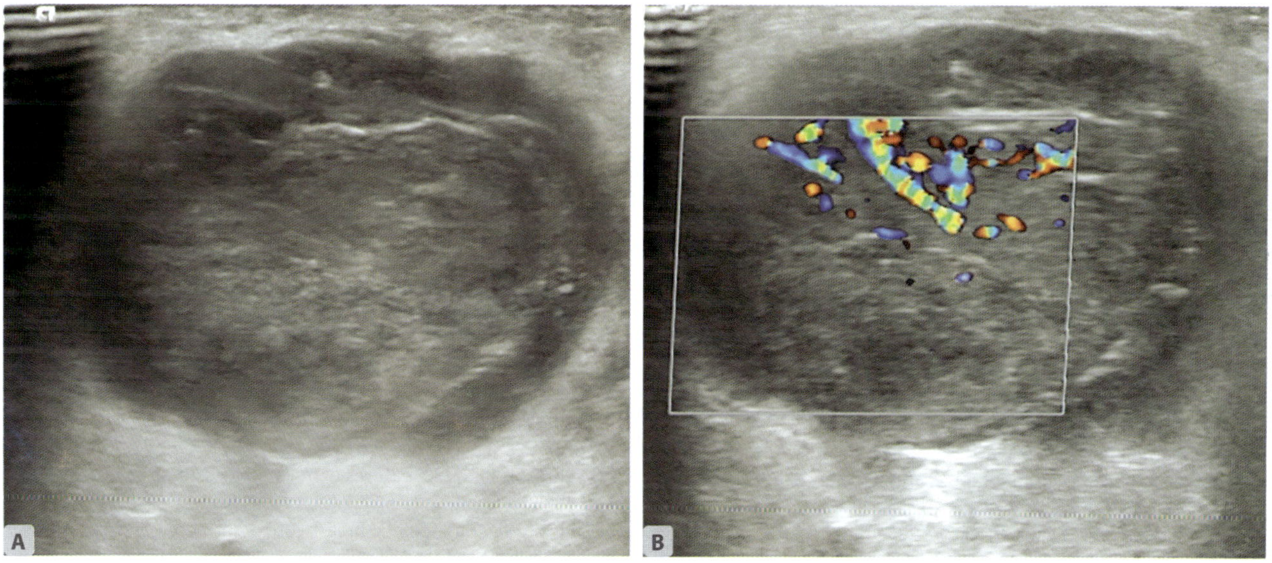

FIGS. 11A AND B: Ultrasonography of breast in an elderly male with generalized lymphadenopathy and painless breast lump, showing a well-defined, lobulated, heteroechoic lesion showing florid internal vascularity. Tissue sampling showed it to be a lymphomatous deposit.

Dermatofibrosarcoma

Dermatofibrosarcoma, also known as spindle cell tumor of the breast, is characterized by a locally aggressive slow-growing mass. Its occurrence is more common in males in the second to fifth decades as compared to females. These lesions appear as ill-defined high-density masses on mammography, and on ultrasonography, they are seen as lobulated echogenic or mixed density masses. Complete surgical resection is indicated as it has high recurrence rates.[12]

Multiple Myeloma

Multiple myeloma involving the breast is very rare, and involvement may be as a part of disseminated disease, or in the form of a solitary plasmacytoma of the breast. Also, the most common cause of a new breast mass in cases of multiple myeloma is carcinoma breast. Myeloma lesions of the breast are well-defined, solid masses that may appear hypoechoic or anechoic on ultrasonography due to good transmission of echoes.

Glomus Tumors

Glomus tumors arise from the specialized neurovascular organ known as the glomus body. Breast is an unusual site of presentation, and very few case reports are available in the literature. These lesions tend to present as chronic breast pain with pinpoint severe tenderness, increasing in cold temperatures. On imaging, they are seen as tender, well-defined, superficially situated hypervascular masses. They are treated by surgical excision. They show high recurrence rates after surgery.

Inflammatory Myofibroblastic Tumor

Inflammatory myofibroblastic tumor, very rarely, involves the breast and has intermediate malignant potential. They present with a nonspecific lump adherent to the skin. Imaging features are nonspecific.

Metastasis

Metastasis to the breast is very rare, and the most common extramammary cancers metastasizing to the breast are from melanoma, carcinomas of the gastrointestinal tract, lung, thyroid, urogenital tract, and prostate. They present as well-defined solid masses, which may show necrosis and dystrophic calcification. On ultrasonography, they are seen as well-defined homogeneously hypoechoic masses with no significant changes in the surrounding tissues.

CONCLUSION

- Though the male breast is rudimentary anatomically and nonfunctional physiologically, a wide spectrum of diseases occurs in the male breast.
- The most common abnormality of male breast is gynecomastia, which is the proliferation of ducts and stroma and classically presents as a soft mobile mass in subareolar location. It is tender and reversible in the acute florid phase but not in the chronic fibrotic phase.
- The dictum is that any gynecomastia must be subareolar, and any mass which is not subareolar does not fit into gynecomastia.
- As in women, there is no lobular proliferation in men; hence tumors of lobular origin like fibroadenoma, phyllode tumors, invasive lobular carcinomas are extremely rare.
- Myofibroblastoma is the only breast mass that occurs more frequently in men than in women.
- Male breast cancer has similar imaging appearance as that in women. It may appear as a taller than wider, spiculated mass, eccentric to the nipple, in contrast to gynecomastia which is central (subareolar). Invasive ductal cancer is the most common subtype. Calcifications are less frequently seen with male breast cancer, but when seen are coarser, and on imaging look like benign calcifications of the female breast.
- For male breast, the rule of thumb is that if imaging appearance is not fitting into normal or benign findings, biopsy should be performed.

REFERENCES

1. Iuanow E, Kettler M, Slanetz PJ. Spectrum of disease in the male breast. Am J Roentgenol. 2011;196:W247-59.
2. Nguyen C, Kettler MD, Swirsky ME, Miller VI, Scott C, Krause R, et al. Male breast disease: pictorial review with radiologic-pathologic correlation. Radiographics. 2013;33:763-79.
3. Draghi F, Tarantino CC, Madonia L, Ferrozzi G. Ultrasonography of the male breast. J Ultrasound. 2011;14:122-9.
4. Popli MB, Popli V, Bahl P, Solanki Y. Pictorial essay: mammography of the male breast. Indian J Radiol Imaging. 2009;19:278-81.
5. Günhan-Bilgen I, Bozkaya H, Ustün EE, Memiş A. Male breast disease: clinical, mammographic, and ultrasonographic features. Eur J Radiol. 2002;43:246-55.
6. Appelbaum AH, Evans GF, Levy KR, Amirkhan RH, Schumpert TD. Mammographic appearances of male breast disease. Radiographics. 1999;19:559-68.
7. Mathew J, Perkins GH, Stephens T, Middleton LP, Yang WT. Primary breast cancer in men: clinical, imaging, and pathologic findings in 57 patients. Am J Roentgenol. 2008;191:1631-9.
8. Yitta S, Singer CI, Toth HB, Mercado CL. Image presentation. Sonographic appearances of benign and malignant male breast disease with mammographic and pathologic correlation. J Ultrasound Med. 2010;29:931-47.
9. Muñoz Carrasco R, Álvarez Benito M, Rivin del Campo E. Value of mammography and breast ultrasound in male patients with nipple discharge. Eur J Radiol. 2013;82:478-84.
10. Yuan WH, Li AF, Chou YH, Hsu HC, Chen YY. Clinical and ultrasonographic features of male breast tumors: a retrospective analysis. PLoS One. 2018;13(3):e0194651.
11. Block WD, Muradali D. Breast cancer in men. Can Med Assoc J. 2013;185:1247.
12. Chen L, Chantra PK, Larsen LH, Barton P, Rohitopakarn M, Zhu EQ, et al. Imaging characteristics of malignant lesions of the male breast. Radiographics. 2006;26:993-1006.

AIIMS-MAMC-PGI's

Comprehensive Textbook of

DIAGNOSTIC RADIOLOGY

AIIMS-MAMC-PGI's

Comprehensive Textbook of DIAGNOSTIC RADIOLOGY

Third Edition

VOLUME 4

- Neuroradiology Including Head and Neck Imaging

Editors

Manavjit Singh Sandhu MD FICR CCST (UK)
Professor and Head
Department of Radiodiagnosis
Postgraduate Institute of
Medical Education and Research
Chandigarh, India

Arun Kumar Gupta MD FAMS
Professor and Head
Department of Radiodiagnosis
All India Institute of Medical Sciences
New Delhi, India

Anju Garg MD
Director Professor and Head
Department of Radiodiagnosis
Maulana Azad Medical College
New Delhi, India

JAYPEE

JAYPEE BROTHERS MEDICAL PUBLISHERS

The Health Sciences Publisher

New Delhi | London

Jaypee Brothers Medical Publishers (P) Ltd

Headquarter

Jaypee Brothers Medical Publishers (P) Ltd
4838/24, Ansari Road, Daryaganj
New Delhi 110 002, India
Phone: +91-11-43574357
Fax: +91-11-43574314
Email: jaypee@jaypeebrothers.com

Overseas Office

J.P. Medical Ltd
83 Victoria Street, London
SW1H 0HW (UK)
Phone: +44 20 3170 8910
Fax: +44 (0)20 3008 6180
Email: info@jpmedpub.com

Website: www.jaypeebrothers.com
Website: www.jaypeedigital.com

Inquiries for bulk sales may be solicited at: jaypee@jaypeebrothers.com

AIIMS-MAMC-PGI's Comprehensive Textbook of Diagnostic Radiology, ***Third Edition (Volumes 1 to 4)*** / *Arun Kumar Gupta, Anju Garg, Manavjit Singh Sandhu*

First Edition: 2016
Second Edition: 2019
Third Edition: 2021
Reprint: **2024**

ISBN: 978-93-90595-55-6

Printed at: Sanat Printers

ASSOCIATE EDITORS

VOLUME 1

Section 1: Genitourinary Imaging

Gaurav Shanker Pradhan DMRD DNB
Director Professor
Department of Radiodiagnosis
Maulana Azad Medical College
New Delhi, India

Alpana Manchanda MD
Director Professor
Department of Radiodiagnosis
Maulana Azad Medical College
New Delhi, India

Sapna Singh MD DNB MNAMS
Professor
Department of Radiodiagnosis
Maulana Azad Medical College
New Delhi, India

Section 2: Advances in Imaging Technology

Sanjay Sharma MD DNB MNAMS FRCR FICR
Professor
Department of Radiodiagnosis
(RP Center division)
All India Institute of Medical Sciences
New Delhi, India

Atin Kumar MD DNB MNAMS FICR
Professor
Department of Radiodiagnosis
(Trauma Centre Division)
All India Institute of Medical Sciences
New Delhi, India

Shivanand Gamanagatti MD MNAMS FICR
Professor
Department of Radiodiagnosis
(Trauma Centre Division)
All India Institute of Medical Sciences
New Delhi, India

VOLUME 2

Section 3: Paediatric Imaging

Ashu Seith Bhalla MD MAMS FICR
Professor
Department of Radiodiagnosis
All India Institute of Medical Sciences
New Delhi, India

Manisha Jana MD DNB FRCR
Additional Professor
Department of Radiodiagnosis
All India Institute of Medical Sciences
New Delhi, India

Devasenathipathy Kandasamy MD DNB FRCR
Additional Professor
Department of Radiodiagnosis
All India Institute of Medical Sciences
New Delhi, India

Priyanka Naranje MD DNB MNAMS
Associate Professor
Department of Radiodiagnosis
All India Institute of Medical Sciences
New Delhi, India

Section 4: Gastrointestinal and Hepatobiliary Imaging

Deep Narayan Srivastava MD MBA FAMS FICR
Professor
Department of Radiodiagnosis
All India Institute of Medical Sciences
New Delhi, India

Raju Sharma MD MAMS FICR
Professor
Department of Radiodiagnosis
All India Institute of Medical Sciences
New Delhi, India

VOLUME 3

Section 5: Chest and Cardiovascular Imaging

Sanjiv Sharma MD
Professor and Head
Department of Cardiovascular Radiology and Endovascular Interventions
CN Centre
All India Institute of Medical Sciences
New Delhi, India

Rashmi Dixit MD
Director Professor
Department of Radiodiagnosis
Maulana Azad Medical College
New Delhi, India

Section 6: Musculoskeletal and Breast Imaging

Mahesh Prakash MD MAMS FIACM FICR
Professor
Department of Radiodiagnosis
Postgraduate Institute of Medical Education and Research
Chandigarh, India

Anindita Sinha MD MAMS
Additional Professor
Department of Radiodiagnosis
Postgraduate Institute of Medical Education and Research
Chandigarh, India

VOLUME 4

Section 7: Neuroradiology Including Head and Neck Imaging

Paramjeet Singh MD FICR
Professor
Department of Radiodiagnosis
Postgraduate Institute of Medical Education and Research
Chandigarh, India

Shailesh B Gaikwad MD FNAMS CCST
Professor and Head
Department of Neuroimaging and Interventional Neuroradiology (CN Centre)
All India Institute of Medical Sciences
New Delhi, India

Vivek Gupta MD DM
Former Professor
Department of Radiodiagnosis
Postgraduate Institute of Medical Education and Research
Chandigarh, India

Ajay Garg MD
Professor
Department of Neuroimaging and Interventional Neuroradiology (CN Centre)
All India Institute of Medical Sciences
New Delhi, India

CONTRIBUTORS

Ajay Garg MD (Radiodiagnosis) Eur Dip in Neuroradiology (EDiNR) Eur Dip in Pediatric Neuroradiology (EDiPNR)
Professor, Department of Neuroimaging and Interventional Neuroradiology
CN Centre
All India Institute of Medical Sciences
New Delhi, India

Ajay Gulati MD MAMS
Additional Professor
Department of Radiodiagnosis
Postgraduate Institute of Medical Education and Research, Chandigarh, India

Ajay Kumar MD
Professor
Department of Radiodiagnosis
Postgraduate Institute of Medical Education and Research, Chandigarh, India

Akshay Kumar Saxena MD DNB FICR
Professor
Department of Radiodiagnosis
Postgraduate Institute of Medical Education and Research, Chandigarh, India

Alpana Manchanda MD
Director Professor
Department of Radiodiagnosis
Maulana Azad Medical College
New Delhi, India

Anil Kumar Pandey MSc PhD
Associate Professor (Medical Physics)
Department of Nuclear Medicine and PET
All India Institute of Medical Sciences
New Delhi, India

Anindita Sinha MD MAMS
Additional Professor
Department of Radiodiagnosis
Postgraduate Institute of Medical Education and Research
Chandigarh, India

Anjali Prakash DMRD DNB MNAMS
Director Professor
Department of Radiodiagnosis
Maulana Azad Medical College
New Delhi, India

Anju Garg MD
Director Professor and Head
Department of Radiodiagnosis
Maulana Azad Medical College
New Delhi, India

Ankur Goyal MD DNB MNAMS
Associate Professor
Department of Radiodiagnosis
All India Institute of Medical Sciences
New Delhi, India

Anmol Bhatia MD FPGI (Paediatric Radiology)
Assistant Professor
Department of Radiodiagnosis and Imaging
Postgraduate Institute of Medical Education and Research
Chandigarh, India

Anuj Prabhakar DNB DM (Neuroradiology)
Assistant Professor
Postgraduate Institute of Medical Education and Research
Chandigarh, India

Anupam Lal MD
Professor
Department of Radiodiagnosis
Postgraduate Institute of Medical Education and Research
Chandigarh, India

Arun Kumar Gupta MD FAMS
Professor and Head
Department of Radiodiagnosis
All India Institute of Medical Sciences
New Delhi, India

Ashu Seith Bhalla MD MAMS FICR
Professor
Department of Radiodiagnosis
All India Institute of Medical Sciences
New Delhi, India

Atin Kumar MD DNB MNAMS FICR
Professor
Department of Radiodiagnosis
(Trauma Center Division)
All India Institute of Medical Sciences
New Delhi, India

Chandan J Das MD DNB MAMS FICR FRCP
Additional Professor
Department of Radiodiagnosis
All India Institute of Medical Sciences
New Delhi, India

Chandrashekhara SH MD DNB MNAMS
Additional Professor
Department of Radiodiagnosis
Dr BRA Institute—Rotary Cancer Hospital
All India Institute of Medical Sciences
New Delhi, India

Chirag Kamal Ahuja MD DM (Neuroradiology)
Associate Professor
Department of Radiodiagnosis and Imaging
Postgraduate Institute of Medical Education and Research
Chandigarh, India

Deep Narayan Srivastava MD MBA FAMS FICR
Professor
Department of Radiodiagnosis
All India Institute of Medical Sciences
New Delhi, India

Devasenathipathy Kandasamy MD DNB FRCR
Additional Professor
Department of Radiodiagnosis
All India Institute of Medical Sciences
New Delhi, India

Ekta Dhamija MD
Associate Professor
Department of Radiodiagnosis
Dr BRA Institute—Rotary Cancer Hospital
All India Institute of Medical Sciences
New Delhi, India

Gaurav Shanker Pradhan DMRD DNB
Director Professor
Department of Radiodiagnosis
Maulana Azad Medical College
New Delhi, India

Gita Devi MD DNB
Assistant Professor
Department of Radiodiagnosis
Postgraduate Institute of Medical Education and Research
Chandigarh, India

Gurpreet Singh Gulati MD
Former Professor
Department of Cardiac Radiology
Cardio-Thoracic Sciences Centre
All India Institute of Medical Sciences
New Delhi, India

Harish Bhujade MD FVIR
Assistant Professor
Department of Radiodiagnosis
Postgraduate Institute of Medical Education and Research
Chandigarh, India

Jyoti Kumar MD DNB MNAMS FICR
Professor
Department of Radiodiagnosis
Maulana Azad Medical College
New Delhi, India

Kartik Ganga MD
Fellow
Department of Cardiovascular Radiology and Endovascular Interventions
All India Institute of Medical Sciences
New Delhi, India

Kirti Gupta MD, Neuropathology Fellowship (St Jude, USA)
Professor
Department of Histopathology
Postgraduate Institute of Medical Education and Research
Chandigarh, India

Kumble S Madhusudhan MD FRCR MAMS
Additional Professor
Department of Radiodiagnosis
All India Institute of Medical Sciences
New Delhi, India

Kushaljit Singh Sodhi MD PhD MAMS FICR
Professor
Department of Radiodiagnosis
Postgraduate Institute of Medical Education and Research
Chandigarh, India

Madhavi Tripathi MD DNB (Nuclear Medicine)
Additional Professor
Department of Nuclear Medicine and PET
All India Institute of Medical Sciences
New Delhi, India

Madhusudhan KS MD MAMS FRCR
Additional Professor
Department of Radiodiagnosis
All India Institute of Medical Sciences
New Delhi, India

Mahesh Prakash MD MAMS FIACM FICR
Professor
Department of Radiodiagnosis
Postgraduate Institute of Medical Education and Research
Chandigarh, India

Manavjit Singh Sandhu MD FICR CCST (UK)
Professor and Head
Department of Radiodiagnosis
Postgraduate Institute of Medical Education and Research
Chandigarh, India

Mandeep Garg MD FRCR
Professor
Department of Radiodiagnosis
Postgraduate Institute of Medical Education and Research
Chandigarh, India

Mandeep Kang MD MAMS FICR
Professor
Department of Radiodiagnosis
Postgraduate Institute of Medical Education and Research
Chandigarh, India

Manisha Jana MD DNB FRCR
Additional Professor
Department of Radiodiagnosis
All India Institute of Medical Sciences
New Delhi, India

Manish Modi MD DM
Professor
Department of Neurology
Postgraduate Institute of Medical Education and Research
Chandigarh, India

Manphool Singhal MD DNB MAMS FICR (India) FSCCT (USA) CMR-fellowship (London) CMR-Certification (SCMR USA and ESCVI France)
Additional Professor
Department of Radiodiagnosis
Postgraduate Institute of Medical Education and Research
Chandigarh, India

Mukesh Kumar Yadav (MD Radiodiagnosis)
Formerly Associate Professor
PGIMER, Chandigarh
Associate Professor
Department of Radiodiagnosis
All India Institute of Medical Sciences (IRCH)
New Delhi, India

Naveen Kalra MD FICR MAMS
Professor
Department of Radiodiagnosis
Postgraduate Institute of Medical Education and Research
Chandigarh, India

Nidhi Prabhakar MD DNB
Senior Research Associate
Department of Radiodiagnosis
Postgraduate Institute of Medical Education and Research
Chandigarh, India

Niraj N Pandey DM
Assistant Professor
Department of Cardiovascular Radiology and Endovascular Interventions
CN Centre
All India Institute of Medical Sciences
New Delhi, India

Niranjan Khandelwal MD Dip NBE FICR FAMS
Former Head
Department of Radiodiagnosis
Postgraduate Institute of Medical Education and Research
Chandigarh, India

Pankaj Gupta MD DNB
Assistant Professor
Department of Radiodiagnosis and Imaging
Postgraduate Institute of Medical Education and Research
Chandigarh, India

Paramjeet Singh MD FICR
Professor
Department of Radiodiagnosis
Postgraduate Institute of Medical Education and Research
Chandigarh, India

Pratik Kumar PhD (AIIMS) Dip RP (BARC)
Professor, Medical Physics Unit
BRA Institute Rotary Cancer Hospital
AIIMS, New Delhi, India

Priya Jagia MD DNB
Professor
Department of Cardiovascular Radiology and Endovascular Interventions
All India Institute of Medical Sciences
New Delhi, India

Priyanka Naranje MD DNB MNAMS
Associate Professor
Department of Radiodiagnosis
All India Institute of Medical Sciences
New Delhi, India

Punit Sharma MD
Former Senior Resident
Department of Nuclear Medicine
All India Institute of Medical Sciences
New Delhi, India

Radhika Batra MD DNB
Associate Professor
Department of Radiodiagnosis
Maulana Azad Medical College
New Delhi, India

Rajat Jain MD DNB FRCR FICR MNAMS
Assistant Professor
Department of Radiodiagnosis
Maulana Azad Medical College
New Delhi, India

Raju Sharma MD MAMS FICR
Professor
Department of Radiodiagnosis
All India Institute of Medical Sciences
New Delhi, India

Rakesh Kumar DRM DNB PhD
Professor and Head
Diagnostic Nuclear Medicine Division
Department of Nuclear Medicine and PET
All India Institute of Medical Sciences
New Delhi, India

Rakesh Kumar Vasishta MD FRCPath
Former Professor and Head
Department of Histopathology
Postgraduate Institute of Medical Education and Research
Chandigarh, India

Rashmi Dixit MD
Director Professor
Department of Radiodiagnosis
Maulana Azad Medical College
New Delhi, India

Sameer Vyas MD DM MAMS (Neuroradiology)
Additional Professor
Department of Radiodiagnosis
Postgraduate Institute of Medical Education and Research
Chandigarh, India

Sanjay Sharma MD DNB MNAMS FRCR FICR
Professor
Department of Radiodiagnosis
(Division at Rajendra Prasad Center for Ophthalmic Sciences)
All India Institute of Medical Sciences
New Delhi, India

Sanjeev Kumar MD
Associate Professor
Department of Cardiovascular Radiology and Endovascular Interventions
All India Institute of Medical Sciences
New Delhi, India

Sanjiv Sharma MD
Professor and Head
Department of Cardiovascular Radiology and Endovascular Interventions
CN Centre
All India Institute of Medical Sciences
New Delhi, India

Sapna Singh MD DNB MNAMS
Professor
Department of Radiodiagnosis
Maulana Azad Medical College
New Delhi, India

Satyam DNB MNAMS
Specialist
Department of Radiodiagnosis
Lok Nayak Hospital and Associated Maulana Azad Medical College
New Delhi, India

Shailesh B Gaikwad MD FNAMS CCST
Professor and Head
Department of Neuroimaging and Interventional Neuroradiology
CN Centre
All India Institute of Medical Sciences
New Delhi, India

Shamim Ahmed Shamim MD (Nuclear Medicine)
Associate Professor
Department of Nuclear Medicine
All India Institute of Medical Sciences
New Delhi, India

Shashi Bala Paul PhD MAMS
Senior Scientist
Department of Radiodiagnosis
All India Institute of Medical Sciences
New Delhi, India

Shivanand Gamanagatti MD MNAMS FICR
Professor
Department of Radiodiagnosis
(Trauma Center Division)
All India Institute of Medical Sciences
New Delhi, India

Smita Manchanda MD DNB MNAMS
Associate Professor
Department of Radiodiagnosis
All India Institute of Medical Sciences
New Delhi, India

Smriti Hari MD MAMS
Professor
Department of Radiodiagnosis
All India Institute of Medical Sciences
New Delhi, India

Sreedhara BC MD FVIR
Assistant Professor
Department of Radiodiagnosis
Postgraduate Institute of Medical Education and Research
Chandigarh, India

Subrat Kumar Acharya DM FNASc
FASc FNA JC Bose Fellow
Former Professor and Head
Department of Gastroenterology
All India Institute of Medical Sciences
New Delhi, India

Sudesh Prabhakar MD DM
Former Professor and Head
Department of Neurology
Postgraduate Institute of Medical
Education and Research
Chandigarh, India

Sudha Suri MD
Emeritus Professor
Department of Radiodiagnosis
Postgraduate Institute of Medical
Education and Research
Chandigarh, India

Surabhi Vyas MD DNB MNAMS
Additional Professor
Department of Radiodiagnosis
All India Institute of Medical Sciences
New Delhi, India

Swati Gupta MD DNB FRCR
Associate Professor
Department of Radiodiagnosis
Maulana Azad Medical College
New Delhi, India

Tulika Singh MD
Additional Professor
Department of Radiodiagnosis
Postgraduate Institute of Medical
Education and Research
Chandigarh, India

Ujjwal Gorsi (MD Radiodiagnosis)
Associate Professor
Department of Radiodiagnosis
Postgraduate Institute of Medical
Education and Research
Chandigarh, India

Uma Debi MD
Associate Professor
Department of Radiodiagnosis
Postgraduate Institute of Medical
Education and Research
Chandigarh, India

Veenu Singla MD
Professor
Department of Radiodiagnosis
Postgraduate Institute of Medical
Education and Research
Chandigarh, India

Vikas Bhatia MD DNB
DM (Neuroradiology)
Assistant Professor
Department of Radiodiagnosis
Postgraduate Institute of Medical
Education and Research
Chandigarh, India

Vineeta Ojha MD DNB
DM Senior Resident
Department of Cardiovascular Radiology
and Endovascular Interventions
All India Institute of Medical Sciences
New Delhi, India

Virendra Jain MD FRCR
Former Senior Resident
Department of Radiodiagnosis
Maulana Azad Medical College
New Delhi, India

Vivek Gupta MD DM
Former Professor
Department of Radiodiagnosis
Postgraduate Institute of Medical
Education and Research
Chandigarh, India

PREFACE TO THE THIRD EDITION

In 1996, a unique venture was jointly initiated by the faculty of Radiodiagnosis, All India Institute of Medical Sciences (AIIMS), New Delhi; Maulana Azad Medical College (MAMC), New Delhi; and Postgraduate Institute of Medical Education and Research (PGIMER), Chandigarh, India, to organize continuing medical education (CME) programs based on a series of imaging courses. An integral part of this endeavour was publishing books covering all organ systems. The aim was to provide state-of-the-art knowledge for postgraduate students as well as the practicing radiologists along with establishing a uniform pattern of teaching in radiology across the country.

The first series of seven imaging courses was successfully completed in the year 2000. A second series of these courses was then initiated in the year 2002 and was completed in 2004. This was also highly successful. The third series of seven extremely popular and successful courses covering all the organ systems and advances in physics was started in 2008 and was completed in 2013. The fourth series started in 2016 and was completed successfuly in 2020.

Every course in each of the series has resulted in publication of a book. These books have been very popular amongst residents as well as among practicing radiologists.

Considering the popularity of these books, the editors, along with publishers, M/s Jaypee Brothers Medical Publishers (P) Ltd, New Delhi, India, had decided to combine the individual course books into three volumes— *"AIIMS-MAMC-PGI's Comprehensive Textbook of Diagnostic Radiology"*. Its first edition was released in 2016.

In keeping pace with newer developments in the field of diagnostic radiology and in order to cater to the contemporary needs of users, the second edition of *"AIIMS-MAMC-PGI's Comprehensive Textbook of Diagnostic Radiology"* was presented in 2019 after a gap of three years. It was anticipated that with such a complete coverage of all the subjects, the users will not have to refer to any other book during their routine learning of diagnostic radiology.

However by the time fourth AIIMS MAMC PGI Imaging course series was near completion in early 2021, it was felt that there is a very strong need for updating of second edition along with addition of new chapters in view of rapid advancement of knowledge in the last few years. So third edition was planned. It was also agreed that in view of increasing size of individual course books and to keep the size of individual volumes of the Textbook handy and managable the whole textbook should be divided into four volumes from its current three volumes.

We are sure that residents and radiologists will find these comprehensive four volumes easy to handle and very useful in day-to-day practice.

We are once again grateful to all the contributors from the three apex academic institutions of India, i.e. AIIMS, New Delhi; MAMC, New Delhi; and PGIMER, Chandigarh, India.

We are thankful to M/s Jaypee Brothers Medical Publishers (P) Ltd, for helping us to make our dream come true.

Arun Kumar Gupta
Anju Garg
Manavjit Singh Sandhu

PREFACE TO THE FIRST EDITION

In 1996, a unique venture was jointly initiated by the faculty of radiodiagnosis at All India Institute of Medical Sciences, Maulana Azad Medical College, New Delhi, and Postgraduate Institute of Medical Education and Research, Chandigarh, India, to organize continuing medical education programs based on a series of imaging courses. An integral part of this endeavor was publishing books covering all organ systems. The aim was to provide state of the art knowledge for postgraduate students as well as the practicing radiologists along with establishing a uniform pattern of teaching in radiology across the country.

The first series of seven imaging courses was successfully completed in the year 2000. A second series of these courses was then initiated in the year 2002 and was completed in 2004. This was also highly successful.

With the great success of the second series, we, the current editors, decided to start a third series of these courses in 2008. Seven extremely popular and successful courses covering all the organ systems and advances in physics were completed in 2013.

Every course in each of the three series have resulted in publication of a book. These books have been very popular amongst residents as well as among practicing radiologists.

Considering the popularity of these books, we, the three current editors, along with publishers M/s Jaypee Brothers Medical Publishers (P) Ltd., decided to combine the individual books published so far into a "*AIIMS-MAMC-PGI's Comprehensive Textbook of Diagnostic Radiology*" with three volumes.

We are very happy to see the end result of this great effort.

We are sure that residents and radiologists will find these comprehensive three volumes easy to handle and very useful in day-to-day practice.

We are once again grateful to all the contributors from the three apex academic institutions of India, i.e. AIIMS, MAMC, New Delhi and PGIMER, Chandigarh, India.

We are thankful to M/s Jaypee Brothers Medical Publishers (P) Ltd., for helping us to make our dream come true.

Niranjan Khandelwal
Veena Chowdhury
Arun Kumar Gupta

ACKNOWLEDGMENTS

We would like to put on record our deep appreciation and gratitude:

To Professors Manorama Berry, Sudha Suri and Veena Chowdhury (Past Editors) the three pioneers who in 1996 took a bold initiative and started a unique teaching course now popularly known as AIIMS-MAMC-PGI's imaging course. By October 2020, four series, each series comprising of seven courses, have been completed. This course series has become extremely popular and every course is followed by the publication of a book which too is highly appreciated and popular.

To Professors Sima Mukhopadhyay, Sushma Vashisht and Niranjan Khandelwal who have been the Editors of past series and who contributed to organizing the earlier courses in their capacity as Heads of Departments.

To all the Associate Editors of the different course books who put in immense effort to bring the books out on time.

To all the Authors who contributed chapters without whom we could not have collected such an outstanding content of teaching and academic material.

To our respective hospitals for giving us the privilege and unique opportunity to work, which enabled us to amass data from patients and document images of diverse diseases that provide the reader with a wide spectrum of knowledge.

Our sincere and grateful thanks to Shri Jitendar P Vij (Group Chairman), Mr Ankit Vij (Managing Director), Mr MS Mani (Group President), Dr Richa Saxena (Associate Director-Professional Publishing), Ms Nedup Denka Bhutia (Development Editor) and Other staffs of M/s Jaypee Brothers Medical Publishers (P) Ltd, New Delhi, India, for their untiring coordination efforts in the production of this book.

We are very proud indeed at the culmination of two decades of these course series, to compile and present them together in the form of these four volumes of "*AIIMS-MAMC-PGI's Comprehensive Textbook of Diagnostic Radiology*".

Arun Kumar Gupta
Anju Garg
Manavjit Singh Sandhu

CONTENTS

VOLUME 1

Section 1: Genitourinary Imaging

Section 2: Advances in Imaging Technology

VOLUME 2

Section 3: Paediatric Imaging

Section 4: Gastrointestinal and Hepatobiliary Imaging

VOLUME 3

Section 5: Chest and Cardiovascular Imaging

Section 6: Musculoskeletal and Breast Imaging

VOLUME 4

Section 7: Neuroradiology Including Head and Neck Imaging

SECTION

7

Neuroradiology Including Head and Neck Imaging

- Evaluation of Plain X-ray Skull: A Systematic Approach
- Normal Anatomy of Brain on CT and MRI
- Normal Cerebral Angiography
- Advances in Neuroimaging Techniques: Computed Tomography
- Advances in Neuroimaging Techniques: Magnetic Resonance Imaging
- Magnetic Resonance Spectroscopy
- Functional MRI
- Imaging and Interventions in Cerebral Ischemia
- Imaging of Subarachnoid Hemorrhage
- Endovascular Management of Intracranial Aneurysms
- Endovascular Management of Arteriovenous Malformations
- Carotid-cavernous Fistulas
- Central Nervous System Infections
- Imaging of White Matter Disease
- Imaging of Epilepsy
- Imaging of Supratentorial Brain Tumors
- Imaging of Infratentorial Tumors
- Sellar and Parasellar Lesions
- Intraventricular Lesions
- Imaging of the Temporal Bone
- Imaging of the Globe and Orbit
- Imaging of the Paranasal Sinuses
- Imaging of the Neck Spaces
- Thyroid Imaging
- Malignancies of Upper Aerodigestive Tract
- Imaging of Skull Base Lesions
- Maxillofacial Imaging: Imaging of Cysts, Tumors and Tumor-like Conditions of the Jaw
- Craniovertebral Junction Anomalies
- Endovascular Management of Craniofacial Vascular Lesions
- Imaging of Head Trauma
- Imaging of Facial Trauma
- Imaging of Acute Spinal Trauma
- Spinal Neoplasm
- Spinal Vascular Malformations
- Imaging of Low Backache
- Localization in Clinical Neurology
- Basic Neuropathology

CHAPTER

181

Evaluation of Plain X-ray Skull: A Systematic Approach

Niranjan Khandelwal, Sudha Suri, Vikas Bhatia

INTRODUCTION

In the past, skull radiograph was considered an essential step in the investigative protocol of a patient suspected to have a neurological disease. With the introduction of computed tomography (CT) and magnetic resonance imaging (MRI), there has been a tremendous decline in the usage of plain films and the indications for skull radiographs have been redefined.[1,2] The major indication for skull radiographs is in the evaluation of skeletal dysplasia, diagnostic survey in abuse, abnormal head shapes, infections and tumors affecting the skull bones, metabolic bone disease, leukemia and multiple myeloma. Abnormalities in skull radiographs may be seen in the form of change in the size, density and shape of the skull, as well as the other defects of the skull. In patients presenting with stroke, epilepsy, dementia or in postoperative cases, skull X-rays generally provide no useful information and MRI or CT is the investigation of choice.[3] In patients of trauma, CT should be the first line of investigation except in patients who suffer from facial and orbital fractures where plain films are helpful in orientation and in medicolegal cases.[4-6] Occasionally, skull X-rays may reveal linear fractures with more certainty than a CT scan.[4] In patients suspected to have intracerebral tumors, posteroanterior (PA) and lateral view of skull may provide additional information like detection of hyperostosis in case of meningiomas, presence of lytic and sclerotic metastasis in neuroblastomas and tram-track calcification in Sturge-Weber syndrome which may compliment the diagnosis on CT. The present chapter will describe the normal roentgen anatomy as seen in the basic views of skull followed by systematic approach to the analysis of the abnormal skull X-rays.[7-9]

An overview of the basic X-rays of skull is shown in **Table 1**.

LATERAL VIEW OF SKULL

A single lateral view of the skull **(Fig. 1A)** is the most common radiographic X-ray examination to be performed. A systematic approach to the examination consists of evaluation of the size and shape of the cranium, the thickness and density of the bones, the sutures, the vascular markings, the base of skull and the cranial cavity.

Size and shape of the skull is determined by examining the relative size of face and cranium. When the skull is longer and has a relatively shorter vertical diameter, it is referred to as *dolichocephalic*. On the other hand, when the vertical diameter is greater, it is termed as *brachycephalic*. The outer table, the inner table and the diploic space of the bones should be carefully examined for presence of any erosion, sclerosis or widening.

The normal sutures in adults are surrounded by a narrow area of increased density, a fact that helps in distinguishing fracture lines from sutures. Sutures are difficult to visualize in newborns but in children older than 3 years, the width of the suture should not be more than 2 mm. Width of the sutures can be best assessed at the top of the coronal suture in the lateral view. To see the sagittal and the lambdoid sutures, PA and Towne's views are performed. Vascular markings are seen along the coronal suture due to middle meningeal vessels. Arterial grooves become narrower as they go distally. They may be confused with fracture lines but the latter are more radiolucent whereas vascular markings have a halo of increased density around them. Posterior branch of middle meningeal artery as it ascends upward and posteriorly sometimes causes a shadow over the temporal bone that should not be mistaken for a fracture. Enlargement of the arterial grooves may occur in meningioma and arteriovenous malformations **(Fig. 1B)**.

Diploic venous channels are extremely variable in position but are generally seen in the frontal and parietal bones. Venous lakes may be seen as round or oval radiolucent areas and should not be confused with destructive lesions of the bone. Besides the arterial and diploic venous channels, the dural sinuses also produce grooves on the inner table of the skull.

The structures along the base of the skull should be carefully examined, in particular the three lines which represent the floor of the anterior cranial fossa. The upper two lines are formed by the roofs of the orbits, which end posteriorly at the anterior clinoid processes. The lower line

TABLE 1: Overview of the skull X-ray views.

View	Patient positioning	Acquisition	Optimum view	Indications/information provided
Lateral view	• Patient seated or standing • Affected side next to the bucky • Interpupillary line perpendicular to film and tube • Mid sagittal plane parallel to film	• Horizontal CR (central ray): ¾" superior to EAM • Vertical CR: ¾ "anterior to EAM	• Entire skull should be on the film • No rotation • Overlapping of ramus of mandible and orbits	• Most common radiographic X-ray of skull • Overview of the entire skull • Sella, clivus, anterior cranial fossa • Calcifications, suture, vascular markings, fractures
Towne view	• Position patients chin bringing the OML (orbitomeatal line) perpendicular to IR (image receptor) • Align midsagittal plane to CR	• Angle the CR 30 degrees • Center at two and a half inches above glabella. To pass through foramen magnum	• Ensure that the skull is straight with no rotation, include the entire skull in the field of view	• Occipital bone, foramen magnum, dorsum sellae, the internal acoustic canals, mastoids and the condyles of mandible
Caldwell view	• Place the patient's nose and forehead against the IR • Flex the neck as needed to align the OML perpendicular to IR • Align the midsagittal plane to the midline of the grid in order to avoid rotation or tilt	• Angle 15 degrees caudal and center as to exit the nasion	• No rotation	• Frontal and ethmoid sinuses • Supraorbital rim fractures
Frontal view	• Place the patient's nose and forehead against the IR • Flex the neck as needed to align the OML perpendicular to IR • Align the midsagittal plane to the midline of the grid in order to avoid rotation or tilt	• Center the CR as to exit the Nasion.	• No rotation	• Skull fractures • Superior orbital fissure • Greater and lesser wings of the sphenoid
Submentovertex view	• Tilt the patient's head back bringing the chin up until the inferior OML is parallel to the IR. • Be aware of any suspected cervical spine injury before performing this view. • Align the midsagittal plane perpendicular to the IR	• CR is perpendicular to the inferior OML, center 1 and a half inch inferior to the mandibular symphysis	• No rotation	• Foramen ovale • Foramen spinosum • Foramen lacerum • Specific situations such as looking for the skull base lesions, middle ear or inner ear lesions, nasopharyngeal masses or oropharyngeal lesions and sinus pathologies
Waters' view	• Patient seated close to bucky • Mentomeatal line perpendicular to film (closed mouth) • Mouth can be opened for sphenoid sinus (cantho-meatal line 35-40 degree to bucky)	• Horizontal CR exit through base of nose • Vertical CR mid sagittal	• Facial bones and sinus on the film • No rotation • Petrous ridges below floor of maxilla	• Sinus diseases • Injury to maxilla and orbit

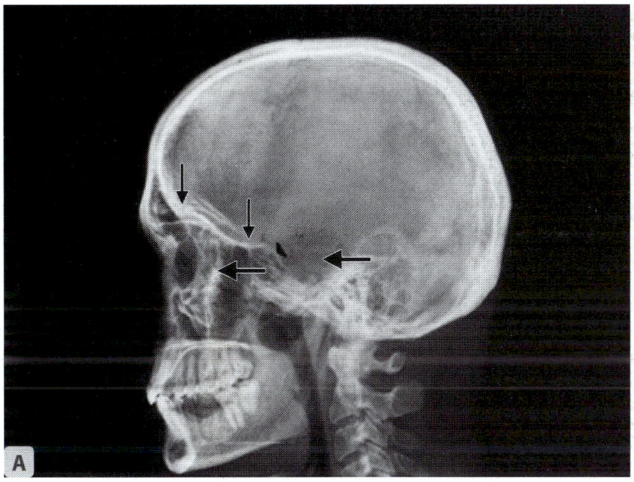

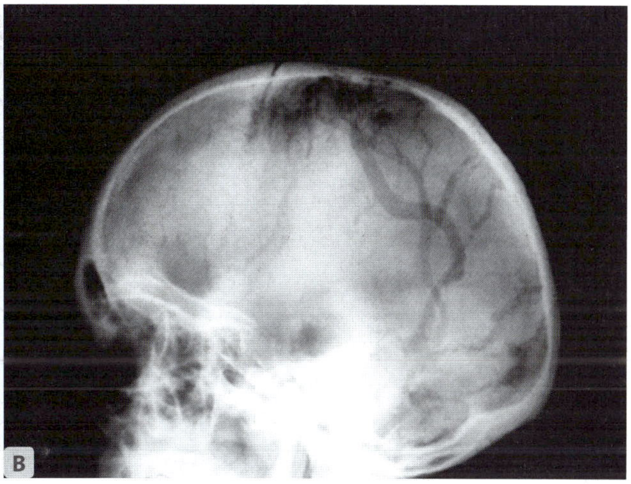

FIGS. 1A AND B: (A) Normal lateral view of skull demonstrates the normal coronal sutures, lambdoid sutures and the vascular grooves due to middle meningeal vessels posterior to coronal sutures. Note the two lines formed by the roof of the orbits ending posteriorly at the anterior clinoid processes. Arrow head marks the tuberculum sellae. Vertical arrows (anterior) show the cribriform plate and the (posterior) planum sphenoidale. Anterior horizontal arrow shows the greater wing of sphenoid bone forming anterior borders of middle cranial fossa. The dorsum sellae (horizontal arrows) with posterior clinoid processes above and the clivus posteriorly are well seen; (B) Lateral view of skull shows multiple dilated vascular markings in the parieto-occipital region in a case of parasagittal meningioma.

is formed anteriorly by the cribriform plate of the ethmoid bone and posteriorly by planum sphenoidale ending at the tuberculum sellae, which marks the superior limit of the anterior wall of the sella turcica. A depression just anterior to the tuberculum sellae is called sulcus chiasmaticus. The roof of the sella posteriorly is formed by the dorsum sellae, which ends in the posterior clinoid processes. Sphenoid sinus is seen below the floor of the sella turcica. The pneumatization of this sinus shows considerable variation. Floor of the middle cranial fossa is formed by the greater wings of the sphenoid on each side, which appear as curvilinear shadows concave outward. These lines serve as a point of reference for locating the temporal lobe of the brain. The dorsum sellae continues as the clivus, which is followed by the occipital bone ending at the anterior margin of the foramen magnum. Clivus is seen to terminate just above the top of the odontoid process of the axis. The normal calcification may be seen in the falx cerebri, petroclinoid ligaments, tentorium, pineal body, habenular commissure and choroid plexus.

FRONTAL VIEW (FIG. 2)

Posteroanterior projection with 15-20° craniocaudal angulation is preferred to straight PA projection as the petrous pyramids are projected below the orbits and the superior orbital fissure as well as greater and lesser wings of the sphenoid are clearly visualized. PA view is also examined for shape of the skull, with special attention to the symmetry of the two sides. The bony landmarks, which require to be carefully examined for any erosions, sclerosis or lack of continuity include crista galli in the midline, planum sphenoidale, floor of the sella, lesser and greater wings of the sphenoid and the three lines of the orbit formed by the palpable superior border of orbit, highest point of roof of the orbit and the sphenoid ridge which represents the floor of the anterior cranial fossa. The floor of the posterior cranial

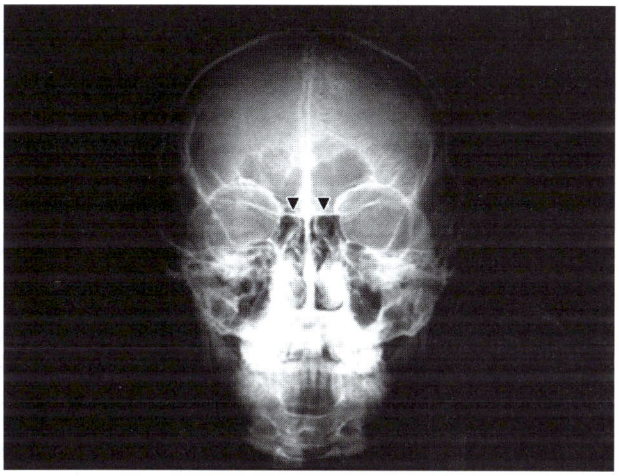

FIG. 2: Posteroanterior (PA) view with 15° caudal angulation demonstrates the dense vertical bony projection in the midline due to crista galli, lesser wings of the sphenoid on both sides joining to form the planum sphenoidale (arrow heads). Floor of sella is faintly visualized in the midline. Oblique line of the orbit is formed by the greater wing of sphenoid in its lower two-thirds and by the frontal bone in its upper one-third.

fossa can also be seen inferiorly. Pacchionian depressions due to arachnoid granulations can be seen in both PA and lateral views as tiny radiolucent areas usually within 2.5-3 cm from the midline. Their margins are well defined superiorly, whereas inferiorly the margins fade away—a feature helpful in distinguishing these from destructive lesions.

TOWNE'S VIEW

Towne's view **(Fig. 3)** is performed by angling the tube 35° caudally from the orbitomeatal line. It is generally performed when pathology is suspected in the petrous pyramids.

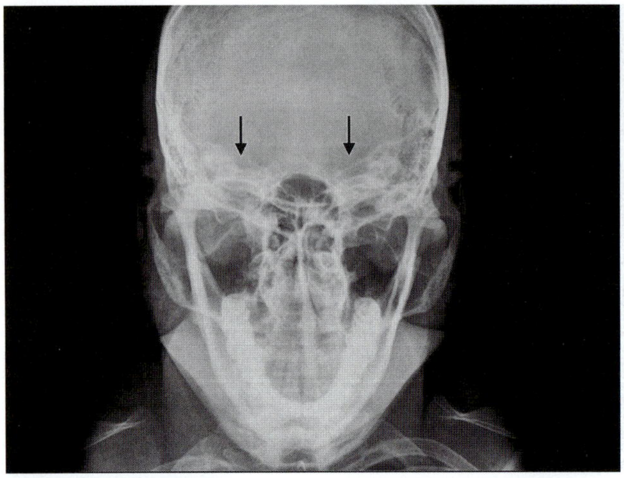

FIG. 3: Towne's view shows foramen magnum in the center with dorsum sellae projecting through it. The parallel lucencies (arrows) on either side represent the internal auditory canals. Further, laterally pneumatized mastoids air cells can also be seen.

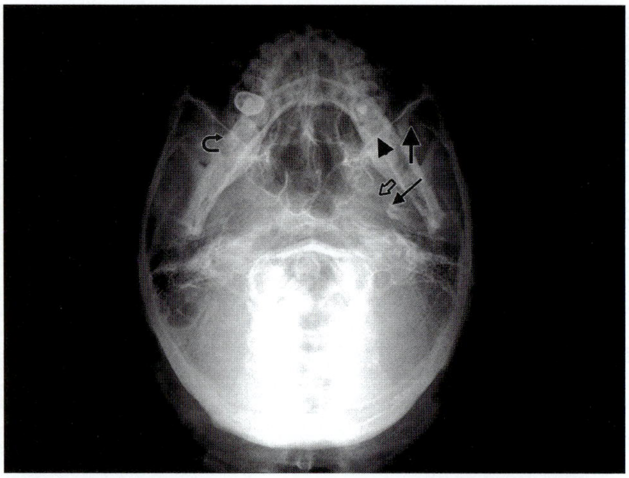

FIG. 4: Basal view of skull shows the nasopharynx, sphenoid sinus and ethmoid sinuses in the midline. Posteriorly odontoid process is seen to project into the foramen magnum posterior to the arch of atlas. Laterally, the foramen ovale (open arrow), foramen spinosum, (long arrow), Eustachian tube posterior to foramen spinosum and the carotid canal are well visualized. Anterolaterally, the three lines formed by the posterior wall of orbit (arrow head), maxillary sinus (S-shaped) (curved arrow) and the anterior wall of middle cranial fossa (thick arrow) (arched shadow with concavity posteriorly) should be looked for in each case. Medial and lateral pterygoid plates are well seen.

This projection also shows the occipital bone, foramen magnum, dorsum sellae, the internal acoustic canals, mastoids and the condyles of mandible.

BASAL VIEW

Basal view **(Fig. 4)** of the skull or the submentovertical view is an infrequent examination and is generally performed in specific situations such as looking for the skull base lesions, middle ear or inner ear lesions, nasopharyngeal masses or oropharyngeal lesions and sinus pathologies. The bony landmarks that should always be identified and carefully examined include three lines, constituted by the lateral wall of the maxillary antrum (S-shaped), the posterolateral wall of the orbit, and the anterior wall of the middle cranial fossa which is arched with concavity pointing posteriorly. The lesser wing of the sphenoid is seen just behind the anterior wall of middle cranial fossa. A transverse dense line in the center represents the anterior margin of sella. The medial and lateral pterygoid processes are projected over the sphenoid ridge. Sphenoid sinuses should be carefully seen as early bone destruction in patients of nasopharyngeal carcinoma or sphenoid sinus carcinoma is well demonstrated in this view.

There are three important foramina seen in the basal view. Foramen ovale lying behind the pterygoid processes gives passage to the third division of the trigeminal nerve, accessory meningeal artery and superficial petrosal nerve. Foramen spinosum lying behind and lateral to foramen ovale transmits the middle meningeal artery. Foramen lacerum is seen anterolateral to the petrous apex and has a well-defined medial margin produced by the internal carotid artery. The Eustachian canal is seen behind the foramen spinosum. The external auditory canal is seen behind the condyle of the mandible. Internal auditory canals and inner ear structures including semicircular canals should be carefully looked for. The clivus and foramen magnum are well seen through which the anterior arch of atlas and odontoid process of axis are seen to project. Jugular fossa and jugular foramen are seen laterally on each side of the junction of petrous portion of the temporal bone and occipital bone.

WATERS' VIEW

It is one of the standard views to study the maxillary and anterior ethmoidal sinuses. Waters' view **(Fig. 5)** is generally performed with the patient in sitting position to facilitate demonstration of any fluid level in the sinuses. Patient is instructed to keep the mouth open with nose and chin touching the cassette in order to visualize the sphenoid sinuses. It is performed by placing the orbitomeatal line at an angle of 35° with the plane of film by either raising the chin or by tilting the tube. It also gives clear picture of the roof of the orbits, destruction of which may be seen in mucocele of frontal sinus and in carcinoma of lacrimal gland.

CALDWELL'S VIEW

Caldwell's view is the best projection for examining the frontal and ethmoid sinuses. Patient is positioned directly facing the cassette in either sitting or prone position with midsagittal plane and orbitomeatal line perpendicular to the film with nose and forehead touching the cassette. Central ray is directed 15° caudally to the nasion.

The various abnormalities that can be detected on the plain skull X-rays can be categorized in the following groups:

- Abnormal density
- Abnormal contour of the skull
- Abnormal intracranial volume
- Intracranial calcification
- Increased thickness of the skull

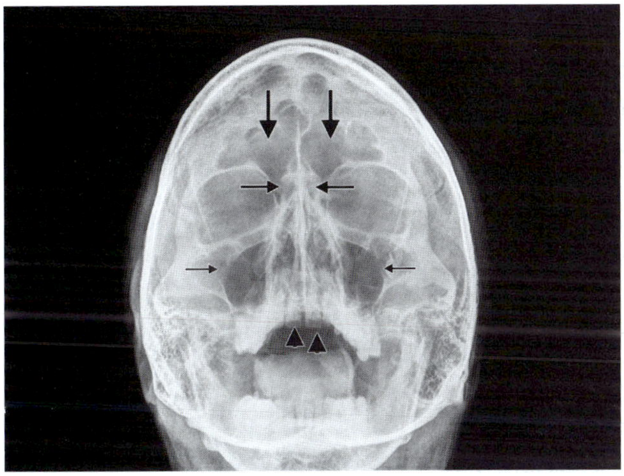

FIG. 5: Waters' view of skull shows bilateral maxillary antrum (lower horizontal arrows), frontal sinuses (vertical arrows), ethmoid sinuses (upper horizontal arrows) and lower margin of sphenoid sinuses (arrowheads).

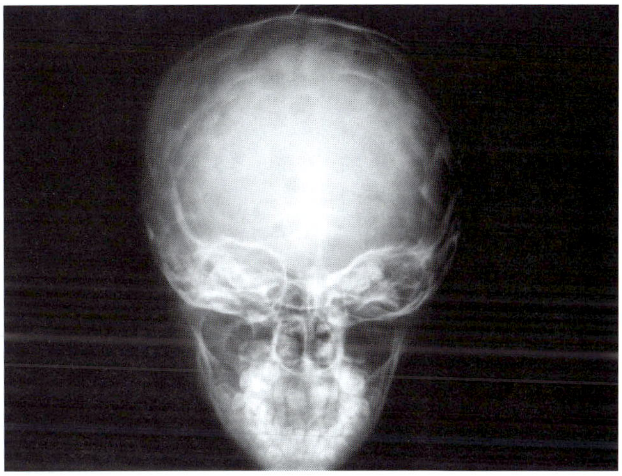

FIG. 6: Craniosynostosis. Anteroposterior (AP) view of skull shows silver beaten appearance due to exaggerated convolutional markings all over the skull vault. None of the sutures is seen.

- Single lucent defect
- Multiple lucent defects
- Sclerotic areas.

Abnormal Density

Generalized reduced density: Thinning of the skull bones with decreased bone density is seen in osteogenesis imperfecta, hypophosphatasia and achondrogenesis. In hypophosphatasia, there is decreased ossification of the skull and vertebrae or as isolated areas of unusually thin calvarial bone. Osteogenesis imperfecta shows increased osseous fragility leading to multiple fractures in addition to decreased density.

Focal reduced density: Focal areas of defective ossification can occur in the lacunar skull where in well-defined lucent areas are seen corresponding to nonossified fibrous bone and the lacunae are bounded by normally ossified bone.

Generalized increased density: It is seen in sclerosing bone dysplasias such as osteopetrosis, and pyknodysostosis. In osteopetrosis increased density is seen in the basal bones initially and later the calvaria becomes dense and thick. The density of facial bones is relatively less dense.

Localized increased density: It may be seen in fibrous dysplasia, osteoma, craniometaphyseal dysplasia, etc.

Abnormal Contour of the Skull

Normal contour of the skull is maintained by sutures, the intracranial contents and normal bone formation. Abnormality in any of these may result in abnormal contour of the skull.

Premature fusion of the sutures, craniosynostosis, is the most common cause of abnormal contour in children. If the suture closes early, the calvarium expands to accommodate the growing brain in the axis of the fused suture. Sagittal synostosis (scaphocephaly) is the most common form of isolated synostosis with M:F = 4:1.[10] It leads to an elongated narrow boat-shaped skull. The closure of both coronal sutures and lambdoid sutures (*turricephaly)* produces a short wide skull with towering head, with bulging temporal areas and shallow orbits **(Fig. 6)**. The recessed supraorbital rims and hypoplasia of the basal frontal bone, gives cloverleaf-like skull appearance.

Plagiocephaly means skewed or oblique head. It results when there is unilateral such as coronal or lambdoid synostosis. Unicoronal synostosis is the second most common form of craniosynostosis, after sagittal synostosis. Two-thirds cases occur in female patients and 10% are familial in nature. In this condition, there is elongation of the orbit, elevation of the lateral portion of ipsilateral orbital rim (the harlequin eye appearance) and tilting of the nasal septum and crista galli toward the affected side. Margins of the affected sutures develop sclerosis. Any decrease or increase in the cerebral volume may result in abnormal contour.

Premature fusion of multiple sutures on one side is associated with signs of raised intracranial tension in the form of increased convolutional markings. The hemicalvarium on the ipsilateral side is smaller than the opposite side. The tables of bones of the skull are thickened and there may be elevation of the petrous pyramid on the same side.

Expansion of the bony calvarium due to the presence of slow growing intracerebral or subarachnoid space occupying lesions such as arachnoid cysts may also result in abnormal contour **(Figs. 7A and B)**. The bony vault bulges outward with thinning of the inner table. Chronic subdural hematomas may also cause expansion of the adjacent calvarium and may even erode the inner table. Calcifications when present facilitate the diagnosis.

Abnormal bone formation such as that occurs in achondroplasia characterized by defective endochondral ossification, results in shortening of the bones of the skull base as these bones develop from cartilage. Since the bones of the vault develop from membranous bones, these remain unaffected. The result is a small foramen magnum and enlarged cranium with frontal bossing and large jaws.

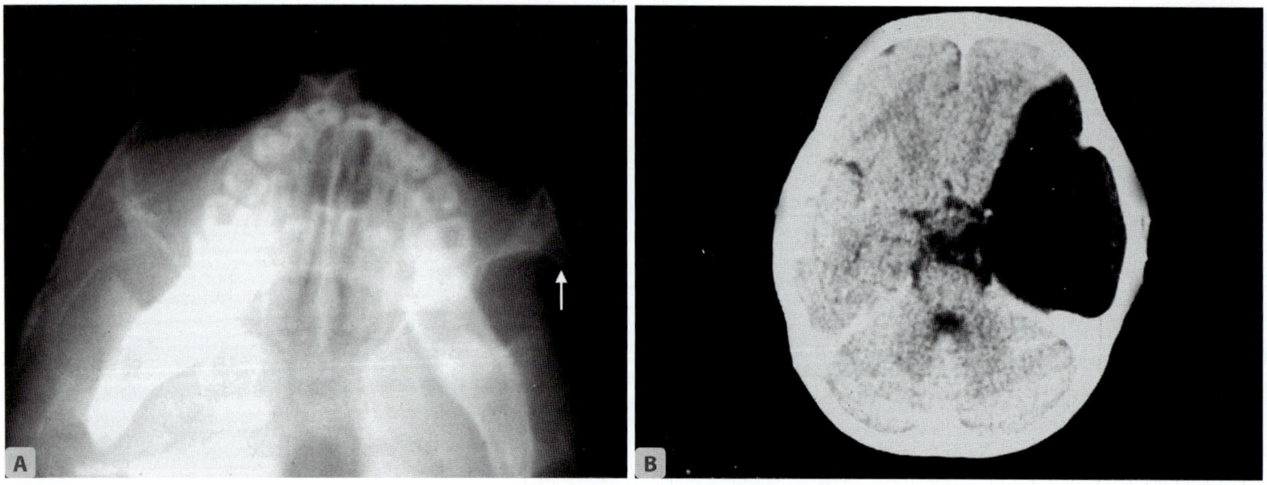

FIGS. 7A AND B: Arachnoid cyst. (A) Basal view of skull shows thinning and ballooning of anterior and lateral walls of the left middle cranial fossa (arrow); (B) Axial CT scan of the same patient shows a large left temporoparietal arachnoid cyst.

Abnormal Intracranial Volume

Size of the calvarium is dependent on the size of the intracranial contents. The most accurate way to determine abnormal cranial volume is to measure the skull directly and compare the measurements to standard for age and body size. A simple method of assessing the size of the skull is to compare the skull vault to the size of the face. At birth, the volume of skull is approximately four times that of face. This ratio decreases to 3:1 by age 2 and 1.5:1 by adulthood.[8]

Enlarged head size may result from hydrocephalus, macrocephaly, hydranencephaly and in pituitary dwarfism. The most common cause of hydrocephalus in children is congenital obstruction of the ventricular system and is associated with raised intracranial tension. Sutures become wide due to expansion of the intracranial contents.

Small skull but otherwise normal contour is characteristically seen in microcephaly associated with mental retardation. Cranial sutures fuse early but this is a result of microcephaly and not the cause. The sinuses are large and the digital or convolutional markings are absent or decreased. It is important to differentiate premature closure of all the sutures from microcephaly with fused sutures. When multiple sutures fuse prematurely, the fusion does not occur simultaneously and the result is an irregular skull due to expansion of the skull in unusual directions to accommodate the brain. Clinically, signs of raised intracranial tension are present. Convolutional markings are exaggerated.

Increased thickness of the skull may result due to early cessation of brain growth or due to cerebral atrophy. Increased width of diploic space due to increased hematopoiesis is seen in hemolytic anemia. Progressive hydrocephalus leads to large bony calvarium and a decreased diploic space. However, if a ventricular shunt is performed and abnormal expansion ceases resulting in arrested hydrocephalus, the cranial sutures close and the inner table of bones of the skull become thicker and the diploic space becomes larger. A history of hydrocephalus and the presence of a ventricular shunt facilitate the diagnosis.

Among the hemolytic anemia producing hyperplasia of the bone marrow, thalassemia causes most marked changes. The diploic space is widened with striking radial striations, the "hair-on-end" appearance **(Fig. 8)**. The paranasal sinuses may also be completely obliterated due to widening of the diploic space of facial bones. Such changes may also be seen in other forms of anemia, such as sickle cell disease, hereditary spherocytosis, but the changes are much less marked.

Radiolucent Areas in Skull

When there is a single lucent lesion, the important considerations that help in deciding its nature are its location, associated soft tissue swelling, table of the bone involved and margins of the lytic lesion, whether sharp, ill-defined or sclerotic. Radiolucent defects in the skull bone may be due to variety of causes, which may be congenital or acquired **(Table 2)**. A sclerotic margin of the lesion sometimes also helps in narrowing down the differential diagnosis **(Table 3)**. Congenital causes may be parietal foramina, anomalous apertures, meningoencephalocele or dermal sinus. The acquired causes include trauma, infections, tumors and histiocytosis.

Bilaterally symmetrical rounded lytic defects located in the posterior parietal bone are characteristic of parietal foramina and are of no clinical significance. Lytic defects due to meningoencephalocele are located in the midline in the frontal or occipital regions and have sharp margins. Associated soft tissue mass clinches the diagnosis. In the first 3 months of life, meningoencephalocele is generally associated with lacunar skull (craniolacunia) **(Fig. 9)**. A *dermal sinus* also occurs in the midline of the skull and may present as a radiolucent defect with a sharp slightly sclerotic border. It is generally associated with a lipoma or a nevus in the overlying soft tissues. These lesions may have an intracranial components which may require a CT scan for demonstration.

Fractures generally occur at the site of injury and may be associated with soft tissue swelling. *Linear nondepressed fractures* may be seen as radiolucent lines and should not be

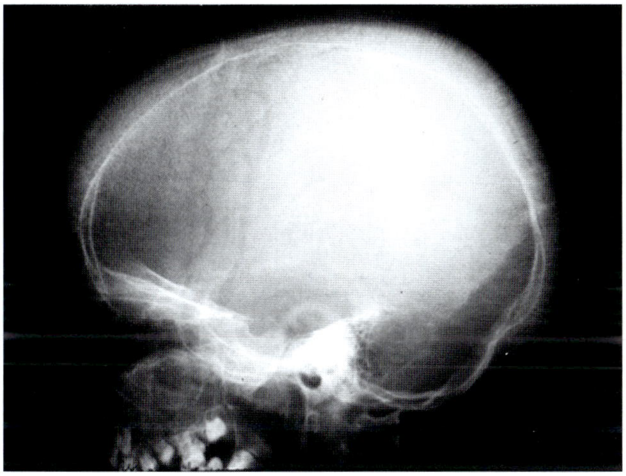

FIG. 8: Thalassemia. Lateral skull radiograph shows widened diploic space with coarsened trabeculae giving "hair-on-end" appearance typical of hemolytic anemia.

TABLE 2: Skull vault lucent areas.
Normal: Parietal foramina, vascular channels, pacchionian granulations, fontanelles
Neoplastic: • Myeloma • Metastasis • LCH (acute phase)
Inflammatory/infective diseases: • Osteomyelitis • TB • Hydatid • Syphilis
Vascular causes: • Hemangioma • Sinus pericranii
Metabolic: • Osteoporosis • Hyperparathyroidism
Miscellaneous: • Leptomeningeal cyst • Burr hole • Intradiploic arachnoid cyst • Neurofibroma • Paget's disease

TABLE 3: Skull vault lucent areas with marginal sclerosis.
• Epidermoid
• Encephalocele/meningocele
• LCH (healing phase)
• Posttreatment metastasis
• Chronic osteomyelitis
• Fibrous dysplasia

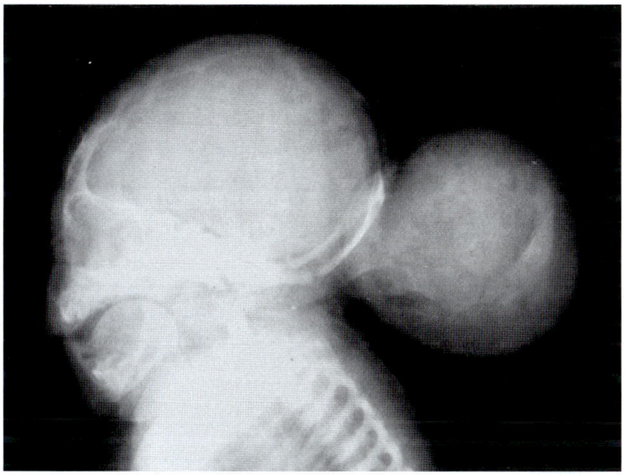

FIG. 9: Craniolacunia. Lateral skull radiograph in an infant shows multiple lucencies with intervening dense areas typical of craniolacunia. Note the associated occipital encephalocele and absence of sutural widening.

confused with sutures or vascular grooves. Fracture lines are nontapering, nonbranching and have sharp borders whereas vascular grooves have ill-defined borders and an undulating course. Sutures are seen in known anatomical positions and have saw tooth edges. *Depressed fractures* generally occur after severe trauma and are considered more serious than linear fractures. Radiologically, the depressed fragment presents as area of increased radiodensity surrounded by a radiolucent zone **(Fig. 10)**. In children, when the dura beneath the suture is torn, the arachnoid membrane herniates through the dura into the bony defect. The pulsations of the brain lead to progressive enlargement of the arachnoid collection resulting in expansion of the fracture line termed as growing skull fracture. The bulging membranes result in the formation of leptomeningeal cyst **(Fig. 11)**.

Infections of the skull are uncommon and generally follow trauma or arise secondary to infection elsewhere in the body. The radiographic appearance consists of mottled irregular lucencies, which have ill-defined borders and are associated with soft tissue swelling of the scalp.

Epidermoid tumors develop from a congenital inclusion of epithelial cells within the calvarium. Radiologically, these lesions present as well-defined lytic lesions, which have sclerotic border and are not necessarily located in the midline such as dermoid **(Fig. 12)**. Intracranial epidermoids may also produce a radiolucent shadow, which may mimick a lytic lesion **(Figs. 13A and B)**.

Malignant lesions such as primary osteosarcoma or metastasis can also produce lytic defects. Osteosarcoma causes gross destruction of the bone with ill-defined margins and soft tissue swelling **(Figs. 14A and B)**. Neurofibromatosis is a rare cause of a lytic defect seen along the suture. This defect is not due to the presence of neurofibroma but is a manifestation of mesenchymal defect. Intracranial mass lesions can also rarely present as lytic areas of the skull.

Eosinophilic granulomas, Hand-Schüller-Christian disease and *Letterer-Siwe disease* all form part of a complex comprising histiocytosis. The severity ranges from mild in eosinophilic granuloma to very malignant course in Letterer-Siwe disease.

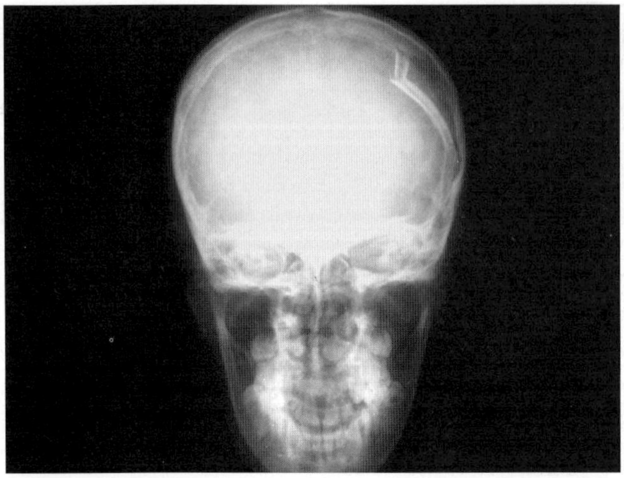

FIG. 10: Depressed fracture. Frontal radiograph shows the parallel dense lines due to depressed bone fragments and associated lucency due to absence of bone.

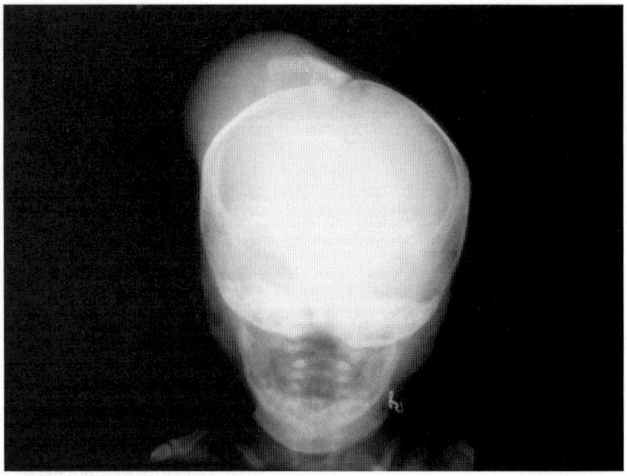

FIG. 11: Growing fracture. Posteroanterior (PA) skull radiographs in a child demonstrate fracture of the right frontal bone with thickening, sclerosis and wide separation of the fracture ends. Note the soft tissue swelling overlying this area.

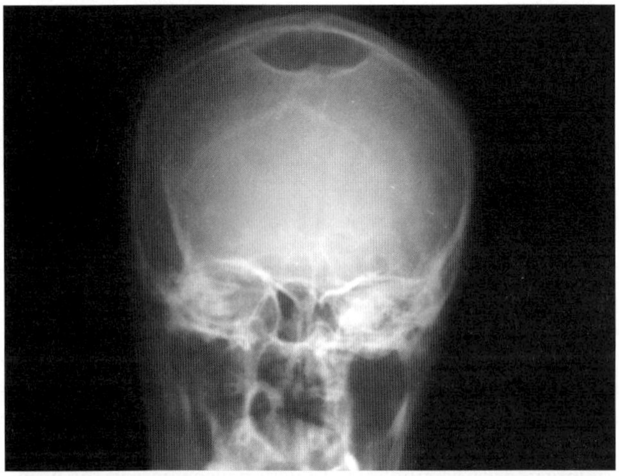

FIG. 12: Dermoid scalp. Skull radiograph shows a well-circumscribed lucency overlying the coronal suture.

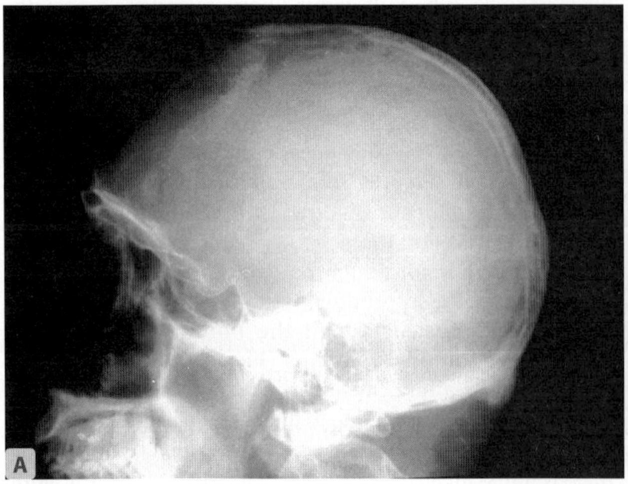

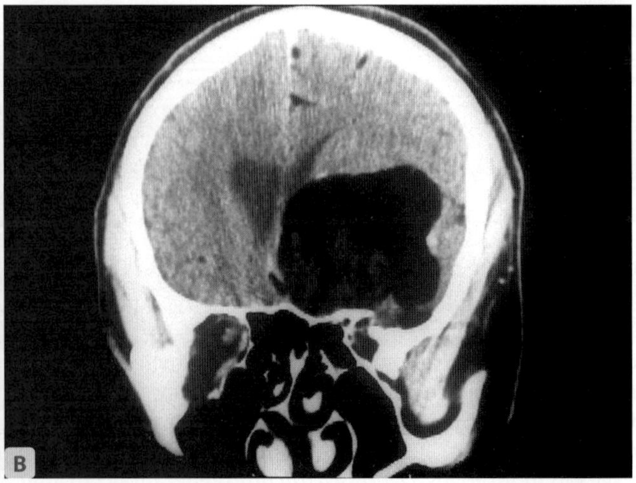

FIGS. 13A AND B: Single lucent lesion. (A) Skull radiograph shows a well-circumscribed lucency overlying the coronal suture mimicking a lytic lesion; (B) Coronal computed tomography (CT) scan in the same patient shows a large hypodense lesion due to epidermoid in the temporoparietal region. No lytic lesion of skull vault is seen.

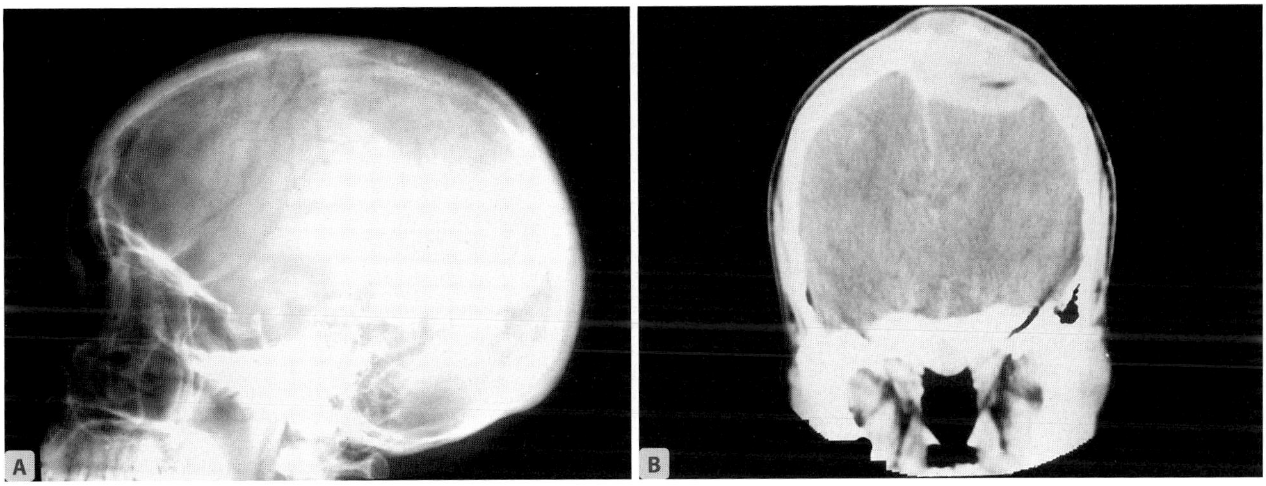

FIGS. 14A AND B: Osteosarcoma. (A) Large lytic area with irregular margin is seen affecting the left parietal bone; (B) Computed tomography (CT) scan of the same patient shows the soft tissue swelling, destruction of the bone and extradural extension of the tumor.

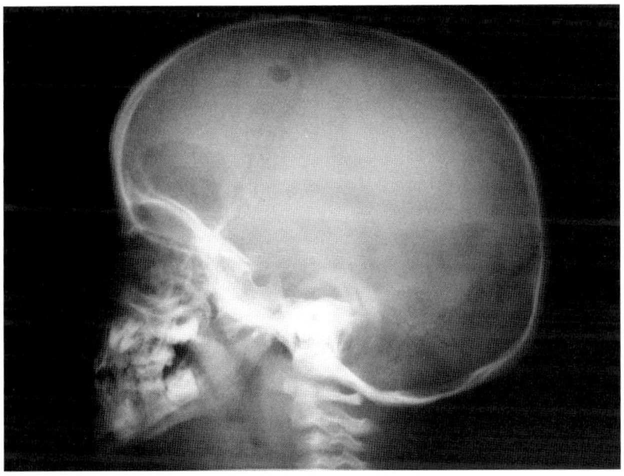

FIG. 15: Eosinophilic granuloma. Lateral skull radiograph shows a single lytic lesion having sharp nonsclerotic border and bevelled edges.

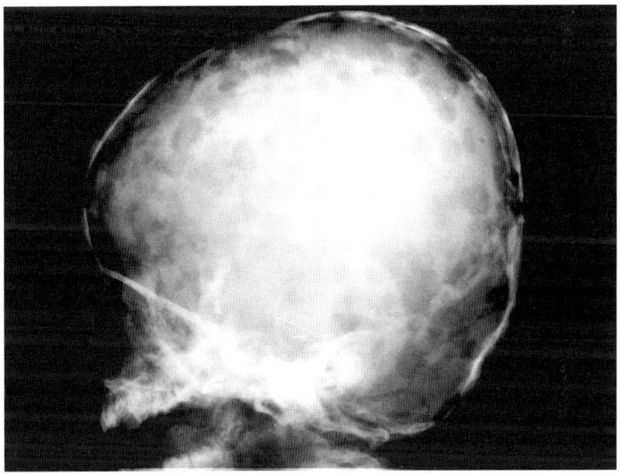

FIG. 16: Histiocytosis (Hand-Schüller-Christian disease). Lateral radiograph of skull shows multiple well-defined lytic lesions of the vault with bevelled edges characteristic of histiocytosis.

A single lytic lesion having sharp nonsclerotic border and bevelled edges is characteristic of eosinophilic granulomas **(Fig. 15)**. Occasionally, a small bone is seen in the center representing button sequestrum. Lytic lesions in the other two variants are larger, multiple and punched out **(Fig. 16)**.

Multiple radiolucent defects in the skull in children may be due to craniolacunia, presence of wormian bones, increased convolutional makings due to raised intracranial tension, histiocytosis and metastasis from neuroblastoma **(Figs. 17A and B)**, leukemia or Ewing's sarcoma. In adults, multiple myeloma **(Fig. 18)**, metastasis and hyperparathyroidism **(Fig. 19)** are the usual causes.

Craniolacunia is due to a defect in ossification of the bones, which develop from membranous tissue. There are multiple radiolucent defects seen all over the cranial vault interspersed with strips of normal bone, which appear dense. Craniolacunia (lacunar skull) by itself is not of much significance, but it is generally associated with myelomeningocele or encephalocele **(*see* Fig. 9)**. Appearance must not be confused with *increased convolutional markings* that result from raised intracranial tension and are seen as multiple radiolucent areas not exceeding the diameter of a finger. Convolutional marking may also be seen in normal children in the frontal and occipital region. Presence of increased convolutional markings in the parietal region should generally be considered abnormal. Wormian bones are seen along the sutures and results due to defective mineralization. Multiple wormian bones are seen in cleidocranial dysostosis, osteogenesis imperfecta, hypothyroidism and pyknodysostosis.

Lytic lesions seen in *multiple myeloma* are punched out, usually associated with osteoporosis and involve the mandible more frequently compared to *metastasis*. However, many times differentiation from metastasis may not be possible on radiological appearance alone. The sclerosis or sclerotic rim is very rare seen in 3% of cases in multiple myeloma and usually occur after therapy.[11] *Hyperparathyroidism* generally results in mottled demineralization **(Fig. 19)** but may sometimes cause multiple well-defined lytic areas **(Fig. 20)**.

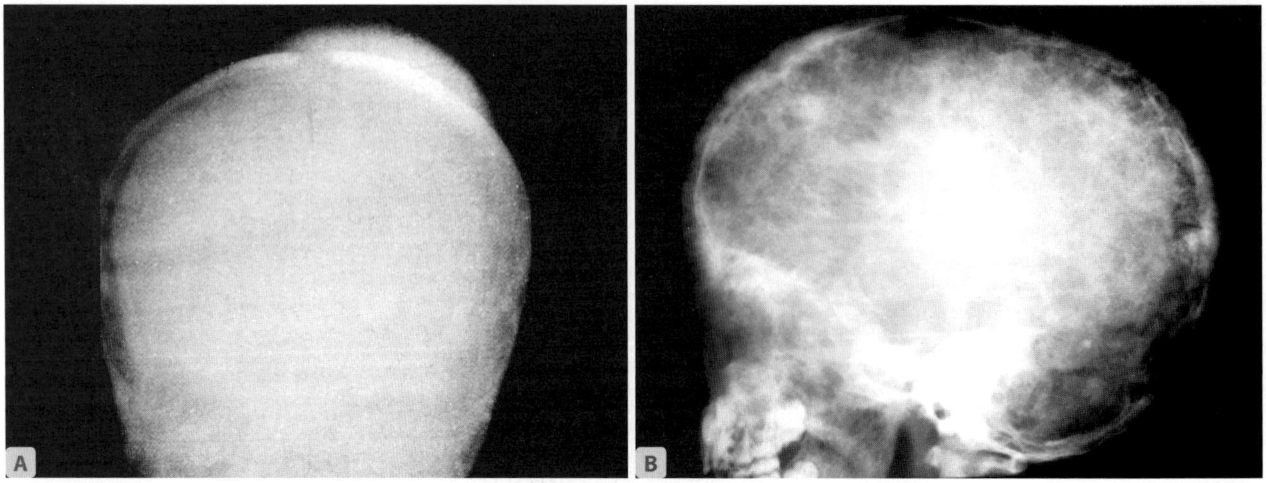

FIGS. 17A AND B: Metastatic lesions of the skull in a child with abdominal neuroblastoma. (A) Sutural metastasis: Frontal skull radiograph shows widening of the sagittal suture with an overlying soft tissue swelling; (B) Diffuse metastasis of skull vault: Lateral skull radiograph shows multiple lytic areas involving both tables of skull and diploic space. Note widening of coronal suture also.

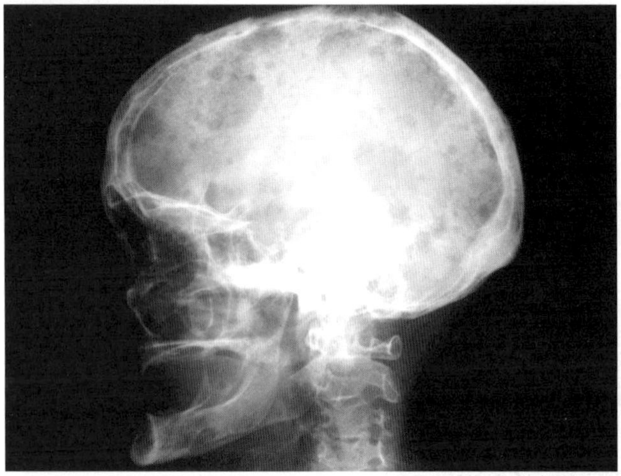

FIG. 18: Multiple myeloma. Lateral skull radiographs shows multiple well-defined punched out lytic lesions affecting the skull vault as well as mandible typical of myeloma.

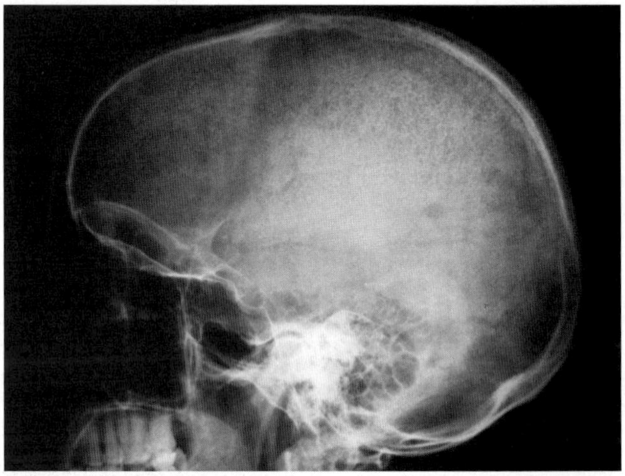

FIG. 19: Hyperparathyroidism. Lateral skull radiograph shows multiple lytic lesions with mottled appearance.

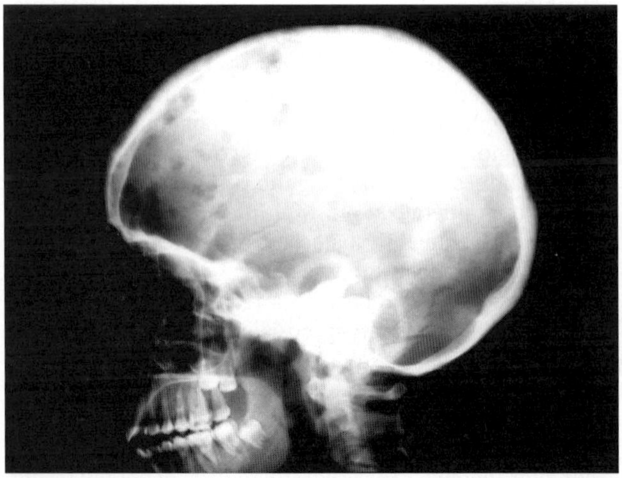

FIG. 20: Hyperparathyroidism. Lateral skull radiograph shows multiple well-circumscribed rounded lytic lesions involving skull vault with bone within bone appearance—an unusual feature of hyperparathyroidism.

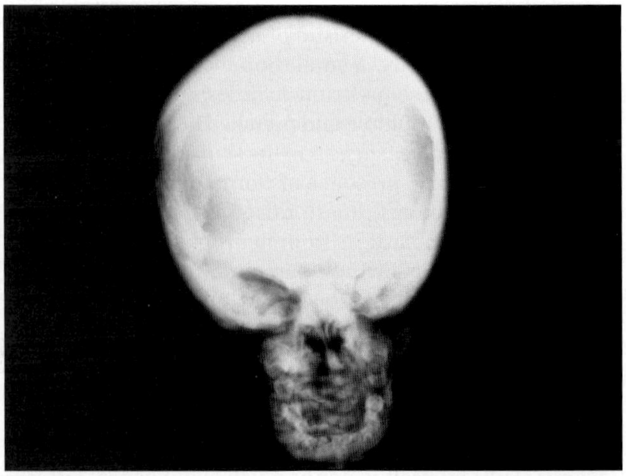

FIG. 21: Osteopetrosis. Frontal radiograph shows diffuse increased density affecting all bones of the skull vault as well as base.

Sclerotic Areas of the Skull

Areas of increased density in the skull may be seen in both normal as well as pathological conditions. Differential diagnosis depends on the localized vs generalized sclerosis **(Table 4)**. Osteopetrosis is a rare condition, which is characterized by diffuse thickening of the skull and face **(Fig. 21)**. Fibrous dysplasia may involve the vault or base of skull. There may be a single lesion or it may be part of syndrome *(McCune-Albright syndrome)* seen in females when it affects multiple bones and is associated with precocious puberty. The lesions are sclerotic with loss of normal trabecular pattern. Mixed types of lesions with sclerotic and lytic areas are also known to occur **(Figs. 22A to C)**. Paget disease in the mixed phase shows marked thickening of the diploic space, particularly the inner calvarial table, causing marked enlargement. The areas of sclerosis may be circular and occur in previous areas of osteoporosis. This pattern often creates focal areas of opacity giving "cotton wool" appearance at radiography **(Fig. 23)**. Multiple hyperostotic lesions affecting the calvarium measuring 5–10 mm in size may be seen in tuberous sclerosis in association with calcified lesion in periventricular region. Thickening of the frontal and parietal bones may occur in rickets due to presence of poorly mineralized bone, which on healing becomes dense. An *osteoma* affecting the skull bones is a benign tumor, which appears as a dense lesion projecting extracranially from the outer table of skull. Osteoma is also the most common benign tumor affecting the sinuses **(Fig. 24)**. Focal areas of hyperostosis are characteristic of *meningioma* **(Figs. 25A and B)**. When the

TABLE 4: Skull vault sclerotic areas.

Generalized sclerosis	Localized sclerosis
• Paget's disease	• Metastasis
• Sclerotic metastasis	• Paget's disease
• Fibrous dysplasia	• Fibrous dysplasia
• Renal osteodystrophy	• Hyperostosis frontalis interna
• Myelofibrosis	• Meningioma
• Chronic hemolytic anemia	• Calcified hematoma
• Bone dysplasias e.g. osteopetrosis, pyknodystosis	
• Prolonged phenytoin treatment	
• Acromegaly	
• Fluorosis	

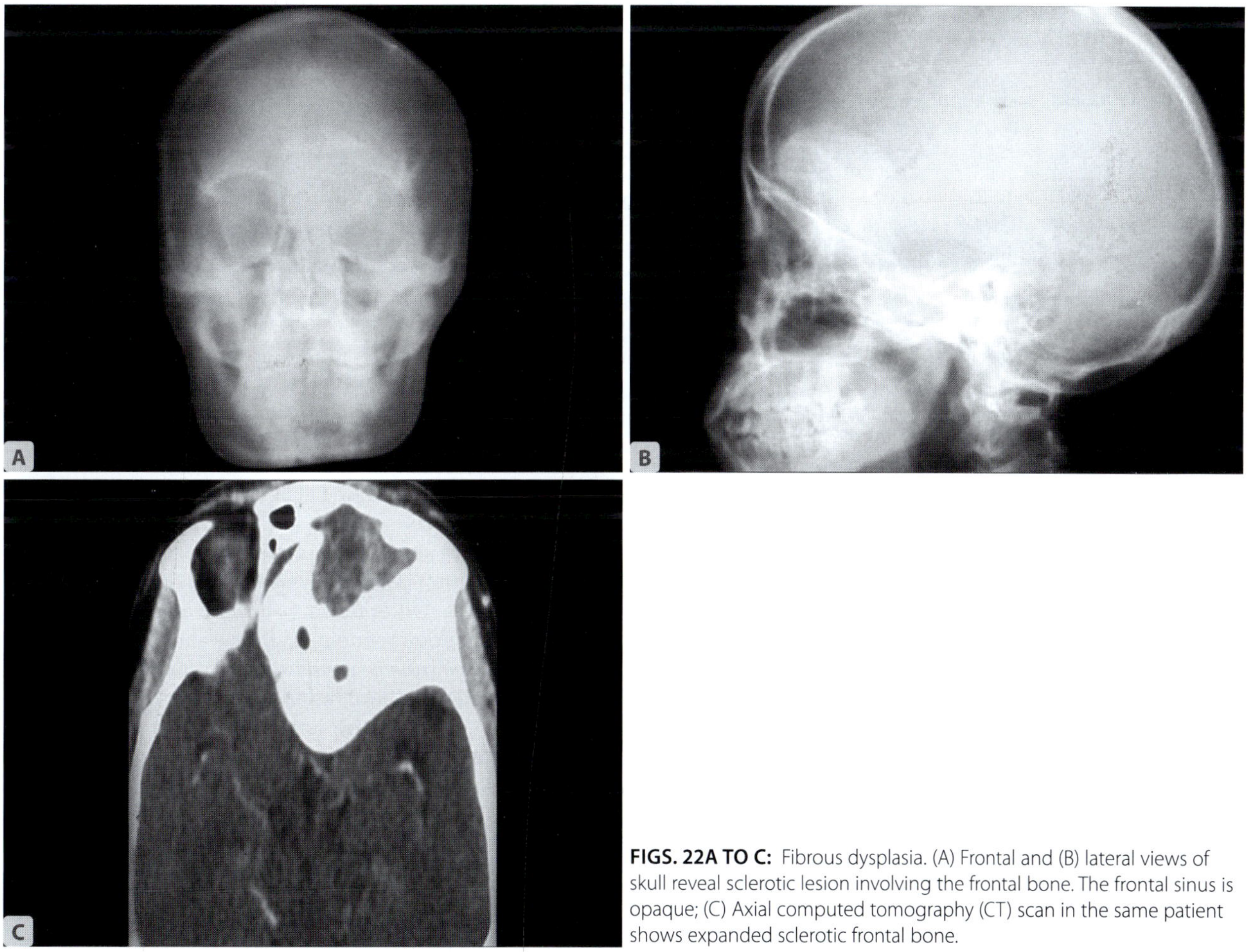

FIGS. 22A TO C: Fibrous dysplasia. (A) Frontal and (B) lateral views of skull reveal sclerotic lesion involving the frontal bone. The frontal sinus is opaque; (C) Axial computed tomography (CT) scan in the same patient shows expanded sclerotic frontal bone.

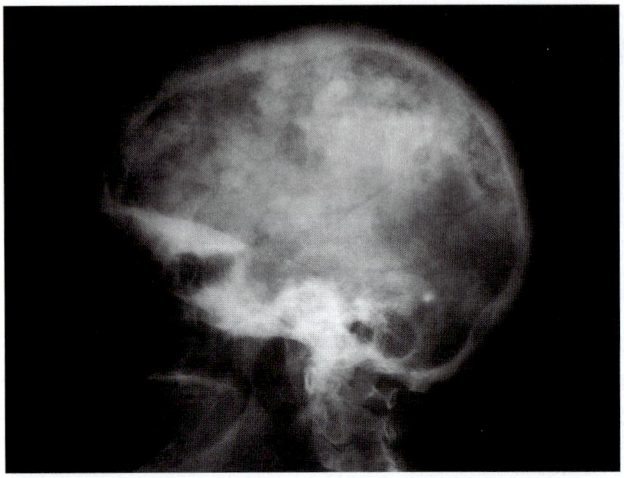

FIG. 23: Paget's disease. Lateral view of skull reveals focal areas of opacities in previous areas of osteoporosis giving "cotton-wool" appearance.

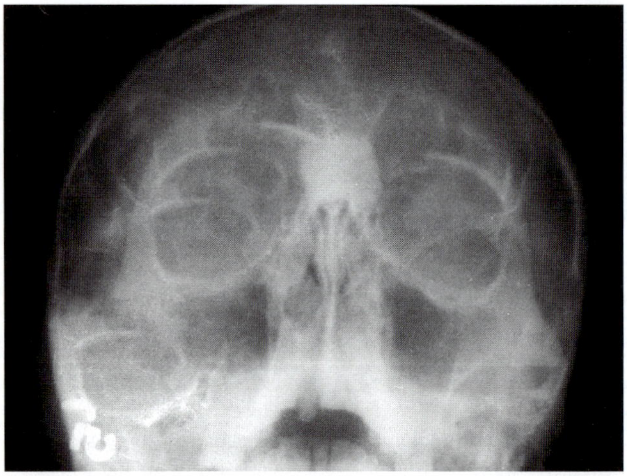

FIG. 24: Osteoma. Waters' view of skull shows osteoma of the frontal sinus.

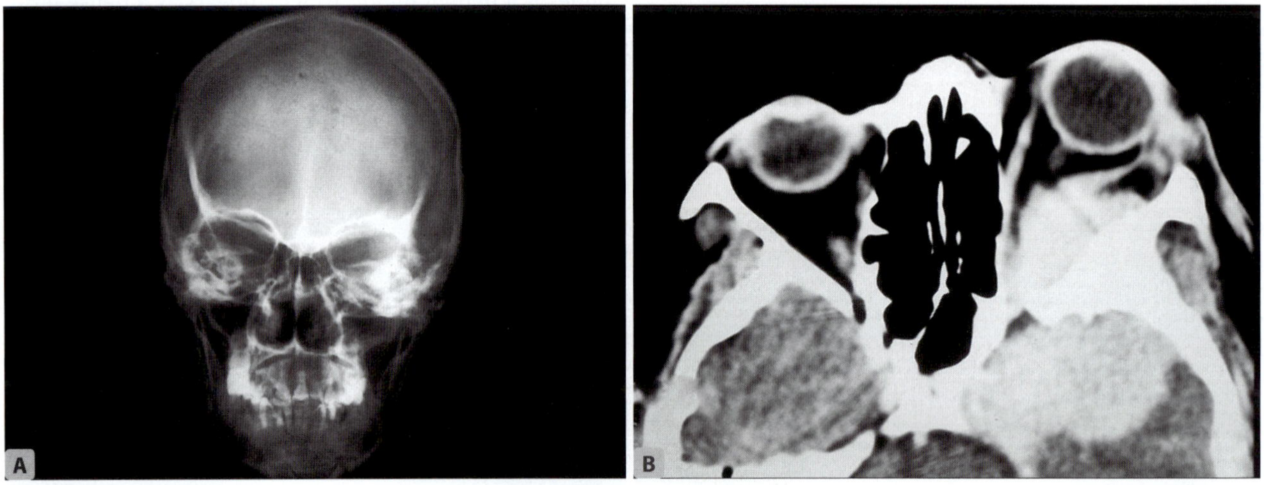

FIGS. 25A AND B: Sphenoid wing meningioma. (A) Posteroanterior (PA) view of skull shows hyperostosis of the left lesser and greater wings of the sphenoid bone typical of meningioma; (B) Contrast enhanced computed tomography (CT) scan in the same patient shows proptosis and hyperostosis of sphenoid wings with enhancing extradural mass due to meningioma on the left side.

hyperostosis affects the frontal bone, in a case of convexity meningioma, it must be differentiated from *hyperostosis frontalis interna* **(Fig. 26)**, the latter is generally seen in elderly females and affects the inner table with sparing of diploic space and does not cross the midline.

Intracranial Calcification

Presence of calcification can provide important clue to the diagnosis in several conditions intracranial calcification can be physiological or pathological **(Table 5)**. Although causes are numerous, some of these conditions have specific appearance, which can be diagnostic.

The most common physiological calcification occurs in the pineal gland. It is seen in the midline approximately 3 cm above and behind the posterior clinoids in the lateral view **(Fig. 27)**. Size of the pineal calcification is most important as any increase in size more than 10 mm is abnormal and raises the possibility of pinealoma.

Habenular commissure calcification has a characteristic appearance and is seen as a C-shaped structure open posteriorly. It lies above and anterior to pineal gland. Choroid plexus calcification is generally bilateral and may be unequal on the two sides. Other normal sites of calcification are the falx and anterior petroclinoid ligaments above the sella.

Tuberous sclerosis is a syndrome comprised of epilepsy, mental retardation and adenoma sebaceum. Multiple hamartomas occur in the brain as well as at other sites such as kidneys. Tumors consist of glial tissue and ganglion cells. In the brain they are usually multiple and are seen in the subcortical, subependymal and basal ganglia regions. Calcification is seen in 50% of the lesions **(Fig. 28)**.

Sturge-Weber syndrome is another important cause of intracranial calcification. Patients present with epilepsy and

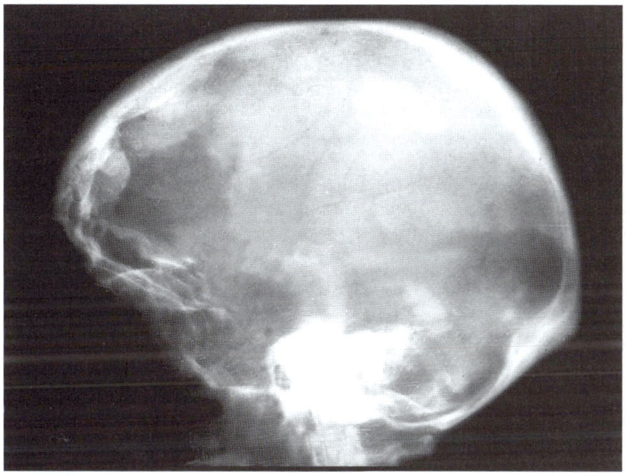

FIG. 26: Hyperostosis frontalis interna. Lateral skull radiograph shows irregular thickening of the frontal bone in an elderly female. The inner table is involved more than the outer table with sparing of diploic spaces.

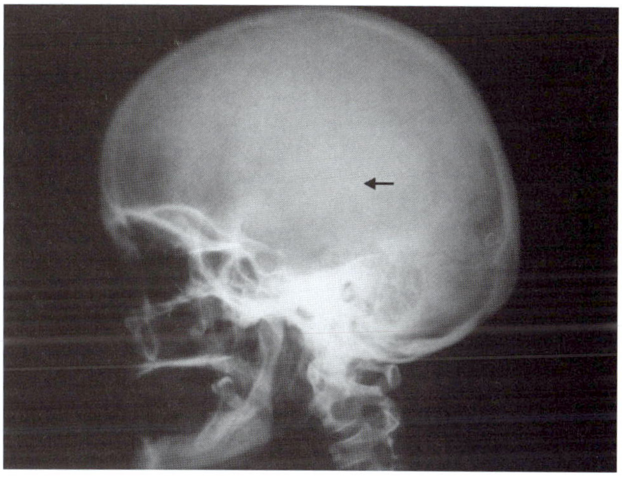

FIG. 27: Lateral view skull shows pineal gland calcification (arrow).

TABLE 5: Causes of intracranial calcification.

Normal intracranial calcification/variants	Abnormal intracranial calcification
• Pineal • Habenular commissure • Basal ganglia • Dentate • Parasellar ligament • Arachnoid granulations • Choroid plexus • Dura	Familial conditions: • Tuberous sclerosis • Sturge-Weber syndrome • Idiopathic familial cerebrovascular calcinosis (Fahr's disease)
	Metabolic causes: • Hypoparathyroidism • Pseudohypoparathyroidism
	Inflammatory diseases: • Cytomegalic inclusion disease • Toxoplasmosis • Rubella • Abscess
	Vascular causes: • Arteriovenous malformation • Intracerebral hematoma • Subdural hematoma
	Neoplasms: • Craniopharyngioma • Astrocytomas • Oligodendrogliomas • Pinealoma

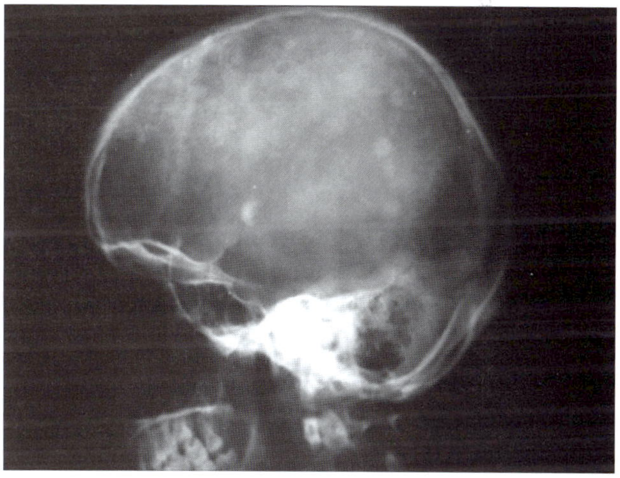

FIG. 28: Tuberous sclerosis. X-ray of skull lateral view showing multiple calcified lesions.

mental retardation and often have cutaneous hemangioma in the distribution of trigeminal nerve on the same side as calcification. Calcification has a typical tram-track appearance and is seen in the cerebral cortex **(Figs. 29A and B)**.

Basal ganglia calcification is an important feature of hypoparathyroidism and pseudohypoparathyroidism. Widespread irregular and punctate areas of calcification, which are diffusely scattered, are characteristic of Fahr's disease. In this condition, patients present with severe growth and mental retardation. The disease is hereditary and is characterized by microscopic deposits of iron and calcium in the basal ganglia, cerebellum and subcortical region. Infections due to toxoplasma and cytomegalovirus are important causes of intracranial calcification in the newborn. Calcifications are multiple and diffusely scattered in the brain parenchyma or paraventricular region. Bacterial infections may progress to cerebral abscess, which may get calcified.

Arteriovenous malformations calcify in 2–25% of all affected patients. Typically, calcification is in the form of an incomplete ring but may be nodular or amorphous. A large arc like calcification seen in the region of pineal gland in a newborn presenting with congestive heart failure and hydrocephalus is characteristic of vein of Galen aneurysm. Intracerebral or chronic subdural hematomas may reveal curvilinear calcification. A variety of tumors may show calcification. In children, suprasellar craniopharyngioma is the most common tumor, which reveals calcification whereas in adults oligodendrogliomas and meningiomas are the common tumors to calcify.

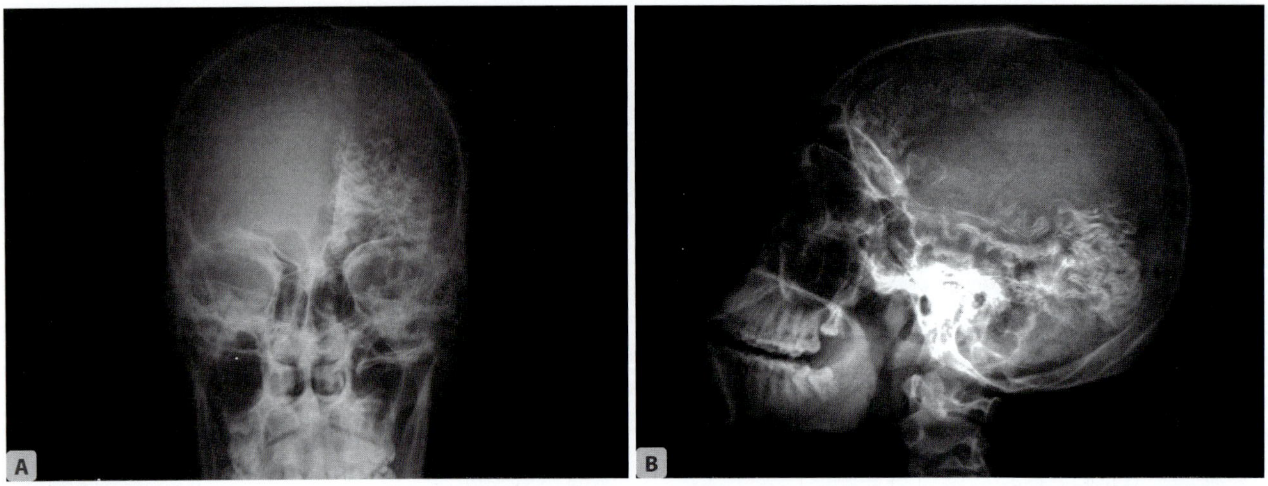

FIGS. 29A AND B: Sturge-Weber syndrome. (A) Posteroanterior (PA) and (B) lateral view of the skull shows gyriform calcification on the left side.

REFERENCES

1. Tress BM. The need for skull radiography in patients presenting for CT. Radiology. 1983;146(1):87-9.
2. Moseley I. Long-term effects of the introduction of noninvasive investigations in neuroradiology. Neuroradiology. 1988;30(3): 193-200.
3. Rastogi SC, Barraclough BM. Skull radiography in patients with psychiatric illness. Br Med J. 1983;287(6401):1259.
4. Taveras JM. Anatomy and examination of skull. In: Interactive Review of Radiology. Lippincotts Williams and Wilkins, 1999.
5. Sanders R, MacEwen CJ, McCulloch AS. The value of skull radiography in ophthalmology. ActaRadiol. 1994;35(5): 429-33.
6. Baker HL Jr. The impact of computed tomography on neuroradiologic practice. Radiology. 1975;116(3):637-40.
7. Taveras JM. The skull. In: Taveras JM, Wood EH (Eds). Diagnostic Neuroradiology, 2nd edition. The Williams and Wilkins Company. 1986.pp.1-65.
8. Gerald B. Systematic radiographic evaluation of the abnormal skull. In: Rabinowitz JG (Ed). Pediatric Radiology. Philadelphia: JB Lippincott Company. 1978.pp.285-313.
9. Butler P, Jeffiree MA. The skull and brain. In: Butler P, Mitchell AWM, Ellis H (Eds). Applied Radiological Anatomy, 1st edition. Cambridge University Press. 2001.pp.17-60.
10. Kirmi O, J Lo S, Johnson D, et al. Craniosynostosis: aradiological and surgical perspective. Seminars in ULTRASOUND CT and MRI. 2009;30(6):492-512.
11. Baur-Melnyk A, Reiser M. Oncohaematologic disorders affecting the skeleton in the elderly. RadiolClin North Am. 2008;46(4):785-98.

CHAPTER

182

Normal Anatomy of Brain on CT and MRI

Paramjeet Singh

INTRODUCTION

An understanding of basic anatomy of the brain is vital to the planning and interpretation of neuroradiologic studies. Modern imaging techniques provide cross-sections of the brain similar to the dissected brain. Computerized tomography (CT) and magnetic resonance imaging (MRI) provides cross-sectional anatomy of the brain. Current MRI scanners and multidetector computerized tomography (MDCT) have expanded the scope of three-dimensional conceptualization of complex brain structures through multiplanar imaging and reconstructions from true volumetric data sets. Better tissue differentiation on MRI allows not only morphological, but also histological information to some extent. Recent advances in functional imaging and diffusion tensor imaging makes understanding of brain anatomy even more important. This chapter reviews the essentials of surface and cross-sectional anatomy of the brain as seen on CT and MRI.

TECHNIQUES AND NORMAL APPEARANCE

General Considerations

Noncontiguous axial CT sections are usually obtained at 15–20° angulation to the orbitomeatal line, while axial MRI sections are generally obtained parallel to it (along bicommissural plane or AC-PC line). MRI, owing to its multiplanar capability allows direct coronal and sagittal sections. However, MDCT scanners and newer MR techniques allow volumetric data acquisitions with reconstructions in desirable planes. T1- and T2-weighted (T1W and T2W) images are routinely obtained on MRI. The T1WI are excellent for showing anatomy while T2WI are highly sensitive in detecting brain pathology (details of MR sequences is beyond the scope of this chapter).

The white matter is hypodense to gray matter on CT. The cerebral white matter appears bright while the gray matter is relatively dark on T1WI. The relationship reverses as white matter becomes progressively darker on increasing the T2-weighting; the crossover occurring in the proton density images. The basal ganglia, red nucleus and putamen appear hypointense on T2WI due to their mineral contents.

The cerebrospinal fluid (CSF) shows low density on CT (0–15 HU) depending on its protein content. The CSF is hypointense on T1WI and extremely bright on T2WI due to its long T1 and T2 relaxation times. The CSF is in constant motion which may occasionally result in flow-related artifacts and loss of signal (flow void), classically seen in the region of cerebral aqueduct. The glomera of the choroid plexus within the lateral ventricles are seen as soft tissue density on CT and show homogeneous enhancement on contrast enhanced CT (CECT). On T2WI the choroid plexus appears heterogeneous due to the presence of calcification and cysts.

Visualization of blood vessels needs administration of iodinated contrast in CT. On MRI, major blood vessels are visualized without contrast administration and appear as flow voids on spin echo imaging or show flow-related enhancement on gradient echo imaging. Flow-related artifacts are often seen in phase encoding direction especially in long TR sequences and should not be mistaken for pathology. Familiarity with normal variations like dilated perivascular spaces is important. Modern MR imaging also provides a good understanding of white matter tracts through diffusion tensor imaging and functional areas of the brain through BOLD imaging.

Except for the intraorbital segment of the optic nerves, the remaining cranial nerves are usually not visualized on CT. On MR, using thin sections and fluid sensitive techniques like SPACE and CISS, the cisternal segments of most of the cranial nerves can be identified.

The inner meningeal layers are not normally visualized on noncontrast MRI and may show no or fine linear enhancement following contrast administration. Major dural folds like falx and tentorium appear hypointense on MRI and enhance after contrast administration along with the venous sinuses within them. Contrast-enhanced MR angiograms are increasingly used for demonstrating vascular anatomy.

The diploic space appears bright on T1WI due to its fat content and is outlined by the low signal intensity compact bones of the inner and outer tables of skull. CT better demonstrates the bony outlines. Similarly, it is superior to MR for visualization of intracranial calcification.

Normal Anatomy of Brain

Figure 1 shows the major subdivisions of brain. Brain consists of three major components.

1. The forebrain (prosencephalon) comprised of two cerebral hemispheres (telencephalon) and thalamus and surrounding gray matter, epithalamus, hypothalamus and subthalamus (diencephalon).
2. The basal ganglia
3. The midbrain (mesencephalon)
4. The hindbrain (rhombencephalon) comprised of cerebellum and pons (metencephalon), and medulla oblongata (myelencephalon).

CEREBRAL HEMISPHERES

Cerebrum consists of two hemispheres which are partially connected with each other through corpus callosum. Each cerebral hemisphere has three borders superomedial, inferomedial and inferolateral. The superomedial border separates the superolateral and medial surfaces, the inferolateral border separates the superolateral and inferior surfaces, and the inferomedial border separates medial surface and inferior surface.

Lateral Surface of the Cerebral Hemisphere (Fig. 2A)

The two cerebral hemispheres are incompletely divided by the interhemispheric fissure. The sylvian fissure (lateral fissure) separates the temporal lobe from the frontal and parietal lobes. Its anterior horizontal and anterior ascending rami extend into the inferior frontal gyrus. The posterior ramus passes backward and upward terminating into ascending and descending rami. The central sulcus separates the frontal from the parietal lobe **(Fig. 3E)**. It originates slightly behind the midpoint between the frontal and occipital poles on the superomedial border and continues obliquely inferolaterally on the lateral surface. Various features on cross-sectional imaging identifying it are upper T or L sign (junction of superior frontal and precentral sulci), lower T sign (identifying inferior frontal sulcus and gyrus), Omega, Epsilon, and Sigmoidal hook signs (shapes of hand motor area or knob), U sign (subcentral gyrus bordering central sulcus inferolaterally), bracket sign (junction of marginal sulcus with interhemispheric fissure), etc. **(Fig. 6N)**.

The frontal lobe is bounded posteriorly by the precentral gyrus, which lies between the central and precentral sulci **(Fig. 3E)**. The precentral gyrus contains the primary motor area with inverse topographic representation of contralateral body parts. The superior frontal sulcus and inferior frontal sulcus divide the frontal lobe anterior to precentral gyrus into superior, middle and inferior gyri **(Figs. 3E, 3F, 5A, 5B, 6H and 5J)**. In front of the precentral gyrus is the premotor area, consisting of posterior part of the superior, middle and inferior frontal gyri. The Broca's area which is concerned with the motor mechanisms of speech also lies at the posterior part of the inferior frontal gyrus in the dominant lobe usually seen at the level of frontal horns on axial sections.

The convexity of the parietal lobe consists of the postcentral gyrus and the superior and inferior parietal lobules separated by the horizontally running intraparietal sulcus **(Figs. 3E and F)**. The postcentral gyrus is located between the central and postcentral sulcus and contains the primary (somesthetic, tactile, thermal and kinesthetic) areas, with body representation corresponding to that in precentral gyrus. The inferior parietal lobule is further subdivided into the supramarginal and angular gyri, which are located around the terminal ascending ramus of the sylvian fissure and the superior temporal sulcus, respectively **(Fig. 3E)**. The temporal lobe is divided into superior, middle and inferior temporal

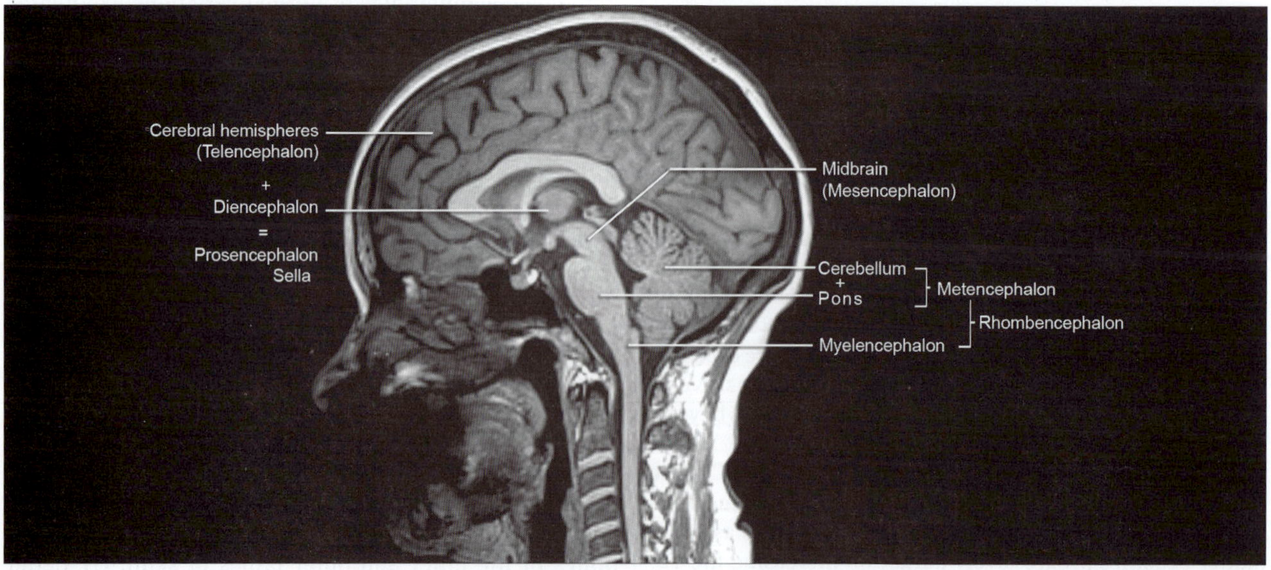

FIG. 1: Midline sagittal image of brain showing embryonal divisions.

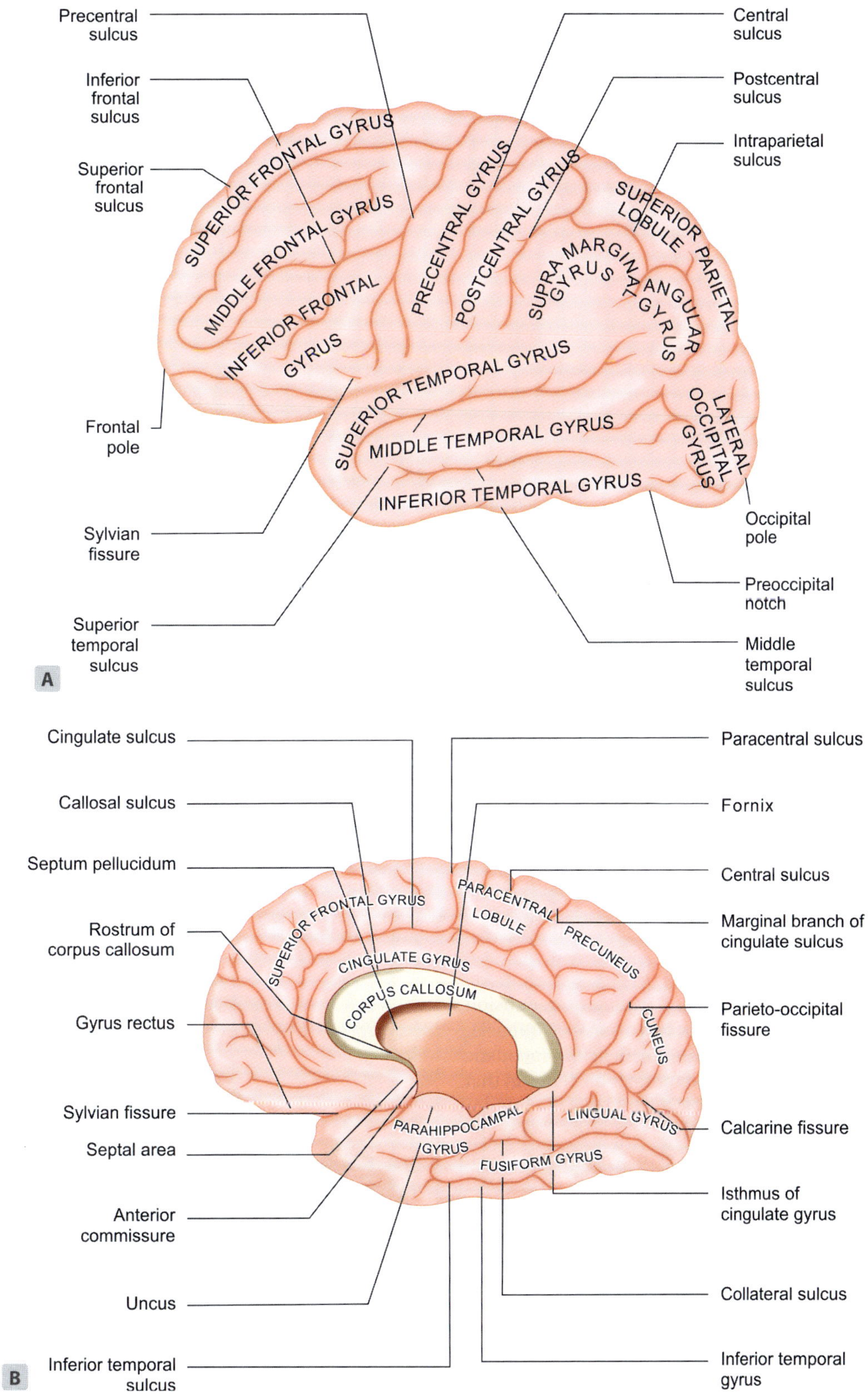

FIGS. 2A AND C *Continued*

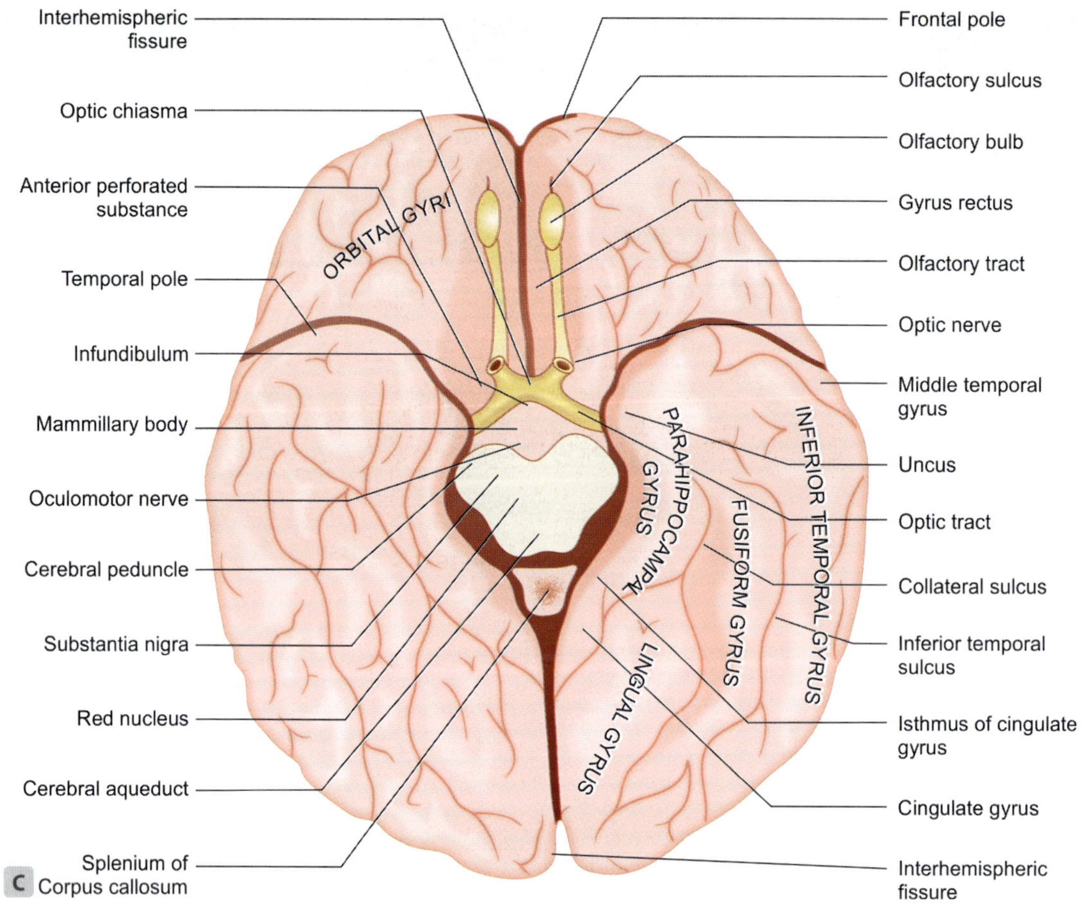

FIGS. 2A TO C: Diagrammatic representation showing anatomy of cerebral hemispheres on the (A) Lateral; (B) Medial; and (C) Inferior surface.

gyri by two horizontally running sulci—the superior and middle temporal sulcus **(Fig. 3F)**. In the dominant cerebral hemisphere at the posterior portion of the superior temporal gyrus lies the Wernicke's area, linked with comprehension of language. A lesion of this area causes sensory aphasia. Another important area is the area for hearing—acoustic area, which is also located in the temporal lobe. It lies in that part of the superior temporal gyrus which forms the inferior wall of posterior ramus of lateral sulcus and is defined as the transverse temporal gyrus (Heschl's gyrus). This is best seen in the coronal sections.

The lateral surface of the occipital lobe consists of the lateral occipital gyri **(Fig. 5I)** (visual associative functions). The preoccipital notch indents the inferolateral border of the hemisphere about 4 cm from the occipital pole. An imaginary line drawn from the superior end of the parieto-occipital fissure to the preoccipital notch marks the boundary between the occipital lobe and the parietal and temporal lobes. Insula (central lobe) is the part of cerebral cortex which lies in the depth of the lateral sulcus. It is formed by portions of the frontal, parietal and temporal lobes **(Figs. 5C and 6H)**.

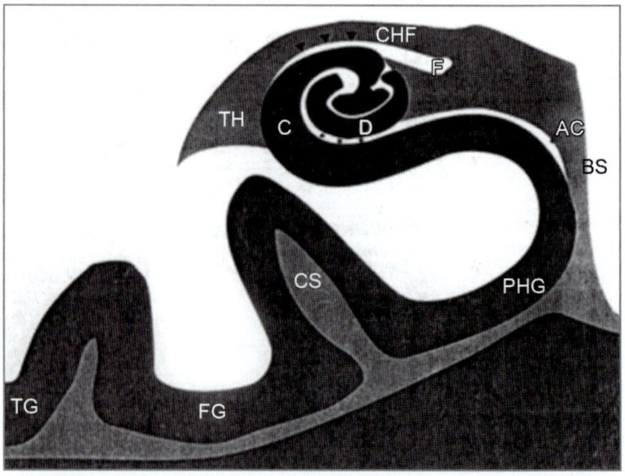

FIG. 2D: Line diagram and corresponding coronal T2 and inversion recovery images of right hippocampus. (AC: ambient cistern; BS: brainstem; C: cornu ammonis; CHF: choroid fissure; CS: collateral sulcus; D: dentate gyrus; FG: fusiform gyrus; F: fimbria; TH: temporal horn; TG: inferior temporal gyrus; PHG: parahippocampal gyrus).

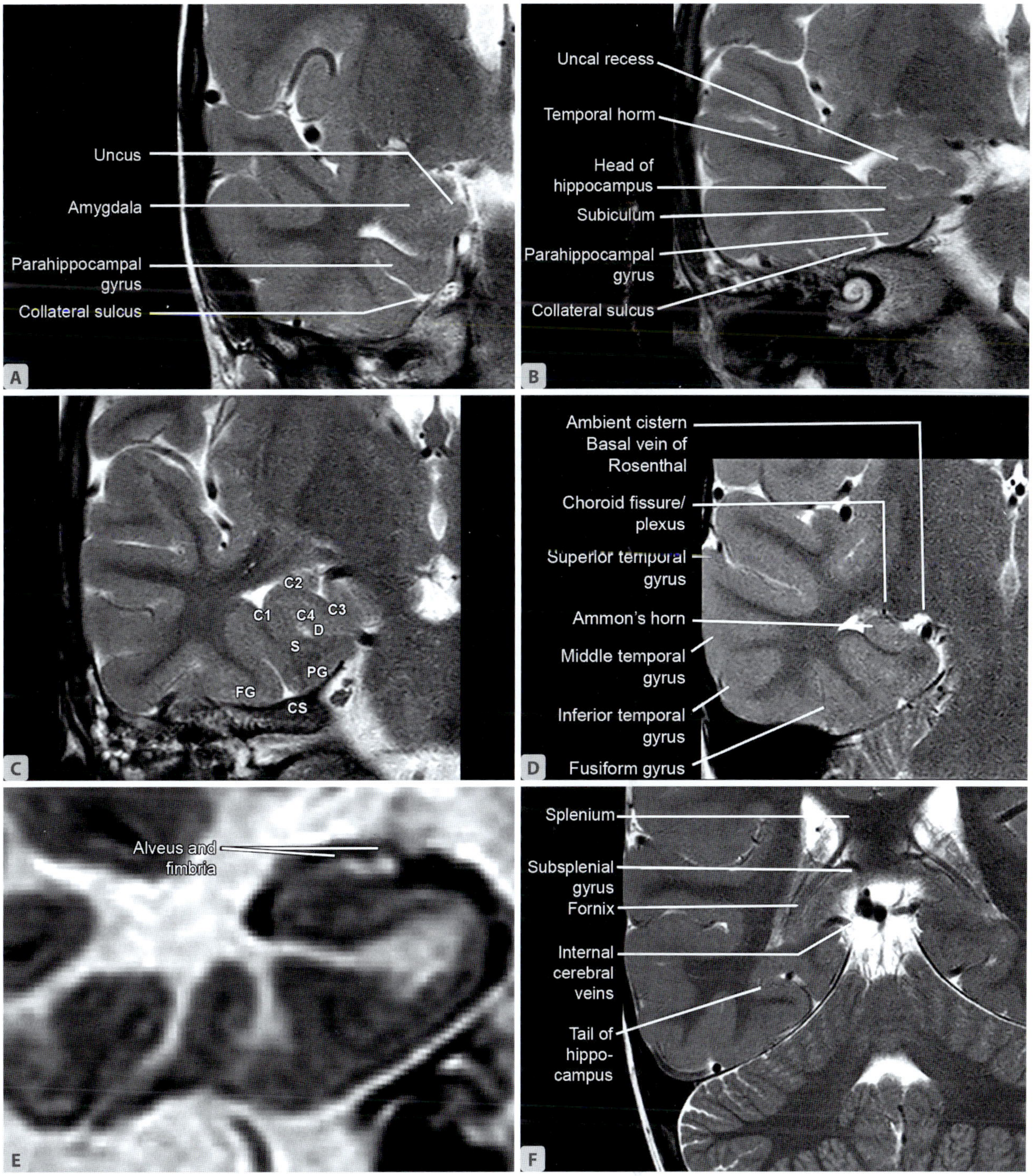

FIGS. 2E (A TO F): (a) At the level of amygdala; (b) At the level of head of hippocampus; (c) Internal anatomy of hippocampus. Sectors of Sommer C1 to C4; (d) At the level of body of hippocampus; (e) T1 image at the level of body of hippocampus; (f) Section at tail of hippocampus. (G: dentate gyrus; PG: parahippocampal gyrus; CS: collateral sulcus; FG: fusiform gyrus).

Medial Surface of the Cerebral Hemisphere (Fig. 2B)

The corpus callosum is a large mass of nerve fibers which connect the cerebral hemispheres and forms most of the roof of the lateral ventricles. It is arbitrarily divided from front to back into rostrum, genu, body, and splenium **(Fig. 3A)**.

The small anterior commissure ventral to the rostrum of the corpus callosum connects portions of the middle and inferior temporal gyri. The two lateral ventricles are separated by septum pellucidum **(Fig. 4C)** which extends from the inferior aspect of the body and genu of the corpus callosum to the superior aspect of the columns of the fornix **(Figs. 5C and D)**.

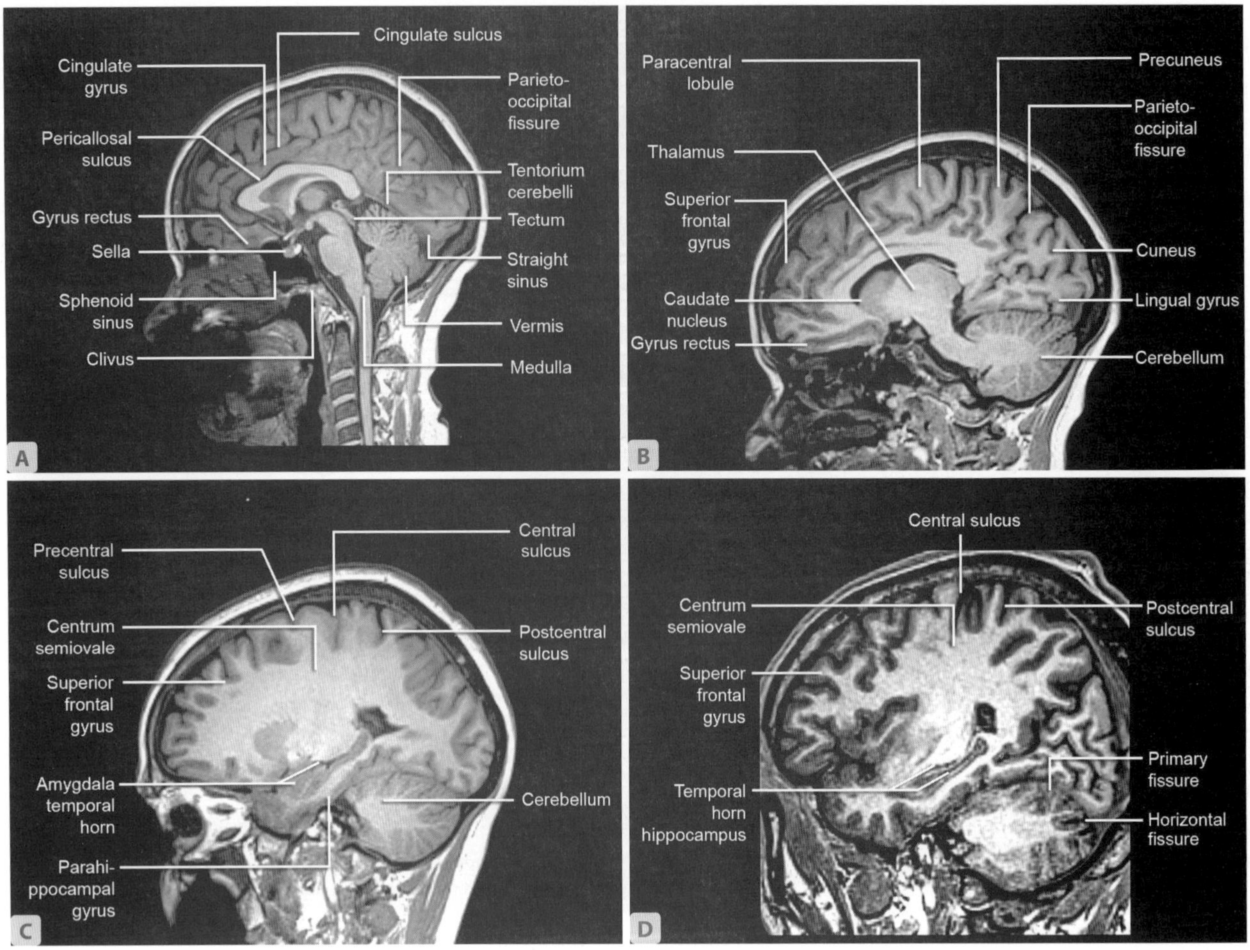

FIGS. 3A TO D: (A) Mid-sagittal MR section shows the entire length of the corpus callosum bordered above by the pericallosal sulcus. Cingulate gyrus and sulcus lie above it. The brainstem divisions, cerebellar vermis and the sellar/suprasellar anatomy are exquisitely shown on this section. The vein of Galen and straight sinus are seen behind the splenium leading to the torcula. A large rounded mass of gray matter within the 3rd ventricle represents interthalamic adhesion. The fornix is seen beneath the corpus callosum. The 3rd and 4th ventricles with the interconnecting aqueduct are well shown in this section. The tectal plate lies posterior to the aqueduct. The suprasellar cistern interpeduncular fossa, quadrigeminal plate cistern and cisterna magna are important cerebrospinal fluid (CSF) spaces identified in this section; (B to D) Parasagittal MR sections. The parieto-occipital fissure marks the boundary between parietal (precuneus) and occipital (cuneus) lobes. The calcarine fissure separates lingual gyrus from cuneus. The central, pre- and postcentral sulci and the related gyri can be followed. The parahippocampal gyrus can be seen following the temporal horn closely. The frontal lobe consists of superior and middle frontal gyri on these sections.

The callosal sulcus separates the corpus callosum from the cingulate gyrus. The cingulate sulcus separates the cingulate gyrus from the superior frontal gyrus anteriorly and the paracentral lobule posteriorly **(Figs. 3A and B)**. The central sulcus is deficient on medial surface and continuations of the precentral and postcentral gyri form the paracentral lobule on medial surface which is limited posteriorly by the marginal branch of the cingulate sulcus and anteriorly by the paracentral sulcus, a direct continuation of the precentral sulcus from the lateral surface. On the medial surface the parietal lobe (precuneus) is separated from the occipital lobe by parieto-occipital fissure **(Figs. 3B and C, 6J and K)**.

The calcarine fissure divides the medial surface of occipital lobe into the cuneus above and the lingual gyrus below **(Figs. 6H and I)**. The calcarine (primary visual) cortex, consisting of portions of the cuneate and lingual gyri lies along the banks of the calcarine fissure deep within the occipital lobe. At the inferolateral aspect of the occipital and temporal lobes lies the fusiform (lateral occipitotemporal) gyrus.

The limbic system is considered a separate lobe by some anatomists. Cingulate gyrus, parahippocampal gyrus, proper hippocampus, paraterminal gyrus and subcallosal area constitute the limbic system. Amygdala, although anatomically distinct, is functionally a part of limbic system. The cingulate gyrus lies above the corpus callosum and continues posteriorly behind the corpus callosum through the isthmus into the parahippocampal gyrus which is separated from the fusiform gyrus by the collateral sulcus. The uncus is the most anterior part of the parahippocampal gyrus which points medially and covers the amygdala which lies superior and anterior to head of hippocampus **[(Figs. 2E (A to F)]**.

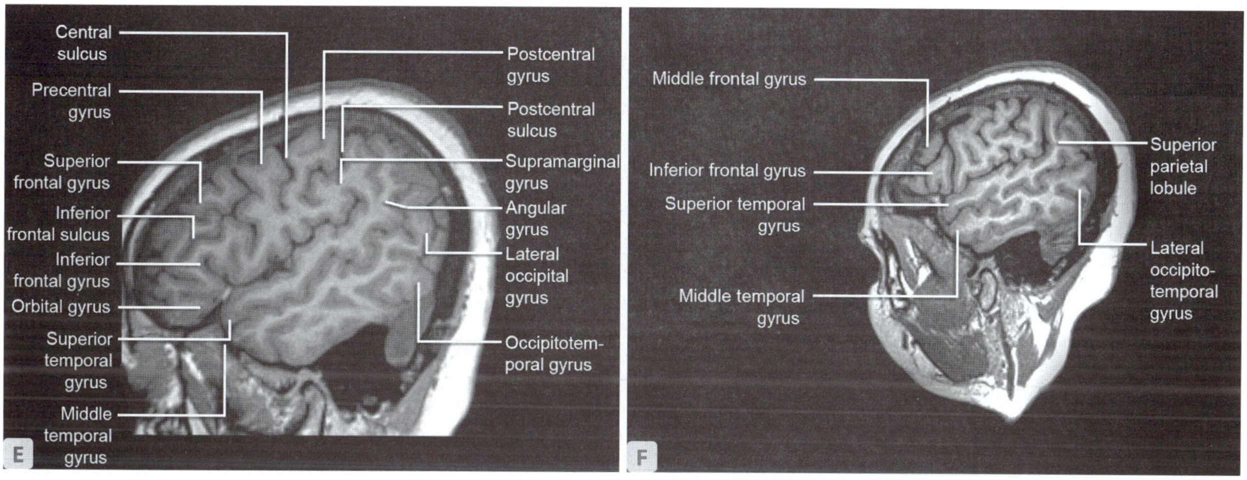

FIGS. 3E AND F: Sagittal MR sections at and lateral to Sylvian fissure. The Sylvian fissure can be traced anteriorly where its anterior ascending and horizontal rami form a V or Y configuration. These divide the inferior frontal gyrus into pars orbitalis, pars triangularis and pars opercularis giving it a characteristic M shape. Posteriorly the fissure ends in ascending and descending rami. The horse-shoe shaped supramarginal gyrus sits atop the ascending ramus. The middle frontal gyrus extends posteriorly to meet the precentral gyrus and the inferior frontal sulcus meets the obliquely coursing precentral sulcus. The central sulcus can be traced inferiorly to the subcentral gyrus. The superior and inferior temporal gyri are identified in the extreme lateral sections.

Understanding of anatomy of hippocampus is important to interpret the MR findings in hippocampal sclerosis in epilepsy. Hippocampus is located on the medial aspect of temporal lobe, superior to the parahippocampal gyrus, bounded superolaterally by the floor of the temporal horn of lateral ventricle. Anteroposteriorly hippocampus is divided into head, body and tail. It is composed of two interlocking U-shaped lamina of gray matter called cornu ammonis and dentate gyrus. The hippocampal fissure separates the subiculum (the superior flat part of parahippocampal gyrus) from the dentate gyrus. Cornu ammonis is connected with gray matter of parahippocampal gyrus through subiculum. The cornu ammonis (Ammon's horn) consists of C1, C2, C3 and C4 sectors of Sommer. White matter tracts extend from cornu ammonis to alveus which lie on the superior surface of hippocampus and converge medially to form fimbria, which in turn is continuous with crus of fornix. Choroid fissure lies superomedial to hippocampus and the ambient cistern lies medially **(Fig. 2D)**.

Inferior Surface of the Cerebral Hemisphere (Fig. 2C)

The lingual and fusiform gyri course through this areas separated by collateral sulcus. The inferior temporal sulcus separates the inferior temporal gyrus from the fusiform gyrus **(Figs. 5I and J)**.

The inferior aspects of the occipital lobe and the temporal lobe sit over the tentorium of the cerebellum.

Olfactory nerve (CN I) originates from nasal mucosa and pierces cribriform plate to enter the cranium. On the inferior (orbital) surface of frontal lobe the olfactory bulb and the olfactory tract over lie the olfactory sulcus which runs in the anteroposterior direction. Area medial to this is called gyrus rectus. Area lateral to olfactory sulcus is divided into four parts by a H-shaped sulcus into anterior, posterior, medial and lateral orbital gyri **(Figs. 5A and B)**.

Optic nerves (CN II) extend from optic disc to optic chiasma and continues posteriorly as optic tracts leading to lateral geniculate body, pretectal nucleus and superior colliculus.

DIENCEPHALON

The diencephalon connects the cerebral hemispheres to the mid brain and is made of thalamus, hypothalamus, subthalamus and epithalamus. The hypothalamus lies within the floor and lateral walls of the third ventricle. It extends from the lamina terminalis anteriorly to the caudal aspect of the mammillary bodies and includes the tuber cinereum which gives rise to the pituitary stalk **(Fig. 6F)**.

Each thalamus is a large mass of gray matter in the lateral wall of the 3rd ventricle. It is bounded laterally by the posterior limb of the internal capsule and ventrally by the hypothalamic sulcus **(Fig. 6G)**. The interthalamic adhesion projecting through the 3rd ventricle forms a medial connection with the opposite thalamus. The dorsolateral margin of the thalamus forms part of the floor of the lateral ventricle. The posterior bulging portion of the thalamus is called the pulvinar **(Fig. 5F)**. It overhangs medial and lateral geniculate bodies.

Ventral to the pulvinar lie the medial and lateral geniculate bodies on each side of midbrain, together called the metathalamus. They relay auditory and visual information to their respective receptor areas of cortex. The subthalamus is bounded by the hypothalamus anteriorly, the internal capsule laterally, and the thalamus above. The subthalamic nucleus integrates and relays connections from the globus pallidus and the thalamus.

The most dorsal division of the diencephalon, the epithalamus, includes the habenular nuclei, posterior

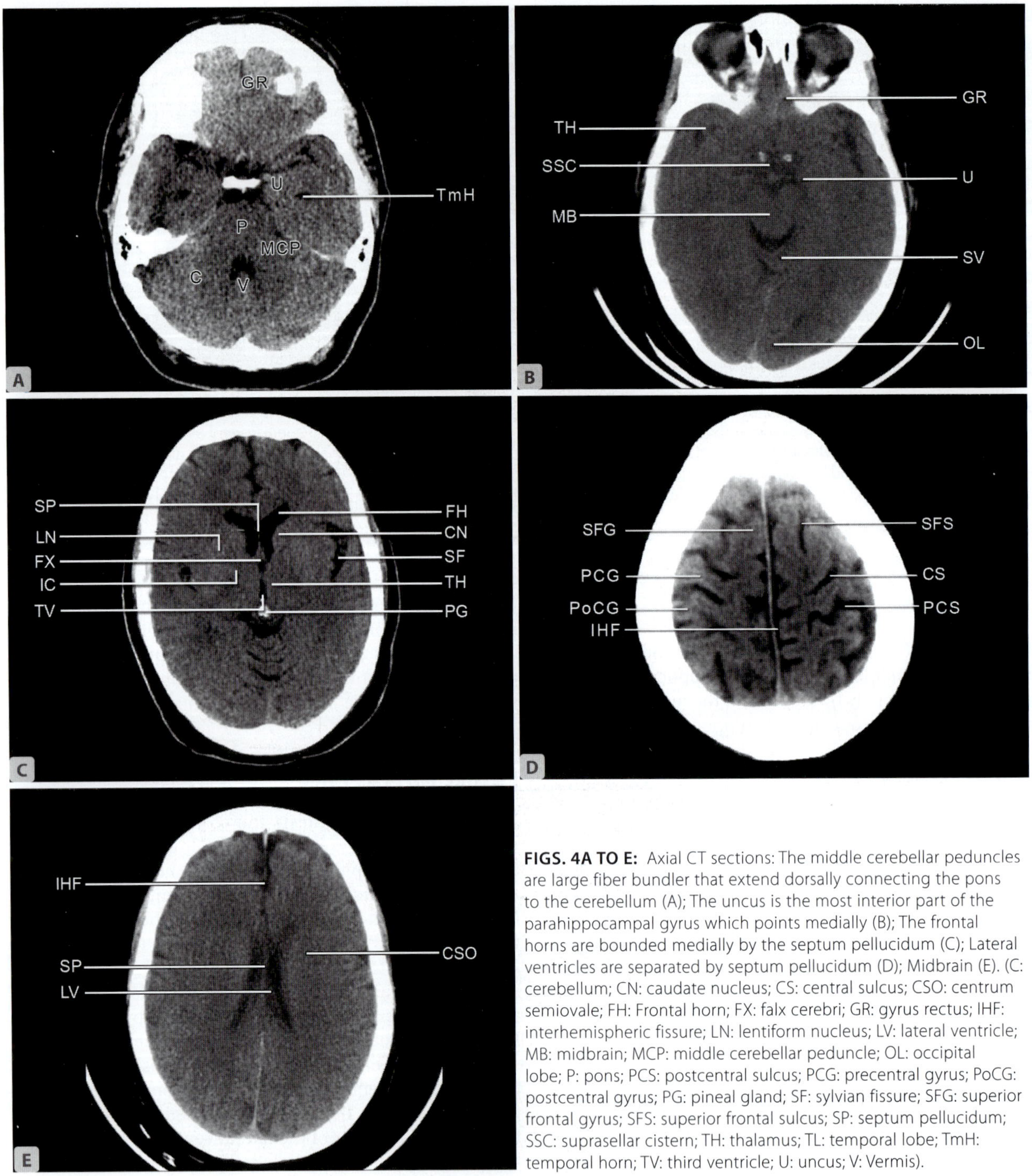

FIGS. 4A TO E: Axial CT sections: The middle cerebellar peduncles are large fiber bundler that extend dorsally connecting the pons to the cerebellum (A); The uncus is the most interior part of the parahippocampal gyrus which points medially (B); The frontal horns are bounded medially by the septum pellucidum (C); Lateral ventricles are separated by septum pellucidum (D); Midbrain (E). (C: cerebellum; CN: caudate nucleus; CS: central sulcus; CSO: centrum semiovale; FH: Frontal horn; FX: falx cerebri; GR: gyrus rectus; IHF: interhemispheric fissure; LN: lentiform nucleus; LV: lateral ventricle; MB: midbrain; MCP: middle cerebellar peduncle; OL: occipital lobe; P: pons; PCS: postcentral sulcus; PCG: precentral gyrus; PoCG: postcentral gyrus; PG: pineal gland; SF: sylvian fissure; SFG: superior frontal gyrus; SFS: superior frontal sulcus; SP: septum pellucidum; SSC: suprasellar cistern; TH: thalamus; TL: temporal lobe; TmH: temporal horn; TV: third ventricle; U: uncus; V: Vermis).

commissure and pineal body. The structure is a part of limbic system.

MIDBRAIN AND BRAINSTEM (PONS AND MEDULLA (FIG. 3A)

The midbrain consists of a smaller dorsal portion the tectum and larger ventral portion, the cerebral peduncles **(Fig. 6F)**. Aqueduct connecting the 3rd and 4th ventricles runs in the center of the junction of the tectum and cerebral peduncles **(Fig. 3A)**. Each cerebral peduncle has a ventral part—the crus and a dorsal part—the tegmentum, separated by substantia nigra. The red nucleus, another pigmented nucleus is located posterior and medial to the substantia nigra on each side. Pars compacta separates the substantia nigra and red nucleus **(Fig. 6L)**. The tectum consists of four rounded prominences—the two superior colliculi and two inferior colliculi or corpora quadrigemina. Each superior colliculus

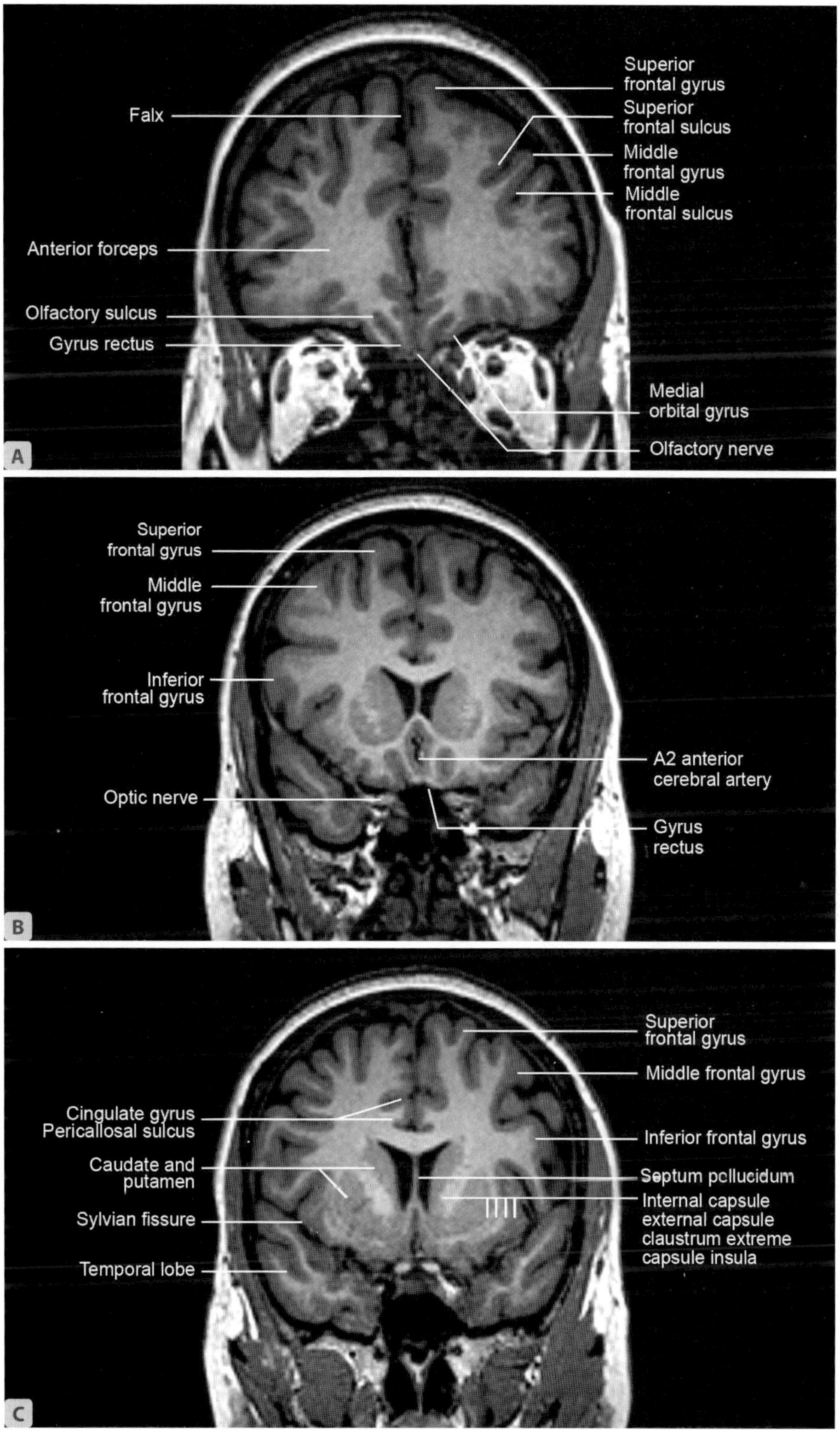

FIGS. 5A TO J: *Continued*

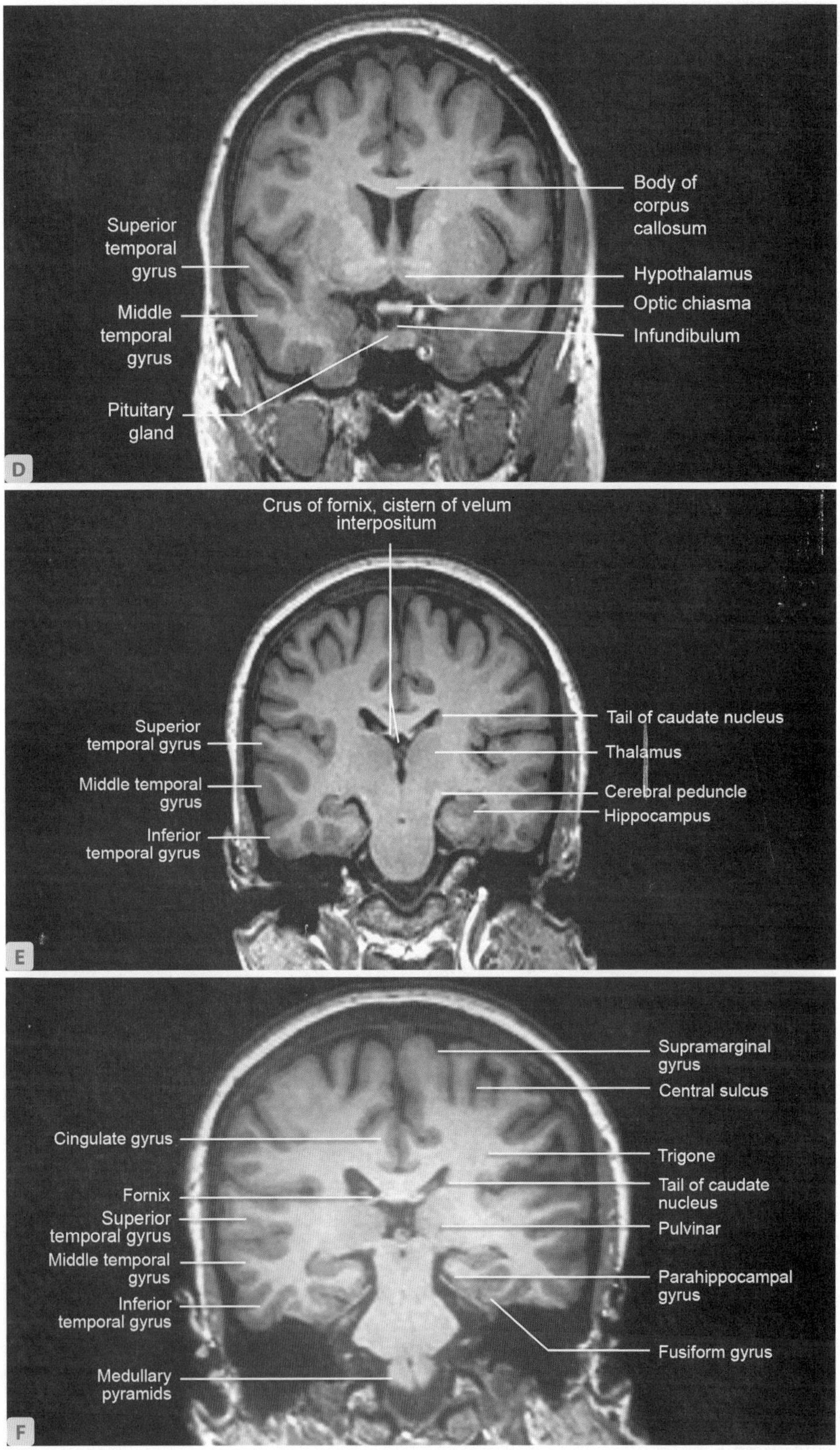

FIGS. 5A TO J: *Continued*

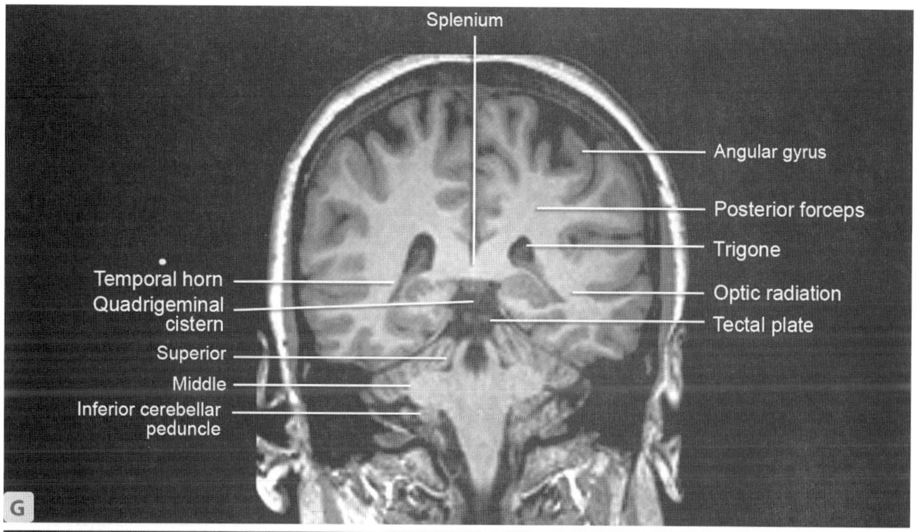

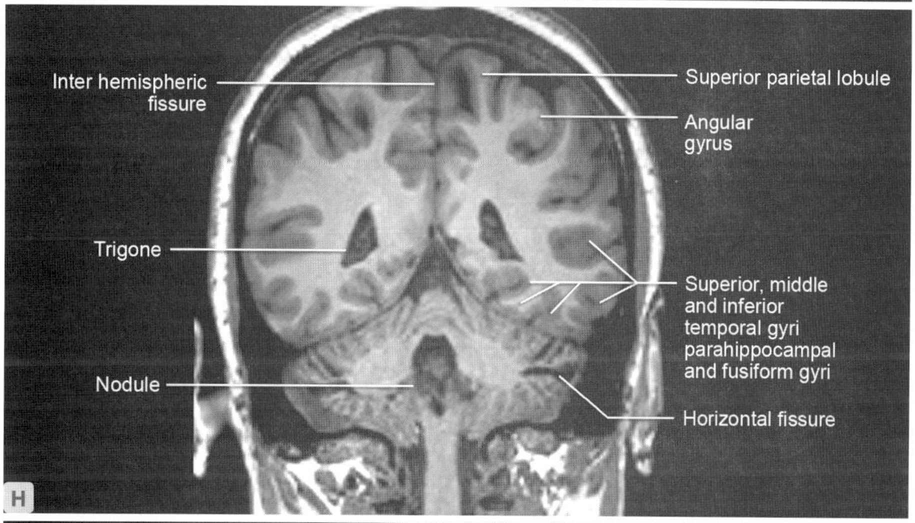

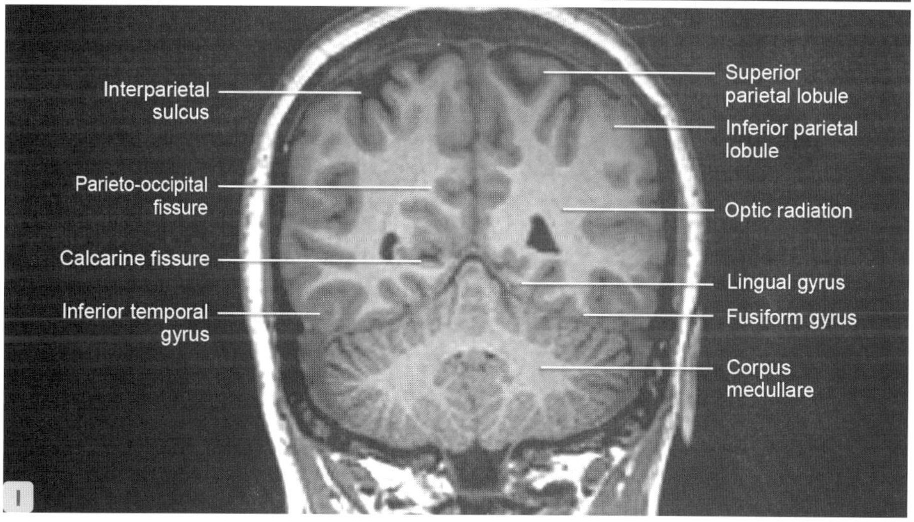

FIGS. 5A TO J: *Continued*

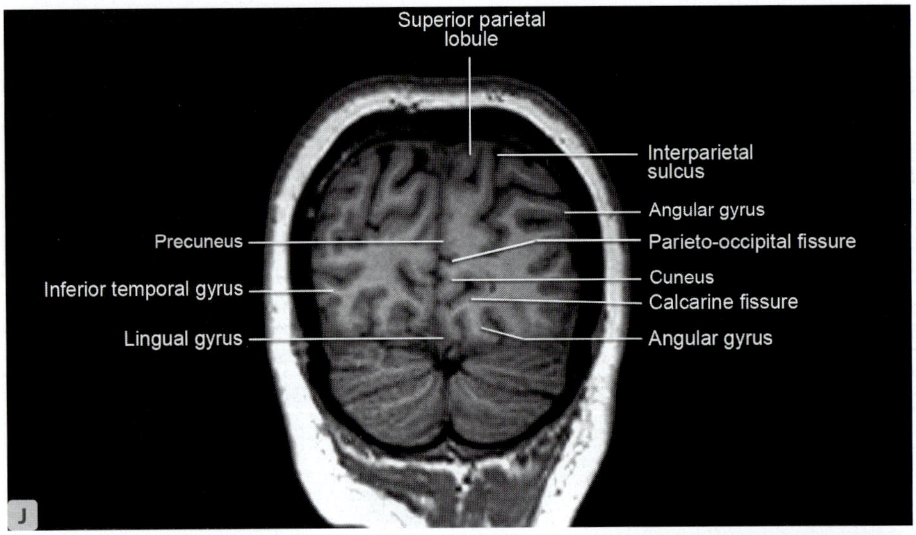

FIGS. 5A TO J: (A and B) Coronal MR sections anterior to the frontal horn. The entire slice contains frontal lobe. The olfactory nerve nestles between the gyrus rectus and medial orbital gyrus on the cribriform plate. (A) The more anterior section shows a continuous interhemispheric fissure which is interrupted by corpus callosum on the more posterior section. (B) The optic strut separates the optic nerve from superior orbital fissure; (C and D) Coronal MR sections through the frontal horn. The frontal horns are outlined by corpus callosum and caudate nucleus. The internal capsule, putamen, external capsule, claustrum and insula can be seen from medial to lateral. The two columns of fornix outline the foramen of Monro with septum pellucidum above it separating the two frontal horns. Optic chiasma can be identified above the pituitary gland and its infundibulum. In the parasellar area, the cavernous sinuses containing third, fourth, fifth and sixth nerves are outlined by low intensity dura; (E) Coronal MR sections at the third ventricle level. Mid third of the lateral convexity is parietal lobe and lower third is temporal lobe. Corpus callosum lies at the bottom of the interhemispheric fissure. The lateral ventricles (with crus fornix on its superior medial part) and third ventricle are seen more inferiorly. The interpeduncular fossa is seen as a CSF space below third ventricle. The tail of caudate nucleus lies on the lateral aspect of lateral ventricle. The medial temporal lobe consists of hippocampus with overlying choroid fissure; (F) Coronal MR sections through the body of lateral ventricle. This section cut through the splenium of corpus callosum with the cingulate gyrus lying just above it. Below it lie the quadrigeminal plate (tectum) and its cistern. The sections pass through the mid brain, pons and medulla. The lateral convexity consists entirely of parietal and temporal lobes; (G and H) Coronal MR sections through the trigone and occipital horns. Superior two-thirds of the lateral convexity of brain at this level consists of superior and inferior parietal lobules. The lower third belongs to the temporal lobe. The inferior surface of temporal lobe consists of parahippocampal, fusiform and inferior temporal gyri; (G) The section through trigones cuts the cerebellar peduncles while; (H) A more posterior section shows the cerebellar hemispheres, vermis and the tonsils; (I and J) Coronal MR sections posterior to the occipital horn. The interhemispheric fissure completely divides the two cerebral hemispheres. The lingual, fusiform and inferior temporal gyri are clearly identified. The precuneus and cuneus are separated by parieto-occipital fissure and between the cuneus and lingual gyrus lies the calcarine fissure.

is connected to the *ipsilateral lateral* geniculate body through the superior brachium, where the optic tract ends. Similarly, the inferior colliculi are connected to the medial geniculate bodies through the inferior brachium thereby connecting it to the auditory cortex **(Fig. 6F)**.

The oculomotor nerves (CN III) exit from the caudal aspect of the interpeduncular fossa **(Fig. 7A)**. The paired trochlear nerves (CN IV) emerge from the dorsal surface of the brainstem caudal to the inferior colliculi, and wrap around the lateral aspects of the midbrain. The ventral and dorsal aspects of the cerebral peduncles are separated by semilunar substantia nigra with red nuclei on its dorsomedial aspect **(Fig. 6L)**.

The pons has a bulging ventral surface with a shallow midline basal sulcus. The middle cerebellar peduncles are large fiber bundles that extend dorsally connecting the pons to the cerebellum **(Fig. 4A)**. Emerging from the lateral aspect of the pons are the trigeminal nerves (CN V) **(Figs. 6D, 7B)**, while the paired paramedian abducens nerves (CN VI) exit ventrally from the pontomedullary junction. The facial nerves (CN VII) and the vestibulocochlear nerves (V III) emerge from the lateral aspect of the pontomedullary junction and pass through the cerebellopontine angle cistern **(Fig. 7C)**.

The medulla oblongata connects the midbrain and the spinal cord. It measures 3 cm in length and 2 cm in width. On the ventral aspect of the medulla the paramedian pyramids form longitudinal protrusions on each side of the ventral median fissure. The paired ventrolateral sulci separate the medullary pyramids and the inferior olives **(Fig. 6A)**. The hypoglossal nerves (CN XII) emerge from the ventrolateral sulci. The rootlets of the glossopharyngeal (CN IX), vagus (CN X) and spinal accessory (CN XI) nerves exit from the dorsolateral sulcus which is located further laterally **(Fig. 7D)**. The paired cuneate and gracilis tubercles form longitudinal ridges on the dorsal aspect of the medulla oblongata just caudal to the fourth ventricles separated by posterior median sulcus.

CEREBELLUM

The cerebellum lies posterior to the pons and medulla. The superior, middle, and inferior cerebellar peduncles connect the cerebellum to midbrain, pons and medulla respectively. The narrowest leaf-like subdivisions of the cerebellar cortex are termed folia. The cerebellum consists of the midline cerebellar vermis connecting the paired lateral hemispheres.

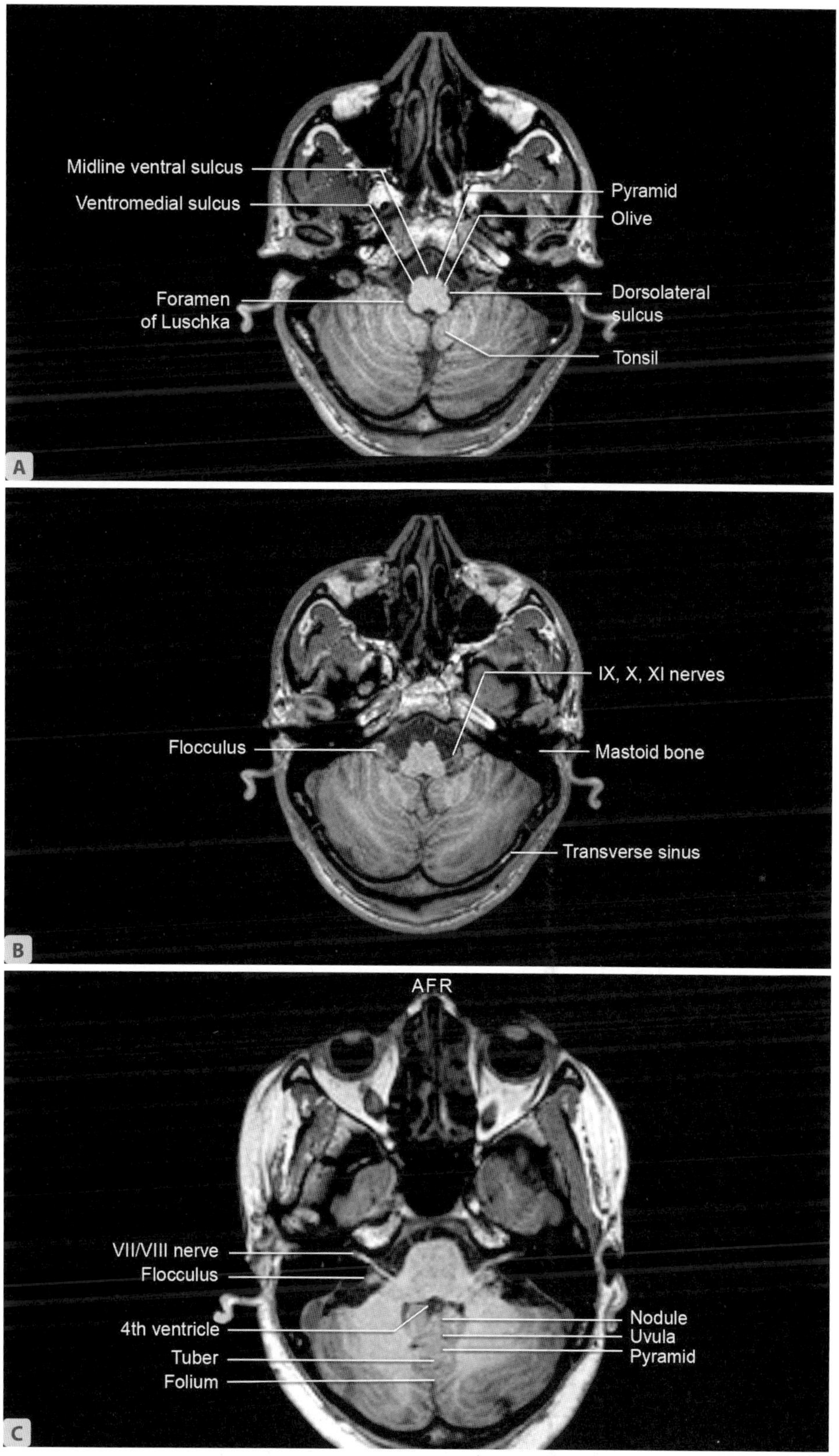

FIGS. 6A TO N: *Continued*

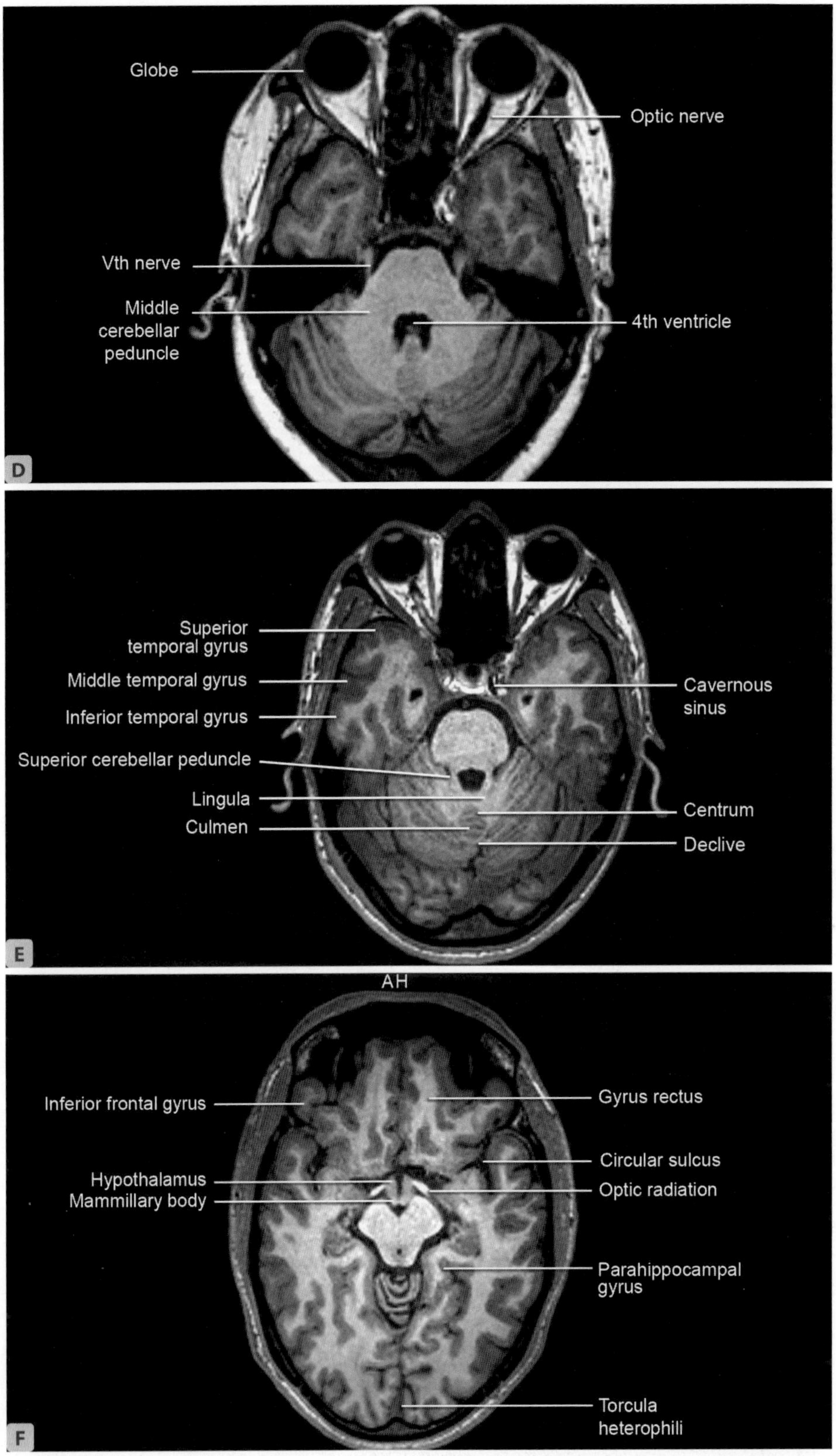

FIGS. 6A TO N: *Continued*

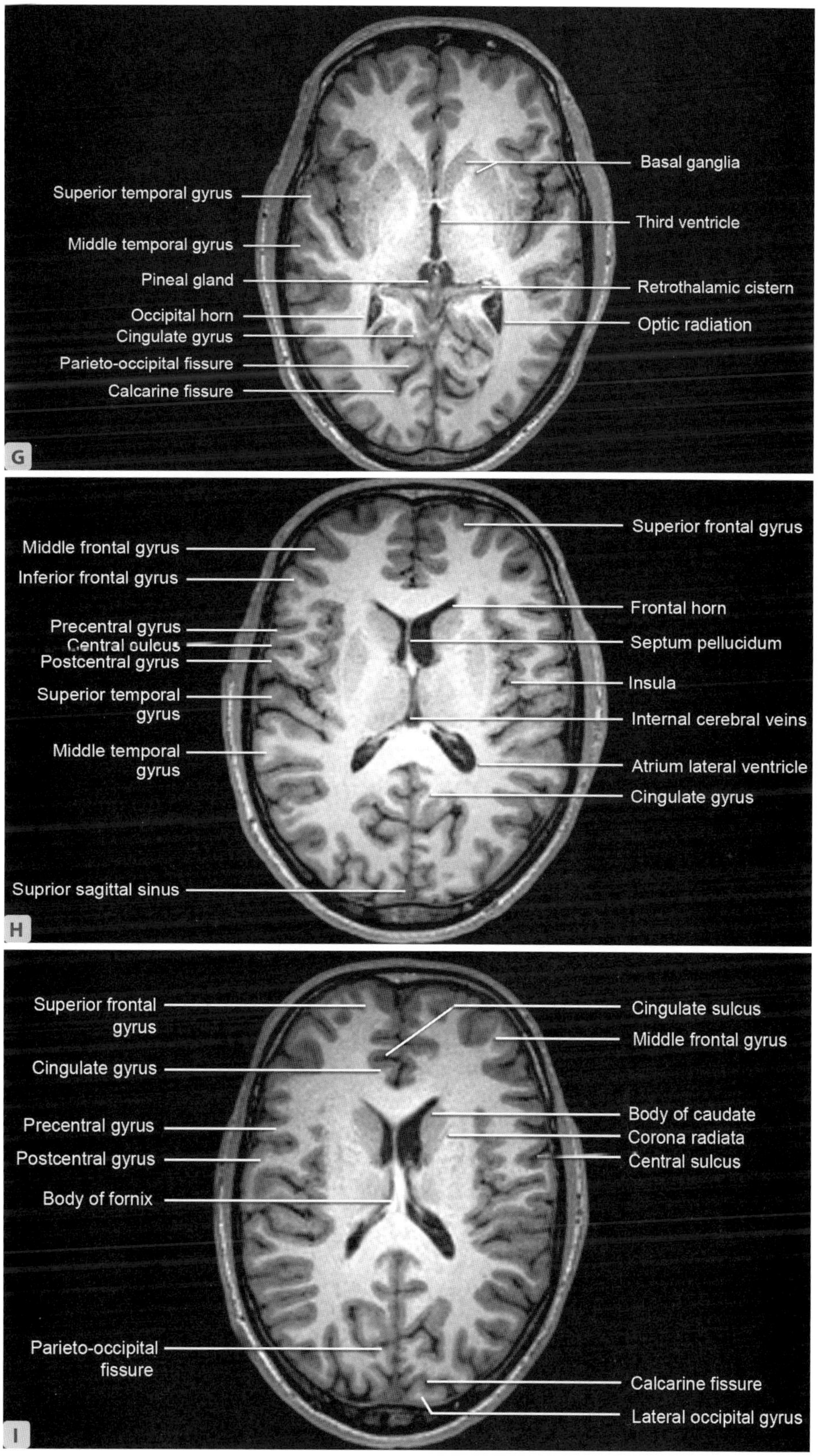

FIGS. 6A TO N: *Continued*

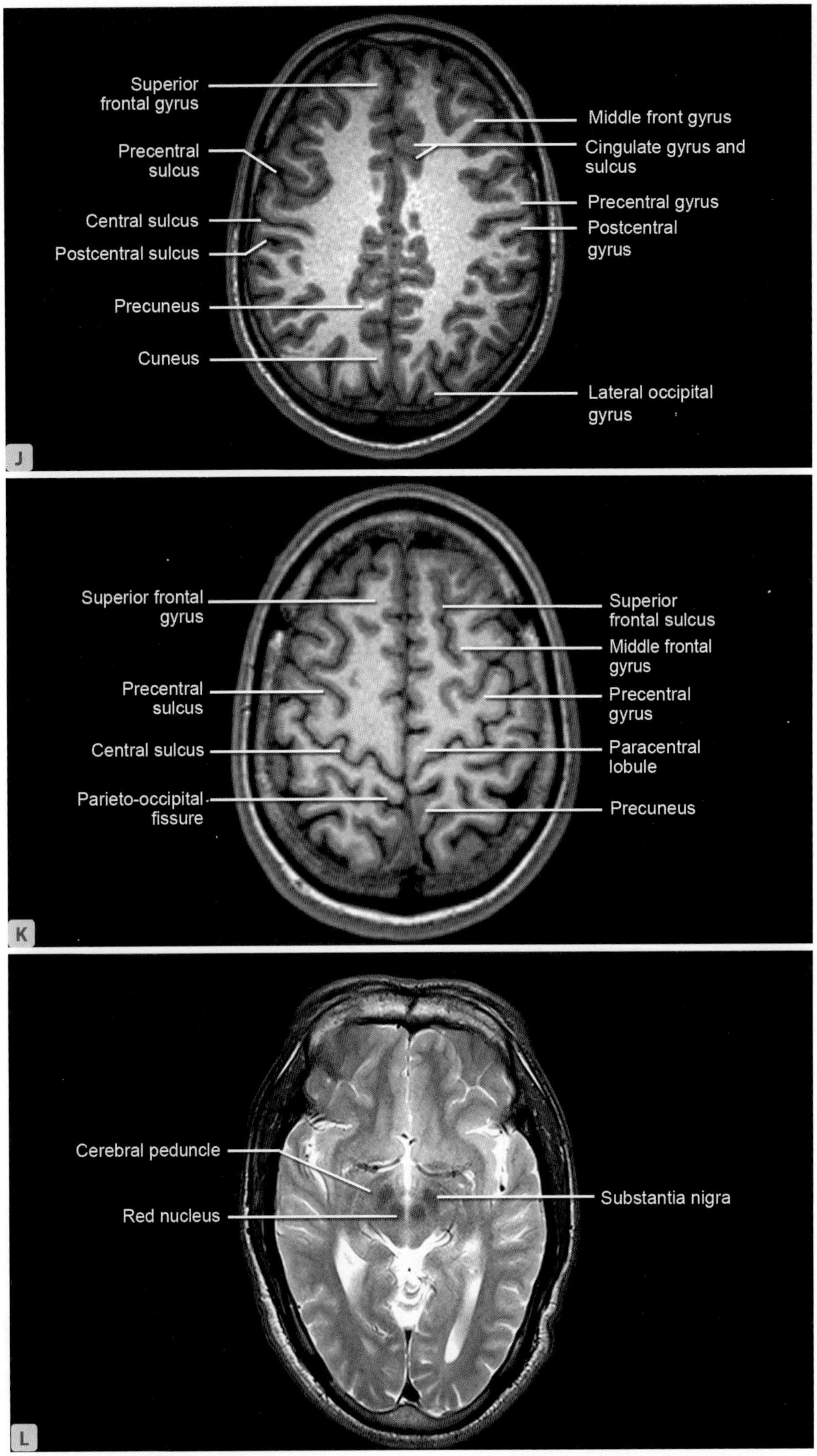

FIGS. 6A TO N: *Continued*

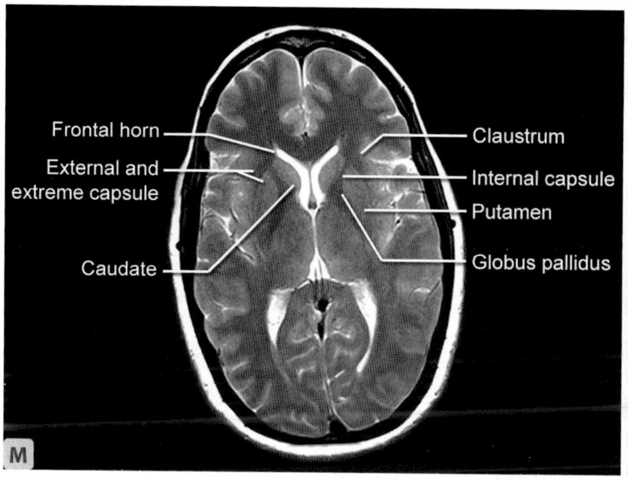

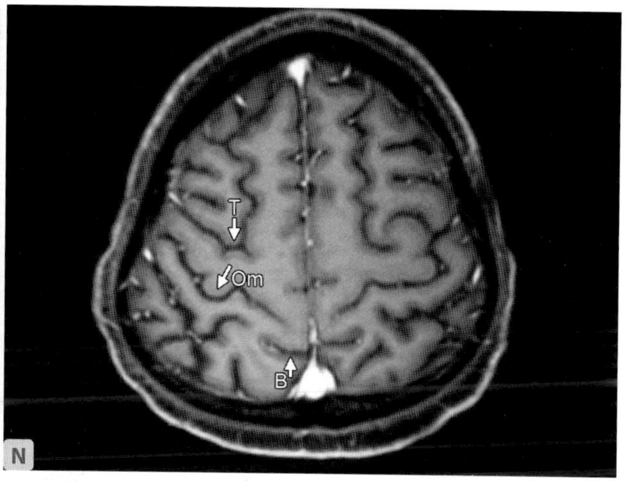

FIGS. 6A TO N: (A) T1-weighted axial MR section at the level of medulla shows the midline ventral sulcus, pyramids and olives separated by ventromedial sulcus. Dorsolateral sulcus is seen posterior to olives. Cerebellar tonsils are seen posterolateral to the medulla. Vallecula is seen posteriorly. Fourth ventricle with foramen of Luschka is seen posterior to medulla; (B) T1-weighted axial MR section at slightly higher level than Figure 2.6A shows the IX, X and XI cranial nerves seen as a common bundle exiting from the dorsolateral sulcus; (C) T1-weighted axial MR section through the pons. Pons is seen in front of the fourth ventricles. The CP angle cisterns lie lateral to the pons. Seventh and eight cranial nerves course through the cistern anterior to flocculus toward internal auditory canals. The inferior vermis and its various divisions are well seen; (D) T1-weighted axial MR section through middle part of fourth ventricle. Middle cerebellar peduncles connecting the pons with cerebellar hemispheres are well seen. Fifth nerves are seen emerging from the lateral surface of pons on both sides. Also seen are globes with optic nerve and lower part of temporal lobes; (E) T1-weighted axial MR section through the midbrain shows the superior cerebellar peduncles, and the parts of superior vermis. Anteriorly the olfactory nerve and gyrus rectus on each side of interhemispheric fissure are seen clearly. The structures of the middle cranial fossa-cavernous sinus, both temporal lobes with superior, middle and inferior temporal gyri, are also seen; (F) T1-weighted axial MR section at the level of midbrain. Inferiorly frontal and temporal lobes are seen separated by sylvian fissure. V-shaped tentorium outlining the superior vermis is seen with quadrigeminal plate and cistern located anterior to it. Parahippocampal gyrus and fusiform gyrus course forward from occipital pole to midbrain. Anterior to midbrain, mammillary bodies, optic radiations and hypothalamus are seen; (G) T1-weighted axial MR section at the level of lower third ventricle shows the basal ganglia, internal capsule, thalami and retrothalamic cistern. Peripherally superior temporal and middle temporal gyri are seen posterior to sylvian fissure. Frontal horns of lateral ventricles are seen anteriorly and occipital horns posteriorly. Pineal gland is seen posterior to the third ventricle. Optic radiations are seen ending in the occipital cortex. Also seen is the Y-shaped parieto-occipital fissure and calcarine fissure, the later forming the lateral boundary of lingual gyrus; (H) T1-weighted axial MR section at the level of mid-3rd ventricle showing various parts of frontal lobe, anteriorly and occipital lobes posteriorly. In the midline genu of the corpus callosum is seen anteriorly connecting the frontal lobes. Septum pellucidum is seen separating the frontal horns of lateral ventricles. Posteriorly in the midline splenium of the corpus callosum is seen forming posterior wall of 3rd ventricle and medial wall of atria of lateral ventricle. Peripherally the central sulcus is seen separating the frontal (precentral) and parietal (postcentral) lobes. The sylvian fissure separates the parietal lobe (post central gyrus) from the temporal lobe (superior temporal gyrus). In the depth of the sylvian fissure, portions of frontal, parietal and temporal lobe form the insula; (I) T1-weighted axial MR section at the superior part of 3rd ventricle shows the superior frontal gyrus and middle frontal gyrus separated by superior frontal sulcus. Body of fornix is seen anterior to 3rd ventricles which separate the lateral ventricles. The other structures seen in Figure 2.6H are also seen; (J and K) T1-weighted axial MR section at supraventricular level show the deep white matter of cerebral hemispheres, the centrum semiovale. The central sulcus characteristically dips posteriorly and leads to paracentral lobule. Posterior to it the precuneus and cuneus are separately seen. Only superior and middle frontal gyri are seen at this level; (L) T2-weighted axial MR section at midbrain level. Semilunar band of pigmented gray matter anteriorly—the substantia nigra, appears hypointense. Another area of hypointensity is seen dorsomedial to substantia nigra called the red nucleus. The substantia nigra and red nuclei are separated by pars compacta; (M) T2-weighted axial MR section at the level of basal ganglia. Slit like third ventricle in midline is flanked by thalamus on each side. The interhemispheric fissure anteriorly separates the two frontal lobes. Medial to the sylvian fissure, lie the insular cortex and external capsule. The caudate and lentiform nuclei with intervening internal capsule lie medially. Globus pallidus appears hypointense in comparison to putamen on T2-weighted images. Claustrum—a strip of gray matter lies between the external and extreme capsule; (N) Localization of central sulcus on axial section. Arrows and corresponding notations indicate upper T or L sign (junction of superior frontal and precentral sulci), Omega sign (shape of hand motor area) and bracket sign (junction of marginal sulcus with inter hemispheric fissure).

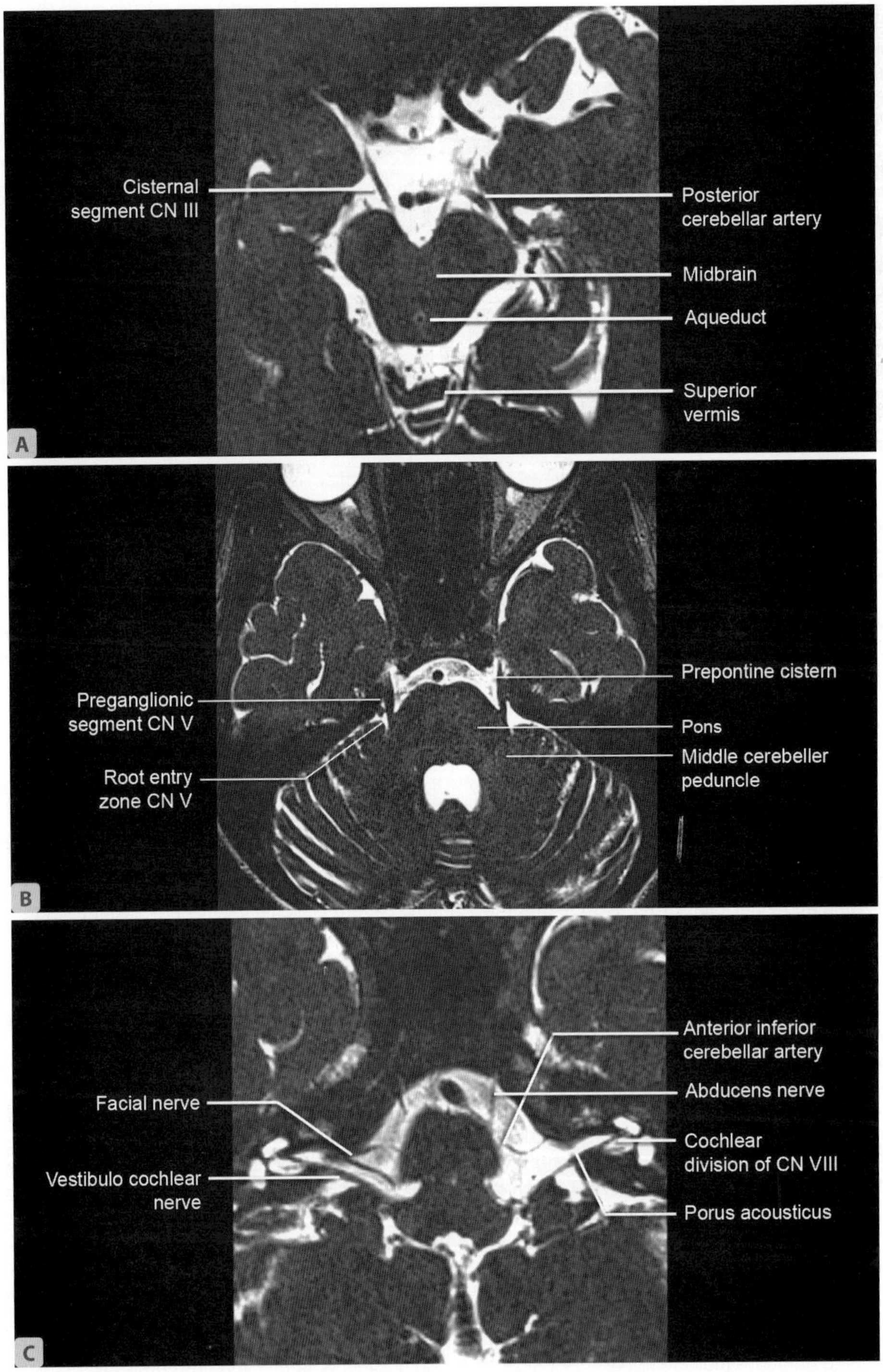

FIGS. 7A TO D: *Continued*

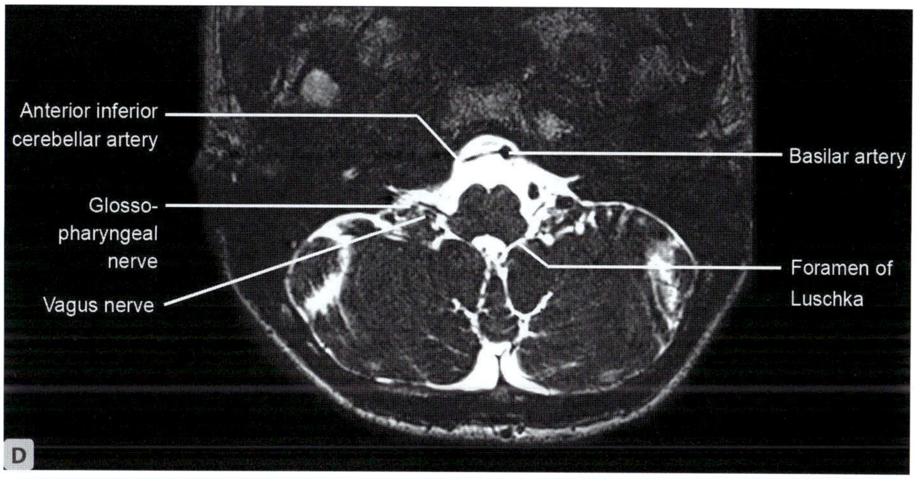

FIGS. 7A TO D: Axial MR cisternography sections using SPACE technique through (A) Midbrain; (B and C) Pons; and (D) Medulla show III, V, VI, VII, VIII, IX and X cranial nerves in relation to brainstem as labeled.

The hemisphere is divided into anterior lobe, middle lobe and flocculonodular lobe by deep fissures named primary fissure and posterolateral fissure **(Figs. 3D and 5H)**. A deep horizontal fissure divides it into superior and inferior halves. Caudal to the inferior vermis and between the cerebellar tonsils is the vallecula **(Fig. 6A)** which communicates with the fourth ventricle through the foramen of Magendie. The superior divisions of the vermis are lingula, centrum, culmen, declive and folium **(Fig. 6E)**. The inferior divisions are tuber, pyramid, uvula and nodule **(Fig. 6C)**. Immediately caudal to the inferior medullary velum is the nodulus of the vermis. The flocculus projects into the cerebellopontine angle cistern ventral to the inferior cerebellar peduncle **(Fig. 6B)**. The deep cerebral nuclei are laterally placed dentate and medially placed paired emboliform, globose and fastigial nuclei.

WHITE MATTER OF BRAIN (FIGS. 8A TO J)

The fiber connections of the cerebral cortex are divisible into three major groups **(Figs. 8A to H)**. Projection fibers are corticospinal, corticobulbar, corticopontine and cortico-thalamic tracts. Association fibers consist of subcortical U fibers, long projection fibers of cingulum, superior/inferior longitudinal fasciculi, uncinate fasciculus and superior/inferior occipitofrontal fasciculi. The commissural fibers interconnecting the two hemispheres are corpus callosum, anterior and posterior commissure, hippocampal/habenular commissures and the hypothalamic commissure. The common central mass of white matter is known as the centrum semiovale **(Fig. 4D)**. Projection fibers passing through the corona radiata converge to form the internal capsule consisting of anterior and posterior limbs and the genu **(Figs. 4C and 6M)**. The brainstem tracts are also well shown **(Figs. 8I to J)**.

The columns of fornix which lie on either side of the foramen of Monro continue posteriorly as body of fornix. It is a C-shaped bundle of white matter forming the roof of III ventricle. Posteriorly it divides into the two crura which continue into the fimbria and alveus of hippocampal formation **(Fig. 2B)**. This is part of limbic system concerned with emotional and sexual behavior and recent memory.

VENTRICLES AND CISTERNS

The ventricular system consists of lateral, third, fourth ventricles and the cerebral aqueduct. The lateral ventricles communicate with the third ventricle by the foramen of Monro while the third ventricle communicates with the fourth ventricle via the aqueduct of Sylvius.

The lateral ventricles consist of frontal horns, body, trigone, occipital and temporal horns. Foramen of Monro defines the junction between frontal horns and body of lateral ventricles and the splenium of corpus callosum arbitrarily separates the body from the trigone. The frontal horns are bounded medially by the septum pellucidum **(Fig. 4C)**, inferiorly and laterally by the head of the caudate nucleus, and superiorly and anteriorly by the corpus callosum. The body is bounded superiorly by the corpus callosum, inferiorly by caudate nucleus and the thalamus, medially by the fornix and laterally by the body of the caudate nucleus **(Fig. 5E)**. The trigone contains large tuft of choroid plexus called glomus **(Fig. 5H)**.

The third ventricle is bounded laterally by the thalami, inferiorly by the hypothalamus **(Figs. 5D and E)**, anteriorly by the anterior commissure and lamina terminalis, posteriorly by the epithalamus and posterior commissure, and superiorly by the cistern of the velum interpositum and body of the fornix. The inferior aspect of third ventricle has downward invaginations called optic, infundibular recesses anteriorly and, suprapineal and pineal recesses posteriorly.

The fourth ventricle is rhomboid in shape and lies between the pons and cerebellum. It communicates above with the third ventricle via the aqueduct and with subarachnoid space through posterior midline foramen of Magendie and posterolateral foramina of Luschka **(Fig. 6A)**.

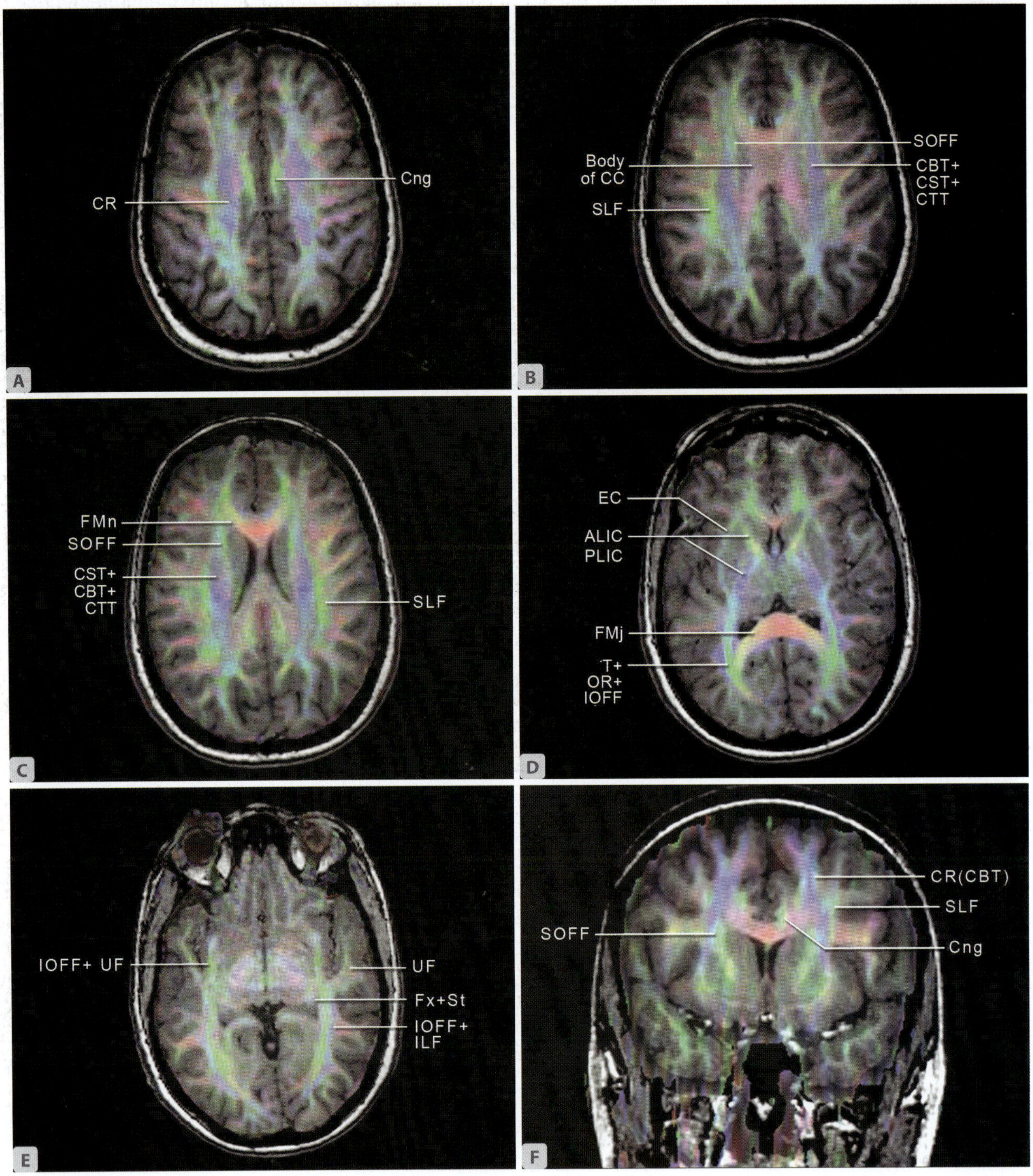

FIGS. 8A TO J: *Continued*

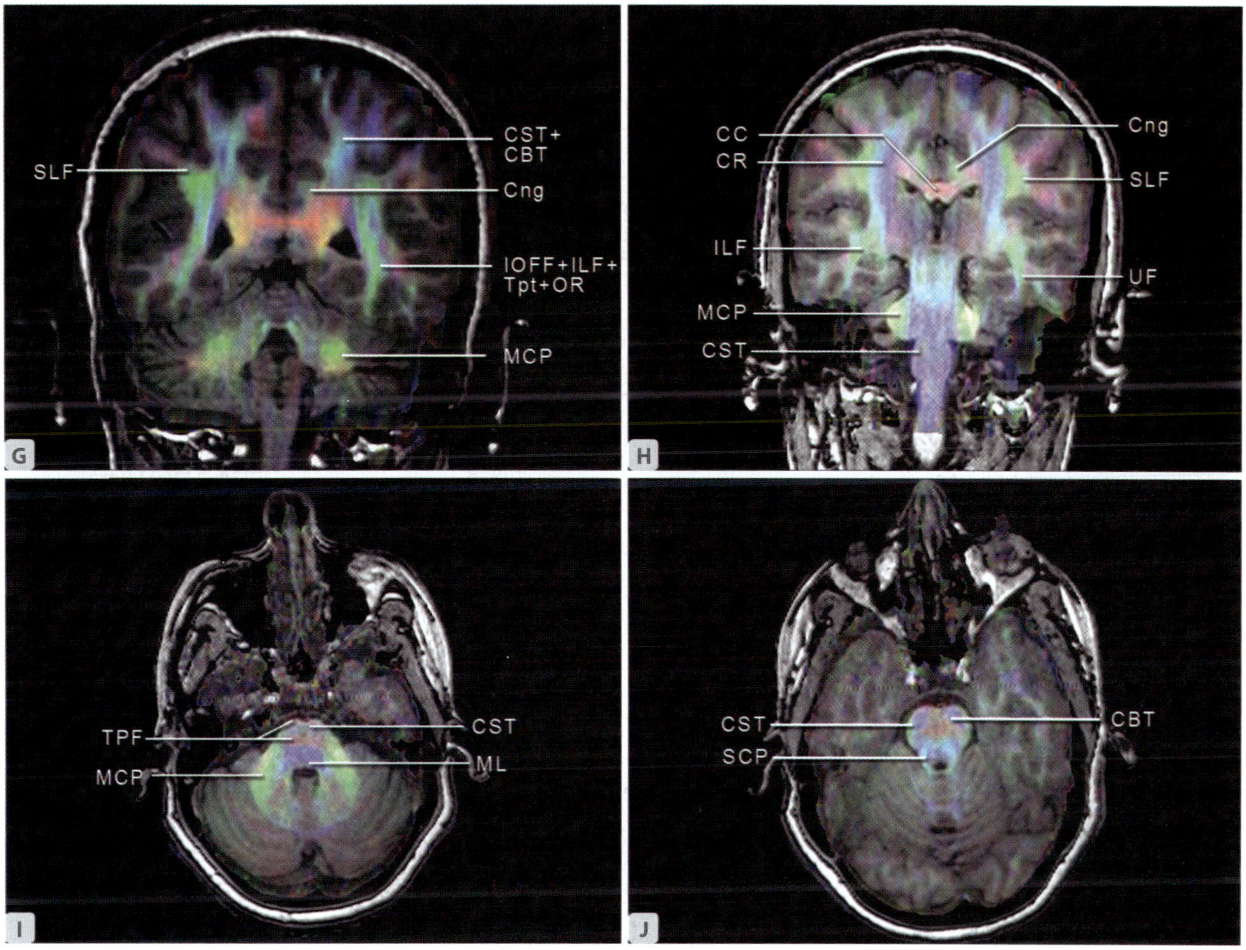

FIGS. 8A TO J: Fractional anisotropy maps superimposed on T1 weighted images of brain showing the white matter tracts. (ALIC: anterior limb of internal capsule; CBT: corticobulbar tract; Cng: cingulum; CR: corona radiata; CST: corticospinal tract; CTT: corticothalamic tract; FMj: forceps major; FMn: forceps minor; Fx: fornix; ILF: inferior longitudinal fasciculus; IOFF: inferior occipitofrontal fasciculus; MCP: middle cerebellar peduncles; ML: medial lemniscus; OR: optic radiation; PLIC: posterior limb of internal capsule; SCP: superior cerebellar peduncle; SLF: superior longitudinal (arcuate) fasciculus; SOFF: superior occipitofrontal fasciculus; St: stria terminalis; TPF: transverse pontine fibers; Tpt: tapetum; UF: uncinate fasciculus).

The major cisterns at the base of the brain are suprasellar cistern, perimesencephalic cistern, prepontine and perimedullary cisterns and the cerebellopontine angle cistern. The suprasellar cistern is a five pointed CSF space, communicating anteriorly with interhemispheric fissure, laterally with Sylvian fissure and posteriorly with perimesencephalic cistern. It contains optic chiasma, internal carotid artery and circle of Willis and pituitary stalk **(Fig. 4B)**. The perimesencephalic cistern consists of interpeduncular, crural, ambient and quadrigeminal plate cisterns lying along the anterior, anterolateral, posterolateral and posterior aspects of the midbrain respectively. The upper end of basilar artery and the III cranial nerve lie within the interpeduncular cistern. Intimately related to the quadrigeminal plate cistern **(Fig. 5G)** are the pineal gland and the vein of Galen. The fourth cranial nerves course in the ambient cisterns around the midbrain.

The cerebellopontine angle cistern **(Figs. 5C, 7B and C)** is bounded medially by the middle cerebellar peduncle and the anteroinferior surface of the cerebellum and laterally by the temporal bone. It contains VII/VIII cranial nerves and anterior inferior cerebellar arteries. Prepontine cistern **(Figs. 7B and C)** lies anterior to the pons and contains basilar artery. The perimedullary cisterns surround the medulla and contain lower cranial nerves (CN IX, X and XI) and vertebral arteries **(Fig. 7D)**. Superior cerebellar cistern lies superior to the cerebellum and contains vein of Galen. The cisterna magna is a CSF space at the posteroinferior aspect of cerebellum and may be sometimes very large in normal people.

BASAL GANGLIA AND ADJACENT STRUCTURES

Basal ganglia represent central gray matter consisting of corpus striatum (caudate nucleus and lentiform nucleus) and claustrum a strip of gray matter lateral to the lentiform nucleus and amygdala at the roof of temporal horn. The caudate nucleus has a larger head anteriorly and a narrow posterior part, the tail, which follows the superolateral border of thalamus and the temporal horn into the amygdala. The lentiform nucleus is wedge shaped and comprised of globus pallidus medially and putamen laterally. External capsule, claustrum, extreme capsule and insular cortex lie lateral to the putamen in that order **(Fig. 5C)**. The internal capsule is bounded anteromedially by caudate head, laterally by lentiform nucleus and posteromedially by thalamus **(Figs. 6G and M)**.

SUGGESTED READING

1. Atlas S (Ed). Magnetic Resonance Imaging of the Brain and Spine, 5th edition. Philadelphia: Lippincott Williams & Wilkins; 2016.
2. Berry M, Standring SM, Bannister LH. Nervous system. In: Susan Standring (Ed). Gray's Anatomy, 41st edition—The Anatomical Basis of Clinical Practice, New York: Elsevier, Churchill Livingstone; 2016.
3. Butler P, Jeffiree MA. The skull and brain. In: Butler P, Mitchell AWM, Ellis H (Eds). Applied Radiological Anatomy, 1st edition. Cambridge University Press. 2001; pp. 17-60.
4. Lee SH, Rao KCVG, Zimmerman RA (Eds). Normal Anatomy in Cranial MRI and CT, 4th edition. New York: McGraw Hill Inc.; 1999. pp.105-37.
5. Patel VH, Friedman L. MRI of the Brain: Normal Anatomy and Normal Variants, 1st edition, Philadelphia: WB Saunders Company; 1997.
6. Scott WR, Hanaway J. Correlative anatomy of the brain. In: Radiology-Diagnosis-Imaging-Intervention, Vol. 3. Philadelphia: JB Lippincott Co.; 1986.
7. Snell RS (Ed). Snell's Textbook of Clinical Anatomy, 7th edition. Boston: Little Brown and Company; 2004. pp. 790-830.

CHAPTER

183

Normal Cerebral Angiography

Shailesh B Gaikwad, Ajay Kumar, Anuj Prabhakar

CEREBRAL ANGIOGRAPHY TECHNIQUE

INTRODUCTION

This is an important albeit invasive procedure wherein most cases of suspected vascular pathologies baring few exceptions are diagnosed. It is a direct examination of the blood vessels that provide not only the information of the vascular anatomy but also the flow dynamics.

Historical Background

Cerebral angiography was first introduced by Moniz. Moniz and Almeida Lima, performed the first cerebral angiography on living human patients in 1927.[1]

Definition

It is the demonstration of the cerebral vascular anatomy by direct injection of the iodinated contrast medium into the vessel.

Six Vessel Angiography

It includes the study of the following vessels:

1. Right internal carotid artery
2. Left internal carotid artery
3. Right external carotid artery
4. Left external carotid artery
5. Right vertebral artery
6. Left vertebral artery.

Indications[2]

- Evaluate intracranial circulation when CT or MR angiography is inconclusive either due to failure to visualize the pathology or patient factors like clips, coils or patient motion.
- Define presence/extent of atherosclerotic vessel disease, especially when information on the presence and nature of collateral supply is needed.
- Define etiology of hemorrhage.
- Define presence, location, and anatomy of intracranial aneurysms and arteriovenous malformations.
- Evaluate vasospasm related to subarachnoid hemorrhage.
- Investigate reversible cerebral vasoconstriction syndrome.
- Define presence/extent of trauma to cervicocerebral vessels.
- Define vascular supply to tumors.
- Define presence/extent of vasculitis.
- Evaluate pulsatile tinnitus or cranial bruit.
- Define presence of venous occlusive disease.
- Perform physiologic testing of brain function and balloon test occlusion.
- Determine presence of intracranial flow for the purpose of documenting angiographic brain death, especially when nuclear medicine blood flow study is inconclusive.
- Evaluate cerebral circulation before or after planned intervention.

Contraindications

There are no absolute contraindications to cerebral angiography.[3] Relative contraindications include:

- Allergy to iodinated contrast agents
- Abnormal renal function
- Coagulopathy
- Local site infection
- Pregnancy.

Patient Preparation

Careful history taking is very important before the procedure. It is advisable to take informed consent from the patient in case of elective procedure and from relatives in case of emergency. Patient should be well hydrated before the procedure. Patient must have passed urine before the procedure. A detailed informed consent should be obtained including specific risks of the procedure. Laboratory parameters that should be evaluated include complete blood cell count, serum creatinine or glomerular filtration rate, prothrombin time and

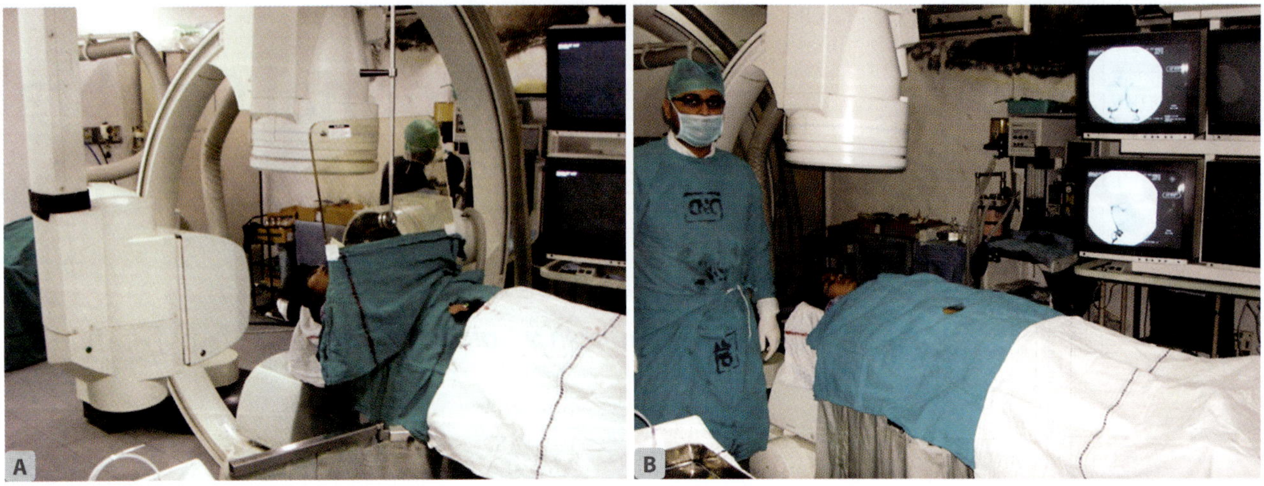

FIGS. 1A AND B: DSA biplane machine with monitors.

international normalized ratio, as dictated by the patients' clinical situation. Anticoagulants should be withheld when possible. Patients should eat nothing by mouth 6 hours before the procedure. The morning insulin dose should be reduced in half. Inguinal region should be shaved and prepared prior to the procedure.[3]

Requirements

- Digital subtraction angiography (DSA) machine **(Figs. 1A and B)**
- Catheterization equipment **(Fig. 2)**
- Disposables.

Catheterization Equipment

Cleaning agents, blade no. 11, puncture needle, vascular sheath, mini-guidewire, various catheters, Terumo guidewire, and syringes.

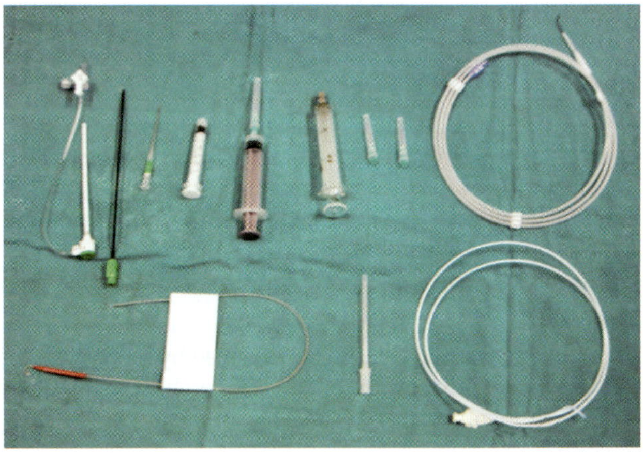

FIG. 2: Instruments required: (left to right) Sheath, dilator, puncture needle, syringes, terumo wire, short guidewire, single puncture needle, catheter.

Site of the Puncture

The common femoral artery (CFA) crosses the pelvic brim at the level of the inguinal ligament, which extends from the spine of the anterior superior iliac crest to the pubic tubercle. It then enters the femoral sheath which is made up of 3 compartments containing the femoral artery laterally and the vein medially. The medial and smallest compartment is called the femoral canal which contains lymphatic vessels and lymph nodes. Lateral to the femoral artery and outside the femoral sheath is the femoral nerve. The CFA represents an ideal site for arterial access and sheath insertion because it is relatively large, is less involved with atherosclerosis, and is readily compressible against the underlying head of the femur.

The ideal site of femoral arterial puncture (not skin puncture) is a point 1 cm lateral to the most medial aspect of the femoral head, midway between its superior and inferior border. Various landmarks have been utilized for identification of the femoral artery:

1. The skin crease may be used as a marker for the underlying inguinal ligament, and an arterial puncture 2 to 3 cm below the midpoint of the skin crease has been used. This technique may be inaccurate in obese patients.
2. A point 2 to 3 cm below the midpoint of a line between the anterior superior iliac spine and pubic tubercle (mid inguinal point) may be used as a site for femoral arterial cannulation **(Figs. 3 and 4)**.
3. Fluoroscopic landmark: The femoral head is identified. skin puncture done at the lower border of the femoral head, with the needle entering the skin at a 30° to 45° angle. Artery puncture is performed at the mid portion of the head of femur in its medial third.
4. Ultrasound-guided femoral arterial cannulation may be performed in obese patients or in those with a weak pulse.

Caudal punctures have an increased risk of hematoma, and pseudoaneurysms as there is lack of underlying bony structure and scaffolding by femoral sheath. High puncture above the inguinal ligament is associated with an increased risk of retroperitoneal hemorrhage due to lack of effective compression and tamponade. Infrainguinal puncture and bleeding may also cause retroperitoneal hemorrhage due to tracking of the blood upward underneath the ligament and into the retroperitoneal space.[4]

Preparation

Sterilize the site first with savlon, then with betadine and with spirit in the last.

Wipe with sterilized gauze piece.

Local Anesthesia

For local anesthesia (LA), give subcutaneous injection of 2% xylocaine without adrenaline. Palpate the artery with index, mid and ring finger of the left hand. Infiltrate 2–3 mL each on the either side of the artery. Care must be taken to not to inject LA into the vessel, before giving injection always check by withdrawing to rule out arterial puncture. Give injection slowly for the patient comfort **(Fig. 5)**.

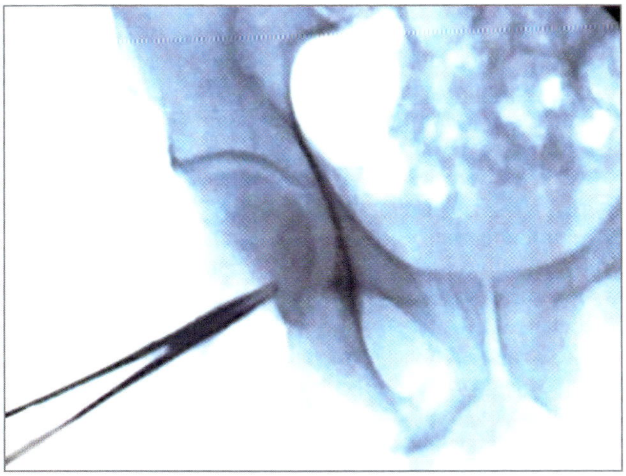

FIG. 3: Marking the site of puncture on fluoroscopy.

Artery Puncture

- Give 3 mm wide and 3 mm deep, superficial skin incision at the puncture site by using 11 no. blade. It is ideal to check the site under fluoroscopy before arterial puncture.
- **Seldinger technique:** Palpate femoral artery by the index, middle and ring finger, of the left hand. Take Medicut (puncture needle with needle inside and plastic cannula outside) in the right hand and advance toward the artery at about 45° angle. Feel the pulse of the artery through the needle in the right hand and as one feels it over femoral artery, enter artery with a jab **(Fig. 6)**. Remove the needle and slowly withdraw the cannula till the jet of the blood is obtained. Rule out venous puncture (blood will not come out in jets). After confirming arterial access introduce a 0.035-inch short J-tip guidewire, and remove the cannula. If resistance is encountered as the guidewire leaves the needle tip, the guidewire should be removed and the needle adjusted to ensure brisk flow. Lowering the hub of the needle before guidewire insertion or slight repositioning either laterally or medially will aid in smooth guidewire advancement. The guidewire must enter smoothly without resistance. Is case excess resistance is felt, the needle and guidewire complex must be removed and a fresh attempt should be made. Finally, introduce arterial sheath over the short guidewire.[4]
- Again check the position of the sheath by withdrawing blood using syringe. Arterial blood will come into syringe in pulsatile manner and with thrust.
- Inject 2500 unit of heparin (0.5 mL) and flush sheath with saline to flush in remaining part of heparin in the sheath lumen.
- Take the desired catheter and start angiography **(Fig. 7)**.

Puncture Technique

It is of two types:

1. Single wall puncture
2. Double wall puncture.

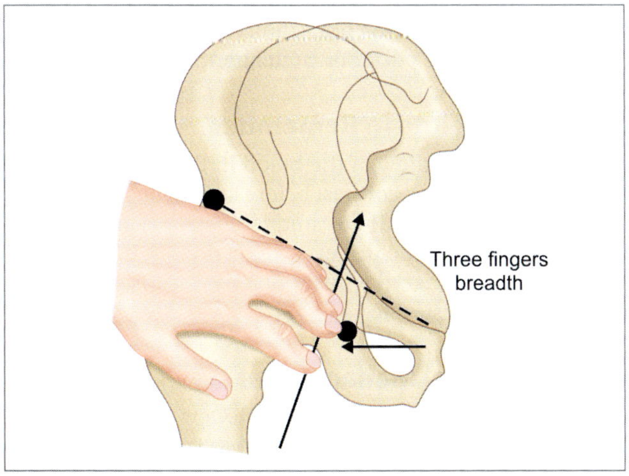

FIG. 4: Localization and palpation of femoral artery.

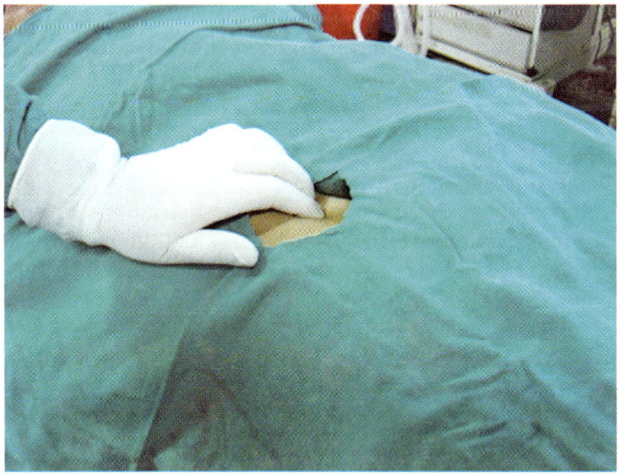

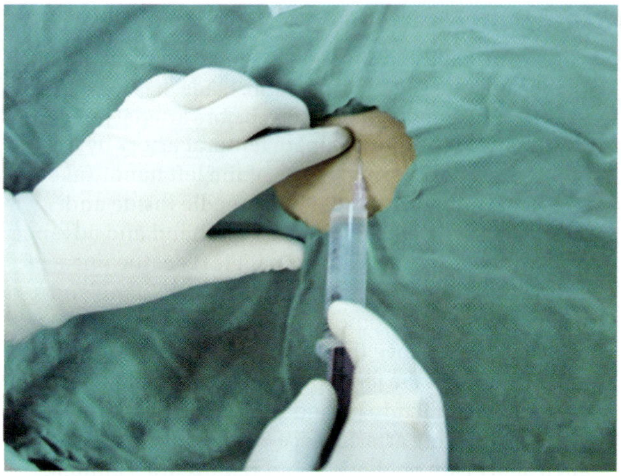

FIG. 5: Infiltrating local anesthetic at the site of puncture.

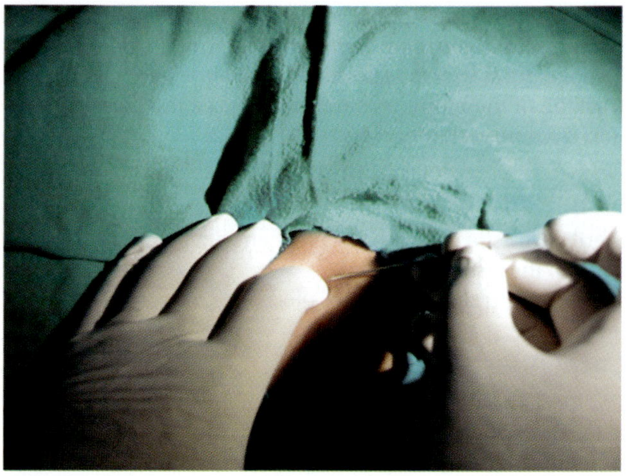

FIG. 6: Arterial puncture.

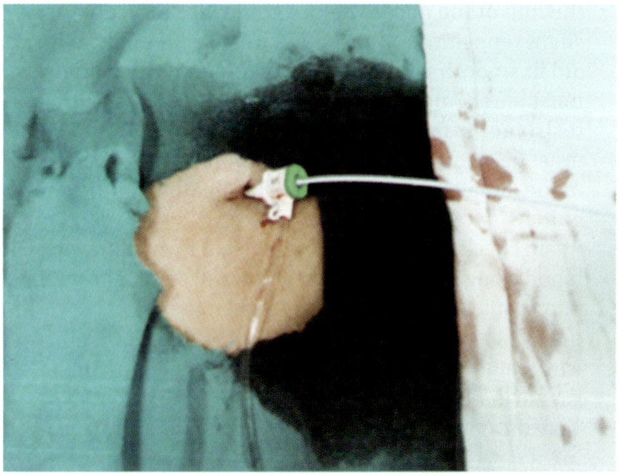

FIG. 7: Placement of arterial sheath.

In single wall puncture technique, only the anterior wall of artery is punctured and in double wall both anterior as well as posterior wall get punctured. Single wall is safe in experienced hands while double wall is safer in inexperienced hand as chances of dissection of artery are higher in single wall technique. In double wall technique the chance of posterior wall hematoma is high. Improper technique can lead to trauma of the vessel regardless of the type of needle used.

Procedure

The aortic arch anatomy will help determine the selection of the catheter. Types I and II arch configurations can be routinely catheterized with an angled catheter, while a reverse curve catheter is generally necessary to select vessels arising from Type III arches. In patients with atherosclerotic vessel disease a hydrophilic 0.035-inch wire with a curved tip such as the terumo wire (Terumo Interventional Systems, Somerset, NJ) is used. The guidewire is advanced into the artery followed by the catheter. As the wire is removed, an inadvertent vacuum effect may occur if the catheter is in a small artery or if the end hole is wedged against the wall of the artery. To prevent inadvertent air embolus, the guidewire should be removed slowly, keeping the catheter hub filled with heparinized saline by dripping or injecting it into the hub while the wire is withdrawn.[3] For Internal carotid artery (ICA) injection, an angled tip catheter and hydrophilic guidewire are needed. If a reverse curve catheter is used for common carotid artery (CCA) catheterization, an exchange of catheters is required over an exchange length guidewire placed in the external carotid artery.

While performing diagnostic angiography for vertebral arteries (VA), the left VA is preferred as it is mostly larger than the right in diameter. The right VA is catheterized only if the left VA is not accessible, right VA pathology is suspected, or when contrast does not reflux into the right posterior inferior cerebellar artery (PICA) on left VA injection. Extra care should be taken when VA injection is performed, as the VA is prone to vasospasm and dissection.[2]

For anterior intracranial cerebral angiography, standard AP Towne's view and lateral projections are used. Oblique images at 45 degrees may separate overlapping arteries. Special views like Stenvers view for middle cerebral artery (MCA) and submental vertex view for anterior communicating artery may be acquired if necessary. For vertebral arteriograms, the standard projections are AP (Towne's view) and lateral projections centered caudally and dorsally to cover the posterior circulation.[3]

Important Points to Remember

Check for free backflow of the blood in the catheter. Inject test amount 2–3 mL of contrast before taking run to check the exact position of the catheter and to check vascular spasm. Instruct the patient before every injection and inform the effect of the contrast like flushing and warm sensation or alteration in the taste, etc.

Postprocedural Management

Before removing the sheath, aspirate few milliliter of the blood to aspirate out any thrombus that could have formed during the procedure. If there is free backflow and if no clots are visible in the aspirate, the sheath can be safely removed. Compress the arterial puncture site which is about 0.5 cm above the skin puncture site (for about 20-min). Compress the actual puncture site with middle finger, compress above it with index finger and below it with ring finger. Puncture site should be clearly visible during compression so that hematoma formation can be avoided. Do not obliterate the pulse, distal pulse should be faintly palpable. Apply steady moderate pressure for 15 minutes, reduce the pressure in next 5-minut. Never remove compression abruptly. After compression feel all distal pulses. If the patient has both an arterial and a venous sheath, the arterial sheath should be removed first and the venous sheath removed 5 minutes later. This technique avoids the risk of arteriovenous fistula formation and also preserves a venous access for medication administration in case of a vasovagal reaction.[4]

Bed rest is recommended for 8 hours after the procedure. The patient is instructed to avoid bending his/her leg. Check groin for hematoma formation. Monitor BP, pulse and neurological status of the patient. If patient is unable to pass urine then catheterize the patient until the patient is able to ambulate.

Complications

Complications may be neurological and non-neurological. Stroke is the main neurological complication. Non-neurological complications are renal failure, arterial occlusions requiring intervention, arteriovenous fistula, and hematoma requiring transfusions or surgical intervention. In a study by Kaufmann et al. 19826 consecutive patients undergoing DSA were retrospectively reviewed. Neurologic complications occurred in 2.63%, with 0.14% of these causing permanent disability. Deaths occurred in 0.06%. Access-site hematoma was the most common complication overall (4.2%). Patients suffering from atherosclerotic vascular disease, subarachnoid hemorrhage and frequent transient ischemic attack were more likely to have complications.[5]

CEREBRAL ANGIOGRAPHIC ANATOMY

ARTERIAL ANATOMY

The brain is supplied by the two internal cerebral arteries, and two vertebral arteries which join to form the basilar artery. The basilar artery divides into two posterior cerebral arteries which along with posterior communicating arteries form the posterior part of circle of Willis. The anterior part of circle of Willis is constituted by both anterior cerebral arteries, anterior communicating artery and internal cerebral arteries.

The internal carotid artery (ICA) is divided into the following segments as per the Bouthillier classification system:[6]

- C1 cervical—CCA bifurcation to entrance of carotid canal
- C2 petrous—extends up to posterior edge of formaen lacerum
- C3 lacerum—extends up to superior margin of petrolingual ligament
- C4 cavernous—extends up to proximal dural ring (anterior clinoid process)
- C5 clinoid—extends up to distal dural ring
- C6 ophthalmic—extends up to just proximal to the origin of Posterior communicating artery (PCom)
- C7 communicating—extends up to ICA bifurcation

ICA on each side enters the cranium by passing through the carotid canal in the petrous temporal bone (petrous segment). Petrous ICA give rise to Vidian artery (artery of pterygoid canal) and caroticotympanic artery which supplies middle and internal ear and occasionally the persistent stapedial artery. At times, the ICA courses posterolaterally than anteromedial (normal course) and presents as pulsatile retrotympanic mass called. Knowledge of this variant is necessary to differentiate it from glomus tympanicum so that hazardous biopsy can be avoided.

The ICA runs within the cavernous sinus to pierce the dura to enter the subarachnoid space adjacent to the anterior clinoid process. The cavernous ICA can be subdivided into ascending cavernous (C5), first posterior genu (C4), horizontal part (C3), second anterior genu (C2) and the rest of cavernous segment (C1). Meningohypophyseal artery arises near junction of C5 and C4. Meningohypophyseal artery branches supply the posterior pituitary, cavernous sinus, clival dura and sometimes III to VI cranial nerves. The horizontal part (C3) extends between first posterior (C4) and second anterior genu (C2). After second genu (C2), rest of the cavernous ICA is called as C1 segment **(Fig. 8)**. The inferolateral trunk arises from C4 segment and supplies the dura of the cavernous sinus and cranial nerves III, IV, V and VI. The superior hypophyseal trunk arises from supraclinoid ICA and supplies anterior pituitary. The ophthalmic artery arises from ophthalmic ICA **(Fig. 9)**. The anterior choroidal artery arises from ICA just above PCom origin which arises posteromedially from communicating segment of ICA. The anterior choroidal artery supplies the choroid plexus

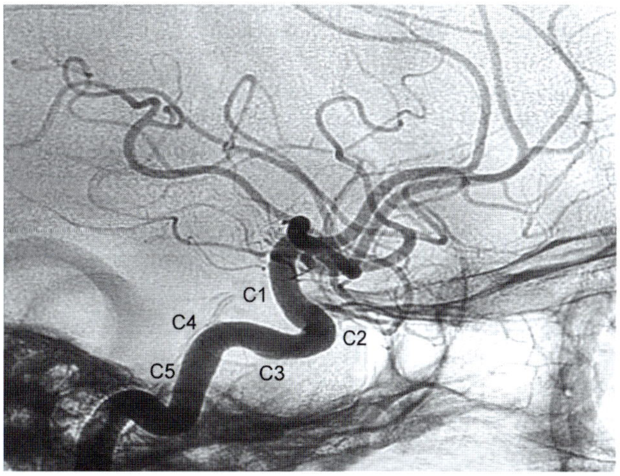

FIG. 8: ICA cavernous segments: Image showing cavernous ICA segments. C5 segment extends from carotid canal opening to first posterior genu (C4), horizontal segment (C3) extends between first posterior genu (C4) and second anterior genu (C2). Rest of cavernous ICA is called (C1).

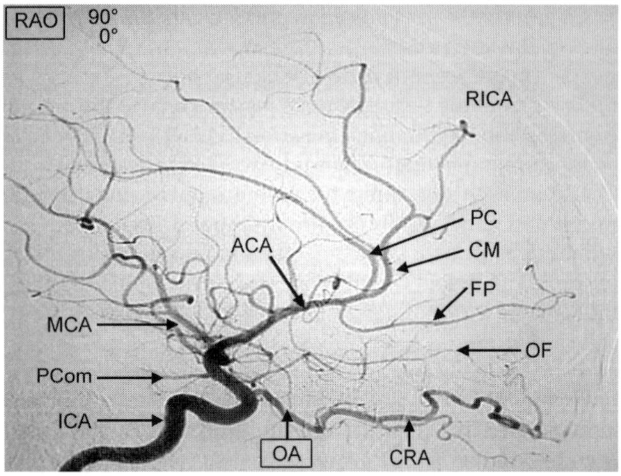

FIG. 9: Anterior circulation lateral view: Selective ICA angiogram lateral view showing different important branches (as annotated). (ICA: internal carotid artery; OA: ophthalmic a rtery; CRA: central retinal artery, PCom: posterior communicating artery; MCA: middle cerebral artery; ACA: anterior cerebral artery; OF: orbitofrontal artery; FP: frontopolar artery; CM: callosomarginal artery; PC: pericallosal artery).

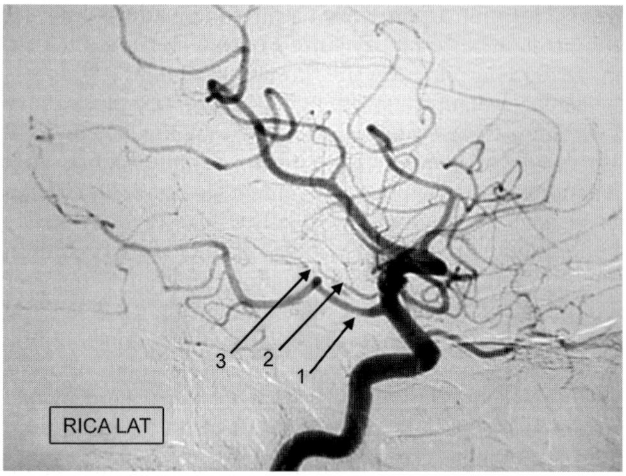

FIG. 10: Lateral ICA angiogram showing fetal PCA (1), anterior choroidal artery (2) and the plexal point (3), the point where artery enters the choroidal fissure.

of the lateral ventricles, medial temporal lobe and some striate branches to deep ganglionic structures **(Fig. 10)**. The PCom runs posteriorly to join the posterior cerebral arteries (branches of basilar artery) to complete the circle of Willis. PCom supplies the deep ganglionic structures including the thalamus.

The anterior cerebral arteries proceed medially within the interhemispheric fissure separated by the falx. Both anterior cerebral arteries are connected by the anterior communicating artery in the midline completing the anterior part of circle of Willis (located in the suprasellar cistern).

Anterior cerebral artery (ACA) is thus divided into three segments. Horizontal (A1) segment which extends from the ACA origin to its junction with the anterior communicating artery (ACom). The medial lenticulostriate arteries arise from A1 segment. A2 segment which extends from the junction of ACom to its bifurcation into pericallosal and callosomarginal arteries. The orbitofrontal and frontopolar arteries arise from A2 segment. The recurrent artery of Heubner which is a lenticulostriate branch may arise from proximal A2 segment and less commonly from A1 segment. A3 segment refers to the cortical branches that supply the anterior two-thirds of medial hemispheric surface and a small superior area over the convexities.

Middle cerebral artery (MCA) is also divided into three major segments. Horizontal (M1) segment: Extends from the origin of MCA to its bifurcation or trifurcation at Sylvian fissure. The lateral lenticulostriate arteries arise from M1 segment and supply the lentiform nucleus, parts of internal capsule and caudate nucleus. Insular (M2) segment: At its genu, the MCA divides into its insular (M2) branches, which loop over the insula and pass laterally to exit from sylvian fissure. Opercular (M3) segment: This gives off branches that emerge from the Sylvian fissure and ramify over the hemispheric surface. The insular and the opercular branches supply the temporal, parietal and variable parts of frontal and occipital lobes **(Figs. 11 and 12)**.

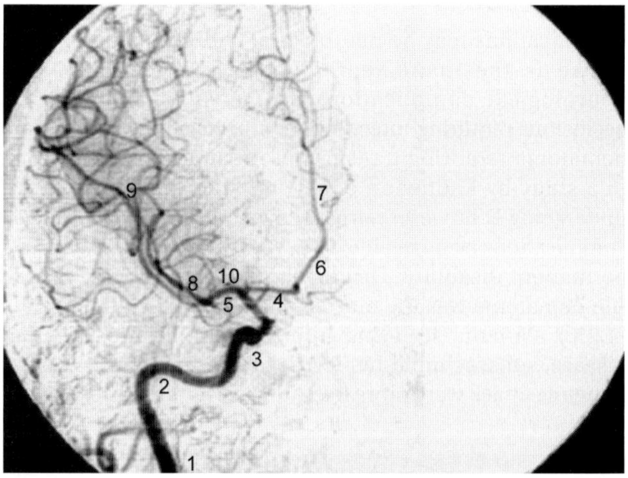

FIG. 11: Right internal carotid artery angiogram PA view. (1: Cervical segment of ICA; 2: Petrous segment of ICA; 3: Cavernous segment of ICA; 4: Anterior cerebral artery (A1); 5: Middle cerebral artery (M1); 6: Anterior cerebral artery (A2); 7: Anterior cerebral artery (A3); 8: Middle cerebral artery (M2); 9: Middle cerebral artery (M3); 10: Lenticulostriate arteries).

The two vertebral arteries (VA) arise from the respective subclavian arteries, course cephalad and enter the cranium through the foramen magnum. These unite in the posterior fossa, usually anterior to the medulla to form the basilar artery. Most of the time vertebral arteries are asymmetrical. In about 60% left vertebral artery is dominant, in 25% right can be dominant and in about 25% both vertebral artery can be symmetrical in size. Left vertebral artery can arise directly from aorta in small percentage.

The intracranial VA gives two major branches: Anterior spinal artery supplying the spinal cord and PICA on each side which supplies choroid plexus of fourth ventricle, medulla, cerebellar tonsils, inferior vermis and parts of cerebellar hemispheres.

Basilar artery (BA) runs anterior to pons in the prepontine cistern and terminates in the interpeduncular cistern by dividing into posterior cerebral arteries (PCAs). In prepontine cistern, it lies within the space marginated by lateral margin of clivus. Any further deviation from these boundaries is considered as dolichoectasia. In addition, the basilar artery gives off anterior inferior cerebellar artery (AICA) and superior cerebellar artery (SCA) on each side, just before bifurcation into posterior cerebral arteries. The anterior inferior cerebellar artery is the first major branch of basilar artery and most of the time (about 70%) arises as single vessel.

AICA courses posterolaterally within the CP angle cistern, whereas SCA curves around the pons and the midbrain just below the tentorial hiatus **(Figs. 13 and 14)**. The AICA supplies the VII, VIII CN, inferolateral pons, middle cerebellar peduncle and anterolateral surface of cerebellum. The SCA supplies the entire superior surface of cerebellum, vermis, deep cerebellar white matter and dentate nuclei. In addition, BA also gives off multiple short and long segment circumflex perforating branches which supply the ventral pons and rostral brainstem.

The PCAs are usually terminal branches of basilar artery but they can arise directly from supraclinoid ICA with hypertrophy of PCom and hypoplasia of ipsilateral P1 segment of PCA called as fetal PCA **(*see* Fig. 10)**. PCA on each side is divided into three major segments. Precommunicating (P1 or peduncular) segment: It extends from the origin of PCA to its junction with the PCom. The posterior thalamoperforating arteries and medial posterior choroidal artery usually arise from P1 segment. Ambient (P2) segment: It courses around the midbrain above the trochlear nerve and tentorial incisura. The lateral posterior choroidal artery and thalamogeniculate arteries arise from the P2 segment.

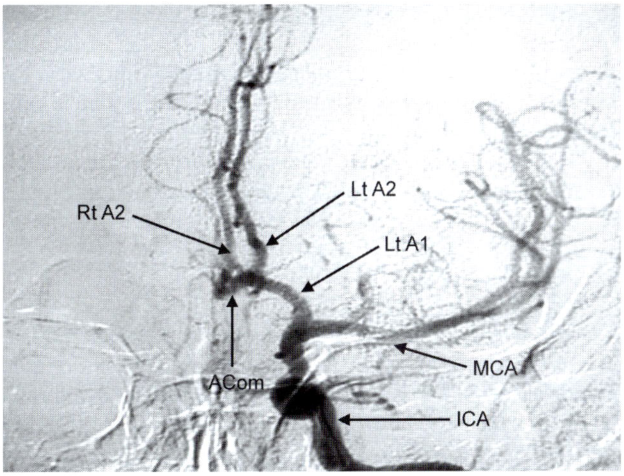

FIG. 12: Left ICA angiogram frontal view revealing ICA bifurcation, MCA, ACA segments and ACom (as annotated).

Quadrigeminal (P3) segment: It runs behind the midbrain in the quadrigeminal plate cistern. The major branches of P3 segment are inferior temporal arteries, parieto-occipital artery, calcarine artery and posterior pericallosal arteries which supply the occipital lobe and posterior part of parietal lobe **(Figs. 13A and B)**.

Venous Anatomy (Fig. 14)

The cerebral venous system is composed of two components, the dural venous sinuses and the cerebral veins.

Dural Sinuses

Superior sagittal sinus (SSS): It is situated in the midline and typically originates near the crista galli anteriorly and extends posteriorly to its confluence with the straight and lateral sinuses at the torcula.

Inferior sagittal sinus is situated in the inferior free margin of the falx cerebri and joins the vein of Galen to form the straight sinus.

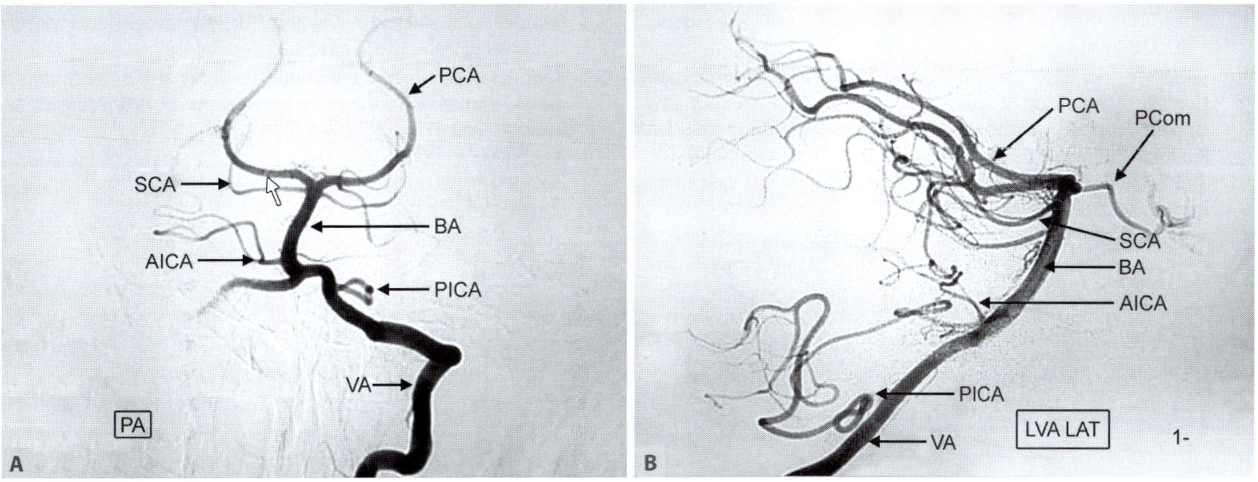

FIGS. 13A AND B: Posterior circulation frontal and lateral view showing the major arteries and their branches. (VA: vertebral artery; BA: basilar artery; PICA: posterior inferior cerebellar artery; AICA: Anterior inferior cerebellar artery; SCA: superior cerebellar artery; PCA: posterior cerebral artery; PCom: posterior communicating artery)

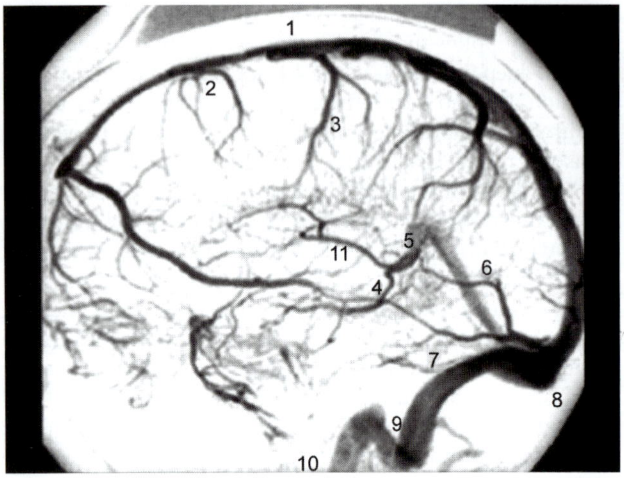

FIG. 14: Right internal carotid angiogram venous phase (lateral view). 1: Superior sagittal sinus; 2: Superior cerebral veins; 3: Vein of Trolard; 4: Basal vein of Rosenthal; 5: Vein of Galen; 6: Straight sinus; 7: Transverse sinus; 8: Torcular herophili; 9: Sigmoid sinus; 10: Internal jugular vein; 11: Internal cerebral vein).

Straight sinus courses backwards to unite with the SSS at the torcular herophili.

Transverse and occipital sinuses: The torcular herophili divides into the transverse (lateral) and occipital sinuses. The transverse sinuses course laterally around the tentorial attachment to form the sigmoid sinuses and drain into the internal jugular veins on either side. The occipital sinus is rudimentary.

Cavernous sinuses: The cavernous sinuses are the largest venous sinuses located in the parasellar region. Its major tributaries are superior and inferior ophthalmic veins. The ICA and 3rd, 4th, 6th, ophthalmic and maxillary divisions of 5th cranial nerves course within each sinus. Both cavernous sinuses communicate with each other, preclival venous plexus, sigmoid sinuses, and jugular bulb (through superior and inferior petrosal sinuses).

Cerebral Veins

These are divided into superficial (cortical) veins and deep veins.

Superficial cortical veins: These are variable in number and enter the SSS near the vertex. The larger veins which may be identified are superficial middle cerebral vein which runs along the sylvian fissure, vein of Trolard which courses from sylvian fissure to SSS and vein of Labbe which courses from sylvian fissure to the transverse sinus.

Deep cerebral veins: The medullary veins originate 1–2 cm below the cortex and course centrally toward subependymal veins which surround the lateral ventricles. The thalamostriate vein and septal vein join near the foramen of Monro to form the internal cerebral vein (ICV). The two ICVs and basal veins of Rosenthal (BVR) join to form the vein of Galen which runs under the splenium of corpus callosum and unites with the inferior sagittal sinus to form the straight sinus which joins the SSS at the torcula.

The major veins draining the posterior fossa are anterior pontomesencephalic vein, precentral cerebellar vein, superior and inferior vermian veins and hemispheric veins.

CONCLUSION

The above chapter was a brief review of the basic anatomy and techniques for cerebral angiography. DSA is the gold standard for detection of vascular pathologies in the brain. Despite its invasive nature and the recent advances in CT, MR technology its importance has not diminished in the current clinical scenario.

REFERENCES

1. Doby T. Cerebral angiography and Egas Moniz. Am J Roentgenol. 1992;159(2):364-4.
2. Wojak JC, Abruzzo TA, Bello JA, et al. Quality Improvement Guidelines for Adult Diagnostic Cervicocerebral Angiography: Update Cooperative Study between the Society of Interventional Radiology (SIR), American Society of Neuroradiology (ASNR), and Society of NeuroInterventional Surgery (SNIS). J Vasc Interv Radiol. 2015;26(11):1596-608.
3. Ahn SH, Prince EA, Dubel GJ. Basic neuroangiography: review of technique and perioperative patient care. Semin Interv Radiol. 2013;30(3):225-33.
4. Bangalore S, Bhatt DL. Femoral arterial access and closure. Circulation. 2011;124(5):e147-56.
5. Kaufmann TJ, Huston J, Mandrekar JN, et al. Complications of diagnostic cerebral angiography: evaluation of 19826 consecutive patients. Radiology. 2007;243(3):812-9.
6. Bouthillier A, van Loveren HR, Keller JT. Segments of the internal carotid artery: a new classification. Neurosurgery. 1996;38(3):425-32; discussion 432-3.

CHAPTER

184

Advances in Neuroimaging Techniques: Computed Tomography

Sameer Vyas, Paramjeet Singh, Niranjan Khandelwal

INTRODUCTION

Computed tomography (CT) technology has significantly evolved over the recent years with technical advancements to increase speed, improve image quality and reduce dose.[1,2] Introduction of spiral (helical) CT scans in 1990 which use slip ring technology allows continuous data acquisition of a volume by 360° gantry rotation during continuous table movement during the scan. The technique reduced slice thickness to submillimeter levels, allowed faster scanning and acquisition of a large volumetric data which can be used to generate thin slices and high resolution reformations of images in any desired plane from very thin isotropic voxels. Nowadays, CT has become valuable diagnostic tool and plays a very pivotal role in current clinical neuro-imaging. Main advantages of the CT include widespread availability, ease of clinical application, and noninvasive nature. There has been several advancement in CT technology, which include multidetector computed tomography (MDCT), dual-energy CT, portable CT, cone beam CT, phase contrast CT and iteractive reconstruction algorithms. Better collimation of the X-ray beams, higher heat capacity of the newer X-ray tubes and increased sensitivity of detector assembly have significantly upgraded the technology.[1]

In this chapter, we will first discuss the recent advances in the CT technology and then will elaborate the neuroimaging applications of CT.

RECENT ADVANCES IN CT TECHNOLOGY

Multidetector Computed Tomography

The introduction of multidetector computed tomography (MDCT) system into clinical radiology has brought a revolution in the field of medical imaging. MDCT are the latest techniques where multiple rows of detectors are used to acquire multiple slices per rotation through interweaving helices (2, 4, 16 up to 320 slices). 1 mm × 20 mm detectors are replaced with arrays of 1 mm × 1.25 mm channels in MDCT which can be arranged in a symmetrical, adaptive or hybrid fashion. MDCT uses high gantry speed (0.5–0.8 seconds) allowing faster imaging and larger volume coverage particularly for CT angiography.[3]

This technology allowed the maturing of traditional CT from plain axial cross-section imaging to a modern real- like three-dimensional (3D) tool with identical spatial resolution along all directions allowing excellent multiplanar reformations and high quality 3D reconstructions. The scan parameters can be manipulated by changing the collimation, detector configuration and reconstruction algorithm.[3] Retrospective data analysis allows flexibility of examination. Simultaneous development of efficient computer systems made possible postprocessing and analysis of enormous data sets.

The two chief benefits of helical or multislice CT are an increase in the speed and defined ability of performance of volume acquisitions.

1. *Increased speed:* Multidetector CT allows high-speed scanning, thinner sections or longer scan ranges. Increased scanning speed leads to less motion artifacts, especially in the cases of children and patients who are critically ill or are in trauma. Since scanning is rapid, more volume can be covered and more data of higher resolution can be acquired for better 3D reconstructions. The contrast requirement is also less compared with standard CT or better images can be obtained with the same amounts of contrast material.
2. *Volume acquisition:* A continuous volume acquisition in a helical CT makes sure that none of the lesions go as miss when a patient respirates or makes a movement. These improved 3D capabilities of multiplanar reformations and exhaustive 3D representations are the prime benefits for volume acquisition. This technology provides best result if the thickness of the chosen section is reduced to the minimum. The utility of volume rendering techniques has risen so much that interpretation of images has progressed from observation of aerial sections to evaluation of real 3D data sets.

Flat-panel Volume Computed Tomography

Flat-panel volume computed tomography is recent development in the CT technology that allows coverage of a large volume per rotation. Fluoroscopic and dynamic imaging is possible with high spatial resolution.[6] It represents combining of different modalities like radiography, fluoroscopy, X-ray angiography, and volumetric CT into one system. Area detectors have replaced the detector rows in this new technology. The flat-panel detector with its wide Z-axis coverage makes the imaging of entire organs possible in a single axial acquisition. Intra-operative and vascular imaging is possible due to its fluoroscopic and angiographic modalities. The flat-panel volume CT is advantageous in comparison to multidetector CT as it allows ultra-high spatial resolution, real-time fluoroscopy, dynamic imaging capabilities, and whole-organ coverage in one rotation.[4] The main limitations of flat-panel volume CT is that it requires a higher radiation dose (needed to achieve a comparable signal-to-noise ratio), lower contrast resolution, and a slower scintillator that slows down the scanning process.

Dynamic Computed Tomography Angiography

Inability to provide any dynamic (i.e. temporal resolved) information was a major limitation of MDCT compared to the gold standard of angiographic, digital subtraction angiography. But this limitation seems to be resolved with the recent introduction of a 320-detector row CT scanner that provides the possibility of dynamic volume scanning (four-dimensional scanning with the fourth dimension being the time).[5,6] Volumetric CT using 320 detector rows enables full brain coverage in a single rotation that allows for combined time-resolved whole-brain perfusion and four-dimensional computed tomography angiography (CTA). Its potential applications in neuroradiology are in stroke, steno-occlusive disease, arteriovenous malformations and dural shunts. The broad coverage enabled by it offers Z-axis c overage allowing for whole-brain perfusion and subtracted dynamic angiography of the entire intracranial circulation. It has the potential of scanning entire organs such as the heart and brain in a single rotation as it provides large maximum detector area that can be used for this scanner, therefore allowing the visualization of dynamic flow and perfusion, as well as motion of an entire volume at very short time interval.

Dual Energy Computed Tomography

Conventional CT demonstrate exquisite anatomic detail with high contrast and spatial resolution whereas Dual Energy Computed Tomography (DECT) provides insights into the material properties of the tissues.[7-9] With DECT, differentiation between tissues that have similar attenuation on conventional CT imaging is possible. The basic principle of DECT is based on that different material show different attenuation (absorption) of energy at varying energy of the incident X-rays (various kVp settings), and this difference in attenuation can be used for tissue characterization. DECT scanners can be performed by sequential acquisition of two separate scans (dual-source CT scanners, one at each energy level, Siemens Healthcare) or fast kV-switching systems (GE Healthcare), or dual-layer detection technology (simultaneous detection of multiple energies by multilayer detectors, Phillips Healthcare).[9] DECT analyzes the changes in attenuation of different materials at 2 disparate energy levels, and subsequently uses a process termed material decomposition to generate monochromatic DECT images. The methodology of image reconstruction varies based on the acquisition method, with single-source fast-kilovoltage switching images constructed from projection space data, whereas dual-source CT (where high-energy and lower-energy acquisitions are not coincident with each other in a helical acquisition) uses image domain material decomposition. DECT minimize the beam-hardening and photon-starvation artifacts, including implanted metal, dense intravenous contrast within central venous structures at the thoracic inlet level, and inherently dense bony structures.

DECT has several useful clinical applications in head and neck imaging for better clinical care, which include atherosclerotic plaque, metal artifact reduction and tumor characterization. Several studies had demonstrated that with DECT, there had been dose reduction or similar dose when compared to single-energy CT. It provides high temporal resolution and enables bone removed CT neuroangiographic images of diagnostic quality. In addition, calcified plaques and surgical clips can be removed by processing the data. Recent studies have reported contrast-enhanced dual-energy CT angiography had high diagnostic accuracy for the detection of intracranial aneurysm as compared with 3D digital subtraction angiography (DSA) at a lower radiation dose.

Cone Beam CT

Standard CT scanners uses the fan-beam geometry of the X-ray, whereas cone beam CT (CBCT) uses X-ray beam which is conical in configuration and enables a volume of tissue to be imaged in a single rotation.[1] By increasing the anode angle in the X-ray tube, there is increase in the cone angle of the X-ray beam. The data of the entire region of interest can captured in a single rotation by rectangular or round two-dimensional (2D) detector. The reconstruction algorithm most frequently used in CBCT is a modified Feldkamp algorithm, which is essentially a 3D adaptation of the filtered back-projection method used in fan-beam 2D reconstructions.

Recent advances in imaging technology have significantly improved the CBCT scanners. These include development of flat-panel detector arrays which are compact, relatively low-cost, high-quality and large-area; better X-ray tubes which are capable of multiple exposures necessary for cone-beam scanning and low-cost computers with processing power sufficient for cone beam image reconstruction in near real time. CBCT is typically implemented as a seat scanner such that the imaging chain is rotated around a vertical axis with the patient seated at the isocenter. The high resolution of flat-panel CBCT is advantageous for many clinical applications in dental imaging, temporal bone imaging, sinonasal imaging, and imaging of implanted devices (e.g., prostheses, endovascular coils, and stents).

Portable CT

Standard CT scanners are stationary and located in the radiology imaging department. The patients are required to travel to a CT suite for imaging, where there is a high-voltage power source with radiation shielding of wall and ceiling. These scanners are not suitable for the patients who are critically ill patients in intensive care units (ICUs) as well as patients undergoing surgery. There is significant higher morbidity (13–71%) in transporting the critically ill patient to the imaging area. The portable CT are used for imaging patients at bedside in ICUs (to minimize movement of critically ill patients) and for perioperative cross-sectional image in operation theatres (to provide fast check on surgical outcome).[10]

Though portable and mobile CT terms are used interchangeably, there is difference between portable CT and mobile CT. Portable CT represents CT system within the hospital that can be moved from place to place whereas mobile CT represents CT system that function as standalone unit, typically in a trailer. There are concerns of scattered radiations for staff and public from ionization radiation arising from the portable scanners in the scanning area (ICUs or operation theaters), as portable system cannot be shielded. Scatter shields on the front and back of the scanner can be used to reduce the scatter dose.

CereTom, produced by NeuroLogica is portable scanner designed specifically for head imaging. It attaches directly to a patient's bed and used for scanning of the head and neck. Though the cost of portable CT is higher than a standard CT scanner, portable head CT are considered to be economically and clinically beneficial in ICUs and operating rooms as the cost of staff personnel and equipment needed for the transport of a patient to and from the conventional scanner exceed in value. Many studies have shown that the portable CT images are of good diagnostic quality and the radiation dose is also near similar to that of standard CT.

Phase Contrast CT

Conventional CT technologies are based on absorption property of the X-ray only; but there are other physical properties of the X-rays penetrating through matter that could potentially contribute to other complementary information. Phase-contrast computed tomography (CT) is non-conventional CT imaging and an X-ray–based experimental imaging modality in which the phase shifts of X-rays passing through matter rather is used to generate tissue contrast.[11] It is based on refraction and interference effects of X-ray imaging, with higher contrast than conventional absorption-based X-ray attenuation. Experiments had shown that suggest that phase contrast CT yields higher contrast in biologic soft tissue than conventional X-ray imaging. The phase-shift information can be gathered with a variety of techniques, including propagation-based, analyzer-based, or crystal interferometer–based methods.

Most of these methods are based on monochromatic, parallel X-ray beams. It requires synchrotron X-ray sources or low-power microfocus X-ray tubes, which have limited availability and hence limits PCCT use in a potential clinical setting. With recent advances in technology, the phase-shift information can also be derived from grating-based phase-contrast CT when conventional X-ray tubes are used, which has lead to potential chances of phase-contrast CT to clinical applications. However, there are still many limitation of PCCT into medical imaging. Clinical applications of the PCCT include atherosclerotic carotid plaque characterization by its capability to differentiate various components of soft plaque, and *ex vivo* breast imaging by demonstrating excellent soft-tissue contrast. Without use of any contrast media, PCCT had shown ductal structures, collagen architecture and the three-dimensional outline of ductal carcinoma.

Advances in Image Reconstruction Algorithms

With the phenomenal advances in CT hardware, there has been significant improvement in the data processing methods, such as reconstruction techniques especially the iterative reconstruction (IR) CT algorithms.[1,12] Analytical approach of filtered back projection (FBP) was standard reconstruction method for diagnostic CT earlier. It was much faster and less perfect method, but has limitations like high image noise, streak artifacts, or low-contrast. These problems have been overcome by development of statistical and model based IR algorithms. By noise reductions in CT image processing, iterative reconstruction (IR) techniques allows substantial reduction in the radiation dose and improve image quality. IR techniques had shown enhanced diagnostic accuracy and artefact suppression. Image reconstruction in iterative reconstruction starts with an image assumption and then compares it to real time measured values while making constant adjustments until the two are in agreement. These algorithms essentially consist of a trial-and-error correction loop that is introduced in the image reconstruction process. Several iterative reconstruction software packages for CT are now commercially available, which includes iDose (Philips Healthcare, Best, Netherlands), ASiR (GE Healthcare, Milwaukee, WI), Adaptive Iterative Dose Reduction (Toshiba, Tochigi, Japan), and IRIS (Siemens, Erlangen, Germany).[1]

COMPUTED TOMOGRAPHY IN NEUROIMAGING

Computed tomography scan has been the workhorse of neuroimaging. It is a cost-effective and quick screening test with established role in cross-sectional imaging of craniospinal trauma, subarachnoid hemorrhage, stroke and evaluation of postoperative patients. In addition, it has a role in those patients in which MRI is contraindicated. The concept of CT imaging was challenged with the advent of MRI; however, with recent technology advancement like multidetector CT, the modality has seen a new resurgence. Many of these CT applications are current standards in clinical practice.

Computed tomography angiography now plays an expanded role in evaluation of subarachnoid hemorrhage by detecting vascular lesions like aneurysms and arteriovenous malformations. These patients are already on the CT table and it only requires and additional few minutes to obtain detailed information about possible causes of the hemorrhage. Most of the surgeons nowadays operate solely on the basis of a CTA exam. With MDCT, spatial resolution is excellent and the results are similar or even superior to angiography. There is an increasing use of the modality in imaging of stroke through CTA of intracranial and neck vessels, venography and CT perfusion imaging. The excellent reconstructions of CT data have also enhanced the utility of CT in neuroimaging, i.e. in spinal trauma and evaluation of craniovertebral junction.

NONCONTRAST CT OF HEAD

Helical CT has not caught on for routine imaging of the neurocranium and axial mode is still used for routine imaging; however, thin-sections obtained on multichannel scans have distinct advantage. Thin sections of the middle cranial and posterior fossa reduce the beam hardening artifacts and improve delineation of the brainstem and temporal lobe. A usual spiral protocol is 5 mm acquisition with thin sections (i.e. 1.5 mm) can be merged into thicker (2.5 mm or more) thus reducing noise and radiation dose. The data may be split back for high resolution reconstructions. Thus, there is now the option of not only axial but also coronal or sagittal images of the brain. The clinical usefulness of this technique, however, has not yet been tested. The technology has affected pediatric neuro applications in many ways. Increased speed has eliminated the need for sedation and a reconstruction of data obtained in least provocative position allows multiplanar depiction of anatomy.

Windowing in the CT is important concept in neuroimaging as changing this will cause significant difference in the appearance of the picture to bring the particular pathology to show particular structures.[13] Windowing helps in changing the grayscale component of a CT by changing the CT numbers. This is also known as gray-level mapping or contrast stretching. Windowing in CT has two components, window level and window width. The window level helps in adjusting the brightness of the image whereas the window width helps in adjusting the contrast. The window width is the measure of the range of CT numbers that an image contains as compared to window level or centre is the midpoint of the range of the CT numbers displayed. Typical window width or level in neuroimaging varies from institution to institution and vendor to vendor. Typical values in neuroimaging consists of for brain parenchyma (WW: 80 WL: 40), for subdural lesions (WW: 150-300 WL: 50-100) and for stroke (WW: 40 WL:40).

CT ANGIOGRAPHY

Catheter angiography; the gold standard for diagnostic neuroangiography, is an expensive and invasive procedure with a morbidity and mortality of 1.5–2%. High spatial resolution for visualization of small and tortuous vessels is required for imaging of vascular anatomy of head and neck region. In addition, to avoid venous enhancement fast acquisition is required. CTA of the craniocervical vessels thus has strikingly benefits from the technology of MDCT. At submillimeter collimation (0.5–0.75), the entire length of the carotids or the cerebral arteries is scanned in a few seconds in pure arterial phase. Finest anatomic detail can be achieved by this isotropic data set providing high quality 2D and 3D renderings of vascular anatomy through different reconstruction techniques.[14,15]

Magnetic resonance angiography (MRA) and color Doppler ultrasound (DUS) are some noninvasive alternatives. The limitations of MRA include motion artifacts, long examination times, loss of signal due to turbulence and in plane saturation leading to exaggeration of stenosis, poor demonstration of calcium and bony landmarks and limitations in evaluating postoperative patients with metallic clips and stents. Color Doppler (CD) is operator-dependent and limited in evaluating the intracranial vasculature.

Computed tomography angiography the current noninvasive modality of choice for neuroangiography, overcomes many of the disadvantages of MRA. It is faster, available in smaller centers, cheaper, sensitive to presence of calcium, displays bony landmarks and can be used in patients with aneurysm clips and other MR incompatible metallic hardware. CTA depends on volume expansion and opacification of blood in the vessel and hence more accurate. Drawbacks of CTA are the use of intravenous contrast and radiation exposure.

Technique

CT angiography evaluates the area from arch of aorta to vertex for cervicocerebral study in one sitting or from C1 to vertex for cerebral angiogram in 15–20 seconds. Typical parameters can be as follows: 120–140 kVp, 200–350 mAs, 1.25 mm cuts with 1 mm overlap, a pitch of 3 for head (1.25 mm/3.75 mm/rev) and 6 (1.25 mm/7.5 mm/rev) for neck and 0.5 second rotation time. 100 mL of contrast is injected at a rate of 4 mL/s by a power injector which can be chased by bolus tracking. When a threshold attenuation of 100 HU is reached as detected by the ROI placed in one of the common carotids, the scan starts automatically. Alternatively, a test bolus method (20 mL), using a single axial section dynamic study at C5 level can be used. An arbitrary delay of 15–20 seconds is also adequate for CTA of brain. A rapid intravenous injection of nonionic contrast, preferably from right hand, via pressure injector with flow rate of at least 3 mL/s achieves a luminal density of 150 HU which is considered to give best results. Higher rates do not offer any significant advantage.[15] The images are reformatted with section thickness of 1.25 mm and overlap of 1 mm at a narrow field of view (120 mm).

Image Processing

There are various display technique for image processing in CT angiography, which include multiplanar reconstructions (MPR), maximum intensity projection (MIP), shaded-surface display (SSD) and volume-rendering technique (VRT).[15,16] MPR allows for viewing of the raw data in any desired plane along the course of the vessel and is good for relatively straight vessels such as the carotid arteries but is not very effective for vascular anatomies which are complex like circle of Willis. MIP images are obtained by projection of imaginary rays through the image data and mapping the maximum attenuation values. The attenuation value, i.e. vessel lumen, calcium and thrombus are well delineated but depth information is totally lost. The degree of stenosis is calculated accurately but there may be overlapping of vessels with bone. Surface shaded display computes all surface connecting neighboring pixels above a particular threshold. Unlike MIP it preserves depth information (displays complex anatomic relationship in region of vessel overlap) but loses attenuation information. It does not show interiors of the vessels, thrombus and wall calcification and as underestimates stenosis. VRT allows integration of all available information through most advanced 3D rendering algorithm. An opacity as well as color is assigned to all the voxels available and VR incorporates all the relevant data into the final resulting image. It overcomes many of the problems seen with MIP and SSD. Since some data loss is inherent with all postprocessing techniques, raw images should be analyzed in all cases.

Applications of CT Angiography

Extracranial Vasculature

Carotid Artery Stenosis

The detection and accurate quantification of carotid artery stenosis is important for appropriate treatment since carotid endarterectomy has a clear benefit in symptomatic patients with high grade stenosis (70–99%) [North American Symptomatic Carotid Endarterectomy Trial (NASCET)]. The gold standard of carotid evaluation has been conventional angiography but the risks associated with it, interobserver variability in interpreting stenosis (up to 7%), a tendency to overestimate stenosis (6%) and limited number of views are some of the limitations. CTA can provide infinite views for accurate estimation of eccentric or irregular stenosis, delineates mural calcium from luminal contrast and prevents inaccuracy in grading stenosis. Magnified axial images with a window setting half way between luminal contrast and wall are considered best to evaluate stenosis followed by MIP and SSD.[17] Length of thickness, thickness of slices presence of calcification and direction of vessel in the imaged volume also affect measurements.[17-19]

It is difficult to assess exact accuracy of CTA in carotid stenosis due to different criteria and parameters used on different machines; however, reported sensitivity for severe stenosis and occlusion has ranged from 88–100%, which correlates well with conventional angiography **(Figs. 1A to D)**. Lee et al. reported 100% accuracy for occlusion, 90% for critical stenosis (90–99%), greater than 95% for severe stenosis (70–89%), greater than 85% for moderate stenosis (50–69%) and 95% for minimal stenosis.[17-19] CTA also has a good correlation of plaque morphology (calcified, soft or ulcerated).

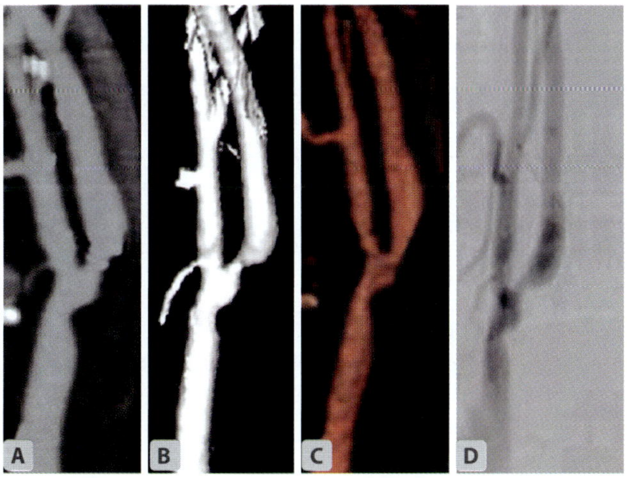

FIGS. 1A TO D: Left common and internal carotid artery stenosis: (A) MIP; (B) SSD; (C) VR and (D) DSA images showing moderate stenosis of distal common carotid and proximal internal carotid artery. The stenosis is not complete.

Computed tomography angiography has a higher accuracy compared to duplex ultrasound (DUS) and is comparable or slightly better than CE MRA (100% vs. 93%) for assessing high-grade stenosis and distinguishing it from complete occlusion. This is crucial, as high-grade stenosis is an indication for carotid endarterectomy whereas complete occlusion is a contraindication to surgery. CTA also provides assessment of the brain parenchyma at the same time.

Dissections

Dissection of carotid or vertebral artery is an increasingly recognized cause of stroke in young is adequately evaluated with CTA and results are comparable to other noninvasive techniques like MRA and CD.[20] Subadventitial dissections, presence of intramural hematoma, stenosis, occlusions and pseudoaneurysms can be picked up.

Computed tomography angiography is not successful for hemodynamic of blood flow. MDCT can simultaneously evaluate the intracranial vasculature for tandem stenosis in same sitting. Polytrauma patients with a high index of vascular injury can also be evaluated by CTA. MDCT provides simultaneous assessment of vascular, soft tissue and vertebral injury in this setting.

Intracranial Vasculature

Aneurysms

Digital subtraction angiography is the gold standard for the evaluation of patients with subarachnoid hemorrhage secondary to suspected aneurysmal rupture, but it is time consuming, invasive and carries a less than 0.1% complication rate of permanent neurological deficit.[15] There is an associated increased risk of rebleed. As shown by some clinical studies, CTA seems suitable in the acute stage after subarachnoid hemorrhage (SAH) as it does not require intra-arterial catheterization, uses short scan times and can immediately follow the initial unenhanced CT examination.[21,22] Yang et al. had evaluated the diagnostic accuracy of CT Angiography for the small intracranial aneurysms by a large cohort study.[23] They demonstrated that CT angiography had high accuracy for detection of small cerebral aneurysms, including those smaller than 3 mm. However the sensitivities of CT angiography were lower for detection of aneurysms smaller than 3 mm and unruptured compared with aneurysms that were 3–5 mm and ruptured.

For diagnosed aneurysms, CTA provides a more detailed analysis of the sac morphology, neck, parent vessel caliber and its spatial relationship with aneurysm, additional vascular relationships and surrounding anatomy (bony and soft tissue landmarks) which helps in finding the appropriate options for treatment (surgical or minimally invasive endovascular) **(Figs. 2 to 4)**.

Computed tomography angiography is also a problem-solving modality in poorly defined aneurysms on DSA and particularly useful for evaluation of paraclinoid aneurysms for their anatomically complex relationships with bony and vascular structures **(Figs. 2A to D)**. CTA is significant in the characterization of giant aneurysms preceeding surgical or endovascular treatment and helps in the detection of pseudoaneurysms. CTA is also indicated in the assessment of postoperative/postintervention status of aneurysm.

Though conventional angiography is more sensitive for small aneurysms, CTA may show small thrombosed aneurysms not shown on DSA.[24] CTA can be very efficient for screening of vasospasm following SAH. It can be a screening technique to detect aneurysms in high-risk group patients such as those with strong family histories, though MRA is currently the modality of choice.

Computed tomography angiography and MRA have been found to be generally equivalent in their ability to detect and characterize aneurysms (>5 mm).[25] CTA however, is superior to MRA, as turbulent flow or slow flow may cause artifactual loss of signal in MRA.

Some drawbacks of CT angiography include bleak visibility of small arteries, difficulty in distinguishing the infundibular dilatation at the origin of an artery from an aneurysm, the kissing vessel artifact, display of venous structures that can simulate aneurysms, inability to identify thrombosis and calcification on three-dimensional images, and beam-hardening artifacts produced by aneurysm clips.

Arteriovenous Malformations

CT angiography though has limited role in intracranial arteriovenous malformations (AVMs), it can visualize the feeding arteries, nidus and draining veins but optimal temporal information regarding arterial and venous phases may not be adequate as compared to DSA.[26] CTA does not possess a high spatial resolution which is required for detecting associated aneurysm, stenosis and small feeding vessels provided by conventional angiography. The major use of CTA today is in the evaluation of the AVM nidus during radiosurgery planning and post-treatment follow-up.[27]

Though any study has not yet compared the roles of CTA and MRA in AVMs yet each modality appears to have its own advantages and disadvantages but flow encoded MR may provide more information in AVM. Embolization material can interfere with delineation of vasculature on MRA but usually is not a problem with CTA.

Tumors

CT angiography can demonstrate vascular encasement by skull-base tumors. It also provides preoperative assessment of the 3D bony and vascular anatomy prior to tumor excision.

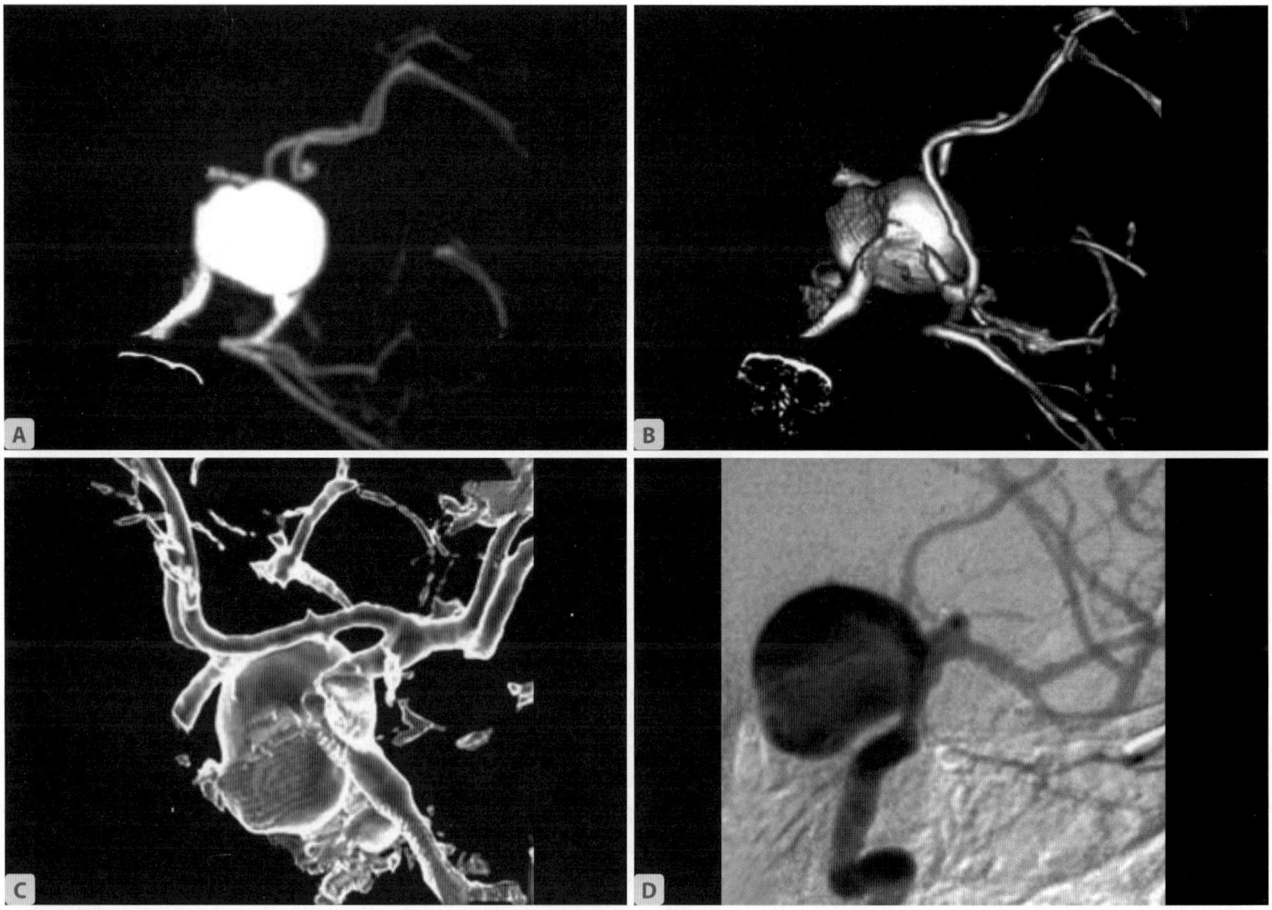

FIGS. 2A TO D: A giant carotico-ophthalmic aneurysm: Maximum intensity projection (A), volume-rendering (B and C) images; and digital subtraction angiography (D). The carotid artery is incorporated into the aneurysm. Postprocessing shows vascular relationship better than DSA.

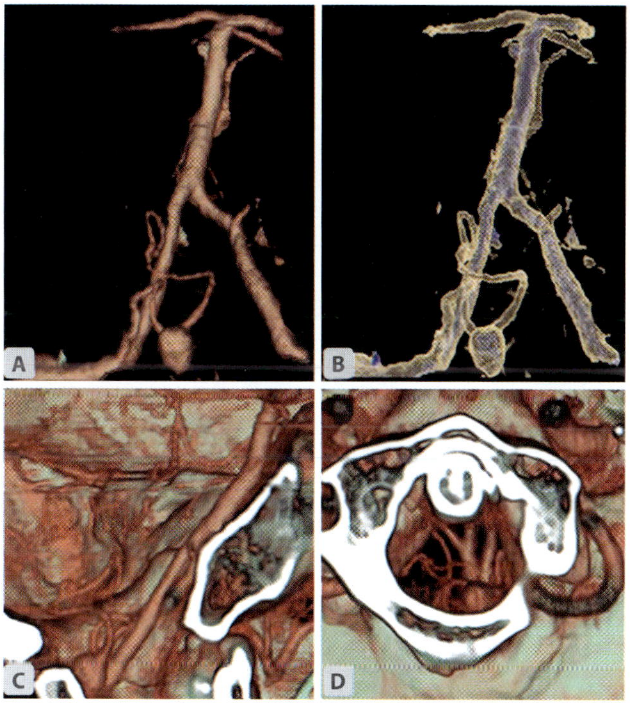

FIGS. 3A TO D: Posterior inferior cerebellar artery (PICA) aneurysm: volume-rendering images (A and B) posterior view showing the aneurysm arising from the left PICA. The relationship with C1 posterior arch was clearly shown (C and D) helping the decision for surgical approach.

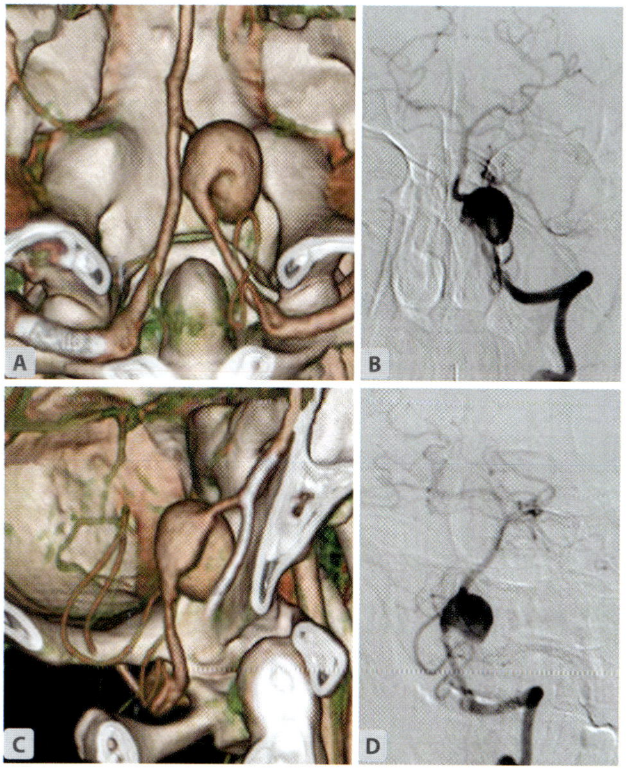

FIGS. 4A TO D: Left vertebral artery aneurysm: Volume-rendering (A and C) and digital subtraction angiography (B and D) showing left vertebral artery aneurysm with complex configuration better shown on computed tomography volume-rendering images.

COMPUTED TOMOGRAPHY PERFUSION

It has been shown that cerebral blood volume when falls below 20 mL/100 g/min synaptic transmission in neurons fails and below 10 mL irreversible cell death occurs. Therefore tissue salvage is possible in areas with lesser degrees of compromise of blood flow. Computed tomography perfusion (CTP) is a rapid means to evaluate cerebral perfusion as there is a linear relationship between the contrast agent concentration and attenuation.[28-34] CTP is based on the central volume principle as per the equation: CBF = CBV/MTT [cerebral blood flow (CBF), cerebral blood volume (CBV), mean transit time (MTT)]. During the first pass of a bolus of contrast, there is a transient increase in attenuation proportional to the concentration of the agent in a given region. Contrast agent-time concentration curves are generated in an arterial and venous region of interest (ROI) (i.e. middle cerebral artery and superior sagittal sinus) and in the area of perfusion abnormality. Deconvolution of this data gives the MTT. Cerebral blood volume (CBV) is calculated as the area under the curve of parenchymal pixel and the arterial ROI. From this CBF can be calculated.[28]

Technique

Usually for anterior circulation stroke, four adjacent 5 mm slices are selected starting at the level of basal ganglia. About 50 mL of a nonionic contrast is injected at a rate of 3 mL/s. Five seconds later a continuous scan is initiated using 80 kVp, 190–200 mA at one second rotation for 50 seconds. The perfusion data is analyzed at a work station to generate color coded CBF, CBV and MTT maps. With the advent of 256 and 320 MDCT, whole brain perfusion CT can be performed which provides access to the entire brain with the administration of one contrast medium bolus so that ischemic region can be identified.[33-34]

Clinical Applications

Acute Stroke

The goal is to identify potentially salvageable tissue for thrombolytic therapy. In a retrospective study, Eastwood et al. found significant difference in CBV, CBF and MTT in symptomatic hemisphere of which MTT was the best indicator for stroke.[30] A 35% decrease in CBF had a good correlation with ischemic penumbra in another study.[30] Early studies do indicate that CTP may enable predication of patients who would benefit from therapy and determine final infarct size.

Cerebrovascular Reserve

In patients with chronic ischemia related to underlying stenotic lesions, the involved territory is maximally vasodilated due to autoregulation and cannot respond to acetazolamide challenge. An increase of 5% in CBF indicates insufficiency and a decrease in CBF indicates higher risk of stroke. CTP has been used to show low CBV and CBF in patients of SAH with moderate-to-severe vasospasm.[31,32]

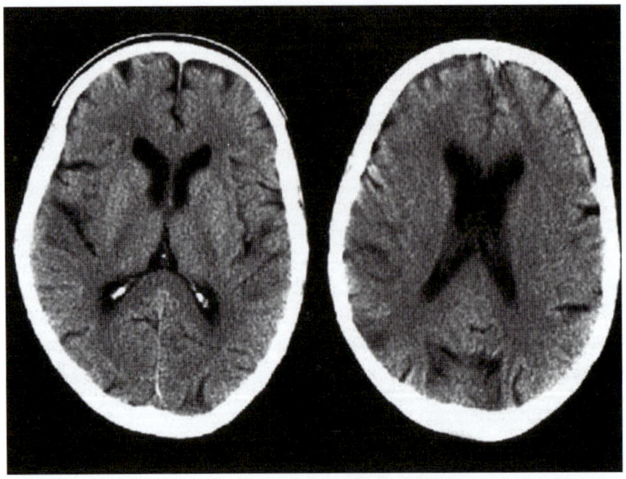

FIG. 5A: Noncontrast CT within 2 hours of stroke showing ill-defined hypodensity in the right parietotemporal region.

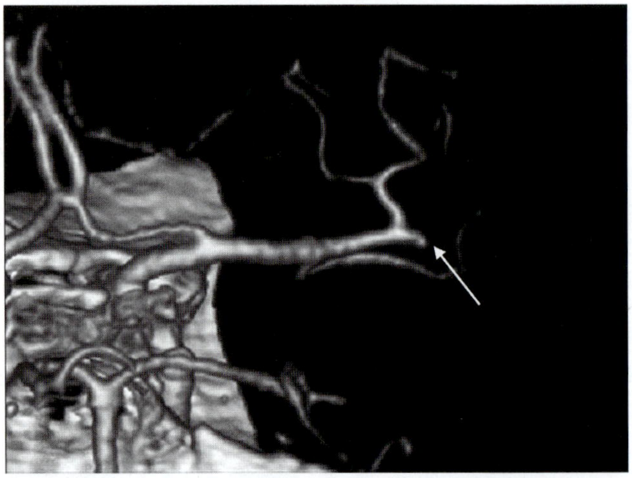

FIG. 5B: Computed tomography angiography in posterosuperior view showing complete occlusion of the inferior division of the right middle cerebral artery (MCA) (arrow).

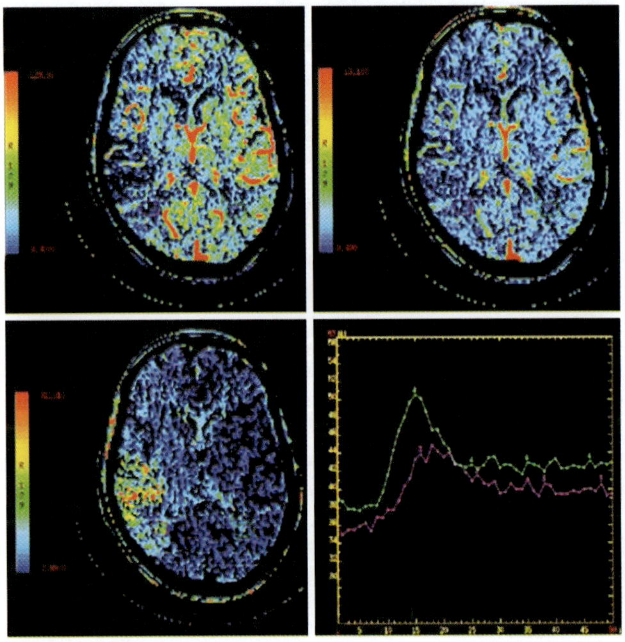

FIG. 5C: Cerebral blood flow, cerebral blood volume and mean transit time maps showing perfusion defect and a large ischemic penumbra. MTT maps shows delayed transit of contrast. Time attenuation curve of penumbra region showing less attenuation compared to normal side.

Tumors

Many studies has shown that modified CTP technique has high permeability surface product (a measure of microvascular permeability) in tumors and may prove advantageous over MR in tumor perfusion studies. CTP can be used for preoperative grading of gliomas and can provide additional information about tumor hemodynamics.[33,34] In addition, perfusion computed tomography (PCT) maps are also useful for surgical biopsy and/or radiosurgery guidance to target the areas of increased CBV which can yield better histology and better response to treatment.

COMPUTED TOMOGRAPHY IMAGING OF ACUTE ISCHEMIC STROKE

Several studies have shown better neurological outcome in patients with acute stroke with thrombolytic therapy which were based on the imaging criteria. Multimodal CT (noncontrast CT, CT Angiography and perfusion CT) allows the assessment of the four Ps (parenchyma, pipes perfusion, and penumbra).[35-40] MDCT provides a 'one-stop-shop' approach for comprehensive noninvasive assessment of acute stroke patients by demonstrating the site of arterial occlusion and hemodynamic status of the brain parenchyma. A noncontrast scan is done to diagnose infarct, determine its extension and rule out hemorrhage. A CTA is an accurate technique for evaluation of vascular patency in acute stroke by allowing comprehensive evaluation of the intra- and extracranial vasculature. A CTA from the aortic arch to the intracerebral vessels helps to detect carotid plaques as possible causes of the event, distinguishes between proximal and distal occlusions of an intracranial artery, differentiates arterial from venous infarct and provides information about hypoperfusion and collateralization of blood flow. Finally, a CT perfusion scan distinguishes between penumbra of hypoperfused and umbra of nonperfused tissue in order to select patients who would benefit from thrombolytic therapy. The above information provides a rational basis on which to choose the optimal treatment for patients with acute stroke **(Figs. 5A to C)**. Due to limited availability of PET, SPECT and Xenon CT, CT and MR perfusion are the two practical choices. MRI imaging with DWI and PWI is equally powerful alternative and both CT and MR techniques are comparable in evaluating the tissue at risk in acute stroke according to a recent study.[40] However, widespread availability of CT in smaller centers is a big advantage.

COMPUTED TOMOGRAPHY VENOGRAPHY

Computed tomography venography allows visualization of the cerebral venous structures and has high sensitivity for depicting the cerebral veins and sinus compared to DSA.[41-43] MDCT venography is a fast, widely accessible, and cost-effective method for evaluating cerebral sinuses in emergency setting. MR venography (MRV) is currently the technique of choice for diagnostic evaluation and follow-up for patient with cerebral sinovenous thrombosis. Studies have shown CTV as comparable to accuracy of MRV in the diagnosis of dural sinovenous thrombosis.[41-43] CT venography overcomes flow-related artifacts (differentiates slow flow from thrombosis) seen on time-of-flight (TOF) MR, takes less time and also helps in distinction of tumors that compress dural sinuses, from those which occlude them. However, CT needs contrast administration and lacks sensitivity of MR in showing venous infarction of brain. Overall, CTV is a reliable alternative to MRV in case MR is contraindicated in such patients or is not diagnostic.

Technique

Computed tomography venography is performed using 100 mL of intravenous contrast injected at the rate of 3 mL/s with power injector. After a scan delay of 40 seconds, 1 mm collimated sections with a pitch of 2:1 are done covering the skull.

Clinical Applications of CT Venography

Cerebral Sinovenous Thrombosis

Dural sinus thrombosis is difficult to diagnose clinically due to varied clinical presentation. The most commonly affected sinuses are the superior sagittal sinus, the transverse sinus and the sigmoid sinus. On CTV, a thrombosed dural sinus is seen as a filling defect and is often associated with contrast enhancement of the walls of the dural sinus as well as abnormal collateral venous drainage and tentorial enhancement **(Figs. 6A to E)**.

Tumors

CTV is also useful for showing venous invasion by meningioma.

MULTIDETECTOR COMPUTED TOMOGRAPHY OF SPINE

Multidetector CT has been a major advancement in imaging of trauma patients to facilitate rapid diagnosis before the patient can be shifted to operation theater. Bony abnormalities are depicted better with MDCT when compared to single slice CT. Current scanners with 16 or more detectors are used to scan from head to below hips using whole body single pass technique. Imaging metallic hardware, which was impossible due to streak artifacts in the single slice helical CT scanning can now be assessed easily with MDCT due to increase in the

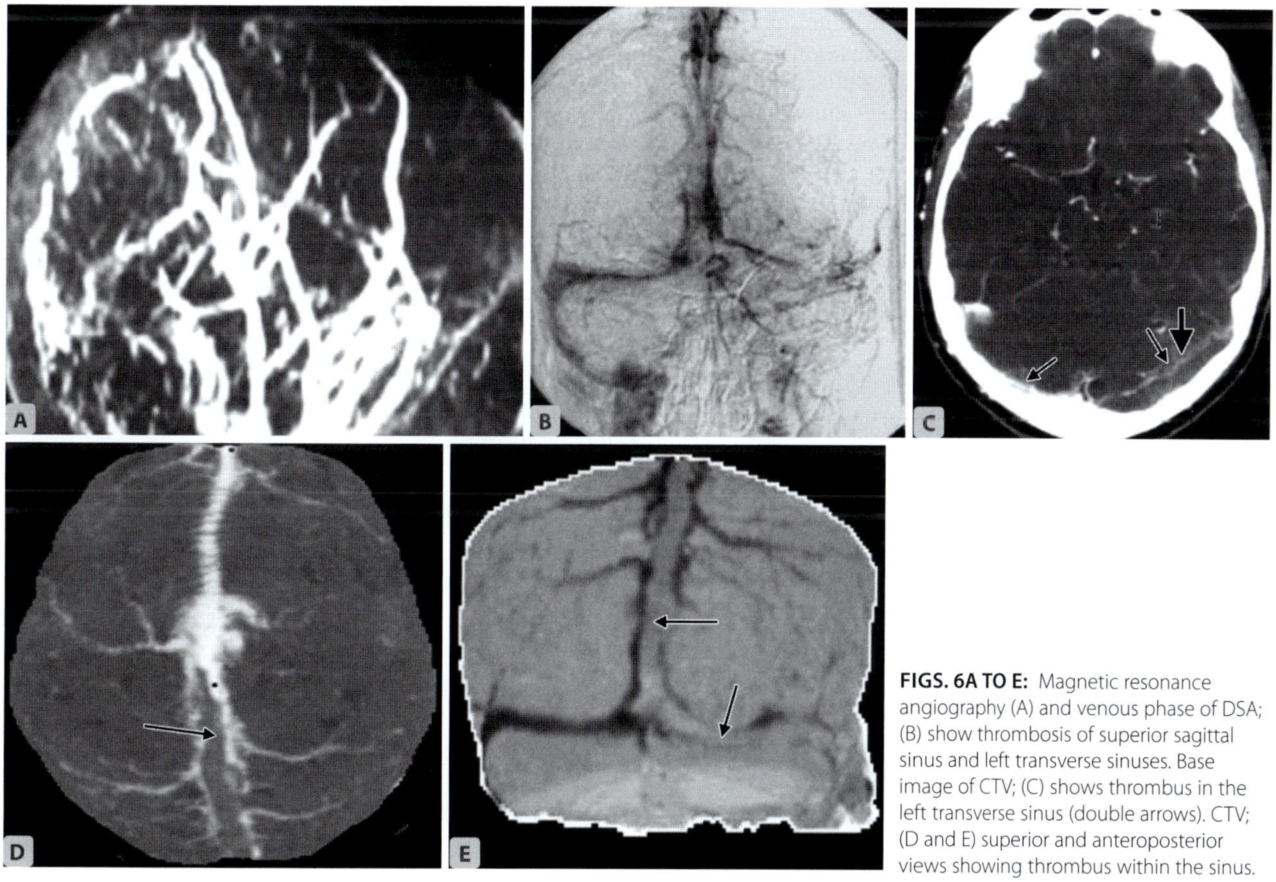

FIGS. 6A TO E: Magnetic resonance angiography (A) and venous phase of DSA; (B) show thrombosis of superior sagittal sinus and left transverse sinuses. Base image of CTV; (C) shows thrombus in the left transverse sinus (double arrows). CTV; (D and E) superior and anteroposterior views showing thrombus within the sinus.

of detector rows.[44] With improvement of isotropic resolutions, multi-planer reformations now enable diagnosis that are not so apparent on axial images, i.e. transverse fractures and fusions. Understanding of complex spatial relationships of bone becomes easier which translates into increased confidence level of the radiologist. While 3D-CT may not add to diagnostic information achieved by use of 2D reformatted image but it does aid the surgeons to plan reconstructive surgery.

Clinical Applications

- *Trauma*
  - *Cervical trauma:* CT is cost effective in patients with closed head injury with high risk of associated cervical spine injury, i.e. in confirming and better depicting the extent of the injuries. MDCT gives excellent reformatted images to identify fractures in horizontal plane that may not be apparent otherwise **(Figs. 7A to C)**. Craniovertebral junction is one area well suited for reformatted images. Any associated vascular injury can also be simultaneously evaluated with CTA.
  - *Thoracolumbar trauma:* Combination of 5–10 mm routine abdominal sections for visceral injuries and plain radiography for lumbar spine fracture is inadequate. In such situations, MDCT due to thinner sections and better reformations is 97% sensitive for detection of unstable fractures as compared to 33% sensitivity of plain radiography.[45]
- *In degenerative diseases of spine:* CT is inferior to MRI for evaluating soft tissue detail. Main advantage of MDCT is to show bony canal, i.e. oblique reformations for foraminal stenosis. MDCT depicts trabecular anatomy in the bone marrow with remarkable clarity and early trabecular destruction by tumors is readily apparent. MDCT complements MR and plain radiographic assessment for marrow infiltrative disorders like multiple myeloma, detects vertebrae at risk for fracture and differentiate benign from neoplastic fractures.[46,47]
- Multidetector CT is also useful in evaluation of postoperative patients for hardware and in assessing progression of healing. The artifacts due to metallic hardware implants can be reduced by various advanced CT techniques. Maximizing the peak voltage and tube current, minimizing the detector collimation and pitch during acquisition can help in reducing the artifacts. Using thin slice reconstruction, thicker slice reformats and 3D-VR techniques are also helpful in reducing the artifacts.[47]
- Numerous vascular conditions like aortic dissection, aortic aneurysm and aneurysm of artery of Adamkiewicz and post-intervention procedures like aortic stent graft placement can endanger the vascular integrity of artery of Adamkiewicz. In these conditions, MDCT angiography of spinal vasculature with adapted brain reconstruction algorithm may provide the details of perfusion and anatomy of artery of Adamkiewicz.[48]
- With multiplanar and 3D reformations, spinal deformities can be assessed in all planes allowing identification of previously unrecognized malformations and better characterization of previously identified deformities. MDCT has a role in depiction of postoperative bony fusions and in patients with indwelling hardware. However, MR still remains the modality of choice to evaluate disc abnormalities and post disc surgery scanning.[46]

RADIATION CONCERNS

Radiation hazard is a major issue as there is a manifold increase in the number of CT examinations performed currently. Helical CT provides a reduction in patient dose over "step and shoot" scans due to short scan times (higher pitch). However, it is known that increasing the pitch does not necessarily decrease the dose as there is an automatic increase in the tube current.[49,50] Further advancement in X-ray tube technology can accomplish decreased dose by modulating the X-ray tube current. The penumbra of the CT beam is a source of wasted radiation. Efforts are on to harvest these for diagnostic information. The organ-specific and shape-specific beam profiles are also being developed like tilted gantries which may reduce radiation to lens.

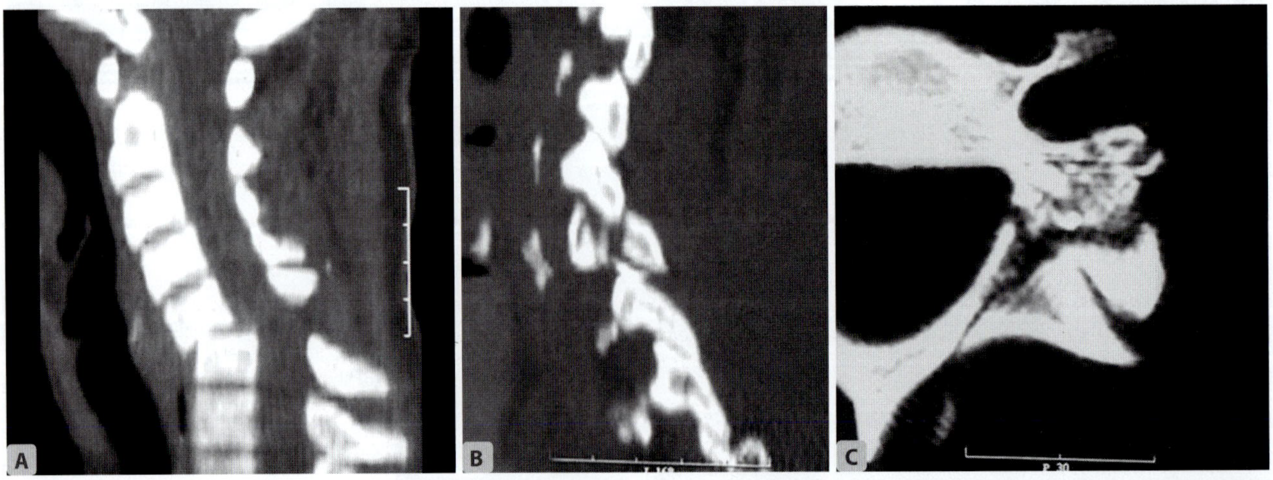

FIGS. 7A TO C: Sagittal reconstructed (A) helical CT images of cervical spine showing malalignment on CT. Parasagittal reconstructed image of CT (B) better shows the fracture and the locked facet. Axial image (C) shows fracture of lateral mass on left side.

3D PRINTING

3D Printing is a technique which helps to generate anatomical models or 3D printed physical models from the volumetric medical imaging data (CT or MRI) with the help of computers.[51,52] This technique primarily consists of three steps, initially image segmentation is done, followed mesh refinement and then 3D printing. These have become more popular and cost effective in medicine due to segmentation algorithms advancement and more accessibility of three-dimensional (3D) printers. The 3D printing can be divided into three groups: extrusion printing, photopolymerization and powder-based printing. Extrusion printing is most common form of the 3D printing and is also known as Fused Deposition Modeling (FDM).[51] In this technique, material is melted and the desired shape is made layer by layer fashion, by depositing via a nozzle.

With the 3D printing, the patient-specific models can be made of various organs in the body (like liver and lungs) and anatomical regions of interest. Now there are open-source post-processing tools for the end-users, which help in segmentation of the anatomical structure or spatial model and then desired final product can be printed with the help of special 3D printers.[52] Physical models or prototypes can be made rapidly from the various virtual datasets of CT or MRI.

CONCLUSION

Extensive technical advances in CT have led to significant improvement in the image quality, speed and reduction in radiation dose. Several CT advancement, like multidetector computed tomography (MDCT), dual-energy CT, cone beam CT, portable CT, phase contrast CT and iteractive reconstruction algorithms have revolutionized the neuroimaging with extensive anatomic coverage and thinner sections. Entire cranial and extra-cranial vasculature can be noninvasively demonstrating with high spatial and temporal resolution. With the recent MDCT scanners, visualization of dynamic flow and perfusion as well as motion of an entire volume at a very short time interval is possible.

REFERENCES

1. Ginat DT, Gupta R. Advances in computed tomography imaging technology. Annu Rev Biomed Eng. 2014;16:431-53.
2. Pelc NJ. Recent and future directions in CT imaging. Ann Biomed Eng. 2014;42(2):260-8.
3. Hu H. Multi-slice helical CT: Scan and reconstruction. Med Phys. 1999;26:5-18.
4. Gupta R, Cheung AC, Bartling SH, et al. Flat-Panel Volume CT: Fundamental Principles, Technology, and Applications. Radiographics. 2008;28:2009-22.
5. Salomon EJ, Barfett J, Willems PW, et al. Dynamic CT Angiography and CT Perfusion Employing a 320-detector Row CT. Klin Neuroradiol. 2009;19:187-96.
6. Brouwer PA, Bosman T, van Walderveen MA, et al. Dynamic 320-section CT angiography in cranial arteriovenous shunting lesions. Am J Neuroradiol. 2010; 31(4):767-70.
7. Hegde A, Chan LL, Tan L, et al. Dual Energy CT and its Use in Neuroangiography. Ann Acad Med Singapore. 2009; 38:817-20.
8. Zhang LJ, Wu SY, Niu JB, et al. Dual energy CT angiography in the evaluation of intracranial aneurysms: Image quality, radiation dose, and comparison with 3D rotational digital subtraction angiography. Am J Roentgenol. 2010; 194:23-30.
9. Ginat DT, Mayich M, Daftari-Besheli L, et al. Clinical applications of dual-energy CT in head and neck imaging. Eur Arch Otorhinolaryngol. 2016; 273(3):547-53.
10. Rumboldt Z, Huda W, All JW. Review of portable CT with assessment of a dedicated head CT scanner. Am J Neuroradiol. 2009; 30(9):1630-6.
11. Hetterich H, Willner M, Fill S, et al. Phase-contrast CT:qualitative and quantitative evaluation of atherosclerotic carotid artery plaque. Radiology. 2014; 271(3):870-8.
12. Geyer LL, Schoepf UJ, Meinel FG, et al. State of the Art: Iterative CT Reconstruction Techniques. Radiology. 2015; 276(2):339-57.
13. Mainali S, Wahba M, Elijovich L. Detection of Early Ischemic Changes in Noncontrast CT Head Improved with "Stroke Windows". ISRN Neurosci. 2014;2014:654980.
14. Westerlaan HE. Gravendeel J, Fiore D, et al. Multislice CT angiography in the selection of patients with ruptured intracranial aneurysms suitable for clipping or coiling. Neuroradiology. 2007;49:997-1007.
15. Kuszyk BS, Beauchamp NJ Jr, Fishman EK. Neurovascular applications of CT angiography. Semin Ultrasound CT MR. 1998;19(5):394-404.
16. Snyder KV, Mokin M, Bates VE. Neurologic applications of whole-brain volumetric multidetector computed tomography. Neurol Clin. 2014;32(1):237-51.
17. Anderson GB, Ashforth R, Steinke DE, et al. CT angiography for the detection and characterization carotid artery bifurcation disease. Stroke. 2000;31:2168-74.
18. Dillon EH, Van Leeuwen MS, Fernandes MA, et al. CT angiography: Application to the evaluation of carotid artery stenosis. Radiology. 1993;189:211-9.
19. Lee A, Boss J, Ngyuyen T, et al. Application of helical computed tomographic angiography in evaluation of carotid artery stenosis. Applied Radiology. 1998;26-30.
20. Link J, Brossman J, Pensclen V, et al. Common carotid artery bifurcation: Preliminary results of CT angiography and color coded duplex sonography compared with digital subtraction angiography. Am J Roentgenol. 1997; 168:361-5.
21. Leclerc X, Godefroy O, Salhi A, et al. Helical CT for the diagnosis of extracranial carotid artery dissection. Stroke. 1996;27:461-6.
22. Zouaori A, Sahil M, Mairo B, et al. Three-dimensional computed tomographic angiography in detection of cerebral aneurysms in acute subarachnoid hemorrhage. Neurosurgery. 1997; 41: 125-30.
23. Yang ZL, Ni QQ, Schoepf UJ, et al. Small Intracranial Aneurysms: Diagnostic Accuracy of CT Angiography. Radiology. 2017; 285(3):941-52.
24. Hope JK, Wilson JL, Thomson FJ. Three-dimensional angiography in the dectection and characterization of intracranial berry aneurysms. Am J Neuroradiol. 1996;17:439-45.
25. Brown JH, Lustrin ES, Lev MH, et al. Characterization of intracranial aneurysms using CT angiography. Am J Roentgenol. 1997;169: 889-93.
26. Barboriak DP, Provenzale JM. MR arteriography of intracranial circulation. Am J Roentgenol. 1998; 171:1469-78.
27. Reiger J, Hoston N, Neuman, K et al. Initial clinical experience with spiral CT and 3D arterial reconstruction in intracranial aneurysm and arteriovenous malformations. Neuroradiology. 1996; 36:245-51.

28. Wintermark M, Reichhart M, Cuisenaire O, et al. Comparison of admission perfusion computed tomography and qualitative diffusion and perfusion weighted magnetic resonance imaging in acute stroke patients. Stroke. 2002; 33:2025-31.
29. Nabavi DG, Cenic A, Craen RA, et al. Assessment of cerebral perfusion: Experimental validation and the initial clinical experience. Radiology. 1999; 213:141-9.
30. Eastwood JD, Lev MH, Azhari T, et al. Perfusion scanning with deconvolution analysis: Pilot study in patients with acute middle cerebral artery stroke. Radiology. 2002; 222:227-36.
31. Wintermark M, Reichhart M, Thiran JP, et al. Prognostic accuracy of cerebral blood flow measurement by perfusion computed tomography, at the time of emergency room admission, in acute stroke patients. Ann Neurol. 2002; 51:417-32.
32. Nabavi DG, LeBlanc LM, Baxter B, et al. Monitoring cerebral perfusion after subarachnoid hemorrhage using CT. Neuroradiology. 2001;43:7-16.
33. Murayama K, Katada K, Nakane M, et al. Whole-Brain Perfusion CT Performed with a Prototype 256–Detector Row CT System: Initial Experience. Radiology. 2009;250:202-11.
34. Ellika SK, Jain R, Patel SC, et al. Role of Perfusion CT in Glioma Grading and Comparison with Conventional MR Imaging Features. Am J Neuroradiol. 2007; 28:1981-7.
35. Srinivasan A, Goyal M, Azri FA, et al. State-of-the-Art Imaging of Acute Stroke. Radiographics. 2006; 26:75-95.
36. Ledezma CJ, Wintermark M. Multi-modal CT in Stroke Imaging: New Concepts. Radiol Clin North Am. 2009; 47(1):109-16.
37. Tomandl BF, Klotz E, Handschu R, et al. Comprehensive Imaging of Ischemic Stroke with Multisection CT. Radiographics. 2003; 23:565-92.
38. Zerna C, Assis Z, d'Esterre CD, et al. Imaging, Intervention, and Workflow in Acute Ischemic Stroke: The Calgary Approach. Am J Neuroradiol. 2016;37(6):978-84.
39. Wardlaw JM. Overview of Cochrane thrombolysis meta- analysis. Neurology. 2001; 57:S69-76.
40. Sunshine J. CT, MR and MR angiography in evaluation of patients with acute stroke. J Vasc Interv Radiol. 2004;15:S47-55.
41. Khandelwal N, Agarwal A, Kochhar R, et al. Comparison of CT Venography with MR Venography in cerebral sinovenous thrombosis. Am J Roentgenol. 2006; 187:1637-43.
42. Linn J, Erlt-Wagner B, Seelos KC, et al. Diagnostic value of multidetector-row CT angiography in the evaluation of thrombosis of the cerebral venous thrombosis. Am J Neuroradiol. 2007; 28: 946-52.
43. Ozsvath RR, Casey SO, Lustrin ES, et al. Cerebral venography: Comparison of CT and MR projection venography. Am J Roentgenol. 1997; 169:1699-707.
44. Buchwalter KA, Rydberg J, Kopecky KK, et al. Musculoskeletal imaging with multislice CT. Am J Roentgenol. 2001; 176:979-86.
45. Rhee PM, Bridgeman A, Acosta JA, et al. Lumbar fractures in adult blunt trauma: Axial and single slice helical abdominal and pelvic computed tomographic scans versus portable plain X ray. J Trauma. 2002; 53:663-7.
46. Crim JR, Tripp D. Multidetector CT of the spine. Semin in US, CT and MRI. 2004; 25:55-66.
47. Ohashi K, El-Khoury GY. Musculoskeletal CT: Recent advances and current clinical applications. Radiol Clinc N Am. 2009; 47: 387-409.
48. Boll DT, Bulow H, Blackam KA, et al. MDCT Angiography of the spinal vasculature and the artery of the Adamkiewicz. Am J Roentgenol. 2006; 187:1054-60.
49. Mahesh M, Scatarige JC, Cooper J, et al. Dose and pitch relationship for a particular multislice CT scanner. Am J Roentgenol. 2001; 177:1273-5.
50. Costello JE, Cecava ND, Tucker JE, et al. CT radiation dose: current controversies and dose reduction strategies. Am J Roentgenol. 2013; 201(6):1283-90.
51. Bücking TM, Hill ER, Robertson JL, Maneas E, Plumb AA, Nikitichev DI. From medical imaging data to 3D printed anatomical models. PLoS One. 2017;12(5):e0178540.
52. Bortolotto C, Eshja E, Peroni C, et al. 3D Printing of CT Dataset: Validation of an Open Source and Consumer-Available Workflow. J Digit Imaging. 2016;29(1):14-21.

CHAPTER

185

Advances in Neuroimaging Techniques: Magnetic Resonance Imaging

Paramjeet Singh, Niranjan Khandelwal, Sameer Vyas

Magnetic resonance imaging (MRI) is probably the most powerful tool in the radiologist's arsenal in diagnosing the brain and spinal pathologies. It has got tremendous role in providing into both the anatomical, pathological and functional aspects of a disease entity. Improvements have been directed toward reducing scan times and improving image quality through developing new pulse sequences, improved receiver coil technology, enhanced gradient performance, use of higher field strength magnets and application of more efficient data processing. Modern ultrafast sub-second sequences virtually freeze the physiological motion. On the other hand, with the advent of diffusion weighted imaging, perfusion imaging, spectroscopy it is now possible to provide an insight into the functional aspect of the disease. With advancement in MRI technology, it has emerged as a powerful tool not only for fast routine scanning, but also establishing its multiparametric applications into studying organ function, metabolism and physiology leading to an integrative approach.

In this chapter, we are going to discuss the hardware improvement in MRI including higher field strength MRI followed by faster scanning techniques and the different sequences exploring functional aspect of disease and finally briefly about the latest exciting developments on artificial intelligence. MR spectroscopy, functional MRI and 3D printing have been discussed in the other chapters in this book.

IMPROVEMENTS IN MR HARDWARE

During last few decades, tremendous improvement has been observed in the MR hardware particularly in the form of evolution of high field MRI. The technical design of magnets operating at 1.5 T has been the subject of an enormous engineering effort and area of research over the last 30 years and evolution of designs over years have led to a high level of performance and efficiency. In the last 15 years we observed similar evolution with 3 T units. Currently further upgradation of magnetic strength is an area of major research.

High field strength MRI: A large number of MR systems operating at a field strength of 3 Tesla (and higher) have been installed worldwide and are gaining acceptance for clinical and research purpose particularly in neuroimaging. The US Food and Drug Administration cleared the first seven tesla (7 T) magnetic resonance imaging device in October 2017 for clinical use. MR scanners with 9.4 T, 10.5 T and 11.75 T are also being used for research purposes in few institutions.

It is an established and well-recognized fact that increasing the static field strength increases the signal detected in MRI.[1-3] It primarily happens through two mechanisms: increasing magnetization and increasing detection efficiency. Spin polarization is produced by most MRI scanners by applying the static field to a spin system that is in thermal equilibrium with its surroundings a phenomenon known as Boltzmann polarization. In this setting, the equilibrium magnetization bears a linear relationship with field strength. The detected signal is proportional to the rate of spin precession, and this leads to a detection efficiency that increases linearly with field strength.[4] The combination of increased magnetization and increased spin detection efficiency leads to an increase in signal strength that is proportional to the square of the applied field. However, to determine the overall advantage of increasing the field strength and, therefore, the operating frequency, it is necessary to consider the frequency dependence of the noise voltages that are inevitably present. The noise voltages are superimposed on the signal voltage and will impair the ability to construct an image from the signal voltage unless the signal to noise ratio (SNR) of the system is sufficiently large. Without going into the complexity of physics it can be commented that the noise voltage is linearly proportional to the Larmor frequency and proportional to the square root of the tissue conductivity. In most tissues, the conductivity increases weakly with frequency, and, as a result, the thermal noise level generally increases slightly faster than linearly with increasing field strength.[5] The advantage of improved SNR can be exploited to increase speed and resolution judiciously, i.e. imaging time can be reduced for a similar SNR as 1.5 T or spatial resolution increased for an equal imaging time on both.[6]

SNR changes linearly with B0. However, in presence of inhomogeneity and changing tissue relaxation, linear increase in SNR may not be possible.[7] Besides the increase in SNR, the other tissue properties or imaging parameters which are also affected at higher field strength include resolution, T1 (in sec), T2* (in sec), apparent T2, sensitivity to susceptibility and spectral resolution in MRSI.[8] Two main advantages of higher field strength are increase in SNR and susceptibility induced contrast. These are especially helpful in functional imaging techniques [fMRI, blood oxygen level dependent (BOLD) contrast], MR spectroscopy and high resolution anatomical imaging (volumetric 3-dimensional imaging) within acceptable acquisition time. High field MRI is clinically very useful for imaging of epilepsy, brain tumors, multiple sclerosis, Alzheimer's disease and psychiatric illness. However, there are many technical challenges and limitations of higher field strength. Technical challenges include increased susceptibility artifacts and specific absorption rate (SAR), and inhomogeneous field (main and radiofrequency). Other limitations include very high cost, and imaging artifacts.

RAPID IMAGE ACQUISITION TECHNIQUES

Ever since the role of MRI has been established in clinical settings, researches are going on to reduce the MR acquisition time and at the same time maintaining high-image spatial resolution, contrast, and quality. The MR imaging techniques that can be employed for rapid image acquisition are discussed below in brief.

Echo-planar Imaging (EPI)

Echo-planar (or Echo volume) imaging is based on acquisition of all of the k-space following a single excitation pulse, and is the most direct approach for rapid image acquisition as well as reduce motion artifacts. EPI may be performed with a series of spin echoes (in which a series of 180-degree refocusing pulses are applied) or with a series of gradient echoes (created by alternating the polarity or direction of the readout gradient). Conventionally, EPI is associated with gradient echo acquisitions, while the spin echo variant is termed fast spin echo (FSE), turbo spin echo (TSE), or rapid acquisition with relaxation enhancement (RARE). Although sampling a different echo for each line in k-space is done in both gradient echo and spin echo approaches, the weighing of the acquired signal is differently. In gradient echo EPI, the different k-space lines have different T2* weightings as the signal is decaying as a function of T2*, while in spin echo EPI, each k-space line has a different T2 weighting as the signal is decaying by the longer T2 time constant. This difference is important with respect to image quality as chemical shift and local magnetic susceptibility artifacts (also known as off resonance effects) can modulate the gradient echo signals. However, these effects can be reduced with spin echo EPI. Other artifact concerns with EPI include ghosting, due to a mismatch in location of the echo center between k-space lines acquired with a positive readout gradient, and those acquired with a negative readout gradient; geometric off-resonance distortions; and fat signal ghosting.

EPI is an excellent tool for many neuroimaging sequences despite its limitations. It has got tremendous utility for functional imaging and diffusion tensor imaging, where the physiologic process under evaluation takes place rapidly (e.g. neuronal activity or blood perfusion) or the method is sensitive to subject motion. On present day MRI scanners, the individual gradient echoes that make up the EPI readout train is separated by temporal gap of less than 2 milliseconds. Thus, 64 to 128 echoes can be acquired following a single excitation pulse in time periods of 100 to 300 milliseconds. Although it is long relative to T2*, this is still short enough making sure there is still a measurable signal at the end of the echo train. Continuing advancements in gradient technology, specifically the rate at which gradients can be turned on and reach their maximum value (slew rate), have been critical to the success of EPI in many neuroimaging applications where precise morphologic information is not strictly necessary.

A simple way to decrease the effects of off-resonance distortions in EPI is to reduce the number of lines acquired following each RF excitation pulse. Multishot EPI divides the number of k-space lines into pieces (e.g. in a four-shot sequence, 128 k-space lines are broken down to 4 sets of 32). The reduced number of gradient echoes significantly reduces the sampling period and, therefore, the T2* weighting across the echo train. This reduces the spatial displacements caused by off-resonance effects by a factor equal to the number of shots used to acquire the k-c plane. Of course, multishot EPI sequences reduce the advantages of EPI, specifically the ability to "freeze" motion.

Fast Spin Echo Imaging

Hennig et al.[9] in the mid-1980s first introduced the spin echo EPI with the publication of the RARE method.[9] It uses RF-generated spin echoes as opposed to gradient echoes and is based on the RF pulse train known as the Carr-Purcell-Meiboom-Gill (CPMG) sequence,[10-12] in which a string of 180-degree pulses separated by intervals of 2τ follow an initial 90-degree excitation pulse. The basic RARE sequence had been modified in the early 1990s to allow for flexible T2 contrast manipulation.[13-17] After these initial modifications, gradually conventional spin echo sequences became replaced with newer versions of the RARE sequence, also referred to as FSE or TSE sequences. Currently, all MR vendors provide both single-shot and multiple shot versions of FSE sequences, under multiple trade names. Generally speaking, the multiple-shot versions of the FSE sequence has completely replaced conventional spin echo sequences which were used as the gold standard for brain lesion detection during the first decade of MR as the FSE sequences can produce comparable T2-weighted tissue contrast and image quality, provided by conventional spin echo imaging in much shorter scan time.[15,18-22] However, FSE has got lesser sensitivity to hemorrhage compared to conventional spin echo sequences[21] while the signal from fat (bright fat phenomenon) is higher in FSE imaging[23,24] as well as MT effects are also higher in FSE compared to conventional spin echo imaging.[25] Despite these limitations, FSE has almost completely replaced conventional spine echo imaging by virtue of reduced scan time.

Gradient and Spin Echo Imaging (GRASE)

The gradient and spin echo imaging can be combined to produce a novel imaging technique that allows rapid image acquisition as well as a unique image contrast. High spatial resolution 3D imaging in a much shorter time is possible with this technique[26] and has been incorporated into perfusion and diffusion imaging sequences.

Steady State Imaging Methods

Simply shortening TR, thereby allowing more data to be acquired in same acquisition time, can lead to acquisition of higher spatial resolution images or higher volumetric coverage. It can also be used to acquire same amount of data in reduced scan time. The technique involves repeated application of identical and, typically low-angle RF pulses with a time separation much less than T1 and T2; thereby not allowing the magnetization to fully relax back to equilibrium prior to each subsequent RF excitation pulse. The process of repeated excitation results in a steady state of magnetization so that the transverse and/or longitudinal magnetization before each RF pulse is constant. Although very rapid imaging is possible with this technique, the signal measured in steady state imaging is significantly less, as the magnetization is not allowed to fully recover and the RF pulses are often less than 30 degrees. Hence it is obvious that while the steady state sequences have very high signal efficiency (signal per unit time), the overall absolute SNR is less compared to conventional methods.

Steady state methods can either be spoiled or nonspoiled. If the transverse magnetization is spoiled before each RF pulse, only the longitudinal magnetization is in equilibrium. Hence, the images acquired in this spoiled situation (termed spoiled gradient, SPGR, or spoiled fast low angle shot, FLASH), show a strong T1 contrast. On the other hand, if the sequence is left unspoiled allowing the transverse magnetization to evolve or to be balanced so that the transverse magnetization is completely refocused prior to each RF pulse and both the longitudinal and transverse magnetizations will be brought into dynamic equilibrium. Images acquired under this condition [termed gradient recalled acquisition in the steady-state (GRASS); fast imaging with steady-state precession (FISP); fast field echo (FFE); reversed FISP (PSIF), or true FISP] have contrast that is a function of T1, T2, and/or T2*. The clinical applications of the gradient echo imaging are predominantly in the characterization of tissue susceptibility characteristics and can be used for demonstration of intracranial calcification and hemorrhages.

Partial Fourier Acquisitions

Echo-planar imaging, FSE and steady state imaging methods although offer rapid image acquisitions, these are frequently associated with a multitude of artifacts and image distortion which makes them incapable of high resolution, high-quality, and motion-free imaging. Hence, alternate approaches based on properties of Fourier transform have been proposed. Zero-padding and partial or half-Fourier acquisition are the main techniques for partial Fourier acquisitions. Zero-padding is the most basic approach and it involves "padding" the original lower-resolution k-space with zeros so as to increase the apparent extent of "acquired" k-space. Zero-padding is commonly associated with Gibbs ringing artifact, which occur due to the sharp boundary in k-space introduced along the border of the acquired k-space data, and the zero-filled portion. Half-Fourier acquisition is based on the fact that conjugate symmetry exists between pairs of points that lie equidistant from the origin of k-space, and on a diagonal line passing through the origin. Hence, only one-half of k-space need be acquired, with the other half synthesized from the acquired data—commonly known as partial or half-Fourier acquisition.[27]

Parallel Imaging

The term parallel imaging encompasses a group of methods which are generally designed to decrease scan time by sub/undersampling k-space data. In order to save scanning time in parallel imaging, some phase encoding lines are not collected. As a result, the field-of-view (FoV) of the image is reduced, which is likely to result into aliasing, or fold-over, artifacts. The term acceleration/reduction factor refers to the amount/factor by which the data is undersampled. For example, the acceleration factor, R = 2 if only half of the normally required data is collected. Parallel imaging reconstruction can be applied in order to remove the aliasing artifacts resulting from the smaller FoV. Parallel imaging can work in either the image domain or in k-space, but the common theme of all of these methods is that they employ the varying spatial sensitivities of a receiver coil array to reconstruct the aliased image.

The salient features of parallel imaging-based sequences are:

- The undersampled data is reconstructed by these the techniques and these are not new imaging sequences.
- Data needs to be acquired simultaneously and independently with multiple receiver channels having different sensitivity profiles.
- Contrast behavior of the underlying imaging sequence generally does not change by the parallel imaging.
- These techniques work either by decreasing the amount of time needed to perform an imaging sequence or increasing the resolution in a given specific measurement time, or combination of the two can be used.
- Main limitation is the reduction in the SNR in the reconstructed image by a factor greater than or equal to the square root of the reduction factor, as R-times fewer data points are acquired.

Currently, parallel MRI methods can be broadly classed based on whether the reconstruction and alias removal is performed in the image domain (e.g. sensitivity encoding, SENSE) or in the k-space domain [e.g. simultaneous acquisition of spatial harmonics (SMASH), generalized autocalibrating partially parallel acquisition (GRAPPA)]. No consensus exists as to which technique is universally superior. The choice may be both vendor- and case-specific. The major

FLOWCHART 1: Various parallel imaging methods.

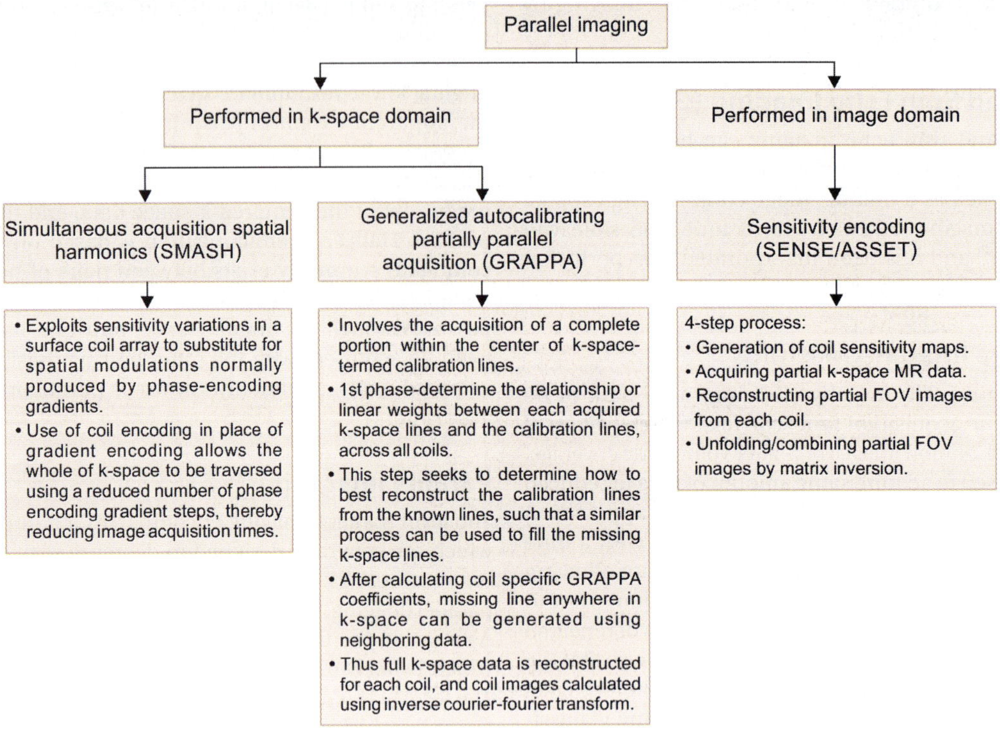

applications of parallel imaging are in MR angiography and dynamic postcontrast imaging.

These parallel MRI methods are summarized in **Flowchart 1**.

Compressed SENSE (CSENSE)

Another technique of reducing the acquisition time came into fray within the last decade known as compressed sensing. The basis of compressed sensing MRI (CS MRI) is image reconstruction from a k-space which is incompletely filled or under sampled.[28-30]

Originally, it was proposed as a general concept to accurately reconstruct a small number of random measurements.[29,30] The concept of CS-MRI was inspired from a similar imaging problem related to transmission and storage of huge volume of imaging dataset generated by modern-day scanners. The solution to this problem was permanently discarding certain data elements and thereby reducing file size—a process known as lossy image compression. Successful compression of medical images can be achieved even at compression ratios from 9:1 to 25:1 using a variety of algorithms, while preserving diagnostic efficacy at the same time. This led Lustig et al.[28] to raise the question that if the images are indeed compressible whether it is necessary to acquire the full dataset at all. Further they proposed that reconstruction of the same image generated from a fully sampled set could be possible from the simple measurement of the compressed information directly from the small number of measurements and it can be achieved by k-space undersampling as MRI measures Fourier coefficients only.

The successful utilization of compressed sensing is team play of data acquisition and image reconstruction. Lustig et al.[28] identified three criteria as being essential to ensure successful image recovery from subsampled data:

- Firstly, once the conversion with a mathematical transformation has been done, the object that is acquired should have a sparse representation.
- Secondly, subsampling of k-space should be done in such a way that incoherent, i.e. noise like artifacts are produced in the image as a result of aliasing.
- Finally, a nonlinear, iterative optimization, that simultaneously enforces a sparse representation of the resulting image, is used for reconstruction of the images, leading to removal of the noise like artifacts, while preserving its consistency to the acquired data.

The role of compressed SENSE in neuroimaging is still an area of research. Major application is in pediatric neuroimaging as it can significantly (~40–50%) reduce the acquisition time thereby reducing the sedation and anesthesia time and at the same time producing images of significant diagnostic quality **(Figs. 1A to H)**. Other potential application is acquisition of high resolution MR angiography images and in vessel wall imaging where images with lesser slice thickness can be acquired at similar time of acquisition using compressed SENSE algorithm.

Multiband or Multiplexed Imaging

Multiband is the latest addition to the suite of rapid MR acquisition methodologies. It aims to excite and acquire data from multiple imaging slices simultaneously.[31,32] Multiband RF pulses, which comprise two or more single-band pulses

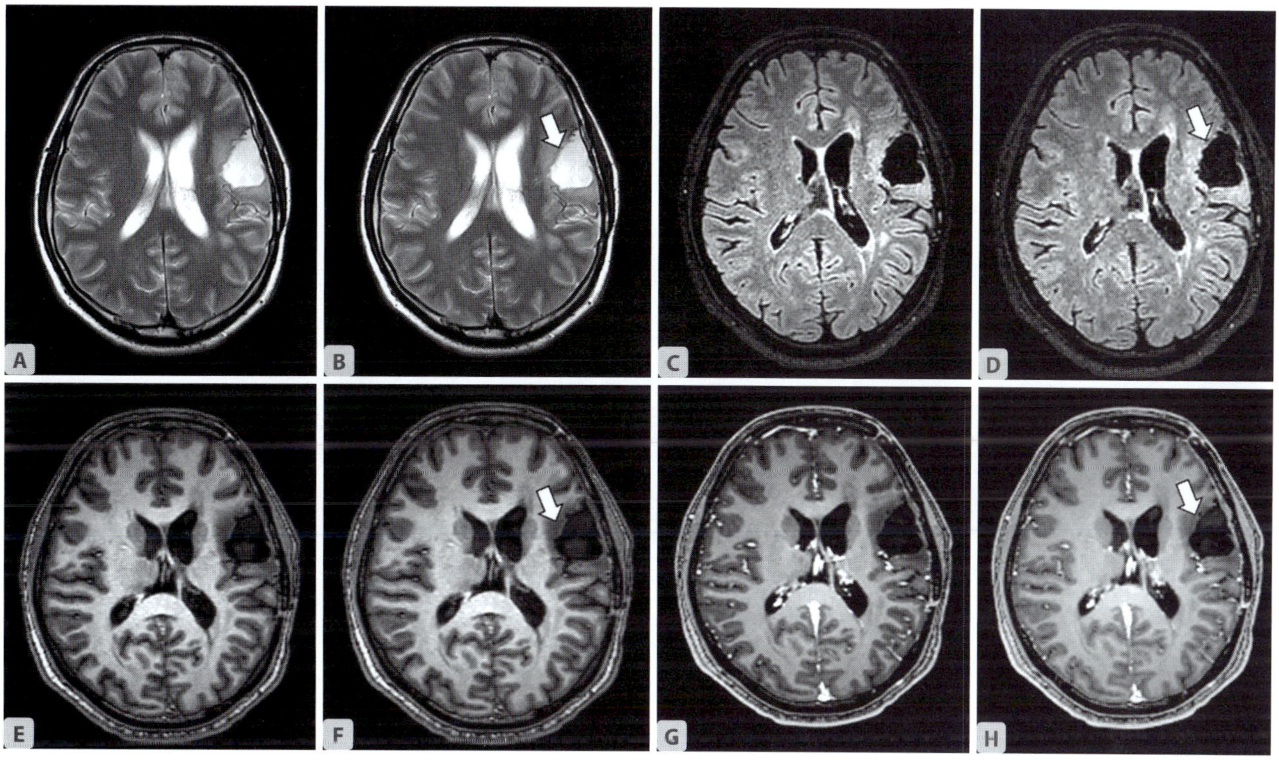

FIGS. 1A TO H: Contrast-enhanced MRI of a 13-year-old male child status postoperative for low grade glial tumor. (A and B) T2 axial sequences of brain acquired with conventional MRI and CSENSE MRI technique with acceleration factor of 2.4 respectively. (C and D) Axial reformatted image of 3D FLAIR sequences acquired with conventional MRI and CSENSE MRI technique with acceleration factor of 8. (E and F) Axial reformatted image of T1-GRE precontrast sequences acquired with conventional MRI and CSENSE MRI technique acquired with acceleration factor of 3.4. (G and H) Axial reformatted image of T1-GRE postcontrast sequences acquired with conventional MRI and CSENSE MRI technique acquired with acceleration factor of 4. Mild blurring of margin of postoperative cavity noted in T2, FLAIR, T1 pre- and postcontrast sequences acquired with C-SENSE (B, D, F and H) shown by arrow.

that each excites specific slices in a conventional 2D multislice acquisition, are used in this technique. To separate the received signal from each slice, parallel imaging methods such as SENSE can be used, provided there are sufficient coil sensitivity variations along the slice direction. Thus, the technique as originally proposed was limited to relatively largely spaced slices. To eliminate this issue, a phase shift can be introduced between excited slices, which can then be readily reconstructed using a phase constrained parallel MRI reconstruction method even in the absence of coil sensitivity differences. Though only developed in 2010, this technique has gained rapid acceptance in neuroimaging research applications particularly in functional MRI and arterial spin labeling (ASL) perfusion. Further, the ability to combine multi-band imaging with in plane SENSE acceleration offers the potential for significant reductions in overall acquisition time in multislice imaging techniques.

ADVANCED MR IMAGING TECHNIQUES

SUSCEPTIBILITY WEIGHTED IMAGING (SWI)

Susceptibility weighted imaging exploits the magnetic inhomogeneity where tissues of higher susceptibility distort the magnetic field and become out of phase from their neighbors at long echo times.[33] Thus, there is signal loss on magnitude images. It is fully velocity compensated high resolution 3D gradient echo sequence that uses magnitude and filtered phase information, separately and in combination to create a new source of contrast. Unlike initial experience with spoiled GRE, with advent of 3T and parallel imaging, it is now possible to image the entire brain with SWI in a short time. Delineation of small vessels particularly veins is exquisite on SWI, due to high T2* of deoxygenated blood. The technique provides additional clinical information in evaluation of traumatic brain injuries, coagulopathic and other hemorrhagic disorders, vascular malformations, cerebral infarctions, neoplasms, and neurodegenerative disorders associated with calcifications or iron depositions.[34]

Interpretation of SWI is dependent on the MR system. The appearance of hemorrhage and calcification in right and left-handed system are opposite to each other and the phase image should be evaluated very carefully for it. **Figure 2** summaries the appearance of hemorrhage and calcification in right and left handed systems.

Quantitative Susceptibility Mapping (QSM)

Quantitative susceptibility mapping is a relatively newer MRI technique that aim to extract the spatial susceptibility distribution of objects or tissues from the measured MRI phase

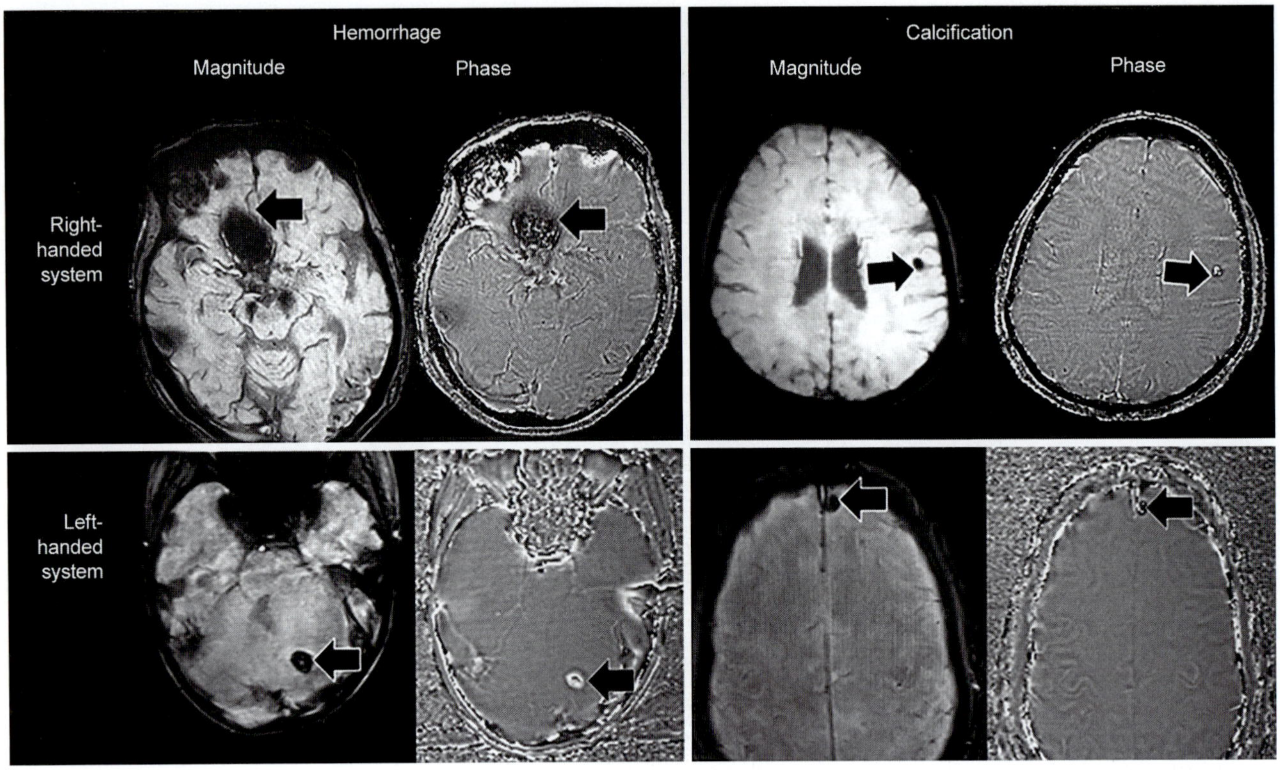

FIG. 2: Appearance of hemorrhage and calcifications (arrows) on magnitude and phase images on SWI in right and left-handed systems.

or local field data by solving a known inverse problem.[35] With the advent of ultra-high field MRI resulting into increased sensitivity to magnetic susceptibility differences, it is now possible to achieve excellent anatomical contrast on T2*-weighted magnitude and phase images. Path-breaking work has been done in last decade for noninvasive quantification magnetic susceptibility in vivo.[35]

Following are the major sources of phase contrast in biological tissue—the heme and non-heme iron content, myelin, calcium and lipid.[36] The phase contrast for deep gray matter structures is dependent chiefly on the amount of iron.[36] The amount of iron deposition is related to aging as well as many neurodegenerative disorders.[36] MR signal magnitude and phase are determined by the level of deoxyhemoglobin, in case of veins in the brain. As deoxyhemoglobin level is directly related to oxygen saturation, it can be used as a surrogate marker of change in blood flow.[36] The cellular composition as well as arrangement may affect the magnetic properties of tissues in cases of white matter structures.[36] Bulk magnetic susceptibility is produced by the integration of the microscopic effects. On the contrary, depending on the geometry and orientation of the object, non-local phase effects are produced by bulk susceptibility. Therefore, although the phase information at any location is directly related to the local magnetic field of the source, it can be spatially distant to the source of susceptibility changes. Such non-local effects can make it difficult to quantify susceptibility changes using phase images.[36] The clinical applications of QSM include anatomical imaging of the human brain, traumatic brain injury, brain tumor, neurodegenerative disease, neurosurgical planning.[35,36]

Susceptibility Tensor Imaging (STI)

The dependence of gradient echo signal phase on the orientation of biological tissues with respect to the main magnetic field can be used to quantitatively determine orientation-independent magnetic susceptibility parameters by a newly developed MR technique known as susceptibility tensor imaging, which bears a conceptual similarity to diffusion tensor imaging (DTI).[37] The principal eigenvectors of the susceptibility tensor can be used for mapping of brain white matter fiber orientations and reconstruction of 3D white matter pathways. Myelin is the main determinant factor of the susceptibility anisotropy, contrary to diffusion anisotropy. Sensitivity of the susceptibility anisotropy of white matter to gadolinium-based contrast agents is another unique feature of STI.

STI has been shown to reproduce anatomical structures comparable to those with DTI while mapping major white matter fiber bundles in mouse brain.[37] In addition, STI, because of its unique sensitivity to oriented lipid molecules, can be a potentially new tool to assess the white matter integrity. In the setting of diseases like fetal alcohol spectrum disorder or multiple sclerosis, myelin formation during development and myelin breakdown in different neural diseases can potentially be studied using STI.[37]

DIFFUSION IMAGING

Diffusion Weighted Imaging (DWI)

Diffusion contrast depends on molecular motion of water. As initially described by Stejskal and Tanner in 1965, spin echo

T2 EPI sequences can be sensitized to random diffusion of water molecules using bipolar gradients of equal magnitude and opposite polarity. The directional nature of net water movement of water in the white matter tracts (anisotropy) is depicted as signal loss on images by application of gradients in three orthogonal directions. This signal loss or diffusion weighting is determined by sequence specific parameter named "b value" (depending on strength, duration and interval of DW gradient) and tissue specific diffusivity factor called "ADC coefficient". Usually a "b value" 1000 sec/mm^2 allows good diffusion weighting in brain but it is used in tandem with a non-zero (20 sec/mm^2) value for calculations. Anisotropic images can be combined to yield isotropic mean diffusivity TRACE images (DWI) which are used for evaluating stroke and other routine purposes. Alternately ADC maps can be calculated to yield true magnitude images. These remove the inherent T2 contrast in these images which cause interpretative problems.[38,39]

The primary use of DWI has been in brain imaging due to its exquisitely unique sensitivity for ischemic stroke. This noninvasive test for cerebral tissue viability came at a vital time when thrombolytic and neuroprotective agents were entering clinical practice. It is a FDI-approved sequence for routine stroke protocol in neuroimaging now. Diffusion changes are detectable within minutes of cerebral ischemia (as early as 20 minutes in humans). This is due to cytotoxic edema (Na^+/K^+/ATPase pump failure) and squeezed extracellular compartment. DWI picks up infarcts with a sensitivity and specificity of 88–100% within 6 hours compared to conventional CT and MRI images which are abnormal only in less than 50% of cases **(Figs. 3A to G)**. Diagnosis of hyperacute infarction within this window period is vital for

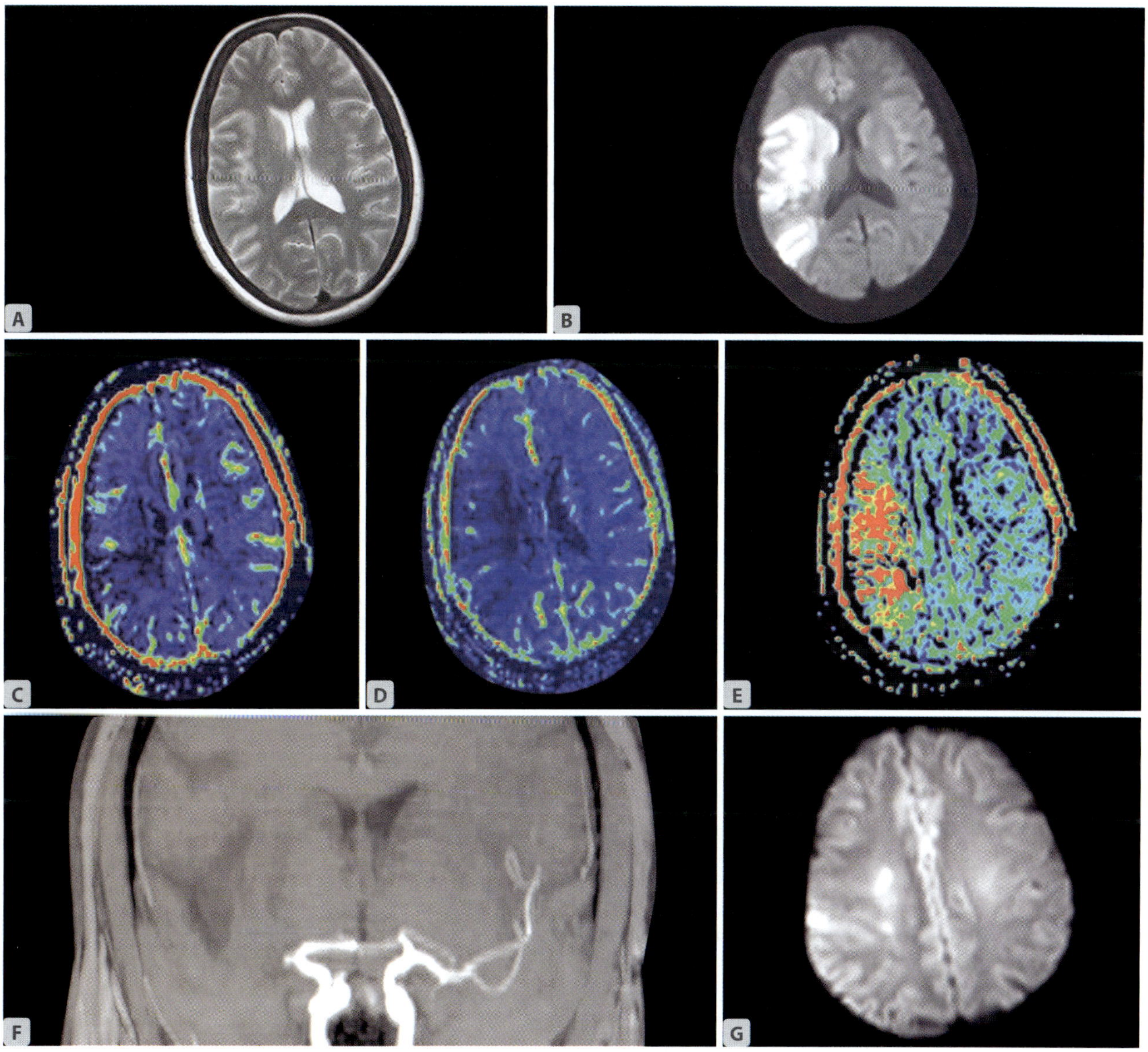

FIGS. 3A TO G: A 42-year-female with acute onset left hemiparesis. (A) T2W image-subtle signal changes along the right insula; (B) DWI–restriction in right MCA territory at the level of basal ganglia. Perfusion maps above the level of basal ganglia show normal color maps of CBV; (C) decreased CBF; (D) and raised MTT; (E) in the right MCA territory; (F) DWI showed no concordant extent of restriction at the corresponding level; (G) suggestive of DWI-PWI mismatch—evolving ischemic penumbra.

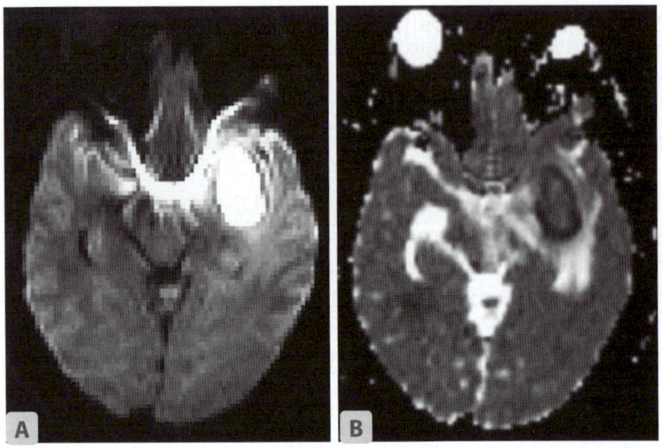

FIGS. 4A AND B: DW (A) and ADC; (B) images show diffusion restriction in the abscess cavity in left temporal lobe (bright on DWI and dark on ADC).

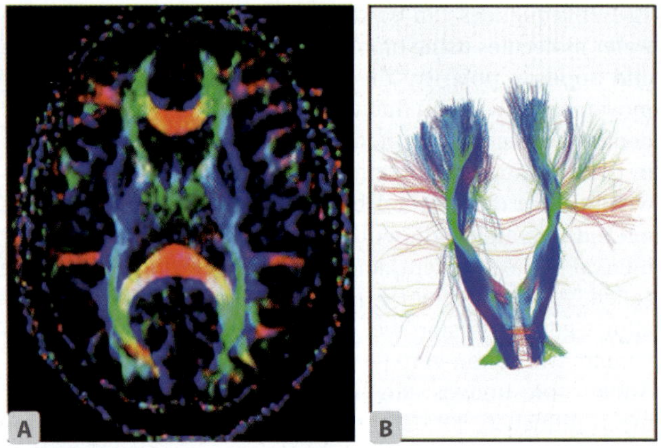

FIGS. 5A AND B: Directionally color coded FA map (A) and fiber tracking; (B) showing corticospinal tracts.

initiation of therapy. Infarcts appear bright on DWI (dark on ADC maps). The reduced ADC persists variably (usually ten days), returns to baseline and then remains elevated subsequently due to ensuing brain softening and gliosis. However, DWI changes may pseudonormalize after natural reperfusion or neuroprotective therapy within 1–2 days. DWI when assessed along with perfusion imaging is a better guide to treatment decisions and clinical outcome. DWI also has a role in the setting of acute on chronic ischemia, neonatal hypoxic injuries and venous thrombosis. More importantly DWI helps excluding stroke in an equivocal clinical setting, i.e. differentiating stroke from multiple sclerosis plaques and from other stroke mimics like vasogenic edema syndromes (hypertensive encephalopathy, eclampsia, meningioma cyclosporine toxicity, etc.) which are not associated with restriction of diffusion.[38]

The other uses of DWI are in diagnosing abscesses **(Figs. 4A and B)**, encephalitides and diffuse axonal injuries. All these conditions show high signal on DWI. It also help in characterizing tumors, i.e. differentiating epidermoids from cysts, by showing restricted diffusion in hypercellular tumors, i.e. lymphoma, malignant meningioma, differentiating necrotic from solid enhancing components, radiation necrosis from recurrent tumor (higher diffusion in necrosis) and postoperative cavity/cystic neoplasms from abscess in operated tumors.[38,39]

Diffusion Tensor Imaging

Dependency of molecular diffusion on the orientation of white matter fiber tracts (anisotropy) can be mapped spatially by acquiring relatively high-resolution DWI.[40] Computer algorithms allow the generation of white matter fiber tract maps from the tensor data. Tensor is a map of directional vectors in 3D space and it is a mathematic construct that describes the properties of an ellipsoid. The data for tensor must be measured along six or more collinear directions by gradients [multidirectional diffusion weighting (MDDW)-6–256 directions]. From this data, diffusion coefficients or eigenvalues along the three principle directions, eigenvectors defining the orientation of fibers and fractional anisotropy (FA) can be calculated **(Fig. 5A)**. Thus, TRACE image (isotropic diffusion), ADC image (pure diffusion contrast from diffusion coefficients), FA maps with and without color codes (directional diffusion) and tensor image (calculated diffusion data with direction and velocity) are the data sets available for analysis from which fiber tracks can be constructed **(Fig. 5B)**.

Quantitative brain maps can be generated coregistering the 3D white matter fiber tracts on the anatomic images using Automated Image Registration Software. 3T due to its high SNR and reduced scan times allows sampling of high number of directions for DTI within an acceptable time. Higher b-values enhance anisotropy effects helping more complex evaluations like fiber tracking and tensor imaging more so for trajectory of crossing fiber. Susceptibility effects can be overcome using PAT, radial imaging or PROPELLER.

Clinical Applications

Diffusion tensor imaging is valuable in assessment of white matter structural integrity and connectivity. Use of DTI has been incorporated by various groups into imaging protocols of stroke, trauma (to study DAI and its long-term effects) and multiple sclerosis (loss of anisotropy in damaged white matter) **(Fig. 6)**. The disruption of fibers can be shown in all the above conditions.[40] It has been used to study brain development and included in a number of psychiatric protocols. The most advanced application is that of fiber tracking along with functional MRI to trace the connectivity of various areas of brain. Studies in schizophrenia have revealed disturbances of anisotropy which reflects possible functional disconnectivity. It can help surgical planning of tumors and when used along with cortical mapping technique, the entire functional unit can be shown. Some studies have also suggested that DTI can differentiate white matter tracts infiltrated with tumors (e.g. in high grade glioma) from those merely displaced (low grade tumor) **(Figs. 7A and B)**.[40,41]

Diffusion Spectrum Imaging

Diffusion spectrum imaging (DSI), first described by Wedeen et al.[42] can be considered as reference standard

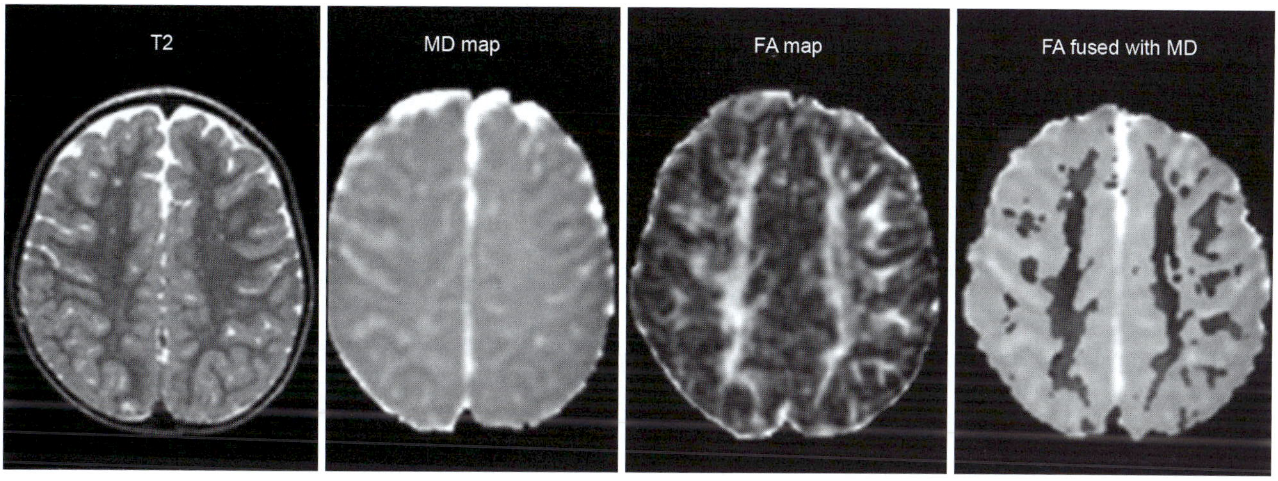

FIG. 6: Patient of multiple sclerosis with white matter subtle lesions on T2. FA data shows severe disruption of white matter anisotropy due to destruction of myelin.

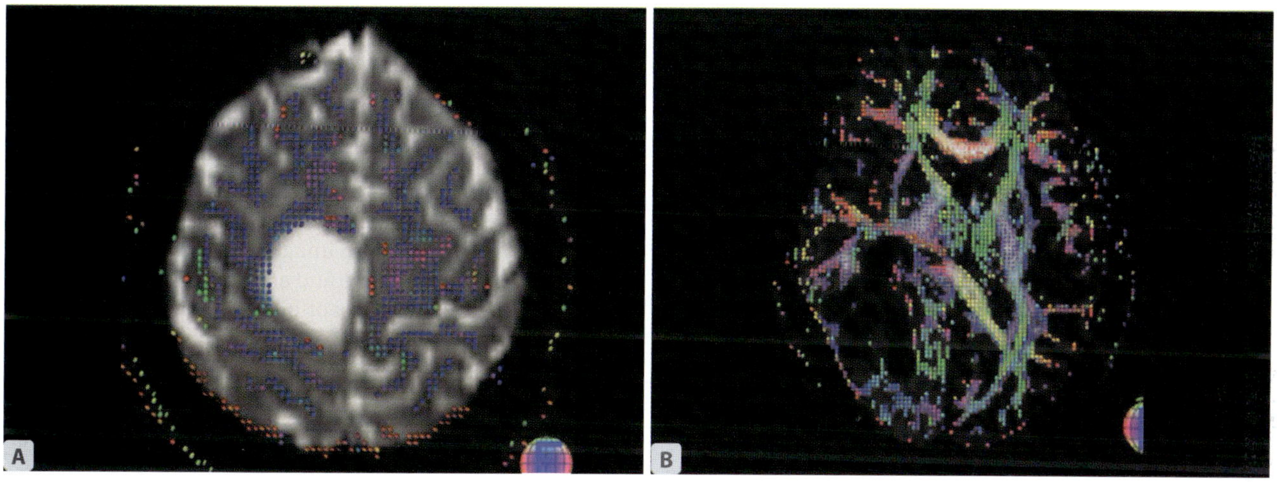

FIGS. 7A AND B: (A) The tensor and anatomy fusion image showing displacement of intact white matter in perirolandic area by the lesion in right high frontal cortex—DNET; (B) Tensor + anatomy fusion image—white matter infiltration by glioblastoma multiforme leading to loss of anisotropy.

of diffusion imaging and is quiet suitable for in vivo application as it is capable of providing sufficiently dense q-space signal sample from which it is possible to derive a displacement distribution with the use of the Fourier transform.[39] A 6-dimensional image of both position and displacement can be obtained with the application of the Fourier transform over q-space in every brain position. Displacement distribution or the probability density function, which describe diffusion at each position, can provide a detailed description of diffusion and excellent resolution of the highly complex fiber organization, including fiber crossings. Diffusion spectrum imaging is generally used for fiber tractography, where only directional information is needed. Hence, by summing the probabilities of diffusion in each direction, probability density function (PDF) is normally reduced to an orientation distribution function.[39]

In DSI, strong diffusion weighting (b-value ~3000–8000 s/mm^2) with large number of diffusion encoding directions. It helps in delineating crossing fibers, which are not resolved by DTI model. The main limitation is long acquisition time.

q-Ball Imaging

q-ball imaging is most common algorithm used for extracting information from high angular resolution diffusion imaging (HARDI). HARDI is based on modeling a 3-dimensional orientation distribution function.[43] The general principle for all these techniques is dense sampling of the signal within a sphere with a constant high b value (>4000 s/mm^2) in q-space.[39] Various algorithms are used to calculate the orientation distribution function is from the resultant data. It helps in depiction of the crossing fibers, and is more clinically applicable. The images acquired with q-ball imaging closely resembles those acquired with DSI.[39] Further validation studies have to be done to determine the image quality for all brain regions and accuracy of fiber tracking with q-ball imaging. Besides q-ball imaging other heuristic methods based on persistent angular structure[44] and spherical deconvolution[45] can also achieve the same purpose.

Diffusion Kurtosis Imaging (DKI)

Diffusion kurtosis imaging is a new imaging technique as extension of the DTI technique which allows the estimation of diffusion as well as kurtosis parameters.[46,47] The DTI model is based on that diffusion occurs in a random unrestricted way and follows a Gaussian diffusion probability distribution function. However, water diffusion in human deviates from that strict Gaussian behavior due to the complexity of tissue and occurs in a restricted way. By incorporating and quantifying non-Gaussianity of water diffusion in tissues in its model, the diffusional kurtosis is a more accurate representation of restricted diffusion than DTI and may give additional biomarkers in various disease states (tissue structure and pathophysiology). DKI uses higher b-values than conventional DWI and gives dimensionless metric of the departure from a Gaussian form called kurtosis. The resulting kurtosis maps are reproducible. The three-dimensional kurtosis angular plots describe tissue-specific geometry for various brain regions and may show the potential of showing multiple fiber structures in a single voxel. Recent studies have shown that diffusion kurtosis imaging can provide information that is complementary of DTI.[46] It has been studied for various pathologies such as brain tumors, degenerative diseases, demyelinating diseases, and cerebrovascular diseases.

Main advantage of DKI is that it allows assessment of the cerebral cortex and basal ganglia which are isotropic structures and is main limitation of DTI. DKI can also improve estimation of the orientation distribution function (ODF) for optimizing white matter fiber tracking and the resolution of crossing fibers.[46]

Readout Segmented EPI-based Diffusion (RESOLVE Diffusion)

While DWI based on single shot echo-planar imaging (ss-EPI) requires less acquisition time, the diffusion weighted image quality in the head and neck regions like orbit, skull bases, temporal bone as well as in spine is often compromised due to the presence of magnetic susceptibility artifacts that can arise due to the presence of air, bone or fat in the vicinity of these structures. In addition two other problems have been encountered with DWI based on ss-EPI namely T2 blurring and long TE.[48] T2 blurring occurs as a result of long data sampling interval during the readout, which leads to broadening of point spread function and blurring of reconstructed image.[48] On the other hand long TE, which results from a combination of the diffusion-encoding gradients and the long data sampling interval, causes low signal to noise ratio (SNR).[48]

In order to address these problems, Porter and Heidemann[48] described a new method of acquiring diffusion-weighted images. This technique involves coupling of readout segmented EPI (rs-EPI), GRAPPA and 2D navigator reacquisition to obtain high resolution diffusion-weighted images. This technique has been popularized by the term RESOLVE (readout segmentation of long variable echo trains) sequence for DWI. This technique offers the advantages of high-quality, high-resolution DWI and DTI with reduced susceptibility and blurring artifacts making it applicable to challenging body regions including brain, skull-base, orbit, spine, breast, pelvis and prostate.[48] Besides that the technique is insensitive to motion-induced phase errors and there is reduced specific absorption rate (SAR) in comparison to turbo spin echo (TSE) based methods.[48]

Contiguous-slice Zonally Oblique Multislice (CO-ZOOM) Diffusion

CO-ZOOM diffusion is another relatively newer technique for high resolution DWI and DTI. Dowell et al.[49] described its application in acquisition of optic nerve and spinal cord DTI. In this sequence, a modified ss-EPI sequence containing a refocusing RF pulse is used in presence of the phase-encoding (rather than slice-select) gradient to acquire the images. Hence it is possible to achieve excitation and refocusing of only a narrow volume; thereby eliminating the problem of signal aliasing associated with narrow FOVs. Two methods for the sequence have been described—for spinal cord cardiac gating is included to reduce the pulsation artifact, whereas inversion recovery (IR) cerebrospinal (CSF) suppression is used in the study the optic nerve in order to eliminate partial volume effects.[49] This technique is considered to be highly useful for diffusion imaging of small structures like spinal cord and optic nerve and achieves high resolution and less distortion due to susceptibility artifacts. Further nerve tracking analyses are also possible with this technique as continuous slices are acquired.

PERFUSION WEIGHTED IMAGING

Perfusion indicates the delivery of blood at the level of the capillaries. It is measured in units of mL/100 gm/minute. Delivery of oxygen and other nutrients to the tissue is closely related to perfusion. Hence measurement of perfusion, an essential physiologic parameter is crucial. The MR perfusion techniques are broadly classified into two groups—those using an exogenous contrast and those not using it.[50] The former includes two methods namely dynamic susceptibility contrast (DSC)—MRI and dynamic contrast enhanced (DCE)—MRI while the latter includes arterial spin labeling perfusion.

DSC perfusion: It measures signal reduction induced in the brain during passage of injected paramagnetic contrast agents which induce magnetic susceptibility effects (T2*).[51] Intravascular compartmentalized contrast produces large magnetic field gradients across the vascular boundaries leading to reduction in T2* and loss of signal which relates to proportion of vascularity. Best results are achieved with gradient based EPI with 2-second sampling rate over a minute. This can be plotted as a time intensity curve or concentration time curve. Integration of area under this curve yields regional cerebral blood volume (rCBV). Similarly mean transit time (MTT), total blood flow (rCBF), time to arrival (TTA) or time to peak (TPP) can also be calculated. High field MR provides better results due to higher SNR, longer T2*, faster scans, parallel imaging and requirement of lower optimal contrast volumes.

DCE perfusion: It depends on the injection of a gadolinium-based contrast agent. Dynamic acquisition of T1-weighted MR images are done before, during, and after bolus injection of a contrast agent. By applying the physical principles of tracer-kinetic modeling, the generated data can be interpreted in terms of physiological tissue characteristics.[50]

ASL perfusion: Brain perfusion can also be measured by spin labeling of arterial water by EPI signal tagging with alternating frequency (EPISTAR, ASL) or other techniques.[52] Two methods of ASL perfusion are described- pulsed ASL (PASL) and pseudocontinuous ASL (PCASL).[53] Pseudocontinuous ASL is method of choice for clinical application as it has high SNR. In this technique, train of short pulses in form of long labeling period (1–2 seconds) is designed to invert the inflowing blood magnetization in an adiabatic or pseudo steady-state manner. Hence it can be considered that blood is being continuously inverted as it flows through a "labeling plane" in the inferior-superior direction. In pulsed ASL, arterial blood is tagged by a short adiabatic inversion pulse (approximately in the order of 10 msec) to invert the blood water instantaneously in a particular region, typically located inferior to the brain. The main limitation of pulsed ASL is that it has low SNR.

Clinical Applications of MRP

PWI in Stroke: Ischemic brain after acute vascular occlusion shows reduced rCBV and elevated MTT and TTP as lack of signal drop after contrast arrival. The ischemic penumbra, i.e. "functionally impaired but not irreversibly damaged" area around an established infarction is identified when areas of PWI and DWI defect are compared. A mismatch; perfusion defect being larger than diffusion abnormality as seen in large arterial occlusion, denotes viable tissue at risk. The neurological deficit will likely to increase in such a situation and needs aggressive treatment. When there is a match between the two (PWI = DWI or PWI < DWI) infarct is presumed stable or already reperfused **(*See* Figs. 3A to G)**. Thus, an MRI stroke protocol should include T2 FSE and FLAIR sections of brain followed by MRA, DWI, PWI and a GRE sequence for hemorrhage. This comprehensive protocol should take less than 15 minutes on a modern state of the art MR scans.[51]

PWI of cerebral tumors: Tumor angiogenesis and vascularity determines biological aggressiveness of the cerebral neoplasms. These can be predicted by MR perfusion imaging. The technique is particularly useful for differentiating tumor necrosis from recurrent tumors (the former being avascular) and assesses response to treatment by antiangiogenetic chemotherapeutic agents (in terms of reduced rCBV post treatment). The rCBV correlates well with histological neovascularity and grades of gliomas. It progresses from lower values in low grade gliomas to high values in glioblastoma multiforme. PWI also acts as a guide in heterogeneous tumors for biopsy from more aggressive areas for appropriate staging. These areas may not necessarily show maximum enhancement on contrast enhanced MR or CT sections. Lymphomas show low vascularity and solitary metastases reduced perilesional contrast activity as compared to gliomas. Another possible role can be in atypical infections and demyelinating lesions mimicking neoplasms. Thus, PWI helps in diagnosing, characterizing and follow-up of brain neoplasms.[51]

ASL perfusion: Clinical applications include early diagnosis of dementia and other neurodegenerative diseases, epileptogenic foci may be identified using ASL in seizure disorder patients and subtle functional changes in psychiatric disorders such as posttraumatic stress disorder or mild traumatic brain injury.[53]

MAGNETIC RESONANCE NEUROGRAPHY (MRN)

With the improvement of MR hardware and newer imaging technique, MR imaging of peripheral nerves is now quite feasible and has become an important adjunct to clinical examination and electrodiagnostic testing in the diagnosis of peripheral neuropathy. With MRN it is now possible to demonstrate the anatomy and pathology of the peripheral nerves in great details.

Role of MRN in Diagnosis of Peripheral Neuropathy[54]

1. Confirmation of clinical suspicion of peripheral neuropathy:
   a. Either by directly demonstrating the nerve abnormality or
   b. By showing the regional muscle denervation changes
2. Assessment of extent of the abnormality in nerve injuries.
3. Evaluation of the disease load in diffuse peripheral nerve lesions, such as hereditary neuropathies and neurofibromatosis.
4. Depiction of the lesions causing nerve entrapment or impingement.
5. Exclusion of the diagnosis of neuropathy by showing normal nerves and regional muscles.
6. To find out incidental lesions in the region of interest mimicking neuropathy symptoms.
7. Providing the image guidance for perineural medication injections.

Interpretation of MRN[54]

The mainstays of MRN are axial T1-weighted and fluid-sensitive fat suppressed T2-weighted images. The following parameters are generally evaluated in MRN-course, caliber and signal intensity (SI) of the nerve, fascicular pattern, size, and perineural fibrosis or mass lesions. The SI of normal nerves is intermediate (similar to muscle) on T1-weighted and intermediate to minimally increased SI on T2-weighted images. In cases of neuropathy, the nerve SI increases tremendously and the nerve may show fluid like SI of the adjacent vessels, on T2-weighted imaging. Various contributory factors are recognized for this signal change, e.g., vascular congestion; blockade of axoplasmic flow, leading to abnormal proximal accumulation of endoneurial fluid; and distal Wallerian degeneration changes. In addition to the nerve injuries, demonstration of denervation related changes in muscle bulk and SI acts as an indirect feature of peripheral neuropathy.

Classification of Nerve Injuries

Seddon et al.[55] classified the nerve injuries in three types:

1. *Neurapraxia—mildest type of injury*: Involve only the myelin sheath around the axon. MRN may show mild T2 hyperintensity with increased bulk of the nerve.
2. *Axonotmesis*: Complete rupture of axon leading to distal Wallerian degeneration with intact epineurium and perineurium. In addition to findings of neurapraxia, MRN may show effacement, enlargement, or disruption of individual fascicles.
3. *Neurotmesis*: It refers to complete disruption of the nerve with complete loss of function. MRN can demonstrate the discontinuity of the nerve directly or fluid in the gap or granulation tissue between the torn nerve endings.

Sunderland[56] further classified nerve injuries into 5 types. While the first and second degree injuries correspond to neurapraxia and axonotmesis, the third-, fourth- and fifth-degree injuries reflect injuries to endoneurium, perineurium and epineurium, respectively. Neuroma, which appears as focal nerve enlargement with a partially or completely effaced fascicular pattern, is commonly found in fourth-degree nerve injuries.

MRN Protocol

The recommended protocol for MRN includes following sequences and can be completed within approximately 45 minutes.

- Axial 2D T1-weighted (3 mm isotropic reconstructions)
- Axial T2 SPAIR (3 mm)
- Coronal 3D STIR SPACE
- T2 SPACE (1 mm)
- 3D DW PSIF [reversed FISP (fast imaging with steady-state free precession)] imaging
- Postcontrast sequences to be used in case of suspected tumor, diffuse peripheral nerve lesions, inflammation, infections.

Future Directions

- DTI has been found to have promising results in demonstration of peripheral nerve imaging in animal models and healthy volunteers. It is possible to calculate ADC, FA and mean diffusivity from DTI besides tractography which is likely to provide more insight into the disease process.
- Whole body MRN though technically challenging to perform can be useful in diseases like neurofibromatosis.
- Gadofluoride M, a newer MR contrast, accumulates in nerves undergoing Wallerian degeneration and disappears with remyelination. By virtue of this property, it has been shown to be useful in demonstrating demyelination and remyelination in animal models.[54]

MAGNETIC RESONANCE ANGIOGRAPHY

Magnetic resonance angiography (MRA) uses inflow effects of blood in 2D and 3D TOF angiography or phase contrast technique in PC MRA. TOF MRA provides satisfactory images of extra and intracranial vasculature and is recommended for screening of aneurysms in asymptomatic patients. TOF MRA suffers from limitations like saturation effects and turbulence-related signal loss. An ultrafast 3D gradient echo version is used for CE MRA which overcomes many of these drawbacks.[57] The short TR nulls fat signal. Being fast, the sequence freezes motion and provides temporal (arterial and venous phases) and spatial resolution. This leads to better visualization of vascular bifurcations, distal vessels and quantification of stenosis and correlates better with other diagnostic modalities. CE MRA needs timing of the sequence with contrast bolus arrival so that data acquisition is in the center of the k-space. This is achieved by rapid contrast infusion with power injector and sequence triggering with test bolus. PAT enabled neurovascular MR coils allow imaging of neck and intracranial vessels at one sitting **(Figs. 8A and B)** and can be used in stroke protocols along with diffusion and perfusion imaging. CE MRA also better evaluates intracranial aneurysms (particularly giant aneurysms) and post coiling follow-up of aneurysms. Improved vessel to background signal, higher visibility of gadolinium, higher resolution, larger FOV, k-space reordering and keyhole techniques on 3 T produces superior quality diagnostic angiograms with improved visualization of smaller vessels **(Fig. 9)**. TOF-MRA using C-SENSE can be an alternative technique to acquire MRA in a shorter time as well **(Figs. 10A to F)**.

Time resolved CE MRA with sub-second temporal resolution and digital substraction has become feasible and initial results are exciting (time resolved imaging of contrast kinetics, or TRICKS).[58] Using parallel imaging, key hole acquisition and CENTRA k-space sampling yields nearly isotropic volume acquisition. This allows direct observation of the fast hemodynamic changes associated with abnormal vasculature of AVM's and directionality of flow in unilateral carotid occlusion syndromes.[59] Generated MIP's show the angio-architecture of AVM in any spatial orientation with enough temporal resolution to differentiate between early arterial, arterial, parenchymal and venous phases **(Figs. 11A to G)**. When the technique fails to show smaller vessels, it can be combined with high spatial resolution MRA.

Degree of stenosis and plaque morphology is important predictors of stroke. High resolution MR imaging is a developing technique. It can characterize atherosclerotic plaques for instability (irregularity and ulceration) with 81% sensitivity and 90% specificity thus facilitating prognosis and decision making of plaque stabilizing therapy.[60]

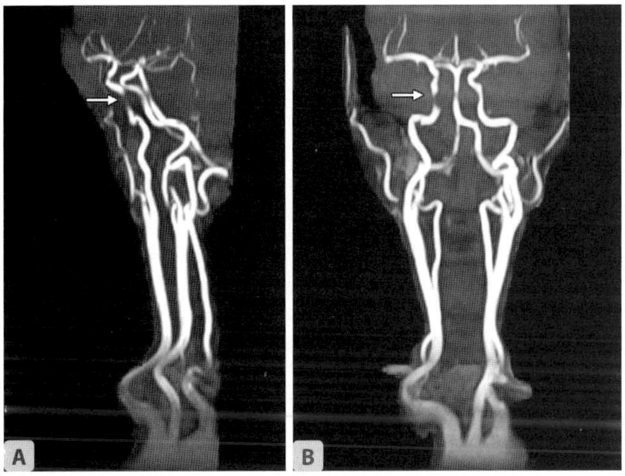

FIGS. 8A AND B: Oblique (A) and AP; (B) views of contrast-enhanced MR angiography of cervicocranial arteries showing a stenotic lesion of the right carotid artery (arrow).

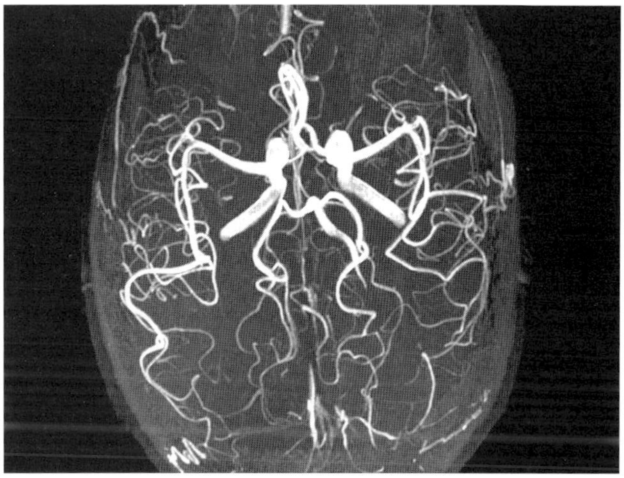

FIG. 9: Time of flight MRA; excellent angiogram due to background suppression and better flow-related signal leading to better distal smaller vessel visibility.

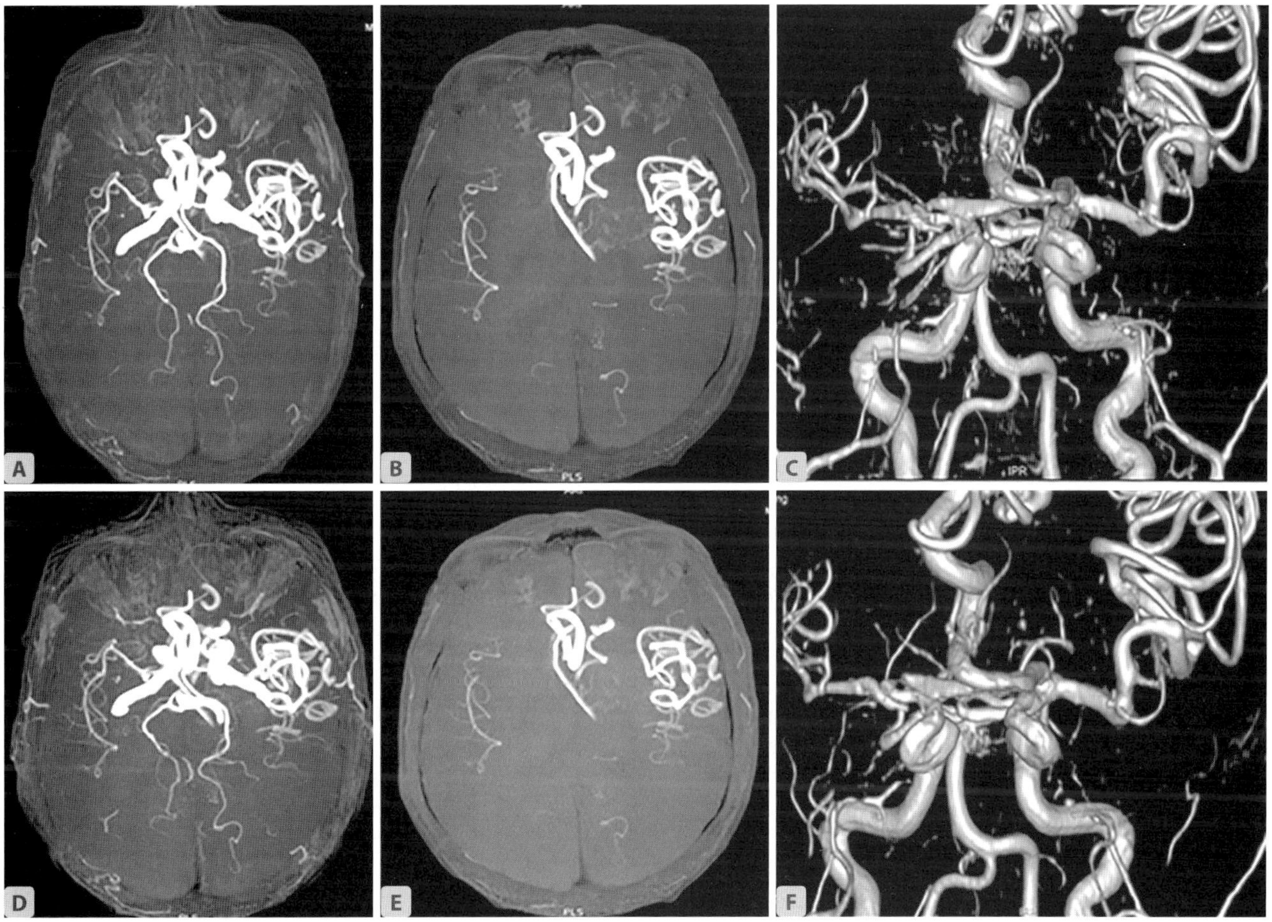

FIGS. 10A TO F: MRA of a 22-year-male patient presenting with headache: (A to C) MRA acquired with conventional technique and (D to F) MRA acquired with C-SENSE with acceleration factor of 3. (A and B) and (D and E) axial maximum intensity projection images and (C and F) volume rendered images. The images showed an arteriovenous malformation in left temporal region with multiple dilated feeding arteries with intervening nidus.

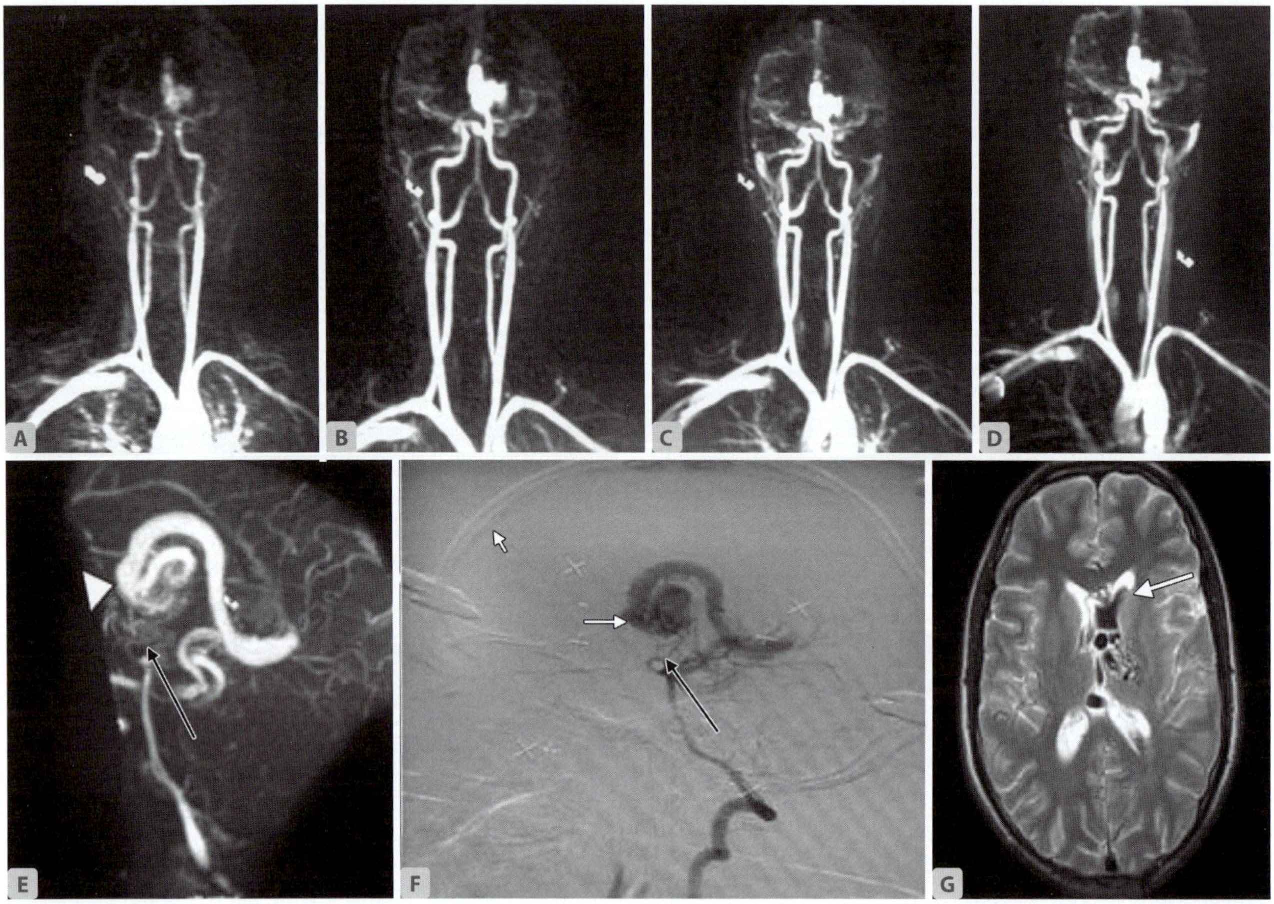

FIGS. 11A TO G: An 18-year-male with left thalamic AVM. (A to D) Sequential arterial, nidus and venous enhancement (white arrows) on time resolved MRA. (E) High spatial resolution MRA—lateral MIP projection with corresponding DSA (F). On DSA left VA run showing feeders (black arrow), nidus and draining veins [white arrowhead in MRA (E) similar to white arrow in DSA (F)]. (G) T2 TSE axial section.

VESSEL WALL MR IMAGING (VW-MR IMAGING)

It is not possible to adequately image the pathology hidden in the vessel wall by conventional imaging techniques like CTA, MRA or DSA which image the vessel lumen. High resolution vessel wall imaging using MRI has been developed over the past decade in order to overcome this pitfall of conventional angiographic modalities. Currently, vessel wall imaging for both intracranial and extracranial vessels has been developed and they are discussed here briefly.

Intracranial Vessel Wall Imaging

Essential technical requirements for intracranial vessel imaging are:[61]

High spatial resolution: By virtue of being extremely thin, the wall of the intracranial vessel is extremely difficult. Normal thickness of wall of the middle cerebral artery or basilar trunk is 0.2-0.3 mm, which is approximately 1/10th of the luminal diameter of these arteries and is smaller than the voxel dimensions currently available. However, as most of the disease condition is associated with wall thickening, the conspicuity of vessel wall increases in disease state. Besides it is possible to suppress the blood or CSF signal in the voxel. 3T is preferred over 1.5 T for VW-MR because of its intrinsically higher SNR. At 3 T for a 2D sequence following parameters are considered standard-voxel size: 2.0 mm × 0.4 mm × 0.4 mm, scan duration-approximately 5-7 min for a 2-4 cm thick section of tissue. For 3D sequence, a 0.5 mm isotropic voxel (range 0.4–0.7 mm) can be used and the coverage time for circle of Willis and 2nd and 3rd order branches typically varies between 7 and 10 minutes.

Multiplanar 2D or 3D acquisitions: The vessel wall need to be visualized in both long and short axis plane for accurate interpretation of VW-MR imaging. One of the approaches for achieving this could be acquisition of the 2D sequence multiple times in orthogonal planes. However, as most intracranial vessels have a curved course rather than straight course. Hence, partial volume averaging can result from the vessel obliquity and curvature, confounding the appearance of the arterial wall. The other approach is to use a 3D (volumetric) sequence and viewing the images in different orthogonal 2D planes. It reduces scan time and provides the option of viewing the arterial wall in any plane of choice. Variable flip angle refocusing pulse, fast spin-echo sequences are generally used for 3D VW-MR acquisitions. The sequence is known by different names from different vendors, e.g. VISTA (volume isotropic turbo spin-echo acquisition; Philips Healthcare, Best, the Netherlands), SPACE (sampling perfection with application-optimized contrasts by using different flip angle evolutions; Siemens, Erlangen, Germany), and Cube (GE Healthcare, Milwaukee, Wisconsin). Despite the advantages of 3D sequences, some groups have found 2D images to have better quality for a particular vessel of interest. Hence, it may be prudent to include both 2D and 3D sequences.

Multiple tissue weightings: Baseline TOF MRA is used for localizing the abnormality. In cases with severe luminal narrowing or dilation, a contrast enhanced MRA may be required because of slow flow leading to signal drop on TOF MRA. T1-weighted vessel wall sequence, before and after gadolinium-based contrast agent administration, is the primary sequence used. Proton density sequence can be used because of its higher SNR compared to T1-weighted sequence; but as vessel wall signal approaches that of CSF on PD images, the vessel wall becomes less conspicuous on PD. The contrast enhancement on PD can also be less prominent compared to T1. A T2-weighted VW-MR sequence is also incorporated in the typical imaging sequence. Fat suppression is generally not required, unless imaging of external carotid branches in scalp needs to image in some specific situation like giant cell arteritis.

Suppression of MR imaging signal in blood and CSF: Suppression of MR signal from blood, CSF or brain parenchyma (if vessel is embedded in the brain parenchyma) is a mandatory prerequisite for good quality VW-MR. Use of spin echo sequences, presaturation bands and double inversion recovery are some of the techniques used to suppress the blood MR signal.

Clinical applications: Intracranial VW-MR imaging is a useful adjunct to conventional imaging in many clinical conditions **(Figs. 12A to D)**. It is especially helpful in characterizing and differentiating between intracranial atherosclerotic plaque, vasculitis, reversible cerebral vasoconstriction syndrome, moyamoya disease, radiation induced arteriopathy and arterial dissection. In addition, it is also helpful to identify symptomatic, nonstenotic disease of the intracranial arteries. Recent studies have shown that is useful for prediction of future behavior of unruptured intracranial saccular aneurysms.[61]

Extracranial Vessel Wall Imaging

High resolution vessel wall MRI for cervical vessels is an important adjunct to ultrasonography and Doppler and CT angiography and has developed significantly over the last decade. Following information can be obtained from cervical VW-MR: (a) the degree of stenosis, (b) total volume of the plaque, (c) component of the plaques, and (d) surface morphology of the plaque, including ulceration and fibrous cap rupture.[62] A number of MR sequences including T1, T2 and PD-weighted sequences, and time-of-flight (TOF) imaging and black- and bright-blood sequences. The characteristics of carotid plaque on MR is summarized in **Table 1**.[62]

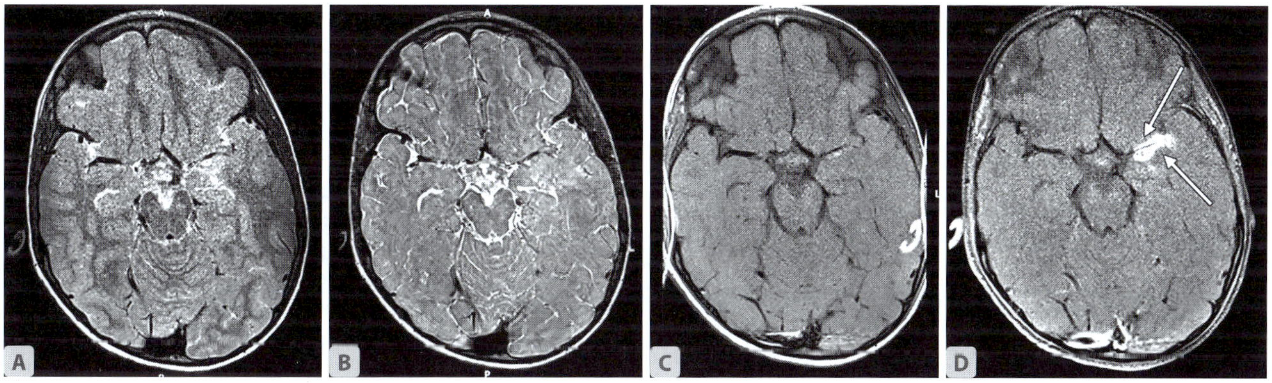

FIGS. 12A TO D: A 7-year-old girl with left middle cerebral artery (MCA) arteriopathy: T2 (A), PD (B) and T1 (C) MR images showing marked narrowing of left MCA with contrast-enhanced T1 MR images showing florid enhancement of the MCA wall (arrows in D).

TABLE 1: Carotid plaque morphology on MRI.

	Plaque Component					
			Hemorrhage			
Sequence	Lipid core	Fibrous tissue	Fresh (<1 week)	Recent (1–6 weeks)	Chronic (>6 weeks)	Calcification
3D TOF	Iso	Iso	Hyper	Hyper	Hypo	Marked hypo
T1W	Iso/hyper	Iso/hyper	Hyper	Hyper	Hypo	Marked hypo
T2W	Hypo	Iso/hyper	Iso/hypo	Hyper	Hypo	Marked hypo
PDW	Iso/hyper	Iso/hyper	Iso/hypo	Hyper	Hypo	Marked hypo
Postcontrast T1-w	Nonenhancing	Enhancing	Nonenhancing	Nonenhancing	Nonenhancing	Nonenhancing

The following reading scheme can be followed for deciding carotid plaque morphology:[62]

1. Calcification: hypointense on all sequences
2. Recent/fresh hemorrhage: hyperintense on T1 and TOF MRA
3. Lipid core: focal decrease in signal intensity from PD weighted images to T2-weighted images.
4. Fibrous component: the remaining areas should be considered as fibrous component.

The plaque inflammation is a risk factor for plaque vulnerability and it is indicated by postgadolinium enhancement. Tissue specific agents like ultra-small superparamagnetic iron oxide particles can be issued for demonstration of plaque inflammation and uptake of these particles is found to be more commonly observed in the carotid plaques of symptomatic patients than asymptomatic patients.[62]

MAGNETIC RESONANCE ELASTOGRAPHY (MRE)

Elastography is radiologist's tool for virtual palpation. It can be used to assess the stiffness of tissues which cannot be palpated clinically, e.g. brain. It is a three step process and includes the following:

- *Firstly,* introduction of shear waves into the tissue under study by an external mechanical driver.
- *Secondly,* a phase contrast MR sequence with motion encoding gradient is used to study the motions.
- *Thirdly,* stiffness maps called elastograms are generated from the measure of displacements.

The role of MRE is well established for different organs of the body particularly liver. The applications of MRE in neuroimaging are relatively new and are discussed briefly. It has been found to be a highly accurate method for measuring brain stiffness. The test-retest repeatability has errors of 1%, 2% and 3–7% for measurement of global stiffness, lobar stiffness and stiffness of subcortical gray matter.[63] It is found that stiffness decreases with age in healthy volunteers and a strong relationship between viscoelasticity and behavioral performance exists. Furthermore, stiffness is found to decrease in diseases like multiple sclerosis and several neurodegenerative diseases including those related to dementia with a variable spatial pattern of stiffness changes observed in different types of dementia. Last but not the least, it is a promising tool for the preoperative assessment of consistency and adherence of intracranial tumors to neighboring tissues and thereby predicts surgical difficulty. Thus, MRE has a potential role in multitude of neurological diseases. However, further studies are required for its validation in the field of neuroimaging.

MAGNETIC RESONANCE FINGERPRINTING

Magnetic resonance fingerprinting (MRF) is a novel approach that does the data acquisition, post-processing and visualization in a completely different fashion.[64] Rather than doing a repeated, serial data acquisition for characterization of individual parameters of interest, MRF uses a pseudo randomized acquisition. In this method, the signals from different tissues have a unique signal evolution or "fingerprint" that is simultaneously a function of the multiple material properties under investigation. A pattern recognition algorithm is used for post processing so as to match the fingerprints to a predefined dictionary of predicted signal evolutions, which can then be translated into quantitative maps of the magnetic parameters of interest. Conceptually MRF is related to compressed sensing[28] and shares some of its benefits. For example, MRF does not suffer from the high sensitivity to measurement errors found in other faster acquisition methods and fully quantitative results can be obtained by MRF within a scanning time which is comparable to that of a conventional qualitative MR scan. Most importantly, while a limited set of parameters can be evaluated at a time using conventional MR techniques, it is possible many MR parameters can be concurrently examined quantitatively using MRF given enough scan time. Thus, MRF opens the door to computer-assisted multi-parametric MR analyses, similar to genomic or proteomic analyses that could detect important but complex changes across a large number of MR parameters simultaneously. When an appropriate pattern recognition algorithm is used, MRF also provides a new and more robust behaviour in the presence of noise or other acquisition errors that may lead to the near complete suppression of deleterious effects stemming from these factors.

CHEMICAL EXCHANGE SATURATION TRANSFER (CEST) MRI

Chemical exchange saturation transfer magnetic resonance imaging is an emerging MR application that has the potential to provide molecular information of different pathologies as well as response to treatment. It is a novel MR technique by virtue of which it is possible to detect certain compounds which are too low to affect the MR contrast in standard sequences or to be detected by MR spectroscopic imaging at typical water imaging resolution.[65,66] For these compounds to be detected, they should be capable of exchanging protons with surrounding water molecules. Water in biological system exists in dynamic equilibrium between free and bound water. By saturating or irradiation of bond water, there is transfer of magnetization between them. Greatly enhanced sensitivity can be achieved as continuous build-up of magnetic saturation of water is possible, by virtue of this property. Thus, CEST MRI has immense potential in providing spectacular image contrast based on specific molecular compositions at relevant millimolar physiological concentrations.[65,66]

On MR imaging perspective, cellular proteins can be divided into two main types; bound proteins, and mobile proteins and peptides. Bound proteins are solid-like macromolecules whose protons have short T2 (~ µs) and are detected by conventional magnetization transfer (MT) contrast. On the other hand mobile protons and peptides have protons having long T2 (~ tens of ms) and can be detected by CEST MRI techniques like amide proton transfer.

Magnetization Transfer

The contrast depending on exchange of magnetization between different tissues (i.e. water pool and macromolecular pool) is called magnetization transfer (MT) contrast. The macromolecules transfer magnetization to water protons leading to a decrease in their relaxation time and loss of signal. Off resonance pulses are added to the routine MR pulse sequences to suppress the macromolecular pool (around 1000–2000 Hz) with subsequent reduction in signal intensity of background tissue in brain.[67]

The effect can be used qualitatively in clinical imaging, i.e. suppression of the background tissue in cerebral MRA for better contrast and small vessel detection, achieve better conspicuity of contrast enhancing lesions and to increase the cord CSF contrast on T2* images of spine. The MT effect can be quantitatively measured from images acquired with and without MT pulse saturation and expressed in form of MT ratio (MTR): Mo – Ms/Mo × 100% where Mo and Ms are signal intensities without and with MT pulse. MTR can be measured at the region of interest or for the entire brain with pixel to pixel coregistration.

Disorders of neural tissue often manifest as reduced MT ratios due to destruction of macromolecules (i.e. myelin). MT has been applied in multiple sclerosis to characterize plaques, determining total lesion load/response to treatment and predict clinical course.[68] It has also been applied for studying myelination in developing brain, SLE, multisystem atrophy, amyotrophic lateral sclerosis, schizophrenia, Alzheimer's disease, etc. It is reliable in differentiating tuberculoma (low MTR) from pyogenic abscess and tumors.[69]

Amide Proton Transfer

Amide proton transfer (APT) is a variant of CEST MRI, and is also known as amide CEST. It is the most popular CEST MRI till date. Proteins and peptides of the tissue are the major known contributors to APT. The main neurological applications reported for APT are the detection of cancer and ischemic stroke.

Clinical Application of APT MRI

Cerebrovascular Stroke

It is possible to identify ischemic regions of brain parenchyma in patients of ischemic stroke.[66] Increase in ATP hydrolysis takes place in setting of decreased cerebral blood flow leading to reduced bicarbonate buffering and local acidosis. This in turn leads to decreased exchange rate of amide protons as the chemical exchange of amide proton is catalyzed in an alkaline environment. This decrease in amide proton exchange leads to a decrease in APT MRI contrast in the ischemic tissue and this can be detected even with a relatively low 0.5 μT saturation power. Compared to the hypoperfused salvageable penumbra, the ischemic core shows much decreased APT. In animal models it has been found that hemorrhagic vs ischemic stroke can also be distinguished by hyperintense vs hypointense APT MRI contrast. Thus, APT can be an important adjunct to anatomical MR imaging, diffusion and perfusion studies in the setting of stroke.

Multiple Sclerosis

Accumulation of mobile proteins in the normal appearing white matter is the neuropathological and biochemical basis of the biochemical neuropathology of multiple sclerosis (MS). APT contrast increases as a result of this protein accumulation and can be detected at 7 T and a moderate 2–3.5 μT saturation power.[66] Furthermore, spectral analysis of the CEST showed increased asymmetry around the amide CEST peak in lesions and normal-appearing white matter in the spine of MS patients compared to healthy white matter in healthy subjects.

Alzheimer's Disease

Reduced mobile protein content related to Alzheimer's disease, can be detected by APT MRI, but it is yet to be translated to clinical studies.[66]

Brain Tumor

APT at 3 T and 7 T magnetic field strengths has been found to have promising role in brain tumor imaging. The histopathological tumor grade bears a positive correlation with APT MRI contrast. APT MRI contrast has been shown to reduce with treatment. Correspondingly, lower APT MRI contrast is generated in pseudoprogression from post-treatment inflammation compared to recurrent glioma. High APT MRI contrast has been more correlated with high-grade gliomas than strongly enhancing imaging regions with gadolinium-based MRI contrast agents.[66]

Intracranial Hemorrhage

High MTR is seen in acute hemorrhages compared to subacute hemorrhages regardless of the underlying pathology and thus can be useful in evaluation of hemorrhagic brain lesions.[70]

gluCEST MRI

It is an extremely difficult task to selectively detect only a single metabolite amidst multitude of metabolites within tissues as the MR frequencies of these metabolites overlap. Fortunately, Glutamate (glu) is an exception showing CEST peak at 3.0 ppm. For glutamate, the chemical exchange occurs for amine group, CEST detection of glutamate is further facilitated by its higher concentration in brain compared to other metabolites.[66]

gluCEST MRI, i.c. the imaging of glutamate with CEST MRI, has been done successfully in healthy brain tissue and the spinal cord. Strong CEST contrast is generated by a 3.6 μT saturation power. The relatively high saturation power is necessary for separation of the MR frequencies of glutamate and water, and the fast exchange rate of the labile protons on glutamate. However, as 7T MRI provides more selective saturation of glutamate than 3T, clinical gluCEST MRI studies have only been performed at 7T scanners.[66]

Strong correlation exists between the gluCEST ratio from gray and white matter to the ratio of glutamate concentration measured with 1H MR spectroscopy. Lateralization of temporal lobe seizure is possible with gluCEST MRI brain study correctly and the findings corroborated with MR spectroscopy. Relative glutamate concentrations in the spinal cord may serve as an additional biomarker for multiple sclerosis, which may complement the mobile protein content measurements made with APT MRI.[66]

POSITRON EMISSION TOMOGRAPHY AND MRI (PET/MRI)

Inability to perform simultaneous data acquisition producing artifacts and exposing the patient to significant radiation are major limitations of PET/CT.[71,72] Moreover, PET/CT has poor contrast in soft tissue as well as in complex anatomical regions like head and neck. An integrated PET/MR scanner (Siemens) which enables simultaneous acquisition of PET and MR imaging was launched in 2010, Munich, Germany.[73] There were many technical and practical hurdles before PET/MR was available for clinical imaging. Firstly, the photomultiplier (PMT)-based PET scanners do not work within or near the magnetic environment of an MR scanner. To overcome this, the developers used avalanche photo diode or silicon PMT-based PET detector systems.[74] Secondly, metallic objects such as surface coils used to get best MR image quality interfere with the gamma rays from PET, causing unwanted attenuation. This can be achieved by modification of surface coils to reduce their metal content. Thirdly, MR data are not readily usable for attenuation correction like PET/CT.[75] Therefore, quantification of PET data was not possible. Various approaches to overcome this problem are currently under investigation.[76]

Applications in Neuroimaging

Besides oncological applications, PET/MRI has got few neurological applications.

- In patients with Alzheimer's disease, PET/MR can be used for the early diagnosis, evaluation of disease progression and therapy response. In addition, morphologic images are essential to exclude other causes of dementia like multi-infarct dementia or normal-pressure hydrocephalus.[77,78]
- Patients with refractory epilepsy despite medical treatment require surgery to resect the epileptogenic focus.[79] For success of surgical procedure structural and functional imaging data is of outmost importance. Therefore, these patients needs to undergo a battery of imaging and non-imaging tests like morphologic MRI, functional MRI, PET, and EEG for correct localization of epileptic focus. The PET/MR will be useful in such patients and data can be obtained using single imaging test in one day rather than multiple imaging tests on different days.

ARTIFICIAL INTELLIGENCE IN NEURORADIOLOGY

Mimicking human cognitive function is the ultimate goal of artificial intelligence (AI). With the advent of AI, the healthcare system is observing a paradigm shift which is enforced by rapid progress of analytics techniques and increasing availability of healthcare data. The AI devices and techniques are broadly classified into two types, machine learning (ML) techniques and natural language processing (NLP) methods.[80] The machine learning techniques analyze structured data such as imaging, genetic and EP data. In the medical applications, the ML procedures attempt to cluster patients' traits, or infer the probability of the disease outcomes. On the other hand, NLP methods natural extract information from unstructured data such as clinical notes/medical journals to supplement and enrich structured medical data. The NLP procedures target at turning texts to machine-readable structured data, which can then be analyzed by ML techniques. The most common types of ML algorithms include neural network, support vector machine (SVM).[80]

Deep Learning

Deep learning has ushered a new era in the ML algorithms. Deep learning is a subset of supervised machine learning method. These techniques use some form of neural network based on their ability to automatically extract relevant features. Deep learning allows constructing an image-classification in shorter time as compared to experts. Rapid development of modern computing enables deep learning to build-up neural networks with a large number of layers, which is infeasible for classical neural networks. As such, deep learning can explore more complex nonlinear patterns in the data. Deep learning is gaining popularity as the data is becoming more complex and the volume of data increases. In the medical applications, the commonly used deep learning algorithms include convolution neural network (CNN), recurrent neural network, deep belief network and deep neural network.[80]

Major Applications of AI in Neuroimaging

Few of the major applications of AI in neuroimaging includes—brain tumor segmentation with MRI, early detection of Alzheimer's disease with fMRI, detection of stroke and possible reduction of gadolinium dose in clinical MR imaging. In fact, US Food and Drug administration (FDA) has granted a de Novo request for the first-ever computer-aided triage and notification platform to identify large vessel occlusion (LVO) strokes in CTA imaging in February 2018. Although the AI technologies are attracting substantial attentions in medical research, the real-life implementation is still unclear due to lack of standards of the safety and efficacy of AI systems.

ACKNOWLEDGMENTS

The authors acknowledge and thank Dr Nirmalya Ray, DM resident in Neuroradiology section of Department of Radiodiagnosis and Imaging, PGIMER, Chandigarh for active involvement and helping in writing the chapter.

REFERENCES

1. Chen CN, Sank VJ, Cohen SM, et al. The field dependence of NMR imaging. I. Laboratory assessment of signal-to-noise ratio and power deposition. Magn Reson Med. 1986;3:722-9.
2. Hoult DI, Chen CN, Sank VJ. The field dependence of NMR imaging. II. Arguments concerning an optimal field strength. Magn Reson Med. 1986;3:730-46.
3. Edelstein WA, Glover GH, Hardy CJ, et al. The intrinsic signal-to-noise ratio in NMR imaging. Magn Reson Med. 1986;3:604-18.
4. Middleton H, Black RD, Saam B, et al. MR imaging with hyperpolarized 3He gas. Magn Reson Med. 1995; 33:271-5.
5. Foster TH. Tissue conductivity modifies the magnetic resonance intrinsic signal-to-noise ratio at high frequencies. Magn Reson Med. 1992;23:383-5.
6. Scarabino T, Nemore F, Giannatempo GM, et al. 3.0 T magnetic resonance in neuroradiology. Eur J Radiol. 2003;48:154-64.
7. Duyn JH. The future of ultra-high field MRI and fMRI for study of the human brain. Neuroimage. 2012;62:1241-8.
8. Balchandani P, Naidich TP. Ultra-high-field MR neuroimaging. Am J Neuroradiol. 2015;36:1204-15.
9. Hennig J, Nauerth A, Friedburg H. RARE imaging: a fast imaging method for clinical MR. Magn Reson Med. 1986;3(6):823-33.
10. Carr H, Purcell E. Effects of diffusion on free precession in nuclear magnetic resonance experiments. Phys Rev. 1954;94(3):630-8.
11. Meiboom S, Gill D. Modified spin-echo method for measuring nuclear relaxation times. Rev Sci Instrum. 1958;29:688-91.
12. Maudsley AA. Modified Carr-Purcell-Meiboom-Gill sequence for NMR Fourier imaging applications. J Magn Reson (1969). 1986;69:488-91.
13. Mulkern RV, Wong ST, Winalski C, et al. Contrast manipulation and artifact assessment of 2D and 3D RARE sequences. Magn Reson Imaging. 1990;8:557-66.
14. Mulkern RV, Melki PS, Jakab P, et al. Phase encode order and its effect on contrast and artifact in single-shot RARE sequences. Med Phys. 1991;18:1032-7.
15. Melki PS, Mulkern RV, Panych LP, et al. Comparing the FAISE method with conventional dual-echo sequences. J Magn Reson Imaging. 1991;1:319-26.
16. Melki PS, Jolesz FA, Mulkern RV. Partial RF echo planar imaging with the FAISE method. I. Experimental and theoretical assessment of artifact. Magn Reson Med. 1992;26:328-41.
17. Melki PS, Jolesz FA, Mulkern RV. Partial RF echo planar imaging with the FAISE method. II. Contrast equivalence with spin echo sequences. Magn Reson Med. 1992;26:342-54.
18. Ahn SS, Mantello MT, Jones KM, et al. Rapid MR imaging of the pediatric brain using the fast spin-echo technique. Am J Neuroradiol. 1992;13(4):1169-77.
19. Constable RT, Smith RC, Gore JC. Signal-to-noise and contrast in fast spin echo (FSE) and inversion recovery FSE imaging. J Comput Assist Tomogr. 1992;16(1):41-7.
20. Jones KM, Mulkern RV, Mantello MT, et al. Brain hemorrhage: evaluation with fast spin-echo and conventional dual spin-echo images. Radiology. 1992;182(1):53-8.
21. Jones KM, Mulkern RV, Schwartz RB. Fast spin-echo MR imaging of the brain and spine: current concepts. Am J Roentgenol. 1992;158:1313-20.
22. Tice HM, Jones KM, Mulkern RV. Fast spin-echo imaging of intracranial neoplasms. J Comput Assist Tomogr. 1993;17:425-31.
23. Hardy PA, Henkelman RM, Bishop JE. Why fat is bright in rare and fast spin-echo imaging. J Magn Reson Imaging. 1992;2(5):533-40.
24. Hiramatsu K, Mulkern RV. A novel method for fat suppression in RARE sequences. Magn Reson Med. 1992;27(1):107-17.
25. Melki PS, Mulkern RV. Magnetization transfer effects in multislice RARE sequences. Magn Reson Med. 1992;24(1):189-95.
26. Feinberg DA, Kiefer B, Litt AW. High resolution GRASE MRI of the brain and spine: 512 and 1024 matrix imaging. J Comput Assist Tomogr. 1995;19(1):1-7.
27. McGibney G, Smith MR, Nichols ST. Quantitative evaluation of several partial Fourier reconstruction algorithms used in MRI. Magn Reson Med. 1993;30(1):51-9.
28. Lustig M, Donoho D, Pauly JM. Sparse MRI: the application of compressed sensing for rapid MR imaging. Magn Reson Med. 2007;58:1182-95.
29. Donoho DL. Compressed sensing. IEEE Transactions on Information Theory. 2006;52(4):1289-306.
30. Candes EJ, Romberg J, Tao T. Robust uncertainty principles: exact signal reconstruction from highly incomplete frequency information. IEEE Transactions on Information Theory. 2006;52(2):489-509.
31. Moeller S, Yacoub E, Olman CA. Multiband multislice GE-EPI at 7 Tesla, with 16-fold acceleration using partial parallel imaging with application to high spatial and temporal whole-brain fMRI. Magnetic Reson Med. 2010;63(5):1144-53.
32. Feinberg DA, Setsompop K. Ultra-fast MRI of the human brain with simultaneous multi-slice imaging. J Magn Reson. 2013;229:90-100.
33. Haacke EM, Mittal S, Wu Z, et al. Susceptibility-weighted-imaging: technical aspects and clinical applications, Part I. Am J Neuroradiol. 2009;30:19-30.
34. Mittal S, Wu J, Neelavalli EM, et al. Susceptibility-weighted-imaging: technical aspects and clinical applications, Part II. Am J Neuroradiol. 2009;30:232-52.
35. Deistung A, Schweser F, Reichenbach JR. Overview of quantitative susceptibility mapping. NMR Biomed. 2017;30(4). doi: 10.1002/nbm.3569.
36. Haacke EM, Liu S, Buch S, et al. Quantitative susceptibility mapping: current status and future directions. Magn Reson Imaging. 2015;33(1):1-25.
37. Li W, Liu C3, Duong TQ, et al. Susceptibility tensor imaging (STI) of the brain. NMR Biomed. 2017;30(4):e3540.
38. Schaefer PW, Grant PE, Gonzalez RG. Diffusion-weighted imaging of the brain. Radiology. 2000;217:331-45.
39. Hagmann P, Jonasson L, Maeder P, et al. Understanding diffusion MR imaging techniques: from scalar diffusion-weighted imaging to diffusion tensor imaging and beyond. Radiographics. 2006;26(Suppl 1):S205-23.
40. Sundgren PC, Dong Q, Go'mez-Hassan D, et al. Diffusion tensor imaging of the brain: review of clinical applications. Neuroradiology. 2004;46:339-50.
41. Bammer R, Acar B, Moseley ME. In vivo MR tractography using diffusion imaging. Eur J Radiol. 2003;45:223-34.
42. Wedeen VJ, Hagmann P, Tseng WY, et al. Mapping complex tissue architecture with diffusion spectrum magnetic resonance imaging. Magn Reson Med. 2005;54:1377-86.
43. Tuch DS, Reese TG, Wiegell MR, et al. Diffusion MRI of complex neural architecture. Neuron. 2003;40:885-95.
44. Jansons KM, Alexander DC. Persistent angular structure: new insights from diffusion MRI data. [Dummy version]. Inf Process Med Imaging. 2003;18:672-83.
45. Tournier JD, Calamante F, Gadian DG, et al. Direct estimation of the fiber orientation density function from diffusion-weighted MRI data using spherical deconvolution. Neuroimage. 2004;23:1176-85.
46. Steven AJ, Zhuo J, Melhem ER. Diffusion kurtosis imaging: an emerging technique for evaluating the microstructural environment of the brain. Am J Roentgenol. 2014;202:W26-33.
47. Fieremans E, Jensen JH, Helpern JA. White matter characterization with diffusional kurtosis imaging. Neuroimage. 2011;58:177-88.

48. Porter DA, Heidemann RM. High resolution diffusion-weighted imaging using readout-segmented echo-planar imaging, parallel imaging and a two-dimensional navigator-based reacquisition. Magn Reson Med. 2009;62:468-75.
49. Dowell NG, Jenkins TM, Ciccarelli O, et al. Contiguous-slice zonally oblique multislice (CO-ZOOM) diffusion tensor imaging: examples of in vivo spinal cord and optic nerve applications. J Magn Reson Imaging. 2009;29(2):454-60.
50. Jahng GH, Li KL, Ostergaard L, et al. Perfusion magnetic resonance imaging: a comprehensive update on principles and techniques. Korean J Radiol. 2014;15:554-77.
51. Cha S. Perfusion MR imaging: basic principles and clinical applications. Magn Reson Imaging Clin N Am. 2003;11:403-13.
52. Wang J, Alsop DC, Li L, et al. Comparison of quantitative perfusion imaging using arterial spin labeling at 1.5 and 4.0 Tesla. Magn Reson Med. 2002;48:242-54.
53. Haller S, Zaharchuk G, Thomas DL, et al. Arterial spin labeling perfusion of the brain: emerging clinical applications. Radiology. 2016;281:337-56.
54. Chhabra A, Andreisek G, Soldatos T, et al. MR neurography: past, present, and future. Am J Roentgenol. 2011;197:583-91.
55. Seddon HJ, Medawar PB, Smith H. Rate of regeneration of peripheral nerves in man. J Physiol. 1943;102:191-215.
56. Sunderland S. A classification of peripheral nerve injuries producing loss of function. Brain. 1951;74:491-516.
57. Sohn CH, Sevick RJ, Frayne R. Contrast-enhanced MR angiography of the intracranial circulation. Neuroimag Clin N Am. 2003;11:599-614.
58. Korosec FR, Frayne R, Grist TM, et al. Time-resolved contrast-enhanced 3D MR angiography. Magn Reson Med. 1996;36:345-51.
59. Taschner CA, Gieseke J, Thuc VL, et al. Intracranial arterio-venous malformation: time-resolved contrast-enhanced MR angiography with combination of parallel imaging, keyhole acquisition and k-space sampling techniques at 1.5 T. Radiology. 2008;246:871-9.
60. Hatsukami TS, Ross R, Polissar NL, et al. Visualization of fibrous cap thickness and rupture in human atherosclerotic plaques in vivo with high resolution magnetic resonance imaging. Circulation. 2000;102:959-64.
61. Mandell DM, Mossa-Basha M, Qiao Y, et al. Intracranial vessel wall MRI: principles and expert consensus recommendations of the American Society of Neuroradiology. AJNR Am J Neuroradiol. 2017;38:218-29.
62. Choi YJ, Jung SC, Lee DH. Vessel wall imaging of the intracranial and cervical carotid arteries. J Stroke. 2015;17:238-55.
63. Murphy MC, Huston J 3rd, Ehman RL. MR elastography of the brain and its application in neurological diseases. Neuroimage. 2017;S1053-8119(17)30821-2.
64. Ma D, Gulani V, Seiberlich N, et al. Magnetic resonance fingerprinting. Nature. 2013;495:187-92.
65. Wu B,Warnock G, Zaiss M, et al. An overview of CEST MRI for non-MR physicists. EJNMMI Phys. 2016;3:19.
66. Jones KM, Pollard AC, Pagel MD. Clinical applications of chemical exchange saturation transfer (CEST) MRI. J Magn Reson Imaging. 2018;47:11-27.
67. McGowan JC. The physical basis of magnetization transfer imaging. Neurology. 1999;53(5 Suppl 3):S3-7.
68. Santos AC, Narayanan S, de Stefano N, et al. Magnetization transfer can predict clinical evolution in patients with multiple sclerosis. J Neurol. 2002;249:662-8.
69. Gupta RK, Hussain M, Vatsal DK, et al. Comparative evaluation of magnetization transfer imaging and in vivo proton MR spectroscopy in brain tuberculomas. Magn Reson Imaging. 2002;20:375-81.
70. Jeong HK, Han K, Zhou J, et al. Characterizing amide proton transfer imaging in haemorrhage brain lesions using 3T MRI. Eur Radiol. 2017;27:1577-84.
71. Chawla SC, Federman N, Zhang D, et al. Estimated cumulative radiation dose from PET/CT in children with malignancies: a 5-year retrospective review. Pediatr Radiol. 2010;40:681-6.
72. Mattsson S, Söderberg M. Radiation dose management in CT, SPECT/CT and PET/CT techniques. Radiat Prot Dosimetry. 2011;147(1-2):13-21.
73. Delso G, Fürst S, Jakoby B, et al. Performance measurements of the Siemens mMR integrated whole-body PET/MR scanner. J Nucl Med. 2011;52:1914-22.
74. Pichler BJ, Judenhofer MS, Catana C, et al. Performance test of an LSO-APD detector in a 7-T MRI scanner for simultaneous PET/MRI. J Nucl Med. 2006;47:639-47.
75. Hofmann M, Pichler B, Schölkopf B, et al. Towards quantitative PET/MRI: a review of MR-based attenuation correction techniques. Eur J Nucl Med Mol Imaging. 2009;36(Suppl 1):S93-104.
76. Zaidi H, Ojha N, Morich M, et al. Design and performance evaluation of a whole-body Ingenuity TF. PET-MRI system. Phys Med Biol. 2011;56:3091-106.
77. Ossenkoppele R, Tolboom N, Foster-Dingley JC, et al. Longitudinal imaging of Alzheimer pathology using [11C]PIB, [18F]FDDNP and [18F]FDG PET. Eur J Nucl Med Mol Imaging. 2012;39: 990-1000.
78. Kenny ER, Blamire AM, Firbank MJ, et al. Functional connectivity in cortical regions in dementia with Lewy bodies and Alzheimer's disease. Brain. 2012;135:569-81.
79. Duncan J. The current status of neuroimaging for epilepsy. Curr Opin Neurol. 2009;22:179-84.
80. Jiang F, Jiang Y, Zhi H, et al Artificial intelligence in healthcare: past, present and future. Stroke Vasc Neurol. 2017;2(4):230-43.

CHAPTER

186

Magnetic Resonance Spectroscopy

Vikas Bhatia, Paramjeet Singh, Niranjan Khandelwal

INTRODUCTION

Nuclear magnetic resonance (NMR) and spectroscopy were introduced as experimental techniques as a method of delineating structure and composition of various physical and chemical materials. Subsequently, it was found to have many applications in medicine and *in vivo* magnetic resonance spectroscopy (MRS) evolved as a new molecular imaging technique to noninvasively determine the metabolites in any given living tissue which are measured as a result of their different chemical shifts or frequencies.[1] Most of the pathologic processes are characterized by metabolic changes earlier than anatomic changes during disease process and after treatment. Thus, MRS imaging provides information which can lead to early diagnosis, treatment plan and response assesment.[2]

MRS is a spectrum which tells us about the chemical and physical properties of a tissue based on the intensity and distribution of energy measured after a certain wavelength or frequency is allowed to interact with the tissue sample.

MR spectra is shown by those nuclei that contain an odd number of protons and neutrons, such as hydrogen-1, carbon-13, fluorine-19, phosphorus-31 as they exhibit a magnetic momentum to interact with the external magnetic field.[3] A major limitation of MRS is that only those metabolites with a concentration of more than 0.1 mM can be detected. However, with the recent development of hardware and localizing techniques, MRS offers a promising future to detect many different metabolites and their role in physiological and pathological conditions.

PRINCIPLE

Basic fundamental principles of magnetic resonance imaging (MRI) and MRS are same.[4] While MRI provides information on anatomy and pathology displayed as visual images, MRS basically obtains chemical information of the region of interest as a spectra which is displayed as numerical values. The simple MRI sequence block contains slice excitation by radio frequency pulse followed by application of slice encoding, phase encoding, and frequency-encoding gradients in mutually orthogonal planes. Whereas, in a classical spectroscopic imaging sequence, the MRS signal is acquired without a frequency-encoding gradient. Thus, acquired MRS signal contains different frequencies that correspond to the chemical shift with no spatial information. The amplitude of chemical shifts of various metabolites depends on the gyromagnetic ratio of the nuclei and intensity of external magnetic field **(Table 1)**. So, at a given external magnetic field, every chemically distinct nucleus shows slightly different resonating frequency—the *chemical shift*—giving rise to separate peaks in the MR spectrum. By the same principle, in a given standard chemical environment increasing the external magnetic field strength transforms into better separation of

TABLE 1: MRS: Properties of nuclei.

Nucleus	Spin quantum number	Natural abundance (%)	Gyromagnetic ratio (MHz/T)	Resonance frequency (MHz) at 1.5T	Resonance frequency (MHz) at 3T
^{1}H	1/2	100	42.6	63.9	127.7
^{31}P	1/2	100	17.2	25.9	51.7
^{19}F	1/2	100	40.1	60.1	120.2
^{23}Na	3/4	100	11.3	16.9	33.8
^{17}O	5/2	0.04	2.0	8.7	17.3
^{7}Li	3/2	92.6	16.5	24.8	49.7
^{13}C	1/2	1.1	10.7	16.1	32.1

signal frequencies of various metabolites in MR spectrum. J coupling or spin-spin coupling is due to interactions with a neighboring nuclear spin and provides additional information.

Spectrum

An MRS provides *in vivo* biochemical information represented spectrum with the peaks in the spectra obtained correspond with various metabolites. The horizontal axis shows resonance frequency as ppm to the total resonance frequency. The vertical axis plots the concentrations or relative signal amplitude of metabolites.

Factors affecting the peak sharpness and line width are:

a. External magnetic field homogeneity
b. Inhomogeneity of the magnetic field due to susceptibility gradient
c. T2 time of the sample.

The spectra obtained are interpretated for the following **(Fig. 1)**:

- Center of the resonance frequency in ppm
- Height of peak
- Line width at half-height
- Area and shape of peak
- Characteristic of the peaks, e.g. single, doublet, triplet.

The display of the MR spectra as per convention include:

- *Up-field* is to the right represents lower frequencies and are shielded.
- *Down-field* is to the left represents higher frequencies and are deshielded.
- *Chemical shifts (in ppm)* is positive going to the left and is negative towards the right.

Zero setting is done by RF of a particular compound, e.g. phosphocreatine for ^{31}P-MRS and tetramethylsilane (TMS) for ^{1}H and ^{13}C MRS (at 4.8 ppm). Since TMS is not seen *in viva* known chemical like NAA at 2.0 ppm is used as chemical shift reference. The ppm scale describes the shifts in hertz from a reference peak divided by frequency of excitation. For example, ^{31}P-MRS acquired at 1.5 T shows resonance frequency at 25.86 MHz and 25.86 Hz is 1 ppm. The ppm scales provides easy comparison of data obtained in different fields.

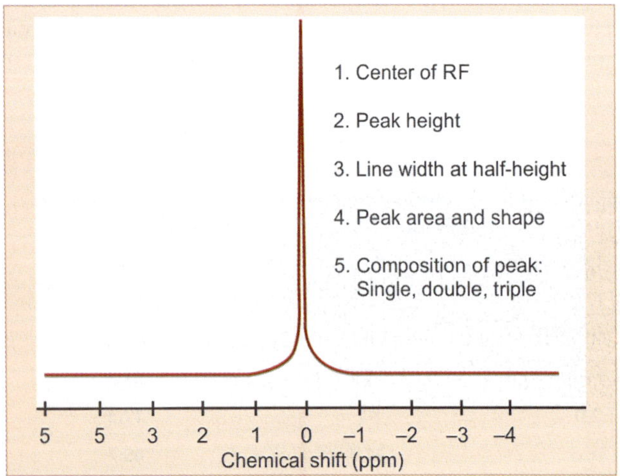

FIG. 1: Parameters for analysis of MR spectrum.

Spectrum and Echo Time

The metabolites and their spectral pattern on proton MRS depend on the time to echo (TE).[5] Various metabolites which are seen on long and short TE are summarized **(Tables 2 and 3)**.

The phenomenon of spin-spin coupling (J coupling) influences the appearance of spectra due to various metabolites obtained at different TE. It is emphasized that the frequency of resonating protons is affected by adjacent electrons and hence various chemical groups within the same molecule resonate at different frequencies. For instance, lactic acid, COOH-CHOH-CH 3, the principle signal is due to CH 3 group at 1.33 ppm. As this group is connected to the CH group, coupling of proton signals is seen: resulting in splitting of CH 3 peak into a doublet with intensity ratio 1:1. Metabolites with doublet peaks (lactate, alanine) are usually seen as positive peaks around TE 280 ms with inversion at TE 140 ms. Triplets (e.g. glutamate/glutamine, aspartate), which have two neighboring protons, are seen at short TE or t intermediate TE). Quartets (e.g. myoinositol) tend to be seen at shortest TE.[6]

TABLE 2: Various metabolites with molecular concentrations.[7]

ppm	Spectral assignment	Approximate concentration mM/kg net wt
0.9–1.3	Macromolecules, amino acids, lipids	<0.5
1.35	Lactate	0.5
1.47	Alanine	<0.3
1.9	Acetate	0.2
2.02, 2.6	N-acetyl aspartate	7–10
2.1/2.5	Glutamate + Glutamine	6–10
2.4	Pyruvate succinate	0.3
3.02, 3.9	Creatine	5–7
3.2	Choline	5–7
3.36	Scylloinositol and taurine	1
3.56, 4.06	Myoinositol, glycine	5–7

TABLE 3: Visualization of metabolites based on TE values.[7]

	Large signals at long TE	Large signals at short TE	Small signals (short or long TE)
Normally present	NAA	Glutamate	N-acetyl-aspartyl-glutamate (NAAG
	Cr	Glutamine	Taurine, ethanolamine
	Cho	Myo-inositol	Glucose
Pathological	Lactate	Lipids	
	Succinate	Macromolecules	
	Pyruvate	Phenylalanine	
	Alanine		
	Glycine		

Observable Biochemicals on MRS

The *in vivo* MR spectroscopy before any postprocessing contains four types of compounds in its spectrum.[8]

1. Water with a concentration of about 40 M between 4.3 and 6 ppm.

   This water signal is required to be suppressed because its signal intensity is about four orders more than other visible metabolites.

2. Lipids, macromolecules, the macromolecules produce a broad signal on the background or are invisible in the MR spectra.
3. Metabolites having concentration >1 mM and molecular weight less than 2000 Da between 0.5 and 4 ppm.

   This is the most important group in clinical MR spectroscopy which comprises of approximately twenty compounds found in ^{1}H MR spectra of humans.

4. Metabolites having concentration <1 mM with molecular weight 2000 Da between 6 and 10 ppm. These are usually not evaluated in clinical MR spectroscopy due to limitation of time and SNR.

Hydrogen 1 (^{1}H-MRS)

Proton is abundantly present in the body and hence most suited for MRS. **Figures 2A and B** shows major spectral peaks from human brain using a 3T MRI system at TE = 135 ms (2A) and TE = 30 ms (2B). **Table 4** shows the major compounds as seen on ^{1}H-MRS with approximate concentration and chemical shift in ppm.

N-acetylaspartate (NAA) peak is seen as major upfield peak on ^{1}H-MRS. It is specifically present in CNS predominantly in mature neurons and axons. It is considered to be a sensitive marker density and viability of neurons.[9] This metabolite is seen in cortex and white matter of fetuses as early as 16 weeks of gestation. During the early years of life, rapid increase in levels of NAA and Cr is seen. After this, levels increase less than 1% a year until reaching adult values by age 16 years. Reduced levels of NAA are seen in pathologies such as degenerative disorders and stroke due to neuronal loss or injury. NAA- glutamate is present only in white matter (not in gray matter) and constitutes a resonance of around 20% near to 2.0 ppm overlapping with the NAA peak.

Choline (Cho) peak is seen at 3.22 ppm and is due to glycerophosphocholine (GPC) and glycerophospho-ethanolamine (GPE) constituting the phospholipid layer of the cell membrane. Raised levels of choline are seen in acute demyelinating lesions due to release of membrane phospholipids during active myelin breakdown. Raised choline is seen in brain tumors due to associated increased cellular density. Infants with active myelination stage also have increased levels of choline as compared to adults.

Creatine (Cr) peak at 3.02 ppm is due to sum of creatine and phosphocreatine and it does not indicate energy state of the cell. Concentration of total creatinine is relative constant throughout the brain with relative resistance to change. These properties make Cr to be used as an internal standard to normalize resonance intensities of other metabolites.

Lactate (lac) peak is formed due to anaerobic glycolysis and seen as doublet at 1.33 ppm.[10] Lactate accumulates when oxidative metabolism is unable to meet energy requirements leading to accelerated anaerobic glycolysis. Certain brain tumors, such as gliomas show elevated concentrations of lactate, because they show increased glycolysis independent of the adequacy of oxidative metabolic pathways. Elevated lactate is also seen in the extracellular environment of necrotic tissue and cysts as well as in areas of ischemic infarction.

Other metabolites such as myoinositol, glutamate/glutamine and glucose, may also be observed. Broad peaks at 0.9–1.3 ppm of lipid may obscure some of the metabolites, contaminate the spectra and need to be separated from lactate peak.[11] The differential diagnostic uses of metabolites of ^{1}H-MRS have been summarized in **Table 4**.[12]

Phosphorus 31 (^{31}P-MRS)

It demonstrates the metabolites involved in the energy metabolism. **Figure 3** shows a typical ^{31}P-MRS spectrum of human brain. The first down-field peak is due to

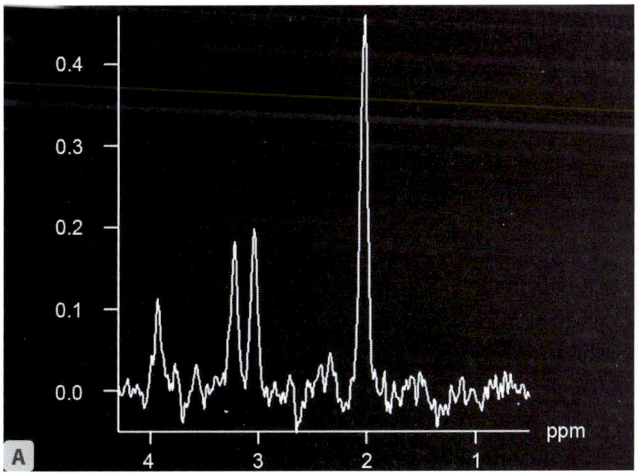

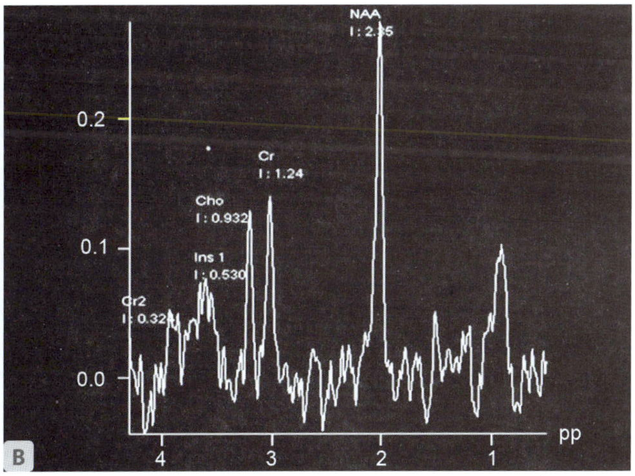

FIGS. 2A AND B: (A) Normal proton ^{1}H-MRS in brain (TE = 135 ms); (B) Normal proton ^{1}H-MRS in brain (TE = 30 ms).

TABLE 4: Differential diagnostic uses of metabolites in MRS.[7]

Metabolite (normal cerebral concentration)	Major resonance peak	Characteristics	Decreased	Increased
1. Creatine (Cr) and phosphocreatine (PCr) (8 mM)	3.0 and 3.9 Singlet	Marker of brain metabolism	• Hypoxic injury • Ischemic injury • Neoplasms • Traumatic insult	Hyperosmolar increasing with age
2. Lactate (Lac) (1 mM: Not visible because of its low concentration)	1.3 Doublet Inverted at TE 144 ms	• Product of anaerobic metabolic activity • Indicates ischemia • Interrupted Krebs' cycle • Inhibition of PDH	Unknown	• Hypoxic/ischemic insult • Hemorrhage • Infections • Neoplasms
3. Myoinositol (mL) (5 mM)	3.5 Multiplet Short TE	• Marker of astrocytes • Regulation of cell volume • Indicates osmotic stress	• Stroke • Tumor • Hypoxia • Hyponatremia • SIADH	• Neonate • Renal dysfunction • DM • Recovery from hypoxic insult
4. N-acetyl aspartate (NAA) (8–9 mM)	2.0 Singlet	• Most prominent upright signal in normal brain tissue • Indicative of normal neuronal function	• Hypoxia • Infants • Ischemic injury • Seizure disorder • Demyelination • Neoplasms • Traumatic insult • Neurodegenerative disorders	• Canavan's disease • Recovery after axonal injury • PMD • Normal developing infant brain
5. Choline (Cho) (1.5 mM)	3.2 Singlet	• Required for membrane synthesis • Increased levels seen after membrane degradation	• Hepatic encephalopathy • Stroke • SIADH • Cryptococcoma	• Traumatic injury • Neoplastic • Ischemic injury • Demyelination • Certain infections • Neonates
6. Lipid	0.9–1.3 Broad peak Short TE	• Indicates pathological process due to liberation of membrane lipids	Not detectable	• Voxel contamination, e.g. scalp • Necrotic neoplasm • Lymphoma • Tuberculoma • Brain abscess • Toxoplasmosis • Traumatic/ischemic insult
7. Glutamine (Gln) and glutamate Glu) (Gln approx 5 mm, Glu approx 10 mm)	2.1–2.6 3.75 Multiplet Short TE	• Marker of astrocytes and increased levels may indicate replacement of neurons by astrocytes	• Traumatic injury • Hyponatremia • SIADH	• Hepatic encephalopathy • Hypoxic injury
8. Succinate	2.4 Singlet	Abscesses with anaerobic metabolism		Succinate > acetate indicative of parasitic abscesses
9. Acetate	1.9 Singlet	Abscesses with anaerobic metabolism		Acetate > succinate indicative of pyogenic
10. Amino acids	0.9 Doublet /triplet Inverted at TE 144 ms	Necessary for protein synthesis		Hypervalinemia Branched-chain ketonuria MSUD Brain abscess
11. Glycine	3.5 Singlet Long TE	Inhibitory neurotransmitter and antioxidant		Pyogenic abscess Hyperglycinemia tumor
12. Alanine	1.5 Doublet/triplet Inverted at TE 144 ms	Produced by transamination of pyruvate in hypoxic tissues		Pyogenic abscess Meningloma Central neurocytoma PNET
13. Trehalose	3.6–3.8	Disaccharide		Fungal infections

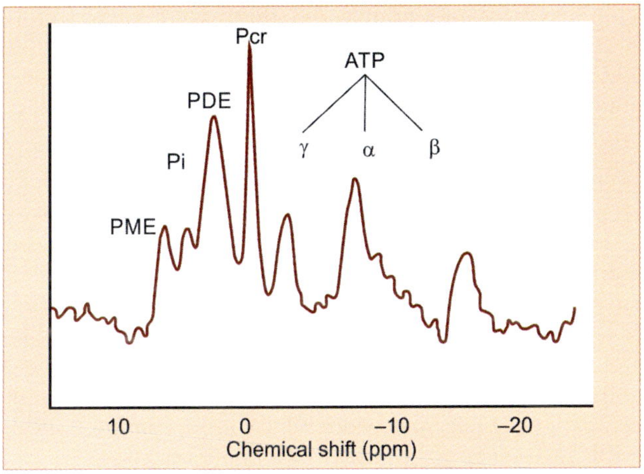

FIG. 3: Normal 31P-MRS of brain.

phosphomonoesters (PME) composed of phosphocholine, phosphoethanolamine and sugar phosphates. It is dependent on metabolic state of the cell. The next peak is due to inorganic phosphate (Pi) composed of monobasic and dibasic inorganic phosphate. In acidosis, there is chemical shifts of Pi towards up-field in contrast to shift of Pi to the down-field in alkalosis and can be used to estimate intracellular pH. The next phosphodiesters (PDE) peak is composed of glycerophosphocholine and phosphoethanolamine followed by phosphocreatine (PCr) peak. Then follows three peaks of ATP – γ, α, β. The β ATP is frequently used to assess ATP concentration.

The other nuclei like 13_{C}, 23_{Na}, 39_{K}, 19_{F}, 7_{Li}, 14_{N}, 15_{N} also exhibit MRS activity and are of research utility at present rather than of clinical significance.[13]

LOCALIZATION TECHNIQUES

The volume of interest when localized precisely leads to a clean spectra that are essential for accurate interpretation of MRS data. There are two types of localization techniques, i.e.(a) by using main magnetic field gradient (B0 field) and (b) by using RF field gradient (B1 field).

B_1 Field Gradient Methods

Surface Coils

Surface coil provides adequate localization of the metabolites insurface tissues close to the coil with good sensitivity. There is inherent inhomogeneity of surface coils. For studies requiring more precise localization or to quantitate metabolites, other localization methods are warranted. Surface spoiling by the use of grid of wires helps alpine eliminating signals from the surface of the tissue with preservation of signal originating from deep layer of the tissue.[14] Inhomogeneity of the surface coils can be used to advantage in localization methods by "rotating frame imaging". By this way, 2D Fourier transformation of the data, sets produces 1D metabolic map where sequential spectra represent greater distance from the surface coil.[15]

B_0 Field Gradient Methods

Static Field Gradient

By using static homogeneous magnetic field over a small volume, ^{31}P-MRS is possible in brain and liver. But this technique is difficult and has limited use.

Slice-selective B_0-gradient Techniques

DRESS

Depth-resolved surface spectroscopy (DRESS) is the simplest gradient localization method. A single plane-selective radiofrequency (RF) pulse is applied to the volume of tissue and data acquisition is done. This method is crude and suffers from lack of information at the center of RF pulse producing baseline artifacts. The sequence can also be used in slice-interleaved multislice mode (SLIT-DRESS). The water suppression is achieved by using a long, low amplitude Gaussian pulse.

3D Localization Methods

Two major localization techniques of the MRS signal are: Single voxel spectroscopy (SVS) and spectroscopic imaging (MRSI) or chemical shift imaging (CSI).

The pulse sequences used in single-voxel spectroscopy are as follows:

a. **STEAM:** The stimulated-echo acquisition mode (STEAM) of localization for ^{1}H-MRS is constituted by three 90° selective pulses, each applied with an orthogonal gradient for slice excitation. This sequence is simple and robust but there is approximately 50% signal loss. It is not suitable for observation of nuclei having short T2 values.[16]
b. **PRESS:** The point-resolved spectroscopy (PRESS) localization consists of a sequence of 90–180–180° pulses which are applied with orthogonal gradient. Unlike STEAM, no signal loss is seen. The PRESS sequence has the disadvantage that it cannot be applied in short TE values (<40 ms). Water suppression is done by using a gaussian pulse preceding the localization pulses. A variant of this sequence is MESA by using binomial (1331) pulse to achieve water suppression followed by a train of three 180–180–180° pulses.
c. **ISIS:** Image selected *in vivo* spectroscopy (ISIS) consists of three inversion pulses and a fourth nonselective pulse. It requires a minimum eight phase cycles to localize the signal. There is minimum loss from T2 relaxation and especially useful for nuclei having short T2 values like ^{31}P.

Chemical shift imaging (CSI): Using phase encoding strategies, it is possible to encode information from multiple voxels simultaneously. Phase encoding can be applied in multiple dimensions. Data are translated to extract chemical shift information from multiple positions using up to 4D Fourier transformations. MRSI has the advantage of obtaining multiple spectra in one data acquisition. The technique requires a larger volume homogeneous magnetic field as compared to than SVS.[4] The vast quantity of data generated with CSI make management, analysis and interpretation of CSI spectra a daunting challenge in the clinical setting.

Figures 4A to F show the various localization pulse sequence methods.

Single Voxel Versus Multivoxel Spectroscopy

Comparative description between the SVS and MRSI is shown in **Table 5**.

As the RF pulses have a nonrectangular profile, the spatial origin of signal in a voxel does not coincide with the rectangular shape of the voxel in MRSI and signal from one voxel is contaminated by signal in others leading to phenomenon known as voxel bleeding. This is more pertinent when interpreting the lipid signals in MRSI, because the lipid signal from the subcutaneous regions such as scalp is about a thousand times in magnitude than the signal of metabolites and can lead to significant voxel bleeding and interference with spectroscopy findings. For the same reason, SVS is usually the method of choice when accurate quantification of metabolites is required where voxel bleeding phenomenon is not significant.[4]

Quantitative Spectroscopy

Measurement of the concentration of metabolites (quantification) is essential to facilitate distinction between normal and diseased tissue and for comparison of results from different laboratories. Quantification relies on calibration of resonance signals with internal or external standard or phantom. The area under a resonance signal is proportional to the number of nuclei, one can find out concentration of an unknown peak. Peak width relates to T2 relaxation. Peak width and height can also be used for quantification.

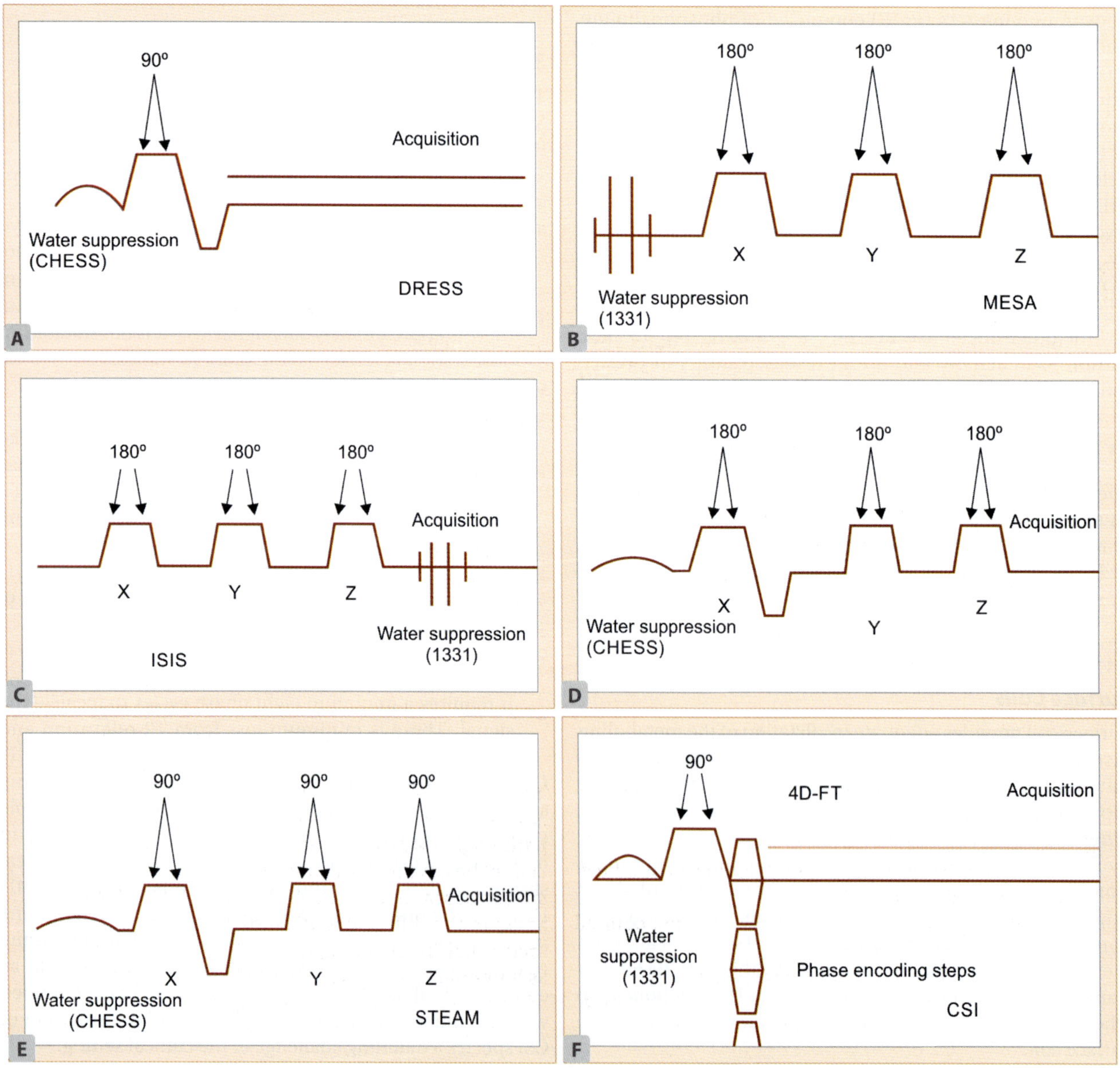

FIGS. 4A TO F: Different techniques of localization in MRS.

TABLE 5: Comparison between SVS and MRSI.[17]

Technique	SVS	MRSI
• TE • Voxel size (cm^3) • Scan times (min) • Shimming • Lipid and water suppression • Processing	• Short or long • 4–20 • 5–10 • Local • Good • Simple processing	• Usually long • 1–4 • 5–30 • Globalized • Worse • Processing time consuming
When to use	• Single focal lesion or diffuse disease • Single query, e.g. abscess vs. tumor • Complementary to MRSI (e.g. different TE in SVS) • Areas close to skull	• Multiple or heterogeneous lesions • Diffuse disease • Comparative assessment of brain regions required
Advantage	• High data quality • Fast • Voxel boundaries better defined • Automatic water reference acquisition • Limited dataset can be used even if aborted early	• Information about heterogeneity of the tissue • Retrospective selection of the ROI can be done in the investigated volume • Smaller voxel volumes used to assess metabolite distribution
Disadvantage	• Selected volume is accurate placement of ROI required at time of investigation • No information on spatial heterogeneity of lesion • No information of normal brain	• More processing required to minimize spectral loss due to insufficient lipid and water suppression • Longer acquisition times • Experienced needed to plan

Data Acquisition and Analysis

The following steps are roughly the guidelines for proper spectral acquisition and analysis:

Voxel positioning: Accurate and proper or pure voxel positioning is essential to acquire good spectra (avoid scalp and CSF). Thin-slice high resolution image acquisition and the best positioning of the voxel within the image is the correct way to achieve best spectral information.

Shimming: Adjustment of the magnetic field homogeneity over the voxel is time consuming. The largest source of variation is due to field inhomogeneity.

Water suppression: The large water signal must be suppressed completely to obtain weaker signal of tissue metabolites. There are three techniques to achieve water suppression:

1. Gaussian chemical shift selective (CHESS) pulses.
2. A narrow band pulse (<50 Hz) is applied prior to localization pulse.
3. Binomial pulse sequence (1331 pulse).

This sequence of RF pulses excite the metabolites of interest and not the water and can be used prior or later to localization pulses.

- Inversion recovery and long echo-times.
- *RF calibration*: The signal strength is optimized by adjusting the amplitude of the pulses.

Averaging: To improve SNR, multiple signals are acquired and average values are recorded.

- Fourier transformation (FT) and phase encoding.
- Baseline correction, curve fitting, relaxation time corrections and normal values in control subjects.
- These steps help in proper quantification and to produce uniformity of spectral studies.

CLINICAL APPLICATIONS OF MRS OF BRAIN

In the last few decades there is phenomenal growth of MRS both *in vitro* and *in vivo* applications. This chapter will focus mainly on the utility of ^{1}H-MRS in neurological disorders; although ^{31}P-MRS is useful in the investigation of mitochondrial diseases. Most centers studying the brain with spectroscopy heavily rely upon ^{1}H-MRS. There are several reasons for this: first, the hardware required for ^{1}H-MRS is the same as that used for conventional brain MRI and ^{1}H-MRS can be implemented on most standard commercial scanners operating at 1.5 tesla without the need for hardware modification that would be required to operate at a frequency other than that used for hydrogen. Second, because the MR is much more sensitive to protons as compared to phosphorus, ^{1}H-MRS provides spatial resolution that is best suitable for examining brain pathology. Third, the information available from changes in the level of NAA as measured by ^{1}H-MRS, provides specific chemical pathologic evidence of neuronal injury, information that cannot be obtained with any other MRS. The goal of clinical spectroscopy is to provide biochemical information to assist in the differential diagnosis when standard clinical images fail. There is a rapid growth of clinical MRS in brain as immobilization of head is relatively easy, close proximity of brain to surface and lack of lipid signals that may contaminate spectra. It is of diagnostic value for evaluating and monitoring the progression of stroke, ischemic injury, brain tumors, epilepsy, white matter disorders, Alzheimer's disease, HIV infection, etc.

Brain Tumors

Both proton and phosphorus spectroscopy provide diverse metabolic patterns in brain tumors. Proton MRS generally shows increased Cho/Cr ratio and lactate level, decreased NAA (or complete absence) and Cr. Cho is generally increased in solid portion of the tumor and decreased in the central necrotic portion. ^{31}P-MRS studies show decreased concentration of all metabolites relative to normal brain reflecting loss of viable tissue. Alkaline pH, increased PME, decreased PDE and P Cr are the typical findings in tumors.[18-22]

The following are the major clinical applications of MRS in patients with brain tumors:

Noninvasive diagnosis and grading of cerebral space occupying lesions.

Grading of Glial Tumors

Spectroscopy findings of astrocytomas reveal elevated choline, reduced Cr and NAA in comparison to the normal brain **(Figs. 5 and 6)**. A higher grade of malignancy is indicated by presence of lactate and lipid peaks reflecting tumor necrosis and hypoxia. Elevated choline peak reflects increased cellularity and membrane synthesis. Localized astrocytomas particularly pilocystic astrocytoma shows raised Cho, low NAA, and presence of a lactate peak—paradoxical findings that are more characteristic of malignant neoplasms than this clinically benign-behaving tumor.[23]

Differentiation between IDH Mutant and Wild Type Astrocytomas

IDH-mutant astrocytoma shows a 2-hydroxyglutarate (2-HG) peak resonating at 2.25 ppm which is not seen in wild type.[24]

Medulloblastoma

Medulloblastomas are characterized by high choline peak, absent or low lipid and taurine peak at 3.4 ppm (relatively specific).[25]

Meningiomas versus GBM

The distinction between an intra-axial GBM and an extra-axial lesion, such as meningiomas is not difficult in the majority of cases, occasionally such distinctions are problematic and in such cases ^{1}H-MRS helps in differentiating them. The spectra from the meningioma show low NAA as well as a alanine peak[26] (Ala) **(Figs. 7A to C)**. Spectra from GBM on the other hand show a different metabolite profile as discussed earlier.

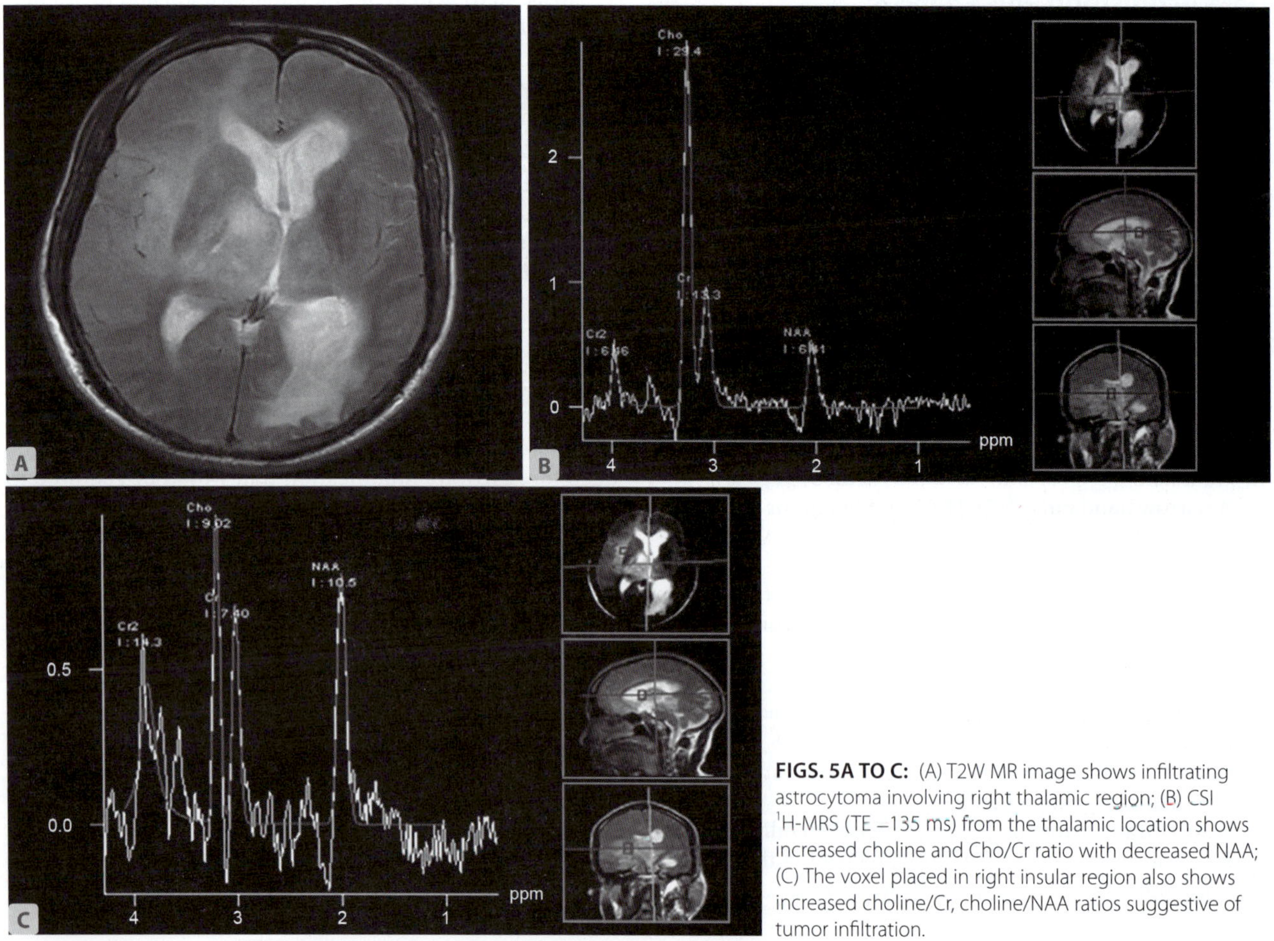

FIGS. 5A TO C: (A) T2W MR image shows infiltrating astrocytoma involving right thalamic region; (B) CSI ^{1}H-MRS (TE –135 ms) from the thalamic location shows increased choline and Cho/Cr ratio with decreased NAA; (C) The voxel placed in right insular region also shows increased choline/Cr, choline/NAA ratios suggestive of tumor infiltration.

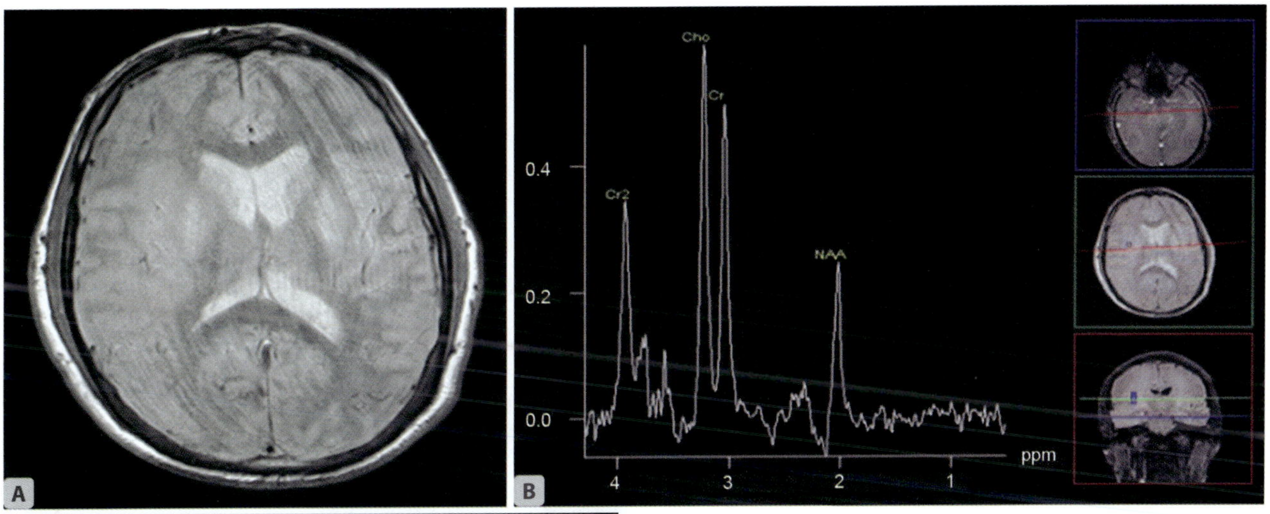

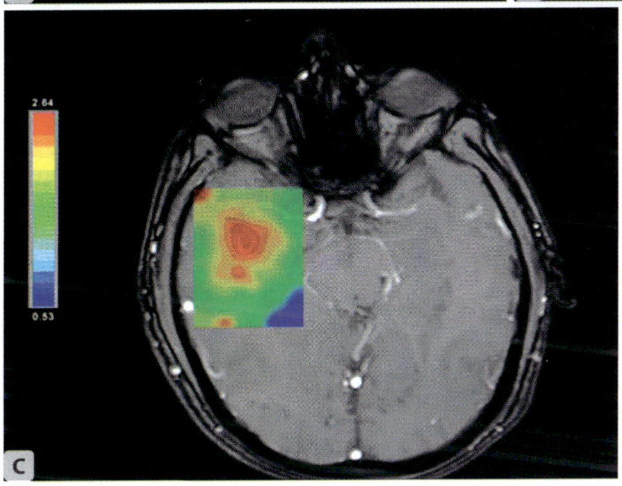

FIGS. 6A TO C: (A) T2W MR image shows ill-defined hyperintense lesion in right insular region; (B) CSI ^{1}H-MRS (TE = 135 ms) from the lesions shows increased choline and Cho/Cr ratio with decreased NAA; (C) Metabolic map shows mapping of choline/NAA ratios with the red-colored areas predicting the yield areas for pathologically higher grade foci of tumor.

Metastases

Spectroscopy findings in metastases show reduction of NAA and Cr with high choline values similar to those of gliomas. They may also contain lipid/lactate peak depending on presence of necrosis. One characteristic that differentiates them from glioma is the defined margins of metastatis, with usually no abnormal spectroscopic findings in surrounding edema. Gliomas on the other hand usually show abnormal spectroscopic findings which can extend beyond the enhancing borders.**(Figs. 8A to C)**.

Lymphoma

These lesions show reduced NAA and high choline with infiltration of adjacent brain. MRS findings may be indistinguishable from gliomas.

Table 6 summarizes the commonly found metabolites in the evaluation of brain tumors.[20]

Tumor Extent (Edema vs. Infiltration)

Spectroscopy can differentiate vasogenic edema from infiltration as in cases of vasogenic edema no abnormal metabolic ratios are seen whereas in cases of infiltration there is demonstrable raised choline and reduced NAA peaks **(Fig. 5C)**. Thus, MRS can aid in depiction of tumor margins for adequate resection and appropriate planning of radiation therapy.[7]

Therapeutic Planning for Gliomas: Utility of Mrs for Identifying Tumor and Predicting Response to Therapy

Metabolite maps from ^{1}H-MRS can be used to suggest regions of higher grade in tumors and to plan stereotactic biopsies and selective tumor resection **(Figs. 6A to C)**. Metabolic changes on chemical profile have also been used to predict chemotherapeutic sensitivity prior to intervention as well as to monitor the response to drug and radiation therapy.

Distinction between Radiation Necrosis and Recurrent Tumor in Postoperative Patients

This is the most common scenario for which MRS is utilized in clinical neuroimaging. This diagnostic dilemma has not been solved by any of the numerous advances in MRI because both of these pathologies are seen as heterogeneous mass lesions with enhancement and edema. MRS has been used to diagnose recurrent tumor, mainly based on relative increases in choline, as opposed to MRS in radiation necrosis, which generally shows low levels **(Figs. 9 and 10)**.[23-25]

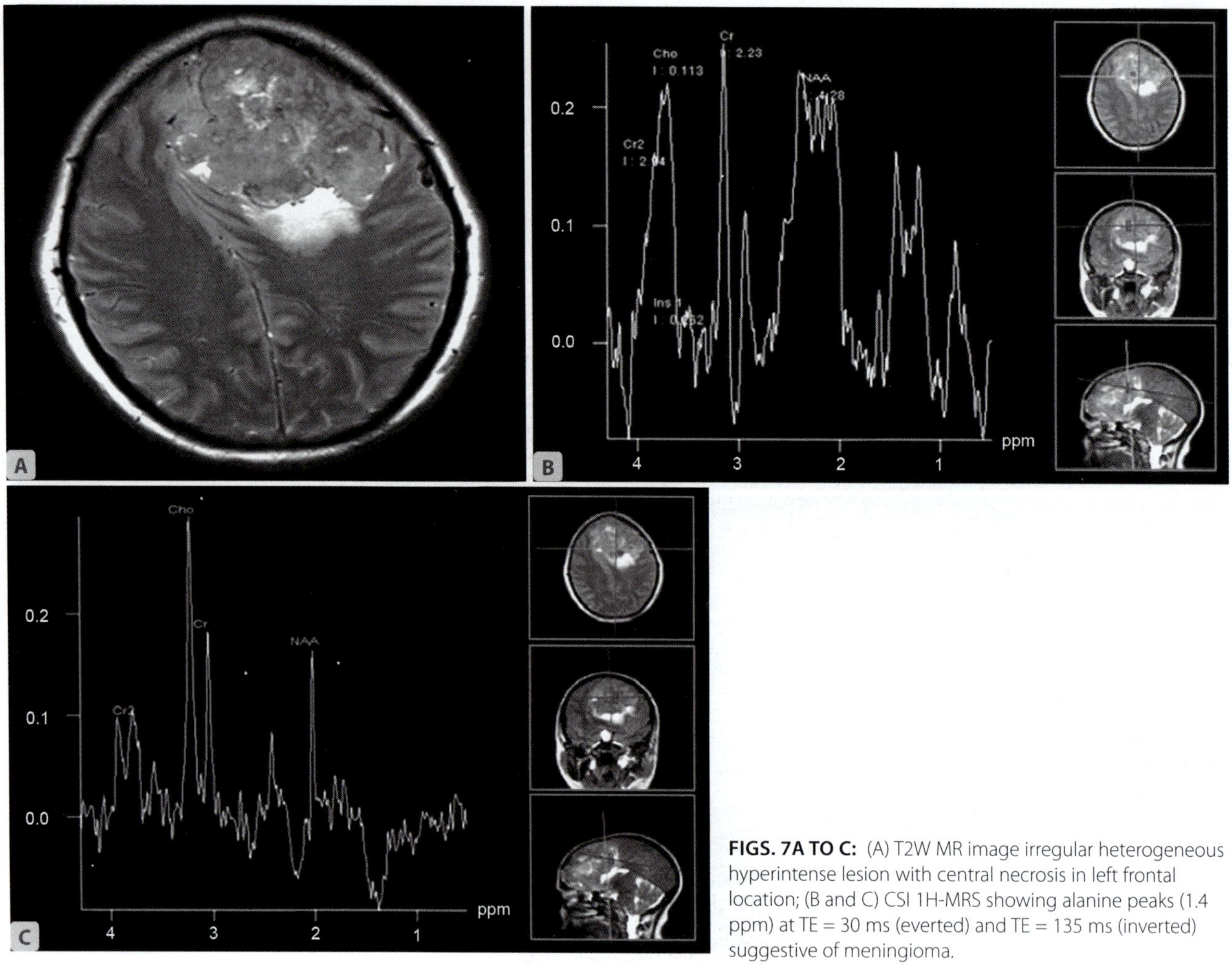

FIGS. 7A TO C: (A) T2W MR image irregular heterogeneous hyperintense lesion with central necrosis in left frontal location; (B and C) CSI 1H-MRS showing alanine peaks (1.4 ppm) at TE = 30 ms (everted) and TE = 135 ms (inverted) suggestive of meningioma.

Differentiation of Intracranial Ring Enhancing Lesions (Table 7)

Necrotic Brain Tumor versus Abscess

Pyogenic brain abscesses shows resonance from amino acids, succinate, acetate and lactate peaks on MR spectroscopy. In contrast, spectra from the necrotic areas of tumors show only lactate peak. The tubercular abscesses and the necrotic tumors both may show lactate levels. But the necrotic high grade tumors significantly elevated Cho/NAA ratios whereas tubercular abscesses show high lipid peaks **(Figs. 11 and 12)**.[26-32]

Pyogenic Abscess versus Tubercular Abscess

Pyogenic brain abscesses show presence of lipid/lactate and amino acid peaks with presence of other metabolites such as succinate and acetate **(Figs. 13 and 14)**, while tuberculous abscesses show only lipid and lactate levels **(Figs. 15A to C)**. Further etiological categorization of pyogenic abscess can also be done by MRS. Aerobic or anaerobic brain abscesses may be differentiated on MRS based on presence of acetate and succinate peaks which are seen only in anaerobic brain abscesses.[29]

Neurocysticercosis versus Intracranial Tuberculoma

It is not always easy to distinguish NCC from tuberculomas based on the CT and MRI findings and MRS may act as a problem solving tool.[33] Evaluation of inflammatory granulomas with ^{1}H-MRS reveals very low level of normal metabolites in NCC with succinate peak **(Figs. 16A and B)** whereas tuberculomas are characterized by prominent lipid resonances due to large lipid fraction present in tubercular bacilli. Lipids are seen in more than 80% of tuberculomas while other nonspecific granulomas and NCC showed lipid in 20% of cases.[33,34] Studies have shown that tuberculomas had prominent lipids, higher choline and reduced NAA and Cr with a Cho/Cr ratio greater than 1 in all tuberculomas as compared to NCC.[35]

MRS IN PEDIATRICS

The metabolic spectra in developing brain are different from those of adult brain, a fact that is important to know before describing the pathological changes in the children.

Low NAA is seen at birth and shows rapid increase during first year with attainment of final values at the age of 3–5 years

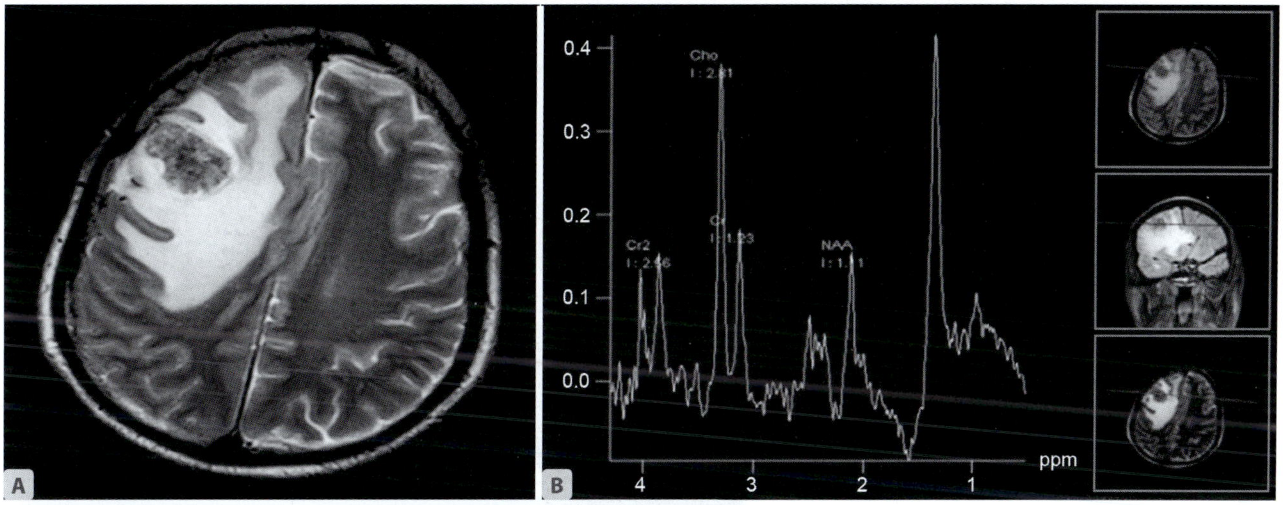

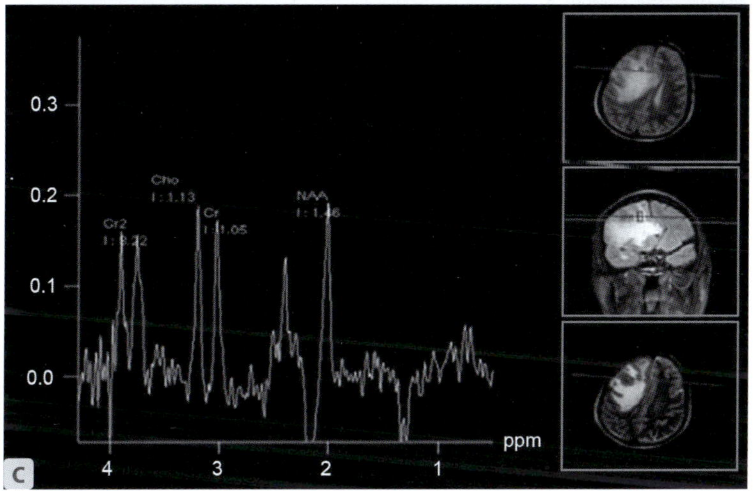

FIGS. 8A TO C: (A) T2W MR image showing heterogeneous lesion with intense perilesional edema in right frontal location; (B) CSI ^{1}H-MRS of the lesion shows marked increase in the Choline/NAA ratios with significant lipid lactate peaks suggestive of metastasis; (C) Voxel placed in perilesional edema shows no Cho/NAA ratio reversal.

TABLE 6: Metabolite patterns in brain tumors

	Major metabolic changes				
Major tumor types	**NAA**	**Cho**	**Cr**	**ml**	**Lip**
Grade II glioma	↓	↑	↓	↑↑/=	-
Grade III glioma	↓↓	↑↑	↓	↑/=	+/-
GBM	↓↓↓	↑↑↑	↓↓	=/↓	++
Lymphoma	↓↓	↑↑↑	↓↓	↓↓	++
Metastasis	↓↓	↑↑	↓↓	↓↓	++
Meningioma	↓↓↓	↑	↓↓	↓↓	+/-

which is correlated with the ongoing neuronal maturation. Choline compounds show a high peak in neonatal age with decrease as cerebral maturation progresses. Myoinositol is the highest peak at 3.5 ppm on spectroscopy of newborn and it rapidly decreases with age.[36]

Prematurity and Birth Asphyxia

In birth asphyxia, there is decrease in PCr/Pi ratio compared to control subjects.[37] Ratio of PCr/Pi below 0.8 is associated with poor prognosis.[38] There is also decrease in Pi/ATP ratio. Increase in lactate/NAA ratio and decrease in NAA level may convey poor prognosis.

Metabolic Disorders and Leukodystrophies

Hepatic encephalopathy is one acquired metabolic disorder that is currently diagnostic with ^{1}H MRS. In this condition, ^{1}H-MRS shows an elevation of glutamine levels and a reduction in choline and myoinositol levels **(Figs. 17A and B)**.

Currently, the MR spectroscopy is not very sensitive *in vivo* to measure the specific metabolite or other markers e.g enzymes, proteins responsible for specific metabolic disorder. However, it can detect the secondary changes that results from these disorder and can help in diagnosis **(Table 8)**. Examples of such situations include:

- Prominent NAA in Canavan's disease **(Figs. 18A and B)**
- Lactate peak in mitochondrial disorders[12]

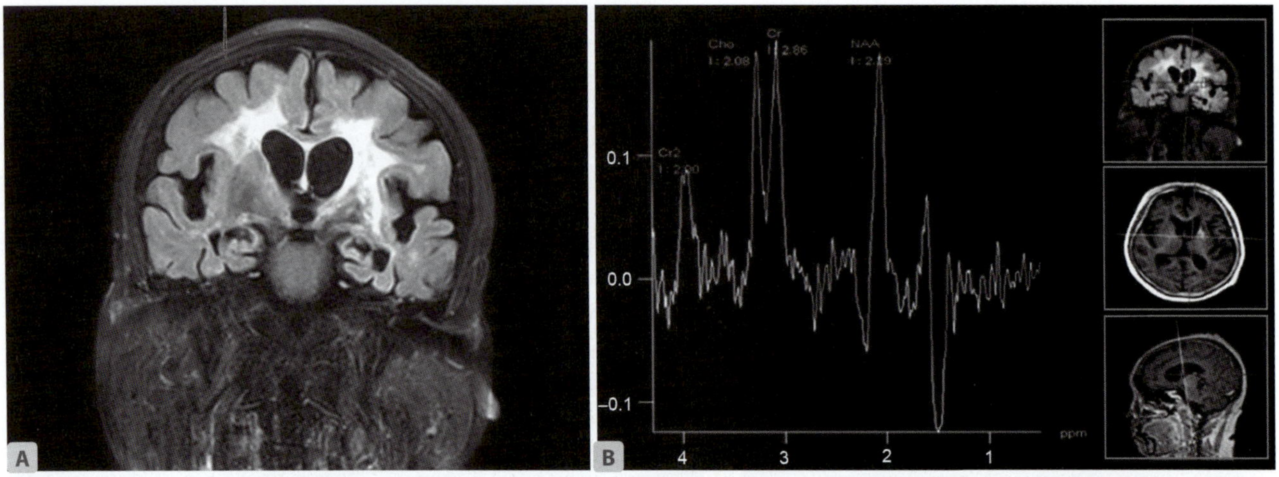

FIGS. 9A AND B: (A) Postcontrast T1W MR image of a postoperative and postradiotherapy of infiltrating astrocytoma showing irregular ring enhancing lesion in the postoperative location; (B) CSI ^{1}H-MRS TE = 135 ms) of the lesion shows marked increase in the Choline/NAA ratios with no significant lactate peaks suggestive of recurrent tumor.

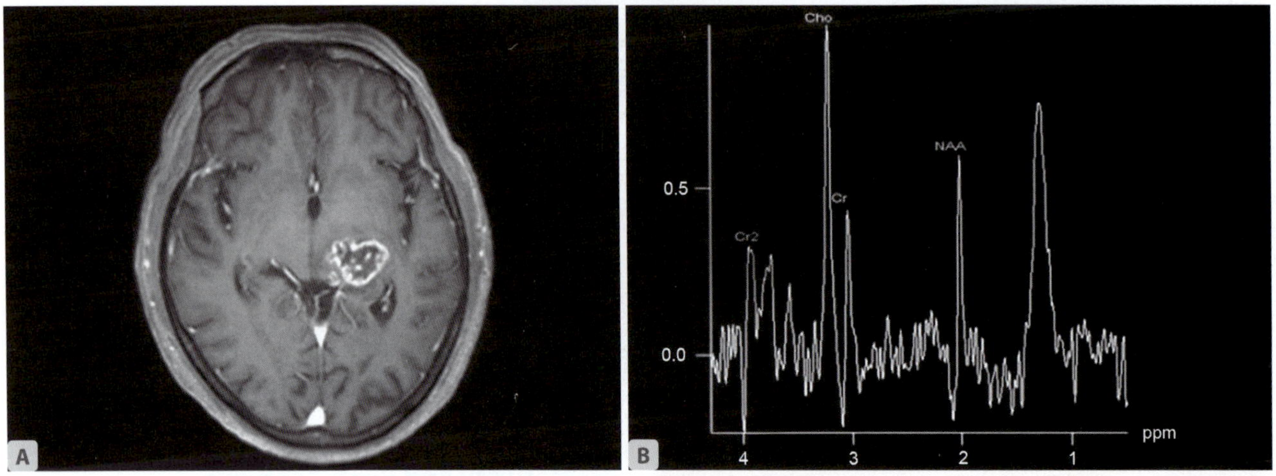

FIGS. 10A AND B: (A) FLAIR image of postradiotherapy of lymphoma showing hyperintense lesions in bilateral periventricular locations; (B) CSI ^{1}H-MRS of the periventricular lesion shows no significant increase in the Choline/NAA ratios with presence of inverted lactate peak.

Patients with PKAN (pantothenate kinase associated neurodegeneration) show spectral broadening due to magnetic inhomogeneity caused by iron deposition in the globus pallidus. Rare metabolic disorders like defective NAA synthesis due to N-acetylaspertase deficiency and defective creatinine synthesis due to arginine: glycine amidinotransferase (AGAT) and guanidino acetate methyl transferase (GAMT) deficiency may not show any signal changes on conventional MR imaging. The spectroscopy in these disorders shows absence of NAA and creatine peaks respectively.[36]

MAGNETIC RESONANCE SPECTROSCOPY IN EPILEPSY

Lateralization in Temporal Lobe Epilepsy

Magnetic resonance spectroscopy can depict the metabolic changes that may precede any definitive imaging changes in the hippocampus in mesial temporal lobe epilepsy which can be seen as normal findings on conventional MRI.[37-40] Such findings are typical for bitemporal lesions or for extratemporal epilepsies. It is also very helpful for lateralization of epileptic focus.[41] There is reduction of NAA and NAA/(Cr + Cho) ratio in the ipsilateral hippocampus. NAA/Cr is also reduced in the ipsilateral frontal lobe in patients with frontal lobe epilepsy. Similarly, ^{31}P MRS shows increase in pH and decrease in Pi in the involved hippocampus or frontal lobe.[22] Alterations of metabolic activity and neuronal integrity persist interictally and make it possible to lateralize the epileptic focus. Therefore, MRSI provides useful information in preoperative planning of epilepsy surgery.[42]

MRS in Neurodegenerative Diseases

Alzheimer's Disease

Alzheimer's disease (AD) is slowly progressive disease with loss of cognitive function and is one of the most common causes of dementia. The diagnosis is usually achieved in autopsy. There is decreased NAA and NAA/Cr in frontoparietal, temporal lobes and hippocampus. Myoinositol is found to be increased in AD but this is nonspecific. The ratio of NAA/Cr is not changed in NPH and therefore can be differentiate from AD. ^{31}P-MRS shows increased PME and decreased PCr in the initial stages of AD. As dementia worsens, the level of PME decreases and the level of PCr increases. ^{31}P-MRS can also distinguish AD from multiinfarct dementia (MID).[43] In MID, there is elevation of P Cr/Pi ratio in both the temporoparietal and frontal regions. Whereas PME and the ratio of PME/PDE are elevated in AD in the temporoparietal lobe. Pi is also elevated in the frontal and temporoparietal regions of AD. These spectral profiles are accurate in distinguish MID from AD in more than 100% cases.

TABLE 7: MRS findings in various ring enhancing lesions.

Lesion	MRS findings
Primary neoplasm/ glioma	Decreased NAA Raised choline Lactate peak 2 hydroxyglutarate at 2.25 ppm in mutant type astrocytoma
Metastasis	Decreased NAA Raised choline Lactate peak Normal spectra in edema
Pyogenic abscess	Lactate lipid peak Amino acid peak Acetate and succinate peak
Tubercular abscess	Prominent lipid peak Lactate peak
Fungal abscess	Variable NAA and choline Lipid lactate peak Amino acids Trehalose peak
Demyelination	Variable findings Increased choline NAA/cr higher than tumors Lactate Glutamate peak
Lymphoma	Raised choline Mild increase lipid/lactate Variably decreased NAA/Cr
Toxoplasma	Lipid lactate peak Suppressed normal metabolites

Amyotrophic Lateral Sclerosis (ALS)

^{1}H-MRS in ALS has demonstrated decreased cortical NAA which was maximal in the motor cortex. The level of NAA has been found to decrease overtime as the disease progresses. Glutamate excitotoxicity has been proposed to be cause of neuronal loss in ALS. ^{1}H-MRS has shown increased signals from glutamate and glutamine in these patients. ^{1}H-MRS findings in patients after treatment with Riluzole (a drug that inhibits glutamate release from presynaptic terminals), the level of NAA increases in these patients which may reflect the reversal of injury.

Idiopathic Parkinson's Disease (IPD) versus Other Parkinsonian Syndromes

In IPD, the primary pathology is thought to be in the substantia nigra and the volume of nigral axonal terminals lost in the basal ganglia are too small to be measured by current MRS techniques and so in IPD, the metabolic resonances do not appear to be changed in the basal ganglia or in the cortex. In contrast, various other parkinsonian syndromes such as progressive supranuclear palsy and multisystem atrophy (MSA) demonstrate significant decreases of NAA/Cho and NAA/Cr in the lentiform nucleus and striatum.

Huntington's Disease (HD)

This condition may affect neurons throughout the brain, but targets initially the cells in the basal ganglia. Studies have shown that in humans NAA/Cho is reduced both in the basal

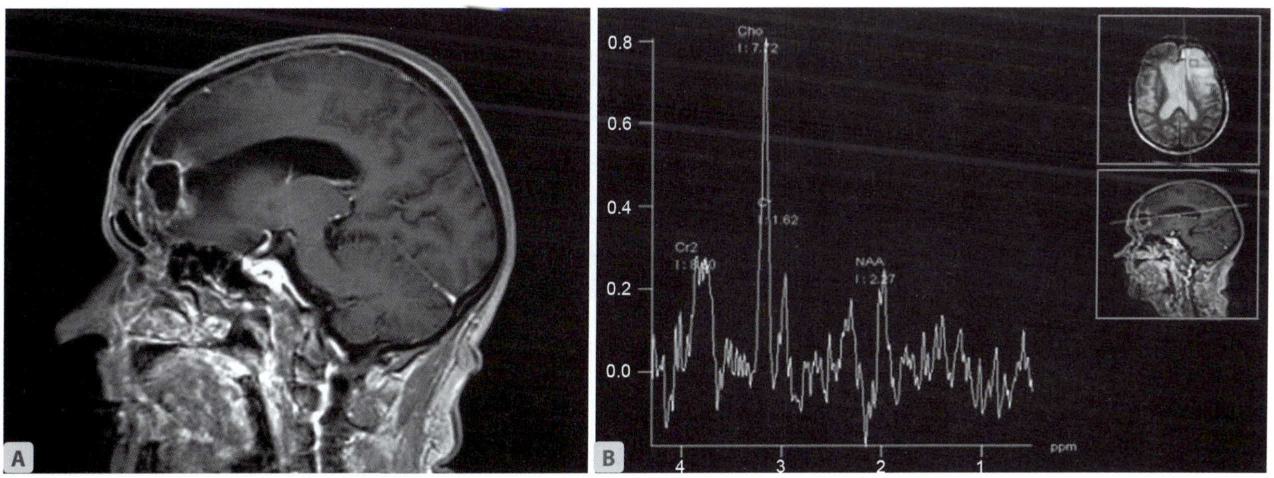

FIGS. 11A AND B: (A) Postcontrast MR image shows ring enhancing lesion in left thalamic location with mass effect—biopsy proven glioma WHO-grade IV; (B) CSI ^{1}H-MRS from the lesion at TE 135 ms shows Cho/NAA. Note the prominent lipid peak that may also be seen in gliomas.

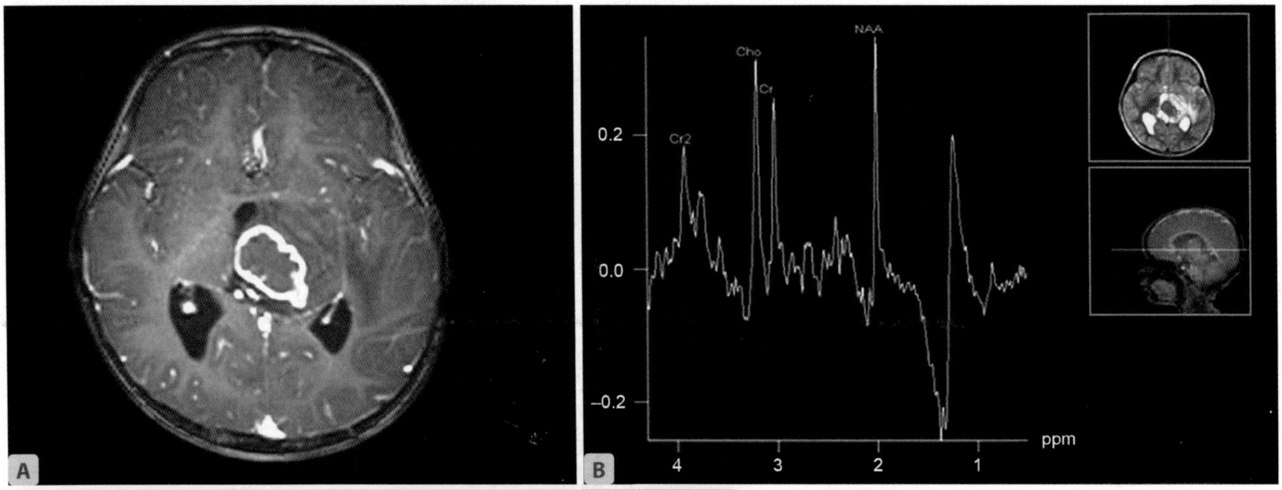

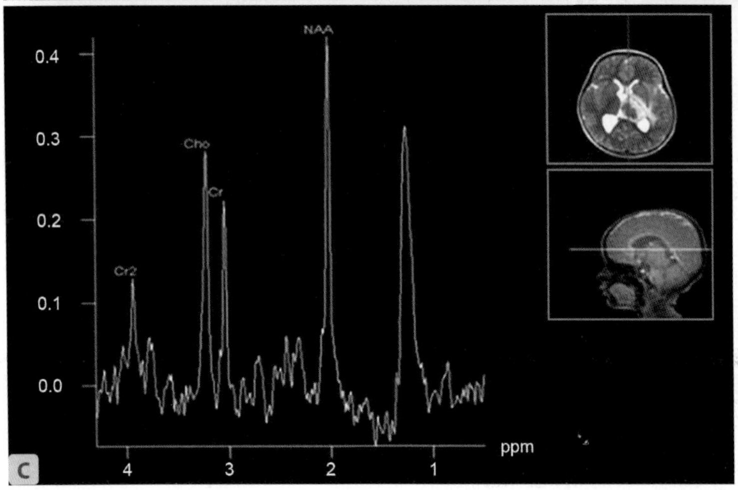

FIGS. 12A TO C: (A) Postcontrast MR image shows ring enhancing lesion in left thalamic location with mass effect; (B and C) CSI ^{1}H-MRS from the lesion at TE 135 ms and 30 ms shows lipid peak that is more prominent at low TE and the lactate doublet.

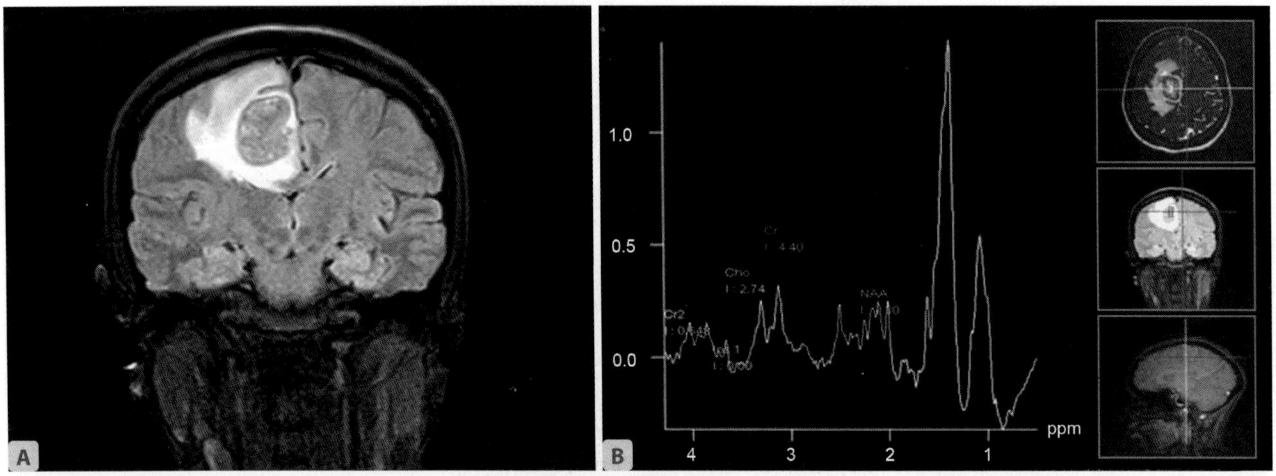

FIGS. 13A AND B: (A) FLAIR image shows heterogeneous ring lesion (pyogenic abscess); (B) CSI ^{1}H-MRS (TE = 30) shows decreased normal metabolites (NAA, Choline, Creatine) and increased amino acids (0.9 ppm), succinate (2.4 ppm) and lipid lactate peaks.

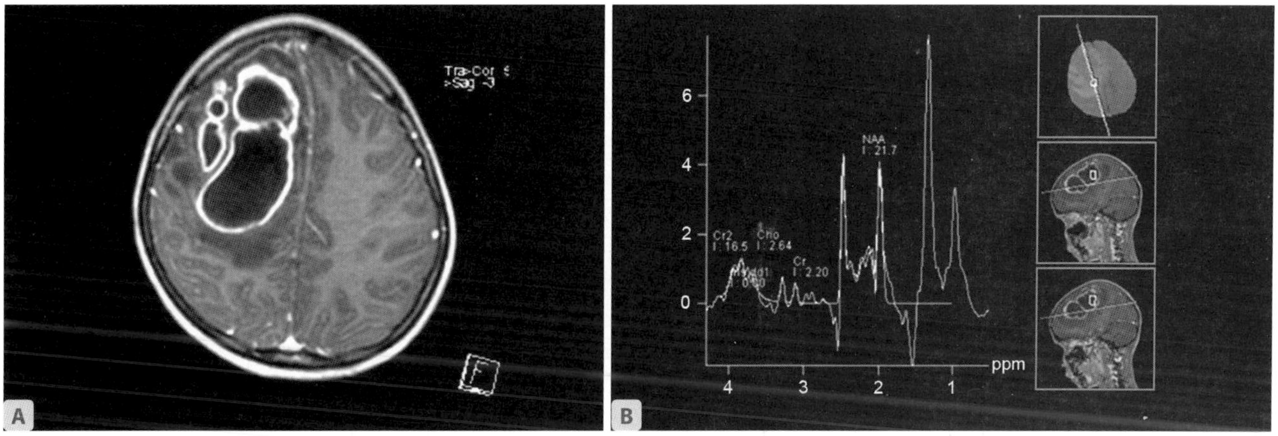

FIGS. 14A AND B: (A) Postcontrast axial images in a 10-year-old male patient show multiple ring enhancing lesions in right frontal lobe; (B) CSI ^{1}H-MRS (TE = 30) shows presence of increased amino acids (0.9 ppm), succinate (2.4 ppm) and lipid lactate peaks (1.3 ppm) s/o pyogenic abscess.

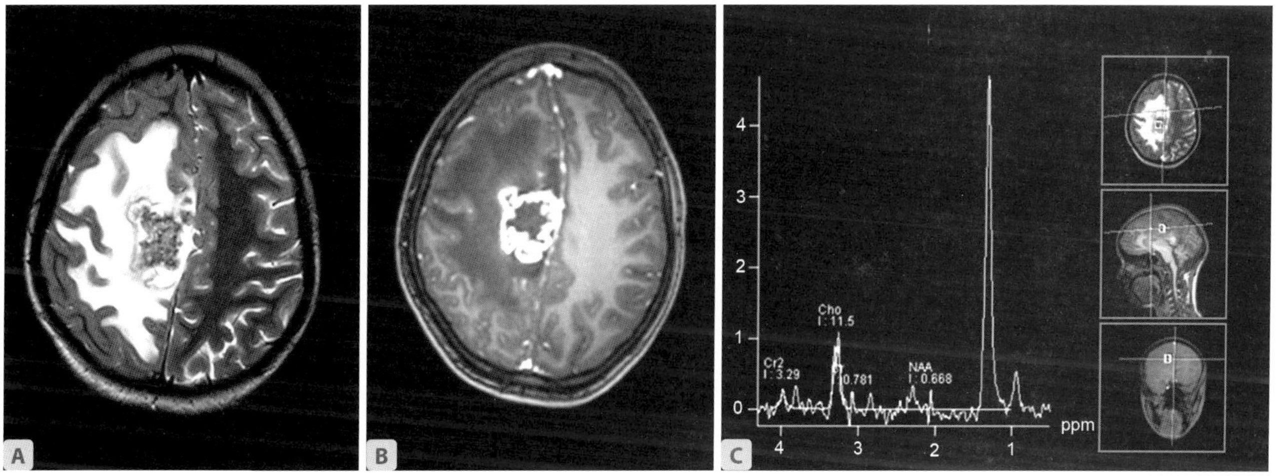

FIGS. 15A TO C: (A) Axial T2w images show heterogeneous hypointense lesion in right frontal lobe with surrounding marked edema. (B) Postcontrast MR image shows ring enhancement; (B and C) CSI ^{1}H-MRS from the lesion at TE 30 ms shows prominent lipid peak. Biopsy came out tuberculosis.

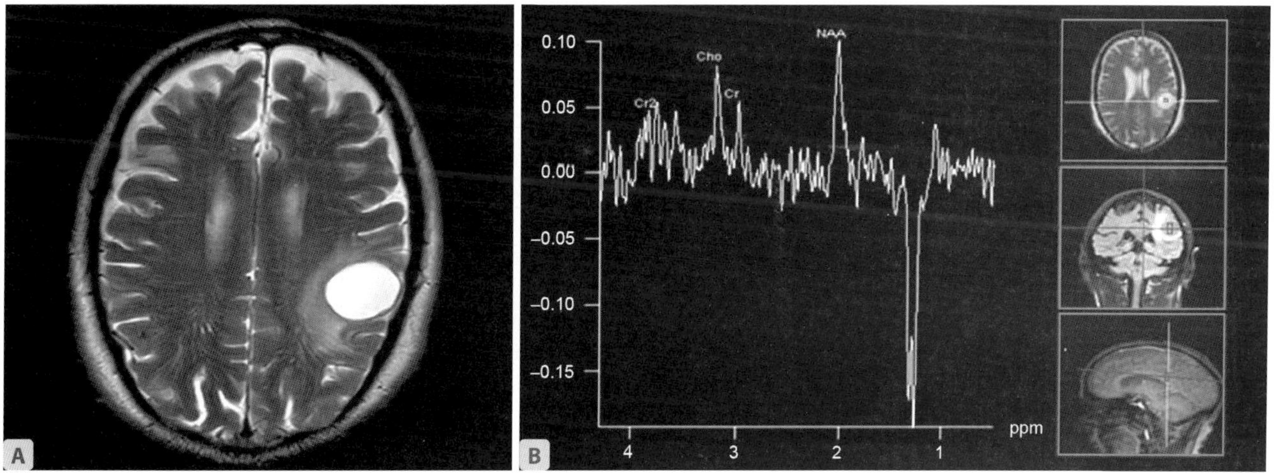

FIGS. 16A AND B: (A) 55-year-old patient with neurocysticercosis. (A) T2 axial MR image shows cystic lesion in left parietal cortex; (B) CSI ^{1}H-MRS (TE = 135 ms) shows lactate peak at 1.3 ppm with decreased normal metabolites.

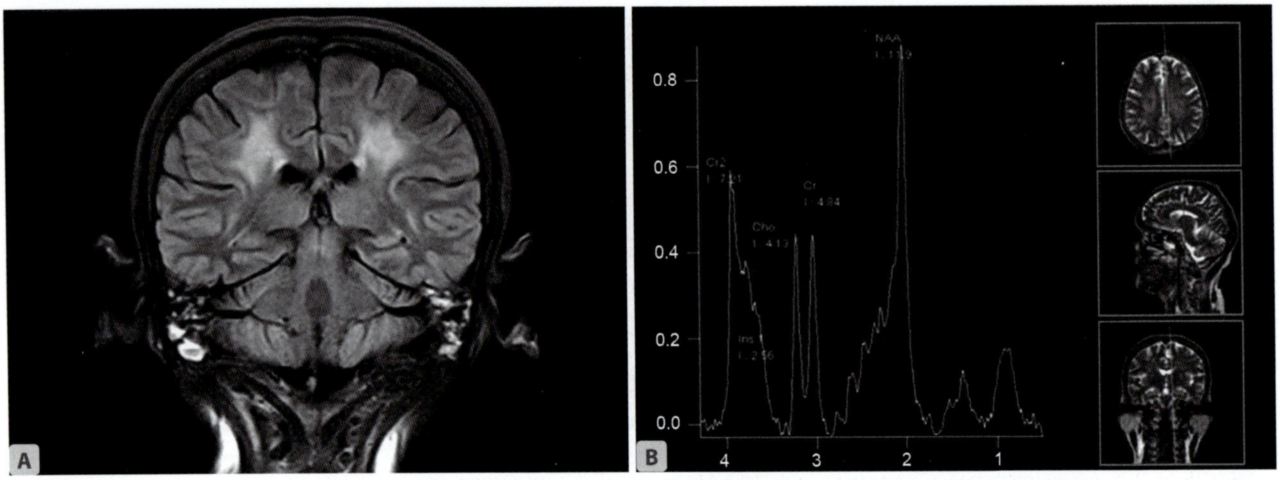

FIGS. 17A AND B: (A) 45-year-old patient with cirrhosis and encephalopathy. (A) FLAIR MR image shows hyperintensities in bilateral centrum semiovale; (B) CSI ^{1}H-MRS (TE = 30 ms) shows glutamate and glutamine peak at 2.5 ppm.

TABLE 8: Spectroscopic findings in hereditary metabolic disorders.

	Cho	Cr	NAA	Lac	Others
(A) Mitochondrial encephalomyopathies					
MELAS	↓	↓	↓	↑↑	
Leigh syndrome	↓	↓	↓	↑↑	
Menkes disease	v	↓	↓↓	↑↑	
SDH complex deficiency	↓	↓↓	↓↓↓	↑↑	suc
(B) Amino acid and organic acidurias					
Phenylketonuria	n	n	n		phe
Nonketotic hyperglycinemia	n	n	n		glycine
Maple syrup urine disease	n	n	↓↓	↑	BCA
Canavan disease	↓	↑	↑↑↑		
Glutaric aciduria type I	n	n	↓↓	↑	
Propionic academia	n	n	↓↓	↑	Glx
Urea cycle defects	↓	↓	↓	↑	Gln
(C) Lysosomal storage disease					
Metachromatic leukodystrophy	↑↑	↓	↓↓↓	↑	
Fucosidosis	n	n	↓	↑	
(D) Peroxisomal disorders					
X-linked adrenoleukodystrophy	↑↑↑	↓↓	↓↓↓	↑	
Adrenomyeloneuropathy	n	n	n		
(E) Leukoencephalopathies					
Alexander disease	↑↑↑	↓↓	↓↓↓	↑↑	
Megalencephalic leukoencephalopathy with subcortical cysts	↓↓	↓↓	↓↓	↑	
Leukoencephalopathy with vanishing white matter	↓↓	↓↓	↓↓	↑	
Leukoencephalopathy with involvement of brain stem and spinal cord and elevated white matter lactate	↑	n	↓↓	↑↑	
Cerebral autosomal dominant arteriopathy with subcortical infarcts and leukoencephalopathy (CADASIL)	n	n	↓↓	↑	
(F) Miscellaneous					
Creatine deficiency	n	↓↓↓	n		
Pelizaeus–Merzbacher disease	n	n/↑	n		

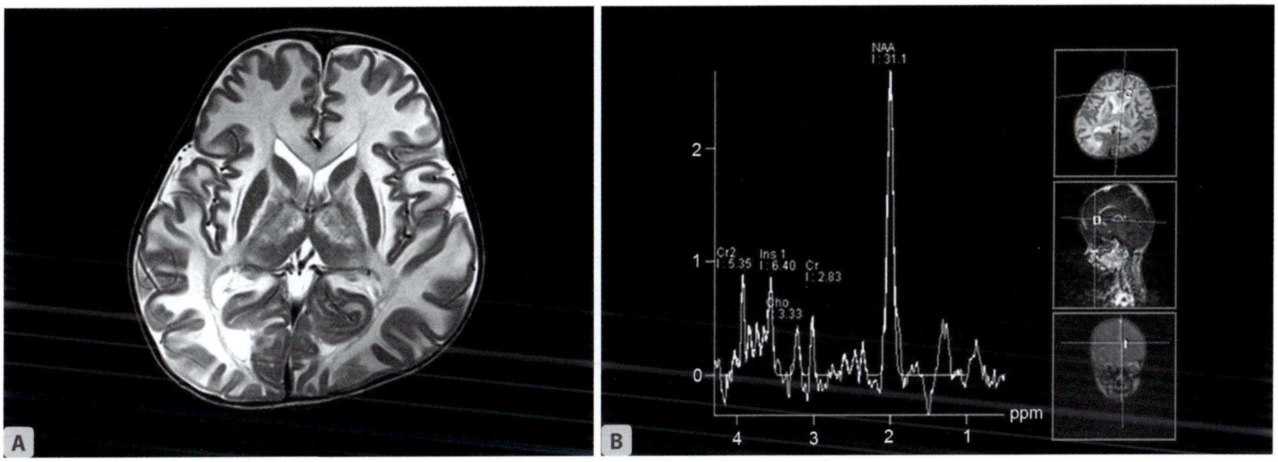

FIGS. 18A AND B: A 2-year-old child with developmental delay. (A) Axial T2-W MR images show extensive high-signal intensity areas throughout the white matter reaching up to the subcortical region, internal and external capsules, and corpus callosum; (B) MR spectroscopy shows raised NAA peak (arrow).

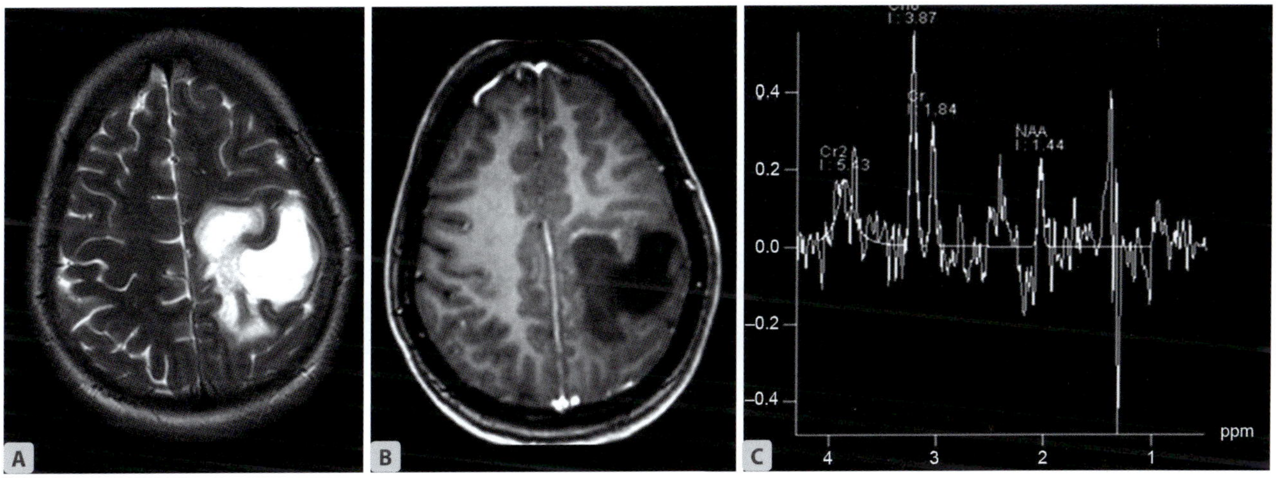

FIGS. 19A TO C: A 35-year-old patient with biopsy proven tumefactive demyelination. (A) T2W MR image shows a large hyperintense areas involving left frontal lobe; (B) T1 postcontrast image—lesion shows peripheral incomplete ring type enhancement; (C) CSI ^{1}H-MRS (TE = 135 ms) from the lesion shows increased choline, decreased NAA, lipid/ lactate peaks at 1.3 ppm and glutamate/glutamine peak at 2.4 ppm.

ganglia as well as in the cortex in patients with symptomatic HD. Although not always found, increase of LA have been observed in the occipital lobes, basal ganglia and frontal lobes of HD patients.

MAGNETIC RESONANCE SPECTROSCOPY IN DEMYELINATING DISEASES

Multiple Sclerosis

^{1}H-MRS shows normal spectrum in hyperacute plaques of MS. In demyelinating plaques, there is elevation of Cho/Cr ratio **(Figs. 19 and 20)**. In subacute to chronic plaques, there is decreased NAA/Cr ratio.[44] Acute active MS plaques (that enhances following Gd DTPA) often show increased lactate, mobile lipids and so called 'marker peaks' in the 2.1–2.6 ppm in region and this help in the differentiation from chronic (irreversible) MS plaques.[45] However, a MRS study in children with acute MS, did not show elevated lipid or lactate level. Inositol which is a marker for astrocyte becomes increased in chronic lesions.[46]

Normal appearing white matter (NAWM) in MS: The NAA/Cr ratio in normal appearing white matter drops one month after the occurrence of an acute lesion in areas distinct from the lesion, it is normalized after 6 months, and drops again, when relapses occur. It correlates well with total lesion load and disability.[47,48] Therefore, NAA or the NAA/Cr ratio is a good surrogate marker for the monitoring of neuroprotection in preclinical therapeutic studies.[49]

Tumefactive demyelination: MRS findings are characterized by reduced NAA, raised choline, lipid/lactate peaks and glutamate/glutamine peaks.

MAGNETIC RESONANCE SPECTROSCOPY IN HEAD TRAUMA

MRS provides a way to evaluate tissue viability following trauma and the results of MRS may provide insight as to how patients should be treated and whether treatment is effective,

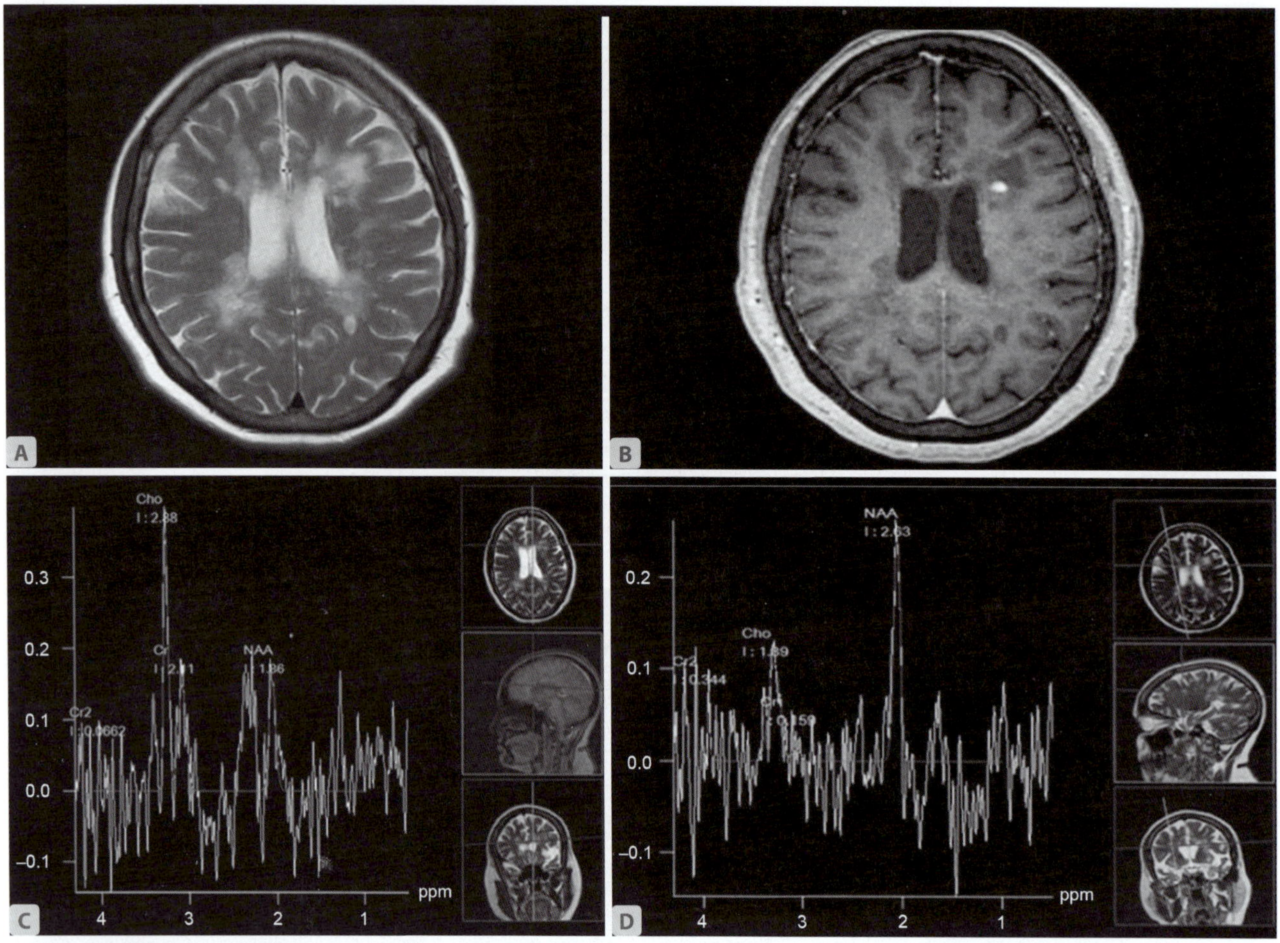

FIGS. 20A TO D: (A) A 30-year-old patient with primary progressive multiple sclerosis. (A) T2W MR image shows multiple hyperintense areas in periventricular location; (B) T1 postcontrast image—lesion in left periventricular location shows enhancement suggestive of acute lesion; (C) CSI ^{1}H-MRS (TE = 135 ms) from the left periventricular lesion shows increased choline and decreased NAA suggestive of acute lesion; (D) CSI ^{1}H-MRS (TE = 135 ms) from the lesion in right periventricular location shows normalized choline and NAA levels suggestive of chronic lesion.

thus helping neurosurgeons make clinical decision. Studies have shown that the injured region had highly increased lactate signal and decreased NAA, Cr and Cho. Increase in lactate is related to ischemia after trauma and decrease of NAA, Cr and Cho is related to edema, which has a dilution effect.[7] A study conducted in the institute to evaluate the role of MR spectroscopy in diffuse axonal injury in patients with head injury who had a grossly normal CT by comparing the metabolic ratios in different regions of the brain in these patients with a control group. The author found that there was a highly significant decrease in both the NAA/Cr and NAA/Cho ratios in the splenium in patients with head injury as compared to the control group **(Figs. 21A to D)**. When the study group was further subdivided according to severity of head injury, there was a highly significant decrease in both the NAA/Cr and NAA/Cho ratios in the splenium in the severely injured groups to whereas the decrease in the metabolite ratios was not significant in the mild on moderately head injured group.

MAGNETIC RESONANCE SPECTROSCOPY IN STROKE

There is loss of NAA and increase in lactate level in the area of infarction and these finding correlate clinically with functional outcome and disability. In ischemic penumbra, there is increase in the lactate level without decrease in NAA. Chronic infarcts often show increased lactate.[50-52]

MAGNETIC RESONANCE SPECTROSCOPY IN PSYCHIATRIC DISEASES

In schizophrenia, there is increase in PCr/ATP and PCr/Pi ratios in the right temporal lobe with decrease in PME in left frontal lobe and elevated PDE and low PCr in both frontal lobes. MRS can also assess lithium levels during treatment. ^{1}H-MRS findings in schizophrenia have been inconsistent

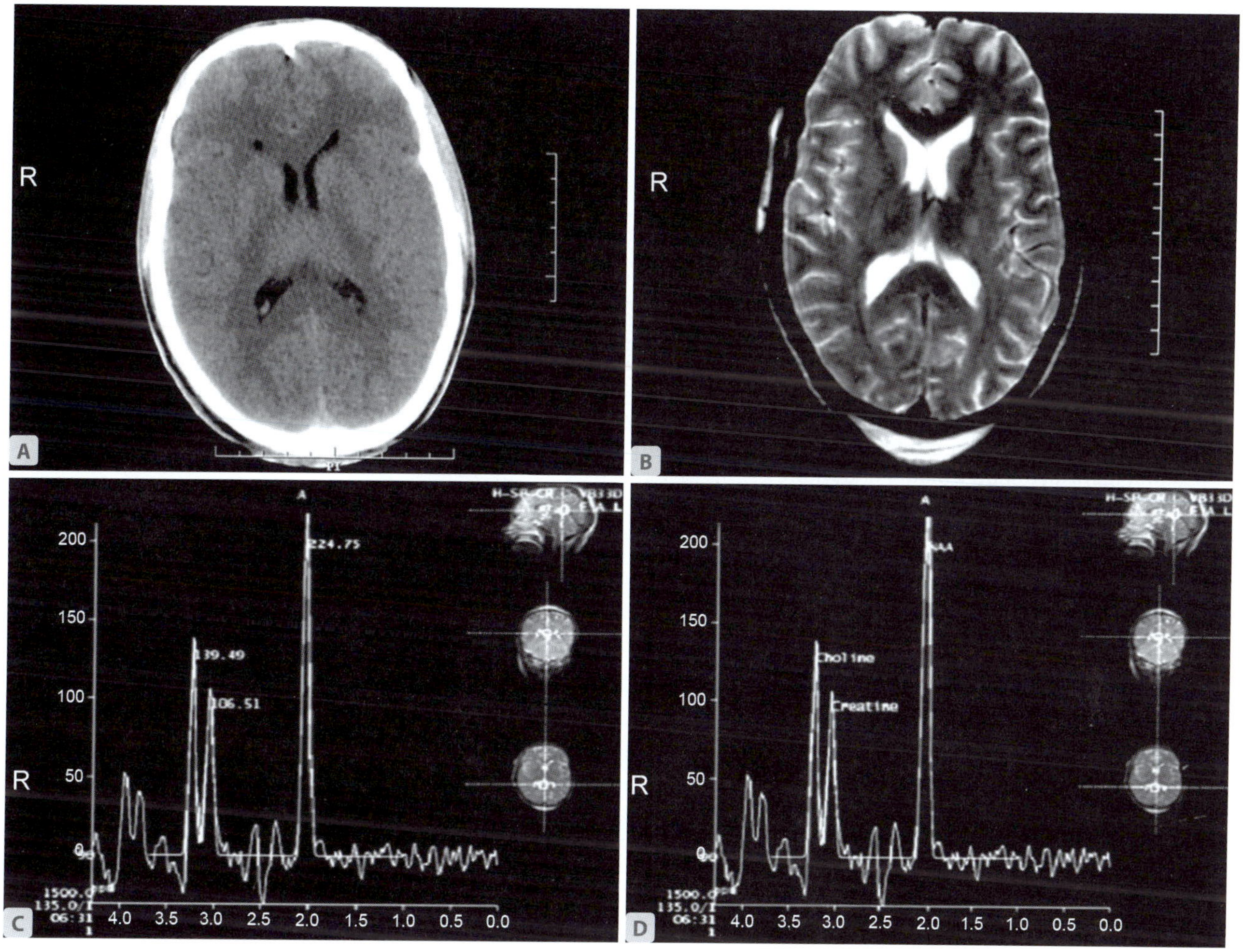

FIGS. 21A TO D: 23-year-old male patient with head injury with (A) Normal NCCT head; (B) Normal MR scan and (C and D) MRS shows decrease in NAA/Cho and NAA/Cr ratios in the splenium.

with some studies finding reduced NAA in various regions of the brain including frontal cortex, dorsolateral prefrontal cortex and temporal cortex. However, low NAA levels in the hippocampus is a more consistent finding.

MAGNETIC RESONANCE SPECTROSCOPY IN HIV/AIDS

It is generally agreed that conventional MRI is not sensitive to the detection of early stages of HIV infection of brain. Neurological disease is found in 30–40% of all AIDS patients and this frequency is increasing as treatment for other complications such as *Pneumocystis carinii* pneumonia have improved.

There is marked reduction of NAA/Cho and NAA/Cr ratios in the regions that appear normal on MRI study in HIV encephalopathy (direct HIV infection). Similar, findings may be seen with gross atrophy of brain in late stage of the disease.

It is observed that Cr resonance is stable overtime on an absolute scale. MRS can also help in the monitoring of drugs that helps in the management of AIDS patients. An important clinical problem in the AIDS patients is differentiating toxoplasmosis from lymphoma. In toxoplasmosis there is a large lipid peak whereas in lymphoma there is increase in Cho/Cr ratio. However, these results are not consistent and atypical spectra are observed in many cases. In PML, there is increase in lactate level. MRS, therefore, provides insights in the neurological problems in AIDS and can help in monitoring the new neuroprotective agents.[53]

CLINICAL SUCCESS

The initial widespread enthusiasm on MRS and MRSI as research methodology useful for clinical applications waned subsequently with many workers terming it as a largely an investigational tool.[1] But MRS does have particular clinical value for the lateralization of seizure focus in temporal lobe epilepsy for preoperative planning.[23] MRS can differentiate radiation necrosis from tumor recurrence, infarct from tumor, lymphoma from PML in HIV patient, monitor treatment response, etc.[20]

Artefacts in MR Spectroscopy

As with other MR sequences, MRS is a very sensitive technique and it is commonly affected by artifacts thereby reducing its diagnostic utility.

Field Inhomogeneity

Field inhomogeneity results in overlapping resonances, reduces the SNR and can result in inadequate water suppression. Broad line widths can result in serious degradation of the quality and interpretation of spectral data. These can result from variety of causes such as improper shimming and the presence of paramagnetic materials (e.g. metallic devices, hemorrhage, or calcifications) and air-tissue interfaces such as mesial anterior temporal and inferior frontal lobes. Iron containing structures such as striatum and substantia nigra also show broader line width.[53, 54]

Remedy

Reshimming or use of high-order shims with repetition of the procedure, or by slightly changing the region of interest slightly may overcome these artefacts.

Inadequate Water and Lipid Suppression

These may occur due to field inhomogeneity or the result of a failed optimization of water suppression pulse flip angles. Spurious water signals can come from outside the voxel in areas of poor field homogeneity degrading the MR spectra. Lipid signals in the scalp are of greater magnitude than metabolites and inadequate suppression can lead to inability to detect lactate and may interfere with NAA signal. Various lipid suppression methods have been described in literature. Adequately placed outer-volume suppression saturation bands may overcome this problem.

Remedy

Repeating the calibration or slightly altering the voxel position can overcome this problem. Spurious water signals can be suppressed using outer-volume suppression saturation bands .[54,55]

Head Motion

Head motion may have a disastrous effect on MRS, with loss of resolution and SNR, lipid and water suppression problems, and erroneous voxel location.

Incorrect Voxel Placement

It is of paramount importance to correctly place the voxel at the region of interest for optimum results. Particularly in follow-up studies it is important that the sectra are recorded from the same location utilizing same technical parameters.

Remedy

Careful radiologist/technician supervision and use of institutional standardized MRS protocols can overcome this problem. Use of automated voxel placement and real time registration of localizer images to standard anatomical templates) may become increasingly used for such studies in future.

Incorrect Protocol

Adequate training and expertise of radiologists/technologists in using a particular choice of protocol for a particular study (e.g. short or long echo time, single- or multi-voxel) has to be encouraged. In general short echo time spectra should be used when compounds such as mI or Glx are required, while multivoxel methods are important for pathologies such as brain tumors. Very small lesions less than 1.0–1.5 cm in diameter may not be evaluated by MRS. Similarly lesions near areas of marked susceptibility may also result in poor spectra.

Out-of-voxel Magnetization

Slice profiles are not usually perfect and there will always be a small amount of residual magnetization originating from outside the voxel particularly from unsuppressed water or lipid signals.

Remedy

These can be minimized by using outer-volume suppression saturation bands and when proper crushing is used in conjunction with an optimum ordering of slice select gradients.[54, 55]

Chemical Shift Displacement Effects

When a slice-selective pulse is applied, the position of the slice depends on the frequency offset and the gradient strength. The voxel position of each metabolite will be slightly different, depending on the chemical shift and the strength of the gradient used. This is more of a problem at higher fields than lower.

Remedy

Use of the highest possible bandwidth RF pulses and high bandwidth saturation pulses to sharpen the edges of the excitation box.[55]

Fast MR Spectroscopy Techniques including Whole Brain MR Spectroscopy

A major limitation of standard MR spectroscopy techniques is long acquisition times, especially with 3D data acquisition. Fast CSI techniques have been shown to significantly reduce data acquisition times. These fast techniques were introduced to reduce the limitations associated with conventional spectroscopy techniques.

Parallel Imaging

These include sensitivity encoding (SENSE), simultaneous acquisition of spatial harmonics (SMASH) and generalized autocalibrating partial parallel acquisition (GRAPPA). In these techniques, multiple receiver coils are used which increases signal sensitivity and spatial encoding by reducing the number of k-space lines and hence accelerating the image acquisition. These can have low SNR for which number of coil elements can be increased.[56-58]

Fast Multivoxel Techniques

A whole brain MRSI can be done by reducing the scanning time and motion sensitivity. Using the time-varying gradients during the readout MRSI can be accelerated. K-space trajectories mostly used in spectroscopic imaging are echo-planar and spiral trajectories reducing the acquisition time.[59]

Spiral MRSI

It is a fast spectroscopic imaging technique that traverses k-space by using spiral trajectories. Oscillating readout gradients are applied in a spectroscopic imaging sequence in two spatial dimensions during the data acquisition resulting in marked reduction in acquisition times. Data is then reconstructed onto a Cartesian k-space and Fourier transformation is applied Spiral MRSI thus leads to shorter imaging time, higher spatial resolution and increased SNR.[60]

Turbo Spectroscopic Imaging (Turbo-MRSI)

Acceleration of acquisition can be done by use of multiple-echo refocusing. It can be combined with parallel imaging techniques such as SENSE to improve SNR these can help in reduction of acquisition times by about eight folds compared to conventional MRSI techniques. Major drawbacks include reduced spectral resolution and SNR.[61, 62]

Echo-planar Spectroscopic Imaging (EPSI)

These techniques have shown improved spatial and temporal resolution compared to typical conventional MRSI. These are particularly useful in whole brain MRSI as these can provide improved spatial and spectral encoding. Modification have been proposed to enhance the acceleration of data collection with use of SENSE-EPSI. These techniques have limitation in the form of contraction of spectral bandwidth and reduced SNR.

Whole Brain MRSI

The whole brain MRSI requires a volumetric echo planar spectroscopy imaging and lipid nulling through an inversion recovery preparation that enables acquisition of spectra from cortical surface and high-speed spectroscopy methods with reduced k-space acquisition and parallel techniques. Major applications have come up in neurodegenerative and psychiatric diseases. It can demonstrate metabolic changes in a larger brain area simultaneously in patients suffering from diseases causing diffuse metabolic changes.[63,64]

FUTURE DEVELOPMENTS

There is tremendous need to improve ease-in-operation, reliability, reproducibility and sensitivity of MRS. MR signals are week and SNR of spectra acquired at 1.5–2.0 T is barely adequate.

One touch MRS protocols where one can choose the position of voxel from the locator images and the system automatically performs all operation including data analysis and baseline correction will be the ideal goal. The plethora of localization technique causes more confusion. There is a need to standardize MRS protocol so as to have a uniform database and reproducibility. Improved instrumentation (3.0T or more) with autoshimming, reduced eddy currents, high SNR may further develop with increase in the use of phased array coils. Further improvements and developments will take place in absolute quantification of metabolites and to produce metabolic images from CSI data. Development of spectroscopic intracellular contrast agents and targeted labels may further improve clinical utility of MRS.

Despite its problems, MRS has a unique ability to noninvasively measure various metabolites in human body. It is a useful addition in basic biochemical research and clinical investigations.[8]

REFERENCES

1. Cousins JP. Clinical MR spectroscopy fundamentals, current applications and future potential. AJR. 1995;164:1337-47.
2. Bolinger L, Insko EK. Spectroscopy: Basic principles and techniques. In: Edelman RR, Hesselink JR, Zlatkin MB. (Eds): Body MRI. Philadelphia: WB Saunders. 1996 pp. 353-79.
3. Matson GB, Weiner MW. Spectroscopy in Magnetic Resonance Imaging. In: Stark DD, Bradley WG (Ed). St Louis: Mosby. 1999;181-211.
4. Skoch A, Jiru F, Bunke J. Spectroscopic imaging: basic principles. Eur J Radio. 2008;67:230-39.
5. Soares DP, Law M. Magnetic resonance spectroscopy of the brain: review of metabolites and clinical applications. Clin Radiol. 2009;64:12-21.
6. McLean MA, Cross JJ. Magnetic resonance spectroscopy: principles and applications in neurosurgery. Br J Neurosurg. 2009;23:5-13.
7. Callot V, Galanaud D, Le Fur Y, Confort-Gouny S, Ranjeva JP, Cozzone PJ. (1)H MR spectroscopy of human brain tumours: a practical approach. Eur J Radiol. 2008;67:268-74.
8. Hajek M, Dezortova M. Introduction to clinical in vivo MR spectroscopy. Eur J Radial. 2008;67:185-93.
9. Birken DL, Oldendorf WH. NAA: A literature review of compound prominent of proton spectroscopy of brain. Neurosci Biobehv Rev. 1989;13:23-31.
10. Rothman DL, Arias MF, Shulman GI. A pulse sequence for simplifying hydrogen NMR spectra of biological tissues. J Magn Reson. 1984;60:430-4
11. Behar KL, Rothman DL, Spencer DD. Analysis of macromolecule resonances in 1H-MRS spectra of human brain. Mag Reson Med. 1994;32:294-8.
12. Gulati S, Shah T, Menon S, et al. Magnetic resonance spectroscopy in pediatric neurology. Ind J Paediatr. 2003;70:317.
13. Trabesinger AH, Meier D, Boesiger P. In vivo H NMR spectroscopy of individual human brain metabolites at moderate field strengths. J Magn Reson Imag. 2003;21:1295.
14. Chen W, Ackerman JJH. Surface coil spin echo localization in vivo via in homogenous surface spoiling magnetic gradient. J Magn Reson. 1989;82:655.
15. Garwood M, Schleich T, Ross BD, et al. A modified rotating frame experiment based on a Fourier series window function: Application to in vivo spatially localized NMR spectroscopy. J Magn Reson. 1985;65:239.

16. Frahm J, Merboldt KD, Hanicke W. Localised proton spectroscopy using stimulated echoes. J Magn Reson. 1987;72:502.
17. Bertoldo D, Watcharakorn A, Castillo M. Brain proton magnetic resonance spectroscopy. Introduction and overview. Neuroimag Clin N Am 2013; 23:359-80.
18. Usenius JP, Kauppinen RA, Vainio PA, et al. Quantitative metabolite patterns of human brain tumors: Detection by1H-NMR spectroscopy in vivo and in vitro. J Comput Assist Tomogr. 1994;18:705.
19. Negendank W. Studies of human tumors by MRS: A review. NMR Biomed. 1992;5:303.
20. Oberhaensli RD, Hilton-Jones D, Bore PJ, et al. Biochemical investigation of human tumors in vivo with phosphorus-31 magnetic resonance spectroscopy. Lancet. 1986;5:8.
21. Fulham MJ, Bizzi A, Dietz MJ, et al. Mapping of brain tumor metabolites with proton MR spectroscopic imaging: Clinical relevance. Radiology. 1992;185:675.
22. Kuesel AC, Sutherland GR, Halliday W, et al. 1H-MRS of high-grade astrocytomas: Mobile lipid accumulation in necrotic tissue. NMR Biomed. 1994;7:149.
23. Smith JK, Castillo M, Kwock L. MR spectroscopy of brain tumors. Magn Reson Imaging Clin N Am. 2003;11:415.
24. Choi C, Raisanen JM, Ganji SK, et al. Prospective longitudinal analysis of 2-hydroxyglutarate magnetic resonance spectroscopy identifies broad clinical utility for the management of patients with IDH-mutant glioma. J Clin Oncol. 2016 20; 34(33):4030-9.
25. Davies NP, Wilson M, Harris LM, Natarajan K, Lateef S, Macpherson L, et al. Identification and characterisation of childhood cerebellar tumours by in vivo proton MRS. NMR Biomed. 2008;21:908-18.
26. Harting I, Hartmann M, Bonsanto MM, et al. Characterization of necrotic meningioma using diffusion MRI, perfusion MRI and MR spectroscopy: Case report and review of the literature. Neuroradiology.2004.46:189.
27. Garg M, Gupta RK, Husain M, Chawla S, Chawla J, Kumar R, et al. Brain abscess: etiological categorization with in vivo proton MR spectroscopy. Radiology. 2004;230:519-27.
28. Gupta RK, Vatsal DK, Husain N, Chawla S, Prasad KN, Roy R, et al. Differentiation of tuberculous from pyogenic brain abscesses with in vivo proton MR spectroscopy and magnetization transfer MR imaging. AJNR J. 2001;22:1503-9.
29. Castillo M, Kwock L, Mukherji S. Clinical applications of MR spectroscopy. AJNR. 1996;17:1-15.
30. Kimura T, Sako K, Gotoh T, Tanaka K, Tanaka T. In vivo single-voxel proton MR spectroscopy with ring like enhancement. NMR Biomed. 2001;14:339-49.
31. Lai PH, Ho JT, Chen WL, Hsu SS, Wang JS, Pan HB, et al. Brain abscess and necrotic brain tumors: discrimination with proton MR spectroscopy and diffusion-weighted imaging. AJNR. 2002;23:1369-77.
32. Jayasunder R, Singh VP, Raghunathan P, et al. Inflammatory granulomas: evaluation with proton MRS. NMR Biomed. 1999;12:139.
33. Cecil KM, Lenkinski RE. Proton MR spectroscopy in inflammatory and infectious brain disorders. Neuroimaging Clinics of North America. 1998;8:863.
34. Pretell EJ, Martinot C, Garcia HH, et al. Differential diagnosis between cerebral tuberculosis and Neurocysticercosis by magnetic resonance spectroscopy. J Comput Assist Tomogr. 2005;29:112.
35. Dezortova M, Hajek M Eur J Radiol. (1)H MR spectroscopy in pediatrics. 2008;67(2):240-921.
36. Cady EB, Costello AM, Dawson MJ, et al. Non-invasive investigation of cerebral metabolism in newborn infants by phosphorus nuclear magnetic resonance spectroscopy. Lancet. 1983;1:1059.
37. Bruhn H, Frahm J, Merboldt KD, et al. Multiple sclerosis in children: Cerebral metabolic alteration monitored by localized proton magnetic resonance spectroscopy in vivo. Ann Neurol. 1992;32:140.
38. Hajek M, Dezortova M, Krsek P. (1)H MR spectroscopy in epilepsy. Eur J Radiol. 2008;67:258.
39. Hugg JW, Laxer KD, Matson GB, et al. Lateralization of human focal epilepsy by 31P magnetic resonance spectroscopic imaging. Neurology. 1993;43:2011.
40. Garcia PA, Laxer KD, van der Grond J, et al. 31P magnetic resonance spectroscopic imaging in patients with frontal lobe epilepsy. Ann Neurol. 1994;35:217.
41. Stefan TH, Ederhart KE, W-Huk BE, et al. Clinical applications of 1H-MR spectroscopy the evaluation of epilepsies. What do pathological spectra stand for with regard to current results and what answers do they give to common clinical questions concerning the treatment of epilepsies. Acta Neurol Scand. 2003;108:223.
42. Pettegrew JW, Moossy J, Withers G, et al. 31P nuclear magnetic resonance study of the brain in Alzheimer's disease. J Neuropathol Exp Neurol. 1988;47:235.
43. Matthews PM, Francis G, Antel J, et al. Proton magnetic resonance spectroscopy for metabolic characterization of plaques in multiple sclerosis, Neurology. 1991;41:1251.
44. Grossman RI, Lenkinski RE, Ramer KN, et al. MR proton spectroscopy in multiple sclerosis. Am J Neuroradiol. 1992;13:1535.
45. Mader I, Rauer S, Gall P, Klose U. (1)H MR spectroscopy of inflammation, infection and ischemia of the brain. Eur J Radiol. 2008;67:250.
46. De Stefano N, Narayanan S, Francis SJ, et al. Diffuse axonal and tissue injury in patients with multiple sclerosis with low cerebral lesion load and no disability. Arch Neurol. 2002;59:1565-71.
47. De Stefano N, Narayanan S, Matthews PM, et al. In vivo evidence for axonal dysfunction remote from focal cerebral demyelination of the type seen in multiple sclerosis. Brain. 1999;122:1933-9.
48. Arnold DL. Evidence for neuroprotection and remyelination using imaging techniques. Neurology. 2007;68:S83-90, discussion S91-6.
49. Graham GD, Kalvach P, Blamire AM, et al. Clinical correlates of proton magnetic resonance spectroscopy findings after acute cerebral infarction. Stroke. 1995;26:225.
50. Barker PB, Gillard JH, van Zijl PC, et al. Acute stroke; evaluation with serial proton MR spectroscopic imaging. Radiology. 1994;192:723.
51. Hugg JW, Duijn JH, Matson GB, et al. Elevated lactate and alkalosis in chronic human brain infarction observed by 1H and 31P spectroscopic imaging (MRSI). J Cereb Blood Flow Metab. 1992;12:734.
52. Paley M. Proton spectroscopy of the human brain. In: Bradley WG, Bydder GM, (Eds). MartynDunitz, London. 1997;309-23.
53. Horská A, Calhoun VD, Bradshaw DH, Barker PB. Rapid method for correction of CSF partial volume in quantitative proton MR spectroscopic imaging. Magn Reson Med 2002; 48: 555-8.
54. Ernst T, Chang L. Elimination of artifacts in short echo time H MR spectroscopy of the frontal lobe. Magn Reson Med 1996; 36: 462-8.
55. Hurd R, Sailasuta N. Elimination of artifacts in short echo proton spectroscopy. 5th Annual Meeting of the International Society of Magnetic Resonance in Medicine; Vancouver, BC, Canada; 1997. p. 1453
56. Pruessmann KP, Weiger M, Scheidegger MB, Boesiger P. SENSE: sensitivity encoding for fast MRI. Magn Reson Med. 1999;42(5):952-62.

57. Sodickson DK, Manning WJ. Simultaneous acquisition of spatial harmonics (SMASH): fast imaging with radiofrequency coil arrays. Magn Reson Med. 1997;38(4):591-603.
58. Griswold MA, Jakob PM, Heidemann RM, Nittka M, Jellus V, Wang J, Kiefer B, et al. Generalized autocalibrating partially parallel acquisitions (GRAPPA). Magn Reson Med. 2002;47(6): 1202-10.
59. Posse S, Tedeschi G, Risinger R, Ogg R, Le Bihan D. High speed 1H spectroscopic imaging in human brain by echo planar spatial-spectral encoding. Magn Reson Med. 1995;33(1):34-40.
60. Block KT, Frahm J. Spiral imaging: a critical appraisal. J Magn Reson Imaging. 2005;21(6):657-68.
61. Martin AJ, Liu H, Hall WA, Truwit CL. Preliminary assessment of turbo spectroscopic imaging for targeting in brain biopsy. AJNR. 2001;22(5):959-68.
62. Stengel A, Neumann-Haefelin T, Singer OC, Neumann-Haefelin C, Zanella FE, Lanfermann H, Pilatus U. Multiple spin-echo spectroscopic imaging for rapid quantitative assessment of N-acetylaspartate and lactate in acute stroke. Magn Reson Med. 2004;52(2):228-38.
63. Maudsley AA, Domenig C, Sheriff S. Reproducibility of serial whole-brain MR spectroscopic imaging. NMR Biomed. 2010;23:251-6.
64. Stagg CJ, Knight S, Talbot K, Jenkinson M, Maudsley AA, Turner MR. Whole-brain magnetic resonance spectroscopic imaging measures are related to disability in ALS. Neurology. 2013;80:610-5.

CHAPTER

187

Functional MRI

Anuj Prabhakar

INTRODUCTION

Functional magnetic resonance imaging (fMRI) is an MRI-based tool that is utilized for analysis and localization of brain function.[1] This technique has enabled neuroscientists to gain valuable insight into the changes that occur while our brain functions. It helps in advancing our knowledge of structural organization in the brain. fMRI is also useful in evaluation of brain function in a wide variety of pathologies and in assessment of the risk of functional compromise after surgery. This chapter provides a brief introduction to the fundamental principles of functional MRI and its applications.

PRINCIPLE OF fMRI AND BOLD CONTRAST

fMRI is useful in evaluation of the eloquent areas of the brain. fMRI technique is usually based upon blood-oxygenation-level dependent (BOLD) contrast. BOLD effect was initially described by Seiji Ogawa. Turner et al. first obtained an echo-planar imaging time series of oxygenation changes occurring in blood with a cat brain during a global oxygenation stress.[2] The BOLD contrast effect was subsequently demonstrated in human subjects in 1992.[3,4] BOLD-fMRI differentiates between active and inactive areas by exploiting the difference in magnetic properties of deoxygenated and oxygenated hemoglobin. This allows the investigator to recognize changes in the local blood flow in the brain. Oxy hemoglobin is diamagnetic in nature while deoxyhemoglobin is paramagnetic and aligns with the magnetic field in the MRI gantry.[1] This paramagnetic nature leads to an increase in field inhomogeneity. This causes a swift dephasing of the local transverse magnetization that reduces the transverse relaxation time (T2*) in the adjacent brain parenchyma.

There is coupling of the local blood flow and neuronal activity in the brain.[5,6] Whenever an external stimulus is provided to the brain there is an increase in the local neuronal activity of the area in the brain associated with that particular task. This leads to an increase in the energy consumption and oxygen utilization within the stimulated area. In order to supply the increased oxygen demand, there is an increase in the regional blood flow and volume. However, the relationship between oxygen demand and blood flow is not linear and paradoxically, the degree of oxygen delivery, outstrips the elevated oxygen requirement. This leads to an increase in the local concentration of oxygenated hemoglobin. There is a commensurate reduction in the amount of deoxygenated hemoglobin in the draining veins, venules and local capillaries. Therefore, the net result of this increase in the neural activity is a reduction in the paramagnetic effect induced dephasing due to deoxyhemoglobin. The T2* signal increases and these changes can be observed using MRI. BOLD fMRI signal changes are small in magnitude and vary between 2% and 5%.[7]

The change in MRI signal secondary to neuronal activation is known as the hemodynamic response function (HRF) **(Fig. 1)**. The BOLD response is delayed by 1–2 s after any stimulus, irrespective of its length. The response has a temporal width of 4–6 s. If the stimulus is sustained for 20 s or longer, it usually reaches a plateau. Some investigators have described an initial fall in the BOLD signal that may last for 1–2 s before the usual increase. A matching transitory boost in deoxyhemoglobin concentration has been seen on optical imaging. There is a poststimulus undershoot that may last for approximately 30 s. Longer stimuli have longer poststimulus undershoot. BOLD response to multiple stimuli is not linear. This means that the response to two stimuli together is less than twice the integrated response of a single activation. Baseline cerebral blood flow (CBF) can also affect the extent of the BOLD effect after a stimulus. For example, if the CBF at baseline is increased by breathing carbon dioxide, the BOLD reaction for a particular task is reduced significantly.[8,9]

ADVANTAGES OF BOLD fMRI

There are many advantages in using fMRI over other conventional imaging methods while studying brain functions:[10]

- fMRI has better spatial resolution (1–4 mm in-plane resolution)
- The temporal resolution (0.1–1 sec) is also higher
- There is no need for radioactive isotopes

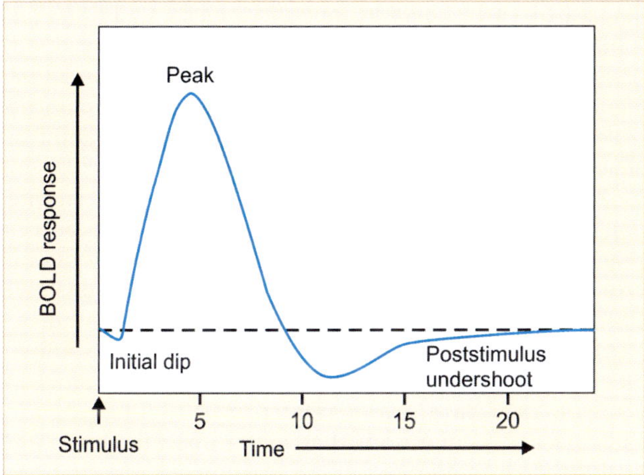

FIG. 1: Hemodymanic response function curve.

- fMRI is a non-invasive technique that can be easily replicated without any significant patient preparation
- The radiologist can acquire both anatomical and functional images in the same session
- There are no significant added costs.

Thus fMRI has become the most commonly used functional brain mapping modality.

LIMITATIONS OF BOLD TECHNIQUE

Susceptibility effects

T2* Gradient recalled echo echoplanar imaging (EPI) sequences are commonly used for BOLD imaging as they allow rapid scanning of the whole brain in a short time frame. However, these sequences are extremely sensitive to intravoxel dephasing. This occurs due to the changes in local magnetic field secondary to the variation in the magnetic susceptibility of different tissues contained within the voxel. Magnetic field gradients are generated which make the protons spin at different frequencies. Dephasing occurs with signal loss. This effect is maximized at areas of air tissue interface like orbitofrontal cortex or the medial and inferior temporal lobes. Activations related to visual and cognitive processing are seen in these areas. Susceptibility effects cause reduction in the sensitivity for this brain activation. Vascular clips, craniotomy hardware or stent grafts also cause significant artifacts during imaging. Another potential source of susceptibility artefacts is the presence of tumor-related hemorrhage in patients undergoing pre operative functional imaging for language or motor function.

Geometric Distortions

EPI sequences are prone to mislocalization of the BOLD signal in the phase encoding direction due to inhomogeneities in the magnetic field, especially if the bandwidth in the phase encoding direction is low. As previously discussed, regions in the brain that are adjacent to the air–soft tissue interface are more susceptible to distortions due to strong local variations in the magnetic field secondary to the susceptibility artefacts. Another source of distortion is the imperfection in linearity of the gradient waveforms. Few strategies may be utilized to correct and reduce image distortions. A field map may be acquired by applying a GRE sequence with 2 echoes at different TE. The field map is calculated by the difference in phase between the images acquired at different TE. This map can be used to map and correct the local field variations. The other technique used in correction of geometric distortion is the point spread function (PSF). Acquisitions using an additional phase encoding gradients are performed to calculate the PSF of each voxel. These PSFs encode the spatial information about the distortion and the overall distribution of intensities from a single voxel. Measuring the PSF allows the distortion in geometry and intensity to be corrected.

Venous Effects

The bold signal is dependent on local vasculature. At 1.5T and 3T BOLD activation may be localized to the adjacent draining vein and venules. This effect increases the likelihood of a false positive activation. It is seen more commonly in areas that are close to large draining veins like the superior sagittal sinus or it's draining cortical veins.

Physiologic Noise and Motion

Normal physiological functions like cardiac activity, respiration or had motion may contribute toward artefacts during acquisition of bold signal especially in resting state fMRI. Various techniques have been developed to mitigate the contribution by these effects to the BOLD signal.

Neurovascular Uncoupling

In a normal individual the activation of neurons and the subsequent hemodynamic changes are coupled in a predictable manner. There are many steps including initial neuronal firing followed by neurotransmitter release at synapses. This is followed by chemical mediator release from interneurons and astrocytes, resulting in vasoconstriction or vasodilatation. In patients who have structural lesions like tumors or arteriovenous malformations, alterations in the hemodynamic response lead to neurovascular uncoupling. This may lead to abnormally decreased or absent BOLD activation. Inadvertent resection of eloquent areas in such cases may cause permanent deficits.[4,7,10]

IMAGING ACQUISITION

BOLD fMRI is acquired using fast imaging read out. T2* weighted imaging is used. EPI sequences allow rapid whole brain coverage. A single-shot EPI technique is able to acquire multiple images at high speed (<100 ms/image). For example, the entire brain can be covered with 28 slices (slice thickness 5 mm) in less than 3 seconds. The TE ranges between 20–40 ms, and TR is between 1000 and 4000 ms. Using shorter TR (<1000 ms) reduces the temporal resolution; however the BOLD signal and the number of slices that can be acquired are also reduced. For this reason it is not generally used in clinical fMRI, which is performed on individual patients and therefore requires the greatest MR signal for both sensitivity and reliability. Single shot EPI is favored over multishot EPI, as it reduces motion artefacts in functionally impaired patients. At our institute the following parameters are used for fMRI in the routine clinical setting: EPI single shot; TR - 2000 ms; TE - 30 ms; Flip angle - 90; FOV - 230*230*140 mm; Voxel size- 3*3*4; Slice thickness - 4 mm; Slice gap - 0 mm; Number of slices- 35; Total scan duration- 5 min 14 sec; 150 dynamics.

fMRI EXAMINATION DESIGN

fMRI experiments are able to identify task evoked signal alteration in a sequence of MR images, and extract areas of activity using statistical analysis.[11] Those areas that show signal changes and correlate with the stimulus that has been applied can be recognized. Subsequently these are compared with the high-resolution T1-weighted anatomical images. Overall, there are two categories of task paradigms: block ('boxcar') designs and event-related designs **(Fig. 2)**. Block design paradigms are the most frequently used because of their simplicity, ease of implementation, and sensitivity. This design consists of repeated presentation of a task for at least 20 seconds followed by an alternate rest condition of similar duration.[3,6,12] The "rest" task must be chosen with care, as it should activate the various neural processes of the stimulus task except for the cognitive process that is being evaluated. The data collected from a block design experiment allow each task condition to be averaged to improve the signal-to-noise ratio (SNR) and then a simple "contrast" can be performed to compare the two conditions. Also, the averaging of BOLD signal over multiple repetitions compensates for any stimuli that may have been missed by the patient. The contrast can be obtained by performing a voxel-wise comparison between the BOLD signals recorded in the active and rest phases using parametric statistical analysis. Currently, most clinical fMRI procedures use block design. Block designs are very useful in clinical fMRI studies because the chief purpose in most clinical settings is to localize and evaluate a focal activated region in the brain rather than define connectivity patterns in the whole brain. The prolonged duration required for each condition in a block design experiment, however, has many inherent design limits. For example, the long duration required for each condition limits the ability to study multiple conditions within the time constraints of a standard scanning session. The ability to extract temporal information about the brain responses is also limited because of the prolonged BOLD response. Excessive repetition of the active and rest phases may cause habituation.

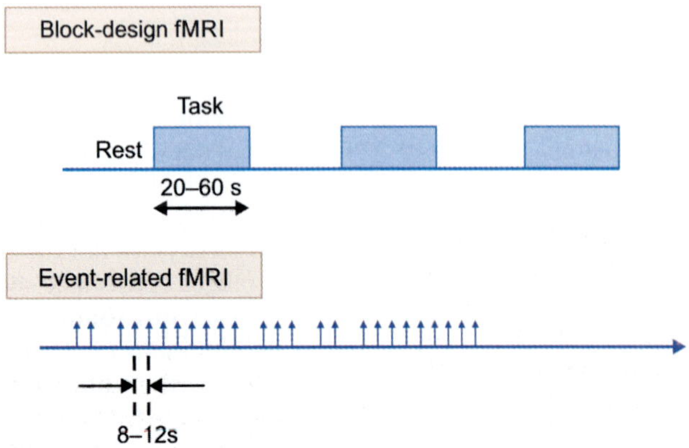

FIG. 2: Illustration showing difference in the technique used for block designs versus event-related paradigms.

Event-related fMRI paradigms utilize very brief stimuli that are presented at random of specific time points **(Fig. 2)**. They can be used to follow the course of neural processing in the brain.[13,14] The differences in the onset of activity produced by different stimuli can also be studied. Furthermore, as the stimuli appear at random time points, they are more statistically robust as compared to blocked designs. Therefore, event-related fMRI paradigms are useful to access questions that center upon the temporal performance of hemodynamic response, any changes that might occur with modification of the experimental context, and differences between various subjects. Event-related approach also avoids the habituation and fatigue that tends to arise in the box car design. Event-related experimental designs are used in most fMRI research on cognition, but their application in the clinical scenario is challenging. Firstly, complicated statistical methods are required to obtain the functional maps, however with increasing processing speed this technique has becoming feasible. Secondly, event-related designs require substantial validation and development prior to clinical use. Nevertheless, event-related designs offer more flexibility and are likely to achieve wider acceptance in the future.

fMRI EXAMINATION TASK PARADIGM

fMRI involves creating a paradigm which is presented to the patient, who is then required to is perform according to the provided instruction. A paradigm is a temporal allocation of stimuli that are used to elicit neuronal activation in a subject. Paradigms include active language, motor or memory tasks and passive auditory, tactile, or visual stimuli **(Figs. 3A and B)**.[15] Finger tapping is a dependable paradigm for localization of the hand activity in the primary motor cortex. A variety of language paradigms like verbal fluency with word generation, sentence comprehension, verb generation and picture naming. The use of multiple language paradigms increases the sensitivity and specificity of presurgical fMRI.[3,16] Verb generation is the most commonly used and probably the most reliable test in the clinical arena. Instructions are simple: given a word think of the associated verb. Most patients understand it well and are compliant once inside the magnet. Various stimulus delivery packages are available in the market, e.g. Cogent (Laboratory of Neurobiology, Wellcome Trust, London, UK;), E-Prime (Psychology Software Tools, Inc.; Pennsylvania, USA), and Presentation (Neurobehavioral Systems, Inc.; California, USA). While presenting the paradigm it is essential to synchronize the stimulus delivery with the MRI sequence trigger. The task may be presented to the subject via an MRI compatible screen in the MRI scanner room, headphones or specially designed goggles.

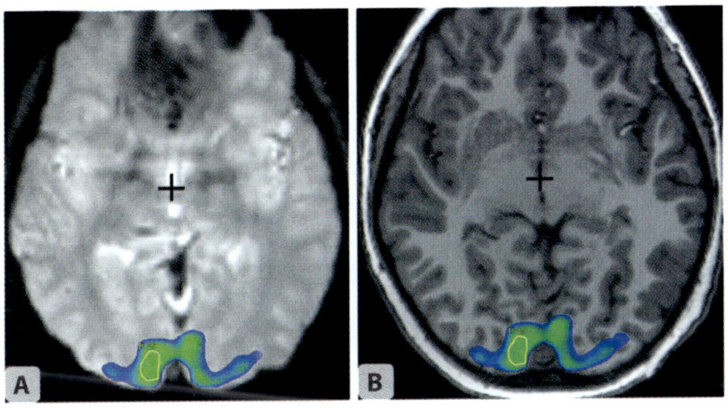

FIGS. 3A AND B: Visual checkerboard paradigm in fMRI: Areas of activation (green blue color) are seen in bilateral occipital cortices superimposed on axial BOLD (A) and T1-weighted (B) images.

POST-PROCESSING AND DATA ANALYSIS

Post-processing of clinical fMRI data generally adopts the approach used in conventional fMRI studies, which includes the following steps:

1. *Realignment*: All BOLD images acquired in a given time series are aligned to each other to correct for motion artifacts. The transformation information utilized in this process may be plotted as a graph. If the plot reveals motion larger than the size of the smallest voxel in any direction at a particular point of time the affected volume/dataset must be removed from the final analysis **(Fig. 4)**.
2. *Slice timing correction*: EPI sequences are acquired slice by slice in two dimensions. Therefore each slice is obtained at a different repetition time. If the statistical calculation is performed using the onset time relative to the first slice only, the delay in acquisition of the last slice will degrade the result of the fMRI scan. Slice timing correction must be performed to prevent this anomalous result.
3. *Coregistration*: In this step the EPI slices are coregistered with a high resolution anatomic scan in a voxel-wise manner. Segmentation of the anatomical image into gray matter, white matter, and cerebrospinal fluid is performed using tissue probability maps. Lastly the segmented images can be co-registered with the functional data.
4. *Normalization*: In clinical research the BOLD signal must be averaged across different subjects. The brain images of each patient are wrapped over the same stereotactic. This enables the researcher to evaluate the functional data from all subjects in a standard space. The most commonly used templates for normalization are the Montreal Neurological Institute (MNI) template, Talairach and Tournoux atlas, ICBM template.[17]
5. *Smoothing*: Smoothing of the fMRI images needs to be done prior to group-level statistical analysis, to superimpose corresponding areas of activity from the different subjects. Smoothening reduces noise and increases SNR. This step also suppresses the effect of anatomical and functional variability among individual subjects during group analysis.[18]
6. Statistical analysis is executed using a general linear model to compare the functional images obtained after performing the above steps to the design paradigm.
7. *Inference and interpretation of results*: Areas of functional activation are obtained after statistical processing. These can be superimposed on structural images or on 3D brain renders.

Clinical fMRI is mostly used for individual subjects and not group analysis. It is not essential to normalize the images. However, motion correction is extremely important in clinical setting. This is performed with rigid body transformation algorithms. Newer techniques for accurate motion correction and reduction of variation due to physiological causes are being developed.[16,19] A flow diagram of the various steps involved in fMRI is given in **Figure 5**.[20]

CURRENT CLINICAL APPLICATIONS OF fMRI

Neurosurgical Planning

The capability to localize functional areas in patients makes fMRI very important in preoperative planning. Presurgical mapping is essential to: (a) to determine hemispheric dominance; (b) to select candidates for awake craniotomy; (c) to guide the intraoperative surgical procedure; and (d) to assess the risk of postoperative neurologic deficits by measuring the distance between the margin of the lesion resection and critical functional structures.[16]

The "gold standard" for localizing foci of activation in the brain is electrical cortical mapping (ECM). ECM has several drawbacks. It is invasive in nature and the procedure takes a lot of time. Only a limited area of the brain is mapped. Another limitation is that the data from ECM is often accessible only during surgery after conclusions as regards to feasibility and surgical approach have already been drawn. The Wada test is another technique that is routinely used prior to epilepsy surgery. The dominant hemisphere for memory and language is recognized by the intra-arterial injection of sodium amytal into bilateral internal carotid arteries.[21] The drug causes temporary anesthetization of the brain tissue. Cerebral dominance for language and memory is determined on the patient's performance during the period of functional disability. The Wada procedure causes significant patient discomfort, and morbidity as compared to functional imaging. fMRI allows the surgeon to assess the functional areas prior to the surgery in a non-invasive manner. This information may be used to make choices regarding the suitability of surgery and the approach. Intraoperatively, it helps to familiarize the surgeon with the functional and structural anatomy within the restricted view available after craniotomy. If intraoperative ECM is still considered essential, fMRI directs the surgeon toward the regions of interest, and shortens the procedure.

The majority of patients with primary brain tumors can perform the various fMRI paradigms. Both motor and language paradigms can be performed. fMRI is highly sensitive in the detection of sensorimotor activation in healthy subjects and is also feasible in patients with lesions around the central sulcus **(Figs. 6A to F)**. Either volitional or passive paradigms

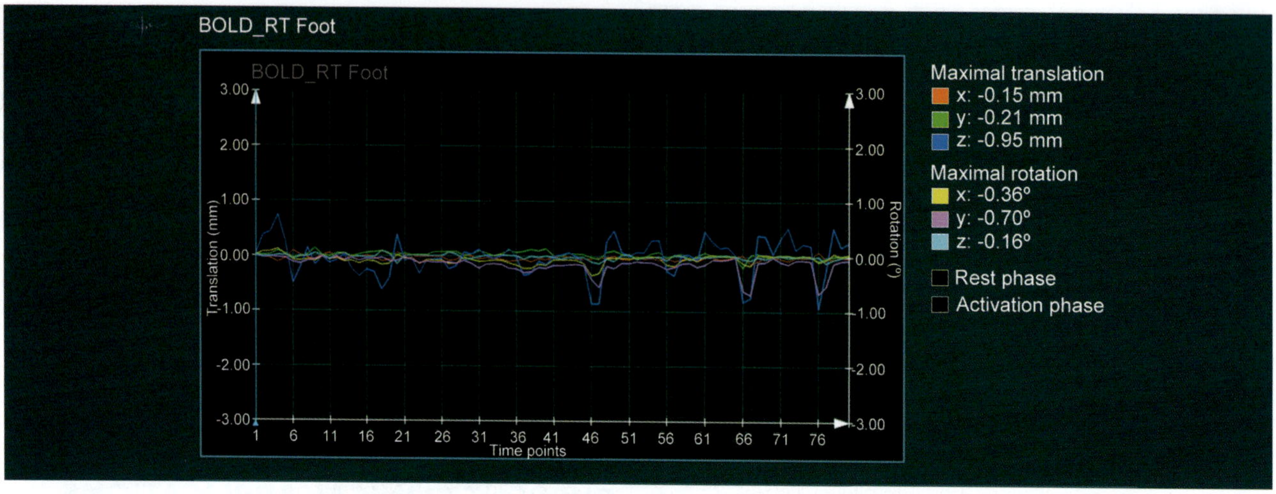

FIG. 4: Motion correction: Graph showing the patients head translation and rotation along all axis during rest and activation phases. If there is excessive motion at any time point, the corresponding EPI volume must be discarded from the final analysis.

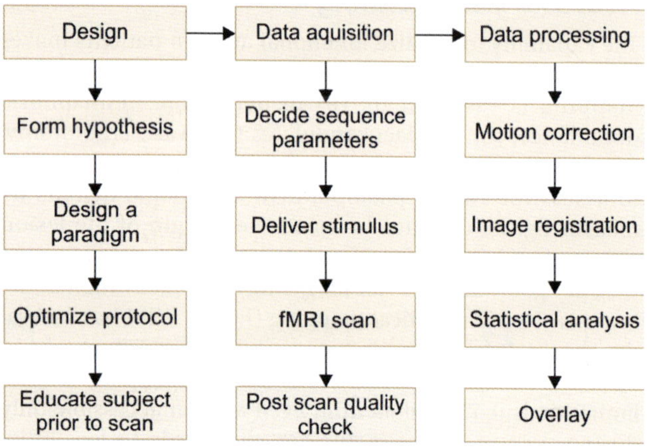

FIG. 5: Flow diagram depicting the various steps necessary for fMRI acquisition and analysis.[20]

may be used. Functional imaging is also useful in identifying functional areas in patients who have significantly distorted anatomy.[22] There is a good quality spatial correlation between motor fMRI and intraoperative ECM results. A distance of 10 mm or more between the functional cortex, as defined with fMRI, and the tumor has been found to be associated with significantly less risk of loss of function postoperatively.[23] The diagnostic performance of fMRI may change according to the grade of the glioma. Bizzi et al. reported higher sensitivity and lower specificity WHO grade II and III gliomas than in glioblastoma multiforme (GBM), particularly for fMRI of language.[24] This was postulated to be due to the neurovascular uncoupling or greater mass-effect seen in GBM. fMRI can also be used to predict deficits and study cortical reorganization.[22]

Epilepsy

Mapping of language and memory functions is possible using fMRI in temporal lobe epilepsy (TLE). This has both preoperative and prognostic significance. Various language paradigms are available to evaluate the Broca's area, Wernicke's area and the anterior temporal lobe language areas. Commonly used tasks include Verbal fluency, semantic decision, and verb generation. Evaluation of hemispheric dominance for language function can also be performed with fMRI using the lateralization index. Language mapping with fMRI has been seen to be more accurate as compared to Wada test in predicting naming ability post-surgery. The likelihood of postoperative preservation of naming function is higher if activation is noted in the left hippocampus during the pre-surgical fluency task, in right TLE patients. On the other hand, left TLE patients, who are more proficient in naming, show more activation in the left frontal lobe during various naming tasks. This suggests that the brain has a compensatory response to epileptic activity. Auditory and visual naming tasks may also help in predicting difficulties during naming after anterior temporal lobe resection.

Verbal or visual memory may be affected in approximately one-third of patients undergoing left or right anterior temporal lobe resection, respectively. Autobiographical, episodic and working memory related networks can be evaluated using fMRI in epilepsy patients. fMRI helps in prognosticating such patients.[25]

Dementia

Functional imaging offers substantial potential to recognize patients with prodromal dementia. The prefrontal cortex and the medial temporal lobe are implicated in working and secondary memory in healthy subjects. An increase in activation has been seen in the prefrontal cortex with increasing memory usage.[26] This is more evident during the initial, learning attempts.[27] Successful recall has been seen to be associated with increased activation.[27] The medial temporal lobe, the hippocampus and the parahippocampal cortex show activation during learning and recall. fMRI studies have revealed that modified patterns of activation in these memory-specific brain regions may be an indicator of brain dysfunction in early-stage dementia and mild cognitive impairment. Such markers may be used in clinical trials of cognition enhancing drugs, as the currently utilized measures

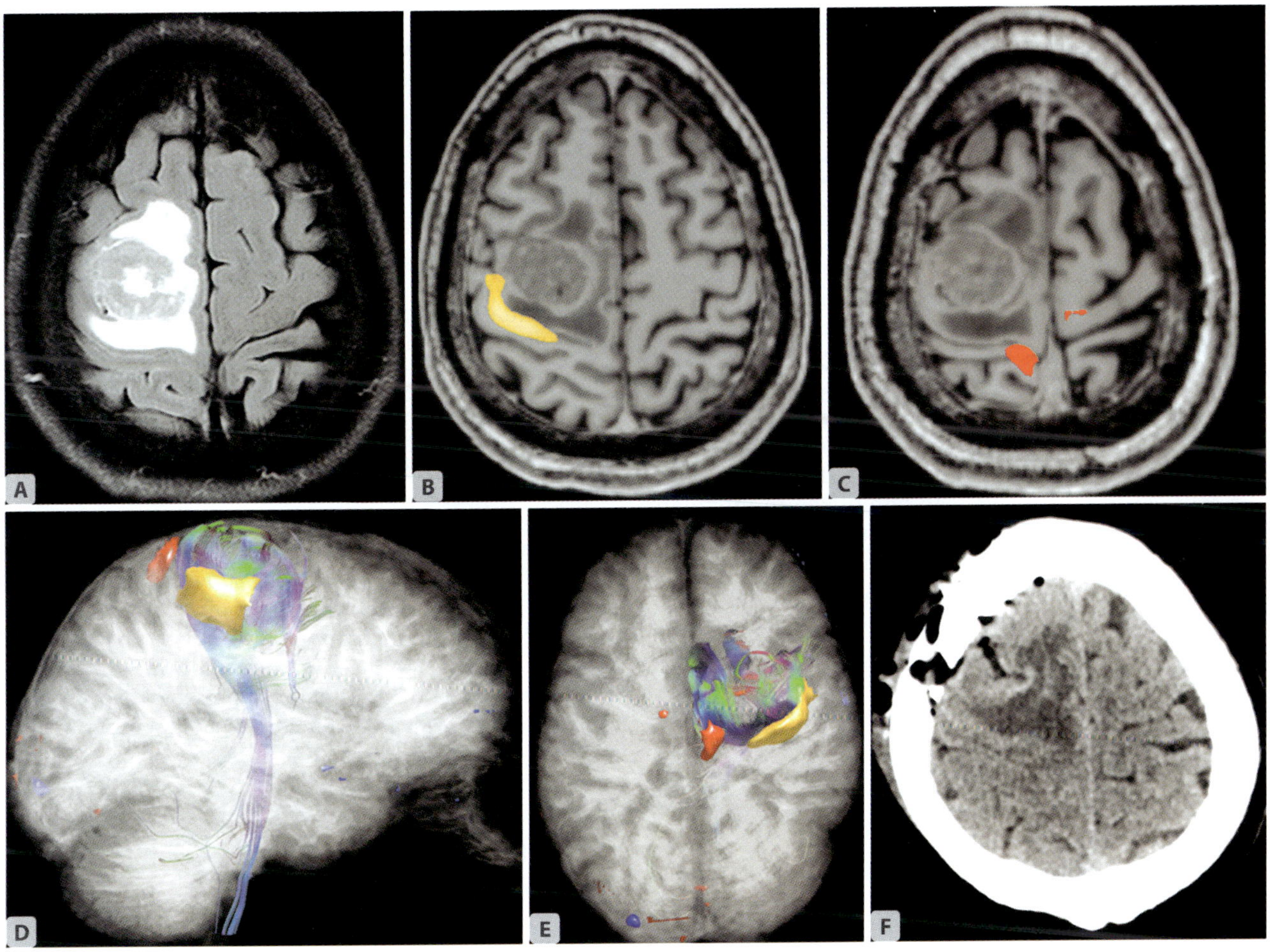

FIGS. 6A TO F: Pre-surgical fMRI: Axial FLAIR image (A) shows a well-defined lesion in the right high frontal region with surrounding edema. The right central sulcus is effaced and displaced posteriorly. Preoperative evaluation of motor area was performed using finger tapping; (B) and foot movement; (C) paradigms. The results were superimposed on axial T1-weighted images. The motor area corresponding to hand motion (orange area in B) has been displaced posteriorly and laterally. The foot motor cortex is also seen along the posterosuperior aspect of the edema. Composite glass brain images; (D and E) with functional and tractography data superimposed give an overview of both with matter tracts (purple, green) and activated areas (orange: hand motor, red: foot motor) surrounding the lesion. Such images allow the surgeons to decide their approach. Postoperative CT; (F) shows the anterolateral approach used in this patient that has spared the motor cortex and white matter tracts.

may be weighed down by measurement error and variability of change with time.

Diminished intensity of activation has been shown in the frontal and temporal regions of patients with Alzheimer's disease. "At-risk" subjects have also shown mixed results in various studies. Both increased and decreased activation have been seen in this group as compared to the control group.[28,29] Increased activation in Alzheimer's or at-risk patients may be explained by compensatory-recruitment of a larger area of the brain as compared to the normal population for the same task. If significant neuronal loss has already occurred, decrease in BOLD activation may be seen, especially in tasks that exceed the patient's compensatory reserve.[28]

Defining Disease Based on Patterns of Brain Function

fMRI could be used to define different "phenotypes" in a particular disease state. This may be especially pertinent in diseases like dyslexia, in which clinical classification is. fMRI studies may also provide an insights into the pathophysiology of the disease process. For example, Eden et al. have demonstrated that there is no activation in the motion sensitive visual cortex when dyslexic patients are presented with a moving stimulus.[30] Subsequent studies have suggested that such insufficiency in the integrity of the cortical magnocellular pathway may serve as a clinical marker in the disorder.[31]

Psychiatric Disorders

Most of the major psychiatric illnesses are characterised by widely distributed disordered neural systems. There is no single brain region associated with a particular mental illness. However, there are a few exceptions. Anterior cingulate cortex hyperactivity has been shown to be associated with major depression. Normalization of activity has been seen after treatment in such patients.[32] In schizophrenia a reduction of activity has been seen in the same area.[33] However, fMRI is not used for individual diagnosis of mental illness in the clinical setting. Resting state fMRI and connectivity analysis are more appropriate for research in psychiatric disorders.

ADVANCES IN fMRI TECHNIQUE

Real-time fMRI Neurofeedback

Real-time fMRI was developed by Cox et al.[34] The main difference between this technique and routine fMRI is in the speed of computation. The post-processing steps in real-time fMRI images are same as those in offline fMRI studies. However, with the advent of faster computer processing, better imaging sequences and algorithms, this process can be performed in a very small time frame. As the data is rapidly analyzed while the subject is in the MRI gantry, the results can be utilized to modulate his/her mental processes. The participants can learn to control multiple areas in the brain. Few studies have been performed which show that various brain areas including cingulate cortex, cingulate cortex, insular cortex, amygdala, motor, premotor and somatosensory cortices, visual and auditory cortex etc. may be controlled in this manner. Real-time fMRI neurofeedback has shown benefit in treatment of diseases like schizophrenia, depression, Parkinson's, tinnitus, and nicotine addiction.[34,35]

Resting State fMRI

Resting state fMRI (RSfMRI) scrutinizes synchronous activations between different areas in the brain that are at distinct locations physically. No external stimulus or task is given to the subject during RS fMRI. The patient lies awake, quietly in the MRI gantry throughout the sequence. The main aim of this technique is to identify the resting state networks. These networks are spatially distinct areas of the brain that are functionally connected with each other. A range of statistical techniques have been developed to identify resting state networks (RSNs) like seed-based analysis, independent component analysis, graph methods, clustering algorithms and multivariate pattern classification.

Various RSNs have been described. The most commonly studied network is the DMN. This network includes precuneus/posterior cingulate, lateral parietal cortex and the mesial prefrontal cortex. Other RSNs include the somatosensory network (primary and higher order motor and sensory areas), visual network (the occipital cortex), auditory network (Heschl gyrus, the superior temporal gyrus, and the posterior insula), language network (Broca and Wernicke areas with prefrontal, temporal, parietal, and subcortical regions), dorsal attention network (intraparietal sulcus and the frontal eye field), ventral attention network (temporoparietal junction and ventral frontal cortex), frontoparietal control network (lateral prefrontal cortex and the inferior parietal lobule) and the cingulo-opercular network (medial superior frontal cortex, anterior insula, and anterior prefrontal cortex). Each of these networks is thought to serve a distinct function.

RSNs have been studied in a variety of disorders such as epilepsy, Alzheimer's, major depressive disorder and schizophrenia.[36] However, RS fMRI is still an experimental tool at present. More research is necessary before it can be used in mainstream clinical practice.

CONCLUSION

Functional MRI is the new frontier for brain research. It gives an insight into brain connectivity, function and complexity. Significant research has been done on fMRI with newer techniques being developed rapidly. Pre-surgical evaluation of language, motor areas has become an essential tool for ensuring best possible patient outcome.

REFERENCES

1. Khanna N, Altmeyer W, Zhuo J, et al. Functional neuroimaging: fundamental principles and clinical applications. Neuroradiol J. 2015;28(2):87-96.
2. Bandettini PA. Twenty years of functional MRI: the science and the stories. NeuroImage. 2012;62(2):575-88.
3. Bandettini PA, Wong EC, Hinks RS, et al. Time course EPI of human brain function during task activation. Magn Reson Med. 1992;25:390-7.
4. Menon RS, Ogawa S, Kim SG, et al. Functional brain mapping using magnetic resonance imaging. Signal changes accompanying visual stimulation. Invest Radiol. 1992;27(Suppl 2):S47-53.
5. Thulborn KR. MRI in the management of cerebrovascular disease to prevent stroke. Neurol Clin. 2008;26(4):897-921, vii-viii.
6. Kwong KK. Functional Magnetic Resonance Imaging with Echo Planar Imaging. Milano: Springer Milan; 1996. pp. 73-90.
7. Zacà D, Agarwal S, Gujar SK, et al. Special considerations/technical limitations of blood-oxygen-level-dependent functional magnetic resonance imaging. Neuroimaging Clin N Am. 2014;24(4):705-15.
8. Buxton RB, Uludağ K, Dubowitz DJ, et al. Modeling the hemodynamic response to brain activation. NeuroImage. 2004;23:S220-33.
9. Tootell RBH, Reppas JB, Dale AM, et al. Visual motion aftereffect in human cortical area MT revealed by functional magnetic resonance imaging. Nature. 1995;375:139-41.
10. Detre JA, Floyd TF. Functional MRI and its applications to the clinical neurosciences. The Neuroscientist. 2001;7:64-79.
11. Bandettini PA, Jesmanowicz A, Wong EC, et al. Processing strategies for time-course data sets in functional MRI of the human brain. Magn Reson Med. 1993;30:161-73.
12. Ogawa S, Tank DW, Menon R, et al. Intrinsic signal changes accompanying sensory stimulation: functional brain mapping with magnetic resonance imaging. Proc Natl Acad Sci. 1992;89:5951-5.
13. Dale AM. Optimal experimental design for event-related fMRI. Hum Brain Mapp. 1999;8:109-14.
14. Rosen BR, Buckner RL, Dale AM. Event-related functional MRI: Past, present, and future. Proc Natl Acad Sci. 1998;95:773-80.
15. Moritz C, Haughton V. Functional MR imaging: paradigms for clinical preoperative mapping. Magn Reson Imaging Clin N Am. 2003;11:529-42.
16. Baciu M, Kahane P, David D, et al. Hemispheric language dominance testing by fMRI in epileptic patients, using a rhyme detection task. NeuroImage. 2000;11:S268.

17. Mandal PK, Mahajan R, Dinov ID. Structural brain atlases: design, rationale, and applications in normal and pathological cohorts. J Alzheimers Dis JAD. 2012;31(03):S169-8.
18. Mikl M, Mareček R, Hluštík P, et al. Effects of spatial smoothing on fMRI group inferences. Magn Reson Imaging. 2008;26(4): 490-503.
19. Bullmore ET, Brammer MJ, Rabe-Hesketh S, et al. Methods for diagnosis and treatment of stimulus-correlated motion in generic brain activation studies using fMRI. Hum Brain Mapp. 1999;7:38-48.
20. Conklin CJ, Faro SH, Mohamed FB. Technical considerations for functional magnetic resonance imaging analysis. Neuroimaging Clin N Am. 2014;24(4):695-704.
21. Sabbah P, Chassoux F, Leveque C, et al. Functional MR imaging in assessment of language dominance in epileptic patients. NeuroImage. 2003;18:460-7.
22. Gabriel M, Brennan NP, Peck KK, et al. Blood oxygen level dependent functional magnetic resonance imaging for presurgical planning. Neuroimaging Clin N Am. 2014;24(4): 557-71.
23. Håberg A, Kvistad KA, Unsgård G, et al. Preoperative blood oxygen level-dependent functional magnetic resonance imaging in patients with primary brain tumors: clinical application and outcome. Neurosurgery. 2004;54:902-15.
24. Bizzi A, Blasi V, Falini A, et al. Presurgical functional MR imaging of language and motor functions: validation with intraoperative electrocortical mapping. Radiology. 2008;248:579-89.
25. Chaudhary UJ, Duncan JS. Applications of blood-oxygen-level-dependent functional magnetic resonance imaging and diffusion tensor imaging in epilepsy. Neuroimaging Clin N Am. 2014;24(4):671-94.
26. Courtney SM, Ungerleider LG, Keil K, et al. Transient and sustained activity in a distributed neural system for human working memory. Nature. 1997;386:608-11.
27. Gabrieli JDE, Poldrack RA, Desmond JE. The role of left prefrontal cortex in language and memory. Proc Natl Acad Sci. 1998;95:906-13.
28. Bookheimer SY, Strojwas MH, Cohen MS, et al. Patterns of brain activation in people at risk for Alzheimer's disease. N Engl J Med. 2000;343:450-6.
29. Small GW, Ercoli LM, Silverman DHS, et al. Cerebral metabolic and cognitive decline in persons at genetic risk for Alzheimer's disease. Proc Natl Acad Sci. 2000;97:6037-42.
30. Eden GF, VanMeter JW, Rumsey JM, et al. Abnormal processing of visual motion in dyslexia revealed by functional brain imaging. Nature. 1996;382:66-9.
31. Demb JB, Boynton GM, Heeger DJ. Brain activity in visual cortex predicts individual differences in reading performance. Proc Natl Acad Sci. 1997;94:13363-6.
32. Temple E, Poldrack RA, Protopapas A, et al. Disruption of the neural response to rapid acoustic stimuli in dyslexia: evidence from functional MRI. Proc Natl Acad Sci. 2000;97:13907-12.
33. Mayberg HS, Brannan SK, Tekell JL, et al. Regional metabolic effects of fluoxetine in major depression: serial changes and relationship to clinical response. Biol Psychiatry. 2000;48:830-43.
34. deCharms RC. Applications of real-time fMRI. Nat Rev Neurosci. 2008;9:20-9.
35. Emmert K, Kopel R, Sulzer J, et al. Meta-analysis of real-time fMRI neurofeedback studies using individual participant data: how is brain regulation mediated? NeuroImage. 2016;124:806-12.
36. Lee MH, Smyser CD, Shimony JS. Resting-state fMRI: a review of methods and clinical applications. Am J Neuroradiol. 2013;34(10):1866-72.

CHAPTER

188

Imaging and Interventions in Cerebral Ischemia

Shailesh B Gaikwad, Anuj Prabhakar

INTRODUCTION

Stroke is characterized as an acute, abrupt onset, central nervous system injury of vascular origin. The term "stroke" encompasses cerebral ischemia/infarcts, intracerebral hemorrhage and subarachnoid hemorrhage. The age adjusted prevalence rate for stroke in our country is 84–262/100,000 for rural areas and between 334–424/100,000 for urban areas.[1] 50–80% of strokes are ischemic in origin. Subarachnoid hemorrhage accounts for 1–7% of stroke cases and intracerebral hemorrhage is found in 7–27% of strokes, thus cerebral infarction is the major contributor towards morbidity and mortality in stroke. There is higher incidence of stroke amongst the younger age group and also among poorer population in India.[1] Imaging plays an important role in not only diagnosis and etiological classification of stroke, but also in its management, especially in the acute setting. A number of modalities may be utilized in imaging of cerebral ischemia and its effects on the brain parenchyma. The management of acute stroke has under gone rapid evolution and an interventional neuroradiologist has become an indispensible in management of acute ischemic stroke. In this chapter we shall discuss the pathophysiology, imaging and the various endovascular techniques that are utilized in these patients.

Pathophysiological Considerations

The cerebral blood flow is maintained by cerebral auto-regulation at a stable level. Under normal circumstances the rate of blood flow in the brain is directed by the cerebral vascular resistance which in turn is decided by the vessel diameter.[2] Auto regulation functions between 60–150 mm Hg mean arterial pressure. The brain is unable to compensate for changes in pressure either below or above this, leading to cerebral injury. When a major cerebral vessel undergoes acute occlusion, there is reduction of cerebral blood flow in the distribution of that particular vascular territory. This leads to a complex sequence of biochemical events that end with death of the involved neural tissue. Normal blood flow to the brain is approximately 50 mL/100 g brain tissue/minute. If the blood flow is reduced below 18 mL, the spontaneous and evoked electrical activity ceases, leading to neurological deficit. Failure of membrane ion homeostasis occurs at 10–12 mL/10 g/minute. Beyond this infarcts develop in the involved parenchyma **(Table 1)**. If the duration of ischemia lasts for more than 30 minutes, cytotoxic edema sets in.[1,3] At the cellular level, local depletion of oxygen or glucose causes a reduction in the production of high energy compounds. 5–10 minutes of complete occlusion may lead to an infarct.[4] Release of excitatory neurotransmitters, oxygen free radicles and apoptosis occur. The ion gradient across cell membranes is lost leading to cytotoxic edema. Cytotoxic edema manifests as focal swelling of the brain parenchyma with effacement of sulci and loss of gray white matter differentiation. Vasogenic edema, that occurs due to extravasation of water through damaged endothelial cells, develops in 3–6 hours and may extend into the white matter.[5] Within 24–48 hours of infarction, in-growth of phagocytic microglial cells occurs with proliferation of new capillaries. These capillaries lack tight junctions, and are permeable to both large molecules and water. This process begins at the periphery of the infarct and proceeds centrally.[6,7] Slowly, the necrotic tissue is removed by the macrophages and the remnant cavities and cysts occupy the infarcted area with glial scar tissue. Over subsequent weeks, complete resorption of necrotic tissue takes place with resultant encephalomalacia and loss of volume.[8]

Significance of a Penumbra

Brain tissue is extremely sensitive to ischemia. In presence of complete occlusion of a major artery, the neuron can remain viable for approximately 2–3 minutes. It is estimated that about 1.9 million neurons die every minute. When the

TABLE 1: Cerebral blood flow (CBF) in the pathophysiology of acute ischemic stroke.

• Normal	CBF - 50–60 mL/100 g/min
• Oligemic State	CBF - 35 mL/100 g/min
• Ischemic State	CBF - 20 mL/100 g/min
• Infarction	CBF - <10 mL/100 g/min

ischemia is incomplete, the injured brain continues blood supply from patent arteries and leptomeningeal collaterals. Therefore, acute cerebral ischemia may result in a central irreversibly infarcted tissue core surrounded by a peripheral zone of potentially salvageable (reversible ischemia) called a "Penumbra" **(Fig. 1)**. The transition from ischemia to irreversible infarction depends on the severity and the duration of reduction of blood supply.[9,10] The penumbra is a dynamic entity and its size is inversely related to the duration of the delay in recanalization. Imaging is currently directed to evaluate the size of the penumbra with the help of multidetector CT and MR imaging.

Etiology

Various systems have been proposed to classify arterial stroke subtypes. The simplest classification system is the ASCO phenotype system. This divides stroke into four subtypes: atherosclerotic, small vessel disease, cardioembolic and others.

Atherosclerotic strokes are the most common subtype of acute arterial stroke. They form approximately 40–45% of cases. Atherosclerotic disease may be intracranial, extracranial, or coronary. The prevalence of these subtypes varies with race and ethnicity. Intracranial atherosclerosis causes upto 30-50% of strokes in Asians.

Large artery infarcts are usually embolic in nature. Emboli arise from thrombi that develop at the site of an "at risk" ASVD plaque. Atherosclerotic plaques are most commonly found at the level of the carotid bifurcation. The cavernous internal carotid artery is the next most common site. The middle cerebral artery is the most frequently occluded intracranial vessel. A gene locus has been identified near TSPAN2 in patient who are susceptible to large artery atherosclerosis.

Small vessel disease represents 15–30% of all strokes. Small artery occlusions, (lacunar infarcts) are defined as lesions measuring less than 15 mm in diameter. They occur when the small penetrating vessels supplying the basal ganglia, thalami, pons, internal capsule and deep white matter are involved. These lesions may be clinically silent or may manifest with severe neurological impairment depending upon the site of infarct. Lacunar infarcts can be embolic, atheromatous, or thrombotic in nature. Most involve penetrating arteries in the basal ganglia/thalami, pons, internal capsule and deep cerebral white matter.

Cardioembolic disease is a cause of 15–25% of major strokes. Myocardial infarction, arrhythmia (most often atrial fibrillation), and valvular heart disease may lead to release of emboli from the heart.

Other is a heterogeneous group that combines strokes with miscellaneous but known etiologies together with strokes of undetermined etiology (cryptogenic stroke).[11]

IMAGING IN ISCHEMIC STROKE

Rowley[12] has emphasized on the assessment of the four Ps—parenchyma, pipes, perfusion and penumbra as summarized in **Table 2**.

Computed Tomography

The three main CT techniques used routinely for acute stroke evaluation are: 1. Noncontrast CT; 2. CT Angiography (CTA); 3. CT Perfusion.

Computed tomography is the initial imaging modality used in a patient presenting with ischemic stroke. Earlier, the main role of CT was to identify intracranial hemorrhage and to rule out other pathologies like neoplasms, that may mimic stroke. However, recent studies have pointed out that CT, in the context of use of thrombolytic therapy, has significant prognostic value in the evaluation of acute stroke patients.[13]

In the hyperacute stage of infarction, changes noticed on CT occur as a result of cytotoxic edema. The latter is seen as reduction in the density of gray matter in the ischemic tissue and obliteration of sulci and gray-white matter differentiation **(Fig. 2)**. In MCA territory infarction, these changes lead to the well-described insular ribbon sign and obscuration of lentiform nuclei due to acute ischemia of lenticulostriate territory **(Figs. 3A and B)**.[14,15] Various studies have reported a sensitivity of 56 to 90% in detection of such changes during initial 3–6 hours of ictus.[9] The extent of these CT identifiable changes at the time of presentation can help in identifying the subgroup of patients who will have a better outcome following

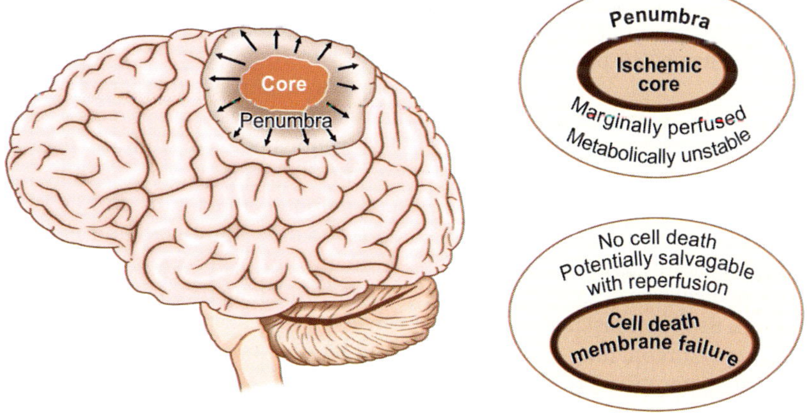

FIG. 1: Schematic diagram of brain involvement in acute ischemic stroke of MCA territory shows central core "representing the irreversible infarcted zone" and surrounded by the penumbra representing reversible ischemic zone if timely thrombolytic therapy is administered.

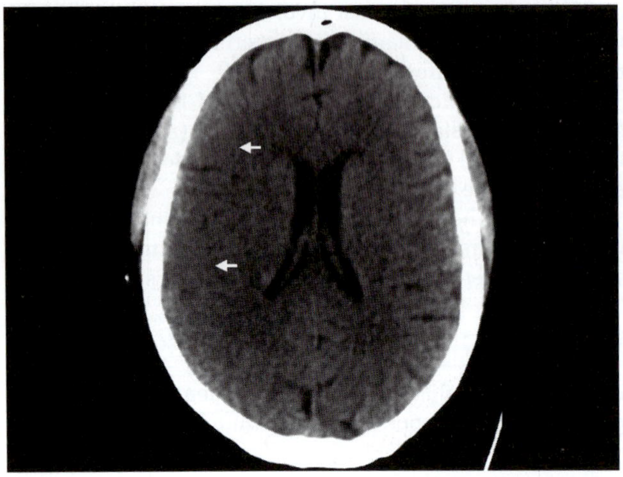

FIG. 2: NCCT head showing effacement of sulci with loss of gray white matter differentiation in the right MCA territory (arrows).

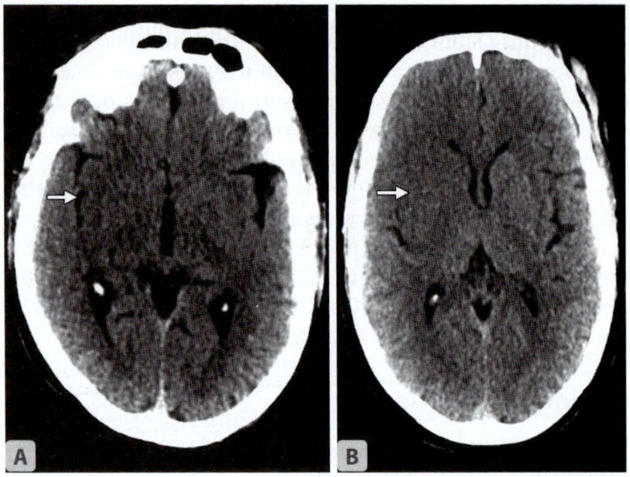

FIGS. 3A AND B: NCCT head showing (A) hypodensity involving the insular ribbon "Insular ribbon sign" (arrow); (B) Obscuration of right lentiform nucleus (arrow).

TABLE 2: Goals of imaging in the evaluation of acute stroke.

• Parenchyma	To evaluate for early imaging features of acute stroke and rule out hemorrhage
• Pipes	To identify an intravascular thrombus in either intracranial or extracranial circulation
• Perfusion	Evaluation of CBF, CBV, MTT
• Penumbra	Assess tissue at risk of infarct if ischemic insult continues without recanalization

thrombolytic therapy.[9] In the early stages, a hyperdense thrombus may be identified within MCA (dense MCA sign) **(Figs. 4A and B)**. [15,16] This may be seen in up to 50% of all cases.[16,17] Narrower window width (~8HU) and center level (~32 HU) settings improve lesion detection as compared to the default CT window. Increased clarity of early CT signs of infarct is associated with increased risk of haemorrhage. Also, involvement of more than 1/3rd MCA territory on NCCT increases the risk of hemorrhage after IV rTPa administration. However, various studies that utilized one-third rule showed that there was poor interobserver correlation.[18] Thus, the Alberta Stroke Program Early CT Score (ASPECTS) was proposed in 2001 to quantitatively assess acute ischemia on CT images by using a 10-point topographic scoring system[19] **(Fig. 5)**.

During the next few days, the density of the infarcted tissue decreases further, associated mass effect increases, and change can be seen in both grey and white matter **(Fig. 6)**. The infarct in acute and subacute stages can usually be easily identified. Sometimes, it may be possible to see a "fogging effect" in the subacute stage. This occurs due to increase in the attenuation of the infarcted tissue to a level approaching that of surrounding normal brain, thereby masking the infarct. This phenomenon is attributed to reopening of capillaries in the region with resultant hyperemia.[5] In the chronic stage; encephalomalacia is seen as area of low density with accompanying loss of volume in the form of dilated sulci and adjacent ventricular system **(Fig. 7)**.

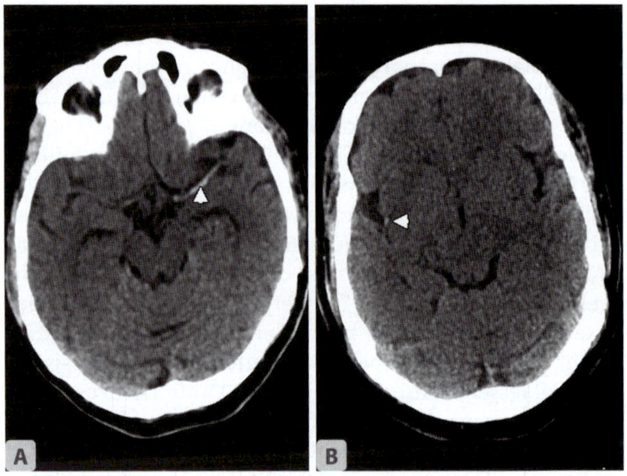

FIGS. 4A AND B: NCCT Head showing the hyperdense MCA sign secondary to an embolus lodged in the MCA (arrow head in A). If the embolus lodges in one of the M2 segmental arteries MCA dot sign is seen (arrowhead in B).

CT Angiography

CT angiography is a recently introduced technique which aims at studying the vasculature by performing rapid sequence computed tomography through the area of interest at the time of maximum opacification of the vessels with an intravenous bolus of contrast **(Figs. 8A to D)**. The data thus acquired can be processed to generate images similar to conventional angiograms.[20] CTA for patients of acute stroke must include both head and neck. The acquisition begins from the arch of aorta and should extend beyond the circle of Willis.[18] An acute thrombus is seen as an abrupt cutoff of the involved vessel without distal contrast opacification **(Figs. 9A and B)**. The thrombus location and extent is associated with subsequent recanalization rates in patients treated with IV TPa. Clot burden score can also be calculated on CTA images. When the CTA does not show occlusion, clot burden score is considered as 10. The intracranial circulation is divided into

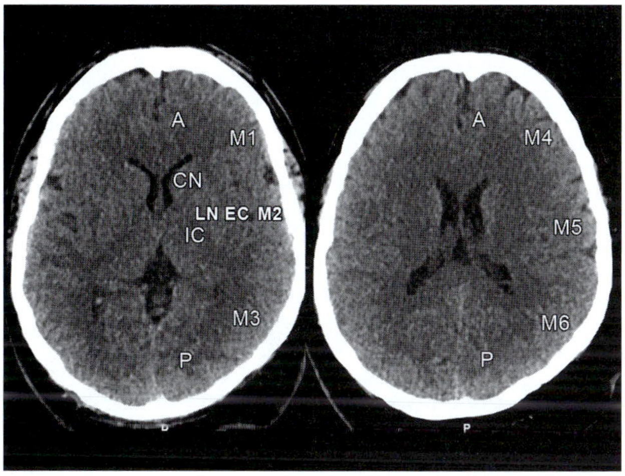

FIG. 5: The ASPECTS is determined from two standardized axial CT cuts, one at the level of the thalamus and basal ganglion and one adjacent to the most superior margin of the ganglionic structures, such that they are not seen. A single point is subtracted for an area of early ischemic change for each of the defined regions. A normal CT scan receives an ASPECTS of 10 points.

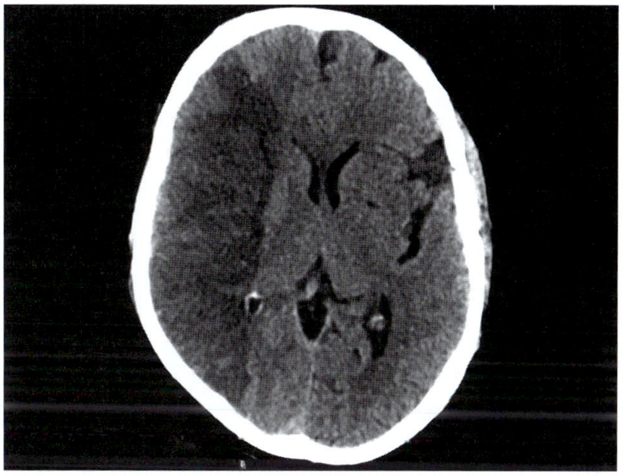

FIG. 6: Acute infarct 2 days after onset of symptoms. A wedge-shaped low density area involving both gray and white matter in the right MCA territory.

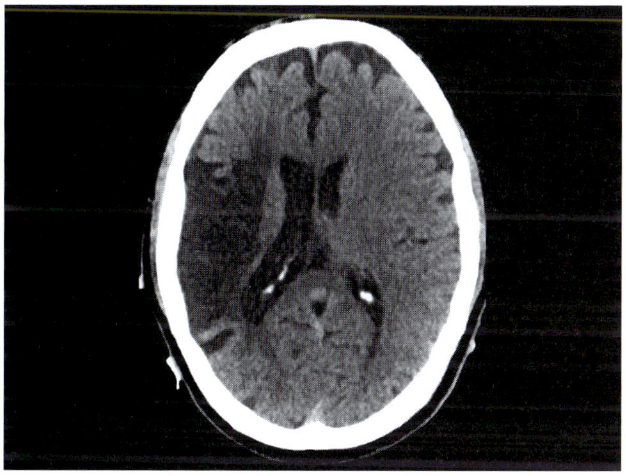

FIG. 7: Chronic infarct—Months to years after a stroke encephalomalacic changes result in volume loss of the affected brain. Calcification is rarely seen in chronic infarction.

the infraclinoid ICA, supraclinoid ICA, proximal M1 segment, distal M1 segment, each M2 branch and the A1 segment. Two points each are deducted if the thrombus involves the supraclinoid ICA, proximal M1 segment or distal M1 segments. One point is deducted if the thrombus involves the either M2 branch, the infraclinoid ICA, or the A1 segment.[21] The distal branches may be reformed through pial collaterals. Multiphasic imaging is essential to evaluate the presence of collaterals.[22] Various collateral scoring systems have been described. The ASTIN/ SIR scoring system is given in **Table 3.**[23] The sensitivity and specificity of CTA for detection of intracranial occlusion is high and varies between 92 and 100 and between 82 and 100% respectively.[24]

ASITN/SIR, American Society of Interventional and Therapeutic Neuroradiology/Society of Interventional Radiology; CTA, CT angiography.[23]

CTA source images (CTASI) can also be utilized to detect ischemic regions. The sensitivity of CTASI and DWI for detection of ischemic regions is similar. DWI is superior at demonstrating smaller abnormalities. In strokes of less than 3 hour duration CTA SI has higher sensitivity to ischemia as compared to NCCT. CTSI also identifies the area that will ultimately undergo infarction as it provides an estimate of cerebral blood volume.

In the extra-cranial circulation CTA is better than ultrasound for differentiating between complete and near complete occlusion. CTA also has 100% negative predictive value for excluding more than 70% stenosis when compared to DSA and functions well as a screening test. A large meta-analysis found CTA to have a sensitivity >90% and specificity >95% for detecting significant lesions compared with DSA.[24]

CT Perfusion Imaging

CT perfusion helps in identifying the tissue at risk. Various parameters are evaluated on CT perfusion. Cerebral blood volume (CBV) is defined as the volume of blood per unit of brain tissue (normal range 4–5 mL/100 g). Cerebral blood flow (CBF) is the volume of blood flow per unit of brain tissue per minute (normal range in gray matter = 50–60 mL/100 g/min). Mean transit time (MTT) refers to the difference between the time at arterial inflow and at venous outflow and time to peak enhancement, depicts the time required from the beginning of contrast injection to reach the maximum concentration within a region of interest.[9] In acute ischemic stroke, the penumbra will show an increase in the MTT with moderately or markedly decreased CBF and normal or increased CBV (80–100% or higher) **(Fig. 10)**, whereas infarcted tissue shows severely decreased CBF (<30%) and CBV (<40%) with increased MTT.[25]

Magnetic Resonance Imaging

Magnetic resonance imaging is more sensitive for detecting acute infarct as compared to CT.[26] During the initial few

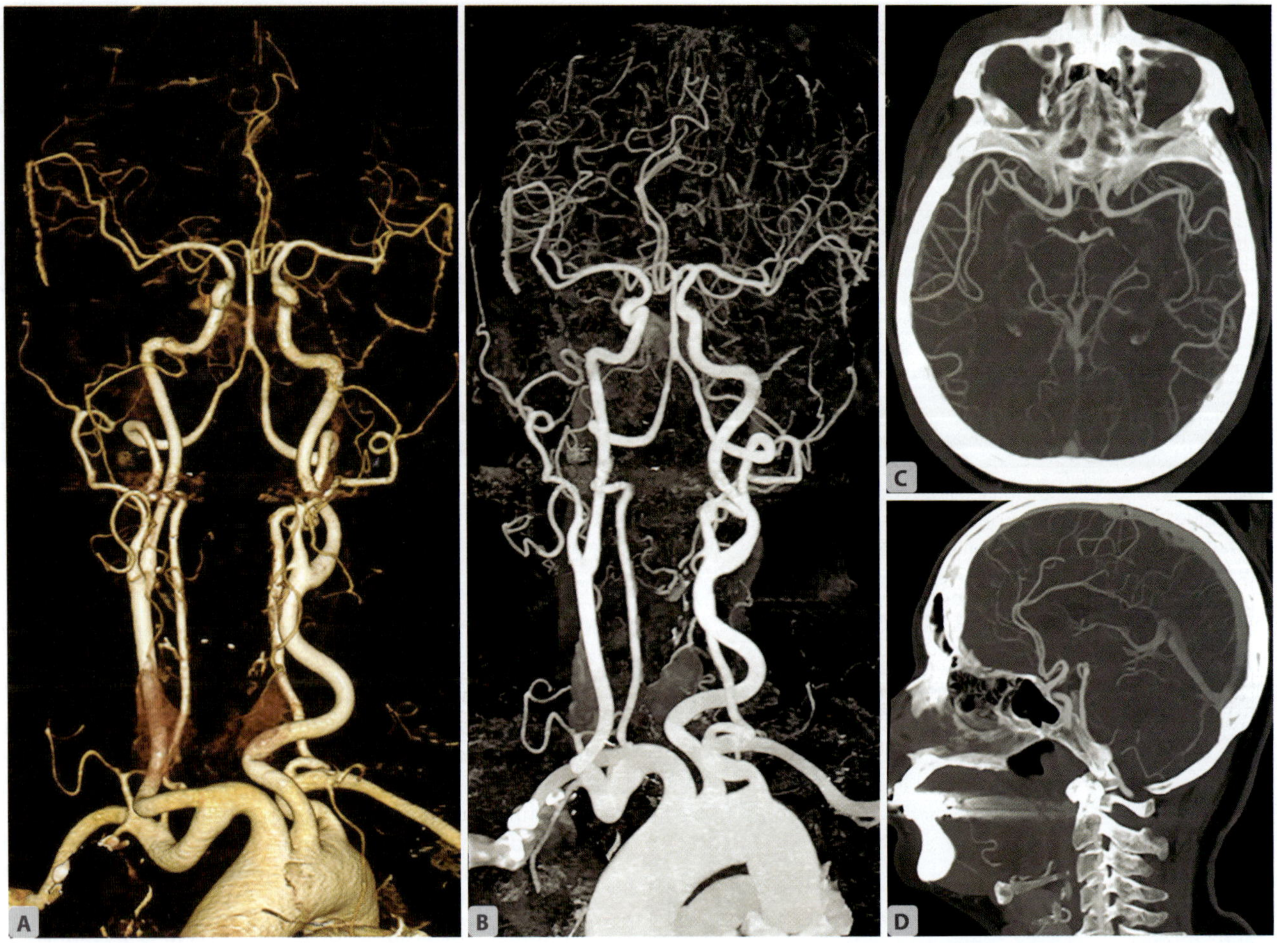

FIGS. 8A TO D: VRT (A), 3D MIP (B) and 2D MIP (C and D) CT angiography images. CTA is able to show the intra- and extracranial circulation in detail.

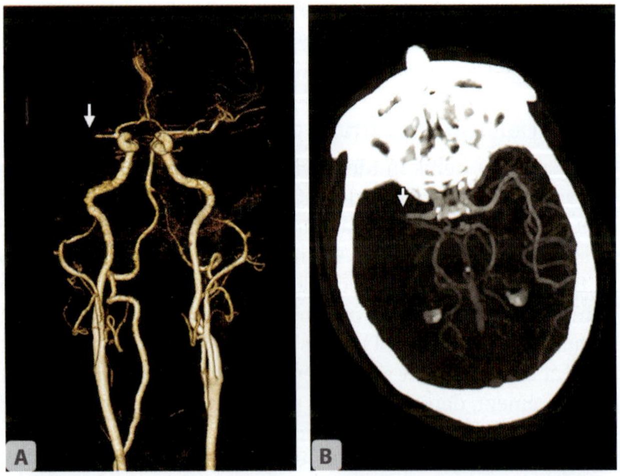

FIGS. 9A AND B: Acute thrombus in right MCA: VRT (A) and MIP(B) images showing abrupt cut off of the M1 segment of right MCA is seen without distal opacification (arrow).

TABLE 3: Modified version of the ASITN/SIR collateral score for dynamic CTA.
• 0—Non-existent or barely visible pial collaterals on the ischemic site during any point of time
• 1—Partial collateralization of the ischemic site until the late venous phase
• 2—Partial collateralization of the ischemic site before the venous phase
• 3—Complete collateralization of the ischemic site by the late venous phase
• 4—Complete collateralization of the ischemic site before the venous phase

hours of ischemia, the findings on MRI are related to vascular occlusion and cytotoxic edema. The sensitivity of apparent diffusion coefficient (ADC) maps and diffusion-weighted imaging (DWI) are very sensitive for the diagnosis of acute stroke. An acute infarct is hypointense on ADC and hyperintense on DWI **(Figs. 11A to F)**. ADC maps may show hypointensity within minutes of stroke onset; however ADC and DWI maps may not be 100 % positive within the first 2–4 hours after stroke onset. Various studies have found a sensitivity of 90–95 % of DWI for diagnosis of hyper acute stroke. Addition of perfusion-weighted imaging improves the

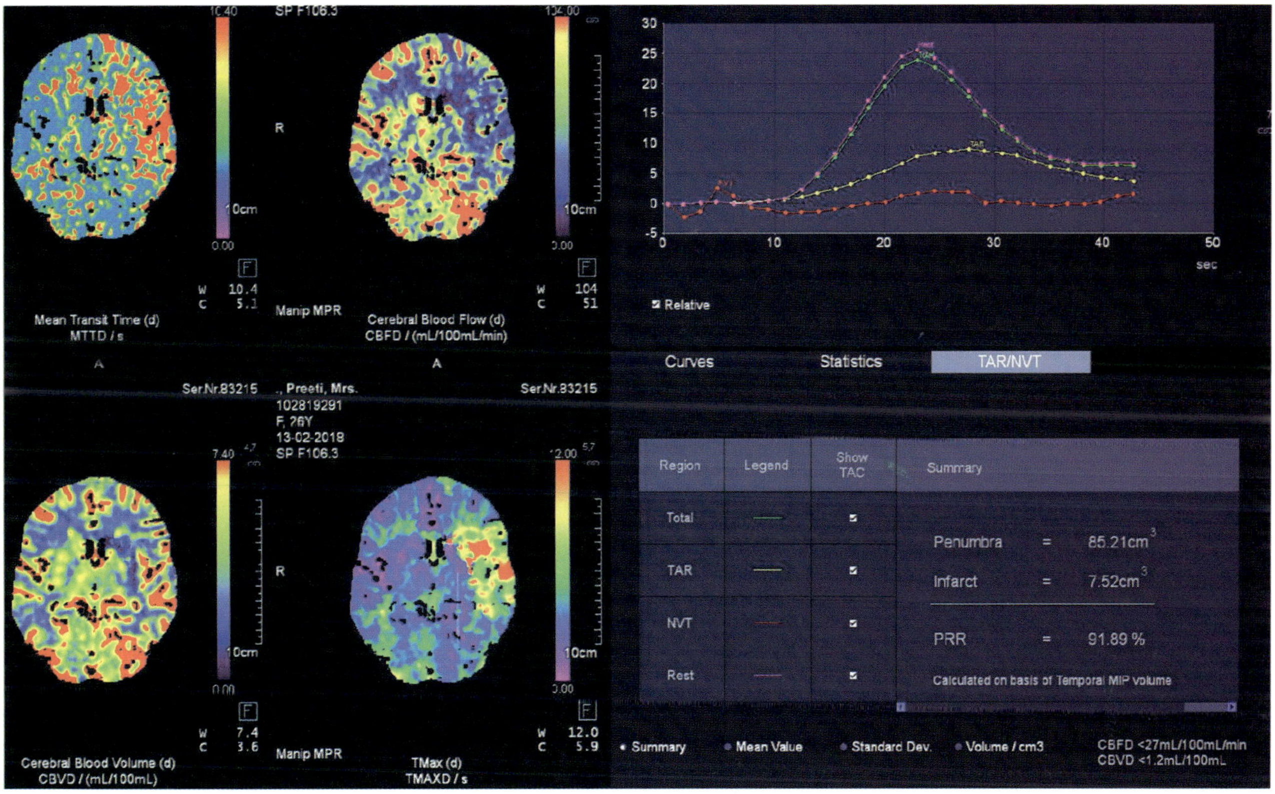

FIG. 10: CT perfusion: Penumbra shows an increased mean transit time with moderately decreased cerebral blood flow and normal cerebral blood volume. The percentage of penumbra can also be calculated.

sensitivity in such cases.[27] "T2 shine-through," may occur at a later stage after infarction and is seen as a bright signal on both DWI and ADC maps **(Figs. 12A and B)**. Hypointensity on ADC is maximum at 2–3 days and persists for 7–10 days. Signal intensity is lowest on DWI 3–4 days after infarction, however hyperintense signal usually persists for about 10–14 days. Pseudonormalization, characterized by normal signal on ADC may be seen on ADC maps approximately 1–2 weeks after stroke onset. The signal intensity, however remains high on T2-weighted images.[28] Restriction on DWI, is secondary to cytotoxic edema and is usually considered irreversible, however partially reversibility has been documented, if early and effective reperfusion is achieved, especially in less than 3 h after arterial occlusion.[29]

Hyperintense signal may be seen on FLAIR imaging after 6–12 hours of symptom onset. A DWI - FLAIR mismatch indicates that the infarct may be less than 6 hours old.[28] Other changes in the brain parenchyma include hyperintensity on T2-weighted images accompanied by subtle mass effect and loss of gray-white matter differentiation on T1-weighted images. These changes are limited to grey matter during the initial few hours. In some cases, hypointensity may be observed on T2-weighted images in the subcortical white matter. The cause for this hypointensity is not clear, but it may be related to presence of iron or free radicals. During next few days, intravascular and overlying meningeal enhancement can be seen in contrast-enhanced studies. The signal alteration and the mass effect become more conspicuous. During the subacute phase, sometimes T2 shortening may be observed in the infarct resulting in almost complete disappearance of the signal alteration observed initially on T2-weighted images. This is the "fogging effect" **(Figs. 13A to C)**. Contrast administration also shows prominent parenchymal enhancement in the infarcted tissue in the subacte phase **(Figs. 14A to D)**.[30] This is followed by resolution of meningeal/intravascular enhancement, reduction in mass effect.

Areas of T1 shortening, indicative of hemorrhage, may be seen in up to 20% of all infarcts.[25,30] T2*-weighted gradient-echo images and susceptibility-weighted images (SWI) may demonstrate areas of abnormal "blooming" in acute intracranial hemorrhage. The "artery susceptibility sign" is also seen on gradient imaging as blooming within the involved vessel. It is considered as MRI correlate of the hyperdense MCA seen on NECT **(Fig. 11D)**. The risk of hemorrhage after IV thrombolysis in patients with microhemorrhages depicted on SWI is unclear; Routine use of MRI to exclude cerebral microbleeds before administration of IV alteplase is not recommended.[31] In the chronic stage, encephalomalacia develops and is seen as focal area of altered signal associated with loss of volume.

As compared to CT MRI offers the capability to differentiate acute from chronic infarcts. Sub-clinical ischemic lesions and infarcts involving the posterior fossa are also better visualized on MRI. There is no radiation exposure and the spatial resolution is better. However MRI is more expensive with limited availability. The test is of longer

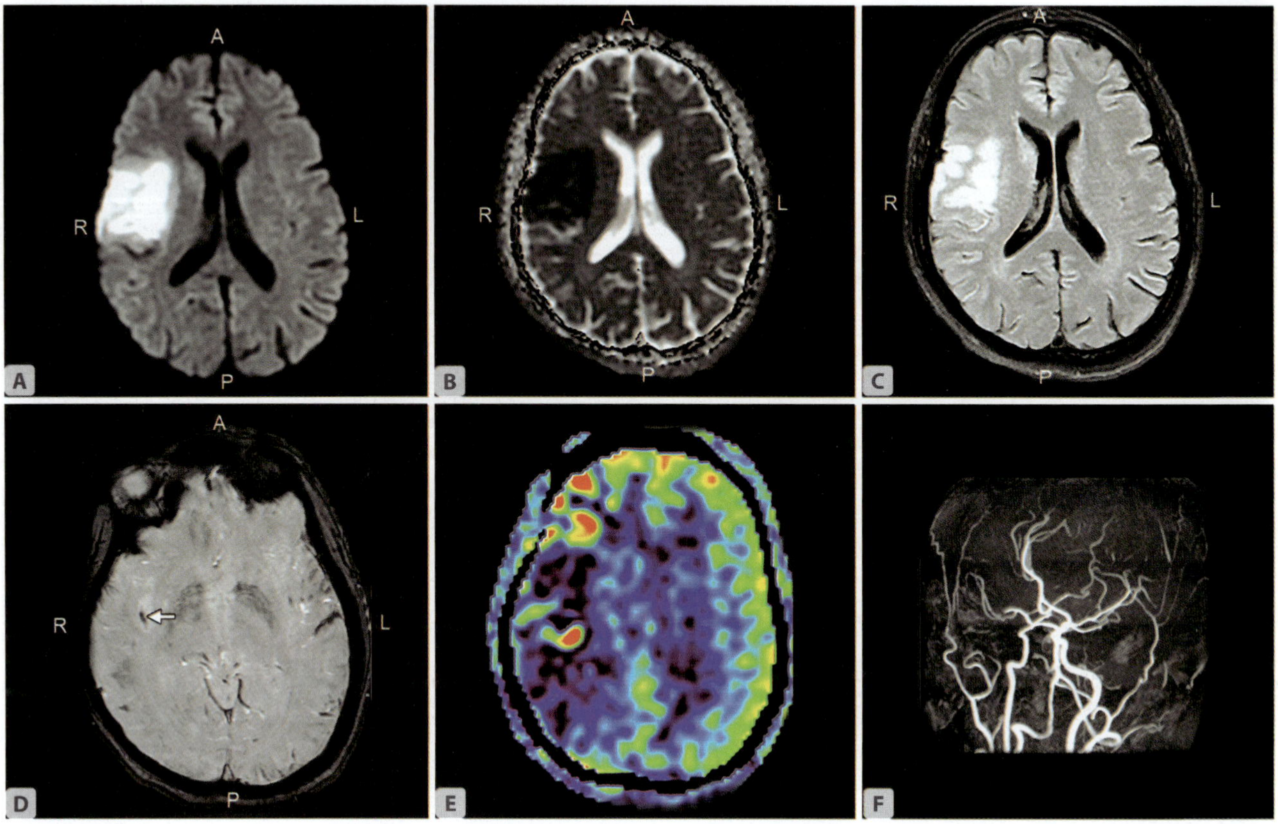

FIGS. 11A TO F: Axial DWI (A), ADC (B), FLAIR (C), SWI (D), ASL (E) and MIP TOF images (F) in a patient presenting with acute right MCA infarct. The lesion is bright on DWI, FLAIR and hypointense on ADC. SWI image is showing the hypointense thrombus within the MCA (arrow). ASL shows hypoperfusion of the involved area. MRA shows loss of normal flow-related signal in the right MCA distal M1 segment.

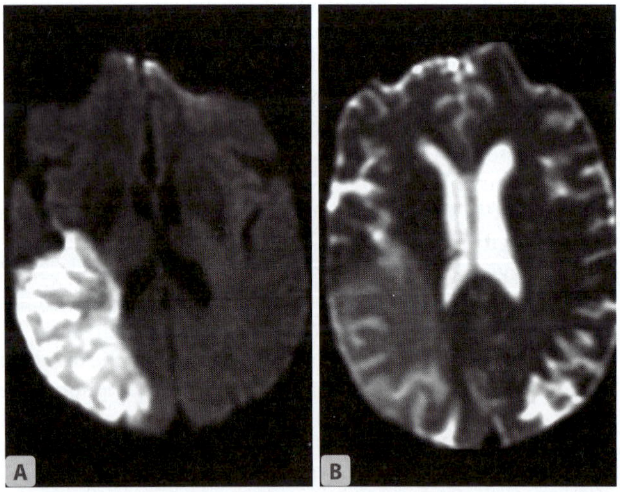

FIGS. 12A AND B: DWI and ADC images showing hyperintense signal - T2 shine-through.

duration as compared to CT and is more vulnerable to motion artifacts. Claustrophobia, metal implants, patient confusion, or cardiac pacemakers are also contraindication for MRI.[24]

Magnetic Resonance Angiography

Magnetic resonance angiography has come up as an effective, noninvasive tool to evaluate the vasculature. There are several different techniques that are available for evaluating intracranial vessels including 2-D time of flight (TOF), 3-D TOF, multiple overlapping thin-slab acquisition, and contrast-enhanced MRA. TOF angiography exploits the fact that the flowing blood continuously replaces the protons present within the vessel at a given point with fresh protons. The sequence is tailored such that the signal can be generated only from the protons in the flowing blood. Due to its simplicity and elegance, TOF technique is most frequently used in assessment of vessels. MRA allows noninvasive assessment of neck vessels as well as large intracranial vasculature.

Intracranial nonenhanced TOF MRA has a sensitivity of 80% to 90% for occlusions and 60% to 85% for stenosis, when compared with DSA or CTA. Although, TOF MRA is useful for identifying proximal large-vessel occlusions, it is not able to reliably identify branch or distal occlusions.[32] MRA has been shown to be better than Doppler US for distinguishing near total stenosis from occlusion of ICA.[33-35] In extracranial carotid disease 2D and 3D TOF MRA has a mean specificity of 88% and a mean sensitivity of 93% in diagnosing 70% stenosis. Contrast-enhanced MRA is more accurate as compared to nonenhanced techniques. It has specificity of 86% to 97% and sensitivitiy of 62% to 91%, when compared with DSA **(Figs. 15A to C)**.[24]

The spatial resolution is still not adequate enough to assess small intracranial vessels on 1.5T systems. However, with 3T MR system, it is now possible to image small intracranial vessels also. Disadvantages of MRA include its

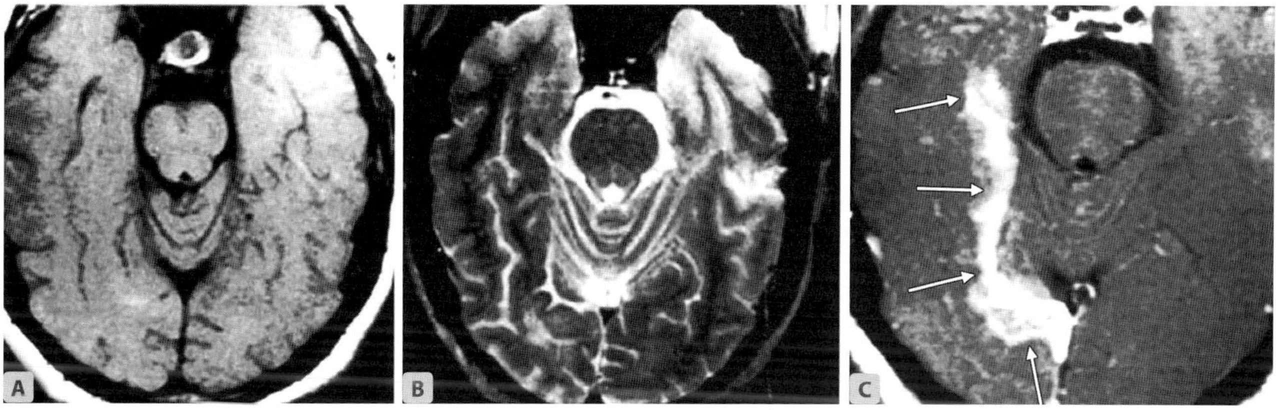

FIGS. 13A TO C: T1-weighted axial section (A) and T2-weighted section; (B) do not show presence of infarct which is seen as an enhanced area; (C) after contrast administration (arrows).

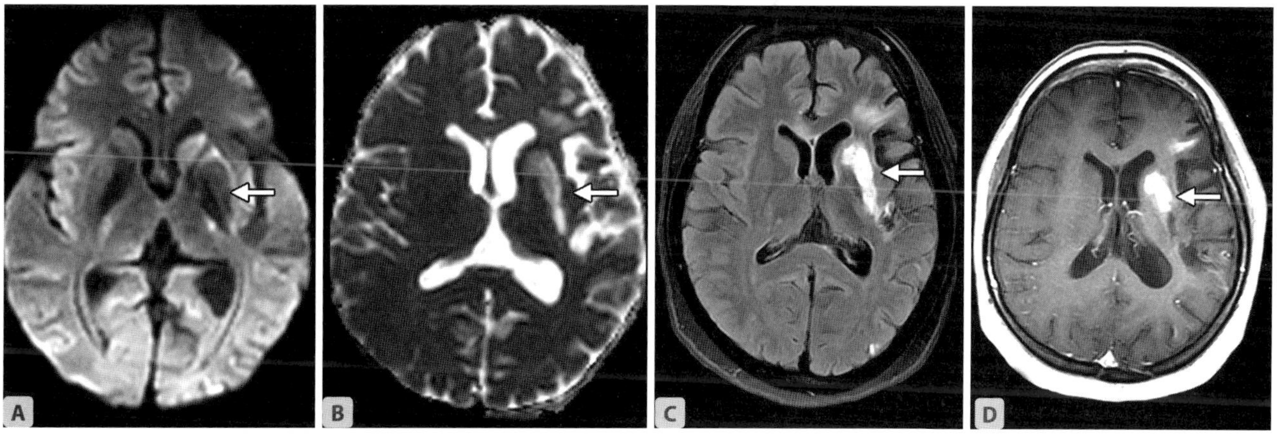

FIGS. 14A TO D: DWI (A), ADC (B), FLAIR (C) and post-contrast T1 (D) images in a subacute left basal ganglia infarct (arrows). The lesion is hypointense on DWI, hyperintense on ADC, FLAIR and is showing post-contrast enhancement.

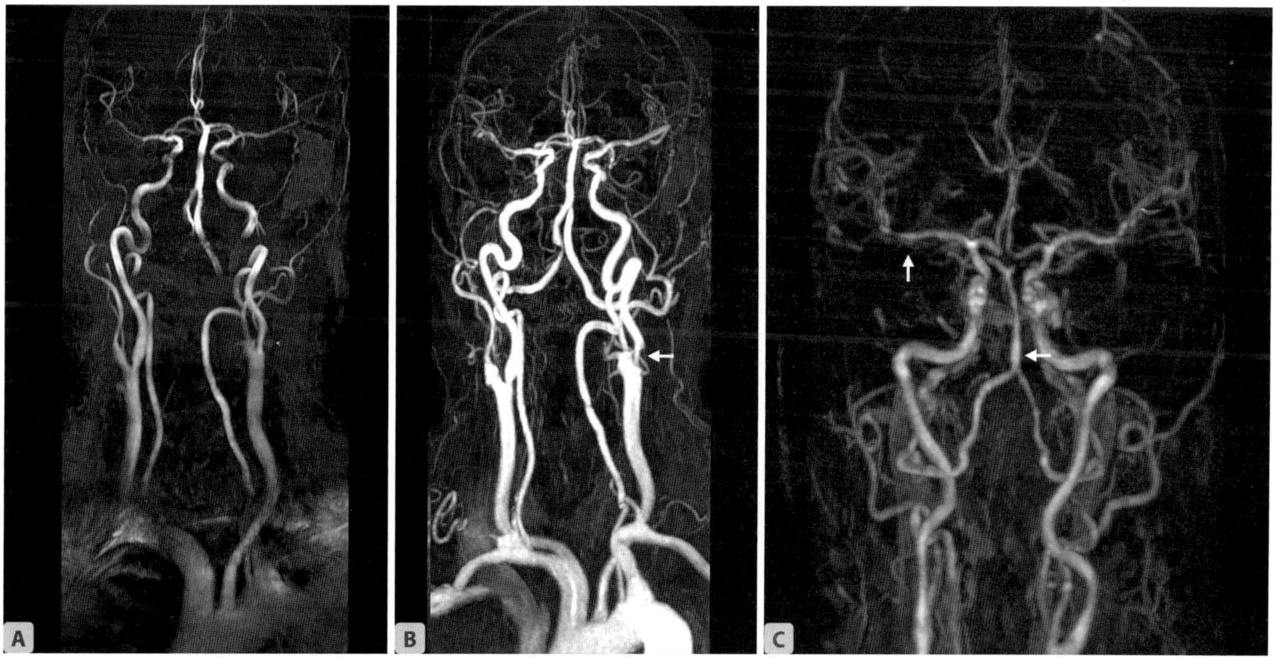

FIGS. 15A TO C: 3D TOF MRA (A), 3D Contrast-enhanced MRA (B) MIP images showing narrowing in left proximal ICA at the carotid bifurcation (arrows). CEMRA is not affected by vessel tortuosity or flow-related phenomena and shows the neck vessels with more clarity. 3D CEMRA MIP projection (C) shows intracranial atherosclerotic narrowing involving the right MCA M1 segment (arrow).

high cost, restricted availability, inability to evaluate small intracranial vessels and susceptibility to complex flow patterns. Additionally, some patients (e.g. claustrophobic, patients with metallic implants) may be unsuitable for MR evaluation and vessels at the root of neck and aortic arch are not so easy to image.

Combination of DWI and Perfusion in Evaluation of Acute Stroke

Perfusion MR is a technique that uses a rapid echo planar MR imaging sequence following the injection of contrast material. PW imaging demonstrates the alteration in physiologic state of the intracranial vasculature immediately after acute vascular occlusion. These changes may be characterized by a variety of qualitative flow-related maps including relative cerebral blood flow (rCBF), relative cerebral blood volume (rCBV) and mean transit time (MTT). Differences in perfusion and diffusion images may indicate the penumbra or the salvagable brain tissue **(Figs. 16 and 17)**. MTT maps show the largest area of abnormality and overestimate the final infarct size. Relative cerebral blood volume maps tend toward underestimation of the final infarct size. However, it has been seen that rCBV maps are closely correlated with changes in infarct size between initial and follow-up DWI maps. A mismatch between initial rCBV map and DWI more often predicts that there will be further extension of the infarct as compared to a mismatch between rCBV map and DWI.[18]

In acute stroke areas that show both diffusion and perfusion abnormalities represent infarcted tissue, while an area that shows only perfusion abnormalities with normal diffusion is likely to represent penumbra. Mismatch may also be seen in patients with symptomatic chronic cerebrovascular disease during challenge testing. In general, complete occlusion involving the proximal artery is more likely to cause a diffusion-perfusion mismatch as compared to distal or lacunar infarctions. In small vessel infarctions, diffusion-perfusion match is less, and the diffusion volume increases only slightly with time. In early reperfusion the diffusion volume may be larger than the perfusion abnormality. The perfusion abnormality may also be absent in early reperfusion.[18]

Carotid Ultrasound

Ultrasound (US) is an inexpensive, noninvasive, widely available tool, which can provide a reliable assessment of extracranial carotid arteries. A complete carotid US study includes a visual assessment of B-mode US image as well as evaluation of flow through the arteries using duplex and color Doppler. Normal carotid artery is visualized on US as two parallel echoic lines separated by an anechoic region.[36] The echogenic wall represents combined thickness of intima and media, and should not exceed 0.8 mm in width.[36] A plaque is seen as a hypoechoic to mildly echogenic eccentric area within the vessel lumen causing variable degree of stenosis. Presence of heterogeneity within the plaque may suggest possibility of hemorrhage, thrombosis, calcification or ulceration of the plaque.[37] US is reported to identify intraplaque hemorrhage with sensitivity and specificity of 90–94% and 75–88% respectively.[38,39] Heterogeneous and irregular plaques are known to be associated with a higher risk of stroke.[40] An ulceration within the plaque appears as a focal defect with sharp or overhanging margins.[41] Addition of color Doppler improves the detection of plaque ulcerations.[36] In addition to its role in atherosclerosis, US is also useful in documenting thickening of carotid arterial wall caused by various vasculitides, e.g. aortoarteritis and to monitor response to medical management in these cases.

Duplex Doppler study of the carotids helps in assessing the velocity of blood flow through the vessel. Normal end diastolic ICA velocity is less than 40 cm/s.[36] In presence of any narrowing of the vessel lumen, velocity of the blood flow at the site of narrowing increases. A number of studies have shown that the increase in the velocity can be used to assess the degree of luminal narrowing.[42-44] The velocity should be measured at or just distal to the site of stenosis

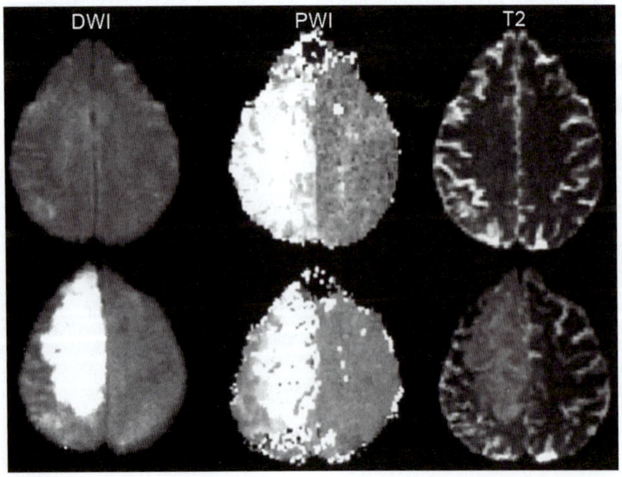

FIG. 16: Diffusion-weighted images and perfusion weighted images showing mismatch in the infarcted areas of the brain.

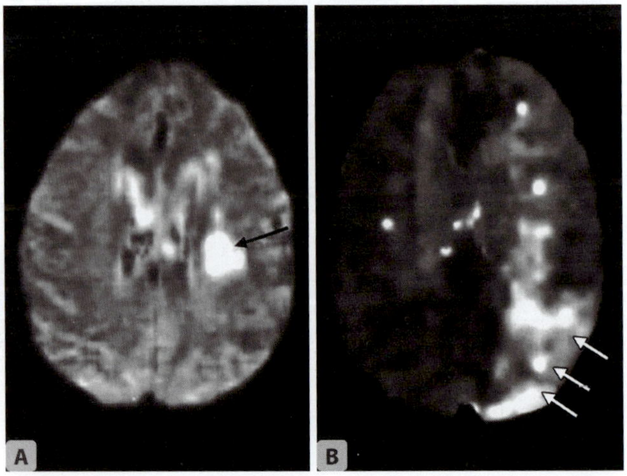

FIGS. 17A AND B: (A) Diffusion-weighted (black arrow) and (B) perfusion-weighted section showing mismatch (white arrows).

as shown on B-mode US or color Doppler study. A number of studies have shown that carotid Doppler can diagnose critical carotid bifurcation stenosis with a sensitivity of 81–94% and a specificity of 78–91%.[33,34,43-45] It is advisable that each center must establish its own criteria for diagnosing critical stenosis.[46] Some of the criteria which have been used in the literature for diagnosing >70% stenosis include peak ICA systolic velocity of >230 cm/s, end diastolic ICA velocity of >100 cm/s and a ratio of peak systolic ICA to CCA velocity of >4.[47]

Color Doppler has become a useful addition to the sonographic evaluation of carotid arteries. Severe stenosis (>70%) with abnormal flow velocities can be easily identified as areas of aliasing with post stenotic turbulence.[41] Color Doppler has high sensitivity for detecting a thin streak of blood flow.[36] The distinction between near total stenosis and vessel occlusion is more accurately made. Another important usefulness of color Doppler is its ability to detect narrowing produced by anechoic plaques, which would otherwise be missed on B-mode US.

The shortcomings of US include its inability to evaluate the intracranial vasculature, chances of missing tandem lesions in ICA higher up in the neck, and inability to assess densely calcified plaques.

Catheter Angiography

It is considered to be the gold standard for vascular studies. The technique allows assessment of vascular lumen of both intra and extracranial **(Figs. 18A and B)** vasculature with unmatched spatial resolution. Unlike MRA and Doppler, artifacts produced by complex flow patterns due to vascular loops or tortuosities do not degrade the technique. However, the procedure is invasive. Even with improvements in catheters, guidewires and contrast media, significant neurological complications may occur in 1–2% of all patients.[48] In spite of these potential risks, catheter angiography remains the investigation of choice in experienced hands for assessment of intracranial vasculature and is used as a problem-solving technique for the larger neck vessels. One limitation of the investigation is its inability to directly visualize the wall of the vessels. The latter information may be useful in certain situations like assessment of calcification in the wall, vasculitis and occult arterial dissections.

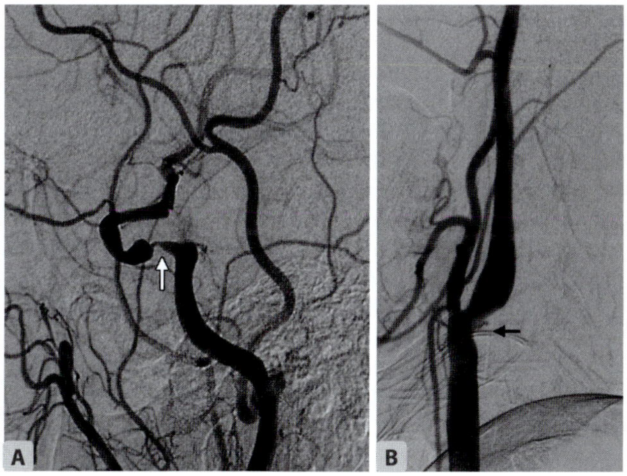

FIGS. 18A AND B: DSA is the gold standard for evaluation of both intra and extracranial circulation. Lateral view of ICA (A) shows narrowing in the petrous segment with reduced distal flow (white arrow). Lateral view of CCA; (B) in another patient shows narrowing with ulceration in the carotid bulb (black arrow).

RECANALIZATION STRATEGIES IN ACUTE STROKE

New therapies are being developed to manage acute ischemic infarction. It is important to distinguish between tissue that has undergone infarction and tissue that is ischemic but will survive despite the reduced perfusion to use these therapies appropriately. Although ischemic tissue may be salvaged successfully, these strategies are associated with risks such as an increased chance of intracranial hemorrhage. Some of the recanalization strategies are discussed in brief.

Intravenous TPA

National Institute of Neurological Disorders and Stroke Study (NINDS trial)

NINDS study showed that there was a benefit of intravenous (IV) tissue plasminogen activator, if it was administered within 3 hours of acute ischemic stroke onset.[49] In this study there was a trend towards an improvement in outcome despite the presence of hypodensity on early CT. The beneficial effects were noted in all stroke subtypes including suspected lacunar infarction. The benefits were sustained at 1 year. There were 12% absolute (30% relative) differences in 2 groups in patients having minimal or no disability at 3 months (32% vs. 44%). Mortality rate of 17% vs. 25% was insignificant and symptomatic intracerebral hemorrhage within 36 hours was reported as 6.4% vs. 0.6%. In both the PROACT II and NINDS trial, clinical outcomes were significantly better in those patients receiving fibrinolytic therapy despite an increase in the rate of intracerebral hemorrhage in the drug group as compared to the placebo group.[50]

The study concluded that despite an increased incidence of symptomatic ICH, treatment within 3 hours improved clinical outcome at 3 months.

ECASS—European Cooperative Acute Stroke Study Trials

In ECASS 1 trial, TPA dose of 1.1 mg/kg (maximum 100 mg) was used, of which 10% of the entire dose was used as bolus. This study showed that there was an increased risk of fatal parenchymal haemorrhage (30% vs. 6.5%) after IV thrombolysis administered within 6 hours (median time of 4 hours) of stroke onset. This unacceptably high risk of ICH may be attributed to various reasons such as: i. increased dose, ii. Increased therapeutic window, iii. Inclusion of large number (17%) of patients who already had unrecognized abnormality on pretreatment CT. This, however, did not statistically affect significant outcome.[51]

The ECASS 2 trial also did not confirm a statistical benefit for IV Alteplase. A dose of 0.95 mg/kg, administered within 6 hours of stroke onset was found to be as safe as that administered within 3 hours. No statistical benefit could be confirmed when compared with a placebo. The extent of hypodensity was found to be a major risk factor for severe hemorrhagic transformation. The ECASS 3 trial demonstrated benefit of IV Alteplase beyond the three hour window that was established in the NINDS trialand extended it upto 4.5 hours.[51]

The 2018 AHA guidelines for the early management of patients with acute ischemic stroke recommend that IV Alteplase (0.9 mg/kg, maximum dose 90 mg over 60 minutes with initial 10% of dose given as bolus over 1 minute) may be given to selected patients who can be treated within 4.5 hours of ischemic stroke symptom onset. Intravenous therapy should be started as soon as possible. Patients who are eligible for IV Alteplase should receive the drug even if endovascular treatment is being considered.[52]

Intra-arterial Therapy

Endovascular treatment for acute stroke includes mechanical thrombectomy or fibrinolysis. The intra-arterial route allows the neuro interventionist to extend the time window available for treatment of acute stroke and to target the large thrombi in the affected vessel directly.

The initial PROACT 1 and 2 trials evaluated the role if intra-arterial recombinant pro-urokinase in patients with acute ischemic stroke of less than 6 hours duration caused by middle cerebral artery occlusion. In the PROACT 1 trial patients with TIMI grade 0 or 1 with occlusion of M1/M2 were included. Recanalization efficacy was assessed at the end of 2 hours infusion and ICH causing neurological deterioration was assessed at 24 hours. Recanalization rates were 58% (partial or complete) vs. 14% for placebo and this difference was significant. Hemorrhagic transformation causing neurological deterioration within 24 hours of treatment was seen in 15.4% in r-proUK group and 7.1% of the placebo arm. Both recanalization and hemorrhage frequencies were influenced by heparin dose. However, neurological outcome was not significant.[53] Similarly, the results of the PROACT 2 trial also showed that arterial recanalization was achieved in 66% of patients who received recombinant prourokinase. Despite an increased risk of early intracerebral hemorrhage in the patients who received recombinant prourokinase (27.8% vs. 5.5% within 24 hours), 90 days mortality rates were not significantly different between the two groups (24% r-proUK vs. 27% control). This was the first randomised acute stroke trial to show a benefit of therapy as long as 6 hours after the onset of stroke.[54] Subsequently, first generation mechanical thrombectomy devices like the Merci retriever and the Penumbra aspiration system were introduced for mechanical thrombectomy. The initial multicenter prospective randomized controlled trials, including IMS 3, MR RESCUE and SYNTHESIS expansion evaluated intra-arterial fibrinolysis with or without first generation embolectomy devices. These failed to demonstrate benefit from endovascular intervention over IV Alteplase. However, there were various drawback and reservations regarding these trials. The imaging of patients enrolled in these trials was not adequate. Also, these studies suffered from a lack of proper selection of patients in the interventional arm. The newer thrombectomy devices were used in only a minority of patients.[55]

MR CLEAN was first randomized trial to demonstrate the benefit of current endovascular therapy combined with medical management over medical management alone for patients suffering from acute anterior circulation ischemic stroke with proximal arterial occlusion that could be treated within a time window of 6 h after stroke onset. A total of 500 patients were included (intervention arm, n = 233; Standard care -IV alteplase, n = 267). Retrievable stents were utilized for 81.5% of the patients in the endovascular group. There was a difference of 13.5% in the rate of functional independence in favor of the intervention (32.6% vs. 19.1%). There were no significant differences in the occurrence of symptomatic intracerebral hemorrhage or mortality.[56]

The DAWN trial was a multicenter prospective open label blinded end point RCT that evaluated 206 patients. It evaluated patients treated between 6–24 hours after stroke. Clinical imaging mismatch was used as the eligibility criteria in selection of patients for mechanical thrombectomy. This trial was stopped early at the first interim analysis. It demonstrated a benefit in functional outcome in the treatment group (mRS score 0–2, 49% versus 13%; adjusted difference, 33%; 95% CI, 21–44; posterior probability of superiority >0.999). This was the first RCT that gave evidence supporting mechanical thrombectomy after 6 hours in selected patients.[52]

The DIFFUSE 3 trial was randomized, multicenter and open-label. The outcome assessment was blinded. All those patients presenting 6–16 hours after symptom onset with remaining ischemic brain tissue that was not yet infarcted were included in the study. The inclusion criteria were proximal ICA or MCA occlusion, initial infarct size at presentation <70 mL, and ratio of the penumbra volume to infarct volume on perfusion imaging of 1.8 or more. These patients were randomly assigned to thrombectomy with standard medical therapy or standard medical therapy alone. The trial was terminated early for efficacy after 182 patients had undergone randomization (92 to the endovascular-therapy group and 90 to the medical-therapy group). It was seen that the functional outcomes in patients who underwent endovascular management, as evaluated on the modified Rankin scale at 90 days, was better as compared to the medical therapy group. The mortality rate at 90 days was 14% in the endovascular-therapy group while the medical-therapy group had 26% mortality rate. There was no significant difference in the frequency of symptomatic intracranial hemorrhage between the two groups (7% and 4%, respectively). The frequency of serious adverse events (43% and 53%, respectively) was also similar. This trial underlined the importance of evaluating the penumbra/core mismatch using CT/MR perfusion imaging in patients who reach the hospital after 6 hours of stroke onset. It also expanded the criteria to identify patients who benefit from mechanical thrombectomy after 6 hours.[57]

As per the 2018 AHA guidelines for acute stroke Patients should receive mechanical thrombectomy if they meet all the following criteria: (1) prestroke mRS score should be between 0 to 1; (2) The occluding thrombus causing symptoms should involve the internal carotid artery or MCA (M1 segment); (3) age ≥18 years; (4) NIHSS score greater than or equal to 6; (5)

ASPECTS greater than or equal to 6; and (6) Groin puncture for endovascular thrombectomy can be performed within 6 hours of stroke onset.[52]

There are no clear guidelines for endovascular management in posterior circulation stroke. Mechanical thrombectomy may be performed for basilar artery occlusion up to 12–24 hours after symptom onset, however a recent analysis of the Basilar Artery International Cooperation Study registry found that severe strokes at presentation treated beyond 9 hours after onset had poor clinical outcome.[58]

Technique

Access is made through a 6-F/8-F sheath. An initial angiogram is performed to assess exact location of occlusion and to assess hemodynamics of cerebral perfusion. Heparin is given in a bolus dose of 5,000 U followed by 1,000 U/hr for 2 hours or until the end of the procedure. A guide catheter is introduced into the affected internal carotid artery. Subsequently, a microcather is advanced into the occluded middle cerebral artery over a 0.14 microguide wire. Both microcatheter and microwire must be navigated across the site of occlusion. A stent retriever is then deployed at the site of the thrombus. This is a cylindrical self-expanding non-detachable stent that is mounted on a wire and deployed via the microcatheter. Once the stent is delivered into the vessel it self-expands within the thrombus pushing the clot against the wall of the artery, reestablishing blood flow to the brain. The stent is kept deployed for a few minutes, thus allowing it to ensnare the thrombus within its tines. The stent, microcatheter and the ensnared thrombus are then pulled out of the vessel while simultaneously aspirating with a 50-cc syringe through the guide catheter **(Figs. 19A to D)**.

Aspiration of the clot may also be performed using the penumbra device. This is a trackable reperfusion catheter with a large inner lumen that is deployed at the surface of the thrombus. A suction pump is used to generate negative pressure that allows the thrombus to be digested.

Various complications like sICH, SAH, IVH, vessel dissection, non-target emboli, vasospasm and stent dislocation may occur during mechanical thrombectomy.[59]

Acute Stroke Imaging Protocol (Flowchart 1)

Based on the experience at our institution and several others in the world, we recommend that whenever acute stroke patients arrive to the hospital within the first 6 hours

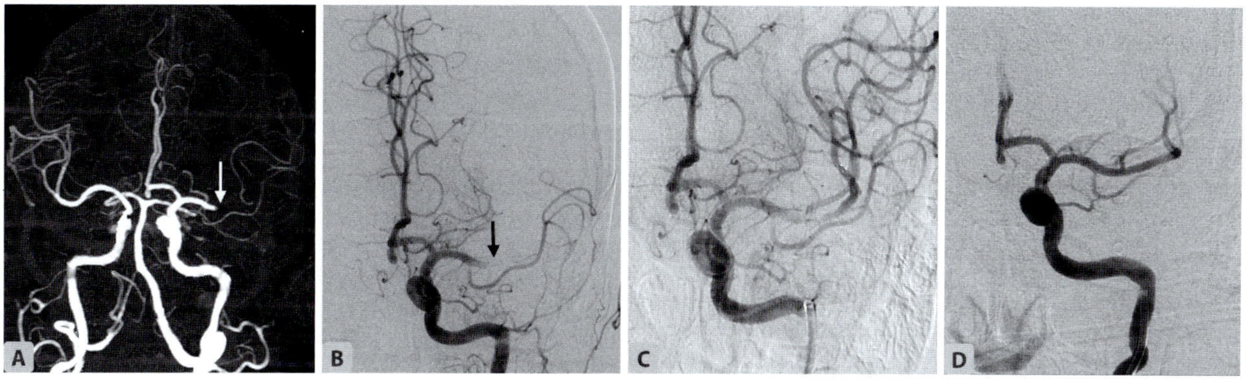

FIGS. 19A TO D: (A) A 55-year-old patient presented with right hemiparesis of 3 hours duration. CTA (A) and DSA; (B) revealed acute thrombus in left MCA M1 segment (arrows). Stent retriever was deployed; (C) and a single pass was taken. Post-procedure DSA; (D) revealed removal of the thrombus with good forward flow.

FLOWCHART 1: Acute stroke management protocol.

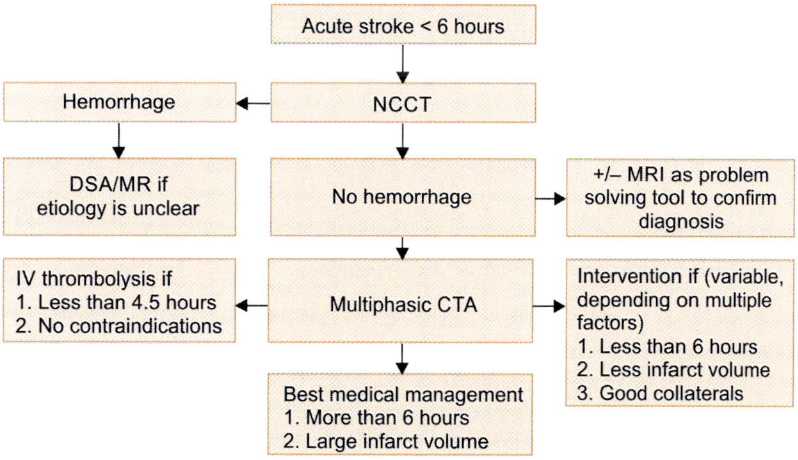

after onset of symptoms, they undergo an unenhanced CT. If NCCT depicts hemorrhage, no thrombolytic therapy is offered. If the CT shows signs of hyperacute infarct or is normal, a CT angiography of the head and neck to identify the site arterial occlusion. Those patients who present within 4.5 hours after the onset of acute stroke are given IV TPA if there are no contraindications for the same. If a large vessel occlusion is seen (ICA, M1 MCA, A1 ACA) on CT angiography the patient is taken up for mechanical thrombectomy. CT/MR perfusion may be performed in patients who are outside the 6-hour time window or in patients presenting with wake up stroke. Such patients may be offered mechanical thrombectomy if significant penumbra is seen on perfusion imaging.

VASCULOPATHIES

Atherosclerotic Vascular Disease (ASVD)

In presence of identifiable risk factors, ischemic stroke in a large number of patients is assumed to be secondary to ASVD. The role of imaging in this group of patients is to identify those patients who can be expected to benefit from intervention by reduction of future risk of stroke. On the basis of trials done so far, this group includes patients with nondisabling stroke in the anterior circulation with >70% stenosis and asymptomatic patients with >80% stenosis according to NASCET technique of stenosis measurement.[43-45] The initial screening is done by a noninvasive techniques, i.e. ultrasound, CTA or MRA. In view of its operator dependence of US, we feel that CTA/MRA should be the initial imaging modalities. Mural calcification, luminal irregularity, vessel stenosis, occlusion and thrombosis may be seen on CTA. Smooth plaques on CTA with extensive coalescent calcification are associated with decreased risk of rupture. A lipid rich core may be seen in larger plaques as subintimal hypodensity. High density subintimal foci are indicative of intra plaque haemorrhage. Both these findings represent an increased risk of plaque rupture. CTA may also reveal ulcerations in the form of contrast filled outpouchings. High resolution MRI can also be used to characterize plaque morphology. Hyperintense signal within the plaque on T1-weighted fat suppressed images represents hemorrhage. Marginal enhancement may occur around the plaque due to neo vascularity and is suggestive of an "at risk"plaque.[41] The MRI imaging appearance of plaque components is given in **Table 4**. Catheter angiography is a useful problem solving tool for confirmation of stenosis, evaluation of intracranial stenocclusive disease, ruling out any tandem lesions and to evaluate the hemodynamics in a patient.[41] Carotid artery stenting/carotid end arterectomy may be performed in selected patients who have significant stenosis at the carotid bifurcation.

Arterial Dissection

Dissection of the internal carotid artery is an important cause of stroke in young patients, responsible for up to 20% of all cases of stroke in young.[61] As a whole, arterial dissection is the cause of stroke in about 3% of all cases. It may be spontaneous or may occur secondary to blunt or penetrating trauma to the vessel. Catheter angiography has been traditionally used for the diagnosis of carotid dissection. Typical findings on angiogram include long segment tapering/narrowing of the cervical ICA extending from just beyond the carotid bulb up to the base of skull.[41] With the development of CTA, MRI and MRA, it is now possible to diagnose arterial dissection noninvasively **(Figs. 20A to C)**.[41,62] Apart from demonstrating luminal changes; wall hematoma can also be directly visualized. Associated pseudoaneurysms, if present, can also be visualized. Catheter angiography is needed only if any additional information is required **(Figs. 20A to F)**.

Aortoarteritis

Aortoarteritis is an important cause of stroke in young and middle-aged female patients in India. Clue to the diagnosis is usually evident in the form of differential limb pulses/blood pressures or hypertension due to renal artery involvement. Catheter angiography is invariably required for complete assessment in these patients as multiple vascular systems are usually involved. By virtue of its ability to visualize arterial wall, ultrasound serves as an excellent modality to document carotid arterial wall thickness and monitor response to medical therapy.

Fibromuscular Dysplasia

This is a non atherosclerotic, non inflammatory arteriopathy affecting medium and large size vessels. It is more common in females and occurs between 20–40 years of age. String of beads appearance, smooth long segment tubular narrowing or asymmetrical diverticulum like outpouchings may be seen.[41]

TABLE 4: MR classification of plaque components.[60]

		T1-weighted	T2-weighted	Proton density–weighted	STIR	Contrast-enhanced T1-weighted
Lipid-rich necrotic core		Iso/hyperintense	Iso/hypointense	Iso/hyperintense	Hypointense	Hypointense
Fibrous tissue		Isointense	Isointense	Isointense	Hyperintense	Hyperintense
Hemorrhage	Fresh	Hyperintense	Hypointense	Hypointense	Hypointense	Isointense
	Recent	Hyperintense	Hyperintense	Hyperintense	Hyperintense	Isointense
Calcification		Hypointense	Hypointense	Hypointense	Hypointense	Hypointense

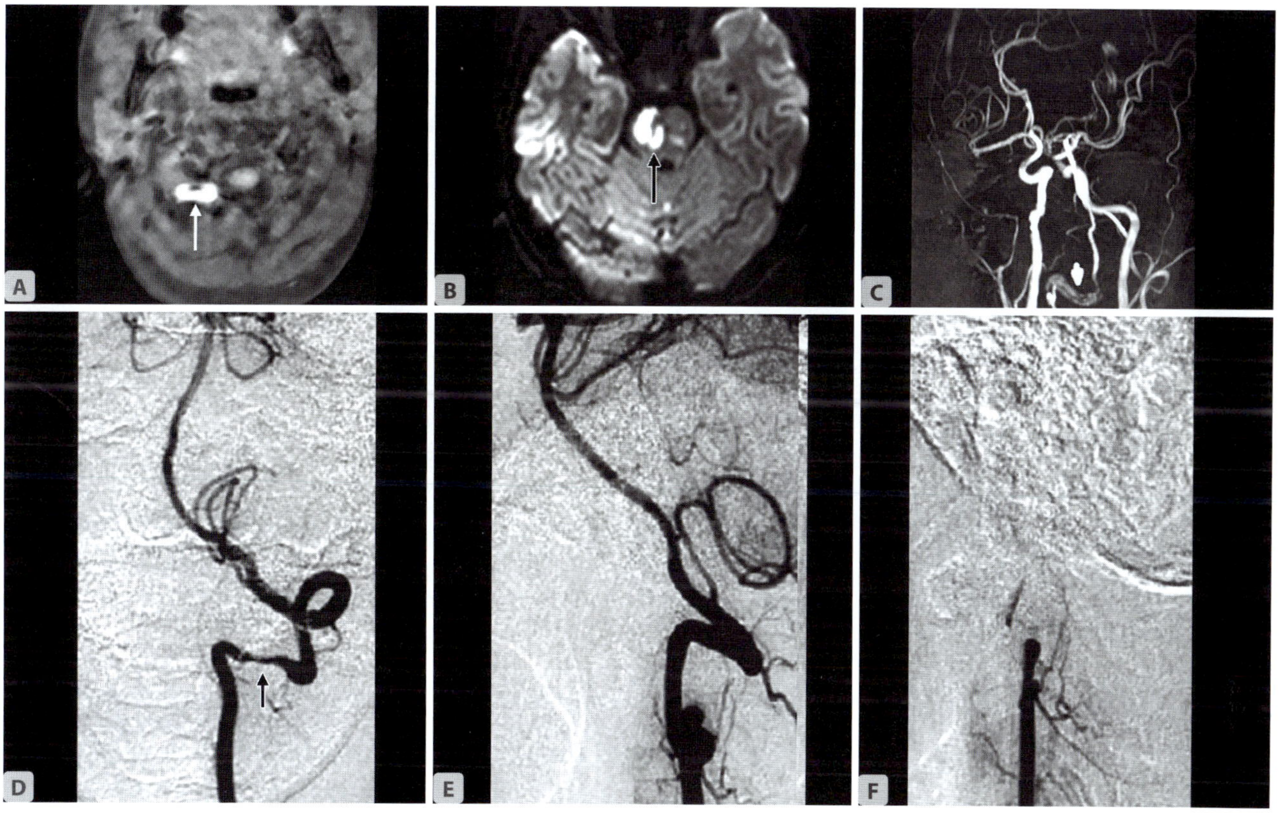

FIGS. 20A TO F: Axial T1 (A), Diffusion (B) and 3D MIP TOF (C) images in a case of right vertebral artery dissection show an eccentric hyperintense hematoma within the vessel wall (arrow, A) with pontine infarct (arrow, B). The right V3 segment shows loss of normal flow related signal (small arrow, C). The hyperintensity seen on TOF images in the right V3 segment is due to hematoma in the dissected segment. Left vertebral artery injection in AP (D), lateral flexion (E) and extension (F) in another patient show left vertebral irregularity and narrowing that is suggestive of dissection (arrow, D). The vessel is patent on flexion however, complete occlusion is noted on extension of neck.

Earlier catheter angiography **(Fig. 21)** was the investigation of choice for diagnosis of FMD for two reasons. One is that due to irregular areas of stenosis and dilatation seen in most cases of FMD, the flow pattern in the vessels is complex.[61] Secondly, FMD is known to be associated with intracranial aneurysms in up to 21-51% of cases. However, current generation CTA enables the radiologist to accurately diagnose FMD in cervicocephalic arteries and can also evaluate the intracranial circulation for aneurysms.[41]

Other Vasculopathies

This is an important, though uncommon, heterogeneous group of conditions, which can present with ischemic or hemorrhagic stroke. The diagnosis may be suggested by the related clinical features, e.g. stroke in young, stroke in the setting of disorders known to cause vasculitis or features suggestive of involvement of other organ systems, e.g. skin, kidneys, etc. Vascular imaging in these patients is needed to reach the diagnosis, to suggest areas suitable for biopsy, and to monitor response to treatment. Catheter angiography is most invariably required to assess the intracranial circulation. Sometimes, however, MRI and MRA may provide sufficient information needed for diagnosis, e.g. in Moya Moya disease particularly in the very young.

RECANALIZATION STRATEGIES IN ATHEROSCLEROTIC VESSEL DISEASE

Carotid Artery Stenting

Carotid artery stenting (CAS) is a minimally invasive procedure for management of carotid artery stenosis. The technique utilized in the North American Symptomatic Carotid Endarterectomy Trial is recommended for the analysis of stenosis. In this, the diameter at narrowest site in the stenotic segment is referenced to the most normal diameter immediately cephalad to the stenosis and not below.[63] The Stenting and Angioplasty with Protection in Patients at High Risk for Endarterectomy trial conducted in North America, favored CAS over CEA in a non-inferiority analysis. There was no difference between the long-term results at the end of 3 years between the CAS and CEA groups. However, this study has been criticized as it was terminated prematurely and most of the patients were asymptomatic. Later, 3 large randomized trials reported results favoring CEA over CAS. These were Stent-Protected Angioplasty versus Carotid Endarterectomy (SPACE), Endarterectomy versus Angioplasty in Patients with Symptomatic Severe Carotid Stenosis (ECASS) and the International Carotid Stenting Study (ICSS). The SPACE trial

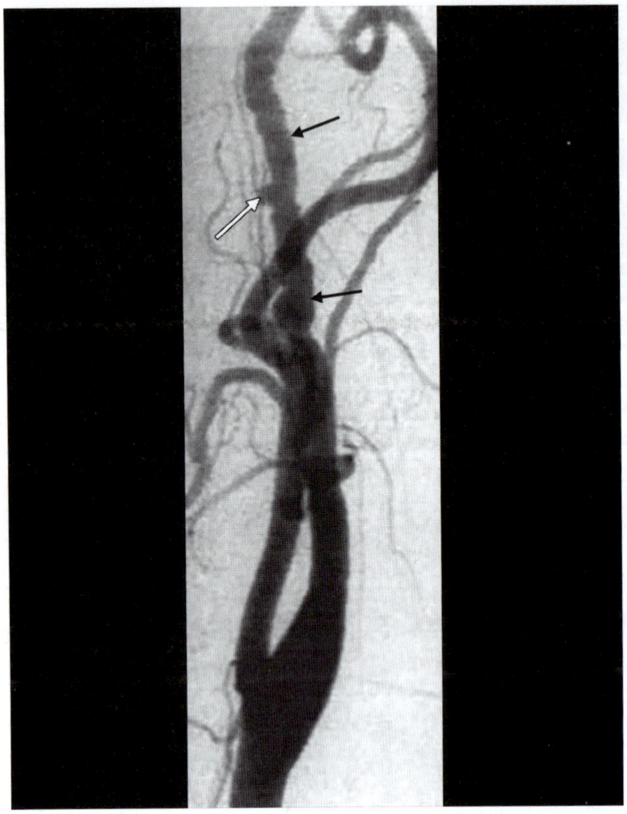

FIG. 21: Case of fibromuscular dysplasia (FMD) showing the string of beads appearance (arrows).

was terminated prematurely as evidence of a significantly higher rate of death or stroke was seen in CAS patients as compared to CEA at 30 days. In the ICSS the rate of stroke, MI or death at 4 months was notably higher in CAS. However, these results showing inferior efficacy of stenting as compared with CEA are considered inconclusive due to certain pitfalls for e.g. EPDs were not required; there was variation in the sort of stent used. Also, dual antiplatelet therapy for CAS was not mandatory in these trials. The Carotid Revascularization Endarterectomy versus Stenting Trial (CREST), a multicenter, randomized trial included 2,502 patients. Both symptomatic and asymptomatic patients were enrolled in this study and assigned to either CAS or CEA. Only one stent type was used in all patients; embolus protection device was compulsory whenever technically feasible and antiplatelet therapy was given in all patients. The treating physicians were strictly evaluated and trained during in the lead-in phase. While evaluating the results significant difference was found between CAS and CEA in the rates of primary end point ($p = 0.51$). It was noticed that rate of stroke during the procedure was higher in the CAS ($p = 0.01$). On the other hand MI was more common during CEA ($p = 0.03$). Women, symptomatic patients and age more than 65 years were found to be associated with higher stroke and death rates in the stenting.[63,64]

TABLE 5: Indications for CAS over CEA.
• Recent history of acute coronary syndrome, cardiac failure or severe left ventricular systolic dysfunction, Myocardial infarction or history of myocardial infarction within the last 6 weeks, severe coronary artery stenotic lesions requiring revascularization
• Severe pulmonary dysfunction
• Recurrent lesions following carotid endarterectomy
• Complete occlusion of the contralateral carotid artery
• History of previous radiation therapy, radical neck surgery, tracheostomy
• Thick, short neck due to obesity or Inability to tilt the head backward
• Paralysis of the laryngeal nerve
• Common carotid bifurcation located in the upper part of the neck (at the level of cervical vertebrae 2–3)
• Lesion is located at the origin or proximal part of the common carotid artery
• Distal internal carotid artery stenosis
• Separated tandem lesions
• Carotid dissection

Best medical management is an essential for treatment for all patients suffering from carotid stenosis. The 2011 American College of Cardiology and American Heart Association (AHA) guideline recommended CAS as an alternative to CEA in average-surgical-risk symptomatic patients when the anticipated risk of periprocedural stroke or mortality is <6% (Class I, B). They preferred CAS to CEA when carotid lesions were anatomically unfavorable (Class IIa, B). They also recommended that CAS may be considered in highly selected asymptomatic patients with ≥60% angiographic stenosis (Class IIb,B). Indications for CAS over CEA are given in **Table 5**.

Contraindications for CAS include unfavorable aortic arch anatomy or a heavily calcified aortic arch or a type 3 aortic arch. Other relative contraindications for which carotid end arterectomy may be preferred include lipid-rich soft plaque, Intraplaque hemorrhage, extensive plaque (>15 mm in length), heavily calcified plaque, thin fibrous cap, a lesion located at a curve or history of severe allergic reaction to iodinated contrast.

Preparation

CAS is generally performed under local anesthesia via trans-femoral route. Sedation is avoided. If general anesthesia is employed, use of intraoperative EEG/brain mapping should be considered. CAS can cause dramatic changes in the patient's hemodynamics, leading to hypotension or bradycardia. Vasoactive medications must be available to treat any hemodynamically significant changes. An arterial line should be placed for invasive hemodynamic monitoring

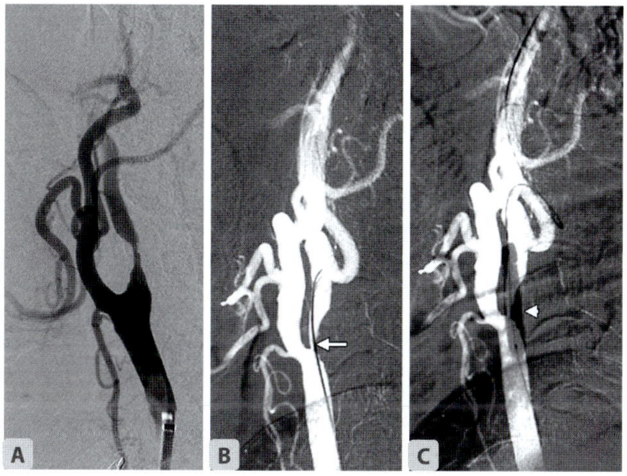

FIGS. 22A TO C: DSA image (A) showing severe ICA stenosis. The stenotic site was crossed by an 0.014 micro guidewire (B, arrow)) and predilatation was performed (C, arrowhead).

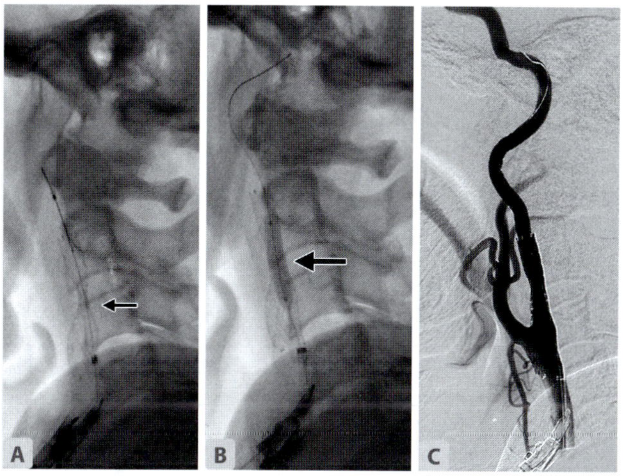

FIGS. 23A TO C: Fluoroscopy images. (A and B) showing stent deployment (thin arrow) and post-stent balloon dilatation (thick arrow). Check DSA (C) reveals normal opening of the stent with good forward flow.

during the procedure. Patients should be on aspirin 150 mg and clopidogrel 150 mg OD for a period of at least 3 to 4 days preoperatively, and these should be continued in the postoperative period. If adequate pretreatment time is not available 300 mg Aspirin + 300 mg Clopidogrel may be administered 2 h prior to CAS. Full sterile precautions should be maintained throughout the procedure as with any invasive procedure.

Technique

The common femoral artery is punctured via the percutaneous route using the Seldinger technique. A short sheath (8F) is then placed over a 0.035 in the wire. Intravenous heparin (70–100 U/kg) is instilled. The Activated clotting time is kept between 250 and 300 seconds. Using an angled catheter with 0.35" guidewire, the common carotid artery is selectively cannulated and mapped. The guidewire is then advanced into the external carotid artery followed by advancement of the catheter into the external carotid artery. Over an exchange length guidewire, a 90 cm shuttle is advanced into the common carotid artery. Dedicated carotid arteriograms are performed in multiple views to identify the lesion. A 0.014 in wire should be used to traverse the lesion. An embolic protection device may be deployed at this point in the straight terminal segment of the ICA . This is followed by pre-dilation using a small profile balloon if the stenosis is severe **(Figs. 22A to C)**. Careful attention must be paid to the patient's hemodynamics during this maneuver. Subsequently an appropriately sized stent is deployed. A self-expanding stainless-steel or nitinol stent is preferred for the carotid artery. Nitinol stents do not undergo foreshortening. They are more flexible and they match the target vessel curvature better as compared to other stents. The length of stent to be utilised depends on the length of the lesion. Usually 20–40 mm length is used. The stent should cover 5 to 10 mm distal and proximal to the area of narrowing. As most carotid stenosis involve the carotid bulb and the proximal ICA, the stent has to be deployed from the ICA into the distal CCA. While sizing the stent a stent-to-artery ratio of 1.1:1 to 1.4:1 for the ICA is considered. For patients with a large size-mismatch between the ICA and CCA, tapered stents can be used. If there is significant residual stenosis after deployment of the stent (>30%), balloon angioplasty may be performed **(Figs. 23A to C)**. The carotid sinus reflex may get activated during post-dilatation, occasionally requiring intravenous atropine or dopamine, depending on the patient's hemodynamic status. Finally, the EPD, if deployed, is removed followed by carotid and a cerebral angiography and removal of catheters and sheaths if the result is satisfactory.

Complications

Complications related to femoral artery access including bleeding, perforation, dissection, thrombosis, and distal embolization may occur. The stent may not deploy properly and can be associated with fracture.

CONCLUSION

CAS has evolved significantly over the past 2 decades. Large studies have shown that CAS, is a safe option for management of carotid artery stenosis in experienced hands. In certain high-risk patients, CAS is already recommended above CEA. Further improvement in technique and hardware, will lead to reduction of perioperative stroke rate. This will enable the CAS to become the standard of care for all patients.

REFERENCES

1. Bell BA, Symon L, Branston NM. CBF and time thresholds for the formation of ischemic cerebral edema, and effect of reperfusion in baboons. J Neurosurg. 1985;62(1):31-41.
2. Markus H. Cerebral perfusion and stroke. J Neurol Neurosurg Psychiatry. 2004;75(3):353-61.
3. Ter Panning B. Pathophysiology of stroke. Neuroimag Clin North Am. 1992;2:389-408.
4. Deb P, Sharma S, Hassan KM. Pathophysiologic mechanisms of acute ischemic stroke: An overview with emphasis on therapeutic significance beyond thrombolysis. Pathophysiology. 2010;17(3):197-218.
5. Taveras JM. Brain vascular disorders. Neuroradiology, 3rd edn. Taveras JM, editor. Maryland: William and Wilkins; 1996.
6. Sage MR. Blood brain barrier: Phenomenon of increasing importance to the imaging clinician. AJR. 1982;138:887-98.
7. DiChiro G, Timins EL, Jones AE. Radionuclide scanning and microangiography of evolving and complete brain infarctions. Neurology. 1974;24:418-23.
8. Einsiedel-Lechtape H, Kleihues P. Pathology of cerebral vascular insufficiency. In: Newton TH, Potts DG, (Eds). Radiology of the skull and brain: Anatomy and pathology. St. Louis: The CV Mosby Co; 1977.
9. Astrup J, Siesjo BK, Symon L. Thresholds in cerebral ischemia:The ischaemic penumbra. Stroke. 1981;12:723–5.
10. Hossmann KA. Viability thresholds and the penumbra of focal ischemia. Ann Neurol. 1994;36:557-65.
11. Osborn A, hedlund G. Arterial anatomy and strokes. In: Brain imaging, pathology and anatomy, 2nd edn. Philadelphia: Elsevier; 2018. pp. 197-252.
12. Rowley HA. The four Ps of acute stroke imaging; parenchyma, pipes, perfusion, and penumbra. AJNR. 2001;22:500-601.
13. Tomandi BF, Klotz E, Handschu R. Comprehensive imaging of ischemic stroke with multisection CT. Radiographics. 2003;23:565-92.
14. Tomura N, Uemura K, Inugami A. CT findings in cerebral ischemia: Obscuration of the lentiform nucleus. Radiology. 1988;168:463-7.
15. Truwit CL, Barkovich AJ, Gean A. Loss of insular ribbon: Another CT sign of acute middle cerebral artery infarction. Radiology. 1990;178:801-6.
16. Leys D, Pruvo JP, Godefroy O. Prevalence and significance of hyperdense middle cerebral artery in acute stroke. Stroke. 1992. 317-24 p.
17. Tomsick T, Brott T, Barsan W. Thrombus localization with emergency cerebral CT. AJNR. 1992;13(1);257-63.
18. Srinivasan A, Goyal M, Azri FA, Lum C. State-of-the-Art Imaging of Acute Stroke. RadioGraphics. 2006; 26(suppl_1):S75-95.
19. Pexman JH, Barber PA, Hill MD, et al. Use of the Alberta Stroke Program Early CT Score (ASPECTS) for assessing CT scans in patients with acute stroke. Am J Neuroradiol. 2001;22(8): 1534-42.
20. Leclerc X, Godefroy O, Provo JP. Computed tomography angiography for the evaluation of carotid artery stenosis. Stroke. 1995;26:1577.
21. Treurniet KM, Yoo AJ, Berkhemer OA, et al. Clot Burden Score on Baseline Computerized Tomographic Angiography and Intra-Arterial Treatment Effect in Acute Ischemic Stroke. Stroke. 2016;47(12):2972-8.
22. Bouchez L, Sztajzel R, Vargas MI, et al. CT imaging selection in acute stroke. Eur J Radiol. 2017;96:153-61.
23. Seker F, Potreck A, Möhlenbruch M, et al. Comparison of four different collateral scores in acute ischemic stroke by CT angiography. J NeuroInterventional Surg. 2016;8(11):1116-8.
24. Jauch EC, Saver JL, Adams HP, et al. Guidelines for the Early Management of Patients With Acute Ischemic Stroke: A Guideline for Healthcare Professionals From the American Heart Association/American Stroke Association. Stroke. 2013;44(3): 870-947.
25. Hoeffner EG, Case I, Jain R. Cerebral perfusion CT: Technique and clinical applications. Radiology. 2004;231:632-44.
26. Bryan RN, Levy LM, Whitlow WD. Diagnosis of acute cerebral infarction: Comparison of CT and MR imaging. AJNR. 1991;12(4);611-20.
27. Simonsen CZ, Madsen MH, Schmitz ML, et al. Sensitivity of diffusion-and perfusion-weighted imaging for diagnosing acute ischemic stroke is 97.5%. Stroke. 2015;46(1):98-101.
28. Allen LM, Hasso AN, Handwerker J, et al. Sequence-specific MR Imaging Findings That Are Useful in Dating Ischemic Stroke. RadioGraphics. 2012;32(5):1285-97.
29. Vilela P, Rowley HA. Brain ischemia: CT and MRI techniques in acute ischemic stroke. Eur J Radiol. 2017;96:162-72.
30. Mathews VP, Whitlow WE, Bryan RN. Cerebral ischemia and infarction. In: Atlas SW, editor. 2nd edn. Philadelphia: Lippincott-Raven Publishers; 1996.
31. Powers WJ, Derdeyn CP, Biller J, et al. 2015 American Heart Association/American Stroke Association Focused Update of the 2013 Guidelines for the Early Management of Patients With Acute Ischemic Stroke Regarding Endovascular Treatment: A Guideline for Healthcare Professionals From the American Heart Association/American Stroke Association. Stroke. 2015;46(10):3020-35.
32. Bash S, Villablanca JP, Jahan R, et al. Intracranial vascular stenosis and occlusive disease: evaluation with CT angiography, MR angiography, and digital subtraction angiography. Am J Neuroradiol. 2005;26(5):1012-21.
33. Mittl RL, Broderick M, Carpenter J P, et al. Blinded reader comparison of MRA and duplex sonography for carotid artery bifurcation stenosis. Stroke. 1994;25:4-10.
34. North American Symptomatic Carotid Endarterectomy Trial: methods, patient characteristics, and progress. Stroke 1991;22:711-20.
35. Pryor JC, Setton A, Nelson PK, et al. Complications of diagnostic cerebral angiography and tips on avoidance. Neuroimaging Clin N Am. 1996;6(3):751-8.
36. Polak JF, O'Leary DH, Kronmal RA. Sonographic evaluation of carotid artery atherosclerosis in the elderly. Relationship of disease severity to stroke and transient ischemic attack. Radiology. 1973;188:363-70.
37. Provenzale JM, Jahan R, Naidich TP, et al. Assessment of the patient with hyperacute stroke: Imaging and therapy. Radiology. 2003;229:347-59.
38. Merritt CRB, El B. The future of carotid sonography. AJR. 1992;158:37-9.
39. Steinke W, Hennerice M, Rautenberg W. Symptomatic and asymptomatic high grade carotid stenosis in Doppler color flow imaging. Neurology. 1992;42(1):131-8.
40. Moneta GL, Edwards JM, Chitwood RW. Correlation of NASCET angiographic definition of 70 to 99 percent ICA stenosis with duplex scanning. J Vasc Surg. 1993;17(1):152-7.
41. Osborn A. Vasculopathy. In: Brain imaging, pathology and anatomy. 2nd ed. Philadelphia: Elsevier; 2018. pp. 277-326.
42. Frught WE, Mattes MA, Van Bemmelen PS. Color flow duplex scanning of carotid arteries. New velocity criteria based on ROC analysis for threshold stenosis used in the symptomatic and asymptomatic carotid trials. J Vasc Surg. 1994;19(5):818-27.

43. Neale ML, Chambers JL, Kelly AJ. Reappraisal of duplex criteria to assess significant carotid stenosis with special reference to reports from NASCET and ESCT. J Vasc Surg. 1994;20:642.
44. Patel MR, Kuntz KM, Klufas RA. Pre-operative assessment of the carotid bifurcation. Can MRA and duplex ultrasonography replace contrast angiography. Stroke. 1995;26(10):1753-8.
45. Kent KC, Kuntz KM, Patel MR. Operative imaging strategies for carotid endarterectomy. An analysis of morbidity and cost effectivenss in symptomatic patients. JAMA. 1995;274:888.
46. Rosovsky MA, Litt AW, Krinsky G. Magnetic resonance carotid angiography of the neck: Clinical implication. Neuroimaging Clin N Am. 1996;6(4):863-74.
47. Tahmasebpour HR, Buckley AR, Cooperberg PL, Fix CH. Sonographic Examination of the Carotid Arteries. RadioGraphics. 2005;25(6):1561-75.
48. Cumming MJ, Marrow IM. Carotid artery stenosis: A prospective comparison of CT angiography and conventional angiography. AJR. 1994;163-517.
49. National Institute of Neurological Disorders and Stroke rt-PA Stroke Study Group. Tissue plasminogen activator for acute ischemic stroke. N Engl J Med. 1995;333(24):1581-7.
50. Del Zoppo GJ, Higashida RT, Furlan AJ. PROACT: A phase II randomized trial of recombinant pro-urokinase by direct arterial delivery in acute middle cerebral artery stroke. Stroke. 1998; 29:4-11.
51. Hacke W, Kaste M, Fieschi C, et al. Randomised double-blind placebo-controlled trial of thrombolytic therapy with intravenous alteplase in acute ischaemic stroke (ECASS II). The Lancet. 1998;352(9136):1245-51.
52. Powers WJ, Rabinstein AA, Ackerson T, et al. 2018 Guidelines for the Early Management of Patients With Acute Ischemic Stroke: A Guideline for Healthcare Professionals From the American Heart Association/American Stroke Association. Stroke. 2018 Jan 1;STR.0000000000000158.
53. Zeumer H, Freitag H-J, Zanella F, et al. Local intraarterial fibrinolytic therapy in patients with stroke: Urokinase versus recombinant tissue plasminogen activator (r-TPA). Neuroradiology. 1993;35:159-62.
54. Furlan A, Higashida R, Wechsler L, et al. Intra-arterial Prourokinase for acute ischemic stroke. JAMA. 1999;282(21):2003-11.
55. Ding D. Endovascular Mechanical Thrombectomy for Acute Ischemic Stroke: A New Standard of Care. J Stroke. 2015;17(2):123.
56. Berkhemer OA, Fransen PSS, Beumer D, et al. A randomized trial of intraarterial treatment for acute ischemic stroke. N Engl J Med. 2015;372(1):11-20.
57. Albers GW, Marks MP, Kemp S, et al. Thrombectomy for Stroke at 6 to 16 Hours with Selection by Perfusion Imaging. N Engl J Med. 2018;0(0):null.
58. Lindsberg PJ, Pekkola J, Strbian D, et al. Time window for recanalization in basilar artery occlusion: Speculative synthesis. Neurology. 2015;85(20):1806-15.
59. Behme D, Gondecki L, Fiethen S, et al. Complications of mechanical thrombectomy for acute ischemic stroke—a retrospective single-center study of 176 consecutive cases. Neuroradiology. 2014;56(6):467-76.
60. Young VEL, Sadat U, Gillard JH. Noninvasive carotid artery imaging with a focus on the vulnerable plaque. Neuroimaging Clin N Am. 2011;21(2):391-405, xi–xii.
61. Provenzale JM. Dissection of the internal carotid and vertebral arteries: Imaging features. AJR. 1995;165:1099.
62. Willinsky R, TerBrugge K, Montanero W, et al. Micro arteriovenous malformations of the brain: Superselective angiography in diagnosis and treatment. AJNR 1992;13(1):325-30.
63. Ahn SH, Prince EA, Dubel GJ. Carotid Artery Stenting: Review of Technique and Update of Recent Literature. Semin Interv Radiol. 2013;30(3):288-96.
64. Noiphithak R, Liengudom A. Recent Update on Carotid Endarterectomy versus Carotid Artery Stenting. Cerebrovasc Dis. 2017;43(1–2):68-75.

CHAPTER

189

Imaging of Subarachnoid Hemorrhage

Niranjan Khandelwal, Vivek Gupta

INTRODUCTION

Bleeding into the subarachnoid space is termed subarachnoid hemorrhage (SAH). It may be spontaneous or traumatic in onset, and may be trivial or massive in volume. Subarachnoid space can be the primary site of bleed or may be secondarily involved by extension of intracerebral hemorrhage (ICH). The causes of spontaneous SAH are:

- Ruptured intracranial aneurysms (75–80%)
- Arteriovenous malformations (AVMs) (5%)
- Cryptic vascular malformations (5–10%)
- Vasculitis
- Blood dyscrasias
- Primary and metastatic brain tumors (<2%)
- Spinal cord AVMs or tumors (<2%)
- Eclampsia (<2%)
- Anticoagulant therapy
- Unknown etiology (7–10%).

INCIDENCE

The incidence of SAH has been estimated to be about 10–28 per 100,000 person-years. However, some recent studies have found it to be much lower in the range of 6–8 per 100,000 person-years.[1] It carries a very high morbidity and mortality.[2,3] Ten percent of patients die before reaching the hospital. About 8% die from deterioration after the initial hemorrhage. Amongst the patients surviving the initial hemorrhage and treated without surgery, re-bleeding is the major cause of death in about 30–38% of cases. Vasospasm kills another 7% and causes severe deficit in another 7%.[2] The 30 days mortality rate for SAH is 46%.[4,5] It is further complicated by intracerebral hemorrhage (ICH) (20–40%), intraventricular hemorrhage (IVH) (15–35%) and subdural hemorrhage (SDH) (2–5%).

CLINICAL FEATURES

Sudden, severe "explosive" headache, vomiting, altered sensorium are common presentations. Usually the headache is described as "worst headache of the life". The usual age of presentation is 55–60 years; 20% of cases during sleep and 50% of patients have warning symptoms.[3] The risk factors are modifiable and non-modifiable. Among the latter group familial predisposition, presence of heritable connective tissue disorders like Ehler-Danlos disease, Autosomal dominant polycystic kidney disease (ADPKD) and Neurofibromatosis-I. Modifiable risk factors are hypertension, cigarette smoking, cocaine abuse, oral contraceptives, alcohol consumption, pregnancy, etc.[2-5]

GRADING SYSTEM OF SUBARACHNOID HEMORRHAGE

The clinical grading is important for estimating prognosis of SAH as well as to assess the operative risk. There are several grading systems and are listed in the Appendix.

DIAGNOSIS

- Lumbar puncture
- Computed tomography (CT)
- Magnetic resonance imaging (MRI)
- Conventional cerebral angiography
- CT angiography (CTA)
- Magnetic resonance angiography (MRA)
- Transcranial Doppler ultrasound.

Lumbar Puncture (LP)

Before the advent of CT, it was the only method to confirm the diagnosis of SAH. Presently, it is indicated only when CT is normal in patients with sudden, severe headache. There is risk of re-bleeding or neurological deterioration after LP and in two studies involving 165 patients with SAH, 17 (10%) patients experienced deterioration in their conditions within 24 hours of LP.[6,7] Opening pressure is usually elevated. Cerebrospinal fluid (CSF) is bloody not clearing with sequential tubes; Xanthochromia is present after 1–2 days of SAH. Presently with the availability of NCCT and MRI it is rare that a LP is required to establish the diagnosis of SAH.

Computed Tomography

Nonenhanced CT is the first step in the investigation of patients with suspected SAH. The probability of detecting hemorrhage is proportional to the clinical grade of the patient and the time after the hemorrhage. Three percent of 1553 patients had normal CT within 24 hours of confirmed SAH.[6] In a prospective series of 100 patients, SAH was detected in all patients within 48 hours of ictus, 85% after 5 days, 50% after one week, 30% after 2 weeks and almost nil after 3 weeks[8] **(Figs. 1A and B)**. Contrast enhanced CT helps in detecting the etiology of SAH, e.g. aneurysms (30–76%), AVMs (98–100%), tumors, etc. The volume and location of SAH on CT gives important prognostic information about vasospasm and outcome after the hemorrhage. In a prospective study, Fisher et al. reported a good correlation between the location and volume of blood and subsequent development of vasospasm. Increasing SAH on CT is associated with worsening clinical grade and poor outcome **(Table 1)**.[9]

CT is also helpful in detecting complications of SAH and surgery including ICH hydrocephalus and infarcts. CT can also predict aneurysm location and the side in more than 70% of cases.

- Bleed in interhemispheric fissure, frontal lobe or septum pellucidum indicates anterior communicating artery (ACoM) aneurysm **(Figs. 2A to C)**.
- Bleed in sylvian fissure or temporal lobe or interpeduncular cistern indicates posterior communicating artery (PCoM) aneurysm.
- Comma shaped bleed in sylvian fissure indicates MCA aneurysm.
- Bleed in interpeduncular cistern and/or brainstem suggests basilar top aneurysm **(Figs. 3A and B)**.

Magnetic Resonance Imaging

Conventional MRI (T1WI and T2WI) is not very sensitive in detecting SAH in acute stage (first 24–48 hours) in which situation CT is the preferred modality. FLAIR sequence has been found to be quite sensitive in detecting acute SAH. Since the application of inversion recovery pulse nulls the signal of CSF on T2 weighted sequence the blood in the subarachnoid space can be seen with a high sensitivity **(Figs. 4A and B)**.[10]

However, with elapsing time in subacute and chronic SAH, MRI is the best modality (>after 48 hours to over 1 month) and can detect hemorrhage even when CSF examination and CT become normal.[8] Standard spin echo (SE: T1, PD, T2) and gradient echo (GE) and susceptibility sequences are used. Contrast enhanced MRI helps in detecting the cause of SAH. MRI had a sensitivity of 95% and in no case CT was positive where MRI had failed.[9] This is because of formation of methemoglobin (usually after 4–5 days) which has paramagnetic properties and hence causes T_1 shortening. With mild SAH, the RBCs may be absorbed before methemoglobin is formed and it may be missed on MRI. GE sequences are especially helpful to observe the products of hemorrhage because of increased sensitivity to magnetic susceptibility. MRI also depicts complications of SAH, i.e. hydrocephalus, mass effect, infarcts, etc. It also helps in determining the etiology of SAH, e.g. aneurysms, AVMs, venous angiomas, tumors, etc. In cases of multiple aneurysms, it may help in determining which aneurysm has ruptured.

Cerebral Angiography

It is considered the gold standard and 4 vessel angiography should generally be performed in all cases of SAH. The role of angiography is to identify the cause of bleed, relationship of the cause to the parent vessel, define collateral circulation and assess vasospasm. Technically adequate angiography is essential. Magnification, subtraction and stereoscopic techniques delineate the cause of bleeding in most cases.

TABLE 1: Modified Fisher grading scale and vasospasm (on CT).

Grade	Features	Risk of vasospasm
1.	Focal/diffuse thin SAH (<1mm)	24%
2.	Focal/diffuse thin SAH (<1mm) with IVH	33%
3.	Thick SAH (>1 mm)	33%
4.	Thick SAH (>1 mm) with IVH	40%

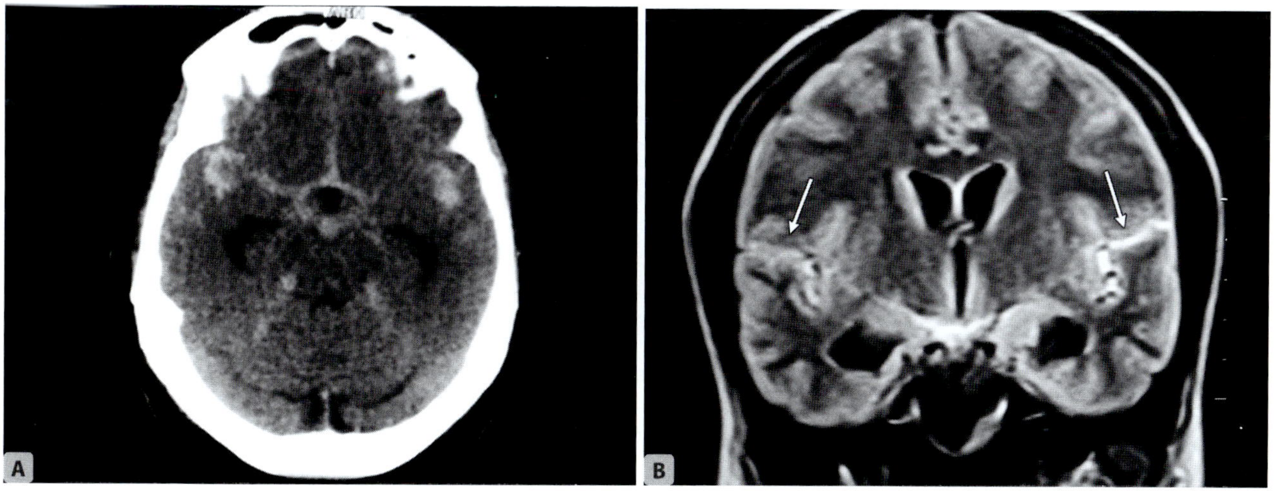

FIGS. 1A AND B: NCCT (A), and MRI–FLAIR (B), (different patients) showing acute subarachnoid hemorrhage (white arrows in B).

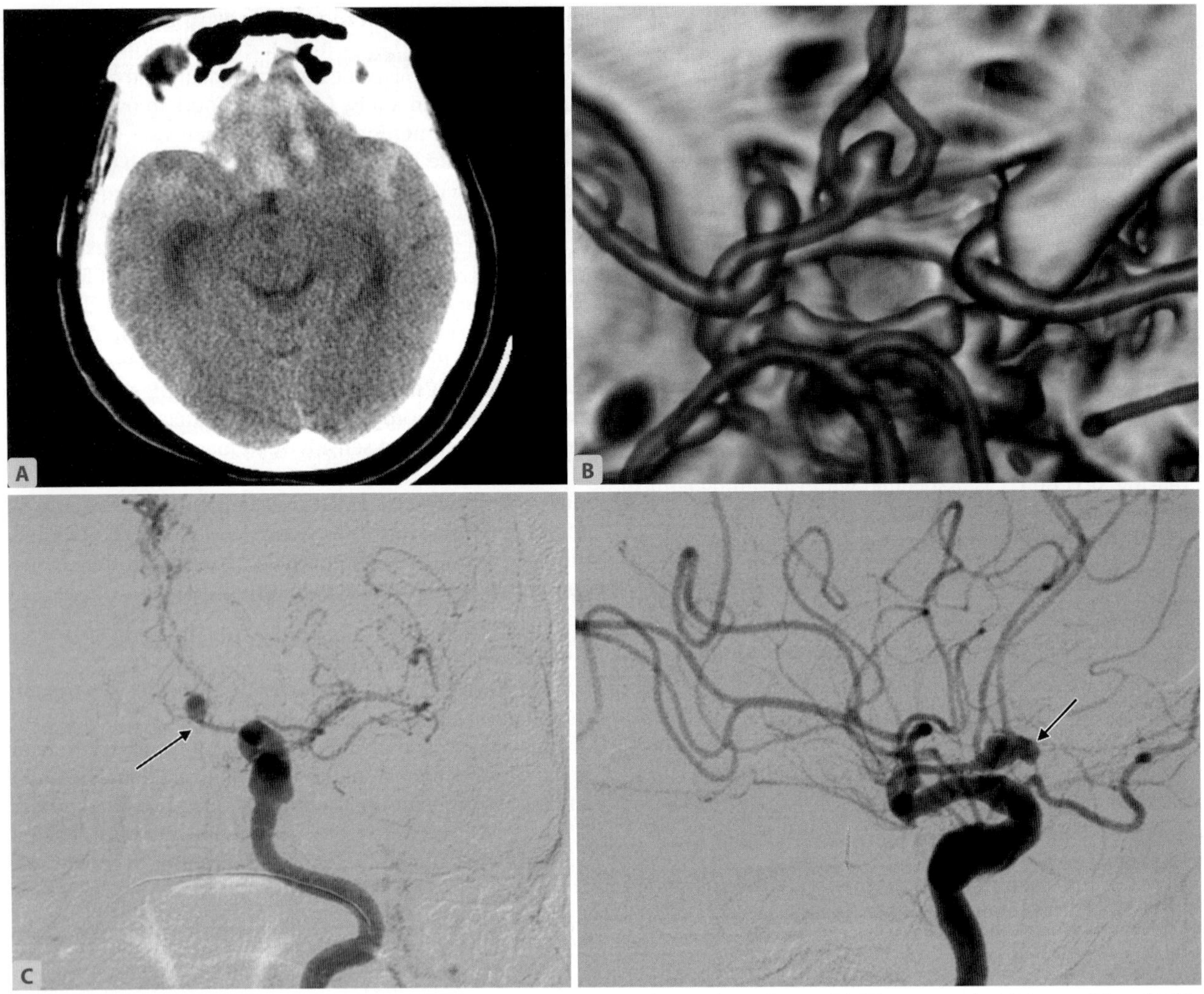

FIGS. 2A TO C: NCCT axial image shows hemorrhage in the anterior interhemispheric fissure (A) CT angiography VR image (B) and DSA AP and lateral views demonstrated anterior communicating aneurysm (arrows) (C).

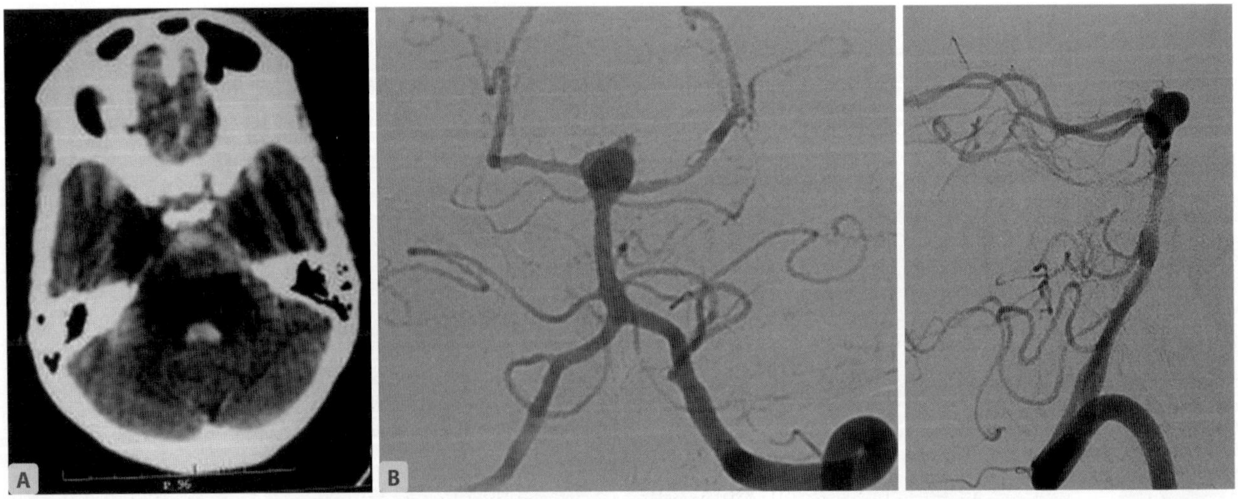

FIGS. 3A AND B: Acute hemorrhage in the prepontine and fourth ventricle (A) on NCCT due rupture of vertebrobasilar aneurysm (B).

Transfemoral catheterization of both internal carotid **(Figs. 5A and B)** and one vertebral artery is generally done. Contralateral vertebral artery catheterization is required if the visualization of the PICA is not seen through reflux. Selective injection of ECA may be required to rule out Dural AVMs. Cross compression study should routinely be done in all case of anterior or posterior communicating artery aneurysms and ICA aneurysm to delineate cross circulation.

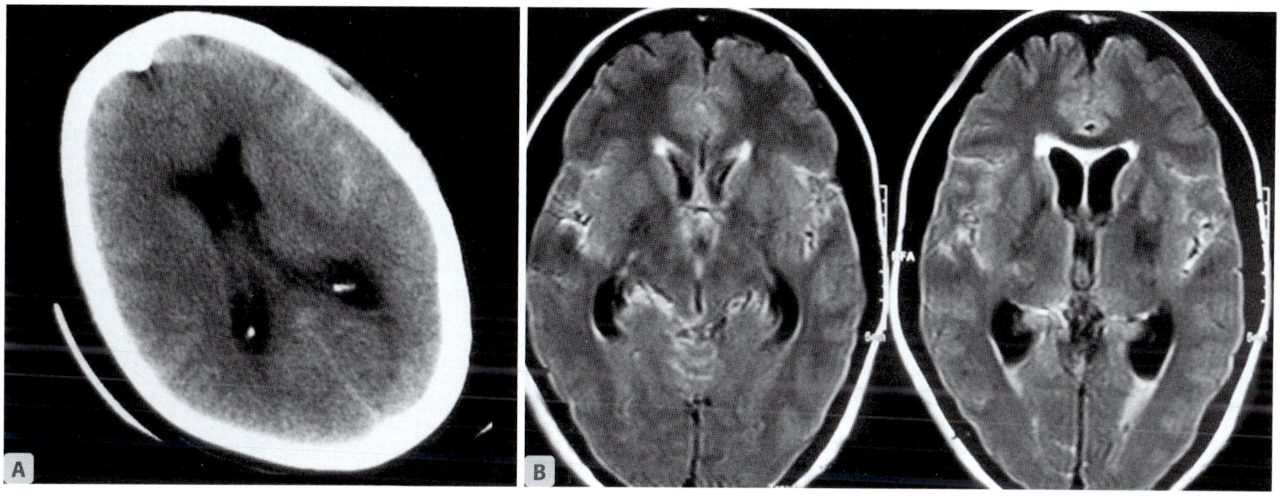

FIGS. 4A AND B: NCCT (A) and FLAIR (B) images to show subarachnoid bleed in bilateral Sylvian fissures (the acute hemorrhage appears hyperintense on FLAIR imaging).

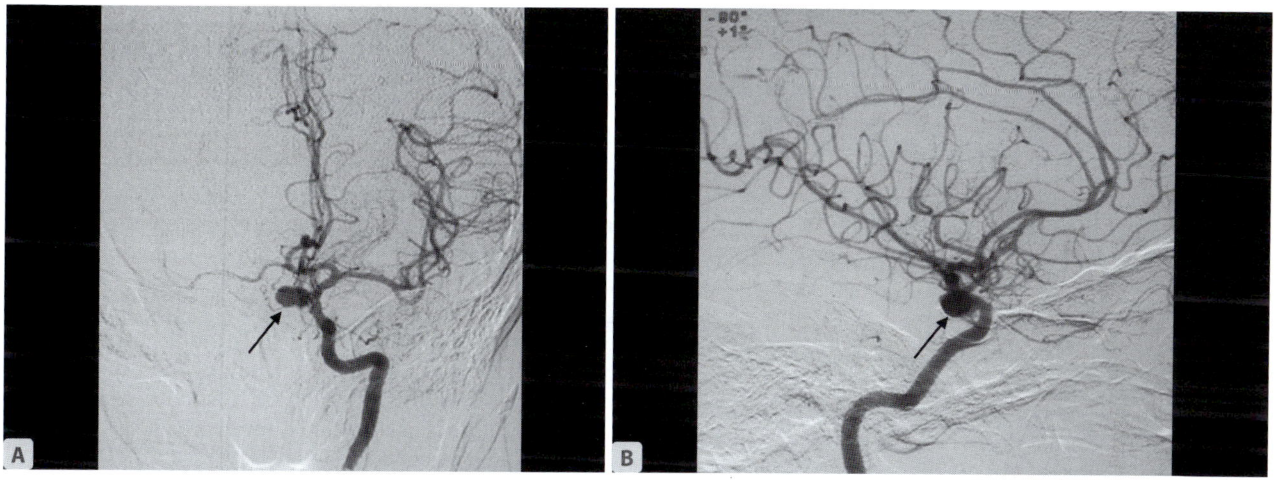

FIGS. 5A AND B: (A) AP and (B) Lateral. Angiographic views of left internal carotid artery showing an ICA aneurysm (arrows).

The angiography should be done as early as possible after ictus. It can be deferred in patients showing rapidly deteriorating neurological status. The risks of angiography are well established. Ischemic events occur in 1.3% of patients in the first 24 hours after angiography. Neurological deterioration occurs in 1.8% of patients between 18 and 72 hours of angiography. Complications are directly related to the volume of contrast, serum creatinine level, number of catheters used, duration of the procedure and the patient's age. Rupture of aneurysm during angiography is rare (0.13%) but carries high mortality **(Figs. 6A and B)**.[11,12] 3D Rotational angiography is a technique in cerebral angiography which gives 3D model of the relevant artery without any bony or venous overlap. Since it can be rotated in any direction and orientation it can give very detailed anatomical information of the involved artery and the aneurysms. To establish the usefulness in detecting arteries less than 3 mm in size (which can be commonly missed on conventional DSA) a review of 350 datasets was done in a recent study. In addition to detecting all the large aneurysms, 94 additional small (<3 mm) aneurysms were detected on 3DRA.[13] This technique can also delineate the aneurysm volume, size, its relations to smaller branches close to neck and incorporation of the vessels **(Fig. 7)**.

CT Angiography (CTA)

With the advent of multislice CT (MDCT), CT angiography has emerged as the alternative to the invasive cerebral digital subtraction angiography (DSA). An increasing number of centers are now treating aneurysms on the basis of findings of CTA with DSA being reserved for the negative cases or cases with diagnostic uncertainty.[14,15]

In a cohort of 223 patients, CTA was safely, effectively and reliably used as a sole modality for planning both operative clipping and endovascular coiling, with an apparent detection rate of 100%.[15] However, it is still to be universally accepted as a standard first line diagnostic test for evaluation for the SAH.

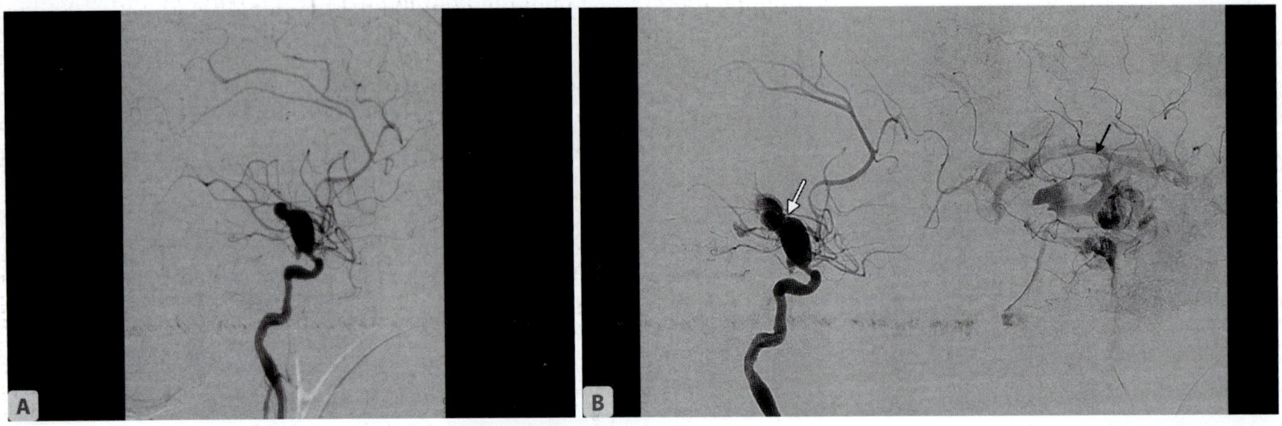

FIGS. 6A AND B: Lateral carotid angiogram shows a complex aneurysm with teat which bleed during angiography. Note the site of bleed (white arrow showing extravasation of contrast) and accumulation of blood in the ventricular system (black arrow).

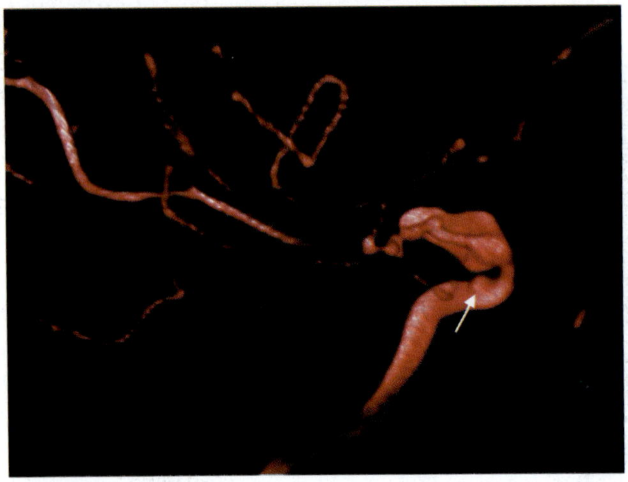

FIG. 7: 3DRA image of right ICA showing a paraclinoid aneurysm. Note a smaller sessile about 3 mm sized aneurysm proximal to it (arrow) which was not seen on DSA.

The advantages of three-dimensional representations of the arteries and their relationship to the surrounding structures are well documented. Additionally the ability to rotate the 3 D images into the identical projection encountered by the surgeon has tremendous advantages. Also, CTA has the ability to characterize the relevant preoperative surgical anatomy such as aneurysmal neck morphology, apical teats, calcification, thrombosis, parent and feeding vessels, diagnosing additional small aneurysms and collateral circulation at the circle of Willis **(Figs. 8 to 10)**.[16] Pitfalls of CT angiography include lack of visibility of small arteries, difficulty differentiating the infundibular dilatation at the origin of an artery from an aneurysm, the kissing vessel artifact, demonstration of venous structures that can simulate aneurysms, inability to identify thrombosis and calcification on three-dimensional images, and beam hardening artifacts produced by aneurysm clips.[17] Now with higher (128/320) slice spiral scanners it is feasible to obtain pure arterial phase images without any venous contamination. Also, it is possible to have high quality images with reconstruction interval of up to 0.24 mm which is close to the spatial resolution of the DSA which is about 0.32 × 0.32.

Standard parameters for the CT angiographic acquisition are 1.00 mm section thickness, 0.5 mm section interval, pitch of 3, and 120 kVp, 240 mAs, and 14.0 cm field of view. Scanning time is approximately 6 seconds for a 64-slice scanner which further reduces in a higher-slice CT. The scanning volume includes from the first cervical vertebra to the vertex. Approximately 80 mL of non-ionic low-osmolar iodinated contrast material is administered intravenously with a power injector at a rate of 4 mL/sec via an 18-gauge catheter positioned in a peripheral vein followed by 20 ml of saline flush (if dual head pressure injector is available). Contrast material is injected and scan initiated at a fixed delay of 16 seconds or a bolus chase technique is used which is more precise in capturing peak arterial phase.

The source images are reconstructed directly into 3 dimensional formats and recorded in maximum intensity projection (MIP), shaded surface display (SSD), volume rendering (VR) or in ray sum projection (projection of the sum of pixel values which is analogous to conventional angiography). The reported sensitivity and specificity of CTA in aneurysms over 3 mm in size are 90.4–95 and 100% respectively in recent studies.[18-20]

In a recent study comparing 64 slice CTA with DSA and 3DRA found sensitivity of 64 slice CTA for aneurysms >4 mm was 100% and for less than 4 mm was 92.3%.[21] In comparison to this, other studies have reported sensitivity of 4/16 slice CTs to diagnose aneurysms 3–4 mm to be in the range of 74–84%.[22-24]

Dual Energy CT

This new technology has made possible tissue differentiation and characterization on CT which was not possible before. This can be used as an added advantage in the work-up of SAH. Dual energy CT can help in removal of aneurysmal clip from the images with much lesser artifacts as compared to conventional CT angiography. Also, bone subtraction while post-processing CTA images is more reliable and

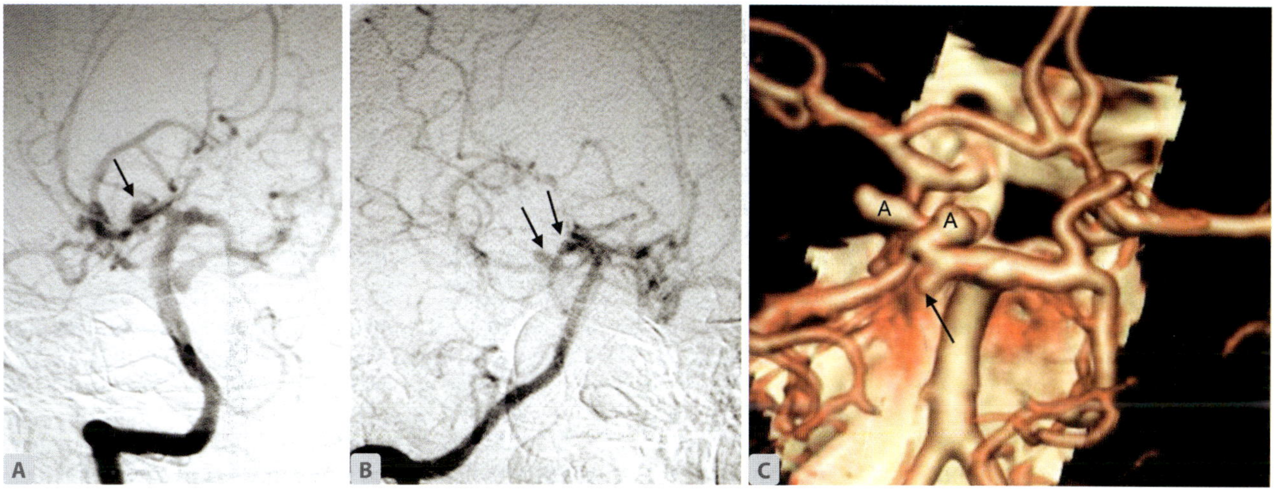

FIGS. 8A TO C: DSA-PA view of posterior circulation showing one right P1-segment aneurysm (A), oblique view showing another PCom. artery aneurysm (B). CTA reconstruction (C), showing an additional third aneurysm (arrow) in the proximal P1 segment not seen on DSA.

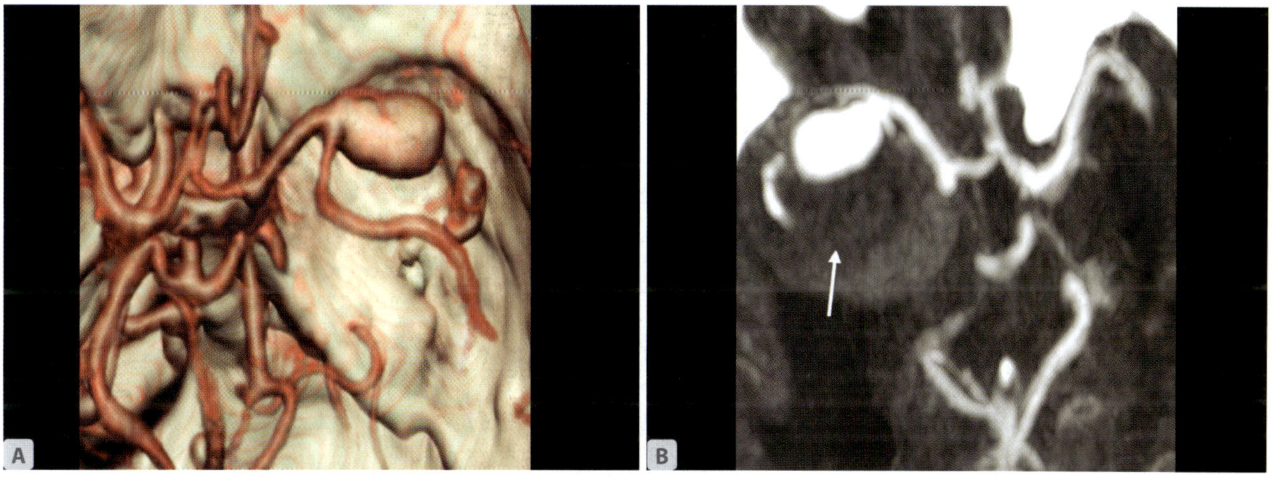

FIGS. 9A AND B: CTA-VR image (A) showing a large MCA aneurysm. However MIP image (B) showing a larger thrombosed portion (arrow) of the aneurysm surrounding the patent central aneurysm.

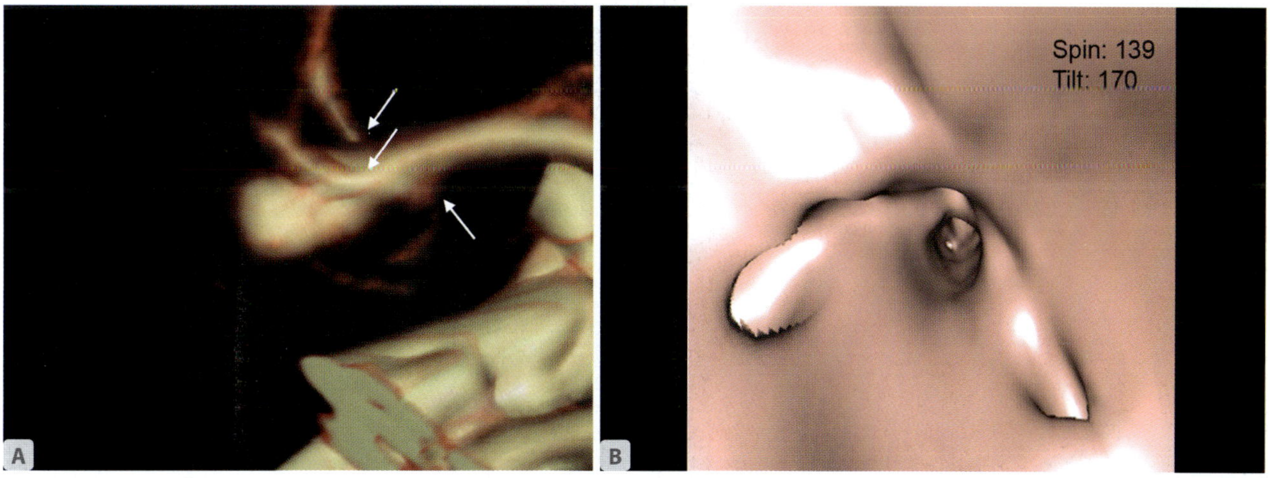

FIGS. 10A AND B: CTA VR image (A) showing multiple vessels arising in close relation to the neck (arrows) whose origins can be seen better on virtual angioscopy (B).

comprehensive as compared to manual or automated/semi-automated algorithms.[25]

Magnetic Resonance Angiography

It is possibly the best noninvasive modality to evaluate the etiology of SAH. The various methods of imaging vascular flow and displaying it in multiple projections with MR are termed magnetic resonance angiography (MRA). The two principle techniques of data acquisition are time of flight (TOF) and phase contrast (PC) in both 2D and 3D planes. Multiple overlapping thin slab acquisition (MOTSA) with or without magnetization transfer has special value in the evaluation of circle of Willis.

A major limitation of time of flight technique is flow artifacts due to turbulent flow and in-plane saturation effects due to slow flow which hinders in the detection of small aneurysms.

The advent of 3D first pass gadolinium-enhanced gradient echo techniques with short repetition times have been shown to be technically superior with lesser artifacts related to flow alterations.[26] Also, MRA is useful as noninvasive tool for the follow-up imaging of coiled aneurysms.[27] Compared with DSA, 3D TOF MRA has sensitivity of 72–97% and specificity of 91–100% in detection of residual flow in aneurysms treated by platinum coils.[28,29] However, this sensitivity goes down significantly for aneurysms size <3 mm **(Figs. 11A to D)**.

Dynamic CEMR may help in detecting small aneurysms or AVMs. Blood oxygen level dependent (BOLD) contrast is a noninvasive functional MRI technique to localize a definable cortical function in relation to the site of AVM nidus as an aid to operative planning. The reported sensitivity and specificity of MRA in detecting aneurysms over 3 mm in size are 90.6 to 96 and 100% respectively in recent studies and are comparable to CTA.[18-20] It is the best screening modality for unruptured aneurysms or AVMs. It is of value in patients with angiographically negative SAH or in renal failure or where contrast injection is contraindicated.

Transcranial Doppler Ultrasound

It is used to study changes in cerebral artery flow velocity after SAH to correlate the onset of clinical vasospasm. Doppler flow velocity is proportional to the blood flow through the artery and inversely proportional to the cross-sectional diameter of the artery. There is rough correlation between angiographic vessels diameter and Doppler flow velocity.[30] Proximal middle cerebral artery (MCA) is normally studied. Mean MCA flow velocity (Normal value 60 cm/sec) of over 120 cm/sec is 100% specific and 59% sensitive, whereas velocity of over 200 cm/sec is 100% sensitive for detection of vasospasm on angiography.[30]

ANEURYSMS

They result from focal degeneration of the arterial wall because of congenital factors which are aggravated by conditions like hypertension and smoking. These are the most common cause of SAH and occur in 1–14% of population. Only <2% occur during childhood.[31] They are of three types: Saccular (out pouching from arterial bifurcation), Fusiform (arterial dilatation) or Dissecting (pseudo-aneurysm) **(Figs. 12A to C)**. The ratio between ruptured versus unruptured aneurysm is 5:3 to 5:6.

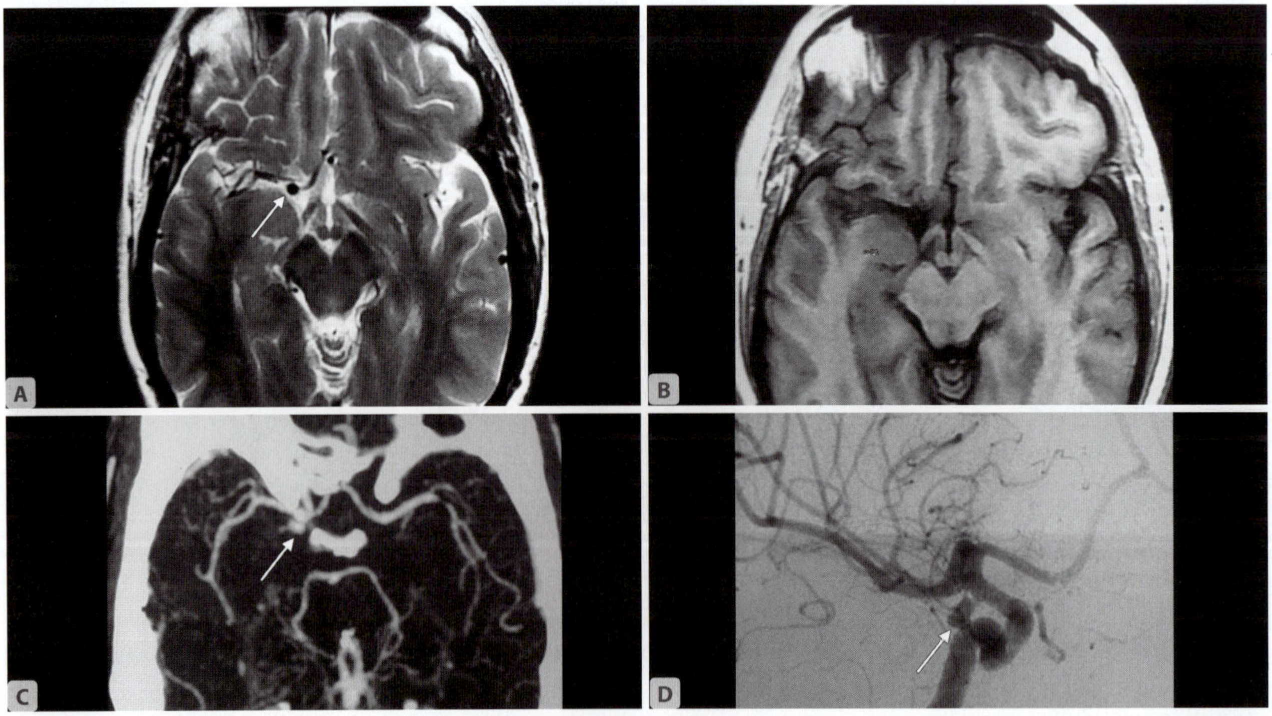

FIGS. 11A TO D: MR T2WI, T1WI (A and B) images showing a small RICA aneurysm (arrow) which was confirmed on CTA and DSA (C and D) to be a PCom. aneurysm.

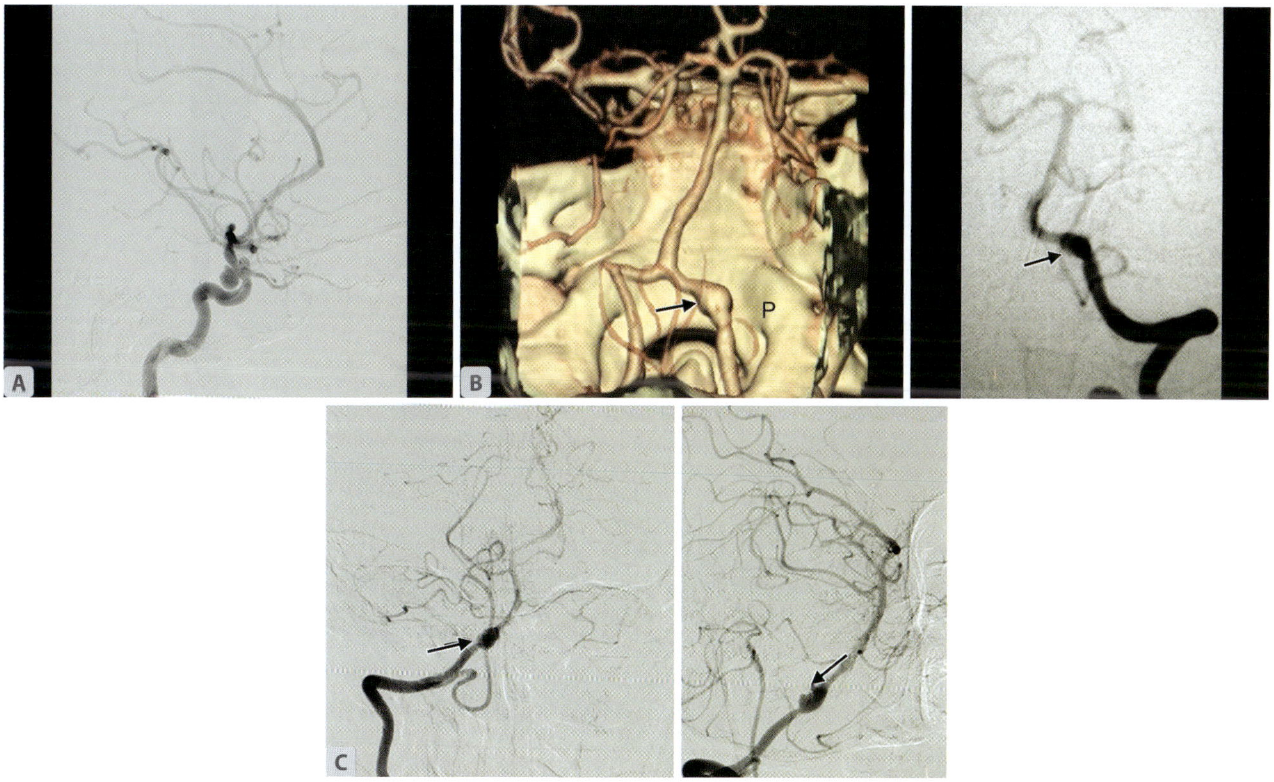

FIGS. 12A TO C: DSA image showing a ICA saccular aneurysm (A), a fusiform left vertebral aneurysm (arrow in B) and a dissecting right vertebral artery aneurysm (arrows in C).

The etiology of aneurysm may be:

- Congenital
- Infection (mycotic aneurysm)
- Trauma
- High flow state (AVM/AVF)
- Neoplasm (primary or metastasis)
- Miscellaneous, e.g. Arteritis, Moya Moya disease, SLE, drug abuse.

Increased incidence of aneurysm is seen in:

- Anomalous vessels (arterial) fenestration persistent trigeminal artery
- Aortic coarctation (8–10%)
- Polycystic kidney disease (10–30%)
- Fibromuscular dysplasia (7–10%)
- Connective tissue disorders (Marfan-Ehler-Danlos)
- High flow status, e.g. AVMs/AVFs
- Familial.

Clinical Presentation

The most common presentation is SAH followed by ICH (20–40%), IVH (15–35%) subdural bleed (2–5%) **(Figs. 13A to C)**. It may present with mass effect and cranial nerve palsy, infarcts, seizures or may be found incidentally on imaging.

Location

About 90–95% of aneurysm are found in carotid circulation, 5–15% in vertebrobasilar circulation and 15–20% aneurysms are multiple. Common locations are anterior communicating artery (30–35%), posterior communicating artery (30–35%) the middle cerebral artery bifurcation (20%), basilar top (5%) and PICA (5%) **(Figs. 14A and B)**.

Multiple Aneurysms

In 15–20% of cases, there may be multiple aneurysm of which 75% have two aneurysms, 15% have three aneurysms and 10% have more than three aneurysms. There is strong female predominance. Aneurysms can be bilaterally symmetrical (mirror aneurysm) or asymmetrical located on different vessels **(Fig. 15)**. In cases of multiple aneurysms, it is important to determine which aneurysm has actually ruptured. Clinical signs alone localize a ruptured aneurysm in only one-third of patients. The imaging findings that are useful to determine the ruptured aneurysms are contrast extravasation (pathognomonic) presence of clot or mass effect on CT/MR and presence of SAH/vasospasm. The size location and configuration of the aneurysm are also helpful: proximally located aneurysm, largest aneurysm and the one having irregular configuration is the most likely the cause of bleed.

Unruptured Aneurysms

The risk of bleeding from unruptured aneurysm is not known and depends primarily on the size of the aneurysm.[32] Since aneurysms are not static and show increase in size on serial angiograms, surgery or interventional occlusion is needed. The critical size above which an unruptured aneurysms should be considered for treatment is debatable and varies from 3 mm–9 mm in various studies.[33] MR is the best modality to follow these patients under observation. In a recent study

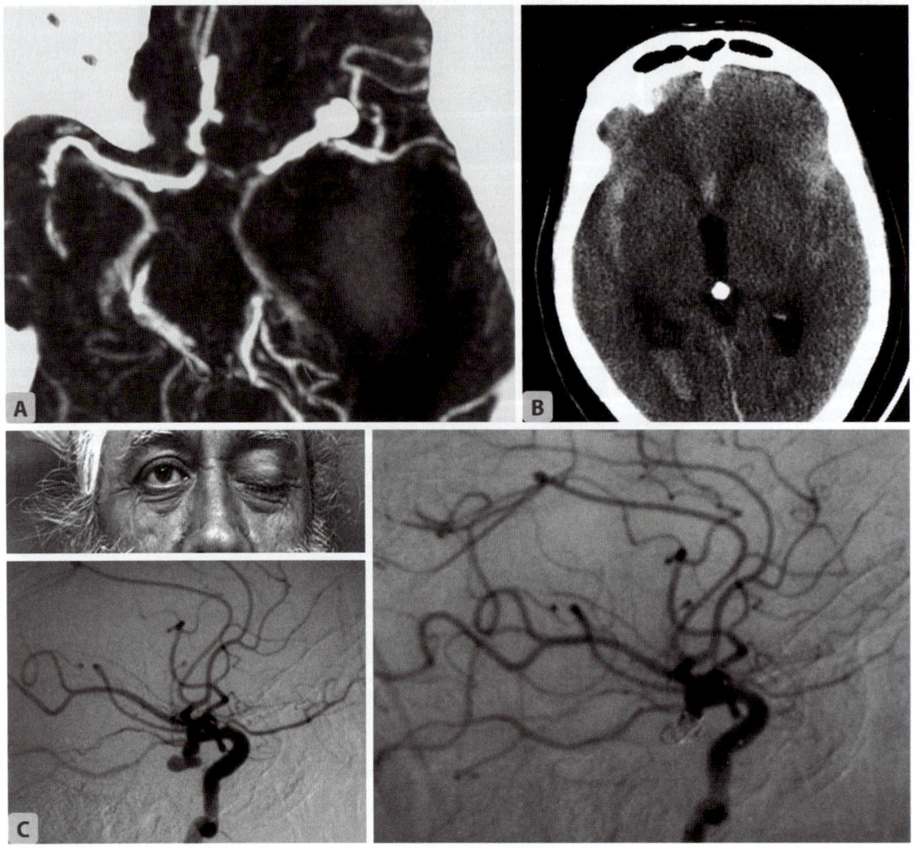

FIGS. 13A TO C: Aneurysm rupture presenting as parenchymal hemorrhage (A) and SAH with intraventricular hemorrhage (B). A nonruptured left PCom. aneurysm presenting with left ptosis (C).

of follow-up of 181 unruptured aneurysms for a median period of 20 years (range- 1–39 years) the cumulative rates of rupture among 142 patients were 10.55% at 10 years and 30.3% at 30 years.[34]

Thrombosed Aneurysms

Partially thrombosed aneurysms have a patent lumen inside a thickened, often partially calcified wall that is lined with laminated clot. The residual lumen and outer rim may enhance strongly on CECT/CEMR. Completely thrombosed aneurysms show variable hyper density on NCCT with no contrast enhancement. On MR, partially thrombosed aneurysms show variable single intensity: an area of flow void surrounded by variable signal intensity, concentric layers with signal void outer rim is a common finding **(Fig. 16)**. Completely thrombosed aneurysm may be hyperintense on T1 and T2WI. It may be missed completely without the use of contrast MRI. Conventional angiography underestimates the size of thrombosed aneurysms and may show only mass effect.

Giant Aneurysms

Aneurysms less than 1 cm in diameter are called small aneurysms, large aneurysms are the ones between 1.0 cm and 2.5 cm. Aneurysms whose diameter exceeds 2.5 cm are termed giant aneurysms **(Figs. 17A and B)**. These usually present in middle aged women with mass effect; SAH does occur but is rare. They are commonly located in the extradural internal carotid artery, proximal MCA or apex of basilar artery. Conventional angiography fails to define the total extent of giant aneurysms because of associated thrombosis and associated extra-aneurysmal parenchymal changes. MRI is best imaging modality to evaluate these lesions.

Mycotic Aneurysms

These are defined an aneurysms that are the result of an infectious process involving the arterial wall and constitute 2–4% of all intracranial aneurysms. These occur in 3–15% of patients of subacute bacterial endocarditis **(Figs. 18A and B)**. The most common location is distal MCA branches (75–80%). They may be multiple (20%).[31,32]

Flow-related Aneurysms

The frequency of aneurysms with AVM has been reported from 2.7%–30%. They can occur in the proximal or distal feeding artery, inside the nidus (8–12%) or in the draining vein of the AVMs **(Fig. 19)**. There is increase in incidence of hemorrhage when AVM is associated with intranidal or venous aneurysm.[31,32]

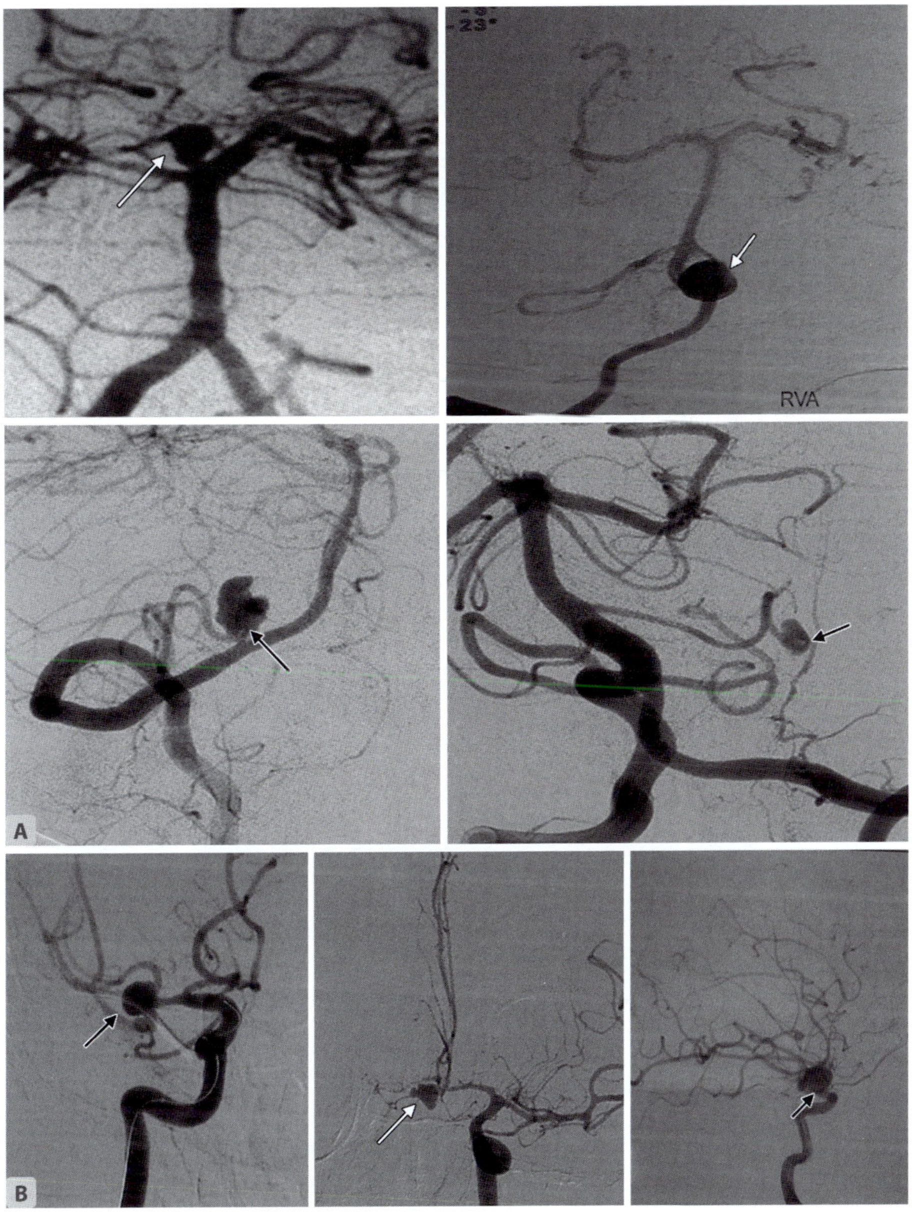

FIGS. 14A AND B: (A) Posterior circulation aneurysms—basilar top (long white arrow), vertebrobasilar junction (short white arrow), PICA aneurysm (long black arrow) and left AICA aneurysm; (B) Anterior circulation aneurysms. A MCA aneurysm (long black arrow), ACom. aneurysm (white arrow) and an ICA aneurysm (short black arrow).

VASCULAR MALFORMATIONS

Vascular malformations are classified into 4 major pathologic types: (A) arteriovenous malformations (AVMs) (B) Capillary telangiectasias, (C) Cavernous angiomas, and (D) Venous angiomas.[35] The overall incidence is from 0.1%–4%.

AVMs can be (A) parenchymal (pial) (B) dural or (C) mixed (pial-dural) type.

Parenchymal AVMs

These are comprised of a complex network of abnormal vascular channels consisting of arterial feeders, the nidus and enlarged veins without an intervening capillary bed and normal brain parenchyma.[35,36] They are usually solitary (98%), but can be multiple (2%), especially in Rendu-Osler-Weber and Wyburn-Mason's syndromes. The common age at presentation is 20–40 years. The presenting clinical features include intracranial hemorrhage (55%), seizures (36%), headache and progressive neurologic deficit (9%). The risk of hemorrhage is 2–4% per year and rebleeding after initial hemorrhage is about 6% in the first year and slowly decreases thereafter.[37] Hemorrhagic complications with AVMs are common when these are peri or intraventricular in location, or have central (deep) venous drainage, or show intranidal aneurysm.

On CT, AVMs are iso to hyperdense and show intense serpiginous enhancement **(Figs. 20A to C)**. Calcification

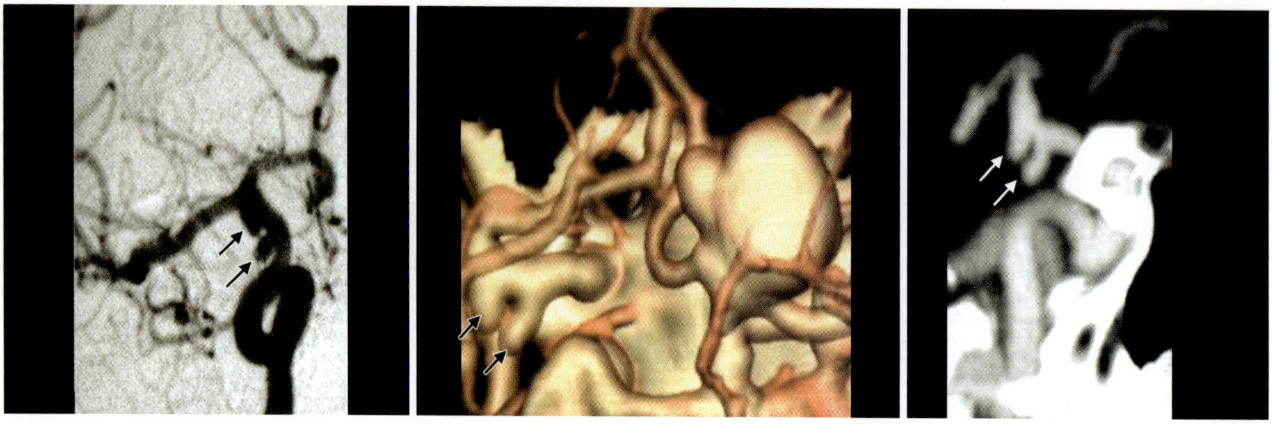

FIG. 15: DSA and CTA images showing two RICA aneurysms (arrows) and a large LICA bifurcation aneurysm.

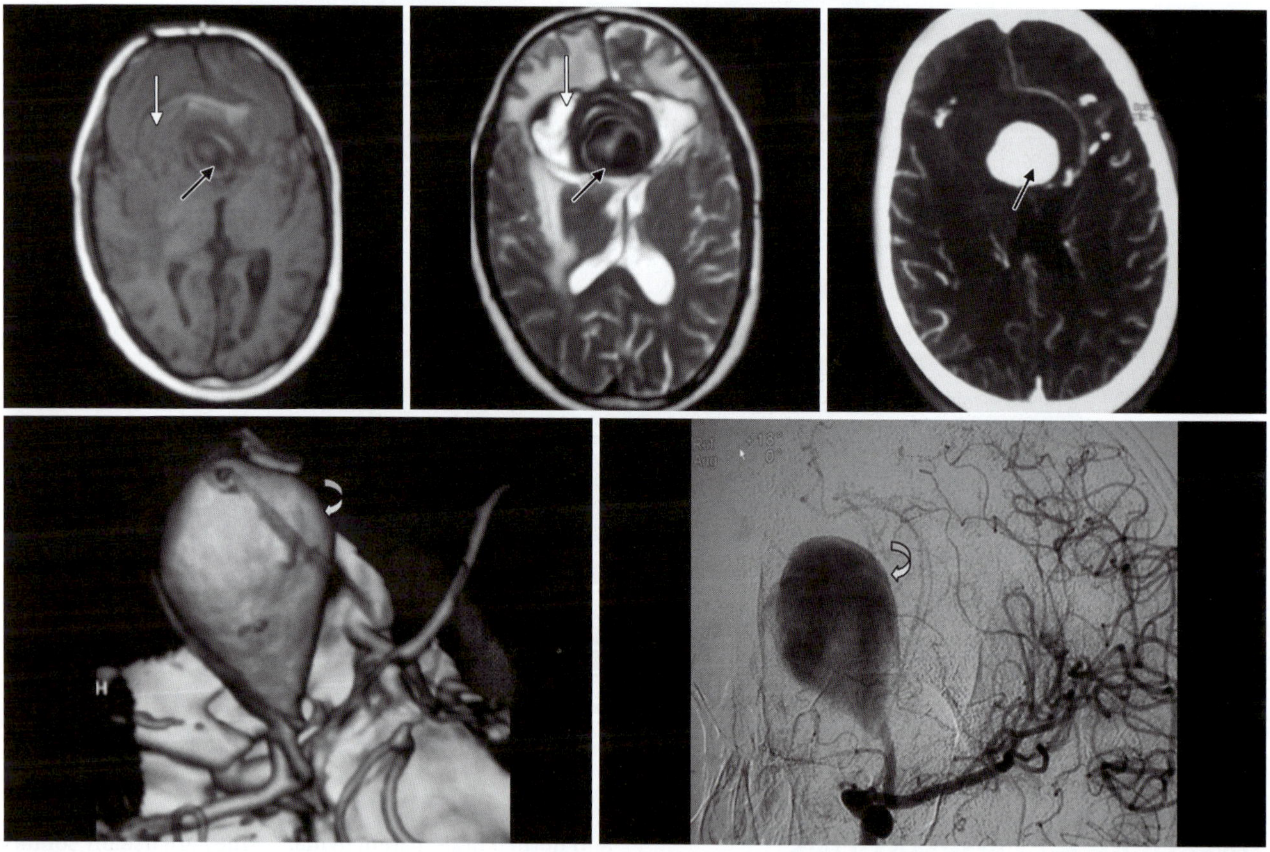

FIG. 16: Partially thrombosed aneurysm seen as a central area of flow void seen on T1WI, T2WI and CTA (black arrows) surrounded by variable signal intensity area seen as isointense on T1WI and hyperintense on T2WI (white arrows). CTA VR and DSA (below curved arrow) images showing it to be a large ACom. artery aneurysm.

is present in 25–30% of cases. Secondary changes such as acute hemorrhage, edema, mass effect and ischemia are readily identified on CT. On MRI, they are usually seen as tightly packed honeycomb of "flow voids" on both T1 and T2 spin echo sequences. The feeding arteries, the nidus or the draining veins may be clearly seen on standard SE or time of flight (TOF) or phase contrast (PC) MRA techniques **(Fig. 21)**. Areas of increased signal may be seen in thrombosed vessels or in vessels with slow or turbulent flow. Hemorrhage in all stages, hypoperfusion because of steal phenomenon atrophy gliosis, mass effect, etc. are better seen on MRI than CT.

Recently with the use of 3T MR systems ultra fast acquisitions have become a possibility. Time resolved contrast enhanced MRA is one such technique which aims at capturing the dynamic information of the AVMs

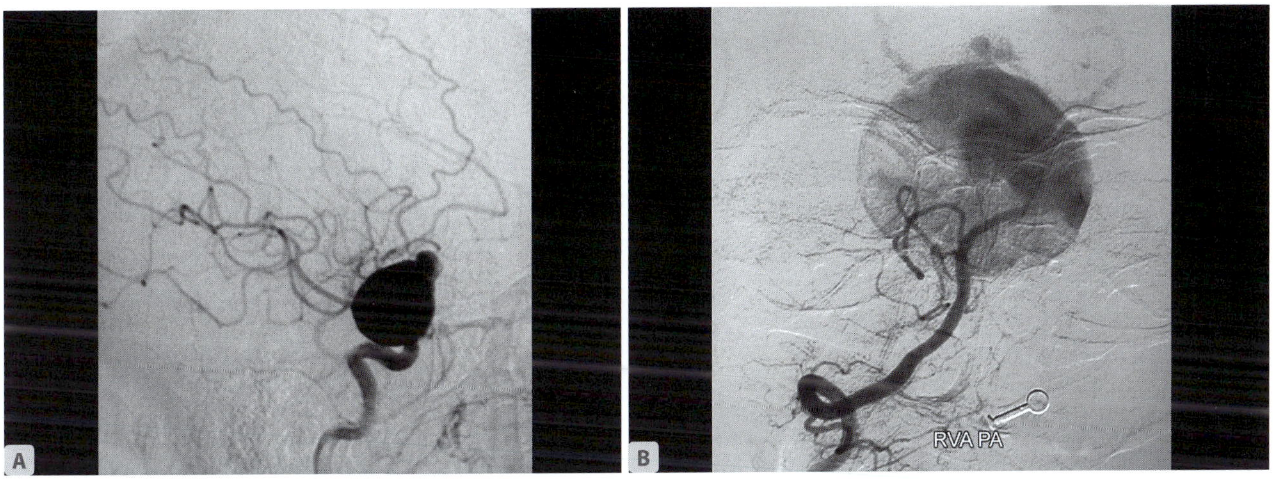

FIGS. 17A AND B: DSA projections showing giant ICA (A) and a giant left PCA (B) aneurysm.

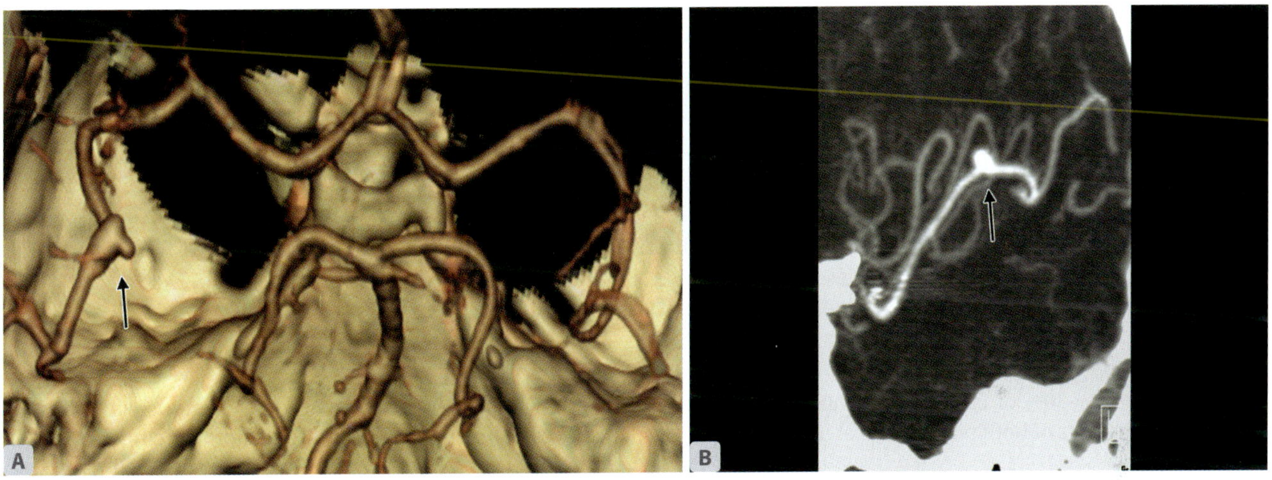

FIGS. 18A AND B: (A) CTA VR and (B) MIP images show an irregular aneurysm (mycotic) in the distal left MCA in a patient of subacute bacterial endocarditis.

in addition to the diagnosis thereby offering an alternative to DSA. By combining parallel imaging, keyhole acquisition and k-space sampling now it is possible to image cerebral AVMs in early arterial phase, late arterial phase, parenchymal and venous phase. Studies have demonstrated a good co-relation of time resolved MRA and DSA in imaging location and number of arterial feeders, size of the nidus and number and type of venous drainage **(Figs. 22A to H)**.[38,39]

Cerebral angiography is the gold standard in the evaluation of AVMs. It demonstrates tightly packed masses of enlarged feeding arteries, the nidus and tortuous draining veins. A flow related aneurysm (arterial, nidal or venous) may be seen in 8–12% of cases. Occasionally, AVM may involve entire lobe with no demonstrable nidus. Thrombosed AVMs may have normal angiogram (cryptic AVM). Occasionally arteries with slow blood flow may be seen till late in capillary phase and rare termed "stagnating arteries."[30]

Dural AVMs

These are abnormal vascular network with thickened dural arteries and veins within the wall of venous sinus without any discrete nidus. Unlike pial AVMs, dural AVMs are acquired secondary to the segmental thrombosis of the dural venous sinus. They usually present with pulsatile tinnitus, bruit, headache, visual impairment or papilledema. CT scan is usually normal except in situations like carotid cavernous fistula (CCF) where there can be enlarged cavernous sinus and dilated superior ophthalmic vein. MRI may also be normal. PC MRA can show the flow direction in the fistula. On angiography, most dural AVMs have multiple feeders from dural branches except in case of fistulae where there is a single dural artery. The dural sinus is usually occluded **(Fig. 23)**.

Mixed Pial and Dural AVMs

When parenchymal AVM is of large size, it may recruit vascular supply from dural branches. Meningeal artery

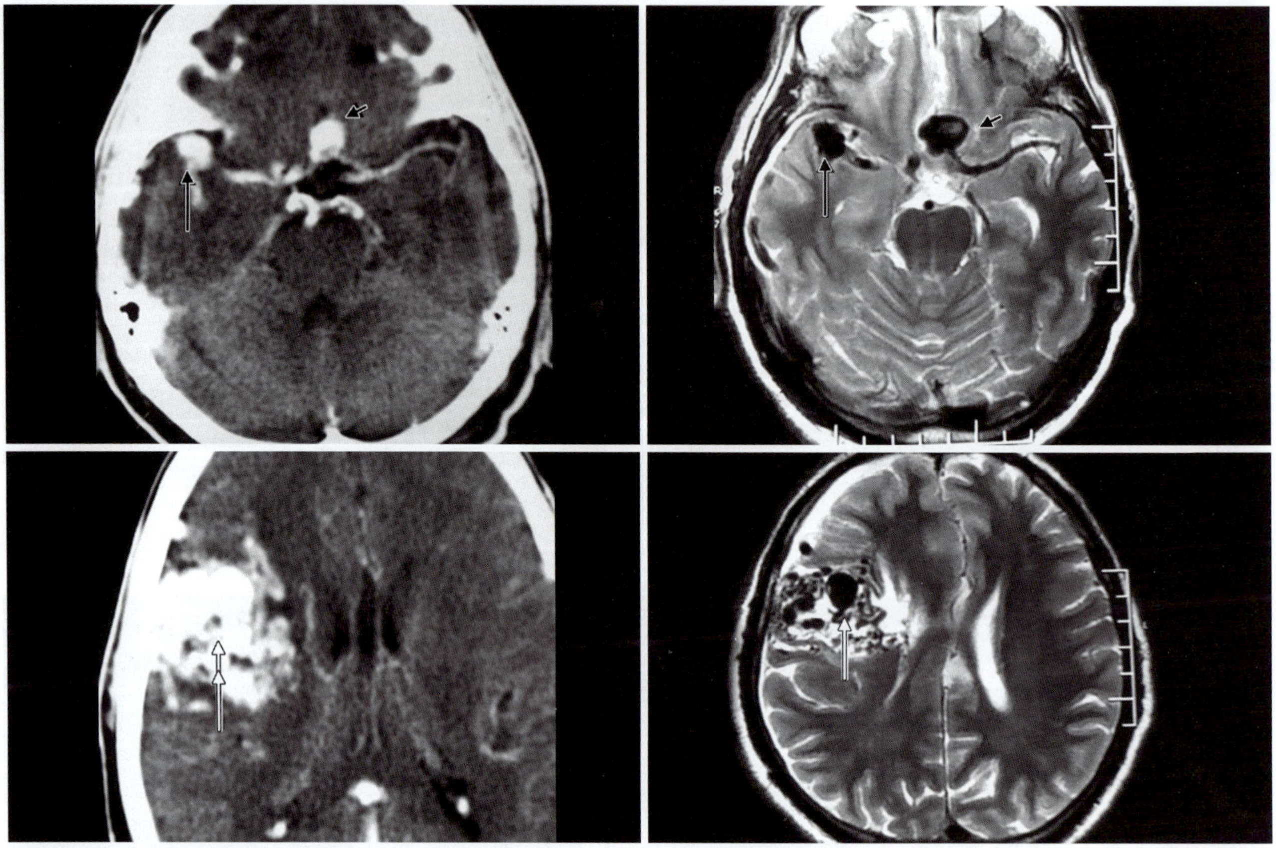

FIG. 19: CT and MR images showing flow-related aneurysms in right MCA (black arrows) and ACom. artery (small black arrow). Also seen is right parietal AVM with intranidal aneurysm (white arrows).

contributes in 15–50% of cases. On imaging, these AVMs show characteristics of both pial and dural AVMs.

CAPILLARY TELANGIECTASIAS

These are nets of dilated capillaries whose walls lack smooth muscle and elastic fibers and have intervening normal brain parenchyma. They are usually multiple and located in the pons, cerebellum or spinal cord. Most lesions are small and clinically silent, discovered incidentally on imaging. CT and MRI are usually normal except for faint increased density on contrast examination. MRI shows the product of hemorrhage as multiple hyperintense foci on T2WI and GE images.

Angiographically also, they are occult; rarely, a faint vascular stain may be seen.

CAVERNOUS ANGIOMAS

Cavernous angiomas are endothelial lined sinusoidal spaces not separated by neural tissues and are discrete multilobulated lesions that contain products of hemorrhage in various stages. They account for 8–16% of all intracranial vascular malformations.[36] The clinical features include seizures (60%), progressive neurological deficit (50%), hemorrhage (20%), hydrocephalus or they may present as incidental findings on routine imaging (50%). They can occur anywhere in the brain; 80% are supratentorial and 20% are infratentorial. On CT, they appear as iso or hyperdense lesions with minimal or no enhancement and show variable calcification. Mass effect or edema is conspicuously absent. On angiography they are "occult". MR shows the most characteristic and diagnostic findings in the form of "popcorn" like lesion with well delineated complex core of mixed signal intensity **(Figs. 24A to C)**. A low signal hemosiderin rim surrounds the lesion which becomes prominent or "blooms" on T2WI or gradient echo images.[31]

VENOUS ANGIOMAS

These are radially arranged dilated anomalous veins that coverage in an enlarged transcortical vein. There is no arterial component or intervening normal brain tissue or evidence of gliosis or hemosiderin. They are the most common vascular malformations found at autopsy and are located in deep cerebral or cerebellar white matter close to ventricle. They are usually solitary but can be multiple. Hemorrhagic complications occur but are rare. Computed tomography is usually normal or may show enhanced tuft of rounded or linear vessels (medullary veins). Magnetic resonance findings are often diagnostic: a stellate tangle of venous tributaries draining into a large dilated anomalous veins. "Flow void" vein is the characteristic findings, especially well seen on CEMR. Cerebral angiography shows normal arterial and capillary phase. Multiple enlarged medullary veins coverage

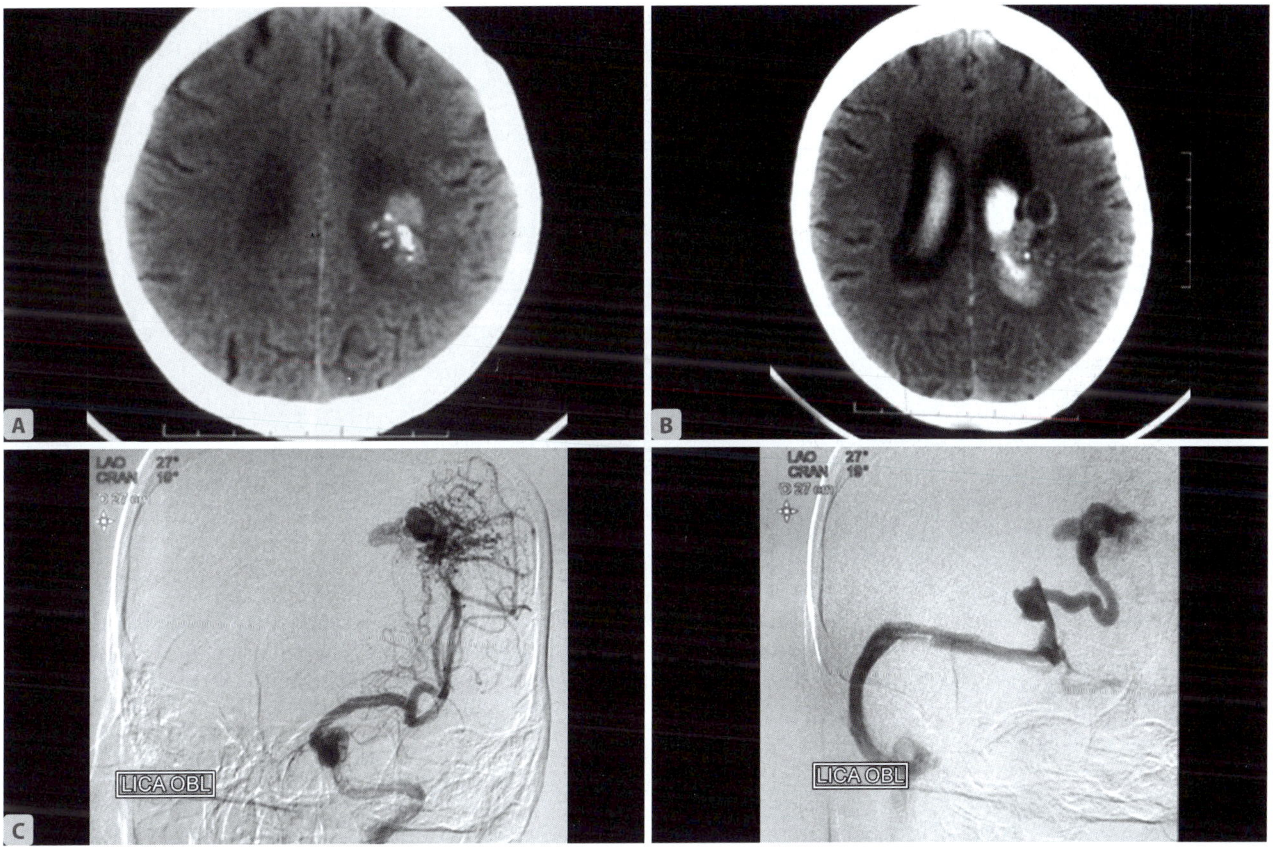

FIGS. 20A TO C: (A and B) Serpiginous hyperdense areas in the left periventricular region with IVH. Carotid angiogram; (C) Oblique projections show the arterial feeder, the nidus and venous drainage into deep venous system.

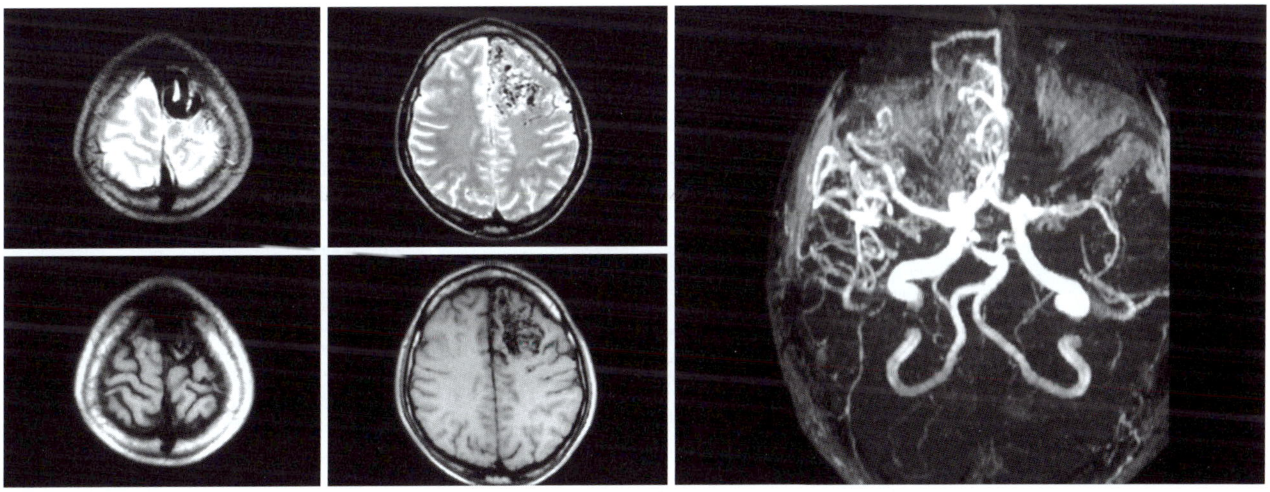

FIG. 21: MR (T2WI, T1WI and MRA) images showing multiple, tortuous flow voids in the left frontal region suggestive of AVM which is seen as bunch of vessels on MRA.

into dilated transcortical vein giving rise to "medusa head" appearance seen in the venous phase **(Fig. 25)**.

Angiographically occult vascular malformations (AOVMs) are 10% of all vascular malformation and are due to:

- Thrombosed AVMs (44%)
- Cavernous angiomas (31%)
- Venous angiomas (10%)
- Capillary telangiectasia (4%)
- Unclassified or mixed angiomas (11%).

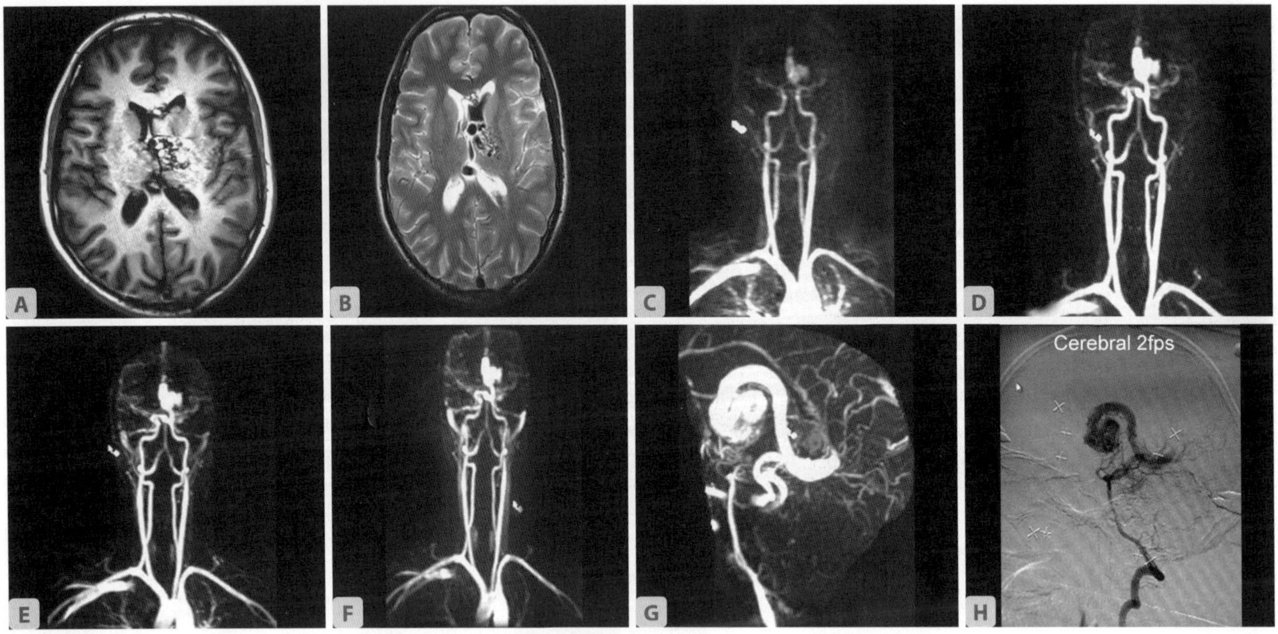

FIGS. 22A TO H: An 18-year-old male with left thalamic AVM T1W and T2WI showing AVM in left basal ganglia and thalamic region (A and B). Sequential arterial (C and D), nidus (E) and venous (F) enhancement on time resolved MRA Coronal projection. High spatial resolution MRA—lateral MIP projection (G) with corresponding DSA (H) –Lt. PCA run image showing feeders, nidus and draining veins.

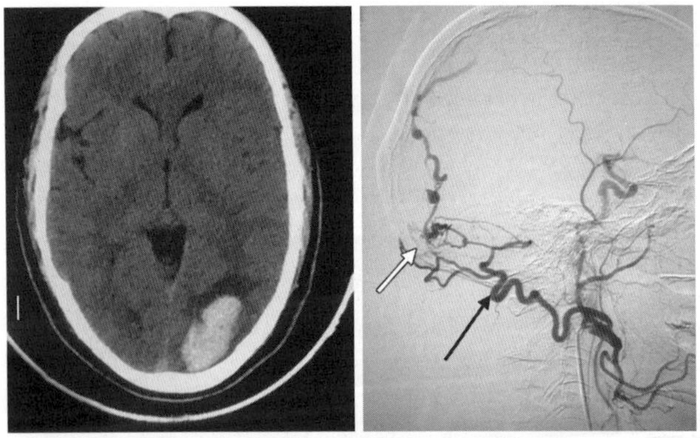

FIG. 23: NCCT image showing acute bleed in left occipital bleed secondary to the dural AV fistula being supplied by the posterior meningeal branch of the left vertebral artery (arrow). Site of the fistula is left sigmoid sinus, marked with white arrow.

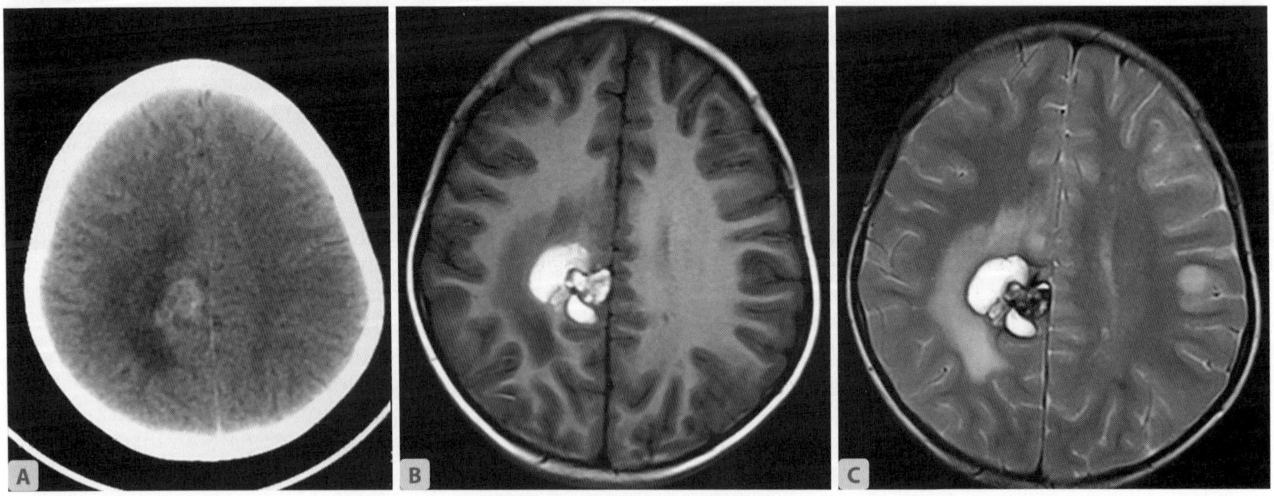

FIGS. 24 A TO C: NCCT, T1- and T2-weighted MR images shows hemorrhagic lesion (with both acute and chronic bleed) with typical "popcorn" appearance with surrounding hypointense rim on T2WI suggestive of cavernous angioma.

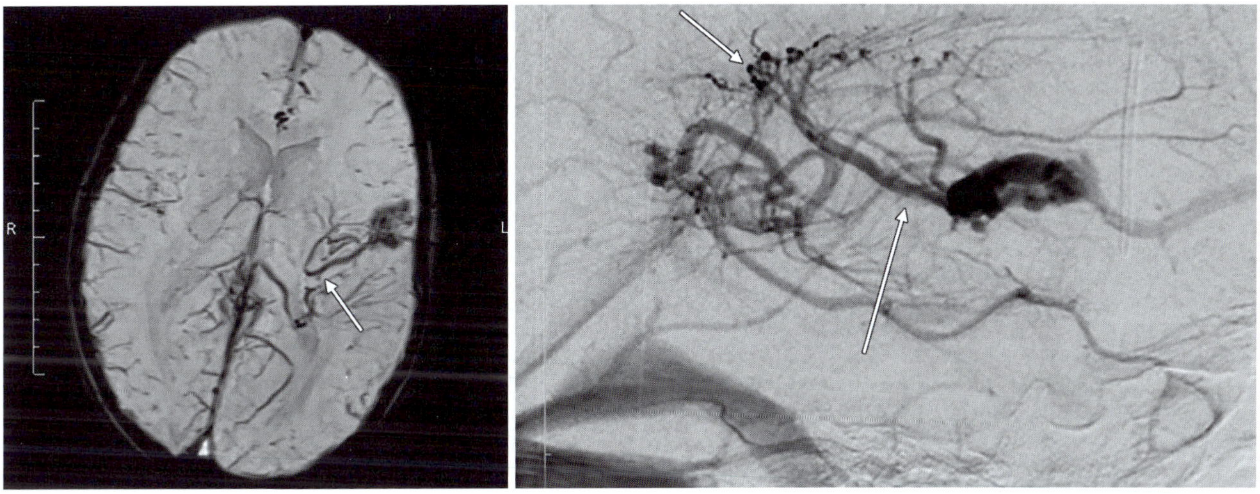

FIG. 25: MRI SWI image showing a prominent transcortical vein (left image). Venous phase of left ICA angiogram showing multiple medullary veins (small arrow) draining into a large vein (large arrow) a typical angiographic picture of venous angioma.

TRAUMATIC SUBARACHNOID HEMORRHAGE

Moderate to severe head trauma may produce SAH and a small percentage show associated aneurysms. "Pseudo SAH" may be seen with severe diffuse cerebral edema where brain becomes very low in attenuation and the circulating blood appears very hyperdense.[31] "Pseudodelta" sign on plain CT may be seen in posterior parafalcine or interhemispheric SAH and should not be mistaken for dural sinus thrombosis.[40]

Subarachnoid Hemorrhage of Unknown Etiology

The incidence of SAH of unknown etiology is about 7–10% of all SAH. The possible causes are:

- *Incomplete angiogram*: 1–2% of aneurysms occur at PICA origin and can be missed, if complete 4 vessels angiogram is not done.
- Obliteration of lesion by the hemorrhage.
- Aneurysm or AVM too small to be visualized.
- Cervical or upper thoracic AVM.
- SAH of nonaneurysmal etiology.

There is risk of rebleed (up to 0.5% per year) and delayed cerebral ischemia. In such cases a repeat angiography is required and is usually done after 6 weeks (may be after 3rd weeks) or till vascular spasm disappears. In a series of 92 cases of negative angiogram in SAH, an aneurysm was demonstrated on a second angiogram in 4 cases and on a third angiogram in 1 case only.[41] In a recent study conducted in the institute in 30 patients of negative DSA, the CTA showed aneurysms in 5 patients where DSA was negative. In one patient repeat DSA at 4 weeks showed small aneurysm (unpublished).

In another review of 61 patients of angiographically negative spontaneous SAH patients was done. In it 18 patients had perimesencephalic pattern of bleed and 34 patients had SAH without any demonstrable cause. Prognosis of both groups was found to be good.[42]

Non-aneurysmal SAH

Perimesencephalic SAH, vasculitis coagulation disorders and trauma are common causes for non-aneurysmal SAH. Perimesencephalic SAH is a distinct benign entity with good outcome and less risk of rebleed or vasospasm than other patients of SAH.

It is possibility due to rupture of small perimesencepalic vein. Cerebral angiography is normal. The criteria that establish the diagnosis on CT or MRI are:[43]

- Epicenter of hemorrhage is immediately anterior to the midbrain with extension into anterior part of ambient cistern or basal part of sylvian fissure.
- Absence of complete filling of anterior interhemispheric fissure.
- No more than minute amount of blood in lateral portion of sylvian fissure.
- Absence of frank intraventricular bleed.
- Repeat panangiography is not indicated in these patients.[31,32]

SUMMARY

The diagnosis of acute SAH can be made on CT but MRI is required in subacute and chronic SAH. There are various etiologies for SAH, the common being rupture of aneurysms and AVMs. Conventional four vessel angiography still remains the modality of choice for defining the location and detailed anatomy of the AVM for surgery, endovascular therapy as well for post-surgical follow-up. CTA and MRA are fast replacing conventional angiography for diagnostic purposes and have comparable specificity and sensitivity.

REFERENCES

1. Menghini VV, Brown RD Jr, Sicks JD, et al. Incidence and prevalence of intracranial aneurysms and hemorrhage in Olmsted Couty, Minnessota, 1965 to 1995. Neurology. 1998;51:405-11.
2. Salis AL, Nibbelink DW, Torner JC (Eds). Aneurysmal subarachnoid haemorrhage : Report of cooperative study: Urban and Schwazzenberg Baltimore – Munich. 1981;370-85.
3. Parkarinen S. Incidence, etiology and prognosis of primary SAH. Acta Neurol Scandina. 1967;48:1-128.
4. Locksley H. Report on the cooperative study of SAH. J Neuosurg. 1966;25:219-39.
5. ICMR, Epidemiological study on SAH in INDIA (1972-75) ICMR Bull, New Delhi, 1987.
6. Patel MK, Clarke MA. Lumbar puncture and subarachnoid haemorrhage. Postgrad Med J. 1986;62:1021.
7. Kasell NF, Toner JC, Haley EC Jr. The international co-operative study on the timing of aneurysm surgery. I overall management results. J Neurosurg. 1990;73:307-25.
8. Van Gijn J, Van Dongen KL. The time course of aneurysmal haemorrhage on computed tomograms. Neuroradiology. 1985;23:153-55.
9. Ogawa T, Inugamia A, Fujita H, et al. MR diagnosis of subacute and chronic subarachnoid haemorrhage. Comparison with CT. AJR. 1995; 165:1257-62.
10. Singer M, Atlas S, Drayer B. Subarachnoid space disease: diagnosis with fluid attenuated inversion recovery MR imaging and comparison with contrast-enhanced T1 weighted images: blinded reader study. Radiology. 1998;208:417-22.
11. Dion JE, Gates FC, Fox AJ, et al. Clinical events following neuroangiography. A prospective study. Stroke. 1987;18: 997-1009.
12. Khandelwal N, Kaur Baljeet, Malik N, et al. Rupture of intracranial aneurysms during angiography. JAPI. 1994;42:76-77.
13. Van Rooji WJ, Sprengers ME, de Gast AN, et al. 3D rotational angiography: the new gold standard in the detection of additional intracranial aneurysms. AJNR. 2008;29:976-79.
14. Vekthuis BK, Van Leeuwen MS, Witkamp TD, et al. Computerized tomography angiography in patients with subarachnoid hemorrhage: From aneurysm detection to treatment without conventional angiography. J Neurosurg. 1999;91:761-7.
15. Hoh BL, Cheung AC, Rabinov JD, et al. Results of a prospective protocol of computed tomographic angiography in place of catheter angiography as the only diagnostic and pretreatment planning study for cerebral aneurysms by a combined neurovascular team. Neurosurgery. 2004;54:1329-42.
16. Wintermark M, Uske A, Chalaron M, et al. Multislice computerized tomography angiography in the evaluation of intracranial aneurysms: A comparison with intra-arterial digital subtraction angiography. J Neurosurg. 2003;98:828-36.
17. Takhtani D. CT Neuroangiography: A Glance at the Common Pitfalls and Their Prevention. AJR. 2005;185:772-83.
18. Harrison MJ, Johnson BA, Gardner GM, et al. Preliminary results on the management of Unruptured aneurysms with magnetic imaging angiography and computed tomography angio-graphs. Neurosurg. 1997;40:947-55.
19. Schwartz RB, Tice HM, Hooten SM, et al. Evaluation of cerebral aneurysms with helical CT: Correlation with conventional angiography and MR angiographs. Radiology. 1994;192: 717-22.
20. Zouaou A, Sahel M, Marro B, et al. Three dimensional computed tomographic angiography in detection of haemorrhage. Neuro Surg. 1997;41:125-30.
21. McKinney AM, Palmer CS, Truwit CL, et al. Detection of aneurysms by 64-section multidetector CT angiography in patients acutely suspected of having an intracranial aneurysm and comparison with digital subtraction and 3D rotational angiography. AJNR. 2008;29:594-602.
22. Dammert S, Krings T, Moller-Hartmann W, et al. Detection of intracranial aneurysms with multislice CT: comparison with conventional angiography. Neuroradiology. 2004;46:427-34.
23. Tipper G, U King-Im JM, Price SJ, et al. Detection and evaluation of intracranial aneurysms with 16-row multislice CT angiography. Clin Radiol. 2005;60:565-72.
24. Yoon DY, Lim KJ, Choi CS, et al. Detection and characterization of intracranial aneurysms with 16-channel multidetector row CT angiography: a prospective comparison of volume rendered images and digital substraction angiography. AJNR. 2007;28:60-67.
25. Postma AA, Das M, Stadler AA, et al. Dual-Energy CT: What the Neuroradiologist Should Know. Curr Radiol Rep. 2015;3(5):16.
26. Parker DL, Goodrich KC, Alexander AL, et al. Optimized visualization of vessels in contrast enhanced intracranial MR angiography. Magn Reson Med. 1998;40:873-82.
27. Leclerc X, Navez JF, Gauvrit JY, et al. Aneurysms of the anterior communicating artery treated with Guglielmi detachable coils: Follow-up with contrast enhanced MR angiography. Am J Neuro Radiol. 2002;23:1121-27.
28. Okahara M, Kiyosue H, Hori Y et al. Three-dimensional time-of-flight MR angiography for the evaluation of intracranial aneurysms after endovascular packing with Guglielmi detachable coils: Comparison with 3D digital subtraction angiography. Eur Radiol. 2004;14:1162-8.
29. Yamada N, Hayashi K, Murao K, et al. Time-of-flight MR angiography targeted to coiled intracranial aneurysms is more sensitive to residual flow than is digital subtraction angiography. AJNR. 2004;25:1154-7.
30. Harders AG, Gillsbach JM. Time course of blood velocity changes related to vasospam in the circle of Willis measured by Transcranial Doppler Ultrasound. J Neurosurgery. 1987;66:718-24.
31. Osborn AG. Intracranial aneurysms. In: Diagnostic neuroradiology. Ed Mosby. 1994;248-329.
32. Atlas SW. Magnetic Resonance Imaging of Brain and Spine. (2nd Edn) Lipincott Raven. 1994;489-556.
33. Wiebers Do, Whiswant JP, Sundt TM. The significance of unruptured saccular aneurysms. J Neurosurg. 1987;66:23-29.
34. Juvela S, Porras M, Poussa K. Natural history of unruptured intracranial aneurysms: probability of and risk factors for aneurysm rupture. J Neurosurg. 2008;108:1052-60.
35. Russell DS, Rubinstein LJ. Pathology of Tumours of the Nervous System, (5th edn) Williams and Wilkins, Baltimore 1989.
36. Graves VB, Duff TA. Intracranial arteriovenous malformations: Current imaging and treatment. Invest Radiol. 1990;25:952-60.
37. Brown RDJ, Wiebers DO, Forbes G, et al. The natural history of Unruptured intracranial arteriovenous malformations. J Neurosurg. 1988;68:352-57.
38. Taschner CA, Gieseke J, Le Thuc V, et al. intracranial arteriovenous malformation: time resolved contrast enhanced MR Angiography with combination of parallel imaging, keyhole acquisition, and k-space sampling techniques at 1.5 T. Radiology. 2008;246(3):871-79.
39. Saleh RS, Lohan DG, Villablanca JP, et al. Assessment of craniospinal arteriovenous malformations at 3T with highly temporally and highly spatially resolved contrast enhanced MR angiography. AJNR. 2008;29:1024-31.
40. Khandelwal N, Malik N, Pathak A, et al. Head Injury: Pseudodelta sign on CT. Australasian Radiology. 1992;36:303-04.
41. Duong H, Meancon D, Tampieri D, et al. The negative angiograms in subarachnoid haemorrhage. Neuroradiology. 1996;38:15-19.
42. Gupta SK, Gupta R, Khosla VK et al. Nonaneurysmal non perimesencephalic subarachnoid hemorrhage: is it a benign entity? Surg Neurol. 2009;71:566-71.
43. Rienkel GJE, Wijdicks EFM, Vermeulen M, et al. Nonaneurysmal perimesencephalic subarachnoid haemorrhage. CT and MR patterns that differ from aneurysmal rupture. AJNR. 1991;12:829-34.

CHAPTER

190

Endovascular Management of Intracranial Aneurysms

Shailesh B Gaikwad

Intracranial aneurysms are localized pathological dilatations of cerebral arteries. They are the most common of the cranial vascular lesion encountered. Rupture of aneurysms is a neurologic event with grave consequences. Rapid advancements in neurointerventional techniques, equipments, and critical care have led to significant reduction in morbidity and mortality particularly in patients with ruptured aneurysm. We attempt to present scenario regarding endovascular treatment of intracranial aneurysms.

The exact prevalence of cerebral aneurysms is not accurately documented and varies widely in the published literature. It is accepted that about 3% to 5% of the population should harbor an intracranial aneurysm. In various adult autopsy studies[1] frequency ranges from 1% to 6%, where as in angiographic series;[2] the incidence of intracranial aneurysms varies from 0.65% to 7%. Berry aneurysms are multiple in about 20% to 30% of cases. Females more commonly harbor intracranial aneurysm with peak prevalence in the fourth and sixth decades. Aneurysms in the pediatric population are rare, accounting for 2% to 4% of all aneurysms. These are generally are found in males and tend to be of larger dissecting variety.[3,4]

Different types of intracranial aneurysms exist. They are classified on their shape, size, location, and cause. Majority of intracranial aneurysms are saccular ones whereas fusiform, dissecting, mycotic and traumatic aneurysms are relatively rare.

PATHOGENESIS

Pathogenesis of intracranial aneurysms remains incompletely understood. For instance, the exact origin of the defect in the parent vessel wall is not established clearly, but it does not seem to be congenital.[5,6] It is believed that intracranial aneurysms result from a combination of hemodynamic stresses and acquired arterial wall degenerative changes, even if inherited diseases may predispose aneurysmal formation by weakening the vessel wall. This idea also is reinforced by the relative rarity of cerebral aneurysms in children.[7]

Hemodynamic Factors

Hemodynamic stress plays the most important role in the development of intracranial aneurysms fact supported by their preferential sites of occurrence at arterial bifurcations and increased frequency in the presence of circle of Willis asymmetry and vascular anomalies such as fenestrations and in cases of high-flow arteriovenous malformations.[8] This hemodynamic stress mainly results in two distinct physical forces.

The impacting force, perpendicular to the vessel wall, corresponds to the inertial force of the bloodstream and can be considered as the local elevation of the pressure at the area where the blood flow impacts.[9] The "wall shear stress", parallel to the vessel wall, caused by the viscous friction of the bloodstream.[10]

Even though impacting forces are important for aneurysm formation, various flow models reveal that their contribution to the rupture of the aneurysms may be less than previously thought. More than hypertension itself, it is the resultant amplification of blood blow and subsequent change of wall shear stress that appears to be main determinant in arterial wall degeneration and subsequent aneurysmal rupture.[11]

Acquired/Degenerative Changes

Several medical conditions are associated with the development of intracranial aneurysms such as systemic lupus erythematosus, Takayasu disease, giant cell arteritis, ADPCKD, Ehlers-Danlos syndrome, Marfan syndrome, fibromuscular dysplasia, neurofibromatosis, pseudoxanthoma elasticum, hereditary hemorrhagic telangiectasia, coarctation of the aorta, and alpha1-antitrypsin deficency.[12-14]

Genetics also plays a role in the formation of intracranial aneurysms. If 2 first-degree relatives in the same family have an intracranial aneurysm with no heritable connective tissue disorder, immediate family members have up to a 17% incidence of harboring an unruptured aneurysm.[15] Furthermore, first-degree and second-degree relatives of a patient with aneurysmal subarachnoid hemorrhage (SAH) are at 4.1- to 6.6-fold increased risk for aneurysmal SAH.[16,17] Therefore, screening is suggested in patients who have 2 or more family members with intracranial aneurysms.

Exogenous risk factors for the development of an intracranial aneurysm formation include cigarette smoking, cocaine use and heavy consumption of alcohol.[17,18] Infections, head trauma and intracranial neoplasms can rarely become primary causes of intracranial aneurysms.

TYPES OF ANEURYSMS

Saccular Aneurysm

True aneurysm with all the layers of arterial wall as its covering. Majority of these aneurysm occur in the anterior circulation (90%), most commonly arising from the circle of Willis. Most common location is anterior communicating artery (35%) followed by the internal carotid artery (30%), including the carotid bifurcation, posterior communicating artery, and ophthalmic artery. The next most common location is the middle cerebral artery bifurcation (20%), followed by the basilar apex (5%). Vertebrobasilar junction, superior cerebellar artery and posterior inferior cerebellar artery account for less than ten percent of intracranial aneurysm.[19,20]

Dissecting Aneurysm

Dissecting intracranial aneurysms are rare, originate from a dissection, which corresponds to a tear through the intima and internal elastic lamina with subsequent intramural hemorrhage.[21] The involved segment can become ectatic in response. Sometimes the tear may extend through the media and the adventitia resulting in pseudoaneurysm formation with or without SAH. Dissecting aneurysms can be acute or chronic. Acute dissecting aneurysms usually present with hemorrhage. Chronic dissecting aneurysms will more often induce compression of the adjacent structures.[22]

Atherosclerotic Aneurysm

Atherosclerotic aneurysms are segmental arterial ectasia caused by atherosclerotic and degenerative changes. They are characterized by an enlarged and elongated course with a circumferential involvement of the parent vessel and lack of a well-defined neck. This gives them a fusiform morphology. Vertebrobasilar circulation is reported to be the most frequent site of occurrence.[23,24]

Mycotic Aneurysm

Infectious (so-called mycotic) aneurysms are rare and account for 2% to 4% of all aneurysms. Most of infectious aneurysms occur in patients with infective endocarditis, the most common causative bacterium being *Streptococcus viridans*, while Aspergillus fumigatus is the most common agent causing fungal aneurysms.[25,26] These are often multiple and located distal to the circle of Willis, because they result from septic emboli in small cerebral arterial branches with resultant inflammation and necrosis.[27] Being fragile in nature, they usually rupture within the first weeks, with high morbidity and mortality.

Traumatic Aneurysm

Account for less than 1% of all intracranial aneurysms, but they represent 5–15% of aneurysms in children. They are pseudoaneurysms, which develop after direct injury or shear of the arterial wall. Injury leads to formation of hematoma that first organizes and then recanalizes. Closed head injuries result in shearing or impaction of the arterial wall against a dural fold and are responsible for distal aneurysms of the pericallosal artery (most common) and the posterior cerebral or the superior cerebellar arteries.[28-30]

CLINICAL PRESENTATION

Subarachnoid Hemorhage

Subarachnoid hemorrhage (SAH) resulting from ruptured cerebral aneurysms with consequent accumulation of blood in subarachnoid spaces. It is the most devastating presentation of cerebral aneurysm.

The patient will present with sever headache, often described as "worst headache of life" associated with varying neurological deficits. Patient with acute SAH may also have varying degree of neurological deficits.

Nonhemorrhagic Neurological Deficits

Aneurysm either due their mass effect or arterial pulsations can produce various neurological deficits. For example, giant cavernous ICA aneurysm can present with ipsilateral third, fourth or sixth cranial nerve palsies. Similarly large supraclinoid or Acom aneurysm may present with vision disturbances due to compression of optic apparatus. Large post fossa dissecting aneurysm may present with symptoms of brain stem compression or hydrocephalus. There is substantial clot burden associated with dissecting aneurysms, which has potential to cause ischemic stroke. Such a scenario is seen with dissecting MCA aneurysm.

Unruptured Incidental Aneurysm

Widespread use of CT and MR imaging has led to significant increase in numbers of intracranial aneurysms discovered incidentally, making the management of patients with unruptured intracranial aneurysms (UIAs) an increasingly relevant. We provide here a brief review of International Study of Unruptured Intracranial Aneurysms (ISUIA) to bring some perspective on this subject **(Table 1)**. The study analyzed 727 patients who had UIAs and no history of SAH (group 1 patients) and 722 patients who had UIAs and a history of SAH from another aneurysm (group 2 patients). Mean follow-up was about 7.5 years.[31]

The rupture rate for patients who had UIAs 7 mm or less in diameter was approximately less 1% per year. Aneurysmal location was important for predicting future UIA rupture, Posterior circulation and the posterior communicating artery aneurysm had greater risk of rupture as compared to anterior counterparts whereas carotid cavernous artery UIAs were associated with least risk.

Even though the above data suggests aneurysm with size less than 7 mm have < 1% annual risk of rupture, majority of ruptured aneurysm that present in our clinical practice are less than 7 mm. This observation compels us to understand the need for providing the patient with extensive preprocedural counseling given procedural risk and risk of future rupture.

TABLE 1: International Study of Unruptured Intracranial Aneurysms (ISUIA) study.

Aneurysm location	<7 mm group 1	<7 mm group II	7–12 mm	13–24 mm	25+ mm
Cav. ICA	0%	0%	0%	3%	6.4%
ACom/MCA/ICA	0%	1.5%	2.6%	14.5%	40%
Post circ. /Pcom	2.5%	3.4%	14.5%	18.4%	50%

Group 1 had no subarachnoid hemorrhage. Group 2 had subarachnoid hemorrhage from a separate aneurysm.

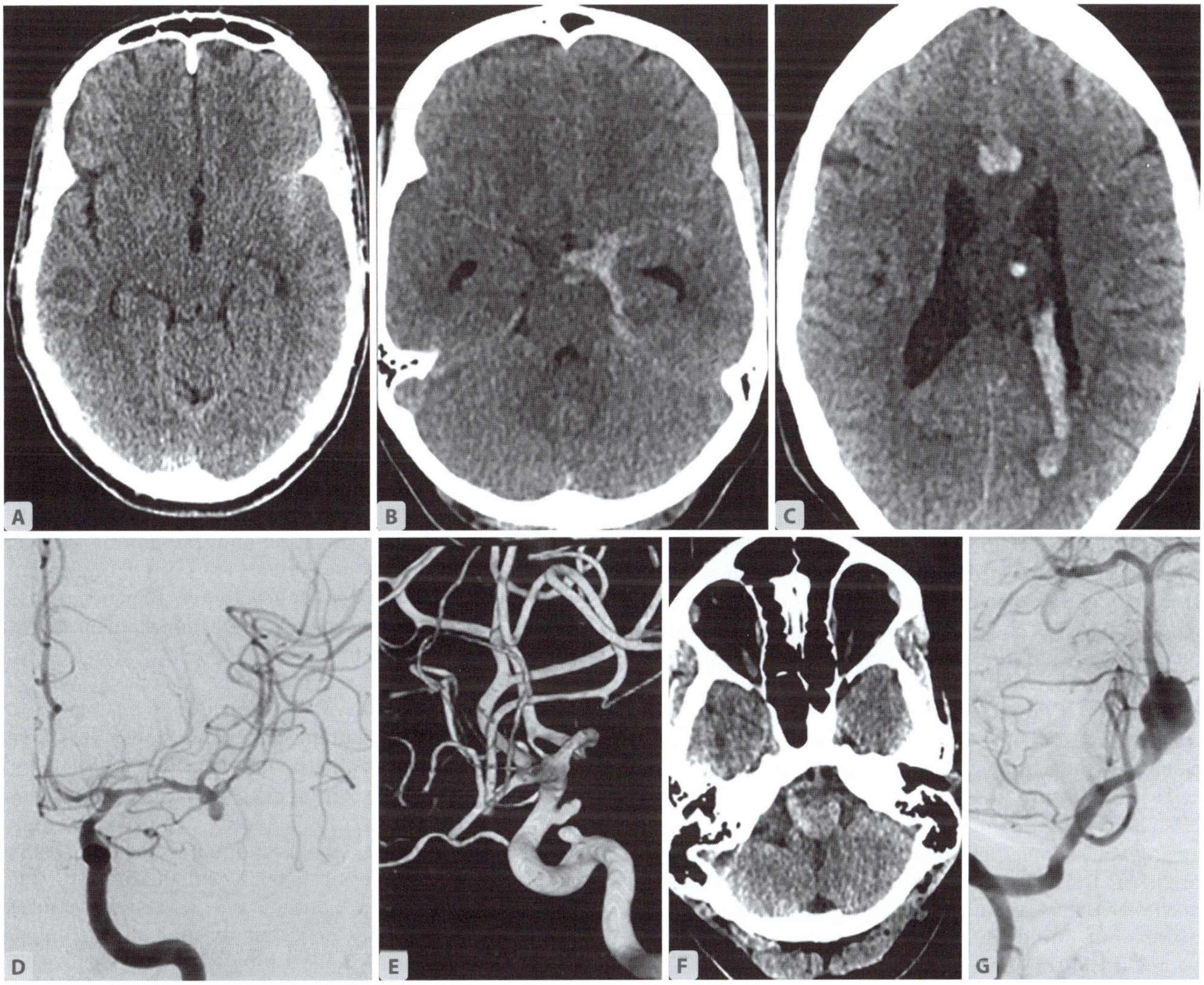

FIGS. 1A TO G: NCCT head in aneurysm. (A to C) show Fischer grade 2 (thin SAH), 3 (thick SAH) and 4 (thick SAH with IVH), respectively. Sentinel hematoma: Angiograms (D and E) of patient in A and B revealed left MCA bifurcation aneurysm and left Pcom aneurysm, respectively. Aneurysm presenting as mass effect: Dissecting vertebra-basilar junction aneurysm (G) compressing the brainstem (F).

DIAGNOSTIC EVAUATION

Whenever SAH is suspected, noncontrast head CT is cornerstone of the diagnosis with very high diagnostic yield. NCCT head not only conforms the diagnosis of SAH, but also provides valuable information regarding ventricular size, status of cerebral parenchyma and suspected location of the aneurysm **(Figs.1A to G)**. NCCT also remains a powerful tool for comparison and follow up.

MR imaging has limited role in evaluation of patient with SAH in emergency. However it is not infrequent for patient to get MRI for headache due to SAH. MRI revels altered signal intensity in sulcal spaces, most apparent on FLAIR images. T2 shortening (blooming) can be noted on gradient images, particularly well on SWI images. Careful attention must be paid so as not confuse cortical vein with surface SAH. MR imaging become important once we are concerned with large or giant aneurysm, where interest lies in assessing parenchymal status. MR vessel wall imaging is sometime done to delineate wall of the aneurysm. This becomes useful in understanding point of rupture and assessing fragility of the wall.

Imaging techniques for intracranial aneurysms include digital subtraction angiography (DSA) both 2D and 3D rotational angiography, multislice computed tomographic (MSCT) angiography, MR angiography, and transcranial Doppler ultrasonography.

Intra-arterial DSA is still the gold standard for evaluation of a patient with a suspected aneurysm, given its high spatial resolution; however with new generation MSCTA has a similar specificity and sensitivity for detecting an intracranial aneurysm, except for aneurysm smaller than 3 mm. The spatial resolution for DSA is 0.2 mm, and about 0.15 mm for 3D-DSA.[32] DSA is an invasive test with about 0.5-1% risk of permanent neurologic complications, whereas there is no risk of neurologic complications with MSCTA or MR angiography.[33,34]

The current spatial resolution of CT angiography is 0.4 to 0.7 mm.[32,35] When compared with DSA as the reference standard, CT angiography has an average reported specificity rate of 96% to 98% (90% to 94% for aneurysms smaller than 3 mm and up to 100% for aneurysms larger than 4 mm) and sensitivity rates of 96% to 98%.[36] The spatial resolution of MR angiography at 1.5 T is on the order of 1 mm. With 3-T scanners, spatial resolution may reach 0.6 mm.[37] When compared with DSA, MR angiography reported specificity rates for detection of intracranial aneurysms ranging from 69% to 100%, with a sensitivity rate of 75% to 100%.[38,39]

As a matter of institute protocol all patient with suspected aneurysm undergo complete cerebral diagnostic angiography. This demonstrate size of the aneurysm and its orientation, length of neck, relationship between the aneurysm and parent artery and the status of rest of intracranial vessels. Some giant and complex aneurysms may require additional physiologic evaluation, including test occlusion and cross compression studies to determine the adequacy of collaterals, there by identifying if a patient can tolerate parent vessel occlusion.

If the first angiogram following SAH is negative, angiography should be repeated 1-2 weeks later. The recent use of 3D DSA has improved the pretreatment delineation of the aneurysm anatomy and of the surrounding vessels, however it could be misleading in presence of close approximation of vessels to the aneurysms.

PREPROCEDURE MANAGEMENT

Patient with acute SAH is an emergency[40] demanding immediate stabilization and management. The initial management is directed at ensuring basic life support. This includes ensuring adequate airway, ventilator, and circulatory support. History and physical examination are obtained to assess possible cause of SAH. Chest radiographs, electrocardiograms, blood work, serum electrolytes, cardiac and liver enzymes, coagulation profile and cross matching of blood is performed.

The clinical picture is classified according to the given algorithms[41] (WFNS: World Federation of Neurological Surgeons[42] and Hunt and Hess grade[43] respectively) **(Tables 2 and 3)**.

TABLE 2: World Federation of Neurological Surgeons (WFNS) grade.

WFNS grade	GCS score	Focal deficit
I	15	Absent
II	14–13	Absent
III	14–13	Present
IV	12–7	Present or absent
V	6–3	Present or absent

TABLE 3: Hunt and Hess grade.

Hunt and Hess Category	Criteria
Grade I	Asymptomatic or minimal headache and slight nuchal rigidity
Grade II	Moderate-to-severe headache, nuchal rigidity, no neurological deficit
Grade III	Drowsiness, confusion or mild neurological deficit
Grade IV	Stupor, moderate-to-severe hemiparesis, early decerebrate rigidity and vegetative disturbances
Grade V	Deep coma, decerebrate rigidity—moribund appearance

Patients are then managed in an intensive care setting, where close observation and frequent neurologic examinations can be done. Patients are kept nil orally until a final therapeutic decision on how to treat the aneurysm is taken. Majority of patients with SAH are hypovolemic, problem compounded by coexisting cerebral salt wasting or SIADH. Large bore IV access, and an arterial line if required is placed. Adequate normal saline with electrolyte supplementation is given with the goal of attaining/maintaining euvolemia. Role of IV dextrose in acute setting is controversial.

Extension of blood into cisterns and/or ventricles incites an inflammatory response and consequent adhesion formation. This hampers normal cerebrospinal fluid (CSF) circulation and results in hydrocephalus, documented in approximately 20–30 % of the cases. Treatment requires augmentation of CSF flow either through placement of external ventricular drain or lumbar drain. Excessive CSF drainage can result in sudden drop of the ICP, which may precipitate rebleeding. Hence drainage bag usually is placed at 18 to 20 cm above the head level. Improvement in CSF circulation not only improves ventricular status but also helps in counteracting development of cerebral vasospasm.[44] Persistent hydrocephalus may require VP shunt.

At authors' institute prophylactic anticonvulsants are currently administered to all patients with acute SAH. Rationale for this stems from the concern that a post SAH seizure could promote rebleeding of the aneurysm.[45]

Management of blood pressure in cases of acute SAH is complex and still slightly controversial. There is strong opinion to treat significantly elevated blood pressure because of increased incidence of rerupture in patients with continuous hypertension following SAH.[22] However moderated increase in blood pressure is a normal physiological response to SAH for maintaining cerebral perfusion. Hence care must be given to fact that sudden or exaggerated drop in blood pressure might precipitate cerebral ischemia due to underlying cerebral vasospasm.

Given high rates of rerupture in ruptured aneurysm, it is imperative that once the patient has been stabilized, next immediate goal should be occlusion of the aneurysm. This can be achieved either through endovascular route or via surgery (clipping). We will now summarize various endovascular methods to treat aneurysm.

ENDOVASCULAR TREATMENT

- *Endosaccular (treatment from within the aneurysm)*
  - Simple coiling without assistance
  - Balloon-assisted coiling
  - Stent-assisted coiling
  - Newer Devices
    - P-conus
    - Pulse Rider
    - WEB
    - Medina coils
- *Endoluminal (treatment from within the parent artery)*
  - Constructive: Parent vessel preserved
    - Flow Diverters
    - Covered Stents
  - Deconstructive: Parent vessel occlusion

SIMPLE COILING

How coiling of a simple aneurysm is done without any adjunctive device **(Figs. 2A to D)**.

Anesthesia

At the authors' institution, each endovascular aneurysm treatment is done under general anesthesia with complete hemodynamic and neurophysiological monitoring. The neuroanesthesiologist takes all necessary steps to avoid exaggerated blood pressure changes (spikes), especially while inducing or extubating the patient. Anesthesia is necessary to not only to maintain immobility but may also herald any intraoperative complication for example, intraprocedure aneurysmal rupture is manifested by immediate hypertension and bradycardia.

Access

Arterial sheath, generally 6F in caliber is introduced via femoral artery. If adjunctive devices are needed larger bore femoral puncture or simultaneous contralateral femoral puncture may be taken. After the sheath is inserted in the groin, 50 international units (IU) of heparin per kilogram is given intra-arterially as a bolus with intent to keep the ACT between 250 and 300 seconds.[43] Protamine sulfate for heparin reversal kept ready in neurointervention suite to be injected in unlikely case of aneurysmal rupture. The usual dose is 10 mg of protamine per 1000 IU of circulating heparin. Anti platelet regimen will be discussed under section on stent-assisted coiling.

Angiogram

A complete cerebral angiogram is performed before treatment with 5F catheter, including injections of the bilateral internal carotid and vertebral arteries. Additional 3D rotational images and cross compression studies are obtained to accurately define the morphology of the aneurysm and status of crossflow/collaterals.

After completion of diagnostic study, for therapeutic procedure a 6F guide catheter is introduced in target artery and positioned in close proximity to the aneurysm. It is necessary for the guide catheter to have a stable position for safe and smooth microcatheter navigation. Guide catheter should always be visible on working road map projection even during advancement of the coil through microcatheter into the aneurysm. Routinely used Guide catheters are the Neuron (Penumbra), Envoy (codman), or Chaperon (microvention). In case of tortuous aortic or neck anatomy Additionally a triple coaxial system consisting of a long sheath (Shuttle: cook) followed by guide catheter can be placed to straighten out the system and provide enhanced stability.[46-48]

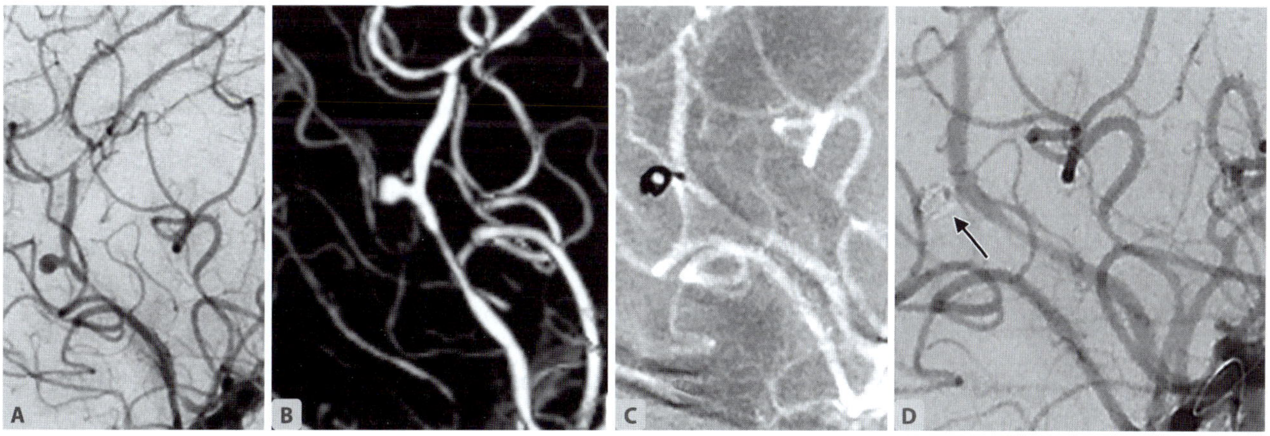

FIGS. 2A TO D: Conventional coiling: LICA angiogram (A) and 3D DSA; (B) reveal DACA aneurysm. Under roadmap; (C) aneurysm is coiled without use of adjunctive device. Control angiogram; (D) showing complete occlusion of the aneurysm (arrow).

Microcatheterization of Aneurysm

Catheterisation of an aneurysm is done via microcatheter-microwire combination under a constant visualization on roadmap. There is hydrophilic coating on outer wall of all microcatheters, which helps in minimizing friction and thus permit distal catheterization into the intracranial circulation. The various microcatheters used are Echelon (eV3), SL-10 (Stryker), Headway-17 (Microvention), etc. Microcatheters are shaped by steam heating of the tip to conform according to anatomy of artery and aneurysm. The ideal microcatheter position is governed by morphology of the aneurysm (shape, size, neck and relation to curve of parent artery). A well-positioned microcatheter should allow stable coil extrusion while maintaining its relation with parent artery and aneurysm.

Coiling

The choice of the coil is governed again by size, shape and neck of the aneurysm. The aim of the first coil or the framing coil is to create a frame or basket for the placement of subsequent coils. The framing coil also acts as bridge across the aneurysmal neck to prevent migrating of additional into the parent vessel. Size of the first coil is determined by largest dimension of the aneurysm. For proper approximation along the aneurysmal sac, the first coil should have largest and longest dimension possible. Well-apposed coil provides sound basket and stability to the subsequent coil mass.

First coil also called as framing coil is usually a 3D coil (complex shaped coil) and subsequent coils (filling coils) are generally helical coils. Under live roadmap keeping good profile of aneurysmal neck, successive coils are introduced into the aneurysm. Additional coils are introduced till they form dense coil mass and aneurysm is no longer opacifying on angiogram.

Once the aneurysm is obliterated, microcatheter is withdrawn slowly. Check angiogram is performed to assess the degree of aneurysm occlusion, patency of parent artery and status of the distal vasculature.

Once the procedure has been completed, femoral artery sheath is removed. Manual compression or closure device can be used to obtain hemostasis. Pressure with fingertips is maintained on the puncture site for usually 30 to 40 minutes if manual compression is used. The patient is then shifted to neuro ICU. Leg is kept immobilized for atleast 6 hours to prevent puncture site complications.[49]

BALLOON-ASSISTED COILING

An aneurysm is considered wide necked when the ratio between the maximum diameters of dome and neck is less than two. The aneurysms then become anatomically unfavorable for conventional coiling as chances of prolapsing of coils in parent artery increases. Moret et al. first described utility of balloon remodeling technique for such aneurysms.[50,51]

The technique consists of inflating a balloon (non detachable) in front of aneurysmal neck during coil placement. The balloon acts as a temporary bridge, allowing coils to be packed into the aneurysm sac without prolapsing into the artery. The coils remain molded within the aneurysm after deflation of the balloon, essentially "remodeling the arterial wall". It is routinely used today to treat wide-necked aneurysms particularly in patients with SAH, thus eliminating stent placement and the use of antiplatelet agents.

To treat wide-necked side-wall aneurysms, the neurointerventionist routinely uses compliant balloons, e.g. HyperGlide (Ev3, Irvine, CA), Ascent (Codman Neurovascular, Raynham, MA) and Scepter C (Microvention-Terumo, Inc, Tustin, CA).

Technique for balloon-assisted coiling **(Figs. 3A to H)** is essentially same as described previously. Under roadmap, first the deflated balloon first is navigated across the neck of the aneurysm. This is followed by catheterization of the aneurysm. The balloon is inflated across the neck of the aneurysm, causing temporary occlusion of the neck and parent vessel. Thus the balloon bridges the neck and allows formation of coil basket. Before the coil is detached, balloon is deflated to test the stability of the coil within sac. If no displacement of the coil loop is observed, the coil is detached. This procedure is repeated multiple times until the aneurysm no longer fills with contrast or has a dense coil mass within the confines of its lumen.

To treat an aneurysm located at arterial bifurcations or aneurysm with arteries arising from its neck, neurointerventionist use extra-compliant low-pressure balloon which conform to the irregularities of any vasculature space. When the balloon is inflated, it y partially herniates into the aneurysm neck or the origin of the arterial branches emerging from the neck of the aneurysm. This configuration secures the parent artery and arterial branches emerging from the neck of the aneurysm during coil placement. Example of extra compliant balloon are hyperform (eV3) and Septor -XC (Microvention).

STENT-ASSISTED COILING

Stent-assisted coiling is done for wide-necked and dysplastic aneurysms that are not amendable with simple or balloon assisted coiling. The stent acts as a scaffold that prevents the coils placed into the aneurysm sac from herniation into the parent vessel. The stent may also reduce the inflow into the aneurysm, promoting stasis and thrombosis of the aneurysm. In addition, the struts of the stent may provide a matrix for the growth of endothelial cells across the neck of the aneurysm.

Initially, balloon-expandable coronary stents were used; however being relatively stiff stents they were difficult to navigate into tortuous intracranial circulation and carried risk of possible rupture of the parent vessel. They were gradually replaced with self-expanding stents.

Self-expanding stents are broadly divided into two types either laser cut or braided. Laser cut stents are Neuroform (Stryker), Enterprise (Codman) and Solitaire (eV3). Braided stents are Leo (Balt Extrusion), and LVIS (Microvention).

Technique of Coiling with Stent Assistance (Figs. 4A to H)

The aneurysm may be coiled by different techniques using stent assistance. We briefly describe four different approaches

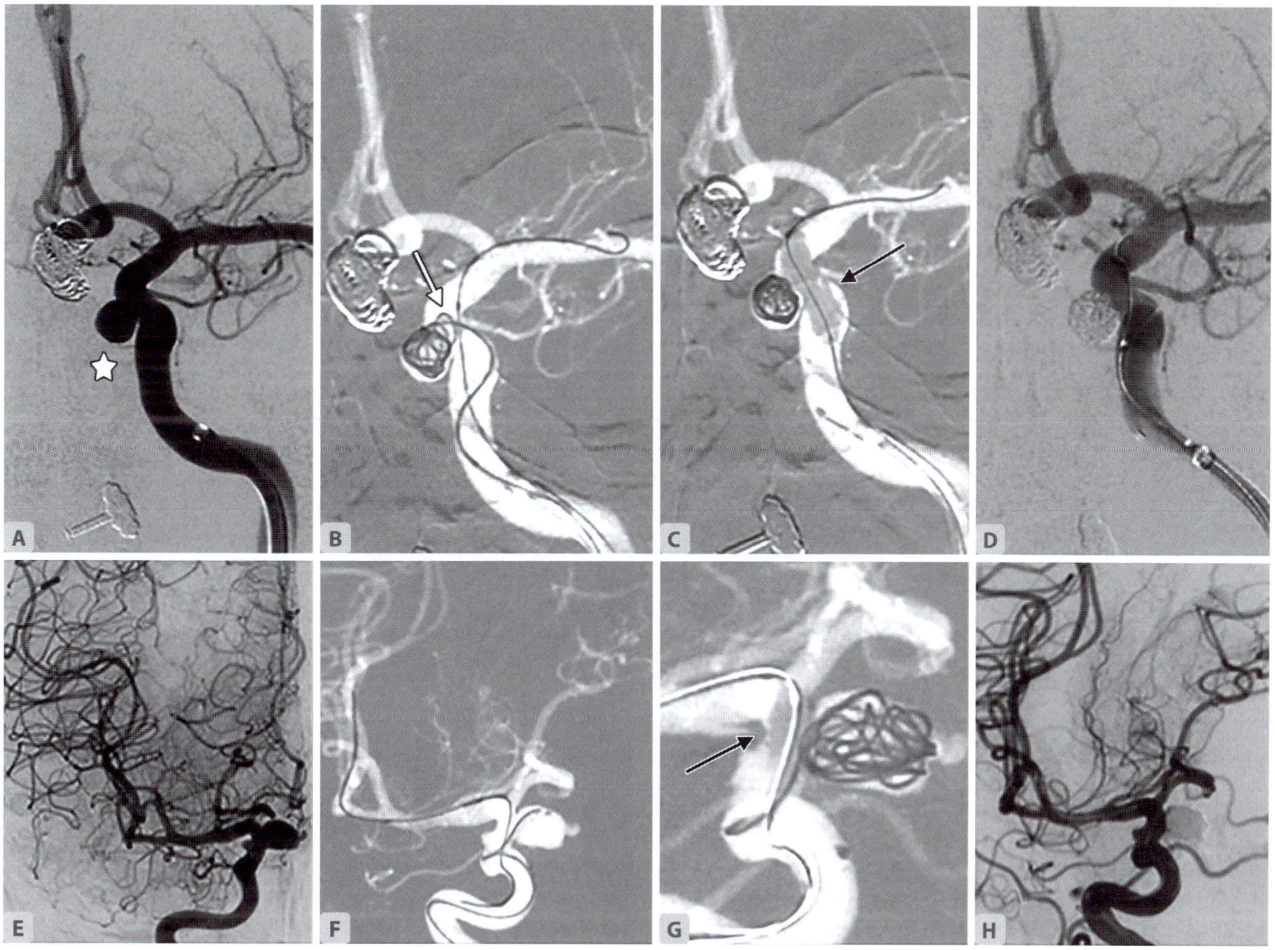

FIGS. 3A TO H: Balloon-assisted coiling: LICA angiogram (A) reveals left carotid cave aneurysm (*). Unassisted coiling; (B) resulted in herniation of coil loops in parent artery (white arrow). After balloon inflation; (C) (black arrow) the aneurysm is remodeled and completely coiled; (D). Another case with wide neck ruptured superior hypophyseal aneurysm; (E) is treated with balloon-assisted (black arrow) coiling; (F and G). Control angiogram; (H) showing complete obliteration of the aneurysm.

for stent assisted coiling. "Jailing the microcatheter", in this technique aneurysm is first catheterized followed by deployment of stent across the aneurysm. This effectively jails the coiling catheter between parent artery and the stent, providing increased stability while coiling. In the second technique stent is first delivered across neck of the aneurysm, followed by placement of coiling catheter into the aneurysm sac through stent struts. Third technique involves coiling of aneurysm by routine balloon assisted manner, then the stent is placed across the neck of the aneurysm with an intention to decrease recanalization by promoting endothelial growth along the stent surface. Final technique also called as stent jack technique, involves partial deployment of a first coil before placement of stent across the aneurysm neck. After complete deployment of the stent, the first coil is detached. This in contrast to jailing technique, which involves only cathe-terization of aneurysm, not coil placement before stent deployment.

It becomes very important for an interventional neuroradiologist to understand anatomy of both aneurysm and parent artery on 3D rotational angiogram. Points to be considered when contemplating size of the stent are length of the neck, dimensions of parent artery at level of aneurysm as well as proximal and distal to the aneurysm. The diameter of the stent is then sized to be about 0.5–1 mm more than diameter of parent artery. Length of the stent is determined by the fact that middle of the stent should be across the aneurysmal neck with at least 5 mm coverage along both proximal and distal aspects of aneurysm neck.

PROTOCOL FOR ANTIPLATELET ADMINISTRATION IN CASES OF INTRACRANIAL STENTING

Stent is a foreign body, thus its placement into the cerebral vessel will incite inflammatory response with consequent platelet activation and clot formation. To prevent this, it is of utmost important to administer optimal antiplatelet agents before placement of an intracranial stent. The optimal dose and treatment regimen, however, has not been determined.

At authors institution dual antiplatelets are administered for at least 3 days prior to the procedure. Aspirin (150 mg/day orally) and clopidogrel (150 mg/day orally) are the drugs used. If a stent needs to be placed on an emergent basis the

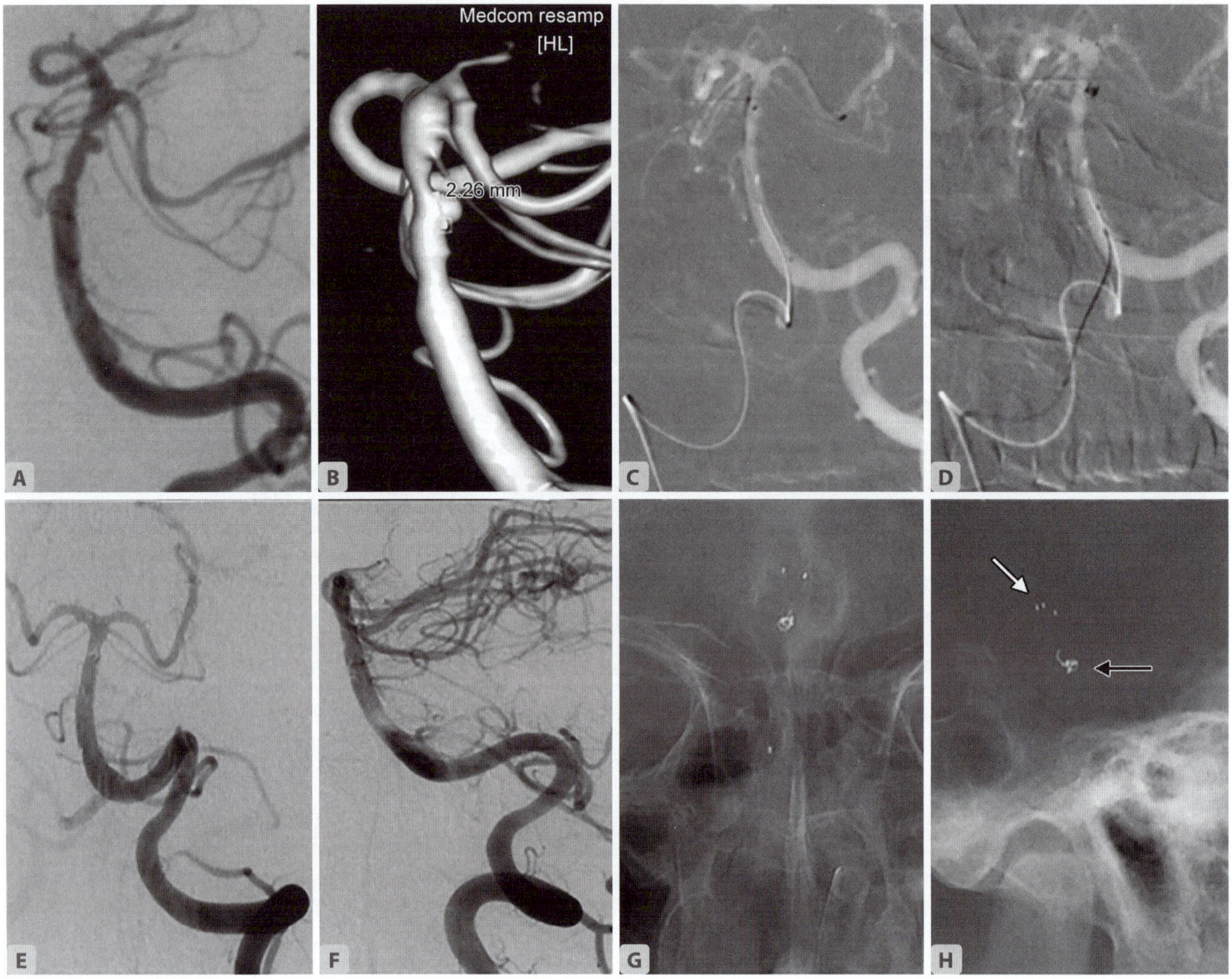

FIGS. 4A TO H: Stent Jack Technique (Stent-assisted coiling). LVA angiogram (A) and VRT image (B) show small dysplastic blister aneurysm in distal basilar artery. Under roadmap (C and D), first coil was partially placed with few loops were seen to be prolapsing into the parent artery, at this point stent was deployed to push the coil loops inside the aneurysm. Control angiogram (E and F) reveals occlusion of aneurysm with patent basilar artery. Native images (G and H) show stent markers (white arrow) and coil loops (black arrow), respectively.

authors will administer dual antiplatelet 3 to 4 hours prior to the procedure. Dose of drugs is clopidogrel (300 mg orally) and aspirin (300 mg orally). If an emergency stent graft **(Figs. 5A to H)** needs to be placed during the procedure in a patient who has not been treated preoperatively with antiplatelet medications, the patient is loaded with abciximab (glycoprotein IIa/IIIb inhibitor) at the dose of 0.25 mg/kg the and subsequently dual antiplatelets are started. Few institutions may keep patient on continuous infusion of abciximab for 12 to 24 hours before shifting to dual antiplatelets.[52]

FLOW DIVERTERS

Over last decade revolutionary devices for treatment of complex aneurysm have appeared in markets called flow diverters.[53] Novelty of these devices lies in the fact that they treat aneurysms from endoluminal rather than conventional endosaccular approach **(Figs. 6A to F)**. Such stent-like devices are designed to reconstruct the parent vessel and to divert flow away from the aneurysm lumen without the use of coils.

Flow diverters are stent like devices has tighter scaffolding, providing a means over which endothelial cells can grow to seal off the neck of the aneurysm. The device promotes thrombus formation within the aneurysm by decreasing the hemodynamic effects within the aneurysm sac, spare side branches and perforators (fill via pressure gradient) promote neointimal remodeling (maintaining outflow in the side branches and perforators) and change the configuration of the parent vessel in relation to aneurysm.[54,55]

Flow diverters are braided stents with high metal coverage and low porosity. They are made of either chromium cobalt or nitinol wires. Number of wires range from 48 to 96. The various flow diverters available in market are Pipeline (Ev3), Silk (Balt), FRED (microvention), SURPASS (Stryker) and p64 (Phenox).

Current indication of flow diverters is wide necked large/ giant intracranial aneurysm (>10 mm) not amenable to other

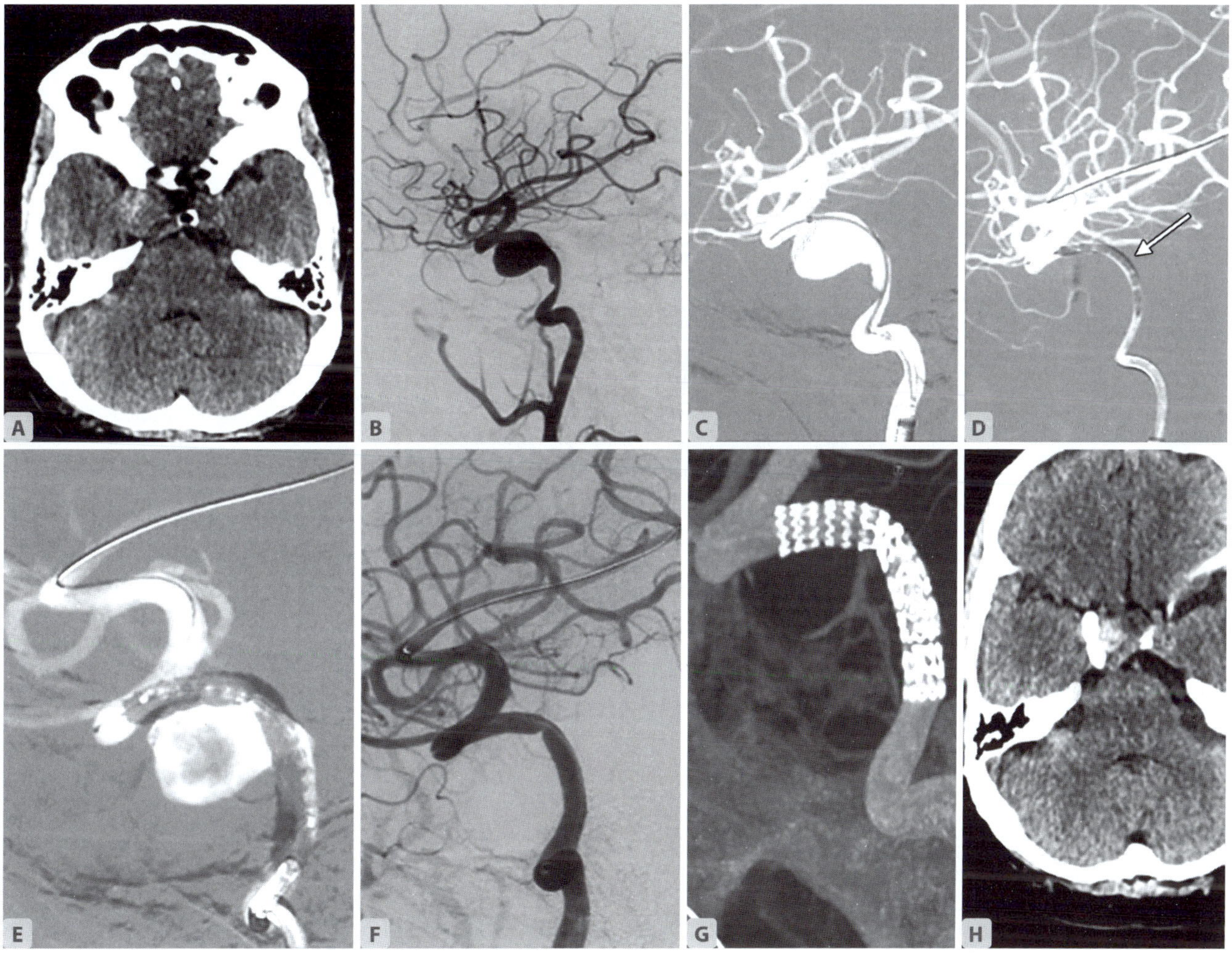

FIGS. 5A TO H: Covered stent placement: NCCT head (A) and RICA angiogram; (B) show partially thrombosed right cavernous ICA aneurysm. Subsequent balloon mounted stent graft (white arrow) (covered stent) is navigated; (C and D) and inflated; (E) across the aneurysm. Control angiogram; (F) shows occlusion of aneurysm with patent ICA. Follow-up CT; (G and H) documents shrinkage of aneurysm with resolution of its mass effect.

endovascular treatment options. However with advancement in their design flow diverters are now also used for blister aneurysms, distal anterior circulation aneurysm and large posterior fossa dissecting aneurysms.[56,57]

Flow diverters are bulky devices with relative difficulty in their deployment across the aneurysm. Hence they are associated with higher incidence of both ischemic and hemorrhagic complications.

PARENT ARTERY OCCLUSION

Sometimes in very complex large dissecting aneurysms, preservation of parent artery may not be possible. In such situations it becomes imperative that parent artery be occluded. This can be done either with concomitant aneurysm occlusion **(Figs. 7A to E)** or as a stand-alone procedure **(Figs. 7F to J)**. The basic idea behind this technique lies in the fact that progression of these aneurysms is directly dependent on direction of the blood flow across them. If we are able to abolish/reverse this flow, the progression of the aneurysm may be arrested and with due passage of time the involved arterial segment will heal. The anatomy of arterial collaterals, competence of COW and possibility of development of new collaterals must be understood when contemplating parent artery occlusion (PAO). In majority of cases prior to arterial sacrifice, a temporary balloon test occlusion (BTO) is done to assess whether the patient can tolerate permanent occlusion of the artery. Once the patient tolerates BTO, parent artery is then occluded either with coils **(Figs. 7A to E)** or detachable balloons **(Figs. 7F to K)**. Possible complications include stroke, non-shrinkage of aneurysm on follow-up and closure of direct anatomical pathway for future intervention. However PAO is a time proven therapeutic option. Elegance of this technique is highlighted by the excellent long-term angiographic and clinical results that are achieved with minimal intervention in complex aneurysms, which are otherwise a challenge to treat.

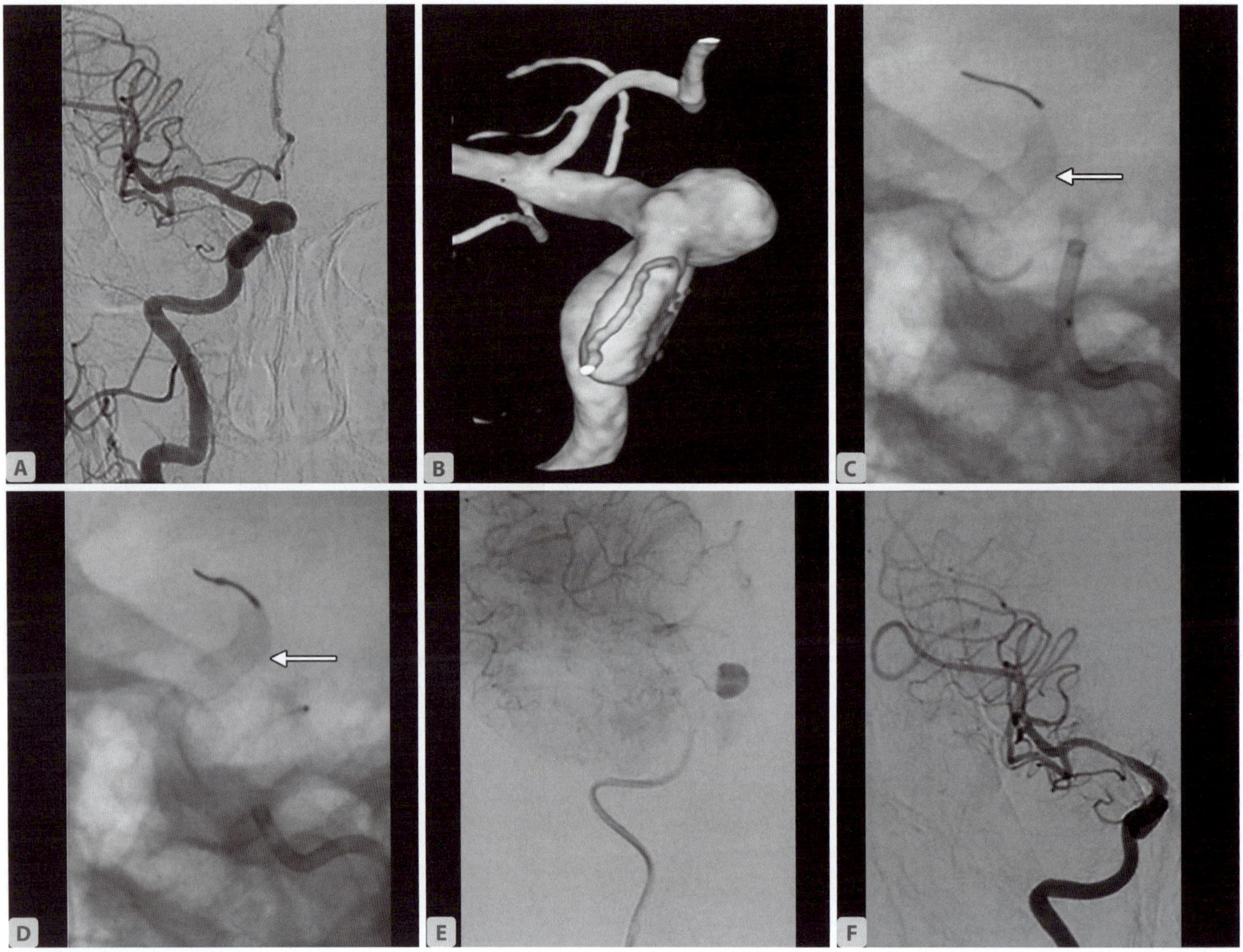

FIGS. 6A TO F: Flow diverter placement. RICA angiogram (A) and VRT image; (B) show wide neck superior hypophyseal aneurysm. Fluoroscopy-spots; (C and D) show deployment of FD (white arrows) across neck of the aneurysm. Control angiogram; (E) showing marked stasis in aneurysm. Follow-up angiogram after 1 year; (F) shows complete obliteration of aneurysm with remodeling of the parent artery.

COMPLICATIONS OF ENDOVASCULAR COILING AND THEIR MANAGEMENT

Alongside the risks, the advantages and disadvantages of endovascular coiling should be weighed against the risk of surgical treatment or a conservative approach before treatment, to determine the best option for the optimal clinical outcome. Patients should be given their full options along with extensive information before treatment. In the case of a ruptured aneurysm this information should be given to the patient's relatives. The information provided must inform patient party in a comprehensive manner about therapeutic options, relative merits and demerits, cost of procedure, goals of treatment and estimated duration of ICU/hospital stay.

Every periprocedural or postprocedural complication needs to be examined thoroughly before corrective actions are taken.

Coil Migration/Malposition

Coil malposition refers to placement of coil outsides the confines of aneurysmal sac. Malposition of a coil usually results from poor coil choice, improper catheter position, or choice of technique not suitable for aneurysm. Most commonly it is a single loop of coil that protrudes into the parent vessel. Single loop plastered along the arterial wall will seldom causes a thromboembolic complication and thus we should refrain from overzealous treatment.

If thrombus forms around the loop of coil, a glycoprotein IIa/IIIb inhibitor can be given at the site of thrombus formation to dissolve the clot. If the coil gas to be removed, one of the retrieval devices like microsnare or retrievable stent must be used **(Figs. 8F to J)**. If coil retrieval is not possible, the loop of coil should be plastered against the vessel wall by placement of intracranial stent.[58]

Stretched Coil

Stretching of a coil is potentially disastrous complication. It requires prompt recognition and remedy. Stretched coil should be suspected if the coil is not responding one-to-one under fluoroscopy with hand movements at the groin, or if difficulty is encountered in repositioning of the coil.

In this situation, the coil and microcatheter should be retrieved together as a single unit from the patient. However if the coil cannot be retrieved, it should be stretched as long

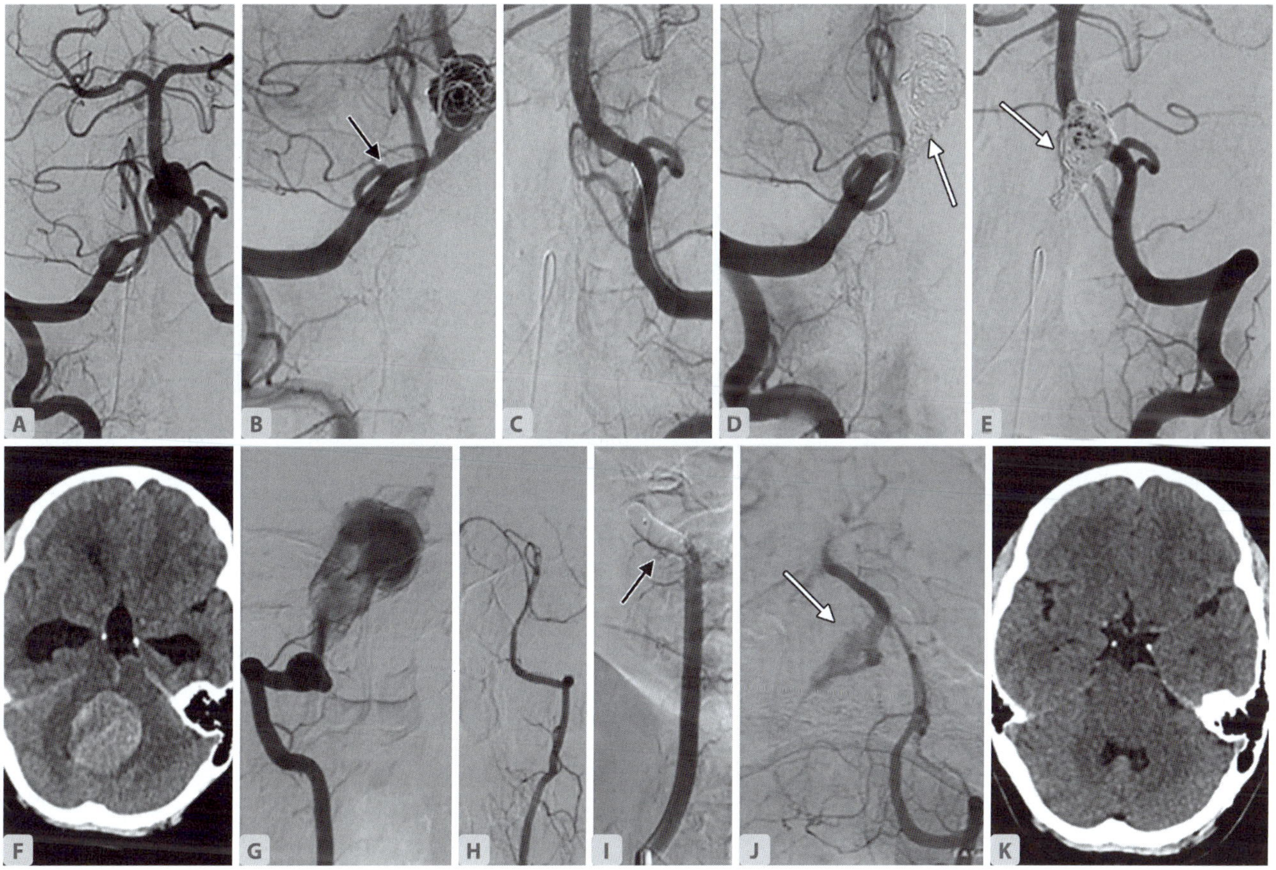

FIGS. 7A TO K: Parent artery occlusion: RVA angiogram (A) reveals vertebrobasilar dissecting aneurysm. It was treated by occlusion of aneurysm and V4 segment of RVA distal to origin of right PICA (black arrow in B) with stent placement from LVA to basilar artery (C). Control angiogram (D and E) revealed occlusion of both aneurysm and parent artery (coil mass marked by white arrows). *Parent artery occlusion with flow reversal:* NCCT head (F) and RVA angiogram (G) reveals large dissecting right V4 segment aneurysm with hydrocephalus. LVA (H) is hypoplastic. After successful balloon test occlusion, RVA (I) was occluded with detachable balloon (black arrow). Postprocedure LVA angiogram (J) reveals reversal of flow in aneurysm (white arrow). Follow-up CT (K) after a year shows resolution of both aneurysm and hydrocephalus.

as possible and positioned either into the external carotid artery or descending thoracic aorta to prevent distal arterial migration. Patient should be kept anticoagulated overnight in the NICU and given an antiplatelet agent. Within span of 6 8 weeks the stretched coil becomes endothelized.

Intraprocedural Rupture of Aneurysm

Intraoperative aneurysm rupture is the most dreaded complication can occur due to fragile nature of the aneurysm wall **(Figs. 8A to E)**. It usually occurs either during aneurysmal microcatheterization or coil placement.[59] When this occurs, there is a rapid severe elevation of the blood pressure.

Given very high mortality with this complication, it is of utmost importance to quickly secure the aneurysm and control blood extravasation into subarachnoid space. Circulating systemic heparin must be immediately reversed with protamine [1 mL (10 mg) protamine per 1000 units of circulating heparin], so that the ACT is less than 150 seconds. If the patient has been placed on dual antiplatelets, an attempt at reversal of platelet inhibition should be made with the infusion of platelets. The blood pressure should also be lowered immediately by pharmaceutical means in an attempt to prevent any further extravasation of blood.[60,61]

If a balloon is present within the parent vessel, this should be carefully positioned and inflated at aneurysmal neck and aneurysm rapidly packed with additional coils. If the microcatheter is within the subarachnoid space, the operator must not panic and remove the microcatheter. Coiling should be performed from the subarachnoid space into the aneurysm.

After the aneurysm is secure, CT of the head should be immediately performed to assess for hydrocephalus and the need for placement of a ventriculostomy catheter.

Rupture of Vessel

Arterial perforation by either microcatheter or microguide wire is rare. This rupture may be self-limiting and seal off spontaneously, or may lead to life-threatening hemorrhage particularly in patients premeditated on antiplatelets. If angiographic leak or life-threatening hemorrhage is identified, permanent occlusion of the vessel may be life-saving. A liquid embolic agent or coils can be used for this purpose.[62]

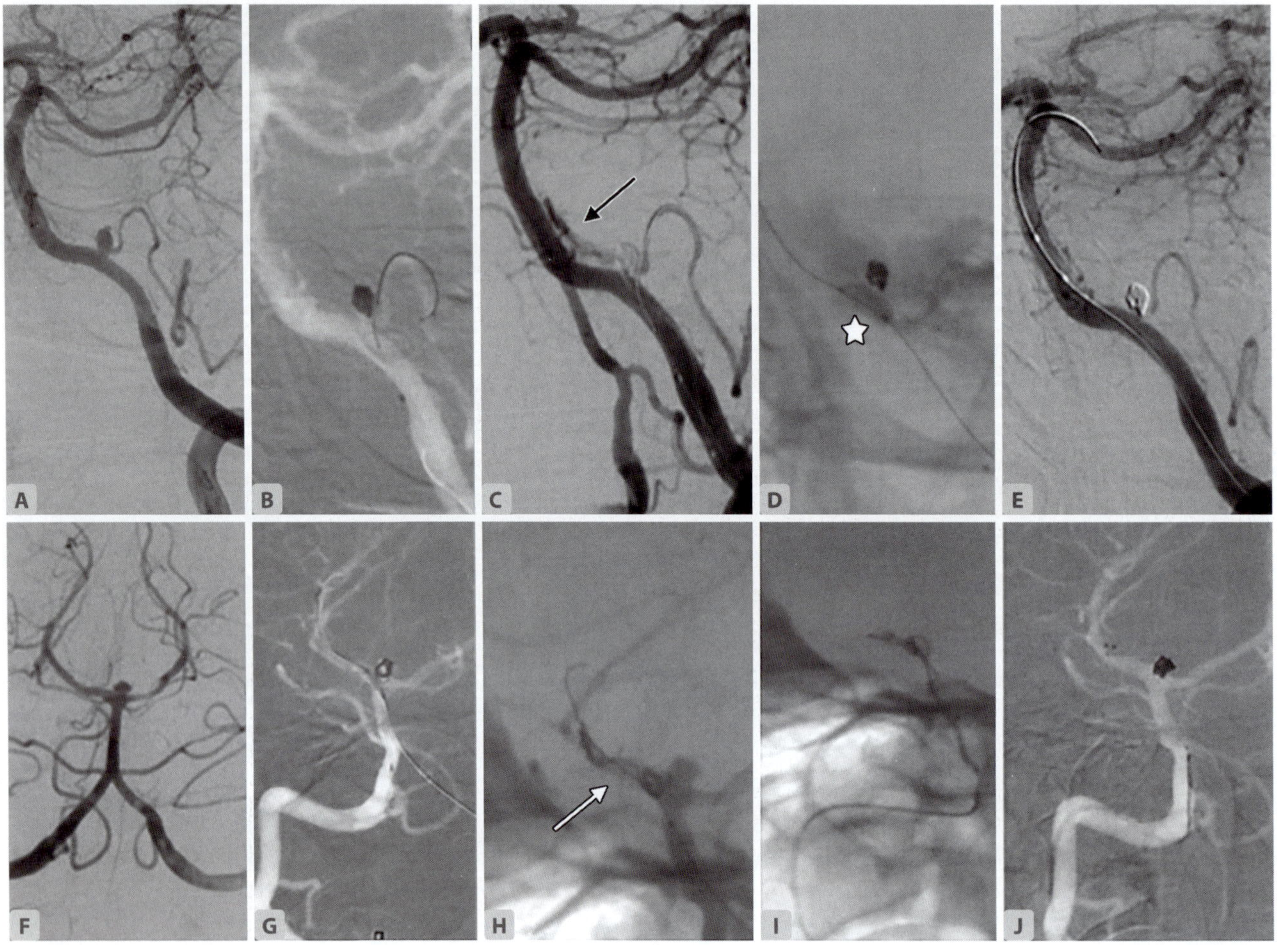

FIGS. 8A TO J: Complications: Intraprocedural aneurysmal rupture. LVA angiogram (A) reveals PICA aneurysm which was coiled with protection of PICA (B). Check angiogram postcoiling (C) shows leak in vicinity of aneurysm (black arrow) suggestive of aneurysmal rupture. Heparin was reversed and balloon inflated across neck of aneurysm (* in D). Control angiogram (E) shows control of contrast extravasation and complete obliteration of aneurysm. *Coil migration:* RVA angiogram (F) shows basilar top aneurysm. Initially balloon assisted coiling was attempted (G). After deflation of balloon (H) detached coil migrated into right PCA (white arrow). It was subsequently retrieved via solitaire stent (I). Finally stent-assisted coiling (J) was done.

Intraprocedural Thromboembolism

A thromboembolic event is probably the most common complication related to endovascular management of an aneurysm. To prevent thrombus formation during the procedure patients are fully anticoagulated so that the ACT range is between 250 and 300 seconds.

If there is evidence of clot formation with or without distal embolization on angiogram, most interventionists prefer local infusion of a glycoprotein IIa/IIIb inhibitor (Abciximab) at site of thrombus formation. At authors' institution, abciximab is administered intra-arterially through the microcatheter at a dose of 2 to 4 mg over 10 to 20 minutes. In case of small emboli with resultant stasis is noted in distal cerebral vasculature, the neuroanesthetic should be asked to escalate the blood pressure in attempt to clear distal emboli and augment pial collaterals. Abciximab has also been shown to be effective in ruptured aneurysms, with no increased risk of bleeding complications.[63]

ANEURYSM TREATMENT COILING VS CLIPPING: WHERE DO WE STAND?

Treatment of intracranial aneurysms is based on their exclusion from the intracranial circulation to prevent bleeding, which can be achieved by surgical or endovascular techniques. In past neurosurgical clipping of the aneurysmal neck was the only effective method of treating a cerebral aneurysm, however with advent of detachable coils by Guglielmi in 1992 endovascular treatment has swiftly transformed into being the primary therapeutic option.

We present couple of studies to bring in the perspective how both the treatment modalities fare when compared to each other.

International Subarachnoid Aneurysm Trial (ISAT)

About 23.7% patients allocated to endovascular treatment were dependent or dead at 1 year compared with 30.6%

allocated to neurosurgical treatment (p = 0.0019). The relative and absolute risk reductions in dependency or death after allocation to an endovascular versus neurosurgical treatment were 22.6% (95% CI 8.9–34.2) and 6.9% (2.5–11.3), respectively. In patients with a ruptured intracranial aneurysm, for which endovascular coiling and neurosurgical clipping are therapeutic options, the outcome in terms of survival free of disability at 1 year is significantly better with endovascular coiling.[64]

Barrow Ruptured Aneurysm Trial (BRAT)

Poor outcome (mRS score >2) was observed in 33.7% of the patients assigned to aneurysm clipping vis-à-vis 23.2% of the patients assigned to coil embolization (OR 1.68, 95% CI 1.08–2.61; p = 0.02). One year after treatment, a policy of intent to treat favoring coil embolization resulted in fewer poor outcomes than clip occlusion.[65]

From the above-mentioned studies it becomes that clinical results with endovascular treatment are better as compared to surgical counterparts. Note should be made that there was higher percentage of patient with complete aneurysm obliteration following surgery in contrast to endovascular coiling. Consequently more patients from endovascular arm required retreatment, however difference in risk of rebleed was statistically insignificant.

With advancement in interventional neuroradiology tools and techniques, complete aneurysmal obliteration is more routinely achieved. There is change in clinical practice favoring endovascular procedure over microsurgical clipping as first choice of treatment in large number of institutes. Although a policy of intent to treat favoring coil embolization resulted in fewer poor outcomes at 1 year, it remains important that high-quality surgical clipping be available as an alternative treatment modality. Treatment of aneurysm needs to tailored for each given case and thereby it is imperative for a centers to offer both treatment modalities

ENDOVASCULAR TREATMENT OF CEREBRAL VASOSPASM

Cerebral vasospasm following aneurysmal SAH is a delayed, reversible narrowing of the intracranial vasculature that occurs most commonly 4–14 days after aneurysmal SAH and can lead to permanent ischemic injury.

Cerebral vasospasm should be suspected in any patient with SAH who develops new onset neurological deficit not attributable to any other cause like seizure, hydrocephalus or hematoma. Patients with Fisher grade 3 SAH have the highest risk of developing symptomatic vasospasm.[66] Transcranial ultrasonography (TCD) can reliably predict the presence of significant cerebral vasospasm when the flow velocities are greater than 200 cm/s or there is a rapid rise in flow velocities as compared to baseline values. Angiography remains gold standard in diagnosing vasospasm. Greater than 50% narrowing in vessel caliber is defined as severe vasospasm, and 25% to 50% narrowing in vessel caliber is defined as mild vasospasm. Plain CT can reveal developing rounded hypodensities, whereas CT perfusion can identify ischemic area at risk of infarction.[67]

Prophylaxis and Medical Treatment for Cerebral Vasospasm

Expectant treatment for cerebral vasospasm following aneurysmal SAH is controversial and varies among institutions. Triple-H (hypervolemia, hypertension, and hemodilution) therapy has been a mainstay of vasospasm treatment for years. Calcium channel blockers, magnesium, HMG-CoA reductase inhibitors (statins), fasudil, thrombolytics and endothelial receptor antagonists have all been used in attempts to prevent and treat vasospasm.[58]

At authors' institute short acting calcium channel blocker namely nimodipine is used as primary pharmacological drug against vasospasm. Drug is given at dose 1 mg (5 mL)/hour as continuous IV infusion and subsequently changed to oral nimodipine tablets 60 mg/4 hourly. The drug is continued at least up to 21 days post SAH. All effort is made to maintain mean blood pressure in range around 90–100 mm Hg, once the aneurysm has been secured. We will emphasize more on endovascular management of cerebral vasospasm.

Endovascular treatment with intra-arterial (IA) infusion of a vasodilator or balloon angioplasty is indicated in patients with symptomatic vasospasm refractory to medical therapy to prevent neurologic deficits referable to the vascular territory of the angiographic vasospasm.

INTRA-ARTERIAL VASODILATOR INFUSION

Calcium Channel Antagonists

Nimodipine is a short acting dihydropyridine derivative, which has proven systemic efficacy in cerebral vasospasm.[68] Nimodipine is administered by diluting 2–6 mg (5 mL = 1 mg) with 75–100 mL of normal saline **(Figs. 9A to D)**. Diluted drug is then administered at a slow continuous infusion over 30–45 minutes. In authors practice maximum dose has never been greater than 6 mg per artery. The main complications of nimodipine include hypotension and bradycardia. It is imperative to maintain blood pressure during and after the procedure. Other CCBs that can be used are verapamil and nicardipine.[69]

Inodilators

Milrinone is a phosphodiesterase III inhibitor that affects cyclic adenosine monophosphate (cAMP) pathways with both inotropic and vasodilatory effects. At authors institution milrinone is administered as slow infusion in 1:4 dilution over 10–20 minutes. Dose ranges from 2–4 mg per artery. Milrinone is now becoming drug of choice at many institutions owing to its no significant effect on blood pressure. Due to its positive inotropic action, potential adverse effect includes tachycardia and arrhythmias. Other phosphodiesterase inhibitor is papeverine.[70,71]

It is important to understand that these drugs have short duration of action, hence repeat procedures are a rule. Patient will generally require multiple session in addition to medical therapy for successfully overcoming period of vasospasm.

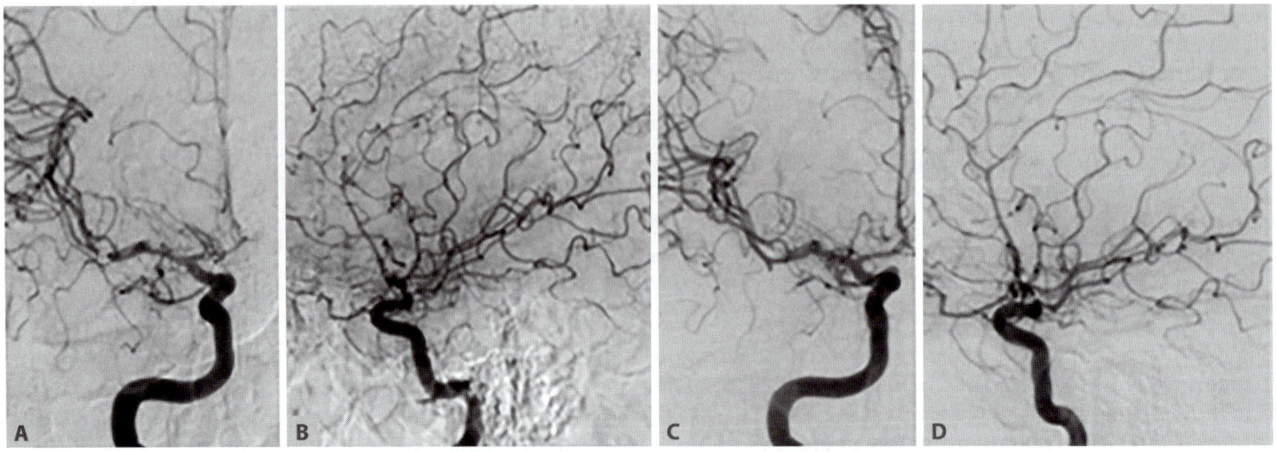

FIGS. 9A TO D: Intra-arterial nimodipine for vasospasm. RICA angiogram (A and B) in postcoiling case show decreased caliber of right supraclinoid ICA, A1 ACA and M1 MCA with attenuation of their distal branches. Postnimodipine infusion (C and D) there is marked improvement in caliber of proximal as well as distal arteries.

TRANSLUMINAL BALLOON ANGIOPLASTY

Contrary to chemical angioplasty (intra-arterial vasodilation), which is more effective for distal arterial spasm, balloon angioplasty is preferred for proximal vessel spasm. Inflammatory changes mediating smooth muscle contraction, changes in the linkage of the protein matrix, and collagen deposition in the vessel wall have all been implicated as a possible cause of blood vessel narrowing in SAH.[72,73]

Transluminal balloon angioplasty (TBA) acts by stretching the vessel wall, leading to morphologic and functional changes in the smooth muscle fibers, resulting in impairment of contractility. At a cellular level it has been shown that there is fragmentation of the collagen matrix and flattening of the endothelial cells, resulting in permanent restoration of vessel diameter.

The typical location for balloon angioplasty is supraclinoid ICA, basilar artery, intradural vertebral artery, A1 ACA and M1 MCA. Balloon angioplasty is generally avoided in vessel with diameter less than 2 mm. Commonly used balloons are either compliant or extra compliant like Hyperglide (eV3) or Secptor (Microvention). Care must be followed when negotiating across the stenotic segment to avoid inadvertent dissection. While perform balloon angioplasty care should be taken not to overinflate, given relatively large volume of these balloons.[58]

Transluminal balloon angioplasty itself has some potential significant risks. These most serious one include vessel rupture and arterial dissection. These balloons can be flow limiting and may cause thrombus formation with resultant stroke. Finally, there is risk of reperfusion injury by restoration of blood flow in ischemic vascular territory.

FOLLOW-UP AND MONITORING

All patients who have undergone an endovascular procedure undergo check angiogram to confirm the aneurysm status after 3–6 months following primary procedure. Aneurysm can re grow secondary to coil compaction, extension of arterial dissection, continued dual antiplatelets or de novo new aneurysm formation. Small neck compactions can be followed up on serial angiograms, whereas larger recurrences require repeat procedure. Follow-up angiogram also assumes importance in modulating and down stepping antiplatelet agent once aneurysm/parent artery is healed. It has been shown that stable occlusions at 6 months, will rarely show recurrences.

CONCLUSION

Advancement in endovascular techniques has revolutionized the treatment of intracranial aneurysm. With further refinement of interventional tools, majority of the aneurysms today can be treated via endovascular route. Clear understanding of the disease, treatment options, available equipment/hardware, possible complications and requirement for follow-up is important is ensuring overall success for any given endovascular procedure is an patient.

ACKNOWLEDGMENT

The author acknowledges Dr Nishchint Jain, DM resident in the Department of Neuroimaging and Interventional Radiology, AIIMS, New Delhi for active involvement and helping in writing the chapter.

REFERENCES

1. Nakagawa T, Hashi K. The incidence and treatment of asymptomatic, unruptured cerebral aneurysms. J Neurosurg. 1994;80:217-23.
2. Winn HR, Jane JA Sr, Taylor J, et al. Prevalence of asymptomatic incidental aneurysms: review of 4568 arteriograms. J Neurosurg. 2002;96:43-9.
3. Krishna H, Wani AA, Behari S, et al. Intracranial aneurysms in patients 18 years of age or under, are they different from aneurysms in adult population? Acta Neurochir. 2005;147: 469-76.
4. Kanaan I, Lasjaunias P, Coates R. The spectrum of intracranial aneurysms in pediatrics. Minim Invasive Neurosurg. 1995;38:1-9.
5. Stehbens WE. Etiology of intracranial berry aneurysms. J Neurosurg. 1989;70:823-31.
6. TerBrugge K. Aneurysm in the pediatric population. Rivista di Neuroradiologia. 1998;11(Suppl 1):54-5.
7. Swietaszczyk C, Maciaczyk J, Tafil-Klawe M, et al. What is the origin of cerebral aneurysms? Przegl Lek. 2004;61:115-9.
8. Strother CM, Graves VB, Rappe A. Aneurysm hemodynamics: an experimental study. Am J Neuroradiol. 1992;13:1089-95.
9. Foutrakis G, Yonas H, Sclabassi R. Saccular formation in curved and bifurcating arteries. Am J Neuroradiol. 1999;20:1309-17.
10. Malek AM, Alper SL, Izumo S. Hemodynamic shear stress and its role in atherosclerosis. JAMA. 1999;282:2035-42.
11. Kondo S, Hashimoto N, Kikuchi H, et al. Cerebral aneurysms arising at nonbranching sites. An experimental Study. Stroke. 1997;28:398-403.
12. Schievink WI. Genetics of intracranial aneurysms. Neurosurgery. 1997;40:651-63.
13. Torner JC. Epidemiology of subarachnoid hemorrhage. Semin Neurol. 1984;4:354-69.
14. Krog M, Almgren B, Eriksson S. Vascular complications in the Elhers-Danlos syndrome. Acta Chir Scand. 1983;149:279-82.
15. Bromberg JEC, Rinkel GJ, Algra A, et al. Subarachnoid haemorrhage in first and second degree relatives of patients with subarachnoid haemorrhage. BMJ. 1995;311:288-9.
16. Schievink WI, Schaid DJ, Michaels VV, et al. Familial aneurysmal subarachnoid hemorrhage: a community-based study. J Neurosurg. 1995;83:426-9.
17. Shinton R, Beevers DG. Meta-analysis of relation between cigarette smoking and stroke. BMJ. 1989;298:789-94.
18. Juvela S, Hillbom M, Numminen H, et al. Cigarette smoke and alcohol consumption as risk factors for aneurysmal subarachnoid hemorrhage. Stroke. 1993;24:639-46.
19. Batjer HH, Kopitnik TA, Giller GA, et al. Surgery for paraclinoid carotid artery aneurysms. J Neurosurg. 1994;80:650-8.
20. Day AL. Aneurysms of the ophthalmic segment: a clinical and anatomical analysis. J Neurosurg. 1990;72:677-91.
21. Endo S, Nishijima M, Nomura H, et al. A pathological study of intracranial posterior circulation dissecting aneurysms with subarachnoid hemorrhage: report of three autopsied cases and review of the literature. Neurosurgery. 1993;33:732-8.
22. Bonneville F, Sourour N, Biondi A. Intracranial aneurysms: an overview. Neuroimaging Clin N Am. 2006;16:371-82.
23. Anson JA, Lawton MT, Spetzler RF. Characteristics and surgical treatment of dolichoectatic and fusiform aneurysms. J Neurosurg. 1996;84:185-93.
24. Schnee CL, Flamm ES. Unusual aneurysms. Neuroimaging Clin N Am. 1997;7:803-18.
25. Corr PD, Wright M, Handler LC. Endocarditis-related cerebral aneurysms: radiologic changes with treatment. AJNR Am J Neuroradiol. 1995;16:745-8.
26. Kurino M, Kuratsu J, Yamaguchi T, et al. Mycotic aneurysm accompanied by aspergillus granulomas: a case report. Surg Neurol. 1994;42:160-4.
27. DiMaio S, Mohr G, Dufour JJ, et al. Distal mycotic aneurysm of the AICA mimicking intracanalicular acoustic neuroma. Can J Neurol Sci. 2003;30:388-92.
28. Holmes B, Harbaugh RE. Traumatic intracranial aneurysms: a contemporary review. J Trauma. 1993;35:855-60.
29. Amirjamshidi A, Rahmat H, Abbassioun K. Traumatic aneurysms and arteriovenous fistulas of intracranial vessels associated with penetrating head injuries occurring during war: principles and pitfalls in diagnosis and management. J Neurosurg. 1996;84: 769-80.
30. Proust F, Callonec F, Bellow F, et al. Tentorial edge traumatic aneurysm of the superior cerebellar artery. Case report. J Neurosurg. 1997;87:950-4.
31. Wiebers DO, Whisnant JP, Huston J III, et al. International Study of Unruptured Intracranial Aneurysms Investigators. Unruptured intracranial aneurysms: natural history, clinical outcome, and risks of surgical and endovascular treatment. Lancet. 2003;362: 103-10.
32. Kallmes DF, Layton K, Marx WF, et al. Death by nondiagnosis: why emergent CT angiography should not be done for patients with subarachnoid hemorrhage. Am J Neuroradiol. 2007;28:1837-8.
33. Schellinger PD, Richter G, Kohrmann M, et al. Noninvasive angiography (magnetic resonance and computed tomography) in the diagnosis of ischemic cerebrovascular disease. Techniques and clinical applications. Cerebrovasc Dis. 2007;24(Suppl 1): 16-23.
34. Willinsky RA, Taylor SM, TerBrugge K, et al. Neurologic complications of cerebral angiography: prospective analysis of 2,899 procedures and review of the literature. Radiology. 2003;227:522-8.
35. Villablanca JP, Rodriguez FJ, Stockman T, et al. MDCT angiography for detection and quantification of small intracranial arteries: comparison with conventional catheter angiography. Am J Roentgenol. 2007;188:593-602.
36. McKinney AM, Palmer CS, Truwit CL, et al. Detection of aneurysms by 64-section multidetector CT angiography in patients acutely suspected of having an intracranial aneurysm and comparison with digital subtraction and 3D rotational angiography. Am J Neuroradiol. 2008;29:594-602.
37. Hacein-Bey L, Provenzale JM. Current imaging assessment and treatment of intracranial aneurysms. Am J Roentgenol. 2011;196:32-44.
38. Wardlaw JM, White PM. The detection and management of unruptured intracranial aneurysms. Brain. 2000;123(Pt 2):205-21.
39. Mallouhi A, Felber S, Chemelli A, et al. Detection and characterization of intracranial aneurysms with MR angiography: comparison of volume-rendering and maximum-intensity-projection algorithms. Am J Roentgenol. 2003;180:55-64.
40. Hunt WE, Hess RM. Surgical risk as related to time of intervention in the repair of intracranial aneurysms. J Neurosurg. 1968;28(1): 14-20.
41. Report of World Federation of Neurological Surgeons Committee on a Universal Subarachnoid Hemorrhage Grading Scale. J Neurosurg. 1988;68:985-6.
42. Adams HP Jr, Kassell NF, Torner JC, et al. Early management of aneurysmal subarachnoid hemorrhage: a report of the Cooperative Aneurysm study. J Neurosurg. 1981;54:141-5.
43. Cognard C, Weill A, Castaings L, et al. Intracranial berry aneurysms: angiographic and clinical results after endovascular treatment. Radiology. 1998;206:499-510.

44. Hasan D, Vermeulen M, Wijdieks EFM, et al. Management problems in acute hydrocephalus after subarachnoid hemorrhage. Stroke. 1989;20:747-53.
45. Rhoney DH, Tipps LB, Murry KR, et al. Anticonvulsant prophylaxis and timing of seizures after aneurysmal subarachnoid hemorrhage. Neurology. 2000;55:258-65.
46. Spiotta AM, Hussain MS, Sivapatham T, et al. The versatile distal access catheter: the Cleveland Clinic experience. Neurosurgery. 2011;68:1677-86.
47. Hauck EF, Tawk RG, Karter NS, et al. Use of the outreach distal access catheter as an intracranial platform facilitates coil embolization of select intracranial aneurysms: technical note. J Neurointerv Surg. 2011;3:172-6.
48. Park MS, Stiefel MF, Fiorella D, et al. Intracranial placement of a new, compliant guide catheter: technical note. Neurosurgery. 2008;63:E616-7.
49. Khaghany K, Al-Ali F, Spigelmoyer T, et al. Efficacy and safety of the Perclose Closer S device after neurointerventional procedures: prospective study and literature review. Am J Neuroradiol. 2005;26:1420-4.
50. Moret J, Cognard C, Weill A, et al. Reconstruction technic in the treatment of wide-neck intracranial aneurysms. Long-term angiographic and clinical results. Apropos of 56 cases. J Neuroradiol. 1997;24:30-44.
51. Aletich VA, Debrun GM, Misra M, et al. The remodeling technique of balloon-assisted Guglielmi detachable coil placement in wide-necked aneurysms: experience at the University of Illinois at Chicago. J Neurosurg. 2000;93:388-96.
52. Blanc R, Piotin M, Mounayer C, et al. Direct cervical arterial access for intracranial endovascular treatment. Neuroradiology. 2006;48:925-9.
53. Fiorella D, Kelly ME, Albuquerque FC, et al. Curative reconstruction of a giant midbasilar trunk aneurysm with the pipeline embolization device. Neurosurgery. 2009;64:212-7.
54. Kallmes DF, Ding YH, Dai D, et al. A new endoluminal, flow-disrupting device for treatment of saccular aneurysms. Stroke. 2007;38:2346-52.
55. Kallmes DF, Ding YH, Dai D, et al. A second-generation, endoluminal, flow-disrupting device for treatment of saccular aneurysms. Am J Neuroradiol. 2009;30:1153-8.
56. Fiorella D, Woo HH, Albuquerque FC, et al. Definitive reconstruction of circumferential, fusiform intracranial aneurysms with the pipeline embolization device. Neurosurgery. 2008;62:1115-20.
57. Nelson PK, Lylyk P, Szikora I, et al. The pipeline embolization device for the intracranial treatment of aneurysms trial. AJNR Am J Neuroradiol. 2011;32:34-40.
58. Gemmete JJ, Pandey AS, Chaudhary N, et al. Endovascular management of intracranial aneurysms. In: Quinones-Hinojosa A (Ed). Schmidek and Sweet Operative Neurosurgical Techniques: Indications, Methods, and Results, 6th edition, Vol. 1. Elsevier; 2012. pp. 1019-27.
59. Doerfler A, Wanke I, Egelhof T, et al. Aneurysmal rupture during embolization with Guglielmi detachable coils: causes, management, and outcome. Am J Neuroradiol. 2001;22:1825-32.
60. Hirai T, Suginohara K, Uemura S, et al. Management of aneurysm perforation during Guglielmi electrodetachable coil placement. Am J Neuroradiol. 2002;23:738-9.
61. Ricolfi F, Le Guerinel C, Blustajn J, et al. Rupture during treatment of recently ruptured aneurysms with Guglielmi electrodetachable coils. Am J Neuroradiol. 1998;19:1653-8.
62. Wada H, Piotin M, Boissonnet H, et al. Carotid rupture during stent-assisted aneurysm treatment. Am J Neuroradiol. 2004;25:827-9.
63. Kwon OK, Lee KJ, Han MH, et al. Intra-arterially administered abciximab as an adjuvant thrombolytic therapy: report of three cases. Am J Neuroradiol. 2002;23:447-51.
64. Molyneux A, Kerr R, Stratton I, et al. International Subarachnoid Aneurysm Trial (ISAT) of neurosurgical clipping versus endovascular coiling in 2143 patients with ruptured intracranial aneurysms: a randomised trial. Lancet. 2002;360:1267-74.
65. McDougall CG, Spetzler RF, Zabramski JM, et al. The Barrow Ruptured Aneurysm Trial. Clinical article. J Neurosurg. 2012;116:135-44.
66. Macdonald LR, Weir B. Epidemiology. In: Cerebral Vasospasm. San Diego (CA): Academic Press; 2001. pp. 17-43.
67. Sloan MA, Alexandrov AV, Tegeler CH, et al. Therapeutics and Technology Assessment Subcommittee of the American Academy of Neurology. Assessment: transcranial Doppler ultrasonography: report of the Therapeutics and Technology Assessment Subcommittee of the American Academy of Neurology. Neurology. 2004;62(9):1468-81.
68. Pickard JD, Murray GD, Illingworth R, et al. Effect of oral nimodipine on cerebral infarction and outcome after subarachnoid haemorrhage: British aneurysm nimodipine trial. BMJ. 1989;298:636-42.
69. Biondi A, Ricciardi GK, Puybasset L, et al. Intra-arterial nimodipine for the treatment of symptomatic cerebral vasospasm after aneurysmal subarachnoid hemorrhage: preliminary results. Am J Neuroradiol. 2004;25:1067-76.
70. Macdonald RL, Weir BK, Young JD, et al. Cytoskeletal and extracellular matrix proteins in cerebral arteries following subarachnoid hemorrhage in monkeys. J Neurosurg. 1992;76:81-90.
71. Pennings FA, Albrecht KW, Muizelaar JP, et al. Abnormal responses of the human cerebral microcirculation to papaverin during aneurysm surgery. Stroke. 2009;40:317-20.
72. Zubkov YN, Nikiforov BM, Shustin VA. Balloon catheter technique for dilatation of constricted cerebral arteries after aneurysmal SAH. Acta Neurochir (Wien). 1984;70:65-79.
73. Zwienenberg-Lee M, Hartman J, Rudisill N, et al. Effect of prophylactic transluminal balloon angioplasty on cerebral vasospasm and outcome in patients with Fisher grade III subarachnoid hemorrhage: results of a phase II multicenter, randomized, clinical trial. Stroke. 2008;39:1759-65.

CHAPTER

191

Endovascular Management of Arteriovenous Malformations

Ajay Kumar, Niranjan Khandelwal, Shailesh B Gaikwad, Chirag Kamal Ahuja, Vivek Gupta

INTRODUCTION

Brain arteriovenous malformations (bAVMs) are uncommon vascular lesions with arteriovenous shunting and a prevalence of about 0.2%–0.8% in general population per year.[1] Classification of arteriovenous malformations AVMs is based on the type of primary defects, such as arterial, arteriovenous, capillary and venous **(Table 1)**. For each of them, different effects on the remaining vascular system can be encountered. Spetzler's classification incorporates the size of the AVM, the pattern of venous drainage, and the "eloquence" of the regions of the brain adjacent to the AVM.[2] Objective assessment of surgical risk is the major aim of this classification, and the risk derived is compared to the assumed natural history of all AVMs as a group.

Brain AVMs are an abnormal connection between the arteries and veins through dysplastic plexiform network of vessels with shunting of blood from arterial to venous side.[3] In the past 15 years, there is a lot of improvement in the understanding of bAVMs, their natural history, angio-architecture, imaging techniques and available treatment modalities. bAVMs can be asymptomatic and incidental finding on imaging or may present clinically with headache, spontaneous ICH (58%), seizures (34%) and neurological deficits (8%).[4-14]

Most common presentation of symptomatic bAVMs is with spontaneous intracranial hemorrhage and the high risk predisposing factors are associated aneurysms, deep venous drainage, deep or posterior fossa location and associated venous stenosis.[15-17] According to large studies by Kim et al.[18] and Gross et al.[19] annual rupture risk for unruptured bAVM was 1.3–2.2% and for ruptured bAVM was 4.5–4.8%. Another important clinical presentation is focal or generalized seizures.[20] The exact etiology for seizures in bAVMs is still unclear. However, some authors propose the role of venous hypertension for seizures.[21,22] The patients with bAVM in temporal location (strong correlation), cortical involvement, larger size and younger age group are at high risk to present with seizures.[23,24] Contrary to this patients with associated aneurysms and posterior fossa location of bAVMs were seen to have less risk for seizures.[25] The occurrence of neurological deficits is rare. The basic mechanism responsible for this is local ischemia/hypoxia either due to arterial steal or venous hypertension.[26,27]

TABLE 1: Primary classification of the brain arteriovenous malformations (Berenstein and Lasjaunias).

Arteriovenous shunts
Single
Micro AV shunts (mAVM or mAVF) Macro AV shunts (compartmented nidus or mAVF)
Multiple (nonfamilial)
Systemic (Wyburn-Mason)
Nonsystemic (multiple separate niduses or separated compartment within one nidus)
Multiple (familial)
Systematized (Rendu-Osler-Weber) Nonsystematized (multiple separate niduses with or without AVF)
Associated vascular variants
Arterial or venous
Secondary vascular changes
Angiogenesis, kinking and dolichoid vessels
Arterial aneurysms, venous ectasias and pouches
Venous and arterial stenoses and thrombosis
External carotid supply
Shunting (remote)
Arterial and venous collateral circulation
Pseudoaneurysms (hematomas)
Secondary morphological changes
Hydrocephalus, cerebral atrophy, cavities
Perivascular ischemia, calcification
Bone hypertrophy
Associated vascular tumors

ANGIOARCHITECTURE/COMPONENTS OF BRAIN ARTERIOVENOUS MALFORMATION

Morphologically AVMs are one of the most complex pathological condition. The central component of AVMs is abnormal/dysplastic tangle of vessels replacing the normal capillary network known as nidus. The nidus can be compact or diffuse depending upon its spread in relation to brain parenchyma. Compact nidus **(Figs. 1A to D)** usually does not have intervening normal brain parenchyma, thus, easier for microsurgery, radiosurgery or embolization. Diffuse nidus **(Figs. 2A to F)** usually have intervening brain parenchyma which poses difficulty in the management by any available treatment modalities.

Another important component of the AVM are arterial feeders. They can be single, multiple and en-passage, latter two poses difficulty in management. However, single feeder are associated with high risk of hemorrhages.[28] Terminal arterial feeders ends into the nidus and are easier for embolization or microsurgery. On the contrary, pseudoterminal feeders supply the normal brain parenchyma distally **(Figs. 3A to I)** and indirect feeders are the smaller branches of major and significant vascular channels that pose great challenge for microsurgery or embolization with high risk of thromboembolic complications and ischemic events

Venous drainage pattern is also equally important for prognostication and management strategies. There can be three patterns of venous drainage—superficial, deep and combined. bAVMs draining into superficial venous system are responsible for less hemorrhagic complications and also associated with better prognosis and management. Apart from venous pattern, the presence of venous stenosis is associated with higher risk of hemorrhage, seizures and neurological deficits.[29]

Along with its complex anatomical morphology another factor peculiar for AVMs is their dynamic nature. Depending on the blood flow rate across the AVM nidus, they can be classified into low, intermediate or high flow lesions. High blood flow rate AVMs poses great difficulty for management by embolization or microsurgery and are also associated with high incidence of failed radiosurgery.

Aneurysms associated with bAVMs are one of the most common causes of spontaneous hemorrhage. Depending up on the location, the aneurysms are classified as pre-nidal/flow related **(Figs. 4A to D)**, nidal/intra and peri-nidal **(Figs. 5 to 7)** and post-nidal/venous varices . Unruptured feeder artery aneurysm (pre-nidal) usually do not warrant any treatment and are believed to regress after nidal obliteration. The aneurysms on any location if responsible for the hemorrhage requires urgent microsurgical resection or embolization on emergent basis to prevent rebleed.[30] Aneurysms unrelated to bAVMs, i.e. in different vascular territory or contralateral hemisphere can be treated as per management strategies for aneurysms.

GRADING/CLASSIFICATION OF BRAIN ARTERIOVENOUS MALFORMATION

The treatment strategies for the bAVM are still unclear and complex in terms of prognostication and choice of available modalities. The Spetzler-Martin (SM) scale (2) is one of the most used and accepted grading system for the treatment planning and prognostication of bAVMs. However, it was developed only for the patients planned for treatment by microsurgical resection.[31] In the recent past advent of newer treatment modalities, i.e embolization and radiosurgery has opened new possibilities in the management protocols of bAVMs with or without rupture. Also with the advent of new embolic materials and endovascular hardware there is an increasing and established role of endovascular management either stand alone or adjunctive to micro or radiosurgery. Apart from the variables used in the SM grading, other components of AVM such as number and diameter of arterial pedicles and draining veins, vascular eloquence and presence of arteriovenous fistulous component also plays important role for the management planning by radiosurgery or embolization. Newer grading scales proposed by Demetrius et al.,[31]

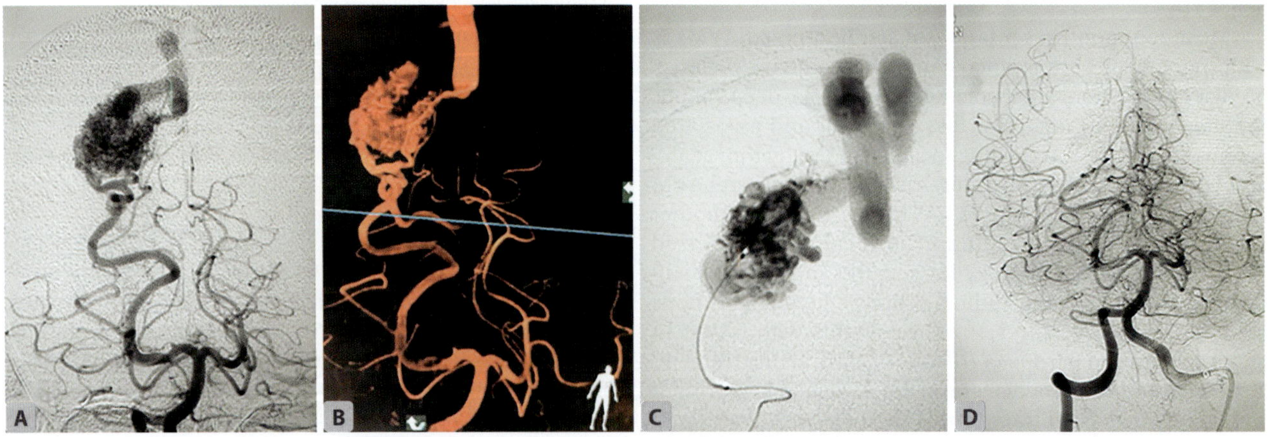

FIGS. 1A TO D: A 27-year-old male presented with severe headache and disorientation and diagnosed to have compact AVM nidus in right parieto-occipital region. Diagnostic DSA with 3-DRA images accurately shows the nidus with PCA feeders and superficial venous drainage (A and B). Complete obliteration of nidus was achieved using PHIL and detachable tip microcatheters (C and D).

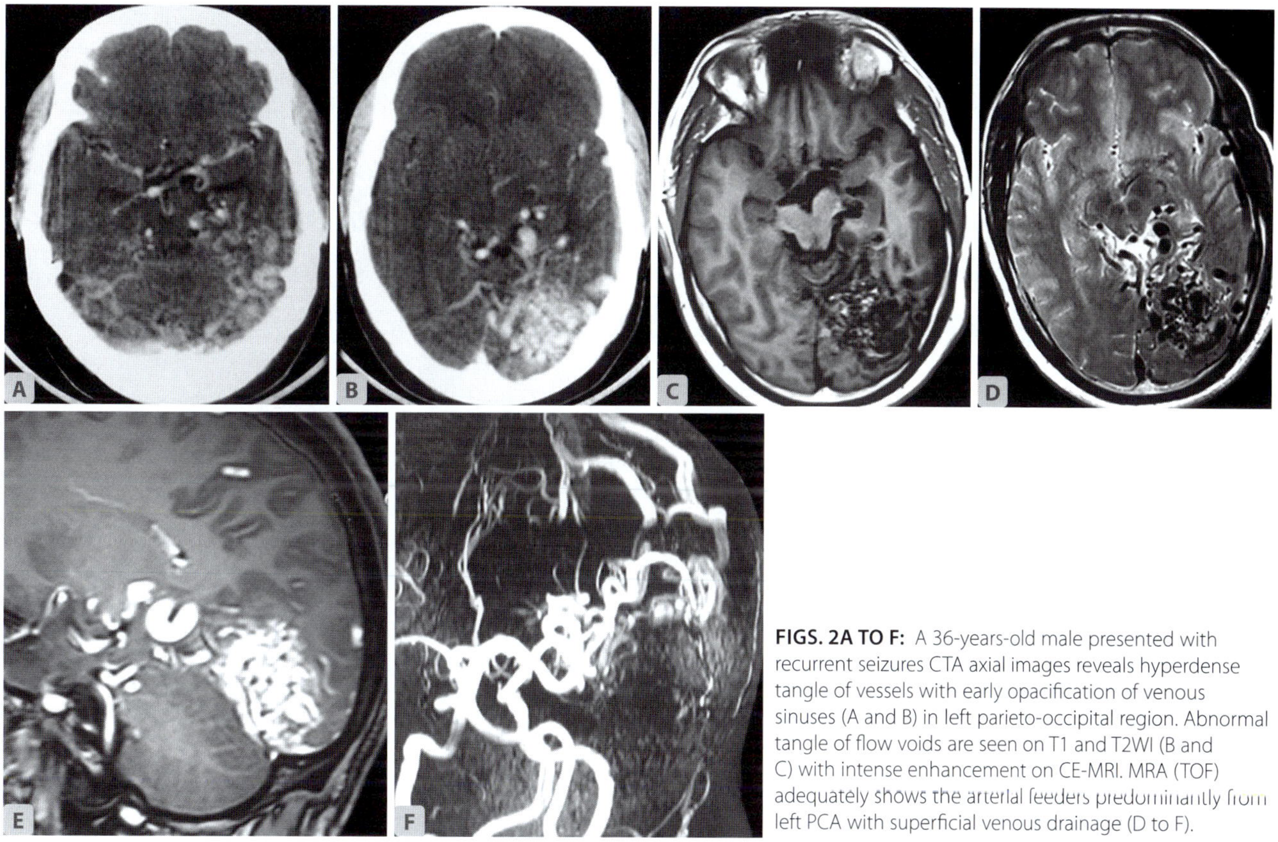

FIGS. 2A TO F: A 36-years-old male presented with recurrent seizures CTA axial images reveals hyperdense tangle of vessels with early opacification of venous sinuses (A and B) in left parieto-occipital region. Abnormal tangle of flow voids are seen on T1 and T2WI (B and C) with intense enhancement on CE-MRI. MRA (TOF) adequately shows the arterial feeders predominantly from left PCA with superficial venous drainage (D to F).

Bell et al.[32] and Buffalo Score of AVM[33] are described in **Tables 2 to 5**. All of these grading scales have point system for different characteristics of AVM and the grade of the AVM can be calculated by adding them up. Higher the scores suggest poorer prognosis and difficulty in management.

IMAGING EVALUATION OF BRAIN ARTERIOVENOUS MALFORMATIONS

Computed tomography (CT) is usually the first line of investigation for the symptomatic bAVMs. Depending upon the findings on non-contrast or contrast-enhanced CT scan the patients can be further evaluated by MRI and digital subtraction angiography (DSA). The primary diagnosis of bAVM can be easily made on CECT and MRI. However, for exact treatment planning, prognostication and follow-up imaging CEMRI and DSA plays important role. bAVMs can represent as incidental imaging finding in the patients of headache and other neurological symptoms undergoing cross-sectional imaging.

Computed Tomography

Noncontrast CT is usually the first investigation in the symptomatic patients. It has high sensitivity for detecting hemorrhage, infarct[34-36] and hyperdensities due to calcification and slow flowing tangle of vessels **(Figs. 3A and B)**. With the advent of multislice technology CT angiography (CTA), thin slice isometric multiplanar imaging can help diagnose the bAVMs with high sensitivity and specificity **(Figs. 2A and B)**. Different bAVM features as-evaluation of arterial feeders, AVM nidus and draining veins can also be assessed easily on CTA. CTA also provides a very good noninvasive imaging tool for the future treatment planning either by microsurgery, embolization or radiosurgery especially in the patients where MRI is contraindicated. There is sufficient literature suggesting that CTA is comparable to DSA in the terms of sensitivity (83.6-100%) and specificity (77.2%-100%) for making the diagnosis and evaluating the other features of bAVMs.[37,38]

4D-CTA is the multiphasic dynamic CTA acquisition algorithm. It is able to diagnose almost all bAVMs however there is suboptimal evaluation of angioarchitecture when compared to DSA. It appears promising noninvasive tool for treatment planning and follow-up imaging for patients of bAVM treated by any of the available modalities.[39]

Magnetic Resonance Imaging

Recent advances in the techniques and acquisition sequences places MRI as key imaging modality for the diagnosis and detailed evaluation of bAVM characteristics. In the pediatric and other patients where the radiation and contrast nephropathy are serious considerations MR imaging plays the central role for the evaluation of suspected brain vascular lesions. The bAVM can be diagnosed as an abnormal tangle of flow voids on basic MR T1W, T2W and FLAIR sequences. The associated hemorrhage and calcification can also be

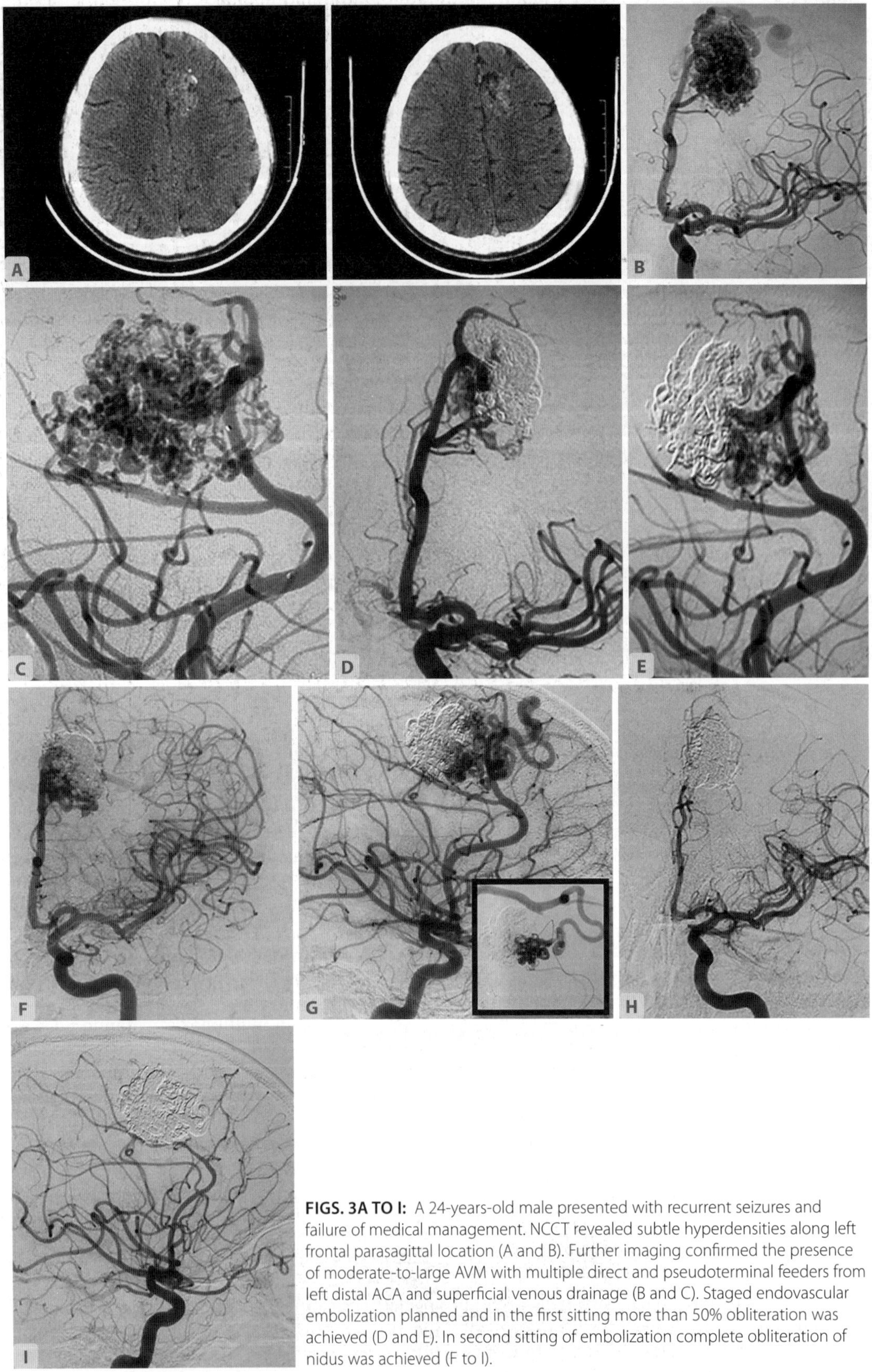

FIGS. 3A TO I: A 24-years-old male presented with recurrent seizures and failure of medical management. NCCT revealed subtle hyperdensities along left frontal parasagittal location (A and B). Further imaging confirmed the presence of moderate-to-large AVM with multiple direct and pseudoterminal feeders from left distal ACA and superficial venous drainage (B and C). Staged endovascular embolization planned and in the first sitting more than 50% obliteration was achieved (D and E). In second sitting of embolization complete obliteration of nidus was achieved (F to I).

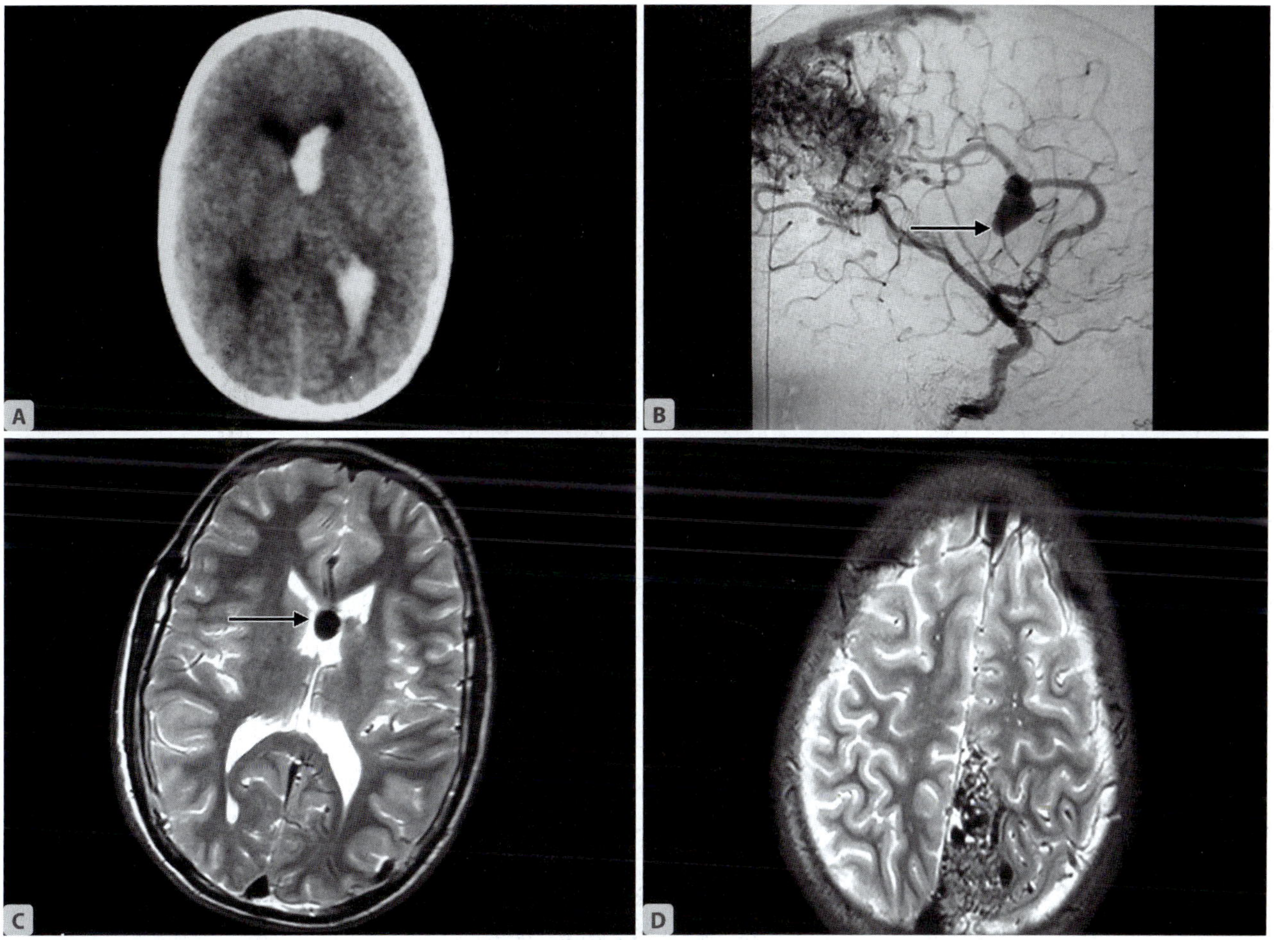

FIGS. 4A TO D: A 17-year-old male presented with severe headache. NCCT shows left IVH (A) with Axial T2WI of MRI depicting pre-nidal aneurysmal flow void projecting into ventricle also confirmed on diagnostic DSA (arrow) along with distal parieto-occipital AVM nidus on both modalities (B to D).

diagnosed on basic sequences along with susceptibility weighted imaging (SWI). MR angiography (time of flight-TOF) gives an adequate idea about the arterial feeders and draining veins **(Figs. 2C to F)**. In the meta-analysis by Josephson et al.[38] MRA was suggested to have high sensitivity (95%, CI 0.80-1.00) and specificity (95%, CI 0.97-1.00) for diagnosis of bAVMs. Even with available advanced MR sequences, there are still some limitations like detecting small arterial feeders (<1 mm), associated aneurysms and AVMs with smaller nidus (<10 mm).[40-42] There is an increasing role of functional MR imaging (fMRI) in the treatment planning and prognostication of the patients presented with symptomatic bAVMs. The findings of fMRI can guide a neurosurgeon for microsurgery, selection of the arterial feeders for neurointerventionist and safe ROI marking during radiosurgery.[43]

Digital Subtraction Angiography

DSA serves as the gold standard imaging modality for the diagnosis and evaluation of bAVMs because of its peculiar ability to assess the dynamicity and role of specific feeder in the AVM nidus. It provides the highest degree of special and temporal resolution.[44-47] The points of concern are its invasive nature, need of operator expertise and experience, radiation risks, use of contrast and risk of some serious vascular and neurological complications.[48] Complete and adequate DSA can accurately evaluate almost all anatomical components (arterial feeder, aneurysms, nidus, shunts, collaterals, draining veins and venous abnormalities) of bAVM.[12,14]

THERAPEUTIC OPTIONS

The treatment of diagnosed bAVM depends upon whether it is symptomatic or asymptomatic and if symptomatic presented with hemorrhage or not. In the present scenario the management options for diagnosed bAVMs include medical management, microsurgery, embolization, radiosurgery and/or combined therapy. The main aim of either modality is to prevent hemorrhage and to ameliorate the symptoms.[23]

Microsurgery

Neurosurgical resection of the bAVM whenever possible remains the only definitive cure. The major aims of microsurgery include complete resection of nidus, evacuation of associated hematoma if present; avoid injury to normal brain parenchyma and careful ligation of the true arterial feeders and draining veins. However indications for the definitive resection are reserved for smaller and superficially located nidus away from eloquent brain parenchyma. Larger

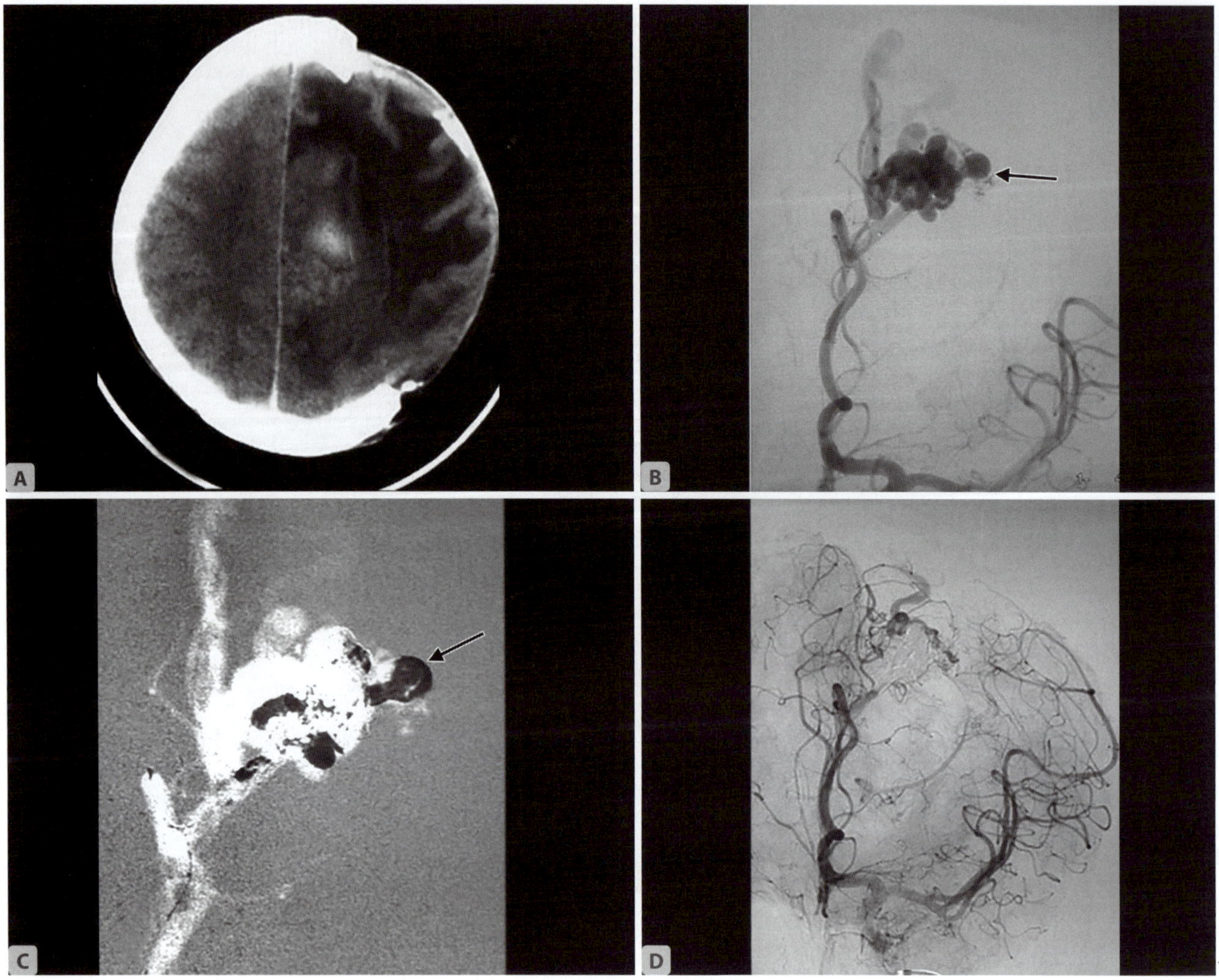

FIGS. 5A TO D: A 18-year-old male had history of sudden unconsciousness with right hemiparesis, large ICH diagnosed on NCCT, undergone emergency decompression craniotomy (A). CTA revealed compact AVM nidus with perinidal aneurysm (arrow) (B). Endovascular embolization with curative intention was performed to obliterate nidus and aneurysm using onyx and 1.5 cm detachable tip Apollo microcatheter (C). Check run post-embolization shows complete obliteration of nidus and aneurysm (D).

complex AVMs requires adjunctive embolization to decrease the size, intra operative hemorrhage and to eliminate weak point in AVM.[23]

Radiosurgery

Radiosurgery as primary modality is usually performed in the patients having high risk for surgery, deep or eloquent location and smaller lesion without weak points. Recent studies suggests that the patients with smaller volumes nidus <12 cm^3 have better treatment outcomes.[49] There are many limiting factors in radiosurgery as radiation necrosis, no significant change in the annual risk of hemorrhage during latency period in comparison with natural history of bAVM and long term cyst formations.[50,51]

ENDOVASCULAR INTERVENTION

Currently the management of bAVM is a multidisciplinary approach and endovascular management serves as an important central role for the same. With the advent of newer techniques, better imaging machines, endovascular hardware and embolic materials, the role of endovascular management is increasing. The endovascular management can be used as a standalone "curative" treatment to eliminate AVMs in selected cases, "palliative" to improve symptoms in cases of larger complex AVMs, "targeted" embolization for eliminating intranidal aneurysms and fistulous components and "adjunct" to radio or microsurgery for larger and complex bAVMs.

Curative Embolization

About 10–20% of patients can be expected to have complete cure by embolization alone using n-butyl cyanoacrylate.[52] Currently with the advent of newer EVOH based embolizing material (onyx and squid) there is significant increase in total obliteration rates up to 51% of all bAVMs. The best results with obliteration rates up to 96% can be achieved in selected cases.[53,54] Most of these AVMs are small in size, with only few feeding arteries **(Figs. 1, 3, 5 and 6)**.

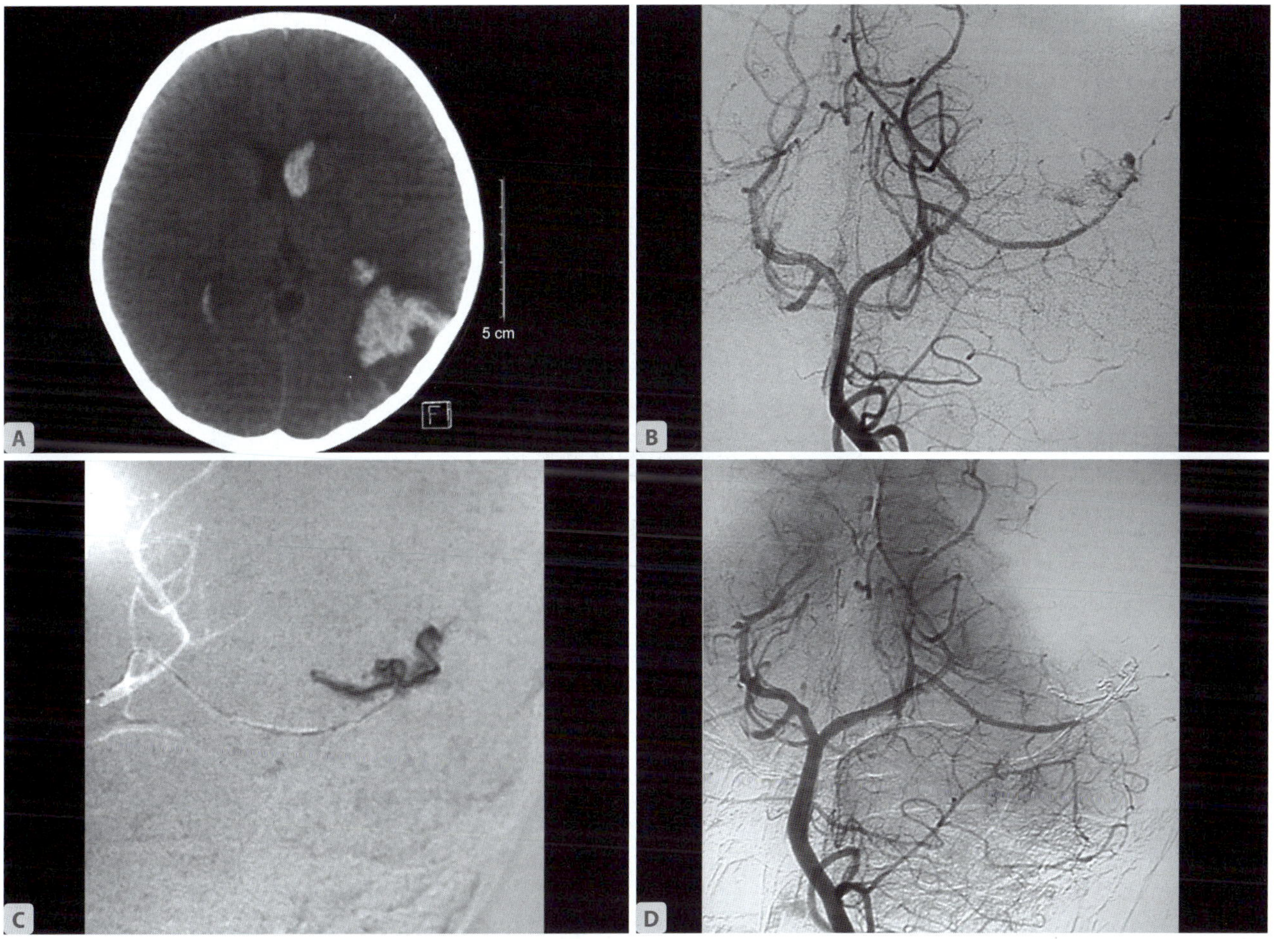

FIGS. 6A TO D: A 3-year old female presented with sudden loss of consciousness, NCCT revealed (A) revealed left parietal ICH with associated IVH. Diagnostic DSA shows small AVM nidus with intranidal aneurysm and having feeder from left posterior cerebral artery (B). Patient taken for endovascular embolization on urgent basis with curative intention, complete obliteration of AVM nidus and aneurysm was achieved (C and D) using onyx 18.

Preoperative Embolization

Preoperative embolization facilitates surgical treatment by reducing the arteriovenous shunt, decreasing the size of feeding arteries and veins and reducing blood loss.[55] High flow direct arteriovenous shunts and areas of the AVM with associated aneurysms should be targeted by embolization. Deep lenticulostriate or posterior cerebral feeder, that may be difficult to access surgically, can also be embolized.

Pre-radiosurgery Embolization

A combination of embolization and radiosurgery may be used for treating AVMs. Embolization can reduce the size of the AVM nidus, making the lesion more amenable to radiosurgery. Areas of nidus that contain aneurysm should be fully embolized to allow added protection from hemorrhage during 1–3 years latency period after treatment before an AVM is cured by radiation **(Figs. 7A to D)**. The fistulous components also needs to be meticulously diagnosed prior to radiosurgery to prevent the failure of treatment as fistulous components are believed to be resistant to radiation treatment.[56,57]

Palliative Embolization

The main aim of the palliative embolization in complex large untreatable bAVMs is to reduce the risk of hemorrhage due to weak points, to diminish the flow across nidus and to further decrease venous hypertension. It is increasingly being realized that potentially reducing the AVM nidus with elimination of fistulous communications effectively accomplishes longer uneventful time period and in many it may ensure a full and unconstrued life.[58,59] Long-term follow-up angiographic studies have shown even the residual lesion in many AVMs to progressively thrombose.

Staging Embolization

Staging embolization is usually done in large malformations or when the delay is expected to let a small feeder enlarge in order to facilitate future catheterization. By staging occlusion of a large AVM, the hemodynamic consequences of rapid elimination of a large shunt are avoided. Normal pressure perfusion breakthrough phenomena are less likely to occur and the ultimate goal is achieved without avoidable risks of embolization **(Figs. 3A to I)**.

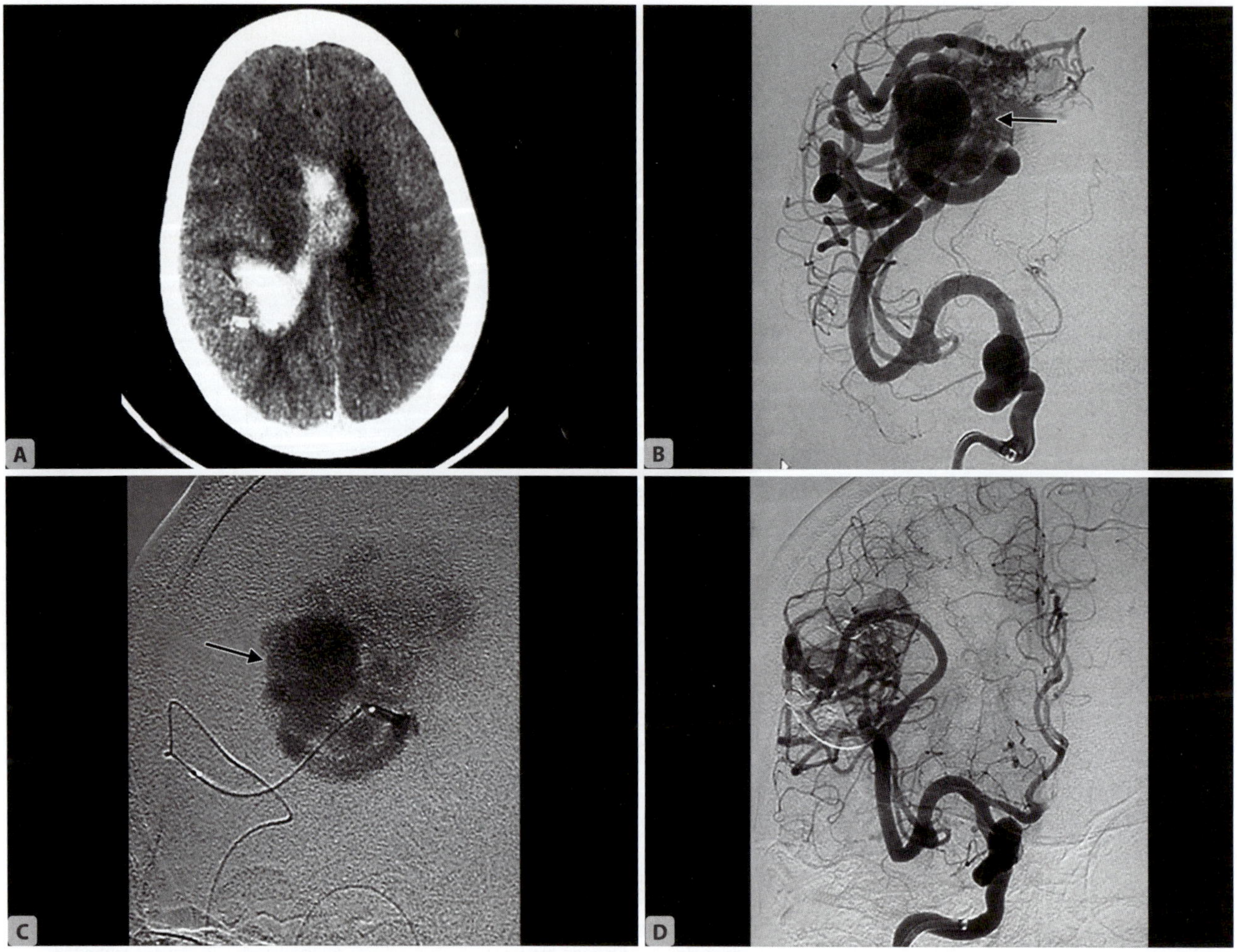

FIGS. 7A TO D: A 50-year-old female presented with sudden severe headache, vomiting and loss of consciousness. NCCT shows large right parietal ICH with extension into lateral ventricle (A). CTA elsewhere revealed AVM with a large perinidal aneurysm (arrow) on the MCA feeder close to nidus (B). Endovascular embolization was planned using onyx and detachable tip micro-catheter (C) adjunct to radiosurgery with the aim to obliterate the aneurysm and decrease the size of AVM nidus. Post embolization check run (D) shows obliteration of aneurysm and part of nidus.

TABLE 2: Spetzler-Martin grading scale for AVMs.

Characteristic	Number of points assigned
Size of AVM	
Small (<3 cm)	1 point
Medium (3–6 cm)	2 points
Large (>6 cm)	3 points
Location	
Non-eloquent site	0 points
Eloquent site*	1 point
Pattern of venous drainage	
Superficial only	0 points
Deep component	1 point

*Sensorimotor, language, visual cortex, hypothalamus, thalamus, internal capsule, brainstem, cerebellar peduncles or cerebellar nuclei

TABLE 3: AVM embocure score (Demetrium et al.).

Value	Definition	Scoring value
Size	Size of AVM nidus	1 (<3 cm) 2 (3–6 cm) 3 (>6 cm)
Arterial pedicles	Number of arterial pedicles feeding AVM	1 (1–3 pedicles) 2 (4–6 pedicles) 3 (>6 pedicles)
Draining veins	Number of draining veins	1 (1–3 draining veins) 2 (4–6 draining veins) 3 (>6 draining veins)
Vascular eloquence	Emergence of small and short arterial pedicles from parent vessel whose injury/occlusion would cause severe neurologic complications	0 (non-eloquent) 1 (eloquent)

TABLE 4: Endovascular grading scale (Bell et al.).

Feature and value	Points
No. of feeding arteries	1
<3	2
≥3, <6	3
≥6	
Eloquence of adjacent areas	
Noneloquent	0
Eloquent	1
Presence of arteriovenous fistula component	
No AVF	0
AVF	1

TABLE 5: Buffalo score of AVM.

Graded feature	Points assigned
Number of arterial pedicles	
1 or 2	1
3 or 4	2
5 or more	3
Diameter of arterial pedicles	
Most >1 mm	0
Most ≤1 mm	1
Nidus location	
Noneloquent	0
Eloquent	1

AVM grade = (number) + (diameter) + (nidus location)

TABLE 6: Characteristics of Liquid embolic agents.

	N-butyl -2 cyanoacrylate (Glue) (Trufil; codman neurovascular)	Ethylene-vinyl alcohol copolymer with dimethyl sulfoxide (Onyx, eV3 Inc)	Precipitating Hydrophobic Injectable Liquid (PHIL; Microvention California)
Availability	Easy	Few places	Near future
Cost	Cheap	Expensive	Expensive
Concentration	Desired	Few specified	Few specified
Compatibility	Most of the catheters	Few selected catheters (For DMSO)	Few selected catheters (For DMSO)
Preparation	With lipiodol	Agitated >20 min	Instant ready to use
Priming	5% dextrose	DMSO	DMSO
Radio-opacity	Lipiodol	Tantalum/Physical form	Iodine chemically bonded
Adhesiveness	High (Depends on concentration)	Low	Low
Polymerization	Depends on conc	Low	Low
Rate of injection	Usually fast	Slow/Fast	Slow/Fast

ENDOVASCULAR HARDWARE

For the endovascular management of bAVM, the hardware to be used are microcatheters (flow related, wire-guided and detachable tip), micro guidewire having longer soft portion unlike wires used for aneurysm treatment and liquid embolic agents (Glue, Onyx, Squid and PHIL). Comparison of the different available liquid embolic agents are given in **Table 6**.

Flow-dependent Catheters

A major advance in the recent past has been the development of the Magic catheter (Balt, Montmorency, France), a variable stiffness design with extremely soft and flexible distal segments. The proximal segment is 3 French, whereas the distal segment varies from 1.8, 1.5 to 1.2 French sizes. In moderate to high flow AVMs Magic or other flow-dependent catheter can be positioned easily within the AVM nidus. Newer catheters come with hydrophilic coating that facilitates rapid, atraumatic and distal catheterizations. Liquid adhesives and thrombi are less likely to adhere to these coated catheters.[60,61] Ultraflow and Marathon (Micro Therapeutics, Inc., Irvine, CA) are also promising micro catheters for AVM cannulation.

Guidewire Dependent Catheters

These include Baltacci (Balt), Tracker-10 (Boston Scientific Target, CA) and Prowler (Cordis Neurovascular, USA). These catheters are available with hydrophilic coating.

Detachable Tip Microcatheters

With the advent of newer detachable tip catheters, the risk of catheter entrapment has been eliminated, hence there is significant increase in the occlusion rate of AVM nidus as per recent literature. In these microcatheters distal 1.5–3 cm segment is detachable from the main micro catheter. Two major available important microcatheters are Apollo Onyx Delivery Micro Catheter (Micro Therapeutics, Inc., Irvine, CA) and Sonic (Balt, Montmorency, France).

EMBOLIC AGENTS

Acrylic Glue

N-butyl-cyanoacrylate (glue) was the main embolic agent for the treatment of bAVM in past. It is readily available and cheap. For visualization and radio-opacity it is mixed with oil based contrast agent lipiodol or tantalum powder. The rate of polymerization, viscosity and penetration depends upon the ratio of its mixture with lipiodol which can be from 10% to >90%. Higher percentage of glue is used for the larger fistulous components. As the rate of polymerization of glue when it comes in contact of ions is very much high, especially with higher concentrations the risk of catheter entrapment is high. The rate of injection of glue is always moderate to high. The catheter must be primed with 5% dextrose to prevent ionic substances from causing premature polymerization in the catheter **(Figs. 8A and B)**.

Onyx/Squid

With the introduction of non-adhesive ethylene vinyl alcohol copolymer embolic agent, onyx (Ev3, Irvine, California), complete obliteration of small and intermediate-sized bAVMs is possible with low complication rate. Onyx consists of EVOH, dissolved in DMSO and mixed with tantalum powder for radio-opacity. When the material comes in contact with an aqueous solution, it precipitates and forms a soft spongy polymer cast. It is available in ready to use vials of 1.5 mL in 3 different viscosities, onyx 18, 20 and 34. The vials must be placed on a mixer and shaken for at least 20 minutes to obtain a homogenous solution.[62] Another EVOH based liquid embolic agent SQUID (emboflu, Switzerland) is also available in different concentrations as SQUID 12, 12LD, 18 and 18LD. The micro catheter needs to be primed with DMSO before using Onyx/SQUID **(Figs. 3, 5 to 7)**.

Precipitating Hydrophobic Injectable Liquid (PHIL)

Recently a newer nonadhesive embolic agent PHIL (Precipitating Hydrophobic Injectable Liquid, Micro-Vention, Tustin, California) was introduced. It is a copolymer dissolved in dimethyl-sulfoxide (DMSO), with chemically bonded iodine for radio-opacity. The PHIL liquid embolic system consists of a sterile, prefilled, 1.0 mL syringe of PHIL liquid embolic agent, a sterile, prefilled 1.0 mL syringe of DMSO, and micro catheter hub adaptors. In comparison with conventionally available EVOH based embolic agents which uses the physical form of tantalum powder for radio-opacity and hence needs to be agitated for 20 minutes, this embolic agent is ready to be used. Another concern with earlier embolic agents were high radio-opacity and streak artefacts due to tantalum powder which hampers the visualization of residual AVM components on follow-up imaging. It is believed that radio-opacity of PHIL is less in comparison with the tantalum powder and lipiodol **(Figs. 1A to D)**.

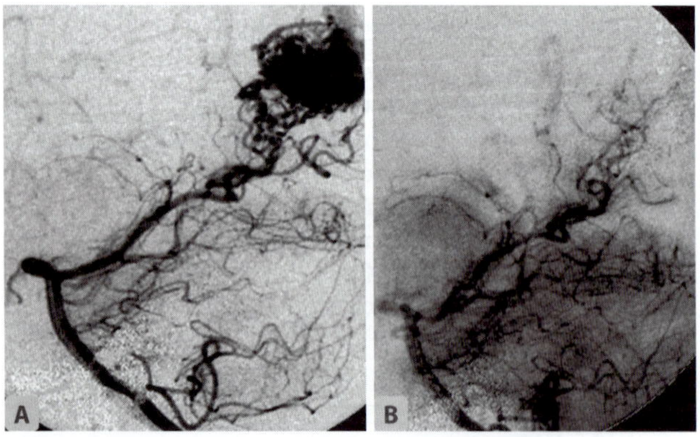

FIGS. 8A AND B: (A) Lateral view of the left vertebral artery shows an occipital AVM. The AVM was embolized with 33% mixture of N-butyl cyanoacrylate and lipoidol; (B) Post-embolization angiogram shows complete ablation of the nidus.

Other Embolic Agents

Microcoils: Detachable microcoils are used for the treatment of high risk/ruptured prenidal or intranidal aneurysms. Another important use of detachable microcoils is to decrease the flow across larger arteriovenous shunts where there is high risk of significant distal migration of liquid embolic agents leading to serious complications.

Complications of AVM Embolization

Complications may occur during or after the procedure itself. These include (i) thromboembolic stroke,(ii) arterial injury producing hemorrhage, (iii) arterial and venous occlusions, (iv) pulmonary embolism. Thrombotic occlusion of normal vessels can be treated by judicious usage of intravenous heparin or intra-arterial thrombolytic agents, such as urokinase. Injecting glue or deploying a coil can treat arterial rupture. Large parenchymal hematomas may be evacuated surgically. After every embolization procedure, a cranial computed tomography must be done to exclude various potential complications at its nascent stage and to obtain a status document. All patients should be closely monitored in an intensive care unit for minimum 24 hours after the procedure to allow for rapid and early intervention for these complications.

DURAL ARTERIOVENOUS FISTULAE

Dural arteriovenous fistulae (DAVFs) are abnormal vascular connections located within the walls of dural sinus or adjacent cortical vein.[63] There is growing evidence to suggest that DAVFs are acquired lesions.[64] The proposed contributing factors are middle ear and intracranial infections, trauma, surgery, and following dural sinus thrombosis.[64] Although the cause and effect relationship between dural sinus thrombosis and DAVF appears well established, it does not exclude other mechanisms for the development of an arteriovenous shunt because most cases of dural thrombosis do not result in a dural fistula.

Classification

Djindjian et al.[64] defined four types, with type 1 draining via the ipsilateral sinus, type 2 draining toward the contralateral sinus, type 3 draining via cortical veins and type 4 with venous ectasia. This classification system allows one to predict the severity of the presenting symptoms and the risk of intra-parenchymal hemorrhage. Modified classification by Cognard has also been proposed (See-appendix—E). Up to 42% of DAVFs with cortical venous drainage were associated with hemorrhage in a series reported by Castaigne.[65]

Radiological Evaluation

Plain skull radiography can sometimes demonstrate enlargement of middle meningeal grooves. CT scan may demonstrate parenchymal edema related to venous hypertension, or intracranial hemorrhage and thrombus in sinus. Contrast-enhanced CT scan can demonstrate serpiginous enhancing parenchymal tubular structures representing the transmedullary veins without any parenchymal nidus. MR imaging may demonstrate brain edema **(Figs. 9A to C)**, infarction and dilated veins.[66] However, CT and MR imaging can both completely miss low grade DAVFs without dilated cortical veins (Djindjian type 1). Selective arteriography **(Figs. 10A to F)** remains the gold standard for the detection and characterization of DAVFs. Bilateral external carotid, internal carotid and vertebral artery studies are mandatory for comprehensive analysis.

Therapeutic Options

Patients with visual loss, hemorrhage or infarction and those with cortical venous drainage require prompt therapy. Djindjian type I fistulae on the other end, can be followed conservatively without treatment.

Compression Therapy

Patients with DAVFs located in the posterior sigmoid or transverse sinus without severe symptoms or high risk angiographic features are ideal candidates for manual compression of the ipsilateral feeding occipital artery behind the mastoid bone.[67]

Transarterial Embolization

Superselective embolization of the ECA feeder vessels to a DAVF can be an effective treatment for certain cases.[68] A variety of agents are available to embolize DAVFs including polyvinyl alcohol (PVA) particles, liquid adhesive agents, such as NBCA. Proximal occlusion of a feeding artery should be avoided because (i) the fistula usually acquires arterial supply from a neighboring collateral vessel and (ii) it interferes with future access when it is needed.

Transvenous Embolization

This method enables placement of coils via a transvenous route under direct fluoroscopic guidance to achieve closure of difficult DAVFs. Development of newer and softer delivery

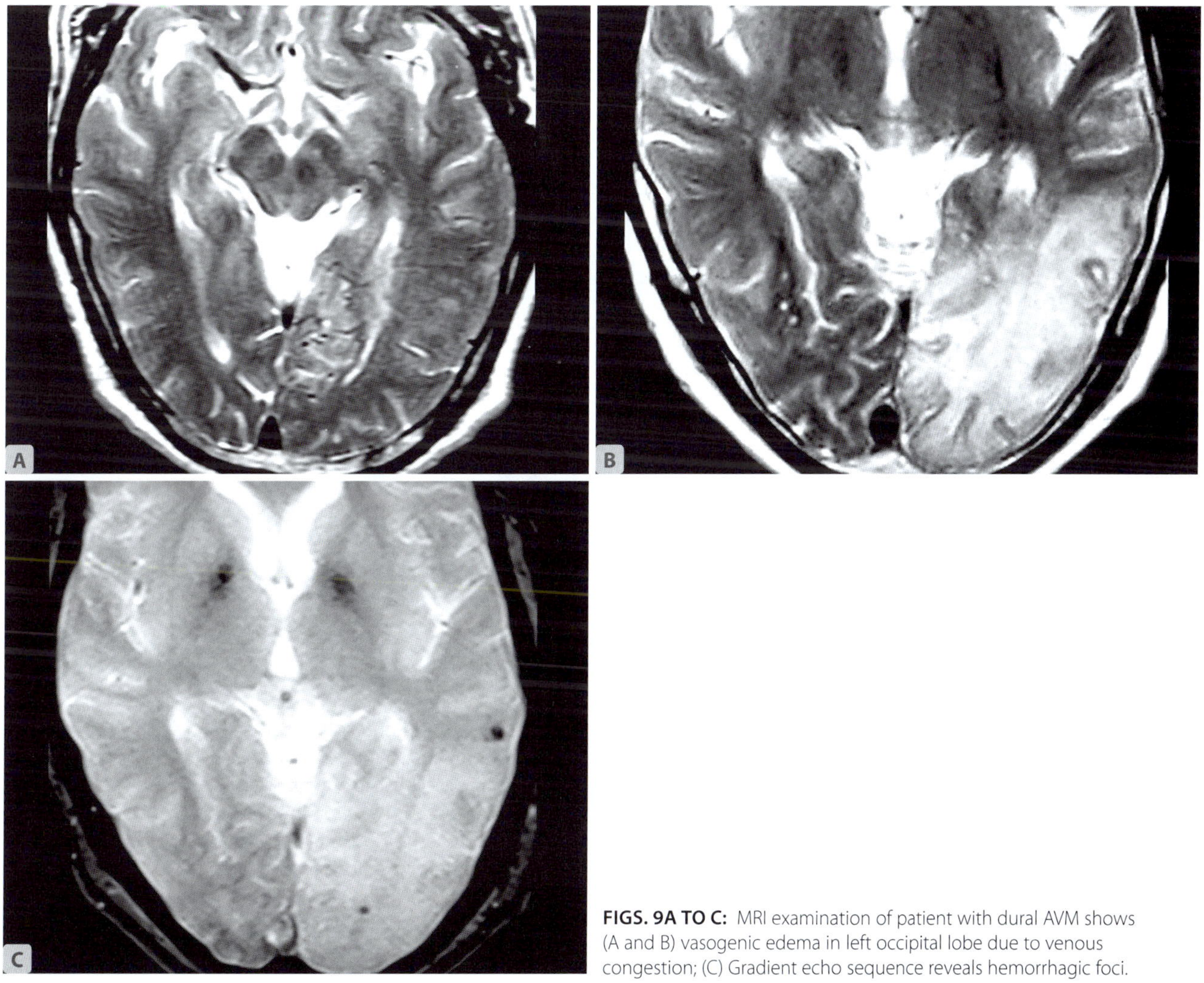

FIGS. 9A TO C: MRI examination of patient with dural AVM shows (A and B) vasogenic edema in left occipital lobe due to venous congestion; (C) Gradient echo sequence reveals hemorrhagic foci.

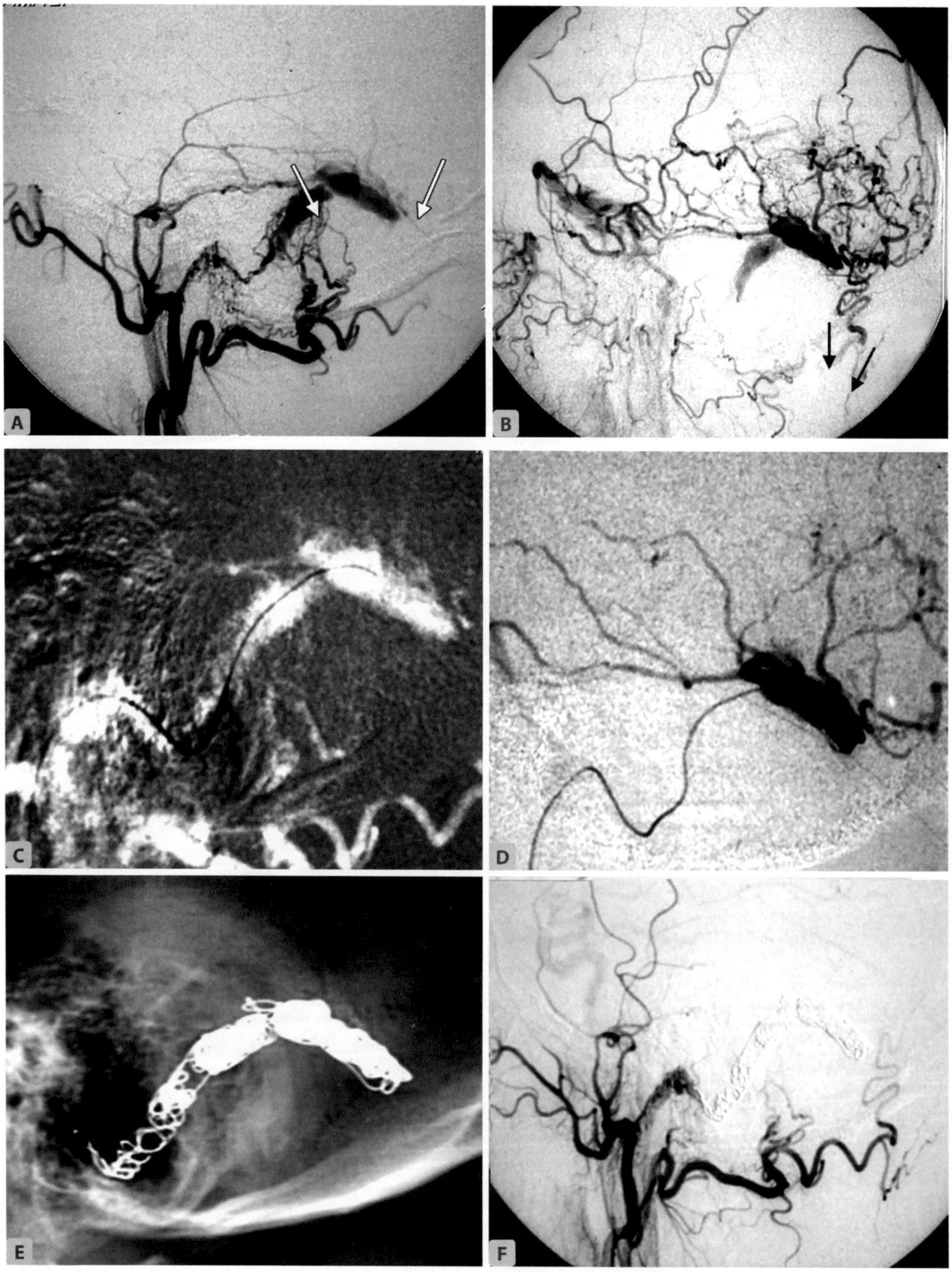

FIGS. 10A TO F: (A) LECA lateral projection shows occlusion of lateral sinus with dural AVF fed by ECA branches; (B) Venous phase with cortical venous reflux. Transvenous occlusion of dural AVFs. Roadmap image (C) showing position of microcatheter in the sigmoid sinus. Angiogram; (D) obtained with microcatheter; (E) Complete packing of the sigmoid sinus with coils; (E) Postembolization ECA angiogram; (F) Showing occlusion of the dural AVF.

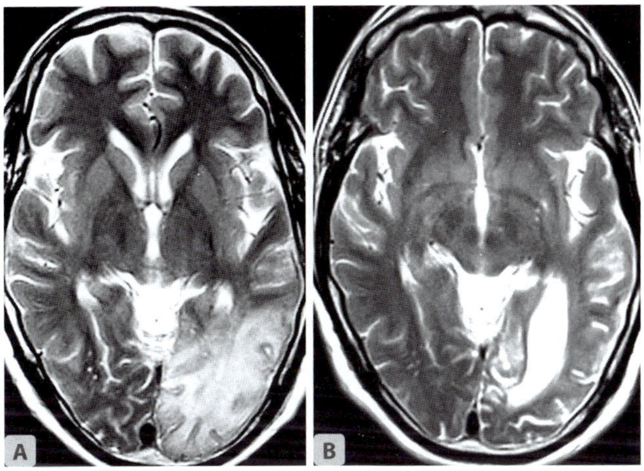

FIGS. 11A AND B: MRI (A) Pre-embolization and (B) post-embolization as in Figures 11.9A to C with significant resolution of edema in the occipital lobe.

catheters have permitted transfemoral access to the venous drainage of many DAVFs allowing coil packing.[69] Only those patients with cortical venous drainage (Djindjian's type 3) should be treated by transvenous route if the sinus is not being used for significant venous drainage of normal brain. Platinum fibered thrombogenic coils with slightly larger diameter than that of the sinus is preferred for packing the fistulous sinus. Follow-up MRI may show regression of brain parenchymal changes **(Figs. 11A and B)**.

Preoperative Embolization

The combination of preoperative arterial and subsequent surgical excision of the DAVF has been shown to be effective in treating complex lesions.[70] Particulate embolic materials are used 1–2 days before the surgical excisions.

CONCLUSION

The endovascular management plays the central role in multimodal treatment strategies of the brain AVMs. Recent advancement in the available angiography machines (flat panel biplane DSA suites), endovascular hardware in the form of detachable tip microcatheters, non-adhesive newer liquid embolic agents and improved skills and experience has presented new possibilities in the treatment of these complex dynamic brain lesions. Ongoing research and increasing literature suggests that endovascular embolization of bAVMs provides safe and effective management options.

ACKNOWLEDGMENTS

The authors acknowledge Dr Vivek Agarwal (DM), resident in the Neuroradiology Division, Department of Radiodiagnosis, PGIMER, Chandigarh for his support in image archival and editing of chapter.

REFERENCES

1. Berenstein A, Lasjaunias P. Surgical Neuro-angiography. New York: Springer-Verlag; 1992. pp.1-266.
2. Spetzler RF, Martin NA. A proposed grading system for arteriovenous malformations. J Neurosurg. 1986; 65:476-83.
3. Dorothea S, Raul G, Sean D L. Endovascular treatment of intracranial arteriovenous malformation. Neurosurg Clin N Am. 2009;20:399-418.
4. Brown RD Jr, Wiebers DO, Torner JC, et al. Frequency of intracranial hemorrhage as a presenting symptom and subtype analysis: a population-based study of intracranial vascular malformations in Olmsted Country, Minnesota. J Neurosurg. 1996; 85:29–32.
5. Brown RD Jr, Wiebers DO, Forbes G, et al. The natural history of unruptured intracranial arteriovenous malformations. J Neurosurg. 1988; 68:352-7.
6. Graf CJ, Perret GE, Torner JC. Bleeding from cerebral arteriovenous malformations as part of their natural history. J Neurosurg. 1983;58:331-7.
7. Arteriovenous Malformation Study Group. Arteriovenous malformations of the brain in adults. N Engl J Med 1999;340:1812-8.
8. Stapf C, Mast H, Sciacca RR, et al New York Islands AVM Study Collaborators. The New York Islands AVM Study: design, study progress, and initial results. Stroke. 2003;34:e29-33.
9. Hartmann A, Mast H, Mohr JP, et al. Morbidity of intracranial hemorrhage in patients with cerebral arteriovenous malformation. Stroke. 1998;29:931-4.
10. Hoh BL, Chapman PH, Loeffler JS, et al. Results of multimodality treatment for 141 patients with brain arteriovenous malformations and seizures: factors associated with seizure incidence and seizure outcomes. Neurosurgery. 2002;51:303-9.
11. Stapf C, Mast H, Sciacca RR,et al. Predictors of hemorrhage in patients with untreated brain arteriovenous malformation. Neurology. 2006;66:1350-5.
12. da Costa L, Wallace MC, Ter Brugge KG, et al. The natural history and predictive features of hemorrhage from brain arteriovenous malformations. Stroke. 2009;40:100-5.
13. Hofmeister C, Stapf C, Hartmann A, et al. Demographic, morphological, and clinical characteristics of 1289 patients with brain arteriovenous malformation. Stroke. 2000;31:1307-10.
14. Stapf C, Labovitz DL, Sciacca RR, et al. Incidence of adult brain arteriovenous malformation hemorrhage in a prospective population-based stroke survey. Cerebrovasc Dis. 2002;13:43-6.
15. Kim H, Al-Shahi Salman R, McCulloch CE, et al. MARS Coinvestigators. Untreated brain arteriovenous malformation: patientlevel meta-analysis of hemorrhage predictors. Neurology. 2014;83:590-7.
16. Gross BA, Du R. Natural history of cerebral arteriovenous malformations: a meta-analysis. J Neurosurg. 2013;118: 437-43.
17. Abecassis IJ, Xu DS, Batjer HH, et al. Natural history of brain arteriovenous malformations: a systematic review. Neurosurg Focus. 2014;37:E7.
18. Kim H, Al-Shahi Salman R, McCulloch CE, et al. MARS Coinvestigators. Untreated brain arteriovenous malformation: patientlevel meta-analysis of hemorrhage predictors. Neurology. 2014;83:590-7.
19. Gross BA, Du R. Natural history of cerebral arteriovenous malformations: a meta-analysis. J Neurosurg. 2013;118: 437-43.
20. Ross J, Al-Shahi Salman R. Interventions for treating brain arteriovenous malformations in adults. Cochrane Database Syst Rev. 2010:CD003436.

21. Fierstra J, Conklin J, Krings T, et al. Impaired peri-nidal cerebrovascular reserve in seizure patients with brain arteriovenous malformations. Brain. 2011;134(pt 1):100-9.
22. Krings T, Hans FJ, Geibprasert S, et al. Partial "targeted" embolisation of brain arteriovenous malformations. Eur Radiol. 2010;20:2723-31.
23. Derdeyn CP, Zipfel GJ, et al. Management of brain arteriovenous malformations A scientific statement for healthcare professionals from the American Heart Association/ American Stroke Association. Stroke.ahajournals 2017;48.
24. Galletti F, Costa C, Cupini LM, et al. Brain arteriovenous malformations and seizures: an Italian study. J Neurol Neurosurg Psychiatry. 2014;85:284-8.
25. Jiang P, Lv X, Wu Z, et al. Characteristics of brain arteriovenous malformations presenting with seizures without acute or remote hemorrhage. Neuroradiol J. 2011;24:886-8.
26. Mast H, Mohr JP, Osipov A, et al. "Steal" is an unestablished mechanism for the clinical presentation of cerebral arteriovenous malformations. Stroke. 1995;26:1215-20.
27. Higgins JN, Kirkpatrick PJ. Stenting venous outflow gives symptomatic improvement in a patient with an inoperable brainstem arteriovenous malformation. Br J Neurosurg. 2013;27:698-700.
28. Lv Xianli, Wu Z et al. Angioarchitectural Characteristics of Brain Arterivenous Malformations with and without haemorrhage. World Neurosurgery. 2011; 76,1/2: 95-99.
29. Alexander MD, Cooke DL, Nelson J, et al. Association Between Venous Angioarchitectural Features of Sporadic Brain Arteriovenous Malformations and Intracranial Hemorrhage. AJNR. Am J Neuroradiol. 2015;36(5):949-52.
30. Ranmos SK, Gardenghi B. Aneurysms Associated with Brain Arteriovenous Malformations. AJNR. 2016;37;1966-71.
31. Lopes DK, et al. Arteriovenous malformation embocure score: AVMES. J Neurointerv Surg. 2016;8(7):685-91.
32. Bell DL, Leslie-Mazwi TM, Yoo AJ, et al. Application of novel brain arteriovenous malformation endovascular grading scale for trans arterial embolization. Am J Neuroradiol. 2015; 36(7): 1303-9.
33. Dumont TM, Kan P, Snyder KV, Hopkins LN, Siddiqui AH, Levy EI. A proposed grading system for endovascular treatment of cerebral arteriovenous malformations: Buffalo score. Surg Neurol Int. 2015;6:3.
34. Byyny RL, Mower WR, Shum N, et al. Sensitivity of noncontrast cranial computed tomography for the emergency department diagnosis of subarachnoid hemorrhage. Ann Emerg Med. 2008;51:697-703.
35. McCormack RF, Hutson A. Can computed tomography angiography of the brain replace lumbar puncture in the evaluation of acute-onset headache after a negative noncontrast cranial computed tomography scan? Acad Emerg Med. 2010;17:444-45.
36. Brazzelli M, Sandercock PA, Chappell FM, et al. Magnetic resonance imaging versus computed tomography for detection of acute vascular lesions in patients presenting with stroke symptoms. Cochrane Database Syst Rev. 2009:CD007424.
37. Delgado Almandoz JE, Schaefer PW, et al. Diagnostic accuracy and yield of multidetector CT angiography in the evaluation of spontaneous intraparenchymal cerebral hemorrhage. Am J Neuroradiol. 2009;30:1213–122.
38. Josephson CB, White PM, Krishan A, et al. Computed tomography angiography or magnetic resonance angiography for detection of intracranial vascular malformations in patients with intracerebral haemorrhage. Cochrane Database Syst Rev. 2014;9:CD009372.
39. Willems Peter WA, Taeshineetanakul et al. The use of 4D-CTA in the diagnostic work-up of brain arteriovenous malformations. Neuroradiology. 2012; 54:123-31.
40. Gross BA, Frerichs KU, Du R. Sensitivity of CT angiography, T2-weighted MRI, and magnetic resonance angiography in detecting cerebral arteriovenous malformations and associated aneurysms. J Clin Neurosci. 2012;19:1093-5.
41. Hadizadeh DR, Kukuk GM, Steck DT, et al. Noninvasive evaluation of cerebral arteriovenous malformations by 4D-MRA for preoperative planning and postoperative follow-up in 56 patients: comparison with DSA and intraoperative findings. Am J Neuroradiol. 2012;33:1095-101.
42. Machet A, Portefaix C, Kadziolka K, et al. Brain arteriovenous malformation diagnosis: value of time-resolved contrastenhanced MR angiography at 3.0T compared to DSA. Neuroradiology. 2012;54:1099-108.
43. Gallagher TA, Nair VA, Regner MF, et al. Characterizing the relationship between functional MRI–derived measures and clinical outcomes in patients with vascular lesions. Neurosurg Focus. 2013;34:E8.
44. Prestigiacomo CJ, Niimi Y, Setton A, et al. Three-dimensional rotational spinal angiography in the evaluation and treatment of vascular malformations. Am J Neuroradiol. 2003;24:1429-35.
45. Neuropathology Group. Medical Research Council Cognitive Function and Aging Study. Pathological correlates of late-onset dementia in a multicentre, community-based population in England and Wales: Neuropathology Group of the Medical Research Council Cognitive Function and Ageing Study (MRC CFAS). Lancet. 2001;357:169-75.
46. Kakizawa Y, Nagashima H, Oya F, et al. Compartments in arteriovenous malformation nidi demonstrated with rotational three-dimensional digital subtraction angiography by using selective microcatheterization. J Neurosurg. 2002;96:770-4.
47. Gailloud P, Oishi S, Carpenter J, et al. Three-dimensional digital angiography: new tool for simultaneous three- dimensional rendering of vascular and osseous information during rotational angiography. Am J Neuroradiol. 2004;25:571-3.
48. Alexander MD, Oliff MC, Olorunsola OG, et al. Patient radiation exposure during diagnostic and therapeutic interventional neuroradiology procedures. J Neurointerv Surg. 2010;2:6-10.
49. Ding D, Yen CP, Starke RM, Xu Z, Sun X, Sheehan JP. Outcomes following single-session radiosurgery for high-grade intracranial arteriovenous malformations. Br J Neurosurg. 2014;28:666-74.
50. Bollet MA, Anxionnat R, Buchheit I, et al. Efficacy and morbidity of arc-therapy radiosurgery for cerebral arteriovenous malformations: a comparison with the natural history. Int J Radiat Oncol Biol Phys. 2004;58:1353-63.
51. Ding D, Yen CP, Starke RM, et al. Outcomes following single-session radiosurgery for high-grade intracranial arteriovenous malformations. Br J Neurosurg. 2014;28:666-74.
52. Yu SC, Chan MS, Lam JM, et al. Complete obliteration of intracranial arteriovenous malformation with endovascular cyanoacrylate embolization: initial success and rate of permanent cure. Am J Neuroradiol. 2004;25:1139-43.
53. Saatci I, Geyik S, Yavuz K, et al. Endovascular treatment of brain arteriovenous malformations with prolonged intranidal Onyx injection technique: long-term results in 350 consecutive patients with completed endovascular treatment course. J Neurosurg. 2011;115:78-88.
54. Van Rooij WJ, Jacobs S, Sluzewski M, et al. Curative embolization of brain arteriovenous malformations with onyx: patient selection, embolization technique, and results. AJNR Am J Neuroradiol. 2012;33:1299-304.
55. Jafar JJ, Davis AJ, Berenstein A, et al. The effect of embolisation with N-butyl cyanoacrylate prior to surgical resection of cerebral arteriovenous malformations. J Neurosurg. 1993;78:60-69.
56. Krings T, Hans FJ, Geibprasert S, et al. Partial "targeted" embolisation of brain arteriovenous malformations. Eur Radiol. 2010;20:2723-31.

57. Brown RD Jr, Wiebers DO, Forbes GS. Unruptured intracranial aneurysms and arteriovenous malformations: frequency of intracranial hemorrhage and relationship of lesions. J Neurosurg. 1990;73:859-63.
58. Batjer HH, Devous MD Sr, Seibert GB, et al. Intracranial arteriovenous malformation: relationships between clinical and radiographic factors and ipsilateral steal severity. Neurosurgery. 1988;23:322–32.
59. Kusske JA, Kelly WA. Embolization and reduction of the "steal" syndrome in cerebral arteriovenous malformations. J Neurosurg. 1974;40:313-21.
60. Kallmes DF, McGraw JK, Evans AJ, et al. Thrombogenicity of hydrophilic and non-hydrophilic microcatheters and guiding catheters. Am J Neuroradiol. 1977;18:1243-51.
61. Mathis JM, Evans AJ, DeNardo AJ, et al. Hydrophilic coatings diminish adhesion of glue to catheter. An in vitro simulation of NBCA embolisation. Am J Neuroradiol. 1997;18:1087-91.
62. Rooij WJ, Jacobs S, et al. Curative Embolization of Brain Arteriovenous Malformations with Onyx: Patient Selection, Embolization Technique, and Result. Am J Neuroradiol. 33:1299-304.
63. Choudhary MY, Sachdev VP, Cho SH, et al. Dural arteriovenous malformations of the major venous sinuses. An acquired lesion. Am J Neuroradiol. 1982;3:13-9.
64. Djindjian R, Cophignon J, Theron J. Embolisation by superselective arteriography from the femoral route in neuroradiology: Review of 60 cases, technique, indications, complications. Neuroradiology. 1973;6:20-26.
65. De Marco KJ, Dillon W, Halbach VV, et al. Dural arteriovenous fistulas: Evaluation with MR imaging. Radiology. 1990;175:193-9.
66. Halbach VV, Higashida RT, Heishima GB, et al. Dural fistulas involving the transverse and sigmoid sinuses: Results of treatment in 28 patients. Radiology. 1987;163:443-7.
67. Vinuela F, Fox AJ, Debrun GM, et al. Spontaneous carotid-cavernous fistulas: Clinical radiological and therapeutic considerations: Experience with 20 cases. J Neurosurg. 1984;60:976-84.
68. Halbach VV, Higashida RT, Hieshima GB, et al. Transvenous embolisation of dural fistulas involving the cavernous sinus. Am J Neuroradiol. 1989;10:377-84.
69. Barnwell SL, Hallbach VV, Higashida RT, et al. Complex dural arteriovenous fistulas: Results of a new combined neuro-surgical and inter-ventional neuroradiology treatment in 16 patients. J Neurosurg. 1989;71:352-8.
70. Panagiotopoulos V, Gizewski E, Asgari S, et al. Embolization of Intracranial Arteriovenous Malformations with Ethylene-Vinyl Alcohol Copolymer (Onyx). Am J Neuroradiol. 2009;30:99-106.

CHAPTER

192

Carotid-cavernous Fistulas

Chirag Kamal Ahuja, Vivek Gupta, Ajay Kumar, Niranjan Khandelwal

INTRODUCTION AND HISTORICAL PERSPECTIVE

Carotid-cavernous fistula (CCF), as the name suggests, is an abnormal communication between the carotid arteries [internal carotid artery (ICA) and/or external carotid artery (ECA)] and the cavernous sinus (CS).[1] It is of two types- direct and indirect. CCF was one of the earliest neurological entities that was recognized and understood by neurophysicians dating back two centuries. Taveras first described it in 1811. Due to unavailability of precise tools to reach the specific site of fistula at that time, it was treated by common carotid ligation for the first time in 1837 followed by internal carotid artery (ICA) ligation in 1847. Dandy and Jefferson are considered pioneers in the surgical treatment of CCFs in the early twentieth century. However, due to proximal occlusion techniques, there was significantly increased incidence of recurrence due to retrograde collateral flow from ophthalmic artery as well as ECA branches. This also resulted in arterial steal resulting in distal ischemia and visual loss. It took decades of thinking in this regard. As a corrective measure, Adson advocated occlusion of ophthalmic artery in addition to ICA (1942). Simultaneously, procedure of muscle embolization of the fistula was also attempted by Brooks[2] with variable results. 1971 marked the modern era of endovascular access routes when Prolo and Hanberry successfully occluded CCFs with *non-detachable balloons* which sacrificed the ICA. Serbinenko's method (1974) of using detachable balloons was a game-changer as it preserved the ICA with complete fistula closure.[3] Latex detachable balloons were subsequently used by Debrun with good ICA patency rates. Mullan achieved fistula closure by cavernous sinus packing with still better ICA patency rates.[4] After the introduction of detachable platinum coils by Guglielmi,[5] cavernous sinus coiling became the standard of care giving excellent results. CCF treatment still evolved further with the availability of liquid embolic material in recent times which can be combined with platinum coils.

ETIOLOGY AND PATHOGENESIS

CCFs can either occur spontaneously, which are more often of the indirect variety (fed by ECA branches), or following closed head trauma associated with basal skull fracture/ rupture of cavernous carotid aneurysm (which leads to direct communication of the ICA with the ipsilateral cavernous sinus[CS], hence referred to as direct type). Other causes of direct CCFs are collagen vascular disorders (Ehlers-Danlos syndrome, Osteogenesis imperfecta, etc.), arterial dissections, direct surgical trauma (iatrogenic), fibromuscular dysplasia, etc.[6,7] Congenital direct CCFs are extremely rare, and only a few cases have been reported.[8] Combined Direct Indirect CCFs have abnormal communication between dural branches of the ICA and/or ECA with the CS. Their etiology is not clear, but they have been noticed following pregnancy, sinusitis, trauma, localized surgical procedures and cavernous sinus thrombosis.

Direct CCFs are postulated to develop secondary to bony fractures which tear the cavernous ICA from its dural attachment or due to shearing strain resulting from sudden change in inertia secondary to acceleration/deceleration.[9] The latter occurs due to fixity of the ICA between the foramen lacerum and anterior clinoid process. Another school of thought contests this hypothesis debating that fractures are not a feature in all CCF cases. These proponents believe that these lesions arise as a result of increased intraluminal pressure of ICA which may occur abruptly as a result of neck flexion or twisting injury which gets transmitted to the weakest arterial point resulting in its rupture within the cavernous sinus.[10] Traumatic CCFs occur mostly in C4 segment of the intracavernous ICA followed by the C3, C2 and C5 segments. Direct CCFs occur more commonly in younger patients. The other mechanism of traumatic CCF is direct injury. A penetrating wound from a bullet, gunshot shrapnel, pellets, a transorbital stab, or a surgical procedure could result in a lesion of the intracavernous ICA.[11,12] Iatrogenic CCFs have been reported as complications of many procedures, including transsphenoidal surgery,[13] microcompression of the Gasserian ganglion[14] and endovascular procedures in which the ICA is perforated with a Fogarty catheter[15] or a guidewire.[16]

The precise pathogenesis of indirect CCFs is controversial. Some authors believe that they arise from rupture of thin-walled dural arteries that normally traverse the CS.[17] Others have proposed that these fistulae are, in fact, collateral anastomoses following cavernous sinus thrombosis that develop in patients prone to venous thrombosis.[18] This partially explains the increased frequency of such fistulae in women, especially in post-partum state.

CLINICAL SYMPTOMATOLOGY

Clinical features of CCFs are similar in nature in both direct and indirect fistulae, except that symptoms and signs are less severe in indirect CCFs because of slow flow shunts. The clinical manifestations of CCFs can be predicted based on the presence of structures in the cavernous sinus and the venous drainage of the sinus. The neural involvement (III, IV, V1, V2, VI) may cause ophthalmoparesis due to involvement of cranial nerves in varying combinations. The symptoms may range from palsy in one gaze (lateral rectus palsy) to complete ophthalmoplegia. With respect to the dominant venous drainage, the symptoms are predominantly localized to the respective drainage site. Venous drainage towards the orbit produces proptosis, chemosis, and arterialization of scleral veins **(Figs. 1A to D)**. The resultant venous hypertension, mass effect, and hemorrhage produce ocular and orbital symptoms. The neural paresis may be exacerbated by thickening of extraocular muscles secondary to venous congestion. The onset of symptoms may be significantly delayed after the onset of trauma and may begin abruptly. Sudden rupture of a cavernous carotid aneurysm has been postulated as a cause, the injury of which would have occurred during trauma. Dominant venous drainage to the inferior petrosal sinus leads to aural symptoms especially tinnitus. Contralateral cavernous sinus drainage through intercavernous anastomosis causes similar symptoms localizing to the other eye. In about 5% of the patients, high venous flow may be retrogradely transmitted to the cortical veins resulting in life-threatening hemorrhages. There may occur brainstem venous congestion resulting in altered consciousness including various other cerebellar symptoms. Another type of symptom which is commonly seen with high-flow direct CCFs is downstream ischemia e.g. transient ischemic attacks (TIA) due to steal of blood away from the intracranial circulation. Even myelopathy due to spinal venous drainage of the fistula is reported.[19] Most direct CCFs are acquired, secondary to trauma, including iatrogenic trauma, or rupture of an intracavernous aneurysm.

Indirect CCFs do not present with abrupt onset of fulminant symptoms due to lesser quantity of shunted blood. A typical patient is a middle aged female presenting with slowly progressive history of orbital pain, congestion and

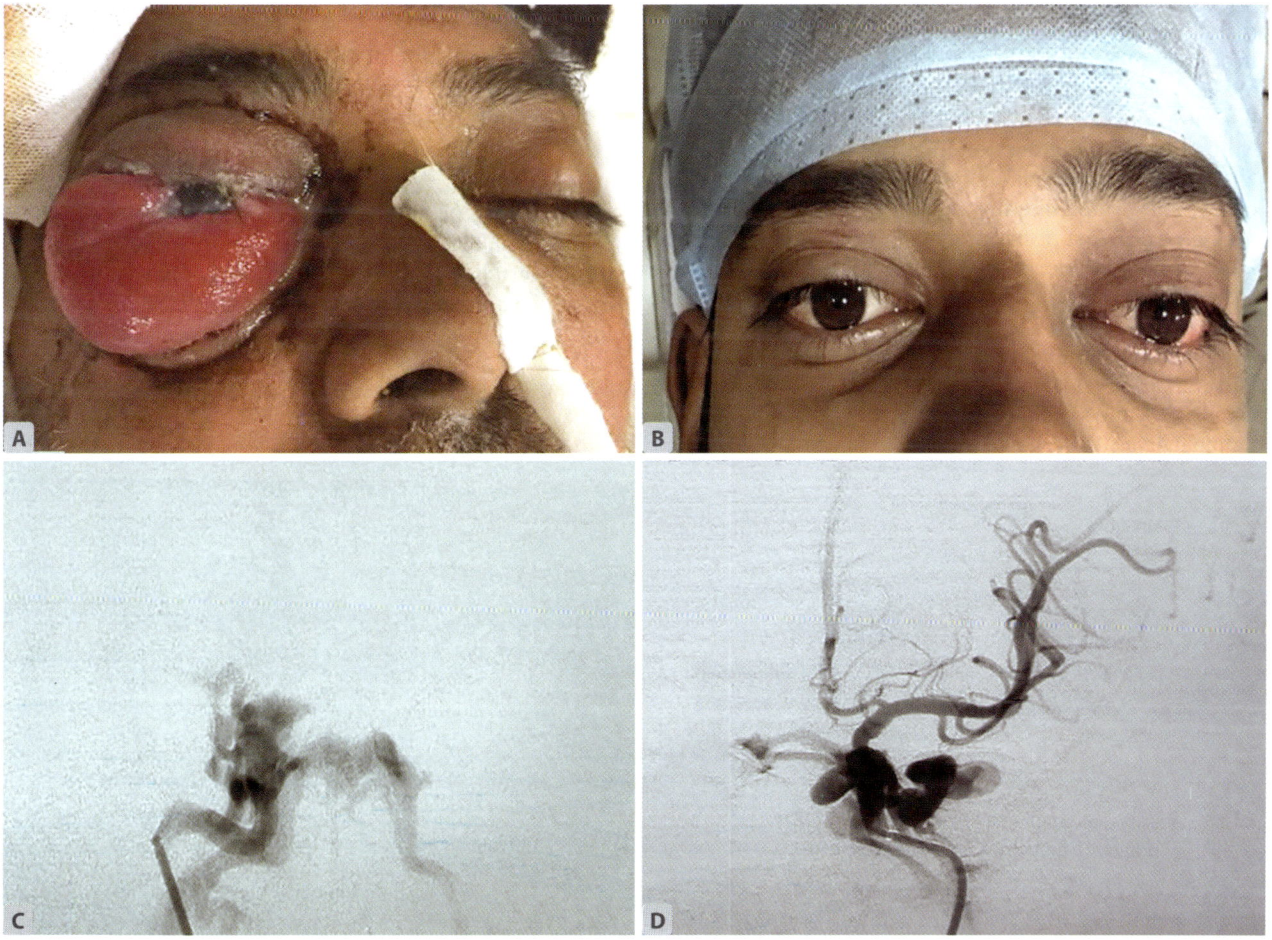

FIGS. 1A TO D: Clinical photograph depicting variable degree of post-traumatic proptosis—severe (A) and mild (B) and the corresponding ICA run showing high flow (C) and low flow states (D).

some degree of restriction of movements. Congestion may not be easily noticeable and hence referred to as 'white-eyed shunt'.[20] There may be increased intraocular pressure with new onset glaucoma. Posterior draining sinus may present as tinnitus. The clinical course may be waxing-waning and some fistulae may occlude due to spontaneous thrombosis. The nature of symptoms including vision loss may not be significantly different between the two groups.[21] However the abruptness and quantum of the symptoms are definitely higher in the direct variety.

Differential Diagnosis

The following need to be considered when the patient presents with ocular signs and symptoms—thyroid disease, idiopathic orbital inflammation (pseudotumor), orbital cellulitis, orbital neoplasms, cavernous sinus thrombosis, Tolosa Hunt syndrome, conjunctivitis, scleritis, episcleritis, etc.

ANATOMY OF INTRACAVERNOUS INTERNAL CAROTID ARTERY AND CAVERNOUS SINUS

Before embarking upon treatment, it is very important to have a thorough knowledge and understanding of the anatomy of the internal carotid artery (ICA) and cavernous sinus (CS).

The cavernous ICA, as the name suggests, runs within the cavernous sinus. The ICA enters the cavernous sinus by piercing the dura as it exits the petrous carotid canal at the skull base across the foramen lacerum. It subsequently has intrasinus course during its cavernous segment beyond which it pierces the dura to enter the subarachnoid space adjacent to the anterior clinoid process. The cavernous ICA can be subdivided into five segments:[22,23] posterior vertical segment (C5), first posterior genu (C4), horizontal segment (C3), second anterior genu (C2) and the ascending vertical segment (C1) **(Fig. 2)**. Meningohypophyseal artery arises near junction of C5 and C4. Meningohypophyseal artery branches supply the posterior pituitary, cavernous sinus, clival dura and cranial nerves III to VI. The inferolateral trunk arises from C4 segment and supplies the dura of the cavernous sinus and cranial nerves III, IV, V and VI.

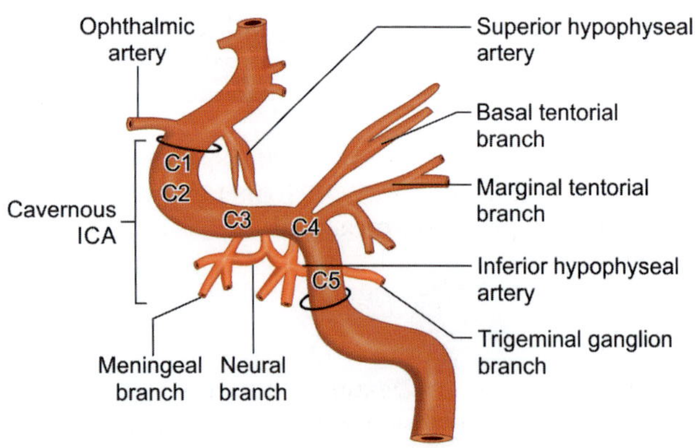

FIG. 2: Pictorial depiction of the segments (C1 to C5) of the cavernous ICA alongwith its branches.

The CS is stuated on either side of the sella turcica and is formed by the folds of the dura. It is not a single venous pouch but is compartmentalized in to smaller caverns, the three main ones being the (i) anteroinferior compartment in relation to the superior and inferior ophthalmic veins and the pterygoid plexus; (ii) the posterosuperior compartment in relation to the superficial middle cerebral vein, the inferior and superior petrosal sinuses, and the contralateral CS through the intercavernous sinus; and (iii) a medial compartment. The CS receives blood flow from the superficial middle cerebral vein, the middle meningeal vein, and the superior and inferior ophthalmic veins. It drains through the superior and inferior petrosal sinuses and the pterygoid plexus **(Fig. 3)**. In the case of a CCF, arterial blood enters the CS at high pressure and flow. The main efferent pathways of this arterialized blood are the inferior petrosal sinus (IPS) and the superior ophthalmic vein (SOV) which are responsible for the patients symptoms.

CLASSIFICATION

CCFs are classified to maintain homogeneity in nomenclature and to prognosticate the disease status. Carotid-cavernous fistulas can be classified based on three criteria:

I. Based on etiopathogenesis—into spontaneous or trasumatic fistulae
II. Based on hemodynamics of blood flow—into high-flow or low-flow fistula
III. Based on angiographic appearance and feeders—into direct or indirect (dural) fistulae.

Based on angiographic findings, Barrow et al.[24] classified CCFs into 4 types: (i) A, (ii) B, (iii) C, and (iv) D.

Type A fistulae—direct shunts between the ICA and the CS. They are usually high-flow fistulae, frequently post-traumatic, may also occur spontaneously from rupture of an intracavernous aneurysm. Type A fistulae have been further divided into three types based on size of fistula[25] on ICA injection.

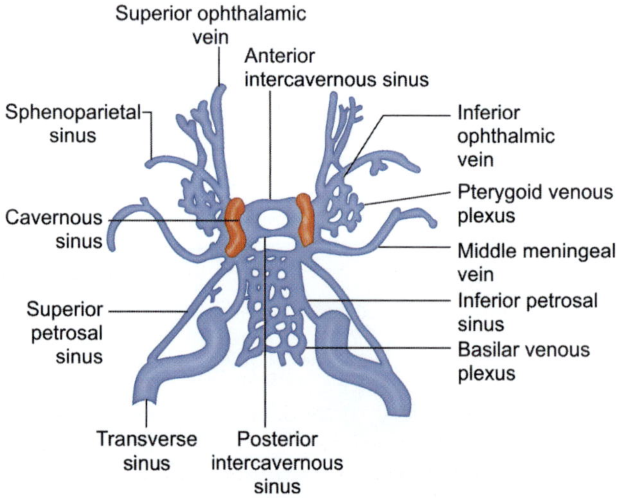

FIG. 3: Pictorial representation of the cavernous sinus anatomy with its drainage connections and tributaries.

Small size: Both anterior cerebral artery (ACA) and middle cerebral artery (MCA) opacified on ICA injection **(Fig. 1D)**.

Medium size: Either ACA or MCA opacified.

Large size: None of the two opacified **(Fig. 1C)**.

Types B, C and D are indirect (dural) shunts, which usually occur spontaneously and generally have slow flow.

Type B: Fistulae between the meningeal branches of the ICA and CS.

Type C: Dural shunts between the meningeal branches of the ECA and the CS.

Type D: Between the meningeal branches of both ICA and ECA and CS.

CCFs have also been classified based on the venous drainage pattern:[26]

Type 1: CCFs with posterior/inferior drainage only.

Type 2: Posterior/inferior and anterior drainage.

Type 3: Anterior drainage only.

Type 4: Retrograde drainage into cortical veins with/without other drainage channels.

Type 5: Direct connection between the ICA and CS.

RADIOLOGICAL EVALUATION

A thorough clinical history and examination often helps us in reaching at a diagnosis of CCF.

The following modalities can be utilized for diagnosis and as part of pre-intervention work-up.

CT Scan

The findings concern the effects rather than the fistula itself. Proptosis is noted on the affected side. There is engorgement of ophthalmic veins alongwith extraocular muscle congestion. A markedly enhancing cavernous sinus, often varicose, is seen bulging outward **(Fig. 4)**. Associated soft-tissue and bony injuries (fractures) may also be seen in the acute stage.[27] CT angiography demonstrates the dilated cavernous sinus. However the rent is often not visible.

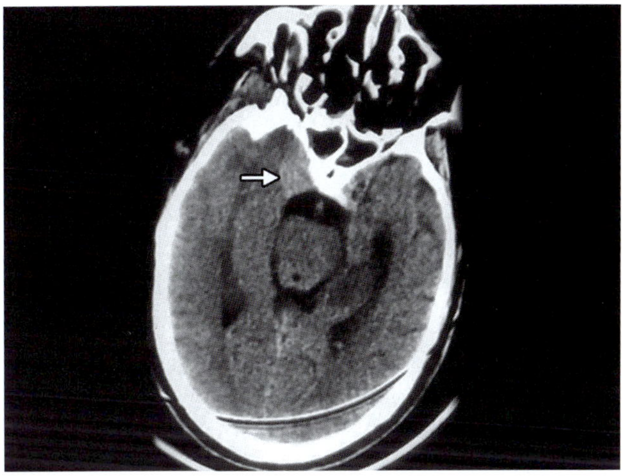

FIG. 4: Axial CT scan shows a prominent right cavernous sinus (arrow) as a manifestation of traumatic CCF.

MRI

The sensitivity of MRI in diagnosing CCF is reasonably high.[28] The features of proptosis, dilated superior ophthalmic vein, orbital congestion, prominent CS point to CCF **(Figs. 5A to C)**. It also helps us in identifying the sequelae of trauma in traumatic fistulae like cerebral contusions, hemorrhages, etc. MRA shows prominent CS and its draining veins (better seen in direct CCF).

Digital Subtraction Angiogram (DSA)

DSA is the gold standard in the diagnosis of carotico cavernous fistula. However it is an invasive modality. Moreover with the advent of multidetector CT scanners and the technique of dynamic CT and MR angiography, DSA is hardly required as just a diagnostic modality. When performed, it demonstrates the CCF and differentiates between a direct and an indirect type. Bilateral ICAs, ECAs and the vertebral arteries must be injected to assess exact site of fistula, its venous drainage and hemodynamic effects. Dangerous angiographic findings include pial venous reflux **(Figs. 6A and B)** and giant CS varix extending intradurally because such signs indicate a higher likelihood of venous rupture and intracerebral or/and subarachnoid hemorrhage. Sometimes in high flow fistula, it becomes very difficult to visualize the ICA rent. We may do a high frame acquisition during ICA injection which may show the fistula in the early frames. However, in a significant subset of cases still, the fistula site remains elusive. A couple of maneuvers have been described which can aid us in identifying the ICA rent.

1. *Mehringer-Hieshima maneuver*: In this maneuver, the ipsilateral common carotid artery (CCA) is compressed manually while taking the ICA run. This prevents the diluting affect of blood coming from below through the CCA and helps in increasing the chance of fistula identification.
2. *Huber/Alcock maneuver*: Herein, manual compression of ipsilateral CCA is done while taking the dominant vertebral artery run.[29] Contralateral ICA run also serves the same purpose. In this case, the blood flows retrogradely from the basilar to involved ICA through the posterior communicating artery or from the contralateral ICA through the anterior communicating artery and lines the outline of the involved ICA and hence the rent **(Figs. 7A and B)**.

In addition, other tests are often performed prior to embolization procedure which include visual acuity, intraocular pressure measurement, fundoscopy and gonioscopy.

INDICATIONS OF TREATMENT

The indications for treatment depends on a number of factors like the patient's general physical condition, severity of the symptoms and the fistula anatomy as the latter decides the treatment modality. As a general rule, type A fistulae almost always require treatment as they rarely

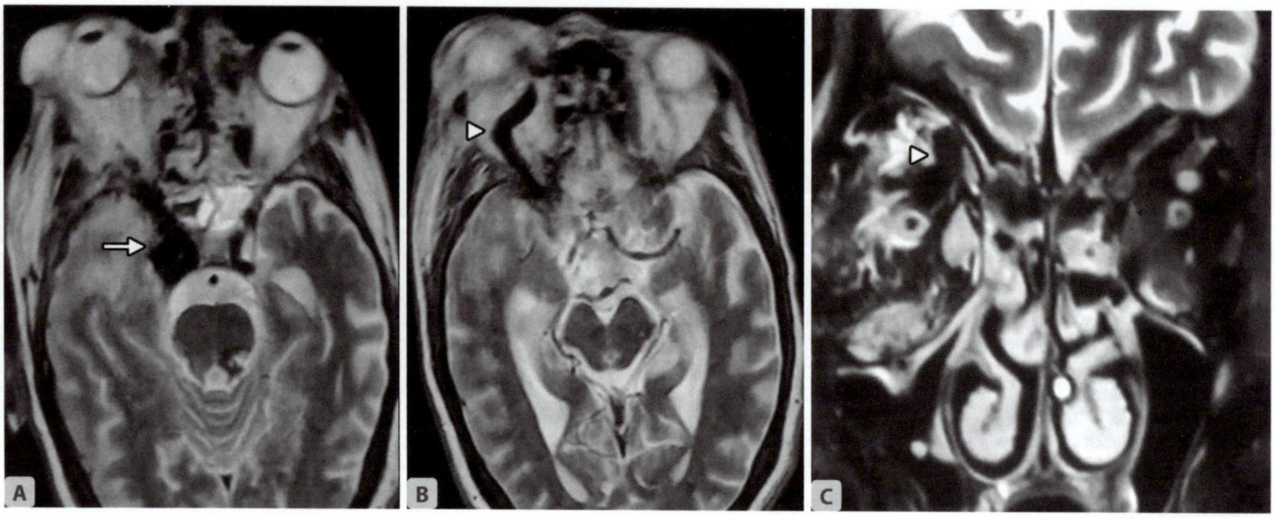

FIGS. 5A TO C: Axial T2 (A and B) and coronal T2-weighted (C) images demonstrating the dilated cavernous sinus (white arrow) and superior ophthalmic vein (arrowhead) in a case of direct caroticocavernous fistula. Note the proptosis, extraocular muscle enlargement and orbital congestion. Note the left superior cerebellar peduncle hemorrhagic contusion.

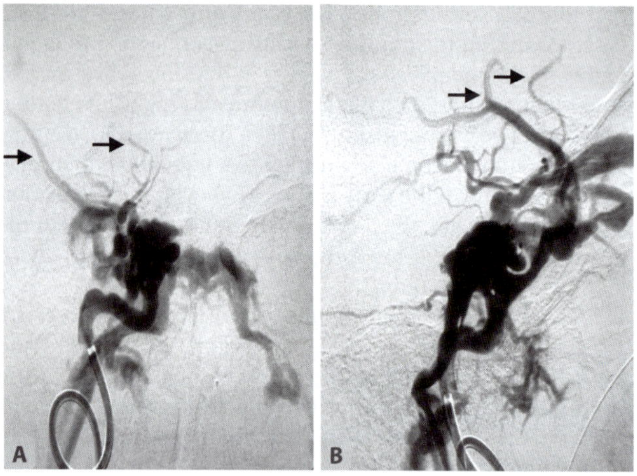

FIGS. 6A AND B: Digital subtraction angiogram frontal (A) and lateral (B) projection showing a high flow direct CCF with non-visualization of the anterior and middle cerebral arteries. A large quantity of blood is being shunted into the cavernous sinus and its drainage routes. Note the poor visualization of the ICA rent and significant cortical venous reflux (arrows) which demand urgent treatment.

resolve spontaneously. Definite indications for treatment are progressive visual loss, uncontrolled glaucoma, intolerable headache/bruit/tinnitus, enlargement of the fistula, epistaxis or signs of cerebral ischemia.[30] Another strong indication is presence of cortical venous reflux which indicates an increased tendency for subarachnoid or parenchymal hemorrhage.

Controversy still exists over the natural history and treatment of indirect CCFs. Several authors have reported that many of these patients will have alleviation of symptoms from spontaneous thrombosis with time, and therefore, treatment should not be instituted. Although indirect dural CCFs tend to be low flow and low-pressure lesions as compared to direct CCFs, follow-up with serial ophthalmologic examinations have shown progressive visual deterioration in such patients. Current recommendation in patients with dural CCFs without rapidly progressive visual deterioration, evidence of abnormal cortical venous drainage, hypoxic ocular changes involving the retina and optic nerve or ischemic keratopathy, is to give a trial of manual carotid artery jugular vein compression therapy first. If patients do not respond to this therapy and continue to have symptoms of visual disturbance, headache, diplopia, and chemosis, then embolization therapy is warranted.

TREATMENT OPTIONS

As discussed in the opening section, the treatment of direct CCF has evolved tremendously over the last century. There are 3 basic methods to manage such patients—conservative, endovascular and surgical. The type of fistula determines the choice of treatment.

Conservative treatment may be attempted in slow flow indirect type fistulae and involves subjecting the patient to a trial of carotid compression.[31] The procedure involves manual occlusion of the affected carotid with opposite hand for 10 seconds three times an hour while the patient is awake. The occlusion time is gradually increased. This maneuver is proposed to induce thrombosis and fistula closure subsequently. Complete resolution of symptoms has been reported in 2–34% of indirect CCF patients. Even without thrombosis, a large number of patients experience significant improvement with conservative treatment alone.

The previous surgical techniques of ligation and proximal embolization have gone out of repute due to the significant risks involved. *Surgical treatment,* in fact, is reserved in only those patients who donot respond to endovascular means.

Endovascular treatment remains an excellent minimally invasive technique which has shown consistently good results over a period of time. The main goal of the treatment is to occlude the fistula without compromising the parent artery. Both arterial and venous access routes are available,

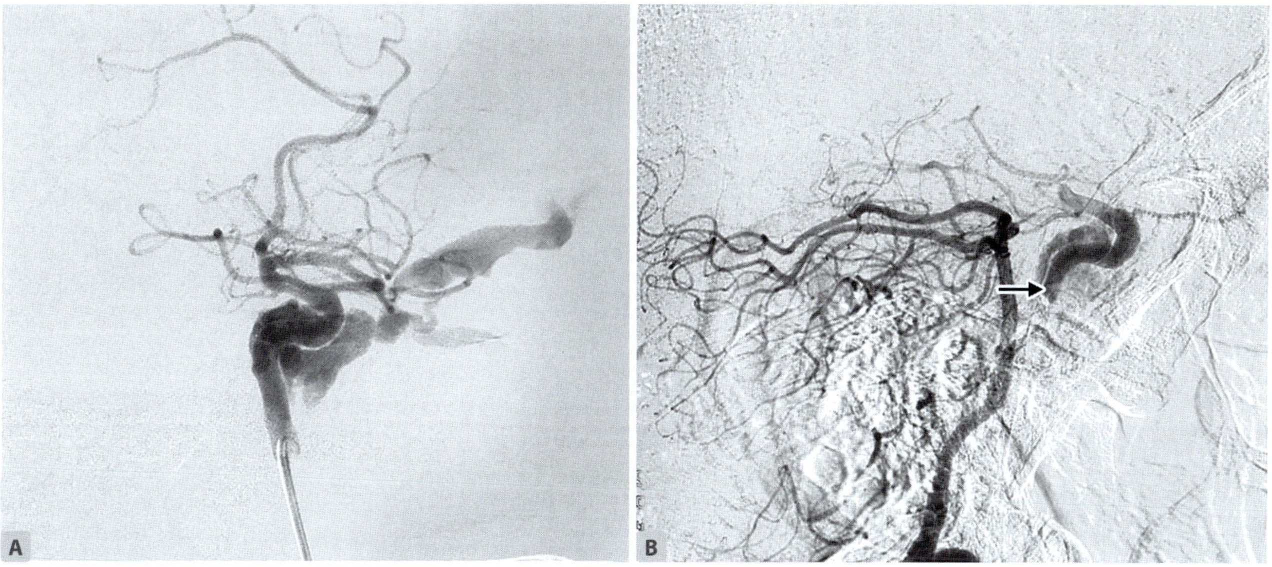

FIGS. 7A AND B: Frontal ICA (A) and lateral verterbal; (B) angiograms in a direct CCF displaying the cavernous sinus opacification simultaneously as that of the internal carotid artery with poor delineation of the rent. Huber maneuver demonstrating the site of rent (arrow) through retrograde flow into the ICA through the posterior communicating artery.

the former has been shown to offer less complications. In polytrauma patients with CCF, the more life-threatening injuries should be addressed prior to embarking upon the fistula closure surgery. Before the surgery is planned and executed, the patients are invariably administered steroid to take care of the inflammation. Additionally, pharmacological treatment is advised for raised intraocular pressure.

ENDOVASCULAR MANAGEMENT

Because the diagnosis is clinical, angiography is usually reserved as the first step of the therapeutic procedure. Local anesthesia with mild sedation is preferred to allow test occlusion of the ICA, but general anesthesia may be necessary in children and uncooperative patients. Anticoagulation is obtained with heparin bolus of 3-5,000 units, followed by 1,000 units every hour in an adult.

The CS is characterized by early filling, which may obscure detection of the shunt; hence, an ICA angiogram with high-speed imaging is necessary. Injection into the vertebral artery (VA) in the lateral view demonstrates retrograde flow into ICA through the posterior communicating artery, moving toward the CCF, if there is a complete arterial steal. If not, compression of the ICA during injection of the VA enhances retrograde flow into the ICA and reveals the exact location of the shunt as described in the previously described maneuvers **(Figs. 7A and B)**. The size of the CS is also an important consideration. Chronic CCFs show progressive enlargement of the CS making the procedure more difficult. Alternatively, a small CS does not necessarily mean easy selective occlusion. Because a small CS corresponds to a small rent and balloon catheterization in such cases may be difficult. Hence, coils may be preferable. The coils can be deployed either through the arterial or through the venous route and the CS is packed close to the rent so that the fistula is obliterated. There have also been reports of stent assisted coiling and covered stents **(Figs. 8A to G)** for fistula closure.[32,33] These options were chosen in cases where the fistula is large or the exact site of the rent is not clear.

The success rates of endovascular management have continued to improve over the last few decades as more experience and expertise has been gained in the field of interventional neuroradiology. Still, as with any neurovascular procedure, complications may occur which include thromboembolic and ischemic events due to catheter, balloon or coil manipulation, injury to the blood vessel, or inadvertent balloon detachment, pseudoaneurysm formation due to balloon deflation or migration and alteration of arterial flow resulting in hemorrhage, edema, or worsening of ocular symptoms.

Tools and Hardware

The tools currently available for use in endovascular treatment include detachable balloons, coils, stents, balloon catheters (for directing microcatheter and coils across the rent), flow diverters, liquid embolics, particles and vascular micoplugs. The optimal and widely practiced treatment of CCFs is embolization by detachable balloons or coils. Since the year 1974 when Serbinenko first reported the use of detachable balloons for occlusion of these fistulae, we have come a long way in devising other embolic agents which are more convenient to use and associated with less complication rates. Of the embolic agents currently available to us in the neurointerventional armamentarium, liquid embolic agents such as N-butyl cyanoacrylate (NBCA) are rarely indicated, whereas particulate agents are not suited to the occlusion of the large arteriovenous shunt of a direct CCF, but have been used for treatment of type B, C, D fistulae.

Extensively used since their inception, balloons are the favored devices for treatment of CCFs[34] because in medium-sized CCFs (which constitute the majority of these fistulae),

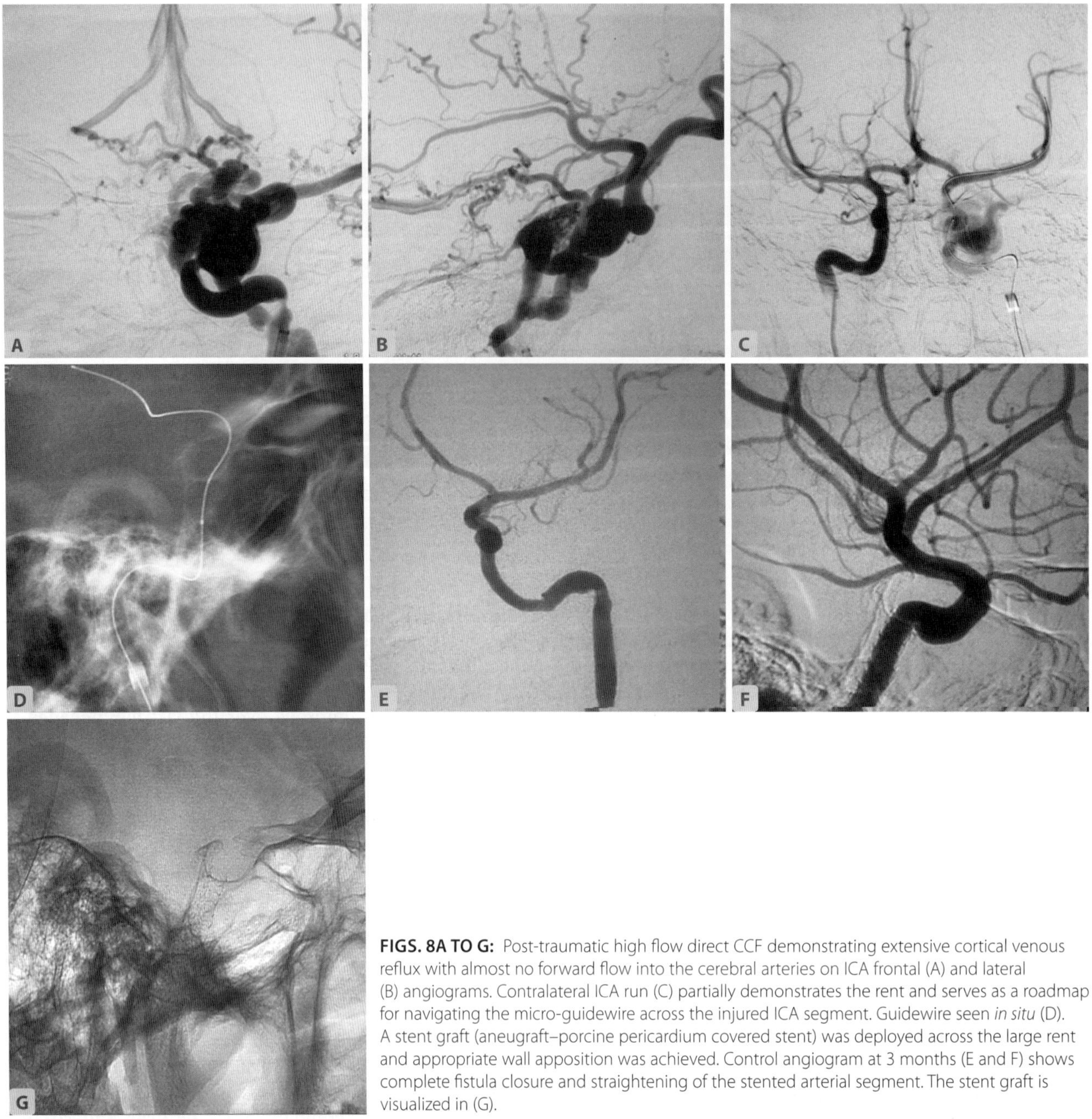

FIGS. 8A TO G: Post-traumatic high flow direct CCF demonstrating extensive cortical venous reflux with almost no forward flow into the cerebral arteries on ICA frontal (A) and lateral (B) angiograms. Contralateral ICA run (C) partially demonstrates the rent and serves as a roadmap for navigating the micro-guidewire across the injured ICA segment. Guidewire seen *in situ* (D). A stent graft (aneugraft–porcine pericardium covered stent) was deployed across the large rent and appropriate wall apposition was achieved. Control angiogram at 3 months (E and F) shows complete fistula closure and straightening of the stented arterial segment. The stent graft is visualized in (G).

a single balloon can occlude the rent while entirely sparing the ICA **(Figs. 9A to F)**. Nycomed-Ingenor (Paris, France) and Balt (Monomorency, France) manufactured latex balloons, some with a self-sealing valve (Gold valve) and others without it. Some interventionists prefer the silicone balloon (Interventional Therapeutics, San Francisco, CA, USA). Most of these balloons were mounted over a microcatheter and a few older ones had to be secured with a hand-made ligature. These balloons are detached by giving traction over the microcatheter. Balloons were available in various sizes and volumes ranging from 0.1 mL to 3 mL.

Metallic coils come in various sizes and shapes and are mostly platinum based, a biocompatible, radiopaque, and nonferromagnetic material. They can be pushed through a microcatheter and on exiting resume their original circular or/helical shape. Some delivery systems allow coils to be retracted into the microcatheter if placement is unsatisfactory. The Guglielmi detachable coils (GDC) (Boston Scientific) are electrically detached **(Figs. 10A to D)**. Coils with controlled detachment, such as GDC, should be used when inadequate placement has a risk of occluding the ICA whereas mechanically detachable coils (MDC), interlocking detachable coils (IDC) or regular coils (cheaper, more thrombogenic and less time-consuming) can be used when there is little risk of migration, as is the case in most transvenous occlusions or in assorted type B, C and D fistulae.

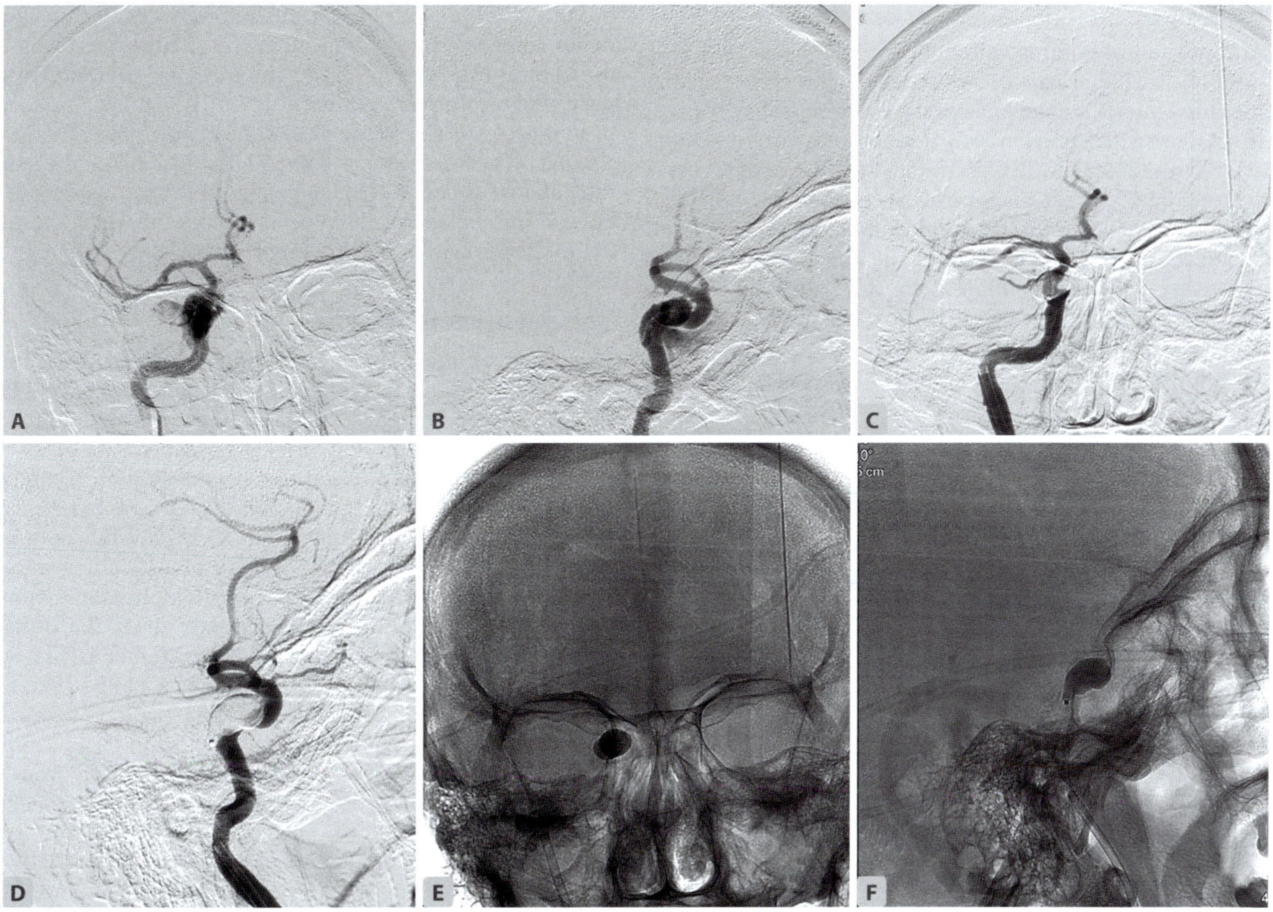

FIGS. 9A TO F: Post-traumatic low flow CCF treated with detachable balloon. Pre- (A and B) and post-embolization (C and D) angiograms displaying fistula closure. The hyperdense balloon is visualized partially within the cavernous sinus across the ICA rent (E and F).

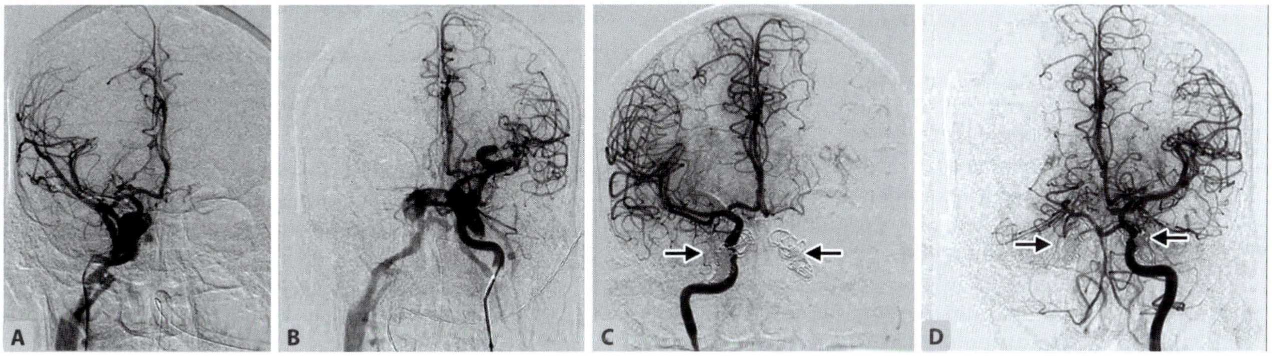

FIGS. 10A TO D: Bilateral traumatic direct CCF treated with endovascular coil embolization. Pre- (A and B) and postembolization (C and D) angiograms revealing complete fistula closure. Note the arrows pointing towards the coil mass.

In recent times, liquid embolic agents like nBCA and 'Onyx', a polymer which precipitates upon contact with blood has been used successfully by some authors both by transarterial as well as transvenous approach.[35-39] Particles like gelfom and polyvinyl alcohol can be used in slow flow indirect fistulae where venous washout is very slow. Flow diverters have been deployed across the rent by few authors[40] with reasonable results.

Transarterial Embolization

Most direct CCFs can be treated by placing a detachable balloon/coils transarterially, through the rent in the ICA wall, and then selectively into the CS, obstructing the fistula while preserving ICA flow. Occasionally, the rents in the ICA are multiple or very large, necessitating carotid occlusion. In children, navigating large size balloons is difficult and hence coil embolization perhaps is preferable.

Procedure

A transfemoral guiding catheter of suitable size (6–9 F) is positioned in the ipsilateral ICA through which the wire/balloon mounted microcatheter or a coaxial assembly is introduced. In a patient with a previously ligated carotid artery, the direct arterial route to the CCF is unavailable, but arterial access is still possible by direct puncture of the cervical ICA or through the anterior or posterior communicating artery.[41] The balloon is guided into the CCF by pushing the microcatheter and, if necessary, by slightly inflating and deflating the balloon to benefit from the preferential flow into the CCF. Once the balloon is in the CS, it is progressively inflated while performing frequent angiographic controls until the CCF is occluded. If there is mild or no ICA stenosis, the balloon is detached, either by gentle traction or by coaxial detachment **(Figs. 9A to F)**. Many large series have described the use of balloons by transarterial approach in CCF with excellent results.[42-44] These series show similar positive results after transarterial balloon embolization of direct CCFs. Overall, cure was obtained in 85–90%, with ICA patency preserved in 59–80% and neurologic complications in 4–5%, of which 2% were permanent. When the CS is large, several balloons may be needed. If coils have been decided to be placed in the CS, the microcatheter tip is guided into the CS and coiling started once a stable position of the tip is reached **(Figs. 10A to D)**. At times when the rent is not easily discernible or it is large, a balloon catheter (hyperglide, scepter C, etc.) may need to be used to outline the parent artery lumen and the rent and for guiding the microcatheter across the rent. Liquid embolic (onyx) may be used at times to complete the CS occlusion by placing the balloon across the rent in the parent artery so that there is no reflux into the ICA and subsequent stroke. Occasionally, there can be extensive skull base fractures leading to CCF on both sides **(Fig. 10A to D)**. In such instances, both the ICAs are individually accessed and the fistulae are embolized by either coils or balloons.

Occasionally, selective balloon occlusion of the CCF is not possible, and the ICA must also be occluded **(Figs. 11A to I)**. ICA occlusion is also mandated when the fistula persists or recurs. A 30-minute balloon test occlusion (BTO) should be done first except in cases of complete cerebral steal from the CCF. Next, both the ICA and the CCF must be occluded, and one must avoid occluding the ICA without occluding the CCF as well. The safest way is to occlude the ICA beyond and proximal to the carotid rent by either detachable balloons or coils. Occlusion of the CCF can be confirmed before balloon detachment by vertebral angiography with a catheter through the contralateral femoral artery. With CCF occlusion, there will be no retrograde flow through the posterior communicating artery into the ICA toward the CCF. When there is extensive damage to the blood vessel with active hemorrhage or a rapidly expanding hematoma of the soft tissues, it is usually not possible to preserve the parent vessel. In these instances, test occlusion across or distal to the tear should first be performed, if possible, to determine the individual tolerance of each patient to occlusion of a major cerebral vessel. Subsequently it may be sacrificed if the patient tolerates the BTO. The presence of underlying persistent primitive trigeminal artery (PTA) has been noticed in two cases of traumatic CCF at our centre over the last 5 years. Whether it was a coincidental finding or it made the patient prone to CCF is debatable. The anatomy in such cases has to be clearly delineated before embarking on the neurointervention procedure **(Figs. 12A to J)**.

Transvenous Embolization

The transvenous approach is indicated only after the transarterial approach fails because of a higher risk of venous rupture and hemorrhage.[45] Because the veins are enlarged and subjected to high flow, they are weaker than arteries and more likely to rupture during catheterization. There is also an increased risk of placing the embolic material at a distance from the fistula itself or redirecting flow into cortical veins. The CCF is accessed through one of its draining veins, generally the IPS **(Figs. 13A to L)** or the ophthalmic vein, whichever seems the easiest to catheterize on the initial angiogram. For IPS access, a guiding catheter is placed into the internal jugular vein at the level of the jugular bulb from a transfemoral venous access or direct cervical jugular puncture. A second possibility is to approach via the superior ophthalmic vein (SOV) and the angular vein from a transfemoral catheterization or if necessary, from a surgically exposed ophthalmic vein.[46] Once the microcatheter has reached the CS, it is guided toward the CCF. Embolization begins with blockage of the venous drainage of the CS, starting with the cortical draining veins if present. Coils are the embolic agent of choice for transvenous embolization, but balloons can be used, if access permits.

Parent Artery Reconstruction

There are instances when the artery needs to be reconstructed. The aim is to exclude the CCF from the circulation. For this purpose, covered stents may be used **(Figs. 8A to G)**. However, dedicated neurovascular covered stents are currently not available. Carotid stent grafts are stiff and not easily maneuverable across the carotid siphon. They find use when there is no other option and artery needs to be preserved. Apart from covered stents, there has been description of deployment of flow diverters with coils/in isolation with favorable results.

Follow-up

The fistula may not be fully embolised. Some angiographic residual flow, if present, is not an indication for an attempt at achieving complete angiographic cure. The goal of treatment is to alleviate the patient's symptoms and not offer a complete cure on angiogram. Follow-up DSA may be done after 3–4 months if there is no significant improvement in patient's symptoms.

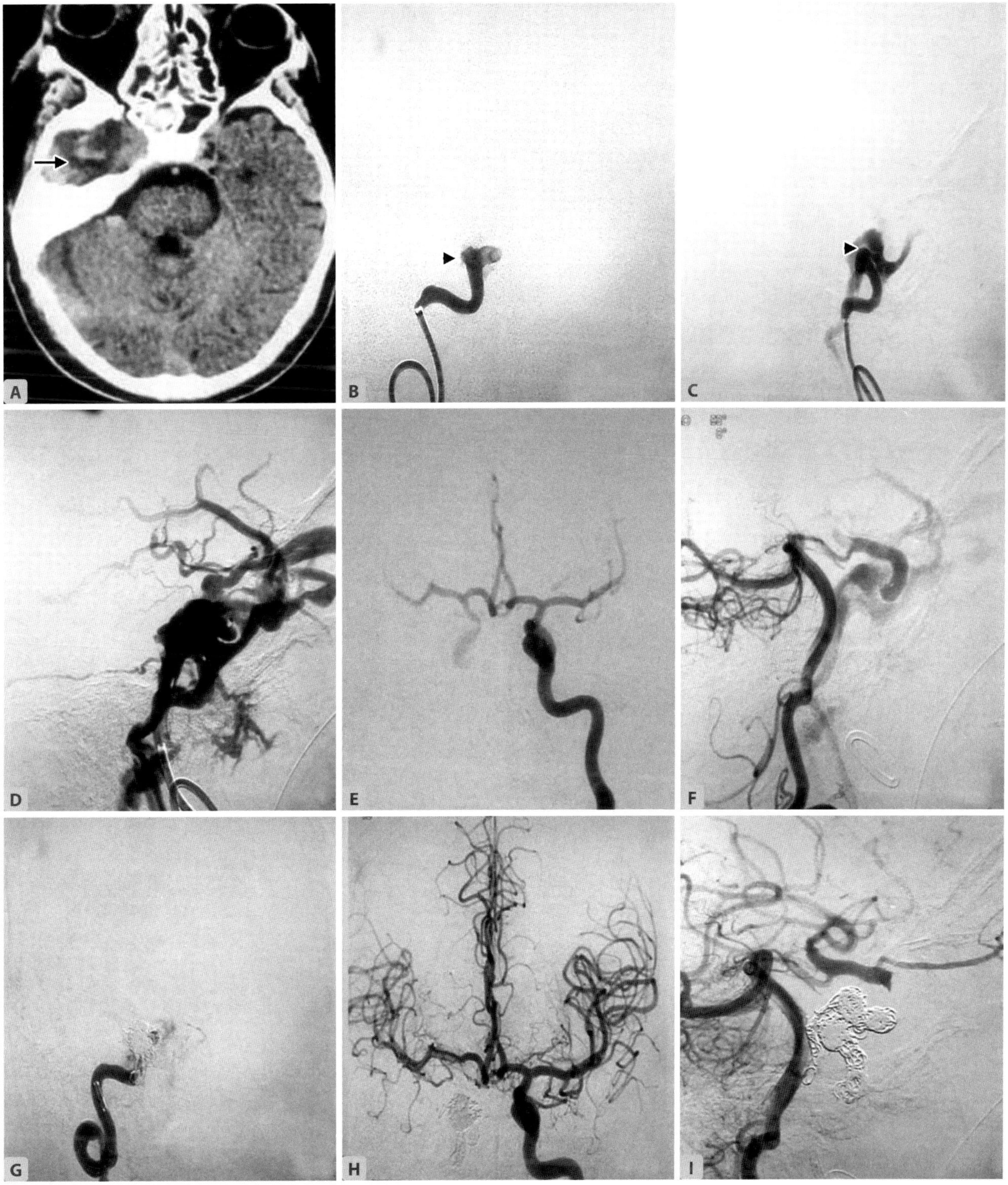

FIGS. 11A TO I: Post-traumatic high flow direct CCF (Barrow type A) showing the temporal contusion (arrow) on computed tomography. Frontal (B) and lateral (C) angiograms demonstrating a large ICA rent (arrowheads) with significant cortical venous reflux and poor downstream cerebral arterial blood flow (D). Contralateral ICA (E) and vertebral angiograms (F) help in delineating the fistula. Endovascular coiling was attempted but there was constant high flow into the cavernous sinus. Balloon test occlusion was performed and the patient was subjected to parent artery occlusion (PAO) (using the sandwich technique across the ICA rent) once the test was tolerated well. Control angiograms following PAO obtained from the ipsilateral ICA (G), contralateral ICA (H) and vertebral artery (I) showed no fistula opacification with good distal flow in the MCA through the anterior and posterior communicating arteries.

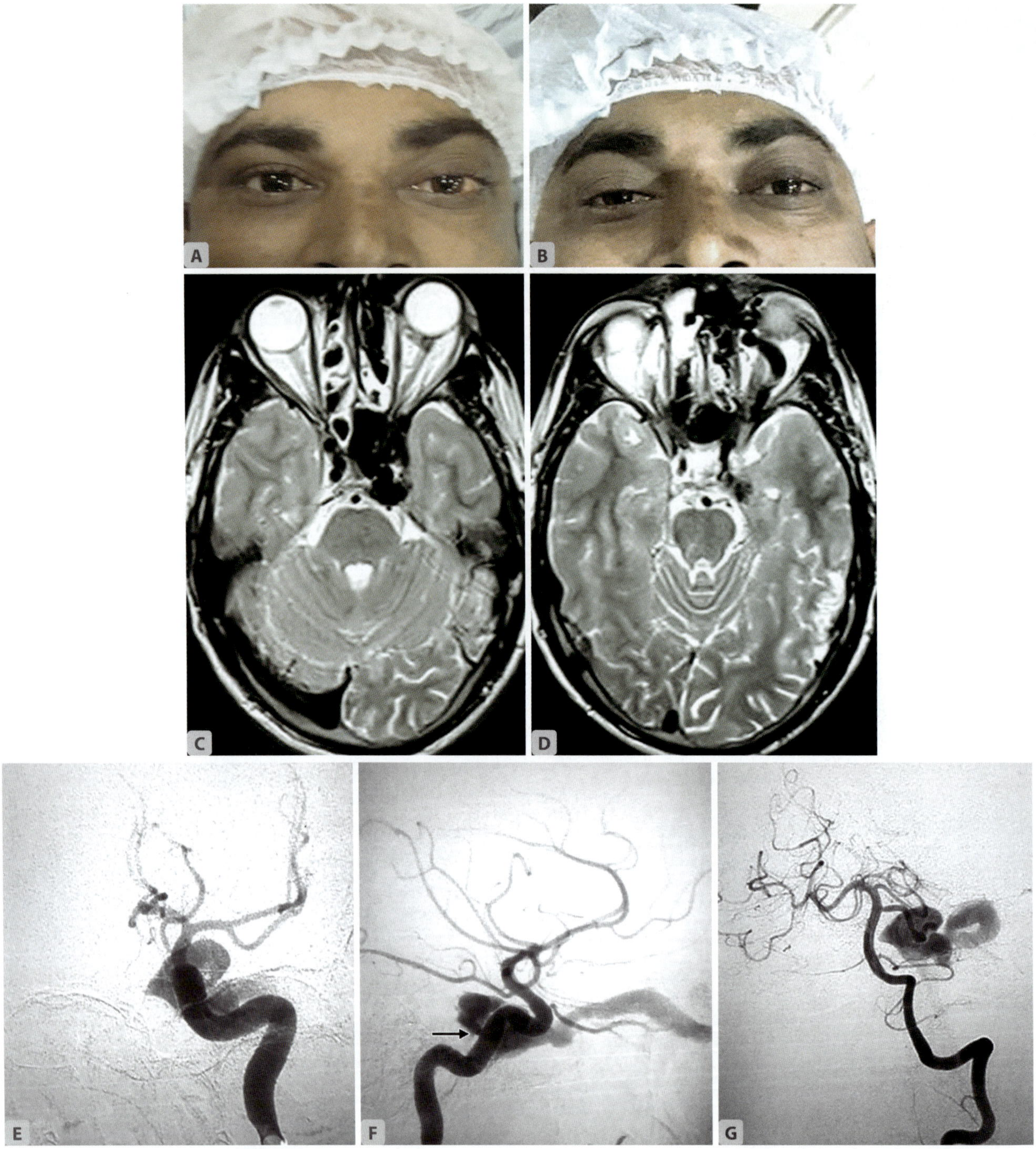

FIGS 12A TO J: *Continued*

CONCLUSION

Interventional neurovascular techniques continue to be at the helm and form the preferred mode of treatment for CCF. The goal of therapy is to occlude the fistulae involving the carotid artery with preservation of the parent vessel. Endovascular coil embolization is the current technique of choice.

ACKNOWLEDGEMENT

The authors acknowledge Dr NK Mishra, former author of this chapter for integral contribution in the revised chapter.

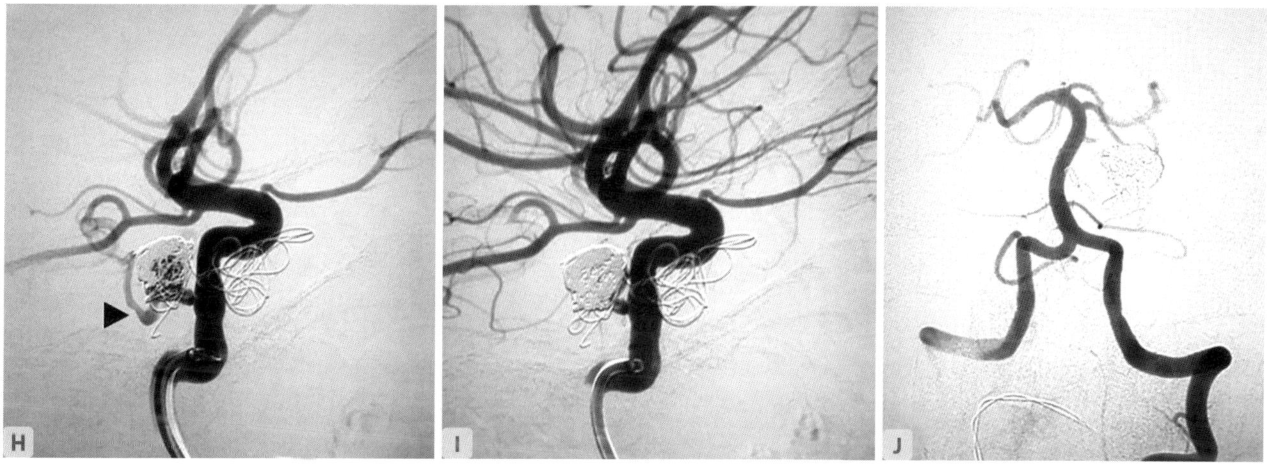

FIGS 12A TO J: Clinical photograph of a patient with traumatic trigeminocavernous fistula prior to (A) and following embolization (B) shows good clinical response. Axial T2-weighted images (C and D) demonstrating the bulky left cavernous sinus with dilated superior ophthalmic vein. Frontal (E) and lateral (F) ICA runs demonstrating the opacification of the cavernous sinus through a small stump (arrow) arising from the C5 segment. Verterbal artery run (G) similarly demonstrates the arterial channel arising from the distal basilar trunk and leading to the cavernous sinus. Following partial coiling of the cavernous sinus close to the rent (H), the persistent trigeminal artery is better visualized (arrowhead). Control angiograms following complete embolization show complete fistula closure with only small stumps on the ICA as well as basilar trunk side (I and J).

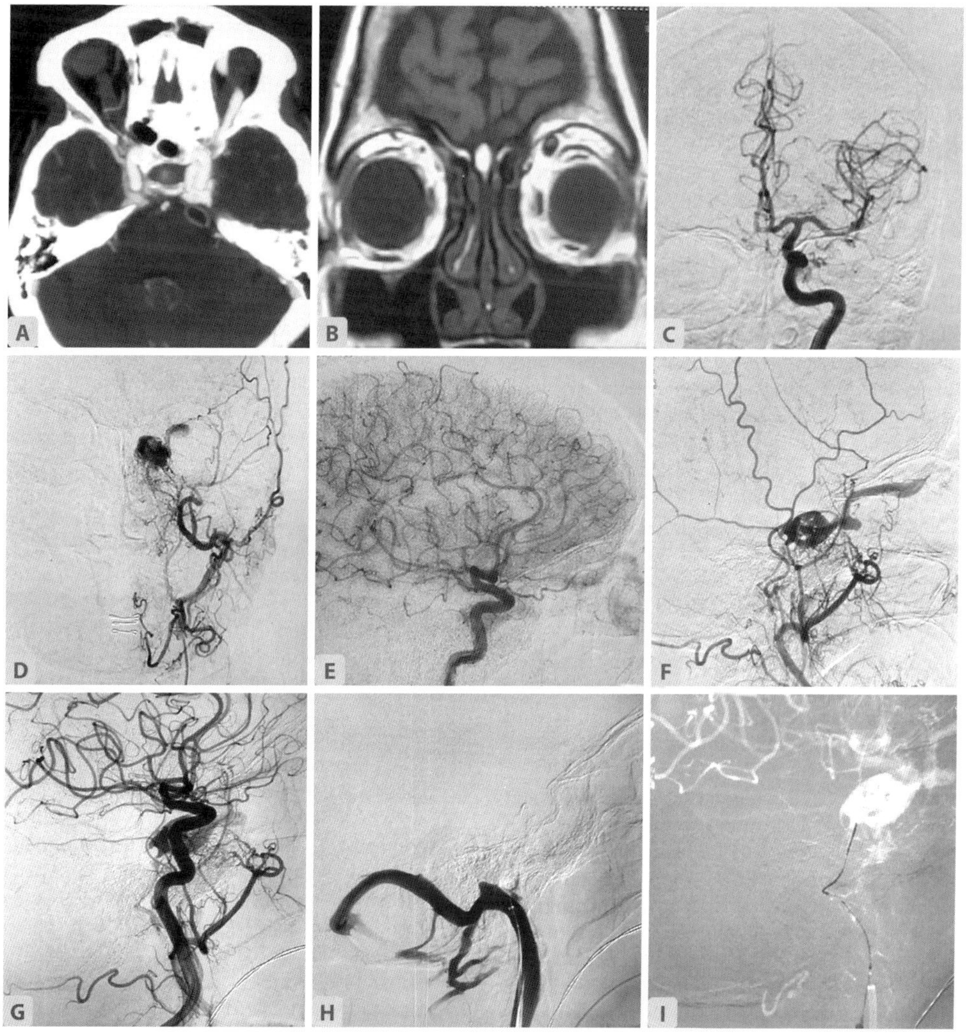

FIGS. 13A TO L: *Continued*

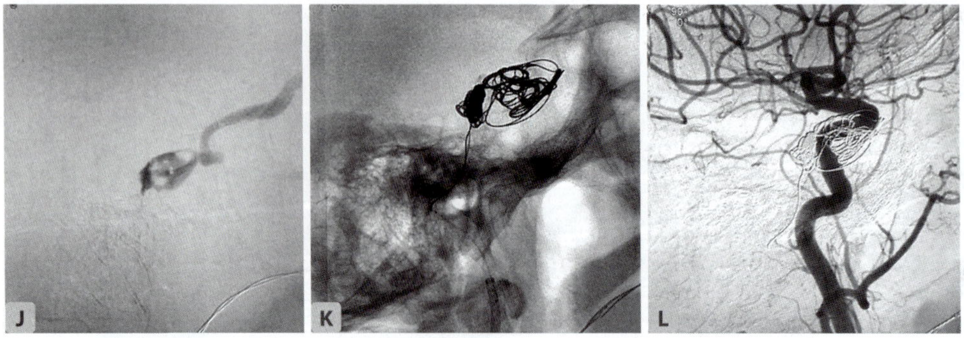

FIGS. 13A TO L: A middle aged female patient presented with long-standing orbital congestive changes. CT angiography (A) shows bulky left cavernous sinus and dilated SOV which was confirmed on coronal T1-weighted MRI (B). Left ICA injection (C and E) shows faint cavernous sinus opacification. The external carotid artery injection demonstrates the venous opacification clearly (D and F), Diagnosis of Barrow type D CCF was made and the patient was subjected to coil embolization through the transvenous route. Preprocedure common carotid angiogram (G) and internal jugular venogram (H) helped in guiding the microcatheter (I). Cavernous sinogram (J) showing the dilated SOV. Progressive coiling of the sinus was done (K) resulting in complete fistula closure as demonstrated on control CCA injection (L) following the procedure.

REFERENCES

1. Pool JL. Carotid-Cavernous Fistula. Arch Neurol. 1967; 16(1):111.
2. Hamby WB. Carotid Cavernous Fistula, Springfield, IL: Charles C Thomas, 1966.
3. Serbinenko FA. Balloon catheterization and occlusion of major cerebral vessels. J Neurosurg. 1974;41:125-45.
4. Mullan S. Treatment of carotid-cavernous fistulas by cavernous sinus occlusion. J Neurosurg. 1979;50:131-44.
5. Guglielmi G, Viñuela F, Briganti F, et al. Carotid-cavernous fistula caused by a ruptured intracavernous aneurysm: endovascular treatment by electrothrombosis with detachable coils. Neurosurgery. 1992;31:591-7.
6. Hirai T, Korogi Y, Goto K, et al. Carotid-cavernous sinus fistula and aneurysmal rupture associated with fibromuscular dysplasia: a case report. Acta Radiol. 1996;37: 49-51.
7. Mitsuhashi T, Miyajima M, Saitoh R, et al. Spontaneous carotid-cavernous fistula in a patient with Ehlers-Danlos syndrome type IV—case report. Neurol Med Chir (Tokyo) 2004;44:548-53.
8. Yamamoto T, Asai K, Lin YW, et al. Spontaneous resolution of symptoms in an infant with a congenital dural caroticocavernous fistula. Neuroradiology. 1995;37:247-9.
9. Parkinson D. Transcavernous repair of carotid cavernous fistula: case report. J Neurosurg. 1967;26:420-4.
10. Helmke K, Kruger O, Laas R. The direct carotid-cavernous fistula: a clinical, pathoanatomical, and physical study. Acta Neurochir. 1994;127:1-5.
11. Lasjaunias P, Berenstein A. Surgical Neuroangioraphy, Springer-Verlag; 1987. pp. 175-234.
12. Bullock R, Van Dellen J. Acute carotid-cavernous fistula with retained knife blade after transorbital stab wound. Surg Neurol. 1985;24:555-8.
13. Ahuja A, Guterman LR, Hopkins LN. Carotid cavernous fistula and false aneurysm of the cavernous carotid artery: complications of transsphenoidal surgery. Neurosurgery. 1992;31:774-9.
14. Revuella R, Nathal E, Balderrama J, et al. External carotid artery fistula due to microcompression of the gasserian ganglion for relief of trigeminal neuralgia. Case report. J Neurosurg. 1993;78:499-500.
15. Flandroy P, Lenelle J, Collignon J, et al. Carotid cavernous fistula associated with Fogarty catheter angioplasty. Am J Neuroradiol. 1988;9:1242.
16. Barr JD, Mathis JM, Horton JA. Iatrogenic carotid-cavernous fistula occurring after embolization of a cavernous sinus meningioma. Am J Neuroradiol. 1995;16:483-5.
17. Newton TH, Hoyt WF. Dural arteriovenous shunts in the region of the cavernous sinus. Neuroradiology. 1970;1: 71-81.
18. Taniguchi RM, Goree JA, Odom GL. Spontaneous carotid-cavernous shunts presenting diagnostic problems. J Neurosurg. 1971;35:384-91.
19. Narita Y, Watanabe Y, Hoshino T, et al. Myelopathy due to large veins draining recurrent spontaneous caroticocavernous fistula. Neuroradiology. 1992;34:433-5.
20. Acierno MD, Trobe JD, Cornblath WT, Gebarski SS. Painful oculomotor palsy caused by posterior-draining dural carotid cavernous fistulas. Arch Ophthalmol. 1995;113:1045-9.
21. Grumann AJ, Boivin-Faure L, Chapot R, et al. Ophthlamologic outcome of direct and indirect carotid cavernous fistulas. Int Ophthalmol 2012;32:153-9.
22. Rhoton AL Jr, Inoue T. Microsurgical approach to the cavernous sinus. Clin Neurosurg. 1989;37:391-439.
23. Dolenc VV. Direct microsurgical repair of intracavernous vascular lesions. J Neurosurg. 1983;58:824-31.
24. Barrow DL, Spector RH, Braun IF, et al. Classification and treatment of spontaneous carotid-cavernous sinus fistulas. J Neurosurg 1985;62:248-56.
25. Chi CT, Nguyen D, Duc VT, et al. Direct traumatic carotid cavernous fistula: angiographic classification and treatment strategies. Study of 172 cases. Interv Neuroradiol. 2014;20(4): 461-75.
26. Thomas AJ, Chua M, Fusco M, et al. Proposal of Venous Drainage-Based Classification System for Carotid Cavernous Fistulae With Validity Assessment in a Multicenter Cohort. Neurosurgery. 2015;77(3):380-5.
27. Chung JW, Chang KH, Han MH, et al. Computed tomography of cavernous sinus diseases. Neuroradiology. 1988;30(4):319-28.
28. Uchino A, Hasuo K, Matsumoto S, et al. MRI of dural carotid-cavernous fistulas: comparisons with postcontrast CT. Clin Imaging. 1992;16:263-8.
29. Huber P. A technical contribution of the exact angiographic localization of carotid cavernous fistulas. Neuroradiology. 1976;10:239-41.

30. Halbach VV, Hieshima GB, Higashida RT, et al. Carotid- cavernous fistulae: indications for urgent treatment. Am J Roentgenol. 1987;149:587-93.
31. Higashida RT, Hieshima GB, Halbach VV, et al. Closure of carotid cavernous sinus fistulae by external compression of the carotid artery and jugular vein. Acta Radiol Suppl. 1986;369:580-3.
32. Archondakis E, Pero G, Valvassori L, et al. Angiographic follow-up of traumatic carotid cavernous fistulas treated with endovascular stent graft placement. Am J Neuroradiol 2007;28(2):342-7.
33. Tiewei Q, Ali A, Shaolei G, et al. Carotid cavernous fistulas treated by endovascular covered stent grafts with follow-up results. Br J Neurosurg. 2010;24:435-40.
34. Debrun G, Lacour P, Vinuela F, et al. Treatment of 54 traumatic carotid-cavernous fistula. J Neurosurg. 1981;55: 678-92.
35. Arat A, Cekirge S, Saatci I, et al. Transvenous injection of Onyx for casting of the cavernous sinus for the treatment of a carotid-cavernous fistula. Neuroradiology. 2004;46:1012-5.
36. Wakhloo AK, Perlow A, Linfante I, et al. Transvenous n-butyl-cyanoacrylate infusion for complex dural carotid cavernous fistulas: technical considerations and clinical outcome. Am J Neuroradiol. 2005;26:1888-97.
37. Baccin CE, Campos CM, Abicalaf R, et al. Traumatic carotid-cavernous fistula: endovascular treatment with Onyx and coils. Interv Neuroradiol. 2005;11:363-7.
38. Luo CB, Teng MM, Chang FC, et al. Transarterial balloon-assisted n-butyl-2-cyanoacrylate embolization of direct carotid cavernous fistulas. Am J Neuroradiol. 2006;27:1535-40.
39. Suzuki S, Lee DW, Jahan R, et al. Transvenous treatment of spontaneous dural carotid-cavernous fistulas using a combination of detachable coils and Onyx. Am J Neuroradiol. 2006;27:1346-9.
40. Iancu D, Lum C, Ahmed ME, et al. Flow diversion in the treatment of carotid injury and carotid-cavernous fistula after transsphenoidal surgery. Interventional Neuroradiology. 2015;21(3):346-50.
41. Garcia-Cervigon E, Bien S, Laurent A, et al. Treatment of a traumatic carotid cavernous fistula: vertebro-basilar approach after surgical occlusion of the internal carotid artery. Neuroradiology. 1988;30:355-7.
42. Lewis AK, Tomsick TA, Tew JM Jr. Management of 100 consecutive direct carotid-cavernous fistulas. results of treatment with detachable balloons. Neurosurgery. 1995; 36:239-45.
43. Higashida RT, Halbach VV, Tsai FY, et al. Interventional neurovascular treatment of traumatic carotid and vertebral artery lesions: results in 234 cases. Am J Roentgenol. 1989;153:577-82.
44. Kendall B. Results of treatment of arteriovenous fistulae with the Debrun technique. Am J Neuroradiol. 1983;4:405-8.
45. Halbach VV, Higashida RT, Hieshima GB, et al. Transvenous embolization of direct carotid-cavernous fistulas. Am J Neuroradiol. 1988;9:741-7.
46. Quinones D, Duckwiler G, Gobin YP, et al. Embolization of dural cavernous fistulas via superior ophthalmic vein approach. Am J Neuroradiol. 1997;18:921-8.

CHAPTER

193

Central Nervous System Infections

Sapna Singh, Gaurav Shanker Pradhan, Anju Garg, Anjali Prakash

INTRODUCTION

Despite advancements in antibiotic therapy, infections of the central nervous system continue to be a major cause of mortality and morbidity. The brain, its surrounding membranes and the subarachnoid space provide an anatomic and functional barrier to the spread of pathogens. However, there are certain structural peculiarities of the central nervous system (CNS).

The factors that account for a unique response of CNS to microorganisms include:

a. Absence of true lymphatics
b. Absence of capillaries in the subarachnoid space.
c. Presence of diploic and emissary veins which provide a direct intercommunication between the intra- and extra-cranial venous system.
d. Differences in the vascular supply between grey and white matter.
e. Deficiency of immunoglobulin and complement making cerebrospinal fluid an excellent culture medium for bacterial growth.

CRANIAL MENINGES AND EXTRA-AXIAL SPACES

The osseous and membranous coverings, that is the pachymeninx (dura) and the leptomeninges (pia-arachnoid), the blood brain and the blood cerebrospinal fluid (CSF) barriers protect the brain from direct spread of infections and disease processes. The pachymeninx or the duramater is a thick tough structure composed of dense connective tissue. The outer layer is highly vascularized and is not of true meningeal origin while the inner dural layer is derived from the meninx. The falx cerebri, the falx cerebelli, tentorium cerebelli are all reflections of the true inner layer of the cranial dura mater.[1] The leptomeninges are constituted by the arachnoid and piamater. The arachnoid is closely apposed to the inner layer of the dura while the piamater covers the cerebral sulci and fissures and carries a vast network of vessels. While the normal parietal duramater is not normally visualized on imaging studies, the normal falx cerebri and tentorium cerebelli may be seen on a normal T1- and T2-weighted MR image as a thin membrane. The epidural space is the space between the dura and the inner table of the skull while subdural space is between the dura and the arachnoid. The subdural space is a potential space containing bridging veins and arachnoid villi. The arachnoid is separated from the pia by the subarachnoid space which contains the CSF.

In normal meninges, enhancement is seen as a thin, markedly discontinuous rim covering the surface of the brain and is most prominent parasagittally. This enhancement is primarily in the dura.[2,3] Thin, linear, well-demarcated and symmetric enhancement may sometimes be seen in the sulci because of enhancing veins.[4] Abnormal meningeal enhancement is asymmetrical, longer and continuous, extends deep into the base of the sulci and is not as sharply demarcated as normal meningeal enhancement **(Table 1)**.

Meningeal enhancement present on more than three contiguous MR images is considered abnormal.[6]

On contrast administration, short segments of enhancing duramater can be visualized on normal MR imaging. Pachymeningeal or dural enhancement occurs along the calvarial contours while enhancement along the cerebral and

TABLE 1: Differences between normal and abnormal meningeal enhancement.[5]

Normal meningeal enhancement	Abnormal meningeal enhancement
Symmetric	Asymmetric
Sharply demarcated	Not well-demarcated
Thin and smooth	Thick, irregular or nodular
Short and discontinuous	Long and continuous
Superficial	Extends deep into the base of sulci
No enhancement in suprasellar cisterns	Enhancement may be seen in suprasellar cisterns
No enhancement of ventricular walls	Enhancement in ventricular walls may be seen

cerebellar sulci and fissures constitutes leptomeningeal or the pial subarachnoid type of enhancement. Enhancement along the brainstem is always of the pial subarachnoid space type. A pachymeningeal or dural enhancement may result from intracranial hypotension, transient postoperative changes, following lumbar puncture, infections, sarcoidosis and even metastasis. Leptomeningeal enhancement which has a gyriform or serpentine appearance is usually associated with meningitis, neoplastic disease and inflammatory diseases (e.g. sarcoidosis).[7] Normal cranial nerves never enhance within the subarachnoid space. Any enhancement of the cranial nerves is always abnormal.

The various infectious agents can be classified as bacterial, viral, parasitic and fungal.

BACTERIAL/PYOGENIC INFECTIONS

Bacteria can reach meninges either by hematogenous route, local extension, direct implantation of microorganisms which is usually due to trauma or by transmission along cranial nerves. Rarely, the infection may be iatrogenic in nature as during cranial surgery or when microbes are introduced with a lumbar puncture needle.

Causative Organisms

The causative bacteria vary according to the age of patient. *Escherichia coli* and group B streptococci are the most common organisms in neonates, Haemophilus influenzae prevails in infants and children, while Neisseria meningitides is most commonly encountered in adolescents and young adults. *Streptococcus pneumoniae* and Listeria monocytogenes are the commonest organisms in the elderly. Eighty percent of the reported cases of meningitis are caused by *H. influenzae, N. meningitides* and *S. pneumoniae.*[8,9] *Klebsiella* and anaerobic bacteria constitute the causative organisms in immunosuppressed or immunocompromised patients.

Pathophysiology

The earliest changes in meningitis begin in the meningeal and cerebral capillaries. The permeability of the blood brain barrier increases resulting in vasogenic edema. The inflammatory mediators in the meningeal exudate and parenchymal hypoxia contribute to cytotoxic edema.[10] The meningeal inflammation then spreads through the basal subarachnoid cisterns and over the cerebral hemispheres which may cause thrombosis of the superficial pial arteries and veins with consequent infarction and resultant focal signs, such as hemiparesis, dysphasia and visual field deficits. The accumulation of inflammatory basilar exudate along the course of nerves through the subarachnoid space results in cranial nerve palsies with the III, VI and VIII cranial nerves being most commonly involved.

Further spread of the inflammation results in ventriculitis which further spreads to involve the walls of the leptomeningeal veins and eventually the substance of the brain resulting in focal meningoencephalitis.

PYOGENIC MENINGITIS

Clinical Features

The clinical findings include headache, photophobia, neck stiffness, irritability and loss of consciousness. The typical triad is of fever, neck stiffness and altered mental status with nearly 100% of patients having one of the three symptoms.[11,12] The cerebrospinal fluid in pyogenic meningitis is turbid with a marked decrease in glucose (<40 mg%) and a marked increase in the protein value (>250 mg%). There is marked pleocytosis with a predominance of polymorphonuclear leukocytes/neutrophils.

Imaging

Cross sectional imaging is neither sensitive nor specific for the detection of meningitis.[13] The role of neuroimaging in meningitis is to identify complications, rule out mimics of meningitis and increased intracranial pressure before lumbar puncture. The earliest positive finding may be slight hyperattenuation with sulcal effacement on a non-contrast CT scan but it may be subtle resulting in a false negative scan. On a fluid attenuated inversion recovery sequence (FLAIR), abnormal hyperintensity may be seen in the sulci due to increased protein content but this again is not a specific finding for meningitis.[14] The sulcal hyperintensity on a FLAIR sequence may be also caused by subarachnoid hemorrhage, CSF pulsations, acute stroke, motion or magnetic susceptibility artifacts and even leptomeningeal carcinomatosis and is hence non-specific **(Table 2)**.[15]

In early meningitis, no abnormality may be detected on imaging. The positive findings on imaging seen later in the course of the disease include leptomeningeal enhancement, enhancement along the fissures or sulci secondary to the presence of brain swelling and inflammatory exudates **(Figs. 1A and B)**. Postcontrast MR imaging is more sensitive than CT in detection of abnormal leptomeningeal enhancement and easily differentiates basal cisternal enhancement from vessels in the region of Circle of Willis. Owing to the inner table of the skull seen as a signal void on MR imaging, enhancement over the cerebral convexities is better seen on MR as compared to CT scanning. Postcontrast T1-weighted magnetization transfer (MT) imaging is superior to the conventional T1-weighted images in detecting meningeal

TABLE 2: Causes of sulcal hyperintensity on FLAIR.[15]
• Subarachnoid hemorrhage
• Meningitis
• Susceptibility/flow artifacts
• CSF metastasis
• Stroke
• Pial angioma
• High inspired oxygen
• Ruptured dermoid

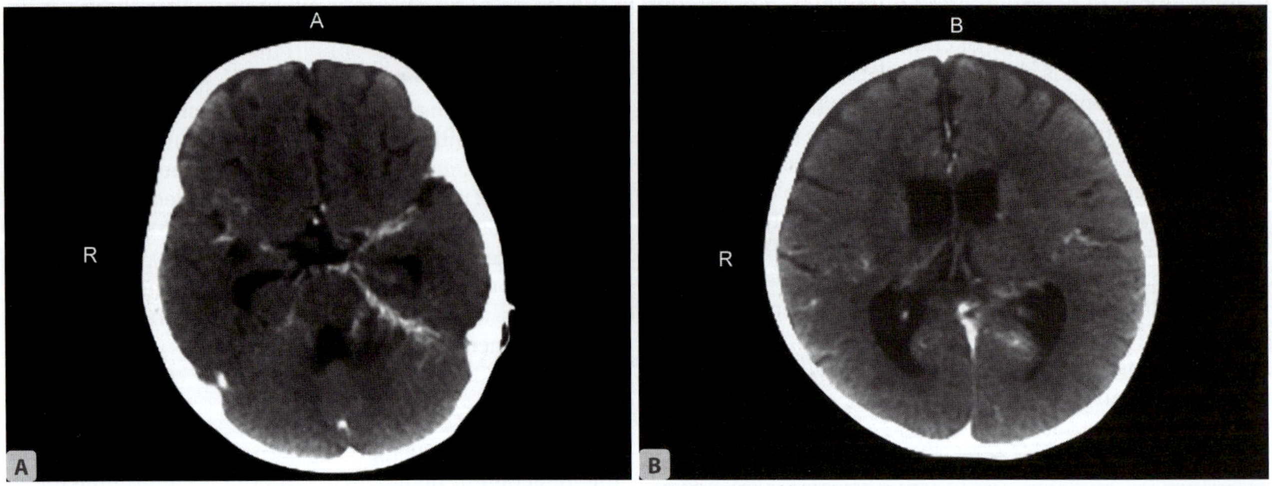

FIGS. 1A AND B: CECT axial scans of the cranium revealing irregular, shaggy enhancement along the tentorium, the basal cisterns and Sylvian fissures with dilated temporal horns and early hydrocephalus—pyogenic meningitis.

enhancement.[16] A differentiation between infective and neoplastic enhancement is important as the two may appear similar on imaging studies. A diffuse, thin, regular sheet like enhancement over the brain surface suggests an inflammatory aetiology whereas an irregular, nodular enhancement favors a neoplastic cause.[4]

Diffusion Tensor Imaging in the Diagnosis of Meningitis

DTI is a relatively new MR imaging technique which provides tissue microstructural information. Fractional anisotropy (FA) and mean diffusivity (MD) are the most commonly used DTI derived metrics. Increased FA values have been reported in both enhancing and non-enhancing cortical regions in pyogenic meningitis.[17,18] The high FA values have been attributed to the diffuse inflammatory activity in meningitis. The orientation of the inflammatory cells in the pia arachnoid causes the high FA values. The high FA values may be used as a surrogate marker of inflammatory molecules in meningitis and DTI has been found to be superior to postcontrast T1W images in the diagnosis of meningitis.

COMPLICATIONS OF BACTERIAL MENINGITIS

There are several complications or alternative manifestations of bacterial meningitis. These are: 1. Hydrocephalus, 2. Extra-axial fluid and pus collections, 3. Cerebritis and abscess, 4. Central nervous system infarction, 5. Cranial nerve involvement, and 6. Ventriculitis.

Hydrocephalus

Hydrocephalus occurs more commonly in children and adults and occurs due to the inflammatory debris blocking the flow and resorption of the CSF.[19] This occurs more commonly at the level of the arachnoid villi. Obstruction at the level of the cerebral aqueduct or the foraminal outflow of the lateral or fourth ventricles due to exudates may also result in hydrocephalus **(Figs. 2A to C)**.[20] A focal parenchymal lesion which compresses ventricular drainage is classified as an extraluminal obstructive type.

The hydrocephalus that develops in cases of meningitis may be irreversible at times inspite of medical treatment, for example, in cases of pneumococcal meningitis, copious amounts of the capsular polysaccharide of the organism produce a gelatinous exudate that leads to arachnoid fibrosis and chronic adhesive arachnoiditis.[21]

Extra-axial Fluid and Pus Collections

Both sterile and infected extra-axial collections may be associated with meningitis. A sterile subdural effusion or hygroma is the most common collection and occurs due to irritation of the pachymeninx by the infectious agent or its products or due to inflammation of the subdural veins with resultant increase in protein and fluid within the subdural space[22] **(Fig. 3)**. Subdural effusions may occur in the H. influenzae meningitis, are usually bilateral and crescent shaped. No specific treatment is required for the effusions, these usually resolve with specific therapy against the infectious agent.[23]

Subdural Abscess/Empyema

Ten to fifteen percent of subdural empyemas are a complication of meningitis. The most common location of subdural empyemas is the cerebral convexities and the interhemispheric fissure. Unenhanced CT scan reveals a crescentic or lentiform extra-axial fluid collection that is slightly denser than cerebrospinal fluid. An overlying peripheral rim of enhancement of varying thickness is identified after intravenous contrast administration **(Figs. 4A and B)**. This rim represents an inflammatory membrane of granulation tissue on the leptomeningeal surface bordering the empyema. Hypodensity with/without contrast enhancement of the adjacent brain parenchyma may also be seen secondary to thrombophlebitis of the bridging draining veins crossing the subdural space resulting in venous occlusion and venous infarction of the involved brain.[24]

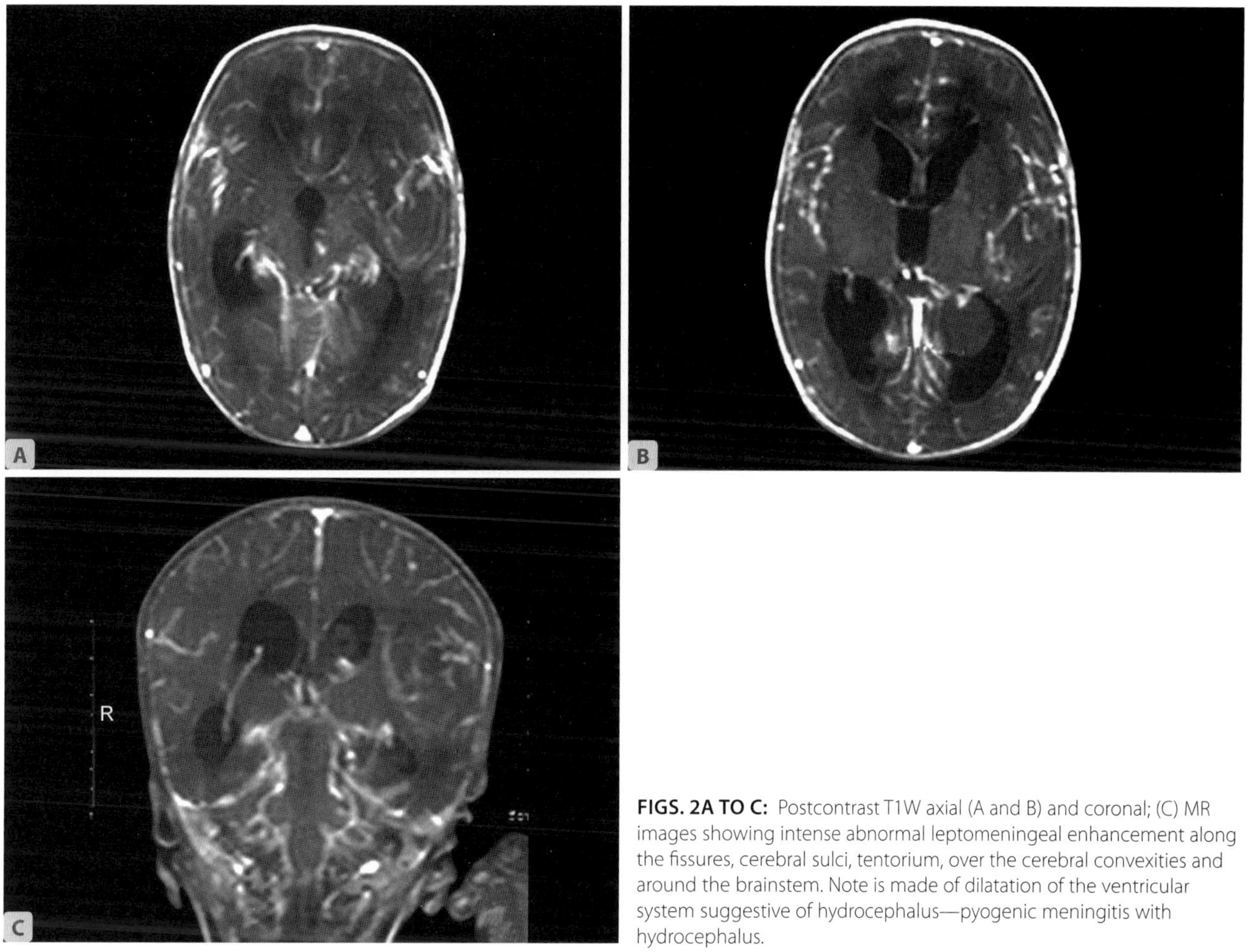

FIGS. 2A TO C: Postcontrast T1W axial (A and B) and coronal; (C) MR images showing intense abnormal leptomeningeal enhancement along the fissures, cerebral sulci, tentorium, over the cerebral convexities and around the brainstem. Note is made of dilatation of the ventricular system suggestive of hydrocephalus—pyogenic meningitis with hydrocephalus.

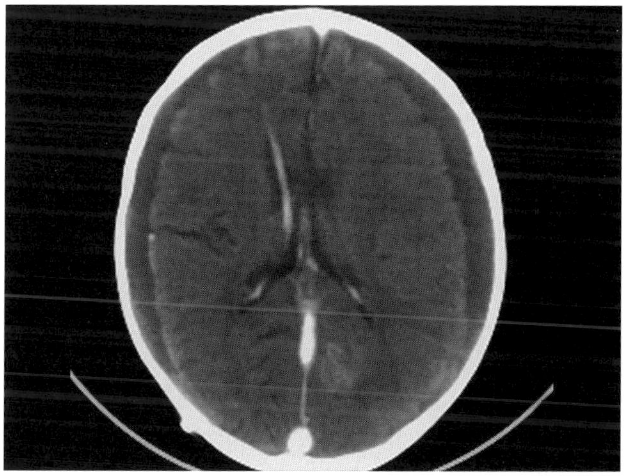

FIG. 3: CECT axial scan of the cranium showing bilateral crescent-shaped concavoconvex extra-axial fluid collections isodense to the cerebrospinal fluid in the parietal region. VP shunt is seen *in situ*—subdural effusions.

MR imaging is considered the modality of choice in the evaluation of subdural empyema.[25] In cases where the findings on CT scanning are equivocal, MR imaging helps differentiate between aseptic subdural effusions and infected subdural empyemas by virtue of the relatively shortened T1 relaxation times of purulent fluid in comparison with otherwise normal cerebrospinal fluid signal within a sterile subdural effusion. Subdural effusions are low-protein collections that are isointense relative to cerebrospinal fluid whereas empyemas are more proteinaceous and have higher MR imaging signal intensities than that of normal cerebrospinal fluid. After intravenous contrast administration, the internal and the external inflammatory membranes of subdural empyemas enhance on MR imaging **(Figs. 5A to C)**. The external membrane often is not appreciated on CT scanning because the adjacent radiodense skull obscures the contrast enhancement. When present concomitant parenchymal changes of edema and venous infarction are best visualized on T2-weighted or contrast-enhanced T1- weighted images. The most helpful imaging technique to identify an empyema

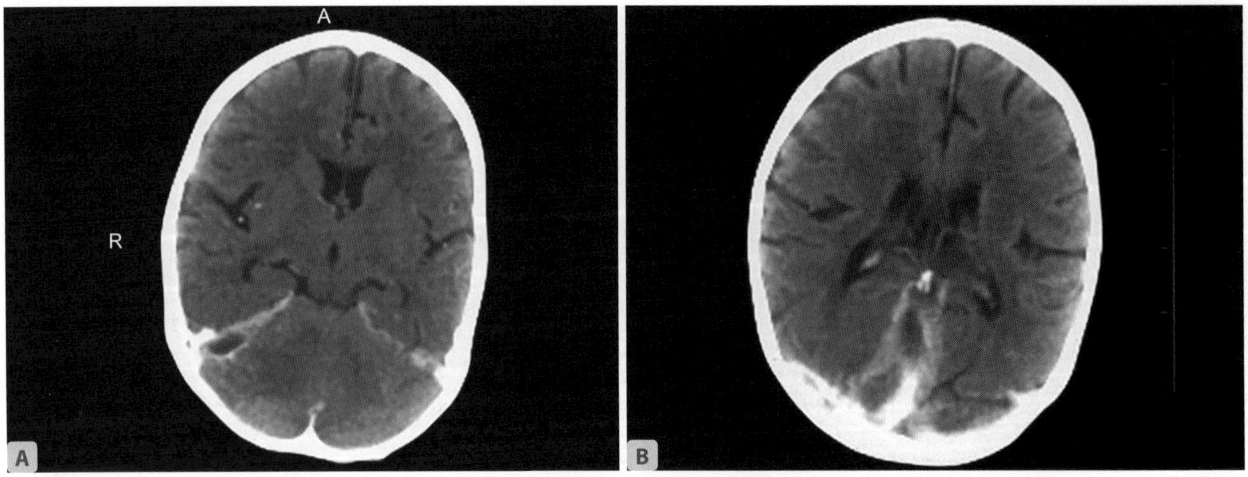

FIGS. 4A AND B: Contrast-enhanced axial CT scans reveal extra-axial collections along the tentorium and the interhemispheric fissure. The collections are crescent shaped with an enhancing rim—Subdural empyemas.

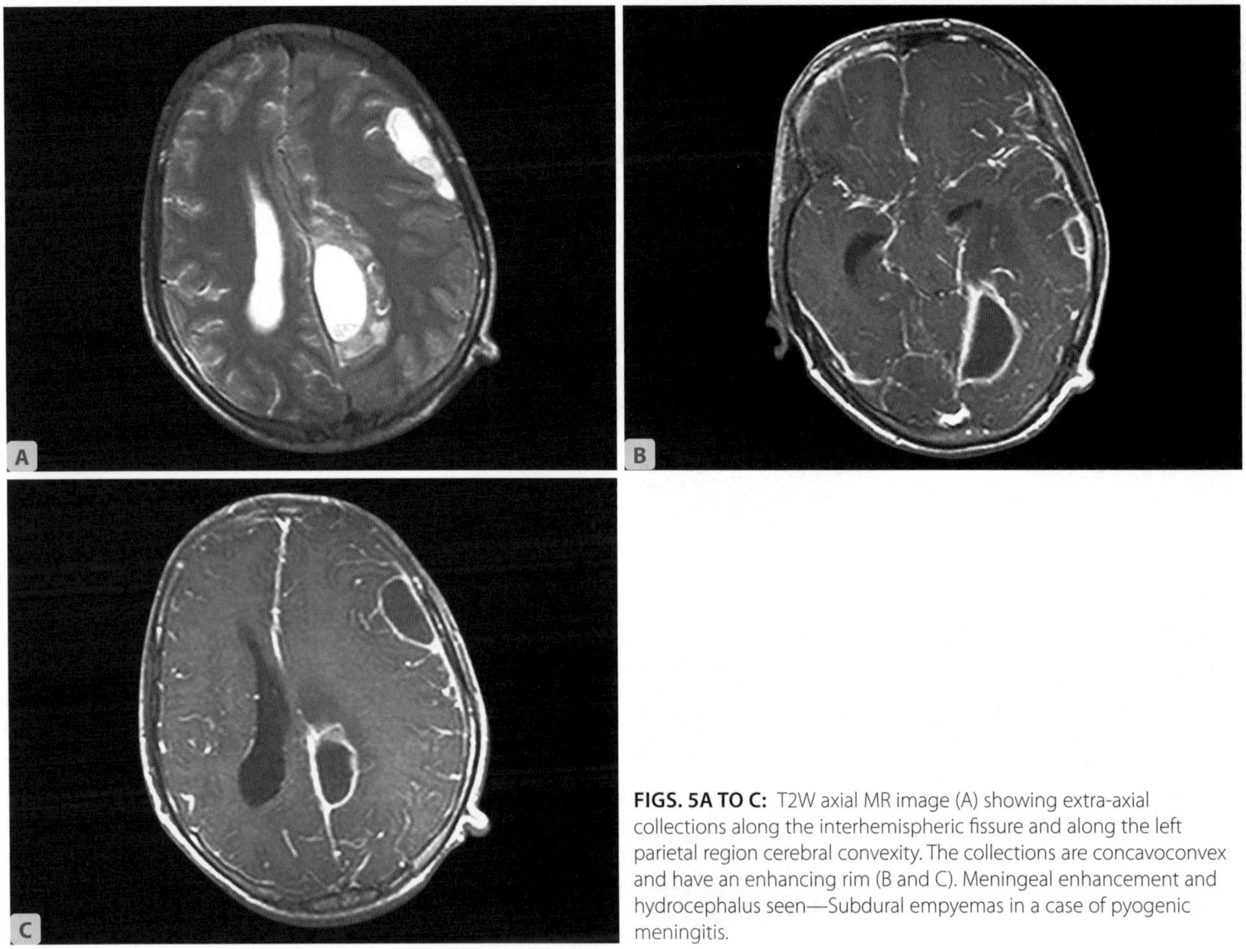

FIGS. 5A TO C: T2W axial MR image (A) showing extra-axial collections along the interhemispheric fissure and along the left parietal region cerebral convexity. The collections are concavoconvex and have an enhancing rim (B and C). Meningeal enhancement and hydrocephalus seen—Subdural empyemas in a case of pyogenic meningitis.

is diffusion-weighted imaging (DWI). Empyemas are very bright on DWI unlike effusions that are dark or only mildly bright **(Figs. 6 and 7)**. Empyemas need to be drained surgically.[26]

Epidural Abscess/Empyema

Epidural abscess associated with meningitis is most frequently seen in cases that result from direct extension of infection from an external source. In infants the extra-axial collections can

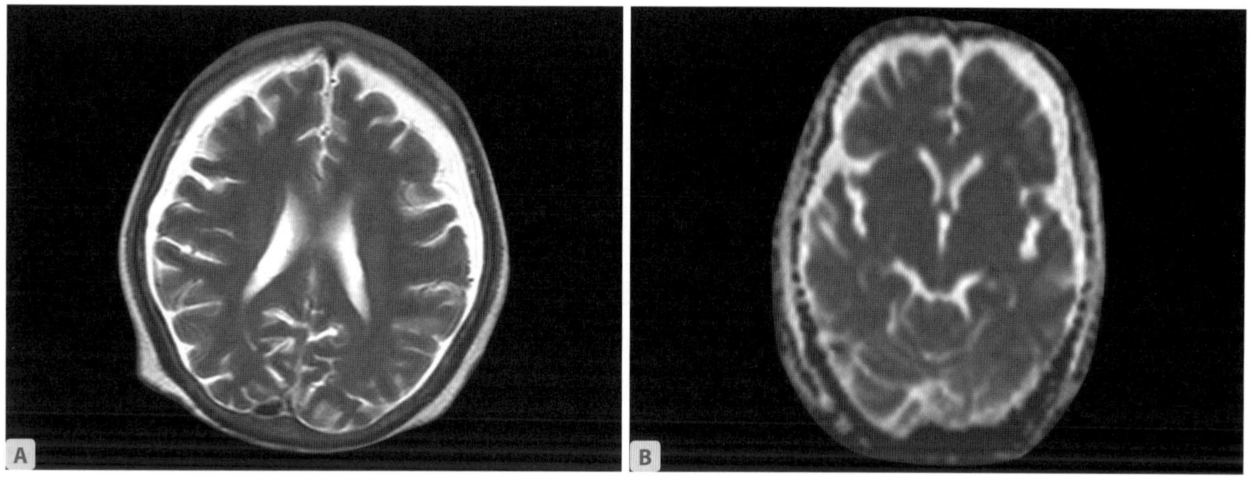

FIGS. 6A AND B: Axial T2W MR image (A) showing bilateral subdural effusions isointense to the CSF. Diffusion-weighted MR image (B) reveals no restricted diffusion.

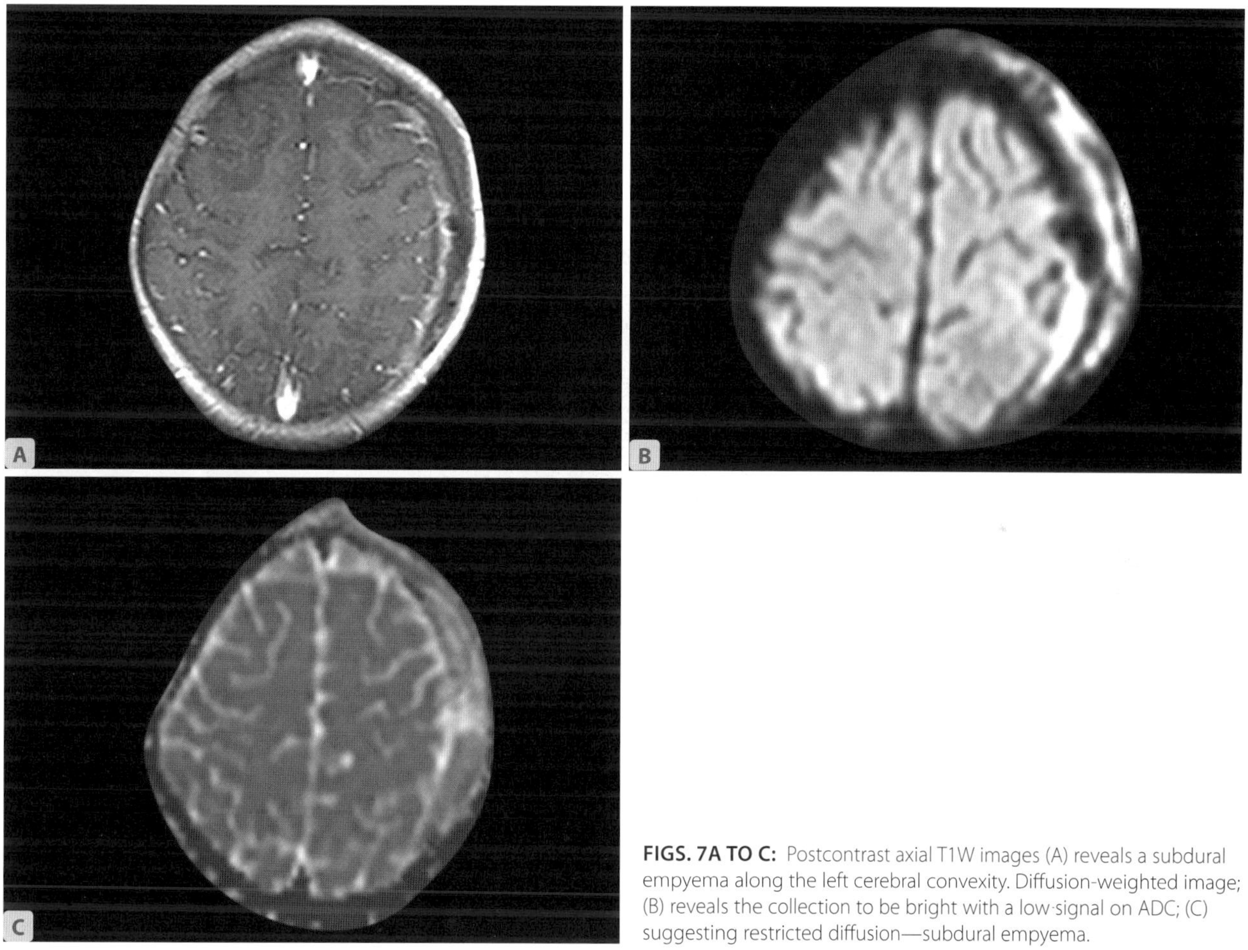

FIGS. 7A TO C: Postcontrast axial T1W images (A) reveals a subdural empyema along the left cerebral convexity. Diffusion-weighted image; (B) reveals the collection to be bright with a low signal on ADC; (C) suggesting restricted diffusion—subdural empyema.

be visualized on sonography as well. As in cases of subdural empyema, the CT density or MR signal intensity within the collection is usually higher than that of normal cerebrospinal fluid. The involved dura mater is thickened and shows marked enhancement after intravenous contrast administration. The dura itself can be detected on MR as a hypointense medial rim separating the fluid collection from the underlying brain parenchyma. The underlying brain parenchyma is usually normal because the dura acts as a strong barrier against further intracranial dissemination. Advanced or untreated cases, however, may eventually spread to the overlying brain by way of retrograde infectious thrombophlebitis.

Cerebritis and Abscess

Cerebritis is an area of acute inflammation in the brain parenchyma which is poorly defined. Though there is an increased permeability of the local blood vessels, there is no neovascularity or angiogenesis. If untreated, cerebritis progresses to abscess formation. A pyogenic brain abscess is a focal area of parenchymal infection containing pus in the center and vascularized collagenous capsule in the periphery.[27]

Brain abscesses can occur by direct extension or hematogenous route. A contiguous focus of infection is usually the cause for a brain abscess, e.g. an abscess in the temporal lobe or cerebellum is the result of chronic otitis media.[28] Chronic sinusitis, untreated dural tears, infections about the face and scalp and dental sepsis constitute the other causative factors for a direct spread. Direct spread occurs through involvement of bone or via emissary veins which are valveless.

The source of a hematogenous brain abscess may be a congenital cyanotic right to left shunt or pulmonary AVM, bacterial endocarditis, pulmonary abscess or intra-abdominal infections[29] **(Figs. 8A to C)**. Hematogenous brain abscesses have a distant focus of infection and show the following features:

- Multiple and multiloculated rather than solitary.
- Location at the corticomedullary junction/gray white matter junction.
- Poor encapsulation.
- Distribution along the middle cerebral artery (MCA)
- High mortality.

About 30% of brain abscesses are reported to be cryptogenic. Brain abscesses may occur secondary to trauma and neurosurgery. Diabetes mellitus, intravenous drug abuse, alcoholism, immunosuppression are the other predisposing factors. In infants and children, congenital malformations, such as meningomyelocele, encephalocele, ectodermal defects are the usual predisposing factors.

The evolution from cerebritis to abscess formation is a continuum. Four stages are involved—the stages of early cerebritis, late cerebritis, early capsule and late capsule formation.[30] In the first 4–5 days, that is, the early cerebritis stage, the organism grows within the parenchyma. The neutrophils migrate to the involved region to destroy the bacteria and edema occurs due to the opening of the blood brain barrier **(Figs. 9A to C)**. Punctate foci of hemorrhage may occur during this stage. Coalescence of the small areas of necrosis to produce a large necrotic focus results in the late cerebritis stage which is seen 7–10 days later. Satellite lesions surrounding the main abscess are seen during this stage. Development of a fibrous capsule to wall off the infection constitutes the early capsule stage which occurs

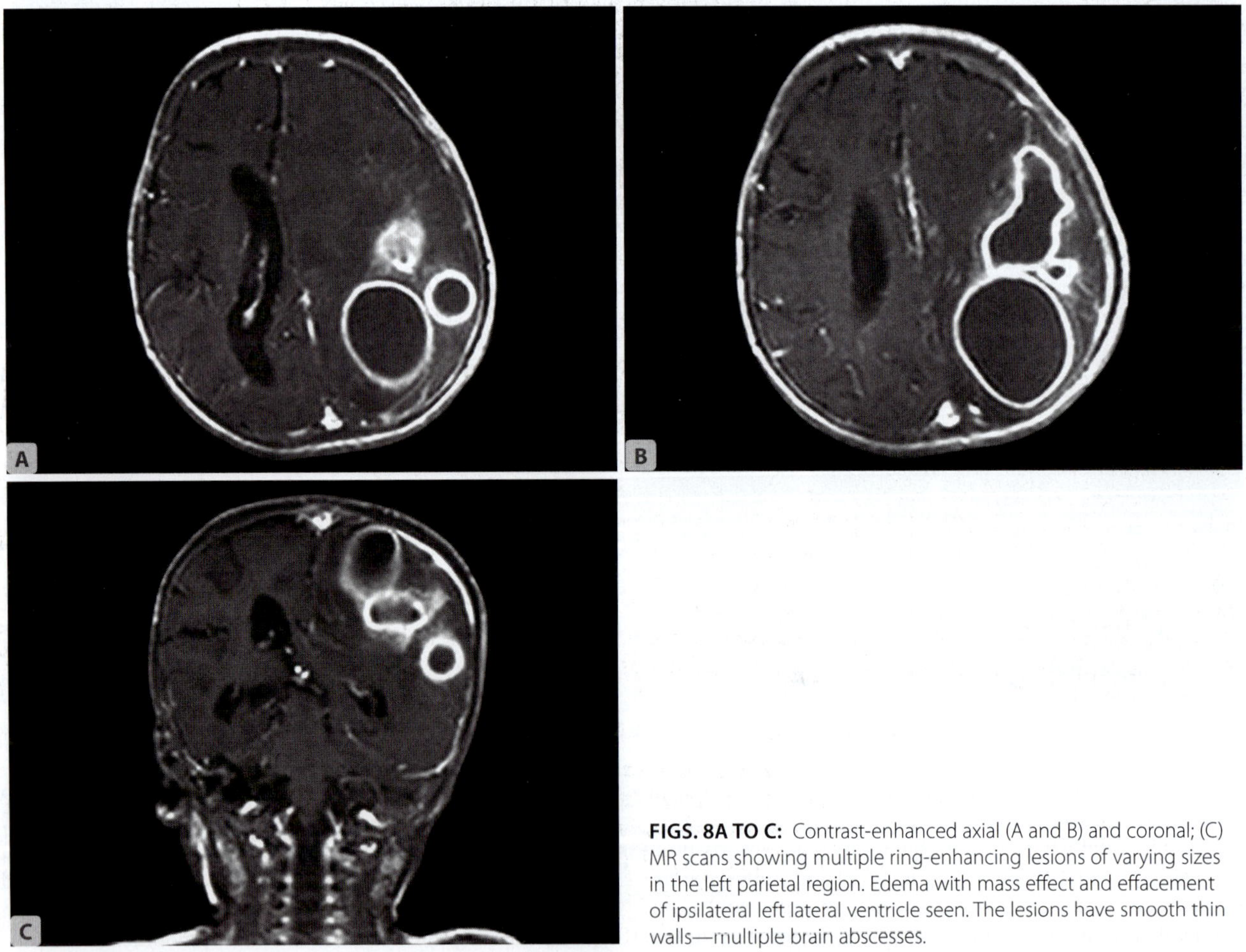

FIGS. 8A TO C: Contrast-enhanced axial (A and B) and coronal; (C) MR scans showing multiple ring-enhancing lesions of varying sizes in the left parietal region. Edema with mass effect and effacement of ipsilateral left lateral ventricle seen. The lesions have smooth thin walls—multiple brain abscesses.

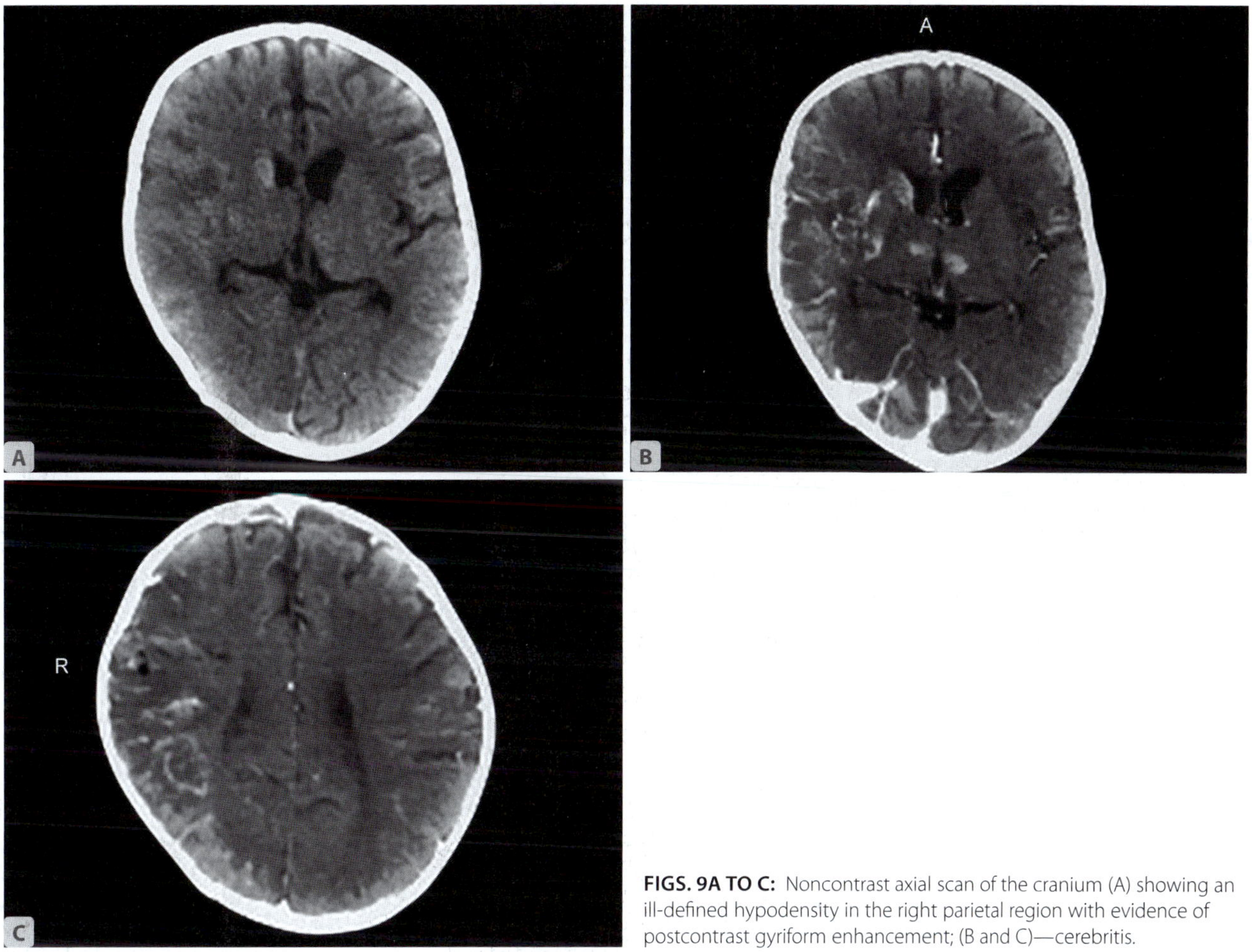

FIGS. 9A TO C: Noncontrast axial scan of the cranium (A) showing an ill-defined hypodensity in the right parietal region with evidence of postcontrast gyriform enhancement; (B and C)—cerebritis.

10–14 days later. Fibroblasts forming the collagenous capsule, liquefaction of central necrotic area and persistence of edema characterize this early capsule stage.[31] In the late capsule stage (>14 days) a gliotic reaction develops at the outer margin of the abscess and there is a decrease in the surrounding edema. It might take 2 weeks to several months for cerebritis to progress to a mature abscess depending on the host's immune response, virulence of the organism and several other factors.

Imaging

In the early stages of cerebritis, a localized hypoattenuation may be seen on a noncontrast CT with variable enhancement on the postcontrast scans. If enhancement is present it is nodular or ring like. When a capsule forms, a round or ovoid area of low density with ring enhancement is seen. The necrotic center of a mature abscess typically shows a low signal on T1 and high signal on T2-weighted MR images while the abscess capsule is typically low signal on the T2-weighted images[32] **(Figs. 10A to F)**. The various constituents of the capsular rim-like collagen, the paramagnetic free radicals produced by the actively phagocytosing macrophages and hemorrhage—account for its marked hypointensity on T2-weighted images. On postcontrast scans enhancement of the capsular rim occurs. The ring enhancement is usually thin and smooth measuring less than 5 mm in thickness. A poorer vascular supply of the white matter as compared to the grey matter of the brain accounts for the thinner medial/ventricular margin of the abscess cavity which may rupture with resultant daughter abscesses in the white matter or ventricle. Daughter abscesses are seen as smaller ring enhancing lesions adjacent to the parent abscess **(Figs. 11A and B)**. Vasogenic edema surrounding the abscess cavity is seen as a surrounding hypointensity on a T1 and hyperintensity on T2W images. Mass effect may be seen **(Figs. 12A and B)**.

Differentiation of a brain abscess from a necrotic neoplasm on imaging can be achieved by the fact that an abscess has a thin, smooth enhancing rim while a neoplasm has an irregular, nodular wall **(Figs. 13A to C)**. The collagen capsule being less developed on the medial/ventricular side of an abscess, presence of daughter abscesses, presence of extra-axial collections, ependymal/meningeal enhancement are features that help differentiate an abscess from a necrotic neoplasm.[33]

MR spectroscopy reveals various amino acid peaks like succinate (at 2.4 ppm), leucine, isoleucine, valine (at 0.85 ppm), glycine (3.5 ppm), alanine (at 1.5 ppm) in case of pyogenic brain abscess. Metabolites like acetate and succinate are of bacterial origin while others result due to death and

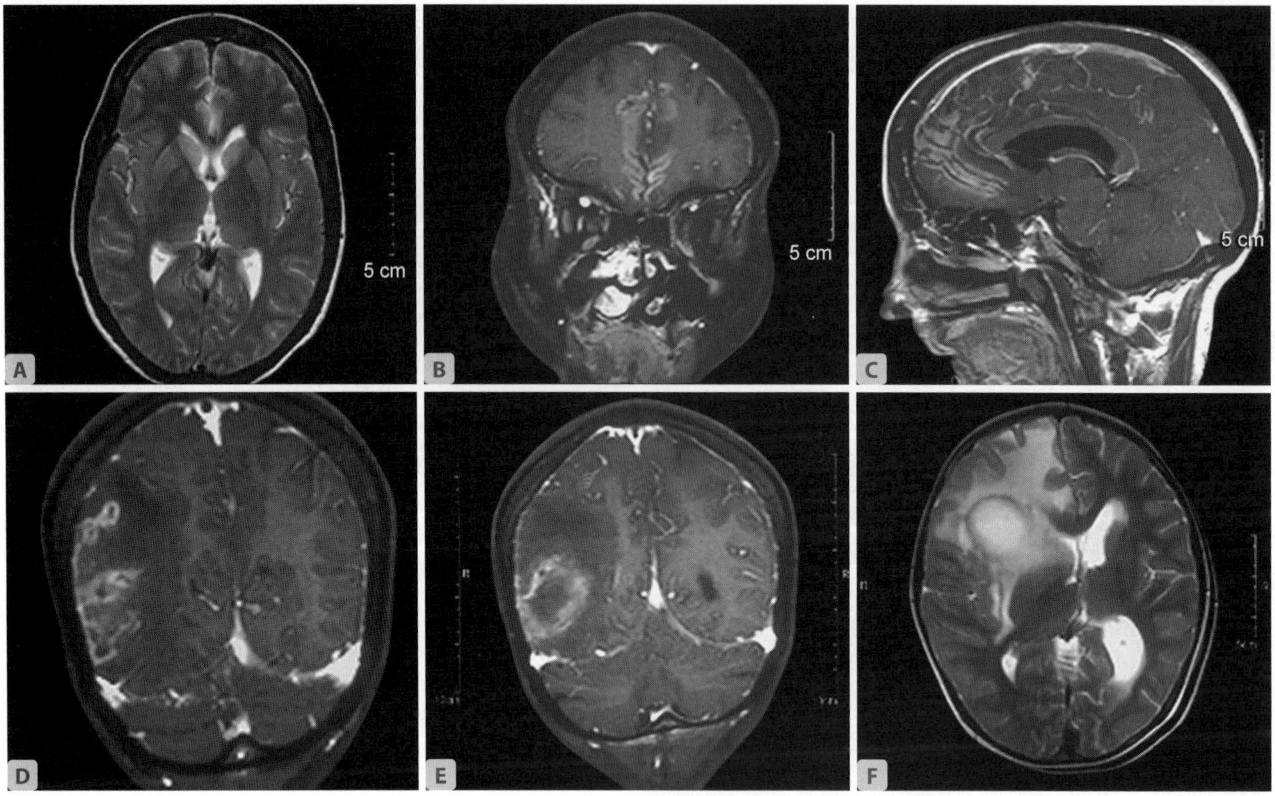

FIGS. 10A TO F: Axial T2W MR image (A) reveals an ill-defined hyperintense signal in the right parietal region. Postcontrast images; (B to D) reveal an irregular gyriform enhancement in the adjacent brain parenchyma—early cerebritis stage. MR image; (E) shows walling of the infection in the late cerebritis stage. Axial T2W MR image; (F) shows the stage of abscess formation with a hyperintense center and a hypointense rim of the collagenous capsule.

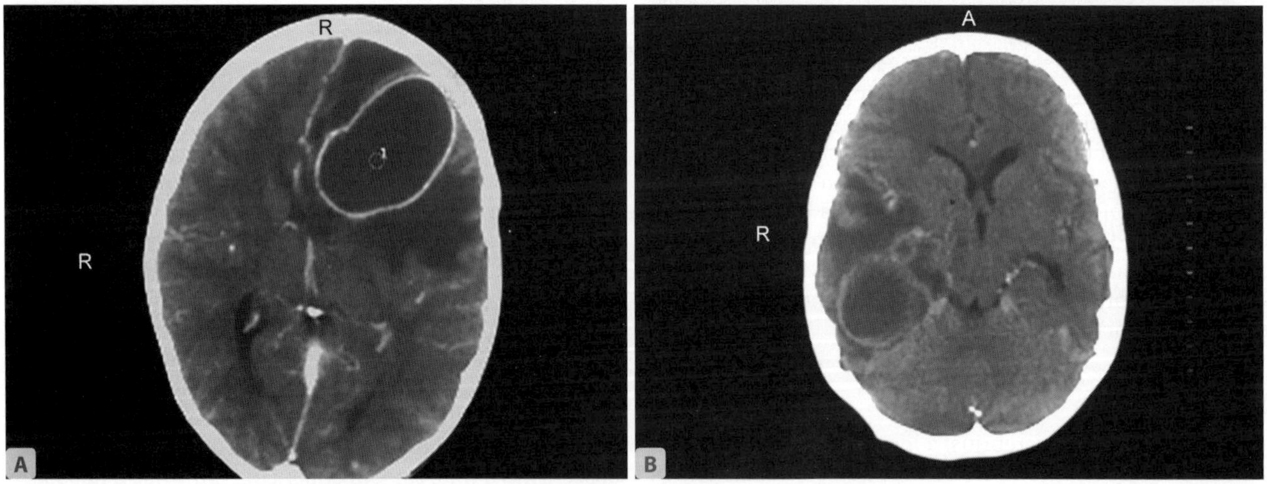

FIGS. 11A AND B: CECT axial scans of the cranium showing a large ring-enhancing lesion with smooth thin walls in a left parafalcine location with extensive vasogenic edema causing effacement of the ipsilateral frontal horn and midline shift to the contralateral side. Adjacent smaller enhancing rings are also seen in another case—brain abscess with daughter abscesses.

degeneration of inflammatory cells and exudate.[34,35] A large amount of proteolytic enzymes are produced by the dead and degenerating inflammatory cells that degrade the proteins to free amino acids. Lactate/lipid peak may be seen in an abscess at 1.3 ppm owing to anaerobic glycolysis. The presence of amino acid peak is considered specific of an abscess and is not seen in a cystic neoplasm.[36]

On diffusion-weighted MR images, the high cellularity and viscosity of pus in an abscess impedes water mobility resulting in a restricted pattern of diffusion with consequent low ADC values.[37] Low ADC values are not observed in cystic necrotic tumors helping in the differentiation of an abscess from cystic neoplasm[38] **(Figs. 14A to D)**. The reported sensitivity of diffusion-weighted imaging in differentiating an

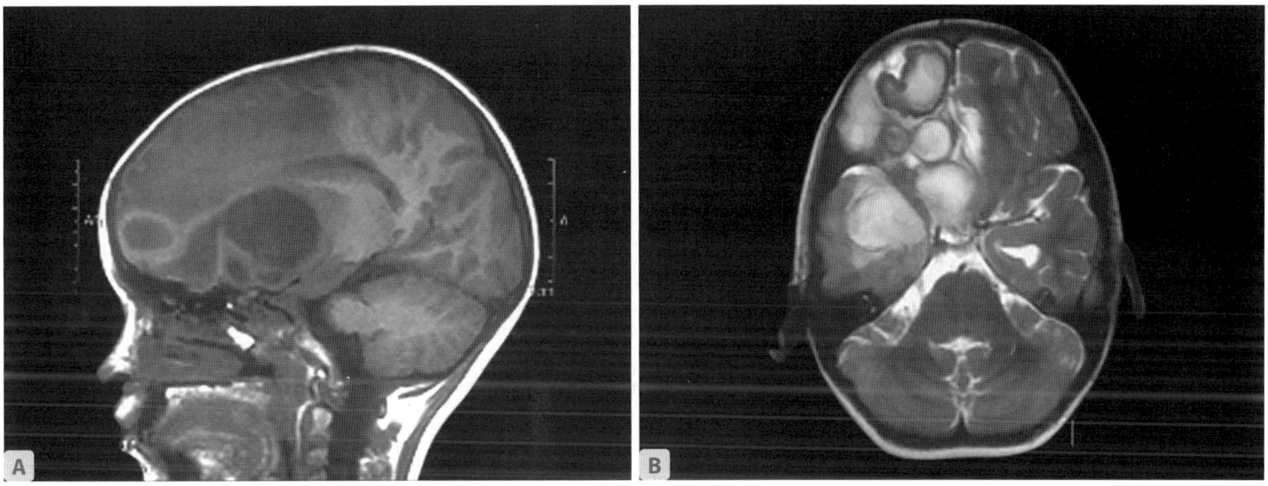

FIGS. 12A AND B: T1W sagittal (A) and T2W axial; (B) MR images showing multiple lesions having a hypointense center on T1 and hyperintense center on T2W images with perilesional edema. The collagenous capsule of the lesions is iso to slightly hyperintense on T1 and hypointense on T2W images. Mass effect on the ipsilateral ventricular system with dilatation of the contralateral temporal horn is seen—multiple brain abscesses.

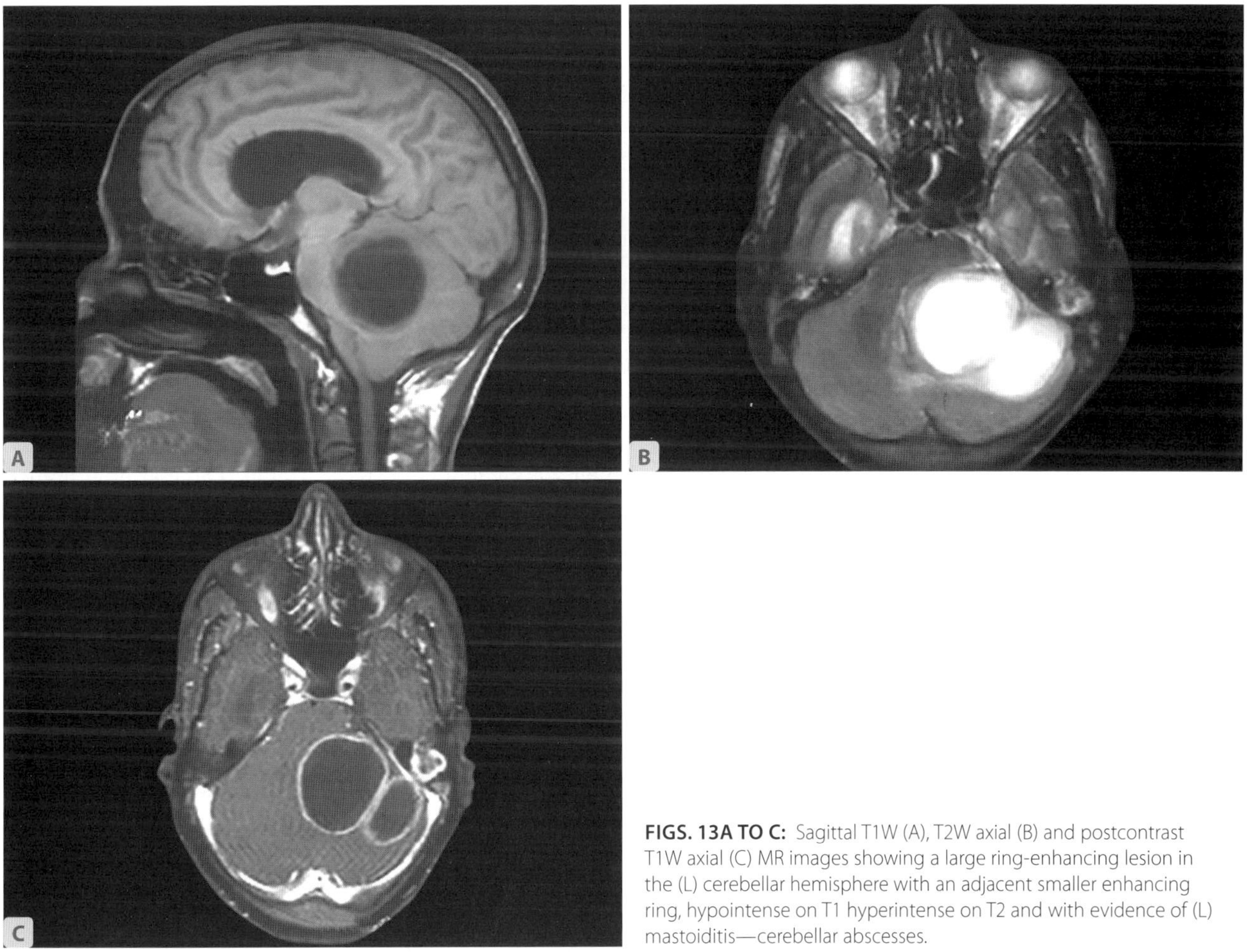

FIGS. 13A TO C: Sagittal T1W (A), T2W axial (B) and postcontrast T1W axial (C) MR images showing a large ring-enhancing lesion in the (L) cerebellar hemisphere with an adjacent smaller enhancing ring, hypointense on T1 hyperintense on T2 and with evidence of (L) mastoiditis—cerebellar abscesses.

abscess from other pathologies is 72-95% while the specificity ranges from 96-100%.[39]

On diffusion tensor imaging (DTI), brain abscess cavity shows regions of increased fractional anisotropy (FA) and low mean diffusivity (Dav) while cystic tumours and neurocysticercosis shows low fractional anisotropy (FA) and high diffusivity (Dav).[40] Dynamic susceptibility contrast perfusion MRI can also help to distinguish an abscess from a neoplasm as an abscess has lower rCBV values compared to a neoplasm. The lower rCBV values are attributed to the

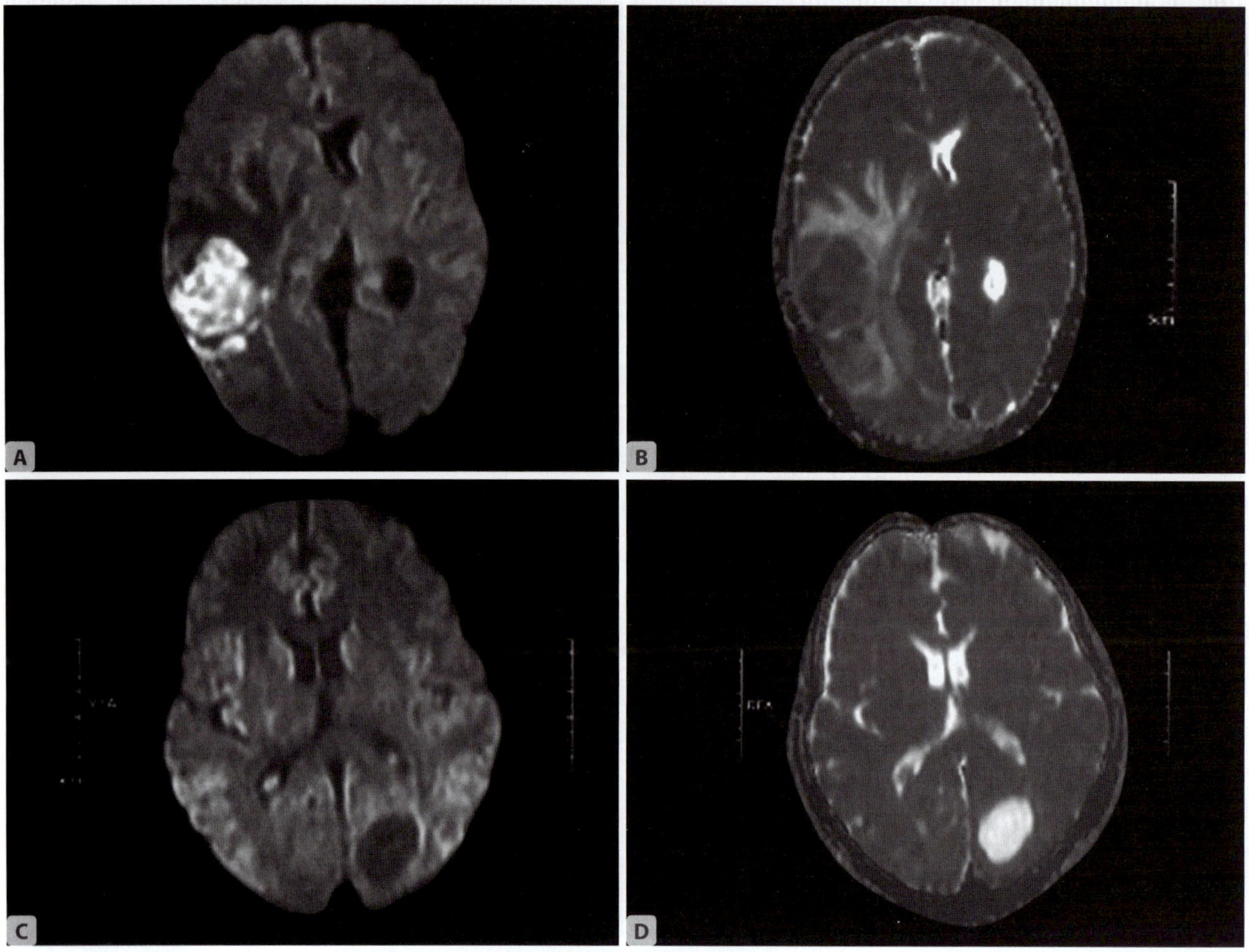

FIGS. 14A TO D: Bright signal on diffusion-weighted images b-1000 (A) and low signal on ADC map; (B) seen in a cerebral abscess while low signal seen on DW images; (C) and high signal on ADC map; (D) seen in a necrotic neoplasm.

presence of mature collagen and decreased neovascularity in an abscess as compared to a neoplasm.[41]

Multiple Brain Abscesses Secondary to Septic Emboli

The causes for septic emboli include cyanotic heart disease, intravenous drug abuse, bacterial endocarditis, etc., **(Figs. 15A to C)**. Small septic emboli may lead to occlusion of small arteries and arterioles while the larger ones may cause hemispheric infarction **(Figs. 16A to D)**. Mycotic aneurysms usually involve peripheral branches of intermediate to small cerebral arteries. The presence of parenchymal and subarachnoid bleed in a patient of abscess/infection should suggest mycotic aneurysm which should be ruled out on MR angiography.[33]

Central Nervous System Infarction

Central nervous system infarction associated with meningitis occurs because of inflammation-induced arterial spasm or because of direct inflammation of the walls of arteries and arterioles resulting in an infectious arteritis. Most infarcts occur in the basal ganglia secondary to involvement of the penetrating lenticulostriate arteries. Large arterial branch occlusions seen in some instances can result in cortical infarction. Cortical veins or dural venous sinuses may also be involved with resultant venous thrombosis and venous infarction of involved central nervous system tissues.[42,43] Venous infarcts are usually bilateral and multiple, involve non arterial territories and tend to occur in the convexities. Areas of hemorrhage are seen in about 25% of cases. On angiography, the spectrum of cerebrovascular changes associated with advanced cases of meningitis and arteritis include:[42,44]

1. Narrowing and spasm of the major arteries at the base of the brain, such as the supraclinoid portion of the internal carotid artery and the A1 and M1 segments of the anterior and middle cerebral arteries.
2. Irregularities or focal aneurysmal dilatations of medium-sized cerebral arteries.
3. Occlusions of the distal branches of the middle cerebral artery with or without retrograde flow.
4. Focal, abnormal parenchymal (i.e. gyral) blush.
5. Marked prolongation of circulation time.
6. Early venous filling.
7. Thrombosis of cortical veins, dural venous sinus or both.

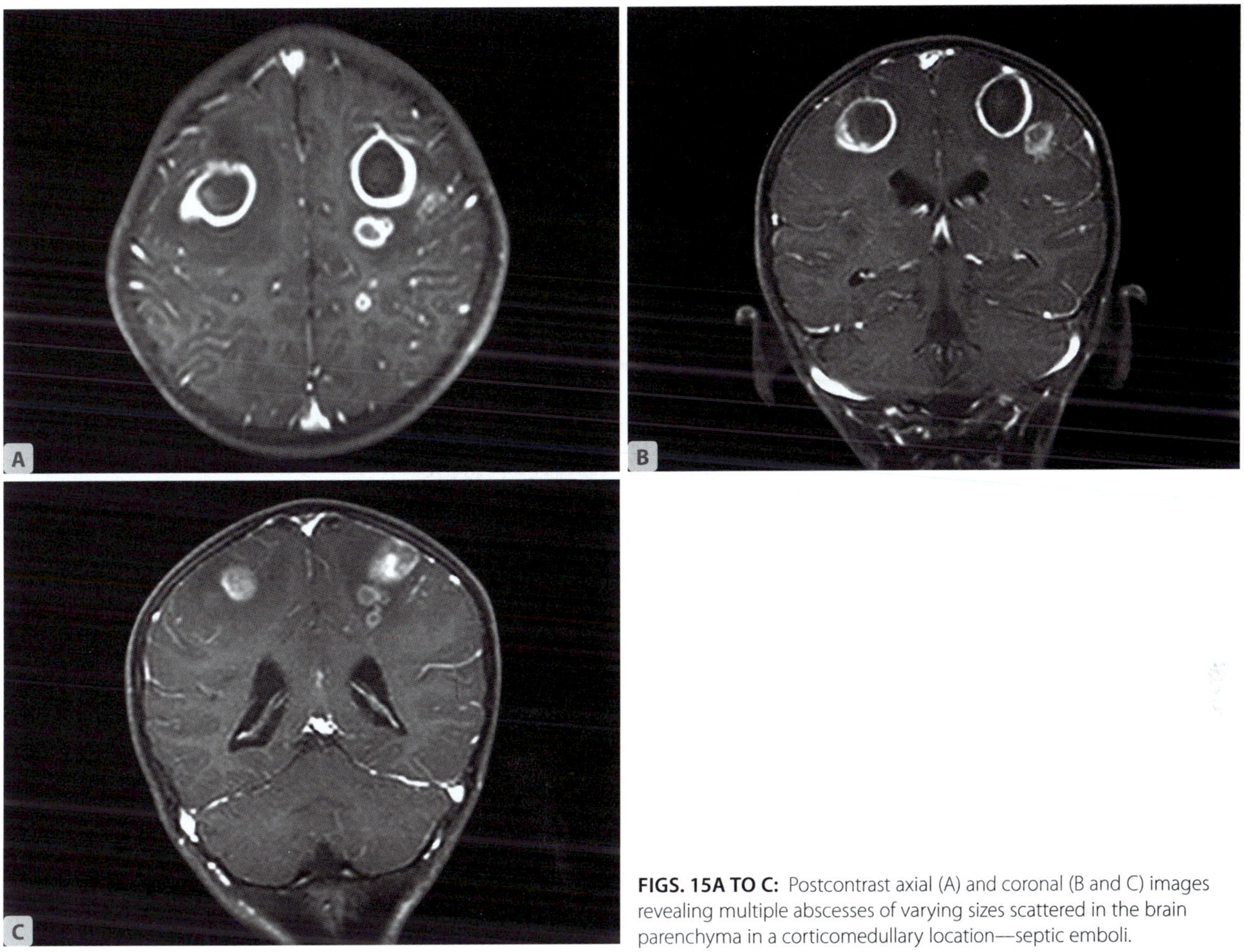

FIGS. 15A TO C: Postcontrast axial (A) and coronal (B and C) images revealing multiple abscesses of varying sizes scattered in the brain parenchyma in a corticomedullary location—septic emboli.

Cranial Nerve Involvement

This occurs due to direct inflammation of the nerve or pressure caused on the nerve by the exudates with resultant stretching. The commonest nerve to be involved is the VIIIth cranial nerve or vestibulocochlear nerve with hearing loss seen in about 30% cases.[5] Hearing loss is usually bilateral, permanent and *Streptococcus pneumoniae* is the commonest causative organism.[45] Other involved nerves include the facial, oculomotor and the optic nerve. Transient palsies of the optic and abducens nerves may be seen due to raised intracranial pressure.

Ventriculitis

Involvement of the cerebral ependyma leads to ventriculitis. Rupture of a parenchymal abscess into the ventricular system, ventricular catheter placement or meningitis may all cause ventriculitis. Cranial sonography is a useful imaging modality for the diagnosis of ventriculitis. Ventricular dilatation, irregular and echogenic ependyma, intraventricular debris are the common findings seen. Intraventricular adhesions and septae seen in about 10% of patients with meningitis are better picked up on sonography than CT. CT and MR may reveal ventricular dilatation, intraventricular debris and periventricular edema seen as hyperintense signal along the ventricular margin on T2W images. Entrapment of portions of ventricles may occur due to adhesions and septae which may result in segmental dilatation. On contrast administration there is diffuse enhancement of the ventricular margin **(Figs. 17A and B)**. Another finding associated with ventriculitis is choroid plexitis. A swollen choroid plexus with ill-defined margins and enhancement on contrast administration constitute the imaging findings[46] **(Figs. 18A and B)**. No calcifications are seen in cases of ventriculitis resulting from pyogenic meningitis unlike those from viral infection. Diffusion weighted images reveal presence of restricted diffusion in the intraventricular debris.

Recurrent Meningitis

Recurrence is seen in about 16% cases of meningitis, the commonest cause is an occult cerebrospinal fluid leak or fistula and the commonest causative organisms include streptococci and gram-negative bacilli[47] **(Figs. 19A to C)**.

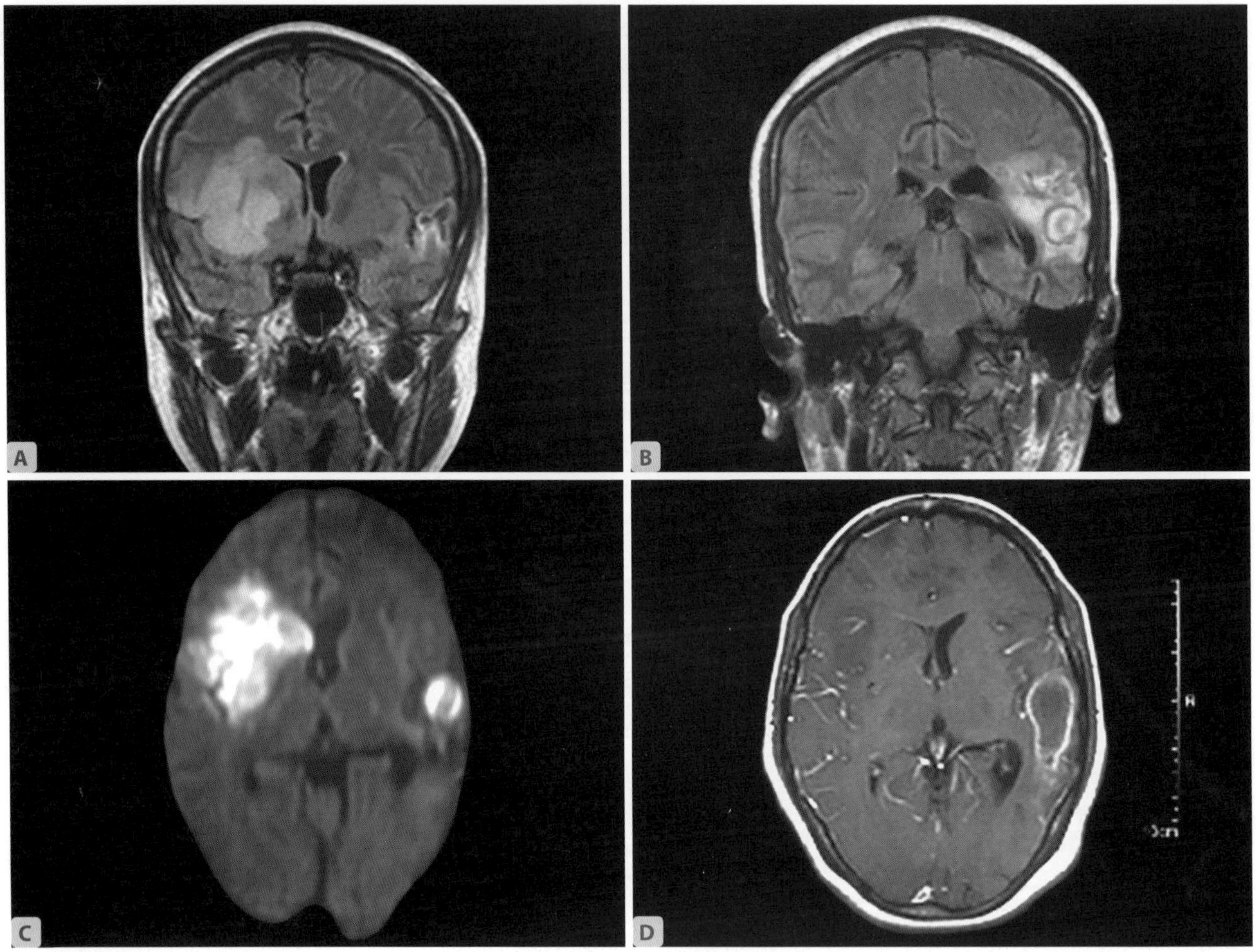

FIGS. 16A TO D: FLAIR coronal (A and B), diffusion-weighted (C) and postcontrast T1W axial (D) MR images showing an area of signal alteration in the distribution of the right MCA territory showing a restricted pattern of diffusion suggestive of infarct. Another lesion showing perilesional edema, a restricted pattern of diffusion and ring enhancement is seen in the left parietal region suggestive of an abscess—septic emboli.

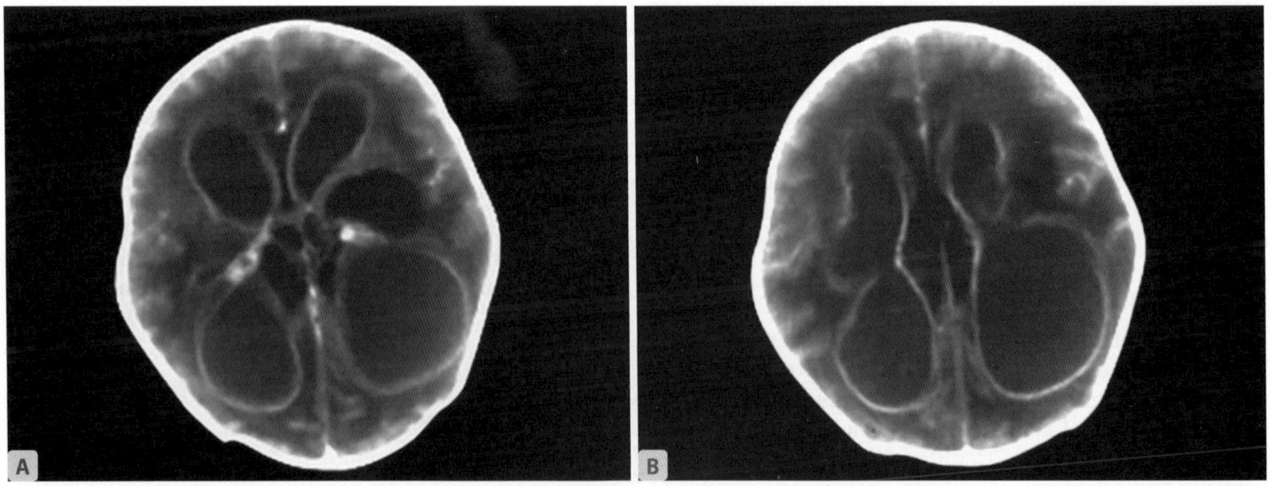

FIGS. 17A AND B: CECT axial scans of the cranium showing massive dilatation of the ventricular system with transependymal edema with diffuse enhancement along the ventricular walls—ventriculitis.

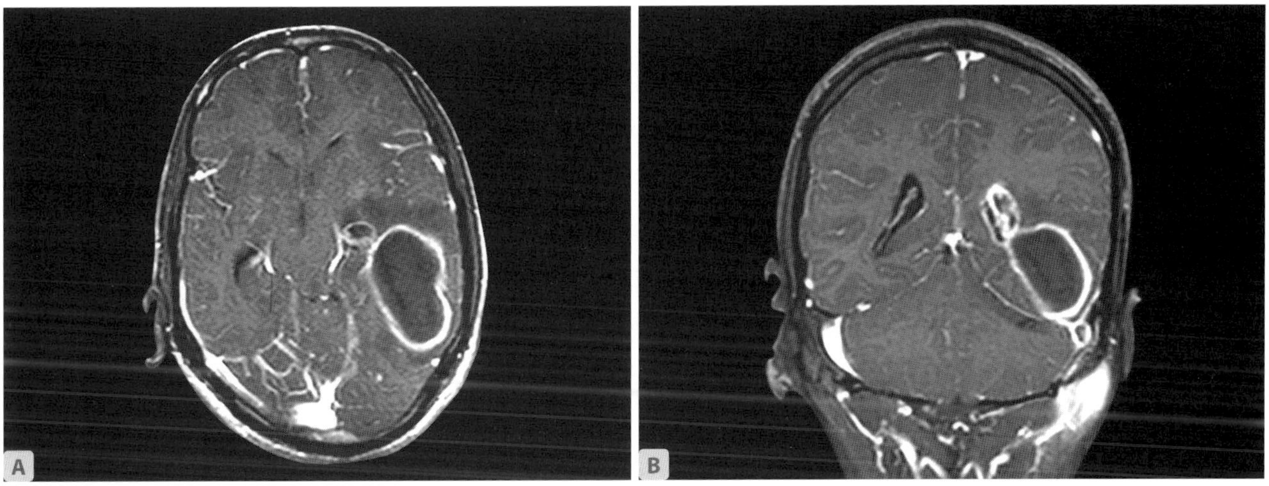

FIGS. 18A AND B: Contrast-enhanced axial (A) and coronal; (B) MR images revealing a large brain abscess in the left parieto-occipital region with enhancing choroid plexus of the left lateral ventricle s/o choroid plexitis. Note is also made of sigmoid sinus thrombosis of the left side and an abscess in the neck (B).

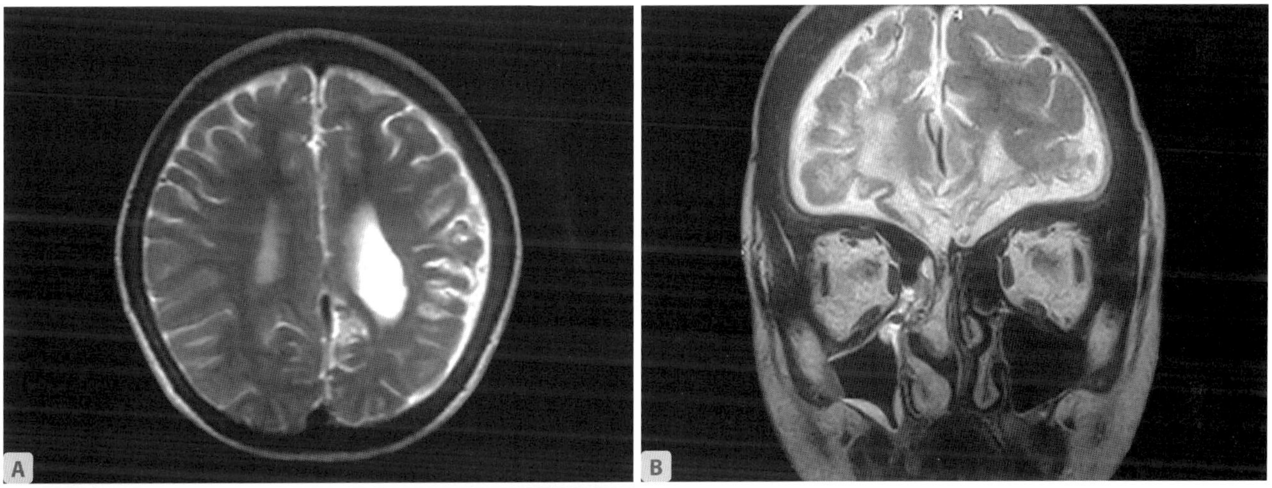

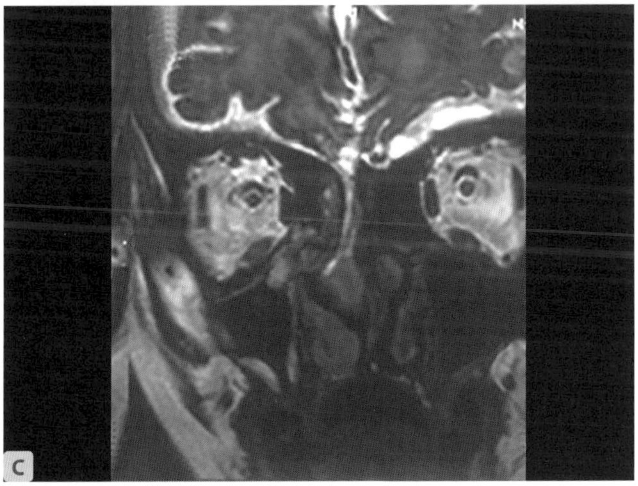

FIGS. 19A TO C: Axial T2W MR (A) showing loss of volume of the brain parenchyma. High resolution T2W coronal; (B) and CISS sequence; (C) reveals the CSF leak/fistula on the right side with defect in the cribriform plate-recurrent meningitis.

GRANULOMATOUS INFECTION

TUBERCULOSIS

The causative organism is *Mycobacterium tuberculosis* which is a slowly dividing facultative intracellular pathogen that has plagued mankind for thousands of years and continues to be the cause of 1.7 million of deaths per year. About 9 million cases of TB are reported every year.[48] The unique feature of this organism to hide and divide in the macrophages (doubling time 15–20 hours) poses a diagnostic challenge and makes administration of therapeutic regimens difficult and time consuming. This is further complicated by the emergence of HIV infection, AIDS and by the multidrug resistant variety. About 5–10% of all patients with tuberculosis and up to 20% of patients with AIDS related tuberculosis have CNS involvement.[49,50]

Pathogenesis

A two step model for the pathogenesis of CNS TB includes: 1. The bacteria reach the oxygen rich CNS via the hematogenous route from a distant focus, e.g. in lungs to establish a subpial or subependymal focus of infection called the "Rich" focus.[51] 2. The Rich focus may rupture into the subarachnoid space or into the ventricular system leading to meningitis.[52] The basal spaces are filled with gelatinous exudates containing chronic inflammatory cells, fibrin and hemorrhage.[53] An initial nonspecific inflammatory response (tuberculous cerebritis) may occur in the beginning. This may then result in granuloma formation. A tuberculous focus may develop into a tuberculoma or abscess in the absence of adequate host immunity.

Tuberculous Meningitis (TBM)

Meningeal tuberculosis is the most common presentation of CNS TB and is seen most frequently in children and adolescents. Children are most vulnerable and more frequently affected by TBM due to their poor immune response to contain bacteria within the lungs. The infection disseminates hematogenously from a distant focal point and the meningeal involvement usually occurs due to rupture of the Rich focus in the subarachnoid space. The primary subpial exudate from the discharging Rich focus is located in the inferomedial surface of the frontal, the anteromedial surface of the temporal lobes, the superior aspect of the cerebellum and the floor of the fourth ventricle. From these sites it disseminates to the interpeduncular cisterns enveloping the optic nerves at the optic chiasma and to the anterior part of the pontomesencephalic cisterns, the ambient cisterns, the suprasellar cisterns and onto the Sylvian fissures. In the later stages, the leptomeningeal process extends to the convexities and to the ependymal surfaces of the ventricles. Within the lateral ventricles, a similar exudate often covers the choroid plexus resulting in choroid plexitis. The exudates surround meningeal and cortical blood vessels inciting inflammation and vasculitis, obstruction of the CSF pathways and obliterative endarteritis leading to infarction.[54]

Clinical Manifestations

Malaise, lassitude, low-grade fever and intermittent headache characterize the insidious prodrome of tuberculous meningitis. The most common clinical manifestation occurs with fever, headache, nausea, vomiting, photophobia and neck stiffness. Cranial nerve palsies of third, fourth and sixth nerves are common. Meningismus, confusion and long tract signs can accelerate into seizures, hemiparesis, hemiplegia, stupor and coma. Cerebrospinal fluid analysis demonstrates lymphocytosis, increased protein levels and decreased glucose level. Identification of *M. tuberculosis* in cerebrospinal fluid by acid-fast methods is achieved in 90% of cases, however, a negative result does not preclude treatment, if there is strong clinical or radiologic evidence of tuberculous disease.

Imaging

Non contrast CT may show obliteration of the basal cisterns by isoattenuating or hyperattenuating exudates. Plaque-like dural thickening may be seen. On contrast administration basal cisternal enhancement is seen **(Figs. 20A and B)**. The objective criteria for abnormal basal enhancement in TBM include:[55]

1. *Contrast filling the cisterns*: The CSF spaces that surround the normal vascular enhancement are obliterated by the contrast medium.
2. *Linear enhancement*: A linear enhancement that is seen in more than two contiguous slices is abnormal as the MCA is too small to be seen in its full horizontal length in more than one slice or as a continuous line.
3. *Double and triple lines*: Two or three lines seen represent enhancement of meninges along the middle cerebral artery.
4. *Y sign*: Pure vessel enhancement is never seen as a Y while meningeal enhancement at the junction of the suprasellar and middle cerebral artery cistern produces the Y.
5. *Ill-defined edge*: The normal vessels always show a sharply marginated enhancement while meningeal enhancement is ill-defined.
6. *Infundibular recess of third ventricle*: No vessel lies in the region and any enhancement along the posterior aspect of the infundibular recess of the 3rd ventricle in suprasellar cistern is abnormal and meningeal.
7. *Join the dots sign*: Vessels in the Sylvian sulcus are seen as separate dots on cross-section. When the dots are joined by linear enhancement it is abnormal.
8. *Nodular enhancement*: Normal meningeal enhancement is smooth and sharply marginated so nodular enhancement is always abnormal.
9. *Asymmetry*: Asymmetry aids recognition of abnormal basal enhancement.

Basal exudative meningitis may extend to the convexities, Sylvian fissures and the tentorium. The Sylvian fissures is a very common site of involvement by tuberculous meningitis.[56] Hydrocephalus may be seen in 45–87% of patients at the time of diagnosis and indicates a poor prognosis.[57,58] Ependymitis may be seen as linear enhancement along the ventricular

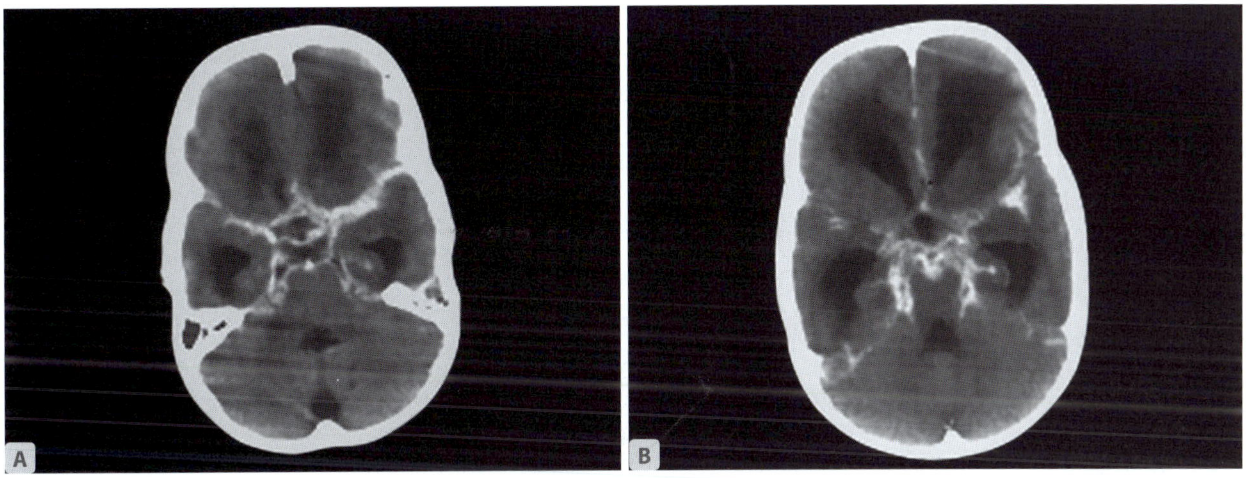

FIGS. 20A AND B: CECT axial scans of the cranium showing dense meningeal enhancement along the basal cisterns, tentorium and the Sylvian cisterns with evidence of hydrocephalus and periventricular ooze—tubercular meningitis.

margin. Infarction is demonstrated on CT as areas of hypoattenuation with loss of gray white matter differentiation. The triad of basal meningeal enhancement, hydrocephalus and infarct increases the specificity of the diagnosis of TBM.

Owing to its multiplanar imaging capability, greater soft tissue contrast and lack of bone artifacts, gadolinium enhanced MR is superior to CT in the detection of meningeal disease and associated parenchymal abnormalities.[59,60] Characteristic thick or nodular enhancement in the basal cisterns is seen in TBM **(Figs. 21A and B)**. Recent advances in neuroimaging of tubercular meningitis.

Magnetization Transfer (MT)

The quantification of MT ratio (MTR) helps in predicting the cause of meningitis. It has been used to differentiate TBM from other causes of meningitis. The abnormal meninges show a hyperintense signal on the precontrast T1 weighted MT images and enhance further on the post contrast T1-weighted MT images. The MTR of the meninges in TBM is lower than that of fungal and pyogenic meningitis but higher than that in viral meningitis.[61] The visibility of the meninges on a pre contrast MT image and low MTR is diagnostic of TBM and differentiates it from other causes of meningitis. It is the high lipid content of the tuberculous bacilli that accounts for the low MTR in TBM.

Ex Vivo Protein MR Spectroscopy

High resolution ex vivo MRS of CSF has shown presence of lactate, acetate, and sugars along with signals from cyclopropyl rings (–0.5 to + 0.5 ppm) and phenolic glycolipids (7.1 and 7.4 ppm) in tubercular meningitis. These metabolites have not been observed with pyogenic meningitis.[33]

COMPLICATIONS OF TUBERCULAR MENINGITIS

Hydrocephalus, cranial neuropathies, focal infarction, focal atrophy and syringobulbia are the complications associated with tubercular meningitis.

Hydrocephalus

Communicating hydrocephalus is more common in tuberculous meningitis than the obstructive type.[62,63] The exudates become thick, adhesive, gelatinous and fibrotic blocking the basal cisterns and CSF circulation and resorption with resultant hydrocephalus. A focal parenchymal lesion may cause mass effect on the cerebral aqueduct or the fourth ventricular foramina causing obstructive variety of hydrocephalus.[64] There may be entrapment of the ventricle by granulomatous ependymitis. A complex type of hydrocephalus can be seen in TB with a combination of communicating (defective absorption) and non-communicating (obstructive) hydrocephalus. It is important to determine the site and type of obstruction because of impending cerebral herniation in case of obstruction and also to determine the optimum treatment option. CSF flow studies done on MR imaging provide qualitative and quantitative information of CSF flow, which help in differentiating the type of hydrocephalus and provides information about the CSF dynamics.

Vasculitis

Intracranial vasculitis, which occurs as a complication of tuberculous meningitis, causes neurological deficits in these patients. In can occur due to a direct invasion of the vessel by the microorganism or extension of adjacent arachnoiditis. It is usually the small arteries or veins that are involved which undergo fibrinoid degeneration resulting in spasm or thrombosis of vessels leading to bland or hemorrhagic infarction. The most commonly involved regions are the basal ganglia, thalamus and internal capsule due to the involvement of the small perforating branches supplying these regions, particularly the lentriculostriate and thalamoperforating arteries.[65] These vessels perfuse the so called "medial tuberculous zone". Vasculitic infarcts are usually bilateral in nature **(Figs. 22A to D)**.

CT shows these vasculitic infarcts as hypoattenuating areas while MR images show them as areas of hyperintense signal with a restricted pattern of diffusion on DW MR images.

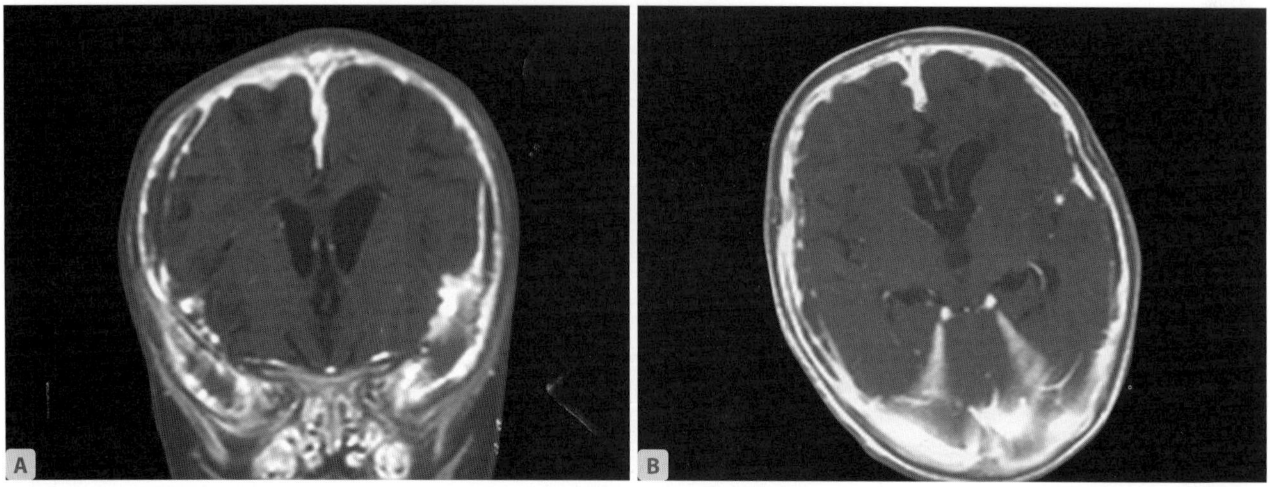

FIGS. 21A AND B: Postcontrast T1W axial (A) and coronal (B) MR images showing diffuse meningeal enhancement along the cerebral convexities, tentorium and the basal cisterns with hydrocephalus—tubercular meningitis.

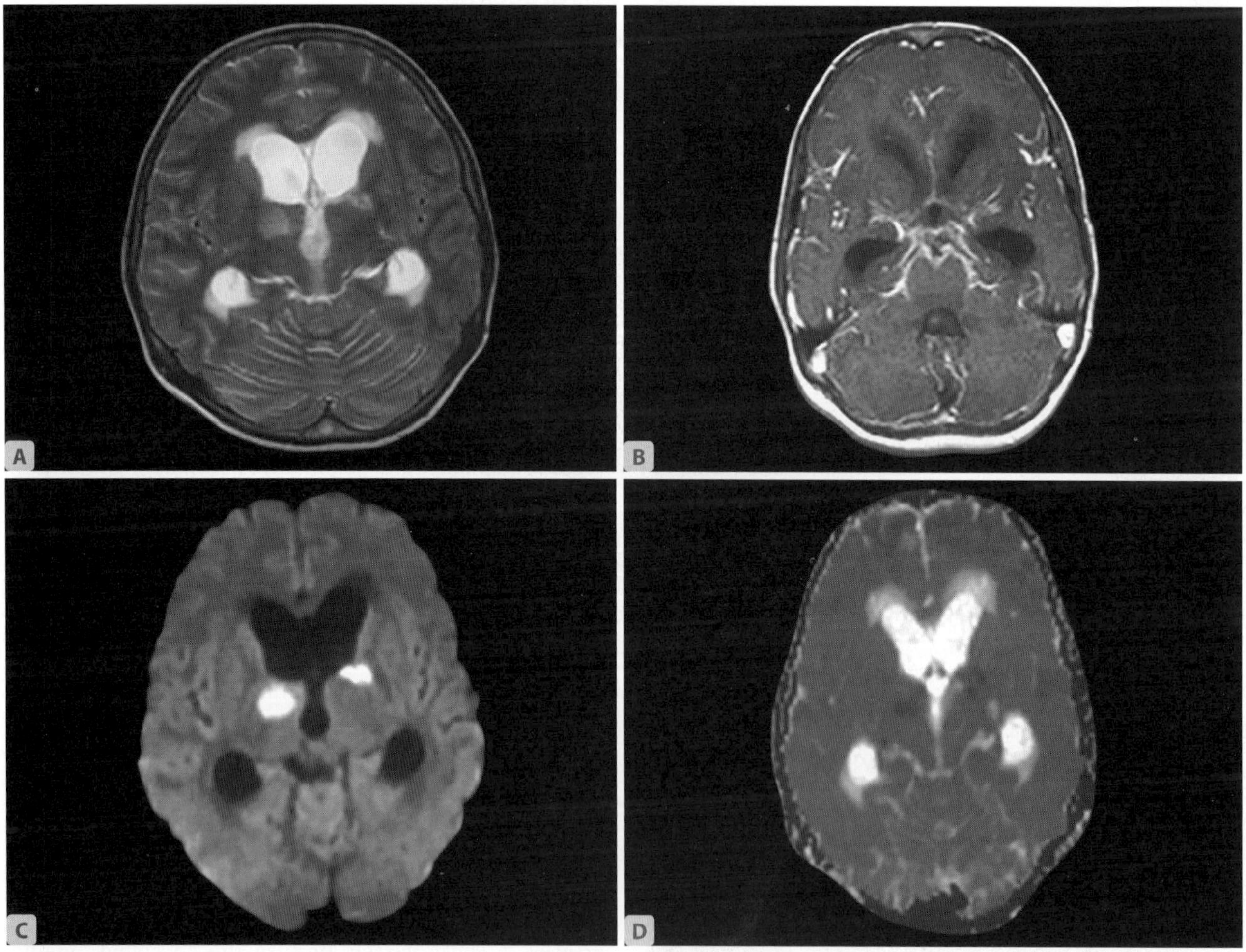

FIGS. 22A TO D: T2W axial (A), T1W postgadolinium axial; (B) diffusion-weighted; (C) and ADC; (D) MR images showing basal cisternal enhancement with hydrocephalus and periventricular ooze suggestive of tubercular meningitis. Areas of signal alteration noted in bilateral basal ganglia showing hyperintense signal on T2W images and increasing hyperintensity on b1000 with hypointensity on ADC maps—bilateral basal ganglia infarcts (vasculitis) in tubercular meningitis.

Cranial Neuropathies

They can occur in 17–40% of patients with CNS TB.[66] The II, III, IV, VI and VII nerves are the most commonly affected cranial nerves in tuberculous meningitis. A vascular compromise may result in ischaemia of the nerve or there may be nerve entrapment caused by the exudates.[67] A direct mass effect on the nerve within the subarachnoid space by a tuberculoma or direct involvement of the cranial nerve nuclei in the brain may be the other causative factors. A permanent loss of function of the nerves can be explained by the fibrotic changes that occur in the late stage. Contrast enhancement may be seen at entry/exit zone of the involved nerve suggesting its involvement. The entire nerve may be thickened and show enhancement.[68] Neuritis/perineuritis may improve with treatment while palsies due to involvement of brainstem nuclei usually do not, hence localization of the cause of cranial nerve involvement is important as it helps in prognostication.

TUBERCULAR PACHYMENINGITIS

Tubercular pachymeningitis can be focal or diffuse. The focal form is known as tuberculoma en plaque and it may mimic other dural based masses like meningioma. On imaging it is hyperdense on non-contrast CT, isointense to brain on T1W image, hypo to isointense on T2W images and shows homogenous enhancement with contrast administration.[69] In the setting of TB elsewhere in the body and a pachymeningeal abnormality, this form should be suspected as it responds well to antitubercular treatment.

PARENCHYMAL TUBERCULOSIS

Parenchymal form of tuberculosis includes tuberculomas, miliary TB, abscess, TB encephalopathy and focal tubercular cerebritis.

TUBERCULOMAS

These usually occur secondary to an infective focus elsewhere in the body and are more common in the pediatric age group than adults. Tuberculomas may occur anywhere in the cerebral hemispheres in the basal ganglia, brainstem or the cerebellar hemispheres. The location is usually corticomedullary junction or periventricular owing to a hematogenous route of dissemination.[70] Tuberculomas can be small or large in size, they can be solitary or multifocal in nature. Rare sites of tuberculomas include the cavernous sinuses, sphenoid sinus, sella turcica, the hypophysis and mastoid air cells.[71,72]

The CT appearance may vary from isodense to hyperdense solid enhancing lesions to ring enhancing lesions with central area of necrosis in cases of caseating granulomas **(Figs. 23A to C)**. A central area of calcification surrounded by a rim of

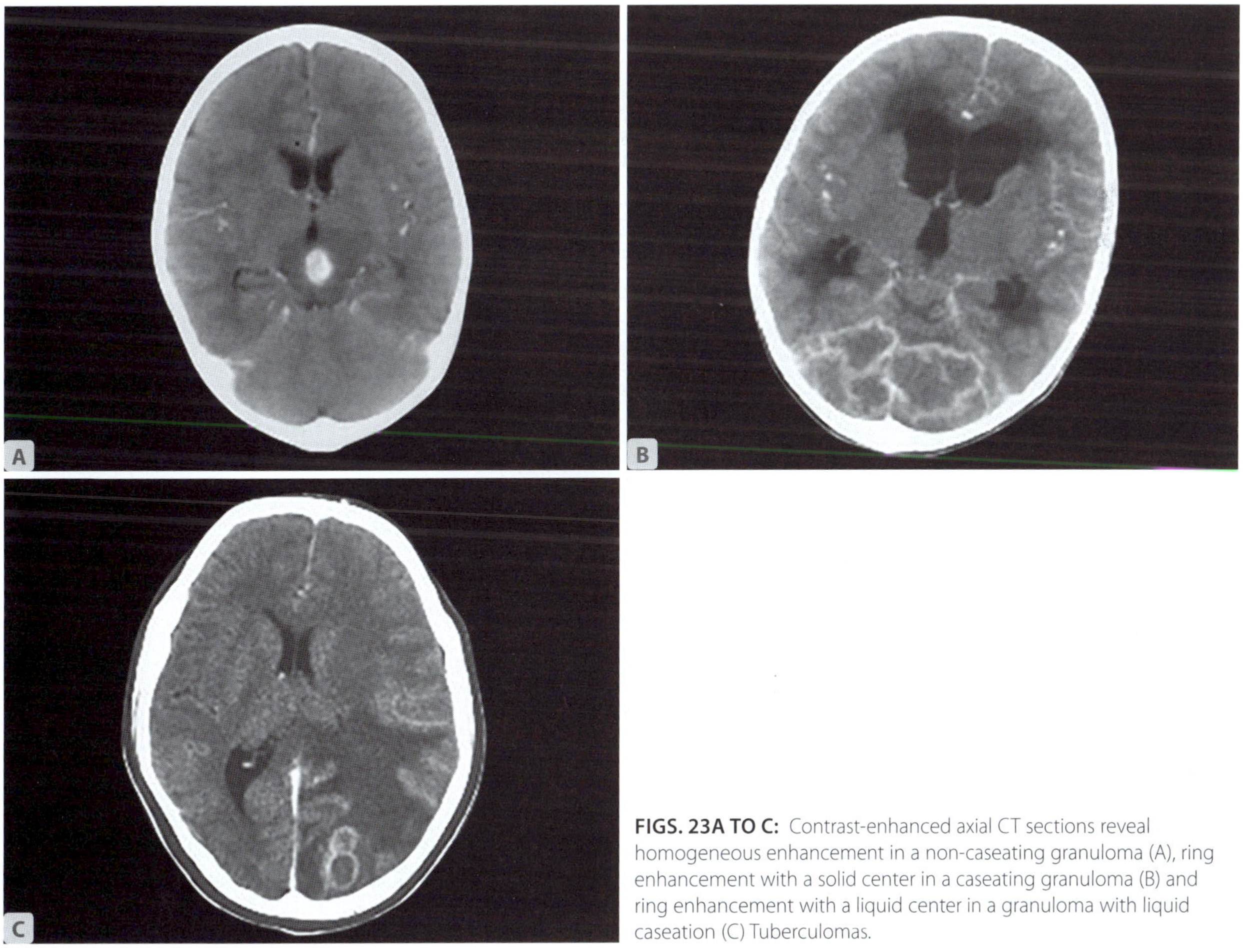

FIGS. 23A TO C: Contrast-enhanced axial CT sections reveal homogeneous enhancement in a non-caseating granuloma (A), ring enhancement with a solid center in a caseating granuloma (B) and ring enhancement with a liquid center in a granuloma with liquid caseation (C) Tuberculomas.

enhancement called the 'target sign' is highly suggestive of a tuberculous infection.[73]

MR features of tuberculomas vary depending on the nature of the granuloma-whether it is non-caseating, caseating with a solid center or caseating with central liquefaction. Non caseating granuloma shows hypointense signal on T1 and hyperintense signal on T2-weighted images. On contrast administration, there is homogenous enhancement of the lesion. Caseating granulomas with a solid centre appear hypointense on T1 and markedly hypointense on T2-weighted images. These granulomas are highly cellular, the compressed glial tissue and granulation tissue in the central core accounting for the cellular density and the marked hypointensity[74] **(Figs. 24A to C)**. Granulomas with central liquefaction show a peripheral hypointense rim on T2 weighted images. The low signal intensity of the capsule is due to the collagen content. Extensive edema and mass effect can be seen around the granuloma specially in the early stages of formation. Rim enhancement on postcontrast images is typically seen[75] **(Figs. 25 and 26)**.

MT Imaging

Precontrast MT T1-weighted images detect the tuberculomas better than conventional spin echo (CSE) images. Lesions which are isointense on both T1 and T2-weighted images may remain undetected and are called CSE invisible lesions. These lesions are detectable on MT images because of the lower transfer magnetization in tuberculomas as compared to the surrounding parenchyma making these lesions visible[61,76] **(Figs. 27A and B)**. Also lower MT ratios are obtained from the outer rim as compared to the inner core. The high lipid content of the tuberculomas contributes to the lower MTR of these lesions.

MR Spectroscopy

Prominent lipid peak at 0.9 and 1.3 ppm is seen in the case of tuberculomas owing to the presence of caseous material[76] **(Figs. 28A and B)**. Differentiation from metastasis and glioma can be achieved by the presence of elevated choline peak in these lesions compared to tuberculomas which show only a prominent lipid peak.

Dynamic contrast-enhanced MRI (DCE MRI) has been performed in tuberculomas and the relative cerebral blood volume rCBV has been correlated with their cellular and necrotic components.

Diffusion Tensor Imaging (DTI)

A decrease in fractional anisotropy (FA), linear anisotropy (CL) and planar anisotropy (CP) while an increase in spherical anisotropy (CS) has been reported in the case of

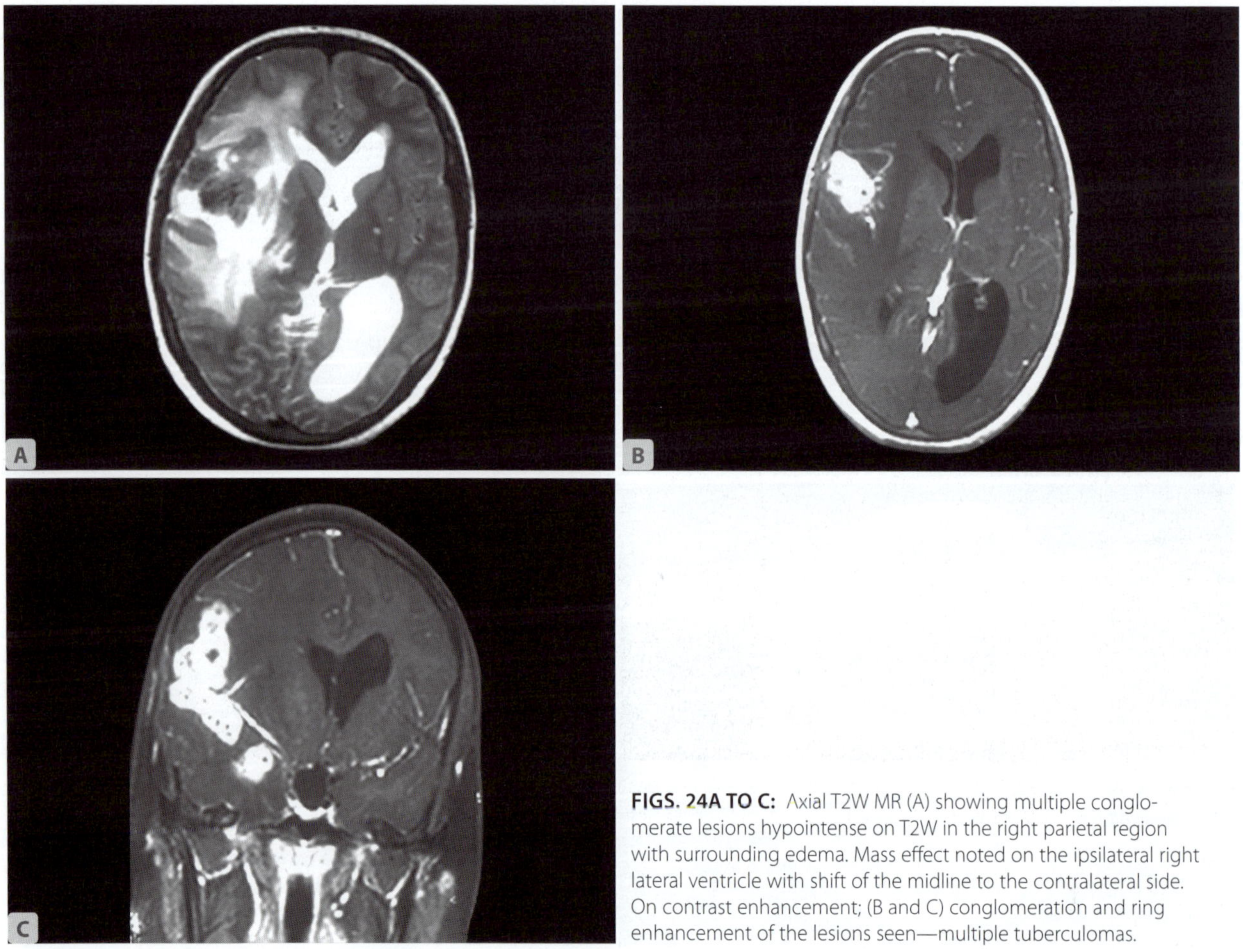

FIGS. 24A TO C: Axial T2W MR (A) showing multiple conglomerate lesions hypointense on T2W in the right parietal region with surrounding edema. Mass effect noted on the ipsilateral right lateral ventricle with shift of the midline to the contralateral side. On contrast enhancement; (B and C) conglomeration and ring enhancement of the lesions seen—multiple tuberculomas.

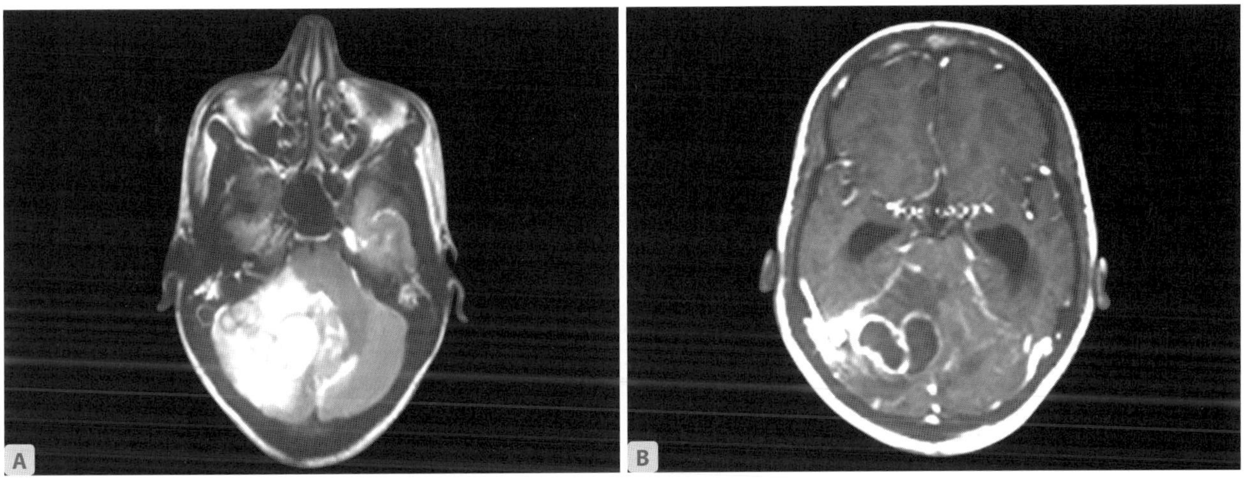

FIGS. 25A AND B: Axial T2W (A) and postcontrast T1W; (B) axial images showing conglomerate round lesions in the right cerebellar hemisphere with surrounding edema. There is attenuation of the fourth ventricle and obstructive hydrocephalus. The lesions show ring enhancement—tuberculomas posterior fossa.

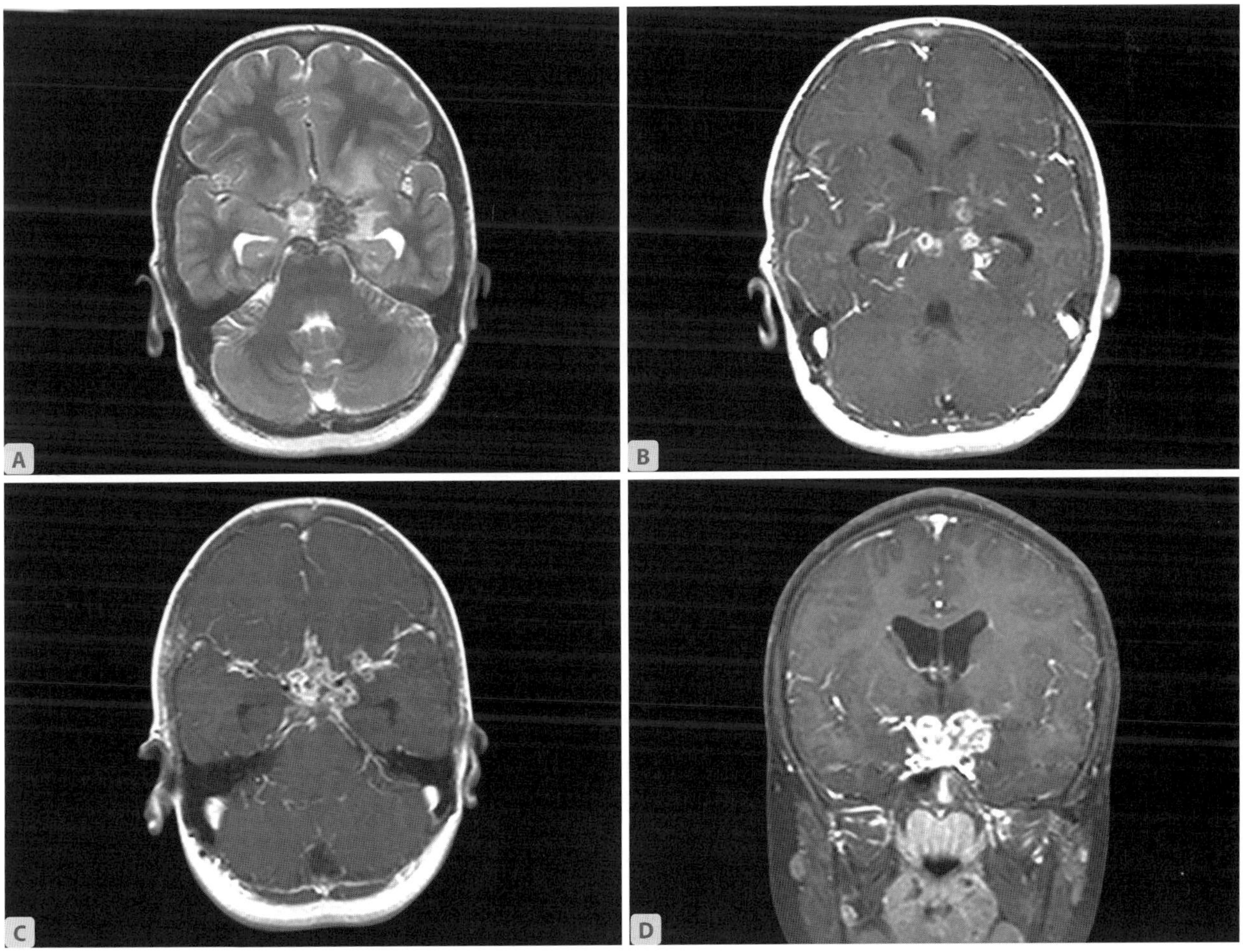

FIGS. 26A TO D: Axial T2W (A) and postcontrast axial; (B and C) and postcontrast coronal images; (D) reveal multiple conglomerate ring enhancing lesions in the suprasellar cisterns with encasement of the optic chiasma—multiple tuberculomas.

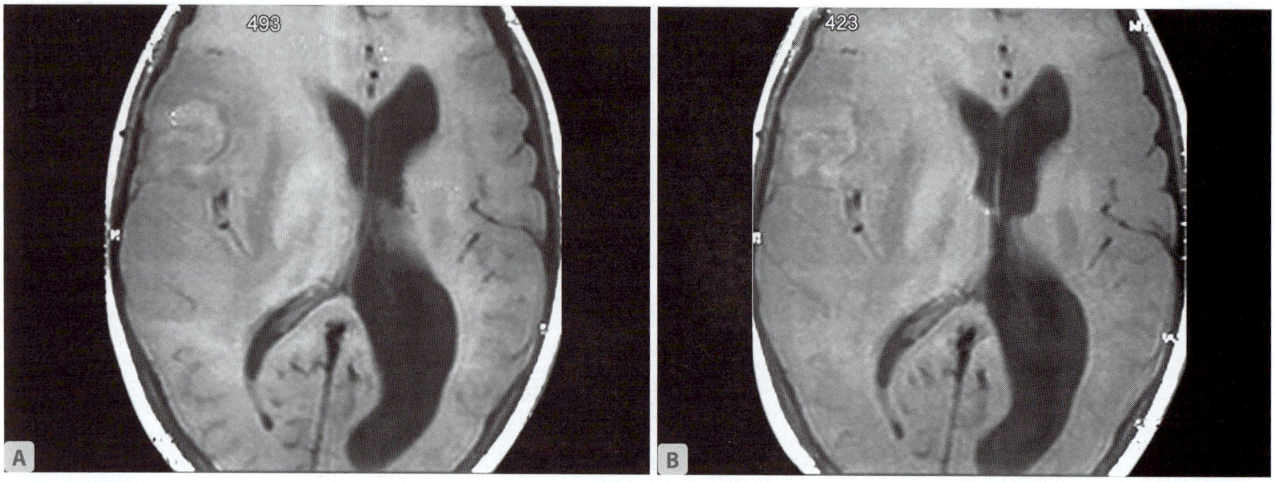

FIGS. 27A AND B: Values taken on axial T1W without MT (A) and with MT; (B) reveal a MT ratio of 14%—multiple tuberculomas with low MT ratio.

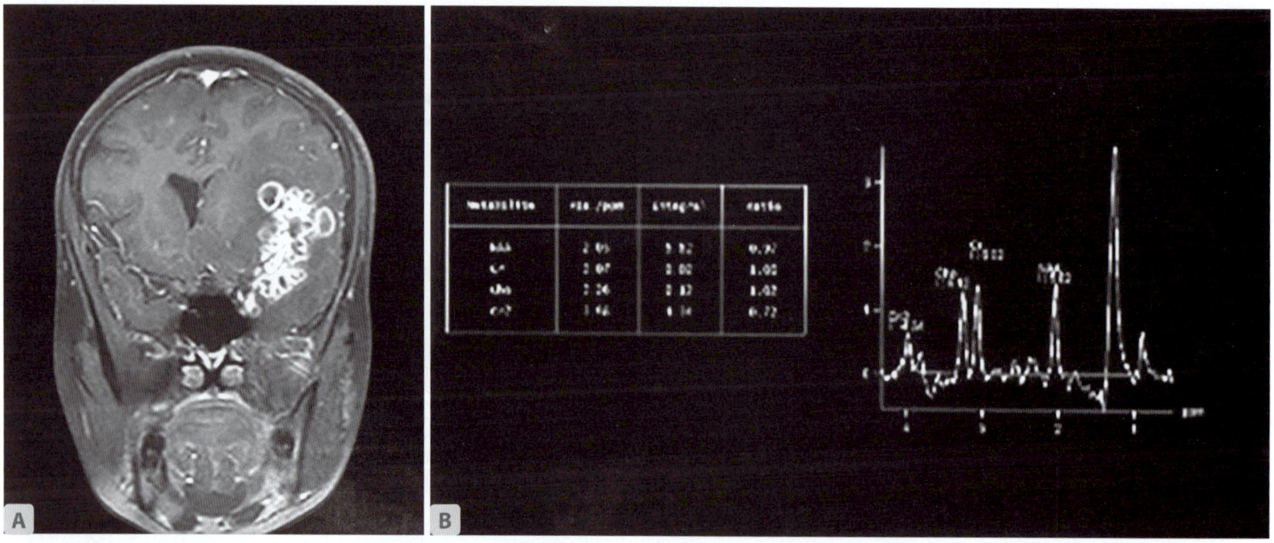

FIGS. 28A AND B: MR spectroscopy image (B) showing a prominent lipid peak at 1.3 ppm in the multiple conglomerate ring-enhancing lesions (A) Tuberculomas.

tuberculomas. These parameters show an increase with antitubercular therapy and hence can be used as a means to follow-up the disease.[77]

Disseminated Tuberculomas (Miliary TB)

Small granulomas (<5 mm) showing high or low signal on T2-weighted images diffusely infiltrating the brain parenchyma form the imaging pattern in disseminated disease[78] **(Figs. 29A to D)**. Gadolinium enhanced MR images which show the lesions as round areas of intense enhancement are best to depict the lesions. These lesions are clearly seen on MT T1W images and MT imaging helps to define the disease load.

TUBERCULOUS ABSCESS

A tuberculous abscess is more common in the elderly or immunocompromised patients and is often indistinguishable from a pyogenic brain abscess or a caseous tuberculoma. Presence of a purulent center rich in tubercle bacilli and absence of giant cell epitheloid granulomatous reaction in the wall distinguishes a tuberculous abscess from a granuloma. According to the Whitner criteria for tuberculous abscess, there should be macroscopic evidence of abscess formation within the brain parenchyma and the abscess wall should have vascular granulation tissue containing acute and chronic inflammatory cells and tubercle bacilli on histology.[79,80]

These occur in less than 10% of patients with CNS TB. On imaging, these are large in size (>3 cm), are multiloculated with smooth, thin enhancing wall, with mass effect and peripheral edema.[81] These are usually solitary with diffusion-weighted imaging showing restricted pattern of diffusion due to the presence of pus[82] **(Figs. 30A and B)**. Differentiation from a pyogenic brain abscess can be done with the help of MR spectroscopy and magnetization transfer MR imaging.[83] A lower magnetization transfer ratio (MTR) in a tubercular abscess as compared to a pyogenic abscess owing to the presence of lipid due to a large number of tubercle bacilli helps in differentiation.[76] Also the presence of amino acid peak (leucine, isoleucine, valine) at 0.9 ppm due to the presence of

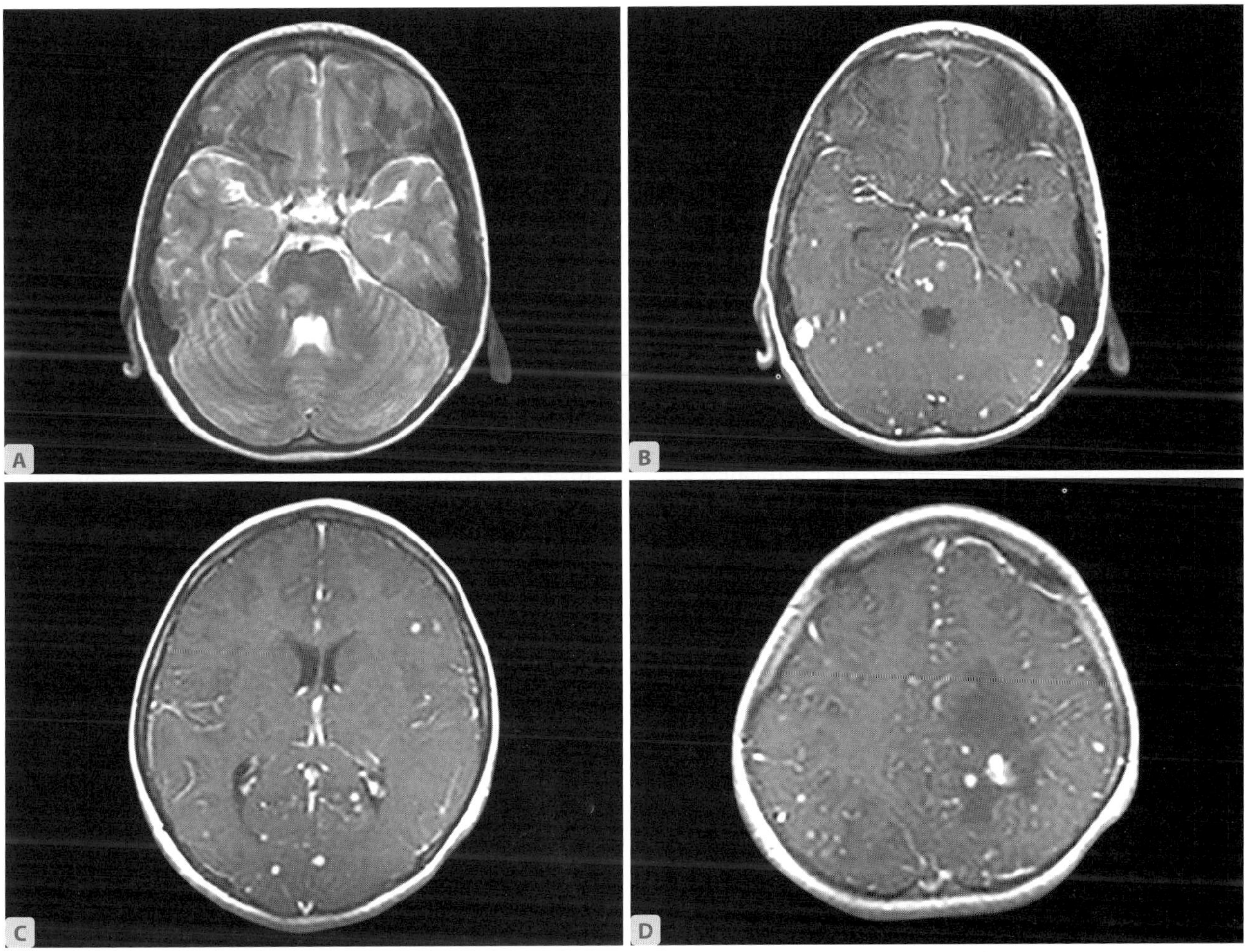

FIGS. 29A TO D: T2W axial MR image (A) showing lesions in the pons, cerebellum with a hyperintense signal. Postcontrast axial images; (B to D) showing intensely enhancing small granulomas in the cerebellum, pons and the cerebral hemispheres. The lesions are numerous and small in size— disseminated tuberculomas.

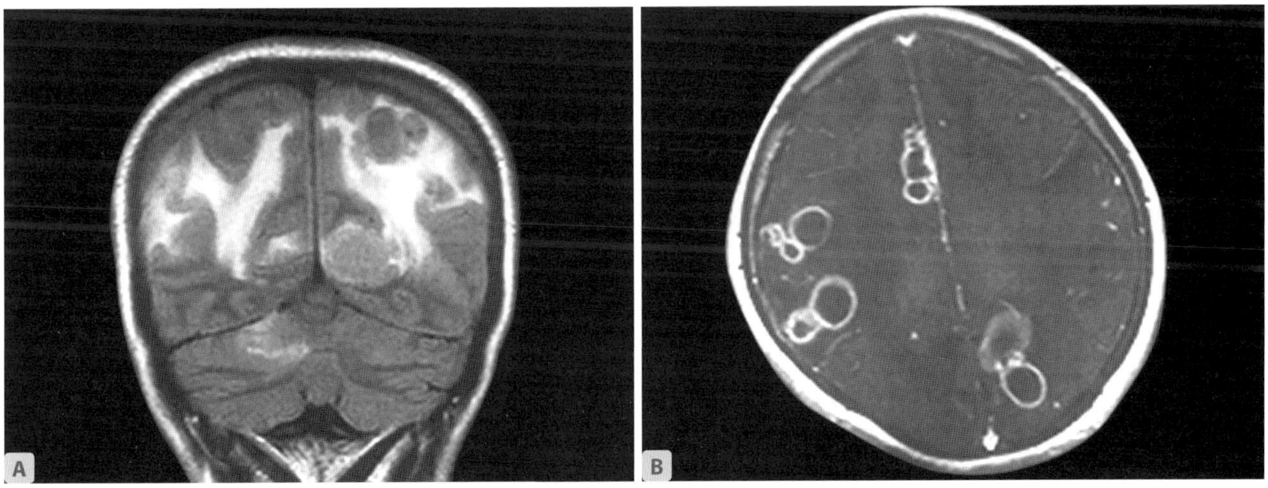

FIGS. 30A AND B: FLAIR coronal (A) and postcontrast axial; (B) images reveal multiple multiloculated lesions with smooth, thin walls seen in bilateral cerebral hemispheres with perilesional edema—multiple tuberculous abscesses.

proteolytic enzymes in a pyogenic brain abscess and absence of amino acid peak in a tubercular abscess further aids in the differentiation. A tubercular abscess may show lipid, lactate and phosphoserine on MR spectroscopy[76] **(Figs. 31A to G)**.

TB ENCEPHALOPATHY

This form usually occurs in infants, pre-school and school age children following pulmonary tuberculosis. It occurs because of an immunologic mechanism with a type IV hypersensitivity reaction to the tuberculous protein mediated by the T lymphocytes. Pathologically, there is loss of myelin, decrease in the oligodendroglia and increase in the astrocytes. There is onset of perivascular demyelination. Imaging shows a diffuse cerebral edema which may be unilateral or bilateral seen as a T2 hyperintense signal. Death usually occurs within 1-2 months of the onset despite antitubercular treatment.[84]

FOCAL TUBERCULOUS CEREBRITIS

This entity has specific clinical, radiologic and histologic manifestations. On histology, multiple caseating and non-caseating granulomas, exudates, Langerhans giant cells and reactive parenchymal changes are seen.[85] A focal gyriform pattern of enhancement is seen on both CT and MR in this entity on imaging.[86]

CNS TB AND AIDS

Tuberculous infections of CNS in AIDS patients follows a rapidly progressive course. Infarction, meningeal enhancement and parenchymal disease are more common in patients with TB who are also HIV infected. However, the differential diagnosis in AIDS patients must include other opportunistic infections and primary or metastatic lymphoma of the CNS.

NEUROSARCOIDOSIS

Involvement of the CNS in sarcoidosis is seen in about 15% of patients. Non caseating granulomas are the histologic hallmark of sarcoidosis. The patterns of CNS involvement by sarcoidosis include—parenchymal, leptomeningeal and meningoencephalitis. The commonest form is leptomeningeal (seen in 40% cases) which is characterized by a circumscribed involvement of the optic chiasma, hypothalamus, the pituitary gland and the floor of the third ventricle. A diffuse involvement and enhancement of the leptomeninges may also be seen, involvement of the cortical sulci, perivascular spaces and basal cisterns distinguish it from dural disease. Postcontrast T1-weighted images are the best to depict the diffuse thickening and enhancement of the leptomeninges. Multiple cranial nerves may also be involved in neurosarcoidosis, the commonest being the facial and optic nerves. A unilateral or bilateral involvement of the cranial nerves can occur which may involve the optic chiasma or the infraorbital portion of the optic nerves.[87] Involvement is usually seen as diffuse thickening and enhancement of the nerves on imaging. The differential diagnosis of this form includes lymphoma and tuberculosis.

Dural involvement by sarcoidosis can be either focal or diffuse. The focal masses appear to be low signal on the

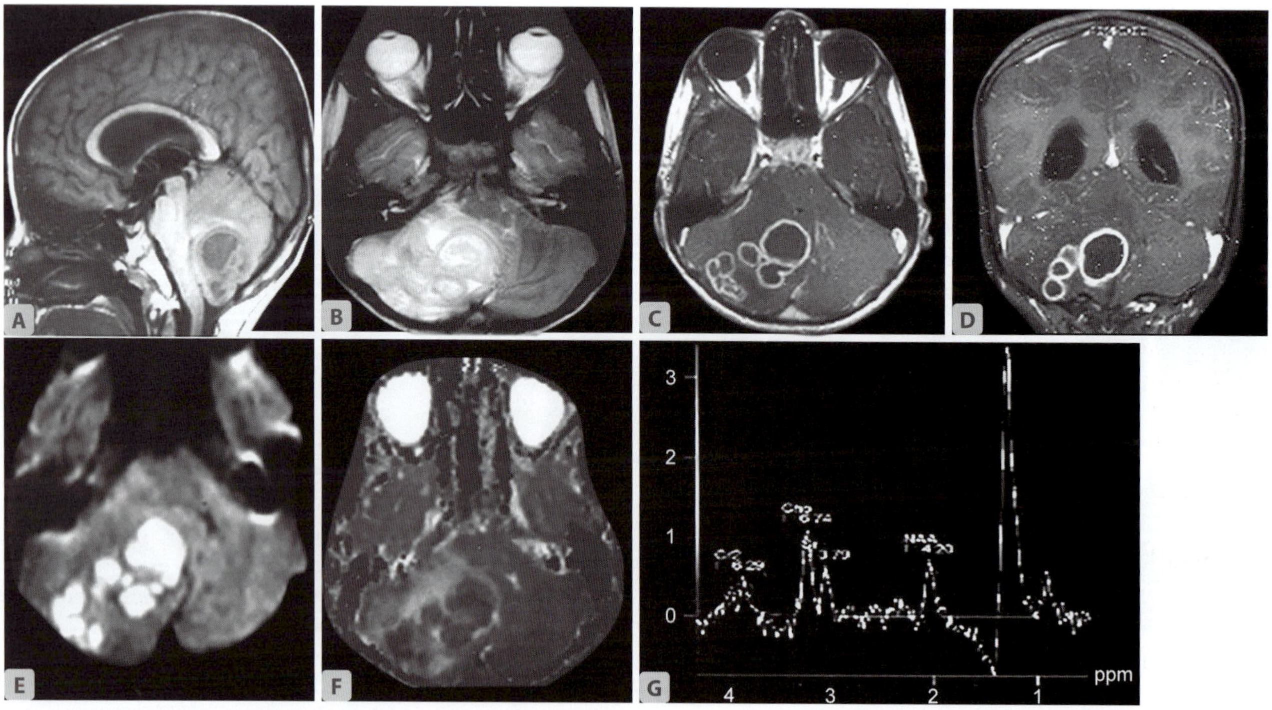

FIGS. 31A TO G: Sagittal T1W (A), axial T2W (B) postcontrast axial; (C and D) images reveal multiple multiloculated ring-enhancing lesions in the posterior fossa with extensive perilesional edema. Diffusion-weighted images; (E and F) reveal restricted pattern of diffusion. MR spectroscopy; (G) shows a prominent lipid at 1.3 ppm—multiple tuberculous abscesses.

T2-weighted images and may mimic a calcified meningioma or very cellular dural metastasis.

The parenchymal form is characterized by multiple granulomas scattered diffusely in the brain parenchyma, iso to hypointense on T1, hyperintense on T2W images and showing intense homogenous enhancement. There is usually little or no perilesional edema around the lesions which resolve significantly following steroid treatment. Another form of parenchymal involvement is multiple periventricular white matter lesions which do not show any contrast enhancement and mimic lesions of multiple sclerosis or those seen in vascular disease. These lesions occur due to involvement of small arteries in the white matter by sarcoidosis.

The meningoencephalitis form is the rarest form and is characterized by nodular and meningeal enhancement. This enhancement usually extends into the parenchyma through the Virchow-Robin spaces.

FUNGAL INFECTIONS OF THE CENTRAL NERVOUS SYSTEM

Fungi are a distinct group of pathogenic organisms which may exist either as yeast form (*Candida, Cryptococcus, Histoplasma, Coccidioides, Torulopsis*) or hyphal form (*Aspergillus, Mucormycosis, Pseudallescheria*). The yeast form or the single celled form being smaller in size usually spreads hematogenously to present as meningitis or granulomas while the hyphal form being the larger form usually involves the parenchyma resulting in cerebritis or encephalitis. Vasculitis, vascular occlusion, septic infarction and aneurysm formation may occur due to invasion of small or medium sized arteries by the large mycelial forms, formed by the coalescence of the yeast or hyphal form.

ASPERGILLOSIS

Aspergillosis is an opportunistic infection which usually involves immunocompromised patients.[88] The predominant form is the hyphal form and this fungus exists in soil, water or decaying vegetation.

The mode of entry is by inhalation of the fungal spores. The infection is initially confined to the pulmonary tree with a resultant hypersensitivity reaction. When the host's defence mechanism are weak a hematogenous dissemination in the body with involvement of the CNS may occur.[89] CNS involvement is in the form of vasculitis/vasculopathy, brain abscess or granuloma formation. A rhinocerebral form may rarely occur caused by the direct extension of disease in the nasal cavity and paranasal sinuses.[90]

MR imaging reveals a characteristic "target like pattern" on the T2W images. *Aspergillus* lesions show a characteristic central hyperintensity surrounded by a peripheral hypo-intensity. The hypointense signal is attributed to increased iron due to fungal elements, hemorrhage and ferromagnetic metals like calcium and manganese resulting from fungal metabolism.[91]

Vasculitis/Vasculopathy

Aspergillus is angioinvasive. The invasive nature of the aspergillosis accounts for the vascular occlusion with resultant infarction which is often hemorrhagic. Focal microhemorrhages occur because of the production of the enzyme elastase by the fungus which digests the internal elastic lamina of arteries. Weakening and digestion of the walls leads to the formation of a mycotic aneurysm. Amongst the fungal infections, aspergillosis is the commonest cause of a mycotic aneurysm. The presence of subarachnoid hemorrhage or mycotic aneurysm formation in immunocompromised patients with suspected fungal infection should prompt instillation of appropriate antifungal therapy.[92] *Aspergillus* has an affinity for the origins of small perforating arteries with consequent sterile infarctions in the basal ganglia, corpus callosum, and thalamus. Thus, infarction of the corpus callosum is highly suggestive of aspergillus infection as this is not the site for pyogenic or thromboembolic infarction.[93] The sterile infarct gets converted into septic infarct as direct extension of fungal elements into the surrounding brain parenchyma occurs when breakdown of brain tissue occurs at sites of infarction.

Cerebritis and abscess formation can occur when the host defense mechanism tries to encapsulate the offending organism **(Figs. 32A to C)**. A restricted pattern of diffusion is seen in an *Aspergillus* abscess due to the high cellularity and viscosity of the pus material.[94] A typical pattern of restricted diffusion "the ring pattern" is seen in *Aspergillus* with the lesion center being hypointense on DWI and the lesion periphery being hyperintense on DWI. Postcontrast scans reveal weak or no enhancement which is an important diagnostic clue. Capsule formation from chronic inflammation and production of granulation tissue can contribute to the weak ring enhancement seen in some cases. A crenated border and non enhancing intracavitary projections also help to differentiate a fungal from a pyogenic or tubercular abscess. The demonstration of α-trehalose peak on MR spectroscopy (3.6–3.8 ppm) in fungal abscess also helps in the differentiation. Meningitis and ventriculitis may manifest as hydrocephalus on imaging and ependymal enhancement is distinctly uncharacteristic.

Rhinocerebral form occurs when infection spreads from the orbit, the paranasal sinuses or base of the skull to the brain. The sinuses have a low signal on both T1- and T2-weighted images owing to the presence of paramagnetic metals within the infectious mass and show evidence of contrast enhancement.[95]

CRYPTOCOCCAL INFECTION

Cryptococcosis is the commonest fungal infection to involve the CNS and the most frequently identifiable fungal infection in AIDS patients.[96] Caused by the fungus *Cryptococcus neoformans*, it is more commonly seen in men (80%). This may be attributed to the fungus thriving in soil contaminated with pigeon droppings and a greater occupational exposure to the fungal spores in men. Inhalation of spores leads to pulmonary disease which is usually subclinical. In the pulmonary tree, the organism forms a highly resistant polysaccharide capsule which may be related to the high carbon dioxide tension present in the lungs. From the lungs, the organism may lodge in the intrathoracic lymph nodes and remain dormant. Any weakening of the host's immune system leads to a reactivation with dissemination occurring to the CNS predominantly.

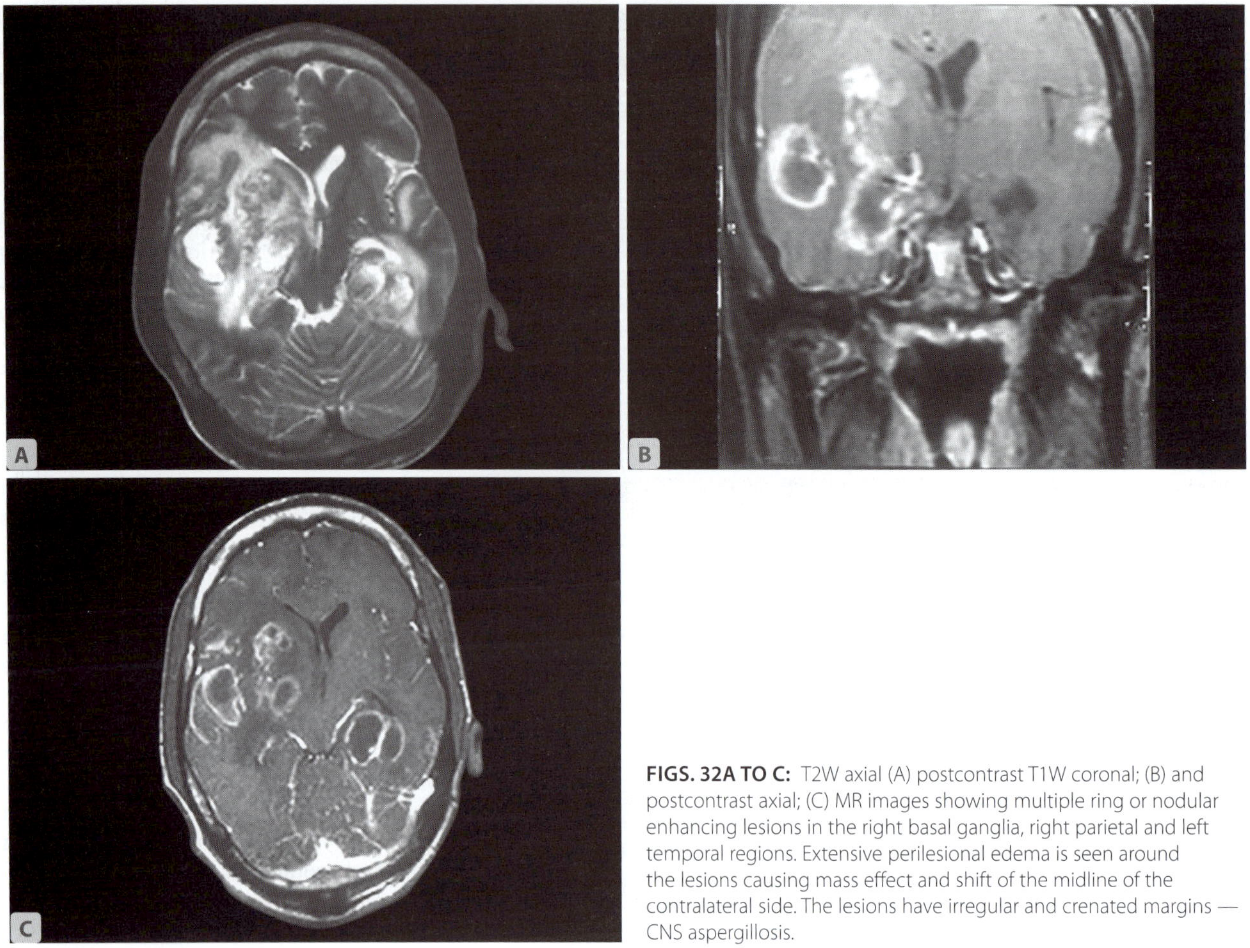

FIGS. 32A TO C: T2W axial (A) postcontrast T1W coronal; (B) and postcontrast axial; (C) MR images showing multiple ring or nodular enhancing lesions in the right basal ganglia, right parietal and left temporal regions. Extensive perilesional edema is seen around the lesions causing mass effect and shift of the midline of the contralateral side. The lesions have irregular and crenated margins — CNS aspergillosis.

The propensity of CNS dissemination is accounted by the absence of anticryptococcal factors in the CSF as compared to serum.[97] Also, the polysaccharide capsule of the fungus is resistant to phagocytosis and confers protection against the host's inflammatory response.

Imaging

On CT, cerebral atrophy and hydrocephalus may be the only positive findings.[98] *Cryptococcus* often causes meningeal disease which is usually basal in location but may not be detected on the postcontrast scans owing to the inability of the host to mount a cell mediated immune response. Hydrocephalus may also not be seen in the immunocompromised patients due to the lack of inflammatory leptomeningeal reaction and paucity of adhesions. Thus imaging findings are often lacking in immunocompromised patients on CT scans.

On MRI, the positive imaging findings include dilated Virchow Robin spaces and cryptococcomas. Dilated Virchow Robin spaces are seen as foci isointense to the CSF, less than 3 mm in size, bilateral and symmetric with a predilection for the basal ganglia and thalamus. These foci are not associated with any mass effect, perilesional edema or contrast enhancement[99] **(Figs. 33A to C)**. These spaces may coalesce producing gelatinous pseudocysts. The perivascular spaces get filled with fungi and mucoid gelatinous material produced by the capsule of the organism. Gelatinous pseudocysts have a classic "soap bubble" appearance and are most commonly seen in the basal ganglia, thalamus and midbrain. These pseudocysts may show restricted diffusion owing to the gelatinous content.

Invasion of the brain parenchyma may result in the formation of chronic granulomas or cryptococcomas. Cryptococcomas are low to intermediate signal on T1 and high signal on T2W images. No enhancement is seen in the immunocompromised/AIDS patients but in the immunocompetent patient some degree of enhancement may be seen. A double dose technique may show the lesions better. These granulomas have also been reported along the ependyma of the choroid plexus and this finding if seen is considered highly specific for cryptococcosis.[100]

MR Spectroscopy in Cryptococcomas

High levels of MR visible α-trehalose have been reported from cryptococcomas. This helps in an early and correct diagnosis and in differentiation from mitotic lesions. Trehalose is a disaccharide found in the fungal wall and identification of multiple signals between 3.6 and 3.8 ppm adds specificity to the diagnosis.[81]

A rare pattern of involvement is multiple miliary enhancing nodules in the parenchyma or leptomeninges

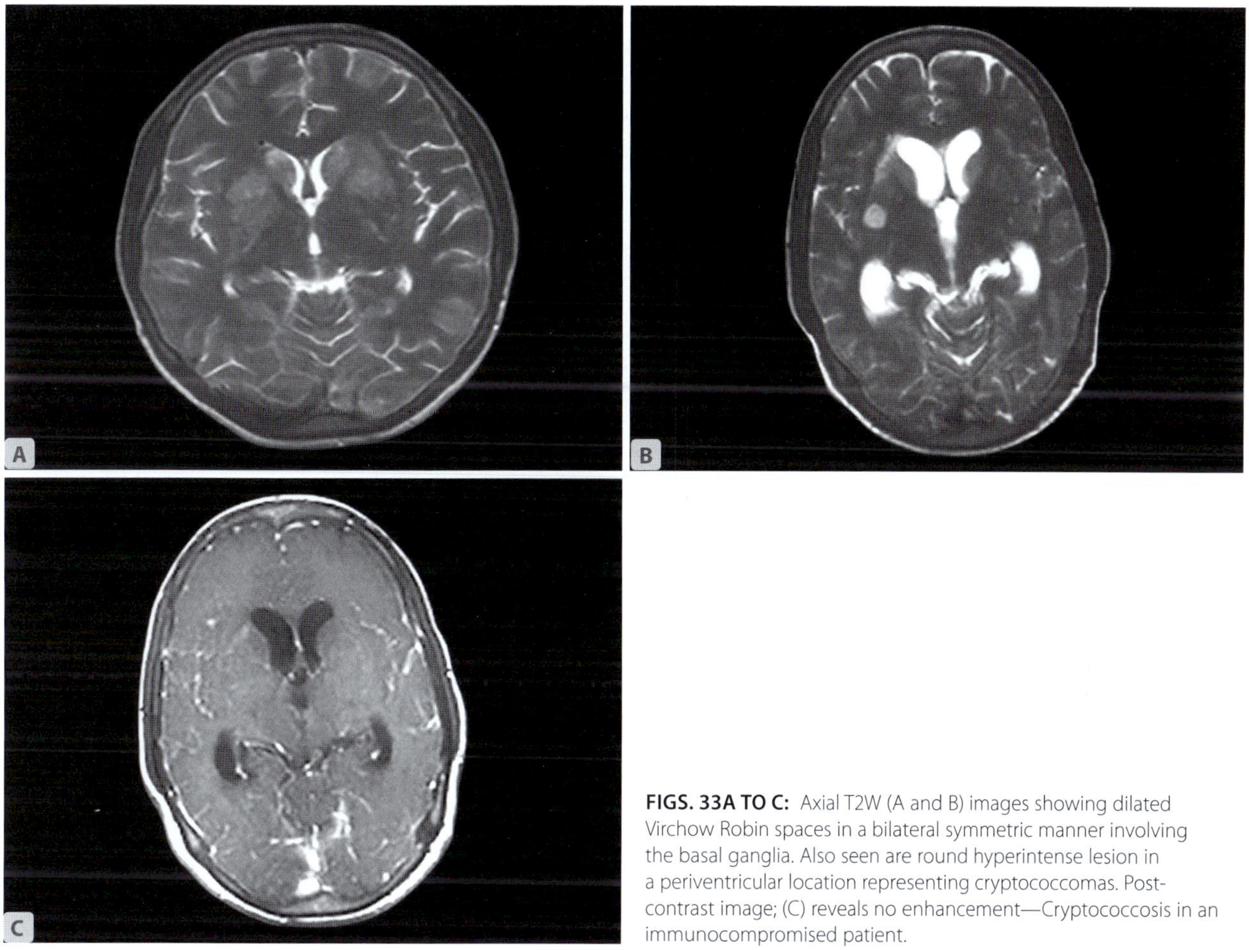

FIGS. 33A TO C: Axial T2W (A and B) images showing dilated Virchow Robin spaces in a bilateral symmetric manner involving the basal ganglia. Also seen are round hyperintense lesion in a periventricular location representing cryptococcomas. Post-contrast image; (C) reveals no enhancement—Cryptococcosis in an immunocompromised patient.

suggestive of granuloma formation. Another uncommon pattern is the involvement of the spinal cord which may be seen as high signal on T2 with or without enhancement.

Diagnosis of cryptococcal infection is easier than other fungal infections because of the following reasons:

1. The yeast can be seen in the CSF
2. Immunologic tests for antigen in blood and CSF are highly sensitive.
3. Infection has a unique appearance on histology.

The diagnosis is usually made by India ink preparation or by fungal culture of CSF.

MUCORMYCOSIS

It is the most aggressive of all fungal infections and those with diabetes are at increased risk. A triad of diabetic ketoacidosis, naso-orbital infection and meningoencephalitis is highly suggestive of the diagnosis. Though diabetes compromises 70% of all cases, sepsis, chronic renal failure, severe chronic diarrhea, severe dehydration constitute the other predisposing factors. Immunocompromised patients or those with a history of renal transplant are also at increased risk.[101] Two forms of the disease are recognized—the rhinocerebral form and the hematogenous form.

Imaging

The rhinocerebral form, which is the more common form occurs when the sinus infection extends into the CNS. The organism may spread via the perivascular and perineural channels through the cribriform plate into the frontal lobe or through the orbital apex into the cavernous sinus[102] **(Figs. 34A to F)**. Direct invasion of the arteries with consequent thrombosis and infarction can occur. The internal carotid artery and the basilar artery may be involved by thrombus formation **(Figs. 35A to C)**. MRI shows nonspecific inflammatory changes involving the paranasal sinuses and the orbits similar to *Aspergillus* infection. The sinuses have a low signal on T2W images owing to the presence of paramagnetic metals like calcium, manganese, magnesium, iron within the fungal mass. A "black turbinate" sign has been describe in mucormycosis.[103] It refers to the non-enhancing mucosa on MRI suggesting infarction of the invaded mucosa. Meningitis may occur in the rhinocerebral form or with central skull base involvement resulting from direct extension of infection.

The hematogenous form is less common and is usually seen in patients with malignancies and intravenous drug abusers. The vascular changes seen are arteritis, ischaemia changes, bland or haemorrhagic infarction and aneurysm formation.[104]

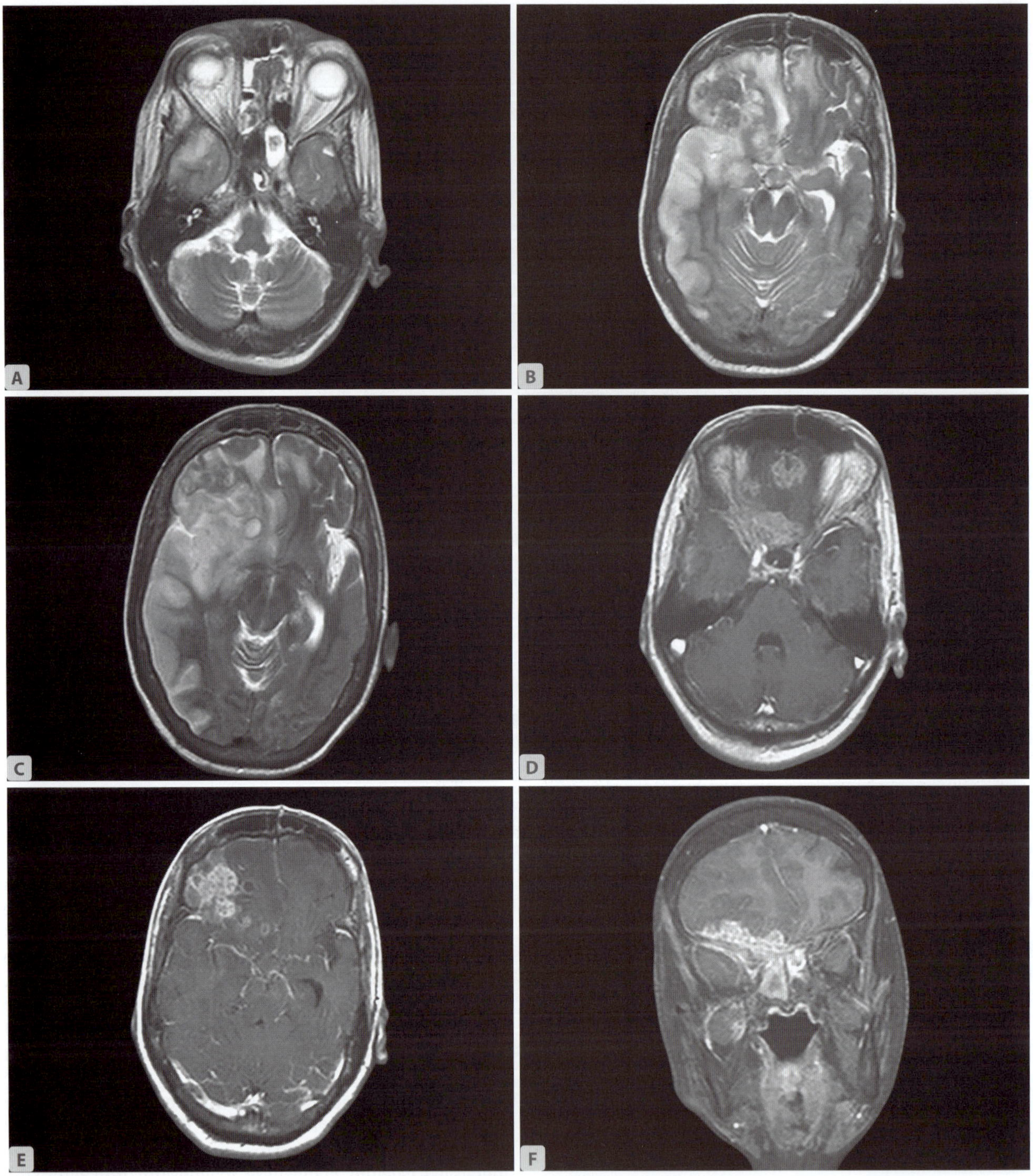

FIGS. 34A TO F: Axial T2W (A to C) images reveal a large area of signal alteration in the right frontotemporoparietal region with mass effect and gyral swelling. Postcontrast; (D to F) images reveal ring enhancing lesions in the basifrontal region, the lesions are hypointense on T2W images. Evidence of sinusitis seen which shows a low signal on T2W images.

CANDIDIASIS

Candidiasis is caused by *Candida albicans* species. These fungi lack a sexual cycle and reproduce by budding or fission. Pseudohyphae predominate though rarely true hyphae may form. The fungus is present as a part of the normal intestinal flora. *Candida* infection occurs when there are disturbances in equilibrium that normally exists within the intestinal flora, such as following antibiotic therapy, chemotherapy and hematologic conditions such as thrombocytopenia. Indwelling catheters, intravenous drug abuse with resulting candidal endocarditis are the other predisposing factors. HIV infection with low CD4 counts (<135 mm^3) is another risk

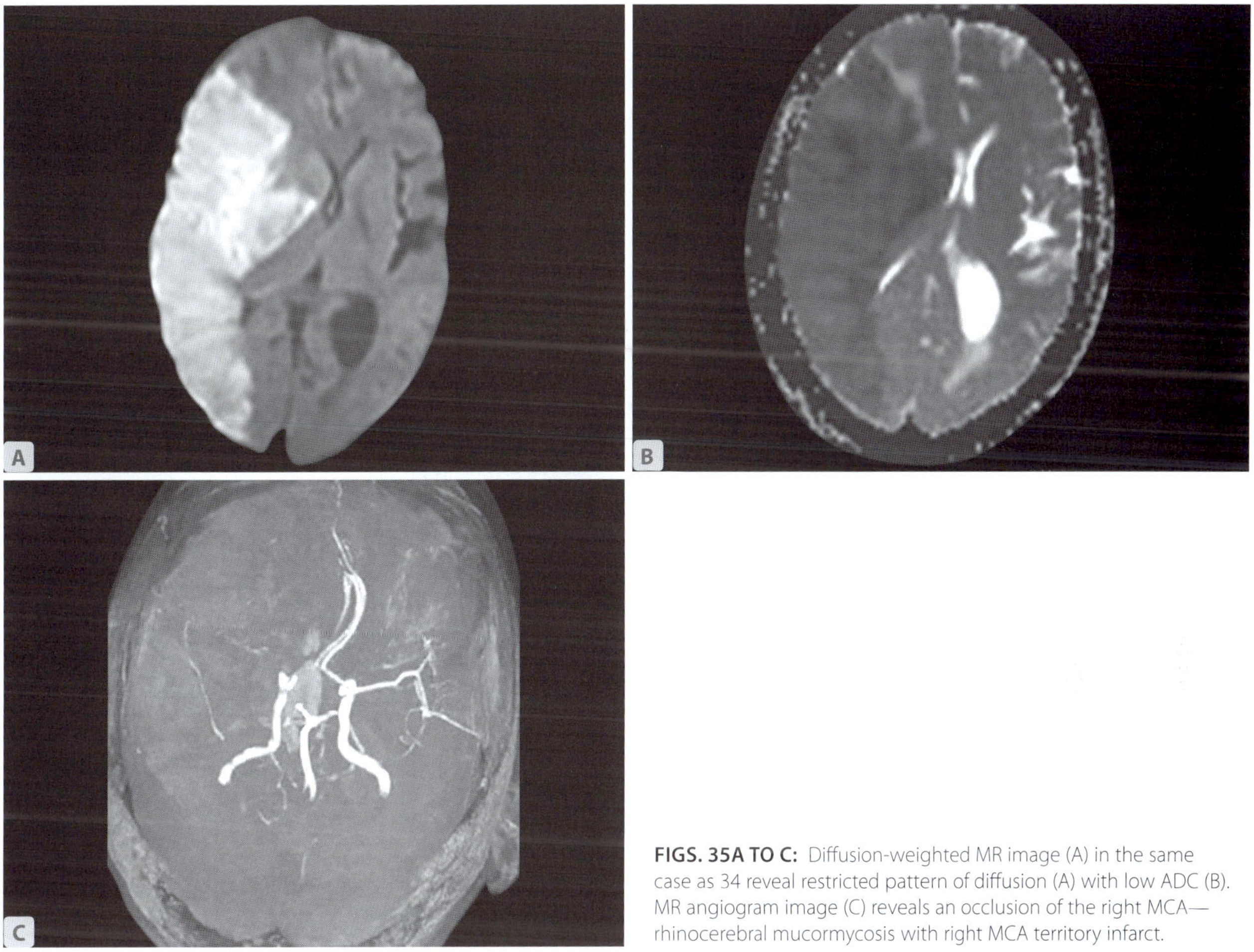

FIGS. 35A TO C: Diffusion-weighted MR image (A) in the same case as 34 reveal restricted pattern of diffusion (A) with low ADC (B). MR angiogram image (C) reveals an occlusion of the right MCA—rhinocerebral mucormycosis with right MCA territory infarct.

factor. Preterm, low birth infants are particularly susceptible to acquire the infection. The infections may be acquired in utero, during passage through an infected genital tract or postnatally. In the disseminated/systemic form of candidiasis the kidneys are the most common affected organs followed by the central nervous system which is involved in about 50% cases.

Imaging

The imaging hallmark is microabscesses which are defined as <3 mm small ascesses diffusely scattered in the brain parenchyma **(Figs. 36A and B)**. Other imaging manifestations include macroabscesses, meningitis, meningoencephalitis, granuloma formation, ependymitis, ischaemia, infarction or mycotic aneurysm formation.[105] Early diagnosis is essential as CNS involvement warrants a different therapy. Fluconazole along with Amphotericin B leads to better prognosis.

COCCIDIOIDOMYCOSIS

The causative organism *Coccidioides immitis*, is a dimorphic yeast found in the soil. The spores produced by this organism are called anthroconidia. These spores are extremely resilient and virulent and may lie dormant in the soil for long periods. Activities like farming and construction may cause a dispersal of the spores which may then be inhaled by the humans resulting in a subclinical upper respiratory inection. An immunocompromised state, diabetes and pregnancy may act as risk factors for dissemination of the infection. The most common CNS manifestation is meningitis which may be associated with cerebritis and hydrocephalus. Granuloma and abscess formation may be the other manifestations with multiple granulomas resembling miliary tuberculosis.[106] Vascular complications can be seen in about 40% of patients with meningitis and include arteritis and infarction. Aneurysm formation and subarachnoid hemorrhage resulting from rupture of the aneurysm are the other manifestations of this infection.

HISTOPLASMOSIS

The most common mode of entry is inhalation of airborne spores. The lung are therefore the most common organ affected and CNS involvement usually occurs in immunocompromised host resulting from a hematogenous spread.

The radiologic findings are similar to other fungal infections such as meningitis, encephalitis, brain abscess and histoplasmoma (granuloma) formation. A miliary pattern and vasculitis has also been described.[107,108] Definitive diagnosis can be achieved by CSF analysis or by brain biopsy.[109]

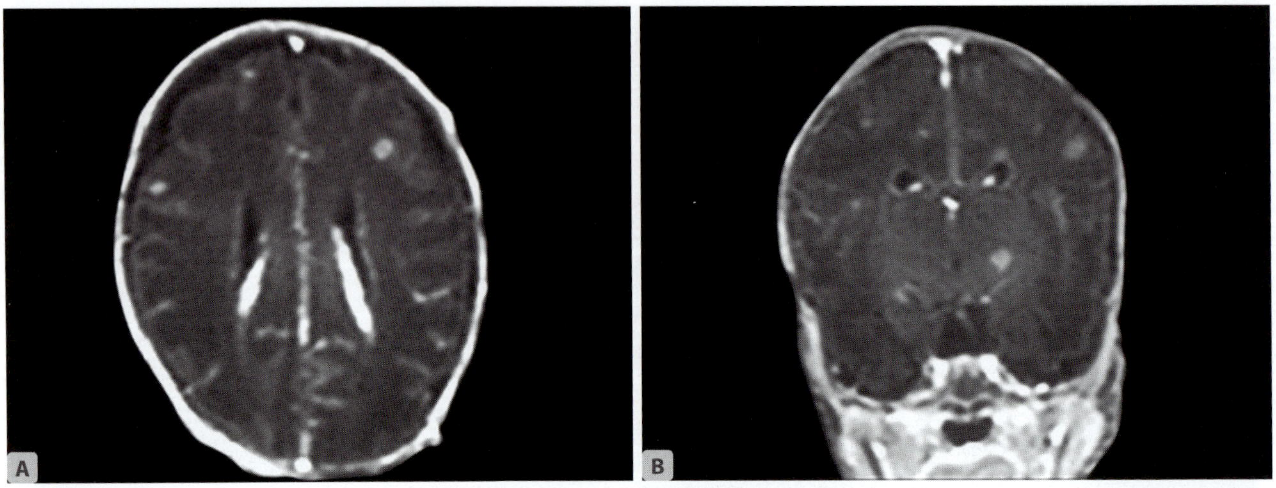

FIGS. 36A AND B: Postcontrast axial images showing multiple microabscesses and nodular enhancing lesions in bilateral cerebral hemispheres—Candidiasis.

NOCARDIOSIS

Nocardia asteroides is actually a bacterial pathogen found in the soil but has traditionally been included in medical mycology. Patients with diabetes, immunocompromised patients, those with a pre-existing pulmonary disease or collagen vascular disease are at increased risk. As the infection is airborne, the primary site of involvement is the lungs and brain involvement occurs secondary to hematogenous spread seen in about 25% of cases. Multiple brain abscesses is the imaging hallmark of the disease. Contrast enhanced CT scan or MRI may show multiple or mutiloculated ring enhancing lesions.

PARASITIC INFECTIONS

NEUROCYSTICERCOSIS

Cysticercosis is the commonest parasitic disease in humans caused by the worm Taenia solium. It is the most common cause of acquired epilepsy throughout the world. Humans are the definitive host when infected with adult tapeworm and the intermediate host when infected with the larval stage/cysticercus. Thus taeniasis is the term used for infection by the adult tapeworm while cysticercosis is an infection by the larval stage. Infected humans excrete the gravid proglottids or eggs in the feces which are ingested by the pig. Pigs acquire cysticercosis as the larva migrate via the circulatory system and get embedded in the muscle where they may persist for many years. Taeniasis is acquired when humans ingest undercooked meat or raw flesh of an infected animal. Humans can also get infected by the larval stage when they accidentally consume T. solium eggs. Once the eggs reach the small intestine, they penetrate the intestinal mucosa to enter the bloodstream and can reach any organ of the body to form cysts. Cysts can be found in the skin, muscles, eyes, heart, and the CNS where they cause neurocysticercosis **(Figs. 37A to D)**.

Clinical Features

CNS involvement occurs in 60–90% of cases with cysticercosis.[110] Patients may be asymptomatic with the neurocysticerci discovered incidentally on imaging. When symptomatic, headache, seizure, diplopia, visual field deficits are the most common neurologic manifestations. At times patients may present with focal neurological deficits and stroke.[111]

Four patterns of cysticercosis in the CNS are recognized-parenchymal, intraventricular, spinal, subarachnoid or a combination of these.

Parenchymal Cysticercosis

The cysts are seen in the parenchyma and basal ganglia owing to the rich vascular supply of these areas. These cysts are usually less than 10 mm in size as the compliance of the brain parenchyma prevents excessive growth of the vesicles.

Escobar classified the cysts into four pathologic states[112] **(Figs. 38A to D)**. In the vesicular stage the larva is seen as a small marginal nodule projecting into a small cyst containing clear fluid. On imaging the vesicular stage is seen as a clearly marginated cyst with thin imperceptible walls with CSF signal intensity and a discrete eccentrically located scolex within. A "dot in a hole" or a "target" appearance may be seen owing to the presence of the scolex which has a soft tissue attenuation or signal intensity distinct from the cyst fluid. No perilesional edema is seen. No contrast enhancement is seen at this stage as there is no immune response by the host.

In the next stage, that is the colloidal vesicular stage, the larva begins to degenerate. This may occur from effects of therapy or from natural death of the scolex with associated disruption of the cyst wall. There is a decrease in the size of the cyst, the cyst fluid becomes turbid, the wall becomes perceptible and thick. There is evidence of substantial perilesional edema and contrast enhancement of the cyst wall owing to the inflammatory reaction caused by the

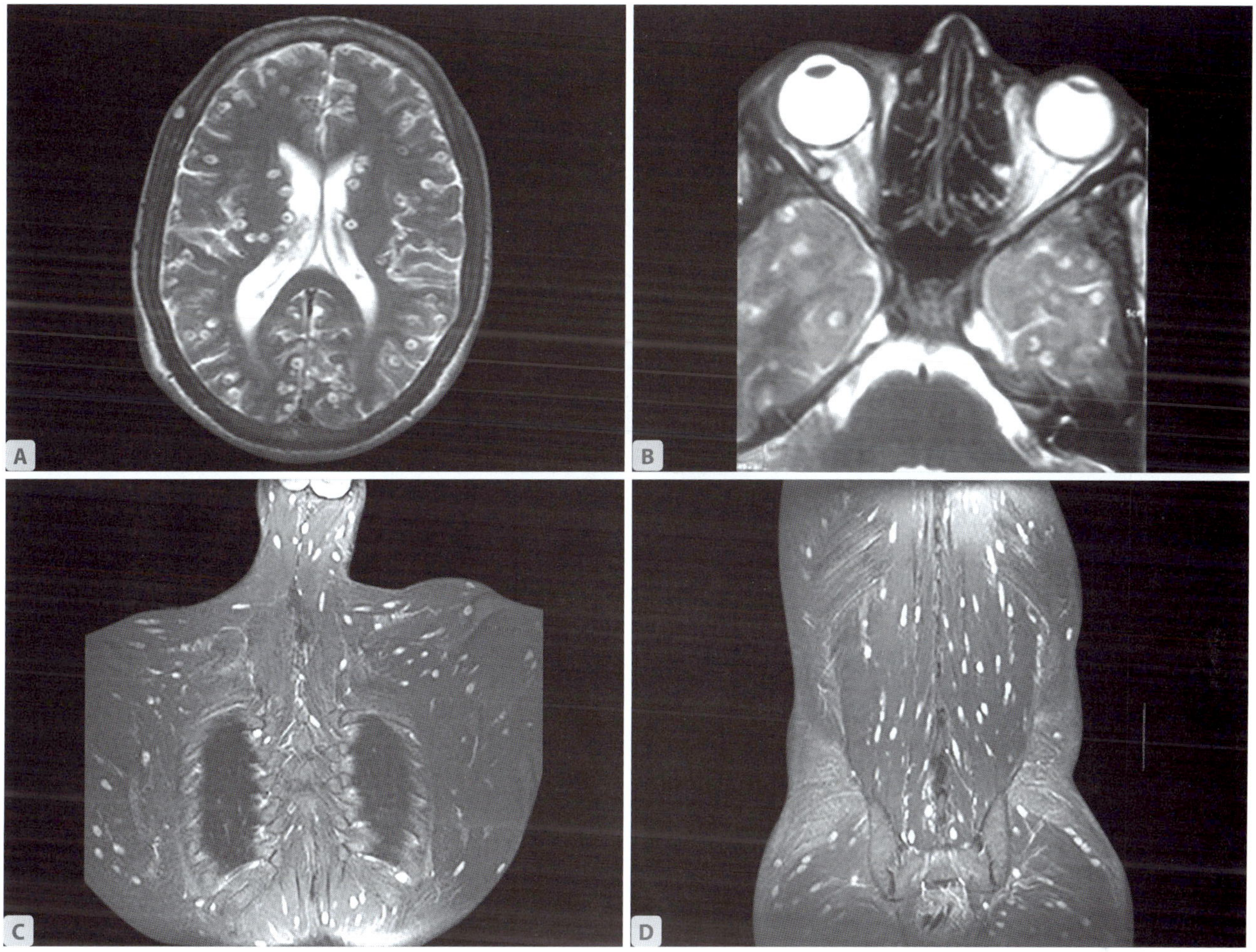

FIGS. 37A TO D: Axial T2W (A and B) images showing multiple small lesions hyperintense on T2W in both cerebral hemispheres, right lateral rectus muscle in the orbit. STIR coronal images (C and D) reveal lesions in the muscles—multiple cysticerci.

degeneration of the larva.[113] On the postcontrast T1W images, a pattern of ring enhancement is seen. The late colloidal vesicular stage is characterized by thick and irregular cyst wall, retraction, moderate perilesional edema and absence of scolex.

The third stage, that is the granular nodular stage, is characterized by further retraction and thickening of the cyst wall with a coarse mineralized scolex. There is near complete resorption of the cyst fluid, the capsule is thick and collagenous and there is a marked decrease in the amount of perilesional edema in this stage.

The fourth or final stage is the nodular calcified stage in which there is shrinkage of the lesion and it is completely mineralized.[114] No perilesional edema or contrast enhancement is seen. On imaging a calcified nodule or a focal area of gliosis is seen. Magnetization transfer ratio (MTR) helps in the differentiation of T2 hypointense lesions of cysticercus (granular nodular stage) from that of tuberculoma. Cysticercus larvae have higher protein and amino acid content and result in higher magnetization transfer ratio as compared to tuberculomas.

On imaging, the cysticercus cysts may be seen in various stages and in transition from one stage to another as the evolution is a dynamic process and no abrupt change occurs from one stage to another. An encephalitic form of cysticercosis can be seen in the pediatric population. This form is characterized by multiple small enhancing lesions along with diffuse cerebral edema[115] **(Figs. 39A to C)**. The increased vascularity and capillary endothelial proliferation adjacent to the cysts accounts for the lesions showing contrast enhancement. The sequelae of the encephalitic form is seen as multiple punctate calcifications scattered in the brain parenchyma representing the nodular calcified stage of the disease.

The cysticercus lesion needs to be differentiated from a tuberculoma on imaging **(Table 3)**.

Intraventricular Cysticercosis

The intraventricular form usually occurs in isolation and is not associated with cysts elsewhere. These are seen most commonly in the fourth ventricle followed by the lateral and third ventricle. These cysts may migrate from one ventricle to another. Obstructive hydrocephalus occurs when the cyst gets entrapped in the aqueduct of Sylvius obstructing the ventricular outflow. Multiple cysts are rare and if found are usually seen in the lateral ventricles.

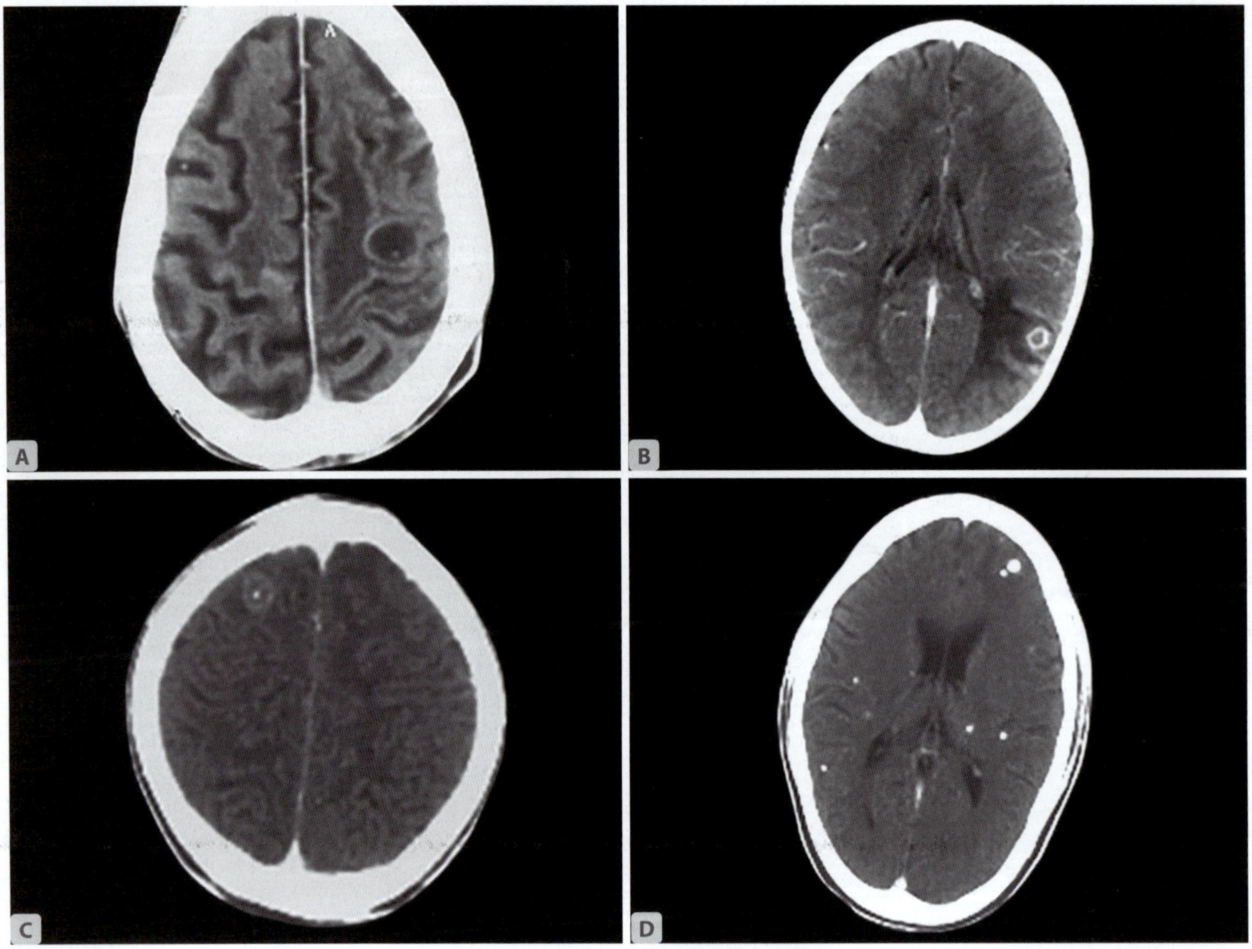

FIGS. 38A TO D: Contrast-enhanced axial CT (A) showing a cyst with fluid similar to CSF attenuation with an eccentrically located scolex in the left parietal region with no contrast enhancement/edema—vesicular stage. Axial CT scan; (B) showing a ring-enhancing lesion with perilesional edema in left parieto-occipital region colloid vesicular stage. CECT axial image; (C) showing a cyst with thick capsule with calcific nodule with no edema—granular nodular stage. CECT axial images; (D) showing calcific foci in bilateral hemispheres—nodular calcified stage.

On imaging, the intraventricular cyst is seen as a high signal intensity mural nodule outlined by the CSF on T1-weighted and FLAIR images.[117] CISS sequence (constructive interference in the steady state) is the best sequence to demonstrate the intraventricular cysticercosis as the cyst wall is clearly delineated on this sequence **(Figs. 40A and B)**. Sagittal T1-weighted imaging is helpful in differentiating a fourth ventricular cysticercus from a dilated fourth ventricle and in showing aqueductal obstruction.

MR imaging is helpful in the preoperative locatization of the cyst and in detecting granular ependymitis seen as ring like or nodular enhancement.[118] The diagnosis of granular ependymitis is important as all these patients require a shunt even after surgical removal of the cyst. Intraventricular cyst may migrate within the ventricular system or into the basal cisterns or subarachnoid space from the ventricles.

Subarachnoid Cysticercosis

The subarachnoid or racemose variety of cysticercosis is seen within the cortical sulci, gyri or within the basal cisterns. Those in the basal cisterns attain a large size owing to the lack of pressure from the adjacent brain parenchyma and characteristically lack a mural nodule. Many theories have been postulated to explain the absence of the scolex in the racemose variety. While Martinez has suggested that the racemose variety is an arrested form in the development of the cyst with the scolex never being formed some have suggested that a disordered proliferation of the cyst wall in the racemose variety accounts for the lack of the scolex.[114,118] A lack of encapsulation in the basal cisterns as compared to the parenchymal forms also has been suggested in the etiopathogenesis. On imaging, large multiple, multilobulated cysts in a basal cisternal location, isointense to the CSF on all sequences, with lack of a mural nodule and leptomeningeal enhancement characterize the racemose variety **(Figs. 41A to C)**.

Cysts located at the cortical sulci are usually small while those located in the Sylvian fissures may grow to large sizes similar to echinococcus infection.

Basilar leptomeningitis, arachnoiditis, mass effect, communicating hydrocephalus and vasculitis may occur in the subarachnoid variety owing to an intense inflammatory response. The walls of the arteries are invaded by inflammatory cells leading to vasculitis and proliferative endarteritis.

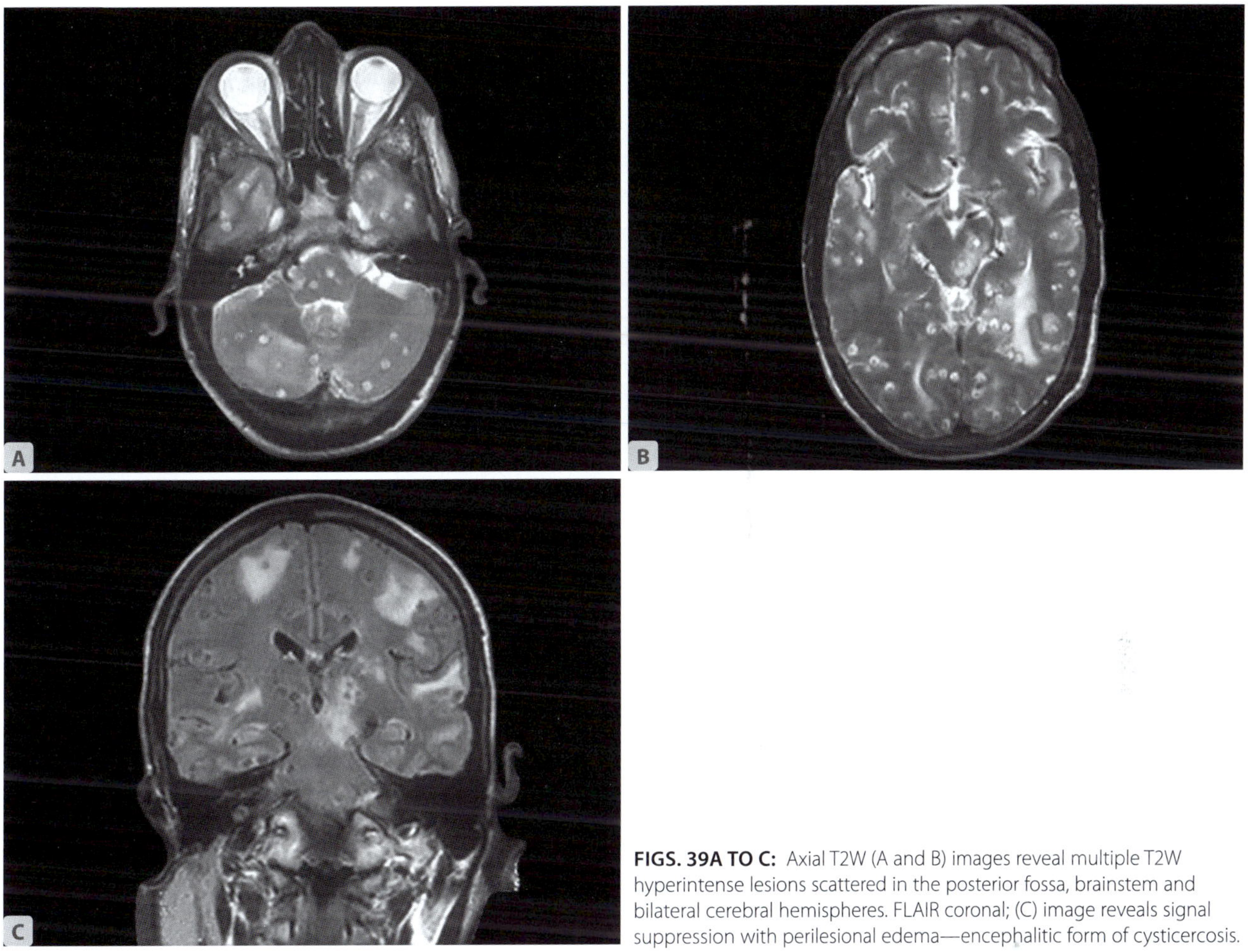

FIGS. 39A TO C: Axial T2W (A and B) images reveal multiple T2W hyperintense lesions scattered in the posterior fossa, brainstem and bilateral cerebral hemispheres. FLAIR coronal; (C) image reveals signal suppression with perilesional edema—encephalitic form of cysticercosis.

TABLE 3: Differences between neurocysticercosis (NCC) and tuberculomas on imaging.[116]

Neurocysticercosis	Tuberculoma
Usually <20 mm in size, cystic	>20 mm in size, solid
Regular in outline	Has an irregular outline
Mild-to-moderate perilesional edema	Extensive/marked perilesional edema
No midline shift seen	Midline shift may be seen
An eccentric scolex may be seen	No scolex seen
May be single/multiple	Usually multiple, may show conglomeration
T2 hyperintense lesions with complete signal suppression on FLAIR sequence	Caseating granulomas with solid centre are hypointense on T2W images. Those hyperintense on T2W images do not show complete signal suppression on FLAIR images
No lipid peak on MR spectroscopy	Lipid peak seen on MRS
High MTR because of protein content	Low MTR because of lipid content

Spinal Cysticercosis

Spinal cysticercus appears as a cystic mass compressing the spinal cord, that is, as an intradural extramedullary cyst or as arachnoiditis.

Orbital Disease

The lesions may involve the globe or the extraocular muscles. The parasitic cysts may be seen in the choroid/retina, in the subconjunctival region. In the muscles, it is the muscle belly which is usually involved and the appearance is that of one or more cysts ("peas in a pod" appearance).

TOXOPLASMOSIS

Toxoplasma gondii is a parasite well known throughout the world. The definitive host is the cat and other Felidae. After ingestion, the organism develops in the epithelial cells of the intestine to form schizonts, gametocytes and oocytes which are shed in the cat's feces. The cat excretes the oocytes for approximately 2 weeks after the primary insult. Human consumption of undercooked, infected meat or contact with infected cat feces can lead to human infection.

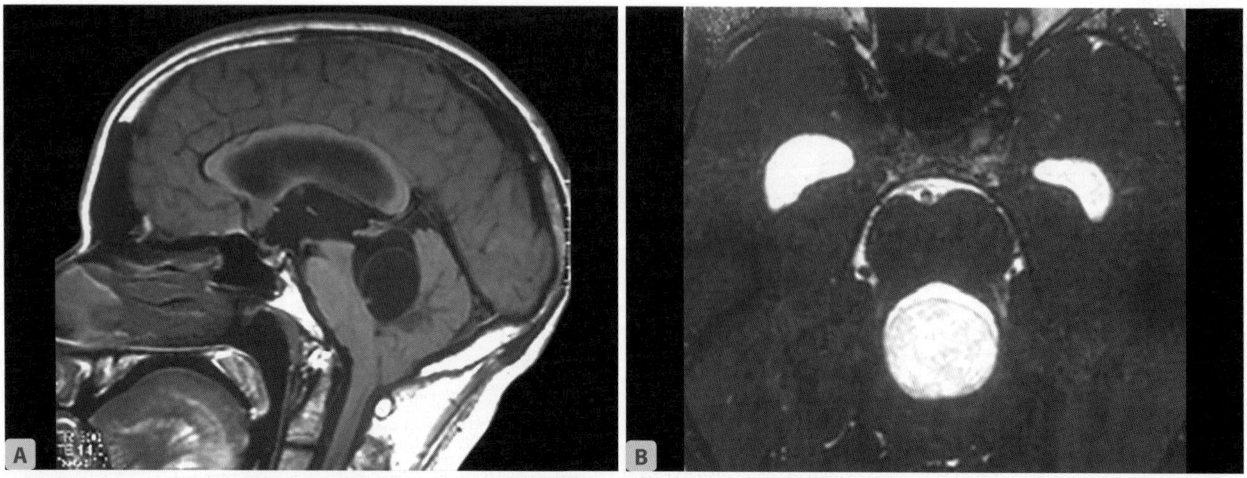

FIGS. 40A AND B: Sagittal T1W (A) and CISS axial; (B) MR images showing a cystic lesion with signal intensity almost similar to CSF in the fourth ventricle with resultant obstructive hydrocephalus—intraventricular cysticercus.

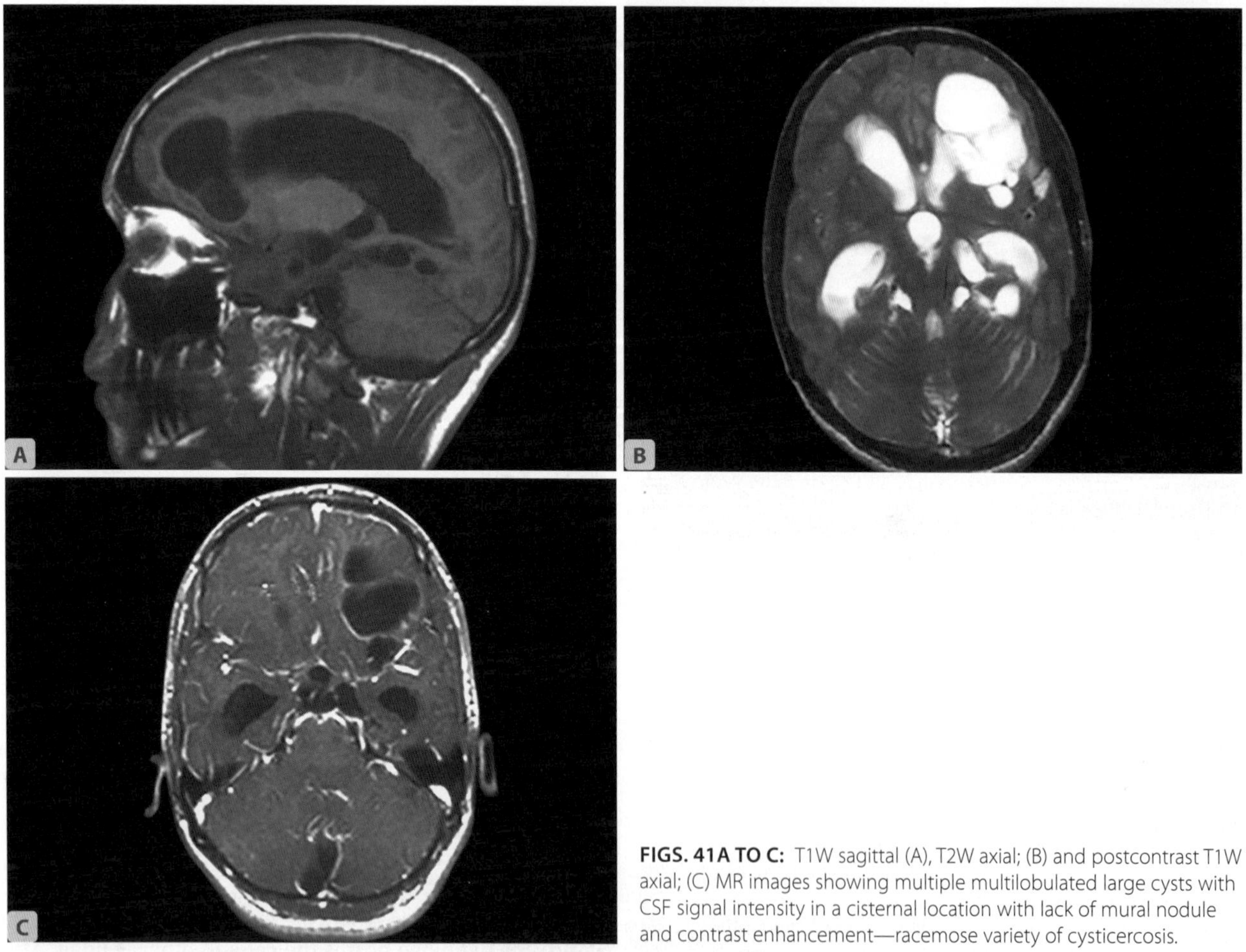

FIGS. 41A TO C: T1W sagittal (A), T2W axial; (B) and postcontrast T1W axial; (C) MR images showing multiple multilobulated large cysts with CSF signal intensity in a cisternal location with lack of mural nodule and contrast enhancement—racemose variety of cysticercosis.

Most toxoplasmosis infections in immunocompetent individuals are subclinical or mildly symptomatic. A minimal number of patients develop symptoms that resemble infectious mononucleosis (i.e. fever, chills, headache, tender lymphadenopathy and fatigue). Rarely, symptoms may be severe and include a maculopapular rash, hepatitis, encephalomyelitis or myocarditis.

Toxoplasmosis is a major cause of encephalitis in AIDS patients. In patients with HIV infection, Toxoplasma encephalitis results in a progressive and often fatal encephalitis if untreated.[119]

Pathologically, parenchymal toxoplasma lesions have three distinct zones: A central zone which is avascular, contains few organisms and demonstrates coagulative necrosis; an intermediate zone which is engorged with blood vessels containing numerous free extracellular and intracellular organisms and has fewer areas of necrosis. The outermost is the peripheral zone with few vascular changes and more encysted organisms with little necrosis. Inflammatory reaction is most intense in the intermediate zone. There is endothelial cell swelling and proliferation with cuffing of venules by lymphocytes, plasma cells and macrophages. *Toxoplasma* lesions do not have capsules. When leptomeningitis is present it only involves the meninges directly adjacent to the areas of encephalitis. Although small vessel thrombosis and necrosis are characteristically associated with lesions, arteritis of large vessels is absent.

Imaging

On noncontrast CT, toxoplasma encephalitis characteristically appears as multiple areas of hypodensity. There is a predilection for the basal ganglia (in 75 to 88%) and the corticomedullary junction and lesions may involve the posterior fossa. Lesions vary in size from less than 1 cm to over 3 cm and there is surrounding mass effect and edema of variable degree. Hemorrhage is uncommon and the presence of hyperattenuating lesions on a non-contrast CT should suggest an alternative diagnosis like lymphoma.

Postcontrast CT demonstrates ring or nodular enhancement **(Figs. 42A to D)**. Ring enhancement is more common with central hypodensity. The rings are usually thin and smooth but may be thick and irregular especially in the larger lesions. Double-dose delayed technique (using 200 mL of intravenous contrast by bolus/drip infusion with delayed scanning at 1 hour) has been found to be extremely effective in detection of these lesions. Double-dose delayed technique permits maximal enhancement and the central portion of ring lesions of toxoplasma may fill in on delayed scans.

The radiologic appearance correlates well with the pathologic findings, with the central hypodensity corresponding to the region of avascular coagulative necrosis. The enhancing ring corresponds to the intermediate zone of intense inflammation and the peripheral zone may appear as edema on neuroimaging studies. Pathologic-radiologic correlation has revealed that the pathologic extent of these lesions is often greater than the area of contrast enhancement evident on CT.

MR imaging reveals multiple ring and nodular enhancing lesions with a predilection for the basal ganglia and the

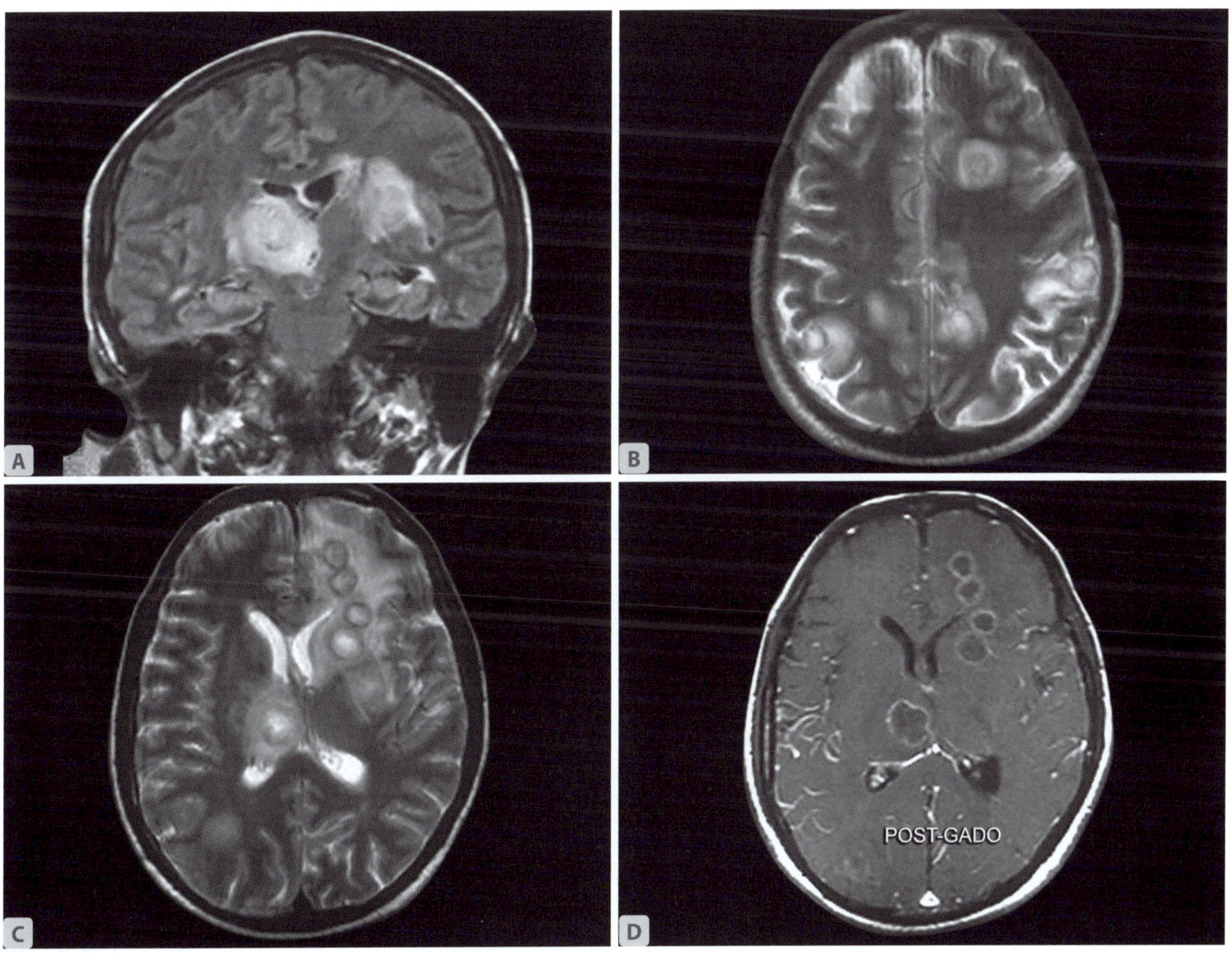

FIGS. 42A TO D: FLAIR coronal (A), T2W axial (B and C) MR images showing multiple lesions in bilateral basal ganglia, left frontoparietal region and right thalamus seen as isointense signal surrounded by a hypointense rim and high signal intensity edema giving the typical 'target' sign. Postcontrast T1W axial (D) MR image reveals ring or nodular enhancement in the lesions—toxoplasmosis.

corticomedullary junction of the cerebral hemispheres. There is some amount of perilesional edema and mass effect. Multiplicity of the lesions is a characteristic imaging finding. On the T2-weighted images, a "concentric target sign" may be seen which is central T2 hypointensity surrounded by alternate concentric bands of hyper and hypointensity. A small enhancing nodule along the lesion margins constitutes an "eccentric target" sign on the post-contrast scans and is considered virtually diagnostic of toxoplasmosis[120] **(Figs. 43A to H)**. This sign is caused by a leash of inflammatory vessels entering the lesion. This sign is seen in 30% cases but is 95% specific.

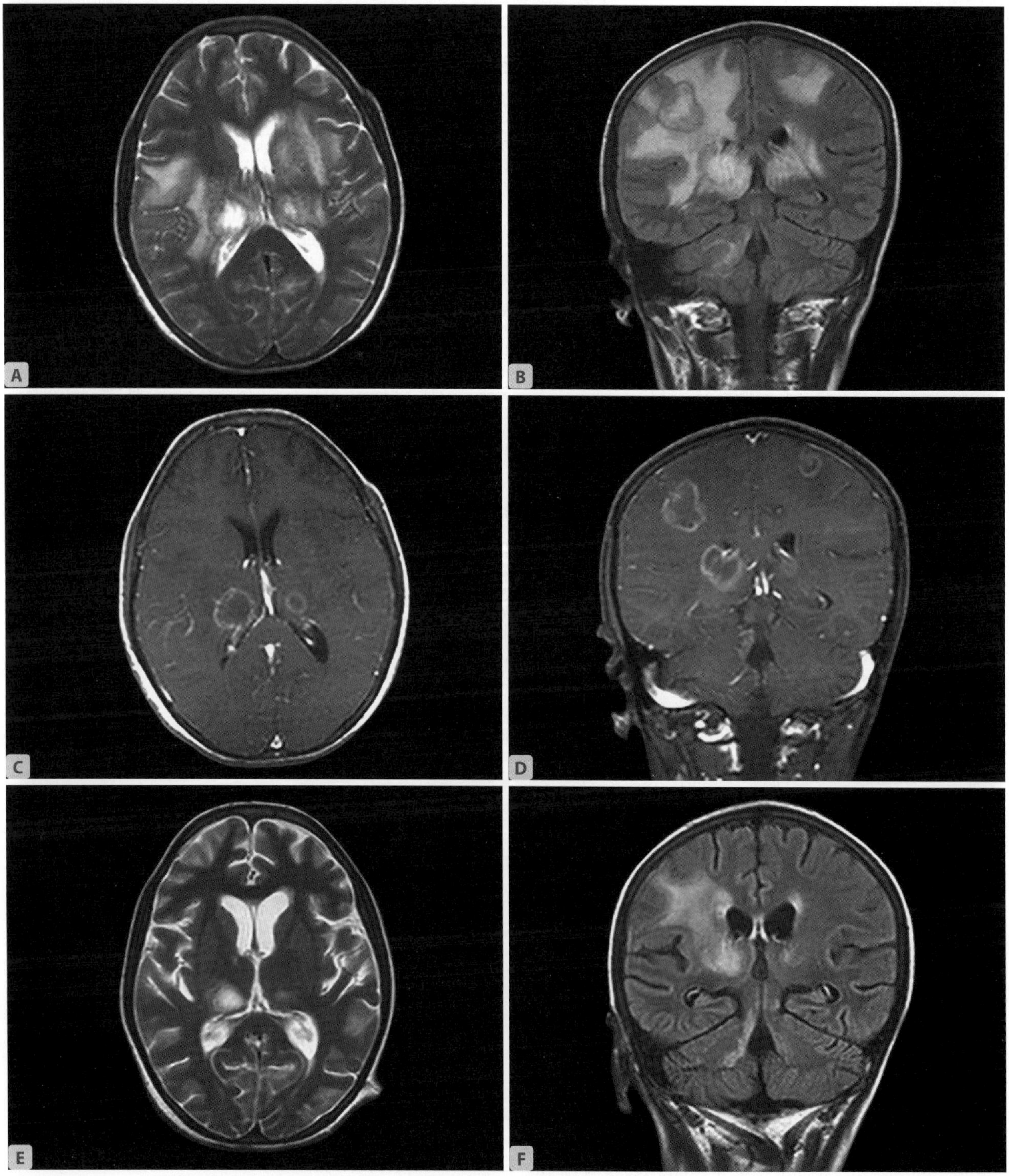

FIGS. 43A TO H *Continued*

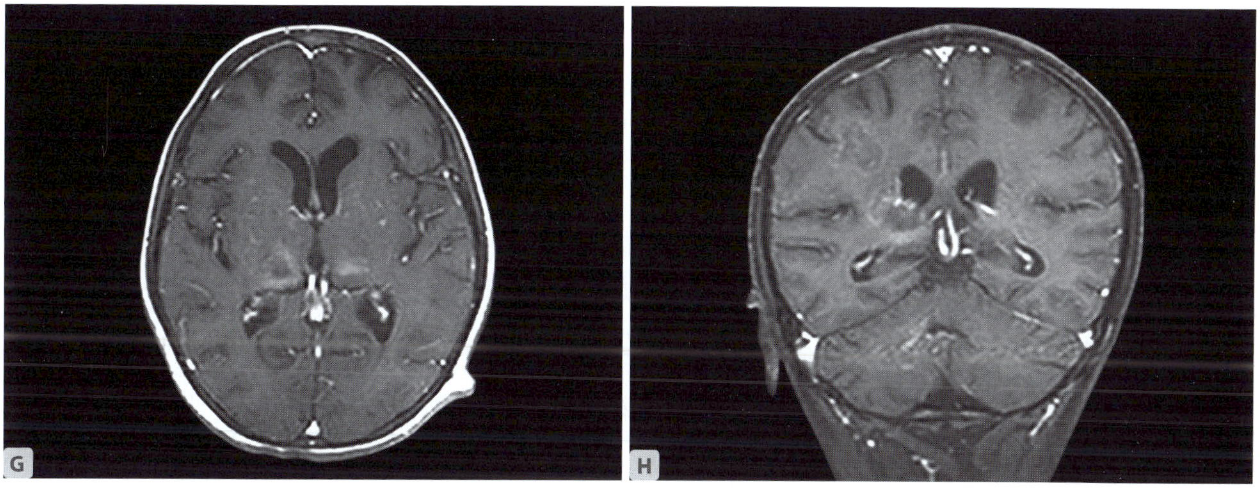

FIGS. 43A TO H: MR images in a case of toxoplasmosis before treatment (A to D) and after treatment (E to H) with sulpha drugs reveals a decrease in the number and size of lesions, a decrease in the amount of perilesional edema and degree of contrast enhancement. An 'eccentric target sign' is well seen in the pretreatment image (D) Toxoplasmosis.

Differentiation of Toxoplasmosis from CNS Lymphoma

It is important to differentiate between the two owing to the difference in treatment and prognosis. A periventricular location in contact with the ventricular/ependymal surface with evidence of subependymal spread and ventricular encasement favours the diagnosis of lymphoma while toxoplasmosis has a predilection for the basal ganglia and the corticomedullary junction. An "eccentric target" sign, absence of corpus callosal or leptomeningeal involvement and marked edema favour the diagnosis of toxoplasmosis while a T2 hypointensity favours the diagnosis of lymphoma. Lymphoma being highly cellular shows a restricted pattern of diffusion while toxoplasmosis does not.[121] On MR spectroscopy an elevated choline peak is seen in lymphomas while toxoplasmosis shows a suppression of all major metabolites with a lipid lactate peak owing to anaerobic glycolysis. An increased uptake on PET imaging favours the diagnosis of lymphoma over toxoplasmosis. Also toxoplasmosis responds to medical treatment while lymphoma does not. If toxoplasmosis is suspected on the basis of clinical and neuroimaging findings, anti-toxoplasma therapy should be given for 2–3 weeks as an empirical treatment. An interval decrease in the size of the lesion is considered to be a sufficient proof for the diagnosis and therapy to be continued. A stable or increasing size of lesion may indicate an alternative diagnosis like lymphoma. Also perfusion MR studies show a much higher regional cerebral blood volume in lymphoma as compared to toxoplasma lesions. The differences are summarized in **Table 4**.

TABLE 4: Differences between toxoplasmosis and CNS lymphoma.

Toxoplasmosis	Lymphoma
Predilection for basal ganglia and corticomedullary junction	Periventricular location in contact with ventricular/ ependymal lining
Lesions are T2 hyperintense	Lesions are T2 hypointense
Ring/nodular enhancement of lesions	Subependymal enhancement, ventricular encasement seen
Corpus callosum not involved	Corpus callosum usually involved
Concentric target or eccentric target signs seen	Absent
No restricted diffusion	Restricted diffusion on DWI
No uptake on PET	↑ uptake on PET imaging
High regional cerebral blood flow on perfusion imaging not seen	Higher regional cerebral blood flow on perfusion imaging seen
Lipid lactate peak on MRS	Choline peak on MRS
Responds to medical treatment	No response to medical treatment

HYDATID DISEASE

The causative organisms are *Echinococcus granulosus* and multilocularis. Humans are intermediate hosts with the definitive host being the dog. Human infection occurs by contact with the definitive host (dog) or by drinking or eating contaminated water or vegetables.

Hydatid disease involves the liver (75%) and the lungs (15–20%) most commonly. CNS involvement is rare and occurs in about 5% cases.[122]

Imaging

The cysts in *E. granulosus* are usually solitary, unilocular and located in the parietal lobe. On imaging, these are seen as large, unilocular cysts with well defined, smooth, thin wall. The cyst fluid is isointense to the CSF on all imaging pulse sequences **(Figs. 44A to D)**. No perilesional edema is seen. No contrast enhancement is usually seen unless the cyst becomes secondarily infected.[123] The capsule of the cyst is seen as a hypointense rim on the T2-weighted images surrounding the hyperintense lesion.[124]

Spinal hydatid cysts are seen in less than one percent of cases and are of five types—intramedullary, intradural, extramedullary, extradural, vertebral and paravertebral. The cysts may occur paravertebrally and then invade the vertebral column and spinal cord. Symptoms usually result from compression of the spinal cord or nerve roots.

E. Multilocularis grows by external budding causing progressive infiltration of the brain parenchyma with resultant multilobulated cystic structure. On imaging these are seen as heterogenous solid, partially solid or cystic masses with calcification. Owing to the calcification, these are hypointense on both T1- and T2-weighted images. Moderate to marked perilesionsal oedema is seen. The enhancement may be heterogenous, ring-like, nodular and cauliflower.[125] Thus oedema and calcification in the wall help it to be distinguished from *E. granulosus.* MR spectroscopy may reveal an elevated succinate level in addition to elevated acetate, glycine and lactate, thus differentiating it from neoplasms.[126] Also, the presence of multiloculated cystic lesions in the liver help it to be differentiated from neoplastic lesions.

CEREBRAL MALARIA

Malaria is caused by the protozoan parasite *Plasmodium. Plasmodium falciparum* infection is one of the most deadly infections. Sequestration of infected erythrocytes in the microcirculation may cause cerebral malaria in 2% of the cases. This may manifest as encephalopathy or coma and is associated with a mortality rate of 15–25%.[127]

MR imaging may reveal cortical infarcts and non-specific white matter hyperintensity on T2-weighted imaging. T2 hyperintense lesions may be seen involving the splenium of the corpus callosum. Hemorrhagic infarctions and multiple punctate petechial hemorrhages may be seen at the gray-white matter junction or in the deep white matter.[128,129]

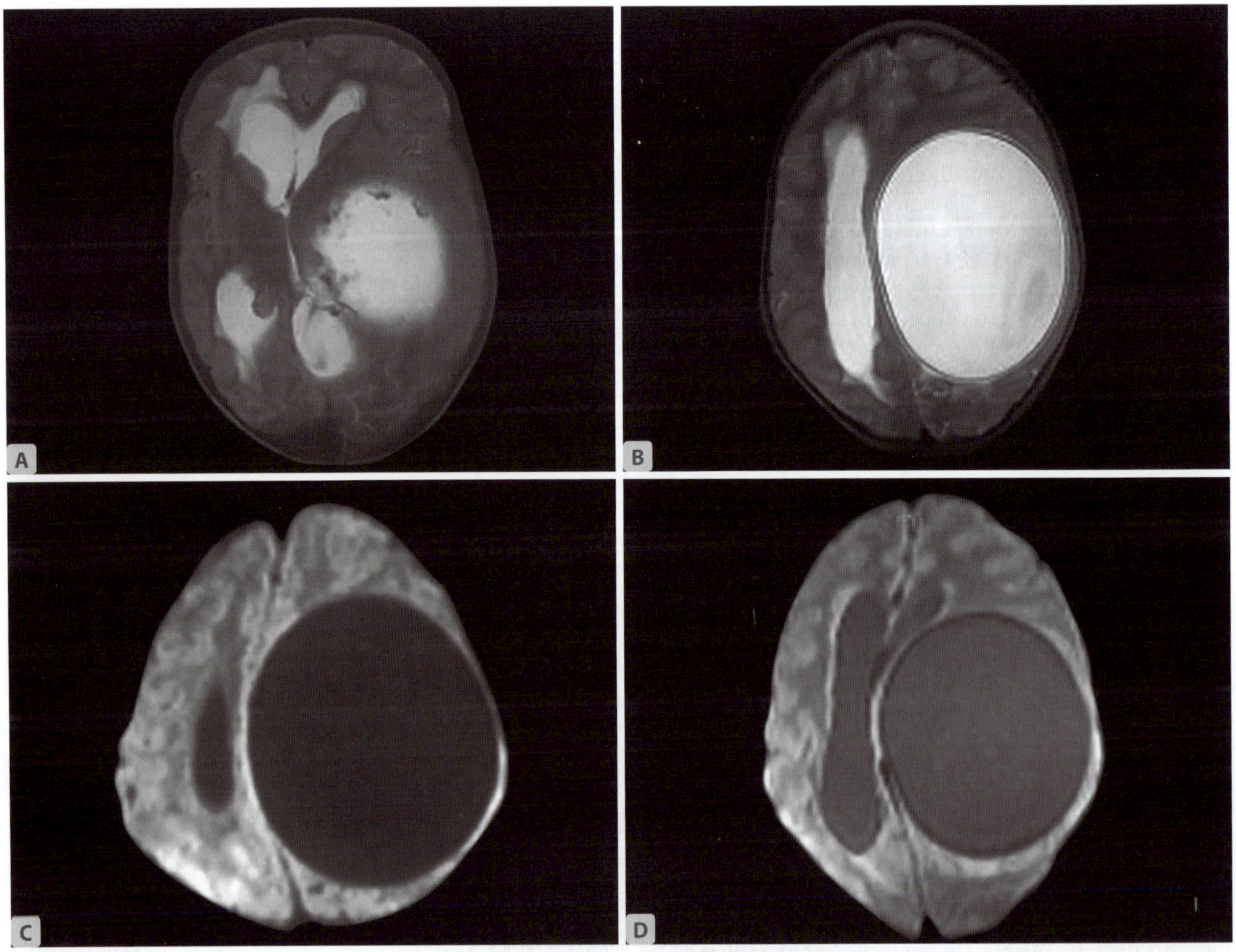

FIGS. 44A TO D: T2W axial (A and B), T1W axial (C) and proton density (D) MR images showing a large well-defined, smooth, thin walled, homogeneous cystic lesion isointense to cerebrospinal fluid on all pulse sequences with no significant edema. Few daughter cysts are seen in the periphery of the large cystic lesion—hydatid cyst.

GRANULOMATOUS AMOEBIC ENCEPHALITIS

Amoeba are free living protozoa. Many of these organisms are non pathogenic but some may cause devastating infection in the CNS, e.g. *Acanthamoeba* and *Balamuthia* species.[130] These infections are seen in the immunocompromised patients and clinical presentation is with headache, altered mental state and focal neurologic deficits. Imaging findings are non specific and may mimic other encephalitis or acute disseminated encephalomyelitis or toxoplasmosis.[131]

PRIMARY AMOEBIC MENINGOENCEPHALITIS

Naegleria fowleri (brain-eating worm) is found in warm fresh water bodies and is thermophilic. Infection is acquired in humans via the nasal cavity following a swimming or diving activity.[132] It is extremely aggressive and usually results in death. Neuroimaging studies are non-specific and a very high index of suspicion is required for the diagnosis.

VIRAL INFECTIONS

HERPES SIMPLEX ENCEPHALITIS (HSV-1) ENCEPHALITIS/ACUTE INFECTIVE ENCEPHALITIS

HSV-1 is the cause of 95% of all herpetic encephalitis.[133] A fulminant haemorrhagic meningoencephalitis, it is the most common cause of fatal encephalitis. High grade fever, an altered mental state, diminished level of consciousness and focal neurologic deficits characterize the clinical picture.

HSV-1 occurs due to reactivation of latent infection. The trigeminal ganglion is the most common site of reactivation. A retrograde transmission of the infection along the trigeminal nerve to the brainstem results in pontine infection/ rhomboencephalitis.

The herpes virus has a predilection for the inferomedial temporal lobes, the insular cortex and the cingulate gyrus.[134] There is a relative sparing of the basal ganglia, a finding that helps to distinguish this disease process from other encephalitis. The occipital cortex, external capsule and the cerebral convexity may also be involved. Infection is unilateral to begin with but soon involves the contralateral side to become a bilateral process. This "sequential bilaterality" is virtually diagnostic of herpes encephalopathy **(Figs. 45A and B)**.

Imaging

CT scan may show symmetric areas of hypodensity involving the limbic system, at times hemorrhagic foci may be seen. Hemorrhage seen in the appropriate clinical setting is highly suggestive of herpes infection.[135] MR images reveal areas of signal alteration in the temporal lobes, inferior frontal lobes, insular cortex and cingulate gyrus **(Figs. 46A to C)**. The signal alteration is seen as hypointense signal on T1 and hyperintense signal on T2-weighted images. There is usually involvement of both grey and white matter. The changes may be seen as early as 48 hours after the onset of symptoms. A gyriform pattern of enhancement seen on the postcontrast scans suggest disease progression.[136] Focal petechial hemorrhages are also better detected on MR imaging as areas of blooming on gradient echo sequences. MR is the modality of choice not only for an early diagnosis but also to monitor response to treatment in cases of herpes encephalitis.

Diffusion-weighted MR Imaging (DWI)

DWI may show the abnormalities much before the conventional MR images **(Figs. 47A to D)**. DWI may reveal a larger number of lesions and more extensive lesions than seen on conventional images and this modality can be used to monitor response to treatment. Facilitated diffusion with high ADC values is seen later consistent with the development of encephalomalacia.

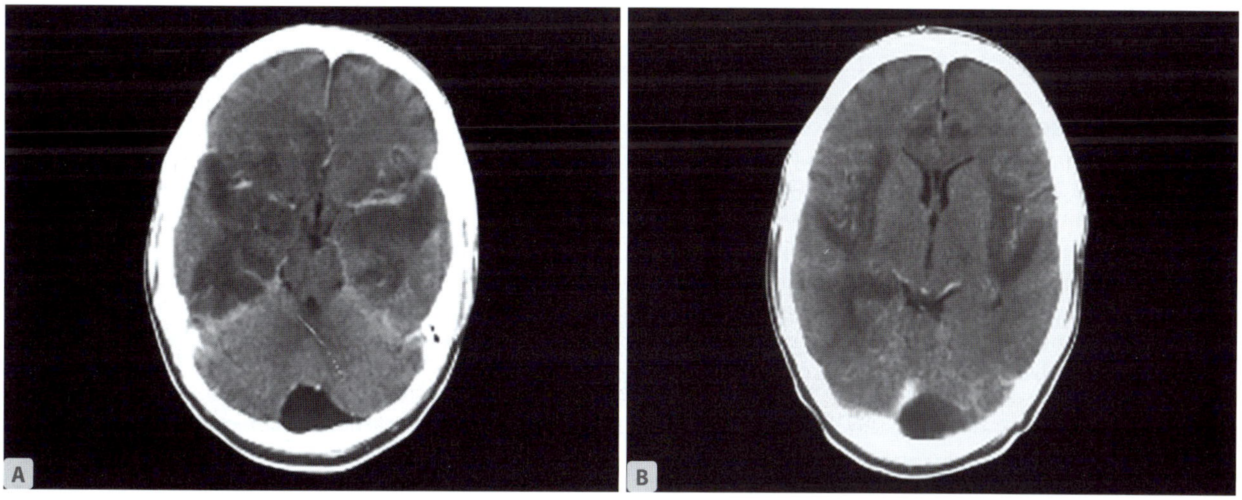

FIGS. 45A AND B: CECT axial scans of the cranium showing bilateral symmetric areas of hypodensity involving the inferomedial temporal lobes,insular cortex and the cingulate gyrus with sparing of the basal ganglia—herpes encephalitis.

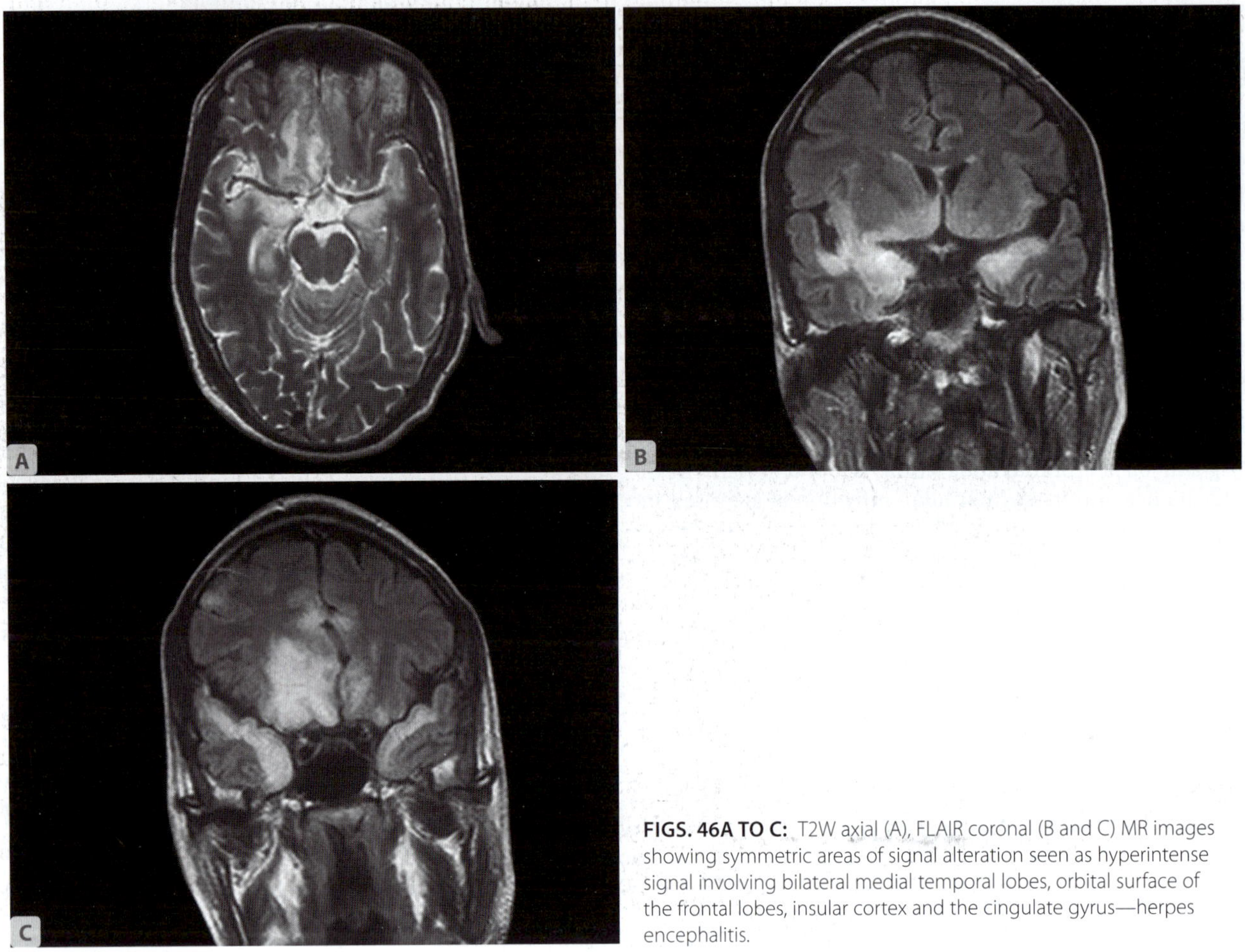

FIGS. 46A TO C: T2W axial (A), FLAIR coronal (B and C) MR images showing symmetric areas of signal alteration seen as hyperintense signal involving bilateral medial temporal lobes, orbital surface of the frontal lobes, insular cortex and the cingulate gyrus—herpes encephalitis.

MR Spectroscopy

A decrease in NAA levels and an increase in choline levels represents the loss of structural/functional activity of the neurons between 2–17 weeks after the onset of the disease. Spectroscopy can be used to predict progression and prognosticate the disease process. An increase of Cho/Cr along with a progressive decrease in NAA/Cr occurs in cases with neurological sequelae in the form of demyelination or neuronal dysfunction.

Differential Diagnosis

Limbic encephalitis has a more protracted and subacute onset (weeks to months). The imaging findings may be indistinguishable from herpes encephalitis. History of an extracranial primary carcinoma and neuronal antibodies in the CSF and serum favor the diagnosis of limbic encephalitis.

HHV-6 encephalitis—This shows an exclusive involvement of one or both medial temporal lobes. Extratemporal involvement and petechial hemorrhages as seen with HSE are not seen with this form.[136,137]

MOLLARET MENINGITIS

It is a rare syndrome seen in young females caused by herpes simplex type 2 virus. It is characterized by recurrent episodes of aseptic meningitis with each episode presenting with fulminant high grade fever, severe headache and signs of meningitis. It can be diagnosed by polymerase chain reaction analysis of CSF. No specific imaging findings are described.[138]

VARICELLA ZOSTER ENCEPHALITIS

Varicella Zoster virus which causes chickenpox (Varicella) and shingles (Zoster) can involve the CNS. The most common manifestation is meningitis with encephalitis being the second most common. In children this infection may present with acute cerebellar ataxia. Diffuse cerebellar swelling with hyperintensity on FLAIR images may be seen on imaging in children. MR may show multiple deep white matter hyperintensities in cases of vasculopathy. Granulomatous angitis involving small cerebral arteries may occur. Cerebral infarction and aneurysm formation may be seen.[139]

JAPANESE ENCEPHALITIS (JE)

JE usually occurs as epidemics in Asian countries specially during the summer season. The clinical presentation is fever, dystonia, tremors, rigidity, seizures often progressing to coma. Seizures are more common in the pediatric population. The disease is a diffuse meningoencephalitis involving both gray and white matter of the cerebral hemispheres, brainstem,

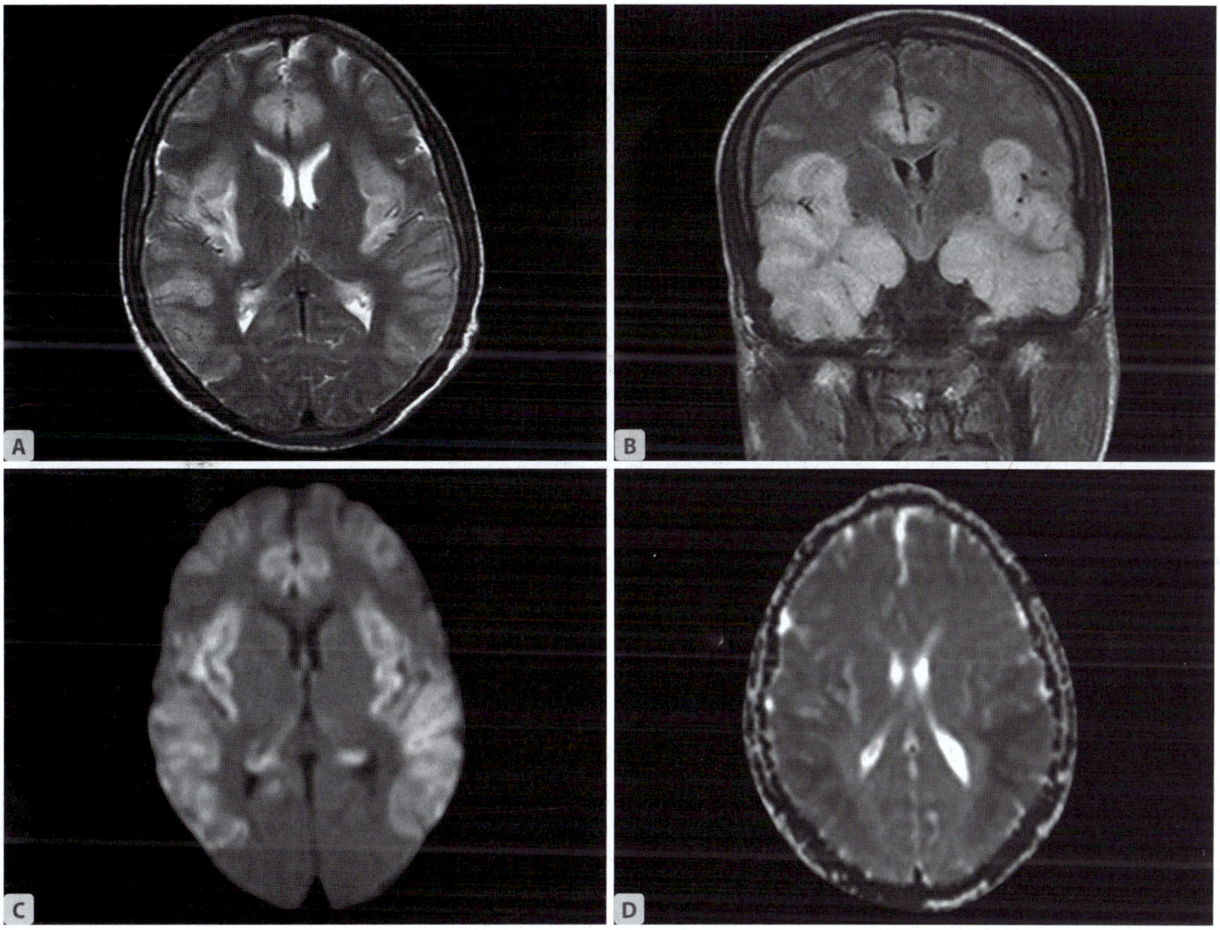

FIGS. 47A TO D: Axial T2W (A) and FLAIR coronal; (B) MR images showing diffuse gyral swelling and areas of signal alteration involving the cingulate gyrus, bilateral insular cortex, bilateral medial temporal lobes and parieto-occipital regions. The areas show evidence of restricted diffusion; (C and D)—herpes encephalitis.

cerebellum, basal ganglia and thalamus. The spinal cord may also be diffusely enlarged particularly the anterior and lateral column.

Imaging

Bilateral and symmetric areas of signal alteration are seen in the thalamus and basal ganglia. This is seen as a hyperintense signal on T2W images and hypointene signal on T1W images. Involvement of the basal ganglia and thalami may occur as an isolated finding without involvement of other regions[140] **(Figs. 48A to C)**. Isolated involvement of the substantia nigra may also be seen. Rarely foci of hemorrhage may occur in the involved regions. Minimal or no enhancement is seen on the post contrast scans. MR spectroscopy shows a decrease in NAA peak, an elevated choline peak at 3.22 ppm and a lactate peak at 1.33 ppm. A definitive diagnosis is established on serology by demonstrating a fourfold rise in antibody titre. However, presence of lesions in the thalamus, basal ganglia and substantia nigra in a patient presenting with encephalitic illness from an endemic zone of JE strongly suggests the diagnosis.

A co-existence of neurocysticercosis and JE has been noted.[141] The reason behind this has been stated to be multiple common factors in the etiopathogenesis of the two disorders. Pigs are the intermediate hosts of *Taenia solium* and act as amplifiers of the JE virus. Common endemicity of the two illnesses caused by poor socioeconomic status, poor hygienic conditions as well as malnutrition is the other factor. The changes of JE have been found to be more pronounced on the side of the cyst and hence NCC may act as an amplifier/ modulator of JE.

Japanese encephalitis needs to be differentiated from herpes encephalitis because antiviral therapy is very effective for herpes while treatment for JE is usually supportive **(Figs. 49A to C)**.

MEASLES ENCEPHALITIS

Measles is caused by the rubeola virus and is an acute highly contagious infection. Three syndromes have been described

Acute Measles Encephalitis (AME)

It is an autoimmune process and presents as renewed fever in patients recovering from measles. A wide variety of neurological symptoms—seizures, altered mental status and

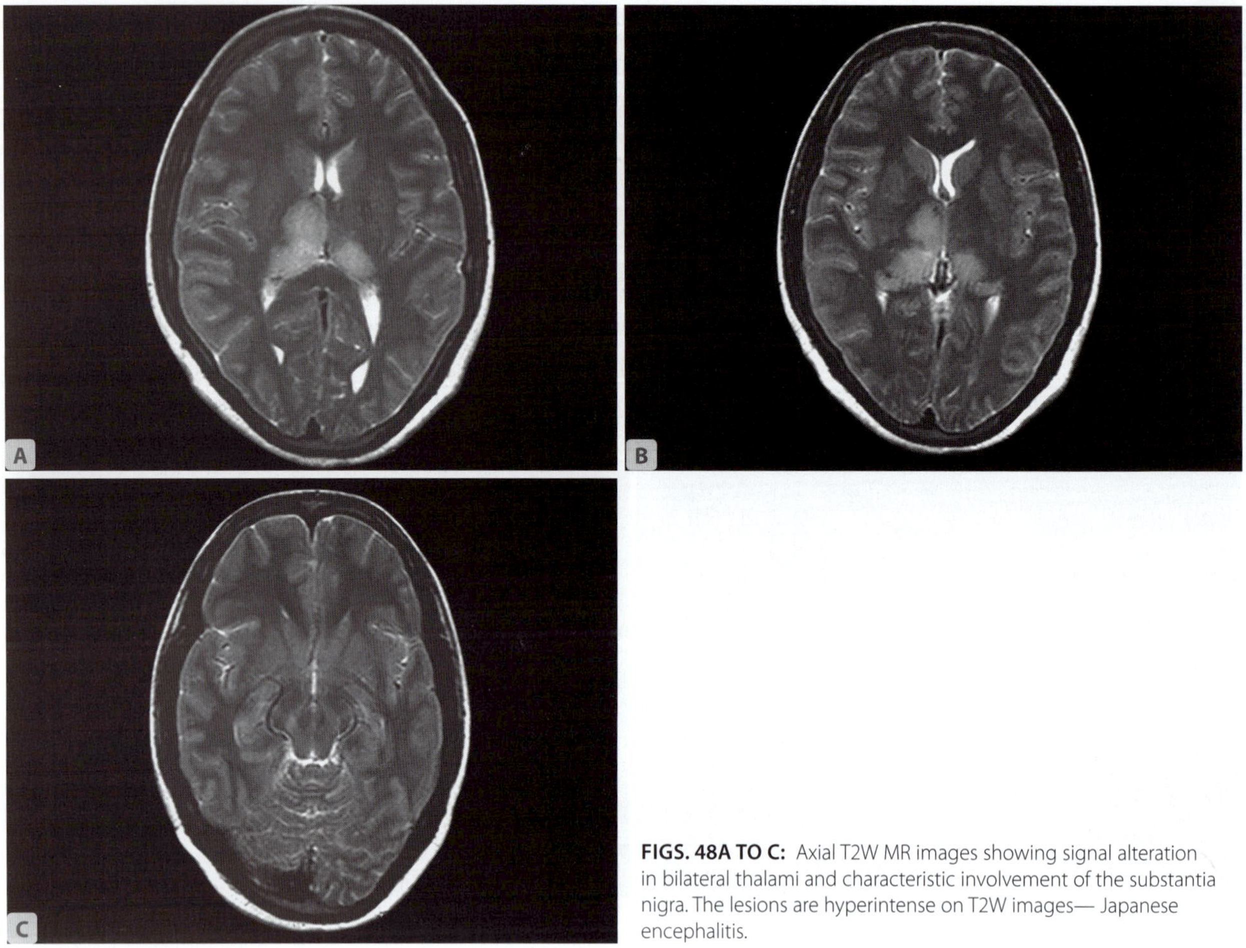

FIGS. 48A TO C: Axial T2W MR images showing signal alteration in bilateral thalami and characteristic involvement of the substantia nigra. The lesions are hyperintense on T2W images— Japanese encephalitis.

focal neurologic signs may be seen during the convalescence period. Though the measles virus is absent during this phase demyelination, hemorrhage, necrosis and vascular damage characterize this phase.

Subacute Sclerosing Panencephalitis (SSPE)

SSPE develops secondary to a previous measles infection early in childhood. The virus remains dormant and becomes active after a decade or so to manifest as SSPE which is invariably fatal.[142] The onset is with mild alterations in behavior in a previously healthy child, followed by myoclonic jerks which become increasingly frequent followed by dementia and coma. The average age of onset is from 9–13 years. An immature immune system that fails to destroy the virus completely has been stated to be the cause for the dormant partially degraded virus that remains in the CNS.

On MR imaging the white matter lesions of SSPE are seen as a predominant involvement of the subcortical white matter with a predilection for the posterior parietal, occipital and temporal region. Lesions may also be seen in the brainstem and cerebellum. The lesions are seen as hypointense signal on T1 and hyperintense signal on T2W images. Diffuse atrophy of the cortex, atrophy of the brainstem and ventricular dilatation may be seen. In long standing disease and severe disease, involvement of the basal ganglia may be seen.

Subacute Measles Encephalitis

This form occurs in an immunocompromised patient with a latent period of 1–7 months. The onset is subacute with a more rapid evolution. However seizures rather than myoclonic jerks is what differentiates SME from SSPE.

MRI shows areas of signal alteration involving the occipital cortical and subcortical regions with some enhancement on the post contrast study.

RABIES ENCEPHALOMYELITIS

It is a fulminant disease and is invariably fatal once clinical symptoms develop. It is caused by a neurotropic RNA virus, the virus being abundant in the saliva of the infected animal which is usually the dog. The virus gets deposited in the bite wounds, replicates in the muscle tissues of the wound and then infects motor neurons. It then gains entry into the CNS via retrograde flow.[143] The rabies virus has a predilection for the brainstem, thalami and hippocampi. An ill-defined hyperintense signal may be seen on the T2W images in these regions. No enhancement or haemorrhage

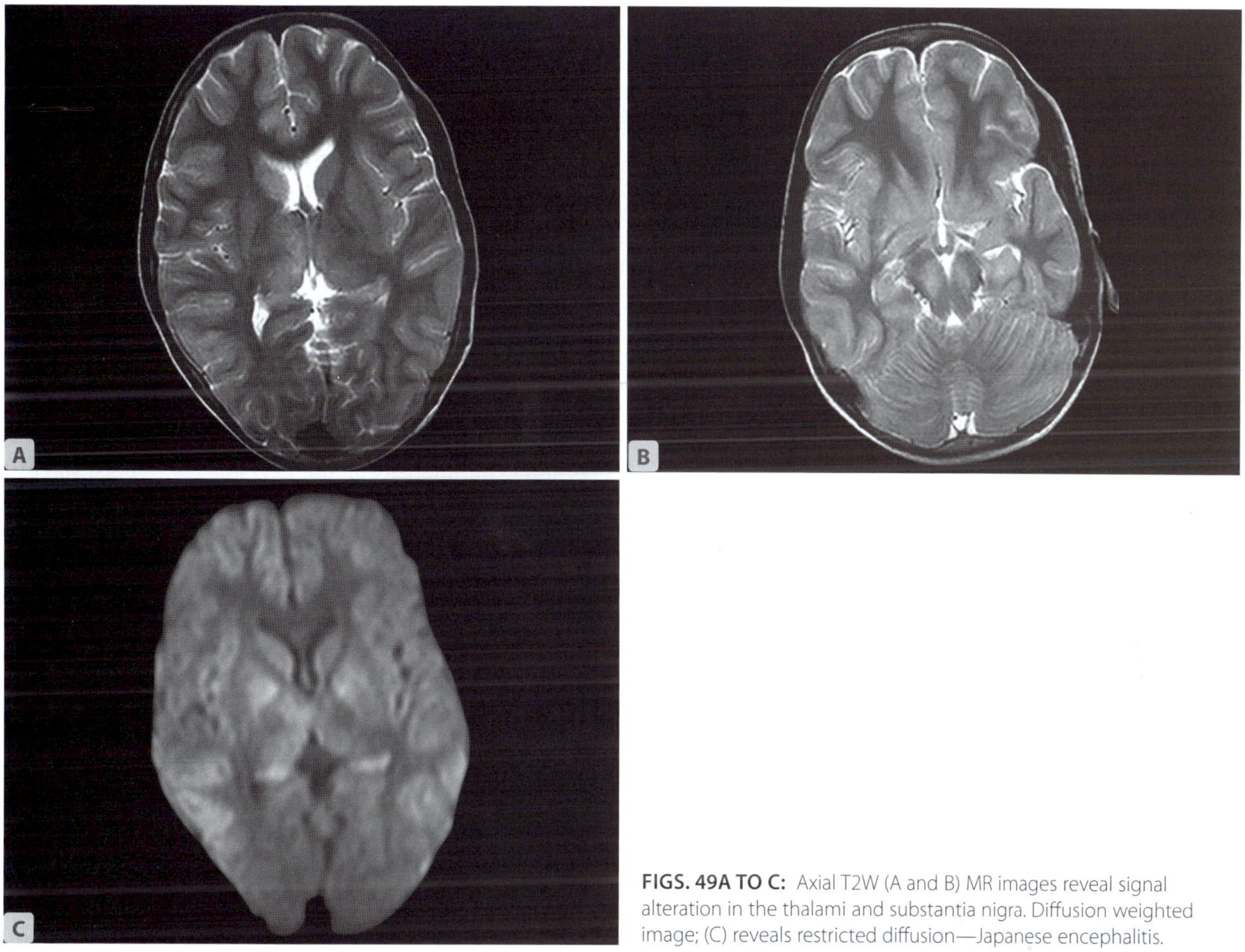

FIGS. 49A TO C: Axial T2W (A and B) MR images reveal signal alteration in the thalami and substantia nigra. Diffusion weighted image; (C) reveals restricted diffusion—Japanese encephalitis.

is seen, features that differentiate it from other viral encephalitis.

RASMUSSEN'S ENCEPHALITIS

Rasmussen's encephalitis is a childhood disease. A viral infection or autoimmune disease involving glutamate receptors with glutamine toxicity have been postulated in the etiopathogenesis. The child presents with severe epilepsy and progressive neurologic deficits. Seizures are usually of the partial motor seizure type and tend to be intractable. The intractable nature of the seizure may make hemispherectomy necessary, if medical therapy is ineffective. The disease tends to affect one hemisphere although bilateral involvement has also been reported.

Early in the disease process, CT and MRI findings may be normal. MRI may reveal focal and progressive atrophy of a hemisphere and hyperintensity in white matter and putamen on T2-weighted images. PET imaging using FDG-18 may show decreased hemispheric activity.

PRION INFECTIONS—CREUTZFELDT-JAKOB DISEASE

Creutzfeldt-Jakob Disease (CJD) is caused by a slow unconventional virus or prion. Prions are proteinaceous infectious particles that contain little or no nucleic acid and evoke no inflammatory response. The age of onset is between 40–80 years with survival being less than a year from the onset of symptoms. Patients typically present with dementia accompanied by confusion and cerebellar ataxia.

CJD is a human spongiform encephalopathy as spongiform changes are seen in the cortical and subcortical gray matter histologically. There is loss of neurons and gliosis. White matter is relatively spared, rarely Wallerian degeneration may be seen. No inflammatory changes are seen.

Imaging Findings

CT of these patients is either normal or diffuse cerebral atrophy may be seen. MRI shows bilateral and symmetric areas of signal alteration in the corpus striatum, that is the putamen and caudate nucleus. No mass effect and no enhancement of the lesion is seen. Lesions may also be seen in the thalamus, basal ganglia, cortical gray matter and occipital lobes. Diffusion weighted images help in an early diagnosis as these show the involved regions as areas of restricted diffusion. DWI has emerged as the most sensitive sequence for the diagnosis of human prion disease. The combined use of FLAIR and DWI improves diagnostic accuracy to 90%.[144] The findings include a restricted diffusion in the cortex, caudate nucleus, putamen and thalamus with a distribution pattern that does not correspond to arterial circulation.[145] Diffuse cerebral atrophy is another characteristic imaging finding that ensues, so rapidly as to result in the formation of subdural hygromas. MR spectroscopy shows decreased levels of NAA reflecting neuronal loss.

ACQUIRED IMMUNODEFICIENCY SYNDROME (AIDS) AND ITS RELATED CNS INFECTIONS

Human immunodeficiency virus (HIV) is a retrovirus that causes AIDS. Two subtypes are recognized HIV-1 and 2. HIV is a neurotropic virus and the commonest pathogen in AIDS patients. Over 40% of untreated AIDS patients develop neurologic manifestations of the disease either by direct invasion of the CNS by HIV virus or by several opportunistic infections like toxoplasmosis, cytomegalovirus, cryptococcosis, progressive multifocal leukoencephalopathy, etc.

CNS infection in AIDS includes:[146]

- HIV encephalitis—most common (60%).
- Toxoplasmosis—commonest opportunistic infection (20–40%).
- Cryptococcosis (5%).
- Progressive multifocal leukoencephalopathy (PML) (1–4%).

Others:

- Tuberculosis (2–18%)
- Neurosyphilis (1–3%)
- Varicella zoster (< 1%)
- CMV encephalitis

HIV ENCEPHALITIS

It is the commonest CNS infection seen in AIDS patients. AIDS dementia complex is seen in 15–20% of HIV patients inspite of highly active antiretroviral therapy (HAART) and usually occurs with CD4 counts of less than 200 cells/μL.[147] it manifests clinically as a progressive dementia characterized by cognitive, behavioural and motor deterioration culminating in death if left untreated.

The lesions are present in the white matter to begin with and progress to involve the cortex and gray matter. Brainstem, cerebellum and spinal cord may also be involved. Demyelination, gliosis, myelin pallor, infiltration with multinucleate giant cells may be seen on pathology.

Imaging

CT may show diffuse cerebral atrophy only. MR is more sensitive in detecting the lesions. MR not only shows diffuse cerebral atrophy but bilateral and symmetric areas of signal alteration involving the deep periventricular white matter and centrum semiovale. The signal alteration is in the form of diffuse, symmetric, confluent areas of hypointensity on T1W and hyperintensity on the T2W images[148] **(Figs. 50A and B)**. No mass effect or contrast enhancement is seen. Gray matter is typically spared initially. The hyperintense lesions correspond to foci of demyelination and vacuolation and the extent of the lesions is proportionate to the neurologic deterioration seen. The frontal lobes are the most common sites to be affected and FLAIR sequence is excellent in the depiction of white matter disease.

MR spectroscopy may reveal metabolic abnormality much before the morphological changes in the form of a decreased NAA and elevated choline peak reflecting neuronal loss and presence of gliosis, macrophages and lymphocytes[149] **(Figs. 51A and B)**. Elevated myoinositol (MI) may be seen early in infection and occurs due to the gliosis. MRS is helpful not only in an early diagnosis of HIV encephalitis but also in monitoring response to treatment.

Magnetization transfer ratio is abnormal in asymptomatic patients and hence can also be used for an early diagnosis. SPECT has also been used in patients suspected of HIV encephalitis, and shows uptake defects in the brain.

Diffusion tensor imaging demonstrates a decrease in both fractional anisotropy and mean diffusivity in the cerebral white matter. This correlates with the neurological findings and DTI picks up changes much before changes are seen on conventional MR.[150]

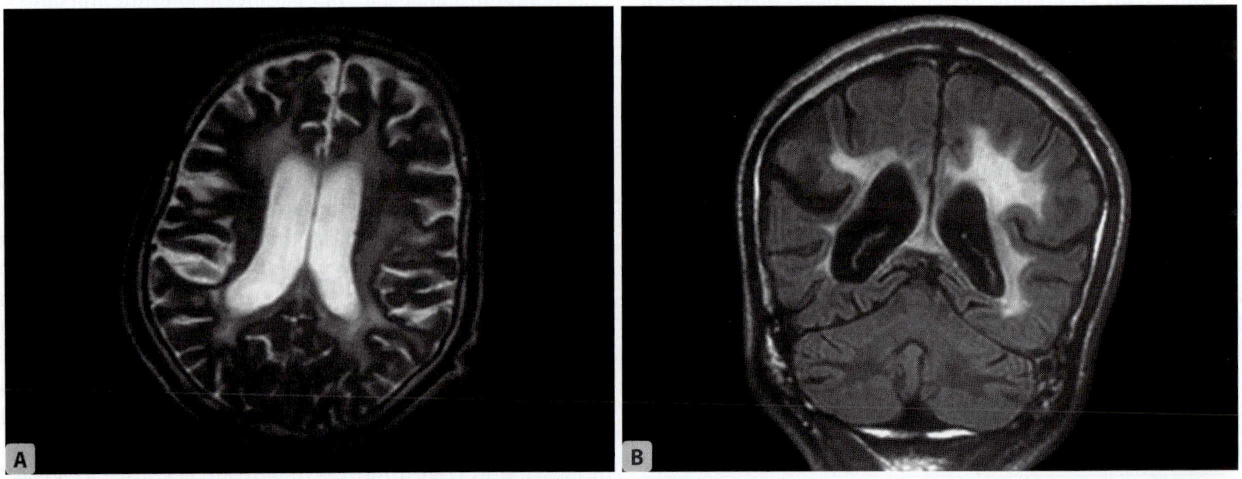

FIGS. 50A AND B: Axial T2W (A) and FLAIR coronal; (B) MR images showing a bilateral diffuse periventricular white matter hyperintensity with sparing of the gray matter with diffuse cerebral atrophy—HIV encephalitis.

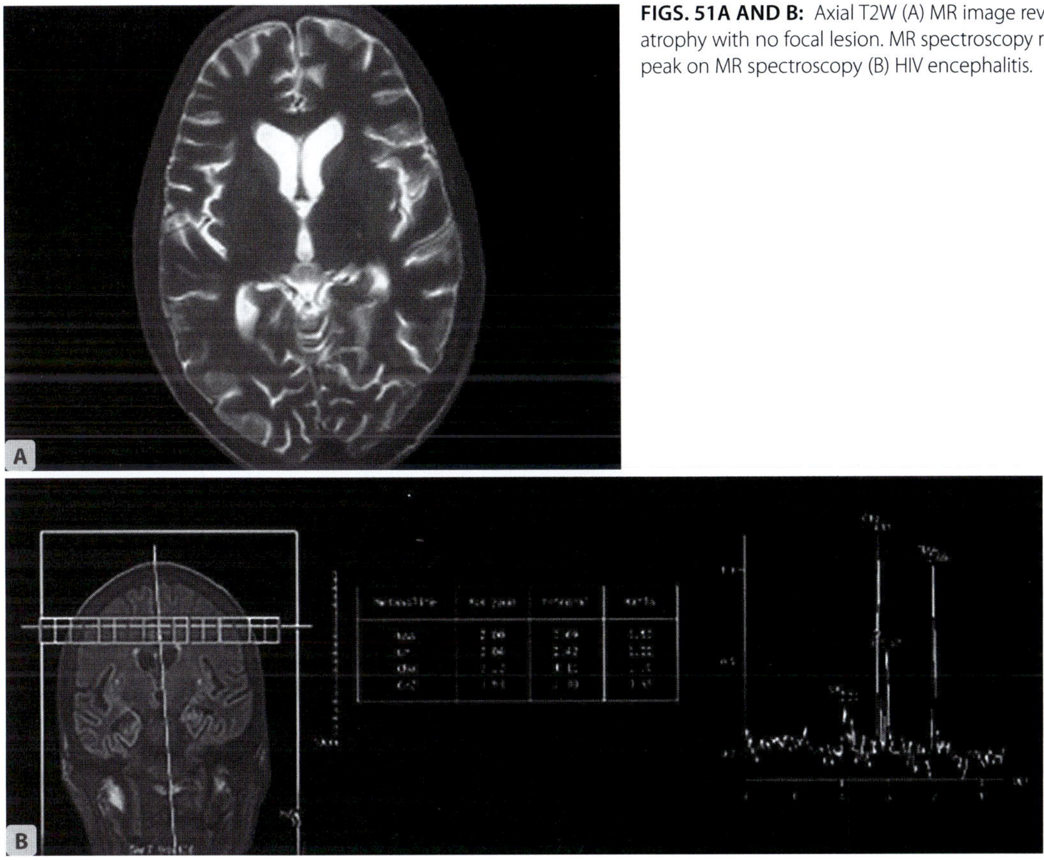

FIGS. 51A AND B: Axial T2W (A) MR image reveals mild diffuse cerebral atrophy with no focal lesion. MR spectroscopy reveals an elevated choline peak on MR spectroscopy (B) HIV encephalitis.

PROGRESSIVE MULTIFOCAL LEUKOENCEPHALOPATHY (PML)

Earlier PML was stated to be seen in immunodeficient states like lymphoproliferative disorders, non-tropical sprue, Whipple's disease, autoimmune disorders and those treated with chemotherapy. However, the strong association of PML with AIDS has now been recognized and 55–85% cases of PML are now attributable to AIDS alone.[151] PML occurs in about 50% of patients of AIDS.

A papovavirus is the causative agent. The JC (John Cunningham) virus, a human polyomavirus, belongs to the papova family of CNS viruses and causes a relentlessly progressive demyelinating disorder. The virus establishes a latency in the bone marrow, kidneys and the CNS becoming reactivated with profound immunosuppressed states or various immunosuppressive drugs such as efalizumab for psoriasis and natalizumab for multiple sclerosis. PML develops in patients of HIV when the CD4 counts are usually below 100.

The target cell for the JC virus is the oligodendrocyte. Cytolytic destruction causes loss of myelin as the primary function of the oligodendrocyte is to form and maintain the myelin sheath. Electron microscopy reveals intranuclear inclusions within the oligodendrocyte corresponding to the JC virus particle (called the spaghetti and meatball appearance), foci of demyelination which enlarge and coalesce over time.[152]

Clinical features of PML are loss of memory, altered mental status, cognitive and speech disturbances, personality change, seizures, headache, vertigo and aphasia. Death occurs within a year of the onset of symptoms.

Imaging

MR is more sensitive than CT in the detection of PML lesions specially for the posterior fossa lesions. The extent and number of lesions are better picked on MR than CT scans. Solitary/multifocal well-demarcated asymmetric lesions are usually seen which are hypointense on T1 and hyperintense on T2-weighted images. It is the subcortical white matter that is predominantly involved with sparing of the deep periventricular white matter **(Fig. 52)**. The lesions become more confluent with disease progression. No mass effect or contrast enhancement is seen. Rarely a faint and peripheral enhancement may be seen.[153] PML lesions usually involve the posterior fossa which is involved in about one third cases with the most common site being the middle cerebellar peduncles. The subcortical lesions follow the gray-white matter interface giving rise to a "scalloped appearance"

The PML lesions need to be differentiated from HIV encephalitis.[152,153] While HIV encephalitis is usually bilateral and symmetrical, PML is multifocal and asymmetric. HIV encephalitis involves the deep periventricular white matter while PML lesions are subcortical in location. "Scalloped"

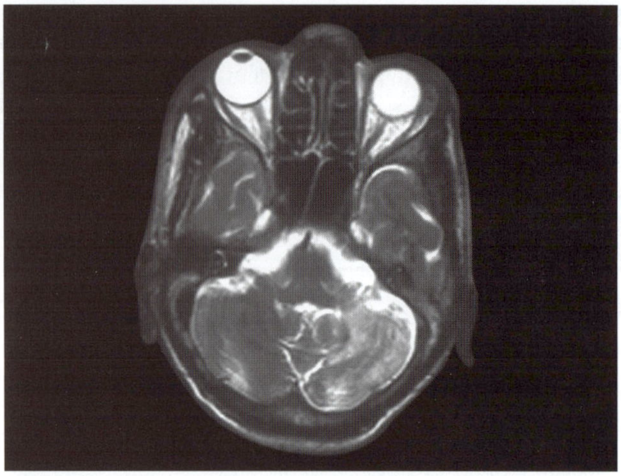

FIG. 52: Axial T2W image in a HIV patient shows a predominantly subcortical lesion in the posterior fossa with no mass effect and along the gray-white matter interface—PML.

TABLE 5: Differences between HIV encephalitis and progressive multifocal leukoencephalopathy (PML).

HIV encephalitis	PML
Presents with global cognitive disturbances	Presents with a focal motor/ sensory deficit
Bilateral and symmetric	Multifocal and asymmetric
Deep periventricular white matter predominantly involved	Subcortical white matter predominantly involved
Not well-defined/sharply defined on T1W images	Well-defined and sharply marginated on T1W images
Scalloped appearance not seen	Scalloped appearance of lesions
Mild reduction of MT ratio	Marked reduction of MT ratio due to its demyelinating nature

appearance and clear demarcations of the lesions on a T1 weighted image favours the diagnosis of PML. HIV encephalitis presents with global cognitive disturbances while PML presents with a focal motor or sensory deficit. PML shows a marked reduction in the MT ratio as compared to HIV encephalitis which is useful in differentiating between the two **(Table 5)**.

In a minority of patients with PML, the institution of HAART can precipitate an immune reconstitution inflammatoty response (PML-IRIS) following recovery of the immune function.[154] PML-IRIS is an acute inflammatory response at the site of the CNS lesions and results in a worsening of the neurological symptoms. Lesions of PML-IRIS may show mass effect and heterogenous enhancement. Thus it is important to consider the clinical context before ruling out PML on seeing an enhancing lesion.

Diffusion-weighted imaging of PML lesions shows a core of low signal intensity with high ADC values while the periphery has a high signal on DWI with low ADC values suggesting restricted diffusion at the more leading edges of the lesion. DWI may thus be used not only for diagnosis but also for monitoring response to HAART and may predict the risk of PML-IRIS.[155,156]

MR spectroscopy demonstrates decreased NAA, increased choline, increased lactate more in the core of the lesion than the leading edge of the lesion where the degree of neuronal loss is less advanced.

NEUROSYPHILIS

The causative organism is Treponema pallidum. It can enter the CNS during primary or secondary syphilitic infection with neurosyphilis developing in 5–10% of untreated cases.[157] The disease became rare after the introduction of penicillin but there has been an emergence again due to the AIDS pandemic. The latent period for different types of syphilis is different. It is <2 years for meningeal, 5–7 years for vascular, 10–20 years for general paresis and 15–20 years for tabes dorsalis. The onset is much earlier in patients with HIV and early forms (meningeal, vascular) may predominate over late forms. The clinical manifestations may range from asymptomatic to headache, confusion, cranial nerve palsies, dementia and focal neurological deficits.

A positive CSF VDRL is specific for neurosyphilis, not very sensitive while a CSF antibody testing is less specific but very sensitive. Histopathology reveals arteritis of the medium and large vessels (Huebner's arteritis). The MCA territory and the perforating vessels are the most commonly involved. Gummas which are granulomas with central necrosis and non-specific white matter lesions may be seen.

Imaging

The imaging findings depend on the form of the disease. Syphilitic meningitis may be thick and nodular like other granulomatous diseases. Vascular neurosyphilis is characterized by medium and large vessel infarcts seen as hyperintense areas showing restricted diffusion in the MCA territory or in the basal ganglia and brainstem because of perforating vessel disease. Angiographic findings may show alternating stenosis and dilatations of vessels within the circle of Willis giving them a beaded appearance. Non-specific white matter changes may be seen as hyperintense foci on T2-weighted images in the deep periventricular and subcortical white matter.

Syphilitic cerebral gummas are usually seen as cortical or dural based mass lesions isointense on T1 and hyperintense on T2 W images mimicking meningioma and dural based metastasis. On contrast administration homogenous enhancement of the lesions may be seen with focal meningeal enhancement adjacent to the lesion. Surrounding vasogenic edema with or without mass effect is seen.[158]

Other findings include leptomeningeal enhancement and cranial neuritis typically of the second and eighth cranial nerves. Bilateral involvement of the medial temporal lobes mimicking herpes encephalitis has also been described.

CYTOMEGALOVIRUS ENCEPHALITIS/ CMV ENCEPHALITIS

Cytomegalovirus is a herpes virus that lies latent in the majority of the population and gets reactivated when the host defense mechanisms are weak. Patients with AIDS (CD4 <50) and those with renal transplant are at the maximum risk of opportunistic infection.[159] Neurologic manifestations may be acute or chronic meningoencephalitis, cranial neuropathies, vasculitis, retinitis, myelitis, brachial plexus neuropathy and peripheral neuropathy. The risk of developing encephalitis increases 10 fold in patients with CMV retinitis. The infection is often unrecognized or subclinical in AIDS patients and CMV often co-exists with other lesions like toxoplasmosis and cryptococcosis.

Two forms of CMV encephalitis are recognized-microglial nodular encephalitis and ventriculoencephalitis. The microglial nodular encephalitis has an extremely rapid and quick course, causes cranial nerve palsies, disorientation and serum electrolyte imbalance such as hyponatremia. The cytomegalovirus ventriculoencephalitis form presents with confusion and lethargy which has a progressive downward course resulting in coma and death in a matter of weeks. This form is a subacute necrotizing infection of the ependyma and subependyma.

The pathologic hallmark of CMV is the "owl's eye", an enlarged cell with a distended nucleus. The cell contains viral inclusion bodies and is surrounded by a halo giving a characteristic appearance.

Imaging

CT is not sensitive in the detection of CMV encephalitis and may show atrophy with low attenuation areas in the periventricular white matter. MR is more sensitive in detecting the changes and may show focal or diffuse areas of high signal on T2W images in the periventricular white matter similar to HIV encephalopathy. An ependymal T2 hyperintensity accompanied with an ependymal and subependymal enhancement on the post-contrast scans is suggestive of CMV infection. Diffusion weighted images may reveal a restricted pattern of diffusion along the ependyma and subependyma which again is diagnostic.[160] A thickened enhancing choroid/retina seen on the fat suppressed post-contrast MR images is suggestive of CMV retinitis which occurs in about 20–40% of the AIDS population.

IMMUNE RECONSTITUTION INFLAMMATORY SYNDROME (IRIS)

This is a T-cell mediated encephalitis that occurs in the setting of treated HIV or autoimmune disease like multiple sclerosis. Several different pathogens have been identified in the setting of IRIS. The most common are JC virus (PML-IRIS), tuberculosis (TB-IRIS) and fungal infections especially cryptoccus (crypto IRIS). There may be a natalizumab associated PML IRIS in patients of multiple sclerosis. Two forms are recognized:

- *Unmasking IRIS*: This occurs when a previously unrecognized opportunistic infection manifests with antiretroviral therapy.
- *Paradoxical IRIS*: This occurs when a patient who has been treated for a recent opportunistic infection deteriorates after initiation of antiretroviral therapy.

The most common presentation of neuro IRIS is clinical deterioration inspite of rising CD4 counts and lower viral loads in a newly treated HIV patient. Patients with neuro IRIS may die within days to weeks, the mortality from PML-IRIS being more than 40%.[161]

Imaging

TB IRIS patients may develop florid TB pseudoabscesses (TB gone wild) and extensive enhancements in the basal cisterns. Bizarre looking parenchymal masses and progressively enlarging enhancing lesions are suggestive of PML-IRIS. This condition needs to be differentiated from non-IRIS associated opportunistic infection as IRIS requires steroids to halt the inflammatory process while non IRIS opportunistic infections require immune restoration.[162] Contrast enhancement with mass effect is highly suggestive of IRIS and should be kept in mind in a patient of PML who shows sudden deterioration following HAART therapy.

DIFFERENTIAL DIAGNOSIS OF RING ENHANCING LESIONS IN THE BRAIN

Various CNS infections, such as an abscess, tuberculoma, neurocysticercus, toxoplasma, cryptococcomas present as ring enhancing lesions. Various other lesions like metastasis, demyelinating plaque, lymphoma also present as ring enhancing lesions in the brain parenchyma. The differential of ring enhancing lesions in the brain are enumerated in **Table 6**.

CONGENITAL INFECTIONS

Congenital infections, as the name implies, are infections acquired in utero through the transplacental route or during birth. Infections acquired during the first 4 weeks of life are called neonatal infections. TORCH is an acronym for the congenital infections—Toxoplasmosis, Others (Syphillis, HIV), Rubella, Cytomegalovirus (CMV) and Herpes simplex virus (HSV) type 2. While others occur via the transplacental route, herpes is most commonly an ascending infection.

TOXOPLASMOSIS

Congenital toxoplasmosis occurs when infection is acquired antenatally. Transplacental infection rates increase with increasing trimester with the infection rate being 20% in the first trimester and 60% in the third trimester.[164] Hydrocephalus, bilateral chorioretinitis and intracranial calcifications form the typical triad found in infants with congenital toxoplasma encephalitis. Mortality rates range from 1 to 5% and children with neurologic symptoms at birth who survive usually have long-term sequelae including developmental delay and seizures.

Toxoplasmosis infection is multifocal and scattered. US, CT and MR scans most often demonstrate calcifications that can involve the periventricular regions, basal ganglia or cerebral cortex **(Figs. 53A and B)**. The size of the calcification has been correlated with the duration of infection. A larger

TABLE 6: Ring-enhancing lesions in the brain parenchyma: Differential diagnosis.[163]

Differential diagnosis	CT	MRI							PET
		T1	T2	Post-contrast	DW1	ADC	MRS	MT ratio	
IMMUNOCOMPETENT									
Neurocysticercosis	Thin regular ring enhancement with eccentric dot sign	Core is hypointense	Core hyperintense with hypointense rim	Ring enhancement, smooth outline	Core dark	High	Variable	Higher due to protein and amino acid	No increased uptake
Tuberculoma with central liquefaction	Irregular outline of ring enhancement	Core is hypointense	Core is hyperintense with hypointense rim	Ring enhancement, irregular outline	Bright due to restriction	Low	Lipid peak	Lower	No increased uptake
Pyogenic brain abscess	Ring-enhancing lesion with thinner medial/ ventricular margin, smooth thin rim, satellite lesions and perilesional edema	Hypointense	Hyperintense	Smooth, thin ring enhancing lesion with thinner medial margin, satellite lesions, edema	Bright	Low	Amino acids, acetate and succinate peaks	Higher than tuberculoma	May show increased uptake
Metastasis	Hypodense lesions with rim enhancement, extensive perilesional edema	Hypointense	Hyperintense, extensive edema	Thick rim or nodular enhancement	Dark	High	Suppressed NAA and elevated choline		Increased uptake
Demyelinating/ tumefactive plaque	Open ring enhancement/ incomplete ring	Hypointense	Hyperintense	Open-rim enhancement thinner at the cortical side	Acute-bright Chronic-dark	Acute-low Chronic-High	Decreased NAA, glutamate peak may be seen	Decreased	Variable depending on phase
IMMUNOCOMPROMISED									
Fungal brain abscess	Hyperdense lesions with thick ring enhancement	Hypointense, show blooming on SWI	Hyperintense core with hypointense rim	Thick rim enhencement	Bright, in an intracavitary projection	Low in projection	Elevate choline peak, suppressed NAA, alpha trehaose at 3.6–3.8 ppm	Higher than tuberculoma	Increased uptake
Toxoplasmosis	Ring enhancement wit central hypodensity	Isointense, predilection for basal ganglia and corticomedullary junction	Central T2 hypointensity surrounded by alternte bands of hyper and hypointensity	Ring and nodular enhancement with perilesional edema, eccentric target sign	Dark	Higher than lymphoma	Lipid and lactate peaks	–	No increased uptake
Lymphoma	Isodense with ring enhancement	Hypointense, predilection for periventricular location/ ependymal surface	Hypointense, lesion crosses the corpus callosum	Intense enhancement, subependymal enhancement and ventricular encasement	Bright	Low	↓ NAA ↑ Choline	–	Increased uptake

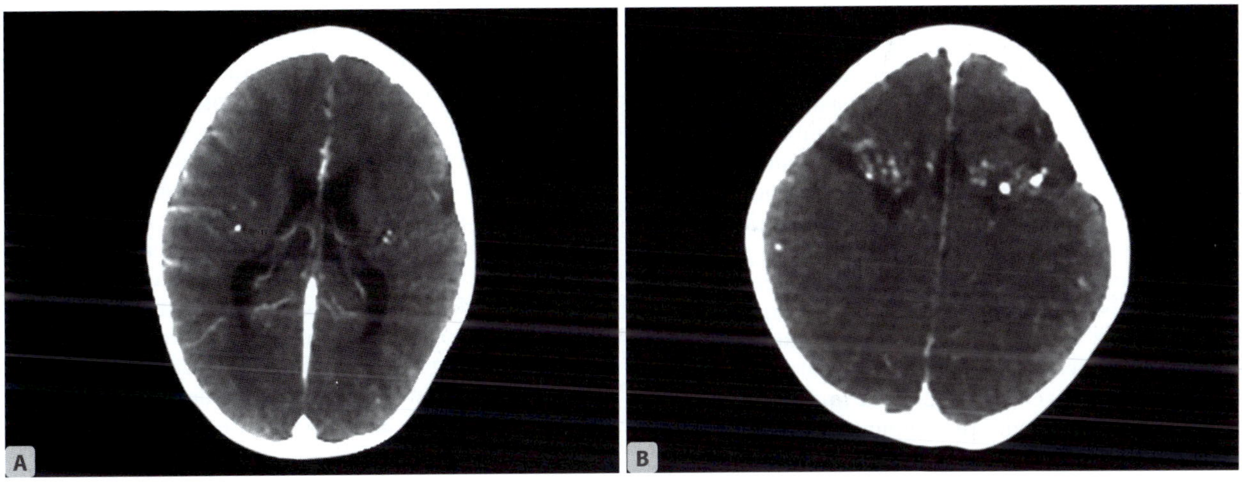

FIGS. 53A AND B: Axial CT sections reveal areas of gliosis with calcification seen in the periventricular regions and peripheral cerebral tissue—congenital toxopasmosis.

size of the calcification is seen in the first and second trimester infections. Hydrocephalus, when present, is secondary to aqueductal stenosis and often has a characteristically marked expansion of the atria and occipital horns resulting from associated tissue loss.[165] Toxoplasmosis causes necrosis but does not result in migrational anomalies. Nonspecific findings include atrophy, encephalomalacia, hydranencephaly or microcephaly.

SYPHILIS

Maternal syphilis poses a threat to the fetus regardless of the stage of the maternal infection. It can result in spontaneous abortion, stillbirth, nonimmune hydrops, premature delivery and perinatal death. Forty percent of congenitally infected infants die during the perinatal period.

Approximately 33% of congenitally infected infants have disseminated infection at birth. Clinical signs of disseminated infection characteristically include long bone periostitis. Other signs consist of hepato-splenomegaly, jaundice, skin rash, persistent rhinitis, lymphadenopathy, meningitis and hydrocephalus. The late manifestations of congenital syphilis appear after 2 years of age. These include orodental, facial and skin deformities, sensorineural hearing loss, hydrocephalus, mental retardation, seizures and hemiplegia.[166]

Cranial imaging findings may show hydrocephalus and enhancement of the leptomeninges. This may extend through the meningeal vessels and the cortical perforators to involve the brain parenchyma and appear on imaging as an enhancing parenchymal mass. Infarction may occur, attributed to the accompanying arteritis or less commonly phlebitis. The cerebral infarction most often involves the middle cerebral artery (MCA) distribution.

RUBELLA

The risk of rubella infection is maximum during the first trimester. Congenital rubella syndrome is characterized by hepatosplenomegaly, congenital heart disease (PDA, pulmonary artery stenosis), growth retardation, ocular abnormalities (cataract, pigmentary retinopathy), jaundice, rash, sensorineural hearing loss and meningoencephalitis. An entity in which the brain is formed but is markedly diminished in size called "microcephalia vera" has also been reported in rubella. Microcephaly in rubella is not caused by a destructive process but is related to an inhibition of progenitor cell multiplication by rubella virus resulting in insufficient generation of astroglia and neurons.

Imaging

Ultrasonography may show nonspecific findings of subependymal cysts in the caudate nucleus and subthalamic regions or echogenic foci in the basal ganglia representing mineralizing vasculitis. CT may show microcephaly and parenchymal calcifications while deep and subcortical white matter lesions, delayed myelination may be seen on MR. Cerebellar hypoplasia and neuronal migration anomalies have been reported.

CYTOMEGALOVIRUS (CMV)

CMV is the commonest cause of congenital infection with CNS involvement seen in about 70% cases. The virus has a predilection for the periventricular subependymal germinal matrix layer. Necrosis of this region followed by calcification accounts for the periventricular calcification seen in these cases. Other sites of involvement include the cerebral cortex, white matter, brainstem, spinal cord and the cerebellum. Disorders of neuronal migration (polymicrogyria, heterotopia), microcephaly, hydranencephaly and porencephaly may also occur. Long-term sequelae such as visual deficits, mental retardation, hearing loss and seizures may occur. CMV is the leading cause of nonhereditary deafness in children.

Imaging

Microcephaly with egg shell periventricular calcification is the imaging hallmark of CMV infection[167] **(Fig. 54)**. On sonography, hypoechoic periventricular ring like zones followed by bilateral periventricular calcifications is specific for CMV. Intracranial calcification is seen in about 40% cases and is typically located in the periventricular areas but may also be seen in the basal ganglia, cortical and subcortical regions. Calcifications are best seen on CT while parenchymal abnormalities like encephalomalacia, migrational anomalies (polymicrogyria, lissencephaly, pachygyria, heterotopia), ventricular enlargement, delayed myelination and subependymal periventricular cysts are better seen on MRI.

The major differential diagnosis of CMV is congenital toxoplasmosis. The calcifications in CMV are generally periventricular while those of toxoplasmosis tend to be peripheral. Microcephaly is seen in CMV while macrocephaly is seen in toxoplasmosis **(Figs. 55A and B)**. Anomalies or cortical development are common in CMV but rare in toxoplasmosis.

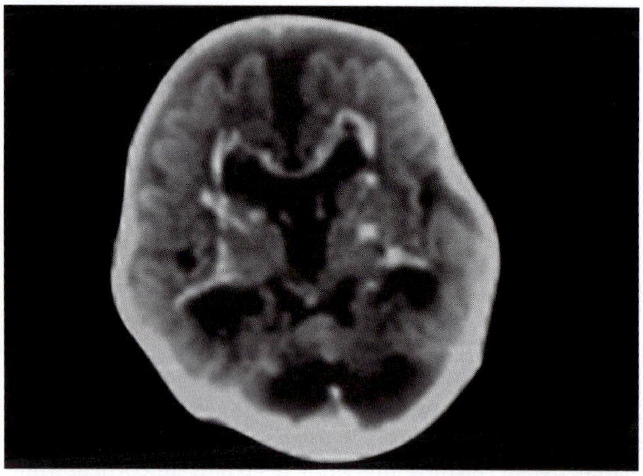

FIG. 54: Noncontrast CT scans of the cranium of a newborn showing hydrocephalus and extensive periventricular calcification. Also seen is calcification in bilateral basal ganglia—CMV.

HERPES SIMPLEX VIRUS (HSV)

HSV is the second most common TORCH infection. In contrast to other TORCH infections most of the HSV infection in neonates are not strictly congenital but occur in the perinatal period. These result from exposure to HSV type 2 genital lesions of the mother at the time of vaginal birth. On CT hypodense lesions may be seen in the periventricular white matter. Finger like areas of increased attenuation within the cortical grey matter along with increased white matter lucency have been attributed to the increased blood flow from cortical infection and has been described as a characteristic imaging finding occurring in the first 3 weeks after presentation. With disease progression, focal necrosis, cystic encephalomalacia, parenchymal calcification and diffuse cerebral atrophy may ensue.

HIV

Mother-to-child transmission of HIV can occur in utero, intrapartum during birth and postpartum via breast milk. The transplacental route accounts for most pediatric AIDS cases and is the major route of infection in infants.

Pathologically multinuclear giant cells and microglial nodules are seen in the basal ganglia, brainstem and the white matter. Perivascular inflammation, demyelination and calcification may be seen, most commonly in the basal ganglia. The infants may be asymptomatic at birth and then develop chronic symptoms over months which include developmental delay, microcephaly, spastic paraparesis and ataxia. However, unlike adults, opportunistic infections like toxoplasmosis and tuberculosis are not seen in the congenital variety.

Imaging

CT may show diffuse cerebral atrophy associated with bilateral low attenuation areas in the white matter with no mass effect or edema. Bilateral and symmetrical calcifications can be seen in the basal ganglia as a result of vasculitis in

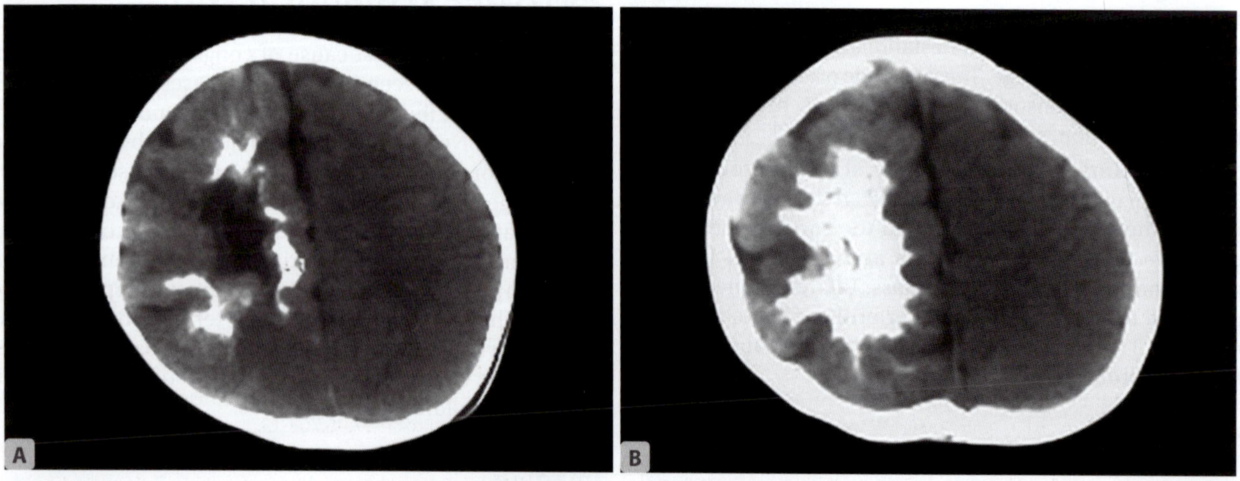

FIGS. 55A AND B: Axial section CT reveal microcephaly with egg shell periventricular calcification (A) and intraparenchymal coarse chunky calcification; (B) Congenital CMV.

which calcium is deposited in and around the small vessels. Calcifications may also occur in the white matter and cerebellum. Rarely haemorrhage may occur in cases where there is severe thrombocytopenia.

MR imaging reveals diffuse atrophy and abnormalities of the white matter. These include delayed myelination and areas of increased signal in the peripheral white matter on proton-density and T2-weighted images without associated mass effect. Cortical spinal tract degeneration and demyelination are also seen in children.

CONCLUSION

The imaging findings seen in CNS infections are variable and challenging. A knowledge of the common patterns seen in the various CNS infections may enable the radiologist to suggest a diagnosis or arrive at a differential diagnosis in equivocal cases. The clinical picture and laboratory testing are of vital importance in making a definitive diagnosis and guiding therapy.

REFERENCES

1. Meltzer CC, Fukui MB, Kanal E, et al. MR imaging of the meninges. Radiology. 1996;20:297-308.
2. Kanamalla US, Ibarra RA, Jinkins JR. Imaging of cranial meningitis and ventricles. Neuroimag Clin N Am. 2000;10:309-31.
3. Farn JW, Mirowitz SA. MR imaging of the normal meninges: Comparison of contrast enhanced patterns on 3D gradient echo and spin echo images. Am J Roentgenol. 1994;162:131-5.
4. Sze G, Soletsky S, Bronen R, et al. MR imaging of the cranial meninges with emphasis on contrast enhancement and meningeal carcinomatosis. Am J Neuroradiol. 1989;10:965-75.
5. Mohan S, Jain KK, Arabi M, et al. Imaging of meningitis and ventriculitis. Neuroimag Clin N Am. 2012;22:557-83.
6. Quint DJ, Eldevik OP, Cohen JK. Magnetic resonance imaging of normal meningeal enhancement at 1.5T. Acad Radiol. 1996;6:463-8.
7. Smirniotopoulos JG, Murphy FM, Rushing EJ, et al. Patterns of contrast enhancement in the brain and meninges. Radiographics. 2007;27:525-51.
8. Hakan T, Ceran N, Erdem I, et al. Bacterial brain abscesses: an evaluation of 96 cases. J Infect. 2006;52:359-66.
9. Xaio F, Tseng MY, Teng LJ, et al. Brain abscess:clinical experience and analysis of prognostic factors. Surg Neurol. 2005;63:442-9.
10. Tunkel AR, Scheld WM. Pathogenesis and pathophysiology of bacterial meningitis. Clin Microbiol Rev. 1993;6:118-36.
11. Ashwal S. Neurologic evaluation of the patient with acute bacterial meningitis. Neurol Clin. 1995;13:549-77.
12. Van de Beek D, de Gans J, Spanjaard L, et al. Clinical and prognostic factors in adults with bacterial meningitis. N Engl J Md. 2004;351:1849-59.
13. Shih RY, Koeller KK. Bacterial, fungal and parasitic infections of the central nervous system-Radiologic-pathologic correlation and historical perspectives. Radiographics. 2015;35:1141-69.
14. Parmer H, Sitoh YY, Anand P, et al. Contrast enhanced FLAIR imaging in the evaluation of infectious leptomeningeal diseases. Eur J Radiol. 2006;58:89-95.
15. Stuckey SL, Goh TD, Heffernan T, et al. Hyperintensity in the subarachnoid space on FLAIR MRI. Am J Roentgenol. 2007;189:913-21.
16. Runge VM, Wells JW, Williams NM, et al. Detectability of early brain meningitis with magnetic resonance imaging. Invest Radiol. 1995;30:484-95.
17. Trivedi R, Malik GK, Gupta RK, et al. Increased anisotropy in neonatal meningitis: an indicator of meningeal inflammation. Neuroradiology. 2007;49:767-75.
18. Yadav A, Malik GK, Trivedi R, et al. Correlation of CSF neuroinflammatory molecules with leptomeningeal cortical subcortical white matter fractional anisotropy in neonatal meningitis. Mag Reson Imaging. 2009;27:214-21.
19. Cabral DA, Flodmark O, Farrell K, et al. Prospective study of computed tomography in acute bacterial meningitis. J Pediatr. 1987;111:201-5.
20. Castillo M. Imaging of meningitis. Semin Roentgenol. 2004;39:458-64.
21. Smith RR. Neuroradiology of intracranial infection. Paediatr Neurosurg. 1992;18:92-104.
22. Rabe EF. Subdural effusion in infants. Paed Clin North Am. 1967;14:831-50.
23. Sze G, Zimmerman RD. The magnetic resonance imaging of infections and inflammatory diseases. Radiol Clin North Am. 1988;26:839-59.
24. Zimmerman RD, Leeds NE, Danziger A. Subdural empyema: CT findings. Radiology. 1984;150:417-22.
25. Weingarten K, Zimmerman RD, Becker RD, et al. Subdural and epidural empyemas: MR imaging. Am J Roentgenol. 1989;152: 615-21.
26. Wong AM, Zimmerman RA, Simon EM, et al. Diffusion weighted MR imaging of subdural empyema in children. Am J Neuroradiol. 2004;25:1016-21.
27. Mathisen GE, Johnson JP. Brain abscess. Clin Infect Dis. 1997;25:763-79.
28. Saez-Llorens XJ, Umana MA, Odio CM, et al. Brain abscess in infants and children. Ped Infect Dis J. 1989;8:449-58.
29. Strong AJ, Ingham HR. Brain abscess. Br J Hosp Med. 1983;30: 396-403.
30. Enzmann DR, Britt RH, Placone R. Staging of human brain abscess by computed tomography. Radiology. 1983;146:703-8.
31. Brit RH, Enzmann DR. Clinical stages of human brain abscesses on serial CT scans after contrast infusion: CT, neuropathological and clinical correlation. J Neurosurg. 1983;59:972-89.
32. Haimes AB, Zimmerman RD, Morgello S, et al. MR imaging of brain abscesses. Am J Neuroradiol. 1989;152:1073-85.
33. Whiteman MLH, Bowen BC, Post MJD, et al. Intracranial infection. In Magnetic resonance imaging of the brain and spine SW atlas, New York: Lippincott Raven. 1996;706-66.
34. Dev R, Gupta RK, Poptani H, et al. Role of in vivo proton magnetic resonance spectroscopy in the diagnosis and management of brain abscess. Neurosurgery. 1998;42:37-43.
35. Demaerel P, Hecke PV, Oostende SV, et al. Bacterial metabolism shown by magnetic resonance spectroscopy. Lancet. 1997;344:1197-202.
36. Martinez-Perez I, Moreno A, Alonso J, et al. Diagnosis of brain abscess by magnetic resonance spectroscopy: Report of two cases. J Neurosurg. 1997;86:708-13.
37. Desprechins B, Stadnik T, Koerts G, et al. Use of diffusion weighted MR imaging in differential diagnosis between intracerebral necrotic tumors and cerebral abscesses. Am J Neuroradiol. 1999;20:1252-7.

38. Ebisu T, Tanaka C, Umeda M, et al. Discrimination of brain abscess from necrotic or cystic tumors by diffusion weighted echo planar imaging. Mag Reson Imaging. 1996;14:1113-6.
39. Lai PH, Hsu SS, Ding SW, et al. Proton magnetic resonance spectroscopy and diffusion-weighted imaging in intracranial cystic mass lesions. Surg Neurol. 2007;68:S25-36.
40. Gupta RK, Hasan KM, Mishra AM, et al. High fractional anisotropy in brain abscesses versus other cystic intracranial lesions. Am J Neuroradiol. 2005;26:1107-14.
41. Holmes TM, Petrella JR, Provenzale JM. Distinction between cerebral abscesses and high grade neoplasms by dynamic susceptibility contrast perfusion MRI. AJR. 2004;183:1247-52.
42. Crain MR, Yuh WT, Greene GM, et al. Cerebral ischaemia: Evaluation with contrast enhanced MR imaging. Am J Neuroradiol. 1991;12:631-9.
43. Harris TM, Edwards MK. Meningitis. Neuroimaging. Clin N Am. 1991;1:39-56.
44. Raimondi AJ, Rocco C. Cerebral angiography in meningococcal inflammatory diseases in infancy and childhood: a study of thirty five cases. Neurosurgery. 1978;3:37-44.
45. Beijen J, Casselman J, Joosten F, et al. Magnetic resonance imaging in patients with meningitis induced hearing loss. Eur Arch Otorhinolaryngol. 2009;266:1229-36.
46. Barloon TJ, Yuh WT, Knepper LE. Cerebral ventriculitis: MR findings. J Comput Assist Tomogr. 1990;14:272-5.
47. Durand ML, Calderwood SB, Weber DJ, et al. Acute bacterial meningitis in adults: A review of 493 episodes. N Eng J Med. 1993;328:21-8.
48. World Health Organization, Global Tuberculosis Control 2014. Geneva, Switzerland: WHO;2014. Available at: http://apps.who.int/iris/bitstreah/10665/137094/1/9789241564809_eng.pdf
49. Bernaerts A, Vanhoenacker FM, Parizel PM, et al. Tuberculosis of the central nervous system:overview of neuroradiological findings. Eur Radiol. 2003;13:1876-90.
50. Berenguer J, Moreno S, Laguna F, et al. Tuberculous meningitis in patients infected with human immunodeficiency virus. N Engl J Med. 1992;326:668-72.
51. Rich AR, McCordock HA. Pathogenesis of tubercular meningitis. Bull John Hopkins hosp. 1933;52:5-13.
52. Dastur DK, Manghani DK, Udani PM. Pathology and pathogenic mechanisms in neurotuberculosis. Radiol Clin North Am. 1995;33:733-52.
53. Leonard JM, Des RP. Tuberculous meningitis. Infect Dis Clin North Am. 1990;4:769-87.
54. Dastur DK, Lalitha VS, Udani PM, et al. The brain and meninges in tuberculous meningitis-gross pathology in 100 cases and pathogenesis. Neurol India. 1970;18:86-100.
55. Przybojewski S, Andronikou S, Wilmshurst J. Objective criteria to determine the presence of abnormal basal enhancement in children with suspected Tuberculous Meningitis. Pediatr Radiol. 2006;36:687-96.
56. Klingensmith WC, Datu J. Tuberculous meningitis of the sylvian fissure. Clin Nucl Med. 1978;3:315-7.
57. Trautmann M, Kluge W, Otto HS, et al. Computed tomography in CNS tuberculosis. Eur Neurol. 1986;25:91-7.
58. de Castro CC, de Baros NG, Campos ZM, et al. CT scans of cranial tuberculosis. Radiol Clin North Am. 1995;33:753-69.
59. Chang KH, Han MH, Roh JK, et al. Gd-DTPA enhanced MR imaging in intracranial tuberculosis. Neuroradiology. 1990;32:19-25.
60. Gupta RK, Gupta S, Singh D, et al. MR imaging and angiography in tuberculous meningitis. Neuroradiology. 1994;36:87-92.
61. Gupta RK, Kathuria MK, Pradhan S. Magnetization transfer MR imaging in central nervous system tuberculosis. Am J Neuroradiol. 1999;20:867-75.
62. Jamieson DH. Imaging intracranial tuberculosis in childhood. Paediatr Radiol. 1995;25:165-70.
63. Kioumehr F, Dadsetan MR, Rooholamini SA, et al. Central nervous system tuberculosis: MRI. Neuroradiology. 1994;36:93-6.
64. Rovira M, Romero F, Torrent O, et al. Study of tuberculous meningitis by CT. Neuroradiology. 1980;19:137-41.
65. Wallace RC, Burto EM, Barrett FF, et al. Intracranial tuberculosis in children: CT appearance and clinical outcome. Paed Radiol. 1991;21:241-6.
66. Torres C, Riascos R, Figueroa R, et al. Central Nervous System Tuberculosis. Top Mag Reson Imaging. 2014;23:173-89.
67. Gupta RK, Kumar S. Central nervous system tuberculosis. Neuroimaging Clin N Am. 2011;21:795-814.
68. Silverman IE, Liu GT, Bilaniuk LT, et al. Tuberculous meningitis with blindness and perichiasmal involvement on MRI. Ped Neurol. 1995;12:65-7.
69. Praharaj SS, Sharma MC, Prasad K, et al. Unilateral meningeal thickening: a rare presentation of tuberculous meningitis. Clin Neurol Neurosurg. 1997;99:60-2.
70. Gupta RK, Kohli A, Gaur V, et al. MRI of the brain in patients with miliary pulmonary tuberculosis without symptoms or signs of central nervous system involvement. Neuroradiology. 1997;39:699-704.
71. Altunbasak S, Baytok V, Alhan E, et al. Suprasellar tuberculoma causing endocrinologic disorders and imitating craniopharyngioma. Paediatr Neurosurg. 1995; 23:328-31.
72. Esposito V, Fraioli B, Ferrante L, et al. Intrasellar tuberculoma: Case report. Neurosurgery. 1987;21:721-3.
73. Bargallo J, Berenguer J, Garcia-Barrionuevo J, et al. The "target sign" is it a specific sign of CNS tuberculoma? Neuroradiology. 1996;38:547-50.
74. Salgado P, Del Brutto OH, Talamas O, et al. Intracranial tuberculoma: MR imaging. Neuroradiology. 1989;31:299-302.
75. Shah GV. Central nervous system tuberculosis imaging manifestations. Neuroimaging Clin North Am. 2000; 10:355-74.
76. Gupta RK, Vatsal DK, Husain N, et al. Differentiation of tuberculous from pyogenic brain abscesses with in vivo proton MR spectroscopy and magnetization transfer MR imaging. Am J Neuroradiol. 2001;22:1503-9.
77. Trivedi R, Saksena S, Gupta RK. Magnetic resonance imaging in central nervous system tuberculosis. Indian J Radiol Imaging. 2009;19:256-65.
78. Patkar D, Narang J, Yanamandala R, et al. Central Nervous System Tuberculosis Pathophysiology and Imaging Findings. Neuroimag Clin N Am. 2012;22:677-705.
79. Whitener DR. Tuberculous brain abscess. Report of a case and review of literature. Arch Neurol. 1978;35:148-55.
80. Farrar DJ, Fiangan TP, Gordon NM, et al. Tuberculous brain abscess in a patient with HIV infection: case report and review. Am J Med. 1997;102:297-301.
81. Luthra G, Parihar A, Nath K, et al. Comparative evaluation of fungal, tubercular and pyogenic brain abscesses with conventional and diffusion MR imaging and proton MR spectroscopy. AJNR Am J Neuroradiol. 2007;28:1332-8.
82. Gupta RK, Prakash M, Mishra AM, et al. Role of diffusion weighted imaging in differentiation of intracranial tuberculoma and tuberculous abscess from cysticercus granuloma—a report of more than 100 lesions. Eur J Radiol. 2005;55:384-92.
83. Saxena S, Prakash M, Kumar S, et al. Comparative evaluation of magnetization transfer contrast and fluid attenuated inversion recovery sequences in brain tuberculoma. Clin Radiol. 2005;60:787-93.
84. Sheller JR, Des Prez RM. CNS tuberculosis. Neurol Clin. 1986;4: 143-58.

85. Garcia-Monco JC. Central nervous system tuberculosis. Neurol Clin. 1999;17:737-59.
86. Ahluwalia VV, Sagar GD, Singh TP, et al. MRI Spectrum of CNS tuberculosis. JIACM. 2013;14:83-90.
87. Post MJ, Quencer RM, Tabei SZ. CT demonstration of sarcoidosis of the optic nerve, frontal lobes and falx cerebri. Case report and literature review. Am J Neuroradiol. 1982;3:523-6.
88. Khoo TK, Sugai K, Leong TK. Disseminated aspergillosis. Am J Clin Pathol. 1966;45:697-703.
89. Young RC, Bennett JE, Vogel CL, et al. Aspergillosis. The spectrum of disease in 98 patients. Medicine. 1970;49: 147-73.
90. Ostrow TD, Hudgins PA. Magnetic resonance imaging of intracranial fungal infections. Magn Reson Imaging. 1994;6:22-31.
91. Cox J, Murtagh FR, Wilfrong A, et al. Cerebral aspergillosis MR imaging and histopathologic correlation. Am J Neuroradiol. 1992;5:1489-92.
92. Ashdown BC, Tien RD, Felsberg GJ. Aspergillosis of the brain and paranasal sinuses in immunocompromised patients: CT and MR imaging findings. Am J Roentgenol. 1994;162:155-9.
93. DeLone DR, Goldstein RA, Petermann G, et al. Disseminated aspergillosis involving the brain: distribution and imaging characteristics. AJNR Am J Neuroradiol. 1999;20:1597-604.
94. Gabelmann A, Klein S, Kern W, et al. Relevant imaging findings of cerebral aspergillosis on MRI: a retrospective case based study in immunocompromised patients. Eur J Neurol. 2007;14:548-55.
95. Zinreich SJ, Kennedy DW, Malat J, et al. Fungal sinusitis: diagnosis with CT and MR imaging. Radiology. 1988; 169:439-44.
96. Mathews VP, Alo PL, Glass JD, et al. AIDS-related CNS cryptococcosis: Radiologic—pathologic correlation. Am J Neuroradiol. 1992;13:1477-86.
97. Igel HJ, Bolande RP. Humoral defense mechanisms in cryptococcosis: substances in normal human serum, saliva and cerebrospinal fluid affecting the growth of Cryptococcus neoformans. J Inf Dis. 1966;116:75-83.
98. Cornell SH, Jacoby CJ. The varied computed tomographic appearance of intracranial cryptococcosis. Radiology. 1982;143:703-7.
99. Andreula CF, Burdi N, Carella A. CNS cryptococcosis in AIDS: spectrum of MR findings. J Comput Assist Tomogr. 1993;17:438-41.
100. Offiah CE, Naseer A. Spectrum of imaging appearances of intracranial cryptococcal infection in HIV/AIDS patients in the anti-retroviral therapy era. Clin Radiol. 2016;71:9-17.
101. Blitzer A, Lawson W, Meyers BR, et al. Patient survival in paranasal sinus mucormycosis. Laryngoscope. 1980;90:635-48.
102. Bergstrom L, Hemenway WG, Barnhart RA. Rhinocerebral and otologic mucormycosis. Ann Oto Rhino Laryngol. 1970;79:70-81.
103. Safder S, Carpenter JS, Roberto TD, et al. The "Black Turbinate" Sign: an early MR imaging finding of nasal mucormycosis. Am J Neuroradiol. 2010;31:771-4
104. Morduchowicz G, Shmueli D, Shapira Z, et al. Rhinocerebral mucormycosis in renal transplant recipients. Rev Infect Dis. 1986;8:441-6.
105. Lipton SA, Hickey WF, Morris JH, et al. Candidal infection in the central nervous system. Am J Med. 1984;76:101-8.
106. Castro S, Bernardes I. Coccidioidal cerebral abscess with peripheral restricted diffusion. J Neuroradiol. 2009;36:162-4.
107. Stone JH, Pomper MG, Hellmann DB. Histoplasmosis mimicking vasculitis of the central nervous system. J Rheumatol. 1998;25:1644-8.
108. Go JL, Kim PE, Ahmadi J, et al. Fungal Infections of the central nervous system. Neuroimaging Clin North Am. 2000;10:409-25.
109. Mathur M, Johnson CE, Sze G. Fungal infections of the Central Nervous System. Neuroimag Clin N Am. 2012; 22:609-32.
110. Stepien L. Cerebral cysticercosis in Poland: clinical symptoms and operative results in 132 cases. J Neurosurg. 1962;19:505-13.
111. Keane JR. Death from cysticercosis: Seven patients with unrecognized obstructive hydrocephalus. West J Med. 1984;140:787-9.
112. Sotelo J, Del Brutto OH, Penagos P, et al. Comparison of therapeutic regimen of anticysticercal drugs for parenchymal brain cysticercosis. J Neurol. 1990;237:69-72.
113. Chang KH, Lee JH, Han MH, et al. The role of contrast enhanced MR imaging in the diagnosis of neurocysticercosis. Am J Neuroradiol. 1991;12:509-12.
114. Martinez HR, Rangel Guerra R, Gonzalez J, et al. MR imaging in neurocysticercosis. A study of 56 cases. Am J Neuroradiol. 1989;10:1011-9.
115. Noujaim SE, Rossi MD, Rao SK, et al. CT and MR imaging of neurocysticercosis. AJR Am J Roentgenol. 1999;17:1485-90.
116. Sharma BB, Sharma S. Neurocysticercosis (NCC) vs central nervous system (CNS) tuberculoma in children: Dilemma over clinicoradiological diagnosis? Open J Pediatr. 2016;6:245-51.
117. Zee CS, Segall HD, Boswell W, et al. MR imaging of neurocysticercosis. J Comput Assist Tomogr. 1988;12:927-34.
118. Zee CS, Segall HD, Apuzzo ML, et al. Intraventricular cysticercal cysts: further neuroradiologic observations and neurosurgical implications. Am J Neuroradiol. 1984; 5:727-30.
119. Ramsey RG, Gean AD. Neuroimaging of AIDS central nervous system toxoplasmosis. Neuroimaging Clin North Am. 1997;7:171-86.
120. Kumar GG, Mahadevan A, Guruprasad AS, et al. Eccentric Target Sign in Cerebral Toxoplamosis-neuropathological correlate to the imaging feature. J Magn Reson Imaging. 2010;31:1469-72.
121. Camacho DL, Smith JK, Castillo M. Differentiation of toxoplasmosis and lymphoma in AIDS patients by using apparent diffusion coefficients. Am J Neuroradiol. 2003;24:633-7.
122. Coates R, von Sinner W, Rahm B. MR imaging of an intracerebral hydatid cyst. AJNR Am J Neuroradiol. 1990;11:1249-50.
123. Turgut M, Benli K, Eryilmaz M. Secondary multiple intracranial hydatid cysts caused by intracerebral embolism of cardiac echinococcosis: an exceptional case of hydatidosis. J Neurosurg. 1997;86:714-8.
124. Nurchi G, Floris F, Montaldo C, et al. Multiple cerebral hydatid disease: case report with magnetic resonance imaging study. Neurosurg. 1992;30:436-8.
125. Senturk S, Oguz KK, Soylemezoglu F, et al. Cerebral alveolar echinococcosis mimicking primary brain tumours. Am J Neuroradiol. 2006;27:420-2.
126. Kohli A, Gupta RK, Poptani H, et al. In vivo proton magnetic resonance spectroscopy in a case of intracranial hydatid cyst. Neurology. 1995,45.562-4.
127. Mohanty S, Taylor TE, Kampondeni S, et al. Magnetic resonance imaging during life: the key to unlock cerebral malaria pathogenesis? Malar J. 2014;13:276.
128. Nickerson JP, Tong KA, Raghavan R. Imaging cerebral malaria with a susceptibility weighted MR sequence. Am J Neuroradiol. 2009;30:85-6.
129. Gupta S, Patel K. Case series: MRI features in cerebral malaria. Indian J Radiol Imaging. 2008;18:224-6.
130. Alkhunaizi AM, Dawamneh MF, Banda RW, et al. Acanthamoeba encephalitis in a patient with systemic lupus treated with rituximab. Diagn Microbiol Infect Dis. 2013;75:192-4.
131. Ranjan R, Handa A, Choudhary A, et al. Acanthamoeba infection in a interhemispheric ependymal cyst: a case report. Surg Neurol. 2009;72:185-9.
132. Mayer PL, Larkin JA, Hennessay JM. Amoebic encephalitis. Surg Neurol Int. 2011;2:50.

133. Corey L, Spear PG. Infection with herpes simplex viruses. N Eng J Med. 1986;314:749-57.
134. Weiner LP, Fleming JO. Viral infections of the nervous system. J Neurosurg. 1984;61:207-24.
135. Baringer JR. Herpes simplex infections of the nervous system. Neurol Clin. 2008;26:657-74.
136. Noguchi T, Yoshiura T, Hiwatashi A, et al. CT and MRI findings of human herpes virus 6-associated encephalopathy: comparision with findings of herpes simplex virus encephalitis. AJR Am J Roentgenol. 2010;194:754-60.
137. Soares BP, Provenzale JM. Imaging of herpes virus infections of the CNS. Am J Roentgenol. 2016;206:39-48.
138. Prandota J. Mollaret meningitis may be caused by reactivation of latent cerebral toxoplasmosis. Int J Neurosco. 2009;119:1655-92.
139. Gliden D, Cohrs RJ, Mahalingam R, et al. Varicella zoster virus vasculopathies: diverse clinical manifestations, laboratory features, pathogenesis and treatment. Lancet Neurol. 2009;8: 731-40.
140. Handique SK, Das RR, Barman K, et al. Temporal lobe involvement in Japanese encephalitis: problems in differential diagnosis. Am J Neuroradiol. 2006;27:1027-31.
141. Singh P, Kalra N, Ratho RK, et al. Coexistent neurocysticercosis and Japanese B encephalitis: MR imaging correlation. Am J Neuroradiol. 2001;22:1131-6.
142. Kipps A, Dick G, Moodie JW. Measles and the central nervous system. Lancet. 1983;2:1406-10.
143. Laothamatas J, Hemachudha T, Mitrabhakdi E, et al. MR imaging in human rabies. Am J Neuroradiol. 2003;24: 1102-9.
144. Ukisu R, Kushihashi T, Tanaka E, et al. Diffusion weighted MR imaging of early stage Creutzfeldt-Jacob disease: typical and atypical manifestations. Radiographics. 2006;26:S191-204.
145. Zeidler M, Sellar RJ, Collie DA, et al. The pulvinar sign on magnetic resonance imaging in variant Creutzfeldt-Jacob disease. Lancet. 2000;355:1412-8.
146. Smith AB, Smirniotopoulos JG, Rushing EJ. Central nervous system infections associated with human immunodeficiency virus infection: radiologic-pathologic correlation. Radiographics. 2008;28:2033-58.
147. McArthur JC, Haughey N, Gartner S, et al. Human immunodeficiency virus associated dementia: an evolving disease. J Neurovirol. 2003;9:205-21.
148. Post MJ, Tate LG, Quencer RM, et al. CT, MR and pathology in HIV encephalitis and meningitis. Am J Roentgenol. 1988;151:373-80.
149. Jarvik JG, Lenkinski RE, Grossman RI. Proton MR spectroscopy of HIV infected patients: characterization of abnormalities with imaging and clinical correlation. Radiology. 1993;186:739-44.
150. Pomara N, Crandall DT, Choi SJ, et al. White matter abnormalities in HIV-1 infection: a diffusion tensor imaging study. Psychiatry Res. 2001;106:15-24.
151. Major EO, Amemiya K, Tornatore CS, et al. Pathogenesis and molecular biology of progressive multifocal leukoencephalopathy, the JC virus induced demyelinating disease of the human brain. Clin J Microbiol Rev. 1992; 5:49-73.
152. Sahraian MA, Radue EW, Eshaghi A, et al. Progressive multifocal leukoencephalopathy: a review of the neuroimaging features and differential diagnosis. EJ Neurol. 2012;19:1060-9.
153. Arbusow V, Strupp M, Pfister HW, et al. Contrast enhance-ment in progressive multifocal leukoencephalopathy: a predictive factor for long term survival. J Neurol. 2000; 247:306-8.
154. Muller M, Wandel S, Colebunders R, et al. Immune reconstitution inflammatory syndrome in patients starting antiretroviral therapy for HIV infection: a systematic review and meta-analysis. Lancet Infect Dis. 2010;10:251-61.
155. Ohta K, Obara K. Lesion extension detected by diffusion weighted magnetic resonance imaging in PML. J Neurol. 2001;248:809-11.
156. Bergui M, Bradac GB, Oguz KK, et al. Progressive multifocal leukoencephalopathy: diffusion-weighted imaging and pathological correlations. Neuroradiology. 2004;46:22-25.
157. Clark EG, Danbolt N. The Oslo study of the natural history of untreated syphilis; an epidemiologic investigation based on a restudy of the Boeck-Bruusgaard material; a review and appraisal. J Chronic Dis. 1955;2:311-44.
158. Brightbill TC, Ihmeidan IH, Post MJ, et al. Neurosyphilis in HIV-positive and HIV-negative patients: neuroimaging findings. Am J Neuroradiol. 1995;16:703-11.
159. Arribas JR, Storch GA, Clifford DB, et al. Cytomegalovirus encephalitis. Ann Intern Med. 1996;125:577-87.
160. Seok JH, Ahn K, Park HJ. Diffusion MRI findings of cytomegalovirus-associated ventriculitis: a case report. Br J Radiol. 2011;84: e179-81.
161. Tan K, Roda R, Ostrow L, et al. PML-IRIS in patients with HIV infection: clinical manifestations and treatment with steroids. Neurology. 2009;72:1458-64.
162. Marzocchetti A, Di Giambenedetto S, Cingolani A, et al. Reduced rate of diagnostic positive detection of JC virus DNA in cerebrospinal fluid in cases of suspected progressive multifocal leukoencephalopathy in the era of potent antiretroviral therapy. J Clin Microbiol. 2005;43:4175-7.
163. Garg RK, Sinha MK. Multiple ring-enhancing lesions of the brain. J Postgrad Med. 2010;56:307-16.
164. Bale JF Jr, Murph JR. Congenital infections and the nervous system. Pediatr Clin North Am. 1992;39:669-90.
165. Diekler C, Dusser A, Dulae O. Congenital toxoplasmosis: clinical and neuroradiologic evaluation of the cerebral lesions. Neuroradiology. 1985;27:125-30.
166. Griffith BP, Booss J. Neurologic infections of the fetus and newborn. Neurol Clin. 1994;12:541-64.
167. Becker LE. Infections of the developing brain. Am J Neuroradiol. 1992;13:537-49.

CHAPTER

194

Imaging of White Matter Disease

Anjali Prakash, Jyoti Kumar, Swati Gupta, Gaurav Shanker Pradhan

INTRODUCTION

The white matter is primarily composed of myelinated axons and support elements, i.e. oligodendrocytes, astrocytes, microglia, and blood vessels. The myelin sheath is formed by the oligodendrocyte. Each oligodendrocyte extends over several cell processes around one or more neighboring axons, forming few segmental myelin sheaths. The myelin sheath is the major structural element in white matter, comprising approximately 50% of the dry weight of the adult brain; thus primary white matter diseases are considered to be diseases affecting myelin and oligodendrocytes. Neuroglial cells, i.e. oligodendrocytes and astrocytes are primarily responsible for the maintenance of the white matter by providing structural and nutritional support of neurons and regulating the extracellular environment. These cells are also important for guiding the migrating neurons during development and are involved in repair of the nervous system.

White matter disease is caused by a pathologic process that prevents the normal formation and maintenance of myelin or that selectively destroys the oligodendrocyte and/or myelin sheath. The disruption of myelin interrupts the efficient transmission of the axonal action potentials, which in turn may be clinically expressed as a neurological deficit. Any process, including metabolic injury or ischemia, that changes the chemical composition of myelin will result in a less stable structure that is more susceptible to injury.[1,2]

White matter diseases may be categorized as inherited or acquired or as demyelinating and dysmyelinating. Primary demyelinating diseases are characterized by loss of normally formed myelin with relative preservation of axons; Multiple sclerosis is the prototype of primary demyelinating disease. Secondary demyelination is demyelination associated with a known etiology or a systemic disorder and with destruction of both axons and myelin. It consists of a group of entities with very diverse etiologies, pathogenesis, clinical presentation and distribution of lesions.[2,3] Dysmyelination is a pathological process characterized by defective formation/maintenance of normal myelin. Many of these disorders or leukodystrophies have a known genetic basis, others however are poorly understood.

Demyelinating Disease: Classification based on Etiology

Autoimmune Causes

- *Multiple sclerosis:*
  - Classic Charcot type
  - MS Variants
  - Acute-Marburg type
  - Diffuse cerebral sclerosis-Schilder type
  - Concentric sclerosis-Balo type
- Neuromyelitis optica-Devic disease
- Acute disseminated encephalomyelitis (ADEM) Classic (acute disseminated encephalomyelitis)
- Hyperacute (acute hemorrhagic leukoencephalitis)

Associated with infectious agents and/or vaccination

- Progressive multifocal leukoencephalopathy (PML)
- Human immunodeficiency virus (HIV) encephalopathy
- Lyme disease
- Subacute sclerosing panencephalitis (SSPE)
- Progressive rubella panencephalitis.

Associated with Vascular Causes

- Small vessel disease
- Cerebral amyloid angiopathy
- CADASIL
- Primary angiitis of the CNS
- Susac syndrome
- Neuro lupus-SLE

Associated with Toxic Metabolic Causes

- Central pontine myelinolysis
- Posterior reversible encephalopathy syndrome (PRES)
- Marchiafava–Bignami disease
- Wernicke encephalopathy
- Vitamin B_{12} deficiency
- Postradiation white matter injury
- Necrotizing leukoencephalopathy following chemotherapy
- Solvent vapor abuse leukoencephalopathy (SVAL)

IMAGING OF WHITE MATTER DISEASES

Magnetic resonance imaging (MRI) has become the standard and, in most instances, the only acceptable imaging modality and it is proven to be far superior to computed tomography (CT) in detecting and demonstrating the extent of abnormality within intracerebral and extracerebral white matter. Conventional MRI is proven to be sensitive for detecting lesions and their changes. However, it is not able to characterize and quantify the tissue damage within and outside these lesions. With the advent of newer MR techniques, including magnetization transfer (MT) imaging, ^{1}H-MR spectroscopy, and diffusion weighted imaging, the ability to detect and characterize disease has increased significantly.[4-6]

Multiple Sclerosis

Multiple sclerosis (MS) is a chronic inflammatory-demyelinating disorder of the CNS characterized pathologically by multifocal areas of demyelination with loss of oligodendrocytes and astroglial scarring. Axonal loss is now being recognized as an important pathological feature.[4] Although the etiology is not clearly understood, MS is considered to be a result of an autoimmune mediated process in which environmental factors (such as exposure to EBV virus) act on genetically susceptible individuals. A strong association with HLA-DR2 class II has been identified. Some authors have proposed a theory of 'Chronic cerebrospinal venous insufficiency' as a cause for MS. It implicates an abnormal CNS venous outflow as a cause of MS.[7-9]

Epidemiology: Multiple sclerosis is one of the most common neurological disorders in the world and the commonest cause of chronic non-traumatic neurological disorders of young adults in the developed world. The prevalence rates of MS have been reported to vary by continent and geographical latitude. The condition is of high prevalence (>30 per 100,000) in northern parts of Europe and North America; medium prevalence (5–30 per 100,000) in southern Europe and southern United States; and Central and South America (10–20 per 100,000); and low prevalence (<5 per 100,000) in Asia and South America.[10] The risk of MS increases in first-order relatives of patients with clinically definite MS as compared to the general population. The presentation of MS typically differs between Asian and western populations. In Asian patients, the opticospinal type of MS is more frequent, an older age group (>35 years of age) is affected, fewer cases are positive for oligoclonal bands and the CSF protein concentration is higher.[11]

The disease onset is usually between 20–40 years of age. Incidence of MS is low in childhood and in the elderly. It is twice as common in females, often with a more favorable prognosis compared to when it affects men. The clinical manifestations of MS are highly variable, but an attack of neurologic dysfunction (e.g., optic neuritis, incomplete transverse myelitis, brain stem or cerebeller syndrome), also referred to as a **clinically isolated syndrome (CIS),**[12-14] heralds the onset of the disease in approximately 90% of patients. **CIS** is the first episode of neurologic symptoms typical of an MS relapse in a person not known to have MS symptoms, which depend on lesion location and extent of tissue destruction. It ranges from mild-to-severe. Common symptoms of an MS exacerbation (relapse or attack) include numbness, tingling, weakness, impaired balance, blurred vision, double vision, vertigo, and bladder or bowel dysfunction. Patients accumulate disability as a result of incomplete recovery from acute exacerbations and/or gradual disease progression.

The clinical course of MS is variable with varying plaque location and disease progression over time. A number of patterns of longitudinal disease presentation have been described.[4] The most common (70% of cases) is a **relapsing-remitting pattern** There is usually an acute episode of worsening, with complete recovery later on ,followed by a relapsing-remitting course. Many of these patients enter a phase where there is only progression of the disease, called **secondary progressive pattern** In some patients there is no clear cut period of remission and the disease follows a progressive course right from the onset—the **primary progressive MS (PPMS)**. Primary progressive MS comprise a minority (10%) of cases. Another variant is called **progressive relapsing MS** which follows a course like PPMS but there are clear acute relapses which may or may not show recovery. In 15–50% of cases, patients have **benign multiple sclerosis** defined as patients who remain functionally active for over 15 years.[15,16]

Radiologically isolated syndrome (RIS)—this subset of patients have MR findings suggestive of MS, but without related symptoms and have a normal neurological examination. One third will develop MS within 5 years whereas 2/3rd will show imaging progression. Patients of RIS who have cervical cord lesions or cortical lesions have a greater likelihood of conversion to MS.[17]

Pathology of MS: Demyelination occurs in discrete perivenular foci, termed plaques, which range in size from a few millimeters to a few centimeters. Each lesion goes through three pathological stages. The early acute stage (active plaque) is of active myelin breakdown. The plaques appear pink and edematous. The subacute stage is characterized by pale colored plaques with abundant macrophages. The chronic stage (inactive plaque) is characterized by gliosis with associated volume loss and plaque becoming grey in color.[18]

Diagnosis of Multiple Sclerosis

Multiple Sclerosis is primarily diagnosed clinically. The criteria for establishing the diagnosis are based on three main principles:

1. Demonstration of demyelinating lesions disseminated in space (DIS)
2. Demonstration of demyelinating lesions disseminated in time (DIT)
3. Exclusion of alternative explanation for the clinical presentation.

The various investigations required apart from clinical history and lack of viable alternative diagnosis, are the presence of oligoclonal bands in CSF, immunoglobulin (IgG) in serum, abnormal visual evoked potentials and MR imaging.[19,20]

MR imaging is the most important paraclinical tool in diagnosing and monitoring MS.[21,22] It was formally included in the clinical workup of patients suspected to have MS in 2001. Acquisition protocols vary widely. A simple protocol recommended is given in **Table 1**.

MR Imaging of Multiple Sclerosis

Distribution and Characteristics of Lesion in the Brain and Spine

The characteristic lesion demonstrated on MRI is the cerebral or spinal plaque and is seen as a T2 hyper intense lesion **(Figs. 1A and B)**. The plaque consists of a discrete region of demyelination with relative preservation of axons. Active demyelination presents as areas of moderate T1 prolongation with mildly indistinct margins due to associated edema. Older plaques are smaller, more sharply defined and lower in signal intensity on T1W1.[23]

Multiple sclerosis plaques have a propensity to affect specific regions of the brain-periventricular white matter, callososeptal interface along the inferior surface of the corpus callosum, cortico-juxtacortical regions and the infratentorial regions. MS plaques are usually round to ovoid in shape, few millimeters to more than a centimeter in diameter **(Figs. 2A and B)**.

Periventricular lesions are oriented perpendicular to the outer surface of the lateral ventricle surrounding the medullary veins that radiate centripetally away from the lateral ventricle. These are the **Dawson's fingers.** These abut the ependymal surface unlike the nonspecific white matter hyperintensities (WMHs) **(Figs. 3 and 4)**. Focal involvement of periventricular white matter in anterior temporal lobe is also typical for MS, rarely seen in other white matter disorders.[23] Small periventricular lesions are best appreciated using FLAIR sequence as it suppress the CSF and makes them more conspicuous **(Figs. 5A and B)**.

The **corpus callosum** is a region that is especially vulnerable to demyelination in MS, possibly due to its intimate neuroanatomic relationship to the lateral ventricular roofs and to small penetrating vessels. Presence

TABLE 1: Recommended sequences—MRI of multiple sclerosis.

Conventional MR sequences used in MS
• Fast spin echo T2W and PD weighted—axial Specially for posterior fossa • FLAIR—axial and sagittal Better visualization of periventricular lesion due to suppression of CSF • Non-contrast T1 Hypointensity of white matter-black hole-axonal loss in chronic plaque • Contrast T1 Enhancement indicates disruption of blood-brain barrier, indicates inflammation • Diffusion-restriction—acute plaque • Scans for comparison must be technically adequate and positioned using specific landmarks
MR findings in multiple sclerosis—brain
• Focal white matter lesion Hyperintense on T2 in following location **Periventricular**—ovoid lesion on axial, triangular on sagittal, often perpendicular to ventricular surface **Callososeptal interface** **Juxtacortical/cortical** **Infratentorial** • Enhancement and diffusion restriction in acute lesion • T1 hypointensity-Acute-excessive edema, chronic-black hole • Basal ganglia and thalamus-T2 hypointensity-iron deposition • Brain atrophy
MRI characteristics of spinal cord lesions typical of MS
• Unequivocal hyperintensity on T2-weighted sequences and visible in two planes (e.g. axial and sagittal) • Size at least 3 mm but less than two vertebral segments in length • Occupy only a part of the cord in cross-section • Focal (i.e. clearly delineated and circumscribed on T2-weighted sequences) • Little or no cord swelling

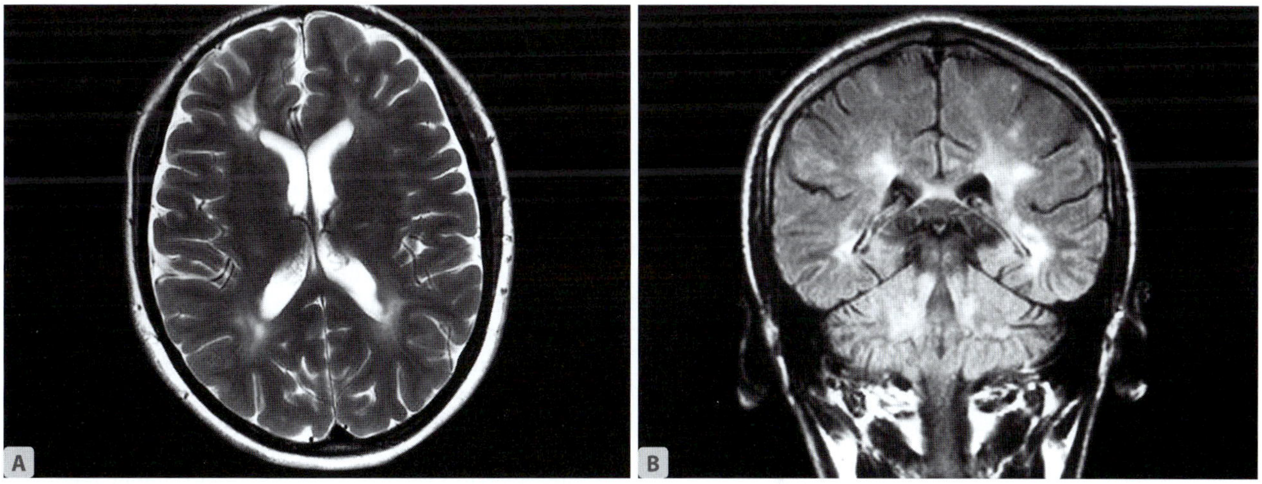

FIGS. 1A AND B: T2W-axial (A) Multiple periventricular hyperintensities seen in a case of multiple sclerosis. In another case, changes are seen in the periventicular location and brachium pontis on FLAIR coronal image (B).

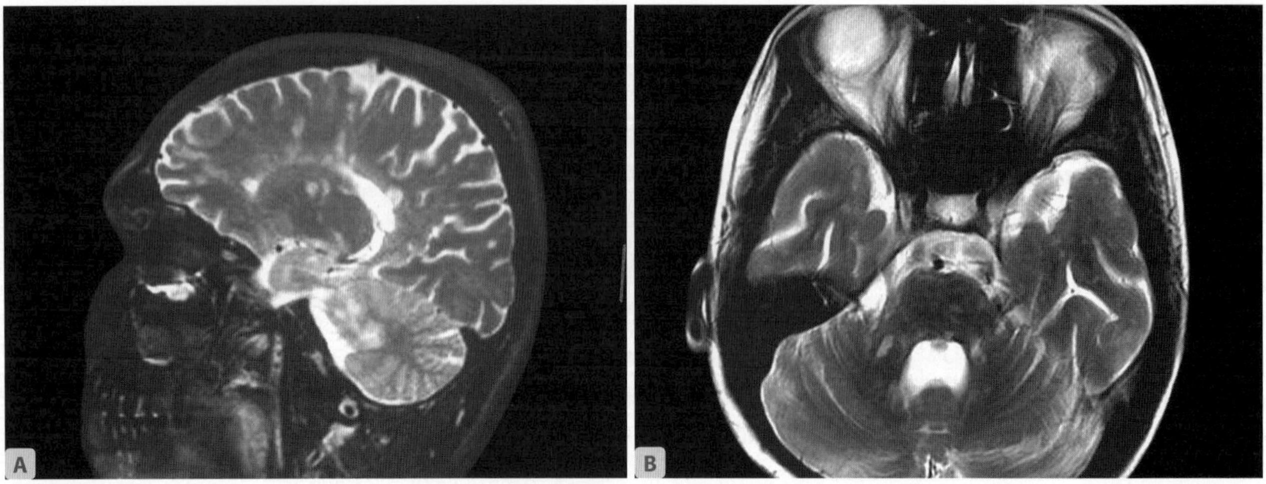

FIGS. 2A AND B: Hyperintense striations are seen in the corpus callosum, middle cerebeller peduncles. T2W sagittal (A), multiple plaques in the brainstem on T2W axial (B) image—a case of multiple sclerosis.

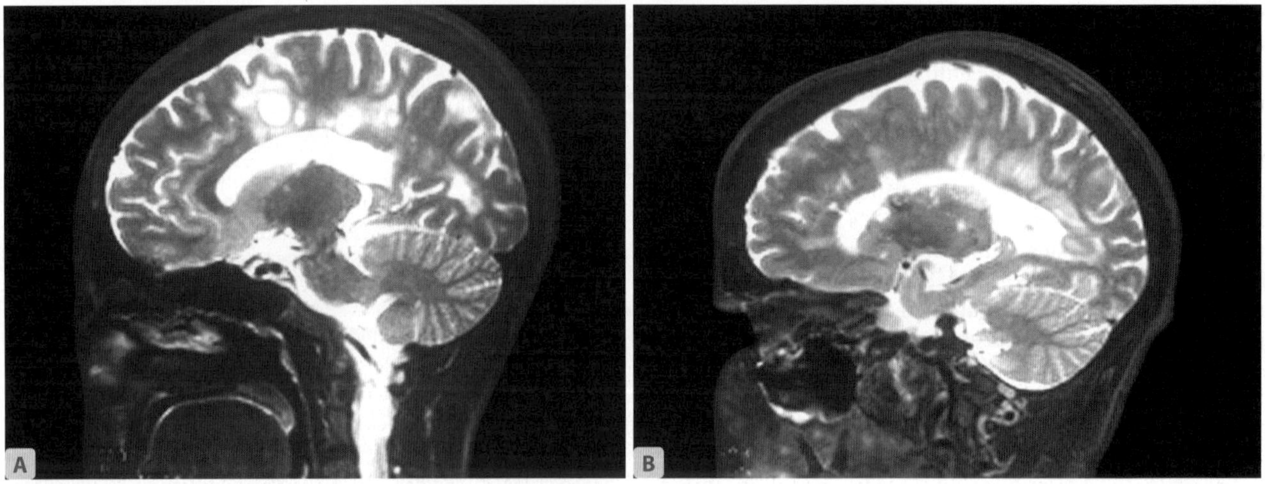

FIGS. 3A AND B: Sagittal T2W images show multiple plaques in the body and splenium of corpus callosum and callosal-septal interface with periventricular extension into centrum semiovale 'Dawson's fingers'.

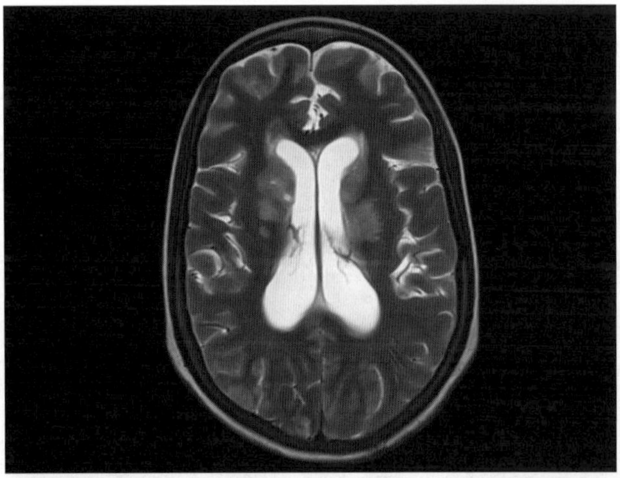

FIG. 4: T2W axial image-multiple hyperintense lesions in the periventricular location, extending almost at a right angle from and touching the ventricular surfaces.

of focal areas of high signal intensity on long TR images in the inferior aspect of the corpus callosum at the junction of the corpus callosum and the septum pellucidum (callosal-septal interface) **(Fig. 6)** is highly sensitive and specific for MS. This area is spared in white matter disease of ischemic origin due to rich collateral supply. In early disease these are focal and discrete and produce the 'dot and dash appearance', best seen on sagittal T2-weighted images **(Fig. 7)**.[24, 25] On T1-weighted images callososeptal interface may have multiple small hypointense lesions (Venus necklace) or the corpus callosum may merely appear thinned.

Juxtacortical lesions involve the subcortical 'U fibers' seen in a majority of patients with MS. These are best appreciated on FLAIR sequences **(Figs. 8A and B)**. Cortical lesions are now recognized in early MS and may precede appearance of classic plaque. These are associated with cognitive impairment and can only be appreciated on 3D double inversion recovery sequence and higher magnetic fields.[26-28]

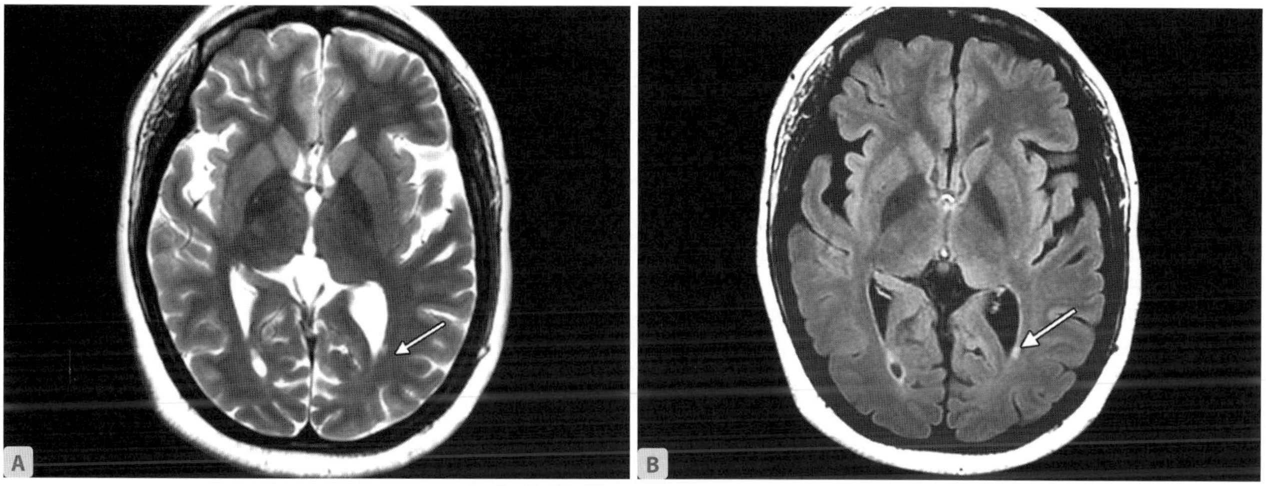

FIGS. 5A AND B: A small hyperintense focus touching the ventricular surface on T2W axial (A), better delineated on the FLAIR axial image (B).

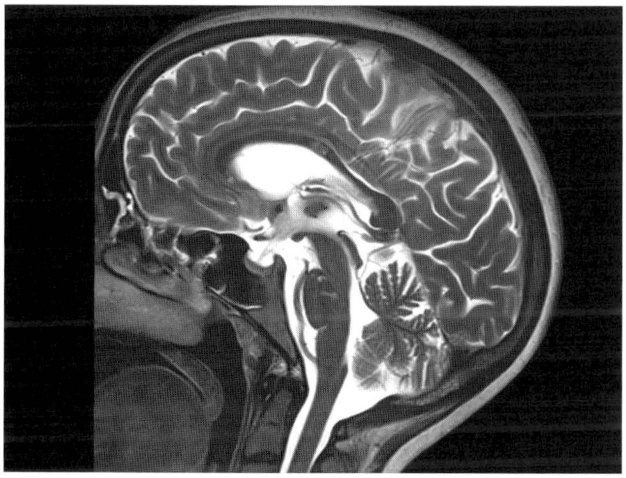

FIG. 6: T2 sagittal FLAIR image shows small plaques in the corpus callosum at the callososeptal interface, periventricular region and in the pons.

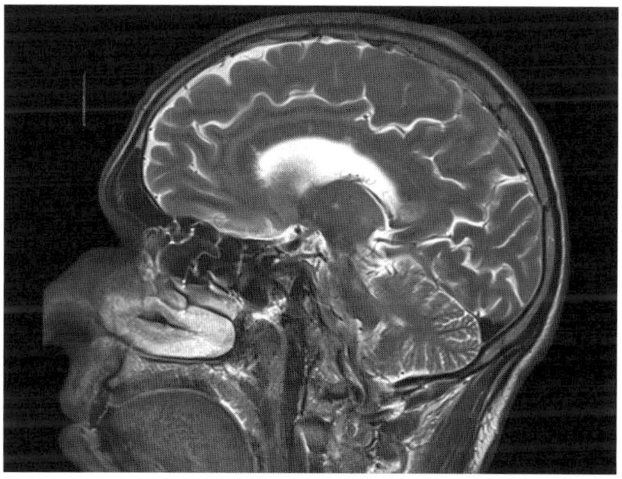

FIG. 7: 'Dot and dash'-small focal and discrete lesions in the corpus callosum in a patient of MS.

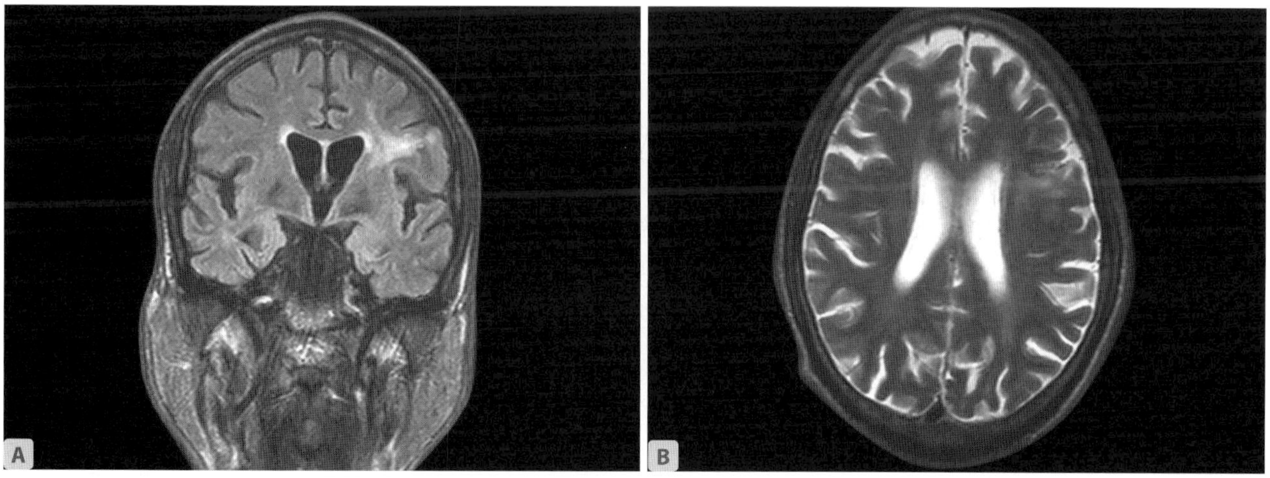

FIGS. 8A AND B: Juxtacortical lesion in a case of MS better appreciated on FLAIR image (A), than the T2W image (B).

In the **infratentorial compartment**, lesions involve the floor of the fourth ventricle, middle cerebellar peduncle and the brainstem **(Fig. 9)**. Contiguous with cisternal or ventricular spaces, these may be seen as patchy, confluent to solitary well defined paramedian lesions or just as a discrete line along the ependymal surface. This peripheral location helps to differentiate them from focal areas of ischemia and infarction where the central white matter tracts are involved. PD/T2 FSE sequences are recommended over SE/FLAIR to image the posterior fossa in patients with MS.

Spinal cord lesions are reported in a high percentage (30–40%) of cases with clinically isolated syndromes and in up to 90% of patients in definite MS.[29] The cervical cord is mostly affected; the lesions are less than 1 or 2 vertebral segments in cranio-caudal dimension, are well defined and occupy less than 50% of cross-sectional area of the cord in axial plane **(Figs. 10A and B)**. The lesion involves the peripheral white matter, the lateral and posterior white matter columns. An acute spinal cord plaque may produce mild-to-moderate mass effect and some cord swelling, though extensive swelling of the cord is uncommon. Active lesions may enhance. The involvement of the spinal cord varies with lesions being multifocal in relapsing remitting MS. Extensive, diffuse abnormalities and cord atrophy are seen in secondary progressive subtype, while there may be more extensive involvement of cord as compared to brain in PPMS.[30,31]

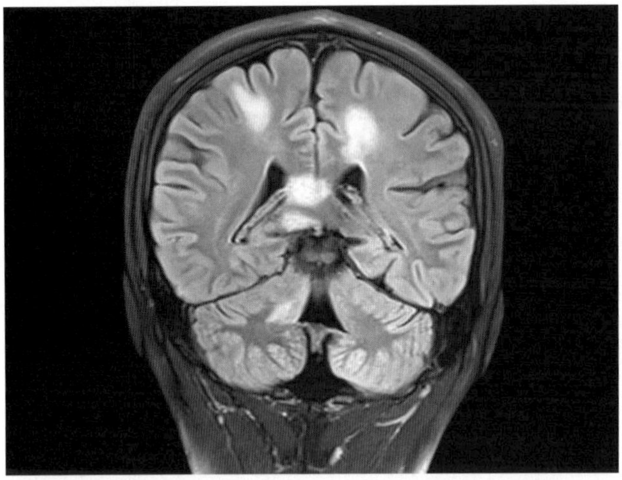

FIG. 9: In a patient of multiple sclerosis multiple T2 hyperintense lesions are seen in corpus callosum, juxtacortical and infratentorial location. Lesion in the middle cerebral peduncle is touching the ventricular surface on coronal FLAIR image.

Optic neuritis may be the only presentation in the initial stage of MS. It is a clinical diagnosis and MR imaging is not required to make the diagnosis. In patients who present initially with optic neuritis, many clinicians believe that the role of MR is to exclude the rarely found alternative cause of the clinical symptomatology aside from optic neuritis and to detect the presence of intracerebral lesions that may indicate MS. Coronal fat saturated T2 images are sensitive to depict signal alteration in optic neuritis. Optic nerve may be thickened, hyperintense and may show intense contrast enhancement. In MS, the optic nerve may show signal abnormalities in the absence of acute attacks of optic neuritis. A positive brain MR at the time of optic neuritis may provide diagnostic criteria for possible MS, if negative, it suggests a low risk for MS.[32]

Atrophy of the brain and spinal cord are seen in patients with multiple sclerosis. This is more severe in progressive form of disease but may also occur early in the disease. Atrophy is an important predictor for development of physical disability. It involves both gray and white matter **(Figs. 11A and B)**. **Basal ganglia** hypointensity is seen in 10–20% of chronic cases and represents heavy metal deposition.

Contrast-enhanced imaging is routinely used to assess inflammatory activity. In the acute inflammatory phase, the lesion may disrupt blood-brain barrier, leading to gadolinium enhancement, which may last for a variable time. Disease activity seen as enhancement is detected more frequently than clinical evaluation of relapses, indicating that most enhancing lesions remain clinically silent. The **enhancement pattern** may be variable within and between patients **(Fig. 12)**.[33,34]

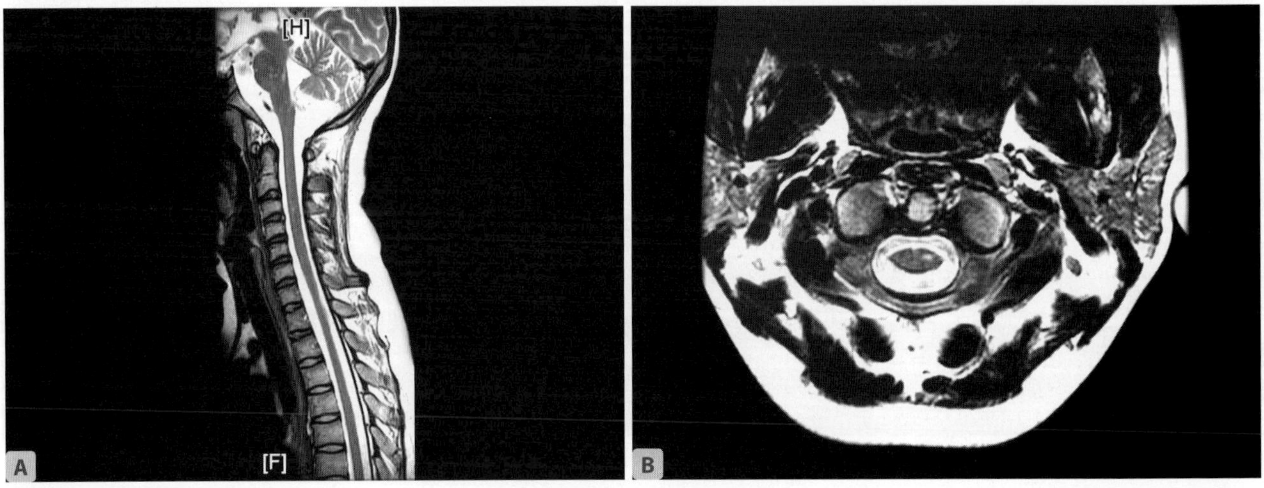

FIGS. 10A AND B: T2W sagittal (A) and axial (B) A tiny speck of hyperintensity is seen in the left lateral aspect of the spinal cord at C3 level. Note that the cord is of normal caliber-MS.

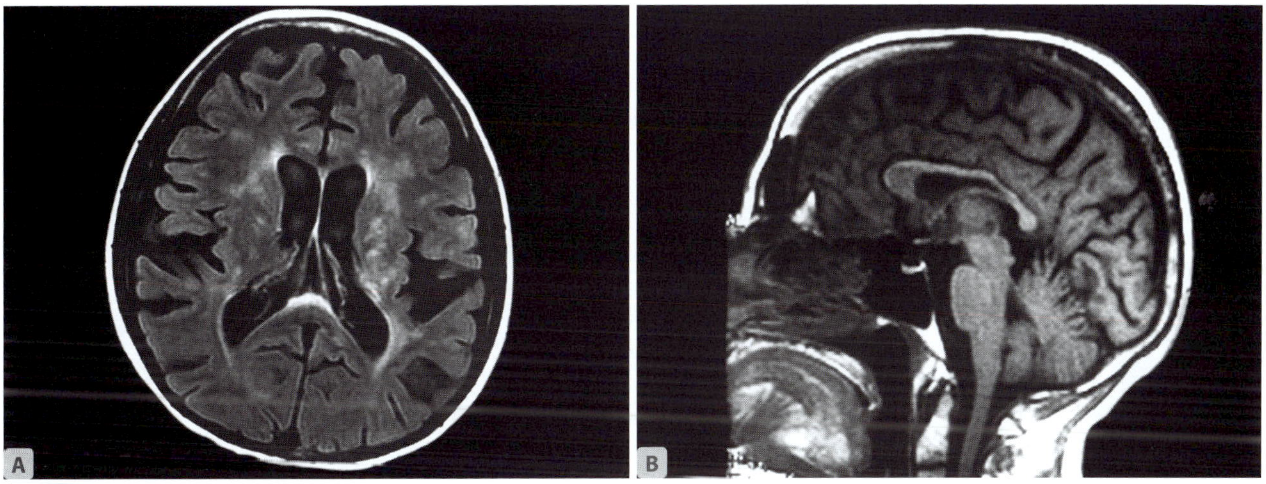

FIGS. 11A AND B: Diffuse cerebral atrophy along with plaques is noted in a case of MS on FLAIR axial image (A), atrophy of the corpus callosum Is noted in another case -T1 axial image (B).

This is suggestive of a heterogenous pathology related to host response. MS plaques may show transient enhancement in acute and relapsing stages of disease. This may be punctate, rim or nodular. Incomplete rim (horseshoe) pattern of enhancement with the open border facing the cortex or basal ganglia in acute stages is a pointer towards inflammatory demyelinating pathology, contrasting to a complete ring in abscess or tumors. Enhancement usually disappears within 6 months; earlier with steroid administration. Persistence of enhancement should be treated with caution as a point against the diagnosis of MS.

Contrast enhancement may be used to add specificity to the finding of multiple hyperintensities on T2-weighted images, because the finding of enhancing along with nonenhancing lesions is seen in MS. In relapsing remitting and secondary progressive MS, enhancement is seen during relapses and correlates with clinical activity. However in PPMS, enhancement does not match the clinical deterioration. High dose of gadolinium and a long post injection delay increase sensitivity in detecting enhancement, especially in the spinal cord.[35]

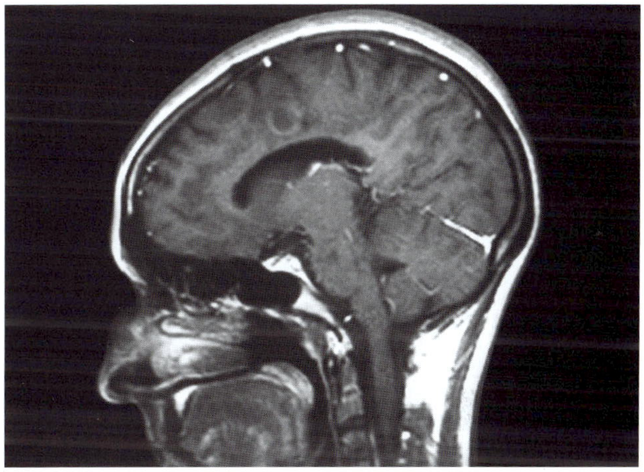

FIG. 12: Contrast-enhanced TIW MR image shows rim enhancement of a plaque, suggesting activity.

Acute or Chronic MS

Acute as well as chronic MS plaques appear hyperintense on PD and T2WI reflecting increased water content with edema, inflammation, demyelination, gliosis and axonal loss being the underlying pathology. Larger lesions may depict a very hyperintense center surrounded by less hyperintense periphery and variable amounts of perilesional edema. Acute MS lesions tend to be larger with fuzzy margins. As resolution occurs they become smaller and more sharply defined, reflecting reduction of edema and inflammation. T2 hyperintensity shrinks over a period of time leaving a smaller lesion which may remain unchanged over years. As the disease progresses the T2 lesion number and volume of T2 lesion increases and is called **T2 load**. This increases in absence of or due to poor response to treatment. The T2 burden is an important measure of abnormal tissue.[36–38]

Most of the MS plaques are hypo- or iso-intense on T1-weighted imaging. These are called '**black holes'** and in acute cases these black holes become iso-intense in a few months, whereas the persisting or chronic black holes correlate with severe demyelination and axonal destruction **(Figs. 13A and B)**.[39] These T1 black holes have relatively reduced MTR, elevated diffusion coefficient and reduced NAA, also indicative of more severe focal injury. Chronicity of T1 hypointense lesion is also based on lack of contrast enhancement **(Figs. 14A and B)**. A T1 hypointense lesion that shows contrast enhancement is an acute lesion, hypointensity being attributable to edema.

A faint peripheral rim of hyper-intensity may surround these T1 hypointensities giving a beveled appearance. T1 hypointensity is an independent predictor of atrophy, disability and disease progression.

Advanced MR techniques in multiple sclerosis: Subtle pathological changes have been described in normal appearing white matter (NAWM) and normal appearing gray matter (NAGM).[40] These represent a significant component of

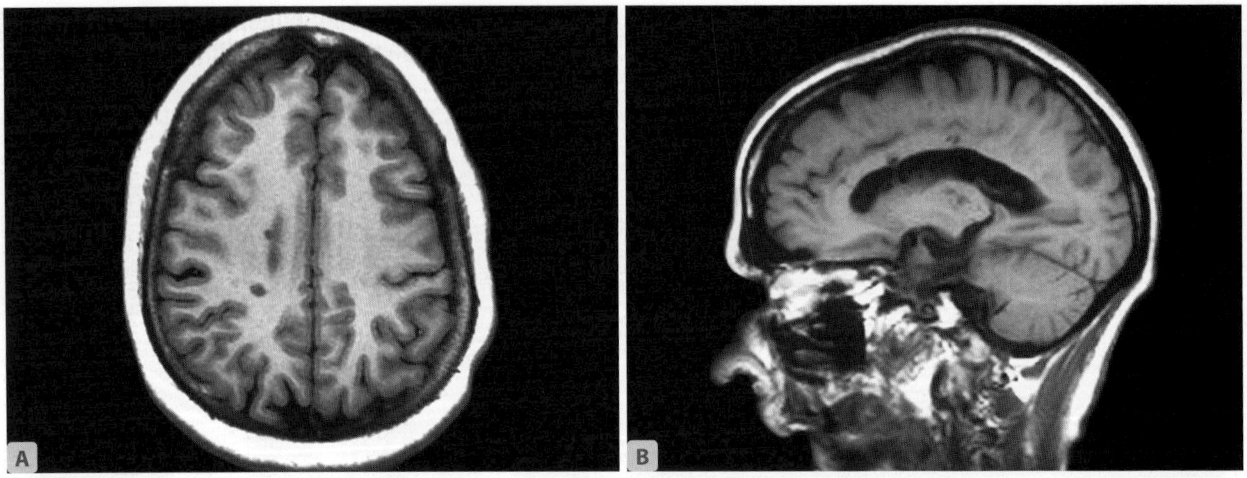

FIGS. 13A AND B: T1W axial image (A) and sagittal image (B) Hypointense well demarcated lesions in right periventricular region and corpus callosum- T1 'black hole'.

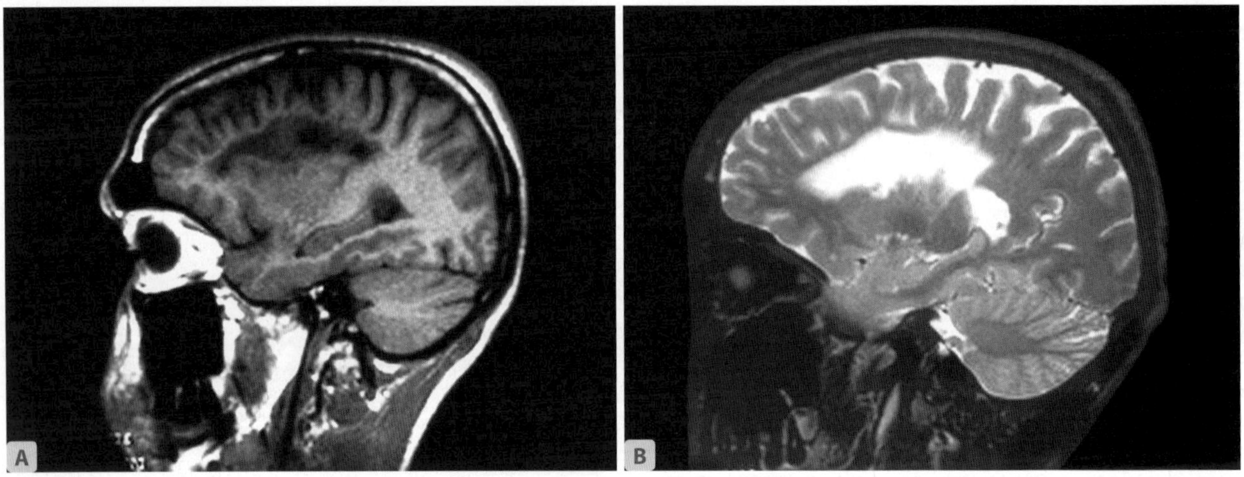

FIGS. 14A AND B: Sagittal T1W MR image (A) shows confluent areas of decreased signal intensity in the periventricular regions and along the callosal-septal interface. Sagittal T2W image (B) shows the same lesions to be hyperintense.

the disease burden and require advanced MR techniques for detection of the same.

Magnetization transfer imaging—is sensitive to the macromolecular environment of cell membrane and tissue. Decreased MTR (magnetization transfer ratio) is noted in NAWM in patients of MS in the absence of visible T2 lesions **(Figs. 15A to F)**. A decrease in MTR parallels enhancement of the lesion, a marker of inflammation. Post treatment these values increase.[41-44]

Diffusion tensor imaging—increased diffusivity is a nonspecific finding and is seen in focal MS lesions and in normal appearing brain tissue in contrast to reduced diffusivity characteristic for cerebral infarction. Acute plaques may be associated with restricted diffusion **(Figs. 16A to F)**. Decreased fractional anisotropy is seen in focal MS lesions. Various studies have correlated damage to a particular white matter tract on DTI with patient symptomatology.[44-51]

MR proton spectroscopy—an alteration in various metabolites has been shown on spectroscopy in both the demyelinating plaque and in NAWM and NAGM. NAA-N acetyl aspartate, a neuronal marker is reduced in focal lesions and in NAWM, the decrease being more pronounced in chronic disease **(Figs. 17A to C)**. Choline, a marker of cell turnover can be increased in acute plaque. Myoinositol and creatine are markers of gliosis and can be increased in acute white matter lesion. Glutamate, an excitatory neurotransmitter increases in focal white matter lesions and in NAWM.[44,52-55]

Functional MR Imaging—studies have shown cortical re-organization on fMRI in patients with MS that varies with stage of disease and correlates with specific symptoms. Brain plasticity has also been demonstrated, explaining the discordance seen between MR findings and patient symptomatology.[56,57]

MR perfusion imaging—Alterations in cerebral perfusion have been seen in patients of MS with increase in CBV in acute lesions, decreased perfusion reflecting microvascular change or injury is detected in NAWM, with increased perfusion preceding development of a new lesion.

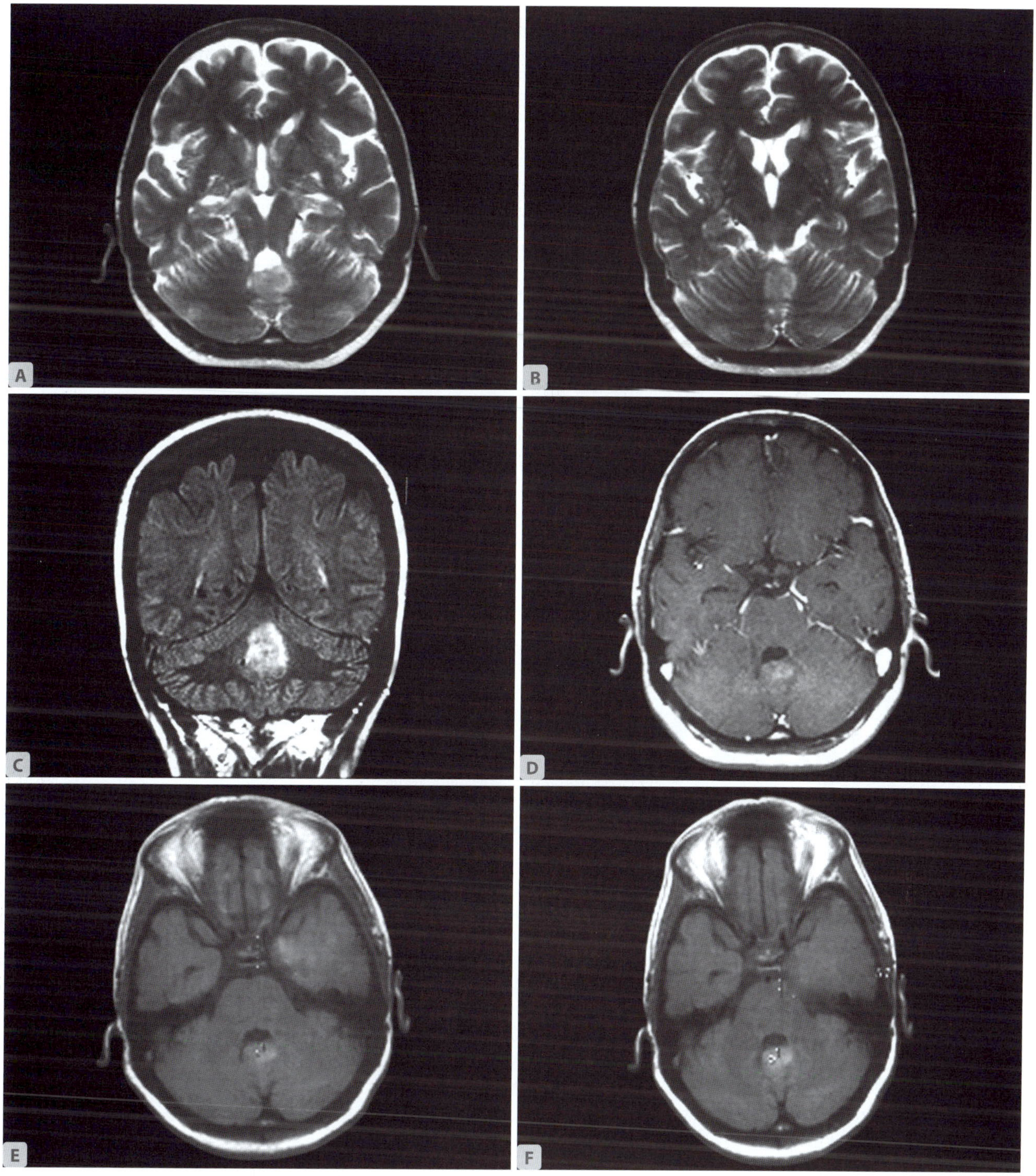

FIGS. 15A TO F: Axial T2WI (A and B) and coronal flair image (C): Poorly marginated hyperintense lesion seen in cerebellar vermis. Small hyperintense areas also seen in periventricular white matter around left frontal horn. The lesion in the vermis shows patchy inhomogenous enhancement (D). Axial T1W without MT (E) and with MT (F) MTR = 15%. Multiple sclerosis-acute plaque.

The reduction in relative CBF and CBV has been shown to correlate with cognitive impairment.[58]

Double inversion recovery (DIR): a new sequence that suppresses both CSF and white matter signal and offers better delineation of the plaques especially in the cortical gray matter.[44,52–55]

7T MRI—Ultra-high Field MR Imaging

One of the main advantages of high field imaging is the high signal intensity to noise ratio, the lesion detection improves, as does the potential to detect cortical lesions. The enhanced T2 effects are also beneficial for perfusion, diffusion and functional MR imaging. Increased detection of cortical

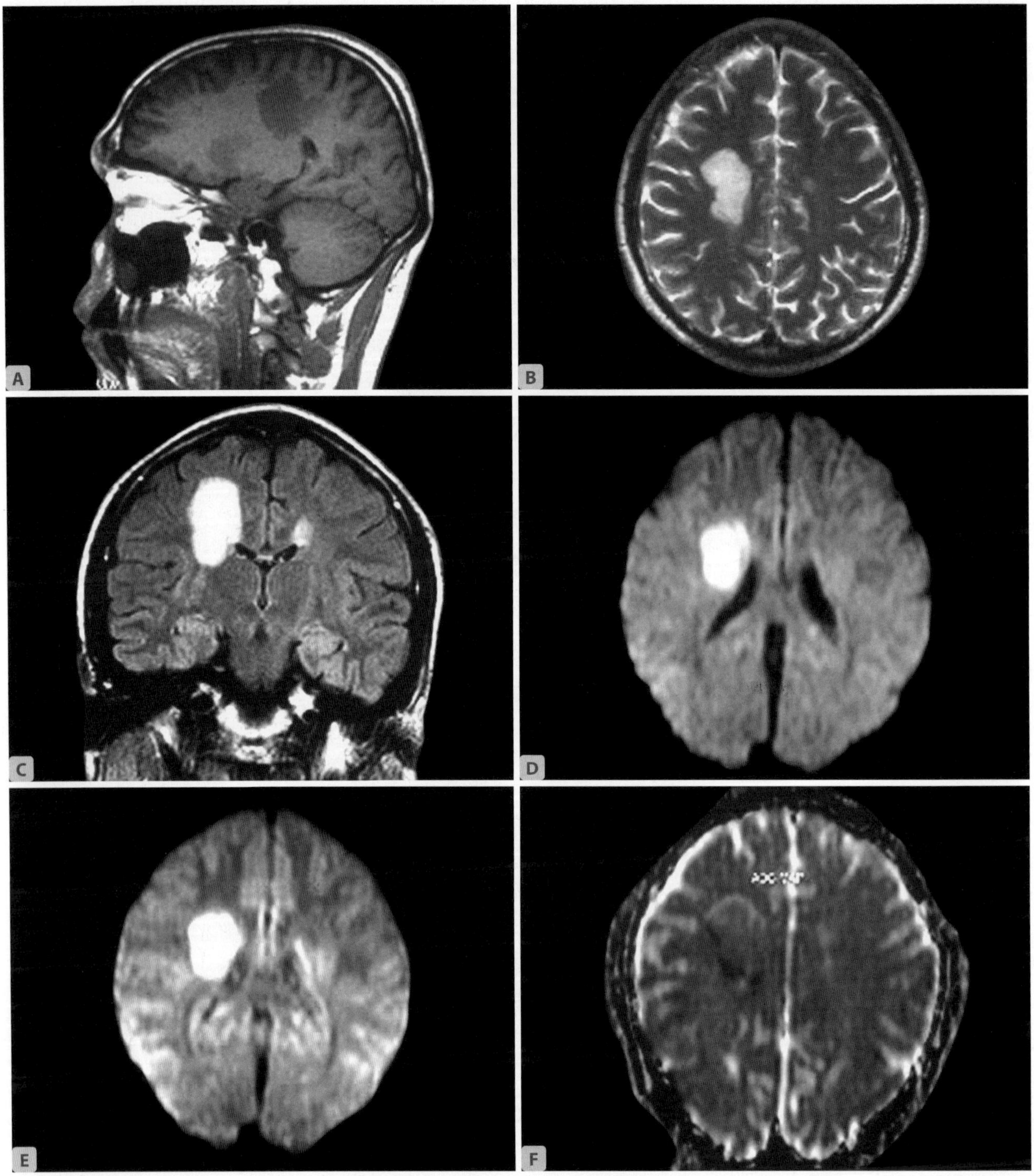

FIGS. 16A TO F: In a case of multiple sclerosis sagittal T1W image (A) shows a large well-defined hypointense lesion in the region of right centrum semiovale which is hyperintense on axial T2W (B). Another small hyperintense focus is also seen in left centrum semiovale region. Coronal FLAIR image (C) shows the lesions to be of high signal intensity. Diffusion-weighted image reveals the lesion to be hyperintense on 'b' = 500. (D) The lesions show increase in signal intensity on 'b' = 1000 DWI (E) ADC map (F) reveals restricted diffusion within the lesions.

abnormalities is seen with the use of ultra high field MR. The perivenular location of the MS plaque has been delineated with high sensitivity on 7T MRI using susceptibility weighted imaging (SWI), this is called the **central vein sign**.[21,44,28] Increased proportion of this finding in the brain may differentiate MS from other neurological diseases such as small vessel disease, migraine SLE etc.

Myelin water imaging: This technique utilizes multiple T2 echoes during a single acquisition. Based on different echo times (TE), it separates the more slowly relaxing intra/

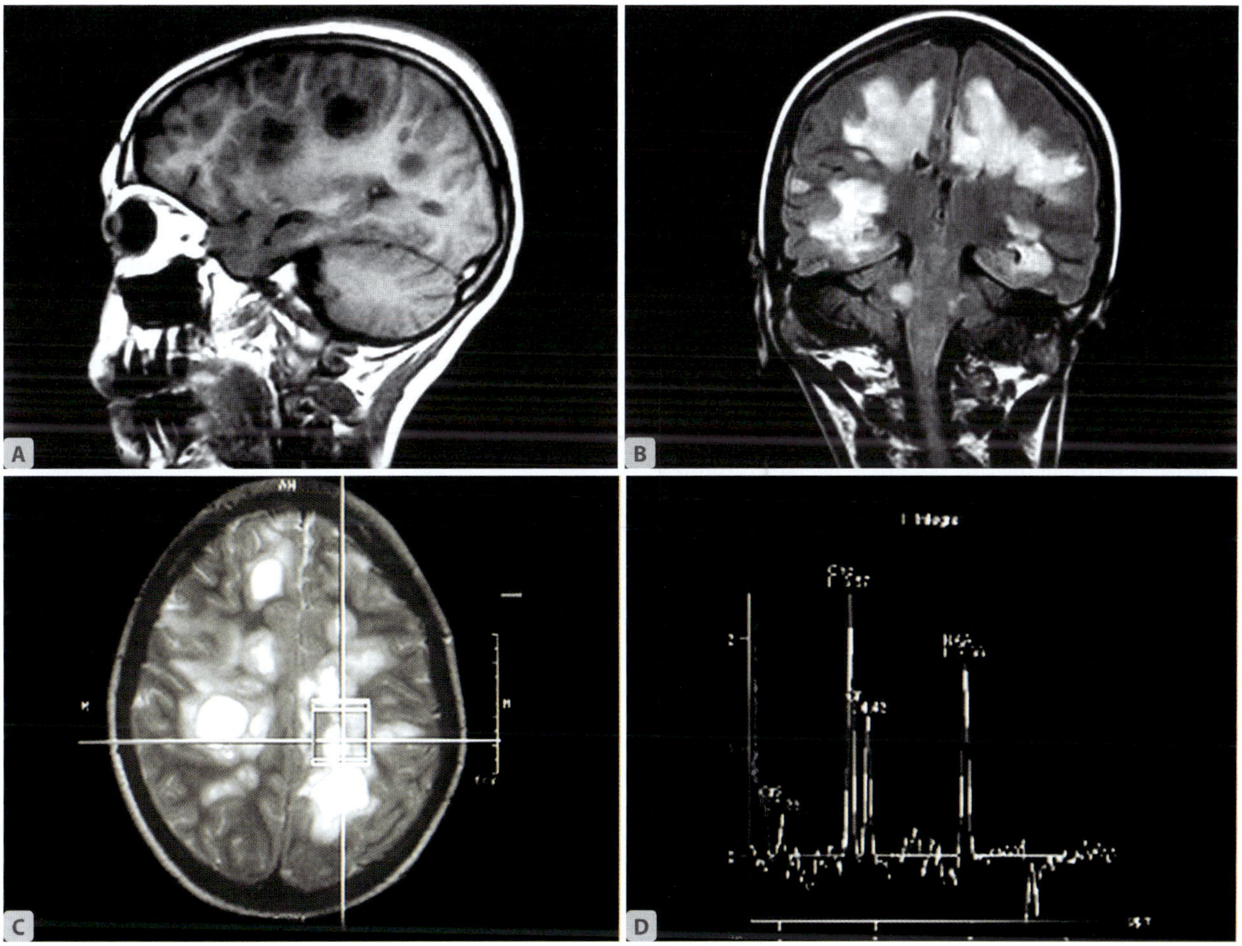

FIGS. 17A TO D: Sagittal T1W (A) shows multiple well-defined hypointense lesions in the deep as well as subcortical white matter in the frontoparieto-occipital regions. Lesions also shows typical 'beveled' or 'lesion within lesion' appearance. FLAIR coronal image (B) and T2 axial image (C) shows multiple hyperintense lesions which appear confluent in the fronto-parieto-occipital white matter. MR spectroscopy (D) reveals reduction of NAA level with marked elevation of choline level and reversal of Cho/Cr ratio. Doublet lactate peak is also noted.

extracellular water compartment from the more rapidly relaxing water trapped between myelin sheaths. The myelin water fraction (MWF) describes the ratio of the myelin water to total water, MWF has been found to be reduced in white matter of patients with MS and also in NAWM.[44,59]

Diagnostic Criteria for Diagnosis of MS

Several criteria have been developed to integrate MR imaging into clinical evaluation to achieve earlier and more accurate diagnosis.

McDonald diagnostic criteria for multiple sclerosis are clinical, radiographic, and laboratory criteria used in the diagnosis of multiple sclerosis. The criteria are named after **Ian McDonald** (1933–2006), a New Zealander neurologist, who devised the original criteria with his international colleagues in 2001. They were originally introduced in 2001,[60] and were revised in 2005,[61] 2010,[62] 2016 (by MAGNIMS[63]) and most recently in 2017.[64]

These criteria apply to individuals experiencing a typical clinically isolated syndrome—CIS. A MS attack (also called as relapse or exacerbation) is defined by McDonald criteria as a patient having reported or objectively observed event typical of an acute inflammatory demyelinating event in the CNS, with a duration of at least 24 hours, without fever or signs of infection. **The criteria are based on demonstration of dissemination in space (DIS), dissemination in time (DIT) and absence of any other viable alternative diagnoses.**

Dissemination in Space on MRI

Dissemination in space requires ≥1 T2-hyperintense lesions (≥3 mm in long axis), symptomatic and/or asymptomatic, that are characteristic of multiple sclerosis in two or more of the four following locations: periventricular (≥1 lesion, unless the patient is over the age of 50 in which case it is better to seek a higher number of lesions), cortical/juxtacortical, infratentorial, spinal cord **(Fig. 18)**.

T2-hyperintense lesions of the optic nerve, such as those in a patient presenting with optic neuritis, are not counted in the 2017 revised McDonald criteria.

Dissemination in Time

- A new T2-hyperintense or gadolinium-enhancing lesion when compared to a previous baseline MRI scan (irrespective of timing).

- Simultaneous presence of a gadolinium-enhancing lesion and a non-enhancing T2-hyperintense lesion on any one MRI scan **(Figs. 19A to C)**.

McDonald Criteria 2017: The following changes were made:

- In patients with a typical clinically isolated syndrome and clinical or MRI demonstration of dissemination in space, the presence of CSF-specific oligoclonal bands allows a diagnosis of multiple sclerosis.
- Symptomatic lesions can be used to demonstrate dissemination in space or time in patients with supratentorial, infratentorial, or spinal cord syndrome;
- Cortical lesions can be used to demonstrate dissemination in space.

The new criteria are expected to speed up the diagnosis of MS, thus enabling early initiation of therapy. In addition, chances of misdiagnosis of MS are expected to reduce. A summary of the criteria is given in the **Table 2**.

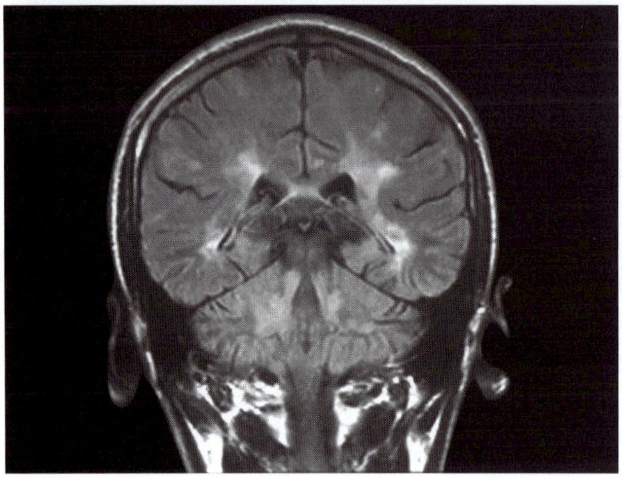

FIG. 18: Coronal FLAIR image depicts multiple hyperintense lesions (>1) in multiple locations-juxtacortical. periventricular and infratentorial-Dissemination in space in MS.

Primary Progressive Multiple Sclerosis

The McDonald criteria also defines the diagnosis of primary progressive multiple sclerosis (PPMS). The diagnosis requires:

- ≥1 year of disability progression which can be determined either prospectively or retrospectively with two of the following:
  - ≥1 T2-hyperintense lesions characteristic of multiple sclerosis in one or more of the following regions: periventricular, cortical or juxtacortical, or infratentorial.

Differential Diagnosis of MS Lesion on MR

The differential diagnosis of lesions with increased signal on T2-weighted images is large. These may be normal variants or truly not primary demyelinating processes, but may simulate MS on MR imaging.

1. **Normal anatomical structures** may potentially mimic MS lesions. Ependymitis granularis represent small areas of denuded ependyma within the lining of the lateral ventricles adjacent to anterolateral angles of the frontal horns with a small amount of CSF seepage adjacent to tips of frontal horns. This should not be confused with periventricular plaque **(Fig. 20)**.
2. **The Virchow Robin spaces** are invaginations of the subarachnoid space into the brain associated with leptomeningeal vessels. These spaces enlarge with age and hypertension as vessels within the space become more ectatic, termed "etat crible".[65] Dilated perivascular spaces occur in characteristic locations, typically in basal ganglia (inferior portion) around the atria, near the anterior commissure, in corona radiata, centrum semiovale and in peri insular region **(Fig. 21)**. They follow the intensity of cerebrospinal fluid. The FLAIR/PDWI sequences are most suited at discriminating perivascular spaces from white matter lesions because the perivascular spaces are isointense to CSF, whereas MS and other lesions are hyperintense.
3. **Ischemic white matter lesions/small vessel ischemic changes**: Incidental white matter hyperintensities are

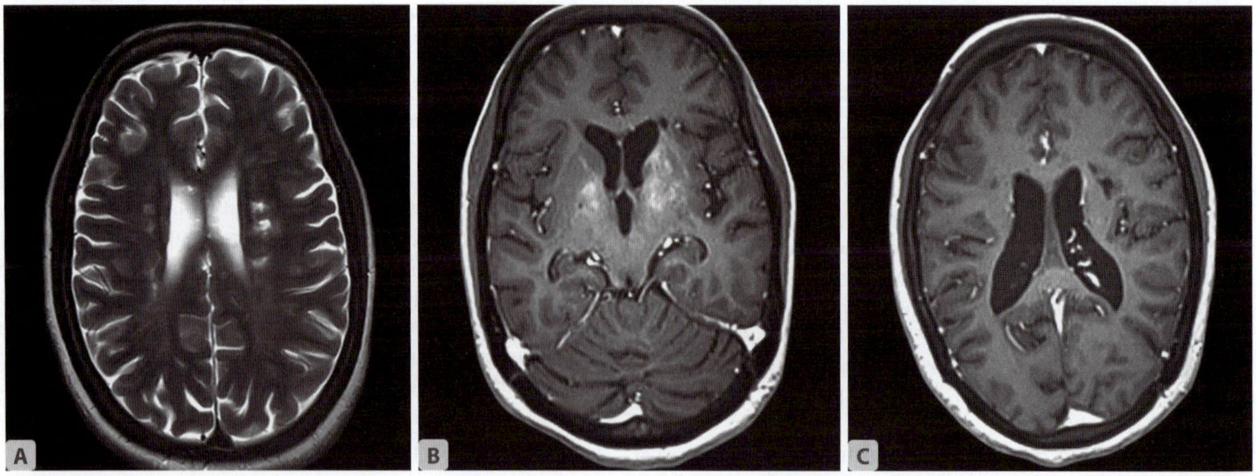

FIGS. 19A TO C: T2W axial image (A), Postcontrast T1WI images (B and C) show enhancing and nonenhancing foci in the same patient—dissemination in time in MS.

TABLE 2: McDonald criteria for the diagnosis of MS (2017).

• Requires elimination of more likely diagnoses • Requires demonstration of dissemination of lesions in the central nervous system in space and time	
Clinical presentation	**Additional criteria to make MS diagnosis**
...in a person who has experienced a typical attack/CIS at onset	
• 2 or more attacks and clinical evidence of 2 or more lesions; OR • 2 or more attacks and clinical evidence of 1 lesion with clear historical evidence of prior attack involving lesion in different location	None. DIS and DIT have been met.
• 2 or more attacks and clinical evidence of 1 lesion	DIS shown by *one* of these criteria: • Additional clinical attack implicating different CNS site • 1 or more MS-typical T2 lesions in 2 or more areas of CNS: periventricular, cortical, juxtacortical, infratentorial or spinal cord
• 1 attack and clinical evidence of 2 or more lesions	DIT shown by *one* of these criteria: • Additional clinical attack • Simultaneous presence of both enhancing and non-enhancing MS-typical MRI lesion, or new T2 or enhancing MRI lesion compared to baseline scan (without regard to timing of baseline scan) • CSF oligoclonal bands
• 1 attack and clinical evidence of 1 lesion	DIS shown by *one* of these criteria: • Additional attack implicating different CNS site • 1 or more MS-typical T2 lesions in 2 or more areas of CNS: periventricular, cortical, juxtacortical, infratentorial or spinal cord AND DIT shown by *one* of these criteria: • Additional clinical attack • Simultaneous presence of both enhancing and non-enhancing MS-typical MRI lesions, or new T2 or enhancing MRI lesion compared to baseline scan (without regard to timing of baseline scan) • CSF oligoclonal bands
...in a person who has steady progression of disease since onset	
1 year of disease progression (retrospective or prospective)	DIS shown by at least *two* of these criteria: • 1 or more MS-typical T2 lesions (periventricular, cortical, juxtacortical or infratentorial) • 2 or more T2 spinal cord lesions • CSF oligoclonal bands

(DT: dissemination in time; CNS: central nervous system; CSF: cerebrospinal fluid; DIS: dissemination in space; T2 lesion: hyperintense lesion on T2-weighted MRI)

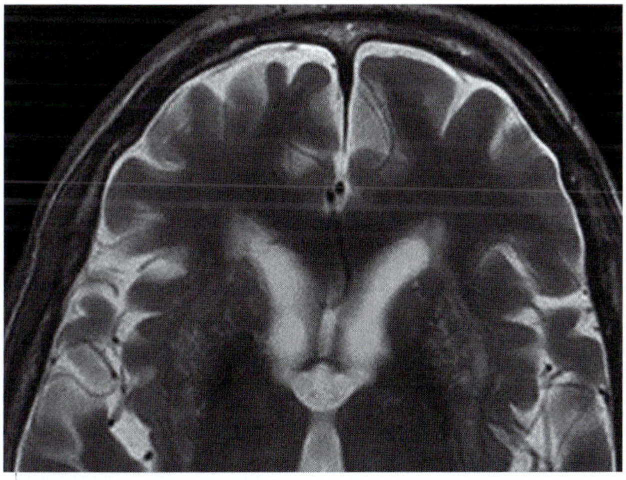

FIG. 20: T2W axial image–Ependymitis granularis at the tips of frontal horns.

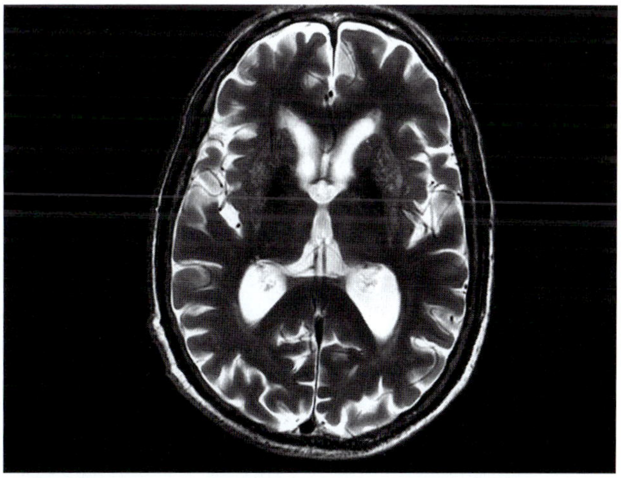

FIG. 21: Virchow-Robin spaces appreciated as multiple pinpoint hyperintense foci in the basal ganglia region on T2W axial image.

seen commonly in the elderly. The prevalence ranges from 11–21% in adults aged around 64 years to 94% at 82 years of age.[66] Foci of hyperintense signal on T2-weighted images, frequently found in subcortical or periventricular white matter in elderly are smoother than the smaller, lobulated ovoid MS lesions **(Figs. 22A to C)**. Corpus callosum and spinal cord involvement is not seen in ischemic changes. MR detects all these changes, but all are not clinically significant. Most lesions are age related, but careful analysis of diffusion images is required to detect acute ischemia.

4. **Vasculitis:** MS lesions can mimic lesions from vasculitides such as SLE.
   MS may involve gray matter in 5–10%. MR is unable to definitively distinguish between these etiologies, although the presence of cortical lesions is suggestive of vasculitis. Therefore, the clinical history, the presence of systemic symptoms, results of laboratory studies and a positive angiogram, all help to differentiate these entities.
5. **Migraine**: Signal abnormalities may be seen in the centrum semiovale, frontal subcortical matter which can extend into deeper white matter at the level of basal ganglia.[67]
6. **ADEM**: This acute demyelinating disease that occurs after a viral infection or a recent immunization bears many similarities to MS in initial clinical presentation, pathological findings and MR appearance. ADEM is a monophasic illness unlike MS. The differences are tabulated in **Table 3**.
7. **Trauma**: Traumatic shear injuries that result from torsional stresses on white matter fiber tracts that occur at the time of high speed acceleration/deceleration brain injury may produce signal abnormalities at gray white matter junction, brainstem and corpus callosum-locations similar to MS. The clinical history of closed head injury plus the presence of associated punctuate hemorrhages clinch the diagnosis.

Treatment of multiple sclerosis: The aim of treatment is twofold: to curtail progression (disease-modifying agents) and to provide symptomatic relief. Immunosuppressant and immunomodulatory drugs are used, and studies have shown a significant decrease in relapse rate and reduction of brain lesion accumulation when therapy is started early.[68-71] Steroids, interferon, monoclonal antibodies and stem cell therapy are all used in the treatment.

There are certain complications, related to treatment.

Progressive multifocal leukoencephalopathy (PML) is seen in patients treated with natalizumab with positive JC virus serology. PML-IRIS, a complication of cessation of natalizumab or treatment for natalizumab-related PML are treated with plasma exchange or immunoabsorption.

Idiopathic Inflammatory Demyelinating Disorders (IIDDs)[72]

They represent a spectrum of CNS disorders that can be differentiated on the basis of severity, clinical course, lesion distribution as well as imaging, laboratory and pathological findings. The spectrum of IIDDs includes monophasic, multiphasic and progressive disorders. The lesions can be localized or multifocal/diffuse variants.

Differential diagnosis—multiple sclerosis
Multifocal T2/FLAIR hyperintensities
• Normal variants-ependymitis granularis, Virchow Robin spaces
• ADEM
• Lyme disease
• Vasculitis- and age related ischemic changes
• Susac syndrome
• CNS manifestations of antiphospholipid syndrome
• Marchiafava Bignami disease (corpus callosum lesion)
Solitary 'tumefactive' MS
• Neoplasm (GBM, metastasis)
• PML/PML-IRIS in natalizumab treated MS
Spinal lesions
• Transverse myelitis
• Spinal tumor

MS is considered the most representative of IIDDs, with others considered as variants or a borderline form of MS.

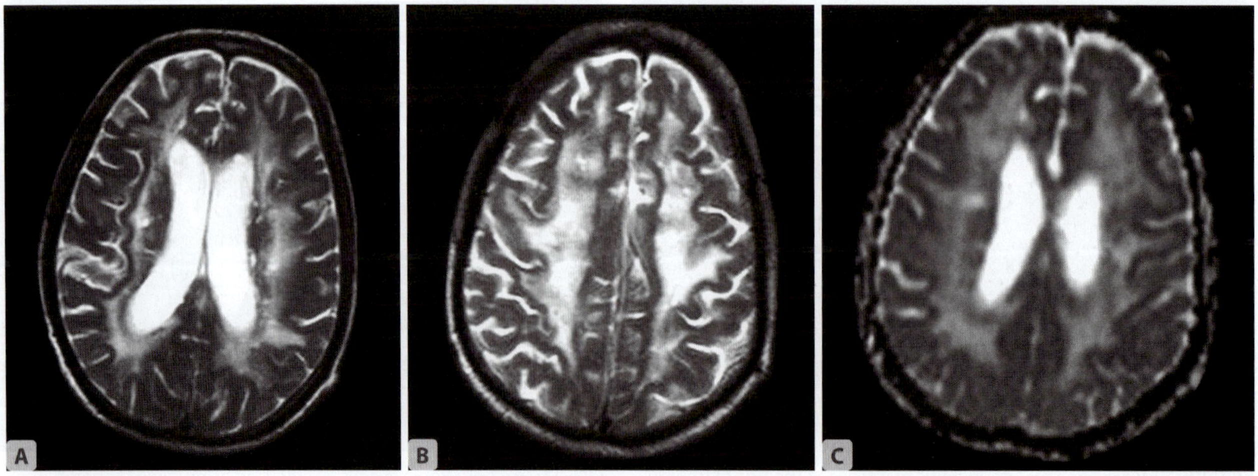

FIGS. 22A TO C: Extensive confluent periventricular and deep white matter hyperintensities on T2WI (A and B) which show facilitated diffusion on ADC map (C) Ischemic changes in an elderly hypertensive patient.

TABLE 3: Differences between multiple sclerosis and ADEM.

Feature	MS	ADEM
Age	>10 years	<10 years
Sex	Female preponderance	No sex predominance
Preceding illness	Usually no	Yes
Encephalopathy	No	Yes
Optic neuritis	Unilateral and common	Bilateral rare
Spinal cord involvement	Partial	Extensive with cord swelling
MRI	Periventricular, callosal	Cortical, deep gray matter Thalamic
T1 black hole	Seen	Not seen
Lesion of different ages	Seen	Not seen
T2 hyperintense lesions	Well circumscribed	Fuzzy margins
Size of lesion-large	Rare	Common
CSF	Oligoclonal bands	Lymphocytosis and increased proteins
Follow-up	New lesions	Monophasic

These are classified on clinical presentation, neuroimaging and CSF abnormalities.

1. *Fulminant/acute IIDDs*: Marburg, Schilder, Balo's concentric sclerosis considered as MS variants.
2. *Monosymptomatic IIDDs*: Isolated optic neuritis
3. *IIDDs restricted to a particular geographic distribution*: Neuromyelitis optica and isolated transverse myelitis

Marburg disease is an acute fulminant disorder with a monophasic rapid progressive course seen in young adults. Mortality is early within weeks or months due to brainstem involvement. It is often preceded by febrile illness and hence is also considered a fulminant form of ADEM. Imaging shows multifocal disseminated involvement with large T2 lesions, which may coalesce and show large cavitating lesions with incomplete ring enhancement.[72]

Schilder disease—myelinoclastic diffuse sclerosis: It is a rare disorder seen in children and young adults. It presents as aphasia and with psychiatric symptoms. There is no prior history of fever or vaccination. MR shows large ring enhancing lesions in both hemispheres, sometimes symmetric and located preferentially in parieto-occipital regions.[72] The lesion rim may show restricted diffusion. Dramatic response, both clinically and on imaging may be noted on administration of steroids. The differential diagnosis includes tumefactive MS, pyogenic abscess, metastasis and glioblastoma.

Balo's concentric sclerosis is a rare aggressive variant of MS seen usually in young adult males. Disease may show a rapid downhill progression or remain relatively benign. The pathological hallmark is concentric ring of myelin destruction and repair in centrum semiovale and corona radiate, resembling an onion ring. MR imaging reflects the same as alternating bands of differing signal intensities (hyper-iso-hypointense) on T2 images. The outer rim or advancing edge of demyelination shows restricted diffusion and may enhance on contrast administration. The center of the lesion may not show layering due to massive demyelination.[72]

Tumefactive or Pseudotumoral IIDDs[73-79]: Tumefactive demyelinating lesion is an acute tumor-like demyelination in which patients present with large (>2 cm) lesions, usually solitary but may be multiple. The solitary lesion is sometimes referred to as **monofocal acute inflammatory demyelination (MAID)**.

The clinical abnormalities in such patients are variable; Focal neurological deficits, seizures may be seen or the symptoms may be very slight even in a patient with a massive lesion. In some instances, there may be a rapid downhill course.

Tumefactive demyelination is most frequently encountered in women, usually young middle age (average onset at 37 years of age). It is not post infective, unlike ADEM. Patients who present with solitary tumefactive demyelinating lesion (TDL) develop MS infrequently though patients with multiple sclerosis can develop similar large tumefactive plaques.

Imaging

MRI: Large demyelinating (T2/FLAIR hyperintense) lesion with relatively less mass effect and edema is seen centered on the white matter and may involve subcortical U fibers. Various patterns have been described-diffusely infiltrative, mega cystic or large 'Balo' like lesion. Half of the TDLs show enhancement, usually in the form of an open ring and the incomplete part of the ring faces the gray matter side of the lesion Low relative cerebral blood volume (CBV) is found in TDLs compared to high grade gliomas. Diffusion imaging shows increase in ADC values similar to necrotic neoplasms. Proton spectroscopy shows an increase in choline and lactate.

Differential Diagnosis

The main imaging differential is a glioma: Clinical and radiological features to differentiate tumor from tumefactive demyelinating lesion are nonspecific. An incomplete ring of enhancement, relative lack of mass effect, and perilesional edema with a lower CBV on perfusion imaging may point towards demyelinating pathology. Biopsy is often required to differentiate the two.

Neuromyelitis Optica (Devic Disease)[80-91]

Neuromyelitis optica (NMO), also known as **Devic disease** and, more recently, **NMO spectrum disorder**, is a severe demyelinating disease of idiopathic nature, possibly of autoimmune etiology. It is caused by autoantibody to the aquaporin-4 water channel. These are found in astrocytes and are related to conduction of water through cell membrane. The antibodies target the region where blood-brain barrier is weakest—the spinal cord and optic nerve. Devic disease was initially considered a variant of MS but is now recognized as a distinct disease.

Epidemiology

Neuromyelitis optica is found in patients somewhat older than those with MS, with an average age of presentation being

41 years, although it can be seen in children and elderly. There is an even stronger female predilection (F:M 6.5:1) than MS. NMO is seen in Asian, Indian and African population.

Clinical Presentation

NMO presents as blindness or paraplegia due to optic neuritis and myelitis which may occur synchronously or metachronously. Optic neuritis is usually bilateral, that some patients present with unilateral optic nerve involvement. It follows a relapsing course though occasionally it may be a monophasic illness.

There is a specific biomarker of the disease, NMO-Immunoglobulin G, which has 90% specificity and 70–90% sensitivity. NMO-IgG is negative in almost all cases of MS and other autoimmune disease.

Criteria have been proposed to diagnose NMO **(Table 4)**. The NMO spectrum includes recurrent longitudinal extensive myelitis, bilateral simultaneous or recurrent optic neuritis. Asian optic-spinal MS, optic neuritis or myelitis associated with lesions in areas like hypothalamus, brainstem and myelitis/optic neuritis associated with systemic autoimmune disease.

Imaging

- **Myelitis**: Cervical spinal cord is usually affected. Involvement of three or more contiguous vertebral segments is seen and is called as longitudinally extensive spinal cord lesion. This pattern differs from MS, with involvement being more extensive in NMO. Central part of cord is involved unlike the peripheral part of the cord in MS **(Figs. 23A and B)**. A heterogeneous appearance of the cord on axial T2 images, described as "bright spotty "lesions may help to differentiate NMO from MS. The lesion appears hypointense on T1WI.Patchy cloud-like enhancement is seen along with thin ependymal enhancement. On sagittal images, lens like enhancement may be seen.
- **Optic neuritis:** Optic nerves appear hyperintense and swollen on T2-weighted sequences and show enhancement. Bilateral optic nerve involvement and extension of the abnormal signal posteriorly as far as the chiasm is particularly suggestive of NMO **(Fig. 24)**. In the chronic stage, there is atrophy of optic nerve.
- **Brain** was initially thought to have no abnormality in NMO but it has been shown that asymptomatic abnormalities may be present in a majority of patients. The lesions are present in areas with high concentration of aquaporin 4-the periependymal region abutting the ventricles, periaqueductal gray matter, hypothalamus and medial thalamus, dorsal pons and medulla. Corpus callosum may also be affected with preferential involvement of splenium; with lesions being larger, edematous and heterogeneous compared to MS. Multiple lesions with heterogeneous signal seen in corpus callosum leads to a marbled appearance. Punctuate lesions resembling MS may be present. Involvement of corticospinal tracts has been seen in a subset of patients. Large hemispheric white matter lesions that respond to steroids are seen in children and in patients from the Far East and Africa. NMO does not involve the cerebral cortex.

TABLE 4: NMO diagnostic criteria.
Essential/required
• Optic neuritis
• Acute myelitis
Plus two or more supportive criteria
• Disease onset MR imaging non-diagnostic for MS
• Contiguous spinal cord lesions on MR ≥3 vertebral segments
• NMO-IgG seropositivity

Differential Diagnosis

The differential diagnosis depends upon the clinical presentation, and in classic cases, the diagnosis can be made with a degree of confidence.

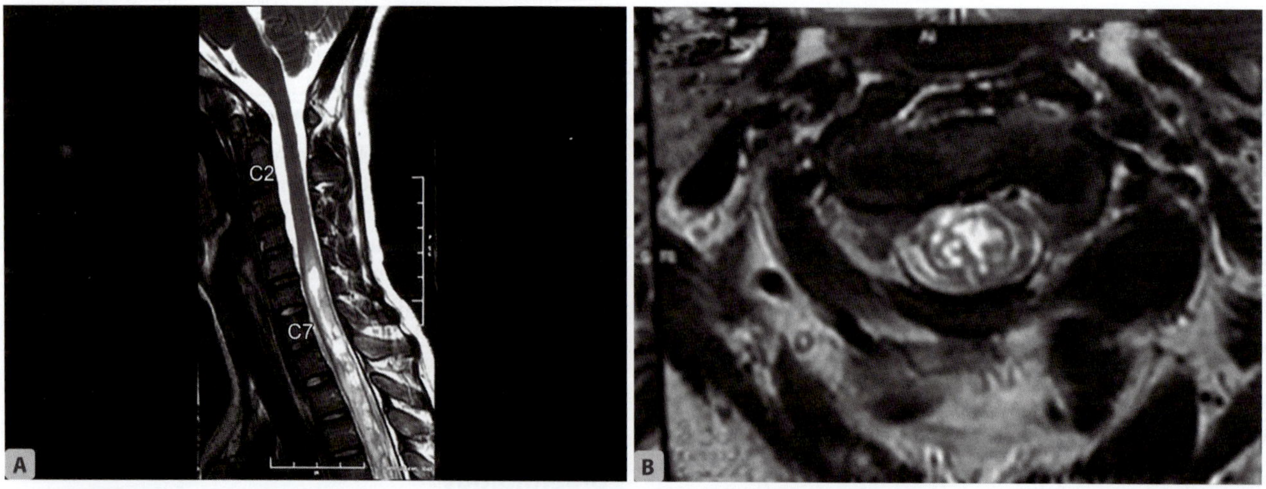

FIGS. 23A AND B: (A) T2W sagittal image of cervicodorsal spine-long segment hypertintensity seen in cervicodorsal cord in a case of neuromyelitis optica. (B) T2W axial image of the spinal cord shows heterogenous hyperintense signal with involvement of entire cross-section of cord in a case of NMO.

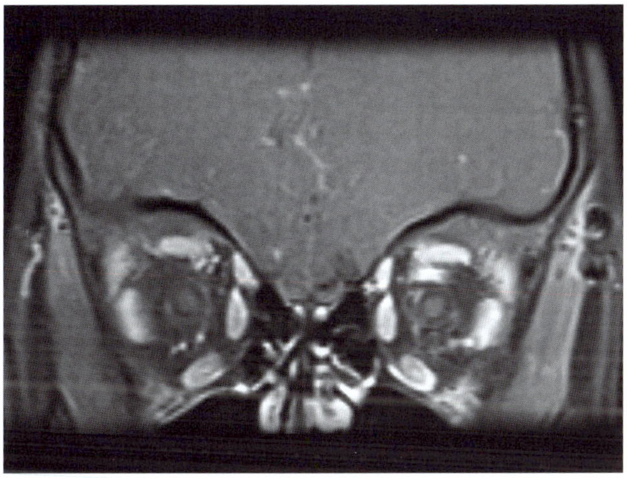

FIG. 24: T1W Post-contrast coronal image with fat saturation shows thickened and enhancing optic nerves on both sides (NMO).

1. For patients with spinal cord involvement, the differential is that of a longitudinally extensive spinal cord lesion which includes idiopathic transverse myelitis.
2. Involvement of the cerebral white matter and corpus callosum has a broad differential depending on the pattern, but the most important differential is Multiple sclerosis. It is important to distinguish NMO from MS as the treatment not only is different but treating a patient with NMO with MS-specific therapies (e.g. beta-interferon or natalizumab) can actually lead to its exacerbation.

Imaging features that favor the diagnosis of NMO over MS are the distribution of lesions—periaqueductal location, absent perivenular orientation of periventricular lesions (Dawson's fingers are not seen in NMO), more extensive involvement of the corpus callosum, larger, more confluent lesions and enhancement of brain lesions that does not show incomplete ring pattern and NMO does not involve the cortical gray matter unlike MS.

Treatment and Prognosis

Treatment of NMO is with immunosuppression (e.g. Anti-CD20 monoclonal antibody rituximab) being the main stay. Patients who relapse have a poorer prognosis with increase in the incidence of blindness and paraplegia.

NMO spectrum disorders
Neuromyelitis optica—Devic disease/syndrome
Other NMO spectrum disorders
• Recurrent longitudinal extensive myelitis
• Bilateral simultaneous/recurrent optic neuritis
• Asian optic—spinal MS
• Optic neuritis or myelitis + specific brain lesions
• Optic neuritis or myelitis + systemic autoimmune disease.

White Matter Diseases Associated with Infections

Viral Encephalitides

The acute encephalitides may be secondary to a known causative agent or may be an autoimmune response to a nonspecific viral illness or vaccination. In such cases, the cerebral hypersensitivity reaction causes the observed clinical and pathologic state, whether the initial offending antigen is a virus, foreign protein, or autoantigen.

Conversely, there are patients with diminished immunity in whom a virus, which normally cannot gain a foothold in the central nervous system, propagates unchecked and results in demyelination.

The glial and neuronal cells may be directly infected or destroyed, as seen in acute encephalomyelitis (ADEM) in which a virus is not isolated from the brain. The subacute encephalitides (i.e. subacute sclerosing panencephalitis and PML) refer to direct infections of the brain that last for months or years and become reactivated years after the primary infections.

ACUTE DEMYELINATING ENCEPHALOMYELITIS

It is also called para-infectious encephalomyelitis. It is triggered by an infection, such as upper respiratory viral infection, measles, mumps or post vaccination for rabies, yellow fever. It is considered as immune mediated myelin destruction. Patients present within a few days or 3 weeks after viral illness/vaccination with fever, headache and decreased level of consciousness varying from lethargy to coma, seizure, and multifocal neurologic symptoms such as hemiparesis, cranial nerve palsies, and movement disorders; behavioral changes like depression, delusions, and psychosis may dominate the symptoms. Unlike multiple sclerosis, symptoms are more systemic rather than focal.

Epidemiology

Acute demyelinating encephalomyelitis (ADEM) presents in children or adolescents (usually younger than 15 years of age). However, cases have been reported in all ages. Winter and spring seasonal peaks in the presentation have been observed in some studies, underlining the upper respiratory infection etiology. Less than 5% of all ADEM cases follow an immunization. Unlike many other demyelinating diseases (e.g. multiple sclerosis or neuromyelitis optica), ADEM has no female predilection.[92]

Pathology

ADEM is thought to occur from cross-reactivity in immunity to viral antigens, triggering a subsequent autoimmune attack on the CNS. In approximately half of confirmed cases, Anti-MOG (myelin oligodendrocyte glycoprotein) immunoglobulin G antibodies can be identified. The pathological hallmark is perivenular inflammation with limited sleeves of demyelination.

Clinical Diagnosis

The diagnosis is clinical. CSF shows lymphocytosis and may show an increase in myelin basic protein. Anti MOG IgG antibodies may be detected. Majority of patients recover completely, while 20% show residual impairment. Mortality ranges from 10–25%. Various patterns of disease evolution have been described.[72,88,93]

Monophasic ADEM is the most common pattern, although, within the episode, individual lesions may be of varying stages of evolution, with different lesions maturing over a number of weeks. In 10% of cases, relapse within the first three months is encountered. Rarely it may show a waxing-waning course over a few months.

Recurrent ADEM is characterized by a second episode occurring more than 3 months after the initial illness and involving the same anatomical area as the original illness.

Multiphasic ADEM—when the subsequent illness involves a different anatomical region.

Progression of ADEM to multiple sclerosis is not uncommon, and has been reported in up to 35% of cases. As fever and infection are well-known triggers for multiple sclerosis, a history of recent infection is identified in clinically isolated syndrome (CIS).

Imaging

Non-contrast CT is usually normal. On administration of contrast punctate lesions with ring enhancement may be seen.

MRI is usually abnormal but normal scans or a delay in appearance of findings may be seen. Clinical improvement often precedes resolution of the MR abnormality, which may continue to evolve while symptoms are regressing. Follow-up MR commonly demonstrates marked decrease in the size and number of lesions, and complete resolution of disease may be seen in response to steroids. No new lesions should appear on MR approximately 6 months from the start of the disease.

Lesions are usually multiple and bilateral but asymmetrical **(Figs. 25A to C)**. ADEM can involve both brain and spine, gray and white matter. T2/FLAIR hyperintensities are seen in the brain parenchyma typically situated in the subcortical location; the thalami and brainstem can also be involved. The size of the lesion may vary from small punctate foci to flocculent cotton ball lesions with poorly defined fuzzy margins **(Figs. 26A and B)**. Large confluent lesions **(Figs. 27A and B)** or occasionally a solitary lesion may be seen. Mass effect is mild, less than expected for the size of involvement. The deep gray matter is usually involved in ADEM **(Figs. 28A and B)**. Corpus callosal involvement can be seen but it does not affect the undersurface, unlike MS. Enhancement may be variable ranging from minimal or intense. Larger 'tumefactive' lesions display incomplete horse shoe enhancement like MS **(Figs. 29A to E)**. Cranial nerves may also enhance in ADEM. Absence of enhancement does not exclude the diagnosis Myelitis is seen in only in 1/3rd of patients. Spinal cord lesion may appear as a swollen confluent lesion resembling transverse myelitis **(Fig. 30)**. Isolated spinal cord lesion without supratentorial involvement is rare.

Severe acute lesions may show restricted diffusion which can be seen as peripherally restricted diffusion; the center of the lesion, although high on T2 and low on T1, does not show restriction on DWI. A nonspecific appearance is seen on proton spectroscopy of a low NAA peak and an elevated lactate peak **(Figs. 31A to C)**.

A rare variant of ADEM is **Acute Infantile bilateral striatal necrosis which** is characterized by enlarged hyperintense basal ganglia, caudate nucleus and internal/external capsules.

Treatment

Treatment consists of methylprednisolone, with immunoglobulin and cyclophosphamide reserved for patients refractory to steroids. Complete recovery within one month is the most common outcome (50–60%), with sequelae (most commonly seizures) seen in a significant proportion of cases (20–30%).

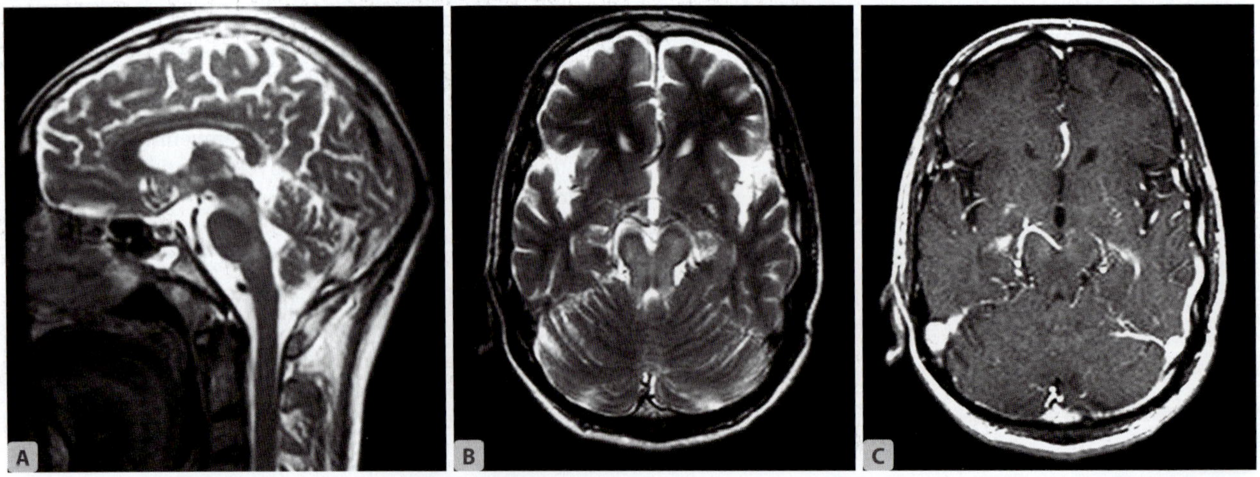

FIGS. 25A TO C: Hyperintensities seen in brainstem on T2W sagittal (A) T2W axial (B) images with subtle enhancement on T1W post contrast image (C) Brainstem encephalitis

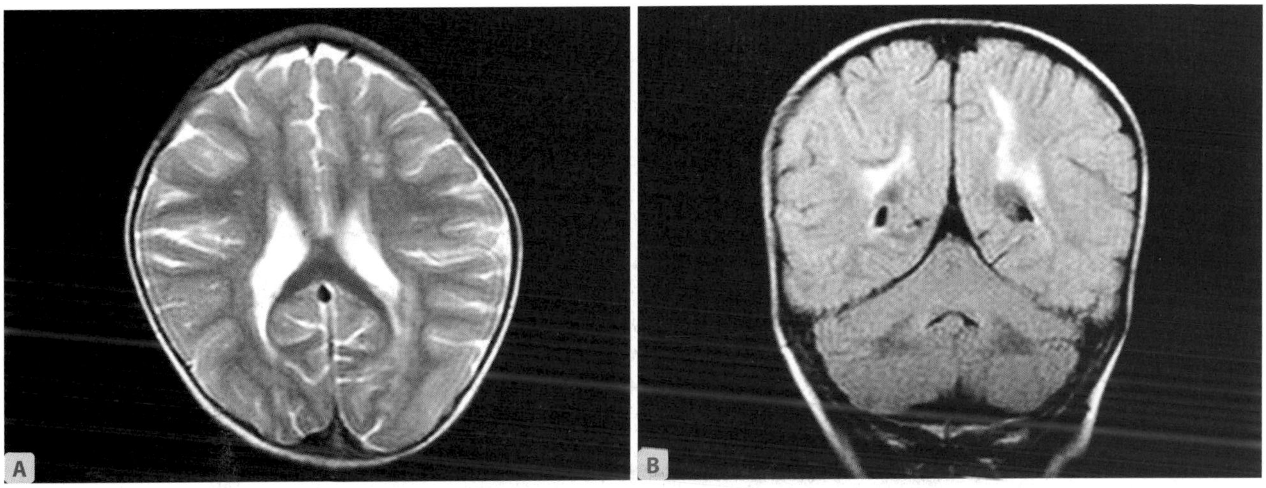

FIGS. 26A AND B: History of viral illness symmetrical white matter hyperintensities seen in T2W axial (A) and FLAIR coronal (B) image in a case of ADEM

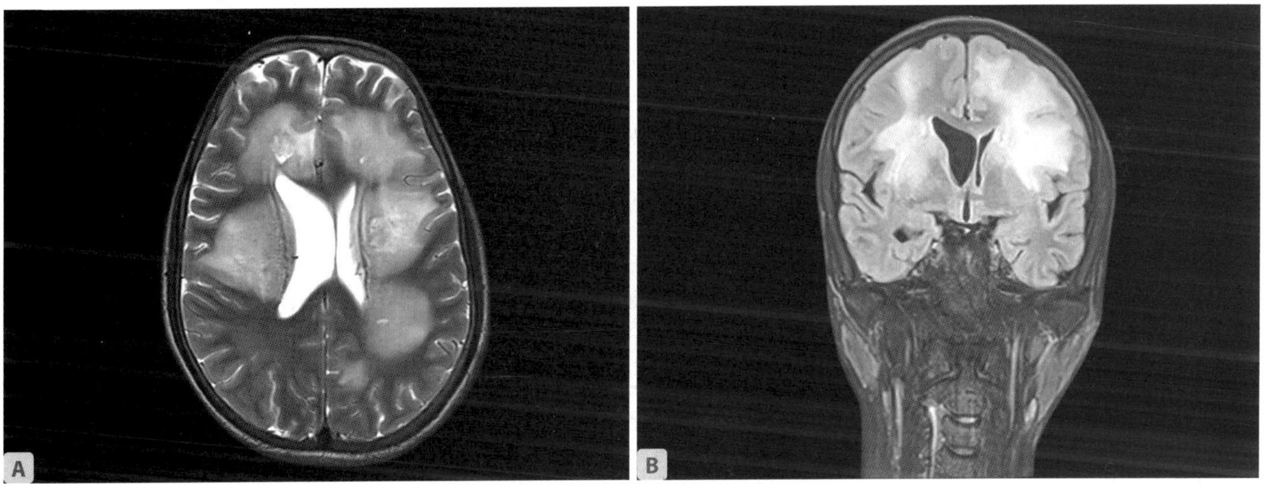

FIGS. 27A AND B: Large confluent hyperintensities seen bilaterally in a patient of ADEM in T2 axial (A) and coronal FLAIR (B) Image.

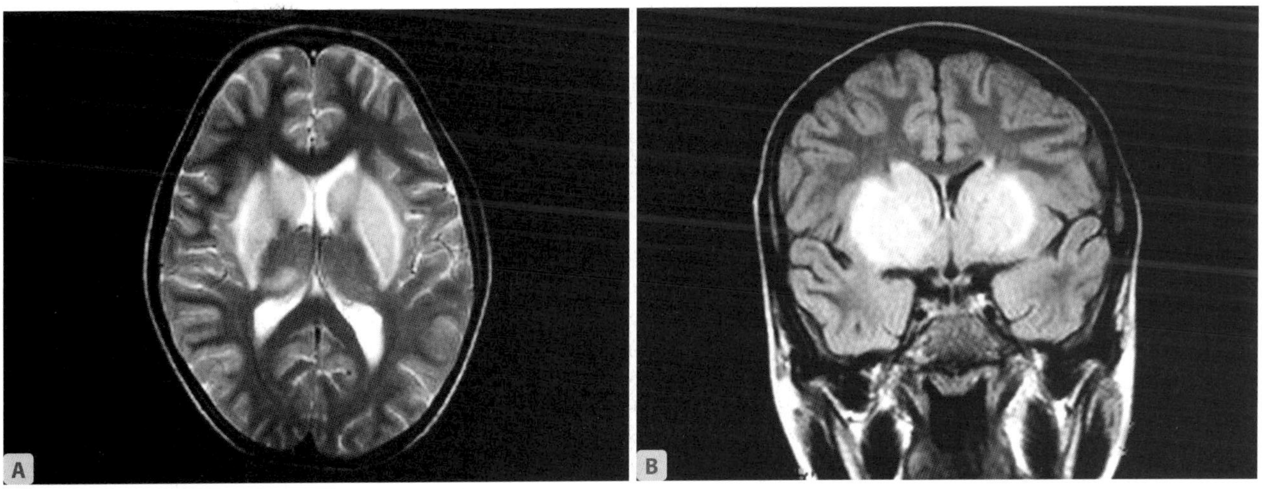

FIGS. 28A AND B: ADEM with predominant basal ganglia involvement. T2W axial (A) and FLAIR coronal (B) image in a patient with recent history of rabies vaccination show hyperintensity in both basal ganglia, right thalamus and cerebral peduncles. Hyperintense foci also seen in subcortical white matter with mild attenuation of right frontal horn.

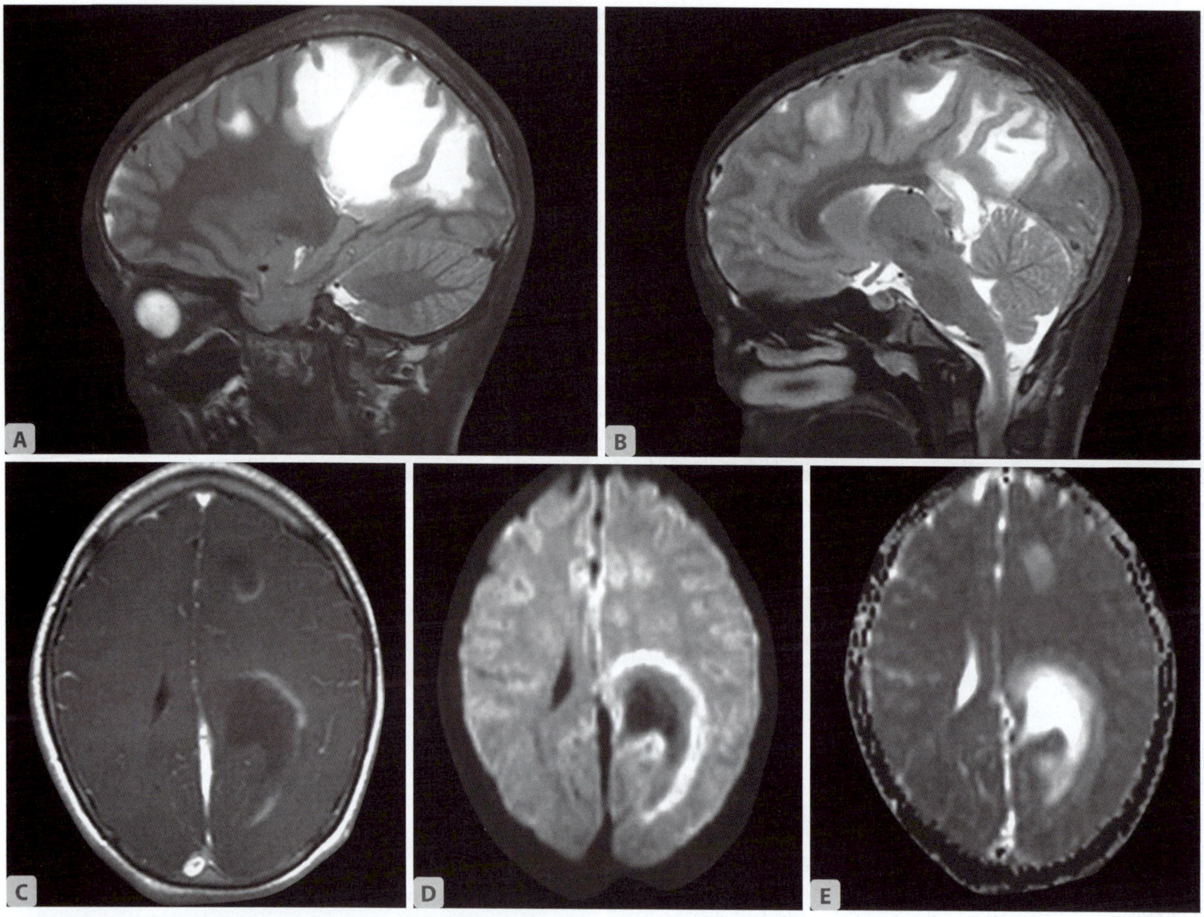

FIGS. 29A TO E: Large tumefactive demyelinating foci are seen in the subcortical location and in corpus callosum (A and B), open ring type of enhancement is seen on post-contrast T1W1 (C) with peripheral restricted diffusion (D and E) acute demyelination in a case of postviral ADEM.

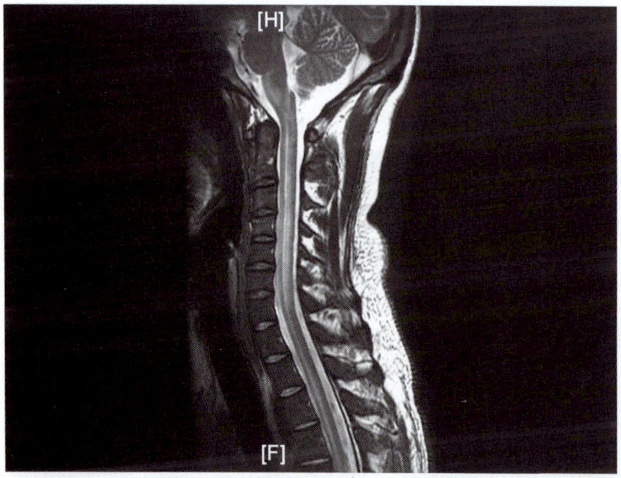

FIG. 30: ADEM-T2W sagittal image shows multilevel involvement of the cord with hyperintensity and mild swelling of the cord.

Differential Diagnosis

- Multiple Sclerosis and variants—the major differentiating features are tabulated in **Table 3**.
- Susac syndrome
- Acute necrotizing encephalitis of childhood—it is a rare condition seen in children less than 4 years of age. Bilateral thalamic involvement hemorrhage, cavitation and post contrast enhancement is seen.
- Acute hemorrhagic leukoencephalitis.

ACUTE HEMORRHAGIC LEUKOENCEPHALITIS

Acute hemorrhagic leukoencephalitis (AHLE), also known **Acute hemorrhagic encephalomyelitis (AHEM)**, or **Weston-Hurst syndrome**, is a very rare form of demyelinating disease. AHLE is a severe fulminant form of ADEM. Histologically it differs from ADEM and is considered as a separate entity. History of flu like illness often precedes the neurological deterioration.[94]

Epidemiology

It is typically seen in young patients, though all ages are affected. Patients present with fever, neck stiffness and progressive neurological deficits, often leading to coma and death in a few days. There is no gender predilection.

Pathology

It is an autoimmune reaction to myelin protein. The brain shows multifocal areas of acute perivascular demyelination and hemorrhage confined to cerebral white matter with

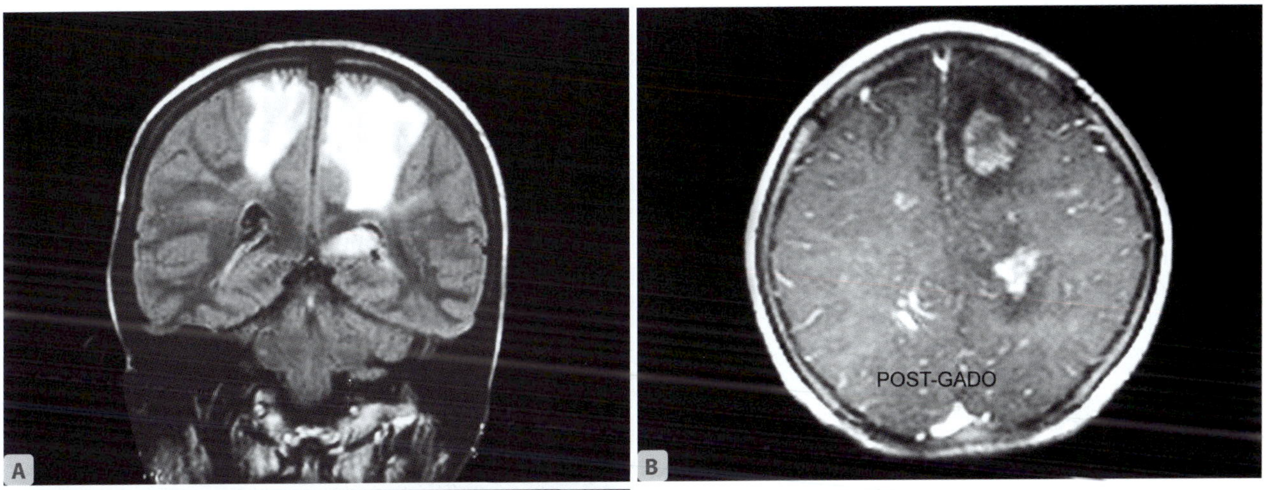

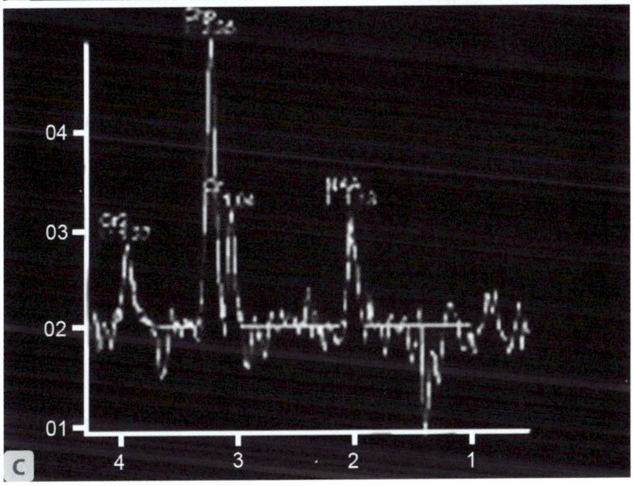

FIGS. 31A TO C: ADEM: Coronal FLAIR image (A) shows confluent hyperintense lesions involving both gray and white matter in the frontoparietal regions. Postcontrast T1W image (B) shows heterogeneous enhancement of the lesions with minimal perifocal edema. MR spectroscopy (C) reveals reduced NAA level, raised choline level with reversal of Cho/Cr ratio. Doublet inverted lactate peak is also noted.

strict sparing of the subcortical U fibers. There is marked cerebral edema and congestion, often with herniation with punctate hemorrhages within the cerebral white matter, not infrequently necrotic. Typically, there is no involvement of the spinal cord.

Imaging

MR-T2* imaging is essential for diagnosis. Hemorrhages are a key finding in AHLE which can range from large, confluent hemorrhages or microbleeds seen on SWI **(Figs. 32A and B)** with extensive mass effect and significant edema. Multifocal, punctate, linear areas of blooming are seen in corpus callosum and extend to the full thickness of hemispheric white matter to subcortical U fibers **(Figs. 33A to C)**. The cortical grey matter is usually spared. About 50% show variable enhancement. Multifocal scattered or confluent hyperintensities of cerebral white matter are seen on T2/FLAIR images but these are non-specific findings.[94]

Treatment and Prognosis

Acute hemorrhagic leukoencephalitis is associated with a very poor prognosis. It is well known to demonstrate an initial good response to steroids with subsequent new onset of symptoms and devastating outcome.

Differential Diagnosis

- **ADEM**: It has a less fulminant course and does not demonstrate characteristic lobar/perivascular hemorrhages of AHLE.
- **Acute necrotizing encephalopathy**: This is a rare complication of viral infection influenza A, B, herpes virus. There are bilateral symmetrical lesions in thalami, internal capsule and tegmentum.[95]
- The petechial hemorrhages seen in AHLE are also seen in other diseases, such as diffuse vascular injury, fat emboli, thrombocytic purpura, sepsis, vasculitis, haemorrhagic viral fever, malaria and rickettsial disease.
- **Acute fulminant MS (Marburg)**: This does not have clinical features of fever and leukocytosis seen in AHLE and no haemorrhages are seen.

Subacute Sclerosing Panencephalitis

Subacute sclerosing panencephalitis (SSPE) results from a slow infection reactivated after an episode of measles.

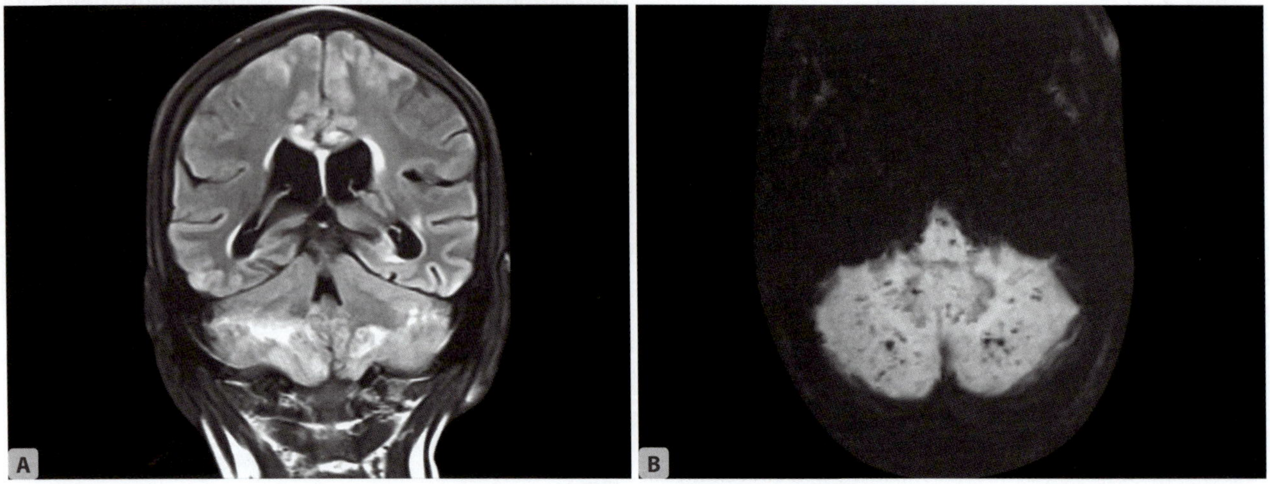

FIGS. 32 A AND B: FLAIR Coronal (A), SWI (B)-Hemorrhagic foci are seen in the cerebeller hemispheres in a case of AHLE. Note is also made of supratentorial involvement. (AHLE: acute hemorrhagic leukoencephalitis)

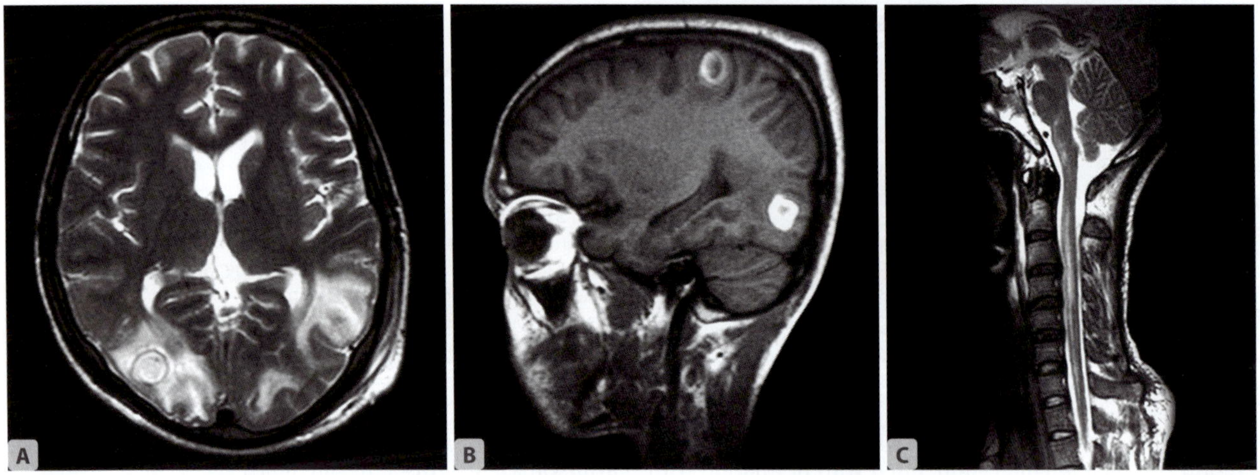

FIGS. 33A TO C: Hyperintensities are seen in parieto-occipital region bilaterally seen on T2W axial (A), with foci of hemorrhage, appreciated on T1W sagittal (B) Mild swelling of the cord with hyperintense signal seen on T2W sagittal (C) hemorrhagic leukoencephalitis.

Clinical features include behavioral changes with progressive myoclonus, ataxia, and seizures. SSPE usually progresses to death in 6 months to 6 years.

Imaging

MRI shows subcortical white matter hyperintensities and extensive symmetrical diffuse periventricular white matter changes, followed by an end stage appearance of marked cerebral atrophy.

Progressive Rubella Panencephalitis

Progressive Rubella Panencephalitis (PRP) is a neurological disorder which may occur in a child with congenital rubella. It is a slow viral infection of the brain characterized by chronic encephalitis, usually manifesting between 8–19 years of age. It is believed to be due to a persistence or reactivation of rubella virus infection. It has an insidious onset with subtle changes in behavior and declining school work, later developing neurological symptoms, develops progressive spasticity, ataxia and seizures. Progressive rubella panencephalitis is characterized pathologically by widespread demyelinating changes in the brain with extensive involvement in the basal ganglia and brainstem. On MRI cerebral atrophy with demyelinating lesions are seen.

Progressive Multifocal Leukoencephalopathy (PML)[96–102]

It is a demyelinating disease secondary to an opportunistic viral infection by the JC virus (John Cunningham virus), a member of the papovaviridae family. This virus is ubiquitous with latent persistence in kidney and cerebrum. In patients who are immunocompromised, JC virus becomes neurotropic with infection and lysis of oligodendrocytes which leads to failure of myelin production. PML is seen in three clinical contexts:

- PML due to immunocompromised state
- *PML-s-IRIS*: Simultaneous development of Immune Reconstitution Inflammatory Syndrome (IRIS) and PML due to immune reconstitution
- *PML-d-IRIS*: Immune reconstitution worsens pre-existing PML.

Epidemiology

Progressive multifocal leukoencephalopathy has a strong association with immunosuppressed states, particularly AIDS, where it typically develops in patients with CD4 counts of 50–100 cells/μL. PML is also seen in patients of collagen vascular disease, in post-transplant patients on immunosuppression, chemotherapy with rituximab for hematological malignancies and patients of multiple sclerosis on natalizumab. PML is one of the classic conditions encountered in immune reconstitution inflammatory syndrome. Patients with idiopathic CD4 lymphocytopenia, systemic lupus erythematosus, cirrhosis, pregnancy have also been diagnosed with PML.

Clinically, PML typically presents with an insidious onset. The most common presenting complaints are motor weakness, followed in frequency by altered mental status, visual disturbances and gait abnormalities. Untreated, it is fatal; with the institution of highly active antiretroviral therapy (HAART) survival improves. PML in natalizumab treated MS cases has high mortality rate.

Pathology

There are multifocal demyelinating plaques involving the subcortical U fibers with sparing of the cortical ribbon and the deep gray matter. The most significant finding is the presence of intranuclear inclusion bodies, which on electron microscopy are viral particles characteristic of papovavirus.

Imaging

Imaging suggests the diagnosis in patients of HIV/AIDS, and is confirmed by presence of JCV antigen in CSF.

The **classic MR appearance of PML** is multifocal areas of ill-defined high signal intensity on long TR sequences within the subcortical white matter. Any lobe may be involved by PML, but the frontal and parieto-occipital locations are most common and thus correlate well with the symptoms of homonymous hemianopia, focal neurologic deficit, and altered mentation. Lesions may be initially small in size but usually progress to larger areas of involvement. A multifocal distribution pattern is seen, which may be unilateral but is more often bilateral and asymmetric **(Fig. 34)**. There is an absence of mass effect. Hemorrhage is uncommon.

The subcortical lesions follow the gray-white interface, resulting in a "scalloped" appearance due to the involvement of subcortical U fibers. This relative sparing of cortical ribbon is called the **"heart of the gyrus"** sign. Individual gyri are thickened by edema of central white matter with conspicuous sparing and margination of the overlying cortical ribbon.

In classical PML there is no significant contrast enhancement which is attributable to the paucity of perivenous inflammation. When enhancement is present, it is faint and peripheral. However ring enhancement is noted in cases of **immune reconstruction inflammatory syndrome (IRIS)** in PML related to natalizumab therapy. On T1-weighted images, PML lesions are usually hypointense to parenchyma and fairly well-demarcated, although early lesions may be isointense. In contrast, HIV- related demyelination is usually isointense on T1-weighted images and is often inapparent.

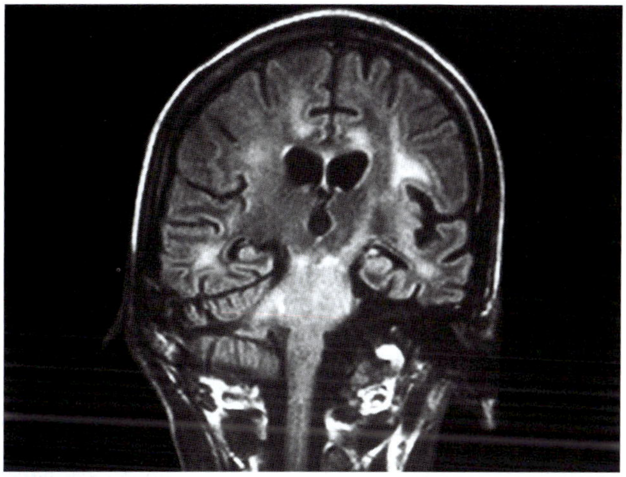

FIG. 34: Coronal FLAIR image: Patchy, asymmetrical white matter hyperintensities predominantly involving subcortical white matter in left cerebral hemisphere. Similar hyperintensities are also seen in pons and midbrain. Diffuse cerebral atrophy is also noted—PML.

TABLE 5: Differences between HIV dementia and PML.

	HIV dementia	PML
Clinical presentation	Memory loss and mental slowing	Focal neurological signs
Course	Several months	Weeks to months
MR findings	Bilateral symmetrical periventricular hyperintensities on T2WI, normal-to-mild hypointensity on T1WI. No enhancement/ mass effect	Focal, unilateral or asymmetrical, multifocal subcortical white matter hyperintensity on T2WI. Mild-to-severe hypointensity on T1WI. Usually no enhancement/mass effect

In advanced PML, smaller, very hyperintense foci may be seen within and surrounding the hyperintense confluent lesion denoting spongy nature of the lesion. There is relatively less mass effect. Acute lesions show diffusion restriction. DTI shows reduced fractional anisotropy suggestive of disorganised white matter structure. Perfusion studies show a decrease in rCBV as compared to normal white matter reflecting its avascular nature.

Differential Diagnosis

- HIV encephalopathy—More symmetric involvement and sparing of subcortical U fibres. The differences are enumerated in **Table 5**.
- Other opportunistic infections—Toxoplasmosis and CMV. Toxoplasmosis is mass like, CMV causes ependymitis and ventriculitis.

Human Immunodeficiency Virus Encephalopathy[103–105]

Neurologic manifestations are the initial manifestations of AIDS in 7 to 20% of patients. White matter changes in HIV have a varied etiology, though may show similar appearance. These can be the result of the primary effects of HIV or due to opportunistic infections (such as cytomegalovirus, toxoplasmosis, JC virus that cause PML and fungi), neoplasms (lymphoma), vascular disease or may be a result of associated metabolic and nutritional disorders.

CNS involvement in AIDS can manifest as acute encephalopathy, subacute encephalitis, acute and chronic meningitis, vacuolar myelopathy and peripheral neuropathy. Among these various forms, subacute encephalitis is most frequently associated with cerebral white matter disease.

HIV-associated dementia (HAD) previously called as **AIDS dementia** complex, corresponds to a neurological clinical syndrome seen in patients with HIV infection. The associated imaging appearance is generally referred to as **HIV encephalopathy (HIE).** HAD, HIE are part of the spectrum of HIV-associated neurocognitive disorders (HANDs). Typically, HIV encephalopathy occurs in patients with advanced immunosuppression and with coexistent systemic diseases.

HIV virus is not only lymphotrophic, but also neurotropic. It replicates in multinucleated giant cells within the central nervous system, resulting eventually in demyelination. This demyelination is characterized by little edema and a lack of inflammation.

The clinical syndrome of HAD comprises of a combination of cognitive, behavioral and motor dysfunction like gait disturbance and tremors. Patients present with inattention and reduced concentration, apathy and dulling of personality, psychomotor slowing, marked motor slowing and ataxia. Prognosis is poor with fatality seen within a year.

Imaging features of HIV encephalopathy, whether by CT or MR, tends to lag behind the pathologic involvement. Generalized atrophy is the most common abnormality that is nonspecific, with a predominantly central distribution. With more severe involvement, CT shows symmetric white matter hypodensity, usually seen bifrontally. There is no contrast enhancement or mass effect. On MR there is greater sensitivity with various patterns seen on T2 and proton density weighted images. These include punctate foci of signal hyperintensity, larger focal and diffuse areas of hyperintensity, and less well-defined patchy areas of hyperintensity. Symmetrical diffuse lesions in periventricular white matter and within the centrum semiovale suggest underlying HIV infection **(Figs. 35A and B)**. There is relative sparing of subcortical region and posterior fossa. Multifocal confluent lesions or diffuse symmetric high signal intensity in the periventricular and deep white matter may be seen as the disease progresses **(Figs. 36A and B)**. Bilateral symmetric increased signal intensity on the long TR sequences has been described in the basal ganglia (caudate and putamen) and thalamus and may also involve the brainstem. Follow-up MR studies after the institution of highly active antiretroviral therapy in patients with the AIDS dementia complex have shown regression or stabilization of signal abnormalities on MR.

A range of decreased MT ratios in areas of high signal intensity as compared with control subjects has been shown. Abnormal MT ratios have also been found in the normal appearing white matter of HIV-positive patients in patients with both PML and HIV encephalopathy. Proton MR spectroscopy studies have shown decreased NAA/Cr, increased levels of choline, and the presence of lactate in normal appearing white matter and regions of white matter with signal abnormality.

LYME DISEASE/LYME NEUROBORRELIOSIS (LNB)

Borreliosis is a multisystem inflammatory reaction caused by a spirochete *Borrelia burgdorferi*. It is transmitted by tick bite and is the most common vector borne disease in the US. Patients initially present with target like rash and flu like syndrome. This is followed by neurological and cardiac abnormalities seen weeks to months later.

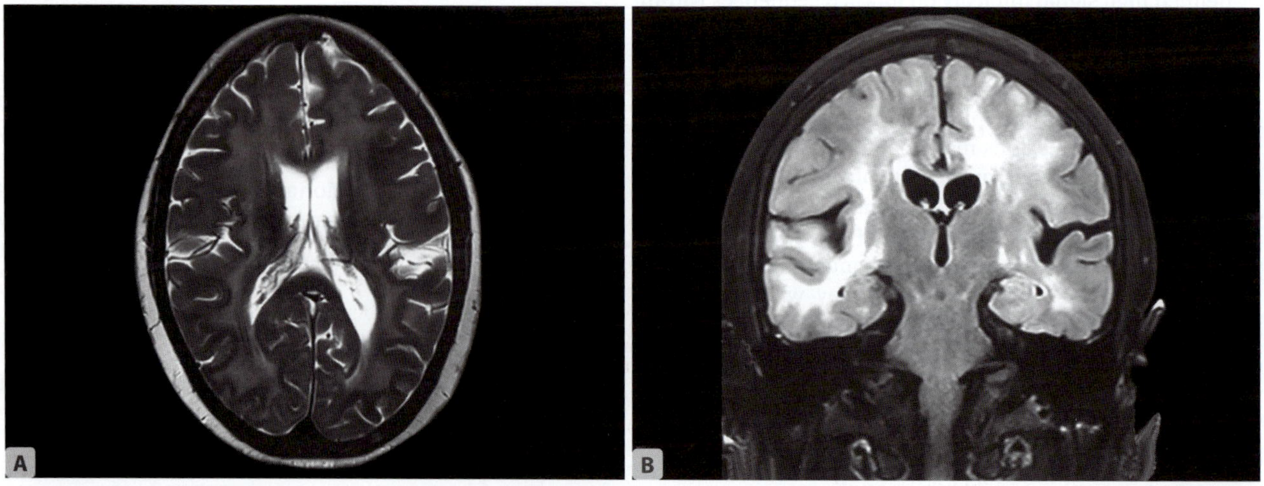

FIGS. 35A AND B: Axial T2WI (A), Coronal FLAIR images (B) show bilateral symmetrical hyperintensities in the periventricular white matter in a case of AIDS-HIV encephalopathy.

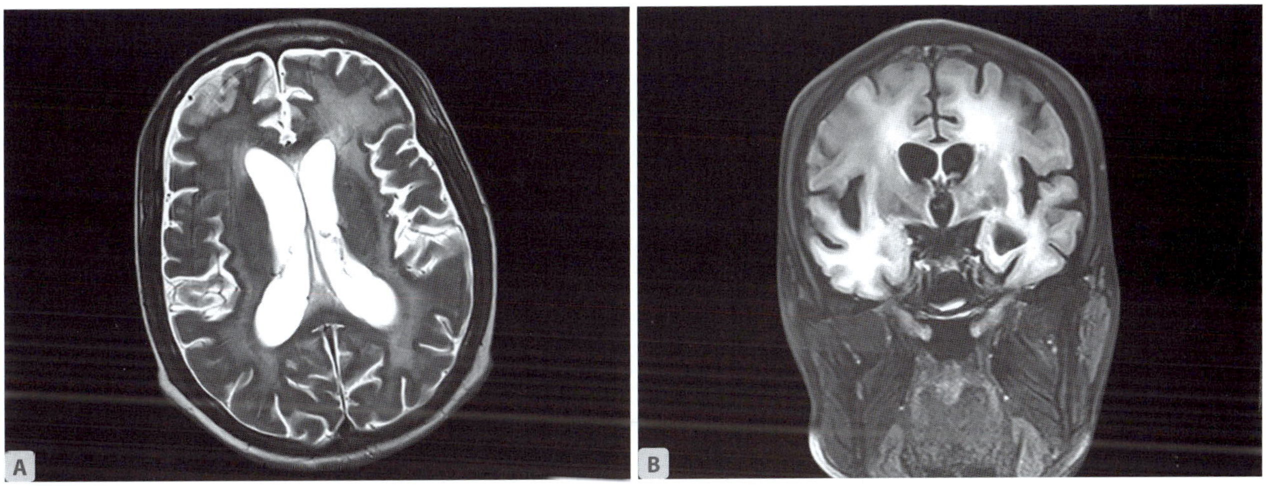

FIGS. 36A AND B: T2W axial image (A) and coronal FLAIR images (B) show bilateral symmetrical hyperintensities in the centrum semiovale with cerebral atrophy in a case of HIV dementia.

Imaging

Multiple T2/FLAIR small (2–8 mm) white matter hyperintensities are seen in the subcortical, periventricular location and Corpus callosum. Variable enhancement is seen. Leptomeningeal enhancement has also been described in LNB. Lyme disease mimics MS due to similarity of site involvement. Cranial nerve involvement most commonly of CN VII, followed by CN III and V is a feature of LNB. Unilateral disease is more common. The altered nerves show uniform contrast enhancement. Spinal cord involvement in rare but may be seen.[106]

Differential Diagnosis

- *Multiple sclerosis*: Involves periventricular white matter. Cranial nerve enhancement is less common in MS. Leptomeningeal enhancement is not seen in multiple sclerosis.
- *Susac syndrome*: Sensorineural hearing loss is a key feature in Susac syndrome.

White Matter Diseases Associated with Vascular Causes

It can be divided into six broad categories:[107]

Type 1: Arteriosclerotic type

Type 2: Cerebral amyloid angiopathy

Type 3: Inherited vasculopathies CADASIL, MELAS (mitochondrial myopathy lactic acidosis, stroke-like episodes)

Type 4: Inflammatory vasculitis—CNS vasculitis encompasses a heterogeneous group of inflammatory disorders that primarily affect the small leptomeningeal and parenchymal blood vessels of the same. Primary angitis of the central vascular system (PACVS), Susac syndrome, connective tissue disorders such as systemic lupus erythematosus and Sjogren syndrome.

Type 5: Venous collagenosis

Type 6: Others—related to radiation.

Type 1: Small vessel disease related to arteriosclerosis: Small vessel disease is the commonest cause of white matter disease and leads to cognitive and physical disability. Multiple nonspecific small hyperintensities seen on T2W/FLAIR involving white matter in subcortical location and deep gray matter are the most frequent presentation of vasculitis. Nonspecific white matter changes range from periventricular caps and rims [periventricular white matter lesions (PVWMLs)] to deep white matter punctuate patchy or confluent lesions. There is a difference in etiology and clinical presentation of white matter lesions. Smooth PVWMLs are due to ependymal loss or differing degrees of myelination in adjacent fiber tracts. These are thought to have a nonischemic origin. Irregular PVWMLs are associated with atherosclerosis. Cerebral microhemorrhages are small (<5 mm) areas of blooming seen on T2*/susceptibility weighted imaging. These are usually not seen on CT or other MR sequences. In patients with chronic hypertension they are found in deep gray matter. Brain atrophy is another manifestation of small vessel disease.

An international task force has drafted a consensus classifying small vessel disease as white matter hyperintensities (WMHs), recent small subcortical infarcts, lacunes, microbleeds and brain atrophy.[108]

White matter hyperintensities (WMHs), are commonly seen in patients above 60 years of age usually in frontal and parietal regions. WMH are further rated as focal, beginning confluent, diffuse confluent, and are seen in basal nuclei, corona radiata and centrum semi ovale—the area of vascular end zones. There is a correlation between WMHs with cognitive, behavioral, gait and urinary impairment.

Recent small subcortical infarcts also known as acute lacunar infarcts are defined as infarcts less than 20 mm. These occur in the territory of perforating arterioles. These acute lacunar infarcts may develop into lacunas which are round/ovoid cavities of 3–15 mm, following CSF signal intensity. Alternately these may develop into WMHs or disappear.

Binswanger's disease (subcortical arteriosclerotic encephalopathy): Binswanger disease, described in 1894 is a demyelinating disease equally affecting men and women generally more than 55 years old. It is associated with hypertension and lacunar infarction.[109] Patients may have acute stroke followed by declining mental status or slow insidious mental status change with psychiatric disturbance, seizures, urinary incontinence and gait changes. MR reveals broad regions of high signal intensity in the white matter of frontal, parietal and occipital regions extending into the centrum semiovale **(Figs. 37A and B)**. The U fibers are spared. Binswanger disease differs from multinfarct dementia because of its distinctive white matter involvement and absence of consistent focal stroke like symptoms.

Type 2: Cerebral amyloid angiopathy (CAA): CAA is one of the manifestations of amyloid disease of the brain. It is caused by accumulation of amyloid protein in the media and adventitia of cerebral small vessels (cortical and leptomeningeal arteries). It shows a preferential involvement of occipital and frontal regions. Advancing age predisposes to the development of CAA; a hereditary form is also known which presents earlier. Patients are usually normotensive. Amyloid disease is typically seen after 55 years of age. There is no gender predilection. Cerebral amyloidosis is not related to systemic amyloidosis.

Gross pathology shows the presence of lobar, corticosubcortical and cortical haemorrhages of different age and sizes. Signs of previous subarachnoid haemorrhage are also seen. The fragility of the vessels due to deposition of amyloid and subsequent inflammation underlines the propensity to bleed and the chronic cerebral hypoperfusion being the cause for leukoencephalopathy.[110]

Imaging

CT: Lobar hematoma with variable peripheral edema is seen. Multiple irregular confluent hyperintensities are noted along with cerebral atrophy; atraumatic convexal subarachnoid hemorrhage may be seen.

MRI: Hematoma is noted which displays age related signal intensity. Focal white matter hyperintensity may be seen. $T2^*$ (GRE, SWI) sequences demonstrate multifocal punctate areas of blooming in leptomeninges. Cortex and subcortical white matter, basal ganglia and cerebellum are relatively spared. The microbleeds associated with CAA lack mass effect, peripheral edema and there is no enhancement, differentiating it from hemorrhagic metastasis. Microbleeds that are associated with hypertension involve basal ganglia, a site not favored by CAA. The radiological findings (Boston criteria) [111] can suggest the diagnosis, but can be confirmed only on postmortem examination.

Type 3: Cerebral autosomal dominant arteriopathy with subcortical infarcts and leukoencephalopathy (CADASIL):[111-114] CADASIL is an inherited non-arteriosclerotic small vessel disease related to mutation in chromosome 19. It is transmitted in an autosomal dominant pattern. It has a prevalence of 2–4 per 100,000, has no gender predilection. It is seen in the 3rd–4th decade of life with young adults presenting with migraines, recurrent ischemic stroke and progressive cognitive impairment.

Imaging

WMHs are noted in the third decade in the temporal pole, a location not seen in other microvascular disease. This progress to involve posterior temporal, frontal and parietal regions, basal nuclei and thalamus. Subcortical U fibers can be involved External capsule and corpus callosum are also involved, these locations being important pointers to the diagnosis of CADASIL. Microbleeds and extension with WMHs are seen as the patient ages.

Type 4: Primary angitis of the central nervous system (PACNS):[115-117] PACNS is a rare idiopathic vasculitis of the brain and spinal cord. It is seen in the 5th–6th decade. Patients present with headache and encephalopathy, stroke and hemorrhages are seen occasionally. CSF is abnormal in majority of the cases, showing elevated inflammatory markers and raised proteins.

Imaging

MRI is abnormal in more than 90% patients and shows multiple cortical, subcortical infarcts, WMHs, hemorrhages, parenchymal and leptomeningeal enhancement. A normal MR study rules out PACNS. Reversible central

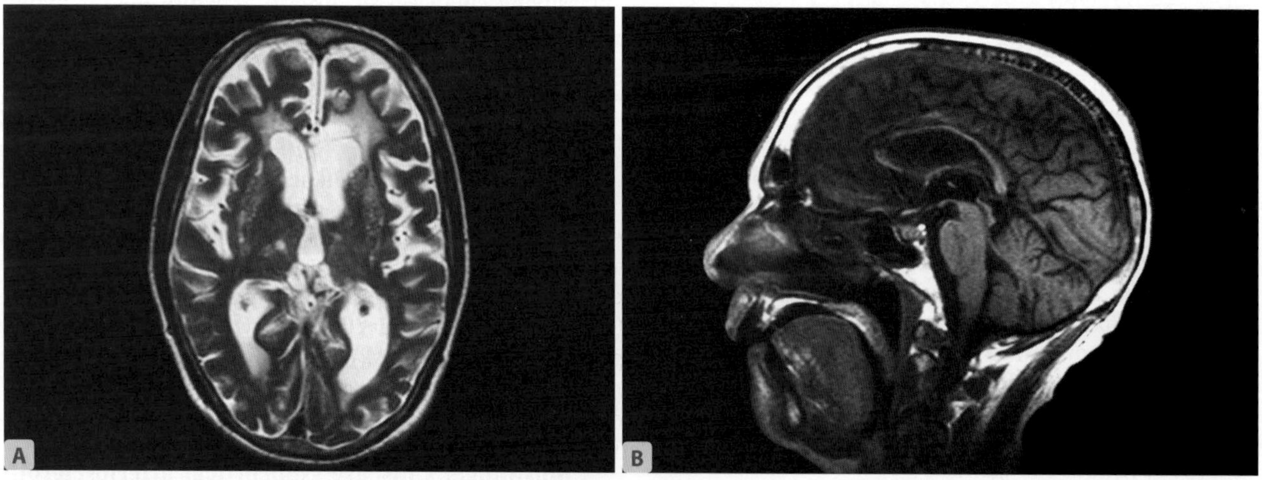

FIGS. 37A AND B: T2W axial image (A) and T1 sagittal image (B). Binswanger's disease. MRI demonstrates bilateral patchy hyperintensities extending from the subcortical region to the ventricular margins. Few lacunar infarcts are seen with evidence of cerebral atrophy.

vasoconstriction syndrome (RCVS) mimics PACNS in its clinical presentation of severe headache, but has normal CSF analysis. Brain biopsy may be required for the diagnosis.

Type 4: Inflammatory Vasculitis

Susac syndrome:[118-124] This is a recently recognized small vessel disease affecting young adults (20–40 years) with a female predominance. Described by **John O Susac,** an American neurologist and neuro-ophthalmologist and his colleagues, it is a vasculitis produced due to antiendothelial antibodies to specific neural vessels. The immune attack causes endotheliopathy that involves cochlea, retina and brain with microinfarcts in these locations.

Patients present with a triad of acute or subacute encephalopathy manifested in a broad spectrum of symptoms, e.g. memory impairment, confusion, behavioral disturbances, ataxia, dysarthria, paranoid psychosis, and headaches, sensorineural hearing loss at low and medium frequencies and visual loss (due to branch retinal artery occlusion). The course is usually self limiting but it may have a relapsing remitting course. It is also known as retino-cochleal-cerebral vasculopathy, RED-M (retinopathy, encephalopathy and microangiopathy) or SICRET (small infarcts of cochlear retinal and encephalic tissue).

Imaging

MRI: Corpus callosum is involved in almost all cases and is considered pathognomic. The middle of the corpus callosum (body and splenium) is involved, without involvement of the callosal undersurface unlike in MS. The roof of the corpus callosum is also frequently involved, resulting in "icicle" or linear "spoke" lesions that look to hang from the roof of the corpus callosum. Lesions have been described as "snow ball" and may involve the entire width of corpus callosum. As the disease progresses lesions become hypointense on T1 (black holes) and there may be atrophy of the corpus callosum signifying severe damage. The lesions are best appreciated on a sagittal view.

Multiple small microinfarcts are seen in the periventricular and deep white matter, centrum semiovale, brain stem as T2/FLAIR hyperintensities. A "string of pearls" appearance due to punctate microinfarcts involving the internal capsule has been described. Contrast enhancement is seen in acute stage. T2 shine through may be seen on DWI.

Differential Diagnosis

- *MS*: callososeptal interface is involved in multiple sclerosis
- *ADEM/Lyme disease*: Middle layer of corpus callosum is not involved. ADEM is usually preceded by viral illness or vaccination.
- Vasculiltis and thromboembolic infarcts—corpus callosum is rarely affected.
- Transient lesions of the splenium—these are seen in many conditions, with sudden stoppage of medication in epileptics being among them. There is no contrast enhancement and restricted diffusion is seen.

SYSTEMIC LUPUS ERYTHEMATOSUS[125-127]

Systemic lupus erythematosus (SLE) is a multisystem autoimmune disorder, affecting respiratory, cardiovascular, gastrointestinal, genitourinary, musculoskeletal and central nervous system when it is termed CNS Lupus or neuropsychiatric SLE (NPSLE).

The peak age of onset is 2nd to 4th decade with female preponderance. Diagnostic criteria have been established by the American College of Rheumatology and include malar rash, renal disease, arthritis, scoliosis etc. NPSLE manifests as psychosis, stroke, epilepsy, headache and cognitive abnormalities.

Imaging

MR may be normal or may show varied abnormality. Multiple small subcortical and deep white matter hyperintensities on T2/FLAIR, cerebral atrophy, infarction, are seen. Diffuse cortical, brainstem lesions and lesions in basal ganglia may be seen and are indicative of vasculitis. Transient enhancement, restricted diffusion and increased perfusion may be seen in acute cases. Dural venous sinus or cortical/deep venous thrombosis may be seen. The **presence of multifocal infarcts and migratory edematous areas are suggestive of CNS lupus.**

Differential diagnosis: Multifocal subcortical and deep white matter hyperintensities are seen in a host of other conditions—arteriosclerosis, multiple sclerosis, susac syndrome, Lyme disease and primary angiitis, etc.

BEHÇET DISEASE

It is a multisystemic, vascular inflammatory disease of unknown origin. Neurological involvement is noted in about a half of these cases and is called Neuro Behçet's disease.[128]

Clinically Behçet's presents as neurocuteneous syndrome, recurrent oral, genital ulcers, aphthous stomatitis, uveitis and arthralgia.

Imaging

MRI: Brainstem and specifically cerebral peduncles are involved in 50% of cases. Other sites of involvement are thalamus, basal ganglia. Circular, linear foci of T2/FLAIR hyperintensities are noted with minimal mass effect and mild to moderate contrast enhancement.

Differential diagnosis: MS, sarcoid and neoplasm form the major differential of Behçet's disease. Oligoclonal bands are not seen in Behçet's disease. Skin lesions are generally absent in sarcoidosis and ACE levels may be elevated in sarcoidosis. Biopsy may be required to differentiate widespread form of Behçet's from gliomatosis/lymphoma. Similar lesions, such as Behçet's are seen in systemic inflammatory diseases such as SLE, antiphospholipid syndrome and Sjögren's disease. Skin lesions are noted in these, but oral and genital ulceration is not seen.

WHITE MATTER DISEASES ASSOCIATED WITH TOXIC METABOLIC CAUSES

Osmotic Demyelination Syndrome (ODS)

Osmotic demyelination syndrome is the new terminology for what was earlier called central pontine myelinosis and/or extra pontine myelinosis. It is seen in hypoosmolar states, where the oligodendrocytes are vulnerable to osmotic changes. It has been considered a pontine lesion, but typically there is extrapontine involvement as well. Isolated pontine involvement is seen in 50% of cases. In 30% of cases there is concomitant extra pontine involvement. In 20–25% of patients white matter demyelination is exclusively extrapontine in the basal ganglia and with hemispheric involvement.[129-132]

Pathology

On gross examination, the classic pontine lesion is seen as triangular or butterfly lesion of symmetric gray discoloration along the midline of the basis pontis. There is edematous demyelination of the central ventral pons, with characteristic sparing of the tegmentum. A rim of normal white matter surrounds the area of demyelination. It is believed that the grid arrangement of descending and crossing tracts in the pons or its vulnerable vascularity leads to the characteristic focality of the lesion.

Clinical features: It is a rare disorder, seen usually in middle aged patients with slight male predominance. The most common cause is rapid correction of hyponatremia, a condition noted in chronic alcoholics or in the setting of malnutrition. Patients on cyclosporine, post liver transplant are also predisposed for electrolyte disturbance. There may be comorbidities such as renal, adrenal or paraneoplastic syndromes predisposing to ODS. The condition is also associated with diabetes and anorexia in paediatric patients. ODS may also be seen in normonatremic patients and independent of changes in sodium level. Clinically osmotic demyelination syndrome presents in a biphasic pattern. The first phase is usually attributable to the underlying electrolyte abnormality, with patients being acutely encephalopathic. Following rapid reversal of this abnormality, the patient transiently improves before progressing onto the classic osmotic demyelination syndrome features 2–3 days later. When pontine involvement is prominent, clinical features consist of pseudobulbar palsy, dysthermia, dysphagia. Patients may recover completely or progress to coma and death.

The clinical diagnosis is often difficult and recognition of the sentity on imaging by the radiologist often prompts a search for electrolyte abnormalities by the physician.

Imaging

CT: Hypo density may be seen in the affected areas.

MRI: Is the modality of choice. It is initially normal on routine sequences. DWI shows restricted diffusion in acute ODS in the lower pons, seen within 24 hours of onset of quadriplegia **(Figs. 38A and B)**. This area shows T2 hyperintensity followed by T1 hypointensity. The characteristic appearance is a symmetric round to oval area of T2 hyperintensity within the base of the pons **(Figs. 39A and B)**. These changes may take up to two weeks to be seen. Peripheral pons as well as corticospinal tracts and transverse fibres are spared leading to a classic trident shaped appearance **(Figs. 40A and B)**. Similar hyperintensity may be seen in basal ganglia, midbrain and subcortical white matter. Usually there is no enhancement but moderate enhancement may be seen in subacute cases.

Differential Diagnosis

- Pontine infarcts are usually asymmetric and involve the surface of pons in basilar perforating artery infarcts.
- Demyelinating disease: MS may involve pons but lesion is usually asymmetric and may show additional lesions in sites such as callososeptal interface.
- Pontine glioma: seen in children and young adults.
- PRES: can involve pons but does not spare the peripheral white matter.

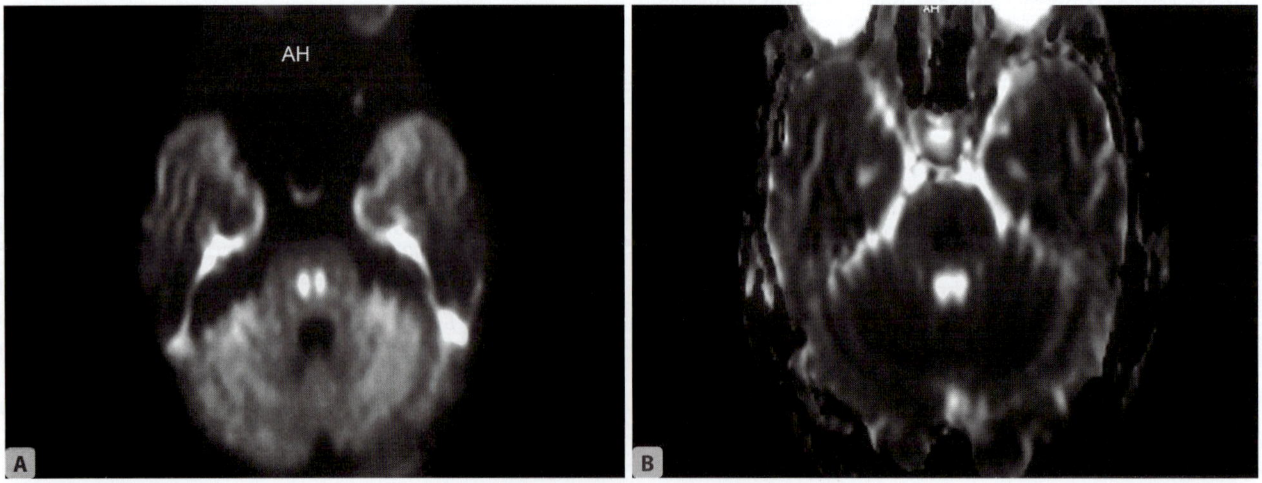

FIGS. 38A AND B: DWI in a suspected case of osmotic demyelination syndrome—restricted diffusion seen in pons signifying acute demyelination.

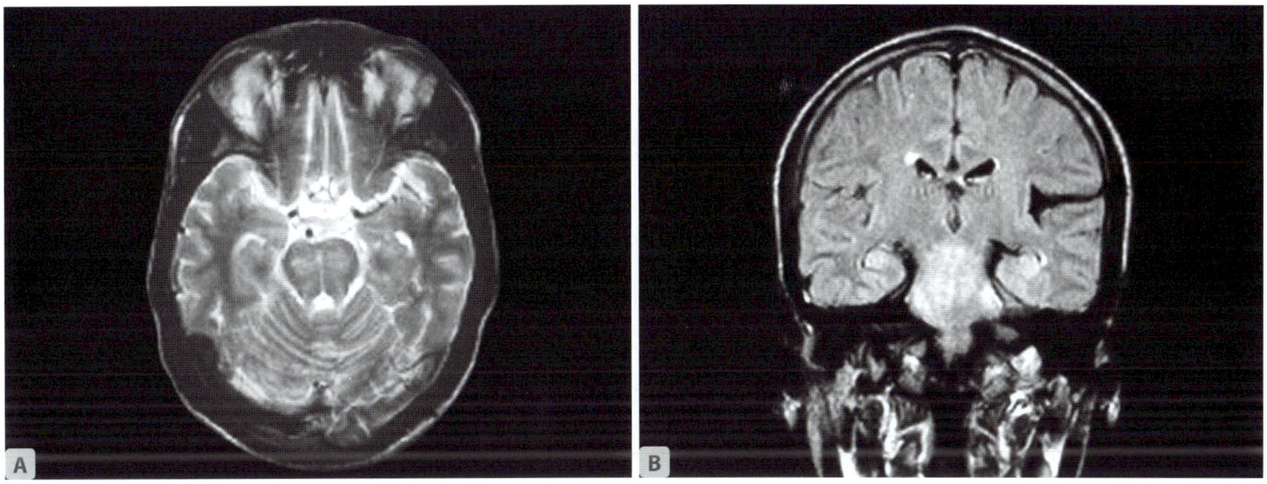

FIGS. 39A AND B: T2W axial image (A) shows increased signal intensity within the midpons, with surrounding rim of normal-appearing pontine parenchyma. Coronal FLAIR image (B) shows patchy area of hyperintensity in the pons—central pontine myelinolysis.

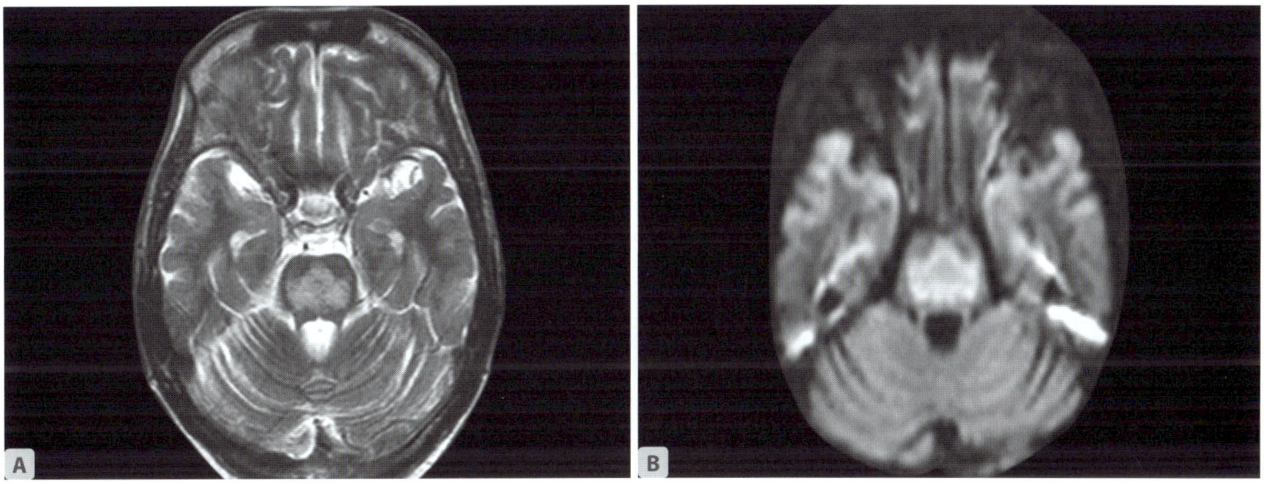

FIGS. 40A AND B: Trident-shaped hyperintensities T2 axial image (A) in the pons with restricted diffusion on DWI (B) in a case of ODS.

- Wilson's disease and mitochondrial disorders may mimic ODS in basal ganglia but pons is rarely involved in Wilson's disease and mitochondrial disorders.

Acute Hypertensive Encephalopathy/ Posterior Reversible Encephalopathy Syndrome (PRES)[133–137]

Hypertension with failed cerebral autoregulation, blood-brain barrier disruption and vasogenic edema are considered the cause for this entity. It was initially described in pre-eclampsia and an acute hypertensive crisis. Other conditions such as thrombotic hemolytic anemia, disseminated intravascular coagulation, use of certain drugs, immunosuppressive therapy have all been implicated.

Patients usually present with single short, grandmal seizure, headache and visual disturbances. Majority of patients have an elevated blood pressure. PRES can also occur in the absence of hypertension or mild hypertension. Severe PRES is a life-threatening complication, if not recognized and treated. PRES usually resolves completely with little or no residual abnormality with rapid institution of treatment. In rare cases disabilities may persist.

Imaging

PRES, as the name implies shows preferential involvement of the parieto-occipital lobes (85–95%) Posterior circulation has comparatively less sympathetic innervation than anterior and hence is less protected from the vasoconstriction mechanism. The frontal lobes are involved in 75–77% of cases and cerebellar involvement is noted in 50–55%.

CT shows subtle patchy cortical/subcortical hypodensity in the parieto-occipital lobes/watershed zones/cerebellum. PRES associated hemorrhages are seen rarely.

MR: shows the classic findings of bilateral parieto-occipital hypointensities on T1 and hyperintensities on T2W/FLAIR. Patchy enhancement may be seen. As the edema is vasogenic and not cytotoxic, DWI is negative except in atypical cases and in children. There is a decrease in rCBV on perfusion MR **(Figs. 41A to D)**.

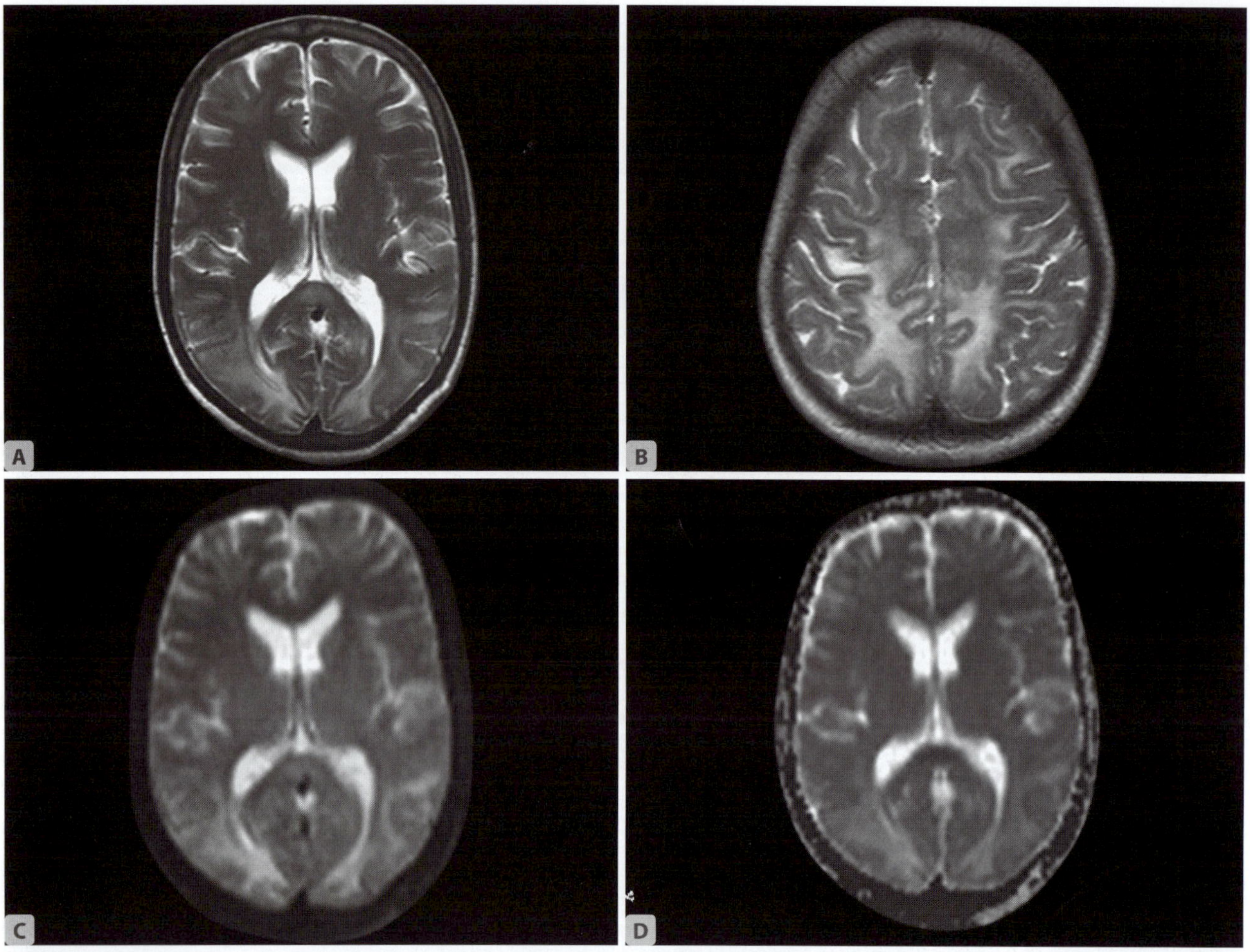

FIGS. 41A TO D: Bilateral symmetrical hyperintensity in the parieto-occipital region on T2W axial images (A and B). No restricted diffusion seen in DWI (C) and ADC map (D)—a case of PRES.

In atypical PRES: There is Involvement of frontal lobes, cortical watershed zones, Basal ganglia, brainstem and cerebellum. Rare site of PRES is spinal cord **(Figs. 42A and B)**.

Differential Diagnosis of PRES

- *Acute cerebral ischemia/infarction*: DWI is positive in infarction. Bilateral PCA distribution infarcts are rare in absence of basilar top thrombosis.
- *Vasculitis*: The lesions in vasculitis are more random and less symmetric.
- *Hypoglycemia*: Affects the parieto-occipital region. Clinical findings of hypoglycemia and lack of hypertension can be used to differentiate the two conditions.
- *Thrombotic microangiopathies*: The distinction may be difficult and is based on clinical/laboratory findings.
- *Reversible cerebral vasoconstriction syndrome*: Convexal subarachnoid hemorrhage may be seen but has a limited distribution to a few sulci.

Ethanol-related Diseases

Chronic Alcoholism

Ethanol adversely affects the vascular, glial and neural tissues and causes myelin degeneration. Nonspecific deep white matter and periventricular demyelinating lesions are seen on MR imaging of chronic alcoholics. Demyelination is the main pathological finding in Marchiafava-Bignami disease and most constant in Wernicke disease.[138]

Wernicke Encephalopathy[139,140]

Wernicke-Korsakoff syndrome: named after Carl Wernicke, a German neurologist and psychiatrist and Sergei Sergeievich Korsakoff, a Russian neuropsychiatrist.

It is related to thiamine deficiency which results in lactic acidosis. Although it is commonly seen in patients with alcohol dependence, nearly 50% of cases occur in non-alcoholics. The underlying pathogenesis in all cases is malnutrition due to any cause resulting in thiamine deficiency.

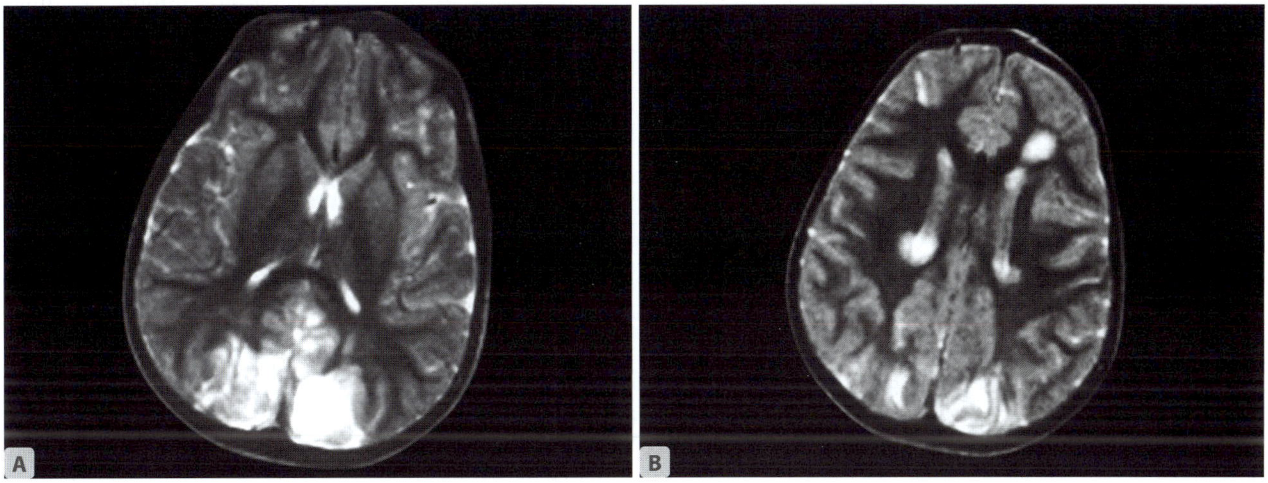

FIGS. 42A AND B: PRES-due to hypertension T2 axial image (A) Typical bilateral symmetric high signal intensity is seen within the occipital white matter with mild swelling of the overlying cortex. Symmetric high signal intensity within the subcortical white matter in frontal-parietal regions (B).

The classical triad of presentation is ocular dysfunction, ataxia, and altered mentation. Untreated, it is fatal and rapid intravenous thiamine replacement can prevent sequelae.

Imaging

MR: In acute phase T2/FLAIR hyperintensity is noted in affected areas—mammillary bodies (which show symmetrical involvement) around the third ventricle, medial thalami, the tectal plate and periaqueductal gray matter. DWI demonstrates diffusion restriction in the involved areas. Strong uniform enhancement of mammillary bodies is pathognomic of Wernicke encephalopathy.

Differential Diagnosis

- Medial thalamic and midbrain involvement is seen in artery of percheron infract but it does not involve the mammillary bodies.
- Leigh disease-mammillary bodies are not invoved.

Marchiafava-Bignami Disease

Marchiafava-Bignami disease (MBD): The disease was originally described in Italian alcoholic patients addicted to crude red wine consumption by Italian pathologists Ettore Marchiafava and Amico Bignami. It is characterized by toxic demyelination of the corpus callosum and frequently, extends to the centrum semiovale. In more recent years, it has been described in other population groups and poorly nourished non-alcoholics. Pathologically, the myelin loss may be striking and accompanied by axonal degeneration. Acute deterioration is common.[141,142]

Imaging

In the acute stage of the disease, the corpus callosum shows diffuse swelling and high signal intensity on the long TR images. In the chronic stage, diffuse atrophy of the corpus callosum and focal necrosis may be seen in the genu, body, or splenium of the central portion of the corpus callosum **(Figs. 43A and B).** Focal hypointensity on T2-weighted images within the corpus callosum has been described, which has been speculated to represent either hemosiderin deposits or lipid-laden macrophages. MR imaging studies have shown that lesions may also be found in the hemispheric white matter. Two cases of MBD have been reported in which FLAIR and diffusion-weighted imaging studies revealed symmetrical hyperintense lesions in the cerebral cortex, particularly in the lateral-frontal regions, in addition to the callosal lesions, which suggests an association of diffuse cortical lesions such as Morel's laminar sclerosis with MBD.

Differential Diagnosis

- Multiple sclerosis-clinical history is different.
- Diffuse axonal injury-involving corpus callosum-history of trauma
- Transient lesions of the splenium of the corpus callosum-related to epilepsy and cessation of antiepileptic medication.

Subacute Combined Degeneration of the Spinal Cord

Vitamin B_{12} (cobalamin) deficiency may affect the central or peripheral nervous system but mainly involves the spinal cord. Subacute combined degeneration (SCD) refers to demyelination and vacuolation found in the posterior and lateral columns of the spinal cord. Patients present with parasthesias, tingling of hands and feet which evolves to ataxic paraplegia and spasticity. Vitamin B_{12} deficiency is a result of pernicious anemia, gastric bypass surgery and malabsorption syndrome.

Imaging

SCD affects the dorsal and lateral columns of the cord and shows increased signal intensity of the affected cord on T2-weighted sequences **(Figs. 44A and B).**[143] This symmetric bilateral high signal within the cord is referred to as inverted V sign.[144] Mild expansion of the cord may be seen, and mild contrast enhancement has been described. There is typically a

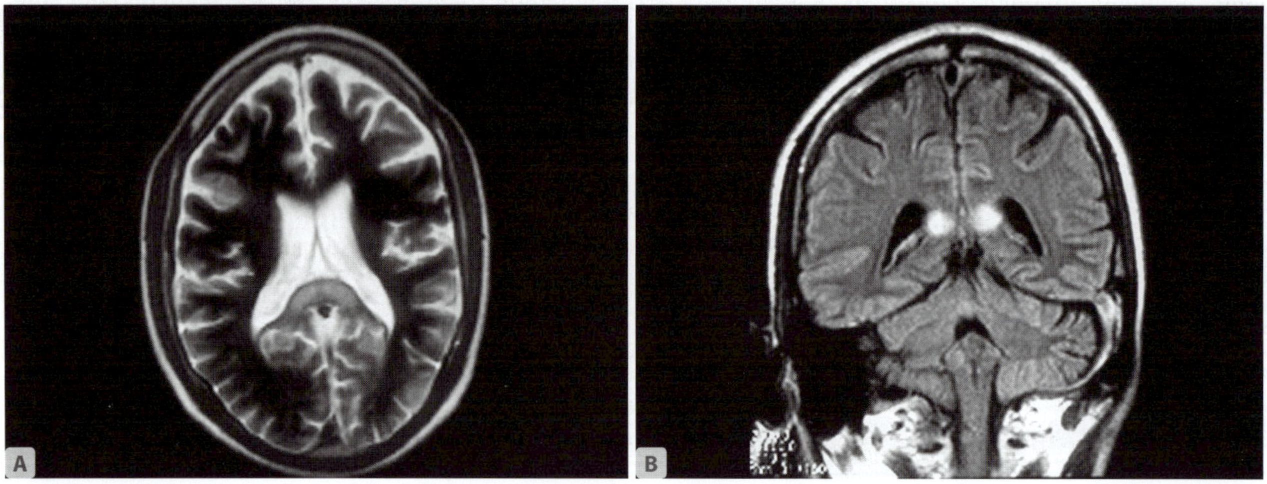

FIGS. 43A AND B: Demyelination seen in the splenium of corpus callosum in an alcoholic patient on T2W axial image (A) and coronal FLAIR image (B)—a case of Marchiafava-bignami disease.

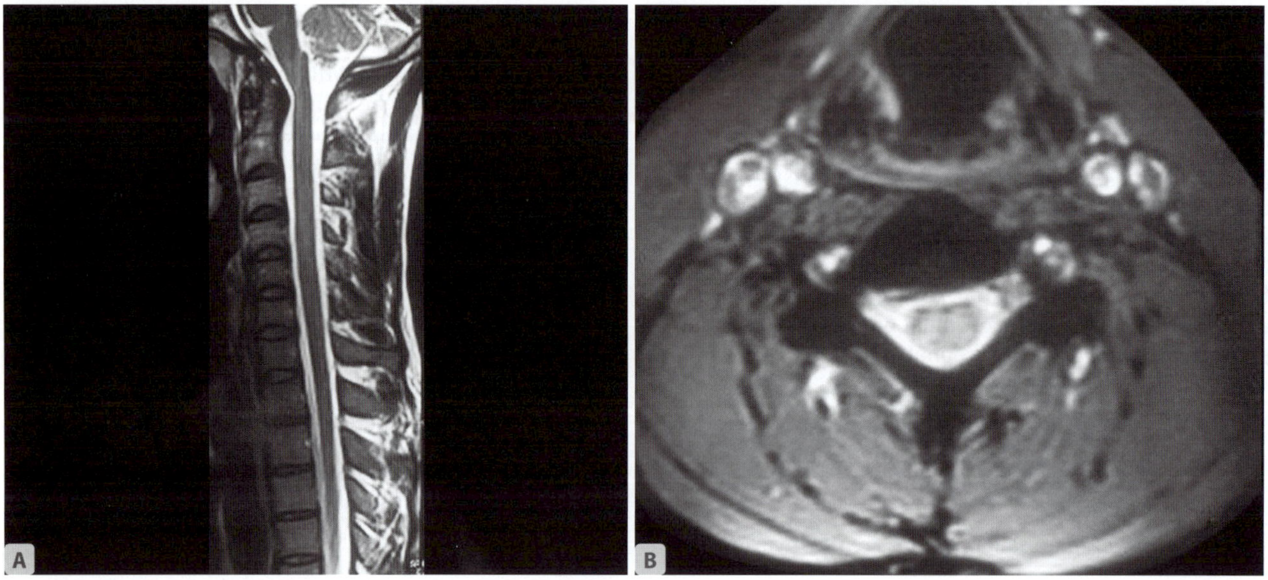

FIGS. 44A AND B: Subacute combined degeneration of the spinal cord (B_{12} deficiency). Sagittal and axial T2W images (A and B) show mild expansion of the cord and increased signal within the dorsal columns of cervical spinal cord.

continuous long segment of signal abnormality confined to the dorsal columns, which may help distinguish this entity from other demyelinating lesions found in the cord that appear patchy in distribution.

Vacuolar myelopathy seen in patients with AIDS may appear similar on imaging, and therefore the clinical history plays an important role in distinguishing these entities. Imaging findings in SCD may resolve after treatment with vitamin B_{12}. MR findings in the brain may reveal areas of high signal intensity on the T2-weighted images in the cerebral white matter that may also resolve after treatment with vitamin B_{12}.

White Matter Diseases Associated with Physical/Chemical Agents or Therapeutic Procedures

There are numerous toxic agents that selectively affect the central nervous system. Specific toxins affect specific vulnerable regions of the brain.

RADIATION INJURY[145-149]

Radiation induced injury to the brain is usually caused by whole brain radiation and with doses of up to 30–40 Gy.

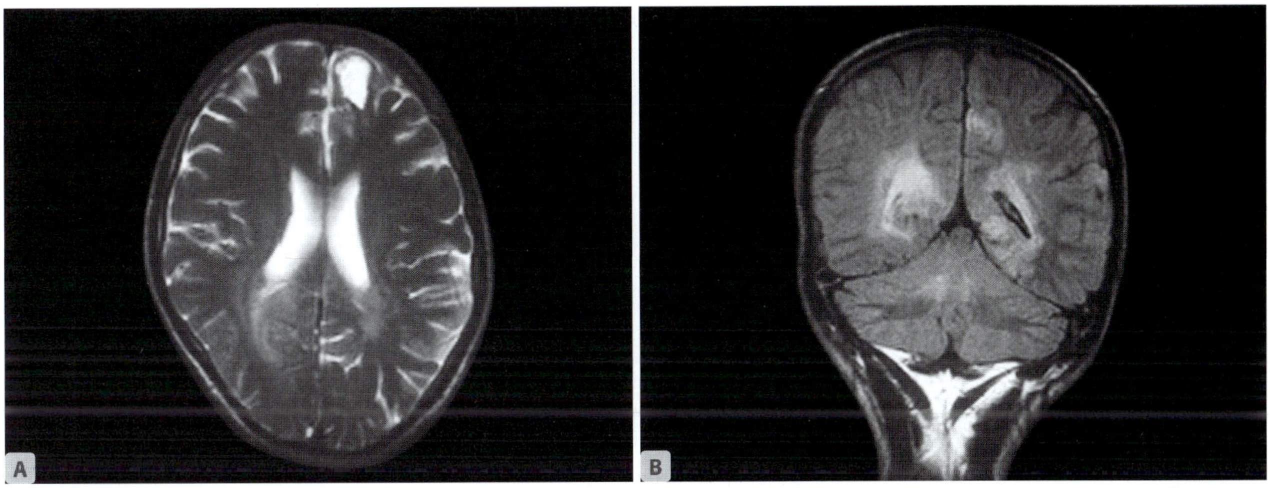

FIGS. 45A AND B: Demyelination following radiotherapy for left frontal lobe astrocytoma. Axial T2W (A) and coronal FLAIR (B) reveal gliosis in left frontal region with poorly marginated subtle hyperintensity in parieto-occipital regions and in the cerebellum.

Associated chemotherapy adds to the risk of radiation injury. It is divided into early and late changes.

Acute radiation injury occurs days to weeks after radiation. This is now rare with use of modern radiation protocols; there can be no changes seen on imaging or transient white matter edema may be seen.

Early radiation injury is noted within 6 months of therapy. Patients may present with cognitive impairment, somnolence. Confluent periventricular hyperintensity is noted which is indicative of transient demyelination. These changes often resolve.

Late delayed injury is seen after 6 months and produce irreversible glial loss noted as necrotizing leukoencephalopathy in deep white matter **(Figs. 45A and B)**. U fibres and corpus callosum are spared. Mass effect and variable enhancement may be seen. The changes depend on total dose of radiation, field size, frequency of dosage and concominant chemotherapy. Various tissues of CNS are affected with oligodendrocytes being most sensitive.

Radiation also predisposes to long term sequlae-vasculopathy (results in ischemic strokes and a moya moya pattern of vasculitis), mineralizing microangiopathy (calcification can be seen in bilateral basal ganglia and subcortical white matter), radiation induced vascular malformation (RIVM)—capillary telangiectasia or cavernomas can be formed. Pediatric patients are at an increased risk. Radiation induced neoplasm are rare, most common being meningioma.

Solvent Vapor Abuse Leukoencephalopathy-Toluene

It is a colorless liquid found in glue, paints and thinner. It is sniffed, huffed or inhaled from a plastic bag. It affects the cerebral white matter and optic nerves. Imaging abnormalities are seen only after several years of abuse. T2/FLAIR hyperintensities are seen in the deep periventricular white matter, centrum semiovale and subcortical areas **(Figs. 46 and 47)**.[150]

Chemotherapy

Various chemotherapeutic drugs such as methotrexate, cytarabine, vincristine have CNS toxicity.

Imaging finding of CNS toxicity include:

Posterior reversible encephalopathy syndrome (PRES)—findings are often atypical with involvement of cerebellum, brainstem and basal ganglia and diffusion restriction with enhancement.

Leukoencephalopathy—confluent T2/FLAIR hyperintensities are seen in periventricular white matter, especially with methotrexate.

Cocaine

Cocaine is sniffed, inhaled or injected. The effects are vascular with patients presenting with spontaneous hemorrhagic strokes due to hypertension. Nearly half of these are associated with rupture of pre-existing aneurysm or underlying vascular malformation. Acute hypertensive encephalopathy-PRES may also be seen.

Differential Diagnosis

- Underlying vascular malformation—unexpected parenchymal hemorrhage in a young adult/middle aged should raise the possibility of drug abuse.
- Embolic infarcts due to heart disease or vasculitis due to any cause (infection, autoimmune, collagen) may appear similar.

Methanol Poisoning

Ingestion of spurious alcohol or accidental ingestion of solvents containing methanol leads to metabolic acidosis due to its metabolite formic acid. It is characterized by headache, visual disturbances and can lead to coma and death. Putamen shows hyperintensity on T2WI **(Figs. 48A and B)**.

Carbon Monoxide Poisoning

It is colorless odorless gas. Poisoning can occur by accident or intentional ingestion. CO attaches to hemoglobin to form

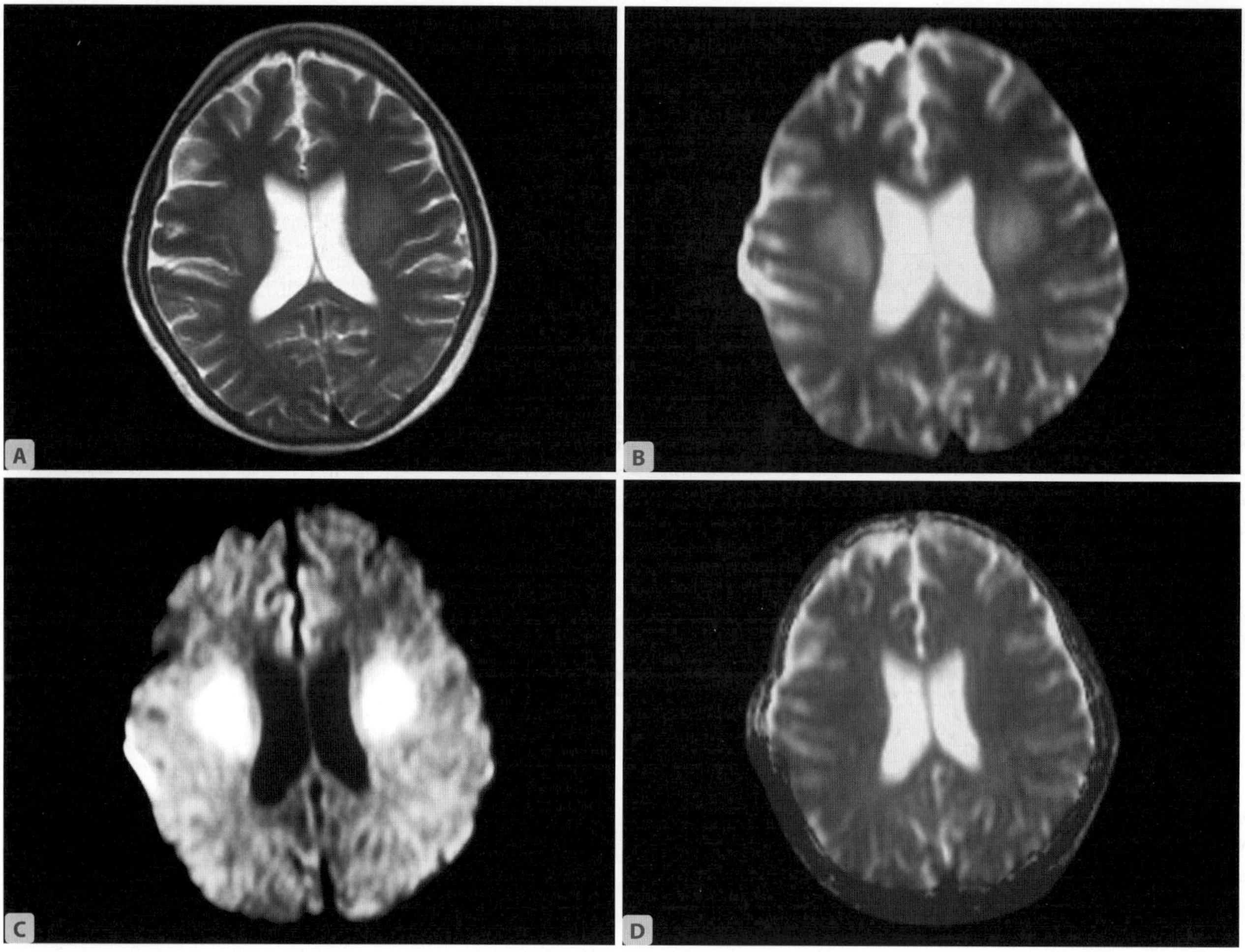

FIGS. 46A TO D: MRI T2 axial image (A) shows hyperintensity in periventricular deep white matter. There is increase in hyperintensity with increase in b values, b = 500 (B) b = 1000 (C) on ADC maps (D) restricted diffusion is seen—toxic demyelination.

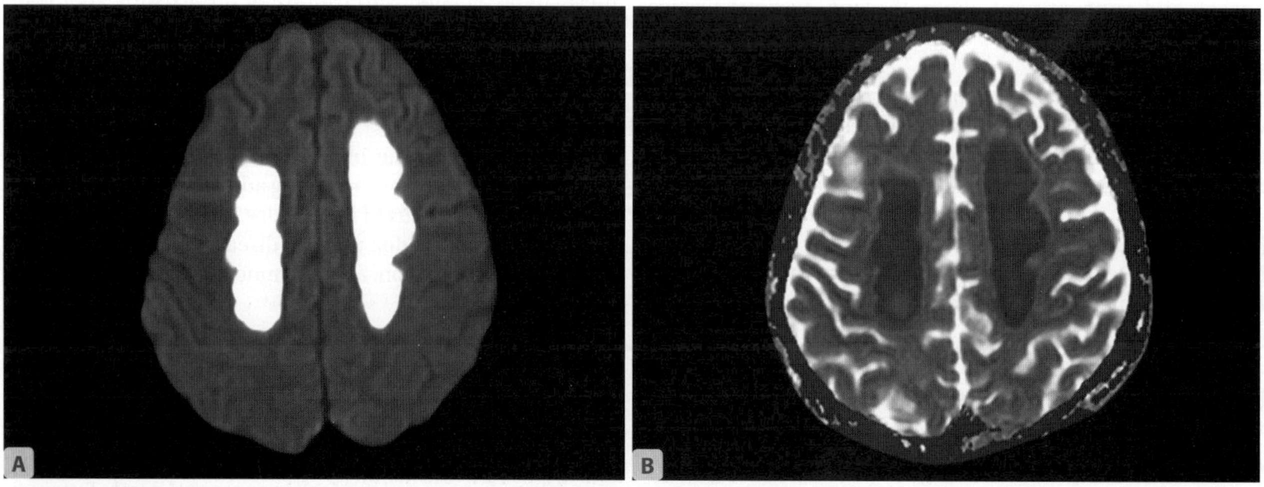

FIGS. 47A AND B: DWI shows restricted diffusion in centrum semiovale in a case of toxic demyelination. Cb = 1000 (A), ADC map (B).

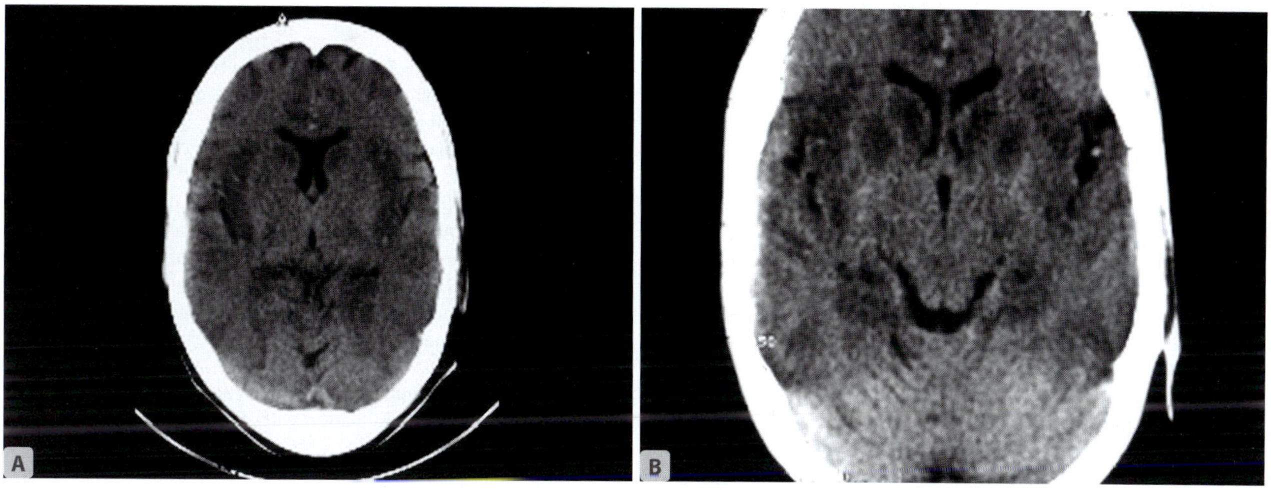

FIGS. 48A AND B: CT scan in a patient with methanol poisoning shows hypodensities within bilateral basal ganglia, subcortical white matter, and insular cortex.

carboxyhemoglobin, reducing its ability to transport oxygen. CO poisoning causes headache, tinnitus, dizziness, loss of consciousness.

Imaging

MR

CO poisoning causes bilateral pallidal necrosis, extending into lenticular nuclei and caudate nuclei which appear hypointense on T1 and hyperintense on T2. There may be involvement of subcortical white matter. Diffusion restriction in basal ganglia may be seen. In patients who survive, the lesions show cavitation and cerebral atrophy. A delayed leukoencephalopathy with extensive bilateral symmetrical confluent areas of hyperintensity on T2/FLAIR may be seen.

Differential Diagnosis: CO Poisoning

- Hypoxic ischemic encephalopathy. HIE affects the entire basal ganglia and hippocampus, rarely only globus pallidus.
- Organophosphorus poisoning- bilateral hemorrhagic pallidal necrosis.
- Wilson disease—involves basal ganglia, midbrain, pons and dentate nucleus.
- Leigh disease affects younger patients; here brainstem and putamen lesions are more common.
- JE-encephalitis preferentially involves the basal ganglia and thalamus.
- Creutzfeldt-Jakob disease—affects caudate nucleus, anterior basal ganglia and cortex. Posteromedial thalamic involvement (pulvinar) is common in CJD and rare in CO poisoning.

Heavy Metal Poisoning

This usually occurs as an occupational health hazard. Manganese poisoning occurs in people working in mining industry or in patients receiving total parenteral nutrition. Manganese gets deposited in basal ganglia and is seen as bilateral global pallidal hyperintensity on T1W images. T2 signal is normal. Mercury poisoning affects people in miners or fish consumers who eat fish from contaminated waters. Mercury accumulates in cerebellar vermis and visual cortex and appears hypointense on T1, iso to hypointense on T2-weighted images.

Amphetamine and Derivatives

There are addictive substances which lead to a short lived feeling of euphoria, increased energy and alertness due to blockage of reuptake of catecholamines. Vascular events such as ischemia, hemorrhage and leukoencephalopathy are noted.[151-153]

Methamphetamine (MA/METH/CRYSTAL) results in both ischemic strokes and hemorrhage. Chronic users show cerebral atrophy, more marked in frontal lobe with nonspecific white matter hyperintensites.

MDMA (Ecstasy)—this is a party drug and causes arterial constriction, vasculitis with acute infarcts.

Benzodiazepine—is frequently prescribed to treat anxiety, insomnia. Overdose can lead to hypoxic encephalopathy, hemorrhagic ischemic strokes.

CONCLUSION

Focal white matter hyperintensities pose a diagnostic challenge as the cause may vary from infectious, inflammatory, neoplastic to nonspecific WMH. A systematic imaging approach including age, history, clinical findings, and pattern of distribution of lesion, enhancement pattern and the use of various MR sequences can help to reach a diagnosis.

REFERENCES

1. Rao, Zimmerman RA (Eds). Cranial MRI and CT (4th edn). New York: Mc Graw Hill; 1999.
2. Nusbaum AO, Kar Ming Fung, Atlas SW. White matter diseases and inherited metabolic disorders. In: Scott W, Atlas (Eds). Magnetic Resonance Imaging of the Brain and Spine (3rd edn). Philadelphia: Lippincott Williams and Wilkins; 2002.
3. Suzuki K, Armao D, Stone JA, et al. Demyelinating diseases, leucodystrophies, and other myelin disorders. Neuroimaging Clin North Am. 2001;11:1.
4. Lakhanpal SK, Maravilla KR. Multiple sclerosis. In: Stark DD, Bradley WG (Eds). Magnetic Resonance Imaging, 3rd ed. St Louls Mo: Mosby; 1999. pp. 1379-402.
5. Jacobs I, Kinkel WR, Polachini I, et al. Correlations of nuclear magnetic resonance imaging, computerized tomography, and clinical profiles in multiple sclerosis. Neurology. 1986;36:27-34.
6. Fillipi M. In vivo characterization of multiple sclerosis and other white matter diseases using magnetic resonance based techniques. Neurology. 2001;248:1019-29.
7. Garaci FG, Marzialis S, Meschini A, et al. Brain haemodynamic changes associated with chronic cerebrospinal venous insufficiency are not specific to multiple sclerosis and do not increase its severity. Radiology. 2012;265(1):233-9.
8. Flynn KC, Flynn Lc, Moster ML. Current thoughts on chronic cerebrospinal venous insufficiency in multiple sclerosis. Curr Opin Ophthalmol. 2011;22(6):463-7.
9. Ghezzi A, Comi G, Federico A. Chronic cerebrospinal venous insufficiency and multiple sclerosis. Neurol Sci. 2011;32(1):17-21.
10. Koch-Henriksen N, Sørensen PS. The changing demographic pattern of multiple sclerosis epidemiology. Lancet Neurol. 2010;9(5):520-32.
11. Fujihara K, Onk BK. MS across continents: challenging our knowledge of MS in Asia and the middle East – Report from 2nd MS Forum Pan – Asian Conference, 19-20 November.
12. Swanton JK, Rovira A, Tintore M, et al. MRI criteria for multiple sclerosis in patients presenting with clinically isolated syndromes: a multicentric retrospective study. Lancet Neurol. 2007;6:677-86.
13. Achten E, Deblaere K. Health technology assessment on the use of magnetic resonance imaging (MRI) and computed tomography (CT) in the diagnosis of multiple sclerosis (MS) and clinically isolated syndromes CIS. European Journal of Radiology. 2008;65:211-3.
14. Montalban X, Tintore M, Swanton J, et al. MRI criteria for MS in patients with clinically isolated syndromes. Neurology. 2010;74(5):427-34.
15. Inglese M. Multiple sclerosis: new insights and trends. AJNR. 2006;27:954-7.
16. Ge Y. Multiple sclerosis: the role of MR imaging. Am J Neuro Radiol. 2006;27:1165.
17. Granberg T, Martola J, Kristoffersen-Wiberg M, et al. Radiologically isolated syndrome. Incidental magnetic resonance imaging findings suggestive of multiple sclerosis-a systemic review. Mult Scler. 2013;19(3):271-80.
18. Sarbu N, Shih RY, Jones RV, et al. White matter diseases with radiologic-pathologic correlation. Radiographics. 2016;36(5):1426-47.
19. Gold Man MD, Cohen JA. Multiple sclerosis. In: Rakel RE, Bope ET (Eds). Conn's Current Therapy. Philadelphia: Elsevier Saunders; 2005. pp. 1057-66.
20. Kornienko VN, Pronin IN. Diagnostic Neuroradiology. Springer Verlag; 2008.
21. Fillipi M, Evangelou N, Kangarlu A, et al. Ultrahigh field MR imaging in multiple sclerosis.J Neurol Neurosurg Psychiatry. 2014;85(1):60-6.
22. Fazekas F, Barkhof F, Filippi M, et al. The contribution of magnetic resonance imaging to the diagnosis of multiple sclerosis. Neurology. 1999;53:448-56.
23. Jackson JA, Leake DR, Schneiders NJ, et al. Magnetic resonance imaging in multiple sclerosis: Results in 22 cases. Am J Neuroradiol. 1985;6:171-6.
24. Gean Marton AD, Venzina LG, Marton KI, et al. Abnormal corpus callosum: a sensitive and specific indicator of multiple sclerosis. Radiology. 1991;180:215-21.
25. Lisanti CJ, Asbach P, Bradley WG. The ependymal 'Dot–Dash' sign. An MR imaging finding of early Multiple sclerosis. AJNR. 2005;26:2033-6.
26. Roosendaal SD, Moraal B, Pouwels PJW, et al. Accumalation of cortical lesions in MS: relation with cognitive impairment. Mult Scler. 2009;15(6):708-14.
27. Filippi M, Rocca MA,Calabrese M, et al. Intracortical lesions: relevance for new MRI siagnostic criteria for multiple sclerosis. Neurology. 2010;75(22):1988-94.
28. de Graaf WL, Kilsdonk ID, Lopez-Soriano A, et al. Clinical application of multi contrast 7T MR imaging in multiple sclerosis: increased lesion detection compared to 3 T confined to gray matter. Eur Radiol. 2013;23(2):528-40.
29. Filippi M, Rocca MA. MR imaging of multiple sclerosis. Radiology. 2011;259(3):659-81
30. Edwards MK, Farlow MR, Stevens JC. Cranial MR in spinal cord MS: diagnosing patients with isolated spinal cord symptoms. Am J Neuroradiol. 1986;7:1003-5.
31. Thielen KR, Miller GM. Multiple sclerosis of the spinal cord: magnetic resonance appearance. J Comput Assist Tomogr. 1996;20:434-8.
32. Smith RR, Edwards MK, Farlow MR, et al. Imaging of optic neuritis using STIR MR. Am J Neuroradiol. 1989;10:905(abstr).
33. Miller DH, Barkhof F, Nauta JJ. Gadolinium enhancement increases the sensitivity of MRI in detecting disease activity in multiple sclerosis. Brain. 1993;116:1077-94.
34. Tas MW, Barkhol F, Van Walderveen MA, et al. The effect of gadolinium on the sensitivity and specifig of MR in the initial diagnosis of multiple sclerosis. Am J Neuro Radiol. 2005;26:2316-9.
35. Silver NC, Good CD, Barker GJ, et al. Sensitivity of contrast enhanced MRI in multiple sclerosis. Effects of gadoliniumdose, magnetisation transfer contrast and delayed imaging. Brain. 1997:120(pt 7):1149.
36. Rovira A, Leon A. MR in the diagnosis and monitoring of multiple sclerosis: an over view. European Journal of Radiology. 2008;67:409-14.
37. Simon JH. Update on multiple sclerosis. Radial Clin N Am. 2006;44:79-100.
38. Lane B. Leucoencephalopathies and demyelinating disease. In: Haaga JR (Ed). Computed Tomography and Magnetic Resonance Imaging of the Whole Body (5th edn), Mosby: Elsiever; 2009.
39. Van Walderveen MA, Kamphorst W, Scheltens P, et al. Histopathologic correlates of hypointense lesions on T1 – weighted spin – echo MRI in multiple sclerosis. Neurology 1998;50:1282-8.
40. Allen IV, Mc Quaid S, Mirakhur M, et al. Pathological abnormalities in the normal appearing white matter in multiple sclerosis. Neurol Sci. 2001;22:141-4.
41. Bozzali M, Rocca MA, Iannucci G, et al. Magnetization transfer histogram analysis of the cervical cord in patients with multiple sclerosis. Am J Neuroradiol. 1999;20:1803-8.
42. Van Buchem MA, McGowan JC, Kolson DL, et al. Quantitative volumetric magnetization transfer analysis in multiple sclerosis: Estimation of macroscopic and microscopic disease burden. Magn Reson Med. 1996;36:632-6.

43. Loevner LA, Grossman RI, Cohen J, et al. Microscopic disease in normal - appearing white matter on conventional MR images in patients with multiple sclerosis: Assessment with magnetization— transfer measurements. Radiology. 1995;196:511-5.
44. Bischof A, Caverzasi E, Cordano C, et al. Advances in imaging Multiple sclerosis. Semin Neurol. 2017;37:538-54.
45. Bammer R, Augustin M, Strasser Fuchs S, et al. Magnetic resonance diffusion tensor imaging for characterising diffuse and focal matter abnormalities in multiple sclerosis. Magn Reson Med. 2000;44:583-91.
46. Basser PJ, Pierpaoli C. Microstructural and physiological features of tissues elucidated by quantitative - diffusion - tensor MRI. J Magn Reson. 1996;111:209-19.
47. Pierpaoli C, Jezzard P, Basser PJ, et al. Diffusion tensor MR imaging of the human brain. Radiology. 1996;201:637-48.
48. Bammer R, Fazekas F. Diffusion imaging in multiple sclerosis. Neuroimag Clin North Am. 2002;12(1):71-106.
49. Nusbaum AO, Tang CY, Wei T, et al. Whole – brain diffusion MR histograms differ between MS subtypes. Neurology. 2000;54:1421-7.
50. Pagani E, Bammer R, Horsfield MN, et al. Diffusion MR imaging in Multiple sclerosis. Technical aspects and challenges. AJNR. 2007;28:411-20.
51. Nusbaum AO, Lu D, Tang CY, et al. Quantitative diffusion measurements in focal multiple sclerosis lesions: Correlation with appearance on T1-weighted MR images. Am J Roentgenol. 2000;175:821-5.
52. Davie CA, Hawkins CP, Barker GJ, et al. Serial proton magnetic resonance spectroscopy in acute multiple sclerosis lesions. Brain. 1994;117:49-58.
53. Arnold DL, Mathews PM, Francis GS, et al. Proton magnetic resonance spectroscopic imaging for metabolic characterization of demyelinating plaques. Ann Neurol. 1992;31:235-41.
54. De Stefano N, Bartolozzi ML, Guidi L, et al. Magnetic resonance spectroscopy as a measure of brain damage in multiple sclerosis. J Neurol Sci. 2005;233:203-8.
55. Tartaglia MC, Narayanan S, De Stefano N, et al. Choline is increased in prelesional normal appearing white matter in multiple sclerosis. J Neurol. 2002;249:1382-90.
56. Fillipi M, Rocca MA, Mezzapesa DM, et al. Simple and complex movement. Associated functional MRI changes in patients at presentation with clinically isolated syndromes suggestive of multiple sclerosis. Hum Brain Mapp. 2004;21:108-17.
57. Filippi M, Rocca MA, Mezzapesa DM, et al. A functional MRI study of cortical activations associated with object manipulation in patients with MS. Neuro Image. 2004;21:1147-54.
58. Law M, Saindane AM, Ge Y, et al. Microvascular abnormality in relapsing – remitting multiple sclerosis: perfusion MR imaging findings in normal appearing white matter. Radiology. 2004;231:645-52.
59. Laule C, Leung E, Lis DK, et al. Myelin water imaging in multiple sclerosis: quantitative correlations with histopathology. Mult Scler. 2006;12(06):747-53.
60. Mc Donald WI, Compston A, Edan G, et al. Recommended diagnostic criteria for multiple sclerosis: guidelines from the international panel on the diagnosis of multiple sclerosis. Ann Neurol. 2001;50:121-7.
61. Polman CH, Reingold SC, Edan G, et al. Diagnostic criteria for multiple sclerosis: 2005 revisions to the McDonald criteria. Ann Neurol. 2005;58:840-6.
62. Polman CH, Reingold SC, Banwell B, et al. Diagnostic criteria for multiple sclerosis: 2010 revisions to the McDonald criteria. Ann Neurol. 2011;69(2):292-302.
63. Filippi M, Rocca MA, Ciccarelli O, et al. MRI criteria for the diagnosis of multiple sclerosis: MAGNIMS consensus guidelines. The Lancet. Neurology. 2016;15 (3):292-303.
64. Thompson AJ, Banwell BL, Barkhof F, et al. Diagnosis of multiple sclerosis: 2017 revisions of the McDonald criteria. The Lancet. Neurology. 2017;17(2)162-73.
65. Kwee RM, Kwee TC. Virchow-Robin spaces at MR Imaging. Radiographics. 2007;27:1071-86.
66. Galluzzi S, Lanni C, Pantoni L, et al.White matter lesions in the elderly: pathophysiological hypothesis on the effect on brain plasticity and treseve. J Neurol Sci. 2008;273(1-2):3-9.
67. Igarashi H, Sakai F, Kan S, et al. Magnetic resonance imaging of the brain in patients with migraine. Cephalagia. 1991;11:69-74.
68. Berger JR. Functional improvement and symptom management in multiple sclerosis: clinical efficacy of current therapies. Am J Manag Care. 2011;17(Suppl 5):S146-53.
69. Brust JC. Current diagnosis & Treatment in Neurology. McGraw-Hill Medical; 2006.
70. McNamara C, Sugrue G, Murray B, et al. Current and emerging therapies in multiple sclerosis: implications for the radiologist, Part 1-mechanisms, efficacy, and safety. AJNR. 2017;38(9):1664-71.
71. McNamara C, Sugrue G, Murray B, et al. Current and emerging therapies in multiple sclerosis: implications for the radiologist, Part 2-surveillance for treatment complications and disease progression. AJNR. 2017;38(9):1772-80.
72. Canellas AR, et al. Idiopathic inflammatory -demyelinating diseases of the central nervous system. Neuroradiology. 2007;49(5):393-409.
73. Cha S, Pierce S, Knopp EA, et al. Dynamic contrast-enhanced T2*-weighted MR imaging of tumefactive demyelinating lesions. AJNR Am J Neuroradiol. 2001;22 (6): 1109-16.
74. Dagher AP, Smirniotopoulos J. Tumefactive demyelinating lesions. Neuroradiology. 1996;38(6): 560-5.
75. Given CA, Stevens BS, Lee C. The MRI appearance of tumefactive demyelinating lesions. Am J Roentgenol. 2004; 182 (1):195-9.
76. Masdeu JC, Moreira J, Trasi S, et al. The open ring. A new imaging sign in demyelinating disease. J Neuroimaging. 1996;6(2):104-7.
77. Paley RJ, Persing JA, Doctor A, et al. Multiple sclerosis and brain tumor: a diagnostic challenge. J Emerg Med. 1989;7(3):241-4.
78. Saindane AM, Cha S, Law M, et al. Proton MR spectroscopy of tumefactive demyelinating lesions. Am J Neuroradiol. 2002;23(8):1378-86.
79. Fallah A, Banglawala S, Ebrahim S, et al. Case Series: tumefactive demyelinating lesions: a diagnostic challenge. Can J Surg. 2010;53(1):69-70.
80. Eckstein C, Saidha S, Levy M. A differential diagnosis of central nervous system demyelination : beyond multiple sclerosis. J Neurol. 2012;295(5):801-16.
81. Wingerchuk DM, Lennon VA, Pittock SJ, et al: Revised diagnostic criteria for neuromyelitis optica. Neurology. 2006;66(10):1485-9.
82. Barnett Y, Sutton IJ, Ghadiri M, et al. Conventional and advanced imaging in neuromyelitis optica. Am J Neuroradiol. 2013. doi:10.3174/ajnr.A3592.
83. Chang KH, Lyu RK, Chen CM, et al. Distinct features between longitudinally extensive transverse myelitis presenting with and without anti-aquaporin 4 antibodies. Mult. Scler. 2013;19 (3): 299-307.
84. Bruna Garbugio Dutra, Antônio José da Rocha, Renato Hoffmann Nunes, et al. Neuromyelitis optica spectrum disorders: spectrum of MR imaging findings and their differential diagnosis. RadioGraphics. 2018;38(1):169-93.
85. Lu Z, Zhang B, Qiu W, et al. Comparative brain stem lesions on MRI of acute disseminated encephalomyelitis, neuromyelitis optica and multiple sclerosis. PLoS One 2011;6(8):e22766.

86. Barnett Y,Sutton IJ,Ghadiri M, et al.Conventional and advanced imaging in neuromyelitis optica. Am J Neuroradiol. 2014;35(8):1458-66.
87. Huh SY, Min JH, Kim W, et al. The usefulness of brain MEI at onset in the differentiation of multiple sclerosis and seropositive neuromyelitis optica spectrum disorders. Mult Scler. 2014;20(6):695-704.
88. Rovira A, Sastre-Garriga J, Auger C, et al. Idiopathic inflammatory diseases of the brainstem. Semin Ultrasound CTMR. 2013;34(2):123-30.
89. Sahraian MA, Radue EW, Minagar A. Neuromyelitis optica: clinical manifestations and neuroimaging features. Neurol Clin. 2013;31(1):139-52.
90. Yonezu T, Ito S, Mori M, et al. "Bright spotty lesions" on spinal magnetic resonance imaging differentiates neuromyelitis optica from multiple sclerosis. Mult Scler. 2014;20(3):331-7.
91. Kister I, Herbert J, Zhou Y, et al. Ultra high field MR (7T) imaging of brain lesions in neuromyelitis optica. Mult Scler INT. 2013;2013:398259.
92. Tenembaum SN. Disseminated encephalomyelitis in children. Clin Neurol Neurisyrg. 2008;110(9):928-38.
93. DeSanto J, Ross JS. Spine infection/inflammation. Radiol Clin North Am. 2011:49(1):105-27.
94. Lee HY, Chang KH, Kim JH, et al. Serial MR imaging findings of acute hemorrhagic leukoencephalitis: a case report. Am J Neuroradiol. 2005;26(8):1996-9.
95. Wong AM, Simon EM, Zimmerman RA, et al. Acute necrotizing encephalopathy of childhood: correlation of MR findings and clinical outcome. Am J Neuroradiol. 2006; 27(9): 1919-23.
96. Mark AS, Atlas SW. Progressive multifocal leucoencephalopathy in patients with AIDS: appearance on MR images. Radiology. 1989;173:517-21.
97. Mader I, Herrlinger U, Klose U, et al. Progressive multifocal leucoencephalopathy: analysis of lesion development with diffusion weighted MRI. Neuroradiol. 2003;45:717-21.
98. Lanska DL. Epidemiology of human immunodeficiency virus dementia. Semin Neurol. 1999;19:105-11
99. Thurnber MM, Thurnber SA, Fleischmann D, et al. Comparison of T2-weighted and fluid – attenuated inversion – recovery fast spin echo MR sequences in intracerebral AIDS – associated disease. Am J Neuroradiol. 1997;18:1601-9.
100. Dousset V, Armand JP, Lacoste D. Magnetization transfer study of HIV encephalitis and progressive multifocal leucoencephalopathy. Am J Neuroradiol. 1997;18:895-901.
101. Berger JR, Major EO. Progressive multifocal leucoencephalopathy. Semin Neurol. 1999;19:223-33.
102. Bag AK, Curé JK, Chapman PR, et al. JC virus infection of the brain. AJNR Am J Neuroradiol. 2010;31 (9):1564-76.
103. Clifford DB, Ances BM. HIV-associated neurocognitive disorder. Lancet Infect Dis. 2013;13(11): 976-86.
104. Smith A, Smirniotopoulos J, Rushing E. Central nervous system infections associated with human immunodeficiency virus infection: radiologic-pathologic correlation1. Radiographics. 2008;28(7):2033-58.
105. Barker PB, Lee RR, McArthus JC. AIDS dementia complex: evaluation with proton MR spectroscopic imaging. Radiology. 1995;195:58-64.
106. Hildenbrand P, Craven DE, Jones R, et al. Lyme neuroborreliosis: manifestations of a rapidly emerging zoonosis. Am J Neuradiol. 2009;30(6):1079-87.
107. Wardlaw JM, Smith EE, Bissels GJ, et al. Neuroimaging standards for research into small vessel disease and its contribution to ageing and neurodegeneration. Lancet Neurol. 2013;128:822-38.
108. Schmidt R, Schmidt H, Haybaeck J, et al. Heterogenity in age related white matter changes. Acta Neuropathol (Berl). 2001;122(2):171-85.
109. Gallasi R, Morrreale A, Montagna P, et al. Binswanger's disease and normal pressure hydrocephlus. Arch Neurol. 1991;48:1156-9.
110. Biffi A, Greenberg SM. Cerebral amyloid angiopathy: a systematic review. J Chin Neurol. 2011;7(1):1-9.
111. Knudsen KA, Rosand J, Karluk D, et al. Clinical diagnosis of cerebral amyloid angiopathy: validation of the boston criteria. Neurology. 2010;74(17):1346-50.
112. Tournier-Lasserve E, Iba Zizen MT, Romero N, et al. Autosomal dominant syndrome with stroke like episodes and leucoencephalopathy. Stroke. 1991;22:1297-302.
113. Chabriat H,Vahedi K, Iba-Zizen MT, et al. Clinical spectrum of CADASIL: a study of 7 families-cerebral autosomal dominant arteriopathy with subcortical infarcts and leukoencephalopathy. Lancet 1995;346(8980):934-9.
114. Singhal S, Rich P, Markus HS. The spatial distribution of MR imaging abnormalities in cerebral autosomal dominant arteriopathy with subcortical infarcts and leukoencephalopathy and their relationship to age and clinical features. Am J Neuradiol. 2005;26(10):2481-7.
115. Salavari C, Brown RD Jr, Calamia KT et al. Primary central venous system vasculitis: analysis of 101 patients. Ann Neurol. 2007;62:442-51.
116. Abdel Razek AAK, Alvarez H, et al. Imaging spectrum of CNS vasculitis. Radiographics. 2014;34(4):873-94.
117. Birnbaum J, Hellmann DB. Primary angiitis of the central nervous system. Arch Neurol. 2009;66(6):704-9.
118. Susac JO. Susac's syndrome. Am J Neuroradiol. 2004;25 (3): 351-2.
119. Demir MK. Case 142: Susac syndrome. Radiology. 2009;250 (2):598-602.
120. Susac JO, Hardman JM, Selhorst JB. Microangiopathy of the brain and retina. Neurology. 1979;29(3):313-6.
121. Gross M, Eliashar R. Update on Susac's syndrome. Curr Opin Neurol. 2005;18(3):311-4.
122. Saenz R, Quan AW, Magalhaes A, et al. MRI of Susac's syndrome. Am J Roentgenol. 2005;184(5):1688-90.
123. Susac JO, Egan RA, Rennebohm RM, et al. Susac's syndrome: 1975-2005 microangiopathy/autoimmune endotheliopathy. J Neurol Sci. 2007;257(1-2):270-2.
124. Buzzard KA, Reddel SW, Yiannikas C, et al. Distinguishing Susac's syndrome from multiple sclerosis. Journal of Neurology. 2015;262(7):1613-21.
125. Goh YP, Naidoo P, Ngian GS. Imaging of systemic lupus erythematosus. Part I: CNS, cardiovascular, and thoracic manifestations. Clinical Radiology. 2013;68(2):181-91.
126. Lalani TA, Kanne JP, Hatfield GA, et al. Imaging findings in systemic lupus erythematosus. Radiographics: a review publication of the Radiological Society of North America, Inc. 24(4): 1069-86.
127. Luyendijk J, Steens SC, Ouwendijk WJ et al. Neuropsychiatric systemic lupus erythematosus: lessons learned from magnetic resonance imaging. Arthritic Rheum. 2011;63(3):722-32.
128. Noel N, Hutié M, Wechsler B, et al. Pseudotumoural presentation of neuro-Behcet's disease: case series and review of literature. Rheumatology (Oxford). 2012; 51(7):1216-25.
129. Gerard D, Healy ME, Hesselink JR. MR demonstration of mesencephalic lesions in osmotic demyelination syndrome (central pontine myelinolysis). Neuroradiology. 1987;29:582-84.
130. Lampl C, Yazdi K. Central pontine myelinolysis. Euro Neurol. 2002;47:3-10.
131. King JD, Rosner MH. Osmotic demyelination syndrome. Am J Med Sci. 2010;339(6):561-7.
132. De Souza A, Desai PK. More often striated myelinosis than pontine? A consecutive series of patients with osmotic demyelination syndrome. Neurol Res. 2012;34(3):262-71.

133. Engelter ST, Petrella JR, Alberts MJ, et al. Assessment of cerebral microcirculation in a patient with hypertensive encephalopathy using MR perfusion imaging. Am J Roentgenol. 1999;173: 1491-3.
134. Senger AR, Gupta RK, Dhanuka AK, et al. MR imaging, MR angiography, and MR spectroscopy of the brain in eclampsia. Am J Neuroradiol. 1997;18:1485-90.
135. Fugate JE, Claassen DO, Cloft HJ, et al. Posterior reversible encephalopathy syndrome: associated clinical and radiological findings. Mayo Clin Proc. 2010;85(50:427-32.
136. Ni J, Zhou LX, Hao HL, et al. the clinical and radiological spectrum of posterior reversible encephalopathy syndrome. A retrospective series of 24 patients. J Neuro Imaging. 2011;21(3):219-24.
137. Bartynski WS. Posterior reversible encephalopathy syndrome, Part 1: fundamental imaging and clinical features. AJNR. 2008;29(6):1036-42.
138. Geibprasert S, Gallucci M, Krings T. Alcohol induced changes in the brain as assessed by MRI and CT, Eur Radiol. 2010;20(6): 1492-501.
139. Zuccoli G, Gallucci M, Capellades J, et al. Wernicke encephalopathy: MR findings at clinical presentation in twenty-six alcoholic and nonalcoholic patients. Am J Neuroradiol. 2007;28 (7):1328-31.
140. Zuccoli G, Pipitone N. MR imaging: an increasingly important tool in the early diagnosis of Wernicke encephalopathy. Am J Neuroradiol. 2012;33(6): E92.
141. Arbelaez A, Pajon A, Castillo M. Acute Marchiafava Bignami disease: MR findings in two patients. Am J Neuroradiol. 2003;24: 1955-7.
142. Johkura K, Naito M, Naka T. Cortical involvement in Marchiafava Bignami disease. Am J Neuroradiol. 2005; 26:670-3.
143. Ravina B, Loevner LA, Bank W. MR findings in subacute combined degeneration of the spinal cord: a case of reversible cervical myelopathy. Am J Roentgenol. 2000; 174(3):863-5.
144. Kumar A, Singh AK. Teaching neuroimage: inverted V sign in subacute combined degeneration of spinal cord. Neurology. 2009;72(1):e4.
145. Chan Y, Leung S, King AD, et al. Late radiation injury to the temporal lobes: Morphologic evaluation at MR imaging. Radiology. 1999;213:800-7.
146. Greene-Schloesser D, Robbins ME, Peiffer AM, et al. Radiation induced brain injury: a review. Front Oncol. 2012;2:73.
147. Vázquez E, Delgado I, Sánchez-Montañez A, et al. Side effects of oncologic therapies in the paediatric central nervous system: update on neuro imaging findings. Radiographics. 2011;31(4):1123-39.
148. Chowdhary A, Spence AM, Sales L, et al. Radiation associated tumours following therapeutic cranial radiation. Surg Neurol Int. 2012;3:48.
149. Brown MS, Stemmer SM, Simon JH, et al. White matter disease induced by high-dose chemotherapy: longitudinal study with MR imaging and proton spectroscopy. Am J Neuroradiol. 1998;19:217-21.
150. Rosenberg NL, Kleinschmidt-DeMasters BK, Davis KA, et al. Toluene abuse causes diffuse central nervous system white matter changes. Ann Neurol. 1988;23:611.
151. Tamrazi B, Almast J. Your brain on drugs: imaging of drug related changes in central nervous system. Radiographics. 2012;32(3):701-19.
152. De Smet K, De Maeseneer M, Talebian YA, et al. Bilateral globus pallidus infarcts in ecstasy use. JBR-BTR. 2011;94(2):93-201.
153. Geibprasert S, Gallucci M, Krings T. Addictive illegal drugs: structural neuroimaging. Am J Neuroradiol. 2010; 31(5):803-8.

CHAPTER

195

Imaging of Epilepsy

Shailesh B Gaikwad, Anuj Prabhakar

INTRODUCTION

As per the International League Against Epilepsy, an epileptic seizure is defined as "a transient occurrence of signs and/or symptoms due to abnormal excessive or synchronous neuronal activity in the brain". Epilepsy is a disease involving the central nervous system that is characterized by any of the following features:

1. Atleast 2 seizures that are unprovoked and occur within 24 hours of each other.
2. One unprovoked seizure and a probability of further seizures similar to the general recurrence risk after 2 unprovoked seizures, occurring over the next 10 years.
3. Diagnosis of an epilepsy syndrome.[1]

The disease afflicts all age groups and socioeconomic strata. It has a significant impact on the quality of life of most patients. The incidence of epilepsy in children varies from 50 to 100 cases per 100,000 persons per year. The highest incidence occurs in the first year of life.[2] Brain imaging is an important part of epilepsy management. Conservative treatment with antiepileptic drugs fails to control seizures in up to one third of the patients. Surgery is helpful in such cases. Presurgical imaging is essential to localize the lesions.

All populations of epilepsy patients do not require imaging. Imaging is useful in the following subsets:[1]

1. Focal seizures that can be localized to a particular part of the brain based on the characteristics of the seizure, abnormalities on the electroencephalogram (EEG), history or examination.
2. Abnormalities in neurological examination like focal deficits, neurocutaneous syndromes or syndromes associated with cerebral malformations.
3. Developmental regression, delay or arrest in children.
4. Children with clinical features suggestive of symptomatic generalized epilepsy syndromes like early Lennox-Gastaut syndrome or infantile spasms.
5. Children younger than two years of age (Those suffering from febrile seizures are to be excluded).
6. Atypical course of seizures.
7. Raised intra cranial pressure.
8. History of status epilepticus.

Imaging is not indicated in:

1. Patients with primary generalized epilepsy
2. Typical absence epilepsy (petit mal)
3. Juvenile myoclonic epilepsy
4. Patients with benign partial epilepsy with either centrotemporal or occipital spikes.
5. Children with simple febrile convulsions.

Rapid advances in the field of imaging have lead to a large number of different imaging techniques that may be utilized to evaluate of a patient with seizure disorder. Imaging techniques may be used to evaluate either the functional or structural substrates of the disease. MRI with nuclear imaging is the main stay of epilepsy imaging nowadays. The primary role of imaging is to detect any form of structural abnormality that might be responsible for seizures.

MRI PROTOCOLS

Patients suffering from chronic epilepsy need to be evaluated using specific imaging protocols which must be tailored to best demonstrate the structural and functional abnormalities. Imaging must be preferably performed at 3T field strength as the image clarity, spatial resolution and contrast resolution are better as compared to 1.5 Tesla MRI scanners.[3] Axial T2, volumetric 3DT1 and 3D FLAIR sequences covering the whole brain are acquired. In order to evaluate temporal lobe sclerosis additional FLAIR and inversion recovery sequences are acquired in the coronal oblique plane that is perpendicular to the hippocampus. The slice thickness in these coronal oblique sections is kept to a minimum (2-3 mm). The entire hippocampus including the head, body and tail must be imaged. Gradient recalled echo and susceptibility weighted imaging are useful to identify small foci of calcification or hemosiderin deposition. Other sequences that may be included in the protocol are diffusion tensor imaging (DTI) and 3D double inversion recovery (DIR). 3D DIR sequence is very sensitive for cortical abnormalities. Non contrast perfusion imaging using pseudo continuous or continuous arterial spin labeling (ASL) is also performed. If a tumor is considered as the cause of epilepsy, a post contrast 3D T1-weighted fast spin echo sequence must be performed to look for enhancement. Specialized sequences like T2* relaxometry and spectroscopy may be performed if necessary.

Structural Lesions in Chronic Epilepsy

The histological findings in patients undergoing surgery for temporal lobe epilepsy reveal mesial temporal sclerosis (50–70%) to be the commonest abnormality, with tumors, developmental abnormalities of neuronal migration and cortical organization, vascular malformations and post-traumatic, inflammatory or ischemic gliosis being found less frequently. A non-specific or normal histological examination is found in 10–25%.

Mesial Temporal Lobe Epilepsy

Mesial temporal lobe epilepsy occurs due to lesions involving the temporal lobe. Hippocampal sclerosis (HS) is the most common pathology affecting the mesial temporal lobe. This is characterized by gliosis and neuronal loss involving the hippocampus. Neuronal pathways undergo reorganization which leads to formation of epileptogenic focus.[4] Hippocampal sclerosis may be associated with a preceding insult like childhood febrile seizures, trauma during birth, perinatal insults, encephalitis. It is the commonest cause of intractable epilepsy. Surgical resection of the anterior temporal lobe and hippocampus has good results in such patients and renders up to 90% of these patients seizure-free. HS affects older children and young adults. Clinically, most patients present with aura and complex partial seizures

The two primary MRI findings of HS are hippocampal atrophy (usually recognized by asymmetry in the case of unilateral atrophy) **(Figs. 1A to C)** and increased T2 signal intensity of the hippocampus.[5] Atrophy of the fornix, mammillary body and widening of the choroid fissure on the ipsilateral side are seen. Other secondary imaging features include temporal horn dilatation, ipsilateral atrophy of the temporal lobe, poor gray-white matter differentiation in the parahippocampus and loss of hippocampal signal on T1-weighted images. These secondary features help in improving the diagnostic confidence when used in conjunction with the primary findings. They may be seen in 40–60% of the cases. However, individually they are not reliable signs. HS does not enhance on post contrast imaging. DWI shows hyperintensity of the involved hippocampus with increased diffusivity on ADC. Spectroscopy shows reduced NAA in the epileptogenic site without any change in choline or creatinine. The reduction in NAA may be seen in the surrounding extrahippocampal and extratemporal regions also.

MR scans done for hippocampal sclerosis may show association with other potentially epileptogenic extrahippocampal abnormalities such as cortical dysgenesis. These are termed as dual pathologies and have been observed in approximately 15% cases undergoing epilepsy surgery. The presence of dual pathologies denotes a poor surgical outcome.

The sensitivity and specificity, for detection of HS using optimized imaging protocols is high (93% and 83%, respectively).[6] Bilateral hippocampal abnormalities **(Fig. 2)** or subtle lesions may be difficult to diagnose. These patients may require volumetric analysis, T2 relaxometry, or MR spectroscopy (increased glutamate ratio). Ictal and interictal single photon emission tomography is used as a complimentary tool **(Fig. 3)**.

MRI IN MALFORMATIONS OF CORTICAL DEVELOPMENT

Disorders of cortical organization and neuronal migration are commonly found in young pediatric epilepsy patients. They are the cause of infantile spasms in up to 40% of the children. Developmental disorders, as a group of epileptogenic abnormalities, are being increasingly recognized with the routine use of MRI during evaluation of investigate patients suffering from refractory epilepsy. The evaluation of these malformations requires close attention to the gray matter, gray-white matter interface, white matter and the periventricular region. Small lesions may require volumetric data acquisition with subsequent 3D reconstruction. Development malformations of the cortex may be classified as:[7]

Group I: Malformations secondary to abnormal cell proliferation or apoptosis

- Microcephaly
- Megalencephaly
  - Polymicrogyria and megalencephaly

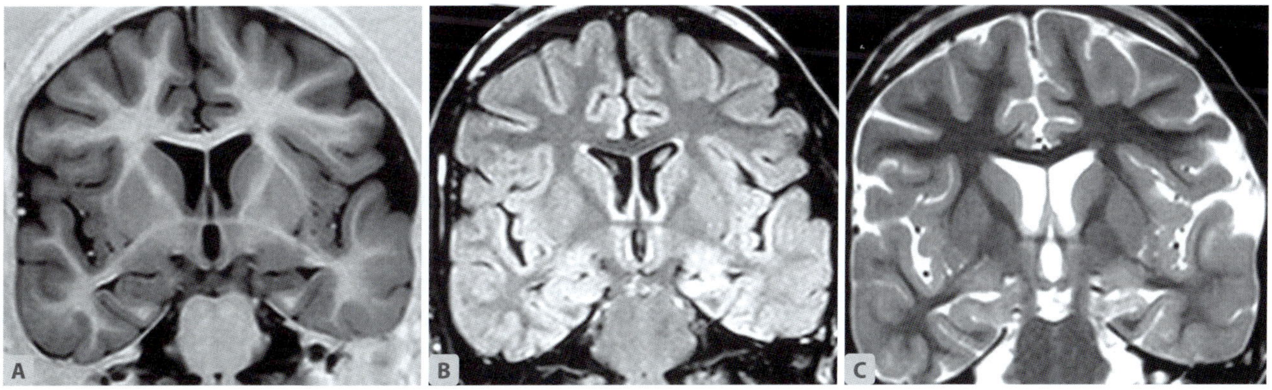

FIGS. 1A TO C: Mesial temporal sclerosis on the left side. (A) STIR sequence with reverse window setting showing loss of volume; (B) FLAIR; and (C) (T2W) sequences showing hyperintense signal in the ipsilateral hippocampus.

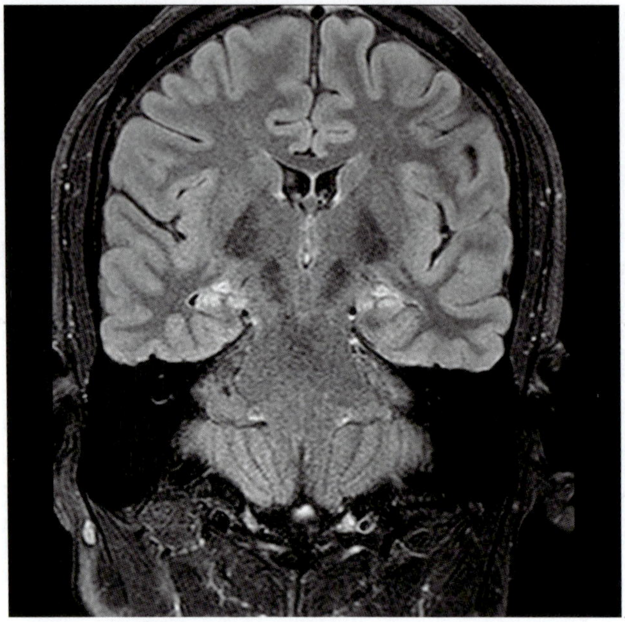

FIG. 2: Volume loss and increased signal alterations in both the hippocampus suggesting bilateral MTS.

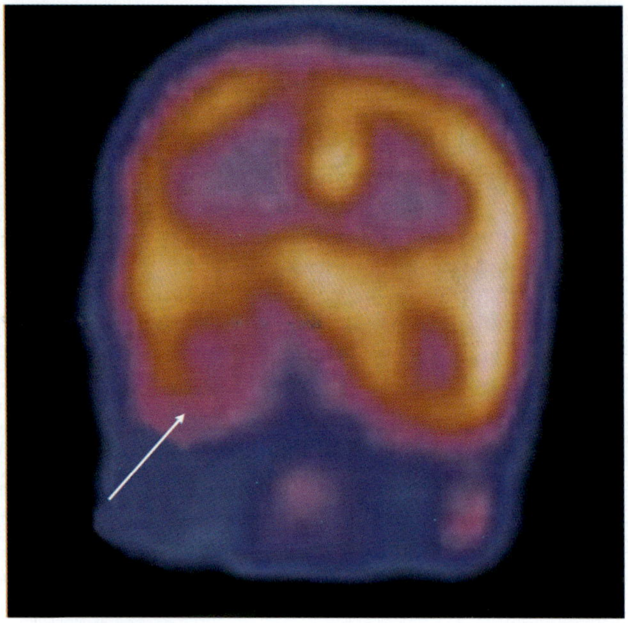

FIG. 3: SPECT (Interictal) shows reduced perfusion in the right mesial temporal lobe.

- Cortical dysgeneses with abnormal cell proliferation
    - Cortical tubers
    - Focal cortical dysplasia 2b
    - Hemimegalencephaly

Group II: Malformations secondary to abnormal cell migration

- Heterotopia
- Lissencephaly pattern
    - Agyria
    - Pachygyria
    - subcortical band heterotopias
- Subcortical heterotopias and sublobar dysplasia
    - Large focal collections of neurons in deep white matter
- Cobblestone malformation
    - Congenital muscular dystrophies

Group III: Malformations secondary to abnormal post-migrational development

- Polymicrogyria
- Schizencephaly
- Fcd (type 1, 3)
- Post-migrational microcephaly.

Focal Cortical Dysplasia

Focal cortical dysplasia (FCDs) are localized areas of malformed gray matter that is not neoplastic. FCDs are a common cause of medically refractory epilepsy in both children and adults. Surgical resection has become an important management option in these patients. However, refractory epilepsy is not seen in all patients harboring an FCD.

Based on the imaging, clinical and histopathological findings FCDs are classified into three types:

Type 1: An isolated lesion showing abnormal layering of the involved cortex that shows persistence of vertical developmental micro columns (type 1a) or the loss of horizontal hexalaminar structure (type 1b). Both patterns of abnormal layering in the cortex may also be seen simultaneously (type 1c). There are no dysmorphic neurons or balloon cells in type 1 FCDs **(Fig. 4A)**.

Type 2: These are also isolated lesions that show both abnormal cortical layering and dysmorphic neurons. Type 2A FCDs **(Fig. 4B)** do not have balloon cells while type 2B **(Fig. 4C)** FCDs show balloon cells.

Type 3: This refers to FCD associated with other lesions. This is considered as a post-migrational disorder secondary to an insult. The cytoarchitectural abnormalities described above may occur along with hippocampal sclerosis (FCD type 3a), epilepsy associated tumors (FCD type 3b), vascular malformations (FCD type 3c) or other epileptogenic lesion (FCD type 3d) acquired in childhood **(Fig. 4D)**.

FCD may be seen as areas of cortical thickening with loss of the normal gray-white interface, T2/FLAIR hyperintense signal, and focal atrophy. FCD type 1a may mild hemispheric hypoplasia without any other visible signal alteration. In many patients MRI may be normal. Mild focal cortical thickening abnormalities in the shape of the gyrus and deep sulci may also be seen.

FCD type 2 presents with a gradient of morphologic changes; ranging from dysplastic lesions that can be easily identified by conventional MRI techniques to minor structural abnormalities, like small areas of discrete cortical thickening and/or blurring of the gray-white-matter interface that often go unrecognized. Sometimes it shows subtle hyperintense T2 signal in the subcortical and deep white matter. FCD type 2a may show only mild discrete changes and without FLAIR hyperintense signal. FCD type 2b shows areas of localized cortical thickening on MRI, blurring of the gray-white-matter differentiation and wedge shaped T2 FLAIR hyperintensity in the subcortical white matter extending to the ependymal

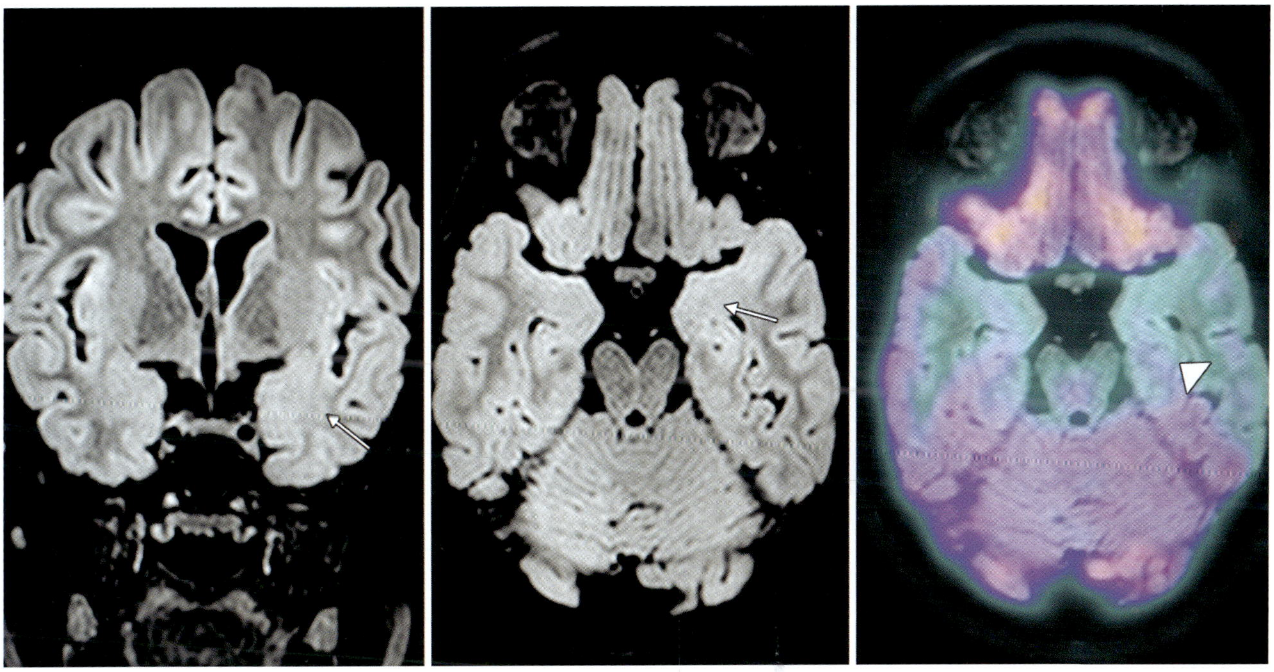

FIG. 4A: FCD type 1: Coronal and axial FLAIR images of patient show hypoplasia of left anterior temporal lobe with blurring of gray-white interface and subtle white matter hyperintensity (arrows). PET-MR fusion shows decreased uptake of tracer within left temporal lobe (arrowhead) as compared to right side.

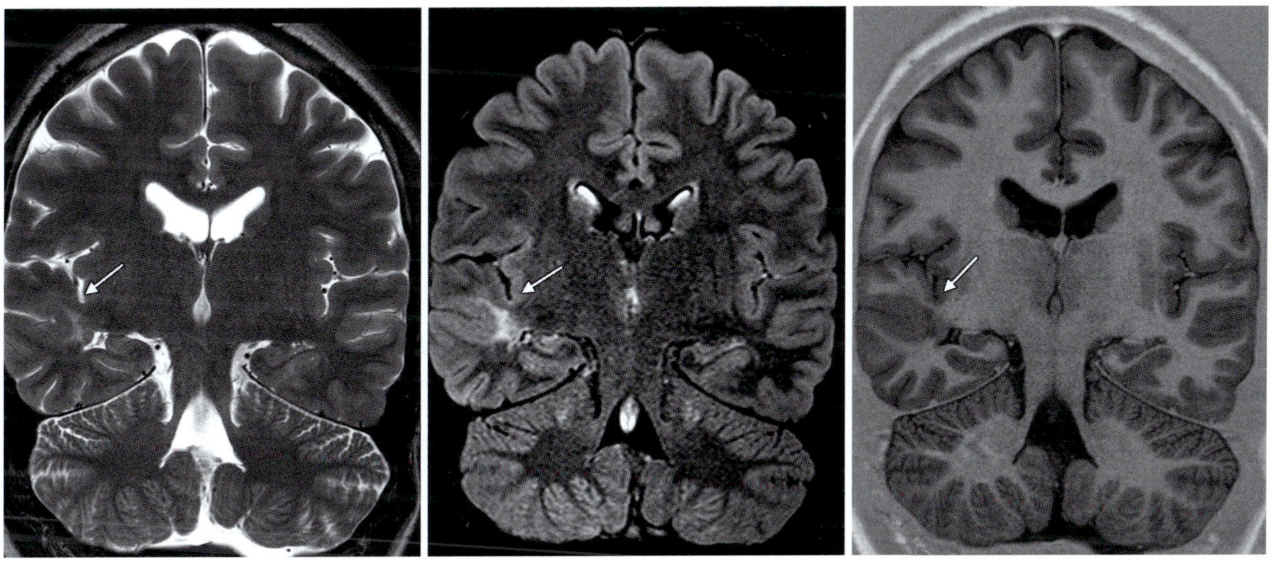

FIG. 4B: FCD type 2A: Oblique coronal T2, FLAIR and IR images of patient show cortical thickening, blurring of gray-white interface and subcortical hyperintensity along right superior temporal sulcus (arrows).

surface of ipsilateral ventricle (transmantle sign) **(Fig. 4C)**. Sometimes the lesion may be localized only to bottom of the sulcus. There is no contrast enhancement.The lesions have increased diffusivity and decreased fractional anisotropy values. NAA: Cr ratio is decreased with elevated Myoinositol on MR spectroscopy. Perfusion (rCBV) is normal or reduced.[8]

Other Disorders of Neuronal Migration and Cortical Organization

Hemimegalencephaly is characterized by hamartomatous growth that may affect either the entire cerebral hemisphere or a part of it. The involved hemisphere shows enlargement with white matter hyperintensity, ipsilateral ventricular enlargement, heterotopias and thickened cortex. It may be associated with areas of heterotopia, polymicrogyria, pachygyria, FCD, and gliosis.[8]

Nodular heterotopia may be periventricular or subcortical depending upon the location of the ectopic neuron clusters. These nodules contain clusters of mature neurons and glial cells that do not show well-defined lamellar organization. These follow gray matter on all sequences and do not enhance on contrast administration.[8]

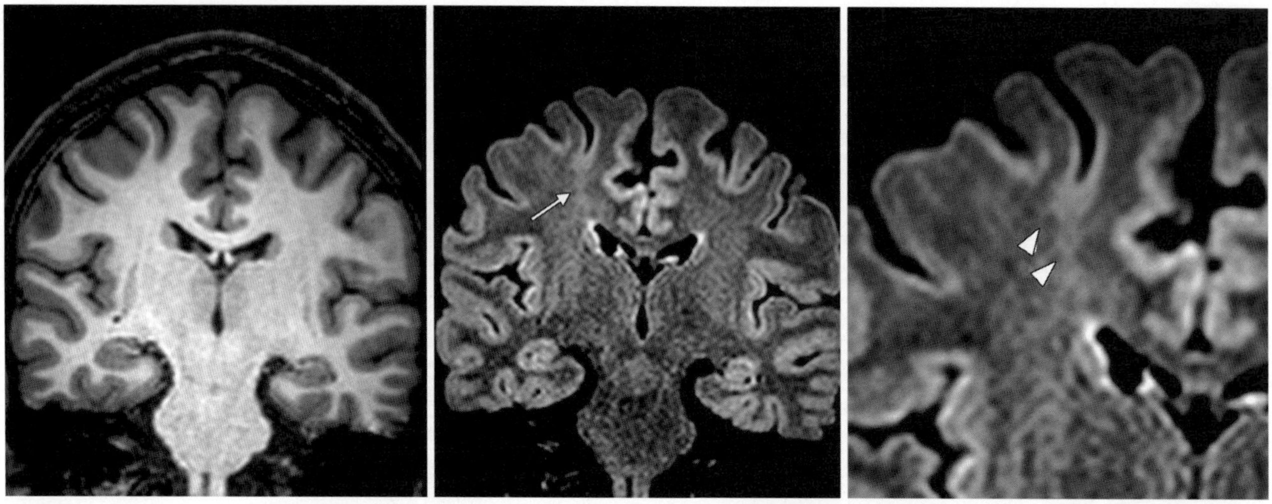

FIG. 4C: FCD type 2B: Coronal T1 and FLAIR images of patient show blurring of gray-white interface and subcortical hyperintensity along right superior frontal sulcus. Increased FLAIR signal tapering from gray-white interface to superolateral margin of right lateral ventricle (arrowheads), typical transmantle sign.

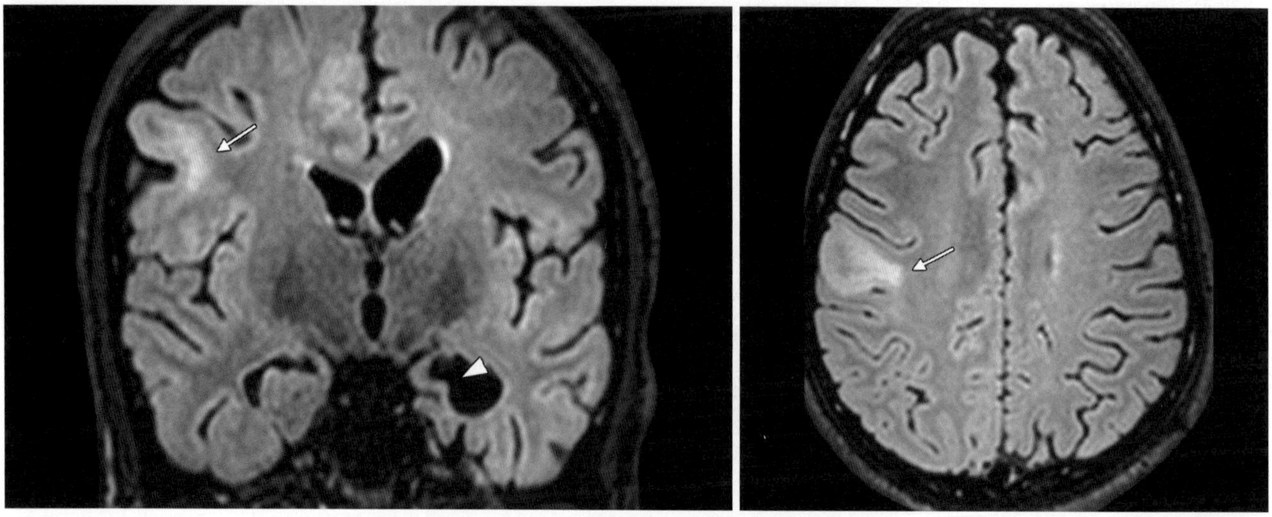

FIG. 4D: FCD type 3D: Coronal and axial FLAIR images reveal cortical thickening, blurring of gray white interface and subcortical hyperintensity along right inferior frontal sulcus (arrows) s/o FCD with left MTS (arrowhead).

Classic lissencephaly incorporates the agyria-pachygyria spectrum. It often has a genetic origin and may be gender linked. This anomaly is characterized by a reduction in the number of sulci and gyri. This manifests as shallow sulci with large gyri and cortical thickening. Near complete absence of sulci with smoothening of the cortex is seen in classical lissencephaly. Subcortical laminar heterotopia (band heterotopia) is characterized by a band of ectopic gray matter that lies below the cortex with intervening normal white matter.[8]

Polymicrogyria most commonly affects the perisylvian region and is a common cortical developmental malformation. It is characterized by a large number of small, prominent convolutions with shallow intervening sulci. The abnormal small gyri give the appearance of thickened cortex on standard thick sections. Polymicrogyria may be associated with other lesions such as callosum agenesis, may or may not lead to epilepsy, and in those patients with epilepsy the seizures are often well controlled with medication.

Schizencephaly refers to CSF containing transcerebral cleft connecting pial and ependymal surfaces, usually lined by polymicrogyric cortex. The lips of the cleft may be closely apposed (closed lip schizencephaly) or widely separated (open lip schizencephaly).

Hypothalamic hamartomas occur due to abnormalities of neuronal migration. These are located between the infundibular stalk and the mammillary body in the tuber cinereum. Pedunculated and sessile subtypes are seen. The pedunculated lesions project into the suprasellar cistern while the sessile lesions arise from the floor of third ventricle and extend into its lumen. Gelastic seizures (ictal laughing fits) are commonly associated with this lesion. The lesions are isointense to normal gray matter on T1-weighted images and iso to hyperintense on FLAIR/T2-weighted images. They do not show any post contrast enhancement.

The imaging algorithm of patients with suspected cortical maldevelopment should include high resolution volume acquisition, high resolution coronal T2 and FLAIR images. Multiplanar reconstructions, thin coronal IR protocols are helpful. Dedicated pulse sequences that generate high gray and white matter contrast are needed with high spatial resolution to detect subtle development malformation. High spatial resolution can be achieved by using the SPGR sequence, use of phased array surface coils and homogenous high field strength magnets.

TUMORS

Brain tumors may cause up to 1–2% of all seizures and 4–6% of partial seizures. Temporal lobe tumors are often slow growing and include gliomas, oligodendrogliomas, dysembryoplastic neuroepithelial tumors (DNETs), and gangliogliomas.

DNETs are known to be associated with partial complex seizures that have an intractable course. Neuro-imaging typically shows predominantly cortical-based, well-demarcated lesion, usually in the temporal lobe or parieto-occipital region. The lesion is hypodense compared to white matter on CT (**Fig. 5**), hypointense on T1WI and hyperintense on T2WI **(Fig. 6)** with variable enhancement following contrast administration. Lack of peritumoral edema and mass effect on midline structures, triangular pattern of distribution and presence of septations are frequently observed.[5] Some lesions may appear as an enlarged gyrus, producing a soap bubble appearance at the cortical margin.[9] Calcification (20%) and scalloping of inner table of skull may be seen **(Fig. 5)**.

Gangliogliomas, the most frequently occurring mixed glioneuronal tumors of the CNS, are more common in the pediatric group and patients usually present with seizures.

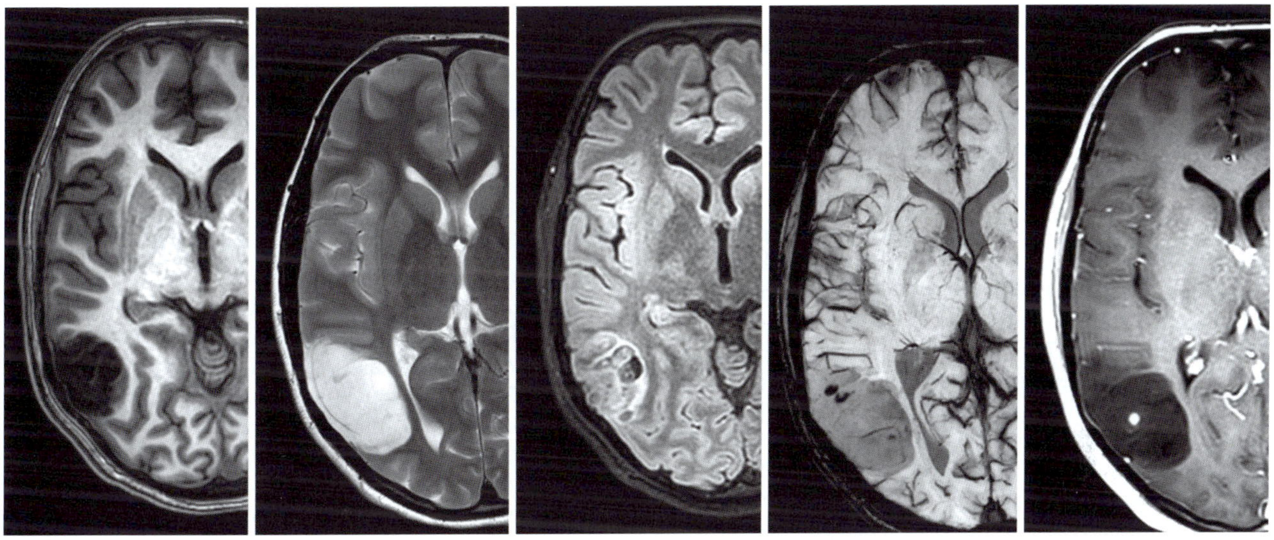

FIG. 5: DNET: T1, T2, FLAIR, SWI and T1 PC show a well-defined cortical-based lesion having "bubbly" appearance in T2 and FLAIR with cystic areas within. SWI shows focal calcification. There is a nodular area of enhancement on the T1 PC image. Note adjacent bone remodeling and no edema.

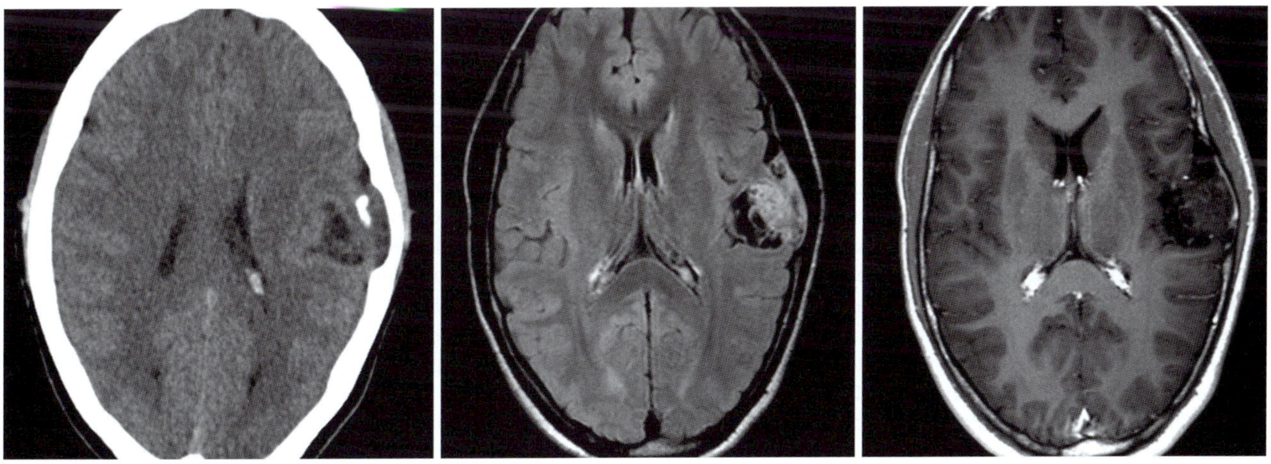

FIG. 6: Ganglioglioma: CT, FLAIR and T1 PC images show a cortical-based solid cystic lesion with calcification. Adjacent bone remodeling is seen. There is no post-contrast enhancement.

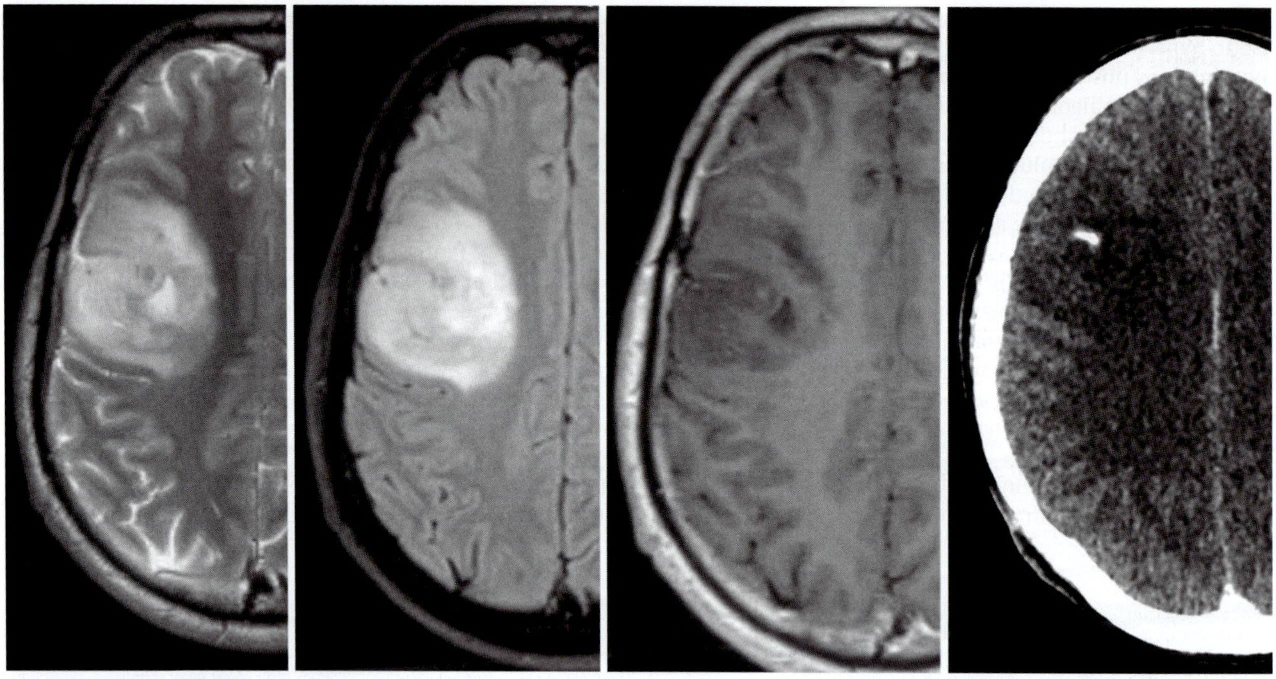

FIG. 7: Oligodendroglioma: T2, FLAIR, T1 PC images show non-enhancing T2/FLAIR hyperintense, T1 hypointense lesion involving gray and white matter with heterogeneity; CT shows a focal calcification.

The temporal lobes are the most common site. Gangliogliomas are characterized on CT scans as hypodense lesions with calcification and a variable contrast enhancement pattern. The MR findings **(Fig. 6)** are nonspecific; the lesions may be iso- to hypointense on T1WI and hyperintense on T2WI.[10] Contrast enhancement was reported in 44% of one series and may have either a nodular rim or solid enhancement pattern **(Fig. 7)**.

Oligodendrogliomas involve the cortex or the subcortical region. They are T1 hypointense, T2/FLAIR hyperintense and show variable enhancement. Foci of increased T1 signal representing intratumoral hemorrhage may be seen. Calcifications are common and may be ring-shaped, shell-like, or nodular **(Fig. 7)**. Dual abnormalities which are usually due to a combination of HS and either glioma, heterotopia or vascular abnormalities, may be present in 8–22% of patients.

Vascular Malformations

Intractable epilepsy due to vascular malformations may be seen in 2–3% of patients. Arteriovenous malformations (AVMs) have are seen on MRI as a cluster of abnormal round or linear signal voids. Cavernous hemangiomas have a higher epileptogenic potential as compared to AVMs.[11] This may be secondary to the greater degree of reactive gliosis in these lesions. Cavernous hemangiomas are seen as circumscribed lesions with a central heterogeneous area of mixed signal intensity secondary to presence of methemoglobin, deoxyhemoglobin and foci of calcification. A complete hemosiderin ring that is hypointense on T2-weighted imaging is seen **(Fig. 8)**. Vascular malformations that are superficial in location with surrounding T2-hyperintensity are more likely to cause seizures as compared to deeper lesions.

Other Lesions Associated with Epilepsy

Insults like trauma, infection or infarction lead to cortical encephalomalacia and gliosis. These lesions may act as epileptogenic foci and are well delineated on MRI. Destructive lesions are also an important source of childhood seizures. Smooth porencephalic cavities form in patients who suffer from an insult during the first 6 months of gestation these cavities are not lined by gliosis. on the other hand, perinatal, post-natal or late gestational injury leads to focal or generalized encephalomalacia. Tuberculomas and cysticercosis are also commonly identified causes of epilepsy in developing countries. MRI may demonstrate the various stages in development of the non-calcified neurocysticercosis lesions. Children with neurocutaneous syndromes, such as Sturge-Weber syndrome **(Figs. 9A and B)** and tuberous sclerosis, are also prone to develop epilepsy.

Congenital infections, like the TORCH group (toxoplasmosis, rubella, cytomegalovirus and herpes simplex), may produce intractable seizures, Lennox-Gastaut syndrome and infantile spasms. Cytomegalovirus infection may also lead to neuronal migration abnormalities.

Rasmussen's encephalitis is chronic encephalitis generally progressive in nature and is characterized by seizures that are refractory to medical treatment. Radiological findings of stable or progressive hemispheric atrophy on serial imaging in a setting of intractable epilepsy with progressive hemiparesis may help to establish the diagnosis **(Figs. 10A to D)**.

Epilepsy occurs in about 20% of children with diplegic and dystonic cerebral palsy, whereas the incidence is 50–80% in the hemiplegic and quadriplegic forms.

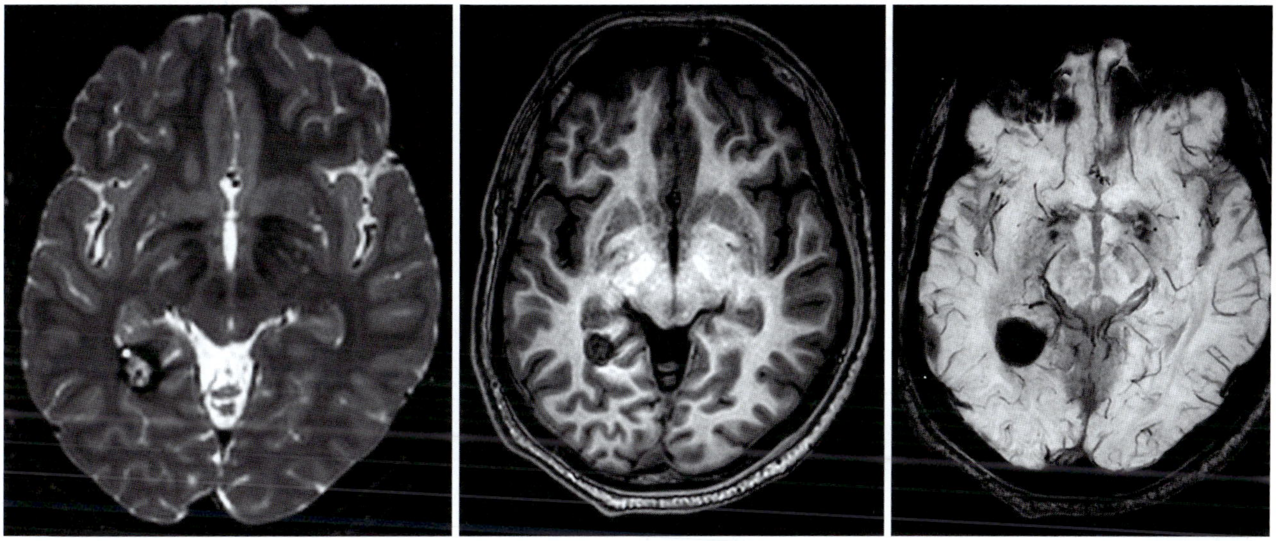

FIG. 8: Cavernoma: T2, T1 and SW images show right temporo-occipital lesion with heterogeneous hyperintense core and a complete hypointense rim. The lesion shows "blooming" on SWI. Core of the lesion is hyperintense due to methemoglobin.

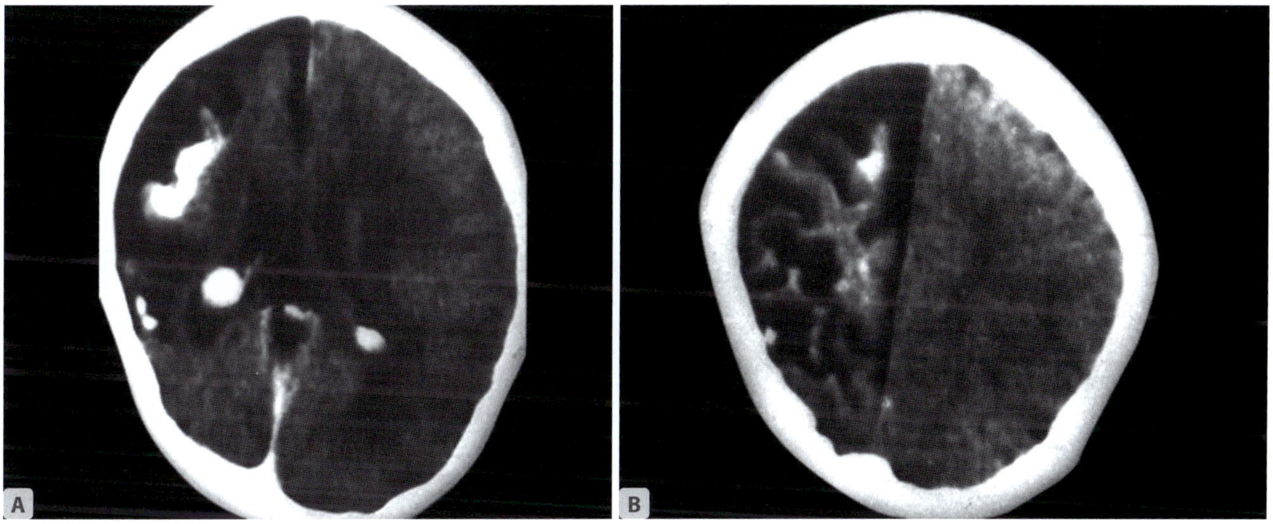

FIGS. 9A AND B: Sturge-Weber syndrome involving right hemisphere with typical tram-track calcification and ipsilateral atrophy.

ADVANCES IN EPILEPSY IMAGING AND MANAGEMENT

Reformatted Images

3D volume data, usually T1-weighted inversion recovery sequences (IR, SPGR, MPRAGE, etc.) and 3D FLAIR are acquired as thin sections (<1.5 mm) can be reconstructed in any desired plane using multi-planar (MPR) and curved-planar (CPR) reconstructions. CPR **(Fig. 11)** is a very useful tool for picking up subtle lesions especially those of focal cortical dysplasias and for clarifying "abnormal" appearing areas on the routine orthogonal sequences.[12]

Quantitative MR Imaging

Volume estimation (MR volumetry) of hippocampi is an established method in epilepsy evaluation.[13] Now, many more techniques of quantitative MR imaging are available, all of them mostly utilizing T1-weighted 3D volume acquisitions. One method is by classifying tissues into categories such as gray matter, white matter, and cerebrospinal fluid, and then segmenting various structures by using manual or automated segmentation techniques, such as artificial neural networks and 3D model-based segmentation techniques. Using this method, volumetric neocortical measurements may provide an objective way to evaluate the extent of resection and its relation to surgical results.

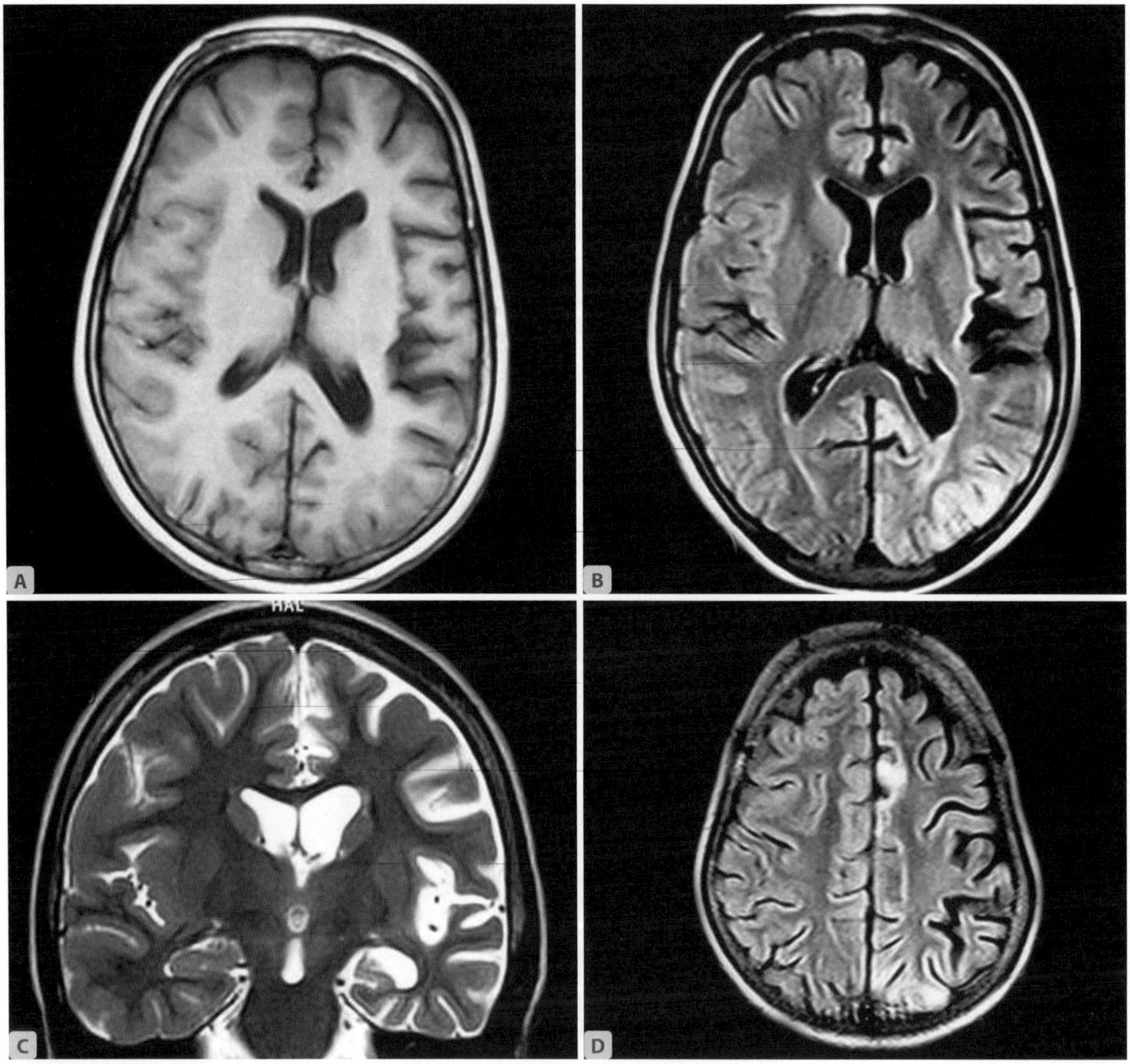

FIGS. 10A TO D: MRI (A) TIW; (C) T2W (coronal); (B and D) FLAIR axial, Rasmussen's encephalitis involving left hemisphere with areas of high signal and atrophy.

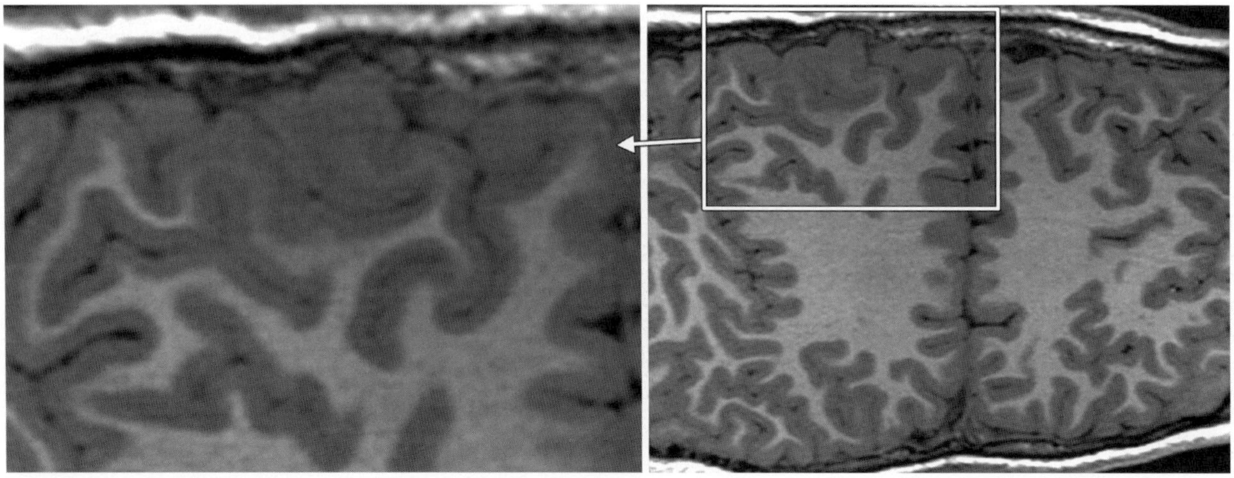

FIG. 11: Curved planar reconstruction of subtle right frontal cortical dysplasia; such lesions are virtually undetectable in routine sequences but well shown on CPR images because they get "opened up".

Another method is voxel-based morphometry, which involves a voxel-wise comparison of the local "concentration" of signal intensity between two groups. Voxel-based morphometry has been used to demonstrate neocortical gray matter reduction, on the same or the contralateral side of seizure focus, and for demonstrating abnormalities in brain parenchyma beyond the visualized lesions. Texture analysis of the 3D T1-weighted images performed using voxel-wise operators has been used to assess focal cortical dysplasias. Voxel-wise operators have been used to model gray matter thickness, to quantify the gray matter–white matter interface to detect its blurring, and to model hyperintense T1-weighted signals within gray matter through intensity measurement of a voxel relative to the threshold intensity between gray and white matter.

Magnetic Resonance Spectroscopy

Magnetic resonance spectroscopy (MRS) is a non-invasive method of evaluating brain metabolites. The role of MRS is in aiding lateralization, detecting bilateral abnormalities and identifying metabolic abnormalities in epileptogenic areas **(Figs. 12A to C)**.[13] Usually, proton (1H) spectroscopy is performed, and can be used to measure N-acetyl aspartate (NAA), choline (Cho) and creatine (Cr) in vivo. Other metabolites useful in epilepsy evaluation are lactate (Lac), myoinositol (mI), and Glutamine and Glutamate (Glx). Both absolute and relative values can be obtained, with neuronal loss reducing NAA levels and gliosis/astrocytosis increasing Cr and Cho levels. Use of the NAA/Cho+Cr signal intensity ratio has been advocated as possibly the simplest and single most useful index of spectroscopic abnormality. Lactate may be raised especially when imaged soon after seizures, and indicate altered metabolism. Myoinositol is raised when there is gliosis and usually reflects irreversible damage to the parenchyma. Glx concentration in gray matter reflects the glutamate concentration in glutamatergic neurons and can be increased even when structural MRI is normal and other metabolite levels are normal on MRS. Abnormal NAA ratios have also been found contralateral to the seizure focus side, which reversed in patients who became seizure free after surgery. Reduction in NAA may relate to neuronal and glial dysfunction rather than absolute neuronal cell loss. In extratemporal epilepsy, the ability of MRS to lateralize seizure focus is less. In a study of patients with frontal lobe epilepsy, MR spectroscopy results enabled lateralization of the seizures in 50% of cases.

T2 Relaxometry (Mapping)

This provides an objective measure of T2 relaxation time. The T2 time is elevated in mesial temporal sclerosis, and abnormal T2 relaxometry is significantly associated with intractable epilepsy. T2 values are elevated ipsilateral to seizure focus, contralateral to seizure focus (to a lesser degree) as well as non-temporal tissues distant from the seizure focus site **(Figs. 13A and B)**.[14]

Diffusion Tensor Imaging

Diffusion tensor imaging (DTI) studies the motion of water at the voxel level and can provide quantitative and reproducible data, e.g. mean diffusivity and fractional anisotropy, to assess the structural integrity of brain tissue. Imaging the preferential direction of water diffusion in the brain allows us to visualize the major white matter tracts and deduce the fundamental basis of cerebral networks. Thus, the effect of epilepsy syndromes on these pathways and the consequences of various therapies can be assessed with this technique. The anisotropy of diffusion in the brain depends on concentration of macromolecules, organelles, density of nerve fibers and glia, fiber diameter, and myelination. In white matter, anisotropy is a result of the parallel structure of axons and their myelin sheaths. Water can diffuse freely along the long axis of the fibers rather than perpendicular to the fiber orientation. Lesions that disrupt the microstructural environment, lead to changes in the anisotropy of the involved brain tissue. This commonly results in reduced anisotropy and increased mean diffusivity.

Diffusion studies can be done in both ictal/peri/postictal and interictal periods.

Ictal/peri-/postictal studies: Seizures generally result in early postictal depression, followed by normalization, and then transient or chronic elevation of mean diffusivity.

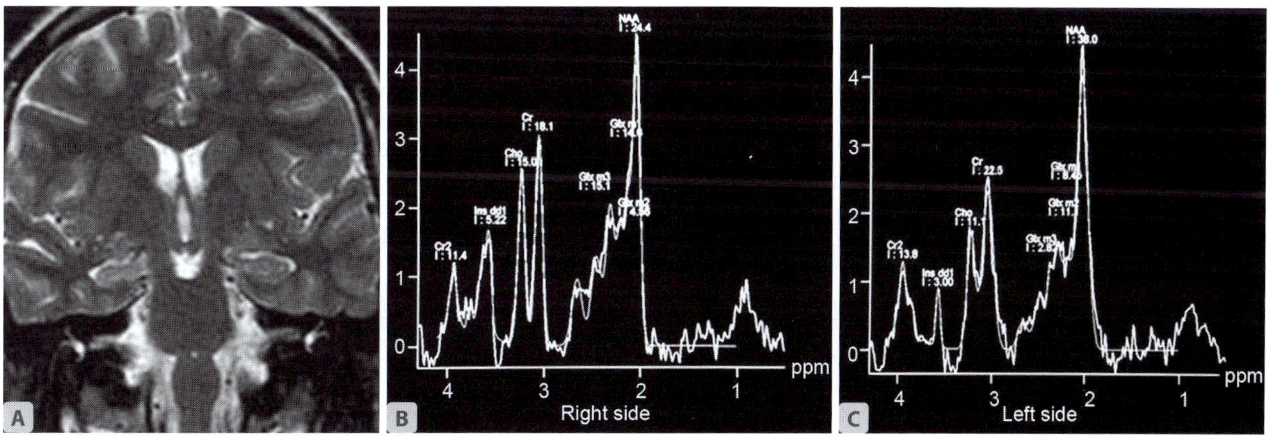

FIGS. 12A TO C: Role of MRS: Minimally increased T2 hyperintensity of right hippocampus (A) but significantly increased Glx/NAA ratio (1.4) of right hippocampus (B) as compared to left side (0.59) (C).

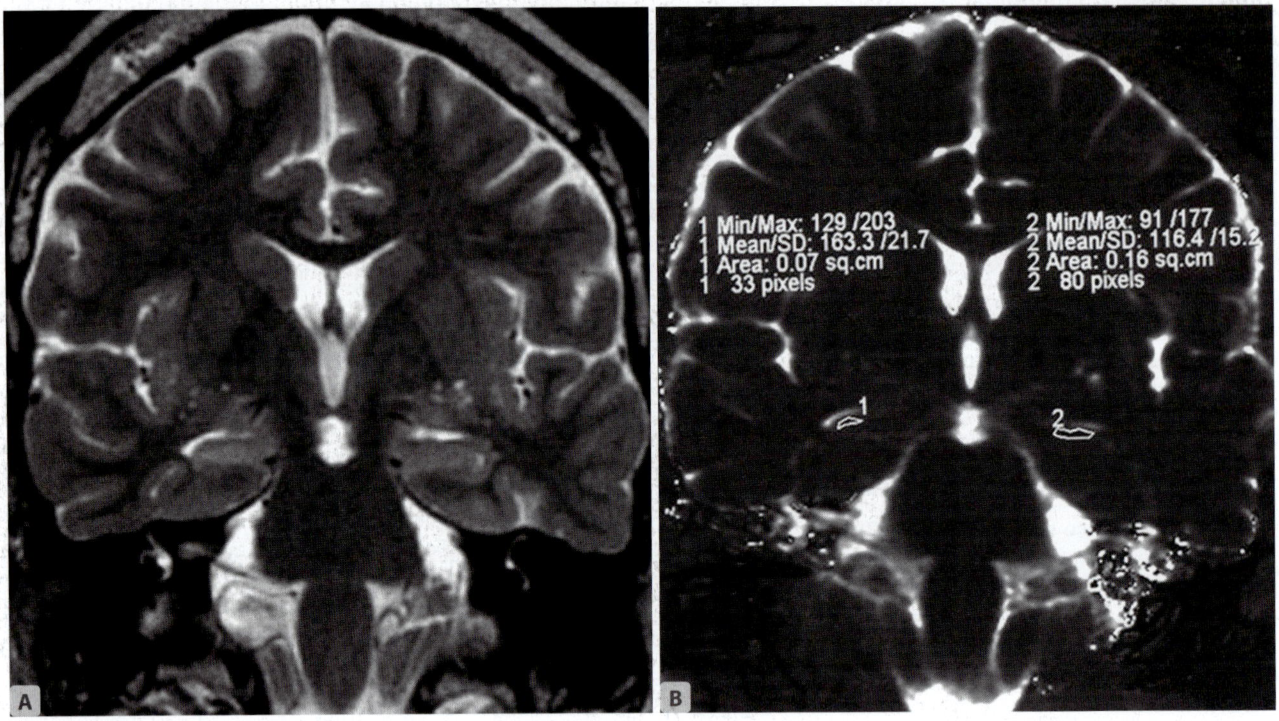

FIGS. 13A AND B: Role of T2 relaxometry: Minimally increased T2 hyperintensity of right hippocampus on T2WI (A) but significantly increased T2 value (B).

The early decline in diffusivity in prolonged seizures is due to cytotoxic edema. Vasogenic edema also has been reported in subcortical white matter. Seizures can trigger breakdown of the blood–brain barrier, which, together with local vasodilatory effects, can give rise to vasogenic edema as well as an increase in intercellular space and diffusivity. Excitotoxic mechanisms eventually lead to cell lysis and death, which result in increased extracellular space and increased diffusion. Diffusion changes often are more widespread, possibly indicating involved networks and secondary spread.

Interictal studies: Diffusivity is increased in diseased hippocampi whether they show increased T2/FLAIR signal or not, or whether they show volume changes or not. Anisotropy also is abnormal in hippocampal sclerosis, but to a lesser magnitude than mean diffusivity changes. Studies of normal appearing tissue have demonstrated bilateral and extratemporal abnormalities, indicative of structural or functional abnormalities that may extend beyond the seizure onset zone. Diffusion tensor imaging also is sensitive to neocortical pathologies that underlie epilepsy. Areas of increased mean diffusivity and decreased fractional anisotropy correlate with abnormalities identified on visual inspection of conventional MRI and also often identify areas of pathology that appear normal on standard MRI. Both diffusion tensor imaging measurements and stereo electroencephalographic recordings have found good spatial concordance between epileptiform activity and diffusivity abnormalities.

Tractography

Diffusion tensor imaging enables the non-invasive in-vivo delineation of white matter tracts **(Figs. 14A to D)**. There are various clinical scenarios were tractography is helpful. Meyers loop is the part of the optic radiation that passes anteriorly into the anterior temporal lobe and then sweeps back along the lateral wall of the ventricle to reach the occiput. Injury to the loop during anterior temporal lobe resection can cause a visual field deficit. Preoperative delineation of the Meyers loop can predict the risk of a visual field defect and thus assist with surgical planning. Similarly, evaluation of the corticospinal tracts and the arcuate fasciculus may be performed if resection of an adjacent lesion is necessary.[15]

Functional MR

Temporal lobe epilepsy (TLE) may be associated with disturbance of language and memory functions. These may be further impaired by anterior temporal lobe resection. Anterior temporal lobe resection in the speech-dominant hemisphere is followed by significant language deficits in up to 40% of patients and often by a decline in verbal memory as well. The main application of functional MR in clinical practice is preoperative localization of the motor strip, language localization and identifying memory laterality in the temporal lobe. While planning surgery for hippocampal sclerosis localization and lateralization of the language and memory functions is essential to minimize the risk of postsurgical deficits and to prognosticate the patients.

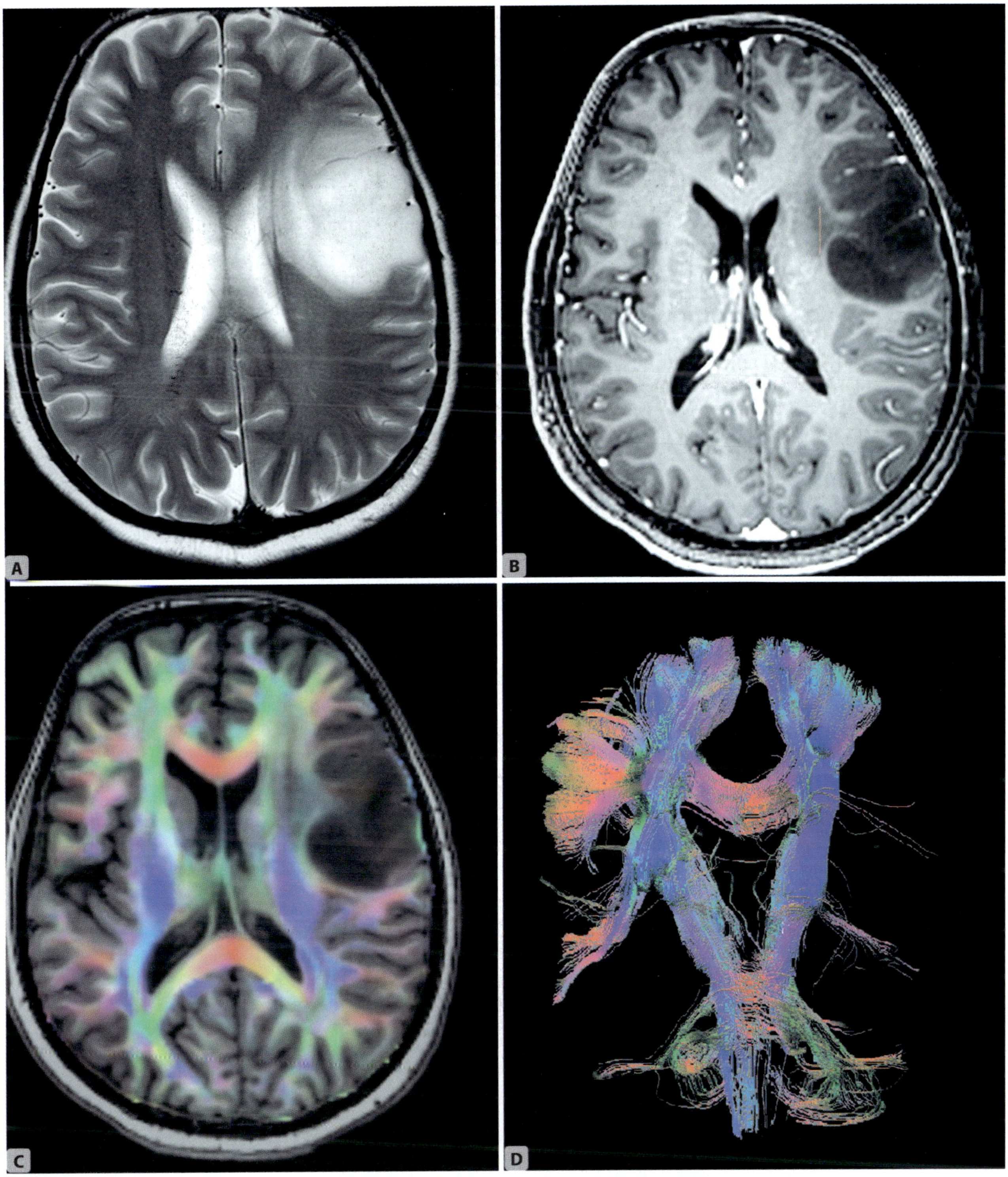

FIGS. 14A TO D: T2 (A), post-contrast T1-weighted (B) images in a 24-year-old female who presented with 3 episodes of seizures, show a non-enhancing T2 hyperintense low grade glioma in the left frontal region. Axial T1/DTI fused image (C) and reconstructed tractography volume image (D) shows infiltration, thinning and displacement of tracts in the left frontal white matter as compared to the right side.

Language

Functional MRI (fMRI) is an essential tool that is used to evaluate the language networks in epilepsy patients. Tasks that activate Broca's area and Wernicke's area are performed by the patient during acquisition of the fMRI. A box car design is commonly used in clinical practice. In this technique discrete blocks of rest and activation follow each other. Various paradigms that may be used include verbal fluency, verb generation, word generation, sentence completion and picture naming. A lateralization index (LI) can be calculated for selected areas of activation in frontal, parietal and temporal lobes. LI is quantitative measure of language dominance (right/left/bilateral). It helps is identifying the dominant lobe for language function and in decision making prior to surgery. Traditionally the Wada test was used for language lateralization. However, the Wada test is invasive and in not available widely. Language lateralization on fMRI has been seen to correlate with results from the intracarotid amobarbital test in 80–90% of patients.[15]

Various studies have shown that the left hemisphere is dominant for language in right handed individuals. Atypical language dominance is seen more in ambidextrous or left handed individuals.[16,17] Individuals who have structural lesions in the left temporal lobe and are left dominant for language are more likely to show atypical language lateralization on fMRI as compared to those with right hemisphere epilepsy suggesting reorganization of the language network. In the absence of reorganization there is a higher risk of postsurgical deficit. Atypical language lateralization in the Wernicke's area is more common in patients with temporal lobe epilepsy. On the other hand, anterior language areas are more likely to be affected in frontal lobe epilepsy **(Figs. 15A to C)**. When cortical resection is essential close to eloquent language cortex, electrocortical stimulation or awake resections are necessary as fMRI is not an adequate modality to mapping the entire eloquent area. Cortical language function can also be localized with transcranial magnetic stimulation and the results fused with the individual's MRI scan.[15]

Episodic Memory

Temporal lobe epilepsy is commonly associated with memory impairment. Temporal lobe surgery can cause further worsening of memory. Activations for verbal memory are seen in bilateral temporal, parietal, and frontal lobes. More activation in the left hippocampus during word encoding has been correlated with better verbal memory in left temporal lobe epilepsy patients. Verbal memory has been seen to decline in 1/3rd of patients after left temporal lobe resection.

Greater right hippocampus activation for face encoding correlates with better visual memory in right temporal lobe epilepsy patients. Visual memory also declines in 1/3rd of right temporal lobe resection patients. Reorganization of networks for verbal and visual memory encoding may occur in hippocampal sclerosis. This suggests that the brain may compensate to some extent for the impaired function of the involved hippocampus.[15]

Motor Function

Motor function can be evaluated in fMRI using finger and foot tapping tasks. Identification of the primary motor cortex is essential prior to surgical resection of lesions in this area and when planning for intracranial electrode implantations **(Figs. 16A and B)**.[15]

Resting State and Connectivity

fMRI studies of functional connectivity using resting state fMRI can be used to investigate the pathophysiological basis of epileptic networks. This may help in predicting the surgical outcome in future. The potential clinical benefit for resting state fMRI has not been established.

Positron Emission Tomography

Interictal FDG-PET is used in presurgical evaluation of intractable epilepsy. It helps to lateralize the epileptogenic focus. Glucose hypometabolism is seen. Although it is widespread, the site of ictal onset is usually located at the area of the most severe hypometabolism within the larger volume. Interictal FDG-PET hypometabolism, when correlated with MR imaging, EEG and clinical data, can be used to lateralize the side of seizure onset, prognosticate the patient for the degree of seizure control after surgery and also help in deciding the placement of intracranial electrodes. Patients in

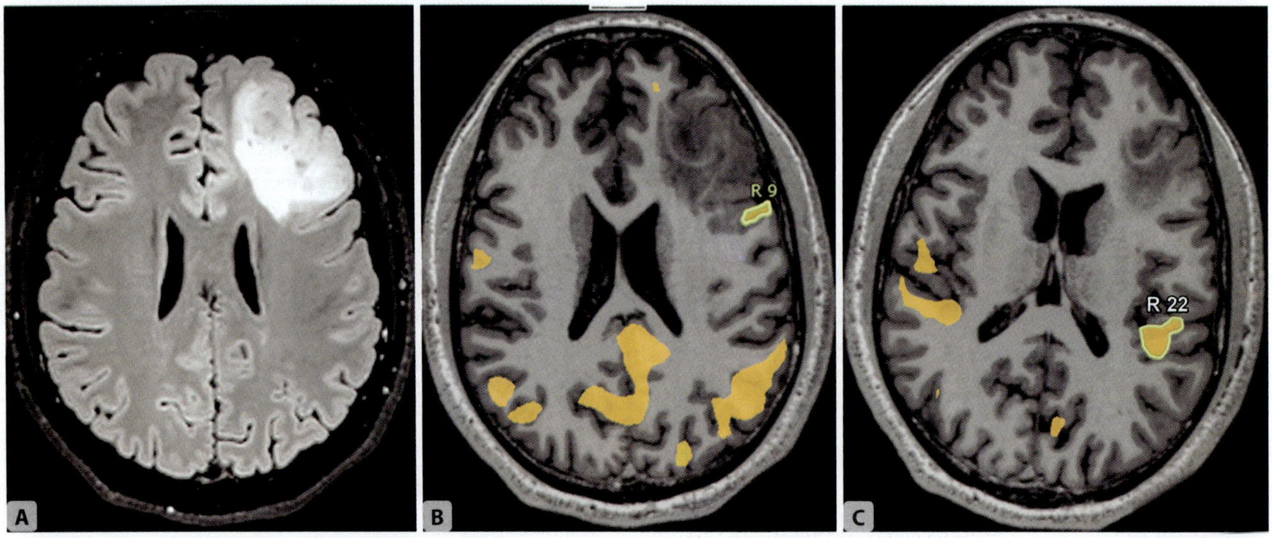

FIGS. 15A TO C: Preoperative imaging in a 35-year-old patient, who presented with focal seizures and headache. Axial FLAIR (A) image shows a hyperintense lesion in the left frontal cortical and subcortical regions. Fused T1/BOLD fMR images for language paradigm in axial plane (B and C) show that the Broca's area (ROI in B) has been displaced posteriorly, while the Wernicke's area (ROI in C) is normal in location.

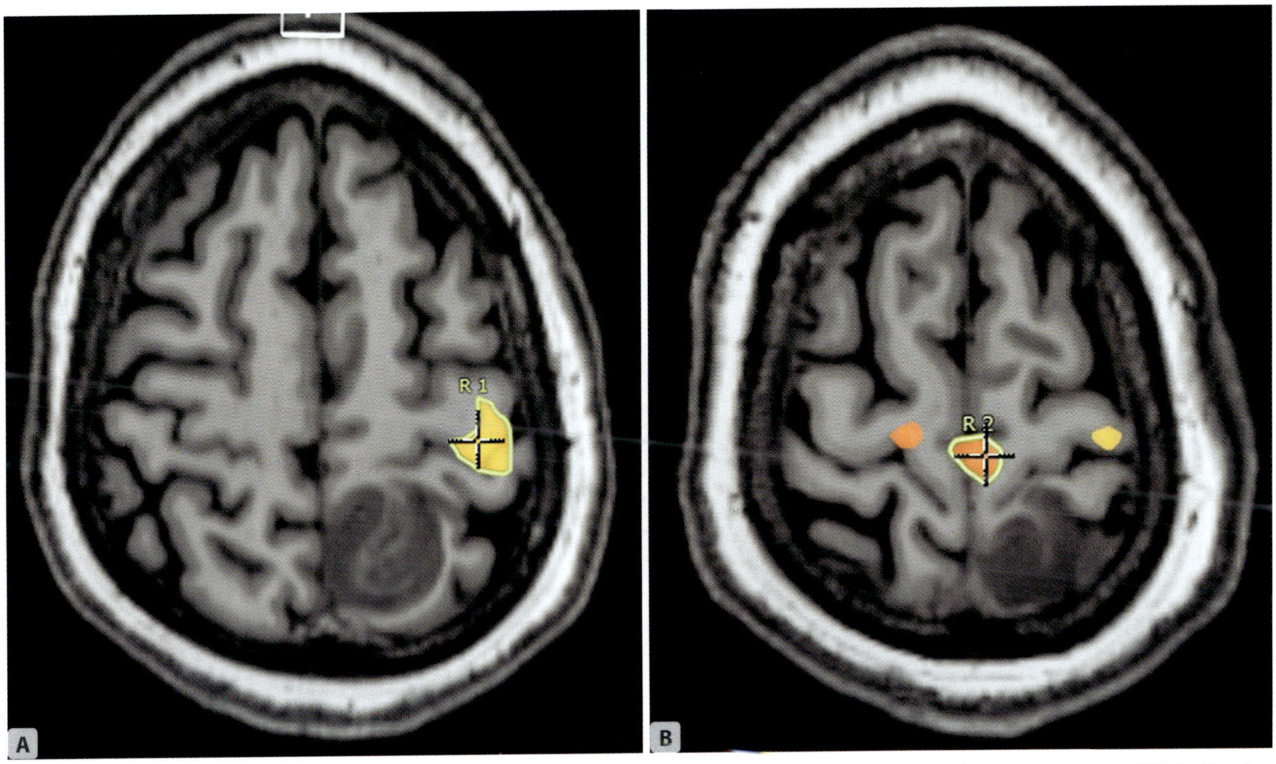

FIGS. 16A AND B: Fused T1/BOLD fMR images for finger tapping (A) and foot movement (B), show activity in the premotor cortex (ROIs in A and B) that is away from the left parietal lesion.

whom the epilepsy focus is localized to the neocortex FDG-PET scans show a large hypometabolic area on interictal imaging, including areas like thalamus and basal ganglia ipsilateral to the involved neocortical site. Also, when a lesion is identified on imaging, the hypometabolic area in the involved neocortex is often much larger than the structural abnormality. The area of hypometabolism, excluding the site of MR imaging-visible structural lesion, usually contains the electrophysiologically defined ictal onset zone. The absence of hypometabolism does not rule out focal epilepsy. Although regional hypometabolism suggests that epileptic discharge may begin within that region, multiple other areas of ictus onset beyond the hypometabolic cortex are not ruled out. It has been seen that severity of hypometabolism in the temporal lobe, correlates with postsurgical outcome for seizure control.

Other PET receptor ligands that have been utilized in the evaluation of epilepsy are ^{11}C-flumazenil/^{18}F-flumazenil and α-^{11}C-methyl-L-tryptophan. In a recent study of patients who suffer from intractable focal epilepsies, decreased ^{11}C-flumazenil uptake was noted in the temporal piriform cortex. This was associated with an increase in the seizure frequency. Increased α-^{11}C-methyl-L-tryptophan uptake has been used to identify the epileptogenic focus in tuberous sclerosis patients with multiple.[15]

Single-photon Emission Computed Tomography (SPECT)

The main role of SPECT studies is as a problem-solving tool. SPECT can localize the site of seizure onset in cases where other imaging modalities are not diagnostic and the physician is unable to identify the epileptogenic site via other non-invasive means also **(Figs. 17A to C)**. The SPECT studies evaluate changes in CBF. Commonly used radiopharmaceuticals include technetium-99m hexamethylpropyleneamine oxime or technetium-99m bicisate. Both of these have rapid first-pass brain extraction. Maximum uptake is achieved 30–60 seconds after IV injection. The SPECT images can be acquired up to 4 hours after the injection therefore combined ictal and interictal examination are performed. The ictal SPECT examination will localize the site of seizure as an area of focal hyperperfusion. The epileptogenic zone will show focal hypoperfusion on the interictal SPECT. The diagnostic yield of ictal SPECT is superior to interictal SPECT alone. Interictal SPECT imaging serves as a reference for evaluation of the ictal SPECT images. Interictal SPECT alone has poor sensitivity with a high false-positive rate in mesial temporal lobe epilepsy. It also has a low diagnostic yield in patients suffering from extratemporal seizures. ictal SPECT imaging has poorer spatial resolution as compared to PET scans. Following image acquisition, the coregistered and normalized interictal images can be subtracted from the ictal images and then coregistered with high-resolution MR images with the aid of computer software. ("subtraction ictal SPECT coregistered to MR imaging" also known as SISCOM). This technique has been shown to reliably indicate the location of the seizure focus, and is superior to visual analysis.

Magnetoencephalography

Magnetoencephalography (MEG) (magnetic source imaging) is a non-invasive modality used in localization of epilepsy **(Figs. 18A to D)**. MEG measures the extracranial changes in the magnetic field that occur perpendicular to the direction

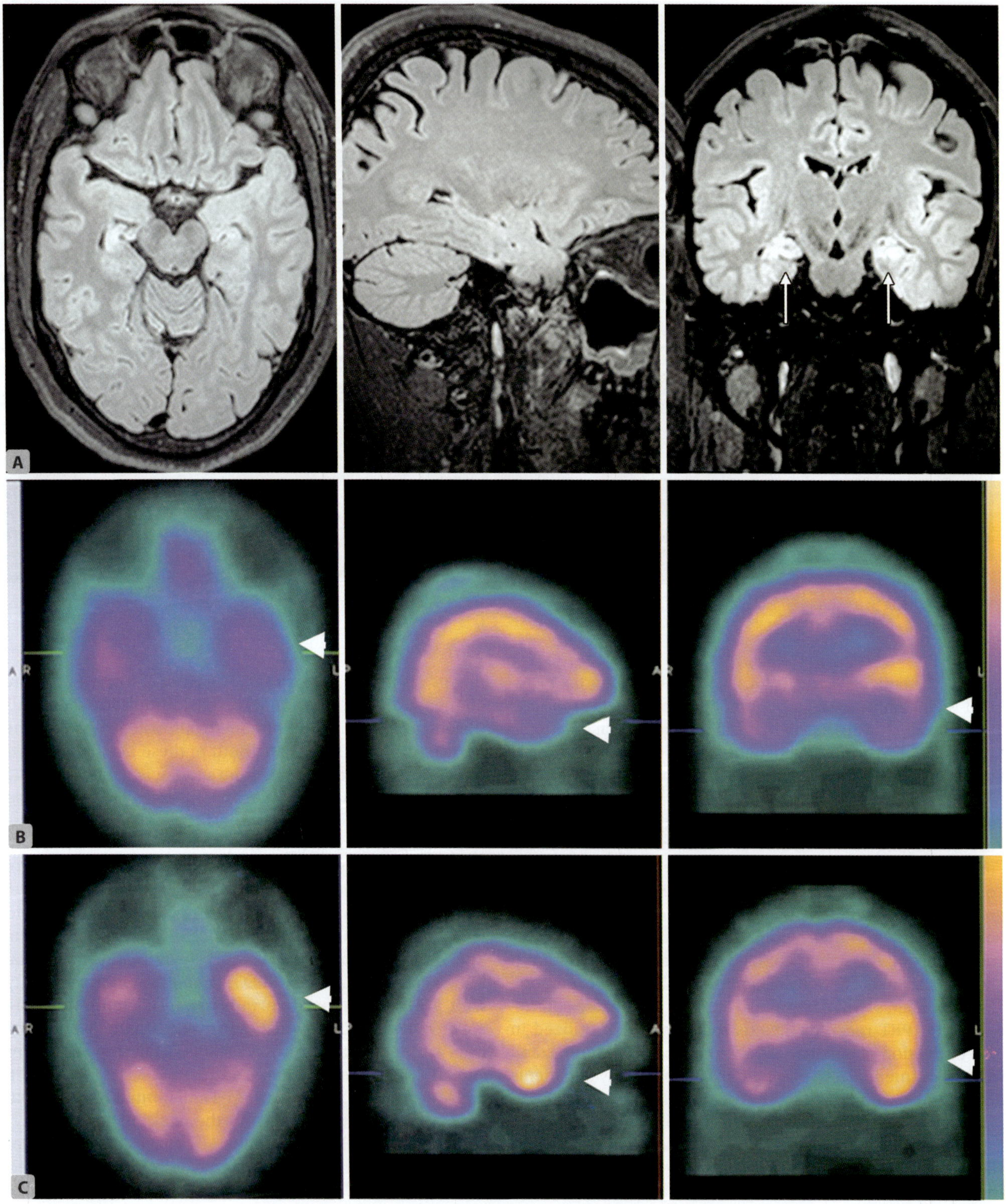

FIGS. 17A TO C: FLAIR MRI (A) and Tc-99m ECD SPECT images (B and C) in a 30-year-old male suffering from complex partial seizures show bilateral hippocampal sclerosis (arrows, A) with interictal hypoperfusion (arrowheads, B) and ictal hyperperfusion (arrowheads, C) in the left temporal lobe, suggesting that the epileptogenic focus is localized to the left temporal lobe.

Courtesy: Dr Madhavi Tripathi, Department of Nuclear Medicine, All India Institute of Medical Sciences, New Delhi, India.

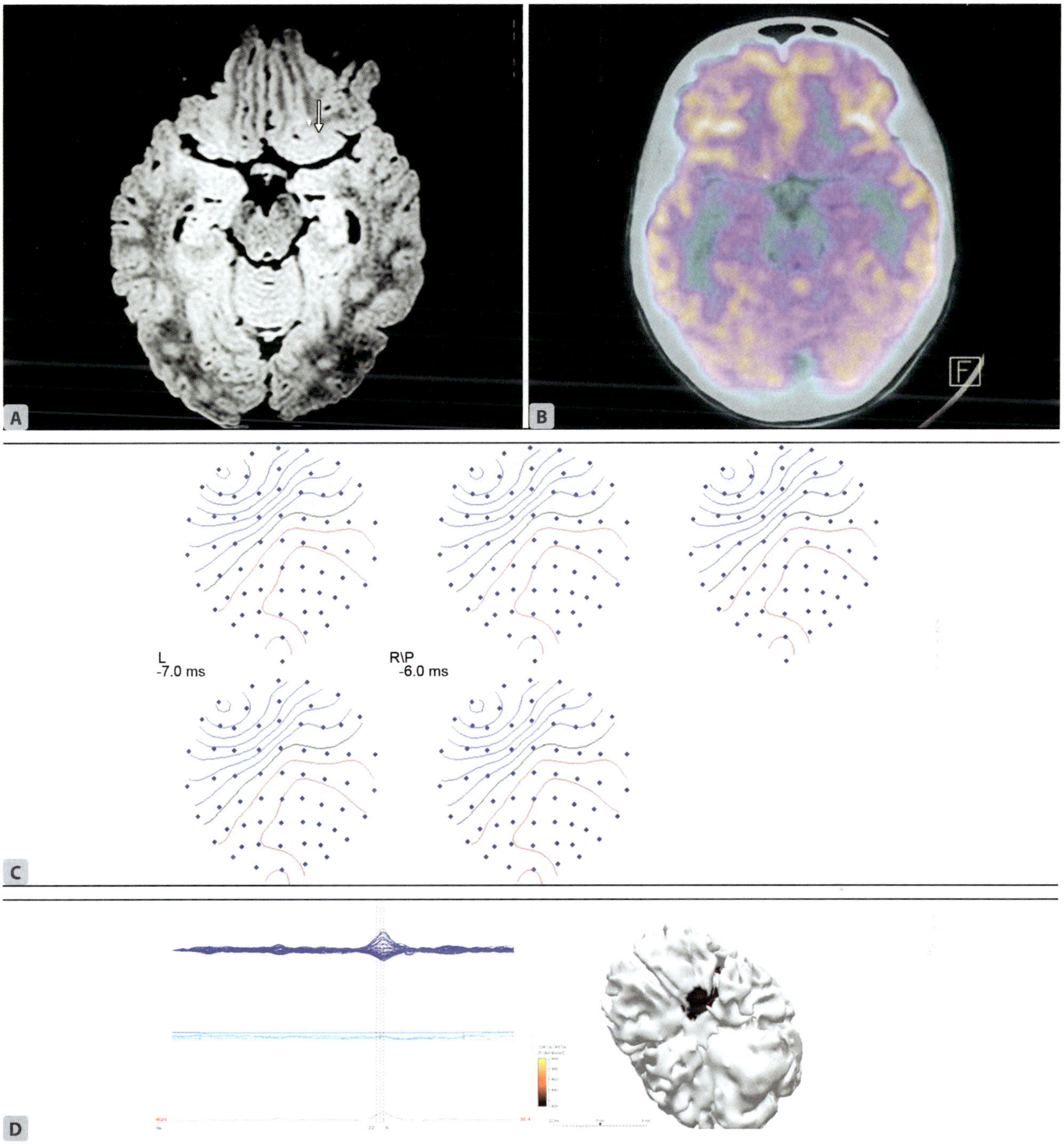

FIGS. 18A TO D: Axial FLAIR (A) image shows subtle cortical thickening in the left basifrontal region with loss of gray-white matter differentiation (arrow). Interictal SPECT (B) shows hypoperfusion in this region. MEG current maps (C) and MEG analysis using CURRY Neuroimaging platform (D) also show localization in the left basifrontal region.

Courtesy: Dr Manjari Tripathi, incharge MEG center; AIIMS-DBT.

of current flow in the apical dendrites. This means that MEG is capable of measuring flow of current tangential to the scalp. This corresponds to activation within the sulci. One of the main advantages of MEG over EEG is that the magnetic fields are not affected by the varying conductivity of the intervening structures like bone and scalp. The spikes that are recorded on MEG have been shown to correlate with invasive monitoring. As MEG records signal from the surface of the brain, it is well suited toward evaluation of neocortical epilepsy. In children who have normal MRI or subtle MR findings, MEG results have been found to predict surgical outcome. Also, in patients who suffer from recurrent seizures after unsuccessful epilepsy surgery, MEG helps in localizing the site of postsurgical epileptiform discharge. This is possible as MEG is affected to a lesser degree by the postoperative changes, cranial defects and gliotic changes. MEG is unable to identify epileptiform discharge from deep areas such as the medial temporal lobe. MEG can also help in pediatric epilepsy by mapping the eloquent cortex. MEG directly measures the electrophysiological changes due to the underlying neuronal activity and has higher temporal resolution compared to fMR.

CONCLUSION

Significant advances have occurred in the presurgical evaluation of epilepsy. It is now possible to utilize multimodality imaging to identify small lesions in the brain. Further advances in MR imaging, for example, 7T MRI scanners will increase the diagnostic accuracy in difficult cases.

REFERENCES

1. Fisher RS, van Emde Boas W, Blume W, et al. Epileptic seizures and epilepsy: definitions proposed by the International League Against Epilepsy (ILAE) and the International Bureau for Epilepsy (IBE). Epilepsia. 2005;46(4):470-2.
2. Nagae LM, Lall N, Dahmoush H, et al. Diagnostic, treatment, and surgical imaging in epilepsy. Clin Imaging. 2016;40(4):624-36.
3. Chavakula V, Cosgrove G. Imaging for epilepsy surgery. Semin Neurol. 2017;37(05):580-8.
4. Cendes F, Andermann F, Gloor P, et al. Atrophy of mesial structures in patients with temporal lobe epilepsy: cause or consequence of repeated seizures? Ann Neurol. 1993;34:795-801.
5. Berkovic SF, Andermann F, Olivier A, et al. Hippocampal sclerosis in temporal lobe epilepsy demonstrated by magnetic resonance imaging. Ann Neurol. 1991;29:175-82.
6. Lee DH, Gao FQ, Rogers JM, et al. MR in temporal lobe epilepsy: analysis with pathologic confirmation. Am J Neuroradiol. 1998;19(1):19-27.
7. Osborn A. Commissural and cortical maldevelopment. In: Osborn's Brain Imaging, Pathology, and Anatomy, 1st edition. Canada: Amirsys; 2013. pp. 1083-113.
8. Cendes F, Theodore WH, Brinkmann BH, et al. Neuroimaging of epilepsy. In: Handbook of Clinical Neurology [Internet]. Elsevier; 2016 [cited March 1, 2018]. pp. 985–1014. Available from http://linkinghub.elsevier.com/retrieve/pii/ B978044453486600051X.
9. Fernandez C, Girard N, Paz Paredes A, et al. The usefulness of MR imaging in the diagnosis of dysembryoplastic neuroepithelial tumor in children: a study of 14 cases. Am J Neuroradiol. 2003;24:829-34.
10. Zentner J, Wolf H, Ostertun B, et al. Ganglio-gliomas: clinical, radiological, and histopathological findings in 51 patients. J Neurol Neurosurg Psychiatry. 1994;57:1497-502.
11. Casazza M, Broggi G, Franzini A, et al. Supratentorial cavernous angiomas and epileptic seizures: preoperative course and postoperative outcome. Neurosurgery. 1996;39:26-32.
12. Bastos AC, Comeau RM, Andermann F, et al. Diagnosis of subtle focal dysplastic lesions: curvilinear reformatting from three-dimensional magnetic resonance imaging. Ann Neurol. 1999;46:88-94.
13. Li LM, Caramanos Z, Cendes F, et al. Lateralization of temporal lobe epilepsy (TLE) and discrimination of TLE from extra-TLE using pattern analysis of magnetic resonance spectroscopic and volumetric data. Epilepsia. 2000;41:832-42.
14. Bernasconi A, Bernasconi N, Caramanos Z, et al. T2 relaxometry can lateralize mesial temporal lobe epilepsy in patients with normal MRI. NeuroImage. 2000;12(6):739-46.
15. Duncan JS, Winston GP, Koepp MJ, et al. Brain imaging in the assessment for epilepsy surgery. Lancet Neurol. 2016;15(4):420-33.
16. Knecht S, Deppe M, Dräger B, et al. Language lateralization in healthy right-handers. Brain. 2000;123(1):74-81.
17. Szaflarski JP, Binder JR, Possing ET, et al. Language lateralization in left-handed and ambidextrous people: fMRI data. Neurology. 2002;59(2):238-44.

CHAPTER

196

Imaging of Supratentorial Brain Tumors

Shailesh B Gaikwad, Ajay Garg

INTRODUCTION

Brain tumors in adults comprise a diverse group of neoplasms that vary in their behavior depending on such factors as cell of origin, site of occurrence, morphology and pattern of spread. The annual incidence of primary intracranial neoplasms is estimated to be 12.3 people per lac population and it is increasing in frequency, however, prognosis of these patients has improved considerably due to recent advances in diagnostic techniques, microneurosurgery, chemotherapy and radiotherapy. Central to the efficacy of these techniques, however, is the ability of the neuroradiologist to diagnose and interpret the growth pattern of these tumors.

This chapter describes various types of brain tumors of supratentorial region in adults with emphasis on imaging features, various modalities used in diagnosis, pitfalls in diagnosis, effect of radiotherapy and important recent advances in imaging of brain tumors. Embryonal tumors have been discussed in chapter on infratentorial brain tumors.

CLASSIFICATION OF SUPRATENTORIAL BRAIN TUMORS (2016)

Classifying brain tumors is valuable, but the conceptual basis for such complex scheme is controversial. The putative histogenic or "cell-of-origin-approach" classification proposed by Bailey and Cushing has been most widely used. In 1993, the WHO ratified a new comprehensive classification of neoplasms affecting the central nervous system.[1]

In 2016 update to WHO brain tumor system classification first time gave the concept of integrated diagnosis taking into consideration the light microscopy findings and molecular genetics[2] **(Table 1)**. The molecular genetics have been found to predict prognosis better than histological grading. Several previously described entities such as gliomatosis cerebri, primitive neuroectodermal tumor have been removed.

DIFFUSE ASTROCYTIC AND OLIGODENDROGLIAL TUMORS

Diffuse astrocytomas and oligodendrogliomas are of different genetic profiles. Diffuse astrocytomas are IDH positive or IDH negative. The term 'NOS' is used when genetic profiling is not done or not available. ODG have genetic hallmark of IDH mutant and 1p/19q co-deletion.[2] IDH mutant gliomas have better prognosis than IDH wild gliomas. Anaplastic astrocytoma, IDH-wild has worse prognosis than GBM, IDH-mutant.

Diffuse Astrocytoma, IDH-mutant/ IDH-wildtype/NOS

These are low-grade WHO grade II gliomas. Genetically they are IDH mutant or wild but negative for 1p-19 q co-deletion. Diffuse astrocytomas constitute 25 to 30% of all cerebral gliomas with peak incidence in fourth decade. These astrocytomas have an inherent tendency for anaplastic transformation. Diffuse fibrillary astrocytoma occurring in the cerebral hemispheres is most common. They are most common in frontal lobe.

Imaging Features

The tumor is hypodense on noncontract CT, hypointense to isointense on T1W and hyperintense on T2W MR imaging **(Figs. 1A to D)**. Enhancement patterns following contrast administration are variable, however, the majority of these tumors demonstrate only minimal and inhomogeneous enhancement. Calcification may be found in 15–20% cases. Up to 10% of diffuse astrocytomas have T2-hyperintense lesion which show more than 50% signal suppression on FLAIR image, a sign known as 'T2-FLAIR mismatch" specific for 1p/19q noncodeleted tumors **(Figs. 2A to C)**.[3]

TABLE 1: Classification of brain tumor[2]
1. *Diffuse astrocytic and oligodendroglial tumors*: • Diffuse astrocytoma, IDH-mutant/IDH-wildtype/NOS • Anaplastic astrocytoma, IDH-mutant/IDH-wildtype/NOS • Glioblastoma, IDH-mutant/IDH-wildtype/NOS • Diffuse midline glioma, H3 K27M-mutant • Oligodendroglioma, IDH-mutant and 1p/19q-codeleted/ NOS • Anaplastic oligodendroglioma, IDH-mutant and 1p/19q-codeleted/NOS • Oligoastrocytoma, NOS
2. *Other astrocytic tumors*: • Pilocytic astrocytoma • Subependymal giant cell astrocytoma • Pleomorphic xanthoastrocytoma • Anaplastic pleomorphic xanthoastrocytoma
3. *Ependymal tumors*: • Subependymoma • Myxopapillary ependymoma • Ependymoma (papillary/ clear cell/tanycytic) • Anaplastic (malignant) ependymoma
4. *Other gliomas*: • Chordoid glioma of third ventricle • Angiocentric glioma • Astroblastoma
5. *Choroid plexus tumors*: • Choroid plexus papillomas • Atypical choroid plexus papillomas • Choroid plexus carcinoma
6. *Neuronal and mixed neuronal-glial tumors*: • Dysembryoplastic neuroepithelial tumors (DNETs) • Gangliocytoma • Ganglioglioma • Anaplastic ganglioglioma • Dysplastic gangliocytoma of cerebellum • Desmoplastic infantile astrocytoma and ganglioglioma • Papillary glioneuronal tumor • Rosette-forming glioneuronal tumor • Diffuse leptomeningeal glioneuronal tumor • Central neurocytoma • Extraventricular neurocytoma • Paraganglioma
7. *Pineal regional tumors*: • Pineocytoma • Pineal parenchymal tumor of intermediate differentiation • Pineoblastoma • Papillary tumor of the pineal region
8. *Embryonal tumors*: • Medulloblastomas, WNT-activated/ SHH-activated/ group 3/ group 4 • Embryonal tumors with multilayered rosettes, C19MC-altered/ NOS • CNS neuroblastoma
Continued
Continued
9. *Tumors of cranial and paraspinal nerve*: • Schwannoma (Cellular/Plexiform) • Melanotic schwannoma • Neurofibroma (Atypical/Plexiform) • Malignant peripheral nerve sheath tumors
10. Meningioma
11. *Mesenchymal, non-meningothelial tumors*: • Solitary fibrous tumor/ hemangiopericytoma • Hemangioblastoma • Ewing's sarcoma
12. *Lymphomas*: • Diffuse large B-cell lymphoma of the CNS • Immunodeficiency-associated CNS lymphoma
13. *Histiocytic tumors*: • Langerhans cell histiocytosis • Erdheim-Chester disease • Rosai-Dorfman disease
14. *Germ cell tumors*: • Germinoma • Embryonal carcinoma • Yolk sac (endodermal sinus) tumors • Choriocarcinoma • Teratoma (mature/ immature) • Mixed germ cell tumors
15. *Tumors of the sellar region*: • Craniopharyngioma • Granular cell tumor of the sellar region • Pituicytoma • Spindle cell oncocytoma
16. Metastatic tumors

Necrosis is not found, but may have cystic degeneration. Edema and hemorrhages are rare.

Progressive malignant transformation is characterized by progressive increase in tumoral necrosis, intratumoral hemorrhage, peritumoral edema and appearance of contrast enhancement. On SWI, areas of susceptibility foci secondary to hemorrhagic foci are usually not seen. On MR perfusion, rCBV values are low.

Anaplastic Astrocytoma, IDH-mutant/IDH-wildtype/NOS

Anaplastic astrocytomas are mixed density/intensity masses with areas of necrosis and cyst formation; blood products from hemorrhage may also be seen, although this is more common in glioblastoma. Mild vasogenic edema of adjacent white matter, mass effect, and more intense irregular enhancement following contrast administration is usually observed. When foci of anaplasia are separated by more low-grade components of the tumor, post-contrast scans may demonstrate multiple separate foci of necrosis or enhancement, thus, mimicking metastatic disease

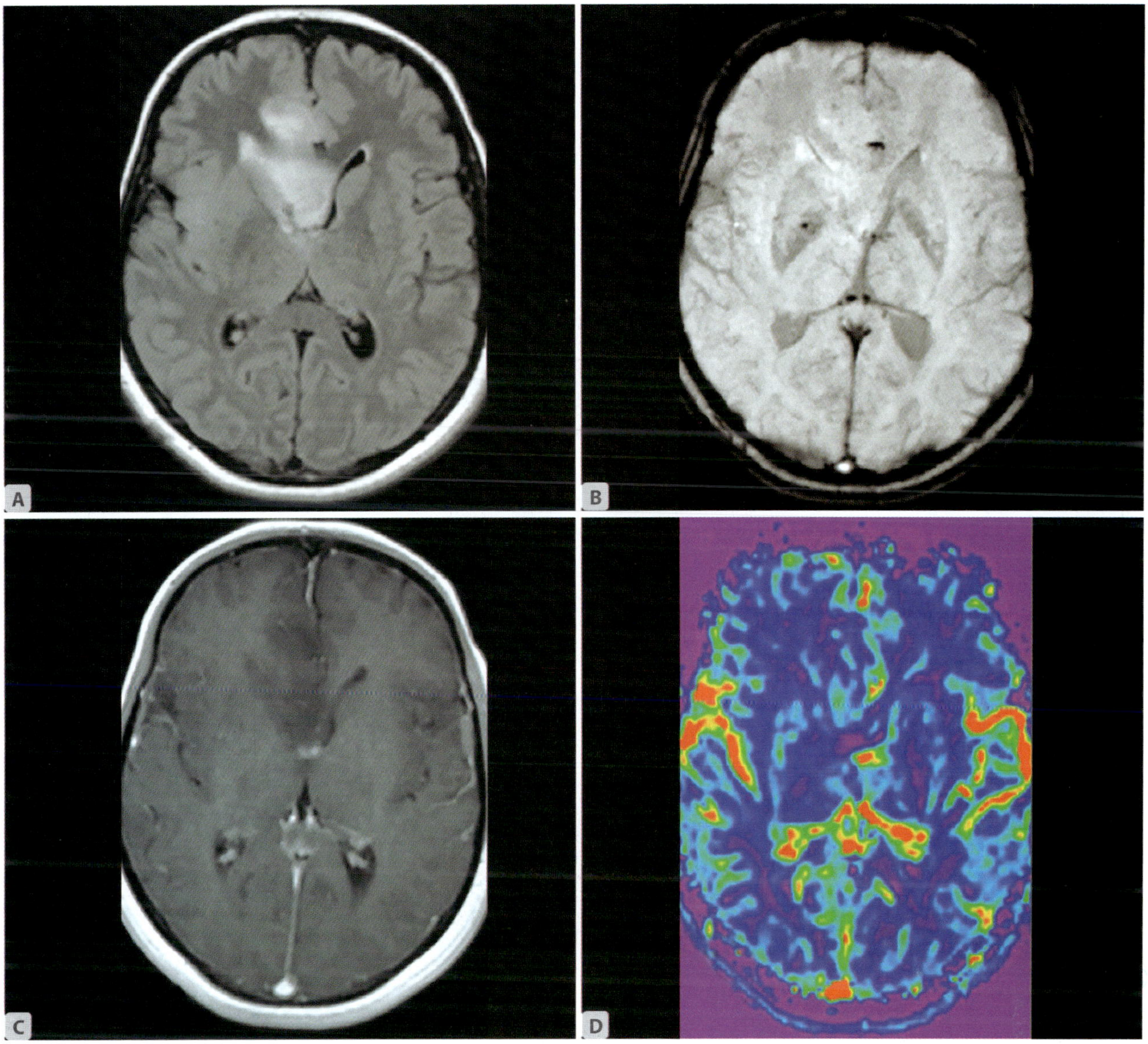

FIGS. 1A TO D: Diffuse astrocytoma: Axial flair (A) shows a well-defined hyperintense lesion in right frontal lobe and adjacent corpus callosum. No hemorrhagic foci are seen on SWI (B). Following contrast administration, no enhancement is noted (C). on DSC perfusion, rCBV maps show low perfusion (D).

or multifocal glioma. On perfusion MRI, these tumors show increased rCBV compared with diffuse astrocytoma **(Figs. 3A to D)**.[4] On MR spectroscopy, increased choline, decreased NAA and decreased myo-inositol is present.

Glioblastoma, IDH-mutant/ IDH-wildtype/NOS

Glioblastoma represent 15–20% of all primary brain neoplasms, and 50% of all astrocytomas. Previously glioblastomas were known as glioblastoma multiforme, but recent WHO classification has dropped the 'multiforme' and these tumors are referred merely as glioblastomas.

Glioblastoma are genetically and imaging phenotypically heterogeneous tumors. The peak incidence is between the ages of 45 and 55 with definite male preponderance. Traditionally glioblastomas have been divided into primary (90%) and secondary (10%); the former arising de novo whereas the later developed from a pre-existing low-grade glioma. Most of the secondary glioblastoma are IDH-mutant, occur at younger age and almost always MGMT methylated. The primary glioblastoma are almost invariably IDH-wild, occur at the older age and have worse prognosis. If IDH status is not known or indeterminate, diagnosis of glioblastoma NOS should be made. Glioblastoma has a predilection for the cerebral white matter especially frontal and temporal lobes and frequently infiltrates into the adjacent lobes and deep structures, such as the corpus callosum. Glioblastoma is an aggressive tumor which spreads locally along the white matter tracts or the ependymal lining of the ventricles into the leptomeninges resulting in seeding of the subarachnoid space. Distant metastasis to lungs, liver and bone have also been reported.

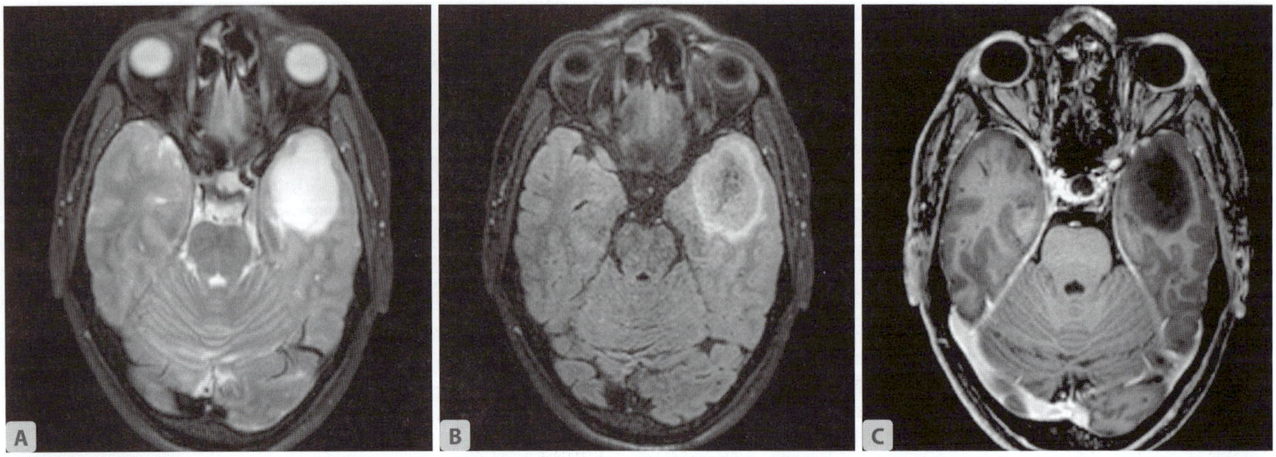

FIGS. 2A TO C: Diffuse astrocytoma in left temporal lobe: The lesion is brightly hyperintense on T2-WI (A) and partial suppression of signal on FLAIR (B): T2-FLAIR mismatch/ No contrast enhancement is seen (C).

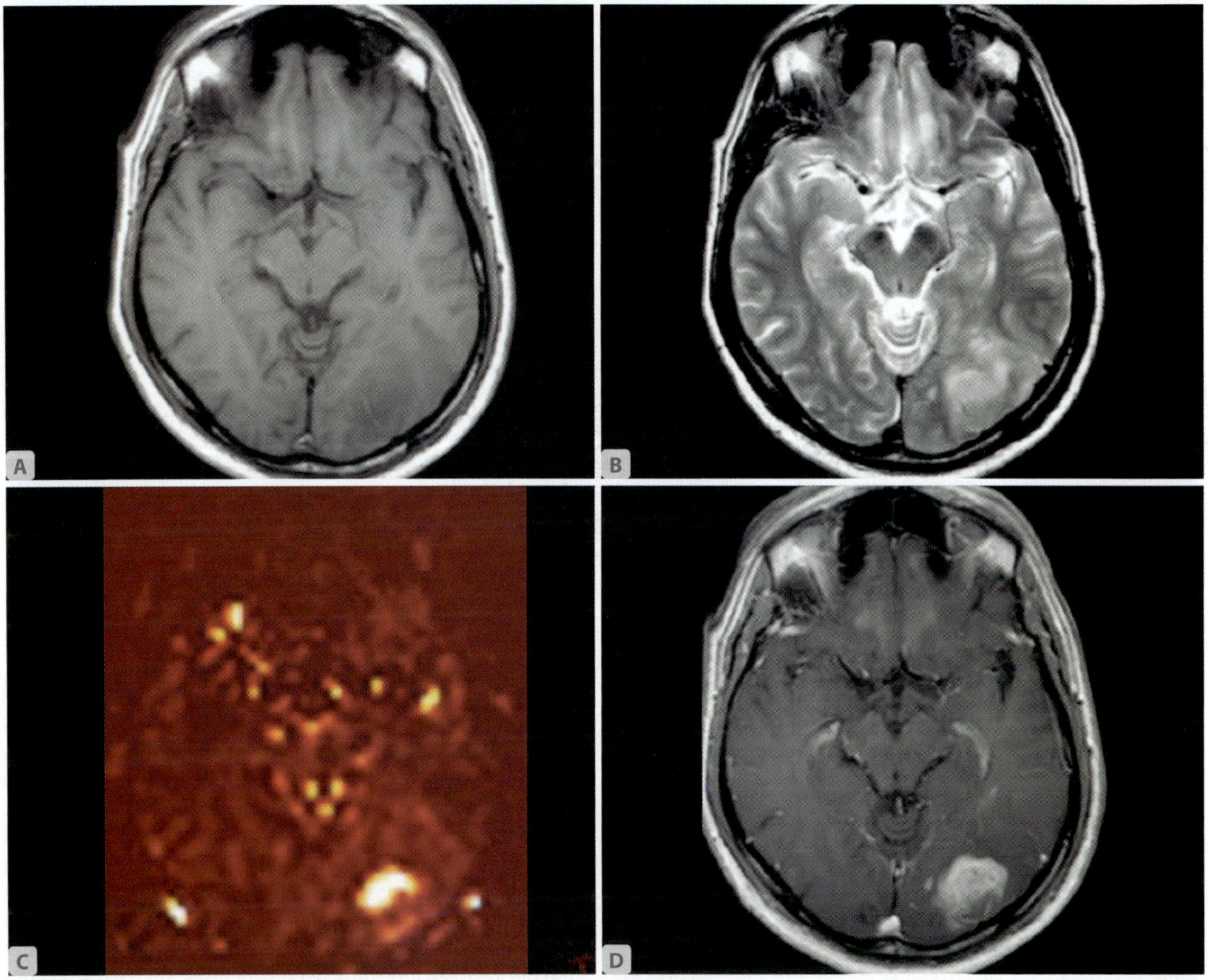

FIGS. 3A TO D: Anaplastic astrocytoma: Axial T1-WI (A) and T2-WI (B) show a left occipital ill-defined lesion, which shows high perfusion in ASL (C) and enhances heterogeneously following gadolinium administration (D).

Imaging Features

Marked intratumoral inhomogeneity is a frequent feature, with focal areas of necrosis or cyst formation producing hypointensity on T1WI and hyperintensity on T2W images **(Figs. 4A to D)**. Focal areas of acute hemorrhage or hemosiderin deposition are often best seen on GRE images, but may produce areas of marked hypointensity on T2WI and less commonly hyperintensity on T1-WI. Identification of blood products may help to differentiate glioblastoma from anaplastic astrocytoma which show bleeds less frequently. SWI are extremely sensitive for detecting blood products. Calcification is rare in de novo primary glioblastomas and are more commonly seen in secondary glioblastoma. Invasion of the cortex, leptomeninges and dura may occur.

Enhancement is almost always seen and usually in the form of thick irregular rim or nodular enhancement surrounded by peritumoral T2- and FLAIR hyperintensity which represents region of tumor cell infiltration and vasogenic edema both in varying proportions **(Figs. 4A to D)**. On angiography large mass with striking tumor blush, contrast stasis and pooling in bizarre vascular channels is noted.

Multiple glioblastomas are also occasionally seen. These have been ascribed to either multifocal origin (when there is a microscopic connection between various foci of the tumor) or a multicentric origin (when there are no connections between the tumors).

Advanced MR imaging techniques like diffusion, perfusion and spectroscopy provide complimentary physiologic information. DWI provide the measure of water diffusion in a voxel. High grade gliomas tend to have areas of high cellularity so lower ADC values. ADC values as a marker of glioma should be interpreted cautiously because of inherent and quite remarkable tissue heterogeneity associated with gliomas. ADC threshold value of 1185×10^{-6} mm^2/s sensitivity (97.6%) and specificity (53.1%) in the discrimination of high-grade (WHO grade III & IV) and low-grade (WHO grade II) gliomas.[5]

MR perfusion imaging evaluate tumor angiogenesis and permeability of blood-brain barrier, which may be predictive of the tumor grade and higher malignant histology **(Fig. 4)**.[6] MR spectroscopy provide metabolic information. One must remember that regional tumor heterogeneity may influence conventional and advanced MRI findings.

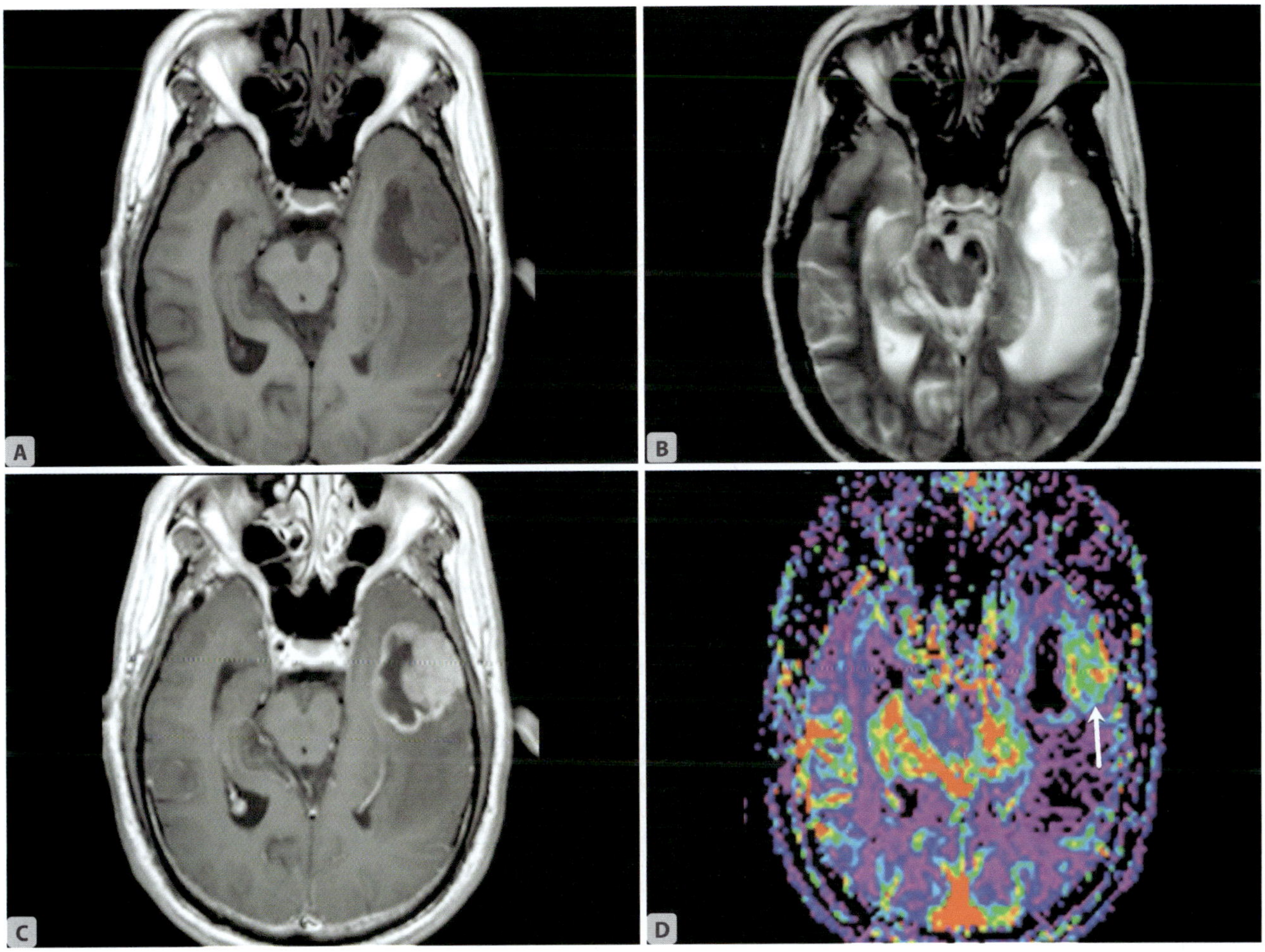

FIGS. 4A TO D: Glioblastoma: Axial T1-WI (A) and T2-WI (B) show a left temporal nodular ring-lesion with perilesional edema. The mass enhances avidly with central necrosis (C). On DSC perfusion rCBV maps, perfusion is high in the solid component of the mass (D).

Diffuse Midline Glioma, H3 K27M-mutant

In 2016 update of the WHO CNS tumor classification, diffuse midline glioma, H3 K27M-mutant is a new entity characterized by a diffuse growth pattern, and a midline location (e.g., thalami, brainstem, spinal cord, and other midline structures, including the third ventricle, hypothalamus, and pineal region) **(Figs. 5A to C)**.[2] The majority of these tumors are high-grade astrocytomas with high proliferative potential.[7,8]

Oligodendroglioma, IDH-mutant and 1p/19q-codeleted/NOS

Oligodendroglioma (ODG) constitutes 5–20% of all cerebral gliomas. IDH-mutation and 1p/19q-codeletion are genetic signature of ODG. The peak age incidence is in the fifth and sixth decades.

Imaging Features

On CT, this tumor appears as a heterogeneous hemispheric mass involving the cortex, usually located in the frontal lobe. The mass is hypo-isodense relative to the gray matter; heavy streaky, ribbon like calcification is seen in 70 to 90% of tumors **(Figs. 6A to C)**. Hemorrhage is present in about 20% of cases with mild edema. Scalloping of inner table of the calvarium is other feature in about 17% of cases. Although cysts are frequent, necrosis or gross hemorrhage may also be rarely seen. Mild to moderate heterogeneous enhancement after contrast administration is common. Most are high grade at time of diagnosis. Contrast enhancement does not necessarily reflect malignant transformation, as in astrocytic tumors. On MR, the tumors have heterogeneously hyperintense signal on T2-WI and typically have indistinct borders **(Figs. 7A to C)** compared to homogenously hyperintense T2 signal and sharp border seen in astrocytomas **(*see* Figs. 2A to C)**.[9]

Anaplastic Oligodendroglioma, IDH-mutant and 1p/19q-codeleted/ NOS

Anaplastic ODG are characterized by more enhancement and increased rCBV values.

OTHER ASTROCYTIC TUMORS

Pilocytic Astrocytoma

These are slow growing WHO grade I CNS neoplasms. It usually presents in the first two decades.[10] These tumors are generally located around the optic chiasma-hypothalamus and optic nerve in the supratentorial region. Cerebral hemispheric pilocytic astrocytomas are rare and present later beyond 20 years of age.

Most PA have BRAF-KIAA1549 fusion gene mutation which is associated with better prognosis.[11] They lack IDH and TP53 mutations. These tumors have strong association with NF1.

Imaging Features

Hemispheric pilocytic astrocytomas present either as a well-defined cystic mass with enhancing mural nodule or solid enhancing lesion on CT and MRI **(Figs. 8A to C)**. About 10% of pilocytic astrocytomas are calcified.

Despite their benign nature, they show intense enhancement and show wide range of choline values in MR spectroscopy. They have low rCBV ratio (<1.5) and characteristic signal intensity curve which overshoots baseline during recovery caused by massive contrast leakage into interstitial space.[12] Angiography demonstrates an avascular mass with displacement of the normal vessels.

Subependymal Giant Cell Astrocytoma

Subependymal giant cell astrocytoma (SGCA) are slow-growing WHO grade I CNS tumors. They are seen in 10 to 15% of patients with tuberous sclerosis complex (TSC). SGCAs probably arise from subependymal nodules in the ventricular wall of patients with tuberous sclerosis.[13] They usually become symptomatic before 20 years of age. These tumors are characteristically located in a lateral ventricle near the foramen of Monro.

Imaging Features

On CT scan, SGCA appears as focal partially calcified mass, iso- attenuated to slightly hypo-attenuated intraventricular

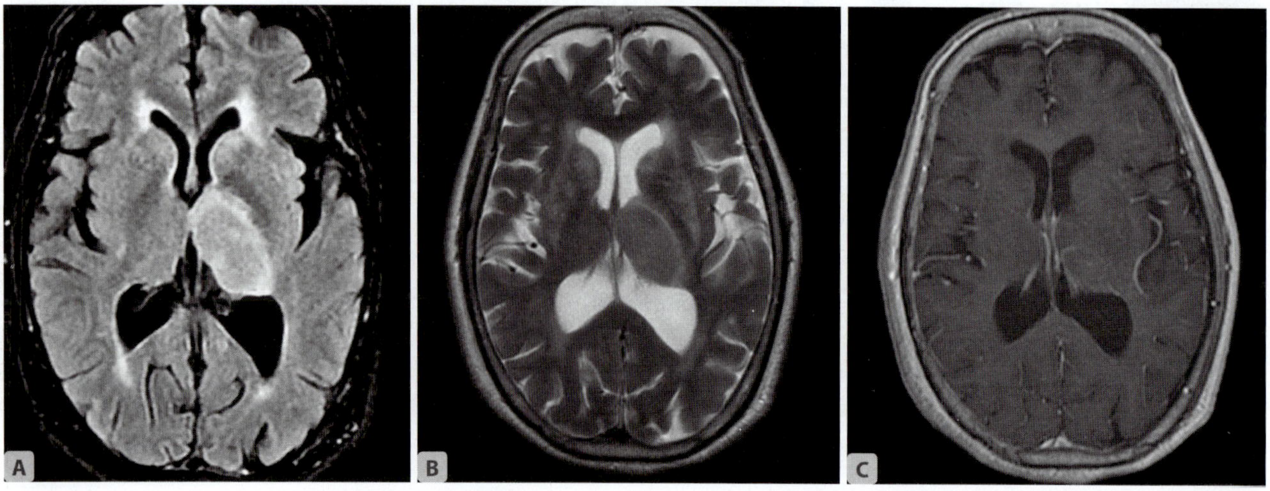

FIGS. 5A TO C: Thalamic glioma: Axial flair (A) and T2-WI (B) show a left thalamic mass, which shows patchy enhancement following contrast administration (C).

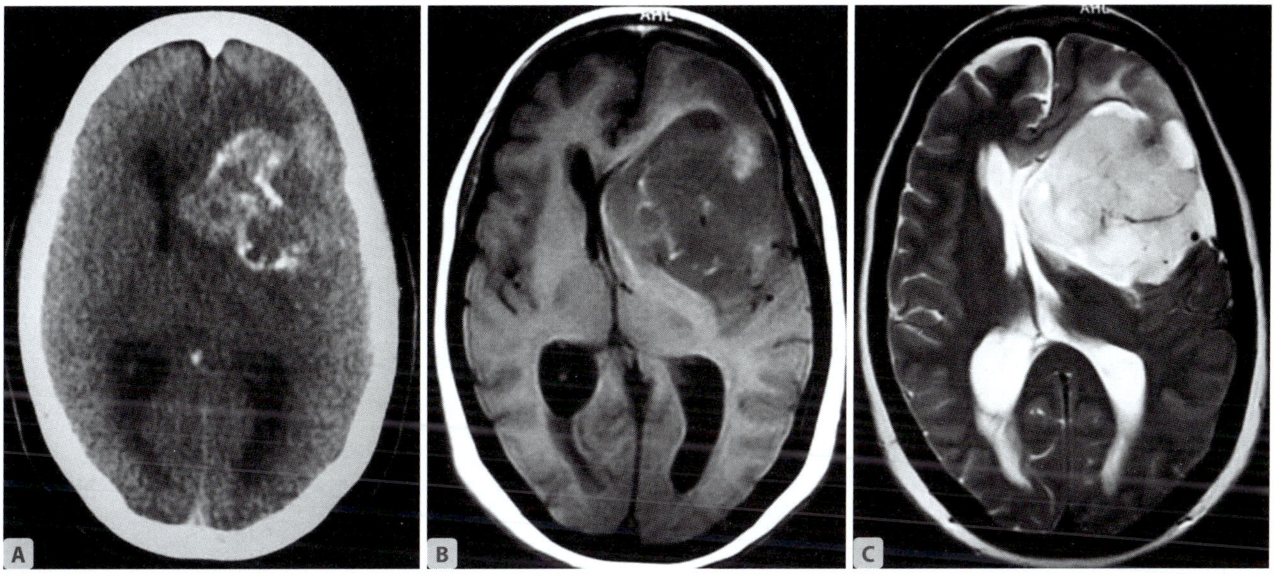

FIGS. 6A TO C: Oligodendroglioma: NCCT (A) shows a left frontal deep white matter and basal ganglion mass with calcification. The mass is predominantly hypointense on T-WI (B) with foci of high signal intensity and heterogeneously hyperintense on T2-WI (C). Minimal perilesional edema is seen.

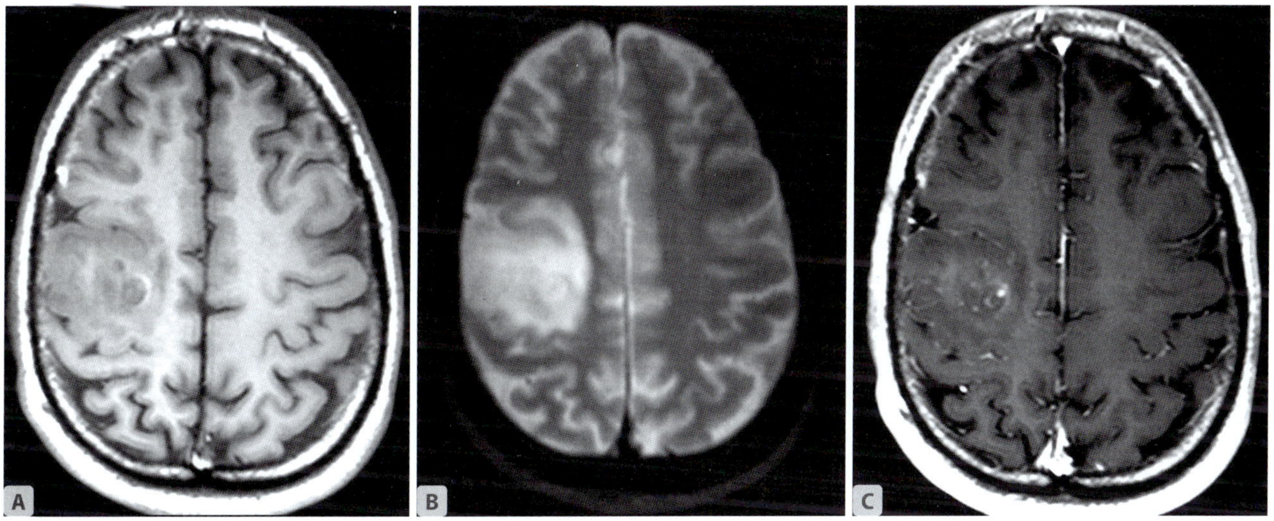

FIGS. 7A TO C: Anaplastic oligodendroglioma: Axial T1-Wi (A) and T2-WI (B) show a right frontal cortical-subcortical mixed signal intensity lesion which show patchy enhancement (C).

mass **(Figs. 9A and B)**. Contrast enhancement is strong but heterogeneous. This enhancement do not distinguish a SGCA from a subependymal nodule, which may also enhance.[14] Growth over serial imaging or symptomatic hydrocephalus may help to differentiate SEGA from subependymal nodule.[15] Co-existing lesions of tuberous sclerosis are usually present. On MR, the tumor exhibits mixed signal intensities on both T1 and T2WI.

Pleomorphic Xanthoastrocytoma (Noninvasive, WHO Grade II)

Pleomorphic Xanthoastrocytoma (PXA) is tumor of children and young adults and usually present with seizures.

Temporal and frontal lobe of young adult is the most common site of involvement. Marked cellular pleomorphism may be noted at histology. In 2016 WHO CNS Tumor classification update, anaplastic PXA (WHO grade III) has been added as separate entity.[2]

Imaging Features

On CT PXAs are typically seen as superficially located solid enhancing nodule, frequently associated with a peripheral eccentric cyst component (50-60%) **(Figs. 10A and B)**.[16] These slow-growing tumor may cause scalloping of overlying calvarium. On MRI, these tumors appear of mixed signal intensity on T1WI. On T2WI both the cystic component and solid components are hyperintense.[17] Peritumoral edema is variable and may be mild to moderate.[18] The solid component shows homogeneous enhancement after intravenous contrast administration **(Figs. 11A to D)**. Extension to leptomeningeal

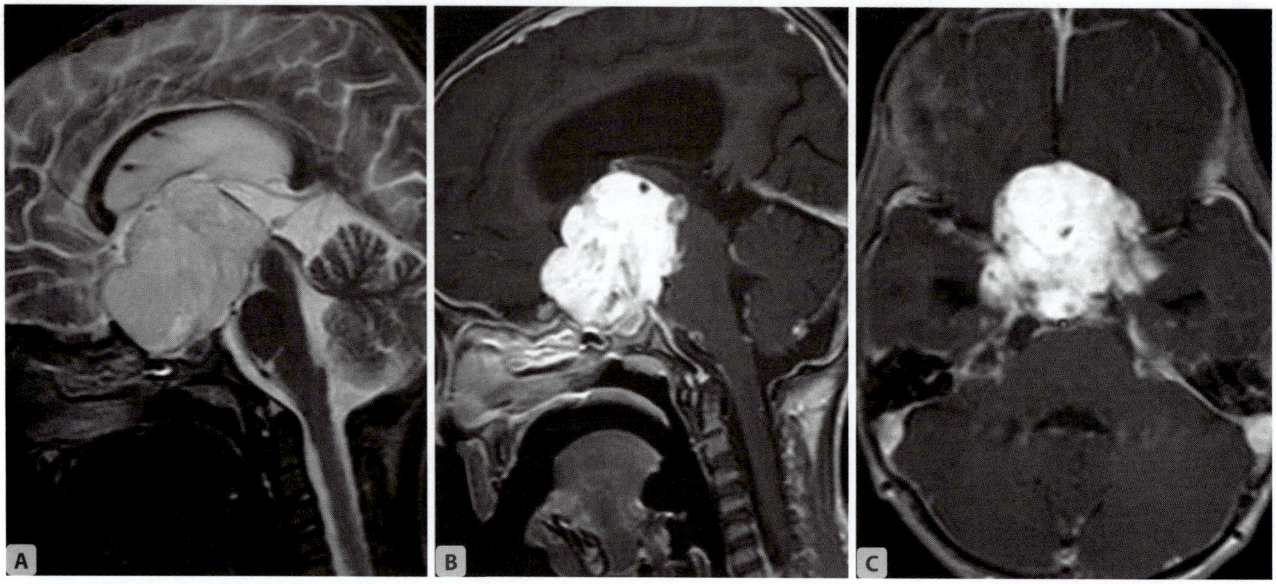

FIGS. 8A TO C: Chiasmal-hypothalamic pilocytic astrocytoma: Sagittal T2-WI (A) shows a hyperintense mass in Chiasmal-hypothalamic region which shows intense contrast enhancement in sagittal (B) and axial (C) T1-WI.

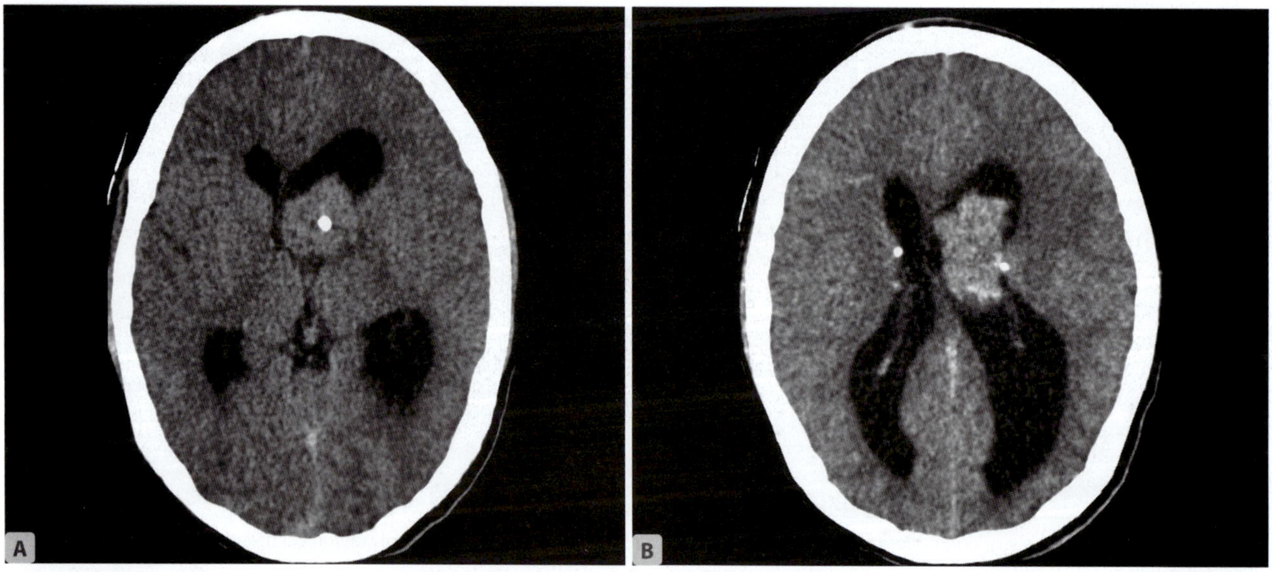

FIGS. 9A AND B: CECT (A and B) show a enhancing mass in region of left foramen of Monro with focal calcification. Also note multiple calcified subependymal nodules (B) along left lateral ventricle suggestive of tuberous sclerosis.

surfaces is present in over 70% of cases.[17] One third may undergo malignant transformation.

EPENDYMAL TUMORS

Subependymoma

Subependymomas are another variant of ependymoma with a significant astroglial component to the tumor; however, they still have characteristic ependymal features. They occur most frequently in the frontal horn of lateral ventricle and inferior fourth ventricle. They are multiple and slow growing. They are common in middle aged and elderly patients.

Imaging Features

On CT and MRI subependymoma, appears as a non-enhancing mass similar to brain with focal areas of cystic degeneration and hemorrhage.[19]

Ependymoma

Ependymomas constitute 2 to 6% of all gliomas. Peak age range is 1–5 years for intraventricular lesions but second small peak occurs in mid-thirties for supratentorial masses. Only 40% of ependymomas are supratentorial where parenchymal location is more common than intraventricular site. It is believed that subependymal neural glia may extend into

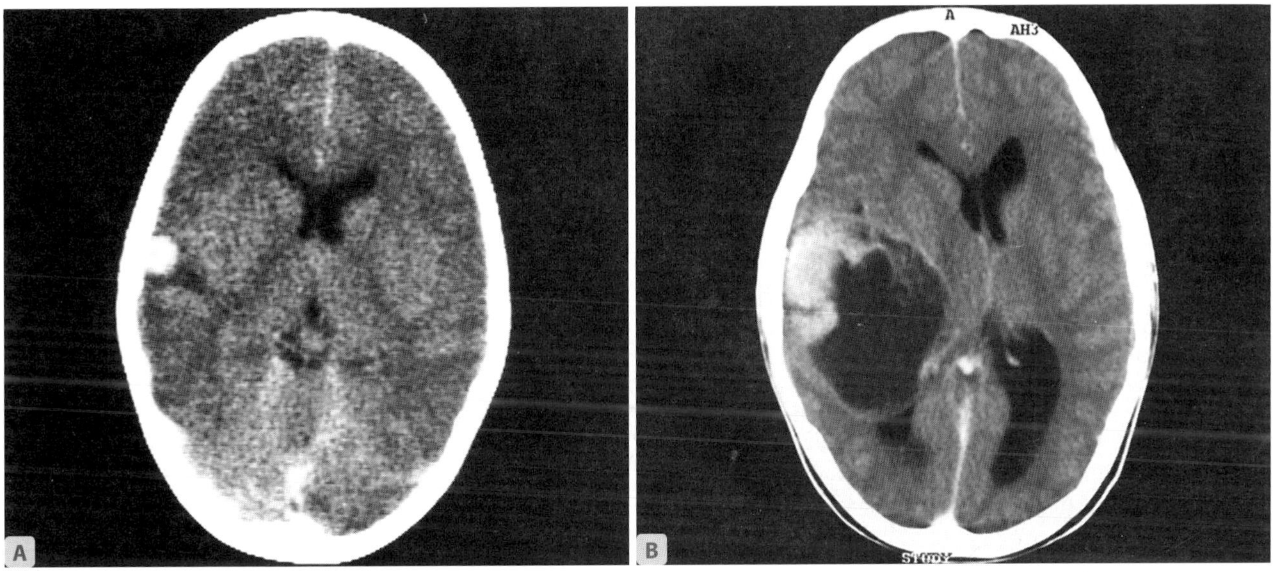

FIGS. 10A AND B: Pleomorphic xanthoastrocytoma. CECT (A) show a enhancing nodule abutting pial surface in right temporal lobe with minimal edema. Three years later, follow-up CECT scan (B) show significant increase in the size of the lesion with cystic component and mass-effect.

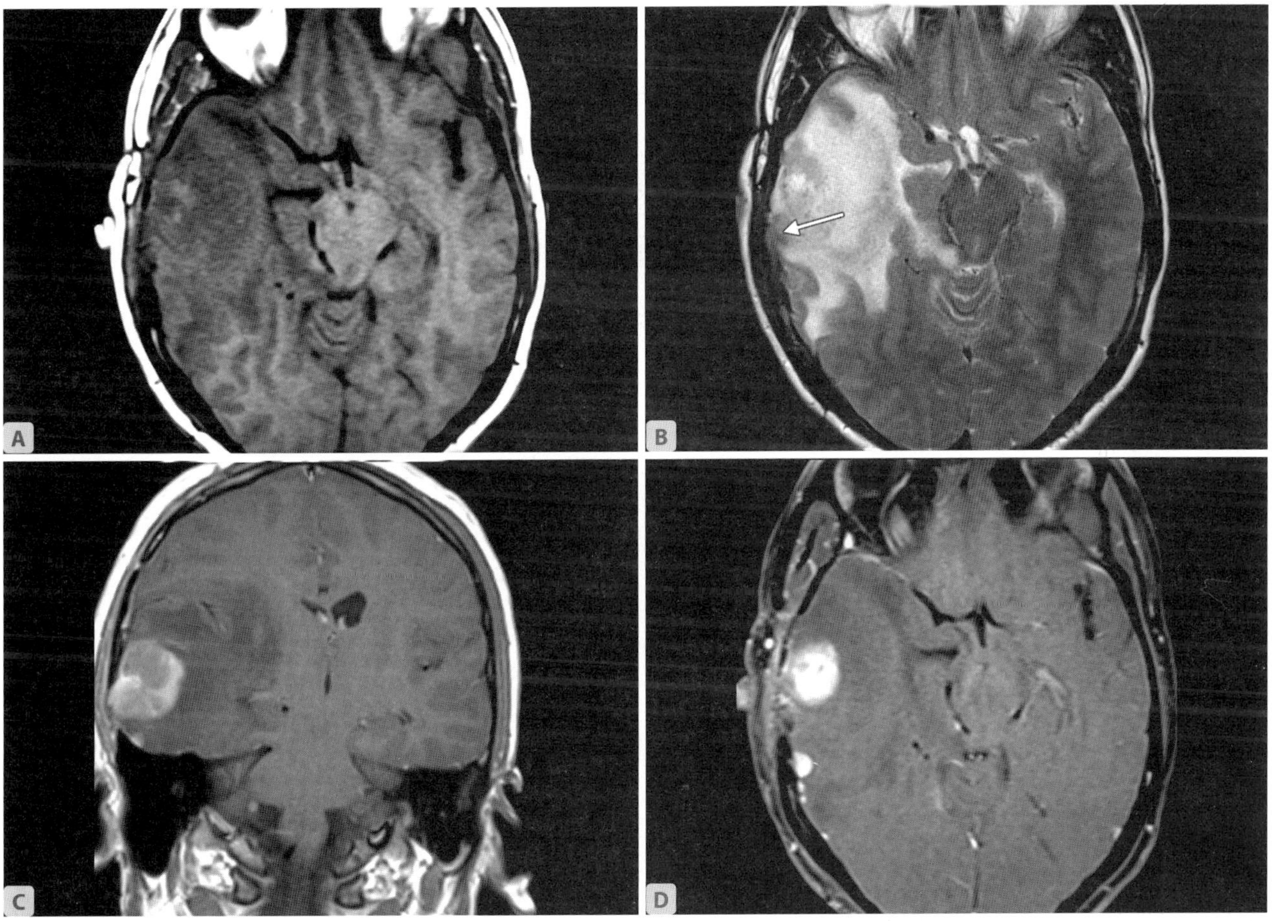

FIGS. 11A TO D: Pleomorphic xanthoastrocytoma: Axial T1-Wi (A) and T2-WI (B) show a mixed signal intensity lesion in right temporal lobe with marked perilesional edema and focal scalloping of overlying bone (arrow in B). The mass enhances avidly (C and D) with enhancement of adjacent leptomeninges (arrow in D).

adjacent white matter leading to ependymal cell rests remote from the ventricular lining.[20] Extraventricular ependymomas are larger than intraventricular ependymomas at time of presentation.

Imaging Features

Ependymomas are multilobulated, well-demarcated, frequently calcified masses that are either intraventricular or juxtaventricular in supratentorial region. On noncontrast CT, ependymomas are isodense with dense punctate calcification in about 50% and hemorrhage may occur.[21] There is mild to moderate enhancement following contrast administration varying from homogenous to inhomogeneous or rim enhancement.[22] On MRI **(Figs. 12A and B)**, the solid component of ependymoma appear hypo- to isointense on T1WI and hyperintense on T2WI. Calcification can be less conspicuous than on CT, whereas cysts and small hemorrhagic foci are better demonstrated on MRI. When calcification, necrosis or blood products are present the tumor appears heterogeneous.[13]

CHOROID PLEXUS TUMORS

Choroid Plexus Papilloma

Choroid plexus papilloma (CPP) are uncommon benign WHO grade I neoplasm. They are commonly seen in children less than 5-year of age and rare in adults. They have predilection for the trigone of lateral ventricle in children and the fourth ventricle in adults.[23]

Imaging Features

On CT, CPP appears as a mottled mass which is isodense to hyperdense on noncontrast scans and usually show homogeneous enhancement. Intratumoral fine, speckled

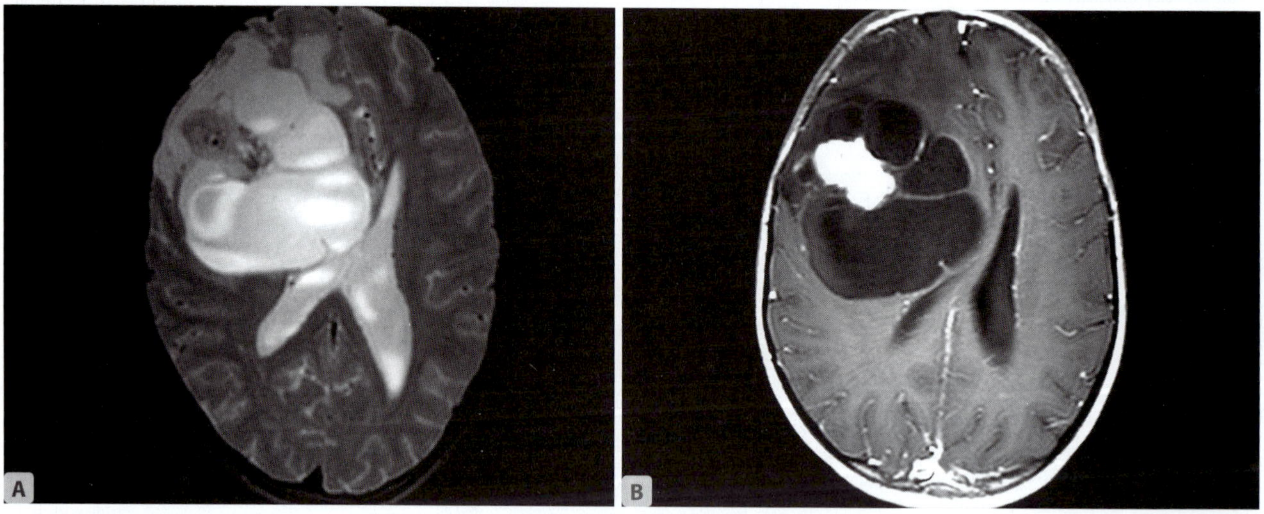

FIGS. 12A AND B: Ependymoma: Axial T2-WI (A) shows a solid-cystic mass in right juxtaventricular region. The solid portion enhances intensely with contrast (B).

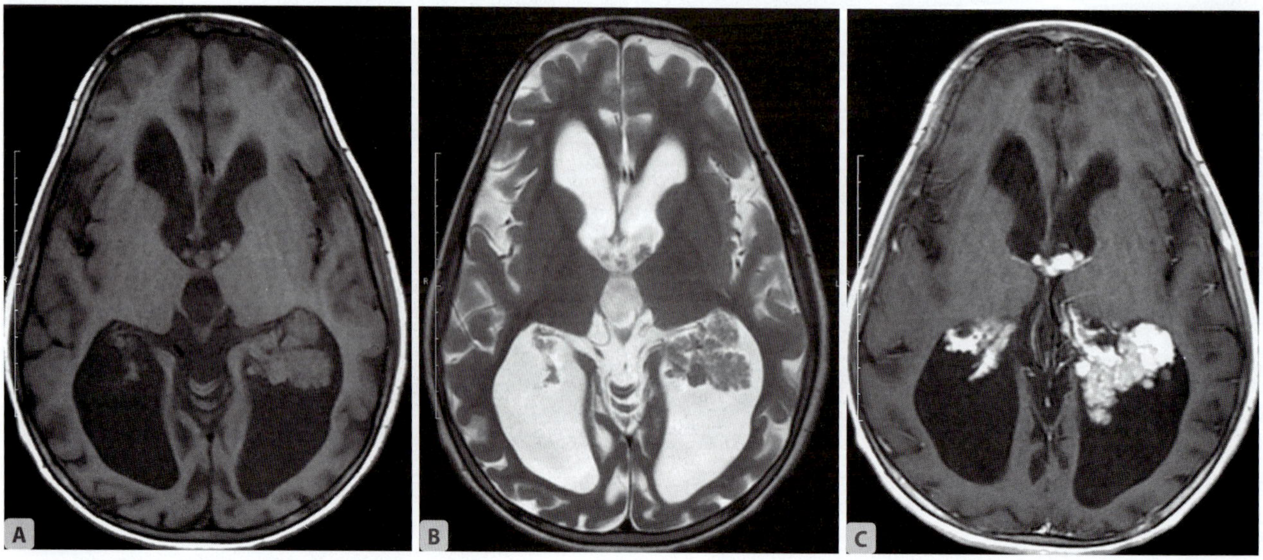

FIGS. 13A TO C: Choroid plexus papilloma: Axial T1-WI (A) and T2-WI (B) show frond-like intraventricular lesion in both lateral ventricles (left larger than right) with hydrocephalus. The lesions are isointense in T1-WI (A) and T2-WI and enhances intensely with contrast (C).

calcification is seen in about 25% of cases. On MRI **(Figs. 13A to C)**, CPPs show lobulations at the peripheral margin (frond-like morphology), masses usually are isointense to brain on T1WI and iso to slightly hyperintense on T2WI. Calcification is not normally appreciated on spin echo pulse sequences. They enhance intensely and homogeneously. Many choroid plexus tumors are attached by a vascular pedicle to the choroid plexus.

All ventricles usually enlarge with trigonal CPPs. Hemorrhage and cyst formation may be seen.

Choroid Plexus Carcinoma

Choroid plexus carcinoma may be difficult to differentiate from CPP on imaging or even on histopathology unless evidence of brain invasion is seen. They occur almost exclusively in young children. Compared to CPP, they show heterogeneous enhancement.

NEURONAL AND MIXED NEURONAL-GLIAL TUMORS

Dysembryoplastic Neuroepithelial Tumor

Dysembryoplastic neuroepithelial tumors (DNET) are benign (WHO grade 1), slow growing mixed glioneuronal tumor. The arise from either cortical or deep gray matter. Children and young adults are commonly affected and present with intractable epilepsy. The "specific glioneuronal element" is characteristic pathological feature. Association cortical dysplasia in seen in up to 80% of cases. Temporal lobe is most common location followed by frontal lobe and caudate nucleus.

Imaging Features

These tumors are hypodense on CT scan, but are slightly denser than CSF. Contrast enhancement or calcification is reported in 20% of cases **(Figs. 14A and B)** MR scans show focal intracortical lesion most commonly located in the temporal lobe.[24] The tumor is hypointense on T1 and hyperintense on T2WI with well demarcated margins and lacks peritumoral edema **(Figs. 15A to D)**. The lesion often follows gyriform pattern. The mass effect is not commensurate with the size of the lesion. Compared with ganglioglioma, DNET is less likely to show enhancement and calcification and 'bubbly' appearance is not seen in ganglioglioma.

Ganglioglioma

Gangliogliomas are usually benign WHO grade I CNS tumors. This tumor has a very high prevalence in patients with chronic epilepsy. It is most common in temporal lobe followed by frontal, parietal and occipital lobes. Grossly and at histology it has been found to be frequently associated with cortical dysplasia. Typically it manifests with cyst and solid enhancing nodule **(Figs. 16A to C)** or a solid mass expanding overlying gyrus. Calcification is found in about 30–40% of cases. Solid non-calcified portion show enhancement in approximately 50% cases.

Central Neurocytoma

Central neurocytoma are WHO grade II intraventricular tumor. They generally occur at young age (range of 17 to 53 years).

Imaging Features

Central neurocytoma appears as inhomogeneous, partially calcified (typically punctate in over 50%) mass; typically located in the lateral ventricles adjacent to the foramen of Monro with broad attachment to the septum pellucidum. Most of the tumors, esp, large one contain multiple small cysts and areas of hemorrhage. Ventricular

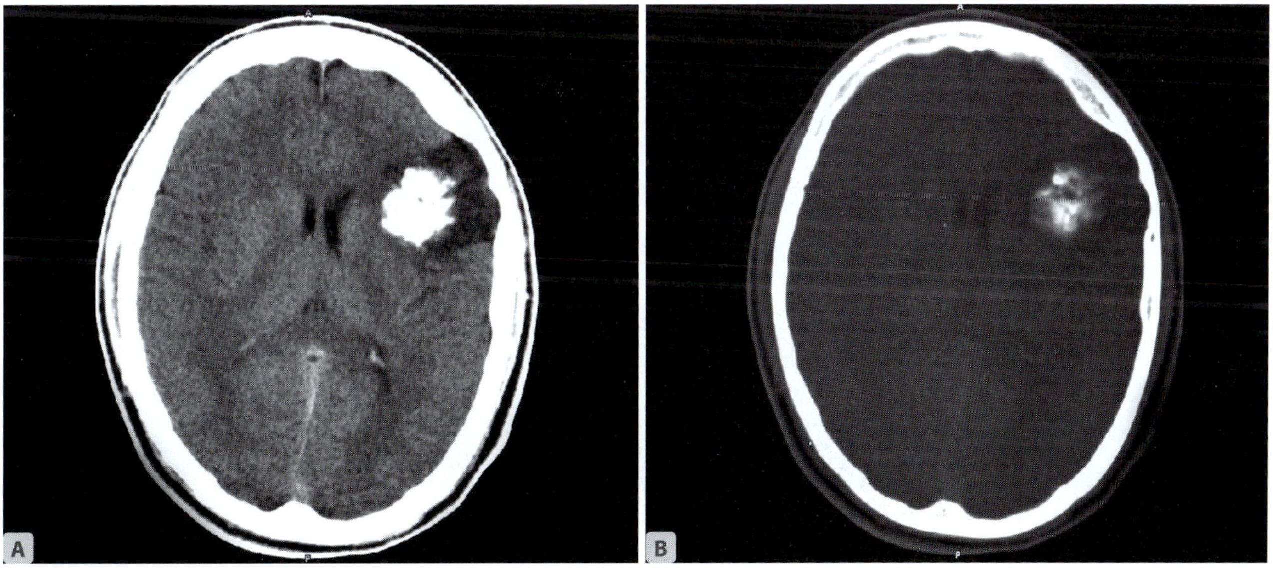

FIGS. 14A AND B: Dysembryoplastic neuroepithelial tumor (DNET): Axial CT (A) shows mixed density lesion in left frontal lobe. The medial portion of lesion is calcified; the lateral portion is hypodense causing scalloping of overlying bone (B). Note that no perilesional edema or commensurate mass effect is seen.

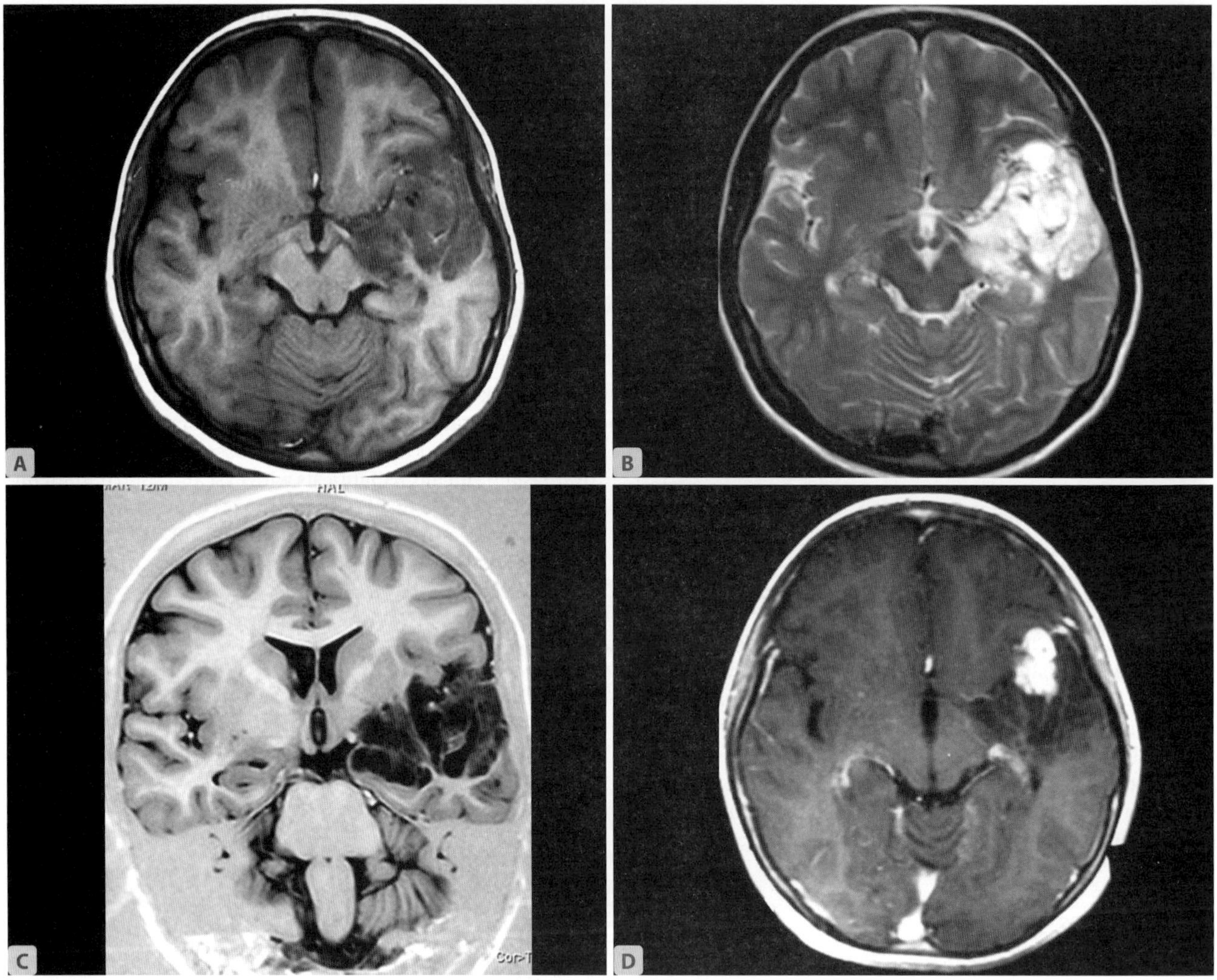

FIGS. 15A TO D: DNET-MRI: Axial T1-WI (A), T2-WI (B) and coronal T1-IR image (C) show a cortical-based lesion in left temporal lobe. The lesion is hypointense on T1-WI (A) and T1-IR image (C) and hyperintense on T2-WI (B) and is following gyriform pattern. Note that no perilesional edema or commensurate mass effect is seen. The anteromedial portion of lesion enhances with contrast (D).

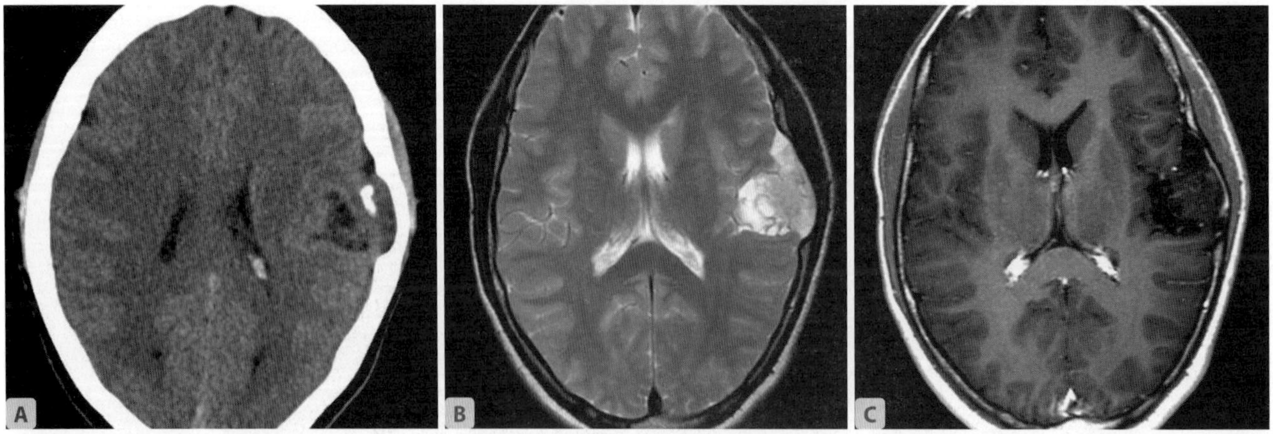

FIGS. 16A TO C: Ganglioglioma: CECT (A) and T2-WI (B) show a solid-cystic lesion in left temporal lobe. On CT, the mass is having focal calcification and causing scalloping of overlying skull. Minimal enhancement is seen following contrast administration (C).

dilation is present in most cases. They show mild-moderate enhancement **(Figs. 17A to C)**. If appropriate staining with immunohistochemical examinations is not performed the lesion will be mistaken for an oligodendroglioma. IDH mutation and 1p/19q co-deletion, genetic signature of oligodendroglioma, are absent.

PINEAL REGION TUMORS

Pineal Germinoma and Teratoma

These account for 55% of all pineal tumors. They are described together as they have common imaging features. On CT, these tumors appear as slightly hyperdense masses which surround and engulf a calcified pineal gland **(Figs. 18A to D)**. On CECT, intense and uniform enhancement is seen in germinomas **(Figs. 19A and B)**. They often have secondary implants in the third ventricular recesses. Diffuse ependymal and subarachnoid spread is common. Teratoma may have heterogeneous appearance because of calcification. On MRI, the germinoma is isointense with cortex on all pulse sequences, and appears homogeneously hyperintense on post Gd T1WI.

Pineal Cell Tumors

Pineal parenchymal tumors represent less than 15% of all pineal region tumors. These are of two types: (i) Pineocytoma, and (ii) Pineoblastoma.

Pineocytoma

Pineocytomas are uncommon slow growing, WHO grade I tumors accounting for only 0.4–1% of all primary brain tumors. Average age of presentation is 34 years. Unlike other pineal neoplasms there is no male predominance.

Imaging Features

They generally appear as well-circumscribed mass with less than 3 cm size. The mass is iso- to hyperdense on NCCT, iso to hypointense on T1WI and hyperintense on T2WI.[25] Following contrast administration, characteristically intense homogenous enhancement is seen. Like other pineal parenchymal tumors, pineal calcification is displaced peripherally. Small cystic tumors may resemble benign pineal cysts on imaging studies.

Pineoblastoma

Pineoblastomas are uncommon malignant WHO grade IV tumors, typically found in young children with slight female predilection.

Imaging Features

On imaging, pineoblastoma appear as large (>4 cm) irregular mass, hyperdense on NCCT, iso to hypointense on T1 and isointense on T2. The diffusion is restricted due to high cellularity.[25] Area of cyst formation and necrosis may be present. The tumor shows intense heterogeneous enhancement. Leptomeningeal spread may be present in 45% of cases **(Figs. 20A to E)**.[25]

TUMORS OF CRANIAL AND PARASPINAL NERVE

Schwannomas and neurofibromas are the commonest tumors arising from the cranial nerves.

Schwannoma (Cellular/Plexiform)

Schwannomas account for 6–8% of primary brain tumors. They are seen in the fourth to sixth decades. These tumors are most commonly seen in relation to VIIIth cranial nerve. The Vth, VIIth IIIrd and VIth cranial nerves are the other nerves which can be affected. On CT, they appear as sharply delineated masses. Smaller lesion show homogeneous enhancement, while larger lesions appear heterogeneous. On MRI 60% of the tumors appear hypointense on T1WI and 34% are isointense. On T2WI these tumors are hyperintense. They enhance after contrast administration.

Neurofibroma (Atypical/ Plexiform)

Neurofibromas are uncommon tumors affecting the cranial nerves, except when associated with the constellation of lesions of neurofibromatosis type I. They are encountered

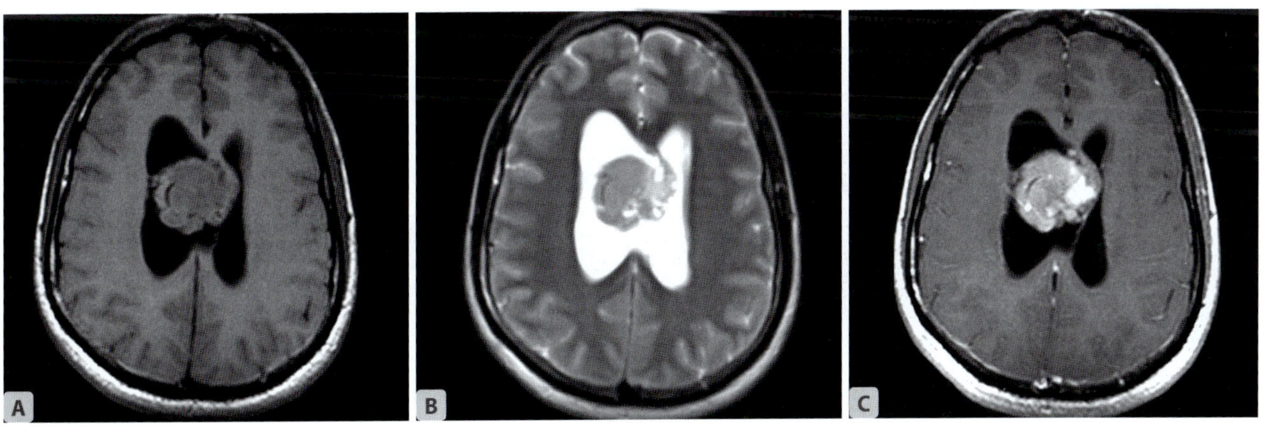

FIGS. 17A TO C: Central neurocytoma: Axial T1-WI (A) and T2-WI (B) show a intraventricular lesion in right lateral ventricle. The lesions are isointense in T1-WI (A) and T2-WI and enhances heterogeneously with contrast (C).

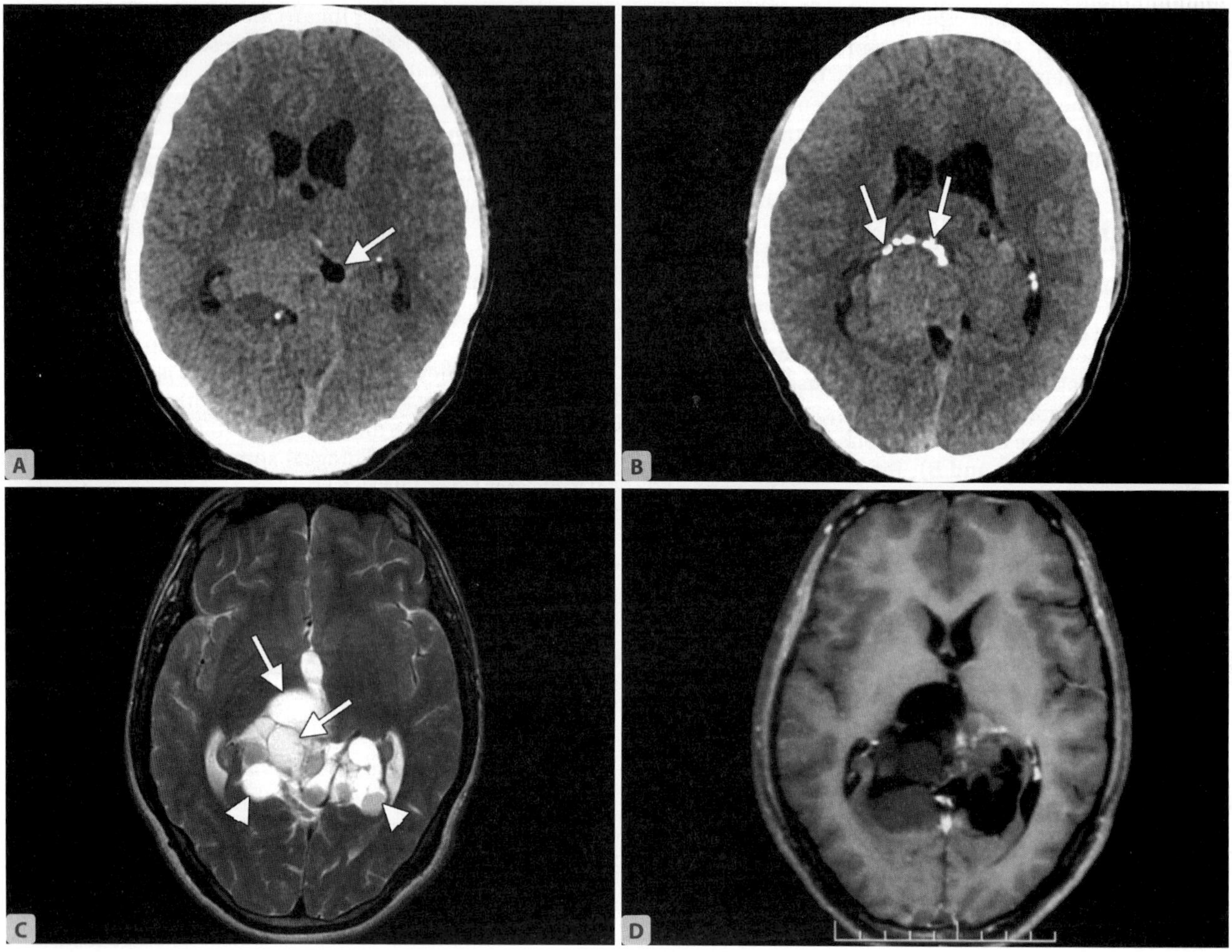

FIGS. 18A TO D: Pineal teratoma: CECTs (A and B) show a mixed-signal intensity lesion in pineal region with foci of fat density (arrow in A) and calcifications (arrows in B). On MRI, T2-WI (C) shows multiple cysts of varying signal intensity **(arrows and arrowheads)**. No enhancement is seen following contrast administration (D).

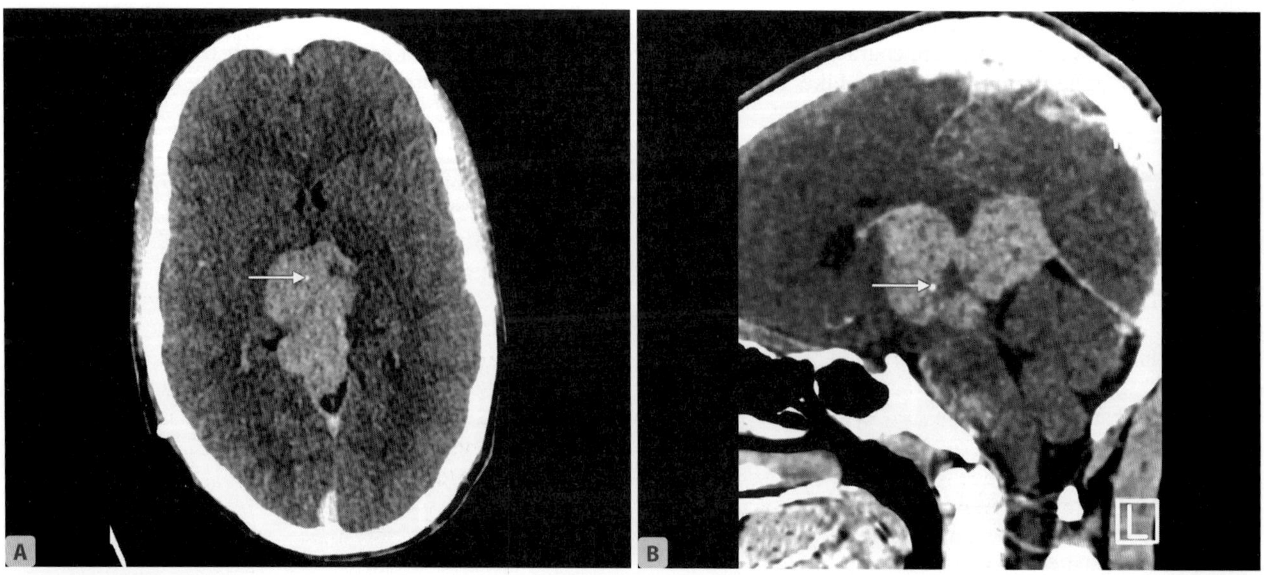

FIGS. 19A AND B: Pineal germinoma. Axial (A) and reconstructed coronal (B) CT show a homogeneously enhancing pineal mass lesion engulfing pineal calcification (arrow in A and B).

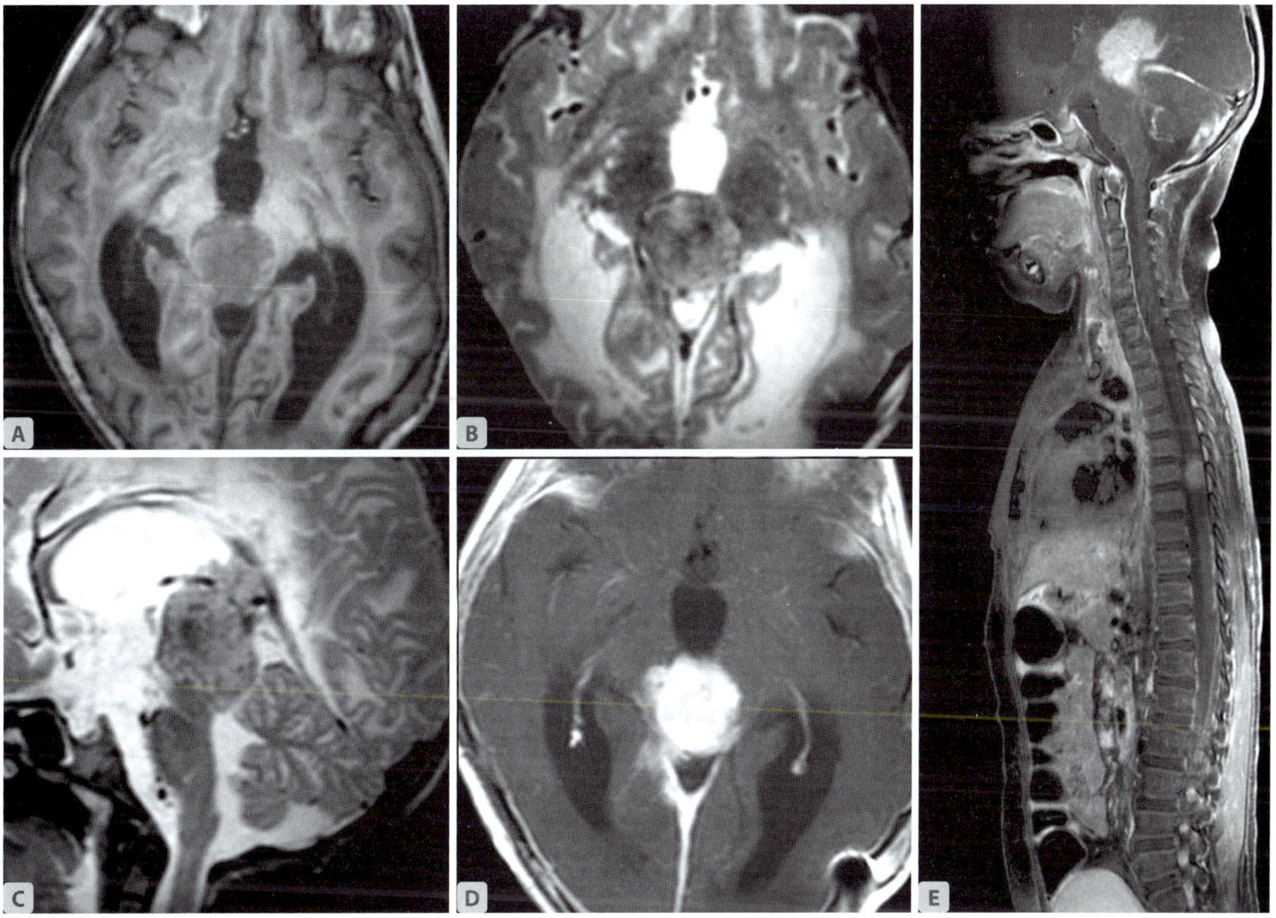

FIGS. 20A TO E: Pineoblastoma: Axial T1-WI (A), T2-WI (B) and sagittal T2-WI (C) show a large ill-defined pineal region mass. The lesions are isointense in T1-WI (a) and T2-WI and enhances intensely with contrast (D), Sagittal T1-WI (E) of spine show multiple leptomeningeal deposits suggestive of CSF dissemination.

in any age group and predominantly affect cutaneous and spinal nerves. In the head and neck the ophthalmic division of the Vth nerve is commonly affected.

On CT, these tumors are poorly delineated. These are infiltrative lesions which shows homogeneous enhancement. On MR they are isointense with muscle on T1WI and hyperintense to muscle on T2WI. Unlike schwannomas they enhance moderately after contrast enhancement.

TUMORS OF THE MENINGES

Meningioma

Meningiomas form 15% of all intracranial tumors, predominantly occurring in 40 to 60 yrs age group with definite female predominance (M:F = 1:2 to 1:4). Most frequent sites are parasagittal (25%) convexity (20%), sphenoid ridge (15–20%), olfactory groove (5–10%), parasellar (5–10%), and posterior fossa (10%). Rarely meningiomas may occur at extracranial sites such as nose, sinus, and orbit (1%). Atypical meningiomas are more common in children than in adults and likely to be malignant than those in adults, and are frequently associated with neurofibromatosis.

Multiple meningiomas have been reported in up to 10% of cases.

Imaging Features

On plain films hyperostosis or erosion of overlying bone, enlarged vascular grooves, tumor calcification and pneumosinus dilatans indicate presence of a meningioma.

On angiography dual vascular supply is common (dural to the central and pial to the periphery of the tumor). Sunburst pattern of enlarged dural feeders in the tumor is characteristic along with prolonged vascular homogeneous stain.

On CT meningiomas are hyperdense in 75% of cases, 90% enhance intensely and uniformly and 20–30% calcify. In 60% of cases peritumoral edema is encountered. Hemorrhage occurs in about 5% of cases. Degenerative parenchymal cysts and trapped arachnoid cysts between the meningioma and adjacent brain may occasionally be found.

On MRI meningiomas exhibit typical features of extra axial tumors. Gray white matter "buckling" or displacement, a cleft or pseudocapsule of CSF and vessels surrounding the mass separating it from brain characterize the extraaxial location of these tumors. The presence of a "dural tail" in 60% of cases on contrast enhanced MRI is highly suggestive but not pathognomonic of meningioma.

It is seen as homogeneously enhancing dural thickening extending from the margin of the meningioma and may be due either to extension of the tumor or to reactive change in the dura. MR imaging is superior to CT in assessing vascular encasement, particularly of the internal carotid arteries in lesions around the skull base. It is also superior in assessing the patency of the venous sinuses, notably the sagittal sinus, which may be invaded by parafalcine meningiomas. 95% of meningiomas show enhancement which is usually homogenous and intense **(Figs. 21A to C)**. Meningiomas tend to be isointense with gray matter on all pulse sequences. Thirty percent to 40% are mildly hypointense on T1WI and mildly hyperintense on T2WI.

Intraventricular meningiomas are usually in the lateral ventricle but can manifest in the third and fourth ventricles. They arise from the arachnoidal cap cell rest within the stroma of the choroid plexus. Although large majority of meningiomas have characteristic imaging features, there are at times lesions that mimic meningiomas. These include schwannomas, gliosarcomas, metastasis, dural vascular malformations associated with venous ectasia, fungal masses and extramedullary hematopoiesis in the skull vault.

MESENCHYMAL, NON-MENINGOTHELIAL TUMORS

Solitary Fibrous Tumor/Hemangiopericytoma

Solitary fibrous tumors/hemangiopericytoma are rare dural masses, histologically identical to solitary fibrous tumors found elsewhere. In the 2016 update to the WHO classification of brain tumors, solitary fibrous tumors of the dura and hemangiopericytomas are considered to be one entity with variable morphology. They are composed of spindle cells thought to be of mesenchymal origin. They usually occur in middle-aged individuals and symptoms depend on the size of the mass and its location.

On imaging, these tumors appear as extra-axial well circumscribed solid masses with intense contrast enhancement thereby mimicking meningiomas **(Figs. 22A to D)**. They are iso-hypointense on T2WI which may suggest diagnosis.

Ewing's Sarcoma

Primary CNS Ewing sarcoma are rare lesions that involve the CNS by extension from dura, bone, or paraspinal soft tissue. The peak incidence is in adolescence.

On MRI, these tumors are well-circumscribed, lobular, homogeneously enhancing masses with broad dural attachments that may be indistinguishable from meningioma.[26]

LYMPHOMA

Primary Lymphoma of the CNS

These tumors account for 1 to 2% of all primary CNS neoplasms. The incidence of these tumors is rising rapidly in both AIDS and non-AIDS patients. Peak incidence is in sixth decade in immunocompetent and in the third decade in immunocompromised patients. Primary malignant lymphoma is a non-Hodgkin's lymphoma that occurs in the brain in the absence of systemic involvement.

CNS lymphoma typically involves deep white matter in the periventricular area (frontal and parietal lobes, basal ganglia, thalami, hypothalamus, and corpus callosum). Believed to arise from periadventitial cells of penetrating arterioles.[27]

Imaging Features

On NCCT, primary CNS lymphomas appear as isodense lesions in two third of cases and hyperdense in remaining one third cases. They may be solitary or multiple in as many as 50% **(Figs. 23A to F)** Have a propensity to extend across the corpus callosum into the opposite hemisphere. Vasogenic edema is usually minimal. Enhancement is homogeneous **(Figs. 23A to F)** in 70% of cases, in AIDS or posterior fossa lesions; ring enhancement is seen in 20% of cases. Calcification is not seen, and hemorrhage is uncommon. On MRI, lymphomas tend to be isointense to gray matter in all spin echo sequences.[28] Intravascular or infiltrative lymphomas may be markedly hyperintense on T2-WI. Restricted diffusion and low ADC

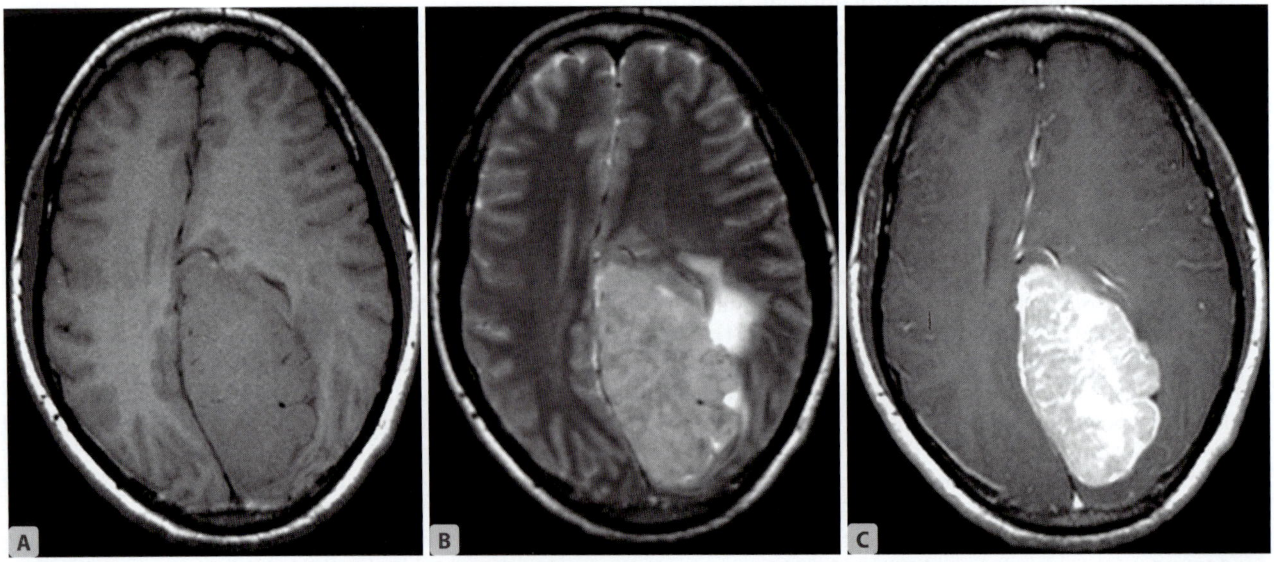

FIGS. 21A TO C: Meningioma: Axial T1-WI (A) and T2-WI (B) show a large extra-axial left parafalcine mass. The lesions are isointense in T1-WI (A) and T2-WI and enhances intensely with contrast (C).

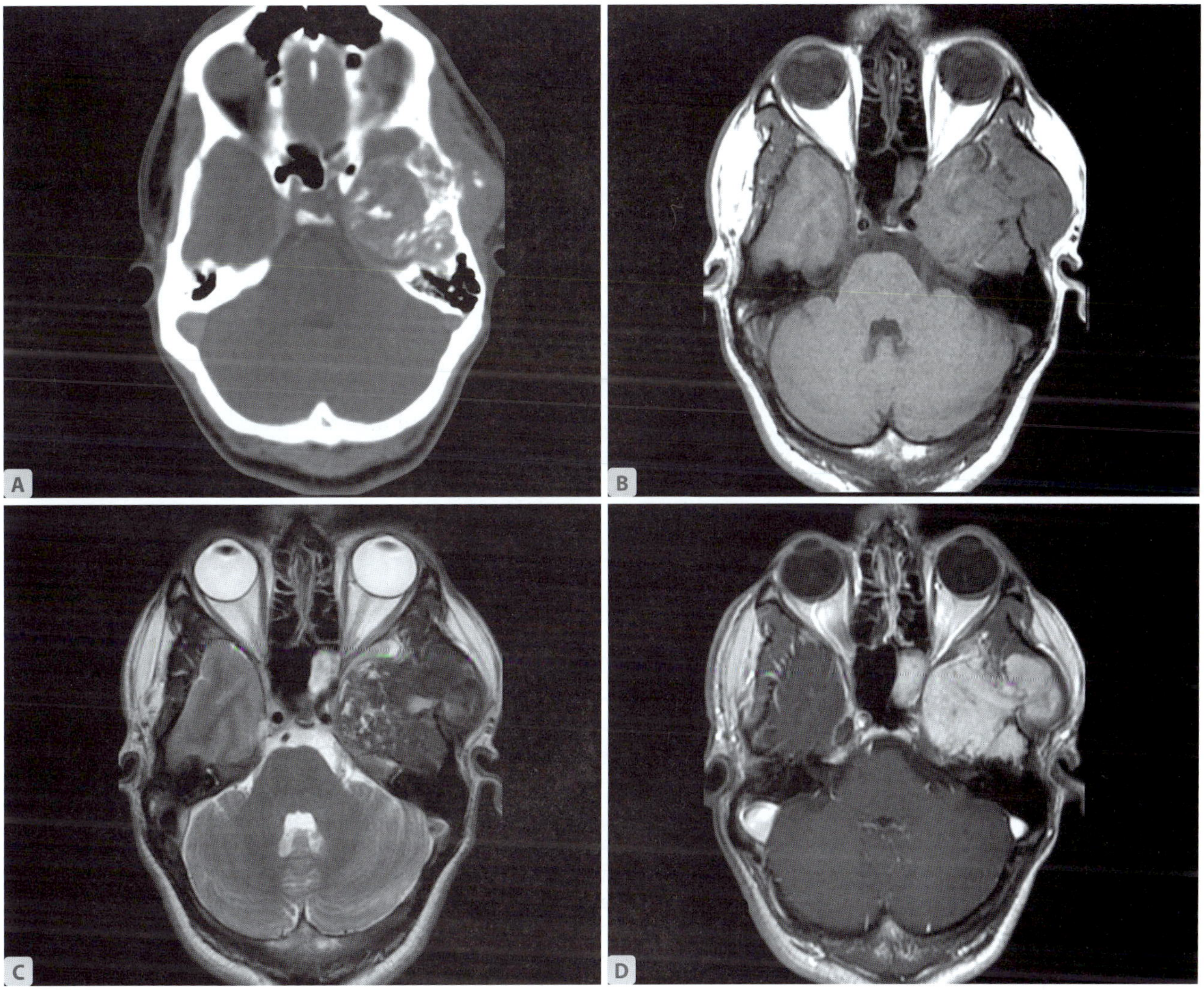

FIGS. 22A TO D: Solitary fibrous tumor: CT bone window (A), axial T1-WI (B) and T2-WI (C) show extra-axial lesion involving left temporal bone. The mass has foci of calcification and extending to scalp. The lesions are isointense in T1-WI (B) and markedly hypointense on T2-WI (C) and enhances intensely with contrast (D).

value on DWI is due to its high cellularity and restricted diffusion matches T2 abnormality. Lymphomas show dense and homogenous enhancement in most immunocompetent patients; ependymal and perivascular enhancement suggest lymphoma. Necrosis, hemorrhage and inhomogeneous or ring enhancement are features of lymphoma in immunodeficiency patients, but may be seen in EBV-positive tumors in immunocompetent patients.[28] Infiltrative and intravascular lymphomas may not enhance.

MR spectral pattern of lymphomas is similar to malignant brain tumors and reveal elevated signals of lipid, lactate, and choline and reduced NAA, creatinine, and myo-inositol signals. Presence of lipids in solid enhancing tumor suggest lymphoma **(Figs. 24A to H)**.[29] MRS can help in differentiating lymphoma from toxoplasmosis, which typically has elevated lactate and lipid signals but absence of the other metabolites in MR.

Differentiation of lymphoma and primary high-grade glial neoplasm is possible using multimodal imaging. Lymphoma tends to have a lower ADC, lower FA and typically lower rCBV. Rarely rCBV in lymphomas may be high, but low ADC values in matching areas of T2 abnormalities and contrast enhancement, and lipid in solid enhancing region help to clinch the diagnosis. Lymphoma tends to show higher rCBV compared with toxoplasmosis.

Cerebral lymphomas are highly radiosensitive and respond dramatically to steroid therapy. Following steroid treatment, restricted diffusion may not be seen.

Immunodeficiency-associated CNS lymphoma

Immunodeficiency-associated CNS lymphoma is seen in organ transplant recipients, patients with congenital immunodeficiency syndrome and patients with AIDS. Incidence of AIDS-related lymphomas is decreasing in patient who receive antiretroviral therapy.[30] Pattern is modified somewhat in AIDS-related lymphoma. Multiplicity seems to be more common. Lymphomas exhibit more aggressive behavior and readily outgrow their blood supply. As a result,

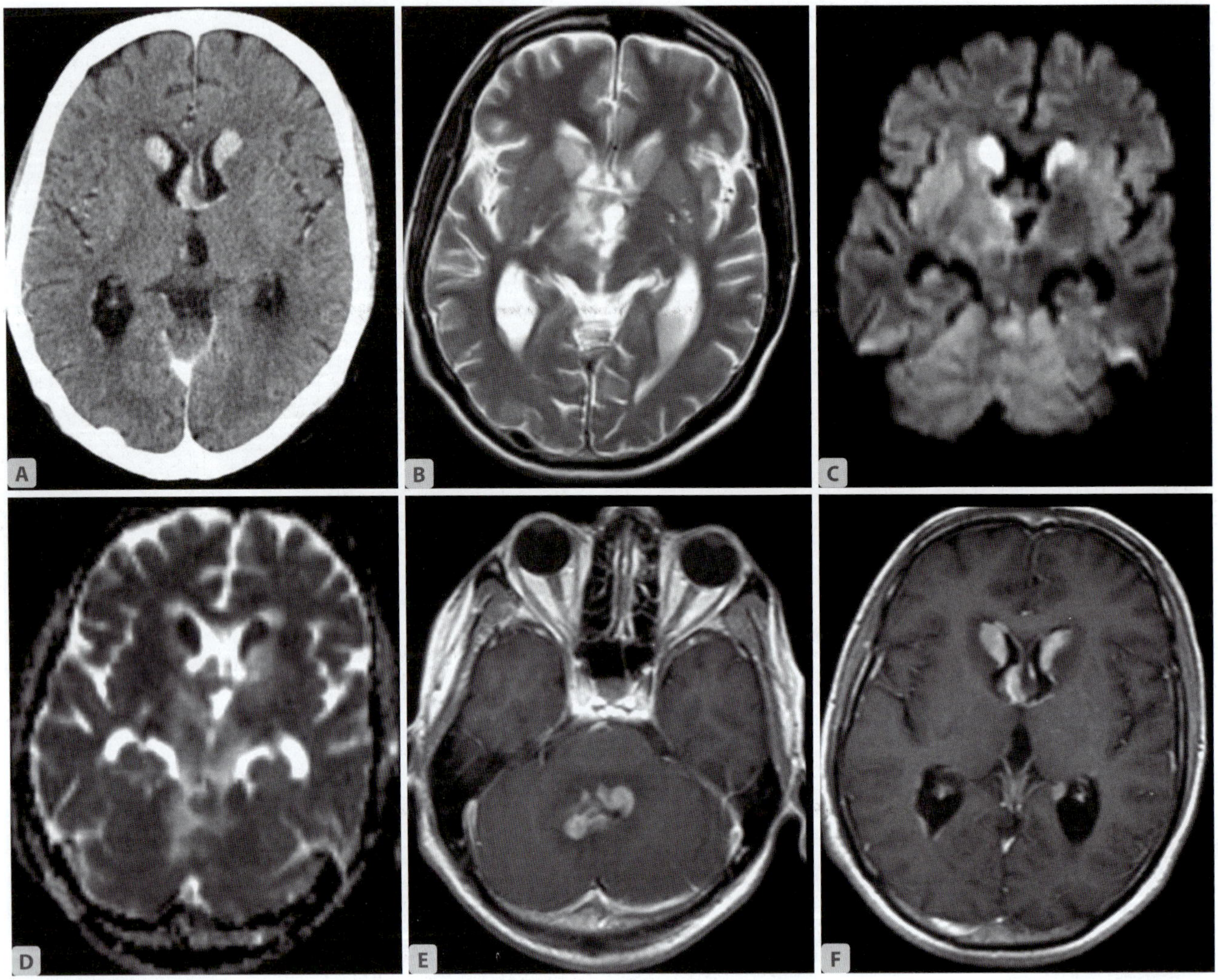

FIGS. 23A TO F: Primary CNS lymphoma: CECT (A) shows multiple enhancing periventricular lesions. These lesions are isointense on T2-WI (B), bright on diffusion trace image (C), dark on ADC maps (D) and enhancing with contrast (E and F). The lesions are distributed in both supratentorial and infratentorial compartment.

central necrosis and ring enhancement are often seen in lymphomatous masses in AIDS patients.

METASTATIC TUMORS

Intracranial metastases may be either parenchymal or extra-axial. Extra-axial metastasis may be epidural, dural or leptomeningeal.

Epidural metastases are nearly always associated with adjacent osseous metastases with spread to the epidural space.

Parenchymal Metastases

Intra-axial metastasis form 13 to 41% of all intra-cranial tumors. Common primary tumors which metastasize to brain are from the lung, breast, melanoma, gastrointestinal tract, and kidney.

More than 60 to 70% metastases are multiple. Solitary (30-40%) are associated with lung and renal carcinomas. Metastases can occur at any site; however, most common site is the gray-white matter junction. The cause of this preferential location is related to abrupt reduction of the diameter of arterioles at this point causing arrest of tumor emboli at this location.

Imaging Features

On NCCT, metastases are usually hypodense and occasionally isodense. Hyperdensity is common and may be due to hemorrhage-especially in secondaries from Choriocarcinoma, melanoma and renal carcinoma, tumor cellularity or contents (melanoma or mucin secreting tumors) and rarely calcification.

Typically, disproportionate and extensive vasogenic edema exists with metastases. CECT reveals cortical

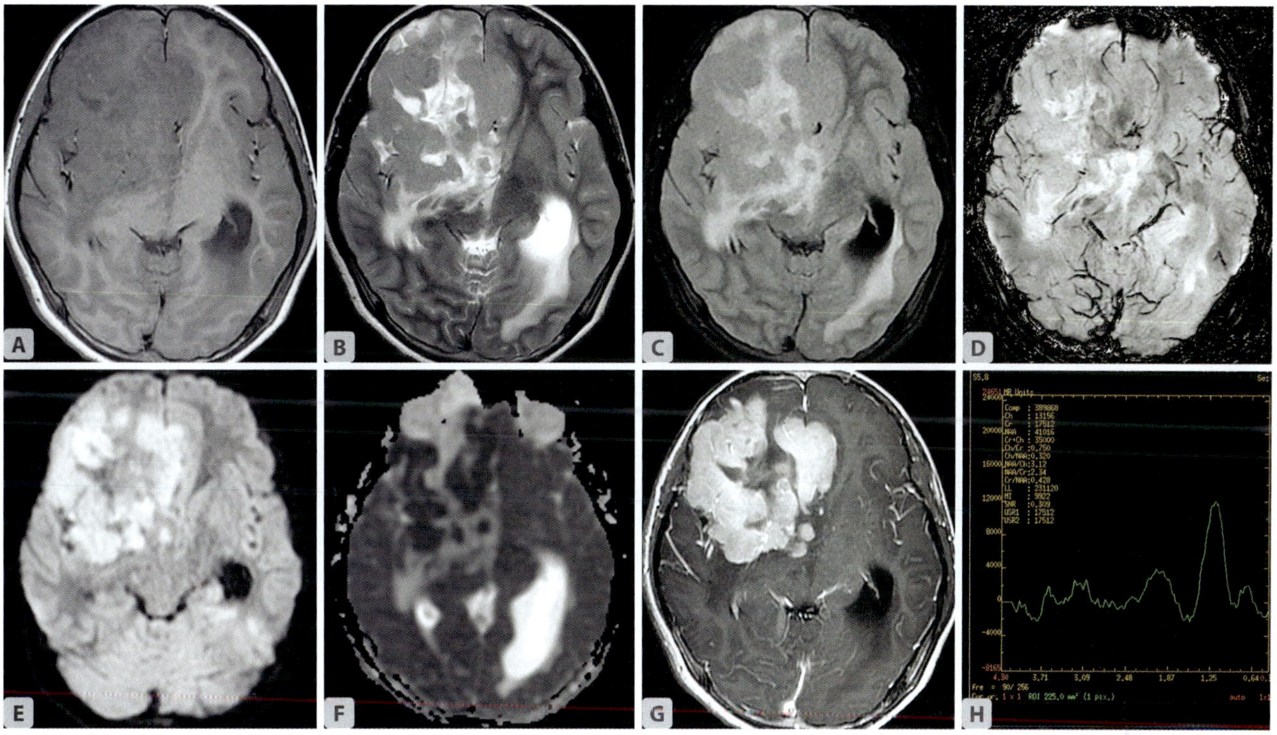

FIGS. 24A TO H: Primary CNS lymphoma. Large T1 (A) and T2 (B) isointense lesion with perilesional edema is present in right frontal lobe (C). No foci of hemorrhages are seen on SWI (D). The lesion is bright on diffusion trace image (E), dark on ADC maps (F) and is enhancing with contrast (G). On MRS from the solid enhancing portion, lipid is seen (H).

metastases and metastases in the white matter that are less than 1 cm in diameter as intense homogenous nodular or ring enhancement with central non-enhancing area caused by cystic degeneration or necrosis. The blood-brain barrier does not exist for metastatic lesions because they recruit their own vascular supply. Contrast-enhanced MRI is the most sensitive modality for detecting cerebral metastases. Metastases are usually hypointense to gray matter and enhance following contrast administration **(Figs. 25A to C)**.

Typical MR spectroscopic features for secondary neoplasms include elevated signals of lipid, lactate, and choline and reduced or absent NAA signal. Primary neoplasms have the propensity to infiltrate surrounding brain tissue; interrogation of areas outside the enhancing portion of the lesion has proved to be promising. The ADC values of metastatic lesions are variable and overlap with those of primary neoplasms. However, it is possible to separate metastasis from primary brain neoplasm by measuring ADC values in the peritumoral regions. Peritumoral diffusion-tensor imaging tends to show lower ADC values in regions of peritumoral "edema" compared with those seen with metastatic disease. Perfusion parameters of metastatic lesions tend to overlap with those of high-grade neoplasms, probably because of their similarity in the degree of angiogenesis. One possible feature that might allow differentiation between secondary and primary neoplasms is that metastatic lesions have lower rCBV measurements outside their enhancing portion, compared with those of the more infiltrative primary neoplasms.

Leptomeningeal Metastases

Leptomeningeal metastases are commonly seen in leukemia, lymphoma, carcinoma of breast, and lung and melanoma. Few primary brain tumors also have leptomeningeal spread pattern like GBM, ependymomas and pineoblastomas. The arachnoid membrane usually provides a barrier to leptomeningeal and parenchymal spread from the dura.

Leptomeningeal involvement is graded as follows:

Type A: Tumor deposited in leptomeninges.

Type B: Minor infiltration into the cortex.

Type C: Edema associated with invasion into the parenchyma.

Type D: invasion into perineural spaces which at times can simulate a benign neurogenic tumor such as-schwannomas.

Imaging Features

Contrast enhanced MR imaging is a more sensitive study than CT and may demonstrate abnormal meningeal enhancement, diffuse or irregular plaque like or nodular deposits along the cortical surface or cisterns.

Dural Metastases

Isolated dural metastases are rare, usually associated with skull lesions and are secondary to hematogenous spread. Sometime solitary focal dural metastases may mimic meningioma. Most common sites of primary are breast, lung, and kidney.

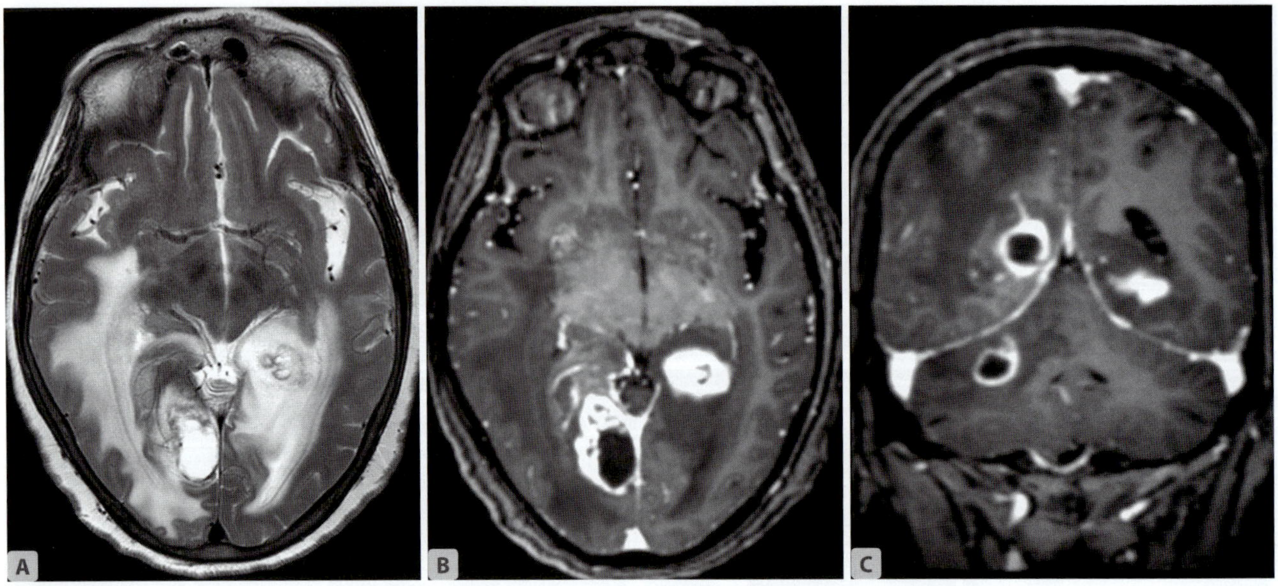

FIGS. 25A TO C: Metastases. T2-WI (A) shows ring lesions in both occipital lobes with marked edema. These lesions enhances with contrast (B and C). Another ring-enhancing lesion is seen in right cerebellar hemisphere.

Calvarial Metastases

CT is still believed by many to be the most sensitive modality for detection of bony calvarial metastases, however, MRI with contrast is superior for detecting subtle intradiploic lesions, for delineating lesion extent and determining involvement of underlying dura or brain. Most common primaries which metastasize to the calvarium are breast followed by lungs, prostate and lymphoma.

CONCLUSION

Supratentorial brain tumors are a diverse group of neoplasms and in this chapter most common neoplasm are covered with stress on their imaging features. There are few recent advanced techniques like diffusion and perfusion MR imaging, MR spectroscopy and positron-emission tomography. These techniques are still evolving and certainly helpful in solving diagnostic dilemmas.

REFERENCES

1. Kleihues P, Burger PC, Scheithauer BW. The new WHO classification of brain tumours. Brain Pathol. 1993;3(3):255-68.
2. Louis DN, Perry A, Reifenberger G, et al. The 2016 World Health Organization Classification of Tumors of the Central Nervous System: a summary. Acta Neuropathol. 2016;131(6):803-20.
3. Lasocki A, Gaillard F, Gorelik A, et al. MRI Features Can Predict 1p/19q Status in Intracranial Gliomas. American Journal of Neuroradiology. 2018.
4. Cha S. Update on brain tumor imaging: from anatomy to physiology. Am J Neuroradiol. 2006;27(3):475-87.
5. Hilario A, Ramos A, Perez-Nunez A, et al. The added value of apparent diffusion coefficient to cerebral blood volume in the preoperative grading of diffuse gliomas. Am J Neuroradiol. 2012;33(4):701-7.
6. Law M, Yang S, Babb JS, et al. Comparison of cerebral blood volume and vascular permeability from dynamic susceptibility contrast-enhanced perfusion MR imaging with glioma grade. Am J Neuroradiol. 2004;25(5):746-55.
7. Aihara K, Mukasa A, Gotoh K, et al. H3F3A K27M mutations in thalamic gliomas from young adult patients. Neuro Oncol. 2014;16(1):140-6.
8. Buczkowicz P, Bartels U, Bouffet E, et al. Histopathological spectrum of paediatric diffuse intrinsic pontine glioma: diagnostic and therapeutic implications. Acta Neuropathol. 2014;128(4):573-81.
9. Johnson DR, Diehn FE, Giannini C, et al. Genetically Defined Oligodendroglioma Is Characterized by Indistinct Tumor Borders at MRI. Am J Neuroradiol. 2017;38(4):678-84.
10. Collins VP, Jones DT, Giannini C. Pilocytic astrocytoma: pathology, molecular mechanisms and markers. Acta Neuropathol. 2015;129(6):775-88.
11. Hawkins C, Walker E, Mohamed N, et al. BRAF-KIAA1549 fusion predicts better clinical outcome in pediatric low-grade astrocytoma. Clin Cancer Res. 2011;17(14):4790-8.
12. Li HM, Hsu SS, Wang JS, et al. Cerebral pilocytic astrocytoma with spontaneous intracranial hemorrhage in adults. J Chin Med Assoc. 2008;71(11):587-93.
13. Shepherd CW, Scheithauer BW, Gomez MR, et al. Subependymal giant cell astrocytoma: a clinical, pathological, and flow cytometric study. Neurosurgery. 1991;28(6):864-8.
14. O'Callaghan FJ, Martyn CN, Renowden S, et al. Subependymal nodules, giant cell astrocytomas and the tuberous sclerosis complex: a population-based study. Arch Dis Child. 2008;93(9):751-4.
15. Rovira A, Ruiz-Falco ML, Garcia-Esparza E, et al. Recommendations for the radiological diagnosis and follow-up of neuropathological abnormalities associated with tuberous sclerosis complex. J Neurooncol. 2014;118(2):205-23.
16. Crespo-Rodriguez AM, Smlrniotopoulos JG, Rushing EJ. MR and CT imaging of 24 pleomorphic xanthoastrocytomas (PXA) and a review of the literature. Neuroradiology. 2007;49(4):307-15.

17. Yu S, He L, Zhuang X, et al. Pleomorphic xanthoastrocytoma: MR imaging findings in 19 patients. Acta Radiol. 2011;52(2):223-8.
18. Moore W, Mathis D, Gargan L, et al. Pleomorphic xanthoastrocytoma of childhood: MR imaging and diffusion MR imaging features. Am J Neuroradiol. 2014;35(11):2192-6.
19. Spoto GP, Press GA, Hesselink JR, et al. Intracranial ependymoma and subependymoma: MR manifestations. Am J Roentgenol. 1990;154(4):837-45.
20. Koeller KK, Sandberg GD, Armed Forces Institute of P. From the archives of the AFIP. Cerebral intraventricular neoplasms: radiologic-pathologic correlation. Radiographics. 2002;22(6):1473-505.
21. Yuh EL, Barkovich AJ, Gupta N. Imaging of ependymomas: MRI and CT. Childs Nerv Syst. 2009;25(10):1203-13.
22. Yanaka K, Kamezaki T, Kobayashi E, et al. MR imaging of diffuse glioma. Am J Neuroradiol. 1992;13(1):349-51.
23. Smith AB, Smirniotopoulos JG, Horkanyne-Szakaly I. From the radiologic pathology archives: intraventricular neoplasms: radiologic-pathologic correlation. Radiographics. 2013;33(1):21-43.
24. Reiche W, Feiden W, Eymann R, et al. Dysembryoplastic neuroepithelial tumor-Neuroradiologic findings in common and uncommon sites. International Journal of Neuroradiology. 1997;3(5):428-34.
25. Dumrongpisutikul N, Intrapiromkul J, Yousem DM. Distinguishing between germinomas and pineal cell tumors on MR imaging. Am J Neuroradiol. 2012;33(3):550-5.
26. Pekala JS, Gururangan S, Provenzale JM, et al. Central nervous system extraosseous Ewing sarcoma: radiologic manifestations of this newly defined pathologic entity. Am J Neuroradiol. 2006;27(3):580-3.
27. Jack CR, Jr., O'Neill BP, et al. Central nervous system lymphoma: histologic types and CT appearance. Radiology. 1988;167(1):211-5.
28. Haldorsen IS, Espeland A, Larsson EM. Central nervous system lymphoma: characteristic findings on traditional and advanced imaging. Am J Neuroradiol. 2011;32(6):984-92.
29. Brandao LA, Castillo M. Adult Brain Tumors: Clinical Applications of Magnetic Resonance Spectroscopy. Magn Reson Imaging Clin N Am. 2016;24(4):781-809.
30. Diamond C, Taylor TH, Aboumrad T, et al. Changes in acquired immunodeficiency syndrome-related non-Hodgkin lymphoma in the era of highly active antiretroviral therapy: incidence, presentation, treatment, and survival. Cancer. 2006;106(1):128-35.

CHAPTER

197

Imaging of Infratentorial Tumors

Ajay Garg

INTRODUCTION

The infratentorial tumors include tumors arising from the brain parenchyma (cerebellum and the brainstem), the cranial nerves, the meninges, or the bone. In addition, head and neck neoplasm can extend into the infratentorial compartment.

In children, 48% of primary intracranial neoplasms are infratentorial in location while in adults infratentorial tumors are uncommon.[1] In pediatric infratentorial neoplasms, medulloblastomas and cerebellar astrocytomas account for one-third each; brainstem gliomas represent another one-fourth and ependymomas account for one-eighth of neoplasms.[1] In adults, most of the infratentorial neoplasms are extra-axial in location; vestibular schwannoma is the most common neoplasm followed by meningioma and epidermoid. Among the intra-axial infratentorial neoplasms in adults, metastases are most common followed by hemangioblastoma and glioma.[2]

Magnetic resonance imaging (MRI) is the imaging modality of choice for the assessment of infratentorial neoplasms as it has better soft tissue contrast, multi-planar imaging capability, and potential to provide complementary physiologic information with diffusion-weighted images (DWI), perfusion MRI and susceptibility-weighted images (SWI).[2] Computed tomography (CT) has better sensitivity to detect subtle calcifications within tumors. Once a mass is identified, it must be localized to the intra-axial or the extra-axial compartment. Extra-axial masses typically have well-defined margins, displace normal brain structures causing enlargement of the ipsilateral cistern and have a Cerebrospinal fluid (CSF)-vascular cleft between an the mass and the adjacent normal brain. On the other hand, intra-axial masses lack such clear cut demarcation and blend into the normal brain; and compress sulci and cisterns.

CLASSIFICATION OF INFRATENTORIAL TUMORS BASED ON TOPOGRAPHY

The diagnostic algorithm to differentiate various infratentorial lesions is most easily formulated using the neuroanatomic classification as a starting point. Then imaging characteristics help to narrow down the differential diagnoses **(Table 1)**.

CEREBELLAR HEMISPHERE AND VERMIS

Medulloblastoma

Medulloblastoma (MB) is a malignant primitive ectodermal tumor and is the most common infratentorial tumor in children, accounting for one-third of childhood pediatric tumors. About three-quarters of MBs occur in children 5–15 years old. In adults, though much less common, MBs usually occur in the 3rd and 4th decades of life. MBs are typically midline infratentorial tumors and the most common location is in the region of the vermis and the inferior medullary velum. Cerebellar hemispheric MBs are less

TABLE 1: Classification of infratentorial tumors based on topography and age.

Location	Age-group	Tumor
Cerebellar hemisphere and vermis	Pediatric	Medulloblastoma, ependymoma, astrocytoma, atypical teratoid/rhabdoid tumor
	Adult	Metastasis, hemangioblastoma, dysplastic cerebellar gangliocytoma, medulloblastoma
Brainstem	Pediatric	Diffuse midline glioma
	Adult	Diffuse midline glioma, GBM
Cerebellopontine angle	Pediatric	Atypical teratoid/rhabdoid tumor, medulloblastoma, ependymoma
	Adult	Vestibular Schwannoma, meningiomas, epidermoid, arachnoid cyst, endolymphatic sac tumor
Fourth ventricle	Pediatric	Medulloblastoma, ependymoma
	Adult	Choroid plexus papilloma, epidermoid, subependymoma

frequent and occur primarily in adults. Approximately 80% of patients with MB present with features of raised intracranial pressure. CSF seeding occurs in 10–30% of patients with MB.

Pathology

Histologically MBs are classified as classic; nodular or desmoplastic; MB with extensive nodularity; or as anaplastic/large cell variants. Over the past 5 years, considerable advances have been made in understanding MB biology[3] and the 2016 WHO update has incorporated histological and molecular schemes into the classification of MBs.[4,5] Based on genomic characterization, MBs can be subdivided into 4 distinct molecular subgroups: wingless (WNT), sonic hedgehog (SHH), group 3, and group 4. These molecular subgroups are more predictive of clinical behavior and outcome than the tumor histology (classic or "variants") or the clinical staging system.[3,4] Distribution of the different molecular subtypes between adult MB (50–60% SHH subgroup, 20–30% group 4 and 10–15% WNT) and pediatric MB (50–60 % group 3 tumors, 10–30% group 4 tumors, 10–15% WNT and 10–15% SHH) are significantly different.[6]

Imaging

Most pediatric MBs arise in the cerebellar vermis and often extend into the roof of the fourth ventricle and the brain stem. On imaging, MB appears as a well-circumscribed fourth ventricular mass. On CT scan, MBs are isodense to hyperdense due to their high cellularity **(Figs. 1A and B)** and show variable enhancement after contrast administration.[7] Approximately 20% of MBs have intratumoral calcification **(Fig. 1B)**. Cystic and necrotic degeneration are most commonly found in adult MBs.

On MRI, typically they are hypointense to isointense on T1- and T2-WI; and show avid contrast enhancement **(Figs. 2A to F)**. The tumors are mostly homogeneous, although some display T2 heterogeneous signal due to the presence of intratumoral cysts, hemorrhage, calcification and necrotic foci.[7] MBs show evidence of restricted diffusion (bright on DWI and dark on ADC maps) in their solid components presumably due to their high cellularity and high nucleus-to-cytoplasm ratio **(Fig. 2D)**[8] Post-gadolinium brain and the spine MR imaging may show evidence of leptomeningeal metastatic spread in 33% of cases at the time of diagnosis or during the course of the disease **(Figs. 3A to C)**.[7] At MR spectroscopy, MBs characteristically show taurine, detectable at short TE, and a high choline peak.[9]

Compared to pediatric MBs, adult MBs are more likely to be located in cerebellar hemispheres and have an atypical presentation with more hyperintense signal on T1-WI, more hypointense signal on T2-WI and inhomogeneous contrast enhancement.[10]

Recently, there have been attempts to predict the molecular subtype of MBs based on imaging phenotype; a new emerging field of imaging known as radiogenomics. This is quite helpful when advanced molecular subtyping is not available. Wingless-type-subgroup MBs are likely to be off-midline tumors arising from the dorsal brainstem and cerebellum around the foramen of Luschka **(Figs. 4A to C)**.[11]

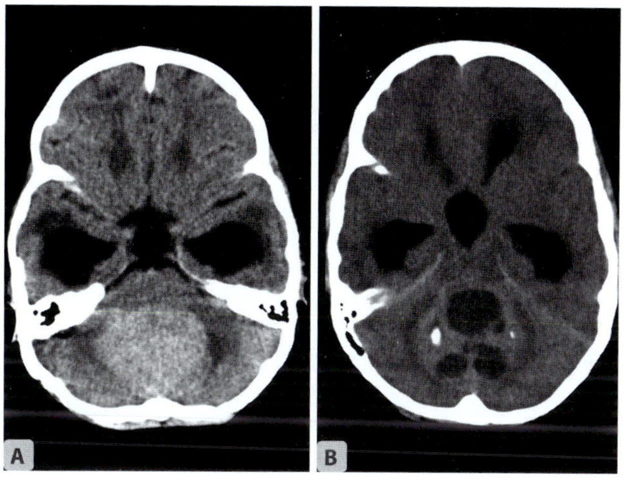

FIGS. 1A AND B: Medulloblastoma: NCCT shows a hyperdense midline mass (A) and midline isodense mass (B) with cystic areas and calcifications.

This subtype of MBs may present as an isolated CP angle mass, a mass in region of foramen of Luschka or as a midline fourth ventricle mass. These tumors are likely to contact the dorsal brainstem. SHH subgroup of MBs typically occurs in adults and appear as off-midline intracerebellar tumors without any contact with the brainstem **(Figs. 4A to C)**. Group 3 MBs are likely to present as midline intraventricular tumors esp. in children with small tumor size and prominent enhancement. In addition, diffuse leptomeningeal spread at the time of first presentation is also more likely to occur in Gp 3 MBs **(Figs. 5A to D)**. Group 4 MBs are likely to present as midline intraventricular tumors which show no or minimal enhancement **(Figs. 6A to F)**.

Ependymoma

Ependymomas are an infrequent group of glial tumors that typically arise from ependymal cells in supratentorial, infratentorial and spinal cord regions. Ependymomas are common tumors in children, comprising 10% of pediatric CNS neoplasms and 15% of infratentorial tumors. The peak age at presentation is 1–5 years, with a smaller peak in adults in their fourth decade. Nearly two-thirds of intracranial ependymomas are present in the infratentorial compartment, arising from the ependymal lining of the fourth ventricle and the foramina of Luschka. Supratentorial lesions can be either intraventricular, typically in the lateral ventricles; or parenchymal. Approximately 60% of these tumors develop infratentorially, 30% supratentorially and 10% in the spinal cord.[12] Infratentorial ependymomas usually present with symptoms of raised intracranial pressure.[13] Cranial nerve palsies are also common, especially involving cranial nerves VI to X.

Pathology

Ependymomas are glial tumors arising from the ependymal lining of the ventricles and the central canal. The WHO classifies ependymal tumors into four types: (1) ependymoma

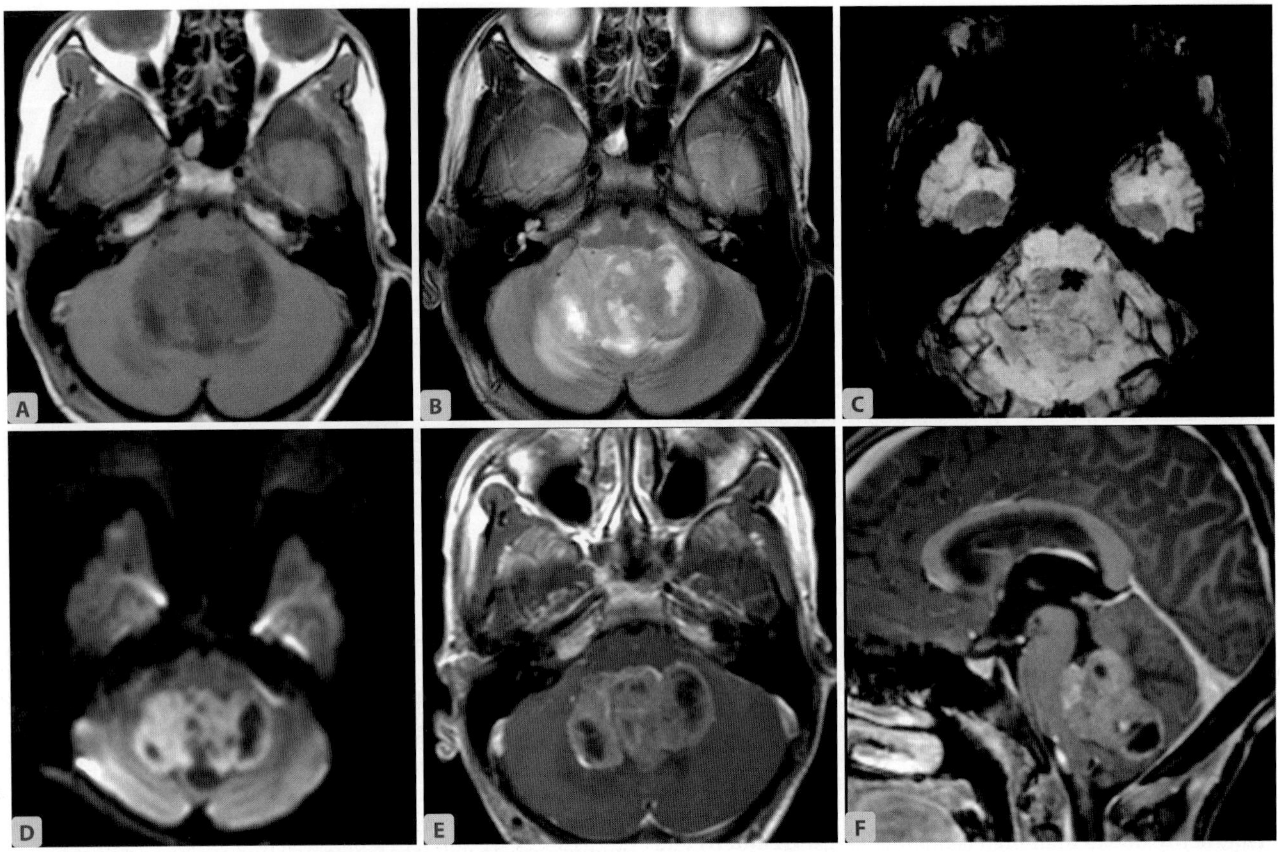

FIGS. 2A TO F: Medulloblastoma: MR scans show a midline vermian mass which is iso-hypointense on T1WI (A) and iso-hyperintense on T2WI (B) having foci of susceptibility on SWI (C). The mass is hyperintense on DWI (D) and hypointense on ADC maps (E) suggesting restricted diffusion. Postgadolinium axial (E) and sagittal (F) T1WI show intense enhancement of the mass.

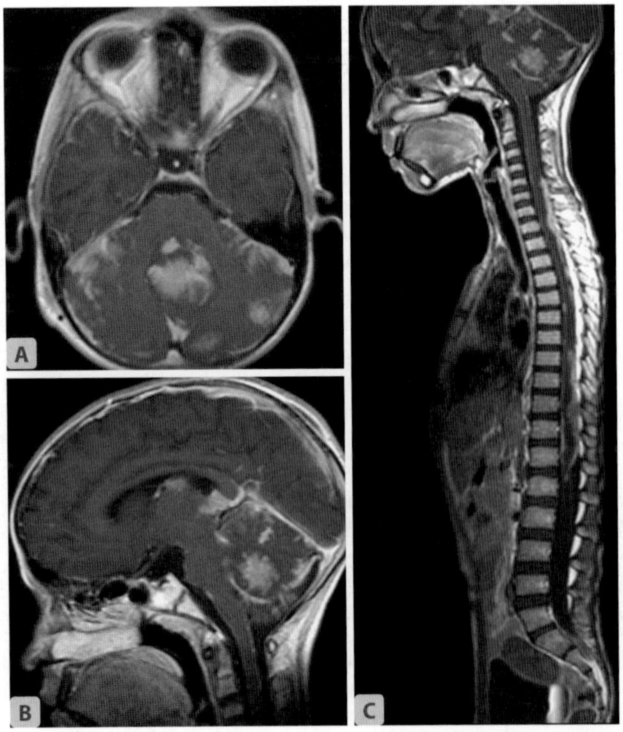

FIGS. 3A TO C: Type 3 Medulloblastoma with leptomeningeal spread: Axial (A) and sagittal (B) T1WIs of brain reveal patchy enhancement within a midline mass and enhancement of the leptomeningeal deposits in bilateral CPA cisterns and cerebellar sulci. Sagittal T1WI (C) of spine show diffuse leptomeningeal deposits in the spinal subarachnoid spaces.

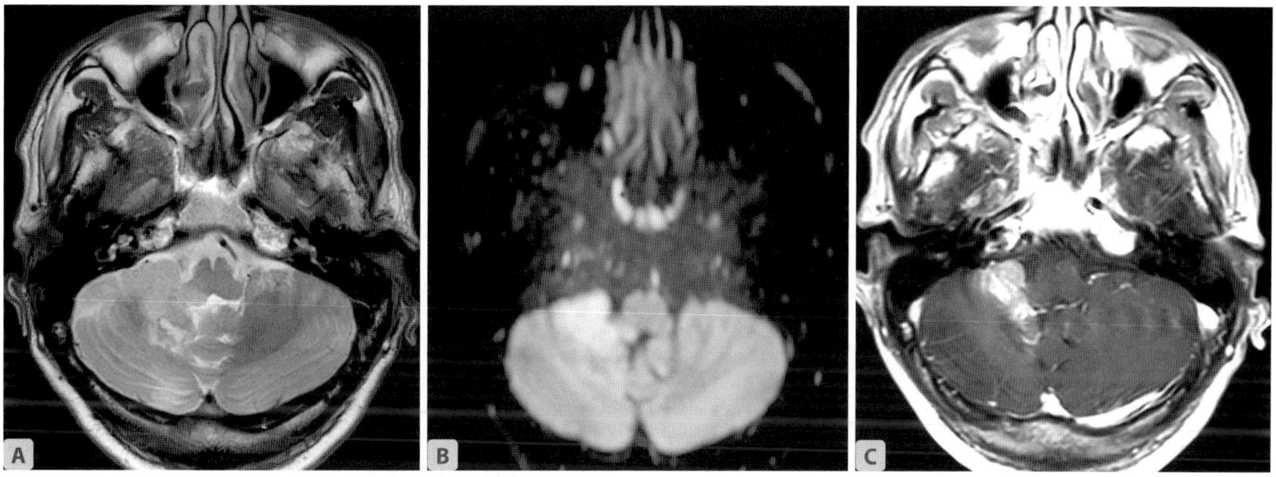

FIGS. 4A TO C: WNT Medulloblastoma: Axial T2WI (A) shows characteristic location in CPA cistern/foramen of Luschka region with involvement of dorsal brainstem, restricted diffusion DWI (B) and intense enhancement following contrast (C).

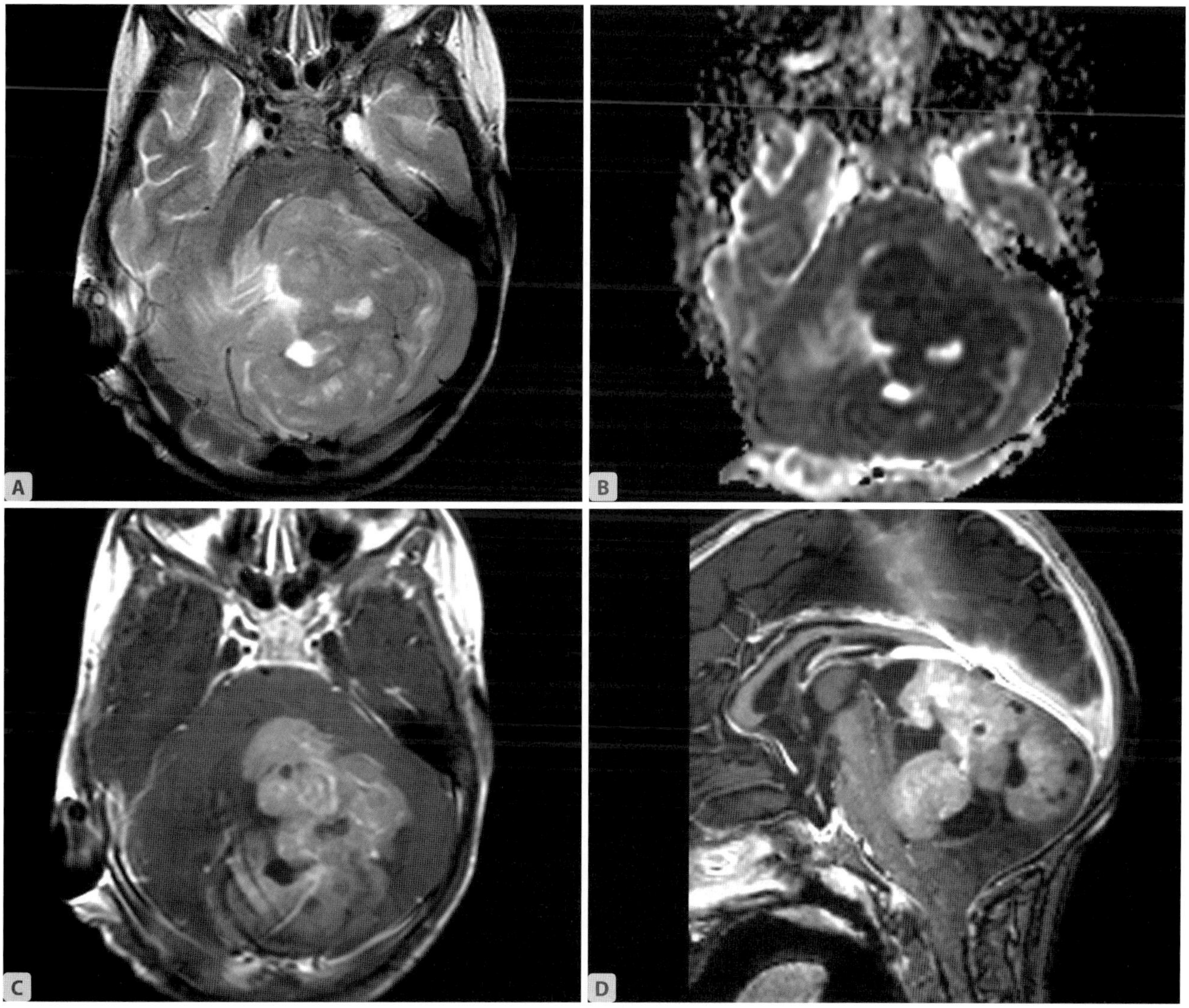

FIGS. 5A TO D: SHH Medulloblastoma: Hemispheric cerebellar tumor isointense on T2WI (A), hypointense on ADC maps (B) and avidly enhancing in axial (C) and sagittal (D) post-gad T1WIs.

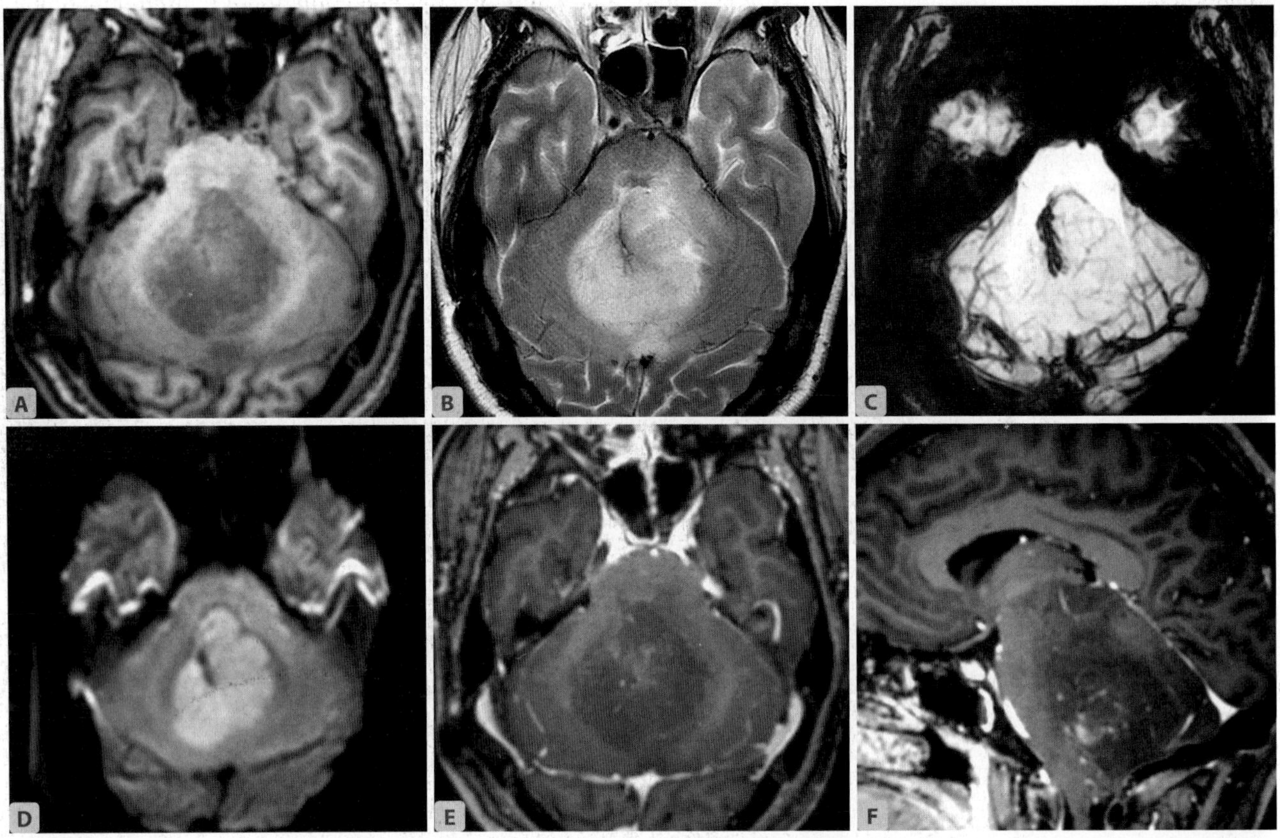

FIGS. 6A TO F: Type 4 Medulloblastoma: MR scans show a midline vermian mass which is iso-hypointense on T1WI (A), iso-hyperintense on T2WI (B), having foci of susceptibility on SWI (C) and hyperintense on DWI (D). Postgadolinium axial (E) and sagittal (F) T1WI show minimal enhancement of the mass.

(grade II), which include variants such as cellular, papillary, epithelial, clear-cell and mixed; (2) anaplastic ependymoma (grade III), (3) subependymoma (grade I), and (4) myxopapillary ependymoma (grade I). Anaplastic ependymomas have a greater incidence of leptomeningeal spread at the time of diagnosis and have poorer prognosis.

Typical gross pathology shows a well-defined lobulated mass with areas of calcification, hemorrhage, and cysts. The tumor cells usually form ependymal rosettes, which are diagnostic but not always present.

Comprehensive genomic studies have divided infratentorial ependymomas into 2 prognostcially different subgroups, PF-A and PF-B.[14] The poor prognostic subgroup (group A), found predominantly in infants, exhibited a CpG island methylator phenotype and transcriptional silencing of the polycomb repressive complex 2, leading to repressed expression of differentiation genes.[14]

Imaging

At CT, ependymomas appear as irregular and lobulated heterogeneous midline intraventricular masses with calcification (up to 45%).[15] At MRI, they appear heterogeneous with T1 hypointensity, T2 iso/hyperintensity and iso-to-hyper FLAIR signal intensity **(Figs. 7A and B)** due to presence of calcification, hemorrhage and cystic changes within the tumor. Following contrast administration they usually show intense mixed heterogeneous enhancement **(Figs. 7C and D)**; however, rarely, ependymomas do not enhance.[16] The presence of calcifications within a lobulated heterogeneous fourth ventricular mass is highly suggestive but not diagnostic of ependymoma. Diffuse leptomeningeal spread is seen in less than 10% of patients at diagnosis when ependymoblastomas (ETANTR) are excluded.[17]

On DWI, ADC of ependymomas is generally intermediate between that of pilocytic astrocytomas and MBs,[18] however, ADC values are not completely reliable in differentiation between various infratentorial parenchymal masses. On Dynamic Susceptibility Contrast (DSC) perfusion MRI, ependymomas typically have markedly elevated perfusion (rCBV) and marked leakiness of contrast with poor return to baseline presumably due to presence of fenestrated blood vessels and an insufficient blood-brain barrier.[19] This behavior, although very characteristic of ependymomas, is not entirely pathognomonic and also may be demonstrated in other tumors, such as embryonal tumors.[20]

Typically, ependymomas show tumor extension through the fourth ventricular outflow foramina; however, this feature is not entirely pathognomonic, as some MBs may also extend through the fourth ventricular exit foramina.[21] The extensions through the foramina in MBs is more bulbous and have more restricted diffusion compared to the thin tongues of tissue and intermediate diffusion in ependymomas. Rarely,

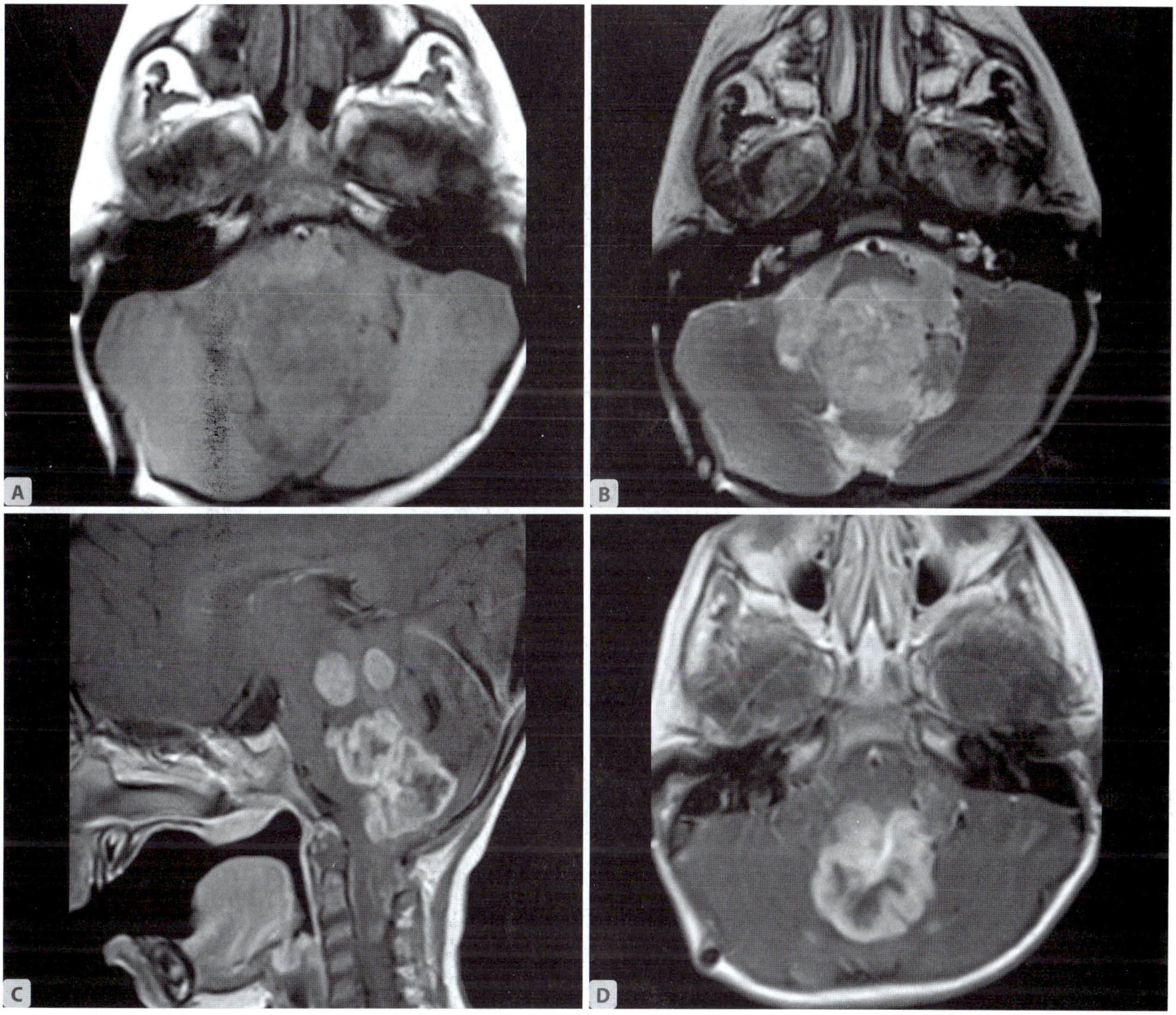

FIGS. 7A TO D: Ependymoma: Axial T1WI (A) and T2WI (B) show a heterogeneous mass filling the fourth ventricle. Post-gadolinium sagittal (C) and axial (D) T1WI demonstrate heterogeneous enhancement. The tumor is creeping anteriorly through foramen of Luschka into CPA cisterns and posteriorly through foramen of Magendie into upper cervical canal.

ependymoma can present as an isolated mass within the cerebellopontine angle, presumably arising from the rests of ependymal cells.

Proton MR spectroscopy typically demonstrates elevated high myo-inositol (MI) levels in classic grade II ependymomas.[22,23]

Treatment for EPN to this date remains maximal-safe surgical resection followed by adjuvant radiotherapy in order to reduce the likelihood of recurrence in the tumor bed.[24] The survival rates have seen limited improvement (~80%) in the last decade, with survivors suffering from the debilitating side effects of radiation induced severe neurocognitive impairment and other radiation-induced complications.

Cerebellar Pilocytic Astrocytoma

Pilocytic astrocytomas (PA) are well-defined, slow growing, WHO Grade I tumors of CNS arising from astrocytic precursor cells. They typically present between 5 and 15 years of age. They generally arise from the cerebellum (60%), hypothalamus-optic chiasma region, brainstem and less commonly from cerebral hemispheres. Classically, cerebellar astrocytoma manifests with waxing and waning headache, truncal ataxia, dysdiadochokinesia are other cerebellar signs. They have an excellent prognosis with 90% of patients having a 10-year survival after total resection.

Pathology

PAs may be vermian or hemispheric in origin. Grossly, the cerebellar PA is usually sharply circumscribed, with a very narrow zone of microscopic infiltration. Approximately 50% of tumors are cystic with an enhancing mural nodule. Enhancement of the cyst wall is possible, but is not pathognomonic.[25] Nearly 40% of tumors are mixed solid with cystic or necrotic components and the rest are purely solid mass lesions. The tumor is supplied by capillaries that lack a complete blood-brain barrier (BBB). It has open tight junction in the endothelial cells with fenestration and therefore differs from low grade astrocytoma. This fact and the lack of BBB is the cause of both intense enhancement, as well as the source of production of the proteinaceous fluid that accumulates in the "cyst" of the tumor.

Imaging

Classically, cerebellar PA appears as a cystic mass with an enhancing mural nodule **(Figs. 8A to C)** or a mixed solid-cystic mass **(Figs. 9A to D)**. Solid portion is hypointense on T1WI (higher than CSF intensity) and hyperintense on T2W1 and show variable enhancement **(Figs. 9A to D)**. Typically diffusion is facilitated in the solid enhancing portion of the tumor in comparison to MB and AT-RT. Peritumoral edema and intratumoral calcifications are usually absent. Hemorrhage can be present but rare **(Figs. 9A to D)**.

MR spectroscopy is quite tricky. Choline is typically very high in pilocytic tumors, despite the benign clinical course for tumors of this type.[22] In addition, Lipids and lactate are also usually demonstrated in the spectra of PAs. Despite being low grade (grade I tumors), PAs may present with high blood volumes on MR perfusion studies. This finding is not related to aggressiveness in these lesions.

Atypical Teratoid/Rhabdoid Tumor

CNS AT/RTs are highly malignant neoplasms which account for 1–3% of all primary CNS tumors in the pediatric population and 6.7% of all primary CNS tumors in children less than 3 years of age.[26,27] Although by definition they contain rhabdoid cells, ATRTs have widely divergent cell populations, including mesenchymal, epithelial, glial, and neuronal cell lines accounting for the "teratoid" descriptor.[28] About two-thirds of ATRTs occur in the cerebellum, typically in the cerebellopontine angle, with invasion of the surrounding structures. About one-fourth are supratentorial and 8% are multifocal.[29] The primary AT-RT of the brain can present between 1 month to 12 years of age (average age 24.5 months), and have with a male predominance (M:F, 3:1).[29]

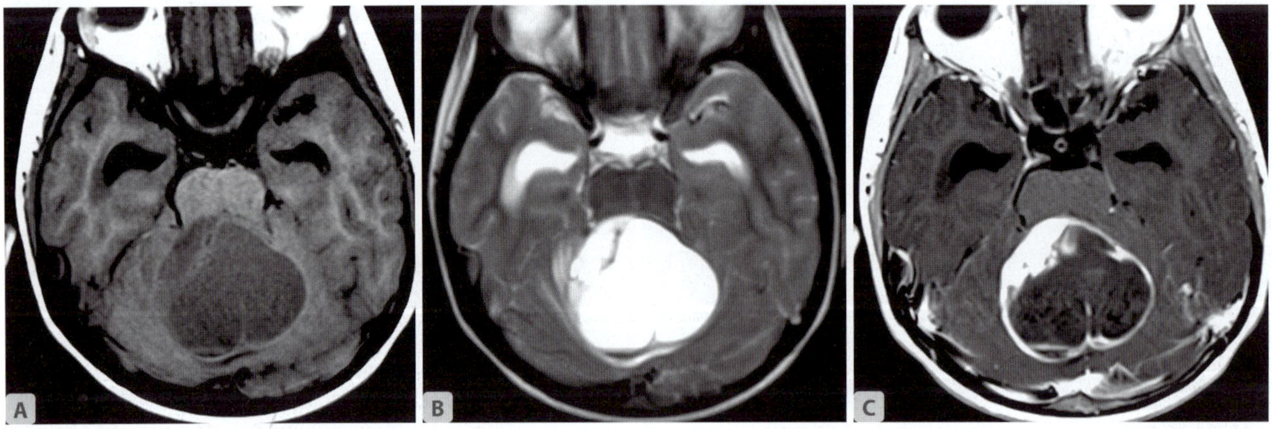

FIGS. 8A TO C: Cystic cerebellar astrocytoma: Axial T1WI (A) and T2WI (B) show a cystic mass with a mural nodule. The mural nodule is hypointense on T1WI (A) and hyperintense on T2WI (B). Following contrast administration, both the mural nodule and cyst wall enhance intensely (C). Note that no vascular flow-voids are seen in and around the mural nodule.

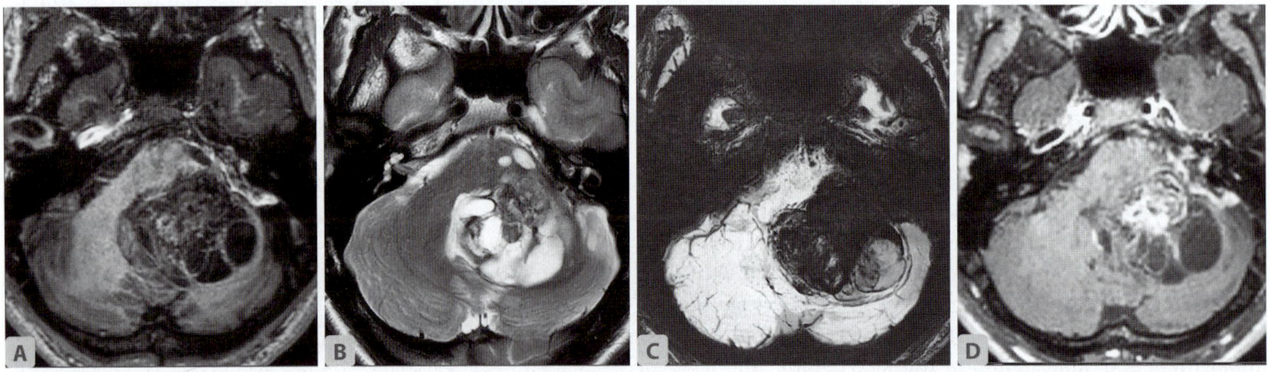

FIGS. 9A TO D: Solid-cystic cerebellar astrocytoma: Axial T1WI (A) and T2WI (B) show a heterogeneous mass in left cerebellum. On SWI (C), evidence of hemorrhage is seen within the mass. Following contrast administration, the mass shows heterogeneous enhancement (D). Note that no vascular flow-voids are seen in and around the mural nodule.

Pathology

Histologically, ATRTs are characterized by rhabdoid cells and are similar to that of other small round blue cell tumors; up to 70% also contain cell fields typical of a primitive neuroectodermal tumor. Necrosis and a high MIB-index are common.

Nearly all ATRTs demonstrate bi-allelic inactivation of SMARCB1 (or INI1) on chromosome 22, whereas a very small percentage show inactivation of SMARCA4 (or BRG1).[30] Having one of these genetic alterations is now formally required for diagnosis.[4]

Imaging

On imaging, lesions are usually large at presentation, with moderate-to-marked surrounding edema. On CT, these tumors are hyperdense or mixed density lesions attributed to the presence of areas of necrosis, cyst formation, hemorrhage and calcification[31] and show varying pattern of enhancement following contrast administration.[32] On MR, they are T1-hypointense, T2-iso to hypointense with restricted diffusion and inhomogeneous enhancement **(Figs. 10A to F)**. These imaging findings overlap with those described for MBs and are likely secondary to high cell density and high nucleus-to-cytoplasm ratio. Diffuse leptomeningeal dissemination is common, hence the spine should also be imaged. MRS shows elevated Cho, reduced NAA and a prominent lipid peak.

The main differential diagnosis for posterior fossa ATRT is MB and both show restricted diffusion. If a posterior fossa tumor occurs in a child less than 3 years of age, located off-midline, has intratumoral blood products and extends to the CPA, it is more likely to be an AT-RT than a MB.[33] Very young children presenting with cranial nerve deficits and masses involving the CPA with restricted diffusion are more likely to have an ATRT.[34]

Hemangioblastoma

Hemangioblastomas are uncommon, slow-growing tumors of CNS (WHO grade 1) that occur in the cerebellum (83–86%), brainstem (2–5%), spinal cord (3–13%) and cerebrum (1.5%).[35] They may occur either sporadically (75%) or as a manifestation of von Hippel-Lindau (VHL) disease in 25% along with retinal angioma, renal cell carcinoma, adrenal pheochromocytoma,

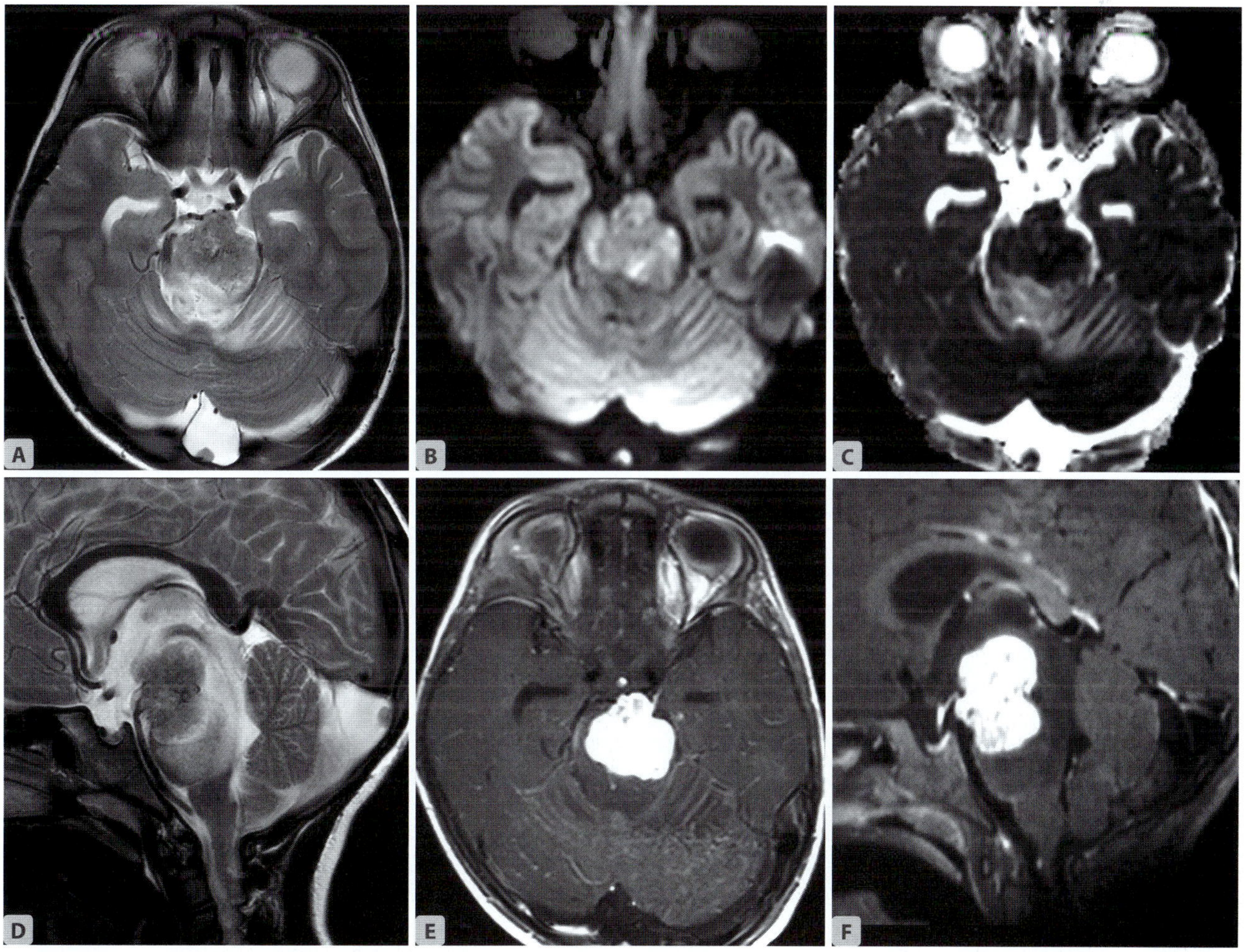

FIGS. 10A TO F: ATRT. A well-defined prepontine mass is seen without any plane between the tumor and the brainstem. The mass is isointense on axial (A) and sagittal (D) T2WI, bright on DWI (B) and dark on ADC maps (C) suggesting restricted diffusion. Post-gad axial (E) and sagittal (F) images show avid contrast enhancement of the mass.

as well as benign cysts in the lungs, liver, kidneys, and pancreas. The hemangioblastomas in VHL disease develop at an earlier age and are often multifocal in 20%.

Pathology

Hemangioblastomas typically appear as well-demarcated masses with smooth margins. The tumor can be either entirely solid (40%) or cystic with a hypervascular enhancing mural nodule with prominent blood vessels (60%). VHL-associated and some sporadic hemangioblastomas are caused by inactivation of the VHL tumor suppressor gene, located on chromosome 3p.

Imaging

On NCCT, hemangioblastoma typically appears as a well-defined, either entirely solid or hypodense cystic lesion with an iso-hyperdense mural nodule. Solid hemangioblastomas appear hyperdense on NCCT and show strong homogeneous enhancement. The iso-hyperdense mural nodule abuts the pial surface and shows strong homogeneous contrast enhancement.

On MRI the cystic component of hemangioblastoma is either iso- or slightly hyperintense relative to CSF on T1WI and hyperintense on T2WI.[35] The nodule is T1 hypointense, T2 hyperintense and enhances avidly following gadolinium administration **(Figs. 11A to D and Figs. 8A and B)**. Vascular flow-voids may be present within and at the periphery of the tumor **(Figs. 11C and D)**. The peritumoral edema is usually minimal or absent. Perfusion MR imaging reveals high rCBV ratios in these lesions (around 11), values significantly higher than those of metastases (around 5) and pilocytic astrocytomas.[36] Cerebral angiography is reserved for preoperative tumor embolization and shows dilated feeding arteries and a prolonged tumoral blush corresponding to the solid portion.[37] The other differential diagnosis of a cyst with enhancing mural nodule in the infratentorial compartment is pilocytic astrocytoma which generally occurs at a younger age, is not associated with intratumoral flow-voids and show less increase in rCBV and permeability.

Metastases

Metastases are the most common infratentorial intra-axial neoplasms in the adult population. They are usually well-defined round masses, often with nodular or ring enhancement (due to central necrosis). Multiple masses are usually seen and help to confirm the diagnosis. However, even if solitary, the lesion is still more commonly metastasis than a primary intracranial neoplasm. In adults, lung and breast carcinoma account for the majority of metastatic disease, followed by melanoma, renal cell carcinoma, thyroid carcinoma, and

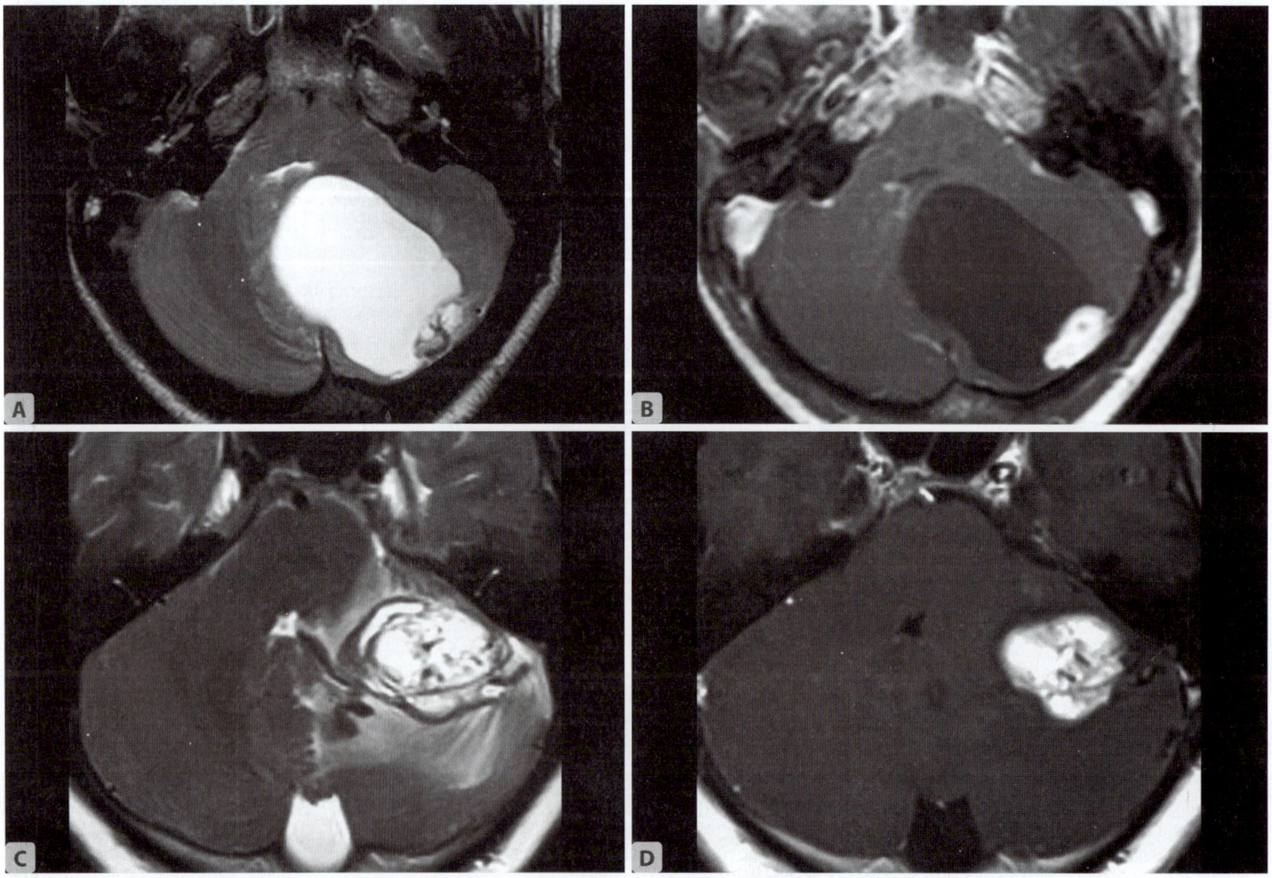

FIGS. 11A TO D: Hemangioblastoma: Axial T2 (A) and post-gad T1(B) show a cystic hemangioblastoma with enhancing mural nodule and vascular flow-voids within the mural nodule (A). Axial T2 (C) and post-gad T1 (D) show a solid hemangioblastoma with intense enhancement, multiple vascular flow-voids and perilesional edema.

gastrointestinal malignancies. Unknown primaries account for 10–15% of patients with brain metastases.

Imaging

Metastases are typically hypodense on CT; they are hypointense on T1WI and hyperintense on T2WI; and show varying pattern of enhancement **(Figs. 12A and B)**. Most metastases have considerable surrounding edema. Metastases with increased T1 signal intensity before contrast administration include melanoma, renal cell carcinoma, lung carcinoma, choriocarcinoma, and gastrointestinal adenocarcinoma (because of the presence of mucin).[38] Metastases with areas of hemorrhage and calcification have variable signal on T2WI. MR spectroscopy shows significantly elevated choline and very low NAA (the presence of NAA in many metastases represents contamination from adjacent tissues due to partial averaging).[39] Lactate and lipids are usually high. The tissues surrounding the enhancing mass usually are normal by spectroscopy (unlike high grade gliomas).

Dysplastic Cerebellar Gangliocytoma

Dysplastic cerebellar gangliocytoma, also known as Lhermitte-Duclos disease, is a rare entity characterized by focal thickening of the folia and loss of normal cerebellar cortical architecture.[40] There is debate as to whether this abnormality is a hamartoma, a malformation or a tumor; if neoplastic, it corresponds to WHO grade I.[41,42] Patients generally present with headache and hydrocephalus. The median age of presentation is in the 4th decade. Most adults, but not children, with dysplastic gangliocytoma have PTEN (phosphatase and tensin homolog) germline mutations.[43] LDD patients should be evaluated carefully to rule out Cowden syndrome, because Cowden syndrome patients have a high incidence of multisystemic cancers and other diseases including breast cancer (25%–50%), nonmedullary thyroid cancer (3%–10%), and endometrial adenocarcinoma (5%–10%).[44] Nowadays, Lhermitte-Duclos disease and Cowden syndrome are included in PTEN hamartoma tumor syndrome (PHTS).

Pathology

Histologically, there is reduced cerebellar white matter and presence of abnormal hypertrophic ganglion cells that superficially resemble Purkinje cells.

Imaging

On CT scan, the lesions are typically hypodense but may be isodense.[42] Calcification may occur but is uncommon.[42] On MRI, the lesion is seen as a focal cerebellar mass typically involving one hemisphere with a highly characteristic folial pattern (also described as laminated, corduroy, lamellar, or striated) **(Fig. 13A)**. The central core of T1 hypointensity and T2 hyperintensity corresponds to the inner molecular layer, widened granular cell layer, and loss of central white matter within the folia; whereas the outer thinner layer on MR images (T1 isointense, T2 iso- to hypointense) corresponds to the outer molecular layer and the leptomeninges.[45] Typically these lesions do not enhance **(Fig. 13B)**.[45] Rarely enhancement may be seen presumably secondary to venous proliferation in the outer portions of the cerebellar cortex and prominent draining veins.[46]

Treatment of symptomatic dysplastic gangliocytoma of the cerebellum is surgical resection.

Embryonal Tumor with Multilayered Rosettes C19MC-altered

A new entity, embryonal tumor with multilayered rosettes (ETMR) C19MC-altered, was recently described in children younger than 4 years.[4] The term, primitive neuroectodermal tumor (PNET), has been removed and they are classified according to the presence of amplification of the C19MC region on chromosome 19 (19q 13.42). The presence of C19 MC amplification results in a diagnosis of ETMRs (ETMR-C19MC-altered). In its absence, the tumor is called ETMR-NOS.

These are usually large masses, more than 5 cm in size at the time of presentation in the supratentorial compartment, but may also be found in the infratentorial compartment. They are well-delineated masses with absent or minimal

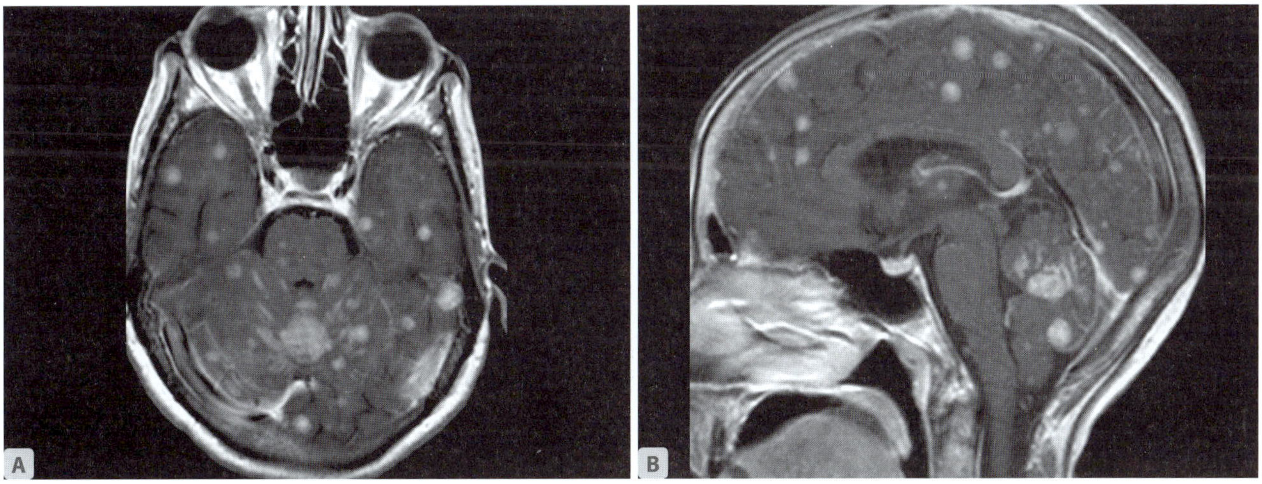

FIGS. 12A AND B: Metastases: Axial (A) and sagittal (B) T1WIs show multiple enhancing nodules throughout the brain parenchyma.

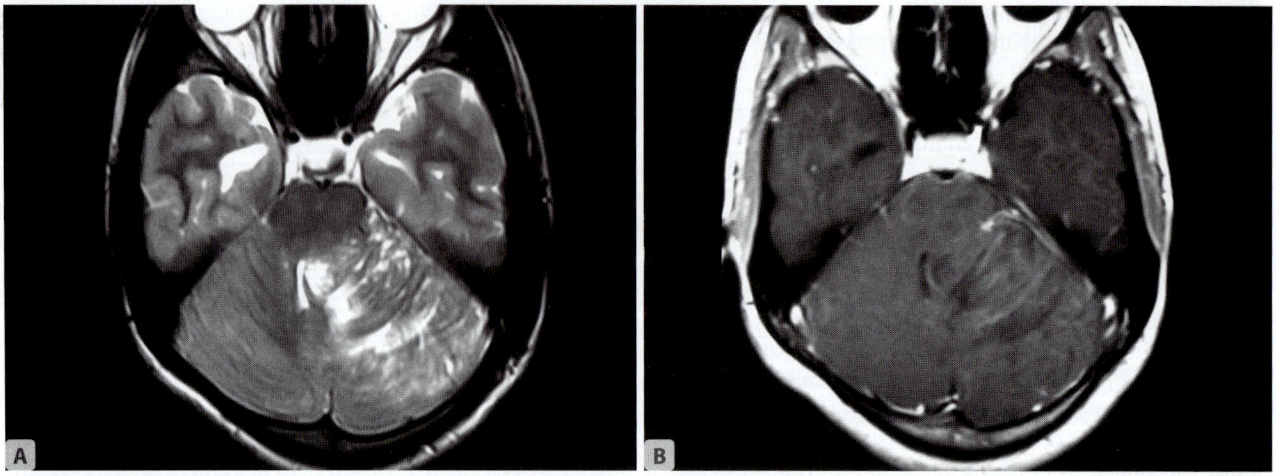

FIGS. 13A AND B: Dysplastic cerebellar gangliocytoma: (A) Axial T2WI shows a cerebellar mass with a striped appearance, composed of alternating hyperintense and isointense bands associated with compression on the 4th ventricle; (B) Contrast-enhanced axial T1WI shows mild enhancement of the mass.

peritumoral edema despite their large size.[47-49] Typically they are heterogeneous isodense to hyperdense masses on CT. Calcifications are seen in 70% of cases.[49] On MRI, the signal on T1/T2 is variable due to the presence of blood products, calcifications, and cystic changes. FLAIR shows areas of necrosis (hyperintense) and cystic components (hypointense).[47] On diffusion-weighted imaging, the tumor shows restricted diffusion presumably due to its high cellularity and nucleus-to-cytoplasm ratio.[47] The solid components demonstrate avid heterogeneous contrast enhancement.[49] Perfusion MRI shows increased relative cerebral blood volume.[49] ETMRs develop subarachnoid dissemination in 40% of cases; thus, the entire neuroaxis should be imaged. The presence of metastases changes management, requiring chemotherapy and increased radiation dose.[47,49] Prognosis is dismal despite radiation therapy.

BRAINSTEM AND CERVICOMEDULLARY JUNCTION

Brainstem Gliomas

Brainstem gliomas are a heterogeneous group of tumors that differ significantly in their growth characteristics, histology, and response to therapy. They represent 10–20% of pediatric CNS tumors and three-fourths of these occur before 20 years of age.[50] In adults, they represent less than 2% of brain tumors and usually occur in younger adults and tend to be of low grade (WHO I or II).

The majority (85%) are composed of high-grade fibrillary gliomas, which arise predominantly in the pons and less frequently in the medulla. There is no sex predilection, and children between 7 and 10 years of age are commonly affected. Multiple cranial nerve palsies, pyramidal tract signs, ataxia and nystagmus are the usual presentation. Except in tectal gliomas, hydrocephalus is uncommon in brain stem gliomas. Diffuse pontine gliomas have the worst prognosis.[51]

Pathology

Brainstem gliomas can be divided into the diffuse brainstem glioma and focal glioma (including dorsal exophytic, tectal, and cervicomedullary).[52]

Recent molecular studies have revealed that diffuse brainstem gliomas in children most likely harbor a highly specific point mutation, K27M, in histone 3.3, 3.2, or 3.1.3–7. In the revised 2016 update of the WHO brain tumor classification, these neoplasms constitute a new entity termed as diffuse midline glioma, H3 K27M-mutant characterized by a diffuse growth pattern, and a midline location (e.g., thalami, brainstem, spinal cord, and other midline structures, including the third ventricle, hypothalamus, and pineal region).[4] The majority of histone H3 K27M-mutant tumors are high-grade astrocytomas with high proliferative potential,[53,54] often with contiguous extension of tumor from the brainstem into the thalami and upper cervical spinal cord.[4,54] Most of these tumors have poor prognosis but exceptions have been reported.

Imaging

MR imaging is useful for diagnosis and localization of the tumor. Diffuse brainstem glioma appears as poorly defined T1 hypointense and T2 hyperintense regions **(Figs. 14A to C)**.[55] Intratumoral heterogeneity is occasionally present, but cysts are not common. The signal changes may extend into the cerebellum and/or the adjacent brainstem. There is often exophytic spread laterally and ventrally with basilar artery encasement. An undulating ventral border of the brainstem on sagittal image may be an indirect clue to the presence of the mass lesion. Contrast enhancement has been reported in approximately one-half of the cases and is often focal and nodular **(Fig. 14C)**. Areas of restricted diffusion may be present, indicating higher cell density and providing targets for biopsy. No significant differences are seen in the characteristics of enhancement, infiltration, or peritumoral

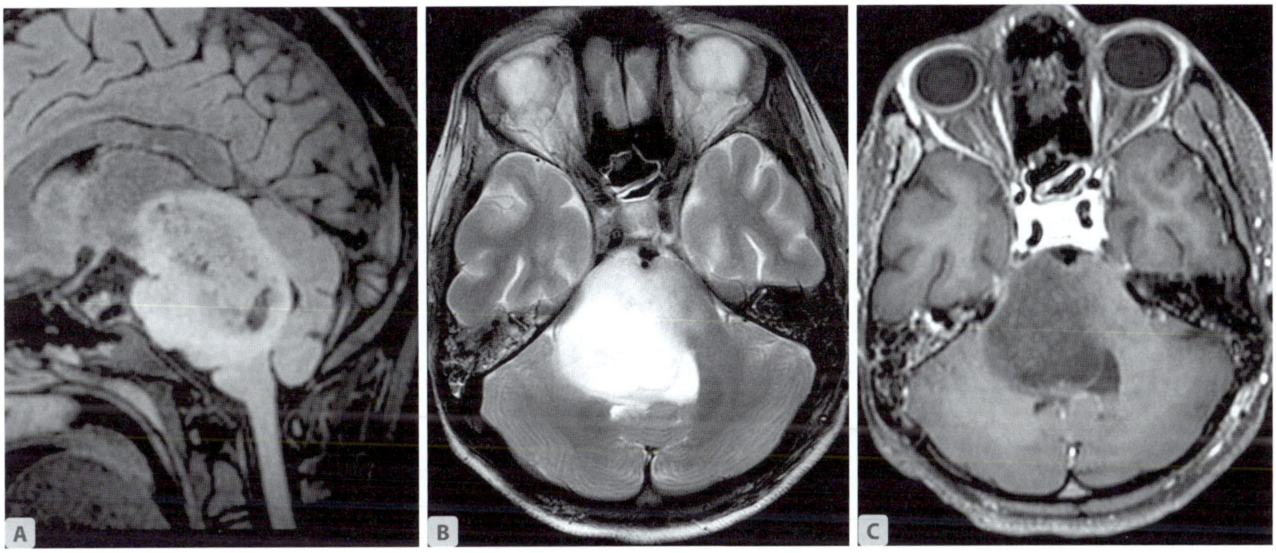

FIGS. 14A TO C: Diffuse midline glioma: Sagittal FLAIR (A) and axial T2WI (B) show diffuse pontine glioma causing expansion of pons and basilar artery encasement. No definite enhancement is seen following gadolinium administration (C).

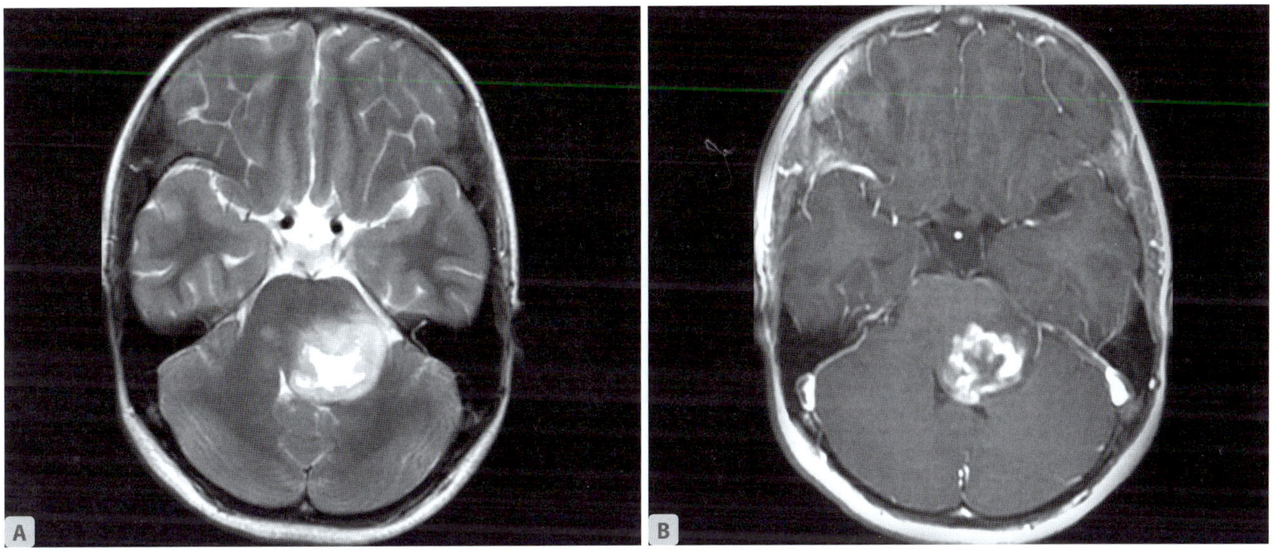

FIGS. 15A AND B: Dorsal exophytic pontine glioma: Axial T2WI (A) shows a hyperintense lesion with central necrosis arising from left brachium pontis and compressing fourth ventricle. The mass shows enhancement around central necrosis (B).

edema in patients with Diffuse pontine glioma with or without the histone H3 K27M mutation.[56]

Focal brainstem gliomas are often well circumscribed and sometimes markedly exophytic. Exophytic component is readily identified on MR, due to its multiplanar imaging capability. The dorsally exophytic lesions are grossly multicystic and often enhance intensely **(Figs. 15A and B)**. The presence of enhancement has not been correlated reliably with type or grade of malignancy.[51] The other subtypes of focal gliomas are tectal plate glioma **(Figs. 16A and B)** and cervicomedullary glioma **(Figs. 17A and B)**.

Ganglioglioma

Ganglioglioma (GG) is another diagnostic consideration for tumors located in the brainstem and upper cervical cord. Infratentorial GGs are less common than supratentorial GGs.[57]

On imaging, infratentorial GGs are typically infiltrative and expansile solid masses with dorsal predominant "paintbrush" enhancement.

Infratentorial GGs are difficult to resect completely and have poor progression-free survival and high mortality, in comparison to supratentorial GGs.[58]

CEREBELLOPONTINE ANGLE AND INTERNAL AUDITORY CANAL

Lesions of the cerebellopontine angle (CPA) are frequent and represent 6–10% of all intracranial tumors. Vestibular schwannomas and meningiomas are the two most frequent lesions and account for approximately 85–90% of all CPA tumors.

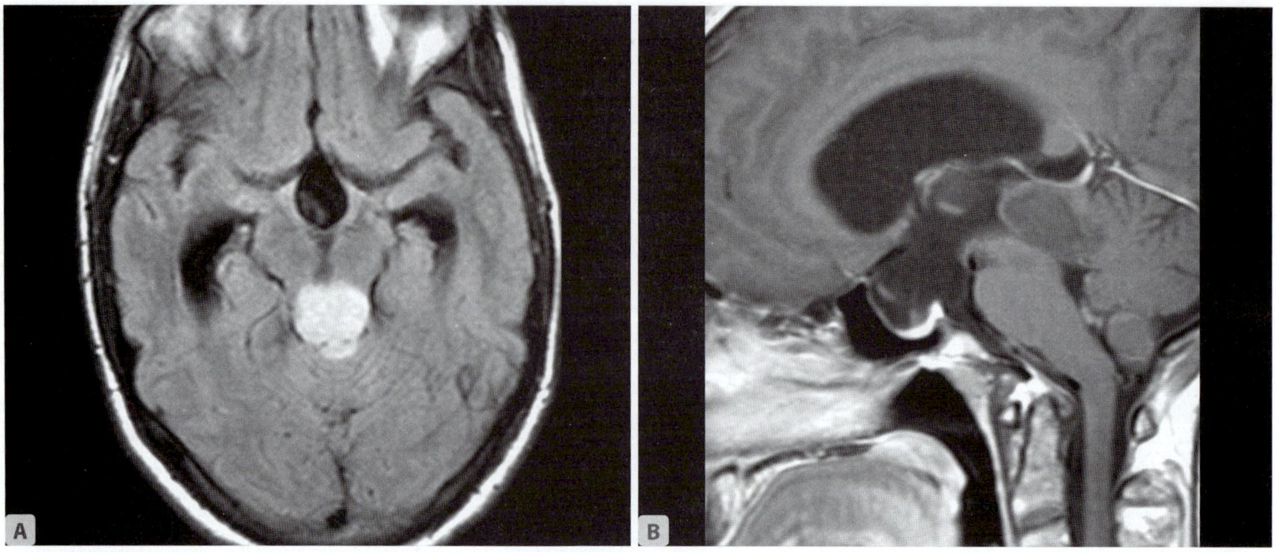

FIGS. 16A AND B: Tectal plate glioma: Axial flair (A) image shows thickening and hyperintensity in the region of tectal plate, compressing the aqueduct and causing proximal hydrocephalus. No enhancement is seen following gadolinium administration (B).

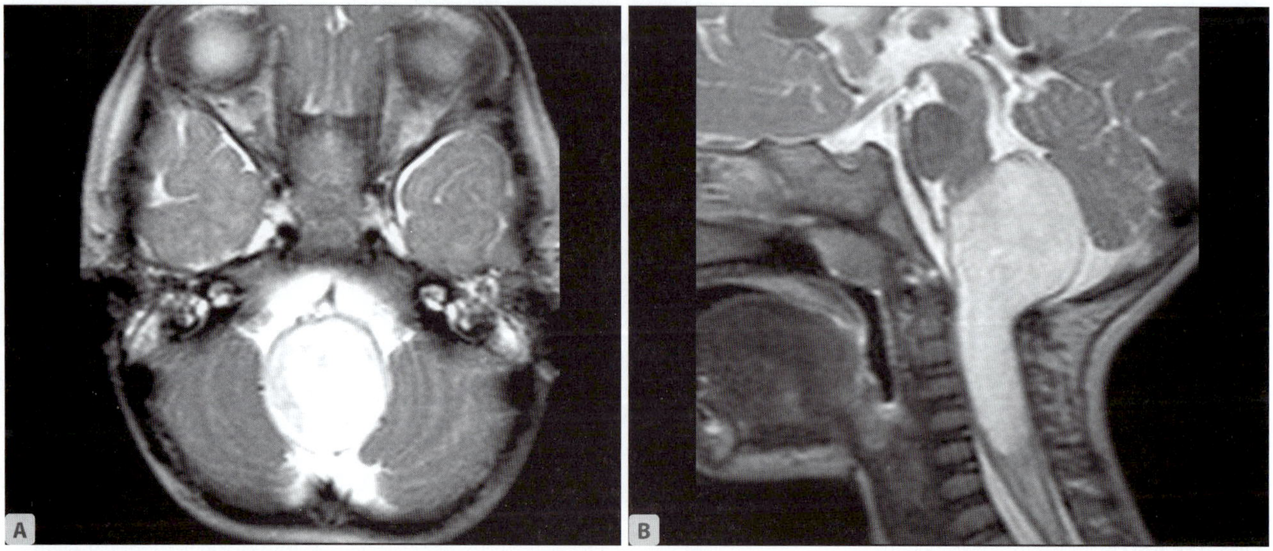

FIGS. 17A AND B: Cervicomedullary glioma: Axial (A) and sagittal T2WI (B) images show an expansile well-defined mass lesion involving medulla and upper cervical spinal cord.

Vestibular Schwannomas

Vestibular schwannomas are Schwann cell-derived tumors that account for nearly 8% of intracranial tumors in adults and 80 to 90% of tumors of the cerebellopontine angle (CPA). Typically they present with adult-onset unilateral sensorineural hearing loss or tinnitus.[59] Bilateral vestibular schwannomas are pathognomonic for neurofibromatosis type 2 (NF2) **(Figs. 18A and B)**. These are generally benign and slow growing tumors with rare malignant degeneration when associated with NF-1.

Pathology

Vestibular schwannomas arise from perineural elements of the Schwann cell and are similar in pathology to other peripheral schwannomas. Histologic examination of schwannomas reveal compact Antoni Type A tissue and loose textured, often cystic, Antoni Type B tissue.

Imaging

On imaging, vestibular schwannomas are seen as enhancing CPA mass lesions with variable extension into the internal auditory canal in most cases, resulting in the description of an "ice-cream cone" tumor. The intracanalicular component often causes widening of the porus acusticus resulting in the trumpeted IAM sign in up to 90% of cases. Purely extracanalicular tumors only abutting the porus acusticus are less common (~20%) and present late with features of mass effect rather than hearing loss. Generally, a small "CSF cap" is present between the intracanalicular component and

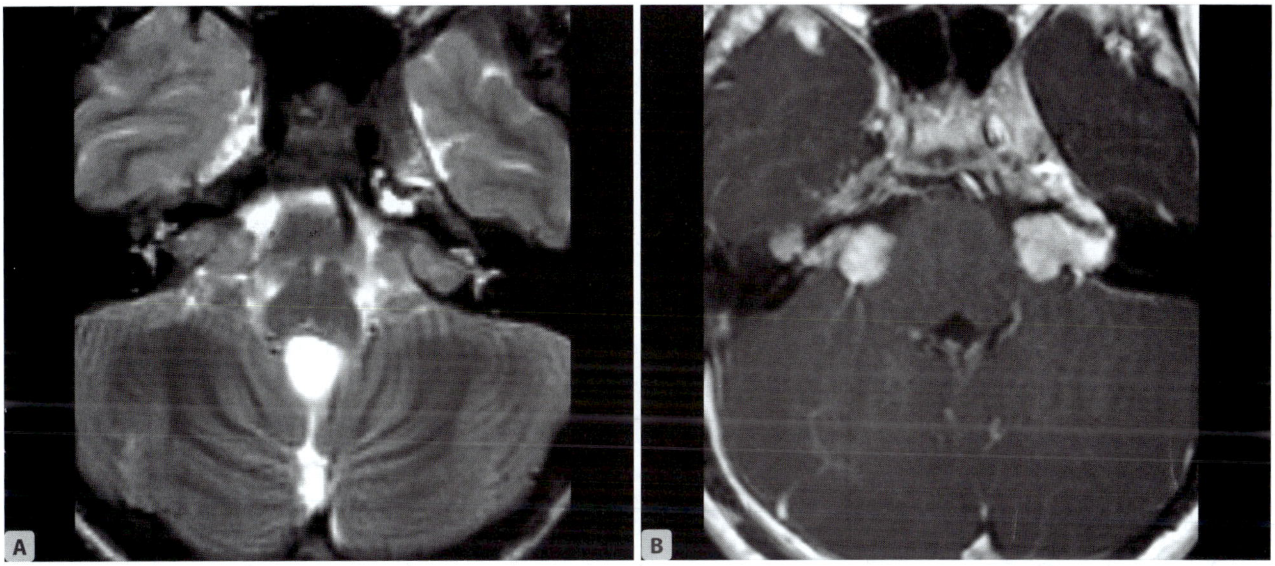

FIGS. 18A AND B: Schwannomas: A patient of neurofibromatosis 2 with bilateral acoustic schwannomas and right facial nerve schwannoma in region of geniculate ganglion. These lesions are isointense on T2WI (A) and shows homogenous enhancement on contrast administration (B).

the cochlea. Sometimes these tumors extend laterally into the middle ear through the cochlea (transmodiolar) or the vestibule (transmacular). Rarely small tumors are limited to the vestibule (intravestibular) or the cochlea (intracochlear) or both (vestibulocochlear).[60]

Degree of IAC widening and the tumor extent ventral and caudal to the IAC on NCCT can predict postoperative hearing loss.[61]

The low T2 acoustic schwannomas have a predominance of the Antoni Type A tissue. Large tumors have predominant Antoni Type B tissue and appear heterogeneous secondary to presence of regions of internal necrosis/cyst formation **(Figs. 19A to F)**. Peritumoral cysts are also associated (7 to 10%) with large lesions-believed to be secondary to elevation and deformation of the leptomeninges. Since the IAC is involved (80%), flaring of the porous acusticus, expansion of the IAC, and an acute angle with the dura can be seen. In vestibular schwannomas, the vestibule may have a low T2 signal intensity, presumably due to increased protein concentration in the perilymph (but not in patients who have CPA meningiomas). Some patients who have vestibular schwannomas larger than 2 cm in diameter demonstrate a tiny area of hyperintensity in the dorsal brain stem on T2WIs at the lateral angle of the fourth ventricular floor. This may represent degeneration of the vestibular nucleus and should not be confused with infarction.

Small tumors typically show homogeneous enhancement, whereas larger lesions more often have heterogeneous enhancement due to presence of hemorrhage and cystic areas. Occasionally, vestibular schwannomas show extension into the cochlea and "dural tails" of enhancement.

The major treatment options for patients with a vestibular schwannoma are surgery, radiation therapy, and observation.

Meningiomas

Meningiomas are extra-axial neoplastic lesions arising from arachnoidal cap cells. Approximately, 10% of all intracranial meningiomas arise in the infratentorial compartment. They are the second most common CPA tumor and account for 10% of CPA masses. They usually arise from the posterior petrous surface or the underside of the tentorium **(Figs. 20A and B)**.

Imaging

On NCCT, meningiomas are frequently hyperdense. Focal areas of calcification are present in up to 25% of cases. A dural tail, the presence of bony reaction, and an obtuse angle with the dura, as well as the centre of the lesion being located away from the IAC, suggest meningioma. Relatively T2 hypointense signal is characteristic of most meningiomas, especially the transitional and fibroblastic varieties.[62] Necrosis and cystic degeneration are uncommon with meningiomas and help to differentiate them from schwannomas **(Figs. 20A and B)**. On SWI, presence of susceptibility foci secondary to hemorrhage suggest schwannoma rather than meningioma. Rarely, meningiomas may originate within the internal auditory canal, or even within the labyrinth. CPA meningioma may extend into the IAC, however canal is often not widened. The presence of a dural tail is suggestive but not pathognomonic of meningioma.

Epidermoid and Dermoid

Epidermoid and dermoid are generally believed to be congenital/developmental masses rather than neoplastic, arising from ectodermal heterotopia. Both cysts have stratified squamous epithelium inner lining, with dermoids having additional mesodermal elements such as hair, sebaceous and sweat glands.

Epidermoids are slightly more common than dermoids and account for 3–7% of CPA masses. They grow very slowly via desquamation and therefore present late in adults despite their congenital etiology. They may become quite large before becoming symptomatic. The CPA is the most common location, followed by the parasellar region.

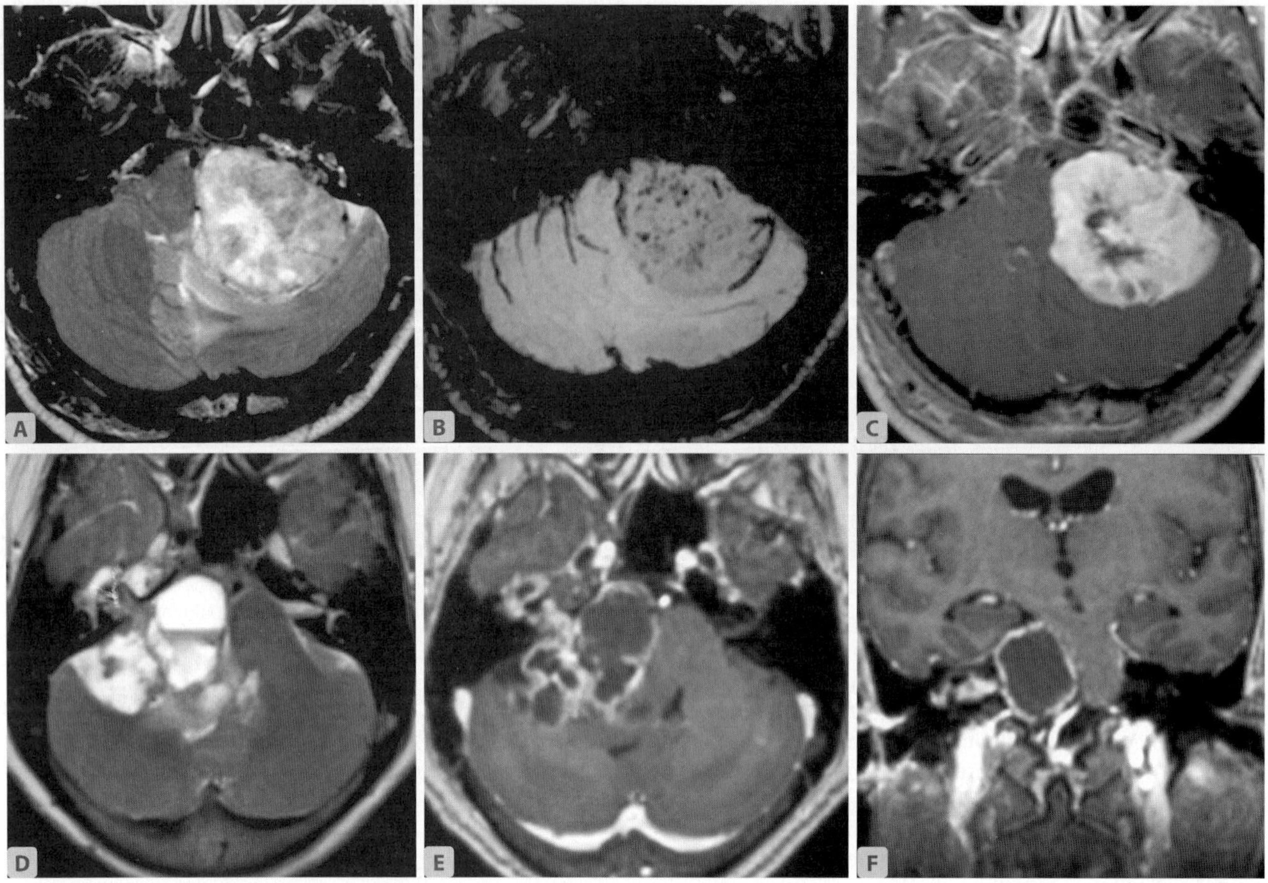

FIGS. 19A TO F: Acoustic Schwannomas: Axial T2 (A) image shows an iso-hyperintense CPA mass with extension into IAC, areas on susceptibility on SWI (B) and heterogeneous enhancement (C). Cystic acoustic schwannomas with multiple septations and fluid-fluid levels on T2WI (D), extension into IAC and heterogeneous enhancement (E and F).

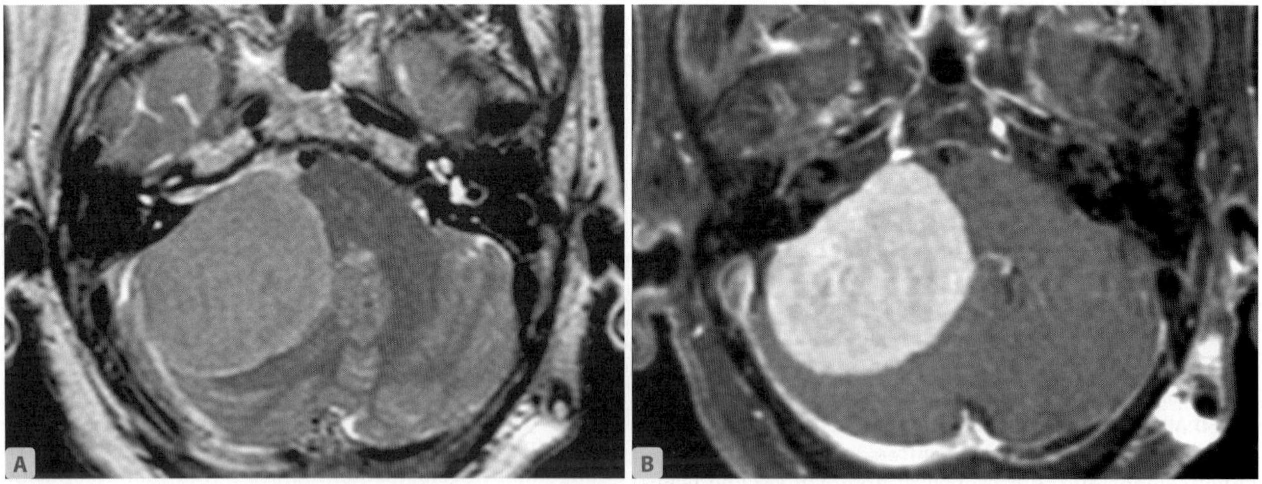

FIGS. 20A AND B: Meningioma: Extra-axial CPA mass with broad dural base, isointense T2 signal (A) and avid contrast enhancement (B).

Imaging

At CT, most epidermoids are non-enhancing hypodense lesions with calcification in up to 25% of cases. Most epidermoids are isointense to CSF on both T1 and T2WI **(Figs. 21A to F)** due to presence of cholesterol in its solid/crystalline state rather than the liquid state. The latter would result in bright T1 signal. The adamantinomatous craniopharyngioma typically contains this type of cholesterol; epidermoids rarely do.[63] Epidermoids often have a lamellated appearance secondary to surface desquamation. Most epidermoids do not enhance, although some minimal rim enhancement occurs in approximately 25% of cases. Malignant transformation of

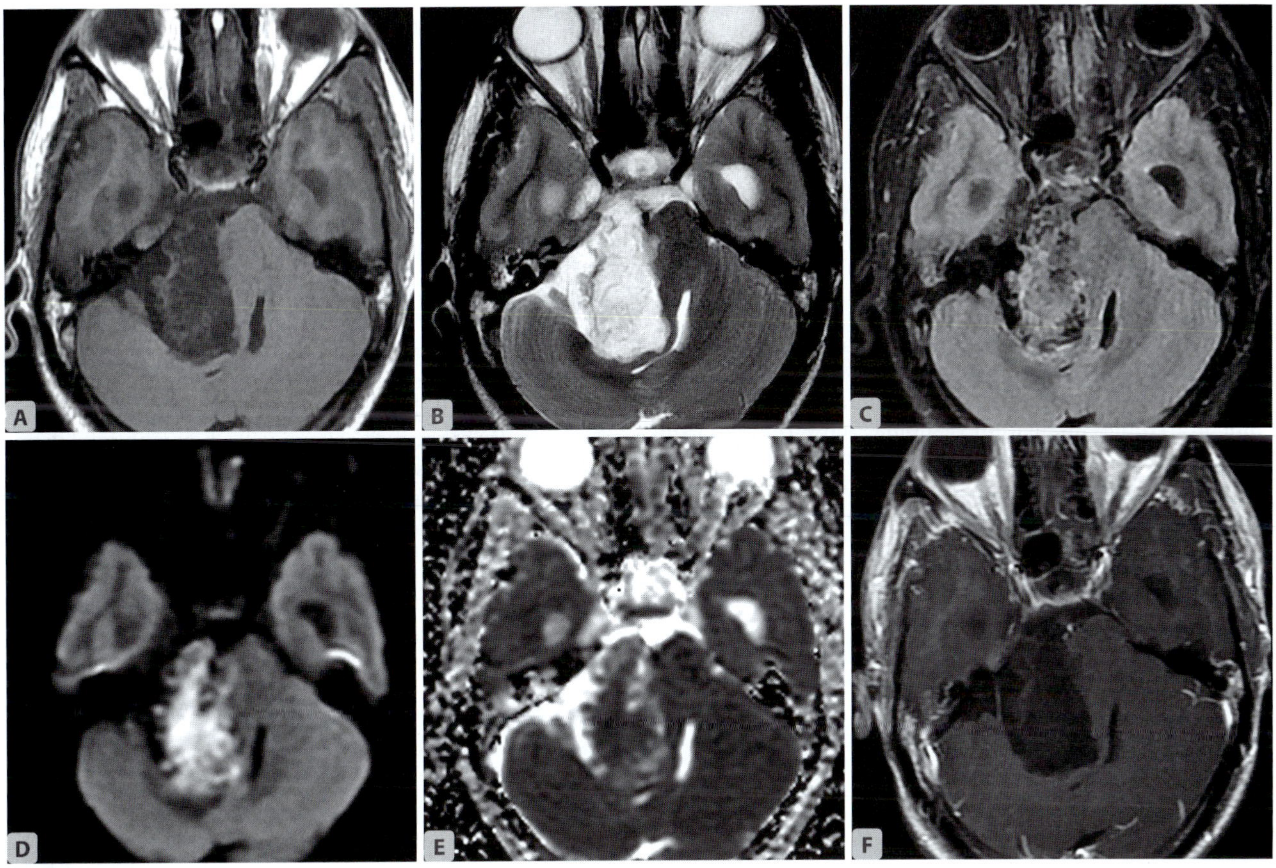

FIGS. 21A TO F: Epidermoid: MR scans show an extra-axial right CPA mass which is hypointense on T1WI (A) and hyperintense on T2WI (B). The mass has little internal heterogeneity on FLAIR images (C); bright on DWI (D) and dark on ADC images (E). No enhancement is seen following gad administration (F).

an epidermoid (squamous cell carcinoma) is rare and shows a significant enhancement. The rare "white epidermoid" is an interesting variant that is hyperdense at CT, hyperintense on T1WI, and hypointense on T2WI. This may be explained by high protein content, hemorrhage or the presence of saponified keratinized debris, and as indicated previously, cholesterol in the liquid state. When epidermoids are hyperintense on T1WI, then they need to be differentiated from dermoids and lipomas. Chemical shift artefact is absent in epidermoids and also a fat saturation pulse sequence will suppress the high signal of dermoids and lipomas, but not of epidermoids.

On FLAIR sequence, epidermoid cysts have mixed iso- to hyperintense signal with poor demarcation **(Fig. 21C)**. On DWI, epidermoids are hyperintense due to restricted diffusion (low ADC), while arachnoid cysts are hypointense due to increased diffusion (high ADC). DWI signal is also useful for detecting postoperative residual epidermoid.[64] The lamellated appearance and the tendency to insinuate rather than displace the surrounding structures are characteristic features of epidermoid.

Like epidermoid cysts, dermoid cysts are congenital ectodermal inclusions but are extremely rare, far less common than epidermoid cysts. Dermoids are midline lesions, occurring in the parasellar, frontobasal region or infratentorial compartment (vermis or fourth ventricle). Dermoids on CT are essentially fat density, extra-axial midline masses that do not enhance on contrast administration. They may be associated with bone defect in nasofrontal or occipital region that indicates the presence of a dermal sinus tract. CT is essential for detection of the calvarial defect, while MR delineates the tumor better. Unruptured cysts are hyperintense, similar to fat on T1WIs and are heterogeneous on T2WI. Chemical shift artefact is present similar to lipomas. However, dermoids are less lobulated than lipomas, and displace blood vessels and neural structures, in contrast to encasement of these structures by lipomas. Growth can lead to rupture of the cyst, causing a chemical meningitis. Imaging findings vary. Fat-like leptomeningeal and intraventricular deposits are diagnostic of a ruptured dermoid cyst.[65]

Arachnoid Cyst

Arachnoid cysts are congenital, benign, intra-arachnoid CSF filled lesions.[65] Mostly these are supratentorial lesions and about 70% are present in the middle cranial fossa[66] anterior to the temporal poles. Infratentorial arachnoid cysts account for only 10% of arachnoid cysts and a vast majority of these are located in the CPA. Typically arachnoid cysts are asymptomatic. However they can compromise cranial nerve functions by stretching them or rarely present with spontaneous or traumatic intracystic hemorrhage.[67]

Imaging

At neuroimaging, arachnoid cyst is hypodense on CT and follows CSF signal intensity on all MRI sequences including DWI, and do not enhance after gadolinium administration **(Figs. 22A to D)**. Complete suppression of signal intensity on FLAIR sequence and the lack of diffusion restriction differentiate arachnoid cyst from epidermoid cyst **(Figs. 22A to D)**.[68]

Facial Nerve Schwannomas

Schwannomas may arise anywhere along the course of the facial nerve from the CPA to the stylomastoid foramen. The facial nerve schwannoma arising in the IAC or CPA may be difficult to differentiate from vestibular schwannoma.[69] The presence of enhancing component extending along the labyrinthine segment of the facial nerve to the geniculate ganglion suggests the diagnosis of a facial nerve schwannoma over a vestibular schwannoma.[70]

Cerebellopontine Angle/Internal Auditory Canal Lipomas

Lipomas represent mesodermal inclusions and are rare CPA/IAC lesions. Characteristically, these lesions are hyperintense on T1WI and show signal suppression on fat-sat images. These should not be mistaken for retained pantopaque (iophendylate) dye when clinical history of previous myelogram may suggest diagnosis.

Metastatic Disease

CPA metastatic disease is rare and may be leptomeningeal or parenchymal (brainstem, cerebellum). Meningeal metastases may be diffuse, nodular or mass-like. Parenchymal lesions are exophytic brainstem or cerebellar hemispheric lesions mimicking CPA masses. With large lesions, it may be difficult to differentiate meningeal from parenchymal metastases. Breast and lung are the most common sources of primary tumors.

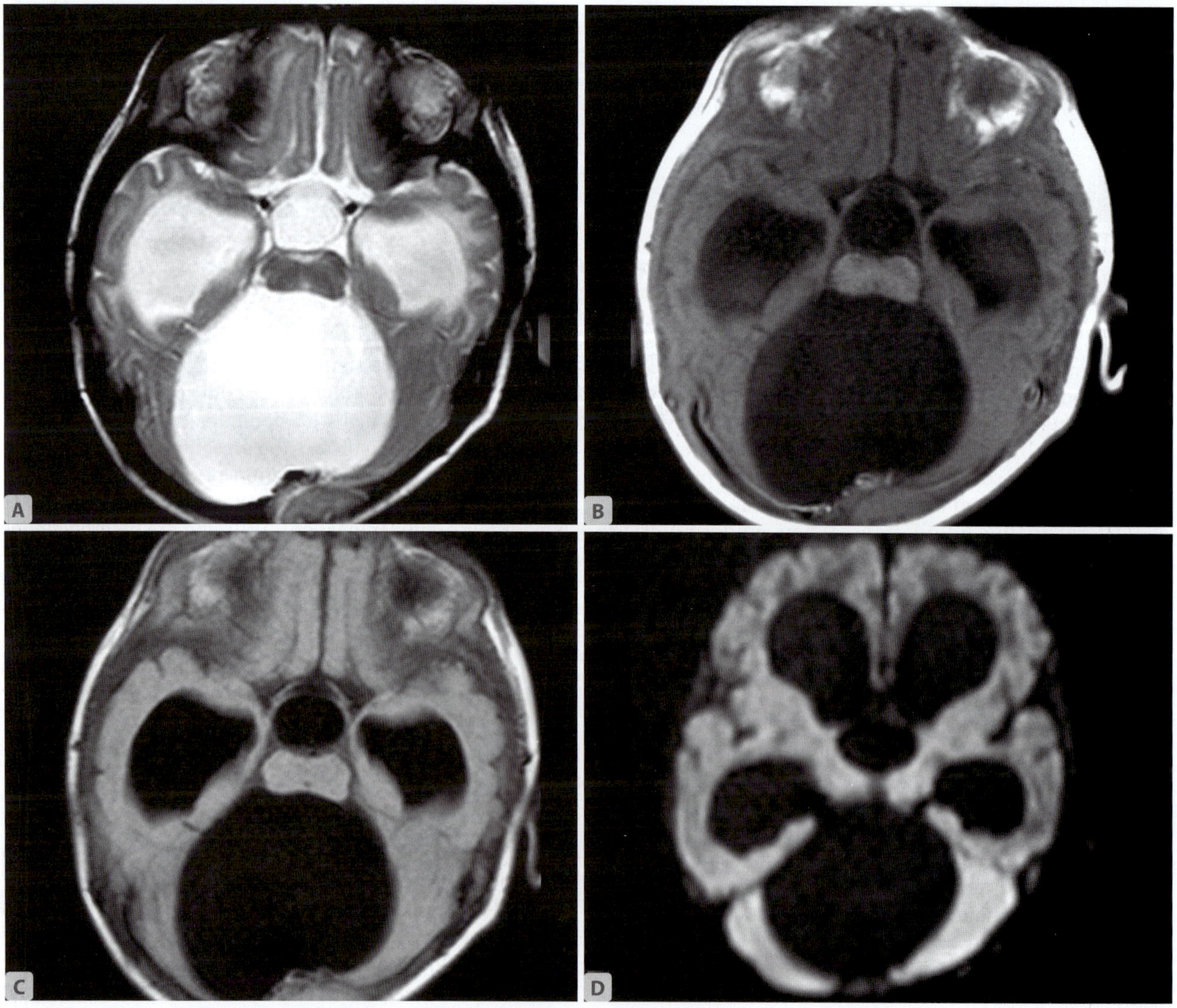

FIGS. 22A TO D: Arachnoid cyst: Axial T2WI shows a well-defined extra-axial cyst in superior cerebellar cistern which is isointense to the CSF on T1WI (A), T2WI (B) and Flair (C). The lesion is dark on DWI (D) suggesting increased diffusion.

Primary Parenchymal Neoplasms

Primary parenchymal neoplasms such as MB, astrocytoma, and ependymoma may rarely have an exophytic component and appear as an isolated CPA mass. One must evaluate different MR sequences in multiple planes to establish an intra-axial component to clinch the diagnosis.

Endolymphatic Sac Tumor

Endolymphatic sac tumors arise from the endolymphatic sac located in the distal portion of the vestibular aqueduct and are papillary adenomatous tumors. These tumors are frequent in von Hippel-Lindau disease,[71] but may also occur sporadically. At CT, the tumor causes destruction of the retrolabyrinthine petrous bone, has geographic or moth-eaten margins, and intratumoral spiculated or reticulated bone **(Fig. 22A)**.[72] At MR imaging, these tumors are heterogeneous on both T1 and T2WIs with foci of hyperintensity due to subacute hemorrhages and hypointensity due to calcification or hemosiderin.[73] Presence of T1- and T2-hyperintense blood-filled cysts and protein-filled cysts may suggest the diagnosis **(Figs. 23A to D and 20A and B)**. Enhancement is heterogeneous after gadolinium administration. Vascular flow-voids are seen within the tumor or peritumoral region in tumors more than 2 cm in size.[74]

FOURTH VENTRICLE

Choroid Plexus Papillomas

Choroid plexus papillomas (CPPs) and choroid plexus carcinomas (CPCs) originate from choroid plexus epithelium. They constitute 5% of supratentorial pediatric tumors and less than 1% of all primary intracranial neoplasms. CPPs are most frequent in the first year of life, and present with hydrocephalus. CPCs make up 30–40% of choroid plexus tumors and occur mostly during the first 5 years of life. Focal neurologic deficit resulting from adjacent brain invasion is a frequent presentation of CPC. Male predominance is seen for both the tumors.

Pathology

The common site of origin for CPP is the lateral ventricles; third and fourth ventricles are rarely involved in children. Fourth ventricle is the commonest site of adult CPP. CPPs are well-defined lobulated masses and cause enlargement of the involved ventricles. Foci of small hemorrhages and calcification may be found. Anaplastic papillomas, frequently invade the brain, and are difficult to differentiate from carcinomas. Metastasis through CSF pathways is common for both anaplastic papillomas and carcinomas.

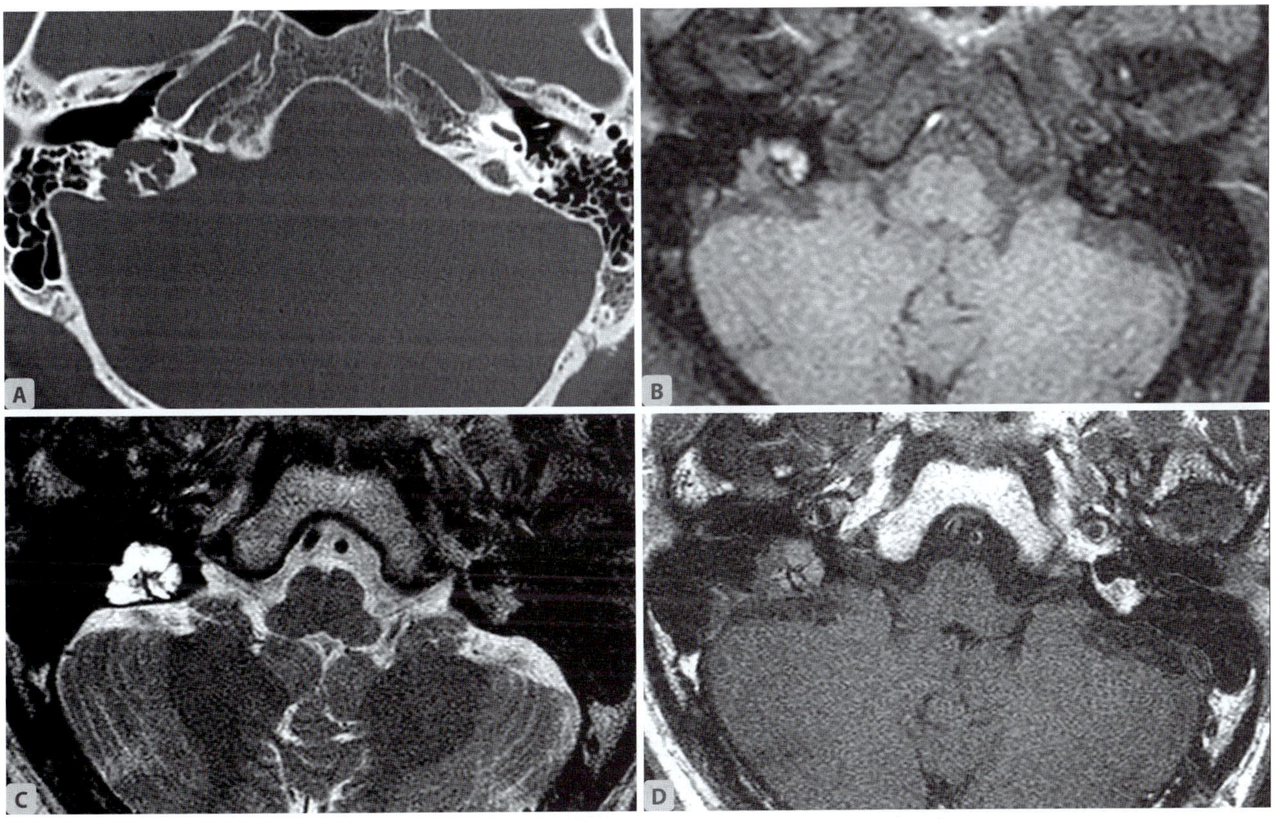

FIGS. 23A TO D: Endolymphatic sac tumor: Axial CT scan (A) shows a well-defined retrolabyrinthine mass in right petrous bone with intratumoral bony spicules. The mass is heterogeneously hyperintense on fat-saturated T1WI (B) and T2WI (C) and shows heterogeneous enhancement (D).

Imaging

CPP are typically isodense to hyperdense on NCCT with occasional foci of calcification **(Figs. 24A and B)**. Homogenous enhancement is seen following intravenous contrast. Anaplastic CPPs invade the ependyma and grow into the surrounding white matter, producing vasogenic edema. They are more irregular in outline and closely resemble CPCs.

Choroid plexus carcinomas are much more aggressive than papillomas, irregular in contour, mixed density on pre-contrast study and show variable enhancement. Cysts and hemorrhage are frequent. They almost always grow through the ventricular wall into the brain with associated edema.

At MRI, CPPs are homogeneous or heterogeneous cauliflower-like tumors. They are usually iso/hypointense on both T1 and T2WI and show avid contrast enhancement, unless the tumor is highly calcified **(Figs. 25A to D)**. Heterogeneous tumors contain areas of low signal intensity due to calcifications, foci of high signal intensity due to intratumoral hemorrhage and vascular flow-voids secondary to feeding vessels.[75] Hydrocephalus is usually associated with CPP; it may be partially explained by CSF hypersecretion by the tumor, but also by fourth ventricle obstruction when the tumor is located in the infratentorial compartment.[76]

Subependymoma

Subependymomas are rare, benign (WHO grade I), slow-growing intraventricular tumors. They usually occur in middle-aged and older individuals with a mean age of 50 years. Fourth ventricle (30-60%) is the most common location followed by lateral ventricles (40–75%).[77] They are commonly identified as an incidental finding. They usually present with hydrocephalus based on critical location and size.[77] Calcifications, hemorrhages and/or micro-vascular proliferation may be present.

Imaging

Imaging findings of subependymoma vary with the location. On CT, fourth ventricular subependymomas demonstrate variable density with calcifications (50–100%) and enhancement (62–92%) in most cases.[77] On the other hand, lateral ventricle subependymomas are more often hypodense, usually do not enhance and less likely to have calcifications (less than 10% of cases).

MRI of fourth ventricular subependymoma demonstrates its origin from the floor of the fourth ventricle and almost always has extension through the foramina of Luschka or Magendie. They are T1 hypo-isointense, T2 iso-hyperintense and almost always demonstrate heterogeneous enhancement. No paraventricular extension is seen in subependymomas, unlike other ventricular tumors.[78] These tumors are very hypometabolic in ^{18}F-FDG PET, which is believed to be secondary to their low cellular density and slow growth.[79]

Rosette-forming Glioneuronal Tumor (RGNT)

RGNT of the fourth ventricle is a rare, benign, mixed neuronal-glial primary brain tumor primarily affecting young adults.[80] It is recognized as a distinct entity since the 2007 WHO Classification of Tumors of the Central Nervous System.[81] RGNT often occupies the fourth ventricle but occasionally it shows cerebellar (vermian) invasion or may involve the aqueduct.[82] Rare extraventricular locations have been reported, including the cerebellar hemispheres, cerebellopontine angles, pineal gland, tectum, thalami, third ventricle, optic chiasm, spinal cord, and a recent case in the septum pellucidum.[80] Symptoms are nonspecific and include headache, gait disturbances, vertigo, and visual disturbances, which develop over months to years. The tumor may be incidentally discovered.[82]

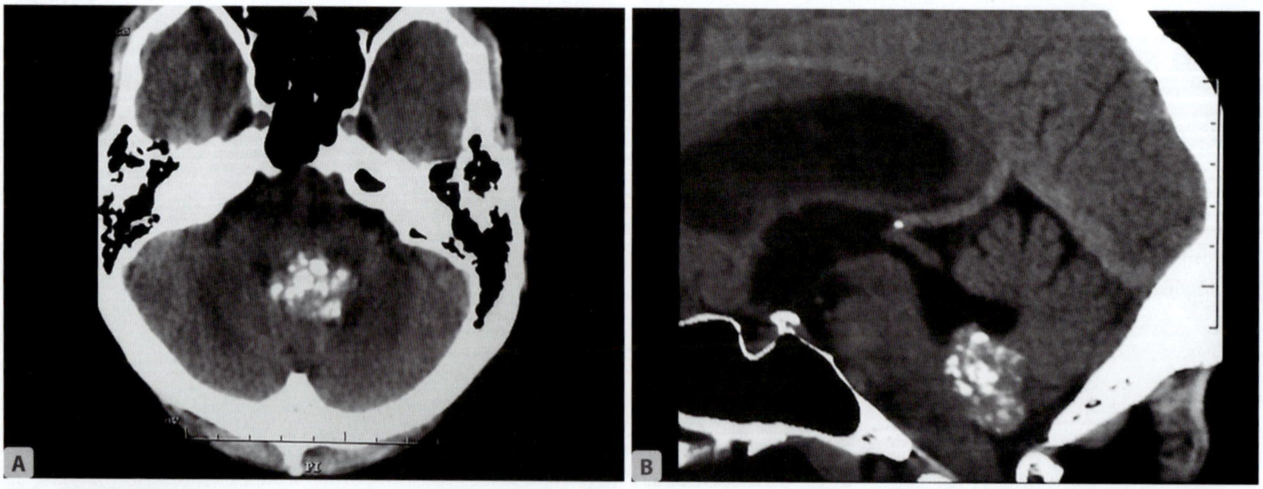

FIGS. 24A AND B: Choroid plexus papilloma—CT. Axial (A) and reformatted sagittal (B) NCCT scan images show a partially calcified mass in the inferior fourth ventricle.

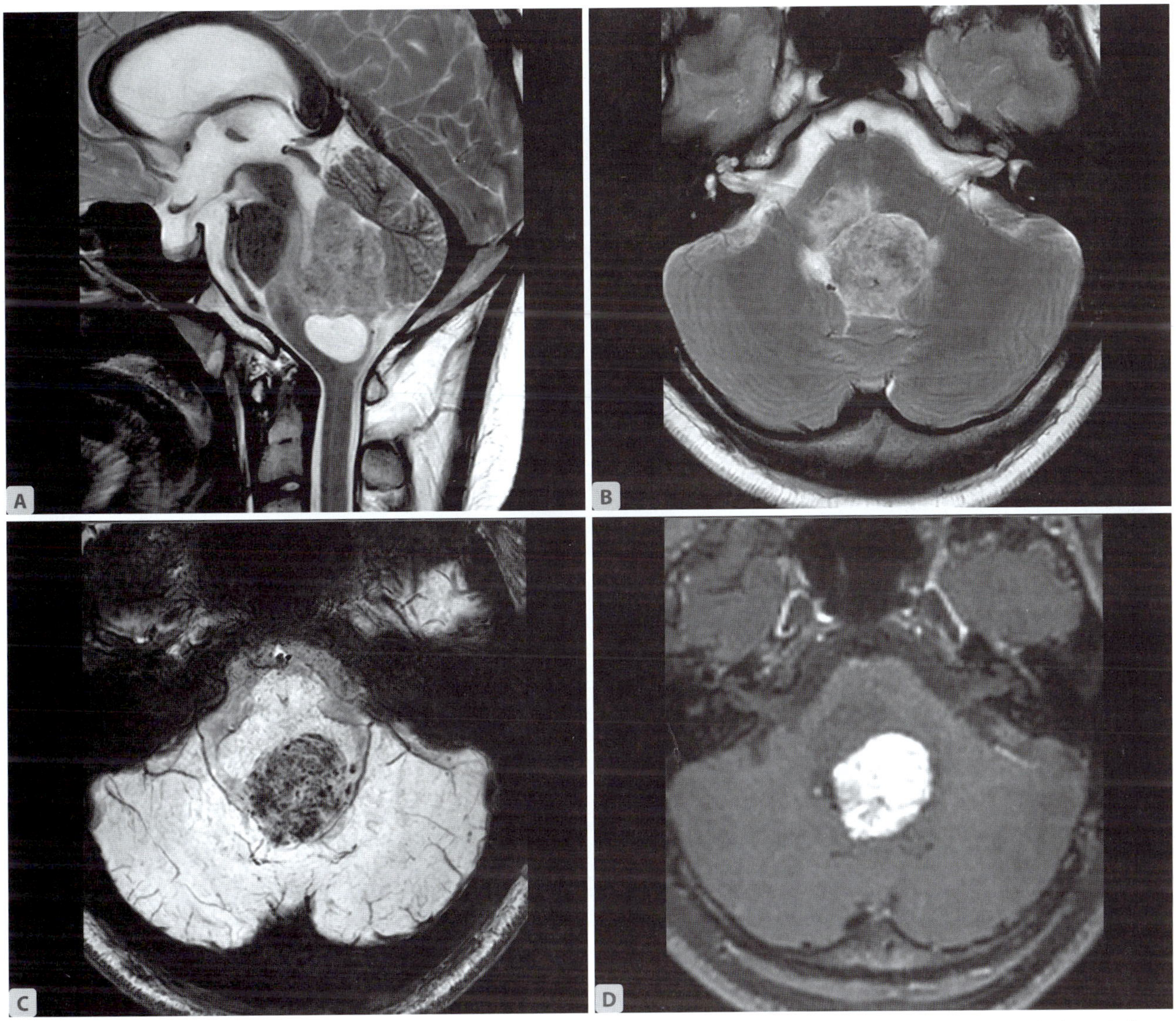

FIGS. 25A TO D: Choroid plexus papilloma—MRI: Sagittal (A) and axial (B) T2-WI show fourth ventricle iso-hypointense mass with hydrocephalus. The mass has foci of susceptibility signal on SWI (C) and shows intense enhancement (D).

Pathology

The defining histopathological feature is a mixed population of neurocytes organized in pseudorosettes and pilocytic astrocytes. Unlike pilocytic astrocytomas, rosette-forming glioneuronal tumors do not harbor alterations in *BRAF*; some may harbor mutations in *PIK3CA* or *FGFR1*.[83,84]

Imaging

RGNT is mostly an enhancing tumor that can display solid, cystic, or mixed features on brain MRI. RGNT is usually T1 isointense or hypointense and T2 hyperintense without any restricted diffusion **(Figs. 26A to F)**. Intratumoral hemorrhage and calcifications (25%) may occur. The diagnosis of RGNT should be considered when a cystic neoplasm of the fourth ventricle/superior vermis is encountered in an adult. RGNT may expand the cortex and involve underlying white matter or be deeply situated abutting the ventricles.

These tumors are usually curable by surgical resection, although rare cases of tumor dissemination throughout the ventricular system have been described.

CONCLUSION

Many neoplastic lesions can occur in the infratentorial compartment of brain. In order to make an accurate diagnosis, radiologists must answer several essential questions: (1) Whether the patient is an adult or a pediatric patient? (2) Whether the tumor is intra-axial or extra-axial? (3) What are the imaging characteristics of the tumor? Apart from the CT scan and conventional MR sequences, advanced MR imaging protocols like DWI, SWI, perfusion and MRS may help to clinch the diagnosis.

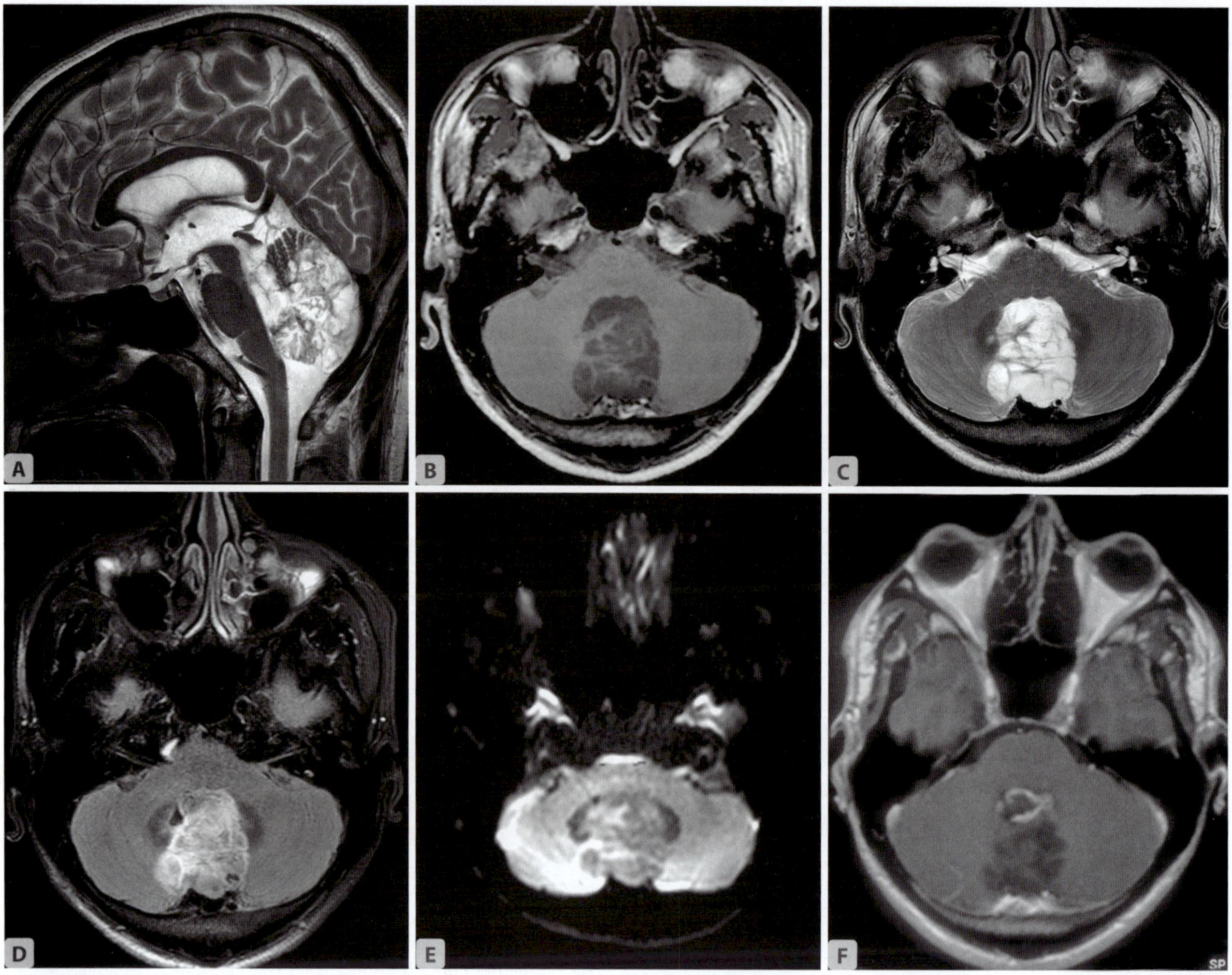

FIGS. 26A TO F: Rosette-forming glioneuronal tumor (RGNT): Sagittal T2-WI (A) shows a midline vermian lesion with extension into the 4th ventricle. The lesion is hypointense on axial T1WI (B), hyperintense on axial T2- (C) and FLAIR (D) images. Note any absence of vasogenic edema. No diffusion restriction is seen on DWI image (E). Post-contrast T1W axial image (F) shows minimal enhancement.

REFERENCES

1. Harwood-Nash DC. Primary neoplasms of the central nervous system in children. Cancer. 1991;67(S4):1223-8.
2. Lizak PF, Woodruff WW. Posterior fossa neoplasms: multiplanar imaging. Semin Ultrasound CT MR. 1992;13(3):182-206.
3. Taylor MD, Northcott PA, et al. Molecular subgroups of medulloblastoma: the current consensus. Acta Neuropathol. 2012;123(4):465-72.
4. Louis DN, Perry A, Reifenberger G, et al. The 2016 World Health Organization Classification of Tumors of the Central Nervous System: a summary. Acta Neuropathol. 2016;131(6):803-20.
5. Wataya T, Hamasaki M, Taylor MD. Molecular subgrouping and characterization analysis of medulloblastomas in a cohort of Japanese patients. No Shinkei Geka. 2015;43(2):117-25.
6. Kool M, Korshunov A, Remke M, et al. Molecular subgroups of medulloblastoma: an international meta-analysis of transcriptome, genetic aberrations, and clinical data of WNT, SHH, Group 3, and Group 4 medulloblastomas. Acta Neuropathologica. 2012;123(4):473-84.
7. Koeller KK, Rushing EJ. From the archives of the AFIP: medulloblastoma: a comprehensive review with radiologic-pathologic correlation. Radiographics. 2003;23(6):1613-37.
8. Kotsenas AL, Roth TC, Manness WK, et al. Abnormal diffusion-weighted MRI in medulloblastoma: does it reflect small cell histology? Pediatr Radiol. 1999;29(7):524-6.
9. Moreno-Torres A, Martinez-Perez I, Baquero M, et al. Taurine detection by proton magnetic resonance spectroscopy in medulloblastoma: contribution to noninvasive differential diagnosis with cerebellar astrocytoma. Neurosurgery. 2004;55(4):824-9; discussion 9.
10. Beier D, Kocakaya S, Hau P, et al. The Neuroradiological Spectra of Adult and Pediatric Medulloblastoma Differ: Results from a Literature-based Meta-analysis. Clin Neuroradiol. 2016.
11. Patay Z, DeSain LA, Hwang SN, et al. MR Imaging Characteristics of Wingless-Type-Subgroup Pediatric Medulloblastoma. Am J Neuroradiol. 2015;36(12): 2386-93.
12. Pajtler KW, Witt H, Sill M, et al. Molecular Classification of Ependymal Tumors across All CNS Compartments, Histopathological Grades, and Age Groups. Cancer Cell. 2015;27(5):728-43.
13. Allen JC, Siffert J, Hukin J. Clinical manifestations of childhood ependymoma: a multitude of syndromes. Pediatr Neurosurg. 1998;28(1):49-55.

14. Witt H, Mack SC, Ryzhova M, et al. Delineation of two clinically and molecularly distinct subgroups of posterior fossa ependymoma. Cancer Cell. 2011;20(2):143-57.
15. Tortori-Donati P, Fondelli MP, Cama A, et al. Ependymomas of the posterior cranial fossa: CT and MRI findings. Neuroradiology. 1995;37(3):238-43.
16. Furie DM, Provenzale JM. Supratentorial ependymomas and subependymomas: CT and MR appearance. J Comput Assist Tomogr. 1995;19(4):518-26.
17. Vanuytsel L, Brada M. The role of prophylactic spinal irradiation in localized intracranial ependymoma. Int J Radiat Oncol Biol Phys. 1991;21(3):825-30.
18. Rumboldt Z, Camacho DL, Lake D, et al. Apparent diffusion coefficients for differentiation of cerebellar tumors in children. Am J Neuroradiol. 2006;27(6):1362-9.
19. Uematsu Y, Hirano A, Llena JF. Electron microscopic observations of blood vessels in ependymoma. No Shinkei Geka. 1988;16(11):1235-42.
20. Brandao LA, Young Poussaint T. Posterior Fossa Tumors. Neuroimaging Clin N Am. 2017;27(1):1-37.
21. Blaser SI, Harwood-Nash DC. Neuroradiology of pediatric posterior fossa medulloblastoma. J Neurooncol. 1996;29(1):23-34.
22. Brandao LA, Poussaint TY. Pediatric brain tumors. Neuroimaging Clin N Am. 2013;23(3):499-525.
23. Harris LM, Davies N, Macpherson L, et al. The use of short-echo-time 1H MRS for childhood cerebellar tumours prior to histopathological diagnosis. Pediatr Radiol. 2007;37(11):1101-9.
24. Merchant TE, Li C, Xiong X, et al. Conformal radiotherapy after surgery for paediatric ependymoma: a prospective study. Lancet Oncol. 2009;10(3):258-66.
25. Fernandez C, Figarella-Branger D, Girard N, et al. Pilocytic astrocytomas in children: prognostic factors—a retrospective study of 80 cases. Neurosurgery. 2003;53(3):544-53; discussion 54-5.
26. Arslanoglu A, Aygun N, Tekhtani D, et al. Imaging findings of CNS atypical teratoid/rhabdoid tumors. Am J Neuroradiol. 2004;25(3):476-80.
27. Jin B, Feng XY. MRI features of atypical teratoid/rhabdoid tumors in children. Pediatr Radiol. 2013;43(8):1001-8.
28. Fuller CE. All things rhabdoid and SMARC: An enigmatic exploration with Dr. Louis P. Dehner. Semin Diagn Pathol. 2016;33(6):427-40.
29. Rorke LB, Packer R, Biegel J. Central nervous system atypical teratoid/rhabdoid tumors of infancy and childhood. J Neurooncol. 1995;24(1):21-8.
30. Hasselblatt M, Gesk S, Oyen F, et al. Nonsense mutation and inactivation of SMARCA4 (BRG1) in an atypical teratoid/rhabdoid tumor showing retained SMARCB1 (INI1) expression. Am J Surg Pathol. 2011;35(6):933-5.
31. Zuccoli G, Izzi G, Bacchini E, et al. Central nervous system atypical teratoid/rhabdoid tumour of infancy. CT and MR findings. Clin Imaging. 1999;23(6):356-60.
32. Agranovich AL, Ang LC, Griebel RW, et al. Malignant rhabdoid tumor of the central nervous system with subarachnoid dissemination. Surg Neurol. 1992;37(5):410-4.
33. Koral K, Gargan L, Bowers DC, et al. Imaging characteristics of atypical teratoid-rhabdoid tumor in children compared with medulloblastoma. Am J Roentgenol. 2008;190(3):809-14.
34. Katz JS, Peruzzi PP, Pierson CR, et al. Cerebellopontine angle tumors in young children, displaying cranial nerve deficits, and restricted diffusion on diffusion-weighted imaging: a new clinical triad for atypical teratoid/rhabdoid tumors. Childs Nerv Syst. 2017;33(5):833-8.
35. Lee SR, Sanches J, Mark AS, et al. Posterior fossa hemangioblastomas: MR imaging. Radiology. 1989;171(2): 463-8.
36. Hakyemez B, Erdogan C, Bolca N, et al. Evaluation of different cerebral mass lesions by perfusion-weighted MR imaging. J Magn Reson Imaging. 2006;24(4):817-24.
37. Abo-Al Hassan A, Ismail M, Panda SM. Pre-operative endovascular embolization of a cerebellar haemangioblastoma. A case report. Med Princ Pract. 2006; 15(6):459-62.
38. Isiklar I, Leeds NE, Fuller GN, et al. Intracranial metastatic melanoma: correlation between MR imaging characteristics and melanin content. Am J Roentgenol. 1995;165(6):1503-12.
39. Smith JK, Castillo M, Kwock L. MR spectroscopy of brain tumors. Magn Reson Imaging Clin N Am. 2003;11(3):415-29, v-vi.
40. Nagaraja S, Powell T, Griffiths PD, et al. MR imaging and spectroscopy in Lhermitte-Duclos disease. Neuroradiology. 2004;46(5):355-8.
41. Nowak DA, Trost HA. Lhermitte-Duclos disease (dysplastic cerebellar gangliocytoma): a malformation, hamartoma or neoplasm? Acta Neurol Scand. 2002;105(3):137-45.
42. Koeller KK, Henry JM. From the archives of the AFIP: superficial gliomas: radiologic-pathologic correlation. Armed Forces Institute of Pathology. Radiographics. 2001;21(6):1533-56.
43. Zhou XP, Marsh DJ, Morrison CD, et al. Germline inactivation of PTEN and dysregulation of the phosphoinositol-3-kinase/Akt pathway cause human Lhermitte-Duclos disease in adults. Am J Hum Genet. 2003;73(5):1191-8.
44. Mester J, Eng C. Cowden syndrome: recognizing and managing a not-so-rare hereditary cancer syndrome. J Surg Oncol. 2015;111(1):125-30.
45. Kulkantrakorn K, Awwad EE, Levy B, et al. MRI in Lhermitte-Duclos disease. Neurology. 1997;48(3):725-31.
46. Awwad EE, Levy E, Martin DS, et al. Atypical MR appearance of Lhermitte-Duclos disease with contrast enhancement. AJNR Am J Neuroradiol. 1995;16(8):1719-20.
47. Chawla A, Emmanuel JV, Seow WT, et al. Paediatric PNET: pre-surgical MRI features. Clin Radiol. 2007;62(1):43-52.
48. Prasad AN. Supratentorial PNET in a young child. Indian J Pediatr. 2011;78(5):613-5.
49. Borja MJ, Plaza MJ, Altman N, et al. Conventional and advanced MRI features of pediatric intracranial tumors: supratentorial tumors. Am J Roentgenol. 2013;200(5):W483-503.
50. Jallo GI, Biser-Rohrbaugh A, Freed D. Brainstem gliomas. Childs Nerv Syst. 2004;20(3):143-53.
51. Fischbein NJ, Prados MD, Wara W, et al. Radiologic classification of brain stem tumors: correlation of magnetic resonance imaging appearance with clinical outcome. Pediatr Neurosurg. 1996;24(1):9-23.
52. Fisher PG, Breiter SN, Carson BS, et al. A clinicopathologic reappraisal of brain stem tumor classification. Identification of pilocystic astrocytoma and fibrillary astrocytoma as distinct entities. Cancer. 2000;89(7):1569-76.
53. Aihara K, Mukasa A, Gotoh K, et al. H3F3A K27M mutations in thalamic gliomas from young adult patients. Neuro Oncol. 2014;16(1):140-6.
54. Buczkowicz P, Bartels U, Bouffet E, et al. Histopathological spectrum of paediatric diffuse intrinsic pontine glioma: diagnostic and therapeutic implications. Acta Neuropathol. 2014;128(4):573-81.
55. Lee BC, Kneeland JB, Walker RW, et al. MR imaging of brainstem tumors. Am J Neuroradiol. 1985;6(2):159-63.
56. Aboian MS, Solomon DA, Felton E, et al. Imaging Characteristics of Pediatric Diffuse Midline Gliomas with Histone H3 K27M Mutation. Am J Neuroradiol. 2017;38(4):795-800.
57. Lindsay AJ, Rush SZ, Fenton LZ. Pediatric posterior fossa ganglioglioma: unique MRI features and correlation with BRAF V600E mutation status. Journal of Neuro-Oncology. 2014;118(2):395-404.

58. Chassot A, Canale S, Varlet P, et al. Radiotherapy with concurrent and adjuvant temozolomide in children with newly diagnosed diffuse intrinsic pontine glioma. Journal of Neuro-Oncology. 2011;106(2):399-407.
59. Moffat DA, Ballagh RH. Rare tumours of the cerebellopontine angle. Clin Oncol (R Coll Radiol). 1995;7(1):28-41.
60. Mafee MF, Lachenauer CS, Kumar A, et al. CT and MR imaging of intralabyrinthine schwannoma: report of two cases and review of the literature. Radiology. 1990;174(2):395-400.
61. Matthies C, Samii M, Krebs S. Management of vestibular schwannomas (acoustic neuromas): Radiological features in 202 cases - Their value for diagnosis and their predictive importance. Neurosurgery. 1997;40(3):469-81.
62. Swartz JD. Lesions of the cerebellopontine angle and internal auditory canal: diagnosis and differential diagnosis. Semin Ultrasound CT MR. 2004;25(4):332-52.
63. Ben Hamouda M, Drissi C, Sebai R, et al. Atypical CT and MRI aspects of an epidermoid cyst. J Neuroradiol. 2007;34(2):129-32.
64. Dechambre S, Duprez T, Lecouvet F, et al. Diffusion-weighted MRI postoperative assessment of an epidermoid tumour in the cerebellopontine angle. Neuroradiology. 1999;41(11):829-31.
65. Osborn AG, Preece MT. Intracranial cysts: radiologic-pathologic correlation and imaging approach. Radiology. 2006;239(3): 650-64.
66. Wester K. Peculiarities of intracranial arachnoid cysts: location, sidedness, and sex distribution in 126 consecutive patients. Neurosurgery. 1999;45(4):775-9.
67. Ikeda H, Deinsberger W, Boker DK. Retroclival arachnoid cyst presenting with spontaneous intracystic haemorrhage—case presentation. Acta Neurochir (Wien). 2000;142(11):1317-8.
68. Dutt SN, Mirza S, Chavda SV, et al. Radiologic differentiation of intracranial epidermoids from arachnoid cysts. Otol Neurotol. 2002;23(1):84-92.
69. Bonneville F, Sarrazin JL, Marsot-Dupuch K, et al. Unusual lesions of the cerebellopontine angle: a segmental approach. Radiographics. 2001;21(2):419-38.
70. Kertesz TR, Shelton C, Wiggins RH, et al. Intratemporal facial nerve neuroma: anatomical location and radiological features. Laryngoscope. 2001;111(7):1250-6.
71. Jensen RL, Gillespie D, House P, et al. Endolymphatic sac tumors in patients with and without von Hippel-Lindau disease: the role of genetic mutation, von Hippel-Lindau protein, and hypoxia inducible factor-1alpha expression. J Neurosurg. 2004;100(3): 488-97.
72. Lo WW, Applegate LJ, Carberry JN, et al. Endolymphatic sac tumors: radiologic appearance. Radiology. 1993;189(1): 199-204.
73. Baltacioğlu F, Ekinci G, Türe U, et al. MR imaging, CT, and angiography features of endolymphatic sac tumors: report of two cases. Neuroradiology. 2014;44(1):91-6.
74. Mukherji SK, Albernaz VS, Lo WW, et al. Papillary endolymphatic sac tumors: CT, MR imaging, and angiographic findings in 20 patients. Radiology. 1997;202(3):801-8.
75. Shin JH, Lee HK, Jeong AK, et al. Choroid plexus papilloma in the posterior cranial fossa: MR, CT, and angiographic findings. Clin Imaging. 2001;25(3):154-62.
76. Pencalet P, Sainte-Rose C, Lellouch-Tubiana A, et al. Papillomas and carcinomas of the choroid plexus in children. J Neurosurg. 1998;88(3):521-8.
77. Chiechi MV, Smirniotopoulos JG, Jones RV. Intracranial subependymomas: CT and MR imaging features in 24 cases. AJR Am J Roentgenol. 1995;165(5):1245-50.
78. Nishio S, Morioka T, Mihara F, et al. Subependymoma of the lateral ventricles. Neurosurg Rev. 2000;23(2):98-103.
79. Mineura K, Shioya H, Kowada M, et al. Subependymoma of the septum pellucidum: characterization by PET. J Neurooncol. 1997;32(2):143-7.
80. Sharma P, Swain M, Padua MD, et al. Rosette-forming glioneuronal tumors: a report of two cases. Neurol India. 2011;59(2):276-80.
81. Hsu C, Kwan G, Lau Q, et al. Rosette-forming glioneuronal tumour: imaging features, histopathological correlation and a comprehensive review of literature. Br J Neurosurg. 2012;26(5):668-73.
82. Kumar M, Samant R, Ramakrishnaiah R, et al. Rosette-forming glioneuronal tumor of the fourth ventricle. Radiol Case Rep. 2013;8(1):740.
83. Ellezam B, Theeler BJ, Luthra R, et al. Recurrent PIK3CA mutations in rosette-forming glioneuronal tumor. Acta Neuropathol. 2012;123(2):285-7.
84. Gessi M, Moneim YA, Hammes J, et al. FGFR1 mutations in Rosette-forming glioneuronal tumors of the fourth ventricle. J Neuropathol Exp Neurol. 2014;73(6):580-4.

CHAPTER

198

Sellar and Parasellar Lesions

Paramjeet Singh, Chirag Kamal Ahuja, Niranjan Khandelwal

INTRODUCTION

Pituitary gland plays a central role in body growth, metabolism and reproductive functions. It is an anatomically complex area where a number of neoplastic, infectious, inflammatory, developmental and vascular pathologies can occur. Pathological lesions of sellar and parasellar region can have profound clinical/endocrinological as well as neurological consequences. The diagnosis often needs multidisciplinary approach using ophthalmological, endocrine, neurological and radiological methods. Cross sectional imaging by computed tomography (CT) and magnetic resonance imaging (MRI), especially the latter, have expanded our understanding of the structure and pathology of this region.

NORMAL ANATOMY AND APPLIED PHYSIOLOGY

The key to imaging interpretation of sellar/parasellar pathology lies in a thorough knowledge of the complex anatomy of nervous, bony, vascular and meningeal structures located in and around this region **(Figs. 1A and B)**. While sella has clearly defined landmarks, the parasellar area includes all structures bordering it.

The sella-turcica is a spherical depression in the superior surface of the sphenoid bone bounded by the sphenoid sinus anteroinferiorly, the paired cavernous sinuses laterally, the suprasellar cisterns and its contents, diaphragma sellae and

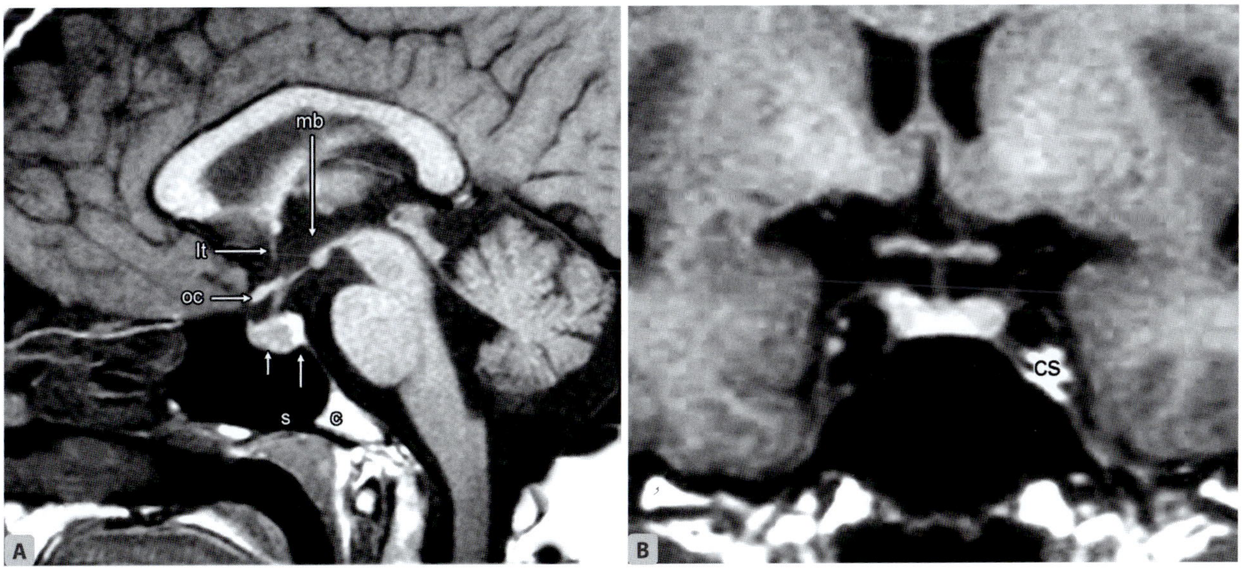

FIGS. 1A AND B: Normal sellar anatomy: T1-weighted (A) sagittal and (B) coronal images showing adenohypophysis (short arrow), posterior pituitary bright spot (long arrow), infundibulum, mammillary body (mb), sphenoid sinus (s), clivus (c), optic chiasma (oc), cavernous sinus (cs) and lamina terminalis (lt). Tuber cinereum is the ridge of tissue between mammillary body and infundibulum.

hypothalamus superiorly and the dorsum sella and brainstem posteriorly.

The cortical bone of sella varies from few microns to several millimeters in thickness, depending upon the degree of pneumatization of the sphenoid sinus. The carotid artery forms a groove on the posterosuperior wall of the sphenoid sinus. The wall between the artery and the sinus may be very thin, even absent in up to one-third of patients, thus making it vulnerable to injury during transsphenoidal surgery. Localized defects in its bony cortex or asymmetry of the sellar floor are common.[1] The bony sella is invested by a reflection of dura, the outer layer of which lines the floor while the inner layer forms a diaphragm at the roof (diaphragma sellae). A central opening in the diaphragm allows the pituitary infundibulum to pass into the sella. Anteriorly, the sellar floor is continuous with the tuberculum sellae and limbus sphenoidale. The dorsum sella demarcates the posterior sellar border.

Cavernous sinuses are two multiseptated, symmetrically paired parasellar venous sinuses with a straight or slightly convex outer wall. The two layers of dura form the roof, outer wall and inner wall of the sinuses. The lateral walls of the cavernous sinuses from superior to inferior contain the cranial nerves III, IV as well as first and second divisions of the Vth nerve (V1 and V2) **(Fig. 2)**. The VIth nerve passes through the sinus below the internal carotid artery (ICA). The ICA has a variable course within the sinus; however, a more medial location of the artery is a normal variation and is surgically important. The artery may actually indent the gland at times and the distance between the arteries may be as little as 4 mm. The ICA exits the sinus at level of anterior clinoid process to give off its supracavernous branches. Meckel's cave housing the Gasserian ganglion lies at the posterior part of the cavernous sinus. The third division of Vth nerve (V3) passes inferior from here to foramen ovale.

The suprasellar cistern is a six pointed expansion of the subarachnoid space containing the optic nerves, optic chiasma and the tracts, circle of Willis and the pituitary infundibulum. The optic chiasma lies 4–6 mm posterosuperior to the tuberculum sellae, however, it may be directly above it (prefixed) or lie more posteriorly above the dorsum sella (postfixed). These variations are important for surgeons. The optic and infundibular recesses are downward invaginations of the third ventricle in relation to its floor.

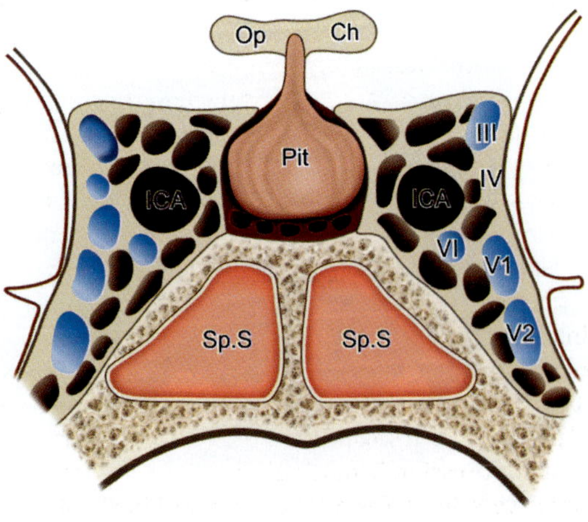

FIG. 2: Pictorial representation of the coronal view of the sella and parasellar (cavernous sinus) region depicting the anatomy and relationship of various structures. (ICA: internal carotid artery; Ch: chiasma; Op: optic; Pit: pituitary gland; Sp.S: sphenoid sinus; III, IV, V1, V2 and VI represent the respective cranial nerves).

The hypothalamus is a layer of tissue extending from the anterior commissure to the posterior commissure and forms the floor and the lateral walls of the third ventricle. The inferior ridge of the tissue from the optic chiasma anteriorly to the paired mammillary bodies posteriorly is called the tuber cinereum. At the lateral margins of the hypothalamus are the optic tracts and the sulci of temporal lobes. The hypothalamus consists of multiple nuclei regulating temperature, water balance, drinking behavior and sexual activity. The hypothalamus and the pituitary gland are functionally and physiologically interlinked contiguous structures and often referred to as the hypothalamic-pituitary-axis (HPA). Release of pituitary hormones is mediated by the hypothalamus. Oxytocin and vasopressin are synthesized in hypothalamus and transported to the posterior pituitary.

The pituitary gland is composed of two anatomically and functionally distinct lobes: the anterior lobe (adeno-hypophysis) and the posterior lobe (neurohypophysis) **(Figs. 1A and B)**. The anterior lobe comprises 75% of the volume of the gland and consists of pars tuberalis, pars intermedia and pars distalis which develop from Rathke's pouch. Pars intermedia which lies between the adeno and neurohypophysis, is a vestigial structure and common site for developmental cysts. The anterior lobe of pituitary is isointense to brain on both T1 and T2WI.[2] It secretes growth hormone (GH), adrenocorticotropic hormone (ACTH), prolactin (PRL), thyroid stimulating hormone (TSH), luteinizing hormone (LH) and melanocyte-stimulating hormone (MSH). The anterior lobe shares a common blood supply with hypothalamus via the hypophyseal portal system, the pathway by which hypothalamic releasing hormones reach this structure. Alternately the hypophyseal arteries, branches of internal carotid supply the stalk and posterior lobe. The venous drainage is to ipsilateral cavernous sinus predominantly and then to petrosal sinuses.

The posterior lobe develops as a downward projection from the neuroectoderm at the base of the brain and along with infundibular stalk, supraoptic and paraventricular hypothalamic nuclei forms the neurohypophysis. Oxytocin and vasopressin synthesized in the hypothalamus are transported to and stored in the posterior pituitary. The posterior lobe appears as a bright spot on T1-weighted images (T1WI) in midline along the dorsum of the sella.[2,3] The anterior lobe of pituitary gland is larger and rounded and appears hyperintense like posterior lobe in newborns and becomes isointense by 4–6 months of life.[3-5]

The dimensions of pituitary gland are extremely variable, particularly its height. The gland undergoes significant changes in size and shape throughout life and this fact must be kept in mind when assessing it for abnormality. A useful guide to the gland's height in relation to age is the "Elster's rule" of 6, 8, 10, 12 **(Table 1)**.[3] On an average, it is 12 mm in width and 8 mm in anteroposterior diameter. The maximal

TABLE 1: Elster's rule for pituitary gland height on MRI.

Age	Maximum allowable height (mm)
Infants and children (either sex)	6
Men and postmenopausal women	8
Women of childbearing age	10
Women in late pregnancy and postpartum	12

TABLE 2: Sellar dimensions on plain radiograph.

Anteroposterior diameter	17 mm (range 5–16 mm)
Depth	13 mm
Width	16 mm (range 10–15 mm)
Area on lateral view	130 sq mm
Volume	1092 cubic mm (mean 599 cubic mm)

height is achieved in adolescent girls and during pregnancy. The pituitary stalk tapers inferiorly and has thickness of 2 mm. It should not exceed the width of the basilar artery or a maximum of 4 mm.

IMAGING MODALITIES

Currently MRI is the examination of choice for sellar and parasellar pathology due to its superior soft tissue contrast, multiplanar capability and lack of ionizing radiation. This allows better demonstration of pathology, relationship of lesions with surrounding structures and tissue differentiation. CT, though less frequently used is a useful examination particularly for showing calcification, bony destruction and surgically relevant bony anatomy (sphenoid septae and pneumatization). Digital subtraction angiography (DSA) is helpful for vascular lesions and to show vascularity of tumors. However, due to its invasive nature, it is hardly used nowadays and instead has been replaced by CT and MR angiographic techniques. In central Cushing's disease, if no adenoma is visible in MRI, inferior petrosal sinus venous sampling may help in lateralizing a microadenoma to guide selective surgical resection.

Plain Radiography

Plain radiography is infrequently requested these days for diagnosing sellar and parasellar pathology. If indicated, lateral view of the skull centered on the sella is the single most important view **(Fig. 3A)**.

The radiographic size of the sella **(Table 2)**[6] in itself is not a sensitive indicator of pituitary gland abnormalities unless distinctive changes of erosion and other bony abnormalities are seen. The empty sella may itself lead to enlargement of size.[1]

The cortical line of sella called lamina dura is a pencil-sharp thin line. When sella becomes enlarged due to intrasellar tumor, it becomes rounded (ballooning; **Fig. 3B**) and extends forward underneath the anterior clinoid processes. The undercutting of the clinoid processes and intact dorsum sella in these cases results in a closed type of sella, characteristic of intrasellar pathology. Posteriorly the loss of lamina dura is first seen at the junction of base of the dorsum and sellar floor. Large intrasellar masses, however, can cause complete destruction of dorsum. Double flooring of sella may also be seen due to intrasellar masses or can be a normal variant. In contrast early involvement of tip of the dorsum or its complete destruction favors a suprasellar mass (open sella from above, **Fig. 3C**).

Suprasellar calcification is seen in cases of craniopharyngioma, meningioma, clival chordoma and vascular lesions. Meningiomas, in addition, may show hyperostosis of the sphenoid bone. Rarely, adenomas may also show calcification on plain radiographs.

Computed Tomography

Computed tomography of sella used to be performed in coronal plane by taking thin (2 mm sections) perpendicular to the sellar floor using high radiation flux. Additional axial sections were required for larger lesions. With the advent of multidetector CT, volumetric data acquisition can be performed and submillimeter thickness excellent quality images can be reconstructed in any plane. Dynamic scanning consists of sequential CT sections obtained at a single level every few seconds after a bolus of contrast which leads to progressive enhancement of the sellar tissue and provides information about differential enhancement of various components helping in the diagnosis of various lesions.

Magnetic Resonance Imaging

The objective of MR is to obtain high contrast spatially resolved images with reasonable signal to noise ratio (SNR). Requirements for spatial detail are to be balanced against SNR and imaging time penalty. It is important to identify the gland separate from the lesion if possible. Coronal and sagittal sections are preferred and acquired using a small FOV (16 × 20 cm), thin slices (3 mm) and high resolution matrix (256 × 512) using T1 spin echo and to a lesser extent T2 fast spin echo sequences. Both dynamic and routine postcontrast images as well as delayed scanning after 30–60 minutes may be combined in one study for optimal imaging. A dose of 0.05–0.1 mmol/kg of gadolinium (Gd) compound is usually adequate.[5] A 3-dimensional Fourier transformation gradient echo or fast spin echo sequence may be used for dynamic study. After injecting a bolus of contrast, 6–8 consecutive sets of coronal images are obtained covering the entire gland (3–5 sections) every 10–12 seconds. Differential rate of enhancement of the normal pituitary from small adenomas help in identifying the latter. Fat suppression is particularly useful in evaluation of postoperative sella. 3 Tesla (MR) imaging has potential for higher resolution imaging particularly for cranial nerves and cavernous sinus, but with penalty of susceptibility artifacts in this region caused by bone air interface.[7]

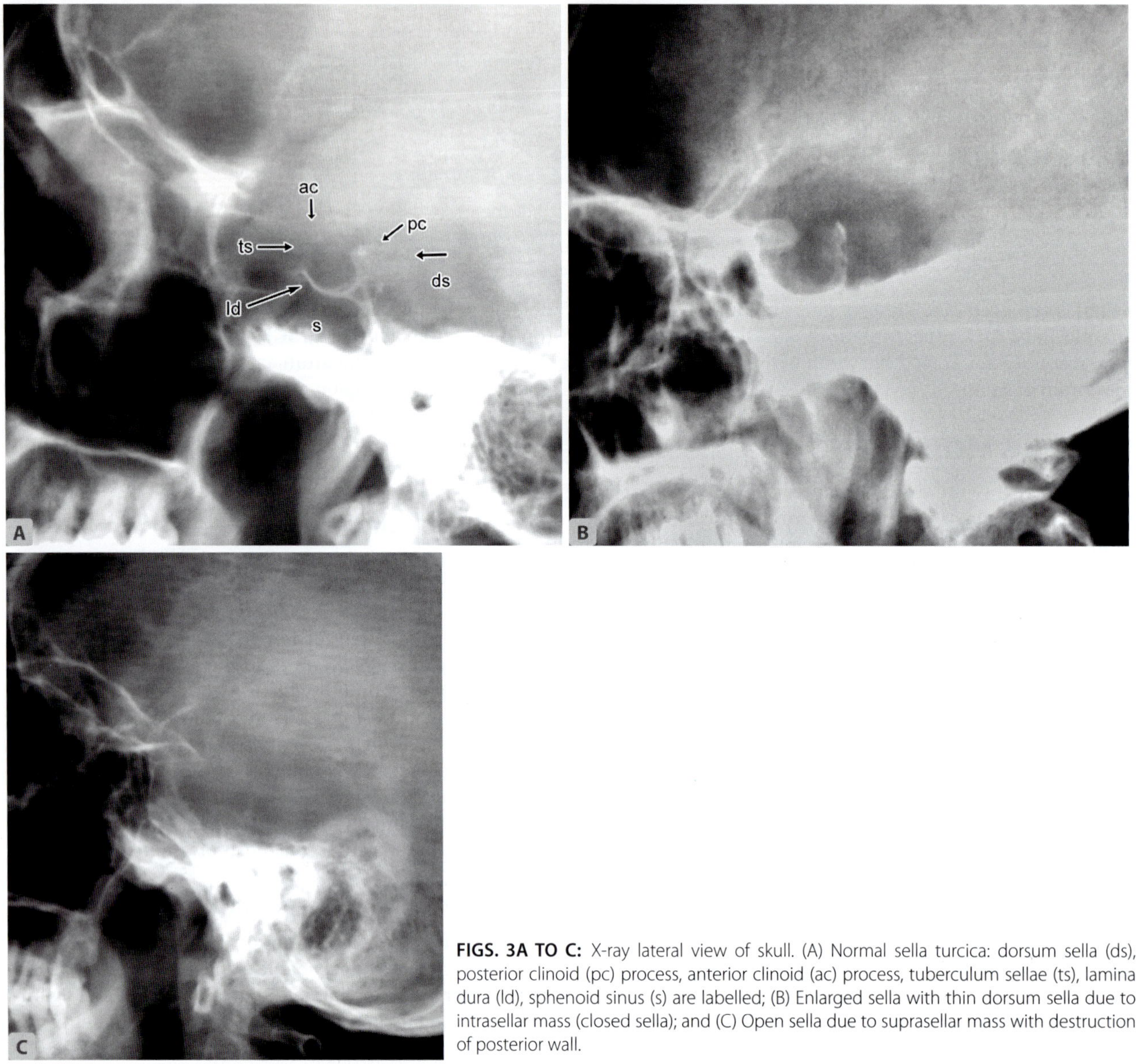

FIGS. 3A TO C: X-ray lateral view of skull. (A) Normal sella turcica: dorsum sella (ds), posterior clinoid (pc) process, anterior clinoid (ac) process, tuberculum sellae (ts), lamina dura (ld), sphenoid sinus (s) are labelled; (B) Enlarged sella with thin dorsum sella due to intrasellar mass (closed sella); and (C) Open sella due to suprasellar mass with destruction of posterior wall.

PATHOLOGY OF THE SELLAR AND PARASELLAR REGION

The lesions in this area may arise from the pituitary gland, infundibulum, adjacent brain, bone, dura, leptomeninges, blood vessels, cranial nerves and the extracranial structures such as nasopharynx and sphenoid sinus. These may be categorized depending on their location (intrasellar, suprasellar and parasellar), the age groups affected, the structures involved (pituitary gland, infundibulum, hypothalamus, cavernous sinus, etc.), predominant tissue character (cystic or solid) or etiology (traumatic, neoplastic, inflammatory, vascular, etc.). The following classification is a rough guide to commonly encountered pathologies, however, there may be considerable overlap with many of the lesions affecting more than one region, structure or age group **(Table 3)**.

TUMORS

Pituitary Adenoma

Adenomas arise from the adenohypophysis and are classified by size and hormonal activity; features that determine their clinical presentation. They are the most common tumors of the sellar and parasellar region in adults and constitute 10–15% of all intracranial neoplasms.[8] By definition, adenomas measuring less than 10 mm are called microadenomas while the larger ones are termed macroadenomas. In general, hormonally active lesions are discovered at a smaller size due to endocrinopathy and consequent clinical symptoms. Nonfunctioning adenomas are usually large at the time of diagnosis when they produce symptoms due to mass effect on surrounding structures. Approximately three-fourths of adenomas show signs of hormone excess while the rest are nonfunctioning tumors.[8] Sometimes these nonfunctioning

TABLE 3: Sellar and parasellar lesions.

Intrasellar masses	Physiological and pathological hyperplasia, micro and macroadenomas, non-neoplastic cyst, craniopharyngioma, meningioma
Suprasellar mass (child)	Craniopharyngioma, hypothalamic glioma, germinoma, arachnoid cyst, tuber cinereum hamartoma
Suprasellar mass (adult)	Macroadenoma, meningioma, aneurysm, metastasis, epidermoid/dermoid
Cystic lesions	Craniopharyngioma, arachnoid cyst, epidermoid, pituitary abscess
Infundibular masses (child)	Pituitary hypoplasia, histiocytosis, germinoma, leukemia
Infundibular masses (adult)	Hypophysitis, sarcoidosis, metastasis/lymphoma, pituicytoma
Parasellar lesion (tumors)	Metastasis, meningioma, schwannoma, lymphoma, chordoma, osteocartilaginous tumors, nasopharyngeal carcinoma, plasmacytoma
Parasellar lesions (vascular and inflammatory)	Sarcoidosis, histiocytosis, infections, fungal, non-fungal, cavernous sinus thrombosis, cavernous sinus hemangioma, aneurysm, caroticocavernous fistula, Tolosa Hunt syndrome

lesions may be discovered incidentally (Incidentalomas). Clinically silent adenomas have been demonstrated in 10% of asymptomatic volunteers.[9] The rest may produce symptoms by compressing adjacent structures, causing various symptoms, i.e. visual field defects (bitemporal hemianopia) due to optic chiasma compression, hypopituitarism due to compression of pituitary gland, cranial nerve deficits due to lateral extension into cavernous sinuses, hydrocephalus/ CSF rhinorrhea due to third ventricular obstruction, or rarely, diabetes insipidus due to mass effect on hypothalamus.

Types of Adenomas

Prolactinomas are the most common functioning adenomas comprising 50% of all adenomas.[5] These tumors clinically present with amenorrhea, galactorrhea and infertility in females and loss of libido and impotence in males. Serum PRL level is usually greater than 100 ng/mL (normal 20 ng/ mL). In case serum PRL level is greater than 200 ng/mL, the cause is nearly always a pituitary adenoma.[10] ACTH secreting adenomas produce early symptoms when they are small,[5] often measuring 1–2 mm in size and thus are difficult to diagnose. However, an ectopic source of ACTH secretion must also be kept in mind in a patient with hypercortisolism. GH secreting tumors are macroadenomas as they are diagnosed late in the course of disease. They produce acromegaly in adults and gigantism in children. Rarely adenomas arise from the thyrotrophs (TSH secreting) or gonadotrophs (FHS and/ or LH secreting). In addition, 10% of secreting adenomas are plurihormonal,[8] the most common combination being the PRL-GH producing adenoma.

Imaging of Adenomas

Imaging is indicated both to confirm the existence of an adenoma and to define its size and location for appropriate surgical or medical therapy. MRI is the preferred modality, though CT is also useful. Reported sensitivity and specificity of noncontrast MRI and contrast enhanced CT are roughly equal varying from 50% to 90%.[3] However, there is no large blinded prospective study comparing CT and MRI in the same group of patients.[5] Overall, T1WI are more reliable for detection of adenomas. The addition of Gd enhancement increases the detection rate of microadenomas by 10%. Postcontrast dynamic acquisition allows evaluation of temporal changes in signal intensity in intrasellar structures and adds additional 5–20% sensitivity over the nondynamic studies for detection of microadenomas (particularly small ACTH secretors and those which are isointense).[10] Signal intensity increases more rapidly and to a greater degree in normal pituitary gland than in microadenoma, however, 3–5 minutes following the contrast administration the signal of the normal gland and the adenoma may become identical **(Fig. 4)**. The maximum contrast difference between the normal gland and the microadenoma occurs at about 30–60 seconds when the distinction between normal pituitary and the adenoma is the best. Microadenomas also demonstrate a slower washout of accumulated contrast that may cause them to appear hyperintense on delayed images (>20 minutes postcontrast). With modern state-of-the-art MRI equipments, more than 90% adenomas should be picked up.[5] The prescribed protocol should be high resolution plain scan which if negative should be followed by contrast- enhanced magnetic resonance imaging consisting of both dynamic scanning and regular postcontrast scan. Certain studies have shown that if the conventional and dynamic contrast imaging is combined with an additional 3D volumetric interpolated breath-hold examination, a spoiled-gradient echo 3D T1 sequence (SGE), the accuracy of identifying microadenomas

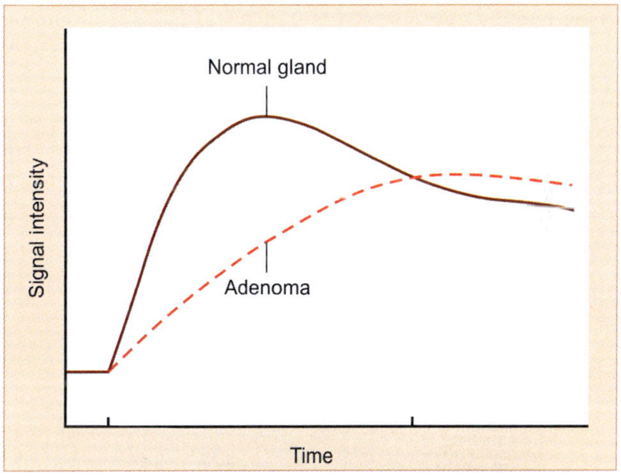

FIG. 4: Enhancement pattern of adenoma and normal pituitary gland shown as time intensity curve. Early and higher degree of enhancement of normal pituitary versus lower and delayed uptake of contrast by the adenoma is noted. After sometime they become isointense as contrast washes out from gland. Later on adenoma may appear hyperintense.

increases significantly.[11] Parasellar extension and invasion of the base of skull are also accurately shown on MRI with dynamic T1 and heavily T2-weighted sequences proving the best. CT scores over MRI in showing subtle cortical involvement, however, this may not be surgically important.[5]

Microadenomas (<10 mm in size) typically appear hypointense compared to the normal adenohypophysis on T1WI (80–90%)[5] and iso to hyperintense on T2WI **(Figs. 5A and B)**. The signal intensity of adenomas and normal gland are comparable to the grey and white matter of the temporal lobe respectively on T1WI. They may sometimes appear hyperintense on T1WI. This is attributable to hemorrhage. Occasionally they may be isointense and can only be detected on enhanced scans (particularly dynamic study) where they stand out as hypointense areas within the enhancing gland **(Figs. 6 and 7)**. On contrast-enhanced CT (CECT) adenomas are seen as discrete, hypodense regions within the enhancing gland **(Fig. 8)**. Imaging has little to offer for differentiating different types of microadenomas; however, the PRL and GH secreting adenomas tend to be located more laterally in the gland and ACTH and gonadotropin secretors tend to be more central **(Figs. 5 and 6)**.[12] Indirect signs for the presence of adenoma include enlargement of gland and a bulge in the gland outline. Tilt of the pituitary stalk and asymmetry of the sellar floor though helpful signs may sometimes occur physiologically due to developmental asymmetry of the brain or stalk insertion. Inferior petrosal sinus sampling may be extremely useful for localizing adenoma and distinguishing Cushing's disease from ectopic ACTH secretion and autonomous adrenal disease when imaging fails to show the site of adenoma. Lateralization of the lesion to either half of the pituitary gland is also possible. However, in larger lesions,

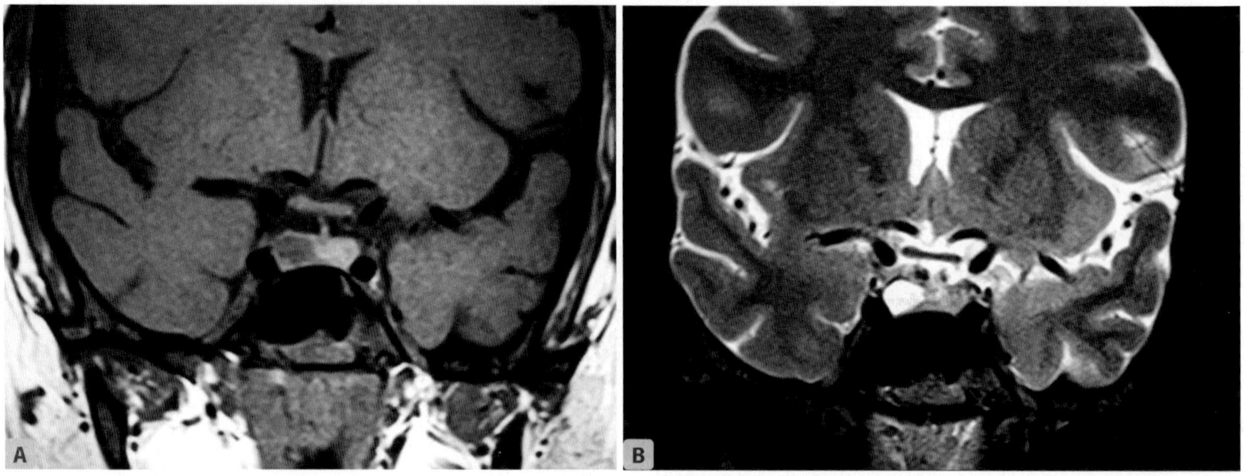

FIGS. 5A AND B: Prolactin secreting pituitary adenoma : T1-weighted coronal image shows hypointense microadenoma on right aspect of the gland (A). Adenoma appears hyperintense on T2WI (B).

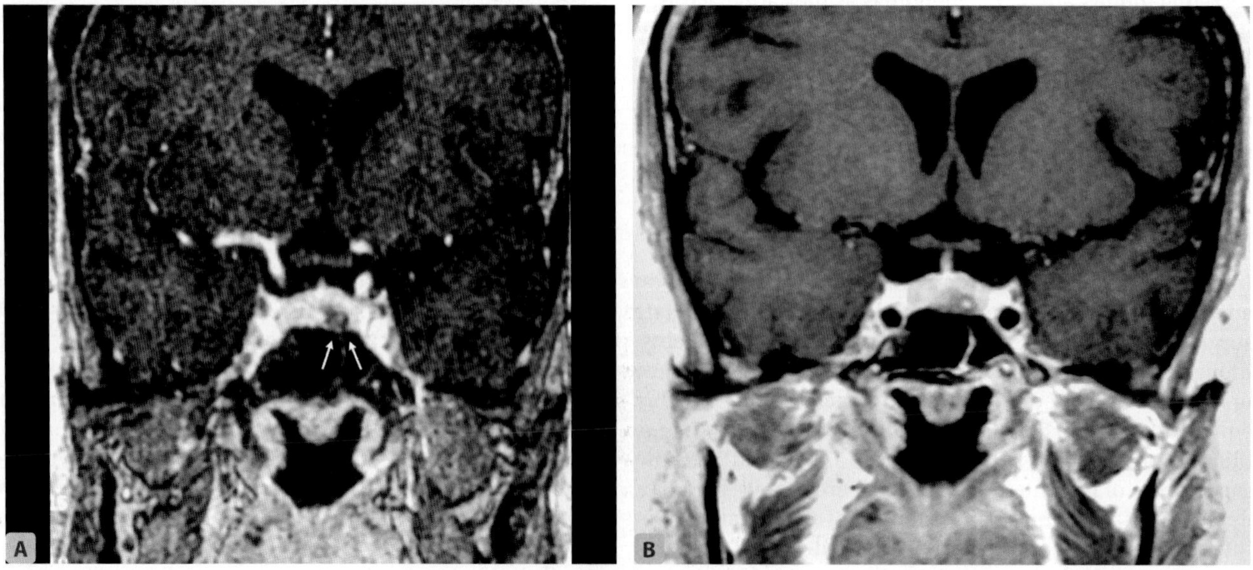

FIGS. 6A AND B: Dynamic CEMR (A) showing a small ACTH secreting adenoma in the central part of the gland (arrows) which is mostly isointense to rest of the gland on routine CEMR, however, a small central area shows higher.

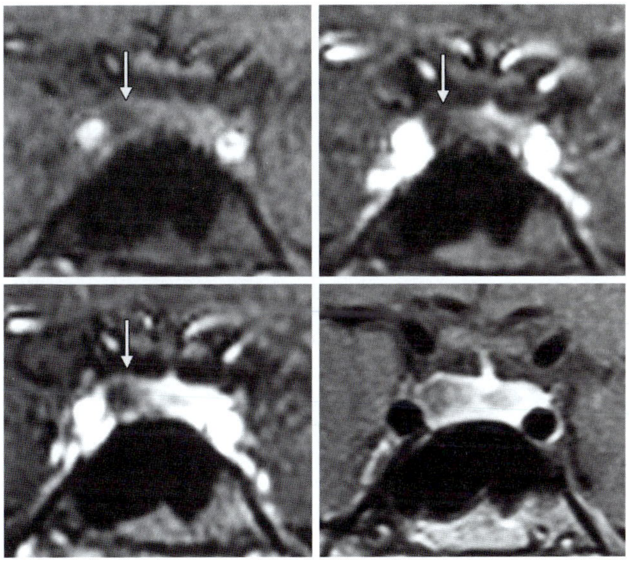

FIG. 7: Consecutive four frames of dynamic CEMR shows progressive enhancement of pituitary gland leading to better definition of microadenoma on the right aspect (arrows). Delayed frame (lower right corner) shows progressive fill in of adenoma.

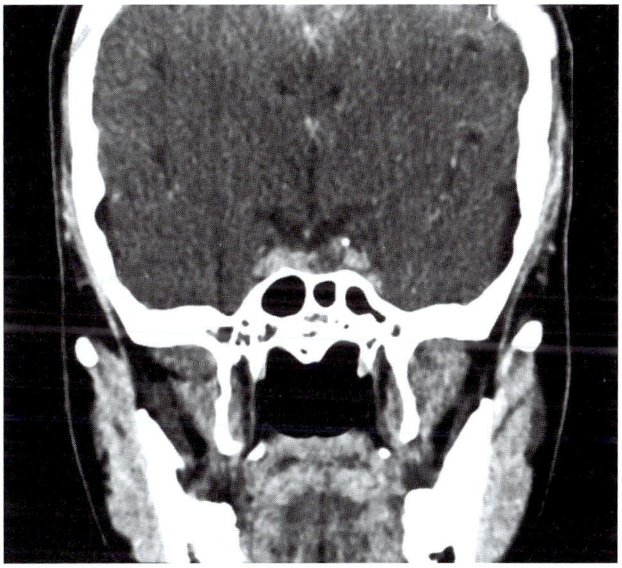

FIG. 8: Adenoma: CECT scan shows a relatively hypodense adenoma within intensely enhancing normal gland.

lateralization may not be accurate due to venous drainage occurring in either direction i.e. both cavernous sinuses.[13,14]

Macroadenomas (>10 mm), being larger, are easier to diagnose. They usually enlarge the sella, erode the sphenoid sinus, encroach upon the suprasellar cistern and may displace the chiasma **(Figs. 9A to D)**. Solid adenomas enhance uniformly, while others may show heterogeneous hypodense areas within it on CECT. Macroadenomas are frequently hyperintense on T2WI. Hyperintense macroadenomas may be soft and necrotic while hypointense lesions may be more fibrous; a finding that may be of help to the surgeon.[5] Apparent diffusion coefficient values on diffusion-weighted imaging may be higher in softer variety.[15] Hemorrhage and necrosis are common particularly following bromocriptine therapy, majority of these being subclinical.[4] In large lesions, residual pituitary tissue may not be visible. Most microadenomas enhance late as compared to the adenohypophysis while macroadenomas enhance early. This reflects the difference in their blood supply. With suprasellar extension, the adenomas acquire a typical "figure-of-eight", appearance.

Early cavernous sinus involvement by adenoma is often difficult to diagnose. The most reliable signs of cavernous sinus invasion are encasement of cavernous carotid arteries, presence of tumor lateral to them, delayed enhancing soft tissue in sinus, a lateral bulge of the outer dura and a serum PRL level of 1,000 ng/mL or more (in case of prolactinomas) **(Figs. 10A and B)**.[3,5] In one study MDCT was found to better delineate the lateral margin of tumor.[15]

MR has been shown to be useful in precisely demonstrating the cavernous sinus invasion. Many grading schemes have been proposed to prognosticate the effect of cavernous sinus extension on the surgical outcomes of these patients. Knosp grading has been widely used and has proven to show good correlation with outcomes.[16] The grading is defined by the relation of carotid lines with the limits of invasion **(Fig. 11)**. These lines pass through supra- and intracavernous parts of ICA in coronal view. There are medial, median and lateral carotid lines. Micko et al.[17] partially revised the classification by bifurcating grade 3 into A and B (marked (*) in **Table 4**). A new classification scheme was proposed by Edal et al.[18] wherein they classified the adjoining invasion in all three planes which was called the SIPAP (superior inferior parasellar anterior posterior) grading.

Atypical Presentations of Adenomas

Their blood supply being marginal, pituitary adenomas may present acutely with infarction and hemorrhage; a condition called *pituitary apoplexy*. However, these events may be silent and only detected at pathology or imaging.[19] Hemorrhage/infarction may be spontaneous or following bromocriptine therapy (in more than half of the treated patients). The gland may show areas which appear hyperdense on noncontrast CT, dark on T2WI (acute blood) or bright on T1WI (subacute blood) **(Figs. 12A and B)**. Massive hemorrhage may have sub-arachnoid/intracerebral extension. Diffusion imaging may show restriction.[20]

Although pituitary adenomas are generally benign slow growing neoplasms, *malignant variants* exist. These tend to infiltrate dura, bone and surrounding structures. As histology and imaging do not allow distinction between the two, the presence of metastatic disease is the only definite clue to diagnosis.[7]

The term *invasive pituitary adenomas* represent an intermediate part of the spectrum. These infiltrate surrounding structures but grow slowly and by definition do not cause metastasis.

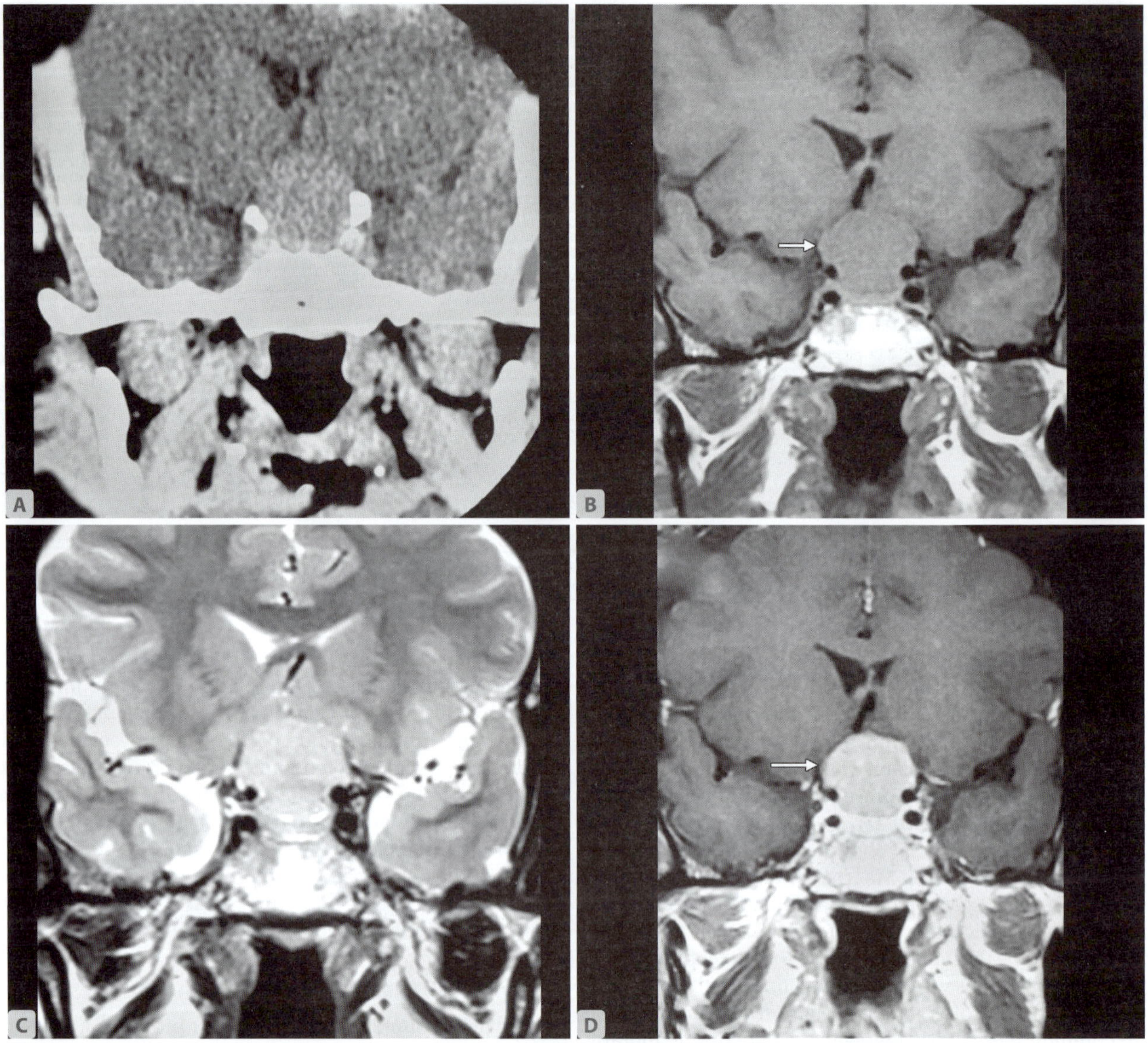

FIGS. 9A TO D: Coronal sections: CECT (A), T1-weighted, T2-weighted and gadolinium enhanced T1-weighted MR images (B to D) show a solid enhancing macroadenoma with suprasellar extension. The optic chiasma is stretched superiorly (arrow).

An aggressive subtype of ACTH producing adenoma is seen in Nelson's syndrome, a condition in which the adenoma enlarges in the absence of regulatory mechanisms after bilateral adrenalectomy.[9]

Ectopic adenomas can arise from infundibulum or in suprasellar cistern from pars tuberalis.

Postoperative Sella

It may be difficult to differentiate residual/recurrent tumor from scarring and a variety of graft materials in the postoperative bed, i.e. fat, gelfoam, muscle, etc. Gadolinium-enhanced scan may be helpful in such cases. It is recommended that postoperative scanning be done 4–6 months after surgery to allow resorption of gelfoam, hemorrhagic material and debris.[21] Comparison with preoperative scans, progressive growth of lesion and correlation with endocrinological markers are important. Development of empty sella, CSF leaks and sinusitis are some of the sequel of surgery.[22] Positron emission tomography potentially appears useful for assessing tumor response to therapy and for differentiating postsurgical changes from recurrent tumors.

Craniopharyngioma

These are benign, slowly growing, locally invasive, hormonally inactive lesions accounting for 2–4% of all intracranial lesions. They are derived from Rathke's pouch. Twenty percent of craniopharyngiomas may be purely intrasellar, while 80% have their epicenter in the suprasellar cistern.[5] Rarely, they may be intraventricular or infrasellar. There is a bimodal age distribution, majority of lesions presenting in the 5–10 years age group with a second small peak in 6th decade.[10] The children usually have features of raised intracranial pressure while visual disturbances and endocrinopathy are the usual presentation in 70–90% of adults. There are two histological

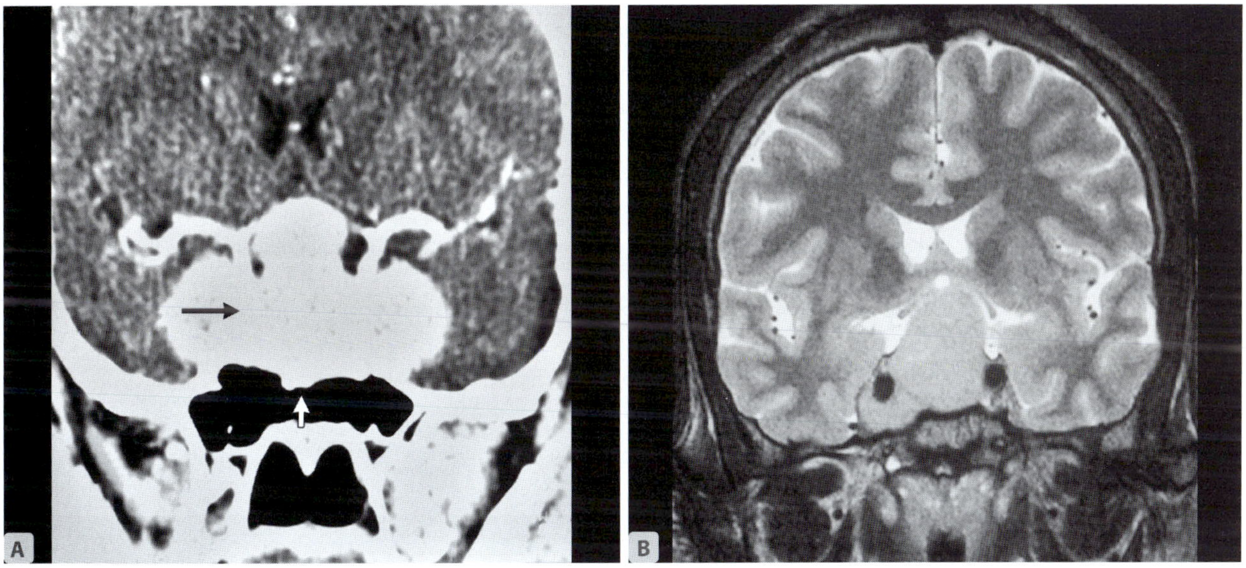

FIGS. 10A AND B: CECT coronal section. (A) Lobulated relatively homogenous macroadenoma with involvement of cavernous sinuses on both sides. Encasement of carotid vessels (black arrow) and erosion of floor of sella (white arrow) can be noted. MR coronal T2 image (B) showing extension of the adenoma into right cavernous sinus.

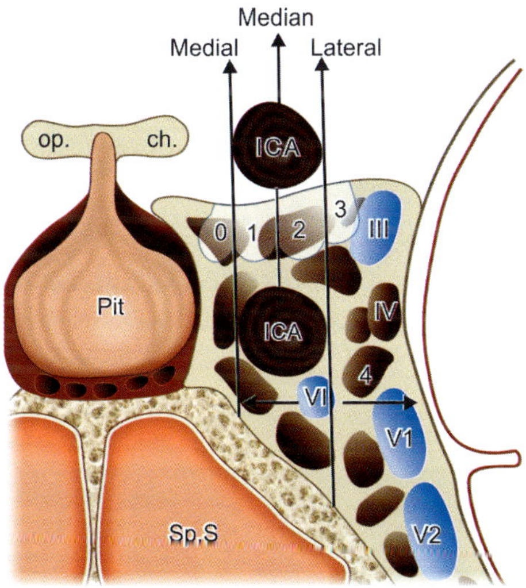

FIG. 11: Pictorial representation of the coronal view of the sella and parasellar (cavernous sinus) region depicting the demarcation of the sinus into three compartments by imaginary medial, median and lateral lines. The numerals 0, 1, 2, 3 and 4 represent the grade of adenoma extension according to Knosp scheme (detailed discussion in the text and table).

subtypes of the lesions-adamantinomatous and papillary types. They are distinct in terms of clinical presentation, imaging features and treatment outcome.[23]

The more common classic form is adamantinomatous type, usually seen in children. They are almost always cystic with small solid component which frequently calcifies (80% cases). Characteristically, these tumors appear as a combination of hypodense (cystic) and hyperdense (calcified) areas on CT. The solid portion appears isodense/isointense to brain on CT and MRI. The cyst fluid contains wet keratin, cholesterol crystals, proteinaceous fluids, hemorrhages and necrotic debris and is likened to *motor oil*. Such cysts appear extremely bright on both T1 and T2-weighted images **(Figs. 13A and B)**. The other cysts may be slightly hyperintense to CSF on T1WI, more so, on FLAIR and may show peripheral enhancement. CT is useful for showing calcification, particularly if the tumor is only a small solid calcified nodule, which may be totally overlooked on MRI **(Figs. 14A to E)**. The adamantinomatous type is more likely to be locally invasive, encase vessels, cause surrounding gliosis and may recur after surgery. Contrast enhancement of the solid portions of the tumor may be seen.[5] Papillary variety of craniopharyngioma seen in adults are solid, often located within third ventricle and do not calcify. They are encapsulated and easily removable and hence have a lesser tendency to recur.[22] Craniopharyngiomas cause fibroinflammatory adhesions with surrounding tissues and tend to recur after surgery.

Pituicytoma

These arise from pituicyte, a glial cell in neurohypophysis and infundibulum and are also called granular cell tumors and myoblastoma. The location is usually posterior intrasellar with suprasellar extension. Size ranges from 1 mm to 2 mm to 4 cm. On CT a hyperdense sellar/suprasellar mass is seen which enhances homogenously. On T1WI, the lesion is iso to hypointense with absent bright spot and on T2 it is usually heterogeneous.[3-5]

Meningioma

Ten percent of meningiomas occur in sellar and parasellar region. The site of origin is commonly tuberculum sella, the other locations being clinoid processes, the dorsum, medial sphenoid wing and cavernous sinuses. Tumors originating from optic sheath, olfactory groove and planum sphenoidale may also extend into supra/parasellar regions.[5] They are

TABLE 4: Knosp grading system for demonstrating invasion of cavernous sinus by pituitary macroadenoma.

Grade	Cavernous sinus extension
0	Adenoma does not extend beyond the medial carotid line
1	Adenoma extends beyond the medial line, but does not reach the median line, so-called "intracarotid" line
2	Tumor extends beyond the median line, but does not extend beyond or tangent to the lateral line
3	Tumor extends beyond the lateral line
3A*	The tumor extends lateral to the lateral tangent of the intracavernous and supracavernous ICAs into the **superior** CS compartment
3B*	The tumor extends lateral to the lateral tangent of the intracavernous and supracavernous ICAs into the **inferior** CS compartment
4	Tumor totally wraps around the intracavernous carotid artery

* Micko et al. revision of Grade 3 into A and B.

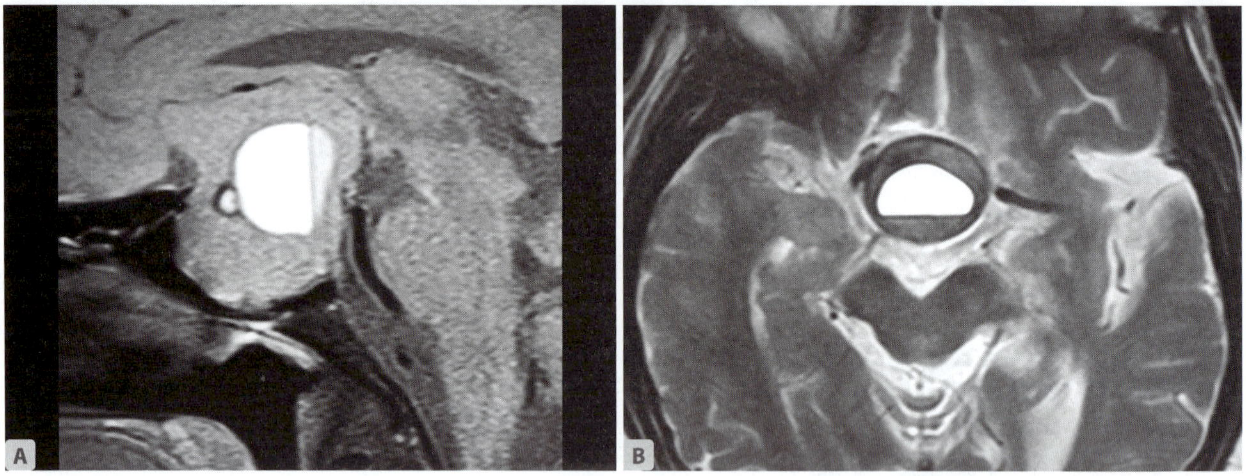

FIGS. 12A AND B: Pituitary apoplexy: T1-weighted sagittal section: Macroadenoma with bright signal with fluid-fluid level within the tumor representing subacute blood (A). T2WI reveals hyperintense blood with a fluid level showing shading in the dependent portions due to settled red blood cells (B).

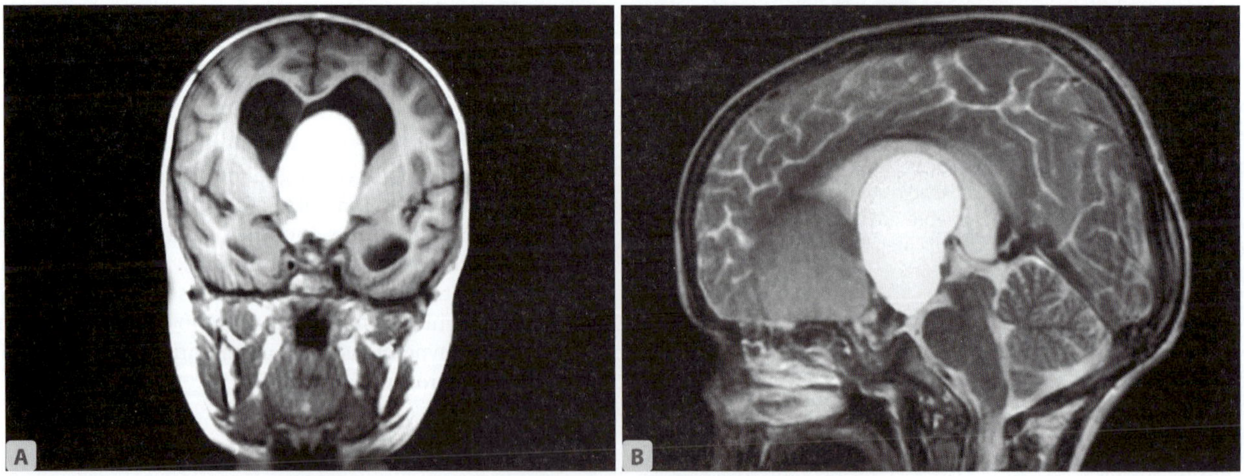

FIGS. 13A AND B: Craniopharyngioma: Hyperintense motor oil cyst on T1 coronal (A) and T2 sagittal (B) MR sections. Differing T2 signal in the cysts can be seen on T2 section (B) with low signal calcification in the immediate suprasellar area.

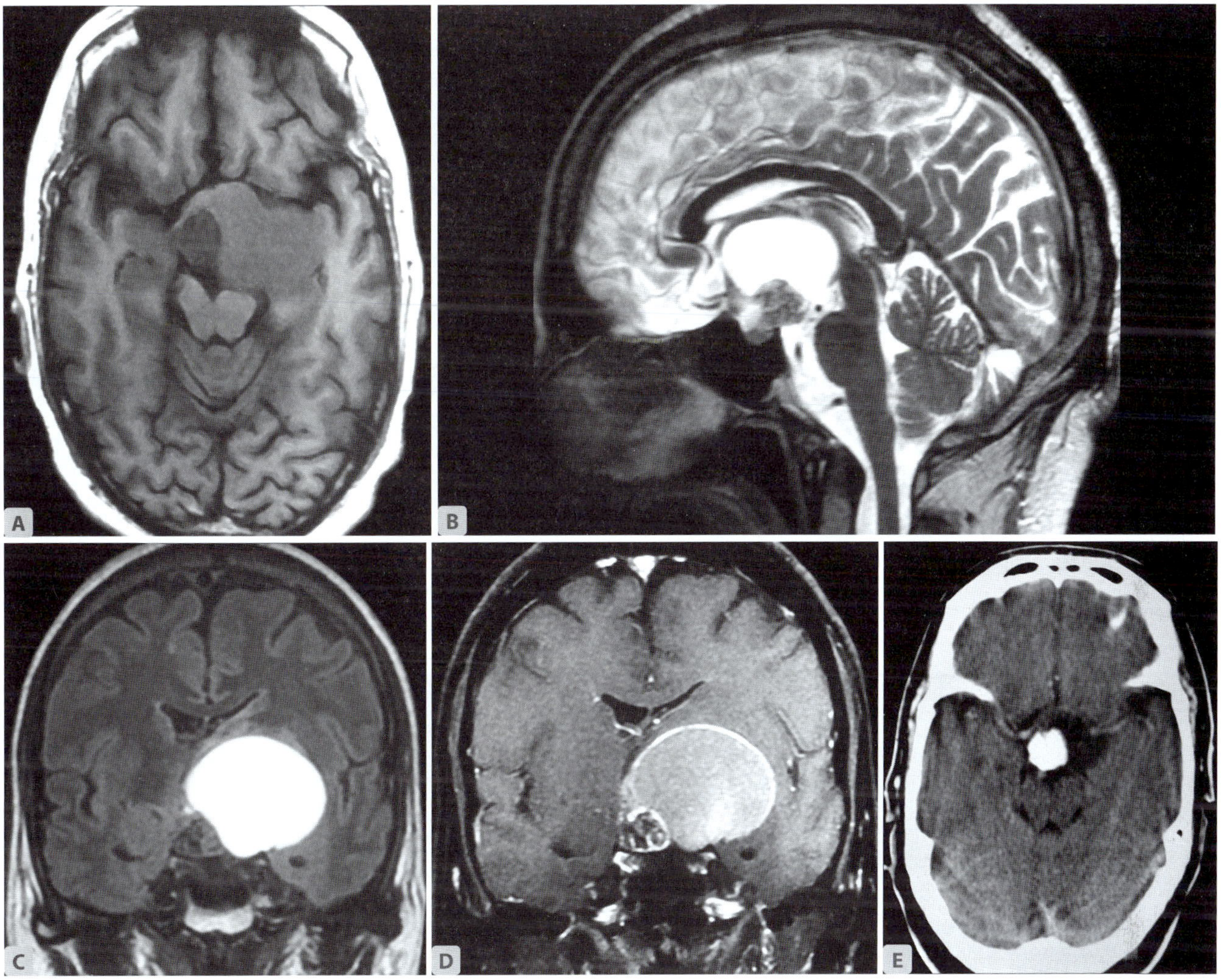

FIGS. 14A TO E: Craniopharyngioma: Axial T1WI (A) and sagittal T2WI (B) show cystic and solid suprasellar mass. Coronal FLAIR (C) shows high signal of the cyst compared to CSF. Enhanced T1WI (D) shows peripheral enhancement of the cyst but calcification is difficult to comment upon which is clearly shown on axial CT (E).

slow growing lesions causing mass effect, i.e. visual loss, ophthalmoplegia or proptosis due to venous congestion at the orbital apex.

On MRI, they are usually isointense to grey matter on T1WI. T2WI images show isointensity in 50% and hyperintensity in 30–40%.[10] Meningiomas show bright contrast enhancement on both CT and MRI **(Figs. 15A and B)**. It is important to differentiate meningioma from adenoma as the surgical approach varies in the two. MR signal intensity and enhancement pattern do not allow this differentiation. However, morphological features like a broad base with dural tail, hyperostosis rather than erosion, calcification (better shown on CT, **Figs. 16A and B**), a cleft demarcating the lesion from brain and pituitary gland, greater propensity for arterial encasement and normal sized sella favor a diagnosis of meningioma. ^{31}P-spectroscopy may show higher phosphate monoester in meningioma vis-à-vis adenoma.

Germinoma and Teratoma

Twenty percent of these germ cell tumors may be seen in suprasellar cistern or pituitary fossa in children and young adults.[24] They may arise here or may be metastatic lesions from a pineal tumor. There is no sex predilection unlike pineal tumors, which have a strong male predominance. Patients present with endocrinopathy, visual field defects, hydrocephalus, etc. as is common to all suprasellar neoplasms. However, diabetes insipidus is the earliest symptom due to invasion of hypothalamus.

Germinomas tend to be large noncapsulated solid lesions, centered on or behind stalk that infiltrate into surrounding structures. They are homogenous lesions without cystic components (unlike craniopharyngioma). On CT they are hyperdense like lymphoma **(Figs. 17A and B)**. On MRI, they are slightly hypointense on T1 and hyperintense on T2WI **(Fig. 17C)**. They show strong contrast enhancement on

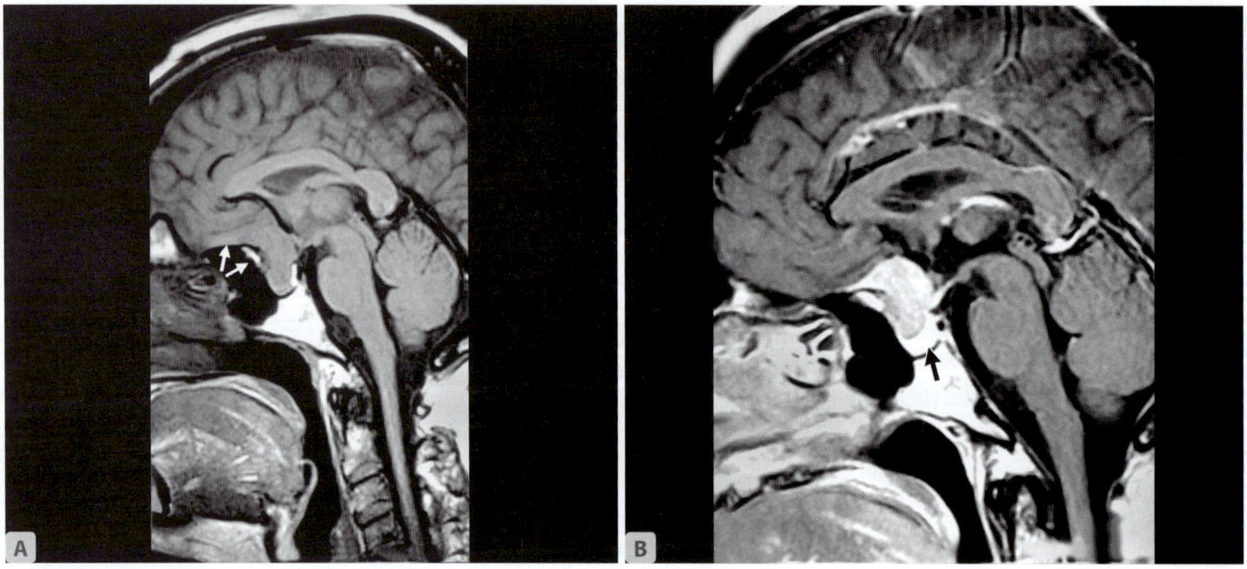

FIGS. 15A AND B: Tuberculum sellae meningioma: T1 sections before (A) and after (B) contrast administration. The broad dural-based tumor is nearly isointense to pituitary gland before contrast but can be easily differentiated from it on early postcontrast images as the gland enhances to a greater degree (arrows).

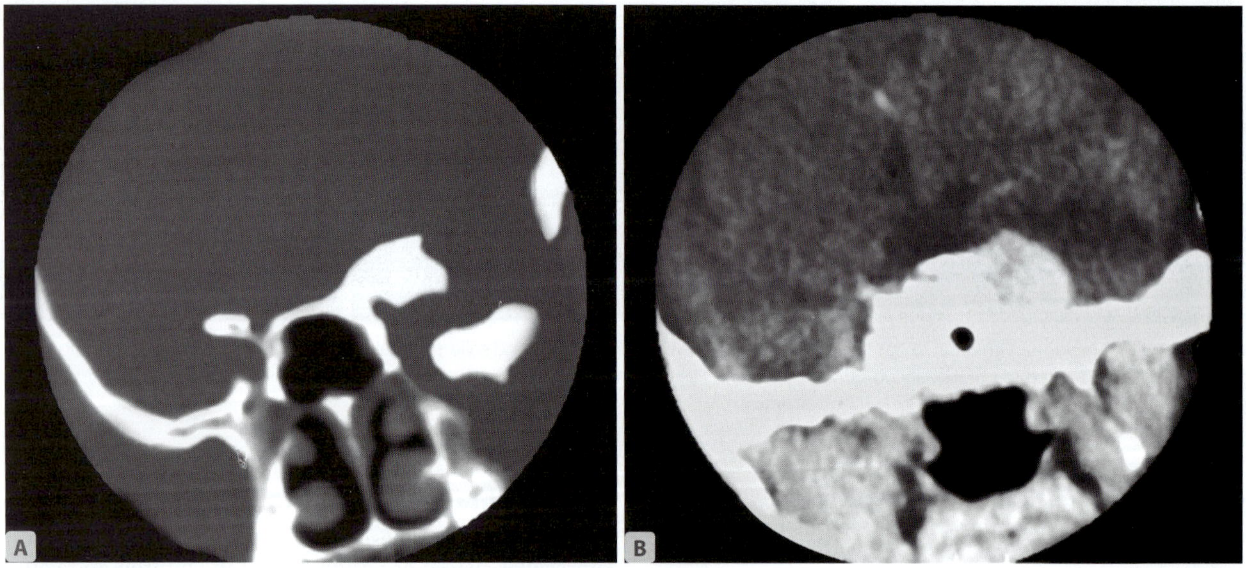

FIGS. 16A AND B: Anterior clinoidal meningioma. (A) Coronal CT bone window and (B) soft tissue window shows hyperostosis of the left anterior clinoid process (A) and associated soft tissue component of the mass (B).

CT/MRI **(Figs. 17D)**. There is also a high tendency of CSF dissemination **(Fig. 17E)**. The posterior pituitary bright spot is often absent. Teratomas show evidence of fat or calcification and are more heterogeneous.[5,24]

Dermoid and Epidermoid Tumors

These are slow growing benign inclusion tumors due to trapping of ectodermal cells during neural tube closure.[25]

Epidermoids are five times more common than dermoids and usually are parasellar in location; the second most common site in the head after the CP angles. They are seen in adults of 20–40 years of age. Dermoids are more common in children,[26] tend to occur in the midline and in posterior fossa but may occur in the suprasellar cistern. Epidermoid cysts are composed of desquamated keratin while the dermoids contain dermal appendages. Both show slow growth, tend to insinuate in the available space and produce symptoms by compression of the adjacent structures. Rarely, chemical meningitis may occur due to rupture. Epidermoids appear heterogeneous and slightly hyperdense to CSF on CT and usually slightly hyperintense to CSF on T1WI **(Figs. 18A to D)**. They rarely enhance but occasionally calcify peripherally.[26,27] FLAIR and diffusion images **(Figs. 18A to D)** are extremely useful in showing these lesions as is CT cisternography.

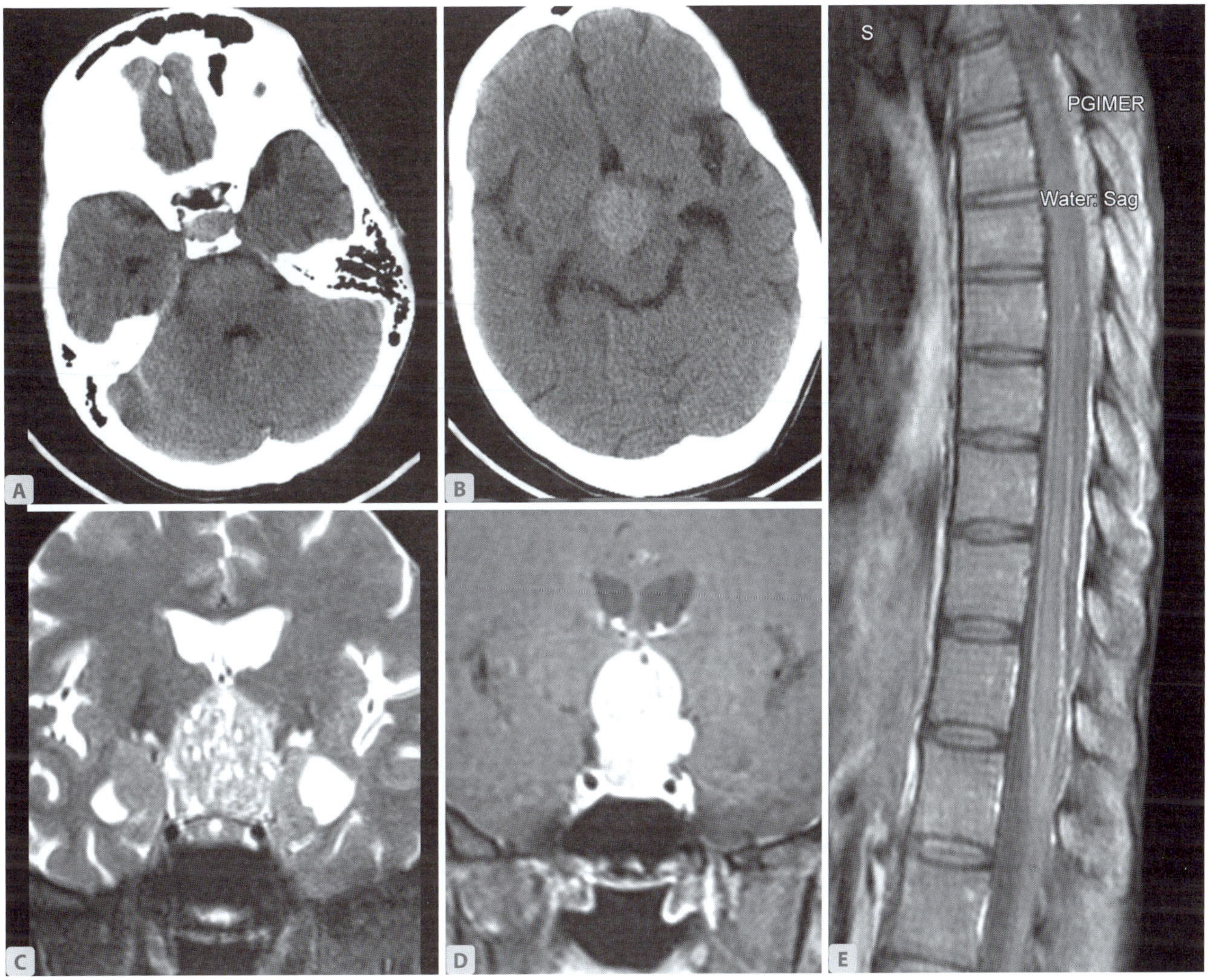

FIGS. 17A TO E: Suprasellar germinoma: A young girl presenting with hypopituitarism was evaluated with noncontrast CT (A and B) which revealed hyperdense sellar-suprasellar mass. Craniospinal MR confirmed the lesion with T2 hypo to isointensity (C) and moderate postcontrast enhancement (D). There was CSF spread in the spinal canal as demonstrated by leptomeningeal enhancement in the dorsal spine (E). She responded to radiotherapy.

Dermoids are more heterogeneous and often show fat density (fat fluid levels sometimes) or calcification. Fat droplets may be visualized in the subarachnoid space in ruptured dermoids. However, epidermoids, dermoids and other purely cystic lesions may be indistinguishable on imaging.

Chiasmatic/Hypothalamic Glioma

Seventy five percent of these tumors occur in first decade of life. This diverse group of neoplasms often present with different behavior and response to therapy and are referred to together as chiasmatic-hypothalamic gliomas. The site of origin is often difficult to decide, as the lesions are usually large when detected and are infiltrative in nature. Neurofibromatosis 1 (NF-1) is present in 20–50% patients with opticochiasmatic lesions. The chiasmatic lesions tend to infiltrate the hypothalamus leading to hypothalamic dysfunction and hydrocephalus. They also tend to infiltrate along the optic tracts, hence the importance of imaging the entire brain.[28] The tumors confined to the chiasma can be differentiated from optic neuritis by clinical presentation or resolution of neuritis on steroids.[5,10,29]

The lesions appear isointense to brain on T1WI and hyperintense on T2WI **(Figs. 19A to D)**. Calcification and hemorrhages are not seen but cystic component can occur. Contrast enhancement is seen in 50% lesions. Lack of serial growth and enhancement differentiate benign hamartomatous NF lesions from glioma.

Hypothalamic gliomas are aggressive and present with hypothalamic dysfunction. Diencephalic syndrome almost always indicates this diagnosis and refers to a clinical state of cachexia in an alert/euphoric child who often has a good appetite.

In general, chiasma/hypothalamic lesions are more aggressive compared to the optic nerve lesions. Lesions arising above 20 years and below 5 years of age also show a more aggressive behavior compared to those arising between

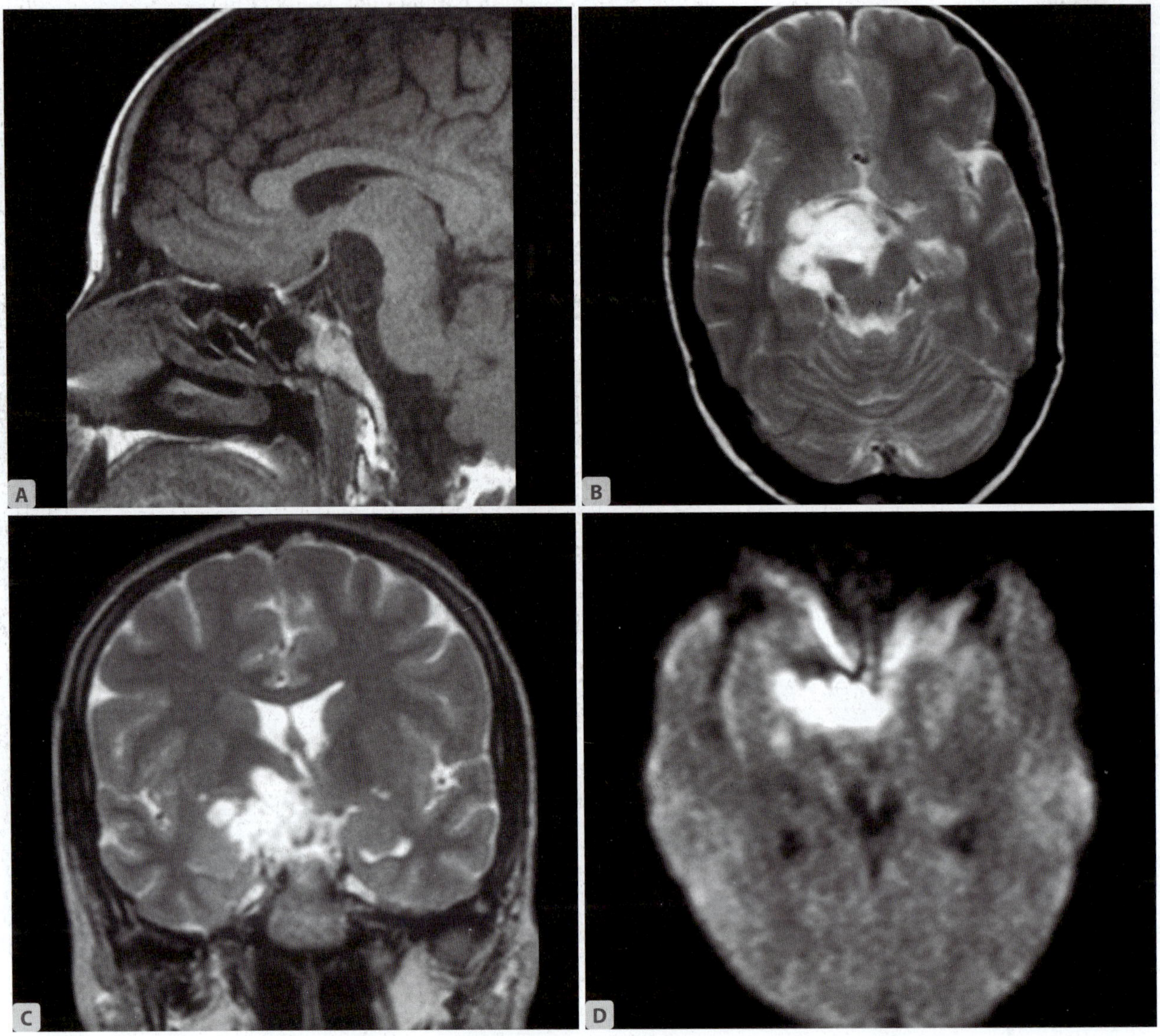

FIGS. 18A TO D: Suprasellar epidermoid appearing slightly hyperintense compared to CSF on T1WI (A), extremely bright like CSF on T2WI (B and C) with a lobulated outline and shows bright signal on diffusion image (D).

5 years and 20 years.[28] Similarly sporadic lesions also are more aggressive.

Schwannoma

Parasellar schwannomas most commonly arise from branches of Vth nerve. The lesions present with sensory deficit, problems of mastication, facial pain or diplopia. Imaging shows asymmetry and expansion of cavernous sinus. They are encapsulated lesions isointense to brain on T1WI and bright on T2WI. They are isodense on CT and enhance strongly. Larger tumors may be heterogeneous with a tigroid appearance. The 3rd to 6th nerve schwannomas follow the course of respective nerves but are rare lesions.

The dumb-bell configuration of Vth nerve schwannoma[30] straddling the petrous apex is characteristic but less common than a Meckel's cave or posterior fossa mass **(Figs. 20A and B)**.

SKULL BASE LESIONS

Primary, secondary and metastatic tumors of the skull base can involve the parasellar area. The primary lesions include chondroma, chondrosarcoma and plasmacytoma. Secondary tumors are often from nasopharynx and paranasal sinuses. Common metastasis comes from lung, breast and prostate primaries. These are difficult to differentiate from chordoma.

Chordoma

They are locally malignant tumors derived from notochordal remnants; 35% of them arise in the clivus (spheno-occipital synchondrosis) though occasionally they may present in Meckel's cave and petrous bone. Mean age of presentation is 20–40 years though no age is exempt. Imaging shows lobular lesions iso to hypointense on T1WI and heterogeneous on T2WI replacing the clival

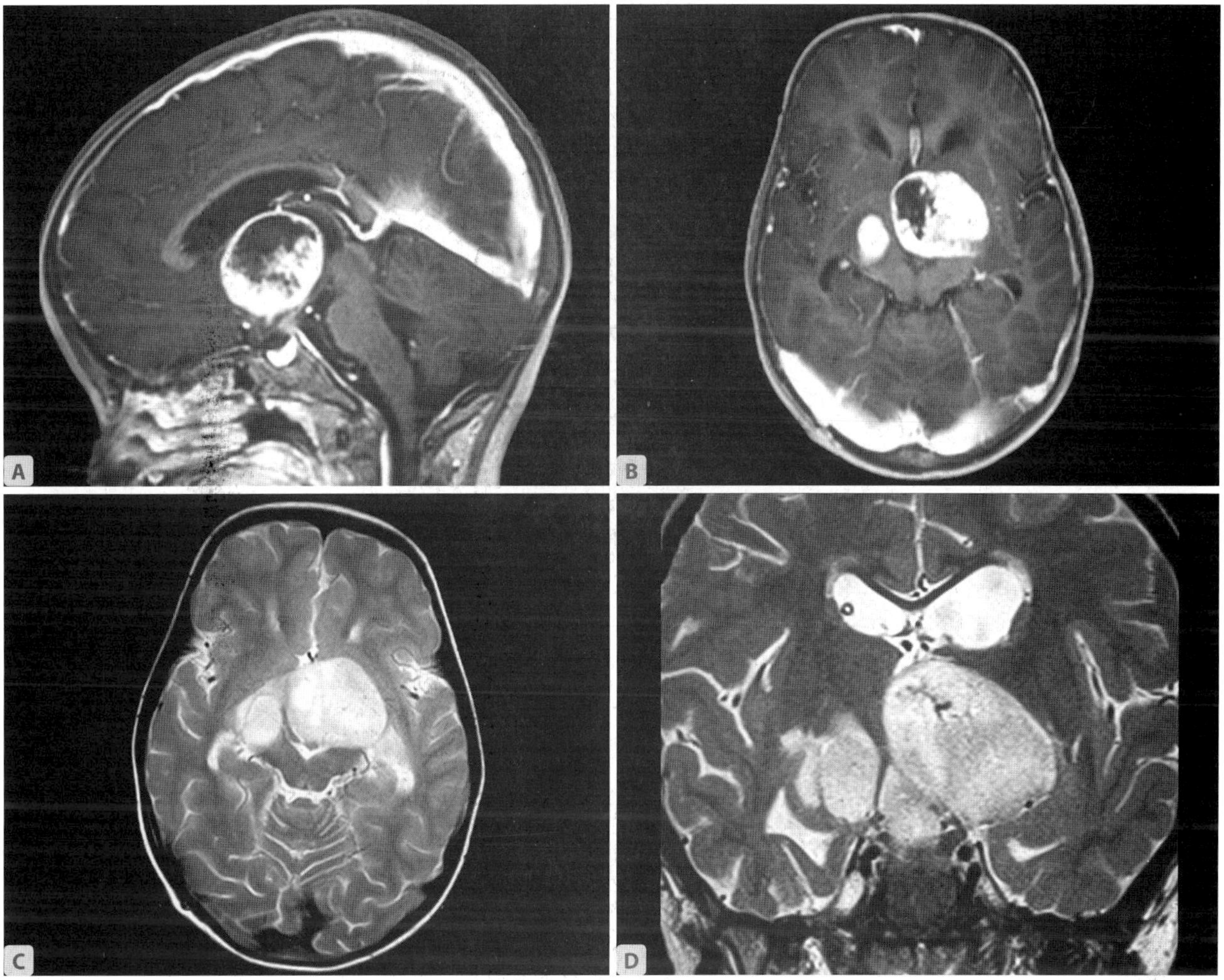

FIGS. 19A TO D: Hypothalamic glioma: The lobulated suprasellar mass shows moderate enhancement on postcontrast T1WI (A and B), is hyperintense on T2WI (C) and is seen to extend along B/L optic tracts (D).

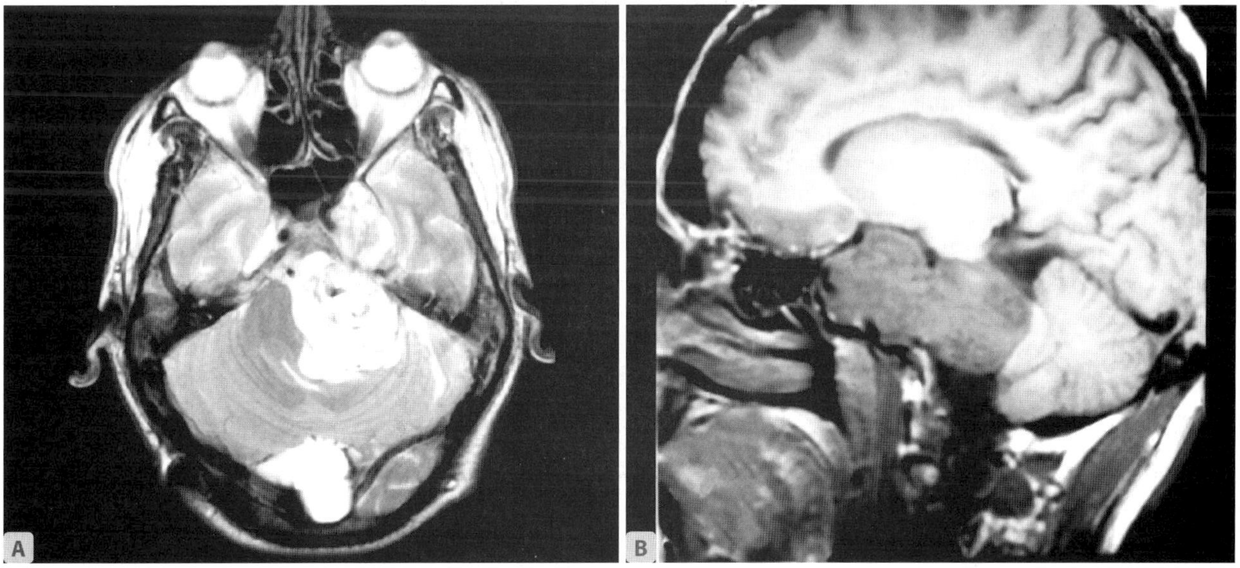

FIGS. 20A AND B: Schwannoma: (A) T2-weighted axial section shows characteristic hyperintense Vth nerve tumor straddling the petrous apex and expanding the left cavernous sinus; (B) T1 sagittal image of another patient shows extension of tumor from posterior to middle cranial fossa.

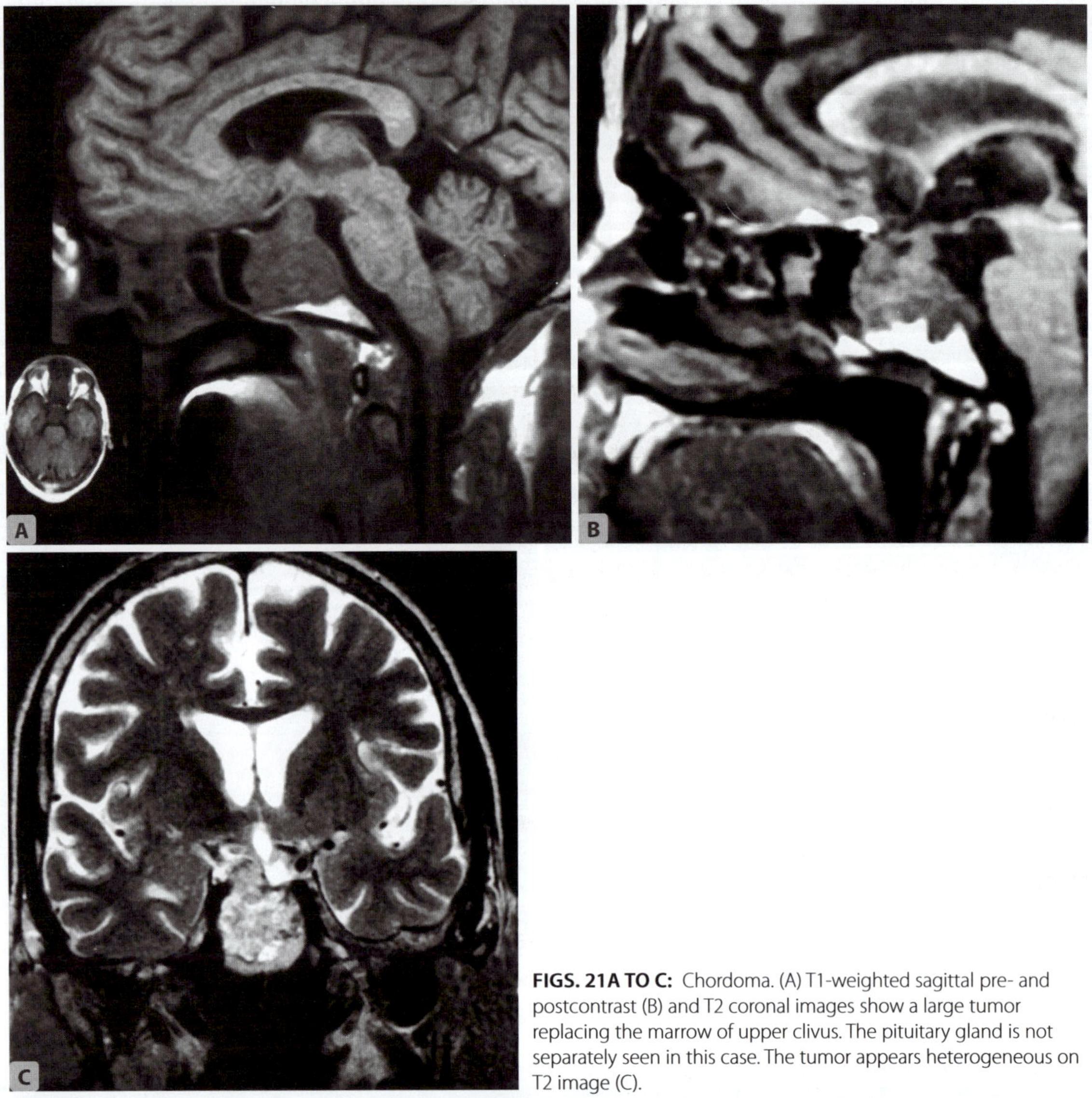

FIGS. 21A TO C: Chordoma. (A) T1-weighted sagittal pre- and postcontrast (B) and T2 coronal images show a large tumor replacing the marrow of upper clivus. The pituitary gland is not separately seen in this case. The tumor appears heterogeneous on T2 image (C).

marrow **(Figs. 21A to C)**.[31] They appear hyperintense on postcontrast studies with septations of fibrous connective tissue. CT shows a destructive mass with fragments of bone and calcification. Localization of the epicenter of the lesion within the clivus and identification of normal or displaced pituitary gland differentiates chordomas from invasive adenomas.[25]

Metastasis

Anterior lobe dysfunction or diabetes insipidus in a patient with known malignancy (carcinomas of lung, GI tract, breast, leukemia/lymphoma and skull base tumors) may indicate pituitary metastasis.[32] However, most of these lesions are detected on autopsy. Presumably, most patients succumb to advanced disseminated malignancy before these lesions produce symptoms. The routes of spread may be hematogenous, by CSF seeding or by direct extension.

Imaging may show an enhancing intrasellar, suprasellar or combined lesion. Although difficult to differentiate from adenoma by imaging, endocrinopathy in a patient with known malignancy, rapid growth/disproportionate invasion and destruction of surrounding structures by a small-sized lesion, a dumbbell shape with constriction at diaphragm in a normal sized sella, associated brain edema and enhancement and thickening of infundibulum suggest the diagnosis of metastasis **(Figs. 22A to C)**.[32]

CONGENITAL AND METABOLIC ABNORMALITIES OF PITUITARY GLAND

Some miscellaneous pathologies of pituitary gland have been grouped here. These either have a developmental basis of origin or are acquired in nature but often have endocrinological and surgical implications.

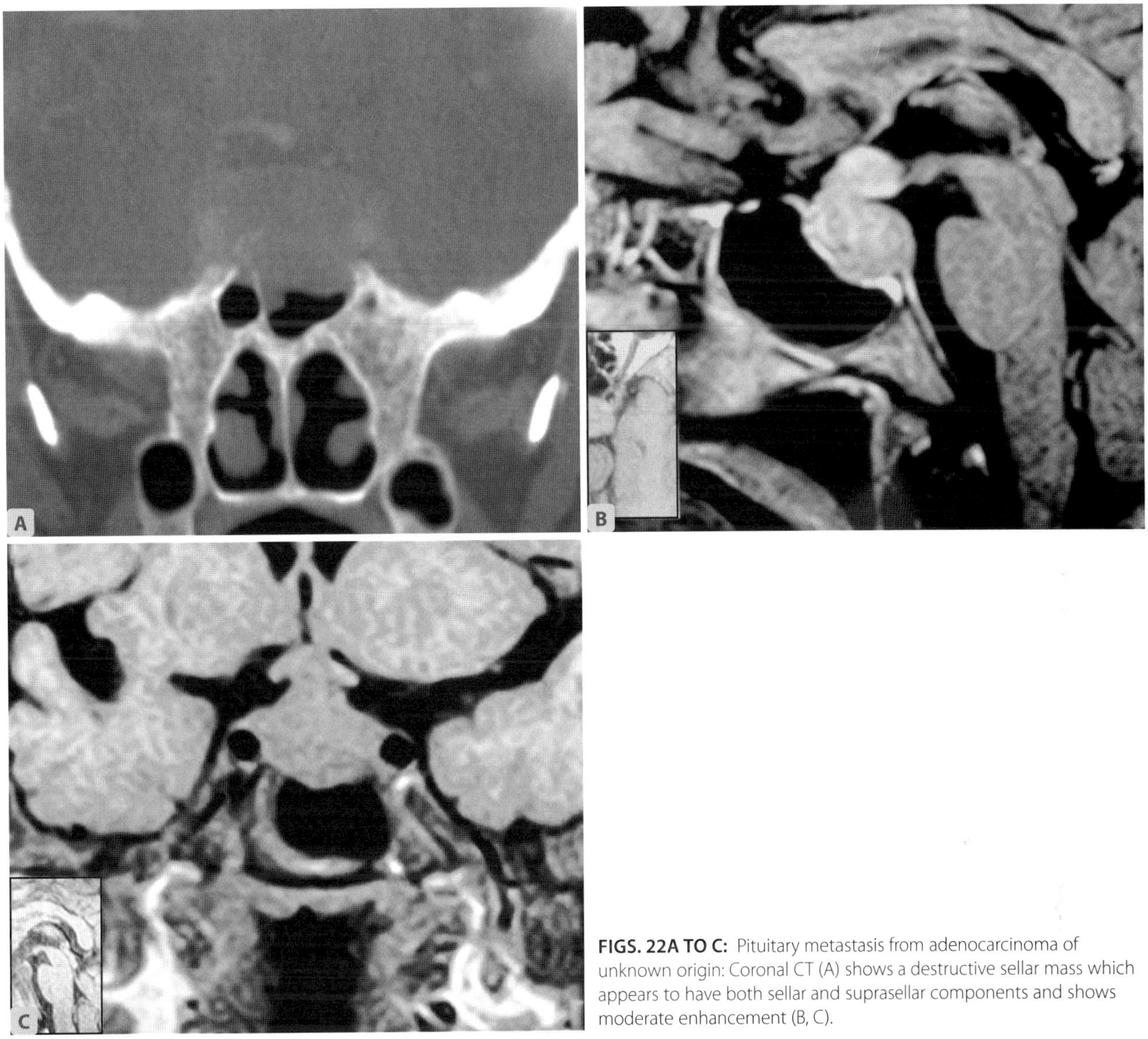

FIGS. 22A TO C: Pituitary metastasis from adenocarcinoma of unknown origin: Coronal CT (A) shows a destructive sellar mass which appears to have both sellar and suprasellar components and shows moderate enhancement (B, C).

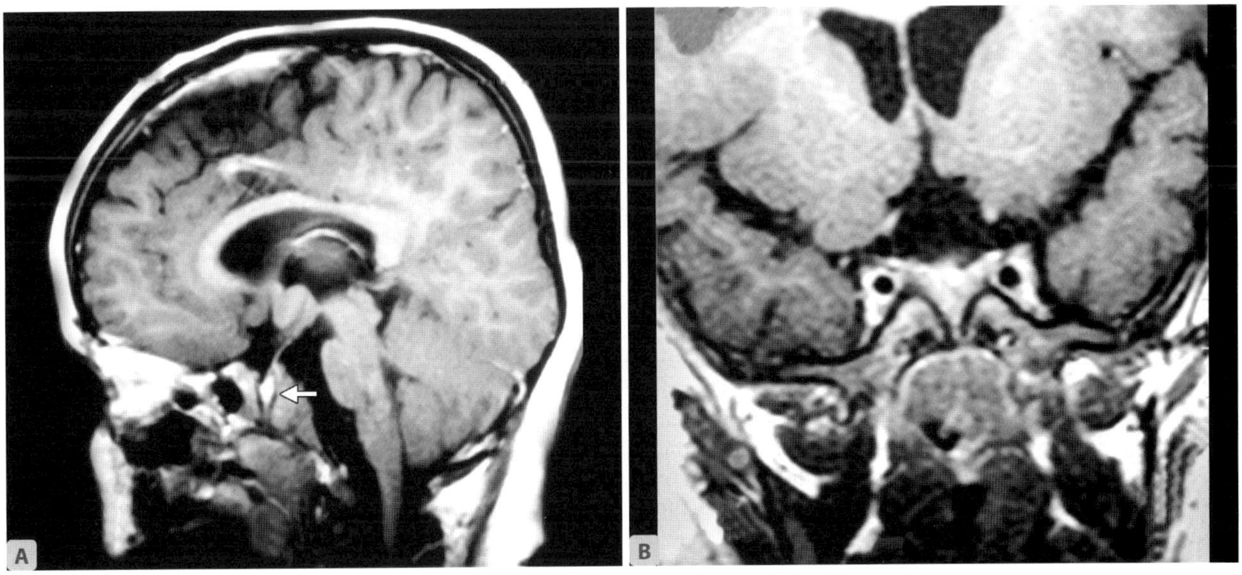

FIGS. 23A AND B: Persistent craniopharyngeal canal. (A) T1 sagittal and (B) coronal sections. A defect in the sellar floor, inferior location of pituitary gland (arrow in A), tubo-mammillary fusion and wide separation of carotid arteries can be observed.

Developmental Anomalies of Pituitary Gland

Persistent hypophyseal canal is a rare congenital anomaly of a skull base defect (craniopharyngeal canal) extending from sellar floor to the nasopharynx (incidence 0.42%). There can be nasopharyngeal extension of the gland, associated hamartomas[33] or duplication of pituitary gland/stalk. The findings on X-ray and CT can be a spur and two widely separated fossae. A duplicated basilar artery with widely separated carotids may be seen. On MRI, thickened tuber cinereum and third ventricular floor (due to tubo-mammillary fusion, **Figs. 23A and B**) or two glands and stalk can be identified. Associated anomalies with larger craniopharyngeal canals include callosal dysgenesis, facial dysmorphism and defects (i.e. frontonasal dysplasia) and various degrees of transsphenoidal meningoencephaloceles presenting as nasopharyngeal masses.

Pituitary Hypoplasia and Congenital Pituitary Deficiency Disorders

This group of deficiency disorders are recognized clinically by growth failure, short stature and occasionally by other anterior pituitary hormone deficiencies.[34] There may be a history of birth trauma, anoxia or associated anomalies of development of midline structures suggestive of a development lesion. The findings are a small pituitary fossa and kissing carotids on CT. On MRI absent or thread like stalk, small adenohypophysis (less than 2 mm high) and ectopic bright spot can be seen **(Figs. 24A and B)**. Associated abnormalities include Chiari I, absent septum pellucidum, ocular and frontal lobe dysgenesis. Absence stalk correlates with multiple hormonal deficiencies and truncated or thin stalk is seen more frequently in isolated GH deficiency.[34] MRI abnormalities may help determine the severity of congenital hormone deficiency syndromes.

Empty Sella

A thin diaphragm, a sellae and a large hiatus in it are responsible for invagination of CSF space into sella leading to empty sella and compression of the gland (primary empty sella). Empty sella may be secondary to surgery and postpartum necrosis too **(Fig. 25)**. This finding may be seen normally in older patients. The symptoms are nonspecific and include memory loss, dizziness and headache. Severe cases may present with CSF rhinorrhea, endocrinopathy or visual field loss due to herniation of optic chiasma into the sella. Imaging typically reveals invagination of suprasellar cistern into the sella compressing the gland against the floor. Typical central position of the infundibulum is a useful sign to rule out a cystic lesion in the suprasellar region.[5]

Diabetes Insipidus

This condition results from lack of ADH. In non-nephrogenic diabetes insipidus, destruction of the ADH producing hypothalamic nuclei, the hypothalamic receptors or the proximal stalk may disrupt the transport of vasopressin via the pituitary stalk to the neurohypophysis. Trauma and operative procedures together account for 50% of cases. Suprasellar/intrasellar neoplasms and granulomatous/inflammatory processes are the other major causes. One-third of all cases are, however, idiopathic.[5,35] The role of imaging in nontraumatic cases is to rule out suprasellar or intrasellar pathology. Stalk transection may be demonstrated on MR.[35] The other consistent observation is lack of visualization of the posterior pituitary bright spot on T1WI irrespective of the cause of diabetes insipidus **(Table 5, Fig. 26)**.[34-36] This bright signal in the posterior lobe is a normal finding due to neurovesicles containing vasopressin in axonal endings seen in 60–98% of normal scans.[2] However, it is important to perform a high resolution thin contiguous section imaging of the gland to avoid false positive results. Patients with psychogenic polydipsia have a normal bright posterior

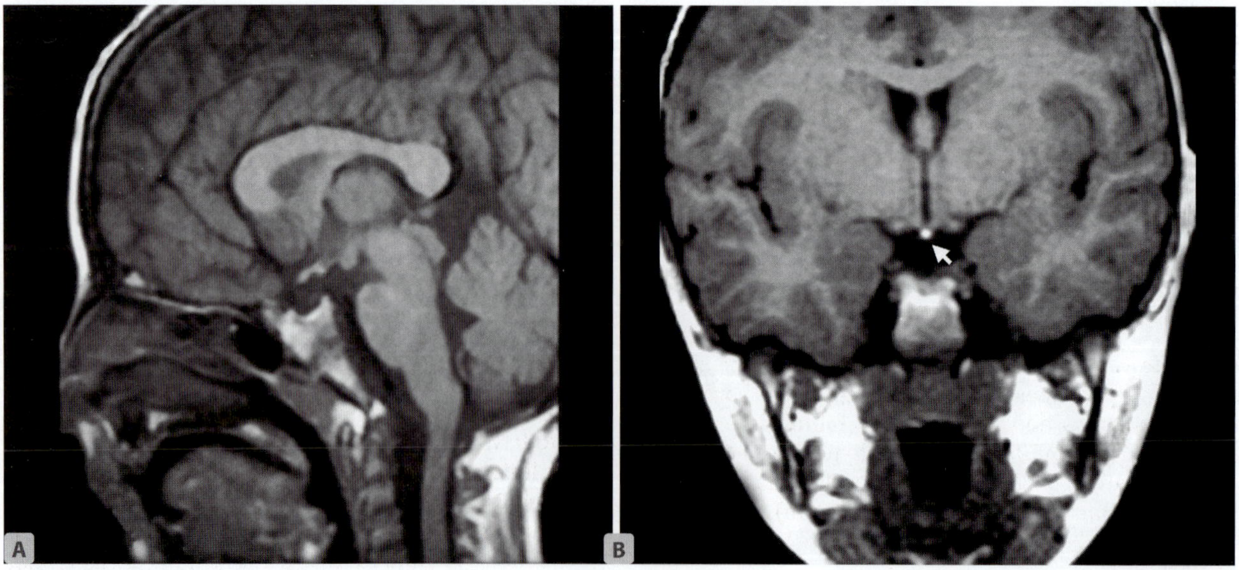

FIGS. 24A AND B: Pituitary hypoplasia in a child with retarded growth. T1 sagittal image (A) shows a small pituitary gland, absent stalk and ectopic bright spot near the hypothalamus [better seen on coronal T1 image (B) arrow].

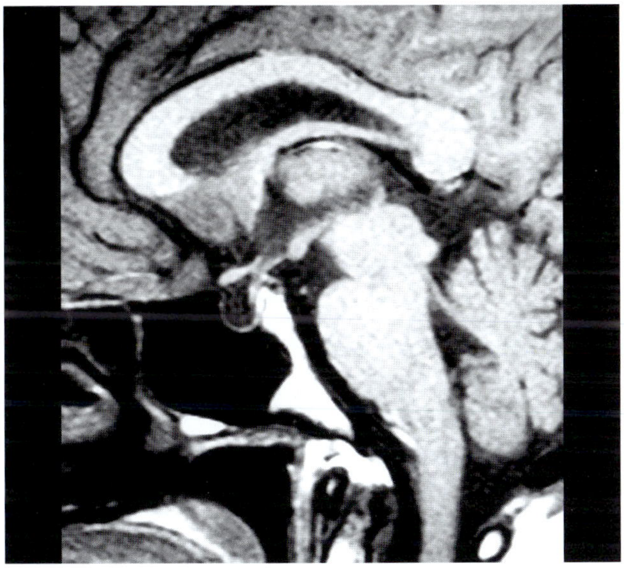

FIG. 25: Empty sella: Pituitary gland is not visualized on this T1 sagittal image, secondary to postpartum necrosis. The stalk is seen extending to the floor.

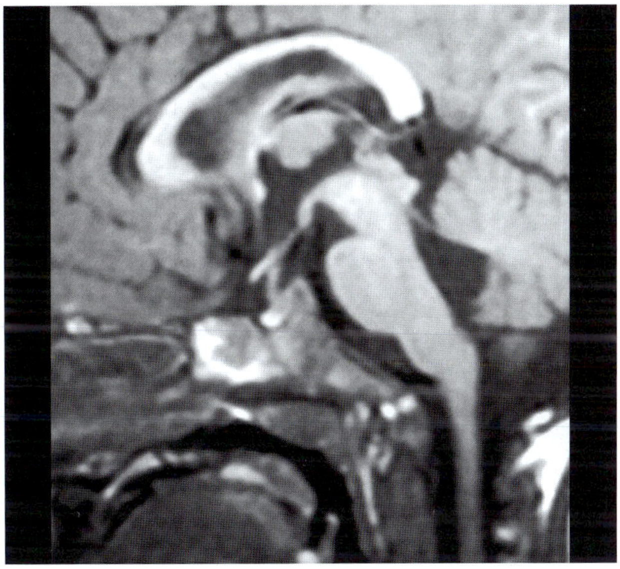

FIG. 26: Diabetes insipidus in a child: Absence of pituitary bright spot on T1 sagittal image with a normal stalk and no other demonstrable intra/suprasellar pathology.

TABLE 5: Central diabetes insipidus.
Etiology
• Trauma or surgery—50% of cases
• Idiopathic—25% of cases
• Craniopharyngioma
• Hypothalamic glioma
• Germinoma
• Granulomatous disease

pituitary as their hypothalamic-neurohypophyseal axis is intact.[35]

Hemochromatosis

Gonadotrophs are particularly susceptible to iron deposition and their dysfunction is reflected in the clinical picture. T2-weighted MR images showing an abnormally dark pituitary gland is the only means of showing iron overload in the pituitary tissue.[37]

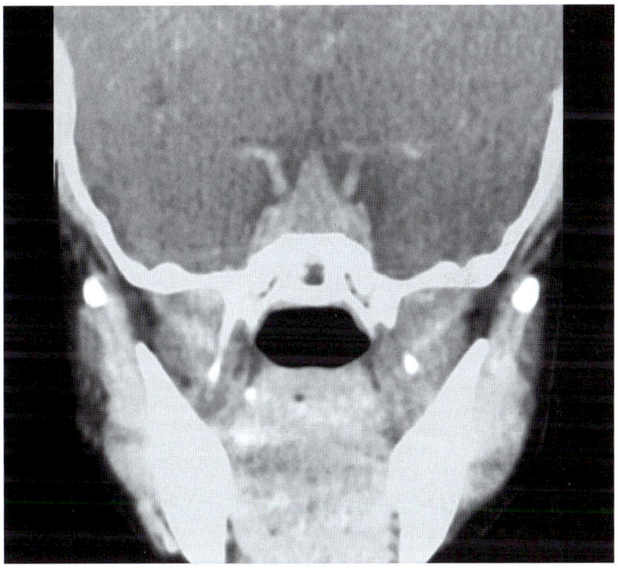

FIG. 27: Pituitary hyperplasia: Diffuse enlargement of the gland on CECT coronal section in a patient of hypothyroidism.

TUMOR-LIKE LESIONS

Pituitary Hyperplasia

Physiological enlargement of the gland can be seen normally (*see* **Table 1**). Glandular enlargement can also be seen in response to exogenous estrogens, extrapituitary hormonally active neoplasms and in end organ failure like primary hypothyroidism due to thyrotroph hyperplasia **(Fig. 27)**. Imaging shows an enlarged homogenously enhancing gland with convex superior margin (size >10–15 mm).

Arachnoid Cysts

Arachnoid cysts are frequent incidental findings in anterior or middle cranial fossae with 15% being juxtasellar.[38] They are usually developmental lesions due to lack of fenestration of membrane of Liliequist. They may also be acquired secondary to adhesions (due to arachnoiditis, trauma and hemorrhage). They are often asymptomatic but may present with hydrocephalus, hypopituitarism or seizures.

Both MRI and CT show a well-defined, nonenhancing cystic lesion with or without remodeling of skull base **(Figs. 28A and B)**. Differential diagnoses include an enlarged third ventricle, craniopharyngioma, epidermoid, Rathke'sand ependymal/parasitic cysts. Enhancement and calcification are usually seen in craniopharyngioma, while signal intensity greater than CSF on T1/proton images and less rounded shape are hallmarks of epidermoid cysts. FLAIR and diffusion

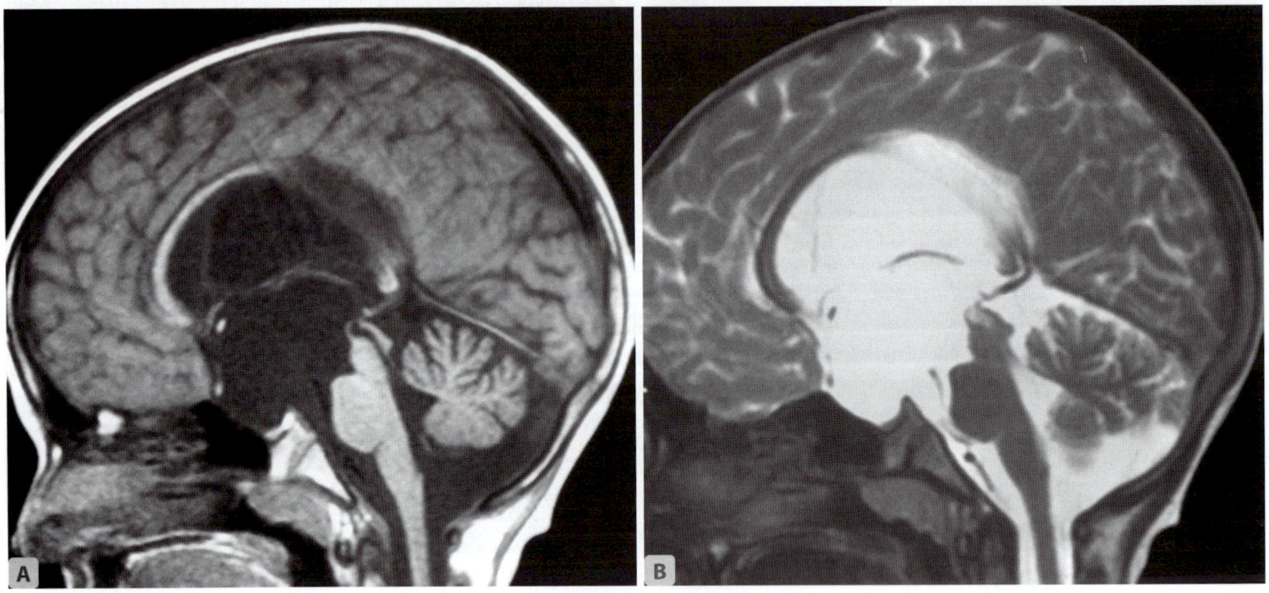

FIGS. 28A AND B: Arachnoid cyst: T1 and T2 sagittal MR images. The cyst appears hypointense on T1 and hyperintense on T2. The sella is normal with normal pituitary gland.

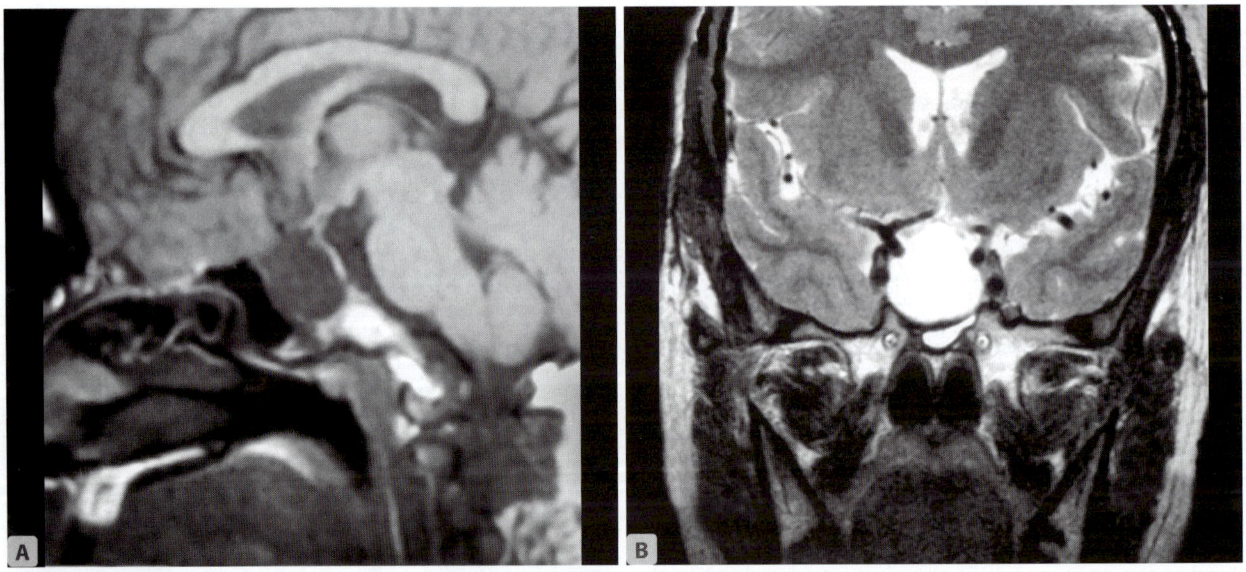

FIGS. 29A AND B: Rathke's cleft cyst: T1 sagittal (A) and T2 coronal (B) MR images. The cyst appears hypointense on T1 and hyperintense on T2 (like CSF). The sella is enlarged and stalk pushed posteriorly.

images characteristically show epidermoids as bright lesions. Arachnoid cysts may extend into the sella and need to be differentiated from empty sella. The key to diagnosis lies in the location of the pituitary stalk which will be displaced in case of arachnoid cyst. The differentiation from other cystic suprasellar lesions may be impossible without histology.[39]

Rathke's Cleft Cysts

This is a common incidental finding at autopsy (11.3% incidence).[40] They form as a result of failure of Rathke's pouch to completely regress. They occasionally become symptomatic due to compression of adjacent structures. The cyst may contain mucoid, serous or cellular debris.[41] Most of the lesions are small, located within the gland in midline or may be large, suprasellar anterior to the stalk and compress pituitary, infundibulum or chiasma.

The imaging findings depend on cyst contents. Mucoid contents may appear hyperintense on T1 and T2WI, thus indistinguishable from craniopharyngiomas. Serous cysts will have features of typical benign cysts (CSF-like intensity) **(Figs. 29A and B)**. Cellular debris may sometimescause a diagnostic problem.[5] However, the lesions only show a faint rim of enhancement. Lack of solid nodular enhancement is a useful differentiating point from necrosed adenomas and along with lack of calcification from craniopharyngiomas.[3,5,25]

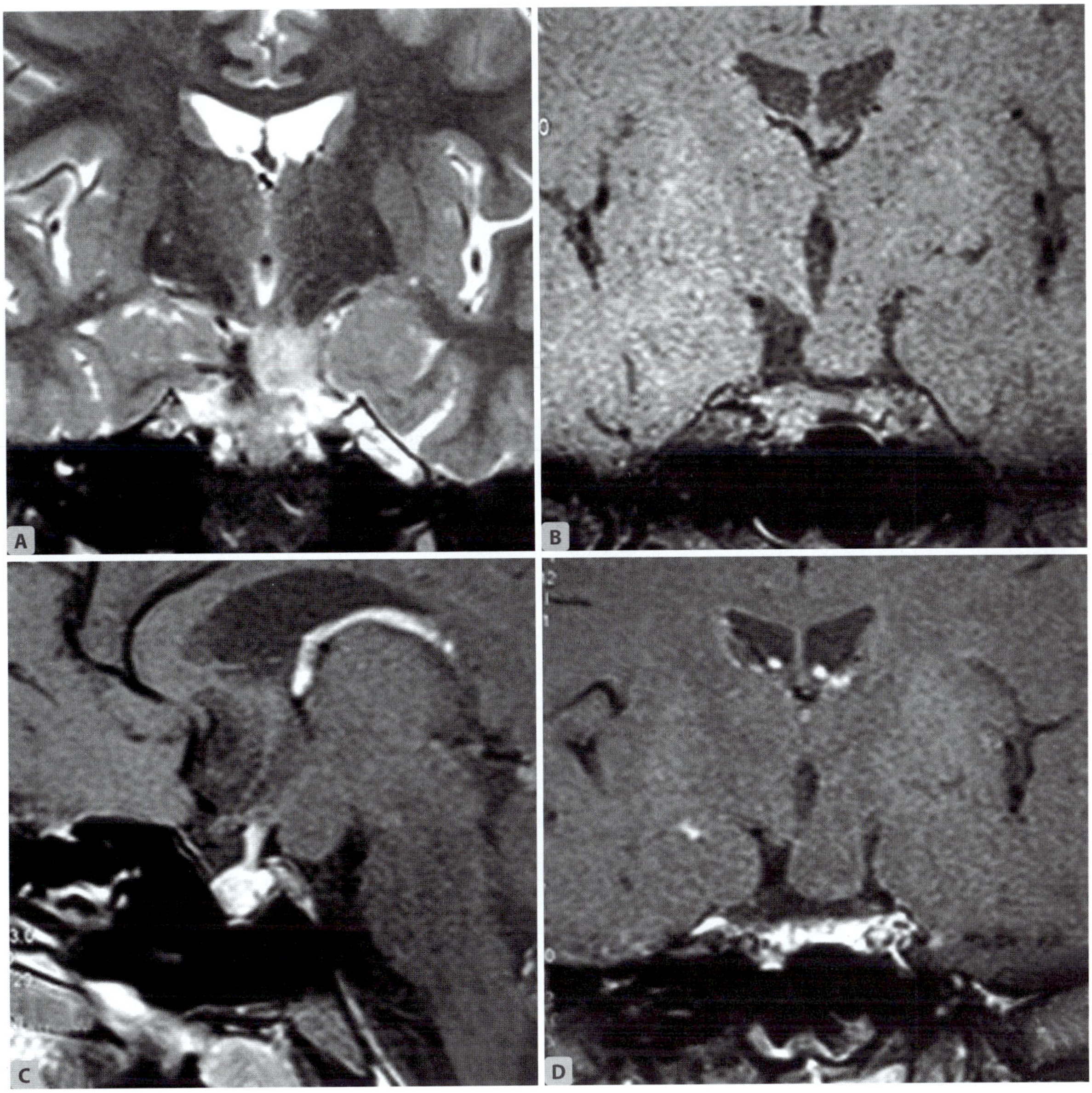

FIGS. 30A TO D: Tuber cinereum hamartoma: Coronal T2 (A) and T1 (B) weighted images reveal a sessile lesion (isointense to grey matter) typically located between mammillary body and infundibulum of pituitary gland. Gadolinium enhanced sagittal (C) and coronal (D) sections show no significant enhancement.

Tuber Cinereum Hamartoma

These are slow growing non-neoplastic heterotopias arising from the tuber cinereum (region between infundibulum and the mammillary bodies).[42] These patients present commonly with precocious puberty [secretion of luteinizing hormone-releasing hormone (LHRH)] and rarely with gelastic seizures (limbic lobe involvement) and mental impairment. On imaging they are sessile, nonenhancing, noncalcified, pedunculated, solid masses isointense to grey matter on T1 and T2WI but may be bright on T2WI **(Figs. 30A to D)**. Clinical history, location and morphology allow a straightforward diagnosis.

INFECTIVE CONDITIONS

Acute infections of hypothalamus and pituitary are rare. Pyogenic, viral, parasitic and tubercular infections, syphilis, candida, toxoplasma and cryptococcosis may affect these structures. A rare but well-described infective pathology is a pituitary bacterial abscess which can occur by hematogenous or direct spread. Infections in up to 30% cases arise in pre-existing lesions like adenoma, craniopharyngioma and Rathke's cleft cyst.[43] Abscesses are ring enhancing hypodense lesions on CT or appear as hypointense masses on T1WI showing bright signal on T2WI images. They are difficult to distinguish from other lesions, particularly adenoma and a

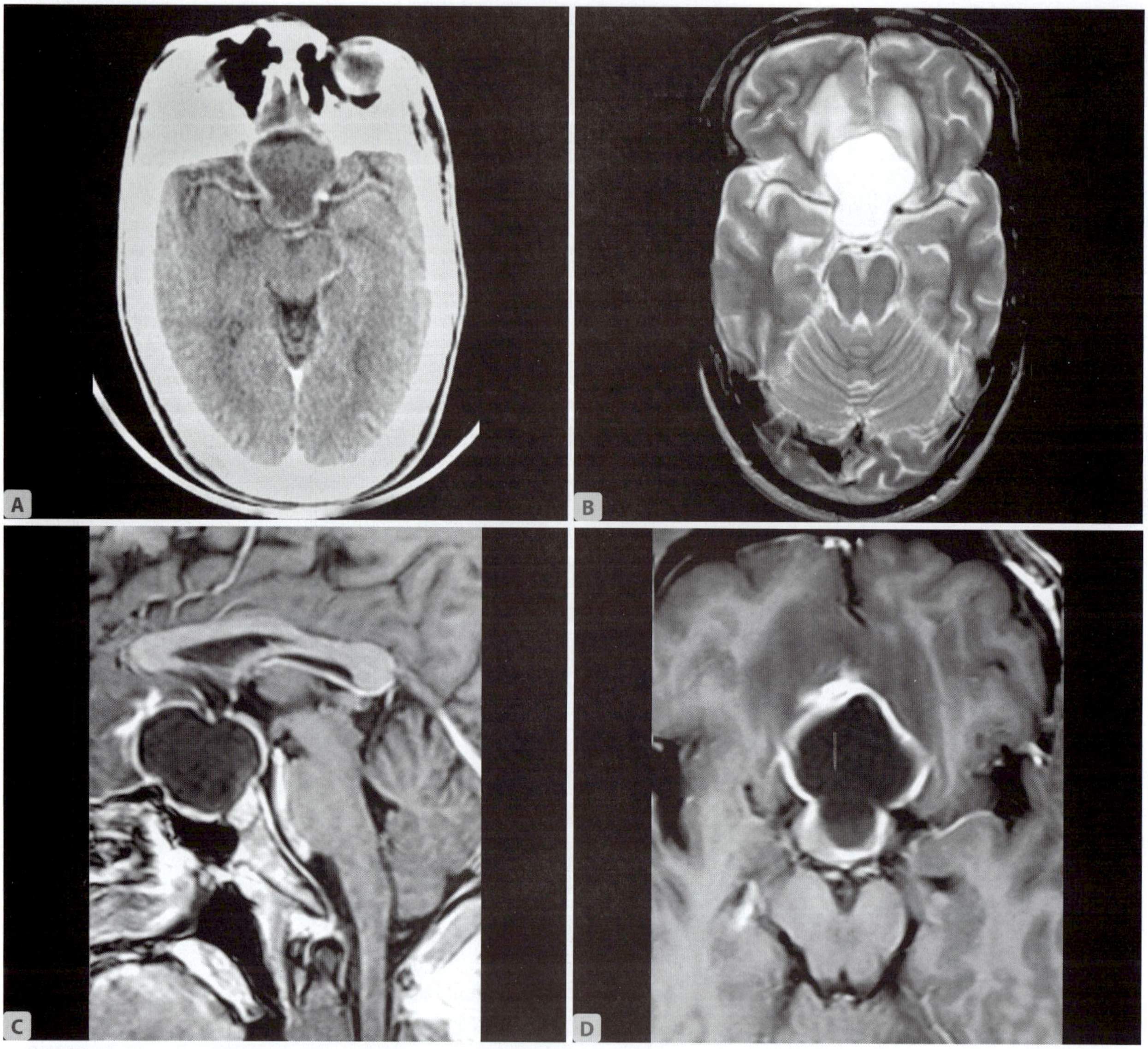

FIGS. 31A TO D: CECT axial (A), MR T2 axial (B), CE MR sagittal and axial (C and D) images show a surgically proven suprasellar tubercular abscess. Note the fluid intensity center, smooth peripheral rim enhancement (C and D) and associated edema in brain (B) indicating an inflammatory lesion.

diagnosis is rarely made preoperatively.[44] Infections in the parasellar region are more common than sellar infections and are usually part of disseminated disease or secondary to sinus infection. Basal meningitis affects this region in tuberculosis and other granulomatous infections. Tuberculosis is a common cause of meningitis and frequently shows thick basal exudates, infundibular involvement, hydrocephalus and brain infarction. Rarely tuberculosis can affect pituitary gland and but isolated tuberculomas or abscesses in the suprasellar cisterns are not uncommon in our setting **(Figs. 31A to D)**. Infections of cavernous sinus spread from a periorbital or paranasal source via the veins. Enhanced scans best show these lesions.

Fungal Infection

Increasing incidence of chronic indolent (granulomas) or fulminant fungal infection of sellar/parasellar region has been observed primarily as part of invasive rhinonasal disease by *Aspergillus* and mucormycosis. Immune compromised and diabetic patients are particularly prone. Paranasal sinus disease with headache, meningitis, altered sensorium, skull base/cavernous sinus or orbital apex syndromes should raise this possibility. Sellar/parasellar area, orbital apex area may show T1/T2 isointense enhancing soft tissue often with concurrent PNS, parapharyngeal space and middle cranial fossa disease **(Figs. 32A and B)**. There may be associated carotid artery aneurysm, brain infarctions, abscesses and orbital involvement.

INFLAMMATORY/GRANULOMATOUS CONDITIONS

Langerhans Cell Histiocytosis

Formerly called histiocytosis X, this is a group of diseases characterized by proliferation of histiocytes.[5] There are unifocal

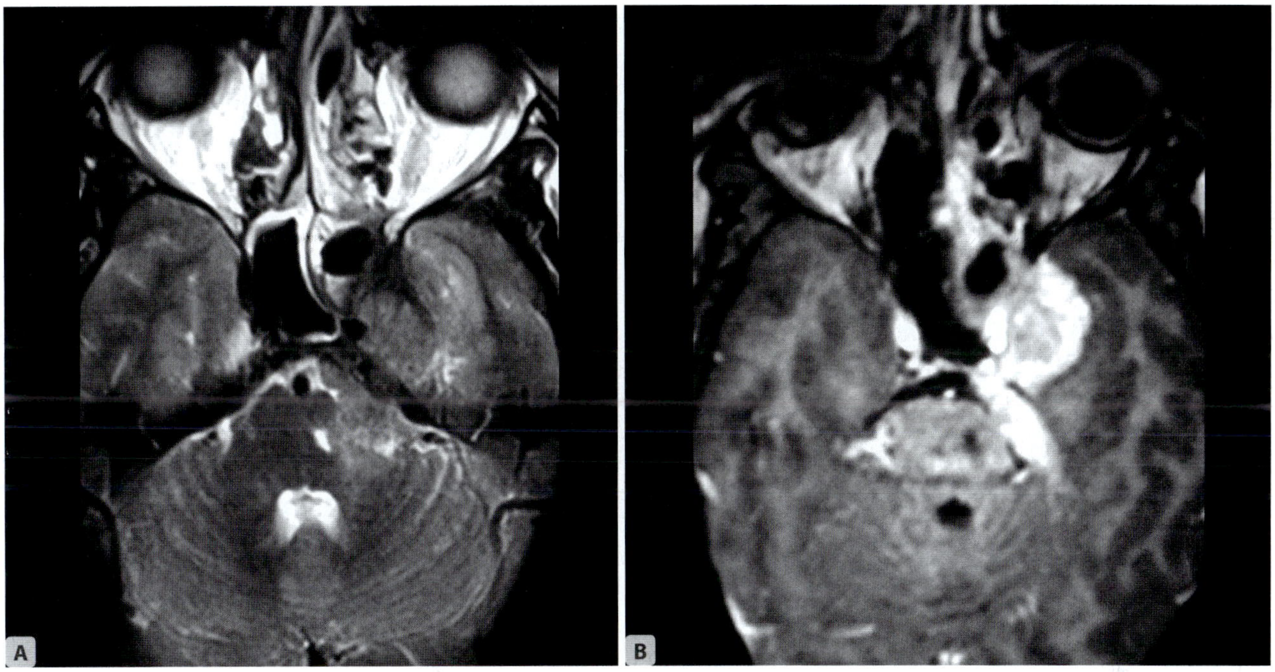

FIGS. 32A AND B: Fungal sinusitis with intracranial extension. Axial T2 (A) and gadolinium enhanced T1 (B) images showing spheno-ethmoid sinusitis with left parasellar and cavernous sinus invasion. Posterior extension into the prepontine and cerebellopontine angle cistern is also noted.

and multifocal forms of this disease. The unifocal disease shows solitary lytic bone lesion. This form spares the hypothalamic pituitary axis. The multifocal form of the disease is recurring, chronic, aggressive and presents in children with classical triad of diabetes insipidus, exophthalmos and lytic bone lesions (Hand-Schüller-Christian disease) due to granulomas in the hypothalamus and pituitary gland.

Computed tomography and MRI show thickening and enhancement of the infundibulum and hypothalamus **(Figs. 33A to D)**.[45] The posterior pituitary bright spot may be absent. The lesions are hyperintense on T2WI.[5] Differential diagnosis includes other suprasellar granulomas. Characteristic bone lesions and classical clinical picture aid in diagnosis of histiocytosis.

Lymphocytic Hypophysitis

This is noninfectious inflammatory process of autoimmune etiology affecting woman in late pregnancy or early postpartum period. The patient may present with severe hypopituitarism or with failure of lactation, headache, visual disturbances, etc. The condition regresses spontaneously with steroids. Pathologically, there is lymphocytic infiltration of the adenohypophysis or less commonly infundibulo-neuohypophysis or a combination of both. Imaging will show an intensely enhancing mass with or without extrasellar component. A thick nontapered enhancing stalk can be seen **(Figs. 34A to C)** as well as diaphragma sellae involvement (periglandular component). Seventy-five percent patients show loss of bright spot. Hence both pre- and postcontrast scans are important. It is differentiated from Sheehan's syndrome by lack of hemorrhage. Physiological enlargement of gland in pregnancy rarely exceeds 12 mm in height and does not show any extrasellar enhancing component.[46] Granulomatous giant cell hypophysitis in middle aged people is another idiopathic inflammatory condition of sellar structures.

Sarcoidosis

This multisystem granulomatous lesion involves the meninges and tracks along perivascular spaces.[47] Five percent patients show neurological findings—frequently cranial nerve palsy and diabetes insipidus. However, since any part of the CNS may be involved, clinical features vary.

Basal meningeal involvement is common in neurosarcoid and best seen on CECT and CEMR.[47] Multiple small nodular or large mass like enhancing lesions or distortion, thickening and enhancement of meninges and cranial nerves may be seen. The pituitary gland infundibulum and hypothalamus may be involved. Multiple scattered parenchymal lesions also suggest a diagnosis of neurosarcoid.[5]

Differential diagnosis is with other granulomatous lesions. Presence of systemic disease in 60% of cases, steroid responsiveness, localized or generalized basal meningeal disease with scattered parenchymal nodules aid in diagnosis of sarcoidosis.

Tolosa–Hunt Syndrome

It is an idiopathic steroid responsive inflammatory lesion of the cavernous sinus causing painful ophthalmoplegia and visual defects. The condition can have recurrent attacks with remissions and is steroid responsive. It is a granulomatous inflammation pathologically similar to orbital pseudotumor which can cause periarteritis of carotid artery. Imaging findings of asymmetric enlargement of cavernous sinus, enhancing soft tissue in the orbital apex and prepontine cistern have been described **(Figs. 35A and B)**.

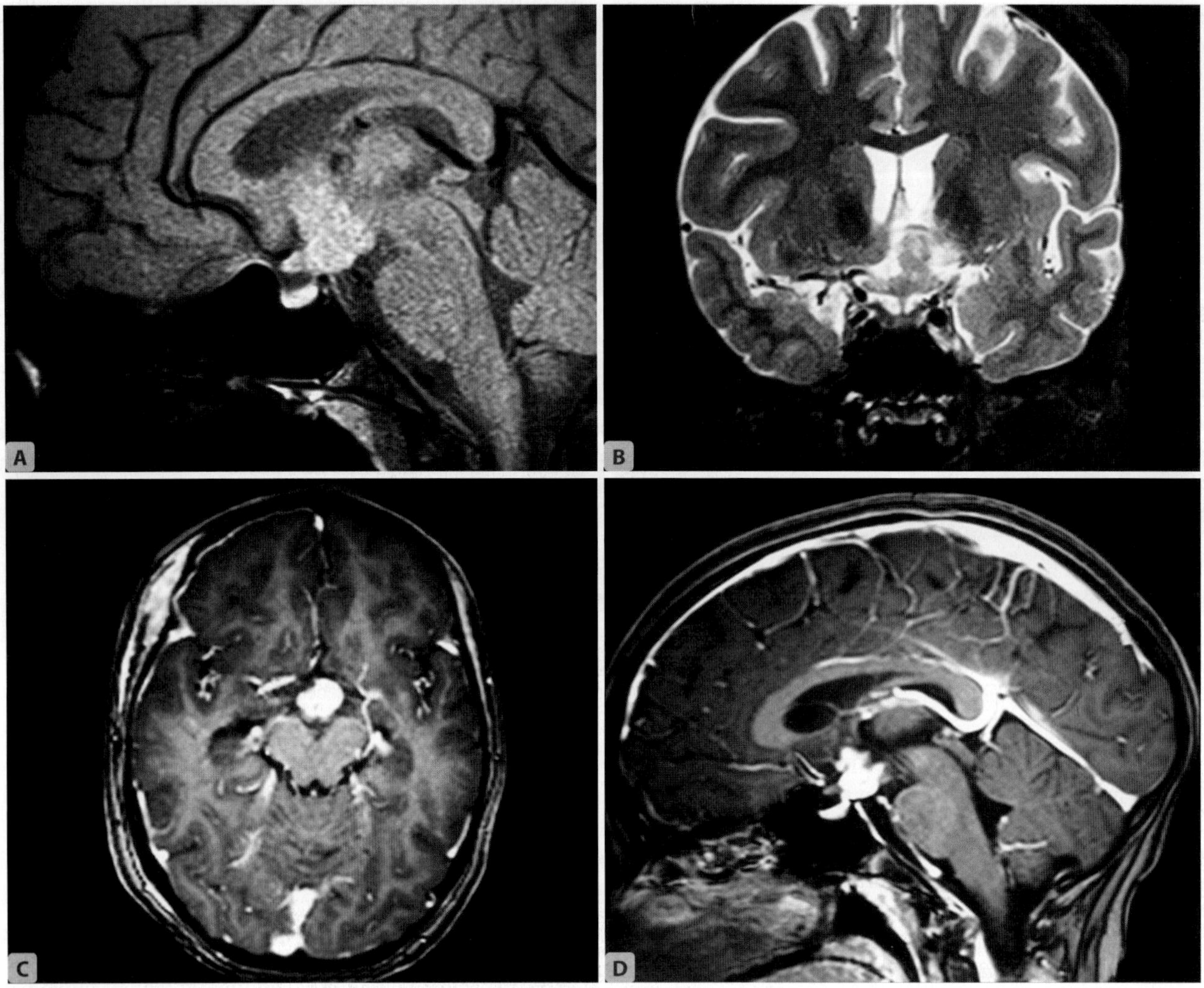

FIGS. 33A TO D: Langerhan's cell histiocytosis: Sagittal T1 WI (A) and coronal T2 WI (B) shows isointense thickening of hypothalamus and infundibulum which is showing strong enhancement (C and D). A bone lesion may be noted in the right frontal area (C).

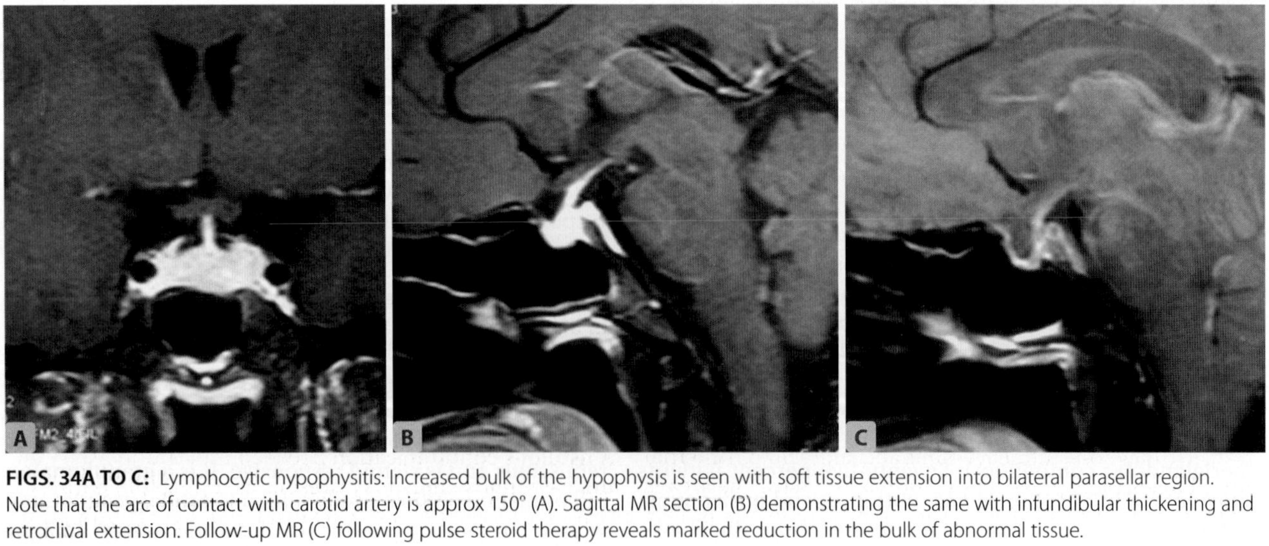

FIGS. 34A TO C: Lymphocytic hypophysitis: Increased bulk of the hypophysis is seen with soft tissue extension into bilateral parasellar region. Note that the arc of contact with carotid artery is approx 150° (A). Sagittal MR section (B) demonstrating the same with infundibular thickening and retroclival extension. Follow-up MR (C) following pulse steroid therapy reveals marked reduction in the bulk of abnormal tissue.

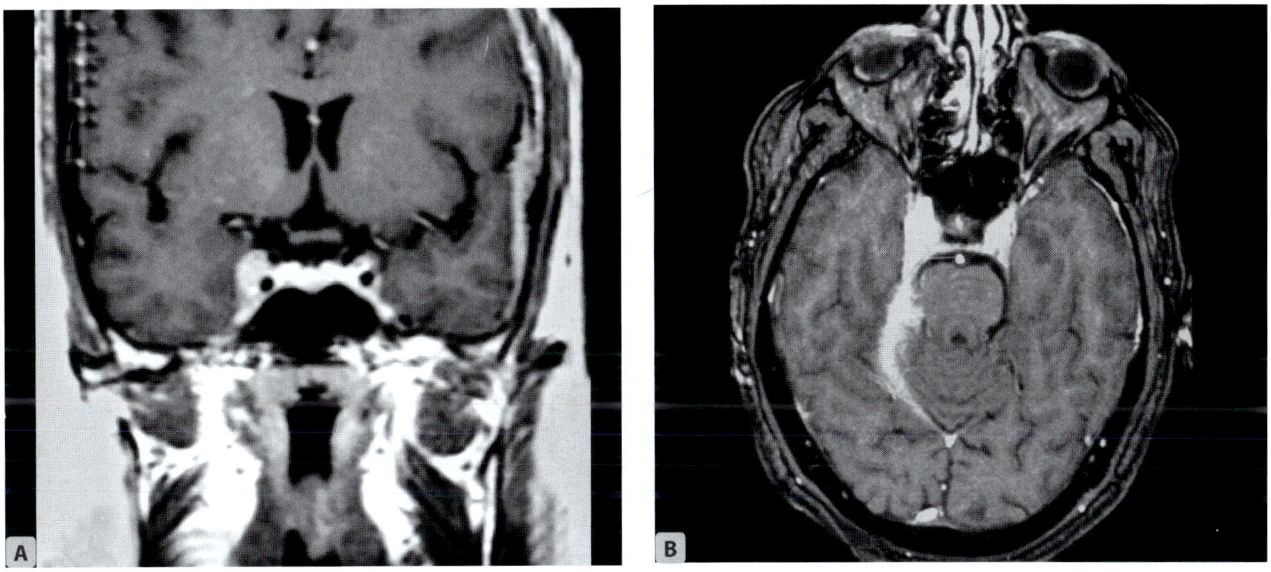

FIGS. 35A AND B: Tolosa-Hunt syndrome: Contrast enhanced T1 coronal (A) and axial GRE image (B) shows abnormal enhancing soft tissue in the region of right cavernous sinus, extending into the tentorium cerebelli in a patient with headache.

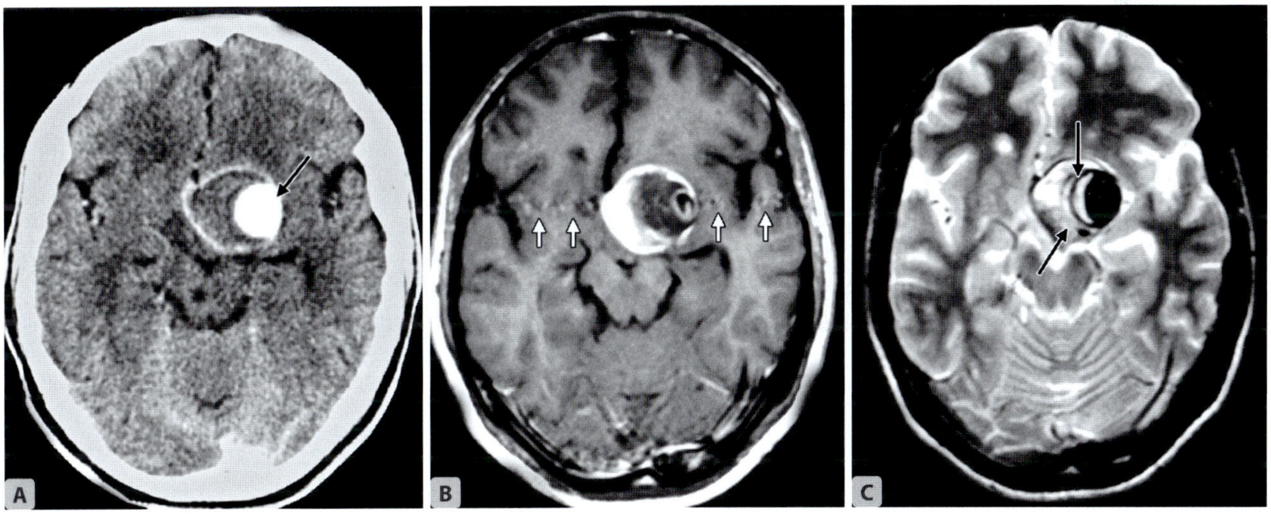

FIGS. 36A TO C: Axial sections CECT (A), T1 SE (B) and T2 FSE (C) show partly thrombosed suprasellar aneurysm arising from left ICA bifurcation. Note layered thrombus (arrows in C) and patent lumen on the left side of the lesion which enhances on CECT (arrow in A). Note pulsation artifacts in phase direction (arrows in B).

The soft tissue typically shows isointensity to muscle on T1 and to fat on T2-weighted images.[48] Similar intensity patterns are also shared by lymphomas, meningiomas and sarcoidosis.

VASCULAR LESIONS

Aneurysms and Vascular Loops

Critical to diagnose, intracavernous and supraclinoid internal carotid aneurysms present as juxtasellar masses. The area is the most common site of giant aneurysms. These may project into the sella and show contiguity with vascular structures, flow void on MRI, strong contrast enhancement and can be easily picked up by CT/CT angiography. Partially thrombosed aneurysms may cause diagnostic difficulty but lamellated thrombus, flow characteristics including artifacts in phase encoding direction, surrounding blood products in various stages of evolution, etc. are distinctive findings of aneurysms on MRI **(Figs. 36A to C)**.[49]

Carotid Cavernous Fistula and Vascular Malformations

A fistulous communication between the carotid artery and the cavernous sinus may present as a pulsatile parasellar lesion due to enlarged arterialized cavernous sinus. Patients present with chemosis, proptosis and visual loss. Presence of flow artifacts, enlarged cavernous sinus and superior ophthalmic vein suggest the diagnosis which is

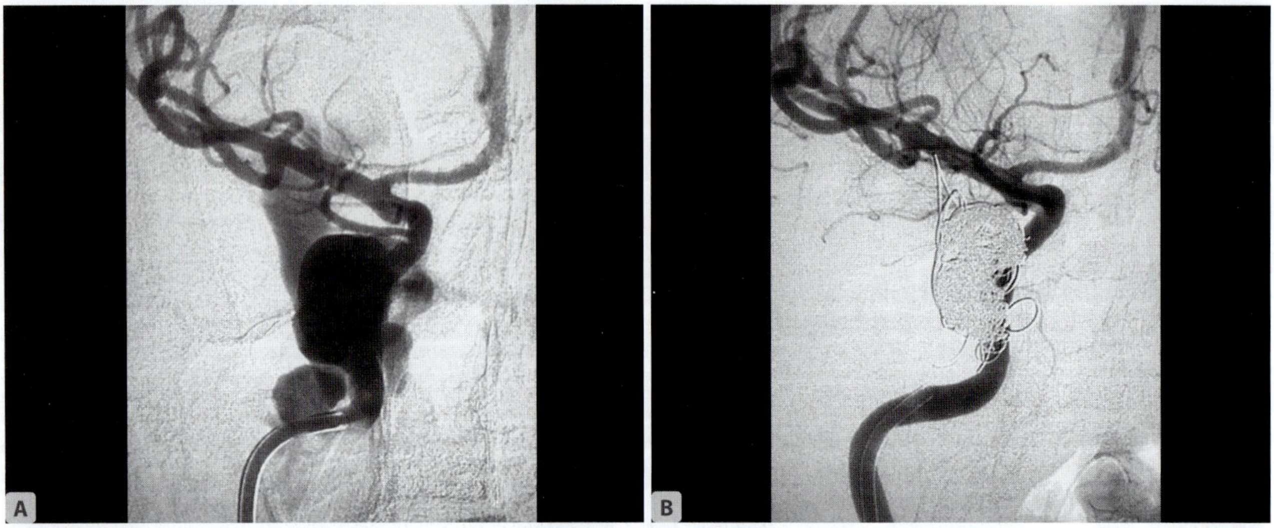

FIGS. 37A AND B: Caroticocavernous fistula (CCF): Digital subtraction angiogram (DSA) of the right internal carotid artery (A) demonstrating immediate opacification of the cavernous sinus through the cavernous ICA segment. Post coil embolization (B) DSA showing complete fistula closure.

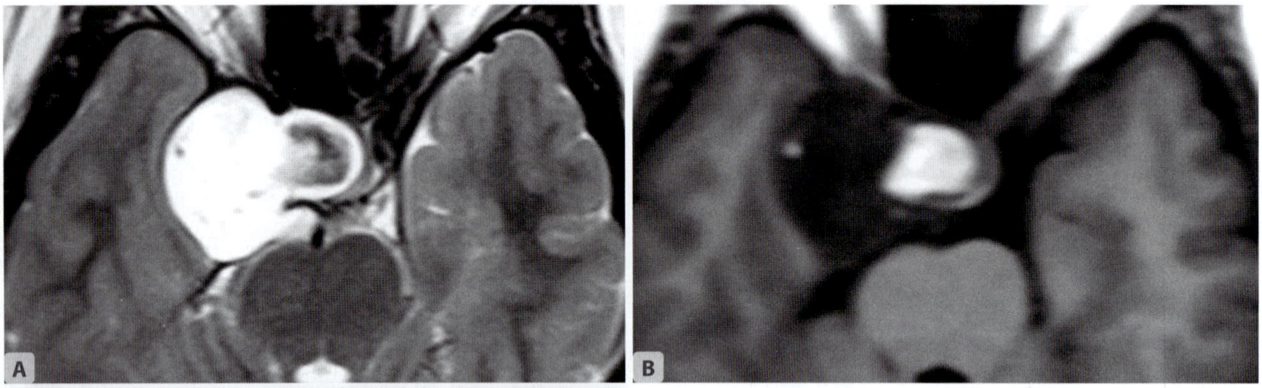

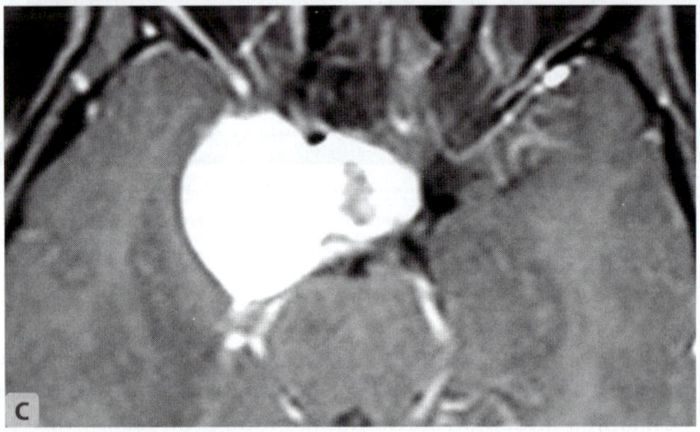

FIGS. 38A TO C: Cavernous sinus hemangioma: Axial T2 (A), T1 (B) and gadolinium enhanced T1 (C) weighted images showing a well-defined right cavernous sinus lesion exhibiting marked T2 hyperintensity and brilliant postcontrast enhancement. Hyperintensity on T1 indicates hemorrhage.

confirmed on an angiographic study. Digital subtraction angiography shows immediate opacification of the cavernous sinus on internal carotid artery (ICA) injection with communication at the level of the cavernous segment of ICA **(Fig. 37A)**. This fistulous communication can be embolized by either detachable balloon or coils **(Fig. 37B)**. Extra-axial cavernous malformations rarely present in supra/parasellar area and should be suspected if an atypical mass with T2 hyperintensity is seen. Cavernous sinus hemangiomas classically show intense T2 hyperintensity with T hypointensity and brilliant enhancement on gadolinium administration **(Figs. 38A to C)**. Dynamic contrast enhanced images show progressive centripetal enhancement of the lesion.

Sheehan's Syndrome

This is a syndrome of postpartum pituitary necrosis in complicated deliveries with clinical and imaging features similar to pituitary apoplexy in the acute phase.[50] However, there is no sellar mass and circulatory disturbances lead to hemorrhage and necrosis of a vulnerable hyperplasic gland secondary to pregnancy related changes.[5,50] The end result may be an empty sella.

CONCLUSION

Though a small zone spatially, the sellar region harbours many structures and hence many pathologies related to these structures. A thorough understanding of its anatomy and structures in its vicinity is of prime importance in formulating an appropriate diagnosis of pathologies in this region. MR has transformed the evaluation of sellar lesions and currently forms the backbone of sellar evaluation. An optimal utilization of the MR techniques helps us in understanding the disease process better. A good correlation of anatomy, clinical symptomatology and imaging (MR) evaluation often clinches the diagnosis.

REFERENCES

1. Latchaw RE, Roppole HMN. Radiographic evaluation of the normal sellaturcica and the pituitary gland. In: Radiology Diagnosis Imaging Intervention, Volume 3. Philadelphia: JB Lippincott Co.; 1986. pp. 1-7.
2. Fujisawa I, Asato R, Nishimura K, et al. Anterior and posterior lobes of pituitary gland, assessment by 1.5T MR imaging. J Comput Assist Tomogr. 1987;11(2):214-20.
3. Elster AD. Imaging of sella: anatomy and pathology. Semin Ultrasound CT MR. 1993;14(3):182-94.
4. Cox TD, Elster AD. Normal pituitary gland: changes in shape, size and signal intensity during the 1st year of life at MR imaging. Radiology. 1991;179(3):721-4.
5. Symons SP, Aviv RI, Montanera WJ, et al. The sella turcica and parasellar region. In: Atlas SW (Ed). Magnetic Resonance Imaging of the Brain and Spine, 5th edition. Philadelphia: Lippincott Williams and Wilkins; 2016. pp. 1120-92.
6. Pressman BD. Pituitary Imaging. Endocrinol Metab Clin North Am. 2017;46:713-40.
7. Pinker K, Ba-Ssalamah A, Wolfsberger S, et al. The value of high field MRI (3T) in the assessment of sellar lesions. Eur J Radiol. 2005;54(3):327-34.
8. Kovacs K, Horvath E, Asa SL. Classification and pathology of pituitary tumors. In: Wilkins RH, Rengachary SS (Eds). Neurosurgery. New York: McGraw-Hill; 1985. pp. 834-42.
9. Hall WA, Lunciano MG, Doppman JL, et al. Pituitary magnetic resonance imaging in normal human volunteers: occult adenomas in general population. Ann Int Med. 1994;120(10): 817-20.
10. Go JL, Rajamohan AG. Imaging of the sella and parasellar region. Radiol Clin North Am. 2017;55(1):83-101.
11. Grober Y, Grober H, Wintermark M, et al. Comparison of MRI techniques for detecting microadenomas in Cushing's disease. J Neurosurg. 2017;28:1-7.
12. Schwartzberg DG. Imaging of pituitary gland tumors. Semin Ultrasound CT MR. 1992;13(3):207-23.
13. Zampetti B, Grossrubatscher E, Dalino Ciaramella P, et al. Bilateral inferior petrosal sinus sampling. Endocr Connect. 2016;5(4): R12-25.
14. Bonnelli FS, Huston J, Carpenter PC, et al. Adrenocorticotropic Hormone-dependent Cushing's syndrome: sensitivity and specificity of inferior petrosal sinus sampling. Am J Neuroradiol. 2000;21(4):690-6.
15. Pierallini A, Caramia F, Falcone C, et al. Pituitary macroadenomas: preoperative evaluation of consistency with diffusion-weighted MR imaging-initial experience. Radiology. 2006;239(1):223-31.
16. Knosp E, Steiner E, Kitz K, et al. Pituitary adenomas with invasion of the cavernous sinus space. A magnetic resonance imaging classification compared with surgical findings. Neurosurgery. 1993;33:610.
17. Micko AS, Wöhrer A, Wolfsberger S, et al. Invasion of the cavernous sinus space in pituitary adenomas: endoscopic verification and its correlation with an MRI-based classification. J Neurosurg. 2015;122:803-11.
18. Edal AL, Skjödt K, Nepper-Rasmussen HJ. SIPAP: a new MR classification for pituitary adenomas. Suprasellar, infrasellar, parasellar, anterior and posterior. Acta Radiol. 1997;38:30-6.
19. Miki Y, Kanagaki M, Takahashi JA, et al. Evaluation of pituitary macroadenomas with multidetector-row CT (MDCT): comparison with MR imaging. Neuroradiology. 2007;49(4):327-33.
20. Ostrov SG, Quencer RM, Hoffman JC, et al. Hemorrhage within pituitary adenomas: how often associated with pituitary apoplexy syndrome? Am J Roentgenol. 1989;153(1):153-60.
21. Rogg JM, Tung GA, Anderson G, et al. Pituitary apoplexy: early detection with diffusion-weighted MR imaging. Am J Neuroradiol. 2002;23(7):1240-5.
22. Steiner E, Knosp E, Herold CJ, et al. Pituitary adenomas, findings of postoperative MR imaging. Radiology. 1992;185(2):521-7.
23. Crotty TB, Sheithauer BW, Young WF, et al. Papillary craniopharyngiomas: a clinico-pathological study of 48 cases. J Neurosurg. 1995;83(2):206-14.
24. Jellinger K. Primary intrasellar germ cell tumors. Acta Neuropathol. 1973;25(4):291-306.
25. Chong BW, Newton TH. Hypothalamic and pituitary pathology. Radiol Clin North Am. 1993;31(5):1147-53.
26. Conley FK. Epidermoid and dermoid tumor: clinical features and surgical management. In: Wilkins RG, Rengachary SS (Eds). Neurosurgery. New York: McGraw-Hill; 1985. pp. 668-70.
27. Takeuchi J, Handa HM, Nagata I. Suprasellar germinoma. J Neurosurg. 1978;49(1):41-8.
28. Hua F, Asato R, Miki T, et al. Differentiation of suprasellar non-neoplastic cysts from cystic neoplasms by Gd-DTPA MRI. J Comput Assist Tomogr. 1992;16(5):744-9.
29. Alshail E, Rutka JT, Becker LE, et al. Opticochiasmatic hypothalamic glioma. Brain Pathol. 1997;7(2):799-806.
30. Yuh WT, Wright DC Barloon TJ, et al. MR imaging of primary tumors of trigeminal nerve and Meckel's cave. Am J Roentgenol. 1988;151(3):577-82.
31. Sze G, Uichanco LS, Brant-Zawadzki MN, et al. Chordomas: MR Imaging. Radiology. 1988;166(1 Pt 1):187-91.
32. Schubiger O, Haller D. Metastasis to the pituitary hypothalamic axis. An MR study of 7 symptomatic patients. Neuroradiology. 1992;34(2):131-4.
33. Kizilkilic O, Yalcin O, Yildirim T, et al. Hypothalamic hamartoma associated with craniopharyngeal canal. Am J Neuroradiol. 2005;26(1):65-7.
34. Fahrendorf G, Bramswig J, Bals-Pratsch M. MR findings in patients with idiopathic panhypopituitarism. Rofo. 1990;152(5): 550-5.

35. Tien R, Kucharczyk J, Kucharcyzk W. MR imaging of the brain in patients with diabetes insipidus. Am J Neuroradiol. 1991;12(3):533-42.
36. Fujisawa I, Nishimura K, Asato R, et al. Posterior lobe of pituitary in diabetes insipidus: MR findings. J Comput Assist Tomogr. 1987;11(2):221-5.
37. Fujisawa I, Morikawa M, Nakano Y, et al. Hemochromatosis of pituitary gland, MR imaging. Radiology. 1988;168:213-4.
38. Wiener SN, Pearlstein AE, Eiber A. MR imaging of intracranial arachnoid cysts. J Comput Assist Tomogr. 1987;11(2):236-41.
39. Gentry LR, Smoker WR, Turski PA, et al. Suprasellar arachnoid cysts: 1. CT recognition. Am J Neuroradiol. 1986;7(1):79-86.
40. Teramoto A, Hirakawa K, Sanno N, et al. Incidental pituitary lesions in 1,000 unselected autopsy specimens. Radiology. 1994;193(1): 161-4.
41. Kucharczyk W, Peck WW, Kelly WM, et al. Rathke cleft cysts: CT, MR imaging and pathological features. Radiology. 1987;165(2): 491-5.
42. Boyko OB, Curnes JT, Oakes WJ, et al. Hamartomas of tuber cinereum CT, MR and pathological findings. Am J Neuroradiol. 1991;12(2):309-14.
43. Domingue JN, Wilson CB. Pituitary abscesses. Report of seven cases and review of literature. J Neurosurgery. 1977;46(5):601-8.
44. Dutta P, Bhansali A, Singh P, et al. Pituitary abscess: report of four cases and review of literature. Pituitary. 2006;9(3):267-73.
45. Tien RD Newton TH, McDermott MW, et al. Thickened pituitary stalk on MR images in patients with diabetes insipidus and Langerhans cell histiocytosis. Am J Neuroradiol. 1990;11(4):703-8.
46. Ahmadi J, Meyers GD, Segall HD, et al. Lymphocytic adenohypophysitis: contrast-enhanced MR imaging in five cases. Radiology. 1995;195(1):30-4.
47. Sherman JL, Stern BJ. Sarcoidosis of the CNS: comparison of unenhanced and enhanced MR images. Am J Neuroradiol. 1990;11(5):915-23.
48. Yousem DM, Atlas SW, Grossman RI, et al. MR imaging of Tolosa-Hunt syndrome. Am J Neuroradiol. 1989;10(6):1181-4.
49. Atlas SW, Mark AS, Fram EK, et al. Vascular intracranial lesions: applications of gradient echo MR Imaging. Radiology. 1988;169(2): 455-61.
50. Sheehan HL, Stanford JP. The pathogenesis of postpartum necrosis of the anterior lobe of the pituitary gland. Acta Endocrinol. 1961;37:479-510.

CHAPTER

199

Intraventricular Lesions

Chirag Kamal Ahuja, Paramjeet Singh, Niranjan Khandelwal

INTRODUCTION

The ventricular system forms an important compartment of the brain with cerebrospinal fluid (CSF) playing the major role of hemodynamic regulation, lubrication and scavenging. It may harbor many different lesions, some of which can be native to it while others may infiltrate from surrounding structures and some even from distant areas through CSF pathways. Intraventricular (IV) lesions can be congenital, inflammatory/infective, traumatic or neoplastic.[1,2] Categorization of IV lesions can often be challenging, especially of the larger ones, as many of these arise in the paraventricular region and efface or grow into the adjoining ventricle. Native IV lesions are fewer in number. There is a predilection of certain lesions for specific age groups and locations. Diagnosis of an IV lesion thus should involve a comprehensive evaluation of the patient's age and clinical symptomatology in addition to imaging findings.[1,3] Tumors constitute the major bulk of intraventricular lesions, though contributing less than 10% of all intracranial tumors.[4] In this chapter, IV lesions are described according to their location within various parts of ventricular system with particular emphasis on the more common lesions.

IMAGING MODALITIES

1. ***Plain skull radiograph***: This may demonstrate calcification within the lesion and evidence of raised intracranial tension. Associated features of syndromic disorders can be seen at times, e.g. cyst-like or sclerotic bone lesions in tuberous sclerosis.
2. ***Plain and contrast enhanced computed tomography (CT)***: CT may aid in lesion characterization and confirm or refute the presence of calcification. Multi detector computed tomography (MDCT) may help in better localization through its multiplanar capability with the help of volumetric data acquisition.
3. ***Conventional ventriculography/CT ventriculography***: These investigations have become obsolete with the advent of magnetic resonance imaging (MRI).
4. ***Magnetic resonance imaging***: It has transformed the way we look at intracranial lesions with its exquisite resolution and multiplanar capability.
5. ***Angiography***: Indicated in vascular malformations and for angioembolization.

A sound understanding of the ventricular lesions requires a thorough knowledge of the anatomy and physiology of the ventricular system. Thus, a brief overview of the ventricles is presented before discussing the various intraventricular lesions.

ANATOMY AND PHYSIOLOGY OF VENTRICULAR SYSTEM

The ventricular system (*Latin*: ventriculus = cavity) is constituted by two lateral and two median ventricles, the latter referred to as the third and fourth ventricles **(Fig. 1A)**. They are lined by ependymal cells and are filled with CSF which has free communication with each other as well as with the extra-axial cisternal spaces through the fourth ventricular outflow tracts. The CSF is produced by the choroid plexus (composed of specialized ependymal cells surrounding a core of capillaries and loose connective tissue) by the process of ultrafiltration and active secretion and flows with a pressure gradient through the ventricles and cisterns before being absorbed by the arachnoid granulations situated in relation to the dural venous sinuses. The lesions in the ventricles can thus, arise per se from within or adjacent to the ventricles or may spread secondarily via CSF or be of hematogenous origin, the latter being extremely rare. Most commonly the lesions are neoplastic in origin, with inflammatory and developmental ones being relatively uncommon. Some lesions can present in the form of diffusely spreading ependymal enhancement along the ventricular margins. These can be either of infective/inflammatory etiology or of neoplastic origin **(Fig. 1B)**. The various intraventricular lesions are described based on their location within the respective ventricles **(Fig. 1C)**. The lesions which are common to all ventricles and can be seen in any of them are mentioned in the box below in the Figure 19.1C. Common lesions in children and adults are tabulated in **Tables 1 and 2**.

Lateral Ventricular Lesions

Neoplasms constitute the major bulk of lateral ventricular lesions.[4] Intraventricular neoplasms constitute one-tenth

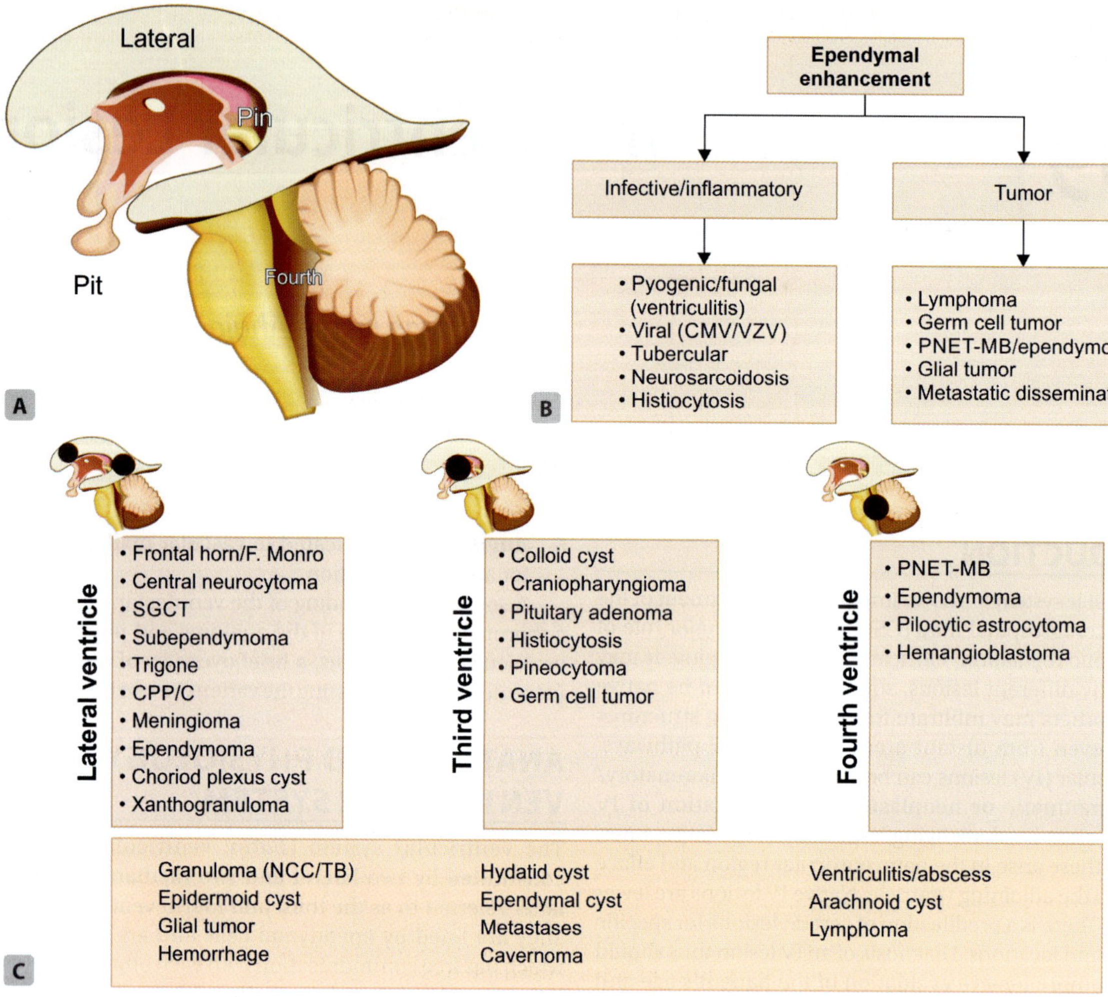

FIGS. 1A TO C: (A) Pictorial diagram of the relationship of the ventricular system with important adjoining structures; (B) Differentials of ependymal enhancement; (C) Distribution of the lesions according to location within the ventricular system. The reverse black box represents lesions common to all ventricles. (CMV: cytomegalovirus; CPP/C: choroid plexus papilloma/carcinoma; FM: foramen of Monro; Pin: pineal gland; Pit: pituitary gland; NCC: neurocysticercosis; PNET-MB: primitive neuroectodermal tumor-medulloblastoma; SGCT: subependymal giant cell tumor; TB: tuberculoma; VZV: Varicella-Zoster virus).

of all central nervous system (CNS) neoplasms.[1,2] About half of these in adults and one-fourth in children are found in the lateral ventricles.[5] The frequency and the type of tumor differs in different parts of the lateral ventricle (e.g. frontal horn, body, atrium, occipital horn). These tumors originate from the cells located within/in the vicinity of the ventricles. The ependymal cells lining the ventricles are the precursors of ependymomas. There is a subependymal plate composed of glial cells just beneath the ependymal lining from which the subependymomas are postulated to arise. Glial cells along with residual neuronal precursor cells line the septum pellucidum from which the central neurocytomas arise. Primary tumors of the choroid plexus (choroid plexus papilloma and carcinoma) originate from the cells of the vascular choroid plexus epithelium. The choroid plexus also contributes to the hematogenous deposition of various metastases. Meningiomas are thought to arise from the trapped arachnoid cap cells forming the arachnoid granulations. There can be secondary ventricular involvement by contiguous extension of lesions from the adjoining brain parenchyma. Apart from neoplasms, the lateral ventricle may harbor a number of developmental, inflammatory and infective lesions, e.g. ependymal cyst, neurocysticercus, hydatid cyst, extension of pyogenic abscess, etc.

In children, intraventricular neoplasms occur more often in the trigone, primarily because certain tumor types that favor the trigonal region have a predilection for occurring in children. Choroid plexus tumors are one of the most common lesions of the lateral ventricle in young children, and the majority occur within the trigone. Ependymomas and low grade astrocytomas [e.g. pilocytic astrocytomas and subependymal giant cell astrocytomas (SGCAs)] occur in the anterior body/trigonal region in older children and young adults. Intraventricular meningiomas typically occur in the trigonal region in older adults. Two non-neoplastic lesions that frequently present as trigonal lesions are choroid plexus cysts and xanthogranulomas, both of which are incidentally detected, benign, typically asymptomatic and are often

TABLE 1: Intraventricular lesions in children.

Lateral ventricle
• Choroid plexus papilloma/carcinoma
• Astrocytoma (low grade)
• Giant cell astrocytoma
• primitive neuroectodermal tumor (PNET)
Foramen of Monro
• Subependymal giant cell astrocytoma
• Astrocytoma
Third ventricle
• Craniopharyngioma
• Astrocytoma
• Histocytosis
• Germinoma
Fourth ventricle
• Astrocytoma
• Ependymoma
• Medulloblastoma

Note: Cysticercal cyst, hydatid cyst, granuloma (TB) can occur in any ventricle.

TABLE 2: Intraventricular lesions in adults.

Lateral ventricle
• Astrocytoma
• Meningioma
• Central neurocytoma
• Subependymoma
• Choroid plexus cyst/xanthogranulomas
• Metastasis
Foramen of Monro
• Astrocytoma
• Central neurocytoma
• Subependymal giant cell astrocytoma
Third ventricle
• Colloid cyst
• Extrinsic masses
• Metastasis
Aqueduct
• Hemorrhage
• Glioma
Fourth ventricle
• Epidermoid
• Arachnoid cyst
• Metastasis

Note: Cysticercal cyst; hydatid cyst, granuloma (TB) can occur in any ventricle particularly during the first two years of life. CPP is a benign tumor but carcinomatous degeneration occurs in up to 20% of patients. The usual presenting symptoms are related to hydrocephalus and increased intracranial pressure.

bilateral. The former are epithelial lined cysts located in the glomus that can be seen in neonates. The latter are choroid plexus masses that typically occur in adults but are occasionally found in children.[6]

Choroid Plexus Tumors

Choroid plexus tumors (CPTs) account for a fifth of all neoplasms occurring in infancy and about 2–4% of all pediatric tumors.[7,8] Half of all arise in relation to the ventricular trigone while the rest occur in relation to the fourth (40%) and third ventricle (10%). Children often present with lateral ventricular masses while adults have an equal distribution between both lateral and fourth ventricles. Syndromic association is also seen sometimes with Aicardi and Li-Fraumeni syndromes. Based on histology, they are divided into choroid plexus papilloma (CPP) (WHO grade I), atypical variant of CPP (WHO grade II) and choroid plexus carcinoma (WHO grade III).

Choroid Plexus Papilloma and its Atypical Variant

It is the most common tumor occurring in the lateral ventricles in the first decade. Their incidence and distribution corresponds to that of all CPTs, mentioned above.[7] Bilateral tumors are rare, accounting for 3–4% of all CPPs. In children, as previously stated they occur more commonly in the atrium of the lateral ventricles in contrast to adults, where these are more frequently seen in the fourth ventricle. On CT the tumor is seen as a well-defined, frond-like mass which is iso or mildly hyperdense to brain. Calcification is seen within the tumor in about 25% cases **(Fig. 2)**. There is usually homogeneous and intense enhancement following contrast administration. Diffuse hydrocephalus involving dilatation of all the ventricles occurs which is usually attributed to the

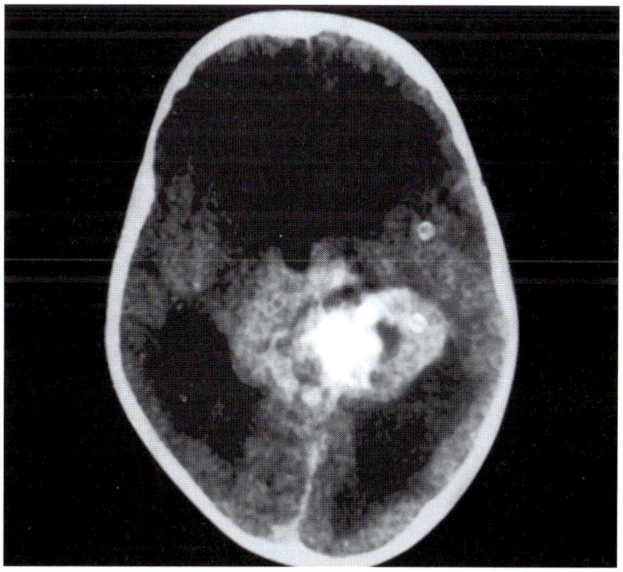

FIG. 2: Choroid plexus papilloma: Plain CT shows hyperdense mass with calcification in the atrium of left lateral ventricle with hydrocephalus.

overproduction of CSF. The ventricular system can also be asymmetrically dilated due to decreased CSF absorption secondary to obstruction of arachnoid granulations following repeated hemorrhage and ependymitis. On MR the tumor is hypo to isointense on T1WI and iso to hyperintense to T2WI[7] **(Figs. 3A to D)**. There is intense homogeneous enhancement after gadolinium administration though heterogeneous enhancement can also be seen when tumor outgrows its blood supply **(Fig. 3D)**. Flow voids can sometimes be seen. Choroid plexus papillomas can transform into carcinomas in 5–15% of cases.[9]

Choroid Plexus Carcinoma

In comparison to papillomas, choroid plexus carcinomas tend to have a more irregular contour. They typically show heterogeneous pattern of enhancement (reflecting necrosis), invasion of surrounding brain and rapid spread along CSF pathways.[10] There is invariably presence of hydrocephalus **(Figs. 4A to D)**. MR spectroscopy demonstrates a high choline peak with elevated lactate.[11]

Astrocytoma

It usually arises in the tissues around the ventricle and invades the lateral ventricle secondarily. The most common site is the thalamus where it can develop into a large mass within the lateral ventricle. The presenting symptoms and signs are dependent on the location and degree of brain infiltration. On CT, the low grade astrocytoma is seen as a poorly marginated low density mass. There is usually minimal mass effect or edema around the lesion. It shows little or no contrast enhancement. The anaplastic astrocytoma and glioblastoma have heterogeneous appearance due to areas

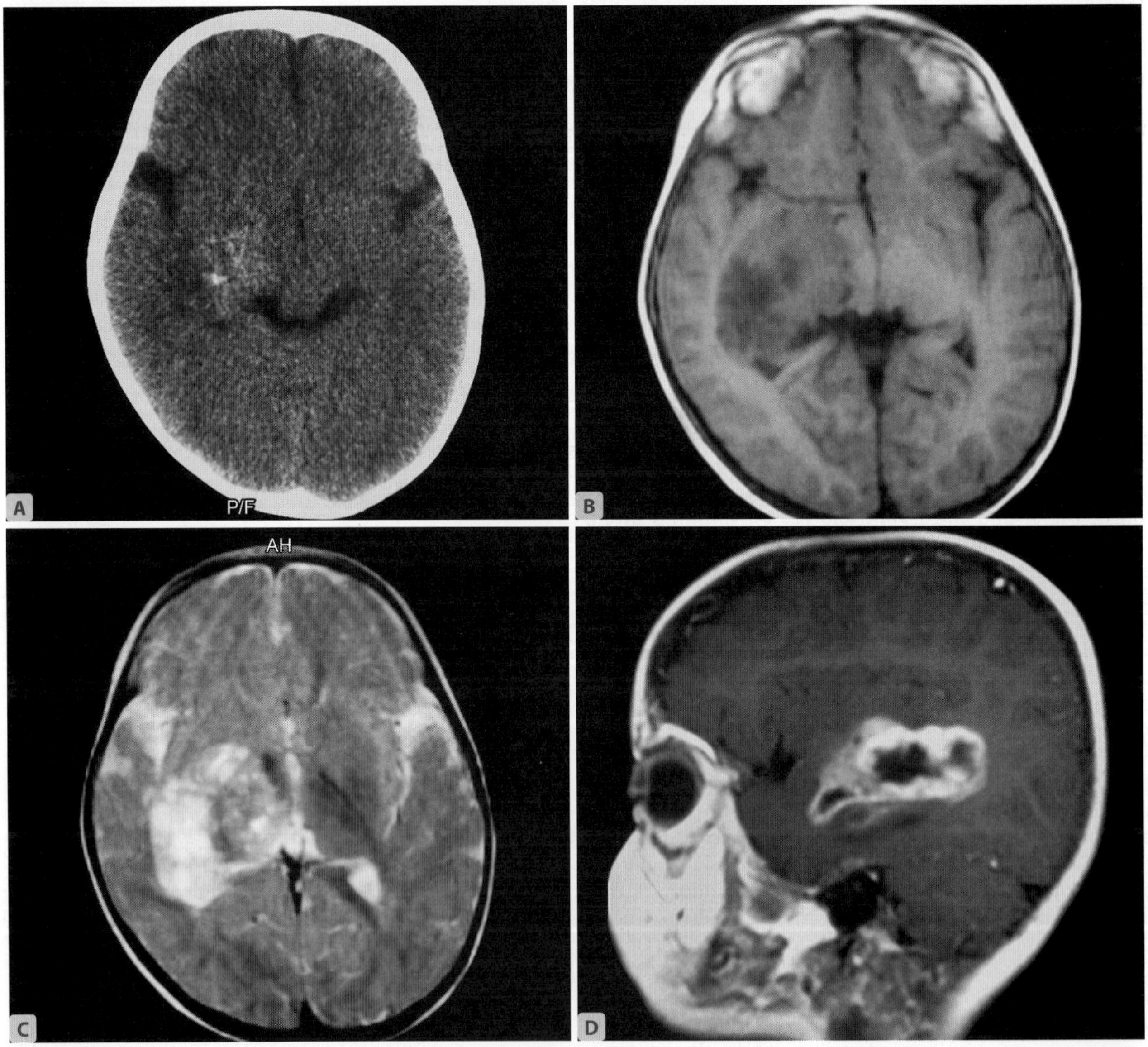

FIGS. 3A TO D: Choroid plexus papilloma: Noncontrast CT (A) shows presence of a relative hyperdense mass with calcific foci in the right temporal lobe which is confirmed to be intraventricular on MRI (B to D) and located in the temporal horn of the right lateral ventricle with peripheral solid enhancement.

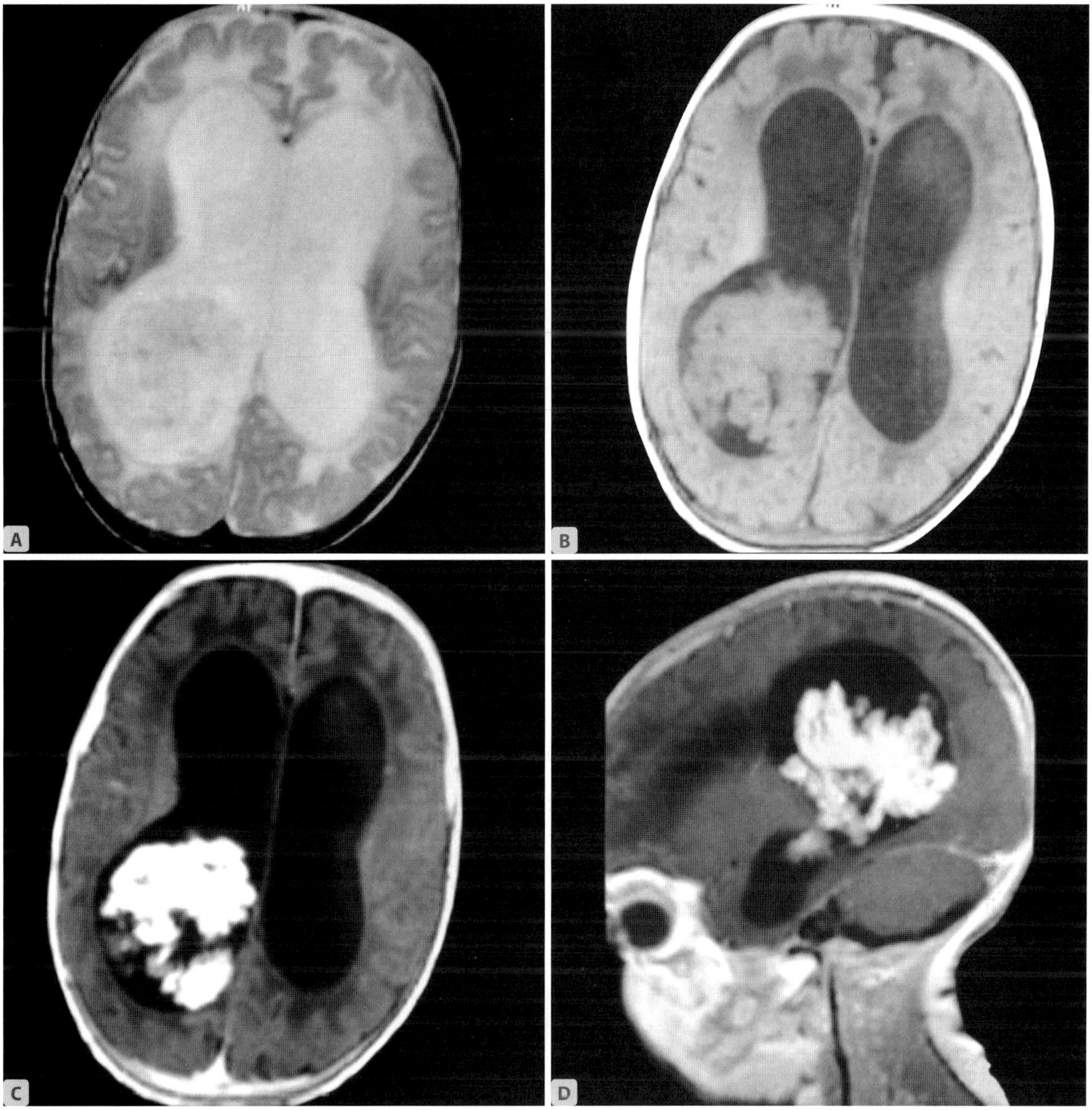

FIGS. 4A TO D: Choroid plexus carcinoma: Axial T2WI (A), T1WI (B), post-contrast axial (C) and sagittal (D) T1W images revealing a lobulated intensely enhancing right lateral ventricular choroid plexus based mass causing hydrocephalus.

of hemorrhage, necrosis or cyst formation[12] (**Figs. 5A and B**). Surrounding white matter edema is more common and there are thick, irregular areas of contrast enhancement. MRI is helpful in the evaluation of degree of differentiation of the astrocytoma. The low grade astrocytoma has a signal pattern lower than normal brain parenchyma. The high grade gliomas and glioblastomas show varied signal intensity with areas of necrosis, hemorrhage, cyst formation and peripheral thick heterogeneous enhancement. MR perfusion and spectroscopy help us to grade the gliomas better with hyperperfusion and significantly raised Choline levels indicative of a higher grade.

Subependymal Giant Cell Tumor

Subependymal giant cell tumor (SGCT) is a circumscribed glioneuronal tumor typically larger than 1 cm, which occurs almost exclusively in patients with tuberous sclerosis (TS). Rarely, it has been reported from patients without manifestations of TS, though these cases may represent somatic mosaicism of the TS gene. It is a slow growing tumor and is discovered either during the course of routine studies in patients with TS or because it causes obstructive hydrocephalus. Rarely, it undergoes malignant change and becomes aggressive. It usually arises in the region of foramen of Monro but can occur anywhere in the ventricles.

SGCT occurs in 10–15% of patient with TS before the age of 20 years in addition to subependymal nodules which are much more commonly seen in these patients **(Figs. 6A and B)**. On CT, SGCT appears as a well-defined mass which is iso to hypodense to cerebral parenchyma. Foci of calcification are common. On MRI, the mass is hypo- to isointense on T1WI and iso- to hyperintense on T2WI with prominent enhancement after IV gadolinium injection.[13] SGCAs are treated only when there is evidence of growth, progressive hydrocephalus, new focal neurologic deficit or symptoms of raised intracranial pressure. Surveillance is recommended every 2 years for patients with TSC2 mutation and every 3 years for the ones with TSC1 mutation, preferably with MRI. Annual follow-up is suggested after SGCT has been diagnosed.

Ependymoma

Ependymomas constitute 3–5% of intracranial tumors.[4] These are commonly seen in children in the posterior fossa (60%) and have a predilection for males. Supratentorial ependymomas are seen in 30–40% cases and are usually parenchymal (>50%). Extraventricular lesions are proposed to arise from embryonic rests of ependymal tissue trapped in the developing cerebral hemisphere. When intraventricular, they usually arise in the trigone of lateral ventricle. They have a variety of histologic patterns varying from well differentiated to aggressive, poorly differentiate ones.[14] The clinical presentation is variable ranging from headache, seizures to focal neurological deficits and are often delayed till these tumors grow into the ventricular system. On CT, ependymomas are iso- to hypoattenuating, may show cystic component (70%), calcification (50%) and rarely hemorrhages. The solid component is iso dense to brain parenchyma with bright enhancement with contrast administration.[15] On MRI, the tumor is iso- to hypointense on T1WI and hyperintense on T2WI. There is usually heterogeneity due to areas of hemorrhage, necrosis and calcification **(Figs. 7A to D)**. With gadolinium administration there is usually moderate to intense enhancement. Diffusion restriction may be seen in highly cellular areas of the tumor. Vasogenic edema may occur in the adjoining white matter. Although ependymoma is a benign tumor, it has a high recurrence rate and can spread through CSF pathways. Thus, imaging of the entire craniospinal axis should be performed at presentation and follow-up.

Meningioma

Intraventricular meningioma is an uncommon tumor and constitutes 0.5–3% of all intracranial tumors.[4] It is more common in adult females. It is a benign tumor (WHO grade I) rising from the arachnoid cap cells trapped within the choroid plexus. Although rare, the meningiomas in children are more frequently intraventricular and malignant, show equal incidence in both sexes and are usually associated with neurofibromatosis 2. The lateral ventricle particularly the atrium, is the most common site (80%) followed by third (15%) and fourth (5%) ventricles.[16] On CT, meningioma appears as a sharply defined, globular mass, iso to hyperdense to brain parenchyma. Calcification is seen in 40–50% cases. It shows diffuse intense enhancement with contrast **(Fig. 8A).** There may be localized or diffuse ventricular dilatation, depending on obstruction to CSF flow. On MRI, it is isointense (60%) or hypointense (40%) on T1WI and isointense (50%) or hyperintense (50%) on T2WI **(Figs. 8B and C)**. There is usually homogeneous and moderate to intense enhancement with IV gadolinium administration **(Fig. 8D)**. Diffusion restriction may be observed in some lesions reflecting high cellular density. High vascularity on perfusion MR is often appreciated with mean rCBV values >3.[17] There is persistence of contrast material within the

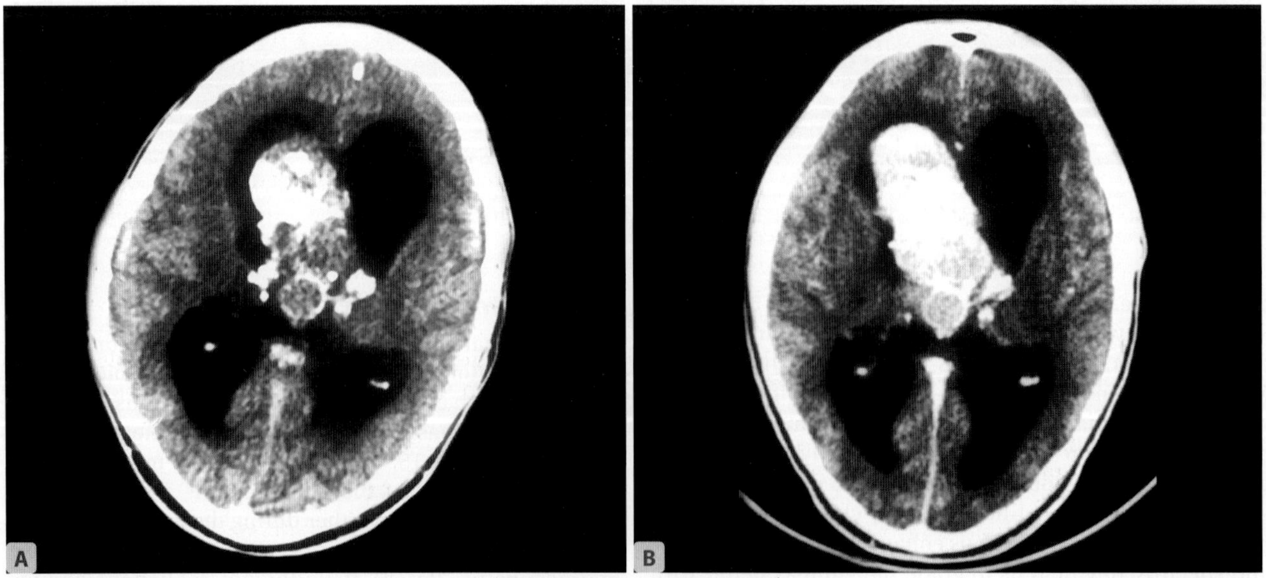

FIGS. 5A AND B: Astrocytoma: Plain (A) and contrast (B) CT show intensely enhancing heterogeneous mass with dense calcification occupying the frontal horn and body of right lateral ventricle.

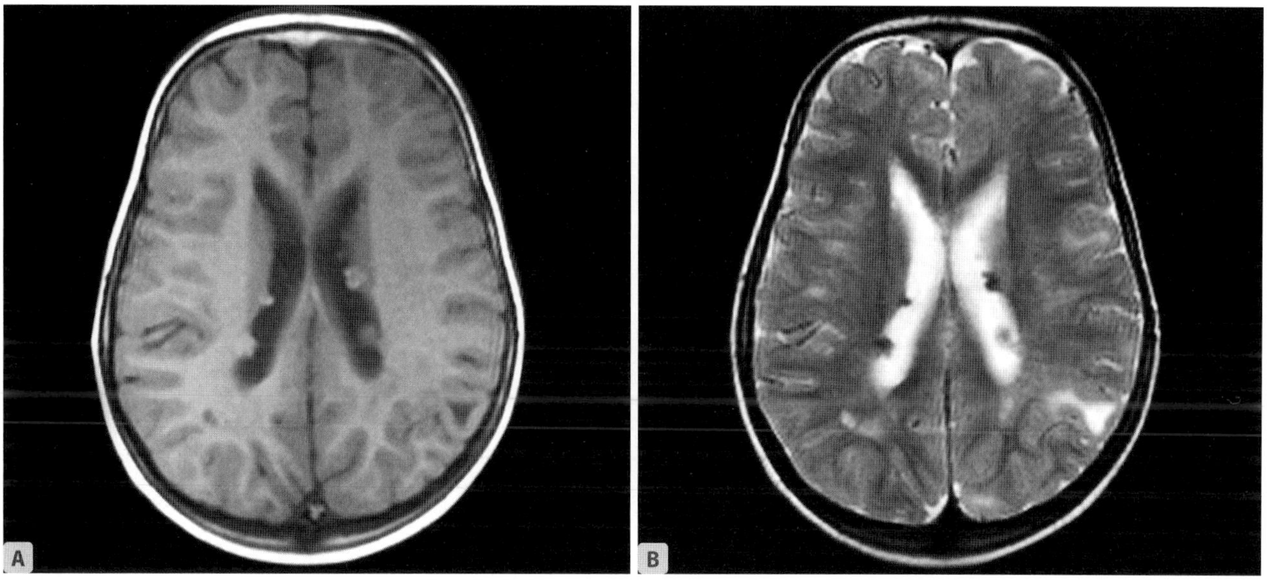

FIGS. 6A AND B: Subependymal nodules in tuberous sclerosis: Axial T1WI (A) and T2WI (B) in a patient of tuberous sclerosis shows presence of multiple small subependymal nodules.

tumor interstitium due to deficiency of blood brain barrier. Proton MR spectroscopy reveals a high choline peak[16] with markedly low NAA and creatine levels. Presence of alanine (doublet at 1.4 ppm) and high levels of glutamate, if seen, are reasonably specific.[18]

Metastases

Intraventricular metastases can develop either due to dissemination by blood (hematogenous route) or CSF. The blood borne metastasis most often involves the choroid plexus in the ventricles due to its direct relationship with the systemic blood supply. The common primary tumors with intraventricular metastases are bronchogenic, breast, renal cell and colon carcinoma in adults and Wilm's tumor, retinoblastoma and neuroblastoma in children.[19] On CT or MRI the choroid plexus metastasis shows expansion of choroid plexus with marked contrast enhancement. Dynamic susceptibility contrast imaging (DSCI) may show elevated rCBV values (>3) in hypervascular tumors (renal and thyroid carcinomas).

The paraventricular spread of tumor can occur along CSF pathways to ventricular ependymal lining and leptomeninges. There may also be infiltration of the subependymal space by a sheet of tumor cells. Such a spread can occur in both primary CNS and systemic malignancies. Malignant astrocytomas are the commonest tumor to show CSF spread followed by ependymomas, medulloblastomas **(Figs. 9A to D)**, pineal tumors and choroid plexus papillomas.[4] The sites involved in order of frequency, are the lateral ventricles, the fourth ventricle, aqueduct and third ventricle. Metastatic deposits are often seen in the recesses such as ventricular horns, supraoptic and interpeduncular recesses of the third ventricle. On CT, these lesions are seen as discrete, iso to hyperdense nodular or sheet like having subependymal rim surrounding a part or the entire ventricle **(Fig. 10)**. On MRI, they appear hypointense on T1WI and hyperintense on T2WI. Melanoma metastasis differs in being hyperintense on T1WI and isointense on T2WI.

Primary CNS Lymphoma

It constitutes 1–1.5% of all primary CNS tumors. There is a male sex predilection and peak incidence is in fifth and sixth decades. There is a sharp rise in the incidence over the past decades with the increasing spread of AIDS.[20] Most primary CNS lymphomas are of the non-Hodgkin's type. Lymphoma rarely presents as a purely intraventricular mass and generally exhibits diffuse subependymal spread (12%). Most commonly, it is seen as well-defined nodular lesion in the subependymal region. There may be extension along the perivascular Virchow-Robin spaces. The imaging findings are reflective of the high cellularity and nucleocytoplasmic ratio in addition to features of blood-brain barrier disruption **(Figs. 11A to F)**. On CT, it appears as iso- to hyperattenuating lesion showing homogeneous or rarely ring-like contrast enhancement. On MRI, it shows variable signal pattern, often isointense on all spin echo sequences **(Figs. 11A and B)**; high cellularity gives a hypointense signal on T2WI. Occasionally it can be hyperintense on T1WI. It shows diffusion restriction **(Fig. 11D)** with low ADC values. Contrast enhancement is usually homogenous **(Fig. 11C)** and bright.[4] MR spectroscopy reveals high choline with low NAA **(Fig. 11E)**. Mean curve analysis of the perfusion data demonstrates blood-brain barrier breach with the curve over-shooting the baseline **(Fig. 11F)**.

Central Neurocytoma

Central neurocytoma is a well-differentiated benign (WHO grade II) intraventricular tumor of neuroepithelial origin, first described in 1982.[21] It is a rare tumor, constituting 0.1%–0.5% of all primary tumors of the CNS and occurs in adults

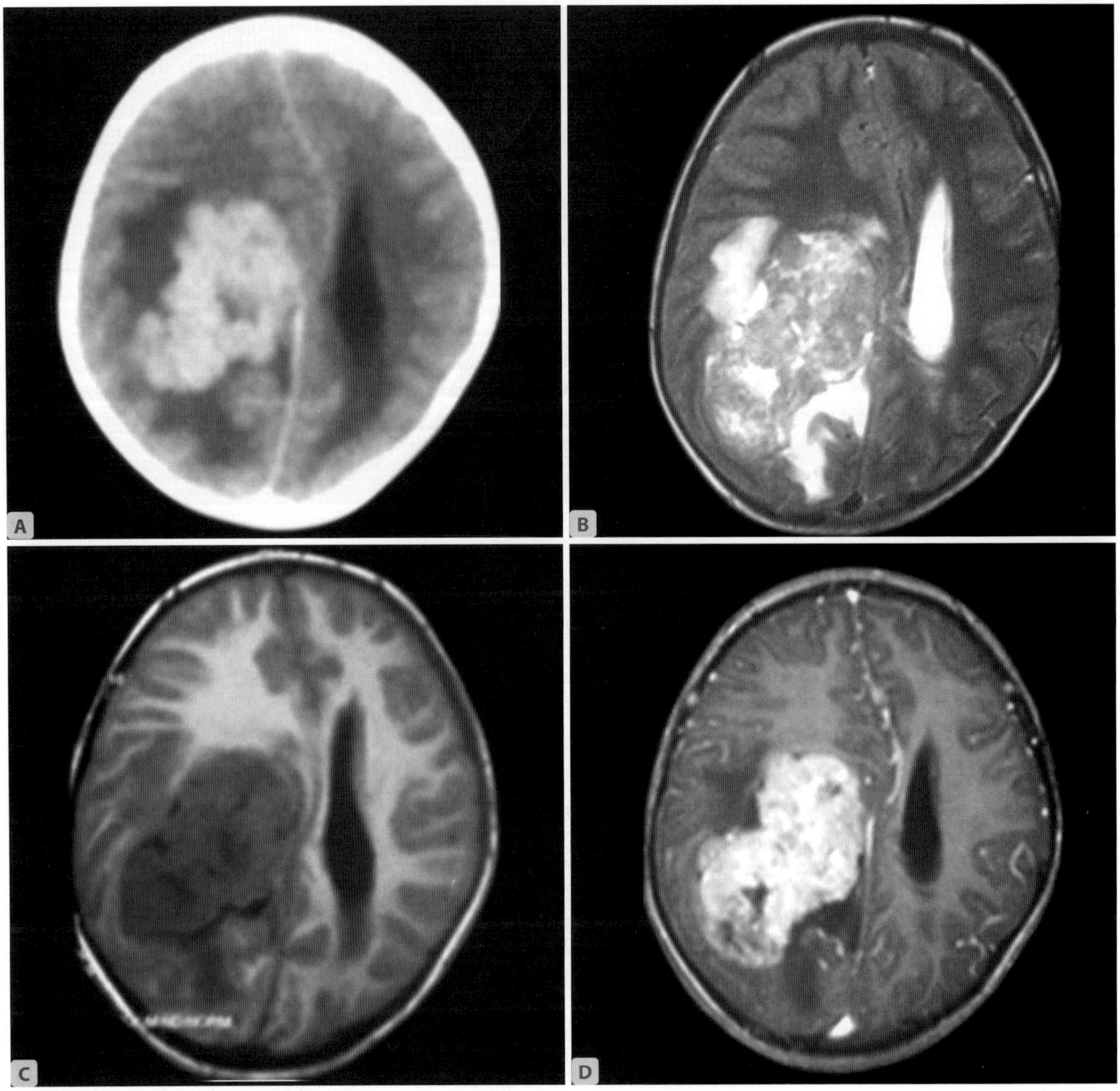

FIGS. 7A TO D: Ependymoma: Axial CT (A) depicting the lobulated moderately enhancing right lateral ventricular mass with adjoining parenchymal edema. Axial T2WI (B), T1WI (C) and contrast-enhanced T1WI (D) demonstrating the lesion character-heterogeneous T2 hyperintense, T1 hypointense with moderate enhancement.

(2nd to 5th decades). The site of origin is usually at or near the midline at the base of the septum pellucidum and usually in close proximity to foramen of Monro. It is quite large at presentation and usually presents due to symptoms of raised intracranial pressure and obstructive hydrocephalus. Neurocytomas are gray friable lesions having solid as well as cystic components, often with amorphous calcification (50%).[22] Gross total excision is usually curative though recurrence is known. Overall it has a good prognosis. Previously these tumors were erroneously classified as "intraventricular oligodendrogliomas (ODGs)" due to their resemblance to ODGs on histopathology. The presence of pineocytomatous rosettes allows their differentiation from ODGs. On CT, they appear as iso to slightly hyperdense masses with cystic changes (giving bubbly appearance) and foci of calcification. Mild-to-moderate enhancement with contrast is seen. On MRI, the tumor shows heterogeneous pattern and there is variable (moderate to strong) enhancement following IV gadolinium administration[22] **(Figs. 12A to D)**. The presence of glycine (3.55 ppm) on MR spectroscopy[23] may help in differentiating it from other similar tumors like ependymoma, subependymoma and oligodendrogliomas. Other differential like heterotopic gray matter can be excluded as the latter neither shows enhancement nor calcification. Meningiomas can be differentiated based on their posterior location in the atrium of lateral ventricle as are choroid plexus tumors.

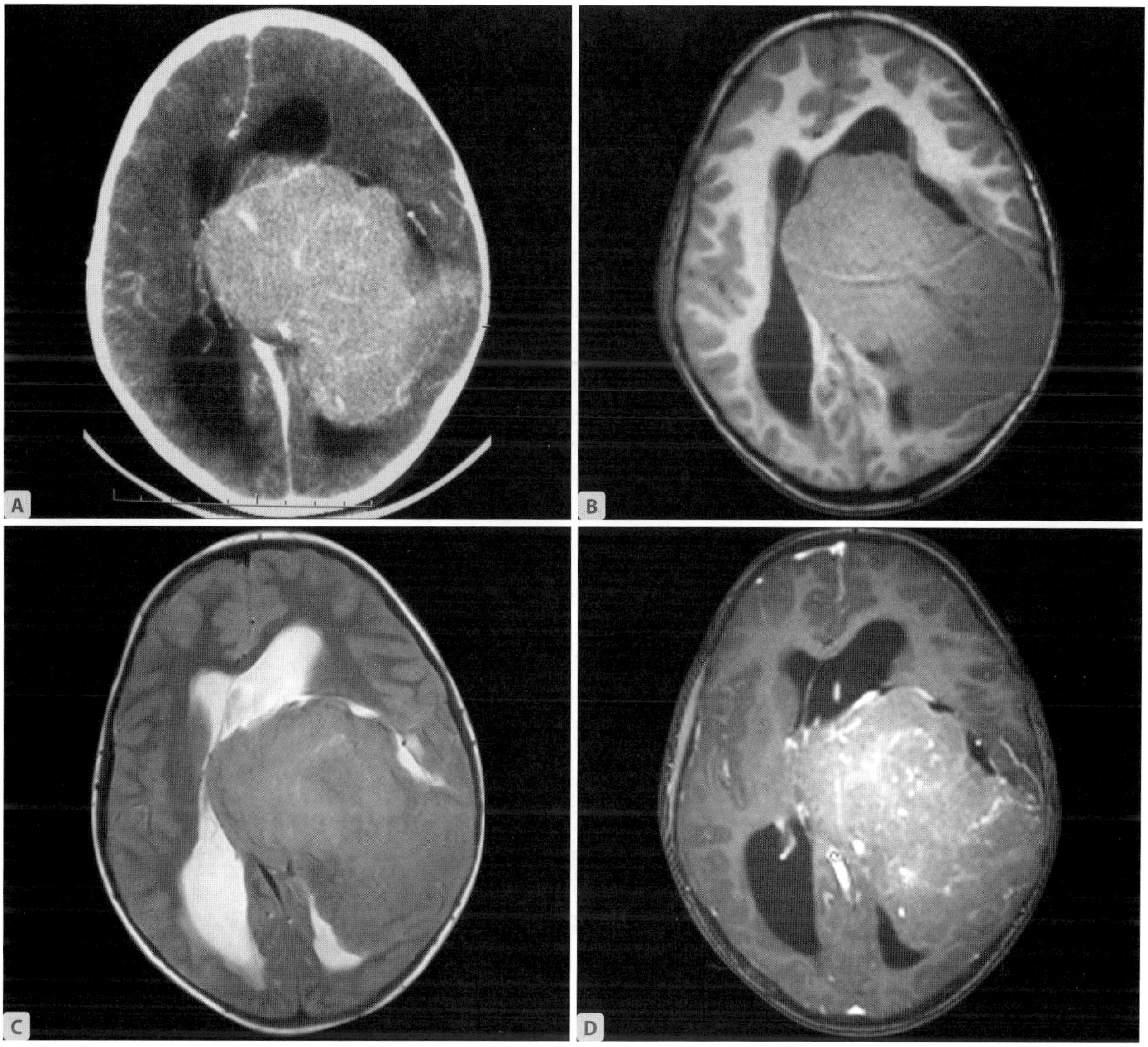

FIGS. 8A TO D: Intraventricular meningioma: CECT (A) shows a well-defined moderately enhancing globular mass in the atrium/body of the left lateral ventricle which is hypointense on T1WI (B), isointense on T2WI (C) with intratumoral vascularity on post contrast T1WI (D). Note the mass effect with mild contralateral midline shift.

Subependymoma

It is a rare benign (WHO grade I) tumor seen in middle-aged and elderly patients. The common site of occurrence is in frontal horn of lateral ventricle or in the caudal fourth ventricle.[24] It typically appears as a well-defined lobular mass. On CT, it appears as an iso- or hypodense lesion with minimal or no enhancement. Calcification is seen occasionally. On MRI, subependymoma is homogeneously hypo to isointense on T1WI and mildly hypointense on T2WI **(Figs. 13A to D)**. Contrast enhancement is typically absent to mild.[24]

Vascular Malformations

Arteriovenous malformations (AVMs) and cavernous angiomas can have some component within the ventricle, particularly those arising in the basal ganglia and thalamus. Lateral ventricle is the most common to be involved but they can occur in any part of the ventricular system.[25] On CT these lesions are seen as heterogeneous areas, with or without calcifications. On contrast administration, abnormal vessels are seen as tortuous high density structures. MRI is superior to CT in demonstrating the feeding vessels the nidus and the serpiginous draining veins which appear as flow voids both on T1WI and T2WI. Digital subtraction angiography (DSA) is the confirmatory study which shows all aspects of the vascular malformations. Four dimensional (4D) CT angiography has been proven to be a noninvasive modality giving excellent details, without the ill-effects of DSA. Subependymal AVMs can be difficult to treat surgically. They are prone to rupture **(Figs. 14A to D)**. Endovascular embolization of the nidus is a minimally invasive method of treating these lesions. Gamma knife radiotherapy can also be offered to these patients.

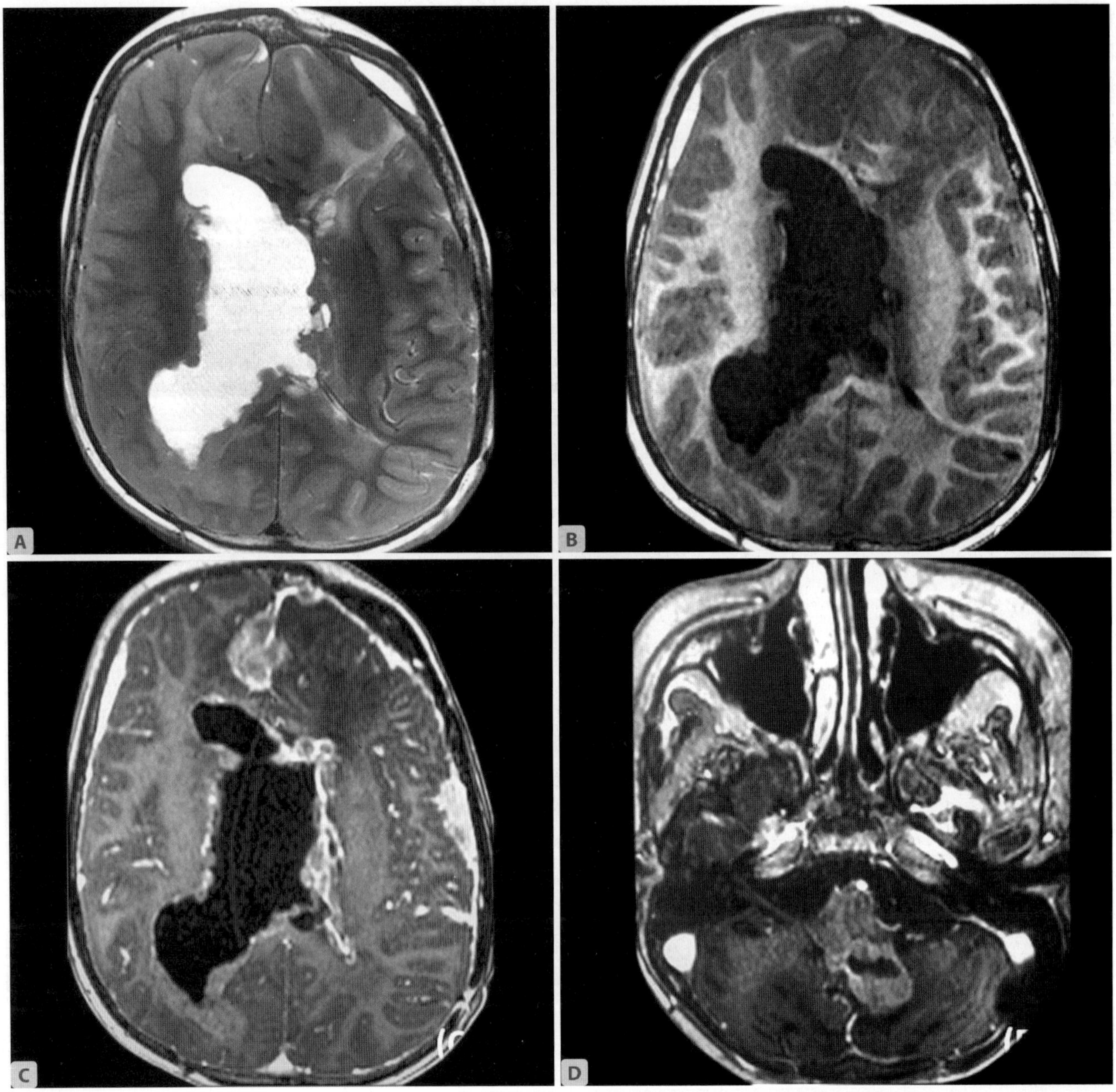

FIGS. 9A TO D: Transependymal and CSF spread of medulloblastoma: Axial T2WI (A), T1WI (B) and post-contrast T1WI (C) revealing diffuse nodular ependymal enhancement with sulcal deposits. Axial post contrast T1WI (D) showing the primary lesion in relation to the fourth ventricle.

Intraventricular blood-fluid levels can occur in cases of intraventricular hemorrhage secondary to rupture of saccular aneurysms or arteriovenous malformations. Other important causes are Moyamoya disease and systemic coagulopathies. Fluid-fluid levels can be seen in severe cases of ependymitis, meningitis or as a result of rupture of parenchymal abscess into the ventricles.

Choroid Plexus Cysts and Xanthogranulomas

Xanthogranulomas are usually discovered incidentally. They are symptomatic only when they cause obstruction at foramen of Monro. Cysts show low density on CT with signal characteristics similar to CSF on MRI.[26] They lack contrast enhancement and show diffusion restriction on DWI. Xanthogranulomas are dense on CT and may show flecks of calcification. The center is often of low attenuation due to fat content. On MRI, these are well-defined partially cystic masses that appear hypo or isointense on T1WI and iso to hyperintense on T2WI and show contrast enhancement.[27]

Sometimes parasitic cysts can also be encountered in the lateral ventricles[28] which may cause obstruction to the CSF flow and may present as hydrocephalus, e.g. neurocysticercosis (NCC) **(Figs. 15A and B)**, hydatid cyst **(Fig. 16)**.

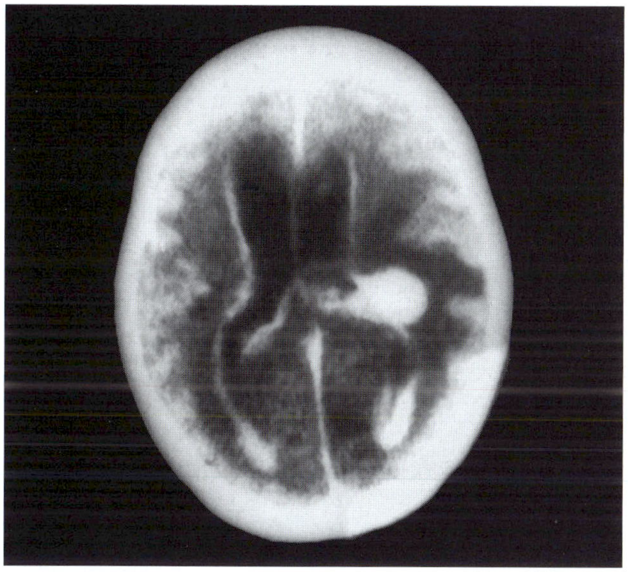

FIG. 10: Metastasis: CECT shows diffuse ependymal enhancement and hyperdense nodule in the left paraventricular region with edema in a patient patient of carcinoma thyroid.

Dermoids

These are uncommon lateral ventricular lesions. On CT, the dermoids are hypodense (fat containing) with presence of calcification. On MRI, the dermoid shows hyperintense foci of fat and areas of signal loss due to calcification on T1WI **(Figs. 17A to C)**. Heterogeneous hyperintensity is noted on T2WI. Contrast enhancement is typically none to mild. Dermoids may show intraventricular rupture with distant spread of fat through CSF. This can lead to chemical meningitis or obstructive hydrocephalus due to blockage of CSF pathways.

Third Ventricular Masses

In children, hydrocephalus is the most common feature of 3rd ventricular masses. The endocrine and visual disturbances are uncommon. Diencephalic syndrome which comprises hyperkinesis and alertness associated with emaciation in infants is the only specific syndrome described with hypothalamic gliomas. In adults mental and behavioral changes, particularly increasing apathy, are common.

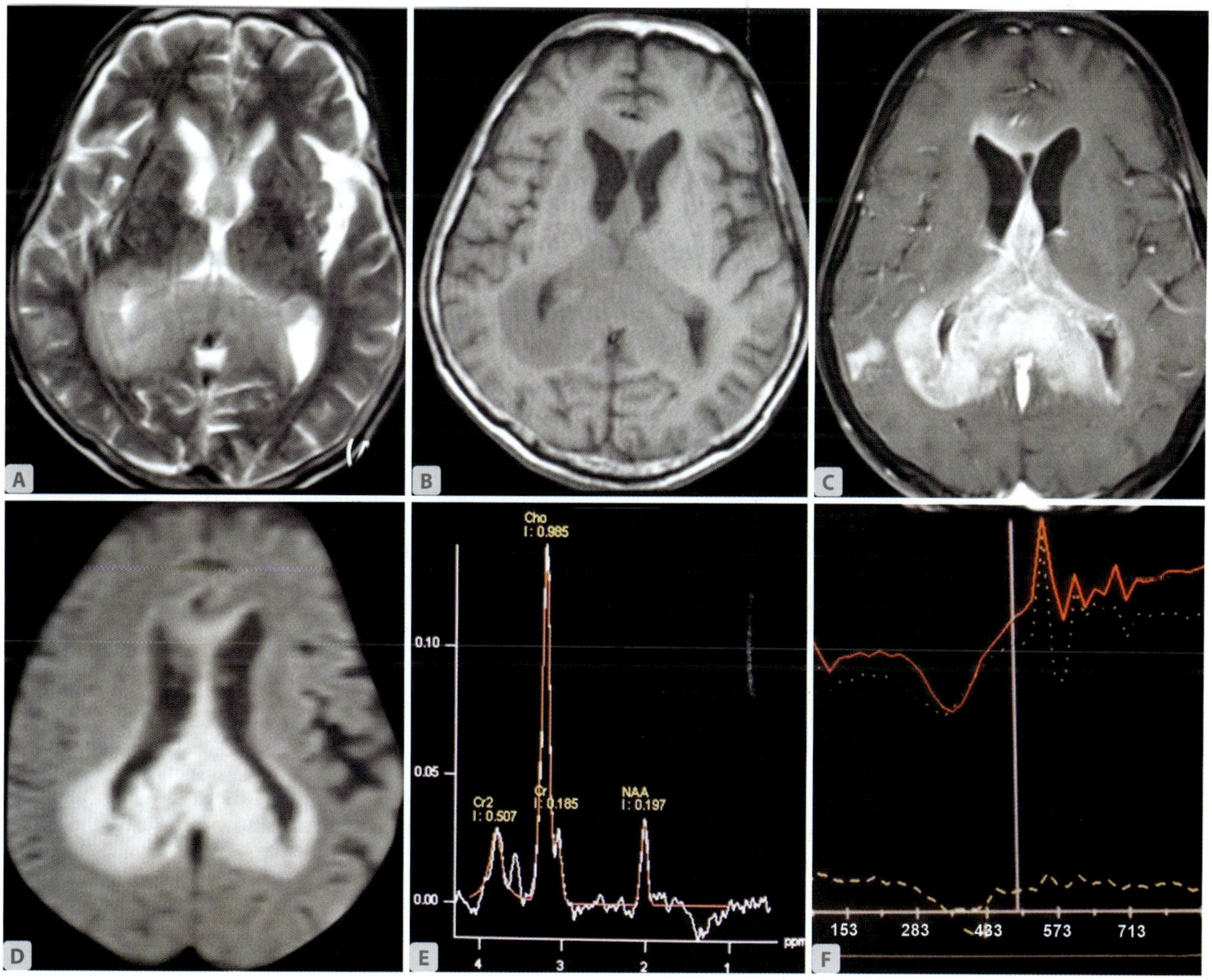

FIGS. 11A TO F: Primary CNS lymphoma: Multiparametric MR depicting the extensive subependymal spread of the lymphomatous lesion having T2 hyperintense (A), T1 hypointense (B), moderate enhancing (C) nature with diffusion restriction (D). MR spectroscopy reveals high choline (E) with upshoot above baseline on mean curve analysis of DSCI due to T1 effect (F).

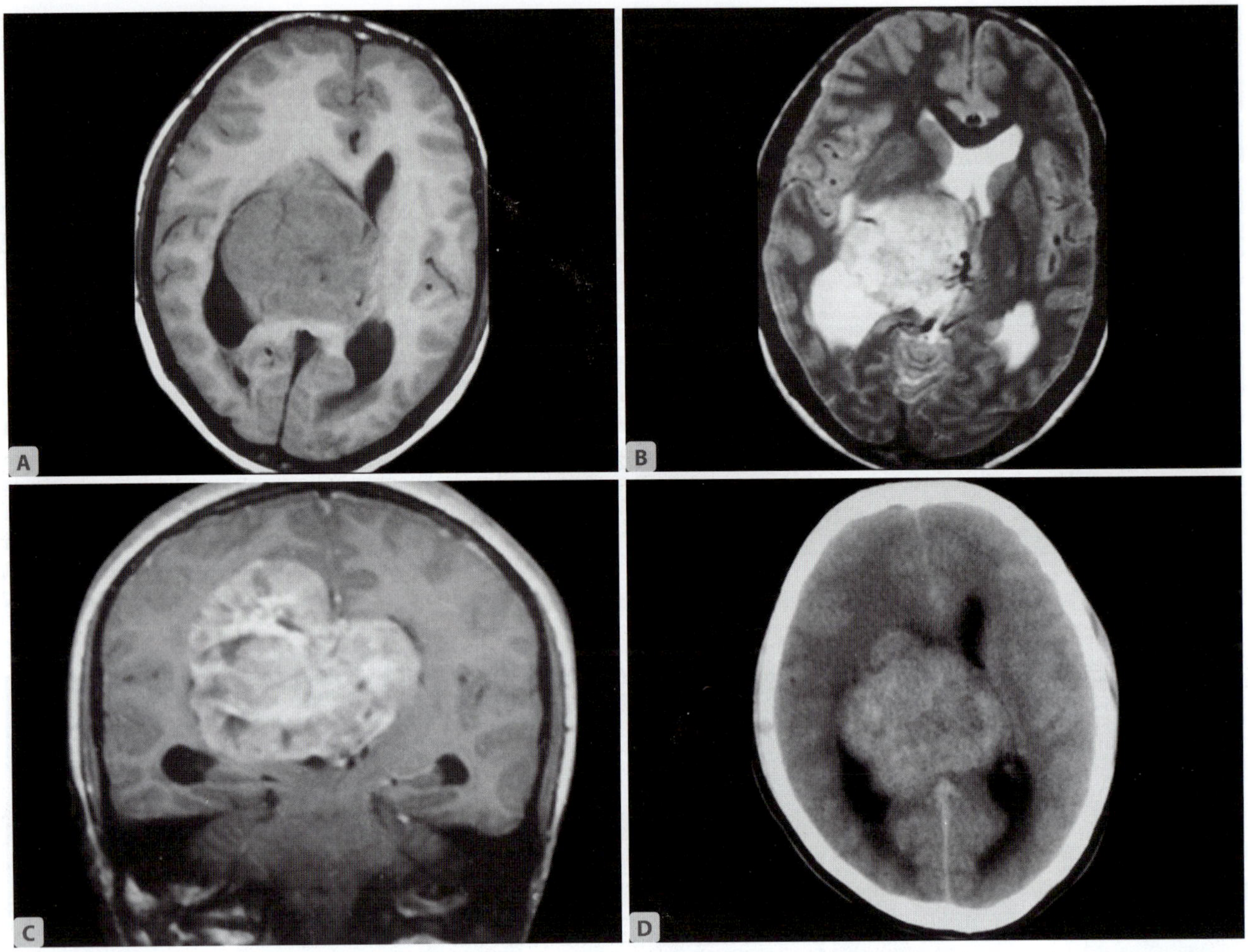

FIGS. 12A TO D: Central neurocytoma: (A) T1 MR image shows intraventricular solid mass attached to septum pellucidum. The tumor shows heterogeneous signal on T2WI (B) and intense contrast enhancement following IV gadolinium (C). (D) CECT shows enhancing intraventricular tumor.

Depending on the parts of the ventricle involved these tumors can be further categorized as anterior or posterior 3rd ventricular masses.

Anterior Third Ventricular Masses

Colloid Cyst

They arise from the roof of the 3rd ventricle at the level of foramen of Monro. They are round to oval lesions and vary in size from few millimeters to several centimeters in diameter. They represent 15–20% of all IV lesions and occur in 3rd to 5th decades of life.[29] Less than 2% of colloid cysts occur in children. Symptoms of intermittent obstruction are common and sudden death due to acute obstruction has been reported.[30] It arises from endoderm rather than ectoderm which is morphologically similar to bronchial and nasal cavity epithelium. On CT, colloid cysts are well encapsulated, homogeneously hyperdense masses (due to intrinsic proteinaceous content) which show little or no contrast enhancement **(Fig. 18A)**. There may be dilatation of lateral ventricles which can be asymmetrical. Hydrocephalus can also be intermittent.[30] Calcification is not a feature. On MR, the signal characteristics of colloid cysts vary widely.[28] The most common appearance is a mass that is hyperintense on T1WI and hypointense on T2WI though it can be isointense on both T1 and T2WI **(Figs. 18B to D)**. Rim enhancement following contrast can be observed. CSF flow artifacts at foramen of Monro can mimic colloid cysts (pseudotumor) on MRI and should be kept in mind while evaluating these lesions.[30] Currently available heavily T2-weighted imaging (e.g. CISS, FIESTA, etc.) helps in better delineating the lesion location and morphological details.

Astrocytoma

In children, the most common type of astrocytoma that arises primarily from ventricular wall is juvenile pilocytic astrocytoma.[31] This differs from the one which arises in cerebellum in that, it rarely shows cystic component. Astrocytoma arising in the hypothalamic or chiasmatic region may extend into the third ventricle. Visual field defects are often the presenting complaints and endocrine disturbances occur late in the course of the disease. Growth hormone deficiency is the earliest endocrine abnormality. Hydrocephalus due to the tumor is rare. Pathologically, it is a low grade-glioma but is usually not resectable. Role

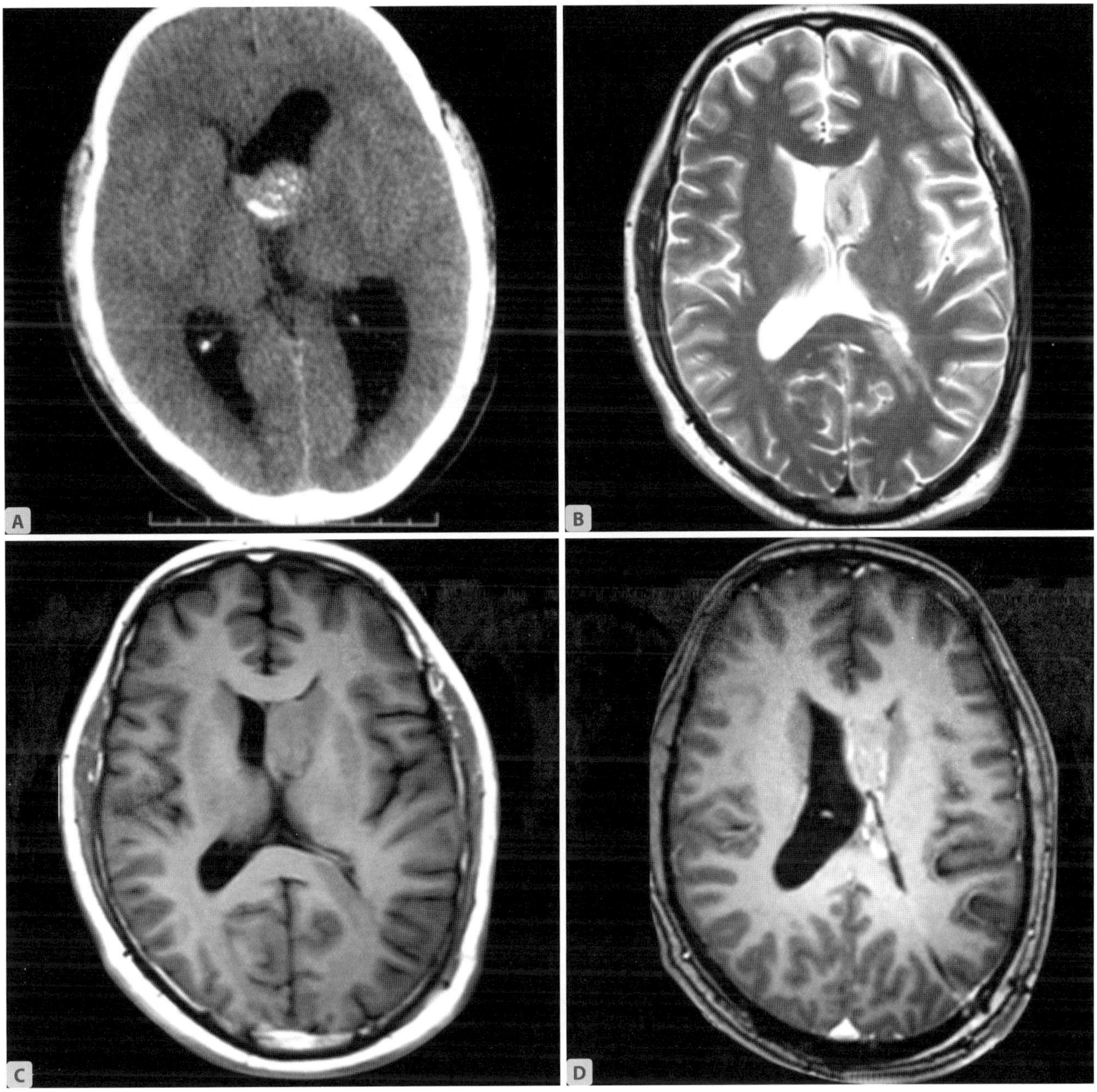

FIGS. 13A TO D: Subependyoma: Hyperdense (A) left frontal ventricular nodular lesion. Axial T2WI (B), T1WI (C) and gadolinium enhanced T1WI (D) showing T2 iso/hyperintensity, T1 isointensity with mild enhancement.

of biopsy is controversial and it is often advocated when the clinical or imaging features are peculiar and suggest a different type of tumor.[28] On noncontrast CT, the tumor is iso to hypodense and shows variable enhancement after IV contrast administration. Calcification and cyst formation are rare. The anatomy is better evaluated on MRI which can show thickened optic chiasm, the floor and walls of the 3rd ventricle with extension of the lesion along the optic tracts. Sometimes, it becomes difficult to distinguish it from craniopharyngioma. Diffusion tensor imaging is important in such cases which reveal altered tensor values along the optic pathways in case of astrocytomas.

Ependymoma

It is rare in the third ventricle. The imaging features are similar to those as seen in other areas.[15]

Germinoma

The tumor that occurs solely in the 3rd ventricle is called "ectopic pinealoma" and rarely occurs in association with the posterior third ventricular germinoma. The clinical triad includes visual loss, loss of libido and diabetes insipidus. Histologically, this tumor resembles seminoma and dysgerminoma. The tumor has the potential to spread via CSF

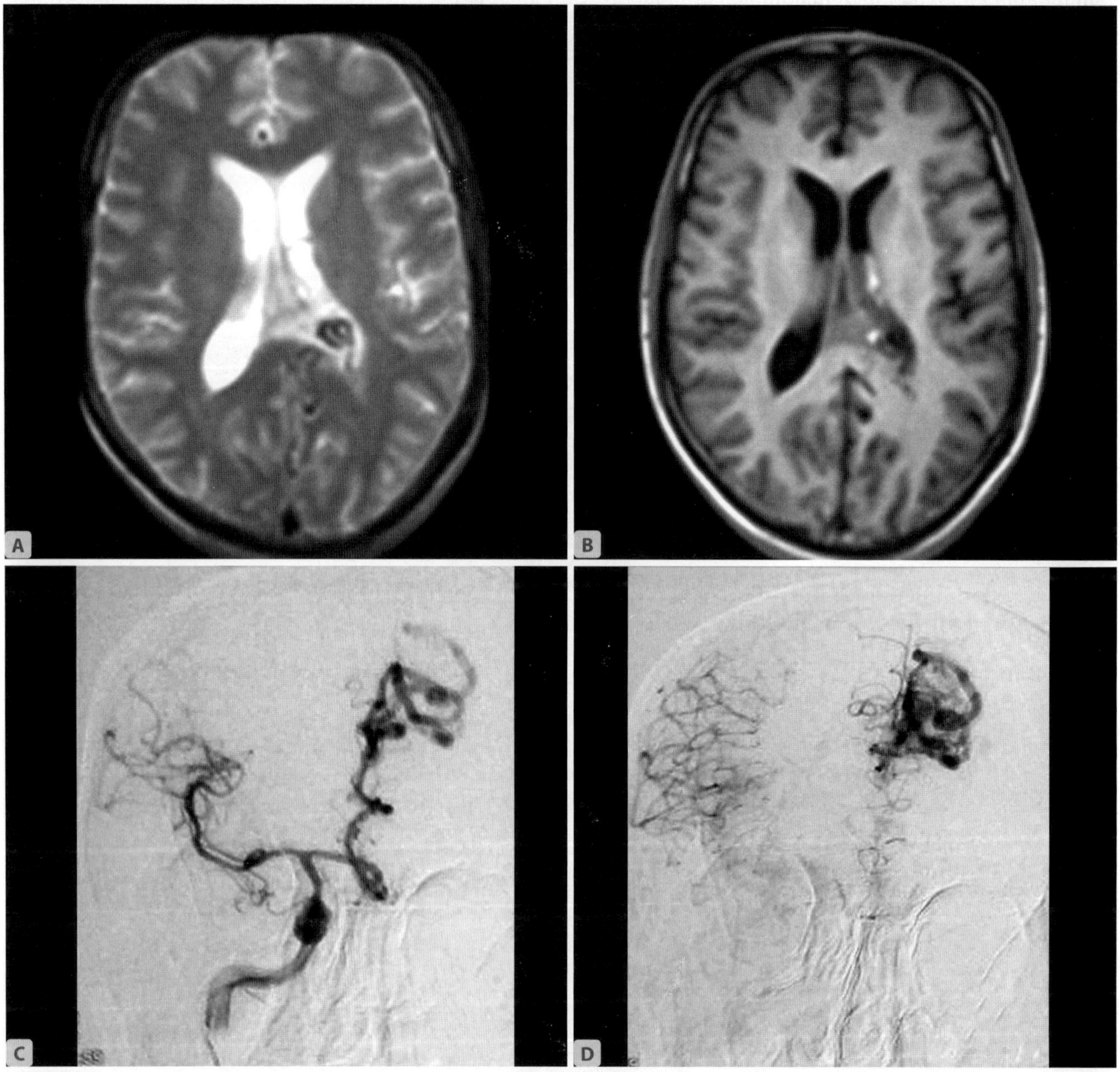

FIGS. 14A TO D: Arteriovenous malformation (AVM): Axial T2WI (A) and T1WI (B) demonstrating left ventricular hemorrhage (mixed signal on T1 and T2). Cerebral DSA frontal (C) and lateral (D) projections depicting the AVM nidus in left parietal lobe as the cause of bleed.

pathways and therefore CSF analysis for tumor cells can be helpful in obtaining diagnosis in some patients.[32]

On noncontrast CT, the germinoma appears as an iso to hyperdense mass with indistinct tumor boundaries. Calcification is rare. It shows uniform enhancement on contrast injection. The tumor shows similar character on MRI with homogeneous enhancement following IV gadolinium administration. Germinomas are very sensitive to radiotherapy **(Figs. 19A to D)**.

Metastases

Isolated metastasis into the 3rd ventricle is very rare and almost always associated with other cerebral metastasis. The imaging features are variable. Most commonly it is hyperdense or hyperintense relative to normal brain with significant edema surrounding the tumor. It shows either a solid or ring-like enhancement following contrast administration. Contrast-enhanced magnetic resonance (CEMR) is the most sensitive modality for defining both the presence and location of metastatic lesions.[4]

Craniopharyngioma

Primary third ventricular craniopharyngioma is extremely rare and is almost always an extension of the craniopharyngioma from the sellar-suprasellar region. There are two peaks of occurrence; the first in young children less than 15 years and the second in the 5th–6th decades. The clinical presentation is growth disturbance and visual field defects in children, and

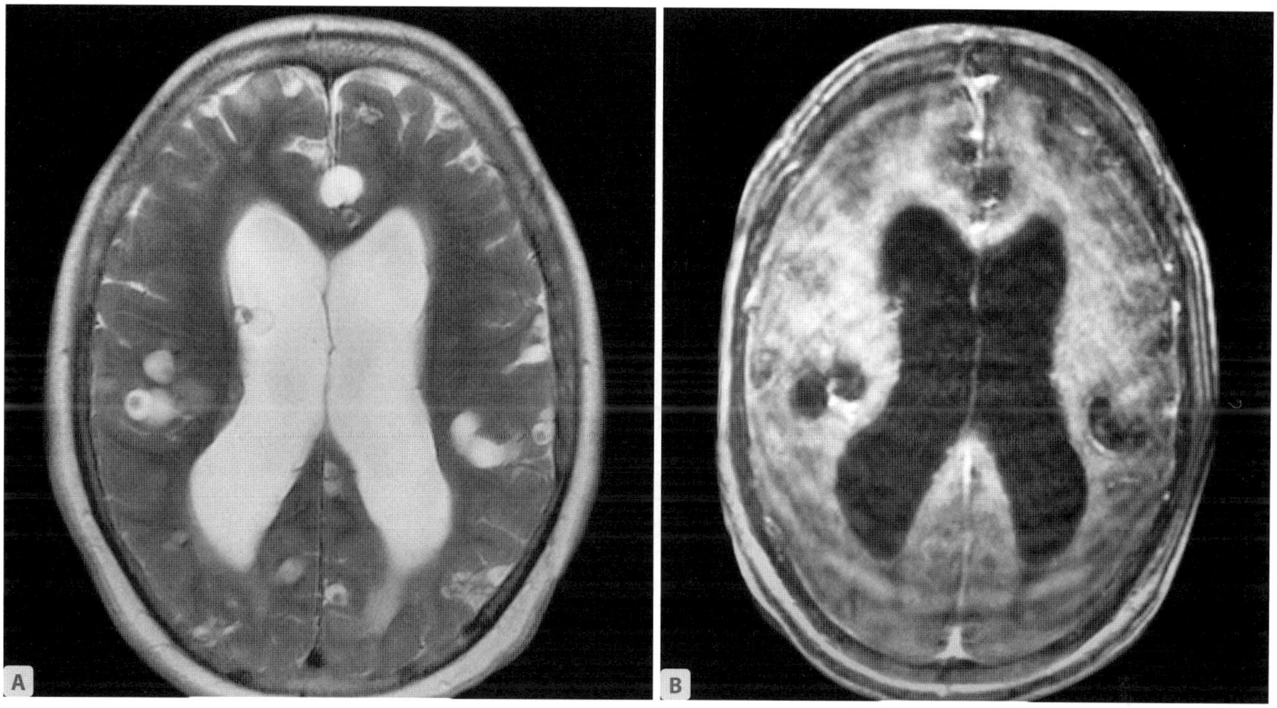

FIGS. 15A AND B: Neurocysticercosis: Axial T2WI (A) and post-contrast T1WI (B) showing multiple cystic lesions scattered in both cerebral hemispheres with one lodged in the right ventricular ependyma. Note the presence of scolices.

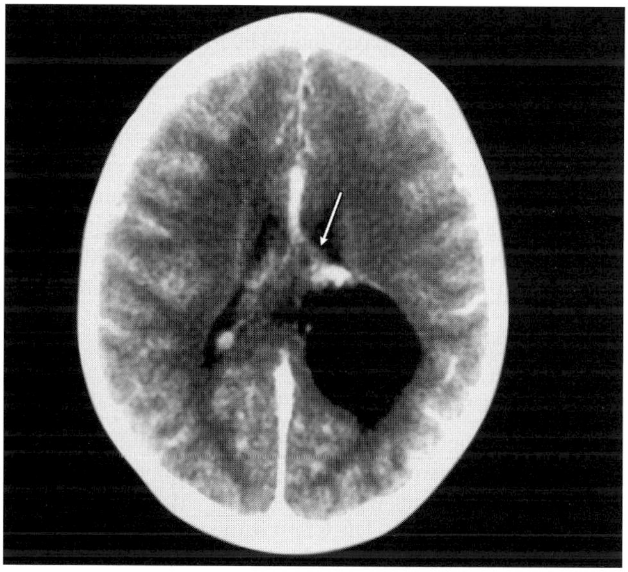

FIG. 16: Hydatid cyst: CECT shows well-defined cystic lesion in the trigone of left lateral ventricle with anteriorly displaced choroid plexus (arrow).

behavioral change or memory disturbance in adults. On CT the tumor shows solid and cystic components in majority of patients. The solid component shows contrast enhancement particularly in children. Calcification is seen in almost all patients in childhood while it is seen in up to 50% of cases in adults. MRI may show T1 hyperintense cyst (motor oil appearance) with heterogeneous enhancement of the solid component **(Fig. 20A to C)**.

Epidermoid and Dermoids

These are uncommon tumors encountered in the anterior 3rd ventricle.[33] They usually present due to obstructive hydrocephalus. On CT, the epidermoid appears as hypodense lesion which does not enhance with contrast administration. Dermoid usually shows the presence of fat and calcification. On MRI, the epidermoid shows signal characters similar to CSF while the dermoid shows hyperintense foci of fat and areas of signal loss due to calcification on T1WI. Both these lesions characteristically displace the brain parenchyma around it rather than invading it. The epidermoid classically shows diffusion restriction **(Figs. 21A to D)**.

Cysticercosis

Intraventricular cysticercosis presents with repeated attacks of meningitis in children and with hydrocephalus in adults. The diagnosis should always be suspected in an endemic area. It is seen in 20–25% of all neurocysticercosis, most commonly in 4th ventricle, foramen of Monro and lateral ventricle **(Figs. 22A and B)**. It can be difficult to diagnose on CT because it shows similar attenuation like CSF. MR is the best imaging modality and T2WI clearly shows the hyperintense cyst in the ventricular wall. It can be of the racemose variety at times and sometimes is not readily differentiated from a tuberculoma. Unilocular cystic forms may often show an eccentric hypointense nodule suggestive of scolex within the cyst on

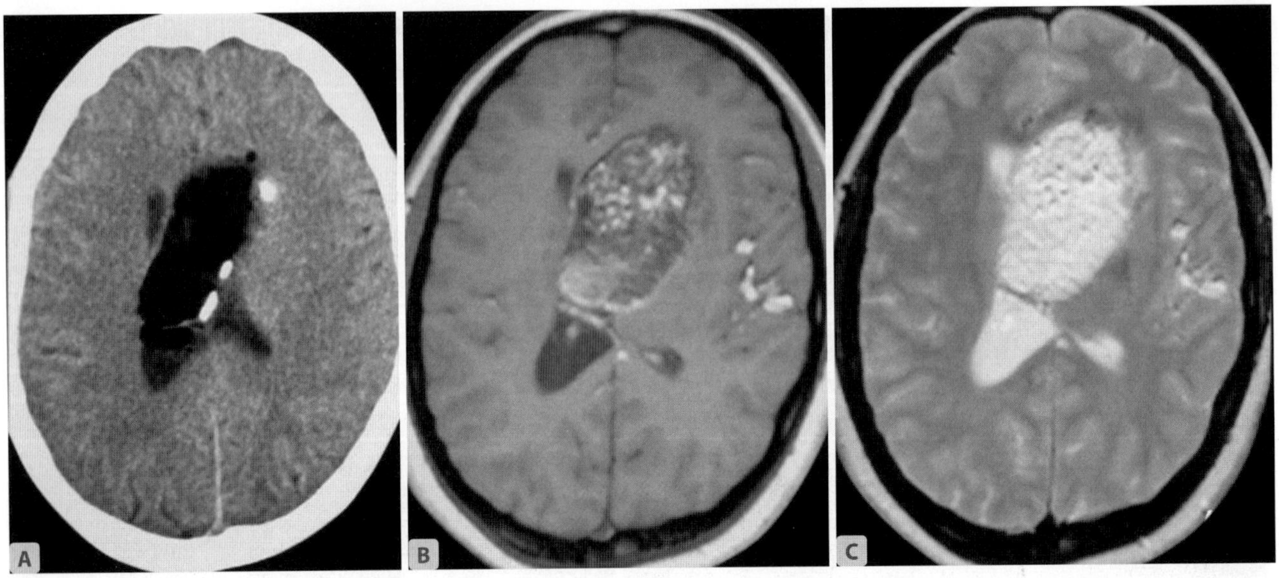

FIGS. 17A TO C: Dermoid: Axial CT (A), T1WI (B) and T2WI (C) showing the fat containing (CT hypodense and T1 hyperintense) left lateral ventricle mass with presence of eccentric calcification causing foramen of Monro obstruction and contralateral lateral ventriculomegaly.

thin T2-weighted sequences [e.g. constructive interference in steady state (CISS)] as previously discussed.

Pituitary Tumor

Pituitary tumors when large can invade the anterior third ventricle and present as anterior third ventricular masses. They can also cause compression of optic pathways. The diagnosis is usually straight forward. There is enlargement and erosion of sella with suprasellar extension.

Posterior Third Ventricular Masses

A variety of structures in and around the posterior third ventricle, including the pineal gland can be the origin of these tumors. The tumors can be astrocytoma of all grades, ependymomas, germinomas, meningiomas, vascular malformations, pineal tumors, metastasis or primary lymphomas. Regardless of the origin, these masses cause obstructive hydrocephalus due to compression of the posterior third ventricle or aqueduct and abnormal eye movements from pressure on, or infiltration of the pretectal area (e.g. Parinaud's syndrome).[28,30,33]

Glial Tumors

Astrocytomas comprise 25% of the mass lesions in the posterior third ventricle. Other gliomas like ependymomas, oligodendrogliomas, or glioblastomas can also occur in this area. There is no significant age or sex predilection. The imaging features are similar to those occurring in other areas of brain.

Germinoma

Germinoma is more common in posterior than anterior 3rd ventricle. It is common in young males and causes precocious puberty. It may lead to Parinaud's syndrome and hydrocephalus. On CT and MRI, it appears as well demarcated, homogeneous soft tissue mass and shows uniform enhancement after IV contrast administration. There is no calcification within the tumor. The tumor spreads through CSF pathway and responds to radiotherapy. Therefore, after obtaining tissue diagnosis (either by stereotactic or open biopsy) the entire neuroaxis should be irradiated.

Teratoma

Mature teratomata are well-differentiated benign tumors with a malignant potential. They are well encapsulated and show no evidence of infiltration of surrounding structures. On CT, teratomas show areas of fat attenuation and calcification or ossification. The solid portion can show some degree of contrast enhancement. On T1WI the fat in the teratoma appears hyperintense. Signal loss due to calcific foci can be seen on both T1WI and T2WI.

Pineoblastoma

It resembles other primitive neuroectodermal tumors (PNETs) (e.g. medulloblastoma) histologically. It is an infiltrative tumor and presents with obstructive hydrocephalus or Parinaud's syndrome. On CT, it appears hyperdense and enhances homogeneously and brightly following IV contrast injection. On MRI, it is hypo or isointense on T1WI and hyperintense on T2WI. Small areas of necrosis, hemorrhage, cyst formation or calcification can be seen. There is typically brilliant enhancement on gadolinium injection. It also shows spread along CSF pathways like germinoma and therefore the entire craniospinal axis should be imaged in such patients.[32]

Pineocytoma

Pineocytoma differs from pineoblastoma in that it contains more differentiated tumor cells and is not as infiltrative

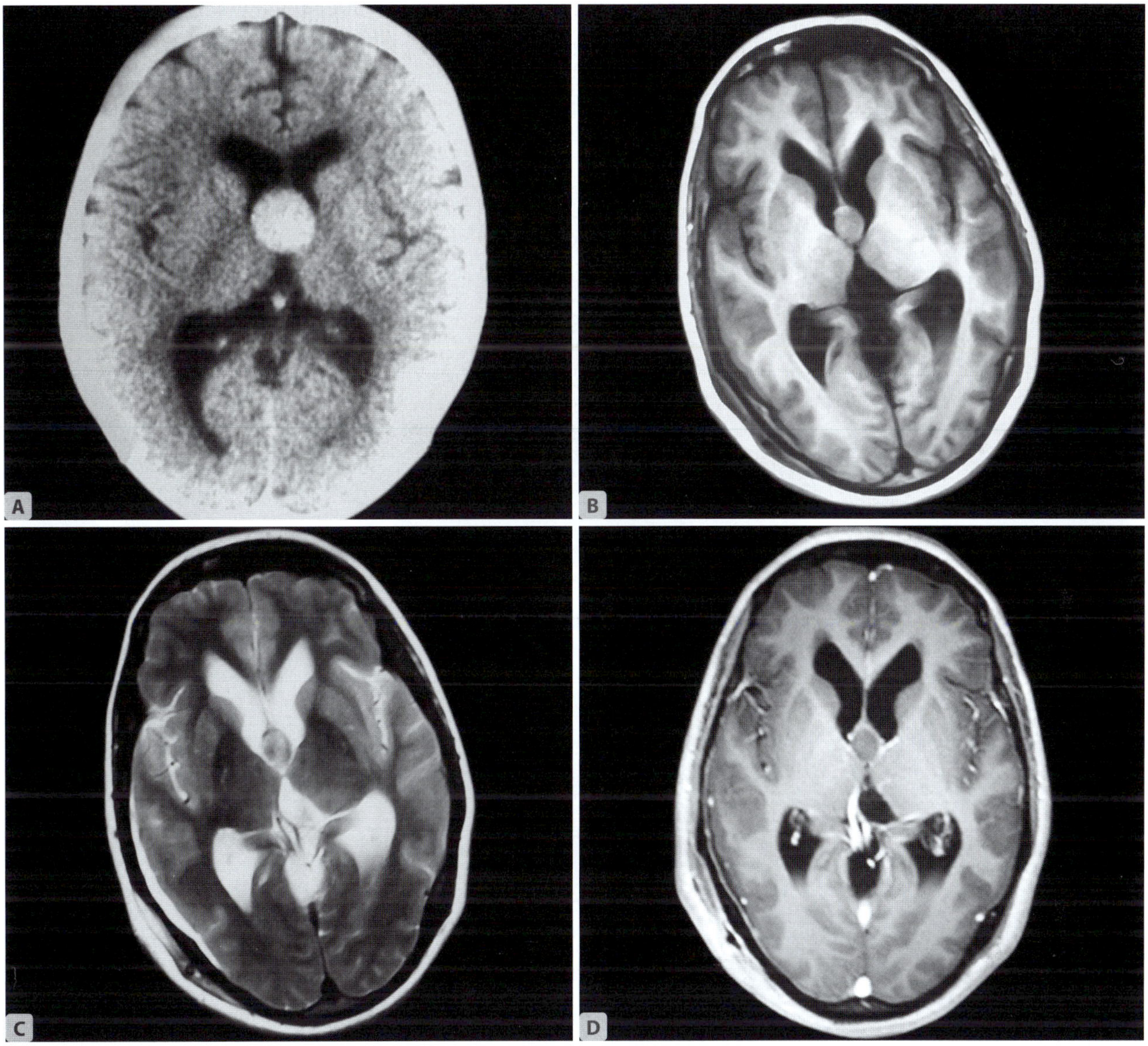

FIGS. 18A TO D: Colloid cyst: Plain CT (A) shows a homogenously hyperdense midline non enhancing globular lesion in the foramen of Monro. MRI in another patient shows a similar lesion which is isointense to gray matter on T1 (B) as well as T2 (C) Weighted sequences showing no post contrast enhancement (D).

(Figs. 23A to C). It can cause hydrocephalus and the imaging features are similar to those of pineoblastoma.[32]

Vascular Masses

Arteriovenous malformations and cavernous angiomas, both can occur in the third ventricle.[25] They present on CT as brilliantly enhancing lesions consisting of serpiginous channels. MRI shows these lesions without contrast injection as serpiginous cluster of signal void seen in a cluster. MR angiography can be useful in delineating the feeding artery or draining veins. Angiography is the definitive investigation and it is almost always required preoperatively. When the feeders are located in surgically inaccessible sites, angioembolization can be attempted as a definitive treatment. Cavernous angiomas classically appear as lobulated "popcorn" shaped lesions having heterogeneous T1 and T2 signal with intense blooming on susceptibility weighted images **(Figs. 24A to C)**.

Fourth Ventricular Masses

Primary fourth ventricular neoplasms are common in children but rare in adults. The pediatric tumors are cerebellar astrocytoma, medulloblastoma, ependymoma and choroid plexus papilloma.[34] In adults, metastases are the most common fourth ventricular neoplasm. Other tumors, such as choroid plexus papilloma, epidermoid, dermoid and hemangioblastomas **(Fig. 25)** are rare. Subependymoma occur in caudal fourth ventricle near the obex. Non-neoplastic masses like arachnoid cysts, vascular malformation, cysticercosis, inflammatory cysts are occasionally seen within the fourth ventricle **(Figs. 26A to C)**. Partially exophytic

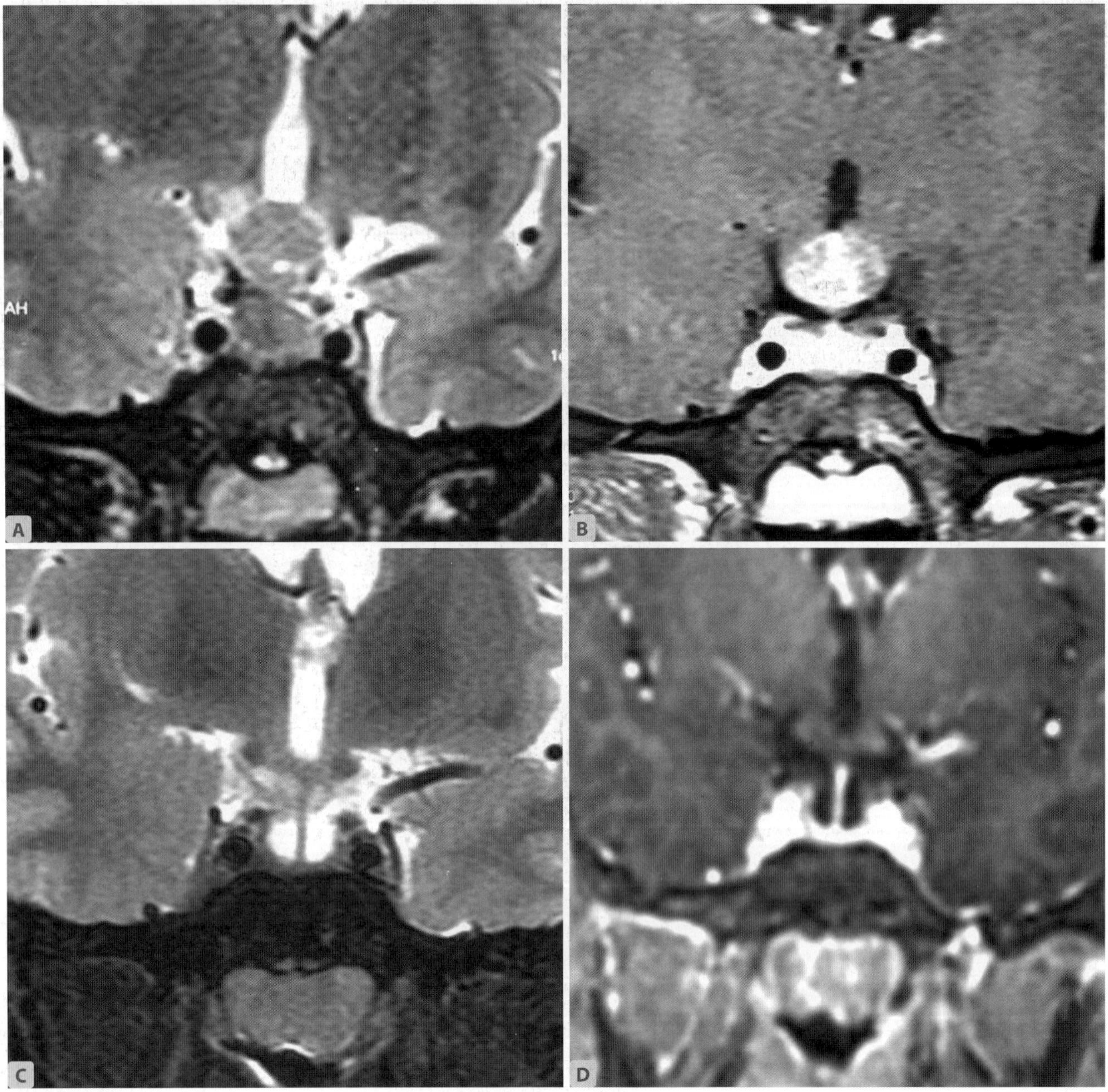

FIGS. 19A TO D: Third ventricular/suprasellar germ cell tumor. Coronal T2WI (A) and post-contrast T1WI (B) showing the T2 isointense homogeneously enhancing third ventricular floor lesion. Corresponding sections (C and D) show complete lesion resolution following radiotherapy.

masses may cause sudden loss of consciousness due to CSF obstruction referred to as Bruns syndrome.[35]

Cerebellar Astrocytoma

It is the most common posterior fossa neoplasm and constitutes 25% of all fourth ventricular neoplasms in children.[34] Histologically majority of the tumors are of pilocytic type. It usually originates from the vermis and extends anteriorly into the fourth ventricle. Rarely, the tumor arises primarily within the ventricle itself. The child usually presents with enlarging head and features of raised intracranial tension due to obstructive hydrocephalus. On CT, the tumor appears as a large lesion with solid (40%) or cystic (60%) components. The cystic mass shows a mural nodule. The nodule is always solitary and isodense with cerebellum on noncontrast scans. The nodule may or may not be calcified. On contrast administration the nodule shows intense, homogeneous enhancement which does not extend beyond the contour of the cyst. The cyst in unilocular and its walls apart from the site of nodule shows no enhancement. This distinguishes it from necrotic astrocytoma in which the cyst is multilocular, has ill-defined mural nodule, the tumor blush extends beyond the contour of the cyst and entire circumference of the cyst wall and the intervening septa also enhance.[36] The solid astrocytoma is round to oval, iso to hyperdense with nearly homogeneous dense contrast enhancement. On MRI, the

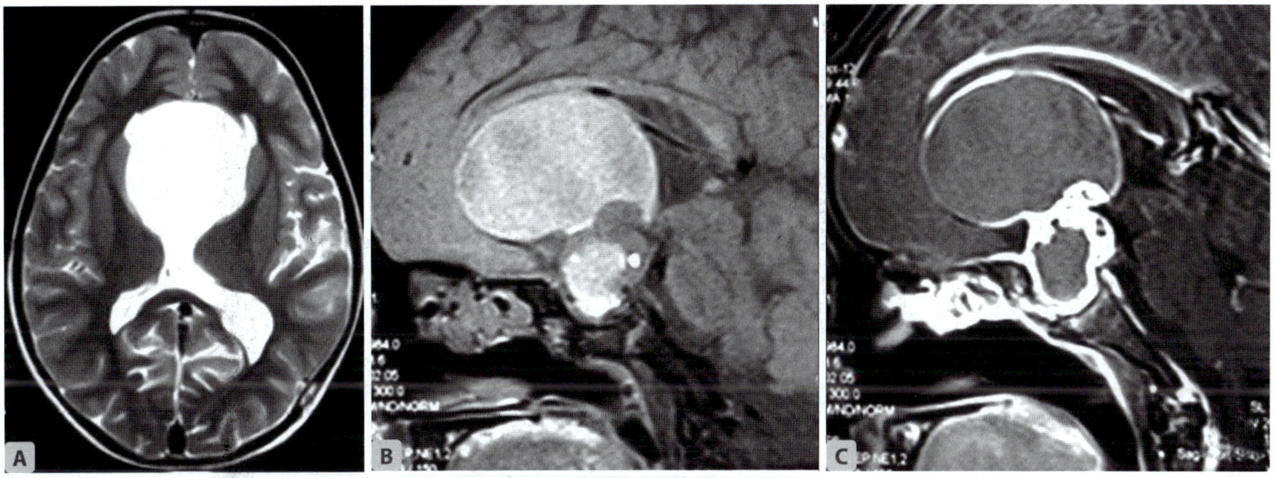

FIGS. 20A TO C: Craniopharyngioma: Large suprasellar lesion invading the anteroinferior third ventricle as shown on axial T2WI (A), sagittal pre (B) and post-contrast (C) T1W images. Note the T1 hyperintense signal in the cyst (motor oil appearance) with peripheral enhancement.

appearance is similar with cystic component being hypo to isointense on T1WI and hyperintense on T2WI. The mural nodule shows intense enhancement with IV gadolinium **(Figs. 27A and B)**.

Medulloblastoma

This primitive neuroectodermal tumor is the second most common posterior fossa tumor constituting one fourth of all posterior fossa tumors in children. Ninety percent of these lesions originate in the inferior vermis and fill the fourth ventricle. The tumor shows dissemination along the CSF pathways in 60–100% cases. This is usually thickest at the skull base and within the sylvian fissures. Spinal cord metastases are also common (12–40%). Dorsal and lumbosacral region is seeded most commonly and the deposits are often multiple. Systemic metastases (15%) can also occur in bones (86%), peritoneum (via shunt) (43%), lymph nodes (30%), and in lung and liver (7%).

On CT, medulloblastoma is usually seen as a large, mildly hyperdense, midline solid mass arising from the inferior vermis. The tumor bulges anteriorly into the fourth ventricle and may extend into adjacent cisterns. Rarely, calcification, hemorrhage and necrosis are seen. On contrast, it shows moderate degree of homogeneous enhancement **(Fig. 28A)**. Typical appearance is seen in only one-third of cases. Cystic changes (65%), isodense mass on plain CT (3%) and absent contrast enhancement (3%) are also encountered. On MR, the typical medulloblastoma fills the fourth ventricle and extends inferiorly through foramen of Magendie into the cistern magna. It appears hypointense on T1WI and shows variable signal pattern on T2WI. Moderate enhancement is typical after IV gadolinium injection **(Figs. 28B and C)**. Due to high tumor cellularity it may show diffusion restriction with low apparent diffusion coefficient (ADC) values **(Fig. 28D)**. Other fourth ventricular tumors like ependymoma and astrocytomas can often be differentiated from it on MRI based on this finding. Hydrocephalus is seen in up to 85% cases.[34]

Ependymoma

It is the third most common fourth ventricular tumor in children. Nearly 50% of posterior fossa ependymomas are located in the fourth ventricle. On CT, the mass is midline and situated within an expanded fourth ventricle and often shows calcification (50%). There is usually moderate enhancement on contrast administration **(Fig. 29A)**. The mass typically extends outward into cerebellopontine cisterns or into the cisterna magna through the fourth ventricular exit foramina **(Figs. 29B and C)**. Hydrocephalus is nearly always seen. The tumor exhibits similar morphology on MRI as hypo to isointense signal on T1WI and intermediate to hyper intense signal on T2WI with heterogeneous post-contrast enhancement.[24]

Table 3 highlights the important points of differences between the most common posterior fossa tumors in childhood.

Brainstem Gliomas

They are the fourth most common posterior fossa tumors in children.[34] About 70% of gliomas in the brainstem are of high grade. The low grade gliomas typically show a dorsal exophytic component that grows into the fourth ventricle. It involves the pons (54%) but can extend inferiorly into medulla, superiorly into thalamus and midbrain and posterolaterally along cerebellar peduncles into cerebellar hemispheres. The imaging features are similar as described in other areas.

CONCLUSION

Intraventricular lesions are histologically distinct but residentially similar lesions. A distinct understanding of their clinical behavior including presenting age, typical location and morphological description is required for reaching at a correct set of differential diagnosis.

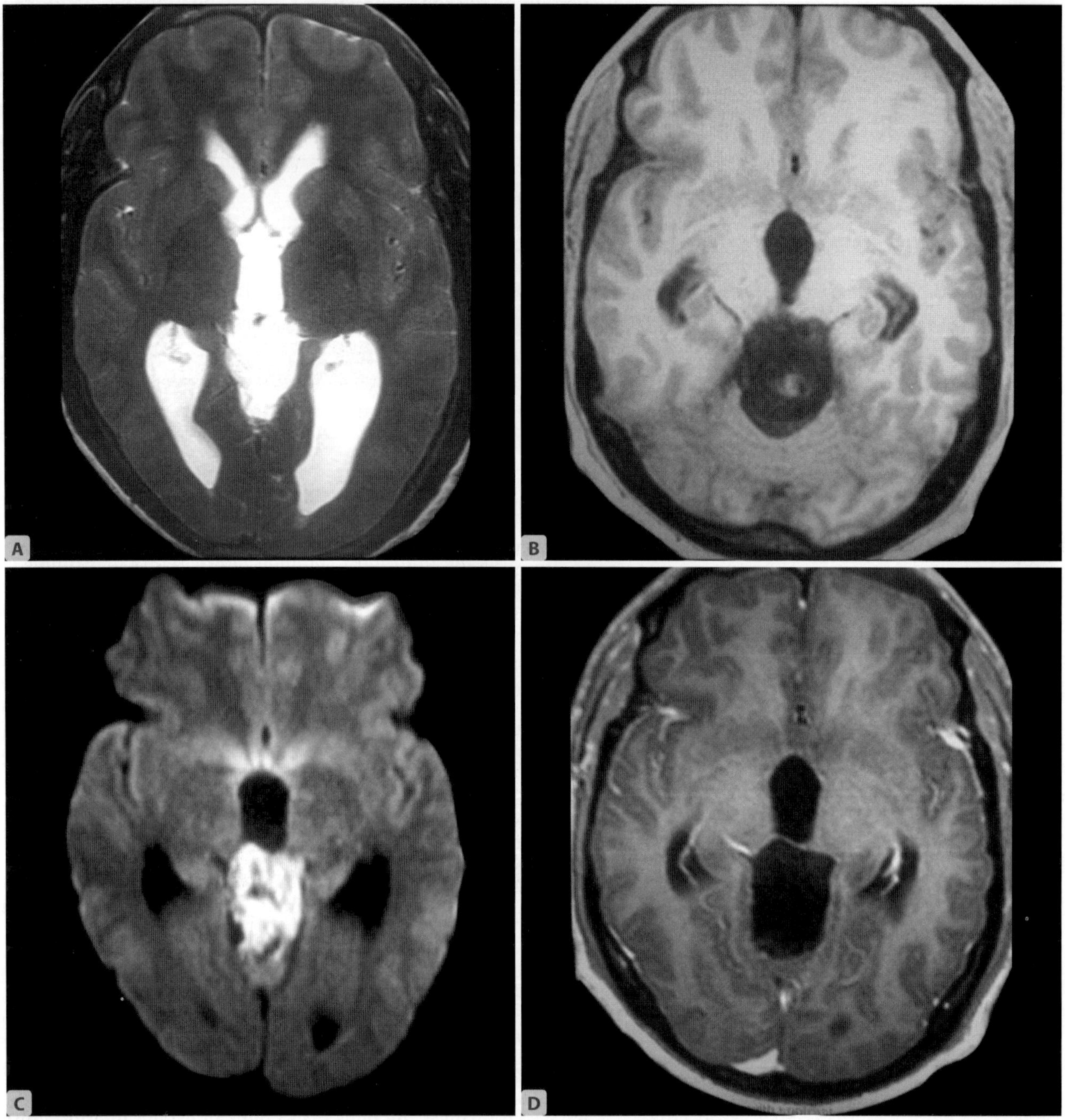

FIGS. 21A TO D: Third ventricular epidermoid cyst: Axial T2WI (A), T1WI (B) showing posterior third ventricular cyst with intense diffusion restriction (C). No post-contrast enhancement seen (D).

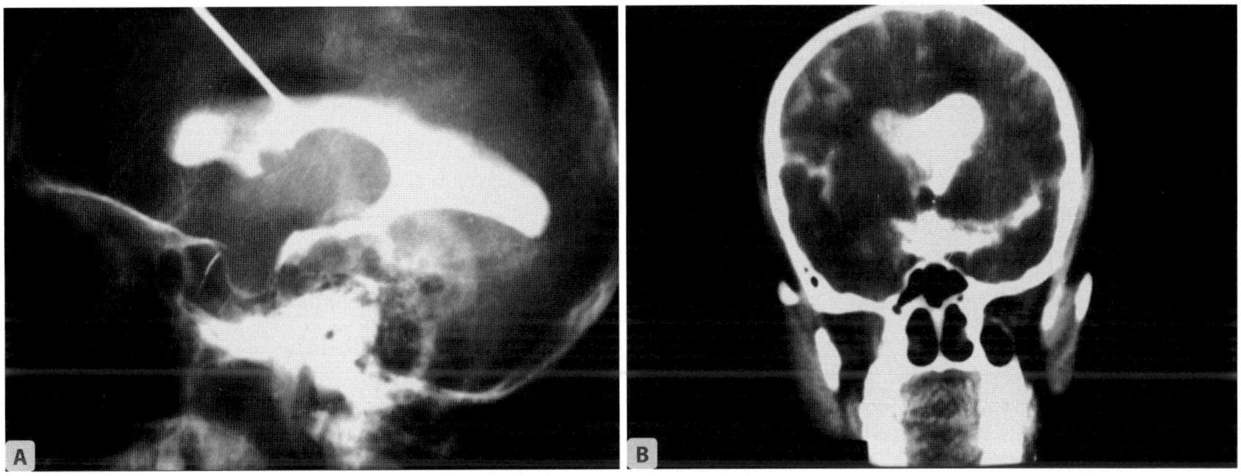

FIGS. 22A AND B: Cysticercosis: Lateral contrast ventriculogram (A) shows well-defined filling defect at foramen of Monro (B) CT ventriculogram confirms the cystic lesion.

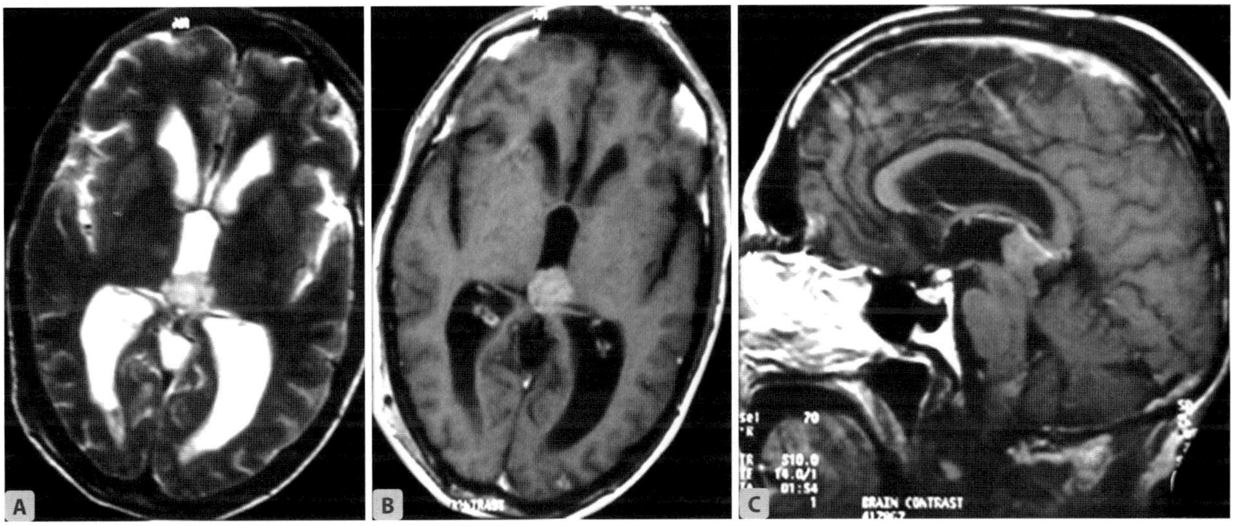

FIGS. 23A TO C: Pineocytoma: Axial T2WI (A), gadolinium enhanced axial (B) and sagittal (C) T1W images showing the posterior third ventricular lesion. Note the origin of the lesion from the pineal gland on sagittal image.

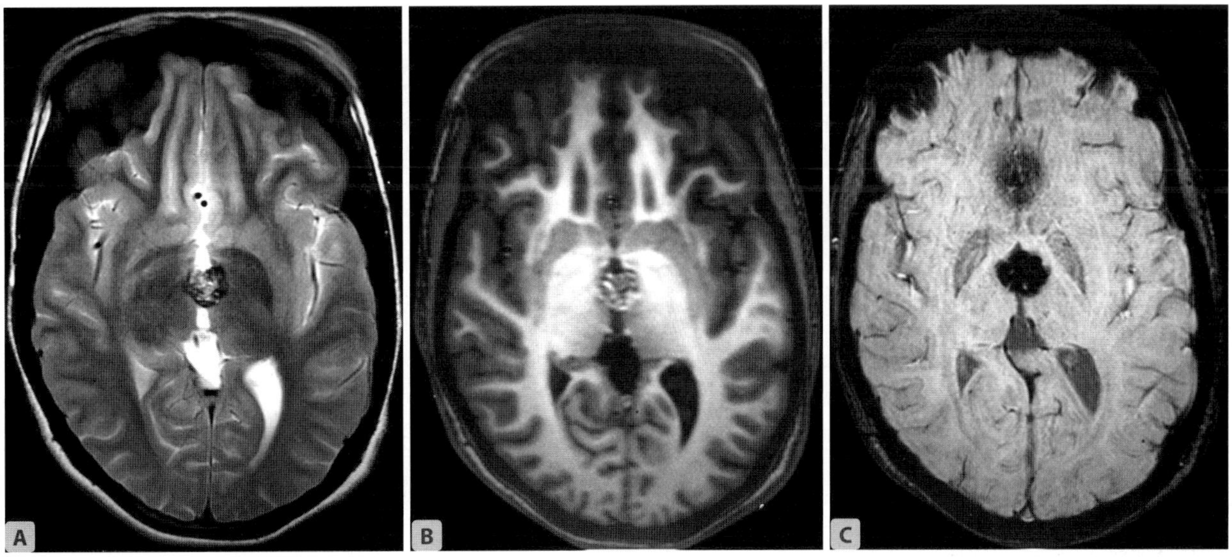

FIGS. 24A TO C: Third ventricular cavernoma: Axial T2WI (A) and T1WI (B) depicting the third ventricular ependymal "popcorn" lesion with blooming on susceptibilty weighted image (C).

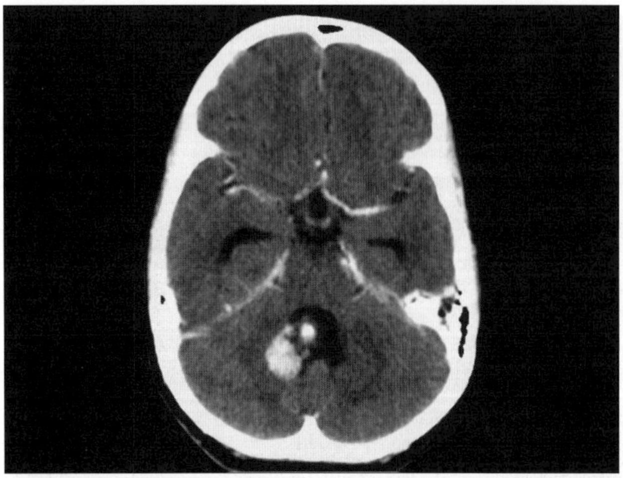

FIG. 25: Fourth ventricular cerebellar hemangioblastoma: Contrast-enhanced CT demonstrating the presence of a cystic lesion with enhancing mural nodule in the fourth ventricle.

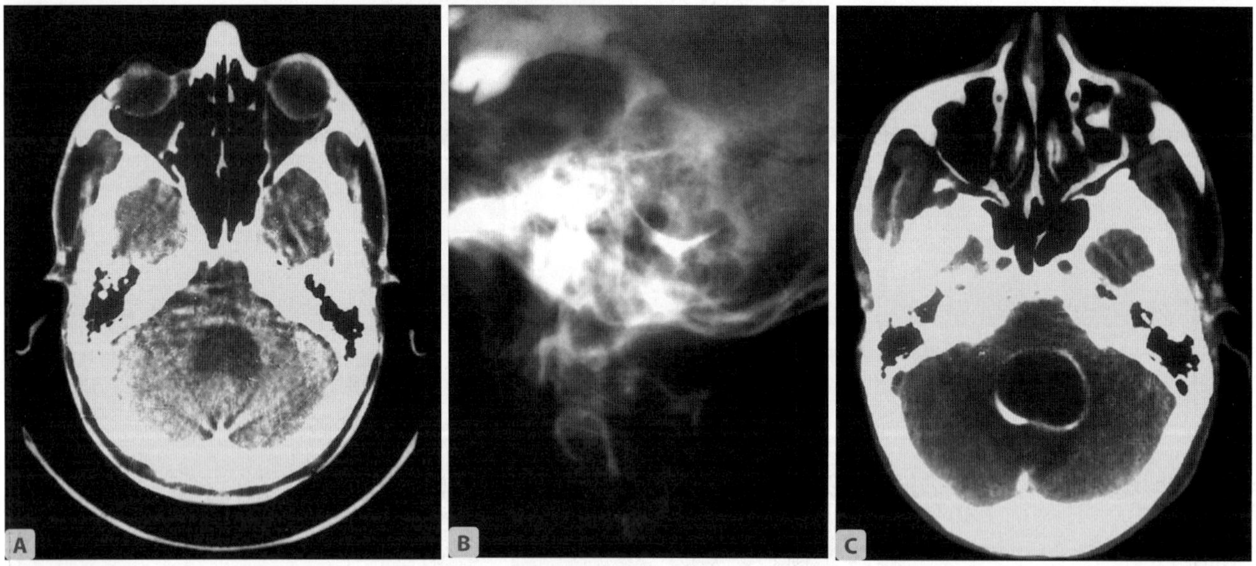

FIGS. 26A TO C: Fourth ventricular cysticercosis: (A) CECT shows dilation of the 4th ventricle, (B) lateral contrast ventriculogram shows well-defined filling detect in the 4th ventricle and (C) CT ventriculogram confirms the findings.

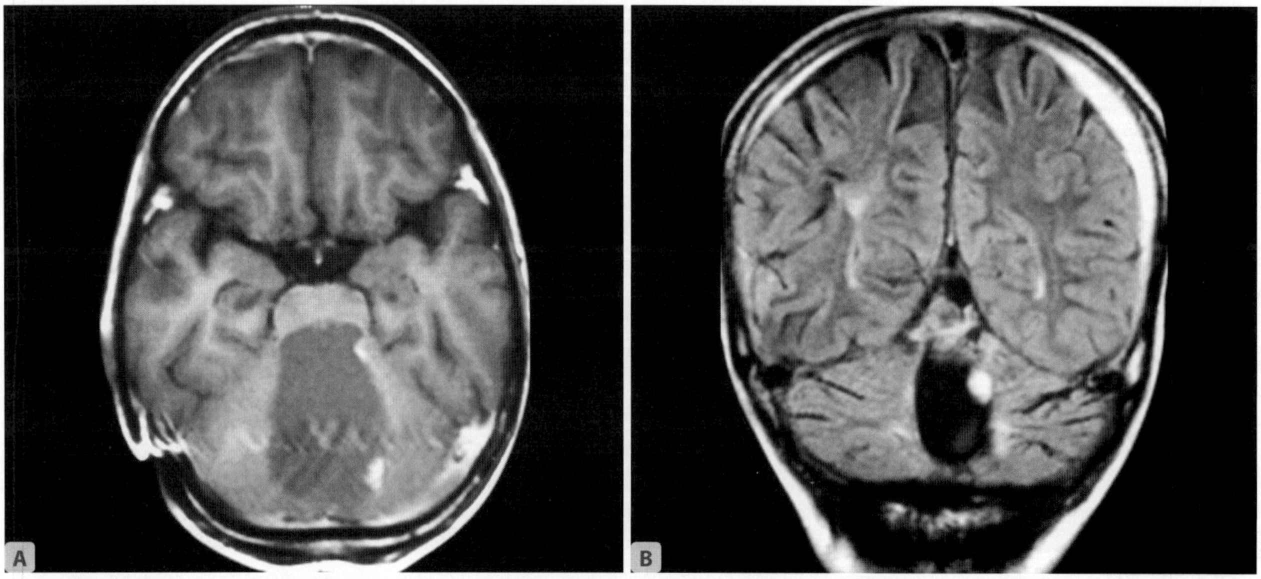

FIGS. 27A AND B: Pilocytic astrocytoma: MRI brain showing a large posterior fossa cystic mass with enhancing mural nodule.

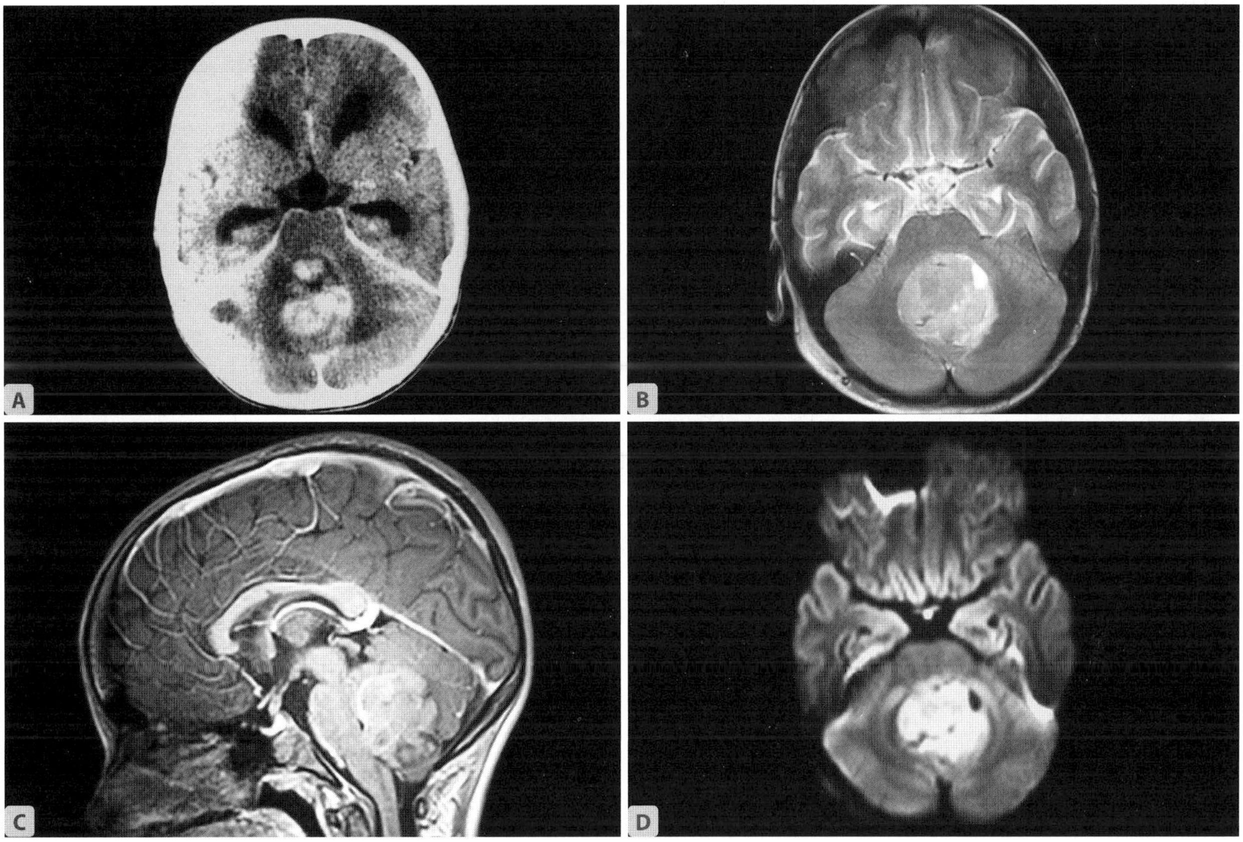

FIGS. 28A TO D: Medulloblastoma: CECT (A) shows a heterogeneously enhancing fourth ventricular mass. MRI (B and C) in another patient shows a similar mass in the fourth ventricle showing diffusion restriction (D) indicating high tumor cellularity.

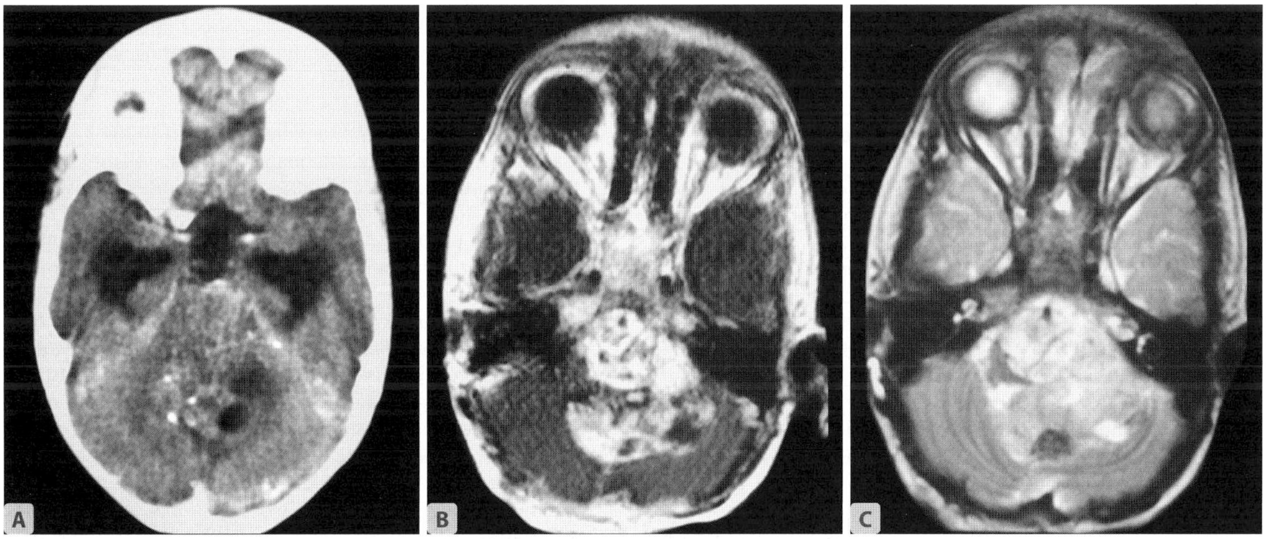

FIGS. 29 A TO C: Ependymoma: CECT (A) showing an ill-defined heterogeneously enhancing fourth ventricular tumor with presence of calcification. MRI (B and C) showing "plasticity" of the tumor with extension through the fourth ventricular outlet foramina into the adjacent cisternal spaces.

TABLE 3: Differences between common posterior fossa tumors in children.

Tumor characteristics	*Astrocytoma*	*Medulloblastoma*	*Ependymoma*
CT	Hypodense	Hyperdense	Isodense
Calcification	~10%	10–15%	40–50%
T1WI	Iso/hypo	Iso/hypo	Iso/hypo
T2WI	Hyper	Iso	Iso/hyper
Post gadolinium	Nodule enhances	Moderate	Mild
Cyst formation	Very common	Rare	Common
Transforaminal spread	No	No	Yes
CSF seeding	Rare	Yes (15–40%)	No

REFERENCES

1. Tien RD. Intraventricular mass lesion of the brain: CT and MRI findings. Am J Roentgenol. 1991;157:1283-90.
2. Waldron JS, Tihan T. Epidemiology and pathology of intraventricular tumors. Neurosurg Clin N Am. 2003;14:469-82.
3. Jelinek J, Smirniothopoulos JG, Parisi JE, et al. Lateral ventricular neoplasms of the brain: differential diagnosis based on clinical, CT and MR findings. Am J Neuroradiol. 1990;11:567-74.
4. Agarwal A, Kanekar S. Intraventricular tumors. Semin Ultrasound CT MR. 2016;37:150-8.
5. Seçer HI, Düz B, Izci Y, et al. Tumors of the lateral ventricle: the factors that affected the preference of the surgical approach in 46 patiens. Turk Neurosurg. 2008;18:345-55.
6. Zuccaro G, Sosa F, Cuccia V, et al. Lateral ventricle tumors in children: a series of 54 cases. Childs Nerv Syst. 1999;15:774-85.
7. Wolff JE, Finlay JL. Choroid plexus tumors. In: Carroll WL, Finlay JL (Eds). Cancer in Children and Adolescents. Sudbury, Mass: Jones & Bartlett; 2009. p. 299.
8. Paulus W, Brandner S. Choroid plexus tumors. In: Louis DN, Ohgaki H, Wiestler OD, Cavenee WK (Eds). WHO Classification of Tumours of the Central Nervous System. Lyon, France: IARC; 2007. pp. 82-5.
9. Coates TL, Hinshaw DB, Peckman N. Pediatric choroid plexus papillomas. MR, CT and pathologic correlation. Radiology. 1989;173:818.
10. Meyers SP, Khademian ZP, Chuang SH, et al. Choroid plexus carcinomas in children: MRI features and patient outcomes. Neuroradiology. 2004;46:770-80.
11. Horská A, Ulug AM, Melhem ER, et al. Proton magnetic resonance spectroscopy of choroid plexus tumors in children. J Magn Reson Imaging. 2001;14(1):78-82.
12. Castillo M, Scatiff JH, Bouldin TW, et al. Radiologic-pathologic correlation: intracranial astrocytoma. Am J Neuroradiol. 1992;13:1609-16.
13. Kumar R, Singh V. Subependymal giant cell astrocytoma: a report of five cases. Neurosurg Rev. 2004;27:274-80.
14. Zamora C, Huisman TA, Izbudak I. Supratentorial tumors in pediatric patients. Neuroimaging Clin N Am. 2017;27:39-67.
15. Swartz GP, Zimemerman RA, Bilaniuk LT. Computed tomography of intracranial ependymoma. Radiology. 1982;143:97-101.
16. Darwish B, Munro I, Boet R, et al. Intraventricular meningioma with drop metastases and subgaleal metastatic nodule. J Clin Neurosci. 2004;11:787-91.
17. Holvek A, Grand S, Boini S, et al. Dynamic susceptibility contrast-enhanced MRI evaluation of cerebral intraventricular tumors: preliminary results. J Neuroradiol. 2010;37:269-75.
18. Vuckovic N, Kozic D, Vulekovic P, et al. MR and MRS characteristics of intraventricular meningioma. J Neuroimaging. 2010;20:294-6.
19. Koeller KK, Sandberg GD; Armed Forces Institute of Pathology. From the archives of the AFIP. Cerebral intraventricular neoplasms: radiologic-pathologic correlation. Radiographics. 2002;22(6):1473-505.
20. Cordoliani YS, Derosier C, Pharaboz C. Primary cerebral lymphoma in patients with AIDS: MR findings in 17 cases. AJR. 1992;159:841-7.
21. Kerkovský M, Zitterbart K, Svoboda K, et al. Central neurocytoma: the neuroradiological perspective. Childs Nerv Syst. 2008;24:1361-9.
22. Kim DG, Chi JG, Park SH. Intraventricular neurocytoma: clinicopathological analysis of seven cases. J Neurosurg. 1992;76:759-65.
23. Shah T, Jayasundar R, Singh VP, et al. MRS characterization of central neurocytomas using glycine. NMR Biomed. 2011;24(10):1408-13.
24. Spoto GP, Press GA, Hesselink JR, et al. Intracranial ependymoma and subependymoma: MR manifestations. Am J Neuroradiol. 1990;11:83-91.
25. Miyagi Y, Mannoji H, Akaboshi K. Intraventricular cavernous malformation associated with medullary venous malformation. Neurosurgery. 1993;32:461-4.
26. Nakase H, Morimoto T, Sakaki T. Bilateral choroid plexus cysts in the lateral ventricles. Am J Neuroradiol. 1991;12:1204-5.
27. Gaskill SJ, Saldivar V, Rutman J, et al. Giant bilateral xanthogranulomas in a child: a case report. Neurosurgery. 1992;31:114-7.
28. Vandesteen L, Drier A, Galanaud D, et al. Imaging findings of intraventricular and ependymal lesions. J Neuroradiol. 2013;40(4):229-44.
29. Lach B, Scheithauer BW, Gregor A, et al. Colloid cyst of the third ventricle: a comparative immunohistochemical study of neuraxis cyst and choroid plexus epithelium. J Neurosurg. 1993;78:101-11.
30. Peraud A, Illner A, Rutka JT. Intraventricular congenital lesions and colloid cysts. Neurosurg Clin N Am. 2003;14: 607-19.
31. Waggenespack GA, Guinto FC Jr. MR and CT of masses of the anterosuperior third ventricle. Am J Roentgenol. 1989;152:609-14.
32. Smirniotopoulos JG, Rushing EJ, Mena H. Pineal region masses: differential diagnosis. Radiographics. 1992;12:577-96.
33. Smith AB, Smirniotopoulos JG, Horkanyne-Szakaly I. From the radiologic pathology archives: intraventricular neoplasms: radiologic-pathologic correlation. Radiographics. 2013;33(1):21-43.
34. Maroldo TV, Barkovich AJ. Pediatric brain tumors. Semin Ultrasound CT MR. 1992;13:412-48.
35. Krasnianski M, Müller T, Stock K, et al. Bruns syndrome caused by intraventricular tumor. Eur J Med Res. 2008:13; 179-81.
36. Favre J, Deruaz JP, de Tribolet N. Pilocytic cerebellar astrocytoma in adults: case report. Surg Neurol. 1993;39:360-4.

CHAPTER

200 Imaging of the Temporal Bone

Vivek Gupta, Niranjan Khandelwal

INTRODUCTION

The temporal bone forms the segment of the cranium which separates the middle cranial fossa from the posterior cranial fossa. It contains the organs of hearing and equilibrium and is in direct relation with the temporal lobe. A number of important vascular and neural structures traverse through this bone.

A number of radiographic views are available which include the standard lateral view of skull, the Towne's view, Law's projection and its modifications, and the Stenver's view. However, with the advent of modern cross-sectional imaging modalities now the X-ray evaluation of the temporal bone has become obsolete. Computed tomography (CT) has revolutionized the imaging of the temporal bone because it is with this modality that axial, coronal and sagittal sections of the dense bone could be obtained and is the mainstay in the imaging of the temporal bone. Reconstructions in virtually any plane is made possible with the advent of multi-detector spiral CT. Magnetic resonance imaging (MRI) essentially complements CT, because of its excellent soft tissue contrast; but the osseous and air-containing structures are suboptimally imaged with this modality.

COMPUTED TOMOGRAPHY TECHNIQUE

Typically, a high resolution matrix (512 × 512) with thin sections (0.6–1.5 mm) and a field of view of 15–20 cm is employed for high resolution imaging in a bone algorithm. Newer high resolution multi-detector spiral imaging can generate isotropic voxels for multiplanar reconstruction making the need for multiple series with direct imaging in several planes unnecessary.

Planes for acquiring (or reconstructing) images are described in relation to the zero degree baseline which is the line extending between the external auditory canal and the inferior orbital rim on a lateral scout film **(Fig. 1)**.[1]

Computed tomography images are usually acquired or displayed in axial or coronal planes. Axial images are acquired in a plane rotated 30° superior to this baseline which is parallel to the lateral semicircular canal, beginning at or just above the external auditory meatus. This section will partly show the basal turn of the cochlea and the round window niche. Sections just above the basal turn of the cochlea will show the incudostapedial region and turns of the cochlea. Sections superior to these will pass through the vestibule and lateral semicircular canal. The internal auditory meatus is visualized at this level, as are the head of malleus and short process of the incus. All three segments of the facial nerve canal can be identified, though the descending portion of the canal appears in cross-section just behind the middle ear cavity. Crura of the stapes can be visualized but the oval window is not adequately demonstrated in these sections **(Figs. 2A to J)**.

Reconstructed coronal images from axial section are oriented 90° to the baseline. With the advent of volumetric data it is no longer required to obtain direct coronal acquisition. However, in the older scanners where volumetric acquisitions are not possible, direct coronal sections are acquired with patient in supine or prone positions. Sections can be acquired with neck extended to the maximum. The

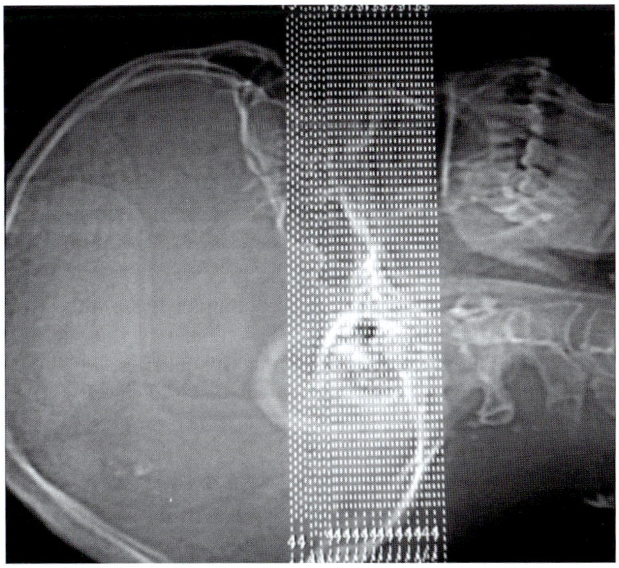

FIG. 1: Lateral topogram with planning for acquiring axial section through the temporal bone.

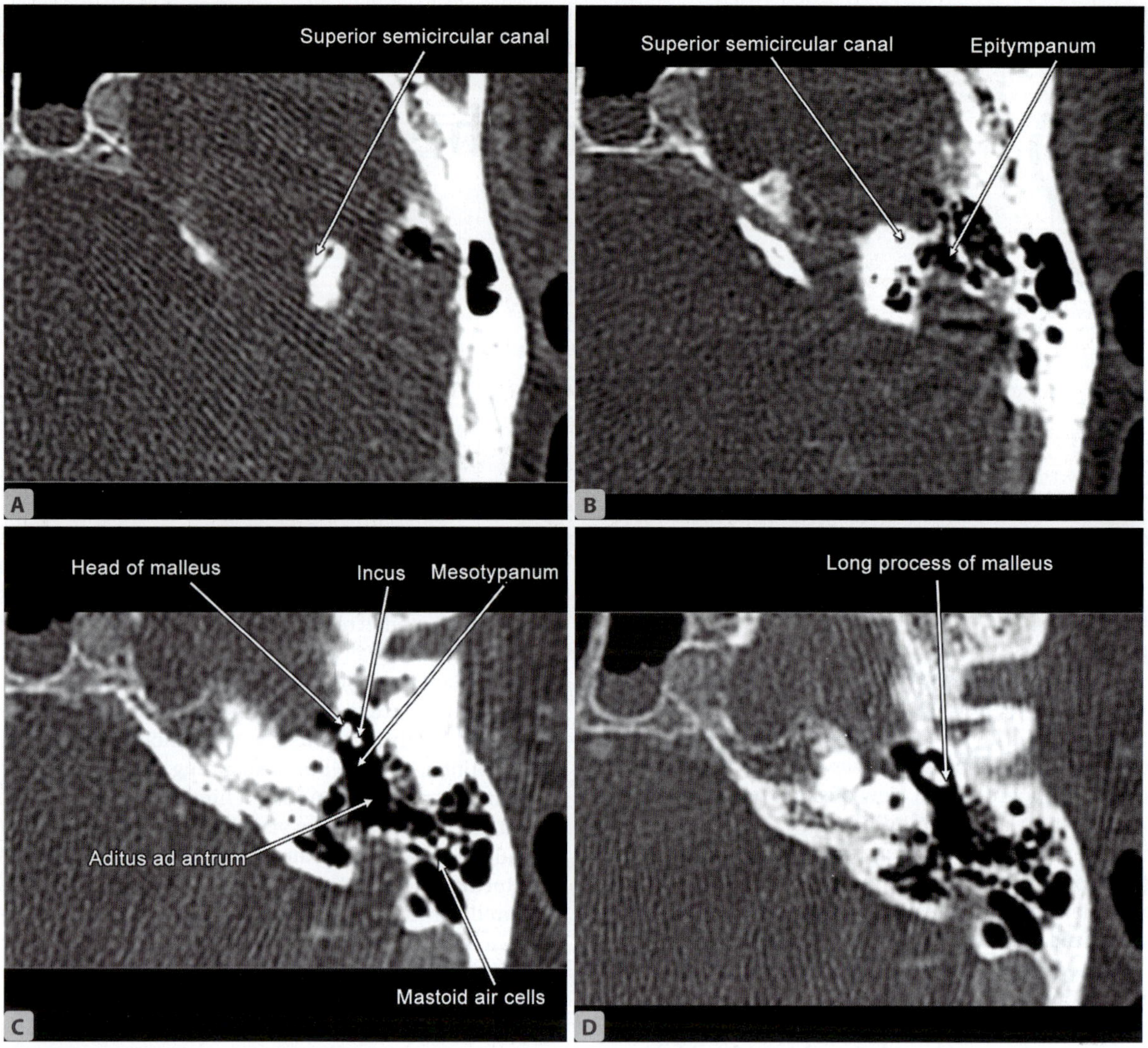

FIGS. 2A TO J: *Continued*

plane is approximately 105° to 120° the baseline which is perpendicular to the lateral semicircular canal. In patients who cannot extend the neck, modified coronal sections can be obtained in a plane parallel to the clivus which is 70° to the baseline.

Coronal sections begin at the level of the carotid canal. The coil of the cochlea forms the bulge of promontory with the oval and round window niches superior and inferior to it. The malleusis best seen in this section. Further posteriorly the vestibule and the semicircular canals can be identified and the internal auditory meatus is well seen in this section. The pyramidal eminence is present at this level, which shows the most prominent segment of the lateral semicircular canals, between the facial recess and sinus tympanicum. The descending facial canal and jugular foramen can be identified in the posterior most sections **(Figs. 3A to C)**.

Sagittal, oblique or curved projections can be reconstructed to obtain images in the plane of the long axis of the temporal bone or in planes parallel to specific areas of interest such as the facial nerve canal. 3D surface reconstructions of the temporal bone or the inner ear structures can be generated to allow studies on models thus obtained.

MAGNETIC RESONANCE IMAGING

Magnetic resonance imaging (MRI) examination is directed towards imaging of fluid containing spaces in the temporal bone, vascular structures and their pathologies and the adjacent brain parenchyma. Basic MR protocols have been recommended[2] which include: (i) whole brain/ head imaging, (ii) high resolution fluid space imaging, (iii) high resolution T1-weighted contrast enhanced imaging with or without fat suppression and (iv) MR angiography.[3]

Routine brain survey includes noncontrast and contrast enhanced T1WI, T2WI fast-echo sequence and a fluid attenuation inversion recovery (FLAIR) sequence. These sequences are especially useful in delineating brainstem demyelination or tumor. Sequences like FLAIR can also be used to differentiate hemorrhage from fat. Three-dimensional constructive interference in steady state

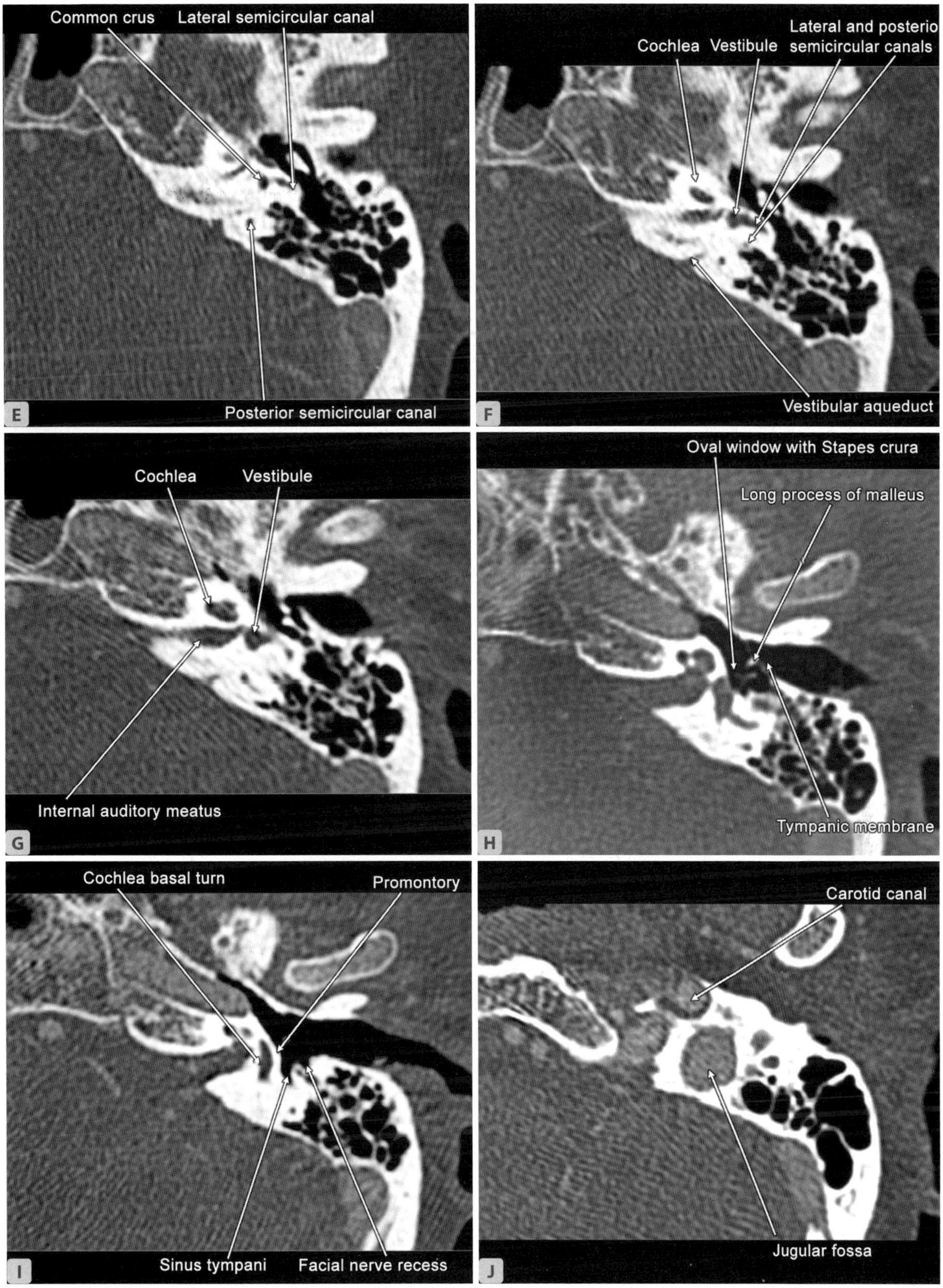

FIGS. 2A TO J: Normal anatomy of temporal bone. Axial high-resolution computed tomography (HRCT) section through the temporal bone superior to inferior.

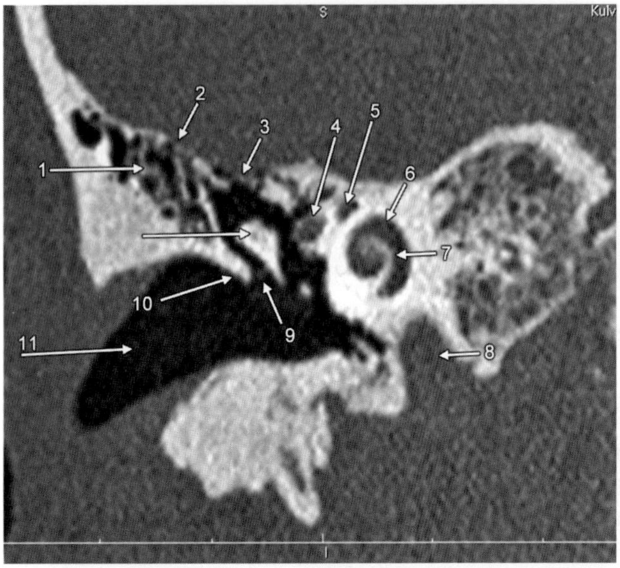

FIG. 3A: Coronal CT image shows: (1) Mastoid air cells; (2) Tegmen mastoideum; (3) Tegmen tympani; (4) Tympanic segment of facial nerve; (5) Labrynthine segment of facial nerve; (6) Basal turn of cochlea; (7) Interscalar septum; (8) Carotid canal; (9) Lateral malleal ligament; (10) scutum; (11) External auditory canal.

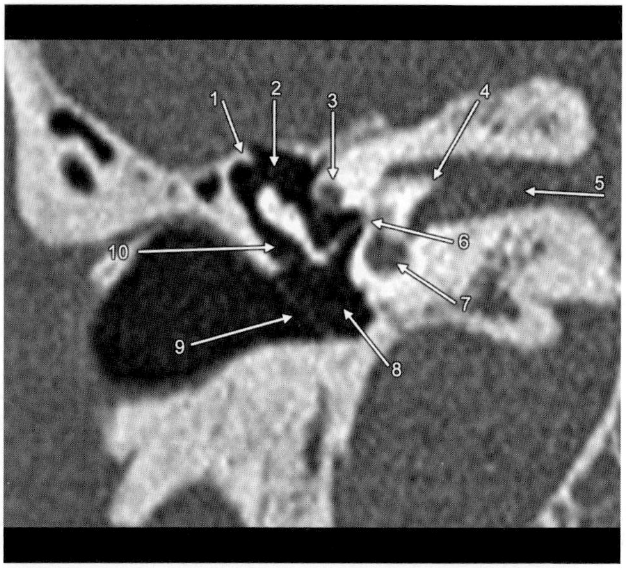

FIG. 3B: Coronal HRCT image. (1) Tegmen tympani; (2) Epitympanum; (3) Tympanic segment of facial nerve; (4) Crista falciformic; (5) Internal auditory canal; (6) Oval window; (7) Vestibule; (8) Hypotympanum; (9) Tympanic membrane; (10) Prussak space.

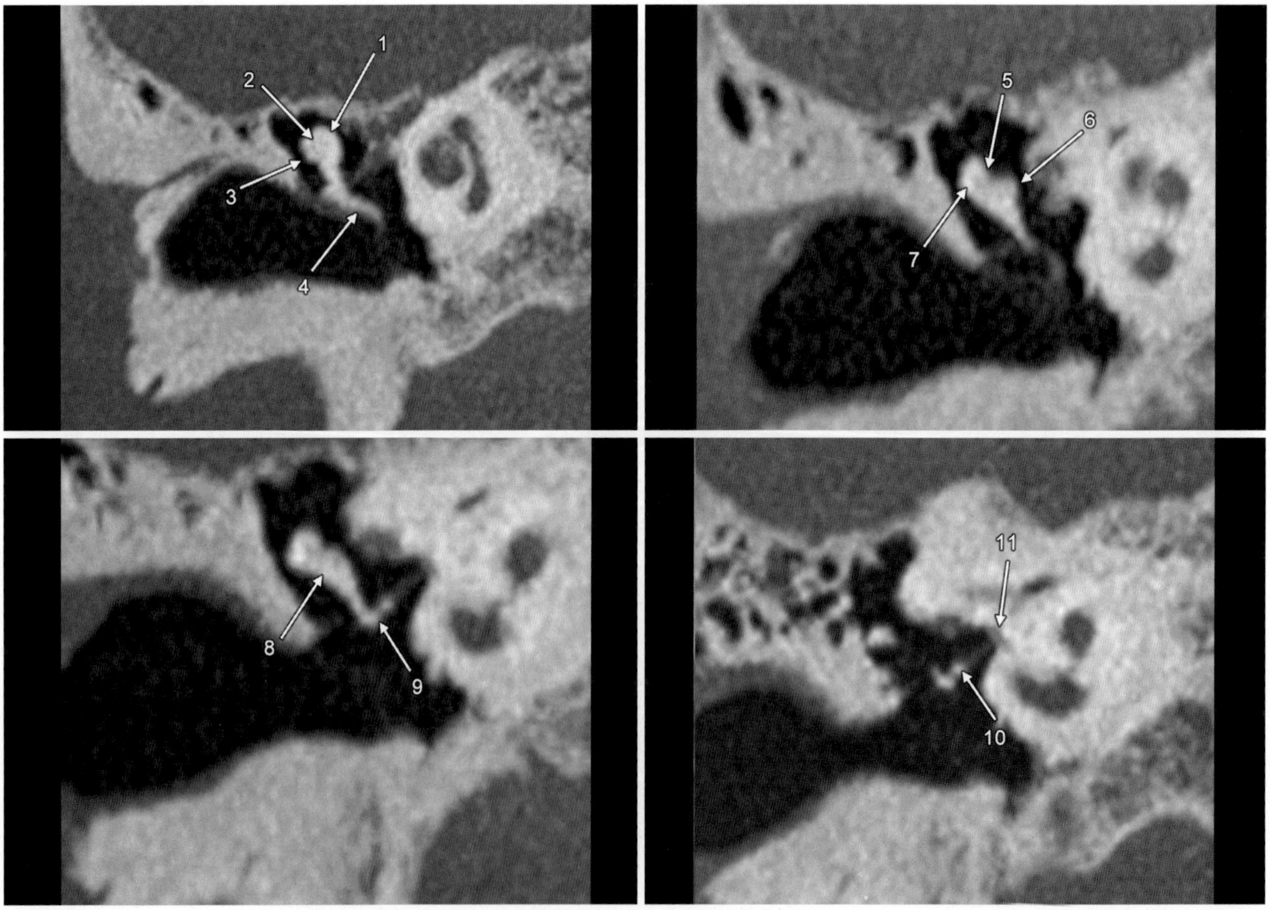

FIG. 3C: Ear ossicles as seen on coronal cuts. (1) Head of Malleus; (2) Malleo-incudo joint; (3) Incus; (4) Handle of Malleus; (5) Articulating surface of Incus; (6) Short limb of Incus; (7 and 8) Body of Incus; (9) Long limb of Incus; (10) Head of Stapes; (11) Oval window.

(3D CISS) sequence is in routine use these days. Since it is a heavily T2 weighted sequence it is especially useful in imaging of structures surrounded by fluid-like seven-eighth nerve complex and membranous labyrinth. It is a 3D sequence and images in any plane can be generated **(Fig. 4A)**. It is important to understand the detailed anatomy and relationship of VII-VIIIth cranial nerve complex once they enter the internal acoustic meatus. On the axial plane the VIIth cranial nerve is anterior to the VIIth cranial nerve in their cisternal segment. Within the IAC, the facial nerve is antero-superior, cochlear nerve is antero-inferior, superior vestibular nerve is posterosuperior and the inferior vestibular nerve is posteroinferior. These relationships are best studied in sagital-oblique plane as shown in **Figure 4B**.

Some authors used another new sequence of 3D variable-flip-angle fast-spin-echo (3D VFA FSE) to image the membranous labyrinth. This technique can be used clinically to reduce susceptibility artifacts and image blurring which may be a problem when small field-of-view (FOV) is used to image temporal bone with sequences which are heavily T2 weighted.[4]

High resolution T1W contrast enhanced images are acquired using a three-dimensional Fourier transformation (3DFT) technique. Fluid spaces have low signal intensity and

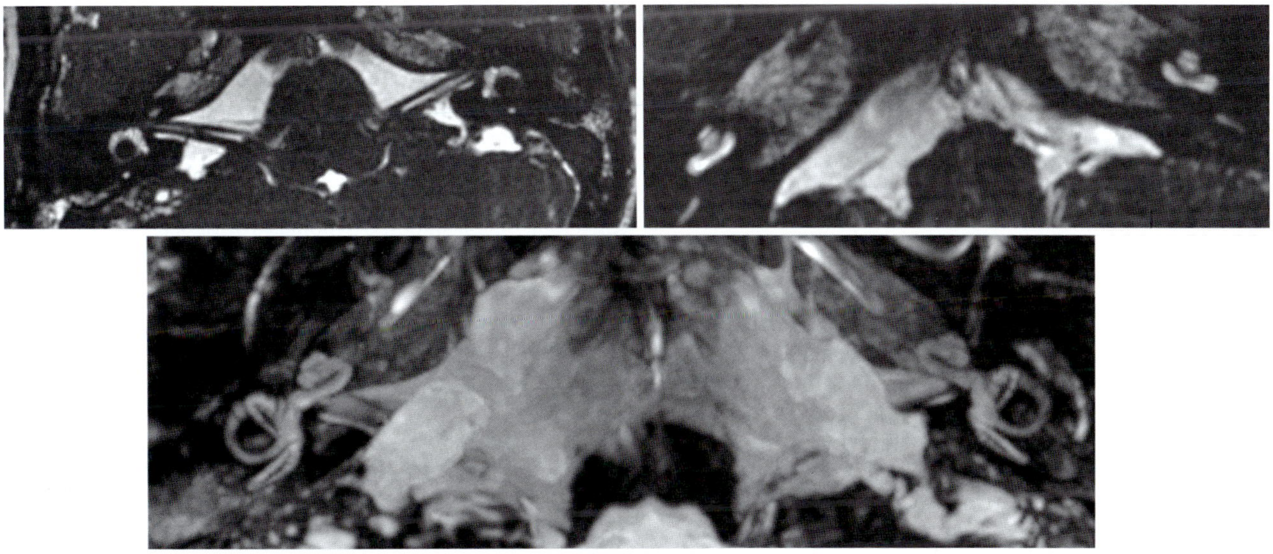

FIG. 4A: Maximum intensity projection (MIP) image of 3D-CISS sequence showing detailed anatomy of inner ear-cochlea (C), vestibule (V), semicircular canals (SC) and VII-VIII cranial nerves (CN).

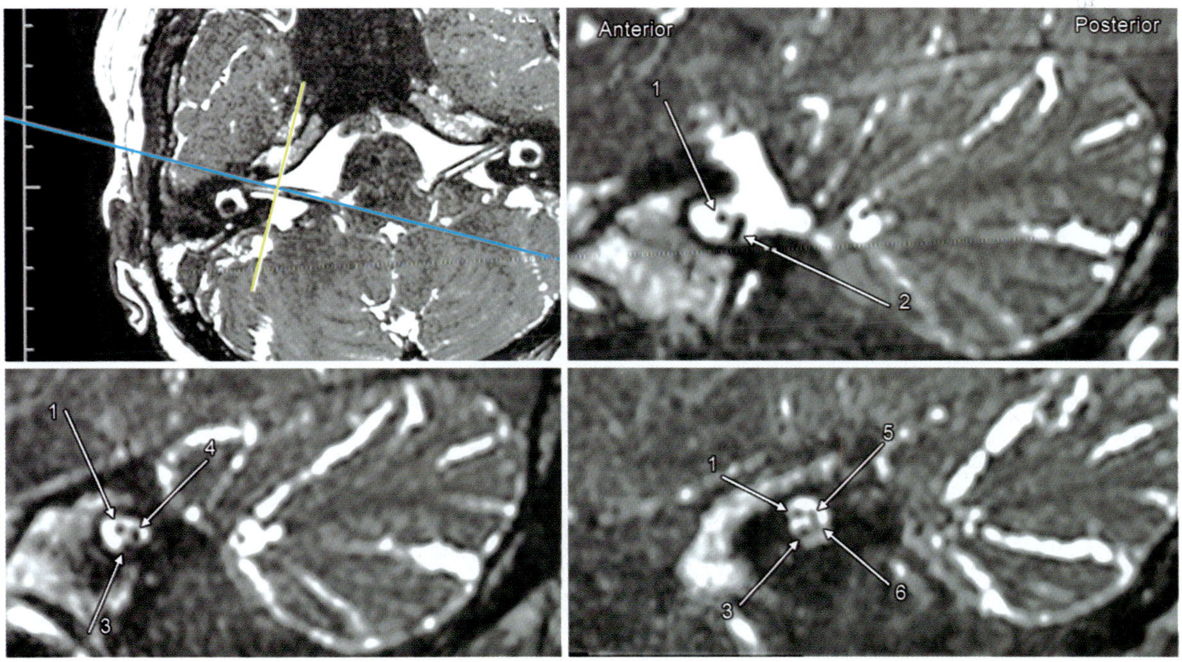

FIG. 4B: (1) Facial nerve; (2) Vestibulocochlear nerve; (3) Cochlear nerve; (4) Vestibular nerve; (5) superior vesibular nerve; (6) Inferior vestibular nerve.

nerves have higher signal intensity on this sequence. This sequence is ideal for identification of subtle changes, such as those seen in vestibulitis or in demonstrating small vestibular tumors. Magnetic resonance angiography is specifically indicated to assess structures around the jugular foramen and internal acoustic meatus and consists of sequence for visualization of arteries and veins in relation to the temporal bone.

CONGENITAL ANOMALIES OF THE TEMPORAL BONE

Congenital anomalies of the temporal bone can be divided into two groups: those involving the external and middle ears and those involving the inner ear. This division can be explained on the basis of development of the temporal bone. The external and middle ear develop from the first and second branchial arches, the first branchial groove and the adjacent mesenchyme. The inner ear develops from the pars optica which develops from auditory vesicle and the adjacent mesenchyme.[2,5,6]

Anomalies of the External and Middle Ear

The external auditory canal may be stenotic or atretic. Both stenosis and atresia of the canal can be associated with small auricles, a condition which is termed as microtia **(Figs. 5A and B)**. Stenosis of the external auditory canal can be diffuse, involving the entire length of the canal, or it can be focal. Severe stenosis of the external auditory canal may be associated with an acquired cholesteatoma due to trapping of epithelial debris in the medial end of the canal.

Bony atresia of the external auditory canal (EAC) is due to aplasia of the tympanic ring. It can be complete or partial, and can be unilateral or bilateral. The canal is replaced by a bony plate called the atresia plate. This anomaly is associated with the fusion of the ossicles with the atresia plate. The neck of malleus is the common segment which fuses with the plate. In certain instances, there may be absence of the short process of the malleus. The middle ear cleft is usually narrow and may be filled with mesenchymal remnants which appear as soft tissue densities similar to fluid on HRCT **(Fig. 6)**.

Anomalous development of the middle ear may be associated with EAC stenosis or atresia. Maldevelopment of the ossicles, their fusion or hypoplasia may be seen. These are associated with anomalous course of the facial nerve or position of the sigmoid sinus. Isolated ossicular abnormalities are rarely seen without coexisting external ear abnormalities. The long process of the incus and stapes are commonly involved in such situations.[6]

Inner Ear Abnormalities

Inner ear abnormalities affect the cochlea, semicircular canals, vestibule and the vestibular/cochlear aqueducts. Radiologically, it is not possible to diagnose the anomalies of the membranous labyrinth because the overlying bony labyrinth may be normal. Amongst the congenital abnormalities of the inner ear, malformation of the semicircular canals is the commonest. Of these, the lateral semicircular canal malformation is most frequent. The most common form of congenital malformation is hypoplasia of the semicircular canal which leads to compensatory enlargement of the vestibule. Aplasia of the semicircular canals is one of the associations of the CHARGE syndrome. A notable recently described anomaly

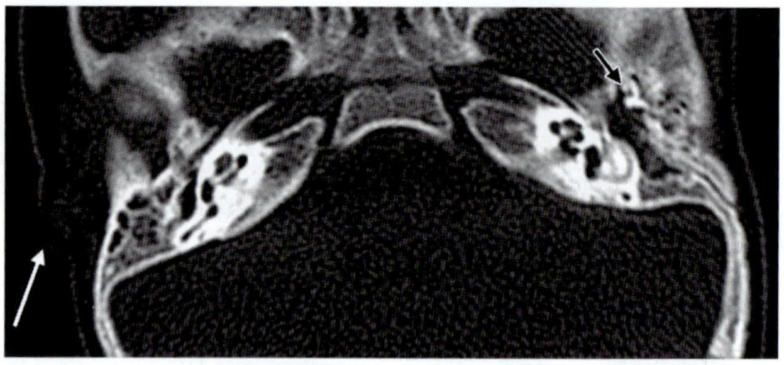

FIG. 6: Axial HRCT section showing the thick atresia plate on the left side (black arrow). The ossicular mass is fixed with the atresia plate. On the right side also the EAC is atretic and rudimentary external ear (white arrow) is seen.

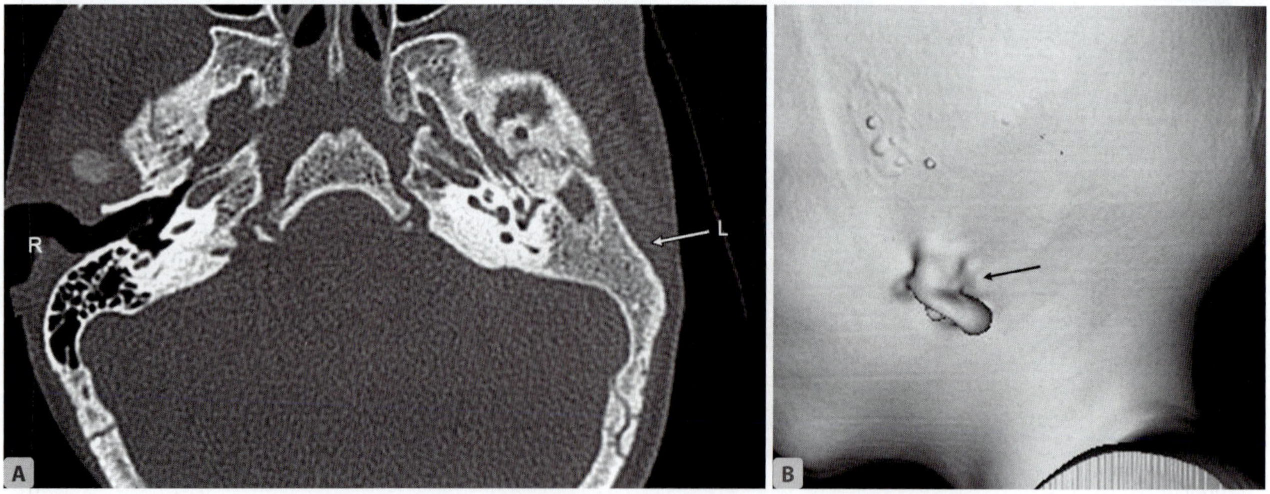

FIGS. 5A AND B: Axial HRCT section showing left external auditory canal atresia (white arrow) and associated microtia (black arrow).

is semicircular canal dehiscence which causes pressure or sound induced vertigo.

Cochlear anomalies are numerous and Jackler et al. have attempted to classify them on the basis of stages of arrested development during organogenesis.[7] According to this classification the cochlear abnormalities can be grouped as follows.

Complete Labyrinthine Aplasia or Michele Aplasia

In this the inner ear is replaced by a small, single, cystic, cavity or several small cavities. This condition on imaging may look like *labrynthitis obliterans*. However, in latter condition since the labyrinth is formed completely but is secondarily obliterated the bulge of promontory as seen on CT is present. The distinction between these two conditions is important because cochlear implant is contraindicated in aplasia.[8]

Common Cavity

A large cystic cavity without any internal architecture is formed due to poor development of cochlea and bony labyrinth. This is associated with poor differentiation of membranous labyrinth as well resulting in severe to profound hearing loss.

Cochlear Aplasia

In this the cochlea fails to form and the other elements of the inner ear may also be malformed.

Cochlear Hypoplasia

This represents a small rudimentary cochlear bud associated with a normal or malformed vestibule and semicircular canal. On CT the height of cochlea is around 6 mm as compared to normal height of about 12–13 mm. Membranous differentiation is affected to a variable degree and is reflected in degree of hearing loss.

Incomplete Partition or Dilatational Defects

This includes the *Mondini's defect*. In Mondini's defect the basal turn of the cochlea is formed, however, the middle and apical turns are replaced by a common cavity or cloaca.[9,10]

Thus instead of having 2.5 turns there are 1.5 turns of the cochlea. It is commonly associated with enlarged vestibular aqueduct; stapes footplate deformity and modiolar defects **(Figs. 7A and B)**. Cystic cochlea lacking all interscalar septae and modiolus has been referred to as *pseudo-Mondini malformation* or cystic cochleovestibular malformation.[11]

Imaging of cochlear implant: cochlear implant is used to restore hearing in select indications of sensorineural deafness. It involves the implantation of the electrode of the cochlear implant in the inner ear. This is achieved via mastoid route, into the middle ear and through the facial recess into the widened round window. The electrode is inserted into the cochlea for about 1½ turn. Pre-procedure, imaging involves the HRCT for evaluation of the bony structures and MRI for establishing the integrity of the hearing pathway including the cochlear nerve. Post-procedure the position of the electrode can be assessed by HRCT evaluation | **(Figs. 8A to D)**.

Congenital Dilatation of the Vestibular Aqueduct

Congenital dilatation of the vestibular aqueduct is the most common cause of congenital sensorineural deafness. Enlargement of the aqueduct to 1.5–2 mm is diagnostic of this condition. This entity is often associated with Pendred syndrome characterized by euthyroid goiter and sensorineural hearing loss.

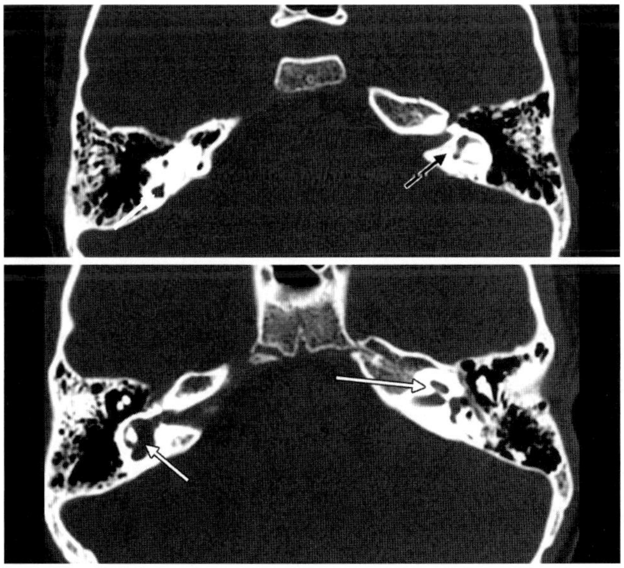

FIG. 7A: Mondini's defect: Axial HRCT images showing dilated vestibule and a large common cavity (white arrows) on right side with absence of cochlear turns. On left side, vestibule (black arrow) and cochlear turn is seen well (long white arrow).

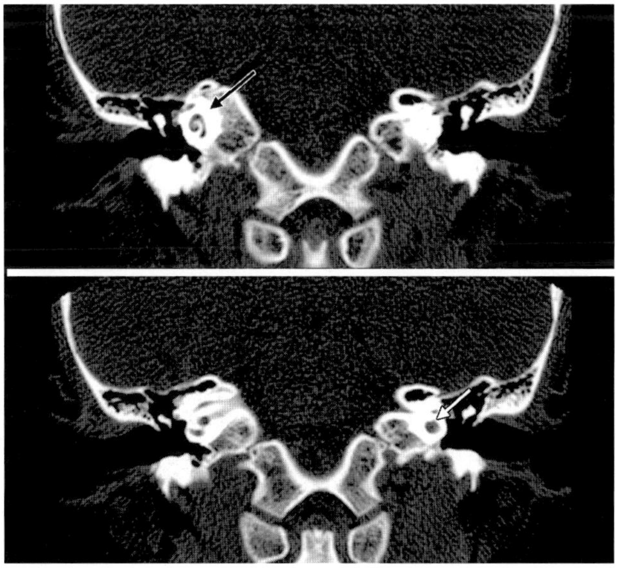

FIG. 7B: Mondini defect: Coronal images showing absence of middle and apical turns of cochlea (white arrow). Note mode of normal cochlear turn on opposite side (black arrow).

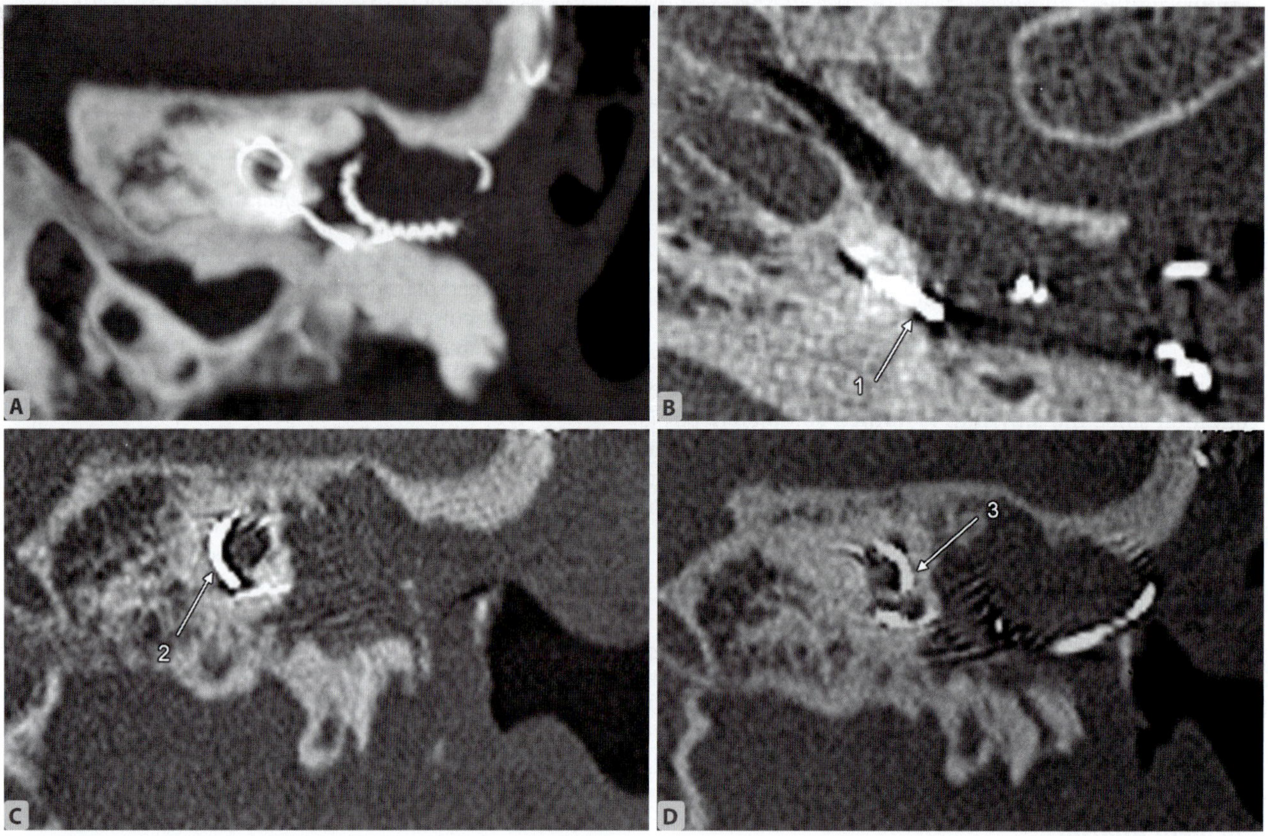

FIGS. 8A TO D: Coronal MIP (A), axial (B) and coronal (C and D) images of HRCT post-cochlear implant. Electrode is seen entering the round window (1) and further into the cochlear basal turn (2) and outer turn (3).

Narrowed vestibular aqueducts less than 0.5 mm are associated with Ménière's disease. Congenital enlargement of cochlear aqueduct may occur. This leads to abnormal perilymph pressure which results in CSF leaks from the oval window during stapedectomy, the eponymous "Stapes Gushers".

Vestibular Anomalies

Most common is absence or dysplasia of lateral semicircular canals.

Internal auditory canals (IAC) may be stenosed or atretic. This is associated with absent cranial nerve VIII. The IAC can be partitioned into two or more separate channels by bony septae.[5]

Vascular Anomalies

Aberrant course of the carotid artery is an important vascular congenital anomaly. The normal carotid canal extends vertically and then horizontally anteroinferior to the cochlea. When the course of the artery is aberrant, the lateral wall of the carotid canal is absent and the canal lays posteroinferior to the cochlea. Therefore, the carotid artery protrudes into the anterior middle ear and has a more lateral and tortuous course than a normal artery.[5]

A persistent stapedial artery is an uncommon vascular anomaly. The artery branches from the infracochlear carotid artery and enters the tympanic facial canal via the stapedial obturator foramen. It usually enlarges the canal and exits the canal at the geniculate ganglion to become the middle meningeal artery.[3-5]

Jugular bulb dehiscence or jugular diverticula are venous abnormalities and are described in the sections on pulsatile tinnitus.

Temporal Bone Fractures

Plain X-ray examination is inadequate in demonstrating temporal bone fractures. In a study, only 17–30% of fractures could be demonstrated on plain X-rays.[12] Diagnosis of fractures is primarily done by CT. MR examination is supplementary in evaluation of temporal bone fractures and is used to evaluate associated intracranial pathologies, e.g. hemorrhage or contusions in the adjacent brain.[12]

Computed tomography examination of the temporal bone consists of routine surveys of the temporal bone by 5 mm thick sections, followed by high resolution scan for assessing the petromastoid complex.[12,13] Fractures of the squamous temporal bone can be easily identified on routine scans. The petromastoid fractures are identified on HRCT and are of two types: longitudinal and transverse.

Fractures of the petromastoid that are parallel to the long axis of the petrous bone are called longitudinal fractures **(Fig. 9)**. There are two subtypes—anterior and posterior.[13] The anterior subtype involves the tegmen, glenoid fossa and

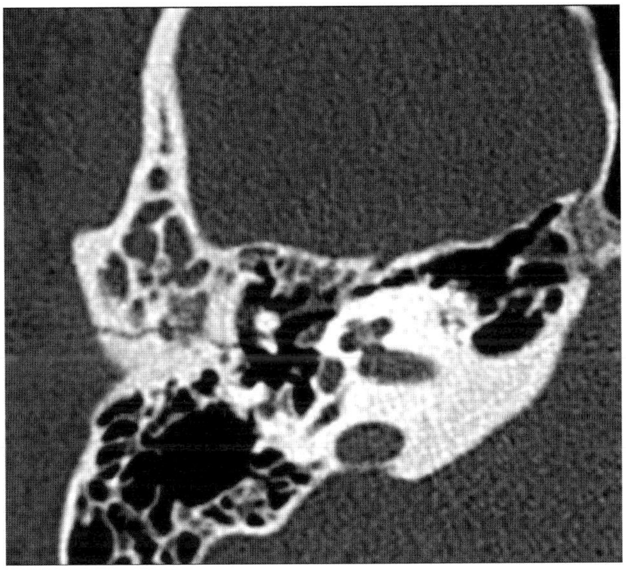

FIG. 9: Longitudinal fracture of the left temporal bone on axial HRCT. The fracture line runs in the long axis of the petrous bone. Ossicular chain was not disrupted and the mastoid air cells are filled with blood which appears as soft tissue density.

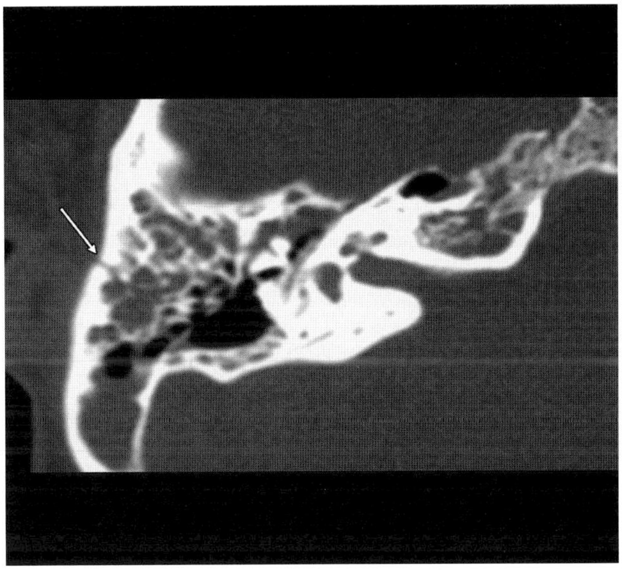

FIG. 10: Axial HRCT section shows a transverse fracture. The fracture line causes disruption of the ice cream cone configuration of the middle ear ossicles. Note blood (soft tissue) in the middle ear and mastoid.

facial nerve together with the squamous temporal bone. The posterior subtype involves the facial nerves, ossicular chain and mastoid. The fractures line passes through the mastoid or along the external auditory canal which is the path of least resistance. The inner ear structures are usually spared, however, as the fracture line passes through the middle ear, there is high incidence of ossicular disruption, the incudostapedial joint being the most common. Tympanic membrane perforation occurs frequently when there is involvement of the external auditory canal. Although, the principle fracture line runs parallel to the longitudinal axis of petrous pyramid, orthogonal fractures convert this seemingly simple injury into more complex lesions. Facial paralysis is found in 10–20% of patients but usually has delayed presentation and is often incomplete.

Transverse fractures are less common than longitudinal petromastoid fractures. They occur perpendicular to the long axis of the petrous ridge **(Fig. 10)**. The etiology of these injuries is thought to be due to a force from the occiput towards the temporal bone and hence is associated with multiple fractures of the skull base. They are of two types, medial or lateral, depending upon the relative position of the fracture line in relation to the arcuate eminence. These fractures commonly involve the bony labyrinth. A 50% of patients may have facial paralysis. The facial nerve can be transected and the resulting deficit can be permanent.[14,15] The bony labyrinth, vestibule and internal auditory canal may be involved resulting in severe vertigo and sensorineural deafness. Complications associated with fractures, such as CSF rhinorrhea or otorrhea, merit an aggressive attempt either by cisternography or noncontrast MR to delineate the site of CSF leak so that attending sequelae can be avoided.[14]

Some authors have proposed a new system of classifying temporal bone fractures as "otic capsule sparing versus otic capsule violating". They believe that this system can be better in predicting the clinical outcome of these fractures.[16]

Inflammatory Diseases of the Temporal Bone

The CT is undoubtedly superior to demonstrate bony abnormalities along with detection and localization of soft tissue masses in inflammatory conditions of the temporal bone. However, MRI offers improved characterization of the soft tissue lesions associated with infections.

Inflammatory Conditions of the External Ear

Otitis externa

It can be diagnosed easily and treated adequately by topical antimicrobial therapy. However, in necrotizing or malignant otitis externa (MOE), imaging studies are required to delineate the extent and spread of the disease. This condition is typically seen in elderly diabetic patients. The most common organism causing MOE is *Pseudomonas*. The infection begins at the junction of the bony and cartilaginous segment of the EAC.[17]

In the early stage, CT shows abnormal contrast enhancement in the region of the external auditory canal. In the late phase, there is increase in the soft tissue thickness with bony destruction **(Fig. 11)**. The aggressive inflammation may rapidly extend into the parapharyngeal space, infratemporal fossa, middle and inner ear, and intracranially in the extradural space. The temporomandibular joint and retroauricular region may be involved. VI, VII, IX, X and XII cranial nerve palsies have been described. Extradural spread in the cranium may lead to sigmoid sinus thrombosis. MRI

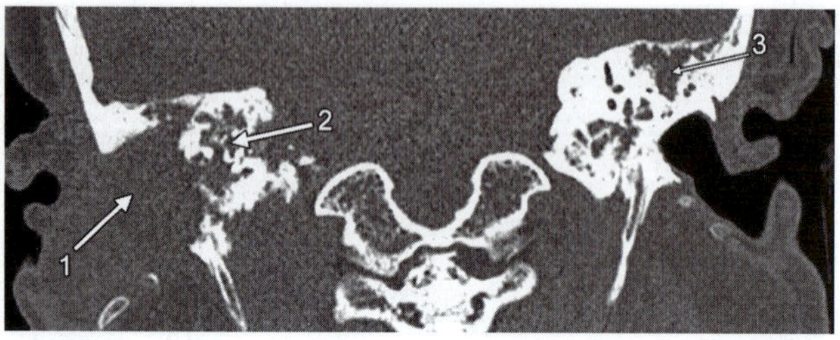

FIG. 11: Right malignant otitis externa causing destruction of the entire external auditory canal with presence of soft tissue (1) at its place with extension and destruction of the mastoid portion of the temporal bone (2). Note is made of the left mastoiditis (3).

TABLE 1: External auditory canal inflammatory conditions.

EAC cholesteatoma	Unilateral, rare, old age, pain and discharge	Soft tissue with erosions
Ketosis obturans	Bilateral, younger age, pain and conductive loss	Soft tissue with widened EAC but no erosions
Malignant otitis externa	Old age, immuno-compromised, severe pain and discharge	Soft tissue with extensive bone destruction

better shows changes in soft tissue and involvement of the retrocondylar fat pad on MRI has been proposed as an early diagnostic finding in patients being evaluated for MOE.[18]

Differential diagnosis includes basal cell carcinoma, squamous carcinoma, adenoid cystic carcinoma, or metastases.

External Ear Cholesteatoma

It arises due to periostitis of the bony canal. The sequestrum resulting from the periostitis embeds into the canal wall and grows through the epidermis to form a cholesteatoma. CT is primarily used to assess the bony erosion and in planning surgical approach. *Keratosis obturans* is a painful condition in which a plug of keratin obstructs the external auditory canal. It is a usually seen in middle aged adults and presents bilaterally. Bone erosion extending into the mastoid or middle ear is similar to the pattern seen with congenital cholesteatomas.[19]

Salient clinical and imaging features of impotant EAC inflammatory conditions are summarized in **Table 1**.

Inflammatory Condition of the Middle Ear

Otitis Media

It is the term given to inflammation of the middle ear. It can be acute or chronic in nature.

Acute Otitis Media

The most common causative organisms of acute otitis media are *Streptococcus pneumoniae*, *Haemophilus influenzae*, and *Moraxella catarrhalis*. The term acute otomastoiditis denotes infection of the middle ear and mastoid. Acute otomastoiditis is diagnosed on CT as opacification of middle ear and mastoid

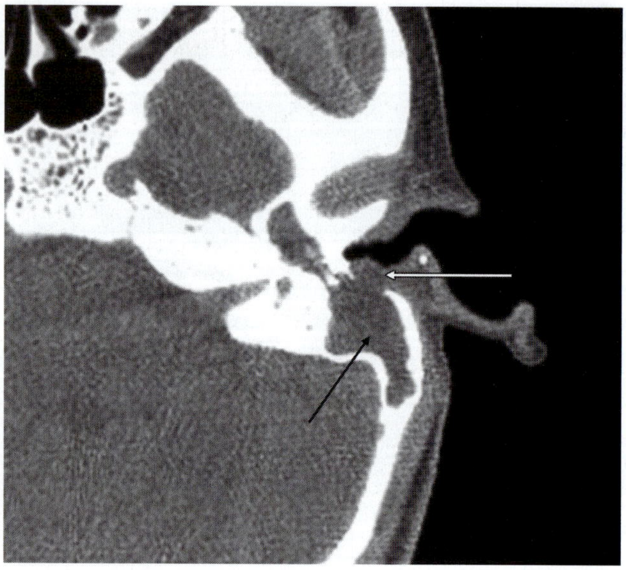

FIG. 12: Complicated acute otomastoiditis. There is evidence of coalescent otomastoiditis (black arrow) with fistulous communication between external auditory canal and mastoid antrum (white arrow).

cells with or without air fluid levels. The bony septae within the mastoid and the mastoid cortex are preserved when there is destruction and/or resorption of bony septate, the term coalescent otomastoiditis is used. Subperiosteal abscesses may form when the retained pus in a closed mastoid erodes through the mastoid cortex. Bezold's abscess is the term given to an abscess formed in the soft tissue of neck when pus discharges from the tip of the affected mastoid. Perisinus, extradural, or parenchymal abscesses can form when the medial cortex of mastoid is breached. A fistula between the external auditory canal forms when pus discharges spontaneously from a breach in the anterior cortex of the mastoid **(Fig. 12)**.

Chronic Otits Media

Acute otitis media frequently progresses to chronic otitis media. It causes either effusion or formation of granulation tissue. If not diagnosed or treated, complications of chronic otits media may result. Inflammatory effusion in the middle ear associated with chronic otitis media is also termed as serous otitis. Presence of air-fluid level in two orthogonal planes helps in diagnosing this condition. However, in many patients opaque middle ear may be present rendering it difficult to diagnose this condition.

Granulation Tissue

It is a common finding in chronic otitis media and is diagnosed when debris is present in the middle ear cavity or in mastoid. On CT, it has variable density and on MRI it usually enhances. However, there is absence of any bony changes or mass effect on both these modalities **(Fig. 13)**.

Cholesterol Granulomas

It is a type of granulation tissue which needs separate mention as this entity can be mistaken for a vascular mass otoscopically owing to its hemorrhagic component. It is

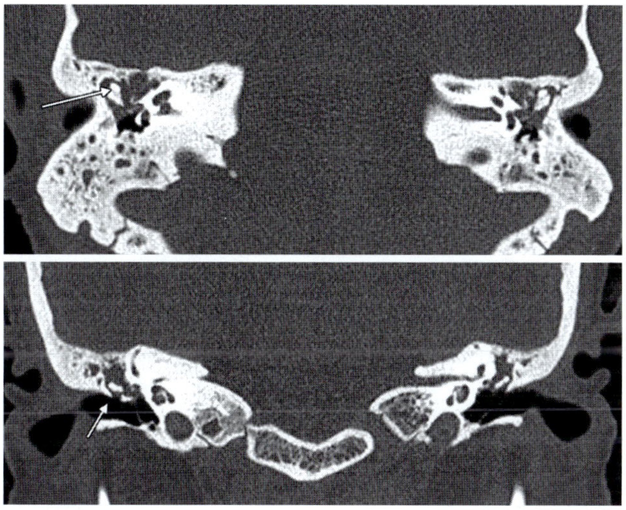

FIG. 13: Bilateral CSOM: soft tissue in the epitympanum likely granulation tissue on both sides without erosion of the ossicles (long arrow) or the scutum (short arrow).

TABLE 2: Inflammatory lesion of the middle ear on MRI.

Lesion	T1WI	T2WI	Post-contrast T1WI	DWI
Granulation tissue	Dark	Bright	Present	No
Cholesterol granuloma	Bright	Bright	No	Variable
Cholesteatoma	Dark	Bright	No	Yes

formed due to foreign body response to the cholesterol crystals in the middle ear. Since it is a type of granulation tissue, the features of mass effect are absent which helps to differentiate it from vascular tumors. Also, presence of history of chronic otitis media helps in the diagnosis.

On MRI, it is hyperintense on all pulse sequences because of extracellular methemoglobin. It can occur anywhere in the middle ear; other common location is petrous apex where it can be seen even without history of chronic otitis media.

The main differentiating features of various important inflammatory lesions seen in middle ear on MR imaging is given in **Table 2**.

COMPLICATIONS

The important complications of otitis media are tympanic membrane retraction, acquired cholesteatomas and ossicular fixation and erosions.

Acquired Cholesteatomas

They are collections of keratinous debris from an ingrowth of stratified squamous epithelium through a perforated tympanic membrane. Acquired cholesteatomas are of inflammatory etiology and are of two types. The more common variety arises from the pars flaccida of the tympanic membrane and the second variety arises from the pars tensa of the tympanic membrane. The former are called attic cholesteatomas and the latter are called sinus cholesteatomas.[20,21]

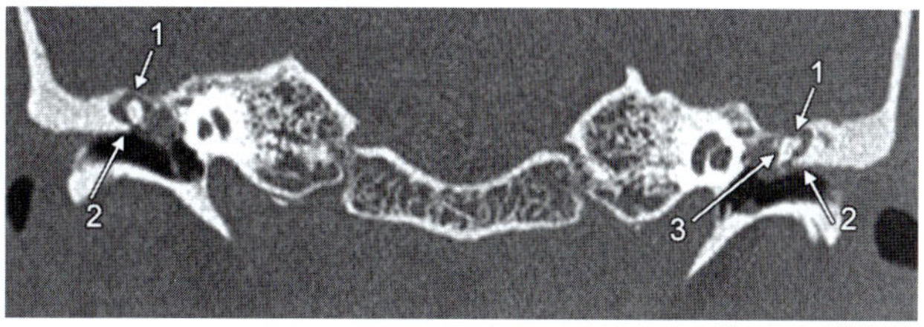

FIG. 14: Case of bilateral acquired cholesteatomas with erosion of Tegmen tympani (1), erosion of scutum (2) and erosion of ossicles (3).

The CT features of cholesteatomas are a nondependent soft tissue mass in typical locations with or without erosions of surrounding bony structures.[22] Attic cholesteatomas are best demonstrated on coronal section while the sinus cholesteatomas are easily identifiable on axial or coronal sections **(Fig. 14)**.

Complete radiographic evaluation of cholesteatomas should include a description of the location of the soft tissue mass, presence of erosion of the margins of the middle ear cavity, status of the ossicular chain and presence of anatomic variants which might affect the surgical approach to the middle ear cavity.[23]

On MRI, the cholesteatomas are hypointense on T1WI and hyperintense on T2WI. They usually do not exhibit any contrast enhancement. However, the peripheral enhancing rim may be seen occasionally. Some authors have advocated delayed MR imaging in cases where differentiation from inflammatory or granulation tissue is doubtful. MRI after 45 minutes following contrast injection may show continued enhancement of inflammatory or granulation tissue and not in cholesteatomas. Also, diffusion weighted imaging has a role as cholesteatomas are hyperintense on $b = 1000/m^2$. In diffusion non-EPI turbo spin echodiffusion sequences give better signal to noise ratio than conventional EPI sequences.[24,25]

The complications of cholesteatomas are disabling and at times life-threatening because there is risk of infection spreading intracranially giving rise to meningitis, otogenic abscesses and sinovenous thrombosis. Ossicular destruction is the most common complication of cholesteatomas.[26,27] The long process of the incus is the most common segment of the ossicular chain which is affected. The other serious complications which should be evaluated are the presence of labyrinthine fistula which occurs when the bone over the lateral semicircular canal is eroded. This diagnosis can be made with confidence when the soft tissue mass is in direct opposition with membranous portion of the labyrinth **(Figs. 15A to D)**.[27]

The facial nerve canal which may be focally dehiscent in normal individual is another important structure which is frequently eroded by aggressive cholesteatomas. Soft tissue masses abutting the horizontal segment of the facial canal with the presence of erosion and with the clinical evidence of facial palsy, suggests that the facial nerve that has been involved by the inflammatory process, is of importance **(Fig. 16)**. Erosion of either the tegmen tympani and the sigmoid sinus plate is a setting for spread of infection into the intracranial cavity.[27,28]

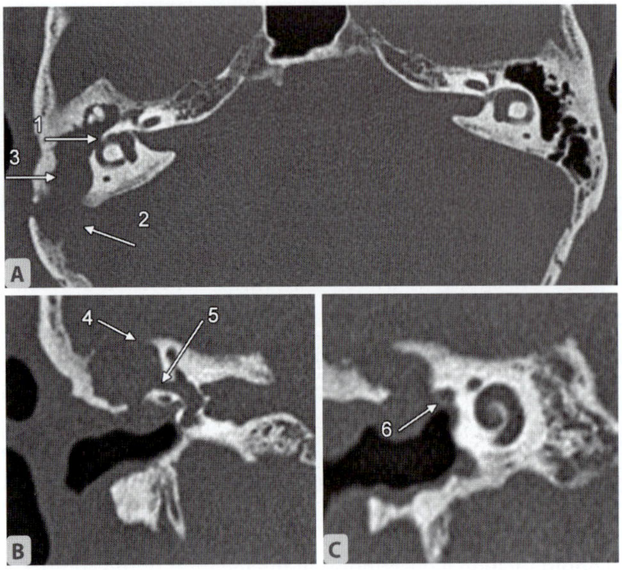

FIGS. 15A TO C: Right CSOM with cholesteatoma: Axial (A) and coronal (B and C) HRCT sections of patient showing fistula between middle ear and lateral semicircular canal (1 and 5) and almost complete erosion of the sinus plate (2) and tegmen tympani (4). Almost the entire mastoid air cells and epitympanum is filled with soft tissue (3). Additionally, there is dehiscence of bony canal of facial nerve in its tympanic segment (6).

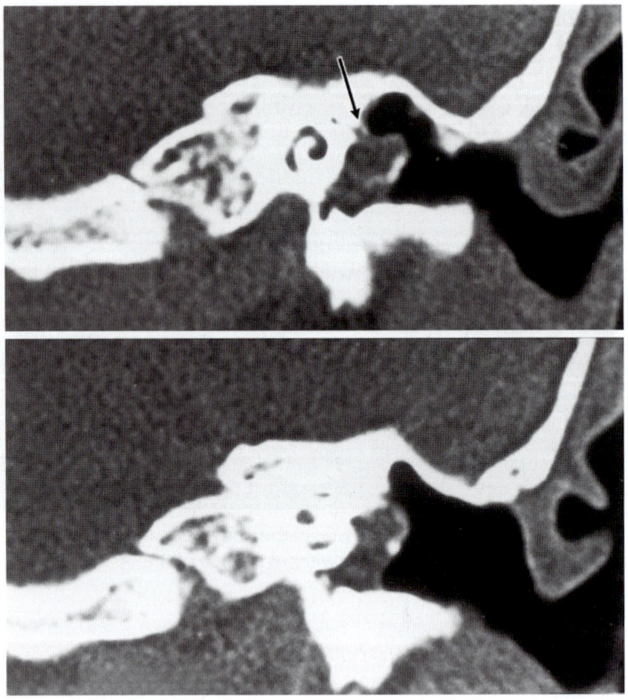

FIG. 16: Facial canal dehiscence due to cholesteatoma: The coronal HRCT shows the facial canal is exposed and the cholesteatoma is adherent to it (arrow).

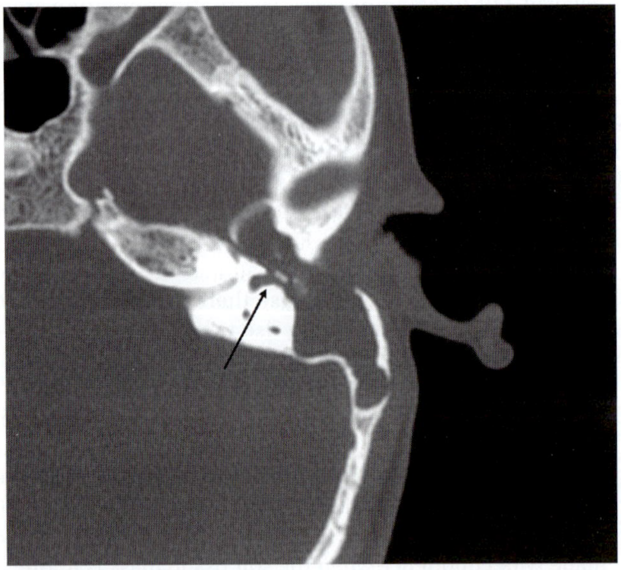

FIG. 15D: Cholesteatoma leading to fistula between lateral semicircular canal and the middle ear cavity (arrow).

OTHER COMPLICATIONS

In children, noncholesteatomatous inflammatory processes affecting the middle ear occur due to eustachian tube obstruction from nasopharyngeal lymphoid hypertrophy. These conditions are broadly termed as tubotympanic diseases. Middle ear effusion, chronic otitis media, granulation tissue, postinflammatory ossicular erosions and ossicular fixation are sequelae encountered in this condition. Middle ear effusions are seen as fluid/soft tissue opacities in the middle ear cavity. There are no erosions of the ossicles. Noninflammatory effusion may be due to a pressure phenomenon and can be seen in patients after air travel in poorly pressurized aircraft.[29]

Ossicular erosions can rarely occur with uncomplicated otitis media. The long process of the incus is commonly affected. Erosions appear as punched out small lytic area on the ossicles. Ossicular fixation occurs due to postinflammatory fibrosis.

Gradenigo's syndrome is a manifestation of petrous apicitis when purulent otitis media is associated with ipsilateral lateral rectus palsy and pain along distributions of the 6th cranial nerve. But the classical presentation of this syndrome is seldom seen. The pathology is explained on the basis of irritation of the 6th cranial nerve as it travels beneath the petroclinoid ligament and irritation of the gasserian ganglion by the inflammatory process in the petrous apex due to disruption of the bony cortex.[29]

Antral cholesteatomas are less common than those found within the middle ear and are diagnosed when a larger than normal smooth walled cavity containing nondependent soft tissue densities are seen within the antrum. These cholesteatomas then erode anteriorly into the external canal or involve the petrous apex via the facial canal.[29]

Inflammatory Conditions of the Inner Ear

Labyrinthitis is the term used to describe inflammation of the membranous labyrinth. Viruses are the most common etiologic agents. But it may also be due to bacterial, luetic or of autoimmune origin. Tuberculous labyrinthitis has also been described.[29]

Labyrinthitis can also be classified as tympanogenic, meningogenic, hematogenic and post-traumatic.

Tympanic labyrinthitis occurs when infection from the middle ear spread to the labyrinth via the oval or round windows, or via a labyrinthine fistula. The latter is commonly associated with cholesteatoma. Infections can travel into the inner ear following surgery and are termed iatrogenic tympanogenic labyrinthitis.

Meningogenic labyrinthitis occurs when infection spreads along CSF spaces via the internal auditory canal or cochlear aqueduct. Labyrinthitis is usually bilateral.

Hematogenic labyrinthitis is caused due to spread of infection by the bloodstream. Viruses, e.g. measles and mumps; syphilis and tuberculosis and other bacterial infections spread by this route.

Post-traumatic labyrinthitis can also occur as a complications of trauma.

Bilateral labyrinthitis leads to profound sensorineural deafness. CT is usually normal in acute and subacute labyrinthitis. Ossification of the fluid-filled labyrinth spaces in late chronic phase appears as areas of increased densities. The best method of diagnosis is by contrast enhanced MR. On the enhancement of cochlea or vestibule is pathognomic for labrynthitis. MR contrast enhanced T1W images show moderate to intense enhancement within the normal fluid-filled structures of the inner ear. Some authors have also advocated use of FLAIR postcontrast images for diagnosing this enhancement.[30]

Usually viral conditions causes subtle contrast enhancement and bacterial especially pneumococcal labrynthitis causes intense enhancement.

A sequela of labyrinthitis is **fibrous obliterans** followed by **labyrinthitis ossification**. It is also called sclerosing labyrinthitis or chronic labyrinthitis.[29] Most common cause of labyrinthitis ossificans is suppurative bacterial labyrinthitis. This condition can also be associated with viral labyrinthitis, advanced otosclerosis, trauma, occlusion of labyrinthine artery, leukemia or following labyrinthectomy. Following suppurative labyrinthitis inflammation leads to fibroblast proliferation within the labyrinth. These fibroblasts differentiate into osteoblasts which lead on to osteoneogenesis and deposition of bone in the labyrinth. The most common site to see fibrosis and new bone formation is the basal turn of the cochlea near the round window niche. Dense sclerosis due to new bone formation is best appreciated on CT. Fibro-osseous changes can be appreciated on high resolution T2W MR images where the normal hyperintense fluid signal intensity of the labyrinth is replaced by intermediate or low signal from the encroaching fibro-osseous material.

It is important to distinguish the changes of labyrinthitis ossifications in the cochlear and pericochlear regions. The cochlear labyrinthitis ossification makes cocheal implantation difficult. A cochlear implant is a multicomponent electronic device which directly stimulates the auditory fibers in cochlea to provide auditory information. Typically the components include a microphone, a speech processor, a transmitter, a receiver and a stimulator. The stimulator wire is placed in the cochlea through the round window to directly stimulate the spiral ganglion cells and the cochlear axons. Placement of a cochlear implant is most effective in patients less than 2 years of age with profound sensorineural hearing impairment in whom hearing aids are not effective or beneficial. Prior to implantation a high resolution temporal bone CT or high resolution T2 MRI study is required to assess the changes in and around the bony labyrinth. Labyrinthine aplasia is an absolute contraindication for an implant. Cochlear labyrinthitis ossificans is a relative contraindication presumably because it can hinder the placement of the stimulator. Other relative contraindications include conditions which may influence the surgical approach, such as aberrant course of the facial nerve, otomastoiditis, fenestral and cochlear otosclerosis and the aberrant course of the internal carotid artery. An ipsilateral brainstem infarct detected on MR scanning of the brain would also be a contraindication for cochlear implantation.[31]

RADIOLOGICAL EVALUATION OF VASCULAR TINNITUS AND VASCULAR TYMPANIC MEMBRANE

Vascular tinnitus is a common complaint pertaining to the ear. The term tinnitus refers to rhythmic sound heard by the patient. This sound may or may not be synchronous with the radial pulse. Nonpulsatile synchronous tinnitus is usually associated with muscular dysfunction, such as myoclonus of the tensor tympani muscle or the palatal muscles. Synchronous tinnitus, also referred to as pulsatile tinnitus is the condition which is of radiological significance. It is classified as objective or subjective. By objective pulsatile tinnitus, authors refer to the tinnitus which is audible to the observing physician as well as the patient, and subjective tinnitus is one which is audible only to the patient. Tinnitus may be caused by extrinsic causes, such as muscular or vascular diseases, or may be due to intrinsic pathologies like vestibulocochlear dysfunction.[31,32]

Causes of Pulsatile Tinnitus[33]

- *Normal vascular variants:*
  - *Arterial variants*: Aberrant/laterally displaced carotid artery, persistent stapedial artery, persistent trigeminal artery, anomalous artery in the stria vascularis of the cochlea
  - *Venous variants*: Large jugular bulb, large emissary veins, idiopathic venous tinnitus, jugular bulb diverticulum.
- *Pathological vascular causes:*
  - *Arterial causes*: Carotid artery dissection, aneurysms of the petrous carotid/anterior communicating artery aneurysms, atherosclerosis, fibromuscular dysplasia, arteritis.
  - *Arteriovenous vascular causes:* Glomustympanicum/glomus jugulare AVMs intracranial arteriovenous malformation, e.g. cerebral AVMs, dural AV fistulas and direct AV fistulas, otosclerosis, Paget's disease

of bone, miscellaneous vascular tumors, such as hemangiomas, jugular meningiomas histiocytosis and cholesterol granulomas.

- *Venous causes:* Pregnancy, anemia, thyrotoxicosis, hypertension, transverse sinus stenosis.

Normal Vascular Variants

Aberrant position of the internal carotid artery is thought to be due to abnormal regression of the cervical ICA during embryogenesis resulting in opening of and enlargement of collateral arteries, such as the anastomosis between the carotid tympanic artery anastomosis between the caroticotympanic artery and the inferior tympanic artery. The aberrant artery, therefore, courses through the middle ear over the cochlear promontory to join the horizontal carotid canal via a dehiscence in the carotid plate. The findings on HRCT are characteristic in that the posterior carotid plate is absent and that the horizontal part of the carotid canal appears to merge with the lateral cochlear promontory. Variations of the jugular bulb include a very high riding jugular bulb. This normal variant is associated with well-defined bony margins of the jugular foramen. When the caroticojugular plate is deficient, the condition is termed as dehiscent jugular bulb. Jugular bulb diverticulum is a finger like extension of the jugular bulb in the cephalad direction. Ecstatic loops of AICA/PICA or tortuous course of vertebral artery going into the internal auditory meatus may cause tinnitus due to compression on the VIII nerve complex **(Figs. 17A and B)**.

Pathological Vascular Causes

Arterial Causes

Dissection of the internal carotid artery can be spontaneous or traumatic. Angiographic appearances include intimal flaps, with or without occlusion. MRI will show loss of flow void which suggest occlusion of the artery. If there is intraluminal hemorrhage, a hyperintense signal will be observed in the affected artery. Petrous carotid aneurysms and AVMs can be detected on digital subtraction angiography (DSA). Atherosclerosis of the carotid artery at times produces pulsatile tinnitus. Atherosclerotic plaques may produce turbulence of carotid flow which manifests as pulsatile tinnitus. Fibromuscular dysplasia (FMD) is a segmental noninflammatory, nonatheromatous vasculopathy. It is seen in 0.5–0.6% of carotid angiograms and autopsies. It is a disease which affects medium-size muscular arteries. Vertebral and renal arteries can also be affected apart from the extracranial arteries. It is associated with intracranial berry aneurysms. Middle-aged females are most commonly affected. Unlike atherosclerotic plaques fibromuscular dysplasia affects the cervical internal carotid arteries at the level of the first two cervical vertebrae. Hence, these patients generally present with symptoms of vascular tinnitus more frequently unlike those with atherosclerosis. The classical angiographic appearance of FMD is the string of beads appearance which is seen in 85% of patients. Successful treatment of FMD by transluminal angioplasty has been reported.[34,35]

Arteriovenous Causes

The diagnosis of cerebral AVMs and dural AV fistulas and direct AV fistulas depends upon the clinical presentation apart from that of pulsatile tinnitus **(Figs. 18A and B)**. Angiography is the gold standard in demonstration of the vascular lesions which may be partly delineated on CT scans and MRI. Paget's disease and otosclerosis are representative bony pathologies associated with neovascularization and AV shunting, resulting in pulsatile tinnitus.[32]

Amongst the group of arteriovenous causes, paraganglionomas or glomus tumors are the typical lesions which require radiographic evaluation.[32] Glomus tumors of the temporal bone are the most common neoplastic cause of pulsatile tinnitus and vascular tympanic membrane. Tumors commonly involve the jugular bulb and/or the tympanic cavity. CT scan will help to delineate whether the lesion is confined within the tympanic cavity or involves the jugular bulb. If the lesion is confined within the tympanic cavity, no further investigation is required **(Figs. 19A and B)**.

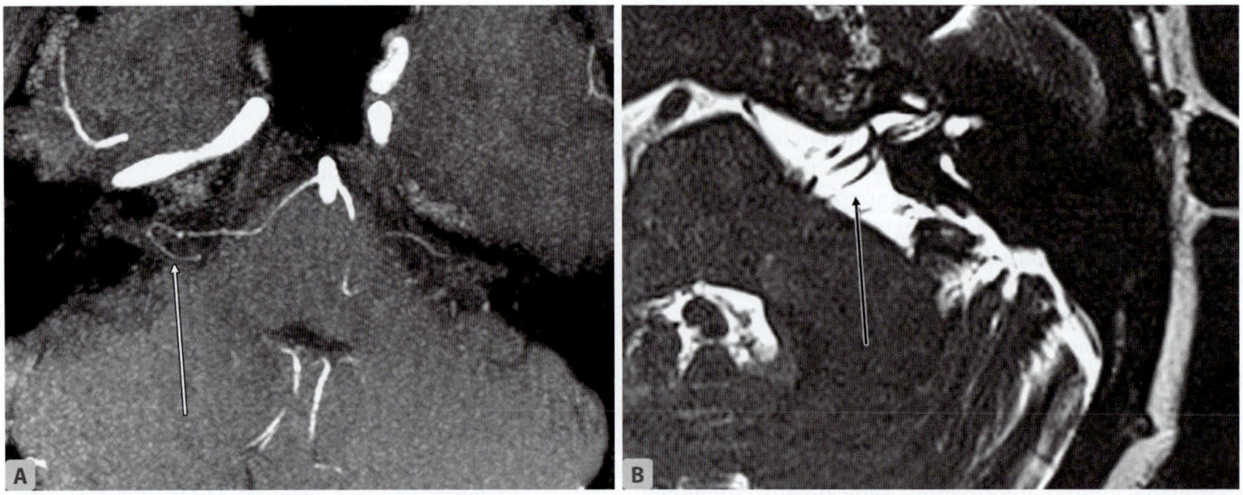

FIGS. 17A AND B: Axial magnetic resonance angiography (MRA) and CISS images showing loops of AICA in the right and left IAC, respectively (arrows).

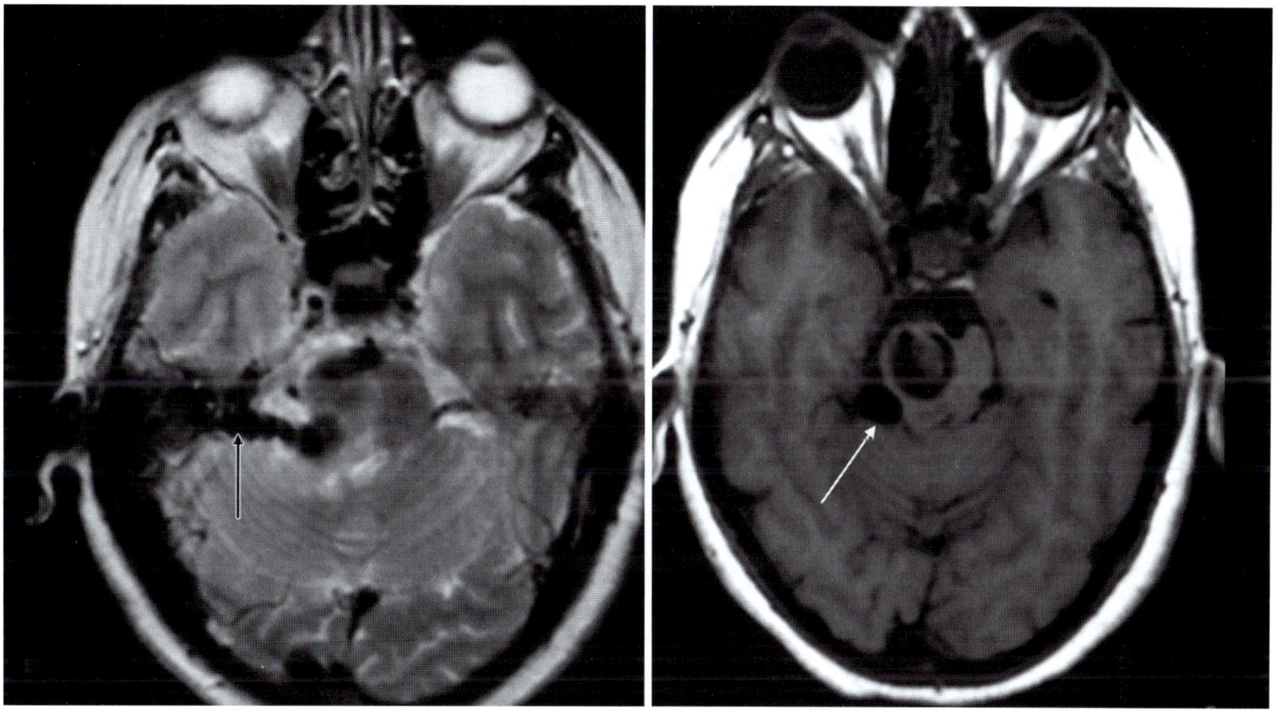

FIG. 18A: Dural AVM as cause of tinnitus: MR T2- and T1WI showing multiple flow voids in the right CP angle region and in pre- and perimesencephalic cistern.

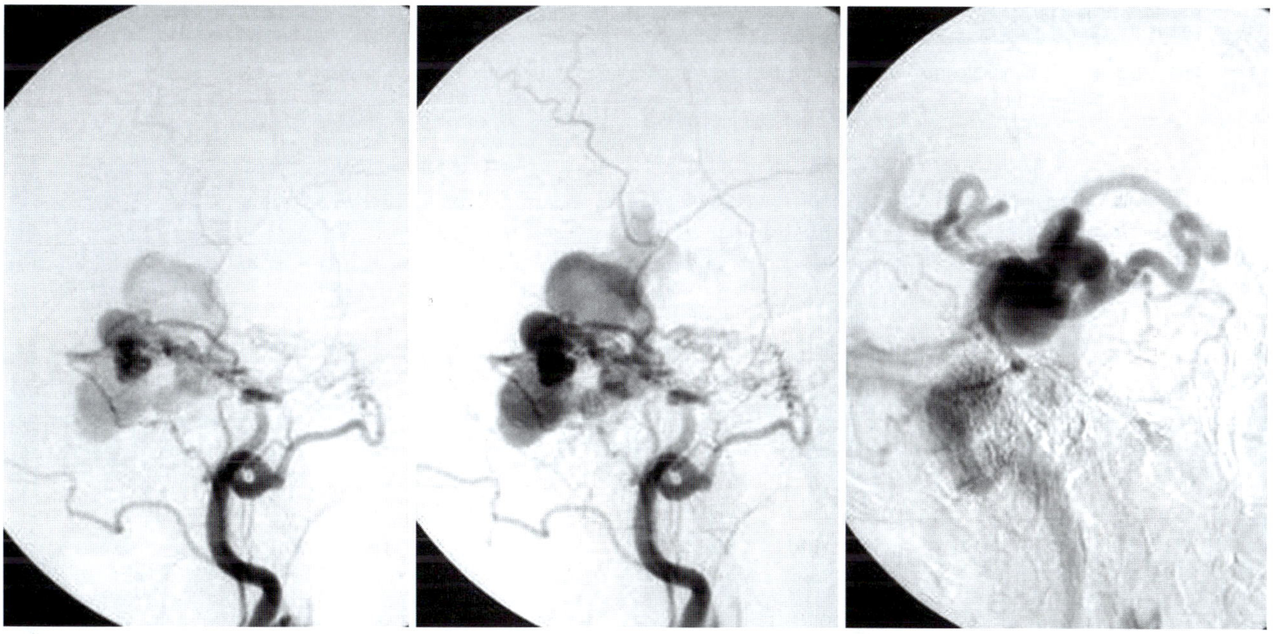

FIG. 18B: DSA images of the same showing a dural AVM being fed by branches of right external carotid artery and draining through ecstatic veins into ipsilateral sigmoid sinus and internal jugular vein (IJV).

If the lesion is seen to extend to involve the jugular foramen and beyond, CT examination is continued up to the carotid bifurcation to see the complete extent of the lesion and to rule out multicentricity. An MR examination will help in assessing the involvement of internal jugular vein. On MR high resolution T1WI, a flow void pattern can be appreciated. On post-contrast T1WI, intense enhancement is seen. Post-contrast MR angiography shows relatively low signal of the tumor with high signal intensity spots inside due to high flow in feeding vessels **(Fig. 20)**.

Venous Tinnitus

Venous tinnitus unlike arterial tinnitus is heard as a continuous murmur accentuated during systole. It is caused

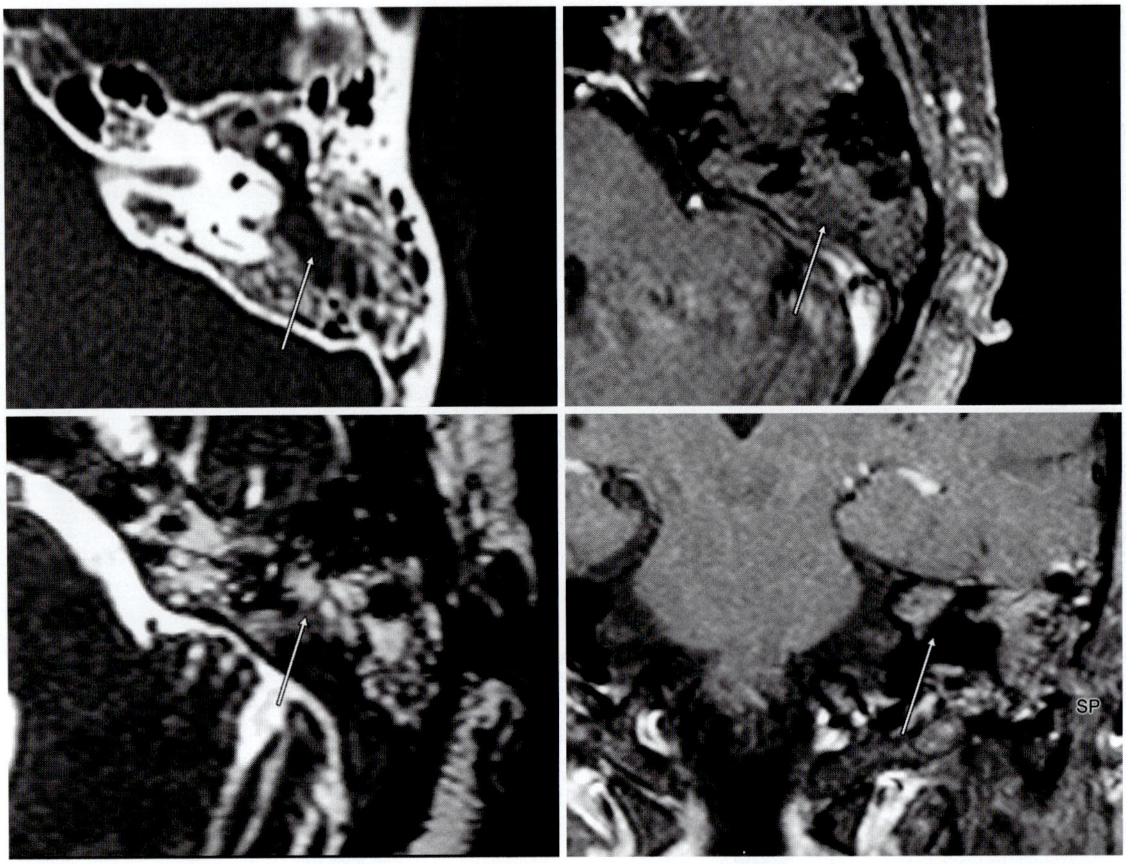

FIG. 19A: Glomus tympanicum: Axial CT, MR images and coronal MR (bottom right) showing a soft tissue within the tympanic cavity suggestive of tumor.

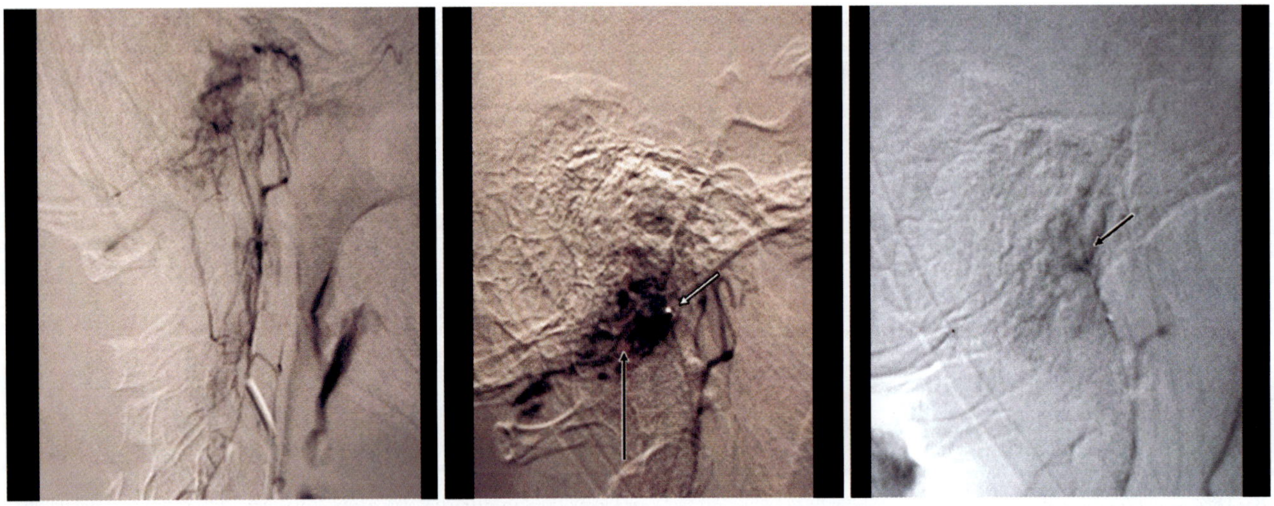

FIG. 19B: Glomus tympanicum: DSA images showing blush in the region of middle ear on ascending pharyngeal artery injection (left), microcatheter injection (tip shown by white arrow) showing intense localized tumor blush (large black arrow) and absence of blush after preoperative embolization (small black arrow).

by turbulent flow in the venous structures around the ear. It is usually heard on the side of the dominant jugular vein which is usually on the right side. A venous hum is physiological and can be elicited in an 80% of pregnant women and in the lower jugular vein in 50% of normal individuals. Venous tinnitus is also observed in patients of thyrotoxicosis, anemia and hypertension.[32]

Venous tinnitus may be the presenting symptom of intracranial hypertension. It is believed that tinnitus in conditions of raised intracranial tension is related to CSF

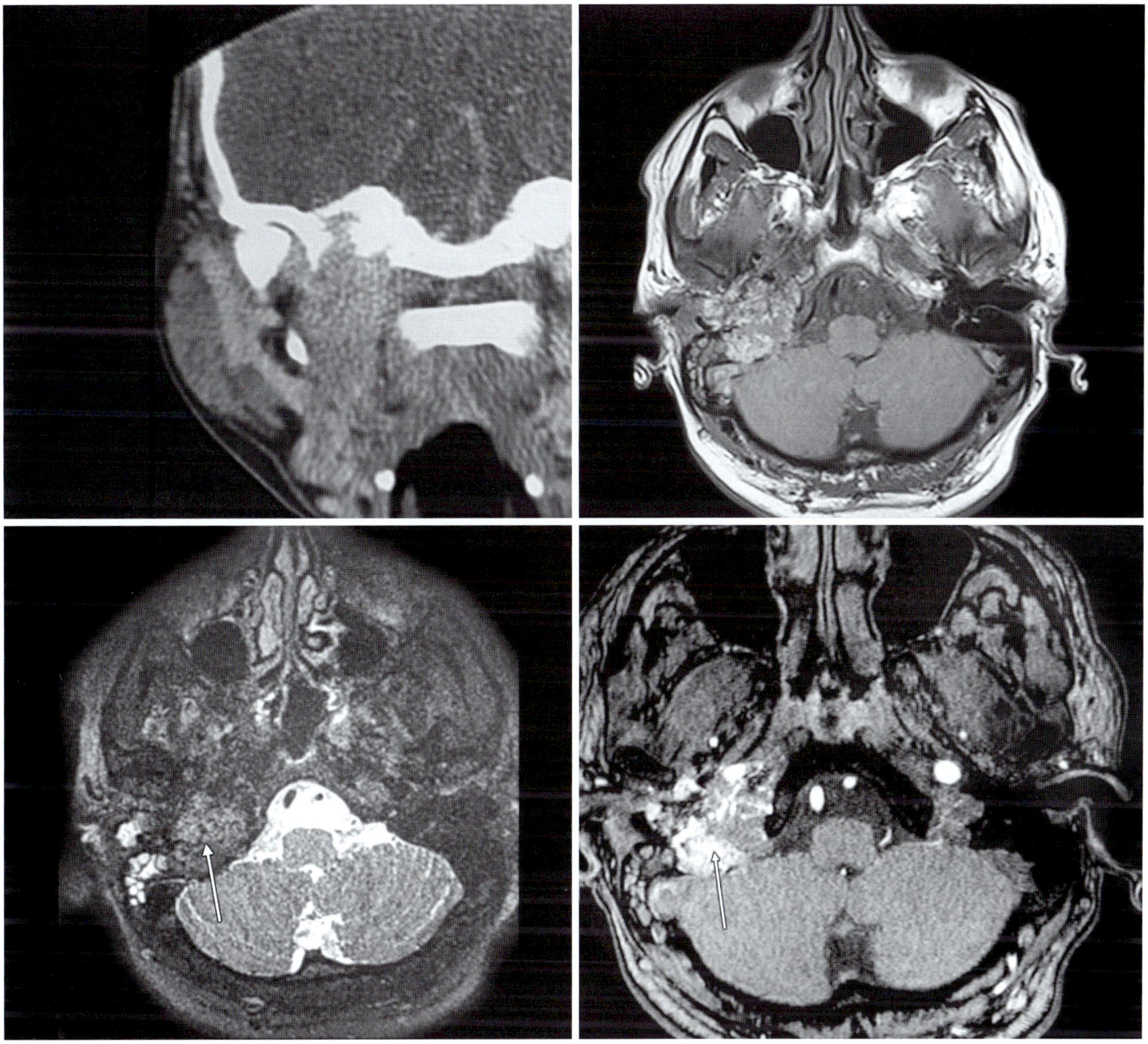

FIG. 20: Glomus jugulare: Contrast-enhanced axial CT, T1WI, T2WI, contrast MRA. All images showing a large mass lesion in the right jugular fossa with typical features of glomus tumor. Note hypointense flow voids on T2WI (black arrow) which are better seen as bright areas on contrast MRA (white arrow).

pressures and compression of dural sinuses by transmitted intracranial arterial pulsations. Raised intracranial hypertension can manifest as pulsatile tinnitus as well. Conditions, such as aqueduct stenosis, Chiari I malformation, pneumocephalus and idiopathic intracranial hypertension can present with tinnitus which can be the role symptoms of the underlying pathology.

Venous tinnitus can also be caused by stenosis of the transverse sinuses. This can be idiopathic and unrelated to dural arteriovenous fistula. A large or exposed jugular bulb or laterally placed sigmoid sinus also has been associated with venous tinnitus.[32]

Otosclerosis

Otosclerosis represents foci of spongy vascular haversian bone in the ivory like endochondral bone of the otic capusle.[36] Otosclerosis is bilateral in up to 90% of patients. It is of two types: cochlear and fenestral. The cochlear variety is rare and presents with sensorineural deafness. CT is the modality of choice in diagnosing this entity. CT diagnosis of cochlear otosclerosis is based upon locating variable sized regions of demineralization. On HRCT, cochlear otosclerosis appears as radiolucent foci in a pericochlear distribution. In very severe cases there is a hypodense ring surrounding the cochlea giving a "double ring sign". In chronic cases mixed dense and lucent foci can be seen around the bony labyrinth. Fenestral otosclerosis presents as similar lesion but they are clustered around the oval and round windows. Fenestral otosclerosis may coexist with cochlear lesions. MR findings of otosclerosis include a ring of intermediate signal intensities in the pericochlear and perilabyrinthine regions on T1WI. Postcontrast T1WI may reveal enhancing pericochlear foci which represent active lesions not detected on HRCT. T2WI may not be useful as early lesions may be missed and chronic lesions may only appear as subtle pericochlear high signal areas. It is important to distinguish cochlear otosclerosis from labyrinthitis ossificans. Labyrinthitis ossificans present as bony encroachment of the membranous labyrinths with progressive loss of the fluid-filled spaces of the labyrinth, unlike otosclerosis which presents as erosions around the labyrinth. Both the conditions are relative contraindication for placement of cochlear implants and are therefore important differential diagnoses.

Fenestral otosclerosis is more common than cochlear otosclerosis. Involvement of the oval window results in stapediovestibular compromise. Plaques of bone formation are present anterior to the oval window and are best seen in the axial HRCT sections. Axial sections also demonstrate narrowing of the oval window, thickening of the stapedial footplate and the annular ligament complex, best seen in the coronal HRCT sections. Prior to surgery, the radiological examination by HRCT is done by taking overlapping sections preferably on a helical scanner. The position of the facial nerve, presence of ossicular fixation, position of jugular vein and internal carotid artery should be meticulously recorded. Differential diagnosis of fenestral otosclerosis include oval window tympanosclerosis and osteogenesis imperfecta.[37]

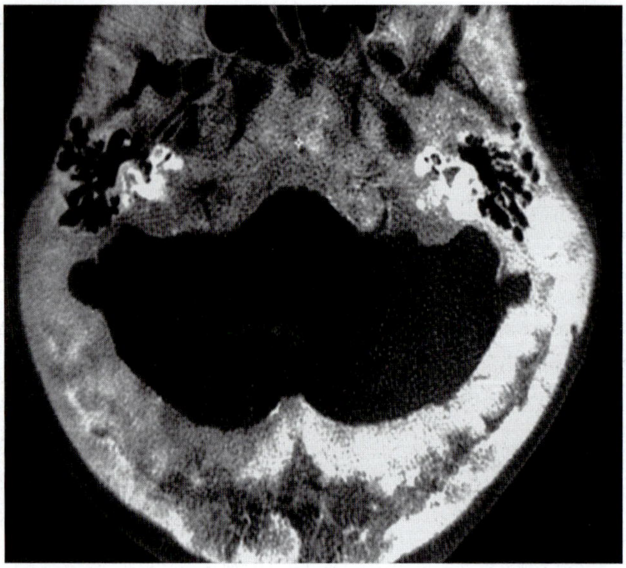

FIG. 21: Paget's disease involving the temporal bone. The bony labyrinth can be partly seen in the mass of thick bone. Both internal auditory canals are obliterated.

DYSPLASTIC CONDITIONS OF THE TEMPORAL BONE

Fibrous dysplasia, osteogenesis imperfecta, Paget's disease and progressive diaphyseal dysplasia are some of the other dysplastic conditions that affect the temporal bone.

Fibrous dysplasia is a disease characterized by progressive replacement of bone marrow by a mixture of disorganized bone matrix and fibrous tissue. CT scan is diagnostic and shows increased bone volume with a ground-glass appearance. Cystic, sclerotic and pagetoid appearance have been described. The cystic lesions contain more fibrous tissue and appear less dense that the predominantly bone containing dense sclerotic variety. Pagetoid variety of fibrous dysplasia contains both fibrous and osseous tissues.[38]

On MR high signal intensity on T1- and T2-weighted spin echo images with strong post-contrast images indicate acute phase of fibrous dysplasia.[39]

Paget's disease is a chronic condition of bone characterized by two phases: the osteolytic phase which is due to resorption of bone by osteoclasts and the osteosclerotic phase where there is increased new bone formation. The new bone is hard and dense **(Fig. 21)**. The petrous apex is the first segment to be affected and the otic capsule is the last to be affected. The calvarium is invariably involved and its characteristic appearance clinches the diagnosis.[38]

Tumors of the Temporal Bone

Primary bone tumors of the temporal bone are numerous and can be classified as carcinomas, sarcomas, metastases, benign epithelial lesions, hematological malignancies and histiocytosis.[40]

Neurogenic tumors of the temporal bone are commonly schwannom as associated with the facial nerve. Hemangiomas and congenital cholesteatomas are other common tumors associated with the temporal bone.[40]

Facial schwannomas can occur in the geniculate, tympanic or mastoid segments of the facial nerve; the geniculate segment being the most frequently involved segment. Symptoms of the tumors depend on the site of involvement hearing loss is present in approximately 70% of cases, followed by slowly progressive facial palsy in nearly 50% of cases.[37] Tumors distally beyond the stylomastoid foramen appear as asymptomatic masses in the neck. Geniculate ganglion schwannomas are the most common variety and they grow silently into the middle cranial fossa until they cause sensorineural deafness or facial nerve dysfunction. Facial schwannomas in the CP angle or internal auditory meatus present with sensorineural deafness.

Facial nerve schwannomas appears as sausage-shaped lesions along the course of the facial nerve with smooth erosion of the facial canal depending on the location of the lesion. Geniculate ganglion lesions cause smooth enlargement of the geniculate fossa, tympanic schwannomas project into the middle ear and the mastoid lesions appears as tubular lesions in the mastoid air cells.

On HRCT, they appear as soft tissue density lesions along the facial nerve. On T1WI, they are intermediate to low intensity lesion which are hyperintense on T2WI. There lesion show uniform contrast enhancement **(Fig. 22)**.

The list of tumors which may present with slowly progressive facial nerve palsy include hemangiomas, hamartomas, meningiomas and epidermoids. In elderly patients spread of parotid carcinomas upward along the facial nerve also needs to be ruled out.

Hemangiomas were considered to be rare tumors of the facial nerve, however, are now considered to be as common as facial neuromas.[41] These subset of tumors along with

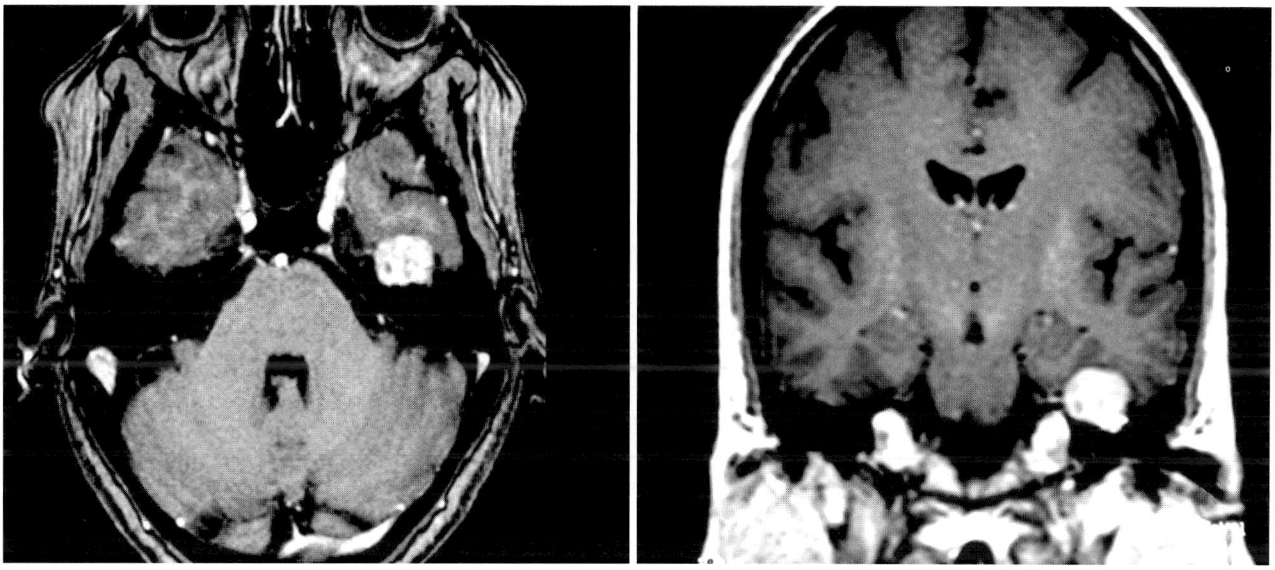

FIG. 22: Facial schwannoma: Axial and coronal contrast-enhanced T1W sections showing the lesion as a uniformly hyperintense lesion consistent with a geniculate facial schwannoma.

vascular malformations are termed intratemporal benign vascular lesions (IBVT). These tumors tend to invade the nerve rather than compress it and present with hemifacial spasm and facial palsy. On CT scan, their presence can be inferred by gas cisternography when in the labyrinthine and geniculate ganglion regions, these tumor cause erosions which are irregular with indistinct margins, give a reticular or "honeycomb" pattern to the eroded bone.[38] Since enhancement after contrast renders them isodense to surrounding bone, this is unnecessary with CT scan. On MRI these lesions are exquisitely delineated. They are isointense to mildly hyperintense on T2WI and markedly hyperintense on T1WI.

Congenital cholesteatoma or epidermoid cysts of the EAC appear as sharply defined mixed density lesions on CT. The core of the lesion may appear hypodense. On MRI, they are hypointense on T1WI images and hyperintense on T2W. These lesions can be also seen in the petrous apex, tympanic cavity or supralabyrinthine region.[41]

Common tumors of the bony external auditory canal are osteoma, and exostoses.[41] Osteoma of the external auditory canal is rare benign lesions which appears as dense pedunculated bony outgrowths from the external auditory canal. They are incidental lesions appearing similar to exostosis which are broad-based expanded bony lesions at or medial to the isthmus of the external auditory canal. Ceruminomas are glandular tumors arising from the apocrine seromucous glands or ectopic salivary gland of the external auditory canal. These are locally invasive tumor and are best treated by en bloc resection. Squamous cell carcinomas are by far the most common malignant tumor of the canal. Lesions appear as aggressive lytic areas of destruction of the walls of bony canal with contiguous spread into the middle ear cavity, temporomandibular joint, parotid gland, or carotid canal. A mass in the external auditory canal which aggressively destroys the adjacent bone suggests the presence of a squamous cell carcinoma. A noncontrast HRCT is the imaging modality of choice to assess the extent of bone destruction. Contrast-enhanced MR may be required for large lesions involving adjacent structures, such as the temporomandibular joint and parotid gland **(Fig. 23)**.[42]

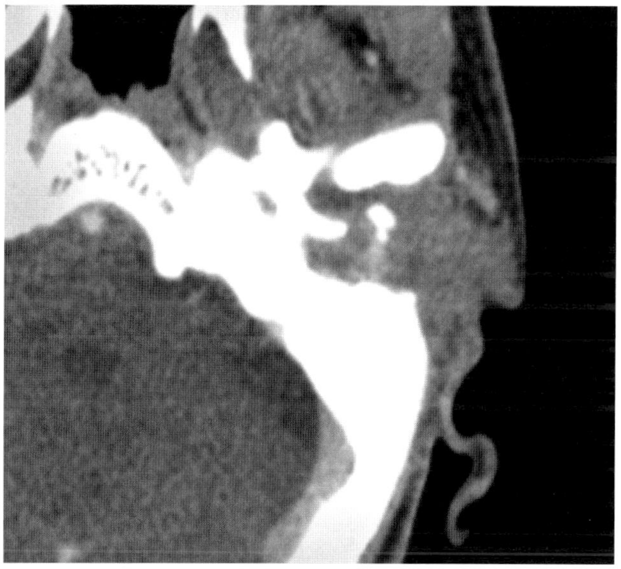

FIG. 23: Squamous cell carcinoma of the external auditory canal: Soft tissue mass fills the canal with partial destruction of the posterior wall of the canal.

REFERENCES

1. Brogan M, Chakeres DW. Computed tomography and magnetic resonance imaging of the normal anatomy of the temporal bone. Semin Ultrasound CT MR. 1989;10:178-94.
2. Eelkema EA, Curtin HD. Congenital anomalies of the temporal bone. Semin Ultrasound CTMR. 1989;10:195-212.
3. Chakeres DW, Augustyn MA. Temporal bone imaging. In: Som PM, Curtin HD (Eds). Head and Neck Imaging, 4th edition. St. Louis Mo: Mosby Year Book; 2003. pp. 1093-108.
4. Lane JI, Witte RJ, Bolster B, et al. State of the Art: 3T Imaging of the Membranous Labyrinth. Am J Neuroradiol. 2008;29:1436-40.
5. Romo LV Casselman JW, Robson CD. Temporal bone congenital anomalies. In: Som PM, Curtin HD (Eds). Head and Neck Imaging, 4th edition. St. Louis: Mosby Year Book; 2003. pp. 1109-72.
6. Swatz J, Faerber EN. Congenital malformations of the external and middle ear: High resolution CT findings of surgical import. Am J Roentgenol. 1985;144:501-6.
7. Jackler RK, Lusford WM, House WF. Congenital malformation of the inner ear. A classification based on embryogenesis. Laryngoscope. 1987;97:2-14.
8. Parry DA, Booth T, Roland PS. Advantages of magnetic resonance imaging over computed tomography in preoperative evaluation of pediatric cochlear implant candidates. Otol Neurotol. 2005;26:976-82.
9. Curtin HD, Vignaud J, Bar D. Anomaly of the facial canal in a Mondini malformation with recurrent meningitis. Radiology. 1982;144:335-41.
10. Curtin HD. Facial nerve canal. In: Vignaud J, Jordin C, Rosen L (Eds). The ear diagnostic imaging CT scanning, tomography and magnetic resonance. Paris: Masson; 1986.pp. 318-33.
11. Rodriguez K, Shah RK, Kenna M. Anomalies of the middle and inner ear. Otolaryngol Clin North Am. 2007;40:81-96.
12. Exadoktylos AK, Sclabas GM, Nuyens M, et al. The clinical correlation of temporal bone fractures and spiral computed tomographic scans: A prospective and consecutive study at a level 1 trauma center. J Trauma. 2003;55:704-6.
13. Swartz JD. Temporal bone trauma. Semin in Ultrasound; CT, MR. 2001;22:219-28.
14. Alvi A, Bereliani A 4th. Trauma to the temporal bone: Diagnosis and management of complications. J Craniomaxillofac Trauma. 1996;2:36-48.
15. Darrouzet V, Duclos JY, Liguoro D, et al. Management of facial paralysis resulting from temporal bone fractures: Our experience of 115 cases. Otolaryngol Head Neck Surg. 2001;125:77-84.
16. Little SC, Kesser BW. Radiographic classification of temporal bone fractures: clinical predictability using a new system. Arch Otolaryngol Head Neck Surg. 2006;132:1300-4.
17. Guy RL, Wylie E, Hickey A, et al. Computed tomography in malignant external otitis. Clin Radiol. 1991;43:166-70.
18. Kwon BJ, Han MH, Oh SH, et al. MRI findings and spreading patterns of necrotizing external otitis: is a poor outcome predictable? Clin Radiol. 2006;61:495-504.
19. Shire JR, Donegan JO. Cholesteatoma of the external auditory canal and keratosis obturans. Am J Otol. 1986;7:361-4.
20. Swartz JD, Goodman RS, Russel KB, et al. High resolution computed tomography of the middle ear and mastoid. Part II: Tubotympanic disease. Radiology. 1983;148:455-9.
21. Swartz JD. Cholesteatoma of the middle ear: diagnosis, etiology and complications. Radiol Clin North Am. 1984;22:15-35.
22. Cody DTR. The definition of cholesteatoma. In: McCabe BF, Sade JM Abramson M (Eds). Cholesteatoma. First International Conference. Birmingham, Ala: Aesculpius Publishers Inc; 1977. pp. 6-9.
23. Sade J. Pathogenesis of attic cholesteatoma: The metaplasia theory. In: McCabe BF, Sade J, Abramson M (Eds). Cholesteatoma. First International Conference, Birmingham, Ala: Aesculpins Publishers Inc; 1977. pp. 6-9.
24. Vercruysse JP, De Foer B, Pouillon M, et al. The value of diffusion-weighted MR imaging in the diagnosis of primary acquired and residual cholesteatoma: a surgical verified study of 100 patients. Eur Radiol. 2006;16:1461-7.
25. De Foer B, Vercruysse J-P, Pouillon M, et al. Value of high-resolution computed tomography and magnetic resonance imaging in the detection of residual cholesteatomas in primary obliterated mastoids. Am J Otolaryngol. 2007;28:230-34.
26. Holliday RA. Inflammatory diseases of temporal bone: Evaluation with CT and MR. Semin Ultrasound CT MR. 1989;10:213-35.
27. Johnson DW, Hinshaw DB Jr, Hasso AN, et al. Computed tomography of local complications of temporal bone cholesteatomas. J Comput Assist Tomogr. 1985;9:519-23.
28. Watts S, Flood LM, Clifford K. A systematic approach to interpretation of computed tomography scans prior to surgery of middle ear cholesteatoma. J Laryngol Otol. 2000;114:248-53.
29. Nemzek WR, Swartz JD. Temporal bone inflammatory disease. In: Som PM, Curtin HD (Eds). Head and Neck Imaging, 4th edition. St. Louis MO: Mosby Year Book; 2003.pp. 1173-242.
30. Sugiura M, Naganawa S, Teranishi M, et al. Three-dimensional fluid attenuated inversion recovery magnetic resonance imaging findings in patients with sudden sensorineural hearing loss. Laryngoscope. 2006;116:1451-4.
31. Witte RJ, Lane JI, Driscoll CL, et al. Pediatric and adult cochlear implantation. Radiographics. 2003;23:1185-200.
32. Lo WWM, Marcel Maya M. Vascular tinnitus. In: Som PM, Curtin HD (Eds). Head and Neck Imaging, 4th edition. St. Louis MO: Mosby Year Book; 2003. pp. 1361-74.
33. Remley KB, Coit WE Harnsberger HR. Pulsatile tinnitis and vascular tympanic membrane: CT, MR and Angiographic Findings. Radiology. 1990;174:383-9.
34. Dufour JJ, Lavigne F, Plante R, et al. Pulsatile tinnitus and fibromuscular dysplasia of the internal carotid. J Otoclaryngol. 1985;14:293-5.
35. Hasso AN, Bird CR, Zinke DE, et al. Fibromuscular dysplasia of the internal carotid artery: Percutaneous transluminal angioplasty. Am J Roentgenol. 1981;136:955-60.
36. Lippy WH, Berenholz LP, Burkey M. Otosclerosis in the 1960s, 1970s, 1980s and 1990s. Laryngoscope. 1999;109:1307-9.
37. Osamu S, Curtin HD, Harro AN, Swartz JD. Otosclerosis and dysplasias of the temporal bone. In: Som PM, Curtin HD (Eds). Head and Neck Imaging Bone, 4th edition. St Louis: Mosby Year Book; 2003. pp. 1245-73.
38. Hullar TE, Lustig LR. Paget's disease and fibrous dysplasia. Otolaryngol Clin North Am. 2003;36:707-32.
39. Casselman JW, De Jonge I, Neyt L, et al. MR in craniofacial fibrous dysplasia. Neuroradiology. 1993;35:234-7.
40. Fisch U, Ruttner J. Pathology of intratemporal tumours involving the facial nerve. In: Fisch U (Ed): Facial Nerve Surgery. Birmingham, Ala: Aesculpius; 1977. pp. 448-56.
41. Marcel Maya M, Lo WWM, Kouvanlikaya. Tumours of the temporal bone and the cerebellopontine angle. In: Som PM, Curtin HG (Eds). Head and Neck Imaging, 4th edition. St Louis MO: Mosby Year Book; 2003. pp. 1275-360.
42. Pulec JL, Deguine C. Squamous cell carcinoma of the external auditory canal. Ear Nose Throat J. 2004;83:9.

CHAPTER

201 Imaging of the Globe and Orbit

Sanjay Sharma, Smriti Hari, Deep Narayan Srivastava, Kumble S Madhusudhan

INTRODUCTION

Radiological evaluation of orbital pathology presents a diagnostic challenge. The aetiologies are diverse and clinical input is often necessary to narrow the diagnostic possibilities. Cross-sectional imaging plays a vital role in detection and evaluation of the disease, supplementing the clinical and ophthalmologic examination in providing information beyond fundoscopy. In this chapter, the imaging features of the more common adult and childhood orbital pathologies are discussed.

NORMAL ANATOMY

The orbit is a lopsided, pear-shaped cavity, wide anteriorly and narrow posteriorly formed by seven interconnecting bones with the optic canal analogous to the stem of the pear. The central axis of the orbit lies approximately 25° to the sagittal plane. It consists of roof, floor, lateral and medical walls and the apex. The roof of the orbit is composed of the orbital process of the frontal bone anteriorly and lesser wing of the sphenoid posteriorly. The lateral wall of the orbit is formed by the greater wing of the sphenoid posteriorly and by the zygomatic process of the frontal bone and frontal process of the zygomatic bone anteriorly. The medial wall of the orbit is formed posteriorly by the lamina papyracea of the ethmoid bone and anteriorly by the lacrimal bone. The floor of the orbit is composed essentially of the orbital plate of the maxilla and is limited posterolaterally by the inferior orbital fissure. The infraorbital groove runs on the orbital floor to reach the infraorbital foramen. Superior orbital fissure is a comma-shaped opening bounded by the greater wing of sphenoid inferolaterally and the lesser wing superomedially. It provides a large communication between the orbit and middle cranial fossa via the cavernous sinus allowing the spread of tumor or inflammation between these two compartments. The inferior orbital fissure lies between the floor and greater wing of sphenoid. It communicates with the pterygopalatine fossa and masticator space. The optic canal lies above and medial to the fissure and is separated from it by the optic strut that connects lesser wing to the body of the sphenoid. The lacrimal gland lies in the lacrimal fossa, a recess of frontal bone anterolaterally within the orbit.

The globe is surrounded by three tissue layers: (1) sclera and cornea, (2) uveal tract (choroids, iris and ciliary body), and (3) retina. The lens and iris divide the globe into anterior and posterior chamber. Optic nerve is about 5 cm long and divided into four segments: intraocular, intraorbital, intracanalicular and intracranial. The subarachnoid space between the dura and pia covering the optic nerve is continuous with the suprasellar cistern. The six extraocular muscles comprise of four recti and two oblique muscles. Thick orbital fascial septum situated anterior to the globe divides preseptal (anterior skin and subcutaneous) from the postseptal (more posterior orbit) compartment.

Radiographic Views

Standard projections for the bony orbit include posteroanterior (PA), lateral and optic foramen view. The patient could be either seated or semi prone. The *PA projection (occipito-frontal)* is obtained with 20° caudad tilt, with the central beam existing at the nasion. In this view, the innominate line is seen crossing the greater wing of sphenoid on the temporal side of the orbit. It has no true anatomical counterpart. For the *lateral view* the mid sagittal plane of the skull is placed parallel to the image receptor with the beam centered at a point 2.5 cm posterior to the outer canthus. In the true lateral projection, the floor of the anterior cranial fossa is superimposed. For *optic foramen view* (Rhese projection), the head rests on cheek, nose and chin, with orbit in center, in a manner that orbitomeatal line is perpendicular, keeping the mid sagittal plane at an angle of 53° to the image receptor, and the orbitomeatal line is raised at 35° from the horizontal. Beam is centered 7.5 cm superior and 7.5 cm posterior to the upper external auditory meatus, emerging at the center of orbit under examination. These orbital radiographs are now less commonly requested. An orbital radiograph is now mainly needed to exclude metallic foreign body prior to MRI.

Ultrasound

It is a widely available non-invasive diagnostic modality for evaluation of ocular and orbital pathology. It is particularly useful in the evaluation of intraocular lesions, especially when the media is opaque. It is useful in differentiating cystic from solid lesions. However, it is limited by the lack of visualization of more deeply placed intraorbital lesions. Both A and B-mode scans are used. A-mode scan is particularly popular with the ophthalmologists. B-mode scan of the globe is done with 7.5–10 MHz, whereas orbit proper is scanned with 5–7.5 MHz transducer. It is carried out after applying coupling gel over the closed eyelids. Both the anterior and posterior chambers of the eyeball are echo-free with the lens present between the two. Posterior to the globe, the echogenic fat is seen with central hypoechoic band representing the optic nerve sheath complex. Colour Doppler evaluation can be combined with the B-scan to evaluate the blood flow in tumors and vascular lesions, or spectral trace obtained from superior ophthalmic vein in patients with carotico-cavernous fistula. Preliminary studies show that the contrast enhanced harmonic imaging could become a powerful tool in the evaluation of perfusion in ocular tumors.[1] Ultrasound biomicroscopy (UBM) uses approximately 50 MHz transducer to produce exceptionally detailed two dimensional gray scale images of the anterior chamber.

Computed Tomography

The newer generation multidetetor row computed tomography represents an important modality offering the advantages of shorter acquisition times, reduced motion artifacts, isotropic resolution, and excellent multiplanar image reconstruction. In addition, postprocessing of axial volumetric data now allows sophisticated 3D volume rendered images that allowing better understanding of the pathology. It provides excellent anatomic detail of the eyeball, extraocular muscles, optic nerve and retrobulbar fat, etc. Volumetric acquisition is routinely performed in contiguous thin (2–3 mm) axial plane,and displayed both in soft tissue and bone windows. The plane of axial orbital imaging is parallel to the infraorbitomeatal line. Intravenous contrast is routinely administered except in the setting of trauma, foreign body or thyroid ophthalmopathy.

Magnetic Resonance Imaging

Magnetic resonance imaging (MRI) has gained widespread acceptance because of its greater sensitivity in characterizing the orbital pathologies with direct multiplanar imaging, higher soft tissue resolution, use of fat suppressed sequences with or without contrast enhancement, T2-weighted images, combined head and surface coils and increasingly faster data acquisition. FLAIR (Fluid Attenuation Inversion Recovery) sequence may be used to suppress the CSF hyperintensity for better evaluation of optic nerve. Compared to CT, MRI has a greater versatility in detecting concomitant intracranial abnormalities. Vitreous body appears aslow intensity on T1 and high intensity on T2-weighted images. Optic nerve and its coverings are hypointense on T1 weighted images and surrounded by high intensity retrobulbar fat. Cerebrospinal fluid (CSF) surrounding the optic nerve can be seen as low intensity sleeve around the optic nerve on T1 and high signal on T2-weighted images. The intracanalicular and intracranial parts of the optic nerve are well evaluated because of lack of bone artifacts. Sequences and plane of imaging must be tailored to suit the clinical requirement. Spin echo T1 and T2-weighted, thin (3 mm) section contiguous (or with small interslice gap) images are acquired in axial, coronal and/or even oblique planes. Applications of MRI are still evolving. Although CT provides good anatomical delineation of structures, MRI has been found to have distinct advantages over CT in certain conditions, e.g. evaluation of hemorrhagic and vascular pathology without the requirement of intravenous contrast, periorbital and orbital apex pathologies. However, it limited by relatively long imaging time and higher cost.

PATHOLOGICAL CONDITIONS

Lesions of the orbit can be broadly subdivided into two groups: Ocular (limited to the globe) and orbital (rest of the orbit excluding globe). The orbital lesions can be further subdivided according to their predominant location in respective spaces. A knowledge of the compartmental localization of the pathological process helps to limit the differential diagnoses **(Table 1)**.[2,3]

OCULAR LESIONS

These comprise a broad spectrum of diseases which include ocular detachment, vitreous hemorrhage, benign and malignant tumors (retinoblastoma, malignant melanoma, choroidal metastases), Coats' disease, persistent hyperplastic primary vitreous (PHPV), intraocular foreign body, parasitic infestation (the commonest being cysticercosis) and congenital anomalies of the eyeball.

Ocular Detachments

Three potential spaces exist-posterior hyaloid space, subretinal space and suprachoroidal space. Only under pathological conditions, when accumulation of fluid or hemorrhage occurs, do these spaces become visible and distinguishable on imaging **(Table 2)**.[4] *Posterior hyaloid detachment* occurs with physiological liquefaction of vitreous in elderly, myopia, PHPV or trauma. It presents on imaging as a fluid-fluid level. *Retinal detachment* is seen as a thin membrane attached to the optic nerve head posteriorly and ora serrata anteriorly, often assuming V or Y shaped appearance due to lifting of retinal leaves by subretinal fluid or hemorrhage. Partial detachment may be seen as a localized area of elevated retina. On CT, mild or focal retinal detachment may not be detected. Any choroidal lesion may produce retinal detachment. It is commonly seen in retinoblastoma in children and neoplasms like malignant melanoma or choroidal hemangioma in adults. *Choroidal detachment* occurs in two distinct forms viz, serous or hemorrhagic, each with different imaging appearances, even though the etiology of both may be similar. It may occur after intraocular surgery, penetrating ocular injury, or inflammatory disorders. Hemorrhagic detachment presents as a lens like configuration, caused by the fixation of choroid by the posterior ciliary vessels. Serous detachment is characterized by a crescent or ring shape, essentially due to ocular hypotony.

TABLE 1: A guide to differential diagnosis.

	Pathological conditions		
Anatomical compartment	Common	Uncommon	Rare
Intraconal	Optic neuritis, papilloedema	Meningioma, sarcoidosis	Lymphoma, hemangioma
Optic nerve	Apical fractures affecting optic nerve Optic glioma, Inflammatory pseudotumor	Metastases	
Others	Cavernous hemangioma, pseudotumor, varices	Lymphangioma, neurofibroma lymphoma, metastasis	Hemangiopericytoma Yolk sac tumor, chondrosarcoma
		Capillary hemangioma	Granular cell myoblastoma
Extraconal	Capillary hemangioma, dermoid Lymphoma, rhabdomyosarcoma	Neurofibroma, metastases	Fibrous histiocytoma
Preseptal space	Cutaneous conditions (xanthelesma etc.), Basal cell cancer	Capillary hemangioma, Dermoid, Lymphoma, Neurofibromas, fibroma	Metastasis, Melanoma
Subperiosteal space	Mucocele, fractures, PNS neoplasms Abscess, osteoma, metastases, Dermoid, epidermoid, Rhabdomyosarcoma, menigioma,	Craniofacial dysplasia Fibrous dysplasia, wegener's granulomatosis Pagets disease, Plasmacytoma	Histiocytosis, sphenoid dysplasia Encephalocele, bone tumors Osteopetrosis
Lacrimal gland	Inflammatory pseudotumor, Dacryoadenitis, abscess	Lymphoma, dermoid, sarcoid Pleomorphic adenoma, carcinoma Sjögren's syndrome	Wegener's granulomatosis, Miculicz syndrome, metastases
Orbital apex and cavernous sinus	Pituitary adenoma, Meningioma, empty sella, craniopharyngioma, arachnoid cyst, optic chiasm glioma	Metastases, Tolosa Hunt syndrome, carotico-cavernous fistula	
Muscles	Endocrine orbitopathy, myositis, Inflammatory pseudotumor	Metastases, wegener's Granulomatosis, acromegaly, Myoblastoma, lithium therapy	
Globe	Foreign body, retinal/choroidal Detachment, scleritis, uveitis	Retinoblastoma, melanoma, Metastases	Lymphoma, hemangioma, PHPV, coats' disease, norie's disease, osteoma, medulloepithelioma

Vitreous Hemorrhage

The vitreous is normally clear and echo-free on ultrasound (US). Vitreous hemorrhage is seen especially in patients with diabetic retinopathyand trauma. On ultrasound acute hemorrhage is seen as scattered, low amplitude echoes on US, which subsequently becomes highly echogenic. Estimation of the extent of vitreous hemorrhage is important to know the prognosis for spontaneous clearing, and planning for vitrectomy in the event of its non-clearance. Normal vitreous is of low attenuation on CT scan but in the presence of vitreous hemorrhage it becomes diffusely hazy.

Retinoblastoma

It is the most common, highly malignant, intraocular tumor of childhood. Over 90% affect children less than 5 years with no sex prediliction. Most common presentation is leucocoria (60%) followed by strabismus (20%). In 25–33% patients the disease is bilateral and represents autosomal dominant pattern of genetic transmission. In bilateral cases there is frequently a family history.[5] Three growth patterns are described: (1) Endophytic-anterior tumor growth from retina into vitreous cavity (simulating endophthalmitis), (2) Exophytic tumor growth into subretinal space, producing secondary retinal detachment (simulating coats' disease), (3) Diffuse tumor growth along the retina appearing as a placoid mass (simulating inflammatory and hemorrhagic conditions). This rare form presents diagnostic difficulties because of its lack of calcification and occurrence outside the typical age group.[6]

Ophthalmoscopy allows diagnostic confirmation of even the smallest tumors, however ultrasound evaluation is complimentary. On US, retinoblastomas are seen as intraocular masses of varying size and mixed echogenicity

TABLE 2: Diagrammatic representation of ocular detachments.

Posterior hyaloid detachment	Retinal detachment	Choroidal detachment	
		Hemorrhagic	Serous
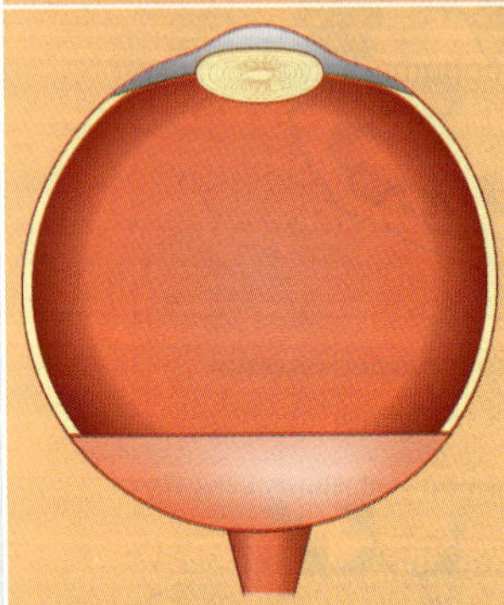	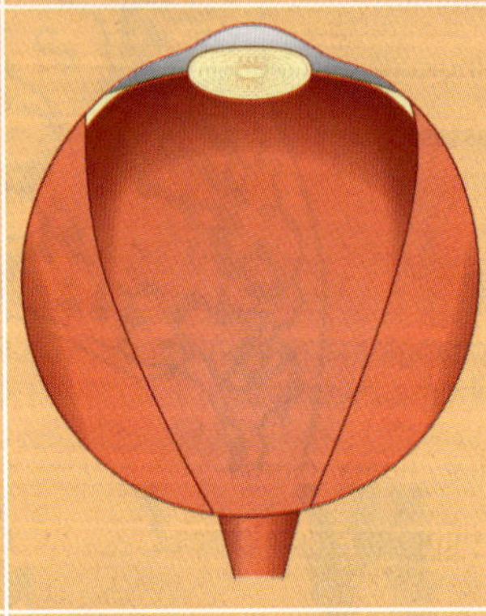	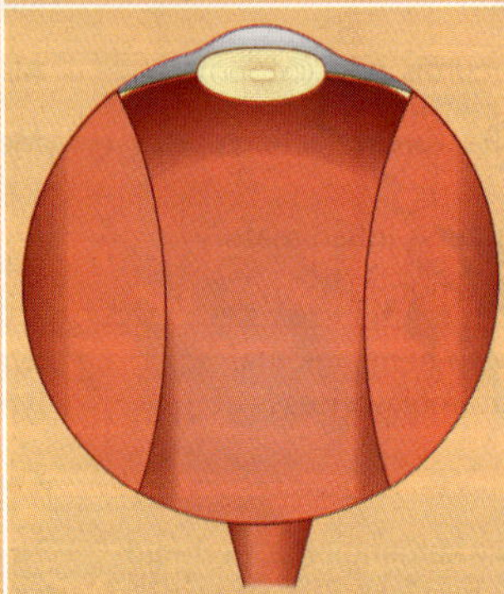	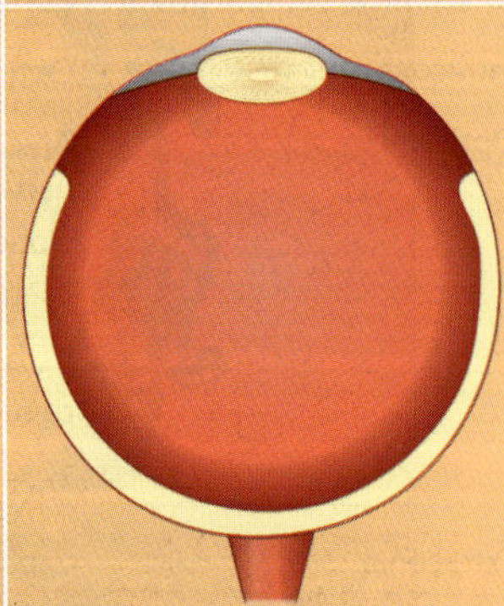
Adults: Macular degeneration *Children*: PHPV	• Subretinal hemorrhage • Choroidal lesion	• Trauma • Intraocular surgery	Ocular hypotony
Fluid-fluid level	• Macular degeneration • Trauma • V-shaped with apex at optic disk	• Contusion • Choroidal inflammation Lentiform	Crescent or Ring

located in the coats of the eyeball with calcification seen in upto 90%.[7,8] The detection of calcification is an important diagnostic criterion. Tumors that are non-calcified may be of low to medium reflectivity. CT scanning better depicts subtle calcification **(Fig. 1)**, delineation of its soft tissue component and intraorbital and/or intracranial extension. However, it is no longer considered a primary modality for the diagnosis of retinoblastoma owing to the radiation risks in small children. On the other hand, MRI has now evolved as a standard tool in the diagnostic assessment of tumor stage (optic nerve spread and extra ocular extension) **(Figs. 2 and 3)** and intracranial involvement. It is also useful in its follow up and differentiating it from other causes of leucocoria. The echoplanar diffusion weighted imaging (DWI) has the benefit of assessing the diffusivity in retinoblastoma, potentially aiding the improved diagnosis of tumors and its follow up on treatment[9] **(Figs. 3A and B)**. However, with its insensitivity to field inhomogeneity and high spatial resolution, the 3D turbo field echo (TFE) with diffusion-sensitized driven-equilibrium (DSDE) MRI technique has been recently shown to better assess the diffusivity in retinoblastomas without geometrical distortion.[10]

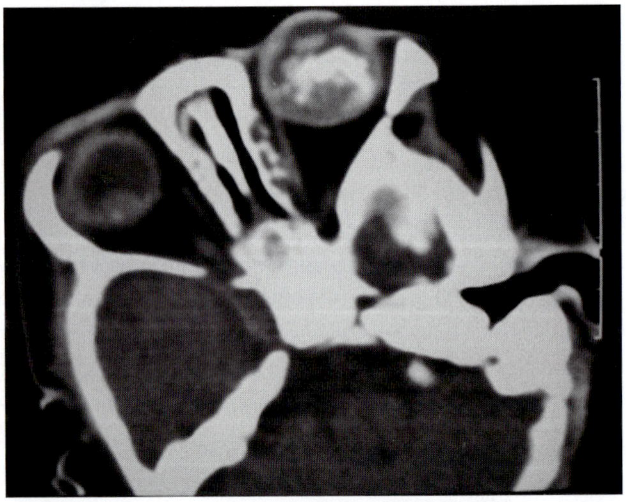

FIG. 1: Retinoblastoma. NCCT shows bilateral calcified intraocular soft tissue masses.

Persistent Hyperplastic Primary Vitreous

The persistent hyperplastic primary vitreous (PHPV) arises when the embryonic hyaloid vascular system fails to regress normally leading to persistence of abnormal segments of primary vitreous. It is primarily unilateral and presents at birth. It is the most common lesion closely resembling retinoblastoma. On ultrasound doppler and MRI a triangular retrolental band of soft tissue extends along the Cloquet's canal from the posterior surface of crystalline lens to the posterior pole of the globe **(Figs. 4A to D)**. It may demonstrate moderate or no enhancement on the administration of intravenous contrast. Computed tomography may demonstrate gravitational layering of high attenuation fluid in retrohyaloid or subrential space, possibly resulting from the presence of hemorrhage or serosanguineous material. The affected eyeball is often small. Absence of intraocular calcification often helps to differentiate PHPV from retinoblastoma.

Although sensitivity of MRI in detecting calcification is inferior to CT, it represents the most important imaging modality in the evaluation and staging of retinoblastoma. This is due to its high soft tissue contrast resolution, enabling simultaneous assessment of spread along the optic nerve and intracranial involvement. Retinoblastoma appears as slightly

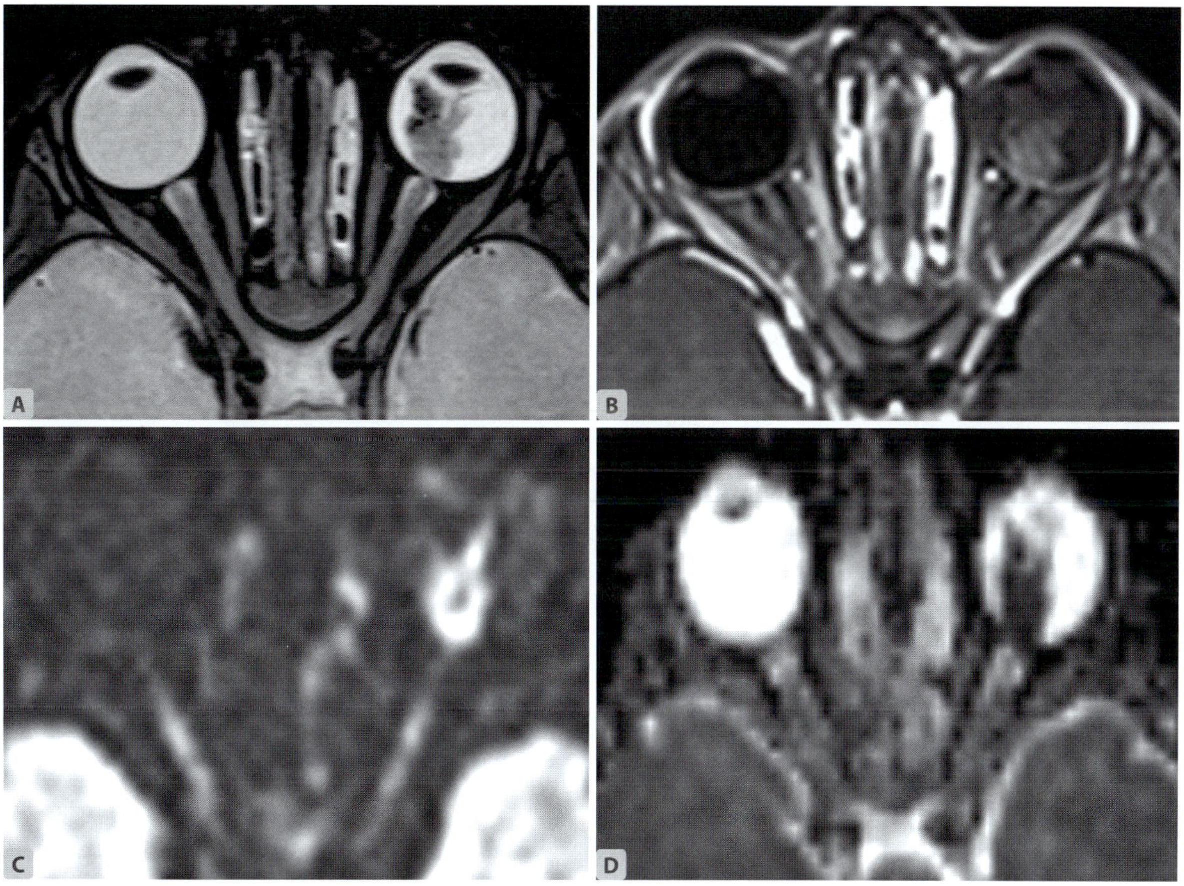

FIGS. 2A TO D: Retinoblastoma. Left intraocular mass is hypointense on T2WI (A) and shows moderate enhancement (B). It exhibits diffusion restriction (C, DWI and D, ADC map). The optic nerve is not involved.

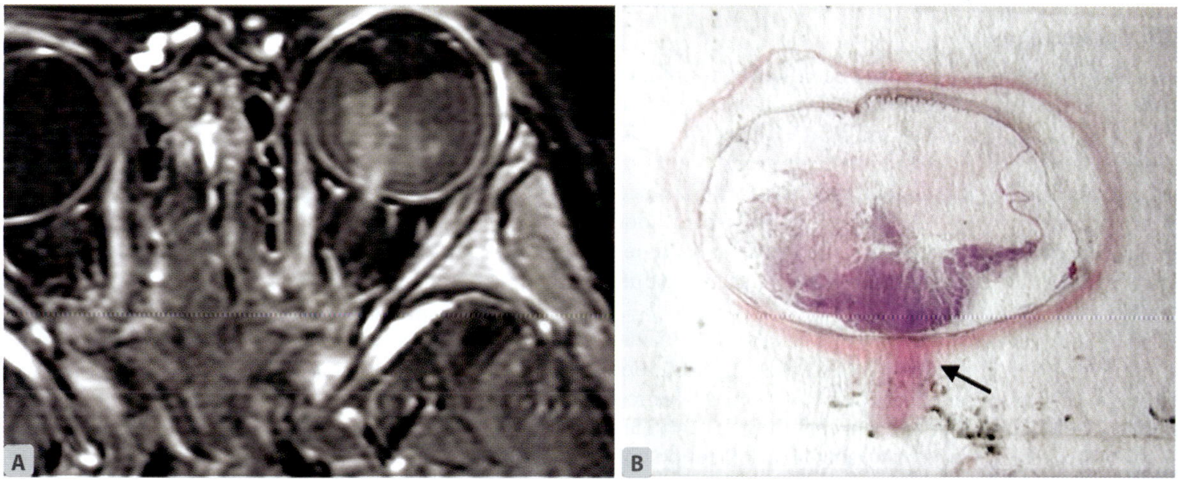

FIGS. 3A AND B: Retinoblastoma involving the left globe (in another child) (A and B). Postcontrast MRI image (A) shows moderate tumor enhancement and postlaminar optic nerve involvement for about 2 mm. Whole mount enucleation specimen (B) confirms early the optic nerve spread (arrow).

hyperintense compared to vitreous on T1 and PD weighted images, with patchy low signal intensity on T2W images.[11] It exhibits moderate to marked contrast enhancement best appreciated in the fat suppressed sequences. The involvement of the optic nerve is best assessed in the postcontrast T1-weighted fat suppressed images and compared with the normal side. It best differentiates patients of retinoblastoma from other causes of leucocoria viz, PHPV and Coats' disease. Less commonly retinal detachment, endophthalmitis, toxocariasis, late stages of retinopathy of prematurity (ROP), choroidal hemangioma, retinal hamartoma, etc. may also be considered.

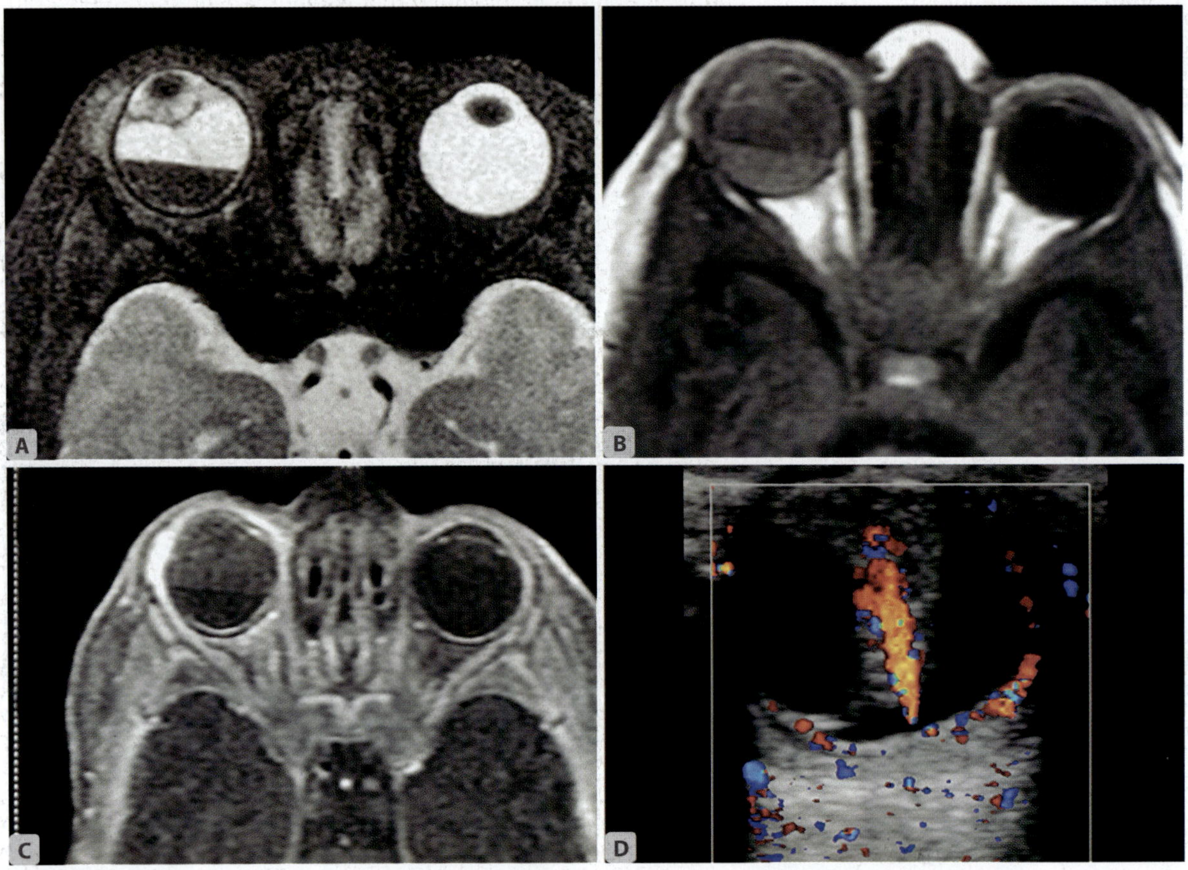

FIGS. 4A TO D: Persistent hyperplastic primary vitreous (right). Axial T2W (A) MRI shows a triangular retrolental opacity with an intraocular linear channel representing embryonic vascular remnant. T1W pre (B) and postcontrast © image shows no mass. Note the posterior hyaloid detachment seen as a fluid-fluid level. Ultrasound Doppler (D) shows a patent vascular channel (another patient).

Coats' Disease

Coats' disease is a primary idiopathic vascular anomaly of the retina, characterized by telangiectasis. The telangiectatic vessels cause leakage of serum and lipid with accumulation of a lipoproteinaceous exudate in the retina and subretinal space. It is almost always unilateral and occurs in boys aged 6–8 years, older than those who have retinoblastoma. It does not generally become symptomatic until retinal detachment occurs, which finally leads to central vision loss and painful glaucoma.

At the early stages the diagnosis is reliably established by Ophthalmoscopy, and CT or MRI provide little additional information. Diagnostic imaging is helpful at a more advanced stage when retinal detachment occurs and is seen on US and CT **(Figs. 5A and B)**. Absence of intraocular calcification does not differentiate Coats' disease from unilateral non-calcifying retinoblastoma. MRI is superior to CT in distinguishing Coats disease from retinoblastoma.[12] The most significant finding on T1, PD and T2-weighted images is the identification of homogenous hyperintensity of subretinal fluid caused by high protein content in comparison to the vitreous body of the opposite eye. Detached V-shaped retina may be seen having a low signal on both T1 and T2-weighted images. Detached retina may show enhancement after intravenous gadolinium, but the subretinal fluid does not. In contrast, retinoblastoma is inhomogenous, moderately hyperintense mass on T1W and PD images, but with hypointense areas on the T2W images. Tumor mass in retinoblastoma shows moderate to marked enhancement after contrast administration in contrast to subretinal fluid in Coat's disease.[13]

Uveal Malignant Melanoma

It is the commonest primary malignant intraocular tumor of adults. The incidence of disease increases with age with mean age at 53 years.[14] The specific diagnostic US, CT and MRI criteria include: collar button (mushroom) shaped intraocular mass which is broad based towards the coats of the eyeball with its dome projecting into the vitreous body. Associated retinal detachment may be seen in a large percentage of patients. Further, choroidal excavation dueto replacement of the choroids by the tumor mass may also be seen.

Ultrasound Doppler imaging may show marked vascularity. MRI is the imaging technique of choice. On MRI the tumor is seen as hyperintense on T1W and hypointense on T2W images **(Figs. 6A and B)**. This unique signal of melanin is due to shortening of both T1 and T2 relaxation times. The factors associated with a poor prognosis include: older patients (60 years), large tumor base diameter, location in anterior uvea and cilliary body, and extraocular extension.[15]

The sites of metastasis include liver, lungs, bone, kidneys and brain.

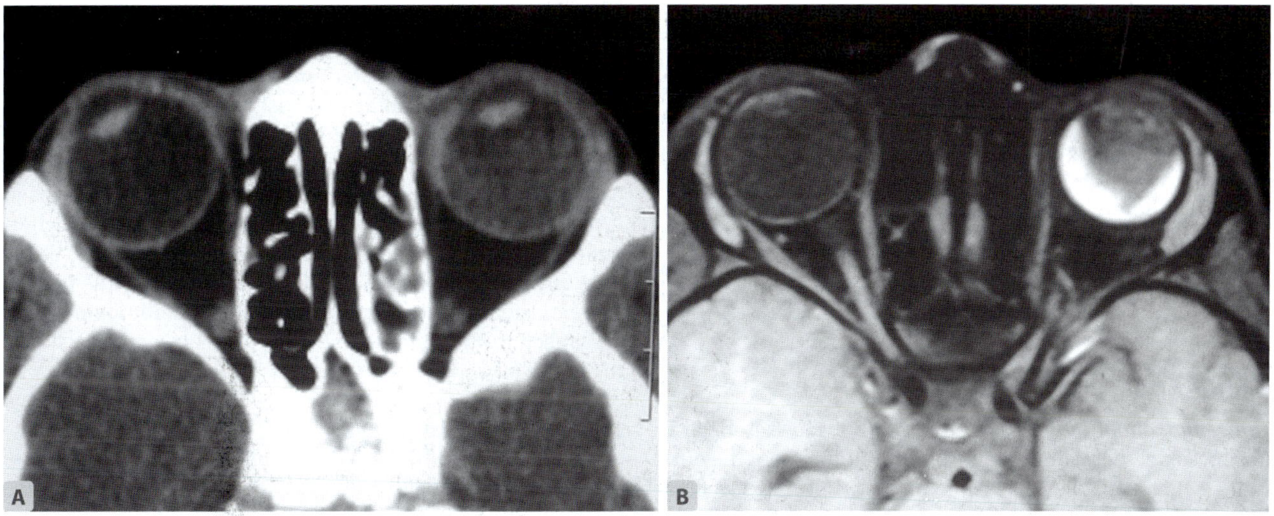

FIGS. 5A AND B: Coats' disease (L). Axial CT (A) and T1W MRI (B) show sub-retinal hemorrhage in the small left globe in a 8-year-old boy. Note that there is no mass or calcification.

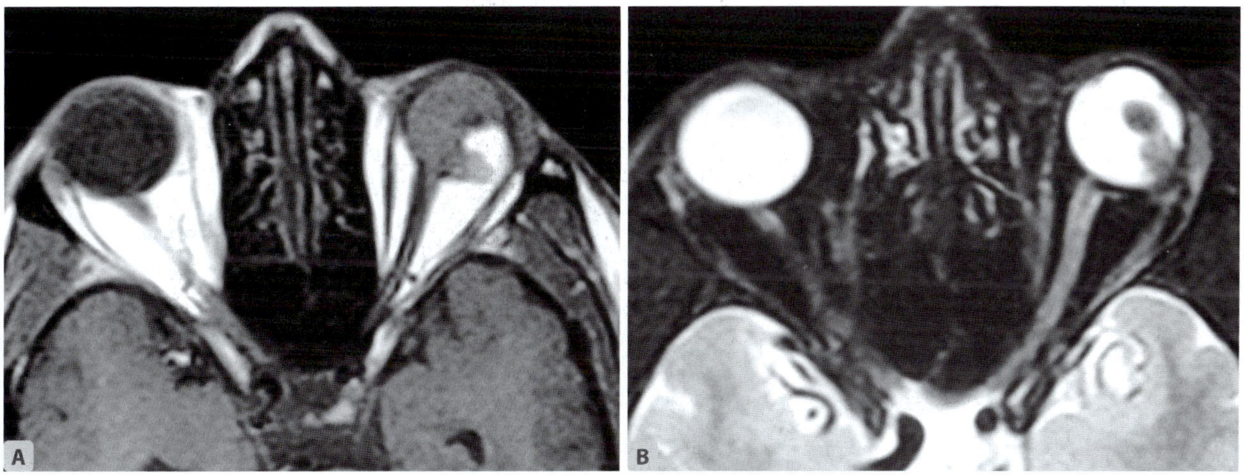

FIGS. 6A AND B: Uveal melanoma involving left globe. MR axial images (A) and (B), showing that the lesion is typically hyperintense on T1W (A) and hypointense on the T2W fat suppressed (B) images.

Choroidal Metastases

The choroid is the most common site of carcinoma metastatic to the eye. The metastatic carcinomas of the choroids are subretinal masses located mainly in the posterior part of the fundus. They are frequently associated with serous retinal detachment. These are relatively flattened or placoid masses and may be multiple. In contrast to the uveal melanoma, these tumors may occur bilaterally or be multifocal and affect both the eyes in about one-third of cases. The common sites of primary tumors are lung, breast, prostate, etc.

Foreign Body

Foreign bodies represent ophthalmic emergencies and require thorough evaluation. It is mandatory to localize a foreign body to define appropriate treatment. Plain radiograph may show presence of radiopaque foreign body. A circular radiopaque marker is sutured to the surface of the eye. Lateral and posteroanterior views are obtained with marker in place to allow reliable measurements. CT is however, the modality of choice for detection of intraorbital foreign bodies, associated brain injuries or facial fractures. In case of wooden foreign body, fresh wood is usually hyperdense on CT whereas dry wood is hypodense, sometimes even indistinguishable from intraorbital fat or air.[16] Glass foreign bodies are hyperdense but without typical streak artifacts of metallic foreign body **(Fig. 7)**. MRI can be useful to differentiate foreign body (generally hypointense) and orbital fat. The patients with suspected metallic-ferromagnetic intraorbital foreign bodies must never be exposed to the high field MRI. A preliminary plain radiograph is customary to exclude its presence. US may be helpful in evaluation of radiolucent intraocular foreign bodies. In addition, the presence of vitreous hemorrhage and retinal detachment may also be assessed. However, in general, US has no significant role in the detection of intraorbital foreign bodies.

Parasitic Infestation

Cysticercosis cellulosae is the most common intraocular parasitic infestation. On US, it is seen as a ring-shaped lesion with a dense nodule representing the scolex **(Fig. 8)**. Cysticerci are usually seen adjacent to the coats of the eyeball. Associated retinal detachment may be seen.[17] CT scan demonstrates the scolex as a pin-head area of increased attenuation. The cyst wall, however, is not seen, presumably due to very low attenuation difference between the fluid in the cyst, vitreous and wall of the cysticercus cellulosae.

Congenital Anomalies

Congenital anophthalmos is a rare condition characterized by absence of globe(s) due to failure of development of the optic vesicle **(Fig. 9)**. No eye is visible on inspection. Extraocular muscles may be well developed. *Microphthalmos* is characterized by a unilateral small eye. This is either isolated or found associated with other craniofacial anomalies. It may be accompanied by a *colobomatous cyst* as a manifestation of failure of the closure of the embryonic optic fissure **(Fig. 10)**. This cyst is generally located inferior to globe and may be a cause of rapidly worsening proptosis mimicking neoplasia.

When congenital anomalies are present, the role of imaging is to rule out associated intracranial abnormalities, or to identify extraocular muscles in a patient who may have to undergo surgery for microphthalmos. However, when anophthalmos is suspected, the presence of cryptophthalmos (eye covered with a layer of skin), a colobomatous cyst or retinoblastoma must be ruled out. When colobomatous cyst is suspected, an orbital cephalocele must always be excluded to choose an appropriate surgical approach.

ORBITAL LESIONS

These can be discussed under the following broad categories: tumors, developmental cysts, inflammatory lesions, endocrine exophthalmos, parasitic infestations, vascular lesions and trauma.

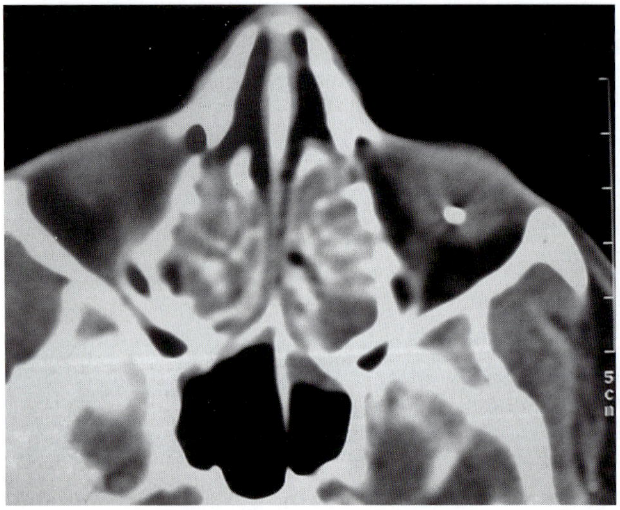

FIG. 7: Foreign body. Metallic intraocular foreign body within the left globe. Note incidental ethmoid sinusitis.

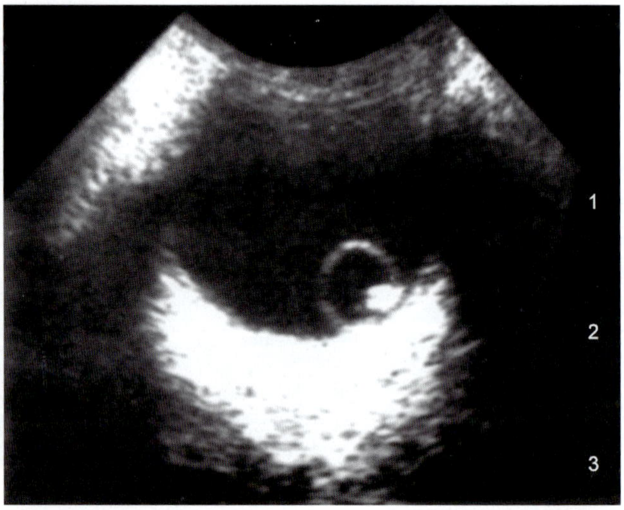

FIG. 8: Intraocular cysticercus. Ultrasound image showing a cyst with a scolex within the left eyeball.

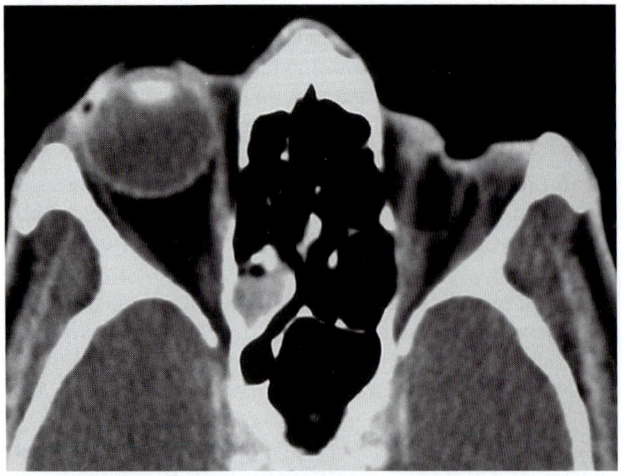

FIG. 9: Anophthalmia (L). Axial CT image shows absence of left globe. Note the intact extraocular muscles, atrophic optic nerve and relatively small bony orbit.

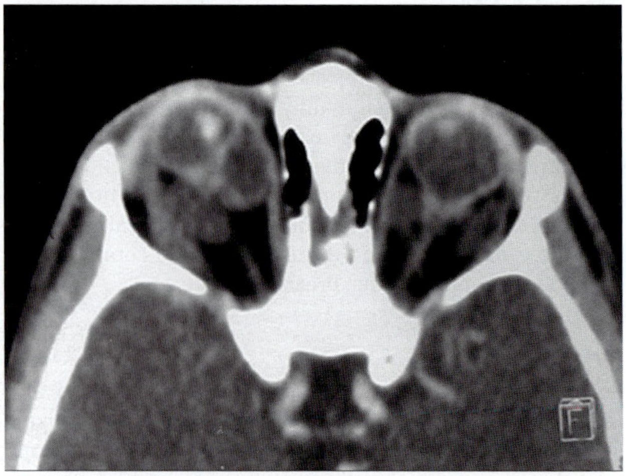

FIG. 10: Bilateral colobomatous cysts. Axial CT shows a bilateral microphthalmia and multiple variable sized intraorbital cysts. The right lens is densely calcified.

ORBITAL TUMORS

Hemangioma

It could be either capillary or cavernous in type. Both are different lesions differing in clinical presentation, location and age of presentation.

Capillary Hemangioma

These are the commonest intraorbital tumors of childhood. They are usually extraconal, situated in the superomedial quadrant with associated cutaneous malformation over the face. They present at birth, grow rapidly in the first year of life and usually regress by 7–10 years of age. They most commonly arise anteriorly, are unencapsulated and less well-defined than the cavernous forms. Intraconal extension also sometimes occurs. On imaging they are slightly hypodense on CT, iso- to hyperintenseon T1 and moderately hyperintense on T2W MR images. Signal intensity is determined by the amount of fibrosis, calcification and hemosiderin deposition after hemorrhage. Flow voids may be identified within and on the surface on T2W images, which is a helpful distinguishing feature from lymphangioma. A prominent arterial supply is usually demonstrable from external or internal carotid circulation.[13]

Cavernous Hemangioma

They are commonest intraorbital tumors in adults, occurring mainly in the 4th and 5th decade of life. Although they usually occur as isolated intraconal masses, these may extend into the extraconal space, may be entirely extraconal or multiple. These are well encapsulated tumors and tend to be round to oval in shape. Histologically, they are composed of large, dilated, vascular channels (sinusoid-like spaces) lined by thin attenuated endothelial cells.[18] They contain relatively stagnant blood and the walls forming the vascular spaces produce large interfaces resulting in either hyperechoic or mixed hypo- and hyperchoic appearance on US. On CT they appear well demarcated, smoothly marginated, homogeneous, rounded, ovoid or lobulated soft tissue masses of increased density with a variable degree of contrast enhancement owing to slow intratumoral circulation. Uncommonly phleboliths may be seen. They are normally iso- to hypointense on T1 and homogeneously hyperintense on T2W image, showing marked enhancement that becomes homogeneous in delayed phase **(Figs. 11A to C)**.[19] Depending upon size of the

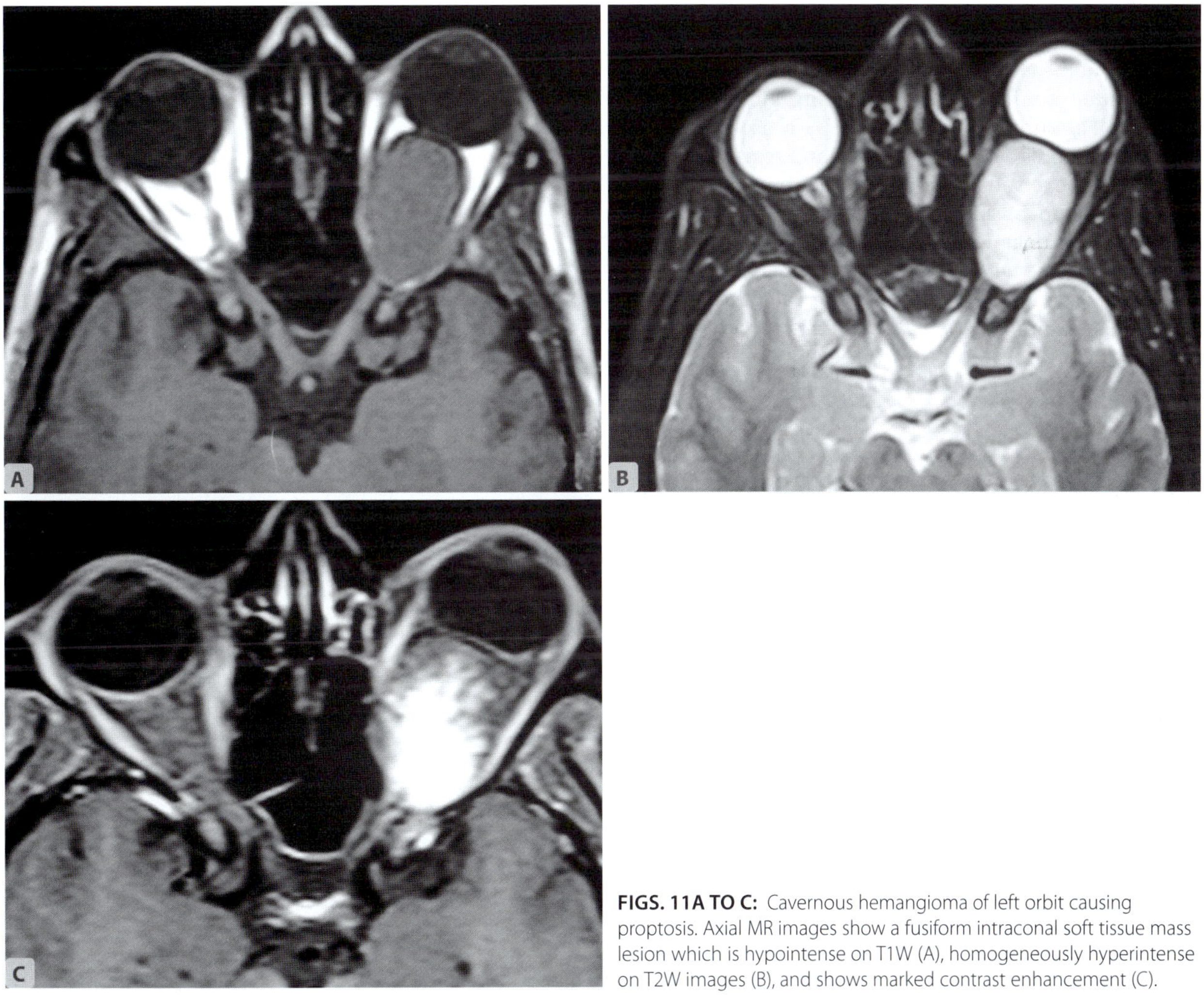

FIGS. 11A TO C: Cavernous hemangioma of left orbit causing proptosis. Axial MR images show a fusiform intraconal soft tissue mass lesion which is hypointense on T1W (A), homogeneously hyperintense on T2W images (B), and shows marked contrast enhancement (C).

lesion, orbital bony expansion may occur. They usually spare the orbital apex.

Lymphangioma

These lesions are unencapsulated and represent hamartomas. Large majority of these lesions are extraconal in location, however these often cross anatomic compartments. They usually present during early childhood. Usual presentation is that of sudden proptosis caused by hemorrhage. On CT and MRI, lymphangiomas appear as irregularly marginated, multilobulated, poorly defined lesions that may be heterogenous and enhance partially. MR is more specific than CT in identifying blood products and showing various components of lymphangioma **(Figs. 12A and B)**. Ultrasound is useful to evaluate the internal architecture of lymphangioma, especially as intralesional sclerotherapy of its macrocystic variants is now becoming an increasingly popular and effective treatment.[20,21]

Lacrimal Gland Tumors

Pleomorphic adenoma (benign mixed tumor) is the most common benign epithelial tumor of the lacrimal gland. The peak age of incidence is between 25 years and 40 years. It is painless and typically develops over many years. These are slow growing and may show fossa formation in the superolateral part of the bony orbit. Most involve the orbital part of the gland and are seen as well defined masses with rounded configuration, displacing and deforming the globe. The tumor is surrounded by a pseudocapsule formed by compressed adjacent tissue and reactive fibrosis. It should be excised without a preceding biopsy and within its pseudocapsule to prevent the risk of recurrence and malignant degeneration. Malignant transformation occurs into an *adenoid cystic carcinoma (malignant mixed tumor)* and is stated to be around 20%. The other primary lacrimal gland tumor is *mucoepidermoid carcinoma*. The morphological criteria on MRI are same as those of CT (smooth outline, round to oval). The tumor is of low signal intensity on T1 and high signal intensity on the T2-weighted images, and frequently heterogeneous. Imaging alone can not distinguish benign from malignant lesions. The presence of calcification and bone destruction suggests malignancy **(Fig. 13)**. Contrast enhancement is moderate to intense. Compared to the globular configuration of the lacrimal gland tumors, the inflammatory or lymphomatous masses show a flattened appearance. Further, in the latter lesions there is almost equal involvement of the palpebral and orbital part of the lacrimal gland.[2]

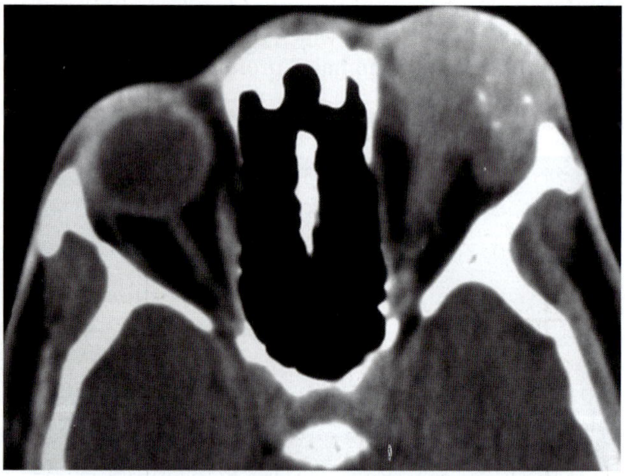

FIG. 13: Malignant mixed tumor of the left lacrimal gland. CECT shows soft tissue mass with calcific foci and remodeling of the adjacent bony lacrimal fossa.

Optic Nerve Glioma

This is the commonest childhood tumor affecting the optic nerve with a female preponderance and largely indolent course. A high association of visual pathway gliomas with neurofibromatosis, amounting to over 50% in some series, has been noted.[22] Two types of neurofibromatosis type I (Von Recklinghausen's disease) and type II (bilateral acoustic

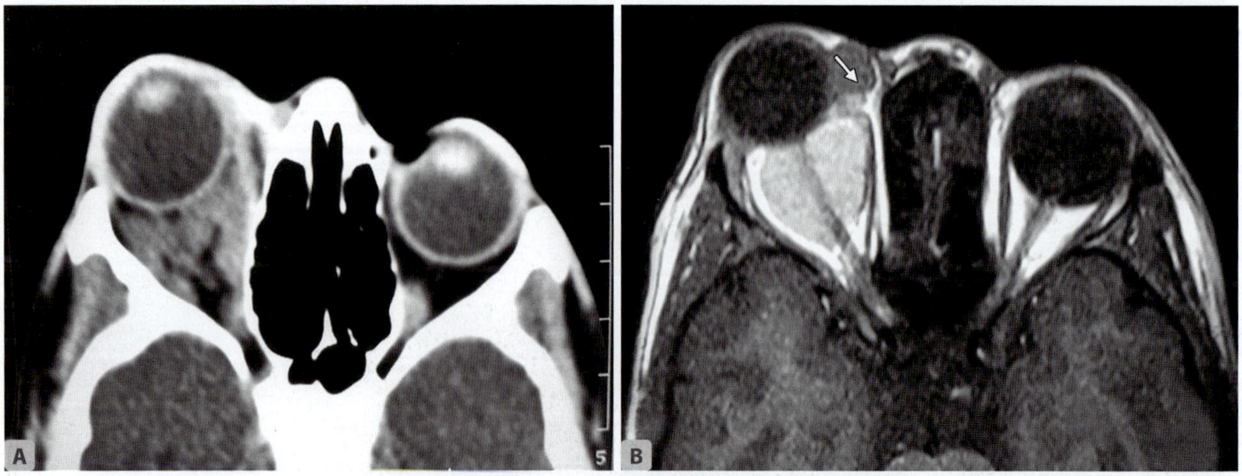

FIGS. 12A AND B: Lymphangioma, right side causing proptosis. Axial CECT (A) and MR image (B), Ill-defined retrobulbar mass involving both intra- and extraconal compartments (A). Axial T1W MR image (another patient), with intraconal mass with small extraconal extension on the nasal aspect. Note that mass is hyperintense and shows fluid-fluid level (arrow) suggesting hemorrhage.

neuromas), have been recognized as distinct disorders, each having a different chromosome linkage.[23] Bilateral optic nerve glioma is almost always a manifestation of neurofibromatosis. The adult form of the tumor is aggressive and associated with high mortality. Fifty percent of those presenting in adulthood will have optic nerve and chiasmatic involvement.[24]

US, CT or MRI may reveal tubular, fusiform or saccular enlargement of the optic nerve **(Fig. 14A)**. Tortuosity of the optic nerve, if seen, goes in favor of optic nerve glioma in contrast to rather straight course of thickened optic nerve in optic nerve sheath meningioma. Contrast enhancement is less intense in optic nerve glioma as compared to optic nerve sheath meningioma. Calcification may be rarely present. MRI permits a better demonstration of involvement of intracanalicular and intracranial part of the nerve **(Figs. 14B to D)** and is a modality of choice. Proton density and T2W images demonstrate homogeneous high signal intensity of the affected nerve compared to the low signal of unaffected contralateral optic nerve. Contrast enhancement is variable.

Meningioma

Second most common tumor of the optic nerve sheath complex is meningioma. These are more common in women and frequently occur in middle age. Symptoms depend on the site of involvement within the orbit and the size of tumor. Orbital meningiomas can be divided into 3 types, sphenoid wing meningioma with extension into the orbit, optic nerve sheath meningioma, and those arising de-novo from arachnoid cell rests in the orbit.

Sphenoid Wing Meningioma

It often results in marked hyperostosis and expansion of the bone. The tumor may extend into the orbit, anterior and middle cranial fossa or extracranially to the temporal fossa. Mass effect from the hyperostotic reaction as well as the soft tissue component compromises the orbital volume causing proptosis. Plain radiography may show sclerosis and thickening of the sphenoid wing. CT and MRI are useful in demonstrating the contiguity between the orbital and intracranial components of orbital meningioma. CT features of a typical meningioma include a well defined smooth outlined mass showing marked contrast enhancement, contiguity with adjacent dura and hyperostosis of adjacent bones **(Fig. 15)**. Bone destruction by an aggressive meningioma may mimic a metastatic or other malignant tumor.

Optic Nerve Sheath Meningioma

Meningioma of the optic nerve sheath arise from arachnoid cells of the dural covering the optic nerve. They are bilateral

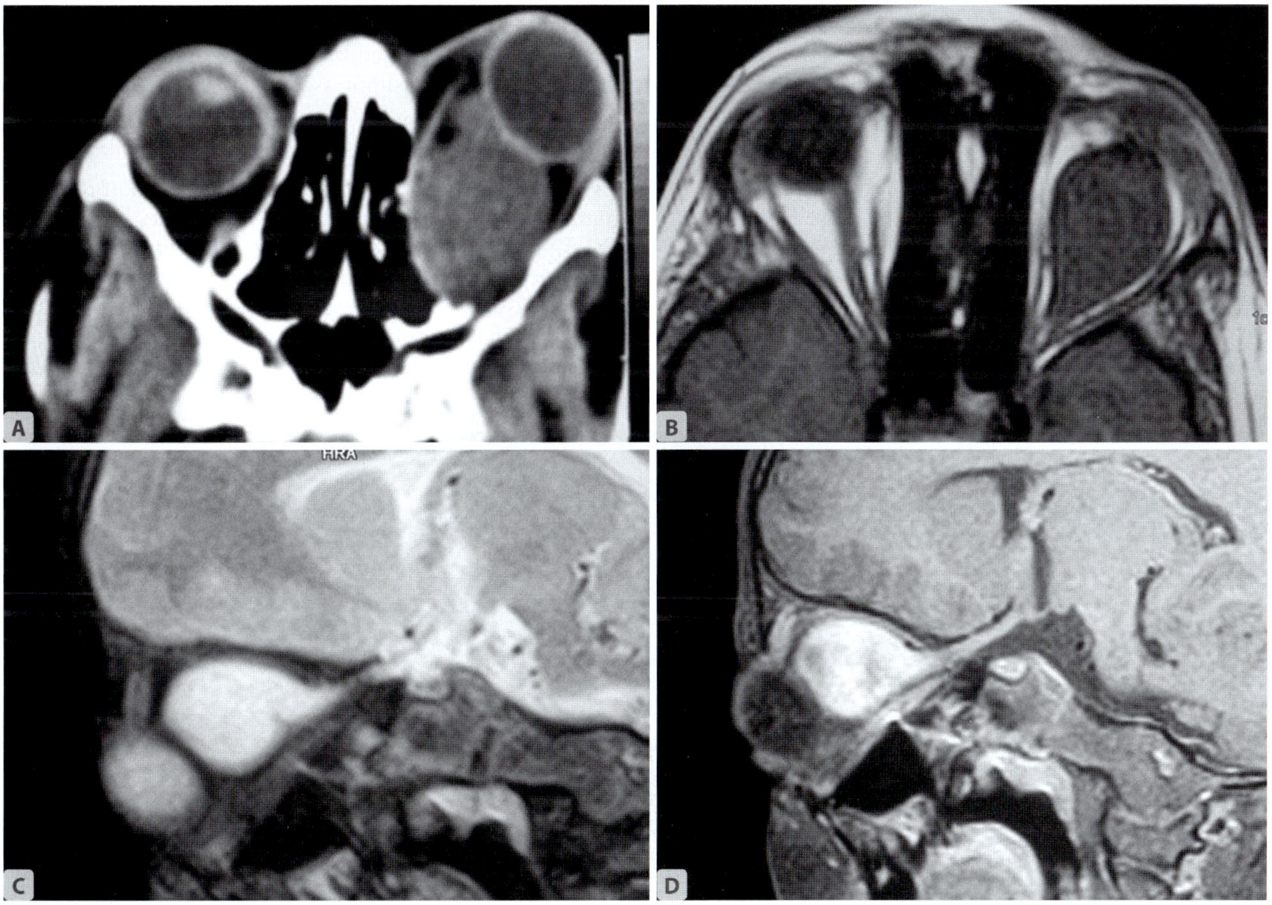

FIGS. 14A TO D: Optic nerve glioma (L). Axial CT (A) shows fusiform intraconal mass causing proptosis and bony expansion. MRI (B, Axial T1W; C, sagittal T2W; D, sagittal postcontrast) shows that the mass is not separate from optic nerve. It is hypointense on T1WI, hyperintense seen on T2WI and shows enhancement.

in about five percent cases, usually associated with NF type 2, radiotherapy or meningiomatosis.[25] These commonly cause diffuse enlargement of the optic nerve sheath complex resulting in a tubular, fusiform or saccular appearance. The difference in density between the tumor and the optic nerve results in a tram track appearance on axial imaging. On the coronal imaging this appears as a 'doughnut sign'. It sign is not specific and has also been described in optic neuritis and pseudotumor. The tumor is isointense to the optic nerve on T1- and T2-weighted images although it may be of low signal intensity on T1 and high signal intensity on T2-weighted images.[26] Fat saturated gadolinium enhanced T1W images provide best lesion demonstration. They usually exhibit marked enhancement following intravenous contrast administration **(Figs. 16A and B)**. Calcification is a common feature of the optic nerve sheath meningiomas and may appear diffuse, coarse or punctuate. The calcification may be tubular in shape along the optic nerve sheath **(Fig. 17)**.

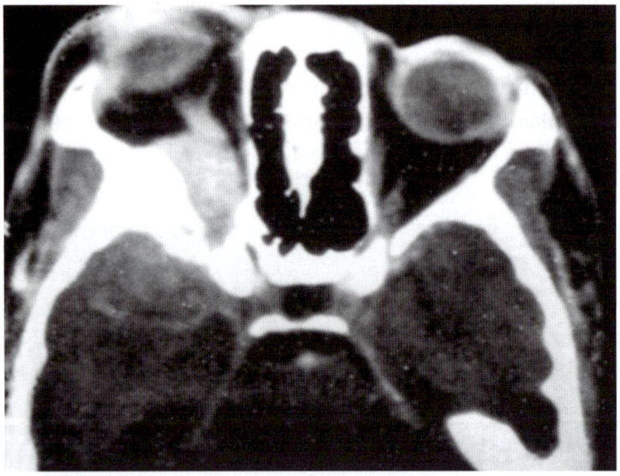

FIG. 15: Sphenoid wing meningioma right orbit. Axial CT scan showing thickening of the greater wing of sphenoid with soft tissue component in the orbit and middle cranial fossa. Right optic nerve appears pushed medially and infiltrated.

Meningioma Arising from Arachnoid Cells Rests within the Orbit

This type is very rare and does not show any characteristic features but is seen as an orbital mass located in any part of the orbit.

Rhabdomyosarcoma

Orbit is the most common location of RMS in children, with 40% of all head and neck tumors occurring here. It is the most common primary orbital malignancy of childhood. The mean age of onset is approximately 6 years. The usual clinical presentation is the rapidly progressive painless proptosis and displacement of the globe or motility disturbance. It is invariably unilateral. The tumor arises in the orbit from extraocular muscles and generally occupies both intra- and extraconal compartments. These are aggressive bone destroying and bone pushing lesions. The most common site of rhabdomyosarcoma (RMS) is considered to be superonasal quadrant of the orbit. Of the head and neck sites, the orbital RMS has a better prognosis presumably because of paucity of lymphatics and confinement by the bony orbit. CT provides information regarding the location, extent of the mass **(Fig. 18)** and presence of bone destruction if any. It is low- to intermediate signal on T1 and bright on T2W images. It exhibits significant contrast enhancement that is more prominent on the fat suppressed images.

Lymphoma

Orbital lymphomas are homogeneous masses of relatively high density and sharp margins more often seen in the anterior portion of the orbit **(Fig. 19)**, retrobulbar area, superior orbital compartment or lacrimal gland. Generally the lesions mold themselves to pre-existing structures such as globe, optic nerve and the bony orbit without eroding the bone or enlarging the orbit.

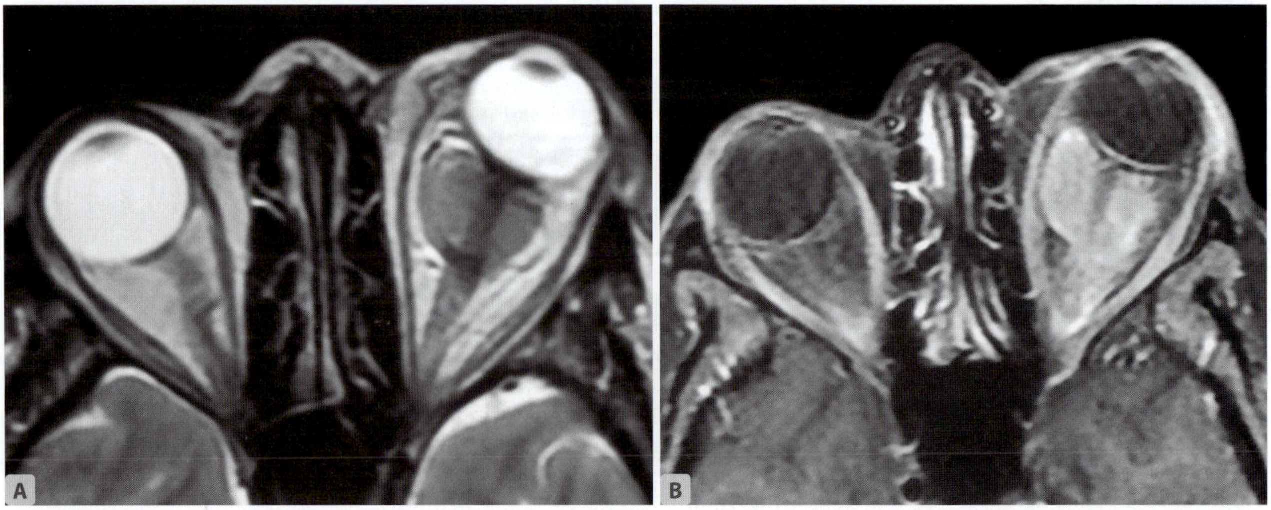

FIGS. 16A AND B: Optic nerve sheath meningioma (L). Axial MRI images that show the mass is hypointense on T2W (A) and shows bright enhancement on T1W postcontrast images (B). It is seen to be centered around the optic nerve.

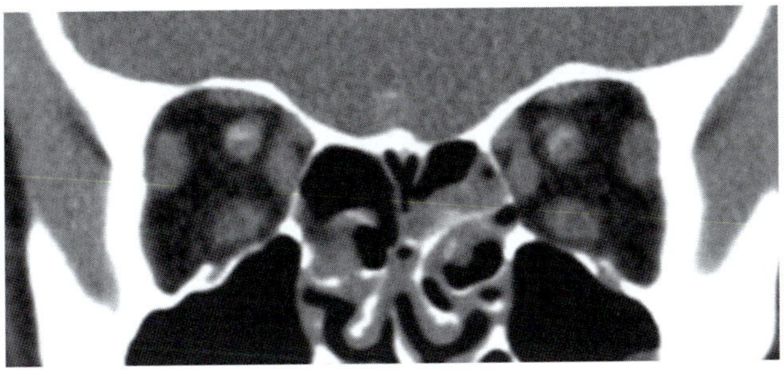

FIG. 17: Bilateral optic nerve sheath meningioma. Ring calcification (Donought sign) of the optic nerve sheaths consistent with neurofibromatosis Type 2.

Majority of orbital lymphomas will eventually have systemic disease, usually non-Hodgkin's lymphomas (NHL). However, rarely will a patient with NHL have orbital involvement during course of their illness. Presentation is usually in adults in the 6th to 7th decade. The signal characteristics are determined by cell packing. It may be low on T1 or and T2-weighted images when packing is dense, or high on T2 where packing is less dense. It shows restriction of diffusion on MRI owing to its marked cellularity. Contrast enhancement is variable. Bilateral orbital masses should raise a suspicion of lymphoma. It may have an appearance identical to that of orbital pseudotumor. Orbital lymphoma responds both to chemotherapy and radiotherapy.[26]

Schwannoma/Neurofibroma

These tend to be extraconal, share similar appearances and nerve involvement and therefore considered together. Schwannoma is more common and comprises upto 6% of orbital masses.[26] Both are benign and slow growing presenting more commonly in adults except neurofibromatosis. Most commonly affected are the sensory branches of ophthalmic division of trigeminal nerve accounting for their superior position in the orbit. Painless proptosis is the commonest presentation. Imaging depends upon the histological characteristics of the schwannomas with Antoni A tumors being more uniform than Antoni B. They are hypointense on T1 and hyperintense on T2-weighted images. Both enhance with contrast. The benign nature of these lesions lead to expansion of bony orbit and remodeling. Plexiform neurofibroma are associated with hypoplasia of the greater wing of sphenoid, and macrophthalmia in neurofibromatosis.[1] Neurofibromas may be distinguished by calcification that is rare in schwannomas.[26]

Orbital Metastases

Orbital metastases are relatively rare. Simultaneous brain metastases may occur in two-thirds, of patients with orbital metastasis. The spread to the orbit may occur by direct extension or through blood borne metastases from a distant primary. In adults, metastases occur from breast, lung, prostate, stomach, etc. In children, the primary sites include neuroblastoma, Ewing's sarcoma and leukemia. The gross morphological pattern of orbital metastatic tumors is variable. These may be infiltrative and poorly defined or may produce a well defined mass. Neuroblastoma is the most common tumor to metastasize to the orbit in infants and young children and bilateral lesions are seen in about 40% of these children.[27] The lesions often show rapid progression with bony and soft tissue components. The bony orbit may be focally or diffusely involved. Bone changes consist of permeative sclerosis, irregular spiculated appearance or irregular destruction **(Fig. 20)**.

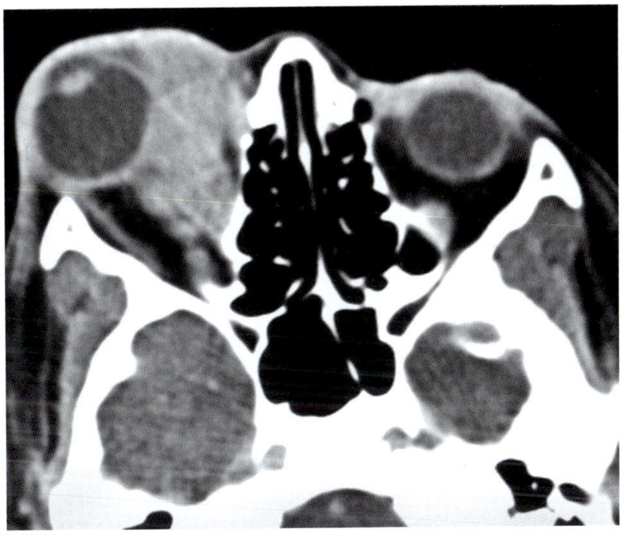

FIG. 18: Rhabdomyosarcoma. Axial CECT showing enhancing soft tissue swelling along the medial quadrant on the right. The mass has both intra- and extraconal components and is causing proptosis.

Developmental Cysts

The most frequent developmental cyst involving the orbit is the dermoid cyst. These cysts are believed to arise from ectodermal elements that get entrapped in developing sutures of the orbital bones. These are most frequently located in the superolateral quadrant of the orbit. Dermoid cysts are lined by keratinizing squamous ephithelium. They contain adnexal structures such as hair and sebaceous glands which contain keratinacious debris and fatty substance **(Fig. 21)**. Contents of dermoid cysts are oily due to presence of secretion of sebum from the sebaceous glands. The slow enlargement of dermoid cysts produces bony changes by expansion and pressure erosion, with thinning and scalloping of adjacent bones. These cysts are usually well marginated, oval, lobulated or dumb bell shaped lesions with cystic or solid components. Specific diagnosis of dermoid cyst can be made when a fat fluid level is demonstrated.

INFLAMMATORY LESIONS

Pseudotumor

Pseudotumor (idiopathic orbital inflammation) is the commonest inflammatory lesion of the orbit. It usually occurs in the middle age and is characterized by the classic triad of proptosis, pain and impaired ocular motility. Children may have constitutional symptoms leading to false diagnosis of orbital cellulitis. It is usually unilateral. Diagnosis is made after

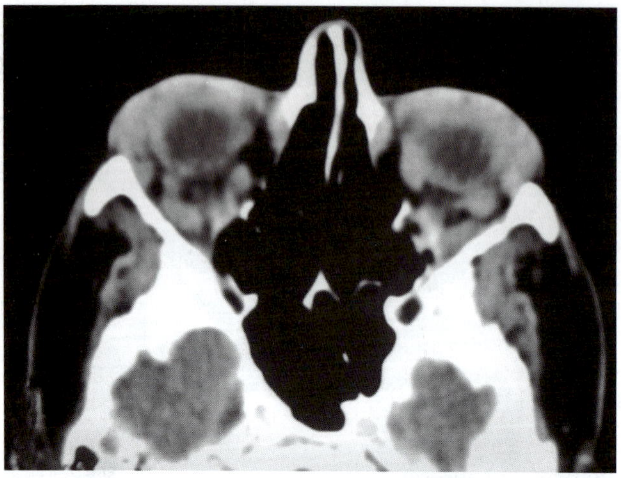

FIG. 19: Lymphoma. Axial CECT of a patient with known systemic Non-Hodgkin's lymphoma shows secondary orbital involvement in form of bilateral preseptal homogeneously enhancing soft tissue swelling.

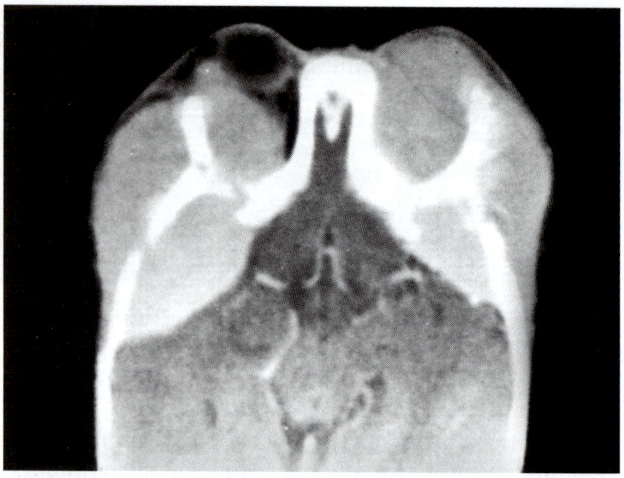

FIG. 20: Metastatic neuoroblastoma. CT shows soft tissue masses occupying both orbits extending into the middle cranial and superficial temporal fossae. The bones show destructive changes and sclerotic bony spiculation.

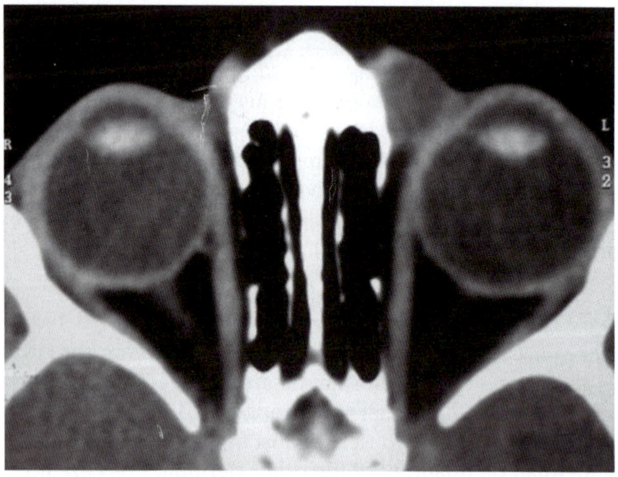

FIG. 21: Inner angular dermoid (L). Axial NCCT image shows a low density (HU-40) mass in relation to the left medial canthus.

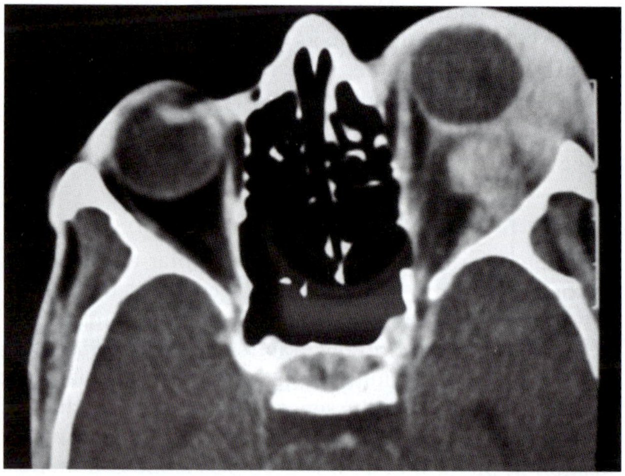

FIG. 22: Pseudotumor. Axial CECT showing a moderately enhancing ill-defined transcompartmental mass involving the left orbit, centered at the lacrimal gland extending to the retrobulbar area and preseptal soft tissues causing proptosis.

exclusion of other pathologies like Wegener's granulomatosis, sarcoid, systemic lupus erythematosus, polyarteritis nodosa, rheumatoid arthritis, lymphoproliferative disorders and metastasis. Associated disorders include fibrosing mediastinitis, retroperitoneal and hepatic fibrosis, Reidel's thyroiditis and cholangitis. Depending upon the site involved, they show varied presentation, the most common being the myositic form in which the affected muscle is enlarged and ill-defined right up to its insertion. The other presentations include lacrimal gland involvement, retrobulbar anteriorly located mass (Tenon's space), posteriorly located mass (apical involvement), focal well circumscribed mass in any part of the orbit, diffuse mass occupying whole of the orbit and multifocal masses involving various intraorbital structures or lacrimal gland **(Fig. 22)**. Sclerosing form presents in a chronic progressive form and is resistant to treatment. Imaging features on CT and MRI are nonspecific. These exhibit some contrast enhancement. It is hypointense to fat on T1 and iso- to hypointense on T2W images. This appearance may help to distinguish pseudotumor from true tumors.[28]

IgG4-related Orbital Disease

This entity is now considered distinct from the orbital pseudotumor. It commonly causes painless swelling of the lacrimal gland(s), extraocular muscles, orbital fat, infraorbital nerve, lacrimal apparatus and lids. It is a systemic condition in which the lesions rich in IgG4+ plasma cells could be present multiple other organs. On MRI the lesions are isointense on T1WI, hypointense on T2WI and enhance following gadolinium administration.[29] FDG-PET imaging is often used for systemic evaluation to locate distant or clinically silent disease.[30] Nearly half of IgG4-related orbital disease (IgG4-ROD) patients will have systemic involvement.[31] There is a well known association between bilateral IgG4-ROD and systemic disease.[32]

Endocrine Orbitopathy

Graves' ophthalmopathy usually affects middle aged women. It may precede systemic disease. It usually causes bilateral muscle enlargement, involving most commonly the inferior rectus followed by the medial rectus muscle and superior rectus complex. Isolated lateral rectus involvement is rare and prompts consideration of alternative diagnoses. There may be increase in volume of intraorbital fat. This combination of extraocular muscle enlargement and increased intraorbital fat produces proptosis. Optic nerve compression due to apical crowding is rare. Muscle belly rather than the insertion is involved **(Figs. 23A and B)**. The tendinous involvement is more suggestive of a pseudotumor. Imaging appearances can be efficiently diagnosed and monitored by with CT, especially in the coronal plane.[26]

Parasitic Cysts

Cysticercosis is the most common parasitic infestation of the orbit. Commonly cysticerci affect the muscles of the orbit resulting in muscle thickening due to inflammatory reaction. In addition, a cystic area representing the cysticercus cellulosae and a nodule representing scolex may be seen **(Fig. 24)**. Muscle thickening due to cysticercus may be confused with a pseudotumor or vice versa.

VASCULAR LESIONS

Caroticocavernous Fistula

The fistulous communication occurs between the carotid siphon and cavernous sinus (direct), or between meningeal branches of internal or external carotid artery and dural veins (indirect) in the vicinity of the carvernous sinus producing congestion of the orbit and globe, pulsatile exophthalmos, bruit and eventually glaucoma and visual loss. It may occur secondary to trauma or spontaneously. Pulsating exophthalmos is the most frequent presenting symptom. CT and MRI depict signs of orbital venous hypertension with an enlarged superior ophthalmic vein and extraocular muscles **(Fig. 25A)**. MRI shows a signal void and in the cavernous sinus superior ophthalmic vein due to arterial flow. The cavernous sinus is enlarged. Digital subtraction arteriography not only demonstrates the fistulous communication **(Fig. 25B)**, but also allows interventional neuroradiological procedures using detachable balloon and/or coil embolization to occlude the site of fistula.

Orbital Varices

True orbital varices are congenital venous malformations in which the afferent and efferent vessels are veins. Most common clinical feature of congenital orbital varices is intermittent proptosis that increases on leaning forward, coughing or straining. US shows dilated intraorbital veins usually with slow flow. On CT and MRI, the varix is seen as a lobulated soft tissue mass that usually tapers towards

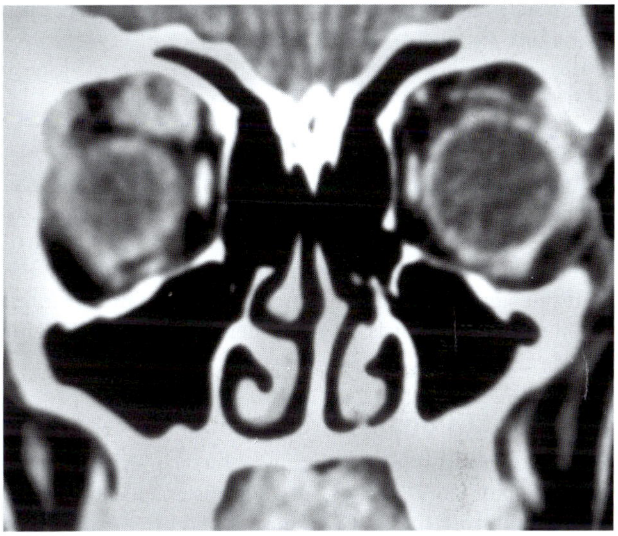

FIG. 24: Orbital myocysticercus. Coronal CT showing a cyst with a scolex and thickened superior rectus muscle in the right orbit.

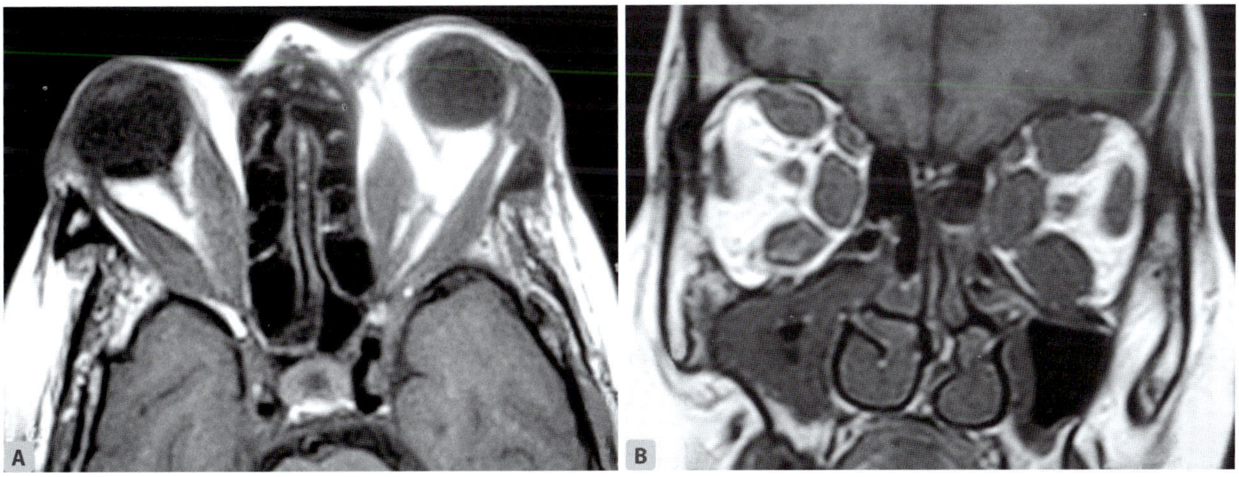

FIGS. 23A AND B: Endocrine exophthalmos. Axial (A) and coronal (B) T1W MR images show thickening of the bellies of extraocular muscle of both orbits, sparing the tendinous insertions.

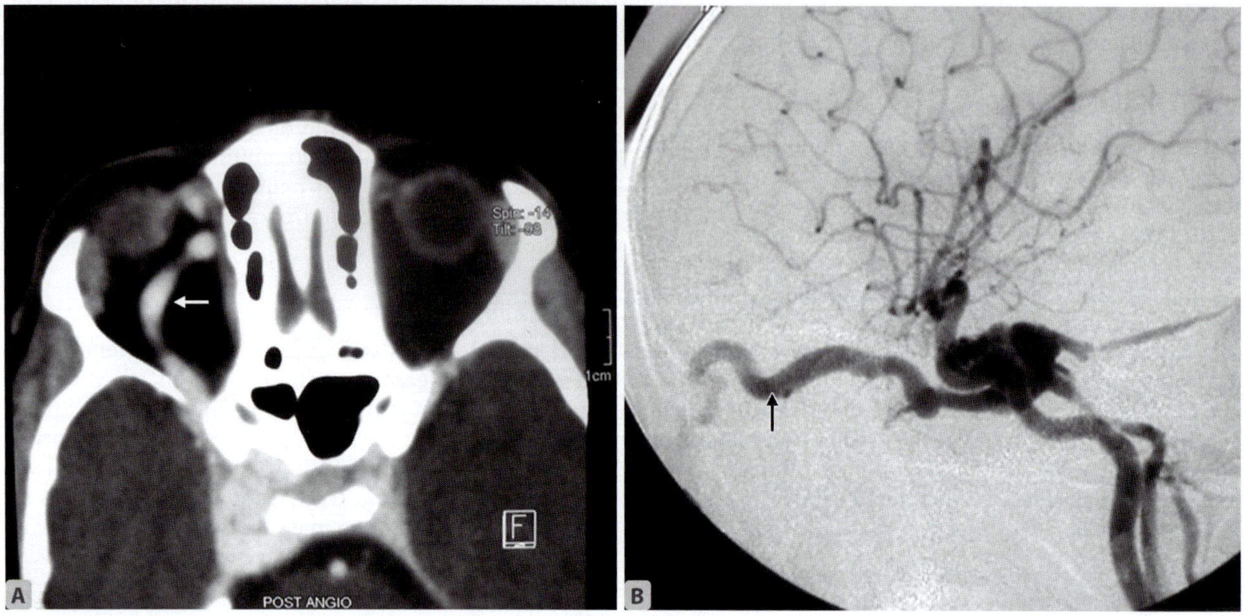

FIGS. 25A AND B: Traumatic caroticocavernous fistula. CECT (A) and right internal carotid angiogram (B) shows dilated superior ophthalmic vein (white arrow) and prominent right cavernous sinus on CT. Angiogram shows direct communication between the internal carotid artery and cavernous sinus with retrograde filling of dilated superior ophthalmic vein (black arrow).

the apex and increases in size during Vasalva maneuver. Calcified phleboliths may be seen in some patients **(Fig. 26)**. MRI depicts the varix as a signal void if associated with rapidly flowing blood. Spontaneous thrombosis is common and the signal intensity depends on the age of thrombus. Orbital phlebography is now considered redundant to define the varices.

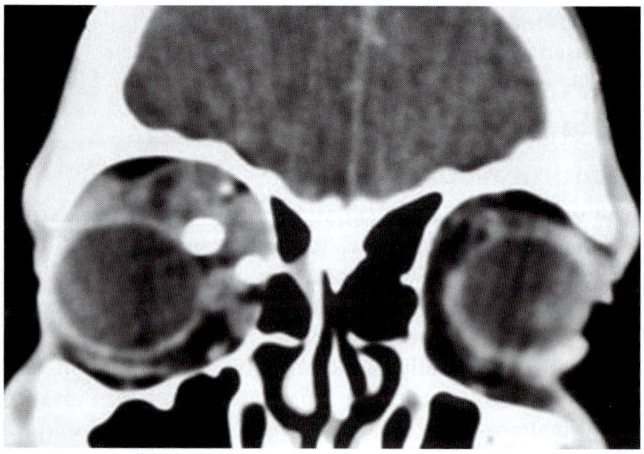

FIG. 26: Orbital varices. Coronal CT image shows tortuous vascular channels with phleboliths superomedial to the right globe.

Osseous Lesions

Bones of the orbit may be involved by dysplasias, primary or metastatic bone tumors, etc. Fibrous dysplasia typically presents during the first two decades of life. It represents both arrested and altered maturation of bone. Alterations in the bone maturation result in replacement of normal bone with immature bone and fibrous stroma. The bone is markedly expanded, encroaches upon and distorts the adjacent structures, e.g. orbits and paranasal sinuses. Lesions of fibrous dysplasia are generally diffusely sclerotic, having a ground glass appearance but may be heterogeneous. Most patients with orbital fibrous dysplasia present with unilateral proptosis. Plain radiography shows characteristic expanded, sclerotic bone often with ground glass appearance. CT better demonstrates these features and exact extent of the lesion **(Figs. 27A and B)**.

Trauma

The orbit may be injured directly or indirectly, both with blunt or penetrating trauma. Injury to the globe may occur as an isolated event. Soft tissue swelling often obscures direct clinical evaluation of the globe. Plain film evaluation of the orbit remains the initial imaging modality; however the lack of soft tissue detail limits its utility for treatment planning. CT is the method of choice in diagnosing traumatic lesions involving the orbit. It shows both bony and soft tissue details, and more clearly defines the location and orientation of displaced bony fragments, foreign bodies and air. A commonly encountered intraorbital fracture, the so called blow out fracture **(Fig. 28)**, occurs when direct

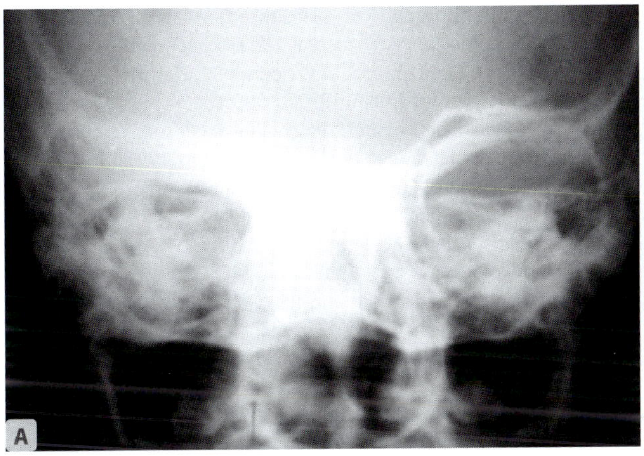

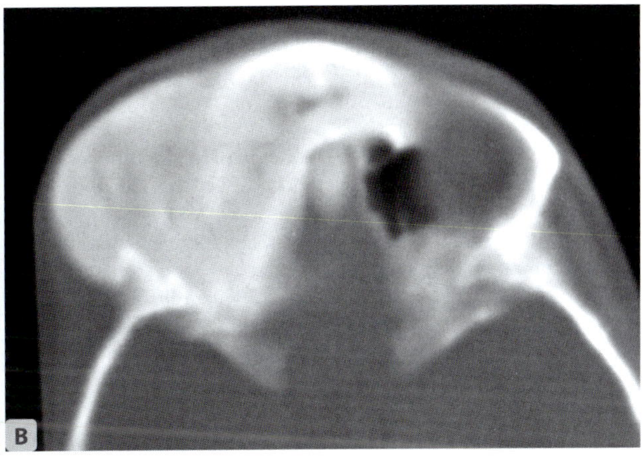

FIGS. 27A AND B: Fibrous dysplasia. (A) Frontal orbital radiograph showing sclerosis of the right orbital and frontonasal region; (B) Axial CT (bone window) shows ground glass haze of the involved bones.

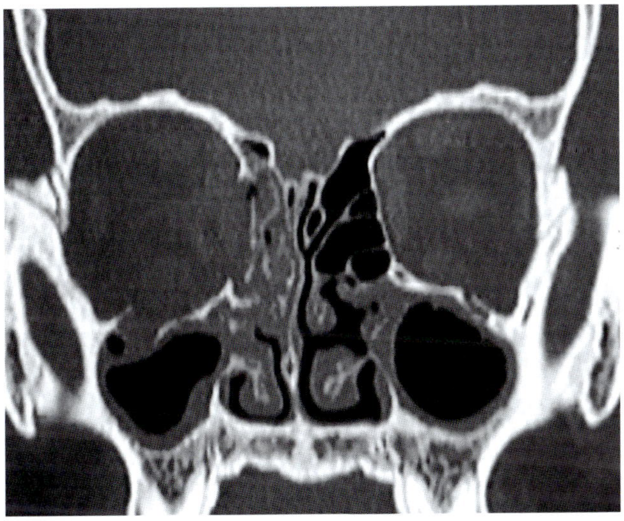

FIG. 28: Blow out fracture. Coronal CT image (bone window) shows fracture of the medial wall and floor of the right orbit. There was no extraocular muscle entrapment on the soft tissue window (not shown).

blunt force is applied to the globe and orbit with disruption of the orbital wall. The floor or medial walls are most often fractured with the orbital rim remaining intact. In patients with optic nerve injury following trauma, thin sections of CT may delineate the injured nerve, apical bony fragments and adjacent hematoma for crucial preoperative assessment. MRI may be complementary to CT scanning in certain patients particularly with injuries involving the globe or optic nerve.[33]

A variety of other injuries occur involving globe, ranging from rupture, dislocation of lens, and vitreous/retrohyloid/ or retro-ocular hematoma. CT provides exact localization of metallic foreign bodies without risk of their dislocation. MRI is contraindicated in the presence of a metallic foreign body but may be useful in detection and localization of a nonmetallic foreign body.[34] Retained foreign bodies may lead to granuloma or abscess formation.

REFERENCES

1. Schlotmann K, Koelwel BF, Hackenberg MD, Gabel VP, Scholmerich J. High frequency contrast harmonic imaging of ophthalmic tumor perfusion. Am J Radiol. 2005;184:574-78.
2. Hosten N, Bornfeld N (Eds). Imaging of the globe and orbit: A guide to differential diagnosis. New York: Thieme Stuttgart, 1998.
3. Mafee MF, Putterman A, Valvassori GE, Campos M, Capek V. Orbital space occupying lesions: Role of computed tomography and magnetic resonance imaging. RCNA. 1987;25:520-59.
4. Muller-Forell WS, Pitz S. Orbital Pathology. In: Muller-Forell WS (Ed). Imaging of orbital and visual pathway pathology. Heidelberg. 2002. pp. 147-340.
5. Zimmerman RA, Bilaniuk LT. Computed tomography in the evaluation of patients with bilateral retinoblastomas. J Comput Tomogr. 1979;3:251-57.
6. Haik BG, Saint Louis L, Smith ME, Ellsworth RM, Abramson OH, Cahill P, Deck M, Coleman J. Magnetic resonance imaging in evaluation of leucokoria. Ophthalmology. 1985;92:1143-52.
7. Vashisht S, Goulatia RK, Dayal Y, Bhargava S. Retinoblastoma: A CT study. IJRI 1986;40:17-21.
8. Char DH, Hedges TR, Norman D. Retinoblastoma. Ophthalmology. 1984;91:1347-59.
9. de Graaf P, Pouwels PJ, Rodjan F, Moll AC, Imhof SM, Knol DL, Sanchez E, van der Valk P, Castelijns JA. Single-shot turbo spin-echo diffusion weighted imaging for retinoblastoma: initial experience. Am J Neuroradiol. 2012;33(1):110-8.
10. Hiwatashi A1, Togao O1, Yamashita K1, Kikuchi K1, Yoshikawa H2, Obara M3, Honda H1. Br J Radiol. 2016;89(1067):20160074. Epub 2016 Sep 16.
11. Mafee MF. The eye. In: Som PM, Curtin HD (Eds). Head and Neck imaging (4th edn.) St. Louis: Mosby. 2003;2:441-527.
12. De Potter P, Shields CL, Shields JA, Flanders AE. The role of magnetic resonance imaging in children with intraocular tumors simulating lesions. Ophthalmology. 1996;103:1774-83.

13. De Potter P, Shields JA, Shields CL, Flanders AE. The role of MRI in children with intra-ocular tumors and simulating lesions. Ophthalmology. 1996;103:1774-83.
14. De Potter P, Shields JA, Shields CL. MRI of the eye and orbit. Philadelphia: Lippincott, 1995.
15. Damato BE, Paul J, Foulds WS. Risk factors of residual and recurrent uveal melanoma after transscleral local resection. Br J Ophthalmol. 1996;80:102-08.
16. Glatt HJ, Custer PL, Barrett L, Sator K. Magnetic resonance imaging and computed tomography in a model of wooden foreign bodies in the orbit. Ophthalm Plast Reconstr. 1990;6:108-14.
17. Kumar A, Verma L, Jha SN, Tiwari HK, Khosla PK. Ultrasonic evaluation of intraocular cysticercosis. Afro-Asian Jour of Ophthalmology. 1989;55:55-6.
18. Ruchman MC, Stefanyszn MA, Flangagan JC, et al. Orbital tumors. In: Gonzalez CA, Becker MH, Flanagan JC (Eds). Diagnostic Imaging in Ophthalmology, New York: Springer – Verlag. 1986. pp. 201-38.
19. Bilaniuk LT. Orbital vascular lesions—role of imaging. Radiol Clin North Am Imaging Ophthal II; 1999;169-83.
20. Barnacle AM, Theodorou M, Maling SJ, Abou-Rayyah Y. Sclerotherapy treatment of orbital lymphatic malformations: a large single-centre experience. Br J Ophthalmol. 2016;100(2):204-8. doi: 10.1136/bjophthalmol-2015-306657. Epub 2015 Jun 17.
21. Patel KC, Kalantzis G, El-Hindy N, Chang BY. Sclerotherapy for orbital lymphangioma—case series and literature review. In Vivo. 2017;31(2):263-6.
22. Bternn J, Jacobiec FA, Housepian EM. The architecture of optic nerve gliomas with and without neurofibromatosis. Arch Ophth. 1980;98:505-11.
23. National Institutes of Health Consensus development. neurofibromatosis. Arch Neural. 1988;45:545-78.
24. Hollander MD, Fitzpatrick M, O'Connor SG, Flanders AE, Tartaglino LM. Optic gliomas. RCNA. 1999;37:59-71.
25. Hodes JE, Sanders M, Patel P, Patchell RA. Radiosurgical management of meningiomas. Stereotact Funct Neurosurg. 1996;6:15-18.
26. Aviv RI, Miszkiel K. Orbital Imaging – Part 2. Intraorbital pathology. Clin Radiol 2005;60:288-307.
27. Rootman J, Chan KW. Neuroblastoma: In rooman J (Ed). New York: JB Lippincott. Diseases of the Orbit. 1988;25.
28. Mombaerts I, Schlingermann RO, Goldschmeding R, Koorneef L. Are systemic corticosteroids useful in the management of orbital pseudotumors? Ophthalmology. 1996;103:521-8.
29. Toyoda K, Oba H, Kutomi K et al. MR imaging of IgG4-related disease in the head and neck and brain. Am J Neuroradiol. 2012;33(11):2136-9.
30. Masaki Y, Kurose N, Umehara H. IgG4-related disease: a novel lymphoproliferative disorder discovered and established in Japan in the 21st century. J Clin Exp Hematop. 2011;51:13-20.
31. McNab A, McKelvie P. IgG4-related ophthalmic disease. Part II: Clinical Aspects. Ophthal Plast Reconstr Surg. 2015;31(3):167-78.
32. Wu A, Andrew NH, McNab AA, Selva D. Bilateral IgG4-related ophthalmic disease: a strong indication for systemic imaging. Br J Ophthalmol. 2016;100:1409-11.
33. Rothman M. Orbital trauma. Seminars in US, CT and MRI 1997;18:437-97.
34. Wilson WB, Dreisbach JN, Lattin DE, Stears JC. Magnetic resonance imaging of non metallic foreign bodies. Am J Ophthal. 1988;105: 612-7.

CHAPTER

202

Imaging of the Paranasal Sinuses

Vivek Gupta, Niranjan Khandelwal

INTRODUCTION

Nose and paranasal sinuses (PNS) are affected by a wide variety of diseases and to diagnose them understanding of the anatomy and physiology of this region is necessary. PNS have been described in ancient text by many people like description of maxillary sinuses by Leonardo da Vinci and of ethmoid air cells by Galen. Later, X-rays remained the mainstay in diagnosing the diseases of the sinuses for many years. Presently the technology has evolved to a point where a virtual tour of the sinuses can be taken to see normal structures and abnormalities. The present chapter deals with all aspects of PNS, from embryology, to development and normal variations followed by infections, inflammations, benign and malignant conditions.

PARANASAL SINUS EMBRYOLOGY

Paranasal sinuses start developing from the primitive choana. At 25–28 weeks of gestation, three projections arise from the lateral wall of the nose and serve as the beginning of the development of PNS. The anterior projection forms the agger nasi. The inferior (maxilloturbinate) projection forms the inferior turbinate and maxillary sinus. The superior projection (ethmoidoturbinate) forms the ethmoidal air cells and their corresponding drainage channels. The middle meatus invaginates laterally to form the embryonic infundibulum and uncinate process and the embryonic infundibulum grows superiorly to form the frontal recess area. The frontal sinus may develop as a direct continuation of embryonic infundibulum and frontal recess superiorly during the 16th week. It can also develop by upward migration of anterior ethmoidal air cells to penetrate the inferior aspect of the frontal bone between its outer and inner tables. The maxillary sinuses are the first to be seen on plain X-rays and are usually aerated at birth. They increase in size till the age of 14 years. The ethmoid sinuses are also aerated at birth but are rarely visible on plain X-rays. They rapidly expand till the age of 4 years with a spurt of growth during adolescence. The ethmoid sinuses are thus a site of infection in childhood sinusitis. The pneumatization of the sphenoid sinus begins by age 2 years. Its growth is slower than other PNS. Pneumatization of frontal sinuses occurs last and is not visualized before 6 years. They grow to adult size by 12–14 years. The osteomeatal complexes (OMCs) are fully developed at birth. The development of sinuses is influenced by dentition.

IMAGING MODALITIES AND TECHNIQUE OF EVALUATION

Conventional Radiography

Standard radiography of the PNS usually consists of four views: (i) Lateral view, (ii) Caldwell view, (iii) Water's view, and (iv) Submentovertex (SMV) or base view. The lateral view demonstrates the frontal, maxillary and sphenoid sinuses. The Caldwell view shows the frontal sinuses and posterior ethmoid air cells. The Water's view shows the maxillary sinuses, anterior ethmoid air cells, inferior orbital rims and orbital floors. The submentovertex view evaluates the sphenoid sinus as well as the anterior and posterior walls of the frontal sinuses.

The findings which are suggestive of bacterial sinusitis on the X-rays are mucoperiosteal thickening, air-fluid level and complete opacification of the sinus **(Fig. 1)**. The X-rays thus have been used based upon above findings as a screening tool for sinusitis. However, there are many studies which question the sensitivity of plain X-rays.[1-3] One such study compared three views (Caldwell, lateral and Water's) with CT scans of the PNS (3 × 3 mm coronal sections). They found that sensitivity was 57–62% and specificity 88% when the X-rays were interpreted by radiologists and were 48–67% and 75–100%, respectively when interpreted by emergency medicine staff members. The wide variation in sensitivity and specificity and interobserver variations makes X-ray evaluation a poor modality even as a screening tool.[4]

Computed Tomography

Computed tomography (CT) is the modality of choice in the evaluation of the PNS and adjacent structures.

Present generation of CT scanners have obviated the need to scan twice in axial and coronal plan. Now, volumetric axial

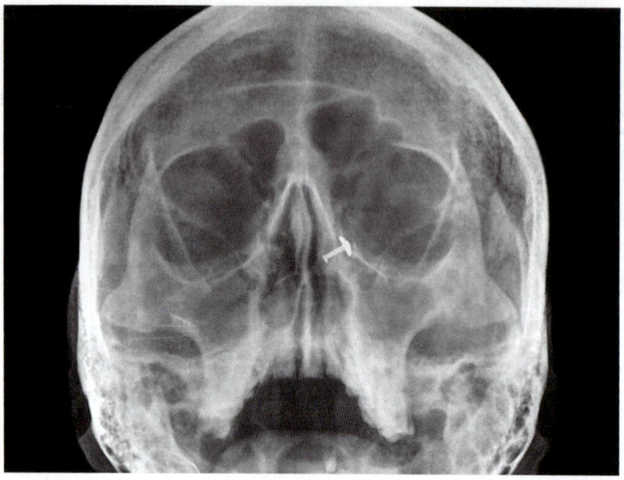

FIG. 1: Plain X-ray (Water's view) showing complete opacification of the bilateral maxillary sinuses.

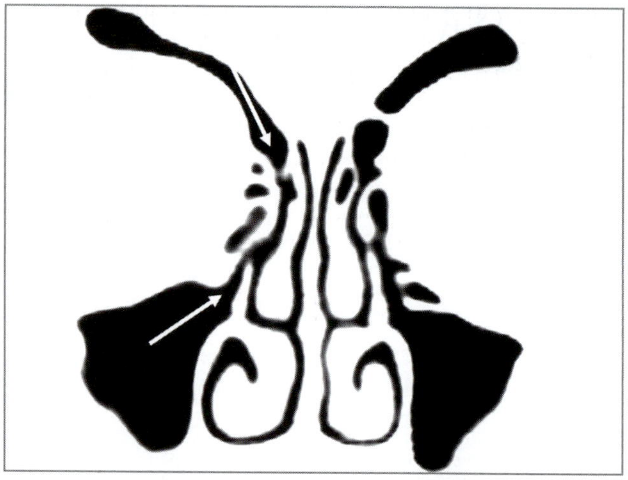

FIG. 2: Paranasal sinuses seen in lung window with clear depiction of osteomeatal complex (OMC) and frontal recess (arrow).

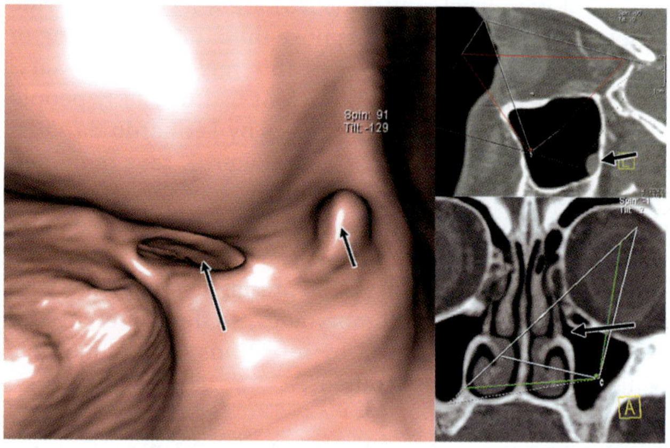

FIG. 3: Virtual sinoscopic image obtained on a 16-slice scanner showing maxillary ostium and infundibulum (long arrows) and a small maxillary polyp (short arrows) on VR, sagittal and coronal images.

scans of the PNS can be one in matter of few seconds and can then be reconstructed automatically into coronal and sagittal orientations. Also, both bone and soft tissue images are reconstructed by the systems.

Positions (if multislice CT is available and thin reconstruction can be done and direct scanning in coronal plane may not be done).

The anatomy is best evaluated in the bone window. The osteomeatal complex may further be studied in lung window **(Fig. 2)** to see for patency of the OM complex and other draining pathways. Since the coronal images closely resemble the view of endoscopy which is frequently employed for diagnosis and treatment. These images are preferred more over axial images. Now, with the advent of contiguous data acquisition, it has become possible to see the sinus anatomy in coronal plane in 3D.[5]

With the improvement in post-processing software and isotropic voxel image acquisition, it is now possible to obtain virtual endoscopic images of the sinus on CT **(Fig. 3)**. In a study exploring this aspect, virtual sinoscopy was done in patients and compared with preoperative fiberoptic endoscopy and intraoperative findings. Significant correlation was found between the findings on virtual sinoscopy, preoperative endoscopy and intraoperative findings.[6]

Sagittal reconstruction adds to the information, especially drainage pathway of sphenoid sinus and posterior ethmoid sinuses and the spread of pathology through them.

Contrast enhancement is not routinely done in the evaluation of sinus pathologies like sinusitis or polyposis. However, it is used if differentiation between inflammation and neoplasms is to be done and if intracranial spread is suspected.

MAGNETIC RESONANCE IMAGING

Magnetic resonance imaging (MRI) has not gained much importance when it comes to routine evaluation of sinonasal diseases, especially sinusitis. There are many reasons for that, bony outlines are not well visualized, sinuses filled with chronic inspissated secretions appear as normally aerated sinuses and also fungal sinusitis in a sinus may give normal signal void like of air on MRI. However, in spite of above mentioned reasons there are certain indications or role of MRI in the sinonasal diseases. MRI has a very important role in evaluating spread of pathology into brain and orbits. Due to its superior soft tissue resolution it can detect even minimal extension into these areas. Also, it is able to differentiate reliably between mucosal hypertrophy, chronic retained secretions and mucoceles.

Postcontrast MRI images are also helpful in differentiating tumors from inflammations. Inflammations enhance peripherally and the tumors show central enhancement.

In a recent randomized study, CT and MRI were compared. They found that Lund–Mackay staging of sinus disease by MRI is closely correlated to corresponding staging based on CT. MRI does not significantly overstage or overclassify patients with sinus disease.[7]

MRI is also particularly suited for the evaluation of the skull base and posterior fossa as these areas are inadequately imaged by CT due to beam hardening artifacts.[8-10]

Routine MRI studies include both coronal and axial images. Sagittal scans are also obtained to image the pathology in planes which are nearly parallel to the axial planes, e.g. palate, orbital floor and skull base. Routine sequences include proton density images (PDI), T1WI and T2WI. Fat suppressed enhanced T1 WI should be routinely employed for evaluation of complicated sinusitis or for suspected neoplastic disease especially when there is orbital or skull base extension or involvement.[11]

NORMAL ANATOMY AND ANATOMIC VARIATIONS[12-14]

Normal Anatomy

Description of the anatomy of this region involves nasal structures, PNS and their draining pathways. In these three areas the delineation of the drainage pathways is most important as their patency or blockage holds the key for treatment.

Nasal Structures

The nasal septum is a midline structure composed of both bone and cartilaginous tissue. Its deviation can cause partial obstruction in the nasal cavities unilaterally or on both sides depending on its shape. The lateral nasal wall has three projections: (i) superior, (ii) middle and (iii) inferior turbinates. These structures divide the nasal cavity into three air passages: (i) superior, (ii) middle, and (iii) inferior meatus.

The inferior turbinate is the lower most projections arising from the lateral nasal bone and extending into the nasal cavity and running posteriorly toward the nasopharynx. These turbinates are frequently enlarged in deviated nasal septum or allergic rhinitis.

The nasolacrimal duct (NLD) is a small tubular structure which runs along the lateral nasal wall and opens into the inferior meatus underneath the inferior turbinate. The NLD runs within a bony canal formed by the maxilla, lacrimal apparatus and inferior turbinate bones.

The middle turbinate lies above the inferior turbinates. Anterosuperiorly, the middle turbinate attaches to the skull base just lateral to the cribriform plate. In its middle third it turns coronally and laterally to insert on the lamina papyracea and posteriorly to the roof of ethmoidal complex. The basal lamella is the portion of the middle turbinate where it attaches to the ethmoid complex and divides it into anterior and middle sinus complex **(Figs. 4 and 5)**.

Draining Pathways

Anterior Draining Pathways

The OMC is the term given to anterior draining pathways and consists of air passages between the frontal, anterior ethmoid and maxillary sinuses.

The components of the OMC include the frontal recess, ethmoid infundibulum, hiatus semilunaris and middle meatus. The frontal sinus, drain via *frontal recess* which is hourglass shaped structure. The frontal recess affords mucociliary drainage of the frontal and anterior ethmoidal sinuses into the middle meatus.

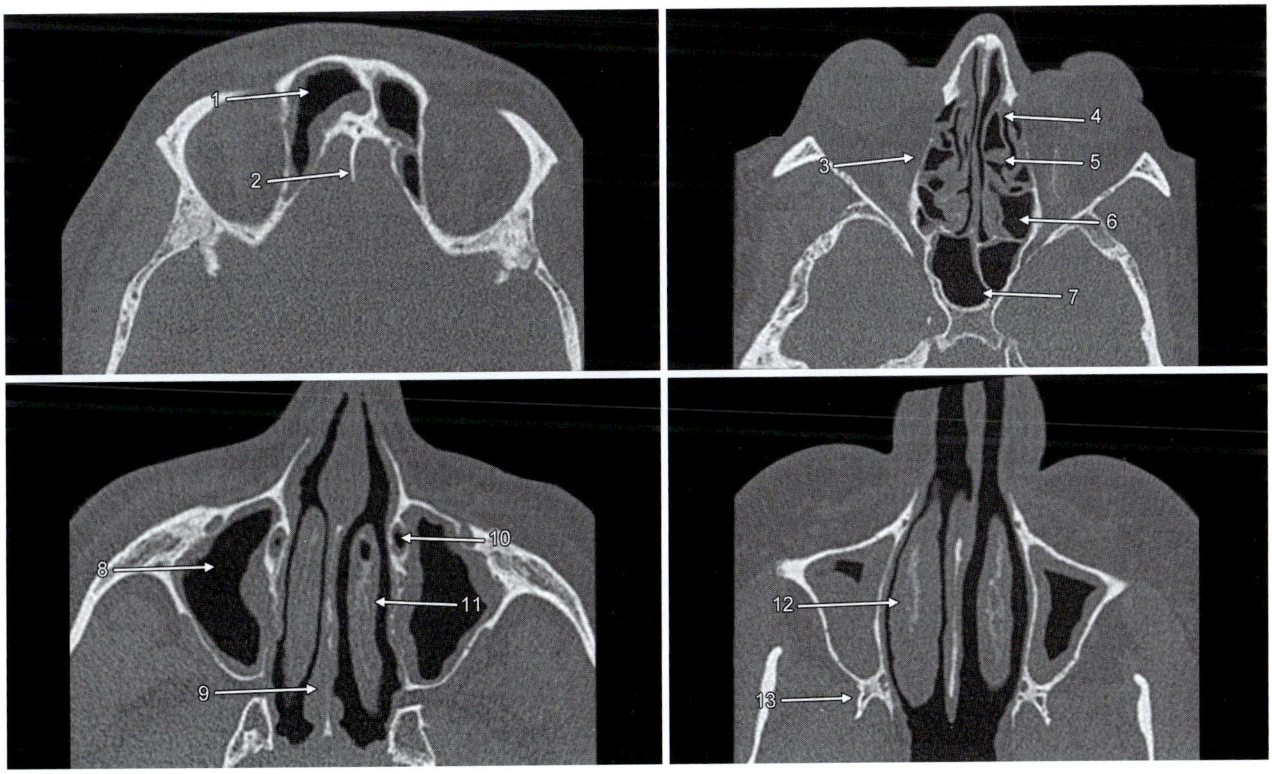

FIG. 4: Axial anatomy. (1) Frontal sinus; (2) Crista galli; (3) Lamina papyracea; (4) Ant ethmoid cells; (5) Middle ethmoid cells; (6) Post- ethmoid cells; (7) Sphenoid sinus; (8) Maxillary sinus; (9) Nasal septum; (10) Nasolacrimal duct; (11) Inferior turbinate; (12) Middle turbinate; (13) Pterygoid plates.

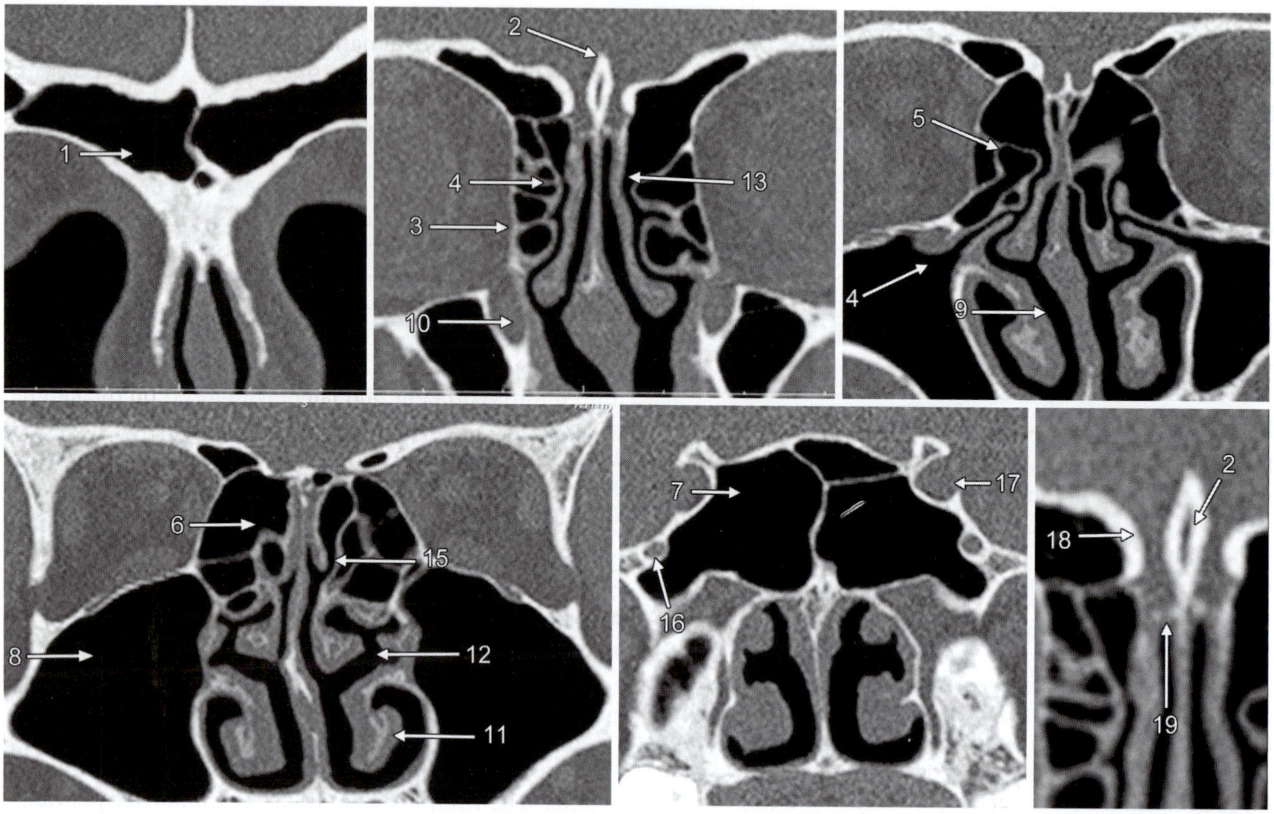

FIG. 5: Coronal anatomy. (1) Frontal sinus; (2) Crista galli; (3) Lamina Papyracea; (4) Anterior ethmoid cells; (5) Middle ethmoid cells; (6) Postethmoid cells; (7) Sphenoid sinus; (8) Maxillary sinus; (9) Nasal septum; (10) Nasolacrimal duct; (11) Inferior turbinate; (12) Middle turbinate; (13) Frontal recess; (14) Infundibulum; (15) Superior turbinate; (16) Optic nerve; (17) Internal carotid artery; (18) Fovea ethmoidalis; (19) Lamina Cribrosa.

The middle meatus is an air space lateral to the middle turbinate and medial to the uncinate process and *ethmoid bulla* (they are largest aerated cells of the anterior ethmoidal complex). The *uncinate process* is a superior extension of the medial maxillary sinus wall. Anteriorly, the uncinate process fuses with the *agger nasi cells* (term given to the most anterior cells in the anterior ethmoidal sinus complex) and the posterior wall of the nasolacrimal duct. Superiorly the uncinate process has a free edge that is separated from the ethmoid bulla by a crevice termed the *hiatus semilunaris.* This hiatus communicates with *ethmoidal infundibulum* which is a short channel starting from the maxillary ostium and leading into middle meatus and is bordered laterally by lamina papyracea and medially by uncinate process **(Figs. 6 and 7)**.

The inferior meatus contains the opening of the drainage channel of the NLD.

Posterior Draining Pathways

It consists of draining pathway of sphenoid and posterior ethmoidal sinuses. The sphenoid sinus drains via an ostium located in its anterosuperior wall. It leads into *sphenoethmoidal recess* which drains the sphenoid sinus along with posterior ethmoidal complex into the superior meatus. This recess lies between anterior sphenoid sinus wall and posterior wall of ethmoid sinus air cells **(Figs. 8A and B)**.

Most of the above-mentioned structures are adequately visualized in coronal plane except for the sphenoethmoidal recess which is seen in sagittal or axial planes.

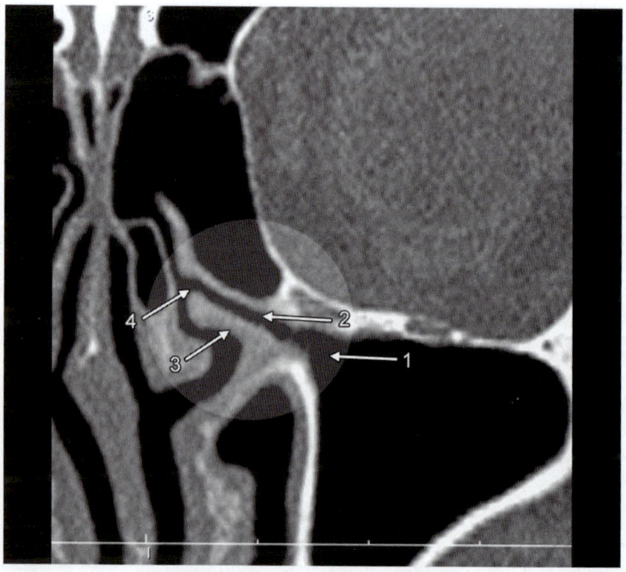

FIG. 6: Osteomeatal complex. (1) Maxillary osteum; (2) Infundibulum; (3) Uncinate process; (4) Hiatus semilunaris.

Anatomic Variations

Certain anatomic variations are common and important. They are frequently associated with chronic inflammatory disease. These variants can obstruct the air passages and thus can give rise to recurrent sinus infections. The most common variations are described in brief.

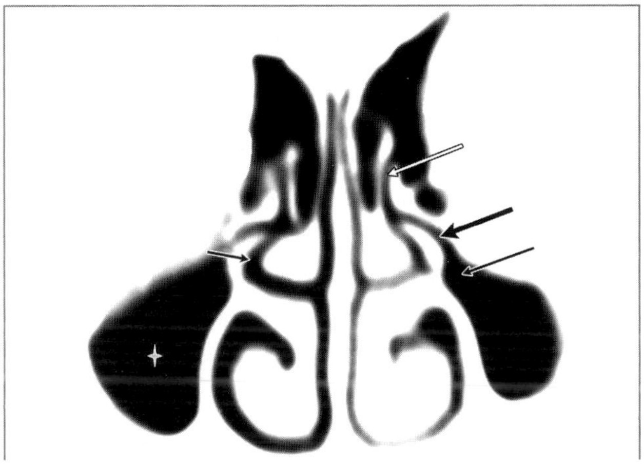

FIG. 7: Coronal section showing anterior draining pathway including frontal recess (white arrow), maxillary ostium (thin black arrow), infundibulum (thick black arrow), middle meatus (short black arrow) and maxillary sinus (star).

Concha Bullosa

This is an aerated middle turbinate. It enlarges to obstruct the middle meatus or even the infundibulum **(Fig. 9)**. It may be unilateral or bilateral. Since the concha is lined with the same mucosa as the rest of the nasal cavity, these cells can suffer the same inflammatory disorders experienced in the PNS. The other normal structures which can be pneumatized are the anterior clinoid processes in conjunction with an extensively pneumatized sphenoid sinus. The crista galli can be pneumatized and may predispose to formation of a mucocele.

Nasal Septum Deviation

It can be asymmetric. The curved septum may compress the middle turbinate laterally and thus narrow the middle meatus. Bony spurs associated with septal deviation may obstruct the OMC.

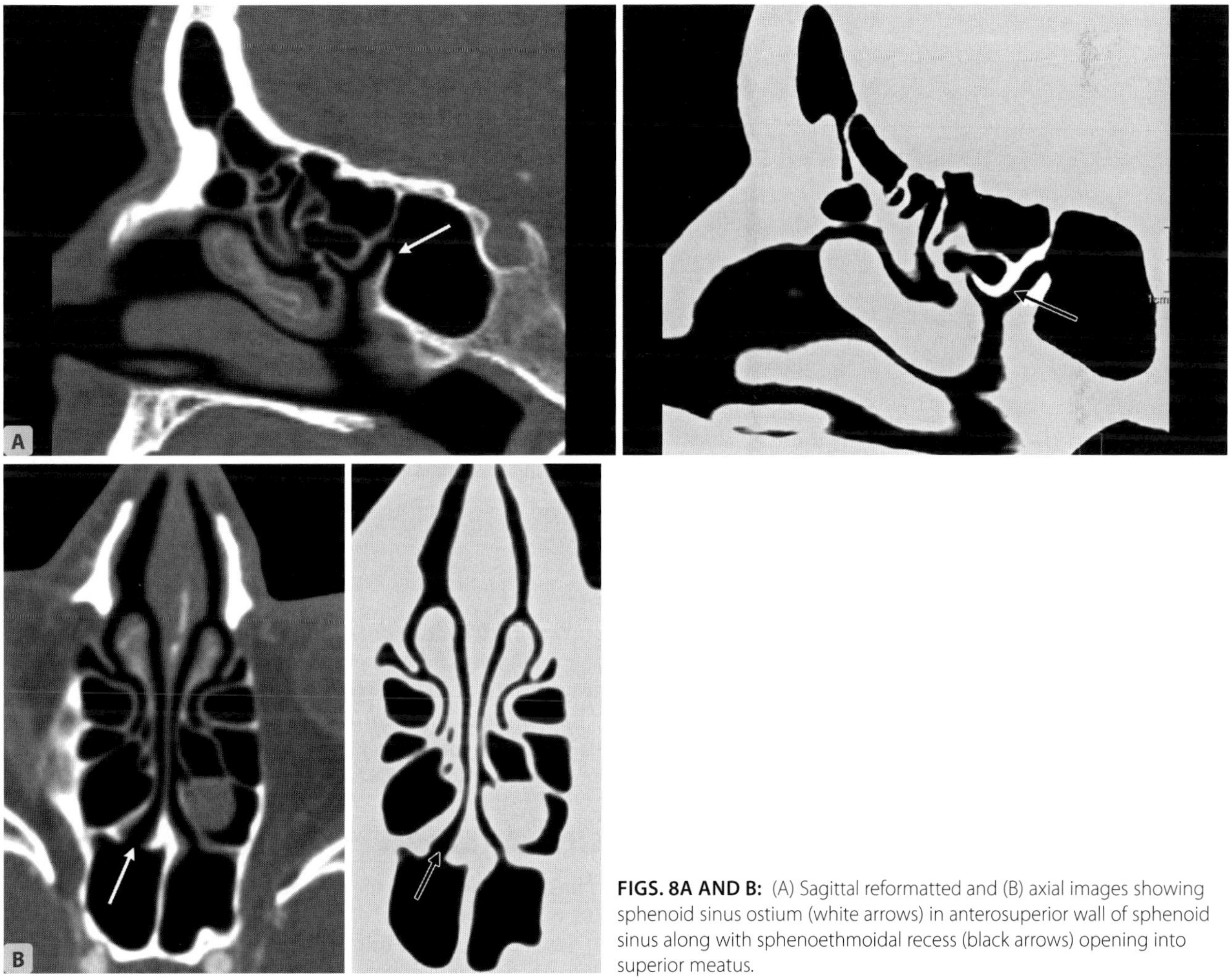

FIGS. 8A AND B: (A) Sagittal reformatted and (B) axial images showing sphenoid sinus ostium (white arrows) in anterosuperior wall of sphenoid sinus along with sphenoethmoidal recess (black arrows) opening into superior meatus.

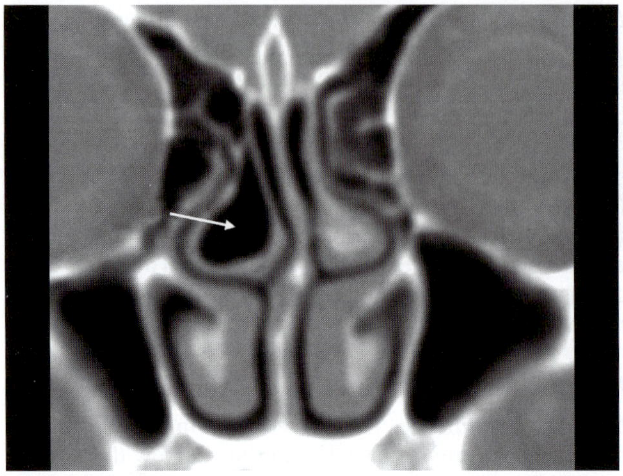

FIG. 9: Concha bullosa (arrow) causing partial obstruction of the middle meatus. Note left DNS.

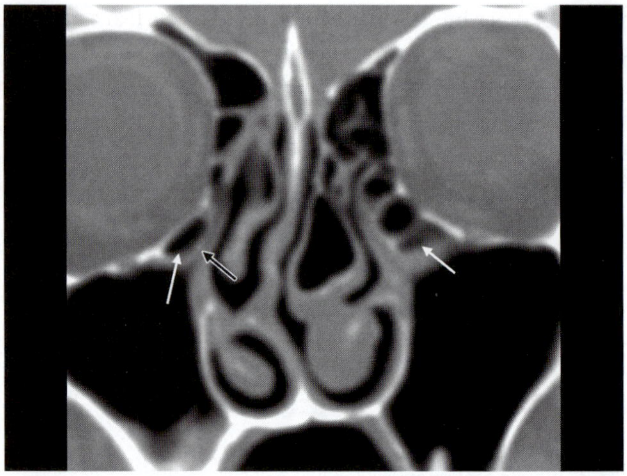

FIG. 10: Coronal CT image showing Haller cells (white arrows) along the roof of the maxillary sinus medially, causing narrowing of the infundibulum (black arrow).

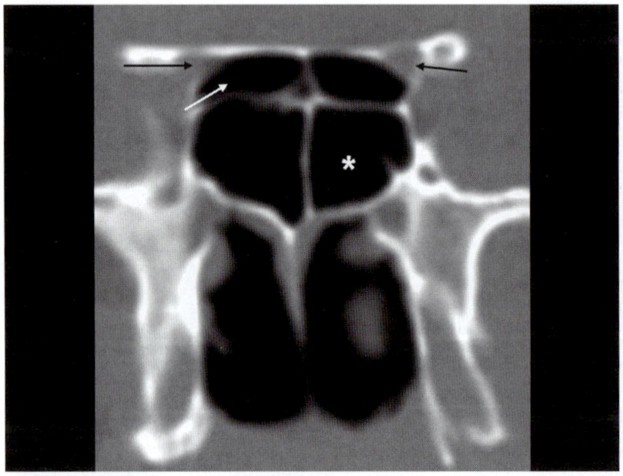

FIG. 11: Coronal CT at the level of sphenoid sinus (asterisk), showing Onodi cells (white arrow) lying superior to the sphenoid sinuses and in close relation to optic nerves (black arrows).

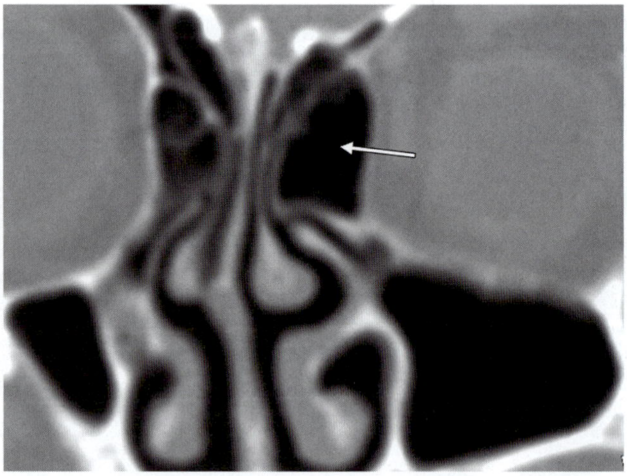

FIG. 12: Ethmoid bulla (arrow) seen on the left side.

Paradoxical Middle Turbinate

The middle turbinate may project laterally rather than medially, thus narrowing the middle meatus.

Variations in the Uncinate Process

The superior "free" edge of the uncinate process may be: (i) deviated medially to obstruct the middle meatus and (ii) inclined laterally to compromise the infundibulum. Fusion with the medial orbital wall may endanger the orbital contents while an uncinectomy is being done.

Haller cells are infraethmoid air cells which extend along the roof of the maxillary sinus. Haller cells may contribute to narrowing of the infundibulum **(Fig. 10)**.

Onodi cells are lateral and posterior extensions of the posterior ethmoid air cells. They extend close to the optic nerves as they exit the orbits **(Fig. 11)**.

Prominent ethmoid bulla is the largest of the ethmoid air cells, and may enlarge to narrow or obstruct the middle meatus and infundibulum **(Fig. 12)**.

SINONASAL REPORTING

It has been observed that the radiology reports of PNS are not very relevant to the operating ENT surgeons before FESS in cases of sinusitis. This is mainly because radiologists are not very well versed about the anatomical variations and or danger points encountered by the surgeon during the FESS.

Thus, it becomes imperative that the radiologists learn about these points and report carry the relevant information.

The points to be included include the information about:

1. Cribriform plate
2. Lamina papyracea
3. Onodi cells
4. Sphenoid sinus pneumatization pattern
5. Ethmoid sulcus

Cribriform plate adjoining the crista galli has Olfactory fossa. Its superior boundary is marked by Fovea ethmoidalis, lateral boundary by Lateral lamella, inferior boundary by lamina cribrosa and medial by crista galli. The deeper the olfactory fossa, more is the chance of injury to the lateral lamella. Since it's the thinnest portion of anterior skull base and its breech can cause CSF rhinorrhea and infections, its status and depth of olfactory fossa needs to be reported **(Fig. 13A)**. Lamina payracea again is very this bony separation between nasal cavity and the orbits. Maintaining its integrity is important during FESS. If it's medially deviated it may get injured during ethmoidectomy. Also, it has close relation with uncinated process.

Onodi cells, are important to report since optic nerve may be passing through it. During posterior ethmoidectomy surgeon may enter these mistaking them for posterior ethmoid cells and nerve injury may result.

Sphenoid sinus lateral wall has intimate relation to the cavernous segment of ICA and optic nerve. Over pneumatization may make the wall thin and chance of inadvertent ICA or optic nerve injury **(Fig. 13B)**.

Lastly, anterior ethmoid artery, a branch of ophthalmic artery lies at supero-medial margin of the orbit at the level of anterio ethmoid air cells. Pneumatization of air cells above and below the sulcus may lead to arterial injury during ethmoidectomy **(Fig. 13C)**.[15,16]

INFLAMMATORY SINUS DISEASE

Acute Sinusitis

Inflammatory sinus is usually caused by superinfection in a previously obstructed sinus. The previously inflamed mucosa becomes edematous leading to obstruction of the ostium of the sinus. Secretions from the sinuses accumulate and form a good culture medium for bacterial pathogens. Viral infections rarely cause sinusitis.[17]

The hallmark of acute sinusitis is an air fluid level on plain X-rays or CT **(Fig. 14)**. It may be associated with shadows of thickened mucosa or may be represented by an opaque sinus. The findings are nonspecific and one of the important differential diagnoses is the presence of fluid in the sinus due to hemorrhage following trauma.

Chronic Sinusitis

Chronic inflammation of the PNS occurs either due to recurrent inflammatory episodes or due to an indolent inflammatory process. Patients usually have a chronic history of headache, retrobulbar pain and may have had previous surgeries which have failed to give relief.[18,19]

Both CT and MRI are used to assess chronic inflammation. However, CT is better in pretherapeutic planning before functional endoscopic sinus surgery (FESS).[20]

MRI can be done post-FESS to see therapeutic response, complications and in patients where dental filling cause artifact obscuring the anatomical details.[21] A recent report in which sinusitis scoring system was used on both CT and MRI images did not find any overstaging or understaging on MRI images. Thus, there is a possibility where MRI may still be used in patients likely to be managed conservatively.[7]

In chronic sinusitis the mucosa is hypertrophic. Polypoid changes can occur with areas of atrophy and fibrosis. If there is superadded acute inflammation due to infections or allergy the mucosa will thicken. It is essential to note the number of sinuses involved and the degree of mucosal thickening within them **(Fig. 15)**.

Sinus secretions in the acute state have a density ranging 10–25 HU, which is slightly higher than water but less than muscle. As the condition becomes chronic, the secretions become more mucoid and CT attenuation values range between 30 HU and 60 HU, and the density equals that of muscle.

Hyperdense secretions on CT may be due to four main causes:[11] (i) inspissated secretions, (ii) fungal sinusitis,

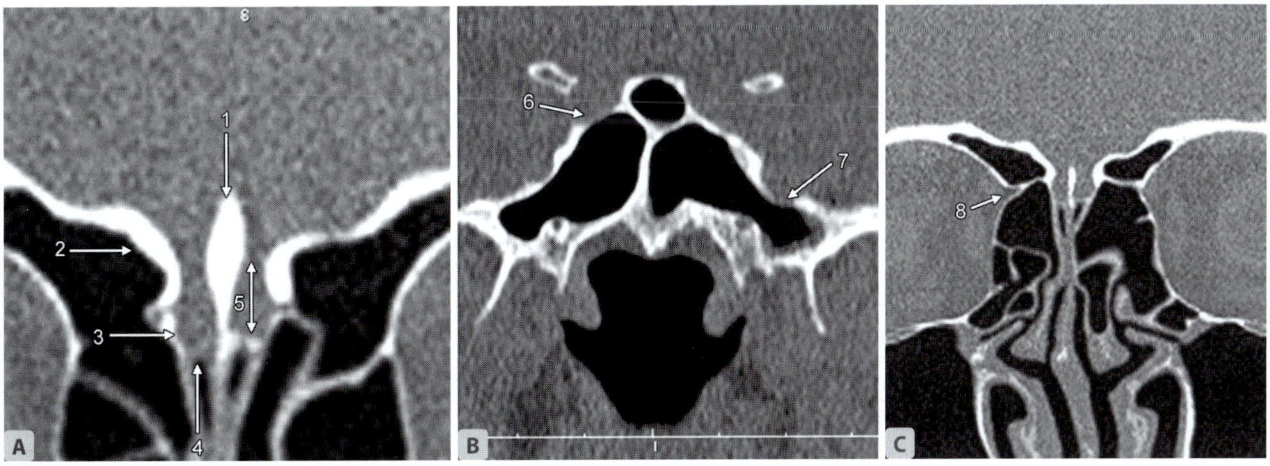

FIGS. 13A TO C: (A) Olfactory fossa bound by fovea ethmoidalis (2), lateral lamella (3), lamina cribrosa (4), crista galli (1), Depth of the fossa (5); (B) Optic nerve (6) and internal carotid artery (7) relation to the sphenoid sinus; (C) Ethmoidal notch (8).

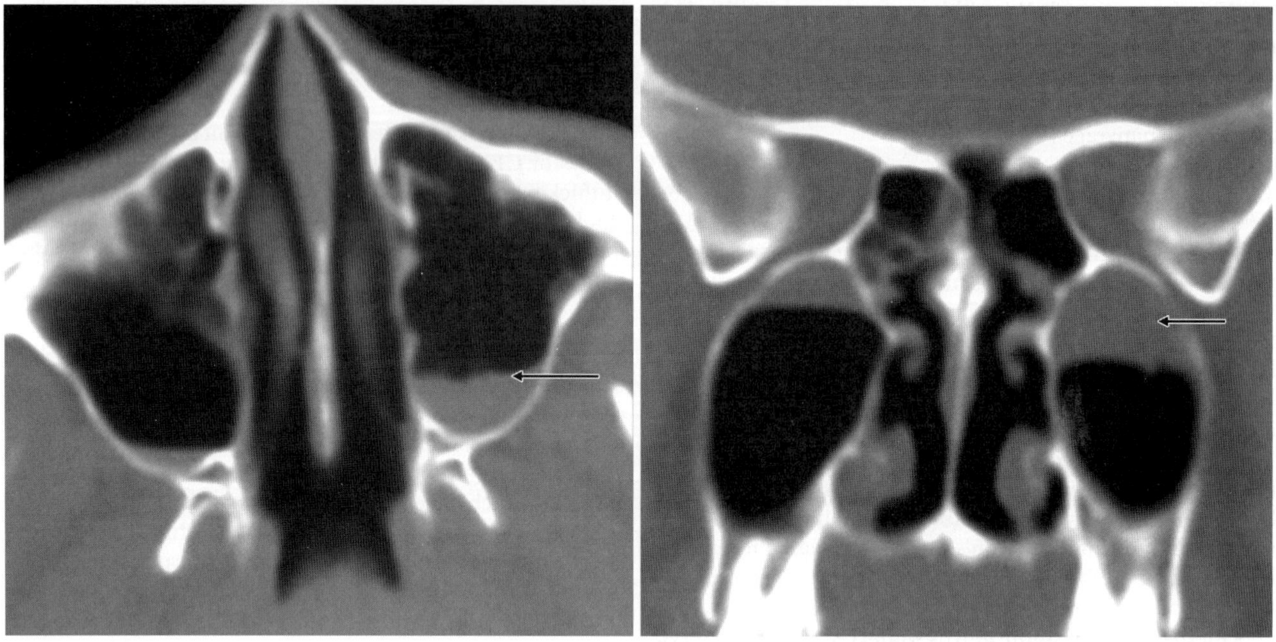

FIG. 14: Axial and coronal CT images showing air-fluid levels (arrows) seen in the dependent position.

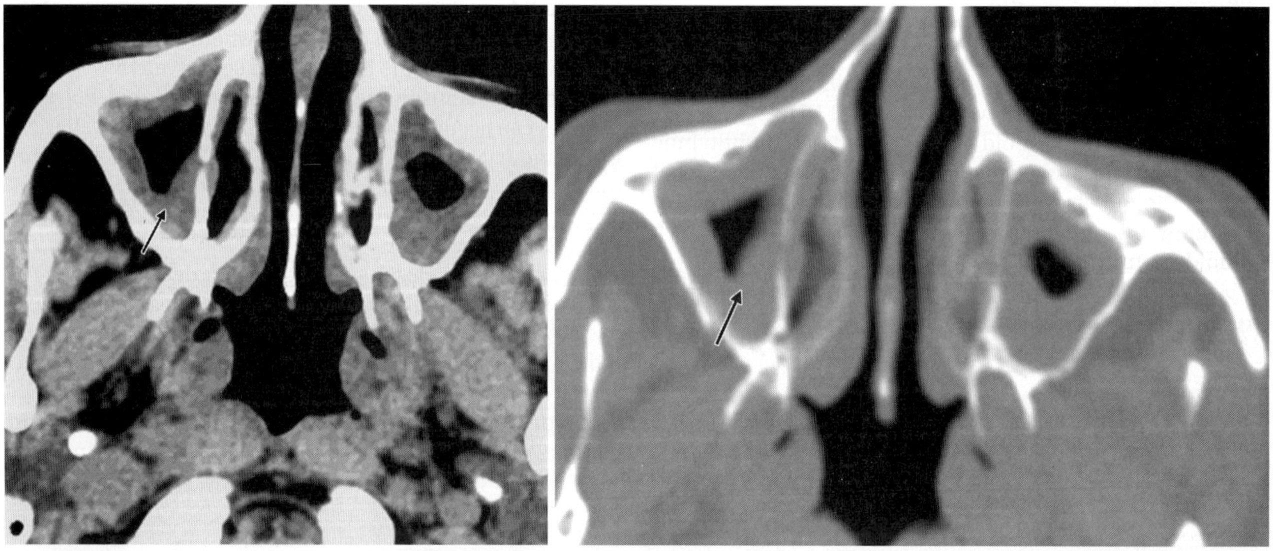

FIG. 15: Axial sections showing diffuse mucosal hypertrophy (arrows) without any significant change in the bones.

(iii) hemorrhage in sinus, and (iv) calcification chronic bacterial sinusitis may occasionally results in a hyperdense sinus on CT, particularly in patients who have very long-standing disease with coexisting cystic fibrosis. The hyperdense sinus often corresponds to the hypointense sinus on T2W MRI images. On MRI, intensity of secretion depend on the relative contrast of water and mucous. The high water content is reflected as low intensity on T1WI and high intensity on T2WI. On MRI appearances of chronic inflammatory sinus secretions vary with the protein content. The intensity on T1WI progressively decreases with the increase in protein content while the intensity on T2WI progressively increases till the protein content is 25% of the secretion following which the intensity decreases till the protein content is 40% of the secretion. This is because all the free water is eliminated from the secretion and macromolecular protein to protein binding occurs. Thus, four intensity patterns on MRI for sinus secretions have been described.[22]

1. Hypointense on T1WI and hyperintense on T2WI in most liquid form (total protein concentration < 9%).
2. Hyperintense on T1WI and hyperintense on T2WI in mild to moderately proteinaceous form (total protein concentration 20–25%).
3. Hyperintense on T1WI and hypointense on T2WI in a highly proteinaceous form (total protein concentration 25–28%).

4. Hypointense on T1WI and hypointense on T2WI when secretion are in a nearly solid (total protein concentration >28%).

On CT scans, the inspissated chronic secretions appear as bright densities whereas on T1WI and T2WI the sinuses show signal voids similar to air. Enhancement of sinuses after gadolinium administration helps diagnose chronic sinusitis **(Figs. 16A and B)**. CT however remains the modality of choice, as it shows both soft tissue and bony changes, and is cost effective and easily available.[22]

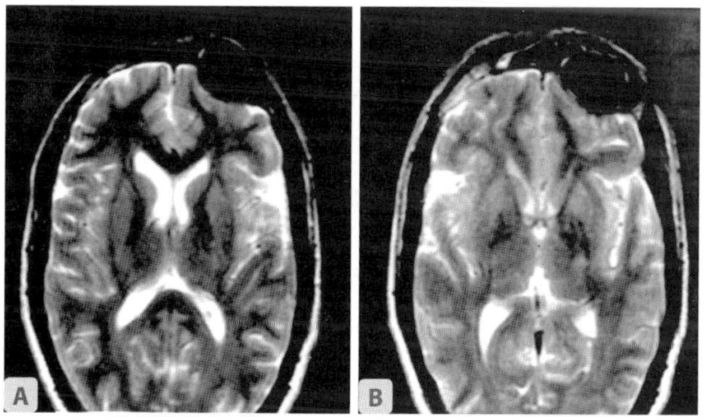

FIGS. 16A AND B: (A) Axial T2WI showing featureless well pneumatized, hypointense frontal sinuses in a diagnosis case of chronic sinusitis; (B) Peripheral rim enhancement of walls of the sinus and enhancement of inspissated secretions characterize the chronic inflammation in these T1W sections.

As the chronic inflammation becomes indolent, changes in the facial bones become evident and these are best seen on CT scans. These include thickening of the facial bones adjacent to the inflamed mucosa and progressive sclerosis in these bones. These changes are due to increased vascularity due to chronic inflammation. Rarely, osteomyelitis may supervene with areas of sequestration and bony rarefaction.

Five patterns of chronic inflammation in the sinuses given by Sonkens et al.[20] give an important insight into the importance of imaging the anterior and posterior draining pathways described before. According to them the patterns are as follows:

1. *Infundibular pattern:* In this the disease is limited to maxillary sinus and corresponding infundibulum and can occur due to mucosal thickening, polyp in that location or Haller cells. Rest of the sinuses are normal.
2. *Osteomeatal unit pattern:* In this the obstruction is in the middle meatus thus causing obstruction and changes in frontal sinus, anterior and middle ethmoid sinus and maxillary sinus. Cause may be mucosal thickening, polyps, concha bullosa, deviated septum or nasal tumor **(Fig. 17)**.
3. *Sphenoethmoidal recess pattern:* In this the sphenoethmoid recess is blocked and changes seen only in ipsilateral sphenoid and posterior ethmoid air cells **(Fig. 18)**.
4. *Sinonasal polyposis pattern:* In this both the nasal cavities and the sinuses are filled with polyps and the resultant chronic inflammatory changes are a mix of above three patterns **(Fig. 19)**.

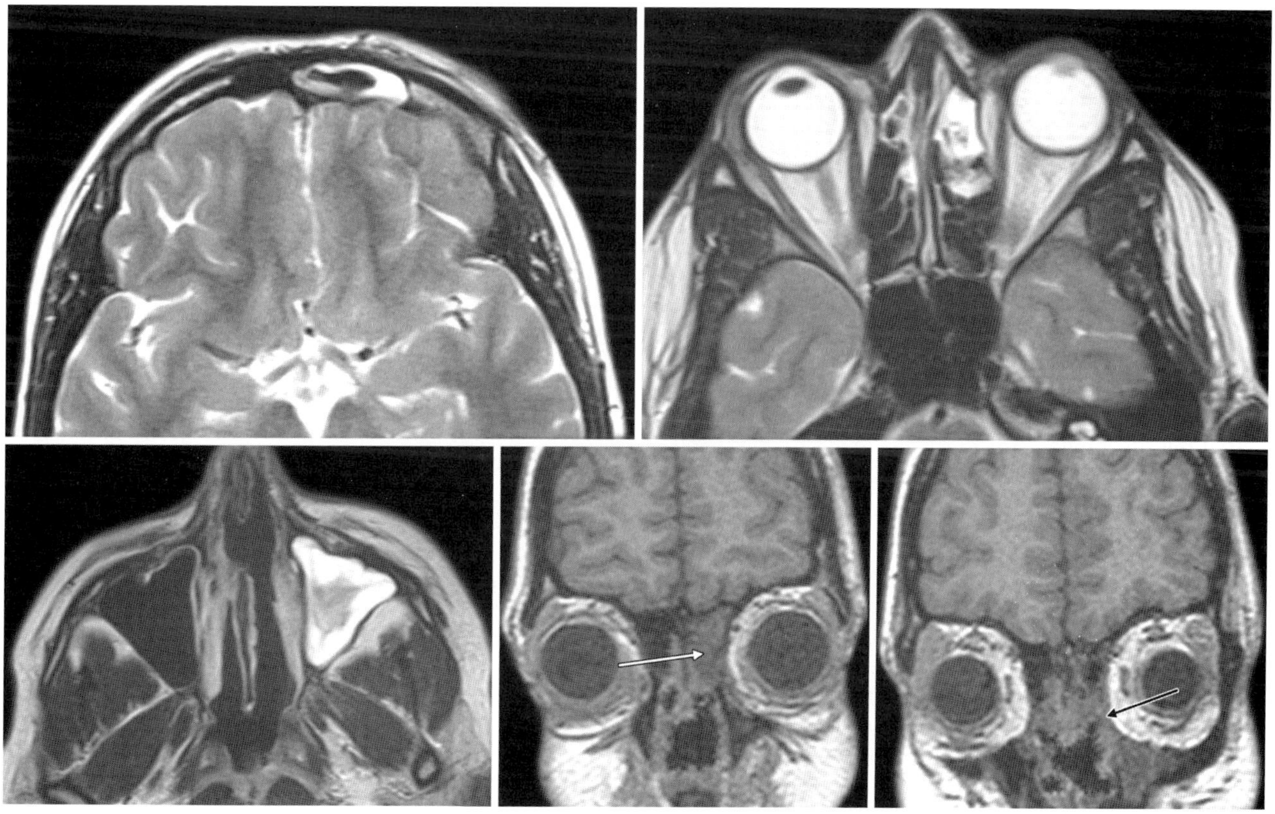

FIG. 17: Osteomeatal pattern of obstruction with involvement of all left sided anterior sinuses due to obstruction at the frontal recess (white arrow) and left OM complex (black arrow).

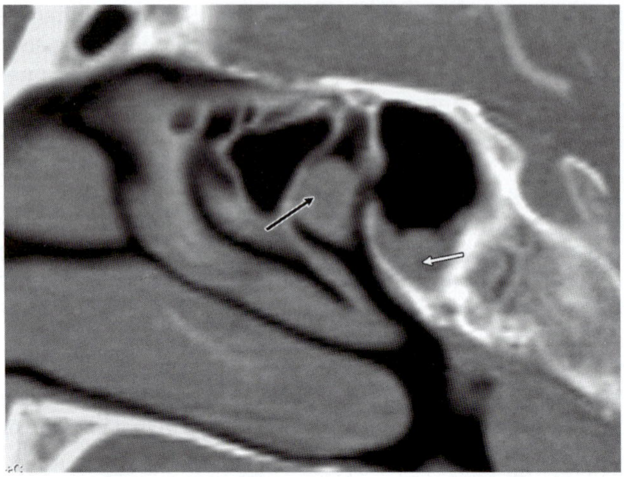

FIG. 18: A polyp in posterior ethmoid (black arrow) is causing partial obstruction of the sphenoethmoid recess causing sphenoid sinusitis (white arrow).

5. *Sporadic/Unclassified pattern:* When no specific kind of obstruction is seen and when mucocele, retention cysts or postoperative changes are there.

Classifying disease under one of these headings can help a surgeon to plan FESS as the rationale behind endoscopic sinus surgery is to restore the flow of sinus secretion via their natural pathways. To revise the anatomy and to systematically read PNS CTs, it is important the following structures are identified first:

- Frontal sinus
- Frontal recess
- Agger nasi cells
- Ethmoid roof
- Ethmoid bulla
- Basal or grand lamella
- Sinus lateralis
- Uncinate process
- Infundibulum
- Maxillary sinus
- Middle meatus
- Nasal septum and nasal turbinates
- Posterior ethmoid sinus
- Sphenoid sinus

Following this evaluation, the orbits and any normal variations are studied. The third step in evaluation involves study of the bony outline of the orbits and to observe areas of erosion or bone thickening.[17]

Post-FESS Scanning

Postoperatively, neither CT nor MRI is accurate in distinguishing fibrosis from inflammation. Both enhance and appear as mucosal thickening. CT is the study of choice in the acute setting of orbital complications after FESS, which usually occurs within 48 hours after surgery. CT is reliable in diagnosing an orbital hematoma, assessing for optic nerve compression or inadvertent resection and also for planning therapy to relieve increased intraorbital pressure.

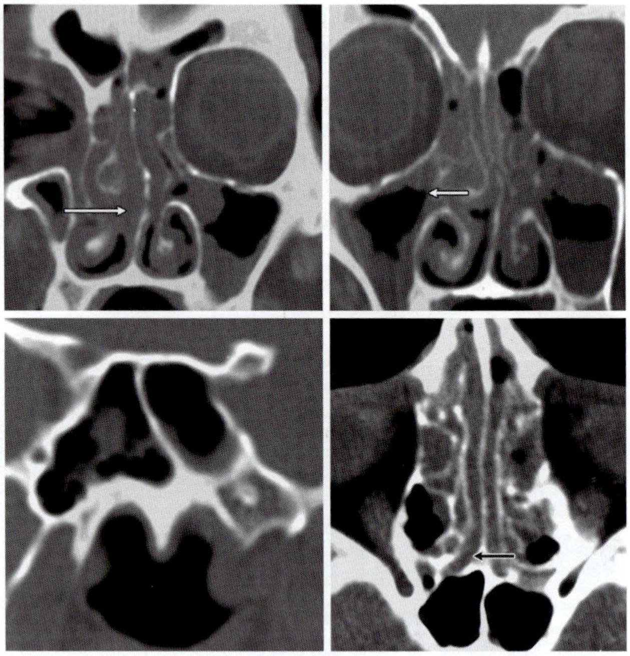

FIG. 19: Extensive nasal polyposis (long white arrow) causing obstruction of anterior (short white arrow) and posterior (black arrow) drainage pathways causing pansinusitis.

Mucocele

Mucocele is a term used for those expanded and remodeled sinuses which are obstructed and contain secretions.[17] About 66% of the mucoceles occur in the frontal sinus, 25% in the ethmoid sinuses and 10% in the maxillary sinus. Sphenoidal mucoceles are rare. When infected a mucocele is termed as a mucopyocele. Radiographically, the sinus is airless, expanded and filled with soft tissue shadows **(Fig. 20A)**. CT appearance is that of an expanded sinus with intact walls, containing mucoid soft tissue densities.[23] The sinus may be remodeled **(Fig. 20B)**. It is essential to note the expanding wall of the sinus and its encroachment upon the orbit, intracranial space, nasal cavities and pterygopalatine fossa, all of which contain important neural and vascular structures.[23,24] MRI appearance depends on the nature of the secretion within the mucocele as in chronic sinusitis. MRI can detect the interface of mucocele with intracranial or intraorbital structures. A peripheral rim enhancement pattern is seen on MRI which is useful for distinguishing mucocele and obstructed secretions form neoplasms such as inverted papillomas on malignancies which may also remodel bone but show solid enhancement[25] **(Figs. 21A and B)**.

Fungal Sinusitis

It may be classified as: (i) allergic fungal rhinosinusitis, (ii) invasive fungal sinusitis, and (iii) noninvasive chronic fungal sinusitis.

Allergic Fungal Rhinosinusitis

It occurs as an allergic response to fungal elements in atopic patients. On CT, diffuse mucosal thickening involving

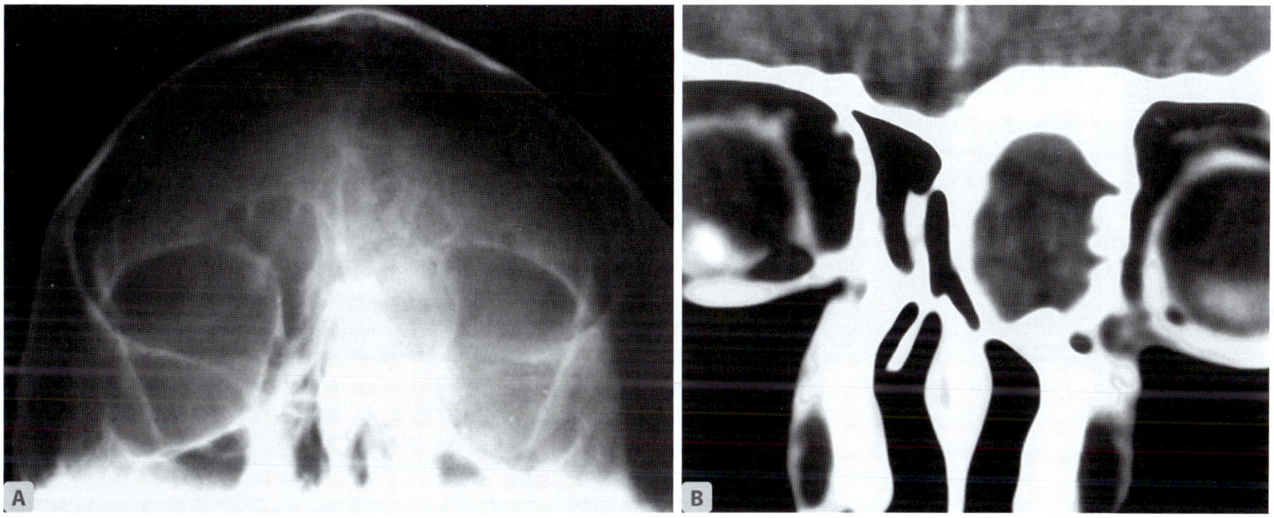

FIGS. 20A AND B: Mucocele of the ethmoid sinus. (A) Plain X-ray Water's view shows an expanded and opaque left ethmoid sinus; (B) Coronal non-contrast CT shows the expanded sinus containing soft tissue densities. The wall of the sinus are thickened but are intact.

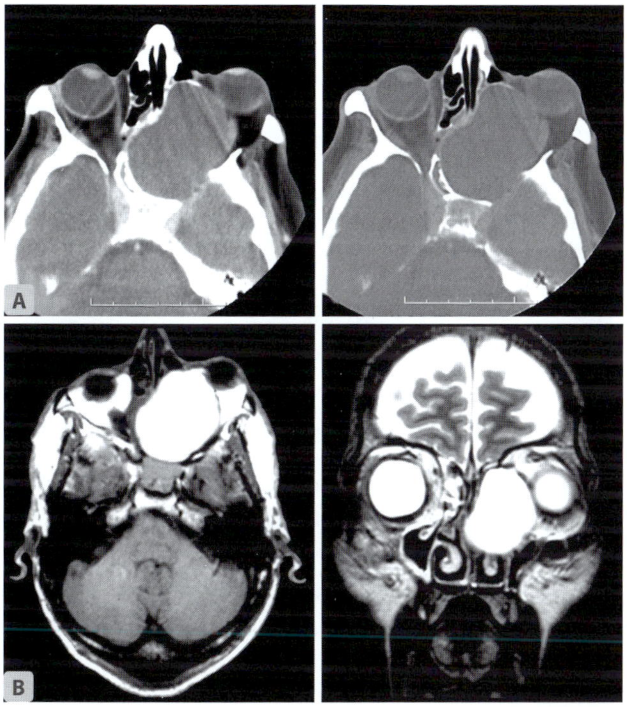

FIGS. 21A AND B: (A) Left-sided ethmoidal mucocele encroaching on the left orbit. Left globe is proposed; (B) T2W MRI axial and coronal sections of the same patient showing hyperintense fluid contents of the mucocele.

multiple sinuses is present. Within the sinus there may be central hyperdense content and peripheral hypodensity. On MRI the central content is usually hypointense on both T1WI and T2WI. Sinus may be expanded with its walls remodeled or rarified **(Fig. 22)**. Bony destruction is usually not seen. Calcification is also a common finding in fungal infections especially with aspergillosis. Central or fine punctate pattern of calcification is characteristic of fungal infection. Many patients may have polyps.

Invasive Fungal Sinusitis

This usually occurs in immunosuppressed individuals and may occur by invasion by the fungus colonizing the sinuses in setting of chronic sinusitis or by inhalation of fungal spores. *Mucor, Aspergillus* or *Fusarium* are the common fungi causing invasive form of sinusitis. On CT, it cause opacification of the sinuses due to mucosal hypertrophy and secretions but the course is fulminant. Also, the bony wall is destroyed early in the course of disease with spread of infection directly into orbits, cavernous sinuses or brain **(Figs. 23A and B)**.

Noninvasive Chronic Fungal Sinusitis

Noninvasive chronic fungal sinusitis or mycetomas may be seen in sinus cavities as a noninvasive ball of fungus which is hyperdense on CT, does not change position on changing head position and may have calcifications. They are usually found in setting of chronic non-resolving sinusitis.

The final diagnosis of the type of fungus however, rests with the pathologist.[17,18,26]

GRANULOMATOUS DISEASES

Actinomycosis,[27] tuberculosis,[28] syphilis, leprosy,[29] rhinoscleroma, rhinosporidiosis, sarcoidosis, Wegener's granulomatosis, midline granuloma, leishmaniasis and yaws are some of the chronic granulomatous diseases which affect the PNS and nasal fossa. As a group, these conditions cause nonspecific findings which include focal erosions and soft tissue masses **(Fig. 24)**. Often the sinuses are filled with fluid-like densities which on multiple examinations are un changing. Involvement of the nasal septum either with erosions or soft tissue thickening is a pointer to such conditions like leprosy **(Fig. 25)**, Wegener's granulomatosis or granulomas due to cocaine abuse. In one study of 28 patients of Wegener's granulomatosis following features were observed—bony destruction, mainly of the nasal cavity, maxillary sinuses and mastoid cells; sclerosing osteitis, mainly of the maxillary sinuses; bony thickening, mainly

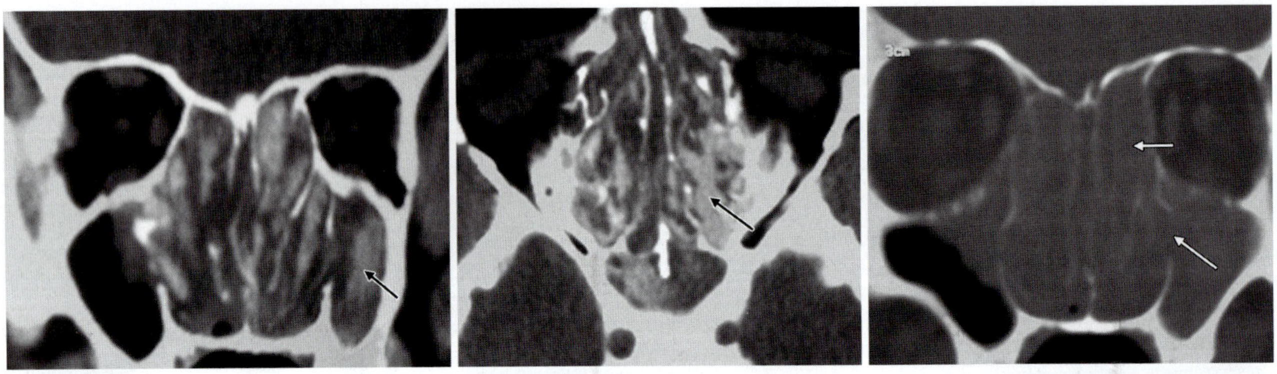

FIG. 22: Allergic fungal rhinosinusitis (AFRS) CT images coronal and axial showing diffuse nasal and sinus mucosal thickening with hyperdensities (black arrows) causing expansion and blockage of the sinuses. On bone window, the ethmoid lamellae and sinus walls are remodeled and eroded (white arrows).

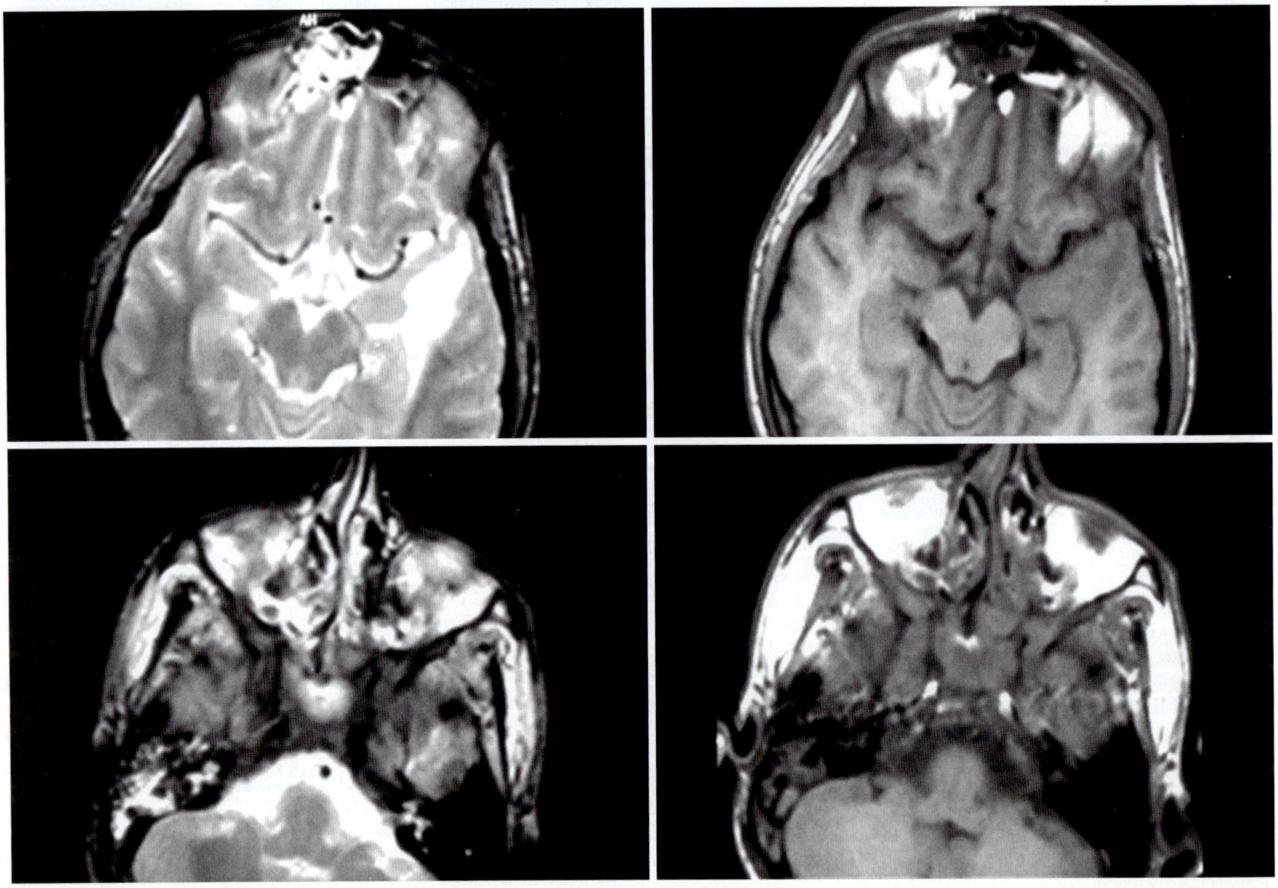

FIG. 23A: Invasive fungal sinusitis: Axial T2WI (left) and T1WI (right) images showing soft tissue in the frontal, ethmoid and sphenoid sinuses which are isointense on T1WI and hyperintense on the T2WI.

of the maxillary sinuses and mastoid cells and mucosal thickening, mainly of the maxillary sinuses. Although these findings were seen frequently still they are nonspecific and need clinicopathologic correlation.[30]

Polyps and Cysts

Polyps appear as well defined dome-shaped homogeneous lesions. If multiple, they trap secretions between their crevices. On CT scan they appear as well defined lobulated lesions, sometimes extending into the nasal cavities **(Fig. 26)**. On MRI, they are of varying intensity depending upon the degree of desiccation within the polyp.

Diagnosis on imaging may be problematic sometimes because the lesion, although benign, may demonstrate aggressive bony destruction on CT. The findings suggestive of polyposis include enlargement of sinus ostia, rounded masses within the nasal cavity, expanded sinuses or portions of the nasal cavity **(Figs. 27A and B)** thinning of bony

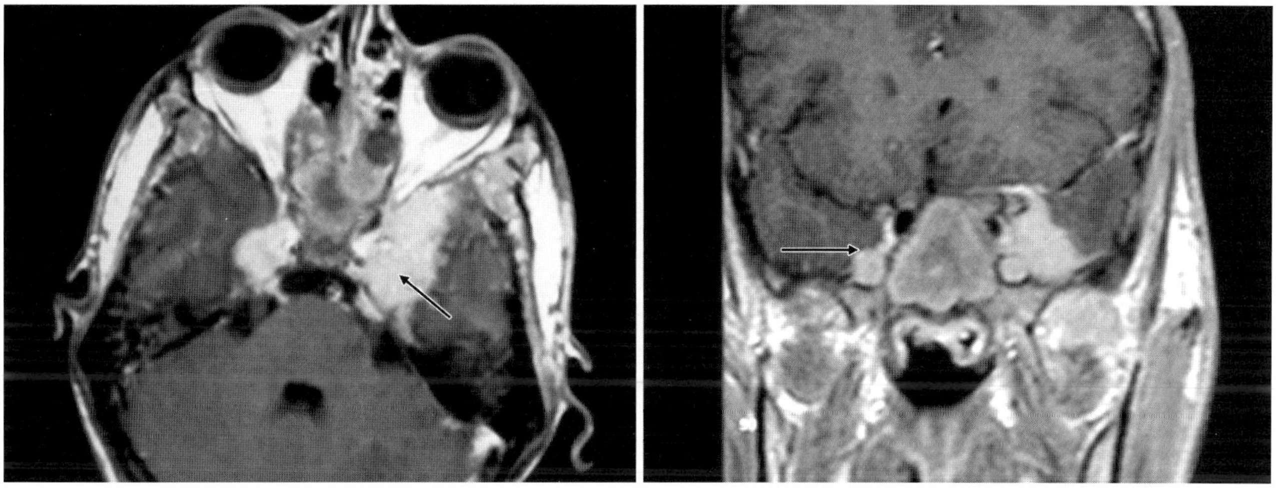

FIG. 23B: Invasive fungal sinusitis: Postcontrast T1WI axial and coronal showing intense enhancement and contiguous extension of the soft tissue from the sinuses into the bilateral cavernous sinuses and temporal lobe (arrows).

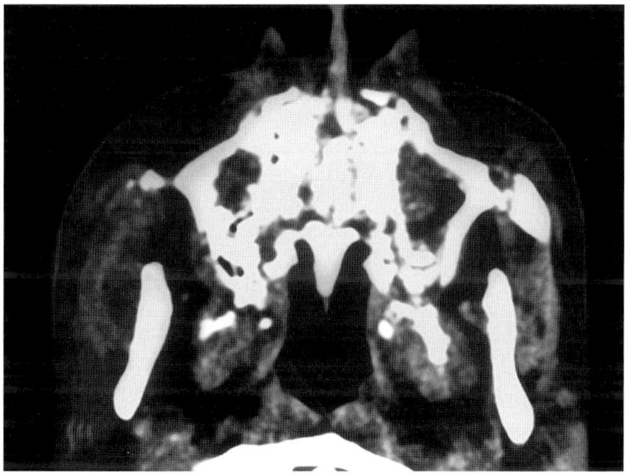

FIG. 24: Actinomycosis of the hard palate and adjacent maxillary antrum. Fragmentation of the palate is present with accompanying soft tissue densities in the maxillary antrum. Similar soft tissues invade the premaxilla and the columella of the nose.

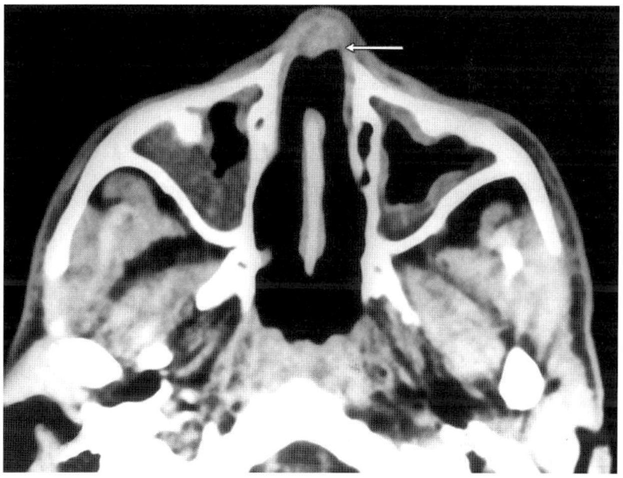

FIG. 25: Leprosy: Destruction of the nasal bones (arrow) and a perforated nasal septum are characteristic changes of lepromatous leprosy.

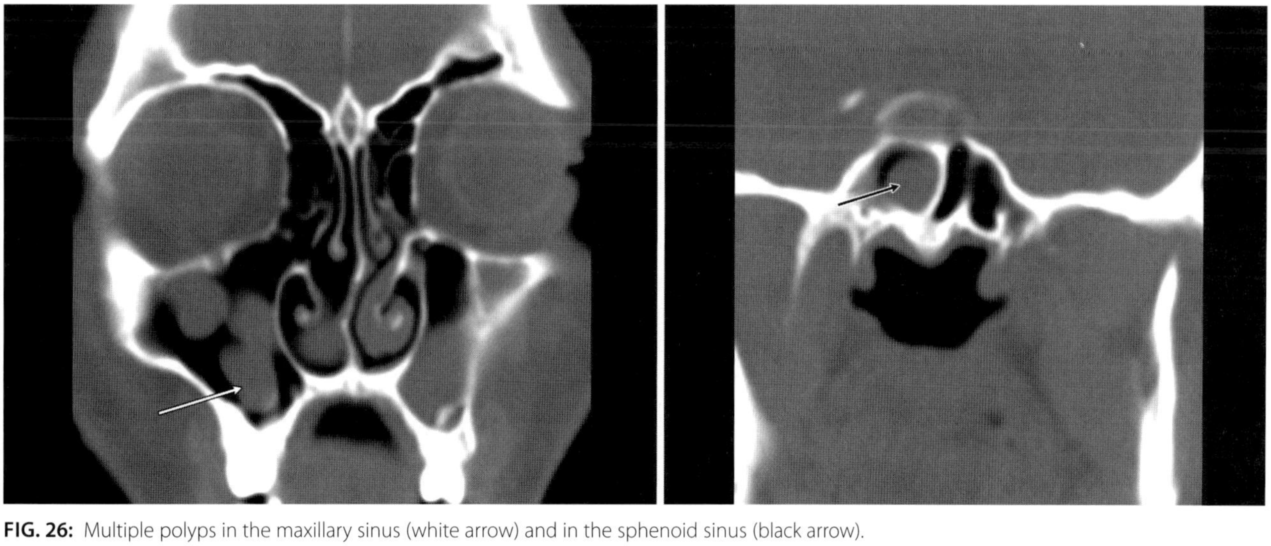

FIG. 26: Multiple polyps in the maxillary sinus (white arrow) and in the sphenoid sinus (black arrow).

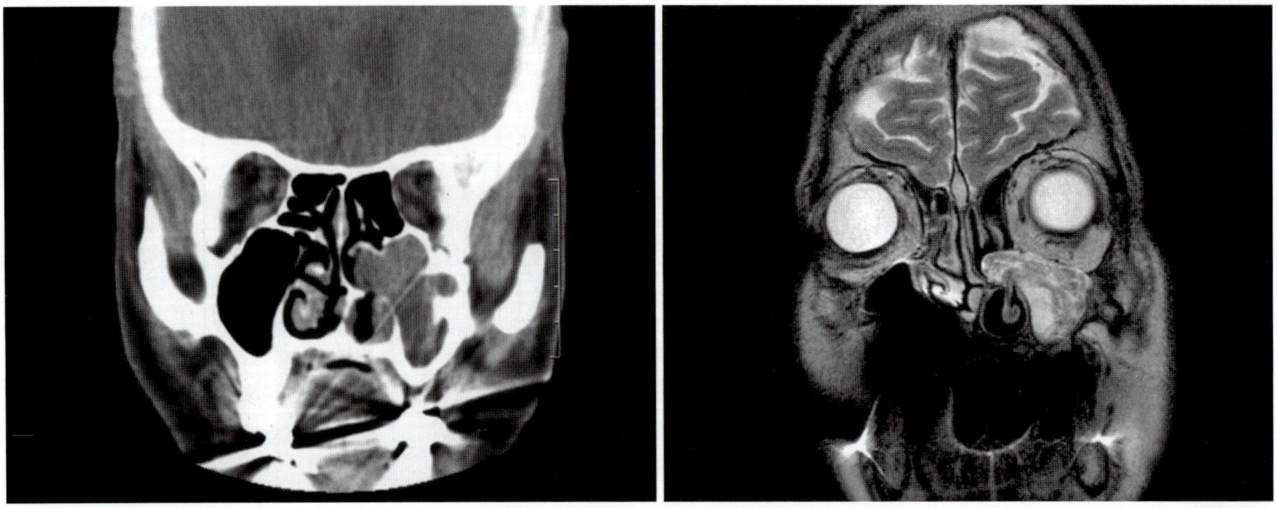

FIG. 27A: Coronal CT image and T2WI MRI image of a left antrochoanal polyps, showing the heterogeneous intensity of the polyps, which widens the ostia enters the nasal cavity and expand the sinus.

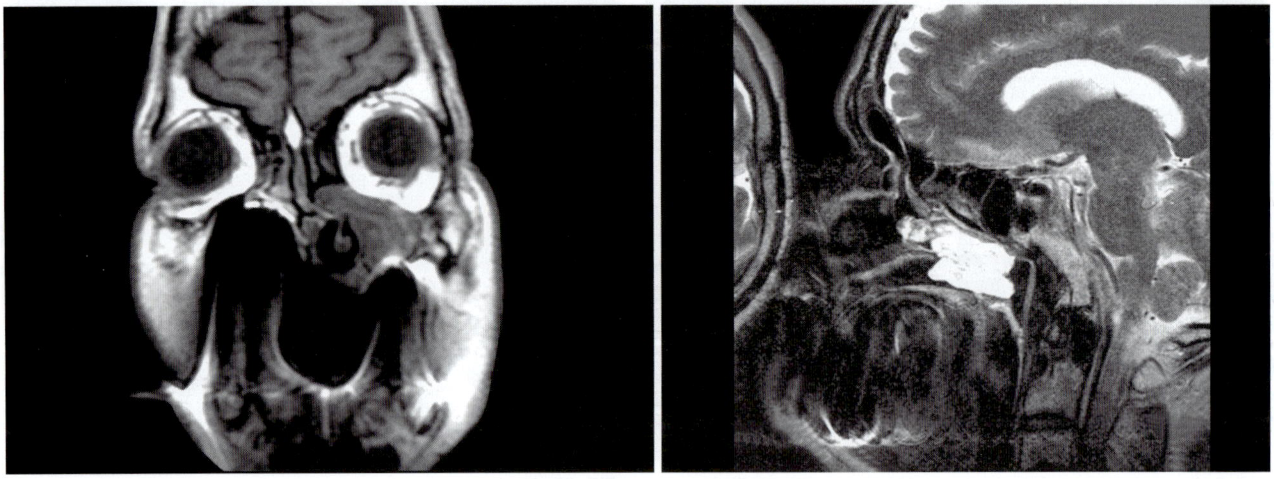

FIG. 27B: Coronal T1WI and sagittal T2WI showing the change in single characterization of the polyps and its extent up to the posterior choana.

trabeculae, and less commonly, erosive bone changes at the anterior aspect of skull base.[11] Retention cysts occur due to obstruction of ducts of the glands in the mucosa. They can be either serous or mucinous. They are indistinguishable from polyps and have similar appearances on CT and MRI.[11,17]

NEOPLASTIC LESIONS OF THE PARANASAL SINUSES

Neoplastic lesions of the paranasal sinus are either of epithelial or nonepithelial origin.

Epithelial Tumors of the PNS

Epithelial tumors are further subdivided into two groups:
1. Tumors of epithelial origin
2. Tumors of salivary gland origin

Tumors of epithelial origin include:
- Papillomas
- Squamous cell carcinoma
- Adenocarcinoma

Tumors of salivary gland origin include:
- Pleomorphic adenoma
- Adenocystic carcinoma
- Acinic cell carcinoma
- Mucoepidermoid carcinoma

Squamous cell carcinomas are the most common epithelial neoplasms of the PNS. They constitute up to 63% of malignancies of this region.[31,32]

Maxillary sinus (25–58%) is most commonly involved followed by ethmoid (10%) and sphenoid and frontal sinuses (1%). The nasal cavity is the site of origin in 25–35% of cases. The industrial workers involved in the production of nickel, chromium, isopropyl alcohol, radium, mustard gas and wooden furniture are at an increased risk to develop this malignancy. Chronic sinusitis and polyposis may predispose to squamous cell carcinomas probably believed to be related to the squamous cell metaplasia of the respiratory mucosal lining of the sinuses.[33,34] Squamous cell carcinoma is twice as common in men than women and occurs in the 6th and 7th decades.[34] Unilateral facial pain and purulent nasal discharge are the most common presenting features of sinonasal carcinoma. Epistaxis and nasal obstruction are other presenting symptoms. If the sphenoid sinus is involved cranial neuropathy may be encountered.

The hallmark of imaging malignancies of the sinonasal cavity is bony destruction, seen in approximately 80% of scans of sinonasal squamous cell carcinomas at initial presentation.[11] Squamous cell carcinomas are hypointense on T2WI and should be distinguished from inflammations which are hyperintense on T2WI. Inspissated inflammatory secretions appear increasingly hypointense on T2WI; however, they retain their homogeneity in contrast to the typical heterogeneous signal intensity of malignant neoplasms.

Maxillary sinus carcinomas appear as destructive lesions which transgress the bony confines **(Fig. 28)** of the sinus and involve the ethmoid sinus, pterygopalatine fossa and infratemporal fossa. Orbital invasion is present in nearly two-thirds of the patients followed by invasion of the pterygopalatine and infratemporal fossa in one-third of the patients. The ethmoid sinus and cheek are involved in roughly a quarter of the patients.[31]

Ethmoid cell carcinomas **(Fig. 29A)** appear as destructive lesions which spread through the fovea ethmoidalis and cribriform plate into the anterior cranial fossa; and from

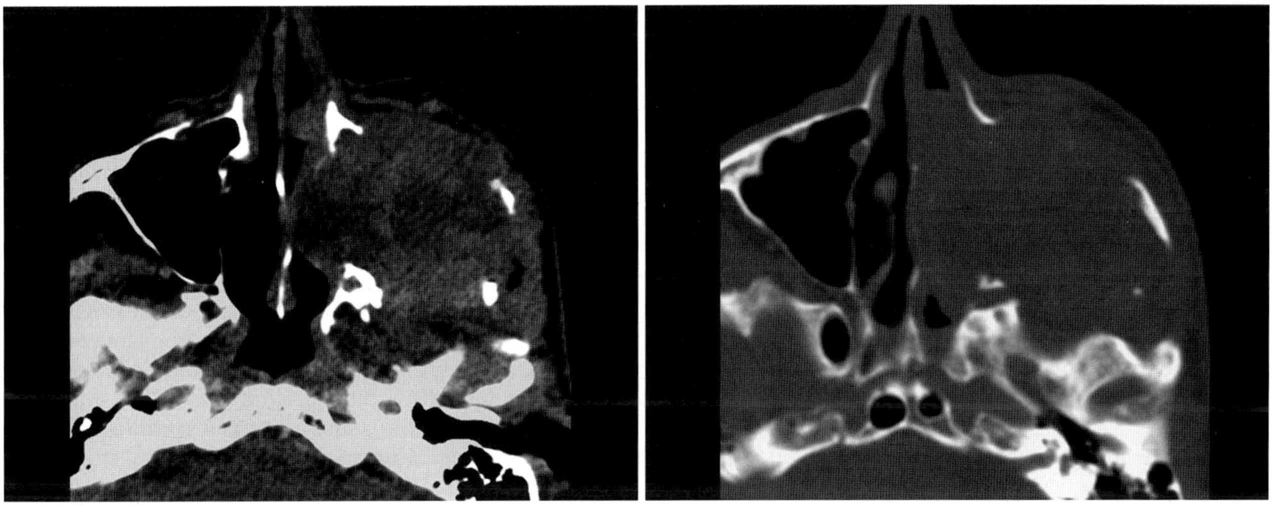

FIG. 28: Squamous cell carcinoma of the right maxillary sinus: Noncontrast CT scan shows soft tissue mass of intermediate attenuation with central necrosis filling the right antrum. The lesion extends beyond the bony walls of the sinus, bone window setting show extensive lytic destruction of the walls.

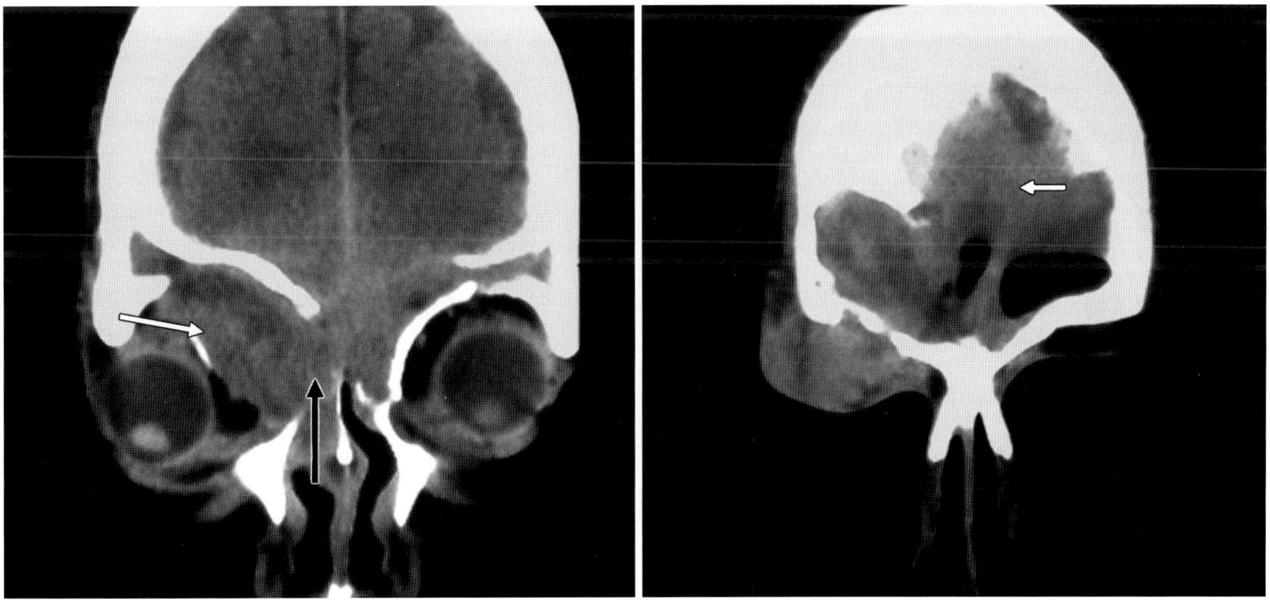

FIG. 29A: Coronal CT showing extensive enhancing ethmoidal soft tissue mass (black arrow) completely filling the sinus with frank bony destruction and extension into right orbit (long white arrow) and frontal sinuses (short white arrow).

the posterior ethmoidal cells into the middle cranial fossa via the superior orbital fissure. Orbital involvements by the carcinomas of the PNS are of some prognostic importance because of considerable morbidity following radiation therapy. These patients may then develop cataract, keratitis and optic nerve atrophy.

Both CT and MRI scans are complementary in assessing the presence, extent and progress following therapeutic intervention. CT scanning is of prime importance, because it is helpful in evaluation of soft tissues, sinus cavities and more importantly involvement of the bones. The posterior wall of the maxillary sinus, the pterygoid plate, pterygopalatine fossa, the cribriform plate, the orbital walls, the sphenoid sinuses, the fossa ethmoidalis and the posterior wall of the frontal sinus are the areas which are of importance because the breach due to the malignant process of any of these structures would indicate the spreads of the lesion beyond the PNS.[35,36]

Squamous cell carcinomas show little contrast enhancement. However, contrast administration is necessitated in CT evaluation of these tumors because it can help to differentiate: (i) fluid from areas of necrosis, (ii) involvement of normal structures from tumors especially in the orbit, and (iii) to delineate intracranial extent of the tumor.[37]

Limitations of CT scan include inability to distinguish between inspissated and retained secretions from tumors, detect involvement of the periorbital structures especially the lamina papyracea and the adjacent structures, and to differentiate soft tissues involvement by tumors versus swelling due to edema.

On MRI, inflammatory tissue and retained secretions can be differentiated with some degree of confidence from tumors as the latter have a higher water content and thus appear to be of high intensity on T2WI and low intensity on T1WI **(Fig. 29B)**. Discontinuous dural enhancement without intervening hypointense epidural margination favors neoplastic invasion.

No dural enhancement and enhancing tissue over 5 mm thick imply neoplasm over reactive changes.[11]

Chow et al.[36] have characterized carcinoma of the nasal cavity and PNS, and have stated that: (1) They are highly cellular tumors with little free water and thus have low to intermediate signal intensity on T1WI and T2WI. They appear as masses of homogeneous signal intensities. (2) Instances where subacute to chronic hemorrhages have appeared within the masses, these will appear as well-defined areas of intermediate to high signal intensities on T1 and T2WI. (3) Necrotic areas within the tumor appear as areas of low to intermediate signal intensities on T1WI and high intensity on T2WI. (4) Intracranial spread of the tumor tends to be broad based and flat despite destruction of the skull base. This is in contrast to the contained, highly polypoidal intracranial surfaces of benign processes like papillomas and polyps. MRI scans with contrast is useful because Gd-DTPA enhancement of tumors is less intense than enhancement of mucosa. In cases where sinuses are obstructed due to inflammation with presence of tumor, mucosal enhancement helps differentiate the obstructed sinus from tumor invasion. The extent of tumor enhancement is directly proportional to the vascularity of the tumor. Gd-DTPA enhancement is also helpful in detecting intracranial extension.

In a study comparing CT and MRI to evaluate extension of tumor, there was no significant difference in staging by either modality. Errors occurred in both modalities and it has been generalized that MRI is more accurate than CT in evaluation of large bony structures and soft tissues, while CT scores over MR in imaging and evaluating fine bony structures.[7] Diffusion weighted MR imaging may help in differentiating malignant lesions from benign lesion. In one study apparent diffusion coefficient (ADC) values of the tumors were found to be significantly lower than benign lesions. Also, the ADC

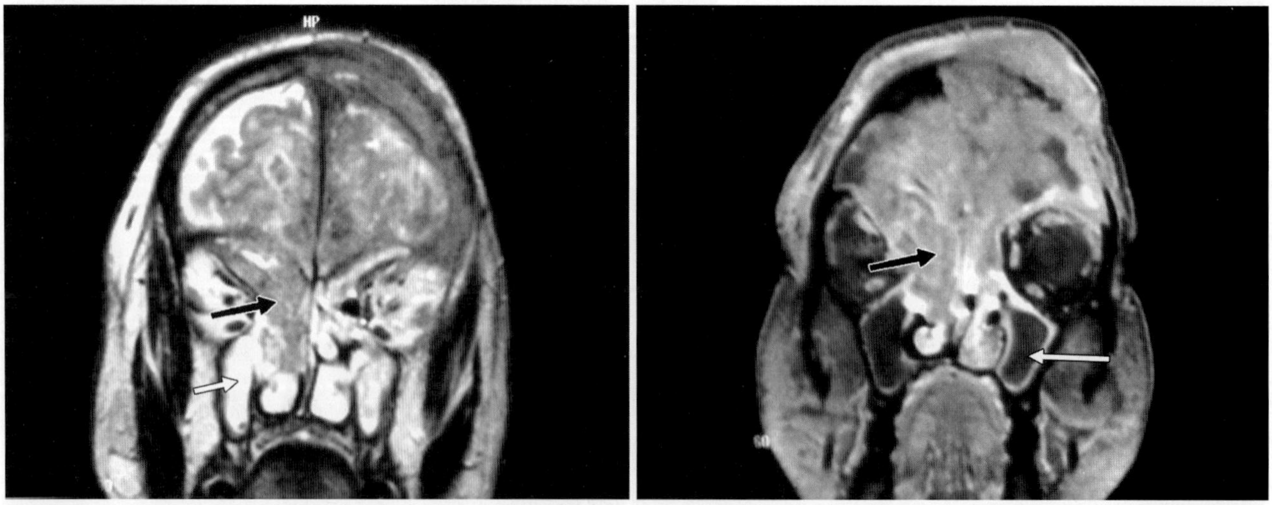

FIG. 29B: Coronal MRI images showing mass to be isointense on T2WI which enhances on post contrast images (black arrows). MRI show extensive lesion with aggressive behavior infiltrating into the right orbit, frontal sinuses and frontal bone diploe. Also seen are intensely bright maxillary sinuses (short white arrow) on T2WI which do not enhance suggestive of postobstructive changes. Note normal thin mucosal enhancement of maxillary sinuses (long white arrow).

values were inversely related to the lesions cellularity.[38] In an another study of 55 patients, the mean ADC value of nasal and paranasal sinus malignant lesions were significantly different from that of benign lesions. Also, there was a significant ADC difference between carcinoma and sarcoma as well as between well differentiated and poorly differentiated malignancies.[39]

Imaging is also important in the assessment of operability of sinonasal tumors. There are the following five general criteria for non-resectability:[32]

1. Distant metastases
2. Optic chiasm invasion
3. Extensive cerebral involvement
4. Bilateral carotid infiltration
5. Very poor general health.

Papillomas arise from the pseudociliated columnar epithelium of the nasal cavity and PNS. They are of three types:

1. Fungiform papillomas
2. Inverted papillomas
3. Cylindric cell papillomas.

Fungiform papillomas constitute 50% of papillomas. The nasal septum is the most common site for fungiform papillomas. They have a verrucous appearance and are not premalignant.

Inverted papillomas constitute 47% of papillomas. They are also called endophytic papillomas. They are unilateral, arise from the lateral nasal wall near the middle turbinate and tend to invade the antrum and ethmoids **(Fig. 30)**. They have a propensity to recur after local resection. They appear typically hyperintense on T2WI. Three to twenty-four percent show malignant transformation.

On MRI, the lesion is typically isointense to muscle on T1WI and is isointense to hypointense on T2WI. A crenated or convoluted enhancement is typical.

Recurrences may be distinguished from postoperative thickening by dynamic enhanced MRI. Recurrent inverted papillomas have earlier and greater enhancement than granulation tissue.

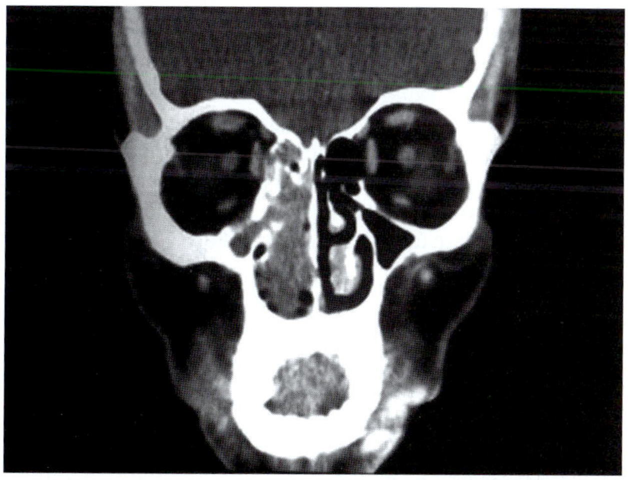

FIG. 30: Inverted papilloma of the right antrum and ethmoids: Non-contrast CT scan shows a hyperdense soft tissue lesion in the right ethmoid and nasal cavity extending into the right antrum. The middle turbinate is destroyed and the septum shows focal erosion. The floor and medial wall of the orbit is eroded at places.

Staging classification for inverted papillomas was proposed by Krause which was later modified by Cannady.[40] The modified Krause staging are as follows:

A. Inverted papilloma (IP) confined to the nasal cavity, ethmoid sinus, or medial maxillary wall.
B. Inverted papilloma with involvement of any maxillary wall (other than the medial wall) or frontal sinus or sphenoid sinus.
C. Inverted papilloma with extension beyond the PNS.

The significance of the staging is that, Stage A lesions may need only endoscopic resection while the more radical approaches reserved for stage B or C lesions.

Cylindric cell papillomas are the rarest of the papillomas and arise from the lateral nasal wall. Imaging findings are nonspecific, lesions vary in appearance as polypoid masses in the nasal cavity to expansile masses causing invasion of adjacent sinuses. Bony margins of nasal cavity are remodeled. Nasal septum is intact.[40,41]

Epithelial Tumors of Glandular Origin

These lesions originate in the minor salivary glands and constitute 10% of all sinonasal tumors. These glands can occur anywhere within the sinonasal cavity; however, the most common site of these glands is within the palate and therefore these lesions can extend into the PNS and nasal cavity from this location. The histological types of tumors in this group are:

- Adenoid cystic carcinoma
- Adenocarcinoma
- Pleomorphic adenomas
- Mucoepidermoid carcinoma
- Acinic cell carcinoma

Amongst these the adenoid cystic carcinoma are the most frequent tumors. This lesion typically causes destruction and remodeling of bone. Adenoid cystic carcinoma characteristically shows perineural and intraneural spread.[17] *Adenocarcinoma* is the name given to the heterogeneous group of neoplasm which does not fit into the classical feature of salivary tumor. They can be subclassified into various morphological subgroups such as mucinous, nonmucinous, clear cell, papillary, tubular and "intestinal type" tumors. These tumors expand bony margins and appear as relatively benign lesions on CT and MRI. High-grade adenocarcinoma invades and destroys bony margins whereas low grade tumors push the margins of bone ahead of them. High-grade adenocarcinomas appear to be of intermediate signal intensity on T2WI because of ill-defined glandular formation and severe nuclear pleomorphism. Low-grade adenocarcinoma appears to have higher signal intensity on T2WI because the cells form small, compact, uniformly glandular patterns.

NONEPITHELIAL TUMOR OF PARANASAL SINUSES

Nonepithelial tumors of the PNS and nasal cavity could be of soft tissue origin (e.g. angiofibroma, hemangioma, hemangiofibroma, hemangiopericytoma), bony/cartilaginous/

odontogenic tissues (e.g. fibrous dysplasia, chondromas myxomas), neuroectodermal origin (e.g. schwannomas and neurofibromas).

Developmental tumors (dermoids, teratomas), metastatic tumors (from the kidneys, lung and GI tract) are also classified into this group. Since this classification contains a wide variety of tumors only common lesions will be described in this section.

Angiofibroma

It is a benign, but locally invasive highly vascular, nonencapsulated neoplasm of the PNS. These tumors always originate near the pterygopalatine fossa. Patients are almost exclusively adolescent males between the ages of 10–20 years. The tumor spreads into the maxillary, ethmoid and sphenoid sinus and also into the infratemporal fossa and nasal cavity. These are highly vascular tumors and are supplied from the internal maxillary and ascending pharyngeal arteries. It can invade the orbit through the inferior orbital fissure or have an intracranial extension via the superior orbital fissure, pterygoid canal and foramen rotundum. On plain X-rays the characteristic sign of anterior bowing of the posterolateral wall of the maxillary sinus **(Fig. 31)** widening of thepterygopalatine fossa and soft tissue density filling the nasopharynx and sphenoid sinus are pathognomonic of this lesion. On plain CT these tumors appear to be slightly isohyperdense on plain scans and show intense enhancement following contrast administration. On dynamic CT the enhancement shows an early peak which characterizes the highly vascular nature of the tumor.

On MRI, these lesions appear as a mass of low to intermediate signal intensity on T1WI and PDI and as intermediate to high signal intensity on T2WI and gradient echo scans. Multiple flow voids within the mass represent vessels within the lesion. There is marked enhancement noted after Gd-DTPA administration **(Fig. 32)**. Imaging studies are required to assess the extent of the tumor, especially when intracranial and intraorbital spread is present.[42] Angiography is necessary to demonstrate: (i) the feeding vessels, (ii) to assess cross circulation from contralateral evaluation of intracranial aneurysms (ECA), and (iii) to assess feeding from the internal carotid artery in cases of intracranial spread and for preoperative embolization. The latter is helpful in reduction of blood loss during surgery.[43]

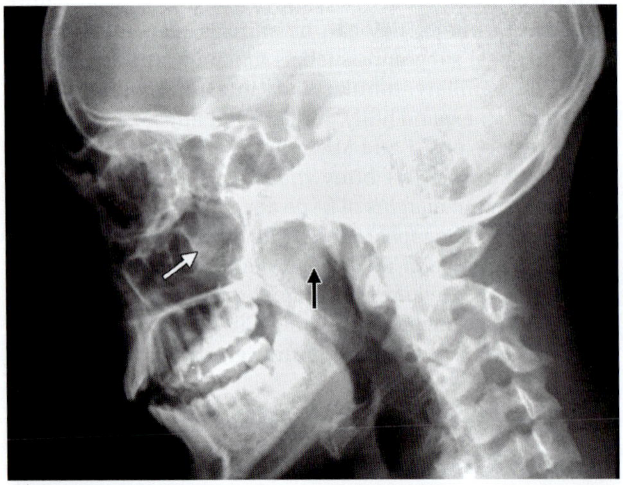

FIG. 31: Angiofibroma lateral X-ray of skull showing anterior bowing (white arrow) of the posterolateral wall of the maxillary sinus due to the angiofibroma (black arrow).

Lymphomas

Forty-seven percent of non-Hodgkin's lymphomas are found in the head and neck; 90% of these are in the cervical lymph nodes. Though the nasopharyngeal region surrounded by the Waldeyer's ring is a potential site of lymphoma, actual involvement of the sinonasal cavity is rare. Lymphomas arising in the nose and PNS are of the non-Hodgkin's type and are seen in cases of disseminated lymphoma. They occur with or without nodal disease. Lesions may be mistaken for sinusitis, polyposis and granulomatous processes. Clinically they may be confused with infection, granulomatous or nonlymphomatous neoplastic processes. On CT and MRI they are seen as bulky masses which show moderate enhancement. The osseous changes include remodeling, expansion, erosion and infiltration of the sinus walls. Primary lymphoma of the paranasal sinus is uncommon. In a study of seven patients of primary maxillary lymphomas, it was found that periantral soft tissue infiltration was the most consistent finding seen in all the patients with some degree of lytic or permeative bony destruction. Mucosal thickening may be mild or in the form of a mass.[44]

Plasmacytoma

Plasma cell neoplasm can be grouped into multiple myeloma, solitary plasmacytoma of bone and extramedullary plasmacytoma (EMP). Of these EMP are the plasma cell tumors which are predominantly seen in the sinonasal region. Only 5% of multiple myeloma cases present with sinonasal lesions. EMP accounts for 20% of plasma cell neoplasm. It is confined to soft tissue and there is no generalized bone involvement or systemic manifestation. It may arise in the sinonasal cavity and nasopharynx, sphenoid sinus, petrous ridge, base of skull and clivus.

Plasmacytoma of the sinonasal tract appears on CT as a well-defined expansile mass. There is associated bone erosion or remodeling. These tumors show moderate to marked enhancement after contrast administration.

On MRI, T1WI reveal a mass of low to intermediate signal intensity and moderate contrast enhancement and T2WI show intermediate to high signal intensity.[43]

Rhabdomyosarcoma is the most common soft tissue sarcoma. Thirty-five to forty-five percent of rhabdomyosarcoma occurs in the head and neck. It primarily affects infants and children. Peak incidence is in the 2–5 years age group with a second peak between 15 years and 19 years of age. Forty-three percent of cases are under 5 years, and 78% of cases are under the age of 12 years. Histopathologically, they are classified as embryonal, differentiated or alveolar. Embryonal rhabdomyosarcoma is the most common type and arises from primitive muscle cells. They have a potential for metastases to lymph nodes. The alveolar rhabdomyosarcoma occurs in older patients in the age range of 15–25 years.

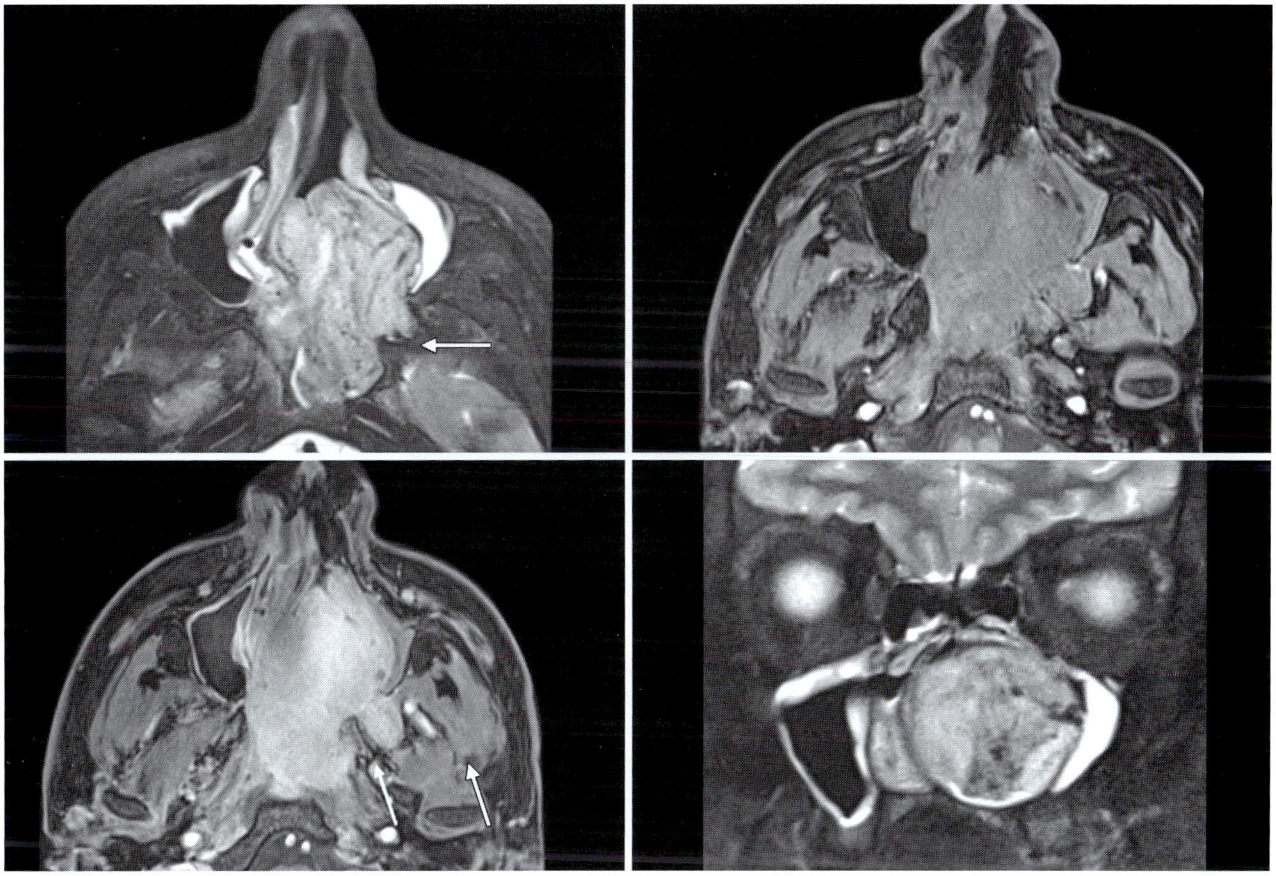

FIG. 32: Nasopharyngeal angiofibroma originating near the pterygopalatine fossa (white arrows) and extending posteriorly into nasopharynx and anteriorly into nasal cavity.

The diagnosis of these two types is difficult. Differentiated rhabdomyosarcoma is the least frequent and most easy to diagnose by histopathology. CT findings are of homogenous soft tissue density mass with moderate enhancement. MRI findings are those of a mass of intermediate signal intensity on all sequences. Bone destruction or remodeling is usually seen.

Olfactory Neuroblastoma (Olfactory Neuroepithelioma/Esthesioneuroblastoma)

It is a rare tumor of neuroectodermal origin that arises from the neural crest. It is located in superior nasal fossa and presents as a polypoid tumor which bleeds profusely when biopsied.

Age incidence has characteristically 2 peaks, the first during 11–22 years and the second in the 50–60 years age group.

Both contrast enhanced CT and MRI are required in the preoperative assessment of these patients to assess intracranial extension into the frontal lobe and dural involvement.

CT imaging shows a homogenous mass with moderate to marked enhancement **(Fig. 33)**. On MRI, they are hypointense to brain on T1WI and hyperintense to brain on T2WI. Sometimes, they may be in homogenous with areas of cystic degeneration. Calcification within these tumors is reported.[10,35,36]

Neurogenic Tumors

Peripheral nerve sheath tumors can be of three types: (i) schwannomas, (ii) neurofibromas, and (iii) neurogenic sarcomas. These tumors usually arise from sensory nerves. In the sinonasal cavity, neurogenic tumors arise from the first and second division of trigeminal nerve and from the autonomic nerves. The olfactory nerve has no Schwann cells. So these tumors cannot arise from this site. Schwannomas are encapsulated, benign, slow growing masses. They are in frequent in nasal cavity, being found in the nasal fossa, maxillary and ethmoidal sinuses. They can be completely excised from the nerve from which they originate.

On CT they appear as well defined, homogenous masses with moderate enhancement after contrast administration. They may be inhomogeneous as well as cystic in appearance occasionally.

On MRI, schwannomas show low to intermediate signal intensity on T1WI and high signal on T2WI with moderate to marked enhancement after contrast administration. They may show varied signal characteristics depending on their

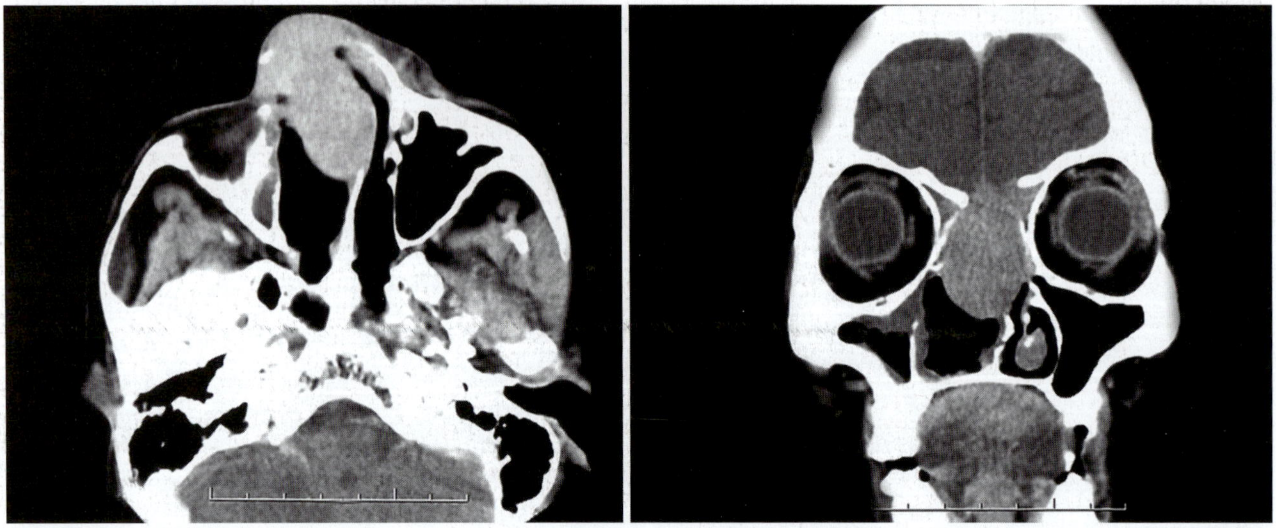

FIG. 33: Olfactory neuroblastoma: Axial and coronal contrast-enhanced CT section showing a uniformly enhanced mass in the right nasal cavity extending from the superior nasal fossa up to the inferior turbinate, the thinned out nasal septum bulges to the left. There is erosion of the right fovea ethmoidalis and the cribriform plate.

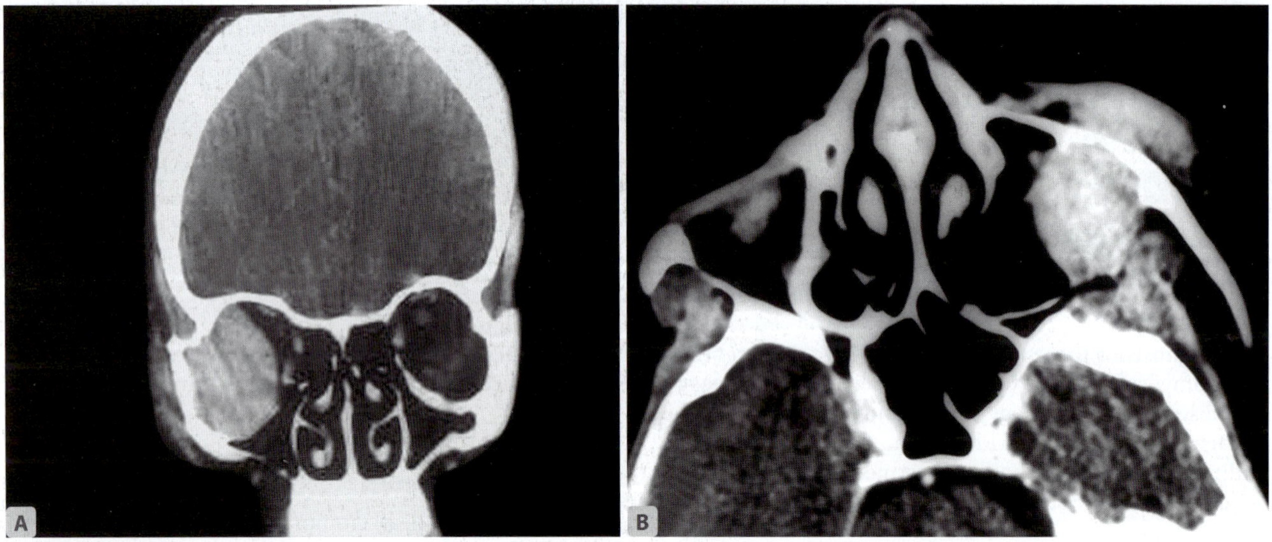

FIGS. 34A AND B: (A) Axial; and (B) Coronal contrast enhanced scan for a neurofibroma. A homogeneous hyperdense soft tissue mass is present in the right temporal quadrants of the left orbit. The orbital walls are remodeled and the lesion projects into the right maxillary antrum and the cheek.

histologic patterns and the presence or absence of cystic as well as cholesterol degeneration. Presence of aggressive bone destruction should be considered as an indication of malignant transformation.[45]

Neurofibromas

Neurofibromas are benign, nonencapsulated nerve sheath tumors. These are seen in the constellation of tumor of neurofibromatosis or Von Recklinghausen's disease.

They have a variable appearance on CT with areas of fatty infiltration and cystic degeneration. Bone remodeling is seen rather than aggressive bone destruction **(Figs. 34A and B)**. On MRI they are usually nonhomogeneous with an intermediate T1WI signal intensity and a higher T2WI signal intensity.[46]

FIBROSSEOUS LESIONS OF CRANIOFACIAL BONES[47,48]

Fibrosseous lesions of craniofacial bones constitute 25% of nonepithelial neoplasm of this region. They are a varied group of pathologic conditions which are difficult to classify. A common denominator to all these lesions is the replacement of the bone with a benign fibrous tissue containing various amounts of mineralized (calcified) structures.

Osteoma

Osteomas are benign lesions which are commonly seen in the skull and facial bones. These tumors are small usually solitary. These are located within the sinus cavity. The most common sinus affected is the frontal sinus followed by ethmoid, maxillary and sphenoid sinus. They are usually silent lesions and found incidentally on plain X-rays. Their radiopacity is determined by the amount of mature bone within them. On CT scans they are seen to arise from the sinus wall. The cancellous bone and fibrous matrix can be distinguished on CT **(Fig. 35)**. On MRI they may be undetected due to absence of any signal from their bony matrix. Multiple osteomas of the skull and mandible are seen in patients of Gardner syndrome. Osteomas may obstruct the outflow of the frontal sinus. Cerebrospinal fluid (CSF) rhinorrhea may be associated with these tumors.

Fibrous dysplasia is an idiopathic skeletal disorder in which medullary bone is replaced by a dysplastic fibrosseous tissue which is composed of woven type of bone with few osteoclasts. Osteoblasts are typically absent except near the area of transition to normal bone. Some authors consider it to be a hamartomatous malformation that presumably results from an idiopathic arrest in the maturation of bone at the woven bone stage.

It is a condition of young adults affecting males and females equally. It can occur at one skeletal site (monostotic) or at multiple sites (polyostotic). Seventy percent of cases are of the monostotic variety, rest being polyostotic. Monostotic fibrous dysplasia does not progress to the polyostotic form of the disease. The process may involve the facial bones, skull bones or both. Polyostotic fibrous dysplasia may be associated with endocrinopathies (3–5% of all cases). This disease if accompanied by skin pigmentations (Café au lait spots) ipsilateral to osseous involvement, and precocious puberty in girls is referred to as Albright's syndrome. Other endocrine disorders that have been identified include hyperparathyroidism, Cushing's syndrome, hyperthyroidism and acromegaly.

The common site in the facial skeleton is the maxilla and mandible amounts to 12% cases of fibrous dysplasia. The most common presentation is with a painless bony swelling causing facial asymmetry. Visual compromise can occur when the sphenoethmoidal complex is involved. Hearing disturbances are present when the temporal bone is involved. The radiographic appearance of fibrous dysplasia is that of diffuse areas of sclerosis termed as ground glass appearance. The affected bones are wide and thick. The lesions if large do not have sharply defined margins. CT appearance of fibrous dysplasia is that of an expanded bone of heterogeneous density. CT attenuation depends on the amount of fibrous tissue and bone present in the affected region **(Figs. 36A and B)**.

On MRI, fibrous dysplasia exhibits an intermediate signal on T1WI and PDWI and heterogeneous hypointense signal on T2WI. With Gd-DTPA the lesions may show moderate to marked contrast enhancement.

Ossifying Fibroma

Ossifying fibroma is a well circumscribed fibrous tumor which ossifies in time. Ossification begins from the periphery of the tumor and progresses to the core. The newly formed bone is of the woven type initially and later matures into lamellar bone. On CT, lesions appear somewhat similar to fibrous dysplasia but have larger areas of unossified fibrous tissues **(Fig. 37)**. They may be indistinguishable from lesions of fibrous dysplasia on histopathological studies. However, these lesions tend to be more aggressive than fibrous dysplasia as they grow inward to involve the orbits nasal cavities and the sinus, leaving the surface contours of bones intact.

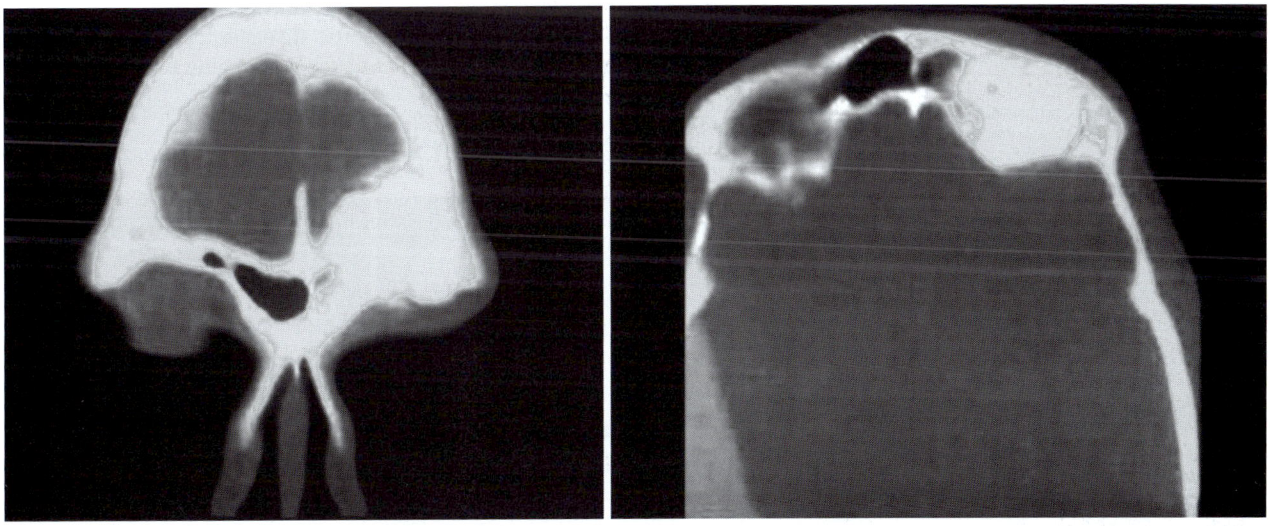

FIG. 35: Osteoma of the left frontal sinus. Axial and coronal CT scans showing a dense bony lesion of the left sinus occupying much of the sinus cavity leaving only a thin rim of air around it.

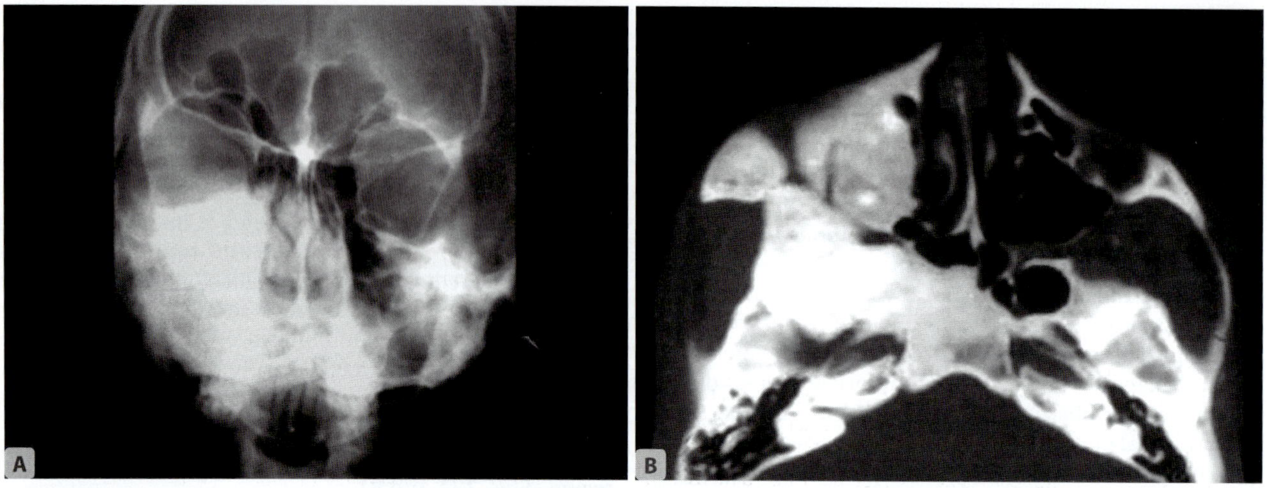

FIGS. 36A AND B: (A) Fibrous dysplasia: Plain X-ray of the skull PA view shows the typical ground glass appearance of the expanded bones of the right side of the face. Note the dimensions of the right orbit are reduced; (B) Axial CT shows the expanded and dense right maxilla, zygoma and sphenoid bones. The right maxillary sinus and the right side of the sphenoid sinus are obliterated. There is relative sparing of the nasal cavities and ethmoids with distortion of the facial contour.

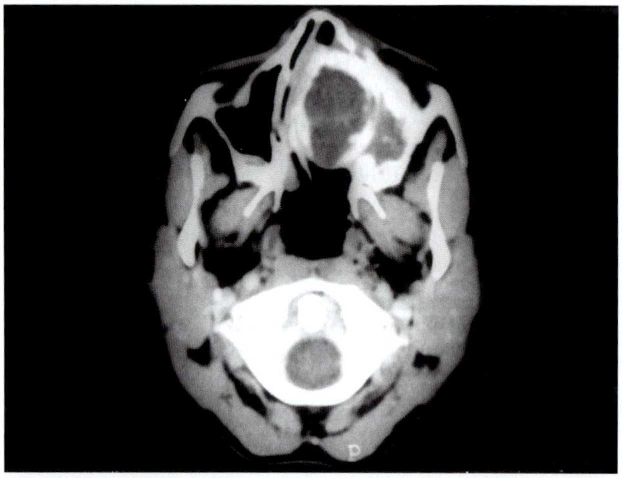

FIG. 37: Ossifying fibroma of the left maxilla: The core of the lesions isodense to muscle, the peripheral zone shows a well ossified structure. The lesion expands toward the median plane, and the facial contour is relatively preserved as compared to fibrous dysplasia (above).

Paget's Disease

Paget's disease affects patients above the age of 50 years. Involvement of the spine calvarium is common and seen in 76% and 65% of cases respectively. Involvement of the facial skeleton is rare. When the sinonasal cavity and orbits are affected signs of neurovascular compromise can develop.

Metastatic lesions to the PNS arise from primaries form the kidneys, lung, breast and GI tract.[49,50] Uncommon primary malignancies metastasizing to the PNS are from the cervix and liver. Clinical presentation is not unlike primary PNS carcinomas as are the imaging findings. Metastases from the breast, lung, GI tract, distal genitourinary tract are aggressive lesions which destroy bony boundaries **(Figs. 38A to C)**. Secondaries from melanoma and renal cell carcinoma appear as enhancing lesions which remodel and destroy sinonasal walls. Multifocal erosion lesions with normal bone are suggestive of metastatic disease; however, a solitary metastatic lesion has nonspecific imaging findings.[11]

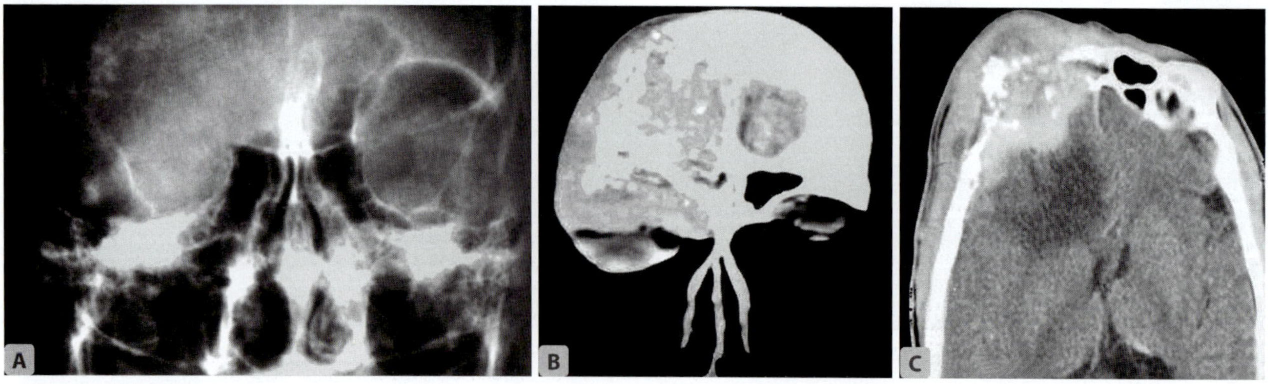

FIGS. 38A TO C: Metastases from carcinoma gallbladder: (A) Detail from X-ray skull shows a soft tissue density lesion causing destruction of the right and superior orbital rim and the bony outline of the right frontal sinus; (B) Coronal contrast enhanced sections show destruction of the frontal bone; (C) Axial sections of the study showing intracranial extension as well as involvement of the soft tissues of the forehead.

REFERENCES

1. Williams JW, Roberts L, Distell B, et al. Diagnosing sinusitis by X-ray: is a single waters view adequate? J Gen Intern Med. 1992;7(5):481-5.
2. McAlister WH, Lusk R, Muntz HR. Comparison of plain radiographs and coronal CT scans in infants and children with recurrent sinusitis. Am J Roentgenol. 1989;153(6):1259-64.
3. Lazar RH, Younis RT, Parvey LS. Comparison of plain radiographs, coronal CT, and intraoperative findings in children with chronic sinusitis. Otolaryngol Head Neck Surg. 1992;107(1):29-34.
4. Burke TF, Guertler AT, Timmons JH. Comparison of Sinus X-rays with computed tomography scans in acute sinusitis. Acad Emerg Med. 1994;1(3):235-9.
5. Gotwald TF, Zinreich SJ, Corl F, et al. Three-dimensional volumetric display of the nasal ostiomeatal channels and paranasal sinuses. Am J Roentgenol. 2001;176(1):241-5.
6. Bisdas S, Verink M, Burmeister HP, et al. Three-dimensional visualization of the nasal cavity and paranasal sinuses clinical results of a standardized approach using multislice helical computed tomography. J Comput Assist Tomogr. 2004;28:661-9.
7. Lin HW, Bhattacharyya N. Diagnostic and staging accuracy of magnetic resonance imaging for the assessment of sinonasal disease. Am J Rhinol Allergy. 2009;23(1):36-9.
8. Lloyd GAS, Lund VJ, Phelps PD, et al. Magnetic resonance imaging in the evaluation of nose and paranasal sinus disease. Br J Radiology. 1987;60(718):957-68.
9. Vogl JJ, Mack MG, Juergens M, Stark M, et al. MR diagnosis of head and neck tumours: comparison of contrast enhancement with triple dose gadodiamide and standard dose gadopentate dimeglumine in the same patient. Am J Roentgenol. 1994;163(2):425-32.
10. Oliverio PJ, Benson ML, Zeinrich SJ. Update on imaging for functional endoscopic surgery. Otolarynaging, 4th editiongol Clin North Am. 1995;28(3):585-608.
11. Grossman RI, Youserm DM. Sinonasal disease. In: Grossman RI, Yousem DM (Eds). Neuroradiology: the Requisites, 2nd edition. Philadelphia: Mosby; 2003.
12. Zeinrich SJ, Albayrams S, Benson ML, et al. Sinonasal cavities: the osteomeatal complex and functional endoscopic surgery. In: Som PM and Curton HD (Eds). Head and Neck Im. St. Louis Mosby-Year Book, 2003.
13. Mafee MF. Preoperative Imaging: anatomy of nasal ethmoid complex for functional endoscopic sinus surgery. Radiologic Clin North Am. 1993;31(1):1-20.
14. Som PM, Brandwein MS. Sinonasal cavities: inflammatory diseases. In: Som PM, Curton HD (Eds). Head and Neck Imaging, 14th edition. St Louis: Mosby Year Book; 2003.
15. Hoang JK, Eastwood JD, Tebbit CL, et al. Multiplanar sinus CT: a systematic approach to imaging before functional endoscopic sinus surgery. Am J Roentgenol. 2010;194(6):W527-36.
16. O'Brien WT Sr, Hamelin S, Weitzel EK. The Preoperative Sinus CT: Avoiding a "CLOSE" Call with Surgical Complications. Radiology. 2016;281(1):10-21.
17. Som PM, Curtin HD. Chronic inflammatory sinonasal disease including fungal infection. The role of imaging. Radiologic Clin North America. 1993;31(1):33-44.
18. Babbel R, Harnsberger HR, Nelson B, et al. Optimization of techniques in screening CT of the sinuses. Am J Neuroradiol. 1991;12(5):849-54.
19. Som PM, Curtin HD. Sinuses. In: Stark DD, Bradley WG (Jr) (Eds). Magnetic Resonance Imaging, 2nd edition. St. Louis: Mosby Year Book; 1992. pp. 1113-34.
20. Sonkens JW, Harnsberger HR, Blanch GM, et al. Hunt S. The impact of screening sinus CT on the planning of functional endoscopic sinus surgery. Otolaryngol Head Neck Surg. 1991;105(6):802-13.
21. Hahnel S, Ertl-Wagner B, Tasman AJ, et al. Relative value of MR imaging as compared with CT in the diagnosis of inflammatory paranasal sinus disease. Radiology. 1999;210(1):171-6.
22. Som PM, Dillon WP, Fullerton GD, et al. et al. Chronically obstructed sinus secretions: observations on T1 and T2 shortening. Radiology. 1989;172(2):515-20.
23. Perugini S, Pasquini U, Menichelli F, et al. Mucoceles in the paranasal sinuses involving the orbit CT signs in 43 cases. Neuroradiology. 1982;23(3):133-9.
24. Osborn AG, Johnson L, Roberts TS. Sphenoidal mucoceles with intracranial extension. J Comput Assist Tomogr. 1979;3(3):335-8.
25. Lanzieri CF, Shah M, Kraun D, et al. Use of gadolinium enhanced MR imaging for differentiating mucoceles from neoplasm in the paranasal sinuses. Radiology. 1991;178(2):425-8.
26. Centono RS, Bentson JR, Mancuso AA. CT scanning in rhinocerebral mucormycosis and aspergillosis. Radiology. 1981;140(2):383-9.
27. Kingdom TT, Tami TA. Actinomycosis of the nasal septum in a patient infected with HIV. Otolaryngol Head and Neck Surgery. 1994;71:675-7.
28. Bath AP, O'Flynn P, Gibbin KP. Nasopharyngeal tuberculosis. J Laryngol Otol. 1992;71:675-7.
29. Sharma VK, Bapuraj JR, Kumar B, et al. Computed tomographic surgery of paranasal sinuses in lepromatous leprosy. International Journal of Leprosy. 1998;66(2):201-7.
30. Lohrmann C, Uhl M, Warnatz K, et al. Sinonasal computed tomography in patients with Wegener's granulomatosis. J Comput Assist Tomogr. 2006;30(1):122-5.
31. Sakai S, Fuchilate H, Hamasaki Y. Treatment policy of maxillary sinus carcinoma. Acta Otolaryngol (Stockh). 1976;82(3-4):172-81.
32. Lund VS, Howard DJ, Lloyd GAS. CT evaluation of paranasal sinus tumor for craniofacial resection. Br J Radiol. 1983;56(667):439-46.
33. Barnes L, Verbin RS, Gnepp DR. Disease of the nose, paranasal sinuses and nasopharynx. In: Barnex L (Ed). Surgical Pathology of the Head and Neck. New York: Marcel Dekker Inc; 1985. pp.403-51.
34. Momose KJ, Weber ALM, Goodman M, et al. Radiological aspects of inverted papilloma. Radiology. 1980;134(1):73-9.
35. Lund VS, Howard DJ, Loyd GAS, et al. Magnetic resonance imaging of paranasal sinus tumor for craniofacial resection. Head Neck. 1989;11(3):279-83.
36. Chow JM, Leonetti JP, Mafee MF. Epithelial tumours of the paranasal sinuses and nasal cavities. Radiological Clinics of North America. 1993;31(1):61-73.
37. Hunink MGM, de Slegte RGM, Gerritsen GJ, et al. CT and MR assessment of tumours of the nose and paranasal sinuses, the nasopharynx and parapharyngeal space using ROC methodology. Neuroradiology. 1990;32(3):220-5.
38. White ML, Zhang Y, Robinson RA. Evaluating tumors and tumorlike lesions of the nasal cavity, the paranasal sinuses, and the adjacent skull base with diffusion-weighted MRI. J Comput Assist Tomogr. 2006;30(3):490-5.
39. Razek AA, Sieza S, Maha B. Assessment of nasal and paranasal sinus masses by diffusion-weighted MR imaging. J Neuroradiol. 2009;36(4):206-11.
40. Cannady SB, Batra PS, Sautter NB, et al. New staging system for sinonasal inverted papilloma in the endoscopic era. Laryngoscope. 2007;117(7):1283-7.

41. Yousem DM, Fellows DW, Kermedy DW, et al. Inverted papilloma evaluation with MR imaging. Radiology. 1992;185(2):501-5.
42. Bryan RN, Serrons RB, Horowitz BL. Radiographic management of juvenile angiofibroma. AJNR. 1981;2(2):157-66.
43. Mafee MF. Nonepithelial tumours of the paranasal sinuses and nasal cavity: role of CT and MR imaging. Radio Clin North Am. 1993;31(1):75-90.
44. Yasumoto M, Taura S, Shibuya H, et al. Primary malignant lymphoma of the maxillary sinus: CT and MRI. Neuroradiology. 2000;42(4):285-9.
45. Derdeyn CP, Moran CJ, Wippold FJ, et al. MRI of esthesioneuroblastoma. JCAT. 1994;18(1):16-21.
46. Jellquist HB, Lundgren J. Neurogenic sarcoma of the sinonasal tract. J Laryngo Otol. 1991;105(3):186-90.
47. Mohammadi-Araghi H, Haery C. Fibrosseous lesions of the craniofacial bones. Radiologic Clinics of North America. 1993;31(1):121-34.
48. Rao VM, El-Noueam KJ. Sinonasal imaging. Radiol Clin North Am. 1998;36(5):921-39.
49. Som P, Norton K, Shugar J, et al. Metastatic hypernephroma to the head and neck. AJNR. 1987;8(6):1103-6.
50. Marchke DA, Mc Culloch TM, Nerad JA. Prostate cancer metastatic to the orbit. Ann Otol Rhinol Laryngol. 1996;105(1):70-1.

CHAPTER

203

Imaging of the Neck Spaces

Rashmi Dixit, Sapna Singh, Radhika Batra, Alpana Manchanda

The neck has a complex anatomy where many critical structures are compartmentalized into a small space. It is divided into various spaces and compartments by arrangement of the superficial and deep layers of the cervical fascia on the basis of pioneering work by anatomists. With the advent of cross-sectional imaging radiologists, clinicians and surgeons have adopted the spatial organization of the head and neck into fascial compartments.

A systematic approach and a sound grasp of this anatomic organization is essential in approaching neck masses. It is important to localize the space of origin or the epicenter of the lesion, which helps generate a differential diagnosis based upon the contents characteristic of each space. Alongwith imaging techniques, clinical history, physical examination and laboratory studies have a very important complementary role to help arrive at the correct diagnosis.[1,2]

This chapter presents a discussion of the various spaces of the neck alongwith the differential diagnosis relevant to that space according to its anatomical contents. Some lesions that are specific to a neck space are discussed alongwith the description of the space and lesions that may be common to various spaces are discussed later in the chapter.

The neck can be divided into two portions anatomically—**suprahyoid and infrahyoid neck**. The suprahyoid neck is the region of the neck that extends from the skull base superiorly to the hyoid bone inferiorly. The infrahyoid neck extends from the hyoid bone superiorly to the thoracic inlet inferiorly.

IMAGING MODALITIES

Plain radiographs were once the mainstay of diagnosis. Fractures, cervical spine abnormalities, airway compromise and calcification are well seen on plain radiographs. Soft tissue radiographs of the neck in the lateral position are used to delineate mass lesions but soft tissue interfaces are often not visualized optimally. Fistulous or sinus tracts are seen on **contrast examinations**.

Ultrasonography performed with a high frequency probe is excellent for visualization of superficial lesions and helps in differentiating solid from cystic lesions. It can also be used to evaluate the vessels of the neck and provides guidance for fine needle aspiration. Sonography is particularly useful in the pediatric age group.

Cross-sectional imaging with **computed tomography** and **magnetic resonance imaging** has greatly extended our understanding of this region. The entire head and neck region from the base of skull to the thoracic inlet is scanned with computed tomography (CT) or magnetic resonance imaging (MRI). Contrast-enhanced studies are performed to assess the vascularity of the lesion and opacify the arteries and veins. High quality three-dimensional reconstructions are useful in evaluating the extent of the lesion. Dynamic maneuvers during the scans are possible due to rapid acquisition by multislice scanners. Such maneuvers include:

a. Phonation (for better visualization of laryngeal ventricle).
b. Modified valsalva (for better visualization of the pyriform sinuses, postcricoid region and the gingivobuccal tumors).
c. Puffed cheek technique (to assess buccal and gingival mucosal involvement and other deeper involvement of oral vestibule).

CT perfusion imaging is a dynamic contrast enhanced technique for quantitative assessment of tissue microcirculation and is a noninvasive tool for the evaluation of microcirculatory changes associated with head and neck carcinomas.[3] A significant increase in blood flow (BF), blood volume (BV) and permeability surface area product alongwith a reduction in mean transit time (MTT) have been found in malignant tumors of head and neck. It can also be used for monitoring treatment response.

While imaging neck spaces on MRI, a combined head and neck coil is used for a comprehensive evaluation of the entire extracranial head and neck evaluating all the nodal masses, a second primary neoplasm and perineural tumor spread. In addition to the conventional contrast-enhanced MR, diffusion-weighted imaging (DWI) may also be performed. DWI is sensitive for detection of tumor recurrence after treatment and also helps in accurate lymph node staging.[4]

Similar to perfusion CT, **dynamic perfusion MRI** offers the potential of visualizing the tumor vascularity. Echo-planar imaging (EPI) or a volumetric interpolated breath-hold examination (VIBE) sequence are used and mean signal intensity versus time curves are plotted. Parameters such as peak time (in seconds), peak enhancement (percent baseline) and washout slope estimate can be obtained.

Proton magnetic resonance spectroscopy (MRS) is another promising technique wherein data can be acquired on the same scanner and with the same coils. Single voxel spin (SVS) echo sequence can be used and it allows detection of the choline signal which is increased in neoplastic tissue. Metastatic nodal disease also shows a higher choline concentration.[5]

PET-CT is useful for assessment of head and neck cancers. It helps to evaluate successful treatment of neoplasms, differentiate between tumor and scar and enables precise localization of the tumor. It also facilitates guided biopsy and allows accurate tissue sampling.[6]

FASCIAL LAYERS OF THE NECK

There are two layers of fascia in the neck, the superficial and deep layers **(Flowchart 1)**. The **superficial cervical fascia** is a thin layer that is comprised mainly of loose areolar connective tissue and adipose tissue. It extends from the head to the thorax and the shoulders to the axilla. It contains the platysma, muscles of facial expression, cutaneous nerves, blood vessels, and lymph nodes.

The **deep cervical fascia (DCF) or fascia colli** is divided into 3 layers **(Figs. 1A and B)**:

The superficial or investing layer of deep cervical fascia is the layer that lies between the superficial cervical fascia and the neck muscles. Anteriorly, it is attached to the hyoid bone and superiorly to the inferior border of the mandible, the mastoid process, the superior nuchal line, and the external occipital protuberance. It invests all the superficial structures of the neck.[7] It splits to enclose the sternocleidomastoid and trapezius muscles and merges posteriorly with the ligamentum nuchae. It splits again between the angle of the mandible and the mastoid process to enclose the parotid gland. Inferiorly, it is attached to the spine and acromion of the scapula, the clavicle, and the manubrium.[8]

The spaces enclosed are: (i) masticator space **(Figs. 2A and B)** (ii) parotid space **(Figs. 3A and B)** (iii) submandibular **(Fig. 4)** and sublingual spaces **(Figs. 5A and B)**.

The middle layer of deep cervical fascia—The extent of this layer ranges from the skull base superiorly to the mediastinum inferiorly and anteriorly from the hyoid bone to the thoracic inlet. It has two divisions: the muscular and visceral. The muscular division encloses the strap muscles—the sternohyoid, sternothyroid, omohyoid, and thyrohyoid. It blends with the superficial layer of deep cervical fascia over the sternocleidomastoid muscle. The visceral division, also known as the *buccopharyngeal fascia* in the suprahyoid neck, encloses the pharynx, larynx, esophagus, trachea, thyroid, parathyroid glands, periesophageal lymph nodes and the recurrent laryngeal nerve. Posteriorly this layer attaches to the prevertebral fascia and fuses with the investing fascia at the lateral margins of the infrahyoid muscles.[9]

The spaces enclosed are: (i) pharyngeal mucosal space **(Figs. 6A and B)** (ii) parapharyngeal space **(Figs. 7A and B)** (iii) retropharyngeal space **(Figs. 8A and B)** and (iv) buccal space.

The deep layer of deep cervical fascia surrounds the deep muscles of the neck and the cervical vertebrae. It extends from the skull base into the mediastinum (to the third thoracic vertebra, it fuses in the midline with the anterior longitudinal

FLOWCHART 1: Cervical fascial layers.

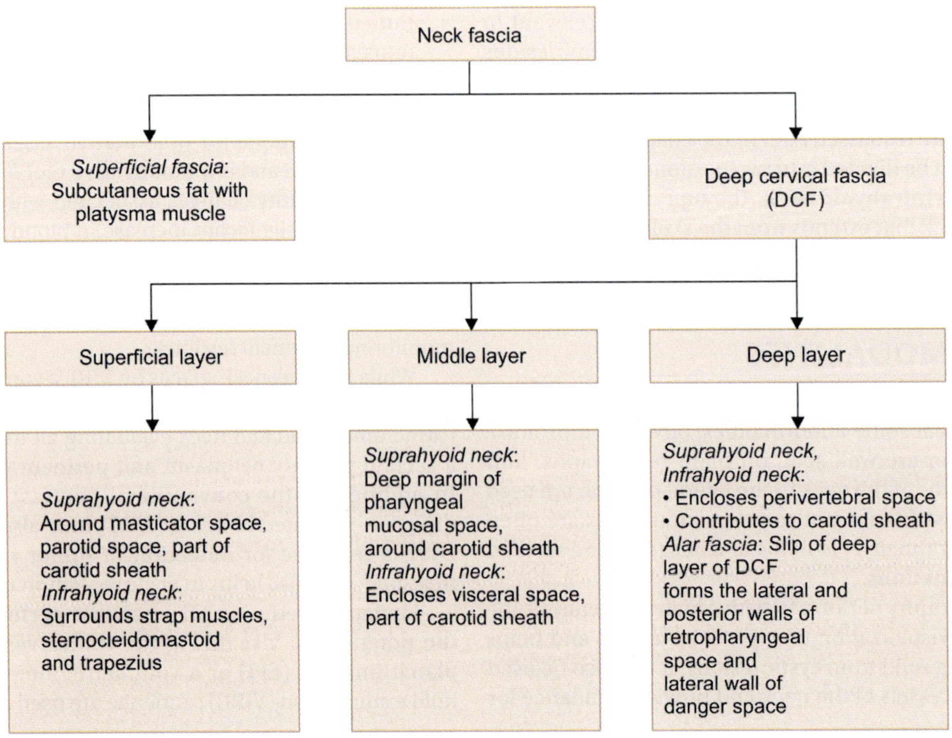

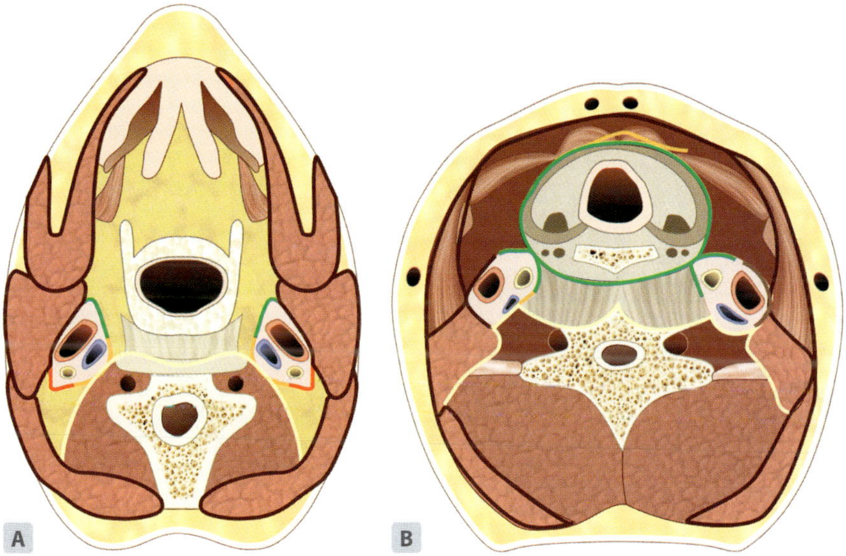

FIGS. 1A AND B: Deep cervical fascia in suprahyoid (A) and infrahyoid (B) neck in axial plane; superficial layer of deep cervical fascia is outlined in red, middle layer of deep cervical fascia is outlined in green and deep layer of deep cervical fascia is outlined in orange color.

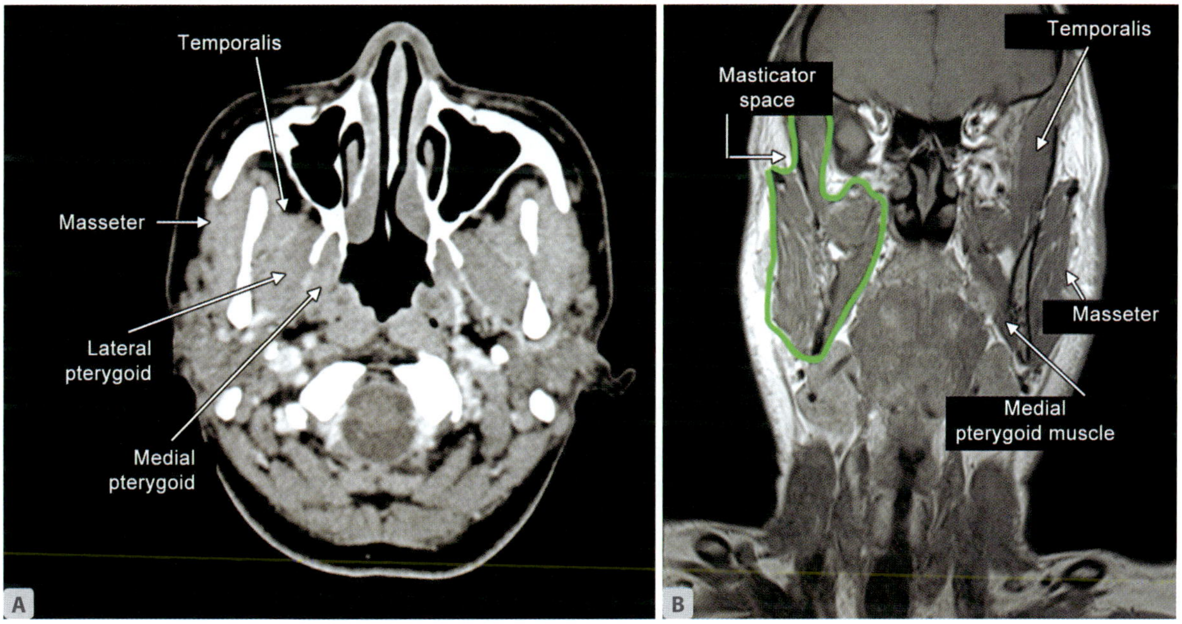

FIGS. 2A AND B: Axial CECT (A) and coronal T1W MR (B) images show the masticator space containing muscles of mastication and ramus of mandible.

ligament in front of T3 vertebral body) and has two divisions: the alar and prevertebral layers. The alar layer contributes to the posterior and lateral walls of the retropharyngeal space and bridges the transverse processes of the vertebrae. The prevertebral layer encircles the paraspinal muscles: the longus colli and longus capitis muscles; the anterior, middle, and posterior scalene muscles; and the levator scapulae. The brachial plexus trunks, phrenic nerve, cervical plexus, vertebral artery and vertebral vein are also surrounded by the prevertebral fascia with the cervical sympathetic trunk fixed into the anterior part of the fascia.[9] The spaces enclosed extend through the suprahyoid and infrahyoid neck. These are the (i) carotid space **(Fig. 9)** (ii) retropharyngeal space (iii) danger space (iv) perivertebral space **(Fig. 10)** and (v) the posterior cervical space **(Fig. 11)**.

Within the infrahyoid neck the three layers of DCF form two additional spaces (i) visceral space **(Figs. 12A and B)** and (ii) the anterior cervical space. **Table 1** lists the various spaces of the neck.

MASTICATOR SPACE

These are paired spaces located in the anterolateral aspect of suprahyoid neck. The superficial layer of DCF splits to

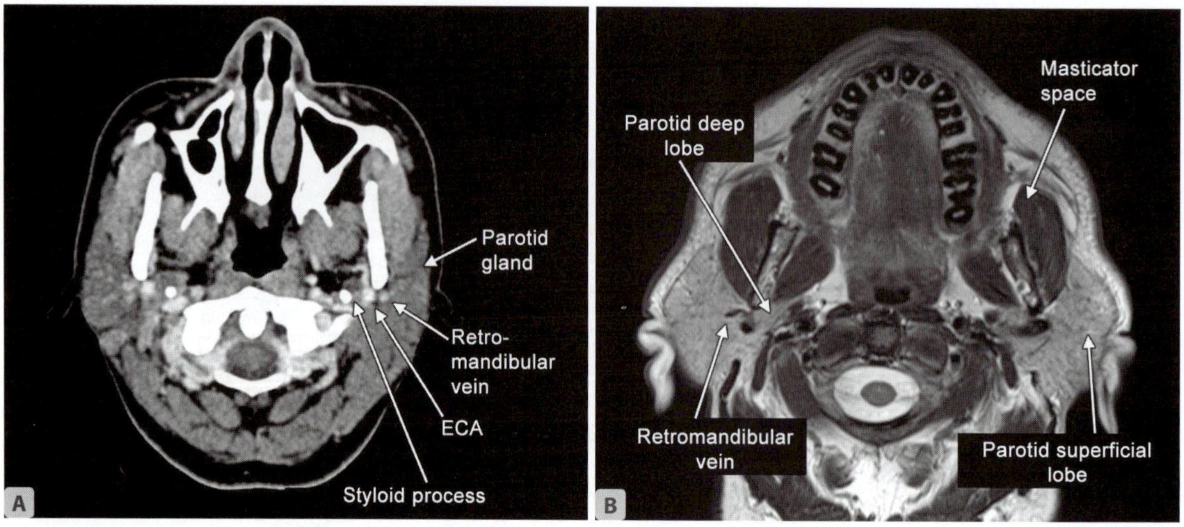

FIGS. 3A AND B: Axial CECT (A) and axial T2W MR (B) images show the parotid space containing superficial and deep lobes of parotid gland, ECA and retromandibular vein.

enclose the muscles of mastication and forms the borders of this space. The masticator space (MS) extends inferiorly to the attachment of the medial pterygoid and masseter muscles to the mandible. Its superomedial margin is at the skull base and includes soft tissues inferior to the foramen ovale. Therefore, any malignancy involving the MS can extend to the cavernous sinus via retrograde perineural extension along the mandibular division of trigeminal nerve (V3).

The **contents (Table 2)** of this space are, therefore, the muscles of mastication (medial and lateral pterygoid muscles, masseter and temporalis), posterior body and ramus of mandible, pterygoid venous plexus and V3 and its branches.[1] **(*see* Figs. 2A and B)**.

The most common **lesions** in the masticator space are dental tumors, cysts and abscesses. Other lesions include osteomyelitis **(Figs. 14A and B)**, nerve sheath tumors, lipomas, vascular lesions such as hemangiomas, lymphatic malformations and rarely pseudoaneurysms. Mandibular and soft tissue sarcomas **(Figs. 15A and B)** can also arise in the masticator space including rhabdomyosarcoma in children.

Mandibular nerve denervation atrophy of the muscles of mastication on one side makes the opposite normal side look like pseudolesion. Accessory parotid gland may appear as a lesion over the surface of masseter muscle. Unilateral or bilateral masseteric hypertrophy may also appear as a pseudomass.[10]

The masticator space is divided by a transaxial plane passing through the notch between coronoid and condyloid process. Disease above this plane is classified as 'supranotch' and below it as 'infranotch' disease. The supranotch compartment includes the lateral pterygoid muscle, tendon of temporalis and upper two-thirds of the pterygoid plates. The infranotch compartment includes the bulk of masseter, medial pterygoid muscle and lower part of the pterygoid plates. This classification is relevant in evaluation of disease spread in oral squamous cell carcinomas. In oral carcinomas, spread of disease above or below the notch has an implication on resectability and good results have been reported in patients with extension of disease below the notch. Therefore, description of disease extension according to this classification by radiologists is useful as infranotch masticator space disease is resectable.[11]

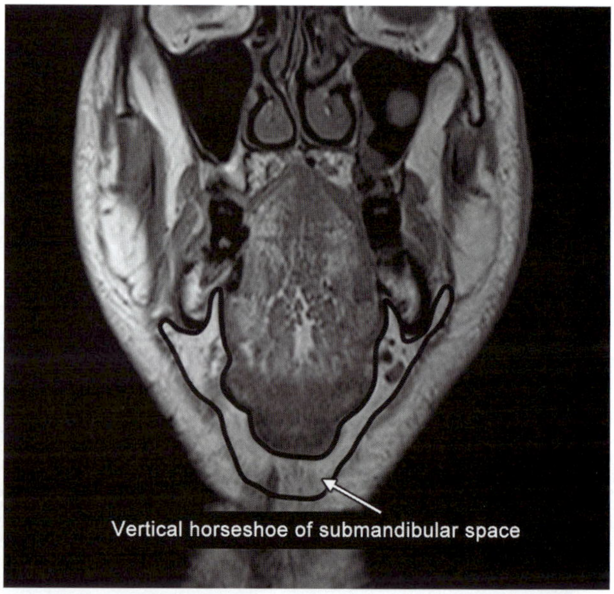

FIG. 4: Coronal T1W MR image showing the submandibular space.

Infratemporal Fossa Versus Masticator Space

Radiologists are familiar with the masticator space while surgeons commonly use the term infratemporal fossa (ITF). However, there is a difference between the two. The ITF contains the medial and lateral pterygoid muscles, the mandibular division of the trigeminal nerve (V3), chorda tympani branch of facial nerve, otic ganglion, internal maxillary artery and pterygoid venous plexus. It lies medial to the inner surface of the vertical ramus of the mandible and

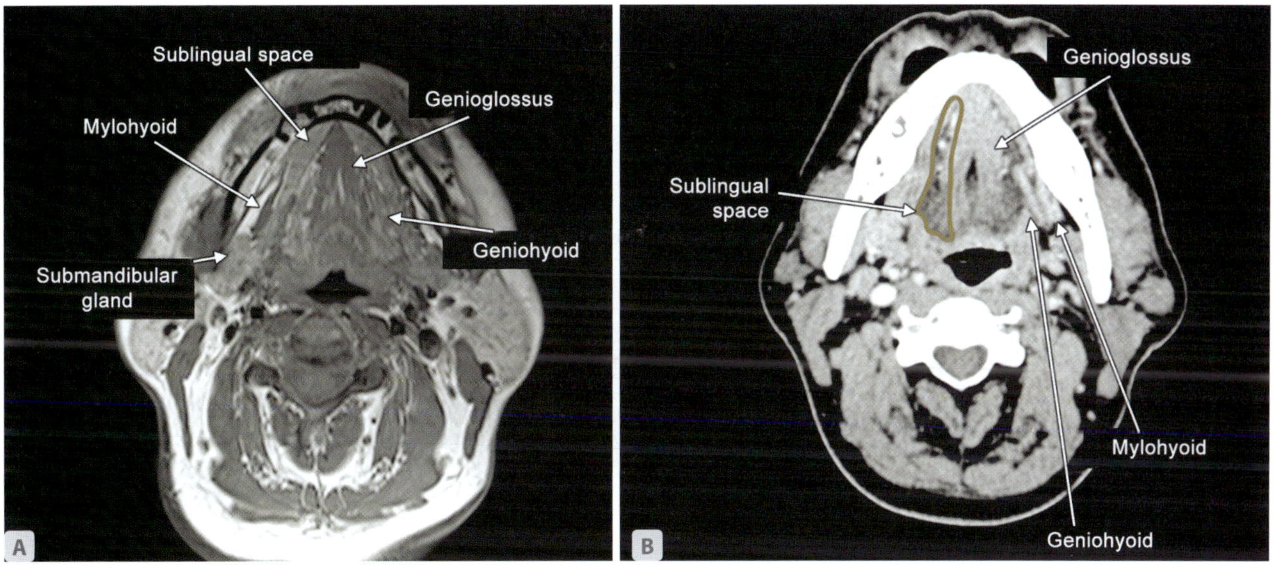

FIGS. 5A AND B: Axial T1W MR (A) and axial CT (B) sections show the normal sublingual space (outlined in brown color in B).

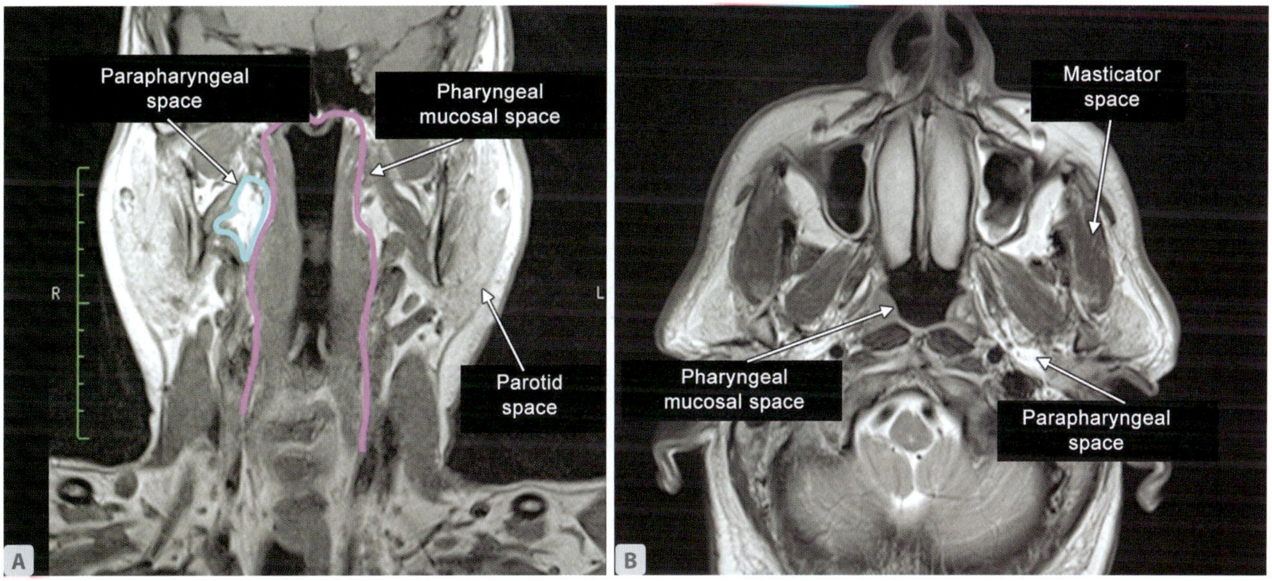

FIGS. 6A AND B: Coronal T1W (A) and axial T2W (B) MR images show the normal pharyngeal mucosal space (outlined in pink) that extends from the nasopharynx to the hypopharynx, the parapharyngeal space (outlined in light blue) lies lateral to the pharyngeal mucosal space.

the zygomatic arch and is not lined by fascia. The ITF contains much of the MS (except masseter), the retroantral buccal fat and the medial part of prestyloid parapharyngeal space (PPS)[11] **(Fig. 16)**.

Its anterior boundary is formed by the posterior surface of the maxilla and the inferior orbital fissure; posterior boundary by the mastoid and tympanic portions of the temporal bone; and superior boundary by the inferior surfaces of the greater wing of the sphenoid and the squamous portion of the temporal bone. The infratemporal fossa communicates with the temporal fossa cranially. The lateral boundary of the infratemporal fossa is formed by the zygomatic arch and ascending ramus of the mandible.[12]

Medially it is bounded by the sphenoid pterygoid process, lateral portion of the clivus, first cervical vertebra and inferior surface of the petrous portion of the temporal bone.[12,13] The lateral lower limit is at the insertion of the medial pterygoid to the mandible and the inferior boundary is the superior limit of the posterior belly of the digastric muscle.

The ITF communicates with the orbit through the inferior orbital fissure, with the middle cranial fossa through the foramina ovale and spinosum, and with the pterygopalatine fossa through the pterygomaxillary fissure.

The incidence of masticator space infections, usually of odontogenic origin is much more common while abscesses in the ITF are uncommon.[14] This is because infective disease

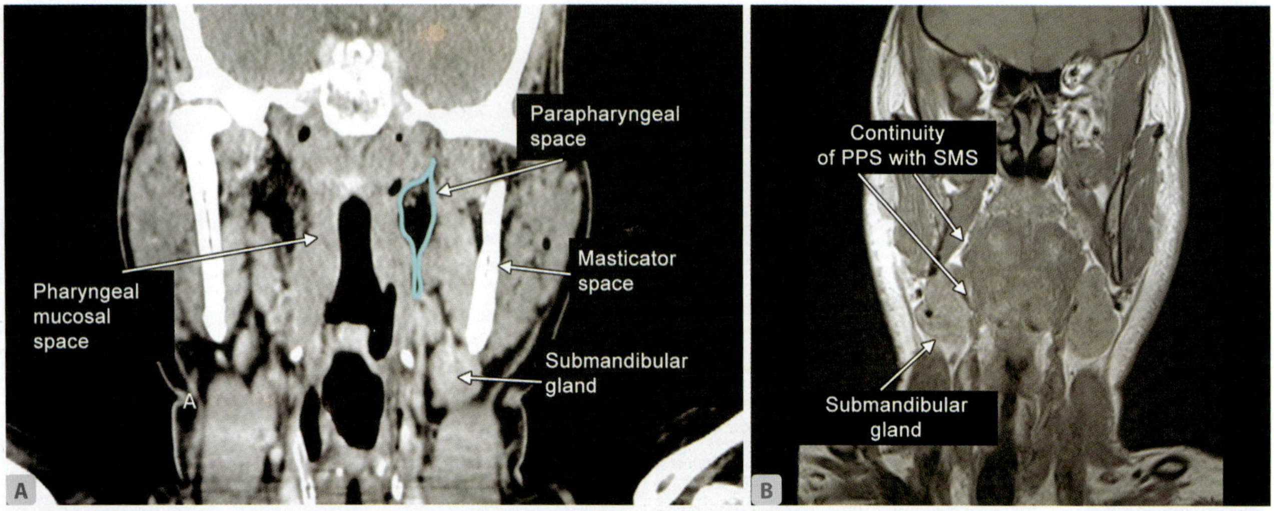

FIGS. 7A AND B: Coronal CECT (A) and coronal T1W MR (B) images depict the fat containing parapharyngeal space in the lateral aspect of suprahyoid neck, continuity of the parapharyngeal space with the submandibular space is seen in B.

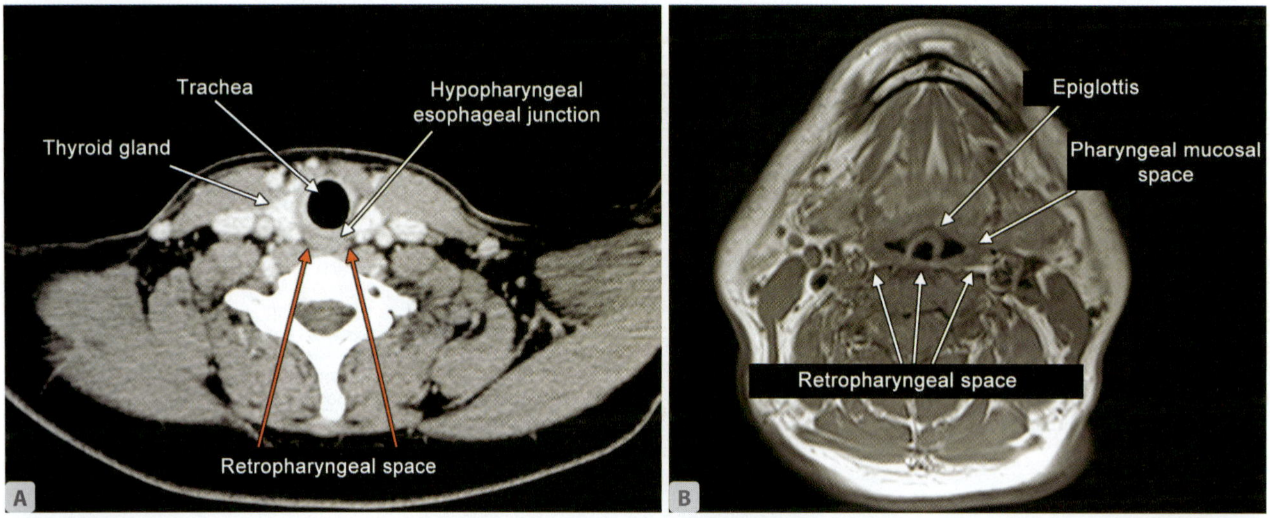

FIGS. 8A AND B: Axial CECT (A) and axial T1W MR (B) images show the fat-filled retropharyngeal space in posterior midline of neck; the carotid space lies lateral and the pharyngeal mucosal space lies anterior to the retropharyngeal space.

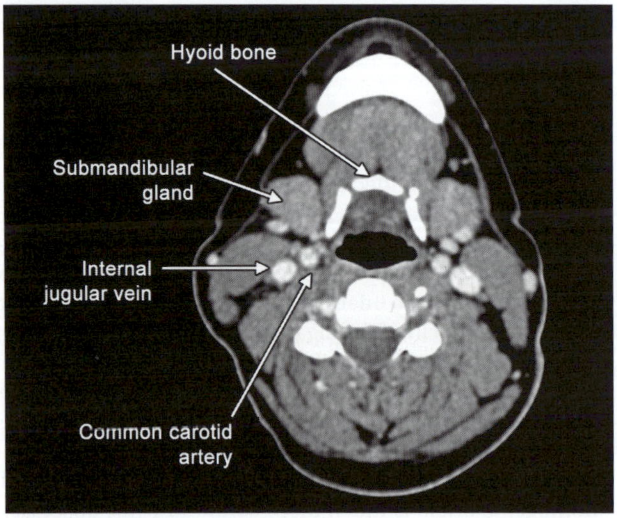

FIG. 9: Axial CECT image shows the carotid space containing the common carotid artery and internal jugular vein with the common carotid artery seen medial to the internal jugular vein.

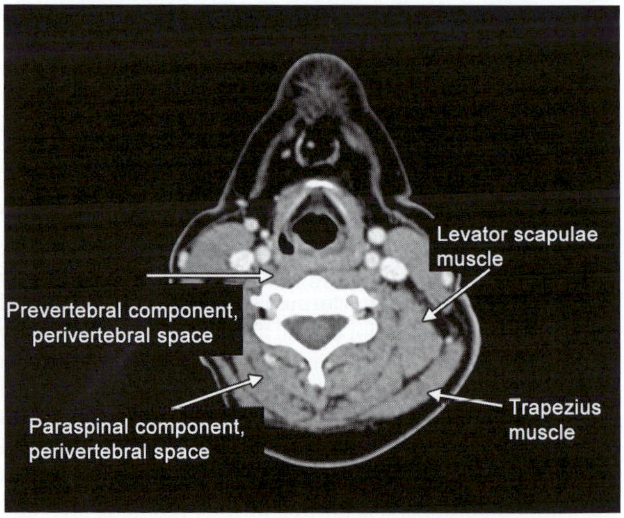

FIG. 10: Axial CECT image shows the two components of the perivertebral space: prevertebral and paraspinal components.

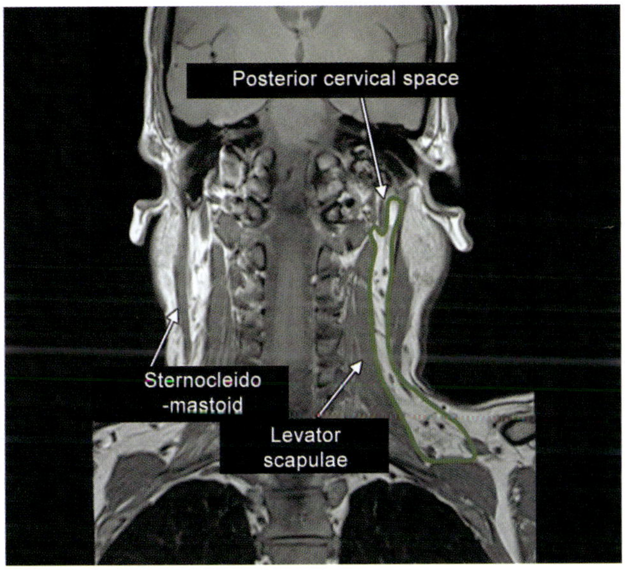

FIG. 11: Coronal T1W MR image shows the posterior cervical space deep to the sternocleidomastoid muscle.

TABLE 1: Spaces of the suprahyoid and infrahyoid neck **(Figs. 13A to D)**.

Suprahyoid neck	Infrahyoid neck	Spaces spanning entire neck
• Masticator space • Parotid space • Submandibular space • Sublingual space • Pharyngeal mucosal space • Parapharyngeal space • Buccal space	• Visceral space • Anterior cervical space • Posterior cervical space	• Retropharyngeal space • Danger space • Perivertebral space • Carotid space

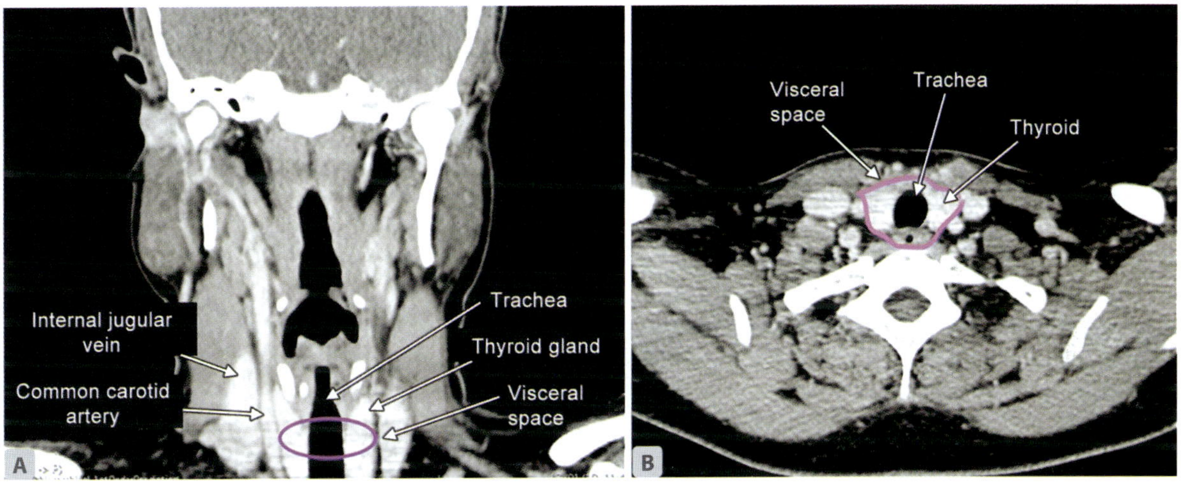

FIGS. 12A AND B: Coronal (A) and axial (B) CECT images depict the visceral space in midline infrahyoid neck (outlined in purple).

TABLE 2: Contents and lesions of the masticator space.

Contents
• Muscles of mastication • Ramus and posterior body of mandible • Mandibular nerve and its branches from foramen ovale to mandibular canal • Internal maxillary artery and its branches
Lesions
• *Mandible:* Odontogenic abscess, osteomyelitis, primary jaw lesions, metastases, myeloma *Muscles of mastication:* Benign and malignant, e.g. hemangiomas and sarcomas, benign masseteric hypertrophy, denervation atrophy, metastases, myositis ossificans • Lymphoma • *Mandibular branch of trigeminal nerve:* Neurogenic tumors, perineural spread of tumor *Secondary extension into MS:* Spread of malignancy from oropharynx or retromolar trigone, inferior extension of intracranial or skull-base lesions

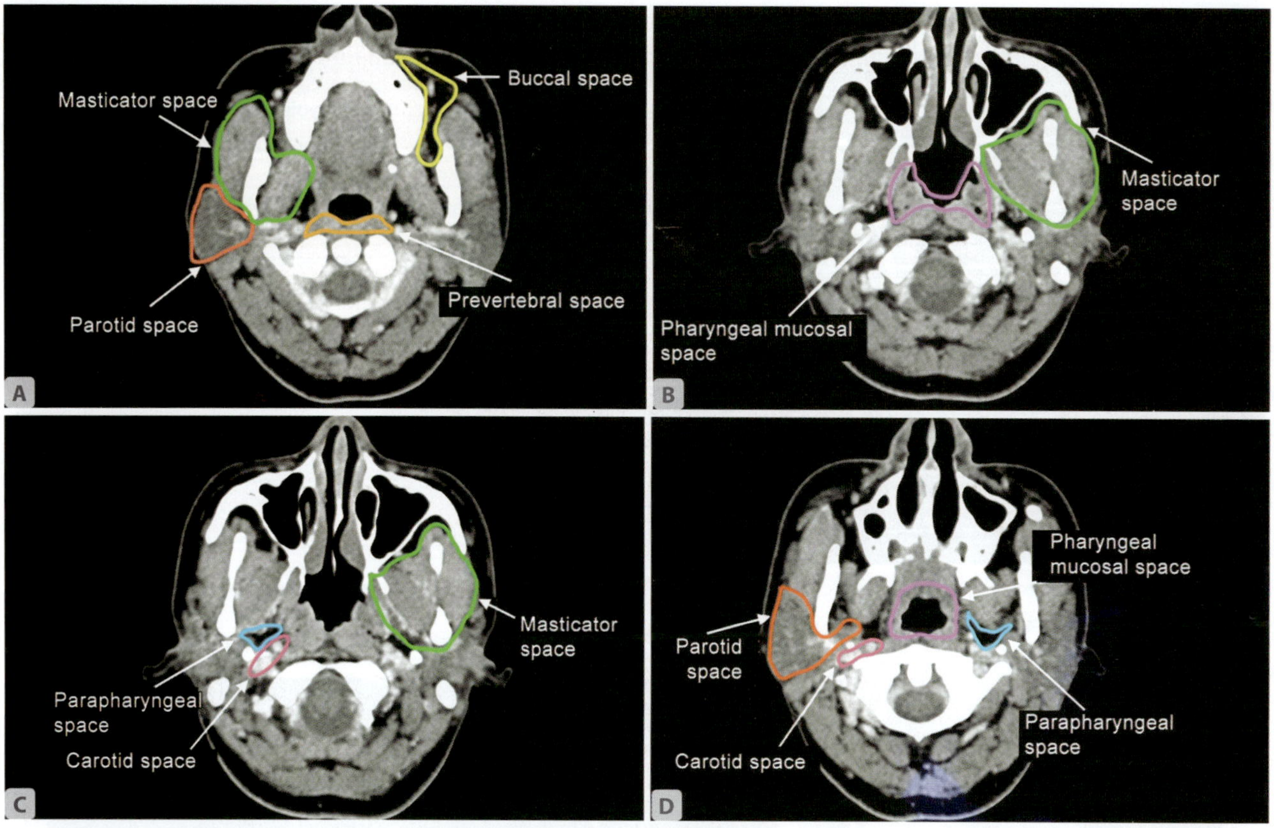

FIGS. 13A TO D: Axial CECT images (A and B) show the various spaces of the neck; masticator space (outlined in green), parotid space (outlined in red), buccal space (outlined in yellow), prevertebral space (outlined in orange) and pharyngeal mucosal space (outlined in pink). Axial CECT images (C and D) show the important spaces including the pharyngeal mucosal space (outlined in pink), parotid space (outlined in red), masticator space (outlined in green) and carotid space (outlined in deep pink); surrounding the parapharyngeal space (outlined in light blue).

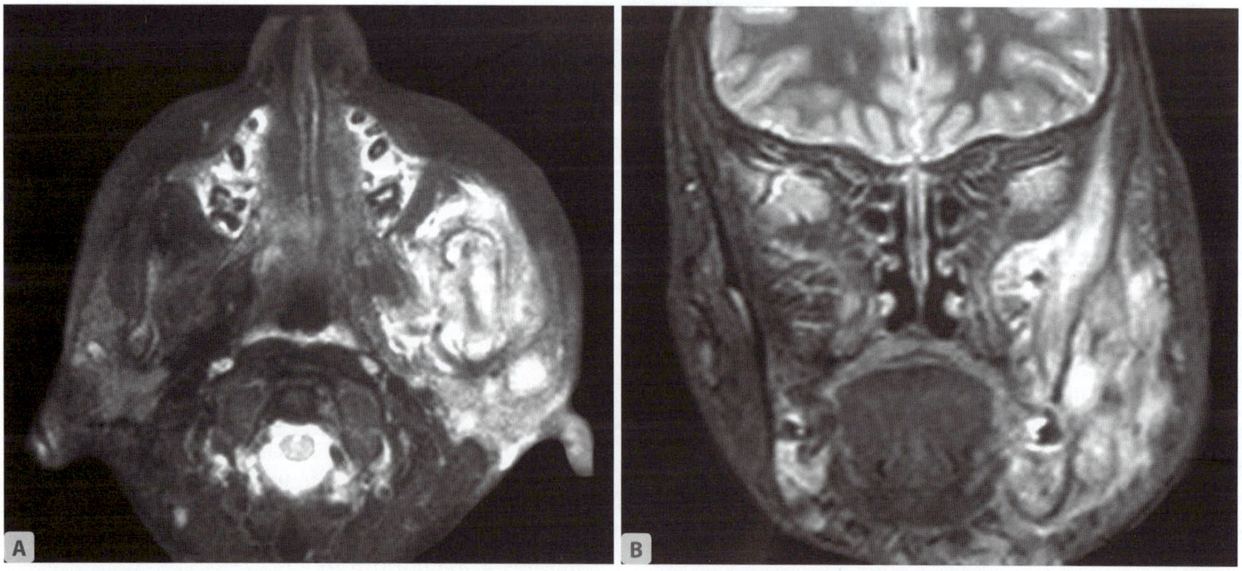

FIGS. 14A AND B: Axial (A) and coronal (B) fat sat T2W MR scans reveal destruction and altered signal of the left hemimandible with soft tissue edema involving muscles of mastication—Osteomyelitis of mandible secondary to odontogenic infection.

processes, especially abscesses tend to be initially confined to fascial lined spaces, while malignancy more commonly spreads across fascial boundaries and hence involvement of the components of a larger compartment like the ITF is more common. Bone erosion is more common with neoplasia than with infections.

The venous drainage of the ITF is by the pterygoid venous plexus, which also anastomoses with the cavernous sinus,

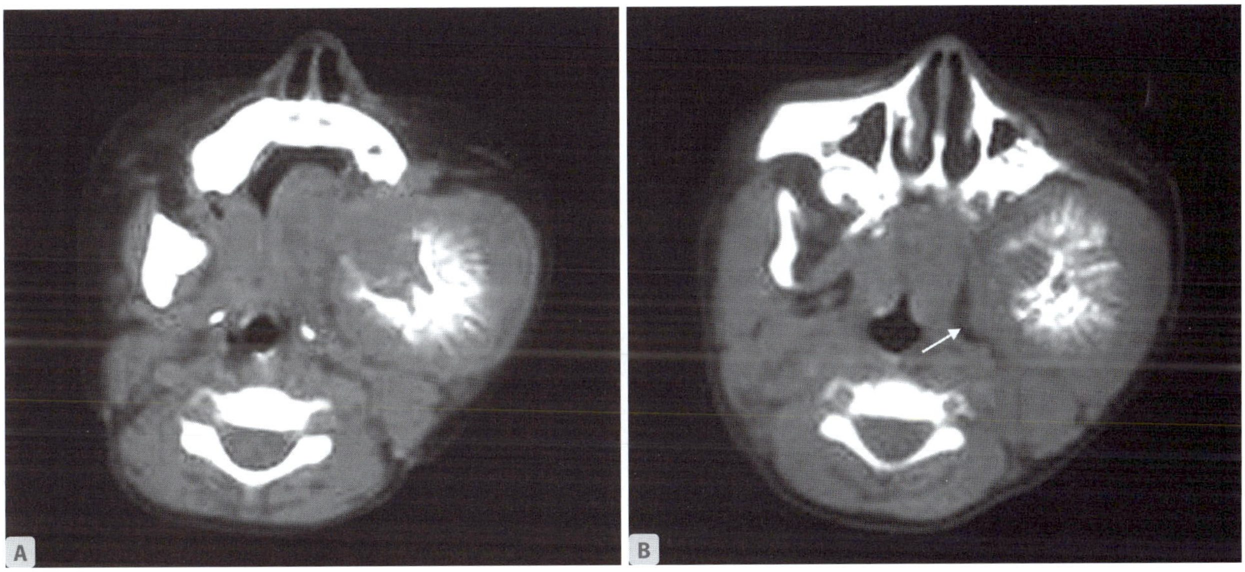

FIGS. 15A AND B: Axial CT scans showing an expansile lytic lesion with spiculated periosteal reaction involving the left hemimandible with a large soft tissue mass, note posteromedial displacement of parapharyngeal fat (arrow in B)—Osteogenic sarcoma of the mandible.

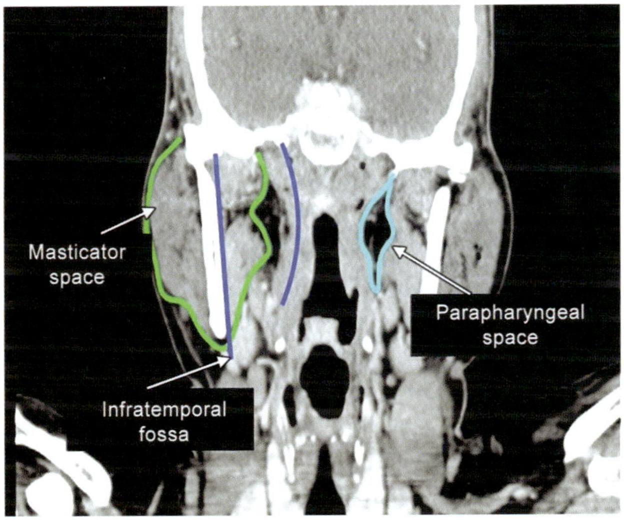

FIG. 16: Coronal CT section shows the relation between the infratemporal fossa (outlined in dark blue), masticator space (outlined in green) and parapharyngeal space (outlined in light blue); note that the infratemporal fossa does not have an anatomical floor.

ophthalmic veins and pharyngeal venous plexus. Therefore, infection in the ITF can extend to involve the orbit and cavernous sinus.

PAROTID SPACE

These are paired lateral spaces in the suprahyoid neck enclosed by the superficial layer of deep cervical fascia. The parotid space (PS) extends from external auditory canal and mastoid tip superiorly to below the angle of mandible. The parapharyngeal space is medial to the parotid space and the masticator space is anterior to it. The posterior belly of digastric muscle separates the upper part of parotid space from carotid space.

The **contents (Table 3)** of this space are the parotid gland, facial nerve, retromandibular vein, branches of the external carotid artery and lymph nodes. The facial nerve divides the parotid gland into superficial and deep lobes **(*see* Figs. 3A and B)**. The facial nerve lies just lateral to the retromandibular vein and maybe difficult to localize on routine imaging, therefore the retromandibular vein is a useful landmark to divide the gland into superficial and deep lobes.

It is important to determine whether a lesion is intraparotid or extraparotid. If 50% or more of the lesion's circumference is surrounded by parotid tissue, it is considered as intraparotid. Intraparotid masses of the deep lobe displace the parapharyngeal fat medially and widen the stylomandibular tunnel.[1,15] Identification of a fat plane between the lesion and the parotid indicates a parapharyngeal space site of origin whereas direct continuity of the mass to the gland indicates a deep lobe parotid origin. It is important to recognize intraparotid lesions of the tail region as excision of these lesions may cause facial nerve injury.

Lesions in the parotid space include benign tumors such as pleomorphic adenomas, Warthin's tumors and less commonly, malignant tumors. The parotid gland may be involved by inflammatory pathology. In children, 50% of parotid lesions are hemangoimas. Other lesions include venous malformations **(Figs. 17A to C)**, calculi, lymphoepithelial lesions associated with HIV, lipomas, first branchial cleft cysts **(Figs. 18A to E)** and rarely schwannomas (from facial nerve).

Tumors of the parotid gland—Majority of the parotid tumors are **benign** (up to 80%). The commonest benign tumor is *pleomorphic adenoma* which is also known as benign mixed tumor. It is commonly seen in middle aged females. Pleomorphic adenoma appears hypoechoic on ultrasound. On CT, it shows smoothly marginated or lobulated surface with homogeneous contrast enhancement. As the size increases, pleomorphic adenoma appears more heterogeneous with foci of necrosis and areas of calcification within **(Figs. 19A and B)**.

TABLE 3: Contents and lesions of the parotid space.
Contents
• Parotid gland • Intraparotid lymph nodes • Facial nerve and its branches • Branches of external carotid artery • Retromandibular vein
Lesions
• *Salivary gland neoplasms:* Pleomorphic adenoma, Warthin's tumor, mucoepidermoid carcinoma, adenoid cystic carcinoma, oncocytoma [most parotid tumors are benign (80%) and around 20–25% are malignant] • *Neoplasms (nonsalivary):* Hemangioma, lipoma • *Vascular malformation:* Venolymphatic malformation • *Infectious/Inflammatory:* Parotiditis, parotid abscess, cellulitis, radiation sialadenitis, lymphoepithelial cysts • First branchial cleft anomaly • *Lymph nodes:* Metastases from skin malignancy (SCC), non-Hodgkin's lymphoma, melanoma • *Facial nerve:* Neurogenic tumors, perineural extension of tumor

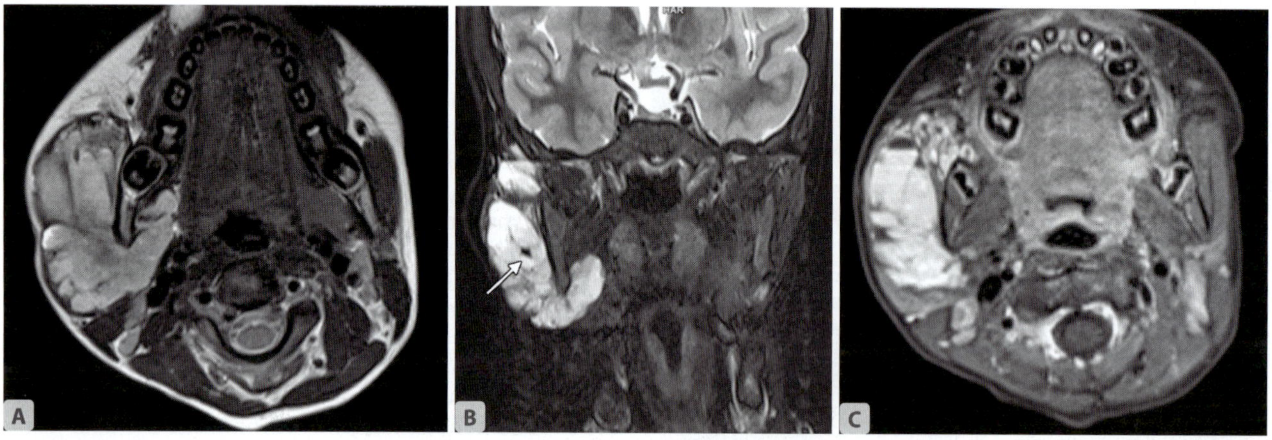

FIGS. 17A TO C: Axial T2W (A), Coronal STIR (B) and axial postcontrast (C) images depict a lobulated lesion involving the superficial and deep lobes of parotid gland, appearing hyperintense on T2W and STIR images with near homogeneous postcontrast enhancement.
A phlebolith is seen in the lesion (arrow in B)—Venous malformation of parotid gland.

It shows very high signal on T2WI, low signal on T1WI and homogeneous postcontrast enhancement on MRI. The lesions are excised as they are associated with risk of malignant degeneration and also for cosmetic reasons. Complete excision is essential as residual tumor can create daughter lesions that are difficult to resect.

Warthin's tumors can present as multifocal masses and are well defined cystic lesions. They often present as slow growing masses in older men. On ultrasound, they show multiple small anechoic areas within. Cystic content of the lesion increases with the size of the lesion. Warthin's tumors are well defined solid cystic structures located in the superficial lobe of parotid or tail region. They may show a mural nodule which is strongly suggestive of the diagnosis. Warthin's tumors appear hypointense on T2WI and show variable enhancement.

Oncocytoma is a rare benign parotid tumor, no specific imaging features are seen on CT and ultrasound, but they show well defined contours on T1WI and appear isointense to the parotid tissue on postcontrast T1WI categorizing it as a "vanishing lesion". *Schwannomas* arising from facial nerve appear as solid enhancing masses that may show cystic degeneration as the size enlarges. Benign tumors are not associated with facial nerve palsy.[16]

Malignant lesions of the parotid include *mucoepidermoid carcinoma* (commonest primary malignancy of the parotid) and *adenoid cystic carcinoma*. Mucoepidermoid carcinoma appears as a well circumscribed hypoechoic lesion with cystic areas within on ultrasound. On CT, enhancement of the solid component is seen and calcification may be present. Mucoepidermoid carcinoma shows areas of low signal intensity on T2WI and may not be seen on postcontrast scans as it appears similar to adjacent parotid tissue. High grade lesions show poorly defined margins, local infiltration and nodal spread **(Figs. 20A to C)**.

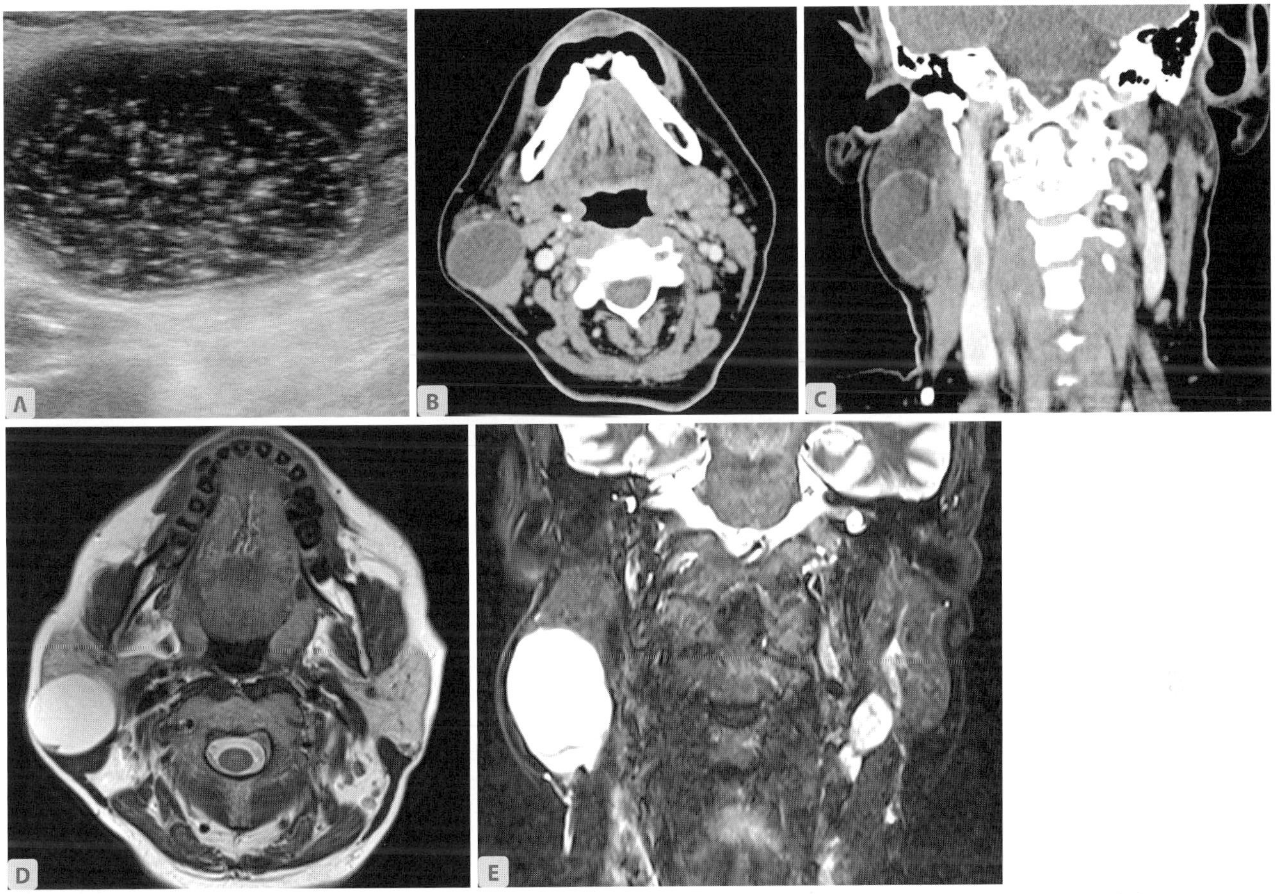

FIGS. 18A TO E: USG (A), axial and coronal (B and C) CECT images show a well-demarcated cystic lesion in the right parotid gland showing multiple internal echoes on USG and few thin septations within, on CECT images. Axial T2W and coronal STIR (D and E) images show a hyperintense lesion with few septations within in right parotid gland—Histopathology proven first branchial cleft cyst in a young patient.

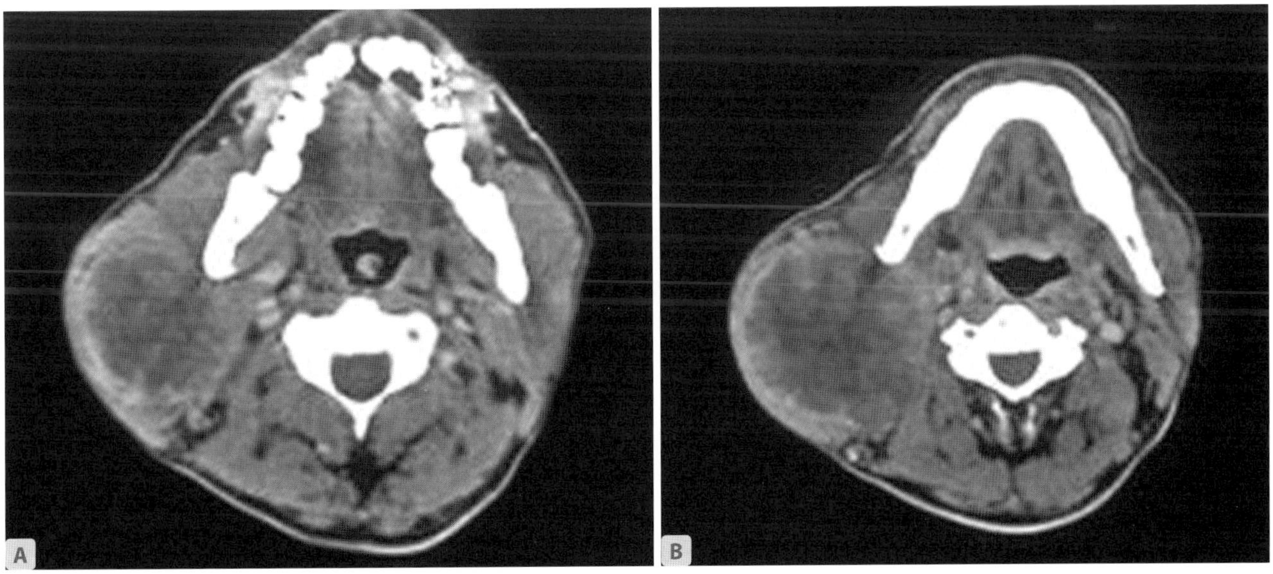

FIGS. 19A AND B: Axial CECT scans show a large, well-encapsulated, hypodense mass in the superficial lobe of the right parotid gland involving the deep lobe and causing displacement of the masseter and sternocleidomastoid muscles. No bony destruction or lymphadenopathy seen—Pleomorphic adenoma of the parotid gland.

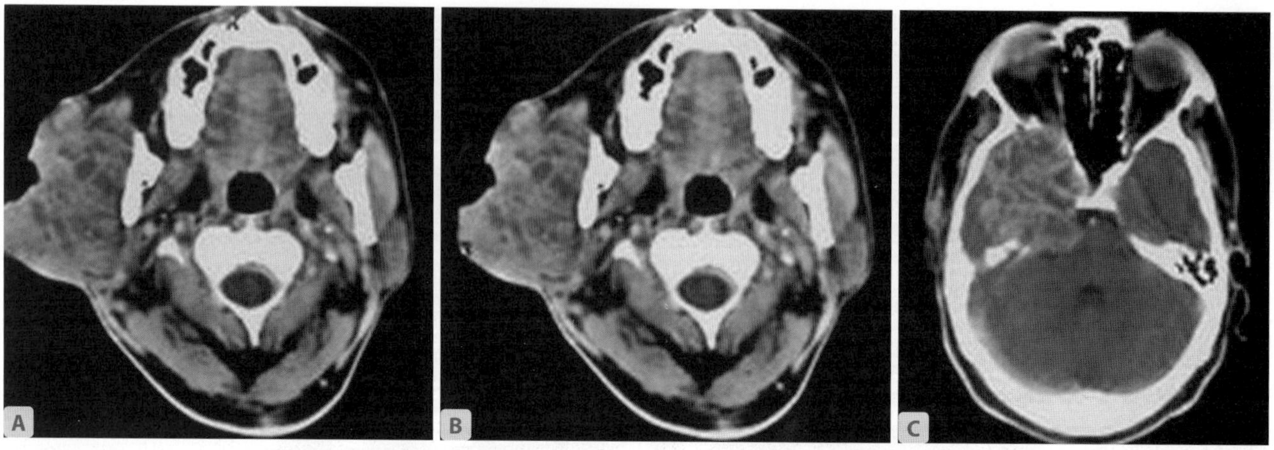

FIGS. 20A TO C: Axial CECT scans show a poorly demarcated ulcerating heterogeneous mass involving the right parotid gland with infiltration of the masseter and sternocleidomastoid muscles (A), multiple hypodense areas s/o necrosis are seen within (B), Intracranial extension into the middle cranial fossa, the right cerebellopontine angle and erosion of the greater wing of the sphenoid bone is also seen (C) mucoepidermoid carcinoma of the parotid gland.

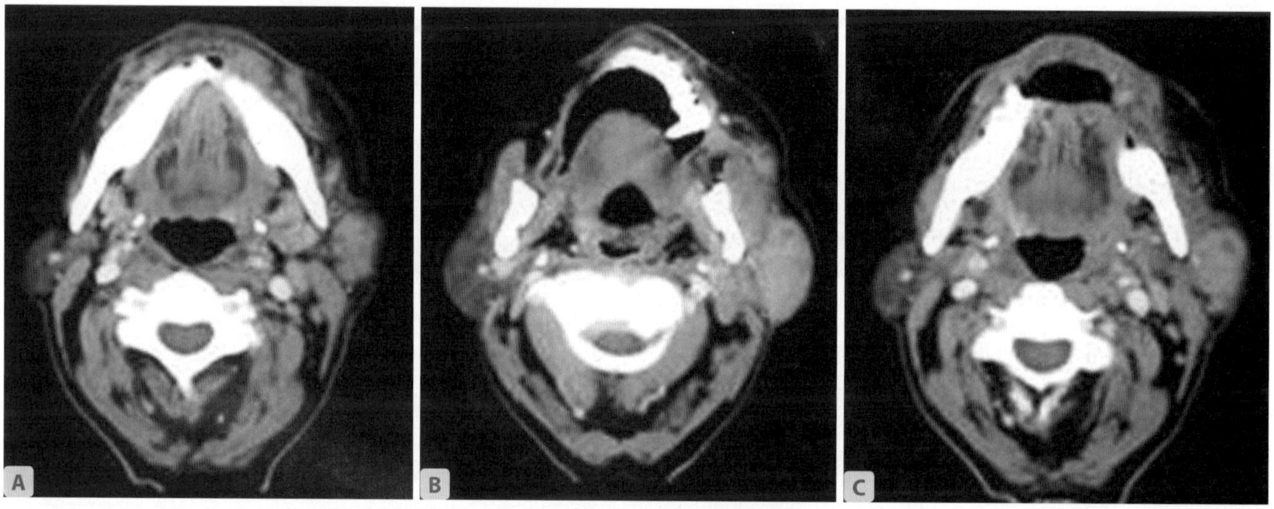

FIGS. 21A TO C: Axial CECT scans showing an enhancing heterogeneous mass involving both the superficial and deep lobes of the parotid gland (A and B) with loss of planes seen with masseter muscle (C) adenoid cystic carcinoma of the parotid.

Adenoid cystic carcinoma shows low signal intensity on T1WI and moderate signal intensity on T2WI, aggressive appearance increases with tumor grade. It has greatest propensity for perineural spread among head and neck cancers and is associated with poor long-term prognosis **(Figs. 21A to C)**.

Sialadenitis—Various conditions can cause inflammatory changes in the salivary glands including infections, ductal obstruction due to calculi or tumor, facial trauma, radiotherapy and autoimmune diseases. Patients present with facial swelling and pain. During the acute phase imaging demonstrates enlargement of the gland with increased enhancement on CT and MRI. Unilateral *infectious sialadenitis* is often due to bacterial infections **(Fig. 22)**.

Bilateral involvement of the glands is seen in viral infection, radiotherapy, HIV infection or autoimmune diseases such as Sjögren's disease and sarcoidosis. Viral sialadenitis is most commonly caused by mumps (*paramyxovirus*). Radiation sialadenitis is seen in patients who receive I-131 therapy for thyroid disease or patients who receive external beam radiotherapy. The glands are swollen, edematous and hypodense in acute phase. In the chronic phase the glands become small and fibrotic, hyperdense on noncontrast-enhanced computed tomography (NCCT) and show increased enhancement on contrast-enhanced CT (CECT).

Sjögren's disease affects female patients in fourth to fifth decades. Acute cases are similar to viral sialadenitis but chronic disease causes atrophic glands with heterogeneous stippled attenuation, multiple small parotid cysts and intraglandular sialoliths. These patients are at a risk of developing lymphoma. A lesion that is hyperenhancing, T2 hypointense and shows restricted diffusion is concerning for development of lymphoma.[17]

Multiple *granulomatous diseases* including tuberculosis, fungal infections and Wegner's granulomatosis can involve the glands with focal or diffuse involvement[18] **(Fig. 23)**.

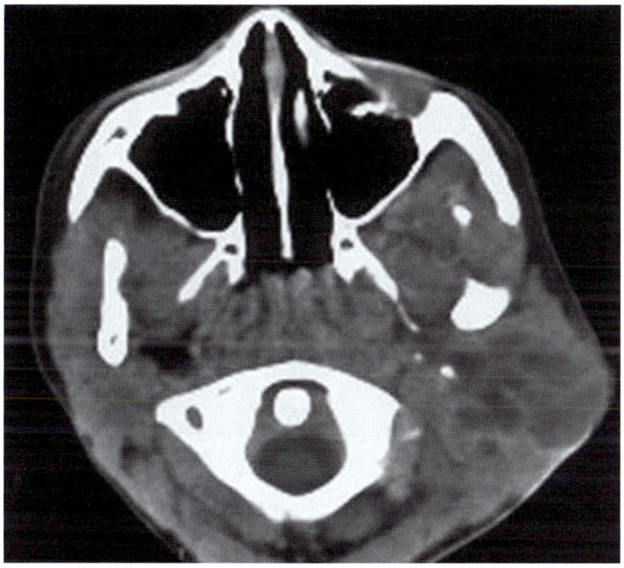

FIG. 22: Axial CECT scan showing enlarged left parotid gland with ill-defined, irregularly marginated hypodense areas within showing mild peripheral rim enhancement—Parotid gland abscess.

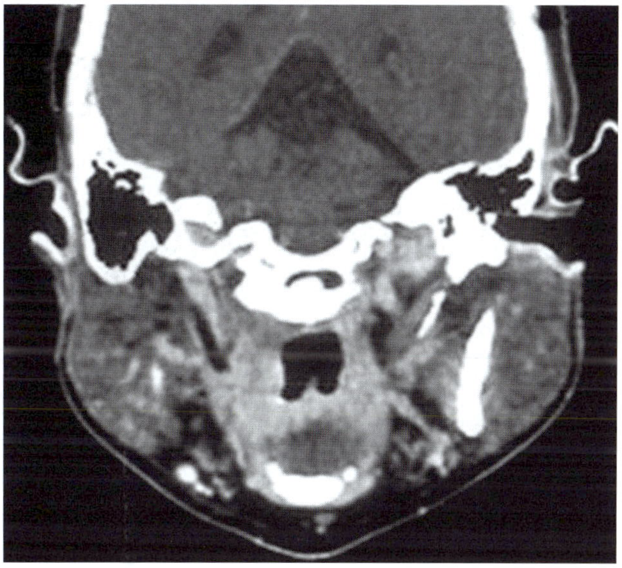

FIG. 23: Coronal CECT image shows enlarged parotid glands bilaterally with heterogeneous appearance of the parenchyma—in a case of granulomatous parotitis.

SUBMANDIBULAR SPACE

The submandibular space (SMS) is a superficial space located inferior to the mylohyoid muscle and above the hyoid bone. It is a vertical horseshoe shaped space and communicates posteriorly with sublingual space and with inferior parapharyngeal space at the posterior margin of the mylohyoid muscle (***see* Fig. 4**).

The **contents (Table 4)** of the submandibular space are the anterior belly of digastric muscle, superficial portion of the submandibular gland, submandibular and submental lymph nodes, facial artery and vein, inferior loop of hypoglossal nerve and fat.

Lesions—Metastatic lymphadenopathy from squamous cell carcinoma of tongue and floor of mouth is the most common lesion of the submandibular space. Other lesions include lymphoma, adenitis, obstructed submandibular duct, salivary gland tumors, spread from odontogenic infections. In children, the most common lesion is second branchial cleft cyst. Congenital and developmental lesions also include thyroglossal cyst, hemangioma, lymphatic malformation, dermoid/epidermoid and diving ranula.

TABLE 4: Contents and lesions of the submandibular space.

Contents
• Anterior belly of the digastric muscle • Superficial portion of the submandibular gland • Submandibular and submental lymph nodes • Facial artery and vein • Fat • Inferior loop of the hypoglossal nerve
Lesions
• *Lymph nodes:* Metastatic disease (most commonly from SCC), lymphoma, adenitis • *Submandibular gland:* Obstructed submandibular duct, salivary gland tumors (around 40–50% of submandibular gland tumors are malignant) • *Infection/inflammation (usually spread from odontogenic infection):* abscess, Ludwig's angina, diving ranula • *Congenital/developmental:* Thyroglossal duct cyst, hemangioma, lymphatic malformation, dermoid/epidermoid, second branchial cleft cyst

Dermoid cysts are composed of epithelial elements but dermoids have skin appendages in contrast to epidermoid. Majority of the cervical dermoid cysts occur in the midline or in paramedian location and are mostly present at birth. They are seen more often in the submandibular space than floor of mouth. Dermoid cysts do not move with swallowing unlike thyroglossal duct cysts. On CT fatty internal elements, mixed density fluid and calcification can be found in dermoid cysts. The admixture of fat globules with fluid can give rise to the typical *sac of marbles* appearance of dermoid cyst.

Sialolithiasis—Approximately 80–90% of salivary gland calculi occur in the submandibular gland and only 10% in the parotid gland. They may be intraglandular or intraductal and can be visualized well on sonography. Associated sialectasia may also be well seen on sialography or sonography. Mucocele formation may also result as a complication of sialolithiasis. The most common cause of salivary inflammatory lesions is calculus disease, especially in the submandibular space (**Figs. 24A and B**), due to the upward secretion of the more mucinous, viscous, and alkaline saliva. Also, the opening of the Wharton's duct (the main salivary duct of the submandibular gland) is narrower than the diameter of the duct.

Calculus disease causes painful glands and is often associated with fever. CT imaging is preferred to MRI for identification of calculi. MR is useful for detecting mandibular infection (osteomyelitis) and to differentiate

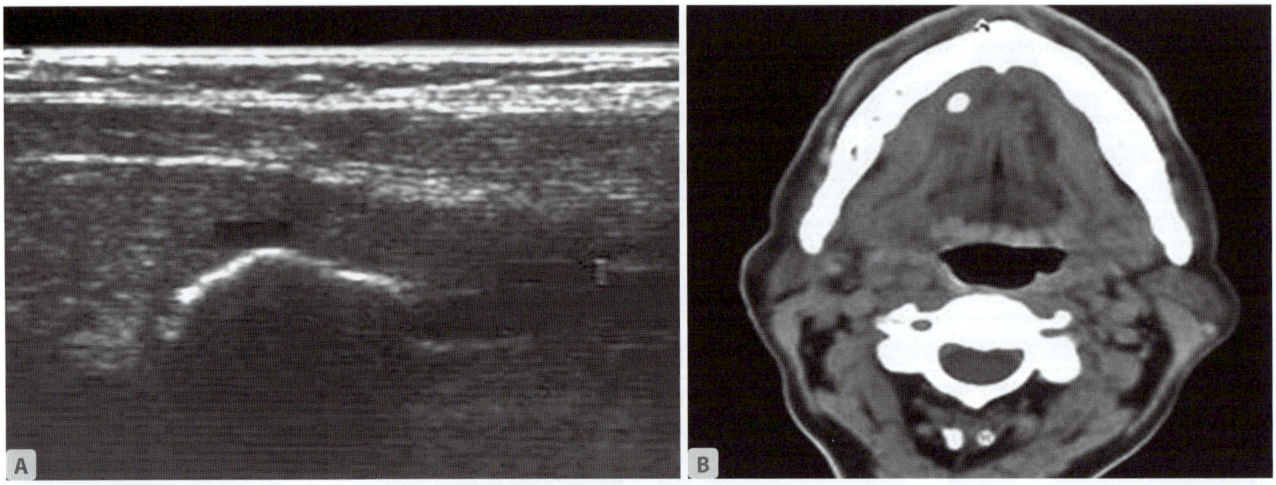

FIGS. 24A AND B: USG showing a dilated right submandibular gland duct with a calculus within (A) a calculus is seen in the floor of the mouth anteriorly in a paramedian location on axial CT scan (B) calculus in Wharton's duct.

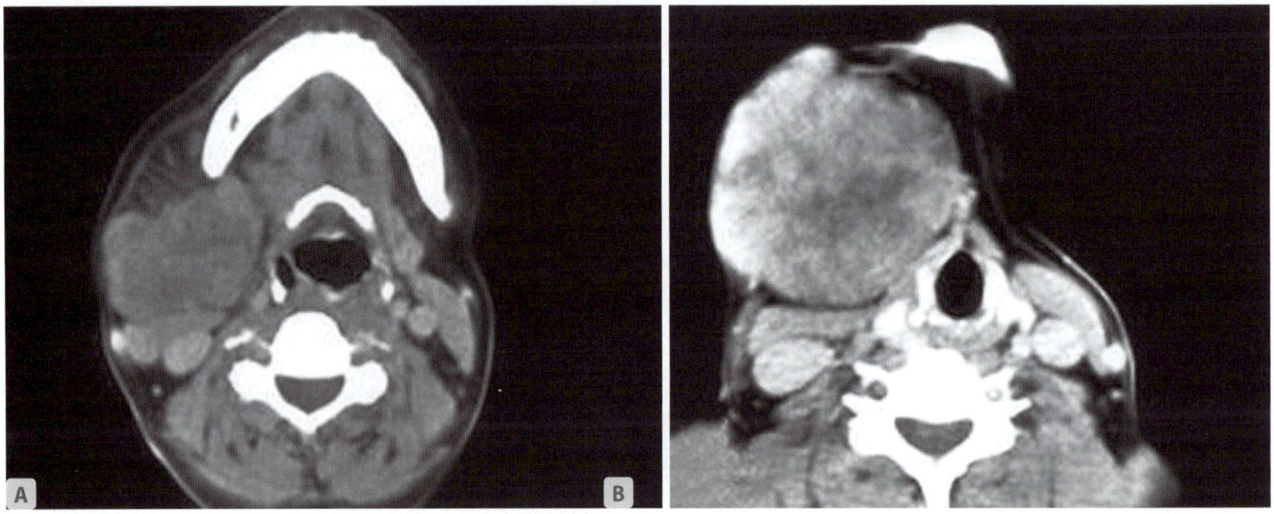

FIGS. 25A AND B: Axial CECT scans showing a bulky heterogeneous mass with patchy contrast enhancement in the right submandibular gland (A) causing displacement of the sternocleidomastoid muscle and attenuation of the right carotid sheath (B) pleomorphic adenoma of the submandibular gland.

between cellulitis/myositis and abscess. MRI demonstrates an enhancing submandibular gland and offers the advantage of MR sialography. Fat infiltration or gland size reduction, compared to the healthy side in MRI may also indicate chronic disease with sialadenitis.

Tumors, such as pleomorphic adenomas can also arise in the submandibular glands **(Figs. 25A and B)**, the imaging features have been discussed in the section on parotid tumors. Adenoid cystic carcinoma is the most common malignant tumor arising from the submandibular gland.

SUBLINGUAL SPACE

It is a tea cup-shaped space located on both sides of the tongue lying superomedial to the mylohyoid and lateral to the midline geniohyoid-genioglossus muscle complex.[19] The mylohyoid sling is formed by the paired mylohyoid muscles, arising from the inner surface of the mandible to insert onto the posterior aspect of the hyoid bone. Medially the paired muscles insert into a fibrous median raphe, forming a muscular sling. The mylohyoid muscle sling separates the sublingual space (SLS) from the right and left submandibular spaces and the midline submental space. The SLS is however continuous with the SMS behind the posterior edge of mylohyoid.

The **contents (Table 5)** of the sublingual space are fat, the anterior extension of the hypoglossal muscle, hypoglossal nerve, lingual artery and vein, sublingual gland and ducts, deep portion of submandibular gland and lymph nodes **(*see* Figs. 5A and B)**. The common **lesions** of the sublingual space include squamous cell carcinoma from the epithelial lining and spread from odontogenic infections. Metastatic lymphadenopathy from squamous cell carcinomas also involves the sublingual space. Other lesions include minor salivary gland tumors, neurogenic tumors, ranula, obstructed submandibular gland duct, dermoid and epidermoid.

Epidermoid cysts typically involve the floor of the mouth incorporating the sublingual, submandibular spaces and the root of the tongue.[20] Epidermoid cysts are composed of epithelial elements and are of fluid density with little or no complex features.

Ranula is an inflammatory lesion of the sublingual space. It is actually a mucous retention cyst that may result from an obstructed sublingual or minor salivary gland or from trauma or retained secretions that may lead to rupture of acini. A ranula usually results from trauma or inflammation of the salivary glands, however rare congenital ranulas have also been described. It may herniate into the submandibular or lower parapharyngeal space through the mylohyoid muscle and evolve into a plunging ranula **(Figs. 26A to C)**. A plunging ranula has a distinct *"tail sign"* within the sublingual space with the bulk of the cyst seen in the submandibular space.

TABLE 5: Contents and lesions of the sublingual space.

Contents
• Fat • Muscles (anterior extension of the hyoglossus muscle) • Hypoglossal nerve • Lingual nerve • Lingual artery and vein • Sublingual gland and ducts • Deep portion of the submandibular gland and duct • Lymph nodes
Lesions
• *Epithelial lining:* SCC—generally secondary spread • *Salivary gland:* Ranula, obstructed submandibular duct, minor salivary gland tumors • *Infection (usually spread from odontogenic infection):* Abscess, Ludwig's angina • *Lingual/hypoglossal nerve:* Neurogenic tumor • *Congenital/developmental:* Lingual thyroid, thyroglossal duct cyst hemangioma, lymphatic malformation, dermoid/epidermoid

Ranula shows high fluid attenuation on CT, the cyst wall may enhance depending upon presence of infection. On MRI, it appears hyperintense on T2WI and may show high signal on T1WI due to high protein content **(Figs. 27A to D)**.

Floor of the Mouth versus Sublingual Space

The floor of the mouth is a term commonly used in surgical literature It is a horizontally aligned U-shaped space situated in the part of the oral cavity lying beneath the tongue. For surgical planning, the floor of the mouth is defined as the space between the mucosal surface and the mylohyoid sling and comprising both structures. Thus, according to the surgical definition, the sublingual space is a part of the floor of mouth. However, in most radiology literature the mylohyoid muscle sling is considered to be synonymous with the floor of mouth and sublingual space is considered as a separate compartment.[19]

PHARYNGEAL MUCOSAL SPACE

The pharyngeal mucosal space (PMS) abuts the skull base along the superior/posterior aspect of the nasopharyngeal roof superiorly and extends to the level of the hypopharynx inferiorly.[16] It is divided into nasopharyngeal, oropharyngeal, and hypopharyngeal segments. The nasopharynx is the part that lies posterior to the nasal choanae and extends from the vault of pharynx superiorly to the soft palate inferiorly. The oropharynx lies posterior to base of tongue, inferior to soft palate and superior to the superior aspect of epiglottis. The hypopharynx lies inferior to the superior aspect of the epiglottis and superior to the cricoid cartilage **(Fig. 28)**.

The retropharyngeal space is posterior to PMS and parapharyngeal space is lateral to it. The middle layer of the deep cervical fascia borders the lateral and posterior deep margins of the PMS, but it is not a truly encircled fascial space as there is no fascia along the surface.

Accurate identification of pathology within the PMS is largely related to the imaging appearance, site of origin, and its effect on the PMS airway. Clinicians can assess the surface of the pharyngeal mucosal surface well, therefore

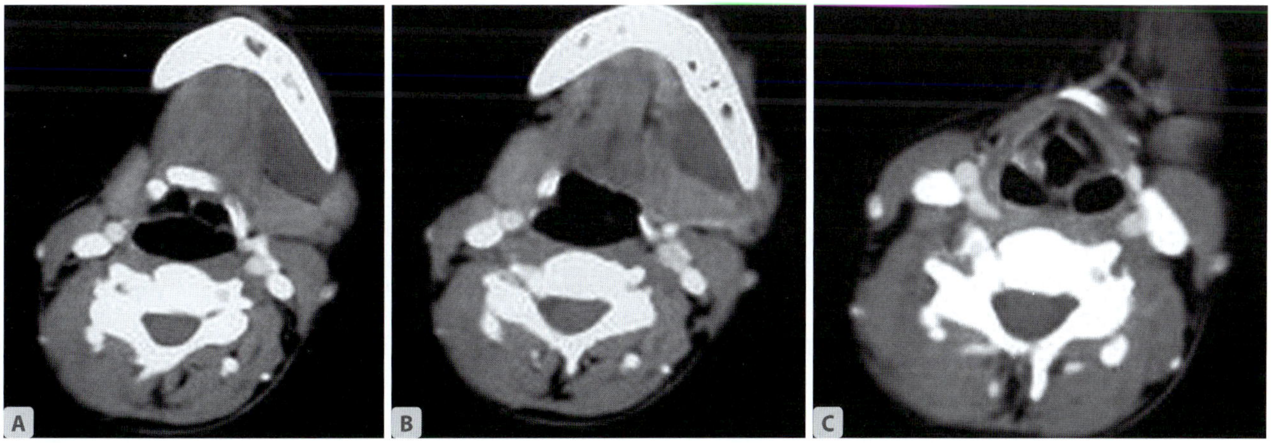

FIGS. 26A TO C: Axial CECT scans revealing an oval, well-defined hypodense lesion with cystic attenuation and smooth walls in the sublingual space on the left side (A and B) extending around the mylohyoid muscle into the submandibular space posteriorly (C) Plunging ranula.

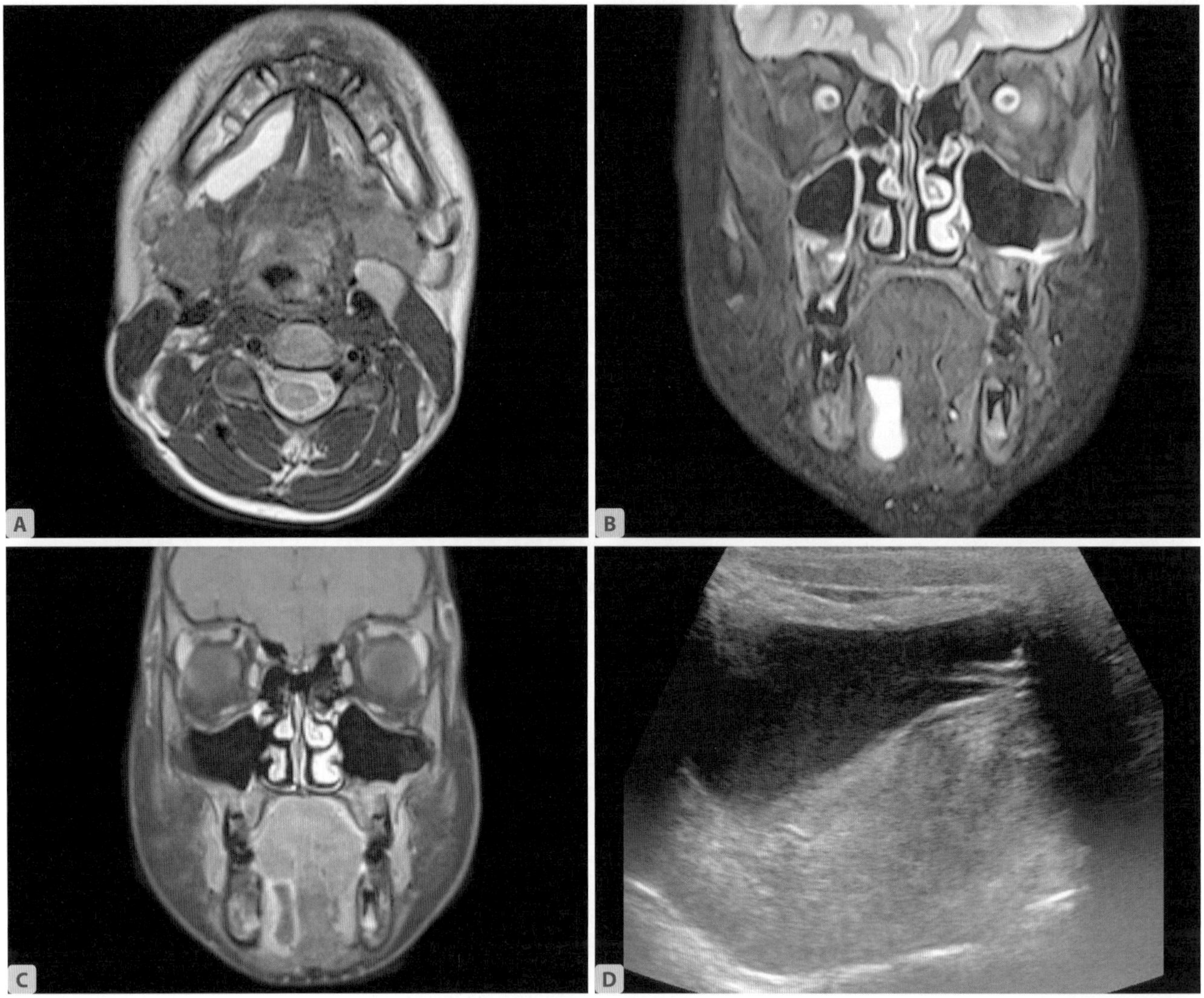

FIGS. 27A TO D: Axial T2W (A), coronal STIR (B), coronal postcontrast T1W (C) and USG (D) images show a cystic lesion in the right sublingual space. It appears markedly hyperintense on T2W and STIR images (A and B) and shows peripheral enhancement (C). On USG (D), it is seen as an anechoic lesion in the sublingual space— Infected simple ranula.

clinical examination and impressions are useful for image interpretation. Asymmetry in the PMS may be misinterpreted as a tumor. A mass which is primary to the PMS will have its center medial to parapharyngeal space, push the parapharyngeal fat from medial to lateral and will disrupt the normal PMS mucosal and submucosal architecture.

The **contents (Table 6)** of this space are the mucosal surface of the pharynx, pharyngeal lymphatic ring and minor salivary glands. **Lesions**—Squamous cell carcinoma (SCC) is the most common malignancy in this location. Cross-sectional imaging helps in guiding treatment decisions in SCC by characterizing the extent of the mass deep to the mucosal surface, invasion into the adjacent spaces and assessing nodal spread. The relationship between the PMS and base of skull is important in the setting of nasopharyngeal carcinoma as it has a propensity for early intracranial spread primarily because of its proximity to the foramen lacerum. Tumors can invade through the foramen's cartilaginous floor and travel along the ICA to invade the cavernous sinus. Nasopharyngeal carcinoma may also spread via perineural tumor spread into the skull base and cavernous sinus. The evaluation of the extent of disease is important for planning of radiotherapy.

Thornwaldt's cyst is a congenital cyst that is seen in the midline in the posterior PMS and is lined by pharyngeal mucosa.[20] Focal adhesion of pharyngeal mucosa to the notochord results in a nasopharyngeal diverticulum. Majority of these cysts are seen as incidental findings on head MRI and the peak incidence is between 15 and 30 years. The patient becomes symptomatic when the intracystic pressure rises consequent to infection with anaerobic bacteria.

CT scan reveals a well-circumscribed, thin-walled cyst located in the midline in posterior nasopharyngeal mucosal space lodged between the prevertebral muscles. Attenuation of the cyst increases as the protein content increases with infection and may mimic a soft tissue mass. On MR the cyst has a T1 signal intensity, which increases from low to high with increasing protein content. The SI is high on T2W images.

Acute tonsillitis is one of the commonest infections that occurs in the pharyngeal mucosal space, especially in young adults. The common causes include viral (*Epstein*

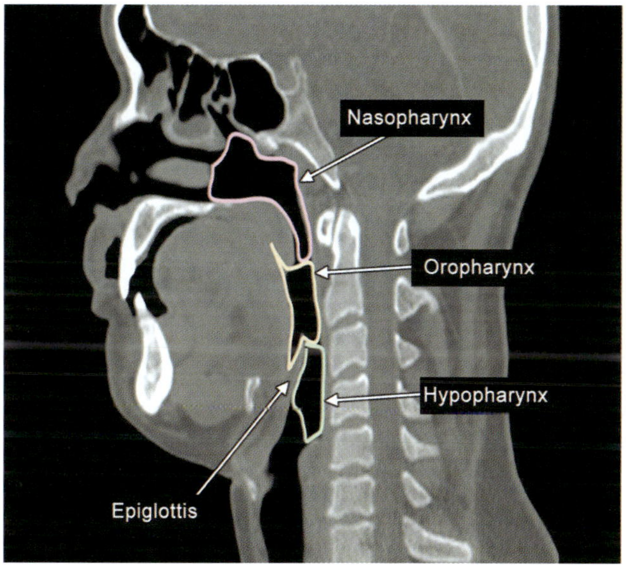

FIG. 28: Sagittal CT image shows the division of the pharyngeal mucosal space into the nasopharynx, oropharynx and hypopharynx.

TABLE 6: Contents and lesions of the pharyngeal mucosal space.
Contents
• Mucosal surface of the pharynx • Pharyngeal lymphatic ring (adenoids, palatine, and lingual tonsils) • Minor salivary glands contained in the submucosa in highest concentration within the hard and soft palate
Lesions
• *Malignant tumors:* Nasopharyngeal carcinoma, oropharyngeal carcinoma (palatine and lingual tonsil), non-Hodgkin lymphoma, minor salivary gland carcinoma • *Inflammatory lesions:* Tonsillar lymphoid hyperplasia, pharyngitis or postradiation change • *Infectious causes:* Tonsillar or peritonsillar abscess • *Musculoskeletal tumors:* Rhabdomyosarcoma, chordoma • *Miscellaneous:* Thornwaldt cyst

Barr virus) and bacterial (*Staphylococcus aureus and Streptococcus species*) infections. The diagnosis is usually clinical and imaging is only required in severe cases to evaluate the extent of disease and associated complications such as presence of abscess. On CT and MRI, acute tonsillitis is seen as enlargement and increased enhancement of the palatine tonsils which may approximate in the oral cavity. A striated enhancement pattern within the tonsils may be seen on postcontrast scans with parallel hypodense streaks within representing edema, cellular debris and trapped fluid. This should not be confused with abscess formation, which requires surgical drainage. Focal hypodense central areas in the tonsils without discernable rim enhancement are also not amenable to drainage.[17]

Abscesses related to tonsillitis may be (i) *peritonsillar abscess* (more common) (ii) *true tonsillar abscess*. In peritonsillar abscess, inflammatory fluid extends into the peritonsillar space. This can result in cellulitis or abscess formation in the parapharyngeal, masticator and retropharyngeal spaces. Peritonsillar abscess can cause airway narrowing by causing midline deviation of the tonsil. In true tonsillar abscess area of liquefaction is contained within the gland and shows rim enhancement.

It is essential to differentiate between *cellulitis* and *abscess* formation as cellulitis can be treated medically and an abscess needs surgical intervention. On CT imaging, abscesses appear as peripherally enhancing, single or multiloculated, low-density masses that conform to fascial spaces. They appear hyperintense on T2WI. Cellulitis can easily spread to adjacent fascial spaces. If a diagnosis of cellulitis is made and the patient shows no response to appropriate antibiotic therapy, a second examination should be performed to ensure that an abscess cavity has not formed.

Lemierre syndrome consists of IJV thrombosis following a primary oropharyngeal infection with development of distal septic emboli, most commonly to the lungs. As imaging findings often precede positive blood cultures, radiologists play an important role in early diagnosis of this entity. *Fusobacterium necrophorum* is almost always the causative organism. Contrast enhanced CT reveals tonsillar and peritonsillar edema and abscess associated with primary site of infection with IJV thrombosis and thrombophlebitis. The infection can spread into the retropharyngeal and perivertebral spaces.[21]

Juvenile nasal angiofibroma is the commonest benign yet locally invasive, noncapsulated, vascular, mesenchymal tumor of the nasopharynx occurring almost exclusively in adolescent boys with mean age of presentation at 15 years. The most common presenting symptom is nasal speech due to nasal obstruction or severe recurrent epistaxis. It is thought to arise near the sphenopalatine foramen at the junction between the nose and the nasopharynx at the root of the medial pterygoid plate. Extra-nasopharyngeal spread is not uncommon at the time of presentation and this occurs to the retroantral region via the pterygopalatine fossa and anterior displacement of the posterior wall of antrum is commonly seen. Lateral extension to the infratemporal fossa occurs through the pterygomaxilla fissure. It may also spread to the orbit through the inferior orbital fissure, to the cavernous sinus and middle cranial fossa through the superior orbital fissure. Inferiorly it can bulge into the oropharynx and oral cavity. Invasion of the sphenoid sinus may be seen in up to two-third of cases implying an internal carotid artery supply whereas the lesion is typically supplied by the ipsilateral internal maxillary and ascending pharyngeal arteries **(Figs. 29A to C)**.

On CT and MR images juvenile angiofibroma appears as a soft tissue mass of variable size. It may be visualized as a small nodule within the sphenopalatine foramen striding the choana or a large, locally aggressive growth extending in any or a combination of directions. Erosion of the pterygoid lamina on CT is probably a pathognomonic sign. On unenhanced CT scans the tumor appears isodense, on MR it displays intermediate signal on T1W and bright signal intensities on T2W images. The extent of the tumor and its characteristics

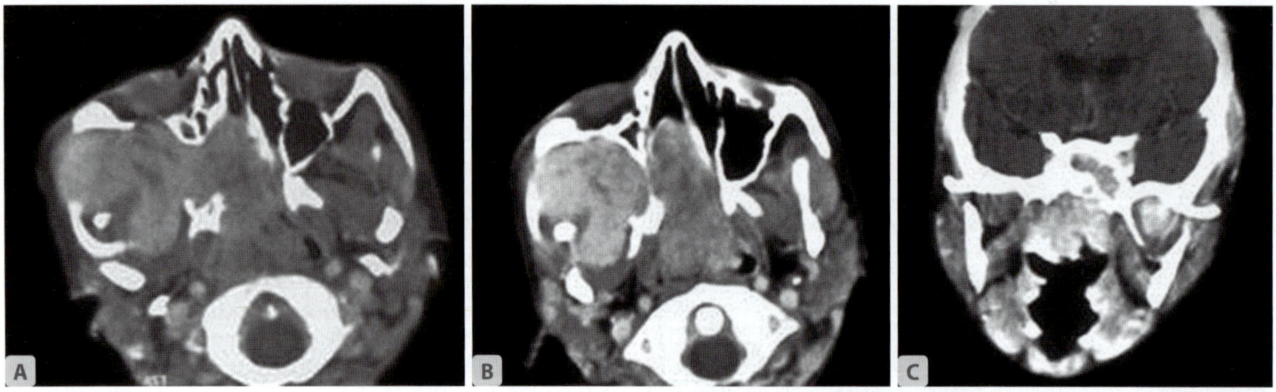

FIGS. 29A TO C: Axial CECT (A and B) and coronal (C) scans showing a large enhancing mass in the nasopharynx extending anteriorly in the nasal cavity pushing the nasal septum medially and encroaching upon/obliterating the contralateral nasal cavity. Widening of the pterygopalatine fossa and anterior bowing of the intact posterior maxillary antral wall is seen. Lateral extension through the pterygomaxillary fissure into the infratemporal fossa is seen. Coronal scan (C) reveals erosion of the floor of the sphenoid sinus with intrasinus extension and erosion of the root of the medial pterygoid plate. No intracranial extension seen—Juvenile nasopharyngeal angiofibroma.

are best evaluated on contrast enhanced scans. Postcontrast scans show intense enhancement with punctate areas of signal void indicating the highly vascular stroma **(Figs. 30A to D)**. The following imaging based grading system of juvenile angiofibroma has been proposed.

Grade I: Tumor confined to nasopharynx.

Grade II: Tumor extending into pterygopalatine fossa or masticator space.

Grade III: Tumor extending into orbit or intracranially.

The high tumor vascularity contraindicates biopsy and preoperative embolization is necessary.

PARAPHARYNGEAL SPACE

The parapharyngeal space (PPS) is located in the suprahyoid neck and is a symmetric crescent-shaped space situated lateral to the pharynx. It is an anatomic recess that was historically separated into the prestyloid and retrostyloid spaces by the tensor veli palatini,[22] styloid process, and associated musculature and ligaments. The anteriorly situated prestyloid compartment is deep to the MS and lateral to the pharyngeal mucosa and medial to the deep lobe of the parotid gland. The posteriorly situated retrostyloid compartment contains the carotid sheath and its contents. The retrostyloid space is now considered a separate carotid space.

The PPS extends from the skull base up to the hyoid bone, however, fusion of the fascial layers and muscle sheaths near the angle of the mandible limits the inferior extent of the PPS. It is encircled by layers of investing fascia laterally, separating it from the MS and PS and by the buccopharyngeal and prevertebral fascia, medially and posteriorly. The PPS does not have a fascial barrier anteriorly and is continuous with the submandibular and sublingual spaces. The lack of anterior border allows the spread of disease from the PPS along the pterygomandibular raphe, which connects the medial pterygoid plate to the lingual surface of the mandible along the posterior margin of the mylohyoid muscle. PPS lesion may present as a mass at the angle of mandible **(*see* Figs. 7A and B)**.

Contents—The PPS contains predominantly fat which can be easily differentiated from other tissue types on imaging. It also contains vascular structures including the maxillary and ascending pharyngeal artery and the pterygoid venous plexus.

Lesions—Primary masses of the PPS are rare, the source is likely minor salivary gland ectopic rests and the commonest tumor arising from these rests is a benign mixed tumor. Identification of a fat plane completely surrounding the lesion localizes the mass to the PPS **(Fig. 31)**.

The importance of PPS is its conspicuity on CT and MRI as well as its direction of displacement by mass lesions of the surrounding suprahyoid neck spaces.

This provides confirmation as to the origin of surrounding pathology as the adjacent mass lesions displace the PPS in specific directions **(Table 7)**.

BUCCAL SPACE

It is situated lateral to the buccinator muscle; medial to the zygomaticus major and anterior to the masseter. The posterior extension of the buccal space is the retroantral fat pad that reaches up to the anterior margin of the masticator space. The buccal space (BS) does not have complete fascial coverings. It is separated from the subcutaneous tissues of the face by the plane formed by the superficial muscles of facial expression and the investing fascia.

The **contents** of the BS include adipose tissue, minor salivary gland tissue, parotid duct, lymph nodes, facial vein, facial and buccal artery, buccal branch of the cranial nerve VII, buccal division of V3.[22] The differential diagnosis for the **lesions** that can occur in this space include SCC (direct extension or nodal metastases), lymphoma, minor salivary gland tumors, lipoma, hemangioma, sarcoma, sebaceous cyst, obstructed duct, cellulitis and abscesses.

RETROPHARYNGEAL SPACE

The retropharyngeal space (RPS) is a midline space bordered anteriorly by the visceral fascia and posteriorly by the prevertebral fascia. It extends from the skull base superiorly

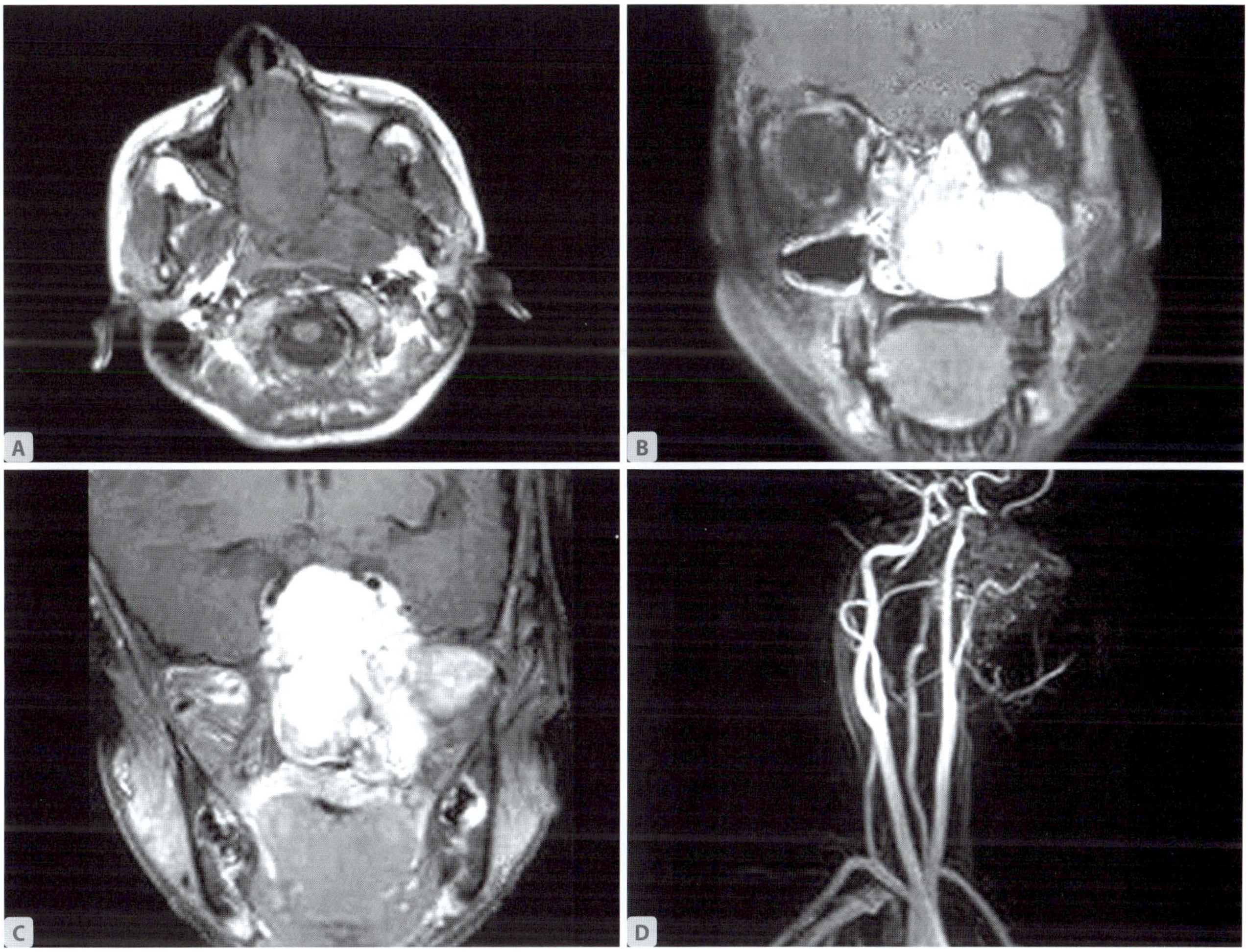

FIGS. 30A TO D: Axial T1W (A), coronal postcontrast T1W (B and C) MR images showing an intensely enhancing lobulated mass in the nasopharynx, the nasal cavity, the pterygopalatine fossa, the infratemporal fossa with erosion of the pterygoid lamina. Extension into the extraconal space of the left orbit, ethmoids and the left maxillary sinus is seen. Superior extension into the sphenoid sinus, and the left cavernous sinus is noted. MR angiogram images (D) show multiple prominent arterial channels suggestive of feeders from branches of left ECA—Juvenile nasopharyngeal angiofibroma.

to the T3 vertebral level inferiorly. In the suprahyoid neck, the PMS is anterior to the RPS while in the infrahyoid neck, hypopharynx and cervical esophagus are anterior to it. The carotid space is lateral to RPS in the suprahyoid and infrahyoid neck **(*see* Figs. 8A and B)**. The alar fascia, which is a thin fascial layer, divides the RPS into two compartments: the anterior and posterior. The posterior compartment is the *"danger space"*. The RPS and danger space cannot be differentiated on imaging.[10] Disease from the RPS can spread into the mediastinum via the danger space.

Contents—The RPS contains mainly fat and retropharyngeal lymph nodes, also known as the nodes of Rouviere (lymph nodes are found only in the suprahyoid RPS).

Retropharyngeal **pathologies** include edema, cellulitis and abscess. Secondary extension into the RPS may result from direct extension of squamous cell carcinoma, tortuous carotid artery, lipoma, hemangioma, diskitis and osteomyelitis from the prevertebral space. Lymph nodal enlargement can be due to reactive adenopathy, suppurative adenitis, metastatic adenopathy and lymphoma. Inflammatory conditions such as IJV thrombosis and longus colli tendinitis can cause edema of the RPS.

A mass in the RPS pushes the prevertebral muscles posteriorly whereas a mass in the prevertebral space lifts the prevertebral muscles anteriorly **(Figs. 32A and B)**. Nodal mass in lateral RPS may mimic a lesion in the carotid space. It is located medial to the carotid space and causes posterolateral displacement of the same.

CAROTID SPACE

These are paired tubular spaces extending along the suprahyoid and infrahyoid neck. Superiorly, the sheath of the carotid space (CS) extends up to the jugular foramen and inferiorly to the aortic arch. Anteriorly, it is bordered by the styloid process and parapharyngeal space, laterally by the anterior belly of the diagastric muscle and parotid space and medially by the lateral aspect of the retropharyngeal space. The CS has nasopharyngeal, oropharyngeal, cervical,

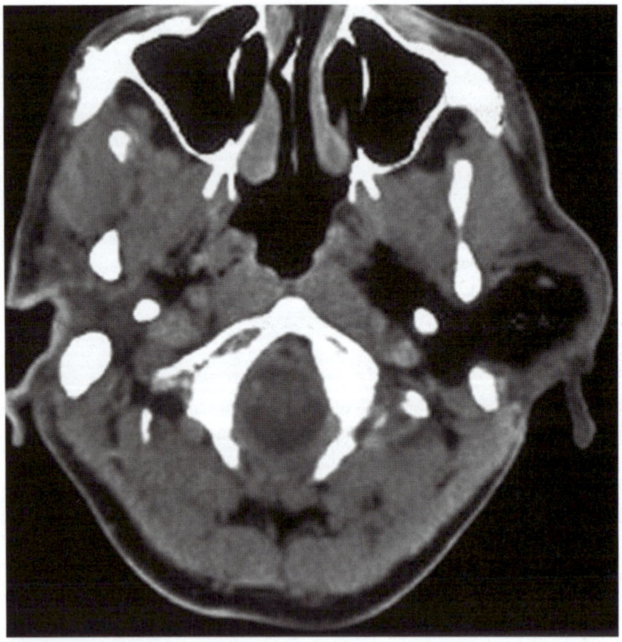

FIG. 31: Axial CECT image showing a well-defined non-enhancing hypodense mass having fat attenuation values within (– 90 HU) in the left parapharyngeal space. The lesion is seen extending superficially between the styloid process and the ramus of the mandible displacing the parotid gland laterally—parapharyngeal lipoma.

TABLE 7: PPS fat displacement pattern by lesions in different neck spaces.

Location of Lesion	Displacement
Pharyngeal mucosal space	Parapharyngeal fat displaced posterolaterally and styloid displaced posteriorly
Masticator space	Parapharyngeal fat displaced posteromedially and styloid displaced posteriorly
Carotid space	Parapharyngeal fat and styloid displaced anteriorly
Parotid space	Parapharyngeal fat displaced anteromedially
Retropharyngeal space	Parapharyngeal fat displaced anterolaterally and styloid displaced anteriorly

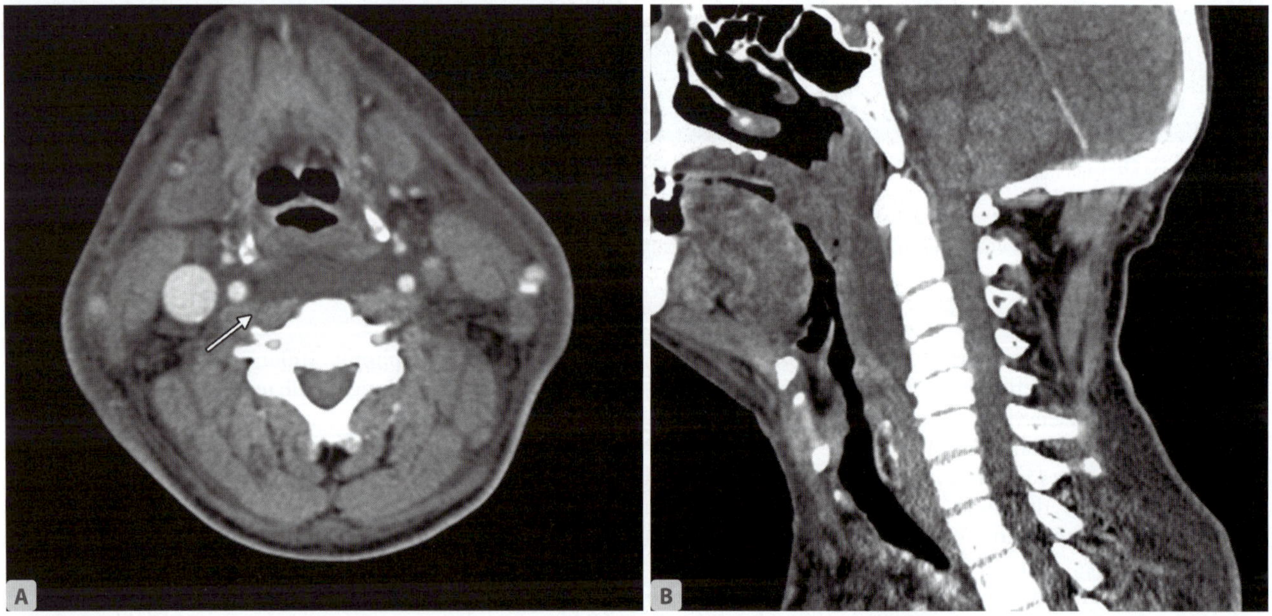

FIGS. 32A AND B: Axial (A) and sagittal (B) CECT images show a hypodense collection in the retropharyngeal space. Note the posterior displacement of prevertebral muscles (arrow in A), localizing the collection to the RPS.

and mediastinal segments. In the suprahyoid neck, the RPS is medial, perivertebral space is posterior, PS is lateral and PPS space is anterior to the CS while in the infrahyoid neck, the visceral space and RPS are medial, perivertebral space is posterior, anterior cervical space is anterior and posterior cervical space is lateral to the CS.

The **contents (Table 8)** of the suprahyoid carotid space include the internal carotid artery (ICA), internal jugular vein (IJV), cranial nerves IX to XII and sympathetic plexus. The contents of the infrahyoid carotid space include the common carotid artery (CCA), internal jugular vein and vagus nerve (X) **(*see* Fig. 9)**.

A lesion primary to the CS is epicentered within the area of CCA/ICA-IJV and posterior to the PPS. It causes anterior displacement of the PPS fat. In addition to anterior displacement of PPS fat, lesions in the nasopharyngeal segment of CS displace the styloid process anterolaterally and lesions in the oropharyngeal segment displace the posterior belly of digastric muscle laterally.

Masses within the CS may arise from or compress the cranial nerves within the space, most commonly detected if cranial nerve X is involved. Glomus jugulare paraganglioma, schwannoma and meningioma[16] are lesions that involve the jugular fossa, therefore, the skull base must be assessed carefully. Displacement of structures within the CS can help as a differentiating factor. Vagal schwannoma and a sympathetic schwannoma have similar imaging appearances but a vagal schwannoma divides the ICA and IJV whereas a sympathetic schwannoma causes displacement of both structures anteriorly.

TABLE 8: Contents and lesions of the carotid space.

Contents
• Carotid artery • Internal jugular vein (IJV) • CNs IX, X, XI, XII and sympathetic chain • Lymph nodes (lateral to carotid space, disease can spread to carotid space).
Lesions
• *Vascular pathology:* Carotid artery—aneurysm, dissection, arteritis; Jugular vein—thrombosis and thrombophlebitis • *Mass lesions:* Neurogenic tumors and paragangliomas • *Lymph nodes:* Neoplastic or inflammatory causes • *Neoplastic causes:* Contiguous or from perineural spread of tumor

Lesions—The commonest pathology in the carotid space is enlarged lymph nodes. Vascular pathology can arise from internal carotid artery or internal jugular vein and includes vessel tortuosity, thrombosis/phlebitis, pseudoaneurysm, dissection and stenosis. Flow related phenomenon of IJV may mimic thrombosis or schwannoma on imaging.

Paragangliomas are slow growing hypervascular tumors arising from neural crest derivatives. They occur at multiple levels within the carotid space including the carotid bifurcation (carotid body tumors), along the nodose ganglia of vagus nerve (glomus vagale tumors) and along the nerves supplying the jugular bulb (glomus jugulare tumors).[23]

Glomus jugulare tumors may present with pulsatile tinnitus. *Glomus vagale* and carotid body tumors often present as a pulsatile neck mass which may be multiple in 3–5% of cases. The nonchromaffin paragangliomas can occur as multifocal lesions especially in patients with a family history of these tumors. Therefore, a study of both the right and the left carotid regions is necessary in these patients. Small tumors are ovoid or spherical while large tumors have a pear or dumb-bell shape with smooth contours.

Paragangliomas are highly vascular tumors that enhance intensely on CT **(Figs. 33A and B)** and MR. On MR these tumors have an intermediate signal intensity on all sequences. Areas of necrosis or hemorrhages give rise to a nonhomogeneous appearance. MRI may also show the typical *'salt and pepper' appearance*. This is present due to multiple serpiginous vascular channels that produce the dark 'pepper'and small hemorrhages that produce focal hyperintensities on T1 the 'salt' appearance. On diffusion weighted MR imaging

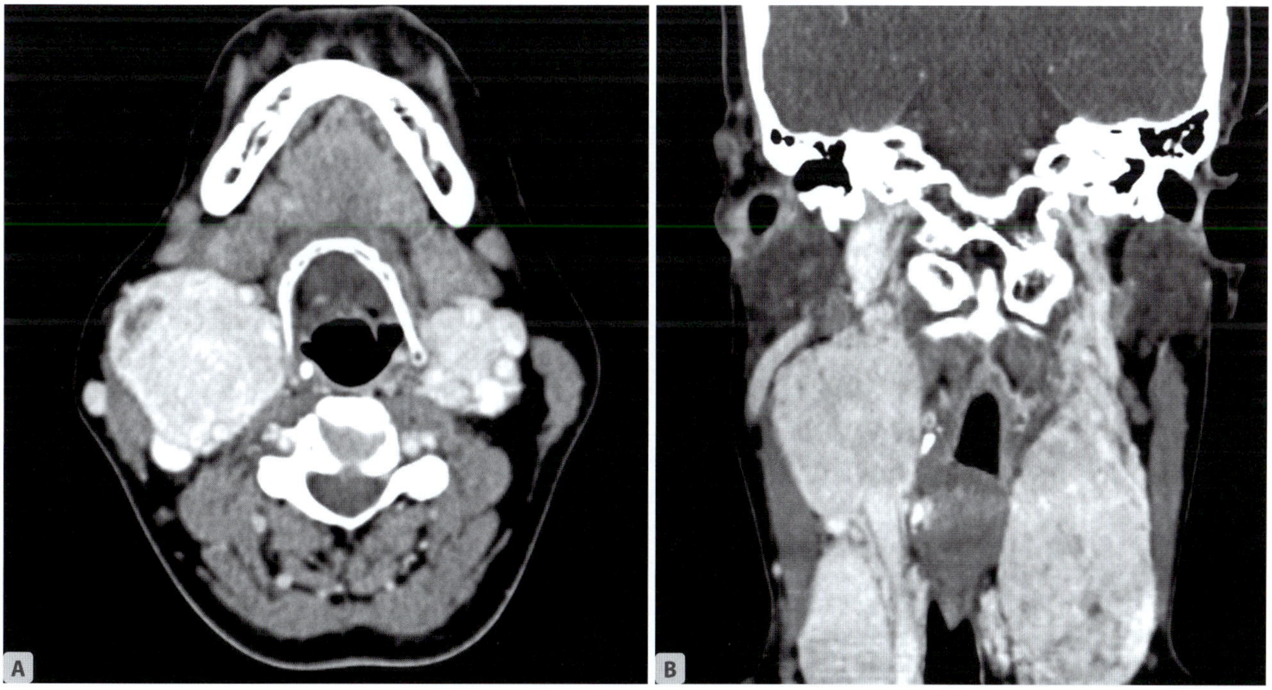

FIGS. 33A AND B: Axial (A) and coronal (B) CECT images show two well-marginated, hyperenhancing solid lesions with lobulated outline in the carotid space on each side—Bilateral paragangliomas.

paragangliomas may show low ADC values, therefore, when dealing with lesions showing lower ADC value in head and neck region, the possibility of paraganglioma should be ruled out before giving a diagnosis of malignancy, especially for those lesions without typical conventional MRI features.[24] Post contrast studies are helpful in identifying small tumors and synchronous lesions. They can be differentiated from schwannomas and neurofibromas on dynamic imaging. Dynamic scanning after 20–25 seconds of contrast injection reveals a sharp filling peak and a rapid washout after 150 seconds.[25] Schwannomas on the other hand do not show early enhancement but enhance intensely in scans obtained after 60 seconds. Angiography may be done in patients with equivocal lesions and for therapeutic embolization. Digital subtraction angiography and reformatted CT angiography/magnetic resonance angiography in case of carotid body tumors show a hypervascular mass splaying the internal and external carotids—the classic *"lyre sign"*.

Glomus jugulare tumor may cause variable erosion of the jugular foramen **(Figs. 34A to E)** and typically produces a permeative pattern of destruction in contrast to a neurofibroma or schwannoma which has a scalloped appearance.

The other differential diagnoses of these vascular lesions include metastasis from primary malignancies like hypernephroma, papillary thyroid carcinomas and melanoma and rare lesions such as extramedullary plasmacytomas, angiosarcomas and hemangiopericytomas. Some hemangiomas may have a similar imaging appearance with flow voids. A key feature for the differential diagnosis is the lack of displacement of adjacent vessels.

Surgical resection is the treatment of choice with preoperative embolization because it decreases operative blood loss.

Neurogenic tumors are the most common carotid space lesions.[26] They can also occur in the masticator space, the parapharyngeal space and rarely the parotid space. The vagus, hypoglossal, or cervical roots may be involved. Two types of tumors (1) *schwannomas* and (2) *neurofibromas* can arise from the nerves in the carotid space.

Schwannomas are the most common tumors originating from the Schwann cells surrounding the nerves. Most commonly the tumor arises from the vagus nerve and less commonly the glossopharyngeal nerve, the ventral and dorsal cervical nerve roots, the cervical sympathetic chain, and the brachial plexus.

A tumor originating from the *vagus nerve* manifests as a mass in the anterior triangle and displaces the internal or common carotid artery anteromedially and the internal jugular vein posterolaterally whereas a tumor arising from the *cervical nerve roots* manifests as a mass in the posterior triangle which may extend into one of the neural foramina of the cervical spine. *Sympathetic chain tumors* demonstrate a constant relationship with the longus colli muscles and lesions of the cervical sympathetic chain as they grow and expand, tend to push the common carotid, or internal and external carotids, anteriorly. *Brachial plexus schwannomas and neurofibromas* in the infrahyoid neck often displace the anterior scalene muscle anteriorly.

Schwannomas are well-encapsulated tumors that do not contain neural or collagen tissue but consists of cellular and myxoid components. The presence of these two

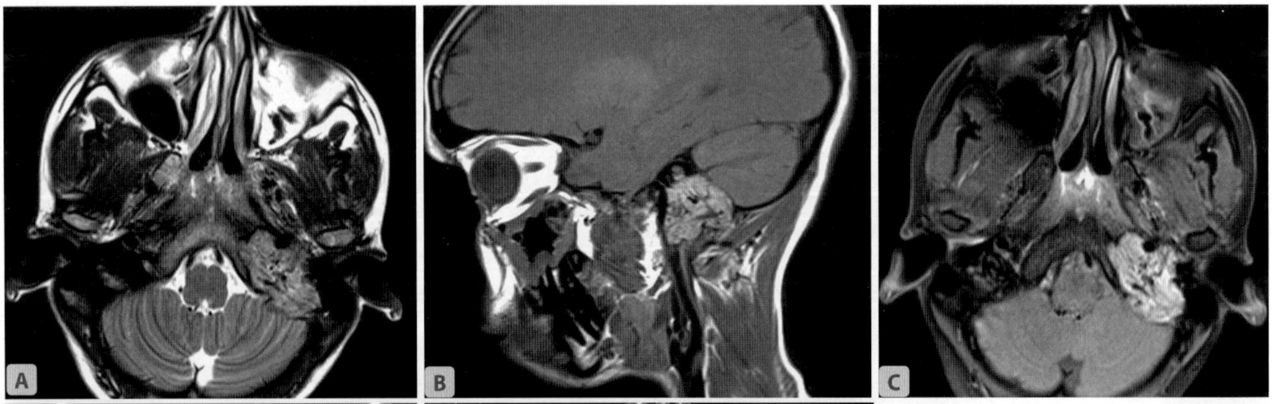

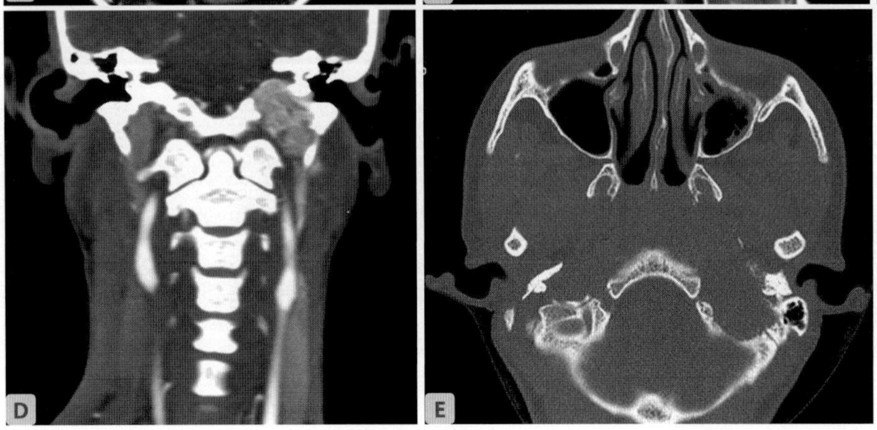

FIGS. 34A TO E: Axial T2W (A), sagittal T1W (B) and axial T1W (C) images show a well-marginated extra-axial lesion with salt and pepper appearance in the left jugular foramen indenting the left cerebellar hemisphere and extending into the left CP angle. Coronal (D) and axial (E) CT images show the hyperenhancing lesion in the left jugular foramen with expansion and destruction of the same—Glomus jugulare tumor.

components differentiates it from a neurofibroma. On CT the tumor is isodense to muscle and displays enhancement. The internal carotid artery is displaced anteriorly and laterally. Hypodense areas due to cystic changes are visualized in 20% of tumors. Fluid-fluid levels may be seen in schwannomas and they must then be differentiated from lymphatic malformations. The fusiform shape is well visualized on sagittal and coronal planes. On MRI the tumor appears hypointense on T1W and hyperintense on T2W. The T2 relaxation time decreases with increasing cellularity of the lesion **(Figs. 35A to D)**.

Avascular schwannomas can be differentiated from paragangliomas due to the absence of flow voids but vascular schwannomas have identical imaging features to paragangliomas. Dynamic scans can reveal the true nature of the lesion and differentiate it from hypervascular lesions. The enhancement of the schwannomas is seen at least two minutes after contrast injection and depicts the equilibrium phase of the contrast agent and the poor venous drainage of the tumor in contrast to paragangliomas which show a rapid filling and rapid wash out.

Neurofibromas are the second type of neurogenic tumors arising in the CS. In contrast to schwannomas these are noncapsulated and contain all elements of the nerve of origin and are continuous with it.[27] Circumferential compression of the involved nerve is seen which is diffusely penetrated by tumor elements and symptoms depend on the nerve involved. Around 10% of patients of neurofibromas have neurofibromatosis and malignant transformation is more common in this group.

The imaging features are dependent on the underlying histology. On CT neurofibromas show low attenuation due to lipid rich schwann and fat cells scattered in the tumor and there is no appreciable contrast enhancement. The low density (near water) on CT is characteristic **(Figs. 36A and B)**. Neurofibromas appear identical to avascular schwannomas on MRI. They have a low SI on T1W and high SI on T2W images with variable enhancement **(Figs. 37A to D)**.

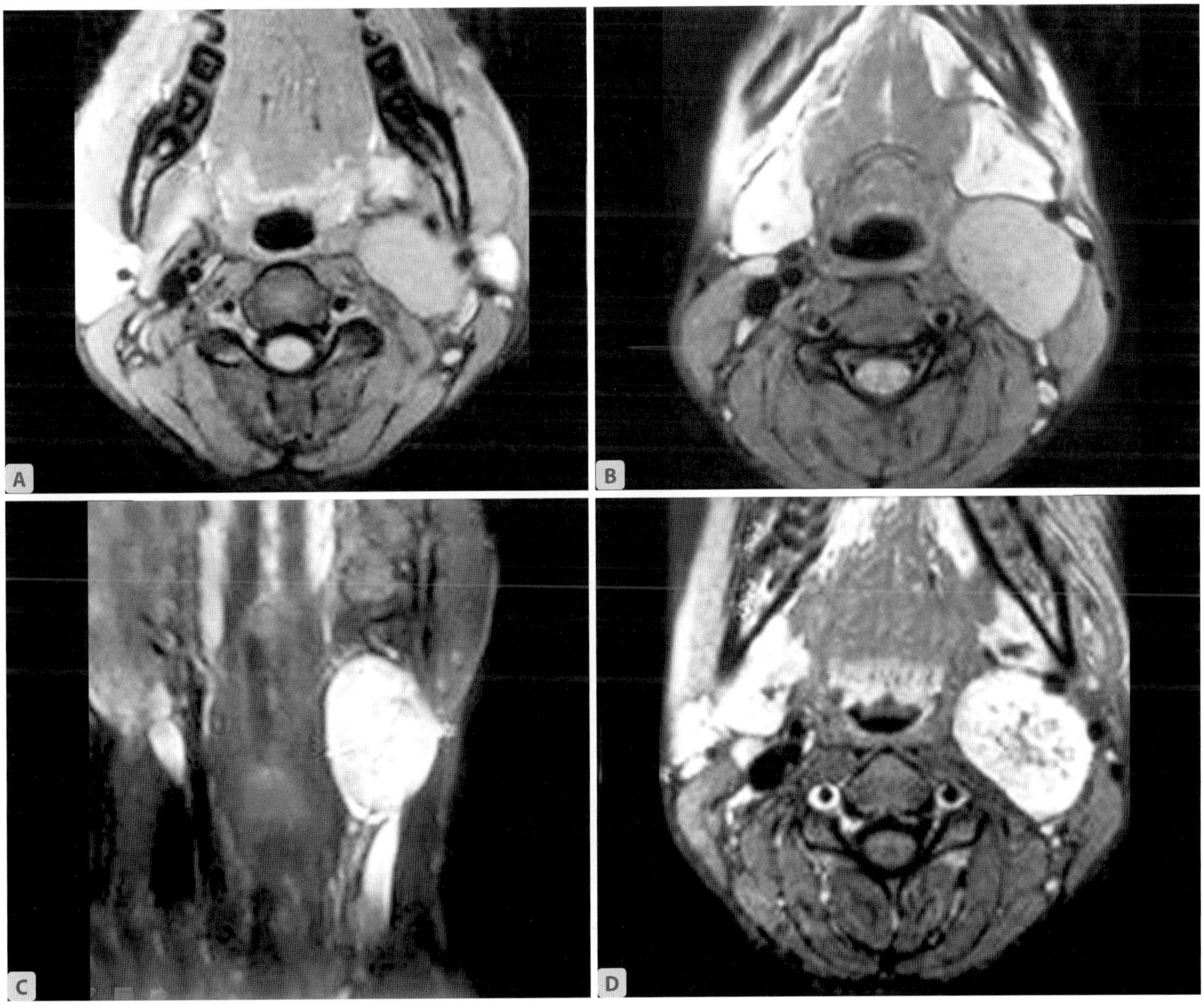

FIGS. 35A TO D: Axial T1W (A and B), coronal STIR (C) and axial postcontrast T1W (D) MR images showing an oval well-marginated lesion in the left carotid space displacing the ICA, ECA anterolaterally with attenuation of the IJV. The lesion is hyperintense with cystic areas on STIR images and shows intense contrast enhancement—Schwannoma.

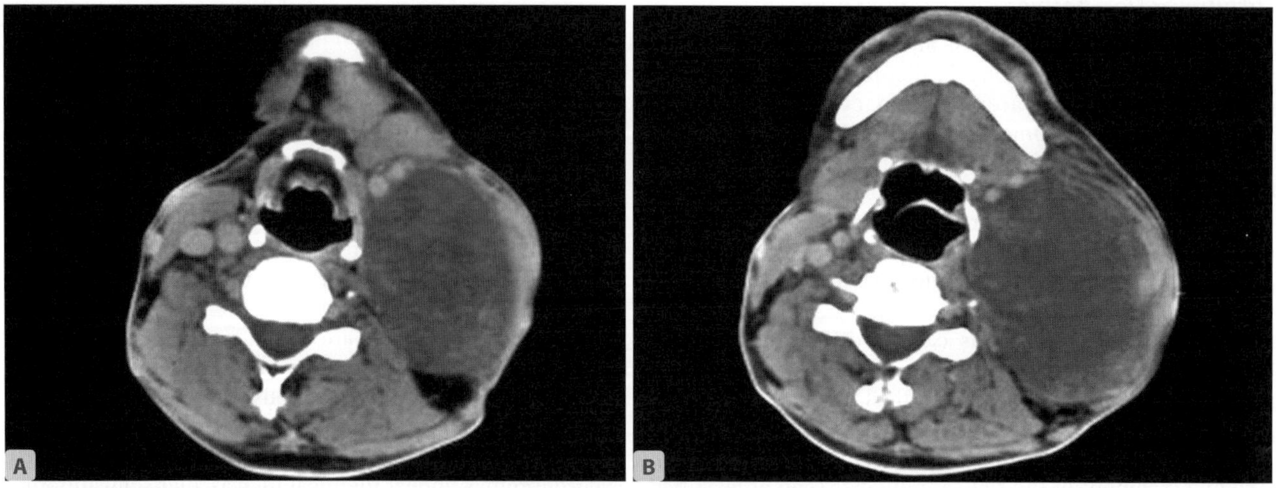

FIGS. 36A AND B: Axial CT scans showing a large well-encapsulated lesion in the left carotid space with displacement of carotid vessels anteriorly. (A) The lesion has a homogeneous low density and shows no significant enhancement (B) Neurofibroma.

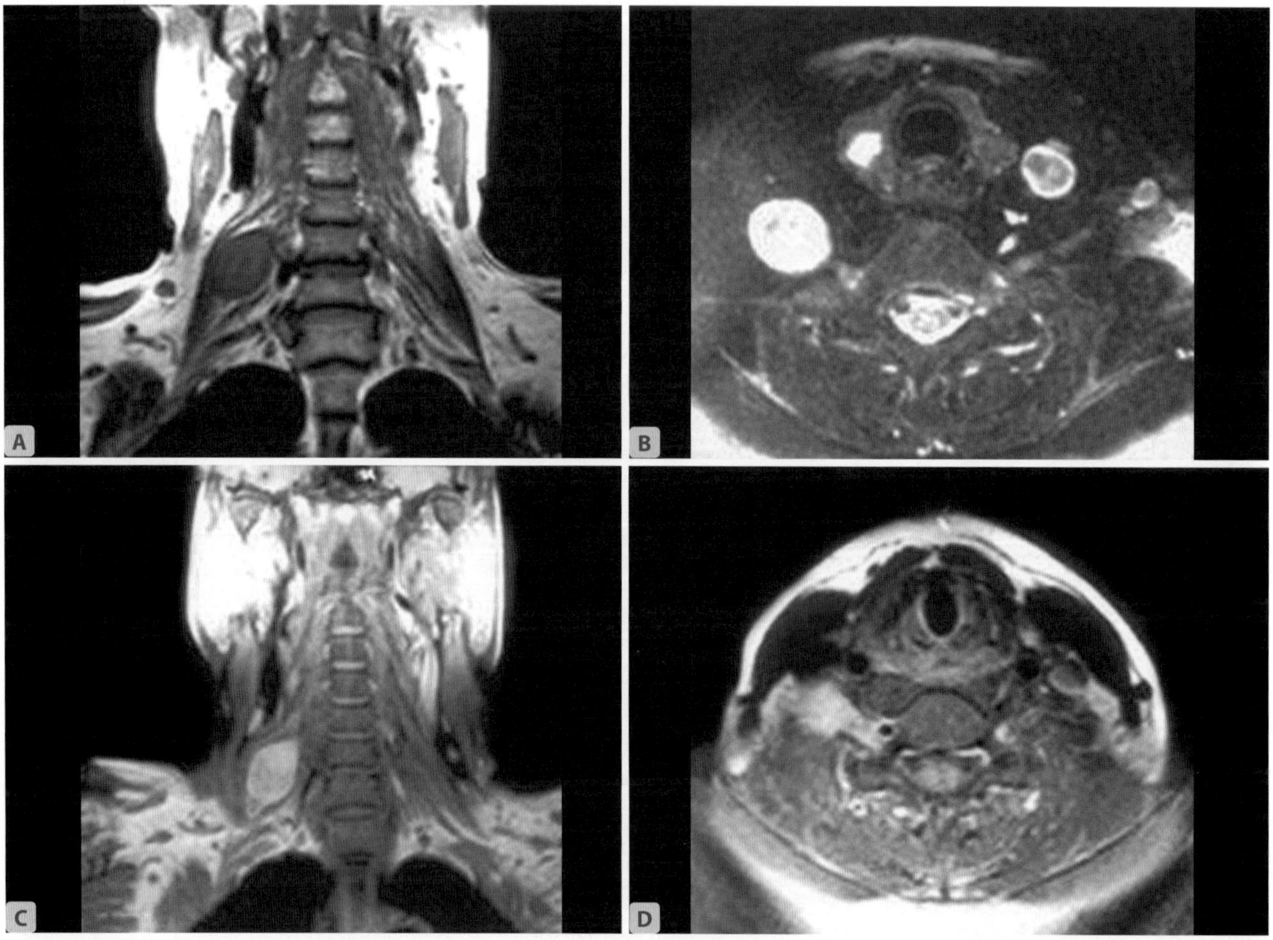

FIGS. 37A TO D: Coronal T1W (A), axial STIR (B), coronal (C) postcontrast and axial (D) postcontrast T1W MR images showing a well-marginated oval lesion in the right carotid space causing anterior displacement of the carotid vessels. The lesion is hypointense on T1, hyperintense on STIR with homogeneous contrast enhancement. Continuity with an enhancing nerve is best seen on the postcontrast coronal images and extension into the right neural foramen is seen—Neurofibroma.

Differentiation between Neurofibromas and Schwannomas

The imaging appearance of peripheral nerve sheath tumors depends on the histologic composition of the tumors and it may not be possible to differentiate between neurofibromas and schwannomas on imaging. However, certain imaging findings may be helpful in distinguishing the two. Neurofibromas may be seen at any age whereas schwannomas most commonly present between 20 and 50 years of age with occasional occurrences in childhood. Neurofibromas are characteristically asymptomatic whereas schwannomas are often associated with pain and tenderness. The pain may be localized or radicular in nature with associated paresthesias. A characteristic finding of neurofibromas is the *"target sign"*. On MRI an area of relatively hypointense central signal with peripheral hyperintense signal is seen on T2-weighted sequences, which is characteristic. NCCT may also be very useful, neurofibromas being hypodense on noncontrast scans as opposed to schwannomas.

Aneurysm of the ICA can present as a mass lesion of the neck. Helpful characteristics for differentiation of aneurysm from schwannomas or other rare tumors are the peripheral calcification and the obliteration of the ICA lumen. CT and MR angiography (MRA) can confirm the diagnosis of aneurysm.

PERIVERTEBRAL SPACE

The perivertebral space (PVS) is a cylindrical space surrounding the vertebral column and extends from the skull base to the coccyx. It is bounded by the deep layer of deep cervical fascia. It consists of the *prevertebral space* and *paraspinal space*. *Prevertebral space* is situated directly behind the retropharyngeal space. The carotid space is anterolateral to the prevertebral space and the posterior cervical space is lateral to it. *Paraspinal space* lies deep to posterior cervical space and posterior to the transverse processes of cervical spine.[21] **(*see* Fig. 10)**

The **contents** of the perivertebral space include prevertebral muscles (longus collis and capitis), scalene muscles, brachial plexus roots, phrenic nerve, vertebral artery and vein and vertebral bodies which lie in the prevertebral PVS. The paraspinal muscles, posterior elements, vertebral column and the proximal aspect of the brachial plexus lie in the paraspinal PVS. The anterior deep layer of deep cervical fascia is tenacious and infections or tumors of the PVS are redirected into the epidural space by this fascia.

The **pathologies** in this space include osteophytes, osteomyelitis, benign and malignant mesenchymal tumors, calcific tendinitis, primary bone tumors, metastases, diskitis, anterior disk herniation, aneurysm, lymphoma, and direct extension of carcinoma of the nasopharynx. The commonest malignancy of the prevertebral space in children is a rhabdomyosarcoma.

Vertebral body involvement is a conclusive sign of prevertebral space involvement. A mass in the prevertebral space proper has its center in the vertebral body or prevertebral muscles and displaces the prevertebral soft tissue. Therefore, a primary prevertebral space mass causes anterior displacement of the RPS and posterior wall of visceral space and lateral displacement of the carotid sheath. A mass from the paraspinal portion has its center in the paraspinal musculature or posterior elements of the vertebrae and displaces the paraspinous muscles and posterior cervical space fat outwards away from the spine.

Prevertebral abscesses represent a significant portion of PVS pathology. Etiologies include tubercular spondylitis, pyogenic osteomyelitis and postoperative infections.

In *tuberculous spondylitis* the inflammation is centered at the disk space which is often associated with partial destruction of the anterior aspect of the vertebral body. This is usually associated with a large paraspinal soft tissue mass that may show calcification **(Figs. 38A and B)**.

Pyogenic vertebral body osteomyelitis presents at the disk space with decreased height, subchondral bony erosions and fragmentation of the vertebral body without well-defined margins. Extension into the epidural space may be seen with both tubercular and pyogenic infections.

Longus colli tendinitis is a condition that needs to be differentiated from infections, it is an inflammatory response to the rupture of calcium hydroxyapatite deposits within the longus colli tendon. Calcification is seen at the longus capitis-colli tendinous insertions usually at C1-C2 levels and is best visualized on CT. Edema is seen in the adjacent retropharyngeal space.[21] On MRI, the calcification appears hypointense and does not enhance. Enlargement of muscle bellies can be seen in longus colli tendinitis, however, presence of the striated appearance of the muscle helps differentiate it from a neoplasm. Absence of lymphadenopathy and preserved bony structures helps differentiate this condition from infectious disease.

INFRAHYOID NECK

This is the region of the neck which extends from the hyoid bone to the thoracic inlet. It is divided into the visceral space, carotid space, retropharyngeal space, posterior cervical space, anterior cervical space and perivertebral space.

VISCERAL SPACE

It is a cylindrical space in the neck in midline enclosed by middle layer of deep cervical fascia. The visceral space (VS) is the largest space of the infrahyoid neck **(*see* Figs. 12A and B)**. The anterior cervical spaces are situated lateral to the visceral space, carotid spaces are posterolateral and the retropharyngeal space is posterior to it.

The **contents** of the visceral space are the larynx, trachea, hypopharynx, esophagus, thyroid and parathyroid glands. The recurrent laryngeal nerve is found in this space. The level VI group of lymph nodes including the paratracheal, prelaryngeal and pretracheal nodes and the infrahyoid strap muscles are also found in this space.

The **pathologies** that can arise in this space can arise from the larynx—laryngocele, squamous cell carcinoma; esophagus—esophageal diverticula, thyroid—colloid cyst, goiter, thyroid carcinoma, thyroglossal cyst; parathyroid—parathyroid adenoma; lymph nodes—metastases and lymphoma.

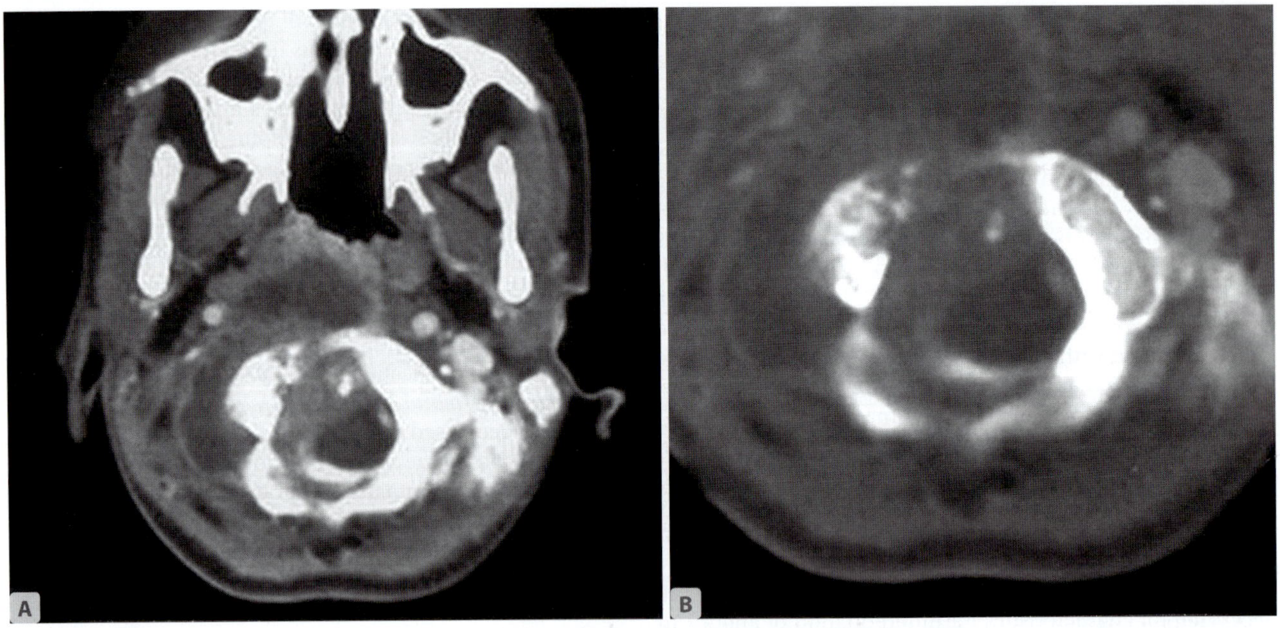

FIGS. 38A AND B: Axial CECT scans showing erosion of the basiocciput, right lateral mass of atlas and the dens with a large prevertebral and paravertebral collection. Note the anterior displacement of prevertebral muscles due to the collection. Caries C1, C2 with prevertebral abscess.

ANTERIOR CERVICAL SPACE

This is a small space situated in the anterolateral aspect of the neck and contains only fat. The anterior cervical space (ACS) lies lateral to the visceral space and anterior to the carotid space **(Fig. 39)**.

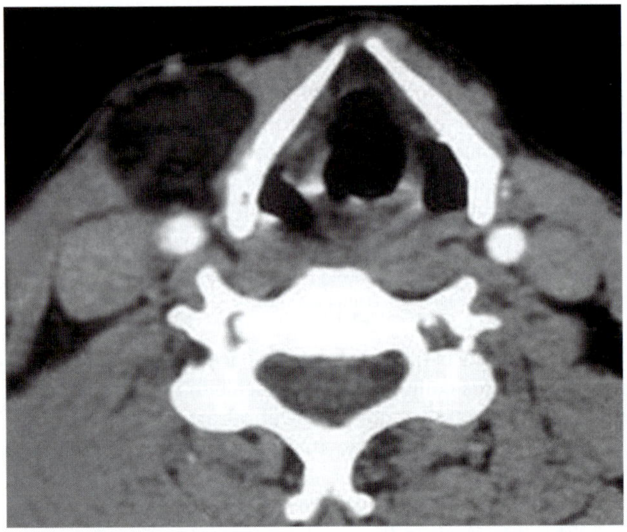

FIG. 39: Axial CECT scan showing a well-defined soft tissue density lesion of fat attenuation values in the anterior cervical space—lipoma.

POSTERIOR CERVICAL SPACE

Posterior cervical space (PCS) is a fat-containing space situated in the posterolateral aspect of the neck and extends from posterior mastoid tip to the clavicle. It lies between the superficial and deep layers of deep cervical fascia. The contents of this space include fat, accessory nerve (cranial nerve XI), spinal accessory lymph nodal chain, pre-axillary brachial plexus and dorsal scapular nerve.

The *posterior triangle* is the region of the neck posterolateral to the sternocleidomastoid muscle and anteromedial to the trapezius muscle. It is divided by the inferior belly of omohyoid muscle into *occipital and subclavian triangles. Occipital triangle* forms majority of the PCS and its boundaries are formed by the sternocleidomastoid muscle anteromedially, trapezius muscle posterolaterally and inferior belly of omohyoid muscle inferiorly. It contains fat, cranial nerve XI, dorsal scapular nerve and spinal accessory nodes. The *subclavian triangle* is the smaller portion of the PCS, it is bound by inferior belly of omohyoid superiorly, sternocleidomastoid anteromedially and trapezius posterolaterally. It contains the third portion of subclavian artery and cervical brachial plexus.[10]

A mass lesion primary to the PCS must be centered within the fat of PCS. It displaces the CS anteromedially, elevates sternocleidomastoid muscle and flattens deeper perivertebral space structures **(Figs. 40 and 41)**.

LESIONS COMMON TO DIFFERENT NECK SPACES

Branchial Cleft Anomalies

Branchial cleft anomalies are thought to arise because of incomplete obliteration of a portion of the branchial apparatus. A **first branchial cleft cyst** arises from the residual embryonic tract that extends from the external auditory canal (EAC) through the parotid gland to the submandibular region and is of two types. Preauricular location is seen with type 1

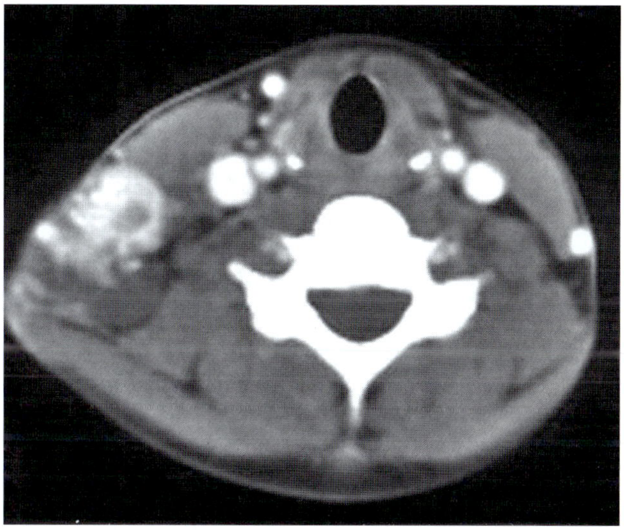

FIG. 40: Axial CECT image shows an ill-defined soft tissue density lesion with intense enhancement posterior to the sternocleidomastoid muscle on the right side—Hemangioma.

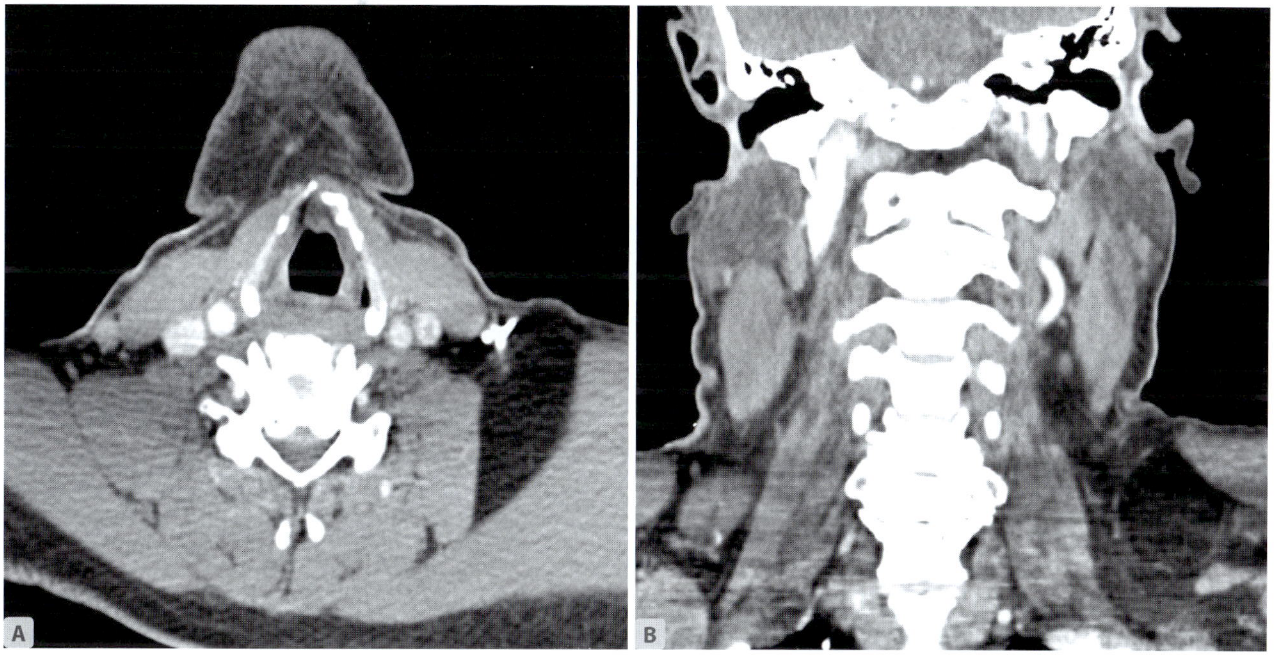

FIGS. 41A AND B: Axial (A) and coronal (B) CECT images show a hypodense lesion of fat density in the posterior cervical space—Lipoma.

cysts while type 2 is periparotid extending from the EAC to the angle of the mandible.

Approximately 95% of branchial cleft anomalies are related to the second branchial cleft, it also represents the second most commonly encountered congenital neck mass after thyroglossal duct cyst. The **second branchial anomaly** may cause fistulas **(Figs. 42A to C)**, sinuses or cysts. It can occur anywhere from the tonsillar fossa to the supracalvicular region. Bailey classified second branchial cleft cysts into four types. Type I are most superficial and lie along the anterior surface of the sternocleidomastoid muscle just deep to the platysma. Type II are seen along the anterior surface of the sternocleidomastoid muscle, lateral to the carotid space and posterior to the submandibular gland.[28] Type III cysts are seen to extend medially between the bifurcation of the internal and external carotid arteries. Type IV is seen in the PMS.

Imaging findings include low echogenicity on US, low attenuation on CT, and variable signal on MR imaging. Thickened enhancing walls are seen on cross-sectional imaging if infection is present.

Third and fourth branchial cleft cysts are rare. Most third branchial cleft cysts are situated posterior to the sternocleidomastoid muscle. Fourth branchial cleft anomalies are usually sinus tracts which arise from the pyriform sinus through the thyrohyoid membrane and descend into the mediastinum.

LESIONS OF VASCULAR ORIGIN

Vascular lesions of the head and neck are common and classified according to system the described by Mulliken and Glowacki[29] into two groups i.e. *vascular malformations,*

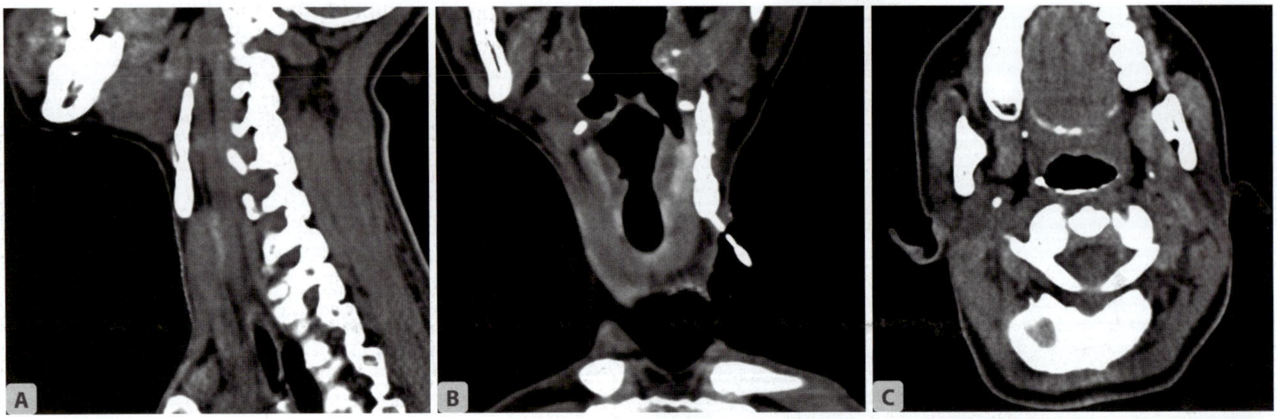

FIGS. 42A TO C: Sagittal (A), coronal (B) and axial (C) images from CT sinogram show a contrast-filled tract in the left side of the neck with internal opening in the tonsillar fossa, pooling of contrast is seen in the pharynx (C) second branchial cleft fistula.

which have normal endothelial cell turnover and *vascular tumors*, with high endothelial cell turnover. Since vascular malformations are not neoplastic, their growth is proportional to body size. Evaluation of the imaging characteristics and clinical presentation is important for correct diagnosis and providing appropriate treatment. There has been confusion with various terms in the past (such as cavernous hemangioma, which actually represent venous vascular malformations), it is important to use more consistent terminology **(Table 9)**.

TABLE 9: New and old terminology for vascular lesions.

New	Old
Hemangioma	Capillary hemangioma
Capillary malformation	Port wine stain
Venous malformation	Cavernous hemangioma
Lymphatic malformation	Lymphangioma, cystic hygroma

Capillary Malformations

Head and neck capillary malformations (CMs) present as a "port wine stain" cutaneous lesion following the dermatomal pattern of the trigeminal nerve in up to 43% of patients. About 3% of patients may have Sturge-Webber syndrome, the association is higher when trigeminal dermatomal pattern is seen.[30,31]

Diagnosis is usually made based on clinical characteristics but imaging can be useful in patients with Sturge-Weber syndrome or with equivocal clinical presentation. Differentials of CMs include superficial hemangioma, venous malformation, and arteriovenous malformation.

CMs are usually located in the dermis and appear isoechoic on high resolution sonography.[32] Doppler signal can be identified in nearly 30%. MRI or CT can be used to evaluate for suspected Sturge-Weber and can also help in the differentiation of CMs from other vascular lesions, which commonly extend deeper into the tissues, may involve bony structures, and have more internal flow. CMs can become darker and more apparent with time in many patients. In these cases, the treatment of choice is laser therapy.

Venous Malformations (VM)

They often present with facial deformity and pain secondary to local inflammatory changes or compressive effects. Up to 50% of head and neck VMs are seen at birth and are soft bluish masses that enlarge with dependent positioning, compression of the ipsilateral jugular vein, and Valsalva maneuvers. Differential diagnosis of VMs includes hemangioma, arteriovenous malformation, mixed vascular malformations, and dermoids.

The hallmark of VMs is the presence of phleboliths, which can be seen in up to 48% of cases.[33,34] On US, they are hypoechoic and heterogeneous with phleboliths appearing hyperechoic alongwith acoustic shadowing. Doppler flow may be seen in up to 37%. Bone changes can include osteolysis, demineralization, hypoplasia, and cortical thickening best seen on CT alongwith phleboliths and variable enhancement. MRI clearly delineates the spatial extent of the lesion. VMs are generally isointense on T1, hyperintense on T2W and show a heterogeneous enhancement pattern after contrast administration. Phleboliths appear as signal voids on both T1WI and T2WI. Rarely, magnetic resonance venography is done when there is suspicion of associated intracranial venous anomalies. On angiography, these lesions have slow flow and arterial supply is often not definitely identified. On direct percutaneous injection, contrast can be seen pooling in dilated venous channels.

Decision to treat VMs depends on the size and functional impact. Conservative management is preferred, if possible. Treatment generally includes percutaneous sclerotherapy with ethanol or sodium tetradecyl sulfate (Sotradecol) with majority of patients being cured or having significant improvement. If the lesion is large and difficult to delineate, sclerotherapy is used in combination with reconstructive surgery. Care should be taken in determining the dose of ethanol given during treatment, particularly when VMs have prominent draining veins as diffuse VMs with high-flow communication to conducting veins or adjacent arteries have increased risk of systemic toxicity and lesion recurrence. Recurrence has been noted to occur in up to 35% of patients.

Lymphatic Malformations (LM)

These generally present as a soft, colorless mass with 70–80% of cases occurring in the head and neck, this being the commonest site in the body. Up to 90% of these lesions are diagnosed by 2–5 years.[35] There are 2 types of LMs, macrocystic (> 1cm) and microcystic (< 1cm) groups. Microcystic LMs are more common and present later than macrocystic LMs, which are mostly present at birth. Macrocystic lesions commonly arise below the mylohyoid in the anterior or posterior triangles of the neck (previously called cystic hygromas). Microcystic LMs generally occur above the mylohyoid in the oral/perioral region and the parotid gland (previously called lymphangiomas).

Differential diagnosis includes venous malformations, mixed malformations, and cystic lesions such as branchial cleft cysts, and thyroglossal duct cysts.

On US, LMs are usually anechoic, microcystic variants appearing hyperechoic; Doppler flow is distinctly uncommon. On CT, these lesions are seen as a low density cystic mass which may be uniloculated or multiloculated and may be poorly circumscribed. In macrocystic lesions with previous internal hemorrhage or infection fluid-fluid levels can be identified **(Figs. 43A and B)**. Simple LMs show absence of contrast enhancement. On MRI, LMs are hypointense on T1WI, hyperintense on T2WI, with no contrast enhancement unlike VMs. Macrocystic LMs show a septated cystic mass appearing T1 hypointense to isointense often heterogeneous due to proteinaceous fluid with fluid-fluid levels. On the other hand, microcystic LMs appear as diffuse hypointensity on T1-weighted imaging and diffuse hyperintensity on T2-weighted imaging. MRI is valuable in preoperative planning and determining lesion extent because LMs can engulf and encase adjacent structures.

LMs located in life-threatening areas such as retropharyngeal LMs require prompt treatment otherwise treatment indications are similar to other VMs. Sclerotherapy is the most common treatment for macrocystic LMs. Microcystic LMs are less responsive to therapy and are typically managed conservatively unless symptomatic, threaten vital structures or for aesthetic reasons. Surgery is the preferred first-line treatment. Whatever the therapy, recurrence rates can be high (especially in microcystic lesions) and more than one procedure is often required.

Arteriovenous Malformations

Arteriovenous malformations (AVMs) are composed of arteries and veins that directly communicate through a central nidus. The lesions are present at birth in 40% of cases but AVMs of the head and neck generally present later in childhood or in adolescence often with cosmetic deformity, skin discoloration, an underlying pulsatile bruit, pain, bleeding, or ulceration.[36] Differential considerations include HM and VM. Color Doppler US helps to characterize these lesions as high flow showing high systolic and diastolic flow, prominent arteriovenous shunting and arterialization of venous flow. CT shows large, dilated, serpiginous enhancing structures, often indistinguishable as arterial or venous in origin. Skeletal involvement, not uncommon, is an additional CT finding.

MRI is integral to determining lesion extent and soft tissue involvement. AVMs are seen as tangled mesh of dilated arteries and veins demonstrating flow void on T1W and T2W echo imaging and hyperintense signal on T2W gradient echo imaging and angiography, indicating rapid flow. T1W postcontrast images demonstrate contrast enhancement of

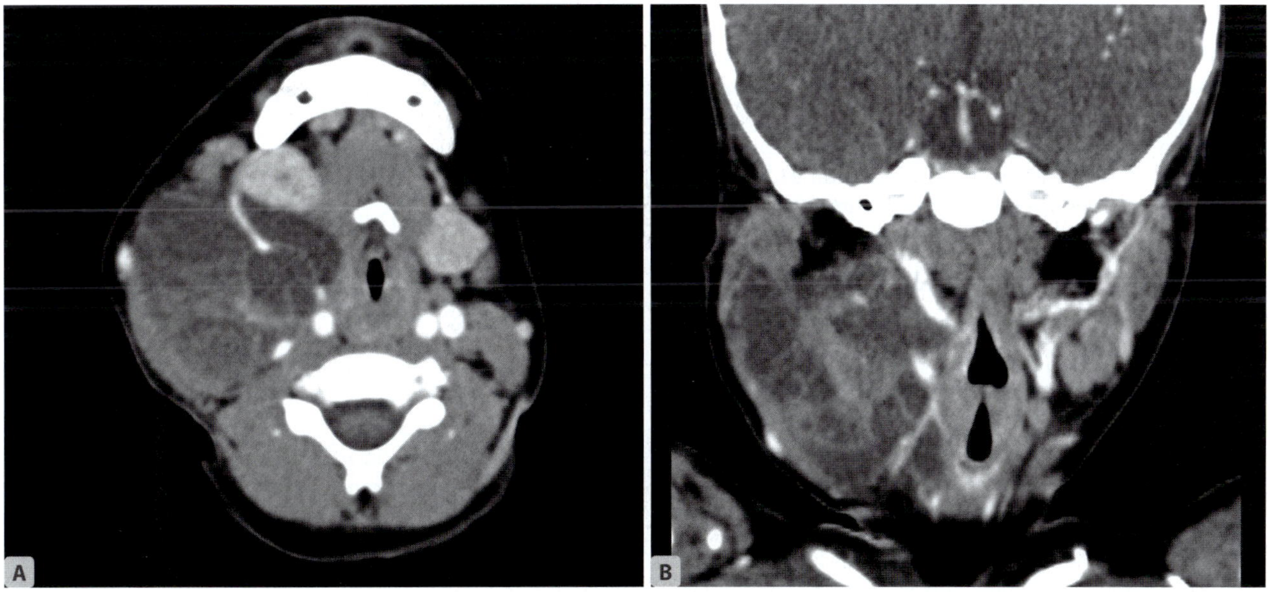

FIGS. 43A AND B: Axial (A) and coronal (B) CECT images show a multiloculated hypodense cystic lesion involving multiple spaces of the neck, displacing the submandibular gland anteriorly and carotid sheath structures posteromedially—Macrocystic lymphatic malformation (cystic hygroma).

multiple vessels with early venous enhancement, AVMs lack enhancement of adjacent soft tissue. Angiography helps in determining extent of the lesion as well as in directing therapeutic embolization. Treatment includes surgical resection, embolization, or combined therapy.

VASCULAR TUMORS

Hemangiomas

Hemangiomas (HM) are benign vascular neoplasms occurring most commonly in the head and neck region. They are divided into *infantile* and *congenital types*. Congenital hemangiomas are further divided into *noninvoluting congenital hemangiomas* (NICH) and *rapidly involuting congenital hemangiomas* (RICH).[36] Infantile hemangiomas (IH) present present postnatally usually by 6 weeks and represent 70% of all hemangiomas. Congenital HMs (30%) are present at birth.

HMs appear as a well-circumscribed mass with variable or heterogeneous echogenicity on gray scale US. They display high vascular flow on Doppler particularly in the proliferative phase seen as flow vessels in and around the mass, with the arterial feeder showing increased color flow, high Doppler shift and low resistance. On NCCT, HMs are isoattenuating to muscle making them difficult to delineate. They however, enhance avidly (especially in the proliferative phase). On MRI, HMs are isointense to slightly hyperintense on T1WI, hyperintense on T2WI, (often being mildly hyperintense to surrounding muscles) with avid contrast enhancement. Adjacent serpiginous flow voids can be seen. MR angiography (MRA) is useful when posterior fossa malformations hemangiomas—arterial anomalies—cardiac defects-eye abnormalities—sternal cleft and supraumbilical raphe syndrome is suspected. In this syndrome, hemangiomas present alongwith cerebral vascular anomalies and other abnormalities. MRA helps to visualize arterial stenosis, agenesis and aneurysms. On catheter angiography, high flow, an arterial blush, and persistent tissue staining is seen.

HM are usually small and self-involuting, hence the first step in therapy is expectant management. When cosmetically bothersome or if associated with compromised function of important structures intervention may be required. The first line of therapy is systemic propranolol, which leads to improvement in 97% of cases, significant improvement mostly occurring during the first week of therapy. In unresponsive cases treatment modalities include surgery, laser therapy, intralesional steroids, or chemotherapeutic agents.

MASSES OF MESENCHYMAL ORIGIN

Lipomatous tumors such as lipoma, lipoblastoma, and liposarcoma are the most common cervical neoplasms of mesenchymal origin. They usually manifest as painless masses, occurring most commonly in the midline of posterior neck or the posterior triangle. Cervical lipoblastoma typically presents as a rapidly growing mass.[37] Liposarcoma is one of the most frequent malignant soft tissue tumors in adults. It should be suspected whenever a large (5 cm) fat containing soft tissue tumor is found especially when it is clinically associated with pain and rapid growth. Well-differentiated liposarcoma displays a hypodense fat density (<–20 HU) mass on CT; the tumor shows signal intensities similar to those of subcutaneous normal fat on MR images. Poorly differentiated liposarcoma displays tissue density on CT and appears hypointense on T1-weighted images, hyperintense on T2-weighted MR images and shows intense early enhancement on dynamic acquisition contrast-enhanced images. Ill-defined borders and nonfatty heterogeneous contents indicate the high probability of malignancy. Other sarcomas that may be present are rhabdomyosarcoma, fibrosarcoma, osteosarcoma, chondrosarcoma, malignant fibrous histiocytoma, leiomyosarcoma, alveolar soft part sarcoma and synovial sarcoma. The imaging findings of these entities frequently are nonspecific.

CERVICAL LYMPHADENOPATHY

Understanding cervical lymph node anatomy, drainage pathways, and common abnormalities is central to interpretation of lymph node pathology. Clinical information along with location-specific approach and knowledge of lymph node morphology in various disease processes can further refine the differential diagnosis.

Cervical lymph nodes can be classified based on anatomic location or described with neoplastic processes using the formal *American Joint Committee on Cancer's (AJCC)* criteria.[10,38] The former differs from the latter in that it includes all lymph nodes and not just those important for surgical planning. Anatomically, various groups and chains of lymph nodes are described. These include:

- **Submental group**: Inferior to the anterior mandible.
- **Submandibular group**: Near the submandibular glands at the angles of the mandible.
- **Parotid lymph nodes**: The intraglandular nodes and within the fascia circumscribing the parotid space.
- **Preauricular nodes**: Within the subcutaneous tissues anterior to the external auditory canal
- **Postauricular nodes**: Posterior to the external auditory canal
- The **retropharyngeal space lymph nodes**: Medial RPS nodes situated in the paramedian RPS and the lateral RPS nodes situated lateral to the prevertebral muscles and medial to the internal jugular vein and internal carotid artery in the lateral RPS.
- The **facial lymph nodes** include multiple nodes named according to location, e.g. mandibular nodes superficial to the mandible, buccinator nodes in the subcutaneous tissues of the cheek, infraorbital nodes below the orbits, the malar nodes at the malar eminence, and the zygomatic nodes anterior to the zygomatic arch.
- The **occipital nodes** within the subcutaneous tissues posteroinferior to calvarium.
- The major nodal chains within the neck can be thought of as 3 linear chains of lymph nodes forming a triangle on each side of the neck. The **internal jugular chain** lies anteriorly surrounding the IJV from the skull base to the thoracic inlet. Posteriorly, the **spinal accessory chain** runs along the spinal accessory nerve in the posterior cervical space. The **transverse cervical chain** lies along

the transverse cervical artery in the supraclavicular fossa and connects the inferior portion of internal jugular and spinal accessory chain.

- The **anterior cervical group** includes the prelaryngeal, pretracheal and paratracheal chains. The prelaryngeal chain is midline and superficial. The pretracheal chain lies in the superficial fascia of the neck external to the strap muscles following the external jugular vein in its course. The paratracheal chain runs in the tracheoesophageal groove in the visceral space of the infrahyoid neck.

Cervical lymph nodes can also be categorized by surgical levels used for cancer treatment planning. These include 7 levels based on surgical landmarks while for imaging, radiologic landmarks are used **(Table 10)**.

Some lymph nodes are not included in the AJCC's surgical classification but are relevant in patient care. These include the parotid, retropharyngeal, occipital, and facial nodal groups.

The term *supraclavicular lymph nodes* is commonly used, however, it is not a defined nodal group and includes parts of both levels IV and VB. Supraclavicular nodes should be identified as they are important in cancer staging. *Virchow node* is a named lymph node that lies within the left supraclavicular fossa.[39]

In evaluation of a neck mass, it is important to differentiate between lymph nodes and other pathologies such as congenital cystic lesions, inflammatory/infective diseases or neoplastic diseases that can mimic a lymph node

TABLE 10: American Joint Committee on Cancer classification of cervical lymph nodes based on level and location **(Figs. 44 to 47)**.

Level I **Ia**: Submental—between anterior bellies of digastric below mandible **Ib**: Submandibular—lateral to anterior bellies of digastric and anterior to submandibular gland
Level II: Anterior cervical lymph node chain. Lymph nodes in the internal jugular chain from the skull base to the level of the hyoid bone. **IIa**; Nodes anterior, medial, or lateral to the internal jugular vein **IIb**: Nodes posterior to the internal jugular vein with a fat plane between the node and the vessel, nodes anterior to posterior edge of sternocleidomastoid
Level III: Nodes along the internal jugular chain between the hyoid bone and the cricoid cartilage
Level IV: Nodes along the lower IJV, from inferior margin of cricoid cartilage to supraclavicular fossa
Level V: Nodes in posterior cervical space corresponding to SAC, lie posterior to posterior margin of sternocleidomastoid in coronal plane **Va**: Level V nodes from the skull base to lower border of cricoid cartilage **Vb**: Level V nodes from lower border of cricoid cartilage to the supraclavicular fossa
Level VI: Nodes in the visceral compartment from the hyoid bone superiorly to the superior aspect of manubrium inferiorly, includes prelaryngeal, pretracheal, paratracheal, tracheoesophageal nodes
Level VII: Nodes in the superior mediastinum, between the carotid arteries, extending from superior margin of manubrium to innominate vein.

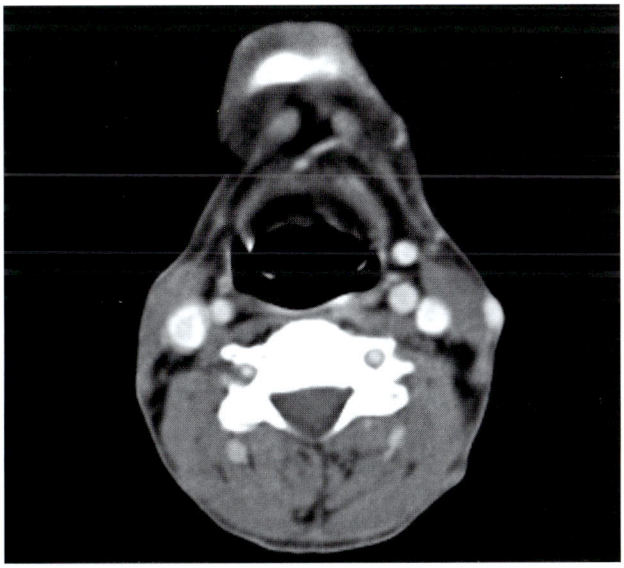

FIG. 44: Axial CECT image showing submental lymph nodes, the nodes are seen between the anterior bellies of digastric, below the mandible (level Ia).

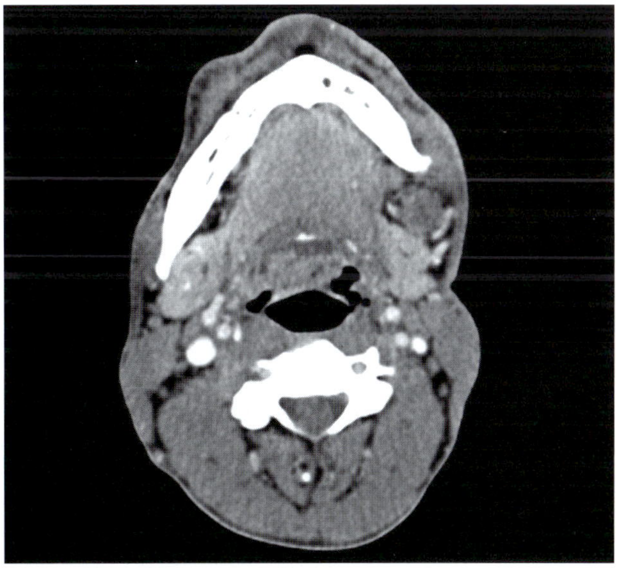

FIG. 45: Axial CECT image shows enlarged necrotic level Ib lymph node (anterior to the submandibular gland) on left side.

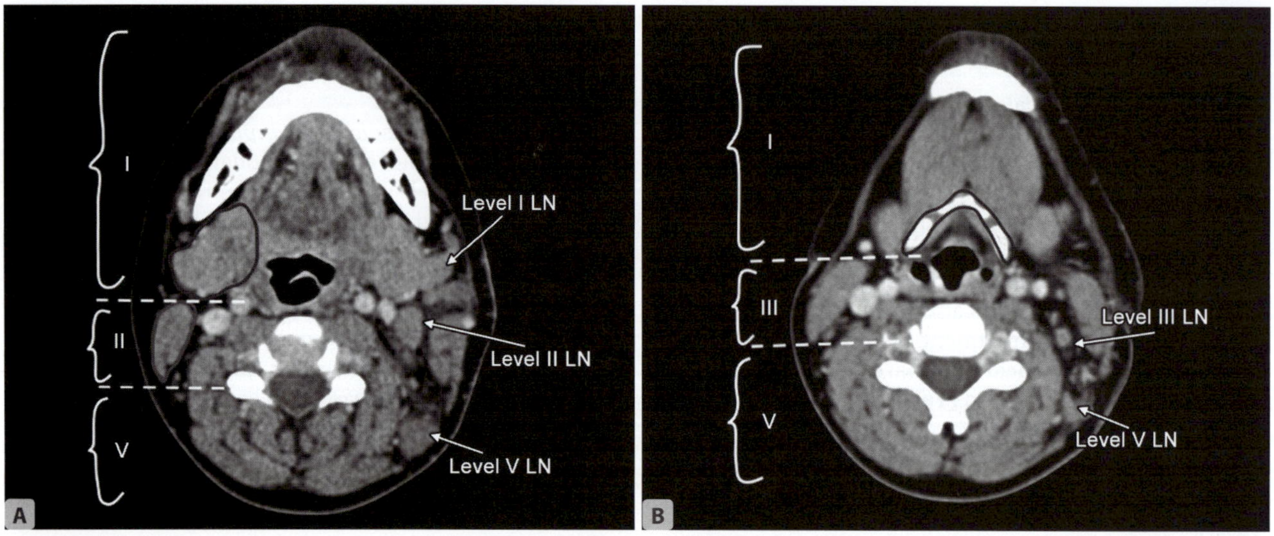

FIGS. 46A AND B: Axial CECT images show enlarged level I, II, III and V lymph nodes on left side in a known case of lymphoma. Level I lymph nodes are anterior to the submandibular gland, level II are posterior to the submandibular gland and level V are posterior to the sternocleidomastoid.

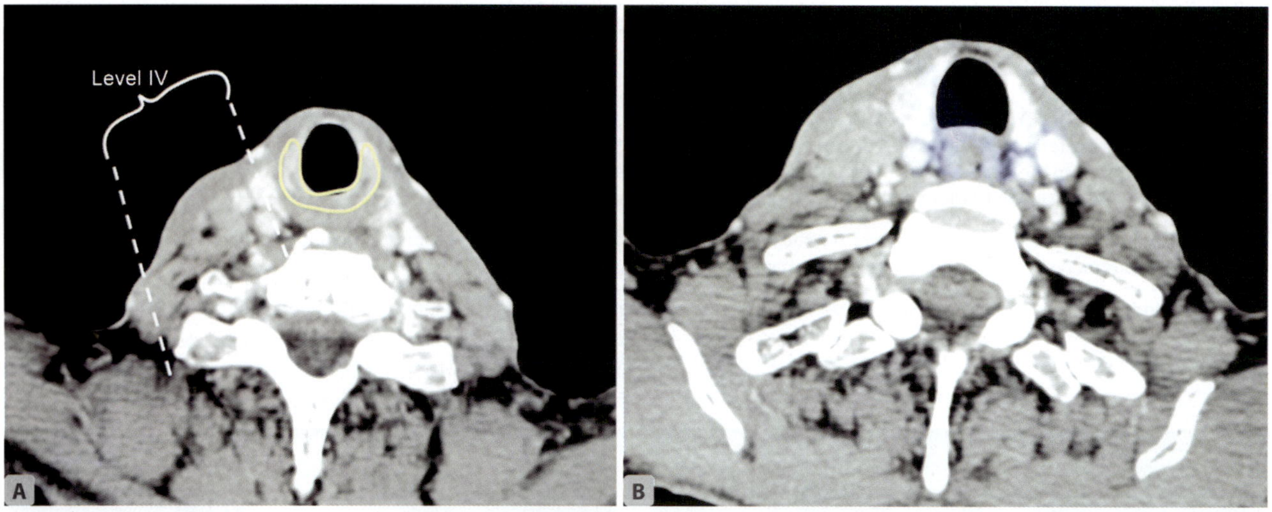

FIGS. 47A AND B: Axial CECT image shows enlarged level IV lymph nodes on right side in a known case of carcinoma larynx, level IV lymph nodes are seen between the inferior margin of the cricoid to supraclavicular fossa.

(Figs. 48A to C). Normal lymph nodes have a central fatty hilum which is continuous with surrounding cervical fat and reniform shape. Lymph node enlargement criteria include a long diameter of more than 15 mm for level I or II nodes, >8 mm for retropharyngeal nodes and >10 mm for other cervical nodes. However, up to 50% of the nodes with malignant deposits measure <5 mm in size.[40] Thus, other important features that should be considered while assessing lymph nodes include configuration, homogeneity, enhancement, fatty hilum and surrounding fat planes.

MORPHOLOGICAL CHARACTERISTICS OF LYMPH NODES

Reactive Lymphadenopathy

Reactive lymph nodal enlargement occurs in response to an antigen or infiltration. It can be acute or chronic and localized or generalized. The causes include drugs, foreign antigens, chemicals and infectious agents. Lymph nodes are enlarged with preserved reniform shape and show mild enhancement

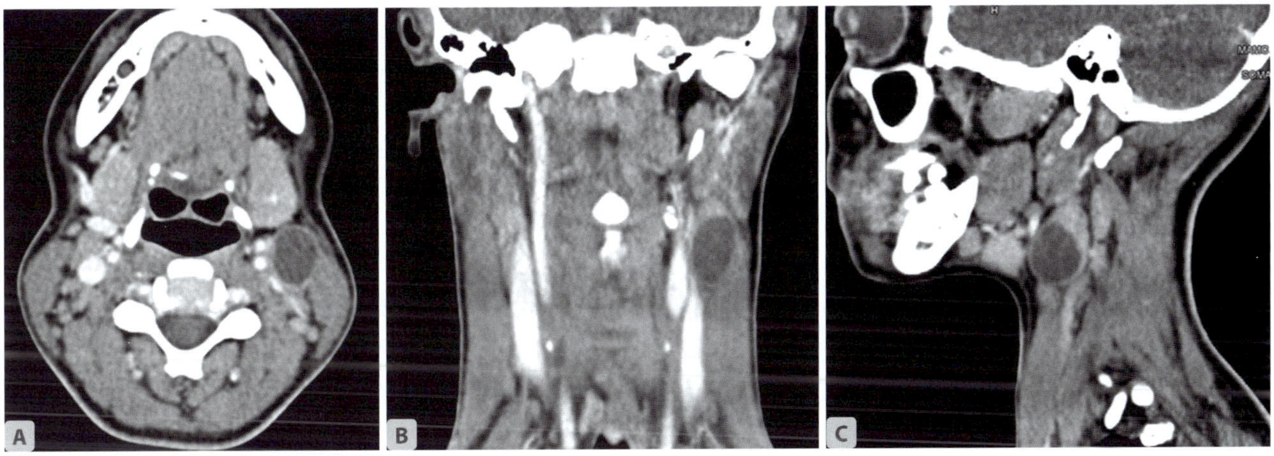

FIGS. 48A TO C: Axial (A), coronal (B) and sagittal (C) CECT images show a necrotic lymph node posterior to the posterior margin of submandibular gland (level II) on left side in a follow-up case of squamous cell carcinoma oral cavity. Note the near cystic appearance of the node.

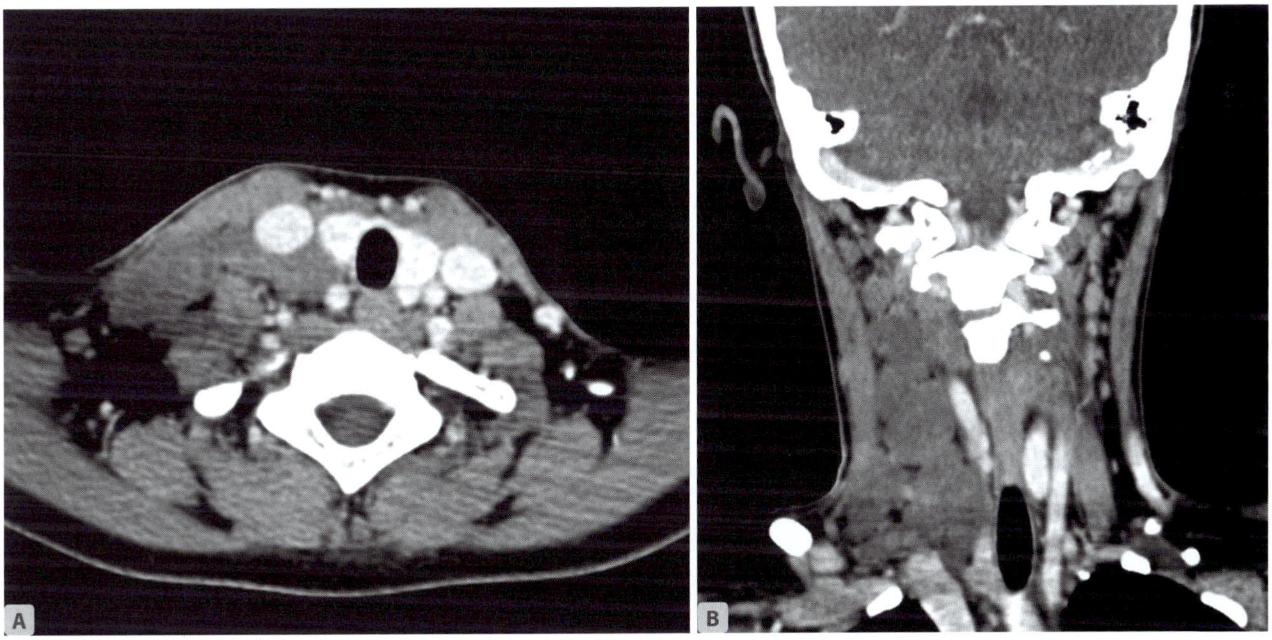

FIGS. 49A AND B: Axial (A) and coronal (B) CECT images show multiple enlarged necrotic lymph nodes (levels II, III, IV, V) on right side, showing conglomeration—Tubercular lymphadenopathy.

with enhancing linear markings. Reactive lymphadenopathy is commonly seen in children following upper respiratory tract infections.

Necrotic Lymphadenopathy

Necrotic lymph nodes show central necrosis due to inadequate vascular supply and can be seen with metastatic disease and necrotizing granulomatous disease like tuberculosis **(Figs. 49A and B)**. The frequency of nodal necrosis increases with metastatic nodal size. Therefore, the detection of nodal necrosis in isolation is most helpful if the necrotic nodes are less than 10 mm and there are no other abnormal nodes.

Contrast enhanced CT shows low central density. On MR, central low signal intensity is seen on T1WI with central hyperintensity on T2WI. Diffusion-weighted imaging can show diffusion restriction, and low apparent diffusion coefficient (ADC) values ($<1.0 \times 10^3$ mm^2/s) can be seen within malignant nodal disease, similar to primary site ADC values. Contrast enhanced MR imaging shows low signal intensity with no enhancement in the central aspect with surrounding enhancement of the part of the lymph nodes that have increased vascular supply. US reveals decreased central echogenicity with increased through transmission, similar to suppurative nodal disease.[41]

If a suspected necrotic lymph node is detected a consideration of tuberculosis and metastatic disease should be kept in mind. Age and smoking history should be taken into account, although some cancers, such as human papillomavirus positive (HPV1) squamous cell carcinomas can occur in younger adults without a smoking history.[42] These are most frequently found in the oropharynx and may be associated with necrotic nodal disease which may mimic cysts.

Suppurative lymph nodes are pus-containing lymph nodes and are also referred to as adenitis, acute lymphadenitis, or intranodal abscess and are commonly seen in children and young adults. The retropharyngeal, jugulodigastric, and submandibular group of lymph nodes are commonly involved. The nodes show similar characteristics as that of necrotic nodes and appear oval to round, cystic and often have poorly defined margins; stranding of the surrounding fat and subcutaneous tissue may be seen. Clinical history may be useful to differentiate between necrotic and suppurative lymphadenopathy.

Calcified Lymphadenopathy

Calcified lymph nodes can be seen with infection, granulomatous disease, or metastatic disease and are best evaluated with CT. Bone windows can help assess the extent of calcification and the configuration. The most important causes of calcified lymph nodes in the neck are tuberculous adenitis **(Fig. 50)** and thyroid cancer, especially metastatic papillary thyroid carcinoma. The configuration of the calcifications within the nodes is similar to the calcifications in the primary lesion helping in determining the site of origin. Lymph nodal calcification may also be seen postradiotherapy.

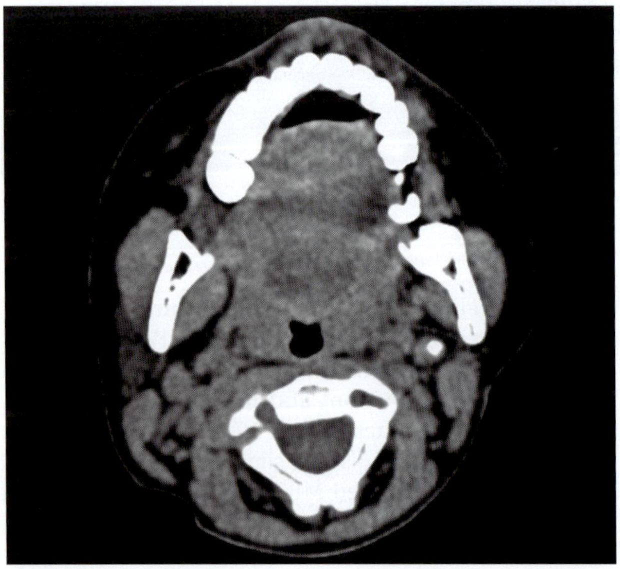

FIG. 50: Axial CT image shows cervical lymph node with a calcific focus within on left side (level II) in a known case of tuberculosis on treatment.

Matted Lymphadenopathy

It is a confluence of nodes that may be associated with surrounding fluid or inflammatory changes. They can be seen with infectious disease such as tuberculosis or metastatic disease. In squamous cell carcinomas, matted lymph nodes are associated with poor prognosis independent of T classification, HPV status, epidermal growth factor or smoking status.

Diffuse Lymphadenopathy

Diffuse lymphadenopathy can be seen with infection, generalized systemic disease or neoplasms. Viral, bacterial sepsis and human immunodeficiency virus adenopathy can cause diffuse nodal involvement. Metastatic disease from lung, breast, kidney and melanoma can metastasize to the head and neck. Non-Hodgkin lymphoma and Hodgkin lymphoma can also cause diffuse cervical lymphadenopathy **(Figs. 51A to D)**. Lymphomas are usually homogeneous on CT and show variable degree of enhancement. On MRI, lymphomas are hypointense to isointense on T1WI and hyperintense on T2WI compared with muscle.

There are a few rare diseases that affect the cervical lymph nodes. *Castleman disease* is a benign lymphoproliferative disorder. Involvement of one or multiple nodal groups can be seen with more than 90% of neck lesions being unifocal.[43] Contrast enhanced CT shows moderate to marked homogenous enhancement. On MRI the nodes are hypointense or isointense on T1WI and hyperintense on T2WI. Branching striations that are hypointense on T2WI are suggestive of Castleman disease, although this is a rare finding.

Kimura disease is another disease of lymph node enlargement also known as eosinophilic lymphogranuloma or eosinophilic hyperplastic lymphogranuloma. It presents with painless unilateral cervical lymphadenopathy or subcutaneous nodules. Parotid or submandibular gland involvement must be present, although the lacrimal gland is rarely involved.

Kikuchi disease, or Kikuchi-Fujimoto disease, is a rare, benign, self-limited disease associated with tender, regional cervical lymphadenopathy and is accompanied by mild fever and night sweats.

Rosai-Dorfman disease, or sinus histiocytosis with massive lymphadenopathy, is another very rare, benign process with proliferation of hematopoietic cells and fibrous tissue often presenting in the head and neck region. Symmetric, painless and bilateral cervical adenopathy is seen.[39]

CONCLUSION

A sound understanding of the anatomy of the spaces and contents of the suprahyoid and infrahyoid neck alongwith a systematic approach is essential for detection and characterization of neck lesions. Alongwith clinical data this helps in accurate diagnosis and providing better care for patients.

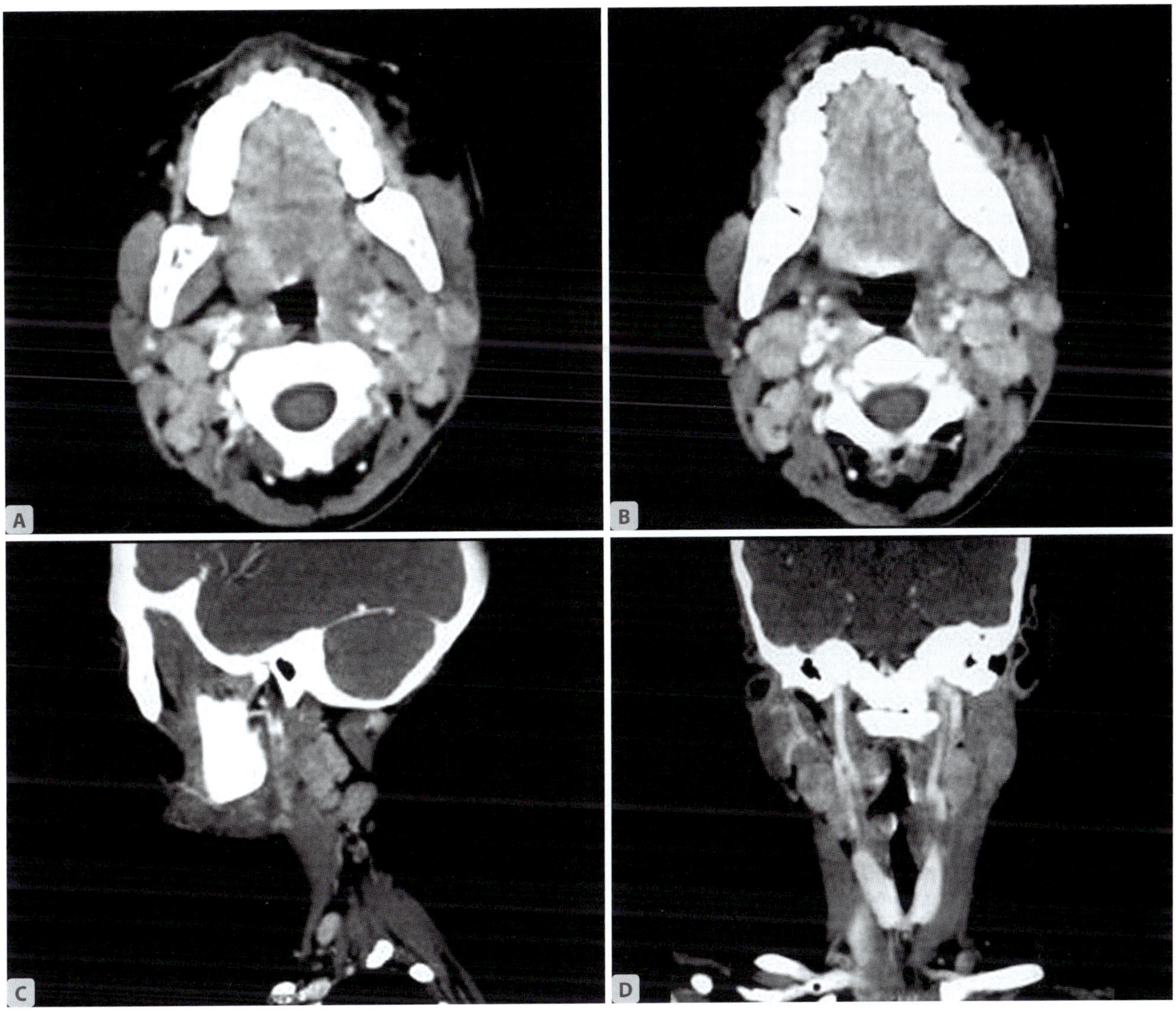

FIGS. 51A TO D: Axial (A and B) sagittal (C) and coronal (D) CECT scans of the neck revealing multiple varying sized round to spherical discrete lymph nodes along bilateral internal jugular veins, posterior triangle of neck and submandibular spaces s/o mitotic etiology—lymphoreticular malignancy.

REFERENCES

1. Bannister LH, Berry MM, Collins P, Dyson M, Dussek JE, Ferguson MWJ. Grays Anatomy. Churchill Livingston: Edinburg, 1995.
2. Carlson GW. Surgical anatomy of the neck. Surgical Clinics North Am. 1993;73:837.
3. Faggioni L, Neri E, Bartolozzi C. CT Perfusion of head and neck tumors: how we do it. AJR. 2010;194:62-9.
4. Chawla S, Kim S, Wang S, et al. Diffusion-weighted imaging in head and neck cancers. Future Oncology. 2009;5(7): 959-75.
5. Bisdas S, Baghi M, Huebner F, et al. In vivo proton MR spectroscopy of primary tumors, nodal and recurrent disease of extracranial head and neck. Eur Radiol. 2007;17:251-7.
6. Fukui MB, Blodgett TM, Snyderman CH, et al. Combined PET-CT in the head and neck. Radio Graphics. 2005;25(4):913-30.
7. Cummings C, Flint P. Cummings otolaryngology—Head and Neck Surgery, 5th edition, revision. Philadelphia: Mosby Elsevier; 2010. pp. 201-8.
8. Brown W, Gleeson M. Scott-Brown's Otolaryngology, Head and Neck Surgery. 7th edition. London: Hodder Arnold; 2008.
9. Warshafsky D, Goldenberg D, Kanekar SG. Imaging anatomy of deep neck spaces. Otolaryngol Clin N Am. 2012;45:1203-21.
10. Harnsberger HR, Glastonbury CM, Michael MA, et al. Diagnositc Imaging. Head and Neck. Salt Lake City (UT): Amirsys Publishing, 2011.
11. Arya S, Rane P, D'Cruz A. Infratemporal fossa, masticator space and parapharyngeal space: can the radiologist and surgeon speak the same language? Otorhinolaryngol Clin: Int J. 2012;4(3):125-35.
12. Oliver ER, Gillespie MB. Deep neck space infections. In: Paul WF, Bruce H, Valerie JL (Eds). Cummings Otolaryngology Head and Neck Surgery (4th edition). Philadelphia, PA: Elsevier Mosby 2005; pp. 202-03.
13. Standring S. Infratemporal and Pterygopalatine Fossae and Temporomandibular Joint. In: Standring S (Ed). Gray's Anatomy: The Anatomical Basis of Clinical Practice, 14th edition. Churchill Livingstone: Elsevier 2011; p. 527.
14. Tovi F, Hertzanu Y, Noyek AM. Infections of the infratemporal fossa: Imaging/clinical correlations. J Otolaryngol. 1991;20(Suppl 3):1-11.

15. Mukherji SK, Castillo M. A simplified approach to spaces of the suprahyoid neck. Radiol Clin North Am. 1998; 36(5):761-80.
16. Gamss C, Gupta A, Chazen JL, et al. Imaging evaluation of the suprahyoid neck. Radiol Clin N Am. 2015;53:133-44.
17. Brucker JL, Gentry LR. Imaging of head and neck emergencies. Radiol Clin N Am. 2015;53:215-52.
18. Rastogi R, Bhargava S, Mallarajapatna GJ, et al. Pictorial essay: salivary gland imaging. Indian J Radiol Imaging 2012;22:325-33.
19. La'Porte SJ, Juttla JK, Lingam RK. Imaging the floor of the mouth and the sublingual space. RadioGraphics. 2011; 31:1215-30.
20. Meuwly JY, Lepori D, Theuman N. Multi modality imaging evaluation of the paediatric neck: techniques and spectrum of findings. Radiographics. 2005;25:931-48.
21. Mills MK, Shah LM. Imaging of the perivertebral space. Radiol Clin N Am. 2015;53:163-80.
22. Meesa IR, Mukherji SK. A simplified approach to the spaces of the suprahyoid neck. Appl Radiol. 2017;46(4):6-14.
23. Win T, Lewin JS. Imaging characteristics of carotid body tumors. Am J Otol. 1995;16:325-8.
24. Yuan Y, Shi H, Tao X. Head and neck paragangliomas: diffusion weighted and dynamic contrast enhanced magnetic resonance imaging characteristics. BMC Medical Imaging. 2016;16:12.
25. Som PM, Brandwein-Gensler MS. Anatomy and pathology of the salivary glands. In: Som PM, Curtin HD (Eds). Head and Neck Imaging, 5th edition. Elsevier Mosby; 2011; pp.2449-609.
26. Colreavy MP, Lacy PD, Hughes J. Head and neck schwannomas—a 10 year review. J Laryngol Otol. 2000;114: 119-24.
27. Chung CJ, Armfield KB, Mukherji SK. Cervical neurofibromas in children with NF-I. Pediat Radiol. 1999-2000;29:353-6.
28. Turkington JRA, Paterson A, et al. Neck masses in children. BJR. 2005;78:75-85.
29. Mulliken JB, Glowacki J. Hemangiomas and vascular malformations in infants and children: a classification based on endothelial characteristics. Plast Reconstr Surg. 1982;69(3):412-22.
30. Hennedige AA, Quaba AA, Al-Nakib K. Sturge-Weber syndrome and dermatomal facial port-wine stains: incidence, association with glaucoma, and pulsed tunable dye laser treatment effectiveness. Plast Reconstr Surg. 2008;121(4):1173-80.
31. Enjolras O, Riche MC, Merland JJ. Facial port-wine stains and Sturge-Weber syndrome. Pediatrics. 1985;76(1):48-51.
32. Eivazi B, Fasunla AJ, Hundt W, et al. Low flow vascular malformations of the head and neck: a study on brightness mode, color coded duplex and spectral Doppler sonography. Eur Arch Otorhinolaryngol. 2011;268(10):1505-11.
33. Berenguer B, Burrows PE, Zurakowski D, et al. Sclerotherapy of craniofacial venous malformations: complications and results. Plast Reconstr Surg. 1999;104(1):1-11.
34. Aspestrand F, Kolbenstvedt A. Vascular mass lesions and hypervascular tumors in the head and neck. Characteristics at CT, MR imaging and angiography. Acta Radiol. 1995; 36(2):136-41.
35. Mathur NN, Rana I, Bothra R, et al. Bleomycin sclerotherapy in congenital lymphatic and vascular malformations of head and neck. Int J Pediatr Otorhinolaryngol. 2005;69(1):75-80.
36. Mulligan PR, Prajapati HJS, Martin LG, Patel TH. Vascular anomalies: classification, imaging characteristics and implications for interventional radiology treatment approaches. Br J Radiol. 2014;87:20130392.
37. Brodsky JR, Kim DY, Jiang Z. Cervical lipoblastoma. Case report review of literature and genetic analysis. Wiley Periodicals. 2007;1055-60.
38. Edge SB, Byrd DR, Compton CC, et al. Lymphoidneoplasms. AJCC Cancer Staging Manual. 7th edition. Salt Lake City (UT): Springer; 2010. p. 599-615.
39. Eisenmenger LB, Wiggins RH. Imaging of head and neck lymph nodes. Radiol Clin N Am. 2015;53:115-32.
40. Chong V. Cervical lymphadenopathy: what radiologists need to know. Cancer Imaging. 2004;4(2):116-20.
41. King AD, Tse GM, Ahuja AT, et al. Necrosis in metastatic neck nodes: diagnostic accuracy of CT, MR imaging, and US. Radiology. 2004;230(3):720-6.
42. Goldenberg D, Sciubba J, Koch WM. Cystic metastasis from head and neck squamous cell cancer: a distinct disease variant? Head Neck. 2006;28(7):633-8.
43. Liang J, Newman JG, Frank DM, et al. Cervical unicentric Castleman disease presenting as a neck mass: case report and review of the literature. Ear Nose Throat J. 2009;88(5):E8.

CHAPTER

204

Thyroid Imaging

Alpana Manchanda, Anju Garg, Jyoti Kumar, Rashmi Dixit

INTRODUCTION

The thyroid is a bilobed butterfly or bow-tie shaped gland located anteriorly in the lower neck. Under or over production of thyroid hormones leading to thyroid dysfunction is relatively common; with blood biochemistry, ultrasonography and radionuclide scintigraphy being the mainstay of investigation and management. Lesions of the thyroid gland arise from a variety of conditions which are usually benign, but may be due to malignancy in a minority. Increasing use of high resolution ultrasonography and cross-sectional imaging like CT and MR Imaging has led to a significant increase in the detection of incidental thyroid lesions. Imaging, especially high resolution ultrasonography is highly sensitive in detecting small nodules, calcifications, septations and cysts, as well as guiding fine needle aspiration (FNA) biopsies and has a major role in the differentiation of a benign lesion from a malignant one.[1]

EMBRYOLOGY

The thyroid gland develops from median and lateral anlages. The median anlage arises in the midline of the oropharynx during the fourth to fifth gestational week and gives rise to follicular thyroid tissue, which secretes hormones. The lateral anlages are thought to arise from the ultimobranchial bodies, which in turn are derived from the fourth and fifth branchial pharyngeal pouches. They give rise to the parafollicular C cells which secrete calcitonin. Fusion of the median and lateral anlages occurs by tenth week *in utero* resulting in the bilobed form of the gland.[2] The thyroid gland originates embryologically in the foramen caecum at the base of the tongue, and migrates to its final location in the anterior lower neck. Knowledge of the typical course of the thyroid primordium during embryologic development is important in understanding the various locations in the path where ectopic thyroid tissue can be found. From its origin at the foramen caecum, the thyroid primordeum first courses anterior to the hyoid bone then loops inferior and posterior to the hyoid and then descends anterior to the thyrohyoid membrane, thyroid cartilage and trachea into the orthotopic location in the infrahyoid neck.[3] This course of descent is represented by the remnant thyroglossal duct, which normally involutes by the 8th week of gestation along which residual thyroid tissue may be found. Descent beyond the normal results in a mediastinal component of the thyroid gland.

Very rare and unusual locations of ectopic thyroid tissue which may be detected within the neck and mediastinum are intralaryngeal, pre-laryngeal, intrapharyngeal, intra-esophageal, intratracheal, intrapericardial, intracardiac, etc. A large majority of mediastinal thyroids are retrosternal extensions of large goiters in the neck.[4]

ANATOMY

The thyroid gland is located in the lower anterior neck in the infrahyoid compartment. It is bounded by the strap muscles anteriorly and the second to fourth tracheal rings and the longus colli muscle posteriorly. The gland is made up of two lobes located lateral to the trachea, each with a superior and inferior pole. The right and left lobes are joined at the midline in front of the trachea by a thin bridge of thyroid tissue called isthmus at the junction of middle and lower one thirds of the gland. The normal dimensions of each lobe of the thyroid is less than 5 × 2 × 2 cm in longitudinal, transverse and anterior-posterior dimension respectively. The gland size varies with patient age, sex and weight and normal weight is between 15 and 35 g. The average thyroid volume in males is 19.6 mL while in females it is 18.6 mL.

An accessory lobe, the pyramidal lobe, may be present in 10–40% of normal population. It originates from the isthmus or the medial aspect of either lobe and extends superiorly along the course of the distal thyroglossal duct.[5] The pyramidal lobe can be regularly seen in younger patients. But it undergoes progressive atrophy in adulthood and becomes invisible.[6] The pyramidal lobe is most commonly recognized in patients with Graves' disease because it is enlarged and easily identified on nuclear scintigraphy.

The thyroid gland is enveloped by portions of the deep cervical fascia which attach the thyroid gland to the larynx and trachea. As a result, the thyroid gland moves with the larynx during swallowing. The entire thyroid gland is in the neck above the level of the clavicles. Sufficient enlargement of the thyroid gland results in its extension to outside the normal volume of the thyroid bed. It grows caudally into the pretracheal space and may even extend to lie in the retrosternal region, anterior to the common carotid arteries and the internal jugular veins. In this location, the thyroid enlargement is referred to as a retrosternal or substernal goiter.

The thyroid gland has a rich vascular supply, being derived from the paired superior and inferior thyroid arteries which are braches of external carotid arteries and the thyrocervical trunk respectively. The thyroidea ima is an inconstant vessel which when present arises directly from the aortic arch and helps supply the inferior thyroid gland. The venous drainage of the thyroid gland is via the superior and middle thyroidal veins which empty into internal jugular vein, and an inferior vein which drains into the innominate vein. The thyroid is innervated by the tenth cranial nerve (vagus) and the cervical sympathetic neural plexus.

ENDOCRINOLOGY

The primary function of the thyroid gland is to synthesize hormones that play a vital role in the regulation of metabolic functions. Triiodothyronine (T_3) and thyroxin (T_4) are two hormones synthesized within the thyroid. They are released from the thyroid in response to a feedback mechanism with the pituitary-hypothalamic axis. The secretion of thyroid hormones is mediated by thyrotropin-stimulating hormone (TSH) secreted by the anterior pituitary gland. Pituitary secretion of TSH, is in turn regulated by thyrotropin-releasing hormone (TRH) secreted by the hypothalamus. T_3 is three to four times more active physiologically than T_4. T_4 is synthesized entirely within the gland while 80–95% of T3 is synthesized by peripheral conversion of T_4. **Table 1** shows the normal reference range of thyroid hormones.

Calcitonin is a hormone produced by the parafollicular (C cells) of the thyroid gland in response to high calcium levels in the bloodstream and helps in regulating calcium and phosphate levels in the blood.

CLINICAL MANIFESTATIONS OF THYROID DISEASE

The spectrum of symptoms of thyroid disease is varied and the clinical manifestations are due to an increased or decreased function of the thyroid gland. **Hyperthyroidism** refers to a sustained thyroid hyperfunction with increase in synthesis and release of thyroid hormone. **Thyrotoxicosis** refers to a clinical syndrome that develops when circulating levels of T_4 and T_3 are markedly increased (TSH is usually suppressed). It is manifested by a multitude of symptoms including warmth, increased heat loss, weight loss, myopathy and increased appetite. Cardiac manifestations are more common in older patients and include tachycardia, palpitations, arrhythmias and cardiomegaly.

TABLE 1: Normal reference ranges of thyroid hormones.

Thyroid hormones		Normal range
Thyroxin	T_4	4.5–12.0 µg/dL
Triiodothyronine	T_3	90–200 ng/dL
Thyroid-stimulating hormone	TSH	0.4–4.5 µIU/mL
Free T_4 (0.03% of T_4)	FT_4	0.7–1 6 ng/dL
Free T_3 (0.4% of T_3)	FT_3	230–420 ng/L

Thyrotoxicosis associated with hyperthyroidism is most frequently seen with Graves' disease (autoimmune thyroiditis) but may also be seen in toxic multinodular goiter (MNG) or a hyperfunctioning adenoma. Thyrotoxicosis not associated with hyperthyroidism (low radioactive iodine uptake) may be related to inflammatory thyroid disease or ectopic thyroid tissue (ovarian strumii).

Thyroid storm may present as a clinical emergency in patients with unrecognized or inadequately treated thyrotoxicosis. It is characterized by hypertension, tachycardia and fever and if unrecognized, may result in death.

Thyroid ophthalmopathy is most commonly seen in Graves' disease and hyperthyroidism. It is more common in women and presents with proptosis secondary to enlargement of the extraocular muscles. A characteristic feature is enlargement of the muscle bellies with sparing of the tendinous insertions. The common patterns of extraocular muscle involvement are enlargement of inferior rectus muscle alone, enlargement of inferior rectus and medial rectus muscles, and enlargement of all of the muscles.[7] Relative sparing of the lateral rectus muscle is usually seen and isolated involvement of this muscle should raise the suspicion of a different disease process such as myositis or pseudotumor.

Hypothyroidism refers to a decrease in synthesis of thyroid hormone (serum TSH is high, while T_3 and T_4 levels are low). Primary hypothyroidism may be secondary to structural or functional derangements of the thyroid gland. In adults it most often results from processes that destroy thyroid tissue such as autoimmune disease or ^{131}I treatment. In children it may be related to enzyme deficiencies, defects in organification or congenital anomalies such as lingual thyroid or thyroid agenesis.

Enlargement of the thyroid gland is most commonly seen in multinodular goiter with other causes of enlargement being neoplastic and inflammatory processes. Many of the secondary manifestations of thyroid disease are frequently responsible for the clinical presentation in patients. The most common effect of glandular enlargement is compression of the adjacent structures such as trachea and esophagus which may result in respiratory distress and dysphagia. Similarly, there may be compression and displacement of the jugular vein and carotid artery. The recurrent laryngeal nerve travels in the tracheoesophageal groove and thyroid lesions that extend to this area may present with vocal cord paralysis.

IMAGING

Plain Radiographs

Soft tissue radiographs of the neck in anteroposterior (AP) and lateral projections show the enlarged thyroid in the pretracheal location, associated calcification within the mass and deviation and narrowing of trachea. The tracheal shift or deviation is appreciated in the AP view while the degree of narrowing is assessed on the lateral view **(Figs. 1A and B)**. This information is important to the anesthetist for intubation prior to surgery. Plain X-rays of the neck and upper chest also demonstrate retrosternal extension of a thyroid mass, and any associated bony destruction.

Nuclear Scintigraphy

Nuclear scintigraphy provides excellent functional information about the thyroid because the radionuclides used to image the gland do so by utilizing some step of hormone synthesis within the thyroid. Thyroid scintigraphy is a reflection of the functional as well as physiological state of the gland and provides information that cross-sectional imaging such as USG, CT or MRI lack. The major role of scintigraphy is in the evaluation of patients with abnormal thyroid function tests, especially hyperthyroidism. It can ascertain if the cause of hyperthyroidism is a diffuse process such as Graves' disease or an autonomously functioning nodule. A patient with hyperfunctioning nodule once identified on scintigraphy does not require tissue sampling.

Scintigraphy of a focal thyroid lesion in euthyroid patients determines if the lesion is "hot" (more uptake than the normal thyroid gland), warm (some activity but not as much as the normal gland) or cold (little or no uptake). A functioning "hot" lesion has an extremely low incidence of malignancy, while the reported risk of malignancy of a non-functioning "cold" lesion ranges from 5% to 25%. The majority (~95%) of the nodules are cold, and advancements in other imaging modalities, especially ultrasonography, has resulted in scintigraphy being less utilized in the evaluation of focal thyroid nodules.[8]

Table 2 lists the various radionuclides used in thyroid imaging.[2,5,8-11]

Nuclear imaging is done with a gamma scintillation camera. The normal thyroid gland shows homogeneous radionuclide uptake and distribution while the isthmus may show slightly less activity than the thyroid lobes.

Thyroid uptake reflects the percentage of the dose given to the patient that is accumulated within the thyroid gland corrected for radioactive decay. Normal 24 hours uptake ranges from 10 to 30%. Several medications and iodine-containing contrast agents used for imaging may temporarily interfere with the organification of iodine, altering radioactive iodine uptake measurements for as long as 6 weeks. The uptake of radioactive iodine may be reduced to one half of the expected one week following the injection of iodinated contrast agent for a CT scan. Also, in more than one third of patients with underlying thyroid disease, temporary changes in thyroid function can occur following injection of iodinated contrast agent.

Hence, if cross-section imaging is necessary in a patient undergoing nuclear scans with iodinated radionuclides, one should perform a CT scan after nuclear scintigraphy, or go for MR imaging instead of CT or perform a non-contrast CT.

Medications which interfere with thyroid function should be withdrawn for adequate period of time prior to nuclear scanning.

Ultrasonography

The superficial location of the thyroid allows excellent visualization and evaluation of its normal anatomy and pathologic condition by high-resolution real-time gray-

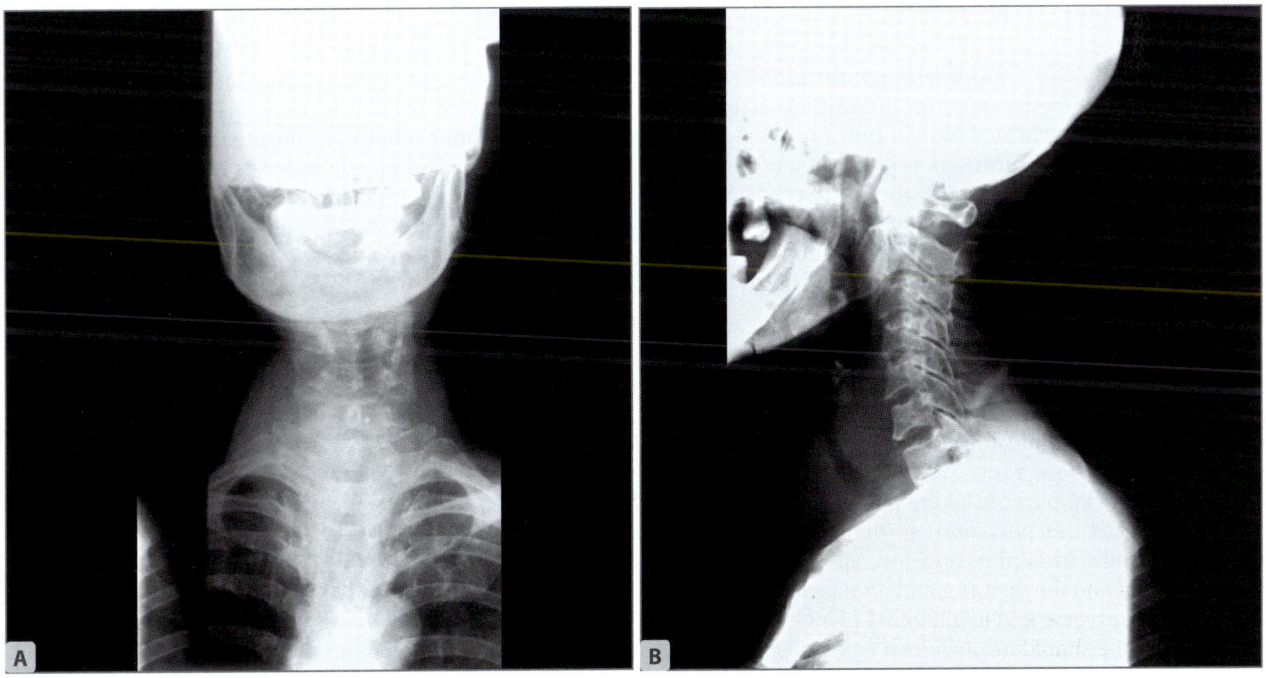

FIGS. 1A AND B: Plain radiographs (A) Anteroposterior; and (B) Lateral view of the neck show a soft tissue opacity in the right lower neck with tracheal deviation to the left with increase in prevertebral space suggestive of retrotracheal extension. Significant narrowing of the trachea is seen opposite C_5-C_6 intervertebral disc space.

TABLE 2: Various radionuclides with their indications used in thyroid imaging.

Radionuclide with half life	Indication	Route of administration	Time of imaging after administration	Remarks
^{99m}Tc pertechnetate $t_{1/2}$ = 6.02hr	Preferred for anatomical evaluation	Intravenous	20 minutes	• Higher dose can be administered. • Permits higher resolution.
^{123}I $t_{1/2}$ = 13.6 hr	• For obtaining 24-hour thyroid iodine uptake. • Gives true assessment of diffuse/focal regions of uptake	Oral	4–24 hours	• Shorter half-life resulting in lower radiation • Better resolution
^{131}I	• In whole body scan. *Diagnostic*: (i) Post-thyroidectomy patients in the operative bed; (ii) To assess for recurrent/distant metastasis; (iii) To detect ectopic thyroid tissue such as struma ovarii. • It is preferred for imaging substernal thyroid as it has high radiation energy (36 KeV) • *Diagnostic and therapeutic*: In the evaluation and treatment of patients with thyroid cancer that concentrate iodine	Oral	24–72 hours	• Limited spatial resolution requires 2–3 sittings for 24 hour scintigraphy. • Is subject to the effects of diet and medicine
^{18}FDG-PET $t_{1/2}$ = 110 minutes	• In the follow-up of patients treated for thyroid cancer due to increased glucose metabolism by malignant tumors. • In metastatic thyroid tumors that do not concentrate radioiodine In the evaluation of patients with rising thyroglobulin levels following thyroidectomy	Intravenous		

scale sonography. As a result it plays an important role in the diagnostic evaluation of thyroid diseases. The advents of high resolution ultrasound and FNA biopsy have decreased the indications for radionuclide thyroid scanning. Ultrasonography is generally the first choice for the evaluation of thyroid morphology because of its sensitivity for small nodule detection. The spatial resolution achieved by ultrasound is of the order of 0.5–1 mm, not achieved by any other imaging method.[6]

Technique

Real-time ultrasound of the thyroid gland is usually performed with high-resolution linear array transducers ranging from 7.5 to 15 MHz.[6] These allow excellent visualization of not only the superficial portions of the gland but also evaluate the deeper structures posteriorly to the level of the spine. With the patient in supine position, the neck is mildly hyperextended and the thyroid gland is imaged in its entirety in both the transverse and longitudinal planes. A small pad placed under the shoulders provides a better exposure of the neck especially in patients with a short, stocky built. Imaging of the lower poles can be improved by asking the patient to swallow, which momentarily raises the thyroid gland in the neck. The carotid arteries and jugular veins are posterior and lateral to the thyroid lobes respectively and provide excellent anatomic landmarks during the examination. The entire gland, including the isthmus, must be examined. The examination should also extend laterally to include the region of the carotid artery and jugular vein to identify enlarged jugular chain lymph nodes, superiorly to visualize submandibular adenopathy, and inferiorly to define any pathologic supraclavicular lymph nodes.

The sternohyoid and omohyoid muscles are seen as thin, hypoechoic bands anterior to the thyroid gland **(Figs. 2A and B)**. The sternocleidomastoid is seen as a larger oval band that lies lateral to the thyroid gland. The longus colli is an important anatomic landmark that is located posterior to each thyroid lobe, in close contact with the prevertebral space. The recurrent laryngeal nerve and the inferior thyroid artery pass in the angle between the trachea, esophagus and the thyroid lobe. On longitudinal scans, the recurrent laryngeal nerve and inferior thyroid artery may be seen between the thyroid lobe and esophagus on the left and the thyroid lobe and longus colli muscle on the right. The esophagus may be seen laterally more on the left side than in the midline and is identified by its target appearance in the transverse plane.

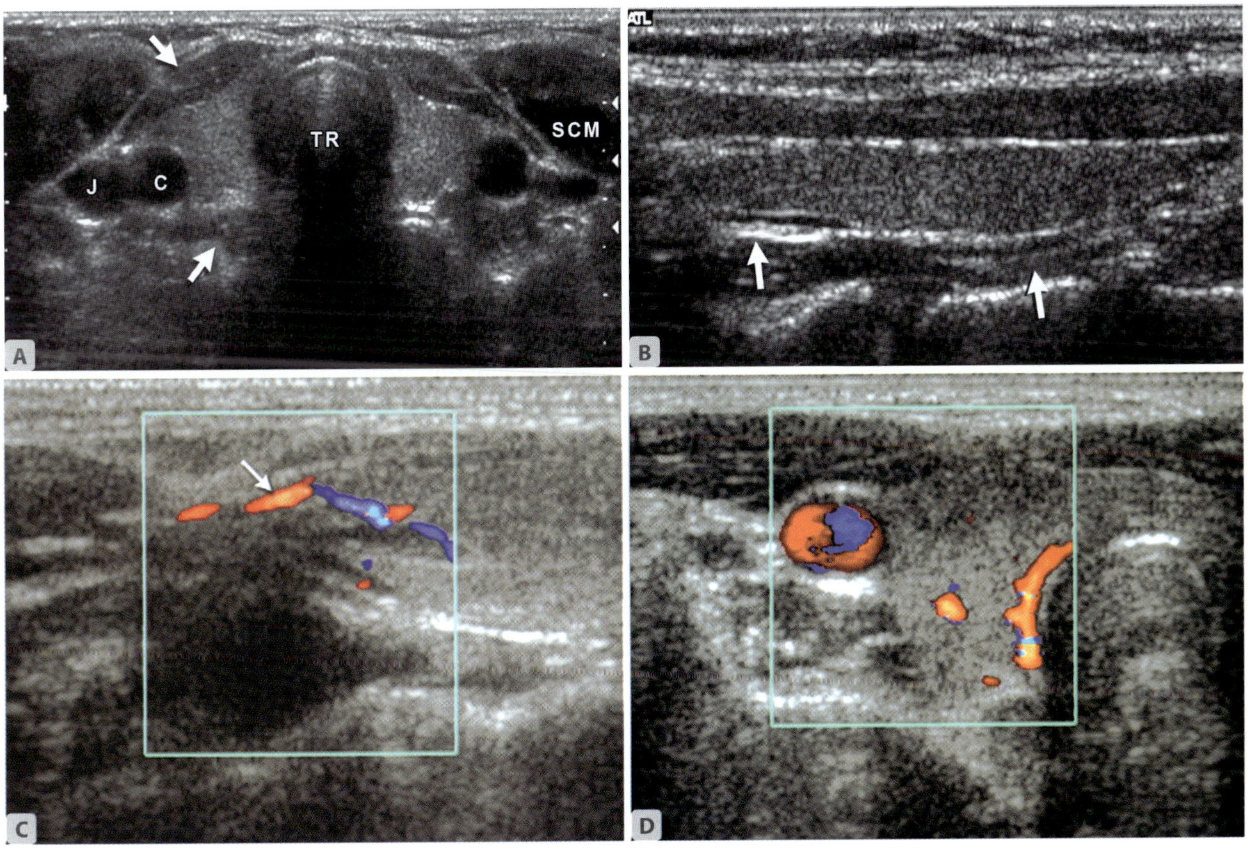

FIGS. 2A TO D: (A) High-resolution sonogram of the normal thyroid gland in transverse section shows homogeneous high level echoes of the parenchyma. The right and left lobes are connected by the isthmus in front of the trachea (TR). The common carotid artery (C) and internal jugular vein (J) are seen posterolaterally in relation to each lobe. The strap muscles are anterior to the thyroid gland while the longus colli is located posterior to each thyroid lobe (arrows).[1] (B) Longitudinal scan showing the thin linear sonolucent recurrent laryngeal nerve (arrow) posterior to the left lobe of the thyroid. CDFI showing the vascularity of the thyroid gland being supplied by (C) superior thyroid artery and (D) inferior thyroid artery. (SCM: sternocleidomastoid muscle).

Appearance

Normal thyroid parenchyma has homogeneous medium to high-level echoes that makes detection of focal cystic hypoechoic thyroid lesions possible. The more hypoechoic a focal lesion is relative to the normal thyroid gland, the higher the likelihood of malignancy. The capsule of the thyroid gland is identifiable by ultrasound and appears as a thin, hypoechoic line that bounds the thyroid lobes. Measurement of the dimensions of the thyroid lobe is an important part of ultrasound examination if diffuse thyroid pathology is suspected.[1] In adults, the mean longitudinal dimension (length) varies from 40 to 60 mm and the mean anteroposterior dimension (depth) is between 13–18 mm. The mean thickness of the isthmus is 4–6 mm. Among the linear parameters, anteroposterior diameter is the most precise and relatively independent measurement that is remarkably constant among individuals. When it is greater than 2 cm, it is suggestive of underlying thyroid pathology that is not sonographically visible, and when it is above 2.5 cm it is considered grossly abnormal.[12]

Ultrasound is an accurate method to use in calculating thyroid volume. Thyroid volume measurements may be useful for determining the size of the goiter, to assess the need for surgery, to permit calculation of the dose of iodine ^{131}I needed for treating thyrotoxicosis and to evaluate the response to suppression treatments. The most common mathematical method to calculate thyroid volume is based on the ellipsoid formula with a correction factor (length × width × thickness × 0.52 for each lobe). By this method the mean estimated error is around 15%.[13] The normal volume in adults ranges from 12 to 15 ± 3 mL. Thyroid volume is found to be larger in patients living in regions of iodine deficiency, and in patients who have acute hepatitis or chronic renal failure, while a smaller volume is seen in patients who have chronic hepatitis or have been treated with thyroxine or radioactive iodine.[6]

The thyroid gland is one of the most vascular organs of the body. The rich vascularity of the gland can be very well seen on Doppler. The superior thyroid artery and vein are found at the upper pole of each lobe. The inferior thyroid vein is found at the lower pole, and the inferior thyroid artery is located posterior to the lower third of each lobe **(Figs. 2C and D)**. Normally the peak systolic velocities in the major thyroid arteries are 20–40 cm/sec and 15–30 cm/sec in intraparenchymal arteries. These are the highest velocities found in blood vessels supplying superficial organs.[13]

Ultrasound also provides guidance for performing FNA/ biopsy thereby obviating the need for an expensive, long and often nondiagnostic workup of a palpable nodule. Evaluation of retrotracheal and mediastinal lesions is difficult by ultrasound because of acoustic shadowing from overlying air or bone.[14] Another limitation of ultrasound is in evaluating for extension of thyroid disease into the soft tissues of the neck or chest.[15]

US Elastography

Ultrasound elastography (USE) is a noninvasive ultrasound based technology which has been developed to evaluate tissue stiffness objectively. It is analogous to manual palpation which is a basic and important method of assessment of thyroid nodules, wherein malignant nodules tend to be harder than benign ones. Conventional ultrasound does not provide any information corresponding to hardness of a nodule. Ultrasound elastography using the technique of **strain elastography** evaluates the degree of distortion of a tissue when an external force is applied and is based on the principle that when compressed, softer parts deform easily compared to harder parts. Elastography has been found to be useful in differentiating malignant from benign thyroid nodules, because malignant nodules are harder than benign nodules as well as surrounding adjacent parenchyma and deform less and exhibit less strain (change in size or shape in response to external compression or stress). **Shear wave or ARFI** (acoustic radiation force impulse) **elastography** is used to evaluate elasticity of tissues quantitatively with stiffer the tissue, the greater is the shear wave velocity (SWV), expressed in m/s. Shear wave elastography has been extensively used in the differentiation of malignant from benign thyroid nodules and also in the evaluation of various diffuse thyroid pathologies.[16]

Cross-sectional Imaging

CT and MR imaging not only provide better delineation of lesions within the thyroid, but also play a critical role in the detection of lymph node metastasis as well as extension of thyroid disease to adjacent tissues in the neck and mediastinum **(Figs. 3A and B)**. Specifically, invasion of paraspinal musculature, esophagus, trachea and carotid sheath structures may be assessed.[17] Cross-sectional imaging is also useful for the evaluation of recurrent disease following treatment of thyroid cancer.

For CT and MR examination, patients are scanned in the supine position with the neck mildly hyperextended when possible, with quiet breathing and suspended swallowing. Contiguous 5 mm thick axial sections are obtained from the level of the base of the tongue superiorly and extend inferiorly into the superior mediastinum to include the aortic arch. When small lesions are being evaluated thin sections (1–3 mm) may be obtained.[15]

On CT the normal thyroid gland is typically seen at or just below the level of the cricoid cartilage.[18] It appears on noncontrast CT as two wedge shaped structures of homogeneous attenuation on either side of the trachea, connected by a narrow isthmus. The normal thyroid gland because of its iodine content has a density of approximately 80 to 100 Hounsfield units on noncontrast CT. It enhances homogenously following intravenous administration of iodinated contrast **(Figs. 4A and B)**. While iodinated contrast may provide additional information about lesions within the thyroid, such contrast will alter radioactive iodine uptake measurements for up to 6 weeks following the study. MR is superior to CT in this regard as MR contrast (gadolinium) does not interfere with iodine uptake or organification by thyroid and hence, may be used in conjunction with scintigraphy.

The role of MR imaging of thyroid has expanded with the development of dedicated surface coils. MRI is best performed with a dedicated surface coil centred over the thyroid gland. Using a surface coil with small field of view allows greater signal to noise ratios and higher resolution than the standard body or head coil. Nodules as small as 4mm size can be detected.[8] Multiple pulse sequences are obtained including non-contrast sagittal, coronal and axial T1-weighted images, as well as axial fast spin-echo T2-weighted

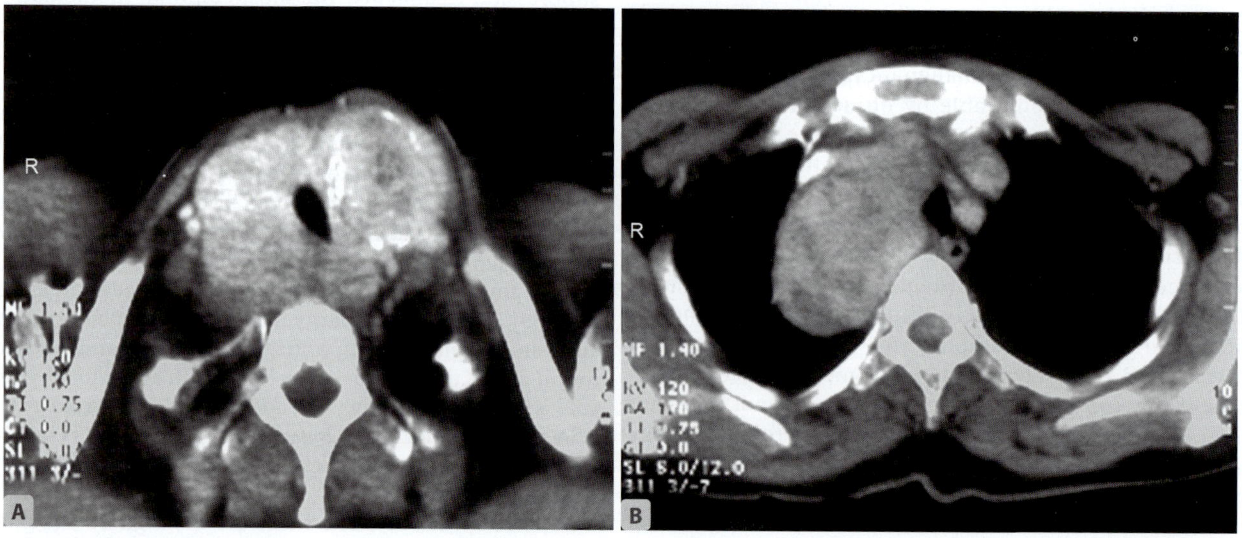

FIGS. 3A AND B: (A) CECT shows enlarged, heterogeneous enhancement of both lobes of thyroid (R > L) with attenuation of tracheal airway. Bilateral carotid sheaths are displaced laterally by the thyroid. However, fat planes are well maintained; (B) Mass shows retrosternal extension.

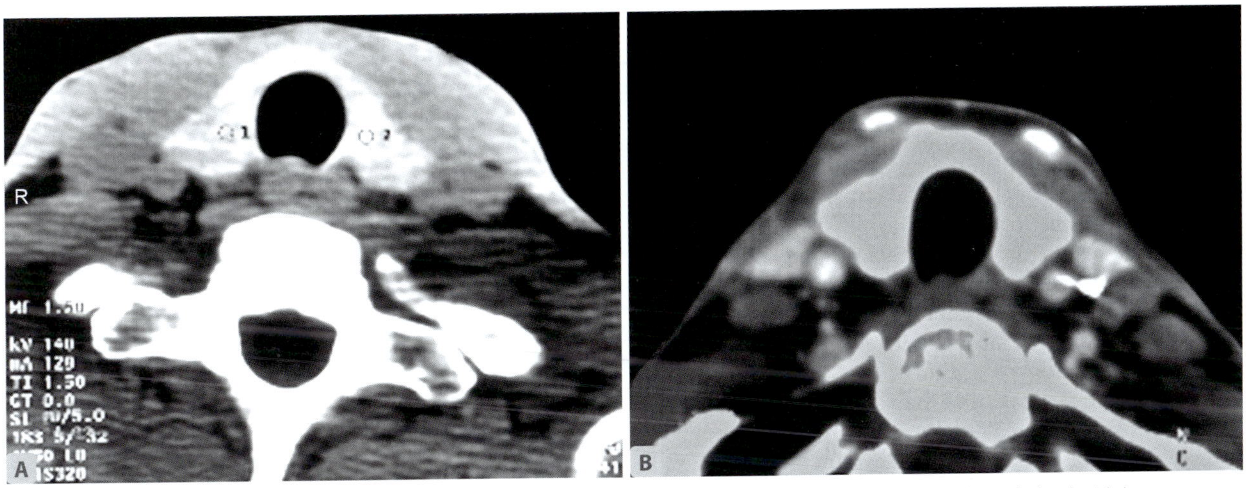

FIGS. 4A AND B: Axial noncontrast and contrast-enhanced sections through the lower neck show the normal thyroid gland with homogeneous enhancement on postcontrast images with normal relation and enhancement of the carotid arteries and jugular veins.

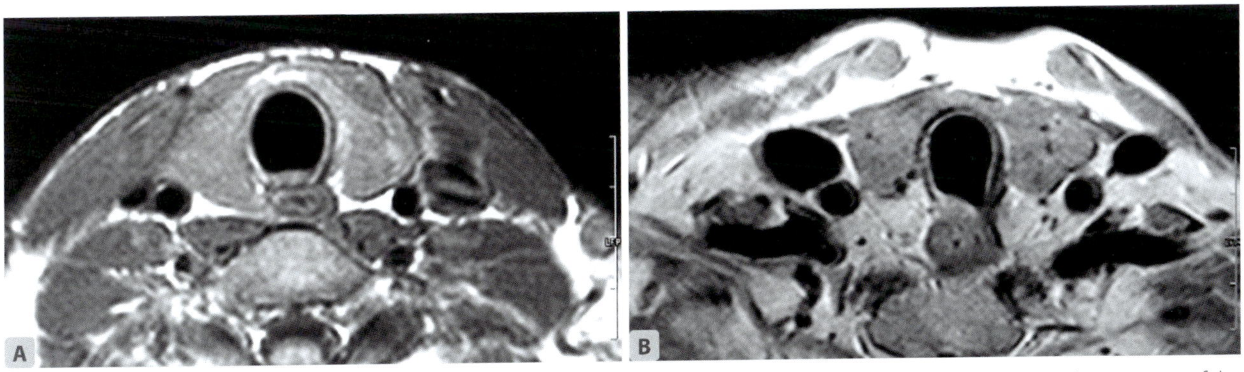

FIGS. 5A AND B: Normal thyroid gland on MR imaging: Unenhanced axial T1- and T2-weighted MR images show the normal appearance of the thyroid gland which is homogeneously hyperintense to the neck musculature. The vessels, carotid artery and jugular vein are seen as signal void posterolateral to the lobes of thyroid.

images with the application of fat saturation. As the lesions may be hyperintense and fat in the neck is hyperintense on T1W and T2W images, fat suppression is necessary to increase the conspicuity of the lesion.[8] Following intravenous contrast administration (0.1 mmol/kg), axial T1-weighted images with fat saturation are usually acquired. On T1-weighted images, normal thyroid gland shows homogeneous signal intensity slightly greater than that of the neck musculature. On T2-weighted images, the thyroid gland is hyperintense relative to the neck musculature **(Figs. 5A and B)**. The normal gland enhances diffusely and homogeneously following contrast administration.

MR imaging provides excellent depiction of the internal parenchyma of the thyroid gland as well as relationship with adjacent structures in the neck and thoracic inlet. It is useful in identifying metastasis to regional nodes, however it is not effective in differentiating benign from malignant causes of lymphadenopathy.[19] MR has also been used to differentiate postoperative recurrence from scar tissue in patients of thyroid carcinoma. On T2-weighed images, postoperative recurrent mass is usually of medium to high signal intensity while scar tissue in the operative bed usually reveals low signal intensity.[20] However, postoperative edema, infection or hemorrhage may simulate a recurrent tumor. MR imaging has been recommended in conjunction with ^{131}I radioisotope scanning for confusing postoperative cases.[21]

PATHOLOGY OF THE THYROID GLAND

Developmental Anomalies

Abnormal development or aberrant caudal descent of the thyroid gland results in a variety of congenital anomalies. Arrest of descent can occur anywhere from the tongue down to the lower neck. The anatomic course of the embryologic thyroid tissue provides a road map for the possible locations of thyroglossal duct cyst and ectopic thyroid as these masses typically occur in lingual, suprahyoid and infrahyoid locations.[3]

Lingual Thyroid

Complete failure of descent of the thyroid gland results in a lingual thyroid at the base of the tongue, in midline. It is the most common type of functioning ectopic thyroid tissue accounting for as much as 90% of reported cases.[3] In such cases up to 75% of patients have no functioning thyroid tissue in the neck.[5] If the tissue at the base of the tongue is not recognized as thyroid and resected, the patient may become acutely and severely hypothyroid.[8]

Nuclear imaging plays a major role in establishing the diagnosis of a lingual thyroid gland as well as determining whether there is normal functioning thyroid tissue in the neck. However, a normal thyroid gland can trap majority of the radionuclide due to which it may be difficult to identify small ectopic rests.[3] On noncontrast CT, lingual thyroid is hyperdense due to its iodine content and on MR imaging it has high signal intensity on T1-weighted and T2-weighted images compared to the tongue musculature with avid enhancement following contrast administration **(Figs. 6A to C)**.

Overdescent of the thyroid may result in ectopic thyroid in the lower neck or mediastinum. Scintigraphy using 99Tc pertechnetate or ^{123}I should be performed when ectopic thyroid is suspected. Other developmental anomalies of the thyroid gland include agenesis or hemiagenesis of one lobe with normal formation of the contralateral lobe and isthmus. In rare occasions, thyroid tissue may be found in remote locations, such as within the heart and within ovarian teratomas (struma ovarii).[5]

Thyroglossal Duct Cyst (TDC)

Incomplete degeneration of the thyroglossal duct (it normally involutes during the eighth to tenth week) may result in a persistent fistulous tract or a thyroglossal duct cyst along the path of migration of the thyroid. **Figure 7** is the schematic representation for the course of thyroglossal duct. Thyroglossal duct cysts are anterior midline cystic neck masses and are commonly occurring congenital masses. They may occur anywhere along the course of the duct but typically occur at or above the hyoid bone. About 15% of thyroglossal duct cysts are at the hyoid bone level, 20% at suprahyoid level and 65% are in infrahyoid location, splaying the strap muscles or are embedded deep within them.[3] Suprahyoid cysts are more likely to be in midline while infrahyoid lesions are paramedian in location.[22] When large, these cysts are detected clinically. Vertical motion of the mass with swallowing or tongue protrusion is highly suggestive of thyroid origin. Small thyroglossal duct cysts are usually occult clinically and may be recognized only when they are secondarily infected or traumatized, or noted incidentally on imaging studies of the neck performed for unrelated reasons.[15] They usually present before 20 years of age and occur four to five times more frequently in females than males.[17]

Imaging Features

Being superficial, thyroglossal duct cyst (TDC) are easily assessed by ultrasound which is the initial investigation of

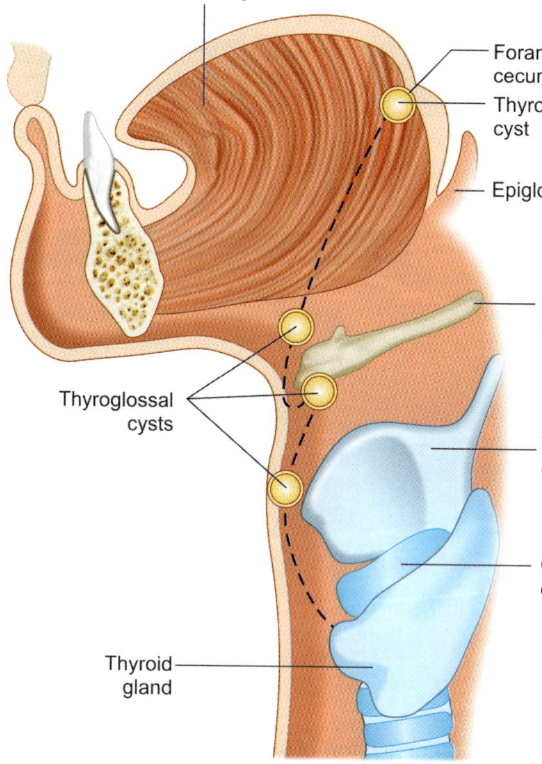

FIG. 7: Schematic diagram showing the course of thyroglossal duct and possible locations of thyroglossal duct cysts from foramen cecum to anterior lower neck.

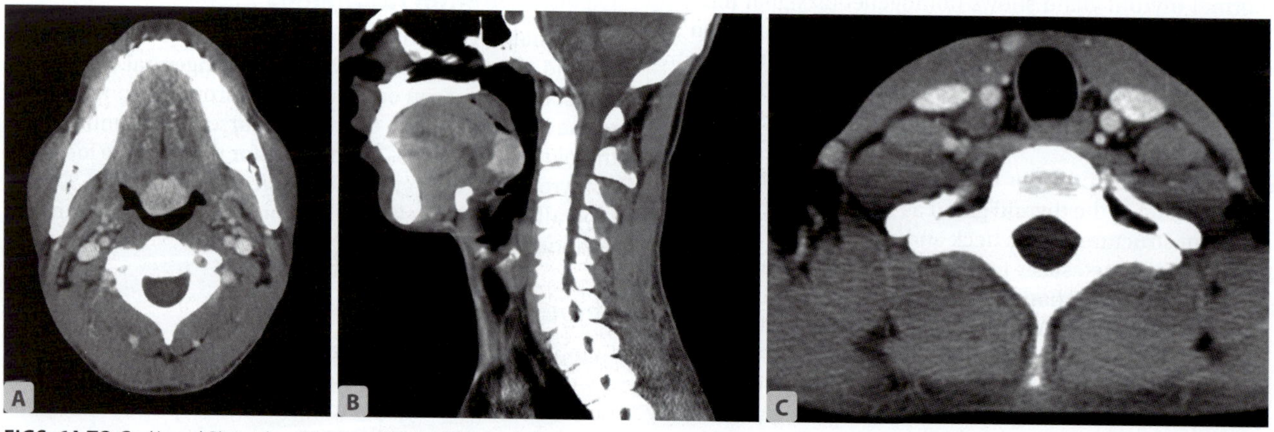

FIGS. 6A TO C: (A and B) Axial and sagittal CECT of the neck shows a well-defined homogeneous markedly hyperdense tissue at the base of the tongue in the midline; (C) Axial CT of the lower neck reveals absence of normal thyroid tissue in the neck. Findings consistent with lingual thyroid.

choice. On sonography, they have typical features of a cyst. They may also show internal echoes when the contents are proteinaceous or get infected. On cross-sectional imaging, uncomplicated thyroglossal cysts are usually well demarcated. Sagittal reconstruction on CT and sagittal MR imaging can help in the detection of TDC and ectopic thyroid tissue as these two masses are typically midline.[3] On CT they are isodense to water **(Figs. 8A and B)**, however, they may be hyperdense when there is high protein content. On MR the intensity is like CSF on T1-weighted and T2-weighted images. If the contents are proteinaceous, cysts become hyperintense on T1-weighted images, but remain intermediate to hyperintense on T2-weighted scans.[15] Enhancement is uncommon in thyroglossal duct cysts unless it has been traumatized or infected. Then, a peripheral rim enhancement or internal septations may be seen.

Nuclear scintigraphy is usually not necessary in the evaluation of thyroglossal duct cysts. Cross-sectional imaging is usually not needed in children because of the clinical presentation of painless midline neck mass that moves on swallowing. Ultrasonography helps to confirm the normal position of the thyroid before surgery. CT or MR is usually performed preoperatively in cases of suspected thyroglossal duct cyst in adults to confirm the diagnosis and to exclude other nodal masses. It is the location of an infrahyoid thyroglossal duct cyst in the strap muscles, and not its signal or attenuation characteristics that allows a definitive diagnosis on imaging.[17] Rarely, thyroglossal duct cysts may undergo malignant degeneration, usually into papillary carcinoma.

On imaging, carcinoma in a TDC should be considered if there is soft tissue in a midline cystic mass associated with irregular calcification, along with a normal thyroid gland. An infected TDC also shows increased density and a thickened wall. A congenital dermoid cyst can appear as a cystic midline mass but can be differentiated from a TDC if fat is detected within the lesion. Also, unlike a thyroglossal duct remnant, a dermoid tumor is usually not closely related to the strap muscles.

DIFFUSE THYROID DISEASE

Several thyroid diseases are characterized by diffuse rather than focal enlargement of the gland. Goiter is the term for the generalized enlargement of the gland and may be seen with hyperthyroidism or hypothyroidism **(Figs. 9A to D)**.

Thyroiditis is infiltration of the thyroid gland with inflammatory cells which may be seen in a disease group of autoimmune, inflammatory and infectious processes. Thyroiditis may be acute and self-limiting or chronic and progressive. Specific conditions commonly produce diffuse enlargement such as chronic autoimmune lymphocytic (Hashimoto's) thyroiditis, colloid or adenomatous goiter and Graves' disease. **Table 3** lists the various diffuse thyroid diseases. Diagnosis of these conditions is usually made on the basis of clinical presentation and laboratory findings of thyroid function, and occasionally by FNAC. Sonography is seldom required and when performed it is the thickness of the isthmus which facilitates the recognition of diffuse thyroid enlargement. The isthmus which is normally only a few millimeters (2–4 mm) thick in anteroposterior dimension, may be up to 1 cm or more in thickness with diffuse thyroid disease.[13]

Each of the types of thyroiditis enumerated has distinctive clinical and laboratory features. Imaging is not important in the initial workup of these patients as the findings in them are usually not distinguishable from other thyroid pathology such as goiter or a neoplastic lesion. However, imaging is useful in patient follow-up and monitoring of the disease.

Diffuse Nontoxic Goiter

Diffuse nontoxic goiter represents diffuse, non-nodular enlargement of the thyroid associated with a euthyroid state. There are two stages in its development. The first stage is hyperplasia characterised by diffuse glandular enlargement and hyperemia. The second stage is colloid involution, which occurs when a euthyroid state is maintained. Over time, most simple goiters progress to multinodular goiters, which may

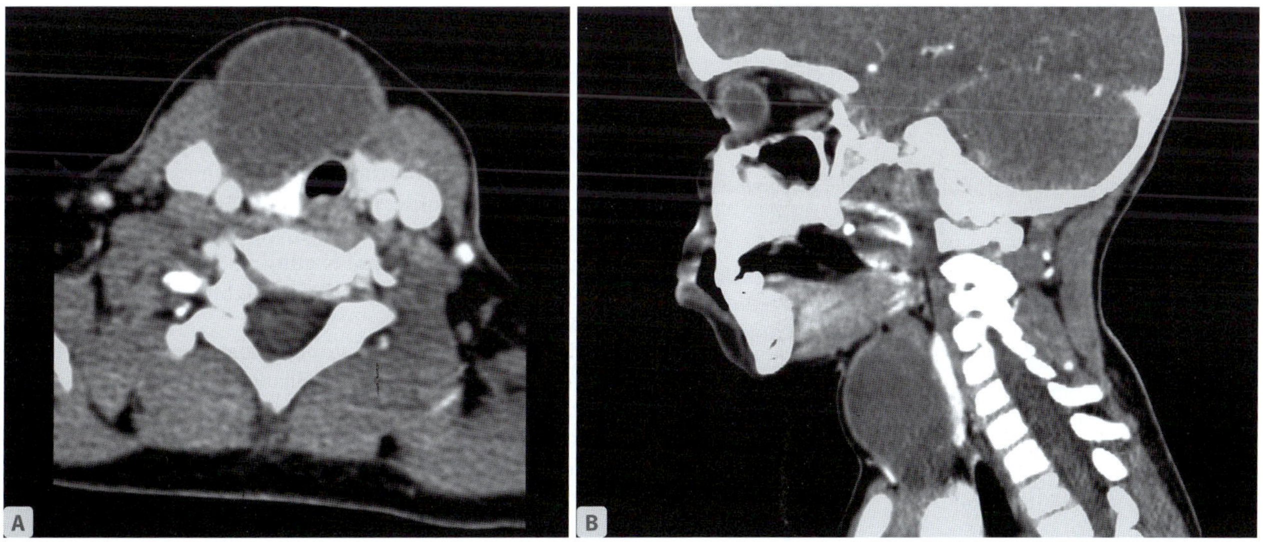

FIGS. 8A AND B: Contrast-enhanced axial CT with sagittal reformation in a 10-year-old child shows a well-defined, rounded lesion of fluid attenuation in the lower neck in the midline anterior to and abutting the right lobe of thyroid: Thyroglossal duct cyst.

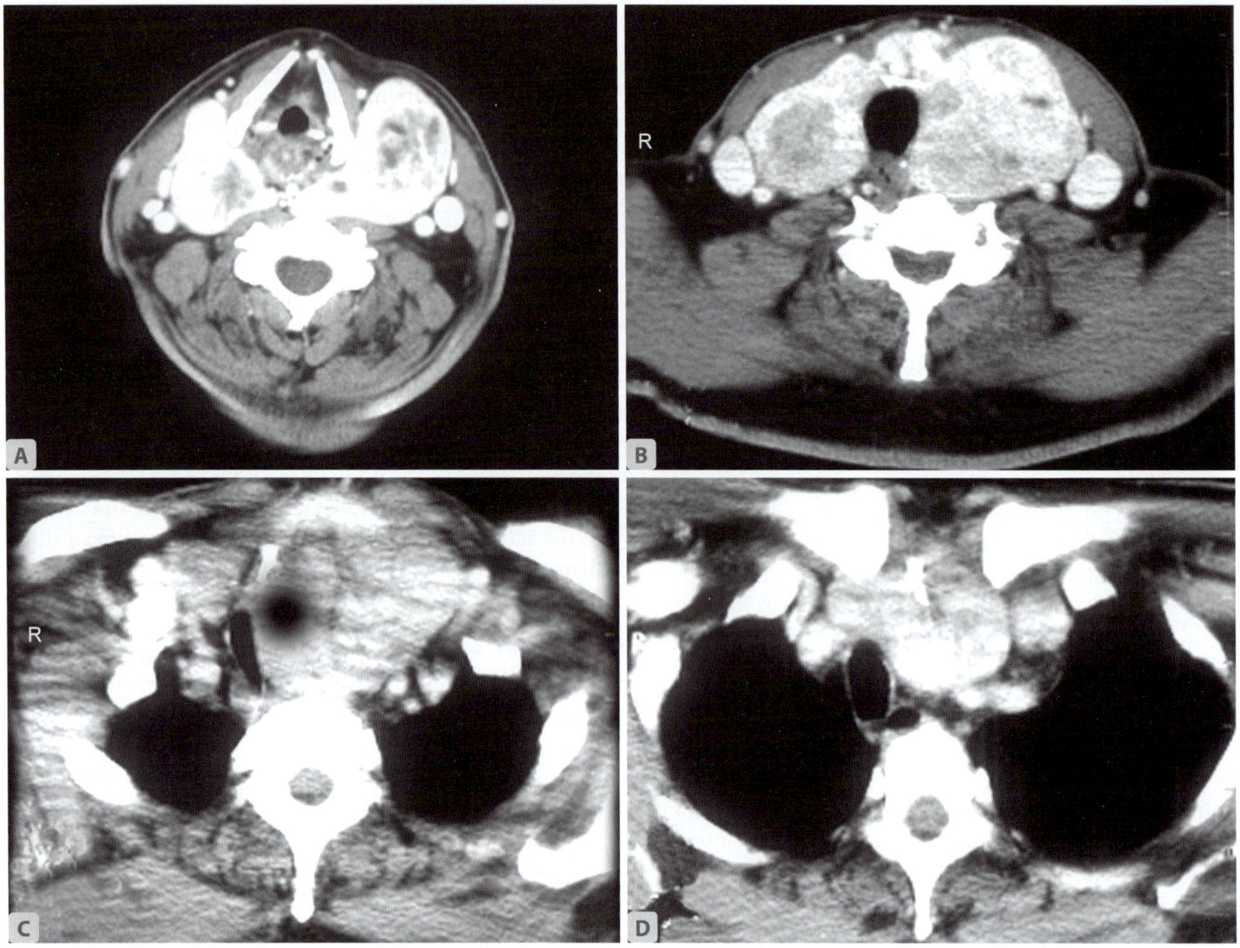

FIGS. 9A TO D: (A and B) CECT showing a densely enhancing thyroid with multiple hypodense nodules in both lobes and isthmus of thyroid. It is seen to extend posteromedially in the retrolaryngeal region; (C and D) The left lobe of thyroid is markedly enlarged, causing attenuation and complete deviation of the trachea to the right. Foci of calcification and necrosis are seen in the gland which extends below the medial end of both clavicles: Multinodular goiter.

TABLE 3: Diffuse thyroid diseases.
• Diffuse nontoxic goiter (Adenomatous or colloid goiter)
• Diffuse toxic goiter (Graves' disease)
• Chronic lymphocytic thyroiditis (Hashimoto's disease)
• Silent painless thyroiditis
• Acute suppurative thyroiditis
• Subacute granulomatous thyroiditis (de Quervain disease)

remain nontoxic or may induce thyrotoxicosis.[2] When 10% or more of the local population has goiter, it is referred to as endemic goiter. These are seen in iodine poor areas, usually away from oceans, with high incidence of goiter as well as anaplastic carcinoma of the thyroid. However, once iodine is introduced in the diet, the incidence of goiter and anaplastic carcinoma decreases while that of papillary carcinoma increases.[8]

Imaging Features

On ultrasonography, a simple goiter appears as diffuse enlargement of the thyroid gland with uniform or variable echogenicity. A heterogeneous appearance may be seen on CT/MRI due to the presence colloid, blood products, calcification or fibrosis in the gland.

Graves' Disease (Diffuse Toxic Goiter)

Graves' disease is a common diffuse abnormality of the thyroid gland and is usually biochemically characterized by hyperfunction (thyrotoxicosis). It is the most common of the autoimmune disorders, with a peak incidence in the third to fourth decades of life, having a female preponderance. Although Graves' disease is autoimmune, it is not really a thyroiditis as it does not have a significant inflammatory component.

In Graves' disease, thyroid autoantibodies bind to the thyrotropin receptor on the follicular cells, stimulating them as though TSH triggered the receptor. This results in constant autonomous function of the thyroid, which results in hyperthyroidism. The diagnosis in confirmed by serological tests for specific autoimmune markers which are elevated.

There is marked enlargement of the thyroid gland without focal nodules. The gland shows diffuse hyperplasia of the follicular epithelial cells with depletion of colloid. Pyramidal lobe may be enlarged. Graves' disease is associated with other autoimmune diseases of the thyroid such as Hashimoto's thyroiditis.[8]

Imaging Features

Radionuclide scintigraphy may be helpful in evaluating patients with suspected Graves' disease and also differentiating it from acute thyroiditis. In Graves' disease, the gland is diffusely enlarged, shows intense homogeneous radiotracer uptake which may be up to 80% in 24 hours (normal is 10–30%). Also, there is concordance between clinical thyrotoxicosis and increased radionuclide uptake in Graves' disease. In contrast, in the acute phase of thyroiditis, though the patient is clinically hyperthyroid, the radionuclide uptake in markedly low (as low as 10%). The uptake generally returns to normal if the gland recovers and the patient becomes euthyroid.

On ultrasound, the gland is diffusely enlarged with a smooth lobular contour. The echotexture is homogeneous without discrete nodules but patchy areas of altered echotexture may be present due to numerous, large intraparenchymal vessels.[6] The parenchyma may be isoechoic or diffusely hypoechoic because of extensive lymphocytic infiltration.

Color Doppler sonography often demonstrates a hypervascular pattern referred to as "thyroid inferno", indicating an acute stage of the process, the severity of which tends to parallel the patient's degree of hyperthyroidism.[8] Spectral Doppler often shows peak systolic velocities to exceed 70 cm/sec which is the highest velocity found in thyroid disease **(Figs. 10A to C)**. Studies have shown that Doppler analysis can be used to monitor therapeutic response in patients with Graves' disease.[23] A significant decrease in flow velocities in the superior and inferior thyroid arteries after medical treatment has been reported.

The CT and MR imaging findings in Graves' disease are nonspecific with the enlarged gland showing intense enhancement. Even though there is an overall increase in iodine content in the gland, the iodine concentration is decreased, due to which the CT density is actually decreased in Graves' disease. Following treatment, the density values may not return to normal.[8]

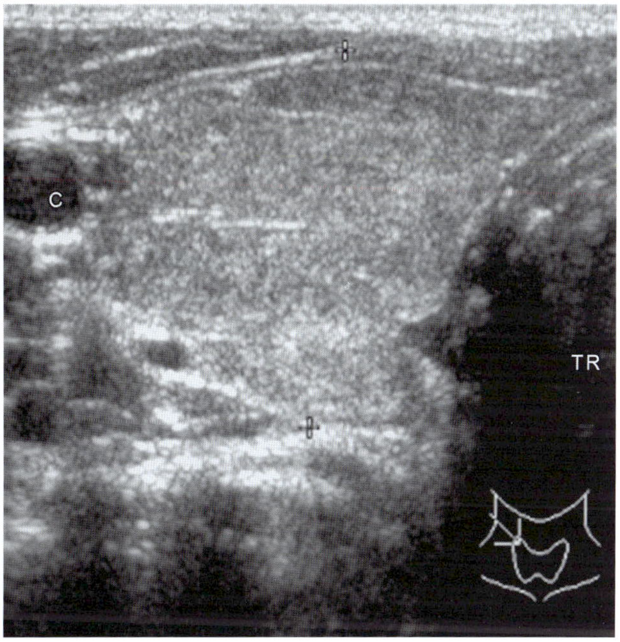

FIG. 10A: High-resolution ultrasound showing mildly enlarged right lobe of thyroid gland (AP diameter 2.27 cm) in a patient of Graves' disease. (C: common carotid artery; TR: trachea).

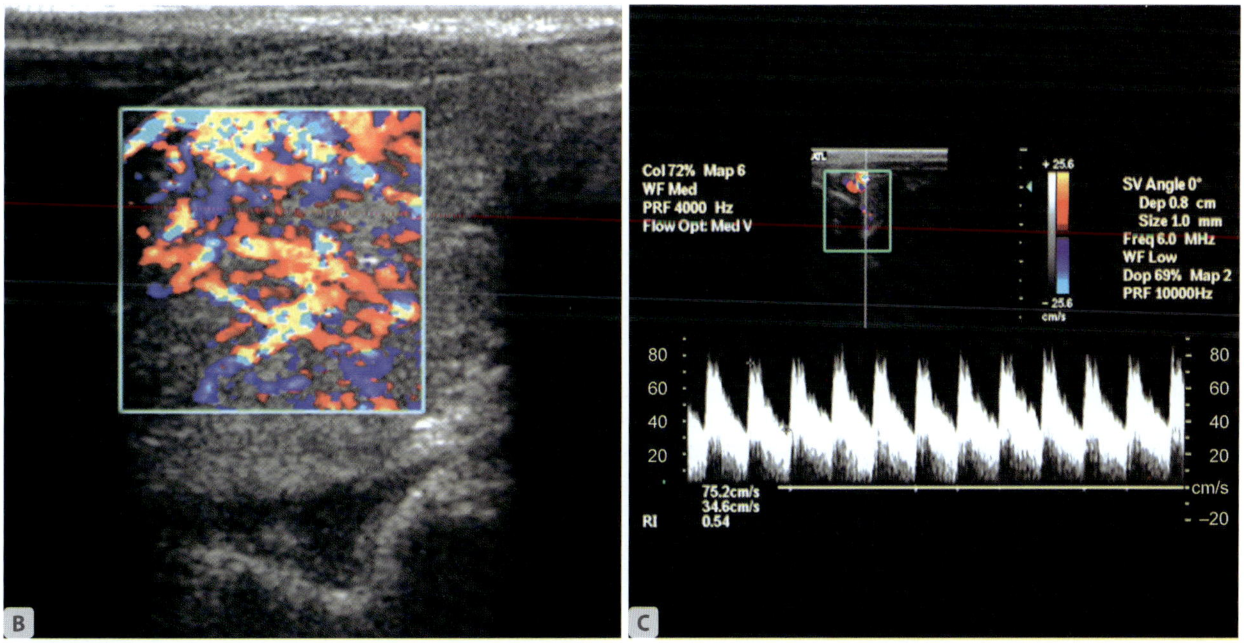

FIGS. 10B AND C: (B) CDFI showing significantly increased intraglandular vascularity in a patient of Graves' disease: Thyroid inferno; (C) Spectral Doppler of the same showing markedly increased peak systolic velocity (75 cm/s).

As the management of Graves' disease and subacute thyroiditis is different, it is important to differentiate the two. The treatment of patients with Graves' disease involves medication to treat the secondary manifestations of hyperthyroidism, radioactive ablation of the thyroid gland or even surgery if necessary, while thyroiditis is treated conservatively with medicines for symptomatic relief.

Chronic Autoimmune Lymphocytic (Hashimoto's) Thyroiditis

Hashimoto's thyroiditis is the most common type of thyroiditis and occurs when patients develop antibodies to their own thyroglobulin. As the disease is an autoimmune process, its diagnosis is based on serology. Antibody titers are usually elevated. It typically occurs as a painless, diffuse enlargement of the gland in young or middle aged women, but in later stages the thyroid may be atrophic.[8] It is often associated with hypothyroidism. It may also be seen in children in whom it is the most common thyroiditis.[5]

Imaging Features

Scintigraphy does not show any typical pattern in Hashimoto's thyroiditis. The uptake of radioiodine or ^{99m}Tc pertechnetate is most commonly heterogeneous and patchy and may be uniformly increased or mildly to severely decreased.[5]

Ultrasonography demonstrates a spectrum of findings in chronic lymphocytic thyroiditis, depending on the duration and severity of disease. The typical appearance is a diffuse, coarsened echotexture, more hypoechoic than the normal thyroid gland. In patients with mild or previously undetected chronic lymphocytic thyroiditis, the gland may be normal with multiple small discrete, irregular hypoechoic micronodules. These nodules range from 1 to 6 mm in diameter and are highly suggestive of chronic lymphocytic thyroiditis with this appearance called "micronodulation"[24] **(Figs. 11A and B)**.

The sonographic appearance of micronodulation has been described to have a positive predictive value of 94.7% in the diagnosis of chronic thyroiditis.[6] Histologically, the micronodules represent lobules of thyroid parenchyma that have been infiltrated with lymphocytes and plasma cells. These lobules are surrounded by multiple linear echogenic fibrous septations which may give the parenchyma a 'pseudolobulated' appearance. Cervical lymphadenopathy may often be present at the lower pole of the thyroid. Both benign and malignant thyroid nodules may co-exist with chronic lymphocytic thyroiditis and FNA is often necessary to establish the diagnosis.

The vascularity on color Doppler imaging is normal or decreased in most patients with the diagnosis of Hashimoto's thyroiditis **(Fig. 11C)**. CT shows an inhomogeneous appearance, while on MR imaging T2-weighted images may show areas of increased signal intensity. Following contrast administration, there may be regions which enhance more than the remainder of the gland.

Ultrasound may be used to follow patients with Hashimoto's thyroiditis to detect occult malignancy. This is because like other autoimmune disorders there is an increased risk of malignancy of non-Hodgkin's lymphoma of the thyroid. Thyroid lymphoma may produce solitary or multiple focal hypoechoic lesions or diffuse disease that may be difficult to distinguish from Hashimoto's thyroiditis. Sonographic features which raise the suspicion of malignancy in Hashimoto's thyroiditis are a large or infiltrating hypoechoic nodule, nodule with microcalcification, development of respiratory obstructive symptoms and/or cervical lymphadenopathy.[8]

The CT and MR imaging findings of thyroiditis are non-specific and hence these are not routinely performed.

The end stage of chronic thyroiditis is atrophy when the gland becomes small with poorly-defined margins and heterogeneous echotexture due to progressive fibrosis. Blood flow signals are absent. Occasionally, discrete nodules may develop when FNAC is needed to establish the diagnosis.[13]

Silent Painless Thyroiditis and Postpartum Thyroiditis

These are two different types of subacute lymphocytic thyroiditis which are usually self-limiting. Patients may present

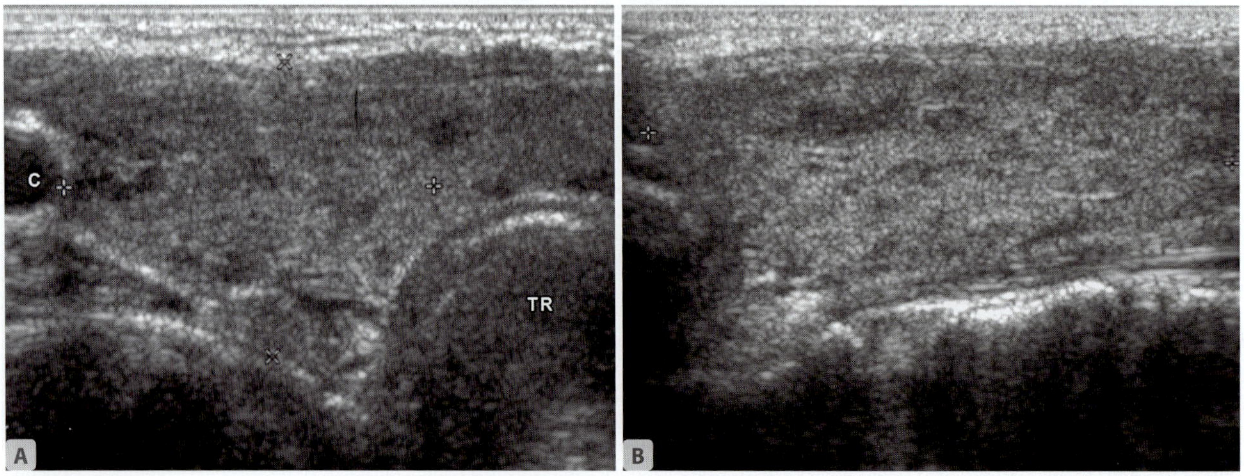

FIGS. 11A AND B: High-resolution sonography of the right lobe of thyroid showing ill-defined hypoechoic foci scattered in the parenchyma. Isthmus measures 5 mm in A-P dimension FNAC: Lymphocytic thyroiditis. (C: common carotid artery; TR: trachea).

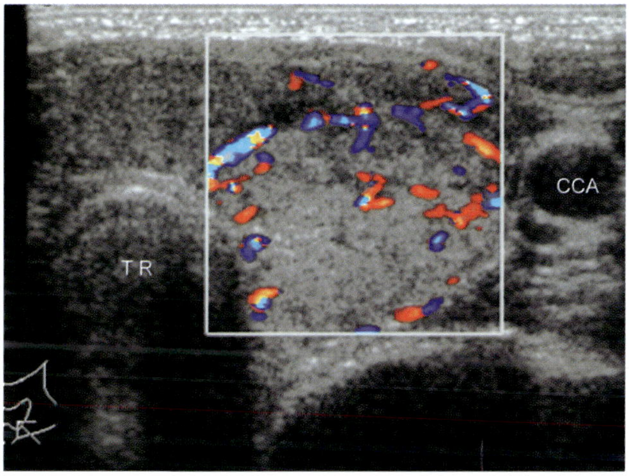

FIG. 11C: CDFI shows normal vascularity in the left lobe of thyroid. (FNAC: lymphocytic thyroiditis).

with goiter, thyrotoxicosis and antithyroid antibodies. When the inflammatory process occurs in the absence of pregnancy, it is termed painless thyroiditis. Postpartum thyroiditis typically occurs 4–6 weeks following delivery in up to 5% of postpartum women and may recur with subsequent pregnancy.[5] It usually resolves after transient hypothyroidism, though some patients may progress to chronic lymphocytic thyroiditis.

Acute Suppurative Thyroiditis

It is an uncommon disease which results from seeding of the thyroid gland by bacterial infection and usually affects children, immunocompromised or debilitated patients. The infection usually develops in the perithyroidal soft tissues. As the disease progresses, focal abscesses may develop. Adjacent soft tissues in the neck may be obliterated due to associated myositis and cellulitis.[25]

Imaging Features

On ultrasound, an abscess is seen as an ill-defined, hypoechoic, heterogeneous mass with internal debris with or without septa or gas. Adjacent inflammatory nodes are often present. On cross-sectional imaging, the affected portion of the gland is enlarged and appears heterogeneous. As thyroid abscesses are rare, any time it occurs in a child, the possibility of a third or fourth branchial cleft cyst must be excluded. On CT, one must rule out a fistula from the pyriform sinus as an etiology of the thyroiditis.[8]

Subacute Granulomatous Thyroiditis (de Quervain's disease)

It is a spontaneously remitting inflammatory disease that usually occurs following a viral upper respiratory tract infection. The peak incidence is in the second to fifth decades of life. Diagnosis is clinical ,with imaging not done routinely.

Imaging Features

Sonographically the gland may appear enlarged and hypoechoic, with normal or decreased vascularity. On noncontrast CT the gland is slightly enlarged with a lower than normal attenuation. Scintigraphy shows a low radioactive iodine uptake that usually reverts to normal as the patient returns to a euthyroid state.

Invasive Fibrous Thyroiditis (Riedel's Struma)

It is the rarest type of inflammatory thyroid disease that is characterized by a fibrosing reaction which destroys the thyroid and extends into the adjacent soft tissues of the neck. The cause of Riedel's thyroiditis is unknown. It is mainly seen in women and usually occurs in the fourth to seventh decades of life presenting with stridor, dysphagia and vocal cord paralysis from recurrent laryngeal nerve involvement. It is the only benign thyroid disease that may cause a recurrent laryngeal nerve paralysis, as the fibrosing reaction encases the nerve. Some cases may be associated with mediastinal or retroperitoneal fibrosis as well as sclerosing cholangitis.[8]

Imaging Features

Ultrasonographic appearance of Riedel's thyroiditis may mimic anaplastic thyroid carcinoma when there is extrathyroid extension of the inflammatory process with encasement of adjacent vessels.[13] This requires an open biopsy to distinguish the two conditions. On ultrasound the thyroid may be hypoechoic and on CT the involved thyroid may be hypodense compared to the normal thyroid. The characteristic MR appearance includes decreased signal intensity on T1-weighted and T2-weighted images, believed to correspond to fibrosis, as well as infiltration of adjacent soft tissues in the neck **(Figs. 12A to D)**.[26] It may spread to encase neck vessels and may obliterate tracheo-esophageal groove.

Miscellaneous Thyroid Conditions

Other inflammatory but rare thyroid conditions include tuberculosis, sarcoidosis, fungal diseases, and opportunistic organisms, especially in patients with acquired immunodeficiency syndrome (AIDS). Amyloidosis and hemochromatosis may replace thyroid parenchyma and may cause decreased signal intensity on T2-weighted MR images.[22] Radiation received from external beam or radioactive iodine therapy may lead to fibrosis and atrophy of the thyroid gland.

NODULAR THYROID DISEASE

Nodular thyroid disease is characterized by the presence of one or more palpable or nonpalpable nodules within the substance of the thyroid gland.[27] Etiology of nodular thyroid disease includes iodine deficiency (endemic), hereditary familial forms and poor utilization of iodine as a result of medication. Approximately 80–85% of nodular thyroid disease is due to hyperplasia of the gland, with women being effected three times more than men.[1] Adenomas and carcinomas are responsible for the rest of the nodular thyroid pathology.

Multinodular Goiter

Multinodular goiter (MNG) is the most common benign pathology of the thyroid with multiple nodules in the thyroid

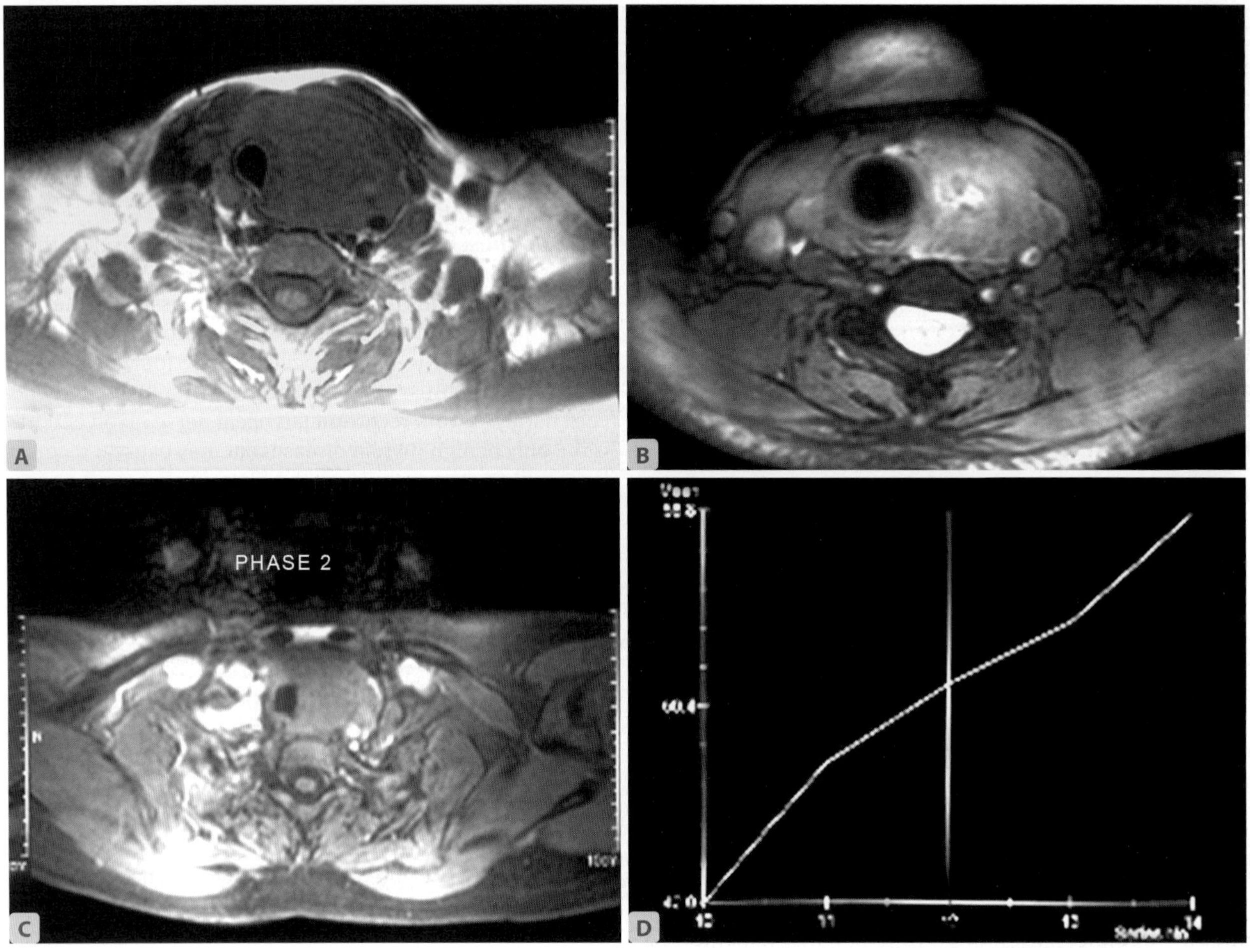

FIGS. 12A TO D: (A) Axial T1W image shows an iso to mildly hypointense nodule in the left lobe and isthmus which is iso to mildly hyperintense on T2W sequence; (B) It is causing tracheal attenuation and displacement to the right with compression of the left CCA and IJV. (C) The lesion is showing mild homogeneous contrast enhancement; (D) The time signal intensity curve reveals a slow persistently rising curve suggestive of a benign etiology. (FNAC: Riedel's thyroiditis).

resulting in an enlarged gland. Glandular enlargement may be asymmetric, involving one lobe more than the other, with or without involving the isthmus. Thyroid goiters may extend substernally and into the anterior mediastinum.

It is characterized by nodularity, focal hemorrhage, focal calcifications, cyst formation, and scarring. Pathologically, the nodules are referred to as hyperplastic, adenomatous or colloid nodules. They appear as complex cystic masses representing colloid, mixed with areas of hemorrhage and necrosis. Dystrophic calcification is a common feature of multinodular goiter and is typically multiple, large and coarse.

Imaging Features

On sonography, multinodular goiter appears as an enlarged gland with multiple nodules of different sizes. Most hyperplastic or adenomatous nodules appear isoechoic compared to the normal thyroid parenchyma, with a thin peripheral hypoechoic halo **(Fig. 13)**. Less commonly, a sponge like or honeycomb pattern is seen **(Fig. 14)**. An ultrasound feature for a benign thyroid nodule that has been described is a "spongiform appearance". This term is used for a nodule containing macrocystic components occupying more than half of the entire volume and has been found to be specific, especially in combination with the feature of isoechogenicity.[28]

The degenerative changes in the nodule are reflected in the sonographic appearance with serous or colloid fluid appearing purely anechoic; hemorrhage appearing as echogenic fluid **(Figs. 15A and B)**; aggregates of colloid typically seen as bright echogenic foci with comet-tail artefacts. Calcification occurring due to the degenerative process may be thin peripheral 'egg shell' type or coarse, seen as highly reflective foci with posterior shadowing scattered throughout the gland.[6]

On CT, the gland is asymmetric in multinodular goiter with multiple low-density areas that reflect regions of hemorrhage, cyst formation, or necrosis. Focal regions of hyperdensity are common, reflecting calcifications, hemorrhage, or colloid. Peripheral or egg-shell-like calcification is considered to be the most reliable feature of a benign nodule, but it is seen only in a small percentage of benign nodules **(Fig. 16)**.[13] On MR imaging, multinodular goiter may show a spectrum of appearances. On T1-weighted images, multiple foci of high

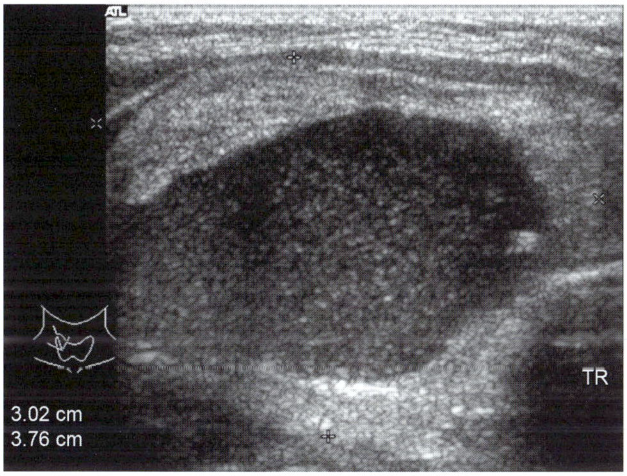

FIG. 13: High-resolution sonography showing a well-defined oval cystic lesion in the right lobe of thyroid with internal echoes within: Benign nodule.

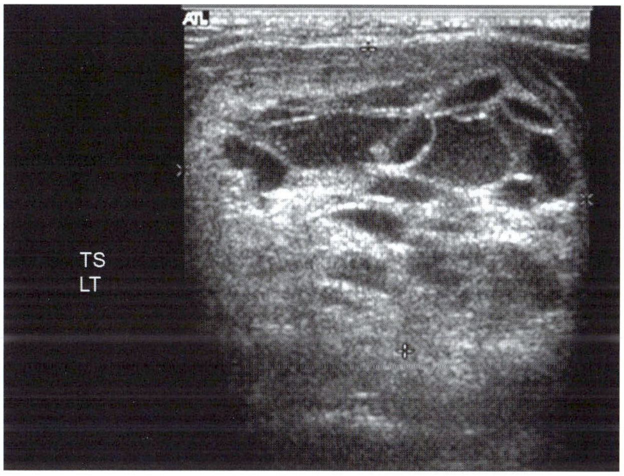

FIG. 14: High-resolution sonography of the left lobe of thyroid reveals a well marginated, multiseptated, cystic lesion. (FNAC: colloid goiter).

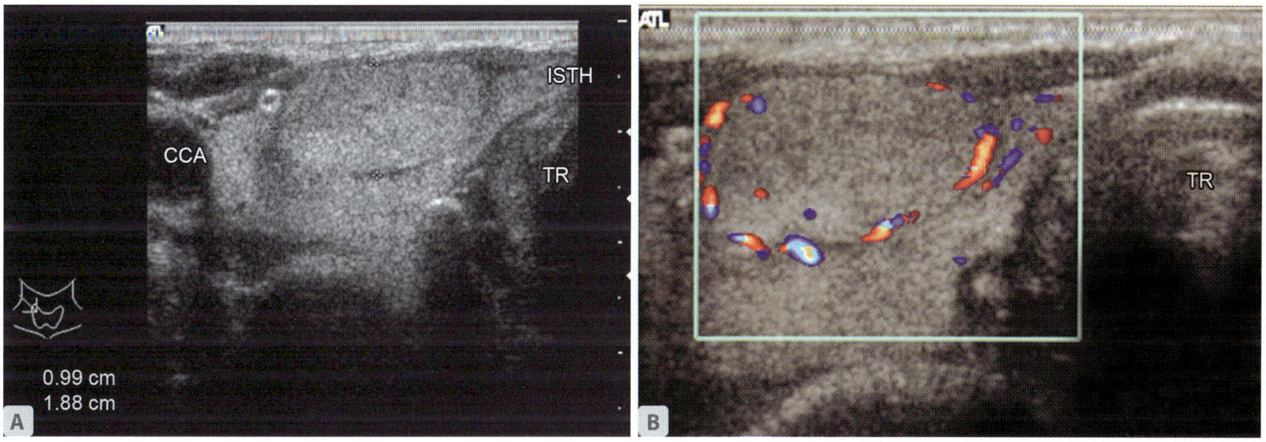

FIGS. 15A AND B: (A) High resolution sonography of the right lobe of thyroid reveals an oval, well-defined isoechoic nodule with thin sonolucent halo around it: Hyperplastic nodule. (TR—trachea, CCA—Common carotid artery); (B) CDFI of a hyperplastic nodule in the right lobe reveals peripheral vascularity.

signal intensity may represent cysts containing colloid or hemorrhage. On T2-weighted images, diffuse heterogeneity is present **(Figs. 17A to D)**.[2] The individual nodules in MNG enhance intensely with contrast on both CT and MRI.[4] Secondary manifestations of goiter such as compression and displacement of the trachea, esophagus and adjacent vessels are best assessed by CT or MR Imaging, which also depict retrosternal and mediastinal extension, if any.

BENIGN NEOPLASMS

Thyroid Adenoma

Thyroid adenomas are true benign neoplasms distinctly separate from the adjacent thyroid parenchyma and encased by a fibrous capsule. They may be functioning or nonfunctioning, but are usually solitary and non-functioning and are most commonly detected in young and middle-aged adults. They are usually less than 3 cm in diameter, have well-defined margins, and may involute, become cystic or

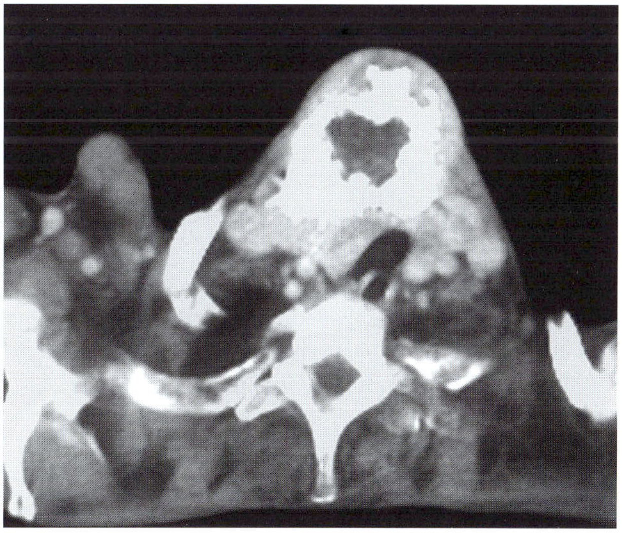

FIG. 16: CT scan showing a nodule in the isthmus of thyroid gland with dense peripheral calcification. Histopathology showed colloid goiter.

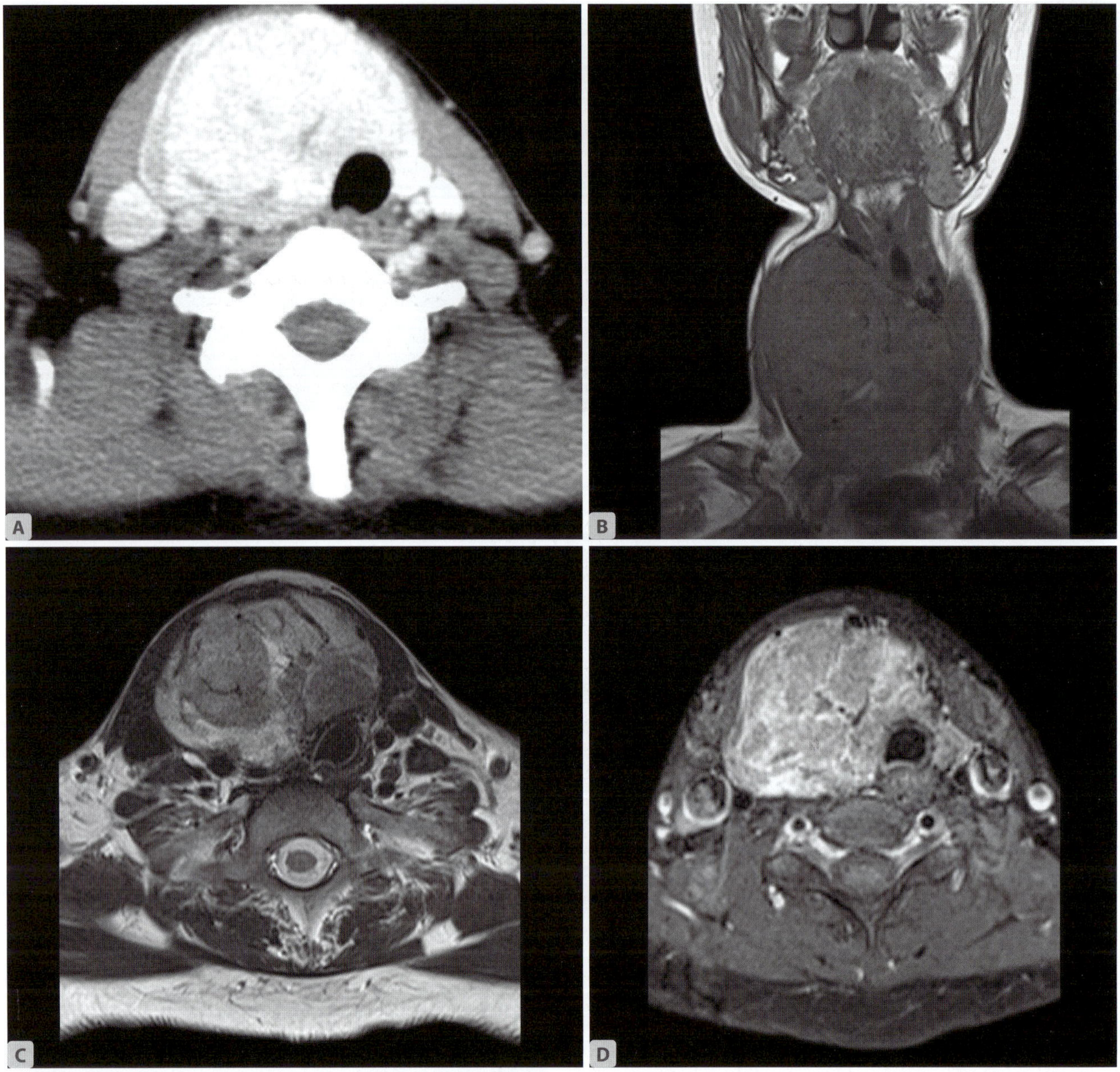

FIGS. 17A TO D: (A) CECT Neck shows markedly enlarged right lobe of thyroid. (B) Coronal T1W and (C) axial T2W images show a well-defined nodule hypointense on T1 and heterogeneously hyperintense on T2W image showing (D) heterogeneous contrast enhancement: Goiter.

may develop internal hemorrhage, necrosis, calcification or fibrosis **(Figs. 18A and B)**.[9]

Benign follicular adenoma is a true thyroid neoplasm that is characterized by compression of adjacent tissues and fibrous encapsulation. Various sub-types of follicular adenoma include the fetal adenoma, Hürthle cell adenoma and embryonal adenoma, each distinguished according to the character and pattern of cell proliferation.

Imaging Features

Most thyroid adenomas are hyperechoic or isoechoic at sonography. Almost 50% of adenomas are isoechoic, but they are often visible because of their hypoechoic peripheral halo.[29] The halo is due to fibrous capsule and blood vessels which can be readily seen by color Doppler imaging. On CT an adenoma may appear solid, or cystic when it has an degenerated. On T2-weighted MR images thyroid adenomas are typically of increased signal intensity, but are often heterogeneous.

FNA cannot generally distinguish follicular adenoma from follicular carcinoma as they have similar cytological features. Only on histopathological examination it is possible to differentiate an adenoma from a carcinoma based on the criteria of vascular and capsular invasion.[29]

MALIGNANT NEOPLASMS

Malignant thyroid neoplasms constitute the most common endocrine cancer.[5] Thyroid carcinoma arises both from

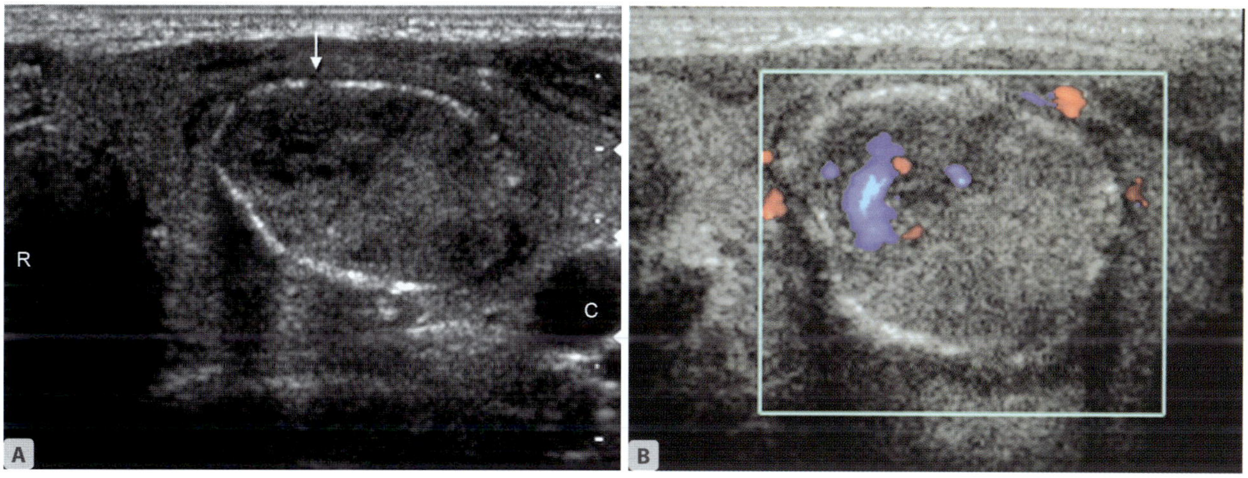

FIGS. 18A AND B: (A) Ultrasound of the left lobe of thyroid showing a well-defined, hypo- to isoechoic nodule with thin peripheral rim of calcification (arrow): Thyroid adenoma; (B) Color Doppler imaging shows both central and peripheral vascularity in a left lobe thyroid adenoma.

follicular and parafollicular C cells. Malignant potential and behavior range from low grade (papillary carcinoma) to aggressive (anaplastic carcinoma). The for major histologic types of thyroid carcinoma includes papillary, follicular, medullary and anaplastic types.

Papillary and follicular carcinomas (including the Hurthle cell variant of follicular carcinoma) are known as differentiated thyroid carcinomas (DTC). They are the most common and account for 88% and 8% respectively of all thyroid malignancies.[30] They originate from the follicular epithelial cells and have an excellent prognosis with 10-year survival rates of greater than 95% and 85% respectively.[31]

Papillary Carcinoma

Papillary carcinoma is the most common type of thyroid cancer. It is a low grade malignancy occurring most commonly in females. They occur in any age with a peak most commonly seen in the third and seventh decade. Histologically, papillary carcinoma may have a spectrum of findings and may be purely papillary, mixed papillary and follicular, or completely follicular. Frequently, papillary carcinoma is multifocal and microscopic in the thyroid gland and is thought to represent intraglandular lymphatic spread rather than multiple synchronous tumors. Papillary carcinoma is associated with risk factors such as exposure to ionizing radiation, especially childhood head and neck irradiation, family history of thyroid cancer.[31]

Imaging Features

Ultrasound is very useful in the evaluation of papillary carcinomas as a high percentage of them are occult and multicentric. Sonographically, 90% of papillary carcinomas are hypoechoic and rarely of mixed or isoechoic echotexture.[32] Fine, punctate, intralesional microcalcifications (Psammomatous) are considered characteristic of papillary carcinomas. Microcalcification are the result of deposition of calcium in Psammoma bodies, which are infarcted papilla that take up calcium into the dying cells. Papillary carcinomas

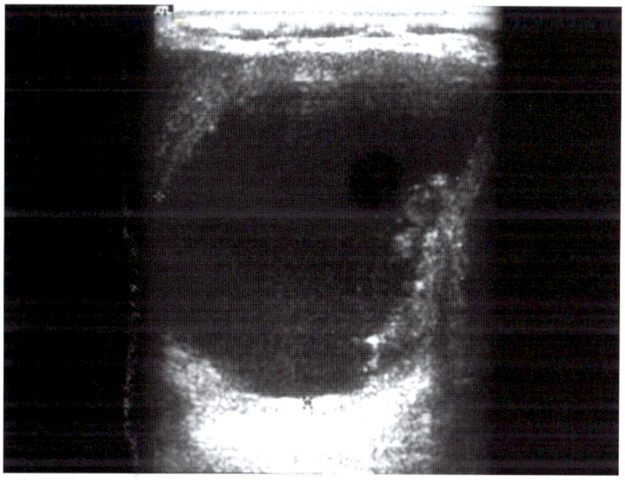

FIG. 19: T-S of right lobe of thyroid on ultrasound showing a predominantly cystic mass with eccentric mural nodularity, punctate calcification: Cystic papillary carcinoma.

are typically centrally vascularized lesions with a chaotic vascular pattern. The irregular vascularization is caused by stenosis, occlusions, aneurysms or arteriovenous shunts of the tumor vessels.[32] Cystic papillary carcinoma, a rare variant consists of a predominantly cystic lesion associated with protruding, mural, solid, hypervascular tissue (excrescences) and microcalcifications **(Fig. 19)**.[33]

Papillary carcinoma has the highest incidence of all the thyroid malignancies for cervical lymph node spread, seen in up to 50% of cases **(Figs. 20A to D)**.[5] However, this does not appear to effect the prognosis. Metastatic lymph nodes are not uncommonly normal in size and may be calcified, cystic, hemorrhagic or may contain colloid.[34] Cystic nodal metastasis are characterized by a thin or imperceptible wall and can be mistaken for benign cysts. They occur in the neck almost exclusively in association with papillary thyroid carcinoma, but occasionally may occur in nasopharyngeal carcinomas.[13] Cystic nodes are different from the necrotic

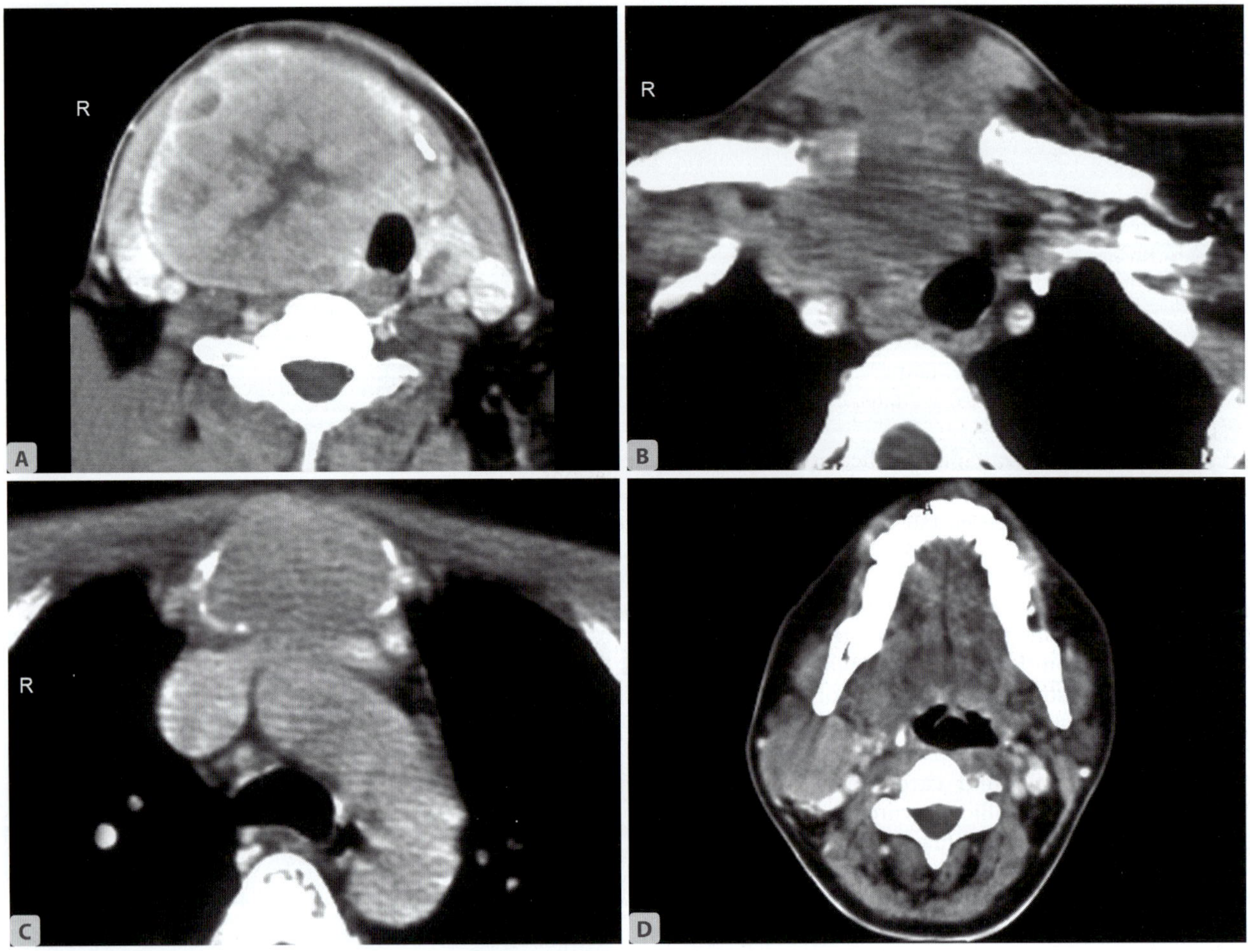

FIGS. 20 A TO D: (A and B) CECT neck showing a large, heterogeneously enhancing mass in the right lobe and isthmus of thyroid causing contralateral displacement of trachea and ipsilateral displacement of carotid sheath vessels. A curvilinear peripheral focus of calcification is seen in the mass along with a small hypodense lesion in the left lobe. CT sections through the upper chest reveals extension of the mass into the thorax with destruction of medial end of right clavicle and (C) expansile lytic destruction of the manubrium. (D) A well- circumscribed metastatic node is seen along the right internal jugular vein: Papillary carcinoma.

nodes frequently seen with metastatic squamous cell carcinoma that have central low density but retain a thick rind of residual lymphatic tissue.[5] In most cases, cystic nodal metastasis show a thickened outer wall, internal nodularity and septations, whereas in younger patients they may appear purely cystic.[35]

Regional nodal metastasis from thyroid cancer occur in the lateral cervical lymph chains (levels II-IV) and central compartment (level VI) in the majority of cases. Occasionally, metastasis may occur in retropharyngeal nodes, usually in the setting of recurrent disease.[8] Hence, any lymph node seen in a patient with papillary carcinoma should raise the suspicion of metastatic disease because of the high rate of lymphatic spread. This is especially true if the node enhances, as these tumours are highly vascular.

Hematogenous spread to the lungs, bones and central nervous system may occur, but this is less common (around 5%) especially in the absence of nodal disease. As papillary carcinomas concentrate radioiodine, scanning with ^{131}I following thyroidectomy may be valuable in detecting residual/recurrent thyroid disease in the operative bed of the neck as well as in detecting distant metastasis. Subsequently treatment with ^{131}I may be instituted. The prognosis for papillary thyroid carcinoma is excellent, with a 20-year survival rate of over 90%.[5]

Follicular variant of papillary thyroid carcinoma (FVPTC) is the second most common variant of thyroid carcinoma after papillary thyroid carcinoma (PTC), accounting for nearly 9–50% of all papillary carcinomas. Sonographic features of FVPTC have been found to be different from the conventional PTC by being larger in size, more round to ovoid than tall in shape, isoechoic or hypoechoic with a hypoechoic halo and the absence of calcification; i.e. having more benign sonographic features. FVPTC have been reported to have a lower incidence of lymph node metastasis and capsular invasion as well as higher rates of lung and bone metastasis as compared to conventional PTC.[36]

Follicular Carcinoma

True follicular carcinomas of the gland comprise 5% of all thyroid tumors. They are well-differentiated or moderately differentiated, relatively low-grade malignancies that are reportedly more commonly seen in the setting of iodine deficiency. They are usually solitary and slightly more aggressive than papillary carcinomas if vascular invasion is present. Women are affected 2–3 times more often than men, with slightly older age group involvement than papillary carcinoma.

There are two variants of follicular carcinoma that differ greatly in histology and clinical course.[13] In the *minimally invasive* form, the tumor often exhibits a capsule indicative of a better prognosis and only the histologic demonstration of focal invasion of blood vessels of the fibrous capsule permits differentiation from follicular adenoma. The *widely invasive* follicular carcinomas are not well encapsulated, and invasion of the vessels and adjacent thyroid is more easily demonstrated. Both the variants of follicular carcinoma tend to spread via blood stream rather than via lymphatics. Distant metastases to bone, lung, brain and liver are more likely than metastases to cervical lymph nodes.

Imaging Features

Follicular carcinoma resemble follicular adenoma on imaging. Ultrasonography of follicular carcinomas demonstrates a hypoechoic mass in approximately 45% of cases and an isoechoic mass in the remainder.[22] Although the diagnosis is strictly histologic, the presence of a nodule with ill-defined borders, heterogeneous internal echoes, a thick irregular capsule, tortuous intranodal and perinodal vessels and sonographic evidence of vascular and extracapsular invasion raises the possibility of malignancy of the tumor.[1]

Power Doppler sonography has been found to be more sensitive and reliable than velocity mode color Doppler sonography in depicting the vascular pattern of intranodular and perinodular vessels, thereby aiding in the differentiation of malignant and benign thyroid nodules.[37] Most of the follicular carcinomas have been found to have a central flow with a moderate increase of intranodular vascularization on Power Doppler sonography (PDS). In contrast, follicular adenomas have been shown to have a predominant peripheral rim of color flow on PDS. However, power Doppler characteristics cannot be used to rule out malignancy as 20% of malignant nodules have been found to have peripheral flow. *Color flow imaging* can show the hemodynamic features of neovascularization such as the presence of penetrating feeding arteries, thereby enabling the differentiation between *follicular adenoma and carcinoma* to be made. The vascularity of each nodule by power Doppler has been graded 0 to 4, in increasing order of flow.

Grade 0—nodule with no visible flow
1—peripheral flow only
2—peripheral with small amount of central flow
3—peripheral with extensive internal flow
4—nodule with central flow only

CT and MR demonstrate a solid mass not dissimilar to papillary carcinoma and are useful for demonstrating invasion of adjacent structures, extension into mediastinum and cervical lymphadenopathy. Like papillary carcinoma, follicular cancers concentrate iodine, and ^{131}I imaging may be useful in the follow-up of these patients. Prognosis for follicular carcinoma is poorer than that for papillary carcinoma. The 5-year survival rate for encapsulated variants is around 90%, while invasive variants have a poorer prognosis.[5]

Hurthle Cell Neoplasms of the Thyroid

Hurthle cell neoplasms (HCN) are poorly understood thyroid tumors and considered variants of follicular thyroid neoplasms. Some consider them distinct from other follicular neoplasms or consider that they should be classified as a sub group of papillary thyroid carcinomas.[38] They represent 3% of thyroid carcinomas. They are also known as oncocytic or oxyphilic neoplasms and are defined as tumors consisting of at least 75% Hürthle cells and a paucity of colloid cells which are thyroglobulin producing epithelial cells. These cells are present in both non-neoplastic and neoplastic thyroid lesions.

Hürthle cell neoplasms have been reported to have a wide spectrum of sonographic appearances from predominantly hypoechoic to hyperechoic lesions and from peripheral blood flow with no internal flow to extensively vascularized lesions. The differentiation between benign and malignant HCNs (adenoma from carcinoma) has been found to be beyond the resolution of sonography and FNAC and diagnosis can only be made by pathological evaluation of resected tumors.

Medullary Carcinoma

Medullary carcinomas of the thyroid are relatively uncommon, and are derived from the parafollicular C cells, which are of neural crest origin. Approximately 80–90% of medullary carcinomas secrete calcitonin which is used as a sensitive indicator of tumor presence and volume. Those medullary carcinomas that do not produce calcitonin have a poorer prognosis. They have a higher mortality rate than well-differentiated papillary and follicular malignancies. Medullary carcinomas are usually solitary lesions. They may invade locally, may spread to regional cervical lymph nodes and may result in hematogenous spread. Distant metastasis most commonly occur to lungs, bones and liver.

Medullary carcinomas occur sporadically, but a familial link is seen in approximately 15% of adult patients.[22] They are inherited as an autosomal dominant trait and comprises a component of the multiple endocrine neoplasia (MEN) syndromes, types IIA and IIB, which include medullary thyroid carcinoma and adrenal phaeochromocytomas. The disease is multicentric and/or bilateral in about 90% of the familial cases.

Imaging Features

On ultrasonographic examination, medullary carcinomas are typically hypoechoic, although focal calcification may cause echogenic foci both at the primary site and within metastatic lymph nodes. The calcifications tend to be more coarse than the calcifications of typical papillary carcinoma. CT and MRI demonstrate a solid mass, are helpful in displaying surgical anatomy and adjacent lymphadenopathy; malignant lymph nodes being seen in approximately 50% of cases **(Figs. 21A to C)**.[9] Unlike papillary and follicular subtypes, medullary carcinoma does not concentrate radioiodine. However, radionuclide specific for neuroendocrine tissue such as ^{131}I meta-iodobenzylguanidine (MIBG) has been used with some success to evaluate primary as well as metastatic medullary thyroid carcinoma.[5]

The prognosis for medullary thyroid cancer is variable. Patients with thyroid cancer in the setting of MEN type IIB tend to have very aggressive tumors that frequently occur at a young age. In contrast, those in association with MEN type IIA have favorable outcomes. The reported 5-year survival rates are around 75%.

Anaplastic Carcinoma

Anaplastic carcinoma of the thyroid is a highly aggressive and rapidly fatal tumor usually presenting in elderly women.It accounts for less than 2% of all thyroid cancers and is often inoperable at presentation. Anaplastic thyroid carcinomas are often associated with papillary or follicular carcinoma. They are more prone to aggressive local invasion of the neck muscles and blood vessels, instead of lymphatic spread. They commonly occur in patients with long standing goiter. These cancers grow rapidly, and compress and invade the aerodigestive tract and vessels.

Imaging Features

On ultrasound, anaplastic carcinomas are usually hypoechoic and often encase or invade blood vessels and neck muscles. Often these tumors cannot be adequately examined by ultrasound because of their large size. On CT, calcification and necrosis are seen in approximately 60 and 75% cases respectively.[39] CT and MR imaging of the neck usually demonstrate more accurately the extent of the disease **(Figs. 22A to D)**. Anaplastic carcinomas do not concentrate radioiodine. Of all the thyroid cancers, anaplastic thyroid cancers carry the worst prognosis, with a 5-year mortality rate of more than 95%.[13]

Primary Lymphoma

Primary lymphoma of the thyroid gland is uncommon. It usually presents in elderly women with a long history of goiter. Patients with Hashimoto's thyroiditis have an increased incidence of developing lymphoma of the thyroid, which is usually of the non-Hodgkin's type.[40]

Patients usually present with a rapidly enlarging thyroid mass and symptoms of obstruction related to compression of the aerodigestive tract.

Imaging Features

Lymphoma typically appears as a solitary, hypoechoic, lobulated mass on sonography with significant enlargement of the gland. The adjacent parenchyma may be heterogeneous due to associated chronic lymphocytic thyroiditis.[13] These tumors are hypodense on CT.[50] On MRI, lymphoma is often

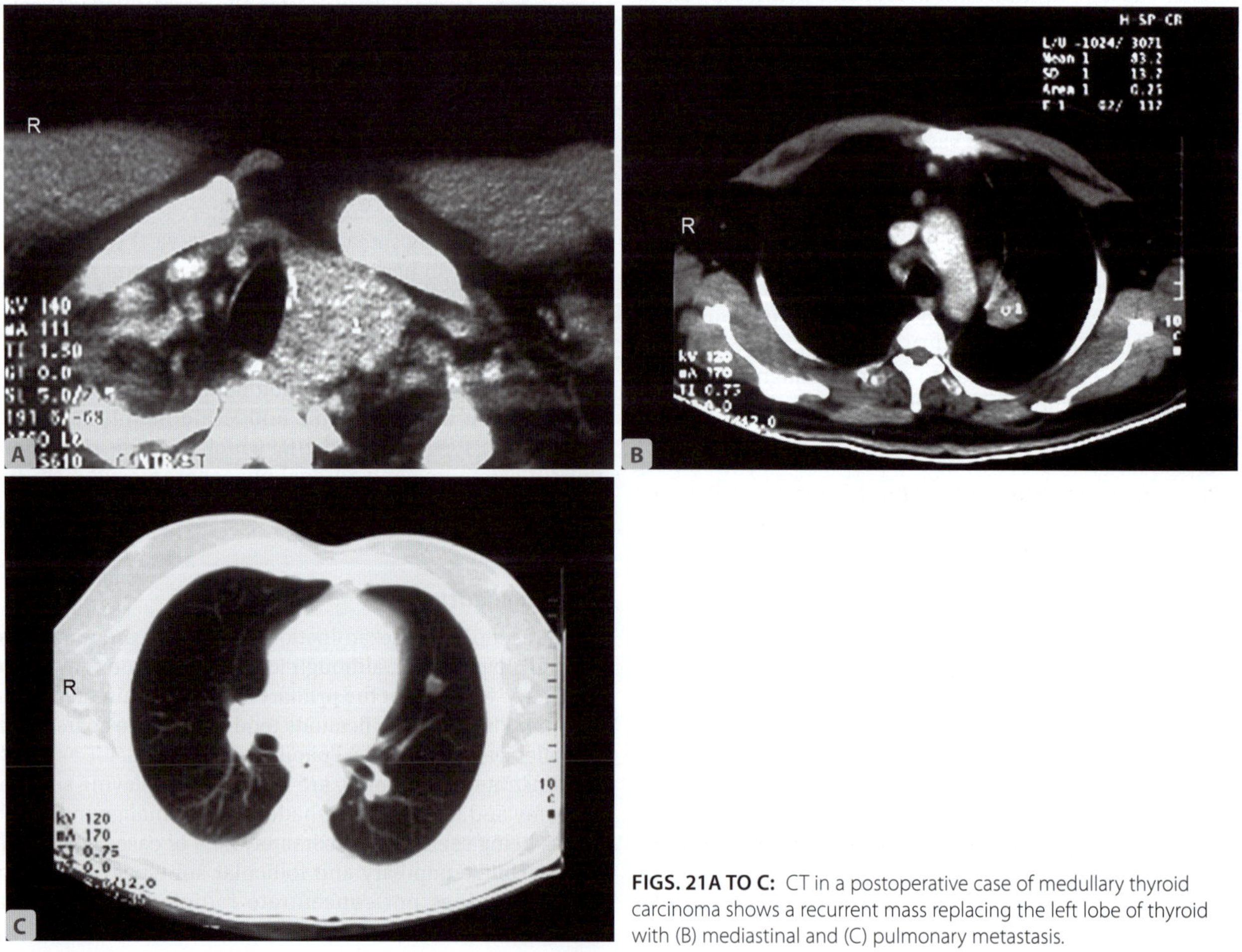

FIGS. 21A TO C: CT in a postoperative case of medullary thyroid carcinoma shows a recurrent mass replacing the left lobe of thyroid with (B) mediastinal and (C) pulmonary metastasis.

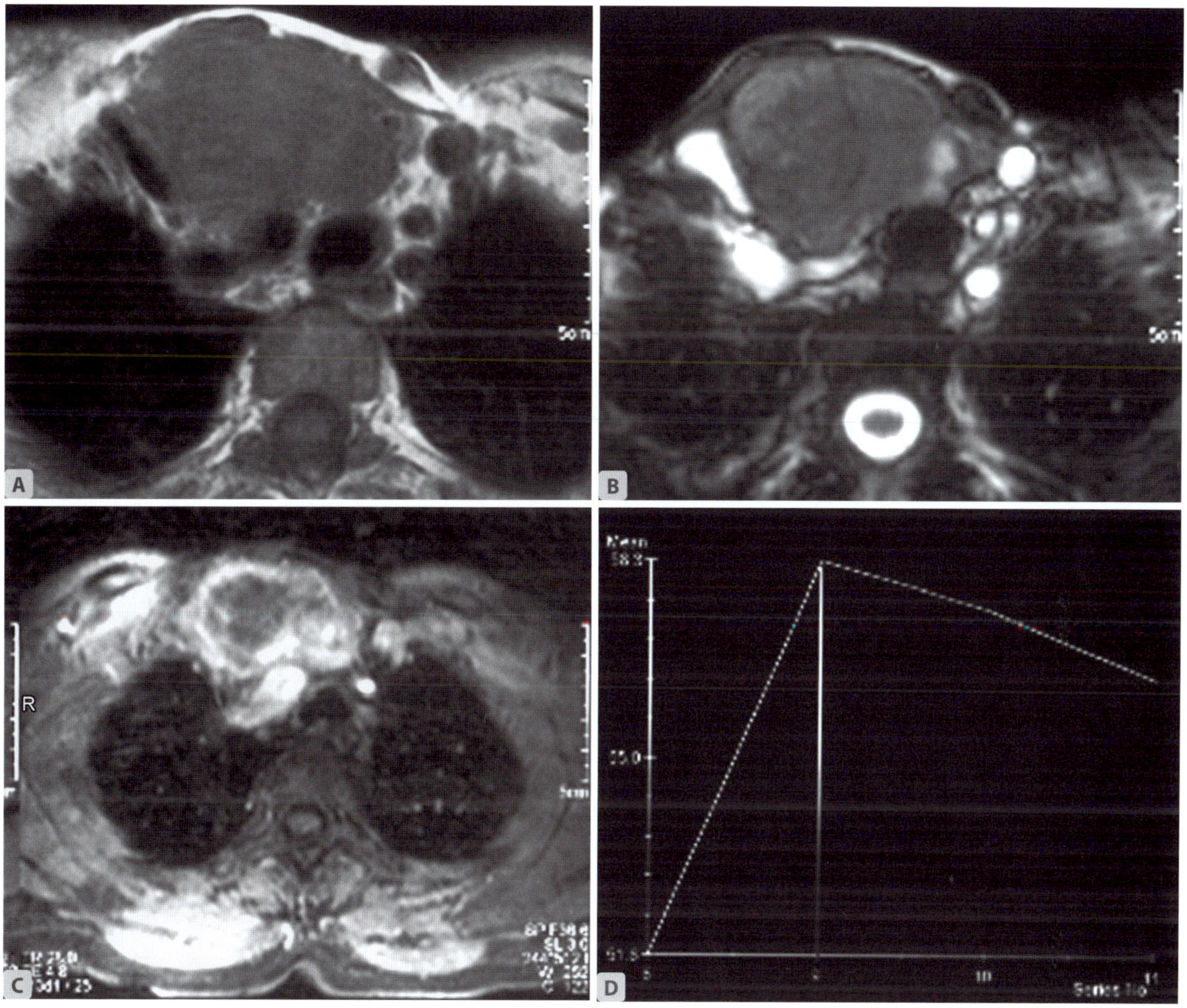

FIGS. 22A TO D: (A and B) T1W and T2W axial images show a hypodense mass in the right thyroid lobe causing deviation of trachea to the left. The mass is causing attenuation and splaying of the strap muscles anteriorly and great vessels posterolaterally; (C) Postcontrast image reveals heterogeneous, intense peripheral enhancement; (D) The time signal intensity curve shows a rapid uptake and washout of contrast: Anaplastic carcinoma.

hyperintense on T2-weighted images and isointense to normal thyroid on T1-weighted images.[41] It enhances less compared to other thyroid tumours.[42] Imaging including MR imaging, cannot reliably distinguish lymphoma from thyroiditis in patients with Hashimoto's thyroiditis.[43] While lymphoma is typically cold on iodine and technetium nuclear scintigraphy, it may show increased uptake on gallium scans.[5] The prognosis is highly variable and depends on the stage of the disease. The 5-year survival rate may range from nearly 90% in early-stage to less than 5% in advanced, disseminated disease.[13]

Metastatic Disease

Metastases to the thyroid gland are relatively rare. The thyroid is a hypervascular organ and the site of haematogenous metastases most commonly secondary to melanoma, carcinoma of the kidney, bronchus and breast **(Fig. 23)**. The appearance of metastatic lesions is nonspecific and may be multifocal.[44] On ultrasound, the echotexture is nonspecific, metastasis from hypernephroma being hypervascular on color Doppler sonography. Metastatic disease should be considered when histology of a resected thyroid mass is atypical.

Preoperative Staging of Thyroid Carcinoma

Thyroid cancer is staged by the AJCC / TNM staging system based on the size/extent of the tumor(T), spread to nearby lymph nodes (N) and the spread to distant sites(M). The extent of local invasion can involve the trachea, larynx, pharynx/esophagus, vascular structures (mainly carotid arteries) and inferiorly up to mediastinum.[45] **Tables 4 and 5** illustrate the TNM staging and the eighth edition of the AJCC/ TNM staging system for thyroid carcinomas.

Preoperative workup involves ultrasonography to detect multifocal disease and lymphadenopathy. CT and MRI are performed if local invasion is suspected.

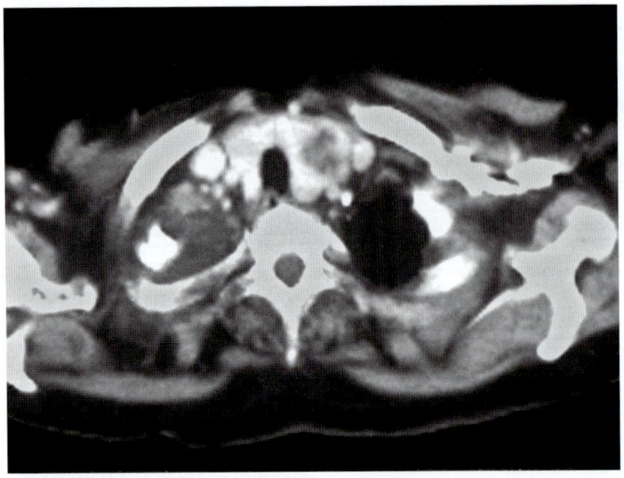

FIG. 23: CT scan in a known case of carcinoma breast showing a hypodense nodule in the left lobe of thyroid. (FNAC: metastatic adenocarcinoma).

Evaluation of Nodal Metastasis on CT/MRI

Papillary carcinoma and medullary thyroid carcinoma are the most common thyroid cancers that metastasise to lymph nodes while nodal metastasis are uncommon in follicular carcinoma. Papillary and medullary carcinoma may first present as nodal metastasis and the primary thyroid nodule may not be seen on CT or MRI due to their small size. Features which suggest that a nodal mass is of primary thyroid origin are its cystic composition, calcification, intense enhancement or proteinaceous/ hemorrhagic content. Lymphatic drainage from the thyroid is extensive and various nodal stations or groups at the highest risk of metastasis are:[45]

- *Central compartment*: Level VII (upper mediastinal lymph nodes)
- *Lateral nodal groups*: Levels II - IV
- Delphian node (or prelaryngeal node) involvement in papillary thyroid cancer is predictive of advanced nodal disease as patients are nine times more likely to have lateral nodal involvement.
- *Lower paratracheal nodes*: Level VI
- Retropharyngeal and retroesophageal nodes

Nodal morphology rather than size criteria should be used when assessing metastatic disease because up to 61% of nodal metastasis maybe < 10 mm in size. **Table 6** depicts the rate of lymph nodal spread and morphological characteristics of lymph nodes of thyroid carcinomas.

MRI has been reported to have an accuracy of 86–94% in detecting local invasion.[4,31] The following findings are suggestive of local invasion on CT /MRI.

- >90° encasement of thyroid cartilage
- 90–180° or more contact with circumference of trachea or esophagus
- Deformity of lumen of trachea, focal mucosal irregularity and thickening—suggestive of tracheal invasion while soft tissue within trachea is highly reliable sign of tracheal invasion
- Invasion of recurrent laryngeal nerve (RLN)which is seen as effacement of fatty tissue in the tracheopharyngeal groove

TABLE 4: TNM Definitions for Papillary, Follicular, Poorly Differentiated, Hürthle Cell, and Anaplastic Thyroid Carcinomas.[45]

	Definition of primary tumor (T)
T category	**T criteria**
TX	Primary tumor cannot be assessed
TO	No evidence of primary tumor
T1	Tumor <2 cm in greatest dimension limited to the thyroid
T1a	Tumor <1 cm in greatest dimension limited to the thyroid
T1b	Tumor >1 cm but <2 cm in greatest dimension limited to the thyroid
T2	Tumor >2 cm but <4 cm in greatest dimension limited to the thyroid
T3	Tumor >4 cm limited to the thyroid or gross extrathyroidal extension invading only strap muscles
T3a	Tumor >4 cm limited to the thyroid
T3b	Gross extrathyroidal extension invading only strap muscles (sternohyoid, sternothyroid, thyrohyoid, or omohyoid muscles) from a tumor of any size
T4	Includes gross extrathyroidal extension into major neck structures
T4a	Gross extrathyroidal extension invading subcutaneous soft tissues, larynx, trachea, esophagus, or recurrent laryngeal nerve from a tumor of any size
T4b	Gross extrathyroidal extension invading prevertebral fascia or encasing carotid artery or mediastinal vessels from a tumor of any size
	Definition of regional lymph node (N)
N category	**N criteria**
NX	Regional lymph nodes cannot be assessed
NO	No evidence of regional lymph nodes metastasis
NOa	One or more cytologic or histologically confirmed benign lymph node
NOb	No radiologic or clinical evidence of locoregional lymph node metastasis
N1	Metastasis to regional nodes
N1a	Metastasis tc level VI or VII (pretracheal, paratracheal, or prelaryngeal/Delphian, or upper mediastinal) lymph nodes; this can be unilateral or bilateral disease
N1b	Metastasis to unilateral, bilateral, or contralateral lateral neck lymph nodes (levels I, II, III, IV, or V) or retropharyngeal lymph nodes
	Definition of distant metastasis (M)
M category	**M criteria**
M0	No distant metastasis
M1	Distant metastasis

- Circumferential encasement of common carotid artery to 270° has been reported to increase the sensitivity and specificity on MRI to 100% and 88% respectively

The presence of vascular and prevascular space invasion (T4b) precludes the patient from any curative surgery.

TABLE 5: Staging protocol for thyroid cancer: Eighth edition of the ajcc/tnm staging system.[45]

Differentiated thyroid cancer				
Age at diagnosis	**T stage**	**N stage**	**M stage**	**Stage group**
<55 yrs	Any T	Any N	M0	I
	Any T	Any N	M1	II
>55 yrs	T1	N0/NX	M0	I
	T1	N1	M0	II
	T2	N0/NX	M0	I
	T2	N1	M0	II
	T3a/T3b	Any N	M0	II
	T4a	Any N	M0	III
	T4b	Any N	M0	IVA
	Any T	Any N	M1	IVB

Anaplastic thyroid cancer			
T stage	**N stage**	**M stage**	**Stage group**
T1-T3a	N0/NX	M0	IVA
T1-T3a	N1	M0	IVB
T3b	Any N	M0	IVB
T4	Any N	M0	IVB
Any T	Any N	M1	IVC

Treatment

Except anaplastic carcinoma, treatment involves total or near total thyroidectomy, central nodal resection and radionuclide ablation.

Recurrent Thyroid Cancer

Rates of recurrence of thyroid cancer range from 7–14%. Patients undergoing thyroidectomy for thyroid cancer require long-term follow-up as in 1/3rd of cases recurrence can occur after more than 10 years after treatment.[46] The most common site of recurrence is the neck mainly to lymph nodes. Recurrence in the chest may be in the form of pulmonary metastasis which are often tiny, i.e. miliary and have an indolent course. Bone metastasis are also common and are seen as expansile lytic metastasis.

Follow up relies on clinical evaluation, TSH monitoring to ensure suppression and serum thyroglobulin measurement (calcitonin levels for medullary thyroid carcinoma). Serum thyroglobulin is used as a marker for recurrent or residual differentiated thyroid cancer. When its levels are increased, neck ultrasound and ^{131}I or ^{123}I scintigraphy is typically obtained. Scintigraphy may be negative in 50–80% of patients when it represents progression to dedifferentiated thyroid cancer. Then, MRI or PET CT has a role in localizing tumor for surgery as well as nodal disease. FDG-PET is frequently positive when radio iodine uptake is negative, and vice versa, as radio-iodine negative tumor represents dedifferentiated disease. A pitfall of PET CT is that thyroid nodal metastasis may be missed because of their small size. However, distant metastasis to lungs and bone can be recognized on PET CT.[31]

TABLE 6: Lymph node characteristics in various types of thyroid carcinomas.

Type of thyroid cancer	Rate of LN metastasis	Lymph nodes morphology
Papillary carcinoma	>75%	Foci of calcification, cystic/necrotic change, increase attenuation (hemorrhage/thyroglobulin)
Anaplastic and medullary carcinoma	>50%	Necrotic change ++
Follicular carcinoma	<20%	Lower incidence of morphological changes in LN

DIFFERENTIATION OF BENIGN AND MALIGNANT THYROID NODULES

High Resolution Gray Scale Ultrasonography

In the past few years, advancements in high resolution gray scale sonography has led to the development of certain ultrasound criteria for differentiating benign from malignant thyroid nodules.[28] Ultrasound features which are predictive of malignant thyroid nodules are:

1. Taller than wide shape
2. Spiculated/irregular margin
3. Markedly hypoechogenic nodule
4. Predominantly solid composition
5. Presence of microcalcification in a predominantly solid nodule (3 fold risk)
6. Macrocalcification in a solid nodule (2 fold risk)
7. Absence of a halo
8. Intranodular vascularity

A taller than wide shape is very specific for differentiating malignant thyroid nodules from benign ones as malignant nodules grow across tissue planes while benign nodules grow parallel to normal tissue planes. A spiculated margin is suggestive of malignancy while an ill defined margin can be seen in both benign and malignant nodules. The reason for an ill defined margin in benign thyroid nodules is that benign nodules are known to be incompletely encapsulated and can also merge with normal tissue. On the basis of echogenicity, there has been a considerable overlap in the echogenicity of benign and malignant thyroid nodules. Marked hypogenicity has been suggested to be a more specific and a more reliable criteria for diagnosing a malignant thyroid nodule than hypogenicity in a broader sense. This is because 50% of the benign nodules and majority of malignant thyroid nodules are found to be hypoechoic.

As regards calcification within a thyroid nodule, it has been found that the presence of microcalcification in a predominantly solid nodule was found to increase the risk of cancer three-fold, while coarse macrocalcifications increase cancer risk two fold compared with predominantly solid nodules without any calcification. There is no clear size criteria for determining whether a calcification is a micro- or macrocalcification, but a cut off of 1 mm has been suggested. Microcalcifications correspond pathologically to calcified psammoma bodies that are typical of papillary carcinoma. Macrocalcifications or coarse calcifications are related to fibrosis and degeneration. Benign nodules have a coarse calcification, especially with a long standing disease. Studies have shown that a combination of the above ultrasound findings provide a better diagnostic accuracy in predicting malignancy in a thyroid nodule than the presence of only one finding.

Various newer imaging techniques have been used in studies for differentiating benign from malignant thyroid nodules.

US Elastography

Various studies have shown significant difference in the SWV of benign and malignant nodules with malignant nodules having a median SWV of 3.0 m/s and benign nodules 2.06 m/s in a study in 2012. ARFI imaging achieved a specificity of 95% using a cut-off of 3 m/s.[47,48] **Figures 24 and 25** depict gray scale images and corresponding shear wave velocities (SWV) of a benign and malignant thyroid nodule.

The use of US- elastography has been found to be a promising technology that can assist in the differential diagnosis of thyroid cancer and in the selection of nodules suitable for FNAC.

Contrast-enhanced Ultrasound for Evaluation of Thyroid Nodules

Contrast-enhanced ultrasound (CEUS) is a noninvasive ultrasound technique that provides macro- and micro-visualization of tissues studied and can assess blood perfusion

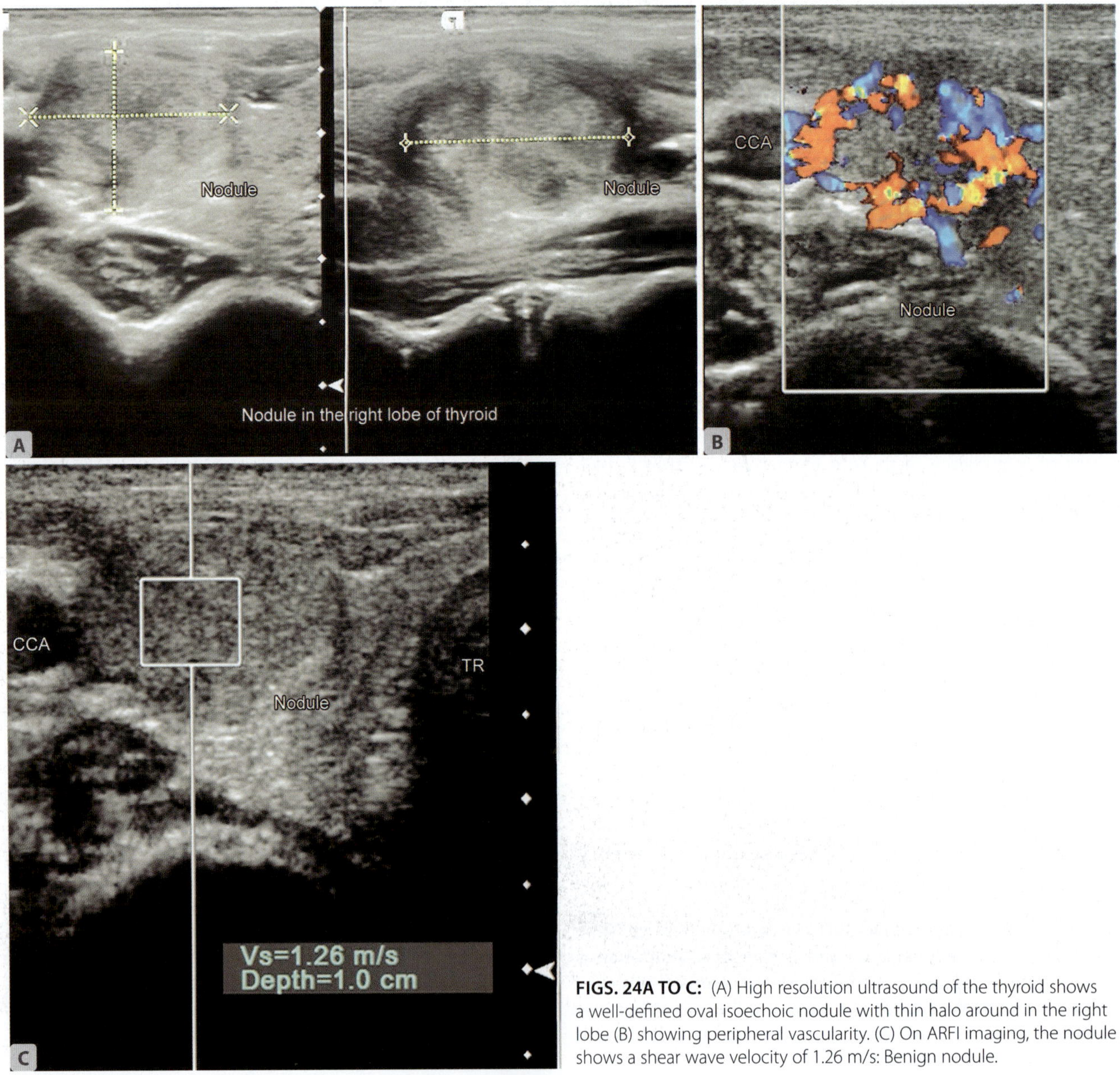

FIGS. 24A TO C: (A) High resolution ultrasound of the thyroid shows a well-defined oval isoechoic nodule with thin halo around in the right lobe (B) showing peripheral vascularity. (C) On ARFI imaging, the nodule shows a shear wave velocity of 1.26 m/s: Benign nodule.

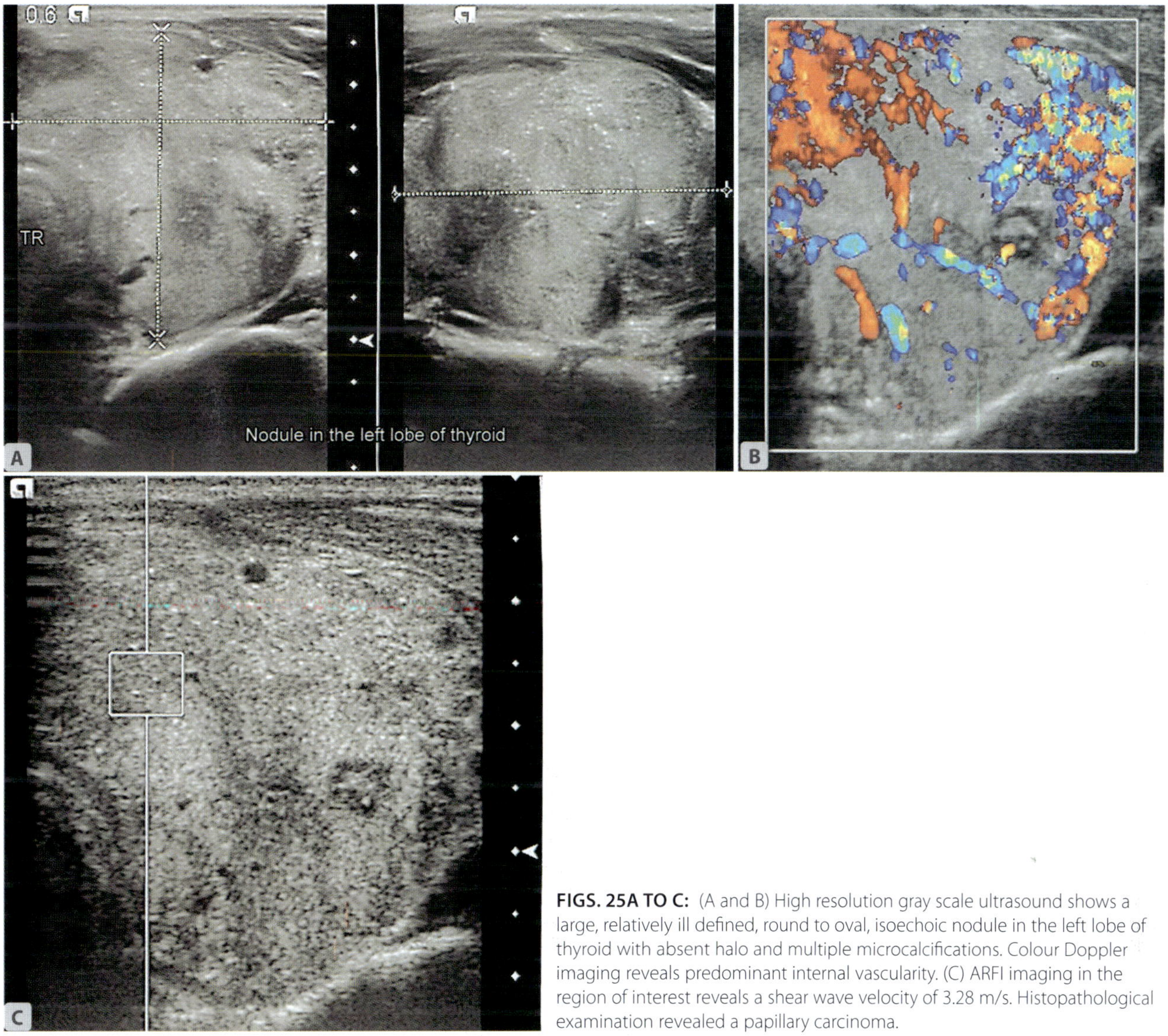

FIGS. 25A TO C: (A and B) High resolution gray scale ultrasound shows a large, relatively ill defined, round to oval, isoechoic nodule in the left lobe of thyroid with absent halo and multiple microcalcifications. Colour Doppler imaging reveals predominant internal vascularity. (C) ARFI imaging in the region of interest reveals a shear wave velocity of 3.28 m/s. Histopathological examination revealed a papillary carcinoma.

of thyroid nodules. Zhang et al. assessed the utility of contrast enhanced ultrasound in the evaluation of thyroid nodules. It was found that the enhancement pattern was different in benign and malignant lesions. In all 104 nodules were scanned with real-time grey-scale pulse inversion harmonic US imaging following intravenous injection of 1.2 ml bolus of SonoVue. Scanning for at least 3 minutes was done and enhancement patterns were classified into one of the 4 patterns—homogeneous, heterogeneous, ring enhancing, and no-enhancement. Ring enhancement was found to correlate highly with benign lesions while heterogeneous enhancement was helpful for detecting malignant lesions.[49]

Diffusion-weighted MR Imaging (DW- MRI)

In recent years, diffusion-weighted MR imaging of thyroid nodules has been performed with the aim of differentiating benign from malignant thyroid nodules. A significant difference in the ADC values of benign and malignant thyroid nodules has been reported, with all benign thyroid nodules having higher mean ADC values compared with malignant nodules. The mean ADC values of malignant solitary thyroid nodules was found to be $0.73 \pm 0.19 \times 10^{-3}$ mm^2/sec and of benign nodules was $1.8 \pm 0.27 \times 10^{-3}$ mm^2/sec.[50] The difference in the ADC values of thyroid nodules is based on the difference in cellularity and histopathologic features of benign and malignant thyroid nodules. Malignant thyroid nodules have increased cellularity and enlarged nuclei as compared with benign ones. This reduces the extracellular matrix and the diffusion space of water protons in the extracellular areas, with a resultant decrease in the ADC values.

Approach to Incidental Thyroid Nodules Detected on Imaging

Incidental thyroid nodules (ITN) or thyroid incidetalomas are one of the most common findings on imaging studies which include the neck. ITN is defined as a nodule identified on an imaging study that was not previously detected or suspected clinically. They are seen in 20–67% of ultrasound studies, up to 25% of contrast enhanced CT scan of the chest and 16–18% of CT and MRIs of the neck.[51]

The malignancy rate of an individual nodule has been found to be low, ranging from 0–9% with a rate as low as 1.2% according to a recent population based case control study[R]. Also, most thyroid cancers are not aggressive in nature, due to which most patients with small thyroid cancers are seen to die with, rather than from, thyroid cancer. There are no reliable signs to indicate that a thyroid nodule detected incidentally on CT and MRI is benign or malignant in the absence of frank local invasion.

If an incidental thyroid nodule has been detected on CT or MRI of the neck, the next investigation is ultrasound due to the higher spatial resolution and better characterization of nodules by sonography.

According to a largest recent retrospective study, the only useful sonographic signs of malignancy reported were microcalcification, solid compostion and a size >2 cm having odds ratios of 8.1, 4.0 and 3.6 respectively.[46]

Due to variability in reporting of ITN on CT and MR imaging, a 3 tiered system of risk categorization for thyroid nodules has been proposed based on patient age, nodule size and suspicious imaging findings as given in **Table 7**.[31,46] A recent study has shown a 46% reduction in ITN work-up with a 3-tiered system compared to a 1 cm size as cut-off size.

TABLE 7: The 3-tiered system of risk categorization for thyroid nodules detected by CT, MRI or PET.

Category	Criteria for categorization	Suggested workup/ recommendation
Risk category 1: Highly suspicious for malignancy	• PET avid thyroid nodule • *Suspicious lymphadenophathy • Extrathyroid spread with or without signs of vocal cord palsy on side of nodule • Lung metastasis	Recommend FNA for nodule of any size
Risk category 2: Indeterminate with risk factors of young age	• **High risk history • Age <35 years	Recommend USG if ≥1 cm in adults Consider USG workup for any size in pediatric patients
Risk category 3: Indeterminate without risk factors	• Age ≥35 years	Consider USG workup if ≥1.5 cm

***Suspicious LN**
- >10 mm short axis (except jugulodigastric which can be up to 15 mm in short axis diameter)
- Nodes with calcification, cystic component or irregular margins

****High risk history**
- History of cancer in one or more relatives
- History of external beam radiation as child, ionizing radiation in childhood/adolescence, previous hemithyroidectomy with thyroid cancer, MEN2/Familial MTC (medullary carcinoma thyroid), associated gene mutation, calcitonin >100 pg/mL

Recommendations for Incidental Thyroid Nodules Detected on CT, MR Imaging and PET Scan (Flowcharts 1 to 3)[51]

With focal metabolic activity in the thyroid on FDG-PET:dedicated thyroid ultrasound and FNA of the PET avid lesion, if the patient has normal life expectancy

Focal activity on other nuclear medicine scans: dedicated thyroid ultrasound if the patient has normal life expectancy

FLOWCHART 1: Incidental thyroid nodule detected on CT/MRI.

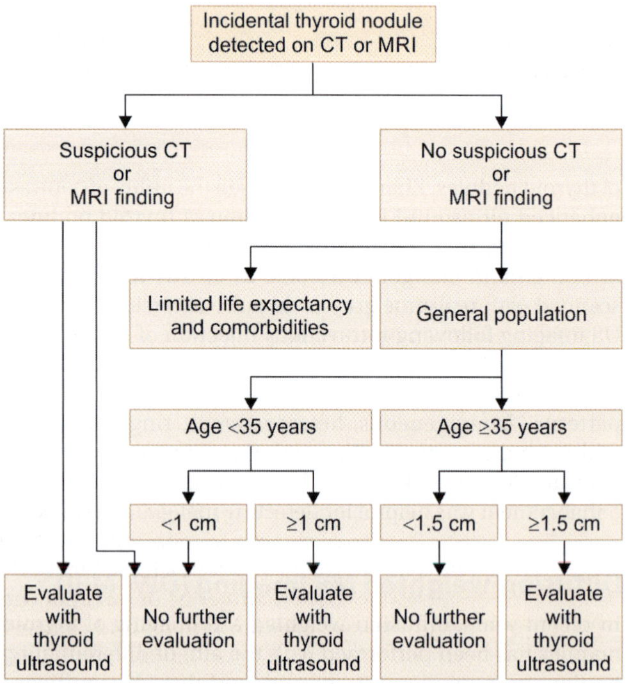

Approach to a Patient with Thyroid Nodule/Nodules

Evaluation of a patient with thyroid nodule consists of *clinical assessment* with complete history, physical examination focussing on the thyroid and for any enlarged cervical lymph nodes. This is followed by *diagnostic evaluation* consisting of

1. High resolution ultrasound of the thyroid
2. Thyroid scintigraphy
3. CT/MRI in case of large nodules/masses to evaluate spread to adjacent structures and for any retrosternal extension
4. FNA (fine needle aspiration) biopsy

Estimation of *serum thyrotropin (TSH)* is the initial evaluation. A low or subnormal TSH is suggestive of hyperthyroidism and requires a *thyroid scintigraphy* with ^{99m}Tc pertechnetate or ^{123}I to determine the functional status of the nodule. If serum TSH is normal or elevated, a radionuclide scan should not be performed as initial evaluation. In the setting of a low TSH, a nodule appears hot or hyperfunctioning and cytological evaluation is not required as hyperfunctioning nodules rarely harbour malignancy.

FLOWCHART 2: Incidental thyroid nodule detected on ultrasound for extrathyroidal structures.

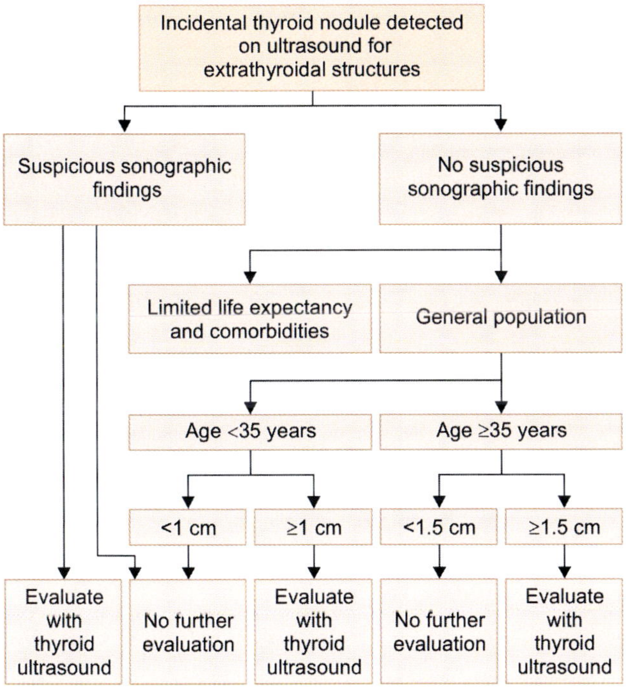

Recommendation: for ITN detected on CT, MRI or extrathyroidal ultrasound

Age <35 yrs: Dedicated thyroid ultrasound if nodule ≥1 cm with no suspicious findings on CT or MRI, with patient having normal life expectancy

Age >35 yrs: Dedicated thyroid ultrasound if nodule ≥1.5 cm with no suspicious imaging findings, with patient having normal life expectancy

FLOWCHART 3: Incidental thyroid nodule detected on 18FDG-PET and other nuclear medicine scans.

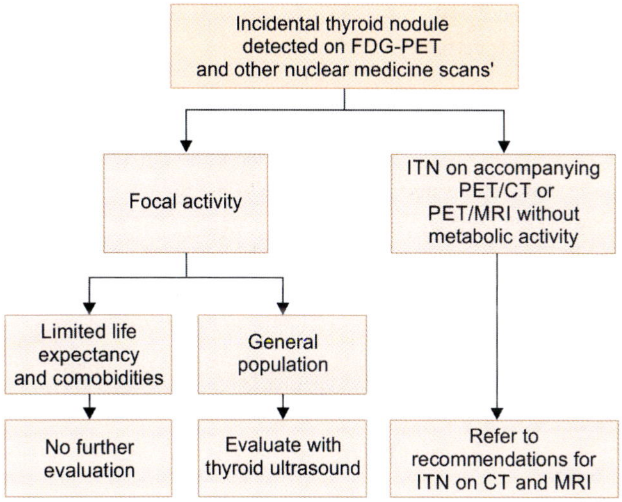

All patients with a nodular thyroid detected clinically should be evaluated with high resolution *ultrasound* to (a) confirm the presence of a mass, (b) determine if it is of thyroidal origin, (c) assess if it is solitary or multiple, (d) characterise the nodule's pattern on the basis of its sonographic characteristics, (e) evaluate for any suspicious cervical lymph nodes whenever a nodule shows features suspicious of malignancy, (f) provide guidance for FNA biopsy.

The American Thyroid Association (ATA) have formulated guidelines for the assessment of thyroid nodules so as to improve inter-and intra-departmental consistency in the assessment of nodules on sonographic evaluation and to facilitate communication with referring clinicians. The ATA guidelines have been last updated in 2015. The recommendations regarding which nodules should undergo fine needle aspiration are based on size and suspicious sonographic features of the nodules. These have been given in **Table 8**.

Fine needle aspiration is an accurate, costeffective investigation and plays an essential role in the evaluation of patients with thyroid nodules. It helps in reducing the number of unnecessary thyroid surgeries in patients with benign nodules and triages patients with thyroid cancer to appropriate surgery. Thyroid nodules which are clinically palpable generally undergo FNA without image guidance. The ATA guidelines recommend ultrasound-guided FNA for those nodules which are: (1) nonpalpable, (2) predominantly cystic, (3) located posteriorly in the thyroid, (4) require a repeat biopsy when a palpation-guided FNA yields an inadequate sample.

The FNA recommendations apply to both solitary and multiple nodules as both have similar risk for malignancy. The sonographic features are considered a better indicator than size in determining which nodule or nodules merit FNA in a multinodular gland.

Guidelines for differentiated thyroid carcinoma (especially papillary)—these may frequently be multifocal, with multiple nodules requiring FNA to ensure appropriate surgical planning. When one suspicious malignant nodule is identified sonographically, a careful assessment to rule out another such nodule is essential as the management for single <1 cm papillary thyroid carcinoma is lobectomy while bilateral cancers require total thyroidectomy.

Flowchart 4 depicts the algorithmic approach to a patient with thyroid nodule [53]

THYROID ULTRASOUND REPORTING LEXICON = THYROID IMAGING REPORTING AND DATA SYSTEM (TIRADS)

Ultrasound is the most commonly used imaging modality for the evaluation of thyroid nodules, with nodules being detected in at least 60% of the population who undergo ultrasonography. However, the percentage which are malignant are relatively low, ranging from 1.6–12%. The sonographic findings described are often not specific in differentiating benign from malignant nodule, and a fine nodule aspiration (FNA) or surgery is required for a definitive diagnosis.

TABLE 8: ATA (2015) guidelines for assessment of thyroid nodules: Sonographic Patterns, Estimated Risk of Malignancy, and Fine-Needle Aspiration Guidance for Thyroid Nodules.[52]

Sonographic pattern	USG features	Estimated risk of malignancy, %	Nodule cut-off size (largest dimension)
High suspicion	Solid hypoechoic nodule or solid hypoechoic component of a partially cystic nodule with one or more of the following features: irregular margins (infiltrative, microlobulated), microcalcifications, taller than wide shape, rim calcifications with small extrusive soft tissue component, evidence of ETE	>70–90	FNA recommended for ≥1 cm
Intermediate suspicion	Hypoechoic solid nodule with smooth margins without microcalcifications, ETE*, or taller than wide shape	10–20	FNA recommended for ≥ 1 cm
Low suspicion	Isoechoic or hyperechoic solid nodule, or partially cystic nodule with eccentric solid areas, without microcalcification, irregular margin or ETE, or taller than wide shape.	5–10	FNA recommended for ≥ 1.5 cm
Very low suspicion	Spongiform or partially cystic nodules without any of the sonographic features described in low, intermediate, or high suspicion patterns	<3	FNA to be considered for ≥2 cm Observation without FNA is also an option
Benign	Purely cystic nodules (no solid component)	<1	No biopsy

*ETE—extrathyroid extension

FLOWCHART 4: Algorithmic approach for evaluation of a patient with thyroid nodule.

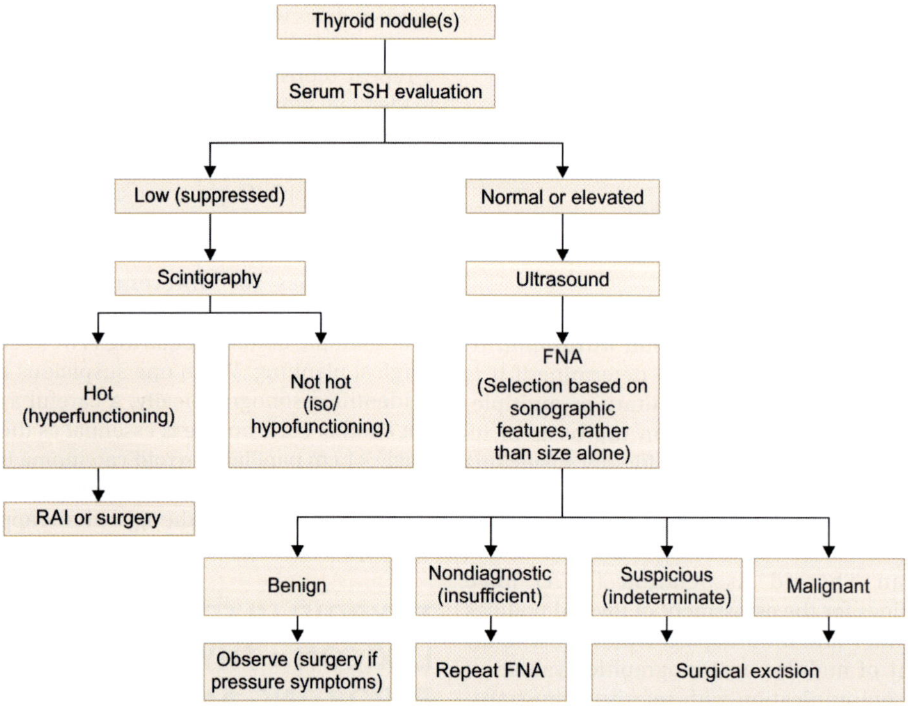

Since 2009, several professional organizations such as the ATA (American Thyroid Association) and the SRU (Society of Radiologists in Ultrasound) felt that the terms used to describe thyroid nodules were poorly defined and inconsistent. They proposed ultrasound based risk stratification to identify which nodules were suspicious and would require a biopsy and sonographic follow-up and which could be safely left alone. This came to be called the Thyroid Imaging, Reporting and Data System (TIRADS), modelled on the BIRADS system of breast imaging. However, these TIRADS classifications came from individual institution, hence; the American College of Radiology (ACR) convened committees to (i) provide recommendation for reporting incidental thyroid nodules (ii) develop a set of standard terms (lexicon) for ultrasound reporting and (iii) propose a TIRADS on the basis of the lexicon.

The White Paper of the ACR–TIRADS Committee was first published in 2015 which describes the consensus process and the resultant lexicon. Ultrasound elastography, though a promising technique for evaluation of thyroid lesions is not incorporated into the ACR-TIRADS.

Table 9 depicts the standard lexicon of the categories of ultrasound features of nodules and the score assigned to them based on their sonographic features.[54]

Points are assigned for all the sonographic features of a nodule, with additional points being awarded to a nodule with a more suspicious feature **(Fig. 26)**. Hence, higher the cumulative score, higher is the TR (thyroid reporting) level and likelihood of malignancy. If multiple nodules (≥4) are present, then, four of the nodules with the highest score are to be scored, reported and followed-up. These need not be the largest nodules.

The ACR-TIRADS does not provide a grade for "normal thyroid gland". The ACR white paper of 2015 which developed a lexicon from descriptive reports has been updated.

TABLE 9: Ultrasound categories of thyroid nodules based on ACR-TIRADS lexicon.

Ultrasound categories	Score
Composition (Choose 1)	
• Cystic or almost completely cystic	0
• Spongiform	0
• Mixed cystic and solid	1
• Solid or completely solid	2
• Cannot be determined due to calcification	2
Echogenicity (Choose 1)	
• Anechoic	0
• Hyper or isoechoic	1
• Hypoechoic (compared to parenchyma)	2
• Very hypoechoic (compared to strap muscles)	3
• Cannot be determined	1
Shape (Choose 1)	
• Wider than tall	0
• Taller than wide	3
Margin (Choose 1)	
• Smooth	0
• Ill-defined	0
• Lobulated or irregular	2
• Extrathyroidal extension	3
• Cannot be determined	0
Echogenic FOCI (Choose 1)	
• None or large comet tail artifact (>1 mm)	0
• Macrocalcification	1
• Peripheral (rim) calcification	2
• Punctate echogenic foci (<1 mm)	3

The ACR-TIRADS white paper of 2017 is a stratified scoring system rather than relying on a pattern-based system. **Table 10** gives the ACR-TIRADS scoring and classification of nodules based on the TIRADS lexicon and recommendation for FNA or follow-up ultrasound based on a nodule's ACR-TIRADS level and its maximum diameter.[55]

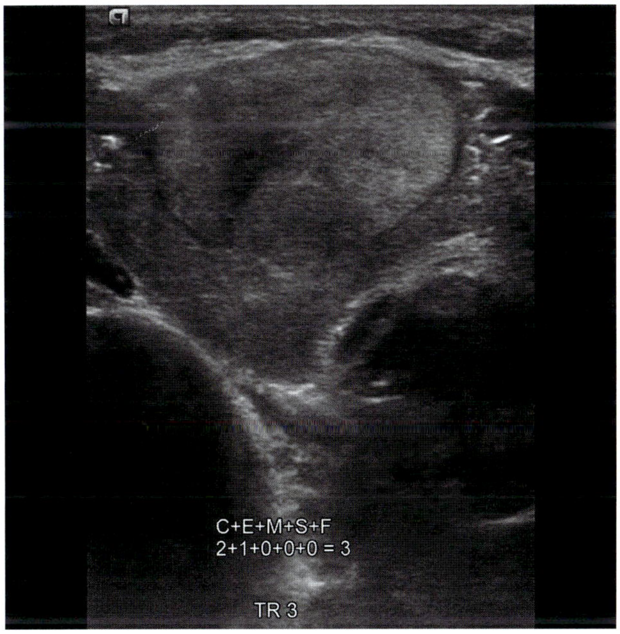

FIG. 26: A well-defined solid (Score 2), isoechoic nodule (Score 1) with smooth margins (Score 0), wider than tall (Score 0) with no echogenic foci within (Score 0) seen in the left lobe of thyroid: TR3 nodule.

TABLE 10: TIRADS scoring and classification.

Scoring	Tirads	Recommendations for FNA	Follow-up ultrasound
0 points	TR 1	Benign, No FNA	—
2 points	TR 2	Not suspicious, No FNA	—
3 points	TR 3	Mildly suspicious FNA if ≥2.5 cm, Follow-up if ≥1.5cm	At 1,3, 5 years
4–6 points	TR 4	Moderately suspicious FNA if ≥1.5 cm, Follow-up if ≥1.0 cm	At 1, 2, 3 and 5 years
>7 points	TR 5	Highly suspicious FNA if ≥1.0 cm Follow-up if ≥0.5 cm	Every year up to 5 years

- ACR-TIRADS recommends FNAC of suspicious lesions (TR 3 – TR 5) with the above size criteria.
- If there are multiple nodules, two of the highest ACR-TIRADS grades should be sampled rather than the two largest.
- Internal enlargement of a nodule on follow-up is considered significant if there is an increase of 20% and 2 mm in two nodules, or a 50% increase in volume.
- Imaging can stop at 5 years if there is no change in size of the nodule

REFERENCES

1. Senchenkov A, Staren ED. Ultrasound in head and neck surgery: Thyroid, parathyroid and cervical lymph nodes. Surg Clin N Am. 2004;84:973-1000.
2. Pawa S, Chowdhury V. Thyroid and parathyroid imaging. In: Berry, Chowdhury, Suri (Eds). Diagnostic Radiology - Advances in Imaging Technology (1st edition); Jaypee; 2000.
3. Zander DA, Smoker RK. Imaging of ectopic thyroid tissue and thyroglossal duct cyst. Radiographics. 2014;34:37-50.
4. Kabala JE. Computed tomography and magnetic resonance imaging in diseases of the thyroid and parathyroid. European Journal of Radiology. 2008;66:480-92.
5. Loevner LA. Thyroid and parathyroid glands: Anatomy and pathology. In: Som PM, Curtin HD (Eds). Head and Neck Imaging (4th edn) Vol 2 Mosby; 2003.
6. Solbiati L, Charboneiu JW, Cantisani V, et al. The Thyroid Gland. In: Rumack CM, Levine D (Eds). Diagnostic Ultrasound. 5th Edition, Volume 1, Elsevier 2013; pp. 691-731.
7. Villadolid MC, Yokoyama N, Izumi M, et al. Untreated Graves' disease patients without clinical ophthalmology demonstrate a high frequency of extraocular muscle (EOM) enlargement by magnetic resonance. J Clin Endocrinal Metab. 1995;80(9):2830-33.
8. Loevner LA. Anatomy and Pathalogy of the Thyroid and Parathyroid glands. In: Som PM, Curtin HD (Eds). Head and Neck Imaging, Volume 1. 5th Edition, Mosby Elsevier 2012, 2611-77.
9. Yousem DM. Parathyroid and thyroid imaging. Neuroimaging Clinics of North America. 1996;6(2):435-59.
10. Feine U, Leitzenmayer R, Hanke J, et al. Fluore 18 - FDG and I131 uptake in thyroid cancer. J Nucl Med. 1996;37:1468-72.
11. Wang W, Larson SM, Fazzari M, et al. Prognostic value of 18F fluorodeoxyglucose positron emission tomographic scanning in patients with thyroid cancer. J Clin Endocrinol Metab. 2000;85:1107-13.
12. Bruneton JN, Livraghi T, Viateau-Poncin J. Thyroid gland. In: Bruneton JN (Ed). Applications of Sonography in Hand and Neck Pathology. Berlin Springer-Verlag. 2002; pp. 1-66.
13. Solbiati L, Charboneau JW, Osti V, et al. The thyroid gland 735-770 Vol I Part IV. In: Rumack CM, Wilson SR, Charboneau JW (Eds). Diagnostic Ultrasound, 3rd edition. Elsevier; 2005.
14. Hopkins CR, Reading CC. Thyroid and parathyroid imaging. Seminars in US, CT and MRI. 1995;16:279-95.
15. Loevner LA. Imaging of the thyroid gland. Seminars in US, CT and MRI. 1996;17:539-62.
16. Moon HJ, Sung JM, Kim EK, et al. Diagnostic performance of gray-scale US and elastography in solid thyroid nodules. Radiology. 2012;262(3):1002-13.
17. Gotway MB, Higgins CB. MR imaging of the thyroid and parathyroid glands. Magn Reson Imaging. 2000;8(1):163-82.
18. Vogi Thomas, Bisdas Sotirios. Cervical Adenopathy and Neck Masses in CT and MRI of the Whole Body: Haaga John R, Dogra Vikram S, Forsting Michael et al (Eds), Fifth Edition Vol I, Mosby Elseiver: 2009; pp. 639-69.
19. Dooms GC, Hricak, Moseley ME, et al. Characterisation of lymphadenopathy by magnetic resonance relaxation times: Preliminary result. Radiology. 1985;691-97.
20. Auffermann W, Clark OH, Thurnher S, et al. Recurrent thyroid carcinoma. Characteristics on MR images. Radiology. 1988;168:753-7.
21. Yousem DM, Scheff AM. Thyroid and parathyroid gland pathology: Role of imaging. Otolaryn Clin N Am. 1995;28(3): 621-49.
22. Larson TC, Smith MM, Chong WK, Martin WH. Thyroid and parathyroid glands in CT and MR imaging of the whole body. In: Haaga JR, Lanzieri CF, Gilkeson RC (Eds). 4th edition Vol I, Mosby. 2003; pp. 663-90.
23. Castagnone D, Rivolta B, Rescalli S, et al. Colour Doppler sonography in Graves' disease: Value in assessing activity of disease and predicting outcome. AJR 1996;66:203-07.
24. Yeh HC, Futterweit W, Gilbert P. Micronodulation: Ultrasonographic sign of Hashimoto's thyroiditis. J Ultrasound Med. 1996;15:813-9.
25. Kawanaka M, Sugimoto Y, Suehiro M, et al. Thyroid imaging in a typical case of acute suppurative thyroiditis with abscess formation due to infection from a persistent thyroglossal duct. Ann Nucl Med. 1994;8(2):159-62.
26. Fontan JP, Carballido FC, Felipe FP, et al. Case report. Riedel's thyroiditis: US, CT and MR evaluation. J Comput Assist Tomogr. 1993;17:324-5.
27. Gharib H. Changing concepts in the diagnosis and management of thyroid nodules. Endocrinol Metab Clin North Am. 1997;26: 777-800.
28. Won-Jin Moon, So Lyung Jung, Jeong Hyun Lee, et al. Benign and Malignant Thyroid Nodules: US Differentiation – multicentre retrospective study. Rad. 2008;247(3):763-70.
29. Gritzmann N, Koischwitz D, Rettenbacher T. Sonography of the thyroid and parathyroid glands. RCNA. 2000;38(5):1131-45.
30. Saeedan MB, Aljohani IM, Elnaas ST. Thyroid Computed tomography imaging: Pictorial review of variable pathologies. Insights imaging. 2016;7(4):601-17.
31. Hoang JK, Branstetter IV, Glastonbury CM. Imaging of thyroid carcinoma with CT and MRI. Cancer Imaging. 2013;13(1): 128-39.
32. Reading CC, Charboneau JW, Hay ID et al. Sonography of Thyroid Nodules: a "classic pattern" diagnostic approach. Ultrasound Q. 2005;21:157-65.
33. Hatabu H, Kasagi K, Yamamoto K, IIda Y, et al. Cystic papillary carcinoma of the thyroid gland. Clin Rad. 1991; 43:121-24.
34. Som PM, Brandwein M, Lidov M, et al. The varied appearance of papillary carcinoma cervical nodal disease: CT and MR findings. AJNR. 1994;15:1129-38.
35. Wunderbaldinger P, Harisinghani MG, Hahu PF, et al. Cystic lymph node metastases in papillary thyroid carcinoma. AJR. 2002;178:693-7.
36. Kim Dae Sik, Kim Ji-hoon, Na Dong Gyu, et al. Sonographic features of follicular variant papillary thyroid carcinomas in comparison with conventional papillary thyroid carcinoma. J Ultrasound Med. 2009;28:1685-92.
37. Miyakawa M, Onoda N, Etoh M et al. Diagnosis of thyroid follicular carcinoma by the vascular pattern and velocimetric parameters using high resolution pulsed and power Doppler ultrasonography. Endocrine Journal. 2005;52(2):207-12.
38. Maizhin ZV, Wiseman SM, Vora P, et al. Hurthle cell neoplasms of the thyroid: sonographic appearance and Histologic characteristics. J Ultrasound Med. 2008;27: 751-7.
39. Takashima S, Morimoto S, Ikezoe J, et al. CT evaluation of anaplastic thyroid carcinoma. AJR. 1990;154:1079-85.
40. Takashima S, Ikezoe J, Morimoto S, et al. Primary thyroid lymphoma: evaluation with CT. Radiology. 1988;168:765-8.
41. Shibata T, Noma S, Nakano Y, Konishi J. Primary thyroid lymphoma: MR appearance. J Comput Assist Tomogr. 1991;15:629-33.
42. Nakahara H, Noguchi S, Murakami N, et al. Gadolinium enhanced MR imaging of thyroid and parathyroid masses. Radiology 1997;202:765-72.
43. Ohnishi T, Noguchi S, Murakami N, et al. MR imaging in patients with primary thyroid lymphoma. Am J Neuroradiol. 1992;13(4):1196-98.
44. Eftekhari F, Peuchot M. Thyroid metastases: Combined role of ultrasonography and fine needle aspiration biopsy. J Clin Ultrasound. 1989;17:657-62.

45. Perrier ND, Brierley JD, Tuttle RM. Differentiated and anaplastic thyroid carcinoma: major changes in the American Joint Committee on Cancer Eighth edition Cancer staging manual. CA Cancer J Clin. 2017;0(0)1-8.
46. Hoang JK, Sosa JA, Nguyen XV, Galvin PL, Oldan JD. Imaging Thyroid disease: Updates, Imaging approach, and management pearls. Radiol Clin N AM. 2015;53:145-61.
47. Zhan J, Diao XH, Chai QL, et al. Comparative study of acoustic radiation force impulse imaging with real-time elastography in differential diagnosis of thyroid nodules. Ultrasound Med Biol. 2013;39(12):2217-25.
48. Liu, BJ, Li DD, Xu Hx, et al. Quantitative shear wave velocity measurement on acoustic radiation force impulse elastography for differential diagnosis between benign and malignant thyroid nodules: a meta analysis. Ultrasound Med Biol. 2015;41(12): 3035-42.
49. Zhang B, Jiang YX, Lin J B et al. Utility of contrast enhanced ultrasound for evaluation of thyroid nodules. Thyroid. 2010; 20(1):51-7.
50. Abdek Razek AAK, Sadak AG, Kombar OR, et al. Role of apparent diffusion coefficient values in differentiation between malignant and benign solitary thyroid nodules. AJNR. 2008;29:563-8.
51. Hoang JK, Langer JE, Middleton WD et al. Managing Incidental Thyroid Nodules Detected on Imaging: White paper of the ACR Incidental Thyroids Committee. J Am Col Radiol. 2015;12: 143-50.
52. Haugen BR, Alexender EK, Bible KC, et al. 2015 American Thyroid Association Management Guidelines for Adult Patients with Thyroid Nodules and Differentiated Thyroid Cancer: The American Thyroid Association Guidelines Task Force on Thyroid Nodules and Differentiated Thyroid Cancer. Thyroid. 2016;26(1):1-133.
53. Bahn Rebecca S, Castro Regina M. Approach to the patient with nontoxic multinodular goitre. J Clin Endocrinol Metab. 2011;96(5):1202-12.
54. Grant EG, Tessler FN, Hoang JK et al. Thyroid Ultrasound Reporting Lexicon: White Paper of the ACR Thyroid Imaging, Reporting and Data System (TIRADS) Committee. J Am Coll Radiol. 2015;12(12 Pt A):1272-9.
55. Tessler FN, Middleton WD, Grant EC, et al. ACR Thyroid Imaging, Reporting and Data System (TI-RADS): White Paper of the ACR TI-RADS Committee. J Am Coll Radiol 2017;14(5): 587-95.

CHAPTER

205

Malignancies of Upper Aerodigestive Tract

Mukesh Kumar Yadav, Ankur Goyal, Ashu Seith Bhalla, Sanjay Sharma

Malignancies of the upper aerodigestive tract (UADT) include a wide range of tumor locations and histology. Majority (~90%) are squamous cell carcinoma (SCCA) or its variants like lymphoepithelioma (carcinoma with lymphoid stroma), spindle cell carcinoma, verrucous carcinoma (low grade) and undifferentiated carcinoma (high grade).[1] Other malignancies include lymphoma, sarcoma and tumors of minor salivary glands. Risk factors for the development of SCCA of the head and neck include tobacco and alcohol use, human papillomavirus or Epstein-Barr virus infection, immunosuppression by HIV infection or transplantation, poor oral hygiene and radiation exposure. The mucosa of oral cavity is derived from ectoderm and tends to be involved by well-differentiated SCCA while the mucosa of pharynx is derived from endoderm and tends to be affected by aggressive SCCA. With declining tobacco use, there has been a steady decline in the incidence of malignancies of the UADT; however, the incidence of human papilloma virus (HPV) associated SCCA of the oropharynx has been rising. In certain cancer registries of the country, oral cancer has surpassed lung cancer to become the commonest malignancy in males.

Computed tomography (CT) and magnetic resonance imaging (MRI) are the primary imaging modalities in head and neck cancers. Most head and neck cancers are diagnosed clinically and primary role of imaging is to define the stage of malignancy. The most recent guidelines for TNM (Tumor, Node, Metastasis) staging are included in the eighth edition of the American Joint Committee on Cancer (AJCC) Staging Manual, published in 2017.[2,3] The indications of imaging are listed in **Table 1**. The commonly used cross-sectional imaging examination is CT/MRI from the skull base to aortopulmonary window; however, for metastatic work-up in advanced disease, whole body positron emission tomography (PET) is employed. Treatment decisions are mainly based on imaging findings. For accurate interpretation of the imaging, the radiologists should be familiar with locoregional anatomy, spread pattern and clinical behavior of the tumors, various treatment modalities and post-treatment imaging appearances. Imaging modalities like ultrasound and CT also enable radiology-guided interventions, especially in sampling of equivocal lesions.

TABLE 1: Role of imaging in head and neck malignancies.
• Staging of the lesion (local extent, nodal status and detection of metastases)—most common indication
• Identifying the lesion in case of clinically occult primary
• Detecting synchronous lesions
• Documenting the local extent of the lesion
• Image-guided interventions (sampling)
• Assessment of response to chemotherapy and radiotherapy
• Follow-up and surveillance of patients

Malignancies of the upper aerodigestive tract shall be discussed under the following headings:

- Oral cavity
- Nasopharynx
- Oropharynx
- Hypopharynx
- Larynx
- Cervical lymph nodes
- Miscellaneous neoplasms
- Post-treatment imaging

ORAL CAVITY

Oral cavity is separated from oropharynx by soft palate, anterior tonsillar pillars and the circumvallate papilla of the tongue. SSCA of oral cavity cancers is more common in males than in females. Very High incidence is observed in India.[4] This is mainly attributed to tobacco and betel chewing. Oral cavity cancer is the most common cancer in males in Ahmedabad and Bhopal. In west, lip is the most common site of oral cancer; followed by oral tongue, floor of mouth, lower alveolus-gingiva, upper alveolus-hard palate and buccal mucosa in that order.[5] In India, gingiva-alveolar, buccal mucosa and tongue cancers are more common. Following are the different sites in oral cavity where malignancy can arise:

- Floor of mouth
- Tongue (excluding the base)

- Lip
- Gingivo-alveolus
- Buccal mucosa
- Hard palate
- Retromolar trigone

Floor of Mouth

Floor of mouth is a space bounded superiorly by under surface of the tongue, laterally by inner mandibular gingiva on both sides and inferiorly by mylohyoid muscles. Paired genioglossus-geniohyoid muscle complex, separated by lingual septum, are located in the central part of floor of mouth and these form the imaging landmark of floor of mouth on axial images **(Figs. 1A and B)**. Hyoglossus muscle can be seen in posterolateral part of floor of mouth where it lies medial and parallel to the mylohyoid. Lingual artery and the hypoglossal nerve are located in the fat medial to hyoglossus muscle. Other contents of floor of mouth include submandibular ducts, sublingual glands and lymph nodes. The space inferior to the mylohyoid muscle is outside the floor of mouth and it is called submandibular space.

Squamous cell carcinoma (SCCA) of floor of mouth commonly arise within 2 cm of anterior midline. With local spread, medially it may involve geniohyoid and genioglossus muscle complex, laterally it involves mylohyoid muscle and subsequently the gingiva and mandible **(Figs. 1A and B)**. Submucosal spread may involve lingual neurovascular bundle, sublingual gland and tongue base. Involvement and obstruction of the submandibular duct leads to enlargement of the ipsilateral submandibular gland.

Oral Tongue

Oral tongue is a muscular structure and consists of two halves which are separated by a midline septum. Intrinsic tongue muscles arranged in various planes and these are not identified separately on imaging. Extrinsic muscles anchor the tongue to floor of mouth and these are named as per their origin and insertion sites. These include genioglossus-geniohyoid muscles near anterior lingual septum and hyoglossus-styloglossus muscles in posterolateral part. SCCA of oral tongue usually arise in middle and posterior third of the tongue at lateral margin or under surface of the tongue **(Figs. 2A and B)**. Early tumors remain localized to the intrinsic muscle of the tongue unilaterally. With local spread, it involves the midline lingual septum and extends across it. Large tumors involve extrinsic muscle of the tongue and floor of mouth. Tumors of posterior part of oral tongue may extend into base of tongue, anterior tonsillar pillar or mandible. On imaging it should be determined if the tumor has crossed the midline lingual septum, extended anywhere outside intrinsic tongue muscles and whether mandible is eroded **(Figs. 3A to D)**. Tongue is richly supplied with lymphatics and large number of patients already have lymph node metastases at the time of initial presentation.[1]

Lip

The lip consists of orbicularis oris muscle. It is covered with thin layer of squamous epithelium. The inside lining of the lip is buccal mucosa. Dry lip is the transition between skin and buccal mucosa. SSCA of the lip most commonly arise at vermilion border of the lip and invade underlying musculature. Subsequently, it may involve buccal mucosa, gingiva and the maxilla or mandible **(Figs. 4A to C)**.

Gingivo-alveolus

Gingiva is the mucosal lining of the alveolar processes of mandible and maxilla. Laterally the gingiva is continuous with buccal mucosa. Medially, the upper gingiva is continuous with mucosa of hard palate while the lower gingiva is continuous with floor of mouth. Tumors arising from gingiva have different patterns of spread depending on whether it is arising from lower or upper gingiva. Lower gingival tumors involve and erode alveolar process of mandible. Lateral spread leads to involvement of the buccal mucosa while with medial or inner aspect spread, these involve floor of mouth. Upper gingival tumors involve

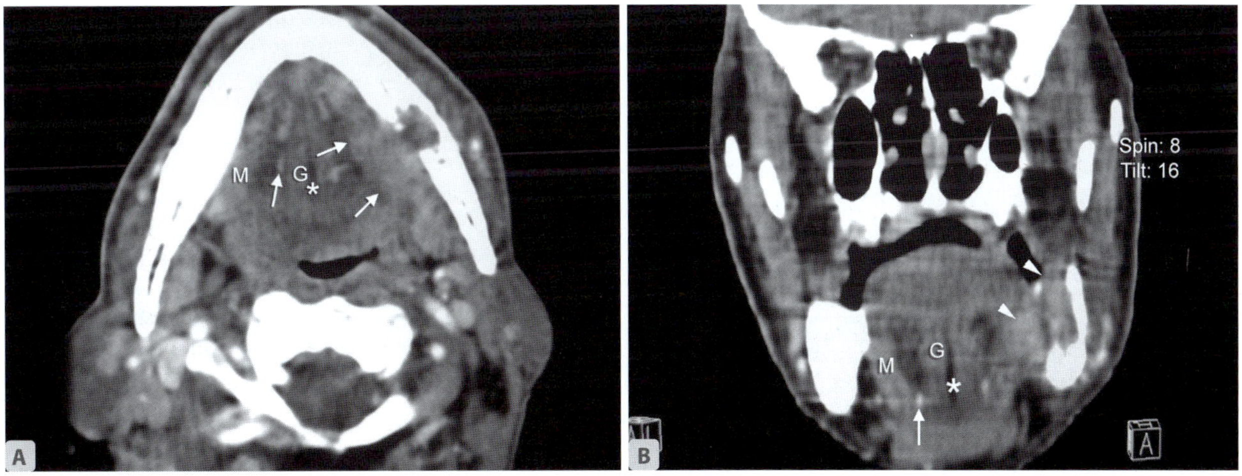

FIGS. 1A AND B: Carcinoma of floor of mouth: Axial (A) and coronal (B) CT show large mass in left floor of mouth (arrowheads) involving mylohyoid and inner cortex of mandible. It is not involving the lingual neurovascular bundle. Normal lingual septum (asterisk), contralateral genioglossus geniohyoid muscle (G), neurovascular bundle surrounded by fat (arrow), and mylohyoid muscles (M).

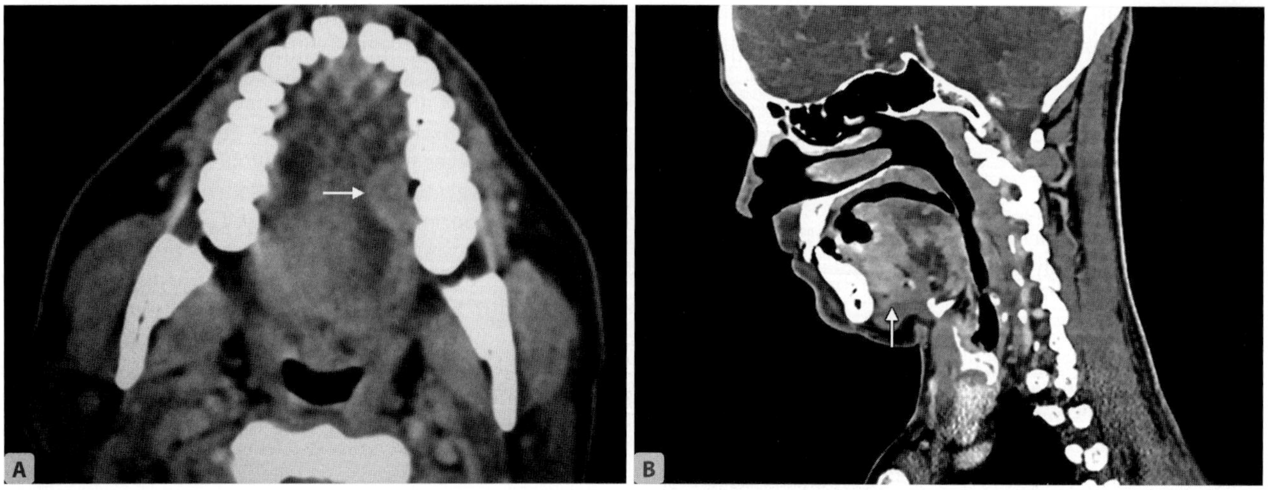

FIGS. 2A AND B: (A) Carcinoma of tongue: CT shows small mass (arrow) located at the left lateral margin of oral tongue; (B) CECT coronal reformatted images showing enhancing mass involving right lateral border in anterior half of the tongue. It is infiltrating the floor of mouth.

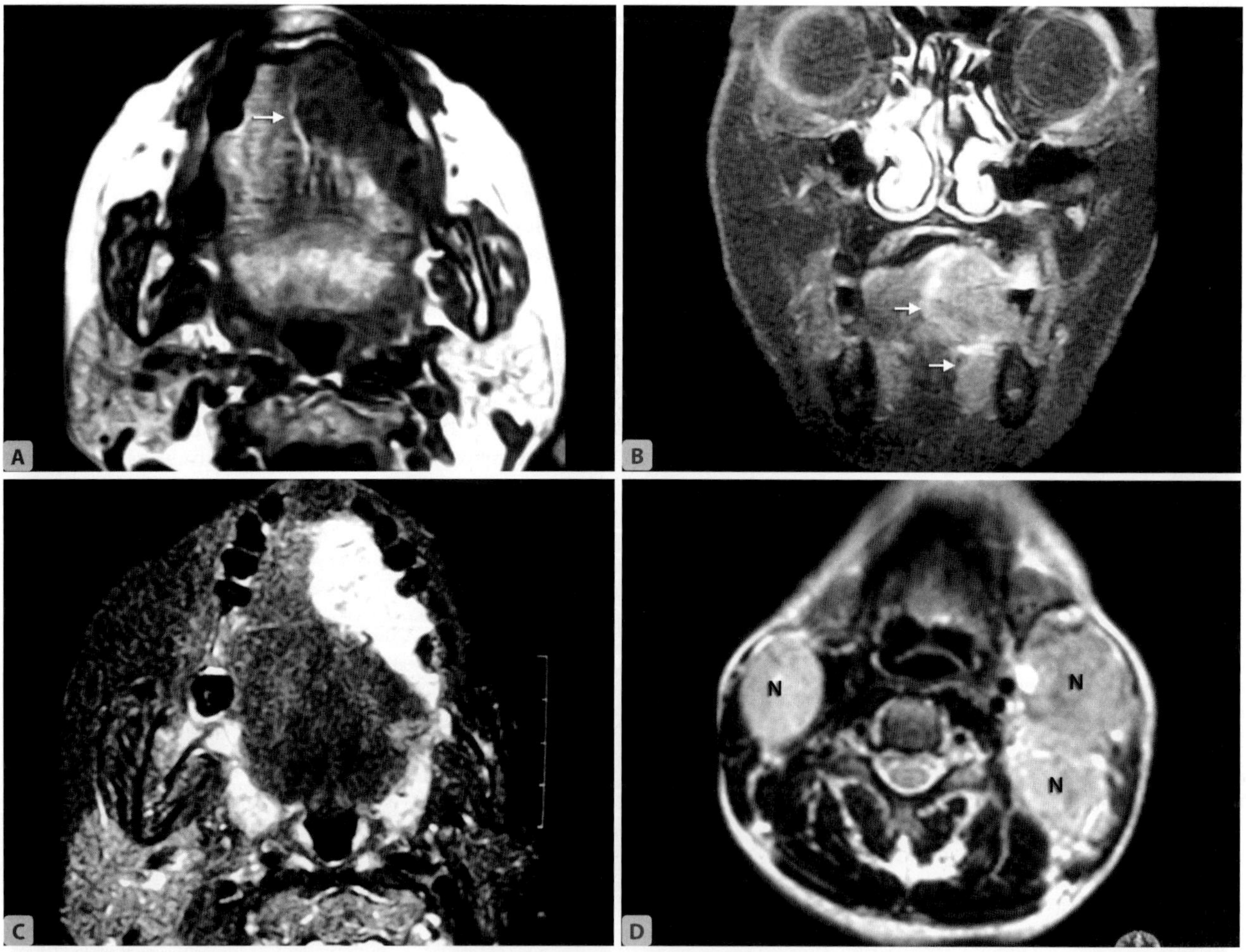

FIGS. 3A TO D: Carcinoma of tongue: MRI shows large mass in left half of oral tongue on T1-weighted (A) and fat suppressed T2-weighted (B) axial images. It abutting and displacing the midline lingual septum (arrows). Fat suppressed contrast-enhanced T1-weighted coronal image (C) shows invasion of lingual septum and extension into floor of mouth. T2-weighted axial image at more caudal level (D) shows multiple bilateral enlarged cervical lymph nodes (N).

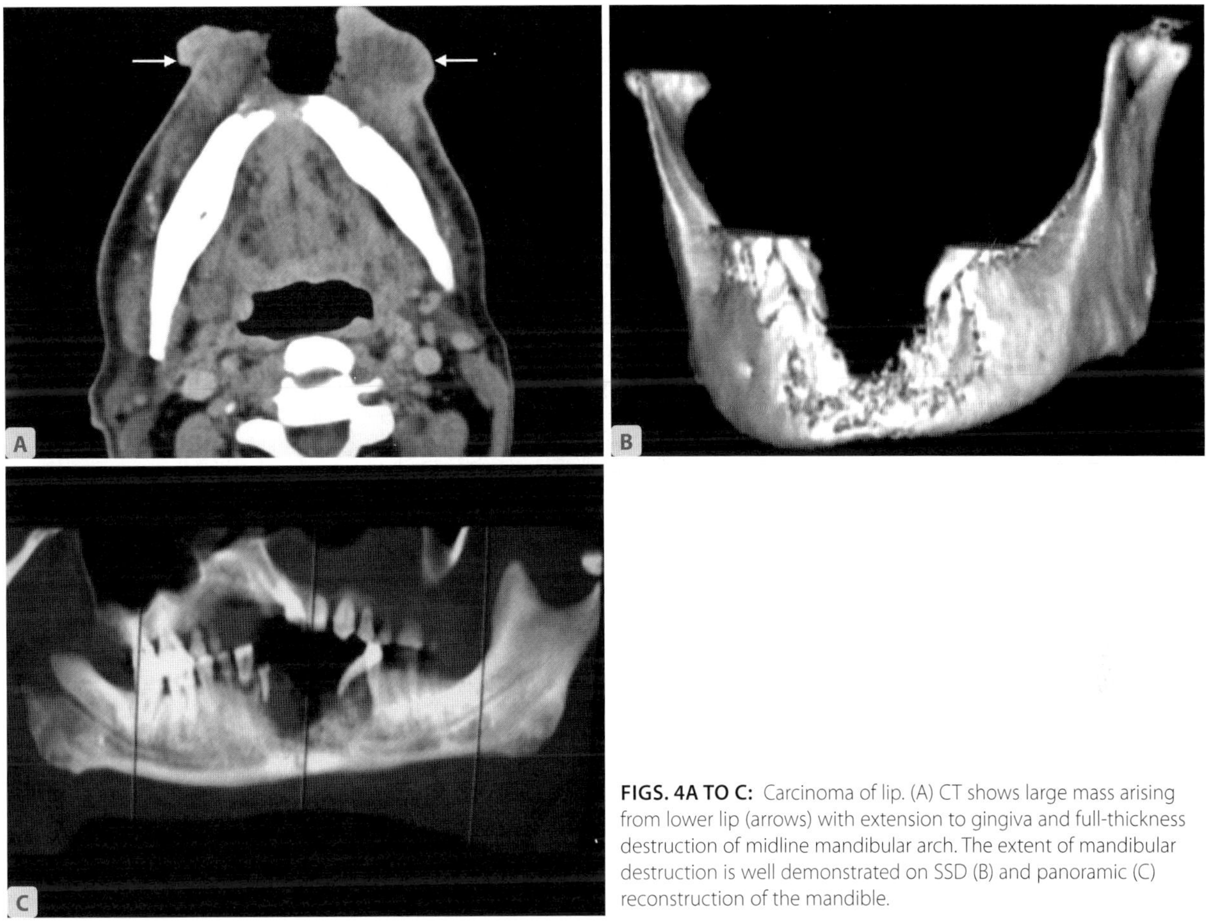

FIGS. 4A TO C: Carcinoma of lip. (A) CT shows large mass arising from lower lip (arrows) with extension to gingiva and full-thickness destruction of midline mandibular arch. The extent of mandibular destruction is well demonstrated on SSD (B) and panoramic (C) reconstruction of the mandible.

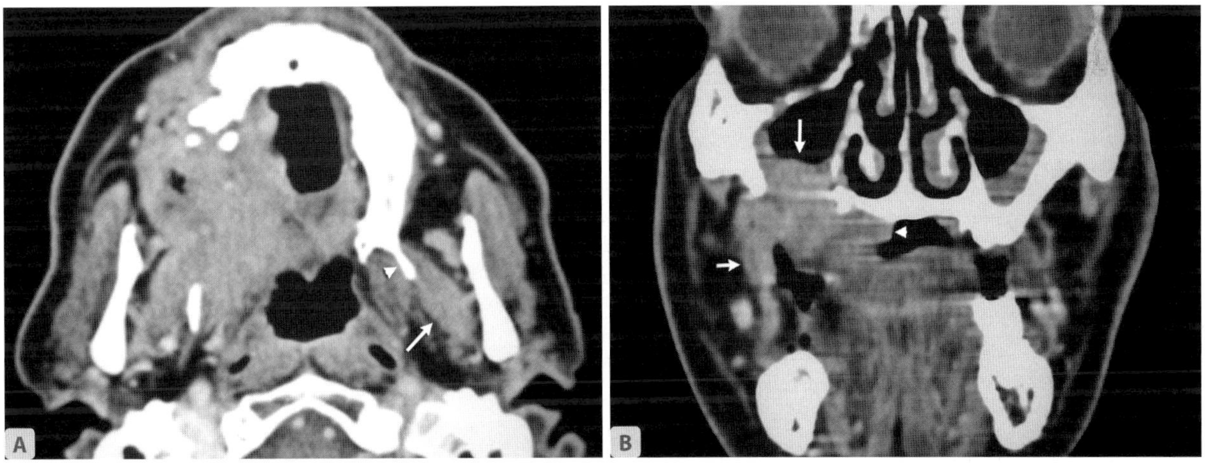

FIGS. 5A AND B: Carcinoma of upper alveolus: (A) CT shows large tumor arising from and destroying right upper alveolus with extension to masticator space. There is destruction of lateral pterygoid plate and invasion and enlargement of lateral pterygoid muscle which can be appreciated if compared with normal contralateral pterygoid plate (arrowhead) and lateral pterygoid muscle (arrow); (B) Coronal image shows extension of tumor to buccal mucosa with thickening of buccinators muscle (small arrow), hard palate (arrowhead) and destruction of floor of the maxillary sinus (large arrow).

mucosa of the hard palate on medial aspect and buccal mucosa on lateral aspect. With further spread, upper gingival tumors involve maxillary alveolar process, hard palate and floors of the maxillary sinus and the nasal cavity **(Figs. 5A and B)**. Coronal images are valuable to assess these areas. Bone involvement makes oral cavity cancer T4 tumor, however, early erosion of tooth socket by a gingival cancer is an exception. With posterior spread, gingivoalveolar tumors involve retromolar trigone and then extend to the masticator space.[6]

Buccal Mucosa

Buccal mucosa is the lining of cheek, inner surface of lips and it is continuous with gingiva via upper and lower gingiva-buccal sulci. Most cancers arise on lateral or buccal surface of the buccal mucosa on the background of leukoplakia. Small tumors are difficult to visualize on imaging. Large tumors are diffuse or ulceroinfiltrative and there spread pattern is similar to gingiva-alveolar tumors **(Fig. 6)**.

Hard Palate

Primary SCCA of hard palate are rare and most are extensions from upper gingival tumors. Primary tumors of hard palate are usually adenocarcinoma of minor salivary gland. These tumors have propensity for early bone erosion and perineural extension along greater and lesser palatine nerves to pterygopalatine fossa, foramen rotundum and the cavernous sinus.[7]

Retromolar Trigone

Retromolar trigone (RMT) is a small triangular areas posterior to the last molar. Primary SCCA of RMT rare and most are extensions of buccal mucosa or gingival tumors. RMT is important because of its strategic location. The pterygomandibular raphe is a band of connective tissue that lies beneath the mucosa of RMT. It extends from hamulus of medial pterygoid plate superiorly to the posterior aspect mylohyoid groove on mandible inferiorly. Pterygomandibular raphe forms a junction of oral cavity, oropharynx and infratemporal fossa. Hence, once the tumor reaches RMT, it gets access to various critical areas. With posterior extension, the tumors enter infratemporal fossa and involve medial or lateral pterygoid muscles. Medially, the tumor may spread to tonsils via superior constrictor muscles **(Fig. 6)**. Superior tumor spread along the pterygomandibular raphe involves skull base and nasopharynx, while inferior spread occurs to the floor of mouth. Mandibular cortex is in close proximity of the mucosa of RMT and hence it is eroded early in cases with tumor at RMT. Inferior alveolar nerve also lies here and can get involved resulting in perineural tumor spread.

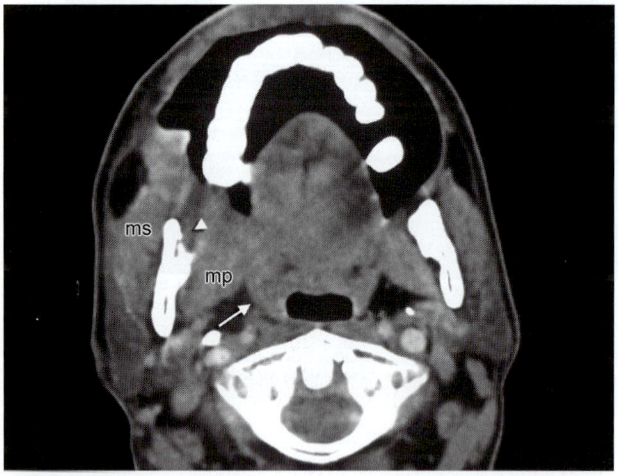

FIG. 6: Carcinoma of buccal mucosa: CT with puffed-cheek maneuver shows polypoid mass in right buccal mucosa. It is extending into right retromolar trigone with erosion of ramus the mandible (arrowhead). There contiguous invasion of pharyngeal wall (arrow), medial pterygoid (mp) and masseter (ms) muscles.

Staging of Oral Cavity Cancers

Staging of oral cavity cancers is based on TNM system of AJCC **(Table 2)**. In the eighth edition, T-stage takes into account the depth of invasion in addition to the size.[2,3] It may be noted that the depth of invasion is different from the tumor thickness since the former does not include the exophytic component, rather assesses only the deep invasion. N stage depends on site and size of the lymph nodes. Another point that has been added in the recent N-staging system is the extranodal spread. Most of the studies on extranodal extension (ENE) of the disease are based on pathological evaluation and imaging (both CT and MRI) are not very reliable. Thus, clinically overt ENE refers to unambiguous cases there is involvement of overlying dermis, invasion of adjacent soft tissues, tethering to adjacent structures or clinical evidence of nerve involvement.[3] Imaging may suggest ENE based on the presence of ill-defined nodal margins and irregularity of the capsule of the node.

TABLE 2: Staging of oral cavity cancers: Overview.

T1	Tumor ≤2 cm and ≤5 mm depth of invasion (DOI)
T2	Tumor ≤2 cm and DOI 5–10 mm OR Tumor 2–4 cm and DOI ≤5 mm
T3	Tumor >4 cm or DOI >10 mm
T4	Advanced local disease
	Moderately advanced: T4a: Invasion of bone, maxillary sinus, extrinsic tongue muscles, skin osf the face OR lip tumor involving inferior alveolar nerve, floor of mouth OR tumor with bilateral tongue involvement and/or DOI >20 mm *Note*: Superficial bone erosion in tooth socket by gingival primary is not T4
	Very advanced: T4b: invasion of masticator space, pterygoid plates, skull base or internal carotid artery (ICA) encasement
N1	Metastasis to single Ipsilateral lymph node (LN) up to 3 cm in greatest dimension, No extranodal extension (ENE)
N2	Sigle/Multiple lymph nodes up to 6 cm
	N2a: Ipsilateral single LN 3–6 cm, No ENE
	N2b: Ipsilateral multiple LNs up to 6 cm, No ENE
	N2c: Contralateral or B/L LNs up to 6 cm, No ENE
N3	*N3a*: Lymph node >6 cm, No ENE
	N3b: Any sized LN with clinically overt ENE present
M0	No distant metastases
M1	Distant metastases
Stage 1	T1, N0
Stage 2	T2, N0
Stage 3	Up to T3 or N1
Stage 4	T4, N2, N3 and M1

Eighth edition of AJCC includes both the pathological/surgical staging as well as clinical stage (based on clinical examination, endoscopy, biopsy and imaging).

Imaging Modalities

CT and MRI are the primary imaging modalities. The role of the imaging in oral cavity cancers is not for the diagnosis but to evaluate extent of the tumor and lymph node involvement. Mere demonstration of the tumor on CT or MRI should not lead to satisfaction and possible overlooking of the important positive and negative imaging findings. Both CT and MRI perform similar in evaluation of most oral cavity cancers. MRI is better for assessment of soft tissue extension of the tumor, however, CT is more accurate for assessment of the bone erosions and lymph node involvement.[8] MRI takes much longer time than CT. Sometimes, this may be problematic, especially in patients with large oral cavity tumors as there is constant pooling and swallowing of the saliva. This degrades the MRI quality.[9] MRI must be performed with contrast enhancement. However, a non-contrast, non-fat suppressed axial sequence is essential to evaluate tumor margins and bone invasion. MRI is a preferred modality in cancer of the oral tongue and floor of mouth as small tumors at these locations may not be visualized on CT. Demonstration and extent evaluation of these tumors better on MRI.[10] MRI is also useful when any oral cavity tumor is extending into the RMT and invasion of other structures, such as pterygoid muscles, is equivocal on CT.[9,11]

SCCA of oral cavity do not enhance significantly when compared with adjacent soft tissues. Hence, small tumors may not be visualized. *Puffed-cheek maneuver* during CT help to identify small tumors which may be seen as asymmetric mucosal thickening, ulceration or the mass **(Fig. 6)**. It also separates buccal mucosa and gingiva and hence, helps to locate the tumor to gingival or buccal side, identify the involvement of upper or lower GB sulcus and submucosal tumor extension beyond it. Bone erosions upstage the oral cavity cancers to T4. These require extensive surgery and mandibular or maxillary resection. Type and extent of the bone resection is also determined by imaging findings. CT images reconstructed with sharp kernel and viewed on bone window are essential to detect and define the extent of bone erosions in oral cavity cancers. 3D reconstruction, MPRs and dental CT software with panoramic and real size zoom CT images provide important information to facilitate surgical decisions **(*see* Figs. 4B and C)**. Coronal images are useful to evaluate hard palate and any tumor extension to the maxillary sinus or floor of the nasal cavity **(Fig. 5)** and hence, these must be assessed in any tumor involving upper gingiva or hard palate.[5]

Oral cavity tumors involving RMT require extensive surgery. Invasion of masticator muscles upstage the tumor to T4 and any involvement of pterygoid muscles must be carefully looked for on imaging. Clinically, presence of trismus is highly specific for the masticator space involvement. Although, limited medial pterygoid involvement at its lower insertion can be resected, tumors involving pterygoid plates or lateral pterygoid muscle are unresectable.

In tumors of oral tongue and floor of mouth, involvement of ipsilateral neurovascular bundle, tumor extension across midline lingual septum and its relationship with contralateral neurovascular bundle must be carefully evaluated on imaging. Any deep invasion along mylohyoid muscle, bone involvement or posterior extension into the base of tongue or deep neck spaces must also be determined.

Treatment

Although small oral cavity cancers are amenable to radiotherapy, surgery is the primary treatment modality. Early oral cavity tumors are not detected on CT and clinical assessment determines the extent of wide local excision. Tumors involving bone or RMT require extensive surgery. Tumor abutting the mandible or with small superficial erosion are subjected to marginal resection in which bony continuity is maintained. With deeper or marrow invasion, segmental resection of the mandible and reconstruction with titanium plate is done. Myocutaneous flap or free flap is used to fill the defect.[12] The decision of marginal versus segmental resection as well as extent of the segmental resection of the mandible depends on imaging findings. Tumors involving upper alveolus or the hard palate require partial maxillectomy.

Floor of mouth cancers are treated with wide local excision using combined transoral and cervical approach. Mandibulotomy is required for tumor extending posteriorly in the base of tongue.[5]

Carcinoma of the tongue with small superficial tumor is treated with wide local excision or radical radiotherapy. Large tumors are treated with partial glossectomy (ipsilateral neurovascular bundle involvement) or total glossectomy (lingual septum and contralateral neurovascular bundle involvement). The latter is functionally crippling and concurrent chemoradiotherapy may be consideredas an alternative.[1]

NASOPHARYNX

Nasopharynx is a cuboid midline fibromuscular structure suspended from the skull base. It is bounded superiorly by sphenoid sinus and clivus, laterally by parapharyngeal spaces posteriorly by prevertebral muscles and anteriorly by nasal choanae. Nasopharynx continues inferiorly into the oropharynx. Two recesses can be normally identified on lateral wall of the nasopharynx; the posterosuperior recess is called the fossa of Rosenmuller. Anterior recess is the site for opening of eustachian tube. It enters in nasopharynx through a defect in pharyngobasillar fascia and this defect is a potential channel for spread of nasopharyngeal cancer to parapharyngeal spaces. Beneath the posterior mucosal surface of nasopharynx lie retropharyngeal and prevertebral spaces. Retropharyngeal lymph nodes are located in retropharyngeal space and these are usually the first lymph nodes to be involved in nasopharyngeal carcinoma.

Nasopharyngeal Carcinoma

Nasopharyngeal carcinoma is most common in China and Southeast Asian countries. In India, it as an uncommon tumor with national age averaged rate of less than 1 case per 100,000 per year, however, much higher incidence is found in some parts of North-East India.[4] Nasopharyngeal carcinoma is more common in males. It usually involves middle aged people but children and adolescents are also frequently affected. Pathological majority of nasopharyngeal carcinomas are undifferentiated and highly aggressive tumors and they have strong association with EBV infection. Unlike most other head and neck sites, well differentiated squamous cell carcinoma is rare in nasopharynx.

Most patients with nasopharyngeal carcinoma present with painless upper cervical nodal mass. Nasal obstruction, epistaxis and otitis media are other presenting symptoms. Facial pain is found in patients with nerve involvement and sore throat in those with oropharyngeal spread. Patients with advanced tumors may also have headache, proptosis, trismus, cranial nerve palsies or painful neck movements.[1] Fiberoptic examination shows tumor in roof or lateral wall of nasopharynx, however, early lesions may not be visible.

Most nasopharyngeal carcinomas arise in fossa of Rosenmuller and spread via submucosal route. Invasion of palatal muscles (levator and tensor veli palatine) occurs early. Dysfunction of these muscles affects normal opening mechanism of eustachian tube. The opening may also be directly obstructed by the tumor. Hence, it commonly results into serous otitis media. On imaging, early nasopharyngeal carcinoma may not be demonstrated or seen as nonspecific bulge or obliteration of fossa of Rosenmuller. Others are seen as mildly enhancing mass confined to nasopharynx **(Fig. 7)**. Advanced tumors then extend along all direction. Lateral spread to parapharyngeal space is the most common direction of spread **(Figs. 8 and 9)**. Subsequently, it involves pterygoid muscles. Tumor involvement of these masticator muscles is prone for mandibular nerve involvement and perineural intracranial extension through the foramen ovale. This is the most common route for intracranial extension in nasopharyngeal carcinoma.[13] Tumor spread in posterior direction involves retropharyngeal space and then prevertebral muscles. In advanced cases, vertebral bodies may also be destroyed. Posterolaterally, the tumors may involve carotid artery and posterosuperiorly, the jugular fossa and posterior cranial fossa. With direct superior spread of nasopharyngeal carcinoma, the tumor erodes skull base in the region of sphenoid sinus, clivus and petrous apex **(Fig. 9C)**. Anterior spread of nasopharyngeal carcinoma extends into nasal cavity, maxillary sinus. From the upper part of nasal cavity, the tumor may extend into pterygopalatine fossa and orbit. Once tumor reaches orbital apex, it can easily gain intracranial access to middle cranial fossa via superior orbital fissure.

Nasopharyngeal carcinoma has very high propensity for cervical lymph node involvement. Up to 75% of the patients have nodal metastases, often bilateral, at presentation.[14] Distant metastases are also common than in other head and neck cancers and these usually occur in bone, lung and liver.[15]

Staging of Nasopharyngeal Carcinoma

Eighth edition TNM staging by AJCC is used **(Table 3)**. T1 tumors are confined to oro-nasopharynx and/or nasal cavity.

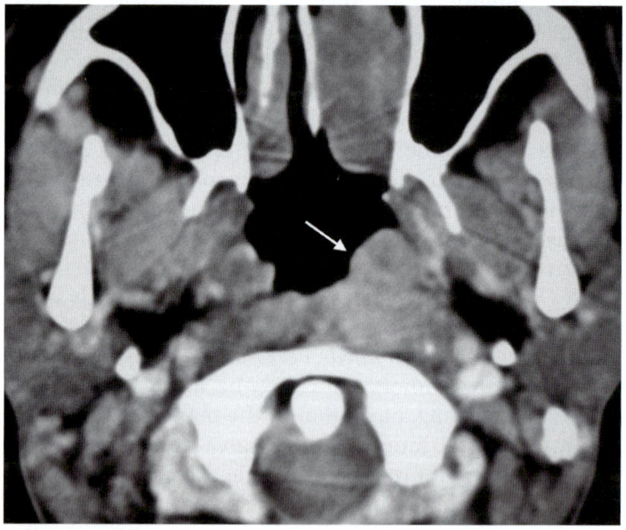

FIG. 7: Carcinoma of nasopharynx: CT shows mildly enhancing mass confined to left posterolateral aspect of nasopharynx.

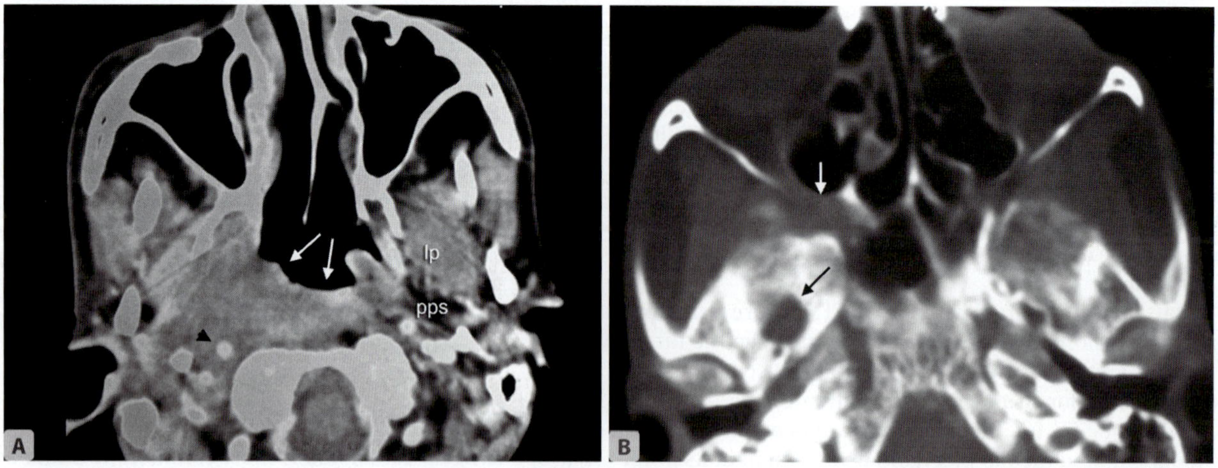

FIGS. 8A AND B: Carcinoma of nasopharynx. (A) CT shows a large nasopharyngeal mass (arrows) extending to retropharyngeal space, obliteration of right parapharyngeal fat space and invasion of right lateral pterygoid muscle. Normal left parapharyngeal space (pps) and lateral pterygoid muscle (lp) are well seen. The tumor is also encasing ipsilateral internal carotid artery (arrowhead); (B) Bone window at the level of skull base shows widening of the right pterygopalatine fossa (white arrow) and foramen ovale (black arrow) suggestive of perineural extension of the tumor.

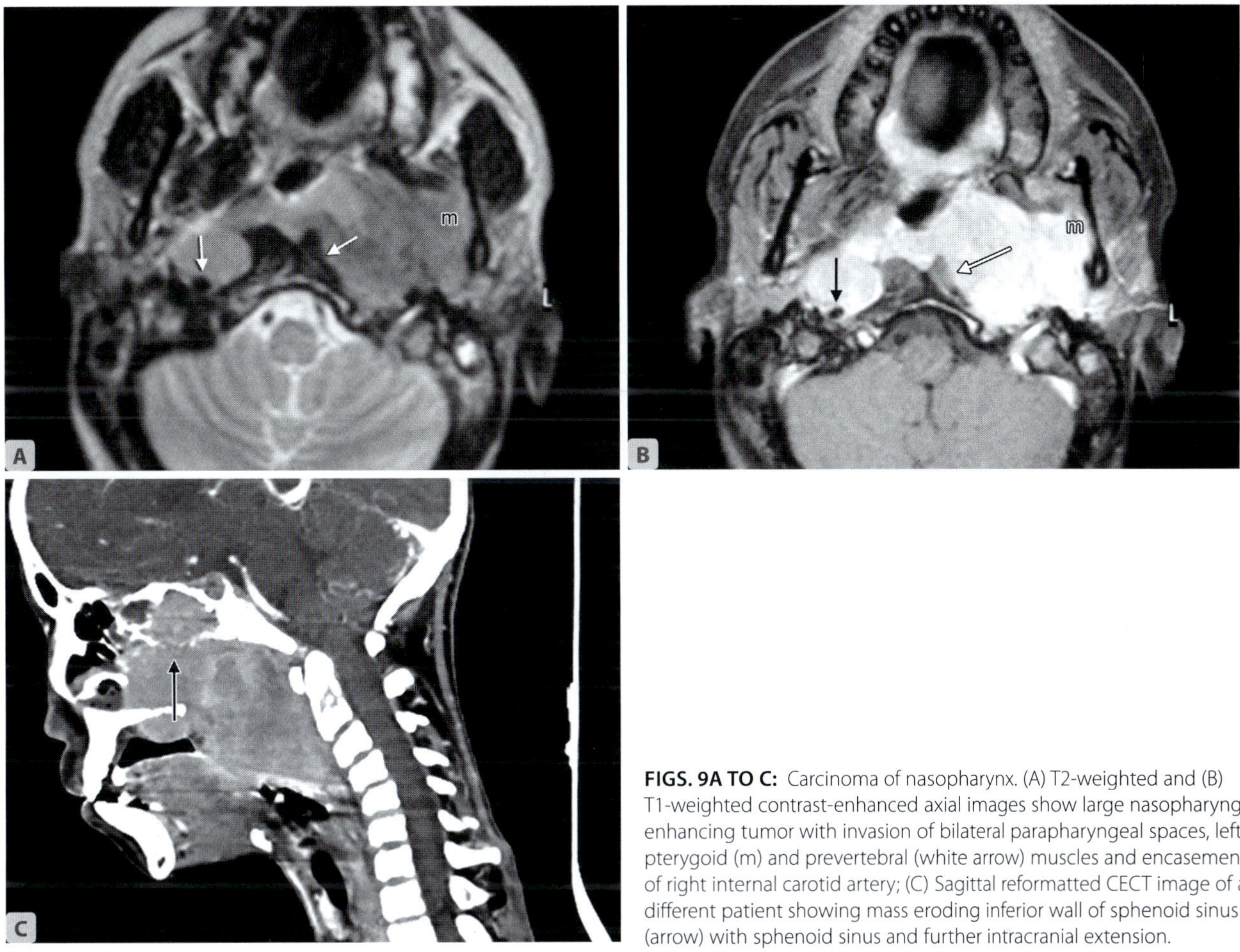

FIGS. 9A TO C: Carcinoma of nasopharynx. (A) T2-weighted and (B) T1-weighted contrast-enhanced axial images show large nasopharyngeal enhancing tumor with invasion of bilateral parapharyngeal spaces, left pterygoid (m) and prevertebral (white arrow) muscles and encasement of right internal carotid artery; (C) Sagittal reformatted CECT image of a different patient showing mass eroding inferior wall of sphenoid sinus (arrow) with sphenoid sinus and further intracranial extension.

TABLE 3: Staging of nasopharyngeal carcinoma: Overview.

T1	Limited to nasopharynx or extends to oropharynx and/or nasal cavity
T2	Parapharyngeal extension and/or involvement of pterygoid, and/or pre-vertebral muscles
T3	Bone invasion (skull base, cervical vertebra, pterygoid plate, paranasal sinuses)
T4	Intracranial extension or involvement of cranial nerves, orbit, hypopharynx, parotid or extension lateral to lateral pterygoid muscles
N1	Ipsilateral cervical LN up to 6 cm (above caudal border of cricoid cartilage) Any side retropharyngeal LN up to 6 cm
N2	Bilateral cervical LN up to 6 cm (above caudal border of cricoid cartilage)
N3	LN more than 6 cm or caudal to caudal border of cricoid cartilage
M0	No distant metastases
M1	Distant metastases
Stage 1	T1, N0
Stage 2	Up to T2, N1
Stage 3	Up to T3, N2
Stage 4	T4, N3 and M1

T2 extend into parapharyngeal tissues. T3 tumors have bony invasion. T4 tumors are those with intracranial extension or involvement of cranial nerves, orbit, hypopharynx, parotid or beyond the lateral pterygoid muscles. Cervical lymph nodal staging for nasopharyngeal carcinoma is different from that of oral cavity cancers. Nodal size of 6 cm is used to differentiate N1 and N2 nodes in nasopharyngeal carcinoma, unlike the criteria of 3 cm for oral cavity cancers.

Imaging Features

Thin section CECT with axial and coronal reconstruction and sharp kernel bone window images are useful. For MRI, pre- and post-contrast fast spin echo sequences are obtained. Both fat suppressed and non-fat suppressed images need to be evaluated. Both CT and MRI are equivalent in staging of nasopharyngeal carcinoma. CT is superior in evaluation of bony erosion and lymph node involvement while MRI better shows perineural intracranial spread along maxillary or mandibular nerves. Along the nerves, it further extends to cavernous sinus and Meckel's cave. The diagnosis of nasopharyngeal carcinoma in children is often made late on because of presence of benign adenoid hypertrophy. It should be remembered that nasopharyngeal carcinoma can occur in children. If any asymmetry of the nasopharyngeal mass is observed, a careful search for any tumor spread outside the nasopharynx should be made on imaging as this suggests the correct diagnosis.[16]

Treatment

Radiotherapy is the standard treatment of nasopharyngeal carcinoma as surgery is not feasible. Patients with advanced disease also receive concurrent chemotherapy. Apart from the nasopharynx, radiation field also includes skull base, infratemporal fossa and adjoin parts of nasal cavity, sinuses and oropharynx. The margin of the radiation field is modified as per the tumor extension into specific areas. 3D CT based conformal treatment planning is normally used. Bilateral neck nodes irradiation up to clavicle is also required in all cases.

OROPHARYNX

Oropharynx extends from soft palate superiorly to the vallecula inferiorly. Anterior margin is a plane formed by soft palate, anterior tonsillar pillars and the circumvallate papilla of the tongue. Posterior pharyngeal wall forms the posterior limit of oropharynx. Laterally, the oropharynx has anterior tonsillar pillar (palatoglossus muscle), posterior tonsillar pillar (palatopharyngeus muscle) and the lymphoid tissue in between these, called as palatine or faucial tonsils. Parts of the oropharynx are soft palate, posterior pharyngeal wall, tonsils and the base of the tongue. Most cancers are SCCA. In India, it is an uncommon malignancy with the national age averaged rate is less than 1.3 per 100,000 per year, except in some parts of North-East India, where higher incidence has been observed.[4] Other tumors of oropharynx include lymphoma involving the Waldeyer's ring, adenocarcinoma, lymphoepithelioma and sarcoma. Submucosal spread of the tumors is common and hence, endoscopy tends to underestimate the tumor spread. Extent assessment and therapeutic decisions are normally based on imaging findings.

Carcinoma of Tonsil

Superficial and small tonsillar tumors, especially those located in the tonsillar fossa may not be visible on CT. Other may just show suspicious tonsillar asymmetry. Larger tumors are seen as ulcerated or infiltrative masses with enhancement similar to normal tonsil on CT[9] **(Fig. 10)**. Fat suppressed post-contrast MRI improves the tumor delineation. Tumors arising from mucosa overlying anterior tonsillar pillar spread along underlying palatoglossus muscle. Superior spread and involvement of the soft palate is common. Subsequently hard palate may also be involved. With further superior spread, tonsillar tumors involve nasopharynx and reach the skull base. Anterior spread of the tumor involves retromolar trigone and pterygomandibular raphe, pterygoid and buccinators muscles. Inferior spread involves the base of the tongue. Posterior tonsillar pillar is rarely a site of origin of SCCA and most are extensions from anterior pillar or tonsillar fossa tumors. The spread is similar; however, inferiorly these may extend to aryepiglottic folds the thyroid cartilage. Tumors arising at the tonsillar fossa between two tonsillar pillars frequently remain occult and may present with cervical nodal metastases. Deep tumor invasion through superior

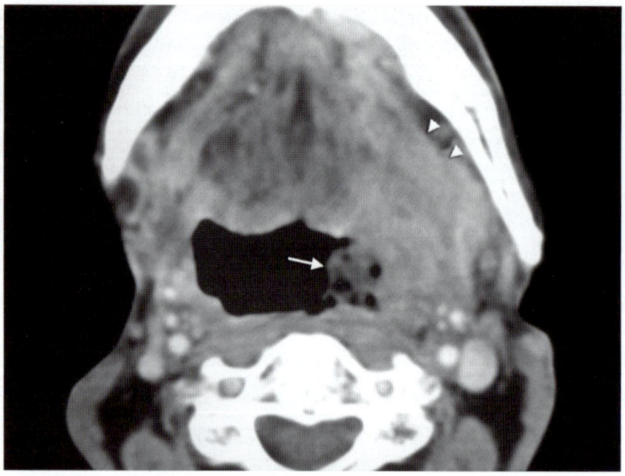

FIG. 10: Carcinoma of tonsil: CT shows ulcerated left tonsillar mass (arrow) with parapharyngeal and base of tongue invasion which is further extending floor of mouth and involving mylohyoid muscle (arrowheads).

constrictor muscle into the parapharyngeal space and then to the skull base is common with tonsillar fossa tumors.[5]

Carcinoma of Soft Palate

Most are SCCA however minor salivary gland type adenocarcinomas (minor salivary gland tumors) are also common, especially in posterior part of soft palate. Soft palate SCCAs are usually well-differentiated or low grade tumors among all pharyngeal cancers and behave more like oral cavity cancers. Carcinomas of the soft palate arise at oral surface and nasopharyngeal surface is rarely involved. Early tumors are difficult to visualize on axial images although it may be seen as asymmetrical thickening of the soft palate **(Fig. 11A)**. Coronal and sagittal CT or MRI is essential to evaluate the tumors involving soft and hard palate **(Figs. 12A and B)**. Soft palate carcinoma commonly spread in anteriorly to hard palate or laterally to tonsillar pillars. Advanced tumors involve nasopharynx, parapharyngeal spaces and the skull base **(Fig. 11B)**.

Carcinoma of Base of Tongue

Posterior-one third of the tongue is called base of tongue. It is the vertically oriented part of the tongue that extends from triangular circumvallate papilla superiorly to the vallecula inferiorly. Lingual tonsils, a lymphoid tissue, lie beneath the mucosa of base of tongue and vallecula and appears isodense to muscles. Most SCCA of base of tongue arise on its lateral aspect. Small cancers of the base of tongue often remain occult and present with neck node metastases **(Figs. 13A and B)**. These may not be clearly visualized on CT or MRI, primarily because of poor contrast enhancement of the tumor, dense muscles of the tongue, isodense lingual tonsils and absence of well-defined fat planes in this region. Larger tumors are seen as asymmetric or bulky contours **(Fig. 14)**. Earliest tumor extension occurs inferiorly to vallecula, which is in anatomical continuity with base of tongue, and then below it into the pre-epiglottic space. Lateral spread form vallecula

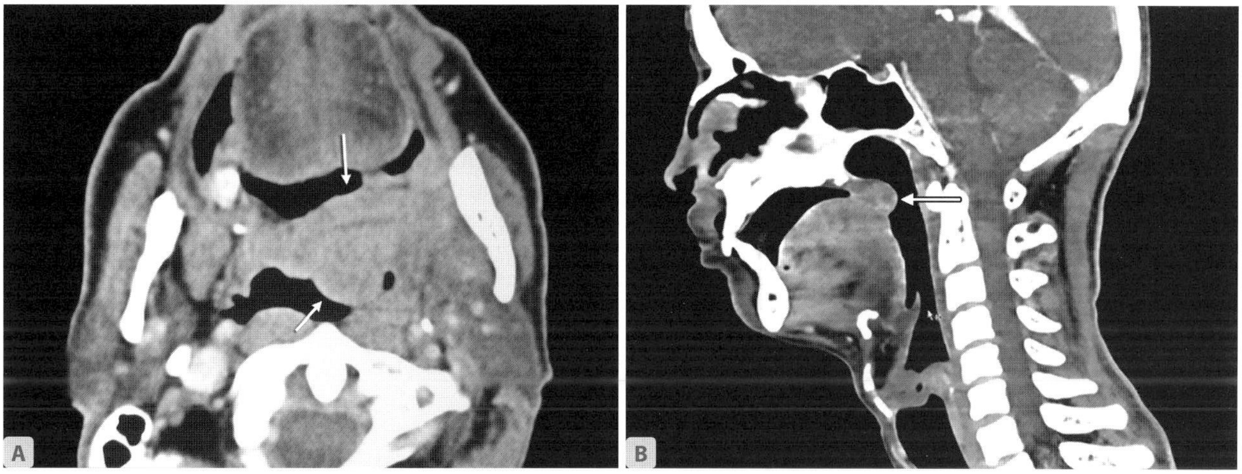

FIGS. 11A AND B: Carcinoma of soft palate. (A) CT shows the tumor as asymmetric bulky thickening of the soft palate on left side (arrows) with left parapharyngeal extension and invasion of left medial pterygoid muscle; (B) Sagittal reformatted image of another patient showing bulbous enlargement of posteroinferior part of soft palate with mild heterogeneous enhancement (arrow).

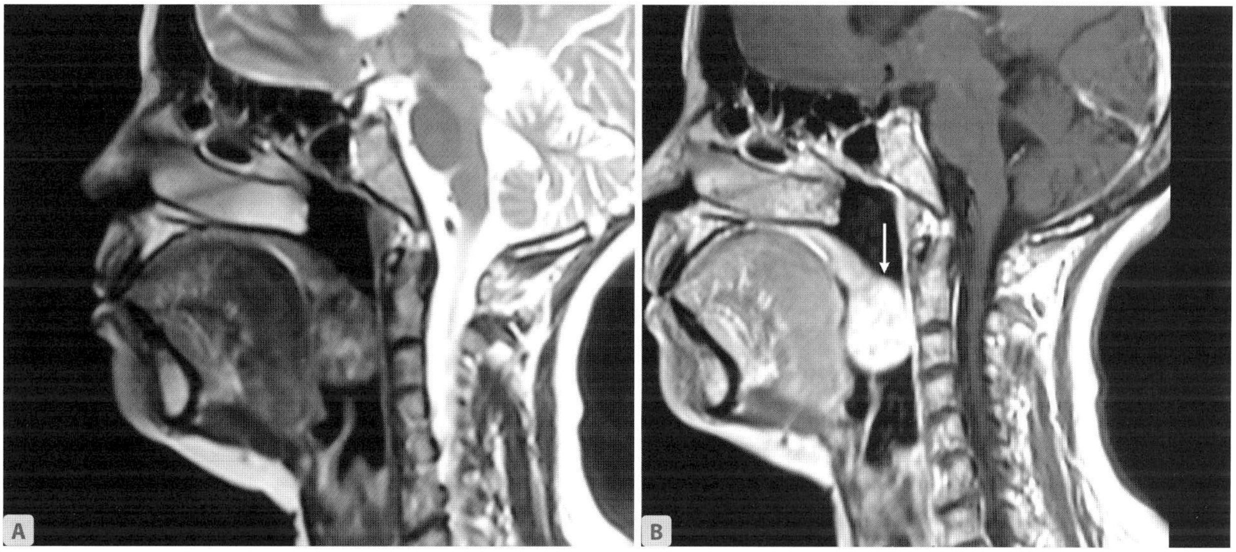

FIGS. 12A AND B: Carcinoma of soft palate. (A) T2-weighted and (B) contrast-enhanced T1-weighted sagittal images show small enhancing tumor (arrows) arising from and limited to the soft palate.

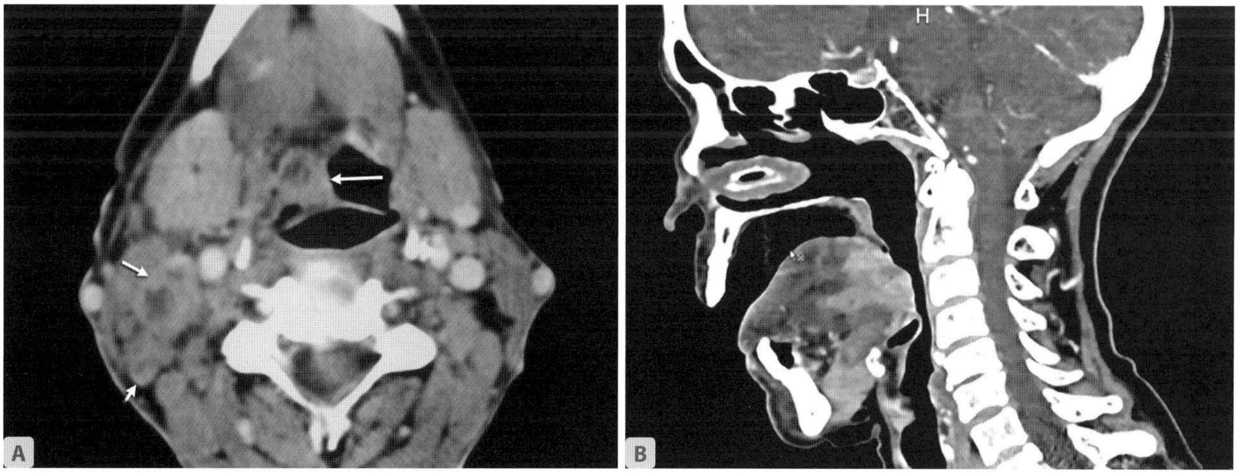

FIGS. 13A AND B: Carcinoma of base of tongue. (A) CT of the patient presenting with left cervical lymphadenopathy shows multiple enlarged necrotic right level II lymph nodes (small arrows). The primary tumor seen in right vallecula (large arrow) was detected on CT; (B) Sagittal image of a different patient showing enhancing mass in posterior third of tongue.

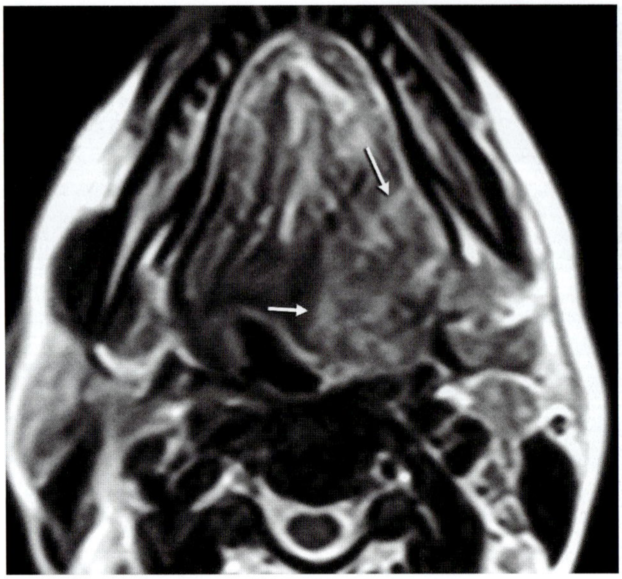

FIG. 14: Carcinoma of base of tongue: T2-weighted MR image shows large tumor in base of tongue on left side with extension to the floor of mouth (arrows).

extends deep into the neck spaces and then rapidly extends to styloid muscles. With further growth to the prestyloid area, it may encase internal carotid artery. Anterior spread of base of tongue carcinoma involves floor of mouth. Obliteration of fat planes around lingual neurovascular bundle is highly suggestive of its encasement and perineural and perivascular spread of the tumor. In base of tongue carcinomas, medial spread across the midline or lateral spread to tonsils are uncommon and occur late in the course of the disease.

Because of the rich lymphatic supply of the tongue and advanced disease stage when patients become symptomatic, most patients of carcinoma of base of tongue have extensive and often bilateral cervical lymph node metastases at presentation.

Staging and Treatment of Carcinoma of Oropharynx

In the latest staging system **(Table 4)**, a new classification has been introduced for HPV-positive oropharyngeal cancers.[4] This was the need of the hour because of their biologically distinct behavior as well as differences in clinical care and

TABLE 4: Staging of oropharyngeal cancers.

T1	Tumor ≤2 cm	
T2	Tumor 2–4 cm	
T3	Tumor >4 cm OR extension to upper surface of epiglottis	
T4	Advanced local disease	
	For p16 negative cancers: Invasion of larynx, extrinsic muscle of the tongue, medial pterygoid, hard palate, or mandible	
	For p16 positive cancers: *Moderately Advanced T4a:* Tumor invades the larynx, extrinsic muscle of the tongue, medial pterygoid, hard palate, or mandible *Very advanced T4b:* Invasion of lateral pterygoid muscle, pterygoid bone, lateral nasopharynx, skull base or ICA encasement	
	For p16 positive tumors	*For p16 negative tumors*
N1	Single/multiple Ipsilateral LNs up to 6 cm	Single ipsilateral LN up to 3 cm, No ENE
N2	Bilateral LNs up to 6 cm	Sigle/Multiple lymph nodes up to 6 cm
		N2a: ipsilateral single LN 3–6 cm, No ENE
		N2b: ipsilateral multiple LNs up to 6 cm, No ENE
		N2c: contralateral or B/L LNs up to 6 cm, No ENE
N3	LN> 6 cm	N3a: LN >6 cm, No ENE
		N3b: LN with clinically overt ENE
M0	No distant metastases	
M1	Distant metastases	
Stage	*For p16 positive tumors*	*For p16 negative tumors*
Stage 1	Up to T2, N1	T1N0M0
Stage 2	Up to T3, N2	T2N0M0
Stage 3	Up to T4 or N3	Up to T3 or N1
Stage 4	M1	T4 or N2 or M1 (further subdivided into A, B and C)

surveillance. HPV-positive oropharyngeal cancers are positive on p16 immunostaining and have better prognosis.

Although early tumors of tonsils or soft palate can be resected with intraoral approach, radical radiotherapy is the primary treatment modality for oropharyngeal tumors. Advanced tumors require concurrent chemoradiotherapy.[1]

HYPOPHARYNX

Hypopharynx is the part of upper aerodigestive tract which lies below and continuous with the oropharynx. Hypopharynx extends from the level of hyoid bone superiorly to the level of inferior margin of the cricoid cartilage. Hypopharynx continues below as the cervical esophagus. Parts of hypopharynx are posterior pharyngeal wall, bilateral pyriform sinuses and the post-cricoid region. The posterior wall of hypopharynx is continuous with posterior wall of oropharynx. Pyriform sinuses are lateral air distended recess created by aryepiglottic folds. Each pyriform sinus is triangular in shape having medial, anterior and lateral walls. The apex or lower tip of the pyriform sinus lies at the level of true vocal cords. At the level of cricoid cartilage, posterior parts of two pyriform sinuses merge to form the post cricoid region of the hypopharynx. Postcricoid region forms the pharyngo-esophageal junction.

Carcinoma of hypopharynx is more common in males. In India, it is more common than naso- or oropharyngeal carcinoma, with age averaged rate ranging from 1 to 6.3 cases per 100,000 per year.[4] Much higher incidence is found in some parts of North-East India, where it is the second most common cancer in males. SCCAs of hypopharynx spread submucosally, often remain clinically silent for long and majority of the patients already have cervical lymph node metastases at presentation.

Carcinoma of Posterior Wall of Hypopharynx

Carcinomas arising at posterior wall of hypopharynx most commonly spread superiorly and inferiorly with submucosal infiltration. With superior spread, these extend into the oropharynx and may also involve posterior tonsillar pillars. Inferior spread involves post-cricoid region and the esophagus. Rarely, the tumor may spread posteriorly into the prevertebral space.

Carcinoma of the Pyriform Sinus

Most SCCA of hypopharynx arise at the pyriform sinus. Apart from endoscopic evaluation, carcinoma of the pyriform sinus can also be demonstrated with barium swallow **(Fig. 15)**. CT or MRI is required for assessment of submucosal extent of the tumor. Adequate distension of the pyriform sinus is essential during imaging. A collapsed pyriform sinus may simulate the tumor and on the other hand, a documented tumor may not apparent on CT or MRI.[5]

Carcinoma of pyriform sinus is seen on CT or MRI as homogenous masses with submucosal spread. Commonly spread in anatomical contiguity into the posterior pharyngeal wall, medially to aryepiglottic fold or inferiorly into the postcricoid region. Tumors on medial aspect of the pyriform sinus involve aryepiglottic fold and then along with it, spread

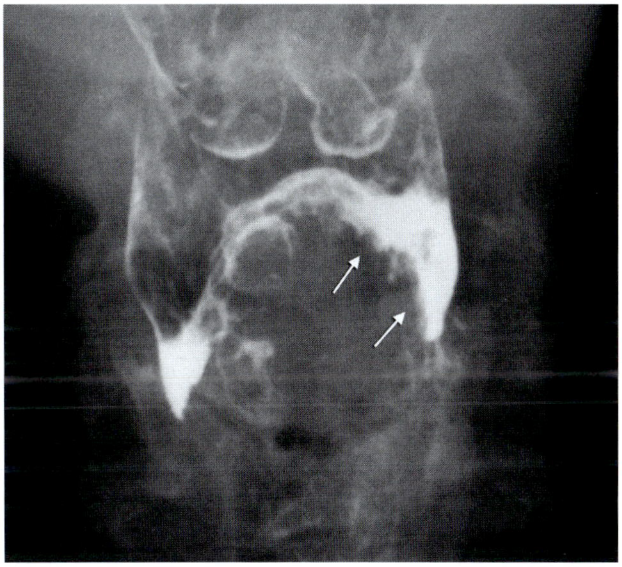

FIG. 15: Carcinoma of pyriform sinus: Barium swallow shows irregularity and narrowing of left pyriform sinus (arrows).

to false vocal cords, paraglottic space and arytenoids cartilage **(Figs. 16A to C)**. With further growth, these may involve epiglottis, pre-epiglottic space and the base of the tongue. Posterior spread of the carcinoma of pyriform sinus involves postcricoid region or posterior pharyngeal wall **(Fig. 17)**. With further posterior submucosal growth along the posterior pharyngeal wall, the tumor extends across the midline to involve contralateral pyriform sinus.

Carcinoma of the Postcricoid

Carcinomas arising at the postcricoid are uncommon. It usually occurs in patients with Plummer-Vinson syndrome (dysphagia, weight loss, iron deficiency anemia and cervical esophageal web). Carcinoma of the postcricoid cause concentric wall thickening and narrowing of the hypopharyngeal lumen. Because of the close anatomical proximity, these usually spread to posterior part of the larynx and involve arytenoids and cricoid cartilages **(Fig. 18)**. Inferior extension of the carcinoma of postcricoid involves cervical esophagus.

Treatment

Radical radiotherapy is the preferred modality of treatment for low volume carcinomas of hypopharynx. Others are treated with surgery and this may include wide local excision and partial or total laryngo-pharyngectomy. Type of the surgery depends on extent of the tumor as depicted on imaging. In hypopharyngeal cancers; important points that need to be determined on imaging include location and submucosal extent of the tumor, extension across the midline, lower margin of the tumor, involvement of apex of the pyriform sinus, cartilage erosion and invasion of prevertebral muscles. Tumor involving apex of the pyriform sinus lies close to true vocal cords and it has high probability of involvement of cricoid and arytenoid cartilages and paraglottic space. Hence,

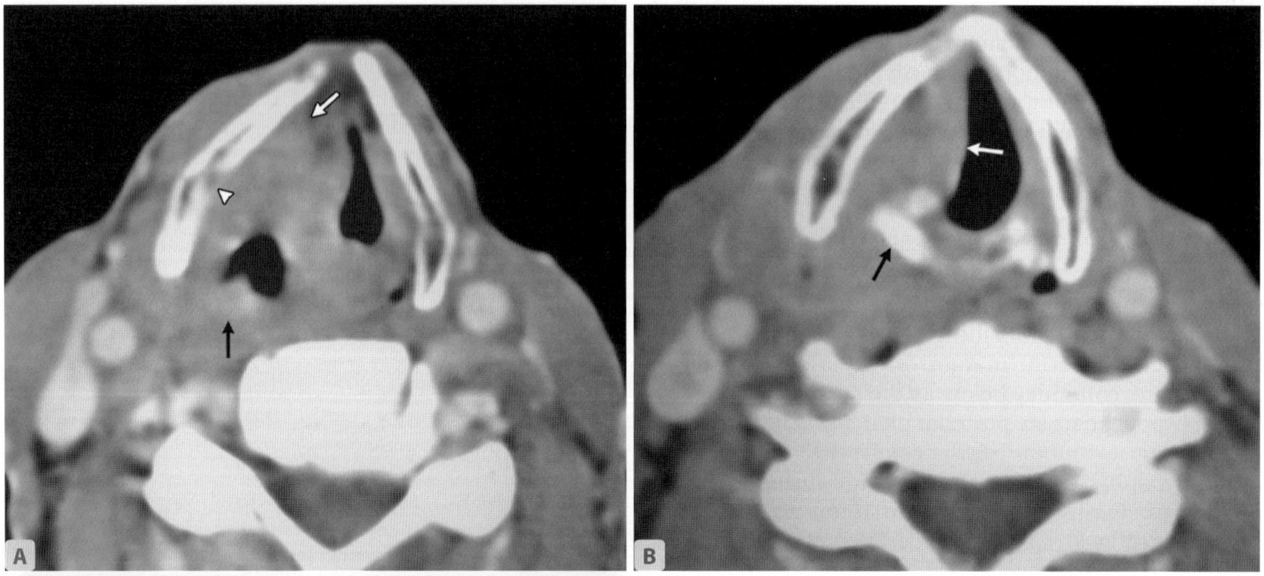

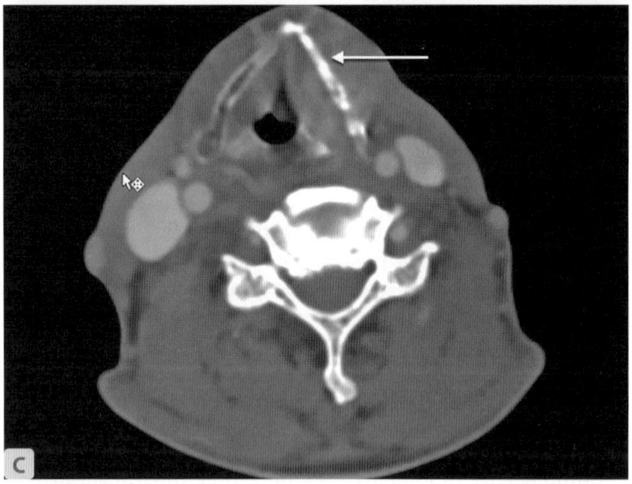

FIGS. 16A TO C: Carcinoma of pyriform sinus. (A) CT shows tumor right pyriform tumor (black arrow) involving aryepiglottic fold and extension to paralaryngeal space (white arrow). Thyroid cartilage invasion is seen as sclerosis of the right thyroid lamina and focal lysis (arrowhead); (B) CT image at caudal level shows extension to paraglottic space and true vocal cord (white arrow). There is sclerosis of arytenoids cartilage suggestive of its invasion (black arrow); (C) CECT image (bone window): The sclerosis of the left side thyroid cartilage is better appreciated on bone window image (white arrow).

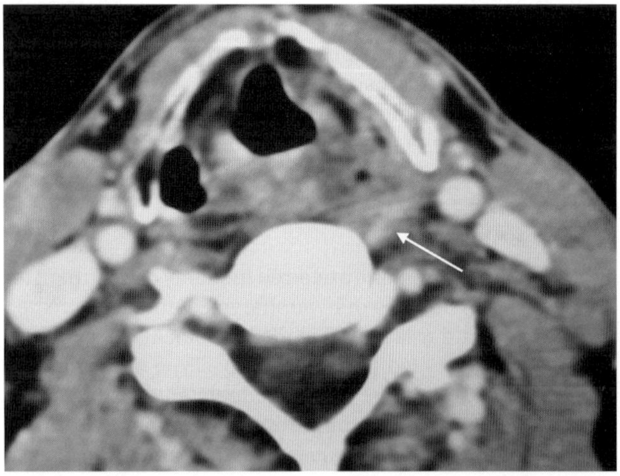

FIG. 17: Carcinoma of pyriform sinus: CT shows left pyriform sinus tumor involving posterior pharyngeal wall and prevertebral muscles (arrow).

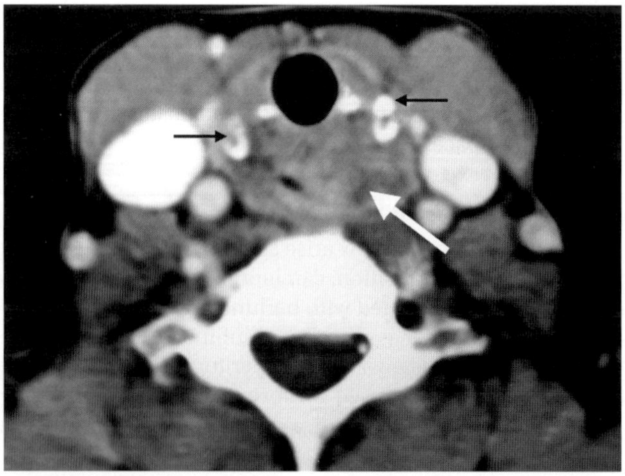

FIG. 18: Carcinoma of postcricoid: CT shows postcricoid tumor (white arrow) with anterior extension to glottis with invasion and sclerosis of cricoid and arytenoids cartilages (black arrows).

such tumors require total laryngo-pharyngectomy. Tumors involving postcricoid or cervical esophagus also require esophagectomy in addition to total laryngo-pharyngectomy. Advanced tumors of hypopharynx are treated with combination of chemotherapy and radiotherapy.

LARYNX

Larynx is made up of mucosal surface and supporting cartilage skeleton. True vocal cords divide larynx into supraglottic, glottis and subglotic compartments. Supraglottis extends from vallecula superiorly to the laryngeal ventricle (space between false and true vocal cords) inferiorly.

Supraglottic larynx includes epiglottis, aryepiglottic folds, false cords and arytenoids process of the arytenoids cartilage. Superior part of the epiglottis has free margins and lower lateral margins have mucosal folds extending from it to the arytenoids cartilages. These are aryepiglottic folds. Inferior continuation of aryepiglottic folds are false vocal cords. Glottic larynx is composed of pair of true vocal cords and cartilages. True vocal cords extend from arytenoid cartilages posteriorly to the anterior commissure. Anterior commissure is composed of mucosa only and measures less than 1 mm on imaging. Arytenoid cartilage is articulated inferiorly to cricoid cartilage and the cricoarytenoid joint allows the movements of the true vocal cords. Subglottic larynx extends from inferior surface of true vocal cords to inferior margin of cricoid cartilage.

Larynx also has several muscles grouped into extrinsic and intrinsic muscles. Extrinsic muscles are elevators of larynx (stylohyoid, mylohyoid, thyrohyoid and digastric) and depressors of larynx (sternothyroid, sternohyoid and omohyoid). Intrinsic muscles are located in vocal cords and adjacent to it and these muscles provide vocal and airway control. Supraglottic and subglottic larynx have rich lymphatic supply, however, glottis has sparse lymphatics.

Carcinoma of larynx is primarily related to smoking. In India, the age averaged rate ranges from 1.4 to 7.5 cases per 100,000 per year.[4] It is the second most common cancer in males in Delhi. Carcinoma of the larynx includes supraglottic, glottic and subglottic cancers. Involvement of both supraglottic and glottis is termed as transglottic cancer. There is separate AJCC tumor staging system for each compartment as outlined in **Table 5**. Nodal staging is same in all.

Supraglottic Carcinoma

These may arise from any mucosal surface of the supraglottic larynx but epiglottis is the most common site of origin. Early tumors of epiglottis are often seen on imaging as midline, well-defined enhancing nodules. With further spread, epiglottic tumors may spread superiorly to vallecula and base of tongue and laterally to aryepiglottic folds, false vocal cords and paralaryngeal fat deep to false vocal cords. Anterior extension of epiglottic tumors involves fat in pre-epiglottic space **(Figs. 19 and 20)**. Early tumors arising from aryepiglottic folds or false cords are also exophytic and confined to the fold of origin. Such early lesions are also called as marginal tumors. With medial or lateral spread, these involve epiglottis and pyriform sinus respectively **(Fig. 21)**.

Any supraglottic carcinoma can directly extend to glottis and involve true vocal cords. The glottic involvement may be anteriorly to anterior commissure or posteriorly to involve cricoarytenoid joint; the later results in fixity of the cord. Further inferior spread to subglottis however, is prevented till late by a fibrous barrier, known as conus elasticus. It extends from cricoid cartilage to medial margins of true vocal cords. Cartilage invasion by supraglottic carcinoma is also a late feature.

In supraglottic carcinoma, deep extension beneath the mucosa is underestimated clinically and can be detected only on imaging. Important submucosal spaces that need to be evaluated on imaging include pre-epiglottic space anterior to epiglottis and paralaryngeal spaces lateral to aryepiglottic folds and false cords **(Figs. 19 and 20)**. These spaces normally contain fat and hence tumor invasion of these spaces can be seen as partial or complete obliteration of fat. Paralaryngeal fat is also continuous with paraglottic space lateral to true vocal cords and via this route; supraglottic cancers can directly involve true vocal cords. Pre-epiglottic space also has rich and bilateral lymphatic drainage and tumors involving this space have high probability of bilateral neck node metastases.

Glottic Carcinoma

True vocal cords are the most common site of laryngeal carcinoma. Most glottis carcinoma arise along the anterior free margin of the true vocal cords. Small lesions result in thickening of the vocal cord on imaging and large lesions may be seen as bulky masses **(Fig. 22)**. With anterior spread, glottis carcinoma readily involves anterior commissure. From here, it may spread to contralateral vocal cord or extend along tendon of the anterior commissure to thyroid cartilage where this tendon is attached. This results in early thyroid cartilage invasion **(Fig. 23C)**. Glottic carcinoma may also arise at the commissure. Posterior extension of the glottis carcinoma involves interarytenoid region (posterior commissure) and cricoarytenoid joint. Glottic carcinoma superiorly spread to ventricle and false vocal cords. It may also extend inferiorly to subglottic region, although it is relatively uncommon **(Figs. 23A and B)**.

Subglottic Carcinoma

Carcinoma primarily arising at subglottic larynx is rare and most are extensions of glottic or supraglottic carcinomas **(Figs. 23A to C)**. Primary subglottic carcinoma is seen as circumferential mucosal thickening of the subglottis. Because of the close proximity, cricoid cartilage invasion occurs early. It may also spread superiorly to involve glottis.

Imaging Protocol

Contrast-enhanced CT or MRI is used for pre-treatment evaluation of the laryngeal carcinoma. Thin section CT images are normallyobtained from the level of skull base to thoracic inlet in a planeparallel to ventricle of the larynx. Ventricle is best seen on the lateral topograms. During scanning, quite breathing is ensured to keep vocal cords away. Breath hold, swallowing or phonation is to be avoided by the patient as it

TABLE 5: Staging of carcinoma of larynx: Overview.

T stage	**Supraglottic tumors**
T1	Limited to one subsite (structure), normal vocal cord mobility
T2	Involvement of more than one subsites or extension outside supraglottis (vallecula, base of tongue, piriform sinus). Vocal cords not fixed
T3	Limited to larynx with fixed vocal cords Any extension to pre-epiglottic space or postcricoid or paraglottic space or inner cortex of thyroid cartilage
T4	*T4a Moderately advanced*: Involvement of outer cortex of thyroid cartilage or extralaryngeal spread (e.g., trachea, soft tissues of the neck including deep extrinsic muscle of the tongue, strap muscles, thyroid, or esophagus)
	T4b Very advanced: Extends to prevertebral space, encases carotid artery, or invades mediastinal structures
T stage	**Glottic tumors**
T1	Limited to one (T1a) or both (T1b) vocal cords with preserved mobility of vocal cords
T2	Extension to supraglottic or subglottis or impaired vocal cord mobility
T3	Limited to larynx with fixed vocal cords or invasion of paraglottic space or inner cortex of thyroid cartilage
T4	*T4a Moderately advanced*: Involvement of outer cortex of thyroid cartilage or extralaryngeal spread (e.g. trachea, cricoid cartilage, soft tissues of the neck including deep extrinsic muscle of the tongue, strap muscles, thyroid, or esophagus)
	T4b Very advanced: Extends to prevertebral space, encases carotid artery, or invades mediastinal structures
T stage	**Subglottic tumors**
T1	Limited to subglottis
T2	Involvement of vocal cords, not fixed
T3	Limited to larynx, vocal cords fixed or invasion of paraglottic space or inner cortex of thyroid cartilage
T4	*T4a Moderately advanced*: Involvement of outer cortex of thyroid cartilage or extralaryngeal spread (e.g. trachea, cricoid cartilage, soft tissues of the neck including deep extrinsic muscle of the tongue, strap muscles, thyroid, or esophagus)
	T4b Very advanced: Extends to prevertebral space, encases carotid artery, or invades mediastinal structures
N	**Stage**
N1	Single ipsilateral LN up to 3 cm, No ENE
N2	Sigle/Multiple lymph nodes up to 6 cm
	N2a: Ipsilateral single LN 3–6 cm, No ENE
	N2b: Ipsilateral multiple LNs up to 6 cm, No ENE
	N2c: Contralateral or B/L LNs up to 6 cm, No ENE
N3	*N3a*: LN> 6 cm, No ENE
	N3b: LN with clinically overt ENE
M	**Stage**
M0	No distant metastases
M1	Distant metastases
Stage grouping	
Stage 1	T1, N0
Stage 2	T2, N0
Stage 3	Up to T3 or N1
Stage 4	T4a or N2 (4a), T4b or N3 (4b) and M1 (4c)

opposes the medial margins of the cord. MRI is performed using dedicated neck coil, short duration sequences and phase encoding gradients in AP direction in order to avoid pulsation artefacts arising from great vessels of the neck. Most laryngeal cancers enhance well on contrast enhanced MR sequences and well demarcated. It is important to note that both CT and MRI may not depict early mucosal cancers.

On CT or MRI, location and size of the tumor should be defined. Any tumor extension to adjacent segments or fat containing spaces, invasion of soft tissues of the neck, exolaryngeal structures or laryngeal cartilage should be documented.

Cartilage Invasion

Cartilage invasion by laryngeal cancers precludes the treatment with radiotherapy as response to radiation is poor in such lesions, chances of recurrence are very high and it

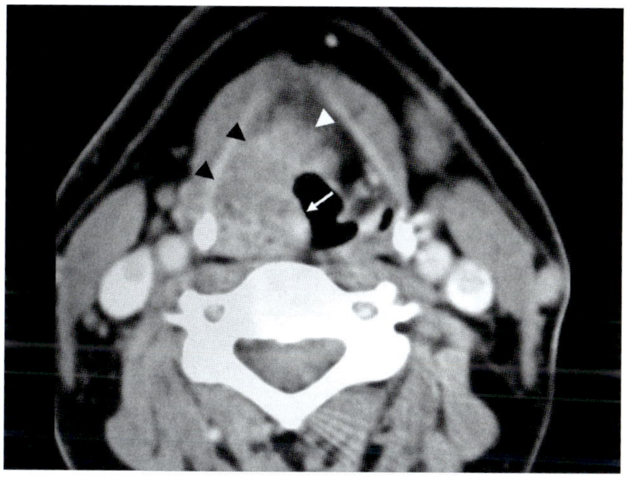

FIG. 19: Supraglottic carcinoma: CT shows epiglottic tumor involving aryepiglottic fold (arrow), paralaryngeal space (black arrowheads) and pre-epiglottic space (white arrowhead).

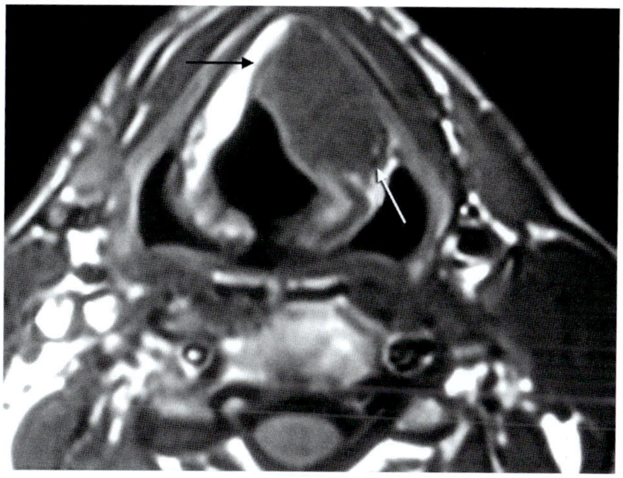

FIG. 20: Supraglottic carcinoma: T1-weighted axial MR image shows hypointense epiglottic tumor extending into and obliterating pre-epiglottic (black arrow) and paralaryngeal (white arrow) spaces.

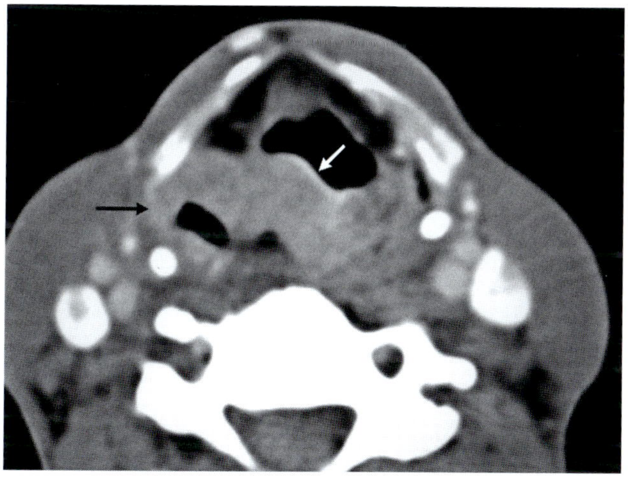

FIG. 21: Supraglottic carcinoma: CT shows right aryepiglottic tumor (white arrow) with extension to the pyriform sinus (black arrow).

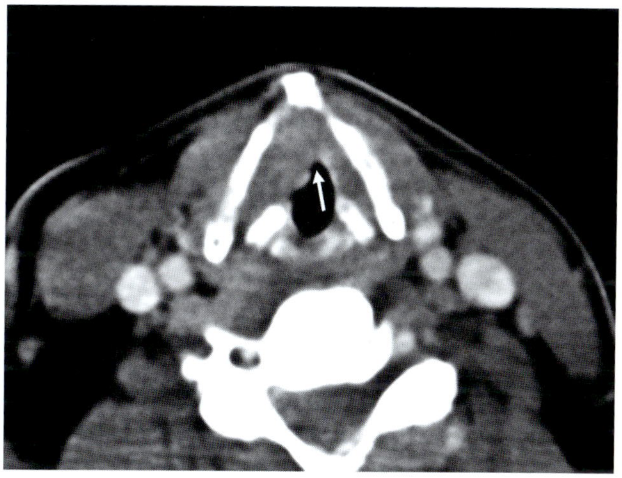

FIG. 22: Glottic carcinoma: CT shows tumor in right true vocal cord with extension to anterior commissure (arrow).

may also induce radiation necrosis of the cartilage.[17] If no other contraindication, extensive surgery is the only option in such tumors. Because of this, cartilage invasion upstages all laryngeal cancers to T4. Cartilage invasion cannot be detected on endoscopy and it must be carefully evaluated on imaging. In adults, normal thyroid, arytenoids and cricoid cartilages have both purely cartilaginous as well as ossified areas with cortex and marrow. However, the pattern of ossification is quite variable in thyroid cartilage and hence, it is the most difficult cartilage to assess for invasion.[18]

On CT, cartilaginous part has soft tissue density while ossified part has bony cortex and medulla. Sclerosis of the cartilage (caused by inflammatory and osteoblastic activities of the tumor) is the earliest CT sign of cartilage invasion, although its specificity is variable. Erosion or frank destruction of the cortex develop subsequently and these are more specific indicators of cartilage invasion by the tumor[19] **(Figs. 16 and 23)**. Presence of tumor on both sides of the cartilage is a reliable CT indicator of cartilage invasion; however, it is seen only in advanced cases. On MRI, non-ossified cartilage has low to intermediate signal intensity on both T1- and T2-weighted images and it does not enhance. Ossified cortex has very low signal intensity while the marrow is hyperintense. Non-ossified cartilage invaded by tumor is hyperintense on T2-weighted images, similar to the tumor signal intensity. Tumor invaded marrow of ossified cartilage appear hypointense on plain T1-weighted images. On contrast administration, the involved part of the cartilage enhances, similar to the tumor. Specificity of MRI for cartilage invasion is lower as abnormal signal intensity or enhancement may also be caused by peritumoral inflammation and edema without actual tumor invasion of the cartilage. However, if these MR abnormalities are absent, cartilage invasion can be reliably excluded on MRI.[18]

Treatment

Radical (definitive) radiotherapy is the preferred treatment for supraglottic carcinomas, as it offers better functional

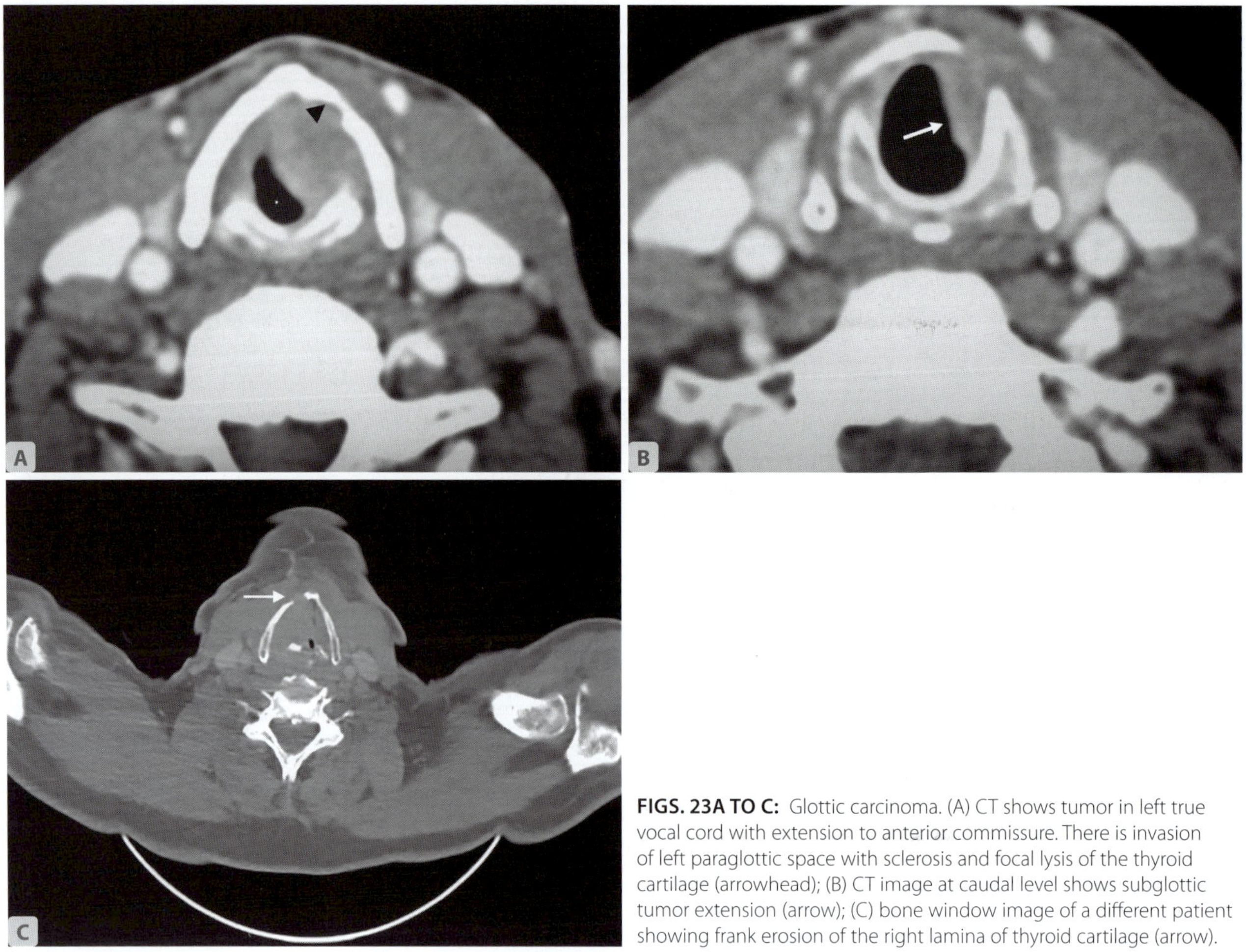

FIGS. 23A TO C: Glottic carcinoma. (A) CT shows tumor in left true vocal cord with extension to anterior commissure. There is invasion of left paraglottic space with sclerosis and focal lysis of the thyroid cartilage (arrowhead); (B) CT image at caudal level shows subglottic tumor extension (arrow); (C) bone window image of a different patient showing frank erosion of the right lamina of thyroid cartilage (arrow).

preservation. Patients with early tumor stage, small (< 6 mL) tumor volume, as assessed on imaging, and absence of cartilage invasion have high chances of cure with radiotherapy.[20] In unfavorable situations, surgery is preferred. Most are amenable to supraglottic laryngectomy. It is a voice preserving procedure and consists of removal of all endolaryngeal structures above the ventricle, including false vocal cords, aryepiglottic folds, epiglottis and hyoid bone. Tumors involving true vocal cords or the cartilage are treated with supracricoid laryngectomy and for advanced tumors, total laryngectomy is required. Cord fixation is an indirect evidence of cricoarytenoid joint involvement. It upstages the tumor to T3 and precludes voice preserving surgery in all laryngeal cancers.

Radiotherapy is also the preferred modality for definitive treatment of early glottic carcinomas as it allows voice preservation.[21] Hemilaryngectomy is the usual surgical procedure early glottic cancers in which affected true vocal cord, ipsilateral false vocal cord and adjacent thyroid cartilage is removed. Supracricoid laryngectomy is performed if there is imaging evidence of invasion of anterior or posterior commissure, contralateral true vocal cord, false vocal cord or paraglottic fat invasion. Patients with advanced tumors may be given neoadjuvant chemotherapy and if they respond well, radiotherapy is subsequently considered. Non-responders may be offered surgery. Supraglotic or glottic tumors which do not respond or recur after radiotherapy are also subjected to salvage surgery.

CERVICAL LYMPH NODES

Cervical lymph node metastasis is the most important prognostic factor in the outcome of patients with carcinoma of head and neck. Regardless of the primary tumor, presence of a metastatic cervical lymph node reduces the 5-year survival by 50% and presence of contralateral lymph node further reduces it to 25%.[22] Risk of distant metastases also depend on the lymph node status; distant metastases are rare in patients with N0 or N1 nodes, but the incidence is above 30% in patients with N3 nodes or any node below the level of thyroid notch.[1]

Site and size of the primary tumor, density of lymphatics in that area, neurovascular infiltration and the histological tumor grade determine the risk of cervical lymph nodes metastases in SCCA of the upper aerodigestive tract. Well lateralized tumors spread to ipsilateral nodal stations. Lesions at the midline or carcinoma of the nasopharynx and tongue, even if well lateralized, may have bilateral lymphadenopathy. AJCC classification is the most widely used system for nomenclature and communication of cervical lymph node locations. It divides the cervical lymph nodes into seven stations on each side **(Table 6)**.

Imaging

Evaluation of cervical lymph nodes is important in patients with head and neck carcinomas as it assesses the prognosis and help to select the appropriate management. Imaging can identify up to 20% of clinically silent metastatic cervical lymph nodes and thus help to choose most appropriate management.[23] Imaging normally use size criteria; lymph node measuring more than 10 mm in short axis or more than 15 mm in long axis are considered to be involved **(*see* Fig. 3D)**. A group of three or more nodes measuring 8-10 mm in tumor drainage area can also be considered involved. Central necrosis in a non-enlarged lymph node, as seen on contrast enhanced CT or MRI is also suggestive of nodal metastasis **(*see* Figs. 13A and B)**. Inaccuracies are common in imaging diagnosis of cervical lymph node metastases. About 16% of CT or MRI negative patients actually have lymph node metastases while 50% patients with imaging positive lymph nodes have no metastases.[24]

TABLE 6: Cervical lymph nodes classification.

Level	Site	Imaging landmarks
I	Submental and submandibular LN	Anterior to submandibular gland, above hyoid
II	Upper jugular	Skull base to hyoid, submandibular gland to posterior margin of sternocleidomastoid
III	Mid jugular	Hyoid to cricoid
IV	Lower jugular	Cricoid to clavicle
V	Posterior triangle	Posterior to sternocleidomastoid
VI	Anterior visceral	Between carotid arteries
VII	Superior mediastinal	Below sternal notch

Perinodal tumor extension is a poor prognostic indicator. Although, it is pathological finding, gross or macroscopic perinodal spread can be seen on CT as a thick, enhancing rim with infiltration of surrounding fat. Such patients have ten times higher chances of recurrence. Invasion of internal carotid artery by nodal mass is also a grave prognostic finding; as such patients cannot be salvaged. On imaging, artery is considered to be invaded if more than 270 degree of the circumference is surrounded by the tumor on CT.

CT and MRI performed for primary tumor evaluation should always include area from skull base to the thoracic inlet. CT is more accurate than MRI, both for detection of metastatic lymph nodes as well as for assessment of perinodal extension.[23] Ultrasound of the neck is generally superior to both CT and MRI in evaluation of cervical lymph nodes, although some found similar accuracies.[25] Apart from the size criteria, various morphological abnormalities seen on ultrasound in enlarged or non-enlarged lymph nodes are also suggestive of metastatic involvement. These include rounded shape, loss of fatty hilum, focal cortical thickening, focal or diffuse hypoechoic areas suggestive of tumor deposits and cystic areas suggestive of necrosis **(Fig. 24)**. Power Doppler may also provide additional findings. A normal lymph node usually shows hilar perfusion. The metastatic lymph nodes may show obliterated hilar vessel, mixed vascularity in entire lymph node or peripheral hypervascularity[26] **(Figs. 24 and 25)**. However, many of these abnormal sonographic features are difficult to demonstrate in small, non-enlarged lymph nodes. In order to improve the negative predictive value of neck ultrasound in clinically N0 neck, smaller size criteria (6 or 7 mm) along with other morphological features can be used. Abnormal nodes are subjected to ultrasound guided FNAC or biopsy. This procedure is very accurate and it can correctly stage the cervical lymph nodes in up to 95% of patients with head and neck carcinoma.[27,28] Newer imaging techniques like contrast enhanced ultrasonography, MRI with superparamagnetic contrast agent, diffusion weighted

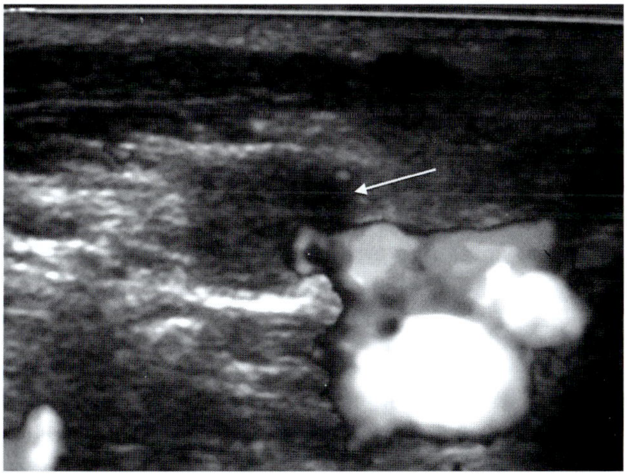

FIG. 24: Cervical lymphadenopathy: Ultrasound of the neck in a patient with tongue carcinoma of pyriform sinus shows a non-enlarged cervical lymph node with obliteration of hilar vessel and peripheral hypoechoic deposit (arrow) suggestive of metastatic involvement.

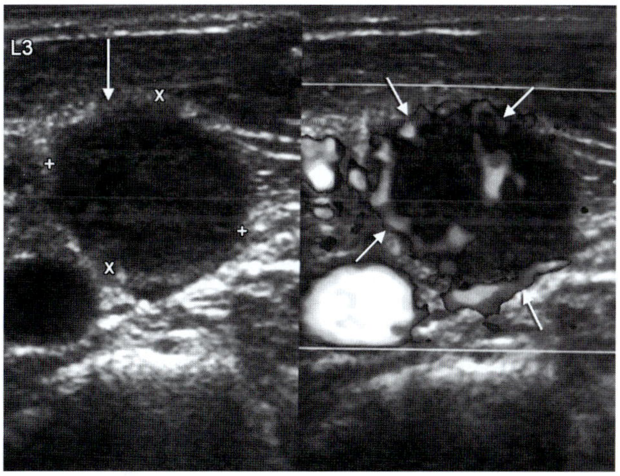

FIG. 25: Cervical lymphadenopathy: Ultrasound of the neck in patient with supraglottic carcinoma shows rounded hypoechoic cervical lymph node (arrow) with fine nodular hypoechoic deposits. Power Doppler shows increased peripheral vascularity (arrows). These features are suggestive of metastatic involvement of the lymph node.

MRI and PET-CT may prove helpful in doubtful cases and to detect metastases in subcentimetric lymph nodes.[29] Sentinel lymph node mapping may also be useful in detection of occult cervical lymph node metastases.[30,31]

Management

Both surgery and radiotherapy are effective in management of cervical lymph nodes. Surgical neck dissection is performed either simultaneously with surgery of primary tumor or electively for patients treated with radiotherapy. This procedure is both diagnostic (for pathological N staging) as well as curative. In a radical neck dissection, superficial and deep cervical fascia with enclosed level I to V lymph nodes are removed along with sternocleidomastoid and omohyoid muscles, internal jugular vein, spinal accessory nerve and the submandibular gland. In modified neck dissection, depending on the type, one or more of these structures are spared. Selective neck dissection is the term used when only selected lymph node levels are removed.[1]

Exact type of management depends on risk, i.e. site as well as pre-treatment T and N stage of the tumor. In clinically N0 neck, patients with small tumors of oral cavity have minimal risk and hence may require follow-up only. With small tumors from intermediate risk sites (oropharynx, larynx) partial neck treatment (selective neck dissection or radiotherapy) may be considered. Some centres use ultrasound of the neck (with or without ultrasound guided FNAC) in clinically N0 patients. If these investigations are negative, no neck treatment is given.[32] Any tumor in high risk areas (nasopharynx, tongue and pyriform sinus) or T4 tumors at any site are subjected to entire neck management; surgery or radiotherapy. In patients with clinically N1 or unilateral N2 lymph nodes, ipsilateral modified neck dissection is performed. If positive, radiotherapy is given to control contralateral subclinical nodes.[1] Patients with advanced nodal disease require both radical neck dissection and radiotherapy, frequently combined with chemotherapy. Lymph nodes which persist or recur after radiotherapy are also treated with surgery.

Cervical Lymphadenopathy with Carcinoma of Unknown Primary Site (CUPS)

Patients frequently present with enlarged cervical lymph nodes positive for squamous cell carcinoma pathologically but with occult primary tumor. In these patients, primary can be located anywhere in head and neck however, nasopharynx, tonsil and base of tongue are the usual primary sites of occult cancer.[33,34] Thorough clinical examination, pan endoscopy and imaging may demonstrate primary site (*see* **Fig. 13A and B**). Location of the lymph node also gives a clue to the likely primary site. Level I nodes are more likely from oropharyngeal or oral tumors while level V are more likely from nasopharyngeal carcinoma. Bilateral lymph nodes raise the suspicion for base of tongue cancers. If the tumor is not visualized on endoscopy and imaging, blind biopsies of nasopharynx or any suspicious site and sometimes, ipsilateral tonsillectomy is performed. If lower cervical or supraclavicular lymph nodes are involved, a lung cancer must also be excluded with CT of the chest. However, despite extensive work-up, the site of origin may remain obscure in up to 50% of patients.[1,34] In all CUPS, the T-stage is taken as T0. For EBV-related disease, N-classification follows that of nasopharyngeal cancers and for HPV-positive disease, N-stage is same as that of p16 positive oropharyngeal carcinomas. In the remaining lesions, N-staging is similar to that of oral cavity cancers and takes into account extranodal extension.

Distant Metastases and Second Primary Tumors

Distant metastases are rare in early, node negative head and neck cancers and hence, routine work up for distant metastases is not required. A chest X-ray may be sufficient. The risk of distant metastases mainly depends on the nodal status as described above. Nasopharyngeal carcinoma has higher risk of distant metastases as compared to other head and neck cancers. Lung is the most common site of distant metastases; other sites are liver and bones. Patients with T4, N3 or any lymph node enlargement below thyroid should be considered for chest CT or PET-CT.[1,35] Patients with SCCA of head and neck also have 10% risk (up to 15% for tonsil or base of tongue cancers) of having second malignancy, either synchronous or metachronous.[7] It may develop in head and neck or elsewhere, such as lung and esophagus.[36]

POSITRON EMISSION TOMOGRAPHY-COMPUTED TOMOGRAPHY

As for other malignancies, positron emission tomography-computed tomography (PET-CT) is increasingly being utilized in head and neck cancers. Normal physiological uptake of FDG is common in lymphoid tissues of Waldeyer's ring, salivary glands and to some extent, mucosa of soft plate and gingiva.

PET is more likely to demonstrate a small tumor in upper aerodigestive tract than CT or MRI and hence, it is frequently used for the search of the tumor in patients presenting with cervical nodal metastases from occult primary. It identifies the primary in up to 70% of patients with occult primary; however, its sensitivity is lower for tonsil and base of tongue carcinomas.[37] In diagnosed cases, CT or MRI is sufficient for local staging and PET does not have a role.[38] PET detects more lymph node metastases than CT.[39] **(Fig. 26)**. However, less than 5 mm lymph nodes cannot be evaluated with PET and hence, it cannot exclude nodal metastases in neck. If distant metastatic work up is indicated, PET is useful to detect metastases as well as synchronous second primary tumors.

PET is highly accurate in detection of recurrences after treatment, both at the primary tumor site and the lymph nodes. PET should not be performed at least for 10 weeks after completion of treatment in order to avoid false positive results from post-treatment changes. After radiotherapy of neck nodes, persistent lymph nodes are worrisome. PET can differentiate between fibrotic and diseased lymph nodes in such situation. Thus, surveillance endoscopies and planned neck dissection can be avoided in PET negative patients.[40]

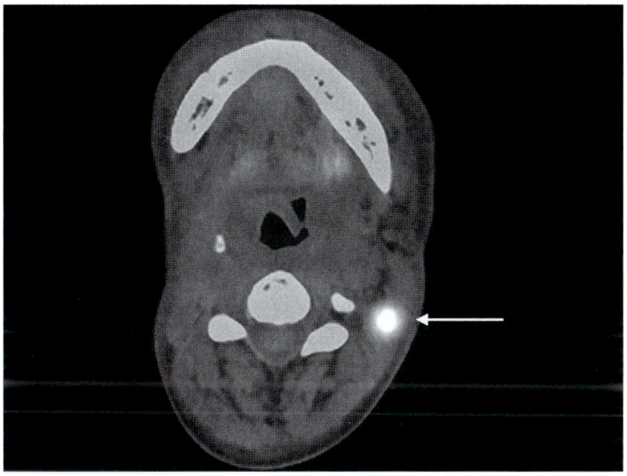

FIG. 26: Follow-up case of nasopharyngeal carcinoma. Small lymph node on left side of neck showing intense uptake on FDG PET (arrow) suggesting metastatic lymph node recurrence.

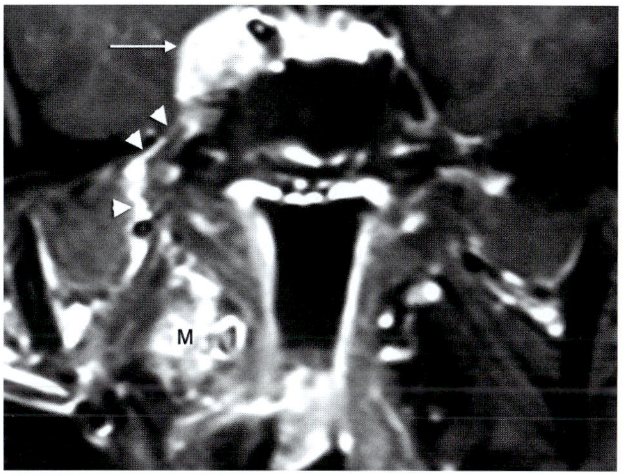

FIG. 27: Perineural tumor extension: Coronal contrast-enhanced T1-weighted MRI of a patient with oral cavity adenoid cystic carcinoma shows tumor invasion of right pterygoid muscles (M) with perineural extension seen as enhancement of thickened mandibular nerve (arrowheads) extending through the foramen ovale to cavernous sinus (arrow).

MISCELLANEOUS TUMORS

Minor Salivary Gland Tumors

These tumors arise in minor salivary glands which are normally located in buccal mucosa, tongue, floor of mouth and oropharynx, apart from sinonasal cavities. Adenoid cystic carcinoma is the most common type and others include mucoepidermoid carcinoma, adenocarcinoma, pleomorphic adenoma and mixed malignant tumors. Minor salivary gland tumors occur in elderly in fifth or sixth decade. Soft palate is the most common site where the incidence is equal to SCCA. Imaging appearances of salivary gland tumors are similar to SCCA; however, cervical lymph node involvement is uncommon.

Adenoid cystic carcinoma is characterized by extensive local invasion and its propensity for perineural spread. Perineural tumor spread is seen on CT as widening of pterygopalatine fossa and foramen rotundum (V2) or that of foramen ovale (V3). V2 involvement is more common in tumors at palate or nasopharynx while V3 involvement is more common with tumors located in oral cavity **(Figs. 8 and 27)**. Direct visualization of nerve involvement is unusual on CT. Contrast-enhanced MRI is more accurate to evaluate perineural spread and intracranial extension and should be performed in all cases of adenoid cystic carcinoma. Mucoepidermoid carcinoma may show cystic areas or calcification within it.

Rhabdomyosarcoma

Rhabdomyosarcoma is the rare malignancy which can involve any part of the body. About 30% of rhabdomyosarcoma occur in head and neck with orbit and nasopharynx as the most common sites. These usually occur in young children but can also affect adolescents and young adults.

On imaging, nasopharyngeal rhabdomyosarcoma appear similar to SCCA. These are seen as large aggressive locally infiltrating tumors with variable contrast enhancement **(Fig. 28)**. Tumor extension to sinuses and skull base erosion are the common findings.[5]

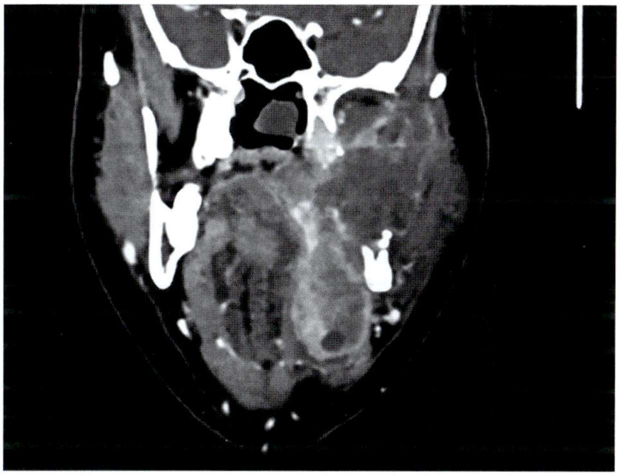

FIG. 28: Coronal reformatted image of a biopsy proven rhabdomyosarcoma patient showing large heterogeneously enhancing locally infiltrating mass lesion with extension into masticator space, parapharyngeal space as well as infratemporal fossa.

Lymphoma

Both Hodgkin's lymphoma (HL) and non-Hodgkin's lymphoma (NHL) can involve cervical lymph nodes and imaging cannot differentiate between nodes of HL and NHL. Lymphoma is the most common diagnosis in young patients presenting with unilateral enlarged neck nodes. Extranodal lymphoma in head and neck is usually NHL and it is more common in elderly. Waldeyer's ring is the most common extranodal site. Other sites of extranodal head and neck lymphoma include sino-nasal cavities, orbit, salivary glands and thyroid.[41] CT is the preferred modality for imaging evaluation of lymphoma and it should also include chest, abdomen and pelvis for baseline staging.

Waldeyer's ring is the lymphoid collection in pharyngeal mucosal space and it consists of nasopharyngeal tonsil (adenoids), palatal (oropharyngeal) tonsils and lingual (base of tongue) tonsils. Large number of patients are asymptomatic. Others have clinical symptoms similar to naso- or oropharyngeal SCCAs and include sore throat, nasal obstruction or hearing loss due to obstruction of eustachian tubes. Unlike SCCA, mucosa over the lesion is usually normal. On imaging, Waldeyer's ring lymphomas are seen as homogenous, mildly enhancing masses which tend to diffusely involve all walls of nasopharynx and spread in exophytic fashion to fill the nasopharynx, nasal cavity or oropharynx **(Figs. 29A and B)**. Invasion of deep structures is absent or minimal.[42] Associated cervical lymphadenopathy is non-necrotic. Primary lymphomas of larynx and oral cavity are extremely rare and have nonspecific imaging findings, similar to SCCA.[43]

POST-TREATMENT IMAGING

Recurrences are detected on endoscopy or imaging. Most recurrences of head and neck cancers appear within 2–3 years which may be local, nodal or both **(Fig. 30)**. Treatment of local recurrence is chemo-radiotherapy. Surgery may be used to resect the nodal recurrence or recurrent tumor confined to nasopharynx. Both surgery and radiotherapy alter the normal imaging appearance of the neck and familiarity with post-treatment changes is essential for accurate response assessment and to prevent misinterpretation of post-treatment changes as residual or recurrent disease.

Post-radiotherapy Neck

Radical (definitive) radiotherapy is the preferred treatment modality for pharyngeal and laryngeal cancers and it involves delivery of high radiation doses. Radiotherapy results in edema and fibrosis and it affects all areas of pharynx, larynx and superficial soft tissues of the neck included in radiation field. Acute effects of radiotherapy are characterized by inflammation, increased capillary permeability of small vessels and lymphatics and interstitial edema. Clinically, acute treatment sequels like sore throat, xerostomia (due to atrophy of salivary glands), mucositis and nausea are common. After 4–6 months, there is sclerosis and fibrosis of the connective tissues, obliteration of small vessels and lymphatics and resolution of the edema. Degree of these changes depends on the total radiation dose. On imaging, thickening of the skin and platysma muscle, enhancement of the mucosa and salivary glands as well as increase density and trabecular thickening of subcutaneous fat is seen in most patients 3 to 4 months after completion of radiotherapy[44] **(Fig. 31)**. In naso-oropharynx, there is thickening of posterior pharyngeal wall and edema of the retropharyngeal space. These changes may resolve or persist for several months. In larynx, radiotherapy also causes symmetric thickening of epiglottis, aryepiglottic folds, and false vocal cords. Such thickening is uncommon in

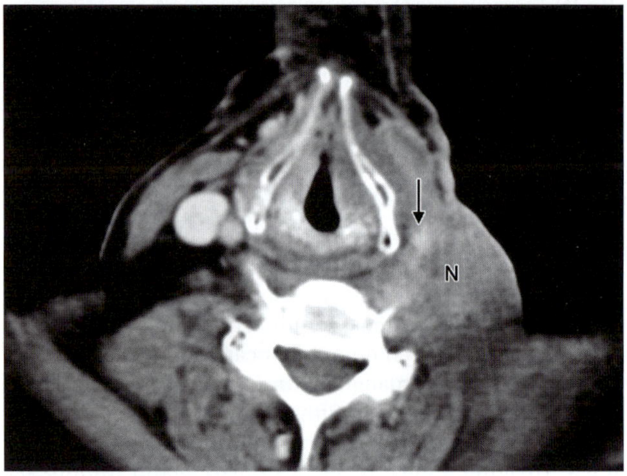

FIG. 30: Lymph nodal recurrence: Follow-up CT of a treated patient of supraglottic carcinoma shows a large ill-defined necrotic left side cervical nodal mass (N) with encasement of the carotid artery. Note the absence of internal jugular vein and the sternocleidomastoid muscle on left side secondary to the modified neck dissection which was performed for the neck treatment.

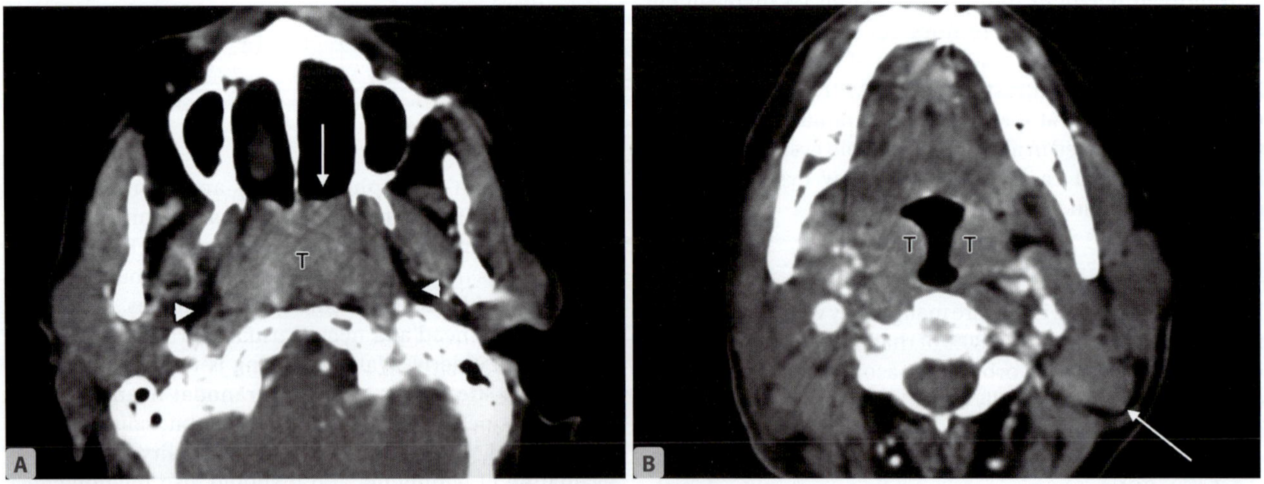

FIGS. 29A AND B: NHL of Waldeyer's ring: (A) CT shows large homogeneous mass filling entire nasopharynx (T) and extending into the nasal choanae (arrow). Note that bilateral parapharyngeal spaces are not involved (arrowheads) in spite of a large nasopharyngeal tumor; (B) CT image at caudal level shows smooth homogeneous enlargement of both tonsils (T) and enlarged left cervical lymph node (arrow).

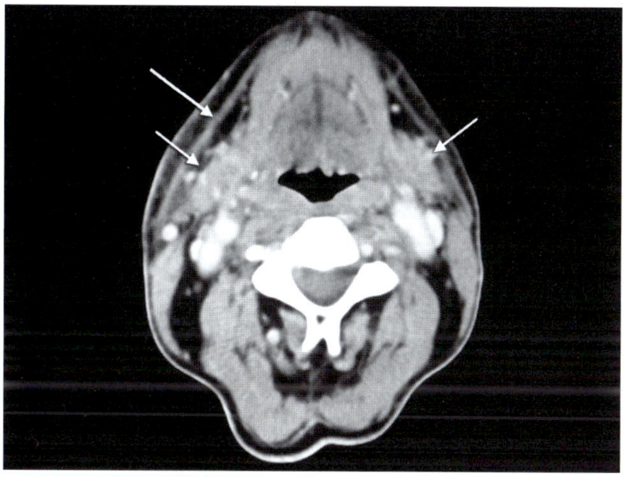

FIG. 31: Post-radiotherapy neck: CT shows diffuse increased density and trabeculations of subcutaneous fat, thickening of skin and platysma muscles (large arrow), atrophy of submandibular salivary glands (small arrows) and symmetric thickening of the pharyngeal wall.

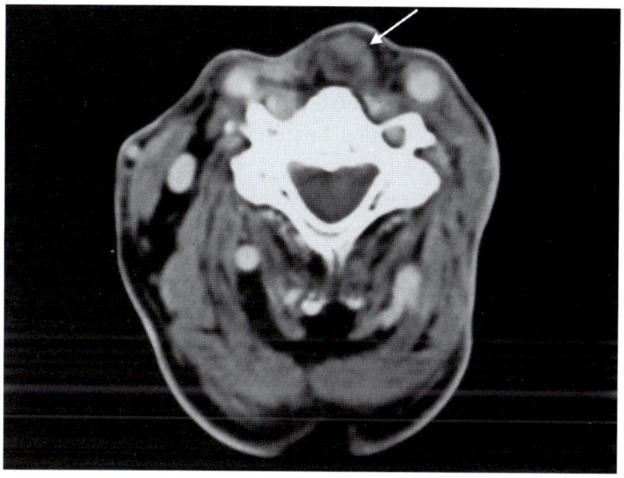

FIG. 32: Post-laryngectomy neck: CT scan after total laryngectomy shows absence of larynx with rounded contour and anterior subcutaneous bulging of the esophagus (arrow).

glottis and subglottis. These radiotherapy changes gradually resolve to variable extent.[45]

Imaging is required to assess the response to the treatment and for follow-up in patients treated with radiotherapy. A baseline post-treatment scan is obtained 3–4 months after completion of radiotherapy. The post-treatment changes and edema have attenuations less than that of muscles and the appearance remain stable on serial imaging. Any high density or enhancing mass or progressively enlarging mass is suspicious for residual or recurrent tumor. Differentiation of recurrence form fibrosis may sometimes be difficult on CT. MRI is useful in such situations but only if the scar is mature, as both tumor and the immature scar tissue are T2 hyperintense and show contrast enhancement on MRI.[46] Diffusion-weighted MRI, perfusion CT and PET-CT may help in differentiating residual/recurrent tumor from post therapy changes. Nasopharyngeal carcinoma is highly radiosensitive tumor and near complete resolution of the tumor is expected after radiotherapy. Persistent, moderately thick nasopharyngeal wall beyond 6 months increases the risk of relapse.[47] In hypopharynx and larynx, near complete resolution of the tumor indicates successful local control whereas less than 50% shrinkage of the tumor or persistent mass measuring more than 1 cm is suspicious for residual disease and biopsy is required. Other cases are indeterminate and require clinical examination and follow-up imaging to determine the stability.[48]

Late Effects of Radiotherapy

Long-term radiation complications include brain necrosis in temporal lobes, trismus due to fibrosis of masticator muscles and atrophy of salivary glands. Uncommon complications of radiotherapy include soft tissue necrosis and osteochondronecrosis. These may occur during radiotherapy or several months after radiotherapy. It may be seen as sclerosis, fragmentation and sloughing of the cartilage or bone, osteomyelitis and fistula formation.[49] On imaging, these findings cannot be reliably differentiated from recurrent tumor. Biopsy is required and if it is negative, a close imaging follow-up is necessary.[18]

Radiation induced tumors are rare and occur several years, at least 5 years, later. Sarcoma is the usual radiation induced tumor. Osteosarcoma is the most common bone sarcoma while malignant fibrous histiocytoma is the most common soft tissue sarcoma. Other radiation induced tumors include meningioma, glioma, thyroid tumors, chondrosarcoma, malignant peripheral nerve sheath tumor and squamous cell carcinoma. Heterogeneous well enhancing mass with bone destruction seen in radiation field, after a latency period of at least 5 years is a useful clue to the diagnosis of radiation induced sarcoma.[50]

Postoperative Neck

Variety of surgical procedures may be employed for the treatment of pharyngeal tumors. Anatomical alterations and depend on type and extent of surgical resection and this information should be available for interpretation of post-operative scans. Postoperative pharyngeal wall is typically thin and smooth. Myocutaneous flap reconstructions are seen as fatty, bulky areas. Neck dissection is a common procedure for the management of cervical lymph nodes and exact postoperative appearance depends on the type of neck dissection procedure.

In total laryngectomy, entire larynx with thyroid and cricoid cartilages and hyoid bone are removed. With no anterior firm structures, pharynx and esophagus are more anteriorly located and appear prominent **(Fig. 32)**. With supraglottic laryngectomy, glottis, cricoid cartilage and contralateral thyroid cartilage are retained. The pharynx is more distended and if not resected, hyoid bone may be seen at the same level as glottis. After hemilaryngectomy, ipsilateral vocal cord, arytenoids cartilage and part of the thyroid cartilages can be seen missing on CT.

Acute postoperative changes (granulation and immature scar tissue) show contrast enhancement on CT and MRI and cannot be differentiated from residual tumor. These changes resolve subsequently. Similar to the post-radiotherapy follow-up, a baseline postoperative scan is obtained and used to compare with subsequent follow-up scans. Recurrent tumor is suspected if there is a progressively enlarging or enhancing mass at the primary tumor site or at the resection margin or appearance of a new lymph node **(*see* Figs. 29A and B)**.

REFERENCES

1. Mendenhall WM, Werning JW, Pfister DG. Treatment of head and neck cancers. In: DeVita VT, Lawrence TS, Rosenberg SA (Eds). Cancer: Principles and Practice of Oncology. 8th edition, Philadelphia, Lippincott Williams and Wilkins 2008;799-877.
2. Huang SH, O'Sullivan B. Overview of the 8th Edition TNM Classification for Head and Neck Cancer.Curr Treat Options Oncol. 2017;18(7):40.
3. Lydiatt WM, Patel SG, O'Sullivan B, Brandwein MS, Ridge JA, Migliacci JC, Loomis AM, Shah JP. Head and Neck cancers-major changes in the American Joint Committee on cancer eighth edition cancer staging manual. CA Cancer J Clin. 2017;67(2):122-37.
4. National Cancer Registry Program three year report of PBCRs 2012-2014. Report of population based cancer registries, Indian Council of Medical Research, New Delhi, 2016
5. Mukherji SK, Fatterpekar G, Chong VF. Malignancies of the oral cavity. In: Brag DG, Rubin P, Hricak H (Eds). Oncologic Imaging, 2nd edition, Philadelphia, WB Saunders Co. 2002;202-31.
6. Kimura Y, Sumi M, Sumi T et al. Deep extension from carcinoma arising from gingival: CT and MR imaging features. AJNR 2002:23;468-72.
7. Ginsberg LE, DeMonte F.Imaging of perineural tumor spread from palatal carcinoma. AJNR 1998;22:14-7.
8. Imaizumi A, Yoshino N, Yamada I, et al. A potential pitfall of MR imaging for assessing mandibular invasion of squamous cell carcinoma in the oral cavity. AJNR 2006;27:114-22.
9. Stambuk HE, Karimi S. Oral cavity and oropharynx tumors. Radiol Clin N Am 2007;45:1-20.
10. Campbell RSD, Baker E, Chippindale AJ, et al. MRI T staging of squamous cell carcinoma of the oral cavity. Radiological pathological correlation. Clin Radiol. 1995;50:533-40.
11. Wiener E, Pautke C, Link TM, et al. Comparison of 16 slice MSCT and MRI in the assessment of squamous cell carcinoma of oral cavity. Eur J Radiol. 2006;24:4371-6.
12. Deo SVS, Purkayastha J, Das DK, et al. Reconstruction of complex oral defects using bi-paddle pectoralis major flap-technical modifications and outcome in 54 patients. Indian Journal of Otolaryngology and Head and Neck Surgery 2003;55:1-9.
13. Sham JST, Cheung YK, Choy D. Cranial nerve involvement and base of skull erosion in nasopharyngeal carcinoma. Cancer 1996;68:422-7.
14. Chong VFH, Fan YF, hoo JBK. MRI features of cervical nodal metastases in metastatic disease. Clin Radiol. 1996;51:103-8.
15. Sham JST, Cheung YK, Chan FL. Nasopharyngeal carcinoma: patterns of skeletal metastases. Br J Radiol. 1990;63:202-07.
16. Stambuk HE, Patel SG, Mosier KM, et al. Nasopharyngeal carcinoma: recognizing the radiographic features in children. AJNR 2005;26:1575-9.
17. Castelijns JA, Becker M, Hermans R. The impact of cartilage invasion on treatment and prognosis of laryngeal cancer. Eur Radiol. 1996;6:156-69.
18. Yousem DM, Tufano RP. Laryngeal imaging. Radiol Clin N Am 2004;14:611-24.
19. Baker M, Zbarin P, Delavelle J, et al. Neoplastic invasion of the laryngeal cartilage: Reassessment of criteria for diagnosis at CT. Radiology 1997;203:521-32.
20. Mancuso AA, Mukerji SK, Schmalfuss I, et al. Preradiotherapy computed tomography as a predictor of local control in supraglottic carcinoma. J Clin Oncol 1999;17:631-7.
21. Mendenhall WM, Werning JW, Hinerman RW, et al. Management of T1 and T2 glottic carcinoma. Cancer 2004;100:1786-9.
22. Som PM. Detection of metastases in cervical lymph nodes: CT and MR criteria and differential diagnosis. AJR 1992;158:961-9.
23. Som PM, Brandwein MS. Lymph nodes. In: Som PM, Curtin HD (Eds). Head and Neck Imaging. 4th edition. St Louis, Mosby 2003;1865-934.
24. Curtin H, Ishwaran H, Mancuso A, et al. Comparison of CT and MR imaging in staging of neck metastases. Radiology 1998;207: 123-30.
25. Casteljins JA, Van Den Brekel MW, Mukherji SK, Lameris JS. Ultrasound of the neck. In: Som PM, Curtin HD (Eds). Head and Neck Imaging. 4th edition. St Louis, Mosby 2003;1935-53.
26. Ahuja A, Ying M. Sonography of neck lymph nodes. Clin Radiol. 2003;58:359-66.
27. Knappe M, Louw M, Gregor KT. Ultrasonography guided fine needle aspiration for the assessment of cervical metastases. Arch Otolaryngol Head Neck Surg. 2000;126:1091-6.
28. DeBondt RB, Nelemans PJ, Hofman PA, et al. Detection of lymph node metastases in head and neck cancer: meta-analysis comprising US, USFNAC, CT and MR imaging. Eur J Radiol. 2007;64:266-72.
29. Sigal R, Vogl T, Casselman J, et al. Lymph node metastases from head and neck squamous cell carcinoma: MR imaging with ultra small superparamagnetic iron oxide particle—results of a phase III multicenter clinical trial. Eur Radiol. 2002;12:1104-13.
30. Ross GL, Soutar DS, Gordon MD, et al. Sentinel node biopsy in head and neck cancer: preliminary results of a multicenter trial. Ann Surg Oncol 2004;11:690-6.
31. King AD. Mutlimodality imaging of head and neck cancers. Cancer Imaging. 2007;7:S37-S46.
32. Nieuwenhuis EJ, Castelijns JA, Pijpers R, et al. Wait and see policy for the N0 neck in early stage oral and oropharyngeal squamous cell carcinoma using ultrasonographically guided cytology: is there a role for identification of sentinel node? Head Neck 2002;24:282-9.
33. Schmalbach CE, Miller FR. Occult primary head and neck carcinoma. Curr Oncol Rep 2007;9:139-46.
34. Cianchetti M, Mancuso AA, Amdur RJ, et al. Diagnostic evaluation of squamous cell carcinoma metastatic to cervical lymph nodes from an unknown head and neck primary site. Laryngoscope 2009;119:2348-54.
35. Loh KS, Brown DH, Baker JT, et al. A rational approach to pulmonary screening in newly diagnosed head and neck cancer. Head Neck 2005;27:990-94.
36. Erkal HS, Mendenhall WM, Amdur RJ, et al. Synchronous and metachronous squamous cell carcinomas of the head and neck mucosal sites. J Clin Oncol 2001;19:1358-61.
37. Dong MJ, Zhao K, Lin XT, et al. Role of fluorodeoxyglucose PET versus fluorodeoxyglucose PET/computed tomography in detection of unknown primary tumor: meta-analysis of the literature. Nucl Med Commun. 2008;29:791-802.

38. Dammann F, Horger M, Berg MM, et al. Rational diagnosis of squamous cell carcinoma of head and neck region: comparative evaluation of CT, MRI and 18FDG PET. AJR 2005;184: 1326-31.
39. Syed R, Bomanji JB, Nagabhushan N, et al. Impact of combined 18F-FDG PET/CT in head and neck tumors. Br J Cancer 2005;92:1046-50.
40. Isle MG, McConkey C, Mehanna. A systematic review and meta-analysis of the role of positron emission tomography in the follow- up of head and neck squamous cell carcinoma following radiotherapy or chemotherapy. Clin Otolaryngol. 2008;33: 210-22.
41. Aiken AH, Glastonbury C. Imaging Hodgkin and non-Hodgkin lymphoma in head and neck. Radiol Clin N Am. 2008;46:363-78.
42. King AD, Lei KI, Richards PS, et al. Non-Hodgkin's lymphoma of the nasopharynx. CT and MR imaging. Clin Radiol. 2003;58:621-25.
43. King AD, Yeun EH, Lei K, et al. Non-Hodgkin lymphoma of the larynx: CT and MR imaging findings. Am J Neuroradiol. 2004;25:12-15.
44. Mukherji SK, Mancuso AA, Kotzur IM, et al. Radiographic appearance of the irradiated larynx. Radiology 1994;193: 141-48.
45. Curtin HD. The larynx. In: Som PM, Curtin HD (Eds). Head and Neck Imaging. 4th edition. St Louis, Mosby 2003;1595-1698.
46. Chong VHF, Fan YF. Detection of recurrent nasopharyngeal cancer. CT vs MR imaging. Radiology 1997;202:453-70.
47. Luo D, Zhou C, Li E, et al. Post radiation CT changes and recurrent nasopharyngeal carcinoma. Chin Med J. 2008;121: 916-22.
48. Hermans R, Parneljer FA, Mancuso AA, et al. Laryngeal or hypopharyngeal squamous cell carcinoma: can follow up CT after definitive radiation therapy be used to detect local failure earlier than clinical examination alone? Radiology 2000;214: 683-87.
49. Hermans R. Imaging of mandibular osteoradionecrosis. NeuroimagClin N Am 2003;13:597-604.
50. Makimoto Y, Yamamoto S, Takano H, et al. Imaging finding of radiation sarcoma of head and neck. Br J Radiol 2007;790-7.

CHAPTER

206

Imaging of Skull Base Lesions

Atin Kumar, Manisha Jana, Priyanka Naranje, Ashu Seith Bhalla

INTRODUCTION

In general, skull base is inaccessible to clinical evaluation. Hence, the clinicians are dependent on the radiological assessment of this region for planning treatment and surgical approach.[1] However, the radiologist needs to be familiar with the complex anatomy of the skull base and also the correct imaging protocols so as to enable him to correctly diagnose and accurately delineate the lesions involving it.

ANATOMICAL DIVISION[2]

When viewed from above, the floor of the calvaria appears to be divided into three naturally contoured regions: (1) the anterior, (2) middle and (3) posterior cranial fossae. However, when viewed from below, the margins between the three fossae are indistinct.

- The anterior skull base is the part of base of skull lying anterior to a line that follows the tuberculum sella, the anterior clinoid processes, the posterior margins of the lesser sphenoid wings and the anterior and superior rim of the greater sphenoid wings.
- The part behind this line is the middle skull base which in turn is separated from the posterior skull base by a line following the spheno-occipital synchondrosis medially and the petroclival synchondrosis and the superior ridge of the petrous and mastoid bones posteriorly and laterally **(Fig. 1)**.

In this chapter, we will discuss the relevant radiological anatomy and the lesions involving each division of skull base separately. However, there may be some lesions like those arising from tissues common to all skull base compartments such as bone, meninges and sinuses which can involve any of the divisions or may diffusely involve the skull base. Some lesions may simultaneously involve more than one division.

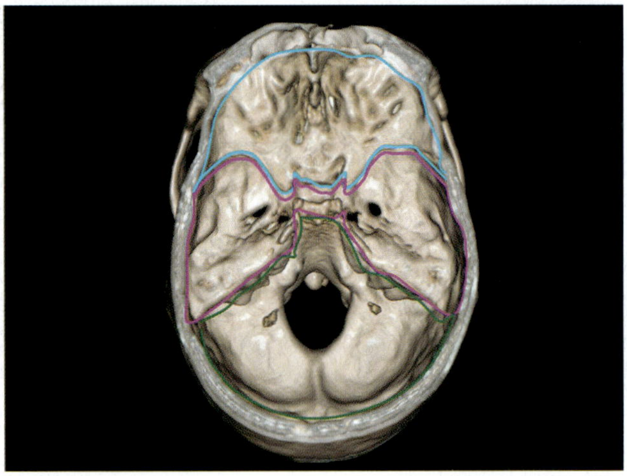

FIG. 1: Surface shaded display CT reconstruction of skull base as viewed from top shows division of skull base into anterior compartment (outlined by blue), middle compartment (outlined by pink) and posterior compartment (outlined by green).

IMAGING TECHNIQUES AND THEIR ROLE

Conventional radiographs of the skull base done in earlier decades have now given way to cross-sectional imaging by CT and MRI. The cross-sectional imaging techniques are useful for localizing the lesion, narrowing the differential diagnosis based on the site of origin, pattern of growth and the imaging features of a given lesion, correctly delineating the lesion margins and its relation to surrounding structures so as to enable treatment planning and are also helpful for follow up of these patients.[3]

CT and MR have a complimentary role in the imaging of skull base and are often used together.[4] CT is the technique of choice for delineation of fine bony details, especially the thin cortical margins of the skull base neurovascular foramina. CT is highly specific in diagnosis of neoplastic as well as non-neoplastic bone lesions, can distinguish aggressive from a benign lesion by delineating the pattern of bone involvement and can depict calcification better than MR. Infectious processes, malignant neoplasms and aggressive rapidly growing lesions lead to permeative and erosive pattern of bone involvement whereas benign slow-growing lesions cause bone expansion and remodeling with cortical thinning.

CT studies of the skull base should be acquired on a multidetector CT scanner with minimum 0.5 mm reconstruction. An acquisition in the axial plane with reconstructions in other planes (coronal and sagittal) should be done. The images should be reconstructed in both soft tissue and high resolution bone algorithm. Contrast imaging should be done in case of evaluation of mass lesions to best assess tumor vascularity, margins, relation to adjacent structures and to obtain perfusion studies which may help to differentiate benign from malignant conditions. Contrast-enhanced images should be evaluated in soft tissue algorithm. However, contrast administration may be obviated if the CT is being done as an adjunct to contrast enhanced MR evaluation.

MR imaging is more sensitive than CT to assess the soft tissue component. It is the modality of choice to detect the intracranial extent including invasion of the dura, leptomeninges, cranial nerves and brain parenchyma. MR imaging is also good for detecting perineural and perivascular spread and bone marrow involvement. Utility of CT and MRI in evaluation of skull base lesions is summarized in **Table 1**.

MR protocol **(Box 1)** should include 3D sequences of a T1-weighted without fat saturation, T2-weighted with fat saturation and balanced steady-state free precession (CISS).[5] The images should be obtained with small field of view, high resolution and isotropic resolution. It should be remembered that skull base has multiple interfaces and hence is extremely susceptible to artifacts from tissue inhomogeneity. Therefore, fat suppression may be a problem sometimes. Contrast administration is required for evaluation of infections, tumors and cranial nerve assessment. A 3D T1-weighted VIBE sequence with fat saturation and 3D CISS sequence should be obtained after contrast. Angiography has a limited role in evaluation of vascular lesions and hypervascular tumors.[6,7]

TABLE 1: Utility of CT and MRI in evaluation of skull base lesions.

CT	MRI
Fine bony details	Assessment of soft tissue component
Walls of skull base neurovascular foramina	Intracranial extension; Invasion of dura, leptomeninges cranial nerves, brain parenchyma
Pattern of bone destruction	Detecting perineural and perivascular spread
Depiction of calcification	Bone marrow involvement

Box 1: MRI protocol for skull base.

Precontrast:
- T1 axial and coronal
- T2 axial and coronal
- 3D T1W sequence without fat suppression (VIBE)
- 3D T2W sequence with fat suppression (STIR SPACE)
- 3D steady-state free precession imaging (CISS)

Postcontrast:
- 3D T1W sequence with fat suppression (VIBE with FS)
- 3D CISS

At our institute it is mainly reserved for interventional procedures like embolization of hypervascular tumors such as juvenile nasopharyngeal angiofibromas, paragangliomas, hemangiopericytomas, etc. Positron emission imaging with FDG is useful in differentiating residual/recurrent neoplasm from post-treatment changes in the follow-up of skull base tumors.

ANTERIOR SKULL BASE

Anatomy

The anterior skull base forms the bottom of the anterior skull, i.e. the floor of the anterior cranial fossa. It is formed by the roof of the nasal cavity and the ethmoid sinuses in the median plane with the roof of the orbits on either side of the median plane. It extends from the posterior wall of the frontal sinus anteriorly to the lesser wing of sphenoid bone posteriorly. The roof of the nasal cavity is formed by the thin cribriform plate of the ethmoid bone which has multiple small perforations transmitting olfactory nerves from the nasal mucosa to the olfactory bulb **(Fig. 2)**. Fracture of this plate (most commonly at the lateral lamella where the anterior ethmoidal artery enters the skull base) either by trauma or by instrumentation during functional endoscopic sinus surgery is a common cause for cerebrospinal fluid (CSF) leaks. The orbital plate of the frontal bone forming the roof of the orbits is comparatively thick and sturdy and relatively resistant to erosions.

Pathology

The anterior skull base may be involved by number of pathologies **(Table 2)** arising from the bones of the skull base proper, exocranially from the sinonasal mucosa, olfactory mucosa and orbit, intracranially from the meningeal coverings, or from the vessels and nerves passing through this region including the olfactory nerve. The involvement can also be secondary to trauma (fractures) or congenital defects leading to cephaloceles. Most of the tumors presenting in this region show similar radiological features. Hence, it is often very difficult to differentiate between them based on

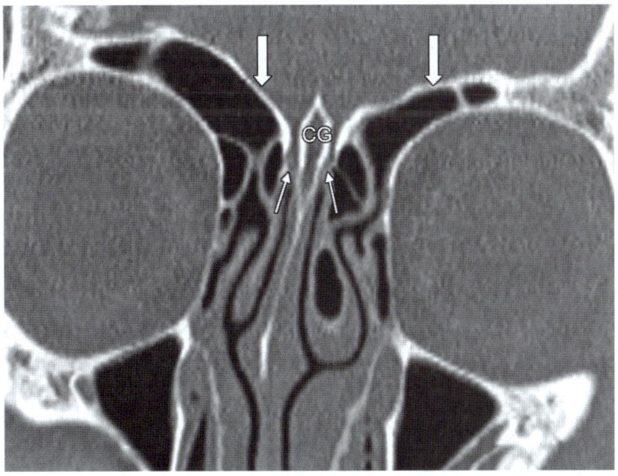

FIG. 2: Coronal CT image of anterior skull base. Crista Galli (CG), cribriform plate (thin arrows), orbital plate of frontal bone (block arrows).

radiology and not possible to give specific diagnosis. The role of imaging should be to comment upon the lesion resectability, bony involvement, invasion of meninges and brain parenchyma, and extension into the orbit and into the neurovascular structures, including the cavernous sinuses. The dural involvement is evident radiologically as thickness of more than 5 mm or nodular thickening whereas brain parenchymal involvement is evident as edema with or without contrast enhancement.[8] Orbital involvement occurs most often through the lamina papyracea. The strong periorbita resists intraorbital invasion for long. However periorbital breach requires orbital exenteration. Involvement of the orbital apex also has serious prognostic implications: tumor reaching orbital apex can also extend into middle cranial fossa via the superior orbital fissure and surgical excision in this region usually requires sacrificing of optic nerve and eye. The nasal cavity and sinus tumors commonly extend across skull base to involve the anterior cranial fossa. In contrast the orbital tumors are rarely seen to breach the orbital roof to involve the anterior cranial fossa.

TABLE 2: Anterior skull base lesions.

Lesions arising from below	
Sinonasal lesions	• Esthesioneuroblastoma
	• Squamous cell carcinoma
	• Adenocarcinoma
	• Adenoid cystic carcinomas
	• Melanoma
	• Lymphoma
	• Sarcomas
	• Juvenile nasopharyngeal angiofibroma
	• Mucocele
	• Other miscellaneous lesions:
	• Sinonasal polyposis, osteomyelitis, fungal sinusitis GPA
Orbital lesions	• Lacrimal gland tumors
	• Neurogenic tumors, lymphoma, sarcomas, metastases
Lesions arising from above	
	• Olfactory groove meningioma
	• Schwannoma
	• Encephalocele
Lesions of the proper skull base	
	• Trauma and CSF leak
	• Osteoma

(GPA: granulomatosis polyangiitis; CSF: cerebrospinal fluid).

Lesions Arising from Below

Sinonasal Lesions

Esthesioneuroblastoma

Also known as olfactory neuroblastomas as they arise in olfactory epithelium. They are similar to other neural crest tumors like neuroblastomas, PNET and small cell lung carcinomas.[9] They have bimodal age distribution affecting in second and fifth decades of life.[10] They appear hyperdense on plain CT and show homogenously enhancing solid mass in the roof of the nasal cavity with possible destruction of the cribriform plate and intracranial extension **(Figs. 3A and B)**. They show intermediate signal intensity on T1- and T2-weighted images on MRI. Larger lesions with intracranial extension may show a specific feature of peripheral tumor cysts at the margins, especially at the interface with brain parenchyma.[11] Calcification may also be seen.

Squamous Cell Carcinoma

Most common epithelial neoplasm of this region. Average age at presentation is 50 years with male predominance.[9] They are aggressive lesions showing bone destruction, intermediate T2 signal (high cellularity), necrosis and hemorrhage and homogeneous contrast enhancement (slightly less than normal mucosa). Contrast enhancement differentiates it from mucoceles which do not enhance.

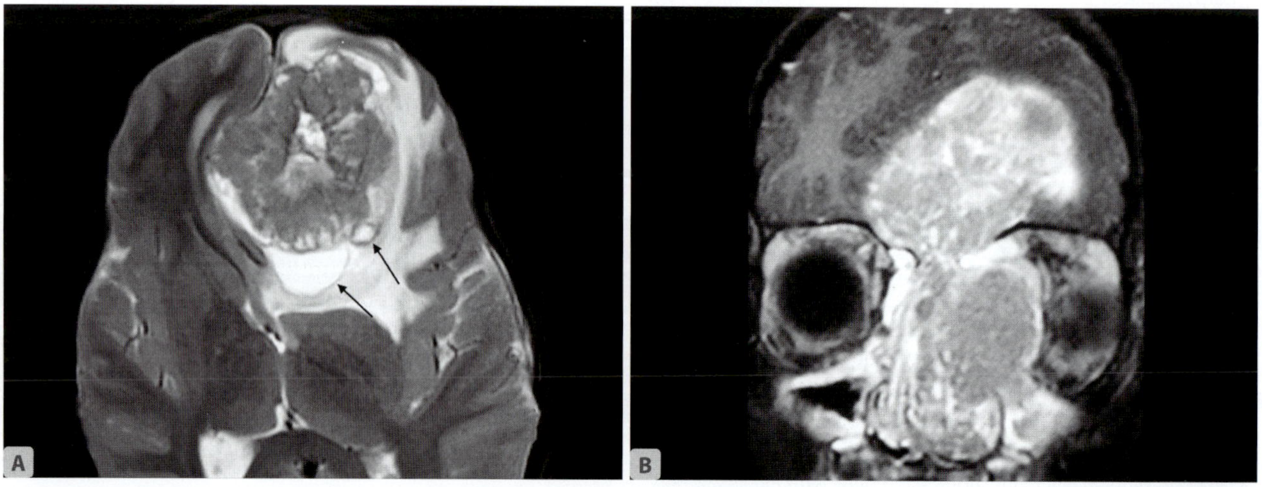

FIGS. 3A AND B: Esthesioneuroblastoma. (A) T2W axial MRI showing a large isointense intracranial extra-axial mass lesion with presence of T2W hyperintense cysts at tumor—brain interface (arrows); (B) Coronal contrast-enhanced MR image reveals avid contrast enhancement of the mass.

Adenocarcinoma

Seen in elderly males. It is difficult to differentiate them radiologically from the more common squamous cell carcinomas but in general, the adenocarcinomas show a less aggressive pattern of bone involvement evident as remodeling and thinning rather than permeative bone destruction.

Adenoid Cystic Carcinomas

These tumors arise from minor salivary glands of the hard palate with spread to involve the paranasal sinuses. They are slow but steady growing lesions which have a strong propensity for perineural spread, trigeminal nerve involvement being most common in this region. These tumors exhibit T2 prolongation with areas of remodeling and destruction.

Melanoma

Presents from fifth to eighth decade with equal preponderance in men and women. Radiological features include bone remodeling, intense contrast enhancement and areas of T1 hyperintensity due to melanin or hemorrhage.

Lymphoma

B cell lymphoma involves paranasal sinuses and presents as bulky expansile mass eroding bones and adjacent soft tissues. T cell lymphoma involves the midline nasal septum with aggressive features of bone destruction in excess of involvement of soft tissues. The differential diagnosis includes granulomatous polyangitis (GPA) and cocaine abuse.

Sarcomas

Rhabdomyosarcoma (pediatric age group), Ewing's sarcoma and chondrosarcoma can also rarely involve the sinonasal region.

Juvenile Nasopharyngeal Angiofibroma

They are benign, highly vascular tumors seen in adolescent males. They arise in the nasopharyngeal region from primitive vascular tissue at sphenopalatine foramen. They are aggressive tumors which infiltrate through foramens and fissures to involve the orbits and intracranial compartment. They involve central skull base more often than anterior skull base.

Mucocele

It is a benign lesion occurring in sinonasal region with frontal sinus more commonly involved than the ethmoidal sinuses. It is formed by obstruction of sinus ostium with resultant expansion of the sinus with secretions. CT confirms the diagnosis. MR may show peripheral enhancement on contrast administration.

Other Miscellaneous Lesions

Sinonasal polyposis, osteomyelitis, fungal sinusitis **(Figs. 4A to D)**, GPA may also extend to involve the anterior skull base after having origin from the sinonasal region.

Orbital Lesions

Lacrimal Gland Tumors

They appear as mass lesions in the superolateral compartment of the orbit anteriorly. They may cause erosion of the orbital roof with subsequent extension into the anterior cranial fossa.

Other Tumors

Rarely neurogenic tumors, lymphoma, sarcomas, leukemic deposits (chloroma) **(Figs. 5A to D)**, metastases arising in orbits may also extend to involve anterior skull base.

Lesions Arising from Above

Olfactory Groove Meningioma

It is the most common intracranial lesion affecting the anterior skull base from above. Radiologically, they appear as well-circumscribed, T1 and T2 isointense, intensely enhancing extra-axial masses with dural tail, with or without calcification **(Fig. 6)**. They may extend exocranially through the cribriform plate. They may also produce characteristic reactive bony sclerosis in the adjacent bone.

Schwannoma

It is a rare tumor at this region which arises from olfactory nerve or from meningeal branch of fifth cranial nerve. On imaging it appears as a benign well-defined lesion with intense contrast enhancement and is difficult to differentiate from olfactory groove meningioma.

Encephalocele

Frontal meningoencephaloceles are rare congenital anomalies that are divided into sincipital and basal types. The sincipital meningoencephaloceles are located anteriorly and are extranasal masses (nasofrontal, nasoethmoidal or nasoorbital) while basal meningoencephaloceles are located posteriorly and usually occur in ethmoid/sphenoid region.[12-14] Imaging by CT or MR help to confirm the diagnosis by noting the skull base defect and the contents of the mass **(Figs. 7A and B)**. Meningoceles have fluid following CSF signal intensity on all sequences while cephaloceles have brain parenchyma following gray matter signal. Correct diagnosis should avert a biopsy.

Lesions of the Proper Skull Base

Trauma and Cerebrospinal Fluid Leak

At the anterior skull base there is dense adhesion of the dura to the bone. Hence fractures of the anterior skull base (most commonly of cribriform plate, fovea ethmoidalis or posterior table of frontal sinus)[15] after trauma also cause dural tear leading to complications of CSF rhinorrhea **(Figs. 8A to C)**, pneumocephalus **(Figs. 9A to C)** and brain herniation. Olfactory nerve injury is also known complication of anterior skull base trauma. Thin section high resolution CT can detect the small defect. Anatomical classification of frontabasal fractures are divided into three types.[16,17]

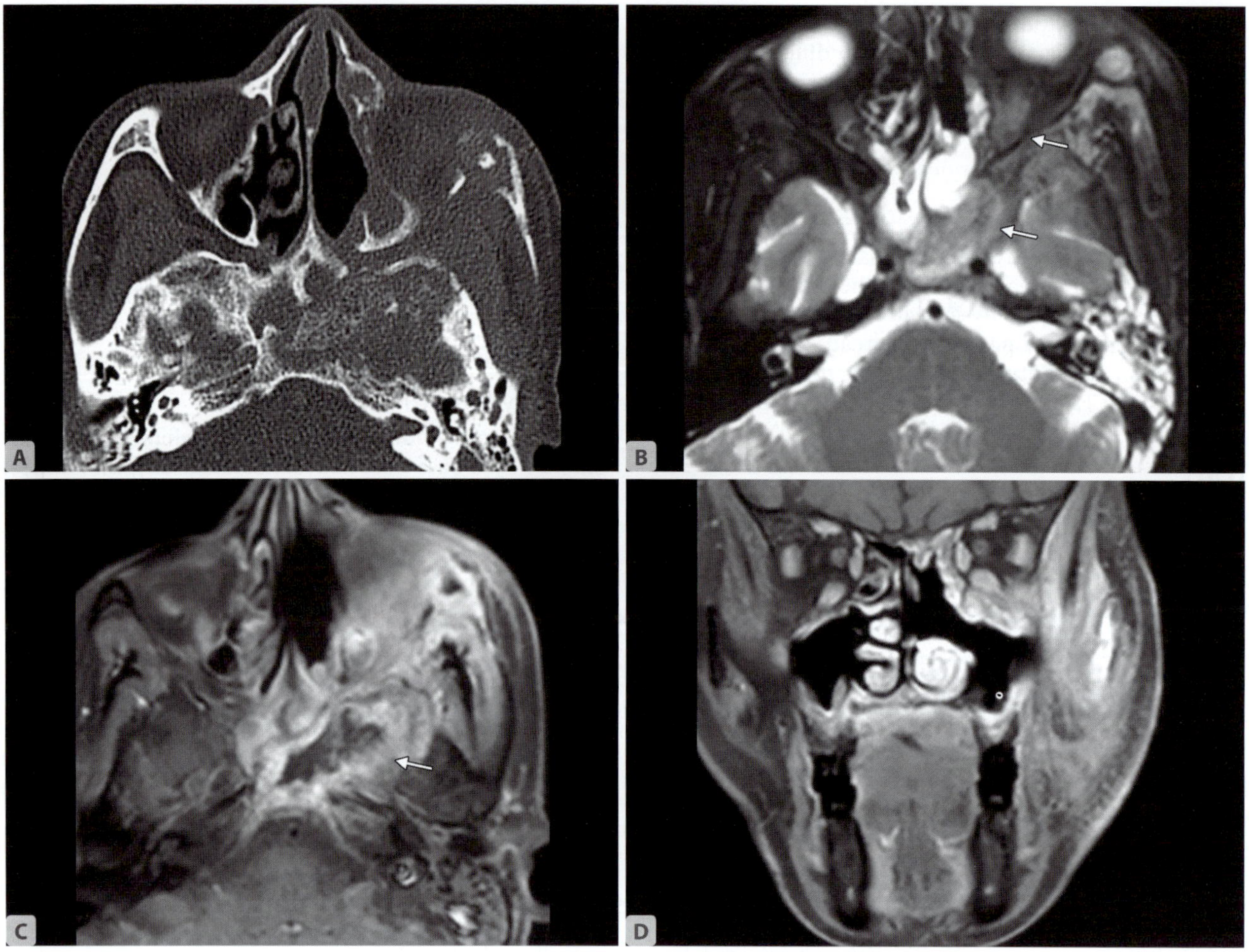

FIGS. 4A TO D: Invasive fungal infection with intracranial extension: Axial CT bone window (A) image shows destruction of the left sphenoid wing, left zygoma and left lateral nasal wall. T2-weighted (B) axial MR image reveals a hypointense mass in left orbital apex and cavernous sinus location (arrows). Contrast-enhanced T1-weighted axial (C) and coronal (D) MR images show a heterogeneous peripheral enhancement of the lesion, and destruction of left side superior and middle turbinates.

Detailed description of it is beyond the scope of this chapter. MRI with cisternography enables differentiating the contents of the herniated tissue. In doubtful cases CT cisternography after intrathecal contrast injection or radionuclide cisternography may help.

Osteoma

Osteomas are benign bone tumors found most commonly in membranous bones of skull and face, commonly within frontal and ethmoidal sinuses. They can be diagnosed on radiograph and confirmed on CT.

MIDDLE SKULL BASE

Anatomy

The middle cranial fossa is limited by the greater wings of sphenoid bone anteriorly and the anterior surface of the petrous bone posteriorly. Cavernous sinus within the sphenoid body forms the medial border whereas the squamous temporal bone forms the lateral border. Sella turcica is a large depression in the body of the sphenoid bone and the sphenoid sinus lies below the sella turcica. The clivus forms the posteromedial boundary. The middle cranial fossa has multiple openings of foramens and fissures which are best demonstrated on CT **(Figs. 10A and B)**. The optic canal passes through the lesser wing of the sphenoid bone to open posteriorly into the middle cranial fossa and transmits the optic nerve and the ophthalmic artery. The superior orbital fissure lies between the lesser wing of sphenoid bone superiorly and greater wing inferiorly and is bordered medially by the sphenoid body. It transmits cranial nerves III, IV, V1, and V2 and the superior ophthalmic vein from the cavernous sinus posteriorly to the orbit anteriorly. Foramen rotundum lies inferior to the superior orbital fissure and transmits the cranial nerve V2 from the cavernous sinus posteriorly to the pterygopalatine fossa anteriorly. The vidian canal, lying between the sphenoid body and the pterygoid process, transmits the vidian nerve and the vidian artery between the foramen lacerum and pterygopalatine fossa. The foramen ovale lies in the posterolateral part of the greater wing and transmits cranial nerve V3 from the middle cranial fossa to the masticator space. The foramen spinosum is a

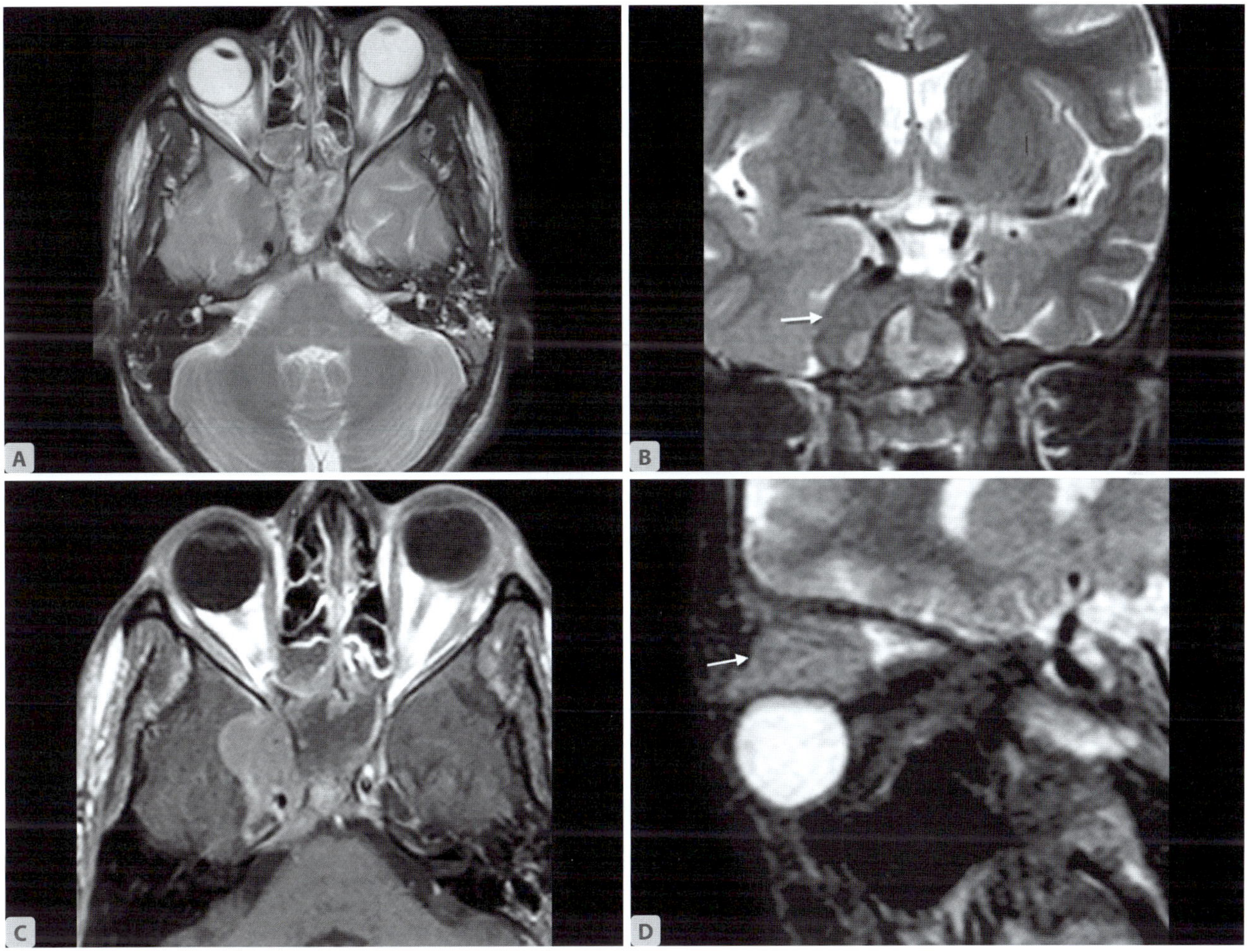

FIGS. 5A TO D: Chloroma in a 40-year-old lady with AML: Axial (A) and coronal (B) T2W MR images show hypointense mass involving right cavernous sinus and parasellar region (arrow). T1W postcontrast MR image (C) shows avid contrast enhancement. Sagittal T2W image (D) of the orbit reveals another deposit (arrow) in the left lacrimal fossa having the same signal intensity.

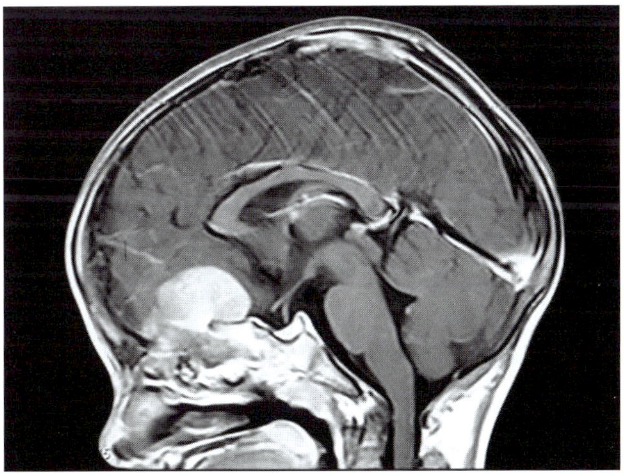

FIG. 6: Meningioma: Postcontrast T1-weighted sagittal MR image shows a homogeneously enhancing dural-based mass at the floor of anterior cranial fossa.

smaller foramen located just posterolateral to foramen ovale and transmits the middle meningeal artery. The cavernous sinus contains the carotid artery and the cranial nerve VI within it and cranial nerves III, IV, V1 and V2 (from superior to inferior) enclosed within the dural leaflet of its lateral wall.

Pathology

The middle skull base may be affected by lesions arising from skull base proper, from the intracranial compartment or from the extracranial compartment. It may also be involved by systemic conditions.

The lesions may extend into the middle cranial fossa from below through the existing foramina in the sphenoid bone or by direct erosion. Spread through these foramina is clinically evident by involvement of the nerves passing through them and is radiologically evident as widening of these foramina. Difference in size of more than 4 mm between the two foramen ovale is considered as abnormal. Foramen spinosum size of

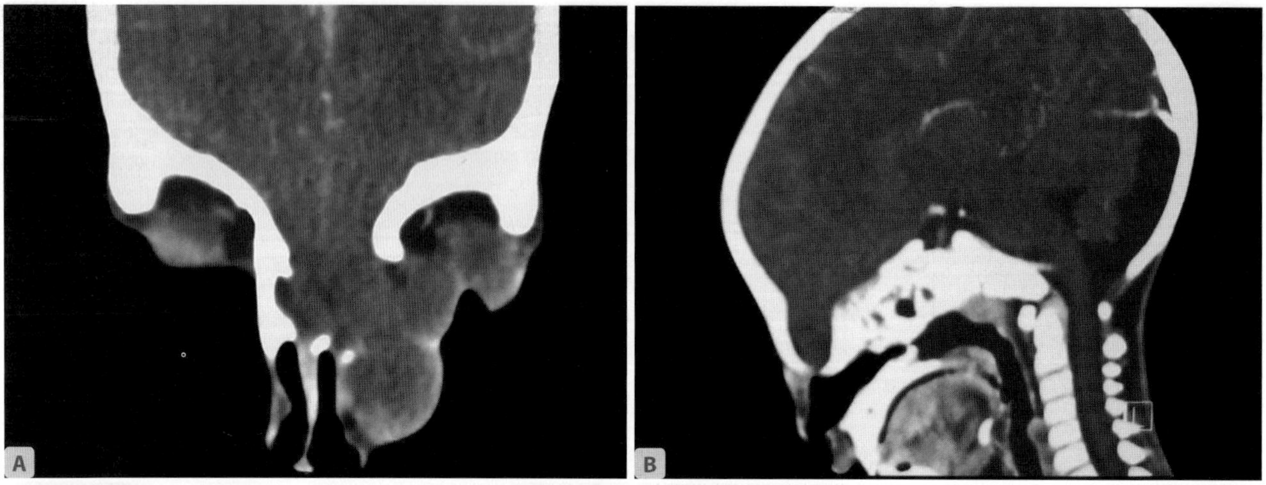

FIGS. 7A AND B: Cephalocele: Coronal MPR (A) and sagittal MPR (B) images of CT show a defect in the floor of anterior skull base on left side with herniation of brain parenchyma downwards.

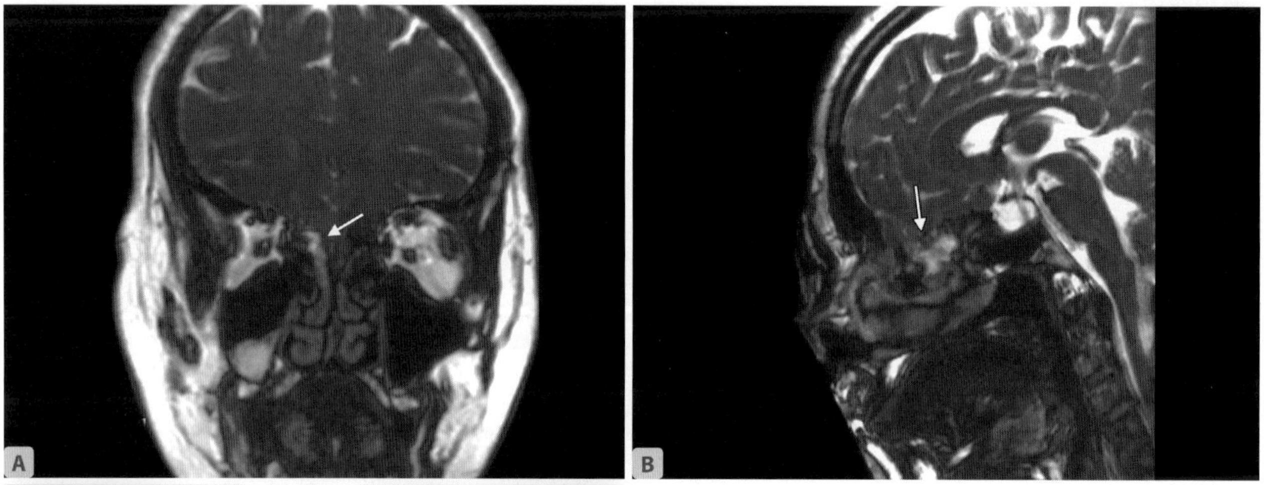

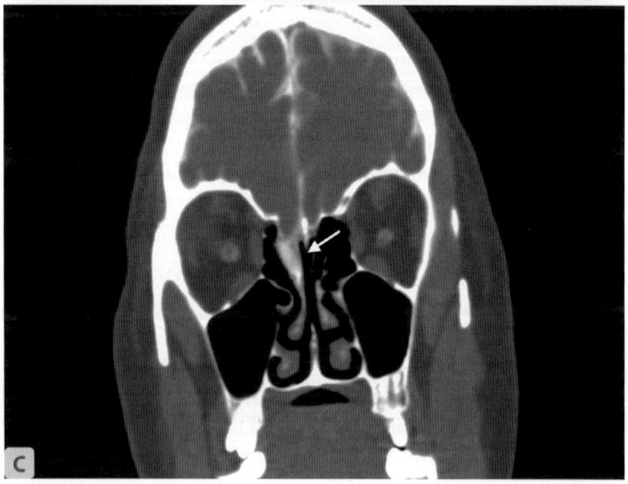

FIGS. 8A TO C: Cerebrospinal fluid rhinorrhea: CISS MR cisternography coronal (A) and sagittal (B) images show a focal defect in right cribriform plate with CSF signal intensity in right ethmoid sinus (arrows) consistent with CSF leak. CT cisternography (C) after instillation of intrathecal contrast, shows constant leaking into the right ethmoid sinus (arrow) below the site of defect.

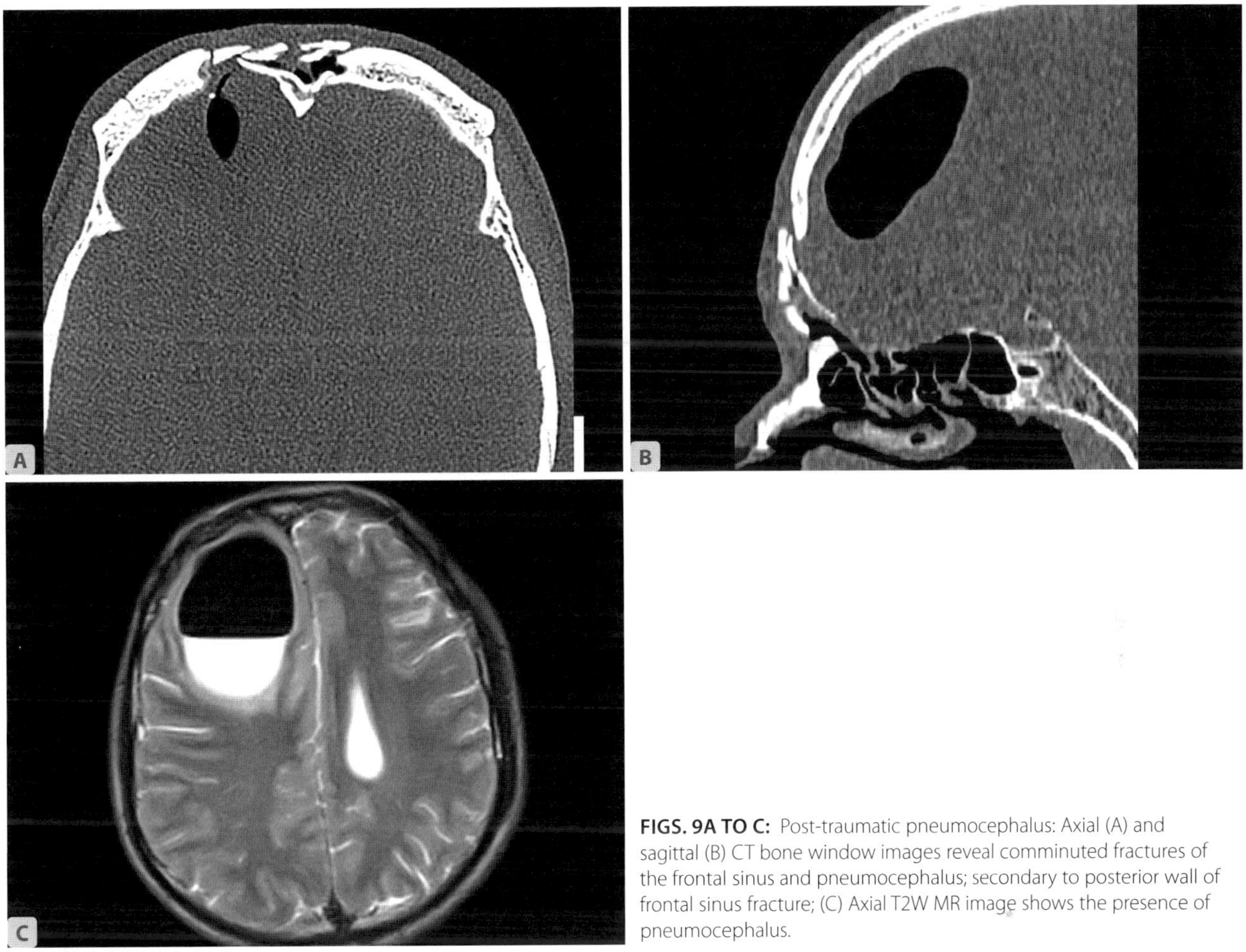

FIGS. 9A TO C: Post-traumatic pneumocephalus: Axial (A) and sagittal (B) CT bone window images reveal comminuted fractures of the frontal sinus and pneumocephalus; secondary to posterior wall of frontal sinus fracture; (C) Axial T2W MR image shows the presence of pneumocephalus.

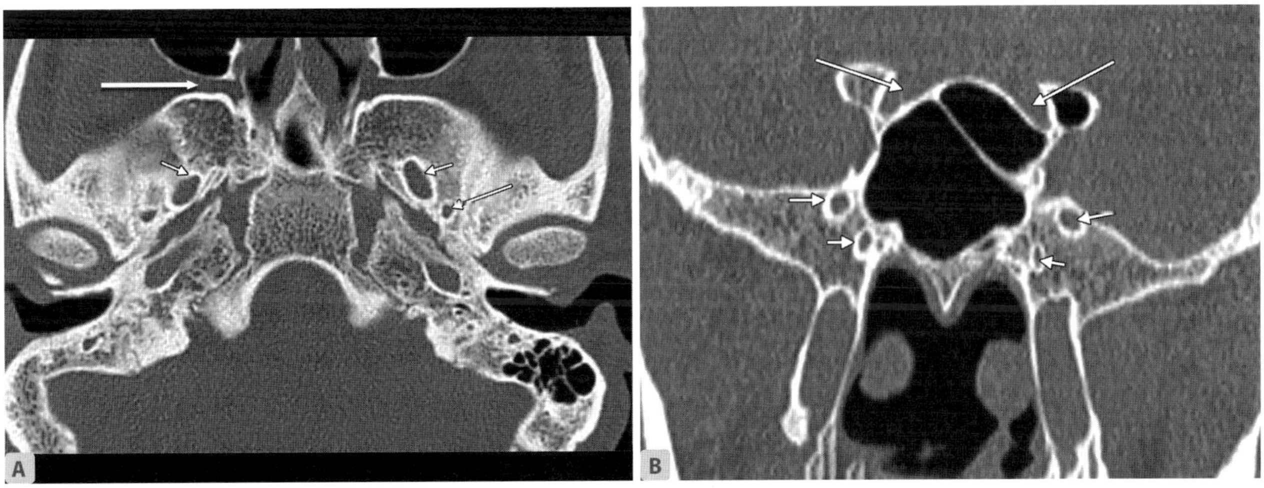

FIGS. 10A AND B: Axial (A) and coronal (B) CT sections through central skull base show foramen ovale (arrows), foramen spinosum (long arrow) and pterygopalatine fossa (block arrow). Coronal CT image (B) reveals foramen rotundum (arrows), vidian canal (short arrows), and optic foramen (long arrows).

more than 5 mm or size difference of more than 2 mm from contralateral side is considered abnormal. It is important to radiologically comment upon involvement of structures which act as contraindications for surgical resection which are summarized in **Box 2**.[18] Imaging signs of cavernous sinus invasion by any mass are described in **Box 3**. Or the purpose of radiologically narrowing down the differential diagnosis of the lesions involving the central skull base, it is useful to subdivide the central skull base into midline sagittal (medial to petroclival fissure), off-midline parasagittal (between petroclival fissure and foramen ovale) and lateral compartments (lateral to foramen ovale) **(Table 3)**.

Midline Sagittal Central Skull Base Lesions

It comprises lesions arising from sphenoid body, sphenoid sinus, clivus, sella turcica and nasopharynx.

Sphenoid Mucocele

As previously described in the frontal and ethmoid sinuses, the sphenoid mucoceles occur due to obstruction of its drainage. It presents as expansion of the sinus with thinning of walls with contained fluid within it which may show T1 hyperintensity on MR due to high protein content. It does not enhance except for a thin enhancing rim of mucosa **(Figs. 11A to D)**. This differentiates it from the rare squamous cell carcinomas originating in the sphenoid sinus.

Box 2: Invasion of following structures is contraindications for surgical resection.

- Cavernous sinus
- Bilateral optic nerves or optic chiasm involvement
- Nasopharynx
- Prevertebral fascia
- Lateral or superior wall of sphenoid sinus

Box 3: Signs of cavernous sinus invasion.[19,20]

- Loss of contrast enhancement
- Bulging of lateral sinus wall
- Compression, stenosis, encasement of cavernous carotid artery

TABLE 3: Middle skull base lesions.
Midline sagittal (medial to petroclival fissure) • Sphenoid mucocele • Clival chordoma • Pituitary macroadenoma • Craniopharyngioma • Meningiomas • Encephaloceles • Nasopharyngeal infections and nasopharyngeal carcinoma
Off-midline parasagittal (between petroclival fissure and foramen ovale) • Peripheral nerve sheath tumors • Perineural spread • Juvenile nasopharyngeal angiofibroma • Cavernous sinus lesions • Chondroid tumors
Lateral compartments (lateral to foramen ovale) • Meningioma • Temporomandibular joint (TMJ) lesions

Clival Chordoma

It is a benign locally invasive neoplasm presenting as expansile lytic lesion with aggressive pattern of bone destruction. It is best seen as replacement of normal bone marrow on T1-weighted MR images with erosion of its cortical margins and heterogeneously hyperintense on T2-weighted images **(Figs. 12A to C)**. It commonly shows areas of hemorrhage, calcification and cystic degeneration. Lobulated pattern of contrast enhancement has been described as a typical feature.[21] The differential diagnosis includes plasmacytoma, metastases and chondrosarcoma.

Pituitary Macroadenoma

Pituitary macroadenomas cause expansion of sella and invade the cavernous sinuses laterally with encasement of the carotid artery. The invasive adenomas may also breach the floor and grow into the sphenoid sinus.[22] The best diagnostic clue is a lesion in the sphenoid bone with the pituitary fossa bulging downwards into the lesion and simulating an empty sella **(Figs. 13A and B)**.

Craniopharyngioma

Craniopharyngiomas are benign neoplasms arising from remnants of pharyngohypophyseal canal or Rathke's pouch and hence can be seen anywhere from the nasopharynx to hypothalamus. They appear as cystic or mixed lesions with calcification and show contrast enhancement of the solid part **(Figs. 14A and B)**. MRI may show T1 hyperintensity of the cystic component due to proteinaceous content.

Meningiomas

In the sellar and parasellar region, the meningiomas arise from planum sphenoidale, tuberculum sella, diaphragm sella or the clinoid processes. Radiological features include a solid T1 and T2 isointense intensely enhancing mass with broad base towards dura, with or without dural tail. The pituitary gland may be seen separately compressed by the mass. Associated findings include pneumosinus dilatans (increased pneumatization of the sphenoid sinus) and hyperostosis with upward blistering of the planum sphenoidale and tuberculum sella. Differential diagnosis includes other causes of dural thickening and enhancement, such as sarcoid, carcinomatous meningitis, lymphoma and granulomatous disease.

Encephaloceles

Encephaloceles or meningoceles may occur into the sphenoid bone or more anteriorly between the ethmoid and sphenoid bones **(Figs. 15A and B)**. CT and MR can show the bony defect with herniated contents.

Other Miscellaneous Lesions

Nasopharyngeal infections and nasopharyngeal carcinoma may spread from below to involve the midline sagittal central skull base.

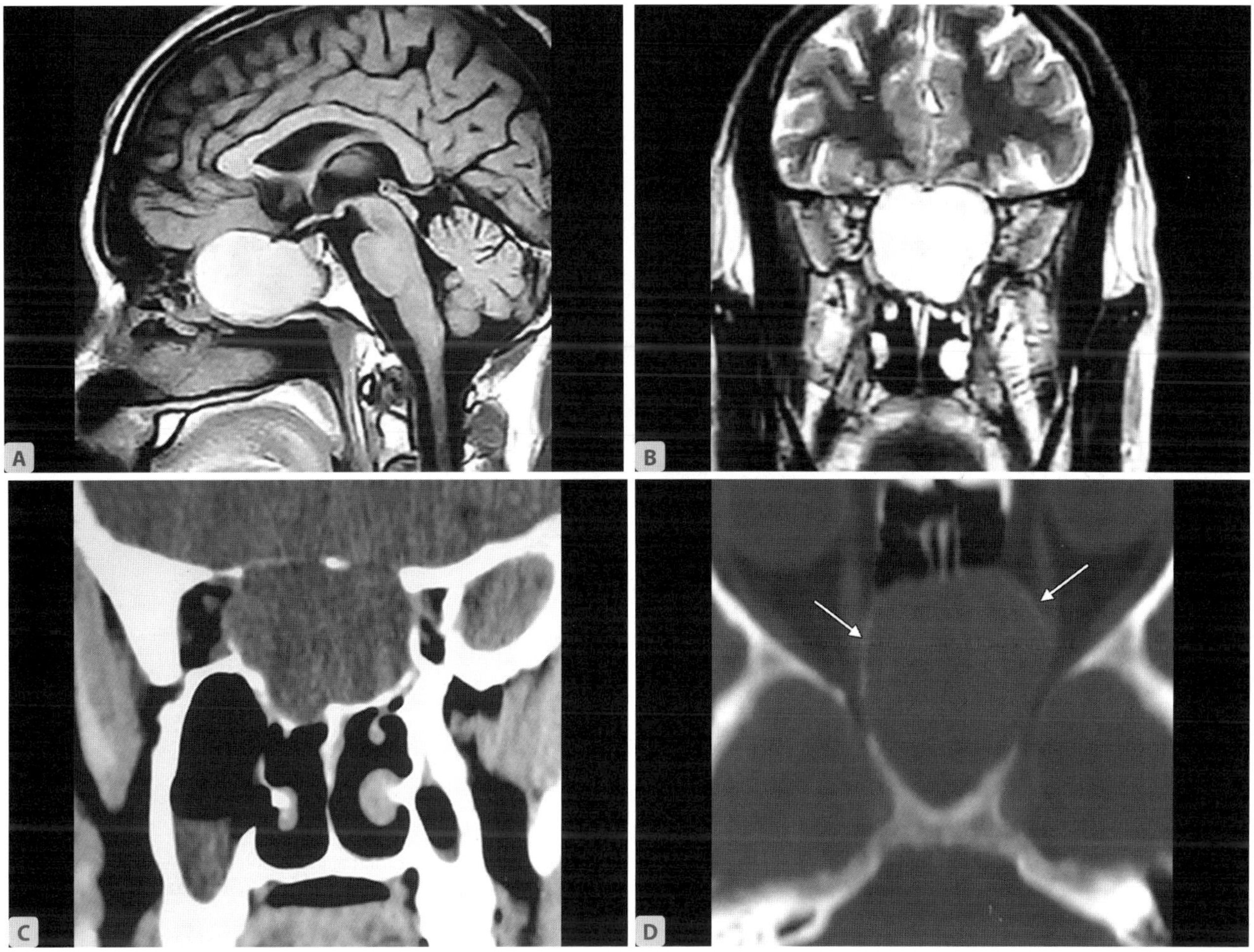

FIGS. 11A TO D: Sphenoid mucocele: T2-weighted sagittal (A) and coronal (B) MR images show expanded fluid-filled sphenoid sinus. Coronal CT soft tissue window reformatted image (C) and axial bone window image (D) reveal bony expansion and thinning (arrows) of sphenoid sinus walls.

Parasagittal Central Skull Base Lesions

It comprises lesions arising from the cavernous sinus, cranial nerves traversing the neural foramina, the greater sphenoid wing and the petroclival synchondrosis.

Peripheral Nerve Sheath Tumors

Schwannomas and neurofibromas can arise from any cranial nerve, most commonly from the trigeminal nerve. Schwannomas show hypointensity on T1-weighted images and intermediate to high signal on T2-weighted MR images with necrosis and intense heterogeneous enhancement after contrast. They remodel the adjacent bone and may cause neural foramina widening if involving the nerve traversing through it. Neurofibromas are more aggressive infiltrative lesions which spread diffusely along peripheral branches and show ill-defined borders.[23] Tumors of the trigeminal nerve often appear as dumbbell-shaped tumors with a middle cranial fossa component within cavernous sinus and posterior cranial fossa component within the Meckel's cave **(Figs. 16A and B)**. Vidian nerve neurofibromas present as soft tissue masses expanding the vidian canal from foramen lacerum posteriorly to pterygopalatine fossa anteriorly.

Perineural Spread

Cranial nerve involvement may be secondary to spread of various malignancies or infectious/inflammatory conditions along the course of the nerve.[24,25] It is commonly seen with squamous cell carcinoma of head and neck region, salivary gland malignancies (most common adenoid cystic carcinoma) and hematological malignancies. MR detects early perineural spread in the form of thickening of nerve, enhancement of nerve and effacement of neuroforaminal fat. Similar features may be seen in neuritis due to infectious conditions like herpes simplex and CMV. CT scan is less sensitive than MR and detects perineural spread in the form of enlargement of the neural foramina, effacement of foraminal fat or indirectly through denervation atrophy of the muscles supplied by the particular nerve.

Juvenile Nasopharyngeal Angiofibroma

As already discussed in the section of anterior skull base, the angiofibroma has propensity to insinuate through various foramina into the skull. It extends into the parasagittal central skull base from the pterygopalatine fossa through the foramen rotundum or the vidian canal and into the orbit through

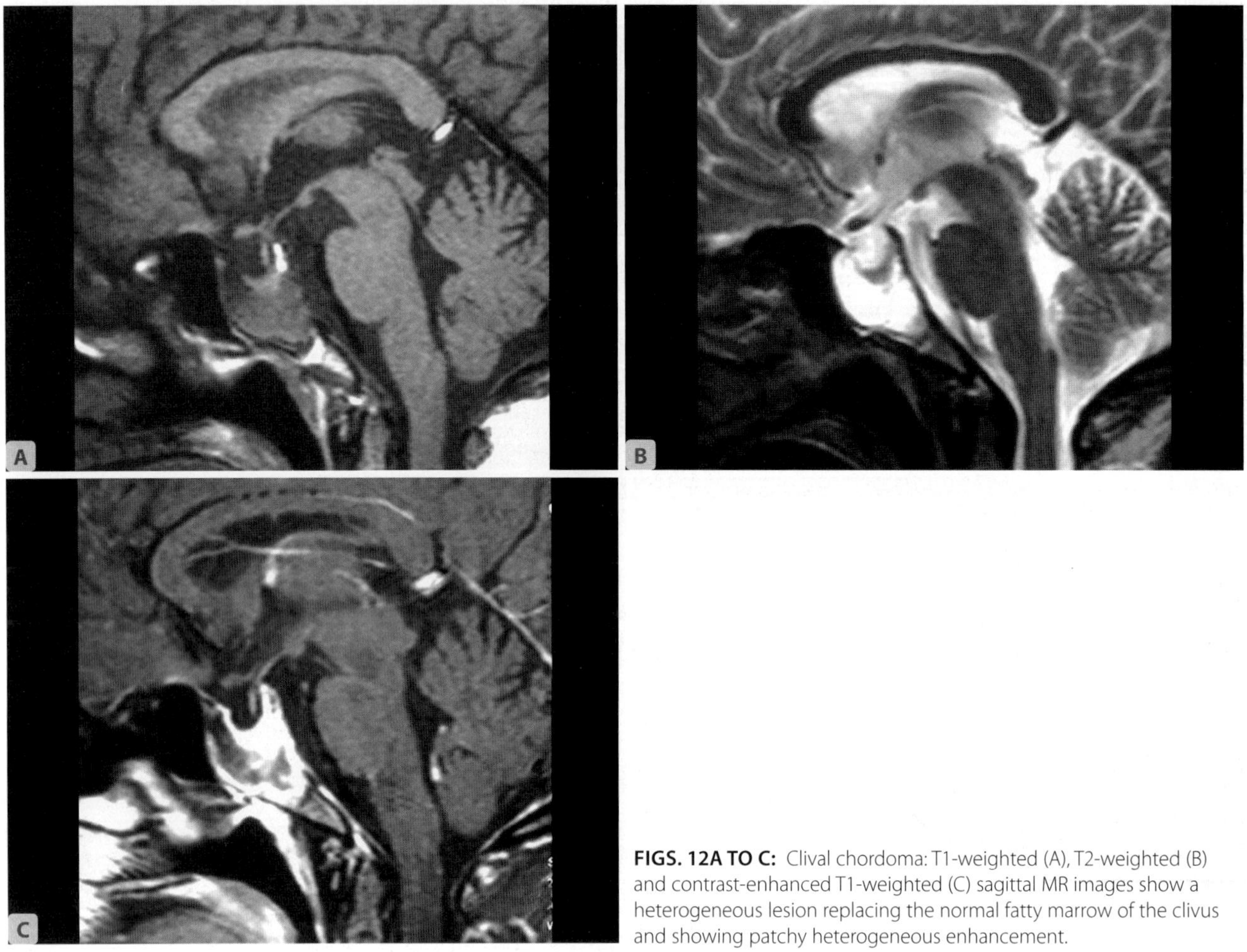

FIGS. 12A TO C: Clival chordoma: T1-weighted (A), T2-weighted (B) and contrast-enhanced T1-weighted (C) sagittal MR images show a heterogeneous lesion replacing the normal fatty marrow of the clivus and showing patchy heterogeneous enhancement.

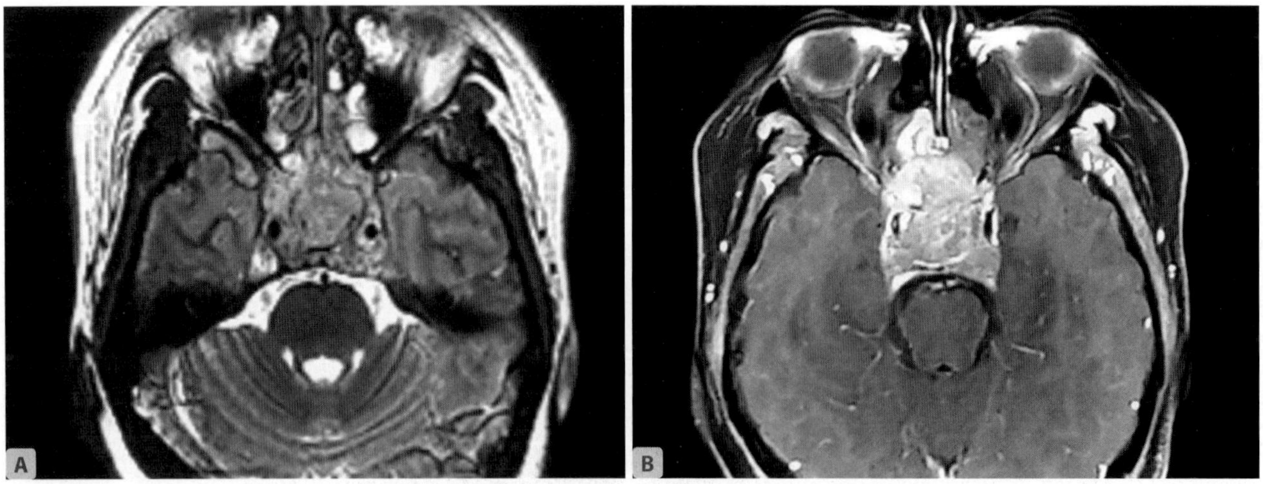

FIGS. 13A AND B: Invasive pituitary adenoma: T2W (A) and postcontrast (B) axial MR images of the sellar region show a soft tissue mass filling the sella, with extension into bilateral cavernous sinuses.

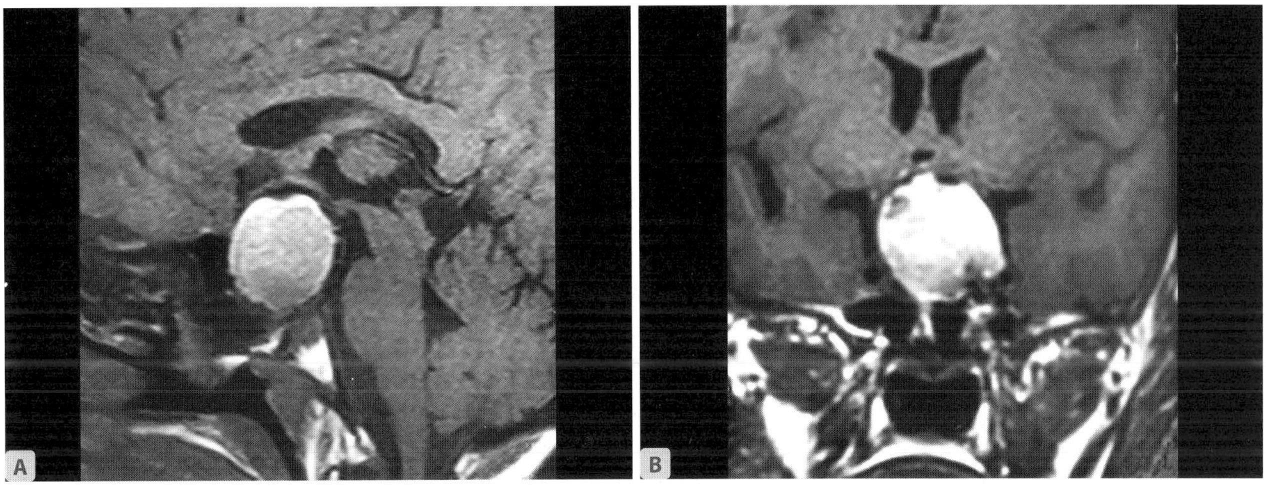

FIGS. 14A AND B: Craniopharyngioma: T1W sagittal (A) and coronal (B) MRI shows a hyperintense mass lesion in the sellar and suprasellar region extending into the sphenoid sinus.

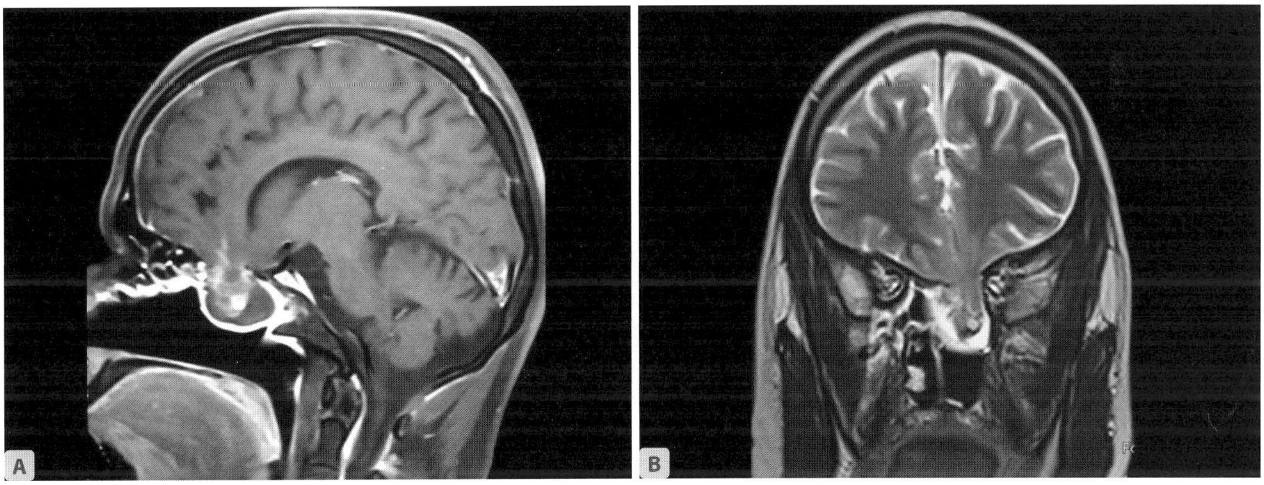

FIGS. 15A AND B: Sphenoid encephalocele: T1W sagittal (A) and T2W coronal (B) MRI show herniation of brain parenchyma into the spheno ethmoid region.

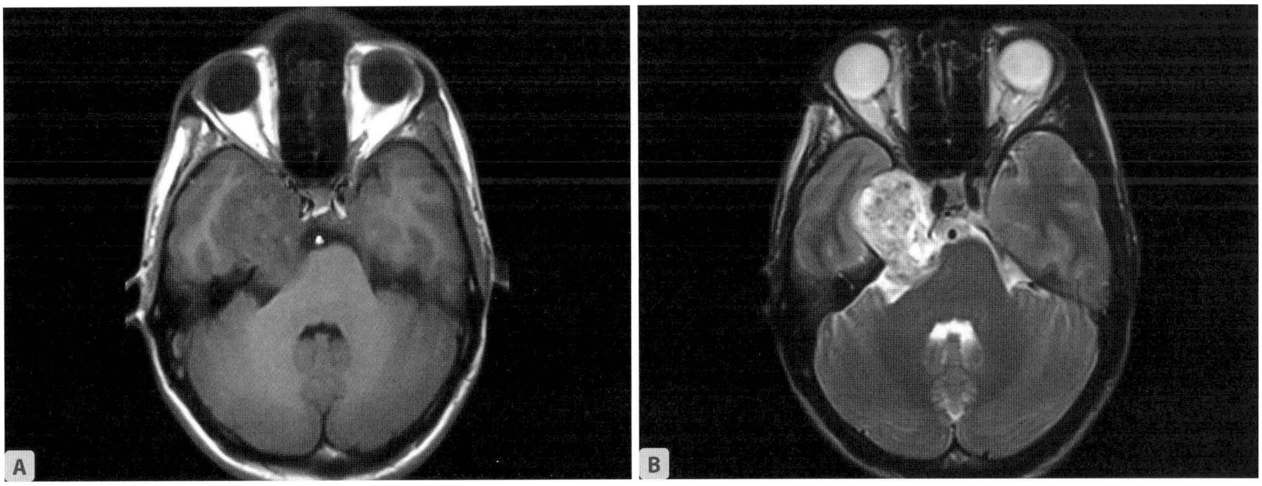

FIGS. 16A AND B: Trigeminal schwannoma: T1-weighted (A) and T2-weighted (B) axial MR images show a dumbbell-shaped heterogeneous mass lesion involving the right cavernous sinus and extending into posterior cranial fossa through the Meckel's cave.

the inferior orbital fissure. They are highly vascular tumors and show 'salt and pepper' pattern on MRI with intense post-contrast enhancement **(Figs. 17A to C)**. Preoperative embolization of these tumors has a significant role in decreasing the hemorrhage and surgical morbidity.

Cavernous Sinus Lesions

The cavernous sinus may be involved by spread of pyogenic or fungal infections originating from paranasal sinuses, nasopharynx and orbits. It will show enlargement of cavernous sinus with or without thrombosis. The cavernous sinus may be involved in addition to orbital apex by inflammatory pseudotumor (Tolosa Hunt syndrome). It is seen on MRI as low signal intensity soft tissue mass on T1- and T2-weighted images which enhances on contrast images and occupies the orbital apex with extension into the cavernous sinus. Cavernous sinus enlargement may also be seen in vascular lesions including carotico-cavernous fistulas, aneurysms and hemangiomas and in meningiomas of the cavernous sinus.

Chondroid Tumors

Chondromyxoid fibromas and chondrosarcomas arise from petroclival synchondrosis. CT depicts the characteristic chondroid type of calcification. Marked high signal intensity on T2-weighted MR images is also a characteristic feature **(Figs. 18A to C)**.

Lateral Central Skull Base Lesions

It comprises lesions arising from the lateral aspect of temporal bone, temporomandibular joint and far lateral aspect of greater sphenoid wing.

Meningioma

Meningiomas commonly arise from the greater sphenoid wing. They may be either en plaque or classic globular. The characteristic MR features include T1 and T2 low signal intensity with intense contrast enhancement and dural tail **(Figs. 19A to D)**.

Temporomandibular Joint (TMJ) Lesions

TMJ infections and tumors including pigmented villonodular synovitis may appear as mass lesions in the region of lateral central skull base.

POSTERIOR SKULL BASE

Anatomy

The posterior cranial fossa extends from the posterior surface of the clivus to the foramen magnum. The posterior skull base consists of the petrous and mastoid parts of the temporal bone and the squamous and condylar portions of the occipital bone. The jugular foramen lies between the

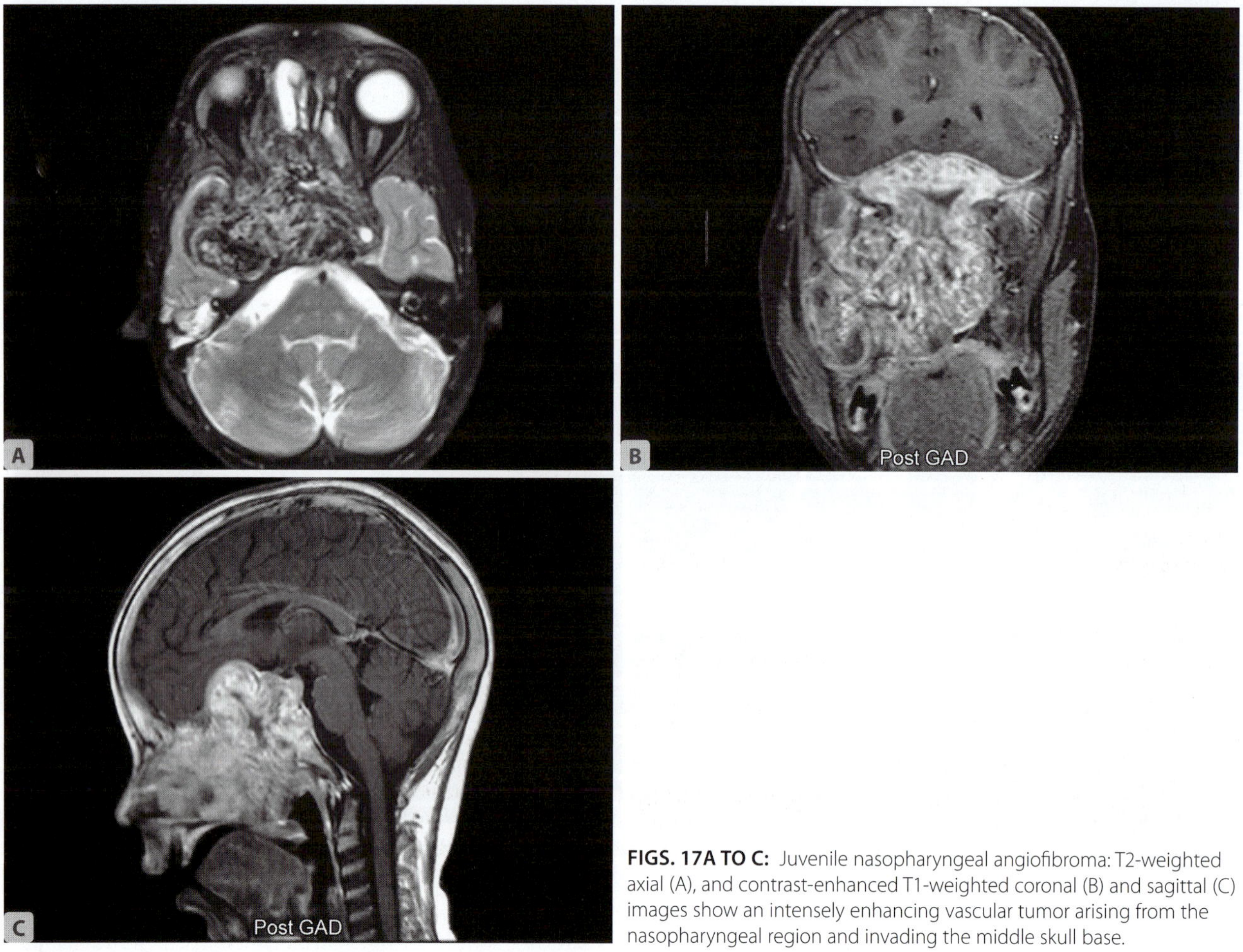

FIGS. 17A TO C: Juvenile nasopharyngeal angiofibroma: T2-weighted axial (A), and contrast-enhanced T1-weighted coronal (B) and sagittal (C) images show an intensely enhancing vascular tumor arising from the nasopharyngeal region and invading the middle skull base.

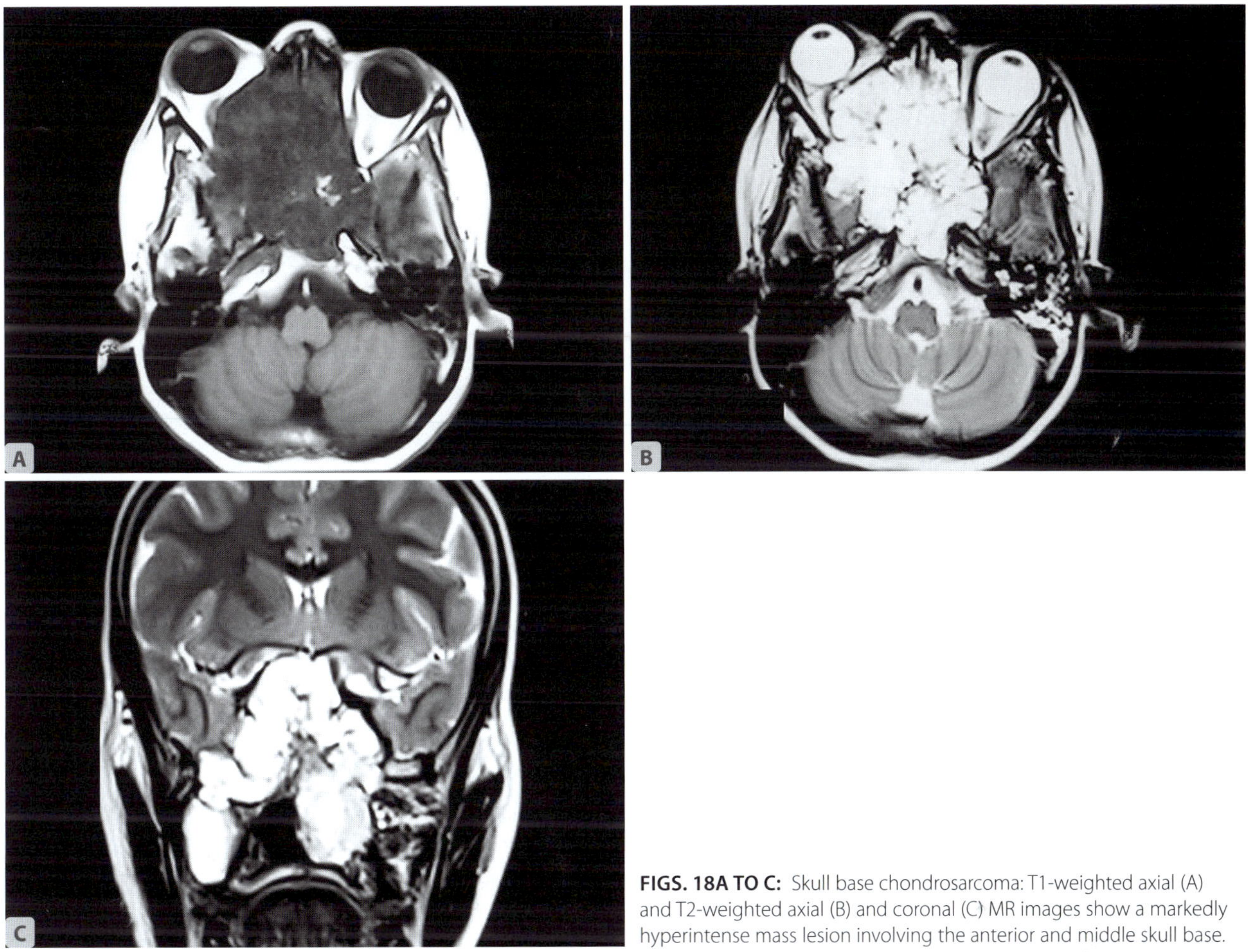

FIGS. 18A TO C: Skull base chondrosarcoma: T1-weighted axial (A) and T2-weighted axial (B) and coronal (C) MR images show a markedly hyperintense mass lesion involving the anterior and middle skull base.

petrous temporal and occipital bones and lies lateral to the hypoglossal canal. The foramen has oblique course through the skull base. It is divided by a fibrous or bony septum into a smaller anteromedial compartment (pars nervosa) and a larger posterolateral compartment (pars vascularis). Cranial nerve IX and inferior petrosal sinus pass through the pars nervosa and cranial nerves X and XI along with jugular vein and posterior meningeal artery pass through the pars vascularis. The foramen magnum lies within the occipital bone.

Pathology

Lesions involving the posterior skull base can be categorized according to the site of origin into jugular fossa lesions, petrous apex lesions and foramen magnum lesions **(Table 4)**.

Jugular Foramen Lesions

Glomus Jugulare Paraganglioma

They are the most common tumors of this region, seen mostly in women in fifth and sixth decades. They are often multiple. It usually arises in the pars vascularis but may extend to involve the pars nervosa. CT shows a permeative 'moth eaten' pattern of bone destruction which distinguishes it from the nerve sheath tumors of this region which produce smooth and scalloped erosions.[26] MR shows the characteristic 'salt and pepper' appearance due to multiple vascular flow voids and foci of subacute hemorrhage interspersed within the lesion. These tumors show intense enhancement on contrast administration. It is important to comment upon the extension into the tympanic cavity if present (glomus jugulotympanicum) as it changes the surgical approach **(Figs. 20A and B)**. Preoperative embolization can significantly reduce the surgical morbidity and mortality.

Nerve Sheath Tumors

Schwannomas and neurofibromas can arise from the cranial nerves traversing the jugular foramina. As described earlier, they tend to cause smooth bone erosions and remodeling rather than frank destruction. On CT they may appear as slightly low attenuation masses due to their rich lipid content. The schwannomas usually show intense postcontrast enhancement with intratumoral cysts in up to 25% of cases but the neurofibromas show variable enhancement.[27] It is radiologically difficult to differentiate between the two.

Lesions Extending into the Jugular Foramen

Perineural spread from malignancies of oral cavity and pharynx can extend to involve the jugular fossa. Glomus vagale arising from the cranial nerve X in the lower part

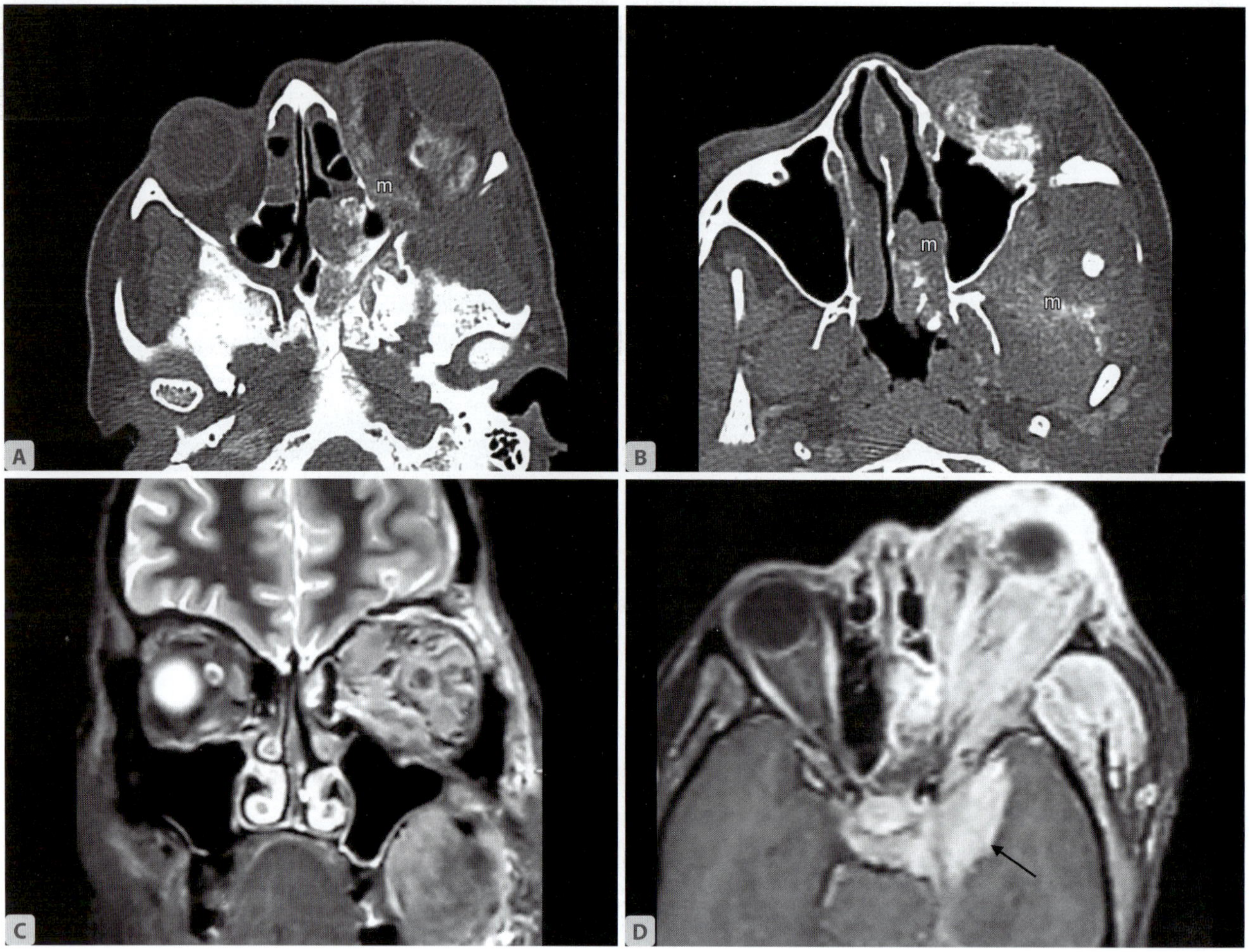

FIGS. 19A TO D: Left sphenoid wing meningioma: Axial CT bone window images (A and B) reveal mass (m) with amorphous calcification involving left infratemporal fossa, left ethmoid air cells and left orbit. T2W coronal MR image (C) shows the mass to be isointense with hypointense areas. Postcontrast T1W image (D) shows avid contrast enhancement of the extracranial soft tissue along with extension to the left cavernous sinus (arrow).

TABLE 4: Posterior skull base lesions.
Jugular foramen lesions
• Glomus jugulare paraganglioma
• Nerve sheath tumors
• Lesions extending into the jugular foramen
• Jugular bulb pseudolesion
• Large or high riding jugular bulb
Petrous apex lesions
• Nonaggressive cystic expansile lesions
• Aggressive appearing solid lesions
Foramen magnum lesions
• Chordoma Chondrosarcoma
• Neurogenic tumors
• Infections and inflammatory processes of the CV junction

may extend up into the jugular foramen causing its expansion. Infections and inflammatory processes arising from adjacent structures like mastoiditis, otitis media and malignant otitis externa can spread to involve the jugular foramen by eroding the intervening bone and may lead to venous thrombosis.

Jugular Bulb Pseudolesion

Abnormal high signal intensity on T1-weighted MR images within the jugular bulb is commonly seen due to the complex flow pattern within a normal jugular bulb. It may be mistaken for a pathology like glomus tumor. It needs to be correctly identified to prevent unnecessary further intervention. It can be recognized as the 'lesion' is not evident on T2-weighted images and MR venogram depicts a normal patent jugular bulb.[28]

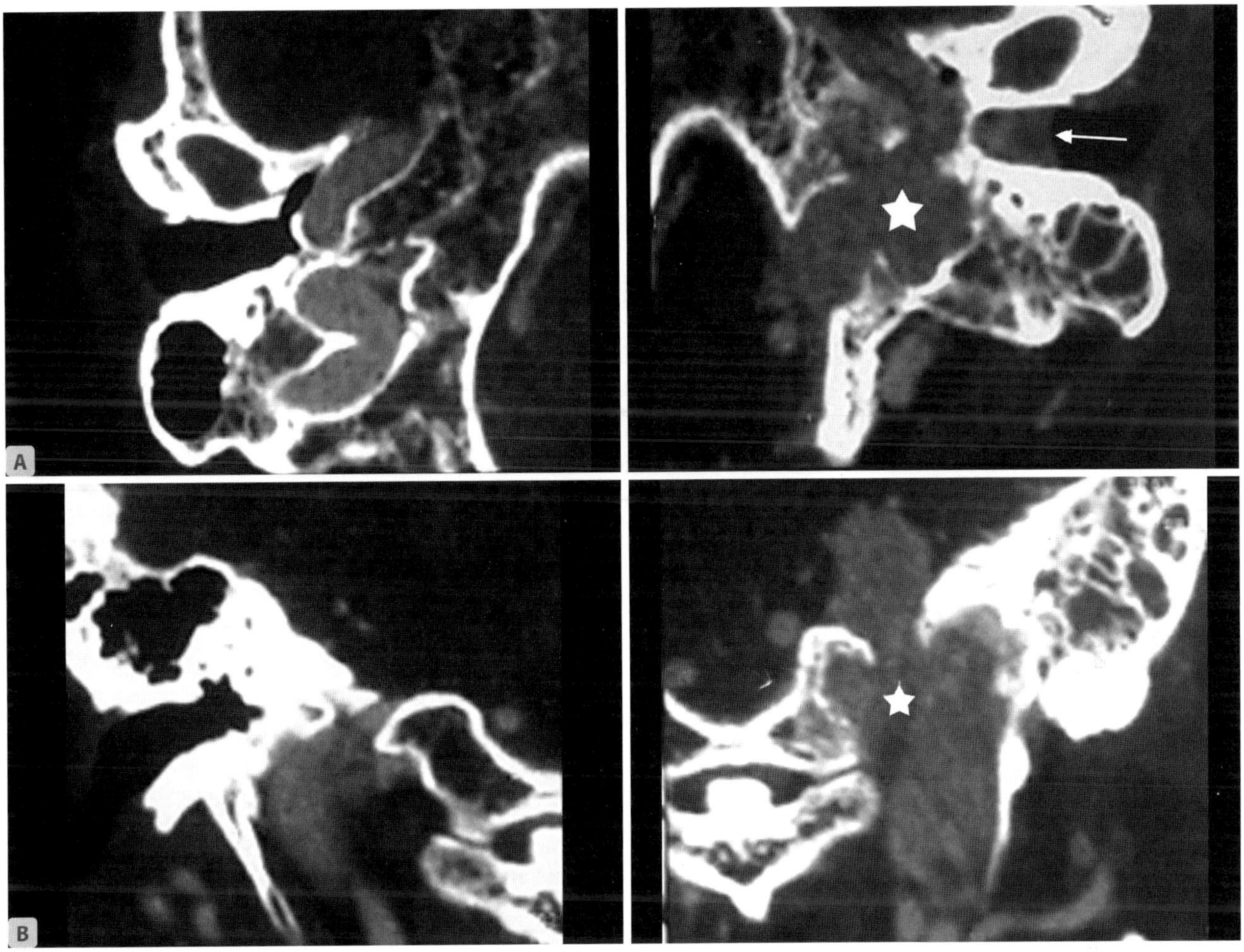

FIGS. 20A AND B: Glomus jugulotympanicum: Axial (A) and Coronal (B) CECT images reveal a hypervascular mass (stars) involving left jugular fossa, middle ear cavity and extending into left external auditory canal (arrow). Note the associated bone destruction.

Large or High Riding Jugular Bulb

Normal variation in size and symmetry of the jugular bulbs is common with right side being dominant. It should not be mistaken for pathology as there is no bony erosion. High riding jugular bulb is defined as a jugular bulb roof extending above the level of inferior margin of the basal turn of the cochlea or the inferior tympanic annulus.[29,30] They are also more common on right side. It may be associated with dehiscence of the superior jugular plate leading to protrusion of the bulb superolaterally into the posterior hypotympanum. It is important to identify these anatomical variations before any surgery for the middle ear or CP angle lesion.

Petrous Apex Lesions

Nonaggressive Cystic Expansile Lesions

Cholesterol granuloma forms secondary to obstruction of a pneumatized air cell with subsequent hemorrhage and cholesterol deposition. It has a characteristic MR appearance of being hyperintense on both T1- and T2-weighted images.[27] CT shows expansion of the bony cortex. No enhancement is seen in the central part. Petrous carotid artery aneurysm can also lead to an expansile lesion in this region with thinning of the walls of the carotid canal. The MR signal changes are dependent upon amount of thrombus within it. Contrast enhancement (if not thrombosed) can differentiate it from cholesterol granuloma. Mucoceles **(Figs. 21A and B)** and arachnoid cysts may also be rarely seen in the region of petrous apex presenting as cystic expansile lesions.

Aggressive Appearing Solid Lesions

Cholesteatomas of the petrous apex are seen as expansile lesions with variable degree of bone destruction.[31] They do not enhance on contrast administration. When no bony destruction is present, they may mimic cholesterol granuloma but can be differentiated on MR wherein the cholesteatomas show low to intermediate signal on T1-weighted images in contrast to cholesterol granuloma which shows high signal on T1-weighted images. Cholesteatoma may also show restricted diffusion.[32] Infection of the petrous apex may be seen in the form of petrous apicitis or a true petrous apex osteomyelitis. The former is caused by extension of otitis media into a pneumatized petrous apex and causes classical Gradenigo's syndrome: triad of otitis media/mastoiditis, severe facial pain in cranial nerve V1 distribution and ipsilateral cranial

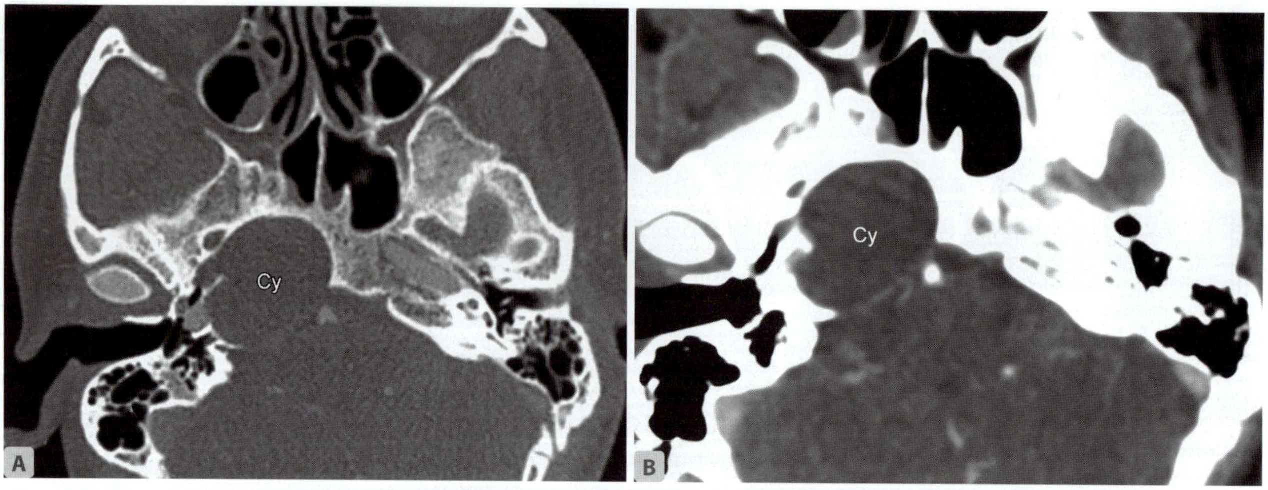

FIGS. 21A AND B: Petrous apex mucocele: NCCT axial bone window (A) and soft tissue window (B) images reveal exapansile low attenuation cystic focal lesion (Cy) at right petrous apex with well corticated scalloped margins.

nerve VI palsy. Imaging shows opacification of petrous air cells with bony erosion and destruction and enhancement of entire petrous apex including the dura on postcontrast MR. Petrous apex osteomyelitis occurs secondary to direct medial extension of malignant otitis externa into a nonpneumatized petrous apex. CT shows bone erosions with sclerosis and MR shows replacement of the normal fatty marrow with enhancement.

Foramen Magnum Lesions

Mass lesions extending into the foramen magnum may have origins from the following structures:

- Bony lesions arising from the clivus-like chordoma and chondrosarcoma which can extend into the foramen magnum causing compression of the medulla and cervical cord.
- Tumors arising from the nerves (neurogenic tumors) and the covering meninges (meningiomas).
- Bony tumors arising from atlas and axis vertebra.
- Infections and inflammatory processes of the CV junction like rheumatoid arthritis and tuberculosis. RA shows evidence of erosion of the dens with pannus causing encroachment of the spinal canal. Tuberculosis will show destruction of the dens with adjacent soft tissue/collections and peripheral enhancement.

DIFFUSE/NON-SITE-SPECIFIC SKULL BASE LESIONS

Skull base may be affected by a variety of systemic conditions, bone tumors, fibro-osseous lesions or infections which are not site-specific and may involve any part of the skull base from anterior to posterior.

Metastases

They usually involve bones with high marrow content so are most commonly seen in the skull base in the region of petrous apex, clivus and sphenoid triangle. They may be lytic (breast, lung, kidney, thyroid and multiple myeloma), sclerotic (prostate) or mixed (breast).[33] CT is the preferred modality to detect them. Diffuse metastases may be difficult to differentiate from Paget's disease or other fibro-osseous conditions.

Fibrous Dysplasia

It is a fibro-osseous lesion arising from skull base seen in children and adolescents. The medullary bone gets replaced by fibro-osseous tissue. CT is the imaging modality of choice for making the correct diagnosis. It initially shows coalescent cystic spaces in the initial phase which progress to the characteristic 'ground glass' appearance with a thin cortical rim and finally a sclerotic late phase **(Figs. 22A and B)**. It shows marked contrast enhancement in the active phase and is nonenhancing in the quiescent phase.[34] CT and MR are also helpful for exact extent of the lesion including depicting the encroachment of the foramina. It appears as low signal intensity lesion on both T1- and T2-weighted images. The lesion spares the cortical bone which helps to differentiate it from Paget's disease.

Paget's Disease

It is seen in adults after 40 years of age. It causes diffuse thickening of the cortical bone and radiologically is seen as bone expansion and sclerosis with coarse bony trabeculae. There is usually associated involvement of skull vault and of the otic capsule which also helps it to differentiate from fibrous dysplasia **(Figs. 23A and B)**.[20]

Skull Base Osteomyelitis

Osteomyelitis of the central skull base is a potentially life-threatening rare condition. Headache may be the only symptom and cranial nerve palsies present later. It is usually seen in patients with underlying diseases such as diabetes mellitus, chronic inflammatory sphenoid sinus disease, corticosteroid use or HIV infection. The diagnosis is difficult to make clinically and therefore is often delayed. The source of infection of the central skull base can be hematogenous or contiguous spread from nearby infective process.

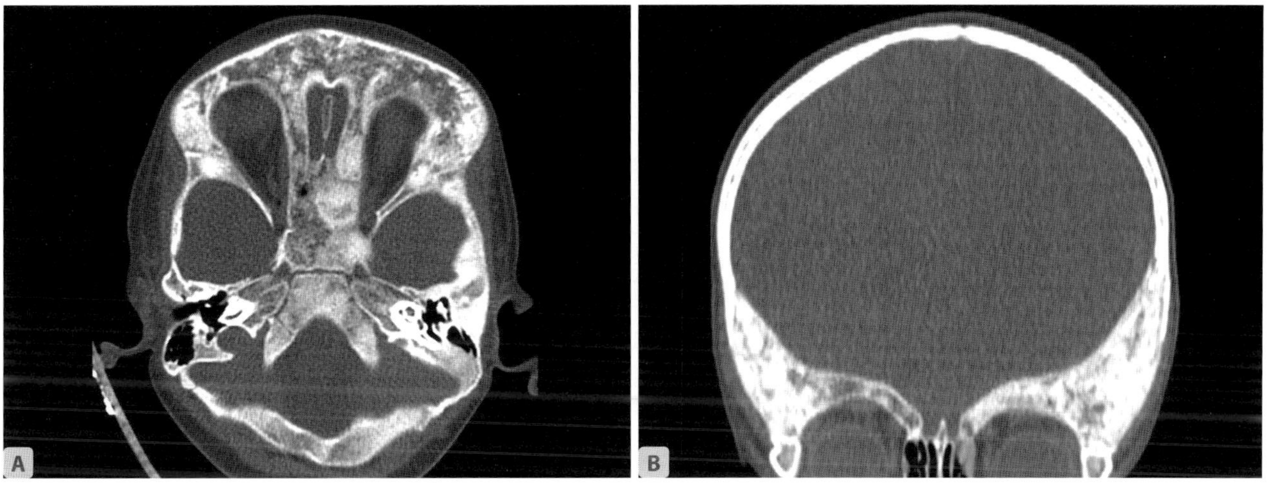

FIGS. 22A AND B: Fibrous dysplasia: Axial (A) and coronal (B) CT images show diffuse involvement of skull base with the characteristic "ground-glass" appearance.

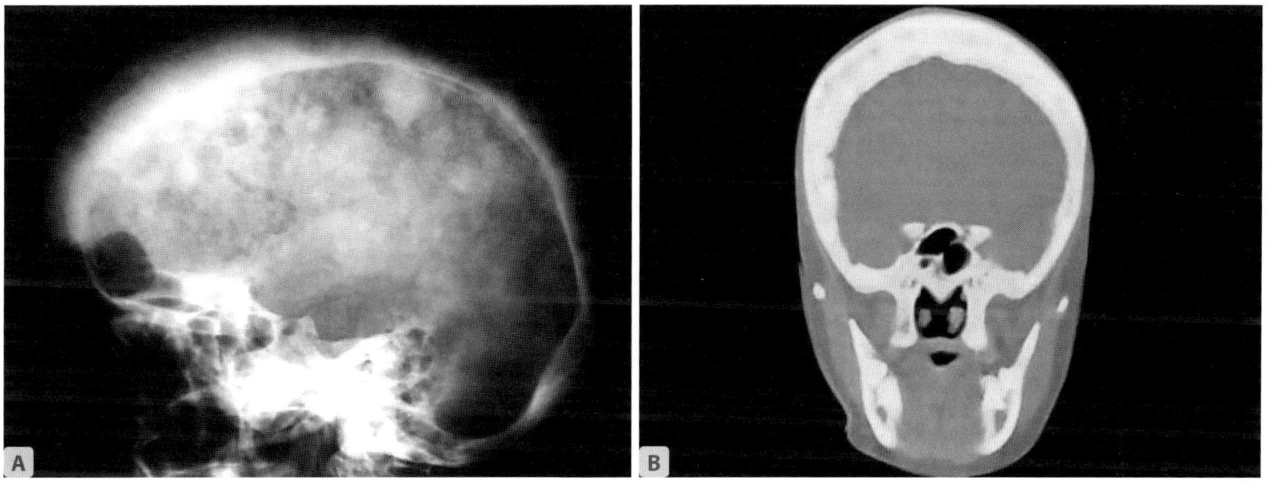

FIGS. 23A AND B: Paget's disease: Lateral skull radiograph (A) and coronal (B) MPR CT images show sclerosis and expansion of the skull bones with involvement of the vault.

The invasive fungal sinonasal infections tend to spread to medial part of central skull base (region of clivus) whereas the otogenic infections and odontogenic infections tend to spread to the lateral aspects of central skull base (region of pterygoid plates and sphenoid wings).[35]

MDCT signs of osteomyelitis are medullary expansion, cortical destruction, periosteal reaction and sclerosis **(Figs. 24A and B)**. The signs of the source of infection may also be noted such as sinonasal disease, otomastoiditis and mandibular osteomyelitis. Soft tissue mass like lesions and fluid colllections may be seen. Surrounding masticator muscles edema (myositis) and overlying fat cellulitis may also be seen. MRI can depict the extent of involvement in the adjacent soft tissues and intracranial extensions with better resolution **(Figs. 25A to D)**. Bony involvement can be seen as T2 hyperintensity and T1 hypointensity within the clival bone, adjacent soft tissue infiltration with obliteration of normal fat planes, abnormal soft tissue in the cavernous sinus, internal carotid artery narrowing or occlusion, abnormal meningeal enhancement and local cerebritis or venous ischemia, abnormal marrow signal intensity around the skull foramina and abnormal soft tissue infiltrating adjacent fat planes.

Tissue sampling is often required for definite diagnosis.

CT and MRI are also helpful in assessing the complications in the form of cranial neuropathy, cavernous sinus thrombosis. septic cavernous sinus thrombosis, meningeal and brain parenchymal extension, epidural and petroclival abscesses.

Miscellaneous Conditions

Osteopetrosis may cause thick and sclerotic skull base appearance with increased tendency to fracture. In children, eosinophilic granuloma may cause punched-out lytic lesions in the skull base. Primary bone tumors like osteosarcoma and osteoblastoma may arise from skull base bones.

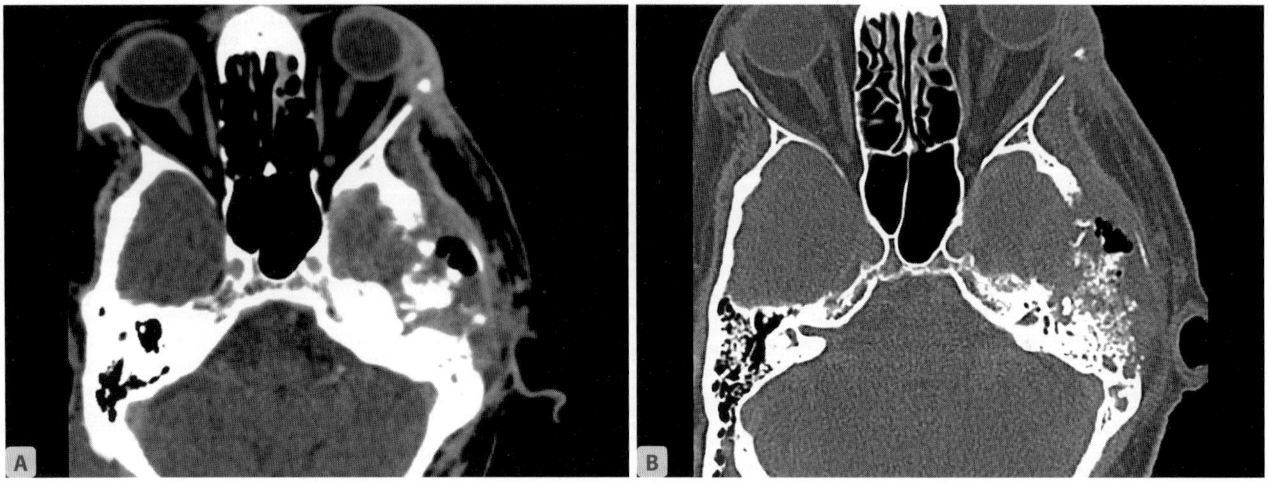

FIGS. 24A AND B: Skull base pyogenic osteomyelitis: Axial CT soft tissue (A) and bone (B) window images reveal permeative lytic bone destruction involving left petrous and mastoid temporal bone, with adjacent soft tissue. Another focus of bone destruction is noted in left lateral orbital wall.

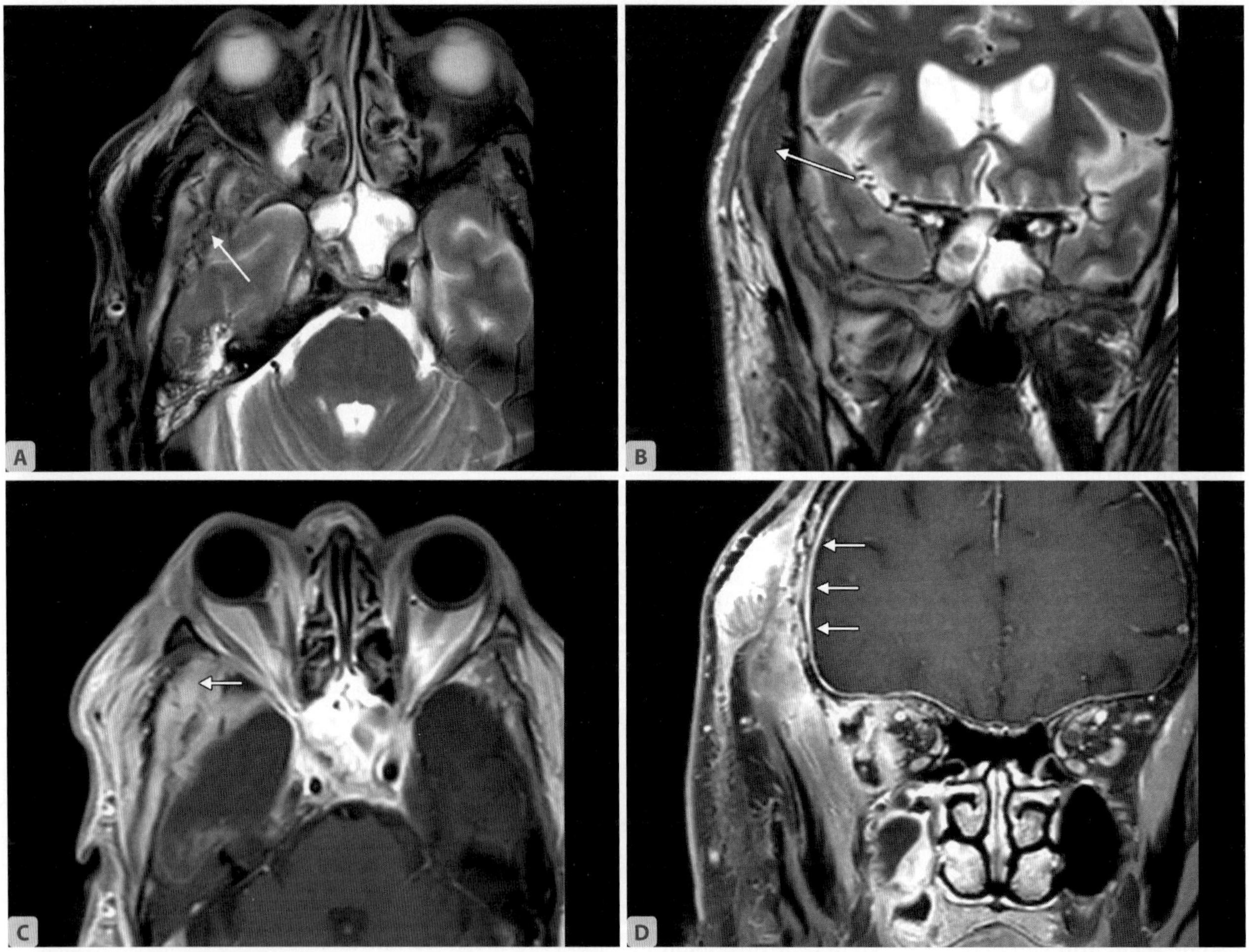

FIGS. 25A TO D: MRI in Skull base pyogenic osteomyelitis: Axial (A) and coronal (B) T2W MR images reveal soft tissue thickening and hyperintensity (arrows) involving right temporal fossa, and altered marrow signal intensity involving right greater wing of sphenoid. Postcontrast T1W images (C and D) show avid contrast enhancement of the soft tissue along the bone (arrows) as well as soft tissues in right orbit and temporal fossa.

CONCLUSION

CT and MRI are the mainstay of evaluation of skull base. MR is more sensitive for evaluation of the soft tissue component, characterization of lesions and their extent whereas CT compliments it by better depicting the fine bony details and the neurovascular foramina. Often, both imaging modalities are used in conjunction. Since the list of lesions involving the skull base is huge, dividing the skull base into three compartments with further subdivision into smaller areas helps in narrowing down the differential diagnosis significantly.

REFERENCES

1. Ginsberg LE, Pruett SW, Chen MY, Elster AD. Skull-base foramina of the middle cranial fossa: reassessment of normal variation with high-resolution CT. Am J Neuroradiol. 1994;15(2):283-91.
2. Policeni BA, Smoker WR. Imaging of the skull base: anatomy and pathology. Radiol Clin North Am. 2015;53(1):1-14.
3. Durden DD, Williams DW, 3rd. Radiology of skull base neoplasms. Otolaryngol Clin North Am. 2001;34(6):1043-64, vii.
4. Borges A. Skull base tumours part I: imaging technique, anatomy and anterior skull base tumours. Eur J Radiol. 2008;66(3):338-47.
5. Blitz AM, Aygun N, Herzka DA, Ishii M, Gallia GL. High resolution three-dimensional MR imaging of the skull base: compartments, boundaries, and critical structures. Radiol Clin North Am. 2017;55(1):17-30.
6. Som PM, Curtin HD. Head and Neck Imaging, Skull Base, 4th edition. St. Louis: Mosby Year Book; 2003.
7. Atlas SW. Magnetic resonance imaging of the brain and spine, 3rd edition. Philadelphia: Lippincott Williams & Wilkins; 2002.
8. Parmar H, Gujar S, Shah G, Mukherji SK. Imaging of the anterior skull base. Neuroimaging Clin N Am. 2009;19(3):427-39.
9. Vrionis FD, Kienstra MA, Rivera M, Padhya TA. Malignant tumors of the anterior skull base. Cancer Control. 2004;11(3):144-51.
10. Morita A, Ebersold MJ, Olsen KD, Foote RL, Lewis JE, Quast LM. Esthesioneuroblastoma: prognosis and management. Neurosurgery. 1993;32(5):706-14; discussion 14-5.
11. Som PM, Lidov M, Brandwein M, Catalano P, Biller HF. Sinonasal esthesioneuroblastoma with intracranial extension: marginal tumor cysts as a diagnostic MR finding. AJNR Am J Neuroradiol. 1994;15(7):1259-62.
12. Kennard CD, Rasmussen JE. Congenital midline nasal masses: diagnosis and management. J Dermatol Surg Oncol. 1990;16(11):1025-36.
13. Rahbar R, Resto VA, Robson CD, Perez-Atayde AR, Goumnerova LC, McGill TJ, et al. Nasal glioma and encephalocele: diagnosis and management. Laryngoscope. 2003;113(12):2069-77.
14. Adil E, Robson C, Perez-Atayde A, Heffernan C, Moritz E, Goumnerova L, et al. Congenital nasal neuroglial heterotopia and encephaloceles: an update on current evaluation and management. Laryngoscope. 2016;126(9):2161-7.
15. Kienstra MA, Van Loveren H. Anterior skull base fractures. Facial Plast Surg. 2005;21(3):180 6.
16. Manson PN, Stanwix MG, Yaremchuk MJ, Nam AJ, Hui-Chou H, Rodriguez ED. Frontobasal fractures: anatomical classification and clinical significance. Plast Reconstr Surg. 2009;124(6):2096-106.
17. Garg A, Prabhakar A. Anterior skull base lesions: Imaging in Clinico Radiological Series: Sinonasal Imaging, 1st edition. New Delhi: Jaypee; 2018.
18. Curtin HD, Chavali R. Imaging of the skull base. Radiol Clin North Am. 1998;36(5):801-17, v-vi.
19. Fischbein NJ, Kaplan MJ. Magnetic resonance imaging of the central skull base. Top Magn Reson Imaging. 1999;10(5):325-46.
20. Borges A, Casselman J. Imaging the cranial nerves: Part I: methodology, infectious and inflammatory, traumatic and congenital lesions. Eur Radiol. 2007;17(8):2112-25.
21. Lufkin R, Borges A, Villablanca P. Teaching atlas of head and neck imaging, 1st edition. New York: Thieme; 2000.
22. Casselman JW. The skull base: tumoral lesions. Eur Radiol. 2005;15(3):534-42.
23. Borges A, Casselman J. Imaging the cranial nerves: part II: primary and secondary neoplastic conditions and neurovascular conflicts. Eur Radiol. 2007;17(9):2332-44.
24. Williams LS. Advanced concepts in the imaging of perineural spread of tumor to the trigeminal nerve. Top Magn Reson Imaging. 1999;10(6):376-83.
25. Borges A. Imaging of the central skull base. Neuroimaging Clin N Am. 2009;19(3):441-68.
26. Ong CK, Fook-Hin Chong V. Imaging of jugular foramen. Neuroimaging Clin N Am. 2009;19(3):469-82.
27. Carvalho GA, Tatagiba M, Samii M. Cystic schwannomas of the jugular foramen: clinical and surgical remarks. Neurosurgery. 2000;46(3):560-6.
28. Chong VF, Khoo JB, Fan YF. Imaging of the nasopharynx and skull base. Magn Reson Imaging Clin N Am. 2002;10(4):547-71, v.
29. Overton SB, Ritter FN. A high placed jugular bulb in the middle ear: a clinical and temporal bone study. Laryngoscope. 1973;83(12):1986-91.
30. Kawano H, Tono T, Schachern PA, Paparella MM, Komune S. Petrous high jugular bulb: a histological study. Am J Otolaryngol. 2000;21(3):161-8.
31. Robert Y, Carcasset S, Rocourt N, Hennequin C, Dubrulle F, Lemaitre L. Congenital cholesteatoma of the temporal bone: MR findings and comparison with CT. Am J Neuroradiol. 1995;16(4):755-61.
32. Aikele P, Kittner T, Offergeld C, Kaftan H, Huttenbrink KB, Laniado M. Diffusion-weighted MR imaging of cholesteatoma in pediatric and adult patients who have undergone middle ear surgery. Am J Roentgenol. 2003;181(1):261-5.
33. Weber AL. Imaging of the skull base. Eur J Radiol. 1996;22(1):68-81.
34. Chong VF, Khoo JB, Fan YF. Fibrous dysplasia involving the base of the skull. Am J Roentgenol. 2002;178(3):717-20.
35. Shama SA. Osteomyelitis of the central skull base: otogenic and odontogenic sources. Multidetector CT study. The Egyptian Journal of Radiology and Nuclear Medicine. 2012;43(4):519-26.

CHAPTER

207

Maxillofacial Imaging: Imaging of Cysts, Tumors and Tumor-like Conditions of the Jaw

Ashu Seith Bhalla, Smita Manchanda, Atin Kumar, Chandan J Das

Maxillofacial imaging represents a diverse area of radiology and includes imaging of dental caries, periodontal tissues, periapical tissues, dental restorations, implants, developmental abnormalities, cysts and tumors, trauma, salivary glands and temporomandibular joints. The application of advanced imaging modalities for these diseases has lead to increased involvement of radiologists in this field. This chapter will focus on evaluation of cysts, tumors and tumor-like conditions of the jaw.

IMAGING MODALITIES

Plain Radiography

Plain radiography remains the mainstay investigation in the evaluation of jaw lesions despite the availability of modern imaging modalities. These radiographs may be intraoral or extraoral **(Table 1)**.

Intraoral Radiographs

Intraoral radiographs **(Figs. 1A and B)** present a detailed view of the teeth and periapical region, however are not useful for lesions larger than 3 cm because of the small film size.[1] Intraoral radiographs include periapical view, which shows individual teeth and tissues around the apices. Two to four teeth are seen in each image with detailed information about the teeth and surrounding alveolar bone. Occlusal radiography refers to a radiographic technique wherein the image receptor (film or digital phosphor plate) is placed in the occlusal plane. Various occlusal views are used depending upon the region of interest. These include the upper standard maxilla for anterior maxilla, upper oblique for posterior maxilla, lower 90° occlusal for evaluating buccolingual expansion of mandible, lower 45° (or anterior) occlusal for anterior mandible and lower oblique for posterior mandible.[2]

TABLE 1: Plain radiographs in maxillofacial imaging.

Plain radiographs
Intraoral: • Periapical • *Occlusal view:* - *Anterior maxilla*: Upper standard maxilla - *Posterior maxilla*: Upper oblique - *Buccolingual expansion of mandible*: Lower 90° occlusal - *Anterior mandible*: Lower 45° (or anterior) occlusal - *Posterior mandible*: Lower oblique
Extraoral: • *Mandible*: Oblique-lateral, PA view • *Maxilla*: Water's view OPG/Panoramic radiography

Extraoral Radiographs

Extraoral radiographs **(Figs. 2A and B)** are primarily used for the larger lesions and to evaluate the skull and facial structures. Commonly used extraoral radiographs include the oblique-lateral view.

Extraoral radiographs were predominantly used before the development of panoramic equipment. In recent years though, due to limitations of panoramic radiographs this view is still useful. Posteroanterior view of the jaw (PA mandible) shows posterior parts of the mandible. It is not suitable however for showing the facial skeleton including maxilla due to superimposition of the base of skull. An occipitomeatal or Water's view may be used for this purpose.[2]

Orthopantomography (OPG)/Panoramic Radiography or Dental Panoramic Tomography

Orthopantomography (OPG)/Panoramic radiography or dental panoramic tomography **(Fig. 3)** is a special technique, for evaluating a broad area with relatively low radiation dose. It is also beneficial for patients who are unable to open their mouths.[1,2] It is an extraoral radiographic technique, which is popular because it is used to examine the upper and lower jaws on a single film and it involves low radiation doses. A number of panoramic systems have been developed that generate tomographic sections of various facial structures such as mid face, orbit, temporo mandibular joints, mandible, and paranasal sinuses.

The major drawback of the technique is that since the resultant film is a sectional radiograph produced by moving equipment, therefore like all other forms of tomography only structures within the section will be in focus. In panoramic

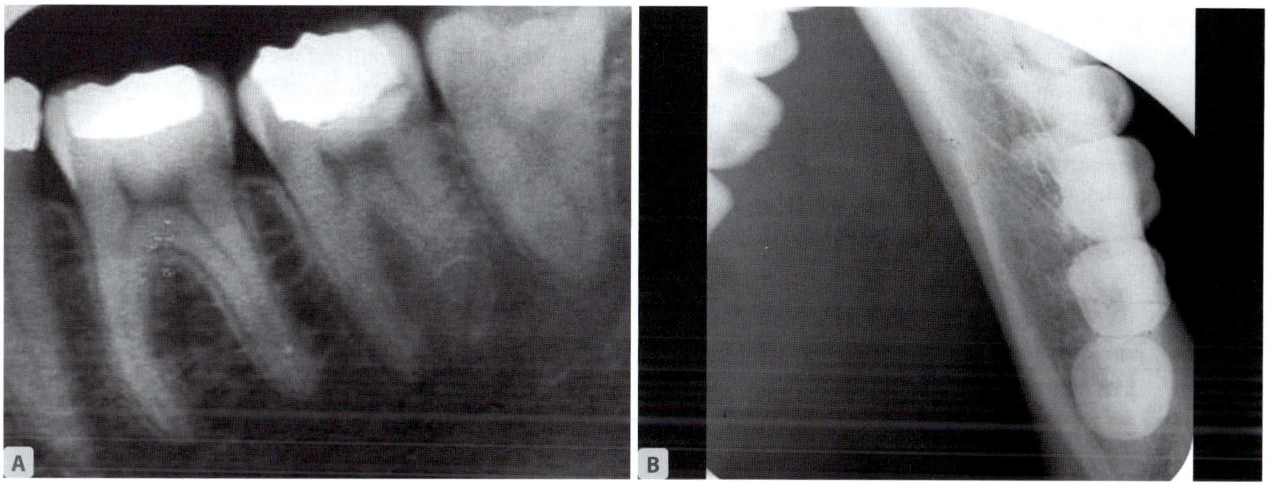

FIGS. 1A AND B: Intraoral radiographs. (A) Periapical view of mandibular molars showing detailed view of three teeth with periapical and interdental tissues; (B) Lower oblique occlusal view demonstrating the posterior mandible. This view is also used for evaluating submandibular gland calculi.

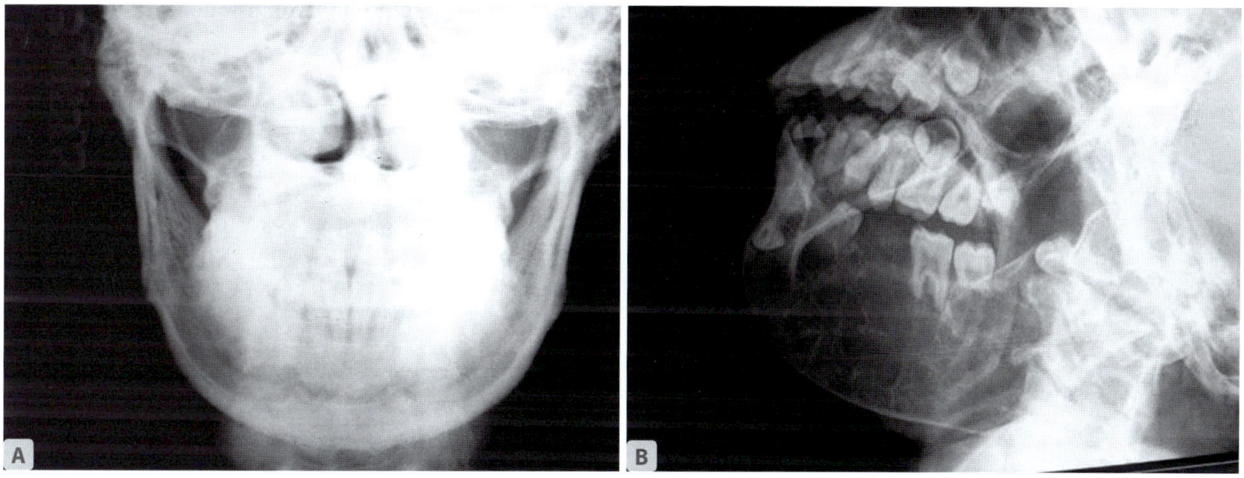

FIGS. 2A AND B: Extraoral radiographs. (A) Anteroposterior view demonstrating the posterior part of the mandible, while the (B) lateral oblique view shows almost the entire hemimandible, except the midline well. Patient in (B) has an odontogenic myxoma.

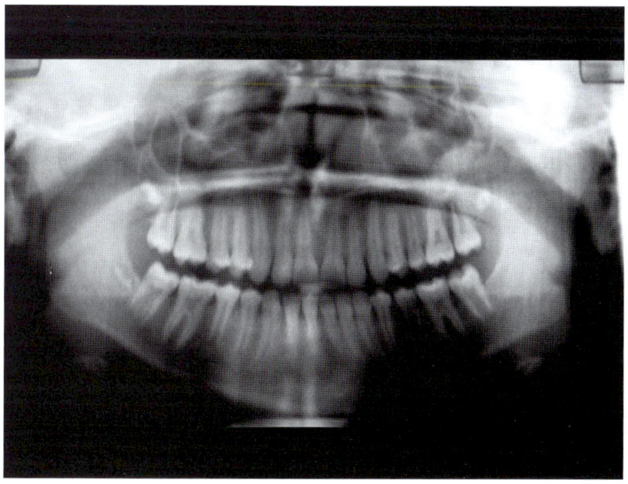

FIG. 3: Panoramic radiograph giving a global view of upper and lower jaws as well as the temporomandibular joints.

imaging, the section or focal trough is nearly horseshoe-shaped aligning to the shape of the dental arches. Image quality is less compared to that obtained using intraoral radiography, irrespective of the image receptor used.[2] Various ghost images and technical artifacts because of patient rotation maybe seen.

Computed Tomography

After plain radiography computed tomography (CT) is the primary modality used in the evaluation of cystic or tumorous jaw lesions. CT is useful in determining the complete topography of these lesions. It aids in evaluating integrity of the bony margins of the lesion, its matrix, proximity of the lesion to vital structures and soft tissue extension.[3] Multislice CT technique using multidetector CT (MDCT) has now become the new standard in radiological imaging, including in head and neck imaging. Because of the shorter examination time due to faster scans, motion artifacts are reduced. Due to the thin-slicing and nearly isotropic multiplanar reconstruction (MPR), examination in only one plane is necessary with MDCT, saving both time and radiation exposure. Various 3D processing and advanced evaluation tools can be used in maxillofacial imaging, as elsewhere in the body **(Table 2)**. Some techniques, which are peculiar to the evaluation of this region, are highlighted.

TABLE 2: Computed tomography in maxillofacial imaging.
Base acquisition: 0.6 mm
Reconstructions: • Standard axial 3 mm in soft tissue and bone windows • Multiplanar reconstructions (MPR): axial, coronal and sagittal planes • Mininmum intensity projections (MIP) • Volume rendered techniques (VRT)
CECT: For all cysts/ tumors
Dental CT Reformatting Programs: Panoramic, Paraxial
Cone-beam CT

Dental CT Reformatting Programs

Dental reformatting programs were basically developed for the preoperative evaluation of dental implants. These are however finding increasing application in the evaluation of a variety of dental and periodontal diseases including cysts and tumors. Dental CT programs are reconstruction techniques that use thin axial images (up to 1 mm) of the mandible and maxilla to reformat a series of multiple cross-sectional and panoramic images **(Figs. 4A to C)**. The axial images should be acquired parallel to the alveolar ridge. The cross-sectional images are used for preoperative implant assessment. The measurements obtained help to determine the size of the implant to be used. The numerous cross-sectional images obtained can be intimidating and need to be closely correlated with the markings on the base axial and reconstructed panoramic image.[4] The panoramic reconstructions are immensely useful in the evaluation of maxillofacial tumors and cysts. Similar to panoramic radiography the relationship of the lesion to the roots of teeth is demonstrated. The relationship to mandibular canal and maxillary antra is exquisitely demonstrated.

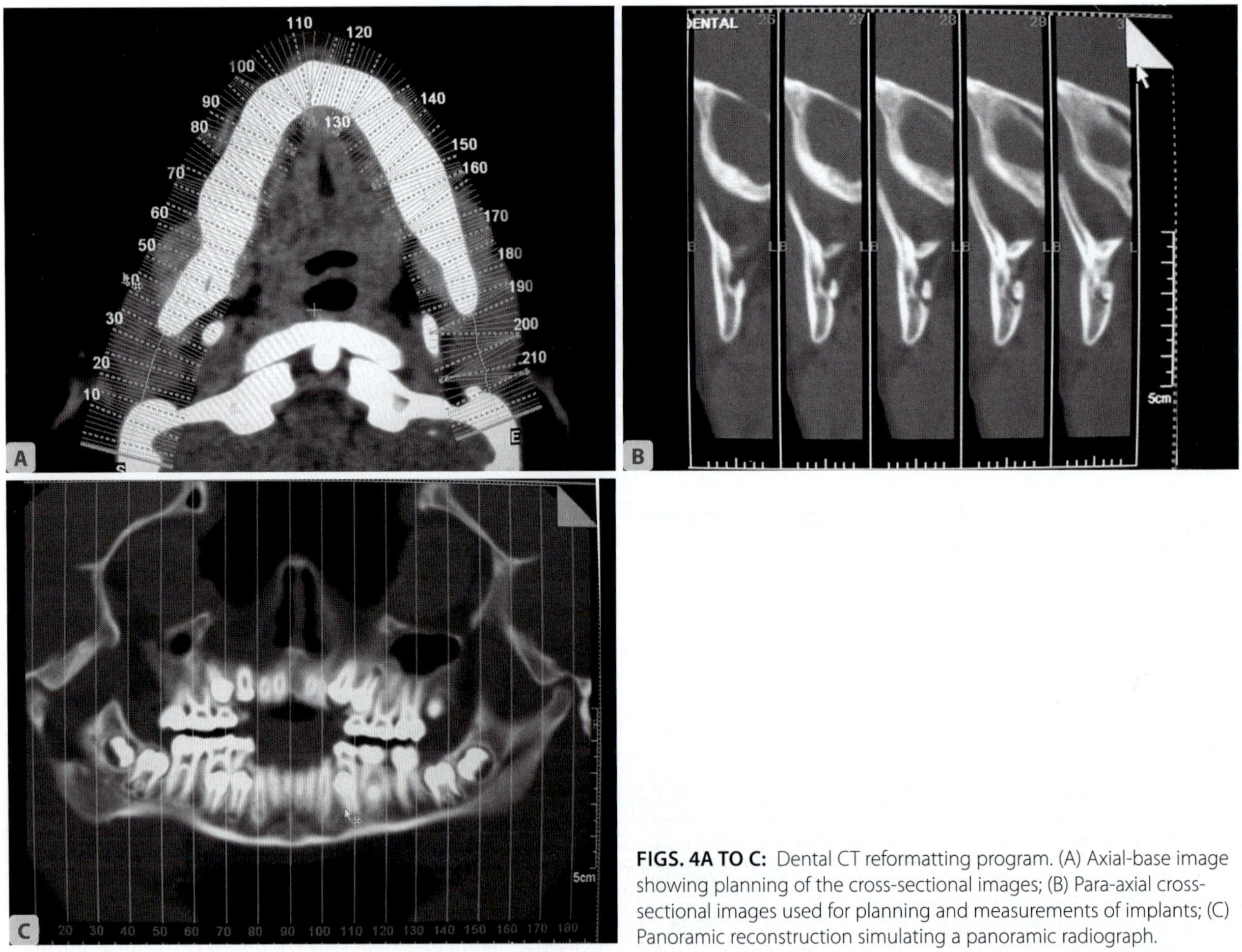

FIGS. 4A TO C: Dental CT reformatting program. (A) Axial-base image showing planning of the cross-sectional images; (B) Para-axial cross-sectional images used for planning and measurements of implants; (C) Panoramic reconstruction simulating a panoramic radiograph.

Cone-beam CT

Also referred to as digital volume tomography cone-beam CT is a low dose CT technology developed specifically for use in dental and maxillofacial region. This equipment uses a cone-shaped X-ray beam vs the fan-shaped beam used in conventional CT. An image intensifier or amorphous silicon flat panel is used as detector. The equipment rotates around the patient acquiring a cylindrical or spherical volume in one rotation. The time taken is approximately 20–40 seconds. The X-ray beam typically has high kV (90–110 kV) pulsed beam to reduce soft tissue absorption. The technique has a small voxel size and hence has high spatial resolution. The computer softwares allow multiplanar reconstruction in axial, coronal and sagittal planes. The advantages of the technique are its low radiation dose, relatively low cost, multiplanar reconstruction and its compatibility with implant and cephalometric planning software. The disadvantage is the need for patient to remain absolutely stationary for 20–40 seconds. Also the soft tissues are not imaged in detail, dental fillings produce streak artifacts and interpretation of panoramic images needs care.[2]

Magnetic Resonance Imaging

Magnetic resonance imaging (MRI) is useful to differentiate cysts from tumors and for evaluating infiltration of the malignant tumors into the bone and surrounding soft tissues, especially for detecting early bone marrow changes of the jaw. However, the differentiation between cysts and tumors requires a contrast-enhanced study.[5]

MRI, unlike CT has the advantage of minimal artifacts caused by heavy metals used for dental fillings. Its major drawback, however, is lack of signal from cortical bone. Hence, it is not effective in identifying calcified portion of the tumor and the cortex of the bone. MR imaging is ideal for the assessment of bone marrow, subtle cortical erosion, and the extent of extraosseous soft tissue component. However, CT remains superior to MRI for the detection of bone destruction and calcification.

MR signal intensities have also been used for evaluating MRI features of cysts of the oral and maxillo-mandibular region **(Figs. 5A to D)**.

Diffusion weighted imaging[6] also has a key role to play in the differentiation of unilocular cystic lesions. It is difficult

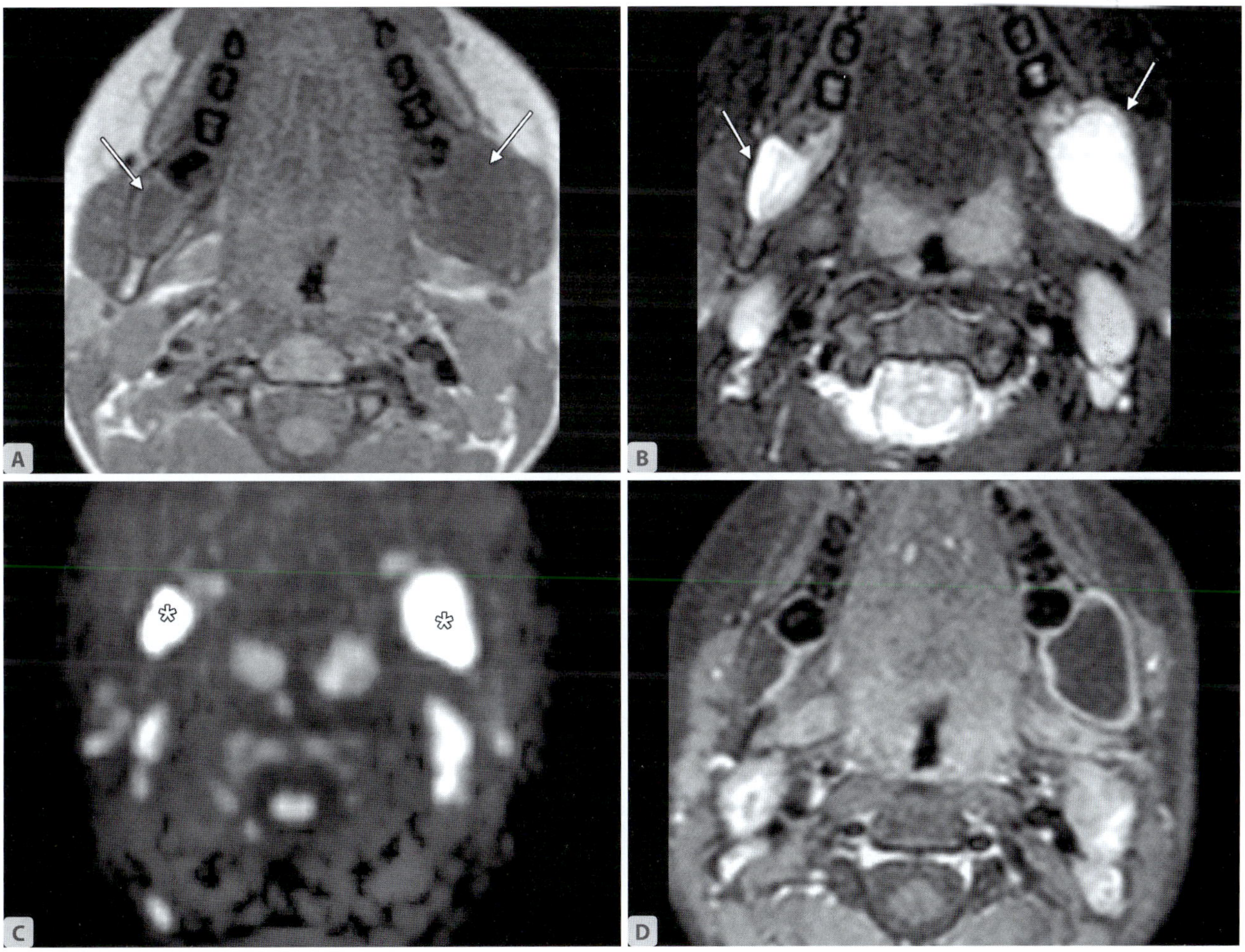

FIGS. 5A TO D: Multiple odontogenic keratocysts MRI: Axial T1WI (A) shows two small, well-defined hypointense lesions in rami of both hemimandible (arrows). These are hyperintense on T2WI (B) and show diffusion restriction in DWI image b value 800 (asterisks in C) . Axial postcontrast T1WI (D) reveals mild enhancement of wall of the lesions.

to differentiate cystic ameloblastoma from keratocystic odontogenic tumor (OKC) on CT and conventional MR sequences. However, OKC **(Figs. 5A to D)** has highly viscous contents and its cystic component shows restricted diffusion (values $<2 \times 10^{-3}$ mm^2 s^{-1} suggestive of OKC).[6]

The superior contrast resolution of MRI helps in the accurate delineation of tumor extent. In addition, the use of a T1-weighted 3D sequence (ultrafast gradient echo) with integrated fat saturation (e.g. VIBE) can accurately demonstrate the inferior alveolar neurovascular bundle. Suppression of the fatty marrow improves the contrast between the neurovascular structures and the surrounding bone. *The reconstructed panoramic image* ***(Figs. 6A and B)*** is an effective alternative to panoramic MDCT images and can be used in patients with contraindications to MRI.[6,7] **Table 3** summarizes the suggested MRI protocol in maxillofacial imaging.[6,7]

CLASSIFICATION

The primary lesions involving the jaw may be either odontogenic or nonodontogenic. Odontogenic cysts and tumors develop during or after the formation of teeth. These lesions could be either cystic or solid and benign or malignant with varying degrees of destructive potential. Most odontogenic maxillomandibular lesions are benign, but some may exhibit aggressive behavior locally.

Secondary involvement of the jaw is seen in neoplastic or inflammatory process involving the soft tissues adjoining the jaw, hematogenous metastases, or part of a systemic disease.[8-10]

In 2017, the 4th edition of the World Health Organization Classification of Head and Neck tumors was published with a number of significant changes.[11,12] The common lesions seen in the maxillofacial region are summarized in **Table 4**.

CLINICAL FEATURES

Usually asymptomatic in the early period, many lesions are incidentally seen on plain radiographs. Most common symptoms are swelling and pain. Swelling may be either intraoral or outside resulting in facial asymmetry. Presence of paresthesia indicates mandibular canal involvement, and is common in malignant lesions. Other presentations include tooth displacement or mobility. Few lesions may present with bleeding or with signs and symptoms of secondary infection. The symptoms have no correlation with benign or malignant disease process.[10]

RADIOLOGICAL FEATURES/APPROACH

Maxillomandibular lesions have a wide range of pathologic descriptions but with similar imaging characters. Many of these lesions have a cyst-like radiographic appearance and can be indistinguishable on imaging. Patient age at presentation, history, and location within the mandible, its internal architecture, border contour, and effect of the lesion on contiguous structures are all taken into consideration before reaching the possible diagnosis. At times, it is difficult to make a definitive diagnosis without biopsy and the role of imaging in such cases is to define the extent and malignant potential. Imaging should help narrow the differential diagnosis and help in guiding patient treatment. Detailed description of the lesion aids in arriving at the differential diagnosis and is also imperative in mapping its extent. The radiological report should detail the features as described in **Table 5**.

ANATOMICAL LOCATION

Some lesions have a predilection for particular sites, whereas others can occur anywhere in the jaw. Systemic disorders (metabolic or endocrine) should be considered if all structures of maxillofacial region appear involved.[1,9]

TABLE 3: Suggested MRI protocol in maxillofacial imaging.
Precontrast sequences: • Axial T1WI • Axial T2WI, coronal and sagittal T2FSWI
Postcontrast sequences: • Post gad axial, coronal T1WI • T1-weighted FS 3D sequence (e.g. VIBE)
Special sequences: Diffusion (b values 0, 500 and 1000)
Advanced reconstructions: Curved MPR (panoramic image)

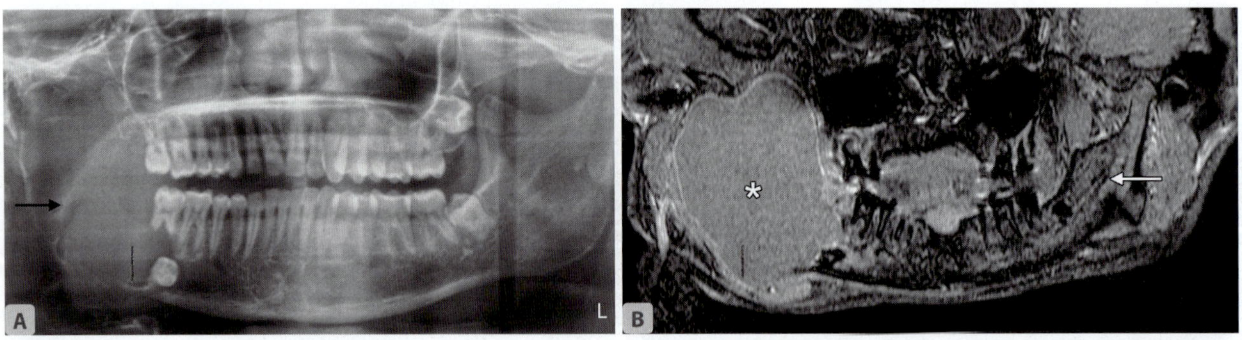

FIGS. 6A AND B: Ameloblastoma. (A) Panoramic radiograph showing large expansile multilocular lesion in the ramus of the right hemimandible (black arrow); (B) Curved multiplanar reformatted image after gadolinium administration shows a hypointense lesion (asterisk) in the right hemimandible with destruction of the right canal. The left inferior alveolar canal was normal (arrow).

TABLE 4: Common odontogenic and maxillofacial lesions[11,12]

Cystic lesions
Inflammatory cysts
• Radicular cyst
• Inflammatory collateral cysts
Developmental cysts
• Dentigerous cyst
• Odontogenic keratocyst (OKC)
• Gingival cyst
• Nasopalatine duct cyst
• Primordial cyst
Solid lesions
Odontogenic tumors
Benign odontogenic tumors
• *Epithelial*:
– Ameloblastoma
– Adenomatoid odontogenic tumor
– Calcifying epithelial odontogenic tumor
• *Mesenchymal*:
– Odontogenic myxoma/myxofibroma
– Cemento-ossifying fibroma
Cementoblastoma
• *Mixed epithelial and mesenchymal*:
– Ameloblastic fibroma
– Odontoma
Malignant odontogenic tumors
• Odontogenic carcinomas
• Odontogenic sarcomas
• Odontogenic carcinosarcoma
Bone and cartilage tumors
• *Benign*:
– Osteoblastoma
– Chondroblastoma
– Osteoma
– Osteoid osteoma
– Chondroma
– Chondromyxoid fibroma
• *Malignant*:
– Osteosarcoma
– Chondrosarcoma
– Mesenchymal chondrosarcoma
Fibro- and chondro-osseous lesions
• Osteochondroma
• Ossifying fibroma
• Fibrous dysplasia
• Cemento-osseous dysplasia
Miscellaneous lesions
• Simple bone cyst
• Aneurysmal bone cyst
• Central giant cell granuloma
• Cherubism
• Solitary plasmacytoma

TABLE 5: Key radiologic descriptors for maxillofacial lesions.

1. *Anatomical location*: – Site – Relation to dentition – Relation to mandibular canal
2. Size
3. Shape
4. Density and Internal architecture
5. Outline/definition/margin
6. *Effect on surrounding structures*: – Teeth – Bone – Soft tissues

Site

In the mandible, majority of the lesions occur in posterior part of mandible or angle as this region has more vascularity. Lesions having a propensity for the anterior mandible include: periapical cemental dysplasia, florid cemento-osseous dysplasia, odontoma, simple bone cyst, central hemangioma, central giant cell granuloma and brown tumor. Midline maxilla may be involved by an incisive canal cyst, central giant cell granuloma, simple bone cyst or hemangioma. Stafne's cyst is typically located inferior to the mandibular canal in posterior mandible (below 3rd molar).

Relation to Dentition

Involvement of only one tooth or a specific part of the tooth is suggestive of odontogenic lesion. For instance, radicular dental cysts develop at the apices of nonvital teeth, whereas dentigerous cysts develop at the crown **(Figs. 7A and B)**. Cementomas occur at the apex of vital teeth.

Non-odontogenic lesions generally have no specific relationship to the dentition or can involve the bone around two or more teeth.

Relation to Mandibular Canal

Relationship of the lesion to the inferior alveolar canal also indicates the origin of the lesion. Lesions above the canal are probably odontogenic, whereas those involving the canal or below it are usually non-odontogenic.

SIZE

Size of a lesion can be expressed in centimeters in two dimensions on a single view (along the axis of the lesion and an axis perpendicular to it). Size may also be expressed in terms of landmarks, e.g. the overlying teeth or mandibular canal. In central lesions it must be mentioned if these cross the midline. Size of the lesion does not help in differentiation between benign and malignant. Some lesions however are

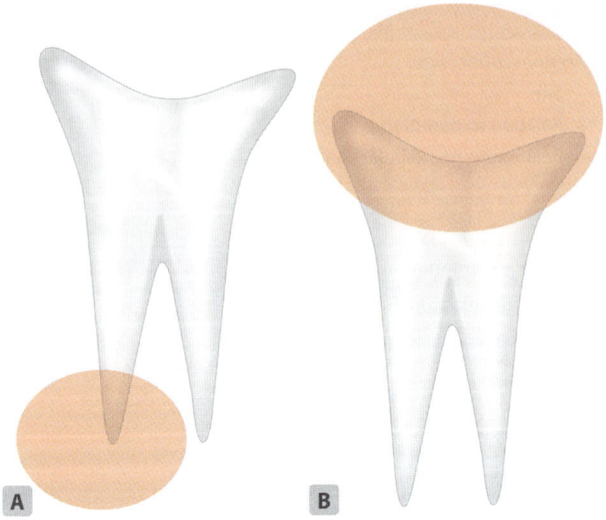

FIGS. 7A AND B: Relationship of cysts to teeth. (A) Periapical lesions: The differential diagnosis of lesions in this location include periapical granuloma, radicular cyst abscess, osteomyelitis, simple bone cyst and periapical cemento-osseous dysplasia; (B) Pericoronal lesions include dentigerous cyst (commonest), ameloblastoma (unicystic), odontogenic keratocyst, calcifying odontogenic cyst (rare).

typically small (2–3 cm, e.g. Stafne's cyst), while others may assume very large sizes (e.g. ameloblastoma).[2]

SHAPE

Shape of a lesion is described as being oval, round, scalloped (or undulating) or irregular. Shape of a lesion may help in the diagnosis, e.g. a radicular cyst is round and unilocular. Odontogenic, keratocyst is oval, growing along the long axis of the mandible. Unequal growth results in scalloped margins. Simple bone cyst typically has irregular margins as it arches between roots of teeth. Irregular margins also suggest an infective or malignant lesion. Whether the lesion is uni or multilocular may also be described under shape of the lesion.[2]

DENSITY AND INTERNAL ARCHITECTURE OF LESION

Radiographically, jaw lesions are often classified according to their radiographic densities on plain radiographs. They can be described as having either a radiolucent, radiopaque or mixed appearance relative to the density of adjacent bone.

The *radiolucent lesions* can be further divided as being well circumscribed or poorly circumscribed.

Well-defined radiolucent lesions include periapical cyst, dentigerous cyst, odontogenic keratocyst, ameloblastoma, simple bone cyst, central giant cell granuloma.

Poorly-circumscribed radiolucent are acute osteomyelitis, primary bone neoplasm and secondary bone neoplasms.

Radiopaque lesions include odontoma, torus, osteoma, osteochondroma, cementoblastoma, and late stages of fibrous dysplasia.

Mixed density lesions are fibrous dysplasia, ossifying fibroma, cemento-osseous dysplasia, chronic osteomyelitis, osteosarcoma.[1,2]

Analysis of internal structure of the lesion is also helpful in narrowing the differential diagnosis, i.e. describing the lesion as being either unilocular/multilocular/honeycomb appearance, thin/thick internal bony trabaculae. Multilocular odontogenic lesions include ameloblastoma and odontogenic myxoma; while non-odontogenic lesions include central giant cell granuloma, hemangioma and rarely aneurismal bone cyst.

The cyst/tumor may be uniformly radiolucent or have calcific radiodensities within or have a ground-glass appearance or be uniformly radiodense. Lesions may also have internal cementum (amorphous calcification) or identifiable dental tissue (dentine or enamel).

OUTLINE/DEFINITION/MARGINATION

In general, lesions with well-defined borders are usually benign, whereas lesions with ill-defined borders represent aggressive, inflammatory or neoplastic processes. A well-defined outline may be further detailed as being punched-out (sharp with no surrounding bone reaction), corticated (surrounding radiopaque bone), sclerotic (non-uniform radiopaque boundary) or encapsulated (surrounding radiolucent line). Similarly a poorly defined margin may blend imperceptibly with the surrounding bone or show "moth-eaten" margins.[2] A benign cyst with secondary infection may mimic a more aggressive lesion.

EFFECT ON SURROUNDING STRUCTURES

The effect of the lesion on surrounding structures, i.e. teeth, bone and soft tissue also needs to be evaluated **(Figs. 8A and B)**.

Teeth

Benign lesions typically cause displacement of teeth without resorption. However, long standing, benign but locally aggressive lesions can cause tooth resorption. Inflammatory and malignant lesions also cause resorption. When lesions occur in young patients, they can result in delayed eruption or disrupted development (abnormal shape or density) of teeth. Loss of lamina dura may also be seen. Malignant lesions may rapidly grow down the periodontal ligament resulting in initial widening and later disruption of lamina dura.[1,2]

Surrounding Bone

Bone expansion in all four directions should be noted, i.e. buccal, lingual, inferior and superior. Areas of cortical perforation should be recorded in the report as they help in guiding management decisions. For mandibular lesions, the thickness and integrity of the inferior cortex is important. On the other hand, for maxillary lesions the superior involvement, i.e. floors of the maxillary antrum, nasal cavity and orbit need to be commented upon. Cortical perforation is seen

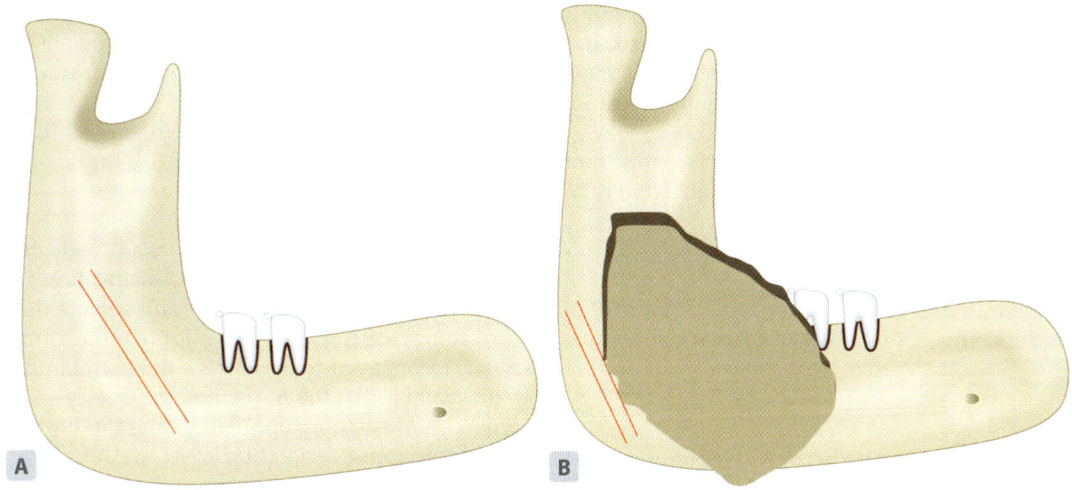

FIGS. 8A AND B: Effect on surrounding structures (A) normal mandible, (B) an expansile aggressive cystic lesion causing displacement of the inferior alveolar canal and erosion of the roots of overlying teeth, as well as tooth displacement.

TABLE 6: Common radiolucent lesions of the maxillofacial region.

Well defined				**Poorly defined**		
Jaw cysts		Solid lesions/tumors		Osteomyelitis	Tumors	
Odontogenic	Non-odontogenic	Odontogenic	Non-odontogenic		Odontogenic	Non-odontogenic
• Radicular cyst • Dentigerous cyst • Odontogenic keratocyst	• Nasopalatine duct cyst • Simple bone cyst • Aneurysmal bone cyst	• Ameloblastoma • Ameloblastic fibroma	• Central giant cell reparative granuloma • Eosinophilic granuloma • Hemangioma • AVM		• Odontogenic carcinoma • Malignant ameloblastoma	• Oteosarcoma • Chondrosarcoma • Fibrosarcoma • Lymphoreticular malignancies

in aggressive inflammatory or malignant lesions. However, focal areas of cortical break may also be seen in benign lesions causing massive osseous expansion, e.g. aneurysmal bone cyst. MDCT with multiplanar reconstruction is superior to plain radiography in this regard.

Involvement or displacement of inferior dental canal and mental foramen needs to be evaluated. Erosion of the cortex indicates involvement. Widening of the inferior alveolar canal may be seen in lesions of vascular and neurogenic origin. Presence of sclerosis or subperiosteal reaction aid in arriving at a diagnosis. Periosteal reaction indicates inflammatory or malignant lesions.

Surrounding Soft Tissues

Extent of soft tissue involvement in aggressive lesions should be detailed including the muscles involved, i.e. masseters and pterygoids.

The further description of the maxillofacial lesions is on the basis of the predominant radiographic appearance (radiolucent, mixed density or radiopaque).

Table 6 summarizes the common radiolucent lesions of the maxillofacial region.

WELL-DEFINED RADIOLUCENT LESIONS

Jaw Cysts

Odontogenic Cysts

Radicular Cyst

Radicular (periapical) cyst is the most frequently seen cyst of the jaw (about 70%).[2] These occur at the apex of a non-vital tooth, particularly upper lateral incisors. A radicular cyst is an inflammatory cyst which is the last step in a chain of events resulting from periapical inflammation secondary to pulpal necrosis in a tooth. Over a period of time, this cyst develops in the bone at the root apex of a carious tooth due to proliferation of the epithelial cell rests of Malassez.[2,10]

Commonly seen in asymptomatic adults between 20 and 50 years of age. These cysts usually measure less than 1 cm, although sizes up to 3 cm may be seen. Plain radiographs reveal round, unilocular, radiolucent lesions in the periapical region with defined, smooth margins and surrounded by a thin rim of cortical bone. There is usually associated caries. The cyst may displace adjacent teeth or rarely cause mild root resorption **(Fig. 9)**. The cyst may cause buccal expansion or displacement of the maxillary antrum. Radicular cysts and periapical granulomas have a similar imaging morphology, and cannot always help distinguish a granuloma from a cyst.[2,9,10,13]

Treatment consists of enucleation of the cyst lining and endodontic obturation (root canal). Tooth extraction may be also required.

Residual Cyst

Cyst, which remains after surgical intervention/removal of the causative root. Thus, most residual cysts are periapical cysts.

Dentigerous Cyst

Dentigerous (follicular) cyst is the most common type of non-inflammatory odontogenic cyst.[14] Impacted tooth is seen with associated pericoronal lucency. It forms within the lining of the dental follicle when fluid accumulates between the enamel epithelium and the crown of the developing or unerupted tooth. Usually seen in adolescents and young adults, and patients are typically pain free.

On imaging, dentigerous cysts appear as well-defined, round or ovoid, smooth, well-defined, well-corticated, uniformly radiolucent, unilocular lesions. These typically are located around the crowns of unerupted teeth, usually third molars and envelope the crown symmetrically **(Fig. 10)**. The roots of the involved teeth are often outside the lesion. The adjoining teeth are displaced and resorbed in about half the cases.[2] They may be large in size and can extend up into the ramus with mandibular expansion. Buccal or medial expansion can be extensive in large cysts causing facial asymmetry or antral displacement. The characteristic features of this lesion are its marked, relatively asymptomatic, expansion and its potential to displace or resorb adjacent teeth.[2,10]

Extremely large dentigerous cysts simulate odontogenic keratocyst or ameloblastoma as they may have undulating borders. Rarely, an untreated cyst may develop an ameloblastoma within its lining referred to as a mural ameloblastoma. However, malignant tranformation is extremely rare.

Treatment includes removal of the entire cyst and associated tooth extraction.

Odontogenic Keratocyst

Odontogenic keratocysts (OKC) has been restored to odontogenic cysts by the WHO Classification[11,12] of Head and Neck Tumors (4th edition) and rejects the previous terminology of Keratocystic odontogenic tumor (KOT). These are believed to arise from the epithelium of dental lamina rather than the normal tooth.[2] The cyst is lined by a parakeratinized lining epithelium and the lumen contains "cheesy" material. Daughter cysts are found outside the primary lesion. Only curettage as the treatment has high recurrence rate of any odontogenic cyst because of the presence of daughter cysts outside the primary lesion.[15] Hence the preferred treatment for these lesions is surgical enucleation, with wide bone margins.

OKC are relatively uncommon and represent approximately 5–15% of all jaw cysts.[10] The age range of these lesions is very variable with the peak during the 2nd to 4th decades of life. Multiple lesions are associated with the basal cell nevus syndrome (Gorlin-Goltz syndrome).

On imaging, OKC may be seen anywhere in the maxilla or the mandible but are most commonly located in the posterior body and ramus of the mandible. OKC are characteristically oval in shape extending along the body of the mandible with relatively little mediolateral expansion. These lesions usually appear as a unilocular, lucent lesions but may be multilocular. Their borders are smooth, scalloped, well-defined and corticated. They are often associated with an impacted tooth **(Figs. 11 and 12)**. Although odontogenic keratocysts in some cases may arise in the lining of primordial cysts without a tooth, while at times they include the crown of the last molar. Such lesions are indistinguishable from dentigerous cysts on

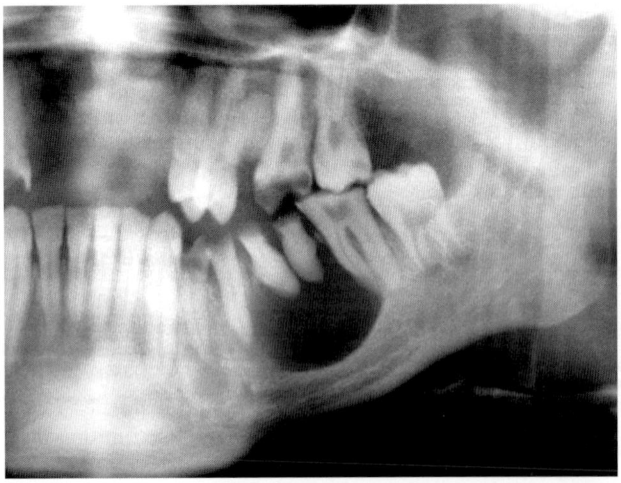

FIG. 9: Radicular cyst: Panoramic radiograph showing a round, well-defined, smooth, unilocular radiolucent lesion located in the periapical region of a grossly carious first molar tooth.

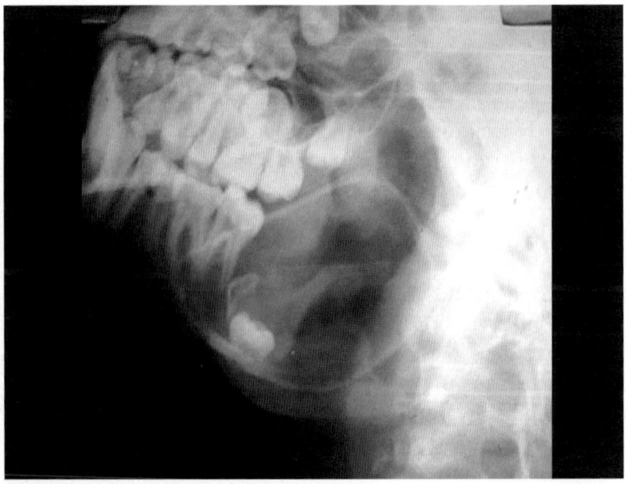

FIG. 10: Dentigerous cyst: Lateral oblique view of mandible show a large expansile, well-defined, ovoid, unilocular, radiolucent lesion surrounding the crown of an unerupted last molar tooth.

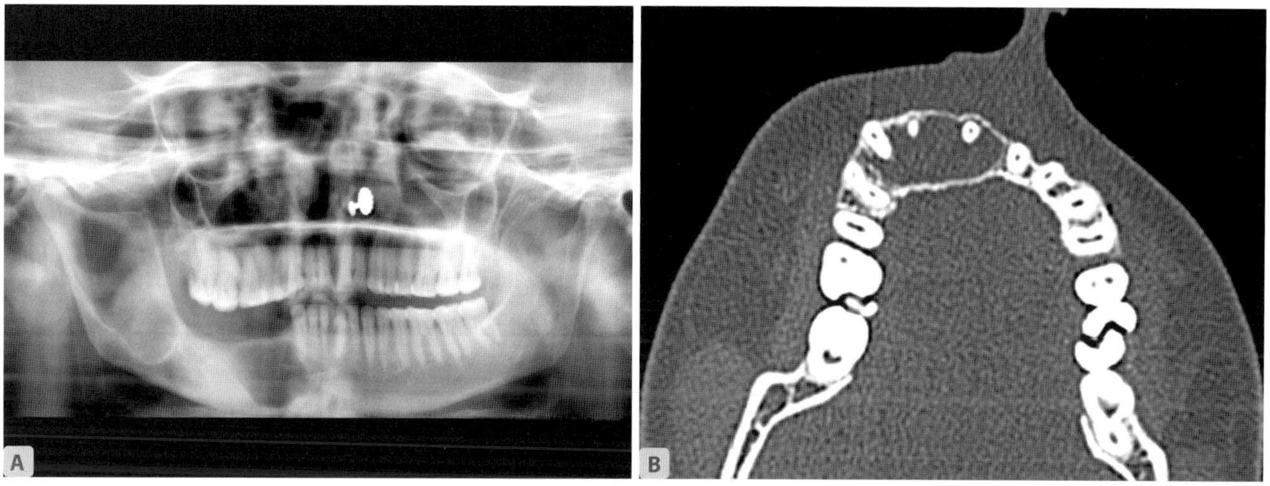

FIGS. 11A AND B: Odontogenic keratocyst. (A) Panorax view of a young adult shows an oval, smooth, well-corticated, unilocular cyst located in the posterior body and ramus of the mandible, extending along the body of the mandible with relatively little mediolateral expansion. Another lesion is present in the body of the mandible on the right side; (B) Axial CT scan of a different patient shows the characteristic ovoid disposition of an OKC with minimal buccolingual expansion.

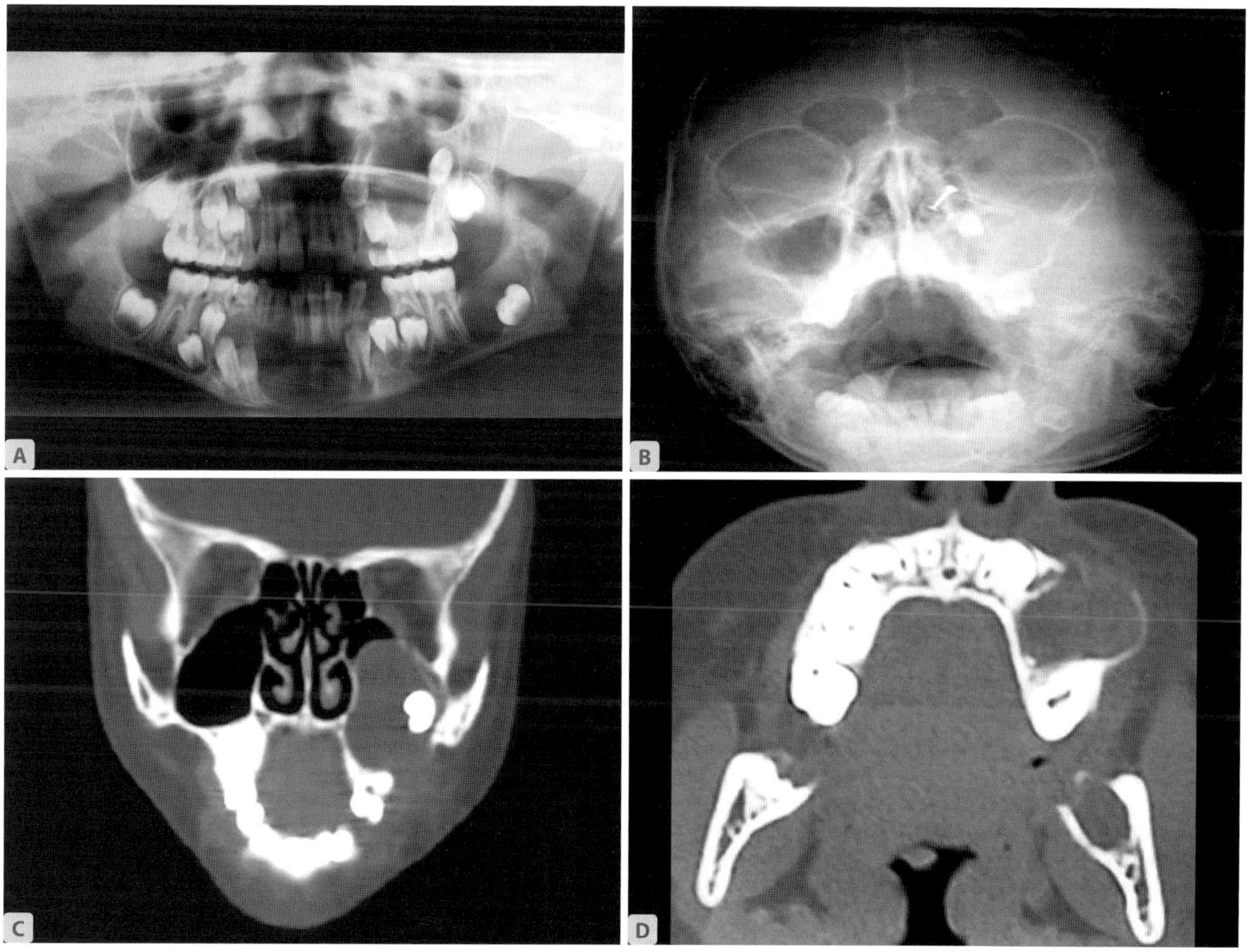

FIGS. 12A TO D: (A) Panorex view of a 12 years old girl with past history of curettage for an OKC shows multiple, recurrent lesions; (B) Water's view shows cranial displacement of a left-sided tooth with apparently opaque maxillary antrum; (C) Coronal CT scan shows a large maxillary cyst displacing and encasing a molar tooth. The maxillary antrum is compressed;[9] (D) Axial CT section reveals both the maxillary and mandibular lesions.

radiography. OKC may show aggressive growth compared to other odontogenic cysts and may have undulating borders and a multilocular appearance simulating ameloblastomas. Odontogenic keratocysts may cause cortical thinning. Adjacent teeth are usually displaced, and occasionally resorbed.[15]

On MRI (***see* Figs. 5A to D**), odontogenic keratocysts have an intermediate to high signal intensity on T1W images and heterogeneous low to high signal intensity on T2W images. On contrast administration OKC show thin rim enhancement unlike tumors such as ameloblastoma, which have solid components. Diffusion restriction of the contents of the cyst is characteristic for OKC.[16]

Primordial Cyst

Primordial cyst is an uncommon cystic lesion, which develops instead of a tooth. Cystic degeneration of the dental follicle before completion of odontogenesis results in primordial cyst. These are well-defined, non-expansile, well-defined radiolucent lesions without an associated tooth.[9]

Non-odontogenic Cysts

Nasopalatine Duct Cyst

A nasopalatine duct cyst (also known as incisive canal cyst) is a non-odontogenic developmental cyst or fissural cyst arising from epithelial remnants of the nasopalatine duct.[16] It is located in the midline in anterior maxilla. It is the commonest nonodontogenic cyst. They are most frequently found at middle age (4th to 6th decades). Their size is variable from 6 mm to several centimetres.[2] These cysts are usually asymptomatic, but at times complain of a swelling in the palate or discharge of mucoid material.

On imaging, they appear as round, ovoid or heart-shaped, well-defind lucent lesion in the anterior maxilla. The margin is well-defined, smooth and a dense rim of cortical bone is often seen along the periphery. The lesion may displace the roots of the central incisor teeth.

Nasolabial or Nasoalveolar Cyst

This lesion too is considered likely to be a fissural cyst arising adjacent to the apex of the incisors just beneath the lip. It may scallop the anterior cortex of the maxilla.[16]

Simple Bone Cyst

A traumatic (simple) bone cyst is an intraosseous pseudocyst because it lacks an epithelial lining. Its cause is not known, though some believe that it develops in response to trauma. These lesions are usually asymptomatic, discovered incidentally in children or young adult.[2,10] They are rare lesions and are usually treated by curettage.

Usually seen in the mandible, particularly anteriorly in the molar/premolar region. On radiography, these appear as typically unilocular, lucent defects between the roots of teeth and with scalloped margins. Mild expansion with cortical thinning may be seen. There is minimal or no displacement of adjacent teeth.

Aneurysmal Bone Cyst

These lesions are rare in the mandible and show imaging characteristics similar to aneurysmal bone cysts elsewhere in the skeleton **(Figs. 13A to D)**.[17]

Lingual Salivary Gland Inclusion Defect

Lingual salivary gland inclusion defect (Stafne's cyst) is a well-defined lucent lesion found on the lingual surface of the posterior body of the mandible. These are usually asymptomatic and seen as incidental findings. On imaging, the appearance is of an oval lucent area just above the inferior border of the mandible and below the mandibular canal. Typical location is anterior to the angle of the jaw and posterior to the third molar **(Fig. 14)**. The border of the defect may be surrounded by an opaque line.[10] No treatment except follow-up is required as it represents an extension of the aberrant lobe of the submandibular gland fat.

Tumors or Tumor-like Conditions

Odontogenic Tumors

Ameloblastoma

Ameloblastomas are benign epithelial neoplasms which arise from various sources of odontogenic epithelium, and constitute about 10% of odontogenic tumors. These tumors show locally aggressive but non-metastasizing behavior. Ameloblastomas may arise from the epithelial lining of dentigerous cysts and are then referred to as mural ameloblastomas.[18]

Ameloblastomas typically present in the 3rd to 5th decades of life but may be seen in younger patients. Patients generally present with a slow-growing, painless mass.[2,10]

Although solid on pathology they are radiolucent on plain radiographs. Most ameloblastomas (about 80%) occur in the ramus and posterior body of the mandible.[11] They have a variable imaging appearance. Typically the lesions are multilocular with distinct internal septae. The closest differential of such lesions is OKC. Lesions may assume a "honeycomb" or "soap-bubble" appearance. Less commonly, ameloblastoma may be unilocular. Their margins are smooth, scalloped, well-defined and corticated but with significant expansion. However, large tumors may have cortical perforation, especially on the lingual side with infiltration of adjacent soft tissues.[2,10] The adjacent teeth are often resorbed, displaced and loosened. Erosion of the roots of adjacent teeth is unique to ameloblastoma and indicates its aggressive nature **(Figs. 15 and 16)**.[9] However, only histopathologic findings can help confirm benignity and the absence of carcinomatous change.[19] Few (about 15%) of ameloblastoma may be unilocular. This form may envelop the crown of a tooth resembling a dentigerous cyst,[1,2] or occasionally the apex of a tooth **(Figs. 17A to D)**.

On CT, ameloblastoma reveal a mixed appearance with cystic areas of low attenuation with iso attenuating solid regions. On MRI, the solid component of the lesion show enhancement on Gd-T1WI and diffusion restriction **(Figs. 18A to D)**.[19,20]

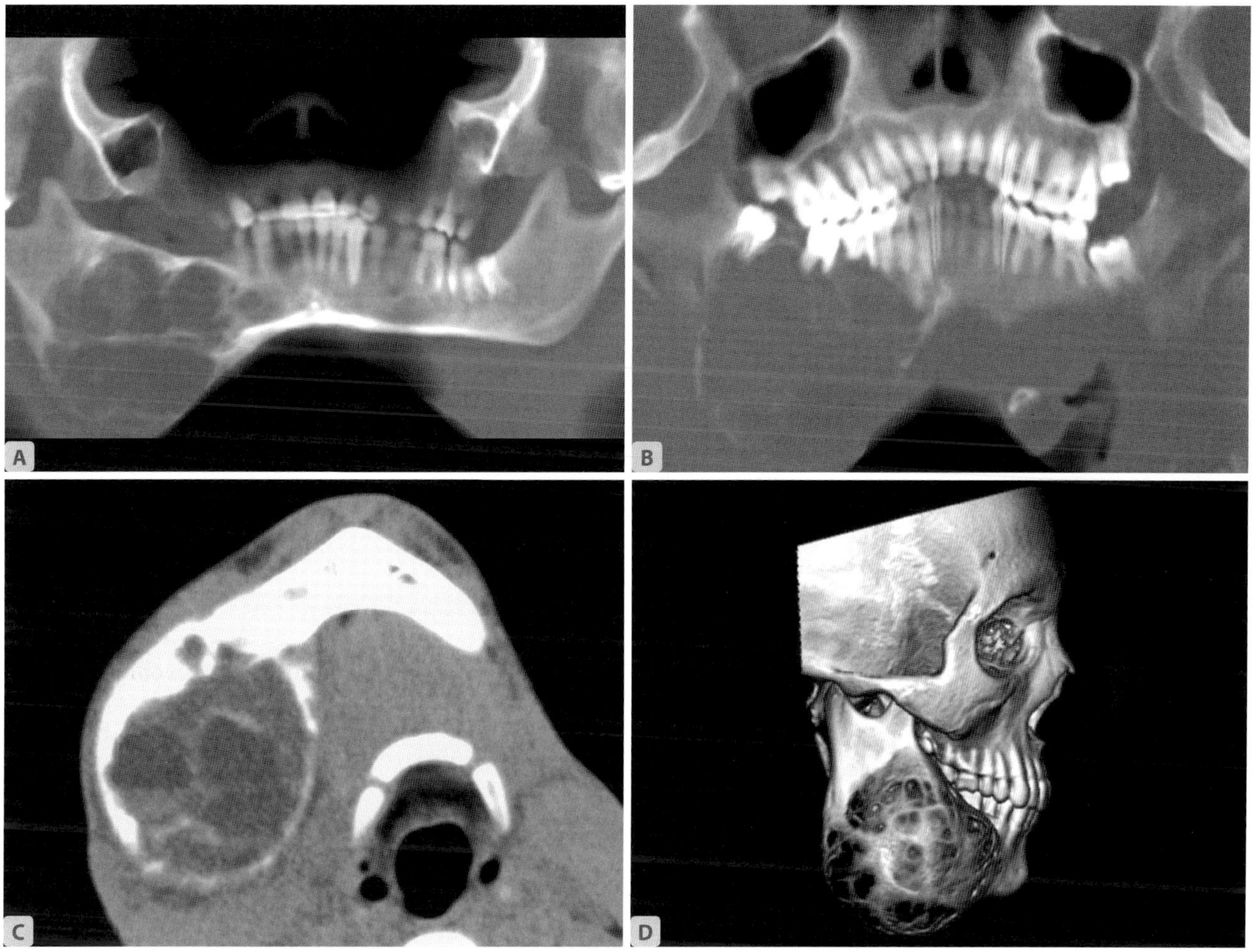

FIGS. 13A TO D: Aneurysmal bone cyst: Posterior to anterior panoramic CT reconstructions (A and B) show a markedly, expansile multilocular radiolucent lesion involving the right hemimandible. Significant cortical thinning is present; (C) Axial CT scan reveals characteristic multiple fluid-fluid levels; (D) VRT image illustrates the expansile, multilocular character of the lesion.

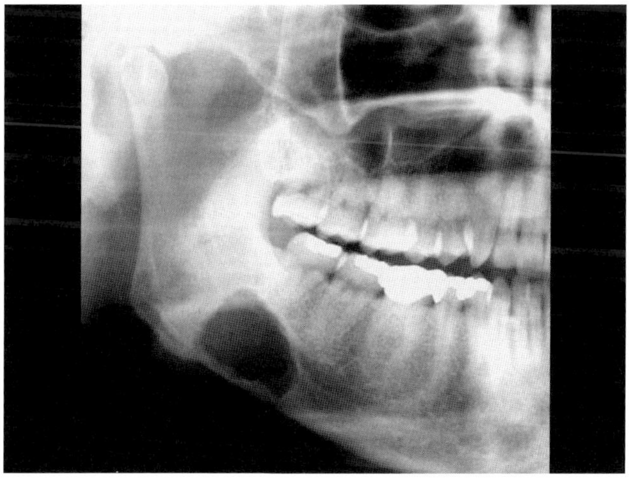

FIG. 14: Stafne's cyst: Lateral oblique view of mandible shows an ovoid, well-defined area of lucency located just above the inferior border of the mandible, anterior to the angle of the jaw and inferior to the mandibular canal.

Treatment of ameloblastoma depends on the extent of adjacent tumor infiltration. Either localized removal of the lesion with wide margins or en bloc resection would be performed.

Ameloblastic Fibroma

Ameloblastic fibroma are rare benign mixed odontogenic tumors arising from both odontogenic epithelium and connective tissue of developing tooth. On imaging, these tumors closely resemble ameloblastomas, but occur in a younger age group (children and adolescents).[2,9]

Non-Odontogenic Lesions

Central Giant Cell Granuloma

Central giant cell granuloma (giant cell reparative cyst) typically occurs in adolescents and young adults. This lesion represents a reactive process rather than a true neoplasm. Histologically, it is composed of fibrous tissue, areas of hemorrhage, reactive bone formation and osteoclast-like

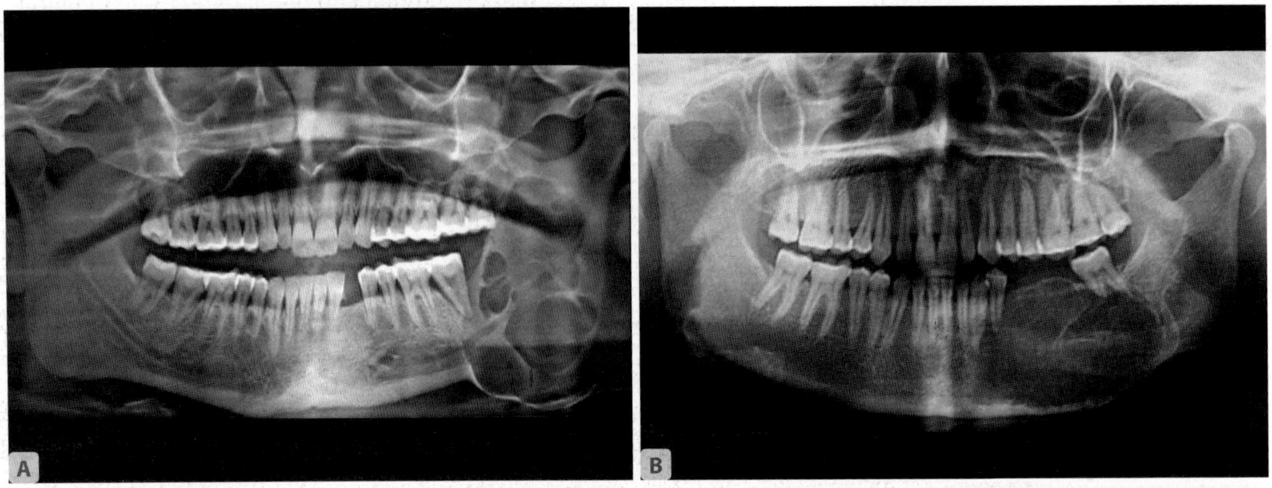

FIGS. 15A AND B: Ameloblastoma. (A and B) Panoramic radiographs of two different adult patients showing multilocular, expansile, smooth, radiolucent lesions located in the ramus and posterior body of mandible adjacent root resorption is seen in (B).

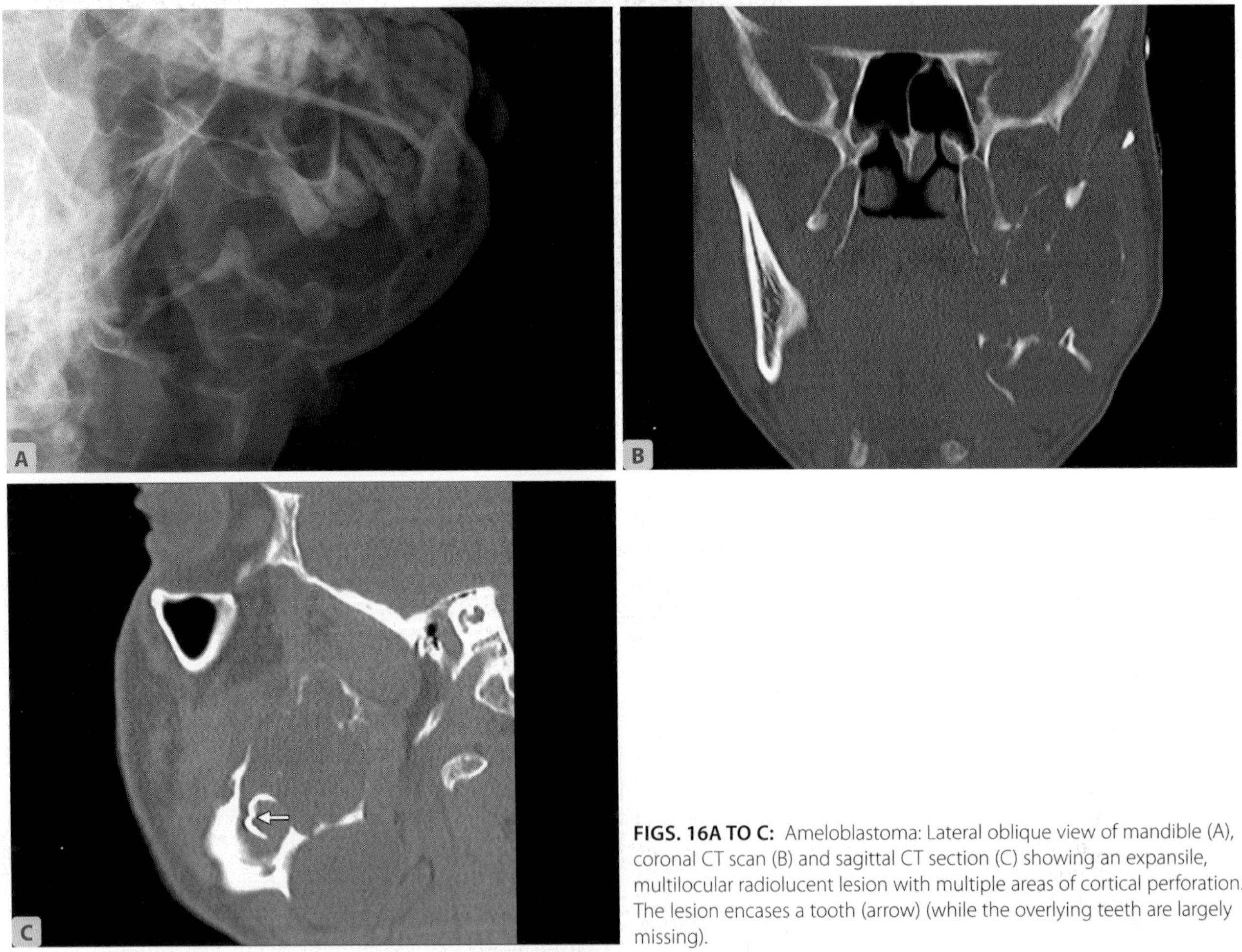

FIGS. 16A TO C: Ameloblastoma: Lateral oblique view of mandible (A), coronal CT scan (B) and sagittal CT section (C) showing an expansile, multilocular radiolucent lesion with multiple areas of cortical perforation. The lesion encases a tooth (arrow) (while the overlying teeth are largely missing).

giant cells.[2] The histologic appearance is similar to that of brown tumor of hyperparathyroidism.[1,21]

These lesions are typically located in the anterior mandible or maxilla, with a tendency to cross the midline. The radiographic appearance is of a radiolucent, multilocular lesion with thin internal septae or sometimes "honey-comb" appearance.[22] Usually well defined because of slow growth, ill-defined borders may be seen in more aggressive lesions. There is uneven osseous expansion causing scalloped borders **(Figs. 19A and B)**. Adjoining teeth are often displaced and less commonly resorbed. On imaging and histopathology, brown tumors of hyperparathyroidism can appear identical.[1,2,10]

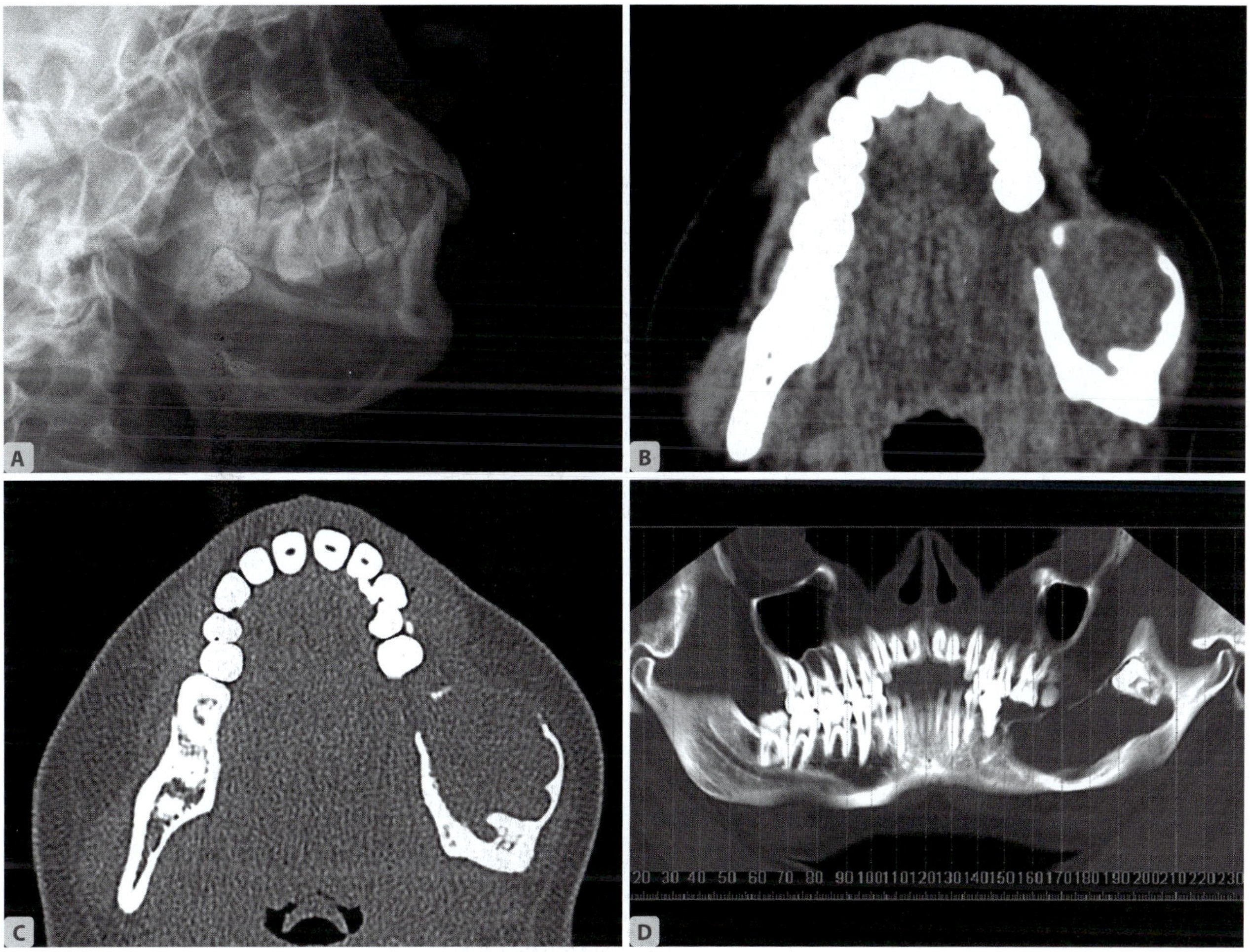

FIGS. 17A TO D: Unicystic ameloblastoma: Lateral oblique view of mandible (A) shows an ovoid well-defined, radiolucent lesion with scalloped borders involving the body and ramus of mandible, encasing an unerupted last molar. Axial CT soft tissue window (B) shows the solid appearance of the lesion, while bone window (C) illustrates areas of cortical perforation. CT panoramic reconstruction (D) exquisitely demonstrates the lesion.

Eosinophilic Granuloma

Eosinophilic granuloma is a benign form of Langerhans'cell histiocytosis, and usually occurr in children or young adults. Multiple or solitary lesions may be seen. Lesions are smooth, well-defined, radiolucent **(Fig. 20)**. Associated floating teeth may be seen due to loss of peri-odontal bone support.[1,2]

Intraosseous Hemangioma

Hemangioma is a rare benign tumor. It is regarded as a developmental malformation (hamartoma), rather than a true neoplasm. It commonly presents in adolescents either with swelling or bleeding. On radiology, these appear as expansile radiolucent lesions with multilocular or "honey-comb" appearance. The thickened trabeculae within the lesion may also give a "spoke-wheel pattern". These often cause displacement of adjacent structures with root resorption **(Fig. 21)**. It is important to suggest the diagnosis on radiology due to their potential to cause bleeding.[2,9]

Arteriovenous Malformation

Arteriovenous malformations refers to abnormal, direct communication between arteries and veins. In the jaw, most lesions occur in the ramus and posterior body of the mandible. These lesions have a potential for causing massive hemorrhage, and extraction of a tooth adjacent to an arteriovenous malformation may result in lethal bleeding. On radiology **(Figs. 22A to C)**, arteriovenous malformations appear radiolucent due to resorption of the adjacent bone. The lesions may be multilocular.[10] They may appear well defined, cyst-like or have erosive margins simulating a malignancy. Angiography is required to confirm the diagnosis and determine its extent and dynamics.

RADIOLUCENT LESIONS WITH ILL-DEFINED MARGINS

Osteomyelitis

While periapical infection causing granuloma and cyst formation is common; osteomyelitis of the jaw bone is rare. It ranges from acute or chronic suppurative to sclerosing osteomyelitis.

Acute suppurative osteomyelitis has no significant early imaging findings. When present, the appearance is of ragged,

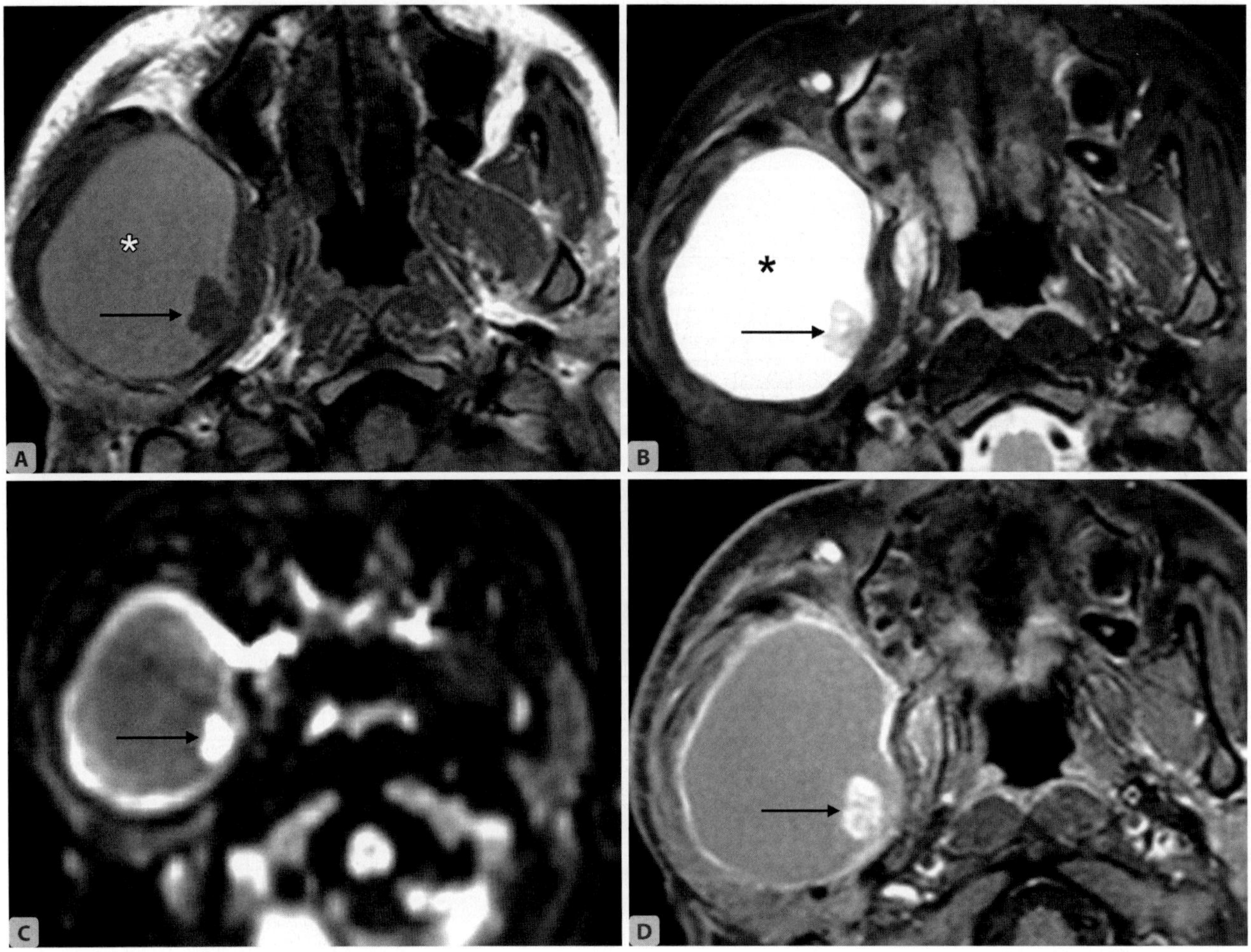

FIGS. 18A TO D: Ameloblastoma MRI (same patient as in Figs. 6A and B): Axial T1WI (A) and T2WI (B) show a large, well-defined cystic mass with hyperintense contents in ramus of mandible (asterix). Note the small eccentric mural nodule (arrows in A and B) showing diffusion restriction (arrow in C) in DWI image b value 800 (C). Axial postcontrast T1WI (D) reveals enhancement of wall of the lesion and the mural nodule (arrow).

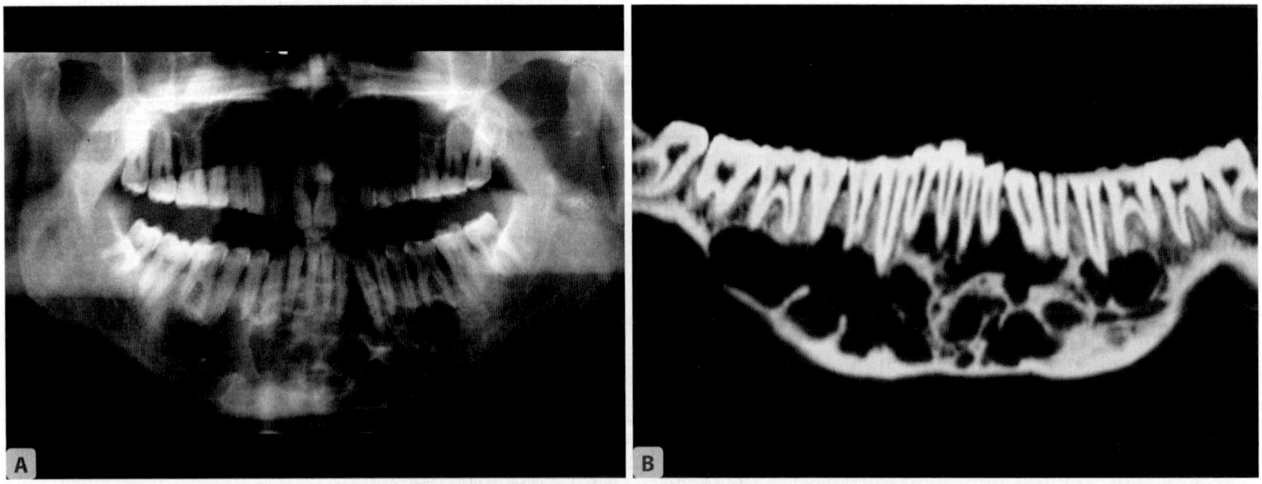

FIGS. 19A AND B: Central giant cell granuloma: Panoramic radiograph (A) and CT panoramic reconstruction (B) show a radiolucent, multilocular lesion with internal septae characteristically located in the anterior mandible, crossing the midline. Adjoining teeth are displaced, not resorbed.

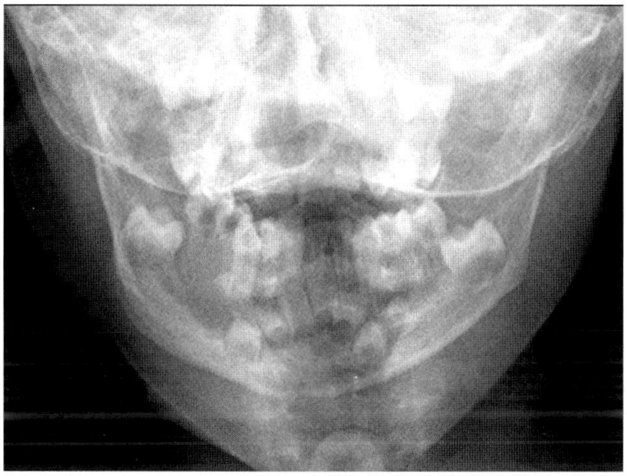

FIG. 20: Eosinophilic granuloma: Panoramic radiograph of a young boy showing a smooth, well-defined lytic lesion involving the right hemimandible.

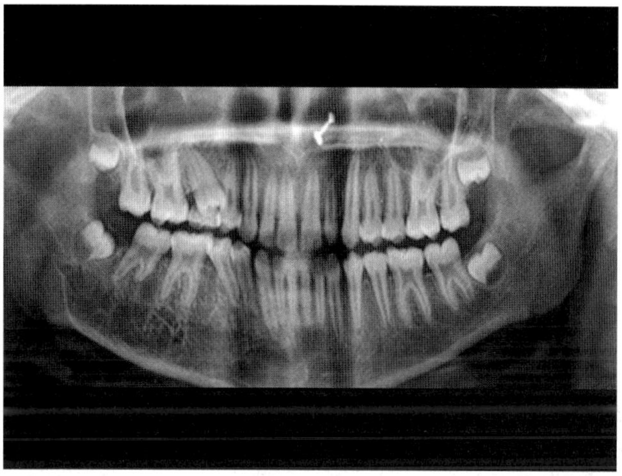

FIG. 21: Hemangioma: A multilocular, mildly expansile radiolucent lesion is seen involving the right hemimandible of a young female. There is displacement of the overlying roots.

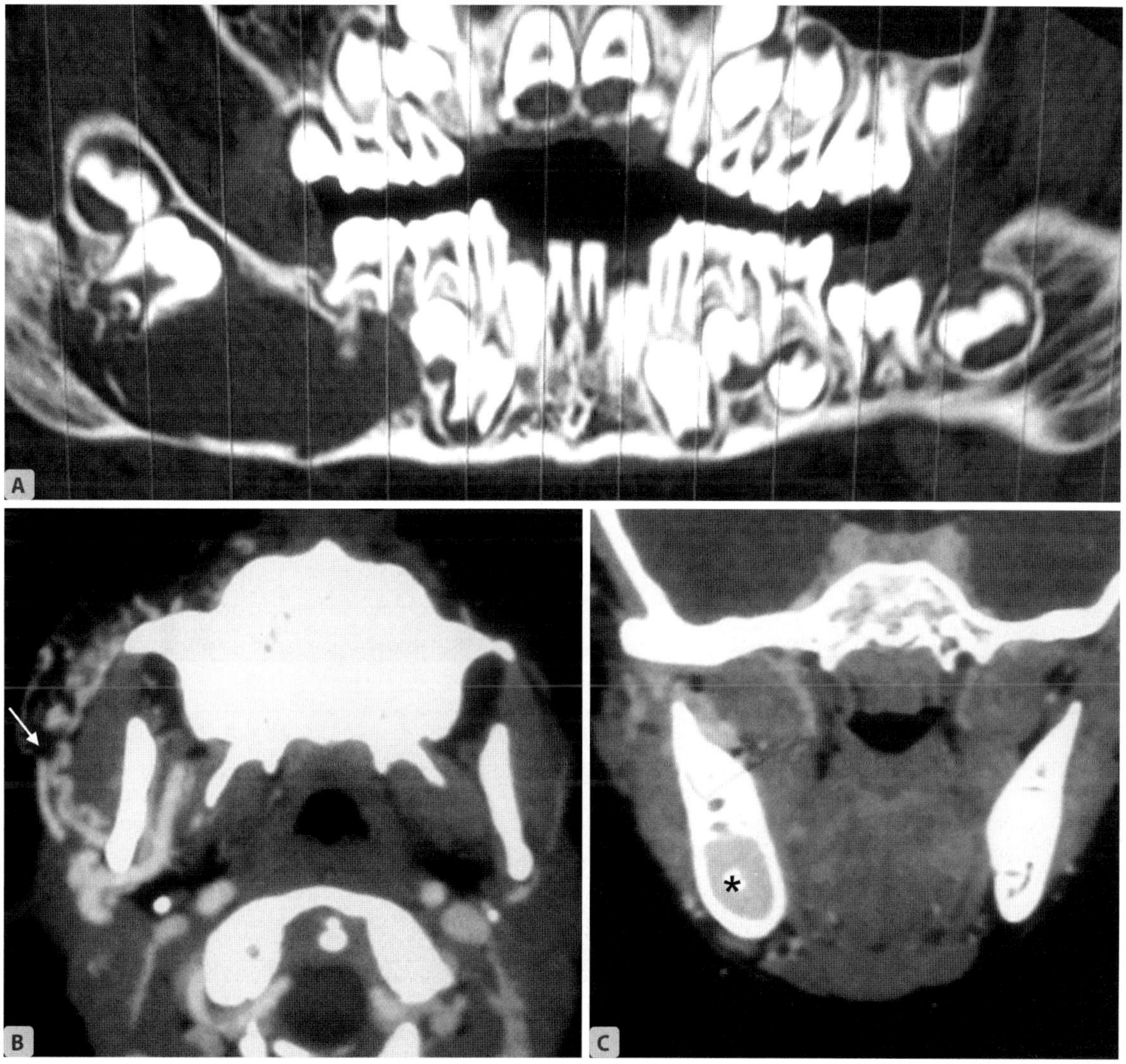

FIGS. 22A TO C: Arteriovenous malformation. (A) Panoramic CT reconstructed image shows well-defined, expansile lytic lesion in the body and ramus of right hemimandible. CECT axial image (B) shows multiple, tortuous vessels in the mandibular space (arrow) and coronal image (C) shows the large, intraosseous ectatic varix (asterix).

patchy or moth-eaten areas of radiolucency, with or without subperiosteal reaction.[2]

Chronic osteomyelitis on the other hand has radiolucent and radiopaque areas and is hence characterized as mixed density lesion. Subperiosteal new bone formation, particularly along lower border of mandible or sequestra may be seen **(Figs. 23 and 24)**.[2,18,23]

Sclerosing osteomyelitis occurs in low-grade infections with bone deposition occurring along the osseous cortex and trabeculae.[9]

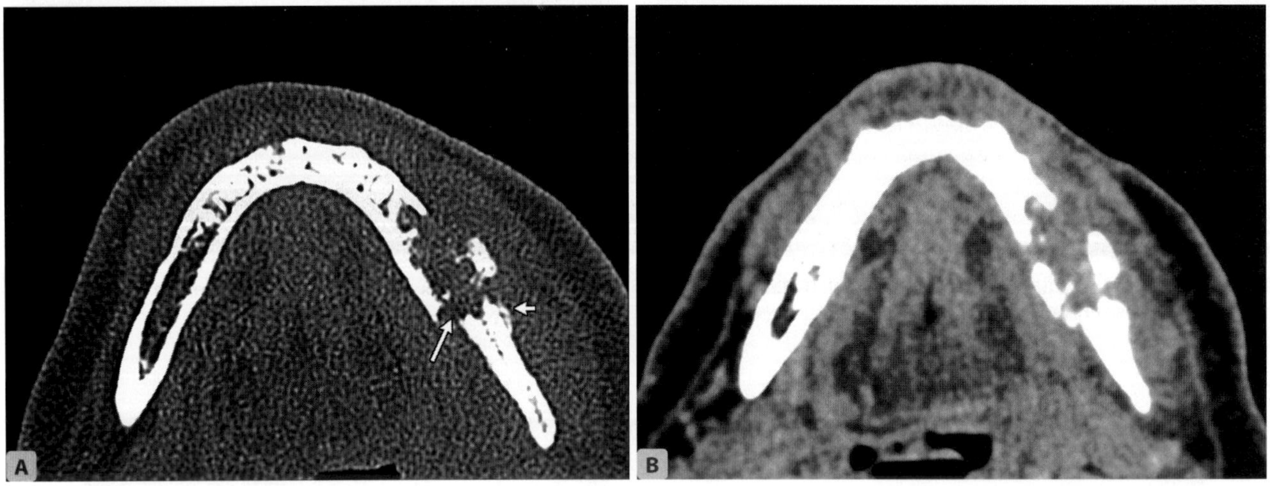

FIGS. 23A AND B: Osteomyelitis: Axial CT scan bone window (A) reveals an irregular lytic defect involving the ramus of left mandible with subtle periosteal reaction (arrow) and pathological fracture (long arrow). Soft tissue window (B) reveals associated inflammation.

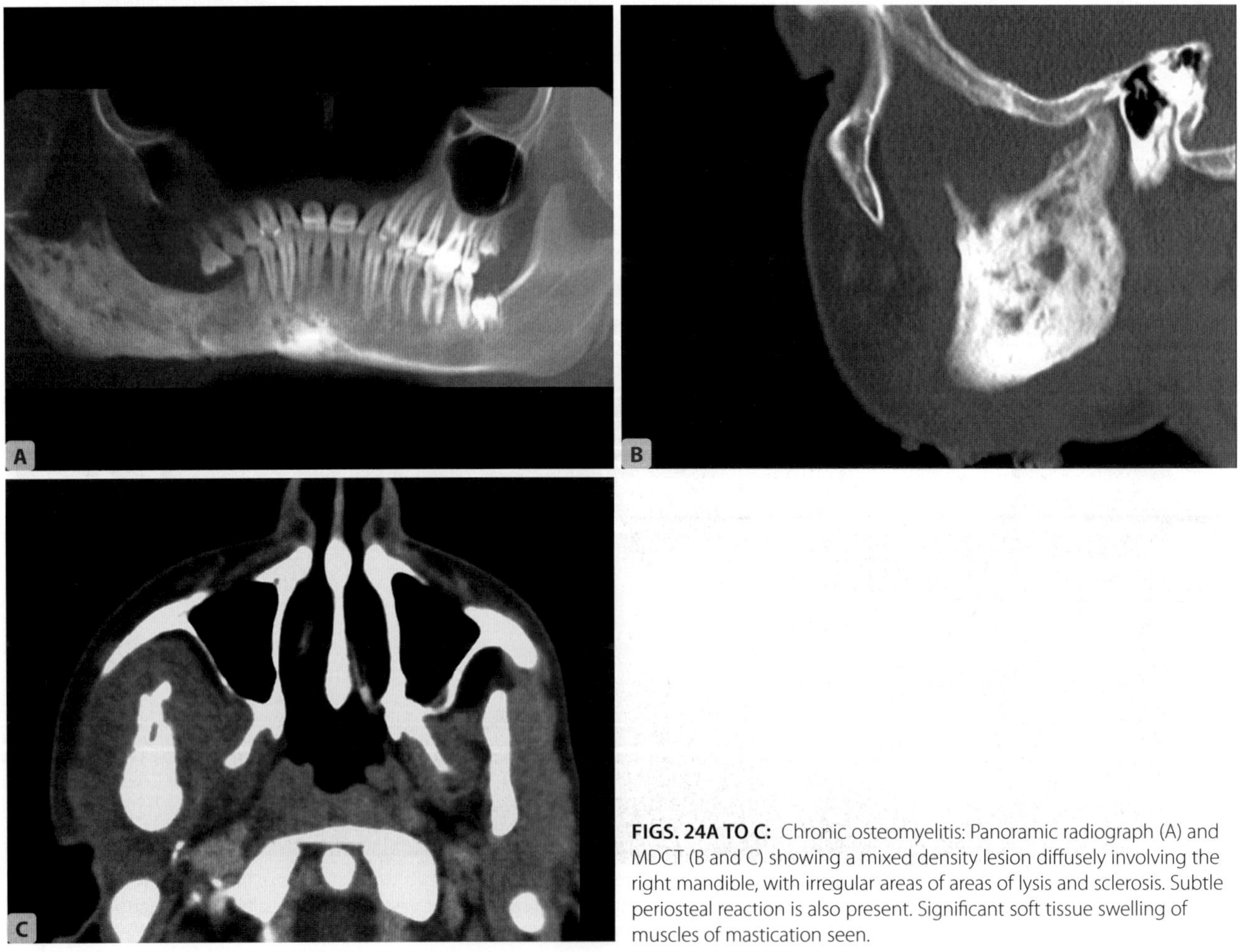

FIGS. 24A TO C: Chronic osteomyelitis: Panoramic radiograph (A) and MDCT (B and C) showing a mixed density lesion diffusely involving the right mandible, with irregular areas of areas of lysis and sclerosis. Subtle periosteal reaction is also present. Significant soft tissue swelling of muscles of mastication seen.

Malignant Tumors

The majority of carcinomas of the mandible are secondary to invasion from the adjoining buccal mucosa **(Figs. 25A and B)**.

Primary Tumors

Odontogenic

Primary odontogenic malignancies are rare and include odontogenic carcinoma and malignant ameloblastoma. Malignant ameloblastoma are very rare and presence of metastases establishes this diagnosis. Few cases of carcinomatous transformation of OKCs have also been reported.[9]

Non-odontogenic Tumors

Various non-odontogenic solid malignant tumors occur in the jaws. Sarcomas such as chondrosarcoma, osteosarcoma, leiomyosarcoma, and fibrosarcoma can occur.

Osteosarcoma

Amongst these osteosarcoma is the commonest, and generally occurs in young adults under 30 years of age. Based on radiological appearance osteosarcomas can be divided into osteolytic, osteosclerotic and mixed lytic-sclerotic types.[2] The osteolytic type presents with an ill-defined, unilocular, ragged area of radiolucency, with no neoplastic new bone formation. The sclerotic and mixed forms on the other hand have variable internal radiopacity with cortical perforation and periosteal reaction, occasionally producing the classical "sun-burst" pattern. Both forms are associated with "spiking" resorption with or without loosening of teeth.[2,9]

Other malignat non-odontogenic primary tumors include chondrosarcoma **(Figs. 26A to C)** and fibro-sarcoma.

Lymphoreticular Malignancies

Lymphoma and leukemia ususlly present as ill-defined osteolytic lesions of varying sizes. Multiple myeloma may also involve the mandible, with or without the typical "punched-out" lesions. The ovoid radiolucent lesions show no osseous expansion but may erode the mandibular cortex **(Fig. 27)**.[9] Patients with multiple myeloma may thus present with "chin numbness" due to involvement of the inferior alveolar nerve.[24]

Metastases

Metastatic disease often involves the jaw, particularly the posterior body and angle of mandible, these being most vascular. Metastasis to the mandible is four times more common than metastasis to the maxilla.[9] Commonly ill-defined radiolucent lesions, blastic metastases may also be seen. The most common primary sites of origin include kidney, lung, and breast.

MIXED-DENSITY LESIONS

Table 7 summarizes the common mixed density lesions of the maxillofacial region.

Odontogenic Lesions

Several benign odontogenic tumors have variable degree of calcification within and present as lesions of variable radiopacity.

Odontogenic Myxoma

Odontogenic myxoma is an uncommon benign neoplasm originating from mesenchymal odontogenic tissue. This tumor has a slight predilection for maxilla. They typically present in young adults and are usually painless. The lesion can be locally aggressive. Unerupted teeth may be associated.

On radiology, odontogenic myxoma typically appear as multilocular radiolucent lesions with fine internal septae giving the so called "tennis-racquet" appearance. Foci of irregular calcification are frequently present within the tumor. Teeth may be displaced with or without root absorption **(Figs. 28A and B)**.[2,10] Treatment is attempt to complete surgical resection because the tumor is infiltrative with high recurrence rates.[10]

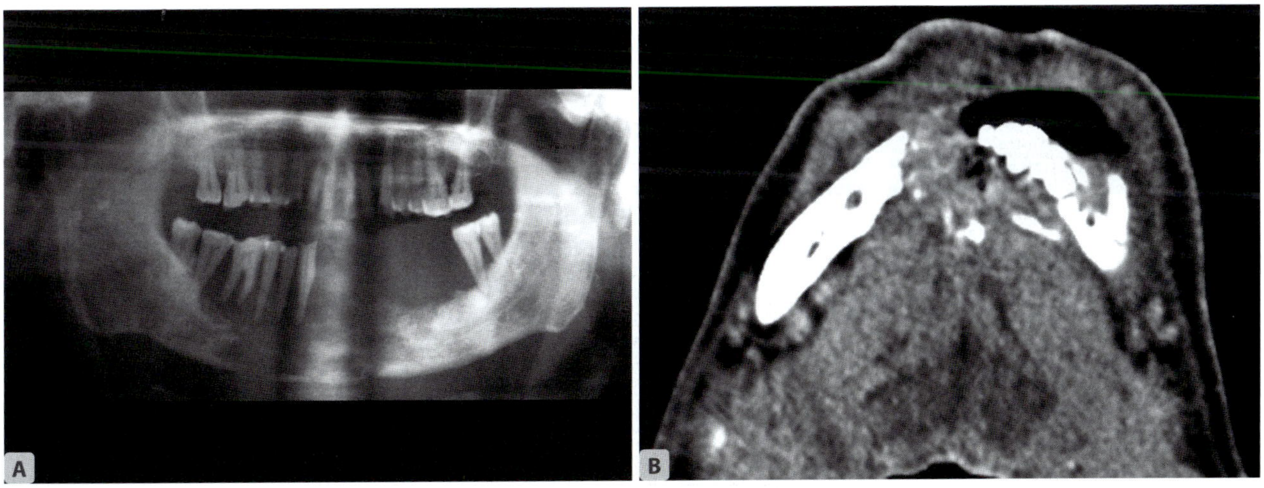

FIGS. 25A AND B: Carcinoma lower alveolus: Panoramic radiograph (A) of an elderly man showing a bulky soft tissue on the left side of the mouth with extensive, ill-defined, permeative destruction of the mandible; (B) CT scan of a different patient revealing an ulcerated buccal mucosa growth with irregular mandibular destruction.

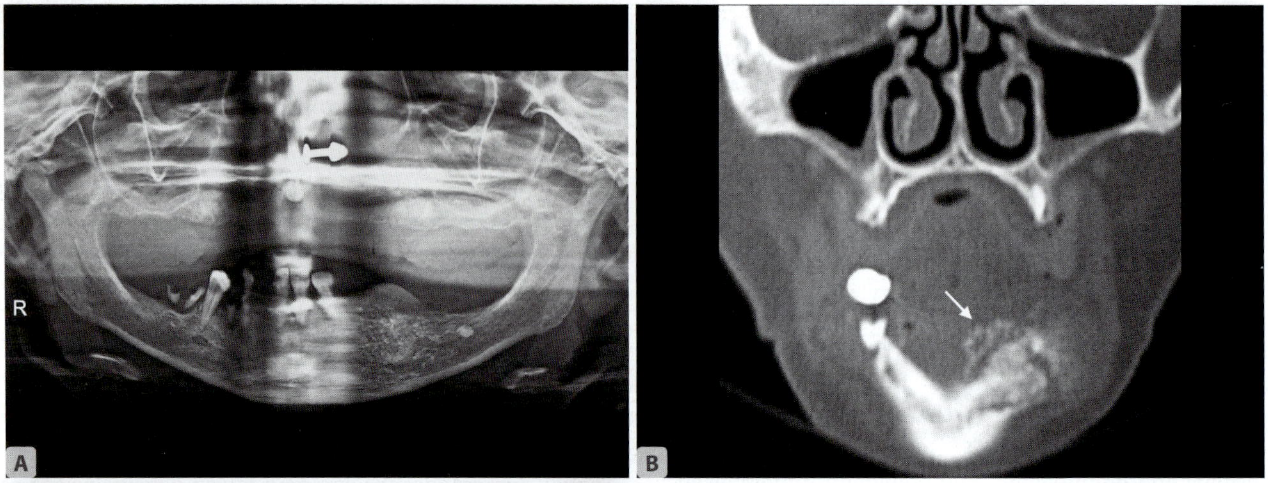

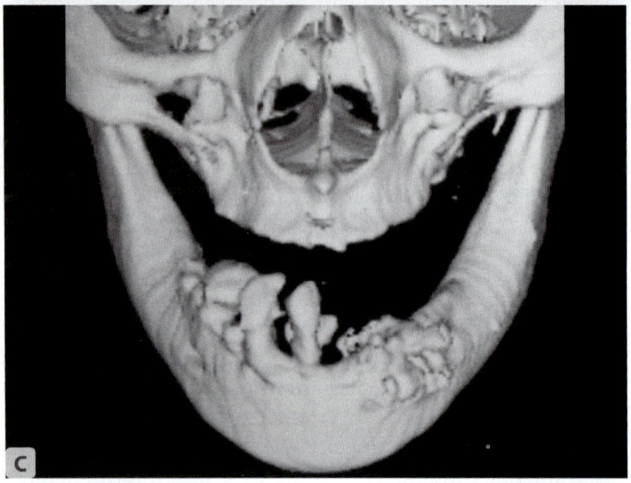

FIGS. 26A TO C: Chondrosarcoma: Panoramic radiograph (A) of an elderly female with a soft tissue swelling overlying the body of left mandible, and a subtle underlying mixed-density lesion. Coronal CT section (B) reveals chondroid pattern of calcification (arrow), cauliflower-like appearance seen on the VRT image (C).

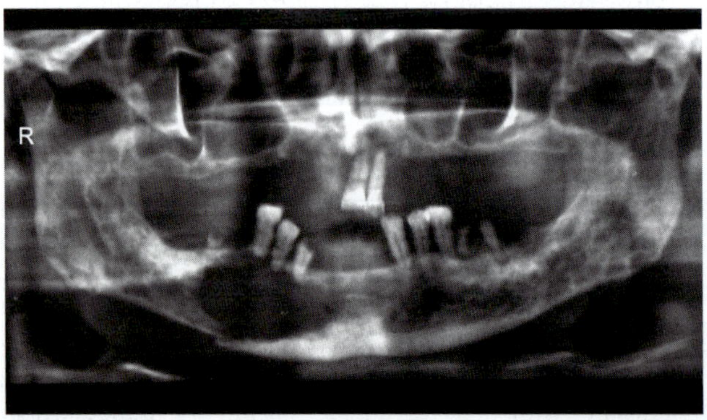

FIG. 27: Multiple myeloma: Panoramic radiograph of an elderly male showing loss of bone density, multiple oval to round rardiolucent lesions scattered throughout and a large lesion in the fracture.

Calcifying Epithelial Odontogenic Tumor

Calcifying epithelial odontogenic tumor (Pindborg tumor) is a rare odontogenic tumor seen in adults, located in molar/premolar region of the mandible. It is composed of epithelial cells in a fibrous stroma. It is a radiolucent lesion with few

TABLE 7: Common mixed density lesions of the maxillofacial region.

Odontogenic	Non-odontogenic
Odontogenic myxoma	Osteoblastoma
Calcifying epithelial odontogenic tumor	Ossifying fibroma
Ameloblastic fibro-odontoma	Fibrous dysplasia
Adenomatoid odontogenic tumor	Focal cemento-osseous dysplasia
	Osteoradionecrosis

scattered calcific densities. Most tumors are associated with the crown of an impacted tooth. The radiodensities are most evident around the crown, giving it the "driven snow" appearance.[2,9]

Ameloblastic Fibro-odontoma

Ameloblastic fibro-odontoma has been questioned in current WHO classification and is believed to be a variant

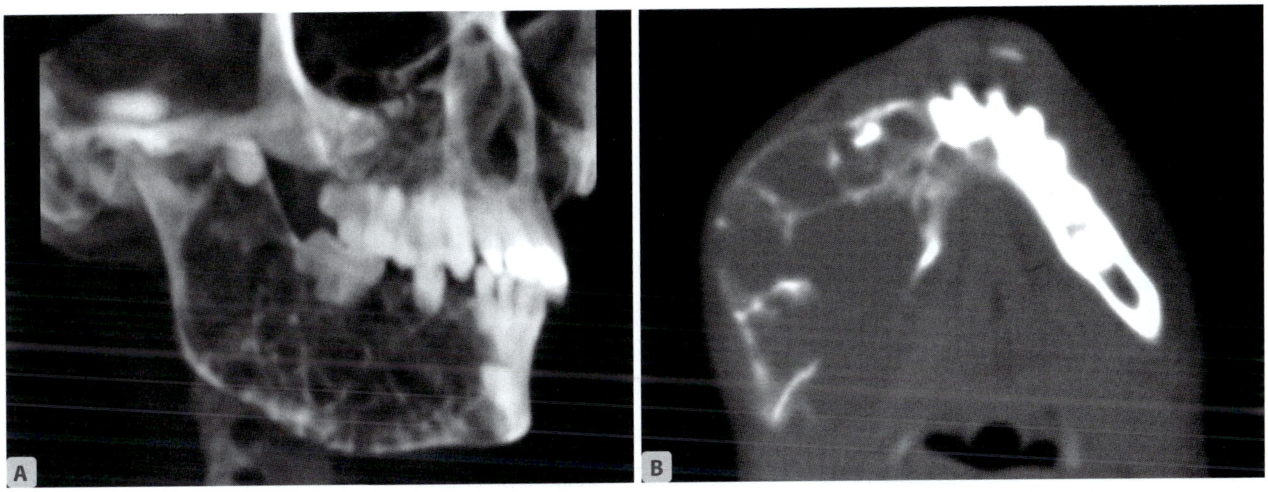

FIGS. 28A AND B: Odontogenic myxoma: VRT image (A) and axial CT scan (B) of a young male reveal an expansile, multilocular lesion with internal septae involving the right body and ramus of mandible. The last molar is displaced cranially. The overlying teeth are splayed with no root resorption.

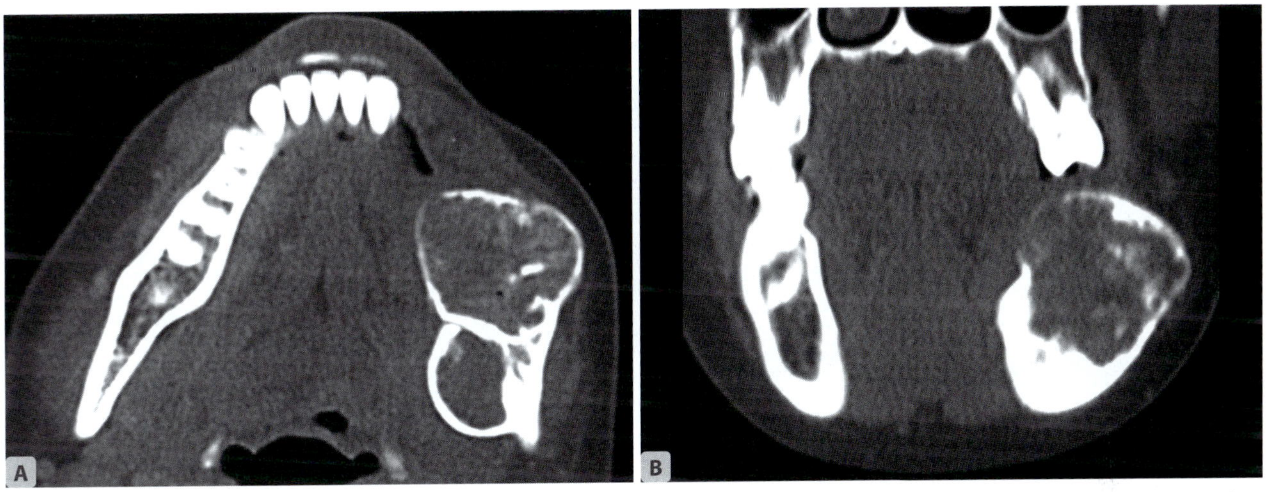

FIGS. 29A AND B: Ameloblastic fibro-odontoma: MDCT axial (A) and coronal (B) of an adult female showing a septated expansile predominantly radiolucent lesion with calcific densities along its periphery and ill-defined radiodensity scattered centrally. Biopsy revealed the lesion as ameloblastic fibro-odontoma.

of odontoma. It has a distinct radiographic appearance of a radiolucent lesion, often associated with an unerupted tooth, and contains enamel or dentine seen as multiple radiopacities **(Figs. 29A and B)**. It may affect children too.[2]

Adenomatoid Odontogenic Tumor

Adenomatoid odontogenic tumor is a rare tumor that is typically seen in young adults, especially girls and young women. Majority are found in the anterior maxilla. The tumors appear as well-defined radiolucent lesions with punctate (snowflakes) calcifications. These tumors can often surround an unerupted tooth, typically more apically on the root than dentigerous cysts.[9]

Non-odontogenic Lesions

Mixed density lesions including chronic osteomyelitis, osteogenic sarcoma and metastases have been previously detailed. *Osteoblastoma* is a rare entity, which can also present as a mixed density or sclerotic lesion.

Osteoblastoma

Osteoblastoma is a rare benign tumor, which infrequently involves the jaws. It is usually either periosteal or medullary and not cortical. The mandible is more commonly affected than the maxilla with most lesions occurring in the body of the mandible. The age group most commonly affected is between 5 and 30 years of age.[25] Lesion is usually of mixed density, however radiolucent and radiopaque lesions have also been described. They are well-circumscribed lesions, usually <12 cm in diameter with internal sclerotic matrix.[26] The associated cortical sclerosis represents the nidus **(Figs. 30A and B)** and should be resected to ensure complete removal.

Other mixed density lesions are benign fibro-osseous lesions, which are discussed below.

Ossifying Fibroma

Ossifying fibroma, previously also known as cemento-ossifying or cementifying fibroma is a fibro-osseous lesion

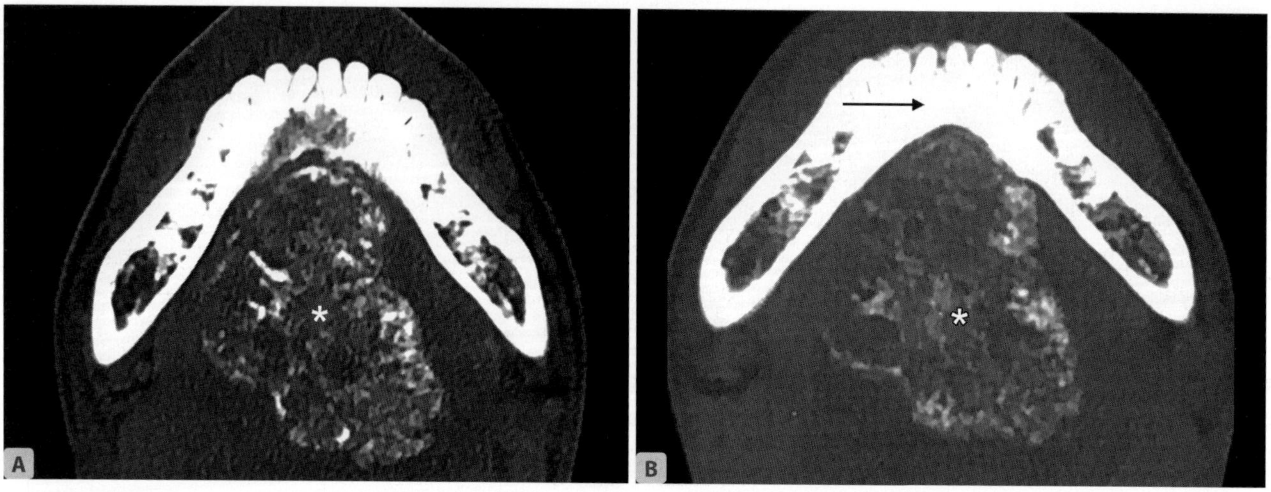

FIGS. 30A AND B: Osteoblastoma. Axial CT images (A and B) of an adolescent male showing a large, expansile, mixed-density lesion in the floor of mouth (asterix in A and B). Note the sclerosis (arrow in B) along the inner margin of the mandible in the midline: the nidus and cause of recurrence in case of incomplete removal.

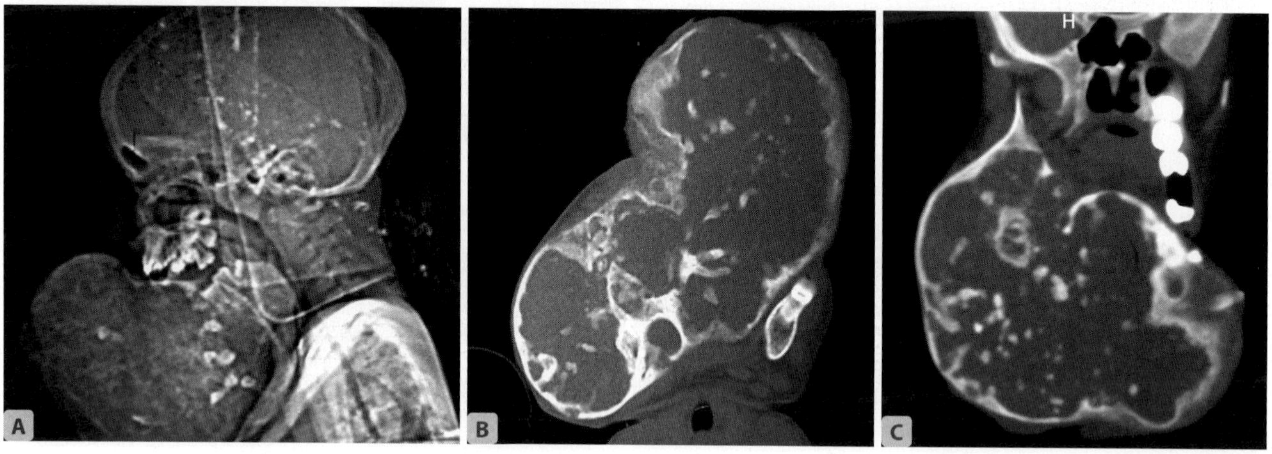

FIGS. 31A TO C: Juvenile ossifying fibroma: CT scout film (A) of a 10 years old male patient reveals a huge mixed-density lesion with caudal displacement of the teeth, involving the mandible; Axial (B) and coronal (C) CT images reveal coalescing radiodensities within. There is massive expansion with bowing of the inferior mandibular cortex, but no thinning. Patient subsequently underwent a difficult resection and reconstruction.

containing fibrous tissue with varying amounts of bony trabeculae. It is typically an encapsulated, well-circumscribed lesion. These lesions grow slowly and symmetrically with resultant bone expansion and facial asymmetry. In the tooth-bearing region, there are two clinicopathologic variants of ossifying fibroma: the odontogenic cemento-ossifying fibroma and the nonodontogenic ossifying fibroma. The juvenile ossifying fibroma variants (trabecular and psammatoid variants) typically occur in the 2nd–4th decades with a female preponderance.[2] Juvenile ossifying fibromas occur in younger patients, can be locally destructive and have a greater tendency to recur.[10]

Ossifying fibroma most commonly affects the posterior mandible, but maxilla is also a less common site. On imaging, early lesions are radiolucent, in the intermediate stage gradually increasing internal, coalescing calcified patches are seen and in the late stages the lesion is predominantly radiopaque.[2,10] The radiopaque lesions may be demarcated from the surrounding bone by a radiolucent line. There is osseous expansion in all dimensions with downward bowing of the inferior mandibular cortex. The adjoining teeth are usually displaced. The differential diagnosis of the lesion varies according to its extent of calcification **(Figs. 31A to C)**. Recurrence of conventional ossifying fibroma is uncommon.

Fibrous Dysplasia

Fibrous dysplasia usually presents in adolescents or young adults. Maxilla (especially posterior maxilla) is more commonly affected than the mandible. The adjoining bones such as zygoma and sphenoid may also be involved. The lesions initially appear radiolucent and gradually become opaque resulting in the classical "ground-glass" appearance **(Figs. 32A and B)**. There is bucco-lingual expansion with encroachment or obliteration of the maxillary sinus. The adjoining teeth are displaced and associated loss of lamina dura may be seen. Involvement of adjoining bones and skull base aids in the diagnosis.[2,18]

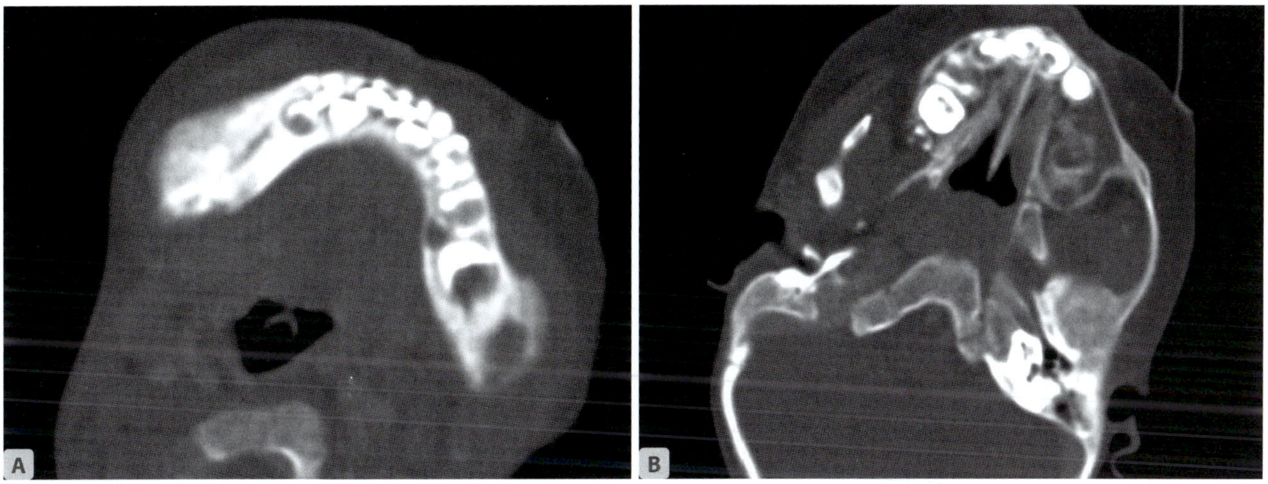

FIGS. 32A AND B: Fibrous dysplasia. (A) Axial MDCT of a 4-year-old girl showing expansion of the mandible with characteristic "ground-glass" opacity. A more cranial section (B) reveals involvement of the left temporal bone.

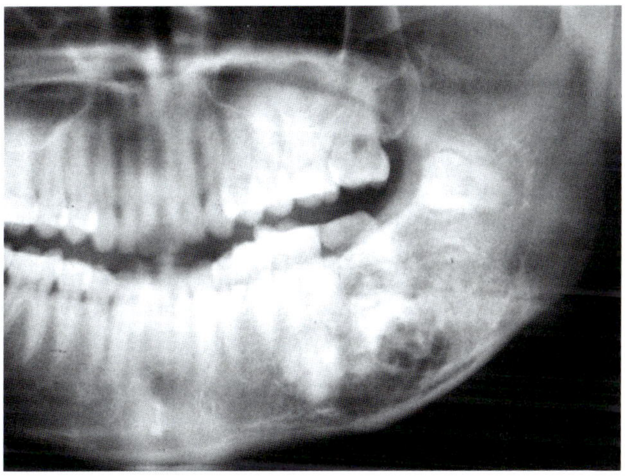

FIG. 33: Cemento-osseous dysplasia: Part of a panoramic radiograph showing a mixed-density lesion in the left hemi-mandible containing amorphous areas of calcification.

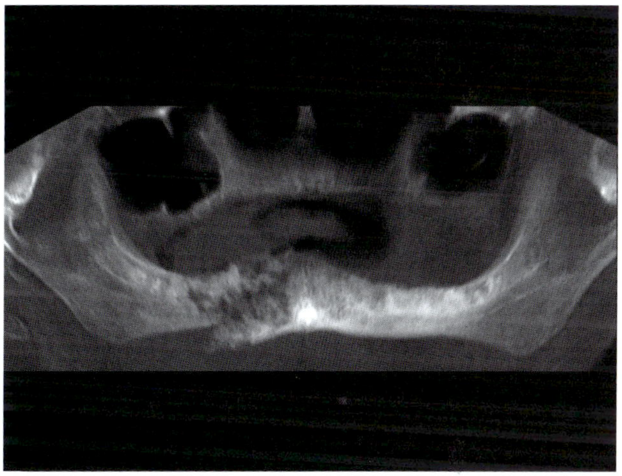

FIG. 34: Osteoradionecrosis of the mandible. Panoramic reconstructed image of CECT face of a 50-year-old male patient of carcinoma tongue (postsurgery and postradiotherapy). Mixed lytic sclerotic density in body of right hemimandible with pathological fracture. Sclerosis is also seen in the body of left hemimandible.

Cemento-osseous Dysplasia

Cemento-osseous dysplasia is a clinicopathologic variant of the spectrum of benign fibro-osseous lesions. These lesions arise exclusively in the tooth-bearing regions of the jaw bones and include three conditions: Periapical osseous dysplasia, focal osseous dysplasia (periapical cementoma), florid osseous dysplasia. These lesions are radiolucent initially (fibrous tissue) and gradually become mixed-density (mineralized tissue). These lesions are generally incidental, asymptomatic radiographic findings. Most variants are localized, small, discrete lesions, more common in the mandible. Florid osseous dysplasia however manifests as diffuse, multi-quadrant mixed lucent-opaque lesions in both the mandible **(Fig. 33)** and the maxilla. The periapical form is characteristically seen as small 5–6 mm lesion at the apices of lower incisor teeth. The teeth are typically viable. Differential diagnosis includes apical periodontitis for small, discrete lucent lesions (carious teeth) and ossifying fibroma for larger lesion.[2,10]

Osteoradionecrosis

Post-radiation therapy, osteoradionecrosis can manifest years later. Imaging appearance varies depending on radiation dose and duration. As with bone elsewhere, radiation results in endothelial cell death and vessel thrombosis. Mixed lytic sclerotic areas are seen with ill-defined borders and enlarged trabecular spaces **(Fig. 34)**. Sequestered bone may be identified within the lesion.[9]

RADIOPAQUE LESIONS

Table 8 summarizes the radiopaque lesions of the maxillofacial region.

Odontogenic Lesions

Odontomes

Odontome is an odontogenic hamartomatous malformation composed of any or all odontogenic tissues in various states of differentiation. It is the most common odontogenic "tumor" (67% of cases).[27]

There are two types of odontomas: complex and compound. Complex odontomes are made of multiple, irregular masses of dental tissue (amorphous calcifications on plain radiographs). Compound odontome contains multiple teeth or toothlike structures. The miniature tooth shape are surrounded by a radiolucent line. Compound odontomes are more common. Most lesions are 1-3 cm in size and may cause malpositioning, impaction or resorption of adjacent teeth. The differential diagnosis of the amorphous odontomes includes focal cemento- osseous dysplasia and adenomatoid odontogenic tumor.[2,10,18]

Cementoblastoma

Cementoblastoma is a rare odontogenic tumor characterized by formation of cementum like tissue in relation to root of a tooth in patients less than 25 years of age. It is characteristically found in association with the apex of the first mandibular molar. These measure up to 2-3 cm. The lesion appears as a round, well-demarcated opaque round or irregular, sunburst mass with a thin radiolucent rim ("golf-ball" appearance) **(Figs. 35A and B)**.[2] It is attached to the root of the tooth, which is often obscured. However, the periodontal ligament space is obscured by the lesion unlike in condensing osteitis.

Non-odontogenic Lesions

Osteoma

Osteomas are slow growing, benign osseous tumors occurring most often in 10–40 years age group.[8] These lesions are found on the skull or facial skeleton. Gardner's syndrome is commonly associated with multiple osteomas. Osteomas may be located within the medullary bone (endosteal) or on the surface (periosteal) **(Figs. 36A and B)**. There are two main types—compact and cancellous. The compact form consists of dense lamellae of bone (ivory osteoma), while the cancellous form comprises of bone trabaculae.[2]

TABLE 8: Common radiopaque lesions of the maxillofacial region.

Odontogenic	Non-odontogenic
Odontomes	Osteoma
Cementoblastoma	Chondroma
	Osteochondroma
	Torus

Chondroma and Osteochondroma

Chondromas and osteochondromas are rare jaw lesions, seen in the region of the condylar head or coronoid process of the mandible. Lesions involving the condylar head cause mandibular deviation to the opposite side and elongation of the face on the affected side.[8] Mushroom-shaped enlargement with restricted mouth opening occurs in lesions involving the coronoid process.[8] On imaging, osteochondromas appear as regular- or irregular-shaped areas of varying radiographic opacity contiguous with the cortex of the involved bone. The imaging morphology is well delineated with CT with 3D reconstructions.[8]

Torus (Exostoses)

Exostoses are developmental abnormalities, which are small irregular overgrowths of bone and are often bilateral. Torus mandibularis is seen on lingual aspects of premolar/molar region of mandible. Torus palatinus is seen on either side of midline on posterior aspect of the hard palate. Usually, two views are required to delineate the lesions.[2]

CONCLUSION

Although the list of tumor and tumor-like lesions in the jaw appears intimidating, familiarity with common lesions and a systematic approach would aid us in often arriving at the diagnosis. In several instances, only a differential diagnosis can be proffered necessitating a biopsy.

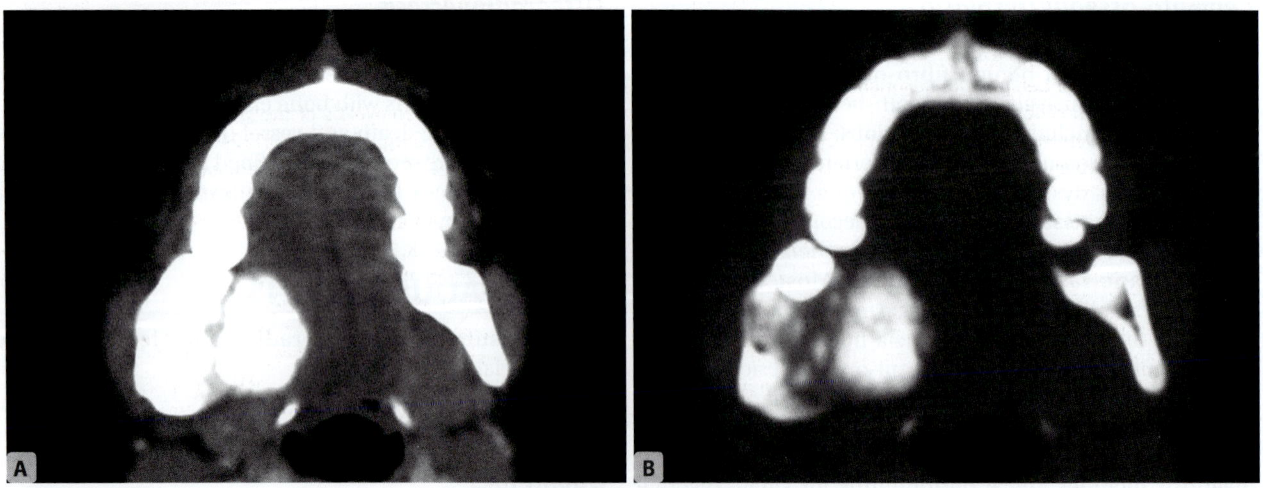

FIGS. 35A AND B: Cementoblastoma: Soft tissue (A) and bone window (B) of axial CT scan of 10 years old girl showing a round, well-demarcated, round, irregular, sunburst radiopaque mass closely related to the adjoining tooth. Biopsy revealed a cementoblastoma.

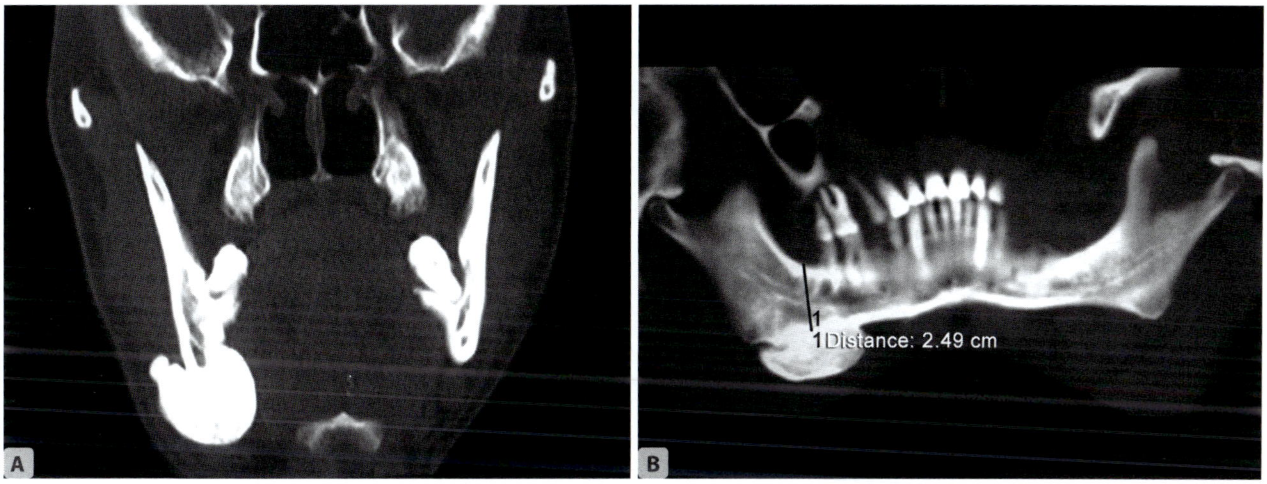

FIGS. 36A AND B: Periosteal (surface) osteoma: Coronal CT (A) and panoramic CT reconstruction (B) of a young male reveal a well-defined radiodense surface outgrowth at the angle of the mandible.

REFERENCES

1. Neyaz Z, Gadodia A, Gamanagatti S, et al. Radiographical approach to jaw lesions. Singapore Med J. 2008;49(2):165-77.
2. Whaites E (Ed). Essentials of Dental Radiography and Radiology, 4th edition. Churchill Livingstone: Elsevier; 2007.
3. Bodner L, Bar-ziv J, Kaffe I . CT of cystic jaw lesions. J Comput Assist Tomogr. 1994;18(1):22-6.
4. Abrahams JJ, Hayt MW, Rock R. Dental CT reformatting programs and dental imaging. In: Som PM, Curtin HD (Eds). Head and Neck Imaging, 4th edition. Missouri, USA: Mosby; 2003. pp. 907-18.
5. Kaneda T, Tohru M. Benign odontogenic tumors of the maxilla and the mandible. Neuroimaging Clin N Am. 2003;13:495-507.
6. Srinivasan K, Bhalla AS, Sharma R, et al. Diffusion-weighted imaging in the evaluation of odontogenic cysts and tumours. Br J Radiol. 2012;85:e864-70.
7. Srinivasan K, Seith A, Gadodia A, et al. Evaluation of the inferior alveolar canal for cysts and tumors of the mandible—comparison of multidetector computed tomography and 3-dimensional volume interpolated breath-hold examination magnetic resonance sequence with curved multiplanar reformatted reconstructions. J Oral Maxillofac Surg. 2012;70:2327-32.
8. DelBalso AM. An approach to the diagnostic imaging of jaw lesions, dental implants, and the temporomandibular joint. Radiol Clin North Am. 1998;36(5):855-90.
9. Dunfee BL, Sakai O, Pistey R, et al. Radiologic and pathologic characteristics of benign and malignant lesions of the mandible. RadioGraphics. 2006;26:1751-68.
10. Scholl RJ, Kellett HM, Neumann DP, et al. Cysts and cystic lesions of the mandible: clinical and radiologic-histopathologic review. RadioGraphics. 1999;19:1107-24.
11. Speight PM, Takata T. New tumour entities in the 4th edition of the World Health Organization Classification of Head and Neck tumours: odontogenic and maxillofacial bone tumours. Virchows Arch. DOI 10.1007/s00428-017-2182-3.
12. El-Naggar AK, Chan JKC, Grandis JR, et al. WHO Classification of Head and Neck Tumours, 4th edition. IARC, Lyon; 2017. pp. 204-6.
13. Weber AL. Imaging of cysts and odontogenic tumors of the jaw. RCNA Radiol Clin North Am. 1993;31:101-20.
14. Mourshed F. A roentgenographic study of dentigerous cysts. Oral Surg Oral Med Oral Pathol. 1967;51:54-61
15. Oikarinen VJ. Keratocyst recurrences at intervals of more than 10 years: case reports. Br J Oral Maxillofac Surg. 1990;28:47-9.
16. Hisatomi M, Asaumi JI, Konouchi H, et al. MR imaging of epithelial cysts of the oral and maxillofacial region. Eur J Radiol. 2003;48:178-82.
17. Roychoudhury A, Rustagi A, Bhatt K, et al. Aneurysmal bone cyst of the mandible: report of 3 cases. J Oral Maxillofac Surg. 2009;67(9):1996-2004.
18. Weber AL, Kaneda T, Scrivani SJ, et al. Jaw: Cysts, tumors, and nontumorous lesions. In: Som PM, Curtis HD (Eds). Head and Neck Imaging, 4th edition. USA: Mosby; 2003.
19. Minami M, Kaneda T, Yamamoto H, et al. Ameloblastoma in the maxillomandibular region: MR imaging. Radiology. 1992;184(2):389-93.
20. Kaneda T, Minami M, Kurabayashi T. Benign odontogenic tumors of the mandible and maxilla. Neuroimaging Clin N Am. 2003;13(3):495-507.
21. Horner K. Central giant cell granuloma of the jaw: a clinico-radiological study. Clin Radiol. 1989;40:622-26.
22. Murphey MD, Nomikos GC, Flemming DJ, et al. Imaging of giant cell tumor and giant cell reparative granuloma of bone: radiologic-pathologic correlation. RadioGraphics. 2001:21: 1283-309.
23. Hudson JW. Osteomyelitis of the jaws: a 50-year perspective. J Oral Maxillofac Surg. 1993;51(12):1294-301.
24. Witt C, Borges AC, Klein K, et al. Radiographic manifestations of multiple myeloma in the mandible: a retrospective study of 77 patients. J Oral Maxillofac Surg. 1997;55(5):450-3.
25. Mardaleishvili K, Kakabadze Z, Machavariani A. Benign osteoblastoma of the mandible in a 12-year-old female: a case report, Oncol Lett. 2014;6:2691-4.
26. Manjunatha BS, Sunit P, Amit M, et al. Osteoblastoma of the jaws: report of a case and review of literature. Clin Pract. 2011;4:e118.
27. Regezi JA, Kerr DA, Courtney RM. Odontogenic tumors: an analysis of 706 cases. J Oral Surg. 1978;36:771-8.

CHAPTER

208

Craniovertebral Junction Anomalies

Niranjan Khandelwal, Vivek Gupta

INTRODUCTION

The craniovertebral junction (CVJ) anatomically denotes the occiput, the first (atlas) and second cervical (axis) vertebral segments, their articulations and connecting ligaments.[1] This is a complex transition between the skull and the upper cervical spine, and the brain and the spinal cord respectively. Collectively, these structures surround and protect the cervicomedullary junction and lower cranial nerves. A knowledge of bony anatomy, embryology and biomechanics of the CVJ helps to understand various anomalies associated with CVJ.[2]

ANATOMY AND EMBRYOLOGY

Skeletal Anatomy (Figs. 1A to D)

Foramen Magnum and the Occiput

The occiput which surrounds the foramen magnum consists of three parts: (1) The squamosal portion (supra-occiput)

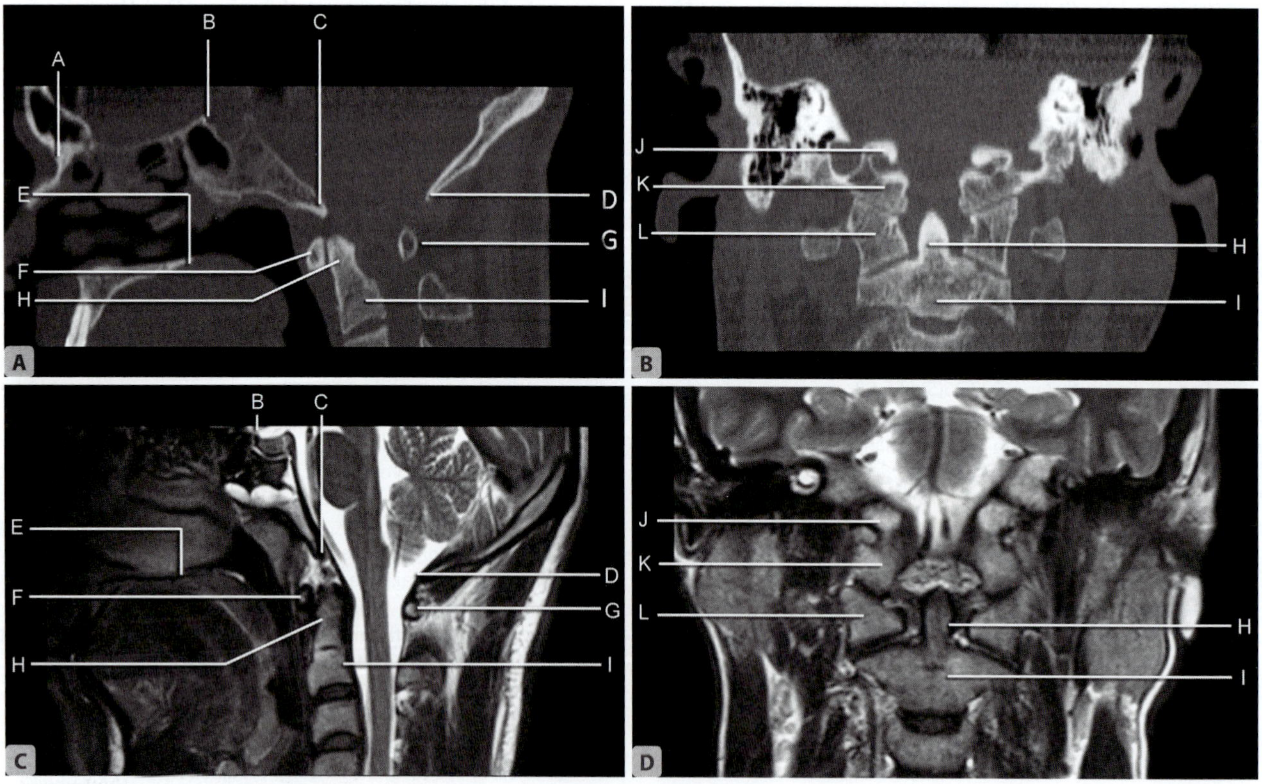

FIGS. 1A TO D: Normal landmarks of craniovertebral junction (CVJ): Midsagittal (A) computed tomography (CT); (B) T2-weighted magnetic resonance (T2W MR) and coronal; (C) CT; (D) T2W MR. (A, nasion; B, tuberculum sella; C, basion (anterior margin of foramen magnum); D, opisthion (posterior margin of the foramen magnum); E, posterior margin of the hard palate; F, anterior arch of atlas; G, posterior arch of atlas; H, odontoid process; I, body of axis; J, jugular tubercles; K, occipital condyles; L, lateral atlas masses).

situated in the dorsal aspect of foramen magnum, (2) The basi-occiput or clival portion located anterior to the foramen magnum, and (3) The condylar part (exo-occiput) that joins the clival parts and the squamosal.[3,4]

Atlas

It is dissimilar to the other cervical vertebrae because it is ring shaped and lacks a vertebral body and spinous process. It consists of two thick lateral masses which are located at the anterolateral part of the ring. A short anterior arch connects it in the front and the long posterior arch at the back. The lateral mass of atlas consists the superior and the inferior articular facets which articulate with occipital condyles and the superior apophysis of the atlas respectively.

It is a ring with pivot-like structure and contains the odontoid process or dens, body of axis, lateral masses, posterior arch and a bifid spinous process. The odontoid process projects cephalad from its articulation with the axis body. The oval facet on the ventral odontoid surface articulates with the dorsal surface of the anterior atlas arch. In the dorsal aspect of the dens is a transverse groove over which the transverse ligament of the atlas passes.[3-5]

The superior and inferior apophysis of the atlas and the superior apophysis of the axis are unique from the rest in that they are located ventral to the spinal nerve exits. The atlantoaxial complex is unique among the intervertebral articulations on account of the horizontal orientation of its lateral facet joints, pivot-like atlantodental articulation and special ligamentous support (alar ligaments and transverse or cruciate ligament).

Ligamentous Anatomy (Figs. 2A and B)

The occipito-atlantoaxial ligaments are arranged in four layers. The most anterior layer is the superior extension of anterior longitudinal ligament known as anterior atlanto-occipital membrane that it attaches to the anterior arch of the atlas. The second layer is formed by the alar ligament and the apical ligament. The paired alar ligaments connect the odontoid with the lateral masses and the occipital condyles. The small apical ligament extends from the tip of the odontoid to the foramen magnum. The cruciate ligament forms the third layer and is seen immediately dorsal to the odontoid process. The transverse portion of the cruciate ligament or the transverse ligament connects both lateral masses of the atlas and passes dorsal to the odontoid, keeping it pressed forward against the anterior arch of the atlas. The most posterior layer is formed by the tectorial membrane which is a superior continuation of the posterior longitudinal ligament.[3-7]

The muscles attached to the cranio-vertebral complex assist in stabilization of the spine and initiate as well as maintain movement of the joints. There is no vascular communication between the base of dens and body of axis. This is important in understanding the etiology of Os odontoideum and formation of a sequestrum with type II odontoid fracture.

Embryology

The bony cranial base is developed by a process of endochondral ossification. The bones of the CVJ are developed from four occipital sclerotomes and the first two cervical sclerotomes. The first two occipital sclerotomes form the basiocciput. The third occipital sclerotome forms the exoccipital bone that forms jugular tubercles. The key sclerotome is the fourth occipital sclerotome termed the pro-atlas. It forms the anterior tubercle of the clivus, the apical cap of the dens, anterior margin of the foramen magnum, occipital condyles, lateral atlantal masses and the superior portion of the posterior arch of the atlas. The first spinal sclerotome forms the anterior arch of atlas, posterior and inferior portion of the C1 arch, odontoid process. The second cervical sclerotome forms the rest of the axis vertebra **(Fig. 3)**.[3-7]

There are two sources of blood supply. First, anterior and posterior descending vessels arise from the vertebral arteries and pass in front and behind the axis and odontoid process. They anastomose in the apical arcade in the region of the alar ligament. These vessels supply small perforators to the body of the axis and odontoid process. Second, the anterior descending artery as well as the apical arcade receives contributions from the carotid and occipital arteries.

A

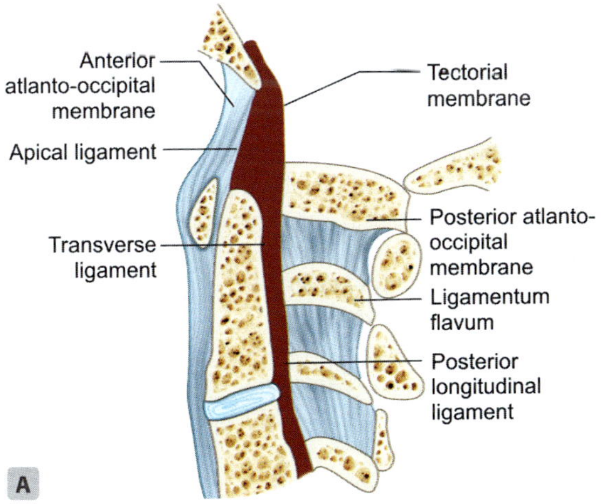

B

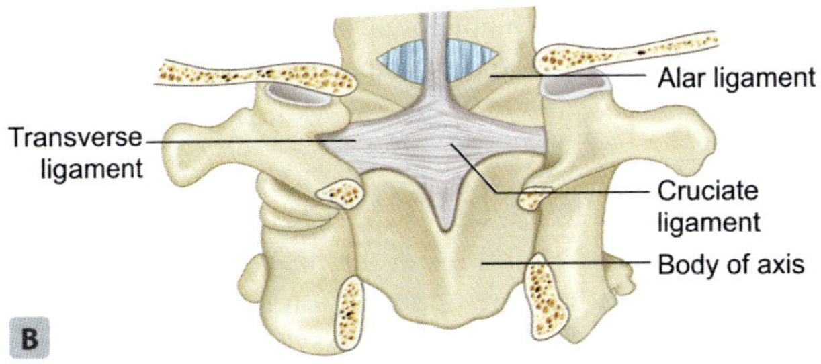

FIGS. 2A AND B: Ligamentous anatomy of craniovertebral junction.

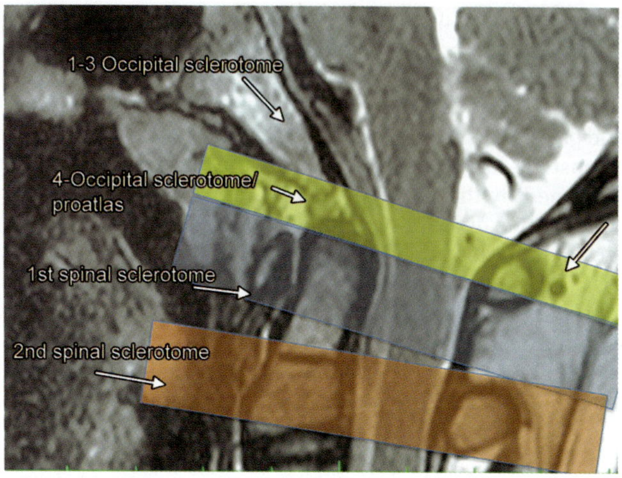

FIG. 3: Occipital and spinal sclerotomes and the development of the CVJ components.

Lymphatic drainage is primarily into the retropharyngeal lymph nodes, and then into the upper jugular deep cervical chain. Thus, a retrograde infection may affect the synovial lining of the CVJ complex.

BIOMECHANICS

Relative motion of the occipitoatlantoaxial region is controlled by the geometry of the surfaces as well as the ligaments and their elastic properties. It functions as a single unit, and the complex allows the necessary range of motion while providing support to the head. Nodding or yes-yes movements occur at the atlanto-occipital joints. Rotatory or no-no movements occur at atlantoaxial joints **(Figs. 4A and B)**. Both occipitoatlantal and atlantoaxial articulations are involved in flexion and extension. The average range of this motion at the occipitoatlantal joint is 13–15°. An additional 10° of motion occurs in the atlantoaxial articulation. Flexion is limited by the tectorial membrane and by contact between the dens and occipital basion.

Extension is restricted by the stretching of tectorial membrane and by bony contact between opisthion and posterior arch of atlas. In the normal adult less than 3 mm of anteroposterior translation occurs between the dens and anterior ring of atlas. This measurement may be up to 5 mm in children younger than 8 years of age. If the transverse component of cruciate ligament ruptures with intact alar ligament, up to 5 mm of displacement may occur.

Rotation of the craniovertebral complex occurs only at the atlantoaxial joint. The articular surfaces of atlantoaxial complex are convex with horizontal orientation so as to allow maximal mobility. Atlantoaxial joint rotation varies from 37° to 42°.[8]

CLINICAL PRESENTATION

In most cases, the symptoms of the pathologic conditions affecting the CVJ become apparent after the compromise of these neural structures. Signs and symptoms are diverse and usually have a subtle beginning; they arise fairly late, progress slowly, remain stationary, and rarely relapse. It may be in the form of dysfunction of the brainstem, cervical spinal cord, cranial nerves, cervical nerve roots or the vascular supply to these structures. Myelopathy is the most common neurological deficit.[2] Sensory abnormalities may be related to posterior column involvement. Lower cranial nerve dysfunction is seen in 20% of children with basilar invagination.[9] Vascular symptoms occur in 15% patients. Neck pain is present in 85% patients typically described as originating in the suboccipital area with radiation to the vertex.[9]

CRANIOMETRY (TABLES 1 AND 2)

Craniometry of the CVJ usesaseries of lines, planes and angles to define the normal anatomic relationships of the CVJ[10] **(Figs. 5A and B)**. These measurements were initially defined on plain X-rays but are now extrapolated to NCCT saggital and coronal images.

CLASSIFICATION OF CVJ ANOMALIES[11,12]

Congenital Anomalies and Malformations of the Craniovertebral Junction

- *Malformations of the occipital sclerotomes including proatlas*:
  - Clivus segmentation anomalies
  - Proatlas remnants around foramen magnum
  - Condylar hypoplasia
  - Assimilation of atlas
- *Malformation of atlas*:
  - Assimilation of atlas
  - Atlantoaxial fusion
  - Aplasia of atlas arches
- *Malformation of axis*:
  - Irregular atlantoaxial segmentation
  - Dens dysplasias
- Ossiculum terminale persistens
- Os odontoideum
- *Hypoplasia-aplasia*:
  - Segmentation failure of C2-C3

Developmental and Acquired Abnormalities of the CVJ

- Abnormalities at the foramen magnum. Foraminal stenosis (e.g. achondroplasia)
- Secondary basilar invagination (e.g. Osteogenesis imperfecta, Hadju-Cheney, Paget's disease, osteomalacia, rickets, rheumatoid arthritis)
- *Atlantoaxial instability*:
  - Down syndrome
  - Ehlers-Danlos syndrome
  - *Errors of metabolism*: Morquio's, Hurlers
  - Trauma
  - *Infection*: Tuberculosis
  - *Inflammatory*: Rheumatoid arthritis, Reiter's syndrome

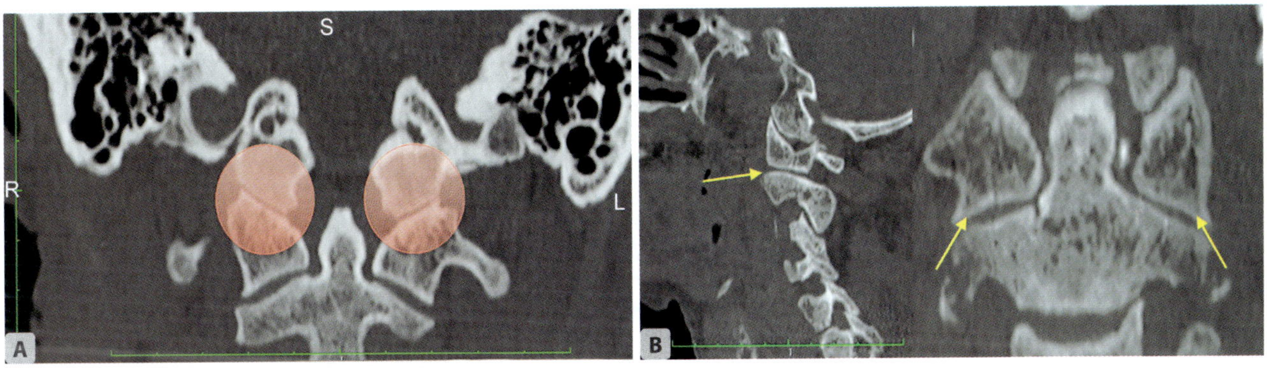

FIGS. 4A AND B: (A) Atlanto-occipital joint; and (B) Atlanto-axial joint.

TABLE 1: Craniometric lines in lateral view.

Synonyms	Definition	Normal measurement	Implications
Wackenheim's line (Clivus canal line)	Line drawn along clivus into cervical canal	Odontoid tip is ventral and tangential to this line	Odontoid process transects the line in basilar invagination or forward position of skull
Chamberlain's line (Palato-occipital line)	Joins posterior pole of hard palate to opisthion	Tip of dens 1 ± 3.6 mm below this line	Odontoid process bisects the line in basilar invagination
McRae's line (Foramen magnum line)	Joins anterior and posterior edges of foramen magnum (Basion to opisthion)	Tip of dens does not exceed this line	When effective sagittal diameter is <20 mm, neurological symptoms occur (Foramen magnum stenosis)
McGregor's line (Basal line)	Hard plate to the lowest point of occipital bone	Tip of dens should not exceed 5 mm above the line	Line position varies with flexion + extension hence not important
Height index of Klauss	Distance between tip of dens and tuberculum torcula line	40–41 mm	<30 mm seen in basilar invagination
Spinolamellar line (Spinous interlaminar line)	Line drawn from interoccipital ridge above and down along the fused spinous process of C2 and C3	Should intersect posterior arch of atlas	If atlas is fused, posterior arch is anterior to the line, posterior compression of spinal cord may occur
Boogard's line	Joins nasion to opisthion	Basion below this line	Altered in basilar impression
Atlanto temporo-mandibular index	Joins superior edge of anterior arch of atlas to the highest point of temporomandibular interspace	30 + 9 mm	<10 mm in basilar invagination
Basion odontoid index (Whooley)	Joins basion to the trip of odontoid process	5 mm in adults up to 10 mm in children (in neutral position)	Measurements altered in both flexion and extension
Basal angle	Angle between the lines drawn from nasion to tuberculum sellae and tuberculum sellae to basion	124–142°	Widening is called platy-basia
Bull's angle (Atlantopalatine angle)	Angle formed by joining the hard palate posteriorly and the line joining mid points of anterior and posterior arches of atlas	<10°	>13° in basilar invagination (BI) 10–13° : tendency to BI
Boogard's angle	Angle between McRae's line and line drawn from dorsum sellae to basion along the plane of clivus	122°	>135° in basilar invagination

- *Tumor*: Osteoblastoma, eosinophilic granuloma, chordoma, neurofibromatosis, metastasis
- Miscellaneous, e.g. Conradi-Hünermann syndrome, fetal warfarin syndrome, fibrous dysplasia
- *Spontaneous atlantoaxial rotatory subluxation*: Grisel syndrome

INCIDENCE

Craniovertebral junction anomalies are seen all over the world, but are common in our country. Exact incidence of these anomalies is not known. In a study over a period of 12 years, they were responsible for 3.03% of total admissions

TABLE 2: Craniometric lines and angles in anteroposterior view.

Synonyms	Definition	Normal	Implications
Fishgold digastric line (Biventer line)	Joins the fossae for digastric muscles on undersurface of skull (Just medial to mastoid process)	Dens tip should not project above this line. Central axis of dens should be perpendi cular to the line	Corresponds to McRae's line on lateral view: may be oblique in unilateral condylar hypoplasia: oblique odontoid suggest paramedian abnormality
Fishgold bimastoid line	Line connecting tips of mastoid process	Runs across atlantooccipital joints, line is 10 mm below digastric line	Odontoid tip may be the line
Schmidt-Fischer angle	Angle of axes of atlanto-occipital joints	124–127° should be measured in plane dens on tomography	Angle is wider in condylar hypoplasia

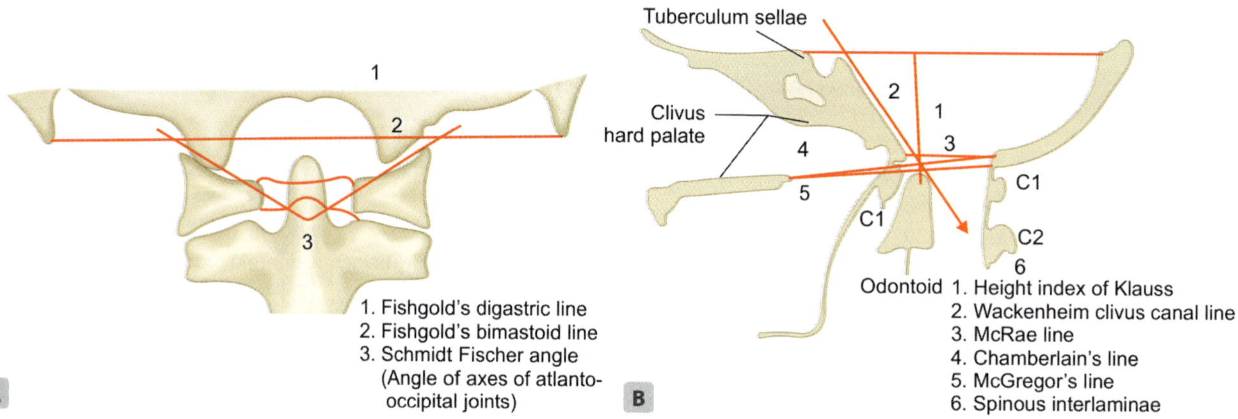

FIGS. 5A AND B: Various craniometric lines in (A) lateral and (B) anteroposterior views.

to the neurology wards.[9] They were the single major cause of cervical cord compression, accounting for nearly half the cases. Therefore, in every patient presenting with high cervical cord compression in our country, the diagnosis of CVJ anomalies must be excluded. Majority of patients are between 11 and 40 years, although the defect is present since birth. There is a male preponderance. Onset is usually gradual. The most common precipitating factor is in the form of trivial trauma to the neck either by a fall or by carrying heavy loads at the back of head.[2,9] Recurrent throat infection and fever may lead to hyperemia and laxity of ligament causing dislocations.

In a recent study of 70 patients with bony CVJ anomalies in our institute, the most common presenting symptom was cervical pain and stiffness (77%) and majority of the patients were in second decade. The common neurological sign was involvement of pyramidal tract (70%). Multiple anomalies are frequently seen. A study of 82 patients with CVJ anomalies in our institute showed congenital atlantoaxial dislocation (AAD) to be the most common (56%) anomaly followed by multiple anomalies (48.8%) the common combinations being AAD with occipitalization of C1, basilar invagination with Chiari malformation and basilar invagination with occipitalization of C1.[13]

NEURORADIOLOGIC INVESTIGATIONS

- *Conventional radiography*:
  - Translateral view of skull including the upper cervical spine (neutral, flexion and extension). These give the points of references for various radiological base lines and angles in assessing atlanto-odontoid distance, anomalies of dens and arches of atlas and axis vertebrae and the soft tissues of neck.
  - Open mouth view—additionally detects dens anomalies and its lateral displacement.
- *Conventional tomography (AP and lateral)*: It defines the CVJ relationship and dimensions (rarely done).
- *Noncontrast CT*: Axial sections show arches of atlas, lateral masses, atlanto-odontoid distance, position of dens and canal diameters. Structures within the canal are indistinguishable without the use of subarachnoid contrast. CT helps to make definitive diagnosis of atlantoaxial rotatory fixation and spatial appreciation of bony fragments in relation to foramen magnum.
- *Three-dimensional CT and reconstruction images*: It helps in understanding the spatial relationships of complex skeletal and traumatic pathology and makes it possible to make a definitive and comprehensive radiographic diagnosis, without additional radiation exposure or significant modification of scanning technique. Little literature is available about its potentials in evaluating CVJ.
- *Conventional MRI*: It provides multiplanar images and is especially helpful in evaluating the brainstem, spinal cord, cerebellar tonsils, syringohydromyelia, cervicomedullary kink and hydrocephalus, etc.
- *Dynamic MRI*: It attempts to combine the advantages of plain films, CT and conventional MRI together. A study

conducted in this institute on the role of dynamic MRI in evaluating the CV-Junction abnormalities in 25 patients revealed the diagnosis of mobile AAD, dynamic nature of spinal canal narrowing and variability in cord compression with changing position of the neck.[14] In neutral position, 81% patients had some degree of canal narrowing out of which 16% patients showed increase in canal narrowing on flexion with half of them having direct cord compression which was not detected in neutral position. Thus, dynamic MRI was able to detect cases where surgical intervention was needed as the cord was being compressed in one of the physiological positions. Dynamic MRI of CVJ attempts to give information regarding the dynamic nature of CVJ abnormalities along with the established advantages of MRI like excellent soft tissue visualization and multiplanar capability. The knowledge of dynamic nature of cord compression is important in planning the management of these abnormalities.

A combination of MRI and either standard radiography or CT is ideal in evaluating most of the CVJ anomalies. In all techniques of investigations, dynamic flexion and extension studies are essential to assess the stability and angular osseous relationships and to provide information related to their reducibility and position of fixation. A recent study was conducted in this institute to compare the role of plain radiographs, linear tomograms, axial noncontrast computed tomography (NCCT) and 3D CT in flexion and extension for CVJ anomalies. It was found that the most common radiological abnormality was bony atlas anomalies (86.7%) followed by AAD (80%) and multiple anomalies (50%). Three-dimensional CT was found either equivalent or superior to plain X-rays and tomograms except in the assessment of foramen magnum dimensions.

SPECIFIC CONDITIONS

Basilar Invagination

It is a developmental defect implying prolapse of the vertebral column into the skull base **(Fig. 6)**. There is a distinct developmental defect of the chondrocranium, often associated with other anomalies of the notochord in the region of the CVJ such as occipitalization of atlas **(Figs. 7A to E)** and Klippel-Feil syndrome.[2] Basilar invagination is also associated with anomalies of development of the epicaudal neuroaxis such as Chiari malformations, syringobulbia and syringomyelia in about 25–30% of cases. Two types of basilar invagination are recognized.[7] In the anterior variety, there is shortening of the basiocciput and the clivus is short and horizontally oriented known as Basi-occiput hypoplasia **(Fig. 8)**. In the paramedian variety, there is hypoplasia of the exoccipital bones and dorsal displacement of the clivus, which is otherwise of normal length.

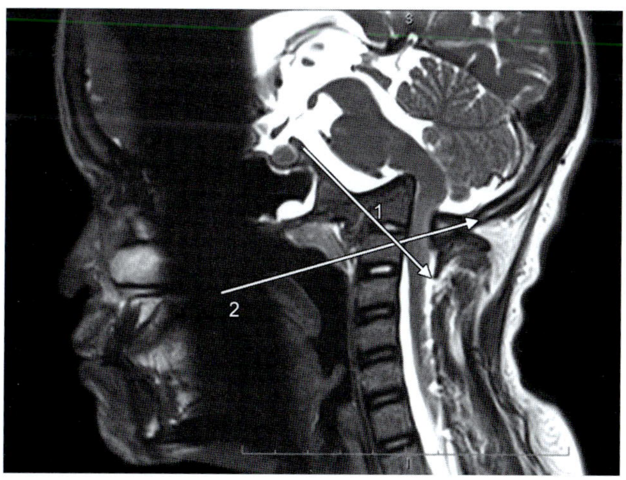

FIG. 6: Basilar invagination with odontoid tip crossing both the clivus-canal line (1) and McGregor's line (2).

Basilar impression refers to secondary or acquired forms of basilar invagination due to softening of the bone as occurs in hyperparathyroidism, rickets, osteomalacia, Paget's disease, Hurler's syndrome, osteogenesis imperfecta, etc. Traumatic basilar impression has also been reported.[15,16] Inflammation and infection producing bone destruction with or without ligamentous instability may also cause basilar impression, e.g. rheumatoid arthritis, tuberculosis, etc. In this anomaly, all three parts of the occipital bone (basiocciput, exoccipital bone, and supraoccipital bone) are deformed. There is abnormal rostral location of clivus-atlas-odontoid complex within the foramen magnum.

Platybasia refers only to an abnormally obtuse basal angle. It is not a measure of basilar invagination, although it may be associated with invagination **(Figs. 9A and B)**. There are no symptoms or signs associated with platybasia alone.

Assimilation of Atlas

Assimilation of atlas represents the most cephalic blocked vertebra encountered in the spine. It is defined as a failure of segmentation between the atlas and skull and occurs in 0.25% of the population.[17] It may be bilateral, unilateral, segmental, or focal **(Figs. 10A and B)**. In most instances, atlas assimilation occurs in association with other abnormalities such as basilar invagination and Klippel-Feil syndrome. Associated congenital anomalies present in 20% of patients, include incomplete clefting of the nasal cartilage, cleft palate, congenital external ear deformities, cervical ribs hypospadiasis and urinary tract anomalies.[18]

A combination of assimilation of the atlas and segmentation failures between the second and third cervical vertebrae results in progressive laxity of the atlantoaxial joint with development of luxation between the atlas and axis in childhood in about 50% of cases. The progressive proliferation of granulation tissue due to instability leads to irreducible compression.

Atlas Arch Anomalies

The most common anomaly in this group is posterior rachischisis, which is present in 4% of the autopsy specimens of adults.[19] Majority of these are midline in location (97%). Posterior arch rachischisis has been reported in 70% of children with myelomeningoceles. It may be associated with atlantoaxial instability.[18]

Congenital defects of the posterior arch of atlas may also be discovered as incidental findings.[7]

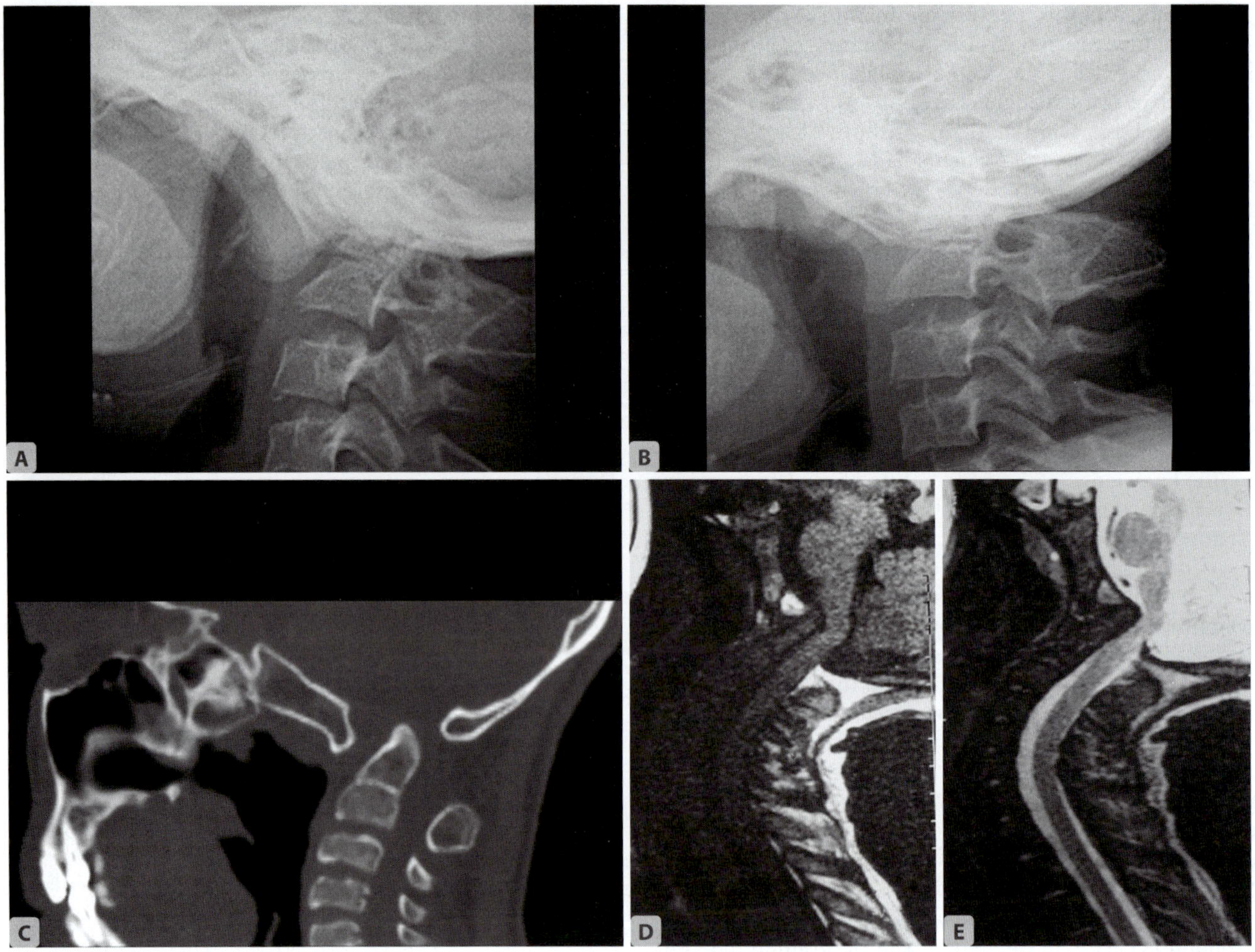

FIGS. 7A TO E: Basilar invagination. (A and B) Lateral cervical X-ray in extension and flexion shows high placed odontoid with narrowed spinal canal. Also note the assimilation of atlas; (C) Noncontrast CT midsagittal maximum intensity projection (MIP) confirms the high placed odontoid and complete assimilation of atlas; (D) T1W and (E) T2W sagittal images show the compression at the cervicomedullary junction.

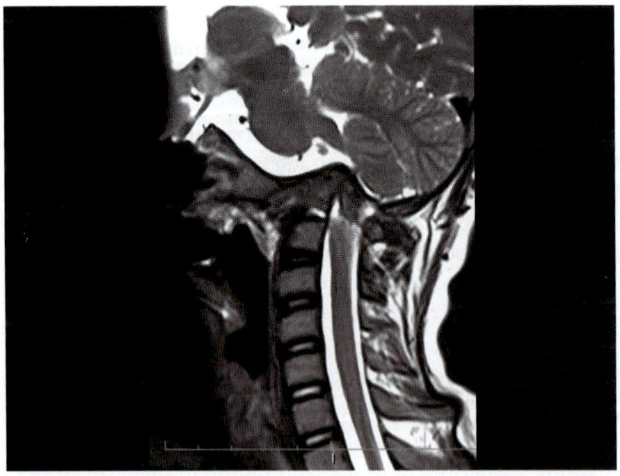

FIG. 8: Basilar invagination (BI) with basi-occiput hypoplasia—clivus is short and clivus-canal angle is typically less than 150°.

Anterior arch rachischisis is very rare and occurs only in 0.1% adult autopsy specimens. It is almost invariably encountered with posterior rachischisis, in case of which the term "split atlas" is applied[20] **(Figs. 11A and B)**.

Malformations of atlas may be confused with Jefferson fracture.[19,21] CT may help in differentiating the two entities. Margins of developmental cleft are smooth with an intact cortical edge with no abnormal soft tissue, whereas fractures have jagged edges or are comminuted and generally associated with soft tissue swelling.[22]

Dens Dysplasias

The odontoid tip normally lies approximately at the level of the superior margin of the anterior arch of atlas. Hypoplasia of the odontoid process **(Figs. 12A to C)** predisposes to atlantoaxial instability, injuries and rheumatoid complications. A hypertrophic odontoid may be viewed as manifestations of the occipital vertebra. Significant vascular compromise on

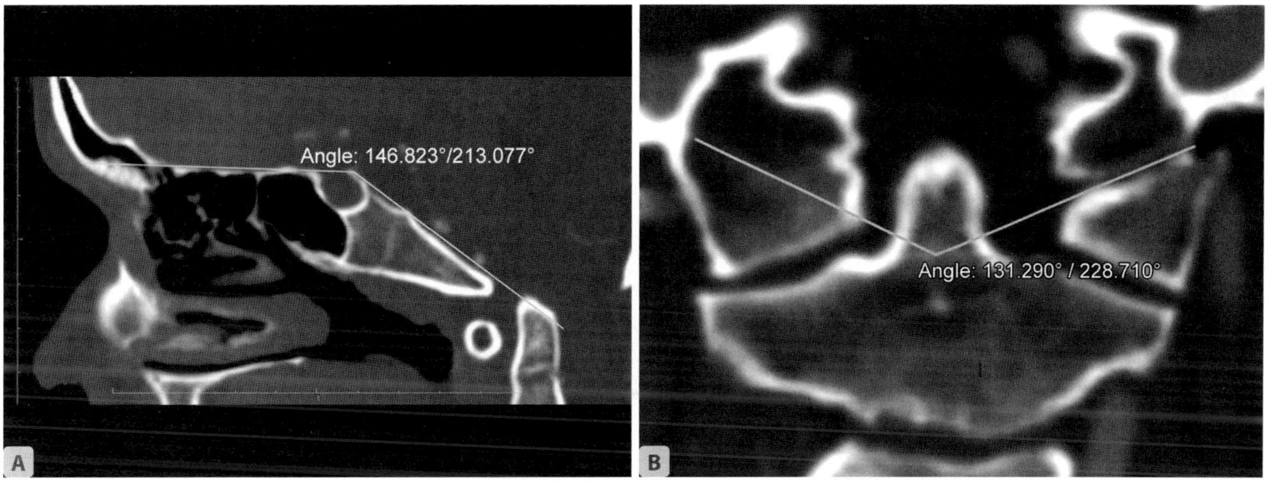

FIGS. 9A AND B: Platybasia may be associated with: Basilar invagination, cord symptoms, clivus-canal angle becomes acute (<150°), Welcher basal angle >140°.

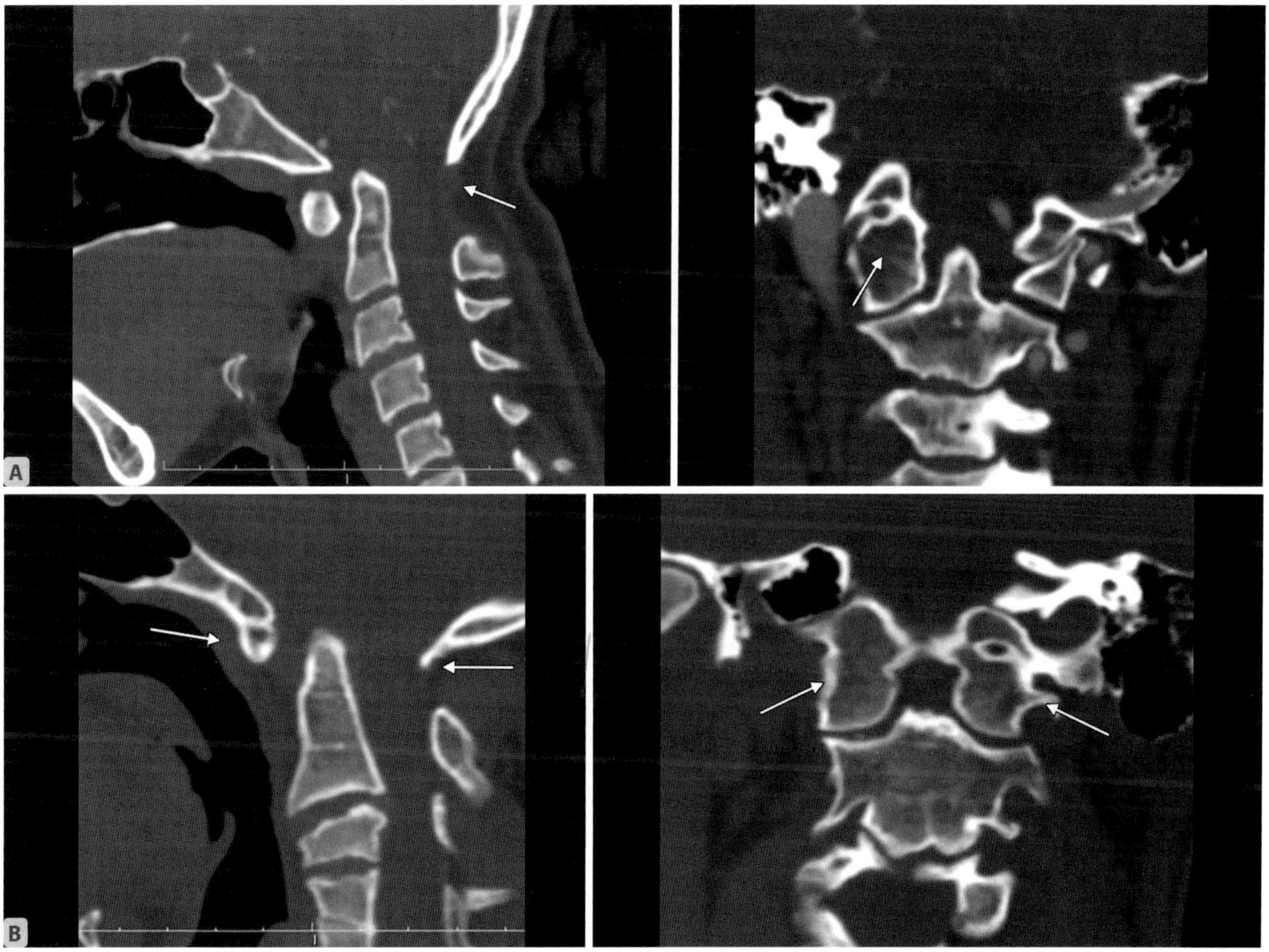

FIGS. 10A AND B: Assimilation of Atlas: Partial assimilation of C-1 With occiput (A). Note (arrows) pointing fusion of posterior arch with occiput and right lateral mass with occipital condyle. Complete assimilation (B) showing fusion of both anterior and posterior arch and lateral masses with occiput.

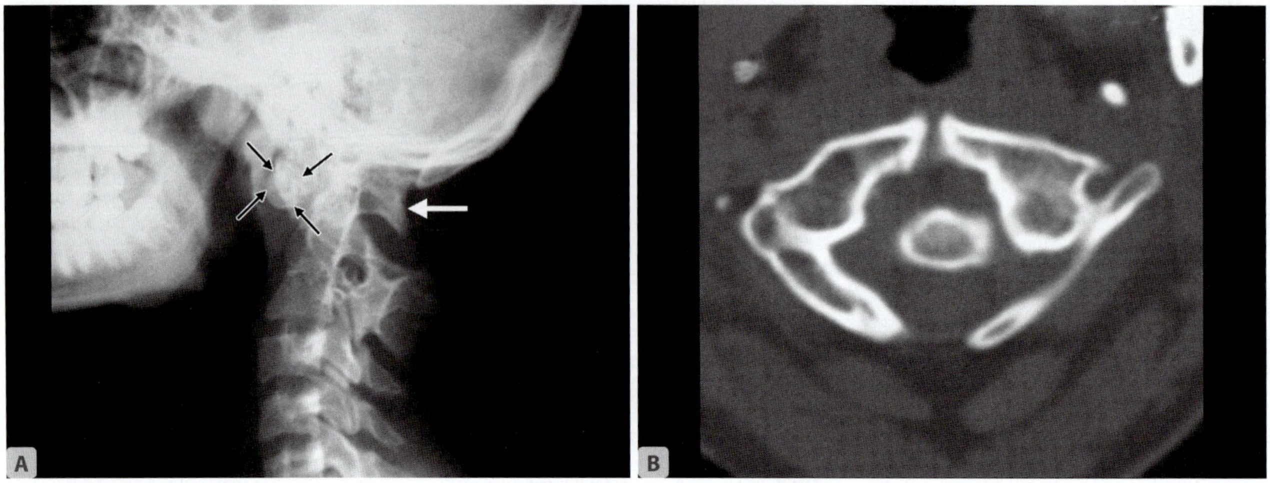

FIGS. 11A AND B: Split atlas. (A) Lateral cervical radiograph shows rounded, hypertrophic anterior arch of atlas without typical cortication (thin arrows) and two posterior atlas arches without visualization of a spinolaminar line (thick arrow); (B) NCCT image show presence of clefts in both anterior and posterior arch of atlas.

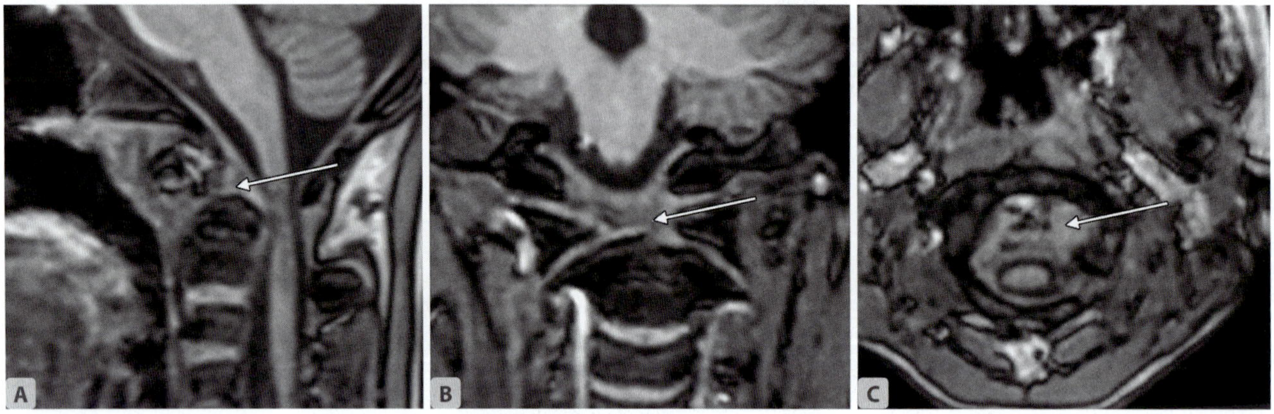

FIGS. 12A TO C: Odontoid hypoplasia—the odontoid process is barely seen and the attachments for the apical and alar ligaments are absent.

stretching and distortion of the vertebral artery may occur with odontoid dysplasias.

Os Terminale

It refers to the nonfused terminal part of the odontoid derived from the centrum of the IVth occipital sclerotome. This apical segment is usually about 12 mm in length, but can be very small. In case of disruption at the interface and if AAD occurs, the remaining part of the odontoid may compress the cervicomedullary region.

Os Odontoideum

This denotes an independent bone seen cranial to the axis in place of the dens, which is hypoplastic. Its most common location is in the position of the normal odontoid tip or near the base of the occiput in the area of foramen magnum, where it may fuse with the clivus. This leads to incompetence of the cruciate ligaments and atlantoaxial instability.[7] Hypertrophy of the anterior arch of C1 is often associated with Os odontoideum **(Figs. 13A to D)**. There are two hypotheses postulated congenital and traumatic in the causation of Os odontoideum. The weight of the current evidence now points to a traumatic etiology in the majority of cases of Os odontoideum.[23]

Two types of Os odontoideum are described: *Dystopic* and *Orthotopic*. In the orthotopic variety, the Os lies in the position of normal dens and moves in unison with the atlas and axis.

In the dystopic variety, the Os lies near the basion or may be fused with the occipital bone and moves in unison with the clivus. The anterior arch of the atlas is hypertrophied and the posterior arch is often hypoplastic. In the orthotopic Os odontoideum, the transverse component of the cruciate ligament is functional as there is movement in unison with atlas and axis. The incidence of Os odontoideum is increased in patients with Down's syndrome, spondyloepiphyseal dysplasia, or Morquio's syndrome. It is important to differentiate Os odontoideum from type II odontoid fracture. CT is the best modality to distinguish these two entities. In Os odontoideum, the upper margin of the body of axis is convex and may be associated with hypertrophy of anterior arch of atlas seen as enlargement, convex posterior border and increased cortical thickness **(Fig. 14A)**.

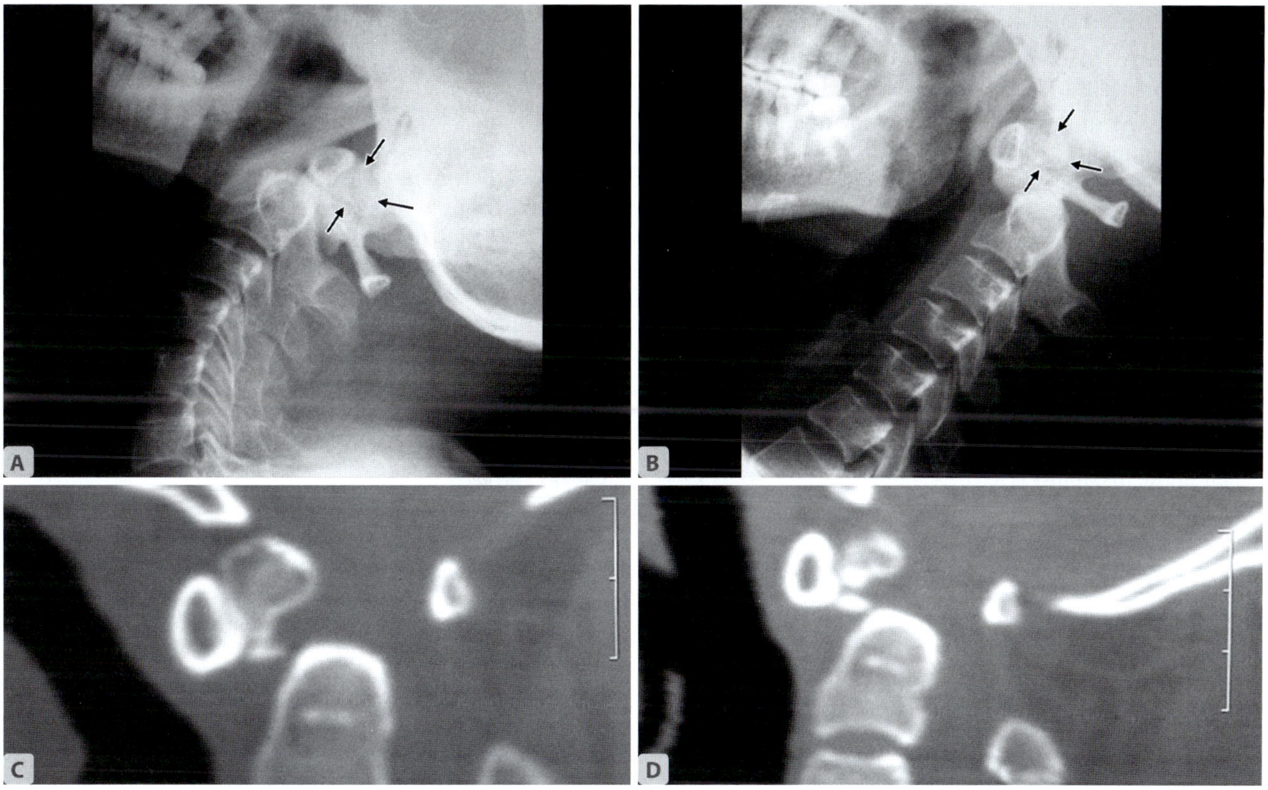

FIGS. 13 A TO D: Os odontoideum. (A and B) Lateral plain radiographs of craniovertebral junction (CVJ) in extension and flexion show the presence of hypoplastic odontoid process and presence of independent osseous structure (arrows) posterior to anterior arch of atlas; (C and D) Sagittal reconstruction CT image confirm the presence of well corticated smooth Os odontoideum and hypertrophied anterior arch of C1. Note a small bony fragment inferior to the Os odontoideum.

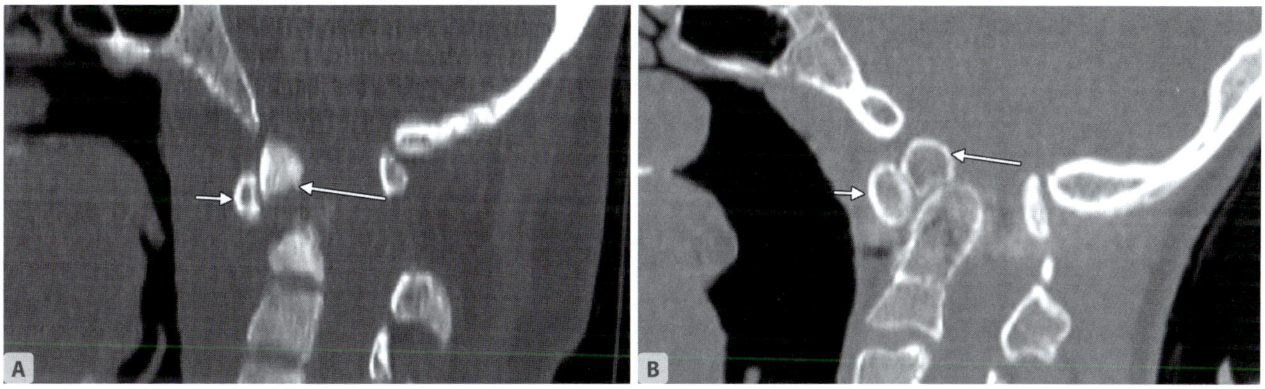

FIGS. 14A AND B: Odontoid fracture (A) and Os odontoideum (B). Small arrows showing normal anterior arch (A) and hypertrophied arch (B); Long arrows showing fracture with no cortex (A) and well corticated surface is Os (B).

In odontoid fracture, the upper margin of axis is flattened with sharp uncorticated margin and normal appearing anterior arch **(Fig. 14B)**.[24,25]

Atlantoaxial Instability

Stability at atlantoaxial area is dependent on integrity of osseous, ligamentous and muscle complex. Instability of atlantoaxial joint can be documented by lateral cervical radiographs done in flexion and extension. The diagnosis of rupture of transverse ligaments and AAD is purely radiological. An atlas dens interval of more than 4 mm in children and more than 3 mm in adults is diagnostic. If more than 5 mm motion of anterior atlantoaxial interval is present, conclusive evidence of instability exists.

The 10–20% of children with Down's syndrome have atlantoaxial instability radiologically, and only 18% of them are symptomatic. AAI or occipitoatlantoaxial dislocations have been reported with upper respiratory tract infection, mastoiditis, partotitis, tuberculosis, gout, seronegative arthropathy, rheumatoid arthritis and following tonsillectomy, adenoidectomy,[19] mastoidectomy and cardiac surgeries.[26]

Classification of AAI

Group I: AAI in combinations with occipitalization of atlas, fusion of C2 and C3. Odontoid is displaced posteriorly.

Group II: AAI due to incompetence of odontoid process (maldevelopment)

Type I: Os odontoideum

Type II: Ossiculum terminale

Type III: Agenesis of odontoid base

Type IV: Agenesis of apical segment Type

V: Agenesis of odontoid.

Group III: Odontoid is seen dislocated posteriorly. There is no abnormality of C1 or odontoid.

Dynamic studies (Flexion and extension) are important not only for the diagnosis but also for the management, i.e. whether the instability is fixed or mobile.[27]

Inflammatory, Arthritic and Infectious Disorders

The most common disorder in this category is rheumatoid arthritis (RA). Other disorders include psoriatic and osteoarthritis, synovial cysts and calcium pyrophosphate deposition disease (CPPD), etc.

Infectious diseases with CVJ involvement are rare and include tuberculosis and fungal infections.

In RA, cervical spine is clinically affected in 44–88% of patients.[28] Three types of abnormalities are seen: (1) AAI (25%), (2) upward migration of odontoid process or cranial settling (8–16%) and (3) rheumatoid granulation tissue or pannus formation around the odontoid process (10–30%). In cranial settling, there is erosion and compression of lateral masses of C1, downward displacement of anterior arch with cranial rotation of posterior arch of C1 resulting in upward migration of dens. The AP diameter of the cervical canal is reduced causing compression. MRI is the imaging modality of choice for the evaluation of rheumatoid pannus. The rheumatoid pannus can be of three types, i.e. hypervascular, hypovascular or fibrous types. On T2W images the hypervascular pannus is hyperintense, whereas hypovascular and fibrous pannus show intermediate and low signal intensity respectively. The hypervascular pannus and the rheumatoid joint effusion, both of which are hyperintense on T2W images can be differentiated by presence of early intense contrast enhancement in hypervascular pannus on dynamic postcontrast studies **(Figs. 15A to E)**. The hypovascular pannus shows delayed enhancement whereas fibrous type of pannus shows no enhancement on postcontrast images **(Figs. 16A to C)**.[29]

Calcium pyrophosphate crystal deposition disease which frequently involves the joints in the appendicular skeleton, has a predilection for anterior atlantoaxial joint. The transverse ligament is usually the site of involvement with presence of retro-odontoid soft tissue. The radiographic findings are usually subtle. The NCCT images show retro-odontoid calcifications and the MRI shows the retro-odontoid soft tissue that is hypointense on both T1W and T2W images with the disruption of transverse ligament at times.[30]

Tuberculosis of atlantoaxial region accounts for less than 1% of all case of spinal tuberculosis.[31] Local neck pain tenderness and restriction of neck movements are the cardinal features.

The disease is divided into three stages:

1. *Stage I*: Retropharyngeal abscess AAD/AAI
   Normal bony architecture
2. *Stage II*: Retropharyngeal abscess ± AAD mild bony destruction
3. *Stage III*: Retropharyngeal abscess ± AAD gross bony destruction

Myelo-CT or MR demonstrates the characteristic radiographic appearance of bony destruction of C1–C2 with increased prevertebral soft tissue.

TRAUMA

As discussed, the continuity of the craniocervical biomechanical is dependent on the integrity of the skull base, atlas, and axis and their attaching ligaments. Initially, most of the trauma patients undergo conventional radiography. However NCCT is now the mainstay in imaging of the trauma for bone and high resolution MRI for the soft tissue. Trauma can cause fractures of clivus, C-1, C-2 vertebrae either in isolation or in combinations. An abnormal distance between the dens or posterior axial line and the basion suggests failure or insufficiency of the alar ligaments, tectorial membrane, or both. Increased atlantoaxial distance, which should be less than 4 mm in children under 9 years of age and less than 3 mm in adults, points to injury of the transverse ligament. On the open-mouth view of the CVJ, the lateral masses of C1 should align exactly with the lateral margins of C2 vertebra. CT with sagittal and coronal reformatted images permits optimal detection and evaluation of fracture and subluxation. The atlanto-occipital and atlantoaxial articulations should be congruent on both coronal and sagittal reformatted images. Fractures of the tip of the dens or of the occipital condyles may be associated with alar ligament insufficiency. Subarachnoid hemorrhage and epidural hematoma may accompany injuries to the craniocervical junction.[32]

The most common bone involved in the fractures of this region is odontoid process. Conventionally, its fractures are classified into three types—Type-I, if there is avulsion of the tip **(Fig. 17)**; Type-II, if there is fracture of the body of the odontoid process **(Figs. 18A to E)** and Type-III if the odontoid process is fractured along with base of C-2.

Magnetic resonance imaging of the cervical spine with fat-suppressed gradient-echo T2W or STIR sequences can display an increased signal intensity in the atlantoaxial and atlanto-occipital joints, craniocervical ligaments, prevertebral soft tissues, and the spinal cord **(Figs. 19A and B)**. Axial gradient-echo MRIs may be prominently useful in assessing the integrity of the transverse atlantal ligament.[33,34]

Conventional radiography and CT findings in AAD include prevertebral soft-tissue swelling, C1-C2 dislocation or subluxation, and widening of the C1-C2 facets. MRI findings consist of prevertebral, interspinous, or nuchal ligament edema as well as facet widening or fluid, possible epidural hematoma, and increased signal intensity of the spinal cord

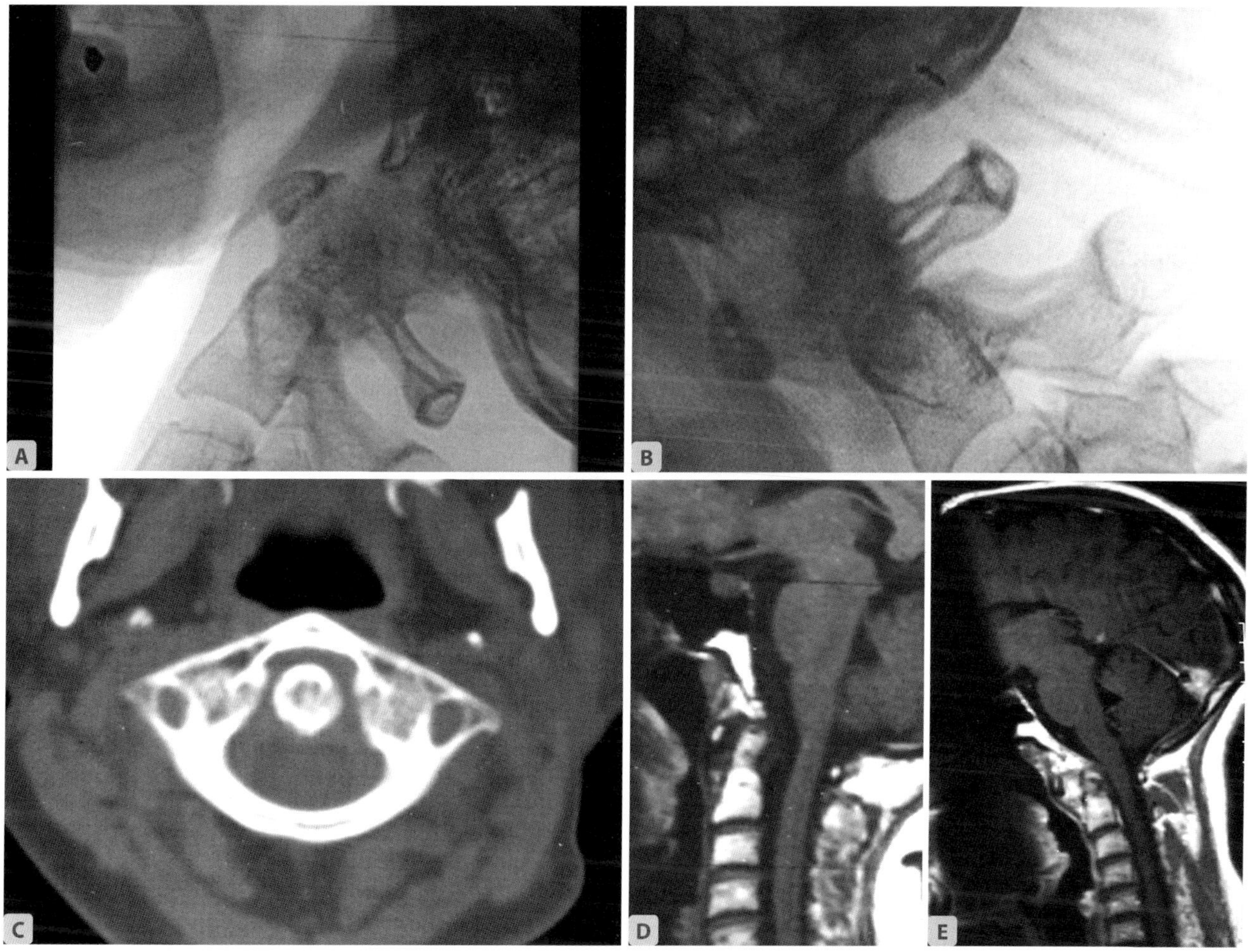

FIGS. 15A TO E: Rheumatoid arthritis of the CVJ. (A and B) Lateral cervical X-rays show minimally increased predental interval in extension position which is more marked in flexion position; (C) CT axial image showing the increased anterior atlantoaxial distance and erosions of odontoid process; (D) Sagittal spin echo precontrast and (E) postcontrast T1W images showing presence of predental hypointense soft tissue that is showing intense postcontrast enhancement.

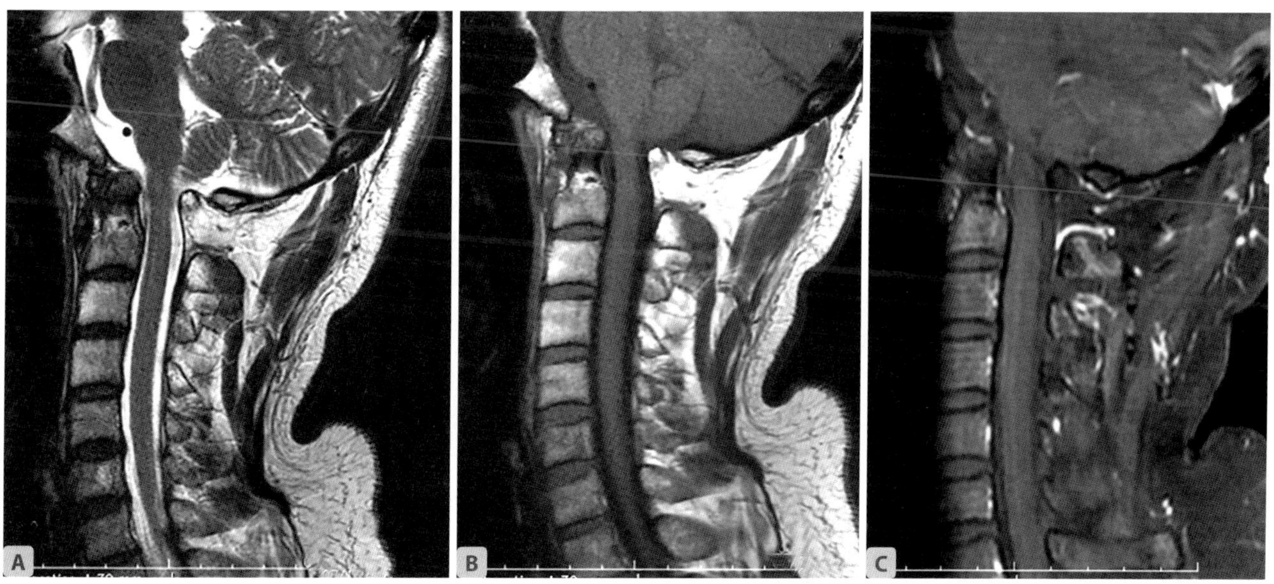

FIGS. 16A TO C: Chronic RA with hypointense soft tissue at the CVJ without any enhancement.

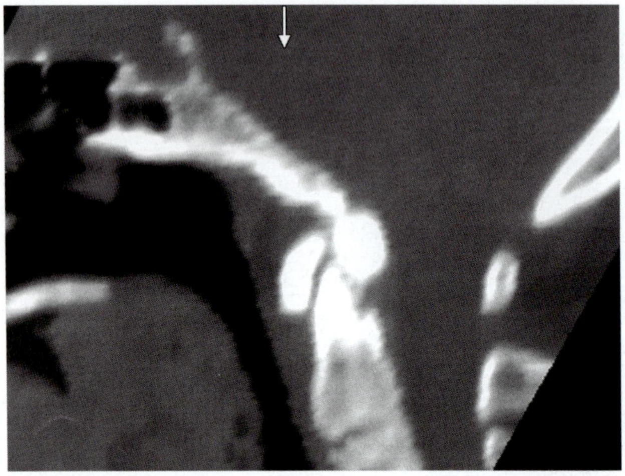

FIG. 17: Type-I odontoid fracture with avulsion fracture of the tip of the odontoid process.

on T2W or STIR images. The various types of CVJ injuries is been discussed elsewhere in this book.

SYNDROMES INVOLVING THE CVJ[35]

Klippel-Feil Syndrome

The classic triad consists of a low posterior hairline, short neck and limitation of neck movement. The syndrome is associated with fused vertebrae (usually C2-3 and C5-6 interfaces), hemivertebra, spina bifida occulta and scoliosis. Along with the vertebral segmentation anomalies, many CVJ anomalies are often present including basilar invagination, atlanto-occipital assimilation, odontoid hypoplasia platybasia, and Chiari I malformation. Associated congenital anomalies include urogenital anomalies, otological anomalies, cleft palate, etc. Syndactyly, Sprengel's shoulder and absence of ulna are common **(Figs. 19A and B)**.

Down Syndrome

Down syndrome or trisomy 21, the most frequent of the chromosomal disorders, is frequently complicated by atlanto-occipital instability (61%) as well as atlantoaxial instability (9–30%). Other observed osseous abnormalities comprise of persistent synchondroses, posterior C1 rachischisis and Os odontoideum.

Arnold-Chiari Malformation

The Arnold-Chiari malformations (ACM), type I through III, are a group of disorders characterized by increasing degrees of hindbrain dysgenesis. Each may be associated with deformities of the CVJ.

Chiari I Malformation

In cases with this disorder the vermis, fourth ventricle and medulla are normal or very slightly deformed. Elongated pointed peg-like cerebellar tonsils are displaced inferiorly through the foramen magnum into the upper cervical spinal canal. A syrinx is present in 20–40% of all patients with Chiari I, which increase to 60–90% in symptomatic patients.

Osseous anomalies are seen in 25% patients in the form of basilar invaginations (25–50%) Klippel-Feil anomaly (5–10%) **(Figs. 20A to C)** and atlanto-occipital assimilation (1–5%).[20]

Presently research is being done to better understand the cause of syrinx formation in patients where there is no direct cord compression. For this researchers have used phase-contrast line MRI to calculate and study CSF flow across Foramen Magnum. During cardiac systole the CSF goes down the spinal canal across the F Magnum and during diastole the reverse happens. This occurs due to relative increase and decrease of the cerebral blood vessels during the cardiac cycle which affects the CSF flow. It has been observed that in majority of these patients there is abnormality of this normal CSF flow **(Fig. 21)**.[36-38]

Chiari II Malformation

This is characterized by herniation of the inferior portions of the vermis, fourth ventricle and medulla into the spinal canal, kinking and displacing normal structures. It is associated with small posterior fossa, low lying transverse sutures, concave clivus and petrous ridges and fenestrate falx. The other associations include myelomeningocele (95–100%), hydrocephalus (90%) syringohydromyelia (50–90%) and segmentation anomalies (<10%).

Chiari III Malformation

This is defined as herniation of the hindbrain associated with occipital encephalocele in combination with many of the features of the Chiari II malformation. MR is the best modality to visualize the various anomalies of ACM.

Achondroplasia

Achondroplasia is the most common of the short-limbed dwarfisms. The radiographic abnormalities involve the regions in which the growth and development occur primarily through enchondral ossification. The foramen magnum is constricted and has a distinct tear drop configuration with obliteration of the surrounding subarachnoid space. Other CVJ abnormalities include odontoid dysplasia, basiocciput hypoplasia, decrease in the basal angle and thickening of the posterior rim of the foramen magnum.

Mucopolysaccharidoses

Mucopolysaccharidoses are inherited lysosomal storage disorders. Abnormalities at the CVJ are a major cause of morbidity and mortality especially in Morquio (type IV) and Hurler (type I) varieties. These include a hypoplastic/dysplastic odontoid process, ligamentous instability, soft-tissue thickening around the dens, and compression of the cord by the posterior atlas arch. The soft-tissue mass around the dens is typically hypointense or isointense on T1W and hypointense on T2W MRIs which may represent nonossified fibrocartilage.

Osteogenesis Imperfecta

Osteogenesis imperfecta, is a hereditary disorder which is the result of a defect in collagen production leading to

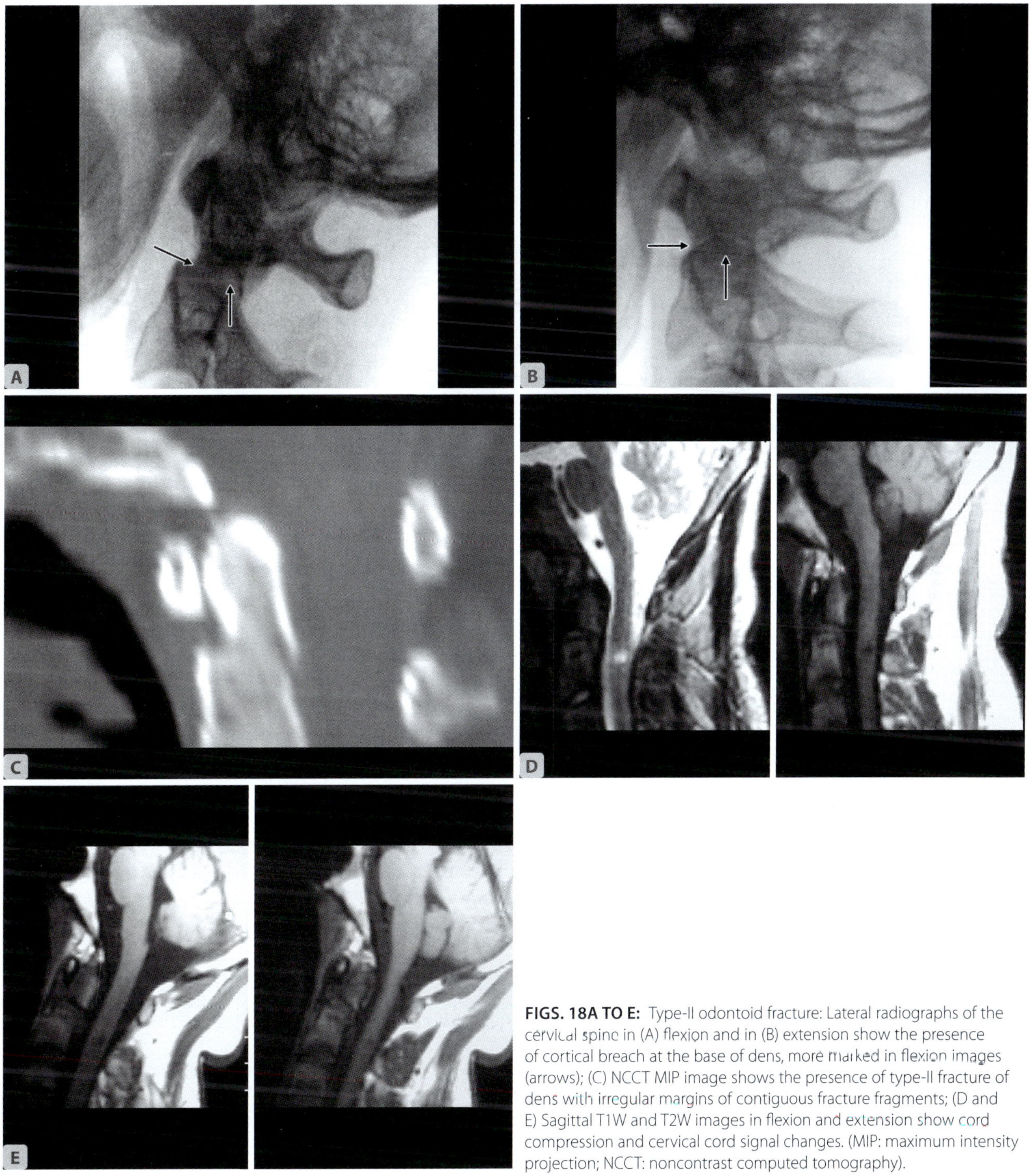

FIGS. 18A TO E: Type-II odontoid fracture: Lateral radiographs of the cervical spine in (A) flexion and in (B) extension show the presence of cortical breach at the base of dens, more marked in flexion images (arrows); (C) NCCT MIP image shows the presence of type-II fracture of dens with irregular margins of contiguous fracture fragments; (D and E) Sagittal T1W and T2W images in flexion and extension show cord compression and cervical cord signal changes. (MIP: maximum intensity projection; NCCT: noncontrast computed tomography).

osteoporosis. Pathology at the CVJ is most commonly seen in type IV, with a prevalent in the range of rare to 25%. The osteoporotic bones result in repetitive microfractures causing infolding of the occipital condyles with elevation of the clivus and the posterior cranial fossa, accompanied by an upward migration of the cervical spine into the foramen magnum (basilar impression).

SUMMARY

There has been renewed interest in the CVJ anomalies with the growth of 3D CT and magnetic resonance. Both the acquired and congenital pathologies are readily diagnosed using these modalities. MR in association with either plain X-rays or 3D CT would be ideal in the evaluation of CVJ anomalies.

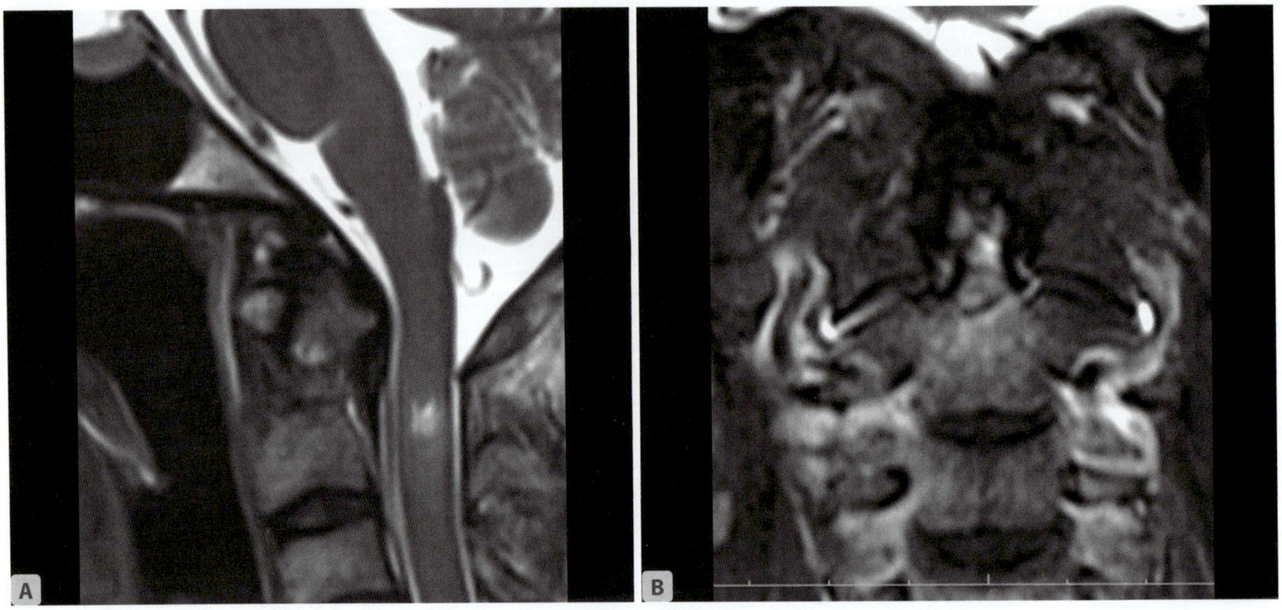

FIGS. 19A AND B: Type-II fracture showing cord contusion on T2WI and marrow edema on the STIR image.

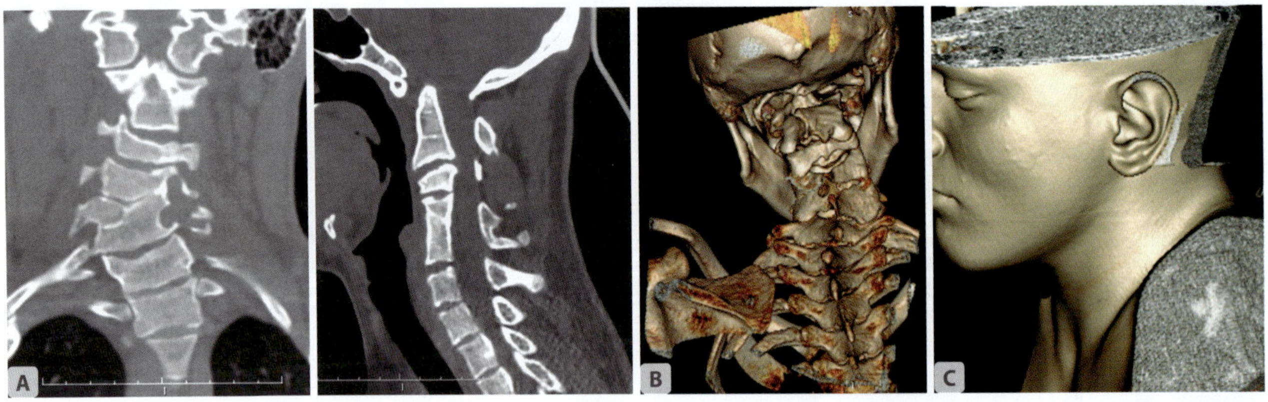

FIGS. 20A TO C: Klippel-Feil syndrome: Young patient showing multiple vertebral anomalies (A), Sprengel's shoulder (B), and short neck (C).

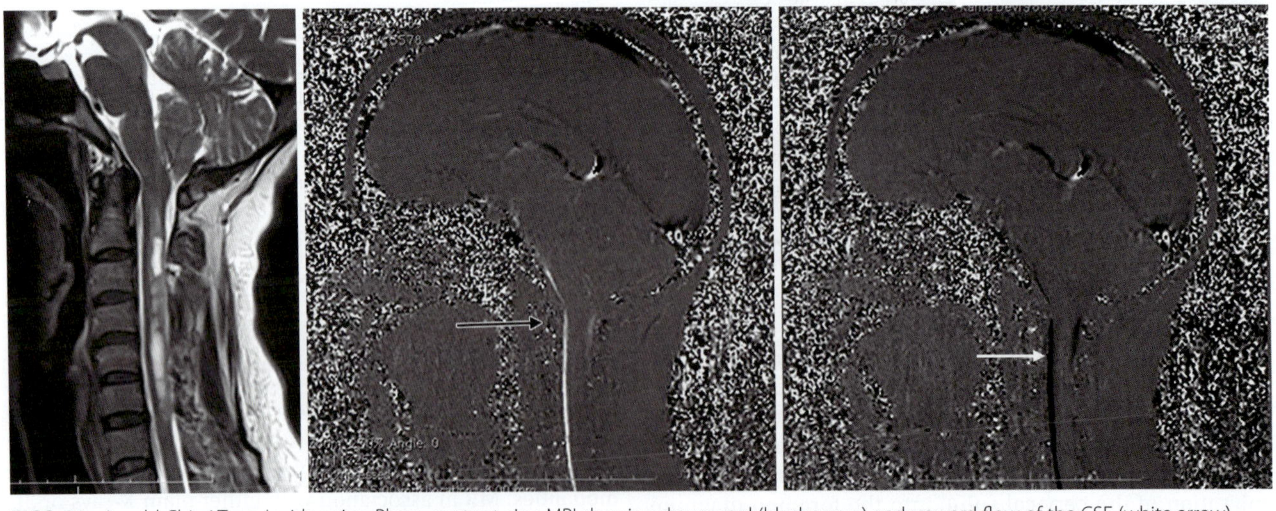

FIGS. 21: Arnold Chiari Type-I with syrinx: Phase-contrast cine MRI showing downward (black arrow) and upward flow of the CSF (white arrow).

REFERENCES

1. Johnson MH, Smoker WR. Lesions of the craniovertebral junction. Neuroimaging Clin N Am. 1994;4:599-17.
2. Menezes AH. Bony anomalies of the craniovertebral junction. In: Pang D (Ed): Disorders of Paediatrics Spine. Raven Press, New York. 1995. pp. 97-100.
3. Menezes AH, Traynelis VC. Anatomy and biomechanics of normal craniovertebral junction (a) and biomechanics of stabilization (b). Childs Nerv Syst. 2008;24:1091-100.
4. Smoker WR. Craniovertebral Junction: Normal anatomy, craniometry, and congenital aomalies. Radiographics. 1994;14:255-7.
5. Menezes AH. Craniocervical developmental anatomy and its implications. Childs Nerv Syst. 2008;24:1109-22.
6. Martin MD, Bruner HJ, Maiman DJ. Anatomic and biomechanical considerations of the craniovertebral junction. Neurosurgery. 2010;66:2-6.
7. Menezes AH. Congenital and acquired abnormalities of the craniovertebral junction. In Youmans Neurological Surgery. WB Saunders. 1996;4:1035-89.
8. Penning L. Normal movements of the cervical spine. AJR. 1978;130:317-26.
9. Sambasivan M. Anatomy of the craniovertebral anomalies. Progress in Clinical Neurosciences. 1988;1:81-100.
10. Dolan KD. Cervicobasilar relationships. RCNA. 1977;15:155-66.
11. Rao VR, Gupta AK. Imaging of craniovertebral anomalies. Progress in Clinical Neurosciences. 1989;2:229-56.
12. Menezes AH. Craniovertebral junction database analysis: incidence, classification, presentation, and treatment algorithms. Childs Nerv Syst. 2008;24:1101-8.
13. Chopra JS, Sawhey IM, Kak VK, et al. Analysis of 82 cases of craniovertebra anomalies. Br J Neurosurg. 1988;2:455-63.
14. Gupta V, Khandelwal N, Mathuria SN, et al. Dynamic magnetic resonance imaging evaluation of craniovertebral junction abnormalities. J Comput Assist Tomogr. 2007;31:354-9.
15. Dilorenzo N, Fortuna A, Guidetti B. Cranio-vertebral junction malformation: clinico-radiological findings, long-term results and surgical indication in 63 cases. Neurosurgery. 1982;57:603-8.
16. Kuroiwa T, Tanabe H, Hasegawa T. Traumatic basilar impression. Surg Neurol. 1995;44:31-2.
17. Mc Rae DL, Barnum AS. Occipitalization of the atlas. AJR. 1953;70:23-46.
18. Smoker WR. Congenital anomalies of the cervical spine. Neuroimaging Clinics of North America. 1995;5:427-49.
19. Dyste GN, Menezes AH. Symptomatic Chiari malformation: an analysis of presentation, management and long term outcome. J Neurosurg. 1989;71:159-68.
20. Zonneveld FW, Lobregt S, Meulen JC, et al. Three dimensional imaging in craniofacial surgery. World J Surg. 1989;13:328-42.
21. Wackenheim A. Occipitalization of the vertebral part and vertebralization of the dorsal part of atlas with insufficiency of the transverse ligament. Neuroradiology. 1982;24:45-7.
22. Gehweiler JA, Daffner RH, Robert SL. Malformation of the atlas simulating the Jefferson fractures. AJNR. 1983;4:187-90.
23. Babak A, Gosselin MP, Fehlings MJ. Os Odontoideum: etiology and surgical management. Neurosurgery. 2010;66:22-31.
24. Holt RG, Helms CA, Munk PL, et al. Hypertrophy of C1 anterior arch: useful sign to distinguish OS odontoideum from acute dens fracture. Radiology. 1989;173:207-9.
25. Menezes AH. Os odontoideum pathogenesis dynamics and management. Paed Neurosurg. 1988;8:133-45.
26. Onerci M, Ogretmenoglu O, Ozcan OE. Atlanto-axial subluxation after tonsillectomy and adenoidectomy. Otolanyg Head Neck Surg. 1997;116:271-3.
27. Gupta SK, Khosla VK, Sharma BS, et al. Cranio-vertebral junction anomalies–PGI Chandigarh experience, In the proceedings of "Cranio-vertebral junction anomalies. The Indian experience". In: Jain VK, Behari S (Eds). 1998. pp. 176-8.
28. Foster HE, Carins RA, Burnell RH. Atlantoaxial subluxation in children with seronegative enthesiopathy and arthropathy syndrome. J Rheumatol. 1995;22:548-51.
29. Stiskal MA, Neuhold A, Szolar H, et al. Rheumatoid arthritis of the craniocervical region by MR Imaging: detection and characterization. AJR. 1995;165:585-92.
30. Kakitsubata Y, Boutin RD, Theodorou DJ, et al. Calcium pyrophosphate dihydrate crystal deposition in and around the atlantoaxial joint: association with type 2 odontoid fractures in nine patients. Radiology. 2000;216:213-9.
31. Khandelwal N, Khosla VK, Malik N, et al. Tuberculous atlanto-axial dislocation. Neuroradiology (Supp). 1991;33:1060-8.
32. Anastasia VD, Alexander B, Julian A, et al. Radiologic spectrum of craniocervical distraction injuries. Radiographics. 2000;20: S237-50.
33. Warner J, Shanmuganathan K, Mirvis SE, et al. Magnetic resonance imaging of ligamentous injury of the cervical spine. Emerg Radiol. 1996;3:9-15.
34. Dickman CA, Memourian A, Sonntag VK, et al. Magnetic resonance imaging of the transverse atlantal ligament for the evaluation of atlantoaxial instability. J Neurosurg. 1991;75:221-7.
35. Smoker WR, Khanna G. Imaging the craniocervical junction. Childs Nerv Syst. 2008;24:1123-45.
36. Linge SO, Haughton V, Løvgren AE, et al. CSF flow dynamics at the craniovertebral junction studied with an idealized model of the subarachnoid space and computational flow analysis. Am J Neuroradiol. 2010;31(1):185-92.
37. Linge SO, Mardal KA, Haughton V, et al. Simulating CSF flow dynamics in the normal and the Chiari I subarachnoid space during rest and exertion. Am J Neuroradiol. 2013 Jan;34(1): 41-5.
38. Ozsoy KM, Oktay K, Cetinalp NE, et al. The role of cine flow magnetic resonance imaging in patients with Chiari 0 malformation. Turk Neurosurg. 2018;28(2):251-6.

CHAPTER

209

Endovascular Management of Craniofacial Vascular Lesions

Ajay Kumar, Niranjan Khandelwal, Chirag Kamal Ahuja

INTRODUCTION

Craniofacial vascular lesions comprise a wide variety of lesions ranging from vascular malformations, arterial and venous injuries to vascular tumors. Due to their heterogeneity, no standardized categorization or classification exists. The workup of these lesions includes an elaborate evaluation of the clinical symptomatology, astute physical examination and appropriate imaging assessment. Magnetic resonance imaging (MRI) currently forms the gold standard for the evaluation of these lesions. Minimally invasive techniques of endovascular and percutaneous interventions have transformed the way these lesions are being treated currently. Interventional radiology can potentially offer cure in certain lesions like slow flow venous malformations, lymphovenous malformations and traumatic vascular injuries. In other lesions like high flow arteriovenous malformation and hypervascular tumors, embolization may be performed prior to surgical excision. The current chapter will discuss these lesions under the heads tabulated in **Table 1**.

TABLE 1: Classification of craniofacial vascular lesions.

• *Hypervascular tumors (tumors with significant vascularity)*: - Juvenile nasopharyngeal angiofibroma (JNA) - Paraganglioma - Meningioma - Esthesioneuroblastoma, etc.
• *Vascular malformation*: - Arterial with or without fistula - Capillary - Capillarovenous - Venous - Lymphangiomas - Hemolymphangiomas

• *Vascular tumors*:
- Hemangiomas
  ▪ Capillary
  ▪ Cavernous
- Hemangiopericytoma
- Hemangioendothelioma
- Kaposi's sarcoma
- Angiosarcoma

Embolization Techniques

Embolization of hypervascular tumors and arteriovenous malformations (AVMs) in the head and neck is a well-established therapeutic modality. Preoperative embolization reduces intraoperative blood loss, shortens surgical time and decreases surgical morbidity and mortality. Furthermore, intraoperative hemorrhage renders incomplete resection of a lesion with an increased risk of recurrence. Embolization as the sole treatment of AVM can be either curative or palliative for symptoms such as pain or mass effect. Treatment of craniofacial vascular lesions assumes a special importance because of their close relationship with the vital structures. Surgical procedure is sometimes extensive and causes esthetic changes and loss of function of important structures. Endovascular interventional techniques offer an alternate mode of treatment either as a definitive therapy or as an adjunct to conventional surgical techniques.[1]

Recent advances in the technology of catheters and guidewire systems have allowed superselective catheterization and targeted embolization. Direct access to many head and neck lesions is possible through percutaneous and intraoral routes and embolization can be carried out under fluoroscopic guidance.[2,3] Injection of the embolic agent with a microcatheter wedged into the nidus may lead to permanent devascularization of an AVM without risk of ischemia of the adjacent normal tissue. Cross-sectional imaging modalities like US and CT have led to further advancement by providing accurate guidance. Open MR units with real time MR imaging (MR fluoroscopy) and availability of MR compatible needles will further increase the scope of treatment in lesions that are poorly visualized by other imaging modalities.

EMBOLIC AGENTS

The choice of embolic agent depends upon the goal of the procedure, the extent of selective catheterization and angioarchitecture of the lesion. These are divided into solid particles or liquid agents by their physical characteristics and into absorbable, nonabsorbable or cytotoxic agents by their biological behaviors **(Table 2)**.[4]

Gelfoam and avitene are collagen-based materials that are reabsorbable and recanalization of the embolized vessel usually occurs within 7–21 days. Gelfoam can be powdered to fine particles to embolize capillary or precapillary bed of tumors whereas the more proximal vessels are embolized by larger particles. It is mixed with contrast medium to allow direct visualization of the embolized vascular bed. It is readily available and easy to use. It is suitable for temporary embolization (e.g. epistaxis, traumatic arterial hemorrhage) and for preoperative tumor embolization to reduce blood loss. But the only shortcoming with gelfoam is that the sizes of particles are not homogeneous.

Polyvinyl alcohol (PVA) particles are similar to collagen-based agents in that they may be mixed with contrast material, injected through the catheter and carried by blood flow into the distal vascular bed. They are nonabsorbable but their irregular shape allows some recanalization. The latter property undermines its advantage as permanent embolic agents especially in AVMs and arteriovenous fistulas (AVFs) where permanent occlusion is essential. It is available in 150–1,000 μm sizes and is suitable in preoperative devascularization. On the contrary to gelfoam, their size is precise and homogeneous.

Detachable balloons and metallic coils are used for the occlusion of large vessels and aneurysms. Detachable balloons can be of silicone or latex type. These can be deflated, repositioned or removed prior to final deployment and therefore offer flexibility in usage. Metallic coil is available in almost any shape and size with or without attached fibers to increase thrombogenicity and can also be custom made. Electrolytically and mechanically detachable coils may also allow repositioning or removal prior to deployment. However, these materials have little role in preoperative devascularization and may even be contraindicated.[4]

Liquid embolizing materials like isobutyl-2-cyanoacrylate (IBCA), n-butyl cyanoacrylate (n-BCA) and ethanol are becoming more popular because they can cause permanent occlusion of the vessels and are easy to handle. NBCA glue is liquid embolic material of choice as it is easily available, cheap, easy to handle and can be prepared in desired concentration (as contrast to onyx). The dangerous drawback is the high risk of catheter entrapment due to its fast polymerization.

Ethanol is a suitable agent when tissue necrosis in addition to devascularization is required specially in venous malformation,[5] in malignant or aggressive tumors. Chemoembolization is an attractive method because of its ability to provide very high concentrations of cytotoxic drugs at the site of tumor which may eliminate the systemic side effects. Time released microcapsules have been developed which have a very promising role in both hypervascular and hypovascular tumors.[4]

Onyx is a less adhesive liquid embolic agent containing ethylene vinyl alcohol copolymer, dimethyl sulfoxide (DMSO) and tantalum. The advantage of onyx is that it is less adhesive and can be injected slowly for a prolonged duration through intra-arterial and direct percutaneous access. Onyx first forms an embolic cast within the vascular structures and then, unlike n-BCA, permeates with each injection following the path of least resistance. This leads to embolization of large area in single sitting through single feeder.

The disadvantages of onyx are high cost, catheter entrapment due to proximal reflux, pain and discomfort during injections and skin discoloration.[6]

TABLE 2: Embolic agents commonly used in head and neck embolization.

Absorbable (biodegradable)
• Gelfoam powder/particles
• Autologous clot
Nonabsorbable (particulate)
• Polyvinyl alcohol foam/particles (PVA)
• Detachable balloons/metallic coils
Nonabsorbable (liquids)
• Isobutyl 1-2 cyanoacrylate (IBCA)
• N-butyl cyanoacrylate (NBCA)
• Onyx
• Cytotoxic agents
• Ethanol (95%)
• Chemotherapeutic agents

PRETHERAPEUTIC EVALUATION

Multidisciplinary approach is the key to optimize the analysis and treatment strategy related to the management of a specific case. A detailed clinical examination and presurgical evaluation is essential. Contrast enhanced CT/MRI provides information regarding the lesion, bone and soft tissue extension and extension to orbit or cavernous sinus.[4]

Doppler examination prior to embolization may be performed whenever it is possible. It gives information about flow dynamics (high/low flow), arterial or venous pattern, lesion architecture and presence of AVFs. It helps in the decision making for percutaneous approach and postembolization follow-up.

Dedicated diagnostic angiography and its detailed evaluation is the most important exercise prior to any attempt at intervention. Superselective catheterization where ever necessary should be performed. These steps determine the contribution of individual vessels to the lesion, ascertain the compartmentalization within the lesion and identify potentially dangerous anastomosis between the vessels supplying the lesion and the internal carotid or vertebral arteries. Determination of compartmentalization is important as different compartments function as hemodynamically independent units. Provocative testing is used to obtain information regarding the adequacy of collateral circulation in cases where it is planned to sacrifice a major vessel or inadvertent occlusion of major vessel is apprehended during the embolization procedure. Provocative testing in the region of interest can be performed by injection of lidocaine through the microcatheter prior to embolization. Lidocaine without preservative (e.g. methylparaben) is used. If the test demonstrates a deficit, then either more superselective catheter position or an embolic material that occludes vessels larger than the vasa nervosa should be used (150–200 μm).[7] A combination of clinical neurologic examination, electroencephalography (EEG) monitoring and blood flow imaging such as positron emission tomography (PET), xenon CT and single-photon emission computerized tomography (SPECT), can be employed to evaluate tolerance of vessel occlusion.[8] Stump pressure monitoring of the vessel proximal to the one planned to be occluded and hypotensive challenge have also been advocated during test occlusion.

IMPORTANT ANATOMIC CONSIDERATIONS

Transarterial embolization in external carotid artery (ECA) territory has major role in endovascular management of epistaxis, skull base tumors and arteriovenous malformation. It appears safe during endovascular embolization in ECA territory than in internal carotid artery (ICA) territory; however there are potential anastomotic routes which can cause significant neurological complication such as blindness or cranial nerve palsies. There are three important regions along skull base which constitute potential anastomoses between ECA and ICA system. The orbital, the petrocavernous and the upper cervical region.

The branches of internal maxillary artery have anastomoses with ophthalmic and petrocavernous ICA. Branches of both ascending pharyngeal and occipital artery have anastomoses with the vertebrobasilar system. Most of these anastomotic channels may not be visualized on routine catheter angiography but may start filling during the course of embolization.

During embolization procedures the penetration capacity of particles (Gelfoam and PVA) is dependent on size. In general, the size of these nonvisualized anastomotic vessels are 50–80 μm therefore particles that are >160 μm will not penetrate these channels. Liquid embolic materials (NBCA and onyx) can open and enter small anastomotic channels and therefore should be used with increased caution. Knowledge of potential anastomotic routes and proper choice of embolic material are crucial to avoid embolic complication to brain and cranial nerves.[9]

POSTEMBOLIZATION CARE

It includes the routine care following diagnostic angiography. Cerebral and/or ophthalmic complications may occur in 0.5–1% of cases and require rigorous treatment like in acute stroke. Postembolization soft tissue swelling occurs within 24 hours and usually resolves spontaneously in a few days; corticosteroids, postural drainage or IV diuretics may help. Skin necrosis, if occurs in skin that is going to be part of the resection, needs no special attention; in other areas grafting may be needed. The need for follow-up angiography will depend upon individual primary problems **(Table 3)**.[10]

NASOPHARYNGEAL ANGIOFIBROMAS

It is the most common benign nasopharyngeal tumor. It occurs almost exclusively in adolescent males, and is rarely reported in females and adults. It is highly vascular, locally invasive and extends into the surrounding compartments like infratemporal fossa, orbit or cranium. The common presenting symptoms are nasal obstruction and recurrent epistaxis. Cross-sectional imaging (CT and MR) demonstrates the complete extent of the tumor. MR is superior to CT because of its ability to demonstrate the extent of local invasion and intracranial extension. Diagnosis is usually made based on clinical features and imaging findings; biopsy is contraindicated because of the risk of uncontrollable bleeding.

TABLE 3: Various lesions amenable to embolization.

• *Preoperative devascularization*: - Nasopharyngeal angiofibroma - Paraganglioma - Meningioma - Schwannoma - Esthesioneuroblastoma - Hypervascular metastatic tumor - Hypervascular soft tissue/bony tumor
• *Definitive therapy*: - Hemangioma - AVM/AVF - Aneurysm/Pseudoaneurysm - Epistaxis

Intrasellar, intracavernous and extra cavernous-intracerebral extension is evaluated using a frontal transorbital projection. Late phase of internal carotid angiogram verifies the patency of cavernous sinus. Surgical removal of tumor is the best therapeutic option, but the limiting factors are intraoperative bleeding, the size of tumor and intracranial extension. Embolization and radiotherapy have been used in such situations as an adjunct to surgery or as a definitive therapy. In view of the risk of secondary neoplastic induction in young patients, radiotherapy is usually reserved for bilateral cavernous sinus involvement, failure of embolization and in situation where adequate surgical or therapeutic angiographic team is not available.

Preoperative embolizations 24–48 hours prior to surgery significantly reduces intraoperative blood loss resulting in better surgical removal.[11,12] The goal of endovascular therapy is to occlude the capillary bed and to devascularize the tumor. Routinely, bilateral external carotid and internal carotid angiograms with cross-compression are performed to evaluate the angioarchitecture of the tumor. The next step involves selective catheterization and embolization of external carotid artery (ECA) feeders to the tumor, starting from the most distal one to avoid the loss of access due to subsequent spasm. In general, distal internal maxillary artery (IMA) is embolized first followed by the accessory meningeal, the ascending pharyngeal and the ascending palatine arteries. Sequential catheterization and embolization of feeding vessels from the opposite side is also done in almost all cases, in the same order.[13] Embolization is performed with gel foam powder or PVA particles (200–250 μm) so as to pack the tumor bed **(Figs. 1A to E)**. This is followed by larger gelfoam particles for temporary occlusion of the feeding artery. This secondary

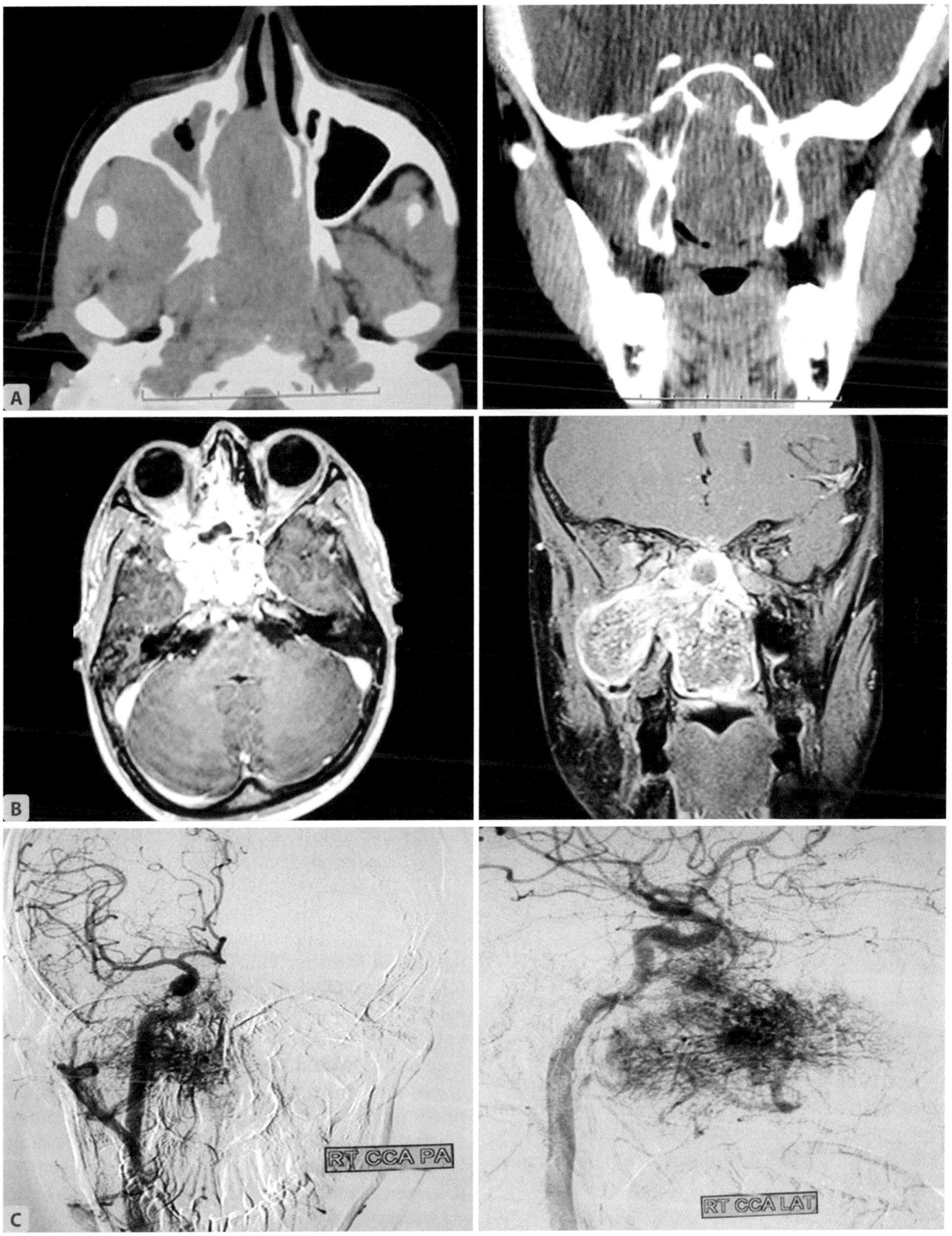

FIGS. 1A TO C: Nasopharyngeal angiofibroma. (A) CECT axial and coronal sections show large nasopharyngeal mass with bone destruction; (B) T1W axial and coronal postcontrast images show intensely enhancing large nasopharyngeal mass with extensions; (C) Right common carotid angiogram show large nasopharyngeal hypervascular mass with tumor blush supplied predominantly by internal maxillary artery (IMA) and partially by internal carotid artery.

embolization produces a transient devascularization of the region adjacent to the tumor, as well as, augmentation of the distal thrombosis within the tumor itself. Intracranial extension or large nonresectable tumors may require the use of liquid agents, e.g. NBCA, alcohol or transient or definitive occlusion of ICA siphon.[14] Direct puncture of the tumor through intraoral or transmandibular route followed by embolization with ethanol or NBCA has been a recent advancement **(Figs. 2A to F)**.

Nasopharyngeal angiofibroma (NAF) has high recurrence rate of 30% or more. Embolization in these patients is feasible only if surgical ligation or prior embolization has not blocked the vascular access. These patients are generally managed by surgery or by radiotherapy.

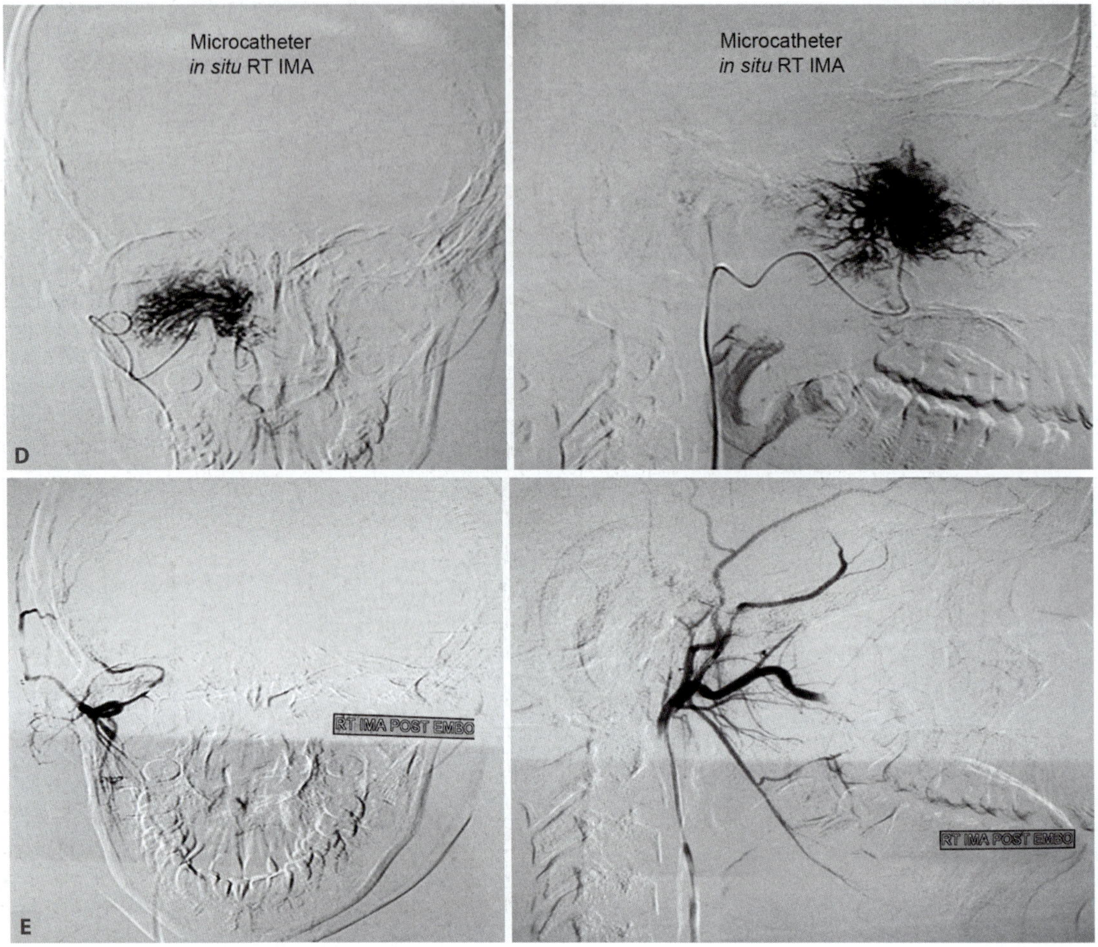

FIGS. 1D AND E: (D) Superselective right IMA angiogram reveals the tumor blush; Preoperative superselective IMA embolization with PVA particles (200–250 μm) was done and postembolization angiogram (E) frontal and lateral projections show almost complete obliteration of tumor bed supplied by IMA.

PARAGANGLIOMA

Paragangliomas (PGs) arise from paraganglion or glomus bodies that form part of the chemoreceptor system. It is also called glomus tumor, chemodectoma, nonchromaffin PG and neurocristopathic tumor. It can be located within or adjacent to the temporal bone (glomus tympanicum and glomus jugulare), carotid bifurcation (carotid body tumor), X cranial nerve (glomus vagale). Laryngeal, nasopharyngeal or orbital PG has been described.

Carotid body tumor and glomus jugulare are the most common PGs encountered in clinical practice. The peak age of presentation is in the 5th decade with a female preponderance (F:M = 2.5–3:1). It is a benign encapsulated neoplasm but can be locally invasive. Familial inheritance of autosomal dominant pattern has also been described. The 30% of the familial forms have multicentric disease which is more common in carotid (15%) and vagal (10%) tumors. Temporal glomus tumors are rarely multicentric (2%) and rarely malignant (3%). Incidence of malignancy is high in carotid (10–15%), vagal (10%) and laryngeal tumors (18%).[4,10]

Pathologically, PG shows sinusoidal stroma with compartments which behave like hemodynamically independent units. The clinical symptomatology is related to the location of the tumor. The tympanic PGs present with pulsatile tinnitus, conductive deafness, VIII cranial N palsy or reddish/bluish bulging of the tympanic membrane. Jugular PGs present with jugular foramen syndrome (Vernet syndrome) which includes paralysis of IX, X and XI cranial nerves. Carotid and vagal PGs present as pulsatile neck masses with or without cranial nerve involvement.

Computed tomography and MRI are usually required to assess the extent of lesion and to rule out other masses mimicking these tumors. On CECT, PGs show a typical intense blush. On MR, the flow void of small vessels within the tumor gives typical pepper pot appearance. Angiography is the most specific diagnostic technique and should always be performed before biopsy is attempted. Typical angiographic features include moderate enlargement of the feeding arteries, an early intense parenchymal blush and rapid venous filling **(Figs. 3A to D)**. In the temporal bone PG, the arteries that should be studied selectively are ipsilateral vertebral, internal carotid, distal ECA, posterior auricular, occipital and bilateral ascending pharyngeal arteries. The late phase of dominant vertebral injection is also necessary for visualization of venous pattern. In cervical PG, the arteries

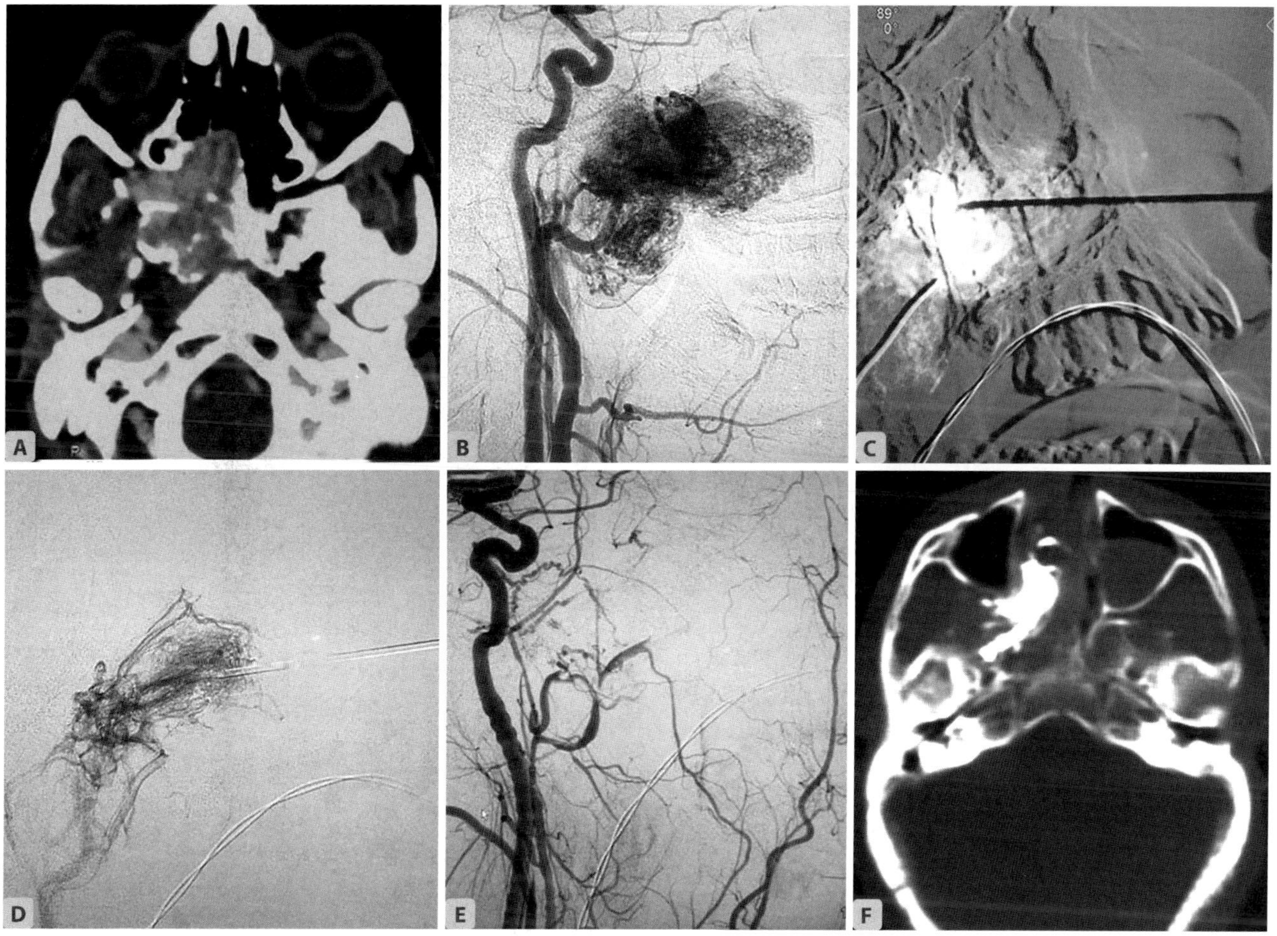

FIGS. 2A TO F: Juvenile nasopharyngeal angiofibroma: Axial contrast-enhanced CT (A) demonstrating the hypervascular nasopharyngeal mass with significant vascularity from branches of right external carotid artery as revealed on DSA (B). Percutaneous transnasal lesion puncture was done under guidance of "smart-mask" (C) followed by a nidogram (D). 60% mixture of n-butyl cyanoacrylate glue was injected under fluoroscopic guidance. Control DSA (E) showing complete lesion embolization. CT scan (F) following the procedure shows hyperdense lipiodol mixed glue within the tumor mass.

that should be studied selectively are ipsilateral vertebral, proximal ICA, facial, lingual, superior laryngeal, carotid body artery, ascending cervical, inferior laryngeal and bilateral ascending pharyngeal arteries. Vagal PG displaces ICA anteromedially whereas carotid PG displaces the ICA posterolaterally.[4]

Embolotherapy is a safe and efficient method to devascularize these tumors preoperatively. It can be used as the sole therapy for inoperable tumors in order to achieve stabilization of growth. In most cases, particulate agents (PVA 140–150 μm) are used to occlude the capillary bed followed by large gel foam particles to promote distal thrombosis **(Figs. 3A to D)**. Liquid agents are used only in the treatment of inoperable tumors and when optimal flow control can be achieved. ICA may be sacrificed where there is encasement of ICA or petrous apex involvement. Provocative testing should be performed prior to such procedures. Those tumors which are supplied by AICA/PICA are usually not amenable to embolization.[15] Embolization can be associated with neurological complications. Ascending pharyngeal artery embolization with liquid agents almost always results in lower cranial nerve palsy and the patient should be informed about the same, prior to the procedure.

Endovascular embolotherapy is considered to be the sole method of preoperative embolization for carotid body tumors. However, recent literature documents that direct percutaneous embolization offers much more important devascularization than endovascular route. The endovascular embolization is often not complete and successful due to high vascularity and numerous tiny feeders from both ECA and ICA system which are not feasible for catheterization even with latest microcatheters. Secondly, there is increased risk of stroke and cranial nerve palsies due to reflux of embolic material into ICA and vertebrobasilar system. Complete devascularization can be achieved using percutaneous embolization with NBCA glue or onyx combined with endovascular microballoon occlusion that offer protection of internal carotid system. Percutaneous onyx appears to be promising than glue.[16,17]

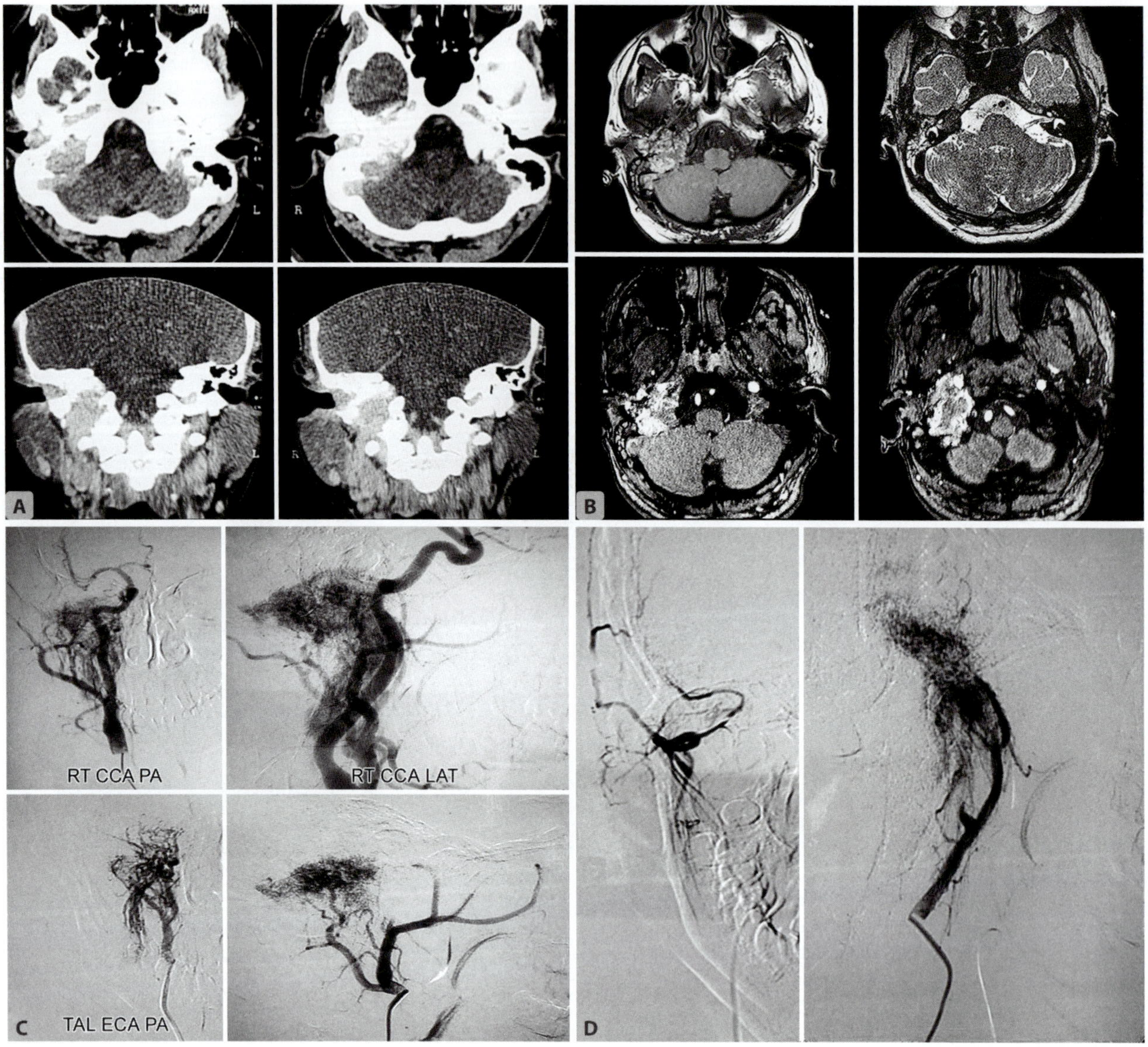

FIGS. 3A TO D: Paraganglioma: (Glomus jugulare) (A) CECT shows brightly enhancing right CP angle mass with bony petrous destruction; (B) T1, T2WI and GRE MR images revealing hypervascular lesion; (C) Selective CCA and ECA injections reveal dense-tumor blush; (D) Selective right ECA and superselective ascending pharyngeal angiogram reveal significant reduction of tumor blush following embolization.

CRANIOFACIAL VASCULAR ANOMALIES

These are complex lesions due to abnormal vasculature and are broadly categorized into vascular malformations and vascular tumors. The original classification of vascular anomalies was given by Mulliken and Glowacki.[18] It was easy to interpret and was used intensively in the clinics but did not correlate with the origin of these lesions. After a series of expert meetings and an intensive understanding of the pathological processes, the International Society for the Study of Vascular Anomalies (ISSVA) came out with the latest classification in 2014 **(Table 4)**.[19]

Vascular Tumor

Hemangiomas

These are benign tumors of endothelial cells and are of two types: capillary and cavernous hemangioma. Capillary hemangiomas are seen in infants and children. They may involute with time. The cavernous hemangiomas are seen in adults and do not exhibit involution. The capillary hemangiomas show strong female predominance (M:F = 1:5) and are present at birth in approximately 30% of patients. They show an initial phase of rapid growth (first 6 months) followed by gradual involution by 7–8 years in more than 95% of patients. Active therapy to increase the rate of involution

TABLE 4: 2014 ISSVA classification of vascular anomalies.

Vascular tumors			Vascular malformations	
Benign	**Locally aggressive**	**Malignant**	**Simple**	**Combined**
Infantile hemangioma	Kaposiform hemangioendothelioma	Angiosarcoma	Capillary malformation (C)	CVM, CLM
Congenital hemangioma	Retiform hemangioendothelioma	Epithelioid hemangioendothelioma	Lymphatic malformation	LVM, CLVM
Tufted hemangioma	PILA, Dabska tumor		Venous malformation (VM)	CAVM
Spindle-cell hemangioma	Composite hemangioendothelioma		Arteriovenous malformation (AVM)	CLAVM
Epithelioid hemangioma	Kaposi's sarcoma		Arteriovenous fistula	
Pyogenic granuloma				

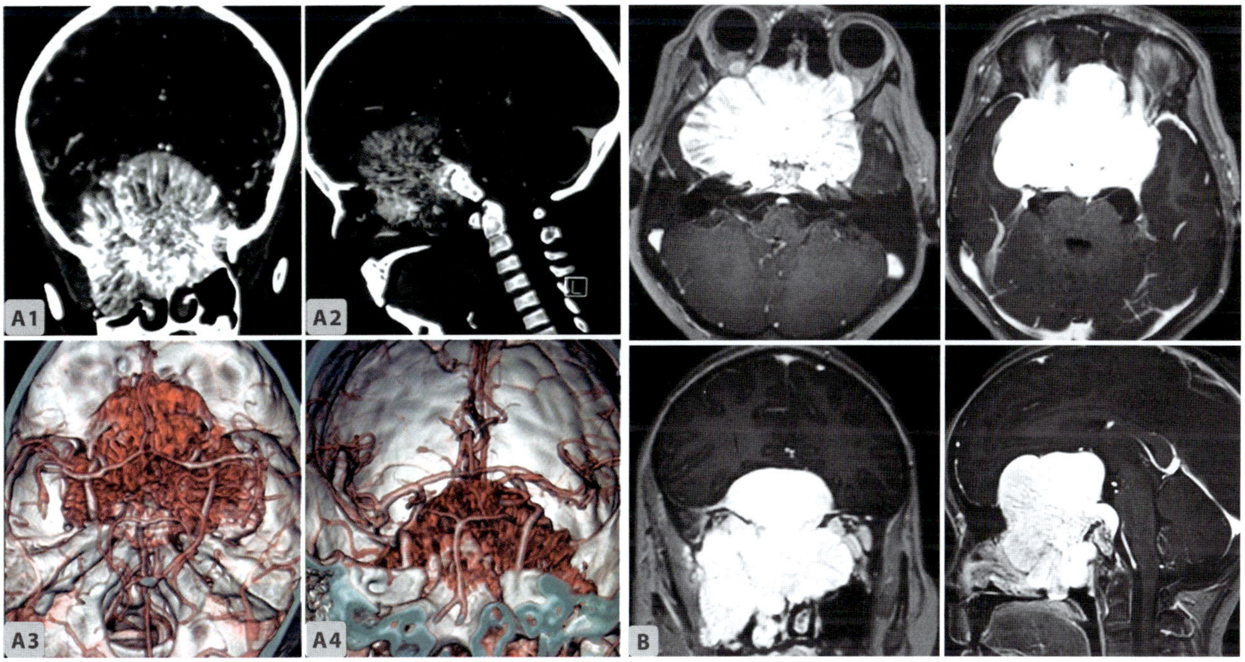

FIGS. 4A AND B: (A1 and A2) CT coronal and sagittal reformatted images showing abnormal rarefaction, trabeculation of skull base predominantly the sphenoid bone; (A3 and A4) CT angiogram VR images cranial and coronal views show large hypervascular base of skull lesion; (B) Postcontrast axial, coronal and sagittal T1W images reveal intense enhancement with intracranial and sinonasal extension.

is indicated in selected patients with functional impairment (orbital, oral, subglottic), complications (hemorrhage, congestive heart failure, hypoprothrombinemia), and in extremely large lesions. Therapeutic embolization has a definite role in these patients as complementary to the natural involutive process.

The angiographic features of capillary hemangioma are mass effect, an organized pattern of arterial supply from adjacent arteries with drainage into dilated superficial veins that empty into normal veins, and parenchymal stains which are often lobulated. AV shunting may be present. Non-involutive cavernous hemangiomas of adults typically appear as soft tissue masses on angiography, and occasionally parenchymal blush and filling of vascular spaces may occur in the late venous phase **(Figs. 4A to C)**.

Vascular Malformations

These are formed by a combination of abnormal capillary, arterial, venous or lymphatic channels with or without shunt. They are almost always present at birth. They are neither proliferative nor potentially involutive. They may remain dormant for years and may result in facial deformity, discoloration or disturbances in orofacial function. They may bleed following trivial trauma or infection. They can exhibit rapid growth with excessive pain. Arteriovenous shunting may sometime result in congestive heart failure.[20]

Vascular malformations of the head and neck often involve multiple contiguous anatomic spaces and encase critical neurovascular structures, making surgical treatment difficult and often unsuccessful. The great majority of vascular lesions in children are treated conservatively until their

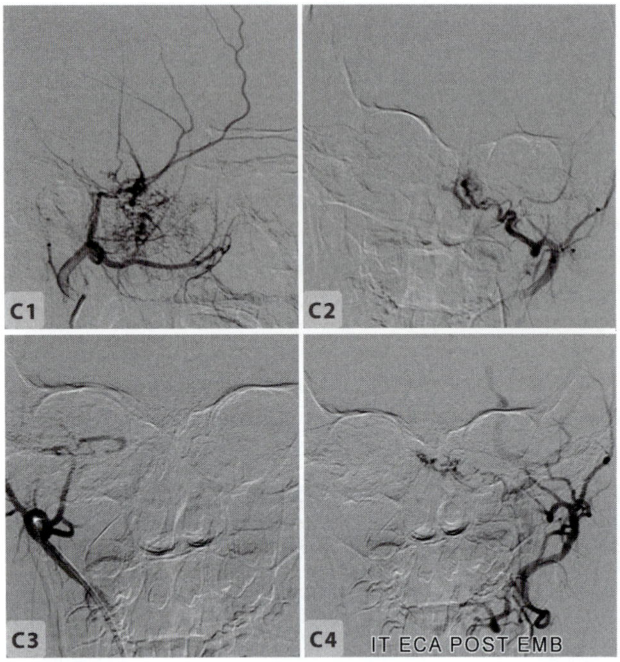

FIG. 4C: (C1 and C2) Primary intraosseus cavernous hemangioma of skull base. Bilateral selective internal maxillary artery angiogram shows tumor blush in early arterial phase with persistence in delayed phase. Postembolization internal maxillary check angiogram shows absence of tumor blush.

complete regression or till maxillofacial maturity is reached. Emergency evaluation is required for subglottic or eyelid hemangiomas, hemorrhagic episodes, severe consumption coagulopathy or heart failure. Angiography is required in cases where therapeutic intervention is planned.

From a therapeutic perspective, one of the most important differentiating characteristics of vascular malformations is their classification as "high-flow" or "low-flow" based on findings at physical examination **(Table 5)**, imaging, or both.[20,21] High-flow lesions are those that contain arteriovenous fistulas (AVFs) and slow flow lesions are those which lack any significant AVFs. MRI is an excellent noninvasive imaging technique for classification of vascular malformations, and it is often used to help therapeutic decision making and to provide follow-up after embolotherapy.[22] High-flow vascular malformations, which produce signal voids on wspin echo (SE) images and high-signal-intensity flow-related enhancement on flow- compensated gradient-echo images, are often treated with embolization via a transarterial approach.[21,23] High-flow lesions are treated by occlusion at the site of fistulous connection with permanent embolic agents **(Figs. 5 to 7)**. Tissue adhesives (NBCA) are used in small fistulas. Platinum coils or detachable balloons are preferred in large fistulas. Alcohol has also been used but the variability in the level of occlusion is a significant problem with this agent. Without superselective catheterization of the nidus, transarterial embolization often results in occlusion of arteries proximal to the arteriovenous connection and of the collateral vessels that are supplied via the rich arterial network that frequently is recruited. Many times combined

TABLE 5: Schobinger classification of arteriovenous malformation.

Stage	Features
I	Cutaneous blush/warmth
II	Bruit, audible pulsations, expanding lesion
III	Pain, ulceration, bleeding, infection
IV	Cardiac failure

endovascular and surgical approaches are used to treat these lesions.

Alternatively, low-flow vascular malformations, which appear predominantly bright on T2-weighted SE images, without evidence of flow void are often successfully treated by a direct percutaneous sclerotherapy using sodium tetradecyl sulfate or alcohol. Slow flow venous malformations can be superficial (subcutaneous or submucosal) or deep (within muscle, bone, etc.). In the superficially located lesions, direct percutaneous puncture is done followed by fluoroscopic-guided injection of contrast material to delineate the exact extent of lesion **(Figs. 8A to C)**. This is followed by embolization using liquid embolic agent such as ethanol. Care is taken to avoid extravasation especially in lesions adjacent to cranial nerves. Large lesion often requires multiple sittings.

Aneurysms

Aneurysms can involve common carotid artery, ICA, ECA, or their branches or vertebral arteries. These aneurysms occur most frequently in the ICA, followed by the vertebral artery and least frequently in the ECA and its branches. Among extradural ICA aneurysms, cavernous segment is most commonly affected (80%) and they are often giant aneurysms. ICA aneurysms are either developmental or traumatic; atherosclerotic and mycotic aneurysms are uncommon. ECA and vertebral artery aneurysms are mostly traumatic. The patients may present with TIA, epistaxis, expanding neck mass, cranial nerve palsies or they may be asymptomatic.

These aneurysms, particularly those near skull base like petrous/cavernous part of ICA are difficult to treat by surgery due to limited access. They are, however, amenable to endovascular therapy with high cure rates. Pretherapeutic evaluation with CTA/MRA is often required to assess the size of aneurysm, the complete extent of trauma and associated complications if any.

There are two approaches of embolization: selective occlusion of the aneurysms and parent artery occlusion. Selective occlusion is the treatment of choice in saccular aneurysms having a narrow neck, which helps to contain the occlusion device within the aneurysm. This is achieved by using conventional fibered platinum coils or the electrolytically detachable coil (e.g. GDC). Fresh traumatic pseudoaneurysms, however, are too fragile to tolerate such manipulation of aneurysms and therefore require parent artery occlusion. Fusiform aneurysms and wide necked saccular aneurysms are also treated by occlusion of parent artery. The occlusion of parent artery is achieved by using

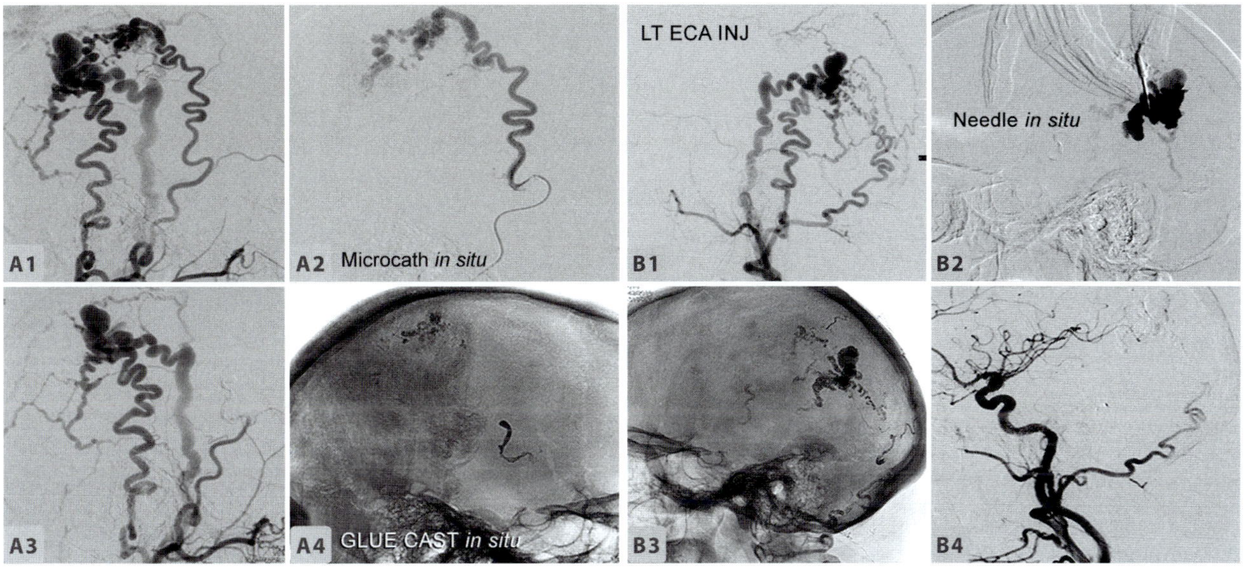

FIGS. 5A AND B: Scalp AVM. (A1) Selective left ECA injection shows dilated tortuous superficial temporal artery branches supplying a large complex AVM with cirsoid aneurysms; (A2) Superselective STA angiogram; (A3) ECA check angiogram after superselective embolization using 50% NBCA glue through STA feeder shows embolization of anterosuperior component of AVM; (A4) Glue cast in the AVM nidus and arterial feeder. Second sitting percutaneous glue embolization; (B1) Post first sitting selective left ECA injection shows superficial temporal and occipital artery branches supplying residual AVM; (B2) Percutaneous intranidal AVM angiogram; (B3) Large glue cast in AVM nidus and distal arterial feeders after percutaneous injection of 60% glue; (B4) Postembolizations CCA check angiogram reveals complete obliteration of AVM nidus and distal most arterial feeders.

detachable balloon (silicone or latex) in large arteries and platinum coils in smaller arteries. The aneurysm is usually trapped by placing a balloon at or just distal to the neck of the aneurysm and another balloon proximal to the first balloon. Caution is taken in preserving circulation to vital tributaries like ophthalmic artery while embolizing ICA aneurysms and PICA while embolizing vertebral aneurysms. Large ICA pseudoaneurysms can also be treated safely with use of covered stent **(Figs. 9A to C)**. A combined surgical and endovascular approach may sometimes be required when provocative testing confirms major functional loss. In these patients, a surgical bypass graft to the distal vessels may be performed in an accessible region, followed by endovascular occlusion of the diseased segment.

MISCELLANEOUS LESIONS

Meningiomas are hypervascular tumors which usually derive their blood supply from dural branches of ECA. A significant contribution can also be from intracranial circulation. Surgery is the treatment of choice in these lesions and embolization is only performed preoperatively for allowing easy resection. Embolization is warranted only in those meningiomas which are at surgically inaccessible sites, e.g. skull base. Small particle (PVA) embolization of tumor bed is done followed by devascularization by embolizing the feeding artery using larger particles like gel foam. The embolization procedure is restricted to external carotid artery branches only.

Occasionally other vascular masses like schwannomas, esthesioneuroblastomas, soft tissue tumor and hypervascular metastatic tumors require embolization. The principle of embolization is similar to that employed for meningiomas.

Epistaxis

Epistaxis is usually self-limiting. However, sometimes, it can be severe and life threatening requiring emergency treatment. Such severe epistaxis usually follows facial trauma, iatrogenic complication, aneurysms rupture, neoplasm, coagulopathies and vascular malformations such as hereditary hemorrhagic telangiectasias. Immediate management includes hemodynamic stabilization, nasal packing with or without electrocautery of bleeding vessels. When these measures fail to control bleeding, angiography and embolization are indicated. The failure rate of surgical ligation of internal maxillary artery (IMA) is as high as 10–15% as the source of bleeding can be elsewhere. Angiography, however, can identify the exact source of bleed and can assist in embolization. Even when the exact site of bleeding is not identified angiographic embolization of the arterial territory of the clinically affected mucosa is usually effective in controlling epistaxis. Super-selective catheterization

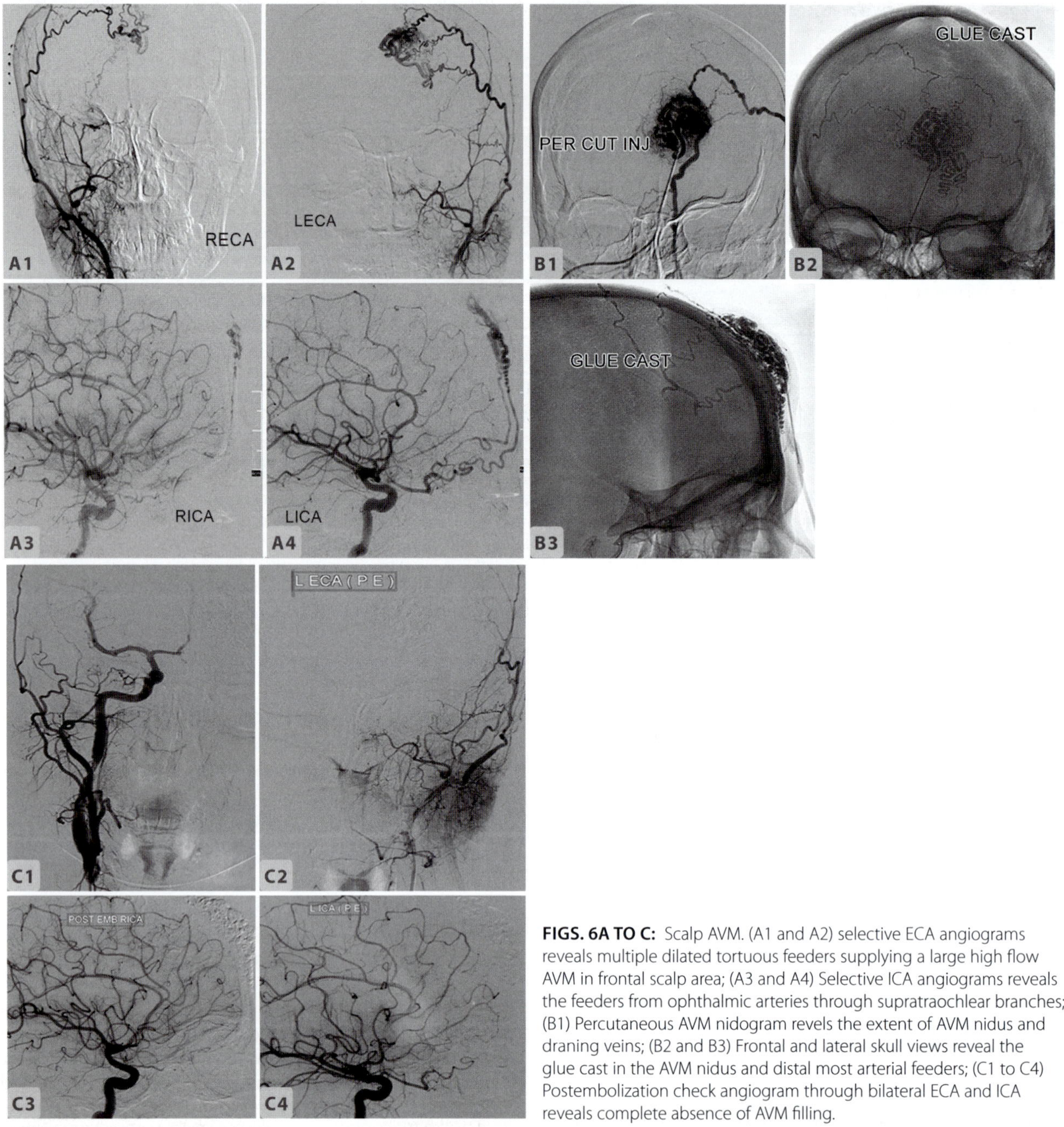

FIGS. 6A TO C: Scalp AVM. (A1 and A2) selective ECA angiograms reveals multiple dilated tortuous feeders supplying a large high flow AVM in frontal scalp area; (A3 and A4) Selective ICA angiograms reveals the feeders from ophthalmic arteries through supratraochlear branches; (B1) Percutaneous AVM nidogram revels the extent of AVM nidus and draning veins; (B2 and B3) Frontal and lateral skull views reveal the glue cast in the AVM nidus and distal most arterial feeders; (C1 to C4) Postembolization check angiogram through bilateral ECA and ICA reveals complete absence of AVM filling.

is done followed by embolization using platinum coils or tissue adhesives (NBCA).[24]

SUMMARY

Endovascular treatment through intra-arterial or percutaneous approach is a safe and cost-effective nonsurgical therapeutic option for the treatment of a variety of non-neoplastic and neoplastic vascular lesions in the craniofacial region. It can be used as a definitive treatment or as an adjunct to surgery. The strategy for selecting the route of embolization and embolic material should be based on clinical and angiographic characteristics. The ongoing improvement in the technique, microcatheters, guidewires and safe embolic agents have widened the scope of endovascular procedures.

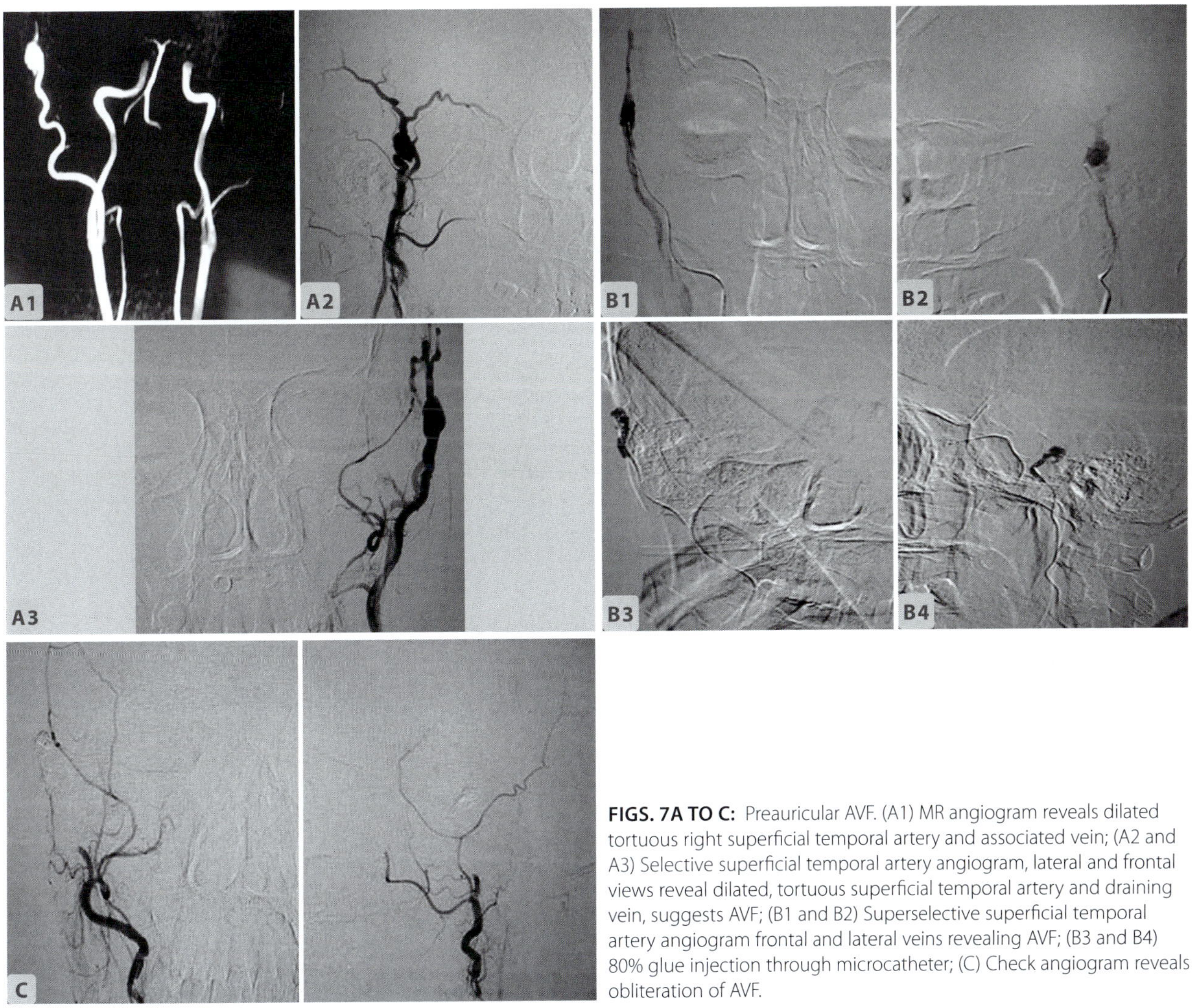

FIGS. 7A TO C: Preauricular AVF. (A1) MR angiogram reveals dilated tortuous right superficial temporal artery and associated vein; (A2 and A3) Selective superficial temporal artery angiogram, lateral and frontal views reveal dilated, tortuous superficial temporal artery and draining vein, suggests AVF; (B1 and B2) Superselective superficial temporal artery angiogram frontal and lateral veins revealing AVF; (B3 and B4) 80% glue injection through microcatheter; (C) Check angiogram reveals obliteration of AVF.

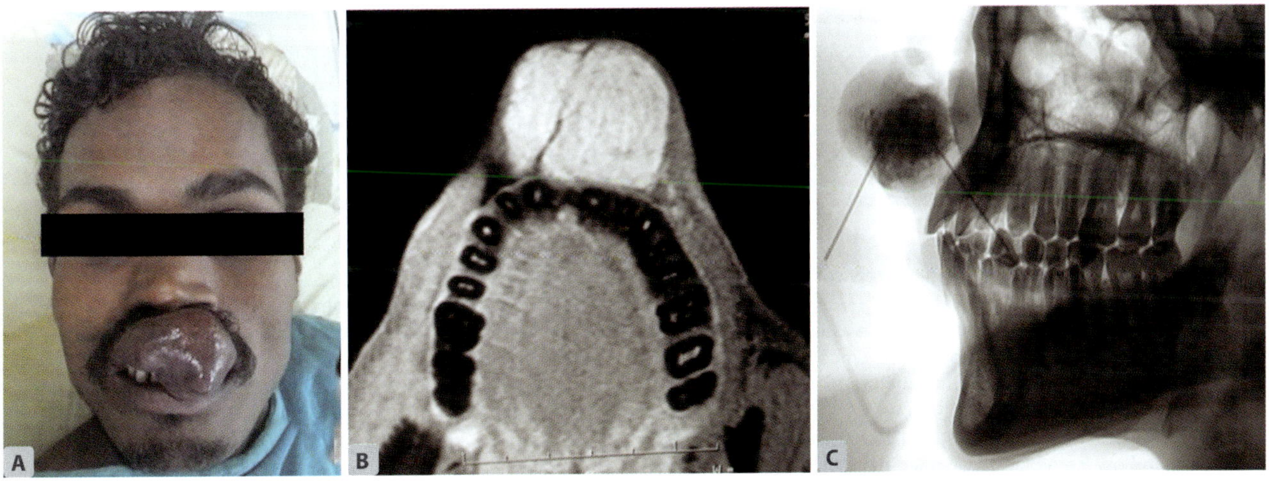

FIGS. 8A TO C: Lip venous malformation: Clinical photograph (A) showing a large upper lip venous malformation. Axial T1W FS (B) image revealing the well-circumscribed exophytic hyperintense upper lip lesion. Fluoroscopy image (C) demonstrating the percutaneous puncture of the lesion followed by sclerosant injection.

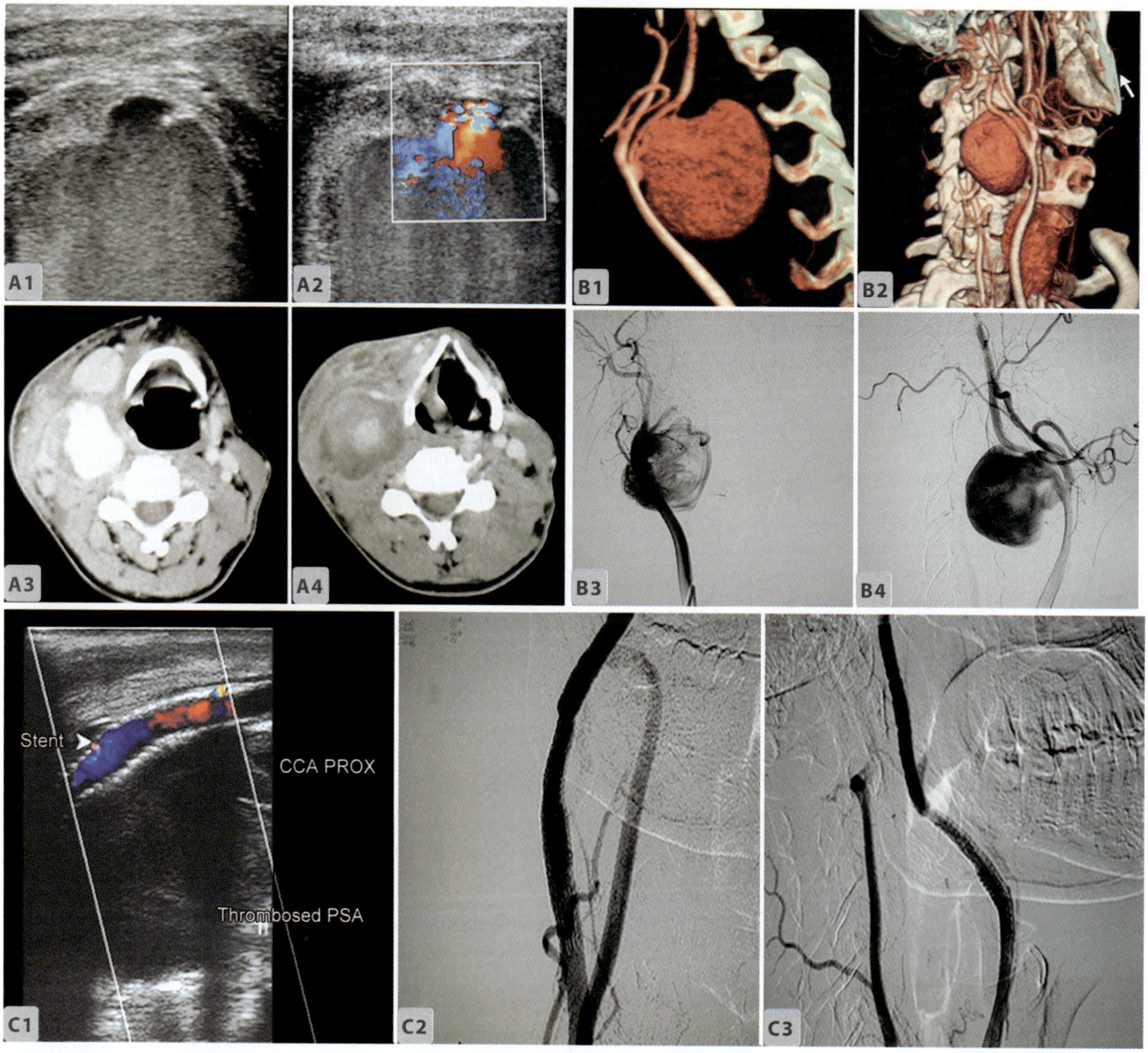

FIGS. 9A TO C: Post-tonsillar biopsy ICA pseudoaneurysm. (A1 and A2) Doppler images reveal large intimal ICA defect with pseudoaneurysm; (A3 and A4) Axial CECT neck sections showing the ICA pseudoaneurysm; (B1 to B4) CT and digital substraction angiogram revealing large pseudoaneurysm arising from proximal ICA; (C1) Post-ICA stenting (covered stent) Doppler USG study reveals absence of flow into the pseudoaneurysm; (C2 and C3) Anteroposterior and lateral angiogram reveals opacification of ICA with obliteration of pseudoaneurysm.

REFERENCES

1. Dion JE. Endovascular treatment of cervicocerebral aneurysms. Semin Intervent Radiol. 1994;11:37-63.
2. Cil BE, Vargel I, Geyik S, et al. Venous vascular malformations of the craniofacial region: preoperative embolization with direct percutaneous puncture and N-butyl cyanoacrylate. Br J Radiol. 2008;81:935-9.
3. Dabus G, Linfante I, Benenati J, et al. Interventional management of high-flow craniofacial vascular malformations: a database analysis and review of the literature. J Neurointerv Surg. 2017;9(1):92-6.
4. Lasjaunias P, Berenstein A. Craniofacial vascular lesions. In: Surgical Neuroangiography. Berlin: Springer Verlag; 1989. pp. 19-45.
5. Horbach SE, Lokhorst MM, Saeed P, et al. Sclerotherapy for low-flow vascular malformations of the head and neck: a systematic review of sclerosing agents. J Plast Reconstr Aesthet Surg. 2016;69(3):295-304.
6. Arat A, Cil BE, Vargel I, et al. Embolization of high flow craniofacial vascular malformations with onyx. AJNR. 2007;28:1409-14.
7. Horton JA, Kerber CW. Lidocaine injection into external carotid branches: provocative test to preserve cranial nerve function in therapeutic embolization. AJNR. 1986;7:105-8.
8. Ebra SM, Horton JA, Latchaw RF, et al. Balloon test occlusion in the internal carotid artery with stable xenon/CT cerebral blow flow imaging. AJNR. 1988;9:533-7.

9. Geibprasert S, Pongpech S, Armstrong D, et al. Dangerous extracranial intracranial anastomoses and supply to cranial nerves: vessels the neurointerventionalist needs to know. AJNR. 2009;30:459-68.
10. Jensen ME. Endovascular treatment of vascular pathology of the head and neck. Semin Intervent Radiol. 1994;11:22-36.
11. Marshall AH, Bradely PJ. Management dilemmas in the treatment and follow-up of advanced juvenile nasopharyngeal angiofibroma. ORL. 2006;68:273-8.
12. Tan G, Ma Z, Long W, et al. Efficacy of preoperative transcatheter arterial embolization for nasopharyngeal angiofibroma: a comparative study. Cardiovasc Intervent Radiol. 2017;40(6):836-44.
13. Davis KR. Embolization of epistaxsis and juvenile nasopharyngeal angiofibroma. AJNR. 1986;7:953-62.
14. Introcaseo JH, Rusell EJ. Interventional neuro-radiologic treatment of head and neck lesions Otolaryng. Clin N Am. 1995;28:563-84.
15. Smith JD, Harvey RN, Darr OA, et al. Head and neck paragangliomas: a two-decade institutional experience and algorithm for management. Laryngoscope Investig Otolaryngol. 2017;2(6):380-9.
16. Firat A, Aytekin C, Boyvat F, et al. Multidisciplinary approach to carotid body paraganglioma: preoperative percutaneous embolization and surgical resection. Turkish Neurosurgery. 2003;13:81-4.
17. Wanke I, Jackel MC, Goericke S, et al. Percutaneous embolization of carotid paragangliomas using solely onyx. AJNR. 2009;30:1594-7.
18. Mulliken JB, Golwacki J. Hemangiomas and vascular malformations in infants and children: a classification based on endothelial characteristics. Plast Reconstr Surg. 1982;69:412-20.
19. Wassef M, Blei F, Adams D, et al.; ISSVA Board and Scientific Committee. Vascular anomalies classification: recommendations from the International Society for the Study of Vascular Anomalies. Pediatrics. 2015;136(1):e203-14.
20. O'Donovan JC, Donaldson JS, Morello FP, et al. Symptomatic hemangiomas and venous malformations in infants, children, and young adults: treatment with percutaneous injection of sodium tetradecyl sulfate. AJR. 1997;169:723-9.
21. Meyer JS, Hoffer FA, Barnes PD, et al. Biological classification of soft-tissue vascular anomalies: MR correlation. AJR. 1991;157: 559-64.
22. Yakes WF, Haas DK, Parker SH, et al. Symptomatic vascular malformations: ethanol embolotherapy. Radiology. 1989; 170:1059-66.
23. Widlus DM, Murray RR, White RI, et al. Congenital arteriovenous malformations: tailored embolotherapy. Radiology. 1988;169: 511-6.
24. Strutz J, Schermacher M. Uncontrolled epistaxis. Arch Otolaryn Head Neck Surg. 1990;116:697-7.

CHAPTER

210

Imaging of Head Trauma

Shivanand Gamanagatti, Atin Kumar, Arun Kumar Gupta, Surabhi Vyas

Traumatic brain injury (TBI) is one of the major causes of mortality and morbidity in the world's population.[1] According to National Center for Injury Prevention and Control, approximately 2% of the entire population of the world currently suffers from disabilities caused by TBI.[2] The etiologies of head trauma vary with the patient age. In the elderly individuals, accidental falls are the most common causes whereas in young individuals, the motor vehicle crashes are common culprits. In children, abuse and neglect are common reasons.

Traumatic brain injury (TBI) is not a single "one and done" event. TBI is an ongoing series of pathophysiologic reactions that extends from the moment of injury for days, months, or even years in to the future. Acute TBI is just the initial triggering insult.

TBI CLASSIFICATION

Broad Classification

- *Primary lesions*: Are the direct result of trauma (Already occurred at the time of presentation)
- *Secondary lesions*: As complications of primary lesions (preventable)
  - *Acute and subacute*: Include cerebral edema, ischemia, and brain herniation
  - *Chronic*: Hydrocephalus, the cerebrospinal fluid (CSF) leak, leptomeningeal cyst, and encephalomalacia.

According to Location of Lesions

- *Intra-axial*: Cortical contusions, intracerebral hematoma, axonal shearing injuries, gray matter injury, and vascular injury
- *Extra-axial*: Epidural, subdural, subarachnoid, and intraventricular hemorrhage.

According to Mechanism

- Open (penetrating)
- Closed (blunt)

According to Clinical Severity (According to Glasgow Coma Scale)[3]

- Minor GCS : 15
- Mild GCS : 13–14
- Moderate GCS : 9–12
- Severe GCS : 3–8

Marshall CT Classification of Head Injury (HI)[4]

A 6 category scheme to classify head injury (HI) based on initial CT scan. It was published in the Journal of Neurosurgery by Lawrence Marshall and colleagues in 1991. It was based on their experience in the pilot phase of the Traumatic Coma Data Bank (TCDB).[5]

An increase in mortality was noted with increasing grade of diffuse injury.

Categories

Diffuse Injury—Type I:

- No CT visible intracranial pathology.

Diffuse Injury—Type II:

- Cisterns present with midline shift 0-5 mm
- No high- or mixed-density lesion > 25 cc.

Diffuse Injury—Type III (swelling):

- Cisterns compressed or absent with midline shift 0-5 mm
- No high- or mixed-density lesion > 25 cc.

Diffuse Injury—Type IV (shift):

- Midline shift > 5 mm
- No high- or mixed-density lesion > 25 cc.

Evacuated Mass Lesion—Type V:

- Any lesion surgically evacuated.

Non-evacuated Mass Lesion—Type VI:

- High- or mixed-density lesion > 25 cc.

This classification grades the severity of the injury as follows: I = normal, II = diffuse injury, III = diffuse injury with swelling, IV = diffuse injury with shift, V = mass lesion surgically evacuated, and VI = mass lesion not operated.

GOALS OF NEUROIMAGING

- To detect the presence of injuries that may require immediate surgical or procedural intervention.
- To detect the presence of injuries that may benefit from early medical therapy.
- To determine the prognosis of patients to tailor rehabilitative therapy or help with family counseling.

IMAGING TECHNIQUES

Plain Radiographs

Skull X-rays are poor predictors of intracranial pathology and should not be performed to evaluate adult TBI.[6-8] Lack of abnormality on skull films does not exclude major intracranial injury.[9] Patients who are at high risk for acute intracranial injury must be imaged by CT. The "scout view" that is obtained with all CT exams can be used as a "pseudo skull film" **(Fig. 1)**. Twenty- five percent of cases with fatal injuries do not demonstrate a skull fracture, although the incidence of intracranial hematomas in patients who have skull fractures is much higher than in those who do not. It is often implied that many skull X-ray films are taken because of medicolegal considerations rather than clinical necessity.[6-8]

Computed tomography (CT), CT is the modality of choice in acute HI. It is easily available, fast, and compatible with equipment for monitoring of vital functions and artificial ventilation. If image is spoiled by motion artifacts, then it is possible to repeat selectively several slices without much time constraints. The acquired CT images can be visualized in bone, soft tissue, and varying window widths (adequate to diagnose subdural hemorrhages) without contrast administration to reveal intra-axial, extra-axial injuries and bone fractures.[10] In addition, CT is usually superior to MR in revealing skull fractures and radiopaque foreign bodies.

The Goal of Imaging is to Identify Treatable Injuries to Prevent Secondary Damage

With modern CT scanners, contiguous 3 or 5-mm sections from the skull base to the vertex can be obtained in less than 10 minutes. Thinner 1- or 2.5 mm sections are used to evaluate the orbits, maxillofacial structures, and skull base. With recent advances in multidetector CT (MDCT), thin cross-sectional slices can be performed which allowed for high-quality three-dimensional reconstruction. Thinner slices also improve the diagnostic accuracy of CT in the evaluation of maxillofacial, orbital, and temporal bone fractures. Intravenous contrast administration should not be performed because it can both mask and mimic underlying hemorrhage.

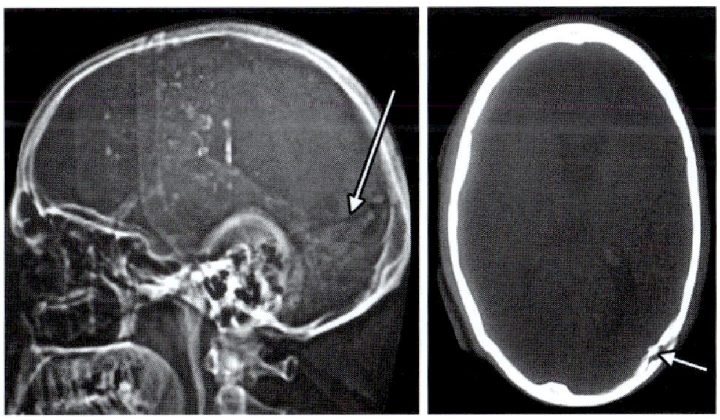

FIG. 1: Lateral topogram (Scout view) of skull obtained during CT scan of head showing linear fracture of parietal bone (arrow) and axial CT section in bone window confirming the presence of fracture in left posterior parietal bone (arrow).

CT images must be reviewed using multiple windows and levels. A narrow window width (W: 80, L: 40) is used to evaluate the brain. A slightly wider window width (W: 150, L: 75) is used to exaggerate contrast between extra-axial blood and the adjacent skull. An even wider window (W: 2500, L: 500) is used to evaluate the osseous structures **(Figs. 2A to C)**.[9]

Perfusion CT (Fig. 3) affords insight into regional brain perfusion alterations due to head trauma, with the major advantages of being able to depict regional heterogeneity. Perfusion CT also offers prognostic information with respect to functional outcome, even as early as at the time of admission. Patients with altered brain perfusion might be considered for more aggressive and early treatment to prevent intracranial hypertension, whereas patients with preserved brain perfusion might benet from less invasive treatment. It might allow clinicians to distinguish between patients with preserved autoregulation (or pseudoregulation) and those with impaired autoregulation.[10,11]

Magnetic resonance imaging (MRI) is recommended for patients with acute TBI when the neurologic findings cannot be explained by CT. MR is also the modality of choice for subacute or chronic injury. MR is usually comparable to CT in the detection of an acute epidural and subdural hematoma.[12,13] However, MR is more sensitive to subtle extra-axial collections, nonhemorrhagic lesions, brainstem injuries, and subarachnoid hemorrhage (SAH) when using fluid-attenuated inversion recovery (FLAIR).[14,15]

Fluid-attenuated inversion recovery imaging improves the conspicuity of focal gray matter abnormalities (e.g. contusions), white matter abnormalities, shear injuries, and SAH by eliminating (or "nulling") the bright cerebrospinal fluid signal **(Fig. 4A)**. Sagittal and coronal FLAIR images are particularly helpful in the detection of diffuse axonal injury (DAI) involving the corpus callosum and the fornix, two areas that are difficult to evaluate on routine T2-weighted images.

Gradient-echo/Susceptibility weighted imaging (SWI) is highly sensitive to local magnetic inhomogeneity caused by the presence of blood. Hemosiderin, a breakdown product of blood, is ferromagnetic. The presence of hemosiderin alters the local magnetic susceptibility of tissue, resulting in areas of signal loss on gradient-echo T2*-weighted images **(Fig. 4B)**. Because hemosiderin can persist indefinitely, its detection on gradient-echo T2*-weighted images allows for improved evaluation of remote injury. However, due to the inherent inhomogeneity adjacent to the paranasal sinuses and mastoid air cells, gradient-echo images are limited in the evaluation of cortical contusions of the inferior frontotemporal lobes.[16,17]

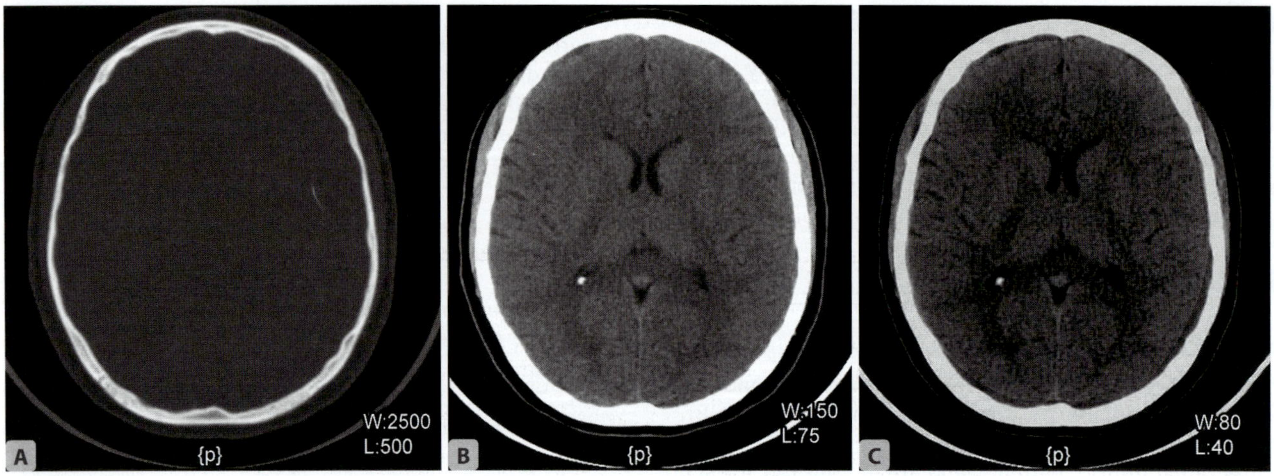

FIGS. 2A TO C: Axial CT images of brain (A to C) to show various window values used to view the CT images.

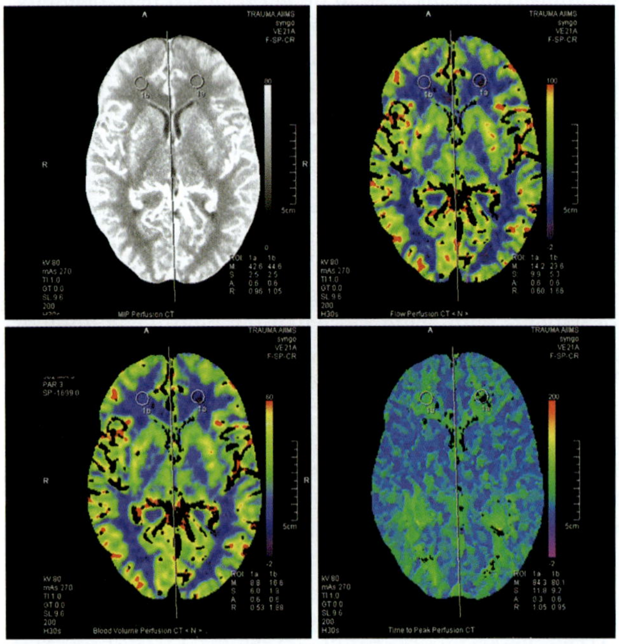

FIG. 3: Axial CT perfusion images showing the various parameters (time to peak, blood volume and flow rate) used to define regional brain perfusion alterations.

Diffusion-weighted imaging (DWI), which measures the random motion of water molecules in brain tissue, has improved the evaluation of TBI. Through its superior sensitivity to foci of acute shearing injury, DWI has especially improved detection of DAI **(Fig. 4C)**. DWI reveals more DAI lesions than fast spin-echo T2-weighted or gradient-echo T2*-weighted images in patients imaged within 48 hours of injury. The apparent diffusion coefficient (ADC), which measures the magnitude of water diffusion averaged over a three-dimensional space, is often reduced in acute DAI. The fractional anisotropy (FA), which measures the preferential motion of water molecules along the white matter axons, is frequently reduced in chronic DAI. Tissue anisotropy is exploited in the new technique of diffusion tensor imaging (DTI).[18-20]

Angiography: Contrast angiography has been the gold standard for diagnosis of vascular lesions. However, MRI, MRA, and CT angiography (CTA) are also growing in use and capability to provide the same information. Unlike conventional angiography that only images the lumen of blood vessels, MRA and CTA can provide information about the arterial walls. CTA offers better resolution and fewer flow-related artifacts than MRA. In addition CT and MRI also provide information about the adjoining brain parenchyma **(Fig. 5)**.

1. Clinical predictors of traumatic neurovascular injuries include a high-velocity mechanism, low Glasgow Coma Scale score, high injury severity score, mandible fracture, complex skull fractures, basilar skull fractures (including carotid canal fractures), scalp degloving, any type of cervical spine injury, and/or TBI with thoracic injuries, and/or thoracic vascular imaging, as well as in patients with penetrating neck injury (class I recommendation).
2. CTA should include arch of aorta till the circle of Willis for all patients with suspected vascular trauma.
3. Significant percentage of traumatic neurovascular injuries is treated by interventional procedures such as coil embolization, stent placement with a less morbidity and mortality.

Advanced Neuroimaging Techniques

Advanced neuroimaging techniques such as diffusion tensor imaging, blood oxygen level dependent (BOLD) functional MRI, spectroscopy and perfusion imaging are useful in recognizing any abnormality in patients with TBI when conventional NCCT and MR imaging findings are normal. These techniques also help in prognostication of patients with intractable symptoms. However, there is no sufficient data available in literature for routine clinical use of these advanced neuroimaging techniques.

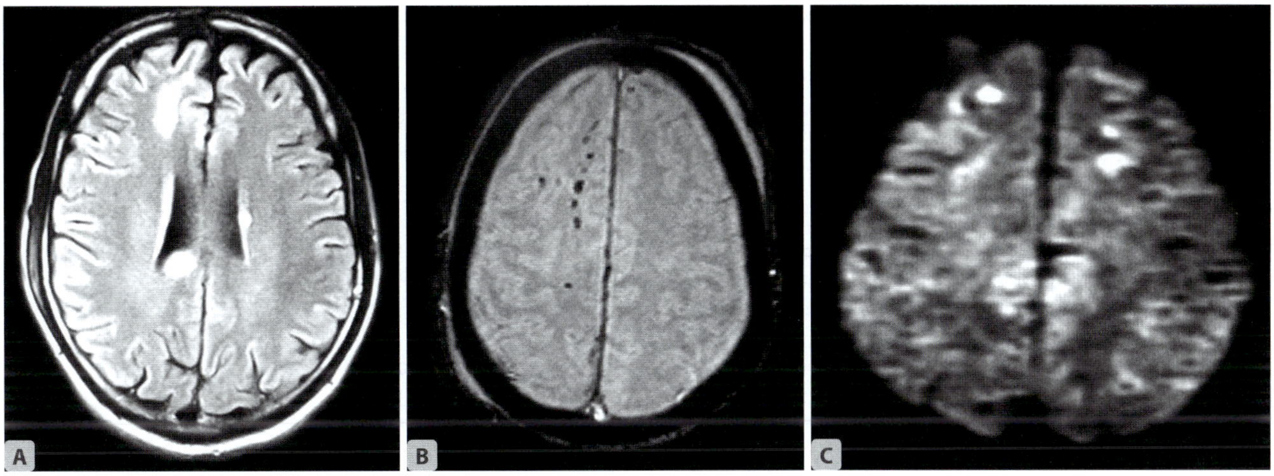

FIGS. 4A TO C: Axial MR images of brain to show the advantages of various MR sequences in detection of different intra-axial lesions (A) FLAIR sequence improves the conspicuity of focal gray matter abnormalities (e.g. contusions), white matter abnormalities; (B) Gradient echo sequence can detect many hemorrhagic foci because of better sensitivity to blood products; (C) DWI sequence improves detection of DAI because of superior sensitivity to foci of acute shearing injury.

Summary of Imaging Recommendations

Modality of sequence	Head injury indication	Recommendation
NCCT head CT	First line acute mild, moderate and severe TBI	Class I
NCCT head CT	Repeat Assessment in Acute TB1 with neurologic deterioration	Class I
NCCT head CT	Judicious use in pediatric mild TB1	Class I
NCCT head CT	Repeat assessment of mild TBI with negative initial NCCT	Class III
CTA of brain	Suspected vascular trauma	Class IIa
Brain MRI without contrast	Acute or subacute TBI, initial or follow/up NCCT is negative with unexplained neurologic findings	Class I
T2* & SWI MRI	Acute, early subacute and chronic stages of DAI	Class IIa
Brain MRI with contrast	Can aid in visualizing subacute brain contusion	Class IIb
Advanced Neuroimaging	Mild TB1 with negative conventional CT and MRI	Class IIb

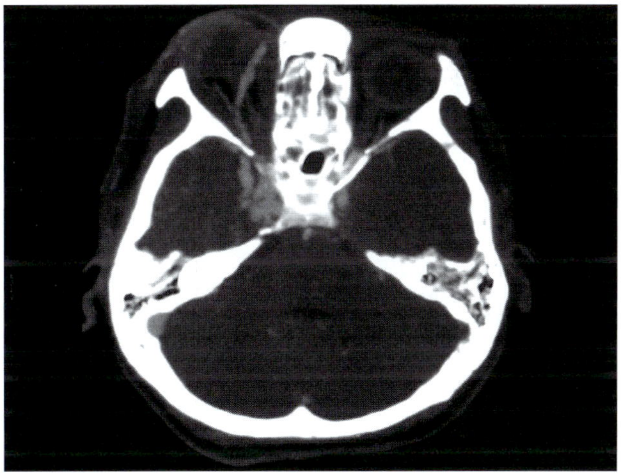

FIG. 5: CT angiography image showing lobulated and enlarged right cavernous sinus with abnormally dilated superior ophthalmic vein suggestive of carotid-cavernous fistula.

Evidence-based Guidelines for Imaging Patients with Head Injury

Suggested guidelines for acute neuroimaging in adult patient with mild TBI (Glasgow Coma Scale score 13–15):[21]

If GCS 13–15, CT recommended if patient has any one of the following:

- *High risk*:
  - GCS remains <15 at 2 hours after injury
  - Suspected open or depressed skull fracture
  - Any clinical sign of basal skull fracture
  - Two or more episodes of vomiting
  - Aged 65 years or older
- *Medium risk*:
  - Possible loss of consciousness
  - Amnesia for period before impact, of at least 30-minute time span
  - Dangerous mechanism (pedestrian versus motor vehicle, ejected from motor vehicle, fall from greater than 3 feet or five stairs)
  - Any transient neurologic deficit
  - Headache, vomiting

  If GCS of 15, patient can be discharged without CT scan if:
- *Low risk*:
  - GCS remains 15
  - No loss of consciousness or amnesia

   - No neurologic/cognitive abnormalities
   - No headache, vomiting

Suggested guidelines for acute neuroimaging in adult patient with severe TBI (GCS 3–8): [21]

- CT scan patient with severe TBI as soon as possible to determine if require surgical intervention.
- If initial scan is normal, but patient has neurologic deterioration, repeat CT scan or consider MRI as soon as possible.
- If initial scan is abnormal, but patient status is unchanged, repeat CT scan within 24–36 hours to determine possible progressive hemorrhage or edema requiring surgical intervention, particularly if initial scan showed:
   - Any intracranial hemorrhage
   - Any evidence of diffuse brain injury
- If initial scan is abnormal, repeat CT scan or consider MRI as soon as possible if GCS worsens
- Consider MRI within first few days if:
   - Suspect secondary injury such as focal infarction, diffuse hypoxic-ischemic injury or infection.

Imaging Guidelines for Pediatric Head Injury

CT Algorithm for Children <2 years

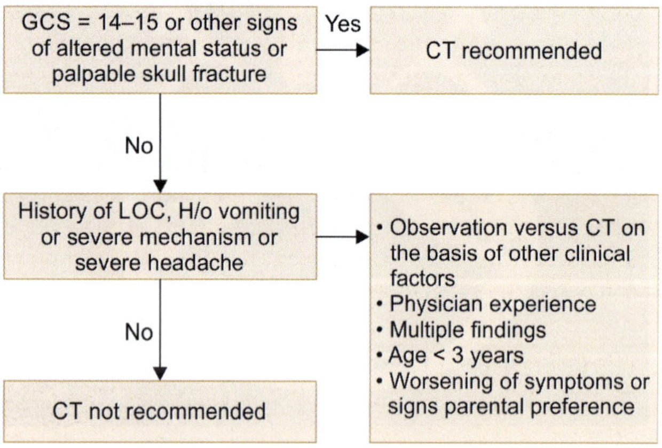

CT Algorithm for Children >2 years

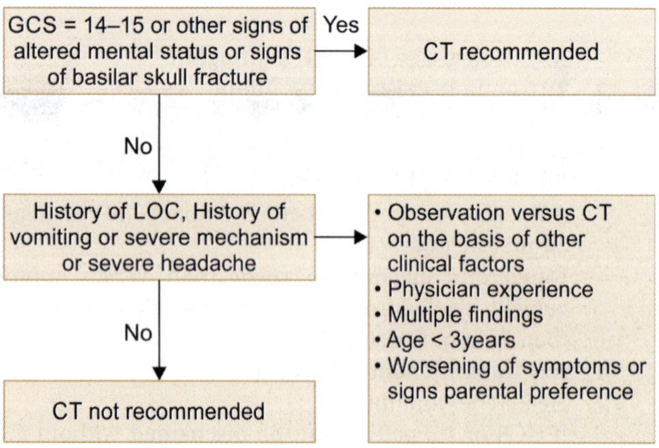

IMAGING FINDINGS

Scalp Injury

While interpreting CT scans of head trauma, begin by looking at the extracranial structures for evidence of soft-tissue injury and/or radio-opaque foreign bodies. Scalp injury provides a reliable indication of the site of impact.

Types of Scalp Injury

- Simple soft-tissue lacerations
- Subgaleal hematoma
- Cephalohematoma
- Residual foreign bodies

The subgaleal hematoma is the most common manifestation of scalp injury **(Fig. 6)**. It is seen as focal soft-tissue swelling located beneath the subcutaneous fibrofatty tissue and above the temporalis muscle and calvarium.[9,23]

Skull Fractures

Types of Skull Fractures

- Linear
- Depressed
- Compound

Non-displaced linear fractures of the calvarium may be difficult to detect on CT when the fracture plane is parallel to the plane of section. Also, isolated linear skull fractures **(Fig. 7A)** usually do not require treatment unless they are associated with an epidural hematoma.

However, the depressed and compound skull fractures are easily detectable on CT **(Figs. 7B and C)**, which require surgical intervention. Depressed skull fractures may be associated with an underlying contusion; therefore, it is

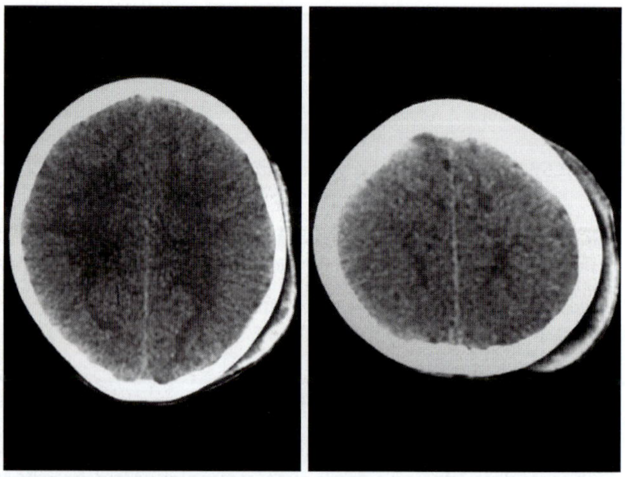

FIG. 6: Axial CT section of brain showing focal soft-tissue swelling located beneath the subcutaneous fibrofatty tissue in left temparoparietal region suggestive of scalp hematoma.

important to have careful look at the subjacent parenchyma **(Fig. 7C)**.

Recommendations

Thin reconstructions (1 mm) and use of bone algorithm is recommended for the evaluation of fractures in the skull base, orbit or facial bones. Thin sections are helpful for evaluating the degree of comminution and depression of bone fragments. MDCT with 3D reconstruction such as volume rendered algorithms can display complex fractures very clearly.[9,23]

Temporal Bone Fractures

When to suspect temporal bone fractures?

- Presence of pneumocephalus,
- Opacification of the mastoid air cells, and
- Fluid in the middle ear cavity should raise the suspicion of a temporal bone fracture.

Thin-sections (1 to 1.5 mm) in axial plane and coronal 3D reconstructions in bone algorithm is recommended for the evaluation of temporal bone fractures.

Types of Temporal Bone Fractures[22] (Figs. 8A and B)

- Longitudinal
- Transverse
- Mixed

Fractures are classified depending on the orientation of fracture line relative to the long axis of the petrous bone. Longitudinal fractures parallel the long axis of the petrous pyramid, and transverse fractures are perpendicular to the long axis of the petrous bone.

Longitudinal temporal bone fractures represent more than 70% of temporal bone fractures.[20] The line of force runs roughly from lateral to medial **(Fig. 8B)**. A fracture line may extend through the facial nerve canal, thereby damaging the facial nerve, designated as cranial nerve (CN) VII. Complications include conductive hearing loss from dislocation or fracture of the ossicles, otorhinorrhea from CSF leak, and facial nerve palsy.

Transverse temporal bone fractures typically result from trauma to the temporal or parietal region and commonly involve fractures of the temporal squamosa or parietal bone. Fracture line passes through the vestibulocochlear apparatus and can cause sensorineural hearing loss and equilibrium disorders **(Fig. 8A)**. Transverse fractures also commonly injure CN VII, because their path often takes them close to the nerve's labyrinthine segment.

Mixed or complex temporal bone fractures involve a combination of fracture planes. They typically result from severe crushing blows to the skull. Patients with mixed temporal bone fractures have a high incidence of associated intracranial injury.

PRIMARY HEAD INJURY LESIONS

Extra-axial Injury[9,23]

- Epidural hematoma
- Subdural hematoma
- Subarachnoid hemorrhage
- Intraventricular hemorrhage

Epidural Hematoma (EDH)

Blood collects in the potential space located between the inner table of the skull and the dura. The developing hematoma dissects the dura from the inner table of the skull, forming an ovoid mass that displaces the adjacent brain. Majority of the EDH are due to arterial hemorrhage and most commonly affected artery is the middle meningeal artery, due to the fracture in the squamous part of temporal bone. In children, EDH can occur due to stretching or tearing of meningeal arteries without fracture. Venous EDHs are less common and can occur due to rupture of venous sinuses.[9,23]

Imaging Features

On CT, the acute EDH appears as a well-defined, hyperdense, biconvex, extra-axial collection **(Fig. 9A)**. It is usually associated with an overlying skull fracture **(Fig. 9B)**. Mass effect with sulcal effacement and midline shift is frequently seen.

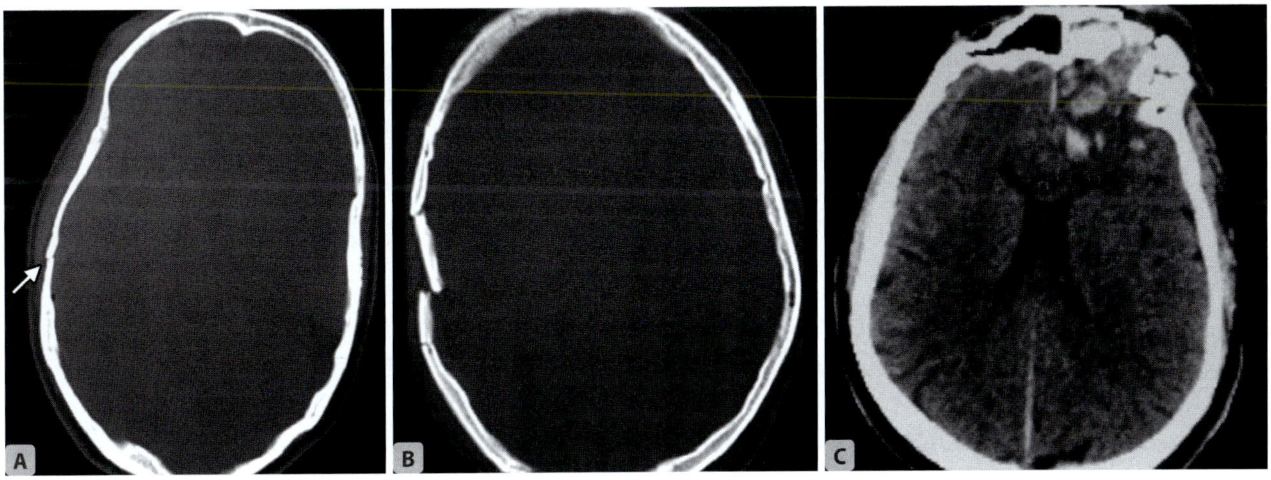

FIGS. 7A TO C: Axial CT sections to show various types of skull fractures. (A) Linear fracture (arrow); (B) Depressed fracture; (C) Compound fracture.

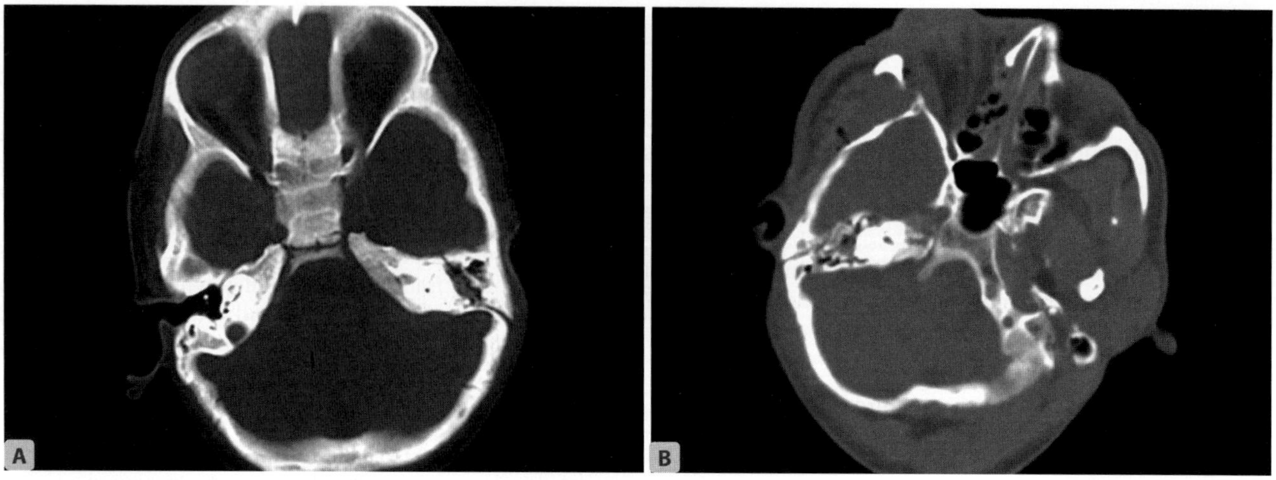

FIGS. 8A AND B: Thin-CT sections (1 mm) in axial plane in bone algorithm showing temporal bone fractures. (A) Transverse fracture; and (B) Longitudinal fracture.

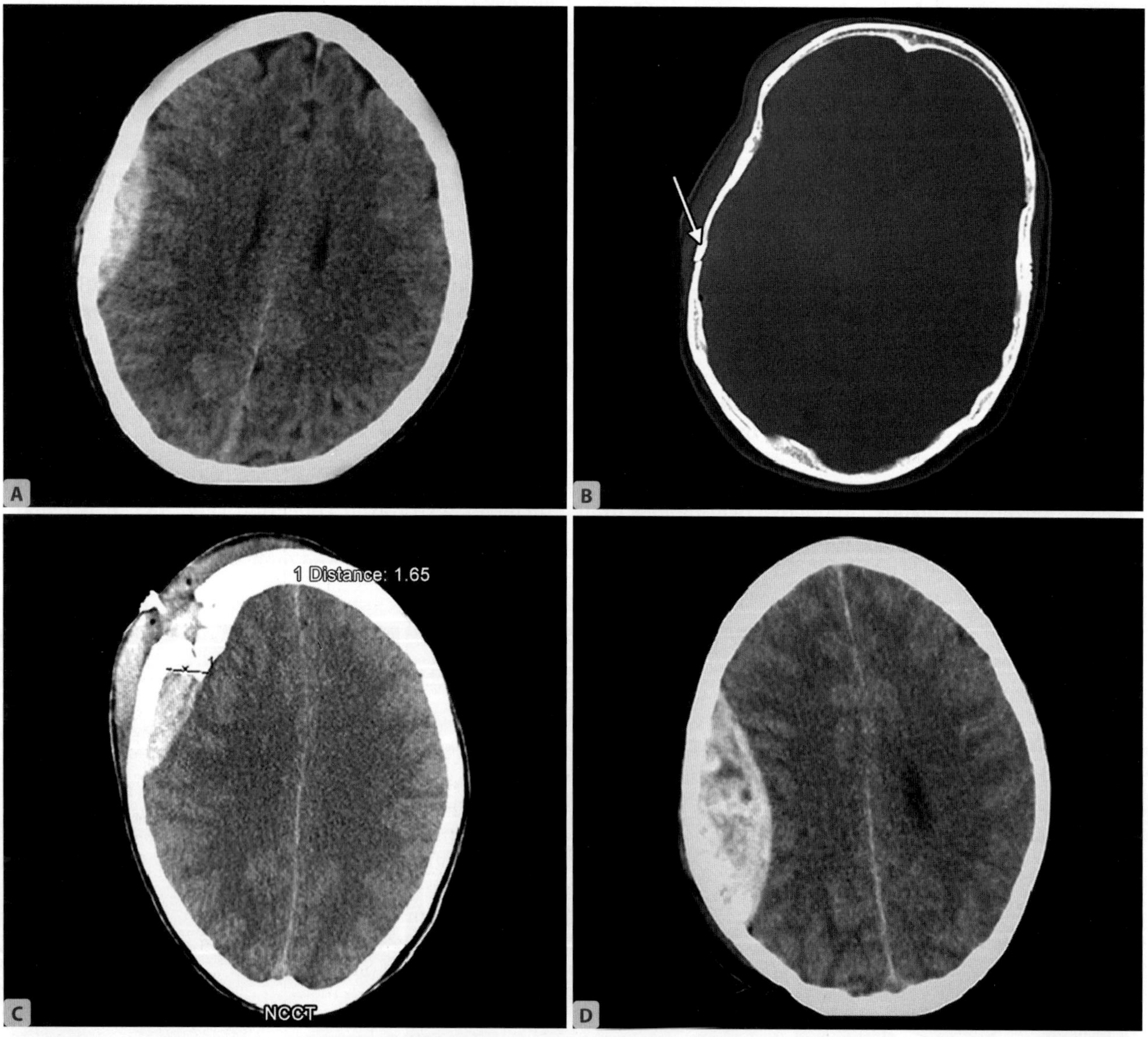

FIGS. 9A TO D: Axial CT images showing features of extradural hematoma. (A) A well-defined, hyperdense, biconvex, extra-axial collection associated with overlying skull fracture (arrow) (B), presence of low-attenuation areas within the hyperdense hematoma called "swirl sign" (D), diameter of hematoma >1.5 cm is an indication for surgery (C).

Because the EDH is located in the potential space between the dura and inner table of the skull, it rarely crosses cranial sutures because the periosteal layer of the dura is firmly attached at sutural margins. However, at the vertex, where the periosteum that forms the outer wall of the sagittal sinus is not tightly attached to the sagittal suture, the EDH can cross midline.[9,23]

Ominous sign: An imaging finding that predicts rapid expansion of an arterial EDH is the presence of low-attenuation areas within the hyperdense hematoma (the so-called "swirl sign"), represents active bleeding **(Fig. 9C)**.[24]

Management[25]

Conservative treatment is persued if:

- Volume of EDH < 30 cm^3
- Midline shift < 5 mm
- Diameter of lesion <1.5 cm

Potential indications for surgery are:

- Size > 1.5 cm **(Fig. 9D)**
- Active bleeding
- Pending herniation
- Corresponding neurological deficit.

In the presence of swirl sign, patient should be carefully monitored for signs of herniation due to expanding hematoma.[24]

Classic Acute Epidural Hematoma
Terminology Blood between dura and skull
Etiology • Skull fracture: 90–95% • Arterial source: 90% (middle meningeal artery) • Venous source: 10%
Pathology • Unilateral, supratentorial (90%) • Dura stripped away from skull • Usually does not cross sutures (exception children) • Does not cross sites of dural attachment
Clinical • 1-4% of head trauma • Most common young adults • M:F = 4:1 • Classic lucid interval in 50% only • Delayed presentation is common • Low mortality of recognized and treated • Small EDHs managed conservatively
Imaging • Hyperdense lens-shaped (biconvex) • *Swirl sign*: Ongoing bleed

Subdural Hematomas (SDH)

Blood collects in between the inner dural layer and the arachnoid. The hematoma dissects in-between these two layers because these layers are not firmly attached, hence SDH are frequently seen along the entire hemispheric convexity from the anterior falx to the posterior falx.

SDHs are generally venous in origin. They usually arise from laceration of bridging cortical veins during sudden head deceleration. SDHs are commonly seen in elderly due to prominent extra-axial space (resulting from cerebral atrophy), which allows an increased motion between the brain parenchyma and the calvarium. Other causes of the SDH include rapid decompression of obstructive hydrocephalus, and injury to pial vessels and pacchionian granulations.[9,23,25]

Imaging Features

On CT, the acute SDH are seen as hyperdense (50–60 HU), homogenous, crescent-shaped, extra-axial collection **(Fig. 10A)**. Most are supratentorial and located along the convexity. They are also frequently identified along the falx and tentorium **(Figs. 11A and B)**.

The density of SDH will progressively decrease due to protein degradation within the hematoma **(Figs. 10A to C)**. Rebleeding during course of a SDH appears as heterogenous attenuation on CT, due to mixture of fresh blood and partially liquid hematoma **(Figs. 12A and B)**. A sediment level or "hematocrit effect" may be seen either from rebleeding or in patients with clotting disorders. The chronic SDH has a low-attenuation value similar to, but slightly higher than, CSF **(Fig. 10C)**.

Challenges During Interpretation[9,23]

1. It can be difficult to distinguish from prominent subarachnoid space in patients with cerebral atrophy. In these patients, intravenous contrast administration can be helpful by demonstrating an enhancing capsule or displaced cortical veins.
2. A small thin convexity SDH can be difficult to appreciate adjacent to the hyperdense skull unless the images are viewed with a "wide window" **(Fig. 13A)**.
3. During the transition from acute to the chronic SDH, an isodense phase occurs, usually between 1 and 3 weeks after the acute event, depending on the patient's hematocrit level, clotting capability, and presence or absence of rebleeding. Recognition of indirect imaging findings **(Fig. 13B)**, such as effacement of sulci, displacement of gray matter with white matter "buckling," and midline shift **(Fig. 14)** on a non- contrast CT scan can avoid this common pitfall.

SDH Evolution on MRI

The MR appearance of a SDH also evolves over time, depending on the biochemical state of hemoglobin **(Table 1)**. The acute SDH is isointense to brain on T1-weighted and hypointense on T2-weighted images. During the subacute phase, when the subdural hematoma may be isodense or hypodense on CT scans, T1-weighted images demonstrate high signal intensity due to the presence of methemoglobin in the subdural collection. The chronic SDH appears hypointense on T1-weighted and hyperintense on T2-weighted images relative to normal brain. The signal intensity of chronic SDH is slightly higher than CSF signal intensity on T1-weighted, FLAIR, and proton-density T2-weighted imaging. Because of its multiplanar capability,

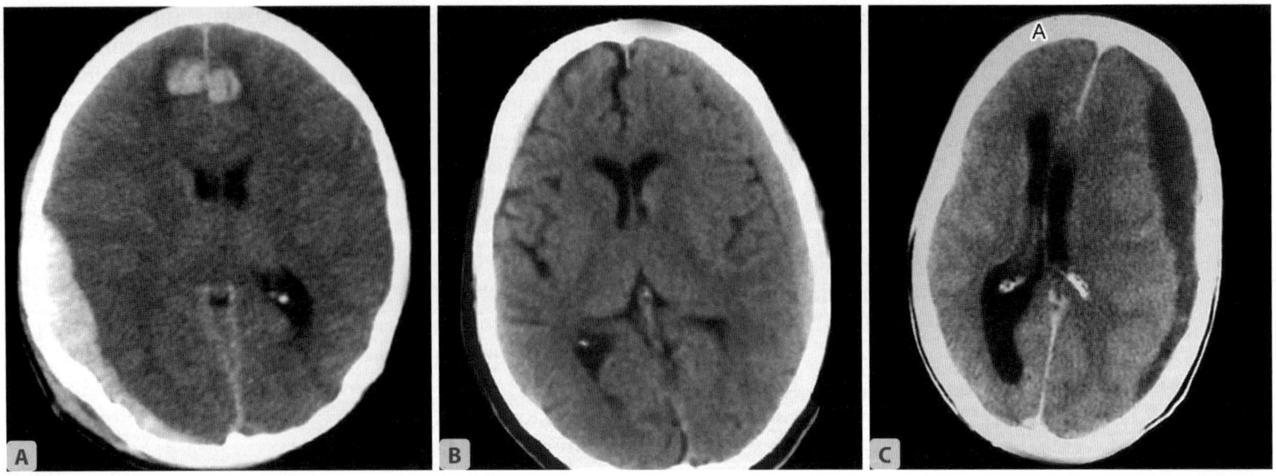

FIGS. 10A TO C: Axial CT images showing various stages of subdural hematoma. (A) Acute SDH seen as hyperdense (50–60 HU), homogeneous, crescent-shaped, extra-axial collection; (B) Subacute SDH seen as isodense (30–40 HU), homogeneous, crescent-shaped, extra-axial collection; (C) Chronic SDH seen as hypodense (10 HU) extra-axial collection.

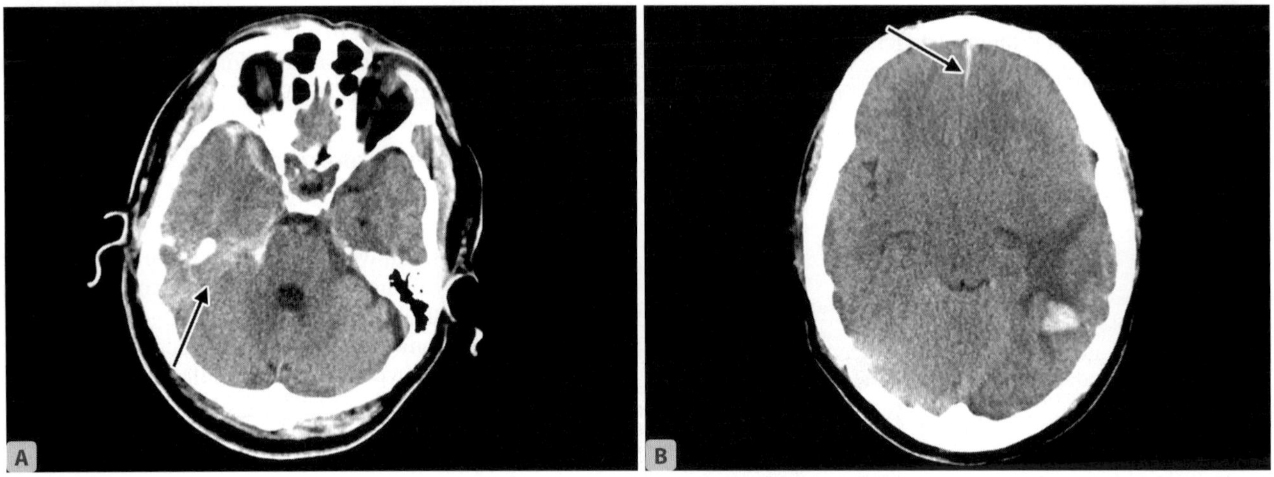

FIGS. 11A AND B: Axial CT section to show SDH along tentorium (arrow) (A) and along falx (arrow) (B).

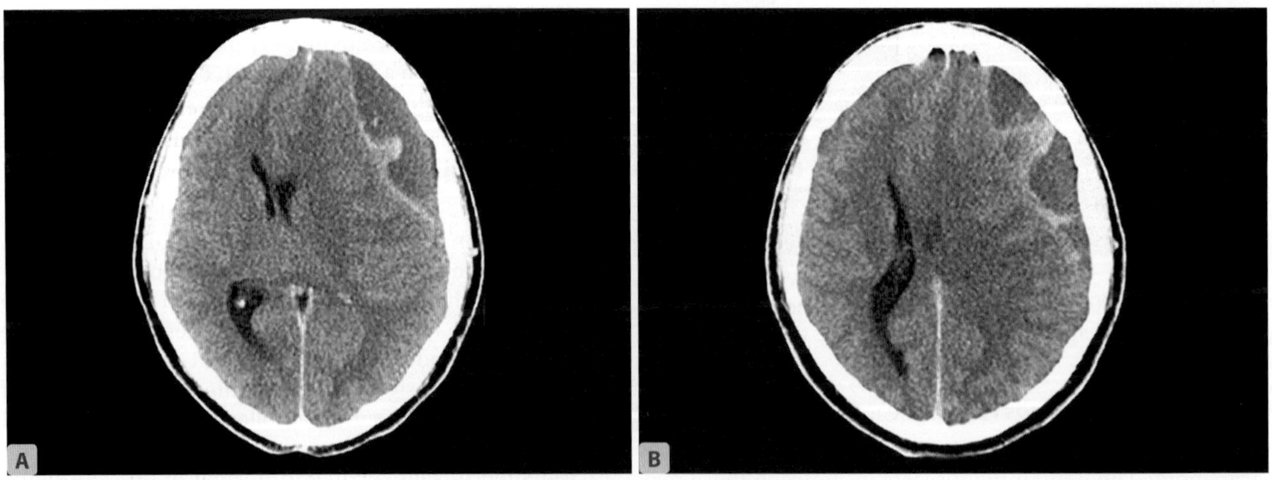

FIGS. 12A AND B: Axial CT section showing heterogeneous attenuation SDH in left frontoparietal region, due to mixture of fresh blood and partially liquefied hematoma due to rebleeding during course of a SDH.

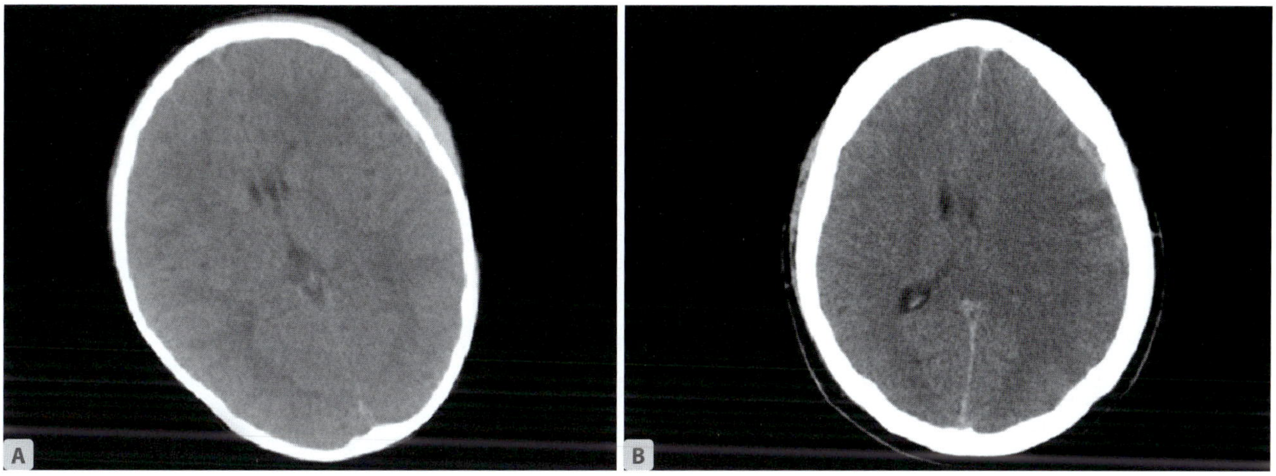

FIGS. 13A AND B: Axial CT images to show technical difficulties in interpretation of SDH. (A) A small thin convexity SDH can be difficult to appreciate adjacent to the hyperdense skull unless the imagesare viewed with a "wide window"; (B) identification of isodense phase of SDH diifficult unless one should look at indirect imaging findings, such as effacement of sulci, displacement of gray matter with white matter "buckling," and midline shift on a non-contrast CT scan to avoid this common pitfall.

TABLE 1: Temporal evolution of ICH.

Biochemical form	Clinical stage	Approximate time of appearance	Intensity on T1WI	Intensity on T2WI
OxyHg in RBCs	Hyperacute	Immediately to first several hours	Isointense	Hyperintense
DeoxyHg in RBCs	Acute	Hours to days	Iso to hypointense	Hypointense
MetHg in RBCs	Early subacute	First several days	Hyperintense	Hypointense
Extracellular MetHg	Subacute to chronic	Days to months	Hyperintense	Hyperintense
Ferritin and Hemosiderin	Remote	Days to indefinitely	Hypointense	Hyperintense

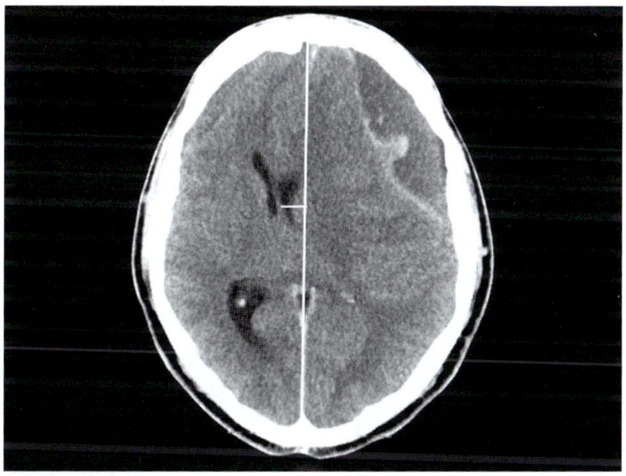

FIG. 14: Axial CT image at the level of septum pellucidum to show technique of measurement of midline shift. Draw a line joining a bone protrusion is located in the anterior section of the skull; (the falx cerebri extends from this point) and another bony protrusion in posterior section of the skull (falx cerebri ends at this point). Another line is drawn perpendicular to the former line from septum pellucidum that gives the exact amount of midline shift.

MR is useful in identifying convexity and vertex hematomas that might not be detected on axial CT scans because of the similar attenuation of the adjacent bone.[9,23,26]

Traumatic Subarachnoid Hemorrhage

Traumatic subarachnoid hemorrhage (SAH) can result from:

- The disruption of small pial vessels;
- Extension into the subarachnoid space by a contusion or hematoma; or
- Diffusion of intraventricular hemorrhage.

SAH is very common with TBI, but it rarely causes mass effect. On CT, SAH appears as linear or serpentine areas of high attenuation that conform to the morphology of the cerebral sulci and cisterns **(Fig. 15)**. Common sites for SAH include the sylvian and interpeduncular cisterns. sometime, "effacement" of sulci due to the presence of intrasulcal SAH may be the only imaging clue of the presence of SAH. In patients who are found unconscious after an unwitnessed event, the detection of SAH in key cisterns (basilar, sylvian, and circle of Willis) may indicate a ruptured aneurysm, rather than trauma. In such cases, contrast-enhanced CT angiography is recommended as the next step in the patient evaluation **(Figs. 16A and E)**.

MR Imaging of SAH

Acute subarachnoid hemorrhage may be more difficult to detect on conventional MR than on CT because it can be isointense to brain parenchyma on routine T1- and T2-weighted images. However, FLAIR has been shown to

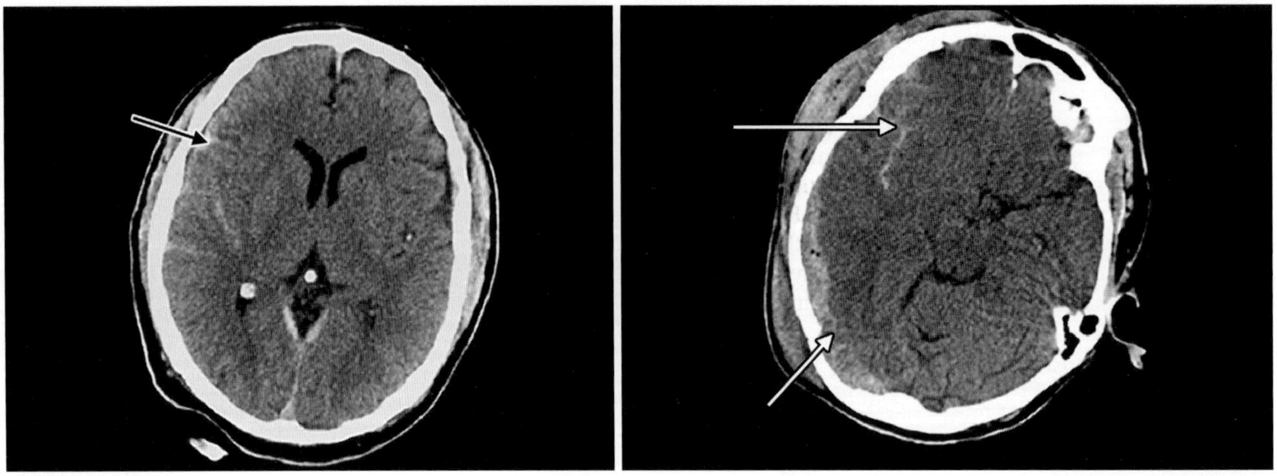

FIG. 15: Axial CT sections showing linear or serpentine areas of high attenuation that confirming to the morphology of the cerebral sulci and sylvian cisterns (Black arrow). *Note:* There is associated SDH along the right occipital region (white arrows).

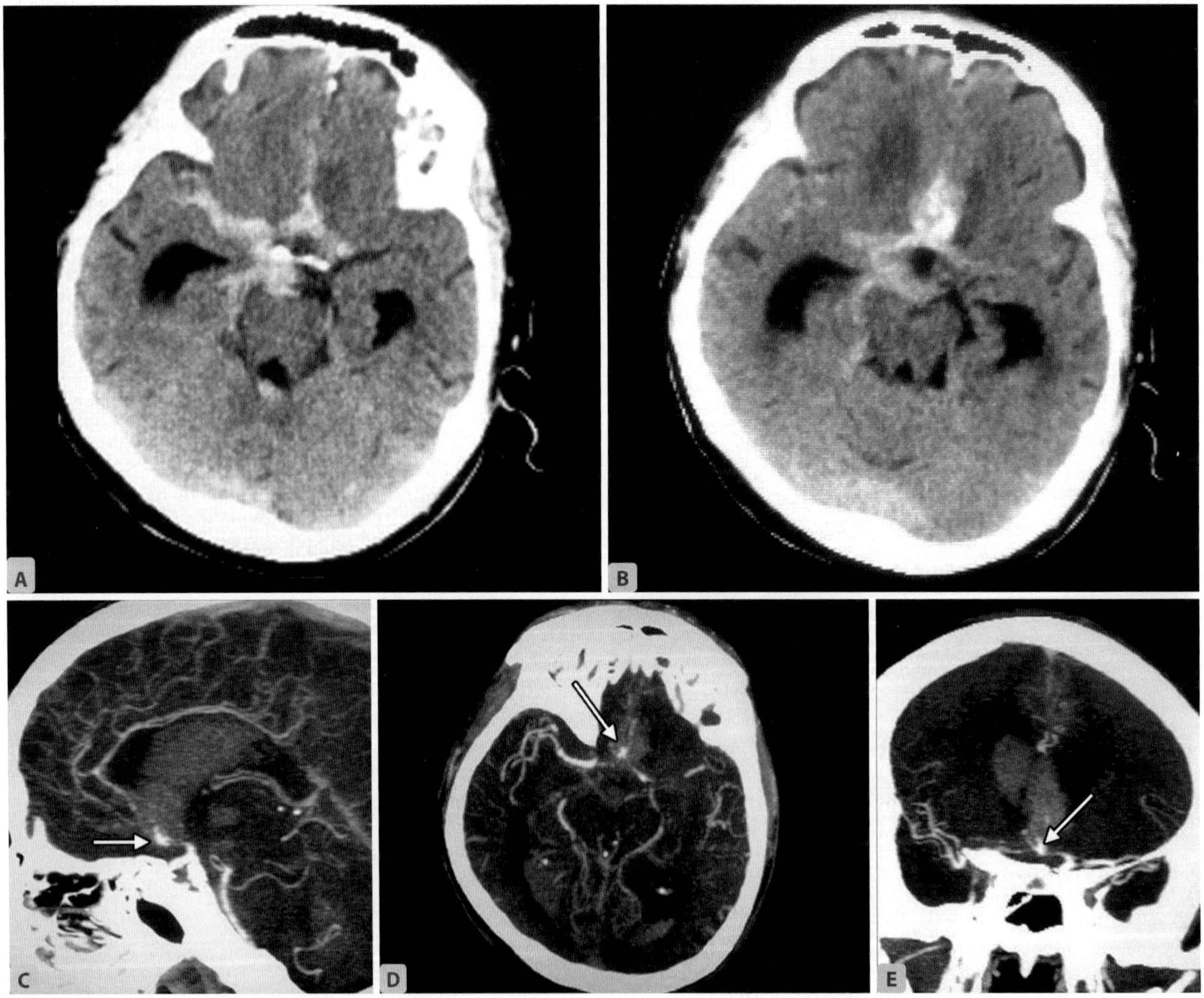

FIGS. 16A TO E: NCCT axial sections showing subarachanoid hemorrhage in basal cisterns (A and B), 3D reformation of CT angiography showing ACoM pseudoaneurysm responsible for subarachanoid hemorrhage (C to E).

be more sensitive than CT in detecting acute subarachnoid hemorrhage.[14] Subacute subarachnoid hemorrhage may be better appreciated on MR because of its high signal intensity when the blood is isointense to CSF on CT. Chronic hemorrhage on MR scans may show hemosiderin staining in the subarachnoid space, which appears as areas of decreased signal intensity on T1- and T2-weighted sequences ("superficial hemo-siderosis"). Hemosiderins are best detected on gradient-echoT2*- weighted images. SAH may lead to communicating hydrocephalus by impeding CSF resorption at the level of arachnoid villi.[9,14,15,23]

Subdural Hemorrhage

Acute SDH (aSDH)

- Second MC traumatic extra axial hemorrhage (SAH>SDH>EDH)
- Crescentic blood collection between dura and arachnoid
  - Supratentorial (95%). bilateral (15%)
  - SDH cross sutures
  - SDH do not cross dural attachments
- CT
  - Hyperdense (60%)
  - Mixed (40%)
  - Isodense acute SDH (anemia—coagulopathy)

Subacute SDH (sSDH)

- Clot organizes. lyses forms neomembranes
- CT
  - Density decreases (1–2HU/day)
  - Isodense with cortex in 7–10 days
  - Look for displaced "dots" of CSF under SDH
  - Gray-white interface "buckled" inward
  - Displaced cortical veins seen on CECT
- MRI
  - Signal varies with clot age
  - R2* and SWI shows bloom ing

Chronic SDH (cSDH)

- Serosanguineous fluid
  - Hypodense on NCCT
  - Rehemorrhage (5–10%)
  - Loculated blood pockets with fluid-fluid levels

Traumatic intraventricular hemorrhage (IVH) can also occur by one of three mechanisms.

- Rotationally induced tearing of subependymal veins along the surface of the ventricles.
- Direct extension of a parenchymal hematoma into the ventricular system.
- Retrograde flow of SAH into the ventricular system via the fourth ventricular outflow foramina (the reverse mechanism in which IVH can extend into the subarachnoid space).

Patients with IVH are at risk for developing both communicating and non-communicating hydrocephalus secondary to obstruction at the level of the arachnoid villi or aqueduct, respectively. They are also at risk of ependymitis from the irritant effects of the blood. On CT, IVH usually appears as CSF-hyperdense fluid level, layering within the ventricular system **(Fig. 17A and B)**. Certainly, tiny collections of increased density layering in the occipital horns may be the only clue to IVH. Occasionally, the IVH may appear "tumefactive" as a cast within the ventricle.[9,23]

Intra-axial Injury

Diffuse axonal injury (DAI) results from rotational acceleration and deceleration forces that produce shearing deformations of brain tissue. Clinically, DAI is characterized by loss or severe impairment of consciousness beginning at the moment of direct impact. DAI in the chronic stage may result in overwhelming cognitive and psychiatric problems.

MRI is clearly superior to CT for detecting DAI, and therefore, provides increased success at explaining neurologic deficits after trauma and predicting long-term outcome. Newer imaging methods, such as DWI and DTI with 3D tractography, have shown potential in improving the detection of white matter injury in both acute and chronic DAI.[26-28]

CT is mostly limited to depicting the small focal hemorrhages associated with axonal shearing injury. Common findings include small, petechial hemorrhages at the gray-white junction of the cerebral hemispheres **(Fig. 18)** and corpus callosum. Unfortunately, only about 20% of DAI lesions contain sufficient hemorrhage to be detectable on CT.

Because of better sensitivity to blood products, gradient-echo T2*-weighted MR demonstrates more DAI lesions than CT **(Fig. 19A)**.[16] Spin-echo T2-weighted MR techniques, especially FLAIR imaging, can detect many nonhemorrhagic foci of DAI but still underestimate the true extent of traumatic white matter damage. On MR, nonhemorrhagic DAI lesions appear as multiple small foci of increased signal on T2-weighted images, DWI images **(Fig. 19B)** and as decreased signal on T1-weighted images within the white matter. Petechial hemorrhage causes a central hypointensity on T2-weighed images and hyperintensity on T1-weighted images as a result of intracellular methemoglobin in the subacute stage.

The conspicuity of DAI on MR eventually diminishes as the damaged axons degenerate and the edema resolves. Residual findings may include nonspecic atrophy, gliosis, or hemosiderin staining, which can persist indefinitely on gradient-echo T2*-weighted images.

The location of the DAI tends to correlate with the severity of the trauma.[26-28]

- **Grade I DAI:** Involves only the peripheral gray-white junctions of the lobar white matter. The parasagittal regions of the frontal lobes and periventricular regions of the temporal lobes are commonly affected **(Fig. 20A)**.
- **Grade II DAI:** Involves both the lobar white-matter as well as the corpus callosum, particularly the posterior body and splenium. The corpus callosum is susceptible to DAI because the falx prevents displacement of the cerebral hemispheres **(Fig. 20B)**.
- **Grade III DAI:** Dorsolateral midbrain (brainstem), in addition to the lobar white matter and corpus callosum are affected **(Fig. 20C)**.

Diffuse Vascular Injury: Diffuse vascular injury (DVI) signifies the most severe form of the diffuse axonal injury

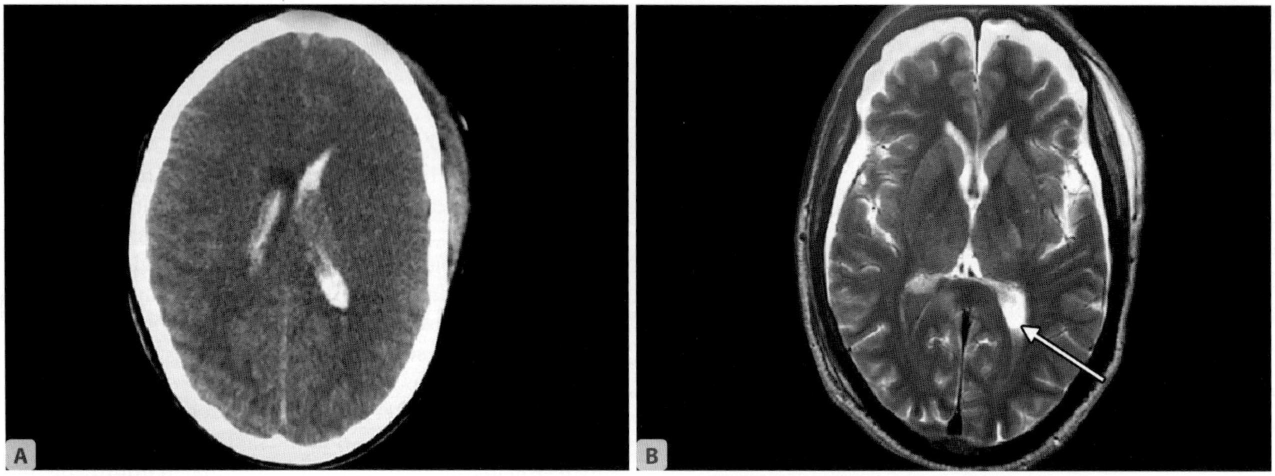

FIGS. 17A AND B: Axial CT and MR sections to show appearances of IVH. (A) Hyperdense (blood) within the bilateral lateral ventricles, (B) CSF-blood fluid level (hyper-hypo intense) layering within the ventricular system (arrow).

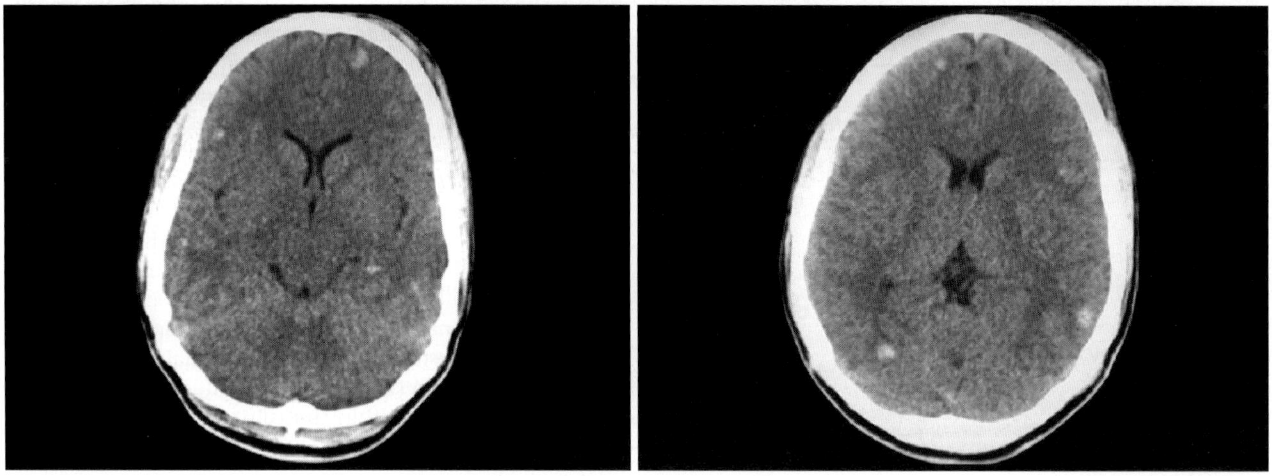

FIG. 18: Axial CT images showing multiple, small, petechial hemorrhages at the gray–white junction of the cerebral hemispheres suggestive of DAI.

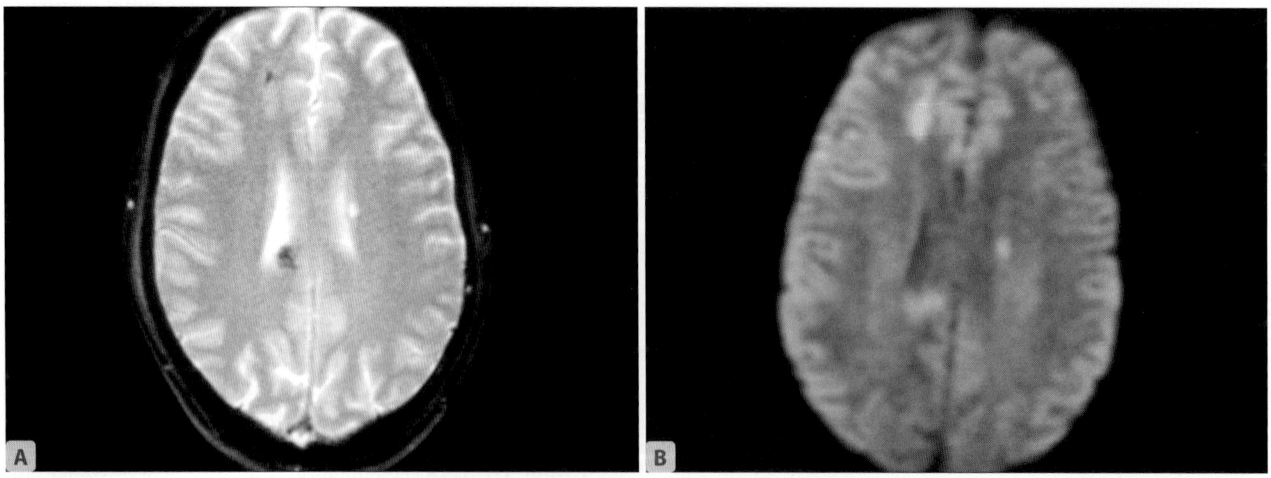

FIGS. 19A AND B: Axial MR images showing features of DAI. (A) Gradient echo sequence showing hypointense foci in carpus callosum and in right frontal lobe (sensitive to detect hemorrhagic DAI lesions due to sensitivity to blood products); (B) DWI image showing multiple small foci of increased signal in both cerebral hemisphere and in corpus callosum (sensitive to detect additional nonhemorrhagic DAI lesions).

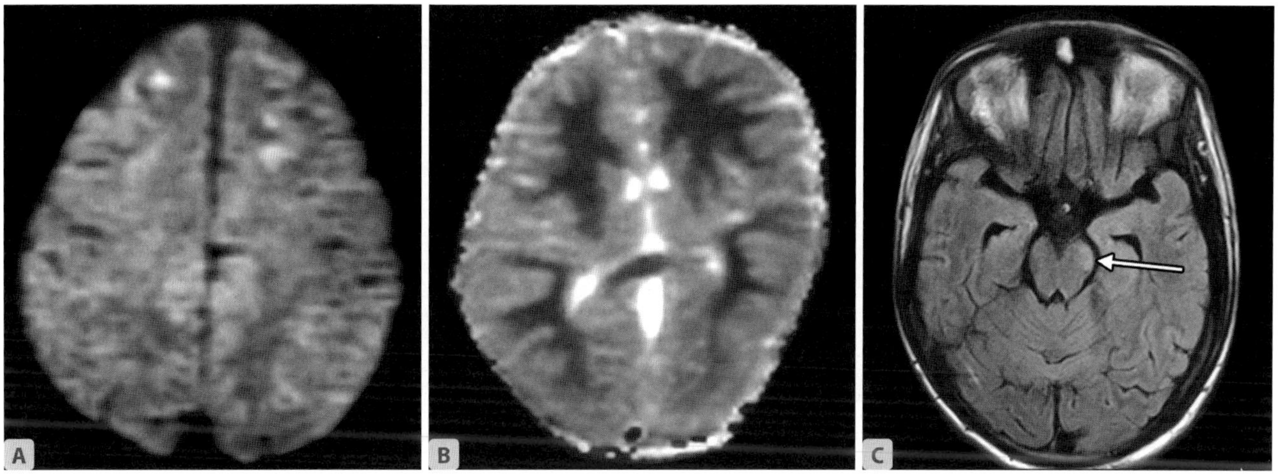

FIGS. 20A TO C: MR images to show types of DAI lesions. (A) Lesions seen at peripheral gray-white junctions of the lobar white matter; (B) Lesions involve both the lobar white-matter as well as the corpus callosum; (C) Lesions involve dorsolateral midbrain (brainstem, arrow).

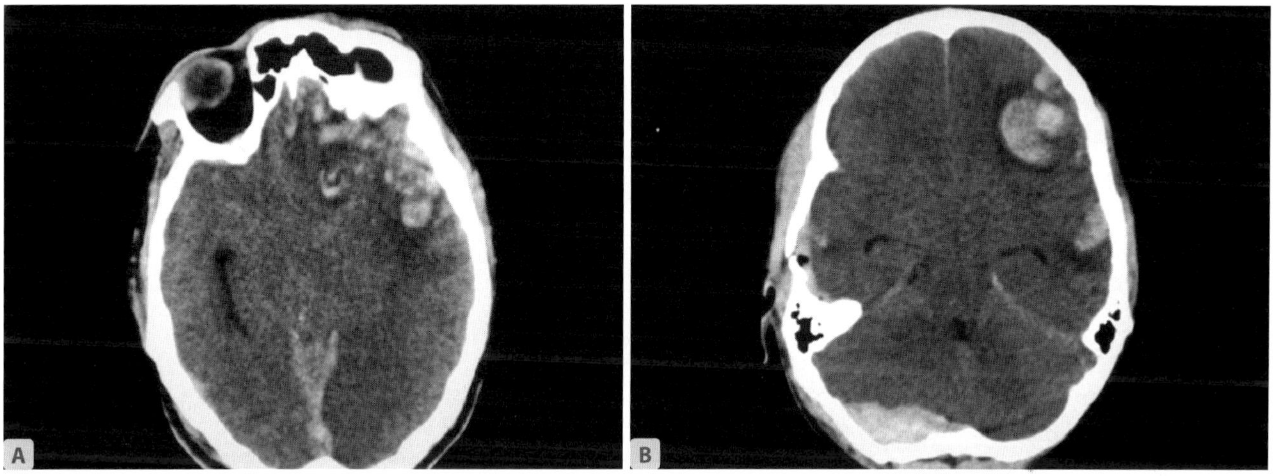

FIGS. 21A AND B: Axial CT sections showing contusions in orbitofrontal lobe (A), temporal lobe (B) involving the superficial gray matter sparing the underlying white matter. *Note:* SDH along tentorium (A) and along right temporo-occipital regions (B).

range. Most of these patients with DVI do not reach hospital or live long ample of time for imaging.

In patients who get imaging done, most conspicuous finding is diffuse brain swelling with effaced sulci and small ventricles. Sometime few small foci of hemorrhage in the white matter and basal ganglia may be identified.

Cortical contusion is a focal brain lesion primarily involving superficial gray matter, with relative sparing of the underlying white matter. Regions of the brain that are in close contact with the rough surface on the inner skull table are commonly affected. These areas include the orbitofrontal and temporal lobes, and less so, the parasagittal convexity. The temporal lobes above the petrous bone or posterior to the greater sphenoid wing, and the frontal lobes above the cribriform plate, planumsphenoidale, and lesser sphenoid wing are commonly affected **(Figs. 21A and B)**. Contusions are associated with a better prognosis than DAI, unless they are accompanied by brainstem injury or significant mass effect. Contusions can also occur at the margins of depressed skull fractures **(Fig. 22)**. The cerebellum is involved less than 10% of the time.[9,23,29]

On CT, non-hemorrhagic contusions are difficult to detect initially until the development of associated edema. Hemorrhagic contusions are more easily identified and appear as foci of high attenuation within superficial gray matter. They may be surrounded by larger areas of low attenuation from the associated vasogenic edema. As the contusion evolves, the characteristic "salt and pepper" pattern of mixed areas of hypodensity and hyperdensity becomes more apparent. Contusions with severe mass effect may require surgical decompression to prevent secondary injury.[9,23]

On MRI, contusions appear as ill-defined areas of variable signal intensity on both T1- and T2-weighted images, depending on the age of the lesions. They are limited to the surface and often have a "gyral" morphology. Hemosiderin from an old contusion leads to decreased signal intensity on T2- and especially T2*-weighted images, especially at higher field strengths. The signal loss can persist indefinitely and serves as an important marker of prior hemorrhage.[29]

The **intracerebral hematoma** is the most common cause of clinical deterioration in patients who have experienced a lucid interval after the initial injury. In contrast to the common

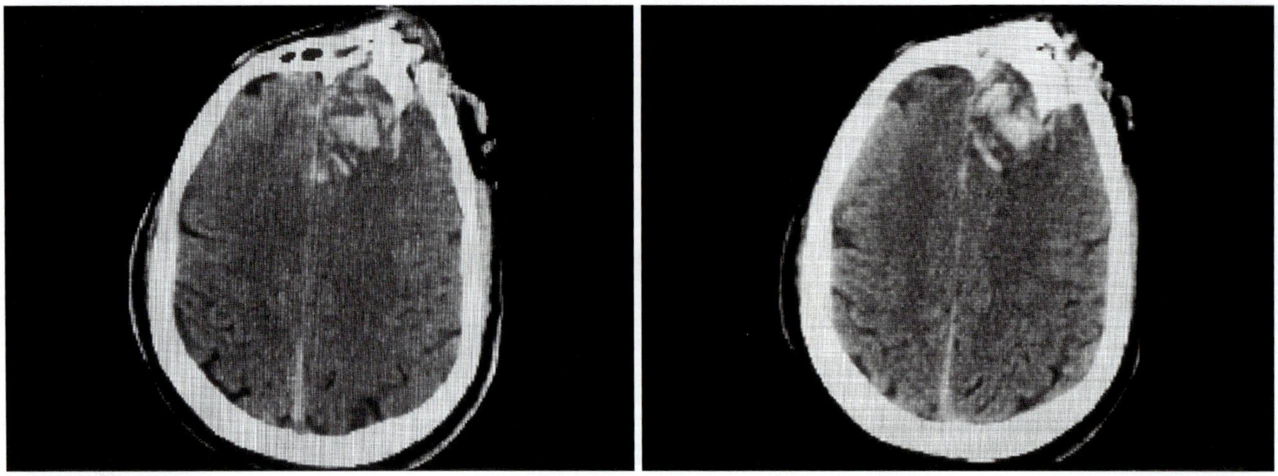

FIG. 22: Axial CT sections showing cerebral contusion in left frontal lobe associated with compound skull fracture.

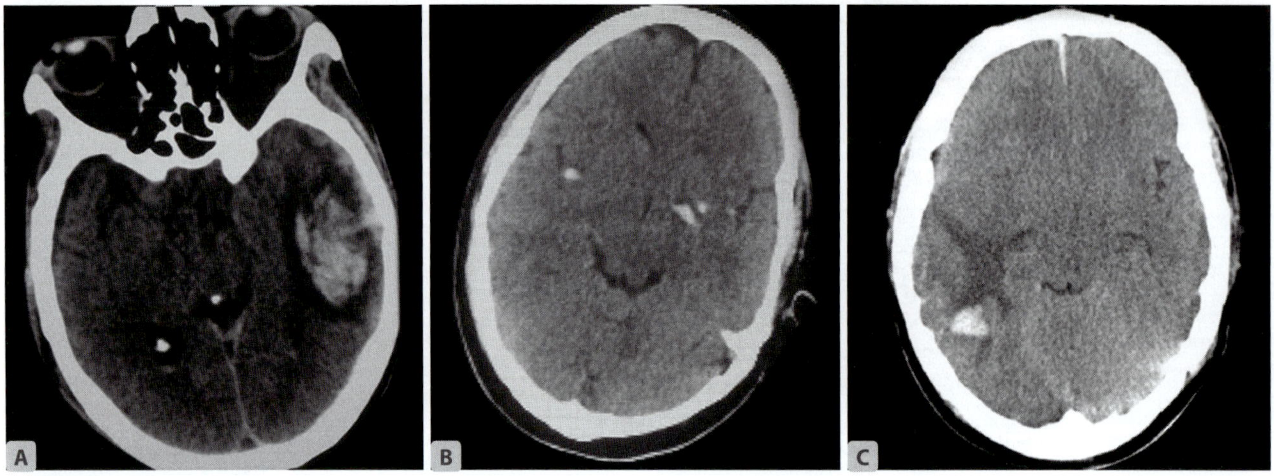

FIGS. 23A TO C: Axial CT sections showing intracerebral hematomas in left temporal lobe (A); basal ganglia (B); and temporo-occipital lobe (C).

contusion described above, the intracerebral hematoma is due to shear-induced hemorrhage from the rupture of small intraparenchymal blood vessels. Because the bleeding occurs into areas of relatively normal brain, intracerebral hematomas tend to have less surrounding edema than cortical contusions. Most traumatic intracerebral hematomas are located in the frontotemporal white matter **(Figs. 23A to C)**. Involvement of the basal ganglia has been described; however, hemorrhage in basal ganglia should alert the radiologist that an underlying hypertensive bleed may be the culprit. Intracerebral hematomas are often associated with skull fractures and other primary neuronal lesions, including contusions and DAI, especially in patients who are unconscious at the time of injury. Symptoms typically result from the mass effect associated with an expanding hematoma. Indeed, delayed hemorrhage is a common cause of clinical deterioration during the first several days after head trauma.[9,23] It is important to differentiate benign hemorrhage from intratumoral hemorrhage **(Table 2)**.

Brain laceration happens when severe injury disrupts the pia mater and factually tears the underlying brain apart. It is usually seen in infants and children due to head trauma associated with child abuse. A "burst lobe" is the most severe form of brain laceration, where in the affected lobe is completely disrupted with surrounding large hematoma formation.

Subcortical (Deep Brain) Injury

Subcortical injuries (SCIs) are traumatic intra-axial lesions that affect deep brain structures such as the brainstem, basal ganglia, thalami, and ventricles. These represent severe form of shear injuries that interrupt axons, tear penetrating blood vessels, and damage the choroid plexus of the lateral ventricles. SCIs are the third most common parenchymal brain injury, after cortical contusions and DAI. On imaging, initial scans may show subtle abnormalities with dramatic increase of findings on follow-up scans. Typical findings include diffuse brain edema with punctate hemorrhages in the deep gray nuclei and midbrain. Bleed within ventricles and choroid plexus are form and may form a "cast" of the lateral ventricles. This condition has to be differentiated from

TABLE 2: Intratumoral hemorrhage versus benign intracranial hematomas.

Intratumoral hemorrhage	Benign hemorrhage
Markedly heterogeneous, related to:	Shows expected signal intensities of acute, subacute or chronic blood, depending on stage of hematoma
• Mixed stages of blood	
• Debris-fluid (intracellular-extracellular blood) levels	
• Edema + tumor + necrosis with blood	
Identification of nonhemorrhagic tumor component	No abnormal nonhemorrhagic mass
Delayed evolution of blood breakdown products	Follows expected orderly progression
Absent, diminished, or irregular ferritin/hemosiderin	Regular complete ferritin/ hemosiderin rim
Persistent surrounding high intensity on long TR images (i.e. tumor/edema) and mass effect, even in late stages	Complete resolution of edema and mass effect in chronic stages

Duret hemorrhage that occur due to descending transtentorial herniation. Duret hemorrhages are typically located within the center of midbrain, whereas SCIs are located dorsolateral.

Pneumocephalus: Pneumocephalus refers to presence of air within the intracranial cavity. In this condition, gas can be found anywhere within any compartment, including blood vessels.

Intracranial air is not normal finding, however it can be an expected and routine finding after brain surgery.

Tension pneumocephalus is a collection of intracranial gas under pressure that causes mass effect on the brain manifests with neurologic deterioration.

Patients with pneumocephalus may be asymptomatic or present with nonspecific headache. Very rarely, neurologic deficit and consciousness disturbances are observed. Most intracranial air resolves spontaneously within a few days after trauma or surgery. Occasionally, air collections increase and may require evacuation with duraplasty especially in case of tension pneumocephalus. On Imaging intracranial air may be seen in any compartment, i.e. epidural, subdural, subarachnoid, intraventricular, or intraparenchymal. It conforms to the shape of that compartment. Pneumocephalus is usually seen in subdural space, and the most common site is frontal location.

Pneumocephalus

Terminology
- Air in any intracranial compartment
- *Tension pneumocephalus*:
  - Air under pressure>>>neurologic deterioration

Etiology
- Surgery (MC)
- Trauma (8–10%)
- Spontaneous (defect in sinus)

Location
- *Epidural*:
  - Unilateral, biconvex
  - May cross midline
  - Does not move with change of position
- *Subdural*:
  - Confluent, Crescentic
  - Bilateral
  - Changes with head position
  - Does not cross midline
- *Subarachanoid*:
  - Discrete spots and dots in sulci, cisterns
- *Intraventricular*:
  - Usually air-fluid levels. frontal horns
- *Intraparenchymal*:
  - Confluent, well delineated

Imaging Features
- CT
  - Extremely hypodense (-1000 HU)
- MRI
  - Signal void
  - Prominent blooming on GRE
  - Alternating dark holes + /- concentric bright rings

Vascular Injury

Vascular injuries are mentioned here because they are causes of both intra- and extra-axial injuries, including the cause of hematomas and subarachnoid hemorrhages. Traumatic vascular injuries include arterial dissection, pseudoaneurysm, and arteriovenous fistula. Arterial injuries are usually related to skull base fractures. Most often injured artery is the internal carotid artery, especially at sites of fixation, where it enters the carotid canal at the base of the petrous bone, and at its exit from the cavernous sinus beneath the anterior clinoid process.

MR findings of vascular injury include: (a) presence of an intramural hematoma, which is best seen on T1-weighted with fat suppression; (b) intimal flap with dissection and (c) absence of a normal vascular flow void secondary to slow flow or occlusion. An associated parenchymal infarction supplied by the injured vessel may also be seen. Conventional angiogram remains the gold standard for confirmation and delineation of the vascular dissection and may also show spasm or pseudoaneurysm formation **(Figs. 24A to F)**. However, magnetic resonance angiography and MDCT angiography serve as important screening tools in the evaluation of patients with suspected vascular injury.[30]

The acquired **carotid cavernous fistula (CCF)** typically results from full-thickness arterial injury. The injury leads to communication between the cavernous portion of the internal carotid artery and the surrounding venous plexus, resulting in venous engorgement of the cavernous sinus **(Figs. 25 and 26)** and its draining branches namely the ipsilateral superior ophthalmic vein and inferiorpetrosal sinus. Skull base fractures, especially those involving the sphenoid bone, should alert the radiologistto search for associated cavernous carotid injury. Another cause of CCF is the rupture of a cavernous carotid aneurysm. On imaging, CCF can present as

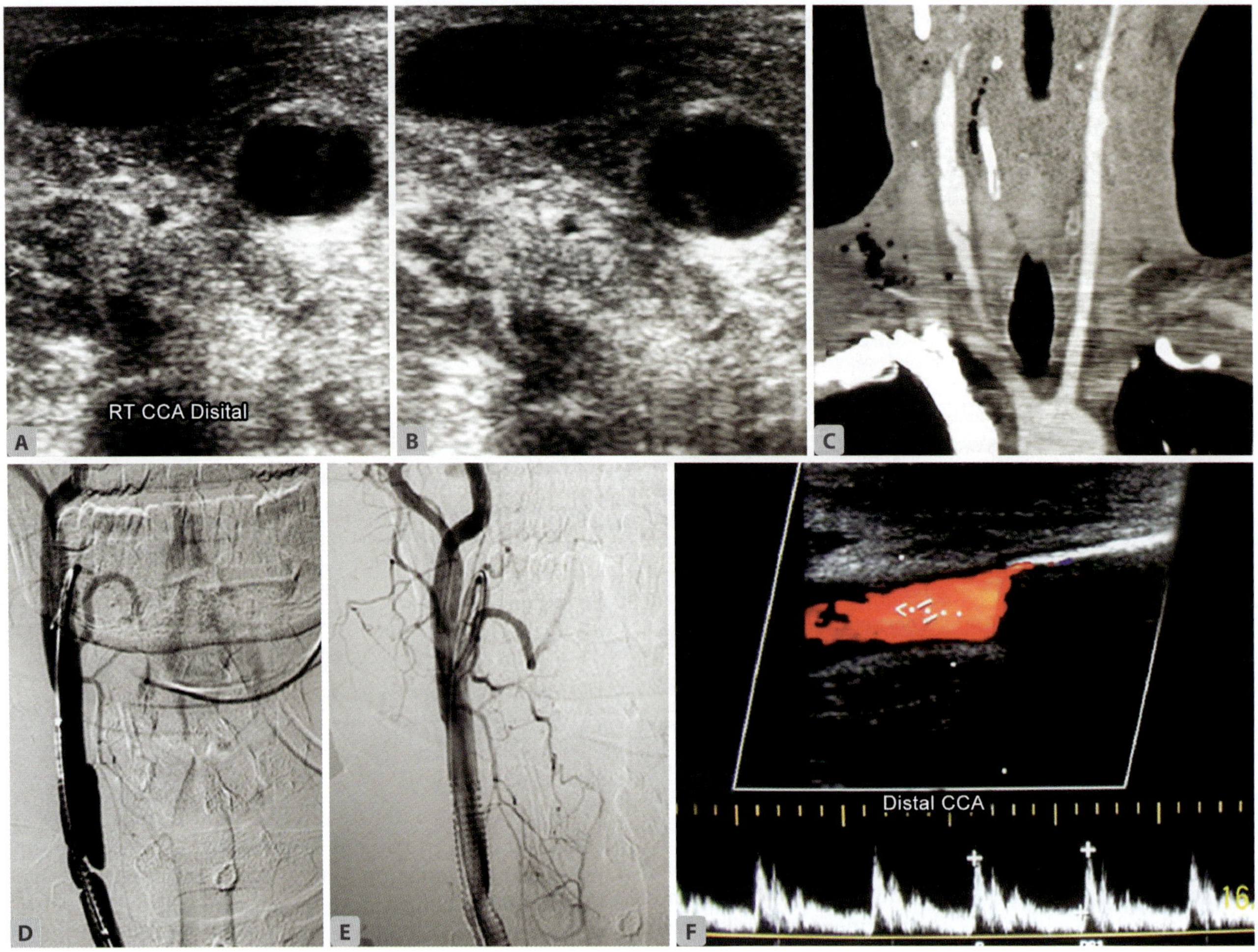

FIGS. 24A TO F: A case of post-traumatic carotid artery dissection with pseudoaneurysm formation. (A and B) Ultrasound images showing intimal flap with dissection; (C) MDCT angiography image better delineation of the vascular dissection and also pseudoaneurysm formation (D) conventional DSA confirming the dissection and pseudoaneurysm formation; (E) DSA image following stent graft insertion to cover the dissection showing complete closure of the dissection flap and patent carotid artery lumen; (F) Follow-up Doppler image showing normal flow through carotid artery and obliteration of dissection flap.

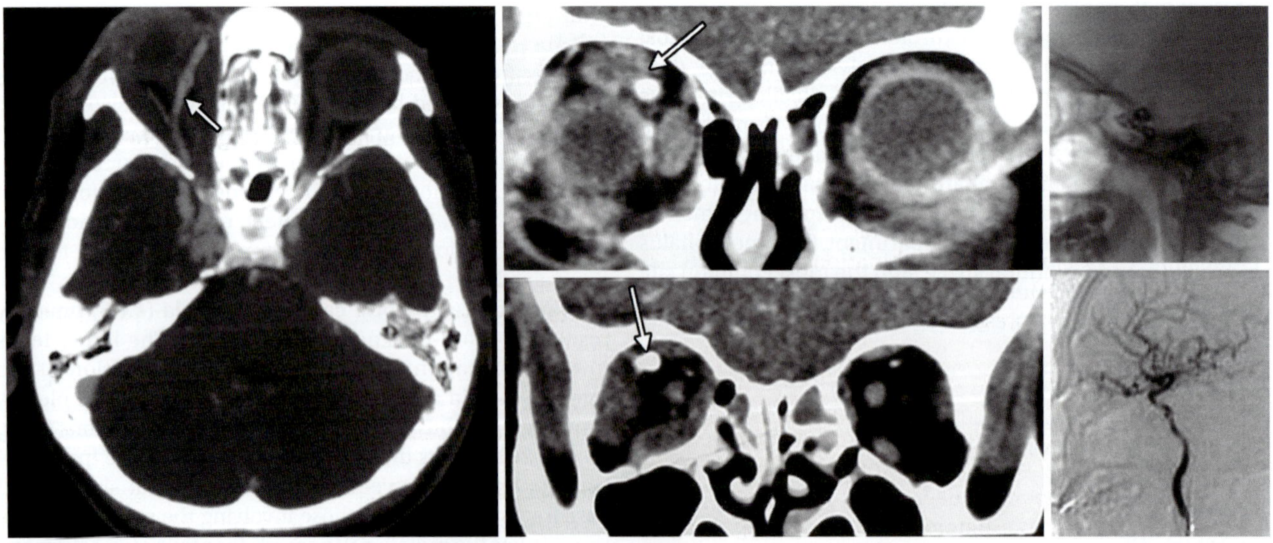

FIG. 25: CT angiography images showing enlarged and lobulated right cavernous sinus with dilated superior ophthalmic vein (arrows) suggestive of carotid cavernous fistula, treated by detachable coils.

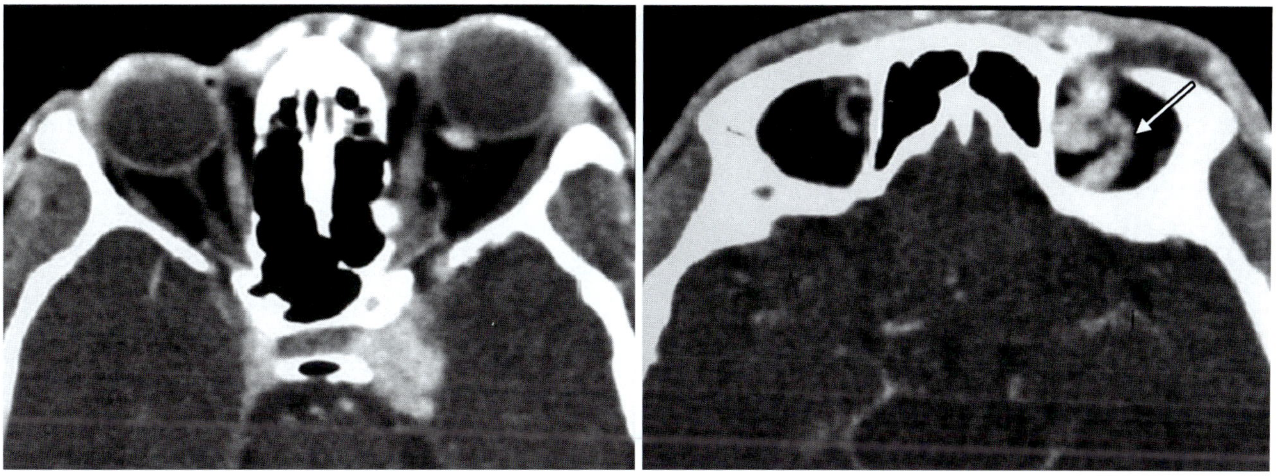

FIG. 26: CT angiography images showing enlarged and lobulated left cavernous sinus with dilated superior ophthalmic vein (arrow) suggestive of carotid cavernous fistula.

an enlarged superior ophthalmic vein, cavernous sinus, and/or petrosal sinus. Other findings include proptosis, preseptal soft-tissue swelling, and extraocular muscle enlargement. The findings may be bilateral because venous channels connect the cavernous sinuses. Again, definitive diagnosis often requires selective carotid angiography with rapid filming to demonstrate the site of communication. Patients can present with findings weeks or even months after the initial trauma.[31] Therefore, a CCF can be overlooked if a detailed clinical history and ophthalmic examination is notperformed.

Types of CCF[31]

Type A: Direct shunt between ICA and cavernous sinus.
Type B: Fistula between meningeal branches of ICA and cavernous sinus.
Type C: Fistula between meningeal branches of ECA and cavernous sinus.
Type D: Fistula between meningeal branches of both ICA and ECA and cavernous sinus.

Treatment of CCF[31]

Direct CCFs rarely undergo spontaneous resolution and, without treatment, eventually cause loss of vision in 80–90% of cases from central retinal vein occlusion orglaucoma.

Endovascular management is the treatment of choice. Direct CCF can be effectively treated by using different therapeutic alternatives such as detachable balloons and detachable coils, alone or in combination with N-butyl-2-cyanoacrylate(n-BCA) or Onyx. Stents have also been used in an attempt to improve preservation of the parent artery while still occluding the fistula.

Indirect fistulas can be cured successfully by transarterial embolization if the blood supply is solely from the ECA territory. Otherwise, the transvenous approach appears to have a higher rate of success with these low-flow indirect lesions, probably due to the decreased resistance imparted upon the small-bore catheters while navigating through tortuous anatomy.

Another traumatic vascular injury is the **dural fistula**, usually caused by laceration of the middle meningeal artery with resultant meningeal artery to meningeal vein fistula formation. The dural fistula generally drains via the meningeal veins; therefore, they rarely lead to the formation of an EDH. Patients are often asymptomatic or present with nonspecific complaints such as tinnitus.

SECONDARY HEAD INJURY

Acute Secondary Changes

1. **Diffuse Cerebral Swelling (edema)** results from
- Increase in cerebral blood volume(hyperemia),
- Vasogenic edema, or
- An increase in tissue fluid (cytotoxicedema).

Imaging features of cerebral edema include effacement of the cerebral sulci and cisterns, compression of the ventricles and loss of gray-white differentiation. The cerebellum and brainstem are usually spared in cerebral edema and may appear hyperdense (On CT) relative to the affected cerebral hemispheres **(Fig. 27)**.

2. **Brain herniation** occurs secondary to mass effect produced by other causes.[9,23]

There are three types of herniation **(Figs. 28A to D):**
1. Subfalcine
2. Uncal
3. *Transtentorial:*
   - Descending
   - Ascending

Subfalcine herniation is the most common form of herniation.

Imaging features include displacement of the cingulate gyrus across the midline under the falx cerebri, compression of the ipsilateral ventricle due to mass effect and enlargement of the contralateral ventricle due to obstruction of the foramen of Monro **(Fig. 28A)**. Due to such displacement, there will be trapping of the callosomarginal branches of the ACA, which may lead to ACA infarction.

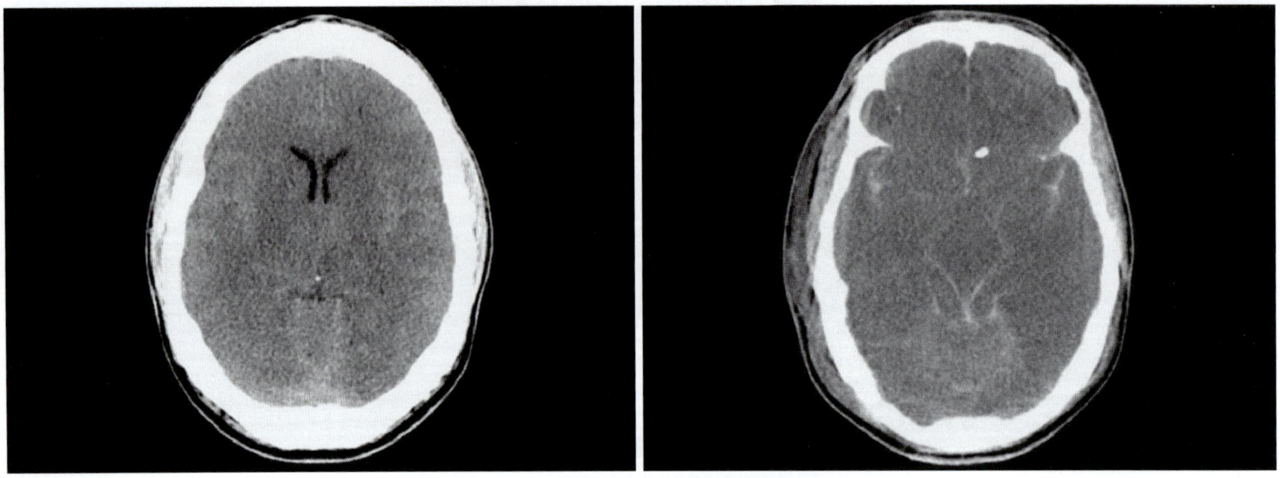

FIG. 27: Axial CT images showing features of diffuse cerebral edema such as effacement of the cerebral sulci and cisterns, compression of the ventricles and loss of gray-white differentiation with relative sparing of cerebellum.

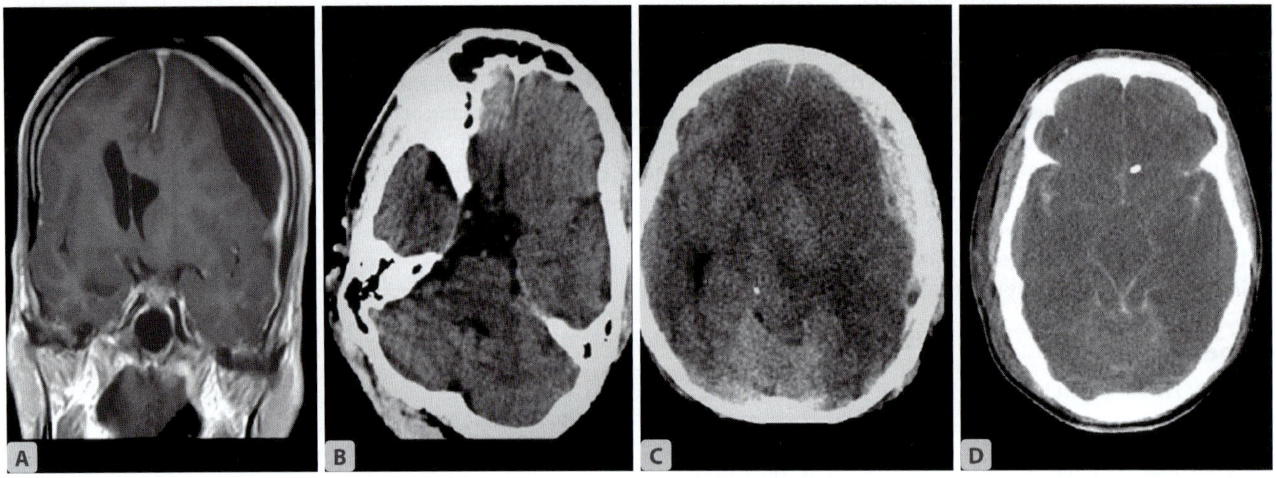

FIGS. 28A TO D: Axial CT images showing various types of brain herniations. (A) Subfalcine herniation; (B) Uncal herniation; (C) Downward transtentorial; and (D) Ascending transtentorial herniation.

Uncal herniation: Imaging features include displacement of the medial temporal lobe over the free margin of the tentorium, effacement of the ambient and lateral suprasellar cisterns. In severe cases, displacement can cause compression of the contralateral cerebral peduncle against the tentorium (Kernohan's notch), leading to peduncular infarction or hemorrhage.

Transtentorial herniation can occur either in upward or downward direction.

Upward herniation typically occurs with large posterior fossa hematomas that displace portions of the cerebellum and vermis through the tentorial incisura. The mass effect of the hematoma can also cause downward herniation of the cerebellar tonsils through the foramen magnum.

Downward herniation of the cerebrum manifests as effacement of the suprasellar and perimesencephalic cisterns. Inferior displacement of the pineal calcification is an additional imaging clue for the presence of downward herniation.

3. **Infarction or ischemia** can complicate TBI as a result of increased intracranial pressure or mass effect on cerebral vasculature by herniation or hematoma. In addition to ACA infarction secondary to the subfalcine herniation described above, uncal herniation and tonsillar herniation can cause ischemia in the territory of the posterior cerebral artery and the posteriorinferior cerebellar artery distributions, respectively **(Fig. 29)**.

Chronic Secondary Changes

1. **Traumatic hydrocephalus** occurs secondary to impaired CSF resorption at the level of the arachnoid villi or secondary to obstruction of the cerebral aqueduct and 4th ventricular outflow by SAH or IVH. Mass effect from cerebral herniation or a hematoma can also cause non-communicating hydrocephalus via compression of the aqueduct and ventricular outflow foramina **(Fig. 30)**.[9,23]

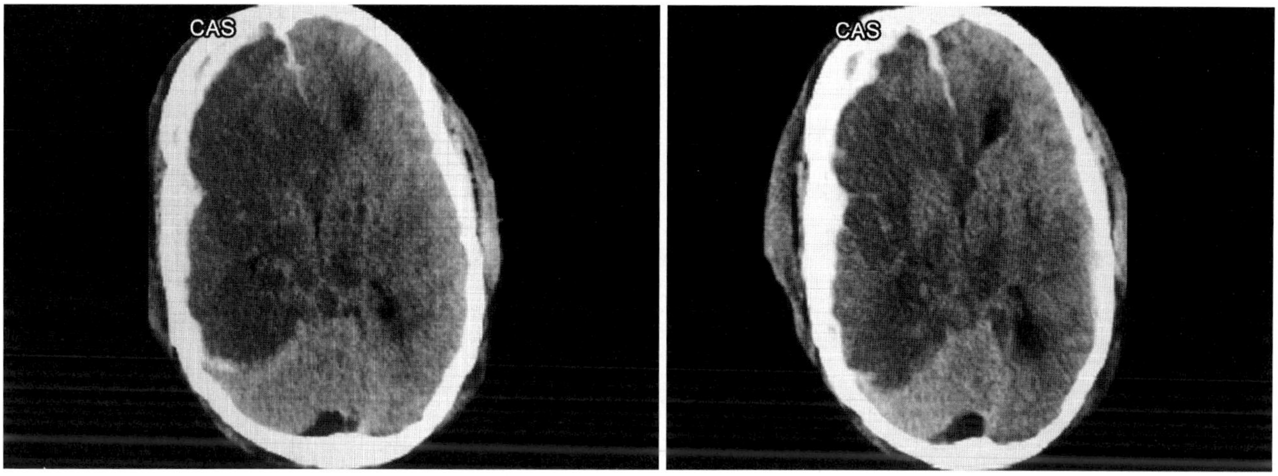

FIG. 29: Axial CT images showing almost near complete infarction of right cerebral hemisphere secondary to increased intracranial pressure following head injury.

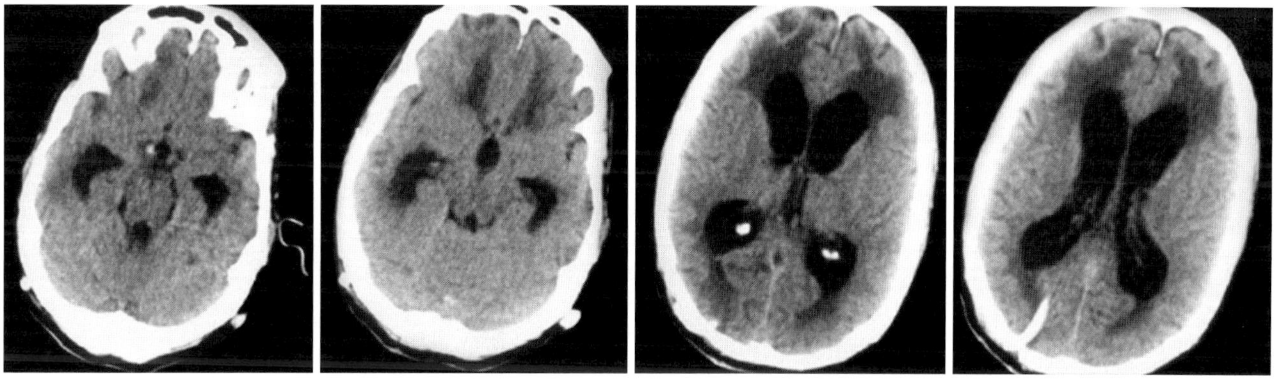

FIG. 30: Axial CT images showing communicating hydrocephalus with periventricular ooze in follow-up scan as a complication of SAH.

2. **Encephalomalacia** is a common, but nonspecific, sequelae of prior parenchyma injury. It may be clinically asymptomatic, but it can also be a potential seizure focus. On CT, the imaging appearance consists of an area of low attenuation with volume loss. It typically follows CSF signal intensity on both CT and MR, except for the areas of gliosis, which appears as low intensity on T1- and high intensity on T2-weighted images. If on imaging encephalomalacia is seen within the orbitofrontal (especially the gyrus rectus) and anteroinferior temporal lobes then it is characteristically due to remote traumatic injury **(Fig. 31)**.
3. **Cerebrospinal fluid (CSF) leak** occurs when there is an osseous and dural defect at the skull base, with direct communication of the subarachnoid space to the extracranial space, usually a paranasal sinus. Recognition of the leak site and source and appropriate treatment are necessary to avoid rhinorrhea or otorrhea, low-pressure headaches, and meningitis, known complications of CSF leak.[32,33]
   - **CSF otorrhea** occurs when there is communication between the subarachnoid space and middle ear in association with a ruptured tympanic membrane.
   - **CSF rhinorrhea** occurs when there is communication between the subarachnoid space and the paranasal sinuses.

About 80% of post-traumatic CSF leaks occur within the first 48 hours after injury, and 95% will manifest within the first 3 months. A small subset of patients will present with rhinorrhea or meningitis decades after the trauma.

Imaging[32,33]

The goals of imaging are
- To confirm the diagnosis
- Evaluate for an underlying cause,
- Localize and characterize the defect site prior to surgical repair, and
- Exclude an associated meningocele at the defect.

Since small skull base defects are now routinely repaired with nasal endoscopy, accurate localization is imperative. CSF leaks are often difficult to localize and a variety of nuclear medicine and cross-sectional computed tomographic and magnetic resonance imaging techniques have been applied to diagnose, localize, and characterize skull base defects responsible for leakage of

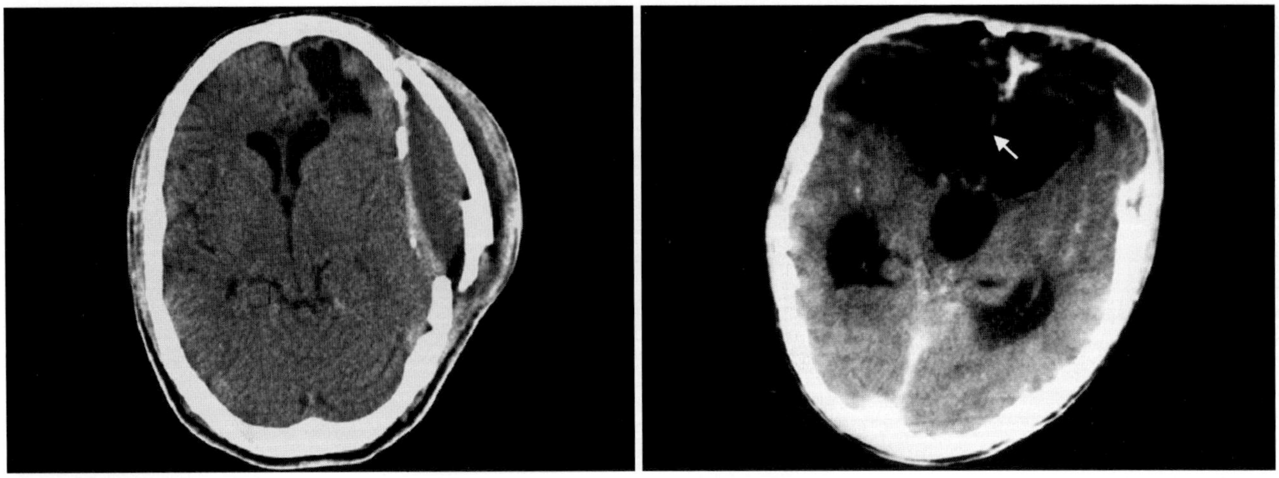

FIG. 31: Axial CT images showing areas of gliosis with exvacuodilatation of ventricles suggestive of encephalomalacia, sequelae of prior parenchyma injury.

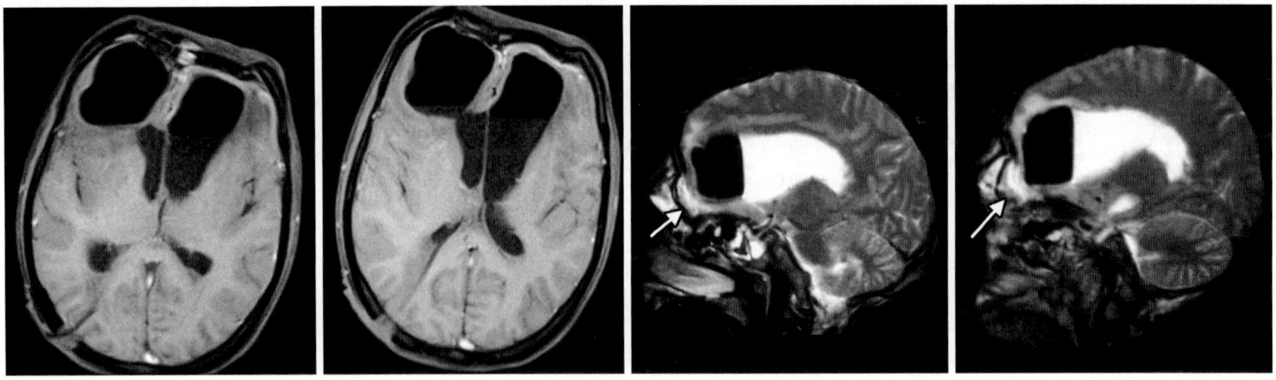

FIG. 32: MR images in multiple planes showing herniation ofbrain parenchyma through the bone defect in anterior cranial fossa (arrows) and air-cerebrospinal fluid level suggestive of communication with paranasal sinuses.

CSF. So far there has been no imaging "gold standard" for the diagnosis of CSF leak.

CT Imaging

The use of CT for evaluation of skull base defects has become a mainstay in the workup of CSF fistula, due to its ability to resolve osseous structures. With the advent of modern thin-section and multidetector CT scanners, smaller defects are visualized with a reported sensitivity as high as 92% and specificity of 100%. The CT findings suggestive of a CSF leak include a skull base bone defect and an air-fluid level or opacification of the contiguous sinus. In the evaluation of temporal bone CT scans, a unilaterally opacified mastoid and middle ear, in the presence of a tegmen defect or fracture through an inner ear structure, is consistent with CSF fistula.

MR imaging techniques offer noninvasive methods of imaginga CSF leak and are indicated to assess possible encephalocele or meningoencephalocele. Herniation of brain parenchyma or meninges through the bone defect may be difficult to differentiate from obstructed secretions on CT scans but is obvious on MR images **(Fig. 32)**.

CT Cisternography

CT cisternography is being used widely for evaluating a possible CSF fistula. This technique traditionally involves obtaining thin-section coronal and axial CT images in both prone and supine positions through the region of interest (maxillofacial or temporal region) both before and after intrathecal contrast material. Approximately 3–10 mL of an iodinated nonionic low-osmolar contrast agent is administered by means of lumbar puncture, and the patient is placed in a Trendelenburg position to opacify the basal cisterns, followed by CT imaging after administration of contrast material. Manoeuvres that provoke an active leak, such as sneezing or head hanging, are performed prior to the CT portion of cisternography. Postcontrast images are then compared with the precontrast images. A positive result involves the presence of a skull base defect and contrast opacification within the sinus, nasal cavity, or middle ear.

MR cisternography typically involves heavily T2-weighted fast spin-echo sequences with fat suppression and subtraction of the adjacent background tissue signal to enhance conspicuity of the fistulous tract, or CSF column. The fast spin-echo sequences have decreased

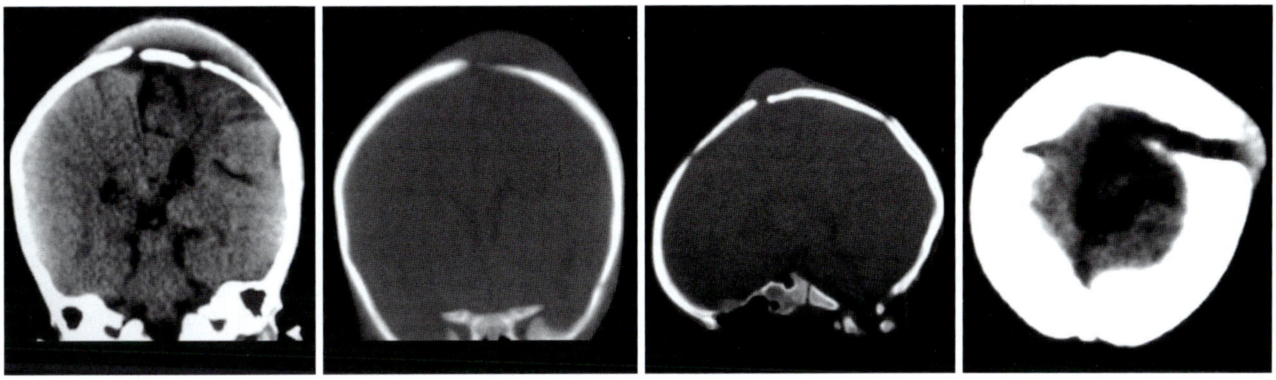

FIG. 33: CT images showing features of leptomeningeal cyst (growing fracture) as evidenced by herniation of subarachanoid space though the fracture line into subcutaneous tissue with underlying encephalomalacia, focal ventricular enlargement.

susceptibility artifacts at the air-bone interface of the skull base, compared with conventional T2-weighted imaging. Images are generally obtained in coronal, axial, and sagittal planes, and, similar to conventional MR, the finding of a contiguous CSF column communicating from the subarachnoid space to the extracranial space and/or the herniation of brain parenchyma and/or meninges, extracranially heralds a positive examination.

4. **The leptomeningeal cyst or "growing fracture"** is usually seen children and are accompanied by tear in the dura in association with a calvarial defect.[34]

Leptomeningeal cysts are usually delayed complications of skull fractures, although they occasionally occur within weeks of trauma. Since the infant skull is highly malleable, the margins of pediatric skull fractures are often inwardly displaced at the time of trauma. Depressed, or transiently depressed, fractures can easily lacerate the underlying dura and severely contuse the adjacent brain. The pia-arachnoid membrane (and occasionally swollen, edematous cortex) can herniate through the dural tear and prevent apposition and healing of the dura. CSF pulsations subsequently fill and enlarge the subarachnoid pouch that extends through the fracture line. The pulsations eventually widen the dural defect and expand the fracture margins. This results in a leptomeningeal cyst that extends from the subarachnoid space into the subgaleal space. CSF pulsations tend to erode the inner table more than the outer one, giving rise to "beveled" edges. The margins of the fracture often show marked resorption and saucerization.

The term "growing fracture" refers to interval widening of the space between the fracture margins on successive skull radiographs or CT scans. CT scans obtained after the development of the leptomeningeal cyst often reveal posttraumatic encephalomalacia, focal ventricular enlargement, and porencephaly because of the prior associated brain injury **(Fig. 33)**.[35]

CONCLUSION

The main aim of imaging in the management of head trauma is to identify treatable injuries so as to prevent secondary brain damage. CT remains the modality of choice in the evaluation of acute head injury, because it is fast, is widely available, and can easily accommodate life-support and monitoring equipment. CT can accurately identify acute hemorrhages, mass effect, midline shift, hydrocephalus, ischemia, and herniation. An advance in CT methods such as CT perfusion offers prognostic information with respect to functional outcome, even as early as at the time of admission. MRI should be used as a problem solving modality and is indicated for patients with acute TBI when the neurologic findings cannot be explained by CT. MRI is also the modality of choice for subacute or chronic injury. An advance in MR methods, such as diffusion-weighted imaging, has improved the neuroradiological evaluation of traumatic brain injury and offers a better understanding of the pathophysiological manifestations of head trauma.

REFERENCES

1. MacDorman MF, Minino AM, Strobino DM, et al. Annual summary of vital statistics—2001. Pediatrics 2002;110(6):1037-52.
2. National Center for Injury Prevention and Control. Injury Fact Book 2001-2002. Atlanta, GA: Centers for Disease Control and Prevention; 2001.
3. Teasdale G, Jennett B. Assessment of coma and impaired consciousness: a practical scale. Lancet 1974;13:81-4.
4. Marshall LF, Marshall SB, Klauber MR, et al. A new classification of head injury based on computerised tomography. J Neurosurg 1991;75(Suppl):S14-20.
5. Kunitz SC, Gross C. A National Traumatic Coma Data Bank. Proc Annu Symp Comput Appl Med Care. 1980;2:1333-9.
6. Bell RS, Loop JW. The utility and futility of radiographic skull examination for trauma. N Engl J Med. 1971;284(5):236-9.
7. Hackney DB. Skull radiography in the evaluation of acute head trauma: a survey of current practice. Radiology. 1991;181(3): 711-14.
8. Masters SJ. Evaluation of head trauma: efcacy of skull lms. Am J Roentgenol. 1980;135(3):539-47.
9. Zee CS, Go JL. CT of head trauma. Neuroimaging Clin North Am. 1998;8(3):525-39.
10. Metting Z, Rödiger LA, Stewart RE, et al. Perfusion computed tomography in the acute phase of mild head injury: regional dysfunction and prognostic value. Ann Neurol. 2009;66(6): 809-16.

11. Wintermark M, van Melle G, Schnyder P, et al. Admission perfusion CT: prognostic value in patients with severe head trauma. Radiology. 2004;232(1):211-20.
12. Gentry LR, Godersky JC, Thompson B, et al. Prospective comparativestudy of intermediate-eld MR and CT in the evaluation of closed head trauma. Am J Roentgenol. 1988;150(3):673-82.
13. Orrison WW, Gentry LR, Stimac GK, et al. Blinded comparison of cranial CT and MR in closed head injury evaluation. Am J Neuroradiol. 1994;15(2):351-6.
14. Noguchi K, Ogawa T, Seto H, et al. Subacute and chronic subarachnoid hemorrhage: diagnosis with fluid-attenuated inversion-recovery MR imaging. Radiology. 1997;203(1):257-62.
15. Woodcock RJ Jr, Short J, Do HM, et al. Imaging of acute subarachnoid hemorrhage with a fluid-attenuated inversion recovery sequence in ananimal model: comparison with non-contrast-enhanced CT. Am J Neuroradiol. 2001;22(9):1698-1703.
16. Akiyama Y, Miyata K, Harada K, et al. Susceptibility-weighted magnetic resonance imaging for the detection of cerebral microhemorrhage in patients with traumatic brain injury. Neurol Med Chir (Tokyo) 2009;49(3):97-9.
17. Topal NB, Hakyemez B, Erdogan C, et al. MR imaging in the detection of diffuse axonal injury with mild traumatic brain injury. Neurol Res. 2008;30(9):974-8.
18. Le TH, Mukherjee P, Manley GT, et al. Automated detection of traumatic white matter injury using voxel-based morphometry of diffusiontensor images: a 3T study with parallel imaging. American Society of Neuroradiology 43rd Annual Meeting, May 23-27, 2005, Toronto, On tario, Canada, Paper 374.
19. Huisman TA, Sorensen AG, Hergan K, et al. Diffusion-weighted imaging for the evaluation of diffuse axonal injury in closed head injury. J Comput Assist Tomogr. 2003;27(1):5-11.
20. Liu AY, Maldjian JA, Bagley LJ, et al. Traumatic brain injury: diffusion-weighted MR imaging ndings. Am J Neuroradiol. 1999;20(9):1636-41.
21. Medina LS, Blackmore CC, Evidence based imaging of Traumatic Brain injury. Evidence-Based Imaging: Optimizing Imaging in Patient Care. Springer Science+Business Media, Eds. New York; 2006.
22. Gentry LR. Temporal bone trauma. Neuroimaging Clin North Am. 1991;1:319-40.
23. Gean AD, Kates RS, Lee S. Neuroimaging in head injury. New Horiz. 1995;3(3):549-61.
24. Al-Nakshabandi NA. The swirl sign. Radiology. 2001;218(2):433.
25. Loftus CM. Neurosurgical Emergencies, 2nd edition. Thieme Medical Publishers, New York; 2008.
26. Arfanakis K, Haughton VM, Carew JD, et al. Diffusion tensor MR imaging in diffuse axonal injury. Am J Neuroradiol. 2002;23(5):794-802.
27. Le TH, Mukherjee P, Henry RG, et al. Diffusion tensor imaging with three-dimensional ber tractography of traumatic axonal shearing injury: an imaging correlate for the posterior callosal "disconnection" syndrome: case report. Neurosurgery. 2005;56(1):189.
28. Adams JH, Graham DI, Gennarelli TA, et al. Diffuse axonal injury in non-missile head injury. J Neurol Neurosurg Psychiatry. 1991;54(6):481-3.
29. Hesselink JR, Dowd CF, Healy ME, et al. MR imaging of brain contusion: a comparative study with CT. Am J Neuroradiol. 1988;150:1133-42.
30. Gentry LR. Head trauma. In: Atlas SW (Ed). Magnetic Resonance Imaging of the Brain and Spine, 2nd edition. Philadelphia: PA, Lippincott-Raven; 1996.pp.611-47.
31. Tjoumakaris SI, Jabbour PM, Rosenwasser RH. Neuroendovascular management of carotid cavernous fistulae. Neurosurg Clin N Am. 2009;20(4):447-52.
32. Bullock R, Soares D. Current imaging of cerebrospinal fluid leaks. West Indian Med J. 2009;58(4):362-6.
33. Lloyd KM, DelGaudio JM, Hudgins PA. Imaging of skull base cerebrospinal fluid leaks in adults. Radiology. 2008;248: 725-36.
34. Husson B, Pariente D, Tammam S, el al. The value of MRI in the early diagnosis of growing skull fracture. Pediatr Radiol. 1996;26(10):744-7.
35. Poussaint TY, Moeller KK. Imaging of pediatric head trauma. Neuroimaging Clin N Am. 2002;12(2):271-94.

CHAPTER

211

Imaging of Facial Trauma

Ajay Kumar, Vivek Gupta, Paramjeet Singh

INTRODUCTION

Imaging of facial trauma requires a thorough knowledge of the regional anatomy and precise imaging techniques. These are required to restore the facial skeleton and prevent disfigurement. The facial skeleton has been described as a honeycomb structure of varying thickness and form, which are protected superficially by strong plate-like bone, so that the deepest and most delicate structures are well protected.

Classification of facial fracture was first described by Rene Le Fort in 1901.[1] He performed a series of macabre cadaveric experiments and described the three facial fractures which bear his name, the concept of which was based on three major levels of inherent facial weakness through which the fracture lines run. Le Fort method of classifying facial fracture was essentially a clinical one. The palpation of fracture margins, the instability of fractured segment, crepitus and plain X-rays provided the indirect evidence of the location of the injury.

The diagnosis of fracture was refined further with the help of plain X-rays and the conventional tomograms. However, the major drawback of this mode of investigation was that it overlooked the evaluation of soft tissues which is also an important aspect in the management of facial fracture.[2]

Computed tomography (CT) scanning not only visualizes the bony injury, but also provided insight into injury of the soft tissues. It also helped to give panoramic access to the entire facial skeleton from its most superficial surface to the intricate depth. The availability of high-spatial resolution and thin-section scanning added to the improvement of diagnosis of lesions of the orbits and its contents, nasoethmoidal region and fractures in children.[3,4] The need for reclassifying facial fractures was thus necessary and in 1980 Gentry et al. gave an extended concept in the imaging of fractures of this region.[5,6]

IMAGING TECHNIQUES

The maxillofacial region represents a complex area for diagnosis especially when it is injured. Most patients with acute maxillofacial trauma do not cooperate for radiographic evaluation and often the situation is further hampered due to associated severe life-threatening injuries, such as injuries to the cervical spine.[7] Tailored radiographic projections and imaging techniques are required to assess the injuries. A systematic approach is thus essential so that all the fractures are delineated and the soft-tissue injuries are adequately demonstrated.

Plain radiography has been the first line of investigation. However, the complexity of the modern high-velocity injuries, the precision required in the diagnosis of fractures as well as the demanding legal aspects of facial injuries highlight the inadequacy and inherent limitations of plain radiography alone as the imaging tool.[8]

Noncontrast CT scan is the modality of choice for the complete evaluation of the osseous and soft-tissue component of facial fractures, the brain and dura. Both axial and coronal sections are done to provide the clinician a complete insight of orientation of fractured segments. Patient cooperation is essential to do direct coronal sections. However, with helical CT overlapping axial acquisitions can be used to reconstruct two- and three-dimensional (3D) views of the facial skeleton. 3D reconstructions are especially useful in treatment planning. This technique enables the surgeon to have a global assessment of the injuries, to locate bony fragments and their relationships when several sites are involved. It enables optimal presurgical planning, indicates the anatomical areas involved and determines the number of fracture lines where miniplates are to be affixed. The display of information in orthogonal planes enhances the perception of malocclusion and comminution and directs the appropriate therapeutic approach. 3D-volumetric evaluation can provide area measurements and volume changes. Measurements of bony landmarks on 3D reconstructions are qualitatively accurate for planning surgery and evaluation of the treatment.[9-12] Dual energy CT (DECT) has shown to be effective in producing significantly improved images in the presence of metal artifacts by using metal suppression techniques.[13]

Although standard CT scanners with three-dimensional dataset are routinely used for maxillofacial trauma, it exposes the patient to a higher radiation dose.[14] A dental CT scanner based on cone beam CT (CBCT) is becoming more popular in diagnosis and treatment planning for maxillofacial trauma because of less radiation dose and its ability to produce accurate three-dimensional imaging.[15,16]

As expected, CBCT offers lower radiation dose compared with standard CT machines: the integral absorbed radiation dose of radiation was less than one-fifteenth that of spiral CT when the exposure condition of the latter was optimized.[17] The radiation dose from CBCT was significantly lower than the lowest dose from conventional CT in terms of effective dose and dose to the lens.[17] Moreover, because of its smaller size, it is possible to install the CBCT scanner in the operative room or physicians' clinic itself which enables the treating physician to assess the adequacy of surgery and immediate appropriate measures for correction.[18] Although the CBCT has found to produce excellent bony details which is comparable to conventional CT, the soft tissue resolution is low because of its inherent low contrast resolution. Hence if soft tissue evaluation is intended, either conventional CT or MRI should be considered.[18]

Magnetic resonance imaging (MRI) has a limited role to play in the assessment of facial fractures since it does not visualize bone directly. MRI is especially helpful in the following situations: (a) in differentiating blood from inflammatory reactions and edema fluid especially, if MRI is performed after 48 hours of trauma. In this situation, such an investigation is directed by those groups of surgeons who wait for several days after trauma before surgical correction as they believe soft-tissue injury will subside and surgery becomes easier, and (b) imaging of injured orbit and its contents can also be better performed on MRI. These fractures of bony orbit can themselves be diagnosed by recognition of the fat invaginating into adjoining paranasal sinuses.[19] MRI is also risky in patients with roadside accidents as there is always risk of metallic foreign body deep inside.

FACIAL BUTTRESSES AND REGIONAL CLASSIFICATION OF INJURIES[5,6]

Le Fort determined the predictable lines of least resistance through which fracture lines run. The forces, which generated these fractures, were small as compared to those of modern day high-velocity injury. Hence, the injuries, which we encounter now-a-days, incorporate the Le Fort fractures together with complex fractures with multiple fracture lines. In keeping with the general concept of plate-like structures, which constitute the facial skeleton; the current analysis of fracture is based on the concept of anatomical buttresses **(Figs. 1 to 4)**.[9]

There are two sagittal buttresses described, on each side of the face. The medial sagittal buttress extends from the maxillary alveolus up to the lateral wall of pyriform aperture and into the medial orbital wall. This buttress comprises of lower maxilla, frontal process of maxilla, lacrimal bone and nasal process of frontal bone. This forms a medial supportive pillar on each of the midline and is termed as the nasomaxillary buttress. The lateral sagittal buttress is formed on each side by the lateral wall of maxilla, body of zygoma orbital process of frontal bone in lateral orbital wall. This is termed as the zygomaticomaxillary buttress. A third buttress called the pterygomaxillary buttress extending from the posterior maxillary alveolus towards the pterygoid plates has also been described.[9] The sagittal group of buttresses also includes a median strut formed by nasal septum. These sagittal buttresses are reinforced by three horizontal buttresses formed by: (1) the floor of the anterior cranial fossa, (2) the orbital floor and zygomatic arches, and (3) the hard palate respectively.

The above two groups of facial supports are in turn strengthened by two conceptualized coronal buttresses. They are called the anterior-coronal buttress and the posterior-coronal buttress. The anterior buttress comprises of the anterior wall of frontal and maxillary sinuses, the nasofrontal process, the zygomaticofrontal buttress and the anterior maxillary alveolar arch. The posterior-coronal buttress comprises of two bilaterally symmetrical walls of maxillary sinus and the pterygoid plates.

Importance of Facial Buttresses[20]

- Buttresses have sufficient bone thickness to accommodate metal screw fixation
- Buttresses are all linked either directly or through another buttress
- Transverse buttresses reduction restores the facial width and vertical reduction restores the facial height
- Buttresses reduction establishes a functional support for teeth and globes.

Table 1 summarizes the components of the facial struts.

CLASSIFICATION OF MAXILLOFACIAL FRACTURES

Facial fractures can be classified by type, location or extension and complexity of the fractures. A detailed system under these different systems is depicted in **Table 2**.

It is evident from **Table 2**, that no single system can describe the complex morbid anatomy of the facial fractures. This is especially true for high-velocity accidents where the injury force acts from multiple directions on the face grossly distorting the anatomy. The traditional and oldest accepted classification of facial fractures of Le Fort merits mention in the modern context. High-impact facial fractures, such as those in automobile accidents, are so extensive and complicated that so-called "pure" Le Fort fractures are unusual. The Le Fort classification can be reworked in the newer framework of buttresses as summarized in **Table 3**. The Le Fort fractures, therefore, can be incorporated in the fractures of the midface **(Figs. 5 and 6)**.

The complexities of the midfacial fractures including Le Fort III need a special mention at this point. These injuries result in distortion of the anatomy in midface causing severe post-traumatic deformities. It is also important to realize that these fractures are often associated with severe intracranial, orbital and paranasal sinus injuries which need special concern in the treatment protocol.[9]

Regional Facial Fractures

Frontal Sinus Fractures

They can result from extensions from calvarial fractures into the frontal sinus or due to direct blows to the forehead.

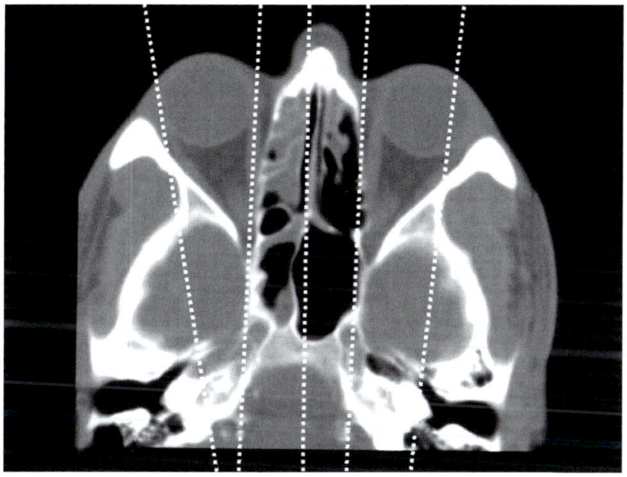

FIG. 1: Axial computed tomography (CT) section at the level of orbits, optic foramen and sphenoid sinus. The midline sagittal strut, parasagittal strut and the lateral sagittal struts are indicated.

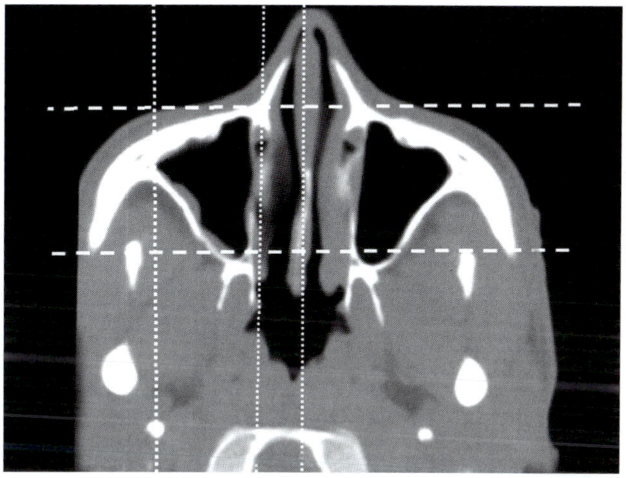

FIG. 2: Axial computed tomography (CT) section at the level of maxillary sinuses with the condyles and pterygoid plates. The anterior and posterior coronal buttress (dashed line) together with the right sagittal buttress (dotted line) are indicated.

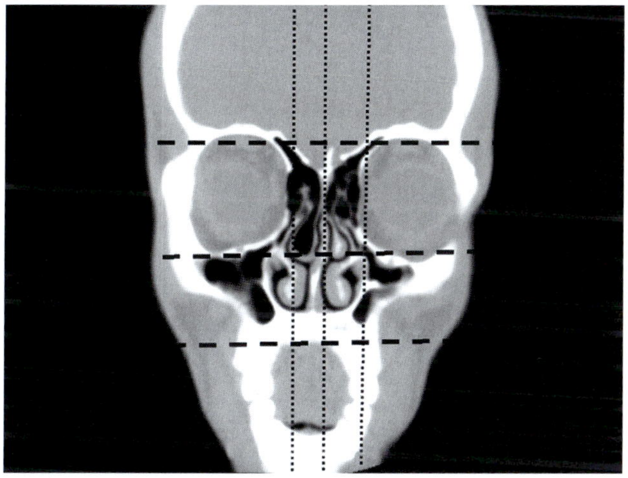

FIG. 3: Coronal computed tomography (CT) section at the level of orbits showing the superior, middle and inferior horizontal struts aligned along the orbital plates, inferior orbital margin and the alveolus. In addition, the position of the sagittal struts are indicated.

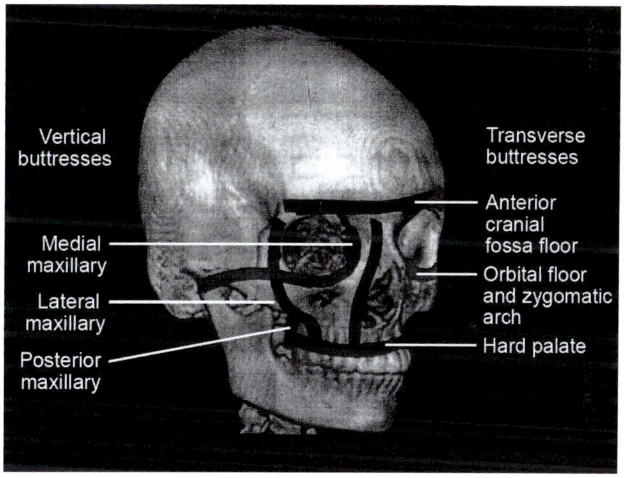

FIG. 4: Diagrammatical representation of facial buttresses system.

TABLE 1: Components of the facial struts.

Superior horizontal	Cribriform plate, ethmoid sinus roof, orbital roof
Middle horizontal	Orbital floor, zygomatic arch
Inferior horizontal	Palate/maxillary alveolus
Midline sagittal	Nasal septum, Vomer
Parasagittal	Medial orbital wall, medial maxillary sinus wall, lateral maxillary alveolus
Lateral sagittal	Lateral orbital wall, lateral maxillary sinus wall
Anterior coronal	Nasal arch, anterior and posterior walls of the frontal sinus, anterior wall of the maxillary sinus, anterior maxillary alveolus
Posterior coronal	Posterior aspect of the maxillary sinus, pterygoid plate

The fractures are described in relation to the anterior and posterior walls of the sinus. The anterior wall of the sinus is most commonly involved resulting in hemorrhage or edema. The sinus appears opaque on plain radiographs. The fracture is best appreciated on lateral views of the skull. They may be obscured on the standard posteroanterior (PA) and Water's projections. CT scan is very helpful to delineate the fractured segments in cases of comminuted fractures **(Figs. 7 and 8)**. It is also helpful to localize injury to the posterior wall of the sinuses and the adjacent orbital palate.

Fractures of the posterior wall of the frontal sinus may result in pneumocephalus. They may also present with cerebrospinal fluid (CSF) rhinorrhea due to tears in the dura of the anterior cranial fossa. Noncomminuted

TABLE 2: Classification of maxillofacial fractures.

Traditional Le Fort classification	• Le Fort I • Le Fort II • Le Fort III		
Based on the type of fracture	• Closed (simple) • Open (compound) • Green stick • Comminuted • Undisplaced • Displaced		
Based on location of fracture	Upper third of the face	• Frontal sinuses (glabella) • Supraorbital ridge • Frontal bone	
	Middle third of the face	• Nasal bones and septum • Naso-orbital area • Zygoma • Zygomatic arch • Orbital floor	
		• *Maxilla*	– Transverse (Le Fort I) – Pyramidal (Le Fort II) – Craniofacial dysjunction (Le Fort III)
	Lower third of the face (mandible)	• Alveolar process • Symphysis • Body • Angle • Ascending ramus • Coronoid process • Condyle • Temporomandibular joint region	
Based on the extent of fracture line	• Limited fracture • Transfacial fracture		

TABLE 3: The Le Fort classification.

Type	Structures involved	Strut
Le Fort I	• Anterior, lateral and medial walls of the maxillary sinuses • Nasal septum • Pterygoid plate	• Parasagittal • Lateral sagittal • Anterior coronal • Midline sagittal • Posterior coronary
Le Fort II	• Nasion (nasal bones, arch, or nasofrontal suture) • Medial orbital wall, lacrimal bone • Orbital floor • Anterior maxillary wall • Lateral maxillary wall • Pterygoid plate	• Anterior coronal • Parasagittal • Middle horizontal • Anterior coronal • Lateral sagittal • Posterior coronal
Le Fort III	• Nasion (nasal bones, arch, or nasofrontal suture) • Medial orbital wall, lacrimal bone • Lateral orbital wall • Zygoma • Pterygoid plate	• Anterior coronal • Parasagittal • Lateral sagittal • Middle horizontal • Posterior coronal

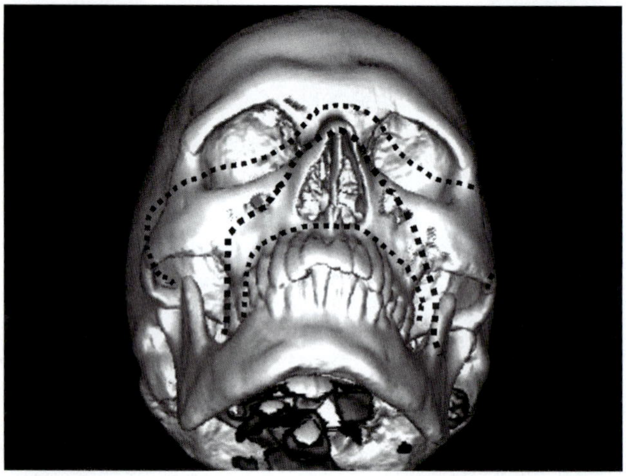

FIG. 5: Fracture lines in the Le Fort I, II and III fractures.

fractures of the frontal sinus involving the anterior wall may be managed conservatively or by relatively simple surgical procedures to restore the contour of the forehead, whereas the more complex comminuted fracture may at times require cranialization of the sinus.[9]

Recognizing nasofrontal outflow tract injuries on CT is of utmost importance as injury to the outflow tract can lead to formation of frontal mucocele and creation of an anaerobic environment leading to subsequent osteomyelitis and possible intracranial extension leading to brain abscess. Such injuries should be strongly suspected on CT if there is involvement of the base of the frontal sinus, the anterior ethmoids, or both.

Nasal Fractures

Nasal bone fractures are amongst the most common facial fractures. About half of these, fractures are isolated nasal pyramid fractures. It is important to differentiate nasal cartilage injuries from nasal bone injuries. Cartilage injuries result from lateral blows to the nose. The nasal cartilages may be depressed with fracture of the ipsilateral nasal bone. Early detection of cartilage injuries is essential as they are often associated with a hematoma which needs to be evacuated. Nasal bone fractures result from anterior blows to the nose **(Figs. 9A to D)**. Such low-velocity injuries result in fractures of the lower third of the nasal bones which are thin. Typically, the nasoethmoid margin is intact.[9]

Central Midface Fractures

The central midface fractures include the naso-orbito-ethmoidal (NOE) fractures, isolated fractures of the maxillary alveolar process and hard palate, and the Le Fort fractures **(Figs. 9 and 10)**.[9]

Naso-orbito-ethmoidal Fractures

They result from a direct impact to the bridge of the nose resulting in fractures of the nasal bones, nasal septum, ethmoid sinuses, frontal process of the maxilla, lamina papyracea, lacrimal bone and the cribriform plate. The NOE fractures are complex because they can be associated with intracranial and orbital injuries and a head and face

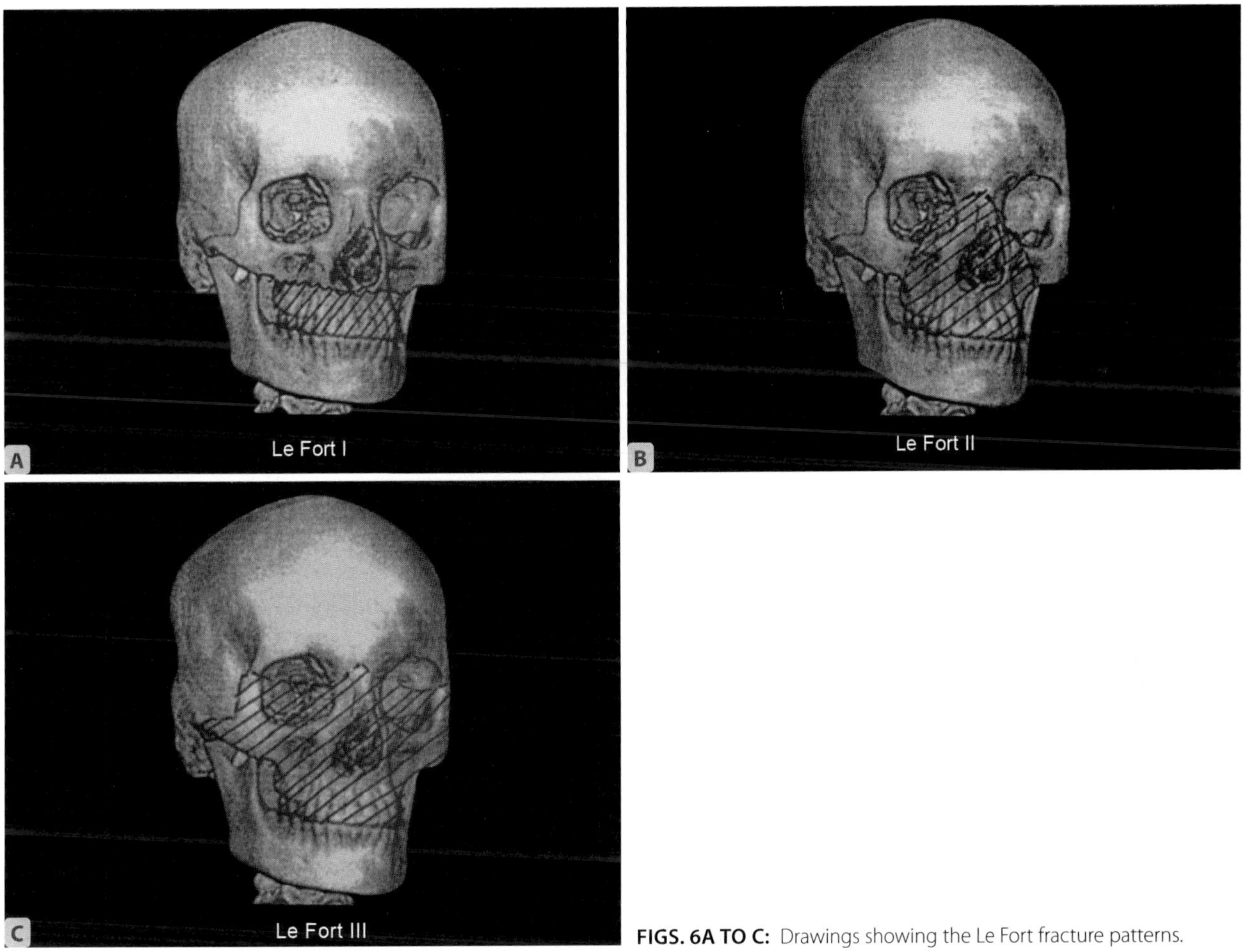

FIGS. 6A TO C: Drawings showing the Le Fort fracture patterns.

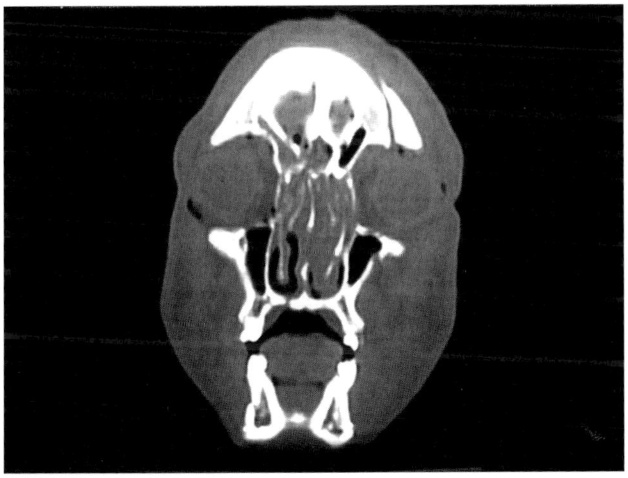

FIG. 7: Computed tomography (CT) three-dimensional coronal reconstruction image shows slightly displaced fracture of left frontal and ethmoid fractures with soft-tissue densities and air specks in orbit and sino-nasal cavities.

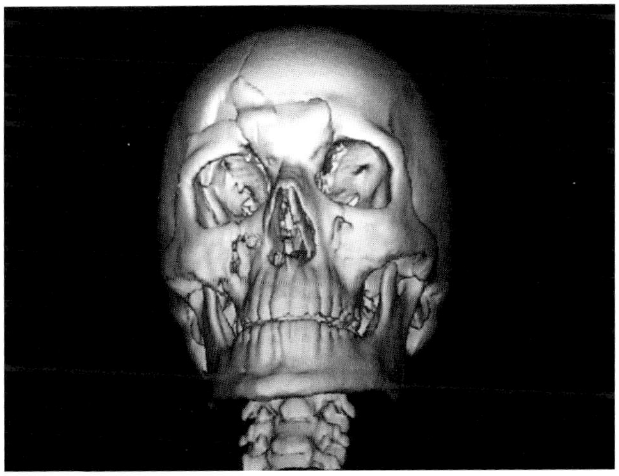

FIG. 8: Three-dimensional volume-rendered image (VRT) reconstruction showing fracture of frontal bone involving superior fracture of frontal bone involving superior orbital margins with right inferior orbital rim fracture.

CT scan is warranted. The floor of the anterior cranial fossa may be fractured in continuation with these structures. The latter fracture may tear the dura resulting in CSF leaks. NOE injuries are divided in three groups according to the degree of injury to the medial canthal attachment using the Manson classification **(Table 4)**.[21] The classification is important from treatment point of view as the most important factor determining the need for surgical correction in NOE fractures is the stability of the bone to which the medial canthal tendon attaches which is generally

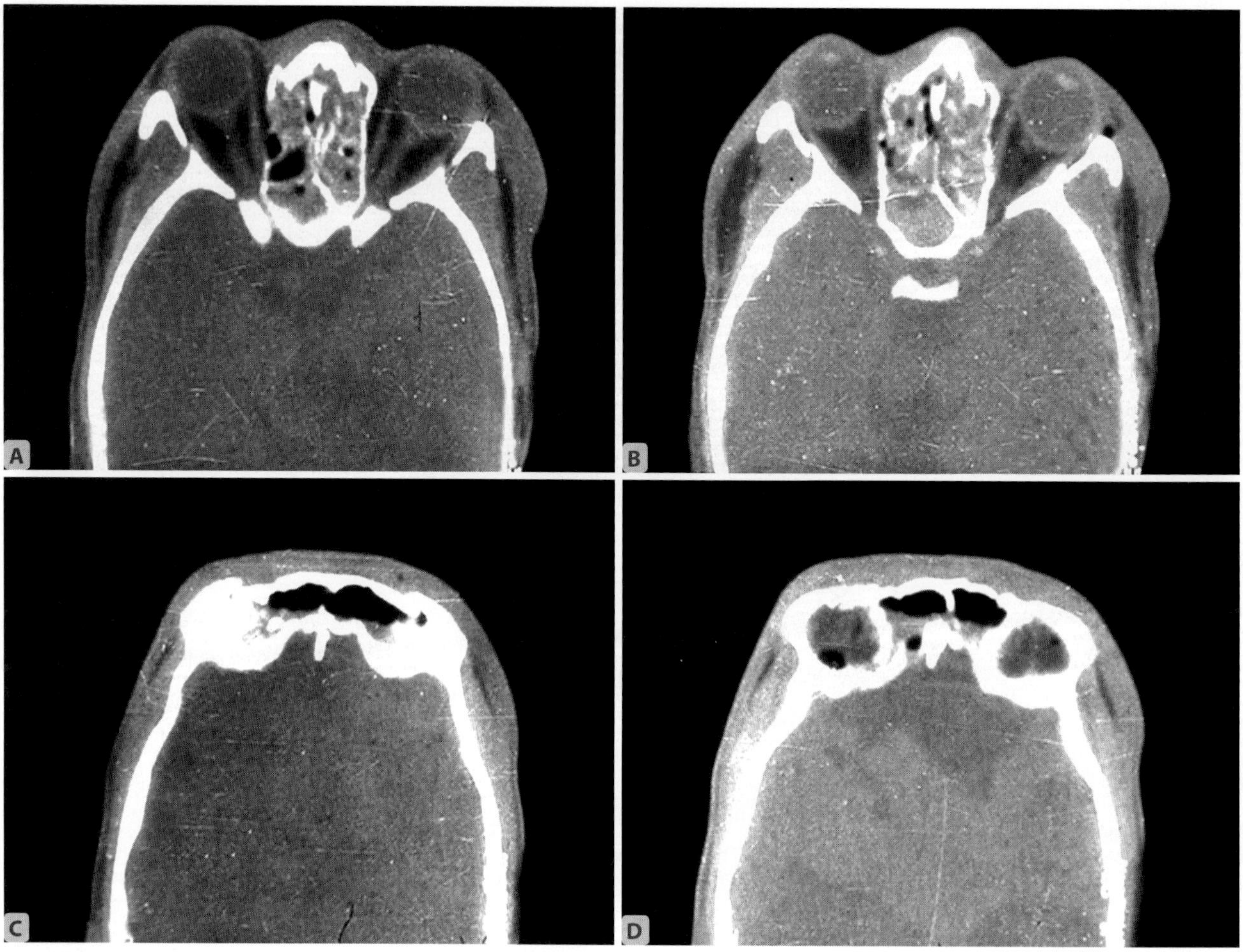

FIGS. 9A TO D: Fracture nasal bones as a result of a direct blow to the bridge of the nose resulting in a depression. Note the accordion-like collapse of the ethmoid bones and a concomitant fracture of the anterior wall of the frontal sinus containing blood.

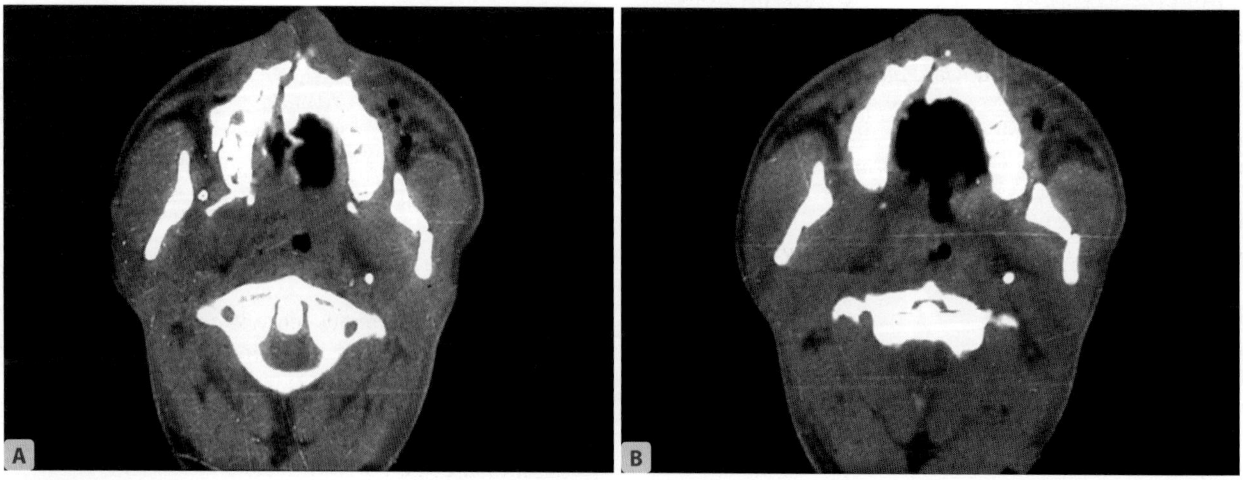

FIGS. 10A AND D *Continued*

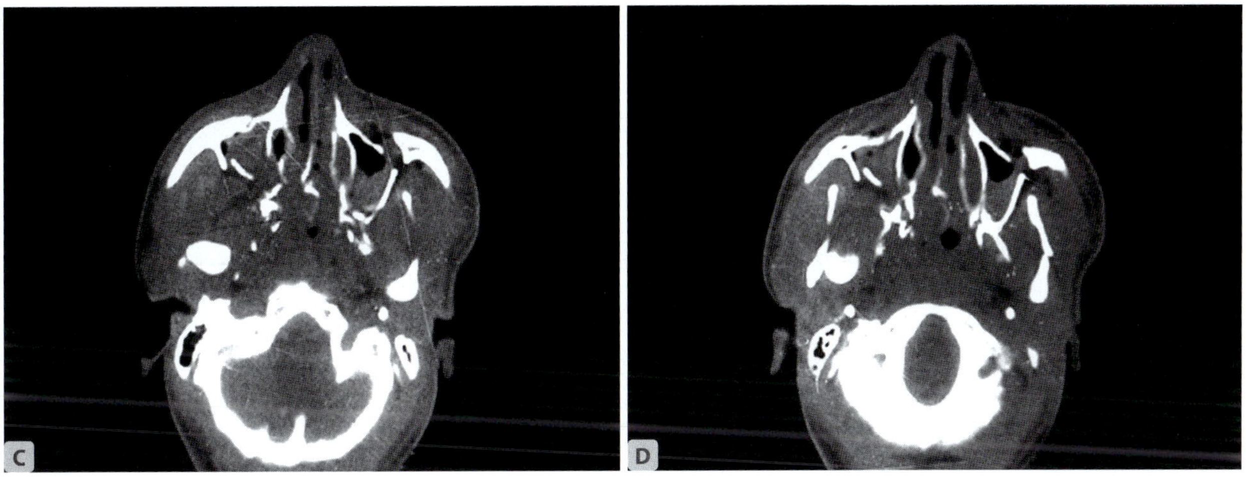

FIGS. 10A TO D: Fracture of the hard palate through the plane of the right palatine foramen as a component of a Le Fort II fracture. Note the fracture of both maxillae.

TABLE 4: Manson classification of naso-orbito-ethmoidal fractures.

Type 1	Single fragment (most common)
Type 2	Comminuted with intact insertion of medial canthal tendon
Type 3	Comminuted with lateral displacement or avulsion of medial canthal ligament (uncommon)

the anterior aspect of medial orbital wall.[22] In addition, the nasolacrimal canal injury is a frequent association of NOE fractures and should be clearly mentioned in CT report as the patients may be asymptomatic in early period but later may develop epiphora or recurrent dacrocystorhinitis.[22]

Isolated Fractures of the Maxillary Alveolus and Hard Palate

They result from a direct upward blow to the mandible which pushes the mandible into the maxilla. The fracture can injure the teeth which can be displaced or devitalized. The hard palate is fractured in the parasagittal plane along the palatine process of the maxilla which is the weakest plane of the hard palate. An axial or oblique blow to the chin or a direct injury to the upper jaw results in these type of fractures.

Le Fort Fractures

- *Le Fort type I fractures*: These fractures extend through the lower nasal septum, inferior walls of the maxillary sinuses and pterygoid plates. This results in palate being displaced posteriorly and malocclusion. There is associated hemorrhage in the maxillary sinuses.
- *Le Fort type II fractures*: These are characterized by fractures through the root of the nose, the lacrimal bones and medial orbital walls, thence on to the floor of the orbits, zygomaticomaxillary suture and the anterior wall of the maxilla. There may be posterior extension towards the inferior edge of the pterygoid plates **(Figs. 9 to 11)**.

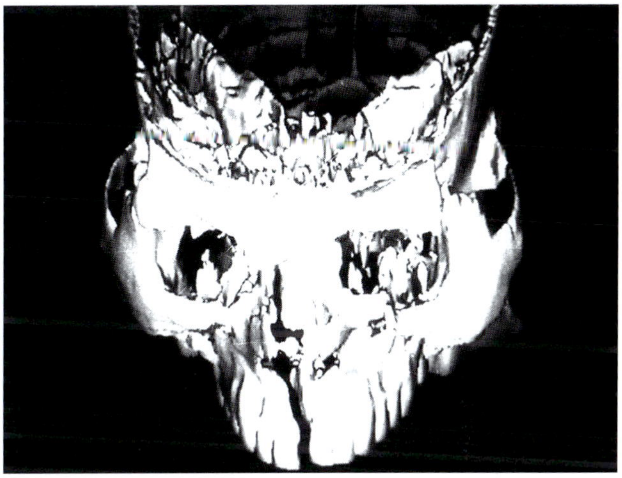

FIG. 11: Three-dimensional (3D) reconstruction of the same patient of Figure 6 showing the involvement of the superior alveolus.

- *Le Fort type III fractures*: These fractures include the entire gamut of injuries included in Le Fort type II fractures with extension into the lateral orbital walls and zygoma. This results in the separation of the entire facial skeleton from the skull base.

There are numerous components in the Le Fort fractures that make classification difficult; however, each of the Le Fort fractures has at least one unique component that is easily recognizable. Therefore, first recognize the unique component as: fracture of lateral margin of nasal fossa indicates Le Fort I, inferior orbital rim (Le Fort II) and zygomatic arch (Le Fort III). Secondly confirm the presence of other fractures which is suspected Le Fort plane.[23] Patient with higher grade Le Fort injuries more frequently need surgical airway. Le fort III injuries have higher chance of requiring neurosurgical intervention and may need immediate intensive care unit (ICU) care.[24]

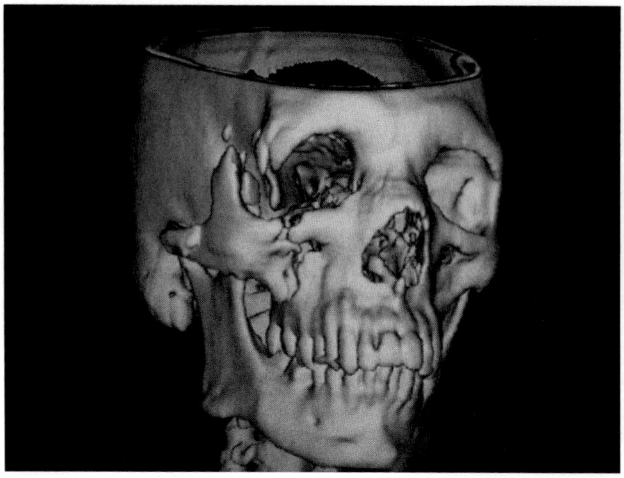

FIG. 12: Trimalar fracture of right zygomatic bone showing three fracture lines which characterize this fracture.

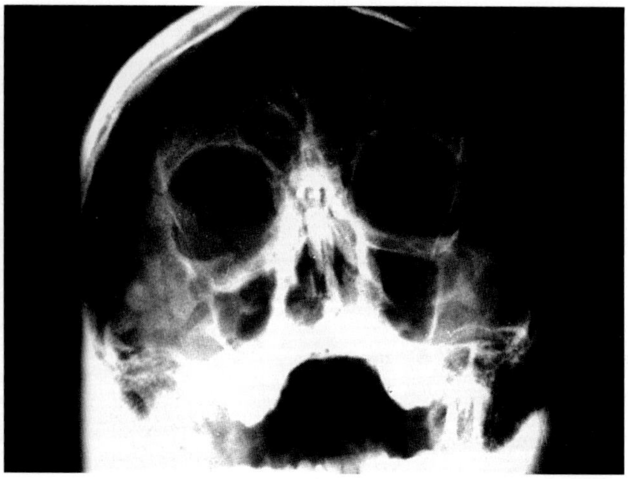

FIG. 13: Blow out fracture of the right orbit showing the fracture of the inferior margin of the orbit in the Walter's view.

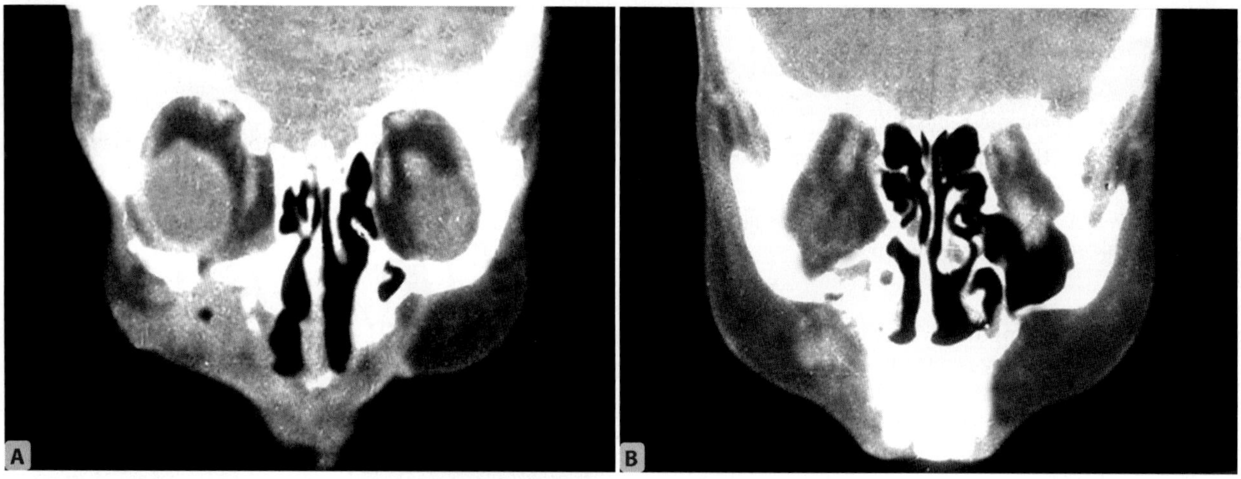

FIGS. 14A AND B: Coronal computed tomography (CT) sections showing the fracture line along the inferior orbital rim and inferior displacement of the globe.

Lateral Midface Fractures

They include the trimalar (zygomatic) fractures, fractures of the zygomatic arch and the zygomaticomaxillary/ zygomaticomandibular fractures. The blowout fractures of the orbits are also included in the fractures of this region.[9]

Trimalar or Zygomatic Fractures

They are so termed because they involve three bony connections of the zygomatic bone namely with the: (1) lateral orbital wall, (2) zygomatic bone and (3) maxilla. The fracture line runs from the lateral orbital wall down to the inferior orbital fissure, along the orbital floor and anterior maxillary wall. The line then turns to involve the lateral wall of the maxilla to end at or near the inferior orbital fissure. These fractures are the second most common fractures of the facial skeleton, the first being fractures of the nasal bone **(Fig. 12)**.

Zygomaticomaxillary Fractures

They include a maxillary component to the zygomatic fracture which includes the hard palate and the pterygoid plates.

The Zygomaticomandibular Fractures

They include fractures of the mandibular condyle or coronoid process in addition to the zygomatic fracture outlined above.[9]

Blowout Fractures of the Orbit

Injuries to the orbital margins result in blowout fractures. Typically, injuries result due to an object larger than orbit. The force of the injury results in the transmission of the vector to the orbital floor. The floor is fractured in the middle third close to the infraorbital canal. Rarely, the inferior orbital rim is fractured resulting in the so-called impure blowout fracture. Herniation of the orbital fat, inferior rectus and inferior oblique muscle into the maxillary antrum may result. Rarely, the fractured fragments may protrude into the orbit impinging on the inferior rectus complex or into the globe **(Figs. 13 to 15)**.[25-27]

Medial Wall Fractures of the Orbit

Imaging is crucial in recognizing these fractures which are often overlooked. CT evaluates these fractures which have been classified into four types:

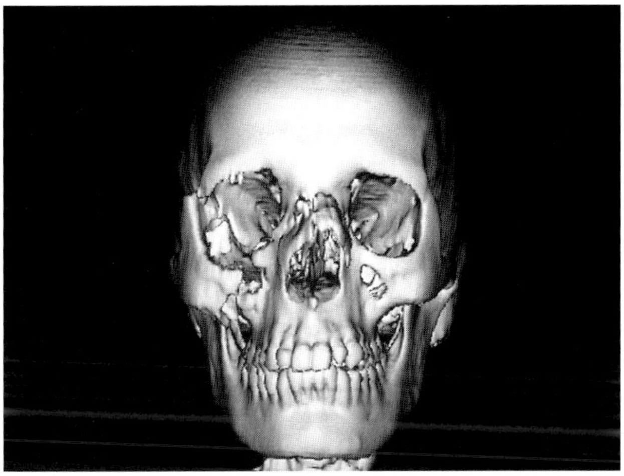

FIG. 15: Three-dimensional (3D) volume-rendered technique (VRT) reconstruction image reveals right orbital fracture involving inferolateral wall (zygomatic bone) with lateral displacement resulting in increased orbital volume.

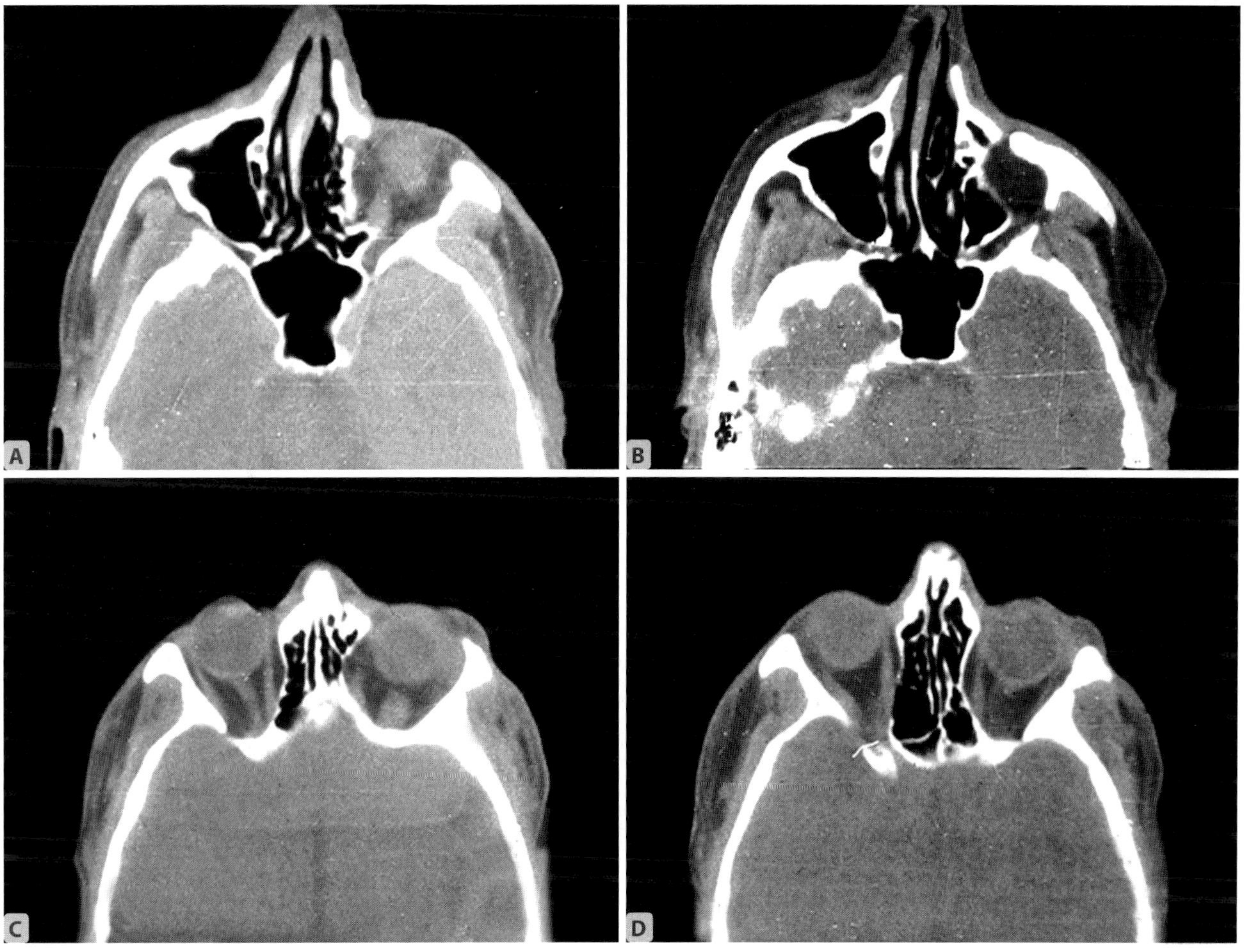

FIGS. 16A TO D: Fracture of the medial wall of the left orbit. The thin lamina papyracea is bowed medially with a resulting increase in the orbital volume. A fracture of the floor of the orbit is present in this axial computed tomography study.

1. Type 1 confined to the medial wall of the orbit
2. Type 2 fracture involves the medial orbital wall and the contiguous floor of the orbit
3. Type 3 is a fracture of the medial wall, orbital floor and the malar bones
4. Type 4 includes medial wall fractures associated with complex midface fractures **(Figs. 13 to 17)**.[23]

An interesting area and often neglected in routine assessment of facial trauma is the nasoethmoidal region and nasolacrimal canal and fossa. Thin coronal and axial

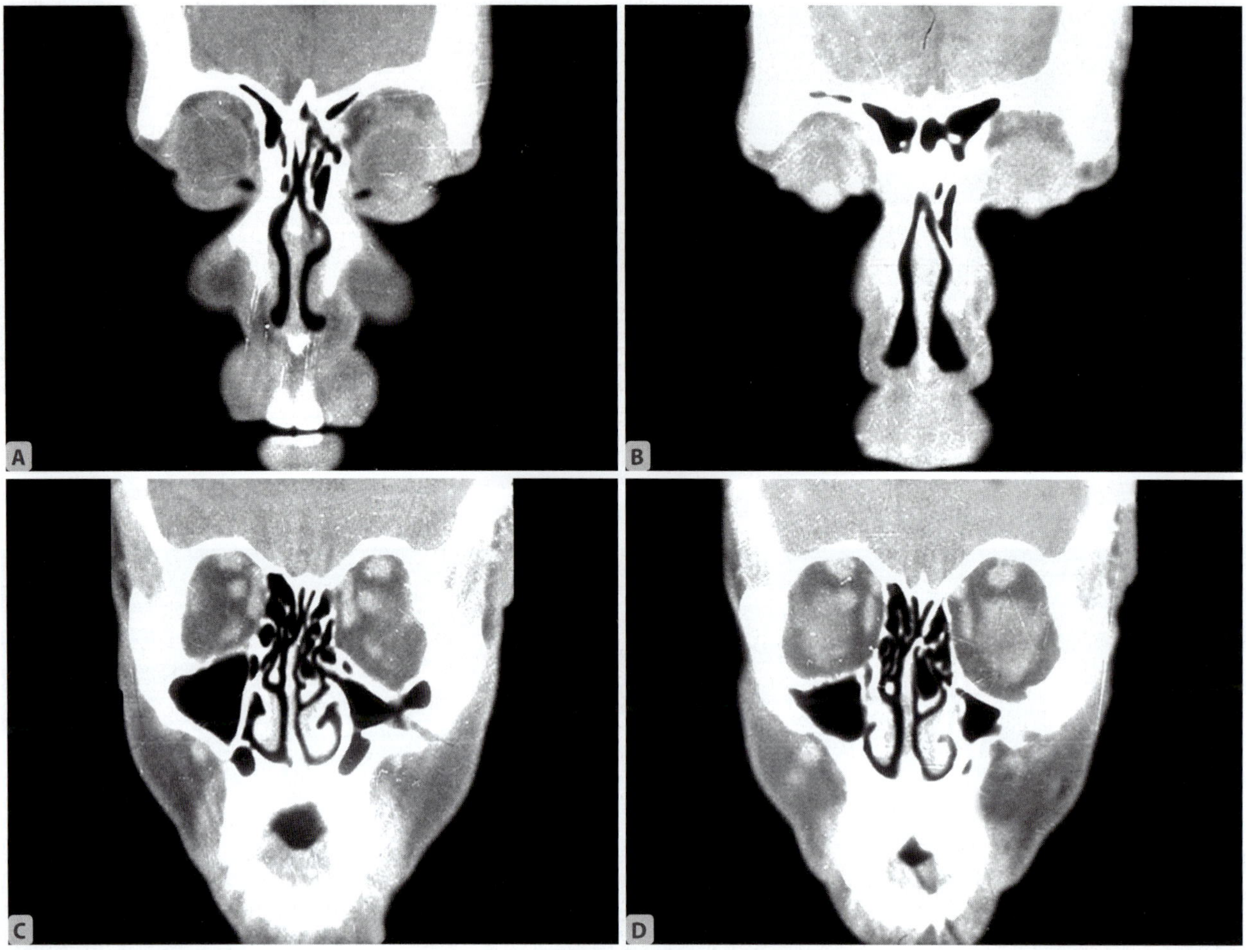

FIGS. 17A TO D: Coronal computed tomography (CT) section of the above patient (Fig. 9), showing the subtle increase in orbital volume. The medial wall fracture cannot be fully appreciated as is the fracture along the orbital floor.

CT sections are essential to image this region. Fractures of this region should be specifically looked for in the medial blow in fractures of the orbit and complications due to this injury avoided.[25,26]

The different types of orbital fractures are also associated with soft tissue injury, injuries to different intra-ocular structures and the optic nerve which are discussed in the Chapter 21.

Mandibular Fractures

Fractures of the mandible are classified according to the site of fracture. They are fractures of the: (a) condyle, (b) coronoid process, (c) angle and body, (d) ramus, and (e) midline fracture of the mandible. This U-shaped bone is likely to fracture at two sites, since it is firmly held at its ends by the capsules of the temporomandibular joints. Fracture of the neck of the condyle of the mandible is most commonly followed by those of the ramus and body **(Figs. 18A and B)**.

The initial radiological investigation for assessment of a mandibular fracture is a panoramic view of the mandible. This investigation will give most of the information regarding the sites of the fractures; however, it may be difficult to obtain in uncooperative patients. In the latter situation, PA views of the skull with oblique views for the mandible are suitable alternatives. Radiological investigations may be tailored to demonstrate fractures at specific site, e.g. intraoral dental views may be required to demonstrate fractures of the teeth and alveolar processes; Towne's view of the skull may be needed to show fractures of the neck of the condyle and rotated PA views may be required to show fractures of the ramus.

Coronal CT scan and 3D reconstructions may be required to demonstrate undisplaced fractures of the ramus and condyle of the mandible.

Skull Base Fractures

The skull base comprises of 7 bones, the paired frontal and temporal bones, and the unpaired ethmoid, sphenoid, and occipital bones. It is divided into anterior, central, and posterior regions, which form the floor of the anterior, middle, and posterior cranial fossae. The skull base fractures are associated with myriad of complications which are summarized in **Table 5**.

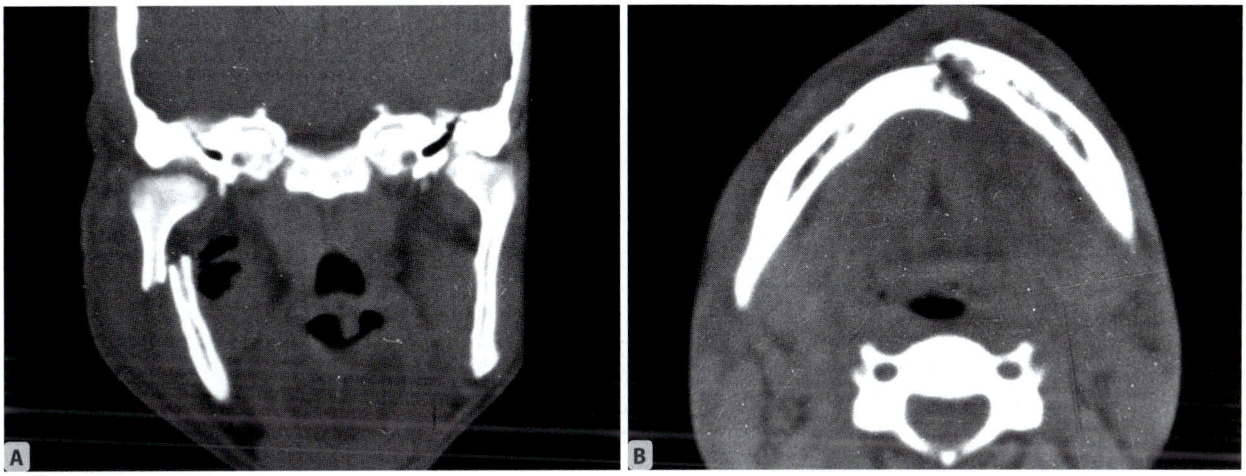

FIGS. 18A AND B: Fractures of the mandible. (A) Coronal computed tomography (CT) section shows fracture of the right condylar process; and (B) The axial CT section shows the concomitant fracture of the body of the mandible.

TABLE 5: Complications associated with skull base fractures.

Site of fracture	Complications
Anterior skull base fractures	• CSF leak and Meningoencephalocele • Orbital Injury • Anosmia (due to CN I injury) • Frontal contusions/hemorrhage
Central skull base fractures	• Vascular injury (Internal carotid artery or basilar trunk)—psedouaneurysm, dissection, laceration or transection, carotid-cavernous fistula and other dural arteriovenous fistula • Nerve injury- CN II, III, IV, V, VI injury, Horner syndrome • Multicompartmental intraparenchymal hemorrhage/contusion, diffuse axonal injury • CSF leak • Anterior middle cranial fossa epidural hemorrhage
Posterior skull base fractures	• Vertebrobasilar injury • Venous vascular injury causing thrombosis • Lower cranial nerve injuries (CN IX to XII) • CVJ and cervical spine injuries
Posterolateral skull base fractures	• Vascular injury (ICA) • Nerve injury-CN VII & VIII injury • CN VII and VIII injuries

(CSF: cerebrospinal fluid; CN: cranial nerve; CVJ: craniovertebral junction; ICA: internal carotid artery).

Anterior Skull Base Fractures

The anterior skull base, formed by the frontal and ethmoid bones, separates the anterior and inferior frontal lobes and olfactory structures within the anterior cranial fossa from the orbits and the sinonasal cavity. Direct frontal trauma often results in anterior skull base fractures, so-called fronto-basal injuries, with the "frontal" component of fractures involving the upper facial third (frontal bone/sinus and superior orbital rim), while the "basal" component of fracture involving the anterior skull base (cribriform plate, ethmoid roofs, and planum sphenoidale).[27] Complications associated with the anterior skull base fractures include orbital injury, CSF leak, meningoencephalocele formation, anosmia (due to cranial nerve olfactory nerve injury) and frontal lobe contusions.[28]

Central Skull Base Fractures

The central skull base, formed by the sphenoid and anterior temporal bones, separates the pituitary gland (within the sella), the cavernous sinuses (including the carotid artery and cranial nerves), the Meckel cave, and the temporal lobes superiorly from the sphenoid sinus anteriorly and inferiorly, and the extracranial soft tissues deep to the skull base inferiorly, including the masticator, parotid, parapharyngeal, and pharyngeal mucosal spaces. Transverse fractures in a coronal plane through the central skull base are common and are usually the result of high velocity lateral impact to the lateral frontal bone, zygoma, temporal, or parietal bone.[27] Extension of frontobasal fractures from frontal impact can occur in a sagittal or oblique fashion through the central skull base with involvement of the sella and sphenoid sinus, and, in some cases, the temporal bone.[28] The management of central skull base fractures are based on the associated complications and it is generally associated with a variety of potentially lethal complications. Associated intracranial injuries like multicompartmental intraparenchymal hemorrhages, contusions and diffuse axonal injuries are common as these are associated with high velocity injury. Injury to the greater wing of sphenoid often causes anterior middle cranial fossa epidural hematoma and are believed to be due to venous injury in sphenoparietal sinus.[29] CSF leaks can occur in association with sphenoid bone fracture although less common than frontobasal fractures.[30] Vascular injuries are most frequently encountered and most dreaded complications of central skull base fractures. Blunt cerebrovascular injury is reported in approximately 1% of all head and facial traumas, with risk increased to 8.5% in the setting of basilar skull fractures.[31-33] The internal carotid arteries are most prone to be involved because of its course through the central skull base and cavernous sinus. However, the basilar trunk is also prone to injury because of its vertical retroclival course.[28] The most common fractures associated with vascular injuries are clival fractures, fractures through the sella/sphenoid sinus, orbital apex fractures, petrous ridge fractures, and occiput and occipital condyle fractures. The vascular injuries include arterial dissection, pseudoaneurysm formation, frank transection or laceration, incarceration (entrapment within fracture line) and dural arteriovenous fistula formation, most notably carotid-cavernous fistula. Cranial nerve injuries may be associated in case of involvement of cavernous sinuses.

Posterior Skull Base Fractures

The posterior skull base is formed by the posterior temporal bone and the occipital bone, and separates the posterior fossa structures, including the cerebellum and brainstem, from the extracranial soft tissues: the posterior nasopharynx, retropharyngeal space, carotid space, and perivertebral space. Most posterior cranial fossa fractures occur as a result of a lateral and/or posterior blow to the occiput, and involve the occipital bone with frequent extension to the petrous temporal bone.[28] Potential complications include associated intraparenchymal hemorrhage and contusions including cerebellar involvement, sigmoid or transverse sinus thrombosis, dural arterio-venous fistula and lower cranial nerve injuries and CSF otorrhea in temporal bone fractures.[28] Associated injury to craniovertebral junction or cervical spine are also frequently encountered.[29]

PEDIATRIC FACIAL FRACTURES

Pediatric patients with facial fractures require a different approach than adults. It has been stressed in literature that routine radiographs may underestimate the most trivial injury. Hence, a CT scan is advocated for complete assessment. A high index of suspicion of maxillofacial trauma should always be maintained, especially in children with multiple traumas. The varying degree of ossification and pediatric dentition will affect the CT images and hence CT parameters should be specifically tailored for children. There are many features of pediatric facial bones which influence radiological features of facial trauma. Pediatric facial bones are elastic and do not fracture as easily as adult bones. The thick elastic periosteum prevents bone displacement resulting in greenstick fractures **(Figs. 19 and 20)**. In pediatric trauma, the fracture of orbital roof is most common and there is strong correlation between the orbital hematomas and orbital roof/naso-orbital ethmoid fractures.[34] Healing of facial fractures is faster in pediatric patients than adults requiring shorter periods of immobilization. Moreover, if the treatment is delayed, the fractures fragments heal and become fixed which prevents any further reduction. Dental deformities or delayed dentition may result, if the growth centers are involved. Since children have fewer teeth to place splints, the treatment plans need to be modified and wire ligatures used frequently in adult fractures are contraindicated, especially in children below 2 years of age.[35]

CLINICAL ASPECTS OF MAXILLOFACIAL IMAGING

There have been major changes in the concepts of surgical management of facial fractures in the last decade. Modern principles of reconstructive surgery lay stress on extensive subperiosteal dissection, exposure of all fracture lines open reduction and rigid fixation. Internal fixation is done by the extensive use of miniplates or microplates with screw. Complex internal fixation schemes using wire sutures and wire suspensions have become obsolete. The use of tissue adhesives, such as N-butyl cyanoacrylate for fixing small thin fragments of bone, have been a novel advance.[9,36,37]

Imaging of a patient with maxillofacial injury should be so complete that the surgeon has a clear delineation of the location of fractures, direction and amount of displacement, and the location of anatomic landmarks (keys) that will help restore the preinjury position of bone.[38] The regional

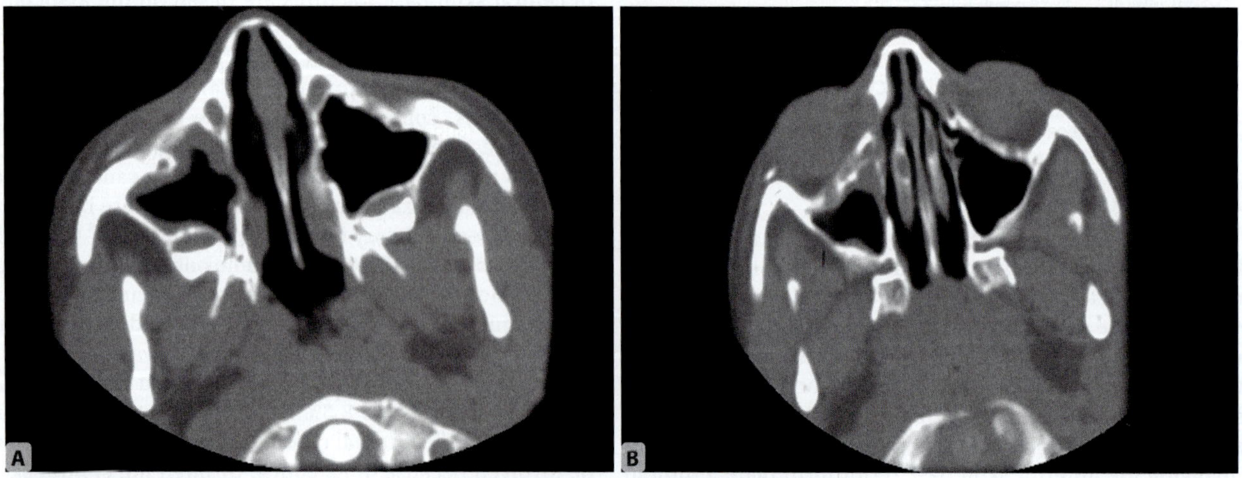

FIGS. 19A AND B: Pediatric facial fractures: Fracture of the inferior and lateral margins of the right orbit in a 6-year-old girl. The fracture appears as a subtle depression in the orbital outline.

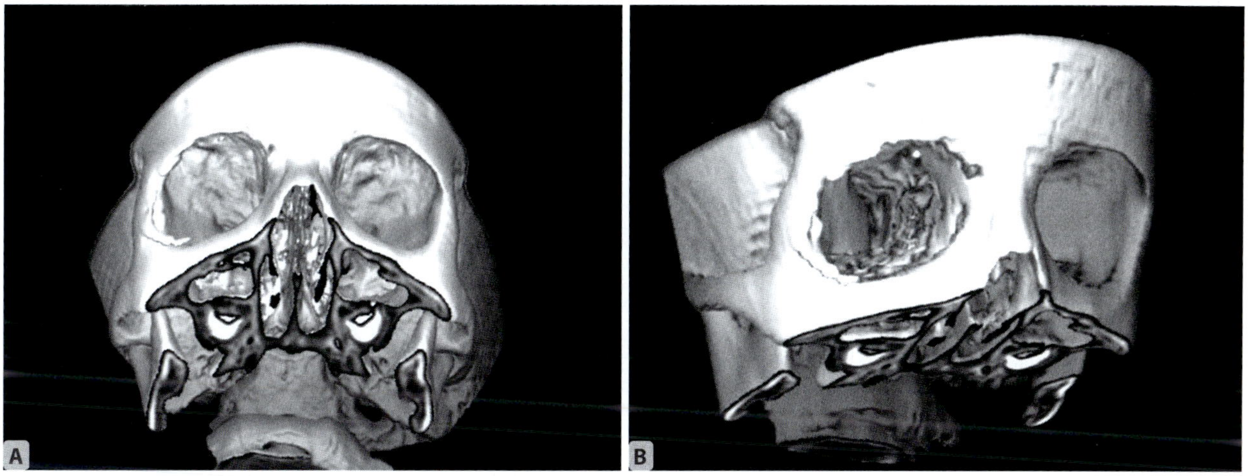

FIGS. 20A AND B: Three-dimensional (3D) reconstruction of the axial computed tomography (CT) of the patient in Figure 15. The fracture line in clearly demonstrated in the reconstructed views.

classification reflects upon the increasing sophistication in the operative management of patients. Surgeons require specific information to accomplish their task in restoring the geometrical symmetry of the face, e.g. in the midfacial fracture. The surgeon would want to restore the vertical dimension of the face in a Le Fort injury which would mean restoration of at least one of the four major buttresses in that region. Together with the corrected dental deformities and mandibular fractures, if any, the preinjury position of the face can be restored. Therefore, the radiologist should understand the morbid anatomy and present to the surgeon both an axial and coronal evaluation so that vertical buttresses can be clearly delineated. In the Le Fort injuries, skull base fractures merit special mention and their presence can influence the prognosis of a seemingly innocuous superficial fracture.[9]

Amongst the more serious complications of facial fractures is infection of the fracture line. Any fracture may be considered to be infected, if the fracture line crosses the alveolus, nasal cavity or any of the paranasal sinuses; or if there is a communication with the associated soft-tissue wound. Demonstration of these fracture lines and fragments should be done with clarity to aid surgical approach to the fractures.[26]

ACKNOWLEDGMENTS

The authors acknowledge Dr Nirmaly Ray, DM resident in the Neuroradiology Division of Department of Radiodiagnosis, PGIMER, Chandigarh for his support in editing of chapter.

REFERENCES

1. Le Fort R. Etude experimental sur les fractures de la machoire superieure. Rev Chir. 1901;25:208-27.
2. Stanley RB. Use of intraoperative computed tomography during repair of orbitozygomatic fractures. Arch Facial Plast Surg. 1999;1(1):19-24.
3. Zilkha A. Computed tomography in facial trauma. Radiology. 1982;144(3):545-8.
4. Bartlett SP, DeLozier JB. Controversies in the management of pediatric facial fractures. Clin Plastic Surg. 1992;19(1): 245-58.
5. Gentry LR, Manor WF, Turski PA, et al. High-resolution CT analysis of facial struts in trauma: 1. Normal anatomy. AJR. 1983;140(3):523-32.
6. Gentry LR, Manor WF, Turski PA, et al. High-resolution CT analysis of facial struts in trauma: 2. Osseous and soft-tissue complications. AJR. 1983;140(3):533-41.
7. Beirne JC, Butler PE, Brady FA. Cervical spine injuries in patients with facial fractures: a 1-year prospective study. Int J Oral Maxillofac Surg. 1995;24(1 Pt 1):26-9.
8. Manson PN. Facial injuries the face—part 1. In: Joseph GM (Ed). Plastic Surgery. Philadelphia, PA, USA: WB Saunders; 1990. pp. 867-89.
9. Som PM, Brandwein MS. Facial fractures and postoperative findings. In: Som PM, Curtin HD (Eds). Head and Neck Imaging, 5th edition. St Louis, MO: Mosby; 2011. pp. 374-438.
10. Lill W, Solar P, Ulm C, et al. Reproducibility of three-dimensional CT-assisted model production in the maxillofacial area. Br J Oral Maxillofac Surg. 1992;30(4):233-6.
11. Cavalcanti MG, Haller JW, Vannier MW. Three-dimensional computed tomography landmark measurement in craniofacial surgical planning: experimental validation in vitro. J Oral Maxillofac Surg. 1999;57(6):690-4.
12. Chen WJ, Yang YJ, Fang YM, et al. Identification and classification in Le Fort type fractures by using 2D and 3D computed tomography. Chin J Traumatol. 2006;9(1): 59-64.
13. Coupal TM, Mallinson PI, McLaughlin P, et al. Peering through the glare: using dual-energy CT to overcome the problem of metal artefacts in bone radiology. Skeletal Radiol. 2014;43(5):567-75.
14. Cavalcanti MG, Rocha SS, Vannier MW. Craniofacial measurements based on 3D-CT volume rendering implications for clinical applications. Dentomaxillofac Radiol. 2004;33(3):170-6.
15. Guerrero ME, Jacobs R, Loubele M, et al. State-of the-art on cone beam CT imaging for preoperative planning of implant placement. Clin Oral Investig. 2006;10(1):1-7.
16. van Steenberghe D, Naert I, Andersson M, et al. A custom template and definitive prosthesis allowing immediate implant loading in the maxilla: a clinical report. Int J Oral Maxillofac Implants. 2002;17(5):663-70.

17. Brisco J, Fuller K, Lee N, et al. Cone beam computed tomography for imaging orbital trauma—image quality and radiation dose compared with conventional multislice computed tomography. Br J Oral Maxillofac Surg 2014;52(1):76-80.
18. Parmar HA, Ibrahim M, Mukherji SK. Optimizing craniofacial CT technique. Neuroimaging Clin N Am. 2014;24(3):395-405.
19. Zimmerman R, Bilaniuk L, Hackney D, et al. Paranasal sinus hemorrhage: evaluation with MR imaging. Radiology. 1987;162(2):499-503.
20. Hopper RA, Salemy S, Sze RW. Diagnosis of midface fractures with CT: what the surgeon needs to know. Radiographics. 2006;26(3):783-93.
21. Manson PN, Markowitz B, Mirvis S, et al. Toward CT-based facial fracture treatment. Plast Reconstr Surg. 1990;85(2):202-12.
22. Uzelac A, Gean AD. Orbital and facial fractures. Neuroimaging Clin N Am. 2014;24(3):407-24.
23. Rhea JT, Novelline RA. How to simplify the CT diagnosis of Le Fort fractures? AJR. 2005;184(5):1700-5.
24. Bagheri SC, Holmgren E, Kademani D, et al. Comparison of the severity of bilateral Le Fort injuries in isolated midface trauma. J Oral Maxillofac Surg. 2005;63(8):1123-9.
25. Schultz RC, Elbel WR. Facial bone fractures. In: Stark RB (Ed). Plastic Surgery of the Head and Neck, Part 3. Philadelphia, PA, USA: Churchill Livingstone; 1987. p. 1039.
26. Burn JS, Chung CH, Oh SJ. Pure orbital blowout fractures: new concepts and importance of medial orbital blowout fracture. Plast Reconstr Surg. 1999;103(7):1839-49.
27. Pelton RW, Rainey AM, Lee AG. Traumatic subluxation of the globe into the maxillary sinus. AJNR. 1998;19(8):1450-1.
28. Baugnon KL, Hudgins PA. Skull base fractures and their complications. Neuroimaging Clin N Am. 2014;24(3):439-65.
29. Gean AD, Fischbein NJ, Purcell DD, et al. Benign anterior temporal epidural hematoma: indolent lesion with a characteristic CT imaging appearance after blunt head trauma. Radiology. 2010;257(1):212-8.
30. Lin DT, Lin AC. Surgical treatment of traumatic injuries of the cranial base. Otolaryngol Clin North Am 2013;46(5):749-57.
31. Berne JD, Cook A, Rowe SA, et al. A multivariate logistic regression analysis of risk factors for blunt cerebrovascular injury. J Vasc Surg. 2010;51:57-64.
32. Mundinger GS, Dorafshar AH, Gilson MM, et al. Blunt-mechanism facial fracture patterns associated with internal carotid artery injuries: recommendations for additional screening criteria based on analysis of 4,398 patients. J Oral Maxillofac Surg. 2013;71(12):2092-100.
33. Feiz-Erfan I, Horn EM, Theodore N, et al. Incidence and pattern of direct blunt neurovascular injury associated with trauma to the skull base. J Neurosurg. 2007;107(2):364-9.
34. Chapman VM, Fenton LZ, Gao D, et al. Facial fractures in children: unique patterns of injury observed by computed tomography. J Comput Assist Tomogr. 2009;33(1):70-2.
35. Kim DB, Sacapano M, Hardesty RA. Facial fractures in children. West J Med. 1997;167(2):100.
36. Venkatramu NK, Khandelwal N, Bapuraj JR, et al. Evaluation of 3DCT in maxilla-facial trauma: surgical correlation (work-in-progress). Ind J Radiol Imag. 1997;7(2):97-102.
37. Schierle HP, Hausamen JE. Modern principles in treatment of complex injuries of the facial bones. Unfallchirurg. 1997; 100(5):330-7.
38. Laine FJ. Maxillofacial trauma. In: Haaga JR, Lanzieri CF, Sartoris DJ, Zerhonni EA (Eds). Computed Tomography and Magnetic Resonance Imaging of the Whole Body, 3rd edition. St Louis, MO: Mosby; 1994. p. 388.

CHAPTER

212

Imaging of Acute Spinal Trauma

Sameer Vyas, Niranjan Khandelwal, Paramjeet Singh

INTRODUCTION

Imaging in acute spinal trauma plays a pivotal role for the diagnosis and treatment of patients by delineating extent, classification and severity of the osseous and ligamentous injury. Spinal trauma occurs with an annual incidence of approximately 15–40 cases per million.[1] It commonly results from motor vehicle accident (most commonly), fall from height, penetrating and sports injuries.[1,2] Most studies had shown a bimodal age distribution and is more common in young adults (approx 80%, <40 years) with a male predominance (80–85%).[3] Spinal cord injuries are seen in about 10–14% of spine fractures and dislocations. The incidence of neurological damage varies with the site of injury (fractures or dislocations), and is seen in approximately 40% of cervical spine, in about 10% of thoracic spine and about 4% of thoracolumbar junction injuries. However, there are no associated fractures or dislocations in about 10% spinal cord injuries. Imaging plays a crucial role in the evaluation of the acutely traumatized patient by providing information that allows timely and appropriate management, thus reducing the morbidity and mortality.

IMAGING INDICATIONS OF THE TRAUMATIC SPINE

Most of the patients presenting with blunt spinal trauma even minor are subjected to radiographs of the spine because of the significant morbidity and mortality associated with the spinal trauma. It is very important to answer these two questions before performing any radiological investigation, Is imaging necessary? And if yes, what is appropriate imaging technique? Several clinical trials have been carried out for improving guidelines and to standardize clinical practice, to help clinicians or radiologists to properly screen and use plain radiographs, to reduce the workload of emergency department and cost of imaging.[2-4] Two clinical decision rules have been developed for the cervical spine injuries. The first rule developed was National Emergency X-Radiography Utilization Study (NEXUS) Low-Risk Criteria (NLC), which tested a five-part decision rule to predict patients with a spinal injury.[4] The NLC concluded that radiography after blunt C-spine trauma is unnecessary, if patients satisfy all five of the following **low-risk criteria**: absence of midline cervical spine tenderness, normal level of alertness, no evidence of intoxication, no abnormal neurologic findings, and no painful distracting injuries. Due to the low specificity of NLC, the Canadian C-spine rule (CCR) was developed subsequently based upon clinical questions. It stated that **low-risk patients** (ambulatory, without midline tenderness or immediate onset of pain, able to attain sitting position, victims of simple rear-end motor vehicle crashes) do not require imaging if they can actively turn their heads 45° in both directions. Similar clinical criteria have been evaluated in the thoracic and lumbar spine. Imaging is however indicated when high risk factors are identified in these patients. These high risk factors are summarized in **Table 1**.

The American college of radiology appropriateness criteria for suspected spine trauma highlights the following points:

- No imaging is required in patients having low risk criteria by NLC/CCR.
- In adults with high risk criteria by NLC/CCR, MDCT is the investigation of choice. The entire spine is usually imaged due to high prevalence of non contiguous multiple injuries.
- However, in children up to 14 years of age radiography is the imaging method of choice due to high radiation dose by a CT scan. Recommended views for cervical spine are: AP, lateral and open mouth and for thoracolumbar spine are AP and lateral.

TABLE 1: Canadian C-spine rule high-risk criteria.

High-risk criteria of CCR
• Age greater than 65 years • Dangerous mechanism of injury (e.g. fall from height >1 metre, high speed motor vehicle accident) • Paresthesia in extremities
Further high-risk criteria
• Altered mental status • Multiple fractures • Drowning or diving accidents • Significant head or facial injury • Rigid spinal disease (i.e. ankylosing spondylitis, DISH)

- MR imaging is method of choice when spinal cord injury, cord compression and/or ligament injury is suspected especially in obtunded patients.
- MRI is also considered in patients with persistent neck pain showing no evidence fracture on CT scan.[5]

Advanced imaging techniques are incorporated more frequently for evaluation of spinal trauma in older patients. It is because the elderly patients undergo a different injury pattern due to associated osteopenia, degenerative changes and ankylosed spinal segments. Low energy mechanism is a common cause of spinal fractures especially in cervical spine. In addition, spinal cord injury is seen in over 20% of cases. CT is excellent to define the full extent of osseous injury; however MRI should also be performed in this subset of patients due to higher incidence of spinal cord and ligamentous injury.[6]

IMAGING MODALITIES

The various imaging modalities for imaging spinal trauma are plain radiograph, tomography, myelography, computed tomography (CT) and magnetic resonance imaging (MRI).[7,8] It is very important to decide the optimal imaging method for the spinal trauma patients depending upon the merits and limitations of each modality.

Plain Radiography

In the current scenario, radiographs are not usually obligatory prior to the CT for acute spinal trauma because a normal radiograph does not exclude an injury and hence a CT is eventually performed if the clinical suspicion of injury is high. Recent studies have shown that MDCT is more effective in identification of thoracolumbar injuries as compared to plain X-ray.[30] The same fact is also supported by the ACR appropriateness criteria as already discussed. However, plain films, is commonly used in the initial evaluation of a patient with spinal trauma. The first and most important radiograph in spinal trauma is the lateral view with cross-table technique.[9,10] This has been reported to be positive in 70–90% of cases. The standard additional views are anteroposterior (AP) open mouth for cervical spine, AP view for thoracic spine and AP and oblique views for lumbosacral spine injury. The most important addition in the routine views of cervical trauma patients has been the cervical trauma oblique view.[11] This is obtained with patient supine and X-ray tube is angled 30–40° from horizontal. This view more often provides a clear visualization of C1 to T1 with an additional 15° cranial tube tilt. A traditional "swimmer's view" is obtained only if "trauma oblique view" is inadequate.[11] The "swimmer's view" usually needs a change in patient's position and is contraindicated in a high suspicion of cervicothoracic injury and is not helpful in obese or muscular patients. The use of flexion-extension radiographs is controversial and can be performed if there is a question of the ligamentous injury. However, they should be performed only in conscious patients who are able to cooperate and only active motion should be applied. Limitations of plain radiography include inability to detect subtle undisplaced fractures, to visualize upper cervical (C1, C2) and cervicothoracic junction and to evaluate nonosseous injuries. At present, CT has replaced plain x-ray as the initial modality for evaluation of spinal trauma at many level 1 trauma centers across the world.[12]

The use of tomography in the evaluation of acute spinal trauma is obsolete with the advent of CT, especially multidetector CT (MDCT). Disadvantages of tomography include need to change position of the patient for lateral tomography and high radiation dose as compared to CT. The role of myelography has significantly reduced since the advent of CT and MRI. It is an invasive procedure and has limited role in present scenario, i.e. patients with contraindication to MRI. There are contrast-related complications and risk of arachnoiditis. Myelography may still be indicated in the evaluation of nerve root avulsions or suspected dural tears.

Computed Tomography

Multidetector CT is the preferred imaging modality for evaluating blunt spinal trauma patients.[13-16] The high quality multiplanar reformations in different planes in MDCT have markedly improved the detection of varied spinal abnormalities like abnormal intervertebral distance, abnormal angulations, subluxations and dislocations which were not well-visualized in axial CT plain radiography or tomography. The advantages of MDCT include larger area coverage, short scanning time, thinner slices and better reconstructions. Thin contiguous axial sections are acquired in helical mode at the site of interest. Other advantages of CT include the ability to assess the spinal canal and impingement by osseous fragments, optimal visualization of vertebral injuries, soft tissue abnormality and associated disk prolapse and imaging without changing patient's position. The disadvantages of CT include incomplete evaluation of horizontal fractures and displacements in the sagittal plane. Multiplanar and three-dimensional (3D) reconstructions help in the evaluation of vertebral alignment and horizontal fractures.[17,18] The spatial information and relationship in complex fractures is better appreciated on 3D images **(Figs. 1A and B)**. Limitations of the CT in spinal trauma include radiation exposure and inability to assess spinal cord injury.

Magnetic Resonance Imaging

The role of MRI in acute spinal trauma is fully established especially in the evaluation of spinal cord, both in correlating the appearances of the spinal cord with the level of neurologic deficit and in identification of parameters predictive of neurologic outcome.[19-22] It is the investigation of choice for assessing injuries to the soft tissue structures including posterior ligamentous complex, spinal cord, intervertebral disks and adjacent muscles. **(Fig. 2)**. Thus, no contraindications assumed, an immediate MR imaging is warranted if CT/neurological symptoms suggest an injury to the neural/ligamentous structures.

According to ACR appropriateness criteria, MRI of spine combined with CT is appropriate in the setting of acute spinal trauma if NEXUS or CCR criteria are met and clinical/imaging (X-ray/CT) findings are suggestive of:

- Myelopathy
- Ligamentous injury
- Mechanically unstable spine

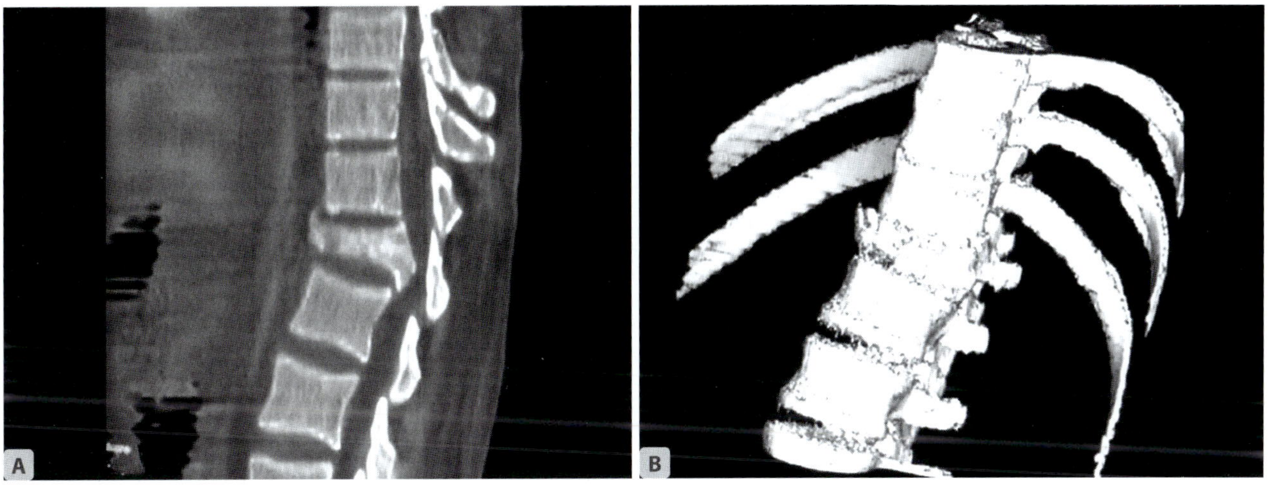

FIGS. 1A AND B: (A) Sagittal reformation of MDCT showing fracture fragments and posterior displacement; (B) 3D CT demonstrating the fractured vertebra.

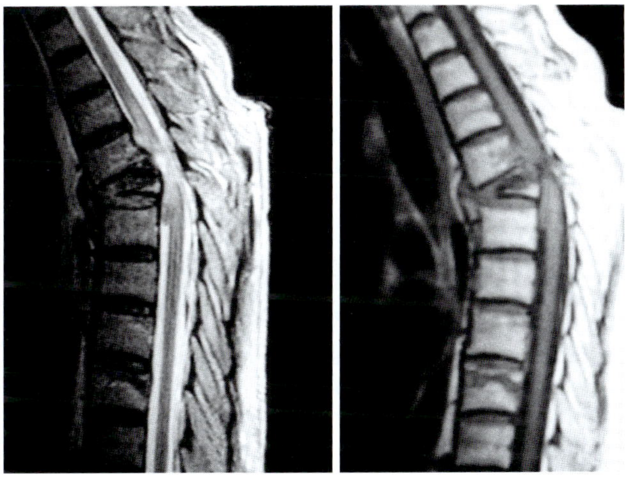

FIG. 2: Sagittal T2- and T1WI MR showing burst fracture of midthoracic vertebra with retropulsed fractured fragment and associated cord changes.

The radiographic or CT findings which suggest ligamentous injury include findings like spondylolisthesis, widening of facet joints/interspinous space or asymmetric disk space widening.

MRI is also used for prognosticating the injury by differentiating the hemorrhagic and non-hemorrhagic cord injury as the former is associated with poorer prognosis.

Both T1- and T2-weighted sequences with a spin echo technique in axial, sagittal and coronal planes are helpful in the assessment of the spinal injury. A spine surface coil is used to improve resolution. T1-weighted images are helpful in the assessment of bony element abnormality while T2-weighted images are more useful for assessment of spinal cord. Cord contusions manifest as hyperintense foci on T2-weighted images and are iso- to hypointense on T1-weighted images. Gradient echo images help to identify the hemorrhagic cord contusions which have prognostic significance. Short tau inversion recovery (STIR) and T2 fat sat images are sensitive for detection of marrow edema which is seen in acute fractures but not in chronic fractures. Appearance of cord hemorrhage varies with the age of hematoma. Patients with predominant edema or contusions show neurological improvement whereas cord hemorrhage has a poor outcome.

Ideally MRI should be done within 72 hours of injury. It is because during this period edema gives T2 hyperintense signal which in turn increases the conspicuity of the ligaments. Later on as the edema subsides, the sensitivity of MRI for detection of injury also reduces.[23]

In addition, the long-term sequelae of spinal cord trauma such as cord transaction, traumatic syrinx, myelomalacia and meningocele are well-delineated with MRI.

The details of MRI imaging for assessing nonosseous injury will be discussed later in this chapter.

The disadvantages of magnetic resonance as compared to CT include its relative inferiority for demonstration of osseous anatomy and fractures and failure to detect the posterior element fractures. In addition, MRI is expensive, not readily available, and patient support and ventilator system should be magnetic resonance compatible.

Advances in Magnetic Resonance Imaging

Diffusion Weighted Imaging

Post-traumatic spinal canal hematoma, though rare, occurs most commonly in cervical spine due to the injury to the epidural venous plexus. Depending on the age of the hematoma, sometimes it becomes difficult to differentiate it from the epidural fat. Hoch et al. have shown that hematoma has fairly obvious hyperintensity on diffusion trace images due to echo planar imaging (EPI) signal artifact.[24] They also show diffusion restriction due to gelatinous nature of the evolving hematoma. It has also been shown that if the cord shows T2 hyperintensity along with low ADC value in acute epidural hematoma, patient may suffer from irreversible compressive cord damage.[25] Role of DWI has also been studied in patients with SCINA as discussed later. Use of DWI is however limited by distortion of the image due to magnetic field inhomogeneity and susceptibility changes due to bones and ligaments of the spine. In addition there is physiologic motion of the cord secondary to respiratory and cardiac motion which further degrades the quality of image.

Diffusion Tensor Imaging

Diffusion tensor imaging assesses the integrity of the white matter tracts in the spinal cord and can detect very early changes in spinal cord injury which are not seen on conventional MR images. Shamuganathan et al. revealed that whole cervical spine DTI parameters in patients with cervical cord contusions were significantly lower and the VR was higher as compared to healthy controls.[26] Greater decrease in ADC and RA values was seen at the site of injury. Thus DTI can be used to document the true extent of injury which otherwise appears normal on conventional imaging. They also concluded that change in DTI parameters correlated with the severity of cord injury and can be used for predicting the severity of cord injury and monitoring recovery following treatment.

CLASSIFICATION OF SPINAL TRAUMA

The spinal trauma can be classified according to the level of injury, severity of injury, mechanism of injury and stability versus instability.[7]

Level of Injury

Cervical spine injury is most common (40–60%) due to excessive mobility and lack of supporting structures. Thoracic spine injury is less common (20%) as the stability is provided by thoracic cage whereas lumbar spine injury is seen in about 20–30%. Most of the thoracic and lumbar injuries are seen at thoracolumbar junction (60% between D12 and L2) as there is transition from immobile to mobile segment and orientation of facet joints from coronal to sagittal. Multilevel injury is seen in about 5–20%.

Severity of Injury

Spinal trauma is minor, when associated with no neurological symptoms and the patient is alert and able to cooperate. Trauma is major, when associated with neurological deficits and the patient is unconscious as well as having multisystem trauma.

Mechanism of Injury

Flexion, extension, rotation, compression, distraction or shear forces may produce damage in isolation or in combination. Ligaments are resistant to compression or distraction but are vulnerable to rotation or shear forces. But the osseous end plates fail when pure compressive or tensile forces are applied to the vertebra. Thus, pure compression or distraction produces fracture whereas rotatory or shear forces result in dislocations.

- Flexion injury results in anterior wedging, vertebral body fractures, posterior longitudinal ligament (PLL) interspinous ligament disruption.
- Hyperextension injury causes fractures of posterior element, anterior longitudinal ligament (ALL) rupture and subluxations. It is common in C-spine.
- Vertical compression (axial load) injury causes burst/compression fractures, lateral element fractures. It is seen in diving and jumping injury.
- Rotation-shearing injury results in lateral mass fracture and facet subluxation.

Stable versus Unstable Fracture

Spinal injuries which can withstand stress without progressive deformity and neurological damage are referred as stable injuries as compared to the injuries where spine is not able to maintain integrity and further damage to spinal cord or nerve root cannot be avoided are reefed to as unstable injuries. Dennis et al. introduced the concept of three columns of spine and concluded that instability requires disruption of at least two of these columns.[27] Anterior column is formed by anterior half of vertebral body, anterior longitudinal ligament and anterior annulus. Middle column is formed by posterior half of the body, posterior longitudinal ligament and posterior annulus. Posterior column is formed by posterior bony complex (pedicles, lamina, articular processes and spinous process) and the posterior ligamentous complex (facet joint capsule, ligamentum flavum, interspinous and supraspinous ligaments). Signs of instability on imaging include widened interspinous distance, increased facet joint distance, disk space narrowing, focal angulation of greater than 11°, vertebral body compression of more than 25% and subluxation of greater than 3.5 mm.

RADIOLOGICAL INTERPRETATION OF SPINAL TRAUMA (ABCS)

The radiographic signs of trauma are as follows:

- *A-Alignment:* Disruption of lines, focal kyphoscoliosis, rotation of spinous process, increased interpedicular distance and vertebral listhesis.
- *B-Bone integrity:* Fracture, anterior wedging, cortical buckling, disrupted posterior vertebral line and disrupted C2 ring.
- *C-Cartilage:* Interspinous/facet joint widening, increased/decreased disk spaces and vacuum phenomenon.
- *S-Soft tissue:* Widening of pre-/paravertebral soft tissue.

NEW RADIOLOGICAL CLASSIFICATION SYSTEMS

The newer classification systems like subaxial injury classification (SLICS) and thoracolumbar injury classification and severity score (TLICS) have included neurologic status of the patient and integrity of posterior ligamentous complex for grading the status of the patient **(Table 2)**. It is contrary to the old radiological classification systems which only considered the location and morphology of the fracture. These newer classifications (TLICS and SLICS) are based on a scoring system that also provides a therapeutic recommendation toward surgical or conservative management. In addition MR imaging has found its way into these classification system which includes evaluation of the posterior ligamentous complex.[5]

TABLE 2: Thoracolumbar injury classification and severity score.

Morphology	0 1 2 3 4	No abnormality Compression Burst fracture Rotation/translation Distraction	Radiograph/CT/MRI
Posterior ligamentous complex	0 2 3	Intact Suspected/indeterminate Injured/disrupted	MRI*
Neurologic status	0 2 2 3 3	Intact Root injury Complete cord/conus medullaris injury** Incomplete cord/conus medullaris injury Cauda equina syndrome	Physical examination
Score	<=3 4 >= 5	Nonoperative treatment Consider conservative or surgical therapy Operative treatment	

*The most reliable sign of PLC injury are disruption of the low-signal intensity black stripe on sagittal T1/T2WI, fluid in the facet capsules or edema in the interspinous regions.

**Contrary to expectation, a higher score (3 points) is allocated to incomplete cord injury and cauda equina syndrome because these patients may experience better outcome from surgical decompression than patients with complete spinal cord injury.

CERVICAL SPINE INJURY

Cervical spine injuries occur predominantly at two levels. One-third fractures occur at the level of C2, and one half at the level of C6 or C7. The most frequent mechanism of injury is flexion, followed by extension, vertical compression and rotation. Injuries of the cervical spine can be divided into injury of upper (C1-C2) and lower (C3-C7) cervical spine.

Upper Cervical Spine Injuries

The upper cervical spine differs both anatomically and functionally from the remainder of the spine. The primary motion is rotation. The bony ring of C1 lacks a body and spinous process and its articulation with C2 is circular and flat. This unique anatomy results in a set of injuries. Upper cervical spine injuries can be divided into dislocations of the cervical spine (occipitoatlantoaxial injuries) and fractures of C1 or C2. Occipitoatlantoaxial injuries occur as atlanto-occipital dislocation or atlantoaxial subluxation.

Atlanto-occipital Dislocation

Traumatic atlanto-occipital dislocation is a rare but fatal injury as it is often associated with spinomedullary transection. The mechanism of the injury is hyperextension and distraction. Plain radiography shows retropharyngeal soft tissue swelling, anterior displacement of basion from its normal position superior to odontoid (distance >12.5 mm on lateral film) and malalignment between spinolaminar line of C1 and posterior margin of foramen magnum. CT demonstrates the above findings clearly particularly with the reformatted images. MRI helps to delineate cord transection that is often associated **(Figs. 3A and B)**.

Atlantoaxial Injuries

Post-traumatic atlantoaxial subluxation is a rare injury. Tears of the transverse ligament or avulsion fractures at the site of insertion allow anterior displacement of C1 relative to C2. The normal distance between dens and posterior margin of C1 in adults is less than 3 mm (less than 5 mm in children). It widens abnormally in flexion. Plain films in flexion and extension or conventional tomography is most helpful in detecting subluxation. Rotatory atlantoaxial dislocation (AAD) may occur following minor trauma or it may develop spontaneously following upper respiratory tract infection. The atlas is rotated more than 45° and the facets are often locked.

Anteroposterior open mouth view shows eccentrically placed dens and no movement following cranial rotation. CT in both resting positions and with maximum rotation to contralateral side is the optimal method of evaluation. There is no change in relationship of C1 and C2 with contralateral rotation in rotatory dislocation whereas in normal healthy subjects or patients with torticollis, the deformity is corrected.

Fractures of the Atlas (C1)

A variety of C1 ring fractures have been described but the most common is that involving posterior arch as it is compressed between the occiput and posterior arch of C2 in extension. Gehweiler and colleagues classified it into five types:

1. *Type I*—fracture of the anterior arch
2. *Type II*—fracture of the posterior arch
3. *Type III*—combined fracture of the anterior and posterior arch (Jefferson fracture)
4. *Type IV*—fracture of lateral mass
5. *Type V*—fracture of transverse process

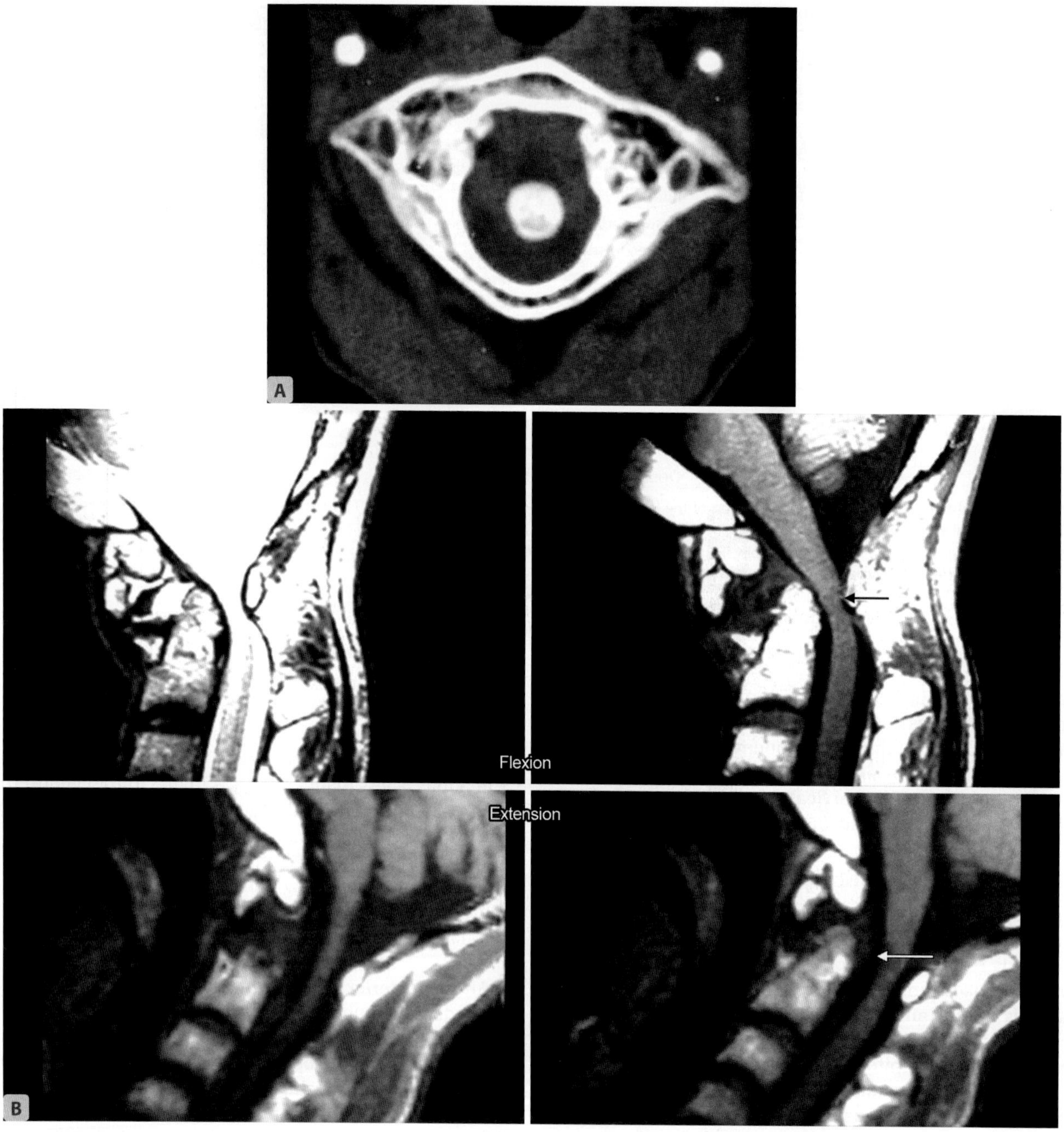

FIGS. 3A AND B: (A) Axial CT showing posteriorly dislocated odontoid process with anterior compression of cord; (B) Sagittal MRI T1 and T2WI in flexion and extension confirm AAD as well as cord compression (maximum in flexion).

Axial compression of C1 results in Jefferson fracture that consists of ipsilateral disruption of both the anterior and posterior arches and it may be unilateral or bilateral. The patient is neurologically intact unless the transverse ligament is disrupted. Plain film or CT shows soft tissue swelling, anterior/posterior arch fracture and lateral displacement of lateral masses of atlas relative to C2.

Vertebral artery injury can be associated with atlas fracture (most commonly with Type V fracture).

Fractures of the Axis (C2)

The Anderson and d'Alonzo classification of odontoid fractures is based on fracture location and has both therapeutic and prognostic significance **(Fig. 4)**. Type I fractures are oblique fractures through the tip of the dens secondary to avulsion of alar ligament (stable). Type II fracture occurs at the junction of dens and body of C2 (nonunion is as high as 36%). Type III is horizontal fracture through the C2 vertebral body (frequently displaced). Odontoid fractures are best

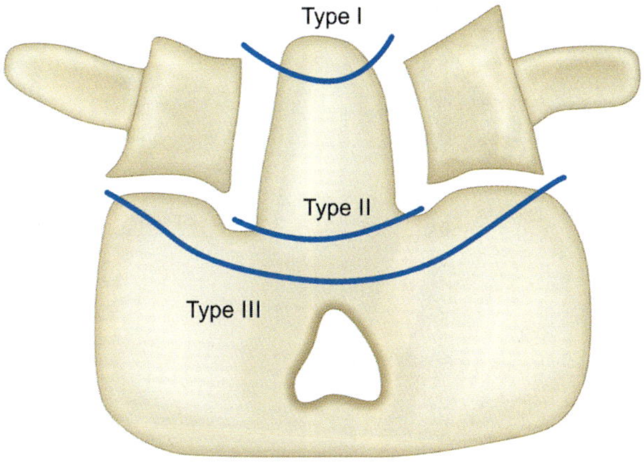

FIG. 4: The Anderson and d'Alonzo classification of odontoid fractures.

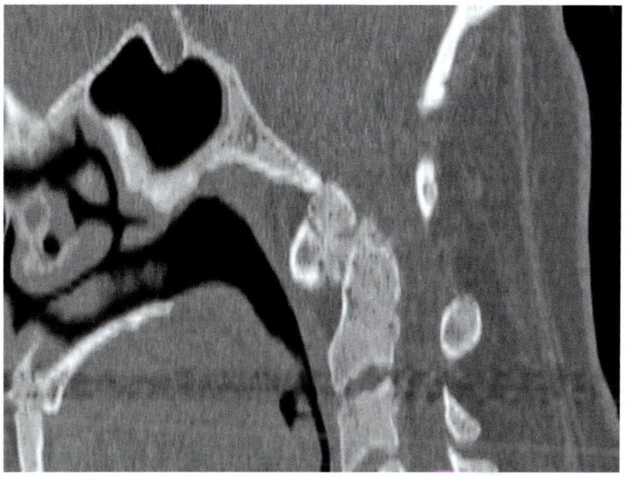

FIG. 5: Sagittal multidetector CT (MDCT) reformation showing fracture of the C2 with anteriorly displaced odontoid.

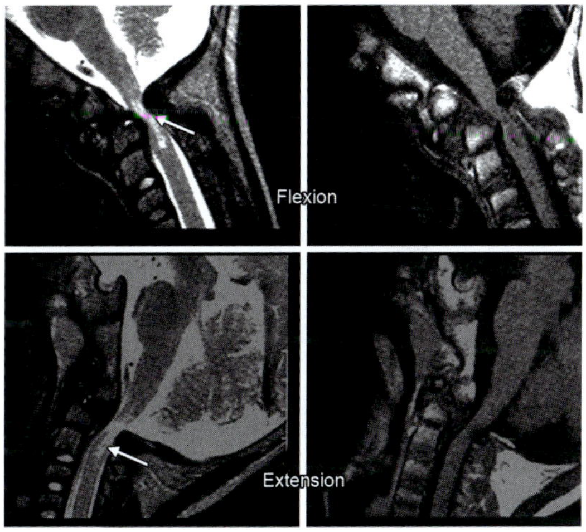

FIG. 6: Sagittal T1- and T2WI in flexion and extension shows Type II odontoid fracture with cord compression and abnormal T2 cord signal (arrows).

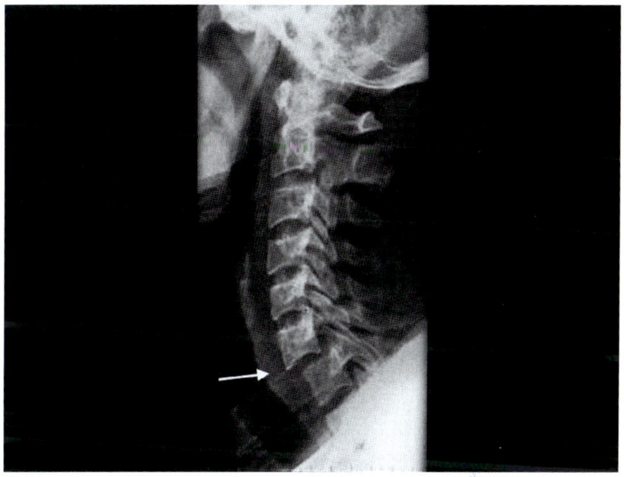

FIG. 7: Lateral view of the C-spine showing anterolisthesis of C6 over C7 with widening of prevertebral space (arrow).

evaluated by open mouth AP view. Since these fractures are mostly horizontal, CT with sagittal and coronal reformats is useful for their detection and characterization.

The most characteristic injury of C2 is the Hangman's fracture that includes bilateral avulsion of neural arches from the vertebral body. In reality this fracture usually involves the pars interarticularis and is referred to as traumatic spondylolisthesis and accounts for 4–7% of all cervical spine fractures. It is classified into three subtypes. Type I is a minimally displaced fracture, Type II is associated with more displacement with involvement of adjacent disk, and Type III includes bilateral facet dislocation with anterior displacement and angulations **(Figs. 5 and 6)**. The lateral view of the cervical spine demonstrates the fracture in more than 90% of patients. There is anterior subluxation of C2 vertebral body and retrolisthesis of the posterior elements of C2 relative to C3. CT is necessary to detect Type I fracture as well as vertebral foramen involvement.

Lower Cervical Spine Injury (C3-C7)

The most frequent mechanism of lower cervical spine injury is flexion and hyperextension.

Flexion injuries are the most common accounting for 50–80% of all cervical spine injuries.[28] C4-C7 vertebrae are affected most commonly **(Figs. 7 and 8)**. Simple wedge compression fracture may involve one or more anterior vertebral bodies without concomitant injury to the posterior vertebral body or posterior bony elements. The clay shoveler's fracture is an oblique fracture of the spinous process of C6 or C7 resulting from avulsion by the supraspinous ligament. The unstable flexion injuries include hyperflexion sprain, bilateral articular facet lock and flexion tear drop fracture. The hyperflexion sprain is a ligamentous injury with disruption of posterior ligamentous complex. Radiographic features are focal hyperkyphosis, mild anterior listhesis, widened apophyseal and interspinous space and narrowed anterior disk space. The facet joint may be subluxated. Flexion/extension views as

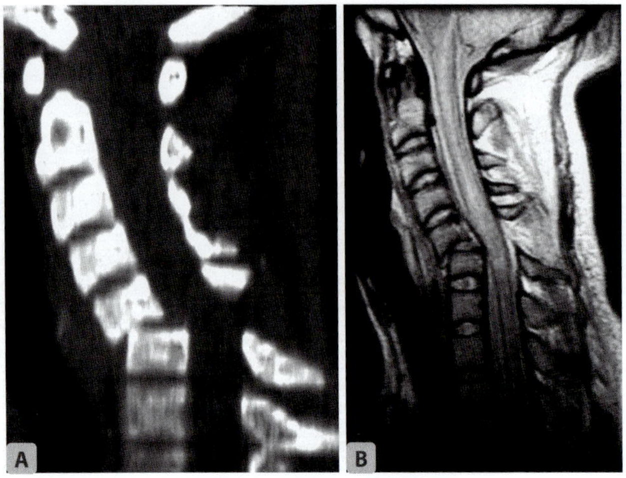

FIGS 8A AND B: (A) CT sagittal reformation showing fracture dislocation of C5 with anterior displacement; (B) Sagittal T2WI confirms the fracture-dislocation but additionally demonstrates cord injury.

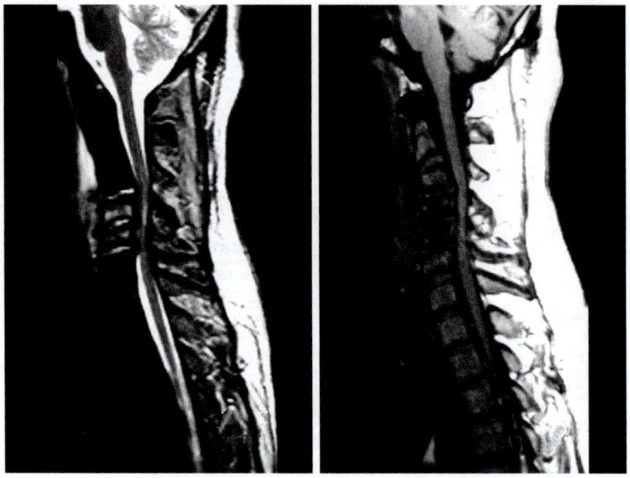

FIG. 9: Sagittal T2- and T1WI in showing altered curvature with marrow signal of the midcervical vertebrae. In addition, cord changes are also seen in the form of abnormal T2 cord signal.

well as delayed images after resolution of muscle spasm are often helpful. Bilateral facet lock is secondary to disruption of posterior and middle columns. This injury is recognized easily on lateral film as anterior subluxation with "bow-tie" sign (oblique position of facet and articular masses). On CT facet dislocation is recognized by the "naked" facet sign where articular surfaces of the apophyseal joints are no longer in apposition.

Flexion tear drop fracture results in acute anterior cord syndrome due to disruption of anterior and posterior ligamentous structures as well as intervertebral disk and apophyseal joints. Radiographically, there is a triangular fragment from anteroinferior corner of the vertebral body (the tear drop), widening of interspinous and interfacet spaces, posterior disk space narrowing, fracture of lamina and focal kyphosis.

Hyperextension injuries include wide spectrum of injuries that may be radiologically occult. In patients with neurologic damage and normal radiographs, hyperextension injury should be suspected. The injuries include hyperextension tear drop fracture, spinal cord injuries secondary to impingement and ligamentous sprain. MRI is the optimal method for evaluation of spinal cord impingement in these patients **(Fig. 9)**.

THORACOLUMBAR SPINE INJURY

Most of the fractures in the adult thoracic and lumbar spine occur near the thoracolumbar junction, about 60% are found between T12 and L2 and about 90% are located between T11 and L4. The increased susceptibility to injury at thoracolumbar junction is due to loss of the stabilizing effect of the ribs and thoracic musculature, change of thoracic kyphotic curve to lumbar lordotic curve and change in orientation of the articular facet joints from the thoracic coronal to lumbar sagittal plane. The thoracolumbar injuries have been classified into hyperflexion compression (wedge) fractures, burst fractures, flexion-distraction (chance type fracture or lap seat-belt type) and fracture-dislocation.

Compression or Wedge Fracture

It is the most common type of injury of the thoracolumbar spine comprising approximately 48% of all fractures. The mechanism of injury is hyperflexion of the spine with the axis of rotation located in the center of the intervertebral disk and represents failure of the anterior column. Flexion compression injuries result in anterior wedge fractures **(Figs. 10 and 11)**. Depression of anterior column is usually less than 50% of focal vertebral height and is usually most prominent at superior endplate. A greater than 50% loss of anterior vertebral body height is frequently associated with posterior ligamentous injury and/or subluxation/dislocation of facet joints. Plain radiograph shows anterior wedging of the vertebral body with or without fracture of anterior bony cortex. Height of posterior bony cortex and interpedicular distance is maintained. In general, anterior vertebral height more than 2 mm shorter than posterior vertebral height indicates a fracture.

Burst Fracture

It comprises approximately 14% of all spinal fractures. The mechanism of injury is axial compression of the vertebral body and represents failure of both the anterior and middle columns. The fractures are usually unstable and frequently associated with neurological deficit **(Figs. 12 to 14)**. Plain radiograph shows a decrease in the height of vertebral body (anterior and posterior), displacement of bony fragment in the spinal canal and vertical fractures involving the pedicle/laminae/spines. Two signs namely posterior bow sign and vanishing line sign have been described recently to diagnose burst fractures. Normally, the posterior cortex is seen as thin white line concave posteriorly. Posterior bow sign occurs when the posterior cortex is deformed and becomes convex. This represents the most posterior aspect of retropulsed fragment. Vanishing line sign occurs when the dorsal cortex is displaced so far back that is no longer visible and becomes obscured by the posterior elements.

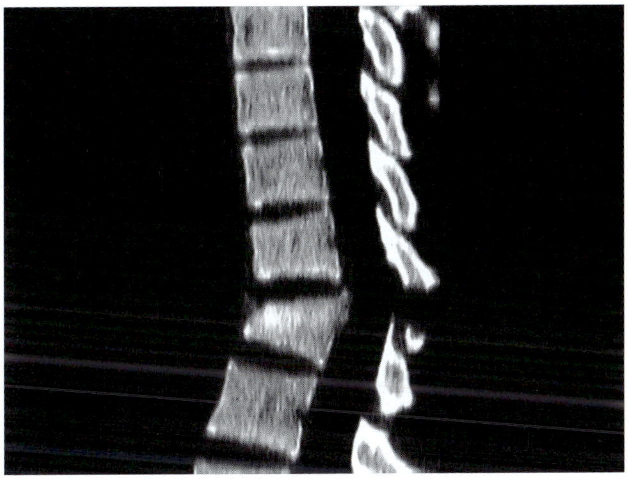

FIG. 10: Sagittal multidetector CT (MDCT) reformat showing wedge fracture of the L1.

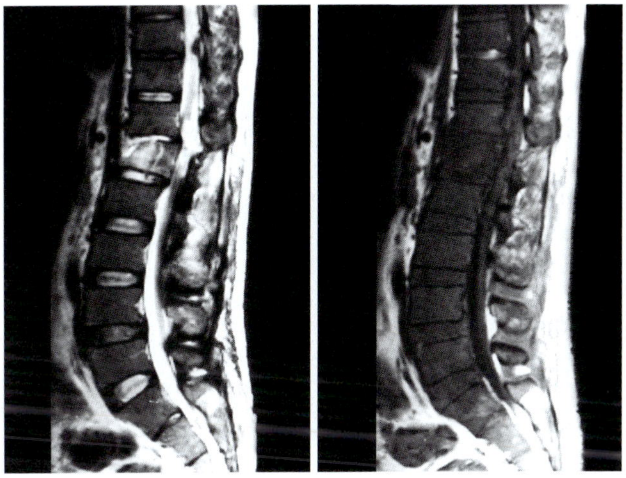

FIG. 11: Sagittal T2- and T1WI showing wedge fracture with altered marrow signal of L1 vertebra.

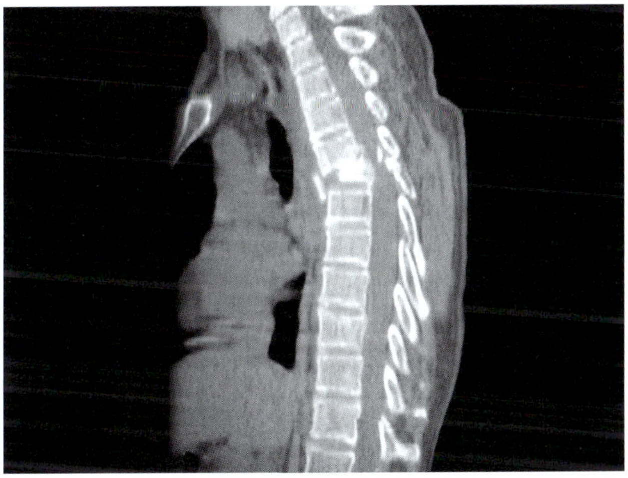

FIG. 12: Sagittal MDCT reformat showing burst fracture of the D5.

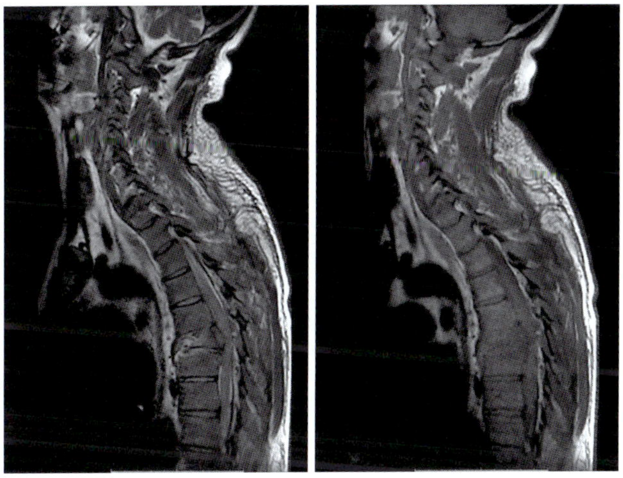

FIG. 13: Sagittal T2- and T1WI showing burst fracture of D6 vertebra with posterior displacement. Note associated ligamentous disruption and cord edema.

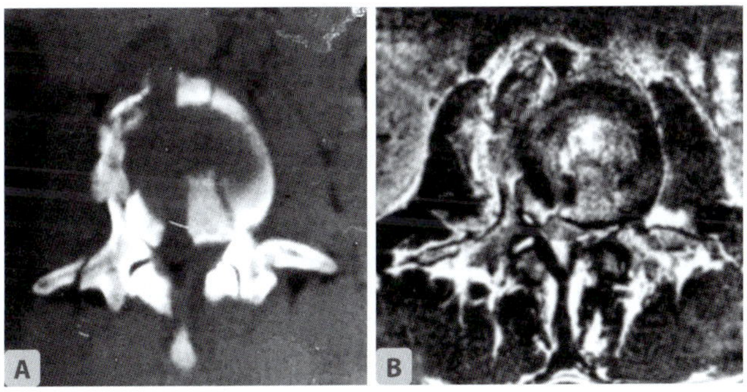

FIGS. 14A AND B: (A) Axial CT; (B) Axial T2WI magnetic resonance show burst fracture of L1 vertebra with narrowing of canal, cord contusion and prevertebral hematoma.

Computed tomography is clearly the best way to evaluate burst fractures. The findings include comminuted fracture of the vertebral body (greatest near the superior aspect), disruption of posterior vertebral body, fracture fragments in the spinal canal and fractures of posterior elements with or without disruption of apophyseal joint. Sagittal or 3D reconstruction clearly shows the retropulsed fracture fragment and the unstable spine. MRI may show the cord changes like cord contusion/hemorrhage, compression of cord as well as soft tissue hematoma/contusion.

Lap Seat-belt Type Fracture or Chance Fracture

The most common variant of flexion-distraction injuries of thoracolumbar spine is the "seat-belt type injury". It represents 10% of all spinal fractures and has a high frequency of neurological deficits. The mechanism of injury is hyperflexion with distraction of the posterior spinal elements and the axis of rotation is located more anteriorly at anterior abdominal wall in contrast to compression or wedge fracture. It is frequently but not always the type of injury associated with the use of lap seat-belt. It represents failure of both posterior and middle columns.

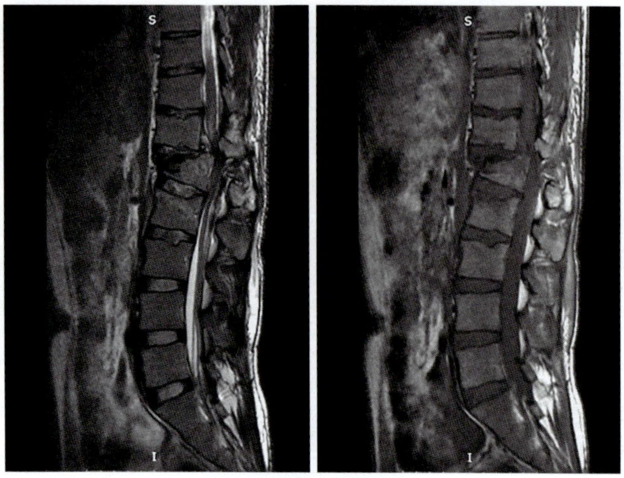

FIG. 15: Sagittal T2WI and T2WI MR images show unstable fracture involving all three columns with associated cord edema.

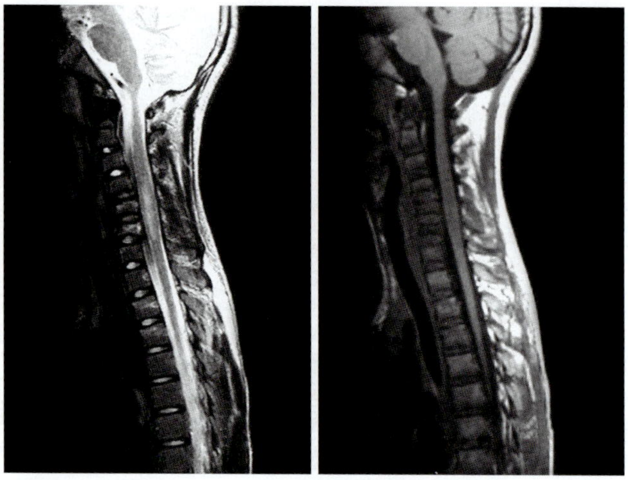

FIG. 16: Sagittal T2 and T1WI showing increased signal intensity within the cervical spinal cord representing intramedullary edema.

Three subtypes of seat-belt type injury have been described. Horizontal disruption pattern may either involve posterior bony elements (Type I chance fracture) or posterior ligaments (Type II Smith fracture). In the third type, the annulus fibroses is torn allowing for subluxation. Plain radiograph shows increase in the distance between the spinous process and horizontal fractures of lamina, pedicles and posterior aspect of vertebral body. There may be apparent increase in the height of the posterior aspect of body or widening of disk space. MDCT with sagittal reconstruction may demonstrate the nature and extent of the injury.

Fracture Dislocation

It comprises approximately 15% of all spinal injuries. The injuries result from violent complex shearing force and there is disruption of all three spinal columns which causes gross instability. There is anterior dislocation with severe hyperflexion injuries and facet joints may be dislocated with flexion rotation injuries **(Fig. 15)**. Plain radiograph shows displacement of vertebral bodies, multiple fractures, locking of articular processes and compression of vertebrae below. CT demonstrates fracture dislocation very clearly as these are recognized by "double rim" sign and "naked facet" sign. When the inferior facet of superior vertebra and superior facet of inferior vertebra are displayed on different images, the facet joint is said to be disrupted and the sign is called "naked facet sign". Reconstructed images demonstrate the degree of canal compromise.

NONOSSEOUS INJURY

Nonosseous injuries in the spinal trauma include injury to spinal cord, intervertebral disk, ligaments and nerve roots.[30,31] In addition, there is formation of spinal epidural hematoma and tears of dura in major spinal trauma.

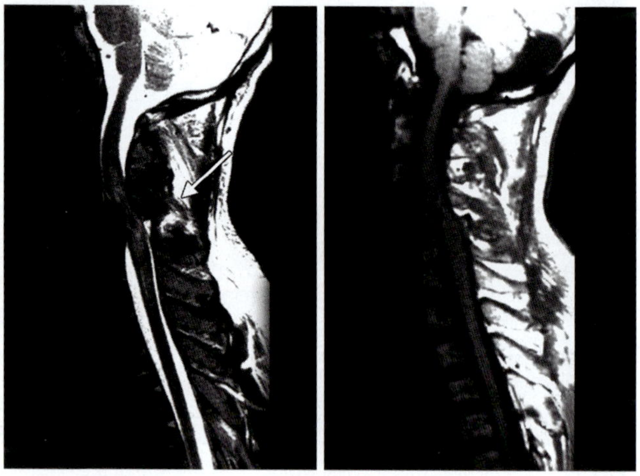

FIG. 17: Sagittal T2- and T1WI demonstrate unstable fracture with fracture-dislocation of C4-C5 vertebrae. Extensive abnormal cord signal on T2WI are consistent with cord contusion. Note also mode of interspinous ligament injury (arrow).

Spinal Cord Injuries

Spinal cord injuries (SCI) can result directly from spinal trauma (fracture or dislocations) or indirectly from compression by displaced bony fragment, hematoma or disk material, or ischemia from damage or impingement of the spinal arteries. MRI can depict the exact location, extent and severity of the injury and cord changes (edema or hemorrhage) **(Figs. 16 and 17)**. Patients with minimal cord changes on MRI have the best outcome followed by those with cord edema.[29]

For assessment of SCI, the best MRI sequences are axial and sagittal T2W and T2*GRE images. The most common MRI finding of SCI are hyperintensity on T2WI involving the cord suggestive of edema and hypointensity on T2/GRE indicating hemorrhage. Presence of hemorrhage on

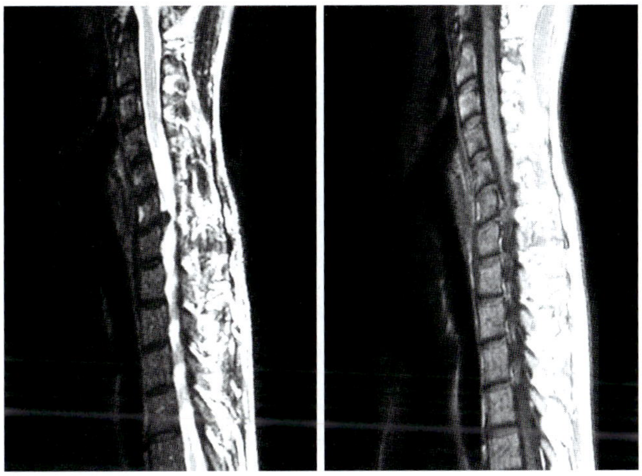

FIG. 18: Sagittal T2- and T1WI showing protrusion of C6-C7 disk into the epidural space with significant neural compromise.

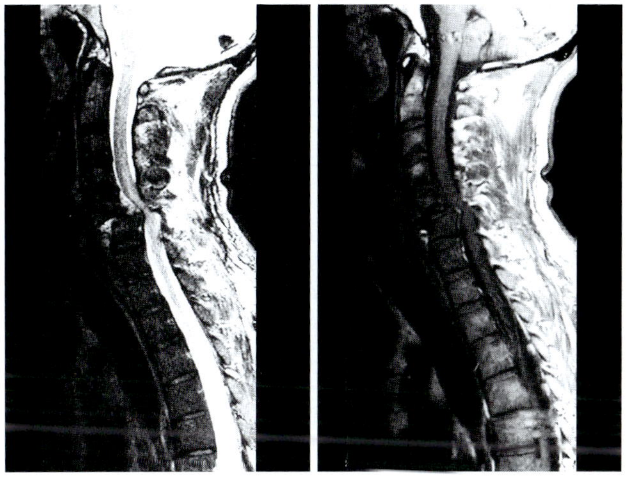

FIG. 19: Sagittal T2- and T1WI showing fracture-dislocation of C5-C6 with discontinuity in the ligaments (ALL and PLL).

MRI is the most important imaging finding associated with poor prognosis, probably explained by the acceleration of the injury cascade due to the presence of iron that potentiates lipid peroxidation. Other findings of prognostic significance are extent of cord hematoma or edema and cord compression by extra-axial hematoma **(Fig. 17)**. In addition, very early detection of spinal cord damage is possible with diffusion-weighted MRI. Resolution of spinal cord edema as demonstrated on follow-up MRI often will correlate with (limited) neurologic improvement. An entity which is more frequently described in elderly patients with hyperextension injury is 'acute traumatic central cord syndrome' in which the patient experiences disproportionately severe upper extremity motor weakness along with bladder dysfunction and sensory loss below the level of injury. This happens due to associated extensive degenerative changes in the elderly patients. The osteophytes or buckled ligamentum flavum along with narrowed spinal canal may result in injury to the central gray matter along with injury to the central portion of the corticospinal tract of the spinal cord.

Intervertebral Disk Injury

It is seen as widening or asymmetric narrowing of disk space, relative hyperintensity of one disk on T2WI, frank protrusion of disk material into the epidural space and dorsal displacement of PLL and epidural venous plexus **(Fig. 18)**.

Disc herniations are commonly seen in association with vertebral fracture dislocation and hyperextension injuries. These are caused due to injury to the annulus fibrosus with resultant herniation of the nucleus pulposus. It is important to identify the disk herniation as undetected herniation can later cause new/worsening cord injury which can result in progressive neurological deficits. Radiologically, however, it is difficult to differentiate a traumatic versus non traumatic disk herniation as appearance is the same. The presence of other post traumatic lesions as the same level can help in differentiating the two entities.

Ligamentous Injury

Spinal ligaments are very essential to maintain the normal vertebral alignment and integrity. Presence of ligamentous injury can convert a stable single column fracture into unstable two column fracture. Recently the TLICS and SLICS classification system have also taken into account the status of the posterior ligamentous complex. Normal ligament of the spine shows low signal intensity in all the sequences. The ligamentous injury can be partial or complete and depends on the mechanism of injury. The partial tear/sprain are the most common variety.

Partial tears are visualized as areas of abnormally high signal areas on T2/STIR images which occur due to associated edema/hemorrhage. Complete tears are seen as complete lack of continuity of fibers associated with increased signal on T2/FLAIR. Hyperextension injuries result in damage to the anterior column ligaments with or without involvement of the ligaments of posterior column depending on the severity of the injury. Conversely, injury to the posterior column ligaments occur on hyperflexion injuries.[23]

ALL and PLL injuries are seen as focal disruption of the hypointense signal on all the sequences **(Fig. 19)** with associated soft tissue edema best seen on STIR. Injury to the ligamentum flavum is best seen in parasagittal image and is usually associated with posterior element fractures. Injuries to the supraspinous/interspinous ligaments are seen as increased signal in the interspinous space and tip of the spinous process especially on STIR sequence.

Epidural and Subdural Hemorrhage

It is a common finding in trauma patient and symptoms depend on the location as well as the severity of compression of the spinal cord. Surgical evaluation is necessary for a favorable outcome. In some scenarios; it becomes difficult to exactly localize the compartment of hemorrhage to epidural or subdural space. 'Curtain sign' may help in differentiating the two if the hematoma is localized anteriroly in the spinal cord. Normally the dura is attached to the posterior longitudinal ligament by the Trolard ligament. Thus the epidural hemorrhage may lift the dura except anteriorly in mid line. Accordingly a subdural hemorrhage will show negative curtain sign.[25]

Nerve Root Avulsion

It is usually seen in cervicothoracic location due to greater degree of mobility of the cervical spine. Complete avulsion of the nerve root can result in pseudomeningocele formation which is pathological collection of CSF. These collections are in communication with the physiological CSF space, however are not covered by dura. These injuries can be easily seen on high resolution T2W sequence e.g, CISS (constructive interference in steady state) or FIESTA (fast imaging employing steady-state acquisition).

Vascular Injury

The incidence of the vascular injury in blunt trauma patients is less than 1%.[2] Vascular injuries should be looked for in patients with otherwise unexplained neurologic deficits, and patients with severe blunt trauma to the neck.[2] Vertebral arteries are more commonly involved as compared to carotid arteries in patients with neck trauma. There is risk of cerebral and cerebellar infarctions especially when the injury is bilateral. Following are the risk factors for vascular injury according to the Denver screening criteria in patients with neck injury:

- C1 to C3 fracture
- Fracture extending into foramen transversarium
- Cervical spine subluxation
- Facial fractures Le fort II and III
- Base of the skull fracture involving the carotid canal
- Expanding neck hematoma
- Diffuse axonal injury

DSA is the gold standard investigation but it carries a minor risk of stroke itself (risk of ~0.5%). CT Angiography is a fast, high resolution technique and is a preferred investigation for detecting vascular injury. A recent clinical review revealed sensitivity of CTA in detecting vertebral artery injury (VAI) to be around 99%.[23]

MR Angiography is also proven to be a valid technique for detecting vascular injury. Most of the vascular injury can be seen as loss of flow void on spin echo sequences associated with wall irregularity. In addition intramural hematoma can be seen as T1 hyperintense periarterial rim with flow void in the patent lumen. This T1 hyperintensity is imparted by the T1 shortening effect of methaemoglobin. In equivocal cases further evaluation can be done by CTA/DSA. However in context of polytrauma patients MRA can be unsuitable due to long scan time as well as safety challenges within the scanning environment.

SUBACUTE AND CHRONIC INJURIES

In the subacute phase following spinal cord injury, MRI often reveals hyperintense signal on T2WI in the white matter tracts above (dorsal columns) and below (lateral columns) the injury level. This Wallerian degeneration is first noticeable on MRI approximately 1 month after trauma. Approximately 1–3 weeks following cord injury, a subacute progressive ascending myelopathy occasionally can be seen, presenting as an enlarged cord with high signal on T2WI several segments superior to the original injury site.

Late sequelae of spinal cord injury include progressive enlargement of an intramedullary or extramedullary cyst, progressive myelomalacia, tethering and adhesions and/ or cord atrophy.

Post-traumatic Syringomyelia

It develops after severe spinal cord injury and is fusiform intramedullary cystic cavitation with an incidence of 3.5–4.3%. Contrary to hydromyelia which is pathologic dilatation of the central canal, it is not lined by ependyma. The pathogenesis of post traumatic syringomyelia is multifactorial and symptoms depend on the location and extent. Arachnopathic scarring plays an important role in its development. Due to altered CSF flow, the lesion may ascend up later, even years after initial insult and can lead to worsening of the neurological status. High resolution T2-weighted images (like CISS) have a role to assess the arachnoid adhesions which facilitate in planning surgical procedures. The disturbance of CSF circulation can also be detected using modern sequences like ECG gated phase contrast imaging which can detect and quantify the altered dynamics of CSF flow.[30]

SPINAL CORD INJURY WITHOUT RADIOGRAPHIC ABNORMALITY

Spinal cord injury without radiographic abnormality (SCIWORA) is defined as "clinical symptoms of traumatic myelopathy with no radiographic or CT features of spinal fracture or instability.[32] Almost 6–19% of spinal injury in children comprises of SCIWORA compared to 9-14% in adults. [32] SCIWORA is most common in children less than 8 years of age probably due to greater head size, weaker neck muscles and higher elasticity of vertebral ligaments. In addition the facet joints are more horizontally oriented which in turn increase the susceptibility to injury. The specific biomechanics of the vertebral column allows for a greater physiological range of motion of the spine without association with fracture. During the excessive motion of the spine, there is temporary occusion of the vertebral artery which leads to ischemic injury to the cord.

In adults SCIWORA mostly occurs as a result of hyperextension forces (e.g. rear end car accident). It is commonly associated with underlying degenerative changes and the level of injury to the cord corresponds to the location of these degenerative changes. Venous congestion in the compressed cord is also believed to be an additional factor.

The most typical presentation of SCIWORA is upper extremity weakness more severe than the lower extremity weakness. MRI is the investigation of choice of spinal cord. Edema **(Fig. 20)** and hemorrhages can be seen using T2 and GRE sequences. The appearance of the hemorrhage on MR will depend on the age of bleed. Bone marrow edema can also be assessed on STIR sequence that cannot be seen on CT. A number of patients however have normal

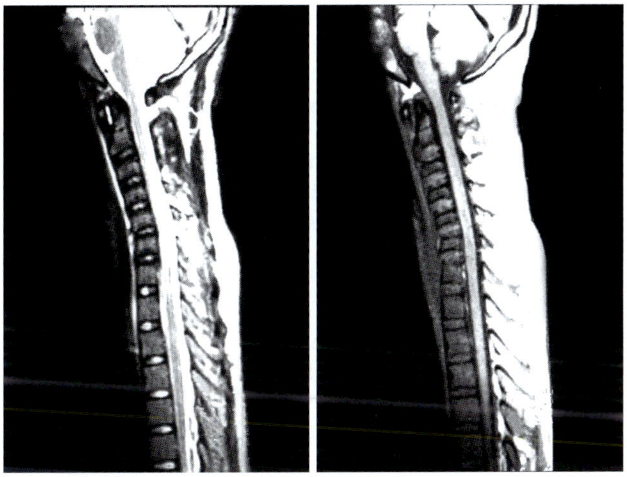

FIG. 20: Sagittal T2- and T1WI demonstrate abnormal cord signal on T2WI suggest cord edema, however, there is no evidence of bony injury.

MRI of the spinal cord but have neurological symptoms. Such patients should be classified as SCIWNA (spinal cord injury without neuroimaging abnormality).[32] In this subset of patients advanced imaging like DWI, DTI can provide vital information. Szwedowski et al. have shown that patients with SCIWNA revealed hyperintense signal on DWI in the areas corresponding to cord injury. In addition DTI can assess the white matter integrity in spinal cord. However the quality of images may be degraded by artifacts due to breathing or pulsatile motion of CSF. In a study conducted in the institute comprising forty patients, SCIWORA contributed to 12% of cases of spinal cord injury.

Whiplash Injury

The term "whiplash" refers to a wide variety of soft tissue neck injuries resulting from multiple causes.[2] Commonly the injury follows a forced hyperextension-hyperflexion of the spine. It can result from rear-end vehicle collision and side- or front-impact collisions. The injury has a wide variety of nonspecific clinical presentations. Common symptoms include neck pain or stiffness, paresthesia, upper extremity pain, jaw pain, and headache. Plausible causes are muscle tears, ligamentous injuries, perineural scarring, discogenic and joint disease, and fractures. Plain radiograph may show abnormal soft tissue or vertebral alignment. CT helps to exclude the presence of fractures or dislocations. MRI is helpful in demonstrating lesion of the ligaments, disks, spinal cord, prevertebral soft tissue and muscles.

OSSEOUS VARIANTS THAT MAY SIMULATE INJURY[33]

Variants of the Atlas (C1)

- *Atlantal clefts:* Most commonly occurs at posterior synchondrosis, however can be seen anywhere within the C1 ring. They occur due to non fusion of ossification center. These clefts show smooth corticated margin differentiating it from fracture. An anterior midline cleft can be formed due to failure of anterior ossification center to form or a bipartite anterior ossification center.
- A normal *groove* is seen along the posterolateral aspect of atlas on both the sides which transmits the vertebral artery and suboccipital nerve (C1). These structures are normally covered by posterior atlantooccipital membrane. Occasionally this membrane can become partially calcified and give an appearance of an apparent bony fragment. On complete ossification, an osseous ring is formed which is known as arcuate foramen.

Variants of the Axis (C2)

Ossific densities cranial to odontoid process: Persistent os terminale, Os odontoideum.

- *Persistent os terminale:* it is a normal secondary ossification center that fuses to the odontoid process by 12 years of age. However, there can be non fusion and is seen as a well corticated ossicle abutting the odontoid tip.
- *Os odontoideum:* It can be mistaken for dens fracture. It has a sclerotic and well corticated margin. It is also associated with hypertrophy of anterior arch of C1. An os odontoideum also has a larger gap between the os and the odontoid process. It usually does not exhibit the expected contour of the upper odontoid process.

Anterior Subluxation of C2 on C3

It is usually seen in children less than 8 years of age. It is caused due to ligamentous laxity and a horizontal orientation of the facet joint.

Variants of C3 through L5 Verterba

- *Anterior wedging of cervical vertbera:* It is a normal finding in young population and is most prominent at C3 level. A difference in height of up to 3 mm between anterior and middle aspects of the vertebral body is considered normal. It should not be confused with compressed fracture.
- *Single linear osseous defect through foramen transversarium:* It likely represents a developmental cleft. A fracture involving the transverse foramen or any ring like structure will likely involve 2 or more locations and are usually displaced fractures. An isolated defect of the transverse foramen is unlikely to be a fracture.
- *Limbus vertebra:* It is due to herniation of disk material between the ring apophysis and the vertebral body. It most commonly occurs in lumbar spine in anterosuperior aspect and is seen as a small triangular bony fragment with smooth corticated margin.
- *Clefts* may occur at several locations due to non fusion of synchondrosis. It may involve pars interarticularis, pedicle, lamina etc.

SUMMARY

There is significant change in imaging spinal trauma over the recent years with advancement in CT (multidetector CT) and MRI technology. When the clinical suspicion of spinal injury is high, MDCT is performed, as it is faster, more accurate and needs less patient mobilization than radiography.

MDCT is an excellent modality in detecting the osseous abnormalities (especially posterior element fractures), spinal alignment and assessment of stability. Early and accurate diagnosis of spinal injury is crucial in better patient management and prevention of neurological deterioration. However, plain radiography remains usually the initial screening modality as it is readily available, portable and inexpensive. MRI is best imaging modality for detection of spinal cord changes (edema and hemorrhage), extradural lesions (disk herniation and epidural hematoma), ligamentous injury and characterizing spinal fractures.

ACKNOWLEDGMENT

The authors acknowledge Dr Shashank Raj, DM resident in the Neuroradiology Division of Department of Radiodiagnosis, PGIMER, Chandigarh for his support in editing of chapter.

REFERENCES

1. Kaji A, Hockberger R. Imaging of spinal cord injuries. Emerg Med Clin North Am. 2007;25:735-50,ix.
2. Bagley LJ. Imaging of spinal trauma. Radiol Clin North Am. 2006;44:1-12.
3. Lali HS, Fehlings MG. Epidemiology, demographics and pathophysiology of acute spinal cord injury. Spine. 2001;26:2-12.
4. Tins B, Cassar-Pullicino V. Controversies in "clearing" trauma to the cervical spine. Semin Ultrasound CT MR. 2007;28:94-100.
5. Wolf M, Weber MA. Neuroimaging of the Traumatic Spine. Magn Reson Imaging Clin N Am. 2016;24(3):541-61.
6. Shah LM, Ross JS. Imaging of spine trauma. Neurosurgery. 2016;79(5):626-42.
7. Pathria MN, Petersirge CA. Spinal trauma. Radiol Clin North Am. 1991;29:847-65.
8. Heinemann U, Freund M. Diagnostic strategies in spinal trauma. Eur J Radiol. 2006;58:76-88.
9. Dalinka MK, Boorstein JM, Zlatkin MB. Computed tomography of musculoskeletal trauma. Radiol Clin North Am. 1989;27:933-43.
10. Kaye JJ, Nance EP. Thoracic and lumbar spine trauma. Radiol Clin North Am. 1990;28:361-77.
11. Abel MS. The exaggerated supine oblique view of the cervical spine. Skeletal Radiol. 1982;8:213-9.
12. Gamanagatti S, Rathinam D, Rangarajan K, et al. Imaging evaluation of traumatic thoracolumbar spine injuries: radiological review. World J Radiol. 2015; 7(9):253-65.
13. Murphey MD, Batnitzky S, Bramble JM. Diagnostic imaging of spinal trauma. Radiol Clin North Am. 1989;27:855-72.
14. Rabassa AE, Guinto FC, Crow WN, et al. CT of the spine: value of reformatted images. Am J Roentgenol. 1993;161:1223-7.
15. Gonzalez-Beicos A, Nunez DB. Role of multidetector computed tomography in the assessment of cervical spine trauma. Semin Ultrasound CT MR. 2009;30:159-67.
16. Bensch FV, Koivikko MP, Kiuru MJ, et al. Measurement of spinal canal narrowing, interpedicular widening, and vertebral compression in spinal burst fractures: plain radiographs versus multidetector computed tomography. Skeletal Radiol. 2009;38:887-93.
17. Blackmore CC, Mann FA, Wilson AJ. Helical CT in primary trauma evaluation of the cervical spine: an evidence-based approach. Skeletal Radiol. 2000;29:632-9.
18. Siberstein M, Tress BM, Hennessy O. A comparison between MRI and CT in acute spinal trauma. Australas Radiol. 1992;36:192-7.
19. Provenzale J. MR imaging of spinal trauma. Emerg Radiol. 2007;13:289-97.
20. Demaerel P. Magnetic resonance imaging of spinal cord trauma: A pictorial essay. Neuroradiology. 2006;48:223-32.
21. Mhuircheartaigh NN, Kerr JM, Murray JG. MR imaging of traumatic spinal injuries. Semin Musculoskelet Radiol. 2006;10: 293-307.
22. Geck MJ, Yoo S, Wang JC. Assessment of cervical ligamentous injury in trauma patients using MRI. J Spinal Disord. 2001;14:371-7.
23. Kumar Y, Hayashi D. Role of magnetic resonance imaging in acute spinal trauma: a pictorial review. BMC Musculoskelet Disord. 2016;17:310.
24. Hoch MJ, Rispoli J, Bruno M, et al. Clinical utility for diffusion MRI sequence in emergency and inpatient spine protocols. Clin Imaging. 2017;45:37-50.
25. Endo T, Suzuki S, Inoue T, et al. Prediction of neurological recovery in spontaneous spinal epidural hematoma using apparent diffusion coefficient values. Spinal Cord. 2014; 52(10):729-33.
26. Shanmuganathan K, Gullapalli RP, Zhuo J, et al. Diffusion tensor MR imaging in cervical spine trauma. Am J Neuroradiol. 2008; 29(4):655-9.
27. Dennis F. The three column spine and its significance in the classification of acute thoracolumbar spinal injuries. Spine. 1983;8:817-31.
28. Jelly LM, Evans DR, Easty MJ, et al. Radiography vs spinal CT in the evaluation of cervicothoracic junction injuries in polytrauma patients who have undergone intubations. Radiographics. 2000;20:251-9.
29. Tewari MK, Gifti DS, Singh P, et al. Diagnosis and prognostication of adult spinal cord injury without radiographic abnormality using magnetic resonance imaging: Analysis of 40 patients. Surg Neurol. 2005;63:204-9.
30. Van Goethem JW, Maes M, Ozsarlak O, et al. Imaging spinal trauma. Eur Radiol. 2005;15:582-90.
31. Sundgren PC, Philipp M, Maly PV. Spinal trauma. Neuroimaging Clin N Am. 2007;17:73-85.
32. Szwedowski D, Walecki J. Spinal Cord Injury without Radiographic Abnormality (SCIWORA)—Clinical and Radiological Aspects. Pol J Radiol. 2014;79:461-4.
33. Carr RB, Fink KR, Gross JA. Imaging of trauma: Part 1,Pseudotrauma of the spine—osseous variants that may simulate injury. Am J Roentgenol. 2012;199(6):1200-6.

CHAPTER

213

Spinal Neoplasm

Ajay Garg

INTRODUCTION

Spinal neoplasms include a wide range of lesions in the spinal cord, the surrounding dural spaces and the spine. Location of the tumor is the most important feature in establishing the differential diagnosis for a spinal lesion, followed by patient's age and gender. Due to the insidious onset of frequently vague symptoms in most spinal neoplasms, clinical presentation is not of much help.

MRI is the imaging modality of choice for evaluation of spinal tumors; helps to classify tumors as intramedullary, intradural-extramedullary or extradural, which is the first step in tumor characterization. Apart from localization, additional imaging features like presence of hemorrhage, degree of edema, extent of the lesion, diffusion characteristics and the enhancement pattern help to narrow down differential diagnosis. This chapter will address the clinical, pathological and imaging characteristics of various spinal tumors to help the reader make a reasonable differential diagnosis.

CLASSIFICATION OF LESIONS

Spinal tumors are classified according to their site of origin into intramedullary, intradural-extramedullary (IDEM) and extradural tumors. This classification provides a convenient and meaningful framework to approach the majority of spinal tumors. Some spinal tumors such as lymphoma have the tendency to traverse these compartments and may not follow this classification.

Intramedullary Tumors

Single: Ependymoma, myxopapillary ependymoma, astrocytoma, ganglioglioma, hemangioblastoma, subependymoma, paraganglioma

Multiple: Hemangioblastomas, metastases, lymphoma

Intradural-extramedullary Tumors

Single: Meningiomas, nerve sheath tumors, intradural metastases, lymphoma/leukemia, paraganglioma

Multiple: Any of the preceding except paraganglioma

Extradural Tumors

Single: Aneurysmal bone cyst, giant cell tumor, osteoblastoma, osteochondroma, chordoma, chondrosarcoma, chondroblastoma, metastasis, hemangioma, solitary plasmacytoma, lymphoma Multiple: Metastatic disease, hemangiomas, multiple myeloma, lymphoma

Epidural lesions: Angiolipoma and angiomyolipoma, epidural lipomatosis, lymphoma.

INTRAMEDULLARY TUMORS

Intramedullary spinal cord tumors account for about 4–10% of all CNS tumors and are rare. These tumors include both glial tumors (ependymoma, astrocytoma and ganglioglioma) and nonglial tumors (such as hemangioblastoma, paraganglioma, lymphoma and metastases).

Intramedullary neoplasms are most often slow-growing masses with vague, nonspecific symptoms. The most frequent presenting symptoms of intramedullary cord tumors are dull, aching back pain and weakness.[1] The pain usually localizes to the involved spinal levels and often worsens at night when lying down.[2] Upper extremity weakness with arm and neck pain is seen with cervical lesions. Sensory levels, spasticity, and gait disturbances predominate with thoracic lesions. Tumors of the lumbar region and conus medullaris present with back pain, radicular symptoms, and bowel and bladder dysfunction. Symptoms tend not to be relieved with rest. Valsalva maneuver frequently amplifies the symptoms.[1] Because of the non-specific nature of symptoms, the clinical diagnosis of intramedullary neoplasms is often delayed.

Ependymomas

Ependymomas are the most common intramedullary neoplasms in adults and generally occur in the cervical region.[3] These are slightly more common in women of 40–50 years of age. Patients with NF2 have increased incidence of these tumors. Most cord ependymomas are of low grade, classified as either WHO grade I or grade II; malignant cord ependymomas are quite rare.[4]

The symptoms are chronic and consist mainly of pain, myelopathy and radiculopathies. Occasionally, these

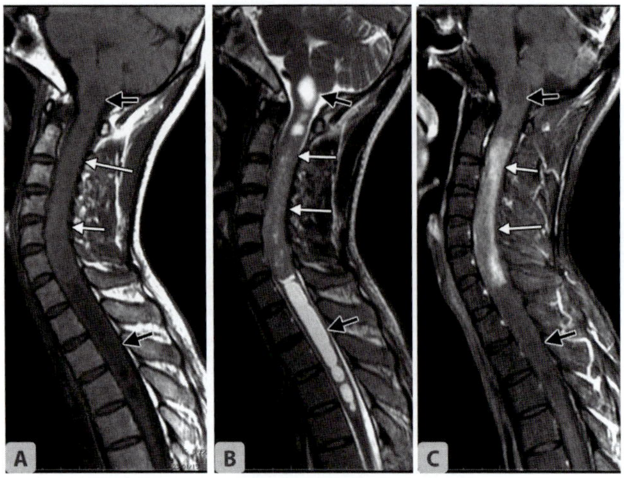

FIGS. 1A TO C: Cervical intramedullary ependymoma. Sagittal T1WI (A) and T2WI (B) show extensive cord enlargement from medulla to D4 level. Except for a cranial and caudal cyst-like area (black arrows in A and B), the mass (white arrows) is nearly isointense relative to the normal spinal cord. Contrast-enhanced sagittal T1WI (C) shows homogeneous enhancement of the oval mass (white arrows, C) extending from C2 to C6. The cranial and caudal cysts (black arrows) show no enhancement of cyst wall suggesting benign cysts.

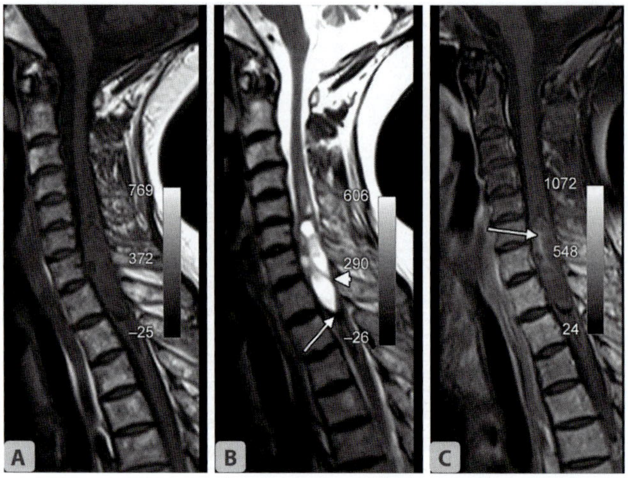

FIGS. 2A TO C: Cervical intramedullary ependymoma. MR imaging reveals a well-defined intramedullary mass extending from C6-D2 with mild cord expansion. The mass is iso-hypointense on T1WI (A) and has mixed intensity on T2WI (B). Note fluid-fluid level within the lesion (arrowhead in b) and hypointense hemosiderin cap at the distal extent of the lesion (arrow in B). Sagittal T1WI (C) shows faint heterogeneous enhancement (arrow).

ependymomas may bleed and produce subarachnoid hemorrhage or hematomyelia, thus producing acute symptoms.

Characteristically, ependymomas have slow growth. So, they compress rather than infiltrate the adjacent spinal cord tissue. Thereby, they have a good cleavage plane that helps in surgical resection.[4] Since these lesions arise from the ependymal cell lining of the central canal, they tend to be central in location.

On MRI, ependymomas are typically central well-circumscribed lesions and tend to produce symmetric spinal cord expansion. Ependymomas typically have both solid and cystic components. The solid component is iso- to hypointense on T1WI and hyperintense on T2WI **(Figs. 1A to C)**. Cysts can be intratumoral or peritumoral (polar). Intratumoral cysts are located within the solid tumor and should be resected along with the tumor as they may contain neoplastic cells.[5] Peritumoral (polar) cysts on the other hand, occur at the superior or the inferior aspects of the tumor and do not need resection as they do not contain neoplastic cells.[4] Similar cysts are also seen with astrocytomas, hemangioblastomas and gangliogliomas and are not specific for ependymomas. Ependymomas show variable contrast enhancement (homogeneous or heterogeneous), but some degree of enhancement is usually seen.[4] In addition, 20% of spinal ependymomas may show a hypointense rim at the periphery of the tumor on T2-WI known as "cap sign", which is related to hemosiderin deposition from intratumoral hemorrhage **(Figs. 2A to C)**.[6] When present, this sign is highly suggestive of an ependymoma.

DTI and DT-FT may show displacement rather than interruption of fiber tracts which confirms the noninfiltrative growth pattern of spinal ependymomas. Unlike in adults, differentiating ependymomas from pilocytic astrocytomas in children by using DTI and DT-FT is difficult.[7]

Clear tumor margins, more uniform enhancement and central location are differentiating features of ependymomas from other intramedullary spinal cord tumors.[3]

Leptomeningeal CSF spread is rarely seen in spinal ependymomas, but when present, it is more commonly associated with higher-grade tumors.

The prognosis in spinal ependymoma depends on the grade of the tumor, degree of surgical resection, and presence or absence of leptomeningeal spread. The 5-year survival rate is approximately 85% when gross total resection is done and approximately 57% with less than suboptimal resection.[8]

Myxopapillary Ependymoma

Myxopapillary ependymomas typically occur at the conus medullaris, cauda equina or the terminal filum level and are the most frequent type of ependymomas in these locations.[9] They tend to occur in the fourth decade of life in adults and rarely between 10 and 13 years of age in the pediatric population. They typically manifest with lower back ache, leg pain, sacral pain, weakness or sphincter dysfunction.

These are believed to arise from the ependymal glia of the filum terminale. Rarely, they are extradural in location, presumably arising from the coccygeal medullary vestige at the distal portion of the neural tube.[10] Multiple lesions may be present in about 14–43% of cases.[9,10] Despite being WHO grade I lesions, CSF dissemination occurs occasionally.

Myxopapillary ependymomas are characteristically lobulated, soft, sausage-shaped masses that are often encapsulated. These are typically T1 isointense and T2 hyperintense relative to the spinal cord **(Figs. 3A to C)**.

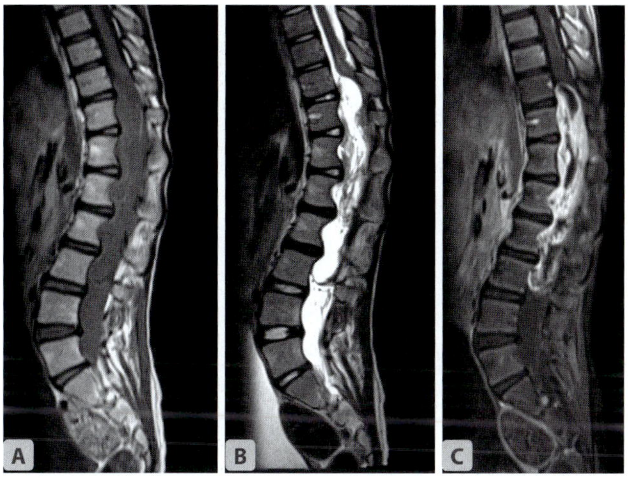

FIGS. 3A TO C: Myxopapillary ependymoma: Sagittal T1WI (A) shows an intradural lesion extending from D10-L3 spinal canal, causing canal expansion with scalloping of posterior margins of vertebral bodies. The mass is of mixed intensity on T2WI (B) and shows intense heterogeneous enhancement (C).

Occasionally, they are T1 and T2 hyperintense presumably secondary to mucin content or hemorrhage. These tumors may show superficial siderosis which is not specific, as it has been reported with other highly vascular spinal tumors. Typically, these show homogeneous enhancement, however may enhance heterogeneously depending the amount of intratumoral hemorrhage. Larger lesions tend to expand the spinal canal (resulting in posterior scalloping of the vertebral bodies) and may extend out of the neuroforamina.

The differential diagnoses of a mass arising in the filum terminale are ependymoma, astrocytoma, nerve sheath tumor, metastases, paraganglioma and hemangioblastoma.

Subependymoma

Subependymoma is a WHO grade I glioma which is a variant of CNS ependymomas.[11,12] It is believed to arise from tanycytes (from the Greek word tanyos—to stretch), cells that bridge the pial and ependymal layers.[11] These tumors present with a slowly progressive clinical course. Pain is the most common symptom, while sensory and motor dysfunctions are less common.

At MR imaging, they appear as well-defined tumors causing fusiform dilatation of the spinal cord. They are located eccentrically within the cord[11] unlike central location of other ependymomas. Enhancement is seen in approximately 50% of cases and non-enhancing tumors present as diffuse symmetric spinal cord enlargement.[11] Edema may or may not be present around the tumor. It may be possible to differentiate ependymomas from subependymomas solely on the basis of MRI findings alone.[11] Rarely, a spinal subependymoma may present as an intradural extramedullary mass lesion, probably arising from leptomeningeal heterotopic glial cells.[13]

Astrocytomas

Astrocytomas arise from the astrocytic glial cells of the spinal cord and represent approximately 30% of spinal cord tumors. They are the most common intramedullary tumors in children and are second only to ependymomas in adults. The cervicomedullary junction and the cervico-thoracic cord are the most common locations, although rarely holocord presentation may occur. Most of the spinal cord astrocytomas arise sporadically, although there is an association with NF 1, particularly for WHO grade 1 pilocytic astrocytomas.

A total of 80%–90% of all spinal cord astrocytomas are low grade and include both fibrillary astrocytomas (WHO grade 2) and pilocytic astrocytomas (WHO grade 1). Most of higher grade tumors consist of anaplastic astrocytomas (WHO grade III), whereas glioblastomas (WHO grade IV) of the cord are uncommon.[4] Spinal cord astrocytomas tend to infiltrate the cord and are, therefore, difficult to resect completely. Hence they have a poor prognosis.[4]

On MR imaging, astrocytomas are classically eccentric within the cord, which demonstrates asymmetric cord expansion. Lesions are usually multisegmental and span fewer than 4 vertebral levels.[2] Pilocytic astrocytomas tend to demonstrate discrete margins, whereas high-grade astrocytomas usually have poorly defined tumor margins due to their infiltrative nature. Tumors can show areas of necrotic-cystic degeneration (60% of cases), can have a "cyst with mural nodule" appearance, or can be structurally solid (about 40% of cases). The solid components are iso- to hypointense on T1WIs and hyperintense on T2WIs **(Figs. 4A to E)**, whereas necrotic-cystic components display higher relaxation times on T1 and T2WIs. The pattern of enhancement can be focal nodular, patchy or diffuse inhomogeneous. The enhancing portions of the tumor do not necessarily define its margins. Up to 30% of intramedullary astrocytomas do not show enhancement.[14] Like ependymomas, they can have intratumoral or polar cysts but hemorrhage is uncommon and, therefore, a "cap sign" is usually absent.[4]

An acute cord lesion in patients with multiple sclerosis (MS) may be virtually indistinguishable from an astrocytoma. MS lesions, however, generally appear more homogeneous than astrocytomas and typically demonstrate a surrounding rim of normal cord intensity, which is less common in astrocytomas.

In adults, DTI and DT-FT often assist in differentiating ependymomas, which displace white matter tracts, versus astrocytomas, which tend to disrupt white matters tracts due to their infiltrative growth pattern. Unfortunately, DTI is less reliable in differentiating these tumors in children because most pediatric astrocytomas are pilocytic, which tend to be circumscribed with discrete margins.[7,15] Non etheless, DTI and DT-FT can still aid preoperative assessment in these patients by determining the degree of resectability. Tumors that displace white matter tracts have well-defined margins and often can be treated with gross total or subtotal resection supplemented with adjuvant chemotherapy.[16] Infiltrative or disruptive patterns indicate a tumor of higher grade, which may preclude resection. These tumors are treated with adjuvant chemotherapy and radiation therapy.

Gangliogliomas

Gangliogliomas are slow-growing benign tumors that are composed of ganglion cells and glial elements.[4] They are

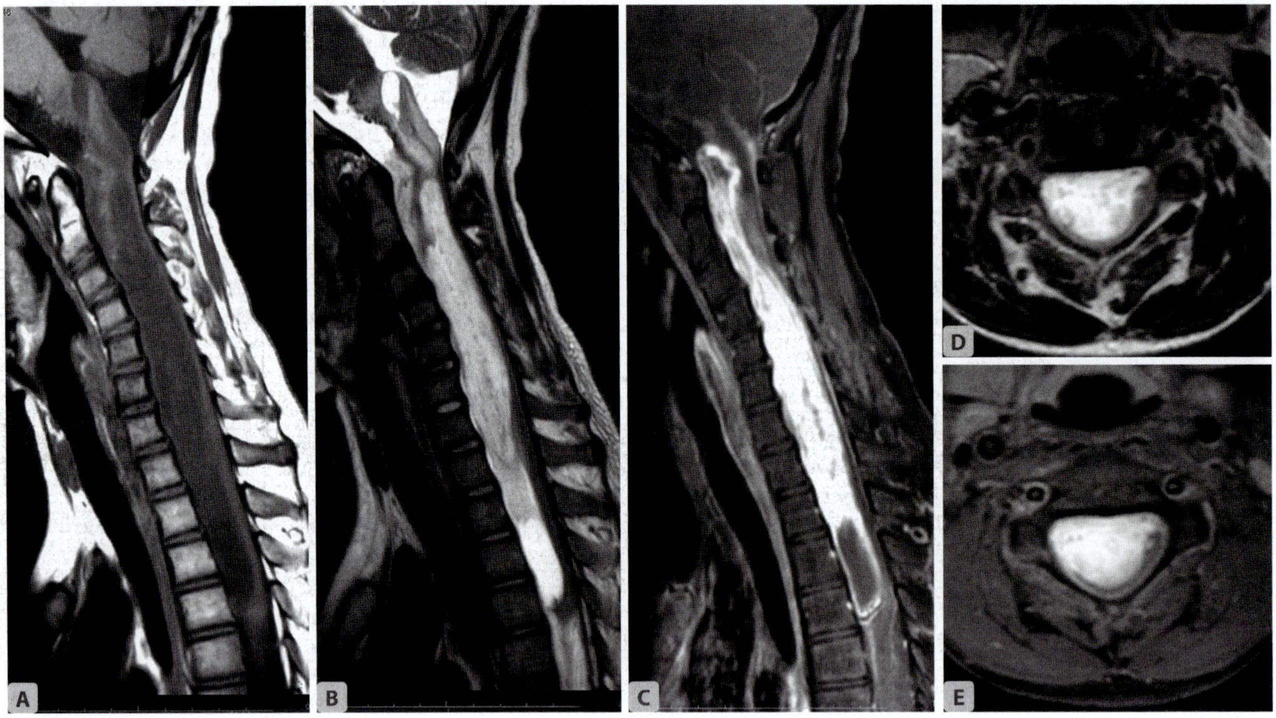

FIGS. 4A TO E: Astrocytoma in a 7-year-old boy. Long segment intramedullary mass lesion in seen extending from lower medulla to T4 vertebral level. The mass is predominantly hypointense on sagittal T1WI (A), hyperintense on sagittal T2WI (B) and show intense enhancement on post-gad sagittal T1WI (C). Axial T2WI (D) and post-gad axial T1WI (E) show eccentric location of the tumor.

the second most common intramedullary tumor following astrocytoma in the pediatric age group (15% of cases). Children between age 1 and 5 years are most commonly affected, like in the case of pilocytic astrocytomas. These neoplasms most commonly occur in the cervical and upper thoracic spinal cord, and occasionally extend up to the medulla. Gangliogliomas tend to be longitudinally extensive occupying an average length of 8 vertebral segments, compared with an average of 4 vertebral segments in length in ependymomas and astrocytomas.[17] Gangliogliomas are perhaps the second most common tumor after astrocytomas to have a holocord distribution. Like astrocytomas, gangliogliomas tend to be eccentrically located within the spinal cord. These tumors tend to have a low malignant potential, but they have a significant propensity for local recurrence.

On imaging, calcification is probably the single most suggestive feature of gangliogliomas. In the absence of gross calcification, the MR imaging appearance of gangliogliomas is highly variable, but certain imaging features may suggest the diagnosis. Gangliogliomas have a mixed signal intensity on T1WI, presumably due to the presence of a dual cell population composed of ganglion cells and glial elements.[17] They are usually T2 hyperintense. Perilesional edema is not as common as seen with ependymomas or astrocytomas. The gangliogliomas usually show patchy enhancement and cord surface enhancement.[17] Tumoral cysts are more common in gangliogliomas than in astrocytomas or ependymomas.[18] Gangliogliomas usually show chronic bony changes, including scoliosis and erosions due to their relatively slow growth; these are rarely seen with ependymomas or astrocytomas.[17]

Surgical resection is the treatment of choice with an excellent 5-year survival rate of 89% following surgical resection.[19]

Atypical Teratoid/Rhabdoid Tumors

Spinal atypical teratoid/rhabdoid tumors (ATRTs) are highly cellular malignant neoplasms of uncertain origin and are very rare. Most cases are seen in children who are less than 24 months old.[20] They may be either intramedullary or intradural extramedullary.

Imaging findings of ATRTs are heterogeneous and variable because of variable degrees of necrosis, hemorrhage, and calcification, mimicking their intracranial counterparts.[21] They show T2 iso-hypointensity and diffusion restriction presumably secondary to the hypercellularity of these tumors.[22] They enhance heterogeneously with gadolinium.[21] Cord expansion and edema are common findings. Diffuse leptomeningeal spread may occur and may be present at the time of diagnosis; therefore, imaging of the entire neuroaxis should be done. Prognosis is poor, and most patients die within 1 year.[23]

Treatment is variable, including surgical resection and/or debulking, chemotherapy, and radiation therapy.[2]

Hemangioblastomas

Hemangioblastomas are benign (WHO grade I) vascular neoplasms of unknown cell origin and account for 1.6 to 6.4% of spinal tumors.[24] Although most of these tumors (75%) are intramedullary, they may involve the intradural space or even be extradural.[4] The thoracic spinal cord is most frequently

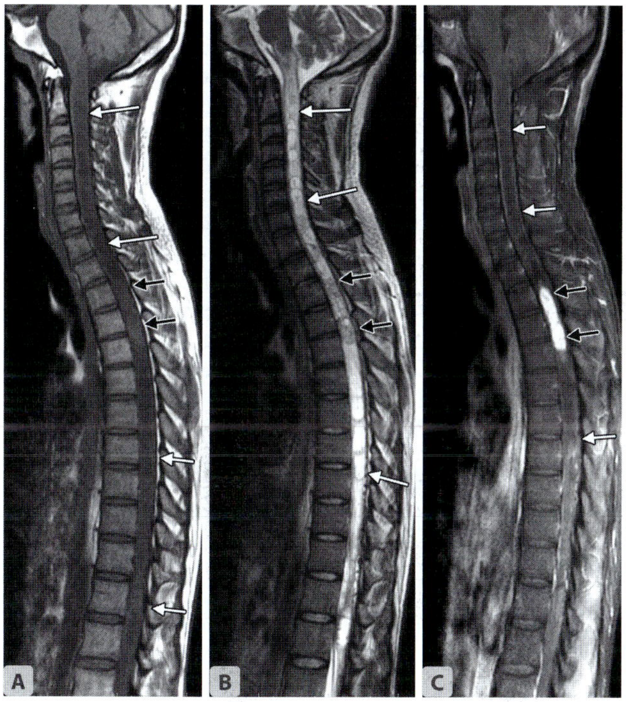

FIGS. 5A TO C: Hemangioblastoma: Sagittal T1WI (A) and Sagittal T2WI (B) show a long-segment syrinx (white arrows) in the cervicodorsal cord. Post-gad sagittal T1WI (C) shows an intensely enhancing pial based lesion (black arrows) at D3-D4 level.

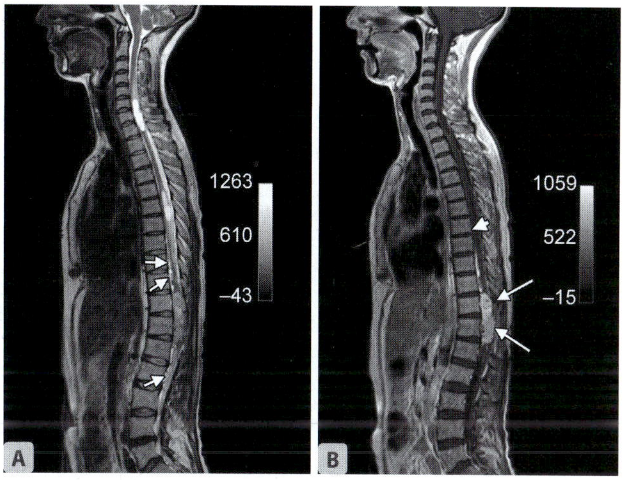

FIGS. 6A AND B: VHL with multiple hemangioblastomas. Sagittal T2WI (A) and post-gad T1WI (B) show cystic hemangioblastomas with enhancing mural nodules (arrowhead in B) in cervicodorsal cord and middorsal cord. In addition, a solid enhancing hemangioblastoma (arrows in B) with multiple intradural flow-voids (arrows in A) is seen in the region of the conus.

involved, followed by the cervical spinal cord. Most spinal hemangioblastomas occur sporadically, but approximately one-third to one-half of cases are associated with von Hippel-Lindau (VHL) syndrome.[25] These neoplasms are slow growing and may present with sensory changes, pain, and motor dysfunction.

MR features of spinal hemangioblastomas vary depending on the size of the tumor.[24] Small (10 mm or less) hemangioblastomas are mostly T1 isointense, T2 hyperintense, avidly enhancing and are located at the surface of the spinal cord, most frequently on it is the posterior aspect. Large hemangioblastomas are T1 and T2 heterogeneous, likely to have associated vascular flow-voids and show heterogeneous enhancement.[24] **(Figs. 5A to C)**. A hemangioblastoma larger than 24 mm is usually accompanied by vascular flow-voids on MR images. On MRI, a tumor is not likely to be a hemangioblastoma if it is 25 mm or more in size without associated vascular flow-voids.[24] Syrinx associated with a spinal hemangioblastoma is usually more extensive than those seen with ependymomas or astrocytomas.[25] When no cystic component is present, extensive edema is typically found. Multiple hemangioblastomas are typically found in patients with von Hippel- Lindau disease **(Figs. 6A and B)** and this necessitates screening of the entire spine and brain. Hemangioblastomas are surgically treated with maximal safe resection.

Key imaging features include a focal pial or subpial enhancing nodule with an intraspinal cyst and enlarged vascular flow voids **(Figs. 6A and B)**.

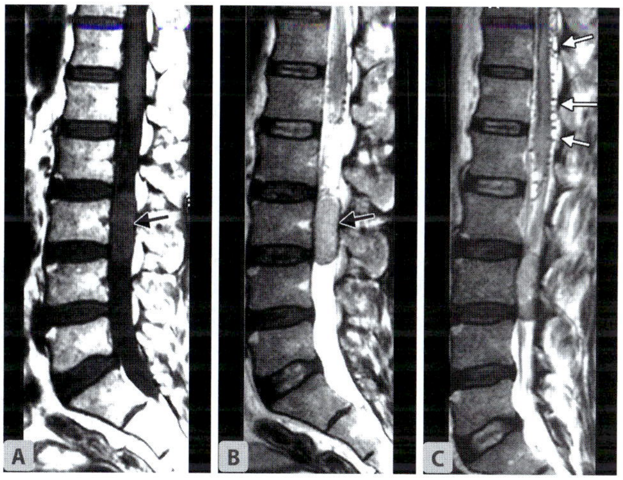

FIGS. 7A TO C: Paraganglioma: Sagittal T1WI (A) and T2WI (B and C) of the lumbosacral spine show an intradural isointense mass at L3 vertebral level. Note multiple vascular flow-voids in the intradural space.

Paraganglioma

Although spinal paragangliomas are rare, they are the third most common primary tumor to arise in the filum terminale (after ependymoma and astrocytoma). On MR imaging, these lesions generally appear as a well-circumscribed mass that is T1 isointense and T2 iso- to hyperintense **(Figs. 7A to C)**.[26,27] Hemorrhage is common (third most common after ependymoma and hemangioblastoma) and a low- signal-intensity rim (cap sign) may be seen on T2WI. After Gd- DTPA administration, heterogeneous and intense enhancement is seen virtually always.[27] Multiple punctate and serpiginous vascular flow-voids may be seen within and around these tumors.[26,27] Associated syringohydromyelia has been reported in some cases.[26]

Intramedullary Lymphoma

Lymphoma of the spine is usually caused by secondary involvement of the CNS from non-Hodgkin's lymphoma (NHL), often presenting with epidural or meningeal disease. Primary spinal cord lymphoma is exceedingly rare, accounting for 1–3% of primary central nervous system lymphoma (PCNSL) which itself constitutes only 1% of all NHLs.[4]

Intramedullary lymphoma can present as a solitary or a multifocal poorly defined enhancing mass. Unlike in the brain, most of the reported cases of spinal cord lymphoma have high signal intensity on T2-weighted images.[2] Multifocality is a characteristic of intramedullary spinal lymphoma, with more than 50% of the cases having multiple sites of involvement, including intracranial lesions. The presence of diffusion restriction can suggest areas of compact cellularity and may provide targets for biopsy.[28] There is no associated syringomyelia. Secondary intramedullary lymphoma of the spinal cord (***see* Figs. 10A to C**) is more common in the cervical and thoracic regions, whereas primary intramedullary spinal cord lymphoma favours both cord and conus regions.[29,30]

Intramedullary Metastases

Intramedullary spinal cord metastases are rare. But, with increasing use of MR imaging, they are being encountered with increasing frequency. These represent approximately 2% of all metastases to the central nervous system; they usually involve the cervical cord. The most common source of intramedullary metastases is lung cancer (>50% of cases). Other primary malignancies include breast cancer, melanoma, lymphoma, leukemia, renal cell cancer, and colorectal cancer.[31] Rarely, intramedullary spinal cord metastasis may be an initial presentation of the malignancy.[4]

Spinal cord metastases are typically small, less than 1.5 cm, enhancing lesions which are spherical or ovoid in configuration, with extensive surrounding edema.[4]

Associated syrinxes, cystic change and hemorrhage are rare and the presence of these findings make the diagnosis of metastasis unlikely.[32] Recently described "rim" and "flame" patterns of enhancement can also be helpful in determining primary vs metastatic disease. Rykken et al.[33] have described the presence of "rim" and "flame" signs, which are more common in cord metastases than primary cord lesions, with sensitivity and specificity of 40% and 97%, respectively. The rim sign is defined as complete or partial rim enhancement more intense than the central portion (**Figs. 8A to C**). The flame sign is characterized as an ill-defined flame-shaped region of enhancement superior and/or inferior to an otherwise well-defined enhancing lesion (**Figs. 8A to C**).

INTRADURAL EXTRAMEDULLARY TUMORS

Intradural extramedullary tumors are located in the spinal subarachnoid space and include benign lesions (such as meningiomas and schwannomas) and metastatic lesions.

Meningiomas

Meningiomas are neoplasms that arise from the meninges of the spinal cord. Spinal meningiomas have a strong female predominance with a peak incidence in the fifth and sixth decades.[34] Childhood meningiomas are rare, commonly of the clear-cell histologic subtype and tend to be more aggressive with higher rates of recurrence and metastasis.[35] Multiples spinal meningiomas are seen in patients with NF-2. Most meningiomas are intradural and only 10% are extradural or dumbbell tumors. Most spinal meningiomas are found in the thoracic spine, followed by the craniocervical junction and the lumbar region.[34] Although most thoracic and lumbar meningiomas are based on the posterior dura, craniocervical ones may be anterior or posterior in location.[36]

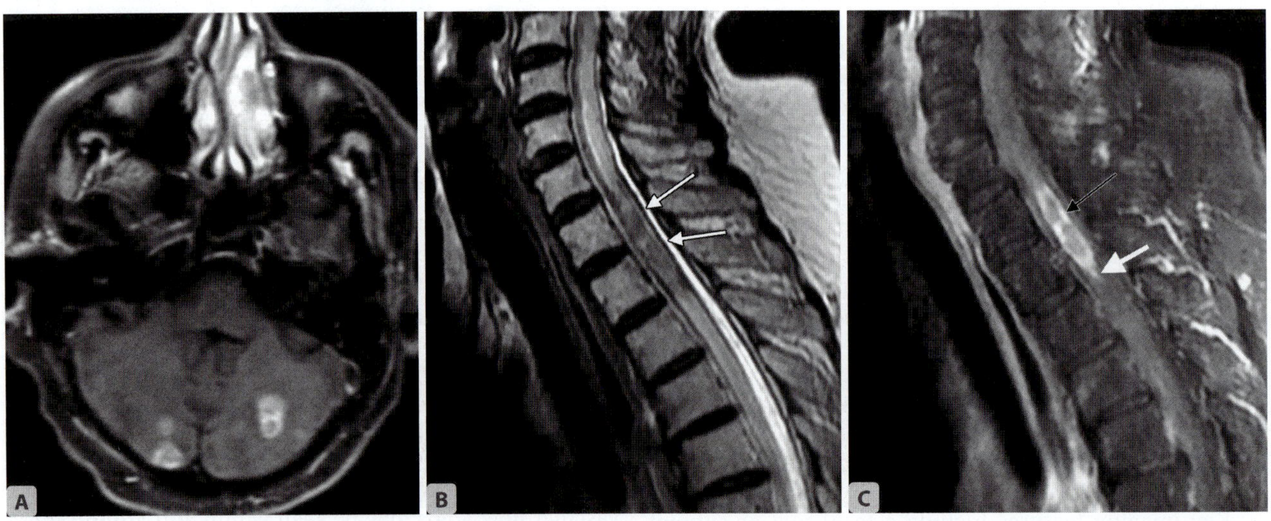

FIGS. 8A TO C: Intramedullary metastases: A 68-year-old lady with metastatic breast carcinoma. Axial post-gad T1WI (A) shows multiple cerebellar metastases. MR imaging of the cervical spine shows an intramedullary spinal cord metastasis at C7-D1 sagittal T2W (B) and post-gad T1W fat-suppressed (C) images. Note the enhancing intramedullary mass with a thin rim of more intense enhancement (rim sign; black arrow, C) as well as the ill-defined flame-shaped regions of enhancement at the inferior margins of the mass (flame sign; white arrow, C).

Typically, these lesions are well circumscribed, isointense to spinal cord on both T1- and T2WI; and display intense homogeneous enhancement following gadolinium administration **(Figs. 9A to C)**.[34] A dural tail may be present which could be secondary to tumor spread or reactive changes in the dura adjacent to the tumor. If they are densely calcified, they show low signal on both T1- and T2WI. CT may show intratumoral calcifications and this finding may aid in distinguishing between meningiomas and nerve sheath tumors, which do not contain calcifications.[36] Occasionally, spinal meningiomas have a plaque-like configuration and may encircle the cord. Meningiomas are primarily treated with surgical resection.

Nerve Sheath Tumors

In this category, most authors include neurofibromas and schwannomas. Strictly speaking, only schwannomas are nerve sheath tumors because neurofibromas arise from proper nerve fascicles. Regardless of this distinction, nerve sheath tumors are the most common spinal tumor. Schwannomas are the most common tumors, while neurofibromas generally occur in association with neurofibromatosis (especially NF-1). Like all nerve sheath tumors (in the absence of NF-1), these tumors tend to arise from sensory nerves (posteriorly in the spine) (Bell Magendie law). Approximately 50% of nerve sheath tumors are intradural-extramedullary (dumbbell-shaped) in location and 50% are purely extradural.[37] Malignant degeneration of neurofibromas may occur in patients with NF-1, but schwannomas rarely undergo malignant transformation.

Neurofibromas and schwannomas present similarly on imaging. They usually are round or fusiform, well-defined masses that can expand the neural foramina (due to extension into the extradural space), erode the undersurface of the ribs, and cause posterior vertebral body scalloping, which is best seen with CT. On MRI, both masses show isointense T1 and hyperintense T2 signal **(Figs. 10A to C)**. However, schwannomas especally large lesions may be heterogeneous on T2WI because of the mixture of Antoni A and B histologies and the presence of necrosis. Sometimes neurofibromas have a central area of lower T2 signal surrounded by peripheral T2 hyperintense signal probably due to a dense central area of collagenous stroma. This is referred to as the "target sign".[38] Localized neurofibromas demonstrate a focal mass, whereas plexiform lesions are multilobulated, often fusiform, masses that extend along nerve fascicles. Plexiform neurofibromas diffusely thicken the involved nerves and consist of numerous smaller lesions.[39] Neurofibromas are bright on short tau inversion recovery (STIR) images. Whole-body MR imaging with STIR is suggested to aid in the assessment of total tumor burden.[40] Schwannomas may hemorrhage and undergo cystic or fatty degeneration, but these findings are rare in neurofibromas. Both may show homogeneous or inhomogeneous enhancement, but schwannomas may have a typical ring or target type of enhancement in which the central portion of the mass remains relatively hypointense after contrast administration. Chronic compression of the spinal cord may result in the formation of syringomyelia.

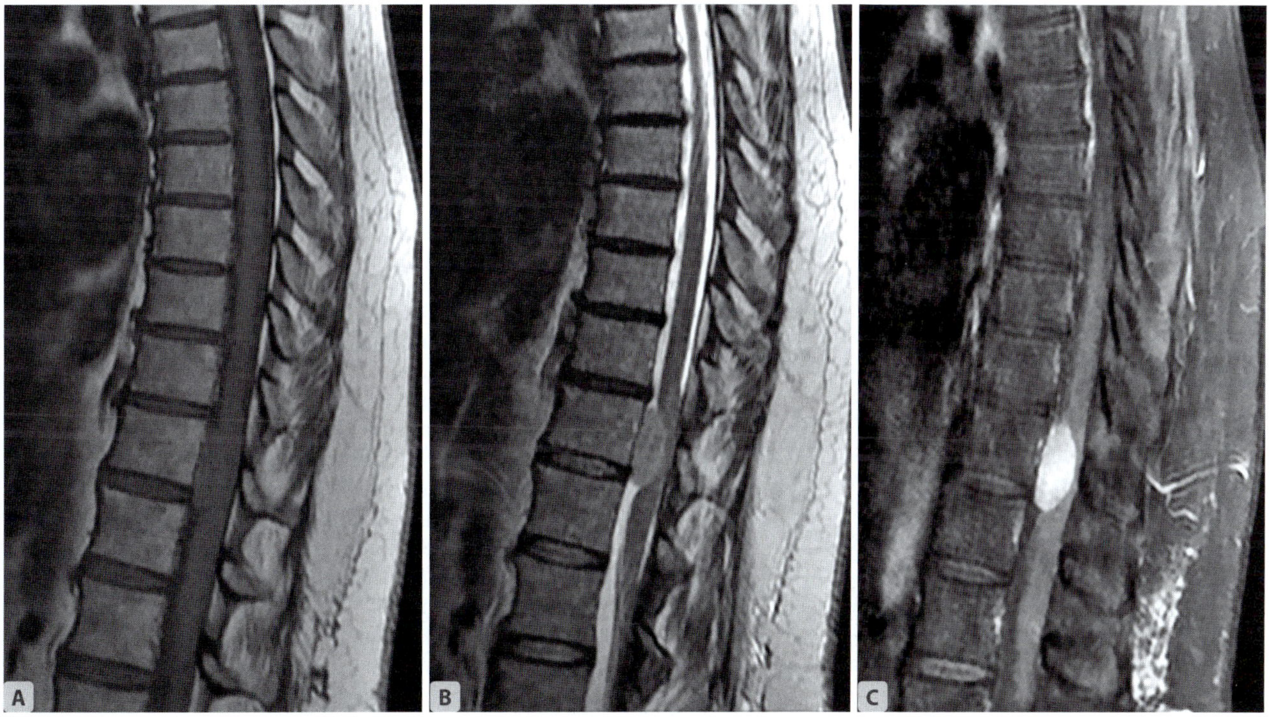

FIGS. 9A TO C: Meningioma: Sagittal T1WI (A) and T2WI (B) of the dorsal spine show an isointense extramedullary intradural mass anterior to the cord. The lesion shows intense enhancement (C) following contrast injection.

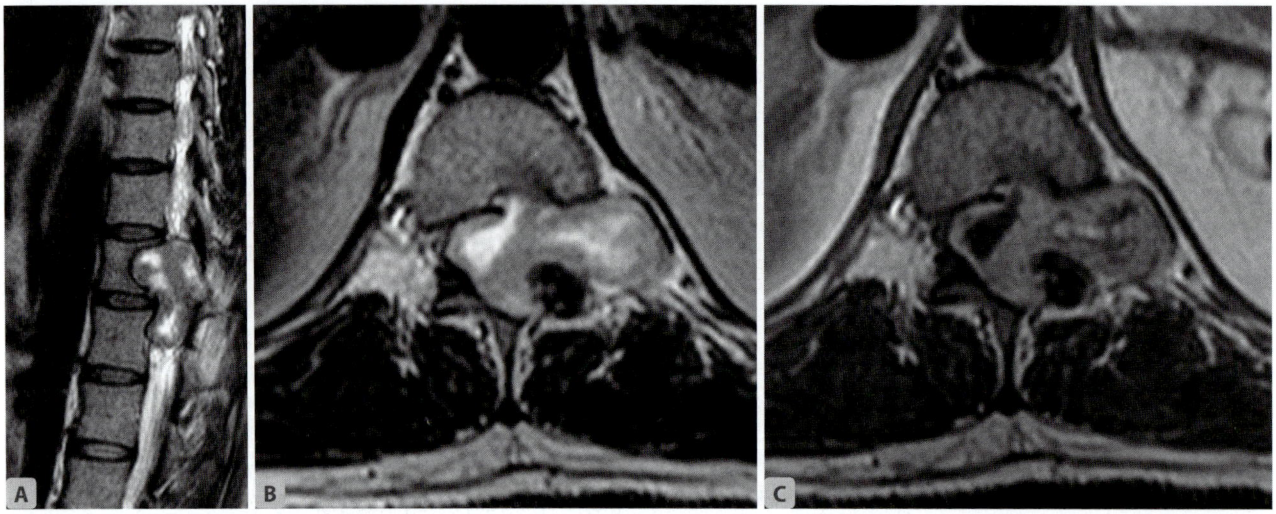

FIGS. 10A TO C: Nerve sheath tumor. Sagittal T2WI (A) and axial T2WI (B) of the spine show an isohyperintense extramedullary intradural mass with extradural extension through left neural foramina. The mass shows heterogeneous enhancement following gad administration (C).

Intradural Metastases (Leptomeningeal Metastases)

Intradural metastases represent metastatic spread of primary malignant tumors into the spinal canal. Tumors of the CNS including medulloblastoma, choroid plexus papilloma and carcinoma, ependymomas, and high-grade gliomas may produce "drop metastases." In addition, primary systemic malignancies; most commonly breast cancer, lung cancer and melanoma, may also present with dural metastasis. The lumbosacral region is the most common location. Gadolinium-enhanced MRI is the imaging modality of choice to assess leptomeningeal spread. These intradural metastatic lesions often appear as small, round, multifocal lesions that enhance and coat the surface of the cord. More diffuse pial enhancement is seen in lymphomatous metastases, breast and prostate metastases.

EXTRADURAL TUMORS

Extradural neoplasms are localized between the osseous structures and dura mater or within the osseous structures themselves.[39] They account for approximately two-thirds of the cases of spinal tumors.[4] They can be classified into primary vertebral osseous tumors, tumors of the epidural space, and extraspinal tumors invading the spinal canal through the intervertebral foramina.

Imaging is used to evaluate the extent of involvement and neural tube compression.[40] Both MR imaging and CT are used to image these lesions because MR imaging allows for superior soft-tissue resolution, whereas CT better depicts the calcified components of lesions and the degree of adjacent osseous involvement.[4]

Multiple Lesions

Metastatic Disease

Spinal metastases are the most common tumors of the spine;[41] develop in approximately 10% of all patients with cancer and are multiple in 90% of cases. In adults, the most common primary tumors are adenocarcinomas of lung, prostate and breast. In children, most vertebral metastases arise from neuroblastoma and Ewing's sarcoma. The most commonly affected regions are the thoracic and lumbar and least commonly, the cervical spine. The metastatic foci may be in the posterior elements or in the vertebral bodies. Symptomatic spinal metastases produce a characteristic clinical syndrome beginning with local back or neck pain. Pain is followed by weakness, numbness and sphincter dysfunction.[41]

Most spinal metastases are lytic. Densely sclerotic metastases are typical (but not pathognomonic) for prostrate and rare cancers such as carcinoid tumors. Although nuclear medicine studies are very sensitive, their specificity is low. Uptake of most tracers requires destruction of cortical bone and thus metastases limited to bone marrow may be missed. Because of this reason, MRI is the imaging method of choice in these patients. Not only does MRI provide information regarding involvement of the bone, but also regarding overt or impending compression of the bone. Metastases to spine generally present as T1-hypointense and T2-hyperintense lesions that replace the normal marrow **(Figs. 11A to D)**. After contrast is given, most metastases enhance. Occasionally, the entire spine is involved by the tumor and its distribution may be so homogenous as to cause the vertebrae to appear normal at first glance (this is particularly true of prostrate metastases). A clue that this is happening is the fact that intervertebral disks appear brighter than bone marrow on T1 images (this is the inverse of what is normal, where the disks are darker than the vertebral body bone marrow on T1 images). By the time of diagnosis, many vertebral metastases have epidural extension.

MRI may be helpful to differentiate between a neoplastic compression fracture and an osteoporotic fracture. In neoplastic compression fracture, there is complete replacement of fatty marrow with neoplastic cells which may also extend beyond the spine. On the other hand, osteoporotic compression fractures may only demonstrate a band of marrow replacement representing edema. There is gradual

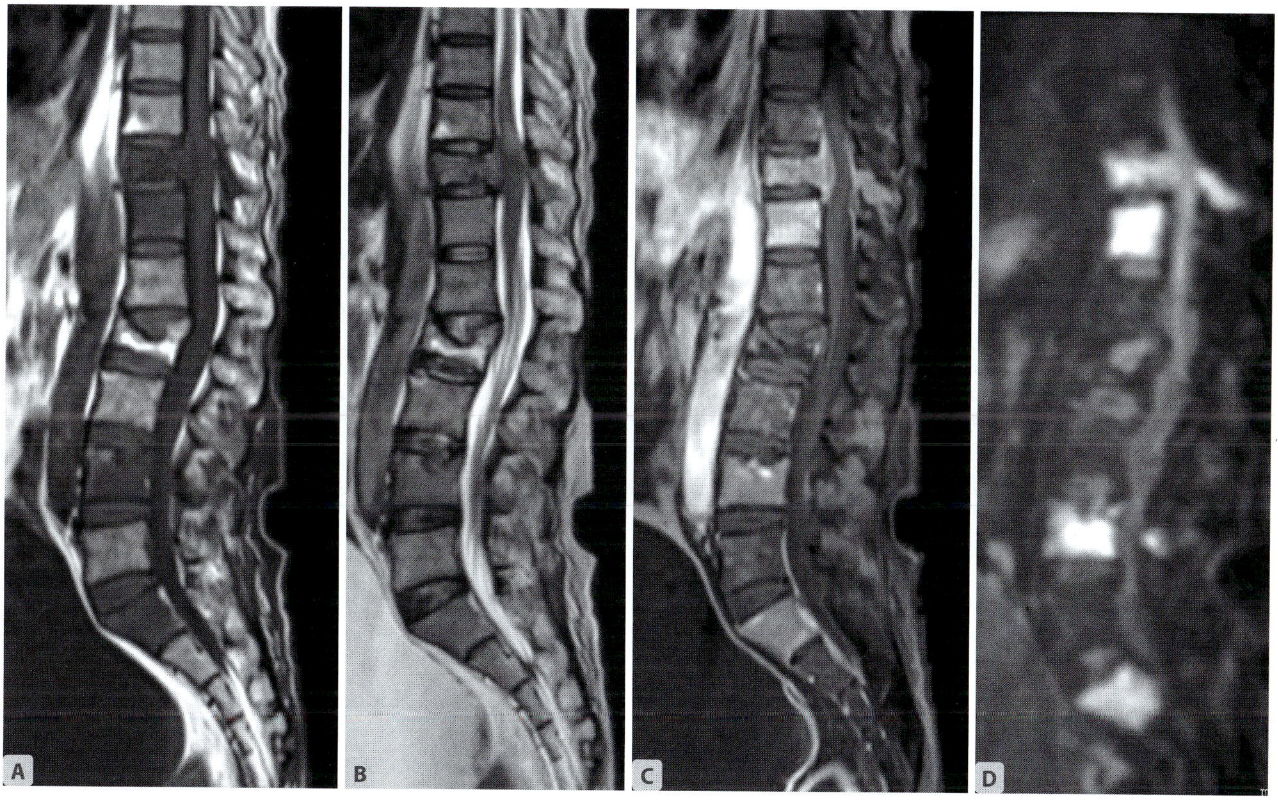

FIGS. 11A TO D: Spinal metastases: Sagittal T1WI (A), T2WI (B) post-gad fat sat T1WI (c) and diffusion-WI (d) show abnormal signal in T11, T12, L4 and S1 vertebral bodies with epidural soft tissue component at D11. These lesion are hypointense on T1 (A) and T2WI (B) and show restricted diffusion (D) and enhance following contrast administration (C). Note benign anterior wedging of L2 vertebrae without any enhancement or diffusion restriction.

return to the normal fatty marrow on follow-up studies. The presence of multiple foci in the spine favors the diagnosis of metastatic disease. Diffusion weighted imaging may be helpful in differentiating benign osteoporotic vertebral body fractures (which have low signal intensity) from malignant ones (which have relatively high signal intensity).[42]

Multiple Myeloma

Multiple myeloma (MM) is a malignancy characterized by monoclonal proliferation of malignant plasma cells. Nearly always, the disease is systemic, but occasionally, it may be isolated (plasmacytoma). In most patients, plasmacytoma is the initial manifestation of the disease and MM develops in most of the cases 5 to 10 years after the initial diagnosis. MM is the most common primary neoplasm of spine with the majority occurring in the thoracic and lumbar spine. Most patients are men, 60 years of age or older. Plasmacytomas are expansile lytic masses that may extend into the epidural space; and may undergo pathological fracture.

On plain film or CT, they usually appear as focal lytic lesions, but often the disease may present innocuously, appearing only as diffuse osteopenia. The lesion may be sclerotic rather than lytic in case of POEMS (polyneuropathy, organomegaly, endocrinopathy, myeloma and skin changes) syndrome. Treated myeloma, after chemotherapy and/or radiation, may also exhibit sclerosis.[43]

MRI is superior to plain radiograph for both, focal and diffuse involvement. On MRI, five different infiltration patterns can be seen: (1) normal appearance of bone marrow despite minor microscopic plasma cell infiltration, (2) focal marrow involvement, (3) homogeneous diffuse marrow infiltration, (4) combined diffuse and focal marrow infiltration, and (5) "salt-and-pepper" pattern with inhomogeneous bone marrow with interposition of fat islands.[44] Typically marrow infiltrations are identified as hypointensities on T1WI, hyperintensities on STIR images and enhancement on gadolinium-enhanced images.[45] Diffuse involvement appears as homogeneous signal reduction on T1WI which enhances after contrast material administration. In general, however, MM is suspected whenever MR images depict an expansile focal mass; multiple focal masses in the axial skeleton; diffuse marrow involvement, particularly at known sites of normal hematopoiesis; or multiple compression fractures in a patient with no known primary malignancy.[45] These imaging features are suggestive but are not pathognomonic for MM and may also be seen in other marrow infiltrative disorders.

Recently, MRI has been used in clinical staging, guiding biopsies[45] and monitoring response to therapy in patients with multiple myeloma. In focal lesions, reduction of signal intensity on T2WI, lack of rim-like enhancement after contrast administration or even a normalization of bone marrow signal on T1 are signs of good response.[44] In diffuse lesions, a patchy reconversion to fatty marrow may be a sign of response to treatment.

Lymphoma

Spinal lymphoma occurs most often between the 5th and 7th decades of life. Most patients have underlying non-Hodgkin's lymphoma. Spinal involvement develops in approximately 2% of these patients and affects mostly the epidural space. Bone lesions are most frequent in the dorsal and lumbar spine and least frequent in the cervical spine. Bony involvement mostly results in osteolytic lesions, but patchy sclerosis and "ivory vertebrae" as well as mixed lytic and blastic lesions are also commonly seen.[46] Vertebral collapse may also occur.

On MRI, lymphoma appears as a nonspecific mass that is hyperintense on T1 images and hypointense or bright on T2 images. The T2 signal characteristics are related to the fact that lymphomas have a high nucleus-to-cytoplasm ratio. For similar reasons, lymphomas have restricted diffusion on DWI.[36] Lymphomas enhance intensely and may compromise the spinal canal, resulting in compression of the spinal cord. Radiation therapy can result in rapid reduction in the size and compressive effects of these lesions so early and accurate diagnosis is of particular importance. Paravertebral soft-tissue masses and gouge defects on the anterior borders of the vertebrae may be seen.

Vertebral Hemangiomas

Vertebral hemangiomas (VHs) are the most common primary bone tumor and are found in over 10% of population in autopsy studies. They are composed of thin-walled capillary-sized to cavernous blood vessels lined by endothelial cells infiltrating the medullary cavity between bone trabeculae. They are most commonly found in the fourth to sixth decades with slight female predominance. They may be solitary (70%) or multiple (30%). The most common locations are the thoracic, lumbar and cervical regions. Most of the hemangiomas arise in the body of the vertebra, but may also involve the pedicles and rarely, spinous processes. The majority of hemangiomas are asymptomatic, but occasionally, they may present as large and aggressive masses destroying a vertebra and producing pain and even compression of the spinal cord. Some hemangiomas enlarge and become symptomatic during pregnancy.

From a strict radiological point of view, VHs can be classified as typical, atypical, and aggressive (also called compressive).[47] The terms "typical" and "atypical" refer primarily to the MR imaging appearance, which is directly correlated with the ratio of fatty to vascular components and interstitial edema. The term aggressive refers to the presence of radiological features such as extension beyond the vertebral body, destruction of the cortex, and invasion of the epidural and paravertebral spaces.[47] Clinically asymptomatic VHs may show "typical" or "atypical" imaging findings, while symptomatic VHs more frequently appear "atypical" or "aggressive."

Typical Vertebral Hemangiomas

At radiography, typical VHs classically have a coarse, vertical, trabecular pattern, (which has been likened to corduroy) presumably a response to stress.[48] At CT, the thickened trabeculae are seen in cross section as small punctate areas of sclerosis, often called the 'polka-dot' appearance **(Fig. 12A)**. On sagittal and coronal reformatted CT images, classical vertical orientation of the thickened trabeculae is seen (the "corduroy" sign). **(Figs. 12B and C)**. The bony cortex is intact and no extraosseous extension is seen. On MRI, typical VHs

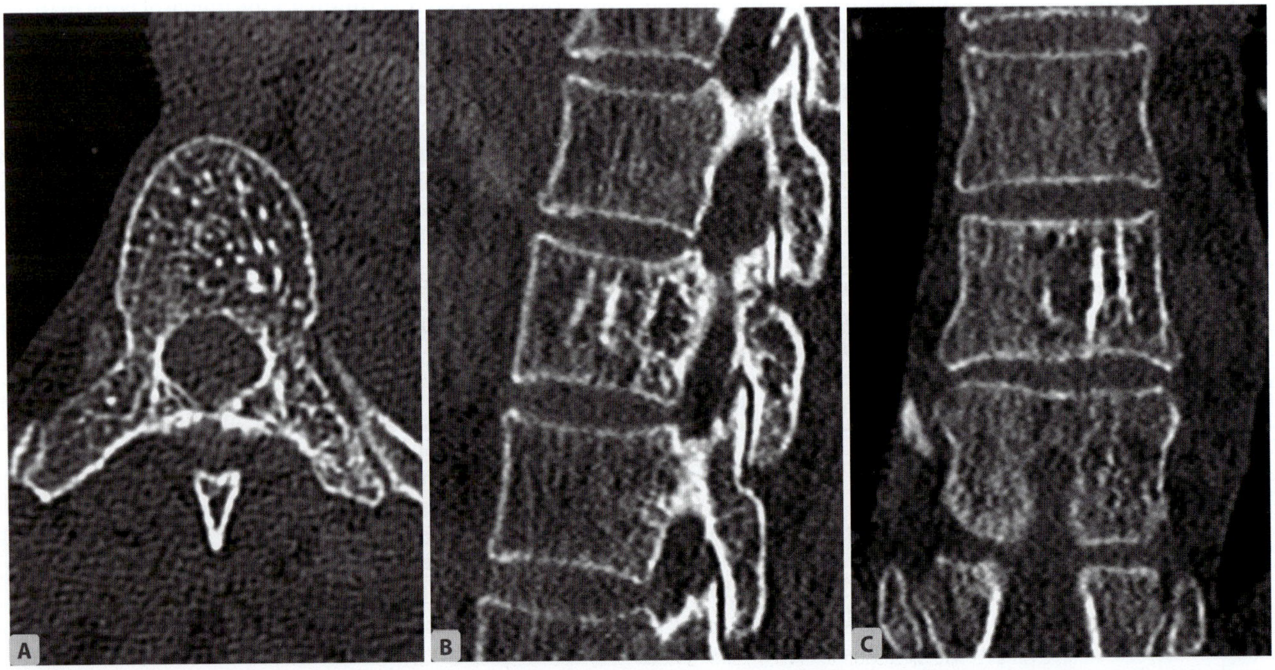

FIGS. 12A TO C: Hemangioma CT. (A) Axial CT of a L3 hemangioma with characteristic "honeycomb" appearance, also described as mottled appearance; Sagittal (B) and coronal (C) reconstructed images show sparse, vertically oriented thickened trabeculae that involve the vertebral body and posterior elements.

appear as well-defined hyperintense lesions on both T1- and T2WI owing to the predominant fatty component and as slightly hyperintense lesions on FLAIR or STIR imaging because of their vascular component. Thickened vertical trabeculae appear as punctate and linear areas of iso- to hypointensity within the hyperintense lesion on T1WI. Variable enhancement is seen in postcontrast T1WI.

Atypical Vertebral Hemangiomas

Atypical VHs have less fatty and greater vascular content. Thus, they appear iso- to hypointense on T1WI and show very high signal intensity on T2W and fluid-sensitive images. Atypical VHs usually show varying degrees of enhancement following gadolinium administration, which is best appreciated on T1W fat-suppressed images. Like typical VHs, thickened vertical trabeculae on CT and MR images is a key feature for diagnosis, though this is more difficult to see in atypical VHs.

Aggressive Vertebral Hemangiomas

Aggressive VHs are more aggressive lesions that are usually made of less fat with more soft tissue hypervascular stroma. Plain radiograph may not detect abnormalities or may show nonspecific findings, such as osteoporosis, poorly defined or expanded cortex, vertebral collapse, pedicle erosion, or vertical trabecular pattern irregularities that are associated with lytic areas of varying size.[6,8] CT may show nonspecific findings such as ballooning[47] and lysis[49] of the cortex or extra-osseous soft tissue extension.[23,24] However, one must look for the typical "polka-dot" sign on axial CT images, even in the more aggressive/destructive lesions, because it can guide the correct diagnosis.

Aggressive VHs are difficult to diagnose by MR imaging as bone is not directly visualized and more aggressive lesions are usually made of less fat with more soft tissue hypervascular stroma. T1WI usually shows hypointense lesions. T2W and fluid-sensitive images usually show areas of very high intensity corresponding to the vascular components of aggressive VHs **(Figs. 13A to D)**.

Some imaging features that might suggest a diagnosis of aggressive VHs include: a maintained vertebral body height, a sharp margin with the normal marrow, intact cortex adjacent to a paraspinal mass, and enlarged paraspinal vessels.[50] The angiographic appearance of VHs is usually characteristic: dilatation of the arterioles of the vertebral body, multiple blood pools in the capillary phase, and intense opacification extending beyond the normal hemivertebral territory throughout the entire vertebral body.[48]

Solitary Lesions

Aneurysmal Bone Cyst

Aneurysmal bone cyst (ABC) accounts for lesser than 1% of all primary bone tumors. Approximately, 20% of all ABCs are located in the spine, particularly in the lower thoracic and lumbosacral regions, where the posterior elements are typically involved. The peak incidence is in the second decade of life with a slight female predominance. Patients complain of back pain and neurologic symptoms resulting from encroachment on the spinal canal.

ABCs may be primary (70%) or secondary. Secondary ABCs may be associated with GCT, osteoblastoma, chondroblastoma, metastases and osteosarcoma. Pathologically, ABCs consist of multiloculated blood-filled spaces, which are not lined by endothelium. Solid components are usually in septations and are composed of fibrous tissue, reactive bone and giant cells. In 5–7.5% of cases, the solid component is predominant.[51]

On plain radiographs, ABCs appear as marked expansile lesions causing bone remodelling. These lesions are centered in the posterior elements, with frequent extension into the vertebral body (75–90% of cases).[52,53] A thin, outer periosteal rim and septations may be seen. Similar to GCT and chordoma, spinal ABCs may also involve adjacent vertebral

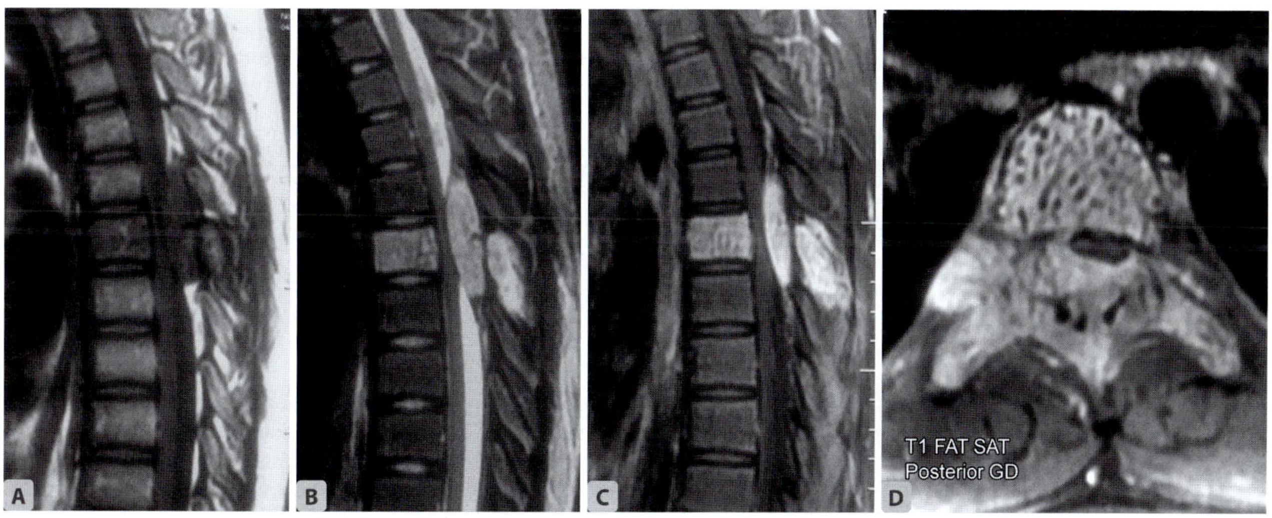

FIGS. 13A TO D: Hemangiomas aggressive: Sagittal T1WI (A) and T2WI (B) of the dorsal spine reveal D4 and D8 hemangiomas. The lesions are hypointense on T1WI and hyperintense on T2WI, suggesting aggressive hemangiomas. Axial T2WI (C) image shows right paravertebral and epidural soft tissue component, (D) compressing the spinal cord.

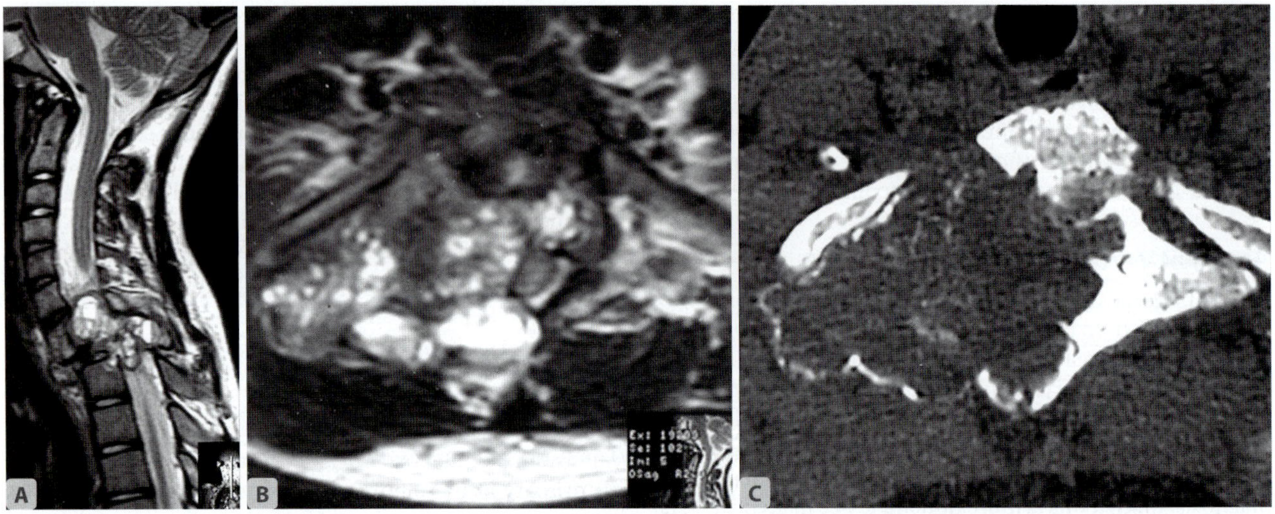

FIGS. 14A TO C: Aneurysmal bone cyst: Sagittal T2WI (A) and axial T2WI (B) of the cervicodorsal spine show and multicystic expansile mass involving the posterior arch, right pedicle and body of the D1 vertebra. The mass contains multiple septae with fluid-fluid levels. The spinal cord is displaced posteriorly and to the left; (C) CT scan shows the thin rim of bone marginating the mass.

bodies, intervertebral disks, posterior ribs and paravertebral soft tissues.[54]

On CT scan, ABCs are eccentric, lytic, expansile, multiloculated lesions that resemble a ''soap bubble'' with a ''blown-out'' appearance **(Figs. 14A to C)**.[55] Cystic spaces with fluid-fluid levels can occasionally be detected on CT scan.[56] Relationship of the tumor with neural elements and fluid-fluid levels are better appreciated with MRI than CT. On MRI, the lobulated lesion is surrounded by a hypointense rim corresponding to an intact, thickened periosteal membrane **(Figs. 14A to C)**.[55] The cystic components vary in appearance on T1 and T2 scans, depending on the age of the blood products and debris within these cysts. Gadolinium contrast enhancement is seen in up to 96% of lesions.[57] and is usually seen within the rim and septations, rather than the cystic spaces.

The presence of fluid-fluid or hematocrit levels is suggestive, but not pathognomic of ABCs. I has also been reported in giant cell tumors, chondroblastomas, fractured simple cysts, fibrous dysplasia and malignant fibrous histiocytomas.[58] The presence of a solid component with diffuse contrast enhancement should raise suspicion for a secondary ABC, although it might also be encountered in the solid variant of ABC.[59]

Endovascular treatment with multiple embolic agents may be done as both, a preliminary procedure to lessen blood loss at surgery and as a stand-alone treatment.[52]

Giant Cell Tumor

Giant cell tumors (GCTs) of the spine are uncommon tumors and account for 3–7% of all GCTs. Spinal lesions occur during 2nd to 4th decades of life and are more frequent in women. Patients present with symptoms of pain (often radicular), weakness and sensory deficits.

Sacrum is the most common site of spinal GCTs.[60] Sacral GCTs are often eccentric and abut or extend across the sacroiliac joint,[35,44] in comparison to a more central location of sacral chordomas. Extra-sacral spinal GCTs are usually located in the vertebral body with or without extension to the posterior elements.[61] GCTs may involve the adjacent intervertebral disks and vertebrae.[62]

Pathologically, GCT is composed of abundant osteoclastic giant cells intermixed throughout a spindle cell stroma. Cystic areas and hemorrhage, with hemosiderin and prominent areas of fibrous tissue with high collagen content are often present.[63] Rarely, GCTs may metastasize and recur, especially with incomplete resection. Approximately 5–10% of GCTs are malignant.[54]

Typically, GCT appears as a lytic lesion with cortical expansion on a radiograph.[26,65] On CT scans, the tumor has soft-tissue density with well-circumscribed margins that may show a thin rim of sclerosis **(Figs. 15A and B)**. GCT shows heterogeneous signal intensity on both T1 and T2WI due to presence of necrosis, hemorrhage, or cystic spaces. Low T2 signal intensity due to presence of hemorrhagic and fibrotic content is often seen. Marrow edema is usually not seen in the absence of a pathological fracture. The lesion enhances after intravenous injection of contrast material.

At bone scintigraphy, GCT may reveal diffusely increased uptake of radionuclide. However, sacral GCTs commonly show the "doughnut" sign of central photopenia and increased peripheral activity. Angiography shows prominent vascularity of these tumors and is often reserved for preoperative embolization.

Osteoid Osteoma

Osteoid osteoma is a benign bone-forming tumor that is characterized by a small radiolucent nidus (usually < 2 cm in diameter). It involves the axial skeleton in 10% of cases.[48] Patients are usually affected between the ages of 10 and 20 years, with a male-to-female distribution of 1.5:2.[61,64] Clinical symptoms include painful scoliosis, focal or radicular pain, gait disturbance and muscle atrophy. Typically, the pain is worse at night and is relieved with aspirin.

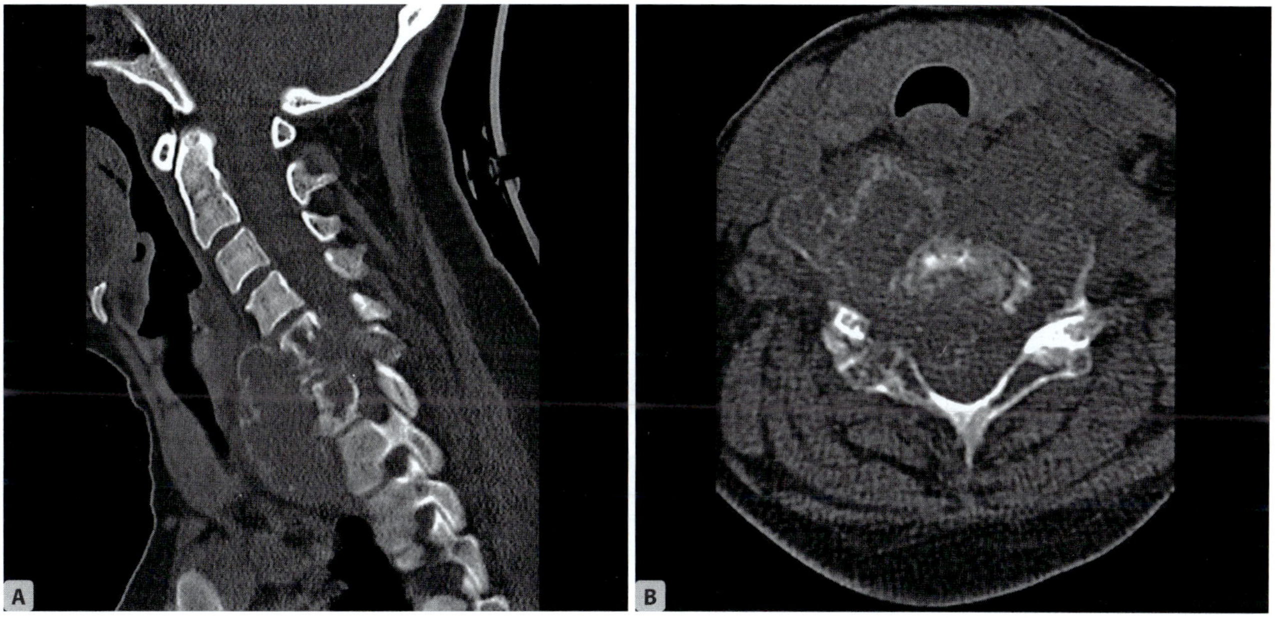

FIGS. 15A AND B: Giant cell tumor of C5 and C6: Sagittal (A) and axial (B) CT scans reveal an expansile lytic lesion centered in the vertebral body with posterior element extension.

The tumor involves the lumbar spine most commonly, followed by the cervical, thoracic and sacral regions.[65] The axial osteoid osteomas are most commonly present in the posterior elements of the vertebra (75%) and are rare in the vertebral body (7%).

Pathologically, the nidus of an osteoid osteoma is a small (<2 cm in diameter), round mass of pink to red tissue of osteoid and woven bone with interconnected trabeculae. The lesion is well circumscribed and may be surrounded by a variable degree of reactive cortical bone.

CT scan is an excellent imaging modality to detect an osteoid osteoma and define its exact location within the bone. CT shows the nidus as a round hypodense lesion surrounded by a hyperdense sclerotic ring **(Figs. 16A to C)**. Calcification within the nidus results in a target appearance of the lesion **(Figs. 16A to C)**. On MR imaging, nidus is generally of a low to iso signal intensity on T1WI, iso to high signal intensity on T2WI and enhances markedly; the surrounding osteosclerotic component results in a hypointense ring. Areas of calcification have low signal intensity on all pulse sequences. On MRI, a small nidus may be obscured by signal changes due to associated surrounding sclerosis, marrow edema and soft-tissue inflammation.[66] Radionuclide bone scans are extremely sensitive in the detection of osteoid osteomas.

Typically, management of spinal osteoid osteoma is complete surgical resection of the nidus. Percutaneous CT-guided removal and percutaneous ablation with a radiofrequency electrode, laser or alcohol are new methods of treatment.[67]

Osteoblastoma

It is classically believed that osteoblastomas differ from osteoid osteomas only in size (>2 cm in diameter). Osteoblastomas occur in young adults, with 90% of cases occurring in the 2nd and 3rd decades of life with a male predominance (2:1). Osteoblastomas present with dull localized pain and neurologic symptoms, including paresthesias, paraparesis and paraplegia.

Osteoblastomas of the spine represent 30–40% of all osteoblastomas and the lesions are equally distributed in the cervical, thoracic and lumbar segments.[68] These most frequently involve the posterior vertebral elements (55% of cases) with frequent extension into the vertebral body (42%).[61,64] Isolated vertebral body involvement in osteoblastoma is rare. Pathologically, the typical osteoblastoma is more than 2.0 cm in diameter. Histologic features resemble to those of osteoid osteoma (interconnecting trabecular bone and fibrovascular stroma), but overall the microscopic pattern is not as well organized as that seen in osteoid osteomas.

Three radiographic patterns have been described with osteoblastoma.[68] In the first pattern, osteoblastoma may resemble osteoid osteoma but is usually larger (>2 cm in diameter). The second pattern appears as an expansile lesion with multiple small calcifications and a peripheral sclerotic rim. This is the most common appearance of spinal osteoblastomas **(Fig. 17)**.[69] The third pattern is the most aggressive pattern and appears as an expansile lesion with bone destruction, infiltration of surrounding soft tissue and intermixed matrix calcification. Interestingly, mineralization within an osteoblastoma may have the radiologic appearance (rings and arcs) of chondroid matrix.

At CT, the lesion shows areas of mineralization, expansile bone remodelling and sclerosis or a thin osseous shell about its margins. MR imaging appearance of osteoblastoma is generally nonspecific, with low- to-intermediate signal intensity seen on T1WI and intermediate-to-high signal intensity seen on T2WI.[68] MR imaging is sensitive to show

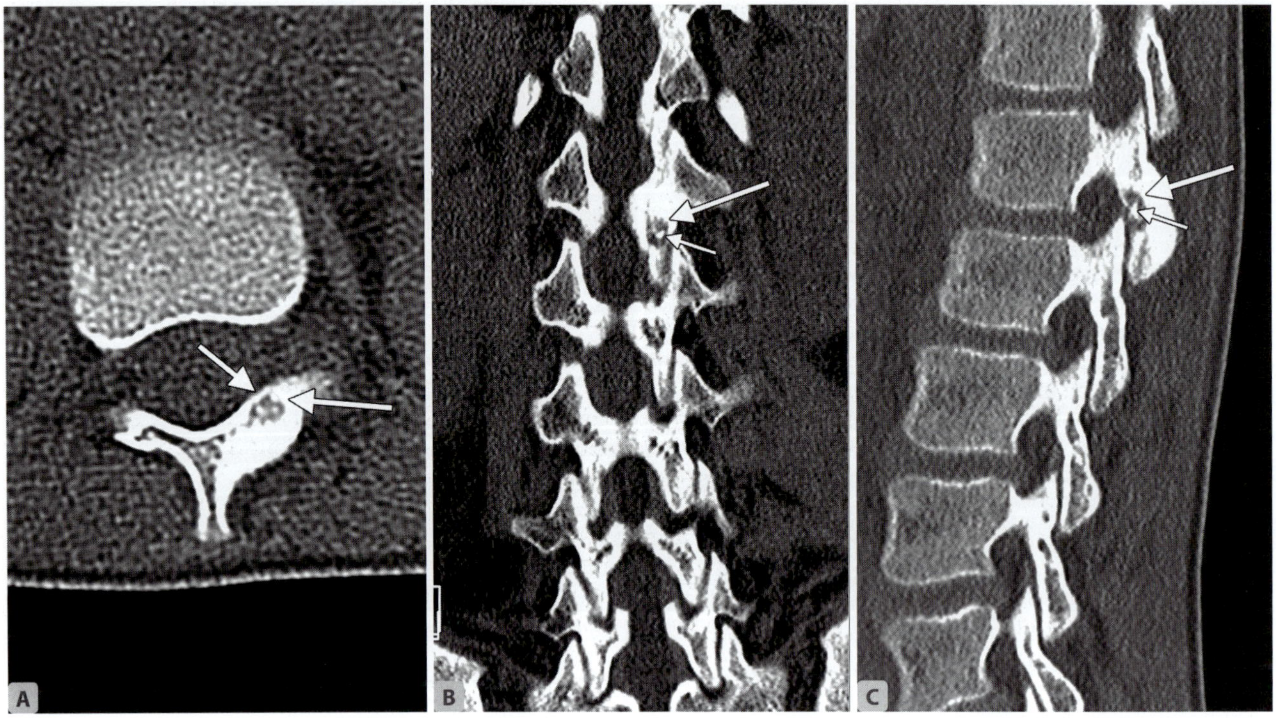

FIGS. 16A TO C: Osteoid osteoma in a 21-year-old man with low back pain: Axial (A), coronal reconstructed (B) and sagittal reconstructed (C) CT scans of lumbar spine show a focal lucency in the left L1 lamina (long arrows) with central mineralization (small arrows) and surrounding sclerosis typical of osteoid osteoma.

relationship of the tumor with neural structures and surrounding soft tissues.[70] Osteoblastomas show marked radionuclide uptake at bone scintigraphy.

Surgical resection is the treatment of choice for spinal osteoblastomas. The recurrence rate is 10–15% and early 50% for conventional and aggressive lesion respectively.[68,71]

Osteochondromas

Spinal osteochondromas are rare, accounting for only 1–4% of solitary exostoses and represent 4% of all solitary spinal tumors.[72] Generally, one spinal osteochondroma is present in 7–9% of patients with hereditary multiple exostoses.[73]

Spinal osteochondromas are often diagnosed during the 3rd and 4th decades of life when solitary and one decade earlier in patients with hereditary multiple exostoses.[72,73] Osteochondromas have a predilection for the cervical spine, particularly C2, though they can occur at all levels of the spine. Most commonly spinal osteochondromas arise from the posterior elements; some may arise from the vertebral body.

Osteochondromas have the composition of a normal bone (cortex and marrow space) with a cartilage cap from which growth occurs. Spinal osteochondromas may be sessile or pedunculated. The lesion is continuous with the marrow and cortex of the underlying bone.[72]

Thin-section CT is the best imaging modality to show pathognomonic marrow and cortical continuity of the lesion to the underlying bone. MR imaging usually shows yellow marrow centrally (T1 hyperintense and T2 isointense) with a low-signal-intensity cortex. The hyaline cartilage cap is often small and thin, with low to isointense signal intensity on T1WI and high signal intensity on T2WI. Marked cartilage cap thickening (>1.5 cm) should raise the suspicion of malignant transformation to chondrosarcoma in adults. Surgical excision of osteochondroma is usually curative.

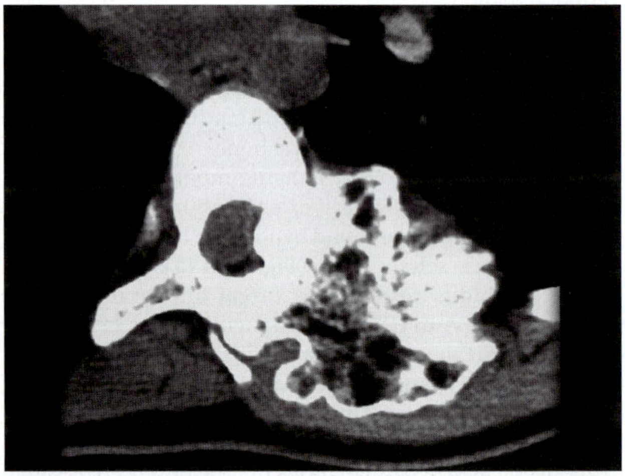

FIG. 17: Osteoblastoma: Axial CT of the dorsal spine reveals an expansile lesion of left pedicle and lamina of D6 vertebra with small foci of mineralized matrix.

Chordoma

Chordoma is a tumor arising from remnants of the primitive notochord and represents 2–4 % of malignant osseous neoplasms.[60] These tumors are almost always midline or paramedian in location. These tumors most commonly occur in the sacral regions (50%), followed by the skull base (35%) and the rest of the spine (15%).[60] Men are affected twice as frequently as women; the mean age of these patients is 50 years, with skull-base chordomas generally affecting a younger population, including children.[60]

Chordomas are slow-growing tumors that are commonly discovered as large masses. Enlarging chordomas tend to involve adjacent vertebral bodies and extend into the adjacent paraspinal tissues and epidural space.[74] Rarely, they can arise solely in the musculature of the perivertebral space.[74]

Pathologically, typical chordomas contain physaliphorous cells; and abundant intracellular and extracellular mucin. The chondroid or osteoid elements replace the mucinous matrix in atypical or dedifferentiated chordomas.[60]

On imaging, chordoma is seen as a destructive vertebral body lesion spanning several segments and sparing the disks with associated soft-tissue component.[75] It may have a "collar button" or "mushroom" appearance and a "dumb bell" shape. About 40% of chordomas are of the mobile spine and up to 90% of sacrococcygeal chordomas contain areas of amorphous calcifications.[55] Most chordomas are iso-or hypointense relative to muscle on T1WI. On T2WI, most chordomas have a high-signal intensity due to the presence of their signature physaliphorous cells (clear cells with intracytoplasmic vacuoles and abundant mucin) **(Figs. 18A to D)**.[60] The focal areas of hemorrhage, calcifications and high protein content of the myxoid and mucinous collections may account for the heterogeneous intratumoural T2 hypointensity and T1 hyperintensity.[55] The fibrous septa that divide the gelatinous components of the tumor appear as areas of low signal intensity on T2WI. T2-hypointense rim due to hemosiderin deposition has been reported in 72% of sacrococcygeal chordomas but is rare in spinal chordomas.[76] Most chordomas show moderate heterogeneous enhancement after gadolinium-injection.[75] Chordomas typically have a poor prognosis due to local recurrence following resection.

Chondrosarcoma

Chondrosarcoma is a malignant neoplasm that represents 10% of all primary bone tumors[77] and is second most common non-lymphoproliferative tumor of the spine. The most common age of presentation is in the fifth decade, with male predominance (M:F 2–4:1). The patient may present with pain, neurological symptoms and a palpable mass. The spine is affected in 3%–12% of cases.[61] Dorsal spine is the most common site, though it can occur at all levels of the spine. Chondrosarcoma may arise from the vertebral body (15% of cases), posterior element (40%), or both (45%).[55] Typically low grade, these neoplasms can arise *de novo* or secondarily from a pre-existing cartilage lesion such as an osteochondroma or an enchondroma.

Radiologically, these tumors appear as destructive lesions in the spine or as a paraspinal mass with calcification.[55] The characteristic chondroid matrix mineralization (rings and arcs) may be evident on radiographs, but are better evaluated with CT. Calcified matrix appears as areas of

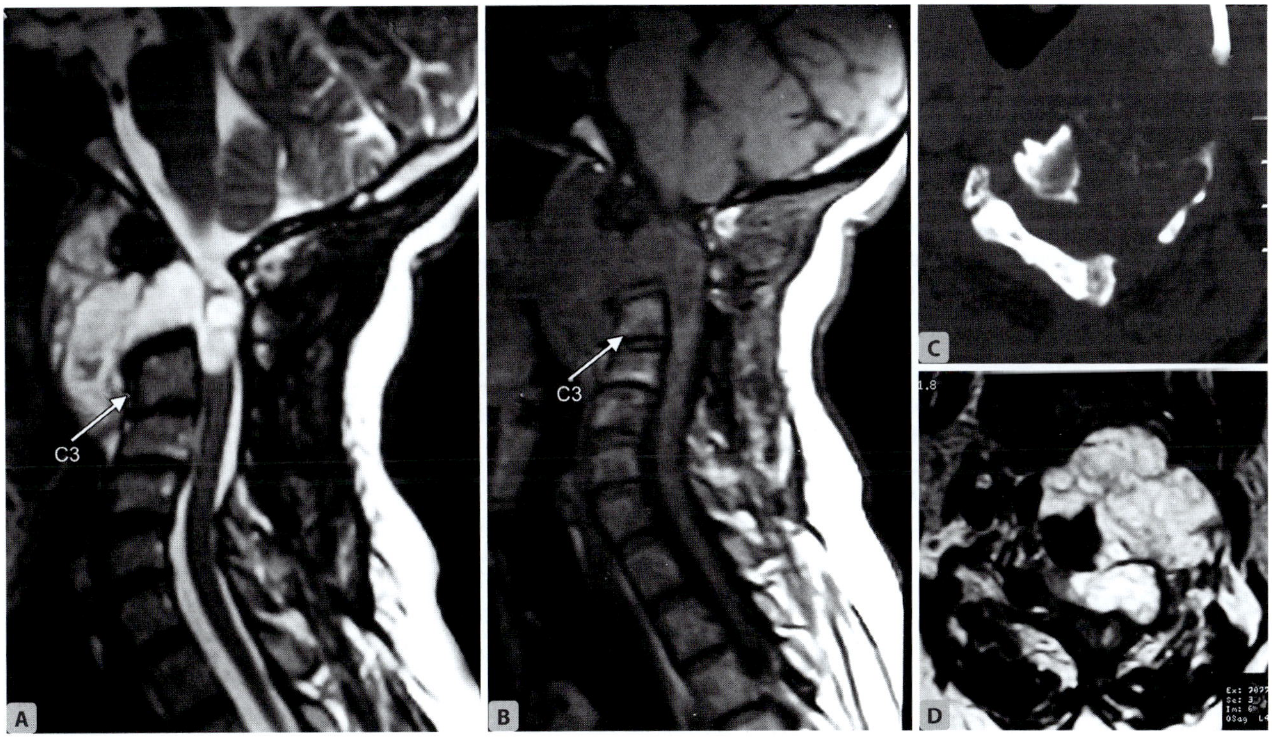

FIGS. 18A TO D: Chordoma: Sagittal T2WI (A), sagittal T1WI (B) and axial T2WI (C) show a mass lesion involving the body of C2 vertebra with a large prevertebral component. The mass is hypointense on T1 (b) and hyperintense on T2 (A and C). Axial CT scan (D) shows lytic destruction of the left half of the C2 vertebra.

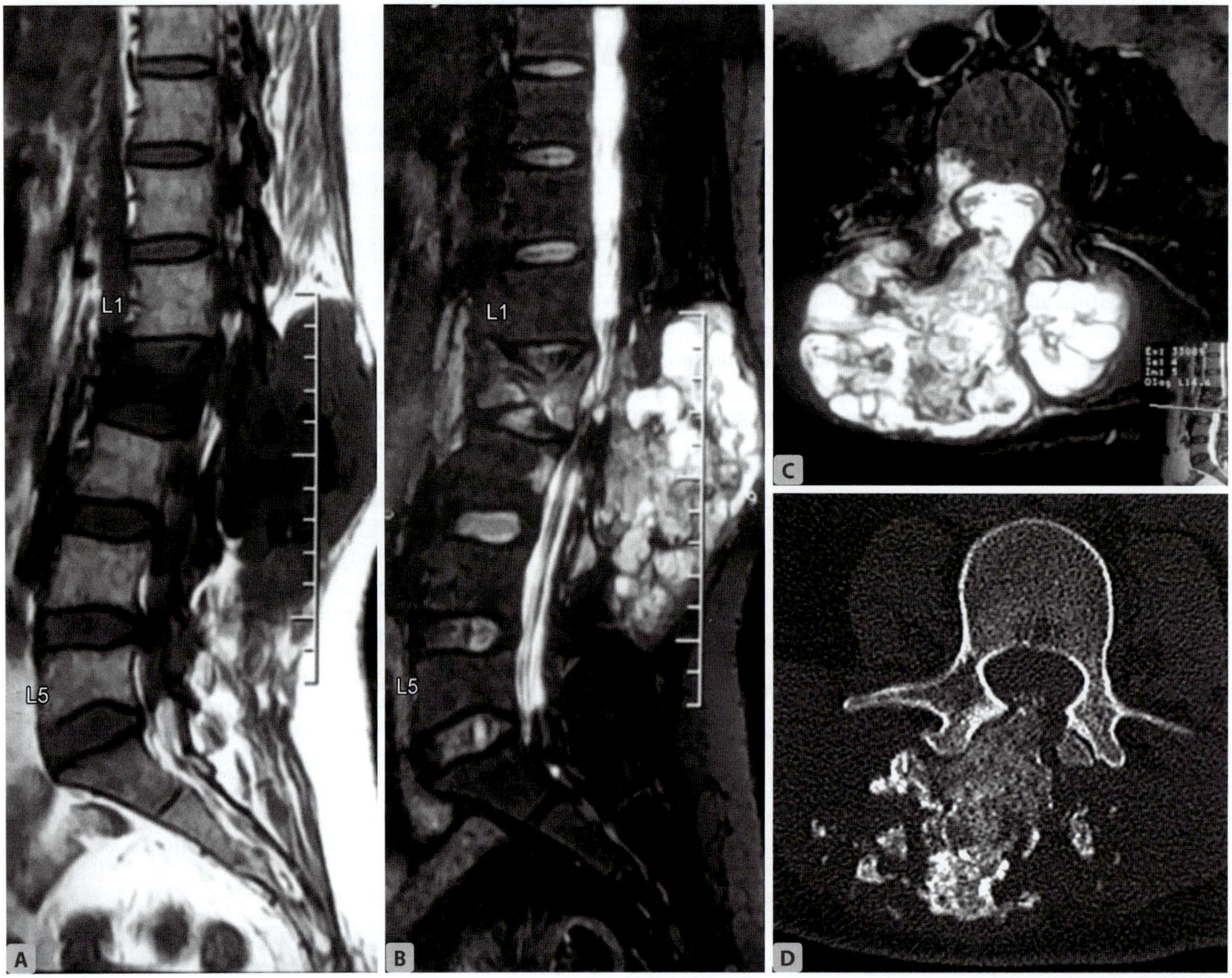

FIGS. 19A TO D: Chondrosarcoma: Sagittal T1WI (A), sagittal T2WI (B) and axial T2WI (C) show a mass lesion involving body and posterior elements of the L2 vertebra. The mass is hypointense on T1 (A) and hyperintense on T2 (B and C). Axial CT scan (D) shows ossification within the mass lesion.

signal voids on MR imaging. Due to the high water content of hyaline cartilage, the non-mineralized portion of the tumor is hypodense on CT scans, low-to-intermediate signal intensity on T1WI and very high signal intensity on T2WI **(Figs. 19A to D)**.[78] Rings and arcs pattern of enhancement is seen at gadolinium-enhanced MR imaging; reflecting the lobulated growth pattern of these cartilaginous tumors. Transdiscal extension has been reported in 35% of cases[79] Chondrosarcoma arising from osteochondroma is seen as thickening of the peripheral cartilaginous cap of more than 1.5 cm. Surgical resection with adjuvant radiation therapy is the treatment of choice for spinal chondrosarcomas.

Fibrous Dysplasia

Fibrous dysplasia (FD) is a developmental anomaly wherein portions of the bone are replaced by fibrous connective tissue and poorly formed trabecular bone. FD affects primarily children and adolescents. FD may present in monostotic or polyostotic forms. Monostotic FD accounts for 80% of cases and tends to occur most often in the ribs, long bones, and skull. Involvement of the vertebral bodies is rare—only occurring in 2.5% of cases.[80,81] Spine involvement is more likely to present in the polyostotic form of the disease. Lumbar spine is most commonly involved in spinal FD. Vertebral body, with or without involvement of pedicles is the most common site of involvement.

Radiographically, spinal FD appears as a decrease in vertebral height. Classic plain radiographic appearance of a ground-glass matrix with definite sclerotic margins is not seen in spinal FD as opposed to FD occurring elsewhere in the body. However, on spine CT scans, "ground-glass" appearance can be seen and is the most common finding. In addition, a mildly expansile lesion with a ''blown-out'' cortical shell or a lytic lesion with a sclerotic rim and a decrease in body height can be seen. On MRI, FD shows variable characteristics, typically intermediate-to-low signal intensity on T1WI and variable signal intensity on T2WI. Benign FD lesions characteristically do not show cortical bone disruption or soft-tissue involvement; hypointense on T1W sequence and have fine well-circumscribed border between the lesion and the normal bone. Malignant transformation, though very rare, should be suspected when there is endosteal or cortical erosion; especially, if there is cortical destruction with associated soft-tissue. FD may be complicated by fractures.

Most lesions are metabolically active and hence show increased uptake on bone scans and increased metabolic activity with PET.

EPIDURAL LESIONS

Angiolipoma

Spinal angiolipomas are rare lesions usually found in the epidural space of the thoracic spine.[82,83] Most patients present in their middle age with slowly progressive symptoms of spinal cord compression. Most of these lesions are found in adults and in the thoracic region. Spinal angiolipomas are typically located in the posterior and lateral aspects of the epidural space. However, infiltrating forms of tumor are generally located in the anterior epidural space.[82,83] On MRI, angiolipomas are predominantly hyperintense on T1WI and inhomogeneous owing to interspersed vascular elements **(Figs. 20A to D)**. A high vascular content is correlated with the presence of large hypointense regions on T1WI. These masses are hyperintense on T2WI.[83] The larger tumors may cause compression of the spinal cord. Intramedullary angiolipomas have rarely been described **(Figs. 21A to D)**.[83]

Epidural Lipomatosis

This entity, although not a tumor, may behave as one and result in compression of neural elements and thus is discussed here. The most common cause of epidural

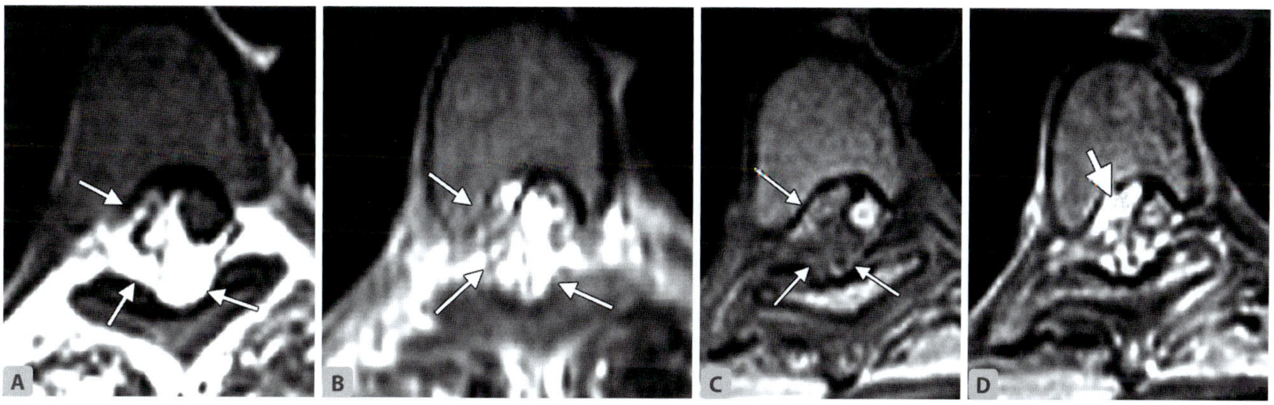

FIGS. 20A TO D: Extradural angiolipoma: Axial T1WI (A) and T2WI (B) show an extradural hyperintense mass (arrows in A and B) displacing the spinal cord anteriorly and to the left side. Axial T1-weighted fat-saturated image (C) showing diffuse, nearly homogeneous decrease in the signal intensity of the mass (arrows in C) suggestive of fatty tissue. Axial T1-weighted post-gadolinium fat-saturation image (D) showing enhancement of the extradural lesion (arrow in D).

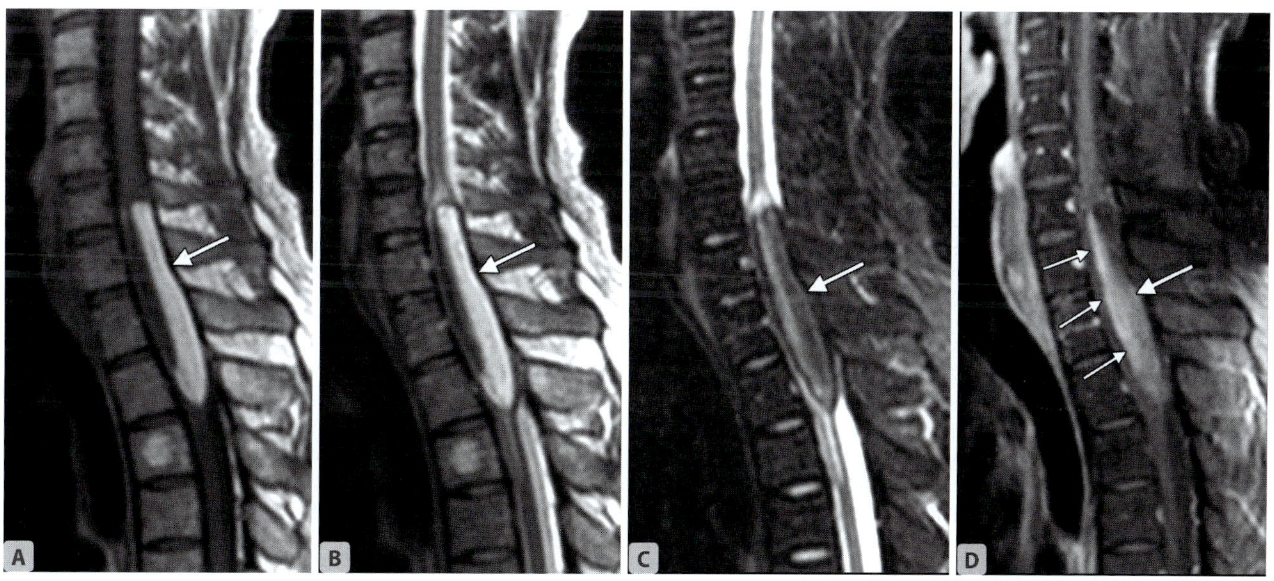

FIGS. 21A TO D: Intramedullary angiolipoma: Sagittal T1WI (A) and T2WI (B) showing the intramedullary angiolipoma. The dorsal component of the mass shows homogeneous high signal intensity, while the ventral component is heterogeneously hyperintense. No vascular flow voids are seen. Sagittal T1-fat-saturated image shows suppression of signal in the dorsal component (C and D).

lipomatosis is prolonged treatment with steroids and rarely endogenous Cushing's syndrome.[84] Epidural lipomatosis may also be seen in morbidly obese patients. In this rare entity, there is hypertrophy of the normal epidural fat, particularly on the dorsal aspects of the thoracic spine and less commonly in the lumbar region. The most common symptom is back pain, but compression of the spinal cord may occur. If the fat grows at the level of neural foramina, radiculopathies may also occur.

The typical MRI appearance of epidural lipomatosis is that of T1 bright excessively thickened epidural fat (>5 to 6 mm) on the posterior aspect of the canal on sagittal images. The subarachnoid spaces are narrowed and the thoracic spinal cord appears thin. The superior and inferior aspects of the lipomatosis taper smoothly and usually extend at least six vertebral segments in length. On axial images, excessive fat is noted on the posterior aspect of the canal, extending laterally. This normal fat does not enhance after contrast administration. On CT, the abnormal fat is of low density and on myelography the fat may compress the canal and result in complete blockage of the passage of contrast. Similar findings are noted when epidural lipomatosis develops in the lumbar region.

CONCLUSION

It is important for the radiologist to be familiar with the imaging characteristics of spinal neoplasms. On the basis of patient's age, lesion location and radiologic appearance, a reasonable differential diagnosis can be arrived for most spinal tumors. A multimodality approach is very helpful to accurately characterize the lesion. It narrows down the differential diagnosis significantly. MR imaging is a particularly useful tool for evaluation of intramedullary neoplasms, whereas CT and MRI are complementary for the evaluation of extradural bony lesions.

REFERENCES

1. Moquin RR, Sandhu FA, Henderson FC. Cystic Intramedullary Neoplasms of the Spinal Cord. Seminars in Spine Surgery. 2006;18(3):168-74.
2. Smith AB, Soderlund KA, Rushing EJ, Smirniotopolous JG. Radiologic-pathologic correlation of pediatric and adolescent spinal neoplasms: Part 1, Intramedullary spinal neoplasms. Am J Roentgenol. 2012;198(1):34-43.
3. Sun B, Wang C, Wang J, Liu A. MRI features of intramedullary spinal cord ependymomas. J Neuroimaging. 2003;13 (4):346-51.
4. Koeller KK, Rosenblum RS, Morrison AL. Neoplasms of the spinal cord and filum terminale: radiologic-pathologic correlation. Radiographics. 2000;20(6):1721-49.
5. Kahan H, Sklar EM, Post MJ, Bruce JH. MR characteristics of histopathologic subtypes of spinal ependymoma. Am J Neuroradiol. 1996;17(1):143-50.
6. Nadkarni TD, Rekate HL. Pediatric intramedullary spinal cord tumors. Critical review of the literature. Childs Nerv Syst. 1999;15(1):17-28.
7. Choudhri AF, Whitehead MT, Klimo P, Jr, Montgomery BK, Boop FA. Diffusion tensor imaging to guide surgical planning in intramedullary spinal cord tumors in children. Neuroradiology. 2014;56(2):169-74.
8. Benesch M, Weber-Mzell D, Gerber NU, von Hoff K, Deinlein F, Krauss J, et al. Ependymoma of the spinal cord in children and adolescents: a retrospective series from the HIT database. J Neurosurg Pediatr. 2010;6(2):137-44.
9. Hallacq P, Labrousse F, Streichenberger N, Lisii D, Fischer G. Bifocal myxopapillary ependymoma of the terminal filum: the end of a spectrum? Journal of Neurosurgery: Spine. 2003;98(3):288-9.
10. Wippold FJ 2nd, Smirniotopoulos JG, Moran CJ, Suojanen JN, Vollmer DG. MR imaging of myxopapillary ependymoma: findings and value to determine extent of tumor and its relation to intraspinal structures. Am J Roentgenol. 1995;165(5):1263-7.
11. Jallo GI, Zagzag D, Epstein F. Intramedullary subependymoma of the spinal cord. Neurosurgery. 1996;38(2):251-7.
12. Sarkar C, Mukhopadhyay S, Ralte AM, Sharma MC, Gupta A, Gaikwad S, et al. Intramedullary subependymoma of the spinal cord: a case report and review of literature. Clinical Neurology and Neurosurgery. 2003;106(1):63-8.
13. Hoeffel C, Boukobza M, Polivka M, Lot G, Guichard JP, Lafitte F, et al. MR manifestations of subependymomas. Am J Neuroradiol. 1995;16(10):2121-9.
14. Seo HS, Kim JH, Lee DH, Lee YH, Suh SI, Kim SY, et al. Nonenhancing intramedullary astrocytomas and other MR imaging features: a retrospective study and systematic review. Am J Neuroradiol. 2010;31(3):498-503.
15. Ducreux D, Fillard P, Facon D, Ozanne A, Lepeintre JF, Renoux J, et al. Diffusion tensor magnetic resonance imaging and fiber tracking in spinal cord lesions: current and future indications. Neuroimaging Clin N Am. 2007;17(1):137-47.
16. Setzer M, Murtagh RD, Murtagh FR, Eleraky M, Jain S, Marquardt G, et al. Diffusion tensor imaging tractography in patients with intramedullary tumors: comparison with intraoperative findings and value for prediction of tumor resectability. J Neurosurg Spine. 2010;13(3):371-80.
17. Patel U, Pinto RS, Miller DC, Handler MS, Rorke LB, Epstein FJ, et al. MR of spinal cord ganglioglioma. Am J Neuroradiol. 1998;19(5):879-87.
18. Dudley RW, Torok MR, Gallegos DR, Mulcahy-Levy JM, Hoffman LM, Liu AK, et al. Pediatric low-grade ganglioglioma: epidemiology, treatments, and outcome analysis on 348 children from the surveillance, epidemiology, and end results database. Neurosurgery. 2015;76(3):313-9; discussion 9; quiz 9-20.
19. Lang FF, Epstein FJ, Ransohoff J, Allen JC, Wisoff J, Abbott IR, et al. Central nervous system gangliogliomas. Part 2: Clinical outcome. J Neurosurg. 1993;79(6):867-73.
20. Bambakidis NC, Robinson S, Cohen M, Cohen AR. Atypical teratoid/rhabdoid tumors of the central nervous system: clinical, radiographic and pathologic features. Pediatr Neurosurg. 2002;37(2):64-70.
21. Moeller KK, Coventry S, Jernigan S, Moriarty TM. Atypical teratoid/rhabdoid tumor of the spine. American Journal of Neuroradiology. 2007;28(3):593-5.
22. Niwa T, Aida N, Tanaka M, Okubo J, Sasano M, Shishikura A, et al. Diffusion-weighted imaging of an atypical teratoid/rhabdoid tumor of the cervical spine. Magn Reson Med Sci. 2009;8(3): 135-8.
23. Rorke LB, Packer RJ, Biegel JA. Central nervous system atypical teratoid/rhabdoid tumors of infancy and childhood: definition of an entity. J Neurosurg. 1996;85(1):56-65.
24. Chu BC, Terae S, Hida K, Furukawa M, Abe S, Miyasaka K. MR findings in spinal hemangioblastoma: correlation with symptoms and with angiographic and surgical findings. Am J Neuroradiol. 2001;22(1):206-17.

25. Baker KB, Moran CJ, Wippold FJ, Smirniotopoulos JG, Rodriguez FJ, Meyers SP, et al. MR imaging of spinal hemangioblastoma. Am J Roentgenol. 2000;174(2):377-82.
26. Faro SH, Turtz AR, Koenigsberg RA, Mohamed FB, Chen CY, Stein H. Paraganglioma of the cauda equina with associated intramedullary cyst: MR findings. Am J Neuroradiol. 1997;18(8):1588-90.
27. Shin JY, Lee SM, Hwang MY, Sohn CH, Suh SJ. MR findings of the spinal paraganglioma: report of three cases. J Korean Med Sci. 2001;16(4):522-6.
28. Lin YY, Lin CJ, Ho DM, Guo WY, Chang CY. Primary intramedullary spinal cord lymphoma. Spine J. 2012;12(6):527-8.
29. Flanagan EP, O'Neill BP, Porter AB, Lanzino G, Haberman TM, Keegan BM. Primary intramedullary spinal cord lymphoma. Neurology. 2011;77(8):784-91.
30. Koeller KK, Smirniotopoulos JG, Jones RV. Primary central nervous system lymphoma: radiologic-pathologic correlation. Radiographics. 1997;17(6):1497-526.
31. Kalaycı M, Çağavi F, Gül S, Yenidünya S, Açıkgöz B. Intramedullary spinal cord metastases: diagnosis and treatment—an illustrated review. Acta Neurochirurgica. 2004;146(12):1347-54.
32. Rykken JB, Diehn FE, Hunt CH, Schwartz KM, Eckel LJ, Wood CP, et al. Intramedullary spinal cord metastases: MRI and relevant clinical features from a 13-year institutional case series. Am J Neuroradiol. 2013;34(10):2043-9.
33. Rykken JB, Diehn FE, Hunt CH, Eckel LJ, Schwartz KM, Kaufmann TJ, et al. Rim and flame signs: postgadolinium MRI findings specific for non-CNS intramedullary spinal cord metastases. Am J Neuroradiol. 2013;34(4):908-15.
34. Yoshiura T, Shrier DA, Pilcher WH, Rubio A. Cervical spinal meningioma with unusual MR contrast enhancement. Am J Neuroradiol. 1998;19(6):1040-2.
35. Rossi A, Gandolfo C, Morana G, Tortori-Donati P. Tumors of the spine in children. Neuroimaging Clin N Am. 2007;17(1):17-35.
36. Van Goethem JWM, van den Hauwe L, Özsarlak Ö, De Schepper AMA, Parizel PM. Spinal tumors. Eur J Radiol. 2004;50(2):159-76.
37. Kyoshima K, Horiuchi T, Zenisaka H, Nakazato F. Thoracic dumbbell intra- and extramedullary schwannoma. Journal of Clinical Neuroscience. 2005;12(4):481-4.
38. Wilne S, Walker D. Spine and spinal cord tumours in children: a diagnostic and therapeutic challenge to healthcare systems. Arch Dis Child Educ Pract Ed. 2010;95(2):47-54.
39. Pilavaki M, Chourmouzi D, Kiziridou A, Skordalaki A, Zarampoukas T, Drevelengas A. Imaging of peripheral nerve sheath tumors with pathologic correlation: Pictorial review. Eur J Radiol. 2004;52(3):229-39.
40. Jaramillo D. Whole-body MR imaging, bone diffusion imaging: how and why? Pediatr Radiol. 2010;40(6):978-84.
41. Perrin RG, Laxton AW. Metastatic spine disease: epidemiology, pathophysiology, and evaluation of patients. Neurosurgery Clinics of North America. 2004;15(4):365.
42. Park SW, Lee JH, Ehara S, Park YB, Sung SO, Choi JA, et al. Single shot fast spin echo diffusion-weighted MR imaging of the spine—Is it useful in differentiating malignant metastatic tumor infiltration from benign fracture edema? Clinical Imaging. 2004;28(2):102-8.
43. Mulleman D, Gaxatte C, Guillerm G, Leroy X, Cotten A, Duquesnoy B, et al. Multiple myeloma presenting with widespread osteosclerotic lesions. Joint Bone Spine. 2004;71(1):79-83.
44. Baur-Melnyk A, Buhmann S, Durr HR, Reiser M. Role of MRI for the diagnosis and prognosis of multiple myeloma. European Journal of Radiology. 2005;55(1):56-63.
45. Angtuaco EJC, Fassas ABT, Walker R, Sethi R, Barlogie B. Multiple myeloma: Clinical review and diagnostic imaging. Radiology. 2004;231(1):11-23.
46. Guermazi A, Brice P, de Kerviler EE, Ferme C, Hennequin C, Meignin V, et al. Extranodal Hodgkin disease: spectrum of disease. Radiographics. 2001;21(1):161-79.
47. Cross JJ, Antoun NM, Laing RJ, Xuereb J. Imaging of compressive vertebral haemangiomas. Eur Radiol. 2000;10(6):997-1002.
48. Laredo JD, Reizine D, Bard M, Merland JJ. Vertebral hemangiomas: radiologic evaluation. Radiology. 1986;161(1):183-9.
49. Gaston A, Nguyen JP, Djindjian M, Le Bras F, Gherardi R, Benhaiem N, et al. Vertebral haemangioma: CT and arteriographic features in three cases. J Neuroradiol. 1985;12(1):21-33.
50. Friedman DP. Symptomatic vertebral hemangiomas: MR findings. Am J Roentgenol. 1996;167(2):359-64.
51. Sanerkin NG, Mott MG, Roylance J. An unusual intraosseous lesion with fibroblastic, osteoclastic, osteoblastic, aneurysmal and fibromyxoid elements. "Solid" variant of aneurysmal bone cyst. Cancer. 1983;51(12):2278-86.
52. Koci TM, Mehringer CM, Yamagata N, Chiang F. Aneurysmal bone cyst of the thoracic spine: evolution after particulate embolization. Am J Neuroradiol. 1995;16(4 Suppl):857-60.
53. Kransdorf MJ, Sweet DE. Aneurysmal bone cyst: concept, controversy, clinical presentation, and imaging. Am J Roentgenol. 1995;164(3):573-80.
54. Diel J, Ortiz O, Losada RA, Price DB, Hayt MW, Katz DS. The sacrum: pathologic spectrum, multimodality imaging, and subspecialty approach. Radiographics. 2001;21(1):83-104.
55. Murphey MD, Andrews CL, Flemming DJ, Temple HT, Smith WS, Smirniotopoulos JG. From the archives of the AFIP. Primary tumors of the spine: radiologic pathologic correlation. Radiographics. 1996;16(5):1131-58.
56. Hudson TM. Fluid levels in aneurysmal bone cysts: a CT feature. Am J Roentgenol. 1984;142(5):1001-4.
57. Mahnken A, Nolte-Ernsting C, Wildberger J, Heussen N, Adam G, Wirtz D, et al. Aneurysmal bone cyst: value of MR imaging and conventional radiography. Eur Radiol. 2003;13(5):1118-24.
58. Tsai JC, Dalinka MK, Fallon MD, Zlatkin MB, Kressel HY. Fluid-fluid level: a nonspecific finding in tumors of bone and soft tissue. Radiology. 1990;175(3):779-82.
59. Suzuki M, Satoh T, Nishida J, Kato S, Toba T, Honda T, et al. Solid variant of aneurysmal bone cyst of the cervical spine. Spine. 2004;29(17):E376-E81.
60. Llauger J, Palmer J, Amores S, Bague S, Camins A. Primary tumors of the sacrum: diagnostic imaging. Am J Roentgenol. 2000;174(2):417-24.
61. Drevelegas A, Chourmouzi D, Boulogianni G, Sofroniadis I. Imaging of primary bone tumors of the spine. European Radiology. 2003;13(8):1859-71.
62. Schwimer SR, Bassett LW, Mancuso AA, Mirra JM, Dawson EG. Giant cell tumor of the cervicothoracic spine. Am J Roentgenol. 1981;136(1):63-7.
63. Aoki J, Tanikawa H, Ishii K, Seo GS, Karakida O, Sone S, et al. MR findings indicative of hemosiderin in giant-cell tumor of bone: frequency, cause, and diagnostic significance. Am J Roentgenol. 1996;166(1):145-8.
64. Flemming DJ, Murphey MD, Carmichael BB, Bernard SA. Primary tumors of the spine. Semin Musculoskelet Radiol. 2000;4(3):299-320.
65. Tourniaire J, Bossard D, Gleize B, Tavernier T, Bochu M. Case report 801: osteoid osteoma of the coccyx. Skeletal Radiol. 1993;22(6):457-9.
66. Houang B, Grenier N, Greselle JF, Vital JM, Douws C, Broussin J, et al. Osteoid osteoma of the cervical spine. Misleading MR features about a case involving the uncinate process. Neuroradiology. 1990;31(6):549-51.
67. Kransdorf MJ, Stull MA, Gilkey FW, Moser RP Jr. Osteoid osteoma. Radiographics. 1991;11(4):671-96.

68. Kroon HM, Schurmans J. Osteoblastoma: clinical and radiologic findings in 98 new cases. Radiology. 1990;175(3):783-90.
69. Kumar R, Guinto FC, Jr., Madewell JE, David R, Shirkhoda A. Expansile bone lesions of the vertebra. Radiographics. 1988;8(4):749-69.
70. Crim JR, Mirra JM, Eckardt JJ, Seeger LL. Widespread inflammatory response to osteoblastoma: the flare phenomenon. Radiology. 1990;177(3):835-6.
71. Lucas DR, Unni KK, McLeod RA, O'Connor MI, Sim FH. Osteoblastoma: clinicopathologic study of 306 cases. Hum Pathol. 1994;25(2):117-34.
72. Albrecht S, Crutchfield JS, SeGall GK. On spinal osteochondromas. J Neurosurg. 1992;77(2):247-52.
73. Barros F TEP, Oliveira RP, Taricco MA, Gonzalez CH. Hereditary multiple exostoses and cervical ventral protuberance causing disphagia. Spine. 1995;20(14):1640-2.
74. Wippold FJ, 2nd, Koeller KK, Smirniotopoulos JG. Clinical and imaging features of cervical chordoma. Am J Roentgenol. 1999;172(5):1423-6.
75. Smolders D, Wang X, Drevelengas A, Vanhoenacker F, De Schepper AM. Value of MRI in the diagnosis of non-clival, non-sacral chordoma. Skeletal Radiology. 2003;32(6):343-50.
76. Sung MS, Lee GK, Kang HS, Kwon ST, Park JG, Suh JS, et al. Sacrococcygeal chordoma: MR imaging in 30 patients. Skeletal Radiology. 2004;34(2):87-94.
77. Sundaresan N, Rosen G, Boriani S. Primary malignant tumors of the spine. Orthop Clin North Am. 2009;40(1):21-36.
78. Mummaneni PV, Rosenberg WS. Spinal chondrosarcoma following adenocarcinoma of the breast: case report. Surg Neurol. 2000;53(6):580-2.
79. Shives TC, McLeod RA, Unni KK, Schray MF. Chondrosarcoma of the spine. J Bone Joint Surg Am. 1989;71(8):1158-65.
80. Fitzpatrick KA, Taljanovic MS, Speer DP, Graham AR, Jacobson JA, Barnes GR, et al. Imaging Findings of Fibrous Dysplasia with Histopathologic and Intraoperative Correlation. American Journal of Roentgenology. 2004;182(6):1389-98.
81. Park SK, Lee IS, Choi J-Y, Cho KH, Suh KJ, Lee JW, et al. CT and MRI of fibrous dysplasia of the spine. Br J Radiol 2012;85(1015): 996-1001.
82. Garg A, Gupta V, Gaikwad S, Deol P, Mishra NK, Sharma MC, et al. Spinal angiolipoma: report of three cases and review of MRI features. Australas Radiol. 2002;46(1):84-90.
83. Samdani AF, Garonzik IM, Jallo G, Eberhart CG, Zahos P. Spinal angiolipoma: case report and review of the literature. Acta Neurochirurgica. 2004;146(3):299-302.
84. Bodelier AGL, Groeneveld W, van der Linden AN, Haak HR. Symptomatic epidural lipomatosis in ectopic Cushing's syndrome. European Journal of Endocrinology. 2004;151(6):765-9.

CHAPTER

214 Spinal Vascular Malformations

Shailesh B Gaikwad

INTRODUCTION

Vascular lesions of the spinal cord are heterogeneous group of disorders with wide spectrum ranging from lesions with simple angioarchitecture such as dural or pial arteriovenous fistula to complex arteriovenous malformations (AVM). Although they are relatively uncommon disorders, they are potentially curable causes of progressive myelopathy hence requiring comprehensive evaluation both clinically and radiologically. Diagnosis of spinal vascular malformations mainly rests on magnetic resonance imaging (MRI), while selective digital subtraction angiography (DSA) is needed for thorough understanding of the disease process, for characterization of its angioarchitecture and planning the therapeutic strategy.

Classification

Classification of vascular lesions of the spinal cord have been confusing in the literature, as there are multiple systems of classifications proposed, with overlapping criteria to classify these disorders.

Genetically spinal cord vascular malformations are classified as three broad categories.

1. Hereditary lesions caused by mutations in vascular germinal cells, e.g. malformations associated with hereditary hemorrhagic telangiectasia (HHT) **(Figs. 1A to E)**
2. Non-hereditary genetic lesions caused by somatic mutations which share metameric links, e.g. spinal AV metameric syndromes (Cobb, Klippel-Trenaunay, and Parkes-Weber syndromes)
3. Isolated sporadic lesions, that are not associated with any genetic links.

In 1993, Anson and Spetzler proposed morphologic classification of spinal cord vascular malformations into the four following morphologic categories, Type I to IV **(Table 1)**.

In 2006, Kim and Spetzler proposed a modified anatomic classification based on anatomic location and type of malformation **(Table 2)**.

In 2002, Spetzler suggested to include spinal artery aneurysms, and tumor and tumor like lesions such as cavernous malformations (cavernomas), hemangioblastomas, which grossly complete the vascular lesions of spinal cord.

T Krings et al, proposed a simple classification scheme to classify vascular malformations of spine. It is based on a simple questionnaire, which is as follows:

1. Is there a shunt? If no—cavernoma
2. If there is a shunt, what is the feeding artery?
   a. If feeding artery is radiculomeningeal artery (RMA)—spinal dural arteriovenous fistula (SDAVF)
   b. If feeding artery is RMA, then what is the nidus architecture?
      i. Glomus type
      ii. Fistulous type—This is further subdivided into micro and macrofistulous form based on the shunt volume.

EXTRADURAL ARTERIOVENOUS FISTULAE (EPIDURAL FISTULAE)

The extradural arteriovenous fistulae, previously called as epidural fistulae, represent an abnormal connection between an artery and the epidural venous plexus (Batson's plexus). This produces engorgement of the epidural plexus and subsequent mass effect upon the spinal cord. Venous drainage can be confined to the epidural space or may reflux into the perimedullary veins. These occur commonly in the thoracic spine. Anatomically they can be further divided into anterior (osteodural) **(Fig. 2)** and posterior **(Fig. 3)** subgroups, depending upon the vein in which the fistula is opening. Rangel-Castilla et al. proposed a sub-classification system of extradural arteriovenous fistulae into three types: A, B1, and B2. Type A fistulae have at least one intradural draining vein, while type B have purely extradural drainage. Type B1 has mass effect on the thecal sac and cord, no mass effect is seen in type B2.

Clinically they present with progressive myelopathy, mainly secondary to mass effect over the cord by engorged epidural veins. Symptoms secondary to congestive myelopathy may be seen if the drainage is seen into the intradural veins. Patients may also present with radiculopathy due to mass effect over nerve roots. Hemorrhage is rare.

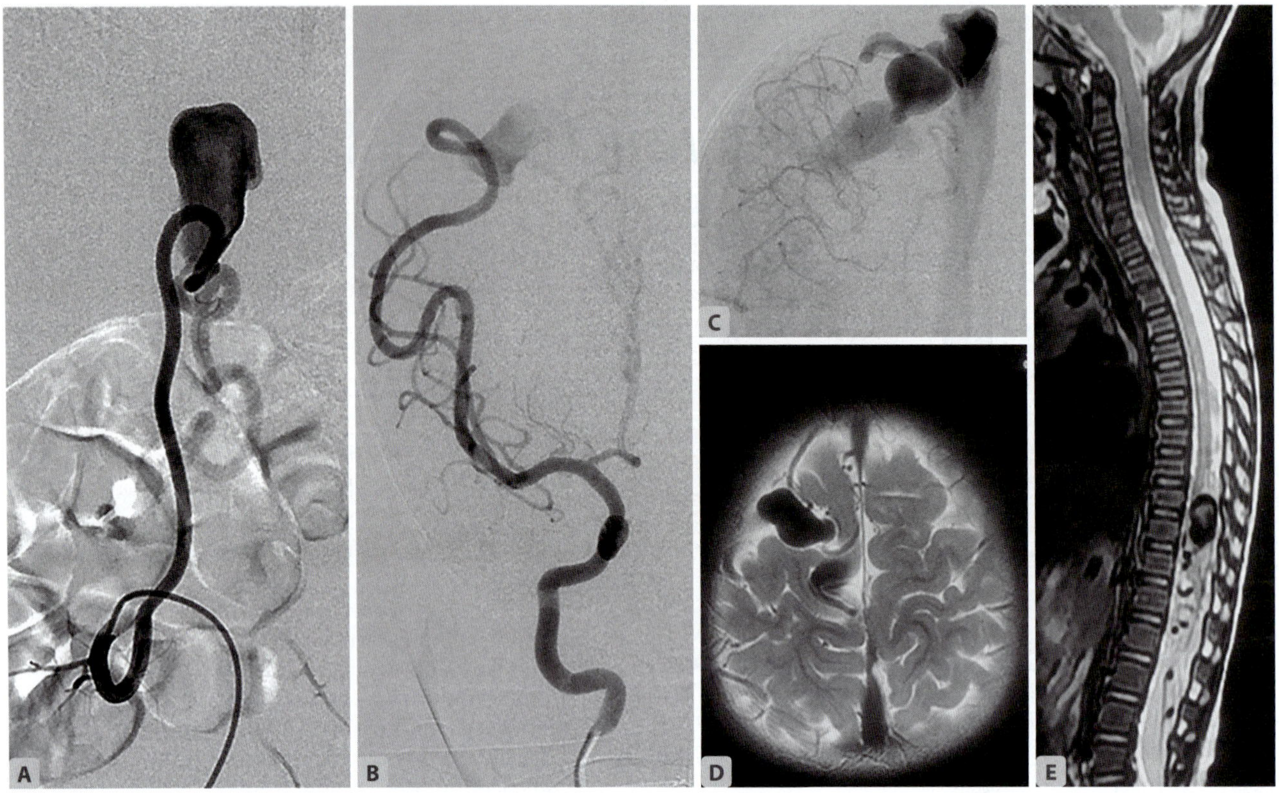

FIGS. 1A TO E: A 6-year-old boy with hemorrhagic telangiectasia (HHT) shows a spinal cord pial macrofistula (SCAVF) fed by radiculomedullary artery (A); Cerebral angiogram of the same child shows a pial AVF fed by right MCA branches with ectatic venous pouch (B and C). MR images showing right frontal and thoracic cord pial AVFs (D and E).

TABLE 1: Anson-Spetzler morphologic classification of spinal vascular malformations (1993).

Anson-Spetzler morphologic classification (1993)		Description
Type I	Spinal Dural AVF (SDAVF)	Radicular artery communicating directly with a dural vein
Type II	Glomus AVM	Intramedullary pial AVM fed by radiculomedullary or radiculopial arteries
Type III	Juvenile or metameric AVM	Complex juvenile metameric AVMs involving multiple compartments (extradural and intradural), along discrete somite levels
Type IV	Spinal cord AVF (SCAVF)	Pial AVF fed by radiculomedullary or radiculopial arteries

TABLE 2: Kim and Spetzler modified anatomic classification (2006).

Types		Other descriptions
Fistulae	Extradural	Osteodural or anterior epidural and posterior epidural fistulae belong to this group
	Intradural dorsal	Classic Type I lesions (SDAVF)
	Intradural ventral	Classic Type IV lesions (SCAVF)
AVM	Extradural-intradural	Classic Type III lesions (juvenile/ metameric AVM)
	Intradural	Classic Type II lesions (Glomus AVM)
	Conus	Conus AVMs

MRI examination reveals engorged epidural veins either anteriorly or posteriorly which may exert mass effect over the cord. Cord signal intensity changes may be present. Adjacent bones, especially vertebral bodies can show osteolysis. Selective DSA shows fistula draining into the epidural venous plexus. On very rare occasions an intradural draining vein may be seen.

These lesions are effectively treated by endovascular means, using liquid embolization agents mainly n-butyl cyanoacrylate (NBCA, glue) or Onyx. In cases were the fistula could not be approached by microcatheter, open surgery can be used. Incomplete occlusion of the fistula actively recruits new feeders, resulting in recurrence.

DORSAL INTRADURAL ARTERIOVENOUS FISTULA (SPINAL DURAL ARTERIOVENOUS FISTULA)

Dorsal intradural AVFs correspond to the classic Type I lesions in the Anson-Spetzler classification. They are the most common type of spinal AV fistula, making up about 70% of all

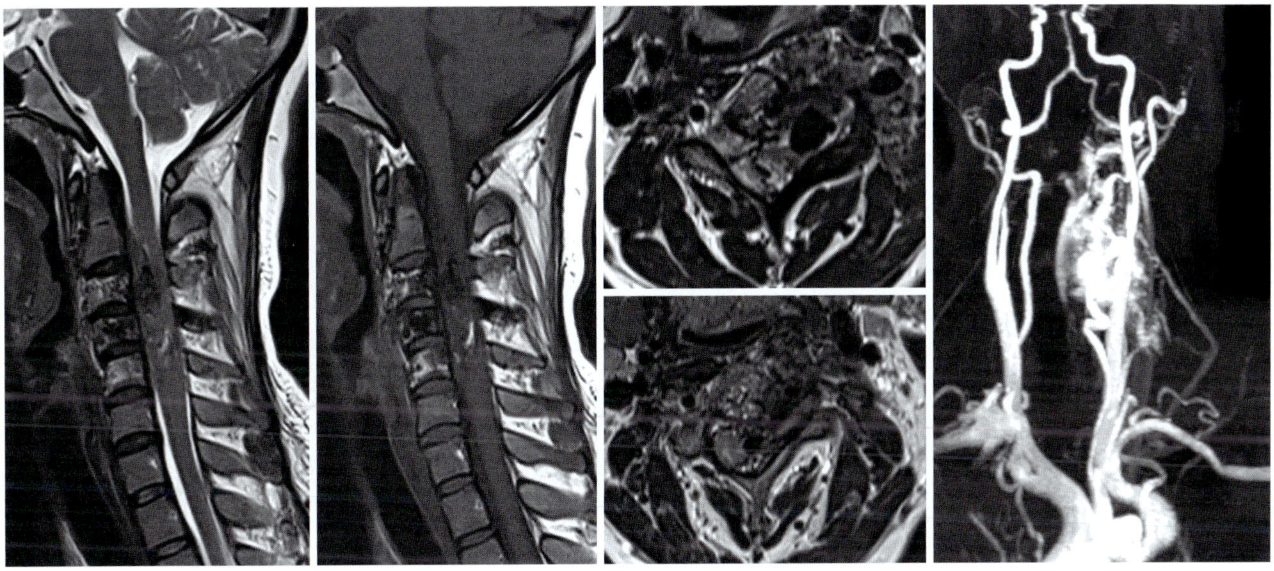

FIG. 2: Anterior epidural fistula. A 24-year-old female patient with paresthesia and quadriparesis. T1 and T2WI shows heterogeneous anterior extradural lesion with areas of hypointensity and hyperintensity s/o hemorrhages. Note extensive osteolysis involving vertebral bodies of C3 to C5. Axial images show extradural location of flow voids with mass effect over the cord. CE MRA images show the fistula fed by branches of left ascending and deep cervical artery.

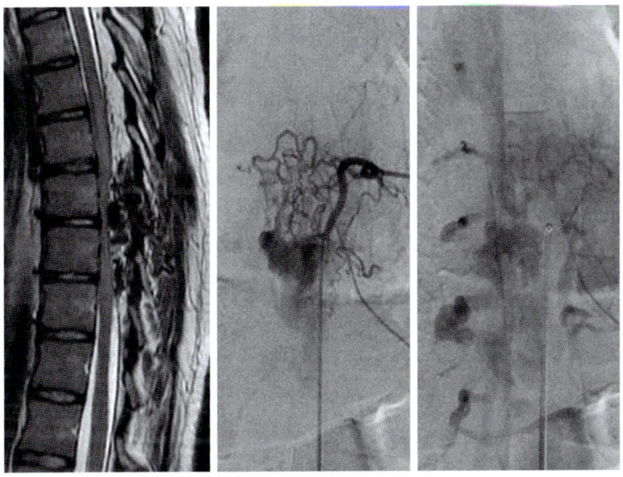

FIG. 3: Posterior epidural fistula. A 26-year-old male patient with paraparesis. T2WI shows multiple vascular flow voids in posterior epidural space, compressing the cord. Selective DSA shows the fistula fed by multiple small arterial feeders from the intercostal artery. Venous phase of the angiogram shows the venous drainage into azygos-hemiazygos system, and not into the intradural veins.

spinal AV malformations. There is a male predominance (M:F - 5:1), and it is usually diagnosed in the 5th to 6th decades of life. They are mostly found in the thoracic and thoracolumbar regions (more than 80%).

SDAVFs are formed by an abnormal connection between one or more radiculomeningeal arteries and the venous outflow. The shunt is located intradurally at the level of the dural sleeve surrounding the nerve root and drains into perimedullary veins. They have slow flow and are grouped into 2 subtypes. Subtype A has a single feeding artery while Subtype B has multiple feeders. Unlike the other spinal vascular malformations, this type of AVF is acquired.

The pathogenesis of SDAVF was first described in 1926 by Foix and Alajouanine. They described a progressive subacute necrotizing myelopathy, now known as Foix-Alajouanine syndrome, and found vascular obstruction, spinal cord necrosis and tortuous and dilated vessels on the surface of the spinal cord. They proposed that spinal cord ischemia is secondary to venous congestion or hypertension, which is the hallmark of this disease. Venous hypertension results in decreased arteriovenous pressure gradient resulting in vascular slowing. This results in progressive venous congestion and edema of the cord parenchyma with progressive symptoms.

Early symptoms of SDAVF are often non-specific which leads to delay in diagnosis. Lower extremity weakness is the most common initial presenting symptom, seen in about half of the cases. Other symptoms seen at presentation, include gait disturbance, paresthesia, back pain and bladder/bowel or sexual dysfunction. Hemorrhage is rare.

MRI is the initial image modality used in the evaluation when SDAVF is suspected. MRI shows increased signal intensity in the cord on T2-weighted images, which corresponds to cord edema which usually spans multiple levels. Dorsal intradural flow voids may be present and are more evident on heavily T2-weighted images or contrast-enhanced T1-weighted images. Selective catheter angiography is the gold standard for diagnosis of SDAVF. It also provides an opportunity for possible endovascular treatment. It usually shows a small low-flow fistula fed by dorsal radiculomeningeal artery draining into intradural veins with venous congestion **(Figs. 4A to F)**.

Conventionally, surgery is used as the main modality of treatment. The target of surgical or endovascular treatment is the arterialized proximal part of the draining vein. After performing a hemi-laminectomy and opening the dura, corresponding dorsal radiculomeningeal artery is followed, as it heads towards the dorsal nerve root. The artery-vein

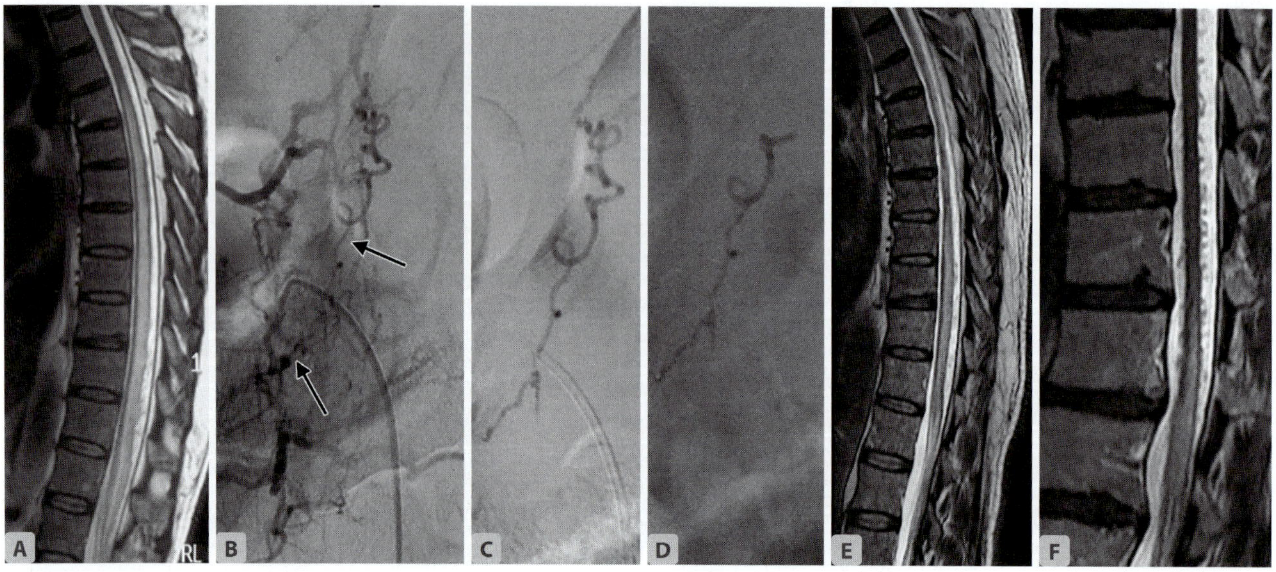

FIGS. 4A TO F: Dorsal intradural AVF (SDAVF). A 52-year-old male with slowly progressive paraparesis, bladder and bowel involvement. (A) Preprocedure MRI showing extensive spinal cord edema and vascular flow voids; (B) DSA and (C) microcatheter run showing fistula (black arrow, down) with draining vein (black arrow, up); (D) Glue cast; (E) Follow-up MRI showing reduction in spinal cord signal changes; (F) MRI of another patient with SDAVF shows spinal cord signal intensity changes and vascular flow voids dorsal to the cord in intradural location.

connection is disrupted by either coagulation, ligation or clipping. Surgery is associated with very low morbidity (2%), with complete occlusion achieved in >98% of patients.

The recent advances in endovascular procedures have given an alternative to surgical treatment of SDAVFs. It is less invasive, and may be performed at the same time as the diagnostic spinal angiogram. Early endovascular procedures used polyvinyl alcohol particles (PVA), however, this had high recanalization rates. Recurrence is less with liquid embolization agents like NBCA and Onyx. Embolization is contraindicated in patients where a radiculomedullary artery arises from the same pedicle as the feeder. Endovascular attempts in such cases may result in spinal cord ischemia and grave neurological deficits. Due to the small size and tortuous anatomy of the arterial feeder, microcatheterization may fail, resulting in need for surgery.

Prognosis after treatment depends on the duration and severity of pretreatment symptoms. Motor symptoms improve better compared with sensory or bladder/bowel symptoms.

VENTRAL INTRADURAL AVF (SPINAL CORD AVF, SCAVF, PERIMEDULLARY AVF)

These lesions correspond to Classic Type IV lesions in the Anson-Spetzler classification **(Figs. 5A to F)**. They are also referred to as perimedullary AVFs or fistulous arteriovenous malformations and are extremely rare, compared with cord AVMs or SDAVFs. They occur in a younger population, commonly presenting in the first and second decade and has no sex predilection.

Ventral intradural AVFs originate from the anterior spinal artery. The fistulous communication lies outside the cord parenchyma and pia matter in the subarachnoid space, anterior to the cord in the midline. Blood flow through these AVFs is very fast and they may have flow-related aneurysms and venous pouches. In contrast to the dorsal types, ventral intradural AVFs are congenital lesions. They can be further subdivided into 3 distinct types based on feeding vessel size, shunt volume and drainage pattern.

1. *Type A:* Small with a single feeder and low shunt volume. The feeding artery and draining vein are not much dilated. Hemodynamic features are similar to dorsal intradural AVFs **(Fig. 6A)**.
2. *Type B:* These are of an intermediate size with a major feeder from anterior spinal artery as well as smaller feeders at the level of the fistula.
3. *Type C:* These are giant lesions with multiple large arterial feeders and massively dilated venous vascular channels and large shunt volumes. Hemodynamic features in this subtype is similar to intramedullary AVMs **(Fig. 6B)**.

SCAVFs were first described by Djindjian in 1977 and later classified as Type IV by Heros. There are no capillaries or nidus between the artery and the venous network. The pathology is similar to dorsal intradural AVFs with venous hypertension. However, the cause of the venous hypertension is due to vascular steal and mechanical compression, than from slow flow and venous congestion. Hemorrhage is more common and occurs in about 20–40% of patients.

Symptoms are produced by vascular steal, mechanical compression from engorged veins or by subarachnoid or intraparenchymal hemorrhage **(Figs. 7A to D)**. Symptoms are usually progressive in nature, with myelopathy the most

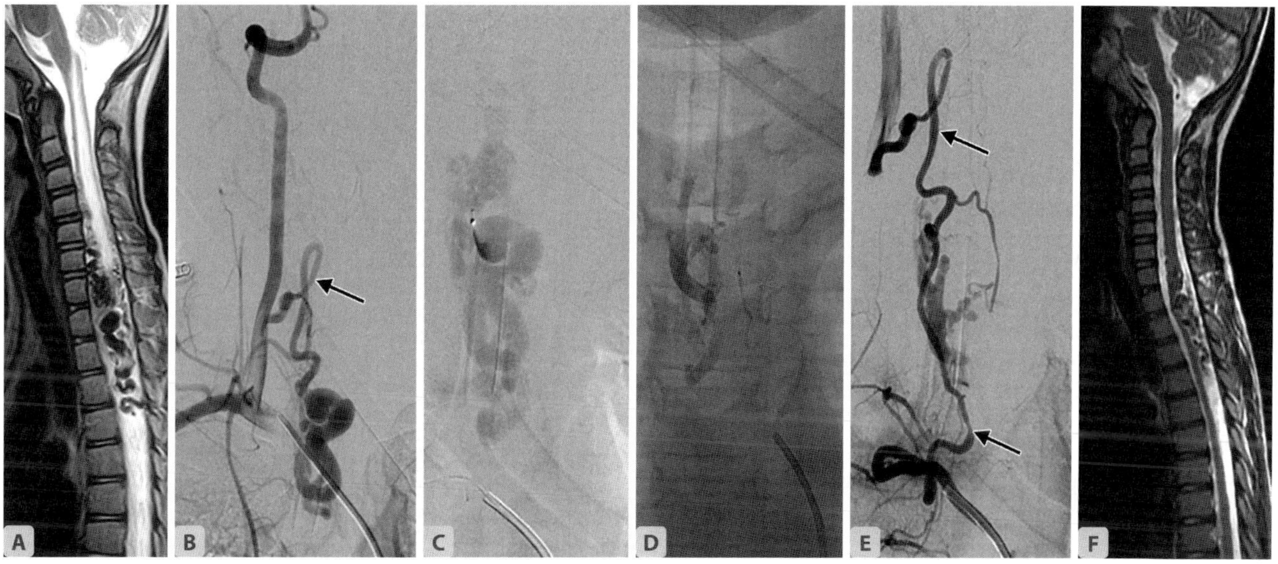

FIGS. 5A TO F: Ventral intradural AVF (SCAVF). A 7-year-old female with acute onset paraparesis. (A) MRI showing multiple dilated vascular flow voids with extensive cord edema; (B) DSA showing macrofistula fed by RMA (black arrow); (C) Microcatheter run; (D) Glue cast; (E) Check angiogram showing preservation of anterior spinal axis (black arrows); Follow-up MR (F) showing decrease in flow voids and resolution of edema.

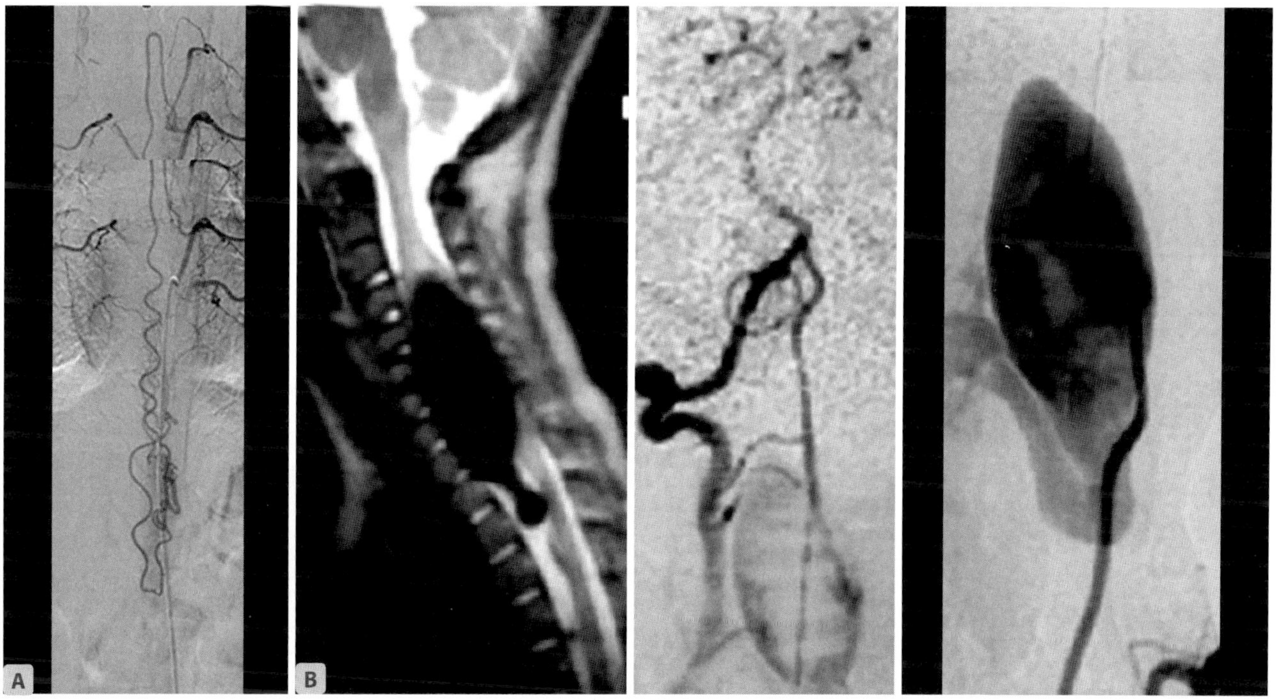

FIGS. 6A AND B: Spinal cord AV fistula (SCAVF). (A) Microfistula. A 8-year-old male with congestive myelopathy. DSA shows single hole fistula fed by radiculomedullary artery. Note the single arterial feeder directly communicating with vein with no intervening nidus. Note the absence of dilatation or ectasia in the venous side; (B) Macrofistula. A 2-year-old male with acute onset quadriparesis and respiratory distress. MRI shows large sac in the spinal canal; compressing the cord. DSA shows macrofistula with a large venous sac, fed by anterior spinal artery and RMA from left superior intercostal artery.

common finding. Cases in which a patient present acutely or an acute exacerbation of baseline symptoms are usually a result of hemorrhage.

MR Imaging is often the initial image modality used to diagnose SCAVFs. T2 prolongation in the cord is seen with flow voids on the ventral aspect of the cord or thecal sac. Hemorrhage may be identified as T1 hyperintense signal.

Treatment depends on the subtype of the ventral intradural AVFs. Types A and B may be treated by surgical or endovascular means, while Type C lesions are almost always treated via endovascular route. Surgery is generally difficult since anterior or anterolateral approach is needed to reach the fistula.

Endovascular embolization with liquid embolic agent, especially NBCA with its rapid polymerization time is generally used to treat these fistulas. Care should be taken to preserve the anterior spinal axis while embolization. Outcome of the patient is generally good if the fistula is occluded and anterior spinal axis is preserved.

EXTRADURAL-INTRADURAL ARTERIOVENOUS MALFORMATIONS (JUVENILE/METAMERIC AVM)

Extradural-Intradural AVMs are rare and complex, and has been called type III, metameric, or juvenile AVM **(Figs. 8)**. They arise from single or multiple somites, having both intra and extradural components. They may also have soft tissue, bone or skin involvement, corresponding to the same metamer as that of the cord. Most often they are diffuse and do not have a nidus. They may also be a part of a syndromic complex such as the metameric angiomatosis (Cobb's syndrome), disseminated angiodysplasia (Osler-Weber-Rendu syndrome), Klippel-Trenaunay syndrome, or Parkes-Weber syndrome. This is a high-flow lesion with multiple feeding and draining vessels.

These type of lesions are commonly seen in adole-scents and young adults who present with pain or progressive myelopathic symptoms from spinal cord compression, venous hypertension, or vascular steal. Intramedullary or subarachnoid hemorrhage could be the initial presenting symptom.

MRI is the modality of choice as it helps to find the extent of the AV malformation and the compartments involved. As the AVM is more extensive, the goal of the treatment should be to avoid morbidity and not complete radiological cure. Targeted approach is needed to specifically focus on selected problems like venous hypertension, obliterating a part of the AVM, which is causing mass effect or occluding the fistulous part of the AVM.

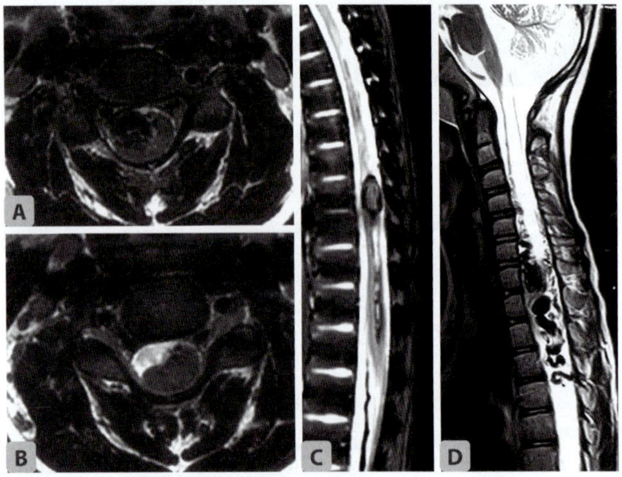

FIGS. 7A TO D: Causes of myelopathy in SCAVF. (A and B) Mass effect; (C) Hematomyelia; (D) Venous congestion.

INTRAMEDULLARY AVM (GLOMUS AVM)

A spinal intramedullary AVM consists of multiple abnormal vessels constituting a nidus with one or more feeding arteries and draining veins. These lesions were previously classified as type II (glomus) AVMs in the earlier classification by Anson and Spetzler **(Figs. 9A to F)**. The nidus may be intramedullary, intra and extramedullary or located in the conus. These lesions are mostly located in the cervicothoracic region. About 20–40% of spinal intramedullary AVMs are associated

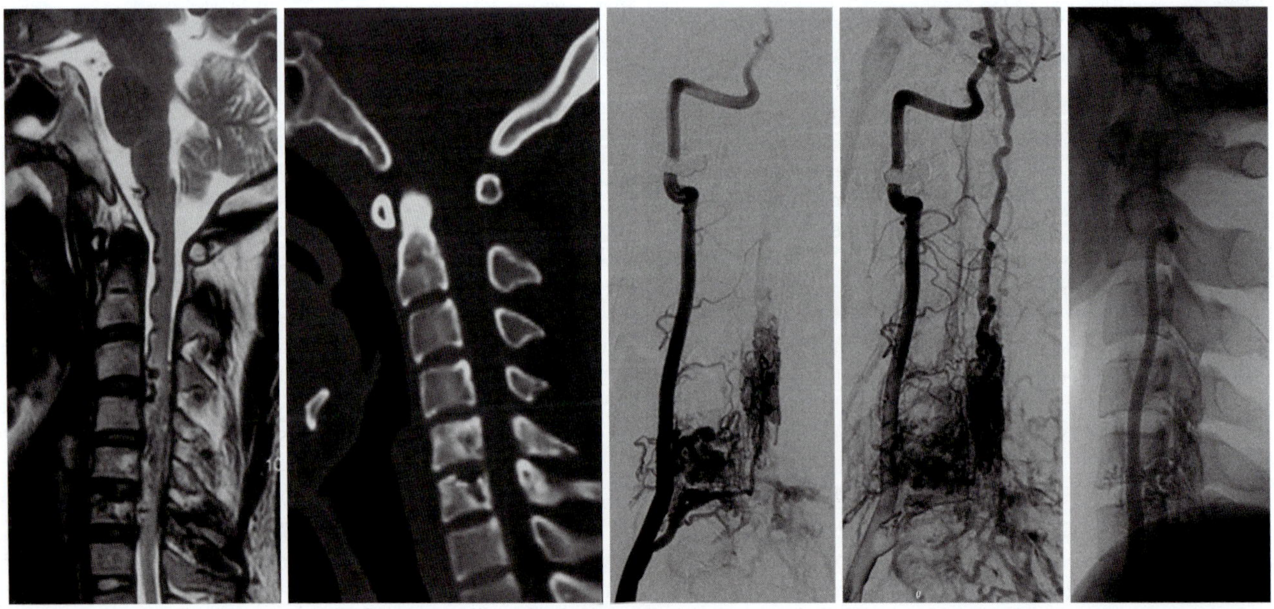

FIG. 8: Juvenilc or metarnerlc AVM. T2W sagittal images show osteodural lesions at C5 and C6 vertebral levels with few vascular flow voids within the cord and a prominent vascular channel anterior to cord. Sagittal CT images show osteolysis of C5 and C6 vertebral bodies. DSA images show an epidural fistula at the level of C5 and C6 vertebral bodies and a spinal cord intramedullary AVM at slightly higher level, corresponding to the same somite. Note the venous drainage into anterior spinal vein, which was seen as prominent vascular channel in T2W image.

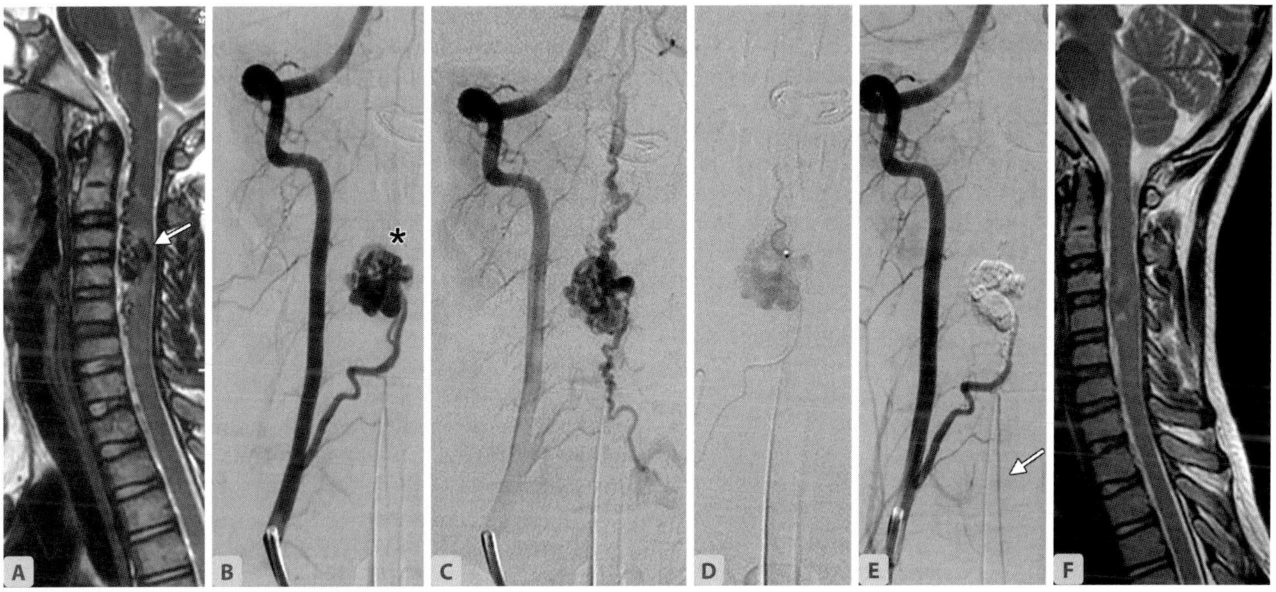

FIGS. 9A TO F: Intramedullary AVM. MRI of a 9-year-old child with acute onset quadriparesis shows cervical cord AVM (arrow, A). DSA showed glomus type of AVM fed by radiculomedullary artery arising from right vertebral artery (asterisk, B), draining into perimedullary veins (C). Microcatheter angiogram after super-selective catheterization shows visualization of only the nidus and draining vein (D). Embolization of the AVM nidus was done with n-butyl cyanoacrylate (glue). Check angiogram showed complete obliteration of AVM with preservation of anterior spinal axis (arrow, E). Follow-up MRI showed complete obliteration of AVM with non-visualization of flow voids (F).

with aneurysms and their presence is related with increased risk of bleeding.

They are more simply classified as compact and diffuse forms (Spetzler). The compact forms were earlier classified as glomus type and the diffuse forms were classified as juvenile AVMs. The juvenile AVMs form a distinct sub-group in that they have an embryological basis for their location.

Patients usually present in the third decade of life. Hemorrhage is seen in up to half of the patients. The risk of re-bleeding in patients presenting with hemorrhage is 10% at one month and 40% at one year. No sex predilection is seen. Non-hemorrhagic manifestations include back pain, radicular pain, motor/sensory deficits, sexual disturbance, sphincter disturbances and bruit.

1. *Hemorrhage:* Half of the patients present with subarachnoid hemorrhage or acute medullary syndrome. These patients present with moderate to severe backache and sudden neurologic deficit.
2. *Venous hypertension:* The arterialized veins have dysplastic walls and are not capable of handling high blood pressure. This may either lead to rupture of vessels, or ischemia secondary to congestion. Symptoms may be positional with squatting or raising the leg above heart level causing exacerbation of symptoms.
3. *Venous thrombosis:* Thrombosis due to venous congestion is seen in low flow AVMs. It predisposes to ischemic damage of surrounding cord parenchyma and hemorrhage.
4. *Vascular steal:* Vascular steal is seen in high-flow AVMs. With limited ability to vasoconstrict, blood is sucked into the AVM and the surrounding normal tissue suffers ischemia.
5. *Mechanical compression:* The nidus and venous pouches can cause compression of the cord. Patient may present with combination of myelopathy or radiculopathy secondary to pressure effect of the AVM.

Magnetic resonance imaging (MRI) and magnetic resonance angiography (MRA) are the first choice of investigation although selective catheter angiography is the gold standard for definitive diagnosis and characterization of these lesions. MR features suggestive of vascular malformations include a serpentine pattern of flow voids and spinal cord signal changes due to venous congestion, myelomalacia, infarction and hemorrhage. MRA is increasingly being used for the diagnosis, localization and characterization of spinal AVMs. The limitations of MRA are difficulty in detecting multiple feeding vessels, low sensitivity for detection of spinal aneurysms, and inability to offer treatment in the same sitting.

Digital subtraction angiography is the gold standard for diagnosis of spinal AVM and characterization of its angioarchitecture. Segmental arteries should be individually catheterized on both sides to avoid missing silent lesions. The information to be sought on DSA includes location, feeding pedicle side and site, type of fistula and location of anterior spinal and posterior spinal arteries in relation to the AVM.

There are three modalities for treatment of spinal AVMs, which includes surgery, endovascular and stereotactic radiosurgery. In some cases, a combination of these treatment modalities may be tried. Although stereotactic radiosurgery is commonly used in cranial AVMs, its use in spinal AVM is only at the research level. Several articles have quoted the effectiveness of radiosurgery of spinal AVMs.

Endovascular therapy is used either primarily or to reduce the size and flow in the lesion before surgery. Super-selective catheterization of feeder arteries rather than the segmental artery helps in preventing ischemic damage to the normal parenchyma thus reducing the chance of neurological deficits. The most commonly used embolic materials for the embolization of spinal AVMs are NBCA and onyx. Factors that favor a successful endovascular occlusion include normal anterior spinal artery separate from the nidus, short distance between the arterial feeders and the nidus, and high flow through the AVM nidus. Occlusion of the nidus may lead to edema of the surrounding cord and neurological deterioration, which is usually a self-limiting condition and the patient recovers in a few weeks. Use of corticosteroids may be helpful in reducing the edema.

CONUS MEDULLARIS AVM

Conus AVMs are a subset of intramedullary AVMs and consists of lesions at the conus with multiple feeding arteries, multiple diffuse niduses and complex venous drainage. They have multiple direct AV shunts that derive from the anterior and posterior spinal arteries. Niduses are usually extramedullary and pial based. Because of the location of these lesions, patients may present with both upper and lower motor neuron symptoms **(Figs. 10A to F)**.

CAVERNOUS ANGIOMAS (CAVERNOMA) OF SPINAL CORD

Cavernomas are intramedullary vascular malformations which is made of dilated thin walled capillaries and sinusoids. There is generally no feeding artery or a draining vein. Cavernomas cause symptoms by acute cord hemorrhage or rarely subarachnoid hemorrhage. They can also present with progressive myelopathy due to repetitive hemorrhages or toxic degradation products of hemorrhage.

On MR imaging, hypointense hemosiderin rim is seen in T2WI and multi-echo gradient images, with a 'popcorn' hyperintense center. Subacute hemorrhage may be detected as T1 hyperintense signal. Usually no enhancement is seen. Cavernomas are angiographically occult **(Figs. 11A to E)**.

Asymptomatic lesions are followed up. Lesions that present with recurrent hemorrhages are best treated with microsurgical removal. As there is no definite feeding artery, endovascular treatment is not a treatment option for cavernoma.

OTHER LESIONS

Although not really vascular malformations, hemangioblastomas and spinal aneurysms are included under vascular lesions of spinal cord classification by Spetzler.

Spinal hemangioblastomas are highly vascular tumors with extensive arterial feeders and draining veins. With its high flow and steal phenomenon, they act like high flow spinal AVM or AVF, and may present with mass effect, venous hypertension, or ischemia secondary to steal. Symptoms of venous hypertension develop if hemangioblastomas drain into perimedullary veins. They appear as T2 hyperintense lesions with adjacent vascular flow voids representing arterial feeders and draining veins. Cystic components are commonly seen. After contrast administration, the solid components of the lesion show intense enhancement **(Fig. 12)**.

Spinal artery aneurysms are extremely rare when not associated with any high flow lesions like AVMs or SCAVFs. When associated with high flow lesions, management of the primary lesion would suffice to remodel and heal the walls of weakened aneurysm wall. In large aneurysms, especially when they have previously ruptures, it is safe to place one or two detachable coils in the aneurysmal sac to prevent re-rupture.

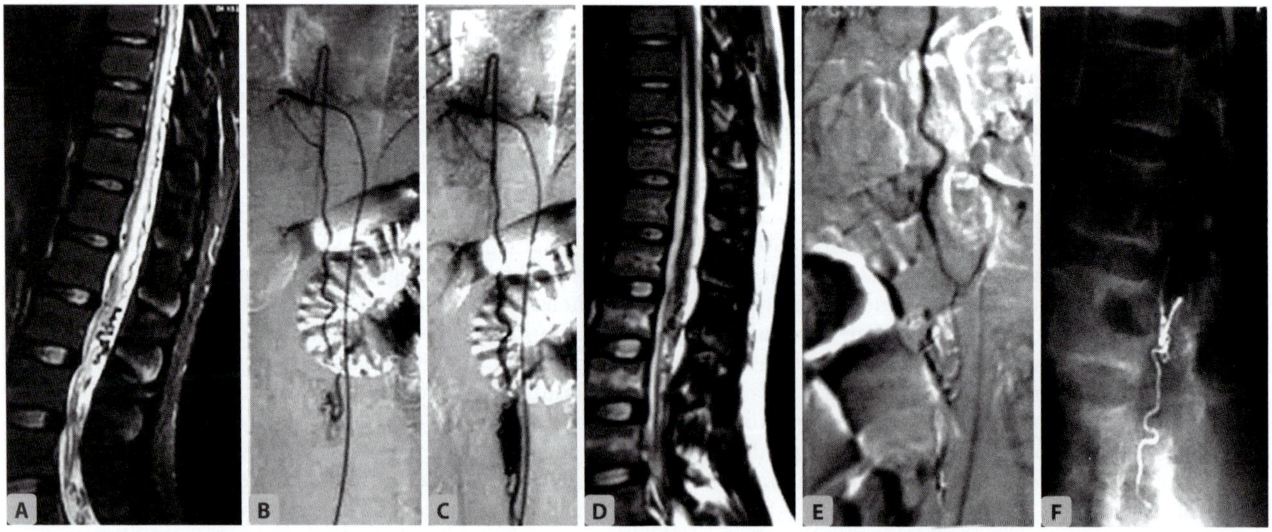

FIGS. 10A TO F: Spinal cord AVM (conus). (A) Sagittal T2W MRI showing the edematous swollen cord and multiple tortuous dilated vascular channels present both anteriorly and posteriorly; (B and C) RD9 injection, showing the enlarged radiculomedullary artery supplying the complex AVM through anterior spinal axis. Post-embolization imaging: (D) T2W sagittal MRI (done on second post-procedure day) showing complete resolution of the abnormal vascular flow voids and decrease in the bright signal and swelling of the cord; (E) Immediate post-embolization RD9 injection showing complete obliteration of the AVM with adequately filling anterior spinal axis; (F) Onyx cast.

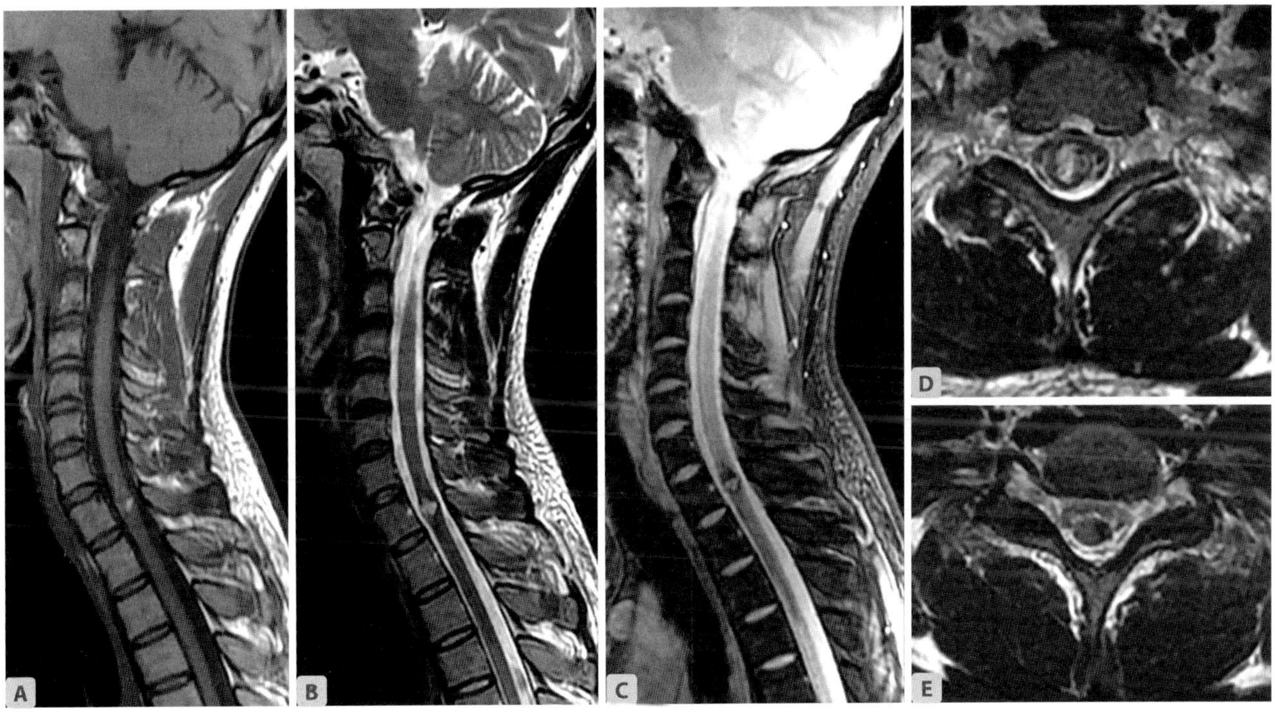

FIGS. 11A TO E: A 26-year-old male patient with acute onset neck pain and neurological deficits; T1 and T2WI (A and B) show a small focal hyperintense lesion in the cord with hypointense rim in T2WI and GRE (B and C); T2W axial images show hyperintense area of subacute bleed with cord expansion and hypointense area of chronic bleed (D and E).

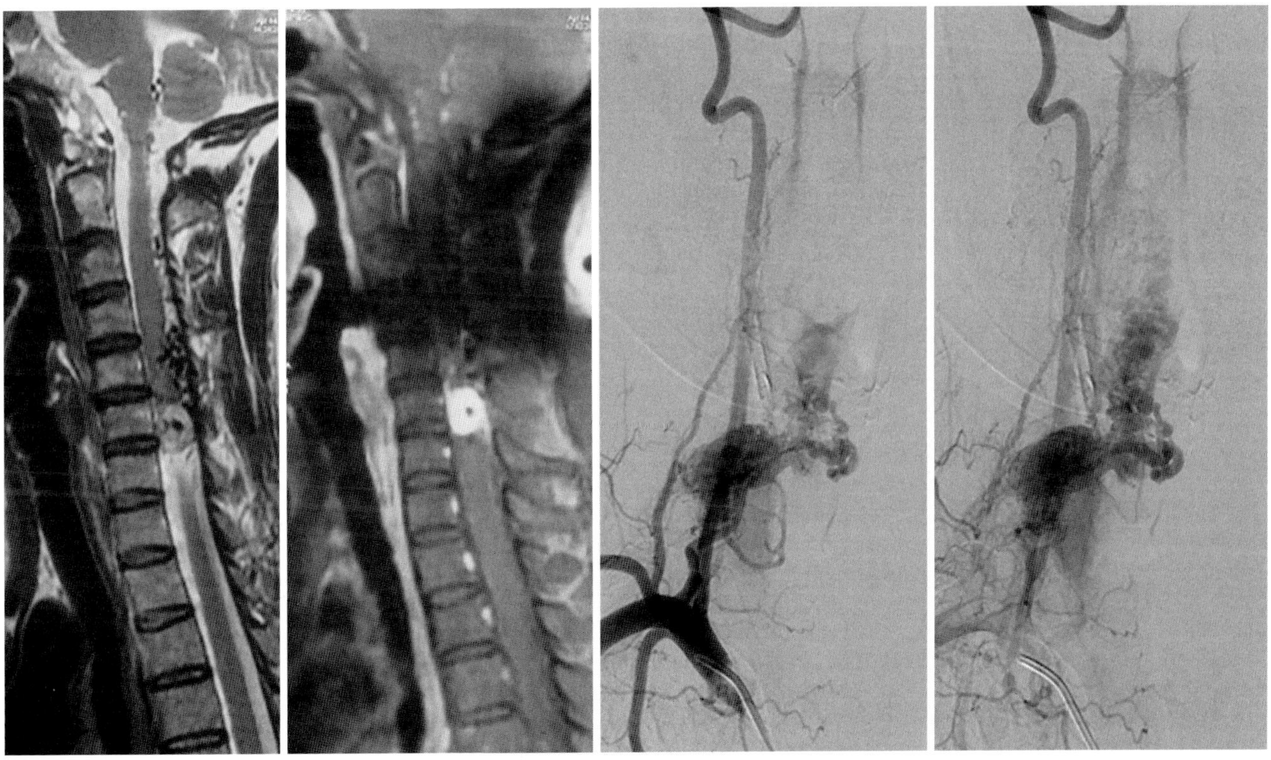

FIG. 12: Hemangioblastoma. Well-defined hyperintense lesion within the spinal canal in T2WI with intense enhancement is seen. Multiple vascular flow voids are seen, predominantly dorsal to cord. DSA shows tumor blush, fed by branches of ascending and deep cervical arteries with venous drainage into perimedullary veins.

CONCLUSION

With a wide spectrum of disorders, along with their varied pathophysiology, it is essential to have a comprehensive idea about identification, classification and treatment of these disorders. It would help in early identification of the disease and avoids misdiagnosis, as it is one of the curable causes of progressive myelopathy.

ACKNOWLEDGMENT

The authors acknowledge and thank Dr Parthiban Bala, DM Resident in Department of Neuroimaging and Interventional Radiology, AIIMS, New Delhi, India, for active involvement and helping in writing the chapter.

SUGGESTED READING

1. da Costa L, Dehdashti AR, terBrugg E KG. Spinal cord vascular shunts: spinal cord vascular malformations and dural arteriovenous fistulas. Neurosurg Focus. 2009;26(1):E6.
2. Gonzalez LF, Spetzler RF. Treatment of Spinal Vascular Malformations.
3. Kim LJ, Spetzler RF. Classification and surgical management of spinal arteriovenous lesions: arteriovenous fistulae and arteriovenous malformations. Neurosurgery. 2006;59(suppl 5):S3-195-201.
4. Krings T. Vascular malformations of the spine and spinal cord: anatomy, classification, treatment. Clin Neuroradiol. 2010;20(1):5–24.
5. Krings T, Geibprasert S. Spinal dural arteriovenous fistulas. Am J Neuroradiol. 2009;30(4):639–48.
6. Nachanakian A, El A, Abou G, Alayw M. In: Tjoumakaris S (Ed). Spinal Dural Arteriovenous Fistulas — Treatable Cause of Myelopathy. Arteriovenous Fistulas - Diagnosis and Management
7. Rodesch G, Hurth M, Alvarez H, Tadié M, Lasjaunias P. Classification of spinal cord arteriovenous shunts: proposal for a reappraisal—the Bicetre experience with 155 consecutive patients treated between 1981 and 1999. Neurosurgery. 2002;51(2): 374–380.
8. Spetzler RF, Kondziolka D, Higashida RT, Kalani MYS, editors. Comprehensive management of arteriovenous malformation of the brain and spine. Cambridge: Cambridge University Press; 2015. 336 p. (Cambridge medicine).

CHAPTER

215

Imaging of Low Backache

Raju Sharma, Shivanand Gamanagatti, Devasenathipathy Kandasamy, Arun Kumar Gupta

IMAGING OF LOW BACK PAIN

Nearly half the adult population in India suffers from back pain, lasting at least 24 hours at sometime every year.[1] The impact of back pain on society is considerable and is associated with an enormous economic burden. Low back pain most commonly affects the 30–50 year age group, with the prevalence peaking during the sixth decade. Young people are more likely to have brief, acute episodes of back pain, whilst chronic pain tends to occur in older people. There is an equal sex distribution. This chapter summarizes the etiology, clinical presentation and radiological investigation of low back pain.

When to Image?

There are many causes of back pain with a complex inter-relationship between anatomical, pathological and psychological factors leading to the eventual clinical presentation. A careful history and physical examination remains the mainstay of initial assessment of back pain. Imaging is not necessary in most cases of back pain because of the high rate of spontaneous remission within 6–8 weeks.[2] Furthermore, the use of early imaging does not appear to alter management in most patients. There are, however, certain features or "red flags" that should suggest serious pathology and prompt early imaging.[3] It is increasingly recognized that plain radiographic evaluation of back pain in the absence of trauma is of limited value, as degenerative changes are very common and sinister pathology may easily be missed.

Indications of a more complicated status, often termed "red flags," include the following:[3]

- Recent significant trauma, or milder trauma, age >50 years
- Unexplained weight loss
- Unexplained fever
- Immunosuppression
- History of cancer
- Intravenous (IV) drug use
- Prolonged use of corticosteroids, osteoporosis
- Age >70 years
- Focal neurologic deficit with progressive or disabling symptoms
- Duration longer than 6 weeks

Four main clinical scenarios:[4]

1. Acute nonspecific back pain, which usually resolves spontaneously within 6–8 weeks. Imaging prior to six weeks does not improve outcome but does increase cost.
2. Chronic back pain without sinister features. This is a very common situation that is usually related to degenerative disease.
3. Back pain with sciatica: A condition usually caused by disk prolapse.
4. Possible serious pathology or cauda equina syndrome, this group encompasses various conditions such as tumor, infection and inflammatory disorders.

Of these conditions, the first two do not usually warrant imaging. In patients suffering from sciatica, the cause is usually a prolapsed disk, and those who have had a failed period of conservative therapy may require imaging. In patients with possible serious pathology, urgent imaging is indicated.

CONDITIONS CAUSING BACK PAIN

The physical causes of back pain can be divided into mechanical conditions such as disk disease and non-mechanical conditions, such as infection, inflammation or neoplasm **(Table 1)**.[4-6] There are also conditions which do not involve the spine, such as abdominal aortic aneurysms and urological conditions that may present with back pain. Due to the complexity of the bony, ligamentous, muscular and neural elements of the back, a specific anatomical diagnosis often cannot be made. Even when radiological investigations show an abnormality, the positive findings may not necessarily relate directly to the back pain. Close clinico-radiological correlation is therefore required.[4-6]

TABLE 1: Causes of low back pain.

Mechanical (95%)	Specific cause
Acquired	Muscular injury Vertebral fracture Facet joint degeneration Disk degeneration Disk herniation Spinal stenosis Pars defects'
Congenital	Transitional vertebra Scoliosis Scheuermann's disease
Non-mechanical (5%)	Infection Neoplasm Spondyloarthropathy
Non-spinal cause	Abdominal aortic aneurysm, renal disease, pancreatitis, psychogenic

IMAGING MODALITIES

The purpose of diagnostic imaging is twofold: first is to provide accurate anatomic information and the second perhaps more important purpose is to affect the therapeutic decision-making process.

Radiographs

Radiographs are recommended when any of the above red flags are present. Lumbar radiographs may be sufficient for the initial evaluation of the following red flags, with further imaging indicated for treatment planning if findings are abnormal or inconclusive.[3,7]

- Recent significant trauma (at any age)
- Osteoporosis
- Age >70 years

The initial evaluation of the LBP patient may also require further imaging if other red flags such as suspicion of cancer or infection are present.

Plain and contrast-enhanced MRI has the ability to demonstrate inflammatory, neoplastic, and most traumatic lesions as well as show anatomic detail not available on isotope studies. Gadolinium-enhanced MRI reliably shows the presence and extent of spinal infection, and is useful in assessing therapy.[7,8] MRI has therefore taken over the role of the isotope scan in many cases where the location of the lesion is known. The isotope scan remains invaluable when a survey of the entire skeleton is indicated (e.g. for metastatic disease).

Magnetic Resonance Imaging, Computed Tomography, Myelography and Myelography/CT

Uncomplicated acute LBP and/or radiculopathy (no red flags) do not warrant the use of any of these imaging studies. The early indiscriminate use of expensive imaging procedures should be avoided. The appropriate use of these imaging procedures is an important challenge. For example, LBP complicated by "red flags" suggesting infection or tumor may justify early use of CT or MRI even if radiographs are negative. The most common indication for the use of these imaging procedures, however, is the clinical setting of LBP complicated by radiating pain (radiculopathy, sciatica) or cauda equina syndrome (bilateral leg weakness, urinary retention, saddle anesthesia), usually due to herniated disk and/or canal stenosis.[3]

Magnetic Resonance Imaging

MRI of the lumbar spine has become the initial imaging modality of choice in complicated LBP, replacing myelography and CT in recent years. Although disk abnormalities are common on MRI in asymptomatic people, acute back pain with radiculopathy suggests the presence of demonstrable nerve root compression on MRI.

However, determining the cause of back pain is complicated as it is often multifactorial and anatomical abnormalities are common in the spine and may not necessarily translate into clinical symptoms. Thus, the use of MRI in nonspecific LBP should be avoided and it should be reserved for the investigation of severe or progressive neurological deficits or for those cases in which serious underlying pathology is suspected. However, it plays a vital role in planning surgical management in cases of radiculopathy and spinal stenosis.[3,7,8]

MRI is particularly efficacious for detecting "red flag" diagnoses, particularly using the short tau inversion recovery (STIR) and fat-saturated T2-weighted fast-spin-echo sequences. MR with contrast is useful for suspected infection and neoplasia. In postoperative patients, enhanced MRI allows distinction between disk and scar when tissue extends beyond the disk space.

MR Protocol for Imaging Patients with Backache[9]

Coils and patient position:

- Phased array spine coils should be used for all spine imaging. Patients are positioned supine in the magnet.

Image orientation:

- Sagittal and axial images are acquired in the lumbar region. In the axial imaging plane, stacked cuts are acquired that cover an entire block of the spine. Acquiring images angled only through the disks is considered inadequate because portions of the spinal canal are not imaged in the axial plane, and sequestered disk fragments and spondylolysis defects are often missed.
- Sagittal images alone are sometimes inadequate to detect a disk fragment that has migrated from the parent disk. Because sequestered disks are a cause of failed back surgery and persistent symptoms, it is important to identify them on MRI by obtaining stacked axial images in addition to sagittal images through the canal.
- In the unoperated lumbar spine, stacked axial images should be obtained from the middle of the L3 vertebral body to the middle of the S1 vertebral body.
- In the postoperative spine, stacked axial images (matched images before and after contrast administration) are obtained by centering at the level of the previous surgery.

- Axial images are often better than sagittal for detecting lesions in the neural foramina. Generally, axial and sagittal planes of imaging are complementary to each other.
- Coronal images may be useful to better define the anatomy in patients with scoliosis.

Pulse sequences and regions of interest:

- T1W and fast T2W images are the standard for sagittal imaging in any segment of the spine.
- Gradient-echo sagittal sequences are used when looking for blood in the cord after trauma to take advantage of the blooming effect.
- A fast STIR sagittal sequence also is useful in trauma patients when looking for ligamentous injury with changes of hemorrhage and edema.
- Gradient echo axial images are used to detect disk disease in the cervical spine, whereas fast T2W axial images are used in the thoracic and lumbar spine for the same indications.
- T1W and FSE T2W images are selected in the sagittal and axial planes for most indications. Slice thickness generally is 3 or 4 mm.
- The fields of view are as small as possible; larger ones are required for sagittal than for the axial imaging planes.
- Phase and frequency encoding gradients should be reversed for imaging the spine in the sagittal plane so that chemical shift artifacts at the diskovertebral interfaces do not obscure pathology in the vertebral body end plates or disks.
- For evaluation of the post-operative spine fast spin echo sequences are better than spin echo sequences and the latter are better than gradient echo sequences. The shortest possible echo time should be used. Increasing band width and decreasing voxel size are useful. The frequency encoding direction should be kept parallel to the long axis of the pedicle screw. Some vendors offer specific metal artifact reduction sequences (e.g. MAVRIK, SEMAC).[10]

Use of gadolinium-based contrast:

- Contrast medium is always used for postoperative spine imaging, suspected infection, tumor, intradural or nontraumatic cord lesions.
- If any abnormality is identified in the epidural space when evaluating for osseous metastases or cord compression, gadolinium is given to show these lesions better.

Standing MR Scanners are available in which the patient can be scanned in weight bearing position. This may sometimes reveal clinically significant pathology like lumbar spine instability, disc disease and spondylolisthesis not detected on the conventional supine MRI. Kinetic MRI can be done in flexion and extension position. It also overcomes the problem of claustrophobia and has some niche indications. However these open scanners use low field magnets and therefore images are of low signal to noise ratio.

COMPUTED TOMOGRAPHY

Computed tomography provides superior bone detail but is not quite as useful in depicting disk protrusions when compared with multiplanar MRI. With the added value associated with high-quality reformatted sagittal and coronal plane images, CT is useful for depicting spondylolysis, pseudoarthrosis, scoliosis, and for post-surgical evaluation of bone graft integrity, surgical fusion, and instrumentation.[3]

CT is useful in detecting tumors like osteoid osteoma. The advent of dual energy CT has further enhanced the role of this modality. Using three material decomposition algorithms virtual non-calcium (VNCa) images can be generated and they can detect marrow oedema and marrow infiltration before osteolytic lesions develop. This can be useful in trauma, spondylodiscitis and in marrow infiltrative disorders like myeloma and skeletal metastasis.[11]

CT is often used to evaluate post-operative spine. There are methods available for metal artifact reduction based on iterative algorithms which should be used to enhance image quality.

Myelography/CT

"Plain" myelography was the mainstay of lumbar herniated disk diagnosis for decades. It is now usually combined with post-myelography CT in problematic cases. The combined study is complementary to plain CT or MRI and occasionally more accurate in diagnosing disk herniation, but it suffers the disadvantage of requiring lumbar puncture and contrast injection.

Discography and CT Discography

When other studies fail to localize the cause of pain, discography may occasionally be helpful. Although the images often depict nonspecific aging or degenerative changes, the injection itself may reproduce the patient's pain, which may have diagnostic value.[12,13]

Isotope Bone Scan

The role of the isotope bone scan in patients with acute LBP has changed in recent years with the wide availability of MRI and especially contrast-enhanced MRI. The bone scan is a moderately sensitive test for detecting the presence of tumor, infection, or occult fractures of the vertebrae but is nonspecific. For spondylolysis or stress fracture in athletes, bone scintigraphy with single photon emission computed tomography (SPECT), followed by limited computed tomography (CT) if scintigraphy is positive, is more sensitive than MRI.

High-resolution isotope imaging, including SPECT, may localize the source of pain in patients with articular facet osteoarthritis prior to therapeutic facet injection.[14] Similar scans may be helpful in detecting and localizing the site of painful pseudoarthrosis in patients following lumbar spinal fusion.

TRANSITION VERTEBRA

In 1917, Mario Bertolotti, an Italian surgeon, was the first to put forward a possible relationship between low back pain and congenital anatomical abnormalities in the last lumbar vertebra, described as "sacral assimilation of the lumbar vertebrae".[15] The presence of a transverse mega-apophysis in a lumbar vertebra with transitional characteristics may be associated with low back pain. Four to seven percent of patients with low back pain have transitional vertebra. Motion between the transitional vertebra and the sacrum is reduced and asymmetrical, resulting in early degenerative changes within the "neoarticulation" or in the normal contralateral facet joint, which gives rise to facet pain. Biomechanical stress transferred to the upper mobile vertebral segment can accelerate the disk degeneration, another mechanism responsible for pain. Lumbosacral transitional disk has reduced height compared with normal lumbosacral intervertebral disks.

If a lumbosacral transitional vertebra (LSTV) is suspected on MRI, the decision of whether it represents a sacralized L5 or lumbarized S1 must be made. Many complimentary imaging findings have been described to identify the transition vertebra. The true nature of the lower vertebral segmentation can be established on conventional radiographs that include the thoraco-lumbar junction so that hypoplastic true ribs may be differentiated from large transverse processes, thus allowing correct identification of the L1 vertebral body. It has been recommended to use a whole spine localizer to count the number of vertebra from C2 with the assumption that there are 7 cervical and 12 thoracic segments which helps in assigning the LSTV.[16]

It has been proposed that the position of the right renal artery may be used to identify lumbar levels on sagittal MRI, because it usually lies closest to the L1-2 disk space and the aortic bifurcation lies at L4. The Iliolumbar ligament can be clearly identified on axial MRI as a single or double hypointense band extending from the transverse process of L5 to the posteromedial iliac crest that also helps in localisation of L5 vertebra. Bone marrow oedema may be seen in the transverse processes of LSTV but has a poor correlation with back pain. The L3 vertebra usually has the longest transverse process which can be used as an additional feature to correctly number the lumbar vertebrae. The identification of vertebral level and transitional vertebra is also important in communicating the correct level of disk abnormalities to the operating surgeon.[16]

SPONDYLOLYSIS AND SPONDYLOLISTHESIS

Spondylolysis is defined as a defect in the pars interarticularis, which appears to be secondary to a stress fracture. A bilateral defect would result in spondylolisthesis (Forward slippage of a vertebra on the one below it) of varying degrees. Most common levels are L4-5 and L5-S1. The prevalence of spondylolysis is low in children and increases with age, there is a high incidence in adolescent athletes. The prevalence in general population is around 5% and commonly affects L5 (~90%) and L4 levels.[17] There is a genetic predisposition to spondylolisthesis, with 30% to 70% prevalence in other family members. Spondylolisthesis may be secondary to stress fracture of bilateral pars in young or may be due to degenerative disease in elders.[18,19]

Spondylolisthesis has been graded as follows, according to forward slippage of a vertebra on the one below it: Grade I (0–25%), II (25–50%), III (50–75%), Grade IV (75–100%).

Imaging

In spondylolysis the aim of imaging is: to detect lysis, distinguish acute and active lesions from chronic inactive non-union, assess bony healing in follow-up of acute lesions, detect listhesis and grade it, and identify spinal and neural foramina stenosis.[20,21]

Conventional radiography is often the first line imaging modality **(Figs. 1A to D)**, and techniques include routine anteroposterior (AP) lateral views and oblique views. Although chronic nonunion may be demonstrated, radiography is unreliable for detection of early and acute lesions. Oblique radiographs of the lumbosacral spine are more sensitive than frontal and lateral radiographs, which may miss 20% of unilateral pars defects.[22] Scotty dog with a collar around the neck is a typical sign described on oblique radiographs representing the break in pars. Bilateral spondylolysis with anterolisthesis of L5 over S1 may show the appearance of Napolean hat on frontal radiographs.

CT is probably the best method for demonstrating spondylolytic defects and may also be used for assessment of healing. Multiplanar reconstruction along the Pars has been utilized successfully for identifying defects, by demonstrating discontinuity in the bony ring of the posterior elements of the vertebra. It may simulate a facet joint giving rise to the "Extra facet sign". However, CT is limited in detection of other pathological processes, and it cannot reliably distinguish between active and inactive lesions.[20,21] Bone scan can be a useful technique to differentiate active stress reaction from inactive disease.

MRI may not depict the bony pars defects; however, it evaluates accurately the degree of slippage **(Figs. 2A to D)**, spinal stenosis, nerve roots, and the associated pathologic disk changes.

A new grading system has been described that utilizes both the morphological information of MRI combined with the presence or absence of marrow edema on fat-suppressed T2W images. This distinguishes between stress reaction and active and inactive spondylolysis.[22,23]

Indications for surgery include worsening pain and progressive listhesis, significant neurologic findings and slippage of more than 50%. Healing is not a feature of developmental spondylolysis, and patients with chronic inactive lysis can usually return to normal physical activities.

Scheuermann's Disease

Scheuermann's disease, also known as juvenile kyphosis, is a disorder that presents with a rigid thoracic or thoracolumbar kyphosis.[24] Its incidence is estimated at 1 to 8%. Scheuermann disease affecting the lumbar region is more painful than the thoracic counterpart.

It was first described in 1920 by Scheuermann, who believed that the endplate irregularity and vertebral wedging was caused by avascular necrosis of the cartilage ring apophysis.[24] Although the etiology is still unknown, it is thought to be related to stress and repeated trauma.

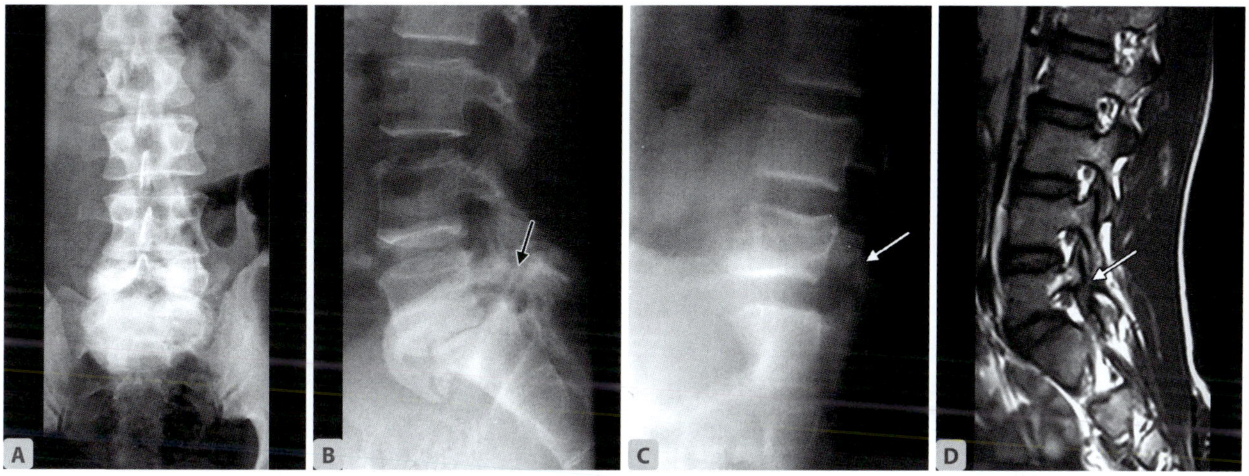

FIGS. 1A TO D: Anteroposterior (A) and lateral (B) radiographs of the lumbosacral spine showing break in the pars interarticularis (arrow) of L5 with grade II spondylolisthesis of L5 over S1. End plate sclerosis and osteophyte formation at L5-S1 levels are also noted. Lateral radiograph of a child (C) showing spondylolysis of L5 vertebra (arrow) and MRI T1 W sequence (D) showing the defect at pars inter-articularis.

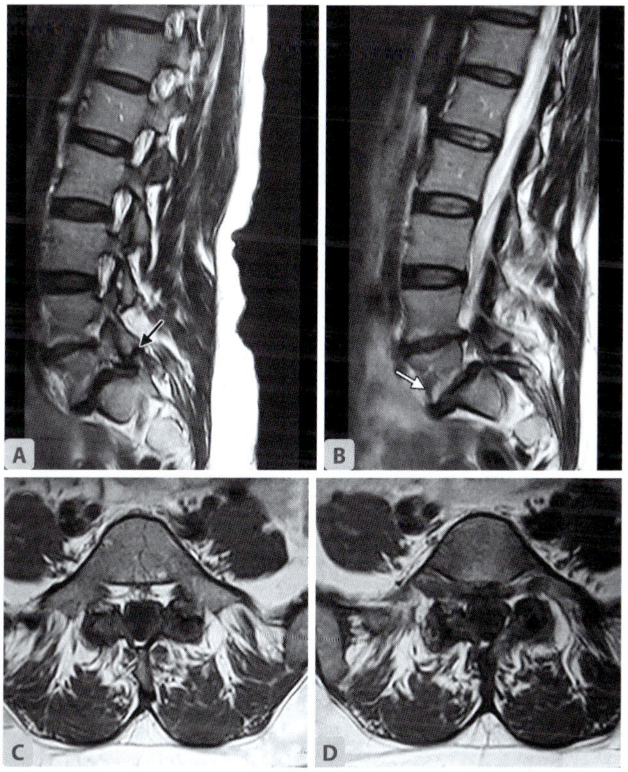

FIGS. 2A TO D: Sagittal T2W (A and B) and axial T1W (C and D) MR images showing spondylolysis seen at L5 (black arrow) with grade II spondylolisthesis (white arrow) of L5 over S1.

A recent study suggests that the presence of a gene defect in the *COL9A3* gene is associated with Scheuermann disease and intervertebral disk degeneration.

Clinical Presentation

Adolescents typically present to medical attention because of cosmetic deformity; adults more commonly present because of increased pain.

Imaging and Diagnosis

The diagnosis of classical Scheuermann's disease is based on involvement of three contiguous thoracic vertebrae with 5° of wedging associated with end-plate irregularity, and a thoracic kyphosis greater than 40°. The diagnosis of lumbar Scheuermann's disease is based on varying degrees of end-plate irregularities and disk narrowing in the lumbar spine or thoracolumbar junction, but with no abnormal kyphosis.[24,25]

Radiographs may show vertebral endplate irregularities, anterior vertebral body wedging, Schmorl's nodes **(Figs. 3A and B)**, and relative narrowing of the disk spaces. MRI **(Figs. 3C and D)** has an important diagnostic role, particularly with severe and painful kyphosis. It demonstrates, with great detail, endplate irregularities, Schmorl's nodes, disk degeneration, disk space narrowing, and anterior wedging of the vertebral bodies. Assessment of vertebral canal is imperative, especially in case of severe kyphosis.[26]

When reporting on radiographs of the lumbar spine with a combination of features such as end-plate irregularity, disk narrowing and Schmorl's nodes, particularly at the thoracolumbar junction, which would usually be recorded as being indicative of Scheuermann's disease, radiologists should avoid the use of this term and report only the anatomical and pathological features seen. The radiological diagnosis of Scheuermann's disease should be restricted to those patients who demonstrate the above features associated with an increased kyphosis of the thoracic spine.[26]

DEGENERATIVE DISEASES OF LUMBAR SPINE

Degenerative Changes in the Anterior Elements

- Degenerative change of the nucleus pulposus
- Annular tears
- Disk herniation

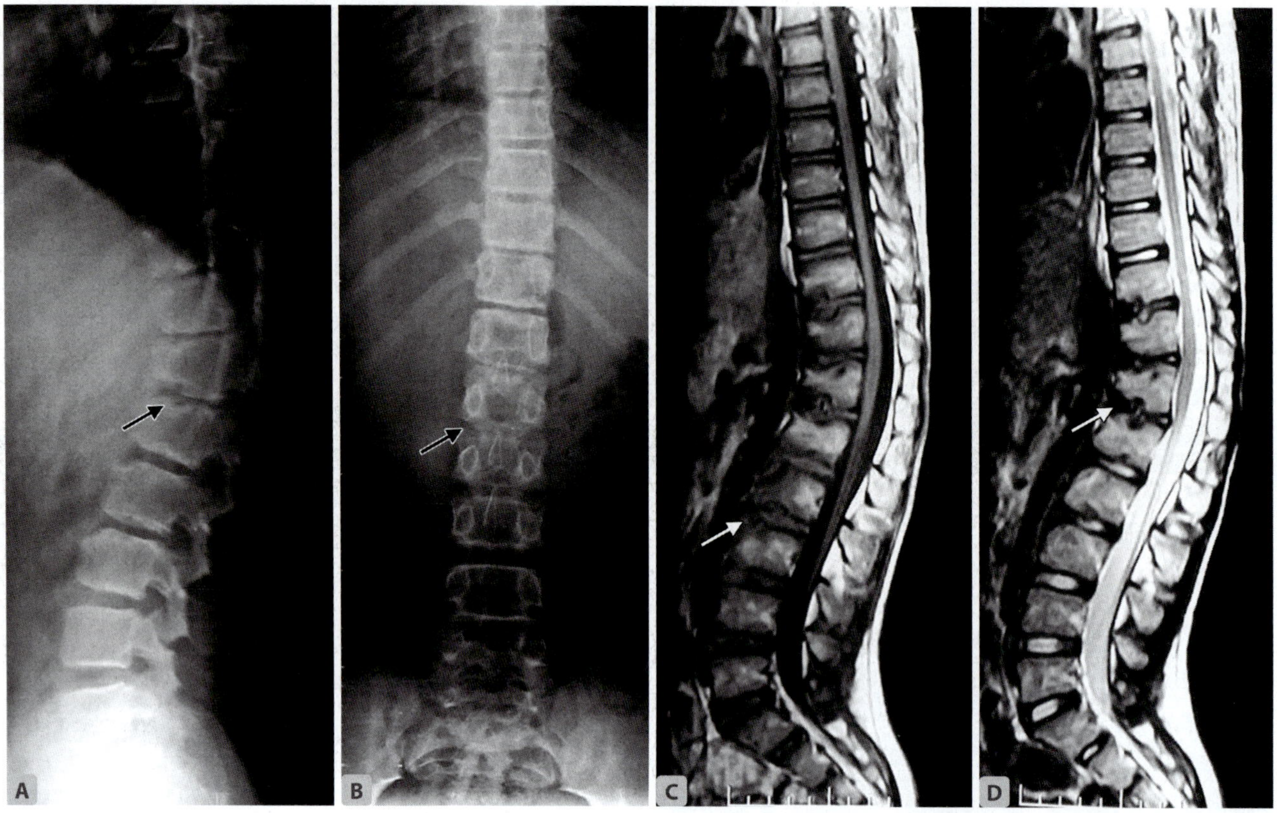

FIGS. 3A TO D: Scheuermann's disease: Anteroposterior (A) and lateral (B) radiographs of the dorsolumbar spine showing end-plate irregularities (black arrow) with decreased disk space at multiple levels and anterior wedging of lower dorsal and upper lumbar vertebral bodies. T1W (C) and T2W (D) MR images of the dorso-lumbar spine showing Schmorl's nodes (white arrow) at multiple levels in the lower thoracic and upper lumbar spine with kyphosis.

- Degenerative end plate changes
- Spondylosis deformans

Degenerative Changes in the Posterior Elements

Degenerative changes of the facet joints.

Complications of Degenerative Spinal Disease

- Scoliosis and kyphosis
- Segmental instability
- Spinal stenosis
- Foraminal stenosis

Presentation

- Degenerative change may present with local back pain, radiculopathy, or myelopathy.
- Degenerative facet arthropathy, degenerative disk disease, degenerative end plate changes, and ligamentous injury are all possible pain generators in the setting of axial back pain.
- Narrowing of the spinal canal or neural foramina can result in myelopathy and radiculopathy, respectively.
- Segmental instability, kyphosis, and scoliosis malalignment that may occur secondary to degenerative disease.
- Imaging of patients who have suspected spine pathology characterizes the level and extent of degenerative changes that may be a source of symptoms.
- Significant morphological changes on imaging are often found in asymptomatic patients without any significant clinical symptomatology, which does not require further evaluation in terms of acquiring electrophysiologic data to determine the significance of anatomic findings seen on imaging studies.

DEGENERATIVE CHANGE OF THE NUCLEUS PULPOSUS

Normal Disk

Intervertebral disks consist of a central gelatinous nucleus pulposus composed of water and proteoglycans. The nucleus pulposus is surrounded by the annulus fibrosus. The inner portion of the annulus is composed of fibrocartilage, whereas the outer fibers are made of concentrically oriented lamellae of collagen fibers. The annulus is anchored to the adjacent vertebral bodies by Sharpey's fibers.

MR Appearance of Normal Disk

On MRI, the normal disk shows low signal intensity on T1W images, slightly lower signal than adjacent normal

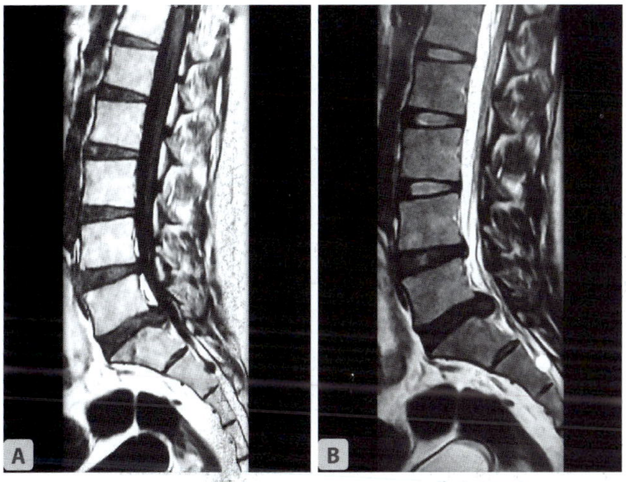

FIGS. 4A AND B: Sagittal T1W (A) and T2W (B) MR images showing normal signal in upper lumbar discs, loss of T2 hyperintensity suggesting dessication in L4 and L5 disks along with disk protrusion at these levels. Incidental perineural cyst is seen at S2 level.

red marrow and very similar to muscle. T2W images show diffuse high signal intensity **(Figs. 4A and B)** throughout the disk except for the outer fibers of the annulus, which are homogeneously hypointense. Distinction between the nucleus pulposus and the inner annulus fibrosus is impossible by MRI.

Normal disks typically do not extend beyond the margins of the adjacent vertebral bodies; however, diffuse extension beyond the margins by 1–2 mm may occur in some histologically normal disks. The posterior margins of disks tend to be mildly concave in the upper lumbar spine, straight at the L4-5 level, and slightly convex at the lumbosacral junction.[27]

Abnormal Nucleus

With aging and degeneration, the intervertebral disks lose hydration, lose proteoglycans, and gain collagen as they become more fibrous. A horizontally oriented fibrous intranuclear cleft develops in the nucleus. MRI shows the intranuclear cleft as a horizontal, low signal intensity line that divides the disk into upper and lower halves on T2W sagittal images. Eventually, there is diffuse decreased signal intensity on T2W images **(Figs. 4A and B)** from the increased collagen content in the nucleus. The disk progressively loses height with increasing degrees of degeneration.[27] There is a five level grading system proposed by Pfirrmann et al. which can be used to objectively evaluate the severity of disk degeneration on T2W spin echo images.[28,29]

Points to Remember

- The term "early degenerative changes" refers to accelerated age-related changes in the disk without evidence of structural failure
- A degenerated disk is a term reserved for those with structural failure combined with accelerated or advanced signs of aging
- Degenerative disk disease is best defined as symptomatic degenerative disk changes
- Many patients exhibit degenerative changes on MR without associated symptoms
- Intervertebral disk height at the lumbosacral junction is variable because of segmentation differences and a decreased disk height at this interspace is not necessarily pathologic.[27]

Annular Fissures

Annular fissure or tear represents a biomechanical failure of the annulus fibrosis and are usually associated with degenerative changes in the nucleus pulposus. The three basic types of annular tears are vertical, radial, and peripheral rim tears, of these radial tear is of practical interest.[30-32] Radial tears involve either part or the entire thickness of the annulus from the nucleus to the outer annular fibers. Radial tears run perpendicular to the long-axis of the annulus and occur more commonly in the posterior half of the disk, usually at L4-5 and L5-S1.[30-32] Radial tears may be source of pain either because the vascularized granulation tissue grows into the tear and causes painful stimulation of nerve endings or the chemical and mechanical irritation to the nociceptive fibers that normally exist in the annulus.

MR Appearance

- Show focal areas of high signal intensity on T2W images or on contrast enhanced T1W images.
- Radial tears may be seen on T2W sagittal images within the posterior annulus as globular or horizontal lines of high signal intensity.
- On axial images, radial tears may be seen as focal areas of high signal intensity that parallel the outer disk margin for a short distance.

Disk Herniation (Abnormalities in Disk Morphology)

It is a nonspecific term used to indicate disk that extends in some abnormal manner beyond the margin of vertebral body. Most surgeons dealing with spine disorders use a more standardized nomenclature that helps to distinguish what are likely to be clinically relevant lesions from lesions that probably are not. Standard nomenclatures used by the orthopedic surgeons include: *Diffuse disk bulge, Broad-based protrusion, Focal disk protrusion, Disk extrusion, and Sequestered disk.*[30-32]

Points to Remember

- A herniation is "focal" if it involves less than 25% of the disk circumference.
- A"broad-based" disk herniation involves between 25% and 50% of the disk circumference.
- Involvement of more than 50% of the circumference of the disk is defined as a "diffuse disk bulge."
- A "disk protrusion" **(Figs. 5A to D)** is defined as a herniation that demonstrates continuity with the adjacent

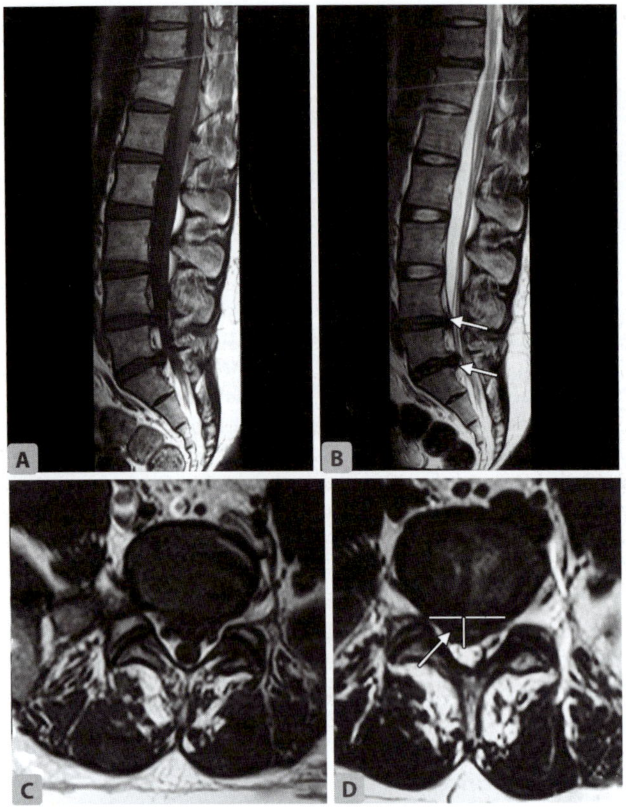

FIGS. 5A TO D: Disk protrusion: Sagittal T1W (A), T2W (B) and axial T1W (C), T2W (D) images showing disk dessication and protrusion at L4-L5 and L5-S1 levels (arrows). The herniated disk has a broad base which is more than its AP diameter, suggesting it is a protrusion. It is causing bilateral foraminal stenosis.

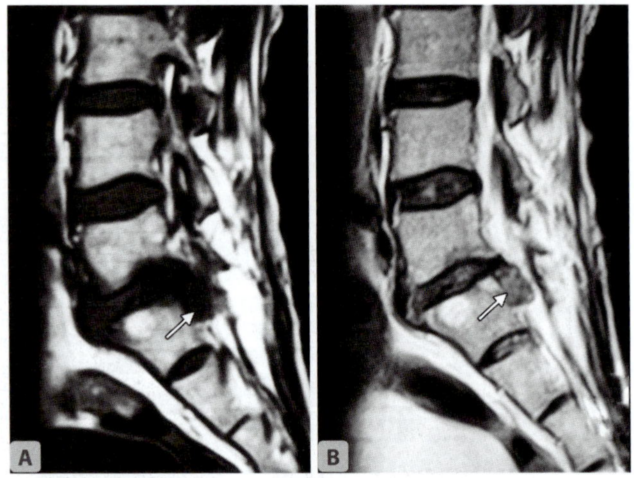

FIGS. 6A AND B: Sagittal T1W (A) and T2W (B) MR images showing disk extrusion at L5-S1 level with caudal migration.

disk. Herniated disk shows anteroposterior < mediolateral diameter.

- If the size of the disk fragment (in any plane) is greater than the width of the base (anteroposterior > mediolateral diameter), it is termed a "disk extrusion" **(Figs. 6A and B)**.
- A"sequestered disc" (free fragment) refers to a disk fragment that has lost all continuity with the parent disk **(Figs. 7A to D)**.

Method of Quantifying the Severity of Disk Disease

- Mild if the anterior epidural fat is not obliterated,
- Moderate if the epidural fat is obliterated and the thecal sac is being displaced, and
- Severe if the cord is being effaced or nerve roots displaced.

Diffusely bulging disk extends symmetrically and circumferentially by more than 2 mm beyond the margins of the adjacent vertebral bodies. This diagnosis is based on axial and sagittal images by comparing the size of the disk with the size of the adjacent vertebral bodies. A segment of disk tissue that projects beyond the margin of the vertebral body but that does not involve the entire circumference of the disk can be called either a focal bulge or a broad-based protrusion.

Disk protrusion is a focal, asymmetric extension of disk tissue beyond the vertebral body margin, usually into the spinal canal or neural foramen. The base (the mediolateral dimension along the posterior margin of the disk) is broader than any other dimension **(Figs. 5A to D)**. Some of the outer annular fibers remain intact, and hence it is referred to as a contained disk. The protruded disk does not extend in a cranial or caudal direction from the parent disk.

Extruded disk is a more pronounced version of a protrusion and often is responsible for symptoms. There is disruption of the outer fibers of the annulus, and the disk herniation usually is greater in its anteroposterior dimension than it is at its base (mediolateral dimension). The extruded disk may migrate up or down behind the adjacent vertebral bodies **(Figs. 6A and B)** but maintains continuity with the parent disk. These also may be referred to as non-contained disks. MRI shows the described contour abnormalities, and because of a significant inflammatory reaction that may occur in response to the extruded disk material, there may be high signal intensity on T2W and contrast-enhanced T1W images in or surrounding the disk. Lumbar disk extrusions that cause radiculopathy but are managed non-operatively have been shown to do well about 90% of the time. Spontaneous reduction in size of disk extrusions and protrusions that were managed conservatively has been well documented with imaging. The regression in disk size may not be the reason for reduction in pain. Much of the pain from extruded disks is probably from the inflammatory response to them rather than from compression of neural elements from the mass effect.

Sequestered disk, when extruded disk material loses its attachment to the parent disk, it is called a sequestered fragment or a free fragment **(Figs. 7A to D)**. These fragments may migrate in a cranial or caudal direction with equal frequency and generally remain within about 5 mm of the parent disk. They may be located between the posterior longitudinal ligament and the osseous spine or extend through the posterior ligament into the epidural space. They almost always remain in the anterior epidural space, but occasionally the fragment may migrate into the posterior epidural space. Rarely, the disk fragment can perforate through the thecal sac to reach the intradural space.

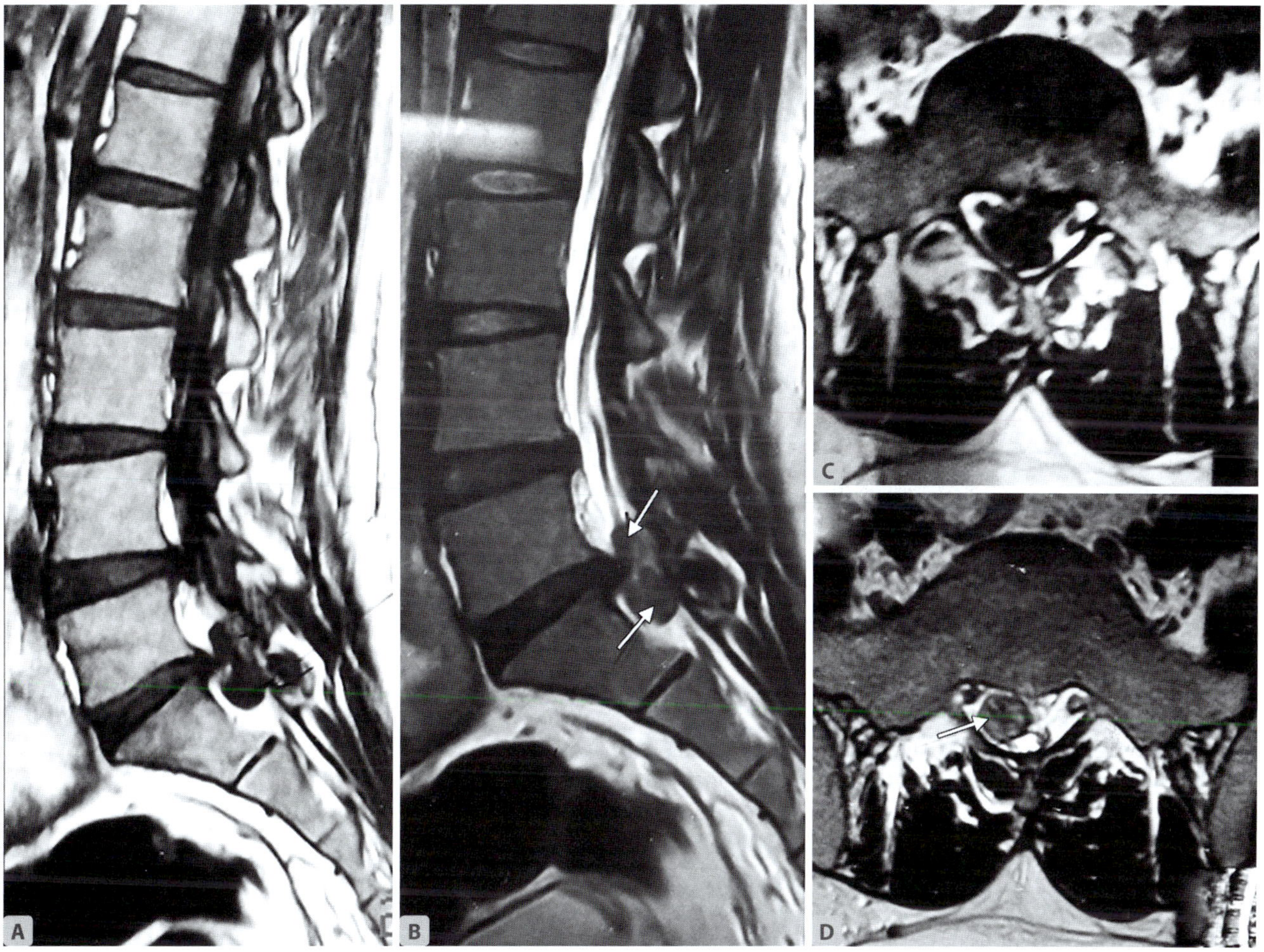

FIGS. 7A TO D: Sequestered disk: Sagittal T1W (A), T2W (B) and axial T1W (C), T2W (D) MR images showing a large herniated fragment of disk (arrow), which is mildly T2 hyperintense, located posterior to S1 vertebral body. This fragment has no attachment to parent disk.

It is extremely important to recognize these fragments because they may be overlooked at surgery. The fragment of disk material that migrates from the parent disk often shows peripheral or diffuse high signal intensity on T2W and contrast-enhanced T1W images, caused by the inflammatory reaction within or surrounding it. Otherwise, a low signal intensity mass resembling the signal of the parent disk is seen. Sequestrations are a contraindication to chymopapain, percutaneous diskectomy, and other limited disk procedures.

Location of Focal Disk Abnormalities

Most of the disk herniation in lower back occurs at L4-L5 or L5-S1 levels. While reporting a focal disk abnormality the size, contour, location and relationship to nerves or other important structures should be described. The location of a focal disk abnormality needs to be conveyed accurately so that the surgical approach can be planned properly and so that it can be determined whether symptoms correlate to the anatomic abnormality seen on MRI. Focal disk abnormalities that remain at the level of the parent disk should be described as being central, left or right paracentral, left or right foraminal, or left or right extraforaminal (also called lateral or far lateral).[30-32]

Significance of Disk Contour Abnormalities

Degenerative Disk Disease can Cause Following Consequences

- Neural compression
- Chemical irritation of nerves
- Osseous abnormalities
- Segmental instability
- Spinal stenosis
- Disk-related compressive myelopathy

Intraosseous Disk Herniations

Disk material not only projects into the spinal canal, but also may directly herniate into the adjacent vertebral bodies through the end plates which are known as a Schmorl's or cartilaginous nodes.

Presentation

These are usually asymptomatic; however traumatic Schmorl's nodes resulting from axial loading forces may be acutely painful. Multiple thoracic Schmorl's nodes can occur in very active teens from axial stresses and result in irregularity of several end plates, loss of disk height, and narrowing of the height of the affected anterior vertebral bodies from fractures, with a resultant kyphosis (Scheuermann's disease).[24,25] An inflammatory, foreign body-type response to intraosseous disk herniation may occur, with vascularization around the disk material and surrounding marrow edema, which may cause severe pain.

Points to Remember

Inflammatory Schmorl's nodes on MRI tend to have large, dome-shaped regions of marrow edema surrounding them; marrow edema is low signal on T1W and high signal on T2W and contrast-enhanced T1W images. A rim of contrast enhancement around the periphery of the Schmorl's node is seen in addition to the surrounding marrow edema. These can have an aggressive look, similar to infection or tumor, and careful evaluation is necessary to make the proper diagnosis.[30-32]

OSSEOUS DEGENERATIVE CHANGES

Vertebral Bodies

The vertebral bodies respond to degenerative changes in the adjacent intervertebral disks in two major ways: (1) formation of osteophytes and (2) marrow changes paralleling the end plates.

Osteophytes

Osteophytes are the excrescences of bone that occur on the upper or lower margins of vertebral bodies. They occur as disks degenerate and bulge, placing traction stresses on Sharpey's fibers, which attach the disks to the vertebral bodies. Osteophytes usually are located anteriorly in the lumbar and thoracic spine, but are commonly anterior or posterior in the cervical spine. MRI of most osteophytes shows low signal intensity cortical margins with fatty marrow that follow the signal of fat on all pulse sequences.

Endplates

The marrow in vertebral bodies adjacent to degenerated disks may change in response to the disk disease. Parallel bands of abnormal signal in the end plates have been divided into three types and are called Modic type 1, 2, or 3 changes. These marrow changes may be focal or diffuse along the end plate but tend to be linear and always parallel to the end plates.[31,32]

- *Type 1*: Decreased signal T1, increased signal T2 (inflammatory tissue)
- *Type 2*: Increased signal T1, follows fat on T2 (focal conversion to fat)
- *Type 3*: Decreased signal T1 and T2 (sclerosis)

Facet Joints

Normal Facet Joints

Are formed by the inferior articular process of the vertebra above articulating with the superior articular process of the lower vertebra. The articular surfaces are covered with hyaline cartilage. The osseous structures are enveloped in a joint capsule lined by synovium; these are true synovial joints. The anterior aspects of the facet joints and the laminae are covered by the ligamentum flavum.

Facet Joint Arthropathy

Degenerative changes of the facet joints manifest as cartilage fibrillation with joint space narrowing, subchondral sclerosis, subchondral cysts, and osteophyte formation that result in overgrowth or hypertrophy of the osseous portions of the joints. Synovial cysts may develop from degenerated spinal facet joints and project either anteriorly (through the ligamentum flavum) or posteriorly from the joints.[31,32]

Symptoms from degenerative changes of the facet joints may result from compression of adjacent neural structures (spinal stenosis) by overgrowth of the bone, inward buckling of the ligamentum flavum, protrusion of synovial cysts into the spinal canal, or the joints themselves being painful.

Imaging Findings

Most of the changes that occur in facet joint arthropathy are bony (sclerosis and joint space reduction) and they are better evaluated on CT scan compared to MRI which can underestimate the severity.[29,33] On the other hand MRI is superior in evaluating marrow edema and effusion.

MRI of degenerative facet joint disease is typical of degenerative changes in any joint (subchondral sclerosis is low signal intensity on all pulse sequences; Synovial cysts are low signal intensity on T1W and high signal intensity on T2W images).

The osteophytes and hypertrophic osseous changes create a rounded and enlarged appearance of the articular processes of the facets on axial images that may cause narrowing of the adjacent spinal canal, lateral recesses, or neural foramina.

Posterior Spinous Processes

Degenerative changes of the spinous processes and intervening interspinous soft tissues is called as kissing spine or Baastrup's disease. On CT scan the features are marginal sclerosis of involved spinous processes with faceted appearance, osteophytes and erosions **(Fig. 8)**. Ankylosis is a late feature. MRI may show marrow edema and hyperintense bursal fluid in the interspinous ligament region.

Spinal Stenosis

Spinal stenosis is narrowing of the central spinal canal, neural foramen, lateral recess, or any combination of these anatomic regions, by soft tissue or osseous structures that impinge on neural elements and may result in symptoms.[34]

Causes

- *Degenerative*:
  - Disk contour abnormalities (bulges, herniations)
  - Vertebral body osteophytes
  - Degenerative spondylolisthesis
  - Facet joint degeneration, osteophytes, synovial cysts
  - Ligamentum flavum buckling

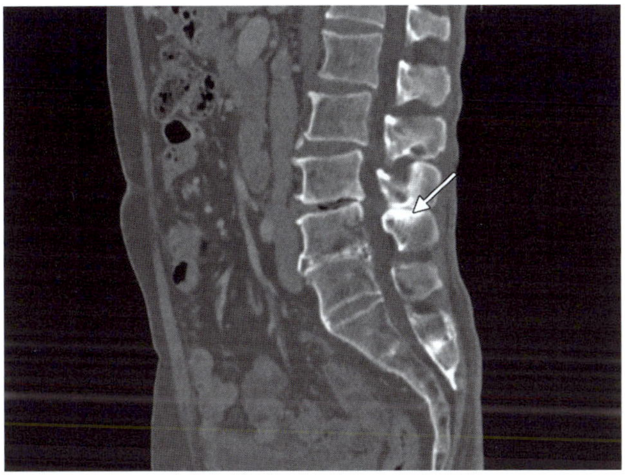

FIG. 8: CT scan of lumbosacral spine in sagittal plane showing reduction of interspinous space between L3-L4 level (arrow) and associated bone sclerosis suggestive of Baastrup's disease.

- *Congenital short pedicles*:
  - Usually requires superimposed degeneration to be symptomatic
- *Any mass arising from bone, disk, or within canal*:
  - Osseous tumor, fracture fragments
  - Spondylolysis, spondylolisthesis
  - Ossification of posterior longitudinal ligament
  - Epidural lipomatosis, hematoma, abscess, tumor, scarring

Symptoms from spinal stenosis are often nonspecific and include back pain, intermittent neurogenic claudication, extremity radiculopathy, pain with hyperextension relieved by flexion, and pain on standing relieved by lying down. The presence of imaging findings of spinal stenosis does not indicate that a patient has symptoms from the stenosis.

Types of Involvement

- Central canal
- Neural foramina
- Lateral recesses

Central Canal Stenosis

Central canal stenosis usually is the result of facet joint osteophytes and inward buckling of the ligamentum flavum posteriorly, with disk bulging anteriorly in the canal. Normally, the central canal and thecal sac are round or nearly round (a plump oval) structures on axial images; if they become flattened ovals or triangular in shape, it indicates central stenosis. Central stenosis can cause edema in the affected nerve roots, or, in the cervical spine, there may be abnormalities of the cord, probably myelomalacia from ischemia at the site of stenosis, which shows high signal intensity on T2W images.[34] Besides the encroachment by the osteophytes, disk bulge and hypertrophied ligamentum flavum, accordion shape of the cauda equina nerve roots is another feature which suggests significant canal stenosis. This appearance is best seen on T2 W sagittal images and it is because of the inability of the roots to slide smoothly during change in posture. There is a lot of variation regarding the imaging criteria used to diagnose canal stenosis. Despite various caveats, size criteria of 10 mm canal diameter is the widely used one. There is a four level grading method proposed by Schizas et al to grade the severity of canal stenosis.[35]

Lateral Recess Stenosis

Lateral recess stenosis usually is caused by hypertrophic degenerative changes of the facet joints, or less commonly by a disk fragment or postoperative fibrosis. Lateral recesses are located on the medial aspects of pedicles. Nerve roots lie in these recesses after leaving the thecal sac, but before entering the exiting neural foramina. There is a neural foramen bordering the upper and the lower margins of a lateral recess. If there is deformity in the shape of the recess, and the descending nerve is displaced or compressed, there is lateral recess stenosis. This space is best evaluated in the axial plane of imaging.

Neural Foramen Stenosis

Neural foramen stenosis occurs as a result of degenerative osteophytes of the facet joints or a foraminal disk protrusion **(Fig. 5D)**, extrusion, or sequestered fragment; a diffuse disk bulge; or postoperative fibrosis. Neurogenic tumors can occur in this location which can mimic a herniated disk **(Figs. 9A to C)**. MRI with contrast can be helpful in differentiating these two entities. Neurogenic tumors usually show iso to mild T2 hyperintensity and enhancement on post contrast images whereas herniated disk does not show any central enhancement.

Narrowing of the neural foramina can be evaluated on sagittal and axial images. On sagittal images, the normal neural foramen has the appearance of a vertical oval. If disk material extends into the foramen, the oval narrows inferiorly, creating a keyhole shape. Axial images may be more accurate for diagnosis because they show more of the extent of each foramen.[34]

Postoperative Changes

The imaging feature of postoperative spine depends on the type of surgery performed, interval after surgery and the basic disease itself. Generally, spine surgery is performed either for decompression or spine stabilization or both. Utility of radiographs are limited to check the positioning of implants and for most of the other indications CT or MRI is the modality of choice in post operative setting. The choice of sequences in MRI will depend on the presence of implant. Even MRI compatible implants cause significant local artifacts and hence the positioning and sequences are optimised to reduce artifacts. Recently, metal artifact reduction sequences have shown significant improvement in image quality.

Failed Back Syndrome

Patients may have persistent, recurrent, or new and different symptoms after surgery of the spine. The reasons for these problems are many and varied. The most common reasons are recurrent or persistent disk extrusions, postoperative

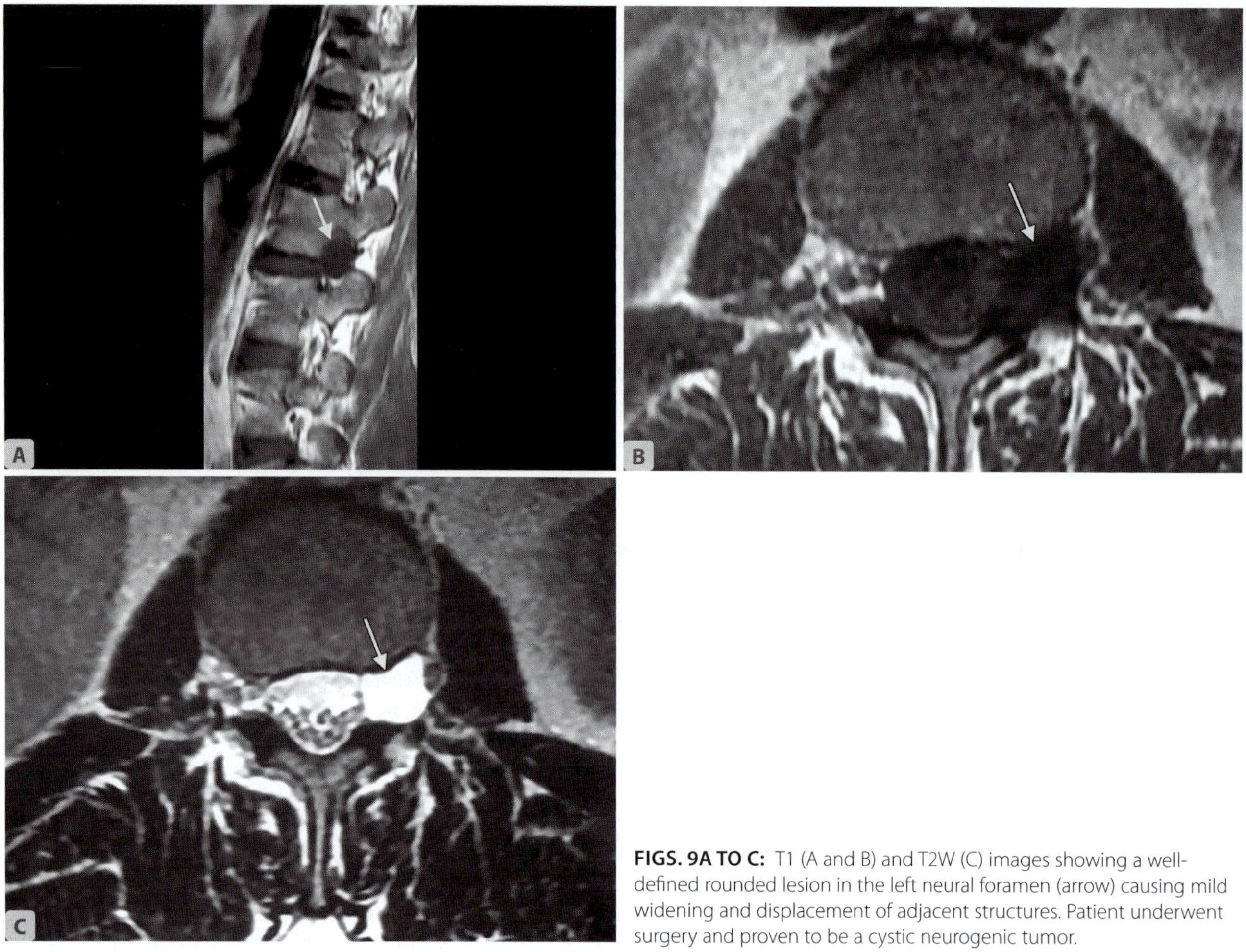

FIGS. 9A TO C: T1 (A and B) and T2W (C) images showing a well-defined rounded lesion in the left neural foramen (arrow) causing mild widening and displacement of adjacent structures. Patient underwent surgery and proven to be a cystic neurogenic tumor.

scarring, spondylodiscitis, arachnoiditis, nerve root damage (neuritis), and inadequate surgery.[36,37]

Distinguishing postoperative scarring (epidural fibrosis) from extruded disk material is one of the most important tasks for radiologists in evaluating postoperative MRI studies. All postoperative spine MRI studies should be done with contrast enhancement to distinguish between these two common causes of symptoms in postoperative patients. Scar tissue that is more than 6 months old enhances diffusely **(Figs. 10A to I)** and early after the intravenous administration of gadolinium (high signal intensity on T1W images). Disk material does not enhance until late, if at all, and usually enhances only peripherally. These rules do not work as well during the first 6 months after surgery, when asymptomatic fibrosis may show peripheral rather than diffuse contrast enhancement that is indistinguishable from an extruded disk. Extruded disk material may be an indication for another operation, whereas there is no benefit from reoperating on a patient with postoperative scarring.[36,37]

Other signs that may help distinguish postoperative scarring from a disk abnormality are that postoperative scarring often has irregular margins; it may not be contiguous with the adjacent disk; and, instead of producing a mass effect on the dural sac, it may cause retraction. Recurrent disk herniations, conversely, usually are contiguous with the disk, have sharp margins, and cause mass effect on the dural sac.[36,37]

Fluid collections in the operative site in the form of hematoma, seroma, pseudomeningocele and abscess, spondylodiskitis and arachnoiditis are the complications which can occur after surgery that can be diagnosed on imaging **(Figs. 11A and B)**.

Postoperative Imaging after Intervertebral Fusion and Instrumentation

Spinal instrumentations have been widely performed using various hardware primarily to maintain the alignment of spine. Interbody devices like mesh and cage are also used to promote fusion. Radiologists should be aware of the type of surgery performed and hardware used to identify the post-operative complications, identify the normal post-operative changes and evaluate the correct placement of implants. The common hardware related complications include implant malpositioning, migration, loosening, fracture and infection. The role of radiograph in this situation is limited and CT scan is a much better modality to show the position and alignment of implants precisely. Role of MRI is to evaluate the spinal cord and nerve roots and to detect infection. Pedicle screw is ideally placed in the center of pedicle parallel to the superior endplate of vertebra. The tip of pedicle screw should not breach the anterior cortex of the vertebral body or in contact with vascular structure. Interbody implants like cage is placed 2 mm from the posterior margin of vertebral body.[10]

Seronegative Spondyloarthropathy

This group of disorders includes ankylosing spondylitis, Reiter's or reactive arthropathy, psoriatic arthropathy and spondyloarthropathy associated with inflammatory disease. They are characterized by rheumatoid factor negative inflammatory arthritis and enthesiopathy affecting the spine and sacroiliac joints. It presents in early to mid adulthood, more commonly in males with symptoms of low backache and stiffness which is worse in the morning. It has a strong association with HLA B27 haplotype. A detailed discussion of this entity is beyond the scope of this chapter and only the salient features are presented.

The disease first affects bilateral sacroiliac joints followed by the thoracolumbar junction and may eventually involve the entire spine. The erosive sacroilitis is best appreciated on a PA view of the pelvis and affects the lower third of the joint. The earliest sign is loss of definition of subchondral bone, and other features are small erosions, widening of joint space, sclerosis and eventually fusion of the joint.[38] Early manifestations of sacroilitis may be better evaluated by CT and MRI. Small erosions are well seen on CT and MRI in the early stage of disease shows T2 and STIR hyperintensity **(Figs. 12A to C)**.[39]

The vertebral bodies show squaring, corner erosions which undergo sclerotic repair. This leads to shiny corner sign

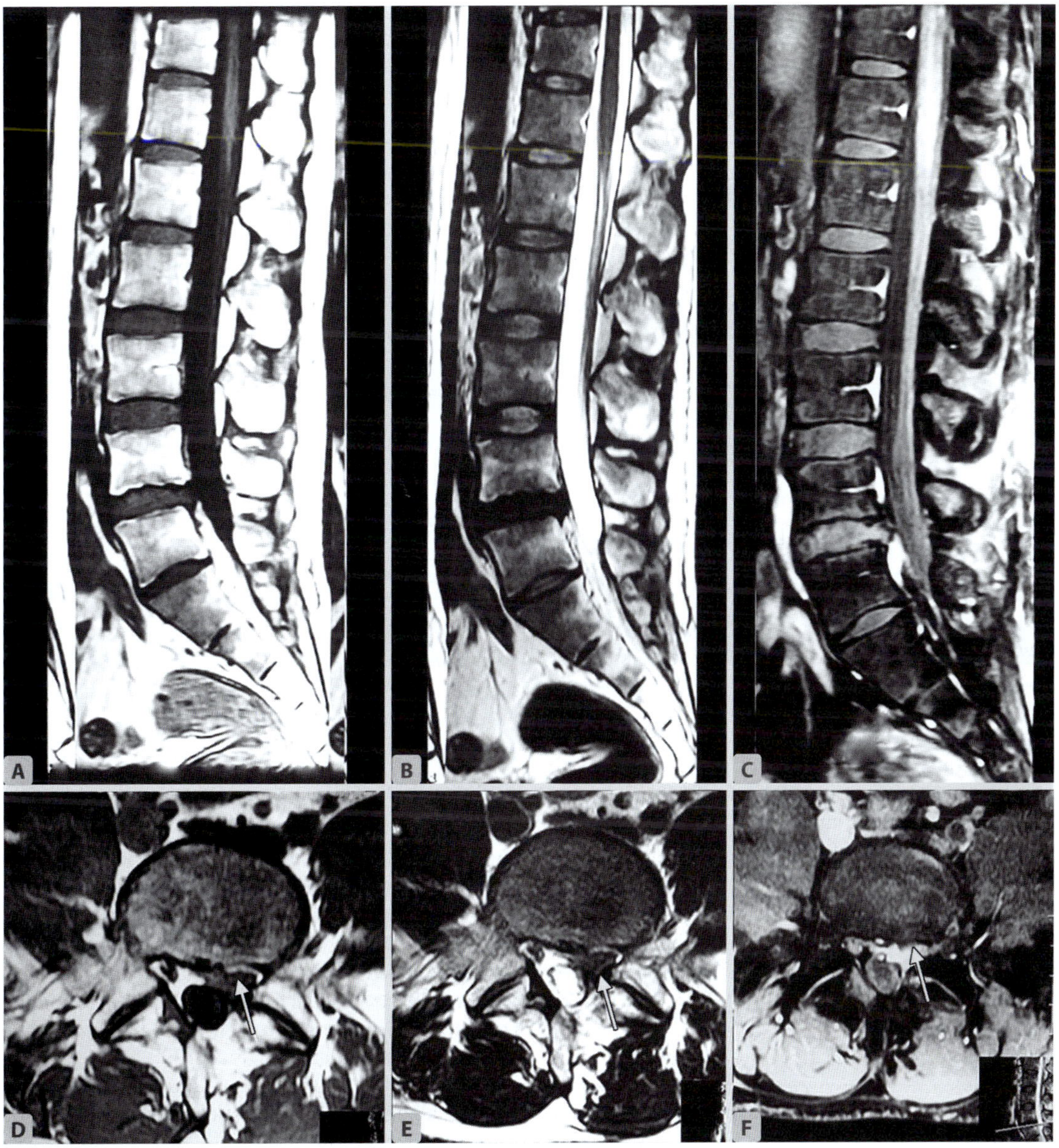

FIGS. 10A TO I: *Continued*

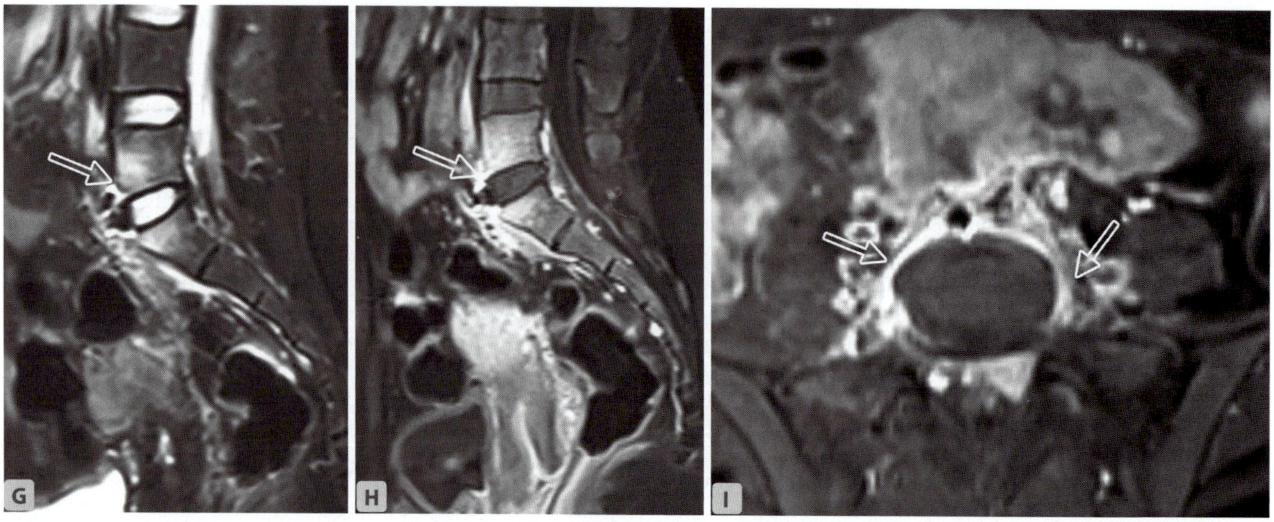

FIGS. 10A TO I: Failed back syndrome: Sagittal T1W (A), T2W (B) and fat-suppressed postgadolinium T1W (C) and axial T1W (D), T2W (E) and fat-suppressed T1W (F) MR images show an intermediate signal mass (arrow) in the left paracentral region of this patient, one year after left laminectomy. Contrast-enhanced images (C and F) show diffuse enhancement of the left paracentral mass, indicating this is scarring/fibrosis, rather than a disk fragment. In another patient who underwent surgery in the lumbosacral region showing T2 hyperintensity (outlined arrow in G) in L5 and S1 marrow with associated soft tissue showing enhancement in postcontrast images (outlined arrow in H and I) suggestive of spondylodiscitis developing after surgery.

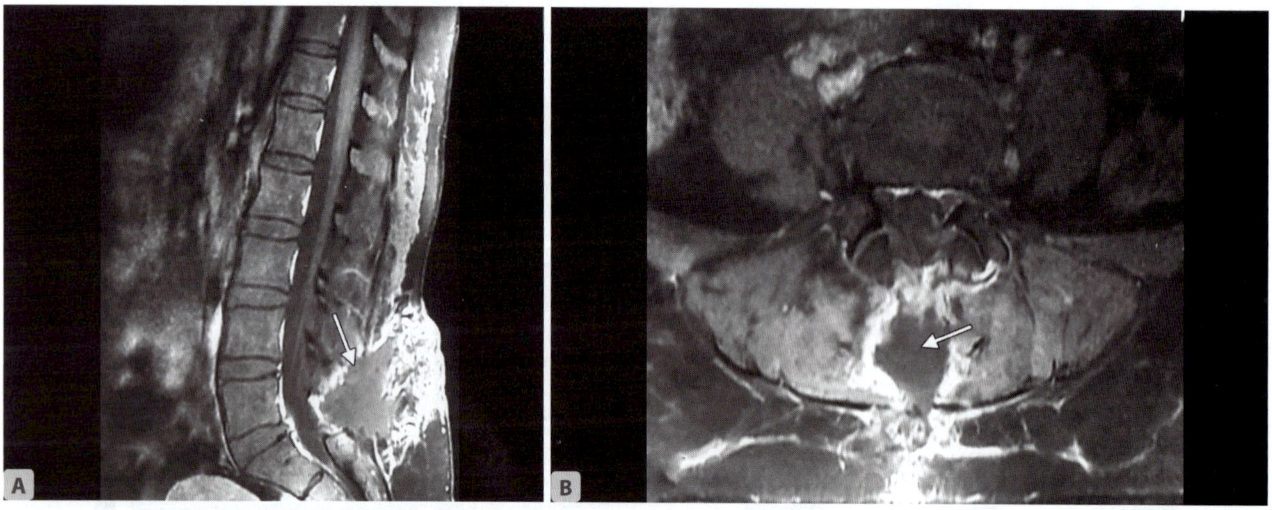

FIGS. 11A AND B: Post-contrast MRI images in sagittal (A) and axial (B) planes in a patient who underwent spinal decompression surgery showing a non-enhancing fluid collection posterior to spine (arrow) with irregular enhancing wall suggestive of abscess.

or Romanus lesion **(Fig. 12C)**. Multilevel syndesmophytes give rise to a bamboo spine appearance. Facet joints are commonly involved and erosions progress to fusion.

Fractures and pseudoarthrosis may occur through the disk or endplate and are referred to as Anderson lesion **(Figs. 13A and B)**. This can mimic infectious spondylodiscitis and the differentiating feature is extension across the posterior elements.[39]

INFECTIONS

Infections of the spine are a common cause of back pain in our country. Infection should be suspected in patients with severe back pain that does not improve with rest, that wakes them at night, and that is associated with a fever. Tuberculosis of the spine is common in India and needs to be kept in the list of differential diagnosis for a wide variety of spinal abnormalities. Conventional radiographs are the initial screening modality when infectious spondylitis is suspected. Compared to MRI and radionuclide scans, radiographs are relatively insensitive early in the course of infection. It takes weeks for destructive changes to become evident.[40] This initial imaging study, however, guides the next diagnostic step.

Tubercular Infection

The spine is the most common site of osseous tuberculous involvement, comprising in most series about 50% of cases.

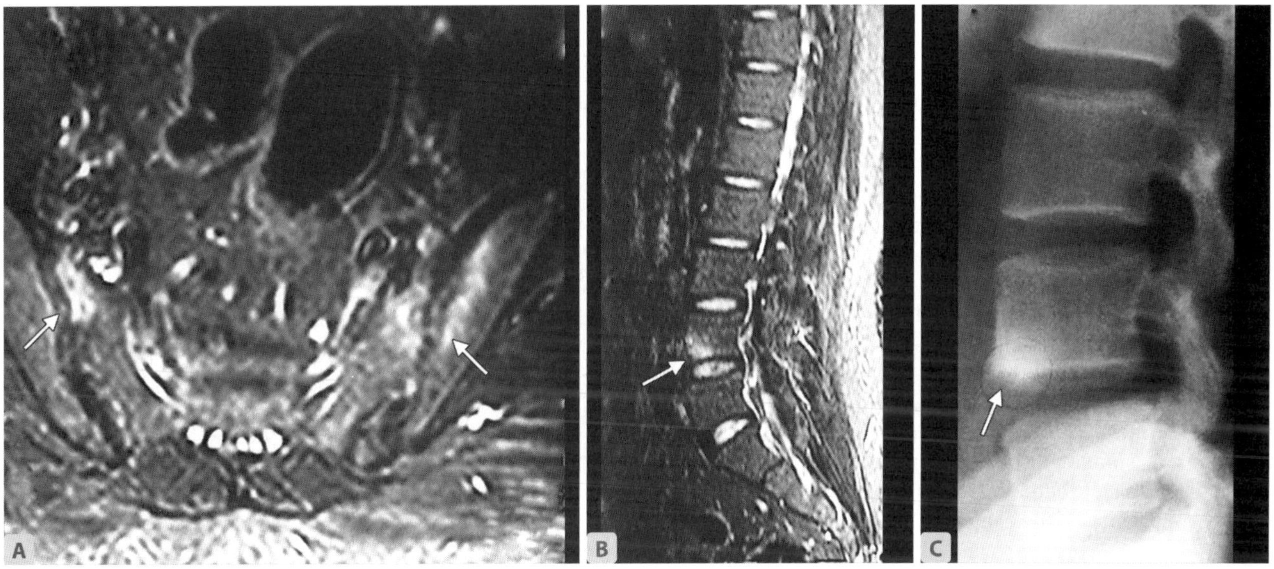

FIGS. 12A TO C: Ankylosing spondylitis: Axial STIR (A) image of bilateral sacroiliac joints and sagittal STIR (B) image of LS spine showing hyperintensity at articular margins of bilateral SI joints (arrows) and at anteroinferior margin of L4 vertebra typical appearance of early spondyloarthropathy. Lateral radiograph (C) of lumbar spine showing anterior corner erosions at the L4 vertebral body. The typical shiny corner sign (or Romanus lesion) is present (arrow).

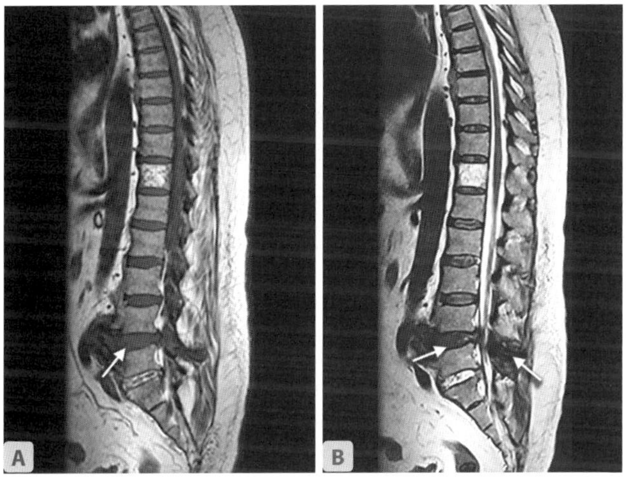

FIGS. 13A AND B: Sagittal T1W (A) and T2W (B) MR image of the thoracolumbar spine showing a fracture through the L5-S1disk which is extending across the posterior elements typical of Anderson lesion (white arrow). Incidental vertebral hemangioma of D12 vertebra is also seen (thick arrow).

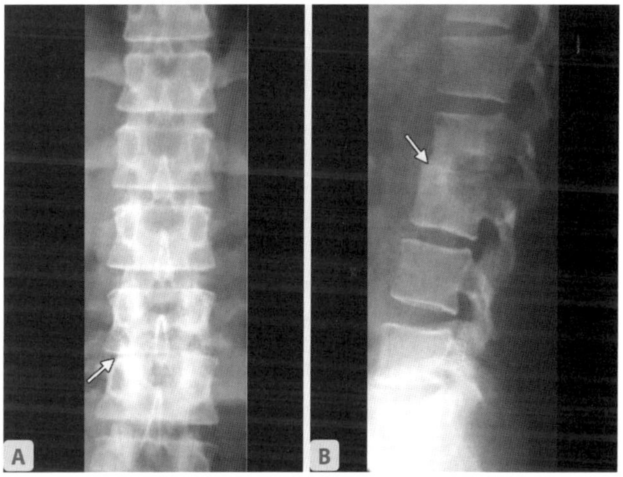

FIGS. 14A AND B: Tuberculosis: Anteroposterior and lateral plain radiographs (A and B) of lumbar spine showing reduced L2-3 disk space (arrow) with indistinct adjacent end plates and lytic lesion centered around the end plates suggestive of infective spondylitis.

Patients present with long-standing and insidious onset of stiffness and local tenderness, with or without constitutional symptoms. The lower dorsal and upper lumbar vertebrae are most frequently affected; cervical and sacral involvement occurs uncommonly. The spread of tuberculosis to the spine is usually by hematogenous route, by perivertebral arterial or venous plexi, or rarely by extension from a paraspinal infection. It is often difficult to differentiate tubercular from pyogenic spondylytis both clinically and on imaging. There are four different patterns of involvement: paradiskal, central, sub-ligamentous and posterior.[40]

Plain film evaluation of the tuberculous spondylodiskitis may demonstrate loss of vertebral height or disk interval, erosions, indistinct margins of end plates **(Figs. 14A and B)** paravertebral masses, and sequestrae. The infection usually begins in the anterior aspect of the vertebral body, adjacent to the vertebral endplate. Focal areas of erosion and osseous destruction in the anterior corners of the vertebral body are typical plain film findings. Involvement of the adjacent intervertebral disk or vertebral body results from penetration of the disk itself or spread of infection beneath the anterior or posterior longitudinal ligament. Contiguous vertebral involvement, destruction of the intervertebral disk and progressive vertebral body collapse result in the characteristic gibbus deformity of the spine commonly associated with spinal tuberculosis.[40] Paraspinal abscess formation may be detected on radiographs as fusiform paravertebral soft tissue masses.

Disk space narrowing may be quite subtle. Over 50% of the trabecular bone is lost before a lesion is conspicuous on plain film; this process may take up to 6 month. In the thoracic spine visualization of a paravertebral abscess requires an adequately penetrated view. In the lumbar spine asymmetry or bulging of the psoas shadow may be detected. Scalloping of the anterior vertebral contour (aneurysmal appearance) is more commonly seen with children. Plain film is limited in evaluation of the posterior arch, particularly in the thoracic spine. No specific or pathognomonic plain film signs distinguish tuberculous from pyogenic spinal infection, and correlation with the clinical picture is important.

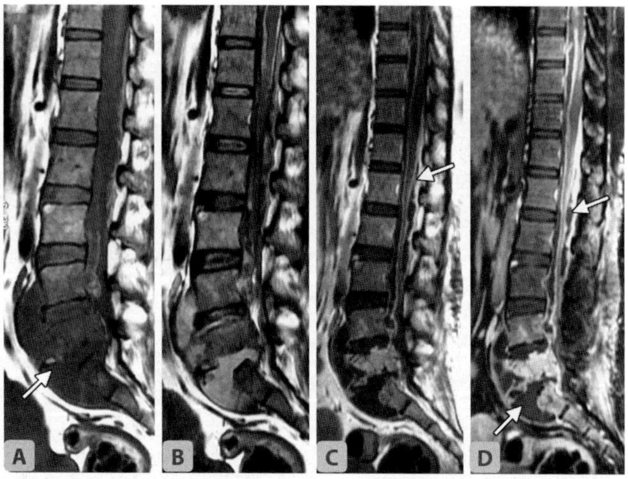

FIGS. 15A TO D: Tubercular spondylitis. Sagittal T1W (A), T2W (B) and postcontrast T1W (C and D) MR images showing destructive lesion involving the L5 vertebra, L5-S1 disk space and adjacent end plates associated with prevertebral soft tissue component which is showing peripheral rim enhancement suggestive of abscess. The abscess is extending into the spinal canal (extradural location) proximally till D12 level (arrow). Leptomeningeal enhancement is also seen.

Computed Tomography Features

Computed tomography (CT) is not a routinely used imaging modality in assessing the tuberculous spondylitis but it may be helpful in assessing the cortical breakdown, destruction of cancellous bone as well as spinal distortion in chronic cases. MDCT using thinnest collimation with multiplanar reconstruction in different planes, can be beneficial to assess the destruction of bone and gibbus/scoliosis deformity of the spine in chronic cases.

One of the major disadvantages of CT as compared to MRI, is difficulty in identifying the early marrow changes of the disease process within the bone. Another disadvantage of CT is its inability to identify subtle epidural soft tissue component due to beam hardening artifact.

However, CT is more sensitive in showing subtle soft tissue calcifications as compared to MRI. Computed tomography is useful for guiding percutaneous drainage of paravertebral abscesses, which are difficult to access under ultrasound guidance.

MR Features

Multiplanar capability and optimal tissue contrast make MR imaging the optimal modality for evaluation of spondylodiskitis.[41-43] The entire spine and canal can be visualized, including the posterior elements. MR imaging has higher sensitivity for early infiltrative disease including end plate changes and marrow infiltration than bone scan and plain films. MR imaging affords excellent definition of epidural, paravertebral, and intraosseous abscesses, and extent of cord compromise. Paravertebral abscesses may be large, and discharge through tracts well seen on multiple planes. The involved vertebrae show hypointense signal on T1-weighted images and heterogeneous increased signal on T2-weighted images. The intravenous administration of contrast improves definition of epidural abscesses and masses, and cord and nerve root compromise **(Figs. 15A to D)**. The abscesses show peripheral enhancement with central necrosis. Acute stage shows inhomogeneous enhancement in areas of marrow infiltration, and enhancing lesion borders. With tuberculous spondylodiskitis, the disk shows signal characteristics seen with pyogenic discitis in at least three quarters of cases, of bright signal on T2-weighted images, decreased signal on T1-weighted images, and enhancement of disk after contrast administration. Disk space preservation, normal signal intensity, and lack of enhancement have been reported in approximately 25% of cases.

In paradiscal variety MRI shows hypointense signal on T1W and high signal on T2W images in the end plate, narrowing of the disk, and large paraspinal and epidural abscesses. In the central type of lesion signal intensity abnormality is confined to the vertebral body and the disk space is preserved. The appearance can be indistinguishable from metastases or lymphoma.[41-45]

Uncommon Patterns

Infection limited to a single vertebral body in the form of osteitis may occur. It is detected late on plain radiographs and is better seen on MRI as a marrow signal abnormality **(Figs. 16A to G)**. Multiple vertebral levels may be involved in a non-contigous manner, manifested on plain radiographs as skip lesions of vertebral body destruction and collapse. The posterior elements of the spine are usually involved secondarily due to spread of infection from the vertebral body. However, isolated involvement of the posterior elements may occasionally occurs **(Figs. 17A to D)**.[43,44]

Response Assessment and Follow-up

There is an increasing move away from surgical intervention towards conservative therapy, percutaneous drainage of abscesses, or both. It is therefore critical to monitor treatment response. MR imaging is a valuable diagnostic tool not only

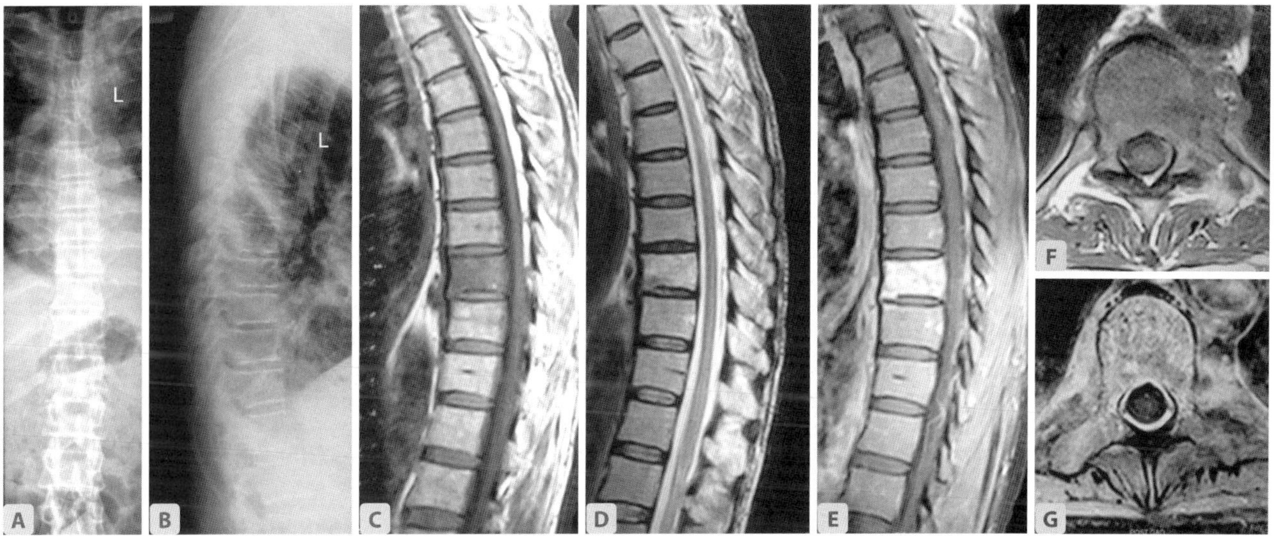

FIGS. 16A TO G: Central tuberculosis: Radiographs anteroposterior (A) and lateral view (B) of the dorso-lumbar spine are normal. Sagittal T1W (C) T2W (D) and postcontrast T1W (E) images and axial T1W (F) and postcontrast images (G) show T1 hypointensity, T2 hyperintensity and enhancement of the marrow of D6 vertebral body with small left paravertebral soft tissue. The height of the vertebra and adjacent disk space is maintained.

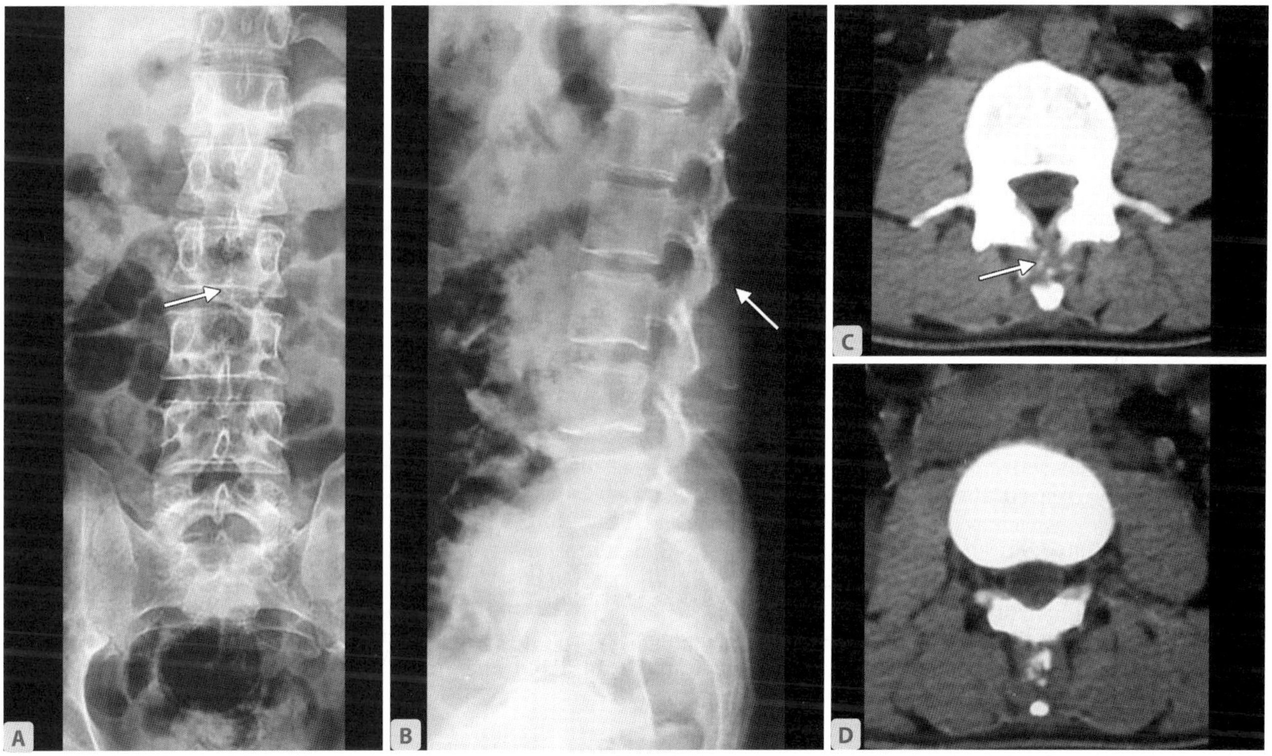

FIGS. 17A TO D: Posterior element TB: Anteroposterior (A) and lateral (B) radiographs of lumbar spine showing non-visualization of the spinous process of L2 vertebra. Axial CT sections (C and D) showing lytic destructive lesion involving the spinous process of L2 vertebra.

for early diagnosis but is also used to effectively monitor treatment response. Particular emphasis should be placed on soft-tissue appearance in the early stages. Progressive reduction in gadolinium enhancement and the eventual loss of all enhancement are useful signs. Later on, fat deposition is a useful sign of healing. Gadolinium enhancement patterns vary and a reduction in gadolinium enhancement is a reliable sign, but an increase does not necessarily denote treatment failure.

Follow-up of patients with tuberculous spondylitis has to be based upon both clinical and radiological findings. Usually there is lag of 2 months for radiological improvement of a lesion to be seen on imaging, as compared to clinical improvement. It takes about 2–3 months to show a radiologically perceptible sclerosis (remineralization), following drug treatment.

MRI done at 2–3 months even in a responsive tuberculous spondylitis may show increased inflammatory response giving false impression of progression of disease. Thus, early MR imaging following the start of drug treatment may be unreliable. However, if MRI findings worsen at 5–6 months of treatment, one should suspect a therapeutically refractory case.

Also, if there is no clinical improvement or there is worsening of spinal abnormality or appearance of a new lesion or failure of healing of ulcer/sinus or dehiscence of wound after 4–5 months of surgery, one should think of either refractory or drug resistant tuberculosis. To label a case as multi-drug resistant tuberculosis, drug resistance has to be demonstrated on tissue sample.

Early Healing

Reduction in amount or degree of gadolinium enhancement of soft tissue (These findings are the best indicators of early healing).

However, progression of bone or disk changes, either an alteration in signal intensity or increasing destruction, during early course of treatment do not indicate failed treatment.

Late Healing

Signs of healed tubercular lesions on follow-up contrast enhanced MRI include complete disappearance of marrow edema, resolution of paravertebral collections and replacement of vertebral body marrow by fat, seen as increased signal on T1-weighted images.

These patients should be monitored for at least 2 years, following the completion of treatment regimen and follow-up MR is performed to show complete resolution of the lesion.

Role of FDG-PET Scan

Active tuberculosis shows increased uptake on FDG-PET scan, but this increased uptake is non-specific. It is also seen in neoplastic as well as other granulomatous diseases like brucellosis. FDG-PET may be requested in patients with equivocal MRI findings or for response evaluation when there are enhancing areas on MRI, after full clinical resolution of the symptoms and completion of ATT. In such situations, increased uptake on FDG-PET supports presence of active infection. FDG-PET also provides a quantitative measurement of the absolute fraction of the injected dose reaching a tissue called the Standard Uptake Value (SUV). SUV values are raised in cases of active tuberculosis.

Differential Diagnosis

Uncommon Infections

Brucellosis is a zoonotic infection, and the most common site of bone brucellosis is the spine. The imaging manifestations closely resemble tubercular spondylitis. Brucellar spondylitis has a predilection for the lower lumbar spine. Features reported in the literature include intact vertebral architecture inspite of diffuse vertebral osteomyelitis, marked T2 hyperintensity and enhancement of the intervertebral disk and facet joint involvement. Gibbus deformities are rare and paraspinal abscesses are smaller than those in tubercular spondylitis. This possibilty should be kept in mind when apparent tubercular spondylitis does not respond to treatment.[42]

Fungal spondylitis caused by organisms like Aspergillus may be seen in immunocompromised hosts and very rarely in immunocompetent patients. The imaging findings mimic pyogenic or tubercular spondylitis and diagnosis is made usually after tissue sampling. T2 hyperintensity in discs is typically lacking in this entity, a fact attribute to the paramagnetic and ferromagnetic elements in fungi.[45]

Non-infectious Diseases that Mimic Spondylodiscitis

Non-infectious inflammatory diseases and degenerative disease may simulate spinal infection. *Discogenic vertebral body degeneration (Modic Type I)* may resemble infectious spondylitis because of the presence of bone marrow edema which has high signal intensity on T2W images. These marrow changes and the associated disk may also enhance on contrast-enhanced images. The lack of increased signal intensity of associated disk on T2W images and the absence of soft tissue abnormality distinguish degenerative changes from infectious spondylitis.[43,44]

Pseudoarthrosis secondary to spinal fracture *(Andersson lesion)* are not an uncommon complication of advanced ankylosing spondylitis. They commonly involve the disk space or juxtaarticular end plate. In pseudoarthrosis subchondral sclerosis and end plate erosion may be seen on radiographs that mimic infectious spondylitis. MRI can help in the differentiation by showing the extension of fracture line across the posterior elements.[43]

Occasionally *Schmorl's nodes* can also mimic infectious spondylodiscitis. The herniation of the disk into the vertebral endplate can incite marrow edema and vascularization which can result in vertebral end plate hyperintensity and enhancement. However, if the bone defect involves only one end plate and the disk does not show diffuse signal abnormality, Schmorl's node rather than spondylodiscitis should be suspected.

Neuropathic spine is seen in patients of diabetes, syringomyelia, syphilis, etc. It most often involves the thoracolumbar junction and lumbar spine. Destructive changes in the vertebral bodies lead to fracture, bone sclerosis, large osteophytes and decreased disk space. The disk space and surrounding marrow show lower T2 signal than in infectious spondylitis. Other distinguishing findings of this entity include facet involvement, osseous joint debris and joint disorganization.

In *neoplastic lesions,* the disk is usually preserved and disk height reduction is rare. The end plates are usually distinct. If posterior elements are involved, neoplastic lesions should be included in the differential.

Other infiltrative granulomatous lesions such as sarcoidosis may show signal intensity abnormalities similar to TB, but diskitis is usually not seen.

Pyogenic Infection

The vertebral infection generally begins adjacent to the endplate, it invades the subchondral bone and extends to the disk. The common causative organism is *Staphylococcus aureus*. This pattern of hematogenous infection gives rise to the classic radiographic picture of infectious spondylitis: destructive changes of two adjacent vertebral bodies and the intervening disk. This is manifested on the radiograph as loss of height of the vertebral bodies and a narrowed disk space. Because of endplate destruction, the disk space may have an apparent increase in height, rather than narrowing. The destructive changes of metastatic tumor have a different pattern. Tumor tends to respect the endplates, extending into the surrounding soft tissues by cortical invasion.

The initial radiographs may be completely normal and the findings typically lag behind symptoms by two to three weeks. The earliest signs include blurring of endplates and decrease in the height of disk space followed by bone destruction in the adjacent vertebrae. Eventually sclerosis supervenes and is a manifestation of a reparative response. Radionuclide scan using Tc99m has an accuracy as high as 90% in patients with more than two days of symptoms.[45-47]

TUMORS

A wide spectrum of tumors can affect the bony spine. Some of them like hemangiomas are common and discovered incidentally. The commonest malignant lesions in the spine are metastases and myeloma. Primary tumors are rare and radiographic and MR features can help to narrow the differential diagnosis.[48]

Benign Tumors

Hemangioma

They are benign vascular lesions, majority of which are asymptomatic and discovered incidentally. They have been reported in up to 10% of all individuals undergoing spinal imaging. Most spinal hemangiomas occur in thoracic spine and are usually confined to the vertebral bodies. They are usually asymptomatic and do not require clinical attention. However, rarely they are aggressive and can grow beyond the vertebral body and may compress the spinal cord or nerve roots.[48]

They show characteristic imaging findings. The radiographic appearance is of prominent vertical striations giving a corduroy cloth or honeycomb appearance. This translates into the polka dot appearance on CT. Thickened trabeculae are surrounded by hypodense fatty tissue. Typical hemangiomas appear hyperintense on both T1 and T2W sequences **(Figs. 18A and B)** and may enhance after contrast administration. The aggressive hemangiomas are hypointense on T1W and bright in T2W scans, may be associated with a paravertebral soft tissue **(Figs. 19A to F)** and resemble metastases or myeloma.[48,49]

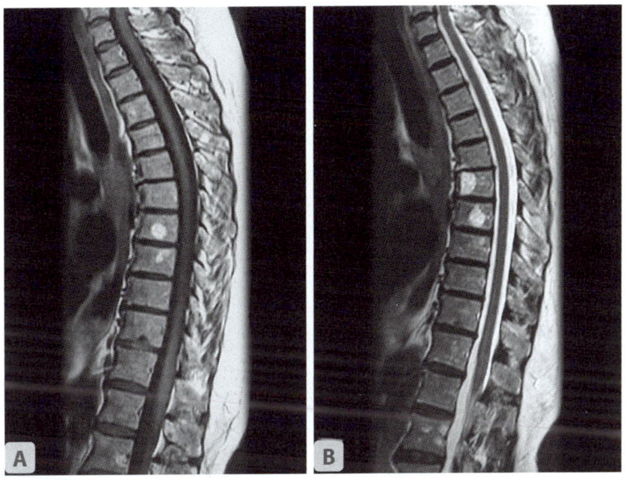

FIGS. 18A AND B: Sagittal T1W (A) and T2W (B) MR images showing lesions involving the vertebral bodies of two dorsal vertebra which are hyperintense on both T1W and T2W images suggestive of vertebral hemangioma.

Osteoid Osteoma

It is a relatively common benign osseous lesion. The peak incidence is in the second decade. It has a tendency to involve the posterior elements and occurs commonly in the pedicle. The lumbar spine is most commonly affected (59%) followed by cervical and thoracic spine.[50,51]

The histological hallmark is a nidus, which is smaller than 1.5 cm. Clinically, the spinal osteoid osteoma presents with a painful scoliosis. The pain is worse at night, and is relieved with aspirin. The lumbar spine radiographs may show scoliosis, concave to the side of the lesion. The central lucent nidus may be obscured by the reactive sclerosis. CT is the modality of choice for a careful search of a nidus **(Figs. 20A to C)**. The nidus is usually a sub-centimeter lytic area with a sclerotic center surrounded by periosteal thickening. Occasionally, vascular channels leading to this lesion may be seen adjacent to the nidus. As with other nonaggressive osteoid lesions, MRI is not indicated. In fact, MR may be misleading, as the nidus is commonly not evident. If visible, it appears as a low signal focus with extensive adjacent marrow and soft tissue edema. The nidus is hypointense on T1W images and hypo to hyperintense on T2W images. Surrounding hyperintensity is reactive host response and involves a much larger area than the tumor. Severe reactive response may lead to a misdiagnosis of malignancy or infection. The lesion is positive on all three phases of a Tc-99m MDP bone scan. The differential diagnosis of osteoid osteoma in the spine includes osteoblastoma which is larger, unilateral absent pedicle, osteoblastic metastases, and stress fracture of pedicle. CT plays a valuable role in distinguishing these entities.[50,51]

The treatment is surgical or image guided percutaneous excision or RF ablation. The entire nidus has to be removed to prevent recurrence.

Osteoblastoma

Osteoblastomas are related to osteoid osteomas and by definition are larger than 1.5 cm in diameter. They are seen in patients in the first to third decades. Up to 40% osteoblastomas are found in the spine. They also have a

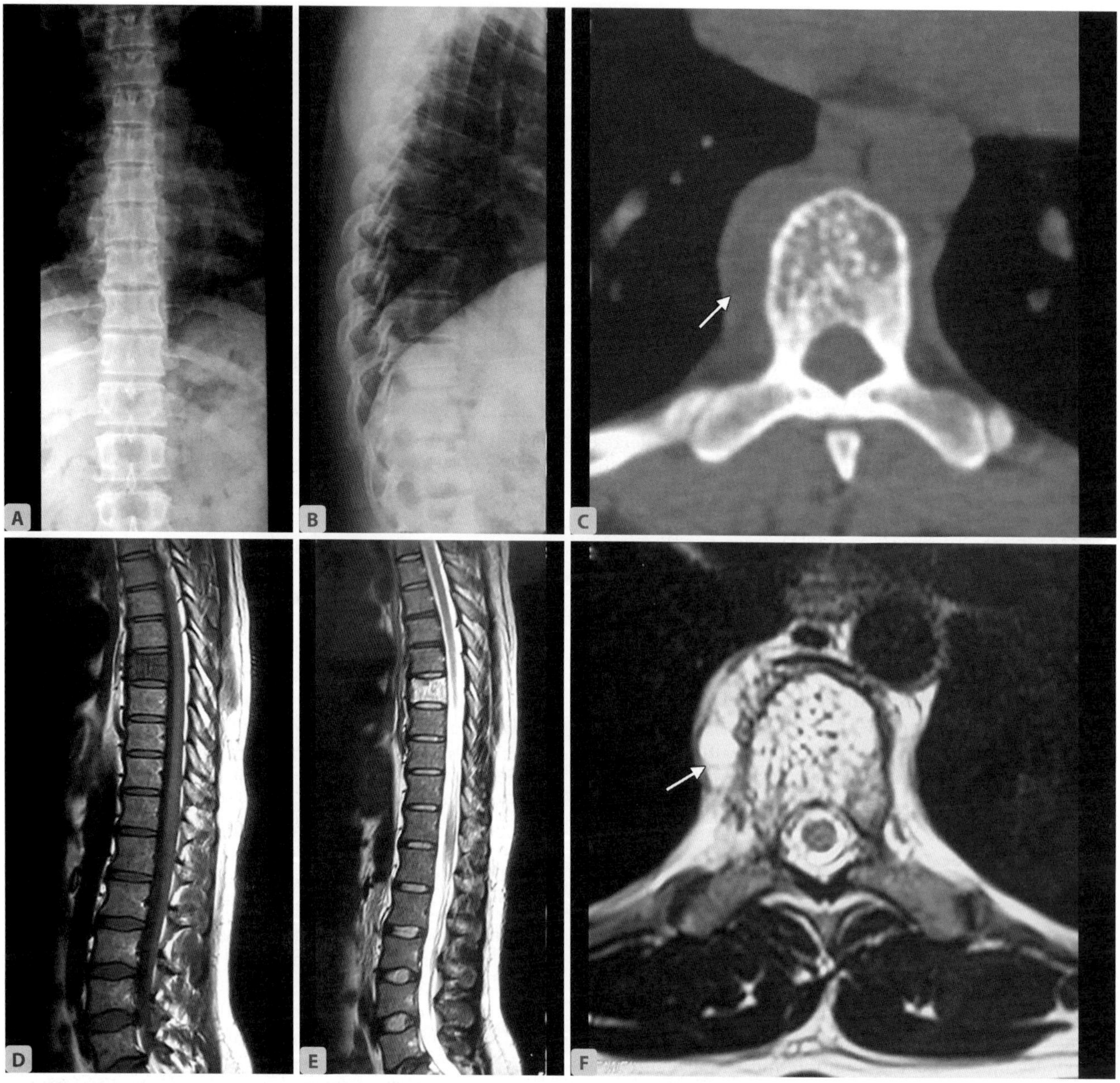

FIGS. 19A TO F: Aggressive hemangioma: Anteroposterior and lateral radiographs (A and B) of dorsolumbar spine show a small right paraspinal mass; Axial CT section (C) of D8 vertebra showing typical polka dot appearance involving the D8 vertebral body associated with right paravertebral soft tissue component (arrow); Sagittal T1W (D), T2W (E) and axial T2W (F) MR images showing lesion involving the vertebral body of D8 which is hypointense on T1W and brightly hyperintense on T2W associated with soft tissue component.

tendency to involve the posterior elements.[48] Radiographs show a lytic, expansile lesion **(Fig. 21A)** in the posterior elements. CT is ideal to show the expansile lesion **(Fig. 21B)** with sclerotic border, which may have foci of calcification representing an osteoid matrix. MRI is usually not required except to show the relationship with the cord and nerve roots. It is T1 hypointense and shows intermediate to high signal on T2W images.[51] Secondary aneurysmal bone cyst may be seen within the lesion and they are T2 hyperintense **(Fig. 21C)** with fluid-fluid levels. Extensive peri-tumoral edema is common and may involve adjacent bones and soft tissues. The differential diagnosis includes osteoid osteoma, aneurysmal bone cyst, infection and metastases.

Aneurysmal Bone Cyst

They are benign lesions with blood filled cavities. They occur in the younger age group within the first two decades of life. The spine is a common location with the lumbar spine ranking second to the thoracic spine. Radiograph shows expansile lesion in the posterior elements **(Figs. 22A and B)** which often extends to involve the vertebral body. CT shows a lesion with balloon like expansion and thinned out cortex, with a non-sclerotic narrow zone of transition. Fluid-Fluid levels with sedimentation of blood products are a typical finding. It commonly extends into the epidural space and causes cord compression. MRI is ideal for showing the cystic spaces **(Figs. 22C and D)** within the lesion separated by septae. Fluid levels of varying signal intensities due to different stages of hemorrhage **(Fig. 22D)** are well seen on MRI.[48,50] On contrast administration only the periphery of the lesion and septae enhance.

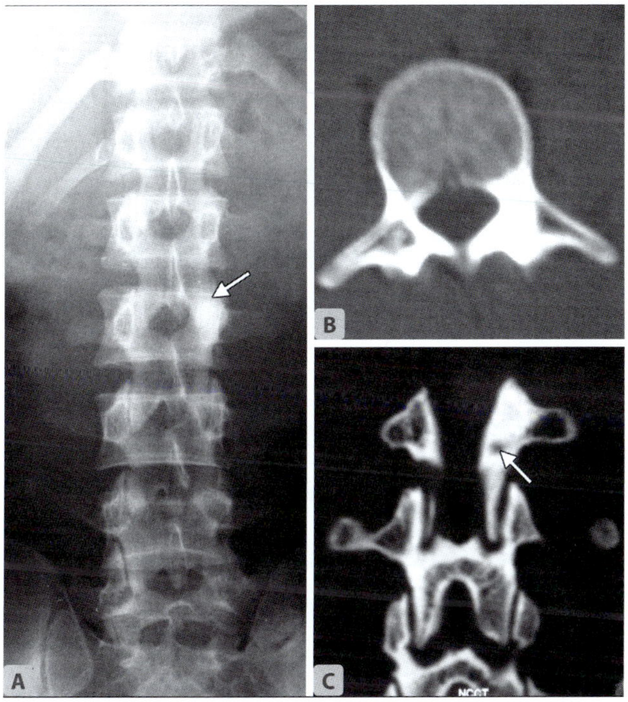

FIGS. 20A TO C: Osteoid osteoma: Anteroposterior radiograph of lumbar region (A) showing sclerotic left pedicle of L2 vertebra (arrow). Axial (B) and Coronal 3D reformatted CT (C) images showing sclerotic lesion involving left pedicle and lamina with small lucent nidus in the centre (arrow).

Giant Cell Tumor

It is an aggressive but benign bone tumor composed of oesteoclastic giant cells. It occurs in mature skeleton commonly in the second to fourth decades. Spine is the fourth most common location for this lesion and majority of spinal GCTs occur in the sacrum.

Radiographs show an ill-defined expansile lytic lesion **(Figs. 23A and B)** with a narrow zone of transition and without a sclerotic border. Sacral lesions can be occult on radiography and may only be picked up on cross-sectional imaging. MRI is ideal for showing the extension into the spinal canal and cord compression. It shows a lesion which is hypointense on T1 and intermediate to high signal on T2W images **(Figs. 23C to E)**. Secondary aneurysmal bone cysts are seen as T2 hyperintense foci within the lesion.[48] The differential diagnosis includes aneurysmal bone cyst, metastases, plasmacytoma and chordoma.

MALIGNANT TUMORS

Chordoma

Chordomas are relatively rare slow growing low grade malignant tumors. They arise from notochord remnants in the centers of the vertebral bodies. They are more common at the cranial and caudal ends of the spine, that is, clivus and sacrum, respectively, but may occur at any level, with 35% arising in the lumbosacral spine. Chordoma is always kept in the differential diagnosis when a midline lesion is seen involving the sacrum.[52] The clinical presentation depends on the location of the tumor. The tumors may present with nonspecific back pain, which may be accompanied with neurological symptoms. It commonly affects patients in the

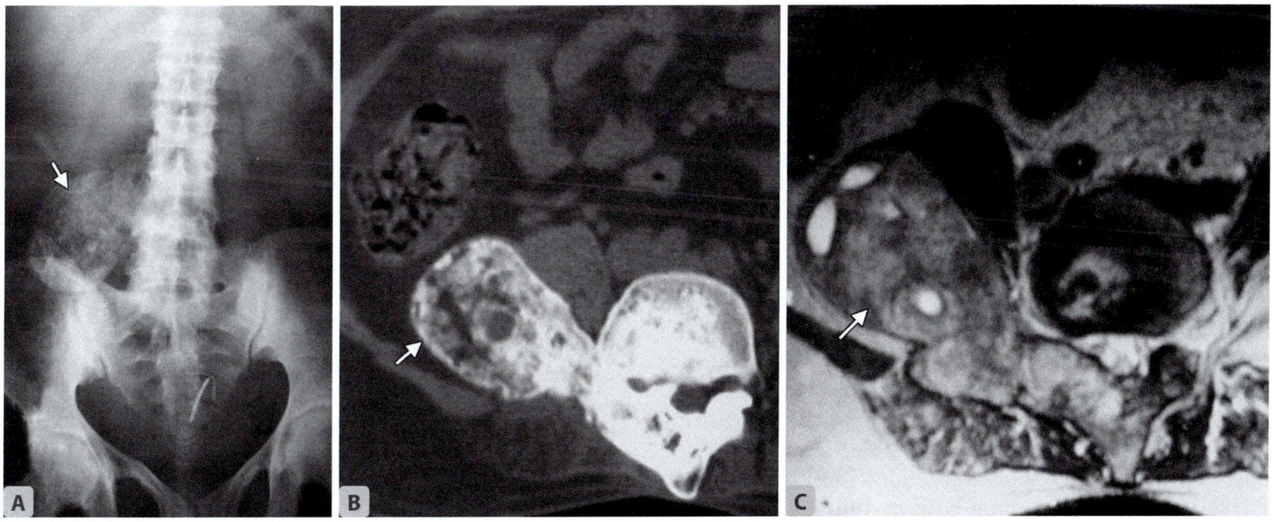

FIGS. 21A TO C: Osteoblastoma: Anteroposterior radiograph of KUB region (A) showing large expansile mixed lytic-sclerotic lesion arising from right transverse process of L4 vertebra (arrow); Axial CT (B) and axial T2W (C) MR images showing large expansile osseous lesion involving the right transverse process and lamina of L4 vertebra (arrow). Hyperintense foci are likely to be due to secondary aneurysmal bone cyst.

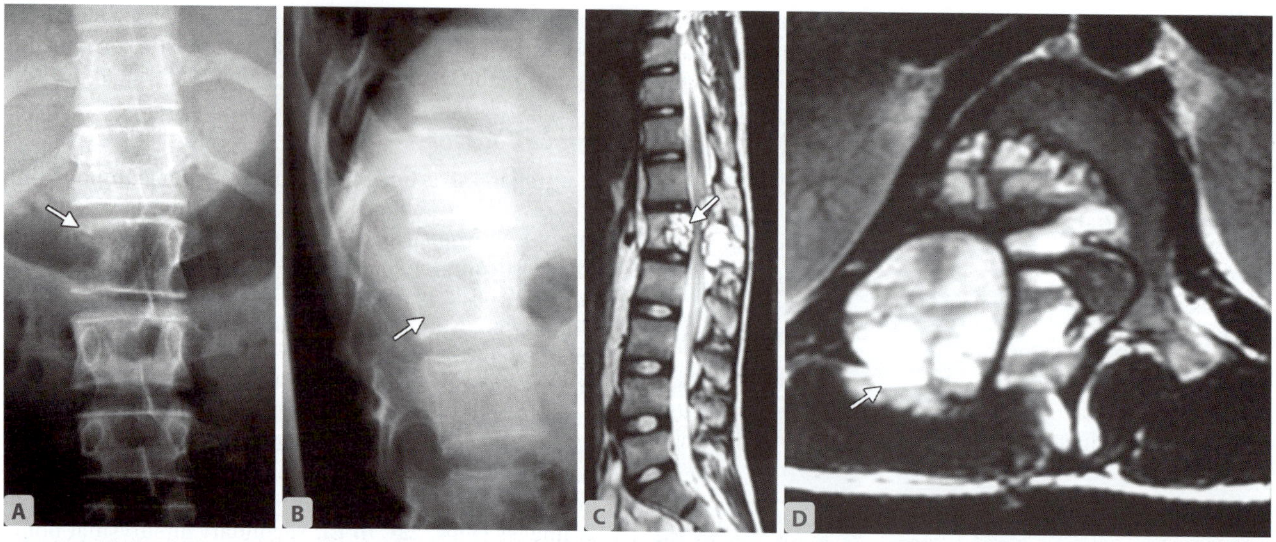

FIGS. 22A TO D: Aneurysmal bone cyst: Anteroposterior (A) and lateral (B) radiographs of lumbar spine showing a lytic destructive lesion involving the posterior vertebral body and right pedicle (arrow). Sagittal T2W (C) and Axial T2W (D) MR images showing hyperintense lesion in L1 posterior vertebral body, right pedicle and lamina with multiple blood fluid levels (arrow).

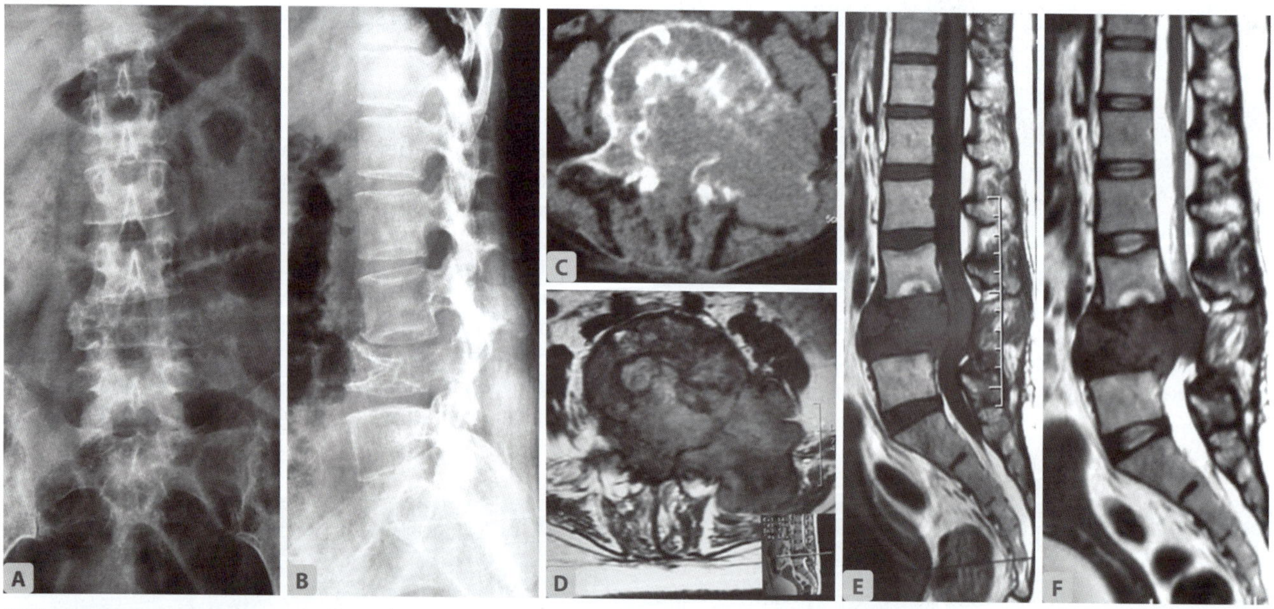

FIGS. 23A TO F: Giant cell tumor: Radiograph anteroposterior (A) and lateral view (B) showing lytic expansile lesion in L4 vertebral body and pedicle with collapse; Axial CT image (C) shows an expansile lesion involving body, pedicle and left transverse process with soft tissue component; Axial T2W (D), Sagittal T1W (E), T2W (F) MR images show collapse L4 with posterior convexity which is hypointense on both T1 and T2W images, with an extradural intraspinal soft tissue component compressing the thecal sac.

third to sixth decades, with no sex predominance. It appears as a lytic lesion on radiography and CT scanning with some amorphous calcification. MRI is the modality of choice for defining the extent of the tumor and its intraspinal extension. This tumor is hypointense on T1W and hyperintense on T2W sequence **(Figs. 24A to D)** with low signal septations.[50,52] Post-contrast images show mild to intense enhancement. These characteristics along with its midline location in an older patient are suggestive of this diagnosis. En bloc resection is the treatment of choice and radiotherapy may play a useful role.

Chondrosarcoma

It is a malignant tumor of connective tissue, characterized by formation of cartilage matrix by tumor cells. Most commonly affects dorsal spine followed by sacrum. Within the vertebra, body and posterior elements are equally affected. Typically they are of large size, at the time of presentation. On imaging, they appear as a lytic mass with chondroid matrix: higher-grade lesions tend to have larger areas without calcifications. CT scan helps in better delineation of extent of the lesion, bone destruction and calcification. MR helps in evaluating

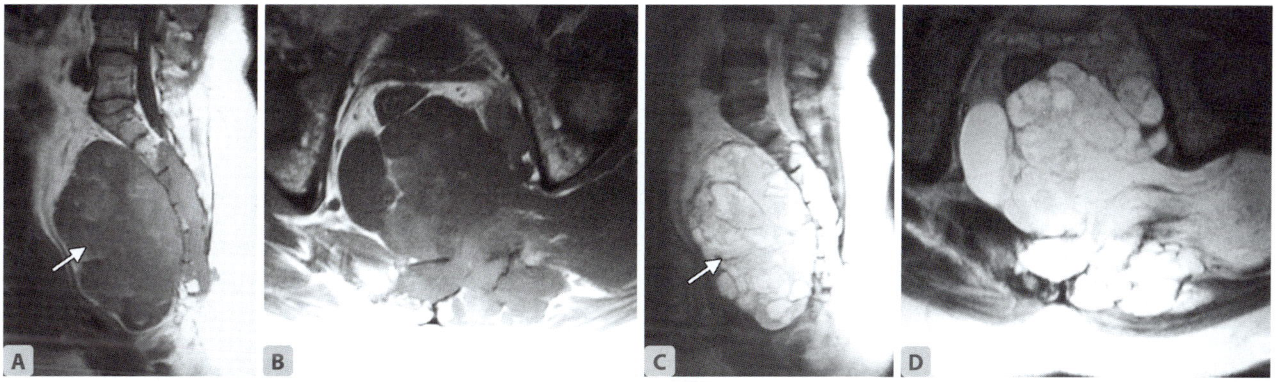

FIGS. 24A TO D: Sacral chordoma: T1W sagittal (A), axial (B), T2W sagittal (C) and axial (D) MR images showing altered signal intensity involving sacrum associated with large soft tissue component (arrow) which is hypointense on T1W and brightly hyperintense on T2W, extending into the sacral spinal canal.

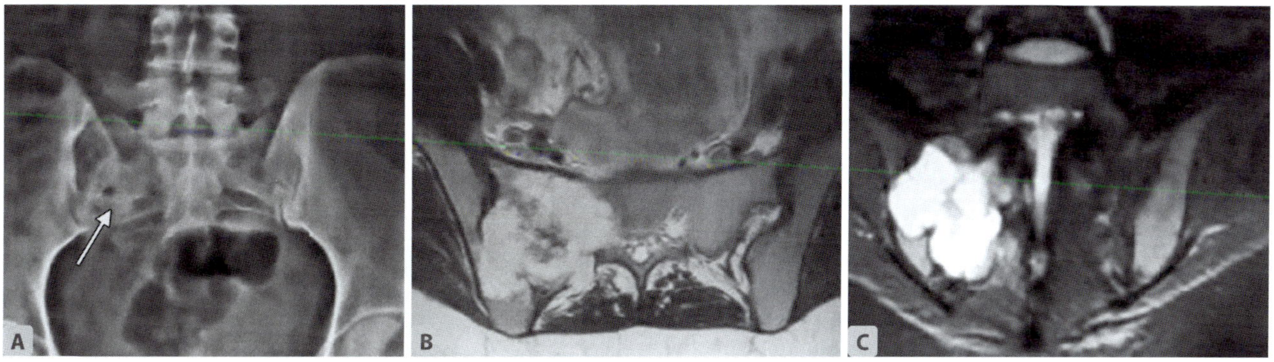

FIGS. 25A TO C: Sacral chondrosarcoma: Anteroposterior (A) radiograph of pelvis showing lytic destructive lesion with central calcification; Axial T2W (B), coronal T2W (C) with fat saturation MR images showing heterogeneous T2 bright lesion involving right half of the sacrum with contiguous extension across the sacroiliac joint.

extent of tumor within bone and degree of extension into adjacent soft tissues.

Differential diagnoses include sacral chordoma. Chondrosarcomas arise off midline, from the sacroiliac joint space cartilage, and display heterogeneous signal intensity on T2-weighted MR images because they consist of both mineralized and nonmineralized chondroid matrix **(Figs. 25A to C)** Chondrosarcomas typically do not contain areas of hemorrhage, a fact that helps differentiate them from chordomas.

Metastases

Skeletal metastases are significantly more common than primary bone tumors. Spinal metastases are common because they occur in hematopoietic active bone marrow, which is predominantly located in the adult spine. Most spinal metastases are found in the thoracic and lumbar regions. They are frequently disseminated via the hematogenous route. Both venous dissemination and arterial dissemination may occur. Batson's plexus of veins, is a major source of spinal metastases, and it connects with venous plexuses inside the spinal canal. Pressure difference in these veins directs tumor cells from the pelvis (prostate) into the lumbar or thoracic vertebral bodies. They frequently invade the vertebral bodies or the pedicles. Metastases can also grow along nervous tissue and thus enter the epidural space inside the spinal canal. The most common sources of vertebral metastases are the breast, lungs, thyroid, kidney, and prostate.[48] As the metastatic lesions grow, they destroy the vertebral body, penetrate through cortical bone, invade the spinal canal, and compromise the neural elements. Cord compression and neurological deficits may also occur when vertebral bodies collapse due to bone destruction.

Radiographs have poor sensitivity for spinal metastases detection. Vertebral bodies can loose upwards of 50% of their density before it becomes detectable in plain films. The vertebral bodies may appear heterogeneous on plain films. This appearance is not specific and can be found in osteoporosis as well. The vertebral bodies' shape, texture, and cortices should be critically observed. Special attention should be paid to the posterior vertebral body wall. The metastatic deposit may be seen as a presence of a lytic or blastic vertebral lesion **(Figs. 26A to D)**. In some patients with metastatic prostate cancer the vertebral bodies may seem completely white. The pedicles should be inspected carefully. They are well seen in posteroanterior views and can be screened rather quickly. Absence, erosion, or sclerosis of

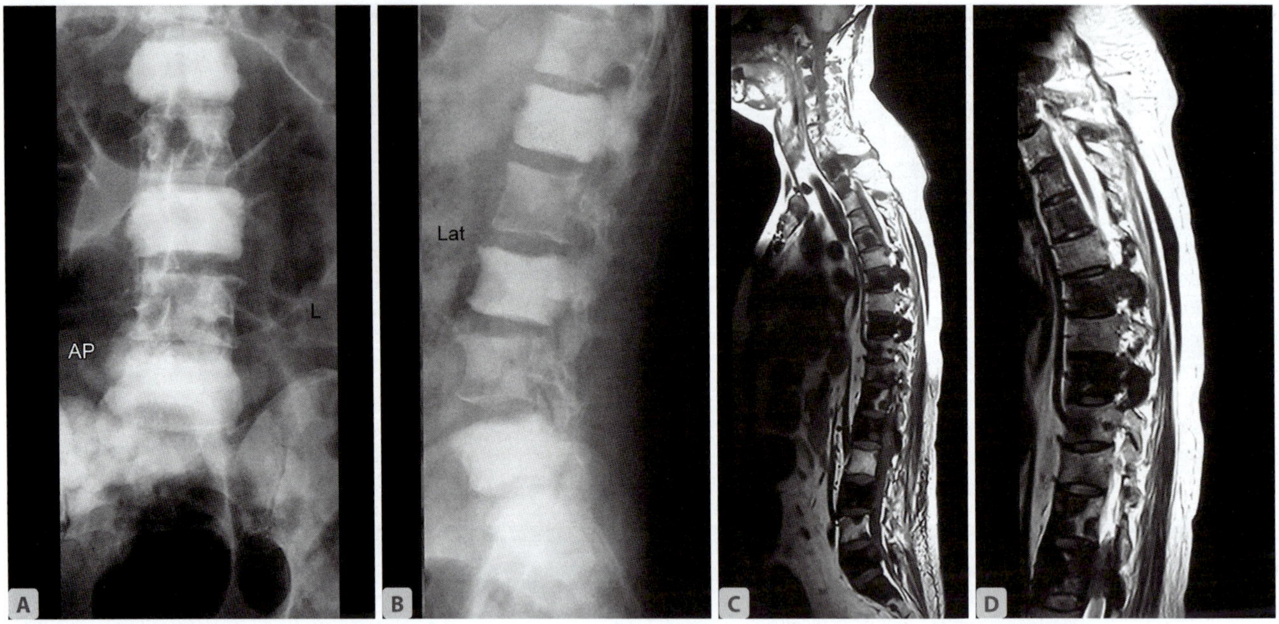

FIGS. 26A TO D: Sclerotic spinal metastases: Anteroposterior (A) and lateral (B) radiographs of lumbar spine showing dense sclerotic lesions involving multiple vertebrae; sagittal T1W (C) and T2W (D) showing lesions hypointense on both T1 and T2 images involving both anterior and posterior elements.

a pedicle may indicate the presence of a bone metastasis at that location.

Bone scan is an efficient and inexpensive tool for detecting skeletal metastases which is sensitive but not specific. Multiplicity of lesions is well-evaluated. False positive scans may be seen in degenerative disease, fracture and infection. Areas of increased activity that may correspond to facet joints or disk spaces are more likely to be due to degenerative changes.

CT can also detect bony metastases and associated soft tissue mass in patients undergoing CT as a part of imaging work up to look for tumor or for staging of known malignancy. MDCT allows excellent sagittal and coronal MPRs **(Figs. 27A and B)** which when viewed on bone window can pick up vertebral metastases.

However, MRI is the most sensitive modality for picking up early vertebral metastases.[48,53] T1W and STIR sagittal sequences of the whole spine **(Figs. 28 to 30)** can be performed and are very sensitive for vertebral deposits and their impact on the spinal canal and the spinal cord. MRI is also very useful to differentiate osteoporotic vertebral collapse from neoplastic collapse. The features are summarized in **Table 2**.

PET-CT scan has emerged as an important tool to image the whole body for the evaluation of metastatic lesions. ^{18}F FDG-PET/CT scan performs better in the evaluation of lytic vertebral metastasis whereas 18F NaF PET/CT scan performs better in the evaluation of sclerotic or mixed lytic sclerotic lesions.

Osteoporotic Collapse versus Neoplastic Collapse

Osteoporotic collapse **(Figs. 31A and B)** is common in the elderly and in post-menopausal women. In the acute

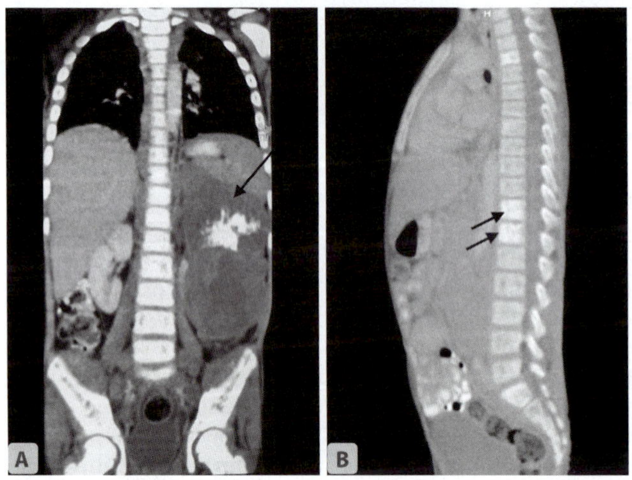

FIGS. 27A AND B: Neuroblastoma with vertebral metastases. Coronal and sagittal 3D reformatted CT images showing large soft tissue mass in left side of abdomen with dense coarse calcification (long arrow) in a child, associated with sclerotic lesions involving multiple vertebrae (small arrows).

setting it may be difficult to distinguish it from malignant collapse, as the presence of edema gives rise to hypointense signal on T1W images and hyperintense signal on T2W and STIR sequences. Majority of the times some fatty marrow signal is preserved, the posterior cortex remains concave and the pedicles are normal. The spectrum of findings are related to the age of the collapse and within three months of injury there is always some restoration of fatty marrow and a linear hypontense band may persist. In chronic fractures return to the fatty marrow signal occurs and at this stage there is no difficulty in distinguishing

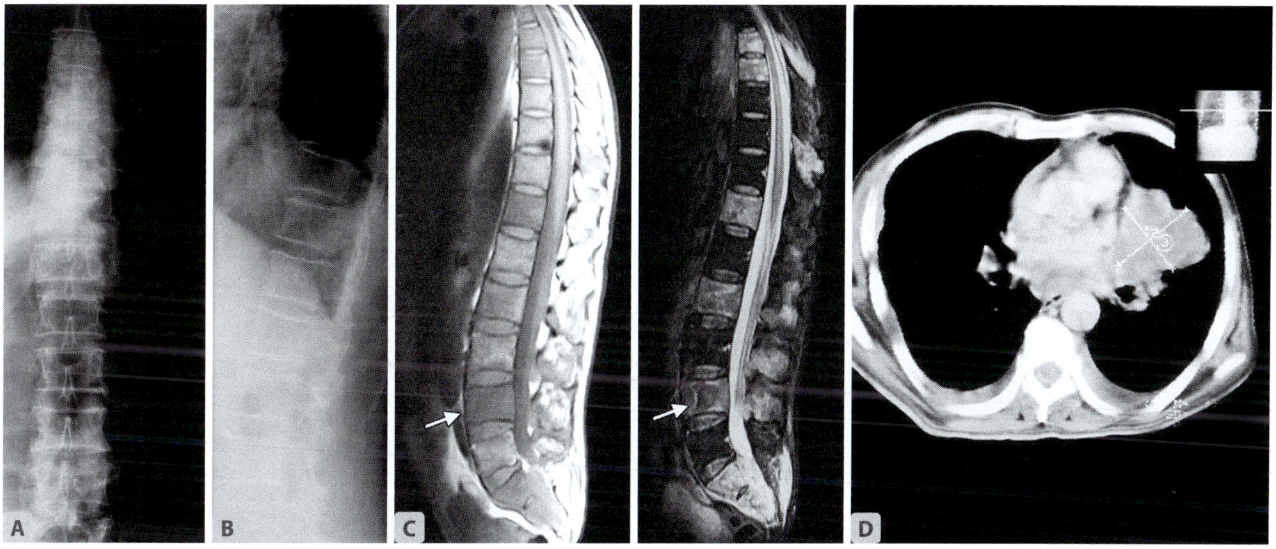

FIGS. 28 A TO D: Vertebral metastases from bronchogenic carcinoma: Anteroposterior (A) and lateral (B) radiographs of dorsolumbar spine show subtle lytic lesions involving pedicles. Sagittal T1W (B), STIR (C) MR images showing multiple lesions (hypointense on T1W and hyperintense on STIR) involving both anterior and posterior elements of vertebrae. Axial CT scan (D) showing large soft tissue mass in left hilar location with bilateral pleural effusion suggestive of carcinoma of lung.

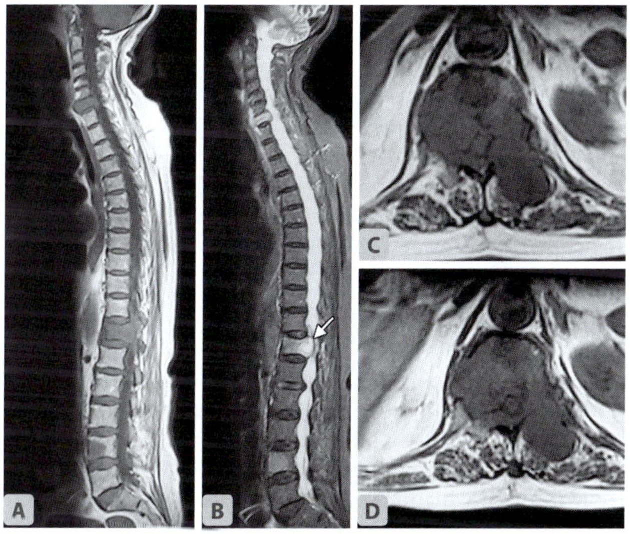

FIGS. 29A TO D: Spinal metastasis: Sagittal T1W (A), T2W (B) MR images showing altered signal intensity (hypointense on T1W and hyperintense on T2W) involving vertebral bodies of multiple vertebrae. Axial T1W (C) and T2W (D) MR images showing involvement of both anterior and posterior elements of vertebra associated with soft tissue component extending into the spinal canal causing spinal canal narrowing. Posterior vertebral margin of the involved vertebrae is showing convex border (arrow).

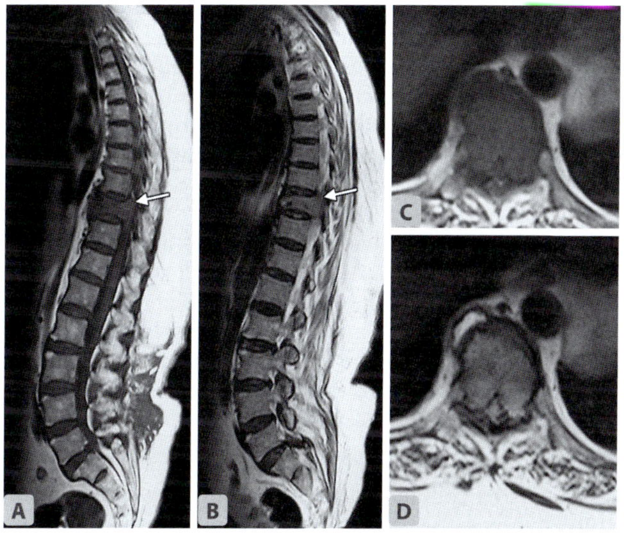

FIGS. 30A TO D: Sagittal T1W (A), T2W (B) MR images show a collapsed D10 vertebra with posterior convexity (arrow). The axial T1W (C) and T2W (D) images show involvement of body and pedicle with extradural soft tissue compressing the cord.

TABLE 2: Features of osteoporotic and neoplastic collapses.

Osteoporotic collapse	Neoplastic collapse
Anterior wedging, height relatively maintained posteriorly	Uniform collapse
Posterior margin flat	Posterior margin convex
Patchy abnormal signal, some fatty marrow present	Uniform replacement of fatty marrow by tumor giving uniform abnormal signal
Fracture line present	Fracture line absent
Absence of extraosseous Soft tissue	Presence of extraosseous soft tissue

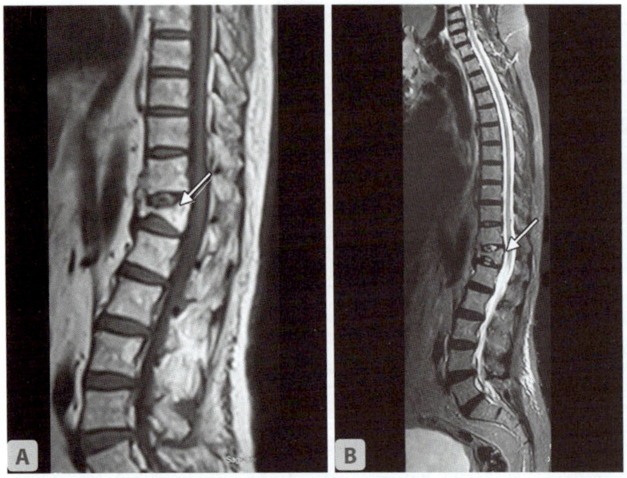

FIGS. 31A AND B: Sagittal T1W (A) and T2W (B) MR images showing near complete collapse with anterior wedging of D12 vertebra with preserved signal intensity (arrow) and straight posterior vertebral margin suggestive osteoporotic collapse.

it from malignant collapse. Multiple lesions of different ages may occur confounding the problem further.[48,54]

Malignant collapse also shows T1 hypointensity and T2 hyperintensity and contrast enhancement.[55] Considering that up to one-third of vertebral collapse in patients with known malignancy are benign the diagnosis is difficult when there is a history of malignancy. The marrow replacement is usually complete, posterior cortex is convex, pedicles are commonly involved and associated soft tissue component may be present.

Recently diffusion weighted MRI has also been used for this distinction. Tumor infiltration will show restricted diffusion whereas osteoporotic collapse will not.

Occasionally central type of tuberculosis involving the vertebral body only without diskal or adjacent vertebral involvement may also mimic malignant collapse.

Multiple Myeloma

It is a plasma cell neoplasm of bone marrow and commonly involves the spine. The imaging appearance in spine is non-specific and mimics metastatic disease. The differential diagnosis is better made on radiographs which in myeloma show osteopenia and typical punched out lytic lesions in the skull vault **(Fig. 32A)**. Occasionally sclerotic lesions may be seen specially in the setting of POEMS syndrome (polyneuropathy, organomegaly, endocrinopathy, myeloma, sclerosis). Myeloma lesions are usually cold on bone scan. MRI is a sensitive screening tool but may be normal even in the presence of proven marrow infiltration. Focal T1 hypo- and T2 hyperintense lesions of variable size **(Figs. 32B to D)** may be seen or there may homogeneously decreased signal may be seen on T1W images which can easily be overlooked. T2W images in the latter group will show hyperintense signal and enhancement will be seen on contrast administration.[48,56]

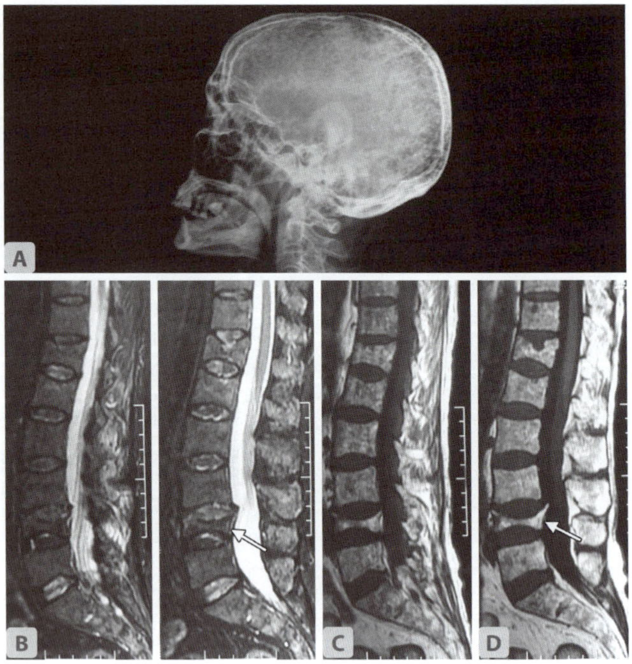

FIGS. 32A TO D: Multiple myeloma: Lateral radiograph of skull (A) showing multiple uniform sized punched out lytic lesions involving the entire calvarium. Sagittal T2W (B) and T1W (C and D) MR images showing patchy focal altered signal intensity involving multiple vertebrae associated with near complete collapse of L4 and partial collapse of D12 vertebrae. Posterior vertebral margin of the collapsed vertebra is straight (arrow) with preserved signal likely due to osteoporosis.

VNCa CT images may become useful in the future for detection of non-osteolytic infiltrative lesions of myeloma.

Lymphoma

Primary lymphoma of bone is a rare entity and spine is the fourth most common location for it. It is usually a Non-Hodgkin lymphoma with a peak incidence in fifth to seventh decade. Secondary lymphomas are far more common and up to 30% of systemic lymphomas have osseous involvement.

Lymphoma in the spine can present as an epidural mass, osseous involvement, lepto meningitis and as an intramedullary mass. In this discussion, we will confine ourselves to osseous lymphoma which is frequently associated with epidural soft tissue masses.

The radiographs show a nonspecific lytic lesion, but it may also be sclerotic. Bone scan shows increased uptake and 67 Gallium scintigraphy has been shown to have a high sensitivity and specificity.[53] MRI shows a lesion which is T1 hypointense and T2 iso to hyperintense, which enhances on contrast administration. The soft tissue mass may show T2 hypointensity due to hyper-cellularity.

Low backache is a very common clinical problem. Majority of patients do not require imaging. It is important to triage patients into chronic nonspecific pain versus those with more ominous pathology who would benefit with imaging. Plain radiographs and MRI play the most useful role and CT and scintigraphy are used as problem solving tools.

REFERENCES

1. Sharma SC, Singh R, Sharma AK, et al. Incidence of low back pain in workage adults in rural North India. Indian J Med Sci. 2003;57(4):145-7.
2. Gilbert FJ, Grant AM, Gillan MG, et al. Low back pain: influence of early MR imaging or CT on treatment and outcome—multicenter randomized trial. Radiology. 2004;231(2):343-51.
3. Davis PC, Wippold FJ, Brunberg JA, et al. ACR Appropriateness Criteria® on low back pain. J Am Coll Radiol. 2009;6(6):401-7.
4. Teh J, Imam A, Watts C. Imaging of back pain. Imaging. 2005;17(3):171-207.
5. Deyo RA, Weinstein JN. Low back pain. N Engl J Med. 2001;344(5):363-70.
6. Borenstein D. Epidemiology, etiology, diagnostic evaluation, and treatment of low back pain. Curr Opin Rheumatol. 1996;8(2):124-9.
7. Jarvik JG, Hollingworth W, Martin B, et al. Rapid magnetic resonance imaging vs radiographs for patients with low back pain: a randomized controlled trial. JAMA. 2003;289(21):2810-8.
8. McNally EG, Wilson DJ, Ostlere SJ. Limited magnetic resonance imaging in low back pain instead of plain radiographs: experience with first 1000 cases. Clin Radiol. 2001;56(11):922-5.
9. Singh K, Helms CA, Fiorella D, et al. Disc space-targeted angled axial MR images of the lumbar spine: a potential source of diagnostic error. Skeletal Radiol. 2007;36(12):1147-53.
10. Bellini M, Ferrara M, Grazzini I, et al. Neuroimaging of the Postoperative Spine. Magn Reson Imaging Clin. 2016;24(3):601-20.
11. Kellock TT, Nicolaou S, Kim SSY, et al. Detection of Bone Marrow Edema in Nondisplaced Hip Fractures: Utility of a Virtual Noncalcium Dual-Energy CT Application. Radiology. 2017;284(3):798-805.
12. Kim HG, Shin DA, Kim HI, et al. Clinical and radiological findings of discogenic low back pain confirmed by automated pressure-controlled discography. J Korean Neurosurg Soc. 2009;46(4):333.
13. Carragee EJ, Lincoln T, Parmar VS, et al. A gold standard evaluation of the "discogenic pain" diagnosis as determined by provocative discography. Spine. 2006; 31(18):2115-23.
14. Dolan AL, Ryan PJ, Arden NK, et al. The value of SPECT scans in identifying back pain likely to benefit from facet joint injection. Rheumatology. 1996;35(12):1269-73.
15. Elster AD. Bertolotti's syndrome revisited. Transitional vertebrae of the lumbar spine. Spine. 1989;14(12):1373-7.
16. Konin GP, Walz DM. Lumbosacral transitional vertebrae: classification, imaging findings, and clinical relevance. Am J Neuroradiol. 2010;31(10):1778-86.
17. Syrmou E, Tsitsopoulos PP, Marinopoulos D, et al. Spondylolysis: a review and reappraisal. Hippokratia. 2010;14(1):17.
18. Beutler WJ, Fredrickson BE, Murtland A, et al. The natural history of spondylolysis and spondylolisthesis: 45-year follow-up evaluation. Spine. 2003;28(10):1027-35.
19. Fredrickson BE, Baker D, McHolick WJ, et al. The natural history of spondylolysis and spondylolisthesis. J Bone Joint Surg Am. 1984;66(5):699-707.
20. Campbell RSD, Grainger AJ, Hide IG, et al. Juvenile spondylolysis: a comparative analysis of CT, SPECT and MRI. Skeletal Radiol. 2005;34(2):63-73.
21. Harvey CJ, Richenberg JL, Saifuddin A, et al. The radiological investigation of lumbar spondylolysis. Clin Radiol. 1998;53(10):723-8.
22. Paajanen H, Tertti M. Association of incipient disc degeneration and instability in spondylolisthesis. Arch Orthop Trauma Surg. 1991;111(1):16-19.
23. Collier BD, Johnson RP, Carrera GF, et al. Painful spondylolysis or spondylolisthesis studied by radiography and single-photon emission computed tomography. Radiology. 1985;154(1):207-11.
24. Scheuermann HW. Kyphosis dorsalis juvenilis. Ugeskr Laeger. 1920;82:385.
25. Blumenthal SL, Roach J, Herring JA. Lumbar Scheuermann's. A clinical series and classification. Spine. 1987;12(9):929-32.
26. Summers BN, Singh JP, Manns RA. The radiological reporting of lumbar Scheuermann's disease: an unnecessary source of confusion amongst clinicians and patients. Br J Radiol. 2008;81(965):383-5.
27. Yu S, Haughton VM, Sether LA, et al. Criteria for classifying normal and degenerated lumbar intervertebral disks. Radiology. 1989;170(2):523-6.
28. Pfirrmann CW, Metzdorf A, Zanetti M, et al. Magnetic resonance classification of lumbar intervertebral disc degeneration. Spine. 2001;26(17):1873-8.
29. Clarençon F, Law-Ye B, Bienvenot P, et al. The degenerative spine. Magn Reson Imaging Clin. 2016;24(3):495-513.
30. Fardon DF, Milette PC. Nomenclature and classification of lumbar disc pathology: recommendations of the combined task forces of the North American Spine Society, American Society of Spine Radiology, and American Society of Neuroradiology. Spine. 2001;26(5):E93-113.
31. Modic MT. Degenerative disc disease and back pain. Magn Reson Imaging Clin N Am. 1999;7(3):481-91.
32. Lee SH, Coleman PE, Hahn FJ. Magnetic resonance imaging of degenerative disk disease of the spine. Radiol Clin North Am. 1988;26(5):949-64.
33. Kalichman L, Hunter DJ. Lumbar facet joint osteoarthritis: a review. In: Seminars in arthritis and rheumatism. Elsevier; 2007. p. 69-80.
34. Modic MT, Masaryk T, Boumphrey F, et al. Lumbar herniated disk disease and canal stenosis: prospective evaluation by surface coil MR, CT, and myelography. Am J Roentgenol. 1986;147(4):757-65.
35. Schizas C, Theumann N, Burn A, et al. Qualitative grading of severity of lumbar spinal stenosis based on the morphology of the dural sac on magnetic resonance images. Spine. 2010;35(21):1919-24.
36. Ross JS, Masaryk TJ, Schrader M, et al. MR imaging of the postoperative lumbar spine: assessment with gadopentetate dimeglumine. Am J Neuroradiol. 1990;11(4):771-6.
37. Ross JS. Magnetic resonance assessment of the postoperative spine. Degenerative disc disease. Radiol Clin North Am. 1991;29(4):793-808.
38. Braun J, Bollow M, Sieper J. Radiologic diagnosis and pathology of the spondyloarthropathies. Rheum Dis Clin. 1998;24(4):697-735.
39. Vinson EN, Major NM. MR imaging of ankylosing spondylitis. In: Seminars in musculoskeletal radiology. Copyright\copyright 2002 by Thieme Medical Publishers, Inc., 333 Seventh Avenue, New York, NY 10001, USA. Tel.:+1 (212) 584-4662; 2003. p. 103-44.
40. Shanley DJ. Tuberculosis of the spine: imaging features. Am J Roentgenol. 1995;164(3):659-64.
41. Moorthy S, Prabhu NK. Spectrum of MR imaging findings in spinal tuberculosis. Am J Roentgenol. 2002;179(4):979-83.
42. Moore SL, Rafii M. Imaging of musculoskeletal and spinal tuberculosis. Radiol Clin. 2001;39(2):329-42.
43. Forrester DM. Infectious spondylitis. In: Seminars in Ultrasound, CT and MRI. Elsevier; 2004. p. 461-73.
44. Ledermann HP, Schweitzer ME, Morrison WB, et al. MR imaging findings in spinal infections: rules or myths? Radiology. 2003;228(2):506-14.
45. Thrush A, Enzmann D. MR imaging of infectious spondylitis. Am J Neuroradiol. 1990;11(6):1171-80.
46. Varma R, Lander P, Assaf A. Imaging of pyogenic infectious spondylodiskitis. Radiol Clin. 2001;39(2):203-13.

47. Carragee EJ. The clinical use of magnetic resonance imaging in pyogenic vertebral osteomyelitis. Spine. 1997;22(7):780-5.
48. Motamedi K, Ilaslan H, Seeger LL. Imaging of the lumbar spine neoplasms. In: Seminars in Ultrasound, CT and MRI. Elsevier; 2004. p. 474-89.
49. Baudrez V, Galant C, Berg BCV. Benign vertebral hemangioma: MR-histological correlation. Skeletal Radiol. 2001;30(8):442-6.
50. Flemming DJ, Murphey MD, Carmichael BB, et al. Primary tumors of the spine. In: Seminars in musculoskeletal radiology. Copyright\copyright 2000 by Thieme Medical Publishers, Inc., 333 Seventh Avenue, New York, NY 10001, USA. pp. 299-320.
51. Ozaki T, Liljenqvist U, Hillmann A, et al. Osteoid osteoma and osteoblastoma of the spine: experiences with 22 patients. Clin Orthop. 2002;397:394-402.
52. Diel J, Ortiz O, Losada RA, et al. The sacrum: pathologic spectrum, multimodality imaging, and subspecialty approach. Radiographics. 2001;21(1):83-104.
53. Nöbauer I, Uffmann M. Differential diagnosis of focal and diffuse neoplastic diseases of bone marrow in MRI. Eur J Radiol. 2005;55(1):2-32.
54. Uetani M, Hashmi R, Hayashi K. Malignant and benign compression fractures: differentiation and diagnostic pitfalls on MRI. Clin Radiol. 2004;59(2):124-31.
55. Tehranzadeh J, Tao C. Advances in MR imaging of vertebral collapse. In: Seminars in Ultrasound, CT and MRI. Elsevier; 2004. p. 440-60.
56. Angtuaco EJ, Fassas AB, Walker R, et al. Multiple myeloma: clinical review and diagnostic imaging. Radiology. 2004;231(1):11-23.

CHAPTER

216

Localization in Clinical Neurology

Manish Modi, Sudesh Prabhakar

LOCALIZATION IN CLINICAL NEUROLOGY

Localization, derived from Latin term locus, is the diagnostic exercise of determining from the signs or symptoms of the patient, what site of the nervous system has been affected by the disease process. Clinical localization has particular relevance to the adequate use of ancillary diagnostic procedures. Current techniques of imaging, electrodiagnosis and other laboratory studies have revolutionized the practice of neurology. However, their use must be integrated with findings of history and neurological examination.

Clinical Diagnosis and Lesion Localization

Clinical diagnosis in neurology requires several steps:

- Recognition of impaired function
- Identification of site of central nervous system (CNS) affected
- Definition of most likely etiology
- Use of ancillary procedures.

Recognition of impaired function depends on a good history and neurological examination. Abnormal neurological findings come in the form of abnormal behavior or cognition, impaired posture or gait, difficulty in movement of face or extremities, and finally the sensory disturbances, including pain.

Neuroanatomy is the key to localization. Neuroanatomy has two broad based aspects: (1) the morphology of the structure, and (2) its "functional representation". Functional representation refers to the function mediated by a given structure of the nervous system. Damage to a structure results in dysfunction in the realm mediated by this structure.

APPROACH TO NEUROLOGICAL DISORDER

Neurological localization and diagnosis is approached in each patient with the following six questions in mind:

1. Is there a disease in the nervous system?
2. At what level(s)?
3. What longitudinal system(s) is (are) involved?
4. Is the process—focal/multifocal/diffuse?
5. What is the lateralization right/left or bilateral?
6. What is the course acute/subacute/chronic? Then further queries like:
   a. Static versus progressive
   b. Relapsing/remitting or monophasic
   c. Onset sudden or insidious

Based on the anatomic-temporal profile, the neurological disorders are broadly grouped into:

- *Degenerative*: Progressive and tend to be chronic and diffuse.
- *Neoplastic*: Progressive, may be subacute or chronic, and tend to be focal or multifocal but may be diffuse (e.g. carcinomatous meningitis).
- *Vascular*: Acute and usually focal but may be diffuse (e.g. subarachnoid hemorrhage).
- *Inflammatory*: Subacute or chronic and tend to be progressive. They may be focal (e.g. abscess), diffuse (e.g. meningitis, encephalitis), or multifocal (e.g. autoimmune disease).
- *Demyelination*: Acute, focal, may be relapsing and remitting.
- *Toxic metabolic*: Diffuse and may have any time course.
- *Traumatic*: Processes are always acute, may be static and improving or progressive, and may be diffuse, focal, or multifocal.
- *Congenital*: Developmental diseases are chronic and typically diffuse, and may be static or progressive.

The present chapter will focus on few important symptoms and signs, which refer to a particular area of the neuraxis and help in clinical localization. The chapter is subdivided into disorders of cranial nerves, motor system, including gait and coordination, sensory system, and finally disorders of higher mental function.

DISORDERS OF CRANIAL NERVES

OLFACTORY NERVE (CRANIAL NERVE I)

Anosmia

Significant olfactory dysfunction has been described with Alzheimer's disease, Lewy body disease, Huntington's chorea, Parkinson's disease, spinocerebellar ataxia, multiplesclerosis. Tumors of sphenoid or frontal bone, pituitary tumors with suprasellar extension, nasopharyngeal carcinoma or giant anterior communicating artery aneurysm can also present with anosmia.

Foster-Kennedy syndrome noted with olfactory groove or sphenoid ridge mass and space occupying lesion of frontal lobe is characterized by:

- Ipsilateral anosmia
- Ipsilateral optic atrophy
- Contralateral papilledema.

Pseudo-Foster-Kennedy syndrome is noted when increased intracranial pressure of any cause occurs in patient who has previous unilateral optic atrophy. However, mostly pseudo-Foster-Kennedy syndrome is due to sequential anterior optic neuropathy or optic neuritis in which optic disk atrophies on the other side.

OPTIC NERVE (CRANIAL NERVE II)

Papilledema: Optic disk swelling, manifested by disk hyperemia, blurring of disk margin, loss of venous pulsations **(Fig. 1)** are usually secondary to raised intracranial pressure and can be manifestation of large number of pathological conditions **(Box 1)**.

Visual Pathway Localization (Fig. 2)

Monocular visual loss is usually caused by lesions affecting retina or optic nerve.

Binocular visual loss is seen in lesions localized to or beyond optic chiasm.

Bitemporal field defects are most often due to a compressive mass lesion affecting the optic chiasm, such as pituitary tumor, suprasellar meningiomas, craniopharyngiomas and gliomas.

Binasal hemianopias are usually due to bilateral intraocular disease of retina or optic nerve. Rarely bilateral compression of lateral chiasma may result in binasal defect.

Homonymous hemianopia appears with lesions in the retrochiasmatic pathways, i.e. optic tract, lateral geniculate body, optic radiations or occipital lobe. A host of diseases like tumors, demyelination, trauma *arteriovenous malformation* (AVM), infections, surgery, etc. can lead to homonymous hemianopia.

Superior homonymous quadrantic defects ("pie in the sky" field defects) result from lesion of temporal loop (Meyer's loop) of optic radiation like space occupying lesion (tumor, abscess, hemorrhage), arteriovenous malformation, infections, infarctions, demyelinating disease, trauma, etc.

Inferior quadrantic defects ("pie on the floor" field defects) occur due to involvement of optic radiations in the depth of parietal lobe.

OCULOMOTOR SYSTEM (CRANIAL NERVE III, IV, VI) (TABLE 1)

Supranuclear Lesions

Disturbance of conjugate gaze may be found in association with midbrain, pontine or cerebral lesions.

Destructive lesion of the motor eye field of the frontal lobe (area 8) causes paresis of the gaze to the opposite side, with deviation of eyes towards the side of the lesion, while an irritative lesion (or an epileptic focus) in this region causes strong, rapid involuntary conjugate deviation of the eye to the opposite side.

BOX 1: Syndromes causing increased intracranial pressure and papilledema.

Primary causes

- Hydrocephalus
- *Mass lesions:* Tumor, hemorrhage, large infarction, abscess
- Meningitis/encephalitis
- Subarachnoid hemorrhage
- Trauma
- High flow arteriovenous malformations with overloading venous return
- Intracranial or extracranial venous obstruction
- Pseudotumor cerebri syndrome

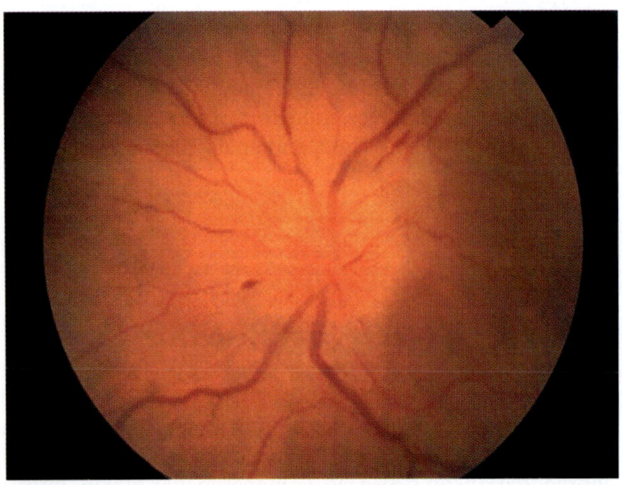

FIG. 1: Fundus photograph showing papilledema.

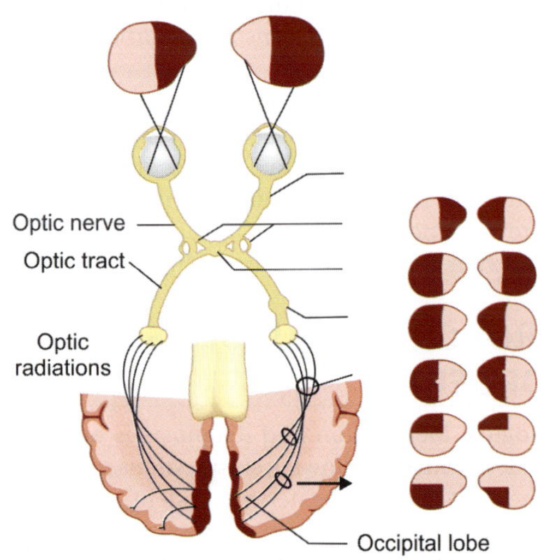

FIG. 2: Visual pathways and field defects.

Parinaud's syndrome is characterized by paralysis of conjugate upward gaze, impairment of convergence. It is seen in lesions at the level of superior colliculi (anterior quadrigeminal bodies), the foretectal region, or the posterior commissure and is found in tumor of pineal glands, encephalitis, multiple sclerosis vascular and other lesions.

Nuclear Lesions

Nuclear involvement of ocular nerves may result from vascular lesions (infarct or hemorrhage), inflammatory lesions, neoplasms, trauma, metabolic disorders, multiple sclerosis, and syringobulbia. There is usually associated involvement of medial longitudinal fasciculus, corticospinal tract, sensory pathways, cerebellar connections, other cranial nerve nuclei, sympathetic pathways, etc.

- *Weber's syndrome:* Caused by involvement of oculomotor nerve as it passes through the cerebral peduncles and produce ipsilateral third nerve paralysis with contralateral paresis of lower face, tongue and extremities.
- *Benedict's syndrome:* Caused by lesion of midbrain involving third nerve as it passes through the red nucleus. It is characterized by an ipsilateral oculomotor paralysis with contralateral ataxia, tremor and hyperkinesias of upper extremity.
- *Nothnagel's syndrome:* There is unilateral oculomotor paralysis combined with ipsilateral ataxia due to involvement of third nerve and brachium conjunctivum.
- *Millard-Gubler syndrome:* There is ipsilateral lateral rectus paralysis, ipsilateral facial paralysis with contralateral hemiplegia.
- *Raymond's syndrome:* Consists of an ipsilateral sixth nerve paralysis and contralateral hemiplegia.
- *Foville's syndrome:* Ipsilateral gaze paralysis, facial paralysis with contralateral hemiplegia. There is contralateral deviation of eyes and head.

Internuclear Ophthalmoplegia

Paralysis of adduction of the contralateral eye, together with variable paresis and monocular nystagmus of the abducting eye. Internuclear ophthalmoplegia (INO) is found in brainstem lesions and is seen with multiple sclerosis, vascular, neoplastic, inflammatory or degenerative lesions

TABLE 1: Localization of lesions of ocular motor nerves.

Location	Symptoms	Signs
Extraocular muscle/ orbit	Eye swelling Monocular vision loss Dry eyes	• Periorbital edema • Conjunctival injection and chemosis • Proptosis • Eyelid retraction • Lagophthalmos (inability to close the eye completely) Lid lag (higher than normal lid position in downgaze) • Von Graefe's sign (dynamic slowing of lid descent during eye movement from upgaze into downgaze) • Optic neuropathy (from optic nerve compression)
Neuromuscular junction	• Fluctuating symptoms • Proximal muscle • Weakness • Shortness of breath • Swallowing difficulty • Worsening at night or with exercise	• Moment-to-moment or visit-to-visit variability • Fatigue of lids or eye elevation with prolonged upgaze • Cogan's lid twitch • Peek sign • Orbicularis oculi weakness • Ptosis and enhanced ptosis
Cranial nerve	Arm and leg weakness	Contralateral hemiparesis: pyramidal tract
Brainstem	• Clumsiness or imbalance • Facial numbness or tingling • Facial weakness	• *Ataxia:* Cerebella peduncle • *Ipsilateral facial sensory loss:* Trigeminal tracts and nuclei • *Upper and lower facial weakness:* Facial nerve fasciculus and nucleus
Cranial nerve Subarachnoid space	Stiff neck Vision loss Headache	• Kernig's and Brudzinski's signs • Papilledema
Cranial nerve	Facial numbness and tingling	Ipsilateral facial sensory loss in the first (V1) and second (V2) trigeminal distributions
Cavernous sinus cranial nerve	Facial numbness and tingling	• *Ipsilateral Horner's syndrome:* Sympathetic fibers • Ipsilateral facial sensory loss in the first (V1) trigeminal distribution
Orbital apex	Eye prominence	Proptosis
Supranuclear	• Arm and leg weakness • Clumsiness or imbalance • Facial numbness or tingling • Facial weakness	• *Contralateral hemiparesis:* Pyramidal tract • *Ataxia:* Cerebellar peduncle • *Ipsilateral facial sensory loss:* Trigeminal tracts and nuclei • *Upper and lower facial weakness:* Facial nerve fasciculus • *Ocular motility:* Saccades affected greater than smooth pursuit; vestibulo-ocular reflexes spared

of the brainstem or compression of latter by neoplasms of the posterior fossa. There are usually symptoms and signs indicating involvement of neighboring centers and pathways.

Infranuclear Lesions

These may be caused by lesions within skull, middle cranial fossa, cavernous sinus, superior orbital fissure or orbit. Involvement in the skull may be produced by meningitis, trauma, subarachnoid hemorrhage, etc.

Cavernous sinus thrombosis consists of ipsilateral ptosis, chemosis, edema of eyelids and orbital tissue, paralysis of third, fourth, sixth cranial nerves, involvement of upper division of trigeminal nerve, and at times papilledema.

In *superior orbital fissure syndrome*, including Tolosa-Hunt syndrome, there is usually painful ophthalmoplegia with or without vision loss. It may also result from sphenoid sinusitis, skull fractures, etc.

Other Disorders of Oculomotor System

- *Nystagmus:* Involuntary oscillation or trembling of the eyeball. It can be congenital or acquired.
  - *Vestibular nystagmus* is caused by either irritation or destruction of semicircular canals, vestibular nerve or vestibular nuclei. It is a fine nystagmus, usually associated with vertigo.
  - *Cerebellar nystagmus* indicates that vestibulocerebellar pathways are affected, i.e. either the vermis or the inferior cerebellar peduncle, though can be seen in cerebellar hemispheric lesions. It is usually a coarse type of nystagmus.
  - Other *central nystagmus* is produced mainly by lesions affecting structures in the region of fourth ventricle or brainstem principally zone between oculomotor nuclei and vestibular nuclei.
  - *Downbeat nystagmus* is seen in brainstem lesions, especially in craniovertebral junction anomalies.
  - *Upbeat nystagmus* is usually caused by lesions of anterior vermis of the cerebellum though can be seen in any brainstem lesion.
  - *See-saw nystagmus,* in which one eye moves upward while the other moves down, is seen in patients with tumors of suprasellar region or anterior third ventricle.
- *Opsoclonus:* Coarse, irregular, nonrhythmic, agitated oscillations of eyes in both horizontal and vertical planes. These have been observed in encephalitis, cerebellar or brainstem disorders, comatose states, metabolic encephalopathies or as part of "paraneoplastic syndromes".
- *Ocular bobbing:* Coarse, synchronous, downward "bobbing" movements of eyes are observed in coma with pontine lesions and is of grave significance.

TRIGEMINAL NERVE (CRANIAL NERVE V)

The fifth nerve may be affected by lesions of brainstem or outside it at different level, by tumor of the cerebellopontine angle, tumors of base of skull, lesions within cavernous sinus, infections of petrous bone, orbital cellulitis, etc.

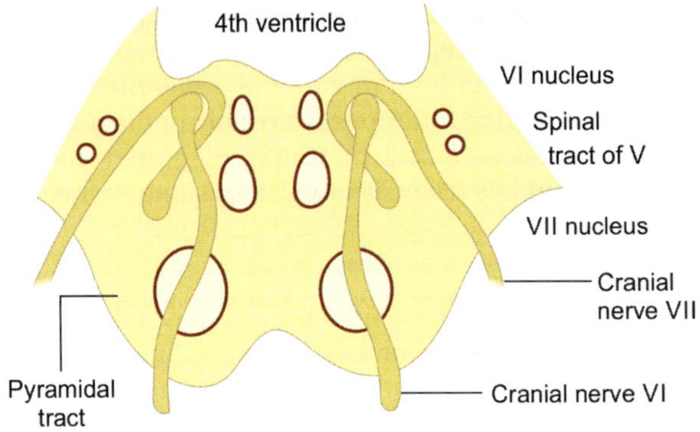

FIG. 3: Facial nerve course in pons.

Trigeminal neuralgia (tic douloureux), characterized by sudden attacks of excruciating, lancinating pain, is usually caused by vascular pressure on the nerve outside the brainstem but can also be a presenting symptom of multiple sclerosis, syringobulbia, herpes zoster and cerebellopontine angle tumor.

FACIAL NERVE (CRANIAL NERVE VII)

Localization of Facial Nerve Lesions (Fig. 3)

Supranuclear Palsy

Supranuclear palsy is the paresis of lower part of the face with relative sparing of upper part. There are two varieties of central facial palsy: (1) Volitional and (2) *emotional* type.

In *volitional palsy*, the involvement is most marked on voluntary contraction (like baring teeth, etc.) while on involuntary contractions such as smiling, crying, etc. There is preservation of function with no evidence of paresis. This variety of volitional palsy is seen in lesions of cortical center in the lower-third of precentral convolution or pathways between this center and nucleus of facial nerve.

In *emotional or mimetic* type of facial palsy, the impairment is most marked on smiling or weeping, though the patient can voluntarily retract his mouth. This type of palsy is considered to be result of deep seated lesion in extrapyramidal, basal ganglia, thalamus, or hypothalamus or frontal lobe lesions anterior to precentral convolution.

Masked facies are seen in Parkinson's disease and other Parkinsonian syndromes. There is loss of associated movements like infrequent blinking and smiling.

Infranuclear Facial Nerve Palsy

It can occur in variety of conditions but the most common is *Bell's palsy*. In this condition, both upper and lower part of face is involved and patient is unable to close the eyes on the affected side. *Bell's phenomenon*, i.e. eyeball turns upward and cornea is hidden, when the patient attempts to close eyes on involved side.

VESTIBULOCOCHLEAR NERVE (CRANIAL NERVE VIII)

Vertigo is a sensation of movement and is often accompanied by feelings of unsteadiness and loss of balance. True organic or vestibular vertigo is usually rotator in type and has been described as *Objective*, if the external objects seem to be rotating around the individual, and as *Subjective*, if the individual himself is rotating. The presence of associated symptoms, like nausea, vomiting, staggering, deviation of eyes, disturbance of balance, tinnitus, hearing loss, effect of change of posture are important clues to localization.

In general, vertigo of *peripheral origin* is usually episodic in character, aggravated by change in posture, and accompanied by nystagmus, which that of *central origin* is more apt to be continuous, less clearly defined and may not be accompanied by nystagmus and there may be evidence of other CNS changes.

Deafness, tinnitus, and vertigo are important presenting symptoms of cerebellopontine angle neoplasms, usually a neurinoma or a neurofibroma.

Partial deafness may be an early symptom of a tumor of *glomus jugulare* (chemodectoma), later there may be tinnitus, vertigo, and involvement of other cranial nerves (facial, vagus and others).

GLOSSOPHARYNGEAL AND VAGUS NERVE (CRANIAL NERVE IX, X)

Lesions of these nerves lead to dysarthria and dysphagia, with associated nasal regurgitation of fluids and nasal intonation of voice. Examination reveals asymmetrical movement of uvula and impaired or absent gag reflex and palatal reflex.

Supranuclear involvement leads to pseudobulbar palsy with associated dysphagia and dysarthria. In this condition, the gag, palatal and jaw jerk reflexes are brisk.

Nuclear involvement occurs in a variety of vascular, demyelinating, neoplastic, degenerative conditions.

Wallenberg's syndrome (lateral medullary syndrome), caused by occlusion of posterior inferior cerebellar artery (PICA) or vertebral artery, leads to acute dysphagia, dysarthria, ipsilateral anesthesia of face, ipsilateral Horner's syndrome, ipsilateral cerebellar hypotonia and asynergy, with contralateral loss of pain and temperature sensation on limbs and trunk **(Fig. 4)**.

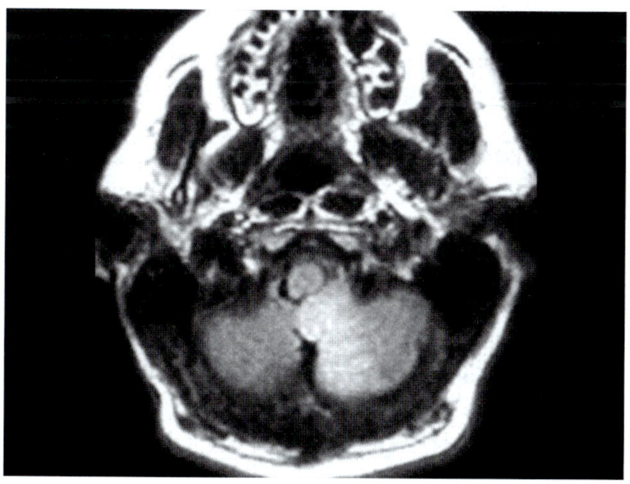

FIG. 4: Magnetic resonance imaging of the brain (T2WI) showing left lateral medullary syndrome.

Infranuclear involvement may follow lesions at the base of skull, jugular foramen or along the course of vagus nerve.

Syndrome of Vernet, caused by lesion at the jugular foramen, is characterized by ipsilateral paralysis of ninth, tenth and eleventh nerves. It is usually of traumatic origin and follows basilar skull fracture; however, vascular or neoplastic lesions may also cause this syndrome.

Syndrome of Villaret is the result of lesion in the retropharyngeal space and results in paralysis of ninth-tenth, eleventh and twelfth nerve and Horner's syndrome.

Palatal Myoclonus

Palatal myoclonus is a rhythmic movement of palate and associated muscles, in frequency of 50–240/min. It probably results from brainstem lesion with interruption of connections between the inferior olivary body, dentate nucleus and red nucleus (*The triangle of Guillain and Mollaret*).

SPINAL ACCESSORY NERVE (CRANIAL NERVE XI)

The lesion of this nerve causes paralysis of sternocleido-mastoid and trapezius muscles.

More commonly hyperkinetic manifestation with tonic or clonic spasm of the muscles is encountered. The muscle contraction of sternomastoid pulls head and occiput to one side and face to opposite side (*Torticollis*).

There are many causes of torticollis: congenital, structural, traumatic and myogenic factors; Klippel-Feil syndrome, rickets, cervical arthritis, spina bifida, trauma, etc. Reflex torticollis may be secondary to vascular lesions, tumor, cervical lymph node metastasis, retrotonsillar abscess, etc. Disorders of extrapyramidal system, especially of the basal ganglia, are probably the most common causes of neurologic torticollis.

HYPOGLOSSAL NERVE (CRANIAL NERVE XII)

This nerve supplies the muscles of tongue. Lesions cause weakness and atrophy of the tongue muscles and may be seen in a variety of lesions in brainstem (neoplasm, vascular, granuloma, multiple sclerosis); within the skull (like meningitis, neoplasm), basilar invagination, Arnold-Chiari malformation; in the hypoglossal canal or in neck (trauma, tumor, vascular lesions).

DISORDERS OF MOTOR SYSTEM

Motor function is a complex process and involves many areas of the CNS, like cerebral cortex, basal ganglia, cerebellum, and reticular activating system in addition to the final common spinomuscular pathway. Lesions of any of the constituent portions of motor system lead to walking difficulty/weakness. The classical features of upper motor neuron lesion versus lower motor neuron are tabulated in **Table 2**.

The examination of motor system involves:
- Inspection for muscle bulk, wasting, fasciculation
- Power for objective weakness
- Tone for any increase or decrease in tone

TABLE 2: Upper motor neuron versus lower motor neuron signs.

Clinical test	Upper motor neuron	Lower motor neuron
Reflexes	Hyper-reflexia	Hyporeflexia
Muscle tone	Increased/spastic	Decreased/flaccid
Fasciculation	None	Present
Atrophy	None	Severe
Babinski sign	Present	Absent

- Tendon reflexes for any attenuated or exaggerated reflexes
- Coordination
- Gait *per se* can give important clue to the localization and diagnosis.

Muscle Bulk

Localized wasting or fasciculation in the weak limb indicates either radicular or anterior horn cell involvement, as well as plexus or nerve involvement. Focal wasting has great localizing value and can be seen in syringomyelia, cord tumors, spondylosis, motor neuron disease, etc.

Power Testing

It is done in individual group of muscles and is graded from Grade 0 (no contraction) to Grade V (normal power), as per Medical Research Council (MRC) grading.

Muscle Tone

It is the resistance to passive movement, when the patient is asked to relax. Tone is a reflex phenomenon and involves alpha motor and gamma efferent fibers. The tone is usually tested by supination-pronation of the forearm; flexion and extension of elbow and dorsiflexion and plantar flexion of wrist joint. In lower limbs, passive flexion and extension of hip, knee and ankle joint is done to assess the tone. Other soft signs of documenting abnormal tone are:

- *Pronator sign*: In the presence of hypotonia with cerebellar lesions, there is tendency of the hands to assume a position of pronation, when the arms are outstretched horizontally.
- *Pronator drift sign*: With eyes closed, the patient holds both arms outstretched in front of him. The elbows should be fully extended, the wrist extended and the hands open with palms up. In the presence of mild hemiparesis (there is mild increase in tone), there may be slow pronation of wrist, slight flexion of elbows and fingers, downward and lateral drift of the hand.

Various pathological conditions can cause either decrease (hypotonia) or increase in tone (hypertonia).

Hypotonia is usually seen in lesions involving spinomuscular level, proprioceptive pathways, cerebellar lesions and choreas.

Hypertonia is caused by interruption of impulses from supraspinal regions. Two types of hypertonia are observed clinically: (1) spasticity, and (2) rigidity.

Spasticity

This is seen with corticospinal lesions. There is *clasp knife* type of resistance, where there is elastic, spring like resistance to stretching at beginning of movement, which continues till certain point and then suddenly the muscle relaxes. Occasionally, spasticity is so marked that the examiner cannot passively move the extremity. The level of corticospinal tract affliction is generally based on associated symptoms and signs.

Extrapyramidal Rigidity

Lesions of extrapyramidal system produces either *lead pipe or cog wheel rigidity*. In this type of hypertonia, there is same degree of resistance in entire range of movement and is seen in both flexor and extensor groups. Often there is intermittent yielding of muscles to stretching.

Rigidity of this kind is seen in Parkinson's disease and other Parkinsonian syndromes. Parkinsonism is characterized by bradykinesia, tremor and rigidity. A large variety of Parkinsonian syndrome produce these symptoms and can be distinguished from Parkinson's disease by a variety of clinical and other diagnostic tests.

- *Idiopathic Parkinson's disease* is characterized by asymmetric onset rigidity, tremor and bradykinesia. Cognition is preserved till late stage and no gross dysautonomia is observed. Usually magnetic resonance imaging (MRI) of brain reveals age-related atrophic change.
- *Multisystem atrophy* is characterized by associated severe dysautonomia, affecting bowel, bladder and postural hypotension. MRI reveals cruciform hyperintensity in pons ("hot cross bun" sign) **(Fig. 5)**.
- *Progressive supranuclear palsy* is characterized by recurrent falls (usually backward), with predominant axial rigidity. There is severe upgaze and downgaze restriction and in later stages lateral gaze restriction is seen. MRI reveals atrophy of the rostral midbrain tegmentum, the pontine base, giving hummingbird appearance on midsagittal view.

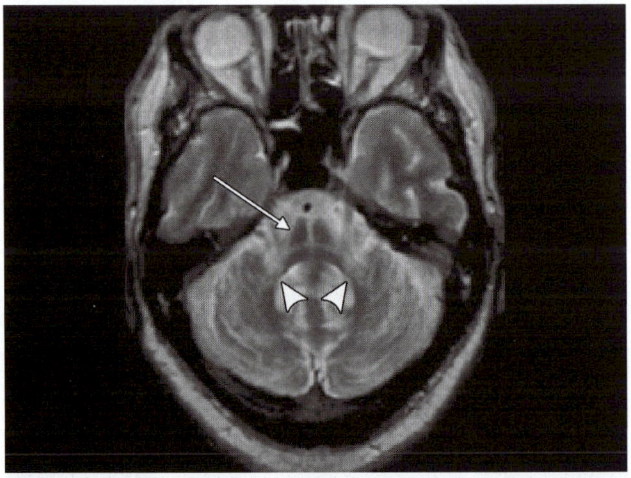

FIG. 5: Magnetic resonance imaging of the brain showing "hot cross bun" sign in *multiple-system atrophy* (MSA).

Reflexes

Reflex action requires a stimulus, a sensory pathway, a link with motor unit, motor neuron and finally, a contractile or other effector element. Any breach in this arc results in an absent reflex. Commonly used tendon reflexes are discussed below.

Biceps Jerk

Press forefinger gently on biceps tendon in antecubital fossa and then strike the finger with the hammer.

Normal Result

Flexion of elbow with visible contraction of biceps muscle.

Segmental Innervations

C5; Peripheral nerve: Musculocutaneous.

Supinator Jerk

Strike lower end of radius 5 cm above the wrist.

Normal Result

Contraction of brachioradialis and flexion of elbow.

Segmental Innervations

C5, C6; Peripheral nerve: Radial.

Triceps Jerk

Strike the triceps 5 cm above elbow, held in midflexed position.

Normal Result

Extension of elbow and visible contraction of triceps.

Segmental Innervations

C6, C7; Peripheral nerve: Radial.

Knee Jerk

Tap the patellar tendon in midflexed position of knee.

Normal Result

Extension of knee and contraction of quadriceps.

Segmental Innervations

L 3-4; Peripheral nerve: Femoral.

Ankle Jerk

Achilles tendon is struck after dorsiflexing the ankle.

Normal Result

Plantar flexion of the foot and contraction of gastrocnemius.

Segmental Innervations

S1; Peripheral nerve: Medial popliteal.

Hoffman Reflex

The terminal phalanx of the patient's middle finger is flicked downwards between examiner's finger and thumb. In hyper-reflexia, the tips of other fingers flex and the thumb flexes and adduct.

Abnormalities of Tendon Reflexes

- *Hyper-reflexia* is usually seen in pyramidal tract lesions but can also be seen in agitation, anxiety and fear.
- *Clonus* indicates marked degree of reflex excitability and usually means pyramidal system disease.
- *Absent reflex* indicates breach in a part of reflex arc either in sensory nerve, root or anterior horn cell, anterior root, peripheral nerve, etc. The other differences in upper versus lower motor neuron lesions are summarized in **Table 2**.
- *Inverted supinator reflex*: When supinator jerk is tested, there is no contraction of brachioradialis or biceps and only exaggerated finger flexion is seen. It indicates cord lesion at fourth or fifth cervical level, as in disk disease, syringomyelia, cervical neoplasm, etc.

Superficial Reflexes

Abdominal Reflexes

Lightly stroking the abdomen from without inwards in all four quadrants of abdomen.

Normal Result

The muscles of the quadrant stimulated contract and umbilicus moves in that direction.

Segmental Innervations

Upper abdominal, T9-10; midabdominal, T10-11; lower abdominal, T11-12.

The abdominal reflexes are usually absent in pyramidal tract lesions, though they may normally be absent in obese individuals and multiparous women.

Cremasteric Reflex

Inner part of thigh is stroked in downward and inward direction.

Normal Result

The contraction of cremasteric muscle pulls up the scrotum and testicle on the side examined.

Segmental Innervations

L1-2.

Anal Reflex

Lightly scratch the perianal skin.

Normal Result

Contraction of external anal sphincter.

Segmental Innervations

S4-5.

Plantar Reflex

Babinski Sign

Extension of great toe with fanning of other toes on striking the outer aspects of foot with blunt key.

Other Important Reflexes

Grasp Reflex

Place first and second finger between the thumb and forefingers of patient's hand and try to draw them lightly away. If grasp reflex is present, the fingers will be held tightly by the patient's hand. It is due to bilateral corticospinal tract involvement, usually seen in neurodegenerative diseases like Alzheimer's disease, multi-infarct state, tumor or vascular accidents in the premotor cortex.

Forced Grasping Reflex

Lightly and repeatedly touching the side of palm results in hand following the stimulus and attempting to grasp it and is usually seen in widespread cerebral lesions. In advanced cases, patient may try to follow the movement of hand (*Groping reflex*).

Sucking Reflex

Touching the corner of mouth produces a sucking movement of the lips and is seen in widespread hemispheric lesions.

Glabellar Tap

Tapping at root of nose is accompanied by synchronous blinking and is commonly seen in Parkinson's disease.

Coordination

For proper coordination, both sensory and motor system should be intact. Various tests used to test coordination are:

Finger Nose Test

Each arm is drawn out to full abduction, with forefinger pointed. Patient is asked to alternatively touch the nose tip with his finger and the examiner's finger. In cerebellar disease, the finger moves to the nose in a wavering side to side or up and down fashion.

Heel-Knee Test

The patient is told to run heel down the front of shin to the top of the foot. In cerebellar disease, the heel overshoots the knee sideways and develops rotating oscillation as it approaches it.

Dysdiadochokinesis

There is failure to efficiently perform rapid alternating movements. Patient is asked to rotate hands rapidly at wrists, holding the forearms vertically, with elbows flexed. In cerebellar disease, the movements will be coarse, irregular and slow.

Past Pointing Test

Patient sits holding his arm forward, so that his fingers touch fingers of the examiner. Then he is asked to lower or raise the arm above head and bring it back to original position. In cerebellar disease, the arm on the side of lesion will deviate outwards towards the side of lesion.

Sensory System

The various modalities of sensation tested in clinical neurology are:

- Pain, light touch and temperature. These are *exteroceptive sensations* derived from sources outside the body.
- Sense of position, passive movement, vibration and deep pain. These are the *proprioceptive sensation* derived from the body itself.
- Stereognosis and graphesthesia are two point of discrimination. These are the cortical sensations.
- It is wise to move from area of impaired sensation to normal sensation, for the change is easier to detect.
- The common patterns of sensory loss with localizing value are:
  - *Total unilateral loss* of all forms of sensation is seen in extensive lesion of thalamus or internal capsule.
  - *Unilateral hyperalgesia* and hyperesthesia follows partial lesions of thalamus.
  - *Crossed hemisensory loss*, on face on one side and body on opposite side, is seen in lesions of medulla (lateral medullary syndrome).
  - *Bilateral loss of all sensations* below a definite level is seen in gross lesion of spinal cord.
  - *Suspended sensory loss*: Impairment of pain and temperature sensation over several segments with normal sensation above and below are seen in intrinsic lesion of the cord, like syringomyelia and intrinsic cord tumor.
  - *Saddle anesthesia*: Impairment of sensation over the lowest sacral segments is seen in cauda equina/conus medullaris lesion.
- Unilateral loss of pain and temperature below a definite level is seen in Brown-Sèquard syndrome of hemisection of cord, as in compression or demyelination.
- *Glove and stocking anesthesia* is seen in peripheral neuropathy.
- *Patchy areas* of sensory loss can be seen in a nerve or radicular distribution.
- *Romberg's sign*: The patient sways from the heels, when the eyes are closed, after making the patient stand with feet opposed. This is characteristic of proprioceptive deficiency (large fiber neuropathy or affliction of dorsal columns).

Gait

At the end of the clinical examination, the patient should be made to walk for few meters. Note the posture of the body while walking, the position and movements of the arms, legs, the distance between feet, the regularity of movement, the ability to maintain a straight course, the ease of turning and stopping. The various gaits of clinical significance are:

- *Dragging of feet*: The patient who drags one foot usually has an upper motor neuron lesion of that leg. In the presence of marked hemiparesis, he will throw the whole leg outwards from the hip, producing the movement called *"circumduction"*. This is usually seen following hemiplegia of any cause.
- *Scissoring gait*: In bilateral upper motor neuron lesions, both feet drag, steps are slow and short, the gait is

stiff legged. The feet tend to cross in "scissor" fashion, most commonly seen in spastic diplegia of childhood.

- *High stepping gait*: The patient raises the foot high to overcome a foot drop; the toe hits the ground first. This gait occurs in lumbosacral root, cauda equina lesions or peripheral nerve lesions causing anterior tibial muscle paralysis.
- *Stamping gait*: The heels tend to strike the floor first and result from loss of position sense, when the patient does not know where his foot is. The abnormality is increased in dark. This is seen in sensory neuropathies or disorders of posterior columns.
- *Shuffling gait*: Movement is a series of small, flat footed shuffles is commonly seen in extrapyramidal syndromes, particularly Parkinson's disease. The steps become quicker as the movement progresses (festination).
- *Gait apraxia*: The gait is irregular and hesitant with small stepped shuffling. The patient may lean backwards rather than forwards. This type of gait is seen in syndrome of normal pressure hydrocephalus (NPH) and can also be seen in multi-infarct states.
- *Ataxic gait*: The patient tends to reel and sway as if drunk and is seen in cerebellar diseases.
- *Waddling gait*: The pelvis is rotated through an abnormally large arc, accompanied by compensatory movements of upper trunk and associated with marked lordosis. This is usually seen in myopathies.
- *Hysterical gaits*: Bizarre gait, which varies from moment to moment and can be altered by suggestion.

DISORDERS OF HIGHER MENTAL FUNCTION

DISORDERS OF SPEECH

Two main types of speech defects are encountered in neurological disorders: (1) Dysarthria and (2) dysphasia (aphasia).

Dysarthria

When the articulation and enunciation of individual words and phrases is distorted, this is dysarthria. Articulation requires coordination of tongue, lips, palate, larynx and muscles of respiration and may be affected by lesions of upper and lower motor neuron, extrapyramidal and cerebellar systems. Various types of dysarthria are:

- *Spastic dysarthria*: This is caused by lesions of bilateral upper motor neuron. The tongue is small and spastic. The speech is slurred, as if the patient is talking from the back of the throat.
- *Rigid dysarthria*: Speech is monotonous, all inflections and accents disappear, and words run into one another. This is a result of extrapyramidal lesion.
- *Ataxic dysarthria*: Speech is irregular, slurred and drunken. The rhythm is jerky, sometimes explosive, staccato or scanning. This is a result of cerebellar disease.
- Weakness of facial, palatal, tongue muscles can also produce dysarthria. There is nasal intonation of speech in bulbar palsy.

Dysphasia

When the patient is failing to put into properly constructed words or phrases the thoughts he wishes to express, even if articulation is adequate, then it is called dysphasia (or aphasia). Evaluation of dysphasia includes assessment of spontaneous speech, comprehension, naming objects, repetition, reading, writing and calculation. Various types of dysphasias are:

- *Broca's aphasia*: Speech is nonfluent with preserved comprehension, poor repetition and naming ability. Usually seen in an infarct in the territory of anterior part of the left middle cerebral artery.
- *Wernicke's aphasia*: Speech is fluent with profoundly affected comprehension, impaired repetition. Naming is poor. The patient produces jumbled string of meaningless words and neologisms. Posterior left middle cerebral artery territory infarction is the most common cause with damage to the posterior third of superior temporal gyrus.
- *Transcortical aphasia*: There is retained repetition with fluent or nonfluent aphasia.
- *Echolalia*: Involuntary repetition of words and phrases spoken by someone else. The lesion lies in the temporo-parietal region.
- *Pure word deafness*: Patient cannot recognize the spoken word. This is due to a lesion in the middle of first temporal gyrus.
- *Pure word dumbness*: This is an apraxic speech defect with inability to articulate. The lesion may be widespread in the left hemisphere. Usually reading, writing, and copying are preserved.
- *Alexia*: Inability to understand written material. There is lesion in left occipital cortex and splenium of corpus callosum. There is associated right homonymous hemianopia and is seen in infarction of posterior cerebral artery.
- *Alexia with agraphia*: The patient cannot read or write spontaneously. The lesion lies in the left angular gyrus and is usually accompanied by nominal aphasia, acalculia, hemianopia and visual agnosia.
- *Agraphia*: Pure writing defect may occur in lesion that lies between angular gyrus and motor area.
- *Acalculia*: Inability to calculate may be seen in lesions of left angular gyrus.

APRAXIA

Inability to carry out well organized voluntary movement correctly despite the fact that motor, sensory, coordinative functions are not significantly impaired. Four types of apraxia are commonly recognized.

1. *Ideomotor apraxia*: Inability to imitate or mime an act involving use of objects. There is lesion between dominant parietal lobe and motor area.

2. *Ideational apraxia*: Carrying out a whole of complex act is defective though execution of different parts of complete act may be normal.
3. *Constructional apraxia*: Inability to make or copy simple designs. The lesion is in the angular gyrus of either hemisphere but when isolated, is usually from nondominant parietal lesions.
4. *Dressing apraxia*: The patient is unable to dress or undress himself in the absence of motor or sensory deficit. The lesion is usually in nondominant posterior parietal lobe lesions.

AGNOSIA

Failure to recognize some object or sound, when the sense by which it is normally recognized remains intact.

Visual Agnosia

The patient is unable to name or describe the use of the objects shown but is able to identify them, when he touches them. The site of lesion lies in second and third occipital gyri and the adjacent subcortical white matter in the dominant hemisphere.

The patient may be unable to find his way around an obstruction or find his way to a given point. This type of visual disorientation is seen in bilateral posteroinferior parietal lesions or in the nondominant hemispheric affliction.

Tactile Agnosia

The patient may be unable to recognize an object, by touching but is able to give its name on seeing. The patient with true tactile agnosia is able to describe its shape, size, texture. The site of lesion is in contralateral supramarginal gyrus or in corpus callosum.

Auditory Agnosia

The patient who is unable to recognize the sound, but can recognize the object on sight or touch, has auditory agnosia. The site of the lesion is in the posterior part of the temporal convolutions of the dominant hemisphere.

PARIETAL LOBE DYSFUNCTIONS

- *Right left disorientation*: Patient is unable to correctly point towards the right or left side of the body in parietal lobe lesion.
- *Autotopagnosia*: Patient is unable to identify any part of the body.
- *Finger agnosia*: Inability to pick out individual digit is termed finger agnosia.
- *Gerstmann syndrome*: It consists of finger agnosia, acalculia, right-left disorientation and agraphia without alexia and is found in lesions of the dominant hemisphere in the region of angular gyrus.
- *Anosognosia*: Complete lack of awareness of opposite half of the body is seen in lesions of parietal lobe of nondominant hemisphere.
- *Sensory inattention*: Bilateral stimulation by visual, auditory or tactile stimuli may result in inattention in one of the fields, though can be appreciated when stimuli are given in individual fields. This phenomenon of inattention is commonly seen in parietal lobe lesion, usually after vascular accidents, or tumor of the contralateral hemisphere.

CONCLUSION

The importance of neurologic examination in the diagnosis of diseases of the nervous system cannot be overemphasized. Neurological examination is a time consuming and tiring exercise for both patient as well as physicians. However, a good history and proper examination can localize the disease process accurately and based on the temporal course of the disease a likely etiology can be postulated. This exercise helps in judicious use of ancillary investigations including radiology.

SUGGESTED READING

1. Brazis PW, Masdeu JC, Biller J. Localization in Clinical Neurology, 5th edition. Philadelphia, USA: Lippincott Williams & Wilkins. 2007.
2. Haerer AF. DeJong's The Neurologic Examination, 6th edition. Philadelphia, USA: Lippincott-Raven. 2005.
3. Hauser SL. Harrison's Neurology in Clinical Medicine. USA: McGraw Hill Professional. 2006.
4. Patten J. Neurological Differential Diagnosis, 2nd edition. New York, USA: Springer-Verlag. 2000.
5. Spillane J. Bickerstaff's Neurological Examination in Clinical Practice, 6th edition. USA: Wiley-Blackwell. 1996.

CHAPTER

217

Basic Neuropathology

Kirti Gupta, Rakesh Kumar Vasishta

REMOVAL OF THE BRAIN FROM SKULL

The most common method of removal of brain from the skull involves a reflection of the scalp followed by the removal of a generous cap of bone using a circumferential saw-cut. The left covering of the brain is called dura. This is the stage at which the superior longitudinal sinus can be tested in two ways: either by opening it or by simply running a fingertip along it and examining any motion of the surrounding blood. When the brain is suspended by the basilar artery, each side of the dura is incised and reflected medially, piercing through the bridging veins with knife or scissors. After dividing the anterior attachment of the falx, the dura is reflected backwards. The frontal lobes are lifted very gently from the base of the anterior cranial fossa, while trying to ensure that the olfactory bulbs remain attached to the brain. The optic nerves, internal carotid arteries (ICA), oculomotor nerves and pituitary stalk are cut neatly across close to the base, when they become visible. The tentorium is uncovered, first on one side then on other, by delicately lifting the temporal lobes; and the attachments of the tentorium to the petrous temporal bones are cut with a sharp knife. As a result of the piercing of the dura, the same cut will separate the roots of the trigeminal, facial and the auditory nerves. In the gap which shows up between the clivus and the pons, the visible abducents nerves are cut. The lower cranial nerves and the vertebral arteries, which are still holding the brainstem down are cut, either with a knife or with long-bladed scissors, without causing any damage to the lower brainstem. This can usually be carried out blind, but cutting as far as possible to each side. After the cutting of vertebral arteries, the lower brainstem and upper cervical cord become visible, thus making it possible to cut across with the knife. After this, a number of bridging veins remain, including the great vein of Galen, which performs the function of draining blood from the deeper cerebral gray matter into the straight sinus. Throughout the whole procedure, the brain should be held by the left hand very carefully, so that the tension and distortion remain at a minimum level. Once it is free, the brain should only be placed with its base upwards in a bucket of a suitable size containing buffered formalin, instead of a flat surface. It is gently suspended by a thread passing through the basilar artery and the ends of the thread are tied to the bucket handle.

REMOVAL OF VENOUS SINUS, CAVERNOUS SINUS AND MIDDLE EAR EXAMINATION

After removal of the brain all abnormalities in the dura at the base of the cranial cavity is noted and the patency of the principal venous sinuses (straight, lateral, sigmoid, superior longitudinal) is examined. A hammer and chisel are used for checking the internal carotid artery (ICA), the ear drums and middle ears. The chisel is applied to the base of the middle cranial fossa and a sharp hit with the hammer then displays the middle ear drum and ICA lying within the carotid canal, which can lead to the wall of the cavernous sinus. In the similar way, after removing the pituitary and the sphenoid sinus the frontal and ethmoidal sinuses are opened and demonstrated.

A vibrating saw is used for removing a square piece of sphenoid block for the cavernous sinus. The portion includes the area around the pituitary fossa containing the parts of ICA, optic tracts, cranial nerves—III, V, VI.

EXAMINATION OF THE BRAIN

After its removal, the brain is fixed in 20% buffered, neutral formalin for the duration of 10–14 days. The fixed brain is then weighed (usually the weight of brain is slightly higher than when unfixed). The normal brain weight ranges from 1,100 g to 1,600 g for males and 1,050–1,500 g for females.

Gross Features to be Noted

- *Meninges*:
    - For exudates
- *Gyri and sulci*:
    - For flattening and narrowing of sulci-cerebral edema
    - Narrowing and thinning of gyri—atrophy
- *Convexities/surface*:
    - *For exudates*:
        - Pyogenic meningitis

- *Enlargement*:
  - Unilateral (space occupying lesion)
  - Bilateral (bilateral lesions, cerebral edema)
- Atrophy of frontal lobes—senile atrophy

- *Base of brain*:
  - *Exudate*:
    - Tubercular meningitis
    - Mucoid—both at base and at convexities (cryptococcal meningitis)
  - *Circle of Willis*:
    - For aneurysm
    - For emboli—in case of stroke the most common sites being the bifurcation of an ICA and the origin of a branch of a middle cerebral artery (MCA)
    - Sites of atheromatous narrowing should be noted
  - Mammillary bodies and optic chiasm-atrophy (alcohol induced)
  - Uncal notching and tonsillar herniation
  - Atrophy of brainstem
  - Cerebellum—cerebellar atrophy
    - Ataxia, chronic debilitating illness.

Slicing of Brain

- *Coronal slicing*: Normally, the first incision separates the hindbrain (brainstem and cerebellum) from the cerebral hemispheres. This should be done with a clean transverse cut across the midbrain, just in front of the third nerve, at right angles to the long axis of the brainstem. The first cut passes through the optic chiasm or mammillary bodies, going through the anterior margin of the thalamus. The anterior part of the cerebrum is then placed to be cut surface down, between a pair of centimeter (or less) guides, and successive slices taken at centimeter intervals or less and laid out, posterior surface upward, with the right side on the right. The same procedure is repeated on the posterior part.
- In the cases which have undergone computerized tomography (CT) scans during their life are preferably sliced at the alternative-horizontal plane because that clearly shows the contrast between the actual and radiographic slices. Usually, the initial cut for horizontal slicing is at level of the upward end of the Sylvian fissure. The slices are spread out, upper surface upward, with right side facing right.
- *Hindbrain dissection*: After serving the midbrain, a clear observation of the occurrence of the transtentorial herniation becomes possible or not. It is visible in the following signs:
  - Excessive grooving of the parahippocampal gyrus, on one side or both, and
  - Lateral compression of the upper brainstem.

    There are two commonly practiced routines for slicing the hindbrain. The first, which is also the most commonly followed, involves cutting through the upper medulla at the level of the lateral apertures (foramina of Luschka) in a plane vertical to the long axis of the medulla, and continuing the cut through the cerebellum. This displays an extremely broad view of the *fourth ventricle*, the dentate nuclei, and the flocculi, uvula and nodulus of the cerebellum. Further cuts are made through the lower part of the specimen, using 5 mm guides or free-hand slices 3–4 mm apart, until it ends. On the other hand, if the interest is intended for the regional differences between areas of cerebellum, the alternate method can be applied. Oblique cuts are made to separate the cerebellum from the brainstem. These cuts pass through the cerebral peduncles ending in the fourth ventricle. These oblique cuts can then be made at right angles to the folia on the upper surface, and a midline cut will display the whole of cerebral vermis. The brainstem is sliced at 3–4 mm intervals as before.

Appearance of the Ventricles

The lateral ventricles may be larger or smaller than normal, or unequal.

Various points to note:

- Whether the ventricles contain blood
- Whether the capaciousness of the subarachnoid spaces between the cerebral sulci and in the basal cisterns is normal or abnormal. If it is more than normal, there is a presumption of cerebral atrophy; but if it is less, a block in the cerebrospinal fluid (CSF) pathway must be looked for
- Whether the dilation of the ventricles affects the ventricular system wholly or partially; and if it is partially affected, whether the difference can be accounted for by local atrophy or tissue destruction.

Choice of Blocks for Histology

There are no strict rules regarding the choice of blocks for embedding, except that at least some should be relevant to the probable diagnosis.

Five standards for brain:

1. The left frontal lobe to include the border zone between anterior and middle cerebral arteries
2. Hippocampus to include the Ammon's nucleus
3. Basal ganglia including globus pallidus, putamen, internal capsule, insular cortex
4. Pons
5. Cerebellum to include the dentate nucleus.

Pediatric Brain Examination

Special and intensive care is required for extracting infants' brains. The tissues of an infant's brain are not only softer and more friable, but the leptomeninges are also fragile. The risk involved in manipulating a soft brain can also be reduced by taking the brain out under water. The brain of an infant can easily be removed by cutting the sutures and reflecting the parietal and frontal bones outwards.

The maturity of the infant brain can be evaluated by weighing it, and by examining the state of development of the cerebral gyri and the extent and distribution of myelination. The same method is followed for slicing of pediatric brain as well as an adult brain.

Points to be noted:

- *Hemorrhages*: Subdural and subarachnoid hemorrhage **(Fig. 1D)**.
- *Congenital malformations*: Common
  - Anencephaly—failure of brain formation
  - Spina bifida occulta
  - Meningocele/meningomyelocele/encephalocele
  - Porencephaly
- Hydrocephalus (HC) characterized by dilated ventricular system **(Figs. 1A to D)**.
  - *Obstructive HC*: Secondary to obstruction within the ventricular system.
  - *Communicating HC*: Secondary to extraventricular obstruction or due to impaired absorption or overproduction of CSF.
  - *HC ex vacuo*: Secondary to primary cortical disease with cerebral atrophy
- Acquired perinatal lesions
- *Germinal matrix hemorrhage*: This is encountered in premature infants. These begin as hemorrhagic infarcts in the involuting subependymal matrix layer of the lateral ventricle. When extensive they produced massive—intraventricular hemorrhagic lesions **(Fig. 1C)**. Smaller lesions are resolved leaving subependymal matrix cysts.
- *Periventricular leukomalacia*: This is encountered more often in the premature infants and consists of focal areas of necrosis in the periventricular white matter. These necrotic foci may undergo mineralization.
  - *Kernicterus*: It refers to heavy bilirubin staining of deep gray nuclei with selective damage to some parts of brain in deeply jaundiced infants **(Fig. 1C)**.
  - *Hypoxia*: Dusky discoloration of central white matter **(Fig. 2)**.

INFECTIONS

While examining a neuropathological case with possibility of a central nervous system (CNS) infection the main aims to be established are:

- The root cause of the infection
- The route taken by the organism to reach nervous system
- The effects of the infection on the nervous system.

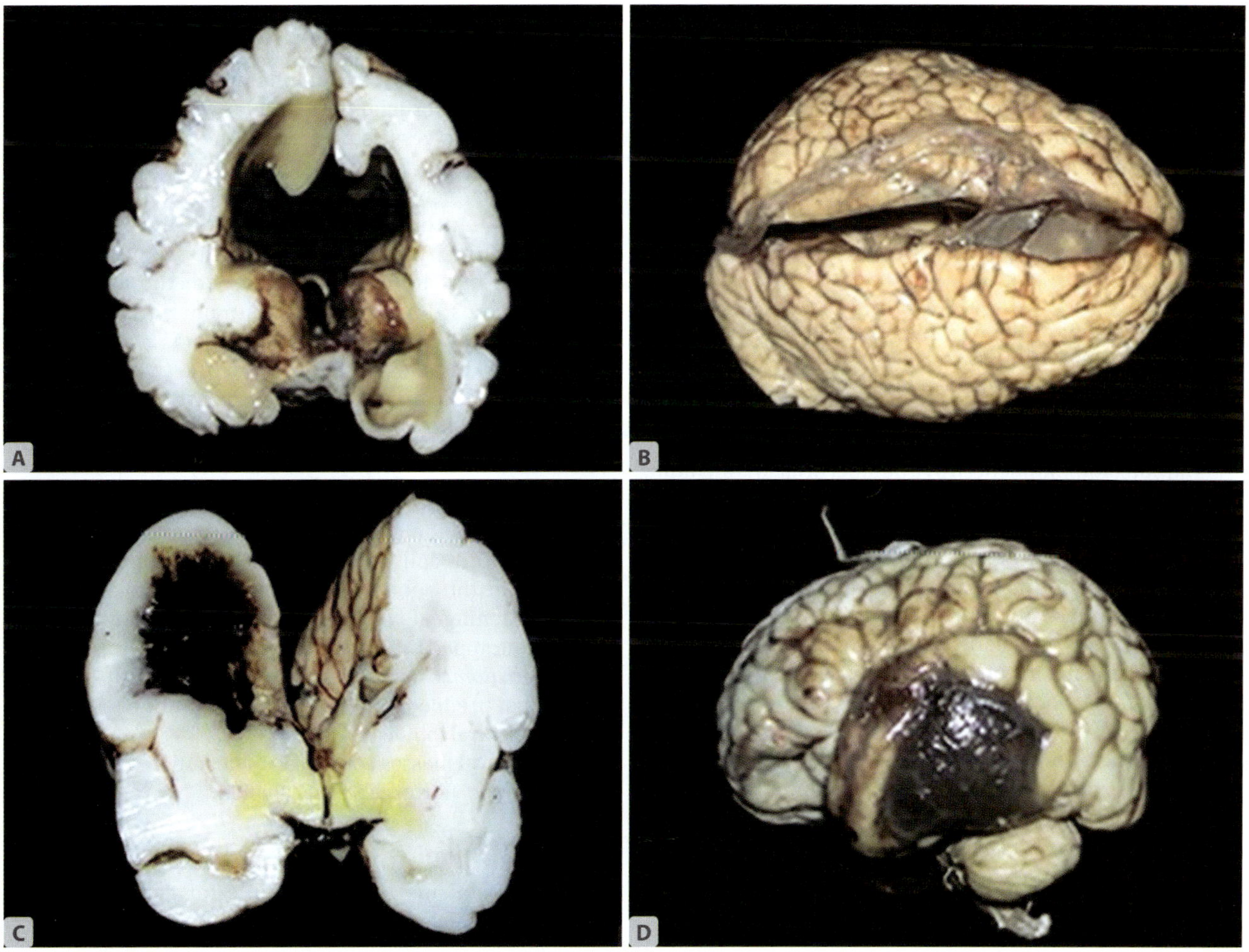

FIGS. 1A TO D: Hydrocephalus. (A) Dilated lateral ventricular system; (B) Superior view of the neonatal brain with hydrocephalus; (C) Intraventricular hemorrhage (left) with kernicterus (bilirubin staining of the thalamus); (D) Patch of subarachnoid hemorrhage over the left temporal lobe.

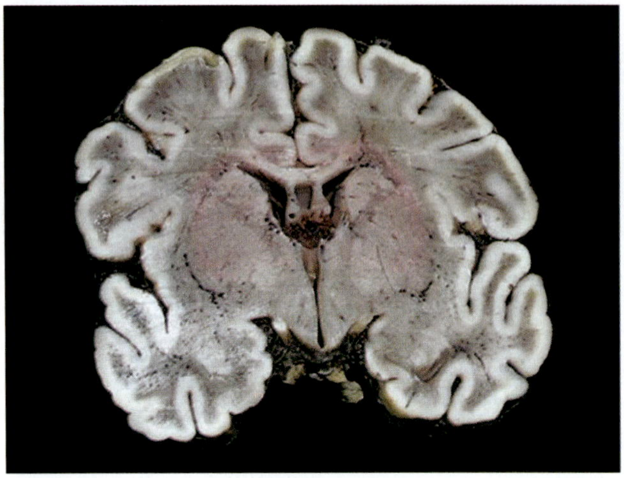

FIG. 2: Coronal slice of a neonatal brain showing marked hypoxic changes with dusky discoloration of the central white matter.

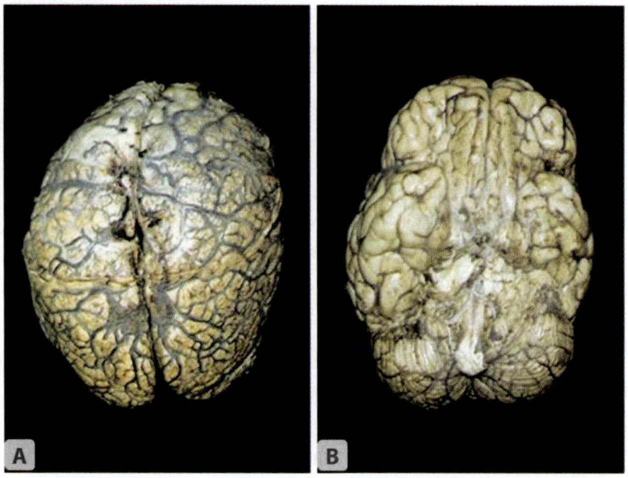

FIGS. 3A AND B: (A) Thick exudates over the surface of the convexities in a case of acute pyogenic meningitis; (B) Organized exudate at the base of the brain in a case of tubercular meningitis.

At autopsy, the following samples are taken:

- CSF samples for:
  - Microscopic examination
  - Culture and sensitivity
- Brain tissue for culture and sensitivity
- Crush smears for organisms, fungal hyphae
- Fresh tissue for PCR especially in case of:
  - Viral infections (1 cm^2 of tissue)
  - Cerebellum, hippocampus: Rabies
  - Temporal lobe: Herpes simplex virus
  - Portion of frontal cortex: Enteroviral encephalitis

Routes of Infection

- Hematogenous from established infection (e.g. osteomyelitis, septic arthritis, endocarditis, bronchiectasis)
- Spread from a nearby focus of infection (paranasal air sinuses, middle ears and bones of skull and spine)
- Penetrating injury.

The outcome is influenced by a number of factors including the virulence of the invading organism, the effectiveness of number of the defenses of the host and the pace of initiating the suitable antibiotic therapy. The CSF provides an excellent culture medium for many organisms to multiply at a rapid speed, it is because it is moderately removed from immune defenses. The low vascularity of the dura makes it difficult to remove organisms in the subdural space. Even antibiotics fail here due to poor penetration unless these are directly instilled.

Less virulent organisms, such as cryptococci and other fungi, and toxoplasmosis, are generally found in very young or elderly and debilitated patients because they have weak immunity, and may evoke little in the way of an inflammatory response.

Consequences of Infection

- Edema, acute, possibly fatal
- Sagittal sinus thrombosis with venous infarction
- Cerebral arterial infarction due to arteritis and HC.

Leptomeningitis

Acute Meningitis

A purulent exudate is readily evident in the subarachnoid space and it may be more marked over the vertex or at the base **(Figs. 3A and B)**. Acute inflammatory cells which are found in the superficial perivascular spaces surround the tiny penetrating vessels present on the walls of the cortex and the brainstem. Cortical and hippocampal neurons also show signs of acute hypoxic changes. The subarachnoid space and leptomeninges contain a neutrophil-rich infiltrate. Fibrin strands can also be frequently seen. Organisms may be demonstrated with the appropriate stains (Gram's, PAS), unless treatment with antibiotics during life has largely eradicated them. There may be adrenal or skin hemorrhages outside the CNS, along with evidence of more prevalent intravascular coagulation.

Tubercular Meningitis (Figs. 3B to 6)

Thick exudates more at the base of the brain with opacity of meninges at the convexities. Microscopically, presence of epithelioid cell granulomas with Langhans' giant cells within the subarachnoid space is the characteristic feature. Meningeal vessels within the subarachnoid space may be entrapped producing arteritis leading to infarcts.

Tuberculomas may be single or multiple.

Sites of predilection— cerebellum, pontine tegmentum and paracentral lobule **(Fig. 5)**.

Round oval masses composed of necrotic, caseous center become cystic, fibrous and get calcified.

Chronic Meningitis

Various organisms are responsible for causing chronic meningitis, which may be accompanied by granulomas or brain abscesses as well. When the inflammatory process in the subarachnoid space persists for duration more than a week or two, secondary effects also start developing in the brain.

- Hydrocephalus

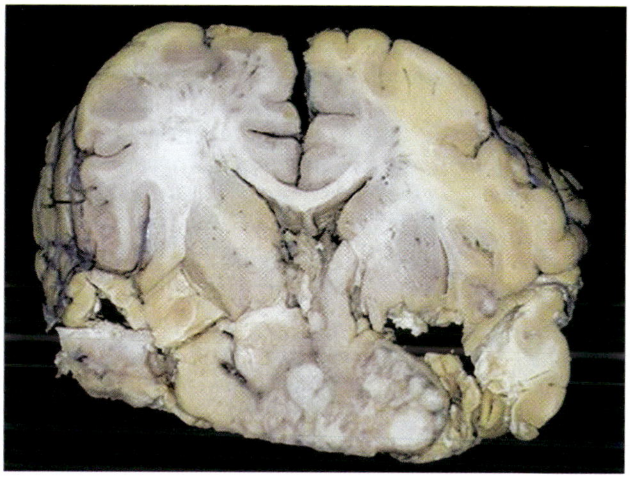

FIG. 4: Thick, organized exudates at the base of the brain with destruction of the bilateral basal ganglia, hippocampus, and optic chiasm in a case of tubercular meningitis.

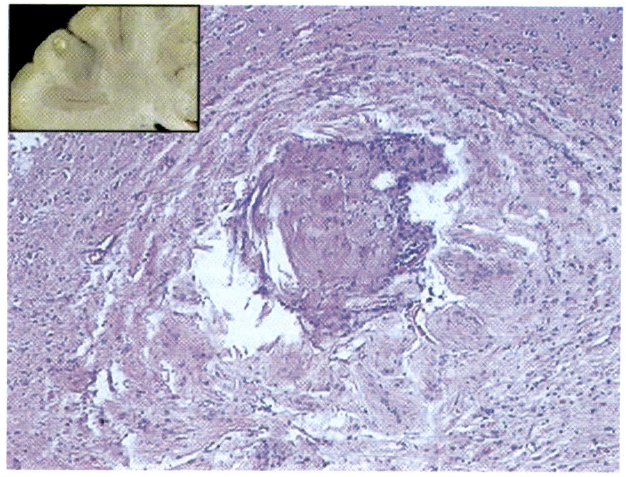

FIG. 5: Tuberculoma at the gray-white junction in the middle frontal gyrus. Microscopically shows a central necrotic focus with minimal inflammatory infiltrate.

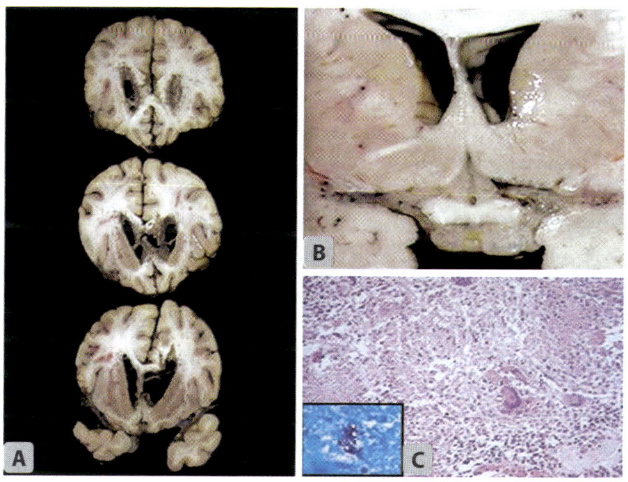

FIGS. 6A TO C: In a case of tubercular meningitis. (A) Ventriculitis with hydrocephalus; (B) Thick exudates at the base of the brain around the optic chiasm; (C) Epithelioid cell granuloma with acid fast tubercular bacilli (ZN stain, inset).

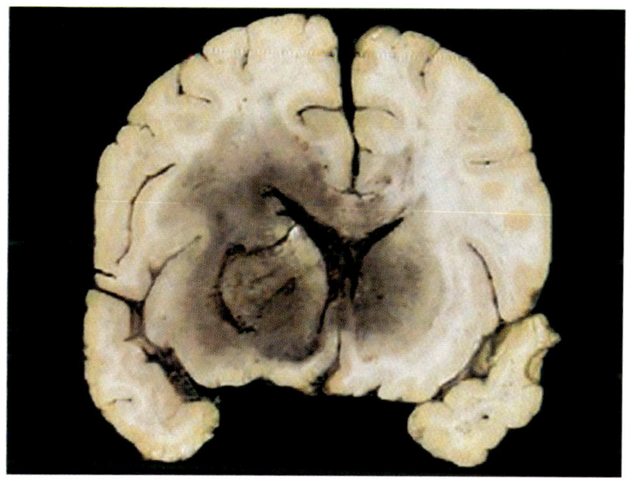

FIG. 7: In a case of fungal meningoencephalitis: Large areas of hemorrhagic necrosis involving the basal ganglia region, corpus callosum and central white matter.

- Multiple cerebral infarcts due to narrowing of, and thrombosis in, arteries affected by endarteritis obliterans, particularly common in fungal infections
- Collagenous thickening of leptomeninges, chiefly at the base
- *Cryptococcus* is liable to produce widened perivascular spaces, particularly in the basal ganglia
- Granulare pendymitis is invariably present in cases of chronic meningitis.

The organisms can themselves be identified with appropriate stains (Gram's for bacteria, Ziehl-Neelsen (ZN) for *Mycobacteria*), periodic acid-Schiff (PAS) and methenamine silver stains for fungi, Giemsa for protozoa).

Fungal Meningitis/Encephalitis

The more common fungi to involve the brain are:

- *Aspergillus*: Commonly in diabetics and produce large areas of hemorrhagic necrosis **(Fig. 7)**.
- *Zygomyces*: Commonly in diabetics and produce largeareas of hemorrhagic necrosis **(Figs. 8A and B)**.
- *Candida: Usually in neonates produce large areas of hemorrhagic necrosis* ***(Fig. 9A)****.*
- *Cryptococcus*: Produces meningitis with basal exudates and because of mucoid capsule gives a "slippery" feel to the brain **(Fig. 9B)**.

Subdural Empyema

It is from a focus of local osteomyelitis or paranasal sinus infection that the pus spreads in the subdural space. There may also be associated acute meningitis.

Brain Abscess

Despite the probability of abscesses cropping up anywhere in the brain, these are most common in the white matter. Those with a local cause have particular sites of predilection.

There may also be multiple, in which case they may be small and easily overlooked, especially when the organisms are blood-borne. At beginning, they consist of a small focus of liquefaction necrosis, or purulent encephalitis. Its expansion leads to the collection of pus in the center which forms a wall around it which composes of glial fibrils. If the abscess is situated near the ependymal surface, it may be incapable of to barring it from penetrating into the ventricle. Bacteria are the organisms most commonly responsible for the brain abscess are bacteria, but there can be involvement of other organisms as well, and these should be considered, particularly if bacterial cultures are not positive.

Purulent Encephalitis Associated with Subacute Bacterial Endocarditis

Septic emboli which arise from the infected heart valves occasionally become the cause of solitary or multiple brain abscesses. They may also block an artery and cause cerebral infarction, which eventually becomes an extension from the septic embolus. If numerous neutrophil polymorphs are found present in and around the edge of an infarct, it should raise the suspicion of the diagnosis, and immediately a Gram stain should be performed to find organisms. A *mycotic aneurysm is also another likely consequence of the presence of septic embolus in the cerebral artery.* It is caused by a local infection and weakening of the arterial wall. This in turn may crack, thus producing brain hemorrhage of the subarachnoid space.

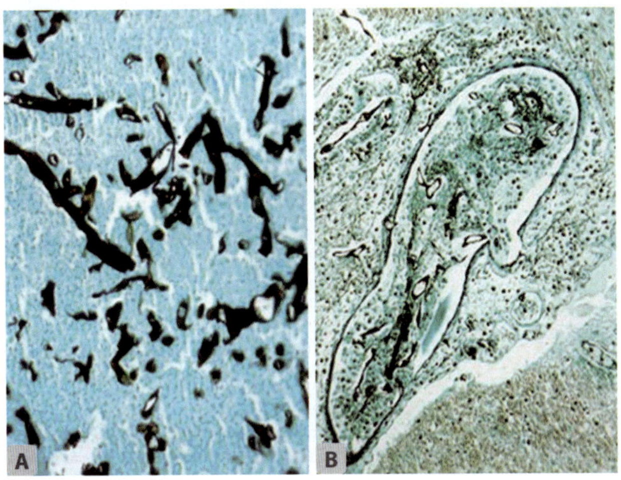

FIGS. 8A AND B: (A) Broad, aseptate hyphae of zygomycetes; (B) Fungal hyphae infiltrating the vessel wall with fibrinoid necrosis (Grocott's stain).

Viral Encephalitis (Fig. 10)

Unlike bacteria and fungi, viruses depend for reproduction on the existence of suitable host cells. Aseptic meningitis due to viral infection is well recognized and relatively common, but generally self-limiting. Enterovirus infection is the most common cause of viral meningitis. Viral encephalitis and myelitis, due to infection of cells of the brain and spinal cord, tend to produce more severe disease, though the extent of the harm incurred is highly variable. The range of viruses pathogenic to nervous system is very wide. Some enter into the blood through bloodstream (e.g. arboviruses), whereas others take a neural route to the CNS after initial replication in extra neural tissues and uptake into peripheral nerves (e.g. rabies). HIV and arboviruses are the most widespread brain infections in the world so far.

Postmortem Examination in Cases of Suspected Viral Encephalitis

Cerebrospinal fluid and samples of serum should be collected for estimating the viral antibody titers. A rise in the serum antibody titer to a particular virus is not a sufficient evidence to declare a virus as the reason for encephalitis. However, with the comparison of antibody titers in CSF with those in serum it is possible to know if intrathecal synthesis of antibody to a specific virus has occurred or not. If it has, this is an indication of the existence of the virus within the CNS, despite the attempts to culture the virus being unsuccessful. In viral encephalitis there is usually also evidence of oligoclonal

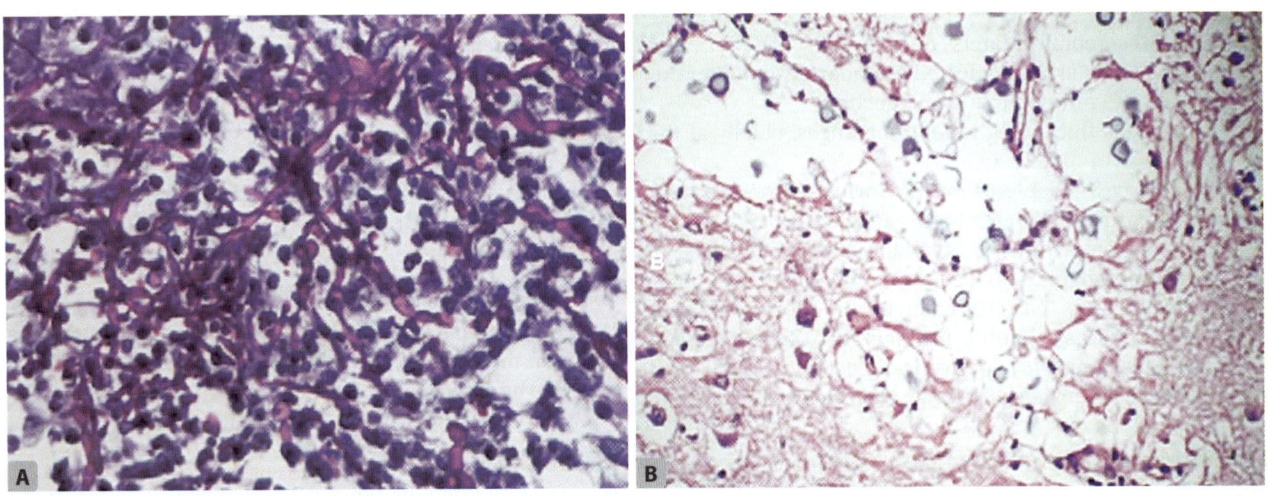

FIGS. 9A AND B: (A) Yeast and pseudohyphae of Candida in a neonatal case of fungal meningoencephalitis; (B) Cryptococci around the perivascular spaces.

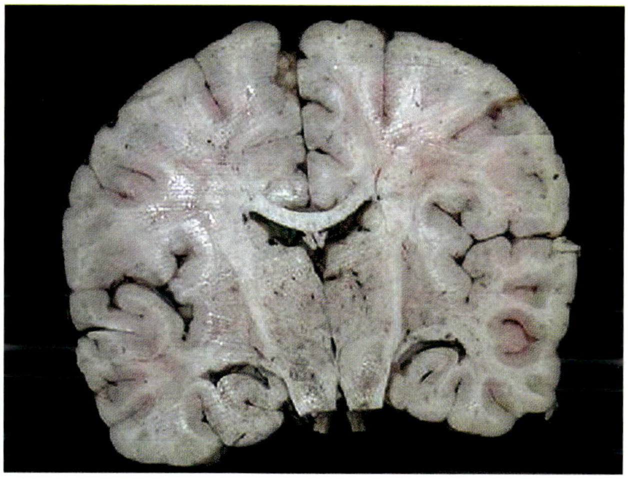

FIG. 10: A case of viral (Japanese B) encephalitis with softening and petechial hemorrhages in the thalami and the midbrain.

immunoglobulin in the CSF. Due to its characteristic of being sensitive and specific, the use of polymerase chain reaction (PCR) to detect specific viral nucleic acid in CSF or brain has become the chosen method for verifying the viral etiology of encephalitis.

Macroscopic Examination of the CNS and the Choice of Blocks for Microscopy

There is a possibility of some generalized swelling and congestion, perhaps with a few petechial hemorrhages on the pial surface. The meninges may be slightly blurred in the acute phase of herpes simplex encephalitis, there is swelling, hemorrhage and softening centered on one or both temporal lobes. If the patient survives until months or years later there is destruction and collapse of same regions. In chronic forms of encephalitis there is likely to be some degree of cerebral atrophy, granular discoloration of the white matter and fibrous thickening of the leptomeninges.

When preparing blocks for microscopy from cases of postmortem, samples should be taken both from areas which appear normal as well as from those which are obviously abnormal, and from transition zones in between. Samples from each major cerebral lobe, hippocampus, basal ganglia, thalamus and several levels of brainstem and cerebellum should be taken. It is necessary to have a wide sampling of the CNS because, although the *type* of damage caused by viral infections tends to be stereotyped, the location and distribution of the damage is often characteristic of particular viruses. The most reliable evidence about the cause of encephalitis appears from culture of a specific organism or detection of specific viral nucleic acid sequences by PCR, and from the use of immune-histological studies or *in situ* hybridization used to detect the presence of specific viral antigens or nucleic acid.

Pathological Features Common to Most Forms of Viral Encephalitis

- Death of cell with neuronophagia
- Perivascular lymphocytic collections
- Microglial nodules
- Inclusion bodies—which contain virus-coded material. Most characteristic are the RNA inclusions that form *Negri bodies*, cytoplasmic inclusions found in neurons in rabies. Round or oval, intranuclear, eosinophilic inclusion bodies, larger than nucleoli, and usually surrounded by a halo of clear nucleoplasm, are found in neurons and oligodendrocyte nuclei in subacute sclerosing panencephalitis (SSPE) and "immunosuppressive" measles encephalitis (Cowdry type A inclusions). They can sometimes be spotted in neurons in herpes simplex encephalitis.

NEUROVASCULAR DISEASES

These are those disorders attributable to pathologic structural and functional modifications of the blood vessels in the central, peripheral and autonomic nervous systems. This term is more encompassing and better than *stroke, or cerebrovascular disease*. Enormous importance should be imparted to the neurovascular diseases as these are the major cause of morbidity and are the third most common cause of death in this country.

Numerous causes can be attributed to the occurrence of a stroke and the following discussion is divided into hemorrhagic and ischemic. The *arterial infarct*s are generally ischemic and are characterized by the involvement of an area corresponding to a territory supplied by a major cerebral artery. The *venous infarcts* are hemorrhagic.

Arterial Infarcts or Territorial Infarcts

The arterial infarcts may be caused by thrombotic or embolic occlusion. The thrombotic infarcts are pale whereas embolic infarcts are hemorrhagic. The pale infarcts may also transform into hemorrhagic infarcts due to re-establishment of circulation.

The three major branches coming of the circle of Willis **(Fig. 11)**, the anterior, middle and the posterior cerebral arteries, provide the vast majority of the arterial blood supply of the cerebral hemispheres. Territorial infarcts in the distribution of the *anterior cerebral artery* are extremely uncommon due to the adequacy of collateral flow through the circle of Willis. Most often these are the result of vasospasm related to rupture of a berry aneurysm on its proximal portion. Infarcts which involve the territory of the *posterior cerebral artery* are either embolic in nature, or are related to the effects of severe transtentorial herniation. Infarcts created by the *MCA* occlusion by embolic or thrombotic episodes manifest as massive strokes **(Fig. 12)**.

Embolic Infarcts

Since the total cerebral blood flow represents about 20% of the cardiac output, emboli are a relatively common cause of infarction. In several clinicopathological studies, embolic infarcts are said to be the most common cause of stroke. Such embolic infarcts may occur in virtually any location in the nervous system, but some locations are more typical. The embolic material rises up the cerebral vessels which bifurcate multiple times leading to the

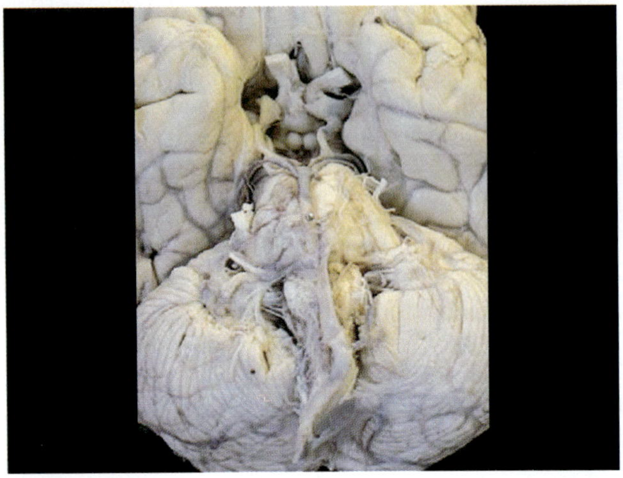

FIG. 11: Circle of Willis at the base of the brain.

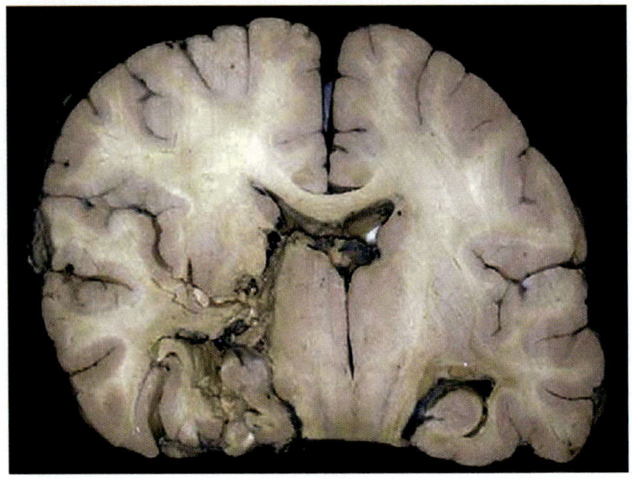

FIG. 12: Ischemic infarct in the region of MCA with softening and breaking down of the left cortical white matter (thalamus and hippocampus). (MCA: middle cerebral artery)

gradual narrowing of the lumina. The embolus finally settles in a vessel that is too small to enable its further travel. In situations with thromboembolism, the clot will rapidly break up into smaller fragments. Attempts to find the embolus by inspection or histologic investigation are mostly unsuccessful. Characteristically, thromboembolic infarcts are multiple and have the tendency of being peripheral in location and have a hemorrhagic appearance to some extent. Since emboli producing such lesions typically originate from either cardiac or carotid sources, they have a tendency of favoring the involvement of the cerebral hemispheres. There are innumerable possible sources for such emboli. In cases of chronic arterial fibrillation, mural thrombi in the auricular appendage of the left atrium may dislodge leading to the embolic infarction in the brain. Another common source of multiple cerebral emboli is from thrombi adherent to the endocardium following myocardial infarction with the formation of a left ventricular aneurysm. Carotid arteries are also a source of cerebral embolization. The carotid arteries, particularly in the region of the carotid bifurcation, are common sites for ulcerative atherosclerosis. Thrombi can form in the region of such lesions, and can embolize, as can fragments of atherosclerotic plaque. The cerebral artery at the center and its branches is the most common vessel to suffer embolic occlusion from an origin in the internal carotid artery. When emboli travel up the vertebrobasilar system, they can readily reach both posterior cerebral arteries, giving rise to bilateral infarcts in this distribution as a consequence of going either to the right or the left as they reach the top of the basilar artery.

Paradoxical embolization of the brain may occur in the situations in which natural filtering capacity of the capillary bed of the lungs has been bypassed, that is, in situations with right to left shunting of blood. Therefore, patients with patent foramen ovale, ventricular septal defects or pulmonary arteriovenous (AV) fistulae are at increased risk for cerebral embolization.

Cerebral Venous Infarcts (Fig. 13)

Thrombosis of one, or more, of major dural sinuses can give rise to the entity of cerebral venous infarcts. Within the system of venous drainage of the cerebral hemispheres, there are numerous interconnecting collateral channels, so one must achieve fairly extensive occlusion of a sinus and its associated major cortical veins, to cause a sufficient degree of interference in cerebral blood flow necessary to induce infarction of the tissues being drained. These causes include women who are taking oral contraceptives or who are postpartum, postoperative patients, hypercoagulable states associated with certain cancers, sickle cell disease, various forms of polycythemia, severe dehydration and cachexia. Local infection can also give rise to such occlusions with the formation of local thrombophlebitis. The resultant occlusion causes a hemorrhagic usually bilateral infarction within the area of drainage of the thrombosed veins.

Lacunar Infarcts

When the brain of elderly patients is being sliced, one commonly comes across small elongated, often multiple, cystic infarcts involving the thalamus, basal ganglia (especially the putamen and globus pallidus) and intervening internal capsule. These are called lacunes or lacunar infarcts and are usually bilateral and multiple. Advanced age, hypertension and diabetes influence the growth of such lesions. Lacunes stand for infarcts that are related to arteriosclerotic pathology in the lenticulostriate arteries arising from the proximal MCA. By definition, lacunes should not exceed 1 cm in their greatest dimension.

Practical Considerations

While evaluating a brain specimen suspected of having an ischemic lesion, the circle of Willis should be examined most carefully, along with its feeding and exiting vessels. Determine the extent and distribution of artherosclerotic

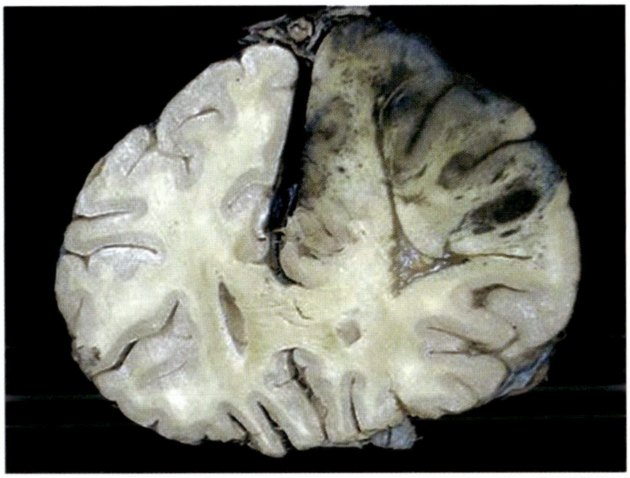

FIG. 13: Venous infarcts: Thrombosed superior sagittal sinus with hemorrhagic infarct involving the right frontal lobe with midline shift, edema and herniation of cingulated gyrus.

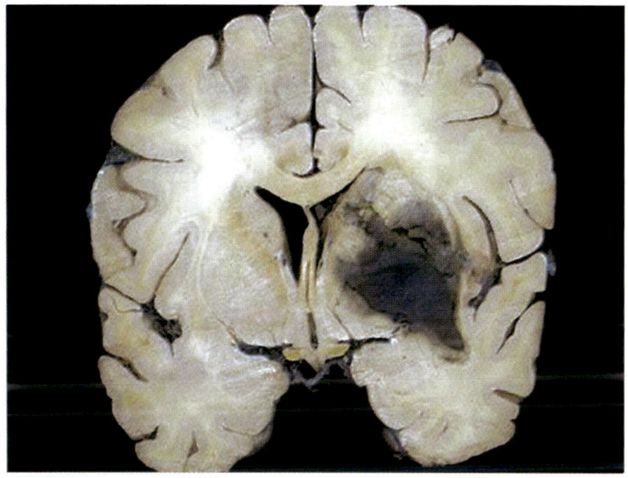

FIG. 14: Hypertensive bleed involving the right basal ganglia region.

lesions, possible occlusion, and for portions that are either incomplete or atretic. Understanding of ischemic stroke in the brain mostly involves a knowledge of the status of the carotid arteries, in particular, the relative patency. The practice of removing the carotid arteries has gone out of favor, leaving the prosector to guess as to what might or might not be present in these extremely important vessels.

Broad guidelines for autopsy on stroke patients:

- Look for extradural or subdural hemorrhage. If present, search for skull fractures.
- In case of SAH, examine circle of Willis and look for aneurysm, AVM, etc. in fresh state.
- Look at carotid siphon, cavernous sinus and dural venous sinuses and remove them if involved.
- Remove carotid arteries and vertebral arteries.
- Look for stenosis, atheroma, thrombosis (serial transverse sections), arterial dissection, etc. Gentle perfusion with water after removal and before cutting gives an idea of blockage.
- Size, site, anatomical location and nature of lesion whether arterial or venous infarct (usually hemorrhagic); single or multiple lesions. Infarcts-central or peripheral. Lesions—single or multiple.
- Observe edema, midline shift, ventricular size, herniation, secondary hemorrhages in pons, secondary infarction and whether hemorrhagic transformation of ischemic infarcts has occurred due to thrombolysis.
- For venous infarct sample the involved venous sinuses, infarcts with overlying thrombosed cortical veins, areas adjacent to look for vascular fibrin thrombi and their age, etc.

Intracranial Hemorrhage

Intracranial hemorrhage may occur as a result of head trauma or it may be spontaneous **(Flowchart 1)**.

The major causes of nontraumatic ICH are as follows:

- Hypertension—common sites are putamen, thalamus, lobar, cerebellum, pons **(Fig. 14)**

FLOWCHART 1: Causes of intracranial hemorrhage.

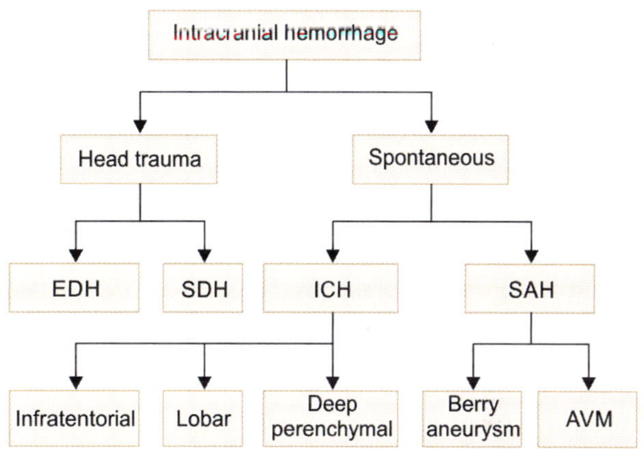

(AVM: arteriovenous malformation; EDH: extradural hemorrhage; ICH: intracerebral hemorrhage; SDH: subdural hemorrhage; SAH: subarachnoid hemorrhage).

- AVM and aneurysms
- Cerebral amyloid angiopathy (CAA)
- Anticoagulant therapy
- Tumors
- Abuse of illicit with licit drugs.

Aneurysm

Subarachnoid hemorrhage is most commonly caused due to rupturing of berry aneurysm. With large aneurysm, a layered thrombus may be found partially filling the inner cavity. Berry aneurysms arise in a very particular geographic pattern of predilection, with approximately 70% of such lesions occurring within 1 cm of the anterior portion of the circle of Willis. Most common sites are the anterior communicating artery, the proximal anterior cerebral artery, the most distal extent of the internal carotid artery, the proximal MCA and the most rostral extent of the posterior extent of the posterior communicating artery.

Arteriovenous Malformations

Arteriovenous malformations may also be the underlying lesion leading to an intracerebral hemorrhage. Usually these represent developmental abnormalities in which arteries have direct communication with veins, without any intervention of a capillary bed. This subjects the veins associated with the malformation of arterial blood pressure directly. Greatly enlarged draining veins may be observed on the vertex lying over such a lesion. After cutting the brain, one can often see with the naked eye many irregular large vascular channel profiles within the hemorrhage. In some cases the arteriovenous malformation is so small that it can be completely eradicated by the hemorrhage. In such cases, identifying the underlying lesion may be quite difficult and require extensive histological sampling. The use of an elastic stain is helpful in visualizing the arterial vascular walls within the pool of blood clot.

Demyelinating Disease and Multiple Sclerosis

Gross Features

- Irregular gray patches on the normally whitish surface of the pons or on the cut surfaces of the upper cervical cord and optic nerves.
- When the brain is freshly incised, sharply demarcated gray or pinkish-gray firm patches (called plaques) can be found on the cut surfaces of cerebral hemispheres (especially subependymal region, angles of lateral ventricles, optic nerves) and spinal cord (mostly at cervical level).
- Chronic plaques are sharply demarcated with smooth edge.

Inherited Metabolic Diseases

In examining cases of inherited metabolic disease it is very important to reserve some fresh tissue for biochemical and genetic study before fixing the remainder of the tissue. Fresh tissue should be taken for electron microscopy.

TUMORS

Postmortem Examination of Brain with Tumor

When examining the CNS in cases with tumors, at the postmortem, the presence of midline shift, softening, necrosis and herniations, as a consequence of intracranial space occupying lesions should be noted. If the tumor caused epilepsy, the brain may show pathological changes associated with this condition, it is very crucial to examine the intracranial viscera very carefully, searching particularly for sources of metastatic deposits. There may also, rarely, be evidence of extracranial spread of primary CNS tumor to other sites.

General Guidelines

- Fresh tissue is snap frozen for rapid intraoperative diagnosis.
- Crush smears may also be prepared from fresh tissue for rapid diagnosis.
- Sampling of adjacent brain is essential to assess the margins and pattern of infiltration.
- Grading as proposed by WHO classification is followed which grades the tumor according to their malignant potential on a scale ranging from I for benign to IV for malignant tumors.
- *Common immunohistochemical stains*:
  - GFAP: Glial fibrillary acidic protein-astrocytic differentiation.
  - Synaptophysin, Neu N for neuronal differentiation.
  - NFP: Neurofilament protein-neuronal differentiation.
  - EMA (epithelial membrane antigen), cytokeratin.
  - Vimentin-mesenchymal marker
  - S-100: positive in choroid plexus tumors
  - CD20, CD3, CD45, CD68, MUM1, bcl2, bcl6- Lymphoid neoplasms
  - MAP-2 (microtubule associated protein)–Neuronal differentiation
  - CD 99: Peripheral PNET/Ewing's sarcoma
  - INI-1, Brg-1: Atypical teratoid rhabdoid tumors (AT/RT)
  - Ki-67: Marker of proliferative index
  - Markers for molecular subtyping/prognostication
  - IDH1 R132H, ATRX, p53: Primary glioblastoma versus secondary glioblastomas
  - H3K27 me3: Midline gliomas enriched for H3K27 trimethylation
  - BRAF V600E: Tumors enriched for *BRAF V600E* mutation
  - LIN 28: Positive in subset of central PNETs
  - YAP1, GAB1, beta-catenin: Molecular subgrouping of medulloblastoma
  - p53—to identify medulloblastoma enriched for *TP53* mutations

WHO Classification of CNS Tumors 2016 Update

For decades, the classification of brain tumors was based on the concept of histogenesis, i.e. the tumors could be classified according to their morphological similarities to the cell of origin. Large scale genomic and transcriptomic studies have significantly improved our understanding of biology and oncogenesis of brain tumors. The 2016 update breaks the century-old tradition of a histological classification and incorporates well-established molecular parameters into the classification of brain tumors. The classification proposes generation of 'integrated' diagnoses which incorporates phenotypic and genotypic classification **(Appendix J)**.

SUGGESTED READING

1. Banerjee AK. Postmortem Examination of the nervous system. Neurol India. 1997;45:120-5.
2. Chhang WH, Kak VK, Khosla VK, et al. Metastatic intracranial tumours : experience and review of literature. Neurol India. 1993;41(2):73-81.
3. Dastur DK, Lalitha VS, Udani PM, et al. The brain and meninges in tuberculous meningitis—gross pathology in 100 cases and pathogenesis. Neurol India. 1970;18(2):86-100.
4. Drlicek M, Bodenteich A, Urbanits S, et al. Immunohistochemical panel of antibodies in the diagnosis of brain metastases of the unknown primary. Pathol Res Pract. 2004; 200:727-34.
5. Gupta K, Salunke P. Molecular markers of glioma: an update on recent progress and perspectives. J Cancer Res Clin Oncol. 2012;138(12):1971-81.
6. Kleinschmidt-DeMasters BK. Central nervous system aspergillosis: a 20-year retrospective series. Hum Pathol. 2002;33(1): 116-24.
7. Louis DN, Perry A, Reifenberger G, et al. The 2016 World Health Organization Classification of Tumors of the Central Nervous System: a summary. Acta Neuropathol. 2016; 131(6):803-20.
8. Murthy JM, Sundaram C, Prasad VS, et al. Aspergillosis of central nervous system: a study of 21 patients seen in a university hospital in south India. J Assoc Physicians India. 2000;48:677-81.
9. Salunke P, Aggarwal A, Gupta K, et al. Large demyelinating lesions: A neurosurgical perspective. Br J Neurosurg. 2012;26(4):490-8
10. Volpe JJ. Brain injury in the premature infant: Overview of clinical aspects, neuropathology, and pathogenesis. Semin Pediatr Neurol. 1998;5:135-51.

Appendices

APPENDIX A: HUNT-HESS GRADING OF SAH

Grade	Description
1	Asymptomatic, or mild headache and slight nuchal rigidity
2	Moderate-to-severe headache, nuchal rigidity, no neurological deficit
3	Drowsy, confused or mild focal deficit
4	Stupor, moderate-to-severe hemiparesis, early decerebrate rigidity or vegetative disturbances
5	Deep coma, decerebrate rigidity

Add one grade for serious systemic disease (e.g. HTN, DM, severe atherosclerosis, COPD) or severe vasospasm on arteriography.
(SAH: subarachnoid hemorrhage)

APPENDIX B: GLASGOW COMA SCALE

Point	Best eye	Best verbal	Best motor
6	-	-	Obeys
5	-	Oriented	Localizes pain
4	Spontaneous	Confused	Withdraw to pain
3	To speech	Inappropriate	Flexor (decorticate)
2	To pain	Incomprehensible	Extensor (decerebrate)
1	None	None	None

APPENDIX C: WFNS SCALE

Grade	GCS	Motor deficit
I	15	Absent
II	14–13	Absent
III	14–13	Present
IV	12–7	Present/Absent
V	3–6	Present/Absent

(WFNS: World Federation of Neurological Surgeons; GCS: Glasgow Coma Scale)

APPENDIX D: COOPERATIVE ANEURYSM STUDY NEUROLOGICAL STATUS SCALES

Status	Signs and symptoms
Status 1	Symptom-free
Status 2	Minor symptoms
Status 3	Major neurologic deficit, but fully responsive
Status 4	Impaired state of alertness, but capable of protective or adaptive responses to noxious stimuli
Status 5	Poorly responsive, but with vital signs
Status 6	No response to shaking, nonadaptive response to stimuli, and progressive instability of vital signs

APPENDIX E: COGNARD CLASSIFICATION OF DURAL ARTERIOVENOUS SHUNTS

I	Venous drainage into dural venous sinus with antegrade flow
IIa	Venous drainage into dural venous sinus with retrograde flow
IIb	Venous drainage into dural venous sinus with antegrade flow and CVR
IIa and b	Venous drainage into dural venous sinus with retrograde flow and CVR
III	Venous drainage directly into subarachnoid veins (CVR only)
IV	Type III with venous ectasias of the draining subarachnoid veins

(CVR: cortical venous reflux)

APPENDIX F: BORDEN CLASSIFICATION OF CRANIAL DURAL AVF

Type I	DAVFs drain into dural venous sinuses without pial reflux
Type II	DAVFs drain into venous sinuses, but show retrograde flow into a pial vein
Type III	DAVFs drain directly into a pial vein (or an isolated dural sinus segment) and are associated with significant venous hypertension

Each type is further characterized by the complexity of the architecture of the arteriovenous shunt into Subtype A, a simple fistula with a direct, single connection between the feeding artery and the draining vein or sinus, and Subtype B, a complex lesion with multiple fistulous connections.

(AVF: arteriovenous fistula)

APPENDIX G: FISHER GRADE OF CEREBRAL VASOSPASM RISK IN SUBARACHNOID HEMORRHAGE

Grade	Appearance of blood on head CT scan
1	No blood detected
2	Diffuse deposition or thin layer with all vertical layers (in interhemispheric fissure, insular cistern, ambient cistern) less than 1 mm thick
3	Localized clot and/or vertical layers 1 mm or more in thickness
4	Intracerebral or intraventricular clot with diffuse or no subarachnoid blood

APPENDIX H: MODIFIED FISHER CT SAH RATING SCALE

Grade 0	No SAH or IVH
Grade 1	Focal or diffuse, thin SAH, no IVH
Grade 2	Focal or diffuse, thin SAH, with IVH
Grade 3	Focal or diffuse, thick SAH, no IVH
Grade 4	Focal or diffuse, thick SAH, with IVH

(IVH: intraventricular hemorrhage)

APPENDIX I: SPETZLER-MARTIN INTRACRANIAL AVM GRADING SCALE

	Score
Size	
0–3 cm	1
3.1–6.0 cm	2
>6 cm	3
Location	
Noneloquent brain area	0
Eloquent brain area*	1
Deep venous drainage	
Absent	0
Present	1

Score = sum of all categories, with lesions graded I to V based upon total sum (e.g. grade I = 1 point).
*Associated with significant neurologic impairment (e.g. language area, motor cortex, others).
From: Spetzler RF, Martin NA, J Neurosurg. 1986;65:476.
(AVM: arteriovenous malformation)

APPENDIX J: WHO CLASSIFICATION OF TUMORS OF THE CENTRAL NERVOUS SYSTEM

Diffuse astrocytic and oligodendroglial tumors	
Diffuse astrocytoma, IDH-mutant	9400/3
Gemistocytic astrocytoma, IDH-mutant	9411/3
Diffuse astrocytoma, IDH-wildtype	9400/3
Diffuse astrocytoma, NOS	9400/3
Anaplastic astrocytoma, IDH-mutant	9401/3
Anaplastic astrocytoma, IDH-wildtype	9401/3
Anaplastic astrocytoma, NOS	9401/3
Glioblastoma, IDH-wildtype	9440/3
Giant cell glioblastoma	9441/3
Gliosarcoma	9442/3
Epithelioid glioblastoma	9440/3
Glioblastoma, IDH-mutant	9445/3*
Glioblastoma, NOS	9440/3

Continued

Continued

Diffuse midline glioma, H3 K27M-mutant	9385/3*
Oligodendroglioma, IDH-mutant and 1 p/19q-codeleted	9450/3
Oligodendroglioma, NOS	9450/3
Anaplastic oligodendroglioma, IDH-mutant and 1 p/19q-codeleted	9451/3
Anaplastic oligodendroglioma, NOS	9451/3
Oligoastrocytoma, NOS	9382/3
Anaplastic oligoastrocytoma, NOS	9382/3
Other Astrocytic Tumors	
Pilocytic astrocytoma	9421/1
Pilomyxoid astrocytoma	9425/3
Subependymal giant cell astrocytoma	9384/1
Pleomorphic xanthoastrocytoma	9424/3
Anaplastic pleomorphic xanthoastrocytoma	9424/3
Ependymal Tumors	
Subependymoma	9383/1
Myxopapillary ependymoma	9394/1
Ependymoma	9391/3
Papillary ependymoma	9393/3
Clear cell ependymoma	9391/3
Tanycytic ependymoma	9391/3
Ependymoma, *RELA* fusion- positive	9396/3*
Anaplastic ependymoma	9392/3
Other Gliomas	
Chordoid glioma of the third ventricle	9444/1
Angiocentric glioma	9431/1
Astroblastoma	9430/3
Choroid Plexus Tumors	
Choroid plexus papilloma	9390/0
Atypical choroid plexus papilloma	9390/1
Choroid plexus carcinoma	9390/3
Neuronal and Mixed Neuronal-glial Tumors	
Dysembryoplastic neuroepithelial tumor	9413/0
Gangliocytoma	9492/0
Ganglioglioma	9505/1
Anaplastic ganglioglioma	9505/3
Dysplastic cerebellar gangliocytoma (Lhermitte-Duclos disease)	9493/0
Desmoplastic infantile astrocytoma and ganglioglioma	9412/1
Papillary glioneuronal tumor	9509/1
Rosette-forming glioneuronal tumor	9509/1
Diffuse leptomeningeal glioneuronal tumor	
Central neurocytoma	9506/1
Extraventricular neurocytoma	9506/1

Continued

Continued

Cerebellar liponeurocytoma	9506/1
Paraganglioma	8693/1
Tumors of the Pineal Region	
Pineocytoma	9361/1
Pineal parenchymal tumor of intermediate differentiation	9362/3
Pineoblastoma	9362/3
Papillary tumor of the pineal region	9395/3
Embryonal Tumors	
Medulloblastomas, genetically defined	
Medulloblastoma, WNT-activated	9475/3*
Medulloblastoma, SHH-activated and TP53-mutant	9476/3*
Medulloblastoma, SHH-activated and TP53-wildtype	9471/3
Medulloblastoma, non-WNT/non-SHH	9477/3'
Medulloblastoma, group 3	
Medulloblastoma, group 4	
Medulloblastomas, histologically defined	
Medulloblastoma, classic	9470/3
Medulloblastoma, desmoplastic/nodular	9471/3
Medulloblastoma with extensive nodularity	9471/3
Medulloblastoma, large cell/anaplastic	9474/3
Medulloblastoma, NOS	9470/3
Embryonal tumor with multilayered rosettes, CI9MC-altered	9478/3*
Embryonal tumor with multilayered rosettes, NOS	9478/3
Medulloepithelioma	9501/3
CNS neuroblastoma	9500/3
CNS ganglioneuroblastoma	9490/3
CNS embryonal tumor, NOS	9473/3
Atypical teratoid/rhabdoid tumor	9508/3
CNS embryonal tumor with rhabdoid features	9508/3
Tumors of the Cranial and Paraspinal Nerves	
Schwannoma	9560/0
Cellular schwannoma	9560/0
Plexiform schwannoma	9560/0
Melanotic schwannoma	9560/1
Neurofibroma	9540/0
Atypical neurofibroma	9540/0
Plexiform neurofibroma	9550/0
Perineuroma	9571/0
Hybrid nerve sheath tumors	
Malignant peripheral nerve sheath tumor	9540/3
Epithelioid MPNST	9540/3
MPNST with perineural differentiation	9540/3
Meningiomas	
Meningiomas	9530/3
Meningothelial meningioma	9531/3

Continued

Continued

Fibrous meningioma	9532/0
Transitional meningioma	9537/0
Psammomatous meningioma	9533/0
Angiomatous meningioma	9534/0
Microcystic meningioma	9530/0
Secretory meningioma	9530/0
Lymphoplasmacyte-rich meningioma	9530/0
Metaplastic meningioma	9530/0
Chordoid meningioma	9538/1
Clear cell meningioma	9538/1
Atypical meningioma	9539/1
Papillary meningioma	9538/3
Rhabdoid meningioma	9538/3
Anaplastic (malignant) meningioma	9530/3
Mesenchymal, Non-meningothelial Tumors	
Solitary fibrous tumor/hemangiopericytoma**	
Grade 1	8815/0
Grade 2	8815/1
Grade 3	8815/3
Hemangioblastoma	9161/1
Hemangioma	9120/0
Epithelioid hemangioendothelioma	9133/3
Angiosarcoma	9120/3
Kaposi sarcoma	9140/3
Ewing sarcoma/PNET	9364/3
Lipoma	8850/0
Angiolipoma	8861/0
Hibernoma	8880/0
Liposarcoma	8850/3
Desmoid-type fibromatosis	8821/1
Myofibroblastoma	8825/0
Inflammatory myofibroblastic tumor	8825/1
Benign fibrous histiocytoma	8830/0
Fibrosarcoma	8810/3
Undifferentiated pleomorphic sarcoma/malignant fibrous histiocytoma	8802/3
Leiomyoma	8890/0
Leiomyosarcoma	8890/3
Rhabdomyoma	8900/0
Rhabdomyosarcoma	8900/3
Chondroma	9220/0
Chondrosarcoma	9220/3
Osteoma	9180/0
Osteochondroma	9210/0
Osteosarcoma	9180/3
Melanocytic Tumors	

Continued

Continued

Meningeal melanocytosis	8728/0
Meningeal melanocytoma	8728/1
Meningeal melanoma	8720/3
Meningeal melanomatosis	8728/3
Lymphomas	
Diffuse large B-cell lymphoma of the CNS	9680/3
Immunodeficiency-associated CNS lymphomas AIDS-related diffuse large B-cell lymphoma EBV-positive diffuse large B-cell lymphoma, NOS Lymphomatoid granulomatosis	9766/1
Intravascular large B-cell lymphoma	9712/3
Low-grade B-cell lymphomas of the CNS	
T-cell and NK/T-cell lymphomas of the CNS	
Anaplastic large cell lymphoma, ALK-positive	9714/3
Anaplastic large cell lymphoma, ALK-negative	9702/3
MALT lymphoma of the dura	9699/3
Histiocytic Tumors	
Langerhans cell histiocytosis	9751/3
Erdheim-Chester disease	9750/1
Rosai-Dorfman disease	
Juvenile xanthogranuloma	
Histiocytic sarcoma	9755/3
Germ Cell Tumors	
Germinoma	9064/3
Embryonal carcinoma	9070/3
Yolk sac tumor	9071/3
Choriocarcinoma	9100/3
Teratoma	9080/1
Mature teratoma	9080/0
Immature teratoma	9080/3
Teratoma with malignant transformation	9084/3
Mixed germ cell tumor	9085/3
Tumors of the Sellar Region	
Craniopharyngioma	9350/1
Adamantinomatous craniopharyngioma	9351/1
Papillary craniopharyngioma	9352/1
Granular cell tumor of the sellar region	9582/0
Pituicytoma	9432/1
Spindle cell oncocytoma	8290/0
Metastatic Tumors	

The morphology codes are from the International Classification of Diseases for Oncology (ICD-O) [742A]. Behavior is coded/O for benign tumors; /1 for unspecified borderline, or uncertain behavior; /2 for carcinoma *in situ* and grade III intraepithelial neoplasia; and /3 for malignant tumors. The classification is modified from the previous WHO classification, taking into account changes in our understanding of these lesions.

*These new codes were approved by the IARC/WHO Committee for ICD-O.

Italics: Provisional tumor entities.

**Grading according to the 2013 WHO Classification of Tumors of Soft Tissue and Bone.

(NOS: not-otherwise specified; MPNST: malignant peripheral nerve sheath tumor; MALT: mucosa-associated lymphoid tissue; CNS: central nervous system; EBV: Epstein–Barr virus).

APPENDIX K: WHO GRADES OF SELECT CNS TUMORS

Diffuse Astrocytic and Oligodendroglial Tumors	
Diffuse astrocytoma, IOH-mutant	II
Anaplastic astrocyloma, IOH-mutant	III
Glioblastoma, IDH-wild type	IV
Glioblastoma, IDH-mutant	IV
Diffuse midline glioma, H3K27M-mutant	IV
Oligodendroglioma, IDH-mutant and 1p/19Q-codeleted	II
Anaplastic oligodendroglioma. IDH-mutant and 1p/19q-codeleted	III
Other Astrocytic Tumors	
Pilocytic astrocytoma	I
Subependymal giant cell astrocytoma	I
Pleomorphic xanthoastrocytoma	II
Anaplastic pleomorphic xanthoastrocytoma	III
Ependymal Tumors	
Subependymoma	I
Myxopapillary ependymoma	I
Ependymoma	II
Ependymoma, *RELA* fusion-positive	II or III
Anaplastic ependymoma	III
Other Gliomas	
Angiocentric glioma	I
Chordoid glioma of third ventricle	II
Choroid Plexus Tumors	
Choroid plexus papilloma	I
Atypical choroid plexus papilloma	II
Choroid plexus carcinoma	III
Neuronal and Mixed Neuronal-glial Tumors	
Dysembryoplastic neuroepithelial tumor	I
Gangliocytoma	I
Ganglioglioma	I
Anaplastic ganglioglioma	III
Dysplastic gangliocytoma of cerebellum (Lhermitte-Duclos)	I
Desmoplastic infantile astrocytoma and ganglioma	I
Papillary glioneuronal tumor	I
Rosette-forming glioneuronal tumor	I
Central neurocytoma	II
Extraventricular neurocytoma	II
Cerebellar liponeurocytoma	II
Tumors of the Pineal Region	
Pineocytoma	I
Pineal parenchymal tumor of intermediate differentiation	II or III
Pineoblastoma	IV
Papillary tumor of the pineal region	II or III
Embryonal Tumors	
Medulloblastoma (all subtypes)	IV
Embryonal tumor with multilayered rosettes, C 19MC-altered	IV
Medulloepithelioma	IV
CNS embryonal tumor, NOS	IV
Atypical teratoid/rhabdoid tumor	IV
CNS embryonal tumor with rhabdoid features	IV

Continued

Continued

Tumors of the Cranial and Paraspinal Nerves	
Schwannoma	I
Neurofibroma	I
Perineunrioma	I
Malignant peripheral nerve sheath tumor (MPNST)	II, III or IV
Meningiomas	
Meningioma	I
Atypical meningioma	II
Anaplastic (malignant) meningioma	III
Mesenchymal, Non-meningothelial Tumors	
Solitary fibrous tumor/hemangiopericytoma	I, II or III
Hemangioblastoma	I
Tumors of the Seller Region	
Craniopharyngioma	I
Granular cell tumor	I
Pituicytoma	I
Spindle cell oncocytoma	I

Source: Louis DN, Ohgaki H, Wiestler OD, Cavenee WK (2016) World Health Organization Histological Classification of Tumors of the Central Nervous System. International Agency for Research on Cancer, France.

APPENDIX L

National multiple Sclerosia society

2017 McDonald Criteria for the Diagnosis of Multiple Sclerosis

ECTRIMS EUROPEAN COMMITTEE FOR TREATMENT AND RESEARCH IN MULTIPLE SCLEROSIS

Diagnosis of MS requires elimination of more likely diagnoses and demonstration of dissemination of lesions in the CNS in space and time. See Lancet Neurology paper* for details.

CLINICAL PRESENTATION	ADDITIONAL DATA NEEDED TO MAKE MS DIAGNOSIS
...in a person with a typical attack/CIS at on onset	(see KEY below for definitions)
• ≥ 2 attacks and objective clinical evidence of ≥ 2 lesions • ≥ 2 attacks and objective clinical evidence of 1 lesion with historical evidence of prior attack involving lesion in different location	None. Dissemination in space (DIS) and dissemination in time (**DIT**) have been met.
• ≥ 2 attacks and objective clinical evidence of 1 lesions	**One** of these criteria: – **DIS:** additional clinical attack implication different CNS site – **DIS:** ≥1 symptomatic or asymptomatic MS-typical T2 lesions in ≥2 areas of CNS: periventricular, juxtacortical/cortical, intratentorial or spinal cord
• 1 attacks and objective clinical evidence of ≥2 lesions	**One** of these criteria: – **DIS:** additional clinical attack – **DIS:** simultaneous presence of both enhancing and non-enhancing symptomatic or asymptomatic MS-typical MRI lesions – **DIS:** new T2 or enhancing MRI lesion compared to baseline scan (without regard to limiting of baseline scan)

Colored text = revisions compared to previous McDonald criteria

KEV: **CIS:** clinically isolated syndrome **CNS:** central nervous system **CSF:** cerebrospinal fluid **DIS:** dissemination in space DIT: dissemination in time T2 lesion: hyperintense lesioin on T2-weighted MRI

*Thompson AJ, et al. Lancet Neurol 2017; online Dec 21,http://dx.doi.org/10.1016/S1474-4422(17)30470-2.

Continued

Continued

2017 McDonald Criteria for the Diagnosis of Multiple Sclerosis (continued)

CLINICAL PRESENTATION	ADDITIONAL DATA NEEDED TO MAKE MS DIAGNOSIS
...in a person with a typical attack/CIS at on onset	(see KEY below for definitions)
• 1 attacks and objective clinical evidence of 1 lesion	**One** of these criteria: – **DIS:** additional attack implicating different CNS site – **DIS:** ≥1 MS-typical symptomatic or asymptomatic MS-typical T2 lesions in ≥2 areas of CNS: periventricular, juxtacortical/cortical, intratentorial or spinal cord **AND** **One** of these criteria: – **DIS:** additional clinical attack – **DIS:** simultaneous presence of both enhancing and non-enhancing symptomatic or asymptomatic MS-typical MRI lesions – **DIT:** by new T2 or enhancing MRI lesion compared to baseline scan (without regard to limiting of baseline scan) – CSF-spcific (i.e. not in serum) oligoclonal bands
...in a person with a typical attack/CIS at on onset	
• 1 progression from onest	**–1** year of disability progression (retrospective or prospective) **AND** **Two** of these criteria: – ≥1 symptomatic or asymptomatic MS-typical T2 lesions (periventricular, juxtacortical/cortical or infratentorial) – ≥ 2 T2 spinal cord lesions – CSF-specific (i.e. not in serum) oligoclonal bands

The international panel on diagnosis of multiple sclerosis was convened under the auspices of the international advisory committee on clinical trials in MS, sponsored by the National MS society and the european committee for treatment and research in multiple sclerosis.

APPENDIX M: INTERNATIONAL LEAGUE AGAINST EPILEPSY (ILAE) CLASSIFICATION OF EPILEPSY

ILAE 2017 classification of seizure types expanded version[1]

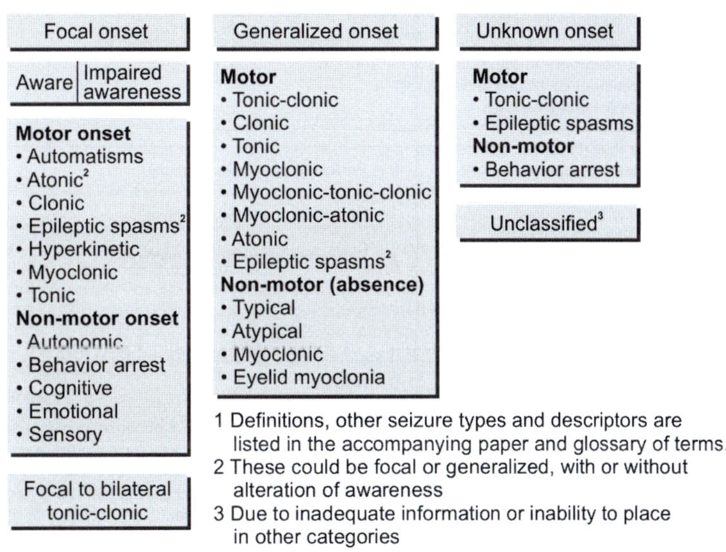

Source: Fisher et al. Instruction manual of the ILAE 2017 operational classification of seizure types. Epilepsia doi: 10.1111/epi.13671.

APPENDIX N: NIH STROKE SCALE

NIH STROKE SCALE

Patient Identification. ___ ___-___ ___ ___-___ ___ ___

Pt. Date of Birth ___ ___/___ ___/___ ___

Hospital ______________________(___ ___-___ ___)

Date of Exam ___ ___/___ ___/___ ___

Interval: [ ] Baseline [ ] 2 hours post treatment [ ] 24 hours post onset of symptoms ±20 minutes [ ] 7-10 days [ ] 3 months [ ] Other ______________________(___ ___)

Time: ___ ___:___ ___ [ ]am [ ]pm

Person Administering Scale ______________________

Administer stroke scale items in the order listed. Record performance in each category after each subscale exam. Do not go back and change scores. Follow directions provided for each exam technique. Scores should reflect what the patient does, not what the clinician thinks the patient can do. The clinician should record answers while administering the exam and work quickly. Except where indicated, the patient should not be coached (i.e., repeated requests to patient to make a special effort).

Instructions	Scale Definition	Score
1a. Level of Consciousness: The investigator must choose a response if a full evaluation is prevented by such obstacles as an endotracheal tube, language barrier, orotracheal trauma/bandages. A 3 is scored only if the patient makes no movement (other than reflexive posturing) in response to noxious stimulation.	0 = **Alert;** keenly responsive. 1 = **Not alert**; but arousable by minor stimulation to obey, answer, or respond. 2 = **Not alert**; requires repeated stimulation to attend, or is obtunded and requires strong or painful stimulation to make movements (not stereotyped). 3 = Responds only with reflex motor or autonomic effects or totally unresponsive, flaccid, and areflexic.	____
1b. LOC Questions: The patient is asked the month and his/her age. The answer must be correct - there is no partial credit for being close. Aphasic and stuporous patients who do not comprehend the questions will score 2. Patients unable to speak because of endotracheal intubation, orotracheal trauma, severe dysarthria from any cause, language barrier, or any other problem not secondary to aphasia are given a 1. It is important that only the initial answer be graded and that the examiner not "help" the patient with verbal or non-verbal cues.	0 = **Answers** both questions correctly. 1 = **Answers** one question correctly. 2 = **Answers** neither question correctly.	____
1c. LOC Commands: The patient is asked to open and close the eyes and then to grip and release the non-paretic hand. Substitute another one step command if the hands cannot be used. Credit is given if an unequivocal attempt is made but not completed due to weakness. If the patient does not respond to command, the task should be demonstrated to him or her (pantomime), and the result scored (i.e., follows none, one or two commands). Patients with trauma, amputation, or other physical impediments should be given suitable one-step commands. Only the first attempt is scored.	0 = **Performs** both tasks correctly. 1 = **Performs** one task correctly. 2 = **Performs** neither task correctly.	____
2. Best Gaze: Only horizontal eye movements will be tested. Voluntary or reflexive (oculocephalic) eye movements will be scored, but caloric testing is not done. If the patient has a conjugate deviation of the eyes that can be overcome by voluntary or reflexive activity, the score will be 1. If a patient has an isolated peripheral nerve paresis (CN III, IV or VI), score a 1. Gaze is testable in all aphasic patients. Patients with ocular trauma, bandages, pre-existing blindness, or other disorder of visual acuity or fields should be tested with reflexive movements, and a choice made by the investigator. Establishing eye contact and then moving about the patient from side to side will occasionally clarify the presence of a partial gaze palsy.	0 = **Normal.** 1 = **Partial gaze palsy;** gaze is abnormal in one or both eyes, but forced deviation or total gaze paresis is not present. 2 = **Forced deviation,** or total gaze paresis not overcome by the oculocephalic maneuver.	____

Rev 10/1/2003

Continued

NIH STROKE SCALE

Patient Identification. ___ ___-___ ___ ___-___ ___ ___

Pt. Date of Birth ___ ___/___ ___/___ ___

Hospital ______________________(___ ___-___ ___)

Date of Exam ___ ___/___ ___/___ ___

Interval: [ ] Baseline [ ] 2 hours post treatment [ ] 24 hours post onset of symptoms ±20 minutes [ ] 7-10 days
[ ] 3 months [ ] Other ______________________________(___ ___)

Contd...

3. Visual: Visual fields (upper and lower quadrants) are tested by confrontation, using finger counting or visual threat, as appropriate. Patients may be encouraged, but if they look at the side of the moving fingers appropriately, this can be scored as normal. If there is unilateral blindness or enucleation, visual fields in the remaining eye are scored. Score 1 only if a clear-cut asymmetry, including quadrantanopia, is found. If patient is blind from any cause, score 3. Double simultaneous stimulation is performed at this point. If there is extinction, patient receives a 1, and the results are used to respond to item 11.	0 = **No visual loss.** 1 = **Partial hemianopia.** 2 = **Complete hemianopia.** 3 = **Bilateral hemianopia** (blind including cortical blindness).	____
4. Facial Palsy: Ask – or use pantomime to encourage – the patient to show teeth or raise eyebrows and close eyes. Score symmetry of grimace in response to noxious stimuli in the poorly responsive or non-comprehending patient. If facial trauma/bandages, orotracheal tube, tape or other physical barriers obscure the face, these should be removed to the extent possible.	0 = **Normal** symmetrical movements. 1 = **Minor paralysis** (flattened nasolabial fold, asymmetry on smiling). 2 = **Partial paralysis** (total or near-total paralysis of lower face). 3 = **Complete paralysis** of one or both sides (absence of facial movement in the upper and lower face).	____
5. Motor Arm: The limb is placed in the appropriate position: extend the arms (palms down) 90 degrees (if sitting) or 45 degrees (if supine). Drift is scored if the arm falls before 10 seconds. The aphasic patient is encouraged using urgency in the voice and pantomime, but not noxious stimulation. Each limb is tested in turn, beginning with the non-paretic arm. Only in the case of amputation or joint fusion at the shoulder, the examiner should record the score as untestable (UN), and clearly write the explanation for this choice.	0 = **No drift;** limb holds 90 (or 45) degrees for full 10 seconds. 1 = **Drift;** limb holds 90 (or 45) degrees, but drifts down before full 10 seconds; does not hit bed or other support. 2 = **Some effort against gravity;** limb cannot get to or maintain (if cued) 90 (or 45) degrees, drifts down to bed, but has some effort against gravity. 3 = **No effort against gravity;** limb falls. 4 = **No movement.** UN = **Amputation** or joint fusion, explain: ________________ **5a. Left Arm** **5b. Right Arm**	 ____ ____
6. Motor Leg: The limb is placed in the appropriate position: hold the leg at 30 degrees (always tested supine). Drift is scored if the leg falls before 5 seconds. The aphasic patient is encouraged using urgency in the voice and pantomime, but not noxious stimulation. Each limb is tested in turn, beginning with the non-paretic leg. Only in the case of amputation or joint fusion at the hip, the examiner should record the score as untestable (UN), and clearly write the explanation for this choice.	0 = **No drift;** leg holds 30-degree position for full 5 seconds. 1 = **Drift;** leg falls by the end of the 5-second period but does not hit bed. 2 = **Some effort against gravity;** leg falls to bed by 5 seconds, but has some effort against gravity. 3 = **No effort against gravity;** leg falls to bed immediately. 4 = **No movement.** UN = **Amputation** or joint fusion, explain: ______________ **6a. Left Leg** **6b. Right Leg**	 ____

Rev 10/1/2003

Continued

NIH STROKE SCALE

Patient Identification. ___ ___-___ ___ ___-___ ___ ___

Pt. Date of Birth ___ ___/___ ___/___ ___

Hospital ________________________(___ ___-___ ___)

Date of Exam ___ ___/___ ___/___ ___

Interval: [ ] Baseline [ ] 2 hours post treatment [ ] 24 hours post onset of symptoms ±20 minutes [ ] 7-10 days
[ ] 3 months [ ] Other ________________________________(___ ___)

Contd...

7. Limb Ataxia: This item is aimed at finding evidence of a unilateral cerebellar lesion. Test with eyes open. In case of visual defect, ensure testing is done in intact visual field. The finger-nose-finger and heel-shin tests are performed on both sides, and ataxia is scored only if present out of proportion to weakness. Ataxia is absent in the patient who cannot understand or is paralyzed. Only in the case of amputation or joint fusion, the examiner should record the score as untestable (UN), and clearly write the explanation for this choice. In case of blindness, test by having the patient touch nose from extended arm position.	0 = **Absent.** 1 = **Present in one limb.** 2 = **Present in two limbs.** UN = **Amputation** or joint fusion, explain: ______________	______
8. Sensory: Sensation or grimace to pinprick when tested, or withdrawal from noxious stimulus in the obtunded or aphasic patient. Only sensory loss attributed to stroke is scored as abnormal and the examiner should test as many body areas (arms [not hands], legs, trunk, face) as needed to accurately check for hemisensory loss. A score of 2, "severe or total sensory loss," should only be given when a severe or total loss of sensation can be clearly demonstrated. Stuporous and aphasic patients will, therefore, probably score 1 or 0. The patient with brainstem stroke who has bilateral loss of sensation is scored 2. If the patient does not respond and is quadriplegic, score 2. Patients in a coma (item 1a=3) are automatically given a 2 on this item.	0 = **Normal;** no sensory loss. 1 = **Mild-to-moderate sensory loss;** patient feels pinprick is less sharp or is dull on the affected side; or there is a loss of superficial pain with pinprick, but patient is aware of being touched. 2 = **Severe to total sensory loss;** patient is not aware of being touched in the face, arm, and leg.	______
9. Best Language: A great deal of information about comprehension will be obtained during the preceding sections of the examination. For this scale item, the patient is asked to describe what is happening in the attached picture, to name the items on the attached naming sheet and to read from the attached list of sentences. Comprehension is judged from responses here, as well as to all of the commands in the preceding general neurological exam. If visual loss interferes with the tests, ask the patient to identify objects placed in the hand, repeat, and produce speech. The intubated patient should be asked to write. The patient in a coma (item 1a=3) will automatically score 3 on this item. The examiner must choose a score for the patient with stupor or limited cooperation, but a score of 3 should be used only if the patient is mute and follows no one-step commands.	0 = **No aphasia;** normal. 1 = **Mild-to-moderate aphasia;** some obvious loss of fluency or facility of comprehension, without significant limitation on ideas expressed or form of expression. Reduction of speech and/or comprehension, however, makes conversation about provided materials difficult or impossible. For example, in conversation about provided materials, examiner can identify picture or naming card content from patient's response. 2 = **Severe aphasia;** all communication is through fragmentary expression; great need for inference, questioning, and guessing by the listener. Range of information that can be exchanged is limited; listener carries burden of communication. Examiner cannot identify materials provided from patient response. 3 = **Mute, global aphasia;** no usable speech or auditory comprehension.	______
10. Dysarthria: If patient is thought to be normal, an adequate sample of speech must be obtained by asking patient to read or repeat words from the attached list. If the patient has severe aphasia, the clarity of articulation of spontaneous speech can be rated. Only if the patient is intubated or has other physical barriers to producing speech, the examiner should record the score as untestable (UN), and clearly write an explanation for this choice. Do not tell the patient why he or she is being tested.	0 = **Normal.** 1 = **Mild-to-moderate dysarthria;** patient slurs at least some words and, at worst, can be understood with some difficulty. 2 = **Severe dysarthria;** patient's speech is so slurred as to be unintelligible in the absence of or out of proportion to any dysphasia, or is mute/anarthric. UN = **Intubated** or other physical barrier, explain:__________________________	______

Rev 10/1/2003

Continued

NIH STROKE SCALE

Patient Identification. ___ ___-___ ___ ___-___ ___ ___

Pt. Date of Birth ___ ___/___ ___/___ ___

Hospital ______________________(___ ___-___ ___)

Date of Exam ___ ___/___ ___/___ ___

Interval: [ ] Baseline [ ] 2 hours post treatment [ ] 24 hours post onset of symptoms ±20 minutes [ ] 7-10 days
[ ] 3 months [ ] Other ______________________________(___ ___)

Contd...

11. Extinction and Inattention (formerly Neglect): Sufficient information to identify neglect may be obtained during the prior testing. If the patient has a severe visual loss preventing visual double simultaneous stimulation, and the cutaneous stimuli are normal, the score is normal. If the patient has aphasia but does appear to attend to both sides, the score is normal. The presence of visual spatial neglect or anosagnosia may also be taken as evidence of abnormality. Since the abnormality is scored only if present, the item is never untestable.	0 = **No abnormality.** 1 = **Visual, tactile, auditory, spatial, or personal inattention** or extinction to bilateral simultaneous stimulation in one of the sensory modalities. 2 = **Profound hemi-inattention or extinction to more than one modality;** does not recognize own hand or orients to only one side of space.	_____

APPENDIX O: MODIFIED RANKIN SCALE (MRS)

MODIFIED RANKIN SCALE (MRS)

Patient Name: ____________________

Rater Name: ____________________

Date: ____________________

Score	Description
0	No symptoms at all
1	No significant disability despite symptoms; able to carry out all usual duties and activities
2	Slight disability; unable to carry out all previous activities, but able to look after own affairs without assistance
3	Moderate disability; requiring some help, but able to walk without assistance
4	Moderately severe disability; unable to walk without assistance and unable to attend to own bodily needs without assistance
5	Severe disability; bedridden, incontinent and requiring constant nursing care and attention
6	Dead

TOTAL (0–6): ______

References

Rankin J. "Cerebral vascular accidents in patients over the age of 60." *Scott Med J* 1957;2:200-15

Bonita R, Beaglehole R. "Modification of Rankin Scale: Recovery of motor function after stroke." ***Stroke* 1988 Dec;19(12):1497-1500**

Van Swieten JC, Koudstaal PJ, Visser MC, Schouten HJ, van Gijn J. "Interobserver agreement for the assessment of handicap in stroke patients." ***Stroke* 1988;19(5):604-7**